EDITORS

MAXWELL M. WINTROBE

B.A., M.D., B.SC. (Med.), PH.D., D.SC. (Hon.), D.SC. (Hon.), F.A.C.P.
Professor of Internal Medicine; Director, Cardiovascular Research and Training Institute; Director, Laboratory for Study of Hereditary and Metabolic Disorders; University of Utah College of Medicine, Salt Lake City

GEORGE W. THORN

M.D., M.A. (Hon.), LL.D. (Hon.), D.SC. (Hon.), M.D. (Hon.), F.R.C.P.
Hersey Professor of the Theory and Practice of Physic; Samuel A. Levine Professor of Medicine, Harvard Medical School; Physician-in-Chief, Peter Bent Brigham Hospital, Boston

RAYMOND D. ADAMS

B.A., M.A., M.D., M.A. (Hon.), D.M.SC. (Hon.)
Bullard Professor of Neuropathology, Harvard Medical School; Chief of Neurology and Neuropathologist, Massachusetts General Hospital, Boston; Director of Kennedy Laboratories of Massachusetts General Hospital; Co-Director of Eunice Shriver Center, Fernald State School; Associate Physician, University Hospital, Lausanne, Switzerland

IVAN L. BENNETT, JR.

A.B., M.D.
Director, New York University Medical Center, New York

EUGENE BRAUNWALD

A.B., M.D.
Professor and Chairman, Department of Medicine, University of California at San Diego School of Medicine, La Jolla; Chief of Medicine, University Hospital of San Diego County

KURT J. ISSELBACHER

M.D.
Professor of Medicine, Harvard Medical School; Physician and Chief, Gastrointestinal Unit, Massachusetts General Hospital, Boston

ROBERT G. PETERSDORF

A.B., M.D. (Associate Editor)
Professor and Chairman, Department of Medicine, University of Washington School of Medicine; Physician-in-Chief, University of Washington Hospital, Seattle

A BLAKISTON PUBLICATION

McGRAW-HILL BOOK COMPANY

New York · St. Louis · San Francisco · Düsseldorf · London · Mexico · Panama · Sydney · Toronto

HARRISON'S
PRINCIPLES
OF INTERNAL
MEDICINE

Library of Congress Catalog Card Number 76-78960

1 2 3 4 5 6 7 8 9 0 COCO 7 9 8 7 6 5 4 3 2 1 0

FOREIGN LANGUAGE EDITIONS

Portuguese (Fourth Edition)—Editôra Guanabara Koogen, Lta., © 1968
Spanish (Third Edition)—La Prensa Medica Mexicana, © 1965
Italian—Casa Editrice Dr. Francesco Vallardi, Societá Editrice Libraria, Spa., Milan, © 1968
Polish—Panstwowy Zaklad Wydawnictw Lekarskich, expected © 1970
Greek—G. Parissianos Medical and Scientific Books, Athens, expected © 1971

This book was set in Caledonia by The Colonial Press Inc., and printed on permanent paper and bound by The Colonial Press Inc. The cover was designed by John Condon; the drawings were done by B. Handelman Associates, Inc. The editors were René Boudreau, Paul K. Schneider, and Diane Drobnis. Eugene Capriotti supervised the production.

NOTICE

Medicine is an ever-changing science. As new research and clinical experience broaden our knowledge, changes in treatment and drug therapy are required. The editors and the publisher of this work have made every effort to ensure that the drug dosage schedules herein are accurate and in accord with the standards accepted at the time of publication. The reader is advised, however, to check the product information sheet included in the package of each drug he plans to administer to be certain that changes have not been made in the recommended dose or in the contraindications for administration. This recommendation is of particular importance in regard to new or infrequently used drugs.

To all those
who have taught us,
and especially to
our younger colleagues
who continue to
teach and inspire us

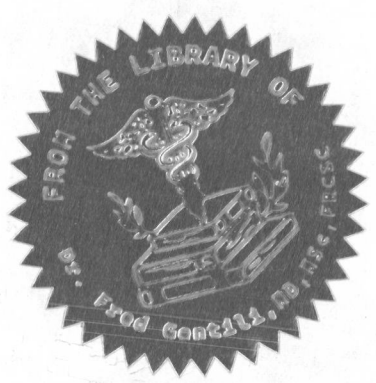

Contributors

AMERICO ABBRUZZESE, M.D.
Clinical Associate in Medicine, Harvard Medical School; Associate in Medicine, Peter Bent Brigham Hospital, Boston.

RAYMOND D. ADAMS, B.A., M.A., M.D., M.A. (HON.), D.M.SC. (HON.)
Bullard Professor of Neuropathology, Harvard Medical School; Chief of Neurology Service and Neuropathologist, Massachusetts General Hospital, Boston.

MENELAOS A. ALIAPOULIOS, M.D., B.S.
Associate in Surgery, Harvard Medical School; Junior Associate in Surgery, Peter Bent Brigham Hospital, Boston.

JAMES C. ALLEN, M.D.
Associate Professor of Medicine and Chief of the Infectious Diseases Unit, State University of New York at Buffalo, School of Medicine, Buffalo, New York.

DAVID H. ALPERS, M.D.
Assistant Professor of Medicine, Washington University School of Medicine; Director, Gastroenterology Division, Department of Internal Medicine, Washington University School of Medicine, St. Louis.

FAYE D. ARUNDELL, M.D.
Clinical Assistant Professor of Dermatology, Stanford University School of Medicine, Stanford, California.

ARTHUR K. ASBURY, M.D.
Associate Professor of Neurology and Associate Director of the Department of Neurology, University of California Medical School at Berkeley, California.

KARL-ERIK ÅSTRÖM, M.D.
Visiting Assistant Professor of Neuropathology, Harvard Medical School; Associate Neuropathologist, Massachusetts General Hospital, Boston.

K. FRANK AUSTEN, M.D.
Professor of Medicine, Harvard Medical School; Physician-in-Chief, Robert Breck Brigham Hospital, Boston.

ROBERT AUSTRIAN, M.D.
John Herr Musser Professor of Research Medicine, University of Pennsylvania School of Medicine, Philadelphia.

HARRY N. BEATY, M.D.
Assistant Professor of Medicine, University of Washington; Head, Division of Infectious Diseases, Harborview Medical Center (King County Hospital), Seattle.

ALBERT R. BEHNKE, B.A., M.D., M.S. (HON.)
Formerly Radiological Medical Director, U.S. Naval Radiological Defense Laboratory, San Francisco.

IVAN L. BENNETT, JR., A.B., M.D.
Director, New York University Medical Center, New York.

DANIEL S. BERNSTEIN, M.D., A.B.
Assistant Professor in Medicine, Harvard Medical School; Senior Associate in Medicine, Peter Bent Brigham Hospital, Boston.

THOMAS C. BITHELL, M.D.
Associate Professor of Internal Medicine and Clinical Pathology, University of Virginia, Charlottesville, Virginia.

DANE R. BOGGS, M.D.
Professor of Medicine; Chief, Hematology Section, Department of Medicine, University of Pittsburgh, Pittsburgh, Pennsylvania.

STUART BONDURANT, M.D.
Robert B. Lamb Professor of Medicine and Chairman, Department of Medicine, Albany Medical College, Albany, New York.

ABRAHAM I. BRAUDE, M.D.
Professor of Medicine; Head, Division of Infectious Diseases, University of California at San Diego School of Medicine, La Jolla.

RALPH W. BRAUER, M.SC., PH.D.
Director, Wrightsville Marine Bio-Medical Laboratory, Wilmington; Professor of Physiology and Pharmacology, Duke University Medical Center, Durham; Visiting Professor of Physiology, University of North Carolina, Chapel Hill.

EUGENE BRAUNWALD, A.B., M.D.
Professor and Chairman, Department of Medicine, University of California at San Diego School of Medicine, La Jolla, California; Chief of Medicine, University Hospital of San Diego County.

THORNTON BROWN, M.D.
Associate Clinical Professor of Orthopedic Surgery, Harvard Medical School; Visiting Orthopedic Surgeon, Massachusetts General Hospital, Boston.

MATTHEW A. BUDD, M.D.
Assistant Professor of Medicine, Harvard Medical School; Associate in Medicine, Beth Israel Hospital, Boston.

GEORGE F. CAHILL, JR., B.S., M.D., M.A. (HON.)
Associate Professor of Medicine and Director, Elliott P. Joslin Research Laboratories, Harvard Medical School; Senior Associate in Medicine, Peter Bent Brigham Hospital, Boston.

EVAN CALKINS, M.D., A.B.
Professor and Chairman, Department of Medicine, State University of New York at Buffalo; Director of Medicine, Edward J. Meyer Memorial Hospital, Buffalo; Attending Physician, Buffalo General Hospital.

CHARLES C. J. CARPENTER, M.D.
Professor of Medicine, Johns Hopkins University School of Medicine; Chief of Medicine, Baltimore City Hospitals, Baltimore.

GEORGE E. CARTWRIGHT, B.A., M.D.
Professor and Head, Department of Medicine, University of Utah College of Medicine, Salt Lake City, Utah.

LEIGHTON E. CLUFF, M.D.
Professor and Chairman, Department of Medicine, University of Florida School of Medicine, Gainesville, Florida.

ROBERT E. COOKE, B.S., M.D.
Given Foundation Professor of Pediatrics and Chairman of

the Department, Johns Hopkins University School of Medicine; Pediatrician-in-Chief, Johns Hopkins Hospital, Baltimore.

LEWIS L. CORIELL, M.A., PH.D., M.D., F.A.A.P.
Professor of Pediatrics, University of Pennsylvania School of Medicine, Philadelphia; Senior Physician, The Children's Hospital, Philadelphia; Director, South Jersey Medical Research Foundation, Camden, New Jersey.

JOHN F. CRIGLER, JR., M.D.
Associate Professor of Pediatrics, Harvard Medical School; Senior Associate in Medicine and Chief, Endocrine Division, Children's Hospital Medical Center, Boston.

EUGENE P. CRONKITE, M.D., D.SC. (HON.)
Chairman, Medical Department, Brookhaven National Laboratory, Upton, New York.

JOSEPH F. DINGMAN, M.D., B.S.
Lecturer in Medicine, Harvard Medical School; Senior Associate in Medicine, Peter Bent Brigham Hospital, Boston.

PHILIP R. DODGE, M.D.
Professor and Chairman of the Department of Pediatrics, Washington University, St. Louis, Missouri.

E. E. EDDLEMAN, JR., B.S., M.D.
Professor of Medicine, University of Alabama Medical College; Associate Chief of Staff for Research and Education, Veterans Administration Hospital, Birmingham.

KENDALL EMERSON, JR., M.D., B.A.
Clinical Professor of Medicine, Harvard Medical School; Physician, Peter Bent Brigham Hospital; Chief of Medicine, Boston Lying-In Hospital, Boston.

KARL ENGELMAN, M.D.
Senior Investigator, Experimental Therapeutics Branch, National Heart and Lung Institute, National Institutes of Health, Bethesda, Maryland.

EDWIN ENGLERT, JR., M.D.
Associate Professor of Medicine and Chairman, Division of Gastroenterology, Department of Internal Medicine, University of Utah Medical Center; Chief, Medical Service, Veterans Administration Hospital, Salt Lake City.

FRANKLIN H. EPSTEIN, M.D.
Professor of Internal Medicine, Yale University School of Medicine, New Haven.

E. HARVEY ESTES, JR., M.D.
Professor and Chairman, Department of Community Medicine, Duke University Medical Center, Durham, North Carolina.

STEFAN S. FAJANS, B.S., M.D.
Professor of Internal Medicine, University of Michigan Medical School, Ann Arbor.

EUGENE M. FARBER, M.D., M.S.
Professor and Executive Head, Department of Dermatology, Stanford University School of Medicine, Stanford, California.

ALVAN R. FEINSTEIN, M.D.
Professor of Medicine and Epidemiology, Yale University School of Medicine, New Haven, Connecticut.

F. ROBERT FEKETY, JR., M.D.
Associate Professor of Medicine; Head, Division of Infectious Diseases, University of Michigan School of Medicine, Ann Arbor.

HARRY A. FELDMAN, A.B., M.D.
Professor and Chairman, Department of Preventive Medicine, State University of New York, Upstate Medical Center at Syracuse, New York.

RICHARD A. FIELD, A.B., M.D.
Professor of Medicine and Director, Division of Endocrinology and Metabolic Diseases, Jefferson Medical College, Philadelphia.

C. MILLER FISHER, M.D.
Associate Clinical Professor of Neurology, Harvard Medical School; Neurologist, Massachusetts General Hospital, Boston.

RUSSELL S. FISHER, M.D., B.S.
Chief Medical Examiner, State of Maryland; Professor of Forensic Pathology, University of Maryland Medical School; Lecturer in Forensic Pathology, Johns Hopkins Medical School; Associate in Public Health Administration, Johns Hopkins School of Hygiene and Public Health, Baltimore.

ALFRED P. FISHMAN, M.D.
Professor of Medicine, Director, Cardiovascular Pulmonary Division, University of Pennsylvania, Philadelphia.

THOMAS B. FITZPATRICK, M.D., PH.D.
Edward Wigglesworth Professor of Dermatology, Harvard Medical School; Chief, Dermatology Service, Massachusetts General Hospital, Boston.

JOHN FOERSTER, M.D.
Assistant Professor of Medicine, University of Manitoba, Winnipeg, Manitoba, Canada.

RICHARD H. FOLLIS, JR., M.D. (DECEASED)
Formerly Armed Forces Institute of Pathology and the Veterans Administration Central Laboratory for Anatomic Pathology and Research, AFIP, Washington, D.C.

EDWARD C. FRANKLIN, M.D.
Professor of Medicine and Head, Division of Rheumatology, New York University School of Medicine, New York.

DONALD S. FREDRICKSON, M.D.
Director of Intramural Research and Chief, Laboratory of Molecular Diseases, National Heart and Lung Institute, National Institutes of Health, Bethesda, Maryland.

LAWRENCE R. FREEDMAN, M.D., B.S.
Associate Professor of Medicine, Yale University School of Medicine, New Haven.

WILLIAM F. FRIEDMAN, M.D.
Assistant Professor of Medicine and Pediatrics; Chief, Divi-

sion of Pediatric Cardiology, University of California at San Diego School of Medicine, La Jolla, California.

ALVIN E. FRIEDMAN-KIEN, M.D.
Associate Professor of Dermatology, New York University School of Medicine, New York.

HARRY W. FRITTS, JR., M.D.
Professor of Medicine, Columbia University, College of Physicians and Surgeons, New York.

GERALD GLICK, M.D.
Associate Professor of Pharmacology and Medicine; Director, Laboratory of Clinical Cardiovascular Pharmacology, Baylor College of Medicine, Texas Medical Center, Houston, Texas.

ROBERT M. GLICKMAN, M.D.
Instructor in Medicine, Harvard Medical School; Assistant in Medicine, Massachusetts General Hospital, Boston.

JOHN R. GOLDSMITH, M.D.
Head of Environmental Epidemiology Unit, California State Department of Public Health, Berkeley, California.

PAUL GOLDHABER, D.D.S.
Dean and Professor of Periodontology, Harvard University School of Dental Medicine, Boston.

J. T. GRAYSTON, M.D.
Professor and Chairman, Department of Preventive Medicine, University of Washington School of Medicine, Seattle.

NORTON J. GREENBERGER, M.D.
Associate Professor of Medicine and Director, Division of Gastroenterology, Ohio State University College of Medicine; Attending Physician, Ohio State University College of Medicine, Columbus.

SHELDON EDWARD GREISMAN, M.D.
Associate Professor of Medicine, University of Maryland School of Medicine, Baltimore.

JOHN F. GRIFFITH, M.D.
Assistant Professor of Pediatrics, Duke University School of Medicine, Durham, North Carolina.

T. R. HARRISON, A.B., M.D.
Professor of Medicine, The Medical College of the University of Alabama, Birmingham, and Distinguished Professor of the University of Alabama.

DONALD H. HARTER, M.D.
Associate Professor of Neurology, Columbia University College of Physicians and Surgeons, New York.

ARTHUR HAUT, A.B., M.D.
Professor of Medicine and Head, Section on Hematology, University of Arkansas School of Medicine, Little Rock, Arkansas.

THOMAS R. HENDRIX, M.D.
Professor of Medicine, Johns Hopkins University School of Medicine, Baltimore.

ALBERT HEYMAN, B.S., M.D.
Professor of Neurology, Duke University School of Medicine, Durham, North Carolina.

ROGER B. HICKLER, M.D.
Lecturer in Medicine, Harvard Medical School; Senior Associate in Medicine, Peter Bent Brigham Hospital; Professor of Medicine, Boston University School of Medicine, Boston; Chief of Medicine, Framingham Union Hospital, Framingham.

PAUL D. HOEPRICH, M.D.
Professor of Medicine and Pathology, School of Medicine, University of California, Davis, California.

EDWARD W. HOOK, M.D.
Henry B. Mulholland Professor and Chairman, Department of Medicine, University of Virginia School of Medicine, Charlottesville.

RICHARD B. HORNICK, M.D.
Associate Professor of Medicine; Head, Division of Infectious Diseases, University of Maryland School of Medicine, Baltimore.

SIDNEY H. INGBAR, M.D.
William B. Castle Professor of Medicine, Harvard Medical School; Associate Director, Thorndike Memorial Laboratory, Boston City Hospital, Boston.

KURT J. ISSELBACHER, M.D.
Professor of Medicine, Harvard Medical School; Physician and Chief, Gastrointestinal Unit, Massachusetts General Hospital, Boston.

ELIZABETH B. JACKSON, A.B.
Formerly Assistant Professor in Medicine, University of Maryland School of Medicine, Baltimore.

LEONARD W. JARCHO, A.B., M.A., M.D.
Professor and Head, Department of Neurology; Associate Professor of Medicine, University of Utah College of Medicine, Salt Lake City.

MICHEL JEQUIER, M.D.
Professor of Neurology, University of Lausanne, Switzerland; Chief of Neurology Services, Cantonal Hospital.

CAROL J. JOHNS, M.D.
Assistant Professor of Medicine, Johns Hopkins University School of Medicine, Baltimore.

JOSEPH E. JOHNSON, III, M.D.
Professor of Medicine; Head, Division of Infectious Diseases, University of Florida College of Medicine, Gainesville.

RICHARD L. KAHLER, M.D.
Associate Professor of Medicine, University of California at San Diego School of Medicine; Head, Division of Cardiopulmonary Diseases, Scripps Clinic and Research Foundation, La Jolla, California.

BYRON A. KAKULAS, M.D., M.R.A.C.P., M.C. PATH.
Lecturer in Pathology, Department of Pathology, School of Medicine, Victoria Square, Perth, Western Australia.

JAN KOCH-WESER, M.D.
Assistant Professor of Pharmacology, Harvard Medical School; Assistant Physician, Massachusetts General Hospital, Boston.

M. GLENN KOENIG, M.D.
Associate Professor of Medicine; Head, Division of Infectious Diseases, Vanderbilt University School of Medicine, Nashville, Tennessee.

RAYMOND S. KOFF, M.D.
Assistant Professor of Medicine, Boston University School of Medicine; Clinical Investigator, Veterans Administration Hospital, Boston.

VERNON KNIGHT, M.D.
Professor of Medicine and Microbiology, Baylor College of Medicine, Houston, Texas.

JOHN H. KNOWLES, M.D.
General Director and Physician, Massachusetts General Hospital; Professor of Medicine, Harvard Medical School, Boston.

STEPHEN M. KRANE, M.D., A.M. (HON.), A.B.
Associate Professor of Medicine, Harvard Medical School; Physician and Chief, Arthritis Unit, Massachusetts General Hospital, Boston.

CARL KUPFER, M.D.
Director, National Eye Institute, National Institutes of Health, Bethesda, Maryland; formerly Professor and Chairman, Department of Ophthalmology, School of Medicine, University of Washington School of Medicine, Seattle.

DAVID P. LAULER, M.D., B.S.
Assistant Professor of Medicine, Harvard Medical School; Senior Associate in Medicine, Peter Bent Brigham Hospital, Boston.

G. RICHARD LEE, M.D.
Associate Professor of Medicine, College of Medicine, University of Utah, Salt Lake City, Utah.

A. MARTIN LERNER, M.D.
Professor of Medicine; Head, Division of Infectious Diseases, Wayne State University School of Medicine, Detroit, Michigan.

BERNARD LOWN, M.D.
Physician, Peter Bent Brigham Hospital; Associate Professor, Harvard School of Public Health, Boston, Massachusetts.

BERNARD LYTTON, M.B., B.S., F.R.C.S. (ENG.)
Yale University School of Medicine, New Haven.

JANET W. McARTHUR, M.D., A.B., M.S., M.B., D.SC. (HON.)
Associate Clinical Professor of Obstetrics and Gynecology, Harvard Medical School; Associate Physician, Massachusetts General Hospital, Boston.

FRED R. McCRUMB, JR., M.D.
Professor of Medicine, University of Maryland School of Medicine, Baltimore.

VICTOR A. McKUSICK, M.D.
Professor of Medicine and Chief, Division of Medical Genetics, Department of Medicine, Johns Hopkins University School of Medicine, Baltimore, Maryland.

GEORGE V. MANN, M.D.
Associate Professor of Medicine and Associate Professor of Biochemistry, Vanderbilt University School of Medicine; Career Investigator, National Heart and Lung Institute, Nashville, Tennessee.

ALEXANDER MARBLE, M.D., M.A., A.B.
Clinical Professor in Medicine Emeritus, Harvard Medical School; Senior Associate in Medicine Emeritus, Peter Bent Brigham Hospital; Senior Physician, Joslin Clinic and New England Deaconess Hospital; President, Joslin Diabetes Foundation, Inc., Boston.

ALBERT I. MENDELOFF, M.D.
Associate Professor of Medicine, Johns Hopkins University School of Medicine; Physician-in-Chief, Sinai Hospital, Baltimore.

JOHN P. MERRILL, A.B., M.D.
Associate Professor of Medicine, Harvard Medical School; Director, Cardiorenal Section, Peter Bent Brigham Hospital, Boston.

EDWARD S. MILLER, M.D.
Associate Clinical Professor in Medicine, University of Colorado School of Medicine, Denver.

JAY P. MOHR, M.D., MAJ MC
Division of Neuropsychiatry, Walter Reed Army Institute of Research, Washington, D.C.

HUGO W. MOSER, M.D.
Associate Professor of Neurology at the Massachusetts General Hospital, Harvard Medical School; Neurologist, Massachusetts General Hospital; Assistant Superintendent, Fernald School, and Co-Director of Eunice Shriver Laboratories.

KENNETH M. MOSER, M.D.
Associate Professor of Medicine and Director, Pulmonary Disease Division, University of California at San Diego School of Medicine, La Jolla, California.

DON H. NELSON, M.D.
Chief of Medicine, Latter-day Saints Hospital; Professor of Medicine, University of Utah College of Medicine, Salt Lake City.

GEORGE NICHOLS, JR., M.D.
Clinical Professor of Medicine, Harvard Medical School; Senior Associate, Peter Bent Brigham Hospital, Boston.

PHILIP S. NORMAN, M.D.
Associate Professor of Medicine, Johns Hopkins University School of Medicine, Baltimore.

JOHN A. OATES, M.D.
Professor of Medicine and Pharmacology, Vanderbilt University Hospital, Nashville.

E. H. O. PARRY, M.D.
Professor and Chairman, Department of Medicine, Ahmadu Bello University, Zaria, Nigeria.

ROBERT G. PETERSDORF, M.D.
Professor and Chairman, Department of Medicine, University of Washington School of Medicine; Physician-in-Chief, University of Washington Hospital, Seattle.

JAMES J. PLORDE, M.D.
Assistant Professor of Medicine and Preventive Medicine, University of Washington School of Medicine, Seattle.

PETER E. POOL, M.D.
Assistant Professor of Medicine, University of California at San Diego School of Medicine, La Jolla, California.

DAVID C. POSKANZER, M.D., M.P.H.
Associate Professor of Neurology at the Massachusetts General Hospital, Harvard Medical School; Associate Neurologist, Massachusetts General Hospital.

EDWARD P. RADFORD, M.D.
Professor of Environmental Medicine, Johns Hopkins University School of Hygiene and Public Health, Baltimore, Maryland.

CHARLES H. RAMMELKAMP, JR., B.A., M.D., D.SC. (HON.)
Professor of Medicine and Associate Professor of Preventive Medicine, Western Reserve University School of Medicine; Director, Department of Medicine and Research Laboratories, Cleveland Metropolitan General Hospital, Cleveland.

T. J. REEVES, M.D.
Professor and Chairman, Department of Medicine, University of Alabama School of Medicine, Birmingham.

WILLIAM H. RESNIK, M.D.
Clinical Professor of Medicine, Yale University; Consultant Physician, Yale–New Haven Hospital; Consultant Physician, Stamford Hospital, Stamford, Connecticut.

JOHN CHARLES RIBBLE, M.D.
Associate Professor of Pediatrics, Cornell University School of Medicine, New York.

CLAYTON RICH, M.D.
Professor of Medicine and Associate Dean, University of Washington School of Medicine; Chief of Staff, Veterans Administration Hospital, Seattle.

EDWARD P. RICHARDSON, JR., M.D.
Associate Professor of Neuropathology, Harvard Medical School; Neurologist and Neuropathologist, Massachusetts General Hospital, Boston.

EUGENE D. ROBIN, M.D.
Professor of Medicine, University of Pittsburgh Medical School, Pittsburgh, Pennsylvania.

DAVID E. ROGERS, M.D.
Professor Medicine, Dean and Vice President for Medicine, Johns Hopkins School of Medicine; Medical Director, Johns Hopkins Hospital, Baltimore.

EUGENIA ROSEMBERG, M.D.
Director of Research, Medical Research Institute of Worcester, Inc., Worcester, Massachusetts.

JOHN ROSS, JR., M.D.
Professor of Medicine; Chief, Cardiovascular Division, Department of Medicine, University of California at San Diego School of Medicine, La Jolla, California.

RICHARD S. ROSS, M.D.
Professor of Medicine and Director, Cardiovascular Division, Johns Hopkins University School of Medicine; Physician, Johns Hopkins Hospital.

JEAN RUBEIZ, M.D.
Assistant Professor of Neuropathology, American University of Beirut, Lebanon.

DAVID C. SABISTON, JR., M.D.
Professor and Chairman, Department of Surgery, Duke University Medical Center, Durham, North Carolina.

FUAD SABRA, M.D.
Professor of Medicine (Neurology) and Neurologist, Department of Medicine, American University of Beirut, Lebanon.

MARIA Z. SALAM, M.D.
Assistant Clinical Professor of Neurology (Pediatric), Harvard Medical School; Clinical Fellow in Neurology, Massachusetts General Hospital, Boston.

JAY P. SANFORD, M.D.
Professor of Medicine; Head, Division of Infectious Diseases, University of Texas—Southwestern School of Medicine, Dallas.

HERBERT A. SELENKOW, M.D., B.S.
Assistant Professor in Medicine, Harvard Medical School; Senior Associate in Medicine and Director, Thyroid Laboratory, Peter Bent Brigham Hospital, Boston.

ARNOLD M. SELIGMAN, M.D.
Professor of Surgery, Johns Hopkins University School of Medicine; Surgeon-in-Chief, Sinai Hospital, Baltimore.

WALTER H. SHELDON, M.D.
Professor of Pathology, Johns Hopkins University School of Medicine, Baltimore.

CHARLES C. SHEPARD, M.D.
National Communicable Disease Center, Public Health Service, U.S. Department of Health, Education and Welfare, Atlanta, Georgia.

LAWRENCE E. SHULMAN, M.D., PH.D.
Associate Professor of Medicine and Director, Connective Tissue Division, Department of Medicine, The Johns Hopkins University School of Medicine, Baltimore.

WILLIAM SILEN, M.D.
Professor of Surgery, Harvard Medical School; Surgeon-in-Chief, Beth Israel Hospital, Boston.

LLOYD H. SMITH, JR., M.D., D.SC. (HON.)
Professor and Chairman, Department of Medicine, University of California, San Francisco Medical Center, San Francisco.

PHILIP J. SNODGRASS, M.D.
Assistant Professor of Medicine, Harvard Medical School; Senior Associate in Medicine, Peter Bent Brigham Hospital, Boston.

EDMUND H. SONNENBLICK, M.D.
Assistant Professor of Medicine, Harvard Medical School; Cardiovascular Division, Department of Medicine, Peter Bent Brigham Hospital, Boston.

WESLEY W. SPINK, B.A., M.D., D.SC. (HON.)
Professor of Medicine, University of Minnesota Hospitals and Medical School, Minneapolis.

EUGENE A. STEAD, JR., B.S., M.D.
Professor of Medicine, Duke University School of Medicine; Durham, North Carolina.

WILLIAM W. STEAD, M.D.
Professor of Medicine, Marquette University School of Medicine, Milwaukee Medical Director, Muirdale Sanatorium, Milwaukee; Chief of Medical Chest Service, Milwaukee County General Hospital, Milwaukee.

JURGEN STEINKE, M.D.
Assistant Professor of Medicine, Harvard Medical School; Senior Associate in Medicine, Peter Bent Brigham Hospital, Boston.

JOHN H. TALBOTT, M.D.
Editor Emeritus, Journal of the American Medical Association, Chicago.

MELVIN L. TAYMOR, M.D., A.B.
Associate Professor of Gynecology, Harvard Medical School; Senior Associate in Surgery, Peter Bent Brigham Hospital, Boston.

LLOYD P. TEPPER, M.D.
Associate Professor of Environmental Health, Department of Environmental Health, University of Cincinnati College of Medicine, Cincinnati, Ohio.

GEORGE W. THORN, M.D., M.A. (HON.), LL.D. (HON.), D.SC. (HON.), M.D. (HON.), F.R.C.P.
Hersey Professor of the Theory and Practice of Physic and Samuel A. Levine Professor of Medicine, Harvard Medical School; Physician-in-Chief, Peter Bent Brigham Hospital, Boston.

WILLIAM A. TISDALE, M.D.
Professor and Chairman, Department of Medicine, University of Vermont College of Medicine, Burlington.

GENNARO M. TISI, M.D.
Assistant Professor of Medicine, University of California at San Diego School of Medicine, La Jolla, California.

ANSGAR TORVIK, M.D.
Assistant Professor of Pathology, Department of Pathology, Ullevaal Hospital, Oslo, Norway.

PHILIP A. TUMULTY, M.D.
Professor of Medicine, Johns Hopkins School of Medicine, Baltimore.

MARVIN TURCK, M.D.
Associate Professor of Medicine, University of Washington School of Medicine; Chief of Medicine, United States Public Health Service Hospital, Seattle.

FRANK H. TYLER, B.A., M.D.
Professor of Medicine, University of Utah College of Medicine, Salt Lake City.

HENRI VANDER EECKEN, H.M., M.D.
Professor of Neurology, Faculty of Medicine, University of Ghent, Ghent, Belgium.

MAURICE VICTOR, M.D.
Professor of Neurology, Western Reserve University School of Medicine; Chief, Neurology Service, Cleveland Metropolitan General Hospital, Cleveland.

ROBERT R. WAGNER, M.D.
Professor and Chairman, Department of Microbiology, University of Virginia School of Medicine, Charlottesville.

HENRY deF. WEBSTER, M.D.
Scientist, National Institute of Neurological Diseases and Stroke, Bethesda, Maryland.

LOUIS WEINSTEIN, M.S., PH.D., M.D.
Professor of Medicine, Tufts University School of Medicine; Lecturer on Infectious Disease, Harvard Medical School; Lecturer in Medicine, Boston University School of Medicine; Chief, Infectious Disease Service, New England Medical Center Hospitals, Boston.

LOUIS G. WELT, M.D.
Alumni Distinguished Professor and Chairman, Department of Medicine, University of North Carolina School of Medicine, Chapel Hill.

JOHN B. WEST, M.D., PH.D.
Professor of Medicine, University of California at San Diego School of Medicine, La Jolla, California.

GORDON H. WILLIAMS, M.D., B.A.
Research Fellow in Medicine, Harvard Medical School; Research Fellow in Medicine, Peter Bent Brigham Hospital, Boston.

MAXWELL M. WINTROBE, B.A., M.D., B.SC. (MED.), PH.D., D.SC. (HON. MANIT.), D.SC. (HON. UTAH), F.A.C.P.
Professor of Internal Medicine; Director, Cardiovascular Research and Training Institute, and Director, Laboratory for Study of Hereditary and Metabolic Disorders, University of Utah College of Medicine, Salt Lake City.

SHELDON M. WOLFF, M.D.
Clinical Director and Chief, Laboratory of Clinical Investigation, National Institute of Allergy and Infectious Diseases, National Institutes of Health, Bethesda, Maryland; Clinical Professor of Medicine, Georgetown University School of Medicine, Washington, D.C.

THEODORE E. WOODWARD, M.D.
Professor of Medicine and Head, Department of Medicine, University of Maryland School of Medicine, Baltimore.

GEORGE W. WRIGHT, M.D.
Head of Medical Research, Department of Medicine, St. Luke's Hospital; Associate Clinical Professor of Medicine, Western Reserve University School of Medicine, Cleveland, Ohio.

RICHARD J. WURTMAN, M.D.
Associate Professor of Endocrinology and Metabolism, Department of Nutrition and Food Science, Massachusetts Institute of Technology, Cambridge.

JAMES B. WYNGAARDEN, M.D., F.A.C.P.
Frederic M. Hanes Professor of Medicine and Chairman, Department of Medicine, Duke University Medical Center, Durham.

ROBERT R. YOUNG, M.D.
Assistant Professor of Neurology, Harvard Medical School; Assistant Neurologist (Clinical Neurophysiologist), Massachusetts General Hospital, Boston.

Preface

It often is asked why prefaces are written and whether they are ever read. In his famous preface to *Cromwell*, Victor Hugo pointed out that one seldom inspects the cellar of a house after visiting its salons nor examines the roots of a tree after eating its fruit. Admittedly, the readers of this book will judge it by the substance of its contents and its style, not by the pretexts offered by its editors. It could be added that if the guest has returned several times, then surely he knows that the cellar is well stocked. Why then a preface to a sixth edition?

This preface is intended to indicate the ways in which the present edition maintains or diverges from, as the case may be, the original objectives of this book. By doing this, it will be possible to present the objectives of this textbook of medicine to readers unfamiliar with earlier editions.

When the first group of editors met together twenty-five years ago, they decided to write a textbook of medicine which would conform to the *clinical method* which they had found most useful both as students and as teachers. It was thought that such a book should recapitulate the steps in the process of thinking by which a physician reaches a diagnosis, these being the recording of the patient's symptoms and signs, the consideration of the various disorders that can give rise to them, and the effective utilization of measures which will support and confirm or alter the first impressions and lead ultimately to a firm diagnosis.

The logical first step consistent with this clinical approach is the consideration of the cardinal manifestations of disease. Patients present themselves with symptoms, not diagnoses. Consequently it is basic to good clinical medicine to appreciate the different causes of various manifestations of disease and to understand how they may be produced. This requires an understanding of physiology and of the ways in which deviations from the normal lead to disorders of one kind or another. For this reason material of fundamental biologic importance was incorporated in the first edition of this book and has been regarded as an essential component ever since.

The revolutionary changes in the curricula of many American medical schools, particularly the abbreviation of the standard courses in the sciences basic to clinical medicine and the substitution of shorter "core" courses, has imposed, we believe, additional responsibilities on the modern teacher of clinical medicine and on the modern textbook of medicine. The student who embarks on his clinical training now, although far more sophisticated in many ways than his predecessor of even one generation ago, may not possess as much understanding of the mechanisms of symptoms and disease processes as is required to deal intelligently with clinical problems. This book recognizes the challenge to education posed by such curricula. Clinical biochemistry and pathophysiology form an integral part of this book but, insofar as possible, are considered within the clinical setting.

The interpretation of symptoms usually is most effectively achieved by proceeding from the general to the particular. Symptoms often can be grouped as syndromes. Syndromes are the consequence of a variety of etiologic factors or disease mechanisms and, if these can be recognized and understood, measures to restore the normal physiologic state can be designed and carried out in a logical, systematic fashion. Furthermore, the method of approaching a diagnosis which is based on an analysis of the symptoms, recognition of the syndrome, and consideration of the various disease mechanisms which may have produced it, ensures consideration of the many possible interpretations of the clinical picture which the patient presents. By pursuing such an approach, it is less likely that a disorder which should be considered will be overlooked.

The plan of this book is consistent with this approach. Following a discussion of the editors' general philosophy regarding the approach to the patient (Part One), certain fundamental matters regarding inheritance and growth are discussed (Part Two), such as the inheritance of human disease (Chapter 4), a subject which is assuming greater and greater importance in clinical medicine. Part Three, Cardinal Manifestations of Disease, discusses the mechanisms whereby various symptoms are produced and outlines an approach to the recognition of the diseases of which they may be manifestations.

Discussion of the cardinal manifestations of disease is not limited to a consideration of symptoms and physical signs. With the increasing availability and sensitivity of laboratory methodology and as the result of the introduction of screening procedures for the early detection of disease, an understanding of laboratory data becomes more essential than ever for the effective practice of medicine. Chapters 64, 65, 66, and 67 have been introduced in this edition to meet these needs and to supplement the discussions of laboratory procedures which will be found throughout the book.

Recognition of the importance of altered immune responses as fundamental mechanisms in the pathogenesis of disease has led to the introduction in this edition of Part Four, Disorders Due to Hypersensitivity and Altered Immune Response, where seven chapters are devoted to this important aspect of clinical medicine.

The remainder of the book is concerned with more specific disorders and disease entities. In all these sections, the syndromic approach is emphasized as much as possible, and the reader will find at the beginning of most of the sections, either in the Introduction and/or in the first chapter, a discussion of the approach to the patient having the type of disease considered in that section.

Treatment is discussed in relation to specific disorders or categories of disease (e.g., Chapter 135, Chemotherapy of Infection, Chapter 266, Principles of Drug Therapy in Cardiac Disorders) and is described in terms which are as specific as possible.

A deliberate attempt has been made to avoid long bibliographies. The references at the end of the chapters are limited, for the most part, to reviews and monographs which contain comprehensive bibliographies, together with older works of historical significance.

With the present edition, two of the original editors, Doctors T. H. Harrison and William H. Resnik, have retired, and their places have been taken by Doctors Eugene Braunwald and Kurt J. Isselbacher. The influence of Doctors Harrison and Resnik is clearly evident in this edition and can confidently be predicted to outlast the lives of all the present editors. Their role in the planning of this textbook was profound, and the present editors are deeply indebted to them. But time, like the science of medicine, moves on, and the reader no doubt will detect the influence of the newer editors. Acknowledgement here also is made of the very effective role which Dr. Robert G. Petersdorf has played as an editor, substituting for Dr. Ivan L. Bennett. He has proved to be a very important member of the team.

Once again the editors take pleasure in expressing appreciation to our many colleagues who have so generously responded to editorial suggestions. We continue to be indebted to numerous friends and colleagues for valuable criticisms. Among these are: Dr. Irwin Arias of New York, Doctors K. Frank Austen, Leon Eisenberg and Seymour Kety of Boston, Dr. Gerald Klatskin of New Haven, Dr. Stephen Robinson of Boston, Dr. Rudi Schmid of San Francisco, Doctors John Butler, Lawrence Harker, E. Donnall Thomas, and Frank Parker of Seattle, and Doctors Dean Ashworth, Arthur M. Brown, Edwin Englert, James Freston, Hiroshi Kuida, Richard Levinson, John Moore, Attilio Renezetti, Joseph Thorne, G. Tikoff, and Theophilus Tsagaris of Salt Lake City.

The preparation of the new edition has been ably facilitated by our several secretarial coworkers. We are especially indebted to Mrs. Beatrice A. Fraser, Mrs. Dorothy Starrett, Mrs. Hilda Gardner, and Miss Clo Flahive of Boston, Miss Pat Jaworsky of Baltimore, Miss Jana Maffey and Miss Doris Williams of Seattle, Mrs. Ethel Taggart Christensen of Salt Lake City, and Mrs. Mary Jackson of San Diego.

M.M.W.
G.W.T.
R.D.A.
I.L.B.
E.B.
K.J.I.
R.G.P.

Contents

SECTION 4   ERRORS OF METABOLISM

PART SIX   DISORDERS DUE TO CHEMICAL AND PHYSICAL AGENTS

SECTION 1   CHEMICAL INTOXICATIONS

SECTION 2   DISORDERS CAUSED BY VENOMS, BITES, AND STINGS

SECTION 3   PHYSICAL AGENTS

SECTION 5   DISORDERS OF THE ALIMENTARY TRACT

SECTION 6   DISORDERS OF THE HEPATOBILIARY SYSTEM

SECTION 7   DISORDERS OF THE PANCREAS

HARRISON'S PRINCIPLES OF INTERNAL MEDICINE

Part One

The Physician and the Patient

Section 1

The Physician and the Patient

1 APPROACH TO THE PATIENT

The Editors

There is no greater opportunity, responsibility, or obligation given a man than that of serving as a physician. In treating the suffering he needs technical skill, scientific knowledge, and human understanding. He who uses these with courage, with humility, and with wisdom will provide a unique service for his fellowman, and will build an enduring edifice of character within himself. The physician should ask of his destiny no more than this; he should be content with no less.

In the practice of medicine the physician employs a discipline which seeks to utilize scientific methods and principles in the solution of its problems, but it is one which, in the end, remains an art. It is an art in the sense that rarely, if ever, can the individual patient be considered the equivalent of an experiment so completely controlled that it is possible to exclude judgment and experience from the interpretation of the patient's reactions. It is an art, too, in the sense that the practicing physician can never be content with the sole aim of endeavoring to clarify the laws of nature; he cannot proceed in his labors with the cool detachment of the scientist whose aim is the winning of the truth, and who, theoretically, is uninterested in the practical outcome of his work. The practicing physician must never forget that his primary and traditional objectives are utilitarian—the prevention and cure of disease and the relief of suffering, whether of body or mind.

THE PATIENT AS A PERSON

The student receives much expert coaching in the methods of physical and laboratory diagnosis, and it is in these areas that he will most easily develop the skills which permit him to be comfortable with the patient. Mastery of the more intangible psychologic aspects of medicine is not so easily acquired, however. The skills essential here depend not simply on instruction but on emotional maturity, manifested by sensitive self-cultivation of the capacity to see deeply and accurately the

problems of another human being. The challenge is further magnified by the fact that the examining physician is himself a human instrument, subject to error arising from events in his own biography. The irritability and exasperation of even the kindest and most conscientious physician may sometimes represent not the legitimate protest at the patient's lack of cooperativeness but a basic and not wholly conscious sense of his own insecurity. The successful management of the patient requires emotional maturity on the part of the physician.

Just as the physical growth of each person depends on an adequate and balanced supply of appropriate foodstuffs, so does emotional growth depend on the receipt of proper psychologic nutrients. Although each individual is born with manifold potentialities determined by his genes, the emotional climate in which he grows and develops will shape his eventual character and abilities just as surely as foodstuffs will shape his physique. Invading bacteria influence multitudinous bodily reactions; so also do the emotions possess the capacity to alter behavior, including certain of the biochemical processes of the body.

Any departure from good health carries a potential threat of physical disintegration or crippling disability, and even the most intelligent and best-informed patient should not be considered immune to forebodings just because he refrains from mentioning them. It is especially important that these fears be borne in mind when dealing with the elderly patient, who is rarely unmindful that "the trap is laid" and death is always near.

The attitude of the patient approaching the doctor must always be tinged, for the most part unconsciously, with distaste and dread; his deepest desire will tend to be comfort and relief rather than cure, and his faith and expectation will be directed towards some magical exhibition of these boons. Do not let yourselves believe that however smoothly concealed by education, by reason, and by confidential frankness these strong elements may be, they are ever in any circumstances altogether absent. (Wilfred Trotter)

In the long development of growth from infancy to adult life, there is a progressive change in social relationships, from one of complete dependence on parent, family, and teacher to one of relative independence. At the same time, the process of maturation requires the partial suppression of egocentric drives to the point that the affairs of other members of one's family and social group assume increasing importance. These trends and their modification during life experience affect the development of personality; and deviations in these natural developments prevent satisfactory social adjustment and result in neuroticism.

Illness constitutes a threat not only to the physical integrity of the individual but also to his status in his social group, a fact that is soon learned by every thoughtful physician. Prolonged invalidism during childhood tends inevitably to leave behind an excessive egocentricity, which may become the basis of a lifelong neurosis. In the adult, illness often enforces a return to a posture of dependency, a change usually accompanied by feelings of apprehension and discouragement, sometimes leading to frank anxiety and depression. It is for these reasons that many adults in positions of responsibility express greater concern about the economic and social implications of their illness than about the illness itself. This explains a number of common psychologic defenses which the patient exercises against illness. He may refuse medical aid; or, if he summons the courage to consult a physician, he may minimize or even fail to mention the very symptom about which he is most deeply concerned. On the other hand, there are individuals whose attainment of maturity has been tenuous and uncertain, so that the position of dependency imposed by illness comes as a welcome relief from adult responsibility. They appear to enjoy illness and to resent anything that menaces their state of invalidism. Lesser degrees of this tendency are to be noted among those who consult the physician at the appearance of every new symptom and who are continuously preoccupied with their past illnesses and operations.

It is not easy to keep these simple facts in mind when examining a draped patient in the relatively neutral domain of the hospital ward or even in the private examining room. There are potent obstacles that stand in the way of the physician's making an adequate study of the patient's emotional life. Organic lesions have a way of compelling attention to themselves, and it is less exhausting to limit one's focus to the sphere of physical disease. More time, energy, and experience are necessary to view the patient as an active participant in an enormous moving pageant which includes the personal eccentricities of his forebears, his own fears and patterns of reaction, as well as the hopes for his children's future. It is not enough to know that poverty, insecurity, and perhaps poor vocational and domestic relations are now keeping the patient unhappily depressed, for all too often it is apparent that present socioeconomic (external) factors are not crucial determinants in the contemporary scene. To explain many of the manifestations of illness, it is necessary to view the patient more deeply as an organism with a vast repository of past experiences dating from the earliest days of life, many of which are vaguely remembered, yet have become the foundation of its cur-

rent system of meeting daily problems. Under the threat of disease, defensive attitudes, which were useful in infancy and childhood but inappropriate in adult life, have a way of reasserting themselves; one of the oldest, the state of readiness for fight or flight (Cannon), may be a precipitating factor in illnesses such as peptic ulcer or hypertension, when called upon too frequently.

The young physician usually finds himself inadequate in his dealings with the patient, for not only does he experience an inevitable sense of insecurity with respect to the patient's problems, but he feels equally uneasy about his newly acquired role of authority and responsibility. Moreover, both he and his older colleague often find it difficult to control their own reactions: disinterest because the patient presents no fascinating problem of organic disease, irritation at his verbosity and lack of clarity and consistency in the recital of the history, annoyance because the patient's illness fails to respond to treatment in the expected manner. The physician can hardly expect to achieve a deep appreciation of the patient's psychologic problems unless he learns to recognize and control his own.

More broadly stated, the physician has a special function in society and should be skilled as a psychologist in human behavior as well as a biologist in human diseases. He brings highly technical knowledge and skills to bear upon the patient's physiologic functioning. He should bring to the suffering patient a quiet humanity, a confidence and security based upon the conviction that all will be done that can be done. The patient must feel that his unique individuality is recognized and appreciated and that his life's problems are meaningful. This is important in patients with well-defined organic disease as well as in the "stress" syndromes largely due to emotional pressures expressed through the body. If we can accept the principle of causality in human behavior, we can, with patience and diligence, learn to fathom some of the patient's motivations even though many of the details very often remain obscure.

Let me see in the sufferer the man alone. . . . Let me be intent upon one thing, O Father of Mercy, to be always merciful to Thy suffering children. (Maimonides)

THE ART OF MEDICINE

Despite the constantly increasing application of scientific methods to the problems of medicine, there remain large areas that are as yet insusceptible of solution by the use of precise methods. To extract the telltale clue from a maze of confusing symptoms, to determine from a mass of conflicting physical signs and laboratory data the ones that are of crucial significance, to know in a borderline case when to initiate and when to refrain from a line of investigation or treatment—the knowledge to accomplish these necessities of medical art is not usually the outcome of laboratory study alone. Involved here are judgments based on "assimilated experience."

Concerning the more personal relations with the patient and the understanding and capacity to peer beyond surface motivations and behavior, no instruction or training can entirely replace an intuitive talent and maturing wisdom. The astute physician will recognize when the casual mention of an apparently trivial complaint is the device for seeking reassurance regarding a feared disorder such as cancer or heart disease. He will at once know or suspect the value of continued probing of the more intimate aspects of the patient's life, and when to overcome a reluctance to discuss them, or to leave them undiscussed, when to express a bright and reassuring prognosis and when and how to utter doubt and caution.

No problem can be more distressing than that presented by the patient with incurable disease, particularly when death is imminent and inevitable. There should be no ironclad, inflexible rule that the patient must be told "everything." Few patients have the courage or faith or stoicism that the advocates of this conviction think they may or should have.

One thing is certain: it is not for you to don the black cap and, assuming the judicial function, take hope away from any patient . . . hope that comes to us all. (William Osler)

The proponents of this principle do not really adhere to their philosophy when they tell the "truth" in such a manner that the kernel of the truth is not conveyed to the patient. How much, for example, is communicated to the patient when the physician says to the patient who has leukemia: "You have more white corpuscles in your blood than is normal, but we found no evidence that any damage has been done." Nor can one conscientiously follow the opposite rule of never telling the patient the truth. How much the patient is to be told will depend on his religious convictions, the wishes of his family, the state of his affairs, and his own desires and character. But even this platitude solves nothing, since it is not merely the recognition of these factors but the physician's wisdom in assessing the relative importance of each that determines how complete a discussion of the facts will best serve the interests of the patient. The younger physician may extract some small measure of consolation from the knowledge that his older and more experienced colleague has no simple and easy formula for meeting the question.

The physician must also be prepared to deal with sentiments commonly experienced at a time of death in the family.

I do not know that I have anything to reproach in my conduct, and certainly nothing in my feelings and intentions towards the dead. But it is a moment when we are apt to think that, if this or that had been done, such event might have been prevented. (Letter to Shelley from Lord Byron on the death of his daughter.)

These words express the feelings of guilt that almost invariably afflict the members of a family when parent or child or spouse has died. The doctor must be prepared to tender what assurance is possible that no fault need be attached to the living.

Somewhat related to this problem is the expiatory attitude of the family when a member becomes gravely or hopelessly ill. The meager resources that may represent the savings of a lifetime of toil may be dissipated in weeks or months in payment for needlessly expensive rooms, private nursing services, and consultations. It is difficult for the physician to oppose these futile gestures too strenuously; they serve more to bring consolation to the family than to assuage the distress of the patient.

Tact, sympathy, and understanding are expected of the physician, for the patient is no mere collection of symptoms, signs, disordered functions, damaged organs, and disturbed emotions. He is human, fearful, and hopeful, seeking relief, help, and reassurance. To the physician, as to the anthropologist, nothing human is strange or repulsive. The misanthrope may become a smart diagnostician of organic disease, but he can scarcely hope to succeed as a physician. The true physician has a Shakespearean breadth of interest in the wise and the foolish, the proud and the humble, the stoic hero and the whining rogue. He cares for people.

CHANGING PATIENT-PHYSICAN RELATIONSHIPS

The patient-physician relationship described above, a relationship which traditionally has been the goal of all physicians, is in danger of deterioration because of the changing setting in which medicine is increasingly being practiced. In many cases the management of the individual patient requires the active participation of a variety of trained professional personnel—not only physicians, but also nurses, dietitians, biochemists, psychologists and physiatrists, and other paramedical personnel. The patient can benefit greatly from such collaboration, but it is the duty of his physician to guide him through his illness; in order to carry out this increasingly difficult task the physician must have some familiarity with the skills and objectives of his colleagues in the fields allied to medicine. He must also be able to interpret their findings not as isolated phenomena but rather as they contribute to the total clinical picture. In giving his patient an opportunity to receive the full benefits resulting from the important advances which have taken place in the health-related sciences, the physician must retain responsibility for the crucial decisions concerning diagnosis and treatment.

The widening scope of medical practice is altering previously existing physician-patient relationships. An increasing number of patients are being cared for by groups of physicians, by clinics, and by hospitals rather than by the single, independent practitioner. There are many potential advantages in the use of such organized medical groups composed of a number of various specialists, but there are also hazards, both to the patient and the physician. The identity of the physician who is primarily and continuously responsible for each particular patient must be clearly defined. It is this physician who must have an overview of a patient's illnesses and who must maintain familiarity with his reaction to illness, to drugs, and to the problems of daily living. In addition, since a number of physicians may, at any one time, contribute to the care of a particular patient, and since both patients and physicians are increasingly mobile, accurate and detailed record keeping assumes progressively greater importance. It is imperative that the physician promptly commit all relevant data obtained from the clinical and laboratory examinations to his patient's permanent medical record. Only in this way can continuity of patient care be provided.

2 APPROACH TO DISEASE
The Editors

HISTORY

The history of an illness should embody all the facts of medical significance in the life of the patient up to the time he consults the physician; but, of course, his most recent diseases attract the most attention, for these, obviously, are the reason he seeks medical advice. Ideally the narration of symptoms should be in the patient's own words, the principal events being presented in the temporal order in which they occurred. Few patients possess the necessary powers of observation and talent for lucid, coherent description. Usually the help of the physician is needed. He must guide them by questions but at the same time avoid influencing them by inserting his own ideas, especially if the patient is suggestible.

Often it happens that a symptom which has greatly concerned a patient possesses little significance as a medical datum, whereas a seemingly minor complaint may be of importance. Therefore the mind of the physician must be constantly alert to the possibility that any event related by the patient, any symptom however trivial or apparently remote, may be the key to the solution of the medical problem.

An informative history is more than an orderly listing of symptoms. Something always is gained by listening to the patient and noting the way in which he talks about his symptoms. Inflection of voice, facial expression, and attitude may betray important clues as to the meaning of the symptoms to the patient. Thus, listening to this recitation, one discovers not only something about the disease but also something about the patient.

With experience one learns the pitfalls of history taking. What patients relate for the most part are subjective phenomena elusively filtered through minds that vary in their background of past experience. Patients obviously differ widely in their responses to the same stimuli. Their remarks are variably colored by fear of disease, disability, and death and by concern over the consequences of illness to their families. And as if these difficulties were not enough, there are the additional ones created by language barriers, by failing intellectual powers which deprive the subject of accurate recall, or by a disorder of consciousness that makes him unaware of his illness. It is not surprising, then, that even the most careful physician may at times despair of collecting factual data; and often he is forced to proceed with evidence that represents little more than an approximation of the truth.

Viewed in another way, the symptom marks, in the patient's mind, a departure from normal health; in the physician's mind, it initiates a process of inductive and deductive reasoning that culminates in diagnosis. In pondering the various possible explanations of a given symptom or clinical state the physician begins a search for other data, elicited by further questioning of the patient and his family, by physical examination, or by special laboratory tests. The symptoms alone sometimes will provide the most certain clue, as in angina pectoris or epilepsy, where physical findings and laboratory data collected between attacks may give no evidence of the existence of heart or brain disease even when it is manifestly present. In most illnesses, however, the history will not be so decisive, though it may still narrow the number of diagnostic possibilities and guide the subsequent investigation.

It is in the taking of the history that the physician's skill, knowledge, and experience are most clearly in evidence. He has learned from experience how to weigh each given symptom, depending on its nature and the context in which it occurs. He knows when to be incredulous and turn to more reliable sources of information, and he never lets his skepticism blind him to an unusual symptom, a manifestation of some new condition that has previously lain beyond the reach of medical knowledge. Moreover, he knows when to press an interrogation more deeply in a search for further details and when to cast about more broadly, realizing that "disease often tells its secrets in a casual parenthesis." And, finally, he knows how to take advantage of the interview in which the history is gathered to obtain the confidence of his patient and to allay apprehension and fear, the first steps in therapy.

The family history, all too often obtained in a routine, cursory fashion, is a leading tool of clinical genetics and can provide important evidence regarding the nature of the patient's complaints. The use of the family history will be discussed further in Chap. 4, but here it may be pointed out that information regarding symptoms like those of the patient which have occurred in blood relatives, or "run in the family," and knowledge of the ethnic origin of the parents and of consanguinity may be exceedingly helpful. The information must be obtained with tact, however, for patients may be embarrassed by such inquiries. Finally it should be emphasized that the best family history is that which is supported by actual examination of other members of the family. Frequently it is found that some physical deviation from the normal, too subtle to be recognized by a lay person, is quite apparent to the trained observer and that a minor deviation in laboratory data assumes significance when evaluated against a family constellation.

PHYSICAL EXAMINATION

Little need be said about the importance of the physical examination, for early in his training the physician learns that physical signs are the objective and verifiable marks of pathology. The physical sign represents a solid, indisputable fact. However, its significance is enhanced when it confirms a functional or structural change already evidenced by the patient's history. At other times, the physical sign may stand as the only evidence of disease, especially in those cases where the history has been inconsistent and confused or is completely lacking.

If full advantage is to be gotten from the physical examination, it must be performed methodically and thoroughly. Although attention has usually been directed by the history to the offending organ or part of the body, nevertheless the examination must extend to all parts of the body. The patient must be literally scrutinized from top to bottom in an objective search for abnormalities that may yield information concerning present and also future illnesses. Unless the examination procedure is systematic, important parts of it may be forgotten, an error against which even the most skilled clinician must guard. The results of the examination, like the details of the history, should be recorded at the time they are elicited and not hours later when they are subject to the distortions of memory. Many inaccuracies in case study stem from the careless practice of writing or dictating notes long after the examination has terminated.

Skill in physical diagnosis is acquired with experience, but it is not merely technique that determines success in eliciting signs. The detection of a few scattered petechiae or a faint diastolic murmur or a small mass in the abdomen is not a question of keener eyes and ears or more sensitive fingers, but of a mind directed by long experience to be alert to these findings. Skill in physical diagnosis reflects a way of thinking more than a way of doing.

All investigations of the body should be regarded as part of the physical examination. The use of various instruments, such as the ophthalmoscope, sphygmomanometer, galvanometer, microscope, or roentgen tube, are mere extensions of the examination to less accessible structures. Proficiency in their use is part of internal medicine. Tests made on fluids or tissues removed from the patient must be selected carefully; even though the physician may not do the tests, he is responsible for the proper collection of the material and for the interpretation of the results.

INSTRUMENTAL AND LABORATORY EXAMINATIONS

The last century has witnessed the introduction of newer methods of instrumental and laboratory investigation of ever-increasing precision and refinement, and inevitably there has been a drift toward reliance on knowledge gained from these special means of study in the solution of clinical problems. It is essential that one always bear in mind the limitations of these newer methods of examination and their proper use in the practice of medicine. By virtue of their impersonal quality and the complexity of the techniques involved in obtaining them, data secured by instrumental and laboratory methods are frequently surrounded by an aura of authority, without heed to the fact that the data are collected by fallible human beings who are capable of committing

errors of technique, or who may misinterpret the most precise evidence. One must not be misled by the "magic of numbers." Too great emphasis may be placed on minor deviations that may yet lie well within the range of normality. These and other possible errors serve to indicate that laboratory data cannot release the physician from the necessity of careful observation and study of the patient. The wise physician is he who understands the merits and limitations of each source of information, whether it be the history, or the physical examination, or the laboratory investigations. Barring those exigencies that make careful study impracticable or impossible, the history and physical examination should be thorough and painstaking, and the special examinations and laboratory tests should be adequate to furnish what additional information may be necessary. In some cases, it will suffice to use merely the simple tests that should be at the disposal of every practicing physician; in the more obscure cases the full resources of the most advanced teaching hospital may be essential for the successful unraveling of the clinical problem. Moreover, the physician should weigh carefully not only the hazards but also the expense involved in every test that he demands. Every procedure that does not have a specific purpose toward contributing to the management of the patient's illness is a pretentious economic waste resulting from ignorance or callousness or plain charlatanism. Scientific study of a clinical problem does not consist merely of filling a patient's record with endless data. Discrimination in the ordering of laboratory procedures and judgment in appraising the risk and expense of a procedure as against the value of the information to be derived from it are among the criteria by which one estimates the manner in which the art and science of medicine have been fused by the physician.

THE CLINICAL METHOD AND THE SYNDROMIC APPROACH TO DISEASE

The steps described above have as their object the collection of accurate data concerning all the diseases to which human beings are subject, namely, all conditions that "limit life in its powers, enjoyment and duration." But much more is required in making a diagnosis. Each datum must be interpreted in the light of the known facts of anatomy, physiology, and chemistry. The synthesis of these interpretations yields information concerning the affected organ or body system. Further, from the vantage point afforded by such an anatomic diagnosis the physician may then turn to other data, such as the mode of onset and clinical course of the illness, and to the results of laboratory tests, in order to ascertain the nature and degree of physiologic impairment and ultimately the cause of the disease.

All these steps comprise the clinical method, which always proceeds in a series of logical steps. The perceptive student will note certain similarities between the clinical method and the scientific method. Each begins with observational data which suggest a series of hypotheses. These latter are tested in the light of further observations, some clinical, others contrived laboratory procedures. Finally, a conclusion is reached, which in science is called a *theory* and in medicine a *working diagnosis*. The modus operandi of the clinical method, like that of the scientific method, cannot be reduced to a single principle or a type of inductive or deductive reasoning. It involves both analysis and synthesis, the essential parts of cartesian logic. The physician does not start with an open mind any more than does the scientist, but with one prejudiced from knowledge of recent cases; and the patient's first statement directs his thinking in certain channels. He must struggle constantly to avoid the bias occasioned by his own attitude, mood, irritability, and interest.

It is particularly in the study of more difficult patients that one observes most clearly the logical order of the clinical method. Anatomic diagnosis regularly precedes etiologic diagnosis. One seldom succeeds in determining the cause and mechanism of a disease before ascertaining which organ has been involved. An intermediate step is syndromic diagnosis. Most physicians attempt consciously or unconsciously to fit a given problem into one of a series of syndromes. The *syndrome*, in essence, is a group of symptoms and signs of disordered somatic function, related to one another by means of some anatomic, physiologic, or biochemical peculiarity of the organism. It embodies a hypothesis concerning the deranged function of an organ, organ system, or tissue. Congestive heart failure, Cushing's disease, and dementia are examples. In congestive heart failure dyspnea, orthopnea, cyanosis, dependent edema, engorged neck veins, pleural fluid, pulmonary râles, and enlargement of the liver are known to be connected by a single pathophysiologic mechanism—failure of the heart, leading to salt and water retention and high venous pressure. In Cushing's disease the moon facies, hypertension, diabetes, and osteoporosis, are the recognized effects of excess corticosteroids acting on many target organs. In dementia deterioration of memory, incoherence in thinking, faulty judgment, etc., are related through a neuroanatomic and a neurophysiologic principle, i.e., all these disordered intellectual functions are related to slow impairment of the function and destruction of the association areas of the cerebrum.

A syndromic diagnosis usually does not indicate the precise cause of an illness, but it greatly narrows the number of possibilities and, thus, suggests whatever further clinical and laboratory studies are required. The derangements of each organ system in human beings are reducible to a relatively small number of syndromes. Diagnosis is greatly simplified if a given clinical problem conforms neatly to a well-defined syndrome. Then one need only turn to a book for a list of the various diseases that may cause it. The search for the cause of an illness that does not conform to a syndrome is much more difficult, for a seemingly infinite number of diseases may then have to be considered. Nevertheless, the principle remains: the clinical method is an orderly intellectual activity which proceeds almost invariably from symptom to sign, to syndrome, and to disease.

3 CARE OF THE PATIENT
The Editors

Enormous strides have taken place during the past few decades in our knowledge of the mechanisms of disease and in the development of powerful and effective treatment agents. The responsibilities of the physician in his management of the patient have correspondingly grown. When little was known about the pathogenesis of a disorder and when, with rare exceptions, practically all the drugs in the huge pharmacopoeias were virtually placebos, when given in the recommended doses, the therapeutic decisions of the physician were seldom of crucial importance. The scientific physician of the time practiced in an era of therapeutic nihilism. He was aware of the worthlessness of most of the drugs that were available to him, and he displayed his skill as a scientific physician by not tampering mischievously with the natural recuperative powers of the body.

Throw out opium, which the Creator himself seems to prescribe, for we often see the scarlet poppy growing in the cornfields as if it were foreseen that where ever there is hunger to be fed there must also be pain to be soothed; throw out a few specifics which our art did not discover and is hardly needed to apply; throw out wine which is a food and the vapors of which produce the miracle of anesthesia, and I firmly believe that if the whole materia medica, as now used, could be sunk to the bottom of the sea it would be all the better for mankind,—and all the worse for the fishes. (O. W. Holmes, 1860)

The discovery during the past several decades of therapeutic agents capable of exerting decisive influence on the course of disease has made it essential that the physician have some understanding of the disturbed functions induced by disease, of the manner of treatment most likely to exert a beneficial effect, and of the risks involved in the proposed therapeutic plan.

Ideally, treatment should strive for the complete restoration of the patient's health, physical and mental.

But medicine contemplates other subjects besides cure. It aims still to postpone the progress of incurable disease and to put off its evil consequences; and, when, they can no longer be postponed, it seeks to render them more tolerable. (Latham)

These goals, which were hardly attainable at the time of Latham, seldom fail to be achieved with at least some degree of success at the present time. Remedies are available. It is the responsibility of the doctor to use them wisely, with due regard for their action, cost, and potential dangers. Every medical procedure, whether diagnostic or therapeutic, contains within it the potentiality of harm, but it would be impossible to afford the patient all the benefits of modern scientific medicine if every reasonable step in diagnosis and therapy were withheld because of the possible risks. "Reasonable" here implies that the physician has weighed the pros and cons of a procedure and has concluded on rational grounds that it is advisable or essential for the relief of discomfort or the cure or amelioration of disease. When the deleterious effects of the physician's action exceed any advantages that could logically have been anticipated, we are justified in designating these effects as *iatrogenic*. It is necessary only to recall the occasionally dangerous or fatal reactions that followed the use of antibiotics given for a trivial respiratory infection, or the gastric hemorrhage or perforation caused by cortisone administered for a mild arthritis, or the fatal homologous serum jaundice that followed needless transfusions of blood or plasma.

It is equally important to consider the harm physicians may do to patients through ill-considered or unjustified remarks. No matter how placid the patient may seem, he approaches the physician with at least some degree of fear and concern. His anxiety can be enhanced by a too serious demeanor, a flippant remark, or an impressive conference. Many persons have been crippled by a cardiac neurosis because the physician expressed a grave prognosis on the basis of a misinterpreted electrocardiogram. The good physician appreciates the fact that he is always in a position to cause injury by his treatment, by his words, and by his behavior.

It is trite to emphasize that the physician must never become so absorbed in the disease that he forgets the patient who harbors it. Nevertheless, this exhortation cannot be repeated too often. As the science of medicine advances, it is all too easy to become so fascinated by the various manifestations of a malady that one disregards the ailing person: his fears, his concerns about his job and the future of his family, the cost of medical care, the specter of economic insecurity, and similar related problems. Treatment of a patient consists in more than the dispassionate confrontation of a disease. It embodies also the exercise of warmth, compassion, and understanding. In the now famous words of Peabody, "one of the essential qualities of the clinician is interest in humanity, for the secret of the care of the patient is in caring for the patient."

THE GROWING ROLE OF PREVENTIVE MEDICINE

There are few areas of medicine which are less dramatic and less appreciated by the patient and by society, but which are of greater importance to a single individual or to an entire population, than is the intelligent practice of preventive medicine. In this aspect of medical practice, the physician deals with individuals or groups who are not overtly ill or whose complaints may be unrelated to the disease process which he wishes to prevent. The increasing use of the periodic physical examination by large companies, unions, other groups, and single individuals and the ready availability of multiphasic screening tests allow the physician to observe and modify disease processes earlier in their course, even prior to their inception. The finding of an elevated arterial blood pressure, blood sugar, serum uric acid or cholesterol in an asymptomatic person provides an unparalleled opportunity to prevent or retard the development of pathologic changes. The physician may, however, need to exert the full prestige of his position to induce an asymptomatic individual to alter his habits or diet or to follow a therapeutic program throughout the rest of his life. However, the compensation for these efforts, in terms of a patient's increased longevity and well-being, is so great that it fully justifies the effort and attention of every physician.

Part Two

Inheritance and Growth

Section 1

Inheritance and Growth

4 INHERITANCE OF HUMAN DISEASE

Victor A. McKusick

Increasingly in recent years the importance of genetics to medicine has come to be appreciated. The relative importance of those conditions in which genetic factors play a leading role has increased as some other etiologic categories of disease, e.g., infectious and nutritional, have become better understood and better treated.

The mutant gene should be considered an etiologic agent. The variability, yet predictability, of the clinical picture in a genetic disorder in which the etiologic agent, a gene, operates from within is very similar to that of an infectious disease in which the etiologic agent invades from the environment. In studying progressive muscular dystrophy of the pseudohypertrophic type, one is not searching for its cause. The cause, a sex-linked recessive gene, is known. It is the mechanism by which the mutant gene produces the clinical manifestations, and methods for interrupting that mechanism, or compensating for it, that are sought by research in muscular dystrophy.

In addition to those conditions for which a single mutant gene in single or double dose is quite directly responsible, and in addition to those disorders which result from chromosomal aberrations, there are many disorders, including some of the commonest affections of man, e.g., atherosclerosis, hypertension, and certain malformations, in which genetic factors and environmental factors collaborate in a complex manner. For a majority of the diseases of man, causation must not be viewed in the rigid sense of a single etiologic agent—a pattern of thinking engendered by the bacteriologic era of medicine—but rather as a nexus, a network of multiple interacting factors among which the genetic factor or factors are always likely to be important. In coronary artery disease, for example, one cannot say that heredity, high-fat diet, cigarette smoking, particular forms of stress, or any other of many postulated factors is *the* cause. The controversy between genetics and environment, nature and nurture, of an early day has now subsided since it is appreciated that both types of factors are important.

The collaboration of heredity and environment is well illustrated by primaquine sensitivity (glucose 6-phosphate dehydrogenase deficiency) in which hemolytic anemia usually occurs only if the genetically predisposed person is exposed to a chemical of a particular type (Chap. 338); and by suxamethonium (succinylcholine) sensitivity (pseudocholinesterase deficiency) in which the genetically predisposed person suffers no obvious ill effects of his defect unless given the agent mentioned as a muscle relaxant in anesthesia.

An important principle of medical genetics is *heterogeneity.* Many genetic disorders which at first were thought to represent single entities have, on close study, been found to consist of two or more fundamentally distinct entities. There are known, for example, to be two types of X-linked hemophilia (Chap. 346), and the genes for these are at loci rather far apart on the X chromosome. Four or five distinct varieties of hereditary intestinal polyposis can be distinguished on clinical grounds. Several recessively inherited varieties of familial goiter are found to result from separate and distinct biochemical defects.

DEFINITIONS. *Congenital* means "present at birth" and is not synonymous with genetic. Genetic factors may or may not be of importance in the cause of individual congenital malformations. On the other hand, hereditary conditions are not necessarily congenital; at least, clinical manifestations may not appear until much later in life. *Hereditary, genetic,* and *heritable* are roughly synonymous. *Familial* and *heredofamilial* were used previously to designate conditions inherited as recessives, i.e., conditions which often occur in multiple siblings with both parents normal. Since a recessive disorder is as genuinely inherited as a dominant one, these terms have little justification. Possibly the only use for the term *familial* is in connection with disorders with a familial aggregation not yet proved to be genetic in basis.

The word *genotype* refers to the genetic constitution of the individual; *phenotype* refers to the outward expression. The phenotype is, of course, what the physician observes, from which he makes deductions about the genotype. The difference is comparable to that between character and reputation—"genotype" and "character" refer to the true nature of the individual, "phenotype" and "reputation" to the apparent nature. *Karyotype* refers to the chromosomal complement of cells. An *ideogram* is a drawing representing the karyotype.

Abiotrophy is a term introduced by Gowers (1902) to describe the behavior of genetic disorders, such as Huntington's chorea and the spinocerebellar ataxias, in which a system functions normally and may be histologically normal up to a stage more or less late in life. The term refers to an inborn defect which leads to premature deterioration of a particular tissue, organ, or system.

SYNDROMES. As with nongenetic conditions, many hereditary disorders have manifold manifestations, the combination of which is referred to as a *syndrome* ("running together"). Genetic syndromes, excluding those like mongoloid idiocy which are due to a chromosomal aberration, appear to be produced by a single mutant gene which has multiple expressions in the phenotype (so-called "pleiotropism") because the protein, enzymatic or other, which is specified by the gene, has wide implications, at least multiple implications, in the economy of the organism. Genetic linkage—the location on the same chromosome of separate genes for each aspect of the syndrome—cannot account for the syndromal relationships observed in clinical medicine.

The investigation of members of a family with regard to a particular disease trait usually begins from a *proband,* or *propositus (-a)*. The proband is the affected person through whom the family is ascertained. The proband is comparable to the *index* case of epidemiologic studies. Often in family studies it is desirable to compare the frequency of a discontinuous trait or the mean level of a biometric trait in the relatives of probands and in the relatives of controls. Data are almost meaningless unless the degree of relationship of the relatives studied is indicated. It means little, for example, to state that 5 percent of the relatives of patients with rheumatoid arthritis have rheumatoid arthritis, but more significance can be attached to the statement that 5 percent of first degree relatives have rheumatoid arthritis. *First degree relatives* are parents, sibs, and offspring; on the average their genetic resemblance to the proband is 0.50, if genetic identity (as in monozygotic twins) is 1.0. *Second degree relatives* are grandparents, aunts and uncles, and grandchildren of the proband; on the average their genetic resemblance to the proband is 0.25.

The aspects of genetics of particular significance to clinical medicine are at least six: (1) cytogenetics, i.e., the study of chromosomes in relation to the phenotype; (2) pedigree patterns, i.e., the behavior in families of single-gene disorders; (3) nature and function of the genetic code; (4) mutation; (5) biochemical aspects of gene action; and (6) the genetics of common disorders (multifactorial inheritance).

CYTOGENETICS IN MAN

It was not until 1956 that the correct chromosome number in man (46) was known and not until 1959 that a microscopically identifiable chromosomal aberration was reported to be the cause of disease in man. These advances were made possible by the introduction of two modifications of technique: (1) the use of colchicine in cell cultures to cause an accumulation of cells in metaphase of mitosis, the stage most favorable for counting the chromosomes; and (2) the use of hypotonic solutions to produce swelling of the nucleus and separation of the chromosomes. The cells studied have been derived from the bone marrow by the usual aspiration technique or from explants of skin or other tissue. Cells grown from the peripheral blood in short-term culture have been particularly useful for family studies and surveys. Use of the mitosis-stimulating properties of phytohemagglutinin is another technique that has facilitated chromosome study. The chromosomes are studied by light microscopy after appropriate fixing and staining (Figs. 4-1 and 4-2).

Mongolism (mongoloid idiocy, Down's syndrome) was found to be characterized by 47 chromosomes, the extra one being one of the smallest autosomes, or nonsex chromosomes (Fig. 4-3). In the *Klinefelter syndrome* it was found that there are 47 chromosomes and a sex chromosome constitution XXY (Fig. 4-4). In the *Turner syndrome* (gonadal aplasia) it was found that there are 45 chromosomes, there being only one sex chromosome, the so-called XO sex chromosome constitution (Fig. 4-5). In both of the latter two cases an abnormality of the sex chromosomes had been suspected because of paradoxic findings on Barr's test of nuclear sex. In the Klinefelter syndrome the subject is ostensibly male but shows the "chromatin-positive" pattern of the normal female; in the Turner syndrome the phenotypic female shows in a majority of cases the "chromatin-negative" pattern of the normal male (Fig. 4-6).

The three conditions above appear to arise through the accident of nondisjunction occurring either during meiosis in one parent (that is, in spermatogenesis or oogenesis) or in the first mitotic cleavage of the zygote. In meiotic nondisjunction both chromosomes of a given pair pass into one cell product rather than separating. Abnormal cells of two types are produced: one with one chromosome too many and one with one chromosome too few. In mongolism the strikingly higher frequency in the offspring of older mothers appears to be due to a higher risk of nondisjunction in older females.

Many other chromosomal aberrations have been discovered. Those which affect the sex chromosomes include XXX, XXXY, XXXXY, XXYY, and XXXX constitutions. Abnormal numbers of X chromosomes are indicated by sex chromatin abnormalities, as indicated in Table 4-1.

The XYY syndrome is of particular significance because the features are, in addition to some degree of mental deficiency, excessive height and behavioral abnormalities leading often to criminality.

Trisomic states (conditions in which, as in mongolism, three chromosomes rather than two of a particular set are present) have been described in which the chromosomes involved are different ones than in mongolism.

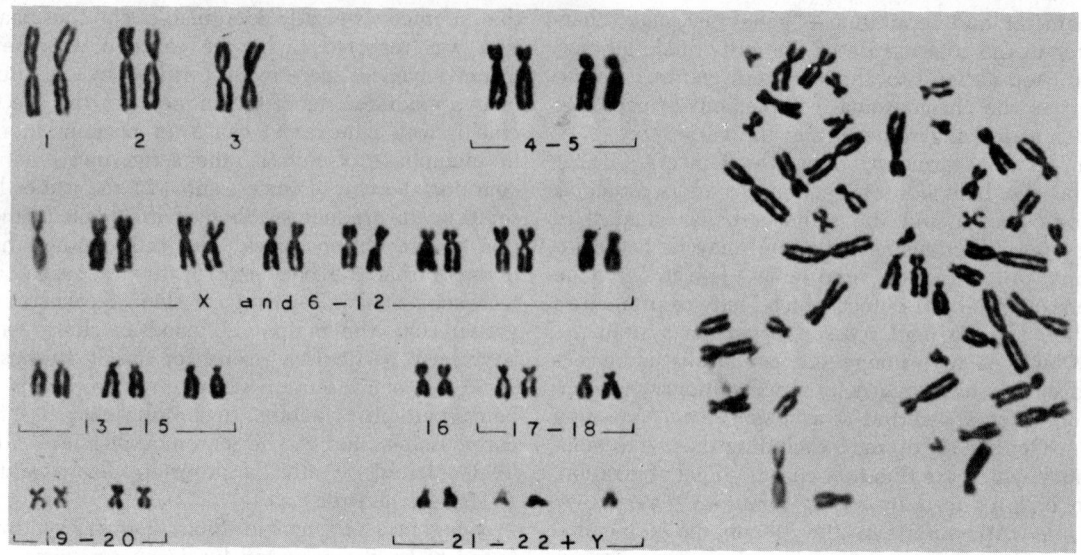

Fig. 4-1. The chromosomes of a normal male. On the right are shown the chromosomes of a single somatic cell in the metaphase stage of cell division. The photographic images of the chromosomes have been cut out and arranged according to descending length and varying arm ratio to form the karyotype shown on the left. The sex chromosomes in this normal male are an X, shown with the 6–12 chromosomes, which it resembles, and a Y, shown near chromosomes 21–22, which it resembles.

Table 4-1. CORRELATIONS OF PHENOTYPE, SEX CHROMATIN, AND SEX CHROMOSOMES

	Sex phenotype	Barr bodies (maximum number per cell)	Sex-chromosome constitution
Normal male......	Male		XY
Testicular feminization syndrome	Female (with testes)		XY
Double Y (or XYY) male..........	Male		XYY
Turner syndrome ..	Female		XO
Normal female	Female		XX
Klinefelter syndrome..........	Male		XXY
Klinefelter syndrome..........	Male		XXYY
Triple X syndrome	Female		XXX
Triple X-Y syndrome..........	Male		XXXY
Tetra X syndrome	Female		XXXX
Tetra X-Y syndrome.........	Male		XXXXY
Penta X syndrome.	Female		XXXXX

The only autosomal trisomies that survive after birth have been those involving chromosome 21 (mongolism), 13, or 18. Nonmosaic autosomal monosomy (only one of a given pair of autosomes is present) must be very rare in living children. About one-fifth of spontaneous abortions show a detectable chromosomal abnormality as the probable "cause" of abortion.

Translocation (displacement of part or all of one chromosome onto another) may be balanced (i.e., a full complement of genetic material is present, although in unusual arrangement), or unbalanced (if excess and/or deficiency of genetic material exists). The most frequent form is probably the D-G translocation which can exist in carriers (with the balanced situation) or in mongoloid idiots (with the unbalanced situation).

Deletion (loss of part of a chromosome) also occurs as the basis of congenital syndromes. The most frequent probably is deletion of part of the short arm of chromosome 5 leading to the *cri du chat* syndrome, so called because of the catlike cry of infants with this abnormality; other features are microcephaly, hypertelorism, and mental retardation.

Mosaicism, with a chromosome abnormality present in only a portion of the cells of the individual, is relatively frequent. It arises through an accident in chromosome mechanics in the early embryo and results in an incomplete or mild form of the syndrome observed with the particular chromosomal abnormality in nonmosaic form.

Estimates of the frequency of selected congenital chromosomal errors are given in Table 4-2.

The relationship of demonstrable changes in the chromosomes to neoplastic disease is under active investigation. In many cases of chronic myelocytic leukemia a con-

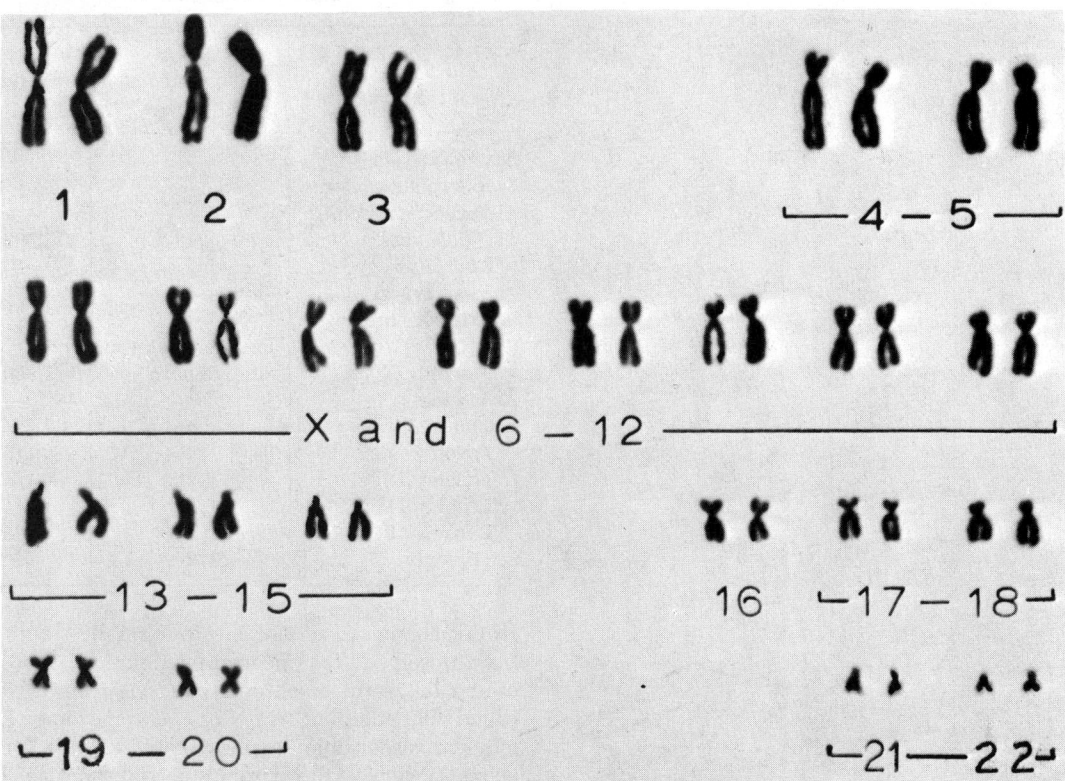

Fig. 4-2. The chromosomes of a normal female. No Y chromosome is present, and two X chromosomes are present with the 6–12 group.

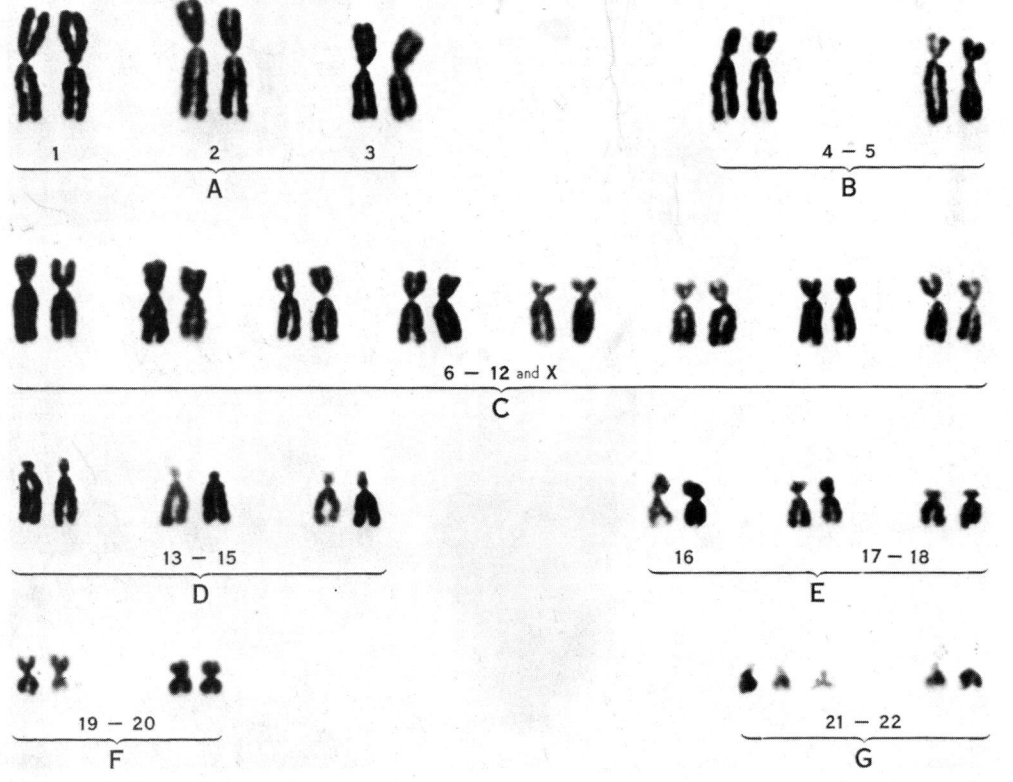

Fig. 4-3. The chromosomes in mongolism. The chromosomal constitution is that of a normal female except for the presence of an extra chromosome in the set numbered 21.

11

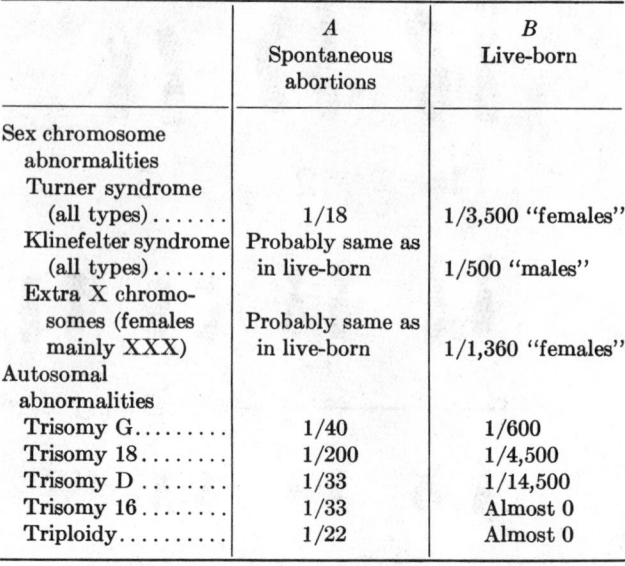

Table 4-2. FREQUENCY OF SELECTED CHROMOSOMAL ABERRATIONS

	A Spontaneous abortions	*B* Live-born
Sex chromosome abnormalities		
Turner syndrome (all types).......	1/18	1/3,500 "females"
Klinefelter syndrome (all types).......	Probably same as in live-born	1/500 "males"
Extra X chromosomes (females mainly XXX)	Probably same as in live-born	1/1,360 "females"
Autosomal abnormalities		
Trisomy G.........	1/40	1/600
Trisomy 18........	1/200	1/4,500
Trisomy D	1/33	1/14,500
Trisomy 16........	1/33	Almost 0
Triploidy..........	1/22	Almost 0

sistent change in one of the four smallest autosomes has been observed. It appears that deletion, or loss, of part of the long arm of chromosome 21, resulting in the so-called Philadelphia (or Ph[1]) chromosome (Fig. 4-7) may be responsible for most cases of this form of leukemia. Whereas the chromosome aberrations leading to abnormalities of sex, soma, and behavior described above are all congenital, the Philadelphia chromosome (which

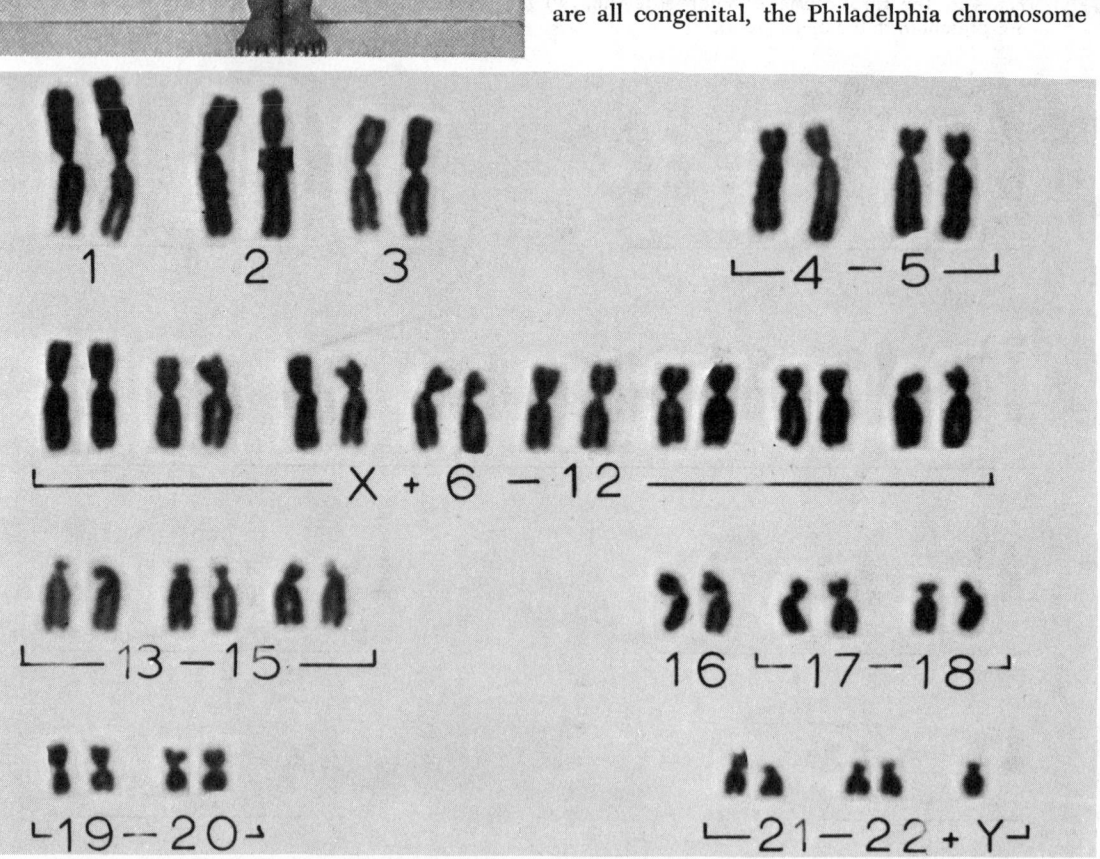

Fig. 4-4. *Upper*, a patient with the Klinefelter syndrome. Note the long legs, gynecomastia, and sparse body hair. *Lower*, the chromosomes in the Klinefelter syndrome. The karyotype is abnormal because of the presence of three sex chromosomes (XXY).

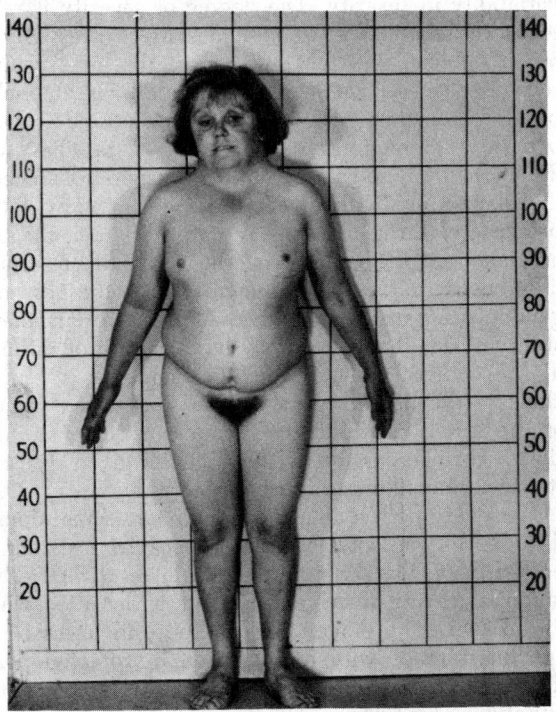

is present only in blood cells) arises in postnatal life through chromosome breakage produced by agents such as radiation and, probably, viruses.

THE BEHAVIOR OF GENETIC DISEASE IN FAMILIES

In accordance with the laws of Mendel, many diseases in man occur in families in a characteristic pattern. These are, for the most part, rare conditions and result from "point mutation" in the genetic material, as will be discussed later. The specific pedigree pattern depends on whether the responsible mutant gene is located on one of the autosomal chromosomes or on an X chromosome. It also depends on whether the effects of the gene are evident in single dose, that is, in the heterozygous state, or whether the gene requires double dosage, or the homozygous state, for its expression. According to the type of chromosome bearing the gene in question, a trait is said to be either *autosomal* or *sex-linked*. Depending on whether expression of the gene occurs in the heterozygous state or only in the homozygous state, a trait is said to be either *dominant* or *recessive*, respectively.

Figure 4-8 presents an idealized pedigree pattern of an *autosomal dominant* trait. Within the limits of chance, half the sons and half the daughters of an affected per-

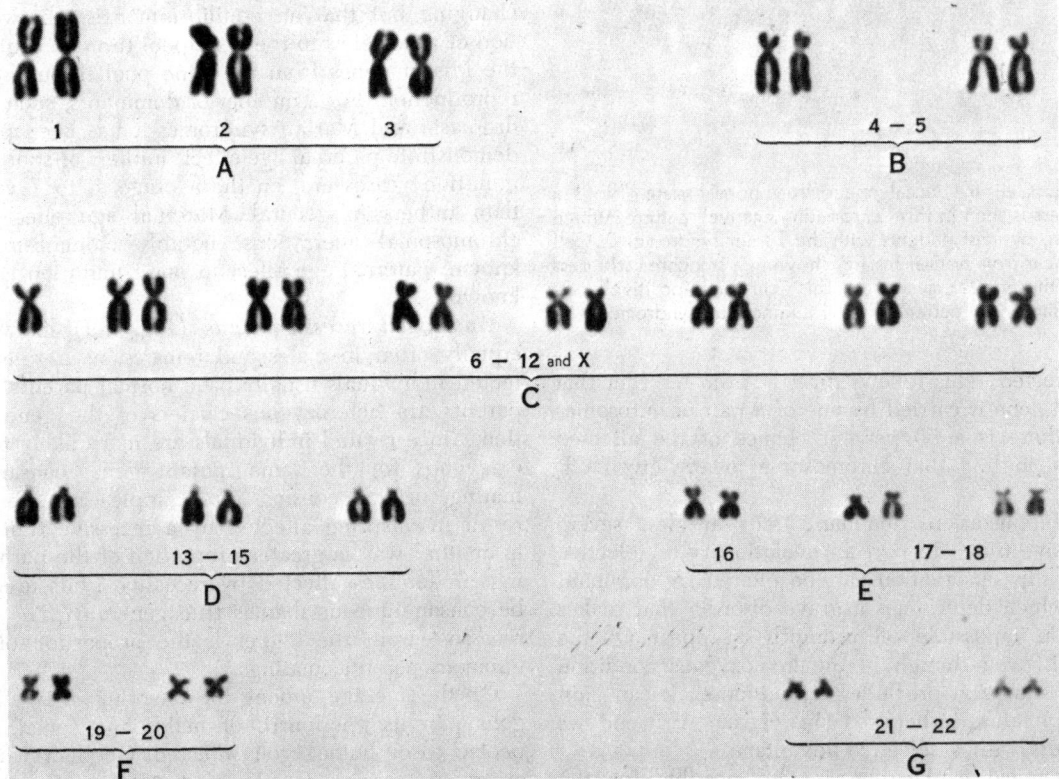

Fig. 4-5. *Upper,* a patient with the Turner syndrome. Note the short stature, broad shieldlike chest with wide intermammary distance, hypoplastic mandible, low-set ears, and webbed neck. Note the scar of the operation for resection of coarctation of the aorta. *Lower,* the chromosomes in the Turner syndrome. Only one sex chromosome, an X, is present.

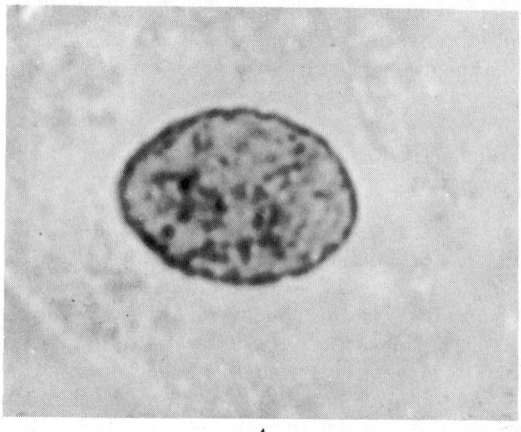

A

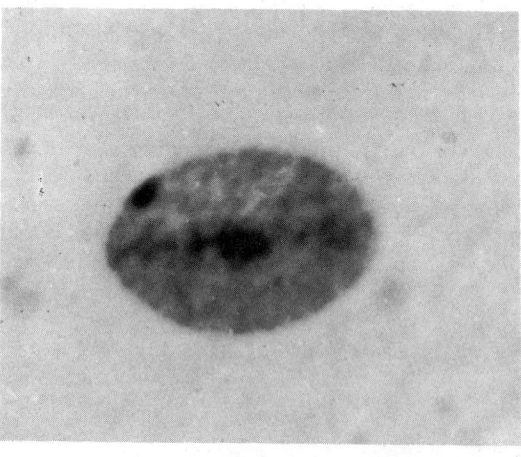

B

Fig. 4-6. *A.* Cell in buccal smear from normal male. No sex chromatin mass is seen in this "chromatin-negative" pattern, which is shown also by most patients with the Turner syndrome. *B.* Cell in buccal smear from normal female, showing a sex chromatin mass adjacent to the nuclear membrane. This "chromatin-positive" pattern is also shown by patients with the Klinefelter syndrome.

Another characteristic of dominant characters is wide variability in severity. The degree of severity is referred to as the *expressivity*. Sometimes the expressivity is so much reduced that the presence of the gene cannot be recognized at all, at least by the methods at one's disposal. When this is the case, the trait is said to be *nonpenetrant*. Sometimes in pedigrees of families with a dominant trait, so-called "skipped" generations occur. In the skipped individual, expressivity is so low that the presence of the gene is not recognizable, i.e., the trait is nonpenetrant in that person. The variability results from differences in the environment and in the rest of the genetic make-up, the *genome*. At least in part the variability of dominant traits may be the result of differences in the "normal" allele which accompanies the mutant allele in the heterozygous affected individual. Evidence of the last is provided when one can demonstrate that sib-sib correlations for behavior of the given disease are stronger than the parent-sibling correlations.

Not every person afflicted with an autosomal dominant disorder has an affected parent because a certain proportion have the abnormal gene as a result of fresh mutation occurring in a germ cell of either the father or the mother. The graver the condition, in terms of average interference with reproduction by affected persons, the larger is the proportion of cases which represent new mutation. This follows from the plausible assumption that the frequency of the particular dominant gene is not changing but that an equilibrium exists between addition of new genes to the gene pool through mutation and the loss of genes from the gene pool through failure of reproduction. For a number of dominants, such as achondroplasia and Marfan syndrome, it has been possible to demonstrate paternal age effect. Fathers of sporadic (new mutation) cases are, on the average, 5 to 7 years older than fathers in general. Maternal age effect in some chromosomal aberrations, notably mongolism, is well known; paternal age effect in point mutation is less well known.

Autosomal recessive traits (Fig. 4-9) likewise occur equally often in males and females, as a rule. The affected individuals usually have normal parents, but both parents are heterozygous carriers of the gene in question. Since related individuals are more likely to be heterozygous for the same mutant gene, consanguineous mating, of first cousins, for example, is more likely to result in offspring affected by a recessive trait. Viewed in another way, a greater proportion of the parental matings in families affected by recessive traits are likely to be consanguineous than is true generally. The rarer the recessive trait, the higher is the proportion of consanguineous parental matings.

On the average, among the offspring of two heterozygous parents one-fourth of males and females are expected to be homozygous-affected. One-half will be heterozygous carriers for the trait, and one-fourth will be homozygous for the normal allele.

Affected sibships can usually be ascertained only through the appearance of one or more affected members. Since there is no way to recognize those matings

son are effected. This follows directly from the fact that the mutant gene is carried by one of a pair of autosomes and that there is a 50 percent chance of the affected parent contributing that chromosome to any given offspring.

As a generalization, dominant traits are less severe than recessive traits. In part an evolutionary or selective reason for this observation can be offered. A dominant mutation which determines a grave disorder that makes reproduction impossible will promptly disappear. On the other hand, even though in the homozygous condition a recessive mutation precludes reproduction, it can gain wide dissemination in heterozygous carriers, if it endows these carriers with a selective advantage.

A biochemical explanation is also possible for the greater severity of recessive traits. One might anticipate a greater derangement when both genes specifying a particular protein, let us say an enzyme, are of mutant type than if only one is mutant.

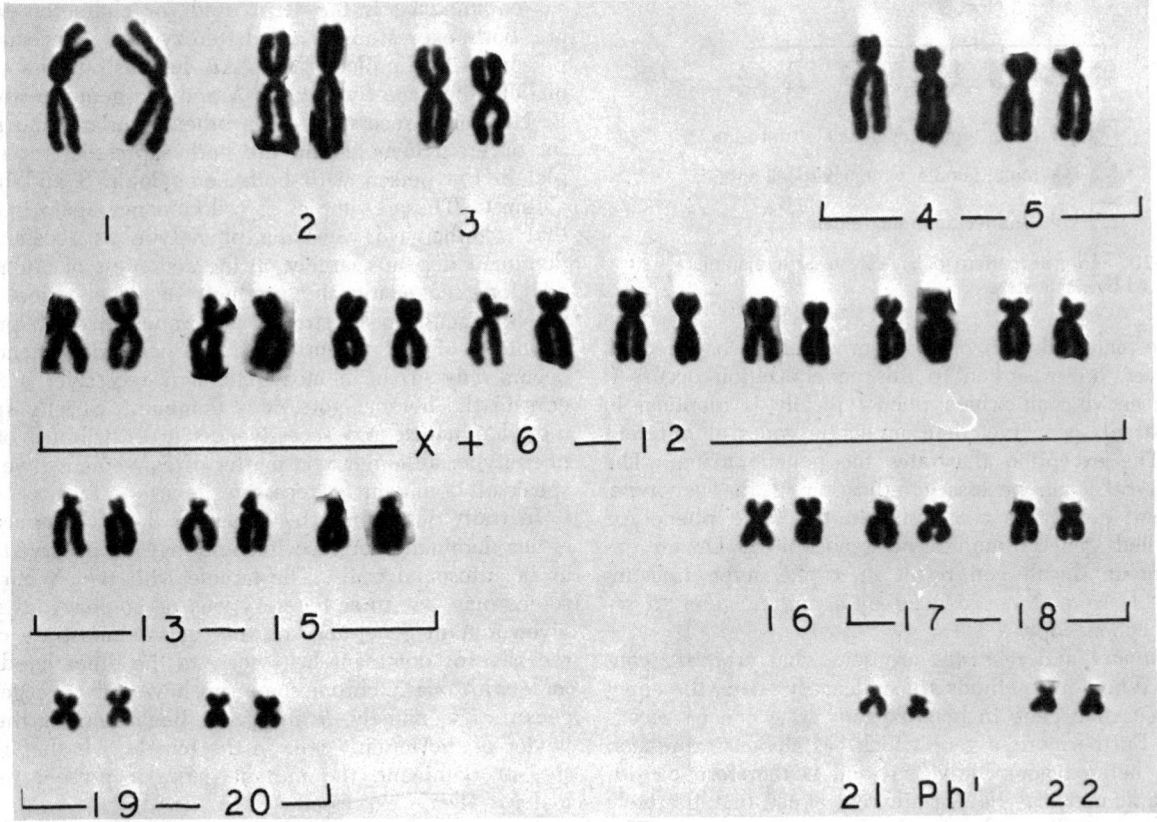

Fig. 4-7. The chromosomes of bone marrow from a female with chronic myelocytic leukemia. One chromosome 21, marked Ph¹ for Philadelphia chromosome, lacks part of its long arm.

of two appropriately heterozygous parents who are so fortunate as to have no affected children, a collection of sibships containing at least one affected child is a biased sample. More than the expected one-fourth of all children in ascertainable families will be affected. Methods for correcting for the so-called "bias of ascertainment" are available.

If an individual affected by a recessive trait marries a homozygous normal person, none of the children will be affected, but all will be heterozygous carriers. If an individual affected by a recessive trait marries a heterozygous carrier, one-half of the offspring are likely to be

affected. A pedigree pattern superficially resembling that of a dominant trait can result. It was previously thought that two genetic forms of alkaptonuria (Chap. 102) exist —one inherited as an autosomal recessive and one as an autosomal dominant. Closer investigation reveals that the apparently dominant form was the same disease as the clearly recessive one. Because of much inbreeding, homozygous affected individuals frequently mated with heterozygous carriers and a quasi-dominant pedigree pattern resulted.

When two individuals affected by the same recessive

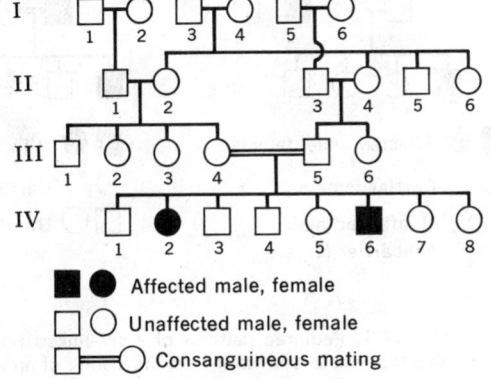

■● Affected male, female
□○ Unaffected male, female
□══○ Consanguineous mating

Fig. 4-8. Pedigree pattern of an autosomal dominant trait.

Fig. 4-9. Pedigree pattern of an autosomal recessive trait.

■● Affected male, female
□○ Unaffected male, female

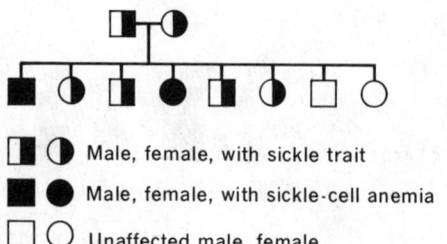

Fig. 4-10. Pedigree pattern of an autosomal intermediate trait as illustrated by sickle state.

disease mate, all their offspring are likely to be affected. However, an exception to this generalization occurs if the recessive trait which phenotypically is identical in two parents is in fact determined by genes at different loci. The exception illustrates the genetic axiom: The phenotype is no necessary indication of the genotype. Different genotypes can result in the same phenotype (so-called genetic mimics or genocopies). Or an environmental insult can result in a phenotype indistinguishable from that produced by a mutant gene (a so-called "phenocopy").

Dominant and *recessive* are somewhat arbitrary concepts. When our methods are sufficiently acute, the effect of a recessive gene in heterozygous state can be recognized. Furthermore, a gene which has obvious expression in the heterozygous individual and is therefore considered dominant may have a different effect, quantitatively and even qualitatively, in the homozygous state. The gene for sickle hemoglobin and the states referred to as sickle-cell anemia and sickle-cell trait illustrate the arbitrary nature of the distinction. If sickle-cell anemia is considered as the phenotype, then the condition is recessive, since a homozygous state of the gene is required. The phenotype sickling, however, is dominant since the gene in heterozygous state is expressed. *Intermediate inheritance* is the term sometimes applied to this type of pedigree pattern (Fig. 4-10).

Codominance is the term used for characters which are both expressed in the heterozygote. For example, persons with the blood group AB demonstrate the effects of both the gene for antigen A and the gene for antigen B. Neither is recessive to the other. Similarly the genes for different hemoglobins are both expressed, for example, in the person with both hemoglobin S and hemoglobin C. These examples of codominance again indicate that whether we view the phenotype as recessive or dominant depends largely on the acuteness of our methods for recognizing the products of gene action. This whole discussion illustrates the importance of precise definition of the phenotype. If the particular phenotype occurs only in the homozygote, it is recessive; if it occurs in the heterozygote, it is dominant. Strictly speaking, dominance and recessiveness are attributes of the phenotype, although as a matter of convenience we may speak of dominant or recessive genes.

In traits determined by genes on the X chromosome, either dominance or recessiveness may be observed, just as in autosomal traits. The female with two X chromosomes may be either heterozygous or homozygous for a given mutant gene, and the trait can demonstrate either recessive or dominant behavior. On the other hand, the male with one X chromosome can have only one genetic constitution, namely, *hemizygous*. Regardless of the behavior of the mutant gene in the female, whether recessive or dominant, the mutant gene, if present in the male, is always expressed.

An important characteristic of sex-linked inheritance, both dominant and recessive, is the absence of male-to-male (that is, father-to-son) transmission of the disease. This is a necessary result of the fact that the male contributes his X chromosome to all his daughters but to none of his sons.

Sex-linked (X-linked) recessive inheritance (Fig. 4-11) is illustrated in a classic manner by hemophilia. The pedigree pattern of an autosomal dominant trait is a horizontal one, with affected persons in successive gen-

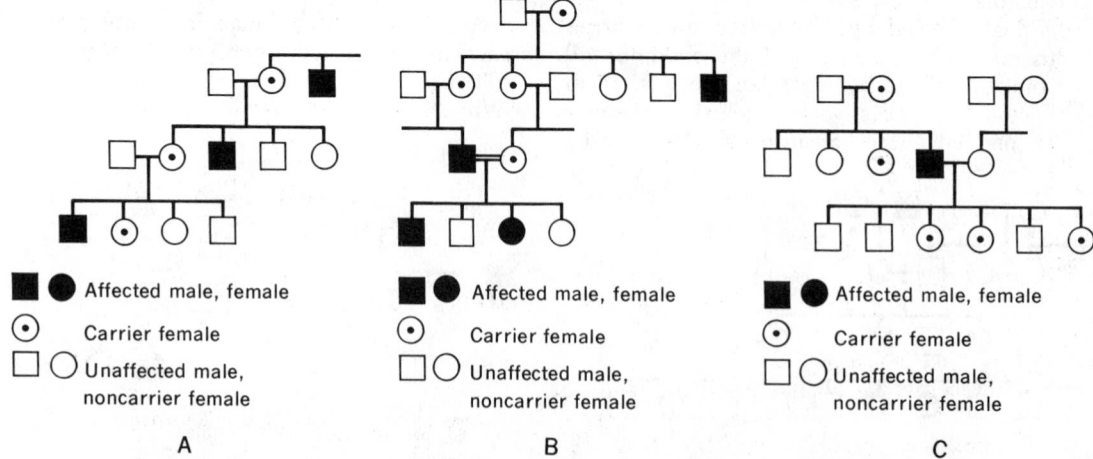

A   B   C

Fig. 4-11. Pedigree patterns of a sex-linked recessive trait. *A.* Note the "oblique" pattern. *B.* An affected female can result from the mating of an affected male and a carrier female, as in the case of a consanguineous marriage shown here. *C.* An affected male mating with a normal, noncarrier female has all normal sons and all carrier daughters.

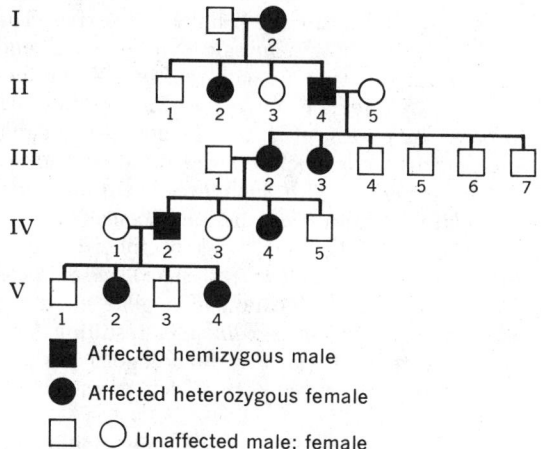

■ Affected hemizygous male

● Affected heterozygous female

□ ○ Unaffected male; female

Fig. 4-12. Pedigree pattern of a sex-linked dominant trait.

erations. The pedigree pattern of an autosomal recessive trait tends to be a vertical one, with affected persons confined to a single generation. The pedigree pattern of a sex-linked recessive character tends to be an oblique one because of transmission to the sons of normal carrier sisters of affected males. Bateson compared this pattern to the knight's move in chess. Tracing sex-linked recessive characters through many generations is often difficult because the patronymic of affected persons tends to change with each generation.

To have hemophilia a female must be homozygous for this recessive gene. She must have received a gene for hemophilia from each parent. Such can occur, and has been observed, when a hemophiliac male marries a carrier female (Fig. 4-11B). As with other recessive traits this homozygous state is more likely to result from consanguineous matings. A hemophiliac female may also occur if a carrier mother is impregnated by a mutant sperm from a normal father, or if the phenotypic female has in fact an XO sex chromosome constitution (the Turner syndrome) or an XY constitution (the syndrome of testicular feminization). (In these comments reference is, of course, made to sex-linked recessive hemophilia A and B and not to other hemophilioid states which occur equally frequently in males and females. Also not considered is the rare possibility that unfortunate lyonization, as described below, in a heterozygous female has resulted in a majority of the cells which produce antihemophilic factor having the mutant-bearing X chromosome as the genetically active one.)

A hemophiliac male can have gotten the hemophilia gene *only* from his mother and can transmit it only to his daughters but to none of his sons. *All* daughters of a hemophiliac male are carriers (Fig. 4-11C).

In man one can enumerate more than sixty other diseases inherited as sex-linked recessives, including such significant entities as primaquine sensitivity (Chap. 338), the Duchenne type of progressive muscular dystrophy (Chap. 376), and agammaglobulinemia (Chap. 69). In some, for example, primaquine sensitivity and nephrogenic diabetes insipidus, a partial defect can be dem-

onstrated in the heterozygous female carrier, and one might prefer to call the inheritance sex-linked intermediate. In another condition, choroideremia, hemizygous males, but only the males, have severe impairment of vision, and from this point of view the disease is a sex-linked recessive; but the heterozygous female carriers show striking changes in the fundus oculi on ophthalmoscopy, even though vision is unaffected.

At least one common trait, colorblindness, is inherited as a sex-linked recessive. It is sufficiently frequent (about 8 percent of white males are colorblind) that the occurrence of homozygous colorblind females is no great rarity.

In sex-linked (*X-linked*) *dominant inheritance* both females and males are affected and both males and females transmit the disorder to their offspring, just as in autosomal dominant inheritance. Superficially the pedigree patterns in the two types of inheritance are similar, but there is a critical difference (Fig. 4-12). In sex-linked dominant inheritance, although the affected female transmits the trait to half her sons and half her daughters, the affected male transmits it to *none* of his sons and to *all* his daughters. Furthermore, in a series of cases females are expected to occur twice as often as males. One of the best studied sex-linked dominant traits is vitamin D–resistant rickets, or hypophosphatemic rickets (Chap. 83). In this condition the hemizygous affected male tends to have more severe clinical involvement than does the heterozygous affected female.

One common trait is inherited as an X-linked dominant: the Xg(a+) blood group. In due course, antisera that directly identify the Xg(a−) blood group will probably be found. These will then be considered co-dominant traits.

Some rare conditions are thought to be inherited as X-linked dominants lethal in the hemizygous male. The characteristics (Fig. 4-13) are (1) occurrence only in females (who are heterozygous for the mutant gene), (2) transmission from affected mother to half her daughters, (3) increased frequency of abortion (male fetus being lost) by affected women. Conditions which appear

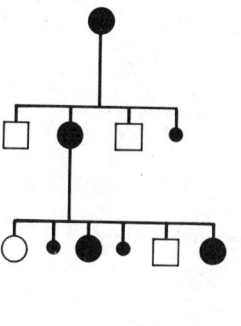

● ○ Affected and unaffected female

□ Unaffected male

● Abortion

Fig. 4-13. Pedigree pattern of a sex-linked dominant trait lethal in the hemizygous male.

to have this mode of inheritance include incontinentia pigmenti, focal dermal hypoplasia, and the orofaciodigital (OFD) syndrome. A male with the last condition was found to be no exception to X-linked dominant, male-lethal inheritance, because in fact he was an instance of XXY Klinefelter syndrome.

Understanding of the behavior of X-linked traits and interpretation of findings in (1) females heterozygous for X-linked genes and (2) persons with an abnormal complement of X chromosomes have been greatly advanced by the *Lyon hypothesis*. There is now good evidence that at an early stage in development one X chromosome of the female becomes relatively inactive genetically (Fig. 4-14). The inactive X chromosome forms the *Barr body*. In each cell it is a random matter whether the X chromosome derived from the mother or that derived from the father is the one that becomes inactive. Once the "decision" is made in a given cell, however, the same X chromosome remains inactive in all descendants of that cell. The adult female is, therefore, a mosaic of two types of cells, those with the mother's X active and those with the father's X active.

The Lyon hypothesis is thought to account for these findings: (1) Heterozygous females tend to vary widely in expression of X-linked recessive genes. As an extreme case, females heterozygous for the hemophilia gene have clinical hemophilia, if most of the pertinent anlage cells destined to produce antihemophilic globulin have the X chromosome with the hemophilia gene active. (2) A mosaic pattern is observed in females heterozygous for traits such as ocular albinism, an X-linked recessive. The fundi in such females show a mosaic of pigmented and unpigmented areas. (3) Persons with multiple X chromosomes, e.g., the XXX female, have two Barr bodies. All X chromosomes in excess of 1 are inactivated (Table 4-1). These persons have much less drastic abnormalities than would be expected with such excess chromosomal material, if relative inactivation did not occur.

Occurrence of the following types of inheritance in man is uncertain: (1) *holandric (all-male) inheritance*, resulting from the possible location of a gene on the Y chromosome, and (2) *partial sex-linkage*, resulting from the location of a gene on possibly homologous parts of the X and Y chromosomes between which crossing over might occur.

Before leaving sex-linked inheritance, one should note the distribution between sex-linked inheritance and sex-influenced (or sex-limited) autosomal inheritance. Baldness appears to be such a sex-influenced autosomal trait. In man baldness is inherited as an autosomal dominant, but in women for baldness to occur the gene must be in homozygous state, that is, in women baldness behaves like a recessive. In women who develop masculinizing tumors of the ovary, baldness can occur if the genotype is proper. As another example, one can imagine a mutant gene whose sole effect was that of preventing lactation in the female. Even though it were located on an autosomal chromosome, it would not have expression in the male. Idiopathic hemochromatosis (Chap. 107) results from the pathologic effects of excessive accumula-

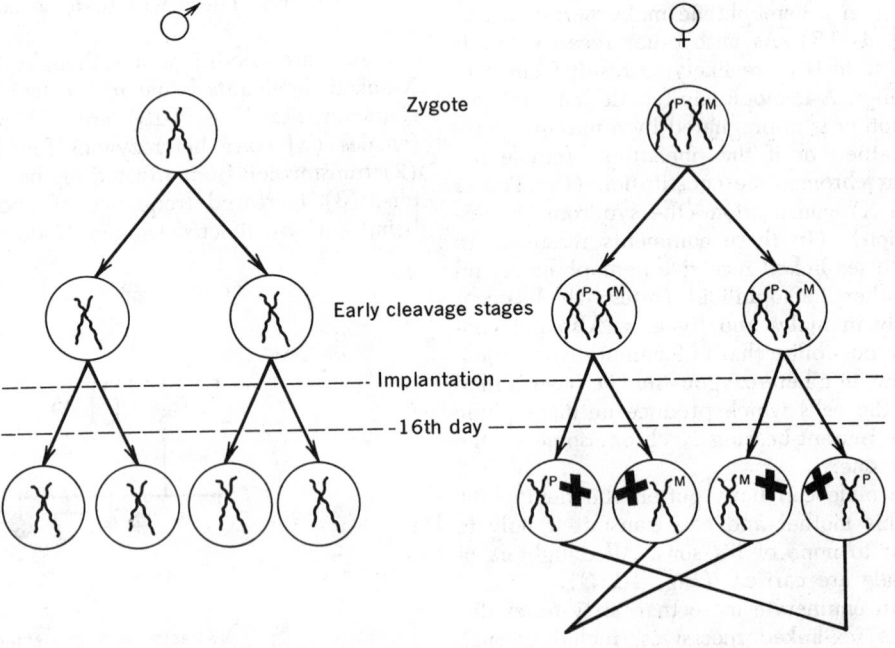

Fig. 4-14. Schematic representation of the phenomenon underlying the Lyon hypothesis. In the normal female, early in embryogenesis (probably soon after implantation) one X chromosome in each cell becomes inactive. Once it has been "decided" whether the maternal (M) or paternal (P) X chromosome will be the inactive one, all descendants of that cell "abide by the decision."

tions of iron within the body, probably as a result of a hereditary defect in the intestinal mechanism regulating iron absorption. Although the inheritance seems to be autosomal dominant, females are rather rarely affected because they have a safety valve on excessive iron accumulation—menstruation and pregnancy.

Note the difficulties in distinguishing sex-linked recessive inheritance from sex-limited autosomal dominant inheritance, if the nature of the disease is such that reproduction of affected males does not occur. The syndrome of testicular feminization (Chap. 97) is an example. The affected individuals are genetic males but, because of endorgan unresponsiveness to androgens, female external genitalia and all the secondary sex characters of the female develop. The affected male does not reproduce and normal females are carriers. The pedigree pattern is precisely that of a sex-linked recessive trait. However, the inheritance can equally well be sex-linked autosomal dominant. In diseases too severe to permit reproduction of affected males—the Pelizaeus-Merzbacher disease (a form of cerebral degeneration), the Duchenne variety of muscular dystrophy (Chap. 376), one variety of gargoylism (Chap. 399)—there is on the basis of pedigree patterns no way to distinguish sex-linked and sex-limited inheritance.

GENETIC COUNSELING. Familiarity with the patterns of disease is useful in diagnosis; if the pedigree pattern is consistent with the mode of inheritance usual for a suspected entity, the diagnosis of that entity is thereby strengthened. Knowing what individuals in a kindred are at risk, one can watch for the earliest signs of hereditary disease.

Furthermore, familiarity with pedigree patterns is essential to genetic counseling. The risk of having an affected child can be stated as 1 in 2 for a person affected by a dominant trait and as 1 in 4 for a couple which has already had a child affected by a recessive disease. For the sister of a male affected by a sex-linked recessive trait the risk of being a carrier is (unless the affected brother represents a new mutation) 1 in 2, of having an affected son one-half of that, or 1 in 4, and the risk of any affected child (considering both sexes) one-half of that, or 1 in 8.

In connection with statements of mendelian risk, it should be made clear to the consultand (person seeking genetic counseling) that the figure is a probability. Parents with one child with cystic fibrosis may take the statement of "1 in 4" to mean that they had their one affected and can now have three children who will be normal. The analogy to tossing coins is useful; with each toss of a true coin the chance of "heads" is 50 percent regardless of the result of earlier tosses. "Chance has no memory."

If a given condition is regularly inherited as a dominant, and if one can be certain that one parent does not have the condition in *forme fruste*, then the risk to later born children is virtually nil. It can be shown that for a rare X-linked recessive disorder of such a nature that the affected males do not reproduce—Duchenne muscular dystrophy is such a condition—about one-third of all cases will be the result of fresh mutation in the X chromosome contributed to the affected male offspring by the mother, and in the other two-thirds of cases the mother will be a heterozygous carrier of the mutation which occurred in an earlier generation. If by chance the carrier female has only one affected son and no affected relative, such as a brother, it is impossible to tell from the pedigree whether she is a carrier or not. Special tests for carrier status for various X-linked disorders have been devised. None is completely discriminatory and probably never can be because of the considerations of the Lyon hypothesis. Screening for heterozygous carriers for X-linked recessives is much more worthwhile than screening for carriers of autosomal recessives. Any X-linked carrier female has a 50 percent chance of having an affected son regardless of the genotype of her husband. An autosomal carrier has a one-fourth chance of having an affected child only if he or she marries another carrier.

Other genetic considerations such as the severity of the disease in question, including its severity in the specific family, must be included in the evaluation. Only the risks should be stated to the persons seeking counsel. The decision as to what action they should follow must be theirs and must take account of factors such as economic status and emotional fortitude. Socially valuable traits partially determined by genetic constitution may be present in the family and outweigh the disadvantage of a mutant gene.

Often the statement of risks is a relief to the persons involved and is not disturbing. For example, a young man with pseudoxanthoma elasticum (Chap. 398), an autosomal recessive trait, was relieved to learn that the likelihood that his children by an unrelated wife would be affected by the severe eye involvement and tendency to hemorrhage is essentially nil. In families affected by a clear-cut, nearly fully penetrant autosomal dominant trait normal persons are sometimes surprised to learn, and considerably relieved, that there is virtually no risk of their offspring being affected.

Genetic counseling in common disorders of multifactor causation presents special problems, which are discussed later.

NATURE AND FUNCTION OF THE GENETIC CODE

The gene is DNA, deoxyribonucleic acid. The function of many genes is to specify the sequence of amino acids that make up a polypeptide chain in a protein, either enzymatic or structural. The code word, or codon, for each amino acid is three-lettered, being spelled in one of four purine or pyrimidine bases: adenine, thymine, guanine, and cytosine (see Table 4-3). The principle of colinearity of the triplet code words in the DNA of the gene and the amino acids in the protein specified by that gene is now well established.

The triplet code for each of twenty specific amino acids is shown in Table 4-3. Messenger RNA (ribonucleic

Table 4-3. THE GENETIC CODE

Second Nucleotide

	A or U		G or C		T or A		C or G		Third nucleotide
A or *U*	**AAA** *UUU* } Phe		**AGA** *UCU*		**ATA** *UAU* } Tyr		**ACA** *UGU* } Cys		A or *U*
	AAG *UUC*		**AGG** *UCC* } Ser		**ATG** *UAC*		**ACG** *UGC*		G or *C*
	AAT *UUA* } Leu		**AGT** *UCA*		**ATT** *UAA* } Stop		**ACT** *UGA* Stop		T or *A*
	AAC *UUG*		**AGC** *UCG*		**ATC** *UAG*		**ACC** *UGG* Trp		C or *G*
G or *C*	**GAA** *CUU*		**GGA** *CCU*		**GTA** *CAU* } His		**GCA** *CGU*		A or *U*
	GAG *CUC* } Leu		**GGG** *CCC* } Pro		**GTG** *CAC*		**GCG** *CGC* } Arg		G or *C*
	GAT *CUA*		**GGT** *CCA*		**GTT** *CAA* } Gln		**GCT** *CGA*		T or *A*
	GAC *CUG*		**GGC** *CCG*		**GTC** *CAG*		**GCC** *CGG*		C or *G*
T or *A*	**TAA** *AUU*		**TGA** *ACU*		**TTA** *AAU* } Asn		**TCA** *AGU* } Ser		A or *U*
	TAG *AUC* } Ile		**TGG** *ACC*		**TTG** *AAC*		**TCG** *AGC*		G or *C*
	TAT *AUA*		**TGT** *ACA* } Thr		**TTT** *AAA* } Lys		**TCT** *AGA* } Arg		T or *A*
	TAC *AUG* Met		**TGC** *ACG*		**TTC** *AAG*		**TCC** *AGG*		C or *G*
C or *G*	**CAA** *GUU*		**CGA** *GCU*		**CTA** *GAU* } Asp		**CCA** *GGU*		A or *U*
	CAG *GUC* } Val		**CGG** *GCC* } Ala		**CTG** *GAC*		**CCG** *GGC* } Gly		G or *C*
	CAT *GUA*		**CGT** *GCA*		**CTT** *GAA* } Glu		**CCT** *GGA*		T or *A*
	CAC *GUG*		**CGC** *GCG*		**CTC** *GAG*		**CCC** *GGG*		C or *G*

The DNA codons appear in boldface type; the complementary RNA codons are in italics. A = adenine, C = cytosine, G = guanine, T = thymine, U = uridine (replaces thymine in RNA). In RNA, adenine is complementary to thymine of DNA; uridine is complementary to adenine of DNA; cytosine is complementary to guanine, and vice versa. "Stop" = punctuation. The amino acids are abbreviated as follows:

Ala = alanine
Arg = arginine
Asn = asparagine
Asp = aspartic acid
Cys = cysteine
Gln = glutamine
Glu = glutamic acid
Gly = glycine
His = histidine
Ile = isoleucine

Leu = leucine
Lys = lysine
Met = methionine
Phe = phenylalanine
Pro = proline
Ser = serine
Thr = threonine
Trp = tryptophane
Tyr = tyrosine
Val = valine

acid), in which the nucleotides are complementary to those of DNA so that it is a negative copy of the DNA, conveys the blueprint for amino acid sequence from DNA on a chromosome in the nucleus to the site of protein synthesis on the ribosomes in the cytoplasm (Fig. 4-15). The code dictionary summarized in Table 4-3 was deduced from studies of the messenger RNA code, in which uridine substitutes for thymine. In addition to ribosomal RNA and messenger RNA, a third type, transfer or soluble RNA, is involved in the assemblage of amino acids into polypeptide chains. The process by which RNA is copied from DNA is called *transcription;* the process by which the RNA-DNA blueprint determines the amino acid sequence of a protein is called *translation* (Fig. 4-15).

The limits of the gene have become clearer. As a functional unit, called by Seymour Benzer the *cistron,* the gene is that portion of DNA responsible for specification of a single polypeptide and a *locus* is physically that portion of the linearly arranged genetic material (DNA)

occupied by the cistron or gene. The alternative forms of the gene which occur at the same locus are called *alleles.* For example, the genes for A, B, and O blood types are multiple alleles at one locus. Within a locus there are many mutable sites. Obviously if the gene at a locus is responsible for specifying all the many amino acids in a complex protein, many base pairs are vulnerable to mutation. This much smaller unit is called by Benzer the *muton.* The genetic unit as revealed by recombination is referred to as the *recon.*

The normal process of development occurs by differential gene action; i.e., by activity of some genes but not of others in particular tissues at particular stages. The mechanism controlling differential gene activity, what switches one gene on and another off at a particular stage, is unknown. Dramatic examples of differential gene function are reflected by the shift from synthesis of embryonic hemoglobin to fetal hemoglobin in the first trimester and from fetal hemoglobin to adult hemoglobin in the first months of extrauterine life.

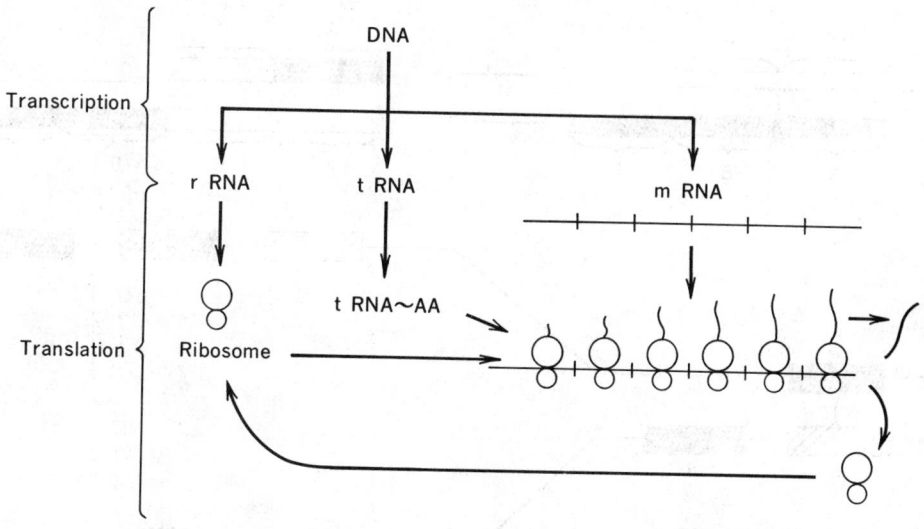

Fig. 4-15. Schema of protein synthesis. (*Courtesy, Dr. Irving M. London*)

MUTATION

This term means change in the genetic material. At least three classes of mutation must be considered. When used without further specification, the term usually refers to "point mutation," that is, change in a single base with substitution of one for another. As seen in Table 4-3, change in DNA from CTT to CAT causes a substitution of valine for glutamic acid in the product protein. This change is the one which occurs in the beta chain of sickle hemoglobin. Similarly, a change from CTT to TTT causes substitution of lysine for glutamic acid, the situation in hemoglobin C. It was first reported that a variant hemoglobin, called Hb I, had lysine (the sixteenth amino acid in the alpha chain) replaced by aspartic acid. Francis Crick insisted, however, that this is not true because change in a single base cannot result in this amino acid substitution. When the matter was re-investigated, it was found that, in fact, glutamic acid is substituted for lysine, a change produced by a single base substitution.

A second class of mutation is that which results in the gross chromosomal abnormalities discussed in the next section. This class includes (1) abnormalities of chromosome number, e.g., missing or supernumerary chromosomes as a result of errors in chromosome segregation during cell division; and (2) abnormalities of chromosome structure, i.e., chromosomal deletions, translocations, inversions, and so on, as a result of chromosome breakage.

A third class of mutation results from nonhomologous pairing and unequal crossing over, as diagrammed in Fig. 4-16. During the meiotic process in gametogenesis, homologous chromosomes pair, but if the matching is not precise, unequal crossing over occurs. The result is either duplication (Fig. 4-16a) of genetic material or deletion. Gene duplication, like the other forms of mutation, has been demonstrably important in evolution. It is

a process by which an organism can experiment with new mutations in one copy of the duplicated gene while retaining an essential function of the original gene. The separate genes that specify the various polypeptide chains of hemoglobin (the beta chain of adult hemoglobin A, the delta chain of adult hemoglobin A_2, the gamma chain of fetal hemoglobin, the epsilon chain of embryonic hemoglobin, and the alpha chain of all four of these hemoglobins) as well as the gene that specifies the single polypeptide chain of myoglobin appear to have evolved from a primordial common ancestral gene through the process of gene duplication and subsequent independent mutation in the separate genes.

Nonhomologous pairing with unequal crossing over also can cause deletion of part of a gene or of part of two contiguous genes. Study of the amino acid sequence in some abnormal hemoglobins suggests that this was the type of mutation responsible, rather than change in a codon which caused a different amino acid to be specified. For example, in hemoglobin Gun Hill five amino acids are missing from the beta chain (amino acids 93 through 97), so that this hemoglobin is only 141 amino acids long rather than 146. Hemoglobin Lepore is another example of mutation due to unequal crossing over. The gene for the beta chain of hemoglobin A and that for the delta chain of hemoglobin A_2 are probably contiguous. In a person with hemoglobin Lepore, the normal beta and delta chains are replaced by a polypeptide chain that has the structure of the delta chain at one end and of the beta chain at the other. As is diagrammed in Fig. 4-16b, a fusion gene specifying a hybrid polypeptide chain of this type could have arisen by unequal crossing over.

BIOCHEMICAL ASPECTS OF GENE ACTION

Biochemical genetics has two parts: One, the chemistry of the genetic material (discussed earlier), had its be-

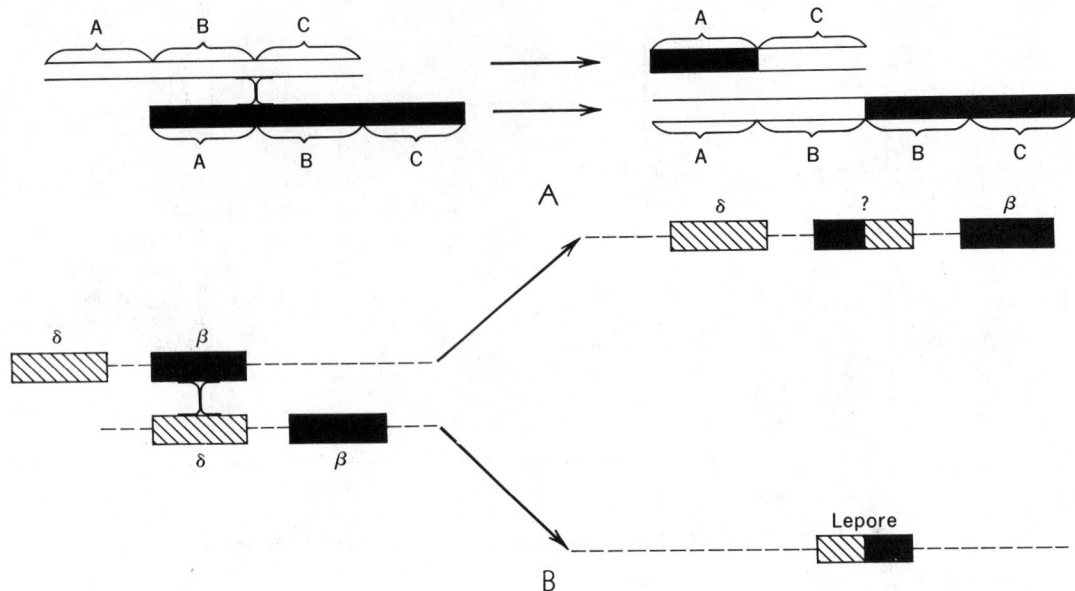

Fig. 4-16. Genetic mutation through nonhomologous pairing and unequal crossing over. *A.* Gene duplication from crossing over between genes. *B.* Creation of a fusion gene through crossing over within a gene, as is thought to have occurred to produce the gene for Lepore hemoglobin.

ginnings with Friedrich Miescher's work on nucleic acid. The second part of biochemical genetics had its origin in the early part of this century, with a physician, Archibald Garrod, and his "inborn errors of metabolism." The disorders he considered were defects in intermediary metabolism resulting from an inherited abnormality of particular enzymes. In its broader implications, biochemical genetics is concerned with the chemical nature of the genetic code and with all the biochemical steps by which that code is translated into an observed characteristic, for example, an inherited disease.

In accordance with the current views, all properties of a protein are a consequence of its amino acid sequence. Probably the proteins specified by genes are not only enzyme proteins but also may be structural proteins, e.g., collagen, or proteins with other functions and properties, such as hemoglobin. The useful concept of "one gene, one enzyme" requires modification to "one gene, one polypeptide," or (see below) "one cistron, one polypeptide."

In the schema outlined earlier, mutation represents a change in the code, that is, a change in the base sequence of DNA. Mutations may be of two types. In "mis-sense" mutations a different amino acid is substituted at a given site in the particular protein, for example, valine for glutamic acid, changing "normal" hemoglobin to sickle hemoglobin. In "non-sense" mutations the change in the base sequence of DNA is such that there is no corresponding amino acid and none of a given protein, e.g., an enzyme, may be found.

The terms borrowed from bacterial genetics, CRM-positive (pronounced "krim-positive") and CRM-negative mutations, correspond to the terms *mis-sense* and *non-sense* mutations, respectively. CRM means cross-reacting material, and in CRM-positive mutations material which

reacts in a normal manner in immunologic tests but is functionally (e.g., enzymatically) ineffective is present. An example of CRM-positive and CRM-negative mutations in man is provided by recessively inherited isolated growth hormone deficiency. Growth hormone is assayed by an immunologic method. Most cases of isolated deficiency have no hormone demonstrable by immunoassay; these are CRM-negative cases. A few have an immunologically demonstrable substance which is apparently ineffective biologically; these are CRM-positive cases.

As stated above, the mutant gene can result in the formation of a different protein or of no protein at all of a given type. If the protein in question is an enzyme, none at all may be formed or an enzyme may be formed which is so impaired in its function that the net effect is the same. In intermediary metabolism such a change can have pathogenetic consequences through any of several mechanisms or through some combination of these. We can represent a hypothetical metabolic process as follows:

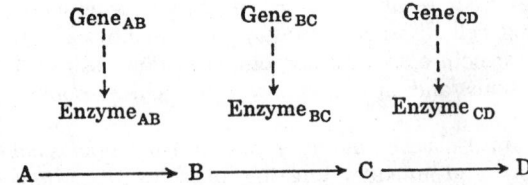

If a mutant form of gene$_{CD}$ results in no formation of enzyme$_{CD}$ or in the formation of functionally defective enzyme, then the effects may be of several types:

1. The disease characteristic may reflect the deficiency of product D:

$$A \longrightarrow B \longrightarrow C \longrightarrow\!\!\!/\!\!/\longrightarrow (D)$$

Albinism (Chap. 104) might be cited as an example; melanin is not formed because of a block in tyrosine metabolism. In several forms of genetic cretinism (Chap. 89), thyroid hormone is not formed because of blocks of this type; in the adrenogenital syndrome (Chap. 98), hydrocortisone is not produced.

2. A metabolite just proximal to the block may accumulate in toxic amounts.

$$A \longrightarrow B \longrightarrow \begin{matrix} C \\ C \\ C \end{matrix} \not\longrightarrow (D)$$

An example is alkaptonuria. Homogentisic acid is not metabolized normally. It is excreted in the urine in large amounts. Furthermore its increase in the body in some way leads to a form of degenerative arthritis.

3. If the reactions in questions are reversible, there may be an accumulation of precursors farther back from the site of block.

$$\begin{matrix} A \\ A \\ A \end{matrix} \rightleftharpoons \begin{matrix} B \\ B \end{matrix} \rightleftharpoons C \longrightarrow (D)$$

An example is the accumulation of glycogen in the form of glycogen storage disease (von Gierke's disease) in which the primary defect involves glucose 6-phosphatase (Chap. 111).

Glycogen $\rightleftharpoons$ glucose 1-phosphate $\rightleftharpoons$ glucose 6-phosphate
$$\not\longrightarrow \begin{matrix}\text{glucose} \\ \text{6-phosphatase}\end{matrix}$$

4. There may be synthesis of products through an accessory pathway which is normally of minor significance.

$$A \longrightarrow B \longrightarrow C \not\longrightarrow (D)$$
$$\downarrow$$
$$X \longrightarrow Y \longrightarrow Z$$

In phenylketonuria, phenylketone products are produced in unusual amounts from phenylalanine, which is not properly metabolized. In hyperoxaluria, an excess production of oxalate may be the result of a defect in the normal metabolism of glyoxylate:

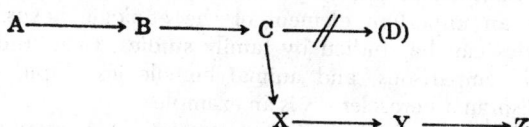

Glycine $\rightleftharpoons$ glyoxylate $\longrightarrow$ formic acid + CO_2

oxalic acid

Undoubtedly these do not exhaust the possible mechanisms of a pathogenetic effect from a mutation in a gene controlling an enzyme.

Metabolic processes are in most instances chains, indeed often networks. A mutation in the genes controlling any of several metabolic steps may lead to the same phenotypic result. Thus, the phenotype is not an indication of the specific genotype. Identical diseases may be produced by mutation of different genes; "genetic mimics," they are called.

A hundred or more disorders have, with varying degrees of reliability, been traced to a deficiency in the activity of a specific enzyme. Almost all behave as recessive traits. Enzyme systems have sufficient margin of safety that the mutant gene must be present in double dose and the deficiency must be complete in order for abnormality to be demonstrable in the phenotype. On the other hand, conditions based on mutation in a gene determining the amino acid sequence of a nonenzymic protein, e.g., hemoglobin, are likely to be dominant in their inheritance pattern. This is because the physical and functional properties of the product protein may be so altered that abnormality occurs even though only about half the product protein is of mutant type. The above principle concerning dominant and recessive inheritance is nicely demonstrated by the methemoglobinemias (Chap. 344), of which dominant and recessive forms exist. The recessive form is due to deficient activity of an enzyme, methemoglobin reductase, of the red cell. The dominant forms have a defect in hemoglobin, these being the several types of hemoglobin M.

The nonenzymic protein which has been subjected to most extensive study is hemoglobin (Chap. 339). Over one hundred mutations in the genes determining the alpha and beta polypeptide chains of hemoglobin have been identified. These mutations have been discovered by finding unitary amino acid changes in variant hemoglobins. Some of the changes involve the same amino acid; e.g., both hemoglobin S and hemoglobin C have a change in the sixth of the 146 amino acids of the beta polypeptide chain. In other variant hemoglobins the change is present in different amino acids of the chain. Understanding of how the particular amino acid substitution alters the function of hemoglobin is steadily increasing.

Another type of process, not strictly enzymatic, by which mutations have pathogenetic effects involves changes in active transport mechanisms in the kidney and elsewhere. Cystinuria (Chap. 102) is an example. Other active transport systems can be cited, such as those involved in the movement of substances such as amino acids across the intestinal mucosa, of substances like bilirubin into and out of the liver cell, and of electrolytes across the muscle cell membrane. All these mechanisms are vulnerable to the effects of mutation in the determinant genes, and diseases for which such mutation is probably responsible can be cited.

Structural genes, i.e., those specifying the amino acid sequence of proteins have for the most part been discussed to this point. "A pile of bricks is not a house," however. Other genes have a controlling role, ensuring an orderly interplay of the structural genes in development and in the adult organism. Mutation can occur also in these controlling genes with resultant disease. The evidence is coming mainly from the study of microorganisms; although a number of disorders of man are suspected to result from mutation in controlling genes, critical evidence is not easily assembled.

The complex machinery of protein synthesis, of which the framework is DNA-RNA-ribosomes, has become more clearly understood in recent years. Of potential therapeutic importance is the demonstration that intermediate steps in protein synthesis can be modified by various measures. It is possible, for example, that although a warped

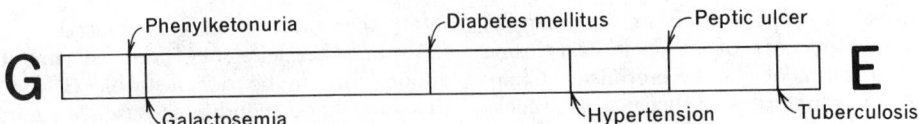

Fig. 4-17. Schematic representation of the spectrum of disease in regard to the relative importance of genetics (G) and exogenous (E) factors in etiology and pathogenesis.

and enzymatically weak protein is formed in a given disorder, the amount synthesized can be increased by some means and the disease abolished or ameliorated.

The Genetics of Common Disorders

All disease is in some degree genetic and in some degree environmental in etiology and pathogenesis. As to the relative importance of endogenous and exogenous factors, disease can be thought of as falling on a spectrum (Fig. 4-17). Near the genetic end (G) are simply inherited disorders such as phenylketonuria and galactosemia, but these are not at the extreme end because exogenous factors, diet in these specific examples, can importantly modify the phenotype. Near the environmental end (E) are infectious diseases but again not at the extreme end because twin and other studies indicate a significant role of genotype in susceptibility.

In the analysis of disorders affecting all systems, two classes of disorders, with regard to the role of genetic factors, are evident: (1) rare, simply inherited disorders (near the G end of the spectrum); (2) common disorders in which genetic factors play some role. Examples in the gastrointestinal system are familial polyposis of the colon and peptic ulcer; in the cardiovascular system, hereditary hemorrhagic telangiectasia and coronary artery disease; in the connective tissue system, Marfan's syndrome, lupus erythematosus; in the eye, retinitis pigmentosa and glaucoma.

The common disorders are, for the most part, multifactorial in causation. The etiology is a nexus in which environmental and genetic factors collaborate in a complex way in determining the disease.

Questions asked in connection with common disease are mainly two: How significant are genetic factors in etiology? By what mechanism does the mutant gene contribute to the pathogenesis?

Methods for evaluating the role of genetic factors in common diseases are mainly six:

1. *Family studies.* If genetic factors are important, a familial aggregation for the disorder should be demonstrable. Familial aggregation can have other than a genetic basis; thus, evidence from family studies is per se not critical.

2. *Twin studies.* Monozygotic twins, because of genetic identity, should show a higher concordance rate (i.e., "both affected") than dizygotic twins show, if genetic factors are significantly involved.

3. *Interracial comparisons.* Races have different frequencies of many genes. If genetic factors are important in etiology, the frequency of common diseases may vary from race to race. A difficulty in interpretation of racial data is the uncertainty of environmental comparability. Races are social as well as biologic entities.

4. *Component analysis.* Whenever a factor is shown to be an important element of the etiologic nexus, its genetics can be studied by family studies, twin studies, racial comparisons, and animal homologies. Lipid metabolism in atherosclerosis is an example.

5. *Blood group and disease association.* A simply inherited trait such as a specific blood group can, in some instances, be shown to occur more frequently with a given common disease than would be expected by chance. Some physiologic peculiarity of the person with that blood group seems to predispose him slightly but definitely to the disorder. The best example is the association between blood group O and peptic ulcer (Chap. 5). Another is the association of non-O and venous thromboembolic disease. Demonstration of association is evidence of a genetic factor in the disorder. Failure to demonstrate association does not exclude the importance of genetic factors.

6. *Animal homologies.* If one has available in animals a disorder seemingly identical to a common disease of man, then one may be able to do breeding experiments and extensive biochemical and physiologic investigations that will throw light on the two questions stated above.

The collaboration of multiple genes appears to be involved in determining stature; i.e., stature is a polygenic trait. Environmental factors, such as nutrition and chronic infectious disease, also influence stature; thus, stature is a multifactorial trait, to use the more general term. When the stature of a large group of persons is plotted, the distribution curve is a "normal," bell-shaped Gaussian

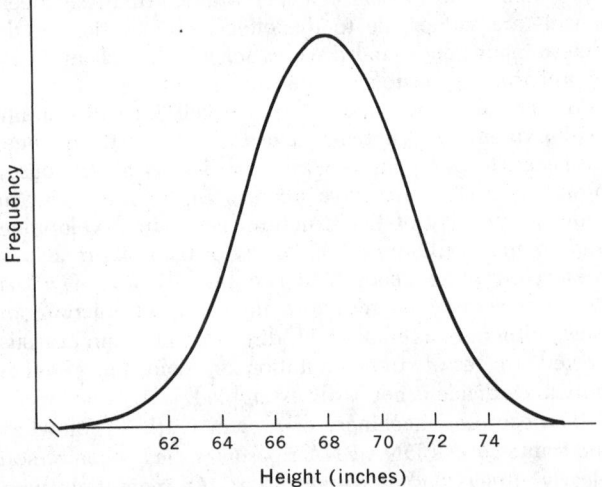

Fig. 4-18. Distribution curve for stature in the southeastern part of England. The mean is 68 in., and the standard deviation 2.6 in. (*Drawn from data analyzed by Cedric O. Carter*)

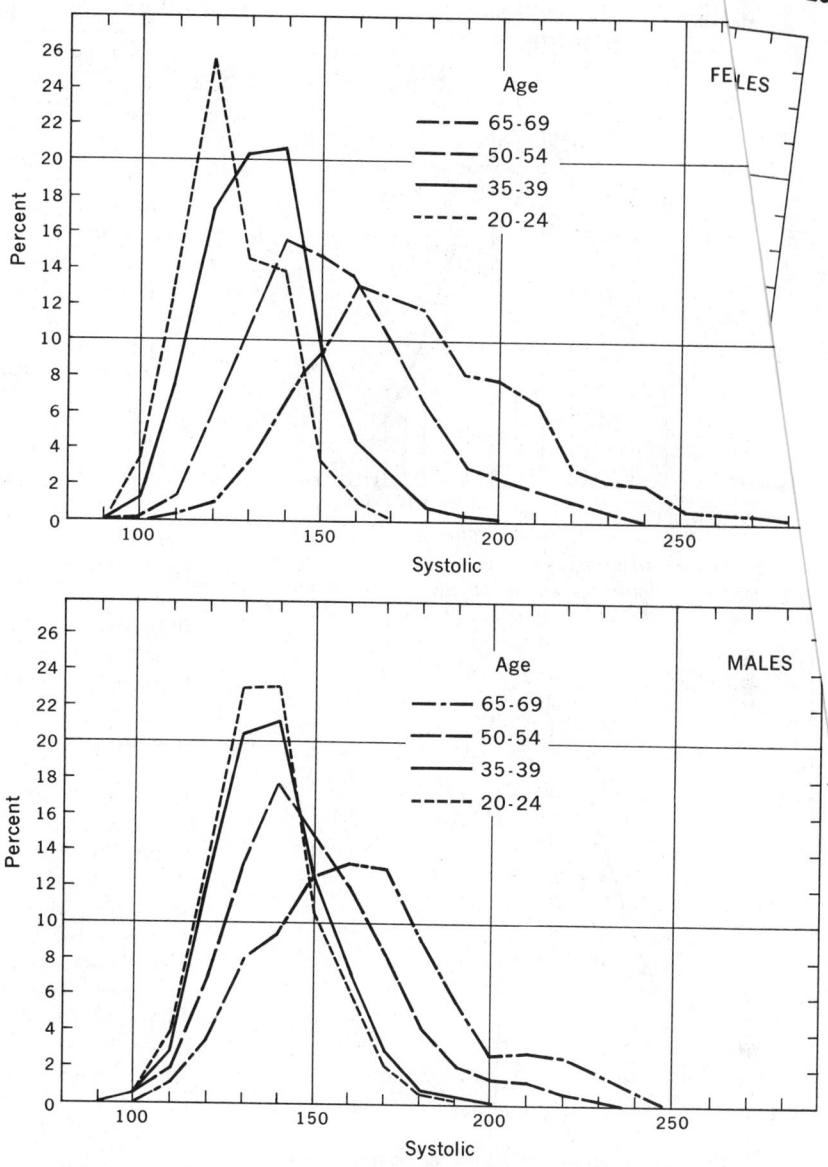

Fig. 4-19. Distribution curves for blood pressure. Normal blood pressure increases with age and is somewhat different in males and females; hence the separate plots. Note that all show positive skew, i.e., a tail at the end of the curve for higher pressures. [Bøe, et al., Acta med. scandin. 157: (suppl. 321), 1957].

one (Fig. 4-18). This suggests that the multiple genes involved in determining a person's height interact in an additive manner. By way of contrast, the distribution curve for blood pressure is "skewed" (Fig. 4-19), suggesting that the multiple genes determining level of blood pressure interact in a multiplicative manner. This conclusion is supported by the fact that if a logarithmic scale is used for blood pressure, the curve is "normalized" (Fig. 4-20). As a corollary to the view that blood pressure is a polygenic trait, essential hypertension is interpreted as the condition present in those persons whose particular assemblage of genes determines a level of blood pressure at the upper end of the distribution curve. What one calls essential hypertension and what one calls normotension are largely arbitrary decisions.

That a rather small number of genes can produce a continuous distribution is indicated by the example shown in Figure 4-21. Stature is assumed to be deter-

mined by two genetic loci on different chromosomes, each with three alleles in frequencies such that an allele (called "−") which decreases stature by 2 in., one (called "0") which determines the average stature of 68 in., and one (called "+") which increases stature by 2 in. have a relative frequency of 1:2:1. Five classes of gametes produced by each sex have the following frequencies (derived from Table 4-4): −−, $\frac{1}{16}$; −0, $\frac{1}{4}$; 00, $\frac{6}{16}$; +0, $\frac{1}{4}$; ++$\frac{1}{16}$. Zygotes formed from random union of gametes in these proportions have four stature genes (two at each of the two loci), and the possible combinations of +, 0, and − alleles found among the zygotes are nine in number. The relative frequencies of these are derived from Table 4-5 and plotted in Figure 4-21. A satisfactory approximation to a normal distribution is obtained, particularly when environmental influences blur the separation of groups. This example illustrates that even in conditions, like essential hyperten-

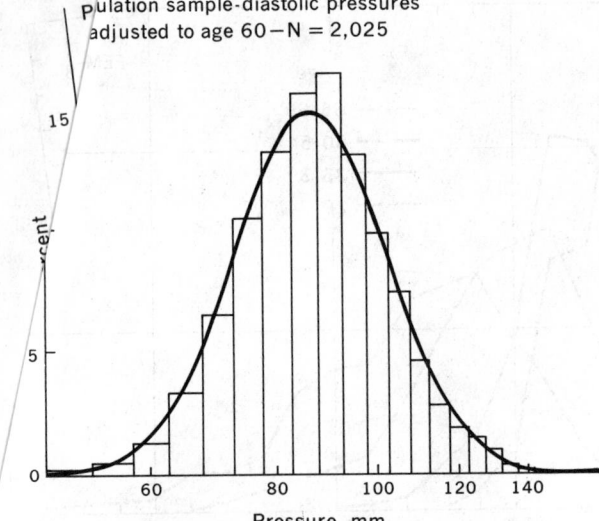

pulation sample-diastolic pressures adjusted to age 60—N = 2,025

Fig. 4-20. An essentially "normal" curve results when adjustment for age and sex differences are made and a logarithmic blood pressure scale is used. (*Courtesy of J. A. Fraser Roberts*)

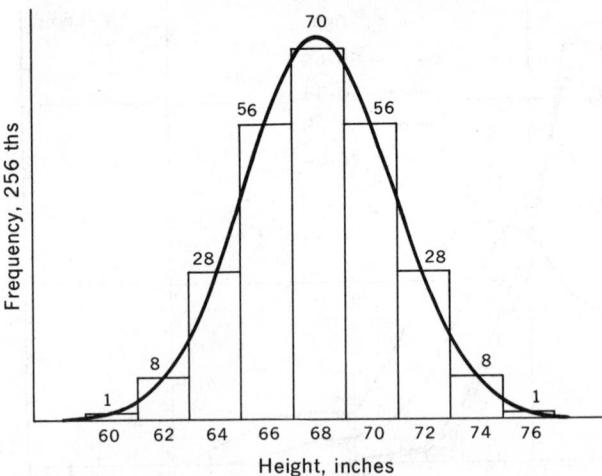

Fig. 4-21. Distribution curve for stature assuming that only two loci, each with three alleles, determine this characteristic. A small number of genes combined with environmental influence can result in a continuous distribution. (*Example from Cedric O. Carter*)

Table 4-4. PROPORTIONS OF EXPECTED TYPES OF GAMETES

		Chromosome 1		
		Allele − 1/4	Allele 0 1/8	Allele + 1/4
Chromosome 2	Allele − 1/4	1/16 − −	1/8 − 0	1/16 − +
	Allele 0 1/2	1/8 0 −	1/4 0 0	1/8 0 +
	Allele + 1/4	1/16 + −	1/8 + 0	1/16 + +

Table 4-5. PROPORTIONS OF EXPECTED TYPES OF ZYGOTES

		Male gametes				
		− − 1/16	− 0 1/4	0 0 6/16	0 + 1/4	+ + 1/16
Female gametes	− − 1/16	60 in. 1/256	62 in. 4/256	64 in. 6/256	66 in. 1/64	68 in. 1/256
	− 0 1/4	62 in. 4/256	64 in. 1/16	66 in. 6/64	68 in. 1/16	70 in. 1/64
	0 0 6/16	64 in. 6/256	66 in. 6/64	68 in. 36/256	70 in. 6/64	72 in. 6/256
	0 + 1/4	66 in. 1/64	68 in. 1/16	70 in. 6/64	72 in. 1/16	74 in. 4/256
	+ + 1/16	68 in. 1/256	70 in. 1/64	72 in. 6/256	74 in. 4/256	76 in. 1/256

sion, which appear to be polygenic, it is worthwhile to search for single-gene determined biochemical and physiologic mechanisms.

REFERENCES

Carter, C. O.: "Human Heredity," Baltimore, Penguin Books, Inc., 1962.

Court Brown, W. M.: "Human Population Cytogenetics," Amsterdam, North-Holland Publishing Company, 1967.

Harris, H.: Molecular Basis of Hereditary Disease, Brit. Med. J., 1:135–141, 1968.

Jink, H. et al.: Venous Thromboembolic Disease and ABO Blood Type, Lancet, 1:539–542, 1969.

McKusick, V. A.: "Human Genetics," 2d ed., Englewood Cliffs, N.J., Prentice-Hall, Inc., 1969.

———: "Mendelian Inheritance in Man. Catalogs of Autosomal Dominant, Autosomal Recessive and X-linked Phenotypes," 2d ed., Baltimore, The Johns Hopkins Press, 1968.

Perutz, M. F., and H. Lehmann: Molecular Pathology of Human Hemoglobin, Nature, 219:902–909, 1968.

Roberts, J. A. F.: "Introduction to Medical Genetics," 4th ed., London, Oxford University Press, 1967.

Rowley, J. D.: Cytogenetics in Clinical Medicine, J.A.M.A., 207:914–919, 1969.

Stanbury, J. B., J. B. Wyngaarden, and D. S. Fredrickson (Eds.): "The Metabolic Basis of Inherited Disease," 2d ed., New York, McGraw-Hill Book Company, 1966.

5 BLOOD GROUPS

J. Foerster and M. M. Wintrobe

Blood groups represent systems of antigenic determinants found on the surface of red cells. These antigens are inherited according to simple mendelian laws and are thought to be the products of allelic or closely linked genes. The major systems of antigens (e.g., ABO and Rh) are inherited independently of each other.

Blood groups are identified by means of specific antibodies occurring in serum, either "naturally," or after immunization with foreign red cells or soluble blood group substances. Chemical characterization of blood group antigens has lagged far behind serologic and genetic studies, and so far only the ABO and Lewis systems have lent themselves to extensive biochemical analysis. The study of the latter systems has been greatly facilitated by the discovery that the antigens in question occur not only as surface components of cells, but are also found in water-soluble form in the tissue fluids and secretions of most people.

THE ABO SYSTEM

The ABO antigens are inherited as simple mendelian characters, the blood group of an individual depending on the presence of two out of the three allelic genes: *A*, *B*, and *O*. The possible genotypic and corresponding phenotypic combinations are listed in Table 5-1. Anti-

Table 5-1. THE ABO BLOOD GROUPS

Phenotype (group)	Genotype	Agglutinogens on red cells	Isoagglutinins in serum
O	*OO*	none	anti-A anti-B
A	$\begin{cases} AA \\ AO \end{cases}$	A	anti-B anti-B
B	$\begin{cases} BB \\ BO \end{cases}$	B	anti-A
AB	*AB*	A and B	none

SOURCE: M. M. Wintrobe, "Clinical Hematology," 6th ed., Philadelphia Lea & Febiger, 1967.

bodies reacting with a particular blood group substance in this system are regularly found in the serum when the corresponding antigen is absent from the red cells. These antibodies were originally thought to occur "naturally," but are now known to arise early in life as a result of exposure to ABO-like polysaccharides occurring ubiquitously in food and other exogenous sources.

In addition to antibodies against A and B antigens, reagents are known which react preferentially with O cells. The antigen defined by these reagents is known as H-substance. Its synthesis is thought to be under the control of an allelic pair of genes, *Hh*, which is inherited independently of the ABO system. Thus the *H* gene in single or double dose gives rise to the H character, and the rare *h* allele, when present in double dose, results in its absence. The H-active material is probably in turn a precursor substance which under the influence of *A* and *B* genes is converted into A and B active substances respectively, thereby accounting for the presence of large quantities of H substance in O individuals.

The capacity to secrete A-, B-, or H-substances in tissue fluids and secretions is controlled by a pair of allelic genes *Sese*. *Se* is considered dominant over *se*, and only homozygous *sese* individuals therefore are nonsecretors of A-, B-, and/or H-substances.

The Lewis system is closely related to the ABO system, although the two allelic genes, *Le* and *le*, which define this system, are inherited independently of the *ABO*, *Hh*, and *Sese* genes. In single or double dose *Le* gives rise to Le^a specific structures; *le* in double dose results in their absence. Le^b specificity, once thought to arise from the activity of an allele of the *Le* gene, is now considered to be an interaction product of *H* and *Le* genes. Most nonsecretors of A, B or H-substances still secrete the Le^a substance, and the secretion of Le^a is therefore considered *not* to be under the control of the *Sese* genes.

The chemical composition of *secreted* ABH and Lewis substances is remarkably similar. They are composed of a carbohydrate moiety which constitutes about 85 percent of the molecule and an amino acid moiety which makes up the remaining 15 percent. The peptide residues are always composed of the same 15 amino acids, and 4 of these, threonine, serine, proline and alanine, make up two-thirds of all the amino acids present. The peptides appear to have structural functions only and are thought to form a firm, spiny backbone to which a large number of relatively short oligosaccharide chains, constituting the blood group substances, are attached at intervals. The carbohydrate moiety of all the ABH and Lewis substances is qualitatively similar in composition. Each contains a methyl-pentose, L-fucose; a hexose, D-galactose; two amino sugars, N-acetyl-D-glucosamine and N-acetyl-D-galactosamine; and a 9-carbon sugar, N-acetyl neuraminic acid. One of these sugars appears to be immunodominant in each of the blood group substances studied.

Cellular blood group substances are much more difficult to isolate, but both A and B active materials have been obtained in water-soluble form. In contrast to the blood group substances found in secretions, these cell-derived extracts are glycolipids. Nevertheless it appears that the oligosaccharide chains which confer blood group specificity on the glycolipid blood group substances of red cells as well as the glycoprotein substances found in secretions are identical, thereby accounting for the similarities in the specificity of antigenic determinants on red cells and on secretions.

The complicated interrelationship between A, B, H, and Lewis substances was clarified considerably when it was recognized that the gene systems controlling these four expressions appear to act sequentially on a common glycoprotein precursor substance. Genetic control presumably comes about through the formation of specific glycosyl transferase enzymes or through some mechanism controlling their function. A simplified version of such a proposed scheme is illustrated in Figure 5-1.

Two precursor chains are recognized on the basis of a $1 \rightarrow 3$ (type I) or $1 \rightarrow 4$ (type II) linkage of the terminal galactosyl unit to the subterminal *N*-acetyl-

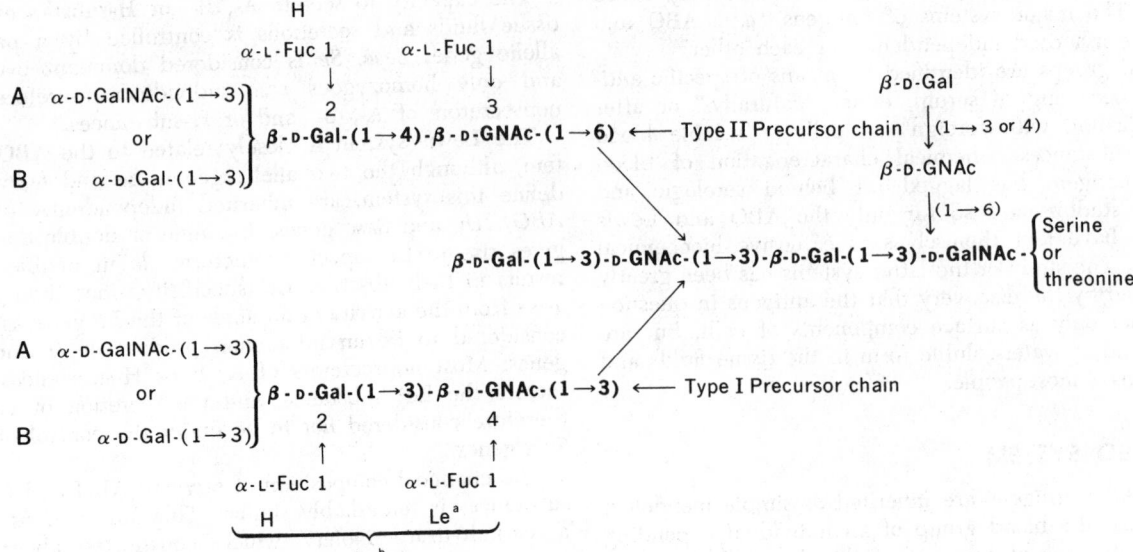

Fig. 5-1. Proposed composite structure of A, B, H, Le^a and Le^b specific blood group substances linked to serine or threonine spines of the polypeptide backbone. Gal refers to galactose; Fuc to fucose; GNAc to N-acetylglucosamine; GalNAc to N-acetylgalactosamine. The numerical notations (e.g., 1 → 4) refer to the respective carbon positions at which linkage occurs. The precursor substance is identified by **Bold Type**; the determinants characteristic of a given blood group substance are in light type and are identified by their appropriate symbols, namely A, B, H, Le^a, and Le^b. The structure shown is a composite which includes all determinants. In individual blood group substances certain residues will be missing; e.g., H, Le^a, and Le^b specific blood group substances lack A and B specific determinants, and Le^a substance also lacks the H specific determinant. See text and references for details. (After K. O. Lloyd, et al., Biochemistry 7:2976, 1968).

galactosamine residue. The latter precursor chain has cross-reactivity with antisera to type XIV pneumococcal polysaccharide.

The transferase controlled by the H gene is thought to add L-fucose in α-linkage to the carbon 2 position of either chain to form an H-active structure. The enzyme controlled by the *Le* gene, also a fucosyl transferase, adds L-fucose in α-linkage to the 4 position of the subterminal N-acetylglucosamine unit in chains of type I only, as chains of type II already are substituted at this position. The resultant structure has Le^a specificity. When both *H* and *Le* genes are present, two fucosyl units are added to adjacent sugars on chains of type I, resulting in a structure which, on the basis of inhibition experiments, is thought to be that of the Le^b determinant.

The presence of the fucosyl unit conferring H specificity to the precursor substance is considered to be essential for the functioning of the transferases controlled by the A and B genes. Thus N-acetyl-D-galactosamine added in α-linkage to carbon 3 of the terminal galactosyl unit confers A-specificity to the H-active precursor substance, whereas addition of D-galactose in identical linkage results in B specificity. The addition of these terminal nonreducing sugars effectively masks the serologic reactivity of the H-active groupings, and the Le^a-active determinants are similarly masked by the substitutions controlled by the A, B, and H genes. The *Se* gene does not bring about structural changes but simply controls the expression of the *ABH* genes for the blood group substances in secretion.

In the case of A substance, differences in the degree of expression of the antigen are well known. Indeed, a spectrum of A exists, extending from the strong A$_1$ to the weak A$_x$ antigen, reflecting a large series of determinant alleles. These differences in A likely represent genetically determined variations in the ability to bind a specific antibody, although the alternate possibility of differences in the number of binding sites per red cell cannot be excluded with certainty. Incomplete expression of blood group antigens also has been noted in rare instances of diseases, such as acute leukemia.

THE Rh SYSTEM

In 1940 Landsteiner and Wiener made the surprising discovery that the sera of rabbits and guinea pigs immunized with the red cells of Rhesus monkeys agglutinated not only the donor erythrocytes but also those of most Caucasian New Yorkers. Those individuals whose red cells were agglutinated by these sera were termed *Rh-positive*, the others, *Rh-negative*. It was subsequently discovered that heterologous antirhesus antibodies do not actually react with red cell antigens presently known to be part of the Rh system, but rather, they react with another antigen (LW) shared by both rhesus and human cells. The original observation did, however, stimulate immediate inquiry into the nature of unexplained intragroup transfusion reactions and incompatibilities between mother and child which result in erythroblastosis fetalis (Chap. 338); and it was found that most of these reactions could be accounted for by antibodies resembling those described by Landsteiner and Wiener.

From this modest beginning has evolved the most complex of human blood group systems, presently characterized by approximately 30 different serologic specificities and an almost unlimited number of complex alleles. Undoubtedly much of the present confusion surrounding this system is related to the fact that chemical definition of these antigens has lagged far behind serologic and genetic studies.

Two systems of nomenclature describing this complex system need to be considered. According to Fisher, the inheritance of Rh antigens is determined by three pairs of closely linked allelic genes. Thus each parent would contribute a set of three Rh genes, C or c, D or d, E or e, each defining a single antigen. A person might therefore inherit CDe from one parent and cde from another, to mention only the two most commonly observed genotypes. This theory also assumes that crossover of linked genes can take place, thereby accounting for the maintenance of the rarer combinations by occasional crossing over from the common heterozygotes. Wiener, on the other hand, postulates a single gene to accommodate a large number of alleles. An equally important part of Wiener's theory implies the existence of several families

Table 5-2. WIENER'S GENE DESIGNATIONS, CORRESPONDING AGGLUTINOGENS AND BLOOD FACTORS, AND FISHER-RACE NOTATIONS

Genes		Frequency among Caucasoids, %	Corresponding agglutinogens	Blood factors present
Wiener	Fisher Race			
r	cde	38.0	rh	hr′,hr″,hr
r'	Cde	0.6	rh′	rh′,hr″
r'^w	C^wde	0.005	rh′^{w}	rh′,rh^w,hr″
r''	cdE	0.5	rh″	rh″,hr′
r^y	CdE	0.01	rh^y	rh′,rh″
R^o	cDe	2.7	Rh$_o$	Rh$_o$,hr′,hr″,hr
R^1	CDe	41.0	Rh$_1$	Rh$_o$,rh′,hr″
R^{1w}	C^wDe	2.0	Rh$_1$^{w}	Rh$_o$,rh′,rh^w,hr″
R^2	cDE	15.0	Rh$_2$	Rh$_o$,rh″,hr′
R^z	CDE	0.2	Rh$_z$	Rh$_o$,rh′,rh″

NOTE: Wiener, in his publications, uses italics for gene symbols and for genotypes, regular type for agglutinogens and phenotypes and boldface type for symbols for blood factors and for the corresponding antibodies used to detect the blood factors in question. Further, to distinguish the symbols for genotypes and phenotypes, the letter "h" is omitted and only superscripts are used in gene symbols.

SOURCE: M. M. Wintrobe, "Clinical Hematology," 6th ed., Philadelphia, Lea and Febiger, 1967.

of antibodies directed against the same Rh determinant (*agglutinogen*), but each having specificity for different aspects of its structure. These structural aspects defined by a given serologic specificity have been termed *blood factors*. According to this scheme, which is outlined in Table 5-2, a given antigenic determinant (agglutinogen) may be recognized by antibodies of heterogeneous specificities directed against any one of its constituent "blood factors." Thus, for example, the presence of the antigenic determinant rh, which is the product of gene r, may be inferred from serologic reactions which are specific for its constituent blood factors hr′, hr″, and hr. Unfortunately the structure of complex antigens, and particularly its mode of synthesis, cannot be derived exclusively from an analysis of agglutination reactions. Confirmation of these assumptions will therefore have to await the structural definition of the antigenic determinants in question.

Other Blood Group Systems

The inheritance of M, N, or MN blood group substances appears to be associated with two allelic genes L^m and L^n. Indeed, it seems likely that the synthesis of MN antigens is similar to that of the ABO system, being the result of sequential, gene-controlled changes in a common precursor substance. This is suggested by the association of both M and N activities with the same macromolecule, by the presence of N activity in M preparations derived from cells of the genotype MM, and the exposure of common specificities in M and N preparations by the removal of N-acetylneuraminic acid. It appears likely that N substance is a precursor of M substance. The chemical nature of M and N substances has been investigated extensively, and it has been shown that carbohydrate units with terminal nonreducing acetylneuraminic acid residues are important constituents of their determinant structures.

The Ss antigens are related to M and N in much the same way as C and c are related to D and d, probably existing as closely linked loci on the same chromosome. Many other antigens such as Hu, He, and Mi are now also known to belong to the MnSs system.

The P blood group system appears to be determined by the three alleles P^1, P^2, and the very rare gene, p, which in double dose results in the absence of P_1 and P_2 antigens. Another determinant, P^k also seems to be associated with the P system but is genetically independent of the P^1, P^2 genes. It has been postulated that the P^k determinant, like the Bombay specificity of the ABO system, results from the absence of a very frequent gene dominant in character. The Tj^a antigen is also known to be part of the P system. Thus, naturally occurring anti-Tj^a antibodies are found in the sera of all pp individuals and react with red cells of P_1, P_2, and P^k phenotype. If anti-Tj^a sera are absorbed with P_2 cells, anti-P$_1$ activity is left behind, confirming the specificity of these reactions. The clinical importance of the P blood group system derives from the fact that antibodies regularly occur in the serum of individuals who lack the corresponding P antigen. Thus, in addition to the anti-P + P_1 + P^k (= anti-Tj^a) antibody found in the sera of pp individuals, anti-P_1 antibody is found in P_2 subjects and anti-P (= anti-P_1 + anti-P_2) antibody occurs in the serum of P^k individuals.

Many other blood group systems have been described (Table 5-3), some of which possess clinical or anthropologic importance because of their high incidence in the population (e.g., Tj^a, Vel, k), difficulties associated with their detection in the laboratory (Kidd), or peculiarities in ethnic distribution (Diego). So-called "private

Table 5-3. BLOOD GROUPS

Name of system	Antigens of major clinical importance	Other identified antigens
ABO, Hh, LEWIS .	A, B, Le^a	H, Le^b
Rh.	D	D^u
	C, c	C^u, C^w, C^x
	E, e	E^u, E^w
MNSs.	S	M, N, s, M_1, M_2, M^g, Mi^a, Vw, Hu, He, U
P.		P_1, P_2, P^k, Tj^a
Kell.	K	k, Kp^a, Kp^b, Js^a, Js^b, K^u, K^w
Duffy	Fy^a	Fy^b
Kidd.	Jk^a	Jk^b
Lutheran.		Lu^a, Lu^b
Ii.		I, i
Diego.		Di^a, Di^b

antigens" (e.g., By, Sw^a, Levay) are of little or no clinical significance, except in the families in which they exist.

CLINICAL SIGNIFICANCE OF BLOOD GROUPS

BLOOD TRANSFUSION REACTIONS. These are of great variety (Table 342-1). Those related to blood group incompatibility are among the most serious. The blood groups A, B, and D (Rh) are involved in by far the greatest majority, perhaps 95 percent of all cases. This is because anti-A and anti-B antibodies occur "naturally," and D is, like A and B, a good antigen to which antibodies are produced readily. The first encounter with ABO incompatible blood may result in a hemolytic transfusion reaction; the first exposure of an Rh-negative person to Rh-positive blood will not, because of the lack of natural (or preformed) antibodies. Such a transfusion may, however, sensitize the individual to the Rh antigens in question, and the resultant antibodies may then lead to a hemolytic transfusion reaction on subsequent exposure to similarly incompatible cells. The Kell system (Kk) also is important because many K-negative persons can be sensitized to K by transfusion. The same holds true for E and c, but the danger is smaller. The remaining blood groups are of comparatively minor clinical im-

portance, although most transfusions are potentially sensitizing. Scarcity of sera and the labor involved make it impractical to type routinely for all the known antigens, but the use of a sensitive cross-match test together with the Coombs test for "incomplete" antibodies is a helpful and essential safeguard.

Blood group incompatibility is responsible for at least one disease, erythroblastosis fetalis (Chap. 338). In addition, the anti-red cell antibodies of some other acquired hemolytic anemias have specificity for blood group antigens, most commonly those belonging to the Rh system. This includes many cases of idiopathic autoimmune hemolytic anemia and certain instances of drug-induced hemolytic anemia, most notably those seen in association with alpha-methyl-dopa therapy.

ABO antigens are also known to act as potent transplantation antigens in man. It has been found, for instance, that graft recipients pretreated with incompatible ABO antigens will reject subsequent skin allografts in a markedly accelerated manner from donors incompatible for the same ABO antigens, whereas skin grafts from ABO-compatible individuals are accorded survival times characteristic of first grafts in nonsensitized individuals. It seems clear, therefore, that matching techniques for organ transplantation must take cognizance of ABO incompatibilities between donor and recipient.

The association of blood groups with certain diseases is a well-documented phenomenon. Thus, gastric carcinoma and pernicious anemia are particularly common in individuals with blood group A, and there is an even closer association between blood group O and duodenal ulceration, especially in nonsecretors. The reasons underlying these correlations are not understood.

MEDICOLEGAL AND ANTHROPOLOGIC IMPORTANCE. The usefulness of serologic examinations in medicolegal and anthropologic work is readily apparent. It has been calculated that, with the ABO system and the two subgroups of A, the MNSs blood groups, P, the Rh system, Lutheran, Lewis, and Kell, the total number of possible different combinations of serologic recognizable phenotypes is 23,616, and the number of genotypes is 972,000. Because of technical and other difficulties, the P, Lewis, Kell, Duffy, and Kidd systems are not recommended for use in problems of parentage or identity, but even without them, when blood of the mother, the child, and the alleged father is available, it is possible to exonerate 51 percent of all men of Western European origin who are wrongfully accused of paternity.

Of additional medicolegal importance is the fact that the antigens A, B, and H are present in the secretions of most individuals and can readily be extracted with aqueous solutions from tissues and organs, especially salivary glands and gastric mucosa. High concentrations of blood group substances can also be found in secretions such as saliva, gastric juice, and semen. As a consequence it is possible to apply blood grouping to the examination of dried stains of these secretions as well as to saline extracts of muscle tissue.

In human genetics and anthropology the blood groups are of the utmost value for a number of reasons. The first is that they are sharply distinguishable "all-or-none" characteristics which do not grade into each other. Then again, they are simple, genetically speaking, and are inherited in a known way according to mendelian principles. Furthermore, they owe nothing to environment in their inheritance, nor are they subject to variations because of natural selection, as is the case, for example, with skin color. Hence, the blood groups are especially fitted to throw light on the moderately remote as well as the recent origins of mankind. Wide differences in frequency in different races have been observed. Consequently the blood groups provide valuable anthropometric measurements.

Considerable and interesting data are being accumulated concerning the ethnologic distribution of the blood groups. Thus the incidence of B has been found highest in certain parts of Asia and declines in all directions from central Asia except for a subsidiary high center in Africa. In the Old World the lowest figures have been found in the Scandinavian countries, and in Australia the gene seems to have been absent until very recent times. A similar complete absence has been found in the living aborigines of North America as well as in the Basques. Group O reaches levels of practically 100 percent among certain Indian tribes in the United States. In the aborigines of America the gene for N is relatively rare, while in those of Australia it is very common. The factor P is much commoner in the blood of American Negroes than in that of American whites. The Rh-negative gene (cde) has been found in 13 to 17 percent of modern inhabitants of Europe and in white inhabitants of America. In the Basques it reaches very high levels (28.8 percent); in contrast, in a study of Eskimo only 1 out of 2,522 was found to be Rh-negative.

REFERENCES

Lloyd, K. O., E. A. Kabat, and E. Licerio: Immunochemical Studies on Blood Groups, XXXVIII, Biochemistry, 7:2976, 1968.

Mollison, P. L.: "Blood Transfusion in Clinical Medicine," 4th ed., Philadelphia, F. A. Davis Company, 1967.

Race, R. R., and Ruth Sanger: "Blood Groups in Man," 5th ed., Philadelphia, F. A. Davis Company, 1968.

Watkins, W. M.: "Blood Group Substances," Science, 152: 172, 1966.

Wintrobe, M. M.: "Clinical Hematology," 6th ed., Philadelphia, Lea & Febiger, 1967.

6 GROWTH AND DEVELOPMENT
Robert E. Cooke

The phrase "growth and development" has acquired a variety of vague meanings, ranging from changes in height to changes in emotional capacity. In this chapter, growth is defined as an increase in size with time, with particular emphasis on accretion of new protoplasm (largely protein and water) as opposed to changes in volume or weight such as might occur with edema. Development is defined as an increase with time in numbers of functions or in complexity of function, with biologic or behavioral aspects, or both, implied in that function.

Growth, as defined here, has two components—increase in cell number and increase in cell size. At various periods in life after conception, particularly early in gestation, increase in cell number may be primarily responsible for growth. During fetal life between 40 and 50 successive divisions take place, with an increase from one cell to 12×10^{12} cells at the time of birth. From birth to adulthood another four divisions occur. Early growth thereby occurs in a geometric progression. Subsequently there is a greater tendency for arithmetic accretion of protein. Numerous attempts have been made to develop equations describing growth. In general an S-shaped curve best fits the data.

In recent years more precise measurement of cell size has been possible by chemical analysis rather than by microscopic observations, including counts of mitotic activity. It has been determined that 6.2 to 7 $\mu\mu$g of DNA characterize most diploid cells. In the absence of polyploidy, measurement of total DNA content of one or more tissues establishes cell number. Protein and DNA analyses on similar samples make possible the calculation of cell size, since the water and protein contents of the body bear a straight-line relationship.

Liver nuclei demonstrate polyploidy under a variety of conditions, and the number and size of these cells cannot be determined readily by these simple analyses; actual counts of nuclei and chromosomes are necessary. Available data indicate that one tissue may differ markedly from another in respect to cell multiplication at various stages of growth. Muscle tends to approximate overall growth changes because it represents at least 40 percent of the total lean body mass. Furthermore, cell multiplication may occur in spurts rather than as a continuous process. Likewise, growth as determined by changes in cell size varies markedly from one tissue to another and from one period of life to another.

The assessment of the growth rate of one tissue or another, or of the whole individual, must be related to the particular biologic age of the individual—i.e., the extent of maturation. In the human being, there is great variation in the onset of adolescence. The peak growth rate in height, for example, may occur anywhere over a 5-year period in chronologic age.

Development, as defined in this chapter, though far more difficult to quantify, also proceeds sporadically and in a nonlinear fashion. The appearance of marked increases in activity of certain enzymes—e.g., tyrosin hydroxylase—corresponds to certain biologic stages but may also exhibit considerable variability in time of peak activity. Likewise, the development of behavioral characteristics, when expressed in terms of norms, proceeds along a fairly smooth curve. However, the individual infant or child exhibits marked variability in rate of progress from one month or year to the next. For example, most infants show a fairly regular sequence of developmental milestones, but it is not unusual to see delays, then spurts; e.g., creeping may be delayed but walking accelerated.

CONTROL OF GROWTH AND DEVELOPMENT

Both phenomena obviously represent the interplay of genetic and environmental factors. Growth rates within a family show much less variability than when compared with those of the general population. Tall parents in general have tall children. However, in a process as complex as growth, many genes are involved, with rates of synthesis of many proteins being controlled by independently segregating genetic loci. It is not surprising, then, that physical size of a population has a normal Gaussian distribution. Environmental factors modify genetic expression considerably, however. Occasional monozygotic twins may differ markedly in size at birth, probably because of circulatory abnormalities. Geneticists some years ago predicted that the average height of the population would decrease because short persons were reproducing at a more rapid rate than the tall. Yet average height may actually be increasing because of environmental factors (possibly nutritional). At least greater growth rates are seen in the first 20 years of life now than in the previous generation.

A clearer understanding of the genetic control of development has come from the demonstration of various molecular forms of cell enzymes. Lactic dehydrogenase (LDH), for example, has been shown to be a variety rather than a single molecular species, with differing electrophoretic mobilities, amino acid sequences, and polypeptide groupings. The distribution of particular isozymes differs from one organ or tissue to another. Particular isozymes are present in varying amounts from one period in life to another. A variety of LDH appears in the testis in the human being and in several animal species only at sexual maturation. The mechanisms for turning genetic action on and off at a particular stage in the development of the individual remain unknown.

Exactly the same principles that apply to control of physical growth and maturation apply to behavioral development. The past tendency to attribute intelligence solely to genetic factors and the present tendency to disregard genetic factors in establishing relative limits for intellectual development are both contrary to the facts.

Gesell and others believed that behavior unfolded in an immutable manner, uninfluenced by experience and determined entirely by the innate potential of the individual. This hypothesis was supported by the fact that normative data collected on large numbers of infants and children indicated a fairly regular pattern for the appearance of a large number of items of behavior indicating cognitive and affective maturation.

Early experience, however, has been shown to alter behavioral development substantially. It has been shown that the longer the exposure to an underprivileged home the greater the fall in intellectual quotient. Children with inferior family and environmental histories, when placed in adoptive homes before the age of two years, despite obviously low IQ scores in the true parents and average but not superior IQ scores in the foster parents, had normal intelligence levels at five years, seven years, and thirteen years of age.

Studies of the intellectual development of twins reared in somewhat different environments show a greater correspondence in comparison with other children in the population but less than twins reared together.

The work of Hebb, Harlow, Riesen, and Piaget has reemphasized the influence of learning experiences on subsequent learning ability. Intelligent behavior results from the acquisition of and exploitation of many programs or schemata for solving problems. The initiative for searching for such programs is dependent on motivation—the genesis of which seems obscure but related in part to previous success or failure.

OPTIMAL GROWTH AND DEVELOPMENT

The possible relationship of longevity to rate of growth raises the issue that the maximal rate of growth may not necessarily be optimal. Much of the experimental data indicate that rate of growth in experimental animals and to an extent in human beings may be influenced by diet. Restriction of intake during gestation and prior to weaning may permanently slow growth despite free access to food thereafter. Increased longevity seemed to be associated with the limited food intake. Only one experiment has been designed to show that aging is probably associated with dietary factors rather than being directly related to accelerated rate of growth. The administration of growth hormone to animals previously subjected to dietary restriction restored growth rate to normal without shortening longevity. Diet, likewise, alters rate of maturation of certain tissues in a manner similar to the aging process. Concentrations of alkaline phosphatase, ATPase, and catalase and histidase increase with age in the rat liver.

The manipulation of diet can produce enzyme patterns in the younger rat comparable to those of a much older animal. Although changes in cell structure, water content, and the like may be responsible for some of these effects, the fact that changes in enzyme activity are in opposite directions lends significance to the findings.

Maximum behavioral development may or may not be optimal, just as with physical growth. Most of the evidence, however, indicates that superior intellectual performance is correlated with good emotional adjustment. Studies of the social success and accomplishments of gifted children negate the lay impression that "genius is tainted with madness." The more favorable environments of such children may be in part responsible for such adjustments. The fact that man has the longest ontogenetic preparatory period permitting opportunities for social training makes possible significant improvement of behavioral development providing the necessary condition for each child can be determined.

MEASUREMENT

The recording of changes in physical size and shape with age is important and a fairly reliable indicator of health. Many systems have been developed to facilitate comparisons with normal children of the same age, body build, weight, and height. The determination of prenatal growth and of premature birth in the past has been assessed primarily in terms of weight; gestational age, although necessarily inaccurate, is being utilized more frequently because of the relatively frequent occurrence of intrauterine growth disturbances. A combination of the two would seem desirable.

The prediction of adult size from measurements during childhood is reasonably accurate, particularly if height and bone age are measured and if parental size is also appreciated. Height at three years shows a better correlation with height at maturity than at any other age. The correlation of childhood measurements with adult height were: birth, 0.77; one year, 0.67; two years, 0.75; and at five years, 0.79. One formula for prediction is that of Weech:

$$H_m = 0.545\,H_2 + 0.544\,A + 14.84 \text{ in.} \quad \text{(boys)}$$
$$H_m = 0.545\,H_2 + 0.544\,A + 10.09 \text{ in.} \quad \text{(girls)}$$

where H_m = height at maturity
H_2 = height at two years
A = average of parents' height

The standard deviation of difference in actual over predicted height is about 1 in.

The assessment of physical development is rapidly being improved. Such determinations as bone age, EEG, enzyme levels, and steroid excretion patterns indicate changes in function and serve to establish biologic age, particularly in the newborn period and at adolescence, when profound functional changes occur.

By the application of multivariate equations utilizing as data measurements of body size, body weight, body water, body chloride, creatinine excretion, cell number, etc., biologic age may be predicted with great precision ($\pm$ 6 to 9 months in a child). Such predictions permit appropriate estimation of the degree of growth failure in relation to change in chronologic and biologic age. Growth failure can be thought of as loss of months or years of growth rather than centimeters or kilograms, thereby permitting better appreciation of the possibilities for and extent of "catch-up" growth.

For the investigator such calculations permit a better understanding of physiologic function in the maturing infant or child so that physiologic function may be properly compared from one child to the next. Unfortunately, accurate prediction of biologic age in the fetus and premature and in the aged is not yet feasible.

The measurement of intellectual development is now being criticized excessively—by modern psychologists especially. The evidence is irrefutable that there is a high correlation between test scores at ages four years and fourteen and school performance, although exceptions occur. Developmental quotients at one year correlate poorly with intelligence quotients in later childhood. However, low developmental scores at six, nine, and twelve months predict serious abnormality in later life with remarkable accuracy.

The major criticism of IQ predictions arises from the attempts of some investigators to attribute intelligence solely to genetic factors. The Gaussian distribution of intelligence test scores has been used as an argument for the genetic basis of intelligence. Unquestionably, there are multiple genetic factors with phenotypic manifestations far removed from primary gene action and, therefore, subject to great environmental alteration. The environmental factors probably have their greatest impact in the first 4 years of life, but, unfortunately, they have not been well characterized. Terms such as "cultural deprivation" and "inadequate stimulation" are used to describe the early environments of many children who later do poorly in school and in employment. The details of such experience that hinder or promote intellectual development in the human infant and child require much elaboration.

ABERRATIONS IN GROWTH AND DEVELOPMENT

Specific disturbances in physical growth and biologic development as well as behavioral development are discussed in other sections of this text. Retarded growth and slow intellectual development far exceed acceleration in frequency. The causes are multiple, and in no way can the terms "growth retardation" or "mental retardation" be considered as an adequate diagnosis. The etiology or pathophysiology leading to retardation must be searched for, even though at present the majority of cases cannot adequately be explained.

If the pathogenetic factor in growth can be ascertained and corrected, remarkable acceleration or catch-up growth may occur. In some cases of congenital heart disease, for example, surgical correction of the defect may lead to an increase in height age of several years occurring in several months. If excessive delay in correction occurs, eventual stature may be stunted.

Experience with correction of defects causing mental retardation is exceedingly limited. However, there are a few examples of young children reared in bizarre circumstances who seemed to have exhibited catch-up development when the biologic and behavioral environment was improved.

REFERENCES

Bloom, B. S.: "Stability and Change in Human Characteristics," New York, John Wiley & Sons, Inc., 1964.

Cheek, D. B.: Human Growth: Body Composition, Cell Growth, Energy, and Intelligence. Philadelphia, Lea & Febiger, 1968.

Riesen, A. H.: Effects of Early Deprivation of Photic Stimulation, pp. 61–85 in S. F. Osler, and R. E. Cooke, "The Biosocial Basis of Mental Retardation," Baltimore, The Johns Hopkins Press, 1965.

Skeels, H. M.: Adult Status of Children with Contrasting Early Life Experiences. A Follow-up study. Monogr. Soc. Res. Child. Develop., 31:1–56, 1966.

Zinkham, W. H., A. Blanco, and L. J. Clowry, Jr.: An Unusual Isozyme of Lactate Dehydrogenase in Mature Testes: Localization, Ontogeny, and Kinetic Properties, Ann. N.Y. Acad. Sci., 121:571–588, 1964.

7 THE DEVELOPMENT OF PERSONALITY

Raymond D. Adams

The term *personality* encompasses all the physical and psychologic traits that characterize man—that distinguish him from all other individuals in his universe.

The notion that every person is a complex of physical peculiarities, determined by inheritance, is accepted as a fundamental datum of biology. One has but to look at resemblances between parent and child to find ample confirmation of it. Only the extent of human variation occasions surprise. Just as no two people are identical, not even monozygotic twins, so too, do they differ in body chemistry or any other quality that one might choose to measure. These qualities, together with certain inherited predilections to disease, explain why any one person may have an unpredictable reaction to a pathogenic agent when a whole population is exposed. Strictly speaking, normal man is an abstraction, just as is a typical case of disease.

But it is in other seemingly nonphysical attributes that man displays the greatest variety of subtle differences. Here reference is made to a patient's variable place on a scale of physical and mental energy, in capacity for effective work, in intellectual power which makes him susceptible to different degrees of training and education, in sensitivity, temperament, and emotional responsivity, in aggressiveness or passivity, in character, and in adaptability to stress. The composite of these qualities and the life experiences which have helped shape them form the basis of the personality structure of man.

The justification for a chapter on this subject in a book which essays to present the principles of internal medicine stems from the fact that major and minor departures from the usual trends in personality development become common sources of medical complaint later in life when they interfere with somatic function, happiness, and effective adaptation in society. As such they fall under the purview of the physician; and if they are sufficiently grave, they demand the attention of the psychiatrist. The recognition of these disorders requires a knowledge of the bases of normal personality development as a frame of reference. The rules and principles underlying these abnormal deviations—the manner in which heritable traits of personality and unfortunate life experiences combine to account for their appearance—comprise psychopathology. These principles have emerged largely from observations of man as a social animal and have been more studied by social than medical scientists; but in the final analysis, personality attributes are as biologic as the reflexes, instincts, emotions, and drives from which they are derived.

THE ROOTS OF SOCIAL BEHAVIOR

Social behavior, like neurologic and psychologic functions in general, depends to a great extent on the development and maturation of the brain, and these are functions of genetic factors and environmental influence. No other organ in the body undergoes such an amazing number of changes from early embryonal to adult life, which explains the unfolding of an infinite array of human behavior, abilities, and mental capacities. The most rapid changes in the brain occur before birth, and they are the least understood because they take place in the remote recesses of the womb, where they are relatively inaccessible to the eye of the physician and scientist. But, unlike all other animals, man then proceeds through a long period of postnatal development. No other creature is more helpless at birth, possibly because the relatively small size of the female pelvic outlet in our species precludes large size and degree of fetal development of the brain. The weight of the brain at different ages reflects this; the ratio of brain weight in adulthood to birth is 3.5 to 4.0 in man and only 2.2 in the chimpanzee. The difference is qualitative as well as quantitative. Whereas the neocortex in general increases fourfold from birth to maturity, the motor areas for hand, tongue, and larynx (the parts subserving manual dexterity and speech) and the suprasensory areas of parietal lobe (concerned with symbolization and thinking) expand proportionately more. The time required for postnatal development provides another dimension, being longer for man than for any other mammal. This extended period of development, so essential to the unfolding of vast human potential, carries with it a liability—an unusually long period of possible exposure to the action of environmental influences that are beyond the control of the individual himself. In a purely evolutionary sense the whole structure of human social organization into family units has as its primary purpose to protect the child in this period while enabling him to realize his full potential through training and education.

Limitations of space allow no more than a few glimpses of the nervous substructure of the prodigious repertoire of behavioral sequences of development. The histologic studies of Conel trace the enlargement of cortical neurones as their dendritic plexuses are elaborated and synaptic surfaces expanded. The observations of Flechsig (verified by Langworthy, Yakovlev, and others) reveal the sequential changes in myelination of the axones of nerve cells in different parts of the brain, which have been shown to proceed in a time-linked orderly fashion. Minkowski, Hooker, Gesell, André-Thomas are other names, famous for their cataloguing of the changing patterns of motility, sensation, and instinctual and emotional drives in early life and their relationship to stages of anatomic development. Reassuring to adults is the finding of Kaes and Rose that brain development continues on into adult years.

The most advanced phases of man's behavior, called *social* because they involve human interaction for their emergence, must be viewed as a continuation of these basic reflex and instinctual patterns. Their progressive elaboration is reinforced by the adaptive processes and the attendant emotions which they engender. Pleasure accompanies behavior demanded by evolution (e.g., the sexual act, so necessary for reproduction), and anxiety and fear guard the organism against conditions leading to maladaptation. But here we begin to see the workings of another principle—that biologic evolution merges with but is finally superseded by cultural evolution. The latter is uniquely human. Man is the only animal with the capacity to change his environment in a systematic fashion. Only he can anticipate the future and plan for it; and, of the advanced primates, man is the only one capable of symbolization and communication by words. It is through language that he becomes capable of thinking through the consequences of an action before attempting it, of abstracting from the concrete to the general, and of perceiving relationships between elements without the necessity of actual manipulation of these elements. Also, language is the agency whereby the experiences of the past generation are transmitted to the next. Thus man builds continuously on his cultural heritage. The growth of our knowledge has become exponential.

THE DEVELOPMENT OF INDIVIDUAL COMPONENTS OF PERSONALITY

As William James once remarked, "The baby, upon entering this world, assailed by sensations from eyes, ears, nose, skin and entrails, all at once, must feel it as one blooming, buzzing confusion." And the ways our complex nervous system brings these to order during development and maturation are nothing short of miraculous.

At the time of birth the human organism is 9 calendar months along his life cycle, and already some degree of individuality has been stamped on him, for no two infants look alike, even though many of the physical characteristics do not become definite until later, being somehow obscured by the delicacy of immaturity. One baby manifestly differs from others in vigor of movement, amount of sleep required, degree of irritability, and strength of instinctual demands. With respect to patterns of behavior, however, at birth he is still virtually a pulp.

Then commences the unfolding of a vast sequence of maturational changes that will transform him from a helpless vegetative state dominated by incretory and excretory activities, with limited capacity to perceive or react to the world about, to a confident, vigorous, intelligent, self-disciplined adult. From the standpoint of postural control, at the age of six months he sits, at twelve to fifteen months he walks, at two years he runs, at six years he may be acquiring the rudiments of athletic prowess or musical skill. In the area of perception he proceeds from the stage of fleeting interest in lights and movement, to which he makes sketchy, wavering ocular responses, to fine discrimination of color, size, and form. At the time of birth he grasps an object reflexly, with eyes wandering or vacantly transfixed, while by six years of age he expertly scans a figure prior to reproducing its form with a crayon. At birth there is only the cry, lacking all modulation and social meaning and marking the lowest level of language; in 2 years it is converted into articulate sounds, intelligible to others as words and already uttered in short sentences, and in 6 years these words take the form of complex syntactic speech by which the child can interrogate adults or inquire in a primitive way about causality. In personality structure, by the age of six he is aware of his identity as a person, occupying a finite part of space, separable from the physical world about, capable of self-assertion and of controlling the behavior of others in ways that foreshadow what he will later be like as an adult.

Each major item in this emergence of an individual from a reflex-dominated organism to one capable of independent decision is age-linked, and the work of André-Thomas and Arnold Gesell and their students have provided us with catalogues of some of the principal postnatal steps. These have been put to the service of neurologic medicine because they faithfully reflect the healthy function of the nervous system at different stages of growth and development. Deviations from normal sensory, motor, reflex, emotional, and social adaptive functions acquire pathologic significance only if they depart from an average standard. The child's neurologic status may thus be expressed as a developmental quotient (DQ). Gesell conceives this trajectory of developmental sequence essentially as an effluorescence of genetically determined events, whereas Piaget looks upon it as a biologic adaptation, a continuous creative interaction between the organism and its environment.

INTELLIGENCE AND COGNITION. Piaget, one of the most critical developmental psychologists of our time, divides the development of intelligence, one of the principal components of personality, into three major periods: *sensorimotor* (birth to two years), *concrete operations* (two to twelve years), and *formal operations* (twelve years through adult life). The sensorimotor period is one in which the congenital sensorimotor schemata and reflex patterns become differentiated from inchoate general behavior, to emerge later as the elementary processes of intelligence. The period of concrete operations is divided into a preconceptual phase (from two to four years) during which symbols are constructed; the intuitive phase (four to seven years) when concepts of space, causality, and time are acquired; and the logical phase (seven to twelve years) in which thought becomes differentiated from perception and action, permitting the classifying, ordering, and numbering of sensory data. The period of formal operations is one of systematization and recombination of the concrete operations, in the course of which the logical steps of abstract thought are mastered.

Facility in the acquisition of these more complex components of cognition is believed also to be determined by genetic factors. Individuals vary widely in their levels of achievement. Binet and many of the so-called "psychometrists" who followed him deduced this fact after devising tests and measuring these functions in a large population. Thus arose the idea of a human trait called *native intelligence,* defined as capacity for purposive behavior and ability to reason and to solve problems; they also found this capacity to be age-linked and expressible as an intelligence quotient (IQ). But their results were obviously contaminated with the effects of verbal skill, education, and scholastic achievement. Moreover, in educable children further statistical analyses of intelligence showed it to be relatively constant from one period to another but to consist not of a single, universal trait but of an aggregate of special abilities. Verbal skill, arithmetic ability, concept of space, speed of learning and memorizing, all essential components of types of intelligent behavior, were found to correlate only roughly with capacity for abstract thought and creativity. The role of intervening experience in the steps of maturation of cognitive function has been emphasized. In fact, it is the richness, complexity, and diversity of stimulation in a favorable social environment that results in the complete functional organization of mind. This is only another way of rephrasing Gesell's idea that "the primary elements in the child's disposition, capacities, and traits are determined largely by heredity but achieved through maturation which requires interaction with environment."

The time course of the cognitive functions of learning, remembering, perceiving, organization of sensory data, solving problems, and pursuing intellectual tasks is of interest. All are well developed by school age. The scheduling of formal education at six years is thus decided by an observed level of nervous organization which allows attentive interest, persistence of effort, the acquisition of written word and number symbols, and tolerance of separation from the family unit. Interestingly, the wide range of differences between individuals, varying from imbecility to genius, becomes increasingly evident as formal education proceeds. Also, many special defects of perception, speech, memory, etc. not earlier manifest in the simple play of the small child, become apparent at this stage when he is forced to compete with others of his age group. Without educational opportunity the natively intelligent mind never realizes its full potentiality.

EMOTIONAL DEVELOPMENT. Much of the child's individuality is undoubtedly attained through the stresses of human relations, which condition and habituate him. It is here that the extensive and pervasive interpenetration of the environment, which completes the patterns of organic growth, becomes apparent. The Freudian formulation of instinctual and emotional development, the most systematic and complete theory yet devised, conceives of emotional development as a series of predictable modifications of the sexual instinct. The latter is defined not merely as the impulse to sexual gratification but more broadly as desire for the pleasure and satisfaction with which such activities are endowed. The energy of sexual impulse, called *libido,* is traced in this scheme back to the earliest sensory pleasures attendant upon the activities of the oral and genital parts of the body. Successively the sexuality of the child expands to include many of the activities of the mother and other members of the same and finally the opposite sex. Powerful repressive forces are exerted upon the sexual impulse by social custom but always with the risk of the energy of sexual drive being displaced to other systems of thought or activities which may then motivate behavior in unexpected ways. Personality development is regarded essentially as a process of sexual maturation, the final purpose of which is to assure procreation and the establishment of the individual as an integral part of a new family. Perversions, arrests, or regressions of this process are thought to be the source of psychopathic and neurotic behavior. This hormic, or motivational, aspect of behavior and the dependence of it on the formation of sexual bonds between infant and mother, family members, and others is confirmed by the studies of monkeys by Harlow. The baby monkey, if deprived of the warmth of social contact with other animals of its kind, grows up to be totally inadequate as a sexual partner, parent, or member of monkey society.

There are many who believe the Freudian emphasis on sexuality takes far too restricted a view of the human personality. While it is true that the tie to the mother can be conceived as a derivative of the nursing act, body contact with mother soon becomes less important than touch, smell, sight, and sound, as a determinative factor in the infant's behavior as he becomes involved in the complex activities of daily care. Perceptual and cognitive maturation enable the infant to relate many initially disconnected and separate experiences to the person who provides them and, thereby, to distinguish the mother from other persons in the environment. Soon many others, such as siblings, father, teacher, etc., begin to figure in special nonsexual ways in his life.

In the formation of the personality, especially the part concerned with feeling and emotional sensitivity, basic temperament and other qualities play a part. Some children by nature tend from the beginning to be happy, cheerful, and unconcerned about immediate frustrations, and others are irritable and difficult. By the third month of postnatal life Thomas and his associates were able to recognize individual differences in activity-passivity, regularity-irregularity, intensity of action, approach-withdrawal, adaptive-unadaptive, high-low threshold of response to stimulation, positive-negative mood, high-low selectivity, and high-low distractability. Ratings at this age were found to correlate well with others made at two years of age and reasonably well with the results of a third examination at five years. Many of these characteristics are presumably genetic but are influenced by the spirit of the environment provided by parents. But, as Cross and his associates have shown, the initial characteristics of the infant also influence parental reaction, just as their behavior influences his.

The more common traits such as the tendency to worry about health and other problems, to be anxious or serene, timid or bold; the power of instinctual drive and need of satisfaction, the sympathy one has for others, the sensitivity to criticism and degree of disorganization resulting from adverse circumstances are presumably traceable to some of the more basic instincts and emotions.

SOCIAL ADAPTATION. Early life requires a long succession of human interactions, first to parents, then to family, other children, and finally to a widening circle of individuals in the classroom, commercial world, and community at large. Capacity to cooperate, to subjugate one's own egocentric needs to those of the group, to lead or be led, appear as modes of response. Qualities of temperament and emotionality such as aggression, passivity, tendency to anxiety, depression, and elation usually are felt and most clearly expressed in relation to individuals in the social environment.

The basis of these social reactions is less clear than that of cognitive qualities of mind and of temperament. The frequency of aggressive behavior in children, for example, is often used as an argument for an innate aggressive instinct. In actuality this is a derived mode of reaction, and such interpretation is an instance of a widespread tendency to explain infantile behavior by a priori assignment of adult motives, assumed on the basis of spurious analogies. In the normal child, aggression usually originates in innate curiosity or takes the form of a defense reaction or a response to frustration and failure, for all of which aggressiveness is a suitable mediator. Its greater frequency in the abnormal child may be correlated with defects in the organism, as in the case of brain injury, and also with resultant distortions in its environment which give rise to faulty identification models. Moreover, the frequency of display of aggressive behavior is a function of the culture in which the child is reared. While encouraged in our culture, where it is recognized as a desirable manifestation of energetic and vigorous action, becoming unacceptable only if assaultive and violent, it may not at all be condoned in other cultures. The capacity for aggression is indeed inherent in the impulse life of man, as it is in all animals, but its frequency of evocation and display are conditioned by other determinants.

The greatest demands and the greatest frustrations in social development are likely to occur during late childhood and adolescence. The child's difficulty is apt to become manifest in his inability to adjust to the exigencies of the classroom. The adolescent is faced with an even greater diversity of environmental challenges. Half emancipated from family ties, he must seek the recognition and respect of his peers. To do this he needs a field for the full exploitations of his power of abstract thought; and for the first time he becomes concerned with what he is and what he will be. In his search for personal identity he becomes more critical of parents and turns increasingly to larger social groups for his sense of belonging. If his relations with his parents have been soundly constructed and if the parents meet his doubts and criticisms with sympathetic understanding, this temporary unsettling of his primary family position leads to a resynthesis of his relations with them on a firm and lasting basis. The development of adult sexual characteristics and the further evolution of psychosexual impulses cause him to experience a bewildering array of new physical sensations. These sensations lead to an upsurge of interest in physical sex and psychologic sensitization to new aspects of interpersonal relationships along this line. The developing ability for abstract conceptualization provides the foundation for advanced education, for scientific study and creativity, and for increasing concern about the basic meanings and values of human existence.

These types of social development continue as long as life continues. As social roles change, as intellectual and physical capacities first advance and later recede, new challenges demand new adaptations. The success of these is enhanced always if started from a solid base of accomplishment in a secure work role, from a position as a stable member of a family unit, and from an acceptable view and philosophy of one's place in life. Conditions which thwart the healthy development of proper attitudes toward health, family, work, and religion often become the sources of maladjustment in later life.

PSYCHOPATHOLOGIC TRENDS AND THEIR SOURCES

The physician faced with countless human problems, no two of which are ever alike, searches among this bewildering kaleidoscope of developmental events for tendencies which indicate the action of pathogenic agencies and the beginnings of social maladjustment. If identified, attempts are made to modify them and to prevent or control, by appropriate measures, their consequences. The assumption that this is possible is the main premise of the entire mental health movement in the United States. The following disturbances should alert the physician to the possibility of psychopathologic deviation:

1. *Sense deprivation and insufficiency of stimulation.* In the earliest period of life sense deprivation appears to be a factor that impairs perceptual development. An animal reared in darkness for several months has been shown to fail to acquire all the natural visual perceptions and visuomotor reactions when later put in light. A human example of this is amblyopia exanopsia, where ocular imbalance has prevented one eye from accommodating and being stimulated in binocular vision. The wandering eye fails to develop as an effective organ despite the integrity of the refractive media, retina, and nervous connections with the brain. Another example is the deaf child who remains mute, or if he speaks, is unable to learn to modulate his own voice in a pleasing fashion. It is doubtful, however, if sensory deprivation has many other effects on man. Human environment is such a busy, noisy, dazzling place that it is hard to imagine sensory deprivation occurring under most conditions of daily life even in the most impoverished circumstances. However, transient derangements in mentation may occur when disease imposes complete quiet in a darkened room or a respirator. Extreme degrees of sensory deprivation, lasting many hours, may disorganize perceptual processes to a degree where illusions and hallucinations may supervene, often with panic. Such depri-

vation psychoses become increasingly frequent in the brain-damaged child and the elderly person, presumably because their adaptive powers are weakened by inadequacy of cerebral mechanisms.

Potentially significant degrees of insufficient stimulation should be suspected in orphans and in families where the mother is absent much of the time or is disturbed by psychiatric illness. Corrective measures involve increased adult contact.

2. *Emotional deprivation.* Emotional deprivation in early life, so clearly pathogenic in the lives of young animals, has been postulated as a cause of mental retardation and neurosis in man. Bowlby's monograph summarizes the literature on this subject and concludes that early separation from mother has persistent and irreversible effects manifest in both intelligence and personality. The work of Goldfarb provides some further documentation of this fact. In comparing two groups of orphaned children (one of which had spent the first 3 years in an orphanage before being placed in a foster home, the second group put immediately in a foster home), he found lower IQ, poorer school performance, and more sociopathic traits in the first group. Skeels and Scogel had earlier observed that orphans given over to the care of affectionate foster mothers early in life raised their IQs from 64 to 91, while the control group had IQs that fell from 86 to 60. However, the fault of all such studies is the difficulty in being sure that the experimental and control groups are comparable and that the psychologic tests, which require a certain degree of activity, maturity, and motivation on the part of the child, are sufficiently accurate in early life and therefore comparable from one time to another. Bowlby's original monograph, which presents well the deleterious effects of maternal neglect, puts too much stress on their irreversibility. Children left alone for long periods during the first year prove to be relatively inactive and disinterested in their environments, but when moved to a more stimulating atmosphere they usually catch up with their more fortunate colleagues. Here it is a mistake to assume that maternal deprivation constitutes a major factor in the causation of definite and permanent mental retardation. Lesser degrees of diminished intellectual stimulation during childhood, lack of encouragement to study, to learn, to excel in school, unquestionably impair intellectual achievement and increase the rate of school failure and drop-out. But these effects are better understood in terms of poor examples being set for emulation, lack of opportunity to acquire self-discipline, lack of satisfying goals, etc.

Children placed early in foster homes and orphanages and those of the lowest social and economic groups are more likely to be subject to the effects of impoverished emotional environment and inadequate motivation. And, these are often the very ones whose innate capacity for adaptation is most limited.

3. *Deprivation of discipline, parental overindulgence and failure of emancipation from family.* Whether unintelligent, thoughtless, cold parents can induce abnormal character in a child is a moot point. The possibility that the child is exhibiting the same inherited traits as the parent cannot be excluded. There is no doubt that the child needs guidance and help in making the transition from a state of helplessness and total dependence to one of independence and capability of effective interaction with its social environment. Certain demanding and difficult items of behavior must be taught by reward and at times punishment in order to keep the behavior within the bounds of acceptability. A vacillating, incomprehensible discipline confuses the child and may result in either epsiodes of violent and assaultive behavior or withdrawal. Many early behavior problems seem traceable to a period of excessive parental dependence. In fact one of the great dangers of any prolonged childhood illness is its tendency to strengthen unduly the ties to parents and to inculcate unnatural concern about health. Lack of firm, intelligent, parental discipline will interfere with adaptive processes in the well endowed as well as the retarded child.

Here the physician must guard against undue criticism of the practices of child rearing. It is easy to find fault with parental care because few parents are well instructed in such matters before having children; and the child may be born when the parents themselves are having problems. The possibility that the parents' behavior may also be conditioned by that of the child must not be overlooked. A jittery, overly active, unhappy baby may cause the frustrated parent to lose patience and neglect him, thus creating a vicious circle. The child with a developmental or other disease, not able to comprehend a complex world, not able to understand the language of the parent, often withdraws from human contact, preferring to deal with simpler objects in the physical world. He often appears out of contact with people and is uncritically labeled *autistic*. Intelligent correction involves helping the parents understand the normal reactions of the growing child and helping the child satisfy his physical and emotional needs in ways that are acceptable to society.

4. *Specific deficits in cerebral function.* Every blemish, every physical abnormality becomes a cross to bear during the formative years, when the child or adolescent seeks tribe approval, but it is the restricted cerebral deficit that dislocates him most consistently. The child with the developmental speech disorder (stammer, stutter, dyslexia, or word deafness) not only stands apart, but the training and education to which his intelligence entitles him are blocked. If forced in his school work beyond the capabilities of his language mechanism, he becomes rebellious and aggressive or gives up completely and withdraws; and not infrequently all social development, which at this age is so completely centered in the classroom, is thwarted. Sometimes the fault is only a delay in language development, which will later correct itself as the mysterious process of cerebral dominance is strengthened.

This latter type of disturbance emphasizes another notable aspect of child development—its unevenness and irregularity. Just as no two humans are ready to walk at the same age, so too are they different with respect to the time of acquisition and stable functioning of language mechanisms and other complex behavioral sequences. The total language repertoire covers a span of 15 to 20 years and is matched in length only by such activities as learning to use numerical symbols, to think, and to reason. Presumably these language and other functions depend on maturation of parts of the brain, and delay often is genetically determined (90 percent of stutterers are males) but exercise and guidance are also necessary for their full development. The tendency among psychiatrists in recent years has been to seek out and attempt to treat the patient's reaction to the frustration caused by these deficits rather than to apply methods of teaching which assist in language development.

Medical action involves the discovery and assessment of the native capacities of the child and helping him to improve them by training and to make a healthy adjustment to any inadequacies thereof.

THE ORIGINS OF PSYCHOPATHY, NEUROSIS, AND PSYCHOSIS

Lack of socialization, of coming to understand the actions, feelings, and needs of other members of one's social group, inability to perceive one's own personality deficits, and extremes of egocentricity, which stand as the central issues in the development of psychoneurosis, are evident by the time adolescence is reached. Indeed, *neurosis* is definable in such terms, and *psychosis* signifies but a more global disorganization of mental function and behavior but again expressed to a maximum degree in disordered social relationships. In later life, the neurotic person habitually attempts to preserve his selfish ways in each newly formed social circle. Being socially unacceptable on this account, conflict situations arise which engender anxiety and depression. The complete detachment of the autistic child, the amorality of the constitutional psychopath, the major deviations of temperament and mood of the hereditary manic-depressive, the characteristic difficulty in thinking and affective relationship of the schizophrenic patient have also declared themselves by the end of childhood and early adolescence. And, now one confronts the key problem: To what extent do neurosis, psychopathy, and psychosis have their roots in the early thwarting or perversion of the natural processes of personality development, and to what degree are they determined by genetic factors?

The answers to these questions cannot be given with finality. Experienced clinicians tend to believe that genetic factors are actually more important than environmental. The discovery that unusually tall males with severe acne vulgaris and aggressive psychopathic behavior have two Y chromosomes is an example of a newly discovered genetic relationship. And then, too, there is the fact that deliberate alteration of the social environment has so far never been shown to prevent a major psychiatric disease, although admittedly the wise counseling of parents has been helpful in the management of children with behavior problems. Children identified as high-risk individuals because of early truancy, conflict with the law, and general social maladjustment, if transferred to a more stable and helpful environment, have, as a group, not turned out better than others who were left alone. Admittedly such investigations are open to many criticisms, and it is for this reason that the mental hygienists have been supported in the United States, even though evidence that their methods are effective is still lacking.

There are other considerations than the development of frank neurosis or psychosis for there are countless unhappy, maladjusted individuals who cannot be included among the psychologically ill. It is with reference to these conditions that one looks for early psychopathologic trends. Adolescent turmoil often seems to stem from unhealthy parent-child relationships, which have engendered excessive dependence or hostility. The result may be either a failure of emancipation or a rejection of family ties and a lasting sense of isolation. Similarly, sexual deviations of adolescent and adult life are often ascribed to lack of early education. The ambivalence of Western society, which evinces interest in sex but then imposes sanctions on its expression, contributes to the problem. Too little is known about the early conditioning that inculcates the traits of masculinity and femininity. Certainly hormonal control plays but a minor part. The basis of homosexuality or sexual perversions is not known. Ignorance of sex and impoverishment of human relations account later for many sexual misadventures.

The sensitivity of the adolescent to the good opinion of his peers renders him psychologically vulnerable to any minor variation in his own physique and to pernicious influences in his social environment. If in addition he should be endowed with limited intellectual and physical capacity, the grounds for persistent and indomitable feelings of inferiority are laid, especially if he is forced to compete in situations which result in repeated failure. The individualization of education and vocational training for such adolescents is essential, both to permit the talented individual to exploit his abilities and to direct the youngster with specific limitations into activities that constructively develop his personality.

It is during the period of late childhood and adolescence, when the psychologic structure is least stable, that transient symptoms, many resembling the psychopathologic states of adult life, are most frequent. Great caution must be exercised lest such temporary maladaptive patterns be misinterpreted. While some of these behavioral disorders represent the early signs of schizophrenia and manic-depressive psychosis, diseases that usually become manifest for the first time around puberty, many of them have a way of disappearing as adult years are reached. One can only surmise that the turbulence of the adolescent period came to be controlled rather late.

CONCLUSION

The internist no less than the psychiatrist must learn to think of his patient in dynamic terms as an organism with a history, with a set of sentiments, attitudes, opinions, and expectations, and with a profound dependence on the forces of his social environment. Assessment of the patient must be as much in terms of his abilities and his disabilities, as in terms of what he is, was, and will be. Clinical diagnosis and treatment are most effective when based on a conception of man that recognizes both the existence of mental diseases and at the same time stresses personality as a series of forces continuously emerging and never fully complete. Developmental disturbances, if global and severe, are usually due to a general structural abnormality of the brain or the effects of disease, whereas maturational delays, related often to inherited predisposition in interaction with social environment and tending to derange nervous function in specific ways (autism, delayed speech and dyslexia, dyscalculia, and uncontrollable or dysinhibited behavior) are not. These latter will be considered further in Chap. 29. The most subtle aberrations in social adjustment, expressed as psychoneurosis and psychosis, will receive separate analysis in Section 10.

REFERENCE

Eisenberg, L.: Normal child development, chap. 38.2 in "Comprehensive Textbook of Psychiatry," A. M. Freedman and H. I. Kaplan (Eds.), Baltimore, Williams and Wilkins Company, 1967.

8 THE AGING PATIENT

The Editors

The clinical phenomena presented under Cardinal Manifestations of Disease depend on pathologic derangements of biologic processes. Only when considered with reference to a time scale in the human life cycle called aging do such biological processes, or morbid derangements thereof, acquire full significance in medicine.

Aging includes the acquired changes which need time for their development and also involutional changes which are as much a part of mammalian life as the autumnal decline of the leaves of deciduous trees. Accumulations of lipofuscins in cells, of cholesterol in the arteries or gall bladder, and of chalk in the cartilages, all require time; hence, they are more advanced in the aged than in the young. Certain changes such as those in the subdeltoid tendon sheath or about the vertebral bodies occur from stress, and the oftener the stress is repeated, the more marked the changes. Hence old persons show more change than younger ones. Involution probably also plays a part in altering the composition of the tissue in all these cases, but age and repeated exposure to a noxious influence are also necessary to evoke clinical evidence of impaired function.

Aging, then, may be defined as the sum of the losses of function and structure of the callosities, scars, and nodular hyperplasias due to "wear and tear" and to involution. Wear and tear includes trauma; infection; overstimulation by emotional, dietary, or other abuses; dietary inadequacies; exposure to inclement weather; or exhausting exertion. Involution may be defined as the physiologic changes in cellular activity leading to the al-

tered structure and functional capacity characteristic of all senescent members of any species. The age at which, in any tissue, involution becomes manifest may show racial as well as familial patterns, varying by years or even decades.

THE MEASURE OF GROWTH AND AGING

The natural length of life is an integral characteristic, built, in some mysterious way, into the organism. The rat is old at 2 years; the rhesus monkey survives for 20 to 25 years; the Galapagos tortoise lives to be 100 years old. Man, like the African elephant, may expect to live for 70 to 75 years. The duration of animal and human life correlates roughly with the size of the brain. Despite all the publicity about medical science lengthening man's life, the change has been only a statistical change brought about by controlling infant mortality and infectious disease. Thereby, more people are enabled to reach the upper limit of life expectancy, but this limit has not been extended. In fact, since Biblical times, when man was said to be allotted three score and ten years, the span of human life has not appreciably lengthened. The clock inevitably runs down for the average person before the seventy-fifth year, and it seems to make little difference whether he lives in a luxurious urban villa or a primitive hut. Only the exceptionally endowed person lives beyond this age.

The disease to which man ultimately succumbs, whether cancer, coronary occlusion, or some other malady, does not greatly alter his predetermined life span. If he were fortunate enough to avoid such conditions, his life would not be lengthened much beyond 10 years. Interestingly, delay in growth by undernutrition early in life has been shown in animals to delay aging and the vulnerability to disease in their senescence. Whether overnutrition has the opposite effect is not known. It also has been observed that whole body irradiation hastens aging and increases susceptibility to disease and death.

To the biologist and physician, death is not the main consideration. What is more meaningful are indices of *vitality*, of resistance to disease, of organ efficiency. In point of fact *senescence* is defined in such terms, i.e., the decline of vitality, the progressive lowering of biologic efficiency, the diminution of the capacity of the organism to maintain itself as an efficient machine. Early loss of certain functions is called *involution*; unexpected, premature decay of any given tissue or cell population has been termed *abiotrophy* (Chap. 4).

The composite of overt bodily changes due to senescence, such as the cessation of bodily growth, wrinkling of the skin, grayness of the hair, loss of teeth, involution of the sexual organs, loss of acuity of the senses, bent posture, weakening of muscular power and coordination, rigidity of the mind, conservative views, and forgetfulness, are known to every observant human. When considered one by one, it is evident that waning vitality or senescence has different times of onset and rates of progress in different organ systems. Measurements of visual and auditory acuity are said to reach their maximum at the age of ten years, and resistance to infection, at fifteen years, whereas intellectual power reaches its peak at twenty-one, and muscular power and coordination at twenty-five. According to Shock, between the ages of thirty and seventy-five, maximum oxygen uptake during exercise decreases 60 percent and maximum ventilation volume, 47 percent. Vital capacity decreases 44 percent, and cardiac output at rest, 30 percent. Kidney plasma flow is reduced 50 percent, glomerular filtration rate 31 percent, and the number of glomeruli in the kidneys, 44 percent. Both adrenal and gonadal activity decrease, basal metabolic rate is reduced 16 percent and the body water content, 18 percent, but the speed of return of blood acidity to equilibrium after exercise declines 83 percent. Brain weight decreases 10 percent, blood flow to the brain, 20 percent, the number of taste buds, 64 percent, the number of fibers in nerves, 37 percent and nerve conduction velocity, 10 percent. It is important, therefore, in the evaluation of the condition of a patient to discriminate between the effects of age and of disease. Diagnostic criteria should be age-linked and cannot be related directly to functional values based on a normal population of young medical students. Likewise, in therapy it is essential to adjust drug dosages to functions which decrease with age, especially cerebral and renal function.

Details concerning changes with age in special organs and tissues will be found in the appropriate sections, viz. nervous system (Chap. 352), skeletal muscles (Chap. 373), kidneys (Chap. 298), and skin and supporting tissues (Chap. 400). From time to time various organs and tissues have been singled out as special targets of the aging process. It is not true, however, that men are "as old as their arteries." Men may die of coronary atherosclerosis before they are old enough to vote; these arteries are diseased, not old. Men are as old as their skins, their scalps, their cerebral cortices, and all their other tissues.

THE CELLULAR BASIS OF AGING

Many mechanisms are presumed to underlie the effects of age on the cellular constituents of various organ systems. Investigative efforts have been directed along a number of lines, viz., (1) the decline in the functional efficiency and finally the deterioration and death of highly specialized, nondividing cells, such as the muscle fiber, neuron, etc.; (2) the failure of the process of mitosis in tissues composed of dividing cells; (3) the accumulation of somatic cell mutations; (4) the progressive alteration of the structural protein, collagen, which constitutes about a third of the body protein; (5) alterations in immune responsiveness and the development of autoimmunologic reactions.

Thus, nerve and muscle cells which cease to divide early and must last the lifetime of the organism are known to have a variable life span. If accidentally destroyed by disease, they are never replaced. Even in the absence of disease, there is a steady outfall which begins about the end of the period of growth and maturation and continues at an accelerated pace into the se-

nium. Functional deficits in organs such as the brain are in large measure to be ascribed to cell loss. Fortunately each organ is endowed with a generous safety factor, a protective excess of cells that must be exhausted before symptoms appear. The extent to which cells begin to falter functionally before their final disintegration is unknown but, in red corpuscles at least, decreasing quantities of certain enzymes have been recorded.

The cytologic events leading to death of nondividing cells are but little understood. In man as well as animals accumulation of lipofuscin in the cytoplasm of these cells is so constant a phenomenon that it can be used as the most reliable cytologic index of age. Called *wear and tear pigment, lipochrome,* or *lipofuscin,* these yellow granules form in the cytoplasm of nerve and muscle cells, being derived in all probability from lysosomes or, possibly, mitochondria. Simultaneous with their formation, the cell diminishes in volume presumably due to loss of other cytoplasmic components such as Nissl bodies (the main cytoplasmic RNA in nerve cells) and mitochondria. Also, the nucleus becomes smaller with infolding of nuclear membrane and alteration of nucleolus. Histochemical stains reveal a depletion of oxidative as well as phosphorylative enzymes. All of these changes have been verified in tissue culture.

Again, alterations occur in the capacity for cell growth and multiplication. Contrary to the original experiments of Alexis Carrel, which showed that cells removed from the animal body and properly sustained and nourished in tissue culture could continue to live and divide forever, Hayflick and his colleagues found that each fibroblast is destined to divide only a certain number of times. Fibroblasts from a human infant divide about 50 times; those of a twenty-year-old, about 30 times; and those from an eighty-year-old person, about 20. Towards the end of the life cycle of the cell, chromosomal aberrations and peculiarities of cell division begin to appear. Only if a special neoplastic type of change takes place with the cells becoming "mixoploid" (50 to 350 chromosomes per cell, many of which are abnormally formed), do cells attain the immortality postulated by Carrel. Male (XY) and female (XX) cells behave alike, whether grown singly or together. Probably leukocytes and liver cells also possess a genetically determined limitation for mitosis.

Hayflick sees the diminishing capacity of cells in vitro to divide as an intrinsic property of the cells themselves, a deterioration of the "genetic program that orchestrates the development of cells." Perhaps with the passage of time the DNA of the dividing cell becomes clouded with an ever-increasing number of copying errors. Depletion with age of certain enzymes involved in the transcription of DNA for the synthesis of proteins may occur. In all events these studies trace the secret of aging in dividing cells back to some obscure degeneration of inherited information-containing molecules in the cell nucleus which provide the final control of cell division. Whether cells in vivo behave differently than cells in tissue culture is not known.

It is important to appreciate that once the fibers of

collagen are laid down, they are not renewed. Labeled constituents of collagen show no "turnover." Aging collagen contracts more strongly when heated (tensile strength and elasticity increase) possibly due to the formation of more H bonds along the sides of the collagen strands between tropo-collagen molecules. The amino acids of aging collagen, particularly hydroxyproline, become less soluble. A diminishing amount of extractable elastin also runs parallel to age, but the change is less marked than in collagen. Chemical analyses have shown the aspartic and glutamic acid components of elastic tissue and amide nitrogen content to increase with age, whereas glycine, proline, and valine decrease.

Little is known regarding the reasons for the cellular changes which occur with age.

It is well recognized that certain diseases are found more frequently in persons of advancing age than in younger ones. Certain types of tumors, vascular diseases of the heart and brain, infections, especially pulmonary ones, and fractures of the hip are well known examples. The reasons, insofar as they are understood, can be best outlined in the various sections which deal with these disorders.

REFERENCES

Birren, J. E.: Human Ageing, a Biological and Behavioral Study, U.S.P.H.S. Publication 986, 1963.

Bourne, G. H., et al.: "Structural Aspects of Aging, "New York, Hafner Publishing Co., 1961.

"Ciba Foundation Colloquia on Ageing," vol. 1. "General Aspects," Boston, Little, Brown and Company, 1955.

Hayflick, L.: Human Cells and Aging, Sci. Am., 218:32, 1968.

Korenchevsky, V., and G. H. Bourne: "Physiological and Pathological Aging," New York, Harper Publishing Company, 1961.

Shock, N. W.: The Physiology of Aging, Sci. Am., 206:100, 1962.

Strehler, B. L.: The Biology of Aging, Am. Instit. Biol. Sci., Publication 6, 1960.

Verzar, F.: The Aging of Collagen, Sci. Am., 208:104, 1963.

Part Three

Cardinal Manifestations and Approach to Disease

Section 1

Pain

9 GENERAL CONSIDERATIONS
Raymond D. Adams and William M. Resnik

Pain, it has been said, is one of "Nature's earliest signs of morbidity." Few will deny that it stands preeminent among all the sensory experiences by which man judges the existence of disease within himself. There are relatively few maladies that do not have their painful phases, and in many of them pain is a characteristic without which diagnosis must always be in doubt. It seems appropriate, therefore, to begin a section on the cardinal manifestations of disease with a discussion of the more general aspects of pain.

The painful experiences of the sick pose manifold problems for the practitioner of medicine, and the student should know something of these problems in order to prepare himself properly for the task ahead. He must be ready to diagnose disease in patients who have felt only the first rumblings of discomfort, before other symptoms and signs of disease have appeared. To cope effectively with problems of this type requires a sound knowledge of the sensory supply of the viscera and a familiarity with the typical symptoms of many diseases. He will be consulted by some patients who seek treatment for pains that appear to have no obvious structural basis, and further inquiry will disclose that worry, fear, and other troubled emotional states may have aggrandized relatively minor aches and pains. To understand problems of this type requires insight into the psychologic factors which influence behavior and a knowledge of psychiatric disease. Next, he must manage the "difficult pain cases," in which no amount of investigation will bring to light either medical disease or psychiatric illness, and it is here that he will sense the need of a sound and assured clinical approach to the pain problem. Finally, he must care for the patients with intractable pain, often from an established and incurable disease, who demand relief either by drug or the "less moderate means of surgery." The possibilities of the latter require a comprehension of the anatomic pathways of pain.

END ORGANS, AFFERENT TRACTS, AND NUCLEI OF TERMINATION OF PAIN PATHWAYS

Pain is now regarded by most physiologists and psychologists as a sensation which depends on its own specific sensory apparatus. The receptors in the skin and deep structures are fine, freely branching nerve endings, which form an intricate network. A single primary pain neurone, with its cell body in the posterior root ganglion, subdivides into many small peripheral branches to supply an area of skin of at least several square millimeters. The cutaneous area of each neurone overlaps with those of other neurones, so that every spot of skin is within the domain of from two to four sensory neurones. These free nerve endings are also found in many of the other specialized sensory receptors in the skin, such as the Krause end-bulbs, the Ruffinian plumes, and Pacinian corpuscles, which may account for the extremes of hot, cold, and pressure sensation becoming painful. However, the whole subject of specific nerve endings for each modality of sensation has been reinvestigated. It appears now that free nerve endings themselves may serve as receptors for other types of sensation. They are the only end organ in the cornea where touch, temperature, and pain are felt.

The sensory nerve fibers for pain course through somatic and visceral nerves, where they are mixed with motor fibers, and they enter the spinal cord and brain stem through the posterior roots and the cranial nerves, respectively. The fibers are of two sizes, one very small, 2 to 4 μ in diameter, with a slow conducting velocity, the other somewhat larger, 6 to 8 μ, with more rapid transmission rates. As the posterior root fibers enter the spinal cord to terminate in the posterior horn of the spinal cord, they divide into two groups. A lateral unmyelinated bundle of thin fibers turns into the substantia gelatinosa where it synapses with (1) many small neurones, whose axons connect with the secondary ascending main neurones in the same and adjacent segments, and (2) more directly, with the large secondary pain neurones themselves. The axons of these small neurones compose the tract of Lissauer. The medial myelinated division synapses with the large secondary sensory neurones in the substantia gelatinosa and the posterior horn of gray matter before ascending in the posterior column. The axones of the secondary sensory neurones ascend for two to three segments and cross through the anterior commissure to take their place as the anterolateral spinothalamic tract. Other pain fibers presumably ascend on the same and opposite side through a chain of short neurones which reside in the gray matter. Some of the nerve cells in the posterior horns send their axones to the central gray matter and to anterior horn cells of the same segment and adjacent segments and subserve such reflex functions as the flexor reflex, of which

Babinski's sign is but a part. The anterolateral spinothalamic tract continues upward to the posterolateral nucleus of the thalamus. This tract lies in the anterior part of the lateral and the anterior funiculi of the spinal cord and passes through the retroolivary part of the medulla and the dorsolateral parts of the pons and midbrain (Fig. 9-1, see also Fig. 9-2). The most superficial fibers are those from the opposite foot and leg and the successively deeper ones from the trunk, arm, neck, and face. Before reaching the thalamus, collateral branches are given off to other segmental structures, such as the reticular formation of the brain stem and the hypothalamus. In addition there appears to be a great diminution in the number of fibers as one pursues the tract upward, which means that many of the ascending fibers are terminating in structures located in the brain stem. The thalamic termination of the spinothalamic tracts along with the secondary trigeminothalamic tracts synapse with the third sensory neurones, which project to the cortex in the parietal lobes. Physiologists are not agreed, however, as to the cortical terminus, for electrical stimulation of the cortex in the conscious human being does not produce a painful sensation but only a tingling as a rule, nor do parietal lobe lesions cause central pain except in rare instances Nearly all pain fibers from the periphery cross to the contralateral half of spinal cord, brain stem, and thalamus, but a few are believed to ascend ipsilaterally, at least for a considerable distance. This point is still being studied.

The pain-sensitive structures in the viscera and integuments of the body, the mechanisms of their excitation, and the peripheral nervous pathways are now fairly well established. The skin and mucous membranes are sensitive to pain, as are also many of the mesodermal tissues. As a means of quick orientation it should be remembered that the facial structures and anterior cranium are the field of the trigeminal nerves; the back of head, second cervical; the neck, third cervical; epaulet area, fourth cervical; deltoid area, fifth cervical; the thumb, sixth cervical; the index finger, seventh cervical; middle finger, eighth cervical; the little finger, first thoracic; the nipple segment, fifth thoracic; the umbilicus, tenth thoracic; the groin, first lumbar; the medial side of knee, third lumbar; the great toe, fifth lumbar; the little toe, first sacral; the back of thigh, second sacral; and genitosacral areas, third, fourth, and fifth sacrals (Figs. 25-1 and 25-2). The first to fourth thoracic nerves are the important dermatomes for the intrathoracic viscera, and the sixth, seventh, and eighth thoracic segments for the upper abdominal orgains (see Figs. 25-1 and 25-2). The student should memorize these facts just as he has the multiplication table.

The stimuli that are effective in arousing the sensation of pain vary to some degree for each tissue. The very existence of pain impulses arising from viscera was debated until it was demonstrated that the adequate stimuli for pain originating in the heart or digestive tract, for example, are different from those which cause pain in the skin. The latter is sensitive to pricking, cutting, and burning, whereas these same forms of stimulation give rise to no distress when applied to the stomach or intestine.

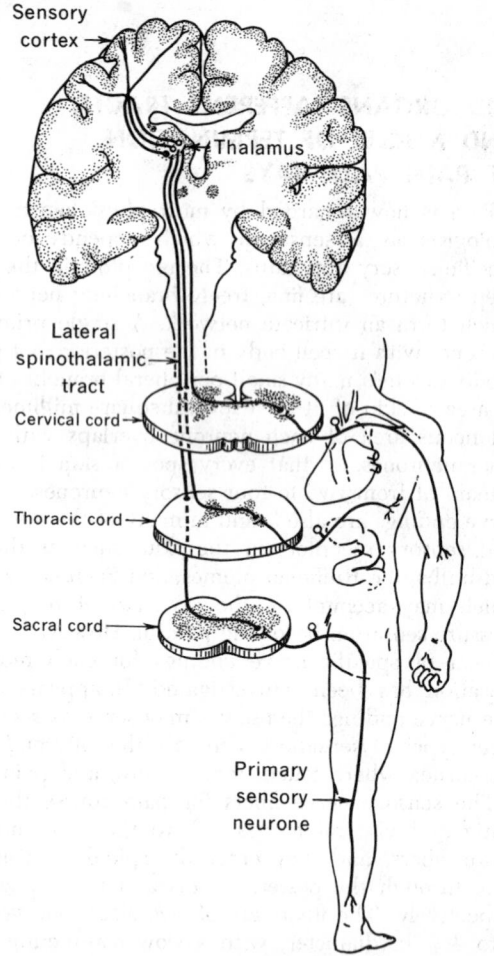

Fig. 9-1. Diagram of pain pathways. Stimuli acting on free nerve endings in the skin, muscles, blood vessels, and viscera give rise to sensory impulses, which are transmitted along the primary sensory neurones into the posterior horn of the spinal cord. The secondary sensory neurones cross to the opposite side of the spinal cord almost immediately, within one or two segments, and combine to form the lateral spinothalamic tract, which terminates in the posterolateral nucleus of the thalamus. The third sensory neurone conveys the impulse from the thalamus to the cortex of the postcentral convolution. Visceral pain fibers, although they pass through the sympathetic ganglions en route to the spinal cord, do not differ from other somatic pain fibers.

Pain in the gastrointestinal tract is produced by local trauma of an engorged or inflamed mucosa, distension or spasm of smooth muscle, and traction upon the mesenteric attachment. Severe pain may be induced in voluntary muscles by ischemia, the basis for the condition known as *intermittent claudication*, and also by the injection of water or irritating solutions. Also, prolonged contraction of muscles is a source of pain. Joints are insensitive to pricking, cutting, or cautery, but the synovial membrane responds to hypertonic saline solution and inflammation. Ischemia, the only proved cause of pain in the heart muscle, is responsible for the pain of angina pectoris and myocardial infarction. Arteries give rise to pain when punctured with a needle, when induced to pulsate excessively, as in migraine, and in certain diseases affecting their walls, such as temporal arteritis. Distortion of cranial vessels by traction, displacement, or distension is a common cause of headache.

PHYSIOLOGY AND PSYCHOLOGY OF PAIN

SUPERFICIAL PAIN. There are distinct differences in the characteristics of pain arising in the skin and that originating in the viscera. The effective stimulus for pain in the skin and superficial structures may be mechanical, thermal, chemical, or electrical. At their lowest levels these stimuli may evoke sensations of touch, pressure, warmth, or cold. Only when they reach a certain intensity, usually approaching tissue destruction, does pain develop, and the resulting experience is thereafter a mixed one, combining pain with the original sensation. Wolff points out that the threshold for burning pain with a thermal stimulus is approximately two thousand times the threshold for warmth. Tissue damage is believed to be a common effect of all pain stimuli, a fact from which our concept of the fundamental biologic or self-preservation value of pain derives much of its plausibility.

The threshold for the perception of pain is defined as the lowest intensity of stimulus which is recognized as pain. It is approximately the same in all persons. The pain threshold is lowered by inflammation of the peripheral nerve endings and is raised by local anesthetics (such as procaine), lesions of the peripheral and cerebral nervous system, centrally acting analgesic drugs, and distraction or suggestion. Neurotic patients in general have the same pain threshold as normal subjects, but their reaction may be excessive or abnormal. The threshold in the frontal-lobotomized patient is undiminished, but he no longer reacts to his pain. The intensity of the pain stimulus bears a roughly quantitative relationship to the reported degree of sensory experience. The ratio between the two is expressed by the Weber-Fechner law, which states that when a series of progressively increasing stimuli is applied, in order for minimal sensory differences to be perceived, the new stimulus must be increased by a constant fraction of the previously effective one.

Pain arising in the skin has a pricking or burning quality and is localized with a high degree of precision. Pricking pain has a more rapid rate of conductivity than burning pain, being transmitted by the larger pain fibers.

Together they constitute the "double response" of Lewis. A painful stimulus to the toe produces first a pricking pain and about 2 sec later a burning pain. Ischemia of the nerve subserving an area of skin, produced by application of a tourniquet, abolishes pricking pain before burning pain.

In the skin, localization of the pain stimulus is achieved by the simultaneous stimulation of multiple overlapping sensory neurones. Analgesia results from the interruption of all sensory neurones, and hypalgesia from the interruption of a few leaving others intact.

DEEP (INCLUDING VISCERAL) PAIN. The existence of visceral pain was long disputed, but it is now generally accepted that pain arising in the viscera does occur, provided that the stimuli are adequate. There is sound evidence that pain from viscera and deep skeletal structures is mediated through a common sensory apparatus and that the character and behavior of both are essentially the same. Hence, when we discuss visceral pain, the same principles will apply to deep skeletal pain. The pain is recognized by the patient as being "deep," i.e., deep to the skin; it is dull and aching in quality (although occasionally burning, as in the heartburn of esophageal disorders and rarely in anginal pain); the double response is absent; the pain is poorly localized and its borders are only vaguely delineated. It is probable that the high threshold and poor localization of deep pain are related, in part at least, to the relatively sparsely occurring sensory endings in the deep structures, in contrast to the closely distributed and overlapping terminals in the skin where pain threshold is low and accurately localized. Probably the most important characteristics are its relatively crude segmental localization beneath the surface of the body and its frequent reference to certain areas of the body. The simplest explanation for these latter phenomena is that suggested by Lewis:

If we suppose that certain tissues are represented in great detail in the sensorium, we can also understand that pain arising in these tissues may be localized with accuracy. But in other tissues having only a massive cerebral representation, localization may be expected to be less accurate. Segmental reference of deep pain may mean no more than that, centrally, the deep tissues supplied by a given cord segment have a general but little detailed representation. Thus, the impulses received whether these are derived from a viscus or from a deep somatic tissue, would tend to awaken very similar sensory impressions, and to be localized over a general sphere having no precise margins. And it may be regarded as natural enough that the general reference should be to regions that are relatively superficial, regions from which we are habitually receiving sensory impressions, and which are endowed with some positional sense.

The above concept implies that when pain originates in a viscus or deep skeletal tissue, the sensorium recognizes and localizes the pain as arising not in the exact region wherein it occurs but roughly in any or all structures innervated by cord segments subserving the affected viscus or deep somatic tissue. The pain appears to be projected toward the body surfaces supplied by these seg-

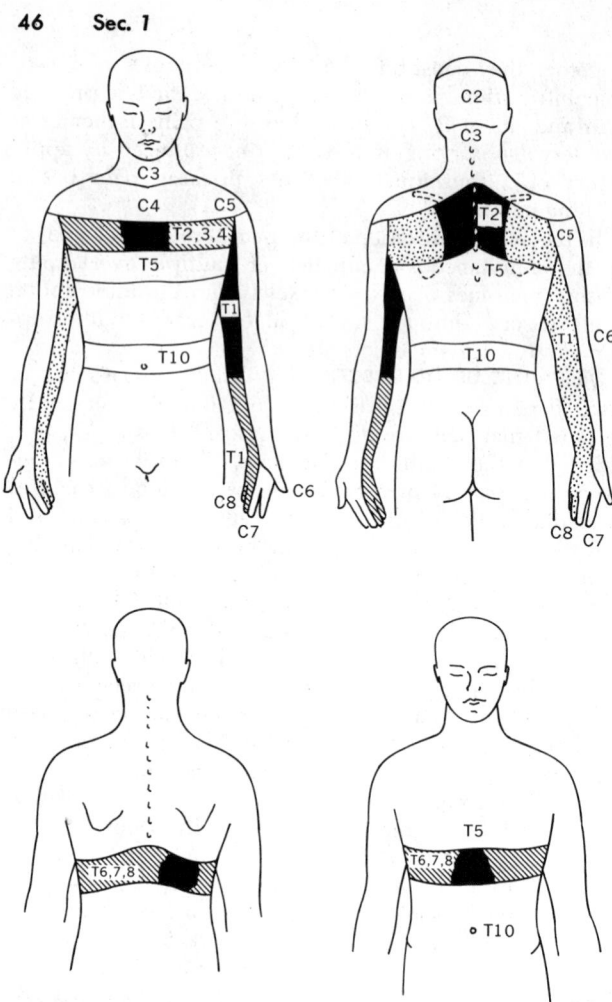

Main sites of sensory experiences

Usual areas of extension

Less common areas of extension

Fig. 9-2. Radiation and sites of reference of cardiac pain (*upper*); gallbladder pain (*lower*).

ments. For example, the sensory fibers from the heart terminate in the first through the fourth thoracic cord segments (possibly in some cases the fifth thoracic); and pain arising in the heart as the result of ischemia is not localized specifically in the region of the heart or in the precise region of the injured myocardium but in those superficial and deep structures whose sensory nerves also end in the first through the fourth thoracic spinal segments (see Fig. 9-2, showing theoretic distribution of heart pain in the first through fourth thoracic segments). Unfortunately, from the standpoint of diagnosis, the same cord segments receive fibers from the aorta, pulmonary artery, esophagus, and skeletal structures, which explains why pain arising in them may resemble that of myocardial infarction.

Referred Pain. All that has been said about segmental localization of deep pain applies also to referred pain, a

term used in clinical medicine to indicate the appearance of pain in a location of the body some distance from the viscus in which the pain originates. According to the hypothesis of Lewis and Kellgren, presented above, the referred pain is an integral part of the phenomenon of visceral pain. Thus, with cardiac pain in which sensory impulses enter mainly the left half of the first through fourth thoracic cord segments, the reference of pain to the arms is explained by the anatomic fact that the first thoracic segment supplies the inner surface of the arm as well as the thorax and heart. Thus it is just as natural for heart pain to appear in the characteristic location in the left arm as it is in the anterior midchest.

This view of visceral and referred pain has an understandable basis in neuroanatomy, for as was said, the thin, slowly conducting pain fibers terminate on small inhibitory neurones in the substantia gelatinosa, whose axones course into several adjacent segments. It is the activation of these neurones that induces a presynaptic depolarization of both large and small pain afferents, raising their threshold of excitation differentially. The unevenness of their inhibitory effects within any given segment might explain why, in the total area bounded by the first through fourth thoracic myotomes, heart pain should so commonly appear only in the anterior midline. It also explains why visceral pain may sometimes overflow into territories completely unrelated to the known innervation of the involved viscus, for example, the appearance of anginal pain in the jaws. Clinical experience teaches us that spread of pain beyond the limits that are "normal" is due in some cases at least to an unusual intensity of pain; thus an anginal pain that is ordinarily confined to the midsternal region (second through fourth thoracic nerves) may spread to the neck and shoulders (third through seventh cervical nerves). In other cases, extension of pain outside the normal boundaries may be due to coexistent lesions in structures with innervation not too distant from the cord segments primarily involved in the cardiac pain. Thus an anginal pain may be localized high in the epigastrium (seventh and eighth thoracic nerves) when peptic ulcer or gallbladder disease is also present. This may be because of summation of stimuli reaching the affected cord segments. It would explain why visceral pains overflowing into neighboring cord segments beyond the limits that are normal for the viscus tend preferentially to wander into higher rather than lower segments. (The inhibitory connections are more numerous in the cephalad structures which have a more abundant representation in consciousness than in caudad ones.)

Deep Skeletal Pain. Since there is sound experimental evidence for the view that visceral pain and deep skeletal pain are mediated through a common deep sensory system, it is not surprising that their characteristics should be similar and that on occasion differentiation between the two may be extremely difficult. Thus a small tear or injury in a lumbar muscle or ligament innervated by the twelfth thoracic or first lumbar nerve may give rise to a pain whose quality and localization, including radiation into the groin and scrotum, are indistinguishable from those of pain caused by renal colic. A similar injury in the right upper rectus muscle may cause a pain that mimics closely the pain of gallbladder colic; and a lesion in a muscle or ligament deep in the chest wall may cause pain with radiation to the left arm, identical in localization with that of angina. Under these circumstances, differentiation of somatic from visceral pain must be made on grounds other than the location and reference of pain.

HYPERESTHESIA, HYPERALGESIA, HYPERPATHIA, AND INVOLUNTARY SPASMS

In the past it has been customary to use the first two of these terms to designate a lowering of the threshold to touch and pain stimuli and the third for a state of pain with a normal or raised threshold but overreaction. The latter may even occur with anesthesia, as in *anesthesia dolorosa*. Any real distinction between these states is ephemeral. Probably only with inflammation is the pain threshold consistently lowered. What is most characteristic of all chronically painful states, and these frequently implicate nerves or central neural structures, is that the part is unusually sensitive to all stimuli, even those which normally do not evoke pain, and the elicited pain is unnatural, radiant, outlasts the initiating stimulus, and is modifiable by fatigue, emotion, etc. One sees listed here many of the characteristics of causalgia, spinal cord pain, phantom pain, zoster neuralgia, thalamic pain, and the like. The explanation currently offered for these states is that at the peripheral as well as central level the system of pain fibres is in equilibrium with other sensory fibers. A kind of inhibition is exerted on the pain system at all times by the small neurones in the substantia gelatinosa, to speak now only of the peripheral nervous system. Since the largest afferent fibers suppress most actively this inhibitory neuronal system, nerve injury, which destroys some of the larger sensory fibers (as happens in herpes zoster and also represents one phase of nerve regeneration after injury) permits overresponse of secondary sensory neurones. According to Melzack and Wall, the small neurones of the substantia gelatinosa constitute a kind of "gate control system," which modulates input. The large, low threshold fibers in a peripheral nerve most effectively activate the gateway cells. This explains the common experience of relieving pain by rubbing, vibration, etc.

Unlike other sensory experiences, pain tends to cause involuntary spasms in the skeletal muscles supplied by the same or adjacent segments of the spinal cord, e.g., spasm of the right upper rectus muscle with a gallstone impacted in the cystic duct or of the pectoral muscles in myocardial infarction.

Pain sensation may be induced by stimulation of the receptors or by irritation of peripheral nerves or roots, and in certain areas of the body it may be abolished by diseases which affect the peripheral or cerebral nervous system or by a surgical procedure which may accomplish the same result. Pain in a circumscribed region may be terminated by section of the nerve which supplies that region (neurotomy) or the spinal roots (posterior rhizotomy); pain in a limb or one side of the trunk may be interrupted by section of the anterolateral spinothalamic tract (lateral spinal tractotomy in the spinal cord or lateral medullary tractotomy in the medulla).

PERCEPTION OF PAIN. The arrival of pain impulses at the thalamocortical level of the nervous system is attended by conscious awareness of the pain stimulus. Clinical study has not informed us of the exact localization of the nervous apparatus for this mental process. It is not entirely abolished by a total hemispherectomy including the thalamus on one side. It is often said that impulses reaching the thalamus create awareness of the attributes of sensation and that the parietal cortex is necessary for the appreciation of the intensity and localization of the sensation. This seems an oversimplification. Probably a close and harmonious relationship between thalamus and cortex must exist in order for a sensory experience to be complete. The traditional separation of sensation (in this instance awareness of pain) and perception (awareness of the painful stimulus) has been abandoned in favor of the view that sensation, perception, and the various conscious and unconscious responses to a pain stimulus comprise an indivisible process.

Although similar to other sensory or perceptive phenomena in certain respects, such as predictable response to given intensity of stimulus, pain differs in other ways. One of its most remarkable characteristics is the strong feeling tone, or affect, with which it is endowed, nearly always one of unpleasantness. Furthermore, pain does not appear to be subject to negative adaptation. Most stimuli, if applied continuously, soon cease to be effective, whereas pain may persist as long as the stimulus is operative and, by establishing a central excitatory state, may even outlast the stimulus.

Stereotaxic surgery by Sweet and Mark on the thalamus in cases of intractable pain permits dissection of the anatomy of the pain experience. Lesions in the terminus of the lateral spinothalamic tract in the posterolateral nucleus abolish pain and temperature sensation in the contralateral side of the body while leaving the patient with all his misery or affect of pain. Lesions in the centrum medianum abolish the painful state without altering pain and temperature sensation. Thus, at this level there must be a balance of inhibitory and facilitatory sensory systems, and one cannot understand intractable pain in terms simply of excitation of chains of neurones.

PSYCHOLOGIC ASPECTS OF PAIN. A discussion of this problem could hardly be complete without some reference to the influence of emotional states or to the importance of racial, cultural, and religious factors on the pain response, especially the overt expressions. It is common knowledge that some individuals, by virtue of training, habit, or phlegmatic character, are relatively stoical and that others are excessively responsive to pain. Rarely one encounters individuals who are totally incapable of experiencing pain throughout their lifetime, not from any lack of sensory endings or peripheral sensory apparatus but from some peculiarity of central reception.

Lastly, it is important to keep in mind the devastating effects of chronic pain. As Ambroise Paré is alleged to have said, "There is nothing that abateth so much the strength as paine." Continuous pain can be observed to have an adverse effect on the entire nervous system. There is increased irritability, fatigue, troubled sleep, poor appetite, and loss of emotional stability. Courageous men are reduced to a whimpering, pitiable state that may arouse only the scorn of a healthy person. They are irrational about illness and may make unreasonable demands of family and physician. This state, which may be termed *pain shock*, once established, requires delicate but firm management. Of course the effect of narcotic drugs often complicates the picture.

CLINICAL APPROACH TO THE PATIENT WITH PAIN AS THE PREDOMINANT SYMPTOM

One of the most frequent errors is to think of pains always in terms of the severe intractable pains of disease, overlooking the fact that there are thousands of other pains which are part of the daily sensory experience of otherwise healthy individuals. To mention but a few, there is the momentary, hard pain over an eye, in the temporal region, or in the ear or jaw, which strikes with alarming suddenness; the more persistent ache which arises in some fleshy part such as the shoulder, neck, thigh, or calf; the darting pain in an arm or leg; the fleeting precordial discomfort that arouses momentarily the thought of heart disease; the breath-taking catch in the side; the cluster of abdominal pains with their associated intestinal rumblings; and the brief discomfort upon movement of a joint. These *normal pains,* as they should be called, occur at all ages, tending to be brief and to depart as obscurely as they come. They acquire medical significance only when elicited by the inquiring physician or when presented as a complaint by the worried patient; and of course they must always be distinguished from the *abnormal pains* of disease.

When pain by its intensity, duration, and the circumstance of its occurrence appears to be abnormal or constitutes one of the principal symptoms of disease, an attempt should be made by careful analysis of it to reach a tentative decision as to its cause and the mechanism of its production. This can usually be accomplished by a very thorough interrogation of the patient in which he is encouraged to relate as accurately as possible the main characteristics of the pain. This is followed by a physical examination and not infrequently by special laboratory tests, of which there has been much refinement in recent years.

LOCATION OF PAIN. When the pain is caused by a superficial lesion, the cause and effect are usually so obvious that no problem is posed. It is the deep lesion, whether involving somatic or visceral structures, that causes trouble, and here exact localization becomes especially important. We have already seen that pain originating from such tissues no longer is sensed as coming from them but is instead roughly segmental, i.e., within the territory of the cord segments innervating the structure. The identification of the segments involved is of value, for it sets the limit on the diagnostic possibilities

that must be considered, i.e., to those structures having a corresponding innervation. Thus an epigastric or subxiphoid pain or one in the opposite region in the back obliges one to search for its cause in all those structures innervated by the sixth through eighth thoracic cord segments, i.e., the esophagus, stomach, duodenum, pancreas, biliary tract, the upper retroperitoneal structures, as well as the deep somatic tissues in this region. Also one must consider the possibility that a lesion in a viscus innervated by spinal segments above or below the sixth through eighth thoracic cord segments may at times be the source of pain that has spread outside its normal boundaries and involved the epigastrium (Fig. 9-2).

PROVOKING AND RELIEVING FACTORS. These factors are of greater value than quality of pain in providing important data concerning its mechanism. Pain related to breathing, swallowing, and defecation focuses attention on the respiratory apparatus, the esophagus, and the lower bowel, respectively. A pain coming on a few minutes after the beginning of general bodily movement and relieved within a few minutes by rest indicates ischemia as the probable cause. Pain occurring several hours after meals and relieved by food or alkali suggests the irritative effect of acid on the raw lining of the stomach or duodenum. Pain that is brought on or relieved by certain movements or postures of parts of the body is usually due to the activity of diseased skeletal structures (bones, muscles, ligaments). Pain that is enhanced by cough, sneeze, and strain is usually radicular in origin or arises in ligamentous structures. Pain that is increased or altered by cutaneous stimuli is due to disease in sensory tracts in the peripheral or central nervous system. These are a few examples illustrating the paramount importance of determining with the greatest possible accuracy the factors that influence the appearance or relief of pain.

QUALITY AND TIME-INTENSITY CHARACTERISTICS OF THE PAIN. These features are of importance. However, too much stress should not be laid on the adjectives that the patient uses to describe his pain. His choice of words will depend, in part at least, on his vocabulary and on what he imagines is taking place. "Crushing" or "squeezing" are commonly employed to describe an anginal pain, and this implication of pressure does have some significance, since the pain may depend on an associated involuntary contraction of the pectoral muscles. Another patient with the same disease, however, may describe the pain as "exploding" or "burning." Far more important than the adjective used is the information that the pain is steady and does not fluctuate. Similarly, the ulcer pain is frequently designated as "gnawing"; but again, the deep, steady quality is more important than the word used to denote it. Gallbladder colic and renal colic are misnomers, if by colic is meant a "paroxysmal abdominal pain due to spasm, obstruction or distension of any of the hollow viscera." *In both these disorders, the pain is steady.* The aching quality of all deep pains is usually characteristic, but there are in addition several other informative attributes. A true colicky pain, one that is rhythmic and cramping, suggests an obstructive lesion in a hollow viscus. If the patient is a woman and has had children, it is a good idea to ask whether her "cramp" resembles the pains she had during childbirth. A pain that is steady and varies little or not at all from moment to moment means that the stimulus to pain is steady and unwavering, as in angina pectoris and peptic ulcer. Thus a pain in the anterior midsternal region whose intensity fluctuates appreciably within the space of a minute or two is not due to angina, even though the history may appear to suggest a relation to exertion. Similarly, a high epigastric pain appearing several hours after a meal and even apparently relieved by food is not caused by an ulcer if the pain fluctuates perceptibly within seconds or a few minutes. The stimulus to ulcer pain does not quickly vary in intensity. A throbbing pain indicates that an arterial pulsation is giving rise to painful stimuli. Sharp, transitory pain is caused by disease of nerve roots or ganglions, as exemplified by tic douloureux or tabes, or by some disorder in a somatic tissue such as a tear of a muscle or ligament; and often there is a background of dull, aching pain. Particularly noteworthy here is the abrupt intensification of the dull ache of root pain by cough, sneeze, or strain which momentarily increases the intraspinal pressure and stretches or alters the position of the root.

MODE OF ONSET OF THE PAIN. This factor is also important. A pain reaching its full intensity almost immediately after its appearance suggests a rupture of tissue. The pain of a dissecting aortic aneurysm often develops in this manner. In fact, the suddenness and the severity of the pain, reaching a peak of intensity within seconds or minutes, sometimes provides the first clue differentiating this type of chest pain from that caused by myocardial infarction. A similarly rapid accession of pain may occur with the rupture of a peptic ulcer.

DURATION OF THE PAIN. This is another important attribute. Anginal pain rarely lasts less than 2 or 3 min or more than 10 or 15 min. Ulcer pain may continue for an hour or more, unless terminated by the ingestion of food or alkali or a tumbler of water.

SEVERITY OF PAIN. In any given disease, the severity of pain is subject to wide variation, and also patients differ in their tolerance to it. Therefore one cannot judge the gravity of an illness by the intensity of the pain. As a rule, pains that completely interrupt work and pleasurable activity, require opiates for relief, enforce bed rest, and awaken the patient from sound sleep are to be taken more seriously than those which have the opposite characteristics.

TIME OF OCCURRENCE. An accurate determination must be made of the time of occurrence. The relationship of ulcer pain to the preceding meal has already been described. Postural aches come after prolonged activity and disappear with rest, whereas arthritic pains are usually most severe during the first movements after prolonged inactivity. The mechanism for this latter phenomenon is not known; nor do we understand why painful lesions of the bone, such as those caused by metastatic cancer, are likely to be most disturbing during the night. It is possible that the occurrence or aggravation of such pains is due to enhanced awareness of painful stimuli at a time when the mind is not distracted by other stimuli; or it may be that the pains are now more easily evoked by unconscious movements made during sleep when protective reflexes are in abeyance.

It should be obvious from these remarks that the full significance of a pain is usually not revealed by any one single characteristic. It is only by combining all these data that one can determine its anatomic site and its mechanism. In general, *the most important and revealing clues are obtained from the answers to the questions: What brings on the pain? What relieves it?* Pain is a subjective manifestation, not a state to be observed or measured. The accuracy of our data depends on the skill with which we frame our questions and on the powers of observation and memory of the person answering them.

Finally the diagnostic value of measures which *reproduce* and *relieve the pain* should be stressed. Not only are they important for diagnosis, but they convince the patient that the physician understands and can control the mechanism of his pain and the illness behind it. Climbing several flights of stairs under the physician's supervision may settle the question of the presence or absence of angina pectoris. An injection of procaine into a tender area in the chest wall or some other skeletal structure with complete disappearance of the pain may establish a skeletal origin and exclude the possibility of visceral disease. Reproducing the distress sometimes caused by aerophagia merely by distending the esophagus or stomach with air, or reproducing the vague but sometimes alarming sensation of pressure in the chest caused by unconscious hyperventilation by having the patient hyperventilate are other examples of how the principle of the reproduction of pain may be usefully employed.

A systematic interrogation of the patient will not lead to accurate diagnosis in every instance, but the habit of searching for the identifying characteristics of pain will enable the physician to increase his skill in this difficult field. Furthermore, after becoming familiar with the customary responses to these questions, he becomes more alert to the anxious, the hysterical, or the depressed patient who while complaining of pain seems incapable of describing any of its details, or unwilling to do so. Instead, there is preoccupation with theories of what is wrong or with the treatments or mistreatments already given. Finally, there will always be cases that defy solution, when the physician can proceed only by repeatedly reexamining the patient, explaining the need for continued observation, and enlisting his aid and forbearance during this trying period. Asking the patient to tolerate a certain amount of pain without the use of powerful analgesics is usually effective, particularly when the possibility of drug addiction is explained to him.

INTRACTABLE PAINS

In the relatively rare circumstances when all manner of investigation has failed to throw light on the cause and mechanism of the pain, demands for pain-relieving surgery may become increasingly insistent. The physician may in desperation turn to measures which are more dangerous than the disease. Here the commonest source of error is to operate unnecessarily on the hysterical patient (see Chap. 370), only to discover too late that each operative procedure leaves a new pain, often at a higher level than the first. Depressive psychosis may masquerade as a painful state, and electric shock therapy may dramatically terminate the illness. Sometimes a half dozen or more operations are unsuccessfully performed on a single patient. The safest rule to follow in these cases is not to use opiates continuously or to recommend operation for the relief of pain unless a reasonable diagnosis has been made. For the pains of metastatic cancer, the thalamic pain of vascular disease of the brain, and other incurable diseases, the relative advantages of the controlled use of opiates versus lateral spinothalamic tractomy or frontal lobotomy must be carefully weighed in each patient. The age of the patient, life expectancy, and mental state are all of importance in selecting the treatment procedure. Too often today an operation on the spinal cord or brain is chosen in preference to narcotics and the controlled use of drugs. Forgotten is the fact that many patients with cancer were formerly kept relatively comfortable and active by the judicious use of morphine and its analogues and were never subjected to costly operations or deprived of any of those qualities of mind and character which are so treasured by their families.

Superficial pain arising in integumentary structures rarely presents a problem in therapy. Acetylsalicylic acid, 0.30 to 0.60 Gm orally every 4 hr, usually suffices. Acetophenetidin may be added. These two drugs are a particularly effective combination when one element of pain is integumentary. Commercial proprietary preparations of these drugs containing caffeine or amphetamine such as A.S.A., Empirin compound, or Edrisal are available in most pharmacies. The caffeine or amphetamine is particularly useful if there is central nervous system depression. When this type of pain is not effectively controlled by nonnarcotic analgesics, codeine should be given. Usually the addition of small amounts (8 to 30 mg) of codeine phosphate to the standard dose of acetylsalicylic acid and acetophenetidin is effective. A preparation containing codeine phosphate 8 to 30 mg, acetylsalicylic acid 0.23 Gm, acetophenetidin 0.16 Gm, and caffeine 0.032 Gm is commercially available (Empirin compound with codeine phosphate). Codeine, 30 to 45 mg every 3 hr, gives maximal analgesia with minimal side effects. Adequate rest and relief of muscle tension should also be encouraged. The application of heat, especially moist heat, is usually beneficial. Occasionally, cold applications are preferred; but with the exception of cooling packs applied to an inflamed, burning skin or to a causalgia, cold is more likely to aggravate than to soothe the painful condition.

Occasionally integumental and deep pains of skeletal structures are of such severity as to require more powerful narcotic analgesics, such as meperidine hydrochloride (Demerol) in doses of 50 to 100 mg orally or intramuscularly, methadone hydrochloride 5 to 10 mg orally or subcutaneously, or dihydromorphine hydrochloride (Dilaudid) 1.0 to 2.0 mg orally or subcutaneously. These drugs are most useful in conditions when sedation is not required. When pain is unusually severe and some degree of euphoria is desired, morphine is the ideal drug. It should be given in doses of 8.0 to 15.0 mg orally or subcutaneously. Frequently a dose as small as 4.0 to 6.0 mg will relieve pain without causing undesirable nausea and vomiting. If the original dose is too small, a second dose of the same or slightly larger size can be given in 2 hr. This divided dose is less likely to induce nausea and vomiting than the larger single dose, because the stimulating effect of the first dose is insufficient to produce these symptoms and the depressant effect which follows reduces the sensitivity of the vomiting mechanism or renders it refractory to the second dose. Since all these narcotic analgesics are, for the most part, detoxified by the liver, they either should not be used or should be given in only half the usual dosage in cases of liver disease, myxedema, adrenal insufficiency, and other states in which the metabolic rate is reduced. Morphine and related narcotic analgesics tend to cause pruritus and therefore should be used with care in patients with skin irritability. The possibility of initiating addiction in susceptible individuals must be carefully evaluated in every instance.

If the patient exhibits mental tension, insomnia, and restlessness, a sedative drug such as phenobarbital or sodium amytal may be given with the analgesic agents. Sedative medication, especially the quick-acting barbiturates, should not be used alone for the control of pain, because they sometimes cause excitement and confusion under these circumstances.

Visceral pain originating in the stomach, gallbladder, intestines, or heart is usually very poorly controlled by the nonnarcotic analgesics. Various combinations of acetylsalicylic acid and acetophenetidin usually prove to be ineffective unless given with sedatives. The narcotic analgesics are the agents of choice, but of course they should never be given until the physician is certain that the relief of the pain will not mask the state of his patient. If sedation is not desirable, and if constipation is a troublesome problem, the newer synthetic analgesics, meperidine in doses of 50 to 100 mg orally or intramuscularly or methadone 5 to 10 mg by mouth or subcutaneously every 4 to 6 hr, are recommended. Like morphine, these drugs are habit-forming, but they do not share with morphine the properties of strong analgesia, sedation, and euphoria. Patients with severe visceral pain who are also anxious or fearful and unable to relax or sleep should be given morphine sulfate in doses of 8 to 15 mg subcutaneously. The well-known spasmogenic effects of morphine are partially counteracted by atropine sulfate, 0.3 to 0.4 mg. Aminophylline, 0.5 Gm intravenously, overcomes much of this undesirable spastic action; a rectal suppository of 0.5 Gm, although less effective, may be substituted.

Intractable pain due to incurable diseases such as metastatic carcinoma is one of the most difficult of therapeutic problems. As a rule, one resorts to narcotic drugs because of their strong analgesic action, and habituation is accepted as the lesser of two evils. An alternative is "pain-relieving surgery." Section of peripheral nerves, the lateral spinothalamic tracts in the spinal cord (cordotomy) or the lateral part of the medulla, stereotaxic thalamotomy, and lobotomy are relatively safe procedures which have advantages in certain cases over the continuous use of opiates.

REFERENCES

Cohen, H.: The Mechanism of Visceral Pain, Trans. Med. Soc. London, 64:35, 1944.

Feindel, W. H., G. Weddell, and D. C. Sinclair: Pain Sensibility in Deep Somatic Structures, J. Neurol., Neurosurg. Psychiat., 11:113, 1948.

Hardy, J. D., H. G. Wolff, and H. Goodell: "Pain Sensations and Reactions," Baltimore, The Williams & Wilkins Company, 1952.

Lewis, T.: "Pain," New York, The Macmillan Company, 1942.

Ryle, J. A.: "The Natural History of Disease," London, Oxford University Press, 1936.

White, J. C., and W. H. Sweet: "Pain, Its Mechanisms and Neurosurgical Control," Springfield, Ill., Charles C Thomas, Publisher, 1955.

10 HEADACHE

John F. Griffith and
Raymond D. Adams

The term *headache* should encompass all aches and pains located in the head, but in common language its application is restricted to unpleasant sensations in the region of the cranial vault. Facial, pharyngeal, and cervical pain are put aside as something different and are discussed here in Chaps. 13 and 355.

Headache, along with fatigue, hunger, and thirst, represents man's most frequent discomforts. Medically speaking, its significance is often abstruse, for it may stand as a symptomatic expression of disease or of some minor tension or fatigue, incident to the affairs of the day. Fortunately, in most instances it reflects the latter, and only exceptionally does it warn of serious disease seated in intracranial structures. But, it is this dual significance, the one benign, the other potentially malignant, that keeps the physician on the alert. Systematic approach to the headache problem necessitates a broad knowledge of the medical and surgical diseases of which it is a symptom and a clinical methodology which leaves none of the common and treatable causes unexplored.

GENERAL CONSIDERATIONS

In the introductory chapter on pain reference was made to the necessity, when dealing with any painful state, of determining its quality, location, duration, and time course and conditions which produce, exacerbate, or relieve it. When headache is considered in these terms, a certain amount of useful information is obtained by careful history, but perhaps less than one might expect.

Unfortunately, physical examination of the head itself is seldom useful.

As to quality of cephalic pain, the patient is rarely helpful in his description. In fact persistent questioning on that point occasions surprise, for the patient usually assumes that the word *headache* should have conveyed enough information to the examiner about the nature of the discomfort. Most headaches are dull, deeply located, and of aching character, a pain recognizable as of the type that usually arises from structures deep to the skin. Seldom is there reported the superficial burning, smarting, or stinging type of pain localized to the skin. When asked to analogize the sensation to another sensory experience, the patient may make some allusion to tightness, pressure, or bursting feeling, terms which then give clue to a muscular tension or psychologic state.

Queries about the intensity of the pain are seldom of much value since they reflect more the patient's attitude toward the condition and his customary way of reporting things that happen to him than the true severity. As usual, the bluff, hearty person tends to minimize his discomfort, whereas the neurotic may dramatize it. Degree of incapacity is a better index. A severe migraine attack seldom allows performance of the day's work. The pain which awakens the patient from sleep at night, or prevents sleep, is also more likely to have a demonstrable organic basis. As a rule, the most intense cranial pains are those which accompany subarachnoid hemorrhage and meningitis, which have grave implications, or migraine and paroxysmal nocturnal orbitotemporal ("cluster") headaches, which are benign.

Data regarding *location* of the headache are apt to be more informative. If the source is in deep structures (extracranial, subdermal, or intracranial), as is usually the case, the correspondence with the site of the pain is fairly precise. Inflammation of an extracranial artery causes pain well localized to the site of the vessel. Lesions of paranasal sinuses, teeth, eyes, and upper cervical vertebrae induce less sharply localized pain but one that is still referred in a regional distribution that is fairly constant. Intracranial lesions in the posterior fossa cause pain in the occipital-nuchal region, homolateral if the lesion is one-sided. Supratentorial lesions induce frontotemporal pains, again homolateral to the lesion if it is on one side. But localization can also be very uninformative or misleading. Ear pain, for example, seldom means disease in the ear, and eye pain may be referred from parts as remote as the occiput or cervical spine.

Duration and *time-intensity curve* of headaches in both the attack itself and the life-profile are most useful. Of course, the headache of bacterial meningitis or subarachnoid hemorrhage occurs usually in single attacks over a period of days. Single, brief, momentary (1 to 2 sec) pains in the cranium are presently uninterpretable and are significant only because they indicate no serious underlying disease. Migraine of the classic type has its onset in the early morning hours or daytime, reaches its peak of severity in a half hour or so, and lasts, unless treated, for several hours up to 1 to 2 days, often terminated by sleep. In the life history a frequency of more than a single attack every few weeks is exceptional. In contrast to this is the nightly occurrence (1 to 2 hr after onset of sleep) over a period of several weeks to months of the rapidly peaking, nonthrobbing orbital or supraorbital pain of cluster headache, which tends to dissipate within an hour. The headache of intracranial tumor characteristically can occur at any time of day or night, interrupt sleep, vary in intensity, and last a few minutes to hours, only to recur later in the day. The life profile is one of increasing frequency and intensity over a period of months. Tension headache, once commenced, may persist continuously for weeks or months, though waxing and waning from hour to hour.

Headache that bears a more or less constant relationship to certain biologic events and also to physical environmental changes may prove to be informative. Premenstrual headaches most typically relate to premenstrual tension during the period of oliguria and edema formation; they usually vanish after the first day of vaginal bleeding. The headaches of cervical arthritis are most typically intense after a period of inactivity, and the first stiff movements are both difficult and painful. Hypertensive headaches, like those of cerebral tumor, tend to occur on waking in the morning, but, as with all vascular headaches, excitement and tension may provoke them. Headache from infection of nasal sinuses may appear, with clocklike regularity, upon awakening and in mid-morning, and is characteristically worsened by stooping. Eye-strain headaches naturally follow prolonged use of the eyes, as in reading, peering for a long time against glaring headlights in traffic, or in watching cinema. Atmospheric cold may evoke pain in the so-called "fibrositic" or "nodular" headache or when the underlying condition is arthritic or neuralgic. Anger, excitement, or irritation may initiate common migraine in certain disposed individuals; this is more typical of common migraine than of the classic type.

PAIN-SENSITIVE STRUCTURES AND MECHANISMS OF HEADACHE

Understanding of headache has been greatly augmented by the observations of surgeons during operations on man. These operations inform us that the following cranial structures are sensitive to mechanical stimulation: (1) skin, subcutaneous tissue, muscles, arteries, and periosteum of skull; (2) delicate structures of eye, ear, and nasal cavity; (3) intracranial venous sinuses and their tributary veins; (4) parts of the dura at the base of the brain and the arteries within the dura mater and piarachnoid; (5) the trigeminal, glossopharyngeal vagus, and first three cervical nerves. The bony skull, much of the pia-arachnoid and dura, and the parenchyma of the brain lack sensitivity. Interestingly, pain is practically the only sensation produced by stimulation of the listed structures.

The pathways whereby sensory stimuli, whatever their source, are conveyed to the central nervous system are the trigeminal nerves for structures in the anterior two-thirds of the skull and the glossopharyngeal, vagus, and first three cervical nerves for those in the posterior third. The central connections through spinal cord and brainstem to thalamus are comparable to those already depicted in Chap. 9.

The pain of intracranial disease is referred, by a mechanism already discussed, to some part of the cranium lying within the areas supplied by the aforementioned nerves (V, IX, X, C-I, II, III). There may be an associated local tenderness of the scalp at the site of reference. Dental or jaw pain may also have cranial reference. The pain of disease in other parts of the body is not referred to the head, although it may initiate headache by other means.

By analysis of several types of headache, Wolfe and his colleagues have demonstrated that most "spontaneous" cranial pains can be traced to the operation of one or more of the following mechanisms:

1. distension, traction, and dilatation of the intracranial or extracranial arteries
2. traction or displacement of large intracranial veins or the dural envelope in which they lie
3. compression, traction, or inflammation of sensory cranial and spinal nerves
4. voluntary or involuntary spasm and possibly interstitial inflammation of cranial and cervical muscles

More specifically, the intracranial mass lesions only cause headache if in a position to deform, displace, or exert traction on vessels and dural structures at the base of the brain, and this may happen long before intracranial pressure rises. In fact the artificial induction of high intraspinal and intracranial pressure by the subarachnoid or intraventricular injection of sterile saline does not result in headache. Some have interpreted this to mean raised intracranial pressure does not cause headache, a conclusion which is called into question by the demonstrable relief of headache by lumbar puncture and lowering the cerebrospinal fluid (CSF) pressure in some patients. Actually, most patients with high intracranial pressure complain of recurrent bioccipital and bifrontal headache, probably due to traction on vessels or dura. As to localization, the pains follow the patterns mentioned above; those deflecting the falx or pressing on superior longitudinal or straight sinuses induce pain behind or above the eye; if the lateral part of the lateral sinus is involved, the pain is felt in the ear. Displacement of tentorium elicits pain felt in the supraorbital region.

Dilatation of the temporal arteries with stretching of surrounding sensitive structures is believed to be the mechanism of most of the pain of migraine. Extracranial, temporal, and occipital arteries, when involved in a peculiar giant-cell arteritis (cranial or "temporal" arteritis), a disease which afflicts individuals over fifty years of age, always give rise to headache of dull aching and throbbing type, at first localized and then more diffuse. Characteristically it is severe and persistent over a period of weeks or months. The offending artery, strangely, is not always tender to pressure, yet section of it, as in biopsy, relieves the pain. Evolving atherosclerotic thrombosis of internal carotid, anterior, and middle cerebral arteries is sometimes accompanied by pain in the forehead or temple; with vertebral artery thrombosis, the pain is postauricular, and basilar artery thrombosis causes pain to be projected to the occiput and sometimes the forehead.

In *infection or blockage of paranasal sinuses,* accompanied usually by pain over the antrum or in the forehead (from the ethmoid and sphenoid sinuses the pain localizes around the eyes on one or both sides or in the vertex or other part of the cranium, especially in disease of the sphenoid sinuses), the mechanism involves changes in pressure and irritation of pain-sensitive sinus walls. Usually it is associated with tenderness of the skin in the same distribution. The pain may have two remarkable properties: (1) When throbbing, it may be abolished by compressing the carotid artery on the same side. (2) It tends to recur and subside at the same hours, i.e., on awakening, with gradual disappearance when the person is upright, and coming again in the late morning hours. The time relations are believed to yield information concerning the mechanism; morning pain is ascribed to the sinuses filling at night, and its relief on arising, from emptying after the erect posture has been assumed. Stooping intensifies the pain by pressure change, as does blowing the nose sometimes; and amphetamine (inhalant), which reduces swelling and congestion, tends to relieve the pain. Some believe that the highly sensitive orifice of the sinus is the source, but more probably, the pain arises in the sensitive mucous membrane of the sinus. However, it may persist after all purulent secretions have disappeared, due probably to a mechanism of blockage of the orifice by boggy membranes and a vacuum or suction effect on the sinus wall (*vacuum sinus headaches*). The condition is relieved when aeration is restored. During air flights both earache and sinus headache tend to occur on descent, when the relative pressure in the blocked viscus falls.

Headache of ocular origin, located as a rule in the orbit, forehead, or temple, is of steady, aching type and tends to follow prolonged use of the eyes in close work. Ocular muscle imbalance is believed to be the mechanism. There is experimental evidence to show that the main faults are hypermetropia and astigmatism (not myopia), which result in sustained contraction of extraocular as well as frontal, temporal, and even occipital muscles. Correction of the refractive error abolishes the headache. Traction on the extraocular muscles during eye surgery and on the iris will evoke pain. Another mechanism is involved in the raised intraocular pressure seen in acute glaucoma or iridocyclitis, which causes steady, aching pain in the region of the eye. When intense, it may radiate throughout the distribution of the ophthalmic division of the trigeminal nerve. As for ocular pain in general, it is important that the eyes should always be refracted, but eyestrain is probably not as frequent as one would expect from the wholesale dispensing of spectacles.

The mechanism of *headaches accompanying disease of ligaments, muscles, and apophyseal joints* in the upper spine, which are referred to occiput and nape of neck on the same side, can be in part reproduced by the injection of hypertonic saline into these structures. Such pains are especially frequent in late life with rheumatoid and hypertrophic arthritis and tend also to occur after whiplash injuries to the neck. If the pain is arthritic in origin, the first movements after being still for some hours are both stiff and painful. In fact, evocation of pain by active and passive motion of the spine should indicate traumatic or other disease to movable parts. The pain of myofibrositis, evidenced by tender nodules near the cranial insertion of cervical and other muscles, is more obscure. There are no pathologic data as to the nature of these vaguely palpable lesions, and it is uncertain whether the pain actually arises in them. They may represent only the deep tenderness felt in the region of referred pain or the involuntary secondary protective spasm of muscles. Characteristically, the pain is steady (nonthrobbing) and spreads from one to both sides of the head. Exposure to cold or draft may precipitate it. While severe at times, it seldom prevents sleep. Massage of muscles and heat have unpredictable effects and relieve the pain in some cases.

The *headache of meningeal irritation* (infection or hemorrhage), which is of acute onset, severe, generalized, deep-seated and constant, and especially intense at the base of the skull and associated with stiffness of neck on bending forward, has been ascribed by some authorities to increased intracranial pressure. Indeed the withdrawal of CSF may afford some relief. But, dilatation and congestion of inflamed meningeal vessels must also be a factor. It seems more probable, therefore, that the pain is due to the chemical irritation of nerve endings in the meninges. The mechanism of the pain, therefore, is probably identical with that occurring in acute inflammatory conditions elsewhere.

Lumbar puncture headache, which is characterized by a steady occipital-nuchal but also frontal pain coming on a few minutes after arising from a recumbent position and relieved within a few minutes by lying down, has as its cause a persistent leakage of CSF into the lumbar tissues through the needle site. The CSF pressure is low (often 0 in lateral decubitus position), and the injection of sterile isotonic saline intrathecally relieves it. The headache is usually increased by compression of the jugular veins and is unaffected by digital obliteration of one carotid artery. It seems probable that in the upright position a low intraspinal and negative intracranial pressure exerts traction on dural attachments and dural sinuses by caudal displacement of the brain. Understandably, then, headache following cisternal puncture is rare. As soon as the leakage of CSF stops and CSF pressure is gradually restored (usually from a few days up to a week or so), the headache disappears. "Spontaneous" low-pressure headache may follow a sneeze or strain, due presumably to rupture of the spinal arachnoid along a nerve root.

The mechanism of the throbbing or steady headache which accompanies febrile illnesses (acute tonsillitis, typhoid fever, malaria, and sandfly fever), located in frontal or occipital regions or generalized, is probably vascular. It is much like histamine headache in being relieved on one side by carotid artery compression and on both sides by jugular vein compression or the subarachnoid injection of saline. It is increased by shaking the head. It seems probable that the meningeal vessels pulsate unduly and stretch pain-sensitive structures around the base of the brain. In certain cases, however, the pain may be lessened by compression of temporal arteries, and in these cases a component of the headache seems to be derived from the walls of extracranial arteries, as in migraine.

PRINCIPLE VARIETIES OF HEADACHE

Innumerable diseases are associated with headache through the operation of some of the aforementioned mechanisms. Usually there is no difficulty in diagnosing the headache of glaucoma, purulent sinusitis, bacterial meningitis, and brain tumor, and a fuller account of these special headaches will be found where these diseases are described in later sections of the book. It is when headache is chronic, recurrent, and unattended by other important signs of disease that the physician faces one of his most difficult medical problems.

The following types of headache should then be considered:

MIGRAINE. There are two identifiable, closely related syndromes, one called *classic* or *typical,* the other, *common* or *atypical.* Positive family history in 80 percent of cases, onset in childhood or adolescence, and early neurologic symptoms such as homonymous hemianopia, paresthesias, aphasia, hemiparesis (present only in classic form), unilateral throbbing pain, sensitivity to light and sound, nausea and sometimes vomiting, and relief by ergotamine are listed as the identifying characteristics of both groups. When all are present diagnosis is easy, but with only one or two there may be uncertainty. Common migraine is more likely to give trouble, especially if the age of onset is later and the attacks are not preceded by neurologic signs, occur with greater frequency, and have less predictable response to ergotamine than classic migraine. Also, if the headache is more clearly provoked by psychologically stressful situations, the possibility of psychiatric illness introduces itself more immediately. Special difficulties are also raised by unusual neurologic manifestations (see Chap. 358).

CLUSTER HEADACHE. This headache is also called *paroxysmal nocturnal cephalalgia, migrainous neuralgia,* and *histamine headache* (Horton). It is characterized by male predominance, uniformly constant, unilateral orbital localization, and onset within 2 or 3 hr after falling asleep (it is infrequent during the waking hours). The pain is usually intense, with lacrimation, blocked nostril then rhinorrhea, and sometimes flush, miosis, ptosis, and edema of cheek, all lasting approximately an hour. It tends to recur nightly for several weeks or a few months (hence the term *cluster*), followed by complete freedom for years. The pain of a given attack may leave as rapidly as it began. Clusters may recur over the years, being possibly more likely in times of stress, prolonged strain, overwork, and with upsetting emotional experiences.

Rarely, the condition may continue for 6, 7, or 8 years. The picture is so characteristic that it cannot be confused with any other disease, though to those unfamiliar with it the possibility of a carotid aneurysm, hemangioma, brain tumor, or sinusitis may be suggested. Appropriate x-rays and carotid arteriography will always exclude such conditions but usually are unnecessary. In the differential diagnosis orbital (nasociliary, supraorbital, Sluder's sphenopalatine) neuralgias must also be considered (see Chap. 355).

In the life history profile the clusters of headache may last for weeks. The clusters may be single or recur two or three times, with years of freedom in between, during which such precipitating factors as alcohol are no longer effective. Often the pain involves the same orbit in each cluster.

The relationship of the cluster headache to migraine remains conjectural. A portion of the cases have a background of migraine, which led to the earlier postulation of migrainous neuralgia, but the majority do not. The family history of migraine, or of cluster headache, is less frequent than in migraine.

TENSION HEADACHE AND VARIOUS OTHER CRANIAL PAINS WITH PSYCHIATRIC DISEASE. The headache is usually bilateral, often with diffuse extension over the top of the cranium. Occipital-nuchal localization is also common. Although described as pain, close questioning may uncover other sensations, viz., fullness, tightness, pressure (as if the head is surrounded by a band or in a vise), on which a nonthrobbing aching pain is engrafted. The onset of a given attack is more gradual than in migraine and not infrequently is added to a pressure ache which lasts unremittingly for weeks or months. In fact, this is the only type of headache that exhibits the peculiarity of being absolutely continuous day and night for long periods of time. Although sleep may be possible, whenever the patient awakens, the headache is present; and the common analgesic remedies have no beneficial effect unless the pain is intense and of aching type.

As to mechanism, the ascription of it to sustained muscle activity, shown by the electromyogram, is only a partial explanation. The continuous pressing quality of milder cephalic sensations at times when the patient is relaxed hardly seems to be attributable to physiologic stimulation and suggests instead that the condition is maintained by focused attention on the head (occasioned by worry and fear of intracranial disease. Moreover, it must be remembered that all types of headache in their late stages may give rise to muscle tension. In contrast to the migrainous patient, whose profile of headache is periodic and lifelong, with tendency to lessen in late adult years, tension headache occurs more often in middle age and usually coincides with anxiety and depression in the trying times of life. Many premenstrual headaches are of this type, and there is an increased incidence of this type of tension headache at menopause.

Psychologic studies of groups of patients with tension headaches have revealed prominent symptoms of anxiety, hypochondriasis, and to a lesser extent, depression. When psychiatric syndromes are searched for headache, it is evident that the majority of patients with anxiety neurosis and other syndromes (hysteria, obsessive-compulsive neurosis, schizophrenia) in which anxiety is a prominent symptom, exhibit this type of headache. With endogenous and reactive depressions it is less frequent, though the incidence is increased in the late-life involutional and hypochondriacal states (see Chap. 369). Migraine and traumatic headaches may be complicated by tension headache.

Other odd cephalic pains, e.g., boring pains, "clavus hystericus," may occur in hysteria and raise perplexing problems in diagnosis. Their bizarre character, persistence in the face of every known therapy, absence of other signs of disease, and the presence of the stigmata of the hysterical personality, provide the basis for correct diagnosis (see Chap. 369).

HEADACHE OF ANGIOMA AND ANEURYSM. Many authorities have declared that a vascular malformation may give rise to periodic hemicranial pain of a type that is indistinguishable from migraine except for its constancy of location (invariably on the same side) in all attacks. The temporal profile of any given attack shows the onset to be sudden or very acute, with the pain reaching a peak within minutes. Neurologic disturbances such as unilateral numbness, weakness, or aphasia tend to occur after the onset of the headache and to outlast it. Should hemorrhage occur, the headache is often extremely severe and localizes more towards the occiput and neck, lasting many days in association with stiff neck. A cranial or cervical bruit and, of course, blood in CSF, establish the diagnosis but it may require verification by arteriography. Other clinicians have denied the relationship of a migrainelike syndrome to angioma or aneurysm, and indeed, entirely adequate statistical data proving or disproving it are wanting. Even appropriate response to ergotamine is not conclusive and may be obtained in angiomatous headaches. Of course, vascular lesions may exist for long periods of time without headache, or the latter may develop many years after other manifestations, such as epilepsy and hemiplegia (see Chap. 351).

TRAUMATIC HEADACHE. Severe, chronic, continuous or intermittent headaches appear as the cardinal symptom of two posttraumatic syndromes, separable in each instance from the headache that immediately follows head injury (i.e., that of scalp laceration and contusion with sanguinous CSF and increased intracranial pressure). The latter lasts several days or a week or two.

The Headache of Chronic Subdural Hematoma. Headache and dizziness of fluctuating severity, followed by drowsiness, stupor, coma, and hemiparesis are the usual manifestations of chronic subdural hematoma. The head injury may have been minor and forgotten by patient and family. The headaches are deep-seated, steady, unilateral or generalized, and respond to the usual analgesic drugs. The typical attack profile of the headache and other symptoms is one of increasing frequency and severity over several weeks or months. Diagnosis is now established by arteriography (see Chap. 358).

Headache of Posttraumatic Nervous Instability. Here, headache is a prominent feature of a complex syndrome comprised of giddiness, fatigability, insomnia, nervousness, trembling, irritability, inability to concentrate, and tearfulness. The pain displays many variations from one day to another and also a highly individualized pattern of localization. Often it centers on the site of injury, where there is also tenderness. Reference to throbbing pain as well as pressure is obtained. Particular importance is attached to its persistence, intensification by mental and physical effort, stooping, noise, bright light, and confusion. The patient looks and acts much like a person in an agitated depression, and indeed, many neurologists believe such a state to be a posttraumatic neurosis or depression. The severity and duration of the headache bear no relation to the magnitude of the injury; some of the worst cases have had minor injuries without loss of consciousness, and major injuries may leave no headache in their wake. Unsettled litigation surely prolongs the discomfort and disability. The observation that histamine may reproduce some of the more severe headaches has suggested to some a vascular origin. Cephalic tenderness and aching pain sharply localized to the scar of the scalp laceration represent in all probability a different problem, raising the question of a traumatic neuralgia. With whiplash injuries to the neck, unilateral retroauricular or occipital pain suggest traumatism of the corresponding nerves (see Chaps. 13 and 358).

HEADACHES OF BRAIN TUMOR. Headache is the outstanding symptom of cerebral tumor. Unfortunately, the quality of the pain has no specific feature. It tends to be deep-seated, nonthrobbing (or throbbing), and aching or bursting. Attacks last a few minutes to an hour or more and occur once or many times during the day. Activity and frequent change in the position of the head may provoke pain, while rest in bed diminishes its frequency. Nocturnal awakening because of pain, although typical, is by no means diagnostic (see above). Unexpected forceful (projectile) vomiting may punctuate the illness in its later stages. As the tumor grows, the pain becomes more frequent, severe, and sometimes is nearly continuous terminally. But there are exceptions, some headaches being mild and tolerable, others as agonizing as that of the headache of bacterial meningitis and subarachnoid hemorrhage. If unilateral, the headache is homolateral to the tumor 9 out of 10 times. Supratentorial tumors are felt anterior to the interauricular circumference of the skull; posterior fossa tumors behind this line. Bifrontal and bioccipital headache, coming on after unilateral headaches, signify the development of increased intracranial pressure.

APPROACH TO THE PATIENT WITH HEADACHE

Obviously very different possibilities are raised by a patient who presents himself for the first time in his life with severe headache and another one who has had recurrent headache over a period of years. The chances of uncovering the cause in the first instance are much greater than the latter, and some of the underlying conditions (meningitis, subarachnoid hemorrhage, epidural hematoma, glaucoma, and purulent sinusitis) are more serious.

In searching for the cause of recurrent headache one should investigate the status of cardiovascular and renal systems by blood pressure and urine examination, eyes (fundoscopic, intraocular pressure, and refraction), the sinuses by transillumination and x-rays, the cranial arteries by palpation (and biopsy), the cervical spine by effect of passive movement and x-rays, and the nervous system by neurologic examination and psychic function by mental status.

Hypertension is, of course, frequent in the general population and is always difficult to prove as a cause of recurrent headaches. Minor elevations of blood pressure may be a result rather than the cause of nervous tension. No doubt severe hypertension with diastolic blood pressures of over 110 mm Hg are regularly associated with headache, and measures which reduce blood pressure can be shown to relieve the headache. But it is the moderate hypertensive when subject to numerous and severe headaches who gives concern. If headache is severe and frequent, there is usually an underlying anxiety or tension state or a common migraine syndrome that is exacerbated by blood vessel disease. The mechanism of the puzzling hypertensive phenomenon of occipital pain, present on awakening in the morning and wearing off during the day, is uncertain.

The adolescent with daily frontal headaches represents a special type of problem. Often their relationship to eyestrain is unclear, and refraction of the eyes and new eyeglasses do not relieve the condition. Anxiety or tension is probably a factor in such cases, but it is difficult to be certain of a causal relationship. Some of the most persistent and inexplicable headaches, which have led to a survey by a battery of diagnostic procedures for tumor, have proven in the end to be depression.

Equally puzzling is the somber, tense adult whose primary complaint is headache, or the migrainous person who in late life or at menopause begins to have daily headaches. Here it becomes important to assess mental status along the lines suggested in Chaps. 18, 30 and 369, looking for evidences of anxiety, depression, and hypochondriasis. The quality and persistence of the headache are suggestive of the possibility of psychiatric illness. Sometimes, a direct question as to the patient's idea of what is the matter may elicit suspicion and fear of brain tumor.

The most worrisome type of patient, in our experience, is the one who has only headache of increasing frequency and severity over a period of months or a year or so. Usually it becomes necessary to resort to a complete neurologic survey, including careful inspection of optic discs and x-rays of skull, electroencephalogram, lumbar puncture, and radioactive-isotope scanning to rule out brain tumor, abscess, or subdural hematoma.

Every elderly person with severe headache of some few days or weeks duration should be considered as a possible case of cranial arteritis. Increased sedimentation rate, fever, and anemia may be conjoined, but only in a minority of cases, unfortunately. The finding of a thickened temporal artery is important, and arterial biopsy establishes the diagnosis and often relieves the pain.

TREATMENT

The most important steps in the treatment of headache are those measures which uncover and remove the underlying disease or functional disturbance.

For the common everyday headache due to fatigue, stuffy atmosphere, or excessive use of alcohol and tobacco, it is simple enough to advise avoidance of the offending activity or agent, and symptomatic therapy in the form of acetylsalicylic acid, 0.6 Gm (in the form of aspirin or Anacin) will suffice. Some patients who invariably have headache when constipated and hypochondriacs who not infrequently suffer incapacitating headache, fatigue, and depression whenever bowel elimination does not meet their expectation, are not easily helped. Certainly, simple explanation, an anti-constipation regimen, and drugs which counteract depression (see Ch. 369) are preferable to the continuous use of analgesics. Premenstrual headache, if troublesome, can usually be helped by the use of a diuretic compound for the week preceding the menstrual period and a mixture of mild analgesic and tranquilizing medications (acetylsalicylic acid, 0.6 Gm and phenobarbital, 30 mg). If the headaches are severe and incapacitating, they should be treated as common migraine (see Chap. 367).

Hypertensive headaches respond to agents which lower blood pressure and relieve muscle tension. Chlorothiazide (Diuril), 250 to 500 mg twice a day, and methyldopa (Aldomet), 250 to 500 mg per day, when combined with a small amount of phenobarbital, 15 mg t.i.d., have given the best results. Meprobamate, 200 mg t.i.d., or chlordiazepoxide HCl (Librium), 5 mg t.i.d., may be administered in place of phenobarbital. For the morning occipital ache a capsule containing sodium nitrite, 30 mg, caffeine sodium benzoate, 0.5 Gm, and acetophenetidine, 0.6 Gm, has been useful. A simplified version is to supply the caffeine in a cup of strong black coffee and to give with it acetylsalicylic acid.

The muscle tension headaches respond best to massage, relaxation, and to a combination of drugs which relieve anxiety (phenobarbital, amobarbital, meprobamate, and chlordiazepoxide HCl) and pain [acetylsalicylic acid, propoxyphene HCl (Darvon) or Percodan]. Stronger analgesic medication may be needed (codeine or meperidine HCl). Psychotherapy is usually not beneficial in this group of patients.

Recurrent vascular headaches (common migraine) and classic migraine should be treated according to the plan outlined in Chap. 367.

The headache of the syndrome of posttraumatic nervous instability requires supportive psychotherapy in the form of reassurance and frequent explanation of its benign and transient nature, a program of increasing physical activity, and drugs which allay anxiety and depression. Tender scars from scalp laceration may be novocainized repeatedly (subcutaneous injection of 5 ml of 1% procaine) with some degree of success. Settlement of litigation as soon as possible works to the patient's advantage.

Heat, massage, salicylates, and indomethacin (Indocin) or phenylbutazone (Butazolidine) usually effect some improvement in those arthritic diseases of the cervical spine which are associated with cervicocranial pain (see Chap. 13).

Corticosteroid therapy is indicated in cranial arteritis to prevent disastrous blindness by occlusion of the ophthalmic arteries and in certain cases of rheumatoid arthritis. The headaches of cranial tumor often respond surprisingly well to large doses of methylprednisolone acetate and like compounds.

In conclusion, it is well to mention the importance of general hygenic measures. Young physicians in particular are apt to seek a specific therapy for each headache syndrome and give little thought to the general health of the patient. We have observed that most of the recurrent and chronic headaches are likely to be more severe and disabling whenever the patient becomes nervous, sick, and tired. A well-rounded diet, adequate rest, a reasonable amount of physical exercise, and a balanced view of the sources of daily anxieties and how to cope with them should be the goal of all therapeutic programs.

REFERENCES

Wolff, H. G.: "Headache and Other Pain," Fair Lawn, N.J., Oxford University Press, 1947.

Friedman, A. P.: "Research and Clinical Studies in Headache," Baltimore: The Wilkins & Wilkins Company, 1967.

Vinken, P. J. and G. W. Bruyn: "Handbook of Clinical Neurology," vol. 5, "Headache and Cranial Neuralgias," Amsterdam North-Holland Publishing Company, 1968.

11 PAIN IN THE CHEST

T. R. Harrison, W. M. Resnik,
T. J. Reeves, and E. Braunwald

The common problem in patients who complain of chest pain involves the distinction of trivial disorders from coronary disease, which is attended by the threat of sudden death. There is little parallelism between the severity of the pain and the gravity of its cause. An incorrect positive diagnosis of a hazardous condition such as angina pectoris is likely to have harmful psychologic and economic consequences. In no field of medicine is accurate diagnosis more important or, at times, more difficult.

The apparently bizarre radiation of pain arising in the thoracic viscera can usually be explained in terms of the known facts concerning nerve supply. These have been considered in Chap. 9. One occasionally sees a patient with extension of pain to a location which cannot be logically explained. In most instances, such an individual will be found to have more than one disorder capable of causing pain in the chest. The presence of the second and often silent condition may affect the radiation of the pain produced by the primary disorder. Thus, when the pain of angina pectoris extends to the back, the patient may be found to have also a significant degree of spinal arthritis. Similarly, the radiation of anginal pain to the abdomen commonly occurs in individuals who have some upper abdominal disorder, such as a hiatus hernia, disease of the gallbladder, pancreatitis, or peptic ulcer. When such instances are excluded, there is only an occasional patient who presents a distribution of pain which cannot be logically explained in terms of the known facts about nerve supply.

The common tendency to assume that the presence of an objective abnormality, such as a hiatus hernia or right bundle branch block, necessarily means that an atypical chest pain arises in the stomach or the heart is to be strongly condemned. Such an assumption is justified only if a careful history indicates that the behavior of the pain is entirely compatible with the site of origin which is suggested by the objective finding.

THE LEFT-ARM MYTH. There is a long tradition, widely accepted by physicians and laymen, that pain in the left arm, especially when appearing in conjunction with chest pain, has a unique and ominous significance as being almost certain evidence of the presence of ischemic heart disease. This is a myth that has neither theoretic nor clinical foundation. From a theoretic standpoint, any disorder involving the deep afferent fibers of the upper thoracic region should be capable of causing pain in the chest, the left arm, both areas, or neither area. Hence a pain of trivial significance arising in skeletal tissues innervated by upper (first to fourth) thoracic nerves would be expected to produce left-arm-area pain. These expectations are exactly in accord with clinical observation. Thus, almost any condition which is capable of causing pain in the chest may induce radiation to the left arm. Such localization is common not only in patients with coronary disease but also in those with numerous other types of chest pain. Although pain due to myocardial ischemia most frequently is substernal and radiates down the ulnar aspect of the left arm (Chap. 271) and is pressing and constricting in nature, the location, radiation, and quality of pain are of less diagnostic significance than is the behavior of the pain, in terms of the conditions which induce it and relieve it.

The majority of individuals also believe that cardiac pain is situated in the region of the left breast and therefore left inframammary pain is one of the common symptoms that brings the patient to seek medical advice. It differs radically from the pain due to myocardial hypoxia, i.e., angina pectoris, in that it is usually a long-lasting, dull ache, occasionally accentuated by sharp stabs. It has no relationship to exertion and may be accompanied by tenderness over the precordium.

Chest pain which occurs after the patient sits down

and upon completion of activity usually is not angina pectoris.

Only the more important or more common conditions listed will be considered in the text.

PAIN DUE TO OXYGEN DEFICIENCY OF THE MYOCARDIUM

PHYSIOLOGIC CONSIDERATIONS OF THE CORONARY CIRCULATION. Pain due to myocardial ischemia occurs when the oxygen supply to the heart is deficient in relation to the oxygen need. The oxygen consumption of this organ is closely related to the physiologic effort made during contraction. It is dependent primarily on three factors: (1) the frequency of cardiac contraction, (2) the tension developed by the myocardium and, (3) the contractile state of the myocardium. When cardiac contractility, arterial pressure, and heart rate remain constant, an elevation of stroke volume produces an efficient type of response because it leads to an increase in the external work of the heart (i.e., in the product of cardiac output and arterial pressure) with little accompanying augmentation of myocardial oxygen requirements. Thus, a rise in flow load causes less increment in myocardial oxygen consumption than does a comparable increase in cardiac work per minute brought about by elevation either of pressure or of heart rate. However, the net effects of these hemodynamic variables depend not on oxygen need alone but rather on the balance between the demand and the supply of oxygen. The heart is always active and the coronary venous blood is normally much more desaturated than that from other areas of the body. Thus the removal of more oxygen from each unit of blood, which is one of the adjustments commonly utilized by exercising skeletal muscle, is already employed in the heart of an individual in the basal state. Therefore, this organ has only one effective means of obtaining the additional oxygen required for greater contractile activity and this is by increase in the coronary blood flow.

It follows, from hydrodynamic considerations, that the flow of blood through the coronary arteries is directly proportional to the pressure gradient between the aorta and the ventricular myocardium during systole and the ventricular cavity during diastole but is proportional to the fourth power of the radius of the coronary arteries. Thus, a relatively slight alteration in coronary diameter will produce a large change in coronary flow, provided that other factors remain constant. In the normal heart, coronary blood flow occurs primarily during diastole, when it is unopposed by myocardial constriction of the coronary vessels. Coronary flow is regulated primarily by myocardial oxygen needs, probably through the release of vasodilator metabolites. Although changes in coronary flow occur with activation of autonomic nerves to the coronary vessels, these alterations result primarily from the effects of these nervous stimuli on myocardial contraction and therefore on the heart's oxygen consumption.

The coronary dilatation which normally occurs during exercise, is impaired in patients with fixed coronary narrowing due to coronary arteriosclerosis. Thus, physical exertion, or any condition which increased heart rate, arterial pressure, or myocardial contractility tends to precipitate anginal attacks by increasing myocardial oxygen needs in the face of impaired oxygen delivery. Bradycardia usually has the opposite effects, and this apparently explains the rarity of angina in patients with complete heart block, even when this disorder is associated with coronary disease.

CAUSES OF MYOCARDIAL HYPOXIA. By far the most frequent underlying cause is organic narrowing of the coronary arteries secondary to coronary atherosclerosis. Less frequently, narrowing of the coronary orifices due to syphilitic aortitis or to distortion by a dissecting aneurysm may be responsible. A drug, such as ergot, which causes constriction of the coronary arteries, may occasionally induce anginal attacks in the absence of organic disease. There is no evidence that vasoconstriction or increased cardiac contractile activity (rise in heart rate or blood pressure, or increase in contractility due to liberation of catecholamines or adrenergic activity) due to emotion can precipitate angina unless there is also structural narrowing of the coronary vessels.

Aside from conditions which narrow the lumen of the coronary arteries, the only other frequent causes of myocardial hypoxia are disorders, such as aortic stenosis, which cause a marked disproportion between the perfusion pressure and the ventricular work. Under such conditions the systolic rise in left ventricular pressure is not, as in hypertensive states, balanced by a corresponding elevation of aortic perfusion pressure, and most of the coronary flow occurs during diastole. Therefore, an increase in heart rate is especially harmful because it shortens diastole more than systole and thereby decreases the total available perfusion time per minute.

Patients with marked right ventricular hypertension may have exertional pain which is, in most respects, identical with that of the common type of angina. It is likely that this discomfort results from relative ischemia of the right ventricle brought about by the increased oxygen needs and by the elevated intramural resistance, with sharp reduction of the normally large systolic perfusion of this chamber.

In persons with *syphilitic aortitis*, angina is not uncommon and the relative roles of aortic insufficiency and of coronary ostial narrowing are difficult to assess. However, the latter factor is absent in patient with rheumatic aortic insufficiency, in whom angina occurs less frequently than in patients with luetic disease. However, angina is frequent and severe in patients with rheumatic aortic regurgitation and stenosis.

The importance of tachycardia, decline in blood pressure, or diminution in arterial oxygen content will be apparent from the above discussion. However, these are precipitating and aggravating factors rather than underlying causes of angina.

THE EFFECTS OF MYOCARDIAL HYPOXIA. The most common of these is anginal pain, which is considered in some detail in Chap. 271. It is usually described as a heavy pressure or squeezing and occurs particularly on walking, especially after meals, on cold days against a wind or uphill. When anginal pain is induced by walking, it forces the patient to stop or reduce his speed. It occurs with anger, excitement, and other emotional states. The exact mechanism of the pain stimulus is still unknown. The evidence that oxygen deficiency is in some way responsible appears to be overwhelming, but the precise mechanism of its action has not been established.

As a rule, myocardial infarction is associated with a pain similar in quality and distribution to that of angina but of great intensity and longer duration. The pain of myocardial infarction is not relieved by rest or by coronary dilator drugs. Occasionally, it is minimal or even completely absent. In such instances, it is possible that preexisting longstanding myocardial ischemia has damaged the nerve fibers which would otherwise conduct the pain impulses.

A second effect of myocardial ischemia is often seen in the electrocardiogram. Most persons with angina have normal tracings between attacks, and the record may even remain normal during the episode of pain. However, in many instances, depression of the S-T segments appears in leads I, II, AVL, or in those from the left precordium during exertion. The finding of deep, ischemic type of S-T segment depressions during an attack of pain with a return to normal after the pain subsides strongly suggests that the pain is anginal in origin. There is strong experimental evidence that such depressions, as well as the elevations which are usually seen in patients with infarction and are observed in a few patients during anginal attacks, are related to alterations in ionic balance (Chap. 260). It appears that the net effect of very severe ischemia is to produce S-T segment elevations, while less marked ischemia has the reverse effect. The value and limitation of electrocardiographic changes occuring after exercise in the diagnosis of angina pectoris are discussed in Chap. 271.

A third effect of myocardial hypoxia is alteration in contraction. It has been shown that the left ventricular end-diastolic pressure may rise during anginal attacks, particularly if they are prolonged. This indicates transient depression of left ventricular function, which is presumably induced by the decreased contractility of the ischemic areas. On auscultation a fourth heart sound is also frequently heard during the anginal episode.

The beneficial effect of nitrites was originally ascribed by Lauder Brunton to reduction in tension in the arteries and thus, presumably, in the heart. Subsequent studies in animals pointed toward absolute increase in coronary flow. However, direct measurements in man suggest that the increase in coronary flow is relative and that the beneficial effects of these agents are dependent on a reduction in the oxygen requirements of the heart.

Another characteristic effect of myocardial hypoxia is liability to sudden death. This may never occur, despite hundreds of anginal episodes. However, it may supervene early in the disease and even in the first attack. When the conducting system is involved, the patient may die from atrioventricular block, with standstill of the ventricle.

However, the usual mechanism is probably ventricular fibrillation, which can often be seen to occur in animals following ligation of a coronary artery.

PAIN DUE TO IRRITATION OF SERIOUS MEMBRANES OR JOINTS

PERICARDITIS. Experimental studies made on man indicate that the visceral and the internal surface of the parietal pericardium are ordinarily insensitive to pain, although when the latter is sufficiently inflamed, painful stimuli may originate from it. The most highly sensitive region is the lower part of the external surface of the parietal layer, and the pain associated with inflammation of the remaining part usually arises in the adjacent pleura. These observations explain why noninfectious pericarditis (that associated with uremia and with myocardial infarction) with relatively mild inflammation is usually painless or accompanied rarely with very mild pain, whereas infectious pericarditis, being nearly always more intense and spreading to the neighboring pleura, is usually associated with typical pleuritic pain (i.e., aggravated by breathing, coughing, etc.). Since the central part of the diaphragm receives its sensory supply from the phrenic nerve, which arises from the third to fifth cervical segments of the spinal cord, pain arising from the lower parietal pericardium and central tendon of the diaphragm is felt characteristically at the tip of the shoulder, the adjoining trapezius ridge, and the neck. Involvement of the more lateral part of the diaphragmatic pleura, supplied by branches from the intercostal nerves (sixth to ninth thoracic), causes pain not only in the anterior chest but also in the upper abdomen and corresponding region of the back, thus sometimes simulating the pain of acute cholecystitis or pancreatitis.

Pericarditis causes three distinct types of pain. By far the commonest is the pleuritic pain, related to respiratory movements and always aggravated by cough or deep inspiration, sometimes brought on by swallowing, because the esophagus lies just beyond the posterior portion of the heart, sometimes by change of bodily position. It is sharper, more left-sided, is frequently referred to the neck or flank, and lasts longer than angina pectoris. This type of pain is due to the pleuritic component of the pleuropericarditis so commonly present in the infectious forms. The next commonest pericardial pain is the steady, crushing substernal pain identical with that of acute myocardial infarction; if the pleuritic component is absent, differentiation on the basis of the pain alone is impossible. The mechanism of this steady substernal pain is not certain, but it is probable that it arises from the highly inflamed inner parietal surface of the pericardium or from the irritated afferent cardiac nerve fibers lying in the periadventitial layers of the superficial coronaries. The third type of pain, one that a priori should appear to be the most common and characteristic, is actually quite uncommon. This pain is synchronous with the heartbeat and is felt at the left border of the heart and left shoulder. Rarely, all three types may be present simultaneously.

The painful syndromes which may follow operations on the heart ("post commissurotomy syndrome"), myocardial infarction, or trauma to the heart are discussed in later chapters (Chaps. 270 through 272). Such pains often but not always arise in the pericardium.

Pleural pain is very common and may be identical with that of pericarditis. However, its sharp superficial quality and its aggravation by each breath readily distinguishes it from the deep dull steady unwavering pain of myocardial ischemia.

The pain resulting from *pulmonary embolism* may resemble that of acute myocardial infarction and in massive embolism it is located substernally. In patients with smaller emboli the pain is located more laterally and is pleuritic in nature. The pain of mediastinitis or of mediastinal emphysema (Chap. 293) usually resembles that of pleuritis but is more likely to be maximal in the substernal region, and the associated feeling of constriction may cause confusion with myocardial infarction. The pain due to *acute dissection of the aorta* is usually extremely severe. It is localized to the center of the chest, lasts for hours, and requires unusually large amounts of analgesics for relief. It often radiates into the back but is not aggravated by changes in position or respiration.

The *costochondral and chondrosternal articulations* are the commonest sites of anterior chest pain. Objective signs in the form of swelling (Tietze's syndrome), redness, and heat are very rare, but sharply localized tenderness is common. The pain may be "neuritic," i.e., darting and lasting for only a few seconds, or a dull ache enduring for hours or days. An associated feeling of tightness due to muscle spasm (see below) is frequent. When the discomfort endures for a few days only, a story of minor trauma or of some unaccustomed physical effort can be obtained. The chronic variety of this discomfort is common in persons with arthritis of the spine and also in patients with ischemic heart disease, but in many instances no associated disorder is found. It should be emphasized that *pressure on the chondrosternal and costochondral junctions is an essential part of the examination of every patient with chest pain*. A large percentage of patients with this disorder, and especially those who also have minor and innocent T-wave alterations (Chap. 260), are erroneously labeled as having coronary disease. The dire consequences of such a mistake have already been emphasized.

Pain secondary to *subacromial bursitis* and *arthritis of the shoulder and spine* may be precipitated by exercise of the local area but not by general exertion. It may be brought out by passive movement of the involved area as well as by coughing.

PAIN DUE TO TISSUE DISRUPTION

Rupture or tear of a structure may give rise to pain that sets in abruptly and reaches its peak of intensity almost instantly. Such a story would, therefore, arouse the suspicion of dissecting aneurysm, pneumothorax,

mediastinal emphysema, a cervical disk syndrome, or rupture of the esophagus. However, the patient may be too ill to recall the precise circumstances, or the pain may be atypical and increase gradually in severity. Likewise, other and more benign conditions, such as a slipped costal cartilage or an intercostal muscle cramp, may produce pain with an abrupt onset.

PAIN DUE TO INCREASED MUSCLE TENSION

This is of two varieties, depending on whether the discomfort arises in skeletal or smooth muscle. The former is very frequent, and the usual causes are discussed later in some detail. A very rare type is *intercostal cramp,* which, except for the location, is identical with the common night cramp in the calves. Here, again, the coexistence of insignificant variations in the electrocardiogram *often* leads to the tragedy of a false positive diagnosis of ischemic heart disease.

It is likely that increased tension in visceral musculature is responsible for the chest pain associated with some esophageal disorders, the splenic flexure syndrome, aerophagia, and diverticulum of the stomach. There is uncertainty whether the same mechanism or pinching of nerve fibers causes the discomfort of hiatal hernia, a disorder that can mimic the pain of myocardial ischemia exactly as regards location, quality, and intensity but not as regards precipitating and alleviating factors.

CLINICAL ASPECTS OF SOME OF THE COMMONER CAUSES OF CHEST PAIN

Some of the features of pericarditis have already been described, and those of the more serious causes of chest pain such as myocardial ischemia (angina pectoris and infarction), dissecting aneurysm, and disorders of the pleura, esophagus, stomach, duodenum, and pancreas are considered in the appropriate chapters dealing with these problems. Here, we are concerned with the discussion of those causes which are not considered in more detail elsewhere.

PAIN ARISING IN THE CHEST WALL OR UPPER EXTREMITY. This may develop as a result of muscle or ligament strains brought on by unaccustomed exercise and felt in the costochondral or chondrosternal junctions or in the chest wall muscles. We mention the upper extremities and especially the left because of the deeply ingrained legend that pain in the left arm has a specific significance in indicting the heart. Other causes are osteoarthritis of the dorsal or thoracic spine and displaced *cervical discs.* Pain in the left upper extremity and precordium may be due to compression of portions of the brachial plexus by a cervical rib or by spasm and shortening of the anterior muscle secondary to high fixation of the ribs and sternum. Finally, pains in the upper extremity (shoulder-hand syndrome) and in the pectoral muscles may, through unknown mechanisms, occur in patients with ischemic heart disease.

Skeletal pains in the chest wall or shoulder girdles or arms are usually recognized quite easily. Localized tenderness of the affected area is usually present, and the pain is sometimes clearly related to movements involving the painful locus. Thus deep breathing, turning or twisting of the chest, and movements of the shoulder girdle and arm will elicit and duplicate the pain of which the patient complains. The pain may be very brief, lasting only a few seconds, or dull and aching and enduring for hours. The duration is, therefore, likely to be either longer or shorter than untreated anginal pain, which usually lasts for only a few minutes.

These skeletal pains often have a sharp or sticking quality. In addition, there is frequently a feeling of tightness which is probably due to associated spasm of intercostal or pectoral muscles. This may produce the "morning stiffness" seen in so many skeletal disorders. The discomfort is unaffected by nitroglycerin but often abolished by infiltration of the painful areas with procaine (Novocain).

When chest wall pain is of recent origin and follows some unusual activity involving the pectoral muscles, it presents no problem in diagnosis. However, *long-standing skeletal pain is frequent in persons who also have angina pectoris.* This association is sometimes coincidental, because both disorders are very common. In other instances, it seems that the coronary disease is responsible for the chest wall pain, the exact mechanism being uncertain but similar to that responsible for the well-known shoulder-hand syndrome. This coexistence of the two different types of chest pain in the same patient is a frequent cause of a confusing history because in the patient's mind the anginal needle may be hidden in the skeletal haystack. Thus every middle-aged or elderly patient who has long-standing anterior chest wall pain merits careful study.

Detailed questioning will sometimes reveal that what was originally thought by the patient to be a single type of discomfort actually comprises two different pains which, though similar in quality and area, differ as regards duration and initiating factors. When the history is inconclusive, the postexertional electrocardiogram may furnish decisive information. However, both false positive and false negative tracings may be obtained, according to whether they are interpreted loosely or critically (Chap. 271). It may thus be necessary to study the pain itself and to learn by direct observations whether exercise alone or postprandial exertion, or even postprandial effort undertaken holding an ice cube, is capable of producing it. Repeated tests may be required, the effects of preceding placebos, as compared to nitroglycerin, on the amount of exertion required to induce the pain being compared. *The confusion created by the presence of innocent skeletal pain impairs the reliability of the history and is probably the commonest cause of errors—both positive and negative—in the diagnosis of angina pectoris.*

Emotional disorders are also common causes of chest wall pain. Usually, the discomfort is experienced as a sense of "tightness," sometimes called "aching," and occasionally it may be sufficiently severe as to be designated a pain of considerable magnitude. Since the discomfort has almost always the additional quality of tightness or constriction and, furthermore, since it is often localized across the sternum, although it may be felt in other areas of the anterior chest, it is not surprising that this type of pain is frequently confused with that of myocardial ischemia. Ordinarily, it lasts for a half hour or more and may persist for a day or less with slow fluctuation of intensity. The association with fatigue or emotional strain is usually clear, although it may not be recognized by the patient until called to his attention. The pain probably develops through unconscious and prolonged increase of muscle tone (as in frowning in the face, or as can be quickly produced in the hand by tightly clinching the fist), often enhanced by an accompanying hyperventilation (by causing a contraction of the chest wall muscles similar to the painful tetany of the extremities). When the hyperventilation and/or the associated adrenergic effect due to anxiety also causes innocent changes in the T waves and S-T segments, the confusion with coronary disease is strengthened. However, the long duration of the pain, the lack of any relation to exertion but association rather with fatigue or tension, and the usual periodic occurrence on successive days without any limitation of capacity for exercise usually make the differentiation from ischemic pain quite clear.

As compared to these two causes (the chest wall muscle and ligament strains and the contraction of the pectoral muscles due to reflex influences, fatigue, or tension) the various other conditions that may cause skeletal discomfort are uncommon and readily recognized after appropriate observation: spinal arthritis, herpes zoster, anterior scalene and hyperabduction syndromes, malignant disease of the ribs, etc.

The several *abdominal disorders* which may at times mimic anginal pain may usually be suspected from the history, which ordinarily will indicate some relationship to swallowing, eating, belching, the expulsion of flatus, etc. Pain resulting from gastric or duodenal ulcer is epigastric or substernal, commences about 1 to 1½ hr after meals and is usually promptly relieved by antacids or milk. Occasionally, as in some patients with hiatal hernia, the gastrointestinal x-ray will be of crucial significance. Rarely, it may be necessary to inflate the stomach or the splenic flexure with air, in order to satisfy both the doctor and the patient that one of these organs is responsible for a tight pain in the lower chest. Roentgenographic examination is also often helpful in differentiating biliary, gastrointestinal, aortic, pulmonary, and skeletal disease pain from angina pectoris. It should be emphasized again that the demonstration of the presence of a coexistent abdominal disorder such as hiatal hernia does not constitute proof that the chest pain of which the patient complains is due to this. Such disorders are frequently asymptomatic and are not at all uncommon in patients who also have angina pectoris.

APPROACH TO THE PATIENT WITH PAIN IN THE CHEST

Most individuals with this complaint will fall into one of two general groups. The first consists of persons with prolonged and often severe pain without obvious initiating factors. Such persons will frequently be gravely ill. The problem is that of differentiating such serious conditions as myocardial infarction, dissecting aneurysm, and pulmonary embolism from each other and from less grave causes. In some such instances, the careful history will provide significant clues, while objective evidence of crucial importance will appear within the subsequent 2 or 3 days. Thus, when the initial examinations are not decisive, a watch and wait policy, with repeated electrocardiograms coupled with measurements of the transaminase, sedimentation rate, etc., will commonly provide the correct answer.

The second group of patients comprises those who have brief episodes of pain, with otherwise apparently excellent health. Here, the resting electrocardiogram will rarely supply decisive information, but records taken after exercise will often reveal characteristic changes (Chap. 271). However, in many instances it is the study of the subjective phenomenon, i.e., of the pain itself, that will lead to the diagnosis. Of the several methods of investigation which are available for such patients, three are of cardinal importance.

A detailed and *meticulous history* of the behavior of the pain is the most important method. The location, radiation, quality, intensity, and, especially, duration of the episodes are important. Even more so is the story of the aggravating and alleviating factors. Thus a history of sharp aggravation by breathing, coughing, or other resporatory movements will usually point toward the pleura, pericardium (because of the associated pleuro-pericarditis), or mediastinum as the site, although chest wall pain is likewise affected by respiratory motions. Similarly, a pain which regularly appears on rapid walking and vanishes within a few minutes upon standing still will usually mean angina pectoris, although here, once again, a similar story will rarely be obtained from patients with skeletal disorders.

When the history is inconclusive, the *study of the patient at the time of the spontaneous episode* will often supply crucial information. Thus the electrocardiogram, which may be normal both at rest and after exercise in the absence of pain, will occasionally demonstrate striking changes when recorded during an anginal episode. Similarly, x-ray of the esophagus or of the stomach may show no evidence of cardiospasm or of hiatal hernia except when the observation is made during the pain.

The third method of study represents the *attempt to produce and alleviate the pain at will*. This procedure is necessary only when doubt exists following the history or when needed for psychotherapeutic purposes. Thus the demonstration that a localized pain, which can be reproduced by pressure on the chest, is completely relieved by local infiltration with procaine will often be of conclusive importance in convincing the patient that the heart is not the site. The discomfort due to distension of the stomach or of the splenic flexure with air is frequently mistaken by the patient, and occasionally by the physician, for pain of cardiac origin. The simple demonstration, by passing a tube to the appropriate area and inflating with air, that the pain can be exactly reproduced may be not only of diagnostic but also of psychotherapeutic value. However, the demonstration that such procedures will reproduce the patient's pain may be misleading in persons who have angina in addition to another disorder. It may, therefore, be necessary to study also the effect of exercise on the pain and on the electrocardiogram.

When, as is not rarely the case, the history is atypical, the correct diagnosis of angina pectoris will often depend in large measure on the response to nitroglycerin. Here, a number of pitfalls should be avoided. If the patient has previously had the drug, careful questioning may be necessary to avoid errors. Thus disappearance after its sublingual administration does not necessarily prove that there is a cause and effect relationship. It is necessary to be certain that the pain vanishes more rapidly (usually within 5 min) and more completely when the drug is used than when it is not employed. A false negative impression concerning the effect of nitroglycerin may be the result of the use of a deteriorated preparation which has been exposed to light. It is thus necessary to be sure that the dosage used is sufficient to induce a pharmacologic effect in the form of a slight flush or a mild pounding headache. In doubtful instances, repeated exercise tests, with and without preceding administration of nitroglycerin, are necessary. The demonstration that the time required for a given exercise to produce pain is consistently and considerably longer when it is undertaken within a few minutes after a sublingual nitroglycerin pill than after a placebo may, in some instances, represent the sole method for accurate recognition of angina pectoris. A completely negative response to such repeated tests constitutes almost conclusive evidence against angina.

SUMMARY

The location of a pain in the chest has little diagnostic import. The concept that radiation from the anterior chest to the left arm necessarily indicates coronary disease as a cause is an old wives' tale. The several thoracic viscera and the chest wall have nerve fibers which pass by a final common pathway to the pain-receptive areas of the brain. One can no more identify the cause of the pain by its location alone than one can hear the ring of a telephone and know the city from which the call originated. Differences in the quality and duration of pain may be of diagnostic value. However, the most important aspect of the history in the diagnosis of *brief and recurrent chest pain is the relationship to various precipitating and alleviating factors.* The observation of the effect of exercise on the electrocardiogram and on the pain is often conclusive. In many instances the study of the effect of nitroglycerin on the amount of exercise required to produce pain is crucial.

In the spontaneously arising pains of long duration, as in myocardial infarction, dissecting aneurysm, pulmonary embolism, acute pericarditis, gallbladder colic, incarcerated hiatal hernia, acute pancreatitis, in all of which the pain may be identical in location, severity, character, and sites of reference, it is often the corollary data, clinical and laboratory, that finally determine the diagnosis.

Reproducing and alleviating the discomfort is not only sometimes of value in establishing the diagnosis but of immense psychologic benefit to the patient when he learns that an apparently mysterious and disturbing disorder can be mimicked and relieved at will.

When, as will occasionally occur, the thorough examination leaves one in doubt, observation over a period of time will often clarify the question, at least to the extent of establishing or excluding the more serious causes of the pain. Under such circumstances the patient should be advised to follow the same exertional and dietary regime which one would advise in any healthy middle-aged person, because this is essentially the same as that advised for a person with minimal myocardial ischemia. At the same time, fear can be alleviated by the reassurance that this regime is aimed not at treatment of an existing condition but at preventing future vascular disease.

REFERENCES

Braunwald, E.: The Determinants of Myocardial Oxygen Consumption, The Physiologist, 12:65, 1969.

Burch, G. E., J. M. Phillips, and N. P. De Pasquale: Cardiac Causalgia, Am. Heart J., 76:725, 1968.

Capps, J. A.: Pain from the Pleura and Pericardium, Assoc. Research Nervous and Mental Disease, Proc. (1942) 23: 263, 1943.

Friedberg, C. K.: Angina Pectoris—Diagnosis, Differential Diagnosis, Prognosis and Treatment, Chap. 19 in "Diseases of the Heart," 3d ed., pp. 734–769, Philadelphia, W. B. Saunders Company, 1966.

Hurst, J. W., and R. B. Logue: Symptoms Due to Heart Disease, Chap. 3 in "The Heart," 1st ed., pp. 47–53, New York, McGraw-Hill Book Company, 1966.

Keefer, C. S., and W. H. Resnik: Angina Pectoria: A Syndrome Caused by Anoxemia of the Myocardium, Arch. Intern. Med., 41:769, 1928.

Keele, K. D.: Pain Complaint Threshold in Relation to Pain of Cardiac Infarction, Brit. Med. J. (Lancet), 1:670, 1968.

Pain and Its Clinical Management, Med. Clinics N. Am., 52: 1–228, 1968.

Prinzmetal, M., and R. A. Massumi: Anterior Chest Wall Syndrome: Chest Pain Resembling Pain of Cardiac Origin, J.A.M.A., 159:177, 1955.

Wehrmacher, William H.: "Pain in the Chest," Springfield, Ill., Charles C Thomas, Publisher, 1964.

Wood, P.: The Chief Symptoms of Heart Disease, Chap. 1 in "Diseases of the Heart and Circulation," 3d ed., pp. 1–25, Philadelphia, J. B. Lippincott Company, 1968.

12 ABDOMINAL PAIN
William Silen

The correct interpretation of acute abdominal pain is one of the most challenging demands made of any physician. Since proper therapy often requires urgent action, the luxury of the leisurely approach suitable for the study of other conditions is frequently denied. Few other clinical situations demand greater experience and judgment, because the most catastrophic of events may be forecast by the subtlest of symptoms and signs. Nowhere in medicine is a meticulously executed detailed history and physical examination of greater importance. The etiologic classification in Table 12-1, although not complete, forms a useful frame of reference for the evaluation of patients with abdominal pain.

The diagnosis of "acute or surgical abdomen" so often heard in emergency wards is not an acceptable one because of its often misleading and erroneous connotation. The most obvious of "acute abdomens" may not require operative intervention, and the mildest of abdominal pains may herald the onset of an urgently correctible lesion. Any patient with abdominal pain of recent onset requires early and thorough evaluation with specific attempts at accurate diagnosis.

SOME MECHANISMS OF PAIN ORIGINATING IN THE ABDOMEN

INFLAMMATION OF THE PARIETAL PERITONEUM. The pain of parietal peritoneal inflammation is steady and aching in character and is located directly over the inflamed area, its exact reference being possible because it is transmitted by overlapping somatic nerves supplying the parietal peritoneum. The intensity of the pain is dependent upon the type and amount of foreign substance to which the peritoneal surfaces are exposed in a given period of time. For example, the sudden release into the peritoneal cavity of a small quantity of *sterile* acid gastric juice causes much more pain than the same amount of grossly contaminated neutral fecal material. Enzymatically active pancreatic juice incites more pain and inflammation than does the same amount of sterile bile containing no potent enzymes. Blood and urine are often so bland as to go undetected if exposure of the peritoneum has not been sudden and massive. In the case of bacterial contamination, such as in pelvic inflammatory disease, the pain is frequently of low intensity early in the illness until bacterial multiplication has caused the elaboration of irritating substances.

So important is the rate at which the irritating material is applied to the peritoneum that a perforated peptic ulcer may be associated with entirely different clinical pictures

Table 12-1. SOME IMPORTANT CAUSES OF ABDOMINAL PAIN

I. Pain originating in the abdomen
   A. Parietal peritoneal inflammation
      1. Bacterial contamination, e.g., perforated appendix, pelvic inflammatory disease.
      2. Chemical irritation, e.g., perforated ulcer, pancreatitis, mittelschmerz
   B. Mechanical obstruction of hollow viscera
      1. Obstruction of the small or large intestine
      2. Obstruction of the biliary tree
      3. Obstruction of the ureter
   C. Vascular disturbances
      1. Embolism or thrombosis
      2. Vascular rupture
      3. Pressure or torsional occlusion
      4. Sickle-cell anemia
   D. Abdominal wall
      1. Distortion or traction of mesentery
      2. Trauma or infection of muscles
      3. Distension of visceral surfaces, e.g., hepatic or renal capsules
II. Pain referred from extraabdominal sources
   A. Thorax—e.g., pneumonia, referred pain from coronary occlusion
   B. Spine—e.g., radiculitis from arthritis
   C. Genitalia—e.g., torsion of the testicle
III. Metabolic causes
   A. Exogenous
      1. Black widow spider bite
      2. Lead poisoning and others
   B. Endogenous
      1. Uremia
      2. Diabetic coma
      3. Porphyria
      4. Allergic factors (C'1 esterase deficiency)
IV. Neurogenic causes
   A. Organic
      1. Tabes dorsalis
      2. Herpes zoster
      3. Causalgia and others
   B. Functional

dependent only upon the rapidity with which the gastric juice enters the peritoneal cavity. *The pain of peritoneal inflammation is invariably accentuated by pressure or changes in tension of the peritoneum,* whether produced by palpation or by movement as in coughing or sneezing. Consequently, the patient with peritonitis lies quietly in bed preferring to avoid motion in contrast to the individual with colic who may writhe incessantly.

The intensity of the tonic muscle spasm accompanying peritoneal inflammation is dependent upon the location of the inflammatory process, the rate at which it develops, and the integrity of the nervous system. Spasm over a perforated retrocecal appendix or perforated ulcer into the lesser peritoneal sac may be minimal or absent because of the protective effect of overlying viscera. As in pain of peritoneal inflammation, a slowly developing process often greatly attentuates the degree of muscle spasm. Catastrophic abdominal emergencies such as a perforated ulcer have been repeatedly associated with minimal or occasionally no detectable pain or muscle spasm in obtunded, seriously ill debilitated elderly patients or in psychotic patients.

OBSTRUCTION OF HOLLOW VISCERA. The pain of obstruction of hollow abdominal viscera is classically described as intermittent, or colicky. Yet, the lack of a truly cramping character should not be misleading, because distension of a hollow viscus may produce steady pain with only very occasional exacerbations. Although not nearly as well localized as the pain of parietal peritoneal inflammation, some useful generalities can be made concerning the distribution of the pain caused by the obstruction of hollow intraabdominal viscera.

The colicky pain associated with obstruction of the small intestine is usually periumbilical or supraumbilical and is poorly localized. As the intestine becomes progressively dilated with loss of muscular tone, the colicky nature of the pain may become less apparent. With superimposed strangulating obstruction, pain may be felt in the lower lumbar region if the obstructing mechanism causes severe traction on the root of the mesentery. Pain arising in the colon is usually perceived in the region involved by the pathologic process.

Sudden distension of the biliary tree produces a steady rather than colicky type of pain, and hence the term "biliary colic" is misleading. Acute distension of the gallbladder usually causes pain in the right upper quadrant with radiation to the right posterior thorax or to the tip of the right scapula, and distension of the common bile duct is often associated with pain in the epigastrium radiating to the upper lumbar region. Considerable variation is common, however, so that differentiation between these may be impossible. The typical subscapular pain of lumbar radiation is frequently absent. Gradual dilatation of the biliary tree as in carcinoma of the head of the pancreas may cause no pain or only a mild aching sensation in the epigastrium or right upper quadrant. The pain of distension of the pancreatic ducts is similar to that described for distension of the common bile duct but in addition is very frequently accentuated by recumbency and relieved by the upright position.

Obstruction of the urinary bladder results in dull suprapubic pain, usually low in intensity. Restlessness without specific complaint of pain may be the only sign of a distended bladder in an obtunded patient. In contrast, acute obstruction of the intravesicular portion of the ureter is characterized by severe suprapubic and flank pain which radiates to the penis, scrotum, or inner aspect of the upper thigh. Obstruction of the ureteropelvic junction is felt as pain in the costovertebral angle, whereas obstruction of the remainder of the ureter is associated with flank pain, which often extends into the corresponding side of the abdomen.

VASCULAR DISTURBANCES. A frequent misconception, despite abundant experience to the contrary, is that pain associated with intraabdominal vascular disturbances is sudden and catastrophic in nature. The pain of embolism or thrombosis of the superior mesenteric artery, or that of impending rupture of an abdominal aortic aneurysm certainly may be severe and diffuse. Yet just as frequently, the patient with occlusion of the superior mesenteric artery has only mild continuous diffuse pain for 2 or 3 days before vascular collapse or findings of peritoneal inflammation are present. The early, seemingly insignificant discomfort is caused by hyperperistalsis rather than peritoneal inflammation. Indeed, absence of tenderness and rigidity in the presence of continuous diffuse pain in a patient likely to have vascular disease is quite characteristic of occlusion of the superior mesenteric artery. Abdominal pain with radiation to the sacral region, flank, or genitalia should always signal the possible presence of a rupturing abdominal aortic aneurysm. This pain may persist over a period of several days before rupture and collapse occur.

ABDOMINAL WALL. Pain arising from the abdominal wall is usually constant and aching. Movement and pressure accentuate the discomfort and muscle spasm. In the case of hematoma of the rectus sheath, now most frequently encountered in association with anticoagulant therapy, a mass may be present in the lower quadrants of the abdomen. Simultaneous involvement of muscles in other parts of the body usually serves to differentiate myositis of the abdominal wall from an intraabdominal process which might cause pain in the same region.

REFERRED PAIN FROM EXTRAABDOMINAL SOURCES AND FROM ABDOMEN TO OTHER AREAS

Pain referred to the abdomen from the thorax, spine, or genitalia may prove a vexing problem in differential diagnosis, because diseases of the upper abdominal cavity such as acute cholecystitis, perforated ulcer, or subphrenic abscesses are frequently associated with intrathoracic complications. A most important, yet often forgotten, dictum is that the possibility of intrathoracic disease must be considered in every patient with abdominal pain, especially if the pain is in the upper abdomen. Systematic questioning and examination directed towards detecting the presence or absence of myocardial or pulmonary infarction, pneumonia, pericarditis, or esophageal disease, the intrathoracic diseases which most often masquerade as abdominal emergencies, will often provide sufficient clues to establish the proper diagnosis. Diaphragmatic pleuritis resulting from pneumonia or pulmonary infarction may cause pain in the right upper quadrant and pain in the supraclavicular area, the latter radiation to be sharply distinguished from the referred subscapular pain caused by acute distension of the extrahepatic biliary tree. The ultimate decision as to the origin of abdominal pain may require deliberate and planned observation over a period of several hours, during which time repeated questioning and examination will provide the proper explanation.

Referred pain of thoracic origin is often accompanied by splinting of the involved hemithorax with respiratory lag and decrease in excursion more marked than that seen in the presence of intraabdominal disease. In addition, apparent abdominal muscle spasm caused by referred pain will diminish during the inspiratory phase of respiration, whereas it is persistent throughout both respiratory phases if it is of abdominal origin. Palpation over the area of referred pain in the abdomen also does not usually accentuate the pain and in many instances actually seems to relieve it. The frequent coexistence of thoracic and abdominal disease may be misleading and confusing, so that differentiation might be difficult or impossible. For example, the patient with known biliary tract disease often has epigastric pain during myocardial infarction, or biliary colic may be referred to the precordium or left shoulder in a patient who has suffered previously from angina pectoris. The explanation for the radiation of pain to a previously diseased area has not been elucidated.

Referred pain from the spine, which usually involves compression or irritation of nerve roots, is characteristically intensified by certain motions such as cough, sneeze, or strain and is associated with hyperesthesia over the involved dermatomes. Pain referred to the abdomen from the testicles or seminal vesicles is generally accentuated by the slightest pressure on either of these organs. The abdominal discomfort is of dull aching character and is poorly localized.

METABOLIC ABDOMINAL CRISES

Pain of metabolic origin may simulate almost any other type of intraabdominal disease. Here several mechanisms may be at work. In certain instances such as hyperparathyroidism, the metabolic disease itself may produce an intraabdominal process such as pancreatitis. Primary hyperlipemia may also be accompanied by severe pancreatitis, which can lead to unnecessary laporatomy unless recognized. C'1 esterase deficiency associated with angioneurotic edema is also often associated with episodes of severe abdominal pain. Whenever the cause of abdominal pain is obscure, a metabolic origin must always be considered. Abdominal pain is the hallmark of familial Mediterranean fever (Chap. 256).

The problem of differential diagnosis is often not readily resolved. The pain of porphyria and lead colic usually are difficult to distinguish from that of intestinal obstruction, because severe hyperperistalsis is a prominent feature of both. The pain of uremia or diabetes is nonspecific, and the pain and tenderness frequently shift in location and intensity. Diabetic acidosis may be precipitated by acute appendicitis or intestinal obstruction, so that if prompt resolution of the abdominal pain does not result from correction of the metabolic abnormalities, an underlying organic problem should be suspected. Black widow spider bites produce intense pain and rigidity of the abdominal muscles and of the back, an area infrequently involved in disease of intraabdominal origin.

NEUROGENIC CAUSES

Causalgic pain may occur in diseases which injure nerves of sensory type. It has a burning character and is usually limited to the distribution of a given peripheral nerve. Normal stimuli such as touch or change in temperature are transformed into, and may precipitate, this type of pain, which is also frequently present in a patient at rest. A helpful finding is the demonstration that cutaneous pain spots are irregularly spaced, and this may be the only indication of the presence of causalgic pain. Even though the pain may be precipitated by gentle palpation, rigidity of the abdominal muscles is absent, and the respirations are not disturbed. Distension of the abdomen is uncommon, and the pain has no relationship to the intake of food.

Pain arising from spinal nerves or roots may be caused by herpes zoster, impingement by arthritis, tumors, herniated nucleus pulposus, diabetes, or syphilis, comes and goes suddenly, and is of a lancinating type. Again it is not associated with food intake, abdominal distension, or changes in respiration. Severe muscle spasm, as in the gastric crises of tabes dorsalis, is common but is either relieved or is not accentuated by abdominal palpation. The pain is made worse by movement of the spine and is usually confined to a few dermatome segments. Hyperesthesia is very common.

Psychogenic pain conforms to none of the aforementioned patterns of disease. Here the mechanism is hard to define, and the most common problem is the hysterical adolescent or young woman who frequently loses an appendix and other organs because of abdominal pain. Ovulation or some other natural event that causes brief mild abdominal discomfort may be maximized as an abdominal catastrophe.

Psychogenic pain varies enormously in type and location but usually has no relation to meals. It is often at its onset markedly accentuated during the night. Nausea and vomiting are rarely observed, although occasionally the patient reports these symptoms. Spasm is seldom induced in the abdominal musculature and if present does not persist, especially if the attention of the patient can be distracted. Persistent localized tenderness is rare, and, if found, the muscle spasm in the area is inconsistent and often absent. Restriction of the depth of respiration is the most common respiratory abnormality, but this occurs in the absence of thoracic splinting or change in the respiratory rate.

APPROACH TO THE PATIENT WITH ABDOMINAL PAIN

There are few abdominal conditions which require such urgent operative intervention that an orderly approach need be abandoned, no matter how ill the patient. Only those patients with exsanguinating hemorrhage must be rushed to the operating room immediately, but in such instances only a few minutes are required to assess the critical nature of the problem. Under these circumstances, all obstacles must be swept aside, adequate access for intravenous fluid replacement obtained, and the operation begun. Many patients of this type have expired in the radiology department or the emergency room while awaiting such unnecessary examinations as electrocardiograms or films of the abdomen. *There are no contraindications to operation when massive hemor-*

rhage is present. Although exceedingly important, this situation fortunately is relatively rare.

Nothing will supplant an orderly painstakingly *detailed history*, which is far more valuable than any laboratory or roentgenologic examination. This kind of history is laborious and time-consuming, making it not especially popular even though a reasonably accurate diagnosis can be made on the basis of the history alone in the majority of cases. The *chronological sequence of events* in the patient's history is often more important than emphasis on the location of pain. If the examiner is sufficiently open-minded and unhurried, asks the proper questions, and listens, the patient will often himself provide the diagnosis. Careful attention should be paid to the extraabdominal regions which may be responsible for abdominal pain. An accurate menstrual history in a female patient is essential. Narcotics or analgesics should be withheld until a definitive diagnosis or a definitive plan has been formulated, because these agents often make it more difficult to secure and to interpret the history and physical findings.

In the examination, simple critical inspection of the patient, for example of his facies, position in bed, and respiratory activity, may provide valuable clues. The amount of information to be gleaned is directly proportional to the *gentleness* and thoroughness of the examiner. Once a patient with peritoneal inflammation has been examined in a brusque manner, accurate assessment by the next examiner becomes almost impossible. For example, eliciting rebound tenderness by sudden release of a deeply palpating hand in a patient with suspected peritonitis is cruel and unnecessary. The same information can be obtained by gentle percussion of the abdomen (rebound tenderness on a miniature scale), a maneuver which can be far more precise and localizing. Asking the patient to cough will elicit true rebound tenderness without the need for placing a hand on the abdomen. Furthermore, the brusque demonstration of rebound tenderness will startle and induce protective spasm in a nervous or worried patient in whom true rebound tenderness is not present. A palpable gallbladder will be missed if palpation is so brusque that voluntary muscle spasm becomes superimposed upon involuntary muscular rigidity.

As in history taking, there is no substitute for sufficient time spent in the examination. It is important to remember that abdominal signs may be minimal but nevertheless exceptionally meaningful if carefully assessed with consistent symptomatology. Signs may be virtually or actually totally absent in cases of pelvic peritonitis, so that careful *pelvic and rectal examination are mandatory in every patient with abdominal pain.* The presence of tenderness on pelvic or rectal examination in the absence of other abdominal signs must not lead the examiner to exclude such important operative indications as perforated appendicitis, diverticulitis, twisted ovarian cyst, and many others.

Much attention has been paid to the presence or absence of peristaltic sounds, their quality and frequency. Auscultation of the abdomen is probably one of the least rewarding aspects of the physical examination of a patient with abdominal pain. Severe catastrophes, such as strangulating small-bowel obstruction or perforated appendicitis, may occur in the presence of normal peristalsis. Conversely, when the proximal intestine above an obstruction becomes markedly distended and edematous, peristaltic sounds may lose the characteristics of borborygmi and become weak or absent even when peritonitis is not present. It is usually the severe chemical peritonitis of sudden onset which is associated with the truly silent abdomen. Assessment of the patient's state of hydration is important. The hematocrit and urinalysis permit an accurate estimate of the severity of dehydration, so that adequate replacement can be carried out.

Laboratory examinations may be of enormous value in the assessment of the patient with abdominal pain, yet with but a few exceptions they rarely establish a diagnosis. Leukocytosis should never be the single deciding factor as to whether or not operation is indicated. A white blood cell count greater than 20,000 may be observed with perforation of a viscus, but pancreatitis, acute cholecystitis, pelvic inflammatory disease, and intestinal infarction may be associated with marked leukocytosis. A normal white blood cell count is by no means rare in cases of perforation of abdominal viscera. The diagnosis of anemia may be more helpful than the white blood cell count, especially when combined with the history.

The urinalysis is also of great value in indicating to some degree the state of hydration or to rule out severe renal disease, diabetes, or porphyria. Determination of the blood urea nitrogen, blood sugar, and serum bilirubin may also be helpful. The serum amylase determination is overrated, since in carefully controlled series where the determination has been done within the first 72 hours, the amylase was less than 200 Somogyi units in one-third of the cases, between 200 and 500 in another one-third, and greater than 500 in one-third. Since many diseases other than pancreatitis, e.g., perforated ulcer, strangulating bowel obstruction, and acute cholecystitis, may be associated with very marked increase in the serum amylase, great care must be exercised in denying an operation to a patient solely on the basis of an elevated serum amylase level. The determination of the output of urinary amylase is probably more accurate than the estimation of the serum amylase in the diagnosis of pancreatitis.

Abdominal paracentesis has proved to be a safe and effective diagnostic maneuver in patients with acute abdominal pain. It is of special value in patients with blunt trauma to the abdomen where evaluation of the abdomen may be difficult because of other multiple injuries to the spine, pelvis, or ribs and where blood in the peritoneal cavity produces only a very mild peritoneal reaction. The gallbladder is the only organ which may continue to seep fluid following accidental perforation, so that the region of this organ must be assiduously avoided. Determination of the pH of the aspirated fluid to ascertain the site of a perforation is misleading, because even highly acid gastric juice is rapidly buffered by peritoneal exudate.

Plain and upright or lateral decubitus x-rays of the abdomen may be of the greatest value. They are usually unnecessary in patients with acute appendicitis or strangulated external hernias. However, in intestinal obstruction, perforated ulcer, and a variety of other conditions, films may be diagnostic. During a search for free air, the patient should be kept in the decubitus or upright position for at least 10 min before the appropriate film is taken lest a small pneumoperitoneum be missed. In rare instances, barium or water-soluble medium examination of the upper gastrointestinal tract may demonstrate partial intestinal obstruction which may elude diagnosis by other means. If there is any question of obstruction of the colon, oral administration of barium sulfate should be avoided. On the other hand, barium enema is of inestimable value in cases of colonic obstruction and should be used with greater frequency where the possibility of perforation does not exist.

Sometimes, even under the best of circumstances with all available auxiliary aids and with the greatest of clinical skill, a definitive diagnosis cannot be established when a patient is evaluated initially. Nevertheless, despite lack of a clear anatomic diagnosis it may be abundantly clear to an experienced and thoughtful physician and surgeon on clinical grounds alone that operation is indicated. Should that decision be questionable, watchful waiting with repeated questioning and examination will often elucidate the true nature of the illness and indicate the proper course of action.

REFERENCES

Cope, Z.: "The Early Diagnosis of the Acute Abdomen," 10th ed., Fair Lawn, N.J., Oxford University Press, 1953.

Fitz, R. H.: Perforating Inflammation of the Vermiform Appendix: With Special Reference to Its Early Diagnosis and Treatment, Trans. Assoc. Am. Physicians, 1:107, 1886.

Glenn, F.: Pain in Biliary Tract Disease, Surg. Gynecol. Obstet., 122:495, 1966.

Holman, E.: The Art of Abdominal Percussion in the Presence of Inflammation, Surg. Gynecol. Obstet., 93:775, 1951.

Lewis, T.: "Pain," New York, The Macmillan Company, 1942.

—— and J. H. Kellgren: Observation Relating to Referred Pain, Visceromotor Reflexes and Other Related Phenomena, Clin. Sci., 4:47, 1939.

Silen, W., M. F. Hein, and L. Goldman: Strangulation Obstruction of the Small Intestine, Arch. Surg., 85:121, 1962.

13 PAIN IN THE BACK AND NECK
Thornton Brown, Michel Jequier, and Raymond Adams

The following remarks concern mainly the lower back, since it is most frequently the site of disabling pain. The lower spine and pelvis, with their many muscular and tendinous attachments, are relatively inaccessible to palpation and also to inspection, even through the medium of x-ray. For want of reliable physical signs and laboratory tests, it is often necessary to depend on the patient's description of his pain, which may not be altogether accurate, and his behavior during the execution of certain maneuvers. Seasoned clinicians, for these reasons, come to appreciate the need of a systematic clinical approach, the description of which will be one of the main purposes of this chapter.

ANATOMY AND PHYSIOLOGY OF THE LOWER BACK

The spine is roughly divisible into two parts: an anterior column of articulated vertebral bodies and intervertebral disks held together by the anterior and posterior longitudinal ligaments and annulus fibrosus which together constitute the supporting pillar of the body; and a posterior segment consisting of pedicles and laminas, fused to form the walls of the spinal canal, which provides protection for the spinal cord.

The stability of the spine depends on two types of supporting structures, the ligamentous (passive) and muscular (active). Active muscular support and movement are contributed by the erector spinae, abdominal, glutei maximus, psoas, and hamstring muscles.

The vertebral and paravertebral structures derive their innervation from the recurrent branches of the spinal nerves. Pain endings and fibers have been demonstrated in the ligaments, muscles, periosteum of bone, outer layers of annulus fibrosus, and synovium of the articular facets. The sensory fibers from these structures and the sacroiliac and lumbosacral joints join to form the sinovertebral nerves which pass via the recurrent branches of the spinal nerves of the first sacral and the fifth to first lumbar vertebras into the gray matter of the corresponding segments of the spinal cord. Efferent fibers emerge from these segments and extend to the muscles through the same nerves. The sympathetic nerves contribute only to the innervation of blood vessels and appear to play no part in voluntary and reflex movement, though they do contain sensory fibers.

The parts of the back that possess the greatest freedom of movement and hence are most frequently subject to injury, are the lumbar and cervical. The majority of their movements are reflex and are the basis of posture.

GENERAL CLINICAL CONSIDERATIONS

TYPES OF LOW BACK PAIN. Of the several symptoms of disease of the spine (pain, stiffness or limitation of movement, and deformity), pain is of foremost importance by virtue of its frequency and its disabling effects. Four types of pain may be differentiated: local, referred, radicular, and that arising from secondary (protective) muscular spasm. One must identify these several types of pain by the patient's description, and here reliance is placed mainly on the character, location, and the conditions which modify them. The mechanism

of the several types of pain has already been described in Chap. 9.

Local pain is caused by any pathologic process which impinges upon or irritates sensory endings. Involvement of structures which contain no sensory endings is painless. The substance of the vertebral body may be destroyed by tumor, for example, without evocation of pain, whereas lesions of periosteum, synovial membranes, muscles, annulus fibrosus, and ligaments are often exquisitely painful. Although painful states are often accompanied by swelling of the affected tissues, this is not apparent if a deep structure of the back is the site of disease. Local pain is steady, sometimes intermittent, of the aching type, and rather diffuse but is always felt in or near the affected part of the spine. Often there is involuntary splinting of the spine segments by paravertebral muscles, and certain movements or postures which alter the position of the injured tissues aggravate or relieve the pain. Firm pressure upon superficial structures in the region of the involved structure usually evokes tenderness which is of aid in identifying the site of the abnormality.

Referred pain is of two types, that projected from the spine into regions lying within the area of the lumbar and upper sacral dermatomes and that projected from the pelvic and abdominal viscera to the spine. Pain due to diseases of the upper lumbar spine is usually referred to the anterior aspects of the thighs and legs; and that from the lower lumbar spine is referred to the gluteal regions, posterior thighs, and calves. Pain of this type tends also to be deep, of aching quality, and rather diffuse. In general the referred pain parallels in intensity the local pain in the back. In other words, maneuvers which alter local pain have a similar effect on referred pain, though not with such precision and immediacy as in "root pain." Pain from visceral disease usually is felt within the abdomen or flanks and may be modified by the state of activity of the viscera. Its character and temporal relationships are those of the particular visceral structure involved, and posture and movement of the back have relatively little effect, either on the local pain or that referred to the back.

Radicular, or "root," *pain* has some of the characteristics of referred pain but differs in its greater intensity, distal radiation, circumscription to the territory of a root, and the factors which excite it. The mechanism is distortion, stretching, irritation, or compression of a spinal root, most often central to the intervertebral foramen. The pain is sharp, often quite intense, and nearly always radiates from a central position near the spine to some part of the lower extremity. It is usually superimposed on the dull ache of referred pain. Cough, sneeze, and strain characteristically evoke this sharp radiating pain, though these maneuvers may also jar or move the spine and enhance local pain. Any motion which stretches the nerve, i.e., forward bending with the knees extended or "straight-leg raising," excites radicular pain; and jugular vein compression, which raises intraspinal pressure and may cause a shift in the position of the root, has a similar effect. The fourth and fifth lumbar and first sacral roots, which form the sciatic nerve, if involved in disease, cause pain which extends mainly down the posterior aspects of thigh, the postero- and anterolateral aspects of the leg, and into the foot, in the distribution of this nerve —so-called "sciatica." Tingling, paresthesias, and numbness or sensory impairment of the skin, soreness of the skin, and tenderness along the nerve usually accompany radicular pain. Also reflex loss, weakness, atrophy, fascicular twitching, and often stasis edema may occur if motor fibers are involved in the anterior roots.

Pain resulting from muscular spasm is usually mentioned in relation to local pain, but it deserves separate consideration. As stated above, muscle spasm is associated with most conditions which result in local pain. Muscles in a state of persistent tension give rise to a dull ache, which Smith-Petersen called "secondary pain." One can feel the tautness of the erector spinae and gluteal muscles and demonstrate by palpation that the pain is localized to them.

Other pains often of undetermined origin are sometimes described by patients with chronic disease of the lower back. In the legs drawing, pulling, cramping sensations (without involuntary muscle spasm), tearing, throbbing, or jabbing pains, feelings of burning or coldness are difficult to interpret and, like paresthesias and numbness, should always suggest the possibility of nerve or root disease.

Since it is often difficult to obtain physical or laboratory confirmation of painful disease of the lower spine, the importance of an accurate history and description of symptoms cannot be overemphasized. Frequently the most important lead comes from the knowledge of the mode of onset and circumstances which initiated the pain. Inasmuch as many painful affections of the back are the result of injury incurred during work or in an accident, the possibility of exaggeration or prolongation of pain for personal reasons, or even hysteria or malingering, must always be kept in mind.

THE EXAMINATION OF THE LOWER BACK. *Inspection* of the spine, buttocks, and legs when standing erect, walking, stooping, and squatting is of value. The patient's resting posture should be noted because faulty posture predisposes to pain in the lumbosacral and sacroiliac regions. With sciatica the lumbar spine is often scoliotic, with the convexity toward the normal side, though the converse may occur. Also, a slight flexion or flattening of the lumbar lordosis is common with acute painful states. The presence of a definite kyphosis usually signifies deformity of one of the vertebral bodies, e.g., fracture. Spasm of paravertebral muscles on one or both sides is often obvious during inspection. One may also notice a hypotonia of the gluteus maximus on the affected side with drooping of the gluteal fold.

The next step in the examination is observation of the spine, hips, and legs during certain motions. During the procedure it is well to remember that no advantage accrues from trying to find out how much the patient can be hurt. Instead, it is much more important to deter-

mine when and under what conditions the pain commences. One looks for limitation of the natural motions of the patient as he disrobes and while he is standing, sitting, and reclining. When standing, the motion of forward bending normally produces flattening and reversal of the lumbar lordotic curve and exaggeration of the dorsal curve. With lesions of the lumbosacral region which involve the posterior ligaments, articular facets, or erector spinae and with ruptured lumbar discs the patient attempts to avoid stretching these structures. As a consequence, the erectores spinae remain taut and prevent motion in the lumbar spine. Forward bending then occurs at the hips and at the lumbar-thoracic junction. With disease of the lumbosacral joints and spinal roots, the patient bends in such a way as to avoid tensing the hamstring muscles and putting undue leverage upon the pelvis. In unilateral "sciatica," with its increased curvature toward the side of the lesion, lumbar and lumbosacral motions are splinted and bending is mainly at the hips; at a certain point the knee on the affected side is flexed to relieve hamstring spasm and tilting of the pelvis, and to slacken the roots and sciatic nerve.

Lateral bending is usually less instructive than forward bending. However, in unilateral ligamentous or muscular strain, bending to the opposite side aggravates the pain by stretching the damaged tissues. Moreover, in lateral disc lesions, bending of the spine toward the side from which the trunk lists is restricted.

In diseases of the lower spine, flexion while sitting can normally be performed easily, even to the point of bringing the knees in contact with the chest. The reason for this is that knee flexion relaxes the hamstring muscles and relieves stretch of the sciatic nerve. The lumbar and lumbosacral joints and the normal curve of the spine need not be altered under these conditions. On the other hand, if the knees are extended, the same impedance of movement noted during forward bending, while standing with the legs straight, is observed.

The study of motions in the reclining position yields the same information as those in the standing and sitting positions, with the difference that there is less pressure on the discs. Passive lumbar flexion is like active forward bending in the standing position. With lumbosacral lesions and sciatica, it causes little pain and is not limited as long as the hamstrings and sciatic nerve are relaxed (knee flexed). With lumbosacral and lumbar spine disease (e.g., arthritis), passive flexion of the hips is free, whereas flexion of the lumbar spine is impeded and painful. Passive straight-leg raising (possibly up to 90° except in those who are congenitally stiff), like forward bending in the standing posture with the legs straight, places the sciatic nerve and its roots, also the hamstrings, under tension, thereby producing pain. It also rotates the pelvis, thus causing lumbar joint pain. Consequently, in diseases of the lumbosacral joints and of the lumbosacral roots, this movement is limited on the affected side and, to a lesser extent, the opposite side. Lasegue's sign (pain and limitation of movement during elevation of the leg when the knee is extended) is but a variation of this test, as are Goldthwait's sign (limited extension at the knee after the thigh has been flexed on the trunk), Lewin's sign (snapping back of the knee into flexion when released), and Bragaard's sign of pain in the opposite leg during straight-leg raising. The evoked pain is always referred to the diseased side, no matter which leg is flexed. In disease of the lumbosacral joints there may also be slight limitation of straight-leg raising, though rarely to the degree seen in disease of the lumbosacral roots.

The motion of hyperextension is best performed with the patient standing or lying prone. If the condition causing back pain is acute, it may be difficult to extend the spine in the standing position. A patient with lumbosacral strain can usually extend or hyperextend the spine without aggravation of pain. If involved in an active inflammatory or other acute process, however, vertical pressure upon these joints will increase the pain. Also, if there is ligamentous strain, no enhancement of pain occurs because the posterior segments of the spine are relaxed during extension. The converse is true if there is strain of extensor muscles, for hyperextension places the muscular attachments to the periosteum under tension. Although disease of articular facets may limit ex-

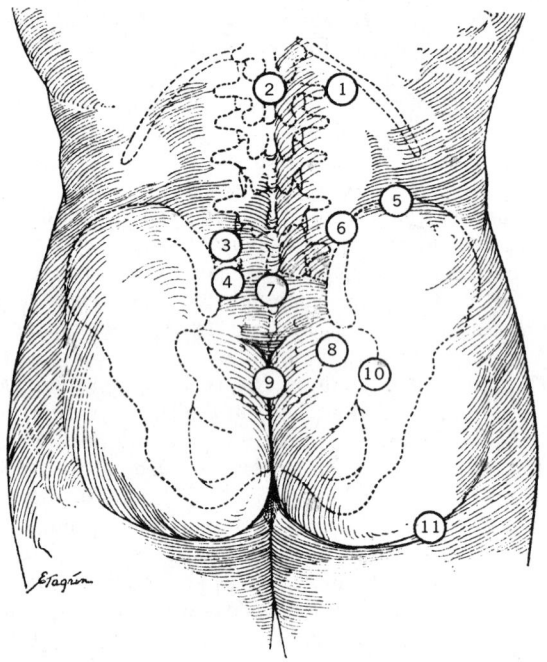

Fig. 13-1. (1) Costovertebral angle. (2) Spinous process and interspinous ligament. (3) Region of articular fifth lumbar to first sacral facet. (4) Dorsum of sacrum. (5) Region of iliac crest. (6) Iliolumbar angle. (7) Spinous processes of fifth lumbar to first sacral vertebras (tenderness = faulty posture or occasionally spina bifida occulta). (8) Region between posterior superior and posterior inferior spines. Sacroiliac ligaments (tenderness = sacroiliac sprain; often tender with fifth lumbar to first sacral disk). (9) Sacrococcygeal junction (tenderness = sacrococcygeal injury, i.e., sprain or fracture). (10) Region of sacrosciatic notch (tenderness = fourth to fifth lumbar disk rupture and sacroiliac sprain). (11) Sciatic nerve trunk (tenderness = ruptured lumbar disk or sciatic nerve lesion).

tension, little or no pain is produced. In lumbar disc disease (except in the acute phase of the illness), extension of the spine is usually tolerated well, though in some patients with a displaced disc fragment situated posterolaterally, pain is evoked by extension rather than flexion. A reversed Lasegue's sign (limitation in the hyperextension of straight leg while in prone position) suggests spinal nerve involvement at the midlumbar level or a lesion of the lumbosacral joint.

Palpation and percussion of the spine are the last steps in the examination. The approach must always be gentle since rough percussion of the designated area of pain only confuses the physician and antagonizes the patient. It is preferable to palpate first those regions which are the least likely to evoke pain. At all times the examiner should know what structures are being palpated (see Fig. 13-1). Localized tenderness is seldom pronounced in disease of the spine because the involved structures are so deep that they rarely give rise to surface tenderness. Mild superficial and poorly localized tenderness signifies only a disease process within the affected segment of the body, i.e., dermatome.

Tenderness over the costovertebral angle often indicates genitourinary disease, adrenal disease (Rogoff's sign), or an injury to the transverse processes of the first or second lumbar vertebra [Fig. 13-1 (1)]. Hypersensitivity on palpation of the transverse processes of the other lumbar vertebras as well as the overlying erector spinae muscles may signify fracture of the transverse process or a strain of muscle attachments.

Upon palpation of the spinous processes and interspinous ligaments any deviation in the anteroposterior or lateral plane must be particularly noted. Such a deviation usually indicates spondylolisthesis. Tenderness of the interspinous ligaments is indicative of disc lesions [Fig. 13-1 (2)].

Tenderness in the region of the articular facets between the fifth lumbar and first sacral vertebras is consistent with a lumbosacral disc disease [Fig. 13-1 (3)]. It is also not infrequent in rheumatoid arthritis.

Rectal and pelvic examination constitute an essential part of the diagnostic study of all cases of low back pain and sciatica.

Upon completion of the examination of the back a search for motor, reflex, and sensory changes (see Syndrome of Ruptured Disc, below), particularly in the lower extremities, should be made.

SPECIAL LABORATORY PROCEDURES. Laboratory tests often aid in diagnosis. Depending on the circumstances, these may include measurement of the serum proteins, phosphatases (alkaline and acid), calcium, phosphorus, uric acid, serum electrophoresis (myeloma proteins), tuberculin, agglutination for Brucella, sedimentation rate, and rheumatoid factor. X-rays should be taken in every case of low back pain and sciatica in the anteriorposterior, lateral, and oblique planes of the lumbar spine (looking for abnormal mobility with disc disease) and at times, the thoracic spine. Stereoscopic or laminographic films may provide further information if the regular x-rays show abnormalities. In many cases of low back pain with neurologic manifestations, examination of the spinal canal with a contrast medium (myelogram) is necessary. This study can be combined with tests of dynamics of the cerebrospinal fluid, and a sample of the fluid should always be removed for cytologic and chemical examination prior to the installation of the contrast medium (Pantopaque, Myodil, or air). Injection and removal of Pantopaque require special skill and should not be attempted without previous experience with the procedure. If done properly, the procedure is harmless. Injection of contrast medium directly into the intervertebral disc (discograms) has recently become popular but is still controversial. The technique of this procedure is more complicated than that of myelographic examination, and the risk of damage to nerve roots or the introduction of infection is not inconsiderable. In the authors' opinion, the results do not warrant the risk involved.

PRINCIPAL CONDITIONS WHICH GIVE RISE TO DISABLING PAIN IN THE LOWER BACK

CONGENITAL ANOMALIES OF THE LUMBAR SPINE

Anatomic variations of the spine are not at all infrequent, and although not of themselves the source of pain and functional derangement, they may be of importance because they dispose to strain by permitting excessive mobility or the adoption of abnormal postures.

There may be a lack of fusion of the laminas of the neural arch—a spina bifida—of one or several of the lumbar vertebras, or of the sacrum. Hypertrichosis or hyperpigmentation in the sacral area may betray the condition, but it may remain entirely occult until disclosed by x-ray. The anomaly induces pain only when accompanied by malformation of vertebral joints or stretching and distortion of nerve roots.

Spondylolysis, another important anomaly, consists of a bony defect in the pars interarticularis, which is replaced by cartilage, permitting a forward displacement of the vertebral body, pedicles, superior articular processes, leaving the laminae, inferior articular processes and spinous processes behind (spondylolisthesis). Although of congenital origin, the first symptoms of disordered function (low back pain radiating to the thighs, tightness of back muscles, and signs of involvement of spinal roots—paresthesias and sensory loss, muscle weakness, and reflex impairment) may not appear until later in life and are often precipitated by an injury.

Articular facets of the vertebras may be set in an unusual plane, either oblique or frontal, rather than the sagittal one as in the normal lumbar spine; there may also be an abnormality of the number of mobile lumbar vertebras (either six or four). The lowest vertebra may be asymmetric in its relation to the sacrum. Although these abnormalities have been blamed for chronic low back pain, large surveys suggest that they bear no relationship to it.

TRAUMATIC AFFLICTIONS OF THE LOWER BACK

Trauma constitutes the most frequent cause of low back pain.

In severe acute injuries, the examining physician must be careful to avoid further damage. In tests of motility, all movements must be kept to a minimum until an approximate diagnosis has been made and adequate measures have been instituted for the proper care of the patient. If the patient complains of pain in his back and cannot move his legs, his spine may have been fractured. His neck should not be flexed nor should he be allowed to sit up. (See Chap. 356 for further discussion of spinal cord injury.)

SPRAINS AND STRAINS. The terms *strain* and *sprain* are used loosely by most physicians. It is probably impossible to differentiate between them. Here we shall use only the word strain. Strain should designate a minor injury which does not produce gross structural damage. The abnormal mechanical force may be acute, as in heavy lifting, or mild and persistent, due to maintenance of an abnormal posture. The latter is often occupational. Rest and relaxation promptly alleviate the discomfort, attesting to the lack of major structural change. What formerly was regarded as sacroiliac strain or sprain is now known to be due to discogenic disease in most instances. This is caused by lifting heavy objects with the spine in a position of imperfect mechanical balance, as when lifting and turning at the same time. Sudden unexpected motion is particularly dangerous.

The diagnosis of lumbosacral and sacroiliac strains with injury of the various structures of the lower back depends upon the description of the injury, the localization of the pain by the patient, the finding of localized tenderness, and the augmentation of pain when tension is exerted on the involved structures by the appropriate maneuvers. The prompt alleviation of the pain by rest and relaxation indicates the existence of a strain. The role of recovery depends on the degree of damage, preexisting disc disease, etc. It may, however, be relieved by local infiltration of an anesthetic agent, a finding which is also helpful in diagnosis.

Sacroiliac strain, once so popular as an explanation of unilateral back pain, is now highly controversial. Because of their irregular surfaces, the sacroiliac bones are interlocked, and joint movement is minimal and is further restricted by strong sacroiliac ligaments. Only violent injury could derange this well-protected and stable joint. Multiple pregnancies close together may be another cause. When the joint is injured, the principal symptom is a localized ache which is made worse by compression of the pelvis. It must be remembered that involvement of a spinal nerve root (fifth lumbar or first sacral) associated with injury to the disk is the more common cause of pain and local tenderness in the area of the sacroiliac joint.

VERTEBRAL FRACTURES. Fractures of the lumbar vertebral body are usually the result of flexion injuries. This is most likely to occur in falls from a height; often the calcaneus is also fractured. Nearly always there is localized tenderness over the fractured vertebra. Spasm of the lower lumbar muscles, limitation of movements of the lumbar spine, and the x-ray appearance of the damaged portion of the lumbar spine (with or without neurologic abnormalities) are the basis of clinical diagnosis. The pain is usually immediate, though occasionally it may be delayed for days, and some patients are found to have had crushed fractures of the vertebral body without being able to recall any traumatic episode.

Fractured transverse processes, which are almost always associated with tearing of the paravertebral muscles, are diagnosed by the finding of deep tenderness at the site of the injury, local muscle spasm on one side, and limitation of all movements which stretch the lumbar muscles. Radiologic evidence provides the final confirmation.

PROTRUSION OF LUMBAR INTERVERTEBRAL DISCS. This condition is now recognized as the major cause of severe and chronic or recurrent low back and leg pain. It is most likely to occur between the fifth lumbar and first sacral vertebras and, with lessening frequency, between the fourth to fifth lumbar, the third to fourth lumbar, the second to third lumbar, and the first to second lumbar vertebras. Almost nonexistent in the thoracic spine, it is next most frequent at the sixth to seventh and fifth to sixth cervical vertebras. The cause is usually a flexion injury, but in a considerable proportion of cases no trauma is recalled. Degeneration of the posterior longitudinal ligaments and the annulus fibrosus, which occurs in most adults of middle and advanced years, may have taken place silently or have been manifested by mild, recurrent lumbar ache. A sneeze, lurch, or other trivial movement may then cause the nucleus pulposus to extrude through the frayed ligament.

The fully developed syndrome of ruptured intervertebral disc consists of backache, abnormal posture, and limitation of motion of the spine (particularly flexion). Nerve root involvement is indicated by radicular pain, sensory disturbances (paresthesias, hyper- and hyposensitivity in dermatome pattern), motor abnormalities (weakness and atrophy, coarse twitching and fasciculation, and muscle spasms), and impairment of tendon reflexes. Since herniation of the intervertebral lumbar discs most often occurs between the fourth and fifth lumbar vertebras and the fifth lumbar and first sacral vertebras with irritation and compression of the fifth lumbar and first sacral roots, respectively, it is important to recognize the clinical characteristics of lesions of these two roots. *Lesions of the fifth lumbar root* produce pain in the region of the hip, groin, posterolateral thigh, lateral calf to the external malleolus, dorsal surface of the foot, and the first or second and third toes. Paresthesias may be in the entire territory or only the distal parts of these territories. The tenderness is in the lateral gluteal region and near the head of the fibula. Weakness, if present, involves the extensor of the big toe and of the foot. Either the knee or ankle reflex may be diminished, but these reflexes are usually unchanged. Walking on the heels may be more uncomfortable than walking on the toes. In *lesions of the first sacral root* the pain is felt in the midgluteal region, posterior thigh, posterior calf to the heel, and the plantar surface of the foot and fourth and fifth toes. Tenderness is most pronounced over the midgluteal region (sacroiliac joint), posterior thigh, and calf. Paresthesias and sensory loss are mainly in the lower leg and outer toes, and weakness, if present, involves the flexor muscles of the foot and toes, abductors of the toes, and hamstring muscles. The ankle reflex is diminished to absent in the majority of cases. Walking on the toes is more uncomfortable than on the heels. With lesions of either root there may be limitation of straight-leg raising during the acute, painful stages.

Low back pain may also be caused by degeneration of the intervertebral disc, without frank extrusion of fragment of disc tissue. Or the herniation may occur into the adjacent vertebral body, giving rise to Schmorl's nodules. In such cases there are no signs of nerve root involvement though the back pain may be referred to the leg.

The rarer *lesions of the fourth and third lumbar roots* give rise to pain in the anterior part of the thigh and knee, with corresponding sensory loss. The knee-jerk is diminished or abolished. An inverted Lasegue sign is positive when the third lumbar root is affected.

The syndrome is usually unilateral. Only with massive derangements of the discs do bilateral symptoms and signs occur, and these may then be associated with paralysis of the sphincters. The pain may be mild or severe. All or part of the above syndrome may be present. There may be back pain with little or no leg pain; rarely leg pain may be experienced without pain in the back. The rupture of multiple lumbar or lumbar and cervical discs is not infrequent, attesting to a basic disorder of the entire disc including the annulus fibrosus.

When all components of the syndrome are present, the diagnosis is easy; when only one part is present, particularly backache, it may be difficult, especially if there has been no accident. Since similar symptoms may occur without demonstrable disc rupture, other diagnostic procedures are required. Plain x-rays usually show no abnormality or at most a narrowing of the intervertebral space or traction spurs, which is indicative of disc degeneration; hence one must resort to Pantopaque myelography. This will reveal in most cases an indentation of the lumbar subarachnoid space or deformity of the root sleeve. Unfortunately, a small ruptured disc may not show, especially at the L-5 S-1 level. The electromyogram is helpful in showing denervation of leg muscles (see Chap. 390). The protein of the cerebrospinal fluid is elevated in some instances.

Tumor of the spinal canal, epidural or intradural, may produce a syndrome similar to that of ruptured disc (see Chap. 356).

ARTHRITIS

Arthritis will be discussed more fully elsewhere. It need only be mentioned that osteoarthritis is much more frequent than rheumatoid and that the latter may take two forms, one in which the spinal involvement is but a part of a generalized arthritis, often with other signs of "connective tissue disease" and the other limited almost exclusively to the spine, sacroiliac joints, and hips (rheumatoid spondylitis or Marie-Strümpell arthritis) (Chap. 390). An extreme form of osteoarthritis in the cervical region, sometimes leading to spinal cord or nerve compression, is called spondylosis (see Chap. 356).

Rheumatoid spondylitis, which often begins with involvement of the sacroiliac joints, induces continuous aching pain and stiffness in the back or in the buttocks and thigh. Fatigue and other systemic manifestations are usually present. Expansion of the chest is limited when the thoracic spine is involved. However, the disease rarely reaches an advanced degree without pain. Acute painful exacerbations are probably due to involvement of the apophyseal joints. The pain is centered in the spine and is worse on movement, especially after the patient has been inactive. Pain during the night or in the early morning hours is another common feature. It may be partially relieved by activity and is often aggravated by seasonal and barometric changes. The effect of salicylates, which usually alleviate the pain to some degree, may be taken as another diagnostic feature. Signs of root involvement may coexist.

Ankylosing spondylitis, a disease closely related to rheumatoid arthritis of the spine, is an important cause of low back pain. The majority of its victims are men, usually in their twenties (onset may be to fifty years). The initial complaint of recurrent low-back pain and stiffness, with or without recurrent sciatic pain, or more vague symptoms (tired back, soreness, aching, or "catches in the back") may precede demonstrable x-ray changes by several years. It differs from rheumatoid spondylitis, which is more frequent in women, affects usually the upper spine (especially cervical), and extends to the whole back; only a third of patients with ankylosing spondylitis develop arthritic changes in the shoulders, hips, knees, and ankles. The aortic valve may become involved, giving rise to insufficiency (spondylitic heart disease). The sedimentation rate is usually elevated, but constitutional symptoms are rare. Recurrent iritis and uveitis are present in approximately 25 percent of patients. X-rays show the sacroiliac and apophyseal joints to be blurred and anterior and lateral spinal ligaments calcified. A therapeutic response to phenylbutazone (Butazolidine) or indomethacin (Indocin) and exercises is also quite characteristic (see Chap. 386). Discogenic disease also figures in the differential diagnosis.

In *osteoarthritis,* by contrast, pain in the spine may or may not be accompanied by the motor, reflex, or sensory changes of root involvement. The pain in the spine is of the same type as in rheumatoid spondylitis and is also accompanied by a sense of stiffness and limitation of movement. It differs slightly in being more clearly aggravated by motion, more readily relieved by rest, and less pronounced at night. Fatigue and systemic symptoms are notably absent. The severity of the pain is not clearly related to the degree of the process as seen in the x-ray. X-ray evidence of the disease in the spine is found in a majority of individuals beyond the age of

fifty as is clicking in the neck on head movement. The presence of such changes should not be accepted as establishing an arthritic source of a severe and progressive pain, since it may be due to a more serious unrelated condition, such as a neoplasm.

Injury may exacerbate the pain of both rheumatoid and osteoarthritis. (See Chap. 390 for further discussion of spondylitis.)

OTHER DESTRUCTIVE DISEASES

INFECTIOUS, NEOPLASTIC AND METABOLIC DISEASES.

Metastatic carcinoma (breast, bronchus, prostate, thyroid, hypernephroma, stomach, uterus), multiple myeloma, and lymphoma are the common tumors which involve the spine; tuberculosis and pyogenic osteomyelitis are the most frequent infections, though brucellosis, typhoid fever, actinomycosis, and blastomycosis are known to occur.

Special mention should be made of the spinal *epidural abscess* (usually staphylococcal), which necessitates urgent surgical treatment. The symptoms are a localized pain, spontaneous as well as on percussion and palpation, often with radicular radiation, and a rapidly developing flaccid paraplegia appearing in a febrile patient.

Destructive lesions of any type may develop silently, i.e., without any pain, as long as they are limited to the osseous tissue. Upon spreading to the periosteum or to the adjacent spinous structures, however, they become the source of much pain of both local and referred type, and often one or more spinal roots are implicated as well, with the typical radicular type being added to the clinical picture. A "spontaneous" fracture may initiate pain. Pain caused by neoplasms of the spine tends to be of aching character and more or less steady, though occasionally waxing and waning. It is especially severe at night, seeming to be only slightly benefited by rest; yet activity during the day also worsens the pain. As the disease progresses, the pain increases in duration and severity. It may then be of a throbbing character. The most important physical finding, which should lead one to suspect a destructive lesion, is an intensification of the pain by jarring the spine, by percussing the spinous processes gently with the fist or a reflex hammer, or by exerting a steady pressure upon these parts. Axial compression (downward pressure exerted on the head or dropping on the heels from the toe position) may also serve to intensify the pain. Nocturnal pain, spinal ache, and percussion sensitivity are also characteristic of Pott's disease and osteomyelitis. The establishment of the cause of the pain is often delayed because the first x-rays may not disclose the lesion. (Nearly a cubic centimeter of bone must be destroyed in a vertebral body before it is visible in an x-ray.) If these are negative, they should be repeated after an interval of a few weeks. Other laboratory data, such as white blood count and smear, sedimentation rate, and electrophoresis of serum proteins, and acid and alkaline phosphatase in the serum are helpful.

In so-called "metabolic bone diseases" (osteoporosis

of either the postmenopausal or senile type or osteomalacia) a considerable degree of loss of bone substance may occur without any symptoms whatsoever. Many such patients do, however, complain of aching in the lumbar or thoracic area. This is most likely to occur following an injury, sometimes of trivial degree, which leads to collapse or wedging of a vertebra. Certain movements greatly enhance the pain, and certain positions relieve it. One or more spinal roots may then be involved. Paget's disease of the spine is nearly always painless. It may lead to compression of the spinal cord. The recognition of these bone disorders is discussed in some detail elsewhere (Chaps. 356 and 381).

REFERRED PAIN FROM VISCERAL DISEASE

The pain of disease of the pelvic, abdominal, or thoracic viscera is often felt in the region of the spine; i.e., it is referred to the more posterior parts of the spinal segment which innervates the diseased organ. Occasionally back pain may be the first and only sign. The general rule is that pelvic diseases are referred to the sacral region, lower abdominal disease to the lumbar region (centering around the second to fourth lumbar vertebras), and upper abdominal diseases to the lower thoracic spine (eighth thoracic to the first and second lumbar vertebras). Characteristically there are no local signs, no stiffness of the back, and motion is of full range without augmentation of the pain. However, some positions, e.g., flexion of the lumbar spine in the lateral recumbent position, may be more comfortable than others.

LOW THORACIC AND UPPER LUMBAR PAIN IN ABDOMINAL DISEASE. Peptic ulceration or tumor of the wall of the stomach and of the duodenum most typically induces pain in the epigastrium (see Chaps. 11, 12, and 314); but if the posterior wall is involved, and particularly if there is retroperitoneal extension, the pain may be felt in the region of the spine. Usually the pain is central in location or is more intense on one side. If very intense, it may seem to encircle the body. It tends to retain the characteristics of pain from the affected organ; e.g., if due to peptic ulceration, it is relieved by food and soda and appears about 2 hr after a meal.

Diseases of the pancreas (peptic ulceration with extension to the pancreas, cholecystitis with pancreatitis, tumor) are apt to cause pain in the back, being more to the right of the spine if the head of the pancreas is involved and to the left if the body and tail are implicated.

Diseases of retroperitoneal structures, e.g., lymphomas, sarcomas, and carcinomas, may evoke pain in this part of the spine with some tendency toward radiation to the lower abdomen, groins, and anterior thighs. A secondary tumor of the ileopsoas region on one side often produces a unilateral lumbar ache with radiation toward the groin and labia or testicle; there may also be signs of involvement of the upper lumbar spinal roots. An aneurysm of the abdominal aorta may induce a pain which is localized to this region of the spine but may be felt higher or lower, depending on the location of the lesion.

The sudden appearance of obscure lumbar pain in a patient receiving anticoagulants should arouse the suspicion of retroperitoneal bleeding.

LUMBAR PAIN WITH LOWER ABDOMINAL DISEASES. Inflammatory diseases of segments of the colon (colitis, diverticulitis) or tumor of the colon cause pain which may be felt in the lower abdomen between the umbilicus and pubis, or in the midlumbar region, or in both places. If very intense, the pain may have a beltlike distribution around the body. A lesion in the tranverse colon or first part of the descending colon may be central or left-sided, and its level of reference to the back is to the second to third lumbar vertebras. If the sigmoid colon is implicated, the pain is lower, in the upper sacral region and anteriorly in the midline suprapubic region or left lower quadrant of the abdomen.

SACRAL PAIN IN PELVIC (UROLOGIC AND GYNECOLOGIC) DISEASES. Although gynecologic disorders may manifest themselves by back pain, the pelvis is seldom the site of a disease which causes obscure low back pain. For the most part the diagnosis of painful pelvic lesions is not difficult, for a thorough palpation of structures by abdominal, vaginal, and rectal examination may be supplemented by methods (sigmoidoscopy, barium enema, pyelography) which adequately visualize all these parts.

Menstrual pain itself may be felt in the sacral region. It is rather poorly localized, tends to radiate down the legs, and is of a crampy nature. The most important source of chronic back pain from the pelvic organs, however, is the uterosacral ligaments. Endometriosis or carcinoma of the uterus (body or cervix) may invade these structures, while malposition of the uterus may pull on them. The pain is localized centrally in the sacrum below the lumbosacral joint but may be more on one side. In endometriosis the pain begins during the premenstrual phase and often continues until it merges with menstrual pain. Malposition of the uterus (retroversion, descensus, and prolapse) characteristically leads to sacral pain, especially after the patient has been standing for several hours. Postural adjustments may also evoke pain here when a fibroma of the uterus pulls on the uterosacral ligaments. Carcinomatous pain due to implication of nerve plexuses is continuous and becomes progressively more severe; it tends to be more intense at night. The primary lesion may be inconspicuous, being overlooked upon pelvic examination. Papanicolaou smears and a pyelogram are the most useful diagnostic procedures. X-ray therapy of these tumors may produce sacral pain consequent to swelling and necrosis of tissue, the so-called "radiation phlegmon of the pelvis." Low back pain with radiation into one or both thighs is a common phenomenon during the last weeks of pregnancy.

Chronic prostatitis, evidenced by prostatic discharge, frequency of urination, and slight reduction in sexual potency, may be attended by a nagging sacral ache; it may be mainly on one side, with radiation into one leg if the seminal vesicle is involved on that side. Carcinoma of the prostate with metastases to the lower spine is another cause of sacral or lumbar pain. It may be present without urinary frequency or burning. Spinal nerves may be infiltrated by tumor cells, or the spinal cord itself may be compressed if the epidural space is invaded. The diagnosis is established by rectal examination, x-rays of the spine, and measurement of acid phosphatase (particularly the prostatic phosphatase fraction). Lesions of the bladder and testes are usually not accompanied by back pain. When the kidney is the site of disease, the pain is ipsilateral, being felt in the flank or lumbar region.

Visceral derangements of whatever type may intensify the pain of arthritis, and the presence of arthritis may alter the distribution of visceral pain. With disease of the spine in the lumbosacral region, for example, distension of the ampulla of the sigmoid by feces or a bout of colitis may aggravate the arthritic pain. In patients with arthritis of the cervical or thoracic spine, the pain of myocardial ischemia may radiate to the back.

OBSCURE TYPES OF LOW BACK PAIN AND THE QUESTION OF PSYCHIATRIC DISEASE

The practicing physician is consulted by many individuals who complain of low back pain of obscure origin. A safe rule is to assume that all of them have some type of primary or secondary disease of the spine and its supporting structures or of the abdominal or pelvic viscera. If the pain is of acute onset and short duration, it may be due to only a minor trauma, a so-called "fibrositis," or some form of articular disease. If it is recurrent, the possibility of a ruptured disc causing an instability of the spine must be considered. If it is severe and progressive, neoplasia, a tuberculous infection, and rheumatoid spondylitis should be kept in mind. Adolescent girls and boys are subject to an obscure form of epiphyseal disease of the spine (Scheuermann's disease) which may cause low back pain upon exercise over a period of 2 to 3 years.

POSTURAL BACK PAIN. Many slender asthenic individuals and some fat middle-aged individuals have discomfort in the back. Their backs ache much of the time, and the pain interferes with effective work. The physical examination is negative except for slack musculature and poor posture. The pain is diffuse in the mid or low back and characteristically is relieved by bed rest and induced by the maintenance of a particular posture over a period of time. Pain in the neck and between the shoulder blades is a common complaint among thin, tense, active women and seems to be related to taut trapezius muscles.

PSYCHIATRIC ILLNESS. Low back pain may be encountered in compensation hysteria and malingering, in anxiety or neurocirculatory asthenia (formerly called neurasthenia), in depression and hypochondriasis, and in many nervous individuals whose symptoms and complaints do not fall within any category of psychiatric illness.

Again it is probably correct to assume that pain in the back in such patients usually signifies disease of the spine and adjacent structures, and this should always be carefully looked for. However, the pain may be exaggerated, prolonged, or woven into a pattern of invalidism or disability because of coexistent or secondary psychologic factors. This is especially true when there is the possibility of personal gain (notably compensation). The patients seeking compensation for protracted low back pain without obvious structural disease tend, after a time, to become suspicious, hostile toward the medical profession or anyone who might question the authenticity of their illness, and uncooperative. One notes in them a tendency to describe their pain poorly and to prefer, instead, to discuss the degree of their disability and their mistreatment in the hands of the medical profession. These features and a negative examination of the back should lead one to suspect a psychologic factor. A few patients, usually frank malingerers, adopt the most bizarre attitudes, such as being unable to straighten up or walking with the trunk flexed at almost a right angle (camptocormia) (see Chap. 370).

The depressed and hypochondriac patient represents a troublesome problem, and a common error is to minimize the importance of anxiety and depression or to ascribe them to worry over the illness and its social effects. The more common and minor back ailments, e.g., those due to osteoarthritis and postural ache, are enhanced and rendered intolerable by the irritable moodiness and self-concern. Such patients are often subjected to surgical procedures, which prove ineffective. The disability seems excessive for the degree of spinal malfunction, and misery and despair are the prevailing features of the syndrome. One of the most reliable diagnostic measures is the response to drugs which alleviate the depression (see Chap. 371).

PAIN IN THE NECK AND SHOULDER

This topic has been discussed to some extent in the chapter on thoracic pain, and further references will be found under Pain in the Extremities.

It is useful to distinguish here three major categories of painful disease—those of the spine, cervical plexus, and shoulder. Although the pains in these three regions of the body may overlap, the patient himself usually can indicate the site of the origin. Pain arising from the cervical spine is nearly always felt in the spine (though it may be projected to the shoulder and arm), is evoked or enhanced by certain movements or positions of the neck, and is accompanied by tenderness and limitations of motions of the neck. Similarly, pain of brachial plexus origin is experienced in and around the shoulder or between the shoulders, is induced by the performance of certain tasks with the arm and by certain positions, and is associated with tenderness of structures above the clavicle. There may be a palpable abnormality above the clavicle (aneurysms of subclavian artery, tumor, cervical rib). The combination of circulatory symptoms and signs referable to the lower part of the brachial plexus, manifested in the hand by obliteration of pulse when the patient takes and holds a full breath with the head tilted back or turned (Adson's test), unilateral Raynaud's phenomenon, trophic changes in the fingers, and sensory loss over the ulnar side of the hand with or without interosseous atrophy, complete the clinical picture. X-rays showing a cervical rib or deformed thoracic outlet or superior sulcus tumor of the lung (Pancoast syndrome) offer confirmation of the diagnosis. Pain, localized to the shoulder region, influenced by motion, and associated with tenderness and limitation of motions (extension, abduction, external and internal rotation), points to tendinitis with calcium deposition of the rotator cuff of muscles surrounding the shoulder joint. Often the term *bursitis* has been used loosely to designate this tendinitis, capsulitis, or muscular tear. Spine, plexus, and shoulder pain all may radiate into the arm or hand, but sensory, motor, and reflex changes always indicate involvement of nerve roots (in disease of the spine), plexus, or nerves.

Osteoarthritis of the cervical spine may cause pains which radiate into the back of the head, shoulders, and arms on one or both sides of the thorax. Coincident involvement of nerve roots is manifested by paresthesias, sensory loss, weakness, or tendon reflex change. Should bony ridges form in the spinal canal (spondylosis), the spinal cord may be compressed, with resulting weakness and atrophy and sometimes sensory disturbances in the arms and spastic weakness and ataxia with loss of vibratory and position sense in the legs. A Pantopaque cervical myelogram reveals the degree of encroachment on the spinal canal and the level at which the spinal cord is affected. The authors have experienced the greatest difficulty in distinguishing spondylosis with or without disc rupture and spinal cord compression from primary neurologic diseases (syringomyelia, amyotrophic lateral sclerosis, or tumor) with an unrelated osteoarthritis of the cervical spine, particularly at the fifth to sixth and sixth to seventh cervical vertebras, where the disc spaces are often narrowed in the adult. A combination of nervous tension with osteoarthritis of the cervical spine or a painful injury to ligaments and muscles after an accident in which the neck is forcibly extended and flexed (e.g., whiplash injury to spine) are extremely vexatious clinical syndromes. If the pain is persistent and limited to the neck, the problem will sometimes prove to have been due to disruption of a disc, but it is often complicated by psychologic factors.

One of the commonest causes of neck, shoulder, and arm pain is disc herniation in the lower cervical region. As with rupture of the lumbar discs, the syndrome includes the aforementioned disorder of spinal function and evidence of neural involvement. It develops after a trauma which may be major or minor (sudden hyperextension of the neck, diving, forceful manipulations, chiropractic treatment, etc.). Virtually every patient exhibits an abnormality in full motion of the neck (limitation and pain). Hyperextension is the movement that most consistently aggravates the pain. With laterally situated disc lesions between the fifth to sixth cervical vertebras, the symptoms and signs are referred to the sixth cervical roots, i.e., pain felt at the trapezius ridge,

tip of the shoulder, anterior upper arm, radial forearm, and often in the thumb; paresthesias and sensory impairment or hypersensitivity in the same regions; tenderness in the area above the spine of the scapula and in the supraclavicular and biceps regions; weakness in flexion of the forearm; diminished to absent biceps and supinator reflexes (triceps retained or exaggerated). With sixth to seventh cervical disc disease and involvement of the seventh cervical root, the pain is in the region of the shoulder blade, pectoral region and medial axilla, posterolateral upper arm, dorsal forearm and elbow, index and middle fingers, or all the fingers; tenderness is most pronounced over the medial aspect of the shoulder blade opposite the third to fourth thoracic spinous processes, in the supraclavicular area and triceps region; paresthesias and sensory loss are most pronounced in the second and third fingers or tips of all the fingers; weakness is in extension of the forearm (occasionally wristdrop is present) and in the hand grip; the triceps reflex is diminished to absent, and the biceps and supinator reflexes are preserved. Cough, sneeze, and downward pressure on the head in the hyperextension position exacerbate pain, and traction (even manual) tends to relieve it.

Unlike lumbar discs, the cervical ones, if large and centrally situated, may result in compression of the spinal cord (central disc, all of the cord; paracentral disc, part of the cord, i.e., Brown-Sequard syndrome). The central disc is often nearly painless, and the cord syndrome may simulate a degenerative disease (amyotrophic lateral sclerosis, combined system disease). A common error is to fail to think of a ruptured disc in the cervical region in patients with obscure symptoms in the legs. The diagnosis of ruptured cervical disc should be confirmed by the same laboratory procedures that were mentioned under lumbar disc.

Metastases in the cervical spine may be very painful, but the problem is not different from that of secondary deposits of tumor in other parts of the spine.

Shoulder injuries (rotator cuff), subacromial or subdeltoid bursitis, the frozen shoulder (periarthritis or capsulitis), tendinitis, and arthritis may develop in patients who are otherwise well, but these conditions are also frequent in hemiplegics or in individuals suffering from coronary heart disease. The pain is often severe and extends toward the neck and down the arm into the hand. The dorsum of the latter may tingle without other signs of nerve involvement. Vasomotor changes also may occur in the hand (shoulder-hand syndrome), and after a time, osteoporosis and atrophy of cutaneous and subcutaneous structures occur (Sudeck's atrophy or Sudeck-Leriche syndrome). These conditions fall more within the province of orthopedics than of medicine and will not be discussed in detail. The physician, however, must know that they can be prevented by proper exercises.

The carpal tunnel syndrome, with paresthesias and numbness in palmar distribution of the median nerve and aching pain which extends up into the forearm, may be mistaken for disease of the shoulder or neck.

MANAGEMENT OF BACK PAIN

A muscular strain is always benign in character, and one may expect full recovery in 2 to 4 weeks. Ligamentous strains, if severe, may last longer, from 6 to 12 weeks. The underlying principle of therapy in both is immobilization in a recumbent position that relaxes and removes pressure from the injured structure. Usually lying on the side with knees and hips flexed is the favored position. If the erector spinae are strained, the optimal position is hyperextension; the same is true of strains of the posterior and sacroiliac ligaments. This position is best maintained by having the patient lie with a small pillow or blanket under the lumbar spine or lie face down. During the acute phase of any injury of this type, application of cold, in the form of an ice bag or cold water bottle (ethyl chloride spray of the skin is said to give dramatic relief at times), is indicated. It reduces the circulation and consequently the swelling. After the third or fourth day, heat is desirable to improve the circulation and to relax protective muscle spasm. Analgesic medication should be given liberally during the first few days [codeine, 30 mg and aspirin, 0.6 Gm, meperidine (Demerol) 50 mg, or morphine 10 to 15 mg]. When ready for ambulation, after some days in bed, the patient may need protection of the injured part, preferably adhesive strapping, in cases of muscle strain, or a belt or brace. Plaster casts should be avoided. Ambulatory treatment is supplemented by corrective exercises designed to strengthen trunk muscles, especially the abdominal, overcome faulty position, and to increase the mobility of the spinal joints. Only if these measures prove inadequate and the patient is partially disabled over long periods of time by an unstable, painful lower back (recurrent lumbosacral backache) should operative intervention be considered.

In the treatment of an acute rupture of a lumbar or cervical disc, complete bed rest is essential and strong analgesic medication is required. Traction is of little value in lumbar disc disease, and it is best to permit the patient to find the most comfortable position. Later, traction, if of any value, keeps the patient confined to bed. In contrast, traction is of great help in rupture of cervical discs. Often the pain subsides after 2 to 3 weeks in bed, and the patient may remain free of pain upon resuming normal activities. He may suffer some minor recurrence of the pain but be able to carry on his usual activities, and eventually he will recover. There is always danger of relapse. To prevent this, mild muscle-strengthening exercises of the spine after the pain has subsided (see Fig. 13-2) and avoidance of activities which favor spine injury (see Fig. 13-3) are recommended. If the pain does not subside after a trial of prolonged bed rest (several weeks) and the myelogram demonstrates a large disc, an operative removal, preferably without spine fusion, should be undertaken. The final decision as to the time and necessity of surgery depends on the duration and gravity of the pain and the neurologic disorder.

For the many patients with back pain who do not fall

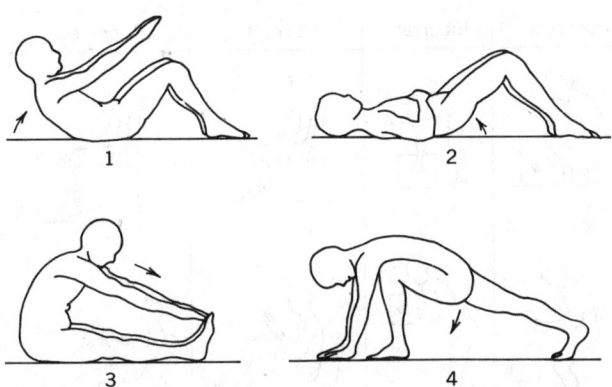

Fig. 13-2. Front of postural instruction sheet. Patient is instructed as follows:

Exercises should be taken on a padded floor. Exercise 3 should be omitted unless otherwise instructed. Start exercises by doing each one ———— times morning and evening, increasing the series one a day until you are doing each one ———— times morning and evening. Exercises are essential in obtaining a proper muscular balance, but a correct posture is acquired only through conscious effort.

Remember—
1. When standing or walking, toe straight ahead and take most of your weight on heels.
2. Try to form a crease across the upper abdomen by holding the chest up and forward and elevating the front of the pelvis.
3. Avoid high heels as much as possible.
4. Sit with the buttocks "tucked under" so that the hollow in the low back is eradicated.
5. When possible, elevate the knees higher than the hips while sitting. This is especially important when driving (driver's seat forward) or riding as a passenger in an automobile.
6. Sleep on your back with knees propped up or on your side with one or both knees drawn up. Bed should be firm.
7. Do not lift loads in front of you above the waist line.
8. Never bend backward.
9. Do not bend forward with knees straight. Always "squat."
10. Avoid standing as much as possible.
Learn to Live 24 Hours a Day without a Hollow in the Lower Part of Your Back

into any one of the above categories, simple measures are beneficial. For the adolescent with a suspicion of epiphyseal disease, restricted activity (avoidance of vigorous sports) for a few months or years and a supporting garment help. Muscle-strengthening exercises and a physical conditioning program are indicated for postural backache (see Fig. 13-2). Spine fusion should be reserved only for the exceptional patient with disabling and persistent pains.

Spondylosis of the cervical spine, if painful, is helped by bed rest and traction; if signs of spinal cord involvement are present, a collar to limit movement may halt the progression and even lead to improvement. Decompressive laminectomy with sectioning of denticulate ligaments is reserved for severe instances of the disease with advancing neurologic symptoms. The shoulder-hand syndrome may benefit from stellate ganglion blocks or ganglionectomy, but the basic treatment is physiotherapy,

| Correct | Incorrect | Correct | Incorrect |

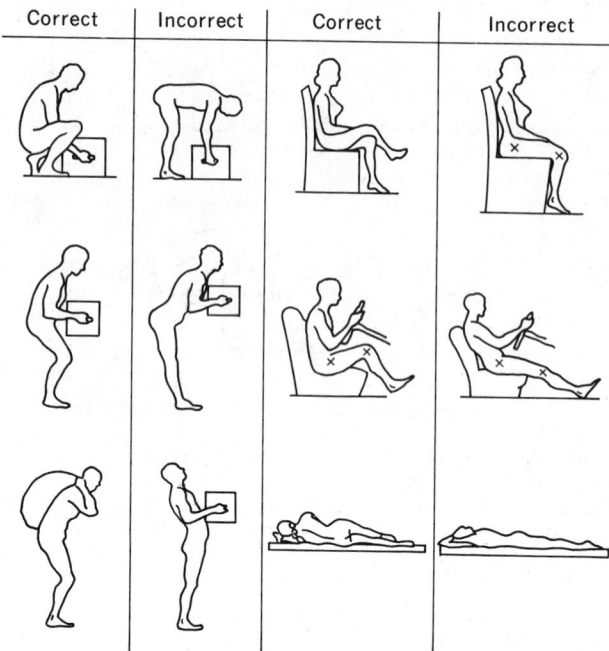

Fig. 13-3. Reverse side of postural instruction sheet showing correct and incorrect methods of lifting, sitting, and sleeping.

with surgical procedures being used only as measures of last resort.

14 PAIN IN THE EXTREMITIES
Eugene A. Stead, Jr.

Pain in the extremities comes from disturbances within the tissues of the extremities or from irritation at any level of the sensory nerve paths serving the extremity, or it is referred from deep somatic or visceral structures.

DISTURBANCES WITHIN THE TISSUES

Any lesion causing inflammation, swelling, ischemia, or destruction of pain-sensitive tissues of the extremity may cause pain. Burns, frostbite, and chemical injuries are painful. Arthritis, cellulitis, abscesses, osteomyelitis and hematomas, tumors, Paget's disease, and bone changes with hyperparathyroidism cause varying degrees of pain. Degeneration of nerves and trauma to nerve trunks are painful. Damage to nerves or to muscles from ischemia is painful.

IRRITATION OF SENSORY NERVES

Involvement of the nerves at any point in their course from the extremity to the spinal cord may cause pain in the extremity. The pain of cervical rib, ruptured intervertebral disk, spinal cord tumor, and tabes dorsalis falls into this group. Central pain from involvement of the spinothalamic tract and thalamus is occasionally seen (see Chap. 9).

PAIN REFERRED FROM DEEP STRUCTURES

The pain of angina pectoris and myocardial infarction frequently radiates to the inner surfaces of the arms. Pain from the hip may be referred to the knee. Pain from the deep muscles of the back or from the vertebras may be the source of pain referred to the extremity.

CAUSES OF PAIN IN THE EXTREMITIES

PAIN FROM TRAUMA, INFLAMMATION, AND SWELLING.
The immediate response to trauma is due to mechanical stimulation of nerve endings. Pain persisting after the injury may result from chemical stimuli produced by the injured tissues. Lewis has described the reactions in skin made hyperalgesic by injury. Needle pricks too light to awaken pain in uninjured skin will arouse a response in a traumatized area. Pain is easily induced by friction or warming, and often by cooling. Distension of the skin by direct stretching or by venous congestion causes pain. If injured skin is rubbed, pain is felt immediately; this subsides and is followed in about 15 sec by a second pain which lasts a minute or more. If the circulation to the part is obstructed, the initial pain is unaltered, but the second pain rises to a greater intensity and persists until approximately 1 min after the circulation is restored. The first pain comes from direct stimulation of sensory nerves, the second from a relatively stable pain-giving substance released into, and held within, the tissue space. The chemical nature of this substance is not known. Skin made hyperalgesic by injury, regardless of the mechanism of the injury, will respond to heat and congestion with burning pain. If this reaction occurs diffusely in the skin of the extremities without obvious cause, the burning pain from warmth and congestion is called *erythromelalgia*.

The injury to the skin caused by heat is well recognized. That prolonged cold will cause tissue damage in many ways comparable to burns is less commonly realized. Prolonged immersion of the feet or prolonged exposure to cold with the feet in wet boots will cause severe tissue damage to the point of gangrene, even though actual freezing does not occur. Freezing, of course, causes tissue damage and may produce gangrene. Fibrosis and ischemic neuritis are common after any form of injury from cold and may cause persistent tenderness and pain.

In bacterial infections, the mechanical factor of rapidly forming edema increases local tissue pressure and causes pain in skin already made hyperalgesic by chemical factors associated with injury. Congestion aggravates the pain, and elevation of the part alleviates it. Less rapid edema formation usually does not cause pain, because the tissues stretch gradually. Patients with cardiac edema complain of heaviness of the legs and occasionally of diffuse tenderness. Edema associated with varicose veins may cause a sense of fullness and dull ache. In acute thrombophlebitis, pain may arise from the involved veins.

It may be aggravated by ischemia secondary to sympathetic vasoconstriction resulting from the sensory stimuli from the inflamed veins. Tumor masses may cause pressure on bone or peripheral nerves.

Arthritis is a common cause of pain in the extremities. When the process is *acute,* as in pyogenic arthritis, gout, and many cases of rheumatic fever, pain is likely to be severe at rest and intensified by the slightest movement. The other signs of inflammation—swelling, redness, and warmth—are pronounced.

In chronic arthritis of the degenerative type, which is especially common in the knees (Chap. 387), pain is usually present only on motion, although there may be minimal discomfort at rest because of local spasm of muscles. Heat and redness are lacking, and swelling may be present or absent. In elderly women with arthritis of the distal interphalangeal joints (Heberden's nodes), pain may be lacking despite striking deformity.

Rheumatoid arthritis (Chap. 386), which is often most pronounced in the hands, is characterized by marked fluctuations in the intensity of the inflammation, and hence of the pain. Prolonged periods of freedom from symptoms other than slight stiffness in the morning and minimal swelling alternate with exacerbations of mild to severe aching, associated with swelling and heat and lasting a few hours to many weeks.

Pain arising in the bones of the extremities is likely to be severe, throbbing, worse at night, and associated with pronounced localized tenderness. Trauma, osteomyelitis, neoplasms, metabolic diseases of bone (Chap. 381), and pulmonary osteoarthropathy are the most important causes.

The syndrome of sore, painful shoulder with superficial and deep areas of exquisite tenderness is common. It frequently begin as wryneck and at times occurs in a number of persons closely associated with one another. Marked spasm prevents abduction of the arm at the shoulder. The entire upper extremity may feel numb and queer. There is no fever. Biopsy of the skin and muscles shows apparently normal tissues. Light freezing of the skin with ethyl chloride or procainization of the superficial and deep tender areas frequently gives dramatic relief of pain, relief which may be permanent. The mechanism of pain production in this syndrome is not known.

PAIN FROM ISCHEMIA, THROMBOSIS, EMBOLISM, AND ARTERITIS. Interference with blood supply may result from obliterative arterial disease or embolus or from arteriolar spasm secondary to stimulation of sensory receptors or nerves. It may be aggravated in polycythemia by the adverse effect of increased viscosity of the blood. The pain may be produced by the action on sensory nerve endings of metabolites accumulating in the muscles or by changes in the nerves themselves.

The sensations produced by ischemia to the extremity are familiar to all. When the blood supply is occluded, the part gradually becomes numb and paralyzed and we say the part has "gone to sleep." If the part is not moved, pain does not develop. The sensation at the end of the fingers becomes dulled in about 12 to 15 min. At that time, light pressure on the fingers may hurt, and stroking the finger tips causes an unpleasant sensation. Later, pain is dulled, and much later, analgesia develops. On release of the arterial occlusion, unpleasant tingling occurs, particularly in the fingers. This tingling is not the result of the inrush of blood into the fingers, because it occurs if blood is released only into the proximal part of the extremity. It results from changes in the main nerves of the arm during recovery. Stroking the fingers accentuates it. The paresthesias produced by the injury and recovery of the nerve from ischemia are similar to·those produced by chronic disease processes involving the peripheral nerves or nerve roots.

If the extremity is exercised while the circulation is completely occluded, a continuous diffuse aching pain develops in the muscles because the sensory nerves are stimulated by the formation of stable metabolites. The pain is present during and between contractions. It is frequently described as a cramp, but the muscles are flaccid. If the contractions are continued, the muscles become tender. On release of the tourniquet, the pain disappears in a few seconds, probably as the result of the carrying away of readily diffusible metabolites.

If the brachial artery at the elbow or the femoral artery at the inguinal ligament is occluded by digital pressure for ½ hr, instead of by application of a cuff, much less change in the circulation occurs, because collateral circulation is not stopped. Loss of sensation does not occur, and on release of the occlusion, the reactive hyperemia is much less intense than with the cuff.

In occlusive vascular disease of the vessels of the legs, a common symptom is pain with tenderness of the muscles which is relieved by rest. It is called *intermittent claudication,* and it represents in the muscles of the extremities the same changes which occur in the heart with angina pectoris. The resting muscle is receiving an adequate supply of blood for normal metabolism. When muscle metabolism is increased by exercise and occlusive vascular disease prevents increase of the blood supply, metabolites accumulate in the muscles and stimulate the sensory nerve endings. The nature of the chemical substances has not been determined. The more severe the circulatory impairment, the less exercise is required to produce the pain and the more slowly the pain disappears on rest.

In occlusive vascular disease, the nerves themselves may become ischemic and cause severe and persistent pain. This pain, in certain instances, is aggravated by dependency because of stimuli resulting from congestion. In addition to Buerger's disease and arteriosclerosis, ischemic neuritis is a prominent symptom in small-vessel involvement of the type seen in periarteritis nodosa.

Embolus or thrombus in the brachial or femoral vessels frequently produces sufficient circulatory impairment to cause pain. The pain in thrombosis is indistinguishable from the pain of embolism. The pains do not occur at the site of occlusion but in the muscles and tissues distal to it. The time of onset of the pain will depend on the temperature of the part, the amount of activity, and the amount of associated vasospasm. If the part is warm and still, the limb may become numb before the muscle pain is produced. Heat applied to a limb with poor circulation may cause gangrene from (1) increased metabolism of tissue without corresponding increase in blood supply or (2) lack of cooling effect of the blood. When heat above body temperature is applied to the skin, the blood normally acts as a cooling system; in the presence of arterial occlusion, local heating causes an immediate rise in temperature of the part. If the part is exercised, the muscle pain occurs early. Twenty-four hours after an embolus has lodged, the vessel wall may be tender because of periarterial inflammation. Occlusion of small blood vessels does not cause pain unless ischemia of muscle or nerve is produced.

Normal skin hurts when warmed after severe exposure to cold. This is a response to direct injury from the cold. The white, cold fingers in Raynaud's phenomenon may be painful. In scleroderma the thickening of the connective tissue combined with spasm of the digital arteries may result in painful ulceration of the fingers and eventual loss of the terminal phalanges.

The pain from ischemia or infection is frequently altered or absent in patients with diabetes because of associated peripheral neuropathy. Whenever a painful-looking lesion of the extremity is treated casually by the patient, neuropathy should be suspected. Tabes dorsalis, leprosy, senile cortical atrophy, and syringomyelia should be considered.

The circulation to the extremities can be greatly modified by overactivity of the sympathetic nervous system. In many instances of injury, inflammation, or thrombophlebitis, sensory stimuli arising in the extremity may produce intense reflex vasoconstriction, and the resulting ischemia may cause diffuse pain. Relief of the vasoconstriction by paravertebral procaine block of the appropriate sympathetic ganglions may cause striking relief of pain. Similarly, sensory impulses arising from ischemic areas after arterial occlusion by an embolus or thrombus may stimulate sympathetic nervous system activity and reflex spasm. Paravetrebral block will relieve the spasm of collateral vessels, and if circulation improves sufficiently, pain will disappear.

PAIN FROM NEUROPATHY, NEURITIS, GANGLIONITIS, AND PRESSURE ON NERVES OR NERVE ROOTS. Involvement of the peripheral nerves frequently causes unpleasant sensations in the extremities. In diabetic neuropathy, numbness may be accompanied by diffuse pains through both lower extremities. Any combination of sensory loss and pain may occur in peripheral nerve damage from infection, poisons, or mechanical factors such as trauma or pressure. Spinal cord tumors and slipped intervertebral disks are common causes of nerve root pain. Inflammation of the dorsal root ganglions results in the syndrome of herpes zoster. The redness and blistering is attributed to antidromic vasodilatation from stimulation of the sensory nerves. Impulses arising in sensory nerves or ganglions and passing peripherally to the sensory end organs are called *antidromic*. Involvement of the dorsal root ganglions, dorsal roots, and adjacent spinal cord produces the lightning pains in the extremities typical of tabes dorsalis. Paralysis from pressure in the axilla may be caused by crutches or by sleeping with the arm thrown over the back of a chair. The latter usually occurs in alcoholic stupor and is called "Saturday night paralysis."

PAIN FROM IMMOBILIZATION, SPASM, AND CRAMPS. Prolonged immobilization of a part results in stiffness of muscles and joints. The muscles tighten and splint the joint, and motion is prevented. An attempt to move the part produces pain. Local infiltration with procaine will frequently allow a great improvement in motility, which may be permanent. Similar spasm occurs after trauma. A painful sprain of the ankle which prevents walking may be relieved in a few minutes by procainization. Even in acute arthritis part of the pain may be secondary to spasm and may respond to curare or procaine, which relax the muscle. In acute poliomyelitis, nonparalyzed muscles may be sore and contracted. Application of hot packs gives relief.

Muscles placed in unusual positions may go into intense contraction and cause severe pain. Cramps in the foot or leg occurring at night are common. They are relieved by forcefully extending the joint so as to stretch the cramped muscles. In nocturnal cramps, pain occurs so quickly that simple ischemia would seem unlikely. They differ from the cramps of arterial disease in that the pain is not brought on by exercise. Painful muscle cramps occur in tetany and in chloride deficiency. Whether the pain of tetany is caused by ischemia from the prolonged contraction or related to damage because of the intensity of the contraction is not known.

Unaccustomed, strenuous exercise causes aching, tender muscles, tendons, and joints. The pain results from low-grade injury to the muscles from repetitive maximal contractions.

GLOMUS TUMOR. Tumor of the glomus, the specialized arteriovenous anastomosis of the skin, produces unusual vasomotor phenomena and radiating pain. It is characteristically a small (a few millimeters in diameter), extremely painful, purplish nodule either in the skin of the extremity or under the nail. Pain is caused by contact or change of temperature and may spread to involve the entire extremity. Why these tumors are so painful is not clear. While most observers have noted an unusually rich nerve supply, others have not found it.

PAIN FROM CAUSALGIA. Pain in the extremity associated with signs of local circulatory dysfunction is seen in nerve injuries after amputations and in persons with coronary arterial disease with or without myocardial infarction. It occurs in the hand-shoulder syndrome. The above conditions have one thing in common: local injury sets up a reaction which at first appears to be the result of sensory stimuli from the injured part. Later changes occur in the peripheral nerves, spinal cord, or central nervous system so that the process continues after the injury has apparently healed.

Classic Causalgia. Injury to any nerve, more commonly the medial or sciatic nerve, may give rise after a few days or weeks to a burning pain. The gross injury to the nerve may have been severe or trivial. The pain will be caused by light friction; deep pressure is less painful.

Heat usually provokes the pain. The skin becomes smooth and glossy and is frequently wet with sweat. It has a red or purplish tint. The temperature of the involved part is usually said to be increased. The pain is frequently relieved by sympathectomy. Causalgic pain may result from the activation of sensory fibers by sympathetic impulses. If injury links the two systems so that leakage of efferent sympathetic impulses into the sensory nerves can occur, most of the clinical phenomena of causalgia, including the relief by sympathetic block, can be explained.

The initiating mechanisms of causalgia are unknown. Several theories have been advanced: (1) The sensitivity of the skin may result from vasodilator substances released by repeated centrifugal impulses arising in the injured area. It is known that stimulation of the paralyzed end of a cut cutaneous nerve results in vasodilatation which may be accompanied by itching and burning pain. (2) The sensitivity of the skin may result from a lack of inhibition of pain and thermal neurones due to loss of large sensory fibers (see Chaps. 9 and 25).

Regardless of the local mechanism, it appears that other mechanisms central to the extremity are capable of continuing the process once the causalgia has been present for some time. At this stage, dorsal root section or sections of the spinothalamic tract may not modify the pain. Chain reactions within the short interconnecting nerves in the spinal cord have been postulated. Paravertebral block or sympathectomy should be done early before these central changes occur and before the patient becomes a drug addict. Because the patient's complaints are so bizarre and because the original injury may be mild, causalgia is frequently mistaken for a compensation neurosis.

Phantom Limb Pain. After amputation of a limb, the patient may complain of pain which he localizes in the removed part. At times this may be caused by a neuroma of the cut nerves or by the faulty construction of the stump. The stump may show vasomotor changes. In most instances, therapy directed toward the stump does not relieve the pain; at times, paravertebral block of the sympathetic ganglions does. The clinical observations suggest that, as in causalgia, pain may begin locally but that changes may take place in the central nervous system which are responsible for its continuation.

Hand-Shoulder Syndrome. Myocardial infarction is frequently complicated by persistent shoulder pain with marked limitation of motion. At times, swelling of the hand and wrist and contraction of the palmar fascia are present. The elbow is not involved. Atrophy of skin and osteoporosis may follow. Similar disturbances in shoulder and hand function have occurred in association with trauma, hemiplegia, herpes zoster, and cervical osteo-arthritis. This syndrome may occur without recognized associated diseases. The exact mechanism of this fairly common syndrome is unknown.

APPROACH TO THE PATIENT

A careful history will usually yield important clues. The pain may be felt in the region of the knee when the disease is in the hip or in the foot when the knee is the seat of the disorder. Pain on first arising in the morning, particularly when associated with stiffness, suggests a disturbance of joints or muscles. When the bone is affected, there is commonly nocturnal aggravation. Pain of throbbing character usually arises in tense tissues with free blood supply, and hence suggests bone as the source. Sharp shooting pain of brief duration, brought on by coughing or sneezing, is common with disorders of the vertebral column or of the posterior nerve roots. Relief of discomfort by elevation suggests venous obstruction; relief by dependency suggests an arterial lesion. Pain ascribed to walking may actually be due to standing and may have its source in the lumbar spine or feet. Pain due to ischemia of muscles is characteristically induced by walking, with latency of onset and of offset. Disorders of joints are likely to be accompanied by pain on local movement, the duration of the discomfort paralleling that of the movement.

The history having suggested the responsible structure, the suspicion is confirmed or disproved by the physical findings and the appropriate special procedures. Since these are mentioned in the later chapters dealing with the disorders of the various systems of the body, they need not be cited here. However, it should be emphasized that x-ray examination, while often invaluable in the case of long-standing disease of the bones, may be entirely negative in the presence of serious skeletal disorders of recent origin. This is especially important in regard to acute osteomyelitis and to the earlier stages of metastatic neoplasms of bone.

REFERENCES

Allen, E. V., N. W. Barker, and E. A. Hines, Jr.: "Peripheral Vascular Diseases," Philadelphia, W. B. Saunders Company, 1946.

Doupe, J. C., C. H. Cullen, and G. Q. Chance: Post-traumatic Pain and the Causalgic Syndrome, J. Neurol., Neurosurg. Psychiat., 7:33, 1944.

Lewis, Thomas: "Pain," New York, The Macmillan Company, 1942.

——: "Vascular Disorders of the Limbs," New York, The Macmillan Company, 1946.

Section 2
Alterations in Body Temperature

15 DISTURBANCES OF HEAT REGULATION

Ivan L. Bennett, Jr. and Robert G. Petersdorf

In health, the body temperature of man is maintained within a narrow range despite extremes in environmental conditions and physical activity. To a lesser but nonetheless remarkable extent, this is true of other mammals as well. An almost invariable accompaniment of systemic illness is a disturbance in temperature regulation, very often an abnormal elevation, or *fever*. In fact, fever is such a sensitive and reliable indicator of the presence of disease that thermometry is probably the commonest clinical procedure in use.

Even in the absence of a frank febrile response, interference with heat regulation by disease is evident. This may take the form of flushing, pallor, sweating, and abnormal sensations of cold or warmth, or it may consist of erratic fluctuations of body temperature within normal limits when a patient is at bed rest.

CONTROL OF BODY TEMPERATURE

The principal source of body heat is the combustion of foods. The greatest amount of heat is generated in the liver and the voluntary muscles. Heat production by muscle is of particular importance because the quantity can be varied according to the need. In most circumstances this variation consists of small increases and decreases in the number of nerve impulses to the muscles, causing unapparent tensing or relaxing. When, however, there is a strong stimulus for heat production, muscle activity may increase to the point of shivering, or even to a generalized rigor.

Heat is lost from the body in several ways. Small amounts are used in warming food or drink and in the evaporation of moisture from the respiratory tract. Most heat is lost from the surface of the body, by *convection* (transfer of heat to a fluid medium, i.e., ambient air), *radiation* (the exchange of electromagnetic energy between the body and the radiant environment) and *evaporation* (passage of water from liquid to gaseous state). Evaporation is particularly important when the ambient temperature exceeds that of the body, when it becomes the major source of heat loss.

The principal method of regulating heat loss is by varying the volume of blood flowing to the surface of the body. A rich circulation in the skin and subcutaneous tissues carries heat to the surface, where it can escape. In addition, sweating increases heat loss by providing water to be vaporized. The sweat, or eccrine, glands are under the control of the sympathetic nerves which in this instance mediate cholinergic stimuli. Heat loss by sweating may be tremendous because as much as 1 liter of sweat per hour may be elaborated.

When the need is for conservation of warmth, adrenergic autonomic stimuli cause a sharp reduction in the blood flow to the surface. This causes vasoconstriction and transforms the skin and subcutaneous tissue into layers of insulation.

The control of body temperature, integrating the various physical and chemical processes for heat production or loss, is a function of cerebral centers located in the hypothalamus. A high decrebrate animal displays a normal temperature if the hypothalamus is left intact. On the other hand, an animal whose brainstem has been sectioned loses ability to control body temperature, which consequently tends to vary with the environment, a condition referred to as *poikilothermia*. Although the centers in the anterior hypothalamus were generally thought to be responsible for heat loss and those in the posterior hypothalamus to control heat conservation, this separation may be an oversimplification. In fact, a new area anterior to the hypothalamus may have important integrating functions in temperature control.

It is probable that the cerebral temperature-regulating centers are affected by more than one kind of stimulus. Experiments on animals show that variation in the temperature of the blood flowing through the brain can cause activation of the appropriate counteracting feedback mechanisms, either for heat loss or for heat production. There is evidence that these centers also may be stimulated by sensory impulses, e.g., the flushing and sweating which may occur after ingestion of highly seasoned food. Furthermore, cutaneous stimuli may exert considerable feedback control on the temperature-regulating mechanisms. Physiologic variations in endocrine function may affect the body temperature; for example, the mean body temperature of women is higher during the second half of the menstrual cycle than it is between the onset of menstruation and the time of ovulation. The sensations of intense heat followed by diaphoresis that characterize the vasomotor instability experienced by some women at the menopause are undoubtedly a result of endocrine imbalance.

A basic problem on which information is needed is why the normal body temperature of warm-blooded animals is in the neighborhood of 98 to 103°F. Animals or human beings whose cervical cords have been severed maintain about the same body temperature, although fluctuations tend to be greater because of lack of neural control. There may be some intrinsic chemical regulating mechanism in the tissues.

Sweating, so important in man, is supplanted by panting and radiation from the body surface in many animals. In the rabbit, for example, the surface of the large ears is of great importance in dissipating heat.

Diseases of many types derange temperature regulation and fever is the result in many animals, but notable exceptions exist. The laboratory mouse responds to most "pyrogenic" stimuli with a profound drop in body temperature, and the rat gives variable responses, sometimes showing an elevation of temperature and sometimes showing a hypothermic response to disease. Furthermore, when mice or rats are maintained at high ambient temperatures, their response to materials known to be pryogenic in man is no longer irregular but is constantly febrile. This is a striking demonstration of the influence of environment and other factors upon the outward expression of the derangement in body temperature control which occurs in disease.

NORMAL BODY TEMPERATURE

It is not practical to designate an exact upper level of normal body temperature because there are small differences among normal persons. There are rare individuals whose temperatures are always elevated slightly above accepted "normal" levels, and there is considerable variation in temperature in a given case. In general, however, it is safe to regard an oral temperature above 98.6°F in a person who has been lying in bed as an indication of disease. An oral temperature above 99.2°F in a person who has been engaged in moderate activity has the same significance. The temperature may be as low as 96.5°F in healthy individuals. Rectal temperature is usually 0.5 to 1.0°F higher than oral temperature. In very hot weather the body temperature may be elevated by 0.5° or perhaps even 1.0°F.

There is a distinct diurnal variation in body temperature in healthy man. Oral readings of 97°F are relatively common on arising in the morning. Body temperature rises steadily through the day, reaches a peak of 99°F or greater between 6 P.M. and 10 P.M., and then drops slowly to reach a minimum at 2 A.M. to 4 A.M. Although it might be postulated that this diurnal variation is dependent upon increasing activity during the day and rest at night, the pattern is not reversed in individuals who work at night and sleep during the day for long periods of time.

The febrile patterns of most human diseases also tend to follow this normal diurnal pattern. Fevers tend to be higher, to "spike," in the evening, and many patients with febrile disease have relatively normal temperatures in the early morning hours.

Severe or prolonged exercise or very hot baths can produce a transient elevation in body temperature, which is quickly compensated for by increased dissipation for the skin and lungs. Such elevations are not properly classified as fevers. Body temperature is somewhat labile in young children, and transient elevations after relatively slight exertion in warm weather are frequently observed in this group.

DISORDERED THERMOREGULATION

All fevers are accompanied by an *increase in heat production,* and abrupt rises after shaking chills may involve as much as a 600 percent increase for a short time. Elevation of body temperature itself increases metabolic activity about 7 percent for each degree Fahrenheit. There is no question, however, about the major importance of *decrease in heat loss* in fevers of any duration. Abrupt rises after severe exertion in healthy individuals are compensated for within a few minutes, but in illness the compensatory mechanism fails and the elevation is sustained. When it is considered that a 10 percent decrease in heat loss will result in a body temperature of 106°F within a few hours, the cardinal role of defective heat loss in fever is more easily appreciated. DuBois has pointed out the existence of a "safety valve" in human adults. When hyperthermia reaches dangerous levels, the mechanisms for heat loss are suddenly activated; consequently, oral temperatures above 106°F are rare in man. While the operation of this cutoff can be spoken of as analogous to the action of a thermostat, there is no evidence to support the existence of any physiologic equivalent of a "thermostat" in the regulation of body temperature; the analogy should not be substituted for a frank admission of ignorance of the basic mechanisms involved.

Deviations of 5°F from the normal body temperature of 98.6°F do not interfere appreciably with most bodily functions. Convulsions are common at temperatures higher than 106°F, and irreversible brain damage, presumably due to protein denaturation (impairment of normal enzymic functions) is common when temperatures of 108°F are reached. Conversely, when temperatures are lowered to 91°F, loss of consciousness occurs, at 86°F poikilothermia sets in, and between 83 and 84°F ventricular fibrillation supervenes.

The systemic symptoms accompanying deviations in temperature are poorly understood. For example at temperatures of 102°F many patients have malaise, drowsiness, weakness, and generalized aches and pains. Many others, however, feel entirely well. Why some individuals are able to tolerate fever so well, while others become markedly ill remains an enigma. Perhaps the inciting stimulus rather than fever per se is the major determinant of systemic complaints.

DISEASES OF THE NERVOUS SYSTEM. Disease of the regulatory centers in the hypothalamus may affect body temperature. Cases have been observed in which there was destruction of the centers controlling heat-conserving mechanisms, with resulting hypothermia. More commonly, cerebral lesions are manifested by hyperthermia; this may occur with tumors, infections, degenerative diseases, or vascular accidents. It is not uncommon in cerebral apoplexy for the temperature to rise to 105 to 107°F during the last few hours before death.

Heat stroke ("sunstroke") is an interesting example of fever due to interference with the controlling mechanism. Here the central mechanisms for cooling seem suddenly to fail and the patient ceases to sweat, despite the fact that his temperature is rising. Some of the highest temperatures ever observed in human beings (112 to 113°F) have been in cases of heat stroke. A temperature higher than 114°F is not compatible with life.

INCREASED HEAT PRODUCTION. Patients with thyrotoxicosis frequently have an elevation in temperature 1 to 2°F above the normal range. This is ascribable to the increased amount of heat produced by an increase in the activity and rate of the metabolic processes. Dinitrophenol, a drug which was formerly used for weight reduction in obese persons, causes elevation of temperature; this too seems to be caused by an increased metabolic activity, produced by some mechanism outside the thyroid.

IMPAIRMENT OF HEAT LOSS. Patients with congestive heart failure often have an elevation of body temperature, between 0.5 and 1.5°F. Perhaps this elevation is caused by impairment of heat dissipation as a result of diminished cardiac output, decline in cutaneous blood flow (with increasing insulation of the central temperature core), the insulating effect of edema, and the increased heat production incident to the muscular activity of dyspnea. On the other hand, patients with congestive heart failure are likely to have other causes of fever, such as venous thrombosis, pulmonary embolism and infarction, myocardial infarction, rheumatic fever, and urinary tract infection. However, since slight fever is so regularly present even in the absence of such complications, the circulatory disturbance may be responsible.

Patients with skin disorders such as ichthyosis or congenital absence of sweat glands may have fever in a warm environment because of inability to lose heat from the surface of the body. Similarly, individuals taking drugs which impair sweating [atropine, propantheline (Pro-Banthine)] may have fever in warm weather.

HYPOTHERMIA. From the clinical standpoint, reduction of body temperature is of far less frequency and importance than is elevation. Daily variation of temperature within the "subnormal" range, i.e., 97 to 98.6°F, is observed in nearly all healthy individuals. The temperature range may be somewhat lower than normal, i.e., 96 to 97.5°F, in patients with myxedema and during the first day or so after critical fall in temperature associated with infectious disease. Oral temperatures below 96°F are rarely encountered, as there is apparently a potent countering mechanism which opposes falls below that level. This barrier may, of course, be broken through exposure to extreme cold. Furthermore, when cerebral function has been impaired, as by alcohol or large doses of sedative drugs, less severe chilling can result in a fall in body temperature. An example of this is the hypothermic temperatures found in vagrants who are found in unheated rooms, railroad yards, and other exposed places after alcoholic debaucheries. The lowered body temperature in shock may be due to impaired cerebral regulation or to inability to produce adequate heat.

One condition in which profound hypothermia may develop is myxedema with coma (Chap. 89). Body temperature in such a patient may gradually sink to 80 to 85°F. Attending personnel may fail to recognize this because the clinical thermometer registers only as low as it has been shaken; hence a series of falsely high readings in the range of 95 to 97°F may be recorded.

REFERENCES

Brengelman, G., and A. C. Brown: Temperature Regulation, pp. 1050–1069 in "Physiology and Biophysics," T. C. Ruch and H. D. Patton (eds.), Philadelphia, W. B. Saunders Company, 1965.

Dubois, E. F.: "Fever and the Regulation of Body Temperature," Springfield, Ill., Charles C Thomas, Publisher, 1948.

Pickering, G. W.: Regulation of Body Temperature in Health and Disease (Lancet), 1:1 and 59, 1958.

16 CHILLS AND FEVER
*Ivan L. Bennett, Jr. and
Robert G. Petersdorf*

In view of the extensive knowledge of physiologic mechanisms controlling body temperature mentioned in the previous chapter, it is surprising that so little is known about the ways in which diseases upset thermoregulation.

Some bacteria, particularly gram-negative species, produce endotoxins which are pyrogenic (Chap. 134, 144), and a few viruses also cause fever when injected into man or animals. Many microorganisms, however, possess no demonstrable pyrogenic toxin, and of course, fever accompanies diseases which do not involve invasion of the body by any known parasite. Omitting disorders which involve cerebral thermoregulatory centers directly, febrile diseases may be grouped as follows: (1) All *infections*, whether caused by bacteria, rickettsias, viruses, or more complex parasites, may cause fever. (2) *Mechanical trauma*, as in crushing injuries, frequently gives rise to fever lasting 1 or 2 days. Not infrequently, however, complicating infection sets in. (3) Most *neoplastic diseases* are associated with fever. In most patients, fever in patients with cancer is related to obstruction or infection produced by the tumor. In some neoplasms, however, particularly cancers of the liver, stomach, and pancreas, fever may be due to the tumor per se, particularly following metastasis to the liver. Hypernephroma can produce hectic fever with daily chills. In lymphosarcoma or Hodgkin's disease, fever may be one of the prominent early manifestations. (4) Many *hematopoietic disorders* are characterized by pyrexia, examples being acute hemolytic episodes and the leukemias. (5) *Vascular accidents* of any magnitude nearly always cause fever, examples being myocardial, pulmonary, and cerebral infarctions. (6) *Diseases due to immune mechanisms* are almost always febrile. These include the collagen diseases, drug fevers, and serum sickness. (7) Certain *acute metabolic disorders,* such as gout, porphyria, and thyroid crisis, sometimes are associated with fever.

PATHOGENESIS OF FEVER

Several hypotheses have been offered to explain disturbed temperature regulation in disease. Some investigators have attributed fever to shifts in body water which interfere with heat production and heat loss. It is true that newborn infants may become febrile when fluid intake is inadequate and that the temperature elevation subsides promptly when fluid is administered. In adults, there are occasional instances of fever associated with extracellular fluid deficit when the ambient temperature is above 90°F. On the other hand, "dehydration" is not ordinarily associated with fever in adults, and the clinical practice of attributing fever to this cause is to be deprecated.

Some have attempted to account for fever on the basis of alterations in endocrine function, with particular reference to the thyroid and adrenals. There is little clinical or experimental evidence to support this idea. Temperature regulation is normal in Addison's disease and in Cushing's syndrome. Body temperature is slightly above normal in thyrotoxicosis and a little low in myxedema, but these differences are entirely in keeping with the metabolic rate and there is no real evidence of impaired thermoregulation in either disease.

There was a renewal of interest in a role of the endocrines in the pathogenesis of fever with the finding that abnormalities of etiocholanolone metabolism exist in some patients with "periodic" fever (Chap. 256). Although administration of progesterone and some of its congeners and of etiocholanolone results in fever in man, there is no evidence that specific steroid fevers (notably etiocholanolone fever) exist.

The common factor in febrile diseases whether or not they are infectious in origin is *tissue injury.* The hypothesis which best fits clinical and experimental observations is that fever results from disturbance of cerebral thermoregulation brought about by a product or products of tissue injury. It has been shown experimentally that inflammatory exudates cause fever when injected intravenously into normal animals, and similar results have been obtained in human subjects. Probably the major source of pyrogenic material is the polymorphonuclear leukocyte, although other cells may also release fever-producing substances.

While considering the pathogenesis of fever, the sequence of events which follows intravenous injection of killed bacteria or of purified bacterial endotoxin is relevant. Figure 16-1 shows a typical human response to injection of typhoid vaccine. Body temperature does not begin to rise until about an hour after injection of the

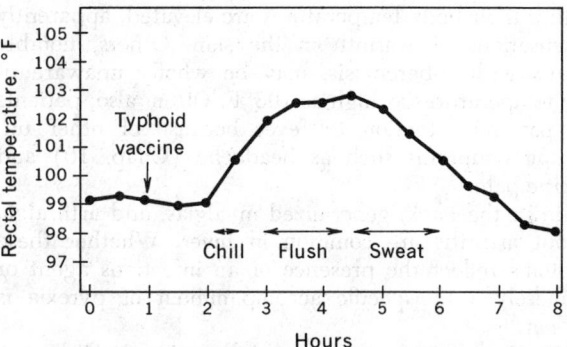

Fig. 16-1. Typical temperature response of a human being to intravenous injection of a comparatively large dose of typhoid vaccine—100,000,000 organisms.

pyrogen. During this interval, the patient notes no discomfort and his appearance is unchanged. Then, rather suddenly, there is malaise, he complains of cold, and within minutes he is burrowing down into the bedclothes, asking for more blankets. He begins to shiver and is soon having a shaking chill which lasts 10 to 20 min. During this time, the skin is pale and cold but rectal temperature rises steeply. After subsidence of the rigor, the patient gradually feels warmer, skin circulation increases, and within 2 hr he is flushed and complains of feeling feverish. After another hour, profuse sweating begins and body temperature begins to return toward normal.

ENDOGENOUS PYROGEN. The pathophysiologic counterpart of these clinical events has been worked out to a large extent in experimental animals. Following its injection, endotoxin is removed rapidly from the bloodstream by the fixed phagocytes of the reticuloendothelial system. At the same time there is, in most species, a profound leukopenia, and these cells are marginated along blood vessel walls. During this period, they appear to be activated to release a fever-producing substance into the circulation. This humoral factor, which has been called *endogenous pyrogen,* is presumably the substance which acts on the thermoregulatory centers to produce fever. Endogenous pyrogen has been found in the bloodstream of animals given endotoxin, antigens (in previously sensitized animals), antigen-antibody complexes, and those with experimental pneumococcal, streptococcal, staphylococcal, and viral infections. Biologically, endogenous pyrogen behaves similarly to sterile inflammatory exudates. It is a low-molecular-weight protein, which is heat-labile and probably basic and may be closely related to lysozomal enzymes. Its biochemical structure has not been worked out, but there is suggestive evidence that it exists in cells in an inactive precursor form. Whether endogenous pyrogen is the sole mediator of fever, or whether some of the agents which incite its release—such as endotoxin—can activate the thermoregulatory centers directly is unknown.

ACCOMPANIMENTS OF FEVER

The perception of fever by patients varies enormously. Some individuals can tell with considerable accuracy whether their body temperatures are elevated, apparently by sensations of warmth in the skin. Others, notably patients with tuberculosis, may be wholly unaware of body temperatures as high as 103°F. Often, also, patients may pay no attention to fever because of other unpleasant symptoms such as headache (Chap. 10) and pleuritic pain.

Pain in the back, generalized myalgias, and arthralgia without arthritis are common in fever. Whether these symptoms reflect the presence of an infectious agent or are merely a nonspecific accompaniment of pyrexia is not clear.

Abrupt onset of fever with a *chill* or *rigor* is characteristic of some diseases and, in the absence of antipyretic drugs, rare in others. Athough repeated rigors suggest pyogenic infection with bacteremia, a similar pattern of fever may occur in noninfectious diseases such as lymphoma and hypernephroma. It is important to differentiate a true chill which is accompanied by teeth chattering or bed shaking from the chilly sensation which occurs in almost all fevers, particularly those in viral infections. In some instances, however, a true rigor occurs in viremia.

Herpes labialis, so-called "fever blister," results from activation of the herpes simplex virus by elevated temperature and occurs frequently in patients undergoing artificial fever therapy. For reasons which are obscure, fever blisters are common in pneumococcal infections, streptococcosis, malaria, meningococcemia, and rickettsioses but are rare in mycoplasma pneumonia, tuberculosis, brucellosis, smallpox, and typhoid.

Delirium can result from elevation of body temperature and is particularly common in patients with alcoholism or cerebral arteriosclerosis.

Convulsions are not infrequent in febrile children, especially those with a family history of epilepsy, although febrile convulsions do not, in general, reflect serious cerebral disease.

CLINICAL IMPORTANCE OF FEVER

The clinical thermometer was one of the first instruments of precision to be introduced into the practice of medicine. Its objectivity and simplicity make it an immensely valuable aid to physical diagnosis. Nowadays we are so accustomed to graphic temperature charts in hospitals and the ready availability of the clinical thermometer for use in the home that we scarcely realize our great dependence upon them. Determination of the body temperature assists in estimating the severity of an illness, its course and duration, and the effect of therapy, or even in deciding whether a person has an organic illness.

A question frequently asked is whether fever is beneficial. There are a few infections of man in which pyrexia appears definitely to be beneficial to the host, examples being neurosyphilis, some gonococcal infections, and chronic brucellosis. Certain other diseases, such as uveitis and rheumatoid arthritis, sometimes improve after fever therapy. In experimental animals some pneumococcal and cryptococcal infections have been influenced in favor of the host animal by raising the body temperature. Aged and debilitated patients with infection may exhibit little or no fever, and this is generally interpreted as a bad prognostic sign. In the great majority of infectious diseases, however, there is no reason to believe that pyrexia accelerates phagocytosis, antibody formation, or other defense mechanisms.

Fever has its detrimental aspects. The greater velocity of all metabolic processes accentuates weight loss and nitrogen wastage. The work and the rate of the heart are increased. Sweating aggravates loss of fluid and salt. There may be discomfort due to headache, photophobia, general malaise, or unpleasant sensation of warmth. The rigors and profuse sweats of hectic fevers are particularly unpleasant for the patient.

In elderly individuals with overt or potential cardiac or cerebral vascular disease, fever may be particularly deleterious.

MANAGEMENT OF FEVER. Since fever ordinarily does little harm and imposes no great discomfort, antipyretic drugs are rarely necessary and may obscure the effect of a specific therapeutic agent and of the natural course of the disease. There are situations, however, in which lowering of the body temperature is of vital importance: heat stroke, postoperative hyperthermia, delirium due to high pyrexia, and shock associated with fever and heart failure. Under these circumstances, sponging the body surface with cool saline or the application of cool compresses to the skin and forehead may be employed. There is no advantage to sponging with alcohol which, because of its pungent odor, makes some patients ill. When high internal temperature is combined with cutaneous vasoconstriction, as in heat stroke or postoperative hyperthermia, the cooling measures should be combined with massage of the skin in order to bring blood to the surface, where it may be cooled. Immediate immersion in a tub of ice water should be considered a lifesaving emergency procedure in patients with heat stroke if the internal body temperature is in excess of 108°F. Cooling blankets which can be set at hypothermic temperatures are a highly effective means for external cooling and have supplanted immersion into ice in most instances.

If antipyretic drugs, such as aspirin (0.3 to 0.6 Gm), are employed to bring about a fall in temperature, the ill effects of the unpleasant diaphoresis, sometimes associated with an alarming fall in blood pressure and the subsequent return of fever, occasionally accompanied by a chill, can be mitigated by enforcing a liberal fluid intake and by administering the drug regularly and frequently at 2- or 3-hr intervals.

The discomfort of a rigor can be alleviated in many patients by the intravenous injection of calcium gluconate. This procedure will stop the shivering and chilliness but has no influence on the ultimate height of the fever. Severe disruptive rigors sometimes need to be abolished with morphine sulfate (10 to 15 mg subcutaneously).

DIAGNOSTIC SIGNIFICANCE OF FEVER

Illnesses of unknown etiology in which fever is a prominent or the only manifestation are frequent. Fever is not an indication of any particular type of disease; it is merely a reaction to injury comparable to alterations in leukocyte count or increased erythrocyte sedimentation rate. In approaching patients with fever, two cardinal diagnostic principles must be kept in mind: (1) Most of the time fever is a manifestation of a common disease, and fever associated with a pulmonary infiltrate is much more likely due to pneumococcal than to pneumocystics pneumonia. (2) The diagnosis of febrile illnesses must occur in the context of the epidemiologic setting. For example, an acute 7-day febrile illness in a soldier in Vietnam is probably due to malaria, scrub typhus, or leptospirosis; in a college student in the United States it may represent infectious mononucleosis or some other viral infection, and in an octogenarian following prostatectomy it is probably an indication of urinary tract infection, wound infection, pulmonary infarction, or aspiration pneumonia. When fever becomes prolonged (2 to 3 weeks) and assumes a central feature in the patient's illness, it is defined as fever of unknown origin, or FUO. The more important probabilities to be considered in dealing with a patient with FUO are discussed below.

FEBRILE ILLNESSES OF SHORT DURATION

Acute febrile illnesses of less than 2 weeks' duration are a common occurrence in medical practice. In many instances they run their courses, progressing to complete recovery, and a precise diagnosis is not made. In most instances, however, it is safe to assume that the illness is of infectious origin. Although short febrile illnesses can be noninfectious, i.e. allergic fevers due to drugs or serums, thromboembolic disease, hemolytic crises, or gout, they are decidedly in the minority.

Most undiagnosed acute febrile infectious diseases are probably viral, since diagnostic methods for bacterial infection are better, and they are rapidly brought under control by the chemotherapeutic agents in common use. It is not practical to carry out tests needed to identify all the known viruses, and furthermore, there must be a considerable number of as yet unidentified viruses pathogenic for man.

The following characteristics, while not restricted solely to acute infections, are highly suggestive that infection is present:

1. Abrupt onset
2. High fever, i.e., 102 to 105°F, with or without chills
3. Respiratory symptoms—sore throat, coryza, cough
4. Severe malaise, with muscle or joint pain, photophobia, pain on movement of the eyes, headache
5. Nausea, vomiting, or diarrhea
6. Acute enlargement of lymph nodes or spleen
7. Meningeal signs, with or without spinal fluid pleocytosis
8. Leukocyte count above 12,000 or below 5,000 per cu mm

None of the symptoms or signs listed is encountered only in infection. Many of these features could be seen in acute myeloblastic leukemia or disseminated lupus erythematosus. Nevertheless, in a given instance of acute febrile illness with some or all of the manifestations listed, the probabilities strongly favor infection, and the patient can be given reasonable reassurance that he will probably recover in a week or two, regardless of a precise diagnosis.

It is desirable of course, to establish an accurate diagnosis, and whatever steps are practicable in the circumstances to establish the cause should be taken. Cultures of the throat, blood, urine, or feces should be obtained *before* institution of antibacterial chemotherapy. Skin and/or serologic tests should be carried out when indicated.

PROLONGED FEBRILE ILLNESSES

Some of the knottiest problems in the field of internal medicine are found in cases of prolonged fever in which the diagnosis remains obscure for weeks or even months. Eventually, however, the true nature of the illness usually reveals itself, since a disease which causes injury sufficient to evoke temperature elevations of 101°F or higher for several weeks does not often subside without leaving some clue as to its nature.

The elucidation of problems of this sort calls for skillful application of all diagnostic methods—careful history, thorough physical examination, and the considered application of good laboratory examinations.

It is obviously not possible or practical in this section to mention all the known entities which may cause prolonged febrile disease, or even to give an adequate discussion of the differential diagnosis of the more frequent ones. Additional details about the manifestations and differential diagnosis of the entities mentioned will be found elsewhere.

INFECTIOUS DISEASES

The infections occupy a less prominent position among the causes of prolonged fever now than formerly, because of the common practice of administering antibiotic drugs to any patient in whom fever persists for more than a few days. Consequently, many infections are at present being eradicated by more or less "blind" therapy, without their nature or location being determined accurately. Nevertheless, patients with infection comprise the greatest percentage in any group of patients with FUO. Furthermore, certain infections do not respond to the usual antibiotic therapy. In general, this does not apply to virus diseases because they tend to run their courses more or less acutely and do not often cause continued illness lasting many weeks or months, irrespective of chemotherapy.

TUBERCULOSIS. (Chap. 174.) This disease proves to be responsible for puzzling febrile disease with surprising frequency, despite the facts that there is a fairly effective therapy and that the simple procedure of chest x-ray is usually sufficient for diagnosis of the commonest clinical form. The drugs given as therapeutic trials may not include those with tuberculostatic activity such as streptomycin or isoniazid. Extrapulmonary forms of tuberculosis may not be easily located, e.g., disease of the bones, deep lymph nodes, genital or urinary organs. Furthermore, the pulmonary lesions of miliary tuberculosis may not be detectable by x-ray until very late in the course of the disease. In considering the possibility of tuberculous infection, the skin test may be of great assistance, since negative reaction to a properly executed skin test rules out the possibility of tuberculosis except in rare instances of overwhelming disease. A positive skin reaction, on the other hand, does not prove that tuberculosis is causing the patient's illness, but in its presence tuberculosis must be kept in mind as a possibility until another cause for the fever is found.

BACTERIAL ENDOCARDITIS. (Chap. 137.) In the classical subacute form of the disease, a heart murmur is nearly always present; therefore, absence of murmur largely eliminated this disease from consideration. The correct diagnosis is likely to be missed in middle-aged or elderly patients, in whom a heart murmur may not be given much weight. For example, an elderly patient with subacute bacterial endocarditis may first present following the occurrence of a cerebral embolus and may be regarded as having had a hemorrhage or thrombosis because of arteriosclerosis. The best clinical practice is to culture the blood of *every* patient who has fever and a heart murmur. Bacterial endocarditis without cardiac murmurs is seen most frequently in intravenous drug users who develop infection on the tricuspid valve, and every such individual who presents with fever should be assumed to have endocarditis until proved otherwise. In addition, antibiotics mask SBE because these drugs often render blood cultures negative until the drugs have been excreted or metabolized. For this reason, patients suspected of having SBE who have received antimicrobials, should have blood cultures taken for several days after administration of the drugs is discontinued.

BRUCELLOSIS. (Chap. 154.) This infection is most unlikely in an American city dweller but has to be considered in farmers, veterinarians, or slaughterhouse workers. Arthralgia and myalgia are common, but actual redness and swelling of joints are rare in this disease. Peripheral leukocytosis is seldom seen in brucellosis. In active febrile disease the blood culture and bone marrow culture frequently are positive, and specific agglutinins are *nearly always* present in the serum.

SALMONELLA INFECTION. (Chaps. 149 and 150.) Although typhoid fever is subject to great variability and may cause fever for several weeks, it should not often be a cause of prolonged fever of obscure origin, since cultures of feces or blood will be positive, and the specific antibodies are detected in the agglutination reaction. Other salmonella organisms may, however, cause prolonged febrile illness, and these may present greater diagnostic difficulty. Routine serologic tests may not be helpful, and antibiotics, including chloramphenicol (Chloromycetin), may not be effective. Repeated culture of the blood or of bone marrow may yield the causative organism. There may eventually be localization of infection in a joint or the pleural cavity from which the etiologic agent can be obtained.

PYOGENIC INFECTION. (Chap. 136.) Chemotherapy often does not succeed in eradicating localized pyogenic infection, and in certain locations inflammation may be relatively asymptomatic. These infections include osteomyelitis of the vertebrae or pelvic bones, subdiaphragmatic, hepatic, perinephric, renal cortical, retropharyngeal, and mediastinal abscesses, cholangitis, bronchiectasis, and pelvic inflammatory disease. The right upper quadrant, pericolonic, periappendiceal, and pelvic regions are particularly prone to sequestration of abscesses. X-ray studies are often helpful, but many times exploratory surgery must be performed to achieve both diagnosis and cure.

AMEBIASIS. (Chap. 240.) Amebic colitis usually evokes symptoms pointing to disease of the colon. Hepatic involvement, on the other hand, may not give a distinctive clinical picture, and prolonged fever may be the principal manifestation. Some assistance may be obtained from a history of dysentery, or from tenderness or enlargement of the liver and elevation of the right leaf of the diaphragm. The complement fixation test has little diagnostic value. Therapeutic trial of an antiamebic drug, such as chloroquine or emetine, which acts on the hepatic form of amebiasis, may be justified.

HISTOPLASMOSIS. (Chap. 188.) This infection is prevalent in the region of the Mississippi Valley of the United States, although in most individuals it is not clinically recognizable. The disease may, however, be manifested as a chronic febrile illness, with localizing manifestations pointing to many organ systems. Fever, leukopenia, anemia, hepatomegaly, and splenomegaly in a person who has resided in a geographic area where histoplasmosis occurs should suggest the possibility. The skin reaction to histoplasmin is often positive but may be negative in disseminated histoplasmosis, which is the form most likely to cause prolonged pyrexia. The complement fixation reaction, on the other hand, is nearly always positive in disseminated disease. The organisms may be demonstrated in biopsy of involved tissue or in bone marrow.

COCCIDIOIDOMYCOSIS. (Chap. 187.) This disease needs to be considered in persons who have traveled through, or resided in, the southwest part of the United States. Clinical manifestations are like those of the various forms of tuberculosis. The coccidioidin skin test and serologic reaction to this antigen are positive.

SCHISTOSOMIASIS. (Chap. 250.) Persons who have lived in the Caribbean islands, in Africa, or in the Far East may have prolonged febrile illness associated with this infestation. Diarrhea, bladder symptoms, cough, hepatosplenomegaly, and anemia are suggestive. Diagnosis is made by finding the ova in feces or urine or in rectal or hepatic biopsy. Salmonella infection, including bacteremia, is common in schistosomiasis and may be responsible for fever.

COLLAGEN DISEASES

Under this term is included a broad spectrum of diseases in which there are histologic evidences of disorders of collagen and the blood vessels. Some of these diseases are particularly important causes of prolonged febrile illness.

DISSEMINATED LUPUS ERYTHEMATOSUS. (Chap. 392.) This disease is by no means rare, being encountered with greater frequency in American hospitals than typhoid fever. The possibility should receive special consideration in a young woman with fever, polyarthritis, low or low-normal leukocyte count, anemia, pulmonary infiltrations or pleural involvement, and hematuria and other evidence of acute nephritis. Behavioral abnormalities, orbital edema, and salivary gland swelling are less common features. The diagnosis can be made with confidence in patients who develop the full clinical picture, or by demonstration of LE cells or a rise in titer of antinuclear factor. The diseases likely to be confused with disseminated lupus erythematosus are rheumatic fever and rheumatoid arthritis.

PERIARTERITIS NODOSA. (Chap. 391.) Features which particularly point to this syndrome are febrile illness in a male of any age, with leukocytosis, eosinophilia, anemia, asthma, peripheral neuritis, arthritis or muscle pain, hypertension, and evidence of renal involvement. Lesions in medium-sized arteries can give rise to the clinical pictures of myocardial infarction, mesenteric embolism, and peripheral vascular disease. There may be a variety of cutaneous eruptions. The only conclusive method of diagnosis is biopsy of a muscle or a skin lesion or of other tissue excised at operation.

RHEUMATOID ARTHRITIS. (Chap. 386.) In its earlier stages there may not be characteristic swelling and deformity of joints but only vague pains in muscles and joints, together with fever, slight anemia, and malaise. Differentiation from rheumatic fever and from disseminated lupus erythematosus may be difficult. Sometimes the diagnosis cannot be made until the more characteristic picture of the disease develops, or the latex test becomes unequivocally positive.

RHEUMATIC FEVER. (Chap. 269.) Fever, with or without muscle and joint pains, may persist for weeks and months at a time. A history of preceding attacks or of an upper respiratory infection before onset of the systemic illness, the presence of a heart murmur, relative tachycardia, and arrythmias or conduction defects are suggestive findings. Significant elevation of the antistreptolysin O titer is present in 80 percent of cases, and other acute phase reactants (antihyaluronidase, antistreptokinase) in the remainder. It may be difficult to differentiate active rheumatic fever with carditis from SLE, rheumatoid disease, bacterial endocarditis, and *atrial myxoma*. This intracardiac tumor may present with fever, arthralgias, peripheral embolic phenomena, and heart murmurs. Cardiac angiography is diagnostic. It is particularly important to consider myxoma in the differential diagnosis because it can be removed completely by open-heart surgical techniques.

HENOCH–SCHÖNLEIN, OR ALLERGIC, PURPURA. (Chap. 245.) There may be fever, joint pains, and evidences of renal and pulmonary involvement. The results of the capillary fragility test and platelet count are normal. Differentiation from lupus erythematosus, rheumatic fever, and acute glomerulonephritis may be difficult. Diagnosis will depend on the finding of hemorrhagic occurrences, usually in the intestinal lumen or in joints.

NEOPLASTIC DISEASES

Fever is a common manifestation of cancer but a very rare accompaniment of benign tumors. In patients in the age range where cancer is common, unexplained fever should always suggest the possibility of neoplasm.

CARCINOMAS AND SARCOMAS. Certain malignant processes seem especially likely to cause fever. Notable are sarcomas involving bone or lymphoid tissue, hypernephroma, carcinoma of the pancreas or stomach, and metastatic cancer of the liver. Occasionally the clinical picture is strongly suggestive of pyogenic infection, with hectic fever, chills, sweats, and marked leukocytosis; and patients have been subjected to laparotomy with preoperative diagnoses such as empyema of the gallbladder, localized peritonitis, or liver abscess.

HODGKIN'S DISEASE. Fever may be the principal symptom and only objective finding early in the course of Hodgkin's disease, especially when the principal involvement is in the abdominal viscera or retroperitoneal regions. Cases with splenomegaly and vague abdominal distress have been confused with typhoid fever. Pel-Ebstein fever is seen in a minority of cases of Hodgkin's disease. The diagnosis of this disorder is made by biopsy.

HEMATOPOIETIC DISEASES

Disorders of blood formation or blood destruction are frequently associated with fever.

LEUKEMIAS. It is not uncommon for acute leukemia to be mistaken for acute infection at the onset. The acute leukemias are nearly always accompanied by fever, sometimes as high as 105°F. The correct diagnosis will be suggested by rapid development of anemia and characteristic changes in peripheral blood and bone marrow. Chronic leukemia, particularly lymphatic, may be characterized by low-grade fever, but because of the typical changes in circulating leukocytes, is not often a diagnostic problem. Both acute and chronic leukemias may be accompanied by infection, which may be responsible for the fever, and before it is assumed that fever in a patient with leukemia is due to the blood dyscrasia, infection must be ruled out by appropriate tests and cultures.

HEMOLYTIC EPISODES. Most of the hemolytic diseases are characterized by bouts of fever. Acute crises of hemolysis may give rise to shaking chills and marked elevations of temperature. The difficulty sometimes encountered in differentiating sickle-cell disease from acute rheumatic fever is well known. The presence of these hemolytic disorders is suggested by the more rapid development of anemia than occurs in other febrile illnesses and by the usual accompaniment of reticulocytosis and jaundice.

Fever is not characteristic of severe anemia due to external blood loss or of the anemia of uremia.

VASCULAR DISEASE

Reference has already been made to the fever of collagen diseases, all of which are accompanied by vascular lesions. In addition, certain other diseases of the blood vessels, not always regarded as being in the same category as the collagen diseases, may cause chronic illness.

TEMPORAL, OR CRANIAL, ARTERITIS. (Chap. 394.) This is a disease of old people, featured by severe aching pain in the temporal area, headache, muscle and joint pains, fever, and leukocytosis. There may be accompanying visual defects or blindness due to involvement of the retinal artery. The temporal or occipital arteries may be inflamed and tender. Diagnosis is not difficult if the superficial arteries are carefully palpated and temporal artery biopsy is performed.

THROMBOEMBOLIC DISEASE. In migratory thrombophlebitis, segments of large veins become inflamed and thrombosed. There is usually local pain and swelling, but sometimes the lesions are cryptic. Symptomless thrombosis of deep calf or pelvic veins may cause prolonged febrile illness as a result of repeated small pulmonary emboli. These emboli may not be manifested by pleuritic pain or hemoptysis, but cough, dyspnea, or vague thoracic discomfort is likely to be present. Careful examination of the legs and repeated examination of the lungs should reveal the diagnosis. Sometimes these patients present with a nephrotic syndrome due to renal vein thrombosis.

MISCELLANEOUS

SARCOIDOSIS. Ordinarily, fever is not characteristic of sarcoidosis, but it is prominent in a minority of cases, especially those characterized by arthralgia, hilar lymphadenopathy, and cutaneous lesions resembling erythema nodosum, or in those with extensive hepatic lesions. Diagnosis is suggested by lymphoid enlargement, ocular lesions, and hyperglobulinemia and is clinched by biopsy of skin, lymph nodes, or liver.

REGIONAL ENTERITIS. Inflammatory lesions of the large and small bowel rarely present as FUO's but an occasional individual who has only fever, abdominal pain, and subtle changes in bowel habits, will be found to have regional enteritis.

DRUG FEVER. (Chap. 73.) This is an important cause of cryptic fever, and a careful history of drug intake should be taken in every patient with unexplained fever. Fever due to allergy to one of the antibiotics may become superimposed on the fever of the infection for which the drug was given, resulting in a very confusing picture. Often fever is due to common drugs including sulfonamides, arsenicals, iodides, thiouracils, barbiturates, and laxatives especially those containing phenolphthalein. Any questions of drug fever can be resolved rapidly by discontinuing all medication. The diagnosis can be further substantiated by giving a test dose of the drug after fever has subsided, but this may result in a very unpleasant or even dangerous reaction.

FAMILIAL MEDITERRANEAN FEVER. (Chap. 256.)

MALINGERING. Rarely, a patient will produce purposeful elevations in temperature. Many methods have been employed to cause the thermometer to register higher than the true temperature. If malingering is suspected, all that is necessary to prove it is to repeat the temperature determination immediately after a high reading has been obtained, with someone remaining at the bedside while the thermometer is in place.

PROLONGED LOW-GRADE TEMPERATURE ELEVATIONS

Not infrequently a patient, while not appearing acutely ill, has been subject to elevation of body temperature above the "normal" level, i.e., his temperature has been in the range of 99.0 to 100.5°F. Prolonged low-grade fever may be a manifestation of serious illness, or it may be a matter of no real consequence. Possibly there are some individuals whose "normal" temperatures are in this range. However, there is no certain way of identifying such individuals. The possibilities to be considered in such cases vary considerably according to the age groups concerned.

In children temperature regulation may be somewhat erratic even up to the age of twelve years. Children may therefore have slight temperature elevations when excited or after exercise. A mother may note that her child's skin feels hot when he has been playing and may find his temperature slightly above normal. Reexamination on subsequent days may reveal the same elevation from time to time. This poses the question whether the "fever" is an indication of disease or of imperfect thermoregulation. If the physical examination reveals no abnormality, if the appetite is good and the child is gaining weight, and if there is no anemia or urinary abnormality, it is fairly safe to advise the parent to cease taking temperatures and forget about "fever." Real harm can be done by restricting the activity of an otherwise healthy child because of misinterpretation of the significance of low-grade fever.

In young adults chronic low-grade temperature elevation cannot easily be imputed to imperfect thermoregulation. Here tuberculosis, brucellosis, rheumatic fever or other collagen disease, as well as many of the conditions mentioned in the preceding section have to be considered. A special problem encountered in females of this age group is *habitual hyperthermia,* and every experienced physician has encountered examples of the syndrome. The patient may have temperatures of 99.0 to 100.5°F regularly or intermittently for years and also usually has a variety of complaints characteristic of psychoneurosis, such as fatigability, insomnia, bowel distress, vague aches, and headache. Prolonged careful study and observation fail to reveal evidence of organic disease. Unfortunately, many of these people go from doctor to doctor and are subjected to a variety of unpleasant, expensive, and even harmful tests, treatments, and operations. The diagnosis of this syndrome can be made with reasonable certainty after a suitable period of observation and study, and if the patient can be convinced of its validity, a real service will have been rendered.

In a patient past middle age even low-grade fever should always be regarded as a probable indication of organic disease. The possibilities to be considered in this age group are the same as those discussed above in the section Prolonged Febrile Illnesses.

RELAPSING AND RECURRENT FEVERS

Occasionally patients are encountered who have recurrent bouts of high fever at more or less regular intervals. The following are among the diseases which have to be considered:

MALARIA. (Chap. 241.) The disease had vanished from the United States almost completely, but Vietnam war veterans constitute an important and sizable reservoir of this infection, as do other persons recently arrived from foreign countries. It is most unusual, however, for malaria to recur after a symptom-free interval of 1 year or more. Seizures recur at 2- or 3-day intervals, or more irregularly in falciparum infections, depending on the maturation cycle of the parasite. Diagnosis depends on demonstration of the parasites in the blood.

RELAPSING FEVER. (Chap. 182.) This disease occurs in the southwest part of the United States, as far east as Texas, and in many other parts of the world. The recurrences are related to some cycle in the development of the parasites. Diagnosis is by demonstration of the spirochetal organisms in stained films of the blood.

RAT-BITE FEVER. (Chaps. 162 and 183.) Two etiologic agents—*Spirillum minus* and *Streptobacillus moniliformis*—can be transmitted by the bite of a rat. Both may cause an illness characterized by periodic exacerbations of fever. The clue as to the diagnosis depends on obtaining a history of rat bite 1 to 10 weeks previous to the onset of symptoms. The cause can be established by appropriate laboratory procedures.

PYOGENIC INFECTION. In rare instances, localized pyogenic infections give rise to periodic bouts of fever separated by afebrile and relatively symptom-free intervals. The so-called "Charcot's intermittent biliary fever," cholangitis with biliary obstruction due to stones, is an example. The febrile attacks are sometimes associated with slight jaundice. There should be a history suggestive of cholelithiasis, and during the attacks tenderness can be elicited in the right upper quadrant. *Urinary tract infection,* with episodes of ureteral obstruction due to small stones or inspissated pus, can also cause recurrent fever.

HODGKIN'S DISEASE. In perhaps 5 to 10 percent of cases, there is seen at some time during the course of the disease the so-called "Pel-Ebstein fever"—bouts of fever lasting 3 to 10 days, separated by afebrile and asymptomatic periods of 3 to 10 days. These cycles may be repeated regularly over a period of several months. In rare instances this periodicity of the fever has been

sufficiently striking to suggest the correct diagnosis before lymphadenopathy or splenomegaly became evident.

DIAGNOSTIC PROCEDURES

When faced with so large a number of possibilities, it is obvious that no single plan can be outlined for the systematic study of every problem in unexplained fever. In any given patient, the history, physical examination, and most importantly, the epidemiologic setting must determine the diagnostic approach. If the features suggest the presence of infectious disease, the main dependence will be upon bacteriologic and immunologic methods, whereas in an obscure febrile disorder in a person in the "cancer age group" the best chance of early diagnosis may lie in x-ray studies and biopsy.

Careful elicitation of the patient's past *history* and the chronologic development of his symptoms may provide important leads. Places of recent residence, contact with domestic or wild animals and birds, preceding acute infectious diseases such as diarrheal illness or boils, contact with persons with tuberculosis, may provide clues to infection. Localizing symptoms may give a clue to an organ system affected by neoplasm or infection.

In the *physical examination,* careful search is made for skin lesions and for petechial hemorrhages in the ocular fundi, conjunctivas, nail beds, and skin. The lymph nodes are carefully palpated, with special attention to the retroclavicular, axillary, and epitochlear areas. The finding of a heart murmur may be important. Detection of an abdominal mass may be the first lead to diagnosis of neoplastic disease. Palpable enlargement of the spleen suggests infection, leukemia, or lymphoma and points away from a diagnosis of cancer. Enlargement of the liver and spleen suggests lymphoma, leukemia, chronic infection, or cirrhosis. A large liver without palpable spleen points to liver abscess or metastatic cancer. The rectum and the female pelvic organs may reveal masses or abscesses and the testicles, teratoma, or tuberculosis. Useful laboratory examinations include cultures of blood, bone marrow, urine, or other body fluids; examination of blood smears for parasites or for evidence of hematologic disorder; tests for hemolysins, LE cells, serologic studies, and antinuclear antibodies. Among x-ray examinations, chest films, which may need to be repeated at intervals, are most useful. Intravenous pyelograms may provide useful clues to disease of kidneys, ureters, or retroperitoneal regions. Lymphangiograms are helpful in the diagnosis of retroperitoneal cancer, abdominal aortograms in renal tumors, abscesses, cysts or pancreatic masses, and cardiac angiograms in atrial myxomas. Gastrointestinal x-rays are of little aid except in regional enteritis. On the other hand, liver scan is the single most useful test in the diagnosis of disease in the right upper quadrant. Lung scans may reveal pulmonary emboli.

Biopsy often is the best means of definitive diagnosis. Bone marrow aspiration may be helpful, not only for the histology of the marrow but also for occasional demonstration of other disease processes such as metastatic carcinoma or granulomas and for culture. Needle biopsy of the liver is a very useful procedure and can be done with reasonable safety. It may be helpful not only with primary or metastatic disease of the liver, but also because the liver may reveal existence of other diseases such as histoplasmosis, schistosomiasis, brucellosis, tuberculosis, sarcoidosis, or lymphoma. Lymph node biopsy is helpful in diagnosis of many diseases, including the lymphomas, metastatic cancer, tuberculosis, and mycotic infections. However, inguinal nodes are notoriously unsatisfactory for biopsy and are too frequently chosen because of their easy accessibility. Axillary, cervical, and supraclavicular nodes are much more likely to yield helpful information, and the node excised need not necessarily be large. Muscle biopsy may be of assistance in the recognition of dermatomyositis, periarteritis nodosa, sarcoidosis, and trichinosis.

Exploratory laparotomy has been advocated as the most definitive diagnostic maneuver in FUO, but is valuable only when other investigations, including history, physical examination, x-rays, and laboratory data, point to the abdomen as a likely source of disease. Blind exploration of the abdomen simply because the diagnosis is obscure is to be deprecated.

THERAPEUTIC TRIALS

It is common practice to give a trial of antibiotic therapy to patients with unidentified febrile disorders. Occasionally this kind of marksmanship is effective, but in general, "blind" therapy does more harm than good.

Undesirable features include drug toxicity, superinfection due to resistant pathogenic bacteria, and interference with accurate diagnosis by cultural methods. Furthermore, a coincidental fall in temperature not due to therapy is likely to be interpreted as response to treatment, with the conclusion that an infectious disease is present. If therapeutic trials are instituted, they should be as specific as possible. Examples are: isoniazid and streptomycin or PAS for tuberculosis; aspirin for rheumatic fever; chloroquine and/or emetine for hepatic amebiasis; penicillin and streptomycin for enterococcal endocarditis, and chloramphenicol for salmonella bacteremia. Shotgun broad-spectrum therapy is contraindicated because it is unlikely to yield useful information and is more likely to be toxic. Similarly, cortisone or ACTH are nonspecific. These drugs have an antipyretic effect and produce euphoria in many individuals, but the apparent improvement induced by these agents tells little about the nature of the underlying disease.

REFERENCES

Atkins, E.: Pathogenesis of Fever, Physiol. Rev., 40:580, 1969.

Geraci, J. E., L. A. Weed, and D. R. Nichols: Fever of Obscure Origin—The Value of Abnormal Exploration in Diagnosis, J.A.M.A., 169:1306, 1959.

Petersdorf, R. G.: The Physiology, Pathogenesis and Diagnosis of Fever, Med. Times, 96:50, 1968.

——, and P. B. Beeson: Fever of Unexplained Origin: Report of 100 Cases, Medicine, 40:1, 1961.

——, and I. L. Bennett, Jr.: Factitious Fever, Ann. Intern. Med., 46:1039, 1957.

Section 3

Alterations in Nervous Function

17 GENERAL CONSIDERATIONS
Raymond D. Adams

The symptoms and signs of nervous disease, which comprise the subject material of this section, are probably the most frequent and the most complex in all of medicine. Naturally, they interest students of neurology and psychiatry, but they are so often found in patients who do not have classifiable diseases of the nervous system that they inevitably become the concern of every physician.

A lucid exposition of the diverse and complex manifestations of nervous disease is difficult, and a certain bias, which will be apparent at once to specialists in this field, is almost unavoidable. The method chosen here is somewhat unconventional and requires a few

words of explanation. The aim has been to bring together all the expressions of disordered nervous function. They are described in some detail, and the most generally accepted explanations from anatomy, biochemistry, physiology, and psychology are offered. No distinction is drawn between relatively simple phenomena, such as motor and sensory paralysis, which are usually based on an easily demonstrated structural change, and the most complex ones, such as anxiety, depression, or paranoia, to which at present no gross or microscopic pathologic changes can be assigned.

An attempt has been made, wherever indicated, to present both the neurologic and the psychologic conceptions of the more complex cerebral phenomena, but the emphasis is on the neurologic because it is more understandable to physicians and surgeons, since the approach is the same as that to all other medical diseases.

NEUROLOGIC (MEDICAL) AND PSYCHOLOGIC CONCEPTIONS OF NERVOUS DISEASE

An understanding of these two conceptions of nervous disease is necessary in order to appreciate current trends in neurology and psychiatry. At the very beginning of this brief exposition of methodology and clinical approach, it should be stated that the terms *neurologic* and *psychologic* do not denote the respective activities of neurologists and psychiatrists. Neurologic means the concepts of medicine applied to the study of nervous disease. They may be and are used by physicians, psychiatrists, and neurologists. Psychologic comprises another set of ideas, largely nonmedical and used by many psychiatrists as well as by neurologists and other physicians. In other words, the conception, the method, or the subject matter does not strictly pertain to any one discipline.

The *neurologic conception* starts with the assumption that all the phenomena of nervous disease are related to a pathologic process within the nervous system. This process may be obvious, like a cerebral infarct or tumor; or it may be impossible to see even with an ordinary light microscope, like the encephalopathy of delirium tremens. In all instances the pathologic process is the result of some physical or chemical change, and the visible lesion may represent only its most advanced and often irreversible stage. The symptoms and clinical signs of nervous disease are the expressions of the activity of the pathologically altered nervous system. These clinical manifestations vary widely and include, on the one hand, the relatively simple, easily elicited, stereotyped objective signs, such as motor paralysis or ataxia, and on the other, the most complex, difficult to evoke, highly individualized, subjective signs, such as hallucination, delusion, or obsessive thought. This is perhaps the most difficult idea for the student to grasp—that there is no necessary difference between "physical" and "mental" or "organic" and "functional" symptoms. To the neurologist, as to other physicians, all these symptoms have their objective as well as their "conscious" or subjective aspects, and the prominence of one or the other should not change our way of looking at them. In either the paralyzed or the delirious patient, something of normal behavior has been lost as a consequence of nervous disease (negative or deficit symptoms), and often something new in his behavior has emerged, presumably because of the unbalanced or unrestrained action of the undamaged parts of the brain (positive symptoms). Some symptoms, like the dementia of general paresis, are understandable largely through the structural alteration of the brain, and the clinical picture is a combination of deficits of function and the activity of intact parts of it. The patient still exhibits behavior and thinking and still responds to his environment. No doubt previous personality structure, educational level, etc., modify the clinical state. Other symptoms, such as a paranoid idea, though believed to be based on a neuropathologic process, are more difficult to analyze, for we cannot easily identify the primary defect nor trace its effects in the patient's reaction. Such symptoms and reactions become more comprehensible when viewed against the background of all previous life experiences, to some of which they may be related. The previous life experiences thus become part of the present illness, but though possibly explaining the content of the nervous symptom and its mode of evolution, they do not explain its occurrence. The neurologic examination becomes merely a device which permits one to sample systematically the activities of the altered nervous system at one moment, and special techniques, particularly refined psychologic methods, may be needed to supplement it. Also, special laboratory procedures, such as biochemical tests of the blood, the electroencephalogram (EEG), the examination of the cerebrospinal fluid, and x-rays, yield additional objective data that cannot be obtained by simple clinical observation. Pathologic study provides the final confirmation of the location and character of the disease. The goal of the neurologic method, or of neuropathology (the laboratory study of nervous disease), is to define the essential pathologic processes underlying disease and to determine their cause and mechanism. A complete theory of a nervous disease should embrace all aspects of it, the anatomic, pathologic, biochemical, and physiologic, as well as psychologic. The method is that of the medical sciences and of medicine itself.

The *psychologic conception of disease* rests on many of the same assumptions as the neurologic concept. For example, it is assumed that in many patients psychologic difficulties are caused by structural changes at the molecular, chemical, or tissue level. They may be due to a genetic or developmental defect, and a lesion may be visualized. But another aspect is emphasized, that the nervous disorder, like the content of the mind, is determined within broad limits by previous life experiences. Certain features of personality, the degree of emotional maturity, and the capacity to adjust adequately to a social situation, which are thought to depend to a considerable extent on learned patterns of reaction, are the sources of pathology. More particularly, aberrations of mental function are regarded as immature and unstable reactions to environmental circumstances, derived, it is believed, from personality inadequacy or traceable to unfortunate experiences in early life. Some of these experiences are easily remembered, i.e., "conscious," others are forgotten, i.e., "unconscious," and can be recalled with difficulty and sometimes only through the free-association method of psychoanalysis. In either case the principal method of approach is to review the patient's autobiography and determine the relationship of the present symptoms to past experiences. The symptoms and signs of mental disease, whether the grandiose delusion of the general paretic or the phobia of a neurotic person, are regarded as responses to a number of stimulus situations acting upon individuals who differ from normal mainly in that they have learned to think and to react emotionally in an abnormal manner. Since their symptoms are often traced to psychic conflicts that have arisen in their personal life, they are in this sense psychogenic. By interview and frank discussion, the physician endeavors to demonstrate these relationships to the patient and thereby to assist him to adjust to them satisfactorily. The ultimate aim of the psychologic study of disease or of psychopathology, which is the scientific study of the psychologic origins of symptoms, is to discover abnormal mental processes and to find their psychologic cause and mechanism. Examples of some of the established mechanisms are conflict, projection, repression, conditioning, and arrest of libido. It is held, particularly by some of the more narrowly trained psychoanalysts, that all psychologic theories of mental disorder must be couched in psychologic terms and that anatomic, biochemical, physiologic, and pathologic terms have no place in such a formulation. In general, the method is that of psychology, and the conception is in line with rationalistic philosophy.

The authors would suggest that each method and each conception of disease has its place in medicine. However, the two methods operate at entirely different levels. In the *diagnosis* of nervous disease the physician's first responsibility is to record accurately all the symptoms and signs obtained in a single examination or a series of them. Here the method is that of any of the medical disciplines. A purely psychologic approach is not of great diagnostic value because eliciting the patient's biography and finding psychologic explanations for his symptoms is a time-consuming procedure and commits one prematurely to a formula of the present illness that may be totally erroneous. In the strict interpretation of nervous disorders both the neurologic and psychologic conceptions come into play; the symptom(s) which appear indicate, upon neurologic analysis, which part of the nervous system has been damaged, but the precise form the symptom takes, especially in complex behavioral derangements, will be divulged by the psychologic study of the premorbid and morbid personality. In *therapy* and in the *management* of many diseases, including those for which there is no known treatment, a detailed knowledge of the patient's personality and his general reactions are, on the other hand, quite indispensable. Success in all fields of medicine depends on the ability to deal with the patient as a troubled individual. Here the psychologic method is of practical value, and the neurologic one often has relatively less to offer. This is a province of medicine where trained psychiatrists may function with great skill. In *theorizing* about disease and in doing *medical research,* however, the neurologic method and concept provide the soundest approach, for they embrace all the methods of medicine and the medical sciences, anatomic, physiologic, biochemical, and neuropathologic, as well as psychologic. Here the psychologic method has limited application, and though it yields useful data about the evolution of symptoms and their content or form, it will probably never explain completely *a disease of the nervous system.*

All that has been said applies to nervous diseases, and thus, from the very beginning, we are confronted by one of the crucial problems of neurology—that of defining a nervous disease. Failure to do this has resulted in great confusion and has been an obstacle to research. The authors propose to define nervous disease as one *in which there is a lesion in the nervous tissue or in which reasonable evidence of an anatomic abnormality or a consistent physical or biochemical disturbance obtains.* This should be distinguished from an abnormal psychologic reaction, which is defined as *a disorder of behavior caused by maladjustment in social relations.* Worry over the loss of a job or the ill health of a child, with all its potential visceral reverberations, would not be classified as a disease. These and countless other daily problems are better looked upon as natural psychologic and physiologic reactions to social problems and dealt with at a psychologic level. A persistent anxiety state without obvious cause in a previously healthy young housewife, on the other hand, would be viewed differently. Most psychiatrists would consider it a reaction to some unconscious conflict, whereas many neurologists might consider it an unexplained socially evoked disorder as mysterious as was hyperthyroidism a century ago. We suggest that anyone who essays to investigate it should do so with a completely open mind and be prepared to review critically any apparently satisfactory explanation, whether psychologic or neurologic. Mania, depression, paranoia, and the several varieties of schizophrenia, which are the major problems of psychiatry, have, unfortunately, an uncertain status. Many experienced psychiatrists would probably agree that they are diseases, rather than deviate ways of living or abnormal psychologic reactions, and that the more comprehensive methods of medicine and the medical sciences offer a more promising approach than does psychology. To the neurologist the major deficiencies in the study of these latter disorders of the nervous system in the past few years have been the relative overemphasis on psychopathology and the neglect of neuropathology, using this term in its broadest sense.

NEUROLOGY AND PSYCHIATRY

All the former has been said to explain the different ways in which neurologists and psychiatrists conceptualize the problems of nervous disease. Actually, the fields of neurology and psychiatry are broad and touch every medical and surgical specialty. Both are concerned with disturbances of behavior, conduct, thinking, and emotional control due to diseases of the brain. In addition, neurology includes as its subject matter many diseases of the nervous system that do not alter the mind, and psychiatry is occupied with countless problems of adjustment in daily life, which are sources of much unhappiness and disability and yet cannot be defined as nervous diseases.

Certain major manifestations of mental illness and of neurologic disease, those most likely to be encountered by general practitioners and internists, will be discussed in the first half of this book, and an attempt will be made to explain them in terms of current anatomic, physiologic, and psychologic theory. A comprehensive account of the major psychiatric and neurologic diseases will be presented in the second half of this book in their appropriate place, with diseases of the nervous system. A systematic discussion of normal personality development will be found in Part 2, Chap. 7. Neurologic disorders will be discussed in sequence, ranging from the most frequent and general symptoms and signs to the most specific.

THE IMPORTANCE OF PSYCHOLOGIC MEDICINE

The magnitude of the field of psychologic medicine can hardly be overestimated, and emphasis on the neurologic method is not intended to depreciate the importance of the psychologic approach. Every physician would agree that illness invariably creates problems for the patient and his family. Some, such as the temporary loss of employment or interruption of normal activities, are relatively minor. Others, such as fear of disability or death, may be so overwhelming as to demand the most thoughtful treatment. The need to understand the patient and his reactions must be taken into account in every medical procedure, even in history taking, where the reliability and validity of symptoms must be evaluated against the background of the patient's personality and his cultural environment. The group of illnesses called the *psychoneuroses* or *neuroses* are known to manifest a wide variety of symptoms that may be confused with those of medical disease.

Of even greater significance is a second large category of diseases of unknown origin (peptic ulcer, mucous colitis, ulcerative colitis, bronchial asthma, atopic dermatitis, urticaria, angioneurotic edema, hay fever, Raynaud's disease, hypertension, hyperthyroidism, amenorrhea and other disturbances of menstruation, enuresis, dysuria, rheumatoid and other forms of arthritis, headache, syncope, and epilepsy) in which a stressful personal problem appears often to be associated with the initial development, exacerbation, or prolongation of symptoms. Three lines of evidence tend to set these *psychosomatic diseases* apart from all others. (1) A large series of observations, made by Cannon, Wolff, Mittelman, Wolf, Cobb, Finesinger, White, Jones, and others, have established the fact that the function of the offending organ is excited and possibly deranged by strong emotions and assuaged by tranquility and feelings of security. (2) A careful analysis of the biographies of patients with these diseases has shown what is believed to be an inordinately high incidence of resentment, hostility, dependence or independence, suppressed emotionality, and inability to communicate matters of emotional concern or to differentiate between reality and subjective falsification (cf., studies of Lindemann, Dunbar, French, and Alexander). (Studies of personality promised at first to show a special group of personality traits to be operating in each disease, but subsequent inquiry indicates that this is not the case.) (3) A search through the biographic data of patients with these diseases has shown relationship between exacerbations of symptoms and the occurrence of frustrating or disturbing incidents; and unsuccessful medical therapy has seemed to result when these emotional factors were neglected.

In the field of psychosomatic disease, despite intensive investigation by psychiatrists in the last 30 years, the reports of which make up an enormous literature, very few facts have been established. Surely it can be said that, like the psychoneuroses, they are "part disturbances" of the personality. But they differ from the psychoneuroses in that (1) they have different symptoms; (2) as a rule they last longer; (3) they have in most instances a known and demonstrable pathologic basis and often a known cause, e.g., allergy in asthma and atopic dermatitis; (4) treatment has been concerned more directly with the relief of symptoms and has tended to be directed by different groups of specialists; (5) the incidence of frank psychoneuroses in this group of patients is no greater than in the population at large, and these psychosomatic disorders are not more frequent in neurotic individuals. No complete proof has thus far been adduced that psychic factors are the primary cause of any of these psychosomatic diseases any more than they are the cause of angina pectoris or exophthalmic goiter. Moreover, the concepts formed about these diseases in recent years, although educationally useful, have not been of great theoretical value. There is no evidence that the therapeutic results obtained by a thoughtful understanding physician, unsophisticated in psychologic theory, are less good than those of the most experienced psychiatrists.

The basic fault in this field of psychologic medicine, as it was in the "somatic medicine" that flourished before and after the First World War, is that one aspect is stressed with too little reference to the other. As pointed out by Wolff in his scholarly exposition of the mind-body relationship, the logical fallacy of such ideas as "psychogenic," "psychosomatic," and "emotional causes of disease" is that they imply a mind acting in opposition to a body.

A third group of illnesses that fall more clearly in the borderland between medicine, neurology, and psychiatry might be termed the *functional overlays of organic disease.* Here under the stress of disease, usually one that is frightening or painful and disabling, an illness of definite organic type becomes complicated by psychologic symptoms which have no direct (causal) relationship to it. At least two patterns of reaction can be discerned: (1) a type of hysterical conversion (cf. Chap. 370) in which some physical symptom such as paralysis, sensory loss, tremor, vomiting, or loss of equilibrium are added to the signs of organic (sometimes neurologic) disease. Inquiry may show that the patient may have exhibited some positive evidence of emotional instability or immaturity in the past, but often this is unclear. The domestic situation may give some clue as to the reason for persistent invalidism. (2) Affective reactions of anxiety or depression (cf. Chaps. 18 and 369), the latter being more frequent and masquerading under the guise of fatigue, insomnia, apathy, and disinterest or suspiciousness. These seem to bear no certain relationship to the nature of the illness, although the fatigue-exhaustion syndrome has been especially frequent after infectious hepatitis, influenza, brucellosis, and Icelandic disease. Again, previous temperament and personality may provide some hint of a natural tendency to anxiety and depression. The separation of the psychologic disturbance from the organic disease assumes importance because the treatment of the two, especially the psychologic one, requires special methods.

An ancient approach to this broad area of psychologic medicine, first suggested by Claude Bernard and ably espoused by Adolph Meyer, regards man as a psychobiologic unit functioning in relationship to his physical and his uniquely social environment. Disease is conceived of as representing a faulty or inadequate adaptation of the organism to the environment. Sometimes the maladaptation can be traced to a single agent in the environment, such as the tubercle bacillus, without which the disease tuberculosis could not develop. In other instances, as in a recurrent infection, the condition is much more complex, indicating a primary physical defect in the individual, such as an agammaglobulinemia. Again, exhaustion from a prolonged stressful situation or malnutrition may have rendered the patient susceptible to the infectious agent. Seldom even in straightforward disease, such as tuberculosis or delirium tremens, can one reduce the problem to a single physical or psychic factor. Hence, it is proposed that a rigid and narrow physical or psychologic approach must be supplanted by this broader, more biologic one, which attempts to weigh each of several factors that make up the equation of disease. At present this is difficult, for all the factors in many diseases, particularly in psychoneurotic and psychosomatic ones, have not been isolated and studied. Until such time as new facts are obtained, the physician must cope with a huge population of patients, as many as 50 percent, who suffer from obscure ailments and diseases, and he is forced to employ inadequate methods of diagnosis and treatment. Fortunately, most of these illnesses are benign and of relatively minor importance, and time and kindly reassurance will alleviate them; some of them represent psychoneuroses that are not disabling. The physician and student must acquire a sensitivity to psychologic problems without becoming so mindful of them that every illness is reduced to a naive psychologic formula. Above all, an open mind should be adopted, one that will permit critical review of all hypotheses in this field and acceptance of only those based on the valid data of controlled clinical observation and scientific experiment.

REFERENCES

Carter, A. B.: The Functional Overlay, Brit. Med. J. (Lancet) 2:1196, 1967.

Cobb, S.: "Emotions and Clinical Medicine," New York, W. W. Norton & Company, Inc., 1950.

Finesinger, J. E.: Psychiatric Components in Medical Disease: Psychosomatic Medicine, New Engl. J. Med., 227:578, 1942.

Masserman, J. H.: "Behavior and Neurosis: An Experimental Psychoanalytic Approach to Psychobiologic Principles," Chicago, The University of Chicago Press, 1943.

Wolf, S., and H. G. Wolff: "Human Gastric Function: An Experimental Study of a Man and His Stomach," Fair Lawn, N.J., Oxford University Press, 1947.

18 NERVOUSNESS, ANXIETY, AND DEPRESSION

Raymond D. Adams

Upon close questioning the majority of patients who enter a physician's office or a hospital will admit to being nervous, anxious, or depressed. Evidently the natural human reactions to the prospect of real or imaginary disease or to the stresses of contemporary social environment are being experienced. If they stand in clear relationship to a stressful situation, e.g., anxiety over pressing economic reverses or grief over the death of a loved one, these states may be accepted as normal, and they become the basis of medical consultation only when excessively intense and uncontrollable or when accompanying derangements of visceral function are excessive. The problem increases in complexity when similar symptoms occur in individuals who are not undergoing immediately stressful or depressing experiences; and any threatening situation, if it exists, is either unknown to the conscious mind of the patient or has been at least partly suppressed. The relationship between social stimulus and the prevailing alteration of mood can then be discovered only by gentle probings by the psychologically sophisticated physician. Once the connection is established and the problem dealt with realistically, the symptoms become understandable and often disappear.

There is still another broad category of nervousness, anxiety, and depression, the significance of which we cannot fully comprehend. These are states in which the individual suffers profound and prolonged anxiety and depression without obvious explanation. Delving into the unconscious mind fails to reveal a plausible psychogenesis. In many such instances a genetic factor appears to operate, and the principal features of the illness and its natural cause are so stereotyped as to indicate a fundamental derangement of the emotional apparatus of the nervous system. These latter states we would categorize as diseases even though they do not possess an established mechanism or pathology.

The problem confronting every physician is to recognize these nervous disorders in all their variations and to decide whether they constitute the nervous reactions of a normal person, a pathologic reaction the psychologic antecedents of which are veiled in the obscurities of the unconscious mind, or a grave occult disease of the nervous system demanding the attention of specialists in psychologic medicine.

In this chapter the cardinal features of these conditions will be described along with current views of their psychologic and physiologic origins; and lines of inquiry that might help determine their significance will be suggested.

NERVOUSNESS

By this rather vague term the lay person usually refers to a state of restlessness and overactivity, tension, uneasy apprehension, or hyperexcitability. But it may also mean other things, such as thoughts of suicide, fear of killing one's child or spouse, a distressing hallucination or paranoid idea, or frank hysterical behavior. Careful questioning as to its exact nature is always necessary.

In its usual signification, a period of nervousness may represent no more than one of the variations to which many otherwise normal individuals are subject. For example, adolescence rarely passes without its period of turmoil as the young person attempts to emancipate himself from his family and to adjust to school work and the opposite sex (cf. Chap. 7). In the female the menses are accompanied by increased tension and moodiness, and of course, the menopause is another critical period. Some individuals claim they have been nervous in all their social relations throughout life, and one should then suspect a psychoneurosis or psychosis even though adjustment to school, family, and work seems to have been adequate. Others come to the physician because of a recent development of nervousness; in this instance one must consider a variety of conditions such as psychoneurosis, psychosis, endocrine disease (e.g., hyperthyroidism), a drug reaction (corticosteroid therapy), or withdrawal reaction from a drug (alcoholic or barbiturate delirium). Some patients complain of nervousness that attends the development of a medical disease; it would appear then to be secondary, i.e., occasioned by fear of disability, dependency, or death.

Nervousness even in its simplest form is reflected in many important activities of the human organism. When it is present, there is often a mild somberness of mood and increased tendency to tears and anger (emotionality). Fatigue that bears no proper relationship to sleep and rest is frequent; and sleep is often troubled, as are eating and drinking habits. The patient subject to headaches often reports these symptoms to have increased in frequency and intensity. All these, then, along with sweating, awareness of cardiac action, queer sensations in the head or giddiness, upset stomach, and frequency of micturition, indicate that the nervous state is inducing some of the same visceral changes that occur with anxiety. Thus, it would appear that nervousness and anxiety constitute a graded series of reactions, anxiety being usually a more intense and protracted nervousness; the underlying cause and mechanisms appear to be essentially the same for both conditions (see p. 369).

THE ANXIETY STATE

Anxiety is "the fundamental phenomenon and central problem of neurosis . . . a nodal point, linking up all kinds of most important questions, a riddle of which the solution must cast a flood of light upon our whole mental life." (Freud) From the viewpoint of the social historian, anxiety is said to be "the most prominent mental characteristic of Occidental civilization." (Willoughby) In these varied contexts anxiety has a broad meaning, more or less equivalent to social and psychologic unrest. In more general psychologic terms it has been defined as "an emotional state arising when a continuing strong desire seems likely to miss its goal." (McDougall)

The more strictly medical meaning of the word *anxiety*, and the one used in this chapter, designates a state characterized by a subjective feeling of fear and uneasy anticipation (apprehension), usually with a definite topical content and associated with the physiologic accompaniments of fear, i.e., breathlessness, choking sensation, palpitation, restlessness, increased muscular tension, tightness in the chest, giddiness, trembling, sweating, flushing, and broken sleep. By topical content is meant the idea, the person, or the object about which the person is anxious. The several vasomotor, visceral, and chemical changes that underlie many of the symptoms and signs are mediated through the autonomic nervous system, particularly the sympathetic part of it, and involve the thyroid and adrenal glands.

Forms of Anxiety

Anxiety manifests itself in acute episodes, lasting a few minutes, or as a protracted state continuing for weeks, months, or even years. In the acute attacks, called *anxiety attacks* or *panics*, breathlessness, palpitation, choking, sweating, and trembling accompany an intense fear of dying, losing one's reason, or committing a horrid crime. In states of chronic anxiety, nervousness, restlessness, irritability, excitability, fatigue, pressure or tension headaches, and insomnia again are the major symptoms, but they tend to be milder and less frightening but by no means less disabling. Discrete anxiety attacks and protracted states of anxiety are not mutually exclusive, though they often occur separately. Episodic anxiety occurring in attacks, without any major disorder of mood or of thinking, is usually classified as an *anxiety neurosis;* the prolonged state of anxiety is called *neurocirculatory asthenia*. These two conditions will be discussed in greater detail in Chap. 369. Anxiety symptoms are a prominent feature in the syndrome of posttraumatic nervous instability (cf. Chap. 358).

Physiologic and Psychologic Basis

The cause, mechanism, and biologic meaning of anxiety have been the subjects of much speculation. The psychologist has come to regard anxiety as anticipatory behavior, i.e., a state of uneasiness concerning something which may or will happen in the future. It is believed to be based on an inherited instinctual pattern (fear); and the occurrence of this emotional state in situations that would not be expected to provoke it could be an example of a conditioned or learned response.

The only well-systematized psychologic theory is that put forth by psychoanalysts, who look upon anxiety as a response to a situation which in some manner threatens the security of the individual. Anxiety is a response to danger, the topical content of which lies in the unconscious mind. It is pointed out that the somatic symptoms of anxiety are similar to those of fear. The postulated danger is internal rather than external; a primitive drive that is not compatible with current social practices has been aroused and can be satisfied only at risk to the individual.

Most psychiatrists accept this theory and believe that psychotherapeutic interviews will disclose the anxiety-provoking stimulus of which the patient is himself unaware. Once insight is gained into the psychodynamic mechanism, the anxiety symptoms are said to subside.

A search for evidences of visceral disease in patients with anxiety has thus far been unrewarding. A reduced capacity for physical work and strong effort has suggested the possibility of a defect in aerobic metabolism, as evidenced by increased oxygen consumption and an excessive rise in blood lactate. Moreover, such patients seem unable to tolerate the physiologic and biochemical effects of work as well as does the average person. Whether these differences are of primary significance or are due merely to lack of training and poor physical condition has not been settled.

A number of endocrinologic studies have been done and have yielded interesting data. The urinary excretion of epinephrine has been found elevated in some individuals; in others, an increase in the urinary excretion of norepinephrine has been noted; in still a third group, normal values for both epinephrine and norepinephrine were obtained. Elmadjian and his associates have observed that aldosterone excretion in patients with anxiety neurosis is two or three times that of normal control subjects. This work has been in part corroborated by Venning, who demonstrated an increase in aldosterone excretion in medical students experiencing fear and anxiety while preparing for examination. The interpretation of these observations is not certain, but it is becoming increasingly evident that prolonged and diffuse anxiety is a pattern of behavior determined by a biochemical abnormality of certain parts of the brain.

Diagnosis of Anxiety

Clinical diagnosis of the anxiety state depends upon recognition of (1) the implicit or subjective disturbance, i.e., the uneasiness and apprehension, and (2) the subjective and more objective vasomotor or visceral changes. The presence of diffuse or more or less circumscribed attacks of autonomic or thyroid and adrenal excitation, *without psychic counterpart*, does not establish the diagnosis of anxiety. Similar autonomic and endocrine discharges may occur with thyrotoxicosis, pheochromocytoma, corticosteroid therapy (usually in large doses), hypoglycemia, and menopause. Penfield has described them also as a manifestation of tumors of the third ventricle (diencephalic autonomic epilepsy), and they have occasionally occurred as a prelude (aura) to a frank convulsive state. When the psychic components of anxiety are fully described by a patient who admits to having visceral manifestations, one must consider as diagnostic possibilities anxiety neurosis, depression, hysteria, psychasthenia,

schizophrenia, or a drug or endocrine psychosis. The differential diagnosis of the anxiety state will be discussed more fully in Chap. 369. The data obtained by history and physical examination, if analyzed carefully, usually permit distinction between pure derangements of autonomic nervous and endocrine systems and true anxiety. One of the commonest sources of error is to mistake an anxious depression for an anxiety neurosis.

DEPRESSION

There are few individuals who do not experience periods of discouragement and despair, and these become manifestly more frequent as modern society increases in complexity, demanding ever greater inhibition of one's impulses and greater conformity to a group. As with anxiety, depression of mood that is appropriate to a given situation in life seldom becomes the basis of medical complaint. The patient then seeks help only when he cannot overcome or control his grief or unhappiness. But, there are numerous instances where he does not fully recognize its cause, and in this respect, the symptoms are viewed as indicative of disease for which help is sought. Thus, depression, like anxiety, may be either a normal reaction or a pathologic state, and the distinction may require searching analysis of the medical data by a discerning physician.

Information about depressions, like knowledge of all psychiatric syndromes, is gained from three sources: the history obtained from the patient; the history obtained from the family or a friend in close contact with the patient; and the findings on examination.

The majority of patients who suffer from depression give a history of "not feeling well," of being "low in spirits," "blue," "glum," "unhappy," or 'morbid." They are vaguely aware that their emotional reactions have changed; activities that were formerly pleasant are no longer so. But it often happens that these patients do not perceive their unhappiness and instead complain of being nervous, worried, fatigued, or unable to think with accustomed efficiency. Pain of obscure origin may be the predominant topic of their conversation, as may any other symptom common in adult life, e.g., tinnitus, dry mouth, burning tongue, arthritis, constipation, pruritus. Multiplicity and persistence of complaint has led to many of these persons being classed as hypochondriacs; and indeed, the most typical examples of excessive preoccupation with symptoms in middle-aged and elderly persons are found in depressed individuals. Since these associated symptoms are so frequent and are often a misleading feature of depression, they will be presented in further detail.

LASSITUDE, FATIGUE, LACK OF ENERGY, POOR APPETITE. A decrease in energy output is a common symptom. The patient complains of being continuously without energy and of tiring out of proportion to the amount of work done. The appetite is usually poor; the patient derives no real enjoyment from eating and may comment, "I only eat to live," "I only eat because I have to." Weight loss is common and probably due to decreased food intake; and the majority of severely depressed patients are constipated. Exceptionally, there is weight gain because of continued food intake and reduced activity. Sexual desire also wanes; complete loss of libido is common.

LOSS OF INTEREST AND INCAPACITY FOR ENJOYMENT. These are noted by both the patient and his family. When formerly the patient found pleasure in his work and was quite capable of doing it well, even the simplest tasks now demand great effort. He feels that he lacks his former efficiency in work and often ascribes this to forgetfulness. However, when one questions his employer, one learns that there has been no impairment of memory or judgment but only a lack of the usual interest in and enthusiasm for work. Also, when the patient's memory is systematically tested, the deficit in memory of which he complains appears as a difficulty in concentration rather than a true memory deficit. This lack of interest and enthusiasm extends also to other activities. Absorbing recreational pursuits now give no pleasure. Cherished friendships are abandoned simply because it is too much of an effort to see people. Irritability is also frequent, and patients who formerly were quite placid and imperturbable find themselves easily irritated by trivial happenings. The noises of children playing about the house are intolerable. However, if the patient is overcritical or harsh with them, he feels guilty and reproaches himself.

WORRY AND DIFFUSE CONCERN. These symptoms are prominent in most cases of depression. Patients find themselves worrying about things that have not happened or feeling apprehensive and fearful about the outcome of some ordinary activity. Incidents that occurred years before may be the objects of concern. For example, the patient may become very much upset and unhappy and may cry about the death of a relative that occurred many years before. He is assailed by pessimistic thoughts and by feelings of inadequacy and unworthiness and is often preoccupied with the possibility of suicide.

INSOMNIA. Almost always present, insomnia manifests itself in several ways. The patient may find it difficult to fall asleep; or he may fall asleep quickly but soon awaken and be unable to return to sleep. Some patients state that they do not awaken during the night but their sleep is restless and unsatisfactory. Usually, when unable to sleep, they cannot remain quietly in bed. Plagued by pessimistic thoughts, they arise, walk about the house, smoke a cigarette, get something to eat, and resort to various measures to induce sleep. Bad dreams or nightmares are common. Occasionally there is excessive sleep, and the patient finds relief from his worries in slumber.

A closely related complaint is that of not feeling rested upon awakening in the morning. Patients frequently state, "I feel more tired upon awakening than I did before I went to sleep." A diurnal variation in mood swing is characteristic. In most patients all symptoms are worse in the morning and improve as the day progresses. Occasionally the reverse is true, and the symptoms are worst in the afternoon or evening.

ANXIETY. A large proportion of depressed patients experience anxiety. There may be anxiety attacks in which the patient becomes tense and apprehensive, perspires freely, and experiences palpitation and labored respiration. These symptoms may occur in discrete attacks or may continue in milder form over a long period of time. There may be crying spells in association with attacks of tenseness and palpitation for reasons not apparent to the patient or to an observer.

NERVOUSNESS. This is another common symptom. Very often depressed patients and psychoneurotic patients state that nervousness is their chief complaint. They may mean by this term a vague, ineffable psychologic state or a feeling of uneasy expectancy or of impending doom, the precise nature of which is uncertain. Again, nervousness may mean tenseness, inner tremulousness, or a diffuse uneasiness. Depressed patients also use "nervousness" to mean a feeling of sadness, with outbreaks of spontaneous weeping.

PAIN. Though it is not generally appreciated, pain may occasionally be one of the earliest, if not the first, manifestations of depression, occurring before other obvious depressive symptoms appear. The pain is often described as "tearing," "pulling," "twisting," "burning," or "clamping" and may be localized or migratory. In one patient it appeared first in the right external auditory canal and then successively in the right chest and shoulder, the left pudendal region, and both lower extremities, starting in the left instep and radiating upward to the left groin, then in the right instep radiating to the right groin. The pain is usually constant from the time of onset. There may be fluctuations in severity, however, with exacerbations which the patient associates with fatigue and emotional disturbances.

The family, in relating the story of the illness, usually can do more than just verify many of the patient's symptoms. They can give a clearer idea of the degree of worry, the extent of disability, the depth of the alteration of emotional reaction, and the distressing effect of the patient's disturbed behavior on others. Moreover, they are often helpful in documenting the time of onset of the illness, the natural fluctuations, and the response to therapy.

SIGNS OF DEPRESSION. Before considering the objective signs on examination, it should be pointed out that the chief abnormalities occur in three domains of psychic function: emotion, ideation, and psychomotor activity. Abnormalities in these three spheres are designated by some psychiatrists as the cardinal signs or "unit symptoms" of the disorder.

The *facial expression* is often plaintive, troubled, pained, or anguished. The patient's attitude and manner betray the prevailing mood of depression, discouragement, and despondency. In other words, the affective response, which is the outward expression of feeling, is consistent with the depressed mood. The patient's eyes during the course of the interview may become tearful, or he may cry openly. At times the immobility of the face will mimic the facies of parkinsonism.

The stream of speech, from which the ideational content is determined, is slow. At times the patient is mute and speaks neither spontaneously nor in response to questions. Again, he may speak very slowly with a long period between his spontaneous utterances, or there may be a long delay between the questions asked by the examiner and the answers given by the patient. The retardation is present regardless of the topic of conversation and is not restricted to certain subjects as it is in the case of emotional blocking (selective retardation) seen in other psychiatric illnesses. At times the flow of speech is accelerated rather than retarded, but still the topical content tends to be restricted to a few subjects, such as the patient's symptoms and his personal problems.

The *motor activity may be decreased* in varying degrees, from slow and deliberate movement even to total cessation as in stupor. Frequently the patient will sit for hours in one place without moving; the slightest movement appears to require great effort. Again, motor activity may be increased to the point of restlessness and agitation, the patient pacing the floor, wringing his hands, and loudly bemoaning his fate.

The *content of speech* varies and is largely conditioned by the past experiences of the patient. Conversation is replete with pessimistic thoughts and fears of cancer or other serious diseases. Expressions of self-depreciation, self-accusation, feelings of unworthiness, inferiority, guilt, a belief that life is not worthwhile, and suicidal preoccupation less often enter the conversation. Although systematized ideas of persecution are not common in depression, the patient often believes he is not liked by his relatives or friends. The patient's reaction to these ideas is usually one of agreement, since he himself feels unworthy and sees no reason for people wanting him around or enjoying his company. In severe depressions some of the ideas expressed by the patient are bizarre and assume the form of somatic and nihilistic delusions. Various parts of the body are said to be "rotting"; there have been "no normal bowel movements for weeks or months"; "all my blood is dried up"; "I am half dead," etc. In severe depressions auditory, visual, tactile, or olfactory hallucinations occur, and as a rule their salient features are consistent with the depressed mood.

Personal and abstract judgment is often pessimistically tinged by the depressed mood. The patient evaluates his illness as a hopeless one and his business as destined for certain failure. His outlook toward the future is pessimistic and hopeless. Insight may be entirely lacking. The patient may insist that he is suffering from malignancy or some incurable disease despite repeated reassurance to the contrary. However, some patients do realize that they are depressed and that their feelings are for the most part determined by this depression.

ETIOLOGY AND MECHANISM. Psychiatrists are not in complete agreement concerning the cause of the depressive syndrome. There are two schools of thought, one of which contends that the depressive reaction has its genesis in hereditary factors, the other, based largely on psychoanalytic theory, considers it to be a psychogenic disturbance brought about by the inability of a rigid personality to adjust its instinctual drives to the demands of the environment. The latter theory, while interesting, has not been substantiated and has not resulted in the development of effective psychotherapeutic measures. Rauwolfia compounds and other agents used to treat nervousness and anxiety may induce a depressive mood, a fact of considerable theoretical importance (cf., Chap. 371).

CLINICAL SIGNIFICANCE. All these symptoms and signs comprise a clinical syndrome of importance because of its frequency and gravity. Errors in diagnosis in our best hospitals are numerous and at times serious. Large numbers of such patients tend to accumulate in the various medical clinics, taking up the time of the medical staff that attempts to give them symptomatic therapy. Here the serious consequences of misdiagnosis lie mainly in the fact that the patient does not receive the appropriate treatment for his depression (see Chap. 371). When anxiety symptoms are prominent, an incorrect diagnosis of anxiety neurosis may be made. This mistake, or the false attribution of depression to some environmental circumstance, may obscure the fact that the illness is in reality an endogenous psychosis, and the patient may unexpectedly commit suicide even while receiving psychotherapy. Again, despondency or depression due to unfortunate life circumstances may be misdiagnosed as an endogenous depression and treated by the more drastic methods of electroshock or powerful antidepressant drugs rather than by supportive therapy.

Depression may occur intermittently in conjunction with all the psychoneuroses and persistently in manic-depressive psychosis and in association with medical and neurologic diseases. Chronic infection, endocrine disorders (hyperparathyroidism, hypothyroidism, or Addison's disease), or neoplasia may at times produce chronic fatigue that is difficult to distinguish from depression.

The most important point to be remembered is that if a patient presents any one of the above symptoms, it is incumbent upon the physician to take a complete history and to examine the mental status in some detail in an effort to determine the existence of a depressive state. Once it is established, since it is but one cardinal manifestation of several psychiatric illnesses, the physician must then undertake a differential diagnosis along the lines suggested in Chap. 369.

TREATMENT OF ANXIETY AND DEPRESSION. See Chap. 369 and 371.

SELF-CONSCIOUSNESS AND PARANOID TENDENCIES

Although the most frequent patterns of abnormal nervous reaction have been described, this chapter would not be complete without brief reference to states of self-consciousness and distrust of others as sources of medical complaint. Not a few adolescents and young adults are assailed by doubts of their adequacy to adapt to social situations. They are timid, shy, unable to think of anything to say ("tongue-tied"), and their embarrassment may be so obvious that others make fun of them. This state may often be traced to simple inexperience, a lack of opportunity to be in social groups, and is corrected in time by further contact with people their own age. A few painful social experiences in the past may have conditioned them to react with panic and fear to a social group. Always the more severe and persistent forms of this so-called "inferiority complex," with a tendency to be overly concerned about and to misinterpret the thoughts and actions of others, should raise the question of a malevolent schizoid trend. Admittedly this is exceptional, however, and not a few individuals, whose nervous reactions are not wholly classifiable, go through life tortured by doubts of their own social competence without ever gaining complete control of themselves and without ever a sign of schizophrenia. They are called *introverted* or *neurotic*. Whether they later become subjects of paranoid reactions and depressions is still a matter of conjecture.

19   LASSITUDE AND ASTHENIA
Raymond D. Adams

The term *weakness* is used by patients to describe a variety of subjective complaints which vary in their import and prognostic significance. Most subjective disorders embraced by this term will be found, on careful questioning, to fall within the following classification:

I. Lassitude, fatigue, lack of energy, listlesssess, and languor. These terms, while not synonymous, shade into each other; all refer to weariness and a loss of that sense of well-being typically found in persons who are healthy in body and mind. Symptoms of this type are present in a large majority of all patients and have little diagnostic specificity. For the sake of brevity this group of complaints will be considered together under Lassitude and Fatigue.

II. Weakness, loss of muscular strength, and asthenia. These may be either persistent or episodic.

A. Persistent weakness: This may be (1) restricted to certain muscles or groups of muscles (paresis, palsy, paralysis) or (2) general, involving the entire musculature, in which instance the term *asthenia* or *myasthenia* is used. Paralysis is discussed in Chap. 21. The generalized type of weakness will be considered below under Asthenia. It is far less common than lassitude and more likely to indicate serious disease.

B. Recurrent weakness: Many patients complain of "attacks of weakness," and careful questioning reveals that a diminished sense of alertness, a feeling of lightheadedness, or a sensation of faintness is the actual symptoms. These complaints are subjectively different from lassitude and asthenia, and the causes are likewise different; such recurrent attacks of weakness are discussed in Chap. 20.

It should be restated that the unqualified term weakness is so vague as to be almost useless and that a sound clinical approach to this problem entails, as the initial step, an analysis of what the patient himself means when he uses this and similar terms.

LASSITUDE AND FATIGUE (Lack of Energy, Languor, Listlessness, Weariness, and Neurasthenia)

Of all symptoms these are among the most frequent and at the same time the most abstruse, More than half of all patients make direct complaint of this group of symptoms or admit their presence when questioned. During the Second World War they figured so prominently in military medicine that the term *combat fatigue* was applied to all acute psychiatric illnesses on the battlefield. Therefore, it behooves every student of medicine to learn as much as possible about these symptoms and their physiologic and psychologic antecedents.

Lassitude or fatigue most commonly refers to a feeling of weariness or tiredness. Patients who complain of this symptom have a more or less characteristic way of describing it. They speak of being "all in," "without pep," having "no ambition," "no interest," or "being fed up." They are inclined to lie down. On close analysis there is a difficulty in initiating activity, and also in sustaining it.

This condition is the familiar aftermath of prolonged labor or great physical exertion, and under such circumstances it is accepted as a physiologic reaction. When, however, the same symptoms or similar ones appear in no relation to such antecedents, they are recognized as being unnatural, and the patient rightly suspects some recently acquired disease.

The physician's first task then is to determine whether his patient is merely suffering from the physical and mental effects of overwork without realizing it. Overworked and overwrought people are everywhere observable in our society. Their actions are both instructive and pathetic. They seem to be impelled by notions of duty and refuse to think of themselves. Or, as is often the case, some personal inadequacy prevents them from deriving pleasure from any activity except their work, in which they indulge as a defense mechanism. Such individuals often experience a variety of symptoms such as weariness, irritability, nervousness, and sleeplessness. The behavior of these individuals and their varied symptomatology are best understood by referring to psychologic studies of the effect of fatigue on normal individuals.

THE EFFECT OF FATIGUE ON THE NORMAL PERSON

According to the most authoritative sources, fatigue has several effects, some explicit, others implicit. These are (1) a series of physiologic changes in many organs of the body, (2) an overt disorder of behavior in the form of reduced output of work, known as *work decrement,* and (3) an expression of dissatisfaction and a subjective feeling of tiredness or weariness in association with a variety of psychologic changes.

Fatigue indicates the presence of changes in the physiologic balance of the body. Continuous muscular work results in depletion of muscle glycogen and accumulation of lactic acid and probably other metabolites which reduce the contractility and the recovery of active muscle. It is said that the injection of blood of a fatigued animal into a rested one will produce the overt manifestations of fatigue in the latter. During fatigue states muscle action is tremulous, and movements become clumsy and cannot be sustained for long without increasing effort. The rate of breathing increases; the pulse quickens; the blood pressure rises and the pulse pressure widens; and the white blood count and the metabolic rate are increased. These reactions bear out the hypothesis that fatigue is in part a manifestation of altered metabolism.

The decreased capacity for work or productivity which is the direct consequence of fatigue has been investigated by industrial psychologists. Their findings show clearly the importance of the motivational factor on work output, whether it be in the operation of an ergograph or the performance of heavy manual labor. Also it appears that there are individual differences in the energy potential of human beings, just as there are differences in physique and temperament. Some people are strong and vigorous from birth, whereas others are weak and lacking in energy.

The subjective feelings of fatigue have been carefully recorded. Aside from weariness the tired person complains of nervousness, restlessness, inability to deal effectively with complex problems, and a tendency to be upset by trivialities. The number and quality of his associations in tests of mental functions are reduced. Behavior tends to be less rational than normal, and the capacity to deliberate and to reach judgments is impaired. The worker physically exhausted after a long, hard day is unable to perform adequately his duties as head of a household, and the example of the tired businessman who becomes the proverbial tyrant of the family circle is well known. A disinclination to try and the appearance of ideas of inferiority are other characteristics of the fatigued mind.

Instances of fatigue and lassitude resulting from overwork are not difficult to recognize. A description of the patient's daily routine will usually suffice; and if he can be persuaded to live at a more reasonable pace, his symptoms promptly subside. Errors in diagnosis are usually in the direction of ascribing fatigue to overwork, chronic infection, or anemia when it actually reflects a psychoneurosis or depression.

FATIGUE AS A MANIFESTATION OF PSYCHIATRIC DISORDER. The great majority of patients who enter a hospital because of unexplained chronic fatigue and lassitude have been found to have some type of psychiatric illness. In former times the term *neurasthenia* was applied to this group of patients, but since fatigue rarely exists as an isolated phenomenon, the current practice is to label such cases according to the total clinical picture. The usual associated symptoms are nervousness, anxiety, irritability, depression, insomnia, palpitation, headaches, breathlessness, inability to concentrate, sexual disorders, and disturbances of appetite. In one series of cases of severe fatigue in a general hospital, 75 percent were diagnosed as anxiety neurosis or tension state. Depression and "psychosomatic disease" accounted for another 10 percent,

and the remainder had miscellaneous illnesses with hysterical, obsessive, or phobic symptoms.

Several features are common to the psychiatric group. The fatigue is frequently worse in the morning. The patient often desires to lie down but finds himself unable to sleep when he does. The feeling of fatigue relates more to some activities than to others; at times certain affairs are prosecuted with great vigor; while even the thought of other activities completely exhausts the patient. A careful inquiry into the circumstances under which the fatigue first occurred or recurs often reveals a specific relationship to certain events. Instances of an acute episode of fatigue coming on during an unpleasant emotional experience, in connection with a grief reaction, or after a surgical operation have been noted. And, finally, the feeling of tiredness extends to mental as well as physical activities. The individual's capacity for sustained mental effort, as in solving problems or carrying on a difficult conversation, is impaired.

Depressing emotion, whether grief from bereavement or a phase of manic-depressive or involutional psychosis, has its characteristic effect on the impulse life and energy of the individual. The initiation of activity is difficult, and the capacity for work is reduced. Lassitude and fatigue are a more prominent feature in many mild depressive illnesses than is the depression of mood. Patients typically complain that everything they do, whether mental or physical, requires great effort, and all their accustomed activities no longer give the usual satisfaction and enjoyment. Sleep is poor, with a tendency to early morning waking. Such individuals are at their worst in the morning, both in spirit and in energy output, and tend to improve as the day wears on. It is difficult to decide whether their fatigue is a primary effect of disease or is secondary to lack of interest.

Many physicians may question whether all patients with chronic fatigue as seen in everyday practice deviate far enough from normal to justify a diagnosis of psychoneurosis or depressive psychosis. Some people because of circumstances beyond their control have no purpose in life and much idle time. They become bored with the monotony of their daily routine. Such conditions are conducive to fatigue, just as optimism or enthusiasm for a new enterprise dispels fatigue. There are other patients who, as far as one can tell, were reasonably healthy and well-adjusted until they met some adversity which aroused fear and worry. They then develop a state which may be classified as simple nervousness or reactive anxiety with the usual lassitude and fatigue, sleeplessness, and difficulty in concentration. Reactions such as these are understandable to everyone who has had "stage fright" or "buck fever." The sense of physical weakness, the utter incapacity to act, the sudden transformation of a normally well-ordered mind into intellectual chaos, and the exhaustion which follows the episode are indelible experiences in the minds of most of us.

PSYCHOLOGIC THEORIES. The significance of lassitude and fatigue in these different life situations and psychiatric illnesses has been the subject of much speculation. Physiologists have remarked on the enervating effect of strong emotion and have argued that a simple prolongation of the emotional experience would provide a rational explanation for all the symptoms of chronic anxiety. This, however, only takes the explanation one step further back and does not account for the patient's being emotionally aroused at a time when there is no explicit stimulus to emotion.

The dynamic schools of psychiatry, particularly the psychoanalytic, have postulated that chronic fatigue, like the anxiety from which it derives, is a danger signal that something is wrong; some activity or attitude has been persisted in too intensely or too long. The purpose of fatigue may be regarded as self-preservation, not merely as a protection against physical injury but also to preserve the individual's self-esteem, his concept of himself. Another hypothesis is that the fatigue is the result of the exhaustion of one's store of energy by the demands of repression. The characteristic situation in which the fatigued patient finds himself is said to be one in which effective behavior is of a type forbidden by the patient's own idea of what is permissible to him as a member of society. Fatigue then is not a negative quality, a lack of energy, but an unconscious desire for inactivity. A reciprocal relationship is believed to exist between fatigue and anxiety. Both are believed to be protective devices, but anxiety is the more imperative. It calls the individual to take some positive action to extricate himself from a predicament, whereas fatigue calls for inactivity. Both fatigue and anxiety operate blindly. The individual does not perceive what it is that must be done or stopped. All this happens at an unconscious level.

Other psychiatrists are not satisfied with the psychoanalytic hypothesis, especially for cases of lifelong weakness and fatigability. They point out that individuals differ basically in energy potential. Certain persons, it is believed, seem endowed with a limited store of energy. The physiologic or psychologic basis for this deficiency is unknown. Eugene Kahn regards it as a constitutional inadequacy and states that at present it cannot be decided whether this is inborn or acquired. Under the heading "Psychopath Weak in Impulse," he describes the individual who has an evident physical inferiority. He is a weakling; his vitality is low. He is unusually susceptible to disease and requires longer to convalesce than the average. Such a person may spend half his life recuperating from illnesses that would not bother a normal person. Vigorous games tire him, and his performance is usually so poor that he takes no interest in sports. Unless born in favorable economic circumstances he earns a meager livelihood. He seeks and accepts subordinate positions and usually cannot establish an independent social position of his own. He gives the impression of weakness of will, dullness, or nervousness, though many such individuals possess an average or superior intellectual endowment. His success is limited by lack of drive and industry. Sexual impulse is also weak, and he may find marriage impossible. He requires medical attention throughout life and, whenever subjected to any unusual stress, is apt to break down and complain of nervousness, lassitude, insomnia, and many other vague symptoms. The physical

inferiority and lack of sexual impulse bring to mind that dwarfs of endocrine origin often show this same deficiency in impulse life, as do also the majority of patients with mental retardation. This weakness in impulse is found in the chronic invalid seen in everyday practice.

It is perfectly obvious that these various psychologic theories are not mutually exclusive. Undoubtedly there are certain individuals whose impulse to activity is weak throughout life, and this deficiency probably is largely, if not exclusively, determined by genetic factors. It is equally clear that boredom, lack of interest, depression of mood, and strong emotion, regardless of the conditions under which they arise, are usually accompanied by fatigue and lassitude. The more chronic varieties of fatigue are probably in most instances related to psychiatric illnesses, and here the proposition that fatigue, like anxiety, is part of a psychologic defense mechanism seems most applicable.

LASSITUDE AND FATIGUE IN CHRONIC INFECTION, ENDOCRINE, AND OTHER MEDICAL DISEASES. Chronic infection is another cause of chronic fatigue, though a much less frequent one. Everyone has at some time or other sensed the abrupt onset of extreme enervation, a tired ache in all the muscles of the body as an acute infection develops, or the listlessness that accompanies an afternoon fever. In chronic infections symptoms of lassitude, fatigue, mental depression, and vague aches and pains are of course more persistent and may even obscure those of the underlying illness. Also, there is often a period of easy fatigability, irritability, and inability to work effectively after a protracted febrile illness. Some diseases, e.g., influenza, brucellosis, and hepatitis, are more likely to be followed by these convalescent symptoms than others. If symptoms of this type are prolonged, it is often difficult, if not impossible, to decide whether they are due to the disease in question or to the presence of chronic anxiety or depression. In many chronic diseases such as infectious hepatitis and brucellosis, neurotic symptoms are often added to those of the original disease, but it is more likely that the primary fatigue state has a biochemical basis.

Metabolic and *endocrine disturbances* (see Chaps. 86 and 373) of various types may produce lassitude or fatigue. The symptom is likely to be extremely marked and to be associated with true muscular weakness. In Addison's disease and Simmonds's disease it dominates the clinical picture. Aldosterone deficiency is another established cause of chronic fatigability (cf. Chap. 92). In persons with hypothyroidism with or without frank myxedema, lassitude is usually pronounced. It is also present in many patients with hyperthyroidism, although often less troublesome than the associated nervousness. Uncontrolled diabetes may be accompanied by excessive fatigability. Hyperparathyroidism, Cushing's disease, and hypogonadism are other instances of endocrine disease in which lassitude may be prominent (see appropriate chapters).

Any type of nutritional deficiency may, when severe, cause lassitude, and in the early stages of the disease this may be the only complaint. Weight loss and the dietary history may be the only objective clues as to the nature of the illness. Most patients who have had a myocardial infarct are left with a sense of fatigue.

Amongst the neurologic diseases in which fatigability is a prominent symptom should be mentioned posttraumatic nervous instability, Parkinson's syndrome, multiple sclerosis, and postapoplectic states. The fatigue in Parkinson's disease may be present for months or years before the neurologic symptoms are recognized. It probably depends on a subjective awareness of the early stages of the motor deficit (akinesia). The majority of patients who have recovered from a stroke complain of persistent fatigue. Relapse in multiple sclerosis may be preceded by inexplicable fatigability, and fever and exposure to environmental heat, even for a brief period, exhaust the patient's energy.

DIFFERENTIAL DIAGNOSIS. Since a large variety of physical and emotional disorders may be accompanied by lassitude, the following discussion is limited to causes likely to be obscure.

When chronic fatigue and lassitude are the presenting symptoms, the commonest cause is a psychoneurosis or depressive psychosis. The basis of diagnosis is the nature of the symptoms and its pervasive effect on both mental and physical function, the associated psychiatric symptoms, usually of anxiety or depression, and the absence of signs of somatic disease. However, since psychic and somatic disorders frequently coexist, it is wise to search for organic disease before concluding that the illness is entirely psychogenic. The clinical examination should be thorough and prompt; unnecessary prolongation of the procedure may aggravate an anxiety state, if present. A careful inquiry should be made for situational factors in the patient's life which could possibly be related to the psychiatric symptoms. If found, measures should be taken to assist the patient to understand how these factors are affecting him. If reassurance that no somatic disease is present and discussion of the patient's problems do not afford relief, a psychiatric consultation is desirable. If the diagnosis is obscure, psychiatric appraisal should be part of the initial examination. Common errors are to mistake a depressive illness in which the leading symptom is chronic fatigue for a psychoneurosis; to fail to recognize the basic energy lack in an "asthenic psychopath" and to attempt to treat him as an individual with a chronic somatic disease or a recently acquired neurotic illness; and to misjudge the relative importance of psychic and somatic factors in a chronic medical disease.

Obscure infections and surgical operations may cause symptoms which closely resemble those of psychoneurosis. Indeed, individuals who have suffered from all three conditions report that the "nuclear" emotional state is similar. As a rule, aches and pains, weight loss, and low-grade fever are more prominent in chronic infection, and anxiety is in the foreground of the neurotic illness. In the United States tuberculosis, subacute bacterial endocarditis, chronic brucellosis, chronic pyelonephritis, subacute infectious hepatitis, or certain parasitic infections such as malaria and hookworm should be considered as a cause of an illness of this type. The status of chronic brucellosis has been especially difficult to evaluate. Unfortunately there is no reliable method (other than blood culture, which is rarely positive in chronic cases) of diagnosing this condition.

Anemia (Chap. 61), when moderate to severe, and regardless of the type, should be accepted as a cause of lassitude. The severity of the symptom is more likely to parallel the hemoglobin level of the blood than the number of erythrocytes. It is the author's impression that mild grades of anemia are usually asymptomatic and that lassitude is ascribed to anemia much too often. *Nutritional deficiency*, combined with anemia, is one of the most frequent causes of lassitude and fatigability in many parts of the world.

The diagnosis of the fatigue and lassitude which accompany endocrine diseases may be difficult. These conditions are relatively rare in comparison to the psychiatric diseases which cause chronic fatigue. One of the most helpful points to keep in mind is that many of these patients are actually experiencing some degree of asthenia as well as fatigue. Details as to the most reliable methods of diagnosis of these rare diseases will be found in later chapters of the book.

Almost any type of chronic *exogenous* or *endogenous intoxication* is likely to be associated with lassitude, which, however, is only rarely the chief complaint. Among the commoner examples are alcoholism, bromism, prolonged ingestion of barbiturates, morphine addiction, and uremia. In these the clue to diagnosis is usually provided by the more troublesome complaints. In patients with acute infections, malignant tumors, and almost any other type of serious disease, other symptoms are in the foreground and are much more likely to be of diagnostic value than is the associated lassitude itself.

Lassitude of sudden onset is likely to be due to (1) an acute infection, (2) a disturbance of fluid balance, especially one producing extracellular fluid deficit, or (3) rapidly developing circulatory failure of either peripheral or cardiac origin. In these various disorders, discussed in detail in later chapters, the subjective manifestation—lassitude—is likely to be accompanied by outspoken objective phenomena, i.e., fever, tachycardia.

GENERALIZED MUSCLE WEAKNESS AND ASTHENIA

As can be judged from the foregoing remarks, the evaluation of lassitude and fatigue involves distinctions between a number of psychiatric and medical diseases; in contrast, the presence of weakness and myasthenia turns one to a rather different class of neurologic diseases which involve nerve and muscle. The symptomatic state of weakness, clearly differentiated from fatigability, is relatively infrequent.

True neural weakness and myasthenia are probably never due to psychologic disorders. Weakness does not attain significant degree in states of anemia, chronic infection, or nutritional depletion, except through the intermediation of some disorder of the neuromuscular apparatus such as a polyneuropathy. This is not to say that the chronically ill and debilitated patient is as strong as a normal healthy individual. Clearly maximal power of contraction and muscle volume are lessened, but the degree of change falls below the threshold of the methods ordinarily used in the examining room and sick bed. In such states the patient's complaints are more likely to center on other aspects of his medical disease, such as lassitude and pain, rather than loss of muscular power.

The proper determination of muscular weakness depends on two lines of inquiry: (1) a history of reduced efficiency in the performance of accustomed duties; (2) actual reduction by clinical tests of *peak power* (maximal single contractions) and endurance of some or all the major groups of muscles. If conducted systematically from head to foot, as outlined in Chap. 373, one may ascertain, by reference to one's idea of normal muscular power for age and sex, whether all the muscles or a given group of them fall below standard. Further, weakness having been demonstrated, the next step is to determine whether there is rapid weakening with continued activity, evinced by tests of sustained contraction of the affected muscles and rapid recovery with rest, as in myasthenia gravis. A series (30 to 60) of maximal contractions of the muscles of a limb, with and without a tourniquet which occludes arterial circulation, will help decide whether the special impairment of contraction that occurs in the biochemical contracture syndromes (cf. Chaps. 377 and 378) or the carpopedal spasms of tetany are present.

Diseases of the peripheral nervous system are among the best-known causes of weakness, and the additional indications of their presence are muscular atrophy, loss of tendon reflexes, and disturbances of sensation, usually in a distal pattern. If all these findings are present, there is no difficulty in distinguishing this class of disease from the myopathies, where the weak muscles may be large (pseudohypertrophic) or small (atrophic) and where reflexes diminish in proportion to the loss of muscular power. A polyneuropathy can further be separated on clinical grounds alone from the true myasthenic states, where failing neuromuscular conduction results in rapid weakening of contraction without associated atrophy, loss of tendon reflexes, or sensory changes. But it is the mild subclinical polyneuropathies that give trouble. In states of chronic renal and hepatic failure one usually finds some degree of weakness, and at autopsy it is found to be based on slight degrees of peripheral nerve degeneration and focal denervation atrophy. Diabetes mellitus, chronic nutritional deficiency, and carcinomatosis are also frequently associated with mild degrees of weakness and atrophy due to a polyneuropathy. In old age a similar picture of motor unit denervation appears in the weak, thin muscles and is due presumably to a degeneration of anterior horn cells and their axones.

Polymyopathies and the myasthenic states are the other principal causes of muscular weakness, either persistent or periodic. Muscular dystrophy in its early stages may occasion only slight weakness in certain muscle groups, and polymyositis has almost identical effects. The former is characteristically familial and its temporal course is slow; the latter has a rapid evolution (in terms of a few weeks) and often is associated with dermatitis (dermatomyositis) and disease of connective tissues or carcinoma. Large doses of corticosteroids given over a period of months or Cushing's disease cause weakness of proximal limb muscles due to segmental degeneration of muscle fibers. In hyperthyroidism and hypothyroidism there are characteristic disturbances of muscle function and size which will be described fully in Chap. 378. Hyperparathyroidism and Addison's disease cause a persistent mild generalized weakness due to some obscure disturbance in the muscle fiber and in adrenal deficiency states, especially in aldosterone deficiency, changes in sodium and potassium levels may interfere with the contraction of the muscle fibers. Many of these and other subtle diseases of muscle can be distinguished by referring to the time course of the disturbance of muscle function and the topography of the muscular affection (cf. Chap. 373).

Not all muscular weakness is due to disease of peripheral nerve or muscle. Central motor disturbances such as early Parkinson's disease or a phenothiazine dyskinesia may induce slowness of muscle action and slight diminution in power without altering the tendon reflexes.

In conclusion, it should be emphasized again that the distinction between lassitude and weakness is of primary importance, for the diseases which underlie these two states are very different. It is usually only in the early stages of a disease causing weakness when one is likely to make mistakes, for as the weakness progresses to frank paresis or paralysis the problem is one which obviously can be analyzed only along the lines described in Chap. 21. Admittedly, the separation of lassitude and weakness is not a sharp one; the former symptom often shades into the latter. Some patients with obvious weakness also complain of fatigue, but very few patients complaining of lassitude are really found to be weak, even though they may use this term to describe their feelings. The elicitation of weakness requires the testing of muscular efficiency. The analysis of fatigue and lassitude requires probing into the psychiatric state as well as the search for medical and neurologic diseases.

The considerations mentioned will lead to an accurate evaluation of the cause of weakness in many patients. Even so, there will remain a group of subjects (unfortunately, not rare) in whom the most exhaustive investigation fails to uncover the cause. In some such individuals time will furnish the answer, but in others recovery will eventually occur without the cause being known.

REFERENCES

Adams, R. D., D. Denny-Brown, and C. M. Pearson: "Diseases of Muscle: a Study of Pathology," 2d ed., New York, Paul B. Hoeber, Inc., 1962.

Walton, J. N.: "Diseases of Voluntary Muscle," 2d ed., Boston, Little, Brown and Company, 1969.

20 FAINTNESS, SYNCOPE, AND EPISODIC WEAKNESS

Raymond D. Adams and
T. R. Harrison

Episodic faintness, lightheadedness or giddiness, and reduced alertness are frequent and vexatious symptoms. The patient may refer to these symptoms as "weak spells" when he actually means loss of vigor, weakness of limbs, or impaired alertness. Any difference between faintness and syncope appears to be only quantitative. Since syncope, though less common, is more definite, it will be considered in greater detail. Those types of episodic weakness, such as myasthenia gravis and familial periodic paralysis, which are associated with striking reduction of muscular strength but not with impairment of consciousness, are discussed in other chapters. Epilepsy, which is also associated with episodic unconsciousness, differs from syncope in most other respects. It is discussed in Chap. 28.

CARDINAL FEATURES OF SYNCOPE

The term *syncope* literally means a "cutting short," "cessation," or "pause," and it is synonymous with swoon or faint. Syncope comprises a generalized weakness of muscles, with inability to stand upright and impairment of consciousness. Abrupt onset, brief duration, and complete recovery within a few minutes are other distinguishing features. Faintness, in contrast, refers to lack of strength, with a sensation of impending faint; it is an incomplete faint. Both faintness and syncope vary somewhat according to their mechanism, but both conform roughly to the following pattern.

The syncopal attack develops rapidly, but it is doubtful whether consciousness is ever terminated with the absolute suddenness of an epileptic seizure. At the beginning of the attack, the patient is nearly always in the upright position, either sitting or standing (the Stokes-Adams attack [cf. Chap. 265] is exceptional in this respect). Usually the warning of the impending faint is a sense of "feeling badly." The patient is assailed by giddiness, the floor seems to move, and surrounding objects begin to sway. His senses become confused, he yawns or gapes, there are spots before his eyes, or vision may dim, and his ears may ring. Nausea and sometimes actual vomiting accompany these symptoms. If the patient can lie down promptly, the attack may be averted without complete loss of consciousness. If he cannot, there is "loss of senses" and falling to the ground. What is most noticeable, even at the beginning of the attack, is a striking pallor or ashen-gray color of the face, and very often the face and body are bathed in cold perspiration. As a rule, the deliberate onset enables the patient to lie down or at least protect himself as he slumps. A hurtful fall is exceptional.

The depth and duration of the unconsciousness vary. Sometimes the patient is not completely oblivious of his surroundings. His senses are confused, but he may still be able to hear the voices or see the blurred outlines of people around him. Again, unconsciousness may be profound, and there may be complete lack of awareness and of capacity to respond. The patient may remain in this state for seconds to minutes or even as long as half an hour.

Shortly after the beginning of unconsciousness, convulsive movements occur in some instances. These usually consist of several clonic jerks of the arms and twitchings of the face. Rarely is there a generalized tonic-clonic convulsion. Usually the person who has fainted lies motionless, with skeletal muscles completely relaxed. Sphincter control is usually maintained. The pulse is feeble or cannot be felt; the blood pressure is low, and breathing is almost imperceptible. The reduction in vital functions, the striking pallor, and unconsciousness simulate death.

Once the patient is in a horizontal position, perhaps from having fallen, gravitation no longer hinders the flow of blood to the brain. The strength of the pulse improves, and color begins to return to the face. Breathing becomes quicker and deeper. Then the eyelids flutter, and consciousness is quickly regained. There is from this moment onward a correct perception of the environment. The patient is nevertheless keenly aware of physical weakness; and if he rises too soon, another faint may be precipitated. Headache and drowsiness, which, with mental confusion, are the usual sequelae of a convulsion, do not follow a syncopal attack.

CLASSIFICATION OF CAUSES OF RECURRENT WEAKNESS, FAINTNESS, AND DISTURBANCES OF CONSCIOUSNESS

The following list is based on established or assumed physiologic mechanisms. Some of the disorders frequently cause episodic weakness but rarely syncope. A few are especially apt to cause syncope associated with convulsive twitchings. These features are indicated in accompanying parentheses. Unless this specific notation is made, it may be assumed that the disorder in question is likely to cause faintness (when mild) and syncope (when severe).

I. Circulatory (deficient *quantity* of blood to the brain—common causes of either faintness or syncope)
   A. Peripheral
      1. Psychogenic (vasovagal-vasodepressor) syncope
      2. Postural hypotension
      3. Increased intrathoracic pressure, e.g., tussive syncope
      4. Other causes of peripheral circulatory failure
        Diseases of autonomic and peripheral nervous system (Chap. 36)
   B. Cardiac (acute cardiac failure, see Chap. 264)
      1. Alterations in rate or rhythm
        a. Bradycardia (sinus, AV block)
        b. Neurogenic (reflex bradycardia) Hypersensitive carotid sinus, vagovagal attacks
        c. Ectopic tachycardias (Chap. 265) (especially ventricular tachycardia and fibrillation)

2. Acute myocardial injury (especially infarction, see Chap. 271)
3. Mechanical hindrance
    a. Aortic stenosis
    b. Chronic pulmonary hypotension
    c. Disorders of pulmonary vessels, e.g., embolism
II. Other causes of weakness and episodic disturbances of consciousness
    A. Chemical (defective *quality* of blood to the brain)
        1. Hyperventilation (faintness common, syncope seldom occurs)
        2. Hypoglycemia (episodic weakness common, faintness occasional, syncope rare)
    B. Cerebral
        1. Cerebrovascular disturbances (cerebral ischemic attacks, see Chap. 357)
        2. Emotional disturbances, anxiety attacks, and hysterical seizures (see Chaps. 369 and 370)

This list of conditions which cause weakness, faintness, and disturbances of consciousness is deceptively long and involved. Close study, however, reveals that the commoner types of faint are reducible to a few simple mechanisms. In order not to obscure the central problem of fainting by too many details, only a few of the commoner varieties likely to be encountered in clinical practice are discussed below.

COMMON TYPES OF SYNCOPE

VASOVAGAL, VASODEPRESSOR (PSYCHOGENIC) SYNCOPE. This is the ordinary faint, and the description already given applies most perfectly to this form of it. The loss of consciousness usually takes place when the systolic pressure falls to 70 mm Hg or below. The pulse is weak or imperceptible, and its rate may be either slowed or slightly increased. Sudden vasodilatation, particularly of intramuscular vessels, is responsible for the fall in blood pressure and the inadequate cerebral circulation. It has been thought to represent a response to an emotional or physical stimulus which would ordinarily call for immediate strenuous physical activity. In the absence of such activity, there is sudden pooling of blood in the muscles, with inadequate venous return, decline in cerebral blood flow, and loss of consciousness. These considerations explain the rarity of vasovagal syncope in the recumbent position or during active muscular exercise, which increases the venous return. However, this explanation is somewhat speculative, and there are surprisingly few studies of this type of syncope.

Vasovagal or vasodepressor faints occur (1) in normal health as a consequence of a strong emotional experience or in conditions that favor vasodilatation, e.g., hot, crowded rooms, especially if the person is tired, hungry, or ill; (2) in anxiety states and neurocirculatory asthenia; (3) during pain; (4) after injury to tissues as a consequence of some combination of shock, pain, and psychologic factors.

POSTURAL HYPOTENSION WITH SYNCOPE. This type of syncope affects persons who have a chronic defect in, or a variable instability of, vasomotor reflexes. The character of the syncopal attack differs little from that of the vasovagal or vasodepressor type. The effect of posture is the cardinal feature of it. Sudden arising from a recumbent position or standing still is the condition under which it usually occurs.

Nature has provided man with several mechanisms by which his circulation adjusts to the upright posture. The pooling of blood in the lower parts of the body is prevented by (1) pressor reflexes which induce constriction of peripheral arteries and arterioles; (2) reflex acceleration of the heart by means of aortic and carotid reflexes; (3) improvement of venous return to the heart by activity of the muscles of the limbs and by increased rate of respiration. A normal individual placed on a tilt table to relax his muscles and tilted upright has a slightly diminished cardiac output, and blood accumulates in the legs to a slight degree. This is followed by a slight transitory fall in systolic blood pressure and then, within a few seconds, by a compensatory rise. Some normal individuals, if tilted on a table, will faint. In them it has been found that at first the blood pressure falls slightly and then stabilizes at a *lower* level. Shortly thereafter these compensatory reflexes suddenly fail, and the blood pressure falls precipitously. This also happens in some of the conditions listed below. In others, e.g., after surgical sympathectomy in diseases of the sympathetic nervous system and in the unusual condition or chronic orthostatic hypotension, the blood pressure never stabilizes after tilting but falls steadily to a level at which cerebral circulation cannot be maintained.

Postural syncope tends to occur under the following conditions: (1) in otherwise normal individuals who for some unknown reason have defective postural reflexes; (2) rarely, as part of a syndrome which comprises chronic orthostatic hypertension, symptoms of peripheral preganglionic autonomic and extrapyramidal disorder; (3) after prolonged illness with recumbency, especially in elderly individuals with flabby muscles; (4) after a sympathectomy that abolishes vasopressor reflexes; (5) in diabetic and other neuropathies, tabes dorsalis, and diseases of the nervous system which cause flabby, weak muscles and paralysis of vasopressor reflexes; (6) in persons with varicose veins because of pooling of blood in the abnormal venous channels; (7) in patients receiving antihypertensive and certain sedative and antidepressive drugs.

In some cases of *chronic orthostatic hypotension*, there is degeneration of preganglionic autonomic neurones with anhydrosis and other symptoms of sympathetic and parasympathetic paralysis (sphincteric disturbances, impotence, lack of tears, lack of saliva, pupillary paralysis) and extrapyramidal disorder (tremor, ataxia, rigidity). The hypotension differs from that already described in that the systolic and diastolic blood pressures fall rapidly as soon as the patient assumes an upright position, but there is no compensatory tachycardia, pallor, sweating, nausea, or other symptoms. The loss of consciousness is usually abrupt and may be attended by confusion. Recumbency restores the circulation of the brain, with a prompt return to consciousness. The pooling of blood in the abdomen and legs does not excite vasoconstriction of peripheral vessels. This is apparently because of the abnormality in the autonomic nervous system. There is also evidence that patients with this type of postural hypotension are deficient in release of norepinephrine and epinephrine. Repeated attacks may result in mental confusion, slurred speech, and other neurologic signs.

Micturition syncope, a condition usually seen in the elderly when they arise from bed at night to urinate, is probably a form of postural syncope. It has been suggested, however, that vasomotor reflexes from the bladder itself play a contributory part.

SYNCOPE OF CARDIAC ORIGIN (CARDIAC SYNCOPE). The occurrence of fainting in patients with a permanently slow pulse was first described by Morgagni and subsequently by Adams and by Stokes. It is today known as the Stokes-Adams syndrome. The heart rate is usually less than 40, and the electrocardiogram shows a transient or permanent atrioventricular block. Rarely, this may be present only during the attack. Usually without more than a momentary sense of weakness, the patient suddenly loses consciousness. This may occur at any time of the day or night, regardless of the position of the body. When the patient is upright, the unconsciousness will develop after a more brief period of asystole than with the recumbent position. According to Engel, 4 to 8 sec of asystole produce coma in the erect position, and 12 to 15 sec are required in recumbency. If cardiac standstill is more than 12 sec, the patient turns pale, falls unconscious, and may exhibit a few clonic jerks. The blood pressure falls rapidly during the period of asystole. With the resumption of the heartbeat, the face and neck become flushed. Longer periods of asystole, up to 5 min, result in coma, ashen-gray pallor giving way to cyanosis, stertorous breathing, fixed pupils, incontinence, and bilateral Babinski signs. Prolonged confusion and neurologic signs due to the relative ischemia of parts of the brain supplied by narrowed, arteriosclerotic arteries may persist in some patients, and permanent impairment of mental function is not unknown. Cardiac faints of this type may recur several times a day. Occasionally the heart block is transitory, and the electrocardiogram taken later shows only evidence of myocardial disease. Another form is that in which the heart block is reflex and due to irritation of the vagus nerves. Examples of this phenomenon have been observed with esophageal diverticula, mediastinal tumors, carotid sinus disease, glossopharyngeal neuralgia, and pleural and pulmonary irritation. However, reflex bradycardia is more commonly of the sinoatrial type than of the atrioventricular type.

Aortic stenosis and, less often, insufficiency dispose to fainting attacks. In rare instances it is due to heart block, but the more frequent mechanism appears to be diversion of blood from the brain to the exercising muscles in a patient who is unable to increase his cardiac output because of the mechanical hindrance. A characteristic clinical feature is that the faint occurs during or immediately after exertion. There may be an initial pallor, weakness,

or lightheadedness, or no warning whatsoever. Unconsciousness may last as long as half an hour and convulsions sometimes occur.

Closely related, and probably also a form of *effort syncope,* is that which occurs in some 20 percent of patients with *primary pulmonary hypertension.* Here exercise leads to dizziness, epigastric distress, and faintness followed by nausea, vomiting, and abdominal cramps. The attacks last from a few seconds to several minutes. Effort syncope in the absence of signs of aortic stenosis should lead to a search for the diagnostic evidence of dilatation of the pulmonary artery, accentuation of pulmonary second sound, or right ventricular hypertrophy. Again the cause of the faint seems to be an impaired cardiac output.

Paroxysmal atrial and ventricular tachycardia cause unconsciousness by interfering with cardiac filling and output. Bigeminal rhythm (Chap. 265) may rarely have the same effect. Most patients who faint because of paroxysmal ectopic tachycardia are aware of the preliminary rapid heart action. Otherwise, the syncopal attack does not differ from the aforementioned types.

A cardiac faint, sometimes fatal, may occur in patients with disease of the coronary arteries. No explanation for death is found at autopsy. Such faints, as well as those occurring during myocardial infarction, may be due to ventricular tachycardia, ventricular fibrillation, heart block, or rarely, to severe pain alone.

CAROTID SINUS SYNCOPE. The carotid sinus is normally sensitive to stretch and gives rise to sensory impulses carried via the intercarotid nerve of Hering (branch of the glossopharyngeal nerve) to the medulla oblongata. Massage of one or both carotid sinuses, particularly in elderly persons, cause a reflex slowing of the heart or even heart block, a fall of blood pressure without cardiac slowing, or an interference with the circulation of the ipsilateral cerebral hemisphere.

Syncope due to carotid sinus sensitivity may be initiated by turning of the head to one side, by a tight collar, or as in a few reported cases, by shaving over the region of the sinus. The absence of such stimuli is of no aid in diagnosis, since spontaneous attacks may occur. The attack nearly always begins when the patient is in an upright position, usually when he is standing. The onset is sudden, often with falling. Clonic convulsive movements are not infrequent in the vagal and depressor type of carotid sinus syncope. Unilateral paresthesias or convulsions have been reported in the central type. The period of unconsciousness seldom lasts longer than a few minutes. The sensorium is immediately clear when consciousness is regained. The majority of the reported cases have been in males.

In a patient displaying faintness on compression of one carotid sinus, it is important to distinguish between the benign disorder, hypersensitivity of one carotid sinus, and a much more serious condition, atheromatous narrowing of the opposite carotid or of the basilar artery (see Chap. 357).

Other forms of vasovagal syncope have been described. Exceptionally intense pain of visceral origin may inhibit cardiac action through vagal stimulation. We have observed instances of cardiac standstill during an attack of gallbladder colic, for example. The patient had been treated for epilepsy for several years despite her statements that pain always preceded loss of consciousness. Weiss has cited other examples, such as esophageal or mediastinal lesions, bronchoscopy, needling of body cavities, etc. Vagal and glossopharyngeal neuralgia are known to occasionally induce a reflex type of fainting. Again the sequence is always pain then syncope—in this instance the pain is localized to the base of the tongue, pharynx or larynx, tonsillar area, and ear. It may be triggered by pressure at these sites. Section of the ninth or tenth cranial nerve relieves the condition. It has been suggested that the cardiovascular effects are attributable to excitation of the dorsal motor nucleus of the vagus via collateral fibers from the nucleus of the tractus solitarius. The rare vertiginous faint which accompanies intense vertigo from labyrinthine or vestibular disease may be another example of reflex vagal stimulation.

TUSSIVE SYNCOPE ("LARYNGEAL VERTIGO"). This condition is rare, but it should be mentioned because it illustrates another mechanism of fainting—that resulting from a paroxysm of coughing. The few patients that the authors have observed have been men with chronic bronchitis. After hard coughing the patient suddenly becomes weak and loses consciousness momentarily. The unconsciousness that results from breath holding in infants is probably similar. Not all the underlying physiologic changes are known. It is said that the intrathoracic pressure becomes elevated and interferes with the venous return to the heart. The Valsalva maneuver of trying to exhale against a closed glottis is believed to produce an identical effect. Episodes of faintness and lightheadedness are not infrequent in pertussis and chronic laryngitis. Exceptionally, some other strong activity, such as laughing, straining at stool, running upstairs, or lifting, may produce a similar syndrome. *Breath-holding* spells of infancy and childhood are probably another example of the Valsalva phenomenon of straining with closed glottis, leading to diminished cardiac filling and reduced output (see Chap. 365).

SYNCOPE ASSOCIATED WITH CEREBROVASCULAR DISEASE. This is infrequent, and when it occurs, there is usually partial or complete occlusion of the large arteries in the neck. The best examples are found in the "aortic arch syndrome" (pulseless disease) where the innominate and common carotid and vertebral arteries have become narrowed. Physical activity, then, may critically reduce blood flow to the upper brainstem, causing abrupt loss of consciousness (cf. Chap. 357). Stenosis or occlusion of vertebral arteries and the "vertebral steal syndrome" is another example. Fainting is said also to occur occasionally in patients with congenital anomalies of the upper cervical spine (Klippel-Feil syndrome) or cervical spondylitis where the vertebral arteries are compromised. Head turning may then cause piercing neck pain, nausea, vomiting, vertigo, visual scotomas, and finally unconsciousness. If one carotid artery is occluded, heavy massage or pressure on the other may cause loss of consciousness, a kind of carotid syncope.

Pathophysiology of Syncope

In the final analysis the loss of consciousness in these different types of syncope must be caused by a change in the nervous elements in those parts of the brain which subserve consciousness. Syncope resembles epilepsy in this respect; yet there is an important difference. In epilepsy, whether major or minor, the arrest in mental function is almost instantaneous and, as revealed by the electroencephalogram, is accompanied by a paroxysm of activity in certain groups of cerebral neurones. Syncope, on the other hand, is not so sudden. The difference relates to the essential pathophysiology—a sudden spread of an electric discharge in epilepsy, and the more gradual failure of cerebral circulation in syncope.

During syncopal attacks, measurements of cerebral circulation (Schmidt-Kety and Gibbs's methods) demonstrate a significant degree of reduction in cerebral blood flow and of cerebral oxygen utilization (cerebral metabolism). Cerebral vascular resistance is decreased. The electroencephalogram reveals high-voltage slow waves, 2 to 5 per sec, coincident with the loss of consciousness. If the ischemia lasts only a few minutes, there are no lasting effects on the brain. If it persists for a longer time, it may result in necrosis of the border zones between the major cerebral and cerebellar arteries.

Conditions Often Associated with Episodic Weakness and Faintness but Not with Syncope

ANXIETY ATTACKS AND THE HYPERVENTILATION SYNDROME. This condition is discussed in detail in Chaps. 18 and 366, and it is necessary here only to state that this disorder is one of the commonest causes of recurrent faintness without actual loss of consciousness, the symptoms *are not relieved by recumbency*, and the diagnosis depends in large measure on reproducing the symptoms by hyperventilation. Two mechanisms are involved in the attacks: the loss of carbon dioxide as the result of hyperventilation and the release of epinephrine. Both mechanisms are said to be initiated by anxiety or allied emotional disturbances. Hyperventilation results in hypocapnia, alkalosis, increased cerebrovascular resistance, and decreased cerebral blood flow.

Of aid in diagnosis, as well as in therapy, is the demonstration to the patient of many of the symptoms of anxiety attack by voluntary hyperventilation for a period of 2 to 3 min and the cautious, slow, intravenous injection, during a period of several minutes, of 0.01 to 0.1 mg epinephrine. However, it must be admitted that the initial symptoms of the attack are not usually reproduced and that in some cases such measures are entirely without demonstrable effect.

HYPOGLYCEMIA. Another frequent cause of obscure episodic weakness is spontaneous hypoglycemia. When severe, the condition is likely to be due to a serious disease, such as a tumor of the islets of Langerhans or advanced adrenal, pituitary, or hepatic disease, in which instances there may be a confusion or even a loss of consciousness. When mild, as is usually the case, hypoglycemia is of the reactive type (Chap. 96) and occurs 2 to 5 hr after eating. The fasting blood glucose is normal. The diagnosis depends largely upon the history and the reproduction by the injection of insulin of a symptom complex exactly similar to that occurring in the spontaneous attacks.

ACUTE INTERNAL HEMORRHAGE. This condition, usually within the gastrointestinal tract, is an occasional cause of syncope. Peptic ulcer is the commonest source of the hemorrhage. When pain is absent, as it often is, and when there is no hematemesis, the cause of the weakness, faintness, or even unconsciousness may remain obscure until the passage of a black stool.

CEREBRAL ISCHEMIC ATTACKS. The attacks which occur in some patients with arteriosclerotic narrowing or occlusion of the major arteries of the brain are all of identical pattern, and indicate a temporary focal deficit in cerebral function. The main symptoms vary from patient to patient and include dim vision, hemiparesis, numbness of one side of the body, dizziness, and thick speech, and to those may be added an impairment of consciousness. The mechanism of this vascular syndrome has not been fully elucidated. Some physicians hold that localized vasospasm is responsible; other ascribe the attacks to small focal vascular lesions. The author's own investigations suggest some other mechanism than either of these. The condition is discussed in Chap. 357.

HYSTERICAL FAINTING. Hysterical fainting, which is rather frequent, usually occurs under dramatic circumstances. These are described in Chap. 370. The attack is unattended by any outward display of anxiety. The evident lack of change in pulse and blood pressure or color of the skin and mucous membranes distinguishes it from the vasodepressor faint induced by a shocking emotional experience. The diagnosis is based on the bizarre nature of the attack in a person who exhibits the general personality and behavior characteristics of hysteria.

Differential Diagnosis

OF SYNCOPE FROM OTHER TRANSITORY NERVOUS DISORDERS. More typical varieties of syncope must be distinguished from other disturbances of cerebral function, the most frequent of which is akinetic or some other form of epilepsy (see Chap. 28). The epileptic attack may occur day or night, regardless of the position of the patient; syncope rarely appears when the patient is recumbent, the only common exception being the Stokes-Adams attack. The patient's color does not usually change in epilepsy; pallor is an early and invariable finding in all types of syncope, except chronic orthostatic hypotension and hysteria, and it precedes unconsciousness. Epilepsy is more sudden in onset, and if an aura is present, it rarely lasts longer than a few seconds before consciousness is abolished. The onset of syncope is usually more deliberate.

Injury from falling is frequent in epilepsy and rare in syncope for the reason that only in the former are protective reflexes instantaneously abolished. Tonic-convulsive movements with upturning eyes are frequent in epilepsy in contrast to syncope, though the same cannot be said of clonic movements of the arms. The period of unconsciousness tends to be longer in epilepsy than in syncope. Urinary incontinence is frequent in epilepsy and rare in syncope, but since it may be observed occasionally in syncope, it cannot be used as a means of excluding this condition. The return of consciousness is prompt in syncope and slow in epilepsy. Mental confusion, headache, and drowsiness are the common sequelae of epilepsy, whereas physical weakness with clear sensorium characterizes the postsyncopal state. Repeated spells of unconsciousness in a young person at a rate of several per day or month are much more suggestive of epilepsy than syncope. It should be emphasized that no one of these points will absolutely differentiate epilepsy from syncope, but taken as a group and supplemented by electroencephalograms (see Chap. 21), they provide a means of distinguishing the two conditions.

OF THE DIFFERENT TYPES OF SYNCOPE. Differentiation of the several conditions that diminish cerebral blood flow is discussed in some detail in Chap. 26, and only a few points need to be repeated here.

When faintness is related to reduced cerebral blood flow resulting directly from a disorder of cardiac function, there is likely to be a combination of pallor and cyanosis, pronounced dyspnea, and distension of the veins. When, on the other hand, the peripheral circulation is at fault, pallor is usually striking but not accompanied by cyanosis or respiratory disturbances, and the veins are collapsed. When the primary disturbance lies in the cerebral circulation, the face is likely to be florid and the breathing slow and stertorous. During the attack a heart rate faster than 150 per min indicates an ectopic cardiac rhythm, while a striking bradycardia (rate less than 40) suggests the presence of complete heart block. In a patient with faintness or syncope attended by bradycardia, one has to distinguish between the neurogenic reflex and the myogenic (Stokes-Adams) types. Occasionally, electrocardiographic tracings will be needed, but as a rule, the Stokes-Adams seizures can be recognized by their longer duration, by the greater constancy of the heart rate, by the presence of audible sounds synchronous with atrial contraction, and by marked variation in intensity of the first sound, despite the regular rhythm (Chap. 265). Clinical diagnosis may at times be difficult or impossible.

The color of the skin, the character of the breathing, the appearance of the veins, and the rate of the heart are therefore valuable data in diagnosis *if the patient is seen during the attack.* Unfortunately, the physician does not have the opportunity to see most of the patients during their "spells" of weakness. Hence he must obtain the proper clues from the patient's story. It is therefore of primary importance that the physician be familiar with the *circumstances* and the *precipitating* and *alleviating* factors in a given episode of weakness or fainting.

The following points are also helpful in the differential diagnosis of syncope:

Type of Onset. When the attack begins with relative suddenness, i.e., over the period of a few seconds, carotid sinus syncope or postural hypotension is likely. When the symptoms develop gradually during a period of several minutes, hyperventilation or hypoglycemia (spontaneous or induced by insulin) is to be considered. Onset of syncope during or immediately after exertion suggests aortic stenosis and, in elderly subjects, postural hypotension. Exertional syncope is likewise occasionally seen in persons with aortic insufficiency.

Position at Onset of Attack. Attacks due to hypoglycemia, hyperventilation, hypertensive encephalopathy, or heart block are likely to be independent of posture. Faintness associated with a decline in blood pressure (including carotid sinus attacks) and with ectopic tachycardia usually occurs only while in the sitting or standing position, whereas faintness resulting from orthostatic hypotension or orthostatic tachycardia is apt to set in shortly after change from the recumbent to the standing position.

Associated Symptoms. The associated symptoms during an attack are important, for palpitation is likely to be present when the attack is due to anxiety or hyperventilation, to ectopic tachycardia, or to hypoglycemia. Numbness and tingling in the hands and face are frequent accompaniments of hyperventilation. Irregular jerking movements and generalized spasms without loss of consciousness or change in the electroencephalogram are typical of the hysterical faint. Genuine convulsions during the attack, although characteristic of epilepsy, may occasionally occur with heart block and with hypertensive encephalopathy.

Duration of Attack. When the duration of the seizure is very brief, i.e., a few seconds to a few minutes, one thinks particularly of carotid sinus syncope or one of the several forms of postural hypotension. A duration of more than a few minutes but less than an hour particularly suggests hypoglycemia or hyperventilation.

SPECIAL METHODS OF EXAMINATION

In many patients who complain of recurrent weakness or syncope but do not have a spontaneous attack while under the observation of the physician, an attempt to *reproduce* attacks is of great assistance in diagnosis. In order to avoid the effects of suggestion, rigid controls must be adopted. Thus, if one wishes to determine whether the attacks in a given subject are hypoglycemic in type and may be reproduced by insulin injection, it is necessary to control the observations by injecting other drugs such as atropine, nitroglycerin, or histamine which evoke subjective symptoms of a different type. When properly controlled, the insulin test is of great value in

the diagnosis of spontaneous hypoglycemia. Without such controls the procedure is useless.

When hyperventilation is accompanied by faintness, the pattern of symptoms can be reproduced readily by having the subject breathe rapidly and deeply for 2 or 3 min. This test is often of therapeutic value also because the underlying anxiety tends to be lessened when the patient learns that he can produce and alleviate the symptoms at will simply by controlling his breathing.

Among other conditions in which the diagnosis is commonly clarified by reproducing the attacks are carotid sinus hypersensitivity (massage of one or the other carotid sinus), orthostatic hypotension, and orthostatic tachycardia (observations of pulse rate, blood pressure, and symptoms in the recumbent and standing positions), and tussive syncope by Valsalva maneuver. In all such instances one should remember that the *crucial point is not whether symptoms are produced* (the procedures mentioned frequently induce symptoms in healthy persons) but whether the exact pattern of symptoms that occurs in the spontaneous attacks is reproduced in the artificial seizures.

Multiple mechanisms of syncope frequently coexist. Combinations of hypoglycemia, hyperventilation, and postural hypotension, or any two of them, are frequent. In order to reproduce exactly the spontaneous symptoms, it may be necessary to have the patient stand and hyperventilate at a time when the blood sugar has been reduced by insulin administration. When tremor, palpitation, and fright are present in the spontaneous attacks, it may be necessary to carry out these procedures in association with the administration of epinephrine. There is great psychotherapeutic value to the patient in knowing that the physician can turn his "spells" on and off at will and, therefore, is not guessing about their cause and significance.

Lastly, the electroencephalogram is helpful in diagnosis. In the interval between epileptic seizures it may show some degree of abnormality in 40 to 80 percent of cases. In the interval between syncopal attacks it should be normal.

TREATMENT

Fainting in most instances is due to a relatively innocent cause. In dealing with patients who have fainted the physician should think first of those causes of fainting that constitute a therapeutic emergency. Among them are massive internal hemorrhage and myocardial infarction, which may be painless. In an elderly person a sudden faint, without obvious cause, should arouse the suspicion of complete heart block, even though all findings are negative when the physician sees the patient.

If the patient is seen during the preliminary stages of fainting or after he has lost consciousness, one should make sure that he is in a position which permits maximal cerebral blood flow, i.e., with head lowered between the knees, if sitting, or lying supine. All tight clothing and other constrictions should be loosened and the head turned so that the tongue does not fall back into the throat, blocking the airway. Peripheral irritation, such as sprinkling or dashing cold water on the face and neck or the application of cold towels, is helpful. If the temperature is subnormal, the body should be covered with a warm blanket. If available, aromatic spirit of ammonia may be given cautiously by inhalation. One should be prepared for a possible emesis. Nothing should be given by mouth until the patient has regained consciousness. Then ½ tsp aromatic spirit of ammonia in a half glass of cold water, or a sip of brandy or whiskey, may be given. The patient should not be permitted to rise until his sense of physical weakness has passed, and he should be watched carefully for a few minutes after rising.

As a rule, the physician sees the patient after the faint has occurred, and he is asked to explain why it happened and how it can be prevented in the future. The prevention of fainting depends on the mechanisms involved. In the usual vasovagal faint of adolescents, which tends to occur in periods of emotional excitement, fatigue, hunger, etc., it is enough to advise the patient to avoid such circumstances. If the patient is sickly, measures to improve general health and circulatory efficiency are useful. In postural hypotension the patient should be cautioned against arising suddenly from bed. Instead, he should first exercise his legs for a few seconds, then sit on the edge of the bed and make sure he is not light-headed or dizzy before he starts to walk. He should sleep with the headposts of the bed elevated on wooden blocks 8 to 12 in. high. A snug elastic abdominal binder and elastic stockings are often helpful. Drugs of the ephedrine group (ephedrine sulfate, 8 to 16 mg) may be useful if they do not cause insomnia. If there are no contraindications, a high intake of sodium chloride, which expands the extracellular fluid volume, may be beneficial.

In the syndrome of chronic orthostatic hypotension special corticosteroid preparations (Florinef acetate tablets, 2 to 4 mg per day in divided doses) have given relief in some cases. Binding of the legs (G suit) and sleeping with head and shoulders elevated are helpful.

The treatment of carotid sinus syncope involves first of all instructing the patient in measures that minimize the hazards of a fall (see below). Loose collars should be worn, and the patient should learn to turn the whole body, rather than the head alone, when looking to one side. Atropine or the ephedrine group of drugs should be used, respectively, in patients with pronounced bradycardia or hypotension during the attacks. Radiation or surgical denervation of the carotid sinus has apparently yielded favorable results in some patients, but it is rarely necessary. Once the possibility has been excluded that the attacks are due to a narrowing of major cerebral arteries, emphatic reassurance is essential for such patients, the majority of whom are under the mistaken impression that strokes or cardiac disease are responsible for the episodes.

The treatment of the various cardiac arrhythmias which may induce syncope is discussed in Chap. 265. The treatment of hypoglycemia will be found in Chap. 96 and of the hyperventilation syndrome and hysterical fainting in Chaps. 366 and 370.

The chief hazard of a faint in most elderly persons is not the underlying disease but rather fracture or other trauma due to the fall. Therefore, patients subject to recurrent syncope should cover the bathroom floor and bathtub with rubber mats and should have as much of their home carpeted as is feasible. Especially important is the floor space between the bed and the bathroom, because faints are common in elderly persons when walking from bed to toilet. Outdoor walking should be on soft ground rather than hard surfaces, when possible, and the patient should avoid standing still, which is more likely than walking to induce an attack.

A number of the topics considered in this chapter are discussed elsewhere in this book. The mechanisms of the circulatory disorders which may cause syncope are considered in Chap. 36. Epilepsy as a cause of recurrent unconsciousness is discussed in Chap. 28. The hyperventilation syndrome is considered in Chap. 366.

REFERENCES

Engel, G. L.: "Fainting," Springfield, Ill., Charles C Thomas, Publisher, 1950.

Gowers, W. R.: "The Borderland of Epilepsy," London, J. A. Churchill, 1907.

21 MOTOR PARALYSIS
Raymond D. Adams

The motor system may undergo dissolution in several ways during the course of nervous disease. In diffuse progressive disorders of the cerebrum there may be disintegration first of the highest, most complex nervous organizations, including learned patterns of volitional movement, and then of more elementary ones. Thus, concepts or memories of specialized, learned movement patterns may be lost while less complicated semivolitional or automatic movements are retained. Later there may be a paralysis of all voluntary movements without change in or with exaggeration of reflexes, as decortication proceeds. In lesions of basal ganglia and cerebellum, volitional movements and normal postures are altered by the presence of abnormal movements (tremor, chorea, athetosis), abnormal postures (dystonia), or incoordination (ataxia). In lesions of the brainstem all volitional movements are abolished on one or both sides of the body with release of certain obligatory postural states (decerebrate) and with normal or enhanced spinal reflexes. In lesions of the spinal cord paralysis of voluntary movement may occur with either increase or abolition of reflex activity. In lesions of peripheral nerves and skeletal muscles all movements, learned, instinctual, automatic, postural, and reflex, are lost, since this is the final common pathway.

These and other impairments of motor function may be somewhat arbitrarily subdivided into (1) paralysis due to affection of lower motor neurones, (2) paralysis due to disorder of upper motor neurones, (3) abnormalities of coordination (ataxia) due to lesions in cerebellum, (4) abnormalities of movement and posture due to disease of extrapyramidal motor system, (5) apraxic or nonparalytic disturbances of purposive movement due to involvement of cerebrum. The first two types of motor disorder and the cerebral disorders of movement will be discussed briefly in the following pages; cerebellar ataxia and extrapyramidal motor abnormalities will be considered in Chap. 22.

DEFINITIONS. The term *paralysis* is derived from two Greek words, *para,* beside, and *lysis,* a loosening. In medicine it has come to refer to an abolition of function, either sensory or motor. When applied to voluntary muscles, paralysis means loss of contraction due to interruption of some part of the motor pathway from the cerebrum to the muscle fiber. Lesser degrees of paralysis are sometimes spoken of as *paresis,* but in everyday medical parlance motor paralysis usually stands for either partial or complete loss of function. The word *plegia* comes from the Greek word meaning stroke; and the word *palsy,* from an old French word, has the same meaning as paralysis. All these words are used interchangeably in medical practice, though it is preferable to use paresis for slight and paralysis or plegia for severe loss of motor function.

Paralysis Due to Disease of the Lower Motor Neurones

Some of the essential facts concerning the anatomy and physiology of this system of motor nerve cells are well known. A few of them deserve brief comment because they explain important clinical phenomena.

Each motor nerve cell through the extensive arborization of the terminal part of its fiber comes into contact with 100 to 200 or more muscle fibers; altogether they constitute "the motor unit." All the variations in force, range, and type of movement are determined by differences in the number and size of motor units called into activity and the frequency of their action. Feeble movements involve only a few small motor units; powerful movements recruit many more units of increasing size. When a motor neurone becomes diseased, as in progressive muscular atrophy, it may manifest increased irritability, and all the muscle fibers that it controls may discharge sporadically in isolation from other units. The result of the contraction of one or several such units is a visible twitch, or *fasciculation,* which can be recorded in the electromyogram as a large diphasic or multiphasic action potential. If the motor neurone is destroyed, all the muscle fibers to which it is attached undergo a profound atrophy, namely, denervation atrophy. For some unknown reason the individual denervated muscle fibers now begin to be sensitive to circulating acetylcholine and contract spontaneously, though they can no longer do so in response to a nerve impulse or as a part of a motor unit. This isolated activity of individual muscle fibers is called *fibrillation* and is so fine that it cannot be seen through the intact skin but can be recorded only as

a repetitive short-duration spike potential in the electromyogram (see Chap. 374).

The motor nerve fibers of each ventral root intermingle as the roots join to form plexuses, and although the innervation of the muscles is roughly metameric, or according to segments of the spinal cord, each large muscle comes to be supplied by two or more roots. For this reason the distribution of paralysis due to disease of the anterior horn cells or anterior roots differs from that which follows a lesion of a peripheral nerve.

All motor activity, even of the most elementary reflex type, requires the cooperation of several muscles. The analysis of a relatively simple movement, such as clenching the fist, affords some idea of the complexity of the underlying neural arrangements. In this act the primary movement is a contraction of the flexor muscles of the fingers, the flexor digitorum sublimis and profundus, the flexor pollicis longus and brevis, and the abductor pollicis brevis. In the terminology of Beevor, these muscles act as *agonists* or *prime movers* in this act. In order that flexion may be smooth and forceful the extensor muscles (antagonists) must relax at the same rate as the flexors contract. The muscles which flex the fingers also flex the wrist; and since it is desired that only the fingers flex, the muscles which extend the wrist must be brought into play to prevent its flexion. The action of the wrist extensors is *synergic,* and these muscles are called *synergists* in this particular act. Lastly the wrist, elbow, and shoulder must be stabilized by appropriate flexor and extensor muscles, which serve as *fixators.* The coordination of agonists, antagonists, synergists, and fixators involves reciprocal innervation and is managed by segmental spinal reflexes under the guidance of proprioceptive sensory stimuli. Only the agonist movement in a voluntary act is believed to be initiated at a cortical level.

If all or practically all peripheral motor nerves supplying a muscle are destroyed, both voluntary and reflex movements are abolished. The muscle becomes soft and yields excessively to passive stretching, a condition known as *flaccidity.* Muscle tone—the slight resistance that normal relaxed muscle offers to passive movement—is reduced (hypotonia or atonia). The denervated muscles undergo extreme atrophy, usually being reduced to 20 or 30 percent of their original bulk within 3 months. The reaction of the muscle to sudden stretch, as by tapping its tendon, is lost. And, finally, it may be demonstrated that the muscle will no longer respond to electric stimuli of short duration, i.e., faradic stimuli, but still does respond to currents of long duration, i.e., to galvanic stimuli. This alteration of electric response is known as *Erb's reaction of degeneration.* If only a part of the motor units in the muscles are affected, partial paralysis or paresis will ensue. The atrophy will be less, the tendon reflexes weakened instead of lost, and the reaction of degeneration may not be obtained. Quantitative testing by determination of strength-duration curves is a means of showing partial denervation, but electromyographic evidence of fibrillations and fasciculations may also be obtained.

The tonus of muscle and the tendon reflexes are now

known to depend on the muscle spindles and the afferent fibers to which they give origin and on the small anterior horn cells whose axones terminate on the small muscle fibers within the spindles. These small spinal motor neurones are called *gamma neurones* in contrast to the large *alpha neurones*. A tap on a tendon, by stretching the spindle muscle fibers, activates afferent neurones which transmit impulses to alpha motor neurones. The result is the familiar brief muscle contraction or tendon reflex. The spindle muscle fibers are then relaxed (unloaded), which terminates the reflex. Thus the setting of the spindle fibers and the state of excitability of the gamma neurones (normally inhibited by the corticospinal fibers and other supranuclear neurones) determine the level of activity of the tendon reflexes and the responsiveness of muscle to stretch. Other mechanisms of inhibitory nature, involving Golgi tendon organs, are brought into play in more powerful stretching of muscle.

Lower motor neurone paralysis is the direct result of physiologic arrest or destruction of anterior horn cells or their axones in anterior roots and nerves. The signs and symptoms vary according to the location of the lesion. Probably the most important question for clinical purposes is whether sensory changes coexist. The combination of flaccid, areflexic paralysis and sensory changes usually indicates involvement of mixed motor and sensory nerves or affection of both anterior and posterior roots. If sensory changes are absent, the lesion must be situated in the gray matter of the spinal cord, in the anterior roots, in a purely motor branch of a peripheral nerve, or in motor axones alone. The distinction between nuclear

(spinal) and anterior root (radicular) lesions may at times be impossible to make. The presence of spasticity in muscles weakened by a spinal lesion points to the integrity of the segments below the level of the lesion.

Paralysis Due to Disease of the Upper Motor Neurones

Several anatomic and physiologic facts concerning the upper motor neurones are worthy of note. It was formerly believed that the corticospinal tract originated from the large motor cell of Betz in the fifth layer of the precentral convolution. However, there are only about 25,000 to 30,000 Betz cells, whereas the pyramidal tract at the level of the medulla contains approximately 1 million axones. This tract must, therefore, contain many fibers that arise not from the giant Betz cells of the motor cortex (area 4 of Brodmann) but rather from the smaller Betz cells of area 4 and the cells of the adjacent precentral area 6) and postcentral cortex (areas 1, 2, 3, 5, 7). Numerous research workers have questioned the premotor, motor, and parietal cortical origin of all the fibers of the pyramid. Some are said to arise in other parts of the cerebrum or basal ganglia, and Brodal and his associates believe that some ascend from spinal cord. The most critical degeneration studies of van Crevel, however, have shown that when areas 4, 6, 1, 2, 3, 5, and 7 are removed in the cat, if one waits several months, all will be found degenerated and none can be traced to other parts of the cerebral cortex. The pyramidal tract is the only long fiber connection between the cerebrum and the spinal cord. At the level of the internal capsule these corticospinal fibers are intermingled with many others destined to end in the globus pallidus, substantia pallidus, substantia nigra, and reticular substance and with others ascending from the thalamus. The fibers to the cranial nerve nuclei become separated at about the level of the midbrain and cross the midline to the contralateral cranial nerve nuclei (Fig. 21-1). These fibers form the corticomesencephalic, corticopontine, and corticobulbar tracts. The decussation of the pyramidal tract at the lower end of the medulla is variable in different individuals. A small number of fibers, 10 to 20 percent, do not cross but descend ipsilaterally as the uncrossed pyramidal tract. Exceptionally, all of them cross; rarely, none. The termination of the corticospinal tract is in relation to nerve cells in the intermediate zone of gray matter, and not more than 10 to 15 percent establish direct synaptic connection with anterior horn cells. These new facts derived from degeneration studies must of necessity modify current views of the anatomy of the pyramidal tract and suggest new interpretations.

The motor area of the cerebral cortex is difficult to define. It includes that part of the precentral convolution which contains Betz cells, but as already mentioned, it probably extends anteriorly into area 6 and posteriorly into the anterior parietal lobe, where it overlaps the sensory areas. Physiologically it is defined as the region of electrically excitable cortex from which isolated movements can be evoked by stimuli of minimal intensity. The

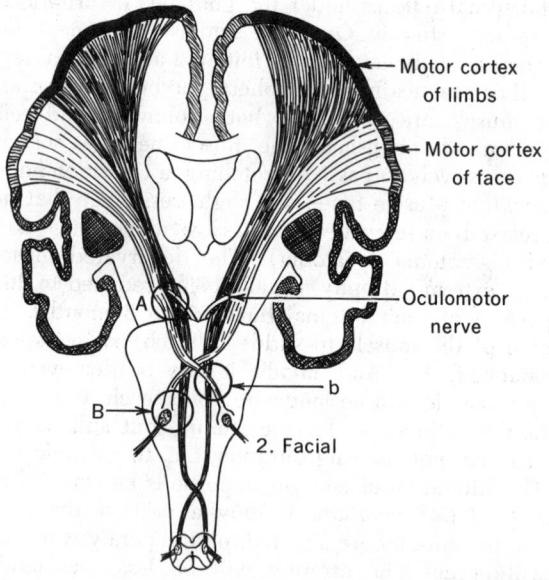

Fig. 21-1. Diagram of the corticospinal and corticobulbar tracts. Lesion at (*A*) produces ipsilateral oculomotor palsy and contralateral paralysis involving face, arm, and leg. Lesion at (*B*) causes ipsilateral facial paralysis of peripheral type and contralateral paralysis of arm and leg. Lesion at (*b*) results in ipsilateral facial weakness of upper motor neurone of central type and contralateral paralysis of arm and leg. (*Bergmann and Staeheln: "Krankheiten des Nervensystems," Berlin, Springer-Verlag, 1939.*)

Motor cortex of limbs

Motor cortex of face

Oculomotor nerve

A

b

B

2. Facial

muscle groups of the contralateral face, arm, trunk, and leg are represented in the motor cortex, those of the face being at the lower end of the precentral convolution and those of the leg in the paracentral lobule on the medial surface of the cerebral hemisphere. These motor points are not fixed but vary somewhat with the conditions of previous stimulation. The parts of the body capable of the most delicate movements have, in general, the largest cortical representation.

Table 21-1. DIFFERENCES BETWEEN PARALYSIS OF UPPER AND LOWER NEURONE TYPES

Upper, supranuclear motor paralysis	Lower, spinomuscular, or infranuclear paralysis
Muscle groups affected diffusely, never individual muscles	Individual muscles may be affected
Atrophy slight and due to disuse	Atrophy pronounced, 70 to 80 percent of total bulk
Spasticity with hyperactivity of the tendon reflexes	Flaccidity and hypotonia of affected muscles with loss of tendon reflexes
Babinski sign	Plantar reflex, if present, is of normal flexor type
Fascicular twitches not produced	Fascicular twitches may be present
Normal reactions to galvanic and faradic current	Loss of faradic reaction, retention of galvanic action (reaction of degeneration)

Area 6, the premotor area, is also electrically excitable but requires more intense stimuli to evoke movements, and the movements produced are more complex than those evoked from area 4. Very strong stimuli elicit movements from a wide area of premotor frontal and parietal cortex, and the same movements may be obtained from several points. From this it may be assumed that one of the functions of the motor cortex is to synthesize simple movements into an infinite variety of finely graded, highly differentiated patterns.

Upper motor neurone paralysis may be due to lesions in the cerebral cortex, subcortical white matter, internal capsule, brainstem, or spinal cord. The distribution of the paralysis varies with the locale of the lesion, but there are also other typical features. Paralysis due to a lesion of the upper motor neurones always involves a group of muscles, never individual muscles, and if any movement is possible, the proper relationships between antagonist, synergists, and fixators are always preserved. The paralysis never involves all the muscles on one side of the body, even in the hemiplegia resulting from a complete lesion of the corticospinal tract. Movements that are invariably bilateral, such as those of the eyes, jaw, pharynx, larynx, neck, thorax, and abdomen, are little if at all affected. The hand and arm muscles suffer most severely, the leg muscles next, and of the cranial musculature only the muscles of the lower face and tongue are involved to any significant degree. Broadbent was the first to call attention to this distribution of

paralysis, and this predilection of certain muscles to paralysis with pyramidal tract disease is referred to as *Broadbent's law.* Paralysis of pyramidal type is rarely complete for any long period of time, and in this respect it differs from the total and absolute paralysis due to a lesion of the lower motor neurones. The paralyzed arm may suddenly move during yawning or stretching, and various other reflex activities can be elicited at all times. However, acute disorders may abolish function in parts of the nervous system distant from the site of the lesion. For example, a sudden lesion of the pyramidal tract in the cervical spinal cord may not only cause paralysis of voluntary movements but also abolish all of the spinal reflexes. This is known as *spinal shock.* It usually lasts but a few days or weeks and is replaced by spasticity of the paralyzed muscles. This phenomenon of *spasticity* is another characteristic of lesions of the upper motor neurones and is due to a release of spinal reflex mechanisms or the release of a "normal component in movement from its natural competitor" (Denny-Brown). Spasticity does not appear immediately after the onset of a sudden lesion but develops gradually over several weeks. In exceptional cases the paralyzed limbs remain flaccid. The spasticity affects some muscle groups more than others. The arm is usually held in a flexed position, and any attempts to extend it encounter resistance, which is maximal at the beginning and then yields (clasp-knife phenomenon). The leg is maintained in an extended position, and passive flexion is resisted. If the limbs are moved to a new position, either flexion or extension, that position is maintained (shortening and lengthening reaction). If patients have suffered paresis due to a lesion of the pyramidal tract, they not infrequently display associated movements upon attempting to carry out a voluntary movement with the weak limb. Attempts to flex the arm may result in involuntary pronation (the pronation phenomenon); or when the hemiplegic leg is flexed, the foot may automatically dorsiflex and evert (Strümpell's tibialis phenomenon). When the patient is asked to make alternating movements with the paretic limb, the healthy limb may mimic these movements (i.e., *mirror movements*).

Table 21-1, modified from Stewart, shows the main differences between paralyses of the lower and those of the upper motor neurones.

APRAXIC OR NONPARALYTIC DISORDERS OF MOTOR FUNCTION

Aside from upper and lower motor neurone paralysis with cerebral lesions there may be loss of purposive movement without paralysis. This is called *apraxia* and may be explained as follows. Many simple actions are acquired by learning or practice. These depend on the formation of movement patterns, particularly those which involve manufacture, i.e., the use of tools and instruments as well as gestures. Once established, they are remembered and may be reproduced under the proper circumstances. Any purposive act may be conceived as occurring in several stages. First, the idea of an act must be aroused in the mind of the patient by an appropriate stimulus situation, perhaps by a spoken command to do something. This idea or concept is then translated into action by excitation of patterns of premotor or motor cortical neurones in proper sequence, which are transmitted to lower centers by the corticospinal tracts. These latter initiate particular movements of individual muscle groups but also modify or suppress the subcortical mechanisms that control the basic attitudes and postures of the body. In right-handed and most left-handed individuals the neural mechanisms for the formulation of an idea of an act (motor schema or image) in response to a spoken command or a verbal stimulus and its reproduction are believed to be centered in the posterior and inferior part of the left parietal lobe, near the angular gyrus; these areas, near the language mechanism, are connected with the left premotor regions for the control of the right hand and with the motor areas of the right cerebral hemisphere through the corpus callosum for the control of the left side.

A failure to execute certain acts in the correct context while retaining the individual movements upon which such acts depend is the main feature of *apraxia*. The most adequate clinical test of motor deficits of this type is to observe a series of self-initiated actions such as using a comb, a razor, a toothbrush, or a common tool, or gesturing, i.e., waving goodbye, saluting, shaking the fist as though angry, or blowing a kiss. These may be called forth by a command or a request to imitate the examiner. Of course, failure to follow a spoken or written request may be due to aphasia that prevents understanding of what is asked, or an agnosia may prevent recognition of the tool or object to be used. But aside from these sources of difficulty there remains a peculiar motor deficit in which the patient appears to understand but has lost his memory of how to perform a given act, especially if called upon for it in an unnatural setting. He is said then to have *ideational apraxia*. Or he may have the idea of what he wants to do or what others command him to do but cannot translate the idea of the sequence of movements into a precise well-executed act. This is called *ideomotor apraxia*. The failure is evident both after spoken command and in requests to imitate the gestures of the examiner. Sometimes these two conditions may be dissociated; the patient, while not aphasic, cannot execute a spoken command but can still imitate the act if it is called forth by gesture. Finally there is a disorder of movement sequences which consists of an inexplicable ineptitude in the use of a part of the body for all actions. This is called *motor* or *kinetic apraxia*. Apraxia may be limited to only one group of muscles, such as tongue or lips as in Broca's aphasia (see Chap. 29). Confused or demented patients may fail entirely to understand what the examiner requests and be unable to perform many self-initiated actions. They have ideational apraxia. If this deficit can be singled out, it reflects a specific loss of certain learned patterns of movement (a "specific amnesia" so to speak, analogous to the amnesia of words in aphasia). The added element of mental confusion tends usually to obscure the disorder.

Thus, ideational apraxia is most often manifest in diffuse or bilateral cerebral lesions; ideomotor apraxia means major hemisphere parietal disease, and the effect is bilateral; left-sided ideomotor apraxia indicates a lesion in the corpus callosum and adjacent white matter of one or other hemisphere; motor (kinetic) apraxia signifies a lesion in the premotor cortex opposite to the affected hand.

The latter lesions (of areas 6 and 8) which leave the more posterior part of the motor and the sensory cortex intact have an added feature in that many voluntary movements, while retained, are slow and awkward. Moreover, grasping and sucking reflexes are manifest. The tendon reflexes are lively, and the plantar reflexes are flexor. In some cases in which basal ganglia are also involved voluntary contractions of hand and foot may persist unduly on tactile stimulation of the palmar and plantar surfaces, so that the patient is unable to release his grip or dorsiflex his foot (*tonic innervation*) voluntarily even after the stimulus is removed. In lesions of the parietal lobe a whole series of aversion or avoidance reactions to sensory stimuli become manifest. For a more complete discussion of the several types of apraxia, see Chap. 30.

Examination Scheme for Motor Paralysis and Apraxia

The first step is to inspect the paralyzed limb, taking note first of its posture and of the presence or absence of muscle atrophy, hypertrophy, and fascicular twitchings. The patient is then called upon to move each muscle group, and the power and facility of movement are graded and recorded. The range of passive movement is then determined by moving all the joints. This provides information concerning alterations of muscle tone, i.e., hypotonia, spasticity, and rigidity. Dislocations, disease of joints, and ankyloses may also be revealed by these same maneuvers. Muscle bulk is then inspected. Slight atrophy may be due to disuse from any cause, i.e., pain, fixation as the result of a cast, or any type of paralysis. A pronounced atrophy usually occurs only with denervation of several weeks' or months' standing.

The tendon reflexes are then tested. The usual routine is to try to elicit the jaw jerk (increased in pseudobulbar palsy) and the supinator, biceps, triceps, quadriceps, and Achilles tendon reflexes. Two cutaneous reflexes are then tested, the abdominal and the plantar reflexes. (The extensor plantar reflex is Babinski's sign.)

If there is no evidence of upper or lower motor neurone disease, but certain acts are nonetheless imperfectly performed, one should look for a disorder of postural sensibility or of cerebellar coordination or rigidity with abnormality of posture and movement due to disease of the basal ganglions (cf. Chap. 22). In the absence of these disorders, the possibility of an apraxic disorder can be investigated by watching the patient's own movements and those called forth by specific command and gesture.

Hysterical paralysis may pose problems. Usually it is

easily distinguished from chronic lower motor neurone disease by the areflexia and severe atrophy that are so characteristic of the latter condition. Diagnostic difficulty arises only in certain acute cases of upper motor neurone disease that lack all the usual changes in reflexes and muscle tone. In hysterical paralysis one arm or one leg or all one side of the body may be affected. The hysterical gait is sometimes diagnostic in itself (see Chap. 23). Often there is loss of sensation in the paralyzed parts and sometimes loss of sight in the eye, of hearing in the ear, and of smell in the nostril on the paralyzed side, a group of sensory changes that is never seen in organic brain disease. The patient should be asked to move the affected limbs; as he does so, the movement is seen to be slow and jerky, often with contraction of both agonist and antagonist muscles simultaneously or intermittently. Hoover's sign and Babinski's combined leg flexion test are helpful in distinguishing hysterical from organic hemiplegia. To elicit Hoover's sign, the patient, lying on his back, is asked to raise one leg from the bed against resistance; in a normal individual the back of the heel of the contralateral leg is pressed firmly down, and the same is true when the patient with organic hemiplegia attempts to lift the paralyzed leg. The hysteric exerts little force with the good leg or will contract it more strongly under these circumstances than as a primary willed action. To carry out Babinski's combined leg flexion test, a patient with an organic hemiplegia is asked to sit up without using his arms; when he does so, the paralyzed or weak leg flexes at the hip, and the heel is lifted from the bed while the heel of the sound leg is pressed into the bed. This sign is absent in hysterical hemiplegia.

DIFFERENTIAL DIAGNOSIS OF PARALYSIS

The diagnostic consideration of paralysis may be simplified by the following subdivisions, which relate to the location and distribution of weakness.

1. *Monoplegia* refers to weakness or paralysis of all the muscles in one limb, whether leg or arm. It should not be applied to paralysis of isolated muscles or groups of muscles supplied by a single nerve or motor root.

2. *Hemiplegia* is the commonest distribution of paralysis—loss of strength in arm, leg, and sometimes face on one side of the body.

3. *Paraplegia* indicates weakness or paralysis of both legs. It is most commonly found in spinal cord disease.

4. *Quadriplegia* indicates weakness of all four extremities. It may result from lesions involving peripheral nerves, gray matter of the spinal cord, or corticospinal tracts bilaterally in the cervical cord, upper brainstem, or cerebrum. *Diplegia* is a special form of quadriplegia in which the legs are affected more than the arms.

5. *Isolated paralyses* refer to weakness localized to one or more muscle groups.

MONOPLEGIA

The physical examination of patients who complain of weakness of one extremity often discloses an unnoticed weakness in another limb, and the condition is actually hemiplegia or paraplegia. Or instead of weakness of all the muscles in a limb, only isolated groups are found to be affected. Ataxia, sensory disturbances, or pain in an extremity will often be interpreted by the patient as weakness, as will the mechanical limitation resulting from arthritis or the rigidity of parkinsonism.

In general, the presence or absence of atrophy of muscles in a monoplegic limb can be of diagnostic help.

PARALYSIS WITHOUT MUSCULAR ATROPHY. Long-continued disuse of a limb may lead to atrophy, but this is usually not so marked as in diseases that denervate muscles; the tendon reflexes are normal, and the response of the muscles to electric stimulation and electromyogram are unaltered.

The most frequent cause of monoplegia without muscular wasting is a lesion of the cerebral cortex. Only occasionally does it occur in diseases which interrupt the corticospinal tract at the level of the internal capsule, brainstem, or spinal cord. A vascular lesion (thrombosis or embolus) is commonest, but of course, a tumor or abscess may have the same effect. Multiple sclerosis and spinal cord tumor, early in their course, may cause weakness of one extremity, usually the leg. As indicated above, weakness due to damage to the corticospinal system is usually accompanied by spasticity, increased reflexes, and an extensor plantar reflex (Babinski's sign), and the electric reactions and electromyogram are normal. However, acute diseases that destroy the motor tracts in the spinal cord may at first (for several days) reduce the tendon reflexes and cause hypotonia (the condition known as *spinal shock*). This does not occur in partial or slowly evolving lesions and occurs only to minimal degree in lesions of brainstem and cerebrum. In acute diseases affecting the lower motor neurones the tendon reflexes are always reduced or abolished, but atrophy may not appear for several weeks. Hence one must take into account the mode of onset and the duration of the disease in evaluating the tendon reflexes, muscle tone, and degree of atrophy before reaching an anatomic diagnosis.

PARALYSIS WITH MUSCULAR ATROPHY. This condition is more frequent than paralysis without muscular atrophy. In addition to the paralysis and reduced or abolished tendon reflexes, there may be visible fasciculations. If completely paralyzed, the muscles exhibit an electric reaction of degeneration and the electromyogram shows reduced numbers of motor units (often of large size), fasciculations at rest, and fibrillations. The lesion may be in the spinal cord, spinal roots, or peripheral nerves. Its location can usually be decided by the distribution of the palsied muscles (whether the pattern is one of nerve, spinal root, or spinal cord involvement), by the associated neurologic symptoms and signs, and by special tests (cerebrospinal fluid examination, x-ray of spine, and myelogram).

Brachial atrophic monoplegia is relatively rare, and when present, it should suggest in an infant a brachial plexus trauma, in a child poliomyelitis, in an adult poliomyelitis, syringomyelia, amyotrophic lateral sclerosis, or brachial plexus lesions. Crural monoplegia is more frequent and may be caused by any lesion of thoracic or lumbar cord, i.e., trauma, tumor, myelitis, multiple sclerosis, etc. It should be noted that multiple sclerosis almost never causes atrophy and that ruptured intervertebral disk and the many varieties of neuritis rarely paralyze all or most of the muscles of a limb. Muscle dystrophy may begin in one limb, but by the time the patient is seen the typical more or less symmetric pattern of proximal limb and trunk involvement is evident. A unilateral retroperitoneal tumor may paralyze the leg by implicating the lumbosacral plexus.

HEMIPLEGIA

This is the most frequent distribution of paralysis in man. With rare exceptions (a few unusual cases of poliomyelitis or motor system disease) this pattern of paralysis is due to involvement of the corticospinal tract.

LOCATION OF LESION PRODUCING HEMIPLEGIA. The site or level of the lesion, i.e., cerebral, capsular, brain stem, or spinal cord, can usually be deduced from the associated neurologic findings. Diseases localized in the cerebral cortex, cerebral white matter (corona radiata), and internal capsule usually evoke weakness or paralysis of the face, arm, and leg on the opposite side. The occurrence of convulsive seizures or the presence of a defect in speech (aphasia), a cortical type of sensory loss (astereognosis, loss of two-point discrimination, etc.), anosognosia, or defects in the visual fields suggest a cortical or subcortical location.

Damage to the corticospinal tract in the upper portion of the brain stem (see Fig. 21-1) may cause paralysis of the face, arm, and leg on the opposite side. The lesion in such cases is localized by the presence of a paralysis of the muscles supplied by the oculomotor nerve on the same side as the lesion (Weber's syndrome) or other neurologic findings. With low pontine lesions a unilateral abducens or facial palsy is combined with a contralateral weakness or paralysis of the arm and leg (Millard-Gubler syndrome). Lesions of the lowermost part of the brain stem, i.e., in the medulla, affect the tongue and sometimes the pharynx and larynx on one side and arm and leg on the other side. These "crossed paralyses," so common in brainstem diseases, are described in Chap. 355.

Rarely, a homolateral hemiplegia may be caused by a lesion in the lateral column of the cervical spinal cord. At this level, however, the pathologic process often induces bilateral signs, with resulting quadriparesis or quadriplegia. If one side of the spinal cord is extensively damaged, the homolateral paralysis is combined with a loss of vibratory and position sense on the same side and a contralateral loss of pain and temperature (Brown-Séquard syndrome).

Muscle atrophy of minor degree often follows lesions of the corticospinal system but never reaches the proportions seen in diseases of the lower motor neurones. The atrophy is due to disuse. When the motor cortex and adjacent parts of the parietal lobe are damaged in infancy or childhood, the normal development of the muscles and the skeletal system in the affected limbs is retarded. The palsied limbs and even the trunk on one side are small.

This does not occur if the paralysis begins after the greater part of skeletal growth is attained (after puberty). In the hemiplegia due to spinal cord injury muscles at the level of the lesion atrophy as a result of damage to anterior horn cells or ventral roots.

CAUSES OF HEMIPLEGIA. In this condition vascular diseases of the cerebrum and brainstem exceed all others in frequency. Trauma (brain contusion, epidural and subdural hemorrhage) ranks second, and other diseases such as brain tumor, brain abscess and encephalitis, demyelinative diseases, complications of meningitis, tuberculosis, and syphilis are of decreasing order of importance. Most of these diseases can be diagnosed by the mode of evolution and the conjoined clinical and laboratory data presented in the chapters on neurologic diseases. For further discussion see Chap. 357.

PARAPLEGIA

Paralysis of both lower extremities may occur in diseases of the spinal cord and the spinal roots or of the peripheral nerves. If onset is acute, it may be difficult to distinguish spinal from neural paralysis, for in any acute myelopathy spinal shock may result in abolition of reflexes and flaccidity. As a rule in acute spinal cord diseases with involvement of corticospinal tracts, the paralysis affects all muscles below a given level; and often, if the white matter is extensively damaged, sensory loss below a particular level (loss of pain and temperature with lateral spinothalamic tracts and loss of vibratory and position sense with posterior columns) is conjoined. Also, in bilateral disease of the spinal cord, the bladder and bowel sphincters are paralyzed. Alterations of cerebrospinal fluid (dynamic block, increase in protein or cells) are frequent. In peripheral nerve diseases both sensory and motor loss tend to involve the distal muscles of the legs more than the proximal ones (an exception is acute idiopathic polyneuritis), and the sphincters are often spared or only briefly deranged in function. Sensory loss, if present, is more likely to consist in distal impairment of touch, vibration, and position sense, with pain and temperature spared in many instances. The cerebrospinal fluid protein may be normal or elevated.

For clinical purposes it is helpful to consider separately the acute and the chronic paraplegias and to divide the chronic ones into two groups, those which occur in infancy and those which begin in adult life.

Acute paraplegia, beginning at any age, is relatively infrequent. Fracture dislocation of the spine with traumatic necrosis of the spinal cord, spontaneous hematomyelia with bleeding from a vascular malformation (angioma, telangiectasis), thrombosis of a spinal artery with infarction (myelomalacia), and dissecting aortic aneurysm or atherosclerotic occlusion of nutrient spinal arteries arising from the aorta with resulting infarction (myelomalacia) are the commonest varieties of sudden paraplegia (or quadriplegia, if the cervical cord is involved). Postinfectious or postvaccinal myelitis, acute demyelinative myelitis (Devic's disease if the optic nerves are affected), necrotizing myelitis, and epidural abscess or tumor with spinal cord compression tend to develop somewhat more slowly, over a period of hours or days, or they may have a subacute onset. Poliomyelitis and acute idiopathic polyneuritis, the former a purely motor disorder with meningitis, the latter predominantly motor but often with minimal sensory disturbances (paresthesias or objectively demonstrated impairment), must be distinguished from the other acute myelopathies and from one another.

In pediatric practice, delay in starting to walk and difficulty in walking are common problems. These conditions may be associated with a systemic disease such as rickets or may indicate mental deficiency or, more commonly, some muscular or neurologic disease. Congenital cerebral disease accounts for a majority of cases of infantile diplegia (weakness predominant in the legs, with the arms minimally affected). Present at birth or manifest in the first months of life, it may appear to progress; but actually it is stationary and only becomes apparent as the motor system develops. Later there may seem to be slow improvement as a result of the normal maturation processes of childhood. Congenital malformation of the spinal cord or birth injury of the spinal cord are other possibilities. Friedreich's ataxia and familial paraplegia, progressive muscular dystrophy, and the chronic varieties of polyneuritis tend to appear later during childhood and adolescence and are slowly progressive.

In adult life multiple sclerosis, subacute combined degeneration, spinal cord tumor, ruptured cervical disk and cervical spondylosis, syphilitic meningomyelitis, chronic epidural infections (fungous and other granulomatous diseases), Erb's spastic paraplegia and motor system disease, and syringomyelia represent the most frequently encountered forms of spinal paraplegia. (See Chap. 356 for discussion of these spinal cord diseases.) The several varieties of polyneuritis and polymyositis must be considered in their differential diagnosis, for they, too, may cause paraparesis.

QUADRIPLEGIA

All that has been written about the common causes of paraplegia applies to quadriplegia. The lesion is usually in the cervical rather than the thoracic or lumbar segments of the spinal cord. If it is situated in the low cervical segments and involves the anterior half of the spinal cord, as in occlusion of the anterior spinal artery, the arm paralysis may be flaccid and areflexic and the leg paralysis spastic (anterior spinal syndrome). There are only a few points of difference between the common paraplegic and quadriplegic syndromes. In infants, aside from developmental abnormalities and anoxia of birth, an inherited cerebral disease (Schilder's disease, metachromatic leukoencephalopathy, lipid storage disease) may be responsible for a quadriparesis or quadriplegia. Congenital forms of muscular dystrophy may be recognized soon after birth and also infantile muscular atrophy (Hoffmann-Werdnig disease).

In adults repeated cerebral vascular accidents may lead to bilateral hemiplegia, usually accompanied by pseudobulbar palsy.

ISOLATED PARALYSIS

Paralysis of isolated muscle groups usually indicates a lesion of one or more peripheral nerves. The diagnosis of a lesion of an individual peripheral nerve is made on the presence of weakness or paralysis of the muscle or group of muscles and impairment or loss of sensation in the distribution of the nerve in question. Complete transection or severe injury to a peripheral nerve is usually followed by atrophy of the muscles it innervates and by loss of their tendon reflexes. Trophic changes in the skin, nails, and subcutaneous tissue may also occur.

Knowledge of the muscular and sensory function of each individual nerve is needed for a satisfactory diagnosis. Since lesions of the peripheral nerves are relatively uncommon in civil life, it is not practical for the general physician to keep all these facts in his memory, and a textbook of anatomy or Chap. 354, the Section on mononeuropathies, should be consulted. It is, however, of considerable importance to decide whether the lesion is a temporary one of conduction only (neuropraxia) or whether there has been a pathologic dissolution of continuity, requiring nerve regeneration for recovery. Electromyography may be of value here.

All the diseases mentioned in the differential diagnosis of monoplegia, hemiplegia, paraplegia, and quadriplegia will be discussed in the chapters on neurologic diseases.

MUSCULAR PARALYSIS AND SPASM UNATTENDED BY VISIBLE CHANGE IN NERVE OR MUSCLE

A discussion of motor paralysis would not be complete without some reference to a group of diseases that appear to have no basis in visible structural change in motor nerve cells, nerve fibers, motor end-plates, and muscular fibers. This group is comprised of myasthenia gravis, myotonia congenita (Thomsen's disease), familial periodic paralysis, disorders of potassium, sodium, calcium, and magnesium metabolism, tetany, tetanus, botulinus poisoning, black widow spider bite, and the thyroid myopathies. In these diseases, each of which possesses a fairly distinctive clinical picture, the abnormality is purely biochemical, and even if the patient survives for a long time, no visible microscopic changes develop. An understanding of these diseases requires knowledge of the processes involved in nerve and muscle excitation and in the contraction of muscle. They will be discussed in Chaps. 377 and 378.

22 TREMOR, CHORIA, ATHETOSIS, ATAXIA AND OTHER ABNORMALITIES OF MOVEMENT AND POSTURE

Raymond D. Adams

In this chapter are discussed the automatic, static, and less modifiable postural activities of the human nervous system. These are believed, on good evidence, to be an expression of the activity of the *older motor system,* meaning, according to S. A. K. Wilson, who introduced this term, the extrapyramidal motor structures in the basal ganglions and brainstem.

In health, the activities of both the old (extrapyramidal) and the new (pyramidal) motor system are blended. The static postural activities of the former are indispensable to voluntary, or willed, movement of the latter.

This close association of the pyramidal and extrapyramidal systems is shown by human disease. Lesions of the pyramidal tract result not only in paralysis of volitional movements of the contralateral half of the body but in the appearance of a fixed posture or attitude in which the arm is maintained in flexion and the leg in extension (predilection type of Wernicke-Mann or hemiplegic dystonia of Denny-Brown). Similarly, decerebration from a lesion in the upper pons or midbrain releases another posture in which all four extremities are extended and the cervical and thoracolumbar spine dorsiflexed. In these released action patterns one has evidence of extrapyramidal postural and righting reflexes which are mediated through bulbospinal and other brainstem structures.

The student may be dismayed to read in current articles trenchant criticism of the validity of the concept of the pyramidal tract and division of motor system into pyramidal and extrapyramidal. Extremists claim the pyramidal tract may be severed in animals and even in men without lasting motor deficits. But it must be remembered that this tract is such a puny thing in most mammals, even in small monkeys, that it can hardly be compared to that of man, and there has yet to be a pathologically proven example in man of complete interruption of this tract with preserved voluntary motor function.

If an oversimplification may be permitted for clarity of exposition, the extrapyramidal motor system may be subdivided into two parts: (1) the striato-pallidonigral and (2) the cerebellar. Disease in either of these parts will result in disturbances of movement and posture without significant paralysis. These two major systems and the symptoms that result when they are diseased are reviewed on the following pages.

THE BASAL GANGLIA: PHARMACOLOGY AND PATHOLOGICAL ANATOMY

As an anatomic entity the basal ganglia have no precise limitation. The list of basal structures originally thought to have some part in motor function, such as the caudate and lenticular nuclei and amygdaloid body, has been greatly expanded by physiologists to include the field of Forel and zona incerta, subthalamic nucleus of Luys, substantia nigra, red nucleus, dentate nucleus of cerebellum, and the reticular formation of the brainstem. The anatomic connections between these structures and other parts of the brain, such as with the cerebral cortex and afferent sensory systems, are too intricate to present

in a textbook of medicine. The reader must refer to a neuroanatomy textbook.

Perhaps the principal new anatomic idea to emerge in recent years is the central position that the *ventrolateral nucleus of the thalamus* plays in the ascending limb of circuits which involve the cortex-pons-cerebellum-dentate nucleus-*thalamus*-cortex, and the cortex-striatum-subthalamic nucleus and substantia nigra-*thalamus*-cortex. Indeed it would seem that all the extrapyramidal motor systems at this level of the nervous system are funneled through the ventrolateral nucleus up to the motor cortex and pyramidal system. Descending pathways to the spinal cord are disputed; probably there are polysynaptic descending systems of fibers through the reticular formation of pons and medulla. It is noteworthy that some of the descending and ascending systems from and to the cortex pass through the internal capsule, hence lesions here and in the cerebral white matter may simultaneously involve both pyramidal and extrapyramidal systems.

A second and most exciting development of recent years has been in the biochemistry and pharmacology of the basal ganglia. In man the substantia nigra, putamen, and caudatum are rich in norepinephrine. Precursors of this substance are shown in the following metabolic pathway:

L—phenylalanine
   hydroxylase
L—Tyrosine
   oxidase
L—Dopa (3–4 hydroxyphenylalanine)—Dopaquinone—Indolquinone—melanin
   decarboxylase
L—Dopamine—homoprotocatechuric acid—homovanillic acid
   oxidase
L—Norepinephrine
   methylase
L—Epinephrine

Dopa is seen to be a step not only in the metabolism of norepinephrine but also of melanin. The former is an important intercellular transmitter substance; the latter is contained in the pigmented neurones of substantia nigra and other brainstem nuclei which degenerate in Parkinson's disease.

This new field of neuropharmacology opened up when it was discovered that prolonged use of tranquilizer medication such as reserpine and chlorpromazine induced Parkinson's syndrome and many other disorders of the extrapyramidal system such as athetosis and other dyskinesias of neck and spinal musculature. Some of these disorders have been permanent, persisting for months and years after the drugs were discontinued; usually they are transitory. Interestingly, reserpine depletes the striatum (putamen and caudate nuclei) of its norepinephrine unless iproniazid is given beforehand or at the same time. The quantity of dopa in the striatum and substantia nigra is diminished in Parkinson's disease. It can be replenished by giving dopa orally or intravenously, with concomitant reduction in extrapyramidal symptomatology.

Some of the most significant facts about clinicopathologic relationships in man are to be found in the writings of a number of famous neurologists. In 1912 S. A. K. Wilson delineated the syndrome of chronic lenticular degeneration, and at about the same time Van Woerkem observed a disturbance of cerebral function in other forms of liver disease. In 1920 Oskar and Cecile Vogt described a number of other motor disturbances associated with lesions limited to the striatum. Lewy was one of the first to describe the pathology of paralysis agitans, and Tretiakoff (in postencephalitic forms) and Hassler (in paralysis agitans) subsequently established the localization of at least part of the lesions in the substantia nigra. The thorough studies of Huntington's chorea by Bielschowsky in 1919 related the choreoathetosis to lesions in the caudate nucleus and putamen. A long series of observations, the most recent ones being those of J. Purdon Martin, have demonstrated the relationship between hemiballismus and lesions in the subthalamic nucleus of Luys.

Unfortunately, many of the classic cases leave much to be desired. In some instances the disease process was of diffuse type, and many other parts of the brain were affected, as in Wilson's hepatolenticular degeneration. Also, lack of quantitative neuropathologic methods hampered progress in the field. Even now the topography of the pathologic findings in several of these diseases (e.g., dystonia musculorum deformans) has not been fully determined.

Table 22-1 presents clinicopathologic correlations accepted by many neurologists; however, there is still much uncertainty as to finer details.

The symptoms that lend themselves best to clinical analysis are akinesia, rigidity, chorea, athetosis, dystonia, and tremor.

AKINESIA

When analyzed along classic neurologic lines, into primary functional deficits and secondary release effects, akinesia stands as the negative or deficit symptom of extrapyramidal disease. By the term *akinesia* one refers to the disinclination of the patient to use an affected part of the body, to engage it freely in all the natural actions of the body. Paralysis, the negative symptom of pyramidal disease, is different in that there is diminution of strength in the part and it cannot be used effectively in the desired movement. In this respect, too, it is unlike apraxia, where movements are lost because of a lesion which erases the memory of the motor schema which combines sequence of movements to form an intended action. The parkinsonian patient exhibits the phenomenon of akinesia most clearly in his extreme underactivity. He sits motionless for long times. In looking to the side he moves his eyes not his head. In arising from a chair he fails to make all the little adjustments needed (putting feet back, putting hands on arms of chair, etc.). Yet he is not weak (paretic) or apraxic. Formerly, akinesia was attributed to rigidity, which could reasonably hamper all movements, but now that stereotaxic surgery can abolish both tremor and rigidity it becomes clear that the motor deficit or akinesia is still there. Strictly interpreted it would appear that, apart from their contribution to the maintenance of postures, the basal ganglia must provide something essential to the performance of the large variety of semiautomatic actions that make up the full repertoire of natural human mobility.

A point of interest is whether akinesia is an invariable manifestation of all extrapyramidal diseases, without which there could be no secondary release effects such as flexion dystonia, athetosis, chorea, and rigidity. The question has no clear answer. While seemingly true of Huntington's and Sydenham's chorea, double athetosis, and Parkinson's disease, one cannot be sure of the existence of either akinesia or paralysis in hemiballismus.

ALTERATIONS OF MUSCLE TONE (SPASTICITY, RIGIDITY, HYPOTONIA)

Already it has been pointed out that muscle tone (the small resistance to muscle stretch offered by healthy muscle) is enhanced in the many conditions that cause a paralysis of voluntary movement by interrupting the corticospinal tract. The special distribution of the increased tone, i.e., greater in antigravity muscles (extensors of leg and flexors of the arm in man), the sudden augmentation of tone with gradual yielding upon quick movement (the

Table 22-1. CLINICOPATHOLOGIC CORRELATIONS

Symptoms	Principal location of morbid anatomy
Unilateral plastic rigidity with static tremor (Parkinson's syndrome)	Contralateral substantia nigra plus (?) other structures
Unilateral hemiballismus and hemichorea	Contralateral subthalamic nucleus of Luys, prerubral area, and Forel's fields
Chronic chorea of Huntington's type	Caudate nucleus, putamen, pallidum (?), and, in some cases, corpus Luysi
Athetosis and dystonia	Contralateral putamen
Cerebellar ataxia, i.e., intention tremor, slowness in starting and stopping alternating, voluntary movements, hypotonia, rebound phenomenon	Homolateral cerebellar hemisphere or middle and inferior cerebellar peduncles, superior brachium conjunctivum (ipsilateral if below, contralateral if above the decussation)
Decerebrate rigidity, i.e., opisthotonos, extension of arms and legs, modification of these postures by turning of head and neck (increased extensor and decreased flexor tone on side toward which head is turned)	Lesion usually bilateral in tegmentum involving red nuclei or structures between red nuclei and vestibular nuclei. Rarely above tentorium in subthalamus
Palatal and facial myoclonus (rhythmic)	Lesion in the central tegmental tract, inferior olivary nucleus, and olivodentate connections.
Diffuse myoclonus	? cerebellar cortex, ? thalami

lengthening reaction or clasp-knife phenomenon), and the absence of resistance upon slow movement, its disappearance in relaxed muscle with "electromyographic silence," and exaggerated tendon reflexes are the identifying characteristics of this spasticity. This type of hypertonus is believed in some instances to be due to hyperactivity of the small gamma motor neurones, resulting in increase in the sensitivity of the spindle muscle fibers to stretch; in other instances it seems clearly related to excessive activity of the larger alpha motor neurones. The "gamma spasticity" is abolished by procaine injection of the motor nerve, which paralyzes the small gamma motor and sensory fibers, leaving the larger ones intact, without weakening the willed contractions of the muscle, whereas the "alpha spasticity" is not affected.

In the state known as *rigidity* the muscles are continuously or intermittently firm, tense, and prominent; and the resistance to passive movement is intense and even, like that noted in bending a lead pipe or in stretching a strand of toffee. Although present in all muscle groups, both flexor and extensor, on the whole, it tends to be more prominent in those which maintain a flexed posture, i.e., flexor muscles of trunk and limbs. It appears to be somewhat greater in the large muscle groups, but this may be merely a question of muscle mass. Certainly the smaller muscles of the face and tongue and even those of the larynx are often affected. The tendon reflexes are not enhanced. Nevertheless, like "gamma spasticity," this rigidity is said to be abolished by procaine, and Foerster had earlier demonstrated that it is eradicated by posterior root section. In the electromyographic tracing, motor unit activity is more continuous than in spasticity, persisting even after relaxation.

A special type of rigidity, first noted by Negro in 1901, is the *cogwheel phenomenon*. When the hypertonic muscle is passively stretched, the resistance may be rhythmically jerky, as though the resistance of the limb were controlled by a ratchet. A number of different explanations of this phenomenon have been suggested. Wilson postulated it might be due to a minor form of the lengthening-shortening reaction, but a more likely explanation is an associated static tremor that is masked by rigidity during an attitude of repose but emerges faintly during manipulation.

Rigidity is prominent in extrapyramidal diseases such as paralysis agitans, postencephalitic Parkinson's syndrome, and some cases of athetosis and cerebral palsy.

The *tension hypertonus of athetosis* differs from both spasticity and rigidity. Strictly speaking, it takes two forms, one which occurs during the involuntary athetotic movement, and another which appears in the absence of any involuntary motion. Clinically these forms of hypertonus are variable from one moment to the next and are paradoxic in that they sometimes disappear during a rapid passive movement or when the limb is passively shaken. The tendon reflexes may be normal or brisk. The lengthening and shortening reactions are absent. This form of variable hypertonus is found in cases of double athetosis and choreoathetosis and in some cases of dystonia musculorum deformans. Usually in Sydenham's and Huntington's chorea a state of hypotonia prevails, sometimes as strikingly as in sensory polyneuropathies and lower motor neurone paralyses.

INVOLUNTARY MOVEMENTS

CHOREA. Derived from the Greek word meaning "dance," chorea refers to widespread arrhythmic movements of a forcible, rapid, jerky type. These movements are involuntary and are noted for their irregularity, variability, relative speed, and brief duration. They are quite elaborate and of variable distribution. In some respects they resemble a voluntary movement in their complexity, yet they are never combined into a coordinated act. The patient may, however, incorporate them into a deliberate movement, as if to make them less noticeable. When superimposed on voluntary movements, they may take on a grotesque and exaggerated character. Grimacing and peculiar respiratory sounds may be other expressions of the movement disorder. Usually they are discrete, but if very numerous, they may flow into one another; the resultant picture then resembles athetosis. They may be limited to a limb or to an arm and leg on one side (hemichorea), or they may involve all parts of the body. Normal volitional movements are, of course, possible, for there is no paralysis, but they too may be excessively quick and poorly sustained. The limbs are often unusually slack or hypotonic. A choreic movement may be superimposed on a tendon reflex, giving rise to the "hung-up reflex." The tendon reflexes tend to be pendular from the associated hypotonia; when the knee jerk is elicited with the patient sitting, the leg swings back and forth four or five times, like a pendulum, rather than one or two times as in a normal person.

Chorea appears in typical form in Sydenham's chorea and was noted also in the acute stages of epidemic encephalitis lethargica. It is a feature also of Huntington's chorea (chronic chorea), where the movements tend more typically to be choreoathetotic. Vascular lesions in the subthalamus, particularly those in and near the subthalamic nucleus of Luys, may result in wild flinging movements of the opposite arm and leg (hemiballismus). As these subside, they become almost indistinguishable from chorea.

ATHETOSIS. This term is from a Greek word meaning "unfixed" or "changeable." The condition is characterized by an inability to sustain the fingers and toes, tongue, or any other group of muscles in any one position. The maintained posture is interrupted by continuous, slow, sinuous, purposeless movements. These are most pronounced in the digits and the hands but often involve the tongue, throat, and face. One can detect as basic patterns of movement an extension and pronation and flexion and supination of the arm, and alternating flexion and extension of the fingers. They may be unilateral, especially in children who have suffered a hemiplegia at some previous date (posthemiplegic athetosis). The movements are slower than those of chorea, but in many cases gradations between the two (choreoathetosis) are seen. Most athetotic patients exhibit variable degrees of motor deficit due in some instances to associated pyramidal tract disease. Discrete individual movements of the tongue, lips, and hand are often impossible, and attempts to perform such voluntary movements result in a contraction of all the muscles in the limb (an *intention spasm*). Variable degrees of rigidity are generally associated, and these may account for the slower quality of athetosis, in contrast to chorea. It must be admitted, however, that in some cases it is almost impossible to distinguish between chorea and athetosis.

Athetosis or choreoathetosis of all four limbs is a cardinal feature of a curious state known as *double athetosis*, which begins in childhood. Athetosis appearing in the first months of life usually represents a congenital or postnatal condition such as hypoxia, kernicterus, or birth injury. Postmortem examination in some of the cases has disclosed a peculiar pathologic change of probable hypoxic etiology, a status marmoratus in the striatum; in others there has been a loss of medullated fibers, a status dysmyelinisatus, in the same regions.

TORSION SPASM OR DYSTONIA. Torsion spasm is closely allied to athetosis, differing only in that the larger axial (trunk, girdle muscles) rather than appendicular ones are involved. It results in bizarre, grotesque movements and positions of the body. The word *dystonia* has been given to these movements but, unfortunately, is also applied to any fixed posture which may be the end result of a disease of the motor system. Thus Denny-Brown speaks of hemiplegic dystonia, the flexion dystonia of parkinsonism, extensor dystonia with retraction of head and arching or twisting of back. If the latter meaning is given, it would be better to speak of athetosis of the trunk as torsion spasms or phasic dystonia, in contrast to fixed dystonia. The former, like athetosis, may show remarkable fluctuations; sometimes the whole musculature of the body may be thrown into spasm by an effort to move an arm or to speak. If mild, the torsion spasm may be limited to the lumbar or cervical muscles or those of one limb and may cease when the body is at rest.

Torsion spasm may be seen in the condition of double athetosis after hypoxic damage to the brain, in kernicterus, and rarely, in Wilson's hepatolenticular degeneration. It is most characteristic of the syndrome designated *dystonia musculorum deformans* but also occurs in other conditions such as the postphenothiazine dyskinesias and Hallevorden-Spatz disease (Chap. 364).

Chorea, athetosis, and torsoin spasm are all closely related. The movements are elaborate and depend for their expression on cortical mechanisms. Paralytic lesions involving the pyramidal tract abolish the involuntary movements. The hypotonia in chorea and some cases of athetosis, the pendular reflexes, and some degree of interference with the natural movements are also reminiscent of the syndrome that follows disease of the cerebellum. Lacking, however, are intention tremor and true incoordination or ataxia.

MYOCLONUS. This term refers to several different motor disorders, some localized, others diffuse. Like chorea, the myoclonic movement is involuntary and arrhythmic, but it is much faster than chorea, being concluded in a few hundred milliseconds. Variations in degree are noteworthy; it may consist of no more than a flick of a single muscle or part of a muscle, but the larger movements always betray its nature, involving as they do a group of muscles. Thus myoclonus can be distinguished from fasciculation. Sensory relationships are another prominent attribute. Flickering light, a series of loud sounds, or abrupt contact with some part of the body may regularly initiate a jerk, sometimes as a direct sensorimotor effect, again through the mechanism of startle. One special variety is evoked by willed movement, presumably through a proprioceptive mechanism. Hence, one may speak of action or intention myoclonus, auditory or visual myoclonus. A series of intense stimuli may recruit a series of myoclonic jerks into a full-blown seizure, as happens often in the familial myoclonic epilepsy syndrome of Unverricht-Lundborg. The pathology of the latter is usually a lipid storage disease or an amyloid nerve cell inclusion.

Familial types of myoclonus may persist in almost pure form or in association with mild ataxia over a period of many years. In the child and adult, herpes simplex encephalitis may present as a confusional state and dementia with myoclonus. In the elderly adult diffuse myoclonus is a prominent symptom in Jakob-Creutzfeld's disease. Intention myoclonus is often a sequela to anoxic encephalopathy. Postsomnolescent myoclonus jerks of arms for 20 to 30 min after a night's sleep is reported by some patients with idiopathic epilepsy. In all these diseases the pathologic changes are so widespread that anatomic localization is impossible. The least degrees of it are seemingly related to diseases of thalamus and cerebellum. Indeed cerebellar incoordination and intention tremor are combined with diffuse myoclonus of action or intention type in several of the aforementioned diseases i.e. lipidoses, and Lafora body type of myoclonus.

The term *myoclonus* unfortunately has also been assigned to a rather different motor phenomenon—that of repetitious, rhythmic clonus of some part of the "branchial cleft" or craniocervical musculature. An example is "nystagmus of the palate" (rhythmic contractions at the rate of 10 to 50 or more per min of soft palate, pharyngeal muscles, vocal cords, facial muscles, and diaphragm). The lesions producing this state, which we would prefer to designate as a form of continuous *bulbar, facial,* or *diaphragmatic clonus,* have been situated in all instances in the central tegmental tract, inferior olivary nucleus, or olivocerebellar tract. Vascular lesions, tumors, and encephalitic processes have all been causative.

The main fault with our concept of myoclonus is that it covers too many motor disorders. When movements are grouped according to their brevity or involuntary nature, one must include the normal dormescent start or jerk of a limb as one falls asleep, and the motor components of a natural startle reaction. The obligatory Moro response also falls within the group, as well as the form of epilepsy known as infantile, or salaam, spasms and the falling spells of the petit mal triad. Metrazol injections cause myoclonus of limbs, which has shown to depend on a lower brainstem (medullary reticular) mechanism.

Another problem arises on the clinical side in distinguishing diffuse myoclonus from other abrupt involuntary movements such as tremors, chorea, and restricted forms of epilepsy (epilepsia partialis continua). Speed of movement, lack of rhythmicity, and relationships to sensory stimulation prove to be the most reliable identifying features of the larger group of myoclonic disorders. There is an advantage in trying to separate the arrhythmic diffuse from the rhythmic restricted form in that each stands as a diagnostic attribute of a whole category of nervous diseases.

TREMOR. This consists of a more or less regular rhythmic oscillation of a part of the body around a fixed point, involving alternate contractions of agonist and antagonist muscles. The rate is usually 3 to 6 beats per sec, but faster frequencies do occur; in any one individual the rate is fairly constant in all affected parts, regardless of the size of the muscle or of the part of the body. Tremors usually involve the distal part of the limbs, the head, tongue, or jaw, and rarely the trunk.

There are many different types of tremor, and only a few are recognized as bearing any meaningful relationship to disease of the extrapyramidal motor system; but since tremors have not been discussed elsewhere, all the different types will be considered here.

Tremors can be classified in several ways. They may be subdivided according to their distribution, amplitude, regularity, and relationship to volitional movement. The following tremors should be familiar to every physician:

Static (Parkinsonian) Tremor. This is a coarse, rhythmic tremor, with an average rate of 4 to 5 beats per sec, most often localized in one or both hands, and occasionally, in the jaw or tongue. Its most characteristic feature is that it occurs when the limb is in an attitude of repose, and willed movement at least temporarily suppresses it. If the tremulous limb is completely relaxed, the tremor usually disappears, but the average patient rarely achieves this state. In some cases the tremor is constant; in others it varies from time to time and with the progress of the disease extends from one group of muscles to another. In paralysis agitans the tremor tends to be rather gentle and more or less limited to the distal muscles, whereas in postencephalitic parkinsonism and hepatolenticular degeneration it often has a wider range and involves proximal muscles. In many cases there is a variable degree of rigidity of plastic type. The tremor interferes with voluntary movements surprisingly little; it is not uncommon to see a patient who has been trembling violently raise a full glass of water to his lips and drain the contents without spilling a drop. The handwriting of these patients is often small and cramped (micrographia). The gait may be of a festinating type (see Chap. 23, Disturbances of Gait). It is the combination of static tremor, slowness of movement, rigidity, and flexed postures without true paralysis that constitutes Parkinson's syndrome (also called amyostatic syndrome).

The exact pathologic anatomy of static tremor is unknown. In paralysis agitans and postencephalitic Parkinson's syndrome, the visible lesions are predominantly in the substantia nigra. In hepatocerebral degeneration,

where this syndrome is mixed with cerebellar ataxia, the lesions are more diffuse. A similar tremor, without rigidity, slowness of movement, flexed postures, or masked facies, is seen in senile individuals. Unlike Parkinson's disease, it does not progress.

Action Tremor. This term refers to a tremor present when the limbs are actively maintained in a certain position, as when outstretched, and throughout voluntary movement. It may increase slightly as the action of the limbs becomes more precise, but it never approaches the degree of augmentation in fine movement of intention tremor. It is easily made to disappear when the limbs are relaxed. Probably the *action tremor* is but an exaggeration of normal or physiologic tremor, which ranges from 6 to 8 per sec, being slower in childhood and old age. More particularly, in adults the tremor is of small excursion, has a frequency of 8 per sec, and is somewhat irregular. The tremor involves the outstretched hand, head, and less often, the lips and tongue, and it interferes little with voluntary movements such as handwriting and speech. This type of tremor is seen in numerous medical, neurologic, and psychiatric diseases and is therefore more difficult to interpret than static tremor. When occurring as the only neurologic abnormality in several members of a family, it is known as *familial* or *hereditary* *tremor*. Familial tremor may begin in childhood, but usually comes on later and persists throughout adult life. Being worse when the patient is under observation, it becomes a source of embarrassment because it suggests to the onlooker that the patient is nervous. A curious fact about familial tremors is that one or two drinks of an alcoholic beverage may abolish them, and they may become worse after the effects of the alcohol have worn off. Similar tremors are seen in delirious states, such as delirium tremens, in the chronic alcoholic patient as an isolated symptom ("the morning shakes"), and in general paretics. An action tremor, usually more rapid than the above, is also characteristic of hyperthyroidism and other toxic states, and a similar tremor is frequently observed in patients suffering intense anxiety. In fact it can be reproduced by injections of epinephrine. Severe action tremor may also accompany certain diseases of the basal ganglia, including parkinsonism.

Intention Tremor. The word *intention* is ambiguous in this context because the tremor itself is not intentional. The term means, instead, that the tremor requires for its full expression the performance of an exacting, precise, willed movement. The term *ataxic tremor* has been suggested because it is always combined with cerebellar ataxia. The tremor is absent when the limbs are inactive and during the first part of a voluntary movement, but as the action continues and greater precision of movement is demanded (e.g., in touching a target such as the patient's nose or the examiner's finger), a jerky, more or less rhythmic interruption of forward progression, with side-to-side oscillation, appears. It continues for a fraction of a second or so after the act is completed. The tremor may seriously interfere with the patient's performance of skilled acts. Sometimes the head is involved (titubation). This type of tremor invariably indicates disease of the cerebellum and of its connections. When the disease is very severe, every movement, even the lifting of a limb, results in a wide-ranging tremor of such violence as to throw the patient off balance. This latter state is occasionally seen in multiple sclerosis, Wilson's disease, and vascular lesions of midbrain and subthalamus.

Hysterical Tremor. Hysterical tremors may simulate any of the aforementioned varieties and are difficult to diagnose. One notable feature is that they usually do not correspond to any of the better known types of organic tremor. Most often they are restricted to a limb and are seldom as regular as the static tremors of paralysis agitans. If the affected limb is restrained by the examiner, the tremor may move to another part of the body. It persists during movement and at rest and is less subject to the modifying influences of posture and willed movement than are organic tremors. This manifestation of hysteria is exceedingly rare.

OTHER INVOLUNTARY MOVEMENTS. There are other abnormalities of movement, about which only a few words can be said. They vary from simple irritative phenomena to complex psychologically related phenomena, such as compulsions.

Spasmodic Torticollis. This is an intermittent or continuous spasm of sternomastoid, trapezius, and other neck muscles, usually more pronounced on one side, with turning or tipping of the head. It is involuntary and cannot be inhibited and thereby differs from habit spasm or tic. This condition should be considered a form of dystonia. It is worse when the patient sits, stands, or walks, and usually contactual stimulation of the chin or of the back of the head partially alleviates the muscle imbalance. Psychiatric treatment is ineffectual. In severe cases muscle sectioning, neurectomy, section of the anterior cervical roots, or cryothalamotomy have given favorable results.

Other Craniocervical Spasms. Blepharoclonus (inability to keep open the eyes), lingual spasms, "spastic" dysphonia, facial spasms, and cervicothoracic spasms are all special varieties of involuntary movement, appearing usually in late middle life and the senium. Facial, cervical, and thoracic spasms have occurred with striking frequency during phenothiazid medication. Transiency, or nonprogressivity, unresponsiveness to psychotherapy, and uncertain amelioration by all pharmacologic agents characterize most of them. Exceptionally, these drug-induced dyskinesias, as they are called (actually athetosis), persist for months or years after the medication is discontinued.

Tics and Habit Spasms. Many individuals throughout life are prone to habitual movements, such as sniffing, clearing the throat, protruding the chin, or blinking, whenever they become tense. The patient admits that the movements are voluntary and that he feels compelled to make them in order to relieve tension; they can be inhibited for a time by an effort of will but reappear when attention is diverted. In certain cases they become so ingrained that the person is unaware of them and unable to control them. Children between five and ten years of age are especially liable to habit spasms. The movements are often purposive coordinated acts which normally serve the organism; it is only their incessant repetition when uncalled for that constitutes a habit. Stereotypy is their main identifying feature. Multiple convulsive tics (*Gilles de la Tourette's disease*) is a more severe form of the same condition. In children it is best to ignore the habit spasm and at the same time to arrange for more rest and a calmer environment. In adults relief of nervous tension by tranquilizing drugs and psychotherapy is helpful, but the disposition to tic formation persists.

Writer's cramp and other so-called "occupational spasms" should be mentioned here if only to indicate their unclassifiable status. Usually a middle-aged man or woman begins to observe upon attempting to write that all the muscles of thumb and fingers either go into a spasm or are in some way inhibited. Usually it is the spasm that interferes, and it may be painful and spread into the forearm or even the shoulder. Sometimes the spasm fragments into a tremor which interferes with the execution of fluid, cursive movements. Although limited to writing, exceptionally it may involve other equally demanding motor acts. At all other times and in the execution of grosser movements the hand is normal. Psychogenesis has been claimed, but careful clinical analysis will disprove it. Many patients learn to write in new ways or to use the other hand though that, too, may be involved. Hypnosis is usually without effect. Liversedge has stated that about half of the patients can be helped by a deconditioning procedure that delivers an electric shock whenever the spasm occurs. His results have not been verified by others. Aside from the spasm there is no other neurologic abnormality.

EXTRAPYRAMIDAL MOTOR DISTURBANCES DUE PRIMARILY TO DISEASES OF THE CEREBELLUM

Isolated lesions in the midline flocculonodular lobe result in grave disturbances of equilibrium. Often the symptoms are exhibited only when the patient attempts to stand and walk. He sways, staggers, titubates, and reels (see under Cerebellar Gait, Chap. 23). There may be no disturbance in coordination and no intention tremor of the limbs. A midline tumor of the cerebellum, such as medulloblastoma, usually produces this syndrome.

Extensive lesions of one cerebellar hemisphere, especially the anterior lobe, cause disturbances of coordination in volitional movements of the ipsilateral arm and leg. This is known as *ataxia*. The movements are characterized by an inappropriate range, rate, and strength of each of the various components of the motor act and by an improper sequence of those components. Electromyographic analysis has shown that ataxia is manifested as a decomposition of movement consisting of abnormal duration and sequences of bursts of contraction and relaxation of agonists and antagonists of a joint, usually a large joint (Carrera and Mettler). This incoordination is also called *asynergia*. The defects are particularly noticeable in acts that require rapid alternation of movements. Slowness in acceleration and deceleration, which is almost invariably present, impedes the performance (dysdiadochokinesis). The direction of purposive movement is frequently inaccurate. Owing to delay in arresting a movement, the patient may overshoot his mark. The antagonist muscles do not come into play at the proper time, possibly because of the hypotonia that is almost always present. This may be demonstrated by having the patient flex his arm against a resistance that is suddenly released. The patient with cerebellar disease will sometimes strike his face because he fails to check the flexion movement (Holmes rebound phenomenon). In movements requiring accurate direction, as the limb approaches its destination it may stop short and then advance by a more or less rhythmic series of jerks and oscillations (intention tremor). In addition to hypotonia, there may be, in acute cerebellar lesions, some slight weakness. Bilateral lesions of the cerebellar hemispheres and midline flocculonodular lobe lead to such a severe disturbance in all movements that the patient may be unable to stand or walk or use his limbs effectively. In addition, there are ocular and speech disturbances, namely, nystagmus, skew deviation of the eyes, and dysarthria. Lesions of the cerebellar peduncles have the same effect as extensive hemispheral lesions. This syndrome due to involvement of one cerebellar hemisphere may be observed in a tumor or abscess or in vascular lesions of the brainstem and cerebellar peduncles. The ataxia tends to be bilateral and symmetric in primary atrophy or degeneration of the cerebellum.

SOME GENERAL FEATURES OF ALL EXTRAPYRAMIDAL MOTOR DISTURBANCES

From the above discussion of many special types of motor disorder the reader must not think that they always appear in pure form. Various combinations occur in diseases. For example, Wilson's disease usually presents with a Parkinson-like picture of tremor, rigidity, slowness of movement, and flexion dystonia of trunk, but exceptionally there is athetosis, tonic innervation, phasic dystonia, and action myoclonus. Hallevorden-Spatz disease may take the form of universal rigidity and flexion dystonia or choreoathetosis. Occasionally the degeneration of Huntington's chorea leads to rigidity rather than choreoathetosis. Pyramidal and various of these extrapyramidal disorders may be associated in patients with cerebral diplegia. Nonetheless certain combinations tend to occur with greater or lesser frequency in certain diseases, as will be pointed out in Chaps. 361, 363, and 364. The benign restricted or localized spasms and twitches are the most obscure disorders with reference to both their pathologic anatomy or physiology.

In broad terms all the extrapyramidal disorders should be viewed in terms of the primary deficit (negative symptom) and the new phenomena (movements, abnormal postures, tremors, etc.) which have appeared. These latter (positive symptoms) are presently ascribed to release from or disequilibrium of the undamaged parts of the nervous system. The clearest negative effect is usually evidenced as an akinesia or disinclination to use the affected muscles. The difficulty in rapid sequences of movement stands as another negative effect both in diseases of basal ganglia and cerebellum. In fact this latter symptom, presenting as a clumsiness, may be the only fault manifest in certain maladroit children. Stress and nervous tension characteristically worsens both the motor deficiency and the abnormal movements in all of these extrapyramidal syndromes, just as relaxation helps the motor performance. All the movement disorders are abolished in sleep.

One of the most remarkable discoveries of recent years, to be credited largely to the pioneering efforts of neurosurgeons (Meyer, Cooper) has been the abolition of tremors, rigidity, and involuntary movements of the limbs by a surgical lesion in the medial segment of the globus pallidus or the ventrolateral nucleus of the thalamus. The effects are contralateral. Usually the lesion has been made by the injection first of procaine (Novocain) and then either alcohol, cooling and freezing (Cooper), or electrocoagulation (White and Sweet and Leksell). The operation has been successful in temporarily alleviating tremor or rigidity (or both) on one side. The procedure is successful in approximately 80 percent of cases of paralysis agitans, and the postural abnormality in dystonia musculorum deformans and double athetosis has responded somewhat less consistently. The operations have been perfected to the point where the mortality rate is less than 1 percent, and the risk of hemiplegia or some other sequel is less than 10 percent. Of course, as the disease progresses, the beneficial effects are lost. The therapeutic procedure indicates that the pallidum and ventrolateral nucleus, probably through their connections with the cerebral cortex (motor cortex and its pyramidal pathway), are essential for the expression of these extrapyramidal syndromes. The indications for these surgical procedures are discussed in Chap. 364.

EXAMINATION AND DIFFERENTIAL DIAGNOSIS

In Chap. 21 the methods of examining the motor system were described at some length, so only a few additional remarks concerning extrapyramidal disorders need be made here. These abnormalities are best demonstrated by seeing the patient in action. If he complains of a limp after walking a distance or of difficulty in climbing stairs, he should be observed under these conditions. Tests of rate, regularity, and coordination of voluntary movement must be sufficiently varied and demanding of the patient's motor coordination to bring out the defect. The physician must cultivate the habit of accurately observing and describing abnormalities of movement and must not be content merely to give the condition a name or to force it into some category such as chorea or tic or myoclonus. The main postures of the body in all common acts should be noted. Aside from the assessment of muscle power and of gait, the usual test applied to the upper limb is to ask the patient to touch the examiner's fingertip and then the tip of his own nose repeatedly (*finger-to-nose test*). In testing the leg the patient is asked to place his heel on one knee and then to run it down his shin and back to the knee (*heel-to-knee-to-shin test*). Finer movements of the hand may be tested by having the patient successively touch each finger to his thumb or pat his thigh rapidly or by having him use tools or handle objects. The performance of rapidly alternating movements such as pronation and supination or opening and closing the hands are valuable tests.

The fully developed extrapyramidal motor syndromes can be recognized without difficulty once the physician has become familiar with the typical pictures. The mental picture of Parkinson's syndrome, with its slowness of movement, poverty of facial expression, and static tremor and rigidity, should be fixed in mind. Similarly, the gross distortions and postural abnormalities of dystonia, whether widespread in trunk muscles or involving only neck muscles, as in spasmodic torticollis, once seen should thereafter be familiar. Athetosis, with its instability of postures and ceaseless movements of fingers and hands; intention spasm; chorea, with its more rapid and complicated movements; and the abrupt movements of myoclonus that flit over the body are other standard syndromes. Characteristic of all is the presence of a mild defect in the voluntary use of the affected parts.

The clinical differences between pyramidal and extrapyramidal disorders are summarized in Table 22-2.

Table 22-2. CLINICAL DIFFERENCES BETWEEN PYRAMIDAL AND EXTRAPYRAMIDAL SYNDROMES

	Pyramidal	Extrapyramidal
Character of rigidity	Clasp-knife effect	Plastic, equal throughout passive movement or intermittent (cogwheel rigidity)
Distribution of rigidity	Flexors of arms, extensors of legs	Flexors of all four limbs and trunk
Shortening and lengthening reaction	Present	Absent
Involuntary movements	Absent	Presence of tremors, chorea, athetosis, dystonia
Tendon reflexes	Increased	Normal or slightly increased
Babinski's sign	Present	Absent
Paralysis of voluntary movement	Present	Absent or slight

Early or mild forms of these conditions, like all medical diseases, may offer special difficulties in diagnosis. Cases of paralysis agitans, seen before the appearance of tremor, are often overlooked. The patient may complain of being nervous and restless or may have experienced an indescribable stiffness and aching in certain parts of the body.

Because of the absence of weakness or of reflex changes, the case may be considered psychogenic or rheumatic. It is well to remember that Parkinson's syndrome often begins in a hemiplegic distribution, and for this reason the illness may be misdiagnosed as cerebral thrombosis. A slight masking of the face, a suggestion of a limp, blepharoclonus (uninhibited blinking of eyes when the bridge of the nose is tapped), a mild rigidity, failure of an arm to swing naturally in walking, or loss of certain movements of cooperation will help in diagnosis at this time. Every case presenting the syndrome of Parkinson or other abnormality of movement and posture in adolescence or early adult life should be surveyed for hepatolenticular degeneration by tests of liver function and split-lamp examination for corneal pigmentation (Kayser-Fleischer ring); if facilities are available, urinary aminonitrogen excretion and copper excretion should be determined.

Mild or early chorea is often mistaken for simple nervousness. If one sits for a time and watches the patient, the diagnosis will often become evident. There are cases, nonetheless, in which it is impossible to distinguish simple nervousness from early Sydenham's chorea, especially in children, and there is no laboratory test upon which one can depend. The first postural manifestation of dystonia may suggest hysteria, and it is only later, when the fixity of the postural abnormality, the lack of the usual psychologic picture of hysteria, and the relentlessly progressive character of the illness become evident, that accurate diagnosis is reached. Another common error is to assume that a bedfast patient who has complained of dizziness, staggering, and headaches and exhibits no other neurologic abnormality is suffering from hysteria. The flocculonodular cerebellar syndrome is demonstrable only when the patient attempts to stand and walk.

REFERENCES

Carrera, R. M. E., and F. A. Mettler: Function of the Primate Brachium Conjunctivum and Related Structures, J. Comp. Neurol., 102:151, 1955.

Denny-Brown, D.: Diseases of the Basal Ganglia and Subthalamic Nuclei," Fair Lawn, N.J., Oxford University Press, 1945.

Martin, J. Purdon, and Ian R. McCaul: Acute Hemiballismus Treated by Ventrolateral Thalamolysis, Brain, 82:104, 1959.

23 VERTIGO AND DISORDERS OF EQUILIBRIUM AND GAIT

*Maurice Victor and
Raymond D. Adams*

The terms to describe sensations of unbalance are often rather ambiguous, and the patient must be carefully questioned. He often uses *dizziness* to indicate not only a sense of rotation but also vague sensory experiences such as unsteadiness, insecurity, weakness, faintness, and light-headedness. Blurring of vision and even petit mal epilepsy may be referred to as dizzy spells. *Giddiness* has almost the same significance, with perhaps more implication of altered consciousness and swaying sensation. *Vertigo* literally means "sense of turning" either of one's body or of the surroundings, a definition which, with a few important qualifications to be mentioned below, is used throughout this chapter. *Equilibrium* refers simply to a state of balance or equipoise in which opposing forces, such as gravity and postural reflexes, exactly counteract each other.

Disorders of equilibrium are suitably considered in connection with dizziness and vertigo because of their frequent conjunction (vertiginous ataxia). Other disorders of equilibrium quite independent of vertigo, e.g., those due to a loss of joint and muscle sense (sensory ataxia) or cerebellar disease (cerebellar ataxia) are also considered briefly in this chapter.

ANATOMIC, PHYSIOLOGIC, AND PSYCHOLOGIC CONSIDERATIONS

Several mechanisms are responsible for the maintenance of a balanced posture and make us aware of the body's position in relation to its surroundings—afferent impulses from the eyes, labyrinths, muscles, and joints relay information about the position of the body in space. In response to these impulses the organism is capable of making fine and rapid postural adjustments to maintain equilibrium, most of which do not demand volitional control. The most important of the afferent impulses are the following:

1. Impulses from the retina and possibly proprioceptive impulses from the ocular muscles, which activate reflexes that influence the position of head and neck.

2. Impulses from the labyrinths, which are highly specialized spatial proprioceptors, whose primary function is to register changes in direction of motion (either acceleration or deceleration) and in the position of the body. The semicircular canals respond to movement and angular momentum, and the otoliths—the sense organs of the utricle and saccule—are mainly concerned with orienting the organism in reference to gravity.

3. Impulses from the proprioceptors of the joints and muscles, which regulate reflex, postural, and voluntary movement. Those from the neck are of special importance in relating the position of the head to the rest of the body.

The cerebellum, the vestibular nuclei, the red nuclei, and other brainstem ganglionic centers are the most important central structures concerned with regulating posture.

Important psychologic phenomena are also involved in the maintenance of equilibrium, namely, those which deal with the relationship between ourselves and the external world. We learn to perceive that portion of space occupied by our body and construct from sensory data a set of integrated sensory experiences called by some neurologists, *the body schema*. The space around our body,

i.e., the external world, is then said to be represented by another schema. Those two schemata are neither static nor independent: they are constantly being modified and adapted to one another; their interdependence is ascribed to the fact that the various sense organs which supply the information on which the two schemata are based are usually simultaneously activated by any movement of our bodies. By a process of learning we see objects as having motion or being still, when we are either moving or stationary. Motion of an object in space is always relative. At times, especially when our own sensory experience is incomplete, we mistake movement of our surroundings for movements of our own body as, for example, the illusion of movement which is experienced in a stationary train when a neighboring train is moving. Hence, in this frame of reference, orientation of the body in space is possible only by the maintenance of an orderly relationship between the body schema and the schema of the external world. As a corollary, disorientation in space or disequilibrium occurs when this relationship is upset.

On clinical grounds, disorders of equilibrium may be divided into three groups: (1) true vertigo; (2) pseudovertigo, or giddiness; and (3) abnormalities of equilibrium without either vertigo or giddiness.

VERTIGO

CHARACTERISTICS. In disorders in which vertigo is a leading symptom, the patient's history assumes special importance in diagnosis, for this symptom may be accompanied by no objective signs. The diagnosis of vertigo is an easy matter when the patient reports that objects in his environment spun around, or his body was turning, or his head was spinning. Very often, however, he is not so explicit. He may state that there was a feeling of to-and-fro or up-and-down movement of the body, usually the head; or he may relate that the floor or walls seemed to undulate or sank or rose up toward him or that he was pulled strongly to one side or to the ground, as though drawn by a strong magnet. This feeling of impulsion is particularly characteristic of vertigo. With milder degrees of vertigo, the patient may have difficulty in describing his symptoms. It may help to ask him whether his present symptoms are similar to the feeling of movement one experiences when coming to a halt after being rapidly rotated. Or, it may be necessary to induce vertigo by rotating the patient rapidly in one direction and have him compare it to his symptoms.

The symptoms of vertigo are usually paroxysmal and of short duration, but at times they may linger for weeks or even months. The chronic state may or may not follow an acute attack; in this latter instance the patient complains of a continuous state of imbalance, of swaying, or a vague sense of movement in the environment.

All but the mildest forms of vertigo are accompanied by varying degrees of nausea and vomiting, nystagmus, headache, and ataxia, as well as by the need to avoid movement of the head. When the attack is at its height, the slightest movement of the head may aggravate the sense of whirling or rotation and of nausea; after the acute symptoms have subsided, vertigo may be evoked only by movement of the head. One form of paroxysmal vertigo (the positional vertigo of Barany) depends entirely on changes in position of the head (see Chap. 355, Diseases of Cranial Nerves).

Stance and gait are almost invariably affected during an attack of vertigo. In exceptionally severe attacks the patient may without warning be thrown to the ground and only then experience vertigo, nausea, and vomiting. Some patients may be so ataxic that they are unable to sit or to stand. In less severe cases the patient may feel unsteady in walking, tending to veer to one side. This type of gait disturbance, which depends on an abnormality of labyrinthine or vestibular function, may be called *vertiginous ataxia*. It is noteworthy that in these circumstances the coordination of individual movements of the limbs is not impaired—a point of difference from most instances of cerebellar disease.

Headache is often associated with vertigo. Loss of consciousness as part of a vertiginous attack rarely occurs and usually signifies another category of disorder, such as syncope or seizure.

DISTINCTION BETWEEN TRUE AND FALSE VERTIGO. It is important to distinguish clearly between true vertigo and a second group of symptoms which do not have the same significance, i.e., *pseudovertigo*. The latter symptoms may be described as a feeling of uncertainty, lightheadedness, or a swimming sensation; or the patient may feel as though he is going to fall or is walking on air. These sensory phenomena are particularly common in psychoneurotic states and in introspective individuals with an overawareness of various body parts. Other peculiar aberrations, for example, a feeling of lengthening of the legs or a sensation as if the ground were receding, may be remarked upon. A feeling of light-headedness is frequently brought about by hyperventilation, and similar symptoms occur in patients with anemia, hypertension, and pulmonary disease, particularly emphysema. In anemia, mild hypoxia is the probable mechanism, and ischemia is probably the cause in emphysematous patients, in whom an attack of coughing may lead to dizziness or even fainting, owing to impaired venous return to the heart (tussive syncope). The dizziness that so often accompanies hypertension is more difficult to evaluate. In some cases it may be due to associated nervousness; in others, it may depend upon transient changes in the intracranial vasculature. *Postural* dizziness is a closely related complaint. Individuals in poor physical condition and many elderly persons, especially if they have cerebrovascular disease, are troubled upon arising from a recumbent or sitting position or after stooping by a momentary giddiness or a swaying type of dizziness with dimming of vision or spots before the eyes. These symptoms last only for several seconds or a minute, during which time the patient may find it necessary to stand still or to steady himself by holding on to a nearby object. There need be no fall in brachial blood pressure at the time of symptom production. The condition may be due to a momentary failure of reflex vasoconstriction in over-

coming the "pooling" effect of gravity upon the circulating blood. This type of dizziness may occur in normal individuals on arising and is more pronounced after a hot bath; it is a frequent complaint in patients convalescing from debilitating illness. A mild syncopal reaction of any type may give rise to similar symptoms and may be described by the patient as "dizziness."

In practice it is not difficult to separate these symptoms from true vertigo; there is not the feeling of rotation nor of impulsion so characteristic of the latter. In addition, the ancillary symptoms of true vertigo, including varying degrees of nausea, vomiting, headache, ataxia, and the need to keep the head immobile, do not occur.

NEUROLOGIC SIGNIFICANCE. A disorder of any of the following structures may give rise to vertigo.
1. Cerebral cortex
2. Ocular muscles
3. Cerebellum
4. Labyrinthine-vestibular apparatus
5. Brainstem

Vertigo may constitute the aura of an epileptic seizure, indicating a cerebrocortical origin. This usually occurs with lesions of the temporal lobe, mainly on the lateral aspect of the middle and posterior portions or at the parietotemporal junction. The patients experience a sensation of movement, either of their body away from the side of stimulation or of the environment in the opposite direction. This type of vertigo lasts for only a few moments before being submerged in the seizure activity. Vertiginous seizures may occur very rarely as a reflex phenomenon, the result of vestibular (e.g., caloric) stimulation.

Ocular disturbances may give rise to vertigo and may even be accompanied by unsteadiness; this occurs most frequently at the outset of an ocular muscle paralysis when the patient looks in the direction of action of the paralyzed muscle. The vertigo is apparently due to a faulty projection of the visual field, the patient being presented with two conflicting images. Some people experience a type of giddiness or uncertainty when wearing bifocal lenses for the first time. The necessity of adapting to an unusual visual environment, as in looking down from a height, may result in a similar sensation. These types of vertigo are usually mild and transient and of relatively little clinical significance.

Whether *lesions of the cerebellum* can produce vertigo seems to depend on what portion of this structure is involved. Thus vertigo may be absent despite large lesions of the cerebellar hemispheres but present if the vestibulo-cerebellar connections are damaged.

For all practical purposes the problem of vertigo resolves itself into deciding whether this symptom has its origin in the labyrinth, in the vestibular division of the eighth cranial nerve, or in the vestibular nuclei and their immediate connections with other structures in the brainstem. A number of features, especially the form of the attack and the associated symptoms, help to make this decision.

Vertigo of labyrinthine origin (aural vertigo) tends to occur in paroxysmal attacks. It has an abrupt onset, is maximal at the beginning, and subsides in a matter of minutes or in an hour or two. Similarly, the nausea, vomiting, pallor, immobility, and ataxia associated with the attack are short-lived. The accompanying nystagmus tends also to be transient and characteristically is rather fine, rotatory, and most pronounced when the eyes are turned away from the offending labyrinth. Occasionally, vertigo of labyrinthine origin may take a more chronic form. However, it seldom continues for more than a few days or weeks, the central mechanisms apparently compensating for the peripheral lesion. Labyrinthine vertigo is frequently associated with deafness and tinnitus, since the pathologic process in the inner ear encroaches on the cochlear apparatus. Labyrinthine vertigo may accompany an ear infection (labyrinthitis) or occur as a cardinal symptom of Ménière's disease, vestibular neuronitis, or Barany's positional vertigo.

Vertigo of acoustic nerve origin, associated as a rule with an acoustic neuroma, is usually mild and intermittent (lasting weeks or months) but it has all the main elements of true vertigo (sense of turning, impulsion, preferred posture, etc.). It may be the initial symptom but more often occurs an interval of time (months or years) after the associated impairment of hearing. Once established, coarse horizontal nystagmus to the side of the tumor and finer nystagmus to the opposite side are demonstrable. Impaired caloric responses and high frequency deafness (without recruitment) confirm the eighth nerve affection. Involvement of adjacent cranial nerves (VII, V, X) and cerebellum (ipsilateral ataxia), the late signs of a cerebellopontine angle mass, facilitates diagnosis.

Vertigo of brainstem origin usually lasts longer than aural vertigo and may disorganize the patient's equilibrium for several weeks or even longer. In these cases, auditory function is usually spared, since vestibular and cochlear fibers become separated soon after entering the brainstem. It is a fairly reliable clinical rule that the combination of auditory and vestibular symptoms occurs only in diseases that involve the inner ear or eighth cranial nerve. Nystagmus which accompanies central lesions tends to be coarse and protracted, is more marked on lateral gaze to one side than the other, and may have a vertical component, particularly on upward gaze. Vertical nystagmus nearly always indicates disease of the brainstem. A demylinative lesion may affect vestibular connections, and this diagnosis should always be considered when a young person has a severe and protracted attack of vertigo without auditory symptoms. Vascular and neoplastic lesions may also give rise to vertigo through involvement of the vestibular nuclei and their immediate connections. In addition, there may be signs of interference with other segmental mechanisms of the lower brainstem or the long sensory and motor tracts that pass through it. These features clearly exclude a labyrinthine or vestibular nerve localization.

Diagnosis

When the patient's complaint is dizziness, it is first necessary to obtain a clear description of the symptoms. The element of rotation or a similar sensation, the sense of impulsion, and the accompanying nausea and vomiting, nystagmus, headache, and ataxia usually distinguish the case of true vertigo from one of giddiness. The latter has no element of rotation or impulsion, and the ancillary manifestations are absent. Although fearful of falling or swooning, the patient can nonetheless walk without difficulty if forced to do so. Smothering and choking feelings, palpitation, trembling, sweating, and a sense of fear or apprehension complete the usual clinical picture of neurotic dizziness. Frequently in cases of recurrent aural vertigo, i.e., *Ménière's syndrome,* symptoms of anxiety and depression may be added to the total clinical picture, which adds to the difficulty of interpretation (see Chap. 355).

If the physician is uncertain whether the patient has true vertigo, it is sometimes helpful to induce these sensations in order that the patient may compare them with his usual attacks. This can be done by having the patient breathe deeply for 3 minutes (which causes giddiness in most persons), stoop over for a minute and then straighten up (postural giddiness), and while standing, turn rapidly in one direction 10 times in order to provoke vertigo. If the patient fails to distinguish these sensations, his history is probably inaccurate and he should be asked to take careful note of his sensations during his next spontaneous attack.

In some cases the attack may be so abrupt and severe that the patient falls immediately to the ground without loss of consciousness. Here the diagnosis of vertigo may be clarified by nausea, vomiting, and dizziness, which almost invariably follow such a fall. If the vertigo has been very mild in degree, it is helpful to elicit a history of disinclination to walk during the attack, a tendency to list to one side, discomfort in sitting or riding in a vehicle, and a preference for maintaining one position fixedly.

A neurologic examination, including tests of ocular movements and nystagmus, cranial nerve function, gait, and coordination of limbs, should be carried out on all patients with dizziness as the presenting complaint. The eardrums should be inspected and hearing tested by the methods indicated in Chap. 24. Vestibular function should also be tested. This is commonly done by irrigating the ear with 5 ml ice water for a period of 30 sec, the head being tilted forward 30° from the body axis, since in this position the horizontal canal is brought into a vertical position. The normal labyrinthine responses consist of falling to the side of the vestibular lesion, past-pointing to that side, and rotary nystagmus on gaze to the opposite side. The nystagmus begins about 20 sec after the irrigation and persists for 90 to 120 sec. The duration of these periods is variable, however, and comparison of the affected and normal labyrinths is more important.

Attempts to reproduce the dizziness should include observation of the patient when his body position is suddenly changed from sitting to recumbency with the neck hyperextended and the head turned first to the right and on the next trial to the left. In Barany's positional vertigo, within 5 to 10 sec after becoming recumbent with the offending ear down, the eyes are seen to jerk in a coarse horizontal nystagmus and the patient feels dizzy. This lasts 10 to 15 sec and the direction of the dizziness is reversed upon returning to a sitting position.

DISTURBANCES OF EQUILIBRIUM (GAIT)

Probably no aspect of equilibrium is more interesting or affords greater opportunity for diagnosis than the analysis of the patient's gait.

The normal gait seldom attracts attention. The body is erect, the head straight, and the arms hang loosely and gracefully at the sides, each moving rhythmically forward with the opposite leg. The feet are slightly everted, and the steps are of moderate length and approximately equal, the internal malleoli of the tibias almost touching one another. With each step there is coordinated flexion of hip and knee and dorsiflexion of foot and a barely perceptible elevation of the hip so that the foot clears the ground. The heel strikes the ground first, and inspection of shoes will show that this part is most subject to wear. In the erect posture, the muscles of greatest importance in maintaining equilibrium are the erector spinae and the extensors of the hips and knees.

When analyzed in greater detail, the requirements for locomotion in an upright, bipedal position can be reduced to the following elements: (1) antigravity support of the body; (2) stepping; (3) an adequate degree of equilibrium; and (4) a means of propulsion. The support of the body is provided by the antigravity reflexes which maintain firm extension of knees, hips, and back muscles, but modifiable by position of head and neck. These reflexes depend on the integrity of the spinal cord and lower parts of the brainstem (pontine transection leads to exaggeration of these antigravity reflexes—decerebrate rigidity). Stepping, the second element, is a basic movement pattern, present at birth, and integrated at the midbrain level. Its appropriate stimulus is contact of the sole with a flat surface and inclination of the body forward and alternately from side-to-side. Equilibrium involves the preservation of balance at right angles to the direction of movement. The center of gravity during the continuously unstable equilibrium which prevails in walking must shift from side to side within narrow limits as the weight is borne first on one foot then the other. Propulsion is provided by leaning forward and slightly to one side and permitting the body to fall a certain distance before being checked by the support of the leg. Here both forward and alternating lateral movements must occur. But in running, where at one moment both feet are off the ground, a forward drive or thrust by the hind leg is also needed. Locomotion may fail in the course of neurologic diseases when one or more of these mechanical principles is prevented from operating, as we shall see.

There are many individual variations of gait, and it is a commonplace observation that the sound of an individual's footsteps, notably his pace and heaviness of tread, may identify him. The manner of walking and the carriage of the body may even provide clues to character, personality, and occupation. Furthermore, the gaits of men and women differ, the steps of women being quicker and shorter and the movement of their trunk and hips more graceful and delicate. Certain female characteristics of gait, if observed in the male, immediately impart an impression of femininity; or male characteristics in the female, one of masculinity.

Since normal body posture and locomotion require visual information (we see where we are going and pick our steps), labyrinthine function, and proprioception, it is of interest to note the effect of deficits in these senses on normal function. A blind man or a normal one who is blindfolded may walk very well. He moves cautiously, to avoid collision with objects, and on smooth pavement shortens his step slightly; with the shortening there is less rocking of the body and he seems unnaturally stiff. A man without labyrinthine function (as happens after prolonged streptomycin therapy) shows a slight unsteadiness in walking and he cannot descend stairs without holding onto a banister. Running is also difficult. Characteristically, he has great difficulty in focusing on a stationary object when he is moving, so that he cannot drive a car. Proof that he is dependent on visual cues comes from his performance blindfolded where he is seen to be unsteady and to stagger to some extent, but usually he does not fall. A loss of proprioception, as in a complete lesion in the posterior columns of the spinal cord in the high cervical region, abolishes for a long time the capacity for independent locomotion. After years of training the patient will still have difficulty in starting to walk and in propelling himself forward. As Purdon Martin has illustrated, he holds his hands in front of his body, bends body and head forward, walks with a wide base with irregular uneven steps but does rock his body. If he loses his balance, he shows no reactions to protect his equilibrium. If he falls, he cannot arise without help, and he cannot get up from a chair. He is unable to crawl or to get into an "all-fours" posture. When standing, if blindfolded, he immediately falls. Thus the postural reactions are demonstrably more dependent on proprioceptive than on visual or labyrinthine information.

When confronted with a disorder of gait, the examiner must observe the patient's natural stance and the attitude and dominant positions of the legs, trunk, and arms. It is good practice to watch the patient as he walks into the examining room, because he is apt to walk more naturally then than during special tests. He should be asked to stand with his feet together, head erect, with eyes first open and then closed. Swaying due to nervousness may be overcome by asking that he touch the tip of his nose with the finger of first one hand and then the other. Next the patient should be asked to walk forward and backward, with his eyes first open and then closed. Any tendency to reel to one side, as in cerebellar disease, can be checked by having him walk around a chair. When the affected side is toward the chair, the patient tends to walk into it; and when it is away from the chair, he veers outward in ever-widening circles. More delicate tests of gait are walking a straight line heel to toe or having the patient arise quickly from a chair and walk briskly and then stop or turn suddenly. If all these tests are successfully executed, it may be assumed that any difficulty in locomotion is not due to disease of the proprioceptive mechanisms or cerebellum. Detailed neurologic examination is then necessary in order to determine which of the many other possible diseases is responsible for the patient's disorder of gait.

The following abnormal gaits are so distinctive that with a little practice they can be recognized at a glance.

CEREBELLAR GAIT. The main features of this gait are *wide base* (separation of legs), *unsteadiness, irregularity,* and *lateral reeling*. Steps are uncertain, some are shorter and others longer than intended, and the patient may lurch to one side or the other. The unsteadiness is more prominent on quickly arising from a chair and walking, on stopping suddenly while walking, or on turning abruptly. If the ataxia is severe, the patient cannot stand without assistance. If lesser in degree, standing with feet together and head erect, with eyes either opened or closed, may be difficult. In its mildest form the ataxia is best demonstrated by having the patient walk a line heel to toe. After two or three steps he loses his balance and must step to one side to avoid falling. Romberg's sign, i.e., marked swaying or falling with the eyes closed but not with the eyes open, is not a feature of cerebellar disease. Compensation may be effected by shortening the step and shuffling, i.e., keeping both feet simultaneously on the ground. The defect in the cerebellar gait is not in antigravity support, steppage, or propulsion but in the co-ordination of proprioceptive, labyrinthine, and visual information in reflex coordination of movements. The abnormality of gait may or may not be accompanied by other signs of cerebellar incoordination and intention tremor of the arms and legs. The presence of the latter signs depends on involvement of the cerebellar hemispheres as distinct from anterior and midline structures; if the lesion is unilateral, they are always on the same side.

Cerebellar gait is most commonly seen in multiple sclerosis, cerebellar hemorrhage, medulloblastoma of the cerebellar vermis, and the cerebellar degenerations. In certain forms of cerebellar degeneration (e.g., the type associated with chronic alcoholism) the disease process reaches a plateau and then remains stable for many years, and the gait disorder, in these circumstances, becomes altered to some extent. The base is wide and the steps are still short, but more regular; the trunk is inclined slightly forward, the arms are held away from the sides, and the gait assumes a somewhat rhythmic quality. In this way the patient can walk for long distances, but he lacks the capacity to make the necessary postural adjustments in response to sudden changes in his position. In this respect, among others, cerebellar ataxia differs from that due to drunkenness (see below).

GAIT OF SENSORY ATAXIA. This gait is due to an impairment of proprioception resulting from interruption of afferent nerve fibers in the peripheral nerves, posterior roots, posterior columns of the spinal cords, or medial lemnisci; it may also be produced occasionally by a lesion of both parietal lobes. Whatever the location of the lesion, the patient is deprived of knowledge of the position of his limbs. The principal features of the resulting

gait disorder are the *uncertainty,* the *irregularity,* and the *stamp* of the feet. Hunt characterized this type of gait very well when he said that the ataxic patient is recognized by "his stamp and stick." When the ataxia is of moderate severity, there is great difficulty in standing and walking, and in advanced cases there is a complete failure of locomotion, although muscular power is retained. The legs are kept far apart to correct the instability, and the patient carefully watches the ground and his legs. As he steps out, the legs are flung abruptly forward and outward, often lifted higher than necessary. The steps are of variable length, and many are attended by an audible stamp as the foot is banged down on the floor. The body is held in a slightly flexed position, and the weight may be supported on the cane that the severely ataxic patient so often carries. The incoordination is greatly exaggerated when the patient is deprived of visual cues, as in walking in the dark. Most patients, when asked to stand with feet together and eyes closed, show greatly increased swaying or actual falling (Romberg's sign). It has been said that a lame man whose shoes are not worn in any one place is probably suffering from sensory ataxia. There is invariably a loss of vibratory and position sense in the feet and legs. Gaits of this type are observed in tabes dorsalis, Friedreich's ataxia, subacute combined degeneration, syphilitic meningomyelitis, chronic polyneuritis, and those cases of multiple sclerosis in which posterior column disease predominates.

HEMIPLEGIC AND PARAPLEGIC (SPASTIC) GAIT. In hemiplegia the leg is held stiffly and does not flex freely and gracefully at the knee and hip. It tends to rotate outward and describes a semicircle, first away from and then toward the trunk (circumduction). The foot scrapes along the floor, and the toe and outer side of the sole of the shoe are worn. One can diagnose the hemiplegic gait by hearing the slow rhythmic scuff of the foot along the floor. The other muscles of the body on the affected side are weak and stiff to a variable degree, particularly the arm, which is carried in a flexed position and does not swing naturally. This type of gait disorder is most frequently associated with vascular disease of the brain.

The spastic paraplegic gait is entirely different from the gait of sensory ataxia, though the two may be combined. Each leg is advanced slowly and stiffly with restricted motion at the knee and hip. The patient looks as though he were wading in water. The legs are extended or slightly bent at the knees and may be strongly adducted at the hips, tending almost to cross ("scissors" gait). The steps are regular and short. Movements of the legs are slow, and the patient may be able to advance only with great effort. An easy way to remember the main features of the hemiplegic and paraplegic gait is by the letter S, which begins each of its descriptive adjectives—spastic, slow, scuffing. The defect is in the stepping mechanism and in propulsion, not in support or equilibrium. Cerebral spastic diplegia, multiple sclerosis, syringomyelia, spinal syphilis, combined system disease, spinal cord compression, and familial spinal spastic ataxia are the common causes of spastic paraparesis.

FESTINATING GAIT. This term comes from the Latin

festinatio, haste, and is appropriate for the gait disorder of both paralysis agitans and postencephalitic Parkinson's syndrome. *Rigidity* and *shuffling*, in addition to *festination*, are the cardinal features of this gait. When they are joined to the typical tremors, rigidity, and slowness of movement, there can be little doubt as to the diagnosis.

The general attitude of the patient is one of flexion; rigidity and immobility of the body are other conspicuous features. There is a paucity of the automatic movements made in sitting, standing, and walking; the head does not turn in looking to one side, the arms are seldom folded, and the legs are rarely crossed. The arms are held stiffly as though in preparation for writing, and the facial expression is unblinking and masklike.

In walking, the trunk is bent forward and the arms are carried ahead of the body and do not swing. The legs are stiff and bent at the knees and hips. The steps are short and the feet barely clear the ground as the patient shuffles along. Once forward or backward locomotion is started, the upper part of the body advances ahead of the lower part, as though the patient were chasing his center of gravity. His steps become more and more rapid, and he may fall if not assisted. This is the festination, and it may occur when the patient is walking forward or backward, taking the form of either propulsion or retropulsion. The defect is in rocking the body from side to side so as to clear the floor and in moving the legs quickly enough to catch the center of gravity in forward propulsion. Other unusual gaits are sometimes observed in the postencephalitic patient. For example, he may be unable to take his first step forward because he cannot lift one foot, or until he hops or takes one step backward; or walking may be initiated by a series of short steps that give way to a more normal gait; occasionally such a patient may run better than he walks.

ATHETOTIC, DYSTONIC, AND CHOREIC GAITS. These are less common than the preceding gait disorders. The athetotic patient is rigid, and his body often assumes the most grotesque postures. One arm may be held aloft and the other one behind the body with wrist and fingers alternately undergoing slow flexion, extension, and rotation. The head may be inclined in one direction, the lips alternately retract and then purse, and the tongue intermittently protrudes from the mouth. The legs advance slowly and awkwardly. Sometimes the foot is plantar flexed at the ankle, and the weight is carried on the toes; or it may be dorsiflexed or inverted. This type of gait is typical of congenital athetosis.

In dystonia musculorum deformans the first symptom may be a limp due to inversion or plantar flexion of the foot or a distortion of the pelvis. The patient stands with one leg rigidly extended or one shoulder elevated. The trunk may be in a position of exaggerated lordosis and the hips are partly flexed, with a tilting forward of the pelvis. Because of the muscle spasms that deform the body in this manner, the patient may have to walk with knees flexed. The gait may seem normal as the first steps are taken, but as the patient walks, one or both legs become flexed, giving rise to the "dromedary" gait. In the more advanced stages walking becomes impossible owing to torsion of the trunk or the continuous flexion of one leg.

In *chorea* the gait is often bizarre. As the patient stands or walks there is a continuous play of irregular "choreic" movements affecting the face, neck, and hands, and in the advanced stages, the large proximal joints and trunk. The positions of the trunk and upper parts of the body vary with each step. There are jerks of the head, grimacing, squirming, twisting movements of the trunk and limbs, and peculiar respiratory noises. The general features of these conditions are described more fully in Chap. 364.

STEPPAGE, DROP-FOOT, OR EQUINE GAIT. This is caused by paralysis of the pretibial and peroneal muscles. The legs must be lifted abnormally high in order for the feet to clear the ground. There is a slapping noise as the foot strokes the floor. The anterior and lateral border of the sole of the shoe becomes worn. The steps are regular and even; otherwise, walking is not remarkable. The steppage gait may be unilateral or bilateral and occurs in diseases that affect the peripheral nerves of the legs or motor neurones in the spinal cord, such as poliomyelitis, progressive muscular atrophy, and Charcot-Marie-Tooth disease (peroneal muscular atrophy). It may also be observed in patients with peripheral types of muscular dystrophy.

WADDLING GAIT. This gait is characteristic of progressive muscular dystrophy. The attitude of the body may be straight, but more often the lumbar lordosis is accentuated. The steps are regular but a little uncertain. With each step there is an exaggerated elevation of the hip, and once the weight is on this hip, it yields to an abnormal degree so that the upper trunk then inclines to that side. This alternation of lateral trunk movements results in the rolling gait, or *waddle*, a term suggested by Oppenheim. The gluteal musculature is weak and inefficient, although leg muscles may appear well developed. Muscular contractures leading to an equinovarus position of the foot may complicate childhood cases, so that the waddle is combined with circumduction of the legs and "walking on the toes."

STAGGERING OR DRUNKEN GAIT. This is characteristic of alcoholic and barbiturate intoxication. The drunken patient totters, reels, tips forward and then backward, threatening each moment to lose his balance and fall. Control over trunk and legs is greatly impaired. The steps are irregular and uncertain. The patient appears stupefied and indifferent to the quality of his performance, but under certain circumstances he can momentarily correct his defect.

The frequently used adjectives *drunken* and *reeling* do not describe aptly the gait of cerebellar disease, except, perhaps, the most acute and severe cases. The intoxicated patient reels in many different directions, unlike the patient with cerebellar disease, and no effort is made to correct the reeling by watching the legs or the ground, as in cerebellar or sensory ataxia. In the drunken patient, despite a wide diversity of excursions of all parts of the body, balance may be exquisitely maintained. In contrast, the patient with cerebellar disease has great difficulty in maintaining his balance if he sways or lurches too far to one side.

HYSTERICAL GAIT. This may take any one of several forms—monoplegic, paraplegic, or hemiplegic. The monoplegic or hemiplegic patient does not lift the foot from the floor while walking; instead, he drags it as a useless member or pushes it ahead of him as though it were a skate. The characteristic circumduction is absent in hysterical hemiplegia, and the typical hemiplegic posture, hyperactive tendon reflexes, and Babinski's signs are missing. The hysterical paraplegic cannot very well drag both legs, and usually he depends on a crutch or remains helpless in bed; the muscles may be rigid with contractures or flaccid. The gait may be quite dramatic. Some patients look as though they were walking on stilts, and others lurch wildly in all directions, actually demonstrating by their gyrations the most remarkable ability to make rapid postural adjustments.

Astasia-abasia, in which the patient, though unable to either stand or walk, retains normal use of his legs while in bed, is nearly always hysterical. When such a patient is placed on his feet, he takes a few normal steps and then becomes unable to advance his feet; he lurches wildly and crumples to the floor if not assisted.

FRONTAL LOBE ATAXIA. Equilibrium and the capacity to stand and walk may be severely disturbed by diseases that affect the frontal lobes, particularly their medial parts. Although this disorder of gait is sometimes spoken of as an ataxia, or as an *apraxia* since the difficulty in walking cannot be accounted for by weakness or loss of sensation alone, it is probably neither. It most likely represents a loss of integration at the cortical and basal ganglionic level of the essential elements of stance and locomotion which were acquired in infancy and are often lost in senility.

The patient assumes a posture of slight flexion, with the feet placed farther apart then normal. He advances slowly, with small, shuffling hesitant steps. At times the patient halts, unable to advance without great effort, although he does much better with a little assistance. Turning is accomplished by a series of tiny, uncertain steps which are made with one foot, the other being planted on the floor as a pivot. The initiation of walking becomes progressively more difficult, and in advanced cases the patient may be unable to take a step or even to stand, and he falls backward.

Some patients are able to make complex movements with their legs, such as drawing imaginary figures, at a time when their gait is seriously impaired. In most cases, however, all movements of the legs are slow and awkward, and the limbs, when passively moved, offer variable resistance (Gegenhalten). An inability to turn in bed is highly characteristic, and may eventually become complete. These motor disabilities are usually associated with dementia, but there need be no parallelism in the evolution of these disorders. Grasping, groping, hyperactive tendon reflexes, and Babinski signs may or may not be present. The end result in many cases is a "cerebral paraplegia in flexion" (Yakovlev), in which the patient lies curled up in bed, immobile and mute, his limbs fixed by contractures in an attitude of flexion. If one frontal lobe is affected, awkwardness of movement appears in the opposite arm and leg, simulating cerebellar ataxia at times except for the absence of intention tremor, pendular reflexes, Holmes's rebound sign, etc.

SENILE GAIT. Elderly persons often complain of difficulty in walking, and examination may disclose no abnormality other than the slightly flexed posture of the senile and short uncertain steps, *marche à petits pas*. Speed, balance, and all the graceful, adaptive movements are lost. The exact nature of this gait disorder is not understood. It may represent no special neurologic defect, but only a general defensive reaction to all forms of defective locomotion. Or, it may represent an early or mild form of frontal lobe ataxia (see above).

REFERENCES

Altmann, F.: Diagnostic Significance of Vertigo. *In* The Vestibular System and Its Diseases. Wolfson, R. J., Ed. University of Pennsylvania Press, Philadelphia, 1966, pp. 353–374.

Citron, L., and Hallpike, C. S.: Observations Upon the Mechanism of Positional Nystagmus of the So-Called "Benign Paroxysmal Type," J. Laryngol. & Otol., 70:253, 1956.

Martin, J. P.: The Basal Ganglia and Locomotion. Ann. Roy. Coll. Med., 32:219, 1963.

Symonds, C.: The Significance of Vertigo in Neurological Diagnosis. J. Laryngol. & Otol., 66:295, 1952.

24 COMMON DISTURBANCES OF VISION, OCULAR MOVEMENT, AND HEARING

Maurice Victor
and Raymond D. Adams

Disturbances of vision and hearing, perhaps more properly considered under diseases of cranial nerves, present so many special problems that they will be dealt with in a separate chapter.

DISORDERS OF VISION

Here the most frequent complaint is blurred, impaired, or distorted vision, and less often, diplopia, ocular pain, irritation of eyes, or inability to keep the eyelids open. It is to be noted that patients do not always distinguish between mild diplopia and a true impairment or diminution of vision in one or both eyes; either condition may be described as blurring or dimming, and there may also be surprising inaccuracy in stating whether one or both eyes are affected. In late childhood and adolescence increasing difficulty in focusing eyes and in seeing clearly usually can be traced to developing myopia, though one must rule out ocular or suprasellar tumors. In the middle years (forty-five to fifty) presbyopia, an almost invariable accompaniment of age, is the usual explanation of this phenomenon; and still later in life glaucoma and cataract are the most frequent causes.

Episodic blindness in one or both eyes merits separate consideration. When it is bilateral and the blind spots are bordered by bright lines and then followed by unilateral headache and nausea, classic migraine is almost invariably the diagnosis. Episodic blindness limited to one eye, lasting a few minutes only but usually recurring (amblyopia fugax), indicates atherosclerosis of the carotid artery with impending thrombosis. Obscurations of vision of minutes' duration attend increased intracranial pressure and papilledema; they often herald permanent blindness and secondary optic atrophy.

Distortions of vision take several forms. The perceived objects may appear too small (micropsia), too large (macropsia), or they may seem to be askew. Such phenomena always suggest a lesion of the temporal lobes. The latter may also be accompanied by complex visual hallucinations (of landscapes, of people, etc.), which actually represent a sensory seizure (see Chap. 28).

ANATOMIC AND PHYSIOLOGIC CONSIDERATIONS

The first neuronal elements in the visual pathway are the rod and cone cells situated in the deepest layer of the retina. The cones are responsible for sharp vision and color discrimination, and they alone are present in the fovea. The rods, which are more sensitive to low intensities of light, predominate in the rest of the retina. Visual impulses are transmitted through the second system of neurones, the bipolar cells, to the ganglion cells, the axones of which form the optic nerve after first perforating the sclera at the optic disk, which has a sievelike structure, the *lamina cribrosa*. The absence of visual end organs at this point accounts for the blind spot in the field of vision. The optic nerve is actually a part of the central nervous system, with glial cells between its fibers but no Schwann cells as in the other cranial and spinal nerves.

The optic nerves extend from the disk to the optic chiasm, where their fibers undergo partial decussation (Fig. 24-1). The rearranged optic fibers continue as the optic tract, which partially encircles the cerebral peduncles and synapses with cells in the lateral geniculate body. From these cells arises the fourth system of neurones, the final visual pathway, comprising the geniculocalcarine tract. These fibers lie close to the wall of the temporal horn of the lateral ventricle. The upper ones take a direct course posteriorly, the lower ones loop forward over the temporal horn of the lateral ventricle into the temporal lobe (Meyer's loop) before they pass posteriorly and join the upper fibers on their way to the calcarine cortex.

The types of visual field defect resulting from lesions in different parts of the visual pathways are shown in Fig. 24-1. A prechiasmal lesion causes either a scotoma (an island of impaired vision within the visual field) or a cut in the peripheral part of the visual field. A small scotoma in the macular part of the visual field may seri-

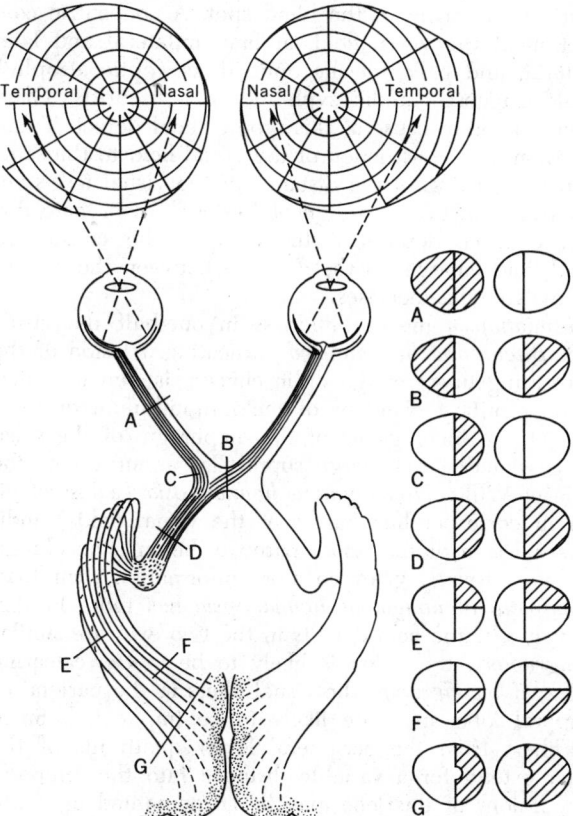

Fig. 24-1. Diagram showing the effects on the fields of vision produced by lesions at various points along the optic pathway. *A*, complete blindness in left eye; *B*, bitemporal hemianopsia; *C*, nasal hemianopsia of left eye; *D*, right homonymous hemianopsia; *E* and *F*, right upper and lower quadrant hemianopsias; *G*, right homonymous hemianopsia with preservation of central vision. (*Homans: "A Textbook of Surgery," Springfield, Ill., Charles C Thomas, Publisher, 1945.*)

ously impair visual acuity. Demyelinative, toxic (methyl alcohol, quinine, and certain of the phenothiazine tranquilizing drugs), nutritional (so-called "tobacco-alcohol" amblyopia), and vascular diseases are the usual causes of scotomas. The toxic states are characterized by symmetrical bilateral scotomas and the nutritional disorders by more or less symmetrical central or centrocecal ones (involving both the fixation point and the blind spot). These scotomas are predominantly in the distribution of the papillomacular bundle, but it is not certain whether the primary effect is on the nerve fibers or the ganglion cells. Vascular lesions, taking the form of hemorrhages or microinfarcts (cytoid bodies) in the retina or infarcts in the optic nerve, cause unilateral scotomas. Demyelinative diseases give rise to unilateral or asymmetric bilateral scotomas. If the lesion is near the optic disk, there may be swelling of the optic nerve head, i.e., papillitis, which can usually be distinguished from papilledema by the marked impairment of vision it produces.

Another common defect encountered on visual field examination is concentric constriction. This may be due to papilledema, in which case it is usually accompanied by an enlargement of the blind spot. A concentric constriction of the visual field, at first unilateral and later bilateral, and pallor of the optic disks (optic atrophy) should suggest chronic syphilitic optic neuritis. Glaucoma is another cause of this type of field defect. Tubular vision, i.e., constriction of the visual field to the same degree regardless of the distance of the visual test stimulus from the eye, is a sign of hysteria. In organic disease, e.g., chorioretinitis, the area of the constricted visual field enlarges as the distance between the patient and the stimulus increases.

Hemianopsia means blindness in one-half the visual field. *Bitemporal hemianopsia*, indicating a lesion of the decussating fibers of the optic chiasm, is due to tumor of the pituitary gland or of the infundibulum or third ventricle, to meningioma of the diaphragm of the sella, or occasionally, to a large suprasellar aneurysm of the circle of Willis. *Homonymous hemianopsia* (a loss of vision in corresponding halves of the visual fields) indicates a lesion of the visual pathway behind the chiasm and, if *complete*, gives no more information than that. *Incomplete homonymous hemianopsia* has more localizing value: if the field defects in the two eyes are similar (*congruous*), the lesion is likely to be in the calcarine cortex; if *incongruous*, the visual fibers in the parietal or temporal lobe are more likely to be implicated. Since the fibers from the peripheral lower quadrants of the retina extend for a variable distance into the temporal lobe, lesions of this lobe may be accompanied by a homonymous upper quadrantic field defect. Parietal lobe lesions may affect the lower quadrants more than the upper.

If the entire optic tract or calcarine cortex on one side is destroyed, there is complete homonymous hemianopsia, including half the field that represents the macula. Incomplete lesions of the optic tract and radiation usually spare central (macular) vision. It must be kept in mind that apparent macular sparing is frequently due to imperfect fixation of gaze. A lesion of the tip of one occipital lobe produces central homonymous hemianopsia because half the macular fibers of both eyes terminate there. Lesions of both occipital poles result in bilateral central scotomas; and if all the calcarine cortex on each side is completely destroyed, there is complete "cortical" blindness. Altitudinal or horizontal hemianopsias are more often due to lesions of the occipital lobes below or above the calcarine cortex than of optic chiasm.

In addition to blindness, i.e., "visual anesthesia," there is another category of visual impairment, which consists of a defect of visual perception, i.e., *visual agnosia*. The patient can see but cannot recognize objects unless he hears, smells, tastes, or palpates them. The failure of visual recognition of words is called *alexia*. The ability to recognize visually presented objects and words depends not only upon the integrity of the visual pathways and primary visual areas of the cerebral cortex (area 17 of Brodmann) but also upon those cortical areas which lie just anterior to the cerebral cortex in the *dominant* hemisphere (areas 18 and 19 of the occipital lobe and the angular gyrus). Visual-object agnosia and alexia re-

sult from lesions of these latter areas or from a lesion of the left calcarine cortex combined with one which interrupts the fibers crossing from the right occipital lobe. These subjects are discussed further in Chaps. 25 and 30.

The optic nerves also contain the afferent fibers for the pupillary reflexes. These fibers leave the optic tract and terminate in the superior colliculi. A lesion of the optic nerve or tracts may abolish the pupillary light reflex; the pupil is dilated and unreactive. Cerebral lesions, on the other hand, leave the pupillary light reflex unaltered. The lack of direct reflex in the blind eye and of consensual reflex in the sound one means that the afferent limb of the reflex arc (optic nerve) is the site of the lesion. A lack of direct light reflex with retention of the consensual reflex places the lesion in the efferent limb of the reflex arc (the homolateral oculomotor nucleus or nerve). Loss of light reflex without visual impairment or ocular palsy (Argyll Robertson pupillary phenomenon) is thought to be due to a lesion in the superior colliculi or periaqueductal region (see below).

Amaurosis refers to blindness from any cause. *Amblyopia* refers to an impairment or loss of vision which is not due to an error of refraction or some other disease of the eye. Hemeralopia and Nyctalopia mean poor twilight or night vision and are associated with vitamin A deficiency and pigmentary degeneration of the retina.

Hereditary diseases account for a significant proportion of cases of congenital or childhood amblyopia. These take the form of anophthalmia, bulbar atrophy (Norrie's disease), hypoplasia of optic nerves, retinitis pigmentosa, often combined with other conditions such as dwarfism polydactyly and gonadal deficiency (Lorain-Moon-Biedl disease), polyneuropathy and deafness (Refsum's disease), vestibulo-cerebellar ataxia and mental deficiency (Hallgren's disease) or mental deficiency alone. Pigmentary degeneration and optic atrophy are also common causes in adult years; some of the former are drug induced.

DIPLOPIA AND STRABISMUS AND DISORDERS OF THE THIRD, FOURTH, AND SIXTH NERVES

Strabismus (squint) refers to an ocular imbalance that results in improper alignment of the two eyes. It may be due to paralysis of an eye muscle; the ocular deviation results from the unrestrained activity of the opposing muscle. It may be due to inequality of tone in the muscles that hold the two eyes in a central position. The former is called *paralytic strabismus* and is primarily a neurologic problem; the latter is *nonparalytic strabismus* (referred to as *concomitant* strabismus if the squinting eye has a full range of movement) and is an ophthalmologic problem. Any type of ocular imbalance causes diplopia for the reason that images then fall on disparate or noncorresponding parts of the two retinas. After a time, however, the patient learns to suppress the image of one eye. This almost invariably happens early in concomitant strabismus of congenital nature, and the individual grows up with a diminished visual acuity in that eye (*amblyopia ex anopsia*).

The oculomotor, trochlear, and abducens nerves innervate the extrinsic and intrinsic musculature of the eye. A knowledge of their origin and anatomic relationships is essential to an understanding of the various paralytic ocular syndromes. The oculomotor nucleus consists of several groups of nerve cells ventral to the aqueduct of Sylvius, at the level of the superior colliculi. The nerve cells that innervate the iris and ciliary body are situated anteriorly in the so-called "Edinger-Westphal nucleus." Below this nucleus are the cells for the superior rectus, inferior oblique, internal rectus, and inferior rectus, in that order from above downward. Convergence is under the control of the medial groups of cells, the nucleus of Perlia. The cells of origin of the trochlear nerves are just inferior to those of the oculomotor nerves. The sixth nerve arises at a considerably lower level, from a paired group of cells in the floor of the fourth ventricle at the level of the lower pons. The intrapontine portion of the facial nerve loops around the sixth nerve nucleus before it turns anterolaterally to make its exit; a lesion in this locality usually causes a homolateral paralysis of both lateral rectus and facial muscles.

All three nerves, after leaving the brainstem, course anteriorly and pass through the cavernous sinus, where they come into close proximity with the ophthalmic division of the fifth nerve, and together they enter the orbit through the superior orbital fissure. The oculomotor nerve supplies all the extrinsic ocular muscles except two —the superior oblique and the external rectus—which are innervated by the trochlear and abducens nerves, respectively. The voluntary part of the levator palpebrae muscle is also supplied by the oculomotor nerve, the involuntary part being under the control of autonomic fibers which also supply the sphincter pupillae and the ciliary muscles (muscles of accommodation).

Although all the extraocular muscles probably participate in every movement of the eyes, particular muscles move the eyes in certain fields. The lateral rectus rotates the eye outward; the medial rectus, inward. The function of the vertical recti and the obliques varies according to the position of the eye. When the eye is turned outward, the elevators and depressors of the eye are the superior and inferior recti; when the eye is turned inward, they are the inferior and superior obliques, respectively. In contrast, torsion of the eyeball is effected by the oblique muscles when the eye is turned outward, and by the recti when it is turned inward.

Accurate binocular vision is achieved by the associated action of the ocular muscles, which allows a visual stimulus to fall on exactly corresponding parts of the two retinas. Conjugate movement of the eyes is controlled by centers in the cerebral cortex and brainstem. Area 8 in the frontal lobe is the center for voluntary conjugate movements of the eyes to the opposite side. In addition, there is a center in the occipital lobe concerned with contralateral following movements. Fibers from these centers pass to the opposite sides of the brainstem, where they connect with lower centers for conjugate move-

ments: those for the right lateral gaze are thought to be in the proximity of the right abducens nucleus; those for the left lateral gaze are near the left abducens. Simultaneous innervation of one internal rectus and the other external rectus during lateral gaze is a function of the medial longitudinal fasciculus. The arrangements of nerve cells and fibers for vertical gaze and convergence are situated in the pretectal areas and paramedian zones of the midbrain tegmentum.

OCULAR MUSCLE AND GAZE PALSIES

There are three types of paralysis of extraocular muscles: (1) paralysis of isolated ocular muscles, (2) paralysis of conjugate movements (gaze), and (3) syndromes of mixed gaze and ocular muscle paralysis.

Characteristic clinical disturbances result from single lesions of the third, fourth, or sixth cranial nerves. A complete third nerve lesion causes ptosis (since the levator palpebrae is supplied mainly by the third nerve), an inability to rotate the eye upward, downward, or inward, a divergent strabismus due to unopposed action of the lateral rectus muscle, a dilated nonreactive pupil (iridoplegia), and paralysis of accommodation (cycloplegia). When only the muscles of the iris and ciliary body are paralyzed, the condition is termed *internal ophthalmoplegia*. Fourth nerve lesions result in an extorsion of the eye and a weakness of downward gaze, so that patients commonly complain of special difficulty in going downstairs. Head tilting, to the opposite shoulder, is especially characteristic of fourth nerve lesions. This maneuver causes a compensatory intorsion of the lower eye, enabling the patient to obtain binocular vision. Lesions of the sixth nerve result in paralysis of abduction and a convergent strabismus owing to the unopposed action of the internal rectus muscles. With incomplete sixth nerve palsies, turning the head toward the side of the paretic muscle may overcome diplopia. The foregoing signs may occur with various degrees of completeness, depending on the severity and site of the lesion or lesions.

Ocular palsies may be central, i.e., due to a lesion of the nucleus or the intramedullary portion of the cranial nerve, or peripheral. Ophthalmoplegia due to a lesion in the brainstem is usually accompanied by involvement of other cranial nerves or long tracts. Peripheral lesions, which may or may not be solitary, have a great variety of causes; the most common are aneurysm of the circle of Willis, tumors of the base of the brain, carcinomatosis of the meninges, herpes zoster, and syphilitic meningitis. The third-nerve palsy that occurs with diabetes is probably due to infarction of the third nerve, and the prognosis for recovery in such cases, as with other nonprogressive diseases of the peripheral nerve, is usually excellent. The points of difference between lesions within and outside of the brainstem are tabulated in Table 24-1, and the various intramedullary and extramedullary cranial nerve syndromes are described in Tables 355-1 and 355-2. See also diagrams in Ch. 357.

When the ocular palsy is slight, there may be no obvious squint or defect in ocular movement; yet the patient experiences diplopia. Study of the relative posi-

Table 24-1. COMPARISON OF LESIONS WITHIN AND OUTSIDE
THE BRAIN STEM

Effect	Lesions within the brain stem	Lesions external to the brain stem
Involvement of multiple contiguous nerves	±	+
Involvement of sensorimotor tracts	+, often "alternating" or crossed sensory or motor palsies	±
Disturbance of consciousness	+	0 (+ late)
Evidence of other segmental disturbances of the brain stem such as decerebrate rigidity, tonic neck reflexes, pseudobulbar palsy	+	0 (+ late)
X-ray evidence of erosion of cranial bones or enlargement of foramens	0	+

tions of the images of the two eyes then becomes the most accurate way of determining which muscle is involved. The image seen by the affected eye is usually less distinct, but the most reliable way of distinguishing the two images is by the red glass test. A *red glass is placed in front of the patient's right eye.* He is then asked to look at a flashlight, held at a distance of a meter, to turn his eyes in various segments of his visual fields, and to state the position of the red and white images. The relative positions of the two images are plotted as indicated in Fig. 24-2.

Three rules aid in the analysis of ocular movements by the red glass test. (1) The direction in which the distance between the images is at a maximum is the direction of action of the paretic muscle. For example, if the greatest separation is in looking to the right, either the right abductor or the left adductor muscle is weak. (2) The image projected farther to the side belongs to the paretic eye. If the patient looks to the right and the red image is farther to the right, then the right abducens muscle is weak. If the white image is to the right of the red, then the left internal rectus muscle is weak. (3) In testing vertical movements, again the image of the eye with the paretic muscle is the one projected most peripherally in the direction of eye movement. One ignores lateral separation at this time. It must be remembered that there are two elevator and two depressor muscles. The responsible muscle may be either one of the obliques or vertical recti muscles. For example, if the maximum separation of images occurs on looking downward and to the left, and the white image is projected farther down than the red, the paretic muscle is the left inferior rectus. If the maximum separation occurs on looking down and to the right, and the white image is lower than the red, the paretic muscle is the left superior oblique. Separation of images on looking up and to the right or left will simi-

larly distinguish paresis of the inferior oblique and superior rectus muscles.

Monocular diplopia may occur and is related to diseases of the lens and refractive media of the eye. Also, paresis of accommodation may produce diplopia for near vision; its cause is unknown.

PARALYSIS OF CONJUGATE MOVEMENT (GAZE). The term *conjugate gaze,* or *conjugate movement,* refers to the simultaneous movement of the two eyes in the same direction. An acute lesion in one frontal lobe may cause paralysis of contralateral gaze. The eyes turn toward the side of the lesion. The ocular disorder is temporary (several days' duration). In bilateral frontal lesions the patient may be unable to turn his eyes voluntarily (oculomotor apraxia) in any direction—up, down, or to the side—but retains fixation and following movements, which are believed to be occipital lobe functions. Gaze paralysis of cerebral origin is not attended by strabismus or diplopia. The usual causes are vascular occlusion with infarction, hemorrhage, and abscess or tumor of the frontal lobe. With certain extrapyramidal disorders, e.g., postencephalitic parkinsonism or Huntington's chorea, ocular movements may be limited in all directions, especially upward. Lesions of the superior colliculus and tegmentum, near the posterior commissure, interfere with voluntary reflex upward gaze, and often movements of convergence as well as the pupillary light reflexes are abolished (Parinaud's syndrome). There also exists a pontine center for conjugate lateral gaze, probably in the vicinity of the abducens nuclei. A lesion here causes ipsilateral gaze palsy, with the eyes turning to the opposite side. Vertical and lateral gaze palsies are combined in the supranuclear ophthalmoplegia syndrome of Steele-Richardson. The palsy tends to last longer than with cerebral lesions and is frequently accompanied by other signs of pontine disease. Fully developed forms of gaze paralysis are readily discerned, but lesser degrees may be overlooked unless one pays special attention to the predominant position of the eyes and tests the ability to sustain conjugate movement.

In skew deviation, a poorly understood disorder of gaze, the eyes diverge, one looking down, the other up. The deviation is constant in all fields of gaze. It may occur with any lesion of the posterior fossa but particularly one in the brainstem. The lesion is on the side of the lower eye.

MIXED GAZE AND OCULAR PARALYSES. These are always a sign of intrapontine or mesencephalic disease. With a lesion of the lower pons in or near the sixth-nerve nucleus, there is a homolateral paralysis of the lateral rectus muscle and a failure of adduction of the opposite eye, i.e., a combined paralysis of the sixth nerve and of conjugate lateral gaze. Lesions of the medial longitudinal fasciculi interfere with lateral conjugate gaze in another way. On looking to the right, the left eye fails to adduct; on looking to the left, the right eye fails to adduct. The abducting eye shows nystagmus. This condition is referred to as *internuclear ophthalmoplegia* and should always be suspected when only adduction of the eyes is affected. If the lesion is in the lower part of the medial longitudinal fasciculi, convergence is intact; if the lesion is in the higher part, i.e., near the oculomotor nuclei, convergence may be lost (anterior internuclear ophthalmoplegia).

NYSTAGMUS. This refers to involuntary rhythmic movements of the eyes; it is of two types, oscillating (pendular) and rhythmic (jerk). In jerk nystagmus, the movements are distinctly faster in one direction than the other; in pendular nystagmus, the oscillations are roughly equal in rate for the two directions, although on conjugate lateral gaze, the pendular type may resemble the jerk type, with the fast component to the side of the gaze.

In testing for nystagmus, the eyes should first be examined in the central position and then during upward, downward, and lateral movements. If nystagmus is monocular (as described below), each eye should be tested separately, with the other one covered. Labyrinthine nystagmus is most obvious when visual fixation is prevented by shielding the eyes; brainstem and cerebellar nystagmus are brought out best by having the patient fixate on a finger. Labyrinthine nystagmus may vary with the position of the head; hence these various tests should be performed with the head in several different positions. In particular, the postural nystagmus of Bárány is evoked by hyperextension of the neck, with the patient in the supine position. Optokinetic nystagmus should be tested by asking the patient to look at a rotating cylinder on which several stripes have been painted or a striped cloth moved across the field of vision.

A few irregular jerks are observed in many normal individuals when the eyes are turned far to the side. These so-called "nystagmoid movements" are probably similar to the tremulousness of a muscle that is contracted maximally. Occasionally a fine rhythmic nystagmus can be obtained in extreme lateral gaze, but if it is bilateral and disappears as the eyes move a few degrees toward the midline, it usually has no clinical significance.

Pendular nystagmus is found in a variety of conditions in which central vision is lost early in life, such as albinism and in various other diseases of the retina and refractive mediums. The syndrome of miners' nystagmus, formerly a common cause of industrial disability, occurs after many years of work in comparative darkness. The oscillations of the eyes are very rapid, increase on upward gaze, and are often associated with vertigo, head tremor, and intolerance of light. *Spasmus nutans* is a specific type of pendular nystagmus of infancy and is accompanied by head nodding and occasionally by wry positions of the neck. The prognosis is good; most infants recover within a few months.

Jerk nystagmus is the commoner type. It may be lateral or vertical, particularly on ocular movement in these planes, or it may be rotary. By custom, the direction of the nystagmus is named according to the direction of the fast component. There are several varieties of jerk nystagmus. When one is watching a moving object—e.g., the passing landscape from a train window or a rotating drum with vertical stripes—a rhythmic jerk nystagmus, *optokinetic nystagmus*, normally appears. The slow phase is a result of visual fixation; the quick phase is compensa-

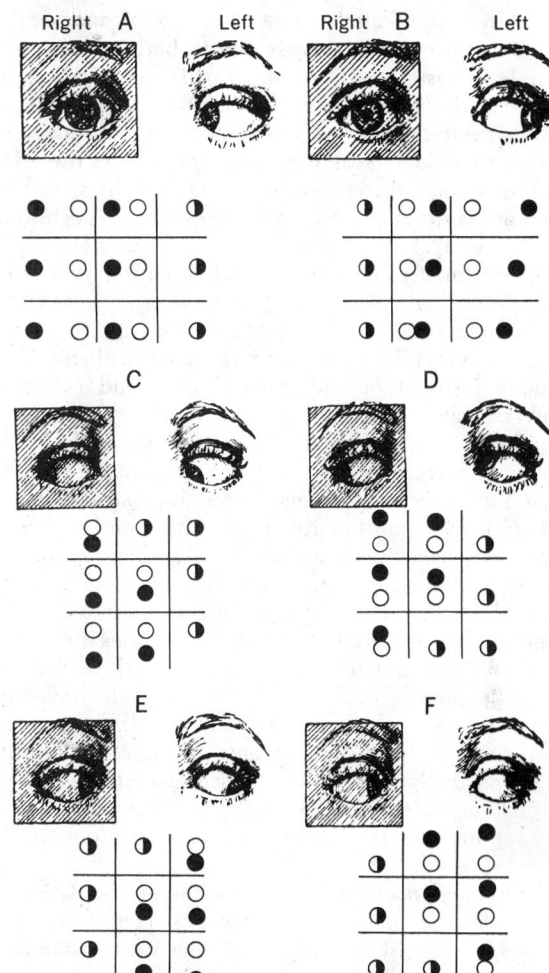

Fig. 24-2. Diplopia fields with individual muscle paralyses. The dark glass is in front of the right eye, and the fields are projected as the patient sees the images. *A.* Paralysis of right external rectus. Characteristic: right eye does not move to the right. Field: horizontal homonymous diplopia increasing on looking to the right. *B.* Paralysis of right internal rectus. Characteristic: right eye does not move to the left. Field: horizontal crossed diplopia increasing on looking to the left. *C.* Paralysis of right inferior rectus. Characteristic: right eye does not move downward when eyes are turned to the right. Field: vertical diplopia (image of right eye lowermost) increasing on looking to the right and down. *D.* Paralysis of right superior rectus. Characteristic: right eye does not move upward when eyes are turned to the right. Field: vertical diplopia (image of right eye uppermost) increasing on looking to the right and up. *E.* Paralysis of right superior oblique. Characteristic: right eye does not move downward when eyes are turned to the left. Field: vertical diplopia (image of right eye lowermost) increasing on looking to left and down. *F.* Paralysis of right inferior oblique. Characteristic: right eye does not move upward when eyes are turned to the left. Field: vertical diplopia (image of right eye uppermost) increasing on looking to left and up. (*Cogan: "Neurology of the Ocular Muscles," 2d ed., Springfield, Ill., Charles C Thomas, Publisher, 1956.*)

tory. With unilateral cerebral lesions, particularly in the parieto-occipital region, there is loss of optokinetic nystagmus when the moving stimulus, e.g., the drum, moves toward the side of the lesion.

Aside from optokinetic nystagmus, lateral and vertical nystagmus are most frequently due to barbiturate intoxication. Jerk nystagmus may signify disease of the labyrinthine-vestibular apparatus. Labyrinthine stimulation or irritation produces a nystagmus with the fast phase to the opposite side. The slow component reflects the effect of impulses derived from the semicircular canals, and the fast component is a corrective movement. Vestibular-labyrinthine nystagmus may be horizontal, vertical, or most characteristically, rotary. Vertigo, nausea, vomiting, and staggering are the usual accompaniments (see Chap. 23). Brainstem lesions often cause a coarse unidirectional nystagmus, which may be horizontal or vertical; the latter is usually brought out on upward gaze and rarely on downward gaze. The presence of vertical nystagmus is pathognomonic of disease in the tegmentum of the brainstem. Vertigo is inconstant, and signs of disease of other nuclear structures and tracts in the brainstem are frequent. Jerk nystagmus of this type is frequent in demyelinative or vascular disease, in tumors, and syringobulbia. Cerebellopontine angle tumors cause a coarse bilateral horizontal nystagmus, with the fast component to the side of the lesion. Nystagmus probably does not occur with cerebellar disease unless the fastigial nuclei and their connections with the vestibular nuclei are involved. The nystagmus that occurs only in the abducting eye and is said to be a pathognomonic sign of multiple sclerosis probably represents an incompletely developed form of internuclear ophthalmoplegia. The movement of the adducting eye (which does not show nystagmus) is impaired.

Convergence nystagmus is a rhythmic oscillation in which a slow abduction of the eyes in respect of each other is followed by a quick movement of adduction. It is usually accompanied by other types of nystagmus and by one or more features of Parinaud's syndrome. Occasionally there is also a jerky retraction movement of the eyes (*nystagmus retractorius*) or eyelids or a maintained spasm of convergence, best brought out on attempted elevation of the eyes to command. These unusual phenomena all point to a lesion of the upper midbrain tegmentum and are usually manifestations of vascular disease or of pinealoma.

Seesaw nystagmus, one eye moving up, the other down, is occasionally observed in conjunction with bitemporal hemianopia. Its mechanism is unknown.

Oscillopsia refers to illusory movement of the environment, in which objects seem to move back and forth, to jerk or to wiggle. It may or may not occur with turning of the eyes and consequent displacement of the image on the retina, and is said to be characteristic of the nystagmus of multiple sclerosis.

ALTERATIONS OF PUPILS

Pupil size is determined by the balance of innervation between the dilator and constrictor fibers. The pupillodilator fibers arise in the posterior part of the hypothalamus, descend in the lateral tegmentum of the midbrain, pons, medulla, and cervical spinal cord to the eighth cervical and first thoracic segments, where they synapse with the lateral horn cells. The latter give rise to preganglionic fibers that synapse in the superior cervical ganglion; the postganglionic fibers course along the internal carotid artery and traverse the cavernous sinus to join the first division of the trigeminal nerve, finally reaching the eyes as the long ciliary nerves. The pupilloconstrictor fibers arise in the nucleus of Edinger-Westphal, join the oculomotor nerve, and synapse in the ciliary ganglion with the postganglionic neurones that innervate the iris and ciliary body.

The pupils are usually equal in size, though if the eyes are turned to one side, the pupil of the abducting eye dilates slightly. Pupil size varies with light intensity; as one pupil constricts under a bright light (direct reflex), the other unexposed pupil does likewise (consensual reflex). Pupillary constriction is also part of the act of convergence and accommodation for near objects.

Interruption of the sympathetic fibers either centrally, between the hypothalamus and their point of exit from the spinal cord, or peripherally, in the neck or along the carotid artery, results in miosis and ptosis (due to paralysis of the levator palpebrae), with loss of sweating of the face, and occasionally enophthalmos (Bernard-Horner syndrome). Stimulation or irritation of the pupillodilator fibers has the opposite effect, i.e., lid retraction, slight proptosis, and dilatation of the pupil. The ciliospinal pupillary reflex, evoked by pinching the neck, is effected through these efferent sympathetic fibers. Abnormal dilatation of the pupils (mydriasis), often with loss of pupillary light reflexes, may result from midbrain lesions and is a frequent finding in cases of deep coma. Extreme constriction of the pupils (miosis) is commonly observed with pontine lesions, presumably because of bilateral interruption of the pupilodilator fibers.

The functional integrity of the sympathetic and parasympathetic nerve endings in the iris may be determined by the use of certain drugs. Atropine and homatropine dilate the pupils by paralyzing the parasympathetic nerve endings, while physostigmine and pilocarpine constrict them, the former by inhibiting cholinesterase activity at the neuromuscular junction and the latter by direct stimulation of the sphincter muscle of the iris. Cocaine dilates the pupils by stimulating the sympathetic nerve endings. Morphine acts centrally to constrict the pupils.

In chronic syphilitic meningitis and other forms of late syphilis, particularly tabes dorsalis, the pupils are usually small, irregular, and unequal; they do not dilate properly in response to mydriatic drugs and fail to react to light, although they do constrict on accommodation. This is known as the *Argyll Robertson pupil.* The exact locality of the lesion is not certain; it is generally believed to be in the tectum of the midbrain proximal to the oculomotor nuclei, where the descending pupillodilator fibers are in close proximity to the light-reflex fibers. The possibility of a partial third-nerve lesion or a lesion of the ciliary ganglion has not been excluded. A dissociation of the light reflex from the accommodation-convergence reaction is sometimes observed with other midbrain lesions, e.g., pinealoma, multiple sclerosis, and diabetes mellitus; in these diseases miosis, irregularity of pupils, and failure to respond to a mydriatic are not constantly present. Another interesting pupillary abnormality is the myotonic reaction, sometimes referred to as *Adie's pupil*. The patient may complain of blurring of vision or may have suddenly noticed that one pupil is larger than the other. The reaction to light and convergence are absent if tested in the customary manner, although the size of the pupil will change slowly on prolonged stimulation. Once contracted or dilated, the pupils remain in that state for some minutes. The affected pupil reacts promptly to the usual mydriatic and miotic drugs but is unusually sensitive to a 2.5 percent solution of Mecholyl, a strength that will not affect a normal pupil. The myotonic pupil usually appears during the third or fourth decade and may be associated with absence of knee jerks, and hence be mistaken for tabes dorsalis.

DISTURBANCES OF HEARING

Tinnitus and *deafness* are frequent symptoms and always indicate disease of the ear or of the auditory nerve and its central connections.

Tinnitus, or ringing in the ears, is a purely subjective phenomenon and may also be reported as a buzzing, whistling, hissing, or roaring sound. It is a very common symptom in adults and may be of no significance, as, for example, the hissing sound due to wax in the external auditory canal or a blocked eustachian tube. On the other hand, it is regularly associated with disease of the eighth nerve, inner ear, or ossicles; severe and prolonged tinnitus in the presence of normal hearing is very rare. If tinnitus is localized to one ear and is described as having a tonal character, such as ringing or a bell-like tone, and particularly if the recruitment phenomenon (see below) is present, it is probably cochlear in origin. Noises described as rushing water or escaping steam point more to disease of the nerve or even the brainstem. Clicking sounds are caused by intermittent contraction of the tensor tympani. A pulsating tinnitus synchronous with the pulse may be related to an intracranial vascular malformation; however, this symptom must be carefully judged, since introspective individuals often report hearing their pulse when lying with one ear on a pillow. Certain drugs such as salicylates and quinine produce tinnitus and transient deafness. Nervous individuals are less tolerant of tinnitus than are more stable persons; depressed or anxious patients may demand relief from tinnitus that has existed for years.

Examination of hearing should always begin with inspection of the external auditory canal and the tympanic membrane. A watch or whispered words are suitable means of testing hearing at the bedside, the opposite ear being closed by the finger. If there is any suspicion of deafness or a complaint of tinnitus or vertigo, or if the patient is a child with a speech defect, then hearing must be tested further. This can be done with the use of tuning forks of different frequencies, but the most accurate results are obtained by the use of an electric audiometer and the construction of an audiogram, which reveals the entire range of hearing at a glance. An auditory recruitment test may also be helpful: the difference in hearing between the two ears is estimated, and the loudness of the stimulus delivered to each ear is then increased by regular increments. In nonrecruiting deafness (characteristic of a nerve trunk lesion) the original difference in hearing persists in comparisons above threshold. In recruiting deafness (as occurs in Ménière's disease) the more defective ear gains in loudness and finally is equal to the better one.

Deafness is of two types: (1) nerve deafness, due to interruption of cochlear fibers, and (2) conduction deafness, due to disease of the middle ear (or occlusion of the external auditory canal or eustachian tube). In differentiating these two types, the tuning fork tests are of value. When the vibrating fork is held several inches from the ear (the test for air conduction), sound waves can be appreciated only as they are transmitted through the middle ear and will be reduced with disease in this location. When the fork is applied to the skull (test for bone conduction), the sound waves are conveyed directly to the cochlea, without the intervention of the middle ear apparatus, and will therefore not be reduced when the disease is confined to the middle ear. With affection of the cochlea or eighth nerve, both air and bone conduction will be reduced or lost. Normally air conduction is better than bone conduction. These principles form the basis for several tests of auditory function.

In *Weber's test*, the vibrating fork is applied to the forehead in the midline. In middle ear deafness the sound is localized in the affected ear, in nerve deafness, in the normal ear. In *Rinné's test* the fork is applied to the mastoid process, the other ear being closed by the observer's finger. At the moment the sound ceases the fork is held at the auditory meatus. In middle ear deafness the sound cannot be heard by air conduction after bone conduction has ceased (abnormal or negative Rinné test). In nerve deafness the reverse is true (normal or positive Rinné test), although both air and bone conduction may be quantitatively decreased. In *Schwabach's test*, the patient's bone conduction is compared with that of a normal observer. In general, high-pitched tones are lost in nerve deafness and low-pitched ones in middle ear deafness, but there are frequent exceptions to this rule.

The common causes of middle ear deafness are otitis media, otosclerosis, and rupture of the eardrum. Nerve deafness has many causes. The internal ear may be aplastic from birth (hereditary deaf-mutism), or it may be damaged by rubella in the pregnant mother. Acute purulent meningitis or chronic infection spreading from the middle ear are common causes of nerve deafness in childhood. The auditory nerve may be involved by tumors of the cerebellopontine angle or by syphilis. Deafness may also result from a demyelinative plaque in the brainstem. A series of genetically determined syndromes which feature a neural type of deafness, some congenital, others progressive, have recently come to light. The most interesting of these are: hereditary deafness with nephritis (Alport's disease); hereditary deafness with goitre (Pendred's disease); hereditary heart disease with deafness

(Jervell and Lang-Nielsen disease); hereditary deafness with renal disease and digital anomalies; hereditary deafness with various combinations of mental retardation, retinitis pigmentosa and polyneuropathy as in Hallgren's disease, Alstrom's disease, Refsum's disease; hereditary deafness with skin abnormalities such as albinism, lentigines, piebaldness, white forelock (Waardenburg's disease), onchydystrophy and pegged teeth, atopic dermatitis, anhydrosis; hereditary deafness with muscular dystrophy. Of the types of conduction deafness hereditary otosclerosis is the most frequent (causes 50 percent of deafness in adulthood); other types are observed with cranial, ear, jaw, and other congenital anomalies (Treacher-Collins disease, Engelman's diaphyseal dysplasia etc.). Hysterical deafness may be difficult to distinguish from organic disease. In the case of bilateral deafness, the distinction can be made by observing a blink (cochleo-orbicular reflex) or an alteration in skin sweating (psycho-galvanic skin reflex) in response to a loud sound. Unilateral hysterical deafness may be detected by an audiometer, with both ears connected, or by whispering into the bell of a stethoscope attached to the patient's ears, closing first one and then the other tube without the patient's knowledge.

REFERENCES

Cogan, D.: Brain Lesions and Eye Movements in Man. Chap. 17 in "The Oculomotor System," M. Bender (Ed.), p. 417, New York, Harper & Row Publishers, Incorporated, 1964.

Pasik, P., and T. Pasik: Oculomotor Functions in Monkeys with Lesions of the Cerebrum and Superior Colliculi, Chap. 3 in "The Oculomotor System," M. Bender (Ed.), p. 40, New York, Harper & Row Publishers, Incorporated, 1964.

Konigsmark, B. W.: Hereditary Deafness in Man, Publication of Dept. of Otology, Johns Hopkins University, 1969.

25 DISORDERS OF SENSATION

*Maurice Victor and
Raymond D. Adams*

Loss or perversion of somatic sensation not infrequently represents the principal manifestation of disease of the nervous system. The logic of this is clear enough, since the major anatomic pathways of the sensory system are distinct from those of the motor system and may be selectively disturbed by disease. An understanding of these sensory disorders depends on a knowledge of applied anatomy, physiology, and the use of special tests designed to indicate the nature of the disordered function and its locality.

Ideally, one should be familiar with the sensory organs in the skin and deep structures, the distribution of the peripheral nerves and the spinal roots, and the pathways by which the sensory impulses are conveyed through the spinal cord and brainstem to the thalamus and parietal lobe cortex. These topics were introduced in Chap. 9,

General Considerations of Pain. Unfortunately, space does not permit a detailed review here of the anatomy of the sensory system nor of its physiology. The interested reader may turn to the references at the end of the chapter. Nor is a final statement on the physiology of the sensory system possible, because our notions about the physiology of receptors and pain are in a state of constant revision. But, the generally accepted views about the cutaneous distribution of sensory spinal roots and peripheral nerves can be obtained from Figs. 25-1 and 25-2.

Disorders of the somatic sensory apparatus pose special problems for the patient. He is confronted with derangements of sensation which may be unlike anything he had previously experienced, and he has few words in his vocabulary to describe what he feels. He may say that a limb feels "numb" and "dead" when in fact he means weakness or paralysis and not a sensory disturbance. Observant individuals may discover a loss of sensation, for example, inability to feel discomfort on touching an object hot enough to blister the skin or unawareness of articles of clothing and other objects in contact with the skin. Or the disease may induce a new and unnatural series of sensory experiences, which are as often a source of complaint as loss of sensation. If nerves, spinal roots,

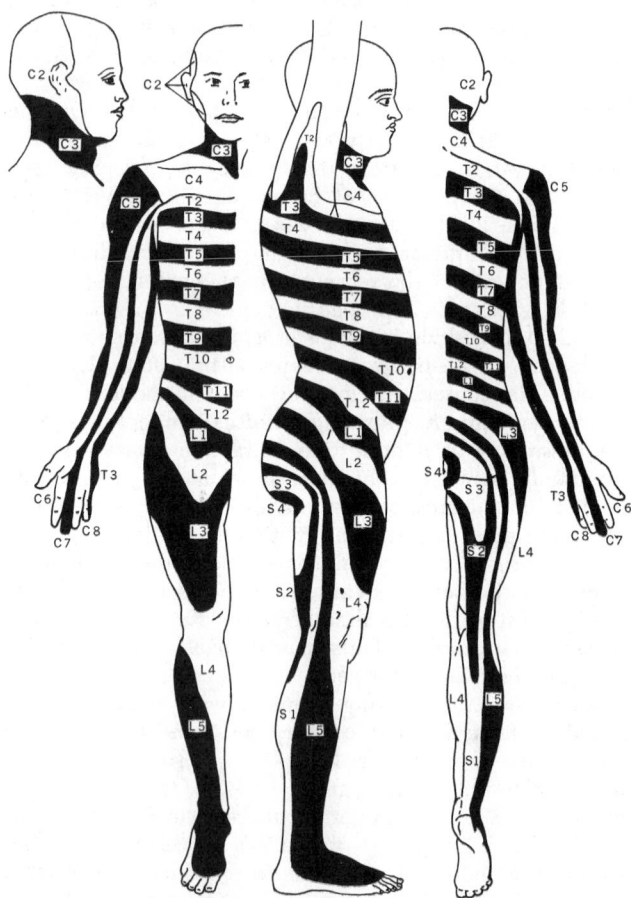

Fig. 25-1. Distribution of the sensory spinal roots on the surface of the body. (Holmes: "Introduction to Clinical Neurology," Edinburgh, E. & S. Livingstone, Ltd., 1946.)

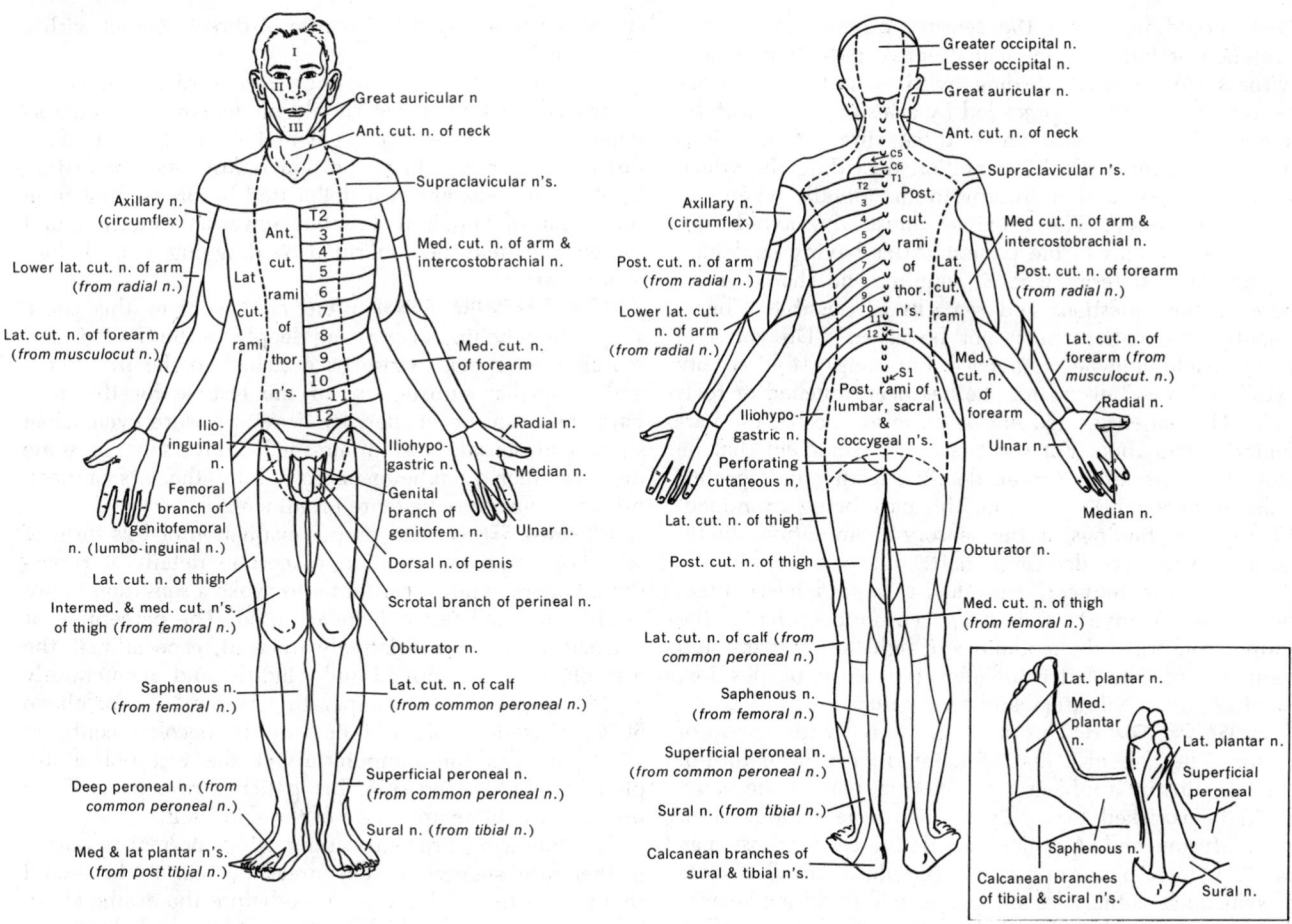

Fig. 25-2. The cutaneous fields of peripheral nerves. (*Haymaker and Woodhall: "Peripheral Nerve Injuries," Philadelphia, W. B. Saunders Company, 1945.*)

or spinal tracts are only partially interrupted, a touch may arouse tingling or pricking (Novocaine feeling), meaning presumably that at least some of the remaining touch and pain fibers are functional but acting abnormally. Similarly, burning and pain may represent over activity of surviving thermal and pain fibers (causalgia). The lesion may be in the peripheral nerve, the lateral spinothalamic tract in the spinal cord or brainstem, or the thalamus. Hyperesthesia or hyperpathia are frequent. Tightness and drawing and pulling sensations, a feeling of a band or girdle around the limb or trunk, are common, with partial involvement of pressure fibers. These abnormal sensations are called *paresthesias*, or *dysesthesias*, if they are unpleasant; and their character and distribution inform us of the anatomy of the lesion involving the sensory system.

EXAMINATION OF SENSATION

The examination of sensation is the most difficult part of the neurologic examination. For one thing, test procedures are relatively crude and inadequate, and at times no objective sensory loss can be demonstrated despite symptoms that clearly indicate the presence of such a

deficit. Also, a response to a sensory stimulus is difficult to evaluate objectively, and the examiner's conclusions depend on the patient's interpretations of sensory experiences. This, in turn, depends on his general awareness, responsiveness, and desire to cooperate, as well as his intelligence, level of education, and the degree of suggestibility and fatigue. At times, children and relatively uneducated persons are better witnesses than more sophisticated individuals who are likely to analyze their feelings too minutely.

The detail in which sensation is tested will be governed by the clinical situation. If the patient has no sensory complaints, it is sufficient to examine vibration and position sense in the fingers and toes, to test the appreciation of pain over the face, trunk, and extremities, and to determine whether the sensory findings are the same in symmetric parts of the body. A rough survey of this sort may detect sensory defects of which the patient is unaware. On the other hand, more thorough testing is in order if the patient has complaints referable to the sensory system, or if there is localized atrophy or weakness, ataxia, trophic changes of joints, or painless ulcers.

A few other general principles should be mentioned.

One should not press the sensory examination in the presence of fatigue, for an inattentive patient is a poor witness. When first dealing with a patient, sensory testing is of necessity preceded by a history and often by a general examination; under these circumstances it is best to aim for a quick orientation regarding the whole sensory system and to return to the details when the patient is rested. The examiner must also avoid suggesting symptoms to the patient. After having explained in the simplest terms what is required, he should interpose as few questions and remarks as possible. Consequently, the patient must not be asked, "Do you feel that?" each time he is touched but simply told to say "yes" or "sharp" every time he has been touched or feels pain. The patient should not be permitted to see the part under examination. For short tests it is sufficient that he close his eyes; during more detailed testing it is preferable to screen his eyes from the part being examined. Finally, the findings of the sensory examination should be accurately recorded on a chart.

Sensation is frequently classified as *superficial* (cutaneous, exteroceptive) and *deep* (proprioceptive); the former comprises the modalities of light touch, pain, and temperature; the latter includes the sense of position, passive motion, vibration, and deep pain.

SENSE OF TOUCH. This is usually tested with a wisp of cotton. The patient is first acquainted with the nature of the stimulus by applying it to a normal part of the body. Then he is asked to say "yes" each time various other parts are touched. A patient simulating sensory loss may say "no" in response to a tactile stimulus. Cornified areas of skin, such as the soles and palms, will require a heavier stimulus than normal, and the hair-clad parts a lighter one because of the numerous nerve endings around the follicle. The patient is more sensitive to a moving stimulus of any kind than a stationary one. The application of the examiner's or preferably the patient's finger tips is a useful method of mapping out an area of tactile loss, as Trotter originally showed.

More precise testing is possible by using a von Frey hair. By this method, a stimulus of constant strength can be applied, and the threshold for touch sensation determined.

SENSE OF PAIN. This is most efficiently estimated by pinprick, although it can be evoked by a great diversity of noxious stimuli. The patient must understand that he is to report the degree of sharpness of the pin and not simply the feeling of contact or pressure of the point or even a special sensation due to penetration of the skin. If the pinpricks are applied rapidly, their effects may be summated and excessive pain may result; therefore, they should be delivered not too rapidly, about 1 per sec, and not over the same spot.

It is almost impossible, using an ordinary pin or needle, to apply each stimulus with equal intensity. This difficulty can be largely overcome by the use of an algesimeter, which enables one not only to give constant stimuli but also to grade their intensity and determine threshold values. Even when the pinpricks are of equal intensity, an isolated stimulus may be reported as exces-

sively sharp, apparently because of direct contact with a pain spot.

If an area of diminished or absent sensation is encountered, its boundaries should be demarcated to determine whether it has a segmental or peripheral nerve distribution or whether sensation is lost below a certain level. Such areas are best delineated by proceeding from the region of impaired sensation toward the normal, and the changes may be confirmed by dragging a pin lightly over the skin.

DEEP PRESSURE SENSE. One can estimate this sense simply by pinching or pressing deeply on the tendons and muscles; no special virtue is attached to the traditional and somewhat sadistic use of the testicle for this test. Pain can often be elicited by heavy pressure even when superficial sensation is diminished; conversely, in some diseases, such as tabetic neurosyphilis, the loss of deep pressure sense may be more prominent.

THERMAL SENSE. The proper evaluation of this form of sensation requires attention to certain details of procedure. One may fail consistently to evoke a sensation of hot or cold, if small test objects are used. The perception of thermal stimuli are relatively delayed, especially if the test objects are applied only lightly and momentarily against the skin. At a temperature below 10°C or above 50°C, sensations of cold or warmth become confused with pain. As the temperature of the test object approaches that of the skin, the patient's response will be modified by the temperature of the skin itself.

The following procedure for testing thermal sensation is therefore suggested. The areas of skin to be tested should be exposed for some time before the examination. The test objects should be large, preferably Erlenmeyer flasks containing hot and cold water. Thermometers, which extend into the water through the flask stoppers, indicate the temperature of the water at the moment of testing. At first, extreme degrees of heat and cold (e.g., 10 and 45°C) may be employed to delineate roughly an area of thermal sensory disturbance; the patient will report that the flask feels "less hot" or "less cold" over such an area than over a normal part. If areas of impaired sensation are found, the borders may be accurately determined by moving the flask along the skin from the insensitive to the normal region. The qualitative change should then be quantitated as far as possible by estimating the *differences in temperature* which the patient is able to recognize. The patient is asked to report whether one stimulus is *warmer or colder* than another and whether a given stimulus is warm or cold, since the cooler of the two may be interpreted as warm. The range of temperature difference between the two flasks is gradually narrowed by mixing their contents. A normal person is capable of detecting a difference of 1° when the temperature of the flasks is in the range of 28 to 32°C. In the warm range he should readily recognize differences between 35 and 40°C and in the cold range, between 10 and 20°C. In many older persons and in others with poor peripheral circulation (especially in cold weather), the responses may be modified in an otherwise normal patient.

The sensation of heat or cold depends not only on the temperature of the stimulus but also on the duration of the stimulus and the area over which it is applied. This principle may be employed to detect slight degrees of sensory impairment; the patient may be able to distinguish small differences in temperature when the bottom of the flask is applied for 3 sec but unable to do so if only the side of the flask is applied for 1 sec. Throughout the test procedure, especially when small temperature differences are involved, the area of sensory disturbance should be continually checked against perception in normal parts.

POSTURAL SENSE AND THE APPRECIATION OF PASSIVE MOVEMENT. These modalities are usually lost together, although in any particular case one may be disproportionately affected.

Abnormalities of postural sensation may be revealed in several ways. When the patient extends his arms in front of him and closes his eyes, the affected arm will wander from its original position; if the fingers are spread apart, they may undergo a series of slow-changing postures ("piano-playing" movements, or *pseudoathetosis*). In attempting to touch the tip of the nose with his index finger, the patient may miss the target repeatedly.

The lack of position sense in the legs may be demonstrated by displacing the limb from its original position and asking the patient to point to his large toe. If postural sensation is defective in both legs, the patient will be unable to maintain his balance with feet together and eyes closed (Romberg's sign). This sign should be interpreted with caution. Even a normal person in the Romberg position will sway slightly more with his eyes closed than open. A patient with lack of balance due to motor disorders or cerebellar disease will also sway more if his visual cues are removed. Only if there is a marked discrepancy between the state of balance with eyes open and closed can one confidently state that the patient shows Romberg's sign, i.e., loss of proprioceptive sensation. Mild degrees of unsteadiness in nervous or suggestible patients may be overcome by diverting their attention, e.g., by having them alternately touch the index finger of each hand to their nose while standing with their eyes closed.

The appreciation of passive movement is first tested in the fingers and toes, and the defect, when present, is reflected maximally in these parts. It is important to grasp the digit firmly at the sides opposite the plane of movement; otherwise the pressure applied by the examiner in displacing the digit may allow the patient to identify the direction of movement. This applies to the testing of the more proximal segments of the limb as well. The patient should be instructed to report each movement as "up" or "down" in relation to the previous stationary position. It is useful to demonstrate the test with a large and easily identified movement, but once the idea is clear to the patient, the smallest detectable changes in position should be tested. The range of movement normally appreciated in the digits is said to be as little as 1°. Clinically, however, defective appreciation of passive movement is judged by comparison with a normal limb or,

if bilaterally defective, on the basis of what the examiner has through experience learned to regard as normal. Slight impairment may be disclosed by a slow response or, if the digit is displaced very slowly, by a relative unawareness that movements have occurred; or after the digit has been displaced in the same direction several times, the patient may misjudge the first movement in the opposite direction; or after the examiner has moved the toe, the patient may make a number of small voluntary movements of the toe, in an apparent attempt to determine its position or the direction of movement.

THE SENSE OF VIBRATION. This is a composite sensation comprising touch and rapid alterations of deep pressure sense. Its conduction depends on both cutaneous and deep afferent fibers, which ascend in the dorsal columns of the cord. It is therefore rarely affected by lesions of single nerves but will be disturbed in cases of polyneuritis and disease of the dorsal columns, medial lemniscus, and thalamus. For this reason, vibration and position sense are usually lost together, although one of them (usually vibration sense) may be affected disproportionately. With advancing age, vibration sense may be diminished at the toes and ankles.

Vibration sense is tested by placing a tuning fork with a low rate of vibration (128 d.v.) over the bony prominences. The examiner must make sure that the patient responds to the vibration and not simply to the pressure of the fork. Although there are mechanical devices to quantitate vibration sense, it is sufficient for clinical purposes to compare the point tested with a normal part of the patient or of the examiner. A 256-d.v. fork can be used for finer testing. The level of vibration-sense loss due to spinal lesions can be estimated by placing the fork over successive vertebral spines.

DISCRIMINATIVE SENSORY FUNCTIONS. Damage to the sensory cortex or to the sensory projections from thalamus to cortex results in a special type of disturbance that affects mainly the patient's ability to make sensory discriminations. Lesions in these structures may disturb postural sense but leave the so-called "primary modalities" (touch, pain, temperature, and vibration sense) relatively little affected. In such a situation, or if a cerebral lesion is suspected on other grounds, discriminative function should be tested further by the following tests.

Two-point Discrimination. The ability to distinguish two points from one is tested by using a compass, the points of which should be blunt and applied simultaneously and painlessly. The distance at which such a stimulus can be recognized as double varies greatly; 1 mm at the tip of the tongue, 3 to 6 mm at the finger tips, 1.5 to 2 cm on the palms and soles, 3 cm on the dorsa of the hands and feet, and 4 to 7 cm on the body surface. It is characteristic of the patient with a lesion of the sensory cortex to mistake two points for one, although occasionally the opposite occurs.

Cutaneous Localization and Number Writing. The ability to localize cutaneous stimuli is tested by touching various parts of the patient's body and asking him to point to the part touched or to the corresponding part on the examiner's limb. Recognition of *number writing*, or of the direction of lines drawn on the skin, also depends on localization of tactile stimuli.

Appreciation of Texture, Size, and Shape. Appreciation of *texture* depends mainly on cutaneous impressions, but the recognition of *shape and size* of objects is based on impressions from deeper receptors as well. The lack of recognition of shape and form, therefore, though frequently found with cortical lesions, may also be present with lesions of the spinal cord and brainstem due to interruption of tracts transmitting postural and tactile sensation. Such a sensory defect, called *stereoanesthesia,* should be distinguished from *astereognosis,* which connotes an inability to identify an object by palpation, the primary sense data being intact. The latter defect is essentially a tactile agnosia and is associated with lesions lying posterior to the postcentral gyrus in the dominant hemisphere. In practice, a pure astereognosis is rarely encountered, and the term is employed where the impairment of tactile and joint sense is of insufficient severity to account for the defect in recognition.

Extinction of Sensory Stimuli and Sensory Inattention. In response to bilateral simultaneous testing of symmetric parts, the patient may acknowledge only the stimulus on the sound side, or he may improperly localize the stimulus on the affected side, whereas stimuli applied to each side separately are properly appreciated. This phenomenon of *extinction* or cortical *inattention* is characteristic of parietal lobe lesions, the symptomatology of which is considered in Chap. 31.

A few other terms require definition, since they may be encountered in reading about sensation. Most of them are pedantic, and it is recommended that the simplest terms possible be used. *Anesthesia* refers to a loss and *hypesthesia* to a diminution of all forms of sensation. Loss or impairment of specific cutaneous sensations is indicated by an appropriate prefix or suffix, e.g., *thermoanesthesia* or *thermohypesthesia, analgesia* (loss of pain) or *hypalgesia, tactile anesthesia* (loss of sense of touch), and *pallanesthesia* (loss of vibratory sense). The term *hyperesthesia* requires special mention; although it implies a heightened receptiveness of the nervous system, careful testing will usually demonstrate an underlying sensory defect, i.e., an elevated threshold to tactile, painful, or thermal stimuli; once the stimulus is perceived, however, it may have a severely painful or unpleasant quality (*hyperpathia*).

SENSORY SYNDROMES

SENSORY CHANGES DUE TO INTERRUPTION OF A SINGLE PERIPHERAL NERVE

These changes will vary with the composition of the nerve involved, depending on whether it is predominantly muscular, cutaneous, or mixed. Since proprioceptive fibers run for at least a portion of their course with the muscular (mainly motor) nerves, and cutaneous sensibility is carried in sensory nerves, each of these sensory systems may be affected separately. In lesions of cutaneous nerves, it is said that the area of tactile anesthesia is more extensive than the one for pain due to greater overlapping of pain fibers.

Because of overlap from adjacent nerves, the area of sensory loss following division of a cutaneous nerve is always less than its anatomic distribution. If a large area of skin is involved, the sensory defect characteristically consists of a central portion, in which all forms of cutaneous sensation are lost, surrounded by a zone of partial loss, which becomes less marked as one proceeds from the center to the periphery. The sense of deep pressure and passive movement is intact because it is carried by muscular nerves. Along the margin of the hypesthetic zone the skin becomes excessively sensitive. A light contact may be felt as a smarting, mildly painful sensation. According to Weddell, this is due to collateral regeneration from surrounding healthy nerves into the denervated region (see Chap. 9).

In lesions involving the brachial and lumbosacral plexuses, the sensory disturbance is no longer confined to the territory of a single nerve and is accompanied by muscle weakness and reflex change.

SENSORY CHANGES DUE TO MULTIPLE NERVE INVOLVEMENT (POLYNEUROPATHY)

In most instances of polyneuropathy the sensory changes are accompanied by varying degrees of motor and reflex loss. Usually the sensory impairment is symmetric, with notable exceptions in some instances of diabetic and periarteritic neuropathy. Since the longest and largest fibers are most affected, the sensory loss is most severe over the feet and legs and less severe over the hands. The abdomen, thorax, and face are spared except in the most severe cases. The sensory loss usually involves all the modalities, and although it is manifestly difficult to equate the impairment of pain, touch, temperature, vibration, and position sense, one of these may seemingly be impaired out of proportion to the others. One cannot accurately predict, from the patient's symptoms, which mode of sensation will be disproportionately affected. The term *glove-and-stocking anesthesia* is frequently employed to describe the sensory loss of polyneuropathy and draws attention to the predominantly distal pattern of involvement. It is an inaccurate term insofar as the border between normal and impaired sensation is not sharp; the sensory loss shades off gradually, and the transition to normal sensation occurs over a variable vertical extent of the limb. In hysteria, by contrast, the border between normal and absent sensation is usually sharp.

SENSORY CHANGES DUE TO INVOLVEMENT OF MULTIPLE SPINAL NERVE ROOTS

Because of considerable overlap from adjacent roots, division of a single sensory root does not produce complete loss of sensation in any area of skin. Compression of a single sensory cervical or lumbar root (in herniated intervertebral disks, for example) causes varying degrees of impairment of cutaneous sensation, however. When two or more roots have been completely divided, a segmental zone of sensory loss can be found in which reduction of pain perception is greater in extent than touch. Surrounding the area of complete loss is a narrow zone of partial loss, in which a raised threshold accompanied by overreaction (*hyperesthesia*) may or may not be demonstrated. The presence of muscle paralysis, atrophy, and reflex loss indicates involvement of ventral roots as well.

THE TABETIC SYNDROME. This results from damage to the large proprioceptive fibers of the posterior lumbosacral roots. It is usually caused by neurosyphilis, less often by diabetic or other types of neuropathy. Numbness or paresthesias and lightning pains are frequent complaints, and areflexia, atonicity of the bladder, abnormalities of gait (Chap. 23), and hypotonia without muscle weakness are found on examination. The sensory loss may consist only of loss of vibration and position sense in the lower extremities, but in severe cases, loss or impairment of superficial or deep pain sense or of touch may be added. The feet and legs are most affected, much less often the arms and trunk.

COMPLETE SPINAL SENSORY SYNDROMES. In a complete transverse lesion of the spinal cord, all forms of sensation are abolished below a level that corresponds with the lesion. There may be a narrow zone of "hyperesthesia" at the upper margin of the anesthetic zone. It is important to remember that during the evolution of such a lesion there may be a discrepancy between the level of the lesion and that of the sensory loss, the latter ascending as the lesion progresses. This can be understood if one conceives of a lesion evolving from the periphery to the center of the cord, affecting first the outermost fibers carrying pain and temperature sensation from the legs. Conversely, a lesion advancing from the center of the cord may affect these modalities in the reverse order.

PARTIAL SPINAL SENSORY SYNDROMES. Hemisection of the Spinal Cord (Brown-Séquard Syndrome). In rare instances disease is confined to one side of the spinal cord; pain and heat sensation are affected on the opposite side, and proprioceptive sensation, on the same side as the lesion. The loss of pain and temperature sensation begins two or three segments below the lesion. An associated motor paralysis on the side of the lesion completes the syndrome. Tactile sensation is not involved, since the fibers from one side of the body are distributed in tracts (posterior columns and anterior spinothalamic) on both sides of the cord.

LESIONS OF THE CENTRAL GRAY MATTER (SYRINGOMYELIC SYNDROME). Since fibers conducting pain and temperature cross the cord in the anterior commissure, a lesion in this location will characteristically abolish these modalities on one or both sides but will spare tactile sensation. The commonest cause of such a lesion is syringomyelia, less often, tumor and hemorrhage. This type of dissociated sensory loss usually occurs in a segmental distribution, and since the lesion frequently involves other parts of the gray matter, varying degrees of segmental amyotrophy and reflex loss may be added. If the lesion has spread to the white matter, corticospinal and posterior column signs will be present as well.

POSTERIOR COLUMN SYNDROME. There is loss of vibratory and position sense below the lesion, but the sense of pain, temperature, and touch are affected relatively little or not at all. This lesion may be difficult to distinguish from an affection of large fibers in sensory roots (tabetic syndrome). In some diseases vibratory sensation may be involved predominantly whereas in others position sense is more affected. It should be stressed that an interruption of proprioceptive fibers may interfere with discriminative sensory function, such as two-point discrimination and recognition of size, shape, and weight, and that impairment of this function may occur with posterior column disease alone. Paresthesias in the form of tingling and "pins-and-needles" sensations or girdle sensations are a common complaint with posterior column disease, and pain stimuli may also produce unpleasant sensations.

THE ANTERIOR SPINAL ARTERY SYNDROME. With occlusion of the anterior spinal artery or other destructive lesions that predominantly affect the ventral portion of the cord, there is a relative or absolute sparing of proprioceptive sensation and loss of pain and temperature sensation below the level of the lesion. Since the corticospinal tracts and the ventral gray matter also fall within the area of distribution of the anterior spinal artery, paralysis of motor function forms a prominent part of this syndrome.

DISTURBANCES OF SENSATION DUE TO LESIONS OF THE BRAINSTEM. A characteristic feature of lesions of the medulla and lower pons is that in many instances the sensory disturbance is crossed, i.e., there is loss of pain and temperature sensation of one side of the face and of the opposite side of the body. This is accounted for by involvement of the trigeminal tract or nucleus and the lateral spinothalamic tract on one side of the brainstem. In the upper pons and midbrain, where the spinothalamic tracts and the medial lemniscus become confluent, an appropriately placed lesion may cause a loss of all superficial and deep sensation over the contralateral side of the body. Cranial nerve palsies, cerebellar ataxia, or motor paralysis are often associated, as indicated in Chaps. 355 and 357.

SENSORY LOSS DUE TO A LESION OF THE THALAMUS (SYNDROME OF DEJÉRINE-ROUSSY)

Involvement of the nucleus ventralis posterolateralis of the thalamus, usually due to a vascular lesion or tumor, causes loss or diminution of all forms of sensation on the opposite side of the body. Position sense is affected more frequently than any other sensory function, and deep sensory loss is usually, but not always, more profound than cutaneous loss. There may be spontaneous pain or discomfort ("thalamic pain"), sometimes of the most torturing and disabling type, on the affected side, and any form of stimulus may have a diffuse, unpleasant, lingering quality. Emotional disturbance also aggravates the painful state. This overresponse is usually associated with an elevated threshold; i.e., a stronger stimulus is necessary to produce a sensation, in spite of the greater discomfort experienced by the patient once the sensation had been evoked. The thalamic pain syndrome may occasionally accompany lesions of the white matter of the parietal lobe.

SENSORY LOSS DUE TO LESIONS IN THE PARIETAL LOBE

There is a disturbance mainly of discriminative sensory functions on the opposite side of the body, particularly the face, arm, and leg. Loss of position sense, impaired ability to localize touch and pain stimuli, elevation of two-point threshold, a general inattentiveness to sensory stimuli on one side of the body, and astereognosis (if the lesion is in the dominant hemisphere) are the most prominent findings. It is generally taught that the primary modalities of sensation (pain and temperature, touch and vibratory sense) are not affected by lesions which are confined to the cerebral cortex, but this statement requires modification. In acute, deep parietal lesions the primary modalities may be abolished, and as was said, it may be followed by the "thalamic pain syndrome," but usually the impairment takes a different form from that due to thalamic lesions. Thus, with cortical lesions, one examination may disclose no sensory abnormalities, whereas the patient's responses may be inconstant and irregular on the next examination. This type of response is often attributed to hysteria. Other features of parietal lobe symptomatology and the differences between dominant and nondominant parietal lobe syndromes will be considered in Chap. 30.

SENSORY LOSS DUE TO SUGGESTION AND HYSTERIA

The possibility of suggesting sensory loss to a patient has already been mentioned. In fact, hysterical patients almost never complain spontaneously of cutaneous sensory loss, although they may use the term *numbness* to indicate a paralysis of a limb. Complete hemianesthesia, often with reduced hearing, sight, smell, and taste, as well as impaired vibration sense over only half the skull, is a common finding in hysteria. Anesthesia of one entire limb or a sharply defined sensory loss over part of a limb, not conforming to the distribution of root or cutaneous nerve, is also frequently observed. Postural sensation is rarely affected. The diagnosis of hysterical hemianesthesia is best made by eliciting the other relevant symptoms of hysteria or, if this is not possible, by noting the discrepancies between this type of sensory loss and that which occurs as part of the usual sensory syndromes.

REFERENCES

Holmes, Gordon: "Introduction to Clinical Neurology," 2d ed., chaps. 8 and 9, Baltimore, The Williams & Wilkins Company, 1952.

Kibler, R. F., and P. W. Nathan: A Note on Warm and Cold Spots, Neurology, 10:874, 1960.

Mayo Clinic: "Clinical Examinations in Neurology," 2d ed., Philadelphia, W. B. Saunders Company, 1963.

Oppenheimer, D. R., E. Palmer, and G. Weddell: Nerve Endings in the Conjunctiva, J. Anat., 92:322, 1958.

Melzack, R., and P. Wall: Pain Mechanisms: A New Theory. Science, 150:971, 1965.

Mountcastle, V. B.: Central Nervous Mechanisms in Sensation. Chaps. 61, 62, and 63 in Medical Physiology, V. B. Mountcastle (Ed.), 12th ed., vol. 2, pp. 1345–1464, St. Louis, The C. V. Mosby Company, 1968.

26 COMA AND RELATED DISTURBANCES OF CONSCIOUSNESS

Raymond D. Adams

The practitioner of medicine is frequently called upon to treat patients whose principal abnormality is an impairment of consciousness, which varies from inattentiveness and simple confusion to coma. In large municipal hospitals it is estimated that as many as 3 percent of total admissions are due to diseases that have caused coma, and although this figure seems high, it serves to emphasize the importance of this class of neurologic diseases and the necessity for every student of medicine to acquire a theoretic as well as a practical knowledge of them.

The terms *consciousness, confusion, stupor, unconsciousness,* and *coma* have been endowed with so many different meanings that it is almost impossible to avoid ambiguity in their usage. They are not strictly medical terms, but literary, philosophic, and psychologic ones as well. The word *consciousness* is the most difficult of all. William James once remarked that everyone knew what consciousness was until he attempted to define it. To the psychologist consciousness denotes a state of awareness of one's self and one's environment. Knowledge of one's self, of course, includes all "feelings, attitudes and emotions, impulses, volitions, and the active or striving aspects of conduct" (English)—in short, an awareness of all one's own mental functioning, particularly the cognitive processes. These can be judged only by the patient's verbal account of his introspections and, indirectly, by his actions. Physicians, being practical men for the most part, have learned to place greater confidence in their observations of the patient's general behavior and his reactions to overt stimuli than in what he says. For this reason when they employ the term *consciousness,* they usually do so in its commonest and simplest signification, namely, a state of awareness of the environment. This narrow definition has another advantage in that the word *unconsciousness* is its exact opposite—a state of unawareness of environment or a suspension of those mental activities by which man is made aware of his environment. To add to the ambiguity, psychoanalysts have given the word *unconscious* a still different meaning; for them it stands for repository of impulses and memories of previous experiences that cannot be immediately recalled to the conscious mind.

DESCRIPTION OF STATES OF NORMAL AND IMPAIRED CONSCIOUSNESS

The following definitions, while admittedly unacceptable to most psychologists, are of service to medicine, and they will provide the student with a convenient terminology for describing the mental states of his patients.

NORMAL CONSCIOUSNESS. This is the condition of the normal individual when fully awake, in which he is responsive to psychologic stimuli and "indicates by his behavior and speech that he has the same awareness of himself and his environment as ourselves." This normal state may fluctuate during the course of the day from keen alertness or deep concentration with a marked constriction of the field of attention to general inattentiveness and drowsiness.

SLEEP. Sleep is a state of physical and mental inactivity from which the patient may be aroused to normal consciousness. A person in sleep gives little evidence of being aware of himself or his environment, and in this respect he is unconscious. Yet he differs from a comatose patient in that he may still respond to unaccustomed stimuli and at times is capable of some mental activity in the form of dreams, which leave their traces in memory. And, of course, he can be recalled to a state of normal consciousness when stimulated.

INATTENTIVE, CONFUSIONAL, AND CLOUDY STATES OF CONSCIOUSNESS. In these conditions the patient does not take into account all elements of his immediate environment. Like delirium, these states always imply an element of sensorial clouding or imperceptiveness. The term *confusional* lacks precision, for often it signifies an inability to think with customary speed and coherence. Here the difficulty is in defining thinking.

An inattentive, severely confused person is usually unable to do more than carry out a few simple commands. His capacity for speech may be limited to a few words or phrases, or he may be voluble. He is unaware of much that goes on around him and does not grasp his immediate situation. A moderately confused individual can carry on a simple conversation for short periods of time, but his thinking is slow and incoherent, and he is unable to stay with one topic. Often he is disoriented in time and place. In mild degrees of confusion the disorder may be so slight that it is overlooked unless the examiner is searching in his analysis of the patient's behavior and conversation. The patient may even be roughly oriented as to time and place and able to speak freely on almost any subject. Only occasional irrelevant remarks betray an incoherence of thinking. Patients with mild or moderately severe confusion may be subjected to psychologic testing. The degree of confusion often varies from one time of day to another and tends to be least pronounced in the early morning. Severe confusion or stupor may resemble semicoma during periods when the patient is drowsy or asleep. Many events that happen to the confused patient leave no trace in his memory; in fact, capacity to recall later events that transpired in any given period is one of the most delicate tests of mental clarity. However, careful analysis will show the defect to be one of inadequate registration and fixation of items rather than a fault in retentive memory.

Some neurologists regard *delirium* as a state of confusion with excitement and hyperactivity, and in some medical writings the terms *delirium* and *confused-cloudy states* are used interchangeably. It is undoubtedly true that the delirious patient is nearly always confused. However, the vivid hallucinations which characterize delirious states, the relative inaccessibility of the patient to other events than those to which he is reacting at any one moment, his extreme agitation and tremulousness, and the tendency to convulse suggest a cerebral disorder of a somewhat different type. The clearest evidence of the relationship of inattention, confusion, stupor, and coma is that the patient may pass through all these states as he becomes comatose or emerges from coma. The author has not observed any such relationship between coma and delirium. These distinctions are drawn with greater clarity in Chap. 30.

At times a patient with certain types of aphasia, especially jargon aphasia, may create the impression of confusion, but close observation will reveal that the disorder is confined to the sphere of language and that behavior is otherwise natural.

STUPOR. In stupor mental and physical activity are reduced to a minimum. Although inaccessible to many stimuli, the patient opens his eyes, looks at the examiner, and does not appear to be unconscious. Response to spoken commands is either absent or slow and inadequate. As a rule tendon or plantar reflexes are not altered. On the other hand, tremulousness of movement, coarse twitching of muscles, restless or stereotyped motor activity, and grasping and sucking reflexes are not infrequent, depending on the way in which disease affects the nervous system. In psychiatry the term *stupor* means a state in which impressions of the external world are normally received, but activity is suspended or marked by negativisim, e.g., catatonic schizophrenia.

COMA. The patient who appears to be asleep and is at the same time incapable of sensing or responding adequately to either external stimuli or inner needs is in a state of coma. Coma may vary in degree, and in its deepest stages no reaction of any kind is obtainable. Corneal, pupillary, pharyngeal, tendon, and plantar reflexes are all absent. With lesser degrees of it pupillary reflexes and ocular movements and other brainstem reflexes are preserved, and there may or may not be extensor rigidity of the limbs and opisthotonos, signs which, as Sherrington showed, indicate decerebration. Respirations are often slow or rapid and may be periodic, i.e., Cheyne-Stokes breathing. In still lighter stages, referred to as *semicoma*, most of the above reflexes can be elicited, and the plantar reflexes may be either flexor or extensor (Babinski's sign). Moreover, pricking or pinching the skin, shaking and shouting at the patient, or an uncomfortable distension of the bladder may cause the patient to stir or moan and his respirations to quicken.

THE ELECTROENCEPHALOGRAM AND DISTURBANCES OF CONSCIOUSNESS

One of the most delicate confirmations of the fact that these states of altered consciousness are expressions of neurophysiologic changes is the electroencephalogram. In the normal waking state the electrical potentials of the cortical neurones are integrated into regular waves of two frequency ranges, from 8 to 15 (alpha rhythm) and 16 to 25 (beta rhythm). These wave forms are established by adolescence, but certain individual differences in general pattern and dominance of alpha waves are maintained throughout adult life. With sleep these cortical potentials slow down and amplitude (voltage) of the individual waves increases. At one stage in light sleep characteristic bursts of 14 to 16 per sec waves appear, the so-called "sleep spindles," and in deep sleep all the waves of normal frequency and amplitude are replaced by slow ones of high voltage (1¼ to 3 per sec). Similarly, some alteration in brain waves occurs in all disturbances of consciousness except the milder degrees of confusion. This alteration usually consists of a disorganization of the electroencephalographic pattern, which shows random, slow waves of high voltage in stages of confusion; more regular, slow, 2 to 3 per sec waves of high voltage in stupor and semicoma; and slow waves or even suppression of all organized electrical activity (isoelectric state) in the deep coma of hypoxia and ischemia, the so-called "brain death syndrome" (see Chap. 363). The electroencephalograms of deep sleep and light coma resemble one another. However, not all diseases that cause confusion and coma have the same effect on the electroencephalogram. Some, such as barbiturate intoxication, may cause an increase in frequency and amplitude of the brain waves. In epilepsy the disturbance of consciousness is usually attended by paroxysms of "spikes" (fast waves of high amplitude) or by the characteristic alternating slow waves and spikes of petit mal. Other diseases, such as hepatic coma, characteristically cause a slowing in frequency and an increasing amplitude of "brain waves" and special triphasic waves. Whether all metabolic diseases of the brain induce similar changes in the electroencephalogram has not been determined. Probably there are differences between them, some of which may be significant (see Chap. 353).

MORBID ANATOMY AND PHYSIOLOGY OF COMA

In recent times there has been some clarification and amplification of earlier neuropathologic observations that the smallest lesions associated with protracted coma are always to be found in the midbrain and thalamus. The essence of more recent neurophysiologic studies, to be found in the writings of Bremer, of Morison and Dempsey, and of Moruzzi and Magoun, is that an ascending series of destructive lesions of spinal cord, medulla, pons, and cerebellum have no effect on the state of consciousness until the level of midbrain and diencephalon (thalamus) is reached. High brainstem transections invariably induce states of prolonged unresponsiveness, whereas stimulation of the upper brainstem reticular formation causes a drowsy or sleeping animal to suddenly become alert and his EEG to change correspondingly. As anesthetic agents abolish consciousness, they are found to suppress the activity of the upper reticular activating system, without interfering, at least at certain levels, with the transmission of specific sensory impulses.

Anatomic studies show the reticular activating system of the upper brainstem to receive collaterals from the specific sensory pathways and to project, not just to the sensory cortex of the parietal lobe, as do the thalamic relay nuclei for somatic sensation, but to the whole of the cerebral cortex. The latter has corticofugal connections which feed back nerve impulses to the reticular formation. Sensory stimulation, it would seem, then, has the double effect of conveying to the brain information about the outside world but also of providing some of the energy for activating those parts of the nervous system on which consciousness depends.

These new data are in line with the older ideas of Herbert Spencer and Hughlings Jackson—that the diencephalon and cerebral cortex always function together as a unit and represent the highest levels of integrative nervous activity, called by Penfield *centrencephalic*. While anatomic details have yet to be worked out and the precise physiology of the reticular activating system leaves much to be desired, being more complicated than this simple formulation would suggest, nevertheless, as a working idea it will make some of the following neuropathologic observations more comprehensible.

The study of a large series of human cases in which coma has preceded death by several days will bring to light two major types of lesion. In the first group a macroscopically visible lesion such as a tumor, abscess, intracerebral, subarachnoid, subdural, or epidural hemorrhage, massive infarct, or meningitis is demonstrable; usually the lesion involves a portion only of the cortex and white matter, leaving much of the cerebrum intact. Rarely, it is located in the thalamus or midbrain, which would make the coma understandable. But in the other instances the coma will always be related to a temporal lobe–tentorial herniation with compression, ischemia, and secondary hemorrhage in the midbrain and lower thalamus or with downward displacement of the brainstem. A detailed clinical record will show the coma to have coincided with these secondary displacements and herniations. Exceptionally, a widespread bilateral damage to the cortex and subcortical white matter will be found—the result of bilateral infarcts or hemorrhages, viral encephalitis, hypoxia, or ischemia—without thalamic or midbrain lesions. In the second group (and this is larger than the first) with no visible lesion seen by the naked eye, often no abnormality is divulged by any technique of pathology. The lesion, here caused by a metabolic or toxic state, is subcellular or molecular. In some instances the grossly normal brain will reveal a demonstrable cellular change under the light microscope which may be characteristic, e.g., hepatic coma. Usually the microscopic lesions are too diffuse for clinico-anatomic correlation. Thus, pathologic changes are compatible with physiologic deductions that the state of prolonged coma correlates with lesions of all parts of the cortical-diencephalic systems of neurones, but it is only in the upper brainstem where they may be small and discrete.

MECHANISMS WHEREBY CONSCIOUSNESS IS DISTURBED IN DISEASE

Knowledge of diseases of the nervous system is so limited that it is not possible to identify all the different mechanisms by means of which consciousness is disturbed. Already several ways in which the mesencephalic-diencephalic-cortical systems are deranged have been identified; there are probably many others.

In a number of disease processes there is direct interference with the metabolic activities of the nerve cells in the cerebral cortex and the central cerebral nuclear masses of the brain. Hypoxia, hypoglycemia, hyper- and hypoosmolar states, acidosis, alkalosis, hyper- and hypokalemia, hyperammonemia, and deficiencies of thiamine, nicotinic acid, vitamin B_{12}, pantothenic acid, and pyridoxine are well-known examples. The intimate details of these underlying biochemical changes have not yet been fully elucidated, but methods are becoming available for their study. The rate of cerebral blood flow can now be determined in human beings with considerable accuracy (Schmidt-Kety method) by measuring the rate of diffusion of inert gases such as N_2O or krypton into the brain, namely, the time required for the gas to reach the same degree of concentration in the jugular venous blood as in arterial blood after a 10-min inhalation of the gas. The normal value of cerebral blood flow (CBF) is 700 to 800 ml per min. The cerebral metabolic rate (CMR — oxygen consumption per minute) can be determined at the same time by measuring the oxygen difference between arterial and jugular blood and multiplying this difference by the rate of cerebral blood flow. Glucose and other nutrients and metabolites can be measured as they enter and leave the brain. Microchemical tests can be done on brain tissues and cerebrospinal fluid (CSF). Normally the brain consumes 3.3 ml O_2 per 100 Gm brain per minute. The relevant point for our discussion is that cerebral metabolism or blood flow are reduced in all the metabolic disorders leading to coma. Oxygen values of below 2.0 ml per 100 Gm are incompatible with an alert state. In hypoglycemia the cerebral blood flow is normal or above normal, whereas the cerebral metabolic rate is diminished, owing to deficiency of substrate. In thiamine and vitamin B_{12} deficiency the cerebral blood flow is normal or slightly diminished, and the cerebral metabolic rate is diminished, presumably because of insufficiency of coenzymes. Extremes of body temperature, either hyperthermia (temperature over 106°F) or hypothermia (temperature below 97°F), probably induce coma by exerting a nonspecific effect on the metabolic activity of neurones.

Diabetic acidosis, uremia, hepatic coma, and the coma of systemic infections are examples of endogenous intoxications. The identity of the toxic agents is not entirely known. In diabetes acetone bodies (acetoacetic acid, β-hydroxybutyric acid, and acetone) are present in high concentration, and in uremia there is probably accumulation of dialyzable toxin, perhaps phenolic derivatives of the aromatic amino acids. In both conditions "dehy-

dration" and serum acidosis may also play an important role. In many cases of hepatic coma, elevation of blood NH_3 to levels five to six times normal has been found. Lactic acidemia and other organic acids may affect the brain by lowering its pH to less than 7.3. The mode of action of bacterial toxins is unknown. In all these conditions the cerebral metabolic rate tends to be reduced, whereas cerebral blood flow remains normal. In water intoxication the membrane excitability of nerve cells is altered by hyponatremia and changes in intracellular K levels.

Drugs such as barbiturates, bromides, dilantin, alcohol, glutethimide and phenothiazines induce coma by their direct suppressive effect on the neurones of the cerebrum and diencephalon. Others such as methyl alcohol, ethylene glycol, and paralydehyde result in metabolic acidosis. Many additional pharmacologic agents have no direct action on the nervous system but lead to coma through the mechanism of circulatory collapse and inadequate cerebral circulation. In toxic and metabolic diseases, although the patient usually approaches coma through a state of drowsiness, confusion, and stupor, and the reverse sequence occurs as he emerges from it, each disease has its special effects manifesting itself by a characteristic clinical picture. This means that the mechanism and topography of the lesion will be different.

A critical decline in blood pressure, usually to a systolic level below 70 mm Hg, affects neural structures by causing a decrease in cerebral blood flow and, secondarily, a diminution in cerebral metabolic rate. If decline in blood pressure is episodic, the corresponding clinical picture is syncope (see Chap. 20). Here the clinical picture is one of physical weakness usually preceding and following the loss of consciousness, the whole process being acute and promptly reversible.

The sudden, violent, and excessive discharge of *epilepsy* is another mechanism. Usually a Jacksonian convulsion has little effect on consciousness until it spreads from one side of the body to the other. Coma immediately ensues, presumably because the spreading of the seizure discharge to central neuronal structures paralyzes their function. Other types of seizure in which consciousness is interrupted from the very beginning are believed to originate in the diencephalon.

Concussion exemplifies still another special pathophysiologic mechanism. In "blunt" head injury it has been shown that there is an enormous increase in intracranial pressure of the order of 200 to 700 lb per sq in., lasting a few thousandths of a second. Either the vibration set up in the skull and transmitted to the brain or this sudden high intracranial pressure is believed to be the basis of the abrupt paralysis of the nervous system that follows head injury. That the increased pressure itself may be the main factor has been suggested by experiments in which raising the intraventricular pressure to a level approaching diastolic blood pressure has abolished all vital functions.

As was pointed out above, large, destructive, and space-consuming lesions of the brain, such as hemorrhage, tumor, or abscess, interfere with consciousness in two ways. One is by direct destruction of the midbrain and diencephalon; the other, far more frequent, is by producing herniation of the medial part of the temporal lobe through the opening of the tentorium and crushing the upper brain against the opposite free edge of the tentorium. Here the mechanism is again mechanical and probably circulatory.

CLINICAL APPROACH TO THE COMATOSE PATIENT

Coma is not an independent disease entity but is always a symptomatic expression of disease. Sometimes the underlying disease is perfectly obvious, as when a healthy individual is struck on the head and rendered unconscious. All too often, however, the patient is brought to the hospital in a state of coma, and little or no information about him is immediately available. The physician must then subject the clinical problem to careful scrutiny from many directions. To do this efficiently, he must have a broad knowledge of disease and a methodical approach to the problem that leaves none of the common and treatable causes of coma unexplored.

It should be pointed out that when the comatose patient is seen for the first time, simple therapeutic measures take precedence over diagnostic procedures. A quick survey should make sure that the comatose patient has a clear airway and is not in shock (circulatory collapse) or, if trauma has occurred, that he is not bleeding from a wound. In patients who have suffered a head injury there may be a fracture of the cervical vertebrae, and therefore one must be cautious about moving the head and neck lest the spinal cord be inadvertently crushed. There must be an immediate inquiry as to the previous health of the patient: whether the patient had suffered a head injury or had been seen in a convulsion, and the circumstances in which he was found. The persons who accompany the comatose patient to the hospital should not be permitted to leave until they have been questioned.

DIAGNOSIS. The temperature, pulse, respiratory rate, and blood pressure are of aid in diagnosis. Fever suggests a severe systemic infection such as pneumonia, bacterial meningitis, or a brain lesion that has disturbed the temperature-regulating centers. An excessively high body temperature, 107 to 110°F, associated with dry skin should arouse the suspicion of heat stroke. Hypothermia is frequently observed in alcoholic or barbiturate intoxication, extracellular fluid deficit, peripheral circulatory failure or myxedema. Slow breathing points to morphine, barbiturate intoxication, or hypothyroidism, whereas deep, rapid breathing suggests pneumonia but may occur in diabetic or uremic acidosis (Kussmaul's respiration) or with intracranial diseases as a central neurogenic hyperpnea. The rapid breathing of pneumonia is often accompanied by an expiratory grunt, cyanosis, and fever. Diseases that elevate the intracranial pressure or damage the brain, especially the brainstem, often cause slow, irregular, or periodic (Cheyne-Stokes)

breathing. The pulse rate is less helpful, but if exceptionally slow, it should suggest heart block or, if combined with periodic breathing and hypertension, an increase in intracranial pressure. A tachycardia of 160 or above calls attention to the possibility of an ectopic cardiac rhythm with insufficiency of cerebral circulation. Marked hypertension occurs in patients with cerebral hemorrhage and hypertensive encephalopathy and, at times, those with increased intracranial pressure; whereas hypotension is the usual finding in the coma of diabetes, alcohol or barbiturate intoxication, or internal hemorrhage, myocardial infarction, dissecting aortic aneurysm, gram-negative bacillary septicemia, and Addison's disease.

Inspection of the skin may also yield valuable information. Cyanosis of the lips and nail beds means inadequate oxygenation. Cherry-red coloration indicates carbon monoxide poisoning. Multiple bruises, and in particular a bruise or boggy area in the scalp, favor cranial trauma. Bleeding from an ear or nose or orbital hemorrhage also raises the possibility of trauma. Puffiness and hyperemia of face and conjunctivas and telangiectasia are the usual stigmas of alcoholism; marked pallor suggests internal hemorrhage. The presence of a maculohemorrhagic rash indicates the possibility of meningococcal infection, staphylococcus endocarditis, typhus, or Rocky Mountain spotted fever. Pellagra may be diagnosed from the typical skin lesions on face and hands. The face may be myxedematous. In pituitary hypoadrenalism the skin is sallow. Excessive sweating suggests hypoglycemia or shock, and dry skin, diabetic acidosis and uremia. Skin turgor is reduced in dehydration. Hemorrhagic blisters will have formed over pressure points if the patient has been motionless for a time.

The odor of the breath may provide clues to the nature of a disease causing coma. The odor of alcohol is easily recognized (Vodka is odorless). The spoiled-fruit odor of diabetic coma, the uriniferous odor of uremia, and the musty fetor of hepatic coma are distinctive enough to be identified by physicians who possess a keen sense of smell.

The next step in the physical examination should give special attention to the status of the nervous system. Although the examination is limited in many ways, careful observation of the stuporous or comatose patient may yield considerable information concerning the function of different parts of the nervous system. One of the most helpful procedures is to sit at the patient's bedside for 5 to 10 min and observe what he does. The predominant postures of the body, the position of the head and eyes, the rate, depth, and rhythm of respiration, and the pulse should be noted. The state of responsiveness should then be estimated by noting the patient's reaction when his name is called and his capacity to execute a simple command or to respond to painful stimuli. The most effective painful stimuli are supraorbital pressure, sternoid pressure, or pinching the side of the neck or inner parts of the upper arms or thighs. By grading these stimuli, one may titrate the response, so to speak, and evaluate both the degree of coma and changes from hour to hour in the course of the disease. Vocalization may persist in stupor and light coma and is the first response to be lost. Deft avoidance movements of parts stimulated, and grimacing are preserved in light coma and substantiate the integrity of corticomedullary and corticospinal tracts.

Usually it is possible to determine whether or not the coma is accompanied by meningeal irritation or focal disease in the cerebrum or brainstem. With meningeal irritation from either bacterial meningitis or subarachnoid hemorrhage, there is resistance to active and passive flexion of the neck but not to extension, turning, or tipping the head. Resistance to movement of the neck in all directions indicates disease of the cervical spine or is part of generalized rigidity. In infants, bulging of the anterior fontanel is at times a more reliable sign of meningeal irritation than stiff neck. A temporal lobe or cerebellar pressure cone or decerebrate rigidity may also limit passive flexion of the neck and may be confused with meningeal irritation.

Evidence of disease of a cerebral hemisphere diencephalon, midbrain, pons, or medulla can be obtained even though the patient is comatose by noting the residual movement, prevailing postures of the body, respiratory rhythm and frequency, and status of cranial nerves. This is of more than passing importance because severe and persistent derangements of these functions are frequent with mass lesions of the brain and rare in metabolic disorders (except in terminal stages). A hemiplegia, in most instances, reflects a contralateral hemispheral lesion and is revealed by lack of restless movements, grasp reflex, and avoidance movements. The paralyzed limbs are slack and remain in uncomfortable positions. If lifted from the bed, they "fall flail." The cheek puffs out in expiration on the paralyzed side, and the eyes are often turned away from the paralysis (toward the lesion). Painful stimuli may provoke a moan or grimace on one side and not the other, reflecting a hemianesthesia. A homonymous hemianopsia in a stuporous patient is revealed by attraction of eyes to visual stimuli presented on one side and not the other.

Of the various tests of brainstem function those which have been most useful are: pattern of breathing, pupillary size and reactivity, and ocular movement and oculovestibular reflexes. As to patterns of abnormal breathing in progressive lesions which reduce the state of consciousness from confusion and inattention to stupor and coma, the earliest abnormality with cerebral lesions is the appearance of posthyperventilation apnea (period of apnea after 5 to 10 deep breaths). Its presence indicates bifrontal disease, wherein lies the mechanism, according to Plum, for activating rhythmic breathing when CO_2 is reduced. In coma due to massive cerebral lesions the rate of respiration increases slightly, and as it progresses an irregularity appears which gives way to the waxing-waning Cheyne-Stokes respiration (CSR). This means that the centers in the midbrain now isolated from the cerebrum are rendered more sensitive than usual to CO_2 (hyperventilation drive); and by intermittently reducing plasma CO_2 to low levels a temporary apnea follows. With midbrain–upper pontine lesions a state of *central neurogenic hyperpnea* (CNH) rather like

Kussmaul breathing, supervenes. Here respirations are increased in rate (up to 100 per min) and in depth, to the extent that respiratory alkalosis may result. The reflex mechanisms for respiratory control in the lower brainstem have in this instance been released, and the threshold of respiratory activation is low. This respiratory drive continues despite low arterial CO_2 tensions and elevated pH. Oxygen therapy (unlike the hyperventilation of pneumonia, pulmonary congestion, etc.) does not modify the pattern. Low pontine-level lesions sometimes cause *apneustic breathing* (where there is a pause of 2 to 3 seconds after full inspiration) or other abnormal patterns, such as short cycle clusters (3 to 4) of respiration without waxing or waning followed by a pause (Biot respirations) or respiration alternans in which a few breaths are omitted from time to time. With lesions of medulla the rhythm of breathing is chaotic, being irregularly interrupted, the breath varying in rate and depth. This has been called "ataxia of breathing," not a very appropriate term. The latter progresses to apnea, as may also CSR or CNR; in fact, respiratory arrest is the mode of death of most patients with serious central nervous disease. As Plum and Fisher both point out, when certain supratentorial brain lesions progress to the point where the temporal lobe and cerebellum herniates, one may observe a succession of respiratory patterns (CSR—CNP—Biot breathing to ataxic breathing) indicating extension of the functional disorder from upper to lower brainstem.

With midbrain lesions the pupils dilate to 4 to 5 mm and become unreactive to light; and with severe destruction of the tissue at this level (anoxic pannecrosis), they will finally dilate widely and not respond. Pontine tegmental lesions cause miotic pupils with only slight reaction to strong light. Thus, the preservation of pupillary light reflexes indicates integrity of the pupillary dilatation and constrictive mechanisms in midbrain. Ciliospinal pupillary dilatation is also lost in brainstem lesions (see Chap. 24). Unilateral Horner's syndrome (miosis, ptosis, exophthalmos, and reduced sweating) may be observed homolateral to a predominantly one-sided lower brainstem lesion, usually medullary. The pupillary reactions are of great importance because drug intoxications and metabolic disorders which cause coma leave the pupils unaffected. Exceptions are glutethimide (Doriden) and deep ether anesthesia where the pupils may be of medium size or slightly enlarged and unreactive for several hours; opiates (heroin and morphine) which cause pinpoint pupils with light reflex so small that it can be seen only with a magnifying glass; and atropine poisoning where the pupils are widely dilated and fixed.

Ocular movements are altered in a variety of ways. In light coma from metabolic abnormalities the eyes rove from side to side in random fashion like the slow eye movements of light sleep. They disappear as brainstem function becomes depressed. Oculocephalic reflexes (doll's eye movements), elicited by briskly turning or tilting the head, with eyes moving conjugately in the opposite direction, are exaggerated. They are not present in the normal person and if elicitable, evidence is obtained of the integrity of the tegmental structures of midbrain and pons which integrate ocular movements, and of the third, fourth, and fifth cranial nerves. Irrigation of each ear with 30 to 100 ml ice water (or just cold water if not completely comatose) will normally cause nystagmus away from the stimulated side (see Chap. 24). In comatose patients in whom the fast corrective "cortical" phase of nystagmus is lost the eyes are deflected to the side irrigated with cold water or away from the side irrigated with hot water. The position is held for 2 to 3 min. These oculovestibular reflexes are also lost in brainstem lesions. If only one eye abducts and the other fails to adduct in the lateral conjugate movement, there is indication of interruption of the medial longitudinal fasciculus (on the side of adductor paralysis). Irrigating both ears with ice water with head extended to 60° will sometimes induce vertical conjugate movements. An abducens palsy (sixth nerve) is reflected by a turning in of the eye due to unopposed action of internal rectus muscle, and oculomotor palsy results in abduction from unopposed action of abducens muscle. The eyes may be held conjugately to one side at all times in a coma—away from the side of the paralysis with large cerebral lesions (looks at the lesion) and toward the side of the paralysis with unilateral pontine lesions (looks away from the lesion). And, during a one-sided seizure the eyes jerk toward the convulsing side of face, arm, and leg (opposite to the irritative focus). The eyes may be turned down and inward (looking at nose) in thalamic and upper midbrain lesion (Parinaud's syndrome, see Chap. 24). Retractory and convergence nystagmus and ocular bobbing [brisk downward movements of both eyes with slow elevation to the original position (two-to-three times a minute)] occur with lesions in midbrain tegmentum and lower pons respectively. The major brainstem structural lesions, including temporal lobe herniation, abolish most, if not all, conjugate ocular movements when producing coma, whereas metabolic disorders do not. Of the intoxications, barbiturates and diphenylhydantoin (Dilantin) are the only common drugs which affect ocular movements, but they leave pupillary reactions intact.

As to the meaning of prevailing postures and movements in the comatose patient it may be said that restless, grasping, picking movements of one arm or arm and leg or all four extremities signify that the corticospinal tract(s) is intact; variable resistance to passive movement (paratonic rigidity) and strong grasping or complex avoidance movements have the same signification and if bilateral, the coma usually is not deep. Focal seizures require intact corticospinal motor system and are seldom seen with massive destruction of a cerebral hemisphere. Often these elaborate forms of semivoluntary movement are present on the "good side" in patients with extensive disease in one hemisphere and probably represent some type of disequilibrium of cortical and subcortical movement patterns. Definite choreic, athetotic, or even hemiballismic movements indicate disorder of subthalamic and basal ganglionic structures, just as they do in the alert patient. *Decerebrate rigidity* with jaw clenched, neck retracted, arms and legs stiffly extended and internally rotated appears in the condition of diencephalic-midbrain

suppression of temporal lobe pressure cone, with hemorrhages and infarction of upper pons and midbrain and with certain metabolic disorders such as hypoglycemia and hypoxia. Occasionally the mechanism of the decerebrate posture is unclear, as with certain bilateral subacute encephalitic, demyelinative and infarctive cerebral lesions. *Decorticate rigidity*, with arm or arms in flexion and adduction and leg(s) extension, signifies higher lesions in cerebral white matter, internal capsules, and thalamus. *Diagonal postures*, opposite arms and legs flexed and extended, probably mean supratentorial lesions; extended arms and flexed legs are probably fragments of decerebrate postures and point to midpontine lesions. *Abolition of all postures and movements* indicates acute bilateral corticospinal interruption, profound coma, and low pontine-medullary lesions involving reticular facilitatory (extrapyramidal) mechanisms.

Lower brainstem reflexes are seldom helpful in the analysis of coma. Only in the most profound metabolic comas and intoxications and in the hypoxemic pannecrosis of the entire brain (brain-death syndrome) are coughing, swallowing, and spontaneous respirations all abolished. Further, the tendon and plantar reflexes give little indication of what is happening. Tendon reflexes may be preserved until late and may be normal or slightly reduced on the hemiplegic side. The plantar reflexes may be absent or extensor. Only in deep coma or in states of decerebrate rigidity will a cerebral hemiplegia not be detected by flaccidity and motionless arm and leg.

A history of headache before or at the onset of coma, recurrent vomiting, and papilledema affords the best clues to increased intracranial pressure. This can be confirmed by lumbar puncture, which is usually safe unless there is a herniation of the temporal lobe through the tentorium or of the cerebellum through the foramen magnum. In the latter instance the cerebrospinal fluid pressure may not reflect intracranial pressure. Papilledema may develop within 12 to 24 hr in brain trauma and brain hemorrhage but, if pronounced, usually signifies brain tumor or abscess, viz., a lesion of longer duration. Multiple retinal or large subhyaloid hemorrhages are usually associated with ruptured saccular aneurysm or hemorrhage from an angioma. Papilledema, with widespread retinal exudates, hemorrhages, and arteriolar changes, is an almost invariable accompaniment of hypertensive encephalopathy. In patients with evidence of increased intracranial pressure, lumbar puncture, although admittedly dangerous because it may promote further herniation, is nevertheless necessary in some instances. See Chaps. 24 and 401 for further discussion of retinal changes.

LABORATORY PROCEDURES. Unless the diagnosis is established at once by history and physical examination, it is necessary to carry out a number of laboratory procedures. If poisoning is suspected, the gastric contents must be aspirated and saved for later chemical analysis. A catheter is passed into the urinary bladder, and a specimen of urine is obtained for determination of specific gravity, sugar, acetone, and albumin content. Urine of low specific gravity and high protein content is nearly always found in uremia, but proteinuria may also occur for 2 or 3 days after a subarachnoid hemorrhage or with fever. Urine of high specific gravity, glycosuria, and acetonuria are almost invariable in diabetic coma; but glycosuria and hyperglycemia may result from a massive cerebral lesion. If bromide or barbiturate intoxication is suspected, it can be verified by special tests for these substances. A blood count is made, and in malarial districts a blood smear is examined for malarial parasites. Neutrophilic leukocytosis occurs in bacterial infections and also with brain hemorrhage and softening. Venous blood should be examined for glucose, nonprotein nitrogen, CO_2, sodium bicarbonate, pH, NH_3, sodium, potassium, chlorides, and Ca. The cerebrospinal fluid must be drawn, and the pressure, presence of blood, white cell count, and results of Pandy's test should be recorded. Bloody cerebrospinal fluid occurs in cerebral contusion, subarachnoid hemorrhage, brain hemorrhage, and occasionally with hemorrhagic infarcts due to thrombophlebitis or arterial embolism. If there is pleocytosis, a stained smear of the sediment should be searched for bacteria, and a rough quantitative sugar determination should be done. The standard cerebrospinal fluid formula in bacterial meningitis is elevated pressure, high white cell count (5,000/20,000), elevated protein, and subnormal sugar values. The fluid should be saved for quantitative tests for sugar and protein, and a bacterial culture and Wassermann reaction should be performed. If the pressure is suspected of being elevated, a number 22 needle should be used. A very high pressure must be slowly reduced by removal of 10 to 15 ml over a period of 15 to 20 min, and urea, mannitol, or other hypertonic solutions should be given intravenously. Also, a corticosteroid may be given to reduce brain swelling over a longer period of time. Jugular compression tests are obviously contraindicated. X-rays of the skull should be obtained as soon as possible after these procedures, preferably on the way from the emergency ward to the hospital room.

CLASSIFICATION OF COMA AND DIFFERENTIAL DIAGNOSIS

The demonstration of focal brain disease or meningeal irritation, with cerebrospinal fluid abnormality, helps in differential diagnosis. The diseases that frequently cause coma can be conveniently divided into three classes, as follows:

Classification of Coma

I. Diseases that cause no focal or lateralizing neurologic signs or alteration of the cellular content of the cerebrospinal fluid
    A. Intoxications (alcohol, barbiturates, opiates, etc.) (Chaps. 118, 119 and 120)
    B. Metabolic disturbances (diabetic acidosis, uremia, Addisonian crises, hepatic coma, hypoglycemia, hypoxia (Chap. 363)
    C. Severe systemic infections (pneumonia, typhoid fever, malaria, Waterhouse-Friderichsen syndrome)
    D. Circulatory collapse (shock) from any cause, and cardiac decompensation in the aged (Chap. 20)
    E. Epilepsy (Chaps. 28 and 368)
    F. Hypertensive encephalopathy and eclampsia (Chap. 357)
    G. Hyperthermia or hypothermia
    H. Concussion (Chap. 358)
II. Diseases that cause meningeal irritation, with either blood or an excess of white cells in the cerebrospinal fluid, usually without focal or lateralizing signs
    A. Subarachnoid hemorrhage from ruptured aneurysm, occasionally trauma (Chap. 357)
    B. Acute bacterial meningitis (Chap. 360)
    C. Some forms of virus encephalitis (Chap. 361)
    D. Acute hemorrhagic leukoencephalitis (Chap. 362)
III. Diseases that cause focal or lateralizing neurologic signs, with or without changes in the cerebrospinal fluid
    A. Brain hemorrhage (Chap. 357)
    B. Brain softening due to thrombosis or embolism (Chap. 357)
    C. *Brain abscess* (Chap. 360)
    D. Epidural and subdural hemorrhage and brain contusion (Chap. 358)
    E. Brain tumor (Chap. 359)
    F. Miscellaneous, i.e., thrombophlebitis, some forms of virus encephalomyelitis (Chap. 361)

With the clinical tests outlined above clearly in mind one can usually ascertain whether a patient with coma falls in one of the above categories. Concerning the group of comas without focal, lateralizing, or meningeal signs, which includes most of the secondary metabolic diseases of the brain, intoxications (both exogenous and endogenous), concussion, and postseizure states, it should be pointed out that a previous neurologic disease may have left residue which confuse the clinical picture. An earlier hemiparesis from vascular disease or trauma may reveal itself in an alcoholic or hepatic coma, uremia, or hyperglycemic encephalopathy. Also, in hypertensive encephalopathy, transitory focal signs may sometimes be present. And occasionally, for no understandable reason one leg may seem to move less or one plantar reflex be extensor in a metabolic coma. In actuality, the diagnosis of postepileptic coma or concussion depends on observation of the precipitating event or indirect evidence thereof; usually the diagnosis is not too long obscure, for another fit may occur and recovery of consciousness, once the seizures cease, is usually prompt. The final determination of the exact toxic or metabolic disorder requires the synthesis of a variety of clinical and laboratory data, which will be described in other parts of the book.

With respect to the comas of group II the signs of meningeal irritation (head retraction, stiffness of neck or forward bending, Kernig and Brudzinski leg flexion signs) are usually elicitable in both bacterial meningitis and subarachnoid hemorrhage. However, if the coma becomes deep, stiff neck may disappear or be absent from the beginning. Here diagnosis is established by CSF examination. In the coma of bacterial meningitis, unless it is associated with brain swelling and cerebellar herniation, the CSF pressure is not exceptionally high (usually less than 400 mm); if the pressure is high, as death approaches there are signs of compression of the medulla with fixed, dilated pupils, arrest of respiration, and fall in arterial blood pressure. Patients in coma from ruptured aneurysms also have high CSF pressure and often a massive hemispheral and ventricular extension of the hemorrhage.

In patients with group III type of coma it is the inequality of sensory-motor disturbances in the two arms and legs and the aforementioned changes in respiratory pattern, pupillary and ocular reflexes, and the remaining postural states that provide clues to serious structural lesions in the segmental brainstem apparatus. As the latter become prominent, they may obscure earlier signs of cerebral disease. It is noteworthy that bilateral cerebral infarction or hemorrhage or traumatic necrosis and hemorrhage may resemble the comatose state of metabolic and toxic diseases, since brainstem mechanisms may be preserved; contrariwise, hepatic, hypoglycemic, and hypoxic coma will sometimes look like the coma of brainstem lesion by causing decerebrate postures. Usually, however, the CSF pressure is elevated and the fluid sanguineous in massive cerebral hemorrhage. Unilateral infarction due to anterior, middle, or posterior cerebral artery occlusion seldom produces more than a stupor or light coma; if bilateral, however, coma may be profound. Evidence of brainstem displacement and temporal lobe herniation is manifested by increased or altered ventilation (CSR, CNH), bilateral Babinski signs, dilated pupil on the side of the lesion, decerebrate postures, dilated pupils, and loss of full ocular movements. The coma itself gives no clue as to the nature of the original mass lesion. The terminal pattern of a descending gradient of diencephalic, mesencephalic, pontomedullary paralysis of nervous paralysis is identical in all. Differential diagnosis must depend on the other data.

An error which must be cautioned against is the diagnosis of irreversible coma (brain-death syndrome) on the basis of complete abolition of all brainstem and cerebral activity and isoelectric (flat) EEG if there is hypothermia or evidence of intoxication. Only with hypoxia and cerebral ischemia can this diagnosis be made securely.

Diagnosis has as its prime purpose the direction of therapy, and it matters little to the patient whether or not we diagnose a disease for which we have no treatment. The treatable forms of coma are drug intoxications, toxemia from systemic infections, epidural and subdural hematoma, brain abscess, bacterial and tuberculous meningitis, diabetic acidosis, and hypoglycemia.

RELATIVE INCIDENCE OF DISEASES THAT CAUSE COMA

There have been only a few attempts to determine the relative incidence of diseases that lead to coma. A report from the Boston City Hospital (Solomon and Aring) includes the largest series of clinical cases but was heavily skewed by the large local problem of chronic alcoholics, which made up 60 percent of all admissions in coma. Trauma (13 percent), cerebral vascular disease (10 percent), poisonings (3 percent), epilepsy (2.4 percent),

diabetes, bacterial meningitis, pneumonia, uremia, and eclampsia followed in that order. In the series of fatal cases studied at the Cook County Hospital (Holcomb), accuracy of clinical diagnosis was not more than 50 percent and did not improve with increasing length of survival (in half the fatal cases the patient died in the first 24 hr and in two-thirds, within 48 hr). Again, trauma, cerebrovascular disease, meningitis, and alcoholism accounted for the majority of cases. In a series of 386 cases of coma of uncertain etiology Plum and Posner observed that approximately 40 percent turned out to be metabolic, 25 percent, drug intoxications, and the remainder to be neurologic disease of supra- or infra-tentorial structures. Diagnostic accuracy was much greater in this recent series than in that of Holcomb.

Of course, figures like these do not provide information concerning coma caused by multiple factors. For example, a patient with a cerebral vascular lesion, old or recent, and diabetes mellitus may lapse into coma during an insulin reaction at a time when there is still sugar in the urine. Only by appreciating the interplay of these several common factors is one likely to reach the correct diagnosis.

The differential diagnosis of diseases that cause focal or lateralizing signs and meningitis will be taken up under the discussions of traumatic, neoplastic, vascular, and infective diseases of the brain.

CARE OF THE COMATOSE PATIENT

Impaired states of consciousness, regardless of their cause, are often fatal because they not only represent an advanced stage of many diseases but also add their own characteristic burden to the primary disease. The main objective of therapy is, of course, to find the cause of the coma, according to the procedures already outlined, and to remove it. It often happens, however, that the disease process is one for which there is no specific therapy; or as in hypoxia or hypoglycemia, the disease process may already have expended itself before the patient comes to the attention of the physician. Again, the problem may be infinitely complex, for the disturbance may be attributable not to a single cause but rather to several possible factors acting in unison, no one of which could account for the total clinical picture. In lieu of direct therapy, supportive measures must be used, and, indeed, it may be said that the patient's chances of surviving the original disease often depend in large measure on their effectiveness.

The physician must give attention to every vital function in the insensate patient. The following is a brief outline of the more important procedures. In order for them to be carried out successfully a well-coordinated team of nurses under constant guidance of a physician is needed.

1. If the patient is in shock, this takes precedence over all other abnormalities. The treatment of shock is discussed in Chap. 36.

2. Shallow and irregular respirations and cyanosis require the establishment of a clear airway and oxygen.

The patient should be placed in a lateral position so that secretions and vomitus do not enter the tracheo-bronchial tree. Pharyngeal reflexes are usually suppressed, and therefore an endotracheal tube can be inserted without difficulty. Stagnant secretions should be removed with a suction apparatus as soon as they accumulate, since they will lead to atelectasis and bronchopneumonia. Oxygen can be administered by mask in a 100 percent concentration for 6 to 12 hr, alternating with 50 percent concentration for 4 hr. The depth of respiration can be increased by the use of 5 to 10 percent carbon dioxide for periods of 3 to 5 min every hour. Atropine should not be given; edema of the lungs and fluid in the tracheo-bronchial passages are not glandular secretions. Furthermore, atropine thickens this fluid and also may disturb temperature regulation of the body. Aminophylline is helpful in controlling Cheyne-Stokes breathing. Respiratory paralysis dictates the use of a positive-pressure respirator or electrophrenic stimulator, but in the author's experience neither has been effective in comatose states in which there is disorganization of respiratory centers.

3. The temperature-regulating mechanisms may be disturbed, and extreme hypothermia, hyperthermia, or an unrecognized poikilothermia may occur. In hyperthermia, removal of blankets and use of alcohol sponges and cooling solutions are indicated.

4. The bladder should not be permitted to become distended. If the patient does not void, a retention catheter should be inserted. If more than 500 ml urine is found in the bladder, decompression must be carried out slowly over a period of hours. Urine excretion should be kept between 500 and 1,000 ml per day. The patient should not be permitted to lie in a wet or soiled bed.

5. Diseases of the central nervous system may upset the control of water, glucose, and salt. The unconscious patient can no longer adjust his intake of food and fluids by hunger and thirst. Salt-losing and salt-retaining syndromes have both been described with brain disease. Water intoxication and severe hyponatremia may of themselves prove fatal. The maintenance of water and electrolytes will be discussed in Chap. 88. If coma is prolonged, the insertion of a stomach tube will ease the problem of feeding the patient and maintaining fluid and electrolyte balance.

6. One should not attempt to forestall the development of bronchopneumonia by the prophylactic use of penicillin and streptomycin or some other broad-spectrum antibiotics; instead, appropriate ones should be administered when the infection occurs. The legs should be examined each day for signs of phlebothrombosis.

7. If the patient is capable of moving, suitable restraints should be used to prevent a possible fall out of bed.

8. Convulsions should be controlled by measures outlined in Chap. 368.

REFERENCES

Fisher, C. M.: Neurological Examination of the Comatose Patient, Acta Neurol. Scand., 1969.

Holcomb, B.: Causes and Diagnosis of Various Forms of Coma, J.A.M.A., 77:2112, 1921.

Plum, E., and J. Posner: "Diagnosis of Stupor and Coma," Philadelphia, F. A. Davis Company, 1966.

Solomon, P., and C. D. Aring: The Causes of Coma in Patients Entering a General Hospital, Am. J. Med. Sci., 188:805, 1938.

27 SLEEP AND ITS ABNORMALITIES
Raymond D. Adams

Sleep, that familiar yet inexplicable condition of repose in which consciousness is in abeyance, is obviously not abnormal; yet there is no absurdity in considering it in connection with abnormal phenomena. There are no doubt irregularities of sleep which approach serious extremes, just as there are unnatural forms of waking.

Inasmuch as sleep is an elementary phenomenon of life and an indispensable phase of man's existence, everyone has had much personal experience of sleep, or the lack of it, and has observed others in sleep. It requires no special knowledge of medicine, therefore, to know something about this condition or to appreciate its importance to health and well-being. Nearly all the great writers of the past have expressed their views on the psychologic and physical benefits of sleep, but probably none with more feeling than Sterne, who has Tristram Shandy remark: "'Tis the refuge of the unfortunate—the enfranchisement of the prisoner—the downy lap of the hopeless, the weary, the broken-hearted; of all the soft, delicious functions of nature this is the chiefest; what a happiness it is to man, when anxieties and passions of the day are over. . . ."

Physicians are often sought by individuals who suffer an illness caused by or accompanied by some derangement of sleep. Most often the problem is one of sleeplessness, but sometimes it concerns peculiar phenomena occurring in connection with sleep.

NORMAL SLEEP

The natural physiologic changes discoverable in sleeping man can be summarized as follows: temperature falls less than 1° but skin temperature rises, only to fall sharply on awakening; BMR reduced 10 to 15 percent; pulse rate slows 10 beats or so; blood pressure falls 10 to 30 mm Hg; sweating increased; gastric, salivary, and lacrimal secretions reduced; intestinal action continues and sphincters are closed; volume of urine diminished; pupils contracted and eyes diverged and turned up; musculature becomes atonic and tendon jerks depressed or absent; Babinski sign present in some persons; breathing deepens and slows, becoming Cheyne-Stokes in some elderly persons; EEG at first shows interruption of alpha rhythm and appearance of slow waves, then sleep spindles of 15 to 18 c per sec and finally delta waves of 2 to 3 c per sec.

More detailed analysis of sleep behavior in recent years has shown that typical slow (EEG) sleep pattern becomes interrupted for brief periods by fast cortical activity. The record looks more like that of an alert person but he remains inactive, his cervical muscles are atonic, and there are at this time rapid eye movements. It is in this period of so-called "paradoxical sleep" (PS) that all dreaming occurs. Paradoxical sleep always bears a certain relationship to slow sleep (SS); it invariably follows it and makes up about 25 percent of the total sleep period. From this discovery it must be argued that sleep behavior is not a unitary function but involves neural organization at more than one level of the nervous system.

Theories as to the anatomic substratum of sleep are numerous. Most of the older ideas about the existence of a sleep center, located somewhere in the walls of the third ventricle, have largely been replaced by a dynamic conception of arousal systems in the reticular activating areas of the upper brainstem and of inhibitory systems from cortex and other regions. Decorticate man, like animals, exhibits natural cycles of sleeping and waking, but paradoxical sleep disappears only when lesions occur in the pontine tegmentum. However, at any level to expect that one nucleus would be responsible for either alertness or sleep would be a gross simplification, for some neurones (e.g., cerebral cortex) are shown to be active during sleep and others not.

The means whereby these systems of neurones are suppressed during sleep is the other great unsolved problem. Over the years fatigue products, acidosis, toxins, and hormones have all had their advocates. Pieron was the first to show that a substance which he called hypnotoxin appears in the CSF of fatigued dogs and when injected into the ventricles of control animals, induces true sleep. And now Monnier has obtained a substance in the dialysate of the blood of sleeping animals that will cause an alert animal to fall asleep. The nature of this substance is unknown. Barbiturates and like soporific drugs act on the upper reticular activating system; tranquilizing drugs which are conducive of sleep by quieting anxiety have their main effects on the hippocampus and cerebral cortex.

Man's sleep pattern is based on daylight living. He learns to adapt all of his activities to the variations in the length of the day. This is a tedious process of conditioning, as every parent knows who struggles to get children off to bed. Temperature, pulse, blood pressure, metabolic rate, amount of physical activity, efficiency of nervous function are all adjusted to wake-sleep pattern. People vary in their capacity to adapt to sudden alteration of their circadian rhythm, with all its biologic nuances, as when moving abruptly to another part of the world, or taking on night work.

The sleep requirement per day and the relative amounts of slow and paradoxical sleep change steadily during the early years of life. The infant sleeps most of the time and gradually, as sleep lessens, adjusts its awake pattern to daylight. Paradoxical sleep at first predominates and then diminishes to 25 percent. By puberty the need of sleep is reduced to 10 to 11 hr, and the adult seldom sleeps more than 7 to 8, the woman needing about an hour more than the man. Slow sleep normally varies in depth; one usually plunges into the deepest sleep within the first hour of going to bed, and as various measurements have shown, sleep lightens after 3 to 4 hours, again becoming somewhat deeper after 5 to 6 hours. Exceptionally, especially in those who work best in the afternoon and night, the deepest sleep comes later in the night and awakening in the morning is difficult. During light sleep many small restless movements are made, often activated by sensory stimuli; each person has his own repertory of them. Kleitman has found that the normal person makes 30 to 60 movements in 8 hr sleep, the duration of movement averaging 8 to 10 secs for a total of about 5 min per night. The febrile patient sleeps with less movement than the normal one.

THE EFFECTS OF LOSS OF SLEEP

Of the conditions making for human efficiency, sleep is one of the most important. Sleep is absolutely essential to normal body metabolism. Experimental animals deprived of sleep will die within a few days, no matter how well they are fed, watered, and housed.

Despite the many studies of the effect of sleeplessness on human beings and animals, we still do not know as much as we should about it. Experiments on human beings have taken the form of enforced abstention from sleep for several days, with tests administered before, and after. One group of psychologists succeeded in keeping their subjects going in a state of apparent wakefulness for more than 200 hr. The surprising result was that on tests such as tapping, aiming at targets, reading letters, and calculation there was no failure of performance even after the loss of two nights' sleep. The sleepless subjects did fail, however, in tasks requiring sustained attention. They could do as well as they normally would on short tests, but on longer ones of the same degree of difficulty they became slow and inaccurate. Another characteristic was sluggishness of attention in shifting from one task or one test item to another. It was difficult for the subjects to redirect their activity; once started on a given line, they could hardly be diverted from it. After 3 days, they could no longer read. Whatever their achievement on the tests, all subjects reported numerous symptoms, such as burning eyes, headache, dazed feeling, nervousness, emotional instability, loss of motor power and coordination, slurred speech, drooping eyelids, and distressing visual hallucinations. In general deportment they were alternately irritable and silly, tending to laugh at anything said to them. There was a progressive decrease in the alpha waves in the EEG.

The reason for the relatively good test performance in the face of these bodily sensations is the ability of the normal individual to compensate. He can "shake himself out of it" and apply himself with an effort that overcomes his deficiencies. The extra effort put forth to remain oriented to the task cannot be maintained without cost. The energy consumed during an arithmetic test, as measured by the metabolic rate, is about three times greater in persons who have lost sleep.

Another surprising finding was that the subjects recovered on less than 35 percent of the sleep that had been lost. Furthermore, the first 8 to 12 hr of sleep is predominantly of the slow type, with very little paradoxical sleep. In other words, the amount of sleep required after the experiment is not equal to the number of hours that they were kept awake. Probably the explanation is that the subjects were not fully awake at all times, and in the latter part of the experiment they may have been half asleep.

A corollary of this hypothesis is that persons who sleep for long periods do not necessarily obtain the maximum benefits from sleep. Sleep may be sound and restful or light and fitful. In sound sleep the psychogalvanic test of skin resistance of the palm is raised, and in poor sleep it remains the same as in the waking state. It has also been found that only in sound sleep does the blood pressure fall. From these fragmentary studies it must be concluded that the value of sleep to the metabolism of the human organism is a function of its depth multiplied by its length, and that long hours spent in bed are no substitute for sound sleep.

Dreaming has been found by Aserinsky and Kleitman to occur always during the period of paradoxical sleep when the electroencephalogram reveals fast waves. This has been shown by awakening the patient when this brain wave pattern appears. Most subjects, if left alone, will awaken without remembering that they have dreamed. Jouvet finds that "paradoxical state" or "dream state" depends on a pontine mechanism.

DERANGEMENTS OF SLEEP

INSOMNIA. The word *insomnia* signifies want of sleep and is used popularly to indicate any interference with the duration or depth of sleep. As every physician knows from practical experience, this is not a disease, but a symptom of many diseases, which differ widely in their nature and gravity. It is associated equally with trivial ailments and with conditions which jeopardize life. The persistence and severity of insomnia are no guide to the diagnosis of the condition on which it depends.

Since insomnia is often a symptom of a minor illness, there is a tendency for the physician to make light of it. Yet few common conditions cause more misery and discomfort to the patient. When deprived of the nightly restoration of his energies, he grows weary and his whole mental and physical vigor is impaired. He seems to exhaust his fund of reserve force. His tolerance of pain, noise, and the countless irritations of everyday life is reduced. This, in turn, reflects itself in his psychologic reaction to all the ordinary symptoms of disease. Also, the capacity for effective work is intimately related to the ability to sleep. In fact, sound sleep is one of the most reliable measures of sound health.

Once there was a tendency to formulate elaborate classifications of insomnia according to the nature of the diseases in each of the different organ systems of the body.

This approach has little to offer because, in the final analysis, the factors operating in all these diseases are relatively few. Most instances of unyielding insomnia are due to (1) the presence of pain and discomfort or (2) anxiety (with muscular tension) and other nervous disorders.

Several types of sensory disorder may cause abnormal wakefulness. The pain of spine and root or peripheral nerve disease may be particularly troublesome at night, and the same is true of abdominal discomfort in a number of gastrointestinal diseases, such as pancreatic carcinoma. Tired, aching, restless legs, which has been described as the "restless leg syndrome" (*anxietas tibialis*) may regularly delay the onset of natural sleep. Excessive fatigue may give rise to many abnormal muscular sensations of a similar nature. *Acroparesthesias,* that peculiar nocturnal tingling numbness of the hands which is so common in women, may awaken the patient nightly, as does also cluster headache, which nearly always occurs 2 to 3 hr after falling asleep.

Insomnia is a frequent complaint of patients suffering from psychiatric disease. Its simplest form is that of a reactive nervous state in which domestic and business worries keep the patient in a turmoil. Also, vigorous mental activity late at night or excitement which leaves the muscles tense counteracts drowsiness and sleep. Under these circumstances there is difficulty in falling asleep and a tendency to sleep late in the morning. Sleeplessness is also commonly recorded in the histories of patients suffering from psychoneuroses and psychoses. In a valuable study of the character of sleep in psychiatric patients Muncie concludes that illnesses in which anxiety and fear are prominent symptoms usually result in difficulty in falling asleep and light, fitful, or intermittent sleep. Also, disturbing dreams, so common in such conditions, may awaken the patient, and he may even try to stay awake in order to avoid them. The sleep pattern is altered, but quality and quantity are little if at all diminished. In contrast, the depressive illnesses, particularly manic-depressive or involutional depression, cause either light sleep in the early part of the night or early morning waking and inability to return to sleep. Quantity of sleep is reduced and nocturnal motility increased, according to the study of Hinton. If anxiety is combined with depression, both the above patterns are observed. In states of mania all types of sleep disorder are known to occur. The sleep rhythm may be totally deranged in acute confusional states and delirium. In the latter the patient may only doze for short periods both day and night. The total amount and depth of sleep in a 24-hr period is reduced. Frightening hallucinations may prevent sleep. The senile and arteriosclerotic patient tends to catnap during the day and then refuse to go to bed at night; his nocturnal sleep is intermittent, and the total amount may be either increased or decreased.

Finally, there are patients who are convinced of the absolute necessity of obtaining sleep of a certain ideal quantity or quality. These are the "sleep pedants" and the "sleep hypochondriacs" of Laudenheimer. They become obsessed with the importance of sleep. Every night they are in a panic lest they remain awake; they cannot sleep because of their anxiety over it. Often they claim to be sleepless the night through, when in fact they are seen fast asleep on more than one occasion. They demonstrate the truth of William McDougall's statement that "peace of mind is an essential preliminary to sleep." Especially interesting is that group for whom insomnia becomes the excuse for all inadequacies and failures in adjustment to the everyday problems of living. Such individuals, although they want to sleep, worry about the loss, and their mental agitation actually opposes sleep.

Whatever the cause may be, the physician should always be on his guard when listening to reports of the amount of sleep lost by victims of insomnia, because they are usually exaggerated. Every individual who has lain awake at night will recall how much longer the time seemed than it actually was. This is an example of an illusion in the perception of unfilled time.

DISTURBANCES IN THE TRANSITIONAL PERIOD OF SLEEP (SOMNOLESCENT STARTS, SENSORY PAROXYSMS, CIRCADIAN RHYTHM, AND NOCTURNAL PARALYSIS). As sleep comes on, it would appear that certain nervous centers may be excited to a burst of insubordinate activity. The result is a sudden start that rouses the incipient sleeper. It may involve one or both legs or the trunk, less often, the arms. If the start occurs repeatedly during the process of falling asleep and is a nightly event, it may become a matter of great concern to the patient. These starts are more apt to occur in individuals in whom the sleep process develops slowly, and it has been observed that they are especially frequent in tense, nervous persons. It is probable that some relationship exists between these nocturnal starts and the sudden isolated jerk of a leg, or arm and leg, which may occur in healthy, fully conscious individuals. It does not appear to be related to epilepsy despite certain superficial resemblances. Disturbances of this nature may be the stimulus for night terrors. These somnolescent starts must be distinguished from flexor spasms of the legs, which occur in individuals who have suffered disease of the pyramidal tracts and from a rare condition known as nocturnal myoclonus in which the legs are involved in brusque flexion or extension movements of such force as to awaken the patient.

Sensory centers may be disturbed in a similar way either as an isolated phenomenon or in association with phenomena that induce motion. As the patient drops off to sleep he may be roused by a sensation that darts through his body. Such sensory symptoms are often in the domain of one of the special senses, especially hearing. A sudden clang or crashing sound disturbs commencing sleep. Sometimes a sudden flash of light occurs as sleep is coming on. A sensation of being lifted and dashed to earth or of being turned is probably a similar sensory paroxysm involving the labyrinthine mechanism.

Curious paralytic phenomena, so distressing to a patient as to cause him to seek medical advice, may also occur in the transition from the sleeping to the waking state. Sometimes in an otherwise healthy individual a state supervenes in the morning in which, although awake, conscious, and fully oriented, he is unable to innervate a single muscle. He lies as though still asleep with eyes closed and is all the while engaged in a struggle for movement. He has the impression that if he could move a single muscle, the spell would instantly vanish and he would regain full power. It has been reported that the slightest cutaneous stimulus such as the touch of a hand may abolish the paralysis. Such attacks are usually transient and of no special significance. They have also been reported to occur during the development of sleep. They may be related to narcolepsy.

NIGHTMARES AND NIGHT TERRORS. Awakening in a state of terror has happened to nearly everyone. Children and nervous adults are especially prone to it. Fevers dispose to it, and it has been said that any upsetting condition of the body, such as a disturbance of digestion, may have a similar effect. Bad dreams, stimulated directly by recent memory of blood-curdling television programs before going to bed, may account for night terrors in children. Some psychologists have drawn a distinction between the nightmare which is merely a terrifying dream and that in which there are visual hallucinations and motor activity. Considering the predominantly visual nature of dreams, it is doubtful if such a separation is valid. Probably any difference is only one of degree.

A night terror is probably always connected with an alarming dream. The victim sits up or jumps out of bed, shouts, or rushes frantically from his room. He is at first unconscious of his surroundings, but usually the intensity of emotional disturbance and the physical activity awaken him. The following morning he may have only a hazy recollection of the experience.

Such phenomena are of little significance as isolated events in childhood but must be distinguished from nocturnal epilepsy. They seldom persist beyond adolescence. If they occur with excessive frequency and continue very long, a relationship to other disturbances, such as psychoneurosis, usually exists.

SOMNAMBULISM AND SLEEP AUTOMATISM. Examples of sleep-walking come to the attention of the practicing physician not infrequently. This condition likewise occurs more often in children than in adults. After being asleep for a time, the patient arises from his bed and walks about the house. He may turn on a light or perform some other familiar act. There is no outward sign of emotion; the eyes are open, and the sleeper is guided by vision, thus avoiding familiar objects. The sight of an unfamiliar object may awaken him. If spoken to, he makes no response; if told to return to bed, he may do so but more often must be led back to it. Sometimes he will mutter strange phrases or sentences over and over. The following morning he usually has no memory of the episode.

Most psychiatrists hold that these are dissociated mental states similar to the hysterical trance and fugue, except that they begin during sleep. Undoubtedly this is true, and sleep walking may be accepted as evidence of a nervous disorder, probably of the psychoneurotic variety. There are nonetheless examples of this in adults who have no other signs of mental illness. One can only regard such a case as an isolated disorder of sleep-waking mechanism. It is probably allied to talking in one's sleep, though the two conditions seldom occur together.

Half-waking somnambulism, or sleep automatism, is a state in which an adult patient, half-roused from sleep, goes through a fairly complex routine such as going to a window, opening it, and looking out, but afterward recalling only a part of the episode. The patient may injure himself during sleepwalking.

NOCTURNAL EPILEPSY. Paroxysmal abnormalities of the brain waves of the type seen in epilepsy tend to occur in epileptic patients during or shortly after the onset of sleep. This characteristic electroencephalographic pattern has been found so frequently in the epileptic patient that the practice of artificially inducing sleep in order to obtain confirmation of epilepsy has been adopted in many laboratories. Of course, it has long been known that epilepsy occurs during sleep.

The sleeping epileptic patient attracts attention to his condition by a cry, violent motor activity, or labored breathing. As in the diurnal seizure, after the tonic-clonic phase, he becomes quiet and falls into a state resembling sleep but from which he cannot be aroused. His appearance depends on the phase of the seizure he happens to be in when first observed. Seizures of this type may occur at any time during the night, and some patients may have all their seizures at night. If the seizure during the night is unobserved, the only indication of it may be disheveled bedclothes, a few drops of blood on the pillow, wet bed linen from urinary incontinence, a bitten tongue, or sore muscles. In some children the occurrence of a seizure is betrayed only by incoherent behavior or a headache, the common aftermath of a convulsive disorder that was unnoticed. Rarely, a patient may die in an epileptic seizure during sleep, presumably from being smothered by bedclothes, aspirating vomitus, or for some more obscure reason.

Other less well-defined types of seizure occur at night. The patient may arise as though in a night terror and perform complex acts. He may be excited and overactive and, if restrained, become combative. After some minutes he is subdued and returns to sleep. The following morning he disclaims all memory of the episode. Probably this does not represent a psychomotor seizure but is instead a night terror. An electroencephalographic study may be helpful in such cases.

Nocturnal jerks of the legs, also called *nocturnal myoclonus,* is another troublesome symptom because it interferes with sleep night after night. Only recently has it been classified as a myoclonic form of epilepsy. It is unaccompanied by all other epileptic manifestations. Anticonvulsant drugs are said to control the condition, though in two cases the author has had better success with an occasional dose of Pantopon. It differs from the restless leg syndrome in that involuntary movements occur.

Epilepsy may occur in conjunction with both night terrors and somnambulism, and the question then arises whether the latter is in the nature of postepileptic automatism. Usually, no such relationship is established.

PROLONGED STATES OF SLEEP AND REVERSAL OF SLEEP-WAKING RHYTHM. Encephalitis lethargica, or "epidemic encephalitis," that remarkable illness which appeared on the medical horizon during the great pandemic influenza following the First World War, has provided some of the most dramatic instances of prolonged somnolence. In fact, protracted sleep lasting days to weeks was such a prominent symptom that the disease was called "sleeping sickness." The patient appeared to be in a state of continuous sleep, or "somnosis," and remained awake only while stimulated. Although the infective agent was never isolated, the pathologic anatomy was fully divulged by many excellent studies, all of which demonstrated a destruction of neurones in the midbrain, subthalamus, and hypothalamus. Patients surviving the acute phases of the illness often had difficulty in reestablishing the normal sleep-waking rhythm. As the somnolence disappeared, some patients exhibited a reversal of sleep rhythm, tending to sleep by day and stay awake at night and Parkinson's syndrome (Chap. 361).

Hypersomnia also occurs in trypanosomiasis, the common cause of sleeping sickness in Africa, and with a variety of diseases localized to the floor and walls of the third ventricle. Small tumors in the posterior hypothalamus and midbrain have been associated with arterial hypotension, diabetes insipidus, and somnolence lasting many weeks. Such patients can be aroused, but if left alone, they immediately fall asleep. Tumors of the brain, in general, show a tendency to cause drowsiness and increased amounts of sleep, but those of the diencephalon more so than any others (e.g., than posterior fossa ones). Traumatic brain lesions and other diseases have been found to produce similar clinical pictures.

NARCOLEPSY AND CATAPLEXY. The term *narcolepsy* has been used rather loosely. According to most authorities, it should refer to peculiar brief recurrent attacks of sleep and not to prolonged or continuous sleep. *Cataplexy* is a sudden brief loss of muscular power evoked by strong emotion, usually laughter. Although a few of the reported cases are doubtless examples of hysteria, there is unquestionably a well-defined clinical entity which bears no relationship to neurosis or any other known psychiatric condition. This will be discussed further in Chap. 366.

SLEEP PALSIES AND ACROPARESTHESIAS. Curious and at times distressing paresthetic disturbances develop during sleep. Everyone is familiar with the phenomenon of an arm or leg falling asleep. The immobility of the limbs and the maintenance of uncomfortable postures without being aware of them permits pressure to be applied to exposed nerves. The ulnar, radial, and peroneal nerves are quite superficial in places; pressure of the nerve against an underlying bone may interfere with intraneural circulation of the compressed segment. If this lasts for half an hour or longer, a sensory and motor paralysis sometimes referred to as *sleep palsy* may develop. This condition usually lasts only a few hours or days, but if the compression is prolonged, the nerve may be severely damaged so that functional recovery awaits regeneration. Unusually deep sleep, as in alcoholic intoxication, or anesthesia renders the patient especially liable to sleep palsies merely because he does not heed the discomfort of an unnatural posture.

Acroparesthesias are frequent in adult women and are not unknown to men. The patient will say that after being asleep for a few hours she is awakened by an intense numbness, tingling, prickling, a feeling of "pins and needles" in her fingers and hands. There are also aching, burning pains or tightness and other unpleasant sensations. At first there is a suspicion of having slept on the arm, but the usual bilaterality and the occurrence regardless of the position of the arms dispel this notion. Usually the paresthesias are in the distribution of the median nerves. Vigorous rubbing of the hands restores normal sensation, and the paresthesias subside within a few minutes, only to return later or upon first awakening in the morning. The condition never occurs during the daytime unless the patient is lying down or sitting with the arms and hands in one position. It may be unilateral but is more often bilateral. It never occurs in the feet. When acroparesthesias are frequent, the hands may at all times feel swollen, stiff, clumsy, slightly numb, and sometimes distressingly painful. Careful examination discloses little or no objective sensory loss, though in some cases touch and pain sensation have been slightly altered in parts supplied by the median nerves. Slight atrophy and weakness of the abductor pollicis brevis and opponens pollicis have been noted, and in a few cases it has been marked (carpal tunnel syndrome). The use of the hands for heavy manual work during the day seems to aggravate the condition, and a holiday or a period of hospitalization may relieve it. It often occurs in young housewives with a new baby or in factory workers who perform a routine skill. Recently it has been demonstrated that there is a compression of the median nerves in the carpal tunnel of the wrist by thickened carpal ligaments, tenosynovitis, bony overgrowth (as in acromegaly), or amyloid deposit (multiple myeloma). The injection of 50 mg hydrocortisone beneath the carpal ligament and the use of Diuril or one of its analogs has given immediate relief in a respectable number of cases. The section of the carpal ligament has nearly always cured recalcitrant cases.

DIAGNOSIS OF DISORDERS OF SLEEP

The diagnosis of the cause of insomnia may be troublesome. The difficulty is usually not with the severe case of insomnia as much as with the chronic one. A common source of error is failure to recognize an underlying psychiatric illness such as anxiety neurosis or depressive psychosis. This failure can be avoided only by having the main symptoms of these illnesses clearly in mind and making particular inquiry concerning them in every case.

Somnolescent starts, somnolescent sensory paroxysms, and night terrors may all be confused with nocturnal epilepsy, but actually the only real problem here is to distinguish between night terrors and epilepsy. This may at times be difficult, if not impossible. The occurrence of other types of seizures, especially if they occur during the daytime, the lack of any display of terrifying emotion,

and the presence of urinary incontinence and tongue biting all indicate epilepsy. Often electroencephalographic confirmation can be obtained.

In the diagnosis of diseases that cause protracted somnolence, a thorough neurologic study, with x-rays of skull, electroencephalogram, and lumbar puncture, must be employed. Diabetes insipidus, signs of pituitary insufficiency, blindness in parts of visual fields, ophthalmoplegia, and sometimes extrapyramidal motor disturbances are helpful in that they indicate disease in areas adjacent to the posterior hypothalamus and midbrain. But, probably the most frequent cause of excess drowsiness is that due to medication which acts either directly on the diencephalon or alters some component of blood, e.g., Na or K, and thereby affects the nervous system.

Sleep palsies must be distinguished from other diseases affecting the peripheral nerves. The onset during sleep, maximal functional disturbance immediately afterward, and steady improvement are the main characteristics. A delay in the appearance of muscular atrophy may be perplexing unless it is remembered that it takes 2 to 3 months for denervation atrophy to develop fully. The syndrome of acroparesthesias is often mistaken for ruptured cervical disk, anterior scalene and cervical rib syndrome, peripheral neuritis, multiple sclerosis, or psychoneurosis. The nocturnal incidence, the localization to the fingers and hands in the median nerve distribution, and the lack of other neurologic signs are diagnostic. A tourniquet around the arm just above the elbow may reproduce the acroparesthetic syndrome.

TREATMENT

In general, there are three varieties of wakefulness. For best management, treatment should be based on the type exhibited by the patient. In younger patients the most frequently observed type of insomnia is the inability to fall asleep. These individuals have become more and more tense during the day and are unable to relax. This type of insomnia usually lasts from 1 to 3 hr, and then the individual sinks into an exhausted, deep sleep which continues through the night. For these patients a quick-acting, fairly rapidly destroyed hypnotic such as secobarbital (Seconal), 0.1 Gm given 15 to 20 min before going to bed, is useful.

The second group consists of patients who are able to go to sleep but who awaken in 2 or 3 hr and lose sleep in the middle of the night. They awaken during the period when sleep normally lightens and some are alternately awake and asleep all the rest of the night. Often these are sick persons with a debilitating or painful illness which generates more pain and restlessness as muscles relax and leave painful areas unsplinted. In others, fever, sweats, dyspnea, or other distressful symptoms develop and demand attention. Frequently, these patients secure relief from pentobarbital (Nembutal), 0.1 Gm given at bedtime. For cardiac patients who have Cheyne-Stokes respiration or moderate orthopnea, a rectal suppository of aminophylline, 0.5 Gm given at bedtime, will frequently relieve the respiratory distress and promote sleep. When pain is a factor in insomnia, acetylsalicylic acid 0.3 to 0.6 Gm, should be given with the sedative. Occasionally, codeine phosphate, 30 mg, may be required when pain is severe.

The third group of insomnia patients consists of those who go to sleep promptly and sleep well most of the night, only to awaken too early in the morning. Most of these individuals are older persons who turn night into day. They go to bed and get up earlier and earlier so that soon they are sleeping during the day and are alert during the night. Into this category also fall those individuals who are under great tension, worry, or anxiety or are overworked and exhausted. These people sink into bed and sleep through sheer exhaustion, but around 4 or 5 A.M. they awake with their worries and are unable to get back to sleep. Most of these patients are benefited by barbital, 0.3 Gm given with fruit juice or milk at bedtime. For debilitated patients the compressed tablets of insoluble material should be crushed to ensure proper absorption or sodium barbital should be substituted. Chloral hydrate, 1.0 Gm given with fruit juice at bedtime, is also effective and may be substituted for barbital if desired.

Patients with serious mental agitation, delirium, or excitement who require prompt, easily controlled, relatively safe sedation should receive whiskey, 30 to 60 ml by mouth, or paraldehyde, 15 to 30 ml by mouth in iced fruit juice, or the same dose of the latter by rectum but diluted with 200 ml physiologic saline solution or 120 ml olive oil. For frankly delirious patients 25 to 50 mg of chlorpromazine (t.i.d.) has been a most helpful medication. Generally, it is wise to avoid barbiturates with highly agitated patients, since occasionally they may precipitate serious mental confusion, excitement, or even manic tendencies. Chloral hydrate, 1.0 to 2.0 Gm by mouth, is also useful in the management of these individuals and frequently proves more satisfactory than the barbiturates.

A word of caution about oversedation is wise in any discussion of sedative drugs. All too frequently they are abused in that they are given when not needed, the dosage is too great, or the wrong preparation is used. These drugs are a common source of constipation, lead to fatigue and lack of energy and strength, and interfere with the patient's recovery from his illness.

When large dosages of quicker-acting barbiturates, 0.4 to 0.6 Gm daily, are given for more than a few weeks, there is real danger of habituation, which once developed, is pernicious in character. Withdrawal, unless accomplished skillfully and in graded steps, may cause serious mental disturbance or precipitate convulsions. The chronic insomniac who has no other symptoms should not be permitted to use sedative drugs as a crutch on which to limp through life. The solution of this problem is rarely to be found in medication. One should search out and correct the underlying difficulty using medication only as a temporary helpful tool. A good book, pleasure in staying awake, and belief that the human organism will always get as much sleep as needed are helpful.

Barbiturate sedatives may be of value in treating night terrors, and if their differentiation from nocturnal epilepsy is impossible, a trial on diphenylhydantoin sodium (Dilantin Sodium) and phenobarbital is indicated. (See Chap. 368 for further information concerning anticonvulsant medication.)

REFERENCES

Kleitman, N.: "Sleep and Wakefulness," Chicago, The University of Chicago Press, 1934.

Kremer, M., R. W. Gilliatt, J. S. R. Golding, and T. G. Wilson: Acroparesthesiae in the Carpel-tunnel Syndrome. Brit. Med. J. (Lancet), II:590, 1953.

Miller, H. R.: "Central Autonomic Regulations in Health and Disease," p. 260, New York, Grune & Stratton, Inc., 1942.

Muncie, W.: "Psychobiology and Psychiatry," p. 104, St. Louis, The C. V. Mosby Company, 1939.

28 RECURRENT CONVULSIONS
Raymond D. Adams

The magnitude of the problem of epilepsy and its importance in our society can hardly be overstated. The statistics of Lennox and Lennox show that at least 1,000,000 persons in the United States are or have been subject to seizures. After apoplexy, epilepsy is the most frequent neurologic disorder. Therefore, the physician must know something of the nature and etiology of this common condition and of the mechanism whereby symptoms are produced.

Epilepsy is an intermittent disorder of the nervous system due presumably to a sudden, excessive, disorderly discharge of cerebral neurones. This was the postulation of Hughlings Jackson, the eminent British neurologist of the nineteenth century, and modern electrophysiology offers no evidence to the contrary. This discharge results in an almost instantaneous disturbance of sensation, loss of consciousness, convulsive movements, or some combination thereof. A terminologic difficulty arises from the diversity of the clinical manifestations. It seems improper to call a condition a convulsion when only an alteration of sensation or of consciousness takes place. The word *seizure* is preferable as a generic term and also lends itself to qualification. Motor or convulsive seizure is therefore not tautologic, and one may speak also of sensory seizures. The word *epilepsy*, which in times past meant the "falling evil," has many unpleasant connotations, and although it is a useful medical term, probably it is best avoided in open discussions until the general public becomes more enlightened.

Epilepsy may begin at any age. It may occur once in the lifetime of an individual or several times a day. Sometimes it is an obvious symptom of a brain disease that also manifests itself in other ways, and at times it is the solitary expression of deranged cerebral function in an individual who otherwise maintains perfect health. The latter is the more frequent circumstance and explains why the convulsive state has for so long been looked upon as a disease entity. However, it is illogical to suppose that a convulsion occurring by itself represents a disease, whereas one occurring in combination with other symptoms is only a manifestation of a disease. The convulsive state must always be looked upon as symptomatic. Use of such epithets as "genuine" or "essential" or "idiopathic" merely point to obscure causation and the more benign nature of the disease.

THE COMMON TYPES OF CONVULSIVE DISORDERS

In a statistical survey of nearly 2,000 patients it was reported that 51 percent of all epileptic patients had had *generalized convulsions;* 8 percent, minor seizures referred to as *petit mal;* 1 percent, *psychic* or *psychomotor seizures;* and the remaining 40 percent, two or even all three types, the most prominent form being psychomotor. Thus psychomotor epilepsy is almost as frequent as grand mal. Although the total number of seizures that had a focal onset was not determined, these data give some notion of the principal forms of the convulsive state in the majority of patients.

THE GENERALIZED CONVULSION (GRAND MAL, MAJOR EPILEPSY)

The term *convulsion* is most applicable to this form of seizure. The patient may sense its possible approach by any of several subjective sensations. For some hours he may feel apathetic, depressed, irritable, or the opposite —unusually alert or even ecstatic. Flatulence, constipation, and headache are other prodromal symptoms, and myoclonic twitches, i.e., sudden movements that affect one or another limb or the trunk, may precede the convulsion by some hours. In approximately half the cases there is some type of sensation or movement of one part of the body before the loss of consciousness or the generalized convulsion. This is called the *aura,* and as will be explained later, it provides the most reliable clue to the location of the underlying disease. The most frequent aura is an epigastric sensation, a sinking or gripping feeling, a strangulation or palpitation. A tingling numbness of the fingers or lips or some other part of the body, a flashing light or panorama, and disagreeable taste or odor are other well-known sensory auras. Clonic twitches, tonic contraction of the muscles of a limb, and turning of the head and eyes are somatic motor auras that at first take the form of focal epilepsy and end in a generalized seizure. They may spread from one part of the body to another in an orderly, predictable sequence. Usually, by the time all one side of the body is affected there is a loss of consciousness. The aura, though truly a warning of the oncoming seizure, is actually the first part of the seizure and not a prodrome. It seldom lasts more than a few seconds.

The generalized convulsion, or *fit,* as it is often called, begins with a sudden loss of consciousness and falling to the ground. The whole musculature is seized in a violent spasm. The contraction of the diaphragm and chest muscles produces a characteristic cry. The eyes turn up or to one side, the face is contorted, the jaw is set, often with biting of the tongue and oozing of saliva or blood from the lips, and the limbs may assume any of several positions. With continued spasm of the respiratory muscles, breathing is impossible, and the color of the skin and mucous membranes becomes dusky or cyanotic. After a fraction of a minute the rigid or tonic state of the muscles gives way to a series of clonic jerking movements. Air begins to enter the lungs in short convulsive gasps, and a bloody froth, a mixture of saliva and blood from a bitten tongue or cheek, forms on the lips. The arms, legs, face, and head jerk violently. After a minute or two the movements become slower, then irregular, and finally cease. The patient then lies relaxed, breathing rather deeply and sweating profusely. There may have been loss of control of urine and occasionally of feces. The state is now one of deep coma, and even the most intense pain evokes no response. Plantar reflexes are often extensor. One or both pupils may not react. After a few minutes the patient stirs and then opens his eyes. His first remarks or questions usually betray mental confusion. For the next several minutes or even hours there is a tendency toward incoherence of thought and drowsiness. Often the patient falls into a deep sleep. Headache is another frequent postseizure or postictal symptom. The patient himself is completely unaware of what has happened or at most remembers only the aura. He may come to his senses in a hospital or other strange place, and his only way of telling that something has happened is by the hiatus in his memory, his disheveled appearance, the bitten tongue, and a soreness of the vigorously exercised muscles. Injury may be sustained during the fall and as a consequence of violent muscular contraction; one or several vertebras may be crushed. Periorbital subcutaneous hemorrhages may reflect the violence of the exertion during the seizures.

Convulsions of this type ordinarily come singly or in groups of two or three and may occur when the patient is awake or asleep. About 5 to 8 percent of patients at some time have a series of seizures without regaining consciousness between times. This is known as *status epilepticus* and demands urgent treatment. Instead of the whole sequence of changes described above, only one part of the seizure may occur; for example, there may be only the aura without loss of consciousness, or the entire spell may consist of a brief loss of consciousness and momentary spasm of the limbs. Anticonvulsive medication abbreviates the seizure.

PETIT MAL (MINOR EPILEPSY, SMALL ILLNESS, L'ABSENCE)

In contrast to the generalized seizure, these attacks are so brief that they are often overlooked. In fact, many patients may have them for years before their true nature is recognized.

The attack comes without warning and consists of sudden loss of consciousness. The person is motionless, and a staring expression of the face and failure to speak or to respond to commands are the only signs of abnormality.

In contrast to grand mal, motor disturbances are conspicuously absent, and at most only a few flickering contractions of the eyelids and facial muscles and jerking of the arms at a rate of three contractions per second are seen. The patient does not fall, as a rule, and he may continue such complex acts as walking or even riding a bicycle during an attack. After 2 to 15 sec or more, consciousness is regained abruptly and fully, and the patient promptly resumes whatever action he was performing before the seizure. To the patient there is only a blank place, an "absence," in his stream of consciousness.

Closely related to petit mal are the *akinetic seizures*, in which the patient suddenly loses consciousness and falls motionless to the ground, and the myoclonic seizure, which consists of a sudden violent contraction of some part of or all the body, often followed by a lapse of posture with falling and loss of consciousness of a few seconds' duration (*generalized myoclonus*). Because of frequent association with petit mal and the similarity of the electroencephalographic pattern, Lennox groups petit mal, the akinetic seizure, and myoclonic seizure into a single entity called the *petit mal triad*.

Episodes of this type are much more frequent in childhood and adolescence. Another characteristic is their great frequency. As many as several hundred may occur in one day. Although benign, they may, if frequent, derange the mental processes so that the patient does poorly in school. Rarely, a series of them in close succession will interrupt consciousness for a longer period of time. This is known as *petit mal status*. *Pyknolepsy* is an almost obsolete term for frequent petit mal during childhood, terminating at puberty. When present as the only type of seizure during childhood, petit mal may give way to or be combined with grand mal, in a majority of cases by the age of sixteen years.

PSYCHOMOTOR EPILEPSY (EPILEPTIC EQUIVALENTS, PSYCHIC VARIANTS, EPILEPTIC MANIA OR DELIRIUM

This differs in several ways from the two types of seizure discussed above. (1) The aura, if it occurs, is often a complex hallucination or perceptual illusion. There may be an unpleasant smell or taste or the revival of a complicated visual scene involving people, dwellings, etc., usually taken from past experiences and resembling a dream. Furthermore, the patient's perception of what is seen and heard and his relationship to the outside world are altered. Objects appear to be far away or unreal (*jamais vu*); or strange objects or persons may seem familiar (*déjà vu phenomenon*). Hughlings Jackson applied the term *dreamy state* to these psychic disturbances. (2) Instead of losing all control of his thoughts and actions, the patient behaves as though he were partially conscious during the attack. He may get up and walk about, unbutton or remove his clothes, attempt to speak, or even continue such habitual acts as driving a car. If he is asked a specific question or given a command, it is evident that he is out of contact with the examiner and does not understand. When restrained, he may resist with great energy and at times can be violent. This type of behavior is said to be *automatic,* presumably because the patient behaves like an automaton. (3) Convulsive movements, when present, are likely to consist of chewing, smacking and licking of the lips, and less often, tonic spasms of the limbs or turning of the head and eyes to one side.

In any given case one or several of these phenomena may be observed. In the series studied by Lennox and Lennox, which numbered 414 cases, 43 percent of patients displayed some of these motor or psychomotor phenomena; 32 percent, the automatic state; and 25 percent, the psychic changes. Because of the concurrence of these three symptom complexes, they have referred to the whole group as the *psychomotor triad*. These types of seizure vary in frequency and duration. Some are very brief, lasting only for seconds, and others continue for hours or days. This calls to mind that the duration of the seizure is an unsatisfactory criterion for classification. Two-thirds of the patients have generalized convulsions at some time in their lives.

In addition to these three major types, the clinicians of the nineteenth century recognized many other special forms of epilepsy, some of which were given descriptive names. The term *tonic seizure* referred to tonic muscle contractions, to the exclusion of phasic qualities. *Epilepsia partialis continua* specified a regular repetitive clonic contraction of one group of muscles, not progressing to a generalized seizure. The terms *focal motor* or *focal sensory epilepsy* were applied to a tonic or clonic movement or a sensation restricted to one portion of the body. *Myoclonic epilepsy* referred to a syndrome of epilepsy and isolated twitches of a muscle or group of muscles, the latter being *myoclonus* (see Chap. 22). Random, arrhythmic myoclonus in a sense might be designated as *epilepsia partialis discontinua et disseminata*. It is usually caused by a more or less diffuse disease of the cerebral and cerebellar cortex and possibly of other parts of the nervous system, such as the thalamus.

In childhood a number of other forms of epilepsy occur, related presumably to the immaturity of the child's nervous system. The seizures of the newborn (*neonatal epilepsy*) are fragmentary and brief. Infantile or salam spasms, i.e., brief flexion of neck and limbs, are peculiar to the age period of six months to three to four years. *Febrile seizures* appear only in the age period of eighteen months to six years. Photic reflex epilepsy is induced by flickering light in childhood and adolescence Chap 365.

It is obvious that the traditional division of seizures into three main general types leaves much to be desired. Whereas petit mal is a more or less homogeneous type, grand mal may represent a phase of generalization of the seizure discharge, regardless of its origin or the initial symptoms of the seizure. Psychomotor epilepsy, as will be evident upon further analysis, is not a uniform syndrome but encompasses a diversity of clinical phenomena. Moreover, careful study of the first symptoms of the seizure and the use of the electroencephalogram have given us a new means of subdividing seizures according to other more significant attributes.

Common Focal Seizure Patterns

The seizure pattern provides information that not only is of great value in determining the topography of the disease causing the convulsive disorder but affords a new basis of classification that will serve until the etiology is discovered. The most definite focal seizure patterns are listed below. They are so helpful in the localization of cerebral lesions that every student of medicine should be familiar with them. These types of epilepsy are often termed *focal* because they can be traced to a circumscript lesion in one part of the brain.

MOTOR SEIZURES (GENERALIZED, CONTRAVERSIVE, FOCAL MOTOR, AND JACKSONIAN SEIZURES)

A lesion in one or other frontal lobe may give rise to a generalized or major convulsive seizure of the type described above, without introductory sensory aura. In some cases there is a turning movement of the head and eyes to one side, simultaneous with loss of consciousness, and in others there are no turning movements. It has been postulated that in both types of seizure, the one with and the one without contraversive movements, the discharge from the frontal lobe spreads rapidly into an integrating center such as the thalamus, with immediate loss of consciousness. In cases with head and eye turning, the discharge is believed to reach area 8 (area for contralateral turning of head and eyes), although it has been found that contralateral turning of the head and eyes can be induced in the experimental animal by stimulation of temporal or occipital as well as of the premotor cortex.

Do most cases of generalized motor seizures (grand mal) of idiopathic type have a frontal focus? Unfortunately, this question cannot be answered at the moment. Such a focus has been found in only a small number of such cases, and these may not be representative of the whole group.

The characteristics of the *Jacksonian motor seizure* are well known. It begins usually with a twitching of the fingers of one hand, the face on one side, or one foot. The movements are clonic and rhythmic; their speed varies. They may occur in bursts, or paroxysms. The disorder then spreads or marches from the part first affected to other muscles on the same side of the body—from the face to the neck, hand, forearm, arm, trunk, and leg; if the first movement is in the foot, the order is reversed. The high incidence of onset in the lips, fingers, and toes probably is related to the greater cortical representation of these parts of the body. The disease process or focus of excitation is usually the Rolandic cortex, area 4 (Fig. 31-1) on the opposite side; in a few cases it has been found in the post-Rolandic convolution. Lesions confined to the premotor cortex (area 6) are said to induce contractions of an arm, face, neck, or all of one side of the body. Perspiration and piloerection, sometimes of the parts of the body involved in a focal motor seizure, suggest that these autonomic functions have cortical representation in the Rolandic area. Some neurologists distinguish focal motor and Jacksonian motor seizures by the absence of a characteristic march in the former, but both have essentially the same localizing significance.

Another type of focal motor epilepsy, the previously mentioned *epilepsia partialis continua*, consists of rhythmic clonic movements of one group of muscles, usually in the face, arm, or leg. These may continue for a variable period of time, minutes to weeks or months. The seizure usually does not march to other parts of the body. Its localizing value has not been settled. Some cases have a lesion in the opposite sensorimotor areas of the cerebral cortex.

SOMATIC, VISUAL, AND OTHER SENSORY SEIZURES

Somatic sensory seizures, either focal or "marching" to other parts of the body on one side, nearly always indicate a parietal lobe lesion. The usual sensory disorder is described as a numbness or a tingling or "pins-and-needles" feeling. Other variations are sensations of crawling (formication), buzzing, electricity, or vibration. Pain and thermal sensations are infrequent. The onset is in the lips, fingers, and toes in the majority of cases, and the spread to adjacent parts of the body follows a pattern determined by sensory arrangements in the postcentral (post-Rolandic) convolution of the parietal lobe. In Kristiansen and Penfield's series the seizure focus was found in the postcentral convolution in 24 of 55 cases; it was central, either pre- or post-Rolandic, in 18, and precentral in 7 cases. One may conclude that this type of sensory phenomenon always indicates a focus in or near the post-Rolandic convolution of the opposite cerebral hemisphere; if localized in the head, the locus is in the lowest part of the convolution, near the Sylvian fissure; if in the foot or leg, the upper part near the superior sagittal sinus is involved.

Visual seizures are also of localizing significance. Lesions in or near the striate cortex of the occipital lobe usually produce a sensation of lights, of darkness, or of color. According to Gowers, red is the most frequent color, followed by blue, green, and yellow. The patient may tell of seeing stars or moving lights in the visual field on the side opposite the lesion. Sometimes they appear to be straight ahead of the patient. Often, if they occur on only one side of the visual field, he believes only one eye to be affected, the one opposite the lesion, probably because the average person is unaware that he has two corresponding visual fields. It is curious that a seizure arising in one occipital lobe may cause momentary blindness in both eyes. It has been noted that seizures in the lateral surface of the occipital lobes (Brodmann's areas 18 and 19) are more likely to cause twinkling or pulsating lights. Complex visual hallucinations are usually due to a focus in the posterior part of the temporal lobe, near its junction with the parietal, and they may be associated with auditory hallucinations. Often the visual images, either those of the hallucination or of objects seen, are distorted and seem too small (*micropsia*) or unnaturally arranged.

Auditory hallucinations are rather infrequent as an initial manifestation of a seizure. Occasionally a patient with a focus in the superior temporal convolution on one side will report a buzzing or a roaring in his ears. A human voice sometimes repeating recognizable words has been noted a few times in patients with lesions in the more posterior part of the dominant temporal lobe.

Vertiginous sensations of a type suggesting vestibular stimulation may be the first symptom of a seizure. The lesion is usually localized in the superior posterior temporal region or at the junction between parietal and temporal lobes. Foerster is said to have evoked a sensation of vertigo by stimulating the parietal lobe, and in one of Penfield's cases the lesion was there. Occasionally with a temporal focus vertigo is followed by an auditory sensation. Giddiness is also a frequent prelude to a seizure, but this has so many different meanings that it is of little diagnostic import.

Olfactory hallucinations are often associated with disease of the inferior and medial parts of the temporal lobe, usually in the region of the hippocampal convolution or the uncus (hence the term *uncinate seizures,* after Jackson). Usually the smell is exteriorized, i.e., projected to someplace in the environment, and is of a disagreeable nature. Gustatory hallucinations have also been recorded in proven cases of temporal lobe disease. Sensations of thirst and salivation may be associated. Stimulation of the upper surface of the temporal lobe in the depths of the Sylvian fissure during neurosurgical operations has reproduced peculiar sensations of taste.

Visceral sensations arising in the thorax, epigastrium, and abdomen are among the most frequent of the auras. They are described as a vague, indefinable feeling, a sinking sensation in the pit of the stomach, and a weakness in the epigastrium or substernal area that rises to the throat and head. In several such cases the seizure discharge has been localized to the upper bank of the Sylvian fissure, but in a few cases lesions were in the upper intermediate or medial frontal areas near the cingulate gyrus. Palpitation and acceleration of pulse at the beginning of the attack have also been related to a temporal lobe focus.

PSYCHIC PHENOMENA

The studies of many neurologists have served to establish the close relationship between psychic changes and the temporal lobe. Disease of either temporal lobe may be accompanied by seizures that have many of the characteristics outlined under Psychomotor Epilepsy. In addition to olfactory and gustatory hallucinations, there are often others of more complex visual and auditory type with feelings of unreality, and partial or complete interruption of consciousness may be observed. Compulsive thought or action may recur in a fixed pattern during each seizure. Automatic behavior or even frank psychoses of many different types, lasting for hours or days, may be induced by seizure discharges or electrical stimulation of the temporal lobe. Masticatory movements are also frequent.

LOSS OF CONSCIOUSNESS

A lapse of consciousness is the initial event in petit mal, which is believed now to represent a disorder of the diencephalon, the so-called "centrencephalic epilepsy." Lesions in the prefrontal regions have been observed to abolish consciousness at the very beginning of the seizure, presumably through the effects on the diencephalon and midbrain structures.

The various motor, sensory, or psychic phenomena may be combined in many different sequences. These presumably indicate the spread of a seizure discharge from one cortical area to another. A flash of light followed by tingling of one side of the body suggests that the epileptic discharge began in the occipital lobe and extended to the somatic sensory areas in the parietal lobe. A smell of something burning, followed by chewing and smacking movements, and then loss of speech would be interpreted as a spread of the seizure discharge from the region of the uncus to the upper parts of the temporal and the inferior frontal lobe. A focal motor seizure followed by a tonic contraction of one side of the body and then turning of the head and eyes contralaterally would indicate a successive involvement of the motor, premotor, and contraversive cortical field for head and eyes. Little is known about the factors that facilitate or inhibit the spread of seizure discharges from one part of the brain to another.

THE EVOCATION OF SEIZURES (Reflex Epilepsy)

For a long time it has been known that seizures could be evoked in susceptible individuals by a physiologic or psychologic stimulus. Approximately 1 in every 15 patients will have remarked that their seizures occur under special circumstances, such as being exposed to flickering light, passing from darkness to light or the reverse, being startled by a loud noise, hearing a series of monotonous sounds or music, touching, rubbing, or hurting a particular part of the body, making certain movements, i.e., eating, reading, carrying out some complex mental task, or being subjected to fright or other strong emotion. The evoked seizure may be focal (beginning often in the part of the body that has been stimulated) or generalized and may take the form of one or a series of myoclonic jerks, a petit mal, or a grand mal. In a few instances *reflex epilepsy,* as it is called, has been due to a focal cerebral disease, such as a tumor, but more often its cause cannot be ascertained. W. Watson has discovered a strong tendency to familial incidence in a variety of myoclonic jerking elicited by photic stimulation (photic epilepsy), and some patients in whom this phenomenon had been noted were unaware of ever having had a seizure. Also of interest in these cases of evoked seizure has been the phenomenon of willfully averting the seizure by undertaking some mental task, e.g., thinking about some distracting subject or counting, or by initiating some physical activity.

Patients of this type suggest to us that epilepsy is a

natural state, a physiologic event resulting from excitation and subsequent inhibition of an injured part of the cerebrum.

PATHOPHYSIOLOGY AND BIOCHEMISTRY OF EPILEPSY

From what has been said about epilepsy it is obvious that a satisfactory theory must account for the following clinical and pathologic data. (1) The majority of demonstrable epileptogenic lesions are situated in or near the cerebral cortex, which suggests that some property of the six-layered neural organization of this structure disposes to this condition. (2) The lesions of any given disease may or may not give rise to epilepsy; some peculiarity of the lesion must, therefore, determine this phenomenon. (3) The epileptic focus, once present, is known to become active, i.e., to discharge, only on occasion, or at least the electrical discharge which attends it only then becomes detectable in the electroencephalogram or expresses itself as an overt seizure. (4) Several events, some of physiologic or psychologic nature and others biochemical, are potent in activating the seizure focus or facilitating its spread. The former include photic and other sensory stimuli; the latter, such agents as pentylenetetrazol (Metrazol), picrotoxin, acetylcholine, excessive hydration, and alkalosis. (5) The seizure discharges upon reaching a certain intensity spread along preformed pathways from their site of origin to other cortical areas and to the diencephalon and brainstem. (6) Some inhibitory process counteracts and ultimately terminates the seizure discharge. (7) In many cases in human beings no cortical lesion has been demonstrated by current neuropathologic methods, and in this group there may be a genetic factor. The evidence on this latter point is not altogether convincing. Certainly, epilepsy and paroxysmal disturbances in the electroencephalogram have been observed in a large series of identical twins. However, the incidence of convulsions among blood relatives of epileptic patients is only two or three times that in the public at large, and a specific genetic pattern has never been established.

Investigations of epilepsy have centered on human cases of focal epilepsy and on experimentally induced focal epileptic lesions in the mammalian cortex. In both man and animal the neurophysiologic analogue to the convulsive seizure in human beings has been identified as a burst of high voltage spike waves, followed by repetitive, self-sustained discharge of electrical activity akin to posttetanic potentiation. This posttetanic potentiation is found so consistently in or near epileptic foci as to be accepted by many as the electrical sign of the epileptic lesion. The afterdischarge, once started, continues at a regular frequency of 10 to 14 per sec. Within a short time (seconds to minutes), the intervals between spikes increase; they tend then to be grouped, and their voltage rises. When the pauses between bursts reach 1/2 sec or more, the afterdischarge ceases altogether and the area of cortex becomes electrically inactive and inexcitable. The basis of the potentiation of the spike discharge is

little understood. Once started, its continuation involves a recycling or feedback process. Cessation indicates a rivalry between two opposing processes, the initial one excitatory, the final one inhibitory. A possible physiologic basis of these two processes has been demonstrated by Eccles at the spinal level. Each motor anterior horn cell, when activated, stimulates through a collateral branch another cell, the Renshaw cell, which is inhibitory in its action and imposes this inhibition on the anterior horn itself. Phillips has noted a similar arrangement between the Betz cells in the cerebral cortex and other interneurones that inhibit the Betz cells. Thus, both anterior horn cells and Betz cells can initiate excitation in another cell via their main axone, which in turn inhibits their own activity. Moreover, on the afferent side of neurone activation each sensory cell from the end organ to the cerebral cortex is monitored by a central descending inhibitory system. And, deafferentation itself is shown to increase the excitability of motor neurones.

The histologic changes in the seizure focus in man and experimental animals have been singularly difficult to interpret. In man epileptogenic foci are found not in gliotic scars but in neighboring intact regions of the brain. Whether the latter contain full populations of nerve cells with all their natural excitatory and inhibitory cortical mechanisms cannot be easily evaluated under the microscope. Golgi preparations are said to show a diminished number of dendritic arborizations and smaller synaptic surface of neurones.

A convulsive seizure could be conceived, therefore, either as an excessive excitation resulting from narrowly focused afferent stimulation on the injured cerebral cortex or as a deficiency of suppressive influences from either the afferent neurones or the special inhibitory neurones of the cortex. Strychnine, one of the most potent agents for discharging neurones and producing seizures, does not facilitate the excitatory postsynaptic potential of motor neurones but, rather, diminishes their inhibitory postsynaptic potentials. Solutions of strychnine, by themselves too weak to have any effect on the cortex, condition it in such a fashion that sensory stimuli conveyed to it will discharge the altered neurones and thus produce convulsive activity. This state of affairs resembles that which prevails in epileptic patients, where a silent, subliminal epileptic focus is discharged by a particular type of sensory stimulus and is restored to its quiescent state by inhibitory neurones.

Since electrical activity is believed to depend on chemical changes (flux of Na, K, Ca, Mg), it is rather to be expected that the effects of these ions would be studied in epilepsy. Hypocalcemia, hyponatremia, and hypokalemia, as well as hypoxia and alkalosis, for example, do increase the seizure tendency, but it is unclear as to whether they play a part in naturally occurring seizures. Also, a search has been made for special excitatory and inhibitory substances in the brain. Acetylcholine is known to be an effective convulsive agent when applied to the animal cortex, and cholinesterase inhibitors, such as isopropylfluorophosphate, likewise produce seizures. Cortical lesions in epileptic patients have been found to contain an increased amount of acetylcholinesterase and in a test tube are unable to "bind" acetylcholine. After a seizure there are increased amounts of acetylcholine in human cerebrospinal fluid. Barbiturates and diphenylhydantoin (Dilantin) are said to act as anticonvulsants because they enhance the acetylcholine-binding power of the cerebral cortex.

With respect to inhibitory substances Florey found that cerebral and spinal cord tissue contain an agent identified as gamma aminobutyric acid (GABA), which if applied to the cortex, blocks excitation of the superficial layer and augments inhibition—an action opposite to that of strychnine. It is formed from glutamic acid, and one of the coenzymes which catalyzes its synthesis is pyridoxine (vitamin B_6), lack of which is known to produce seizures in animals and man. Metrazol and picrotoxin are said to act by preventing the inhibitory effect of GABA. The action of GABA as an intrinsic anticonvulsant has not been fully explored. Given intravenously, it is said to protect animals against chemically induced seizures; others have not confirmed this effect.

A number of metabolic changes have been measured during a generalized convulsion. Presumably they are secondary. Oxygen utilization by the cerebral cortex increases, and of course, the violent generalized motor activity and arrest of respiration produce a hypoxia. CO_2 production in the convulsant brain is increased, and there is a relative acidosis. In the postseizure period cerebral vessels are dilated, and the oxygen content of the cerebral tissue increases. Hypoxic encephalopathy may occasionally complicate a prolonged motor seizure or status epilepticus and give rise to a postepileptic encephalopathy (neuronal loss in some cortical layers, hippocampus, and cerebellum).

Although high-amplitude activity of a group of neurones represents the "functional unit of epilepsy," it is the spread of this electrical potential to other parts of the nervous system that characterizes the whole convulsive seizure both clinically and electroencephalographically. The spread of these discharges proceeds along preformed pathways, i.e., via the uncinate fibers to adjacent cortical fields, via the corpus callosum to corresponding parts of the contralateral cerebral hemisphere, or along corticothalamic and thalamocortical pathways to the diencephalon and reticular formation. Some of the metabolic factors listed above may facilitate this spread. Little is known about agents that interfere with the spread of the seizure discharge. Acting on the assumption that the spread of seizure discharge is responsible for many of the undesirable features of the seizure, the corpus callosum has been sectioned in animals and human beings, and although the results were not conclusive, the seizures usually remained unilateral. The anticonvulsant activity of phenobarbital and diphenylhydantoin is believed to be mainly in preventing the spread of seizure discharges rather than in suppressing the epileptic focus.

Certain occurrences in the seizure, such as the cry, the motor activity, and the sensory experience, may be regarded as the direct manifestations of the seizure discharge in the brain. From the more general neurophysiologic point of view, they are excitatory. Others, like the lapse of consciousness of petit mal, are inhibitory. Electrical stimulation of the brain through the intact skull, as in electroshock convulsions for the treatment of depression or by the application of electrodes on the surface of the brain, is observed to produce the same changes. This initial outburst lasts for only a brief period of time and is often followed by a total or subtotal paralysis or inhibition of cerebral function. Similarly a focal motor seizure, for example, may result in suppression of activity in motor areas and a temporary paralysis of the involved muscles (Todd's postepileptic or exhaustion paralysis). The loss of consciousness that follows a generalized motor seizure, in contradistinction to that of petit mal, is probably due to a postexcitatory paralysis of either diencephalic or midbrain structures. Vital functions may also be arrested, but usually for only a few seconds. In rare instances, however, death may occur owing to a cessation of respiration, derangement of cardiac action, or some unknown cause. The automatic behavior so characteristic of psychomotor epilepsy appears in some instances to be a direct stimulatory effect in the temporal lobe and in others is a postexcitatory, inhibitory, or paralytic effect.

The electroencephalogram provides a delicate proof of Hughlings Jackson's theory of epilepsy—that it is an excessive, disorderly discharge of cortical neurones. At the onset of the focal seizure this is registered in or near the focus as a series of spikes or sharp waves interrupting the normal alpha and beta waves. The clinical spread of the seizure has its electroencephalographic equivalent in the extension of the abnormal electrical waves; and with generalization of the seizure (grand mal) the entire electroencephalographic recording surface of the brain exhibits spikes of high voltage. Petit mal is accompanied by a characteristic cold wave–spike complex occurring simultaneously in all cortical leads and presumably taking origin from a diencephalic focus. At first there was thought to be a characteristic electroencephalographic picture for psychomotor epilepsy, but further studies have not confirmed this. The postseizure state, sometimes called *postictal disturbance of cerebral function*, also has its electroencephalographic correlate in random generalized slow waves; with recovery the electroencephalogram returns to normal. If the electroencephalographic tracing is obtained during the interval between seizures, it is abnormal to some degree in approximately 40 percent of fully conscious and 75 percent of sleeping patients.

The electroencephalographic changes are discussed in Chap. 353.

DISEASES CAUSING SYMPTOMATIC EPILEPSY

In the list of diseases of the nervous system with which every physician must be familiar, a few stand apart by reason of their tendency to produce recurrent convulsions. The seizures are said to be symptomatic in contrast to the large majority of cases in which epilepsy is idiopathic. The physician must distinguish by the usual clinical and laboratory methods the different diseases that may cause, accompany, or precipitate convulsions.

DISEASES LOCALIZED IN THE CEREBRAL HEMISPHERES

Almost any type of cerebral lesion may cause seizures; on the other hand, no cerebral lesion is invariably accompanied by them. In patients with cerebral lesions the seizures are usually focal, leading in most instances to a generalized convulsion of grand mal type; less commonly they are of the petit mal type.

CEREBRAL TUMORS. They give rise to seizures in 35 to 60 percent of cases; in approximately 10 percent of all cases of tumor the seizure is the initial symptom. The nearer the tumor is to the excitable motor cortex, the greater is the likelihood of seizures. Tumors of the cerebellum and brainstem are seldom associated with any of the types of seizures described above, but they may cause episodes of decerebrate rigidity, i.e., opisthotonos and extension of all four extremities, sometimes called *tonic cerebellar fits.*

CEREBRAL TRAUMA. Trauma may cause seizures immediately after the injury, i.e., within hours or days, or after an interval of several months or years. In the former case seizures are rare; in the latter they vary in incidence, being more frequent in the severer grades of head injury. Uncomplicated concussion results in epilepsy in only about 0.5 percent of cases, which is about the expected frequency in the population at large, whereas with penetrating injuries, the incidence rises to approximately 20 percent and some figures have been as high as 40 percent. The average interval between the head injury and the first seizure is about 9 months, with a range of 6 months to 2 years or longer. The frequency of seizures varies from patient to patient; as years pass they tend to become less frequent.

CEREBROVASCULAR DISEASES. Although seizures occur at the time of the hemorrhage or infarction in a small percentage of cases, it has been said that vascular disease is rarely responsible for recurrent convulsions. This is true of atherosclerotic thrombosis and lacunar state and all types of brainstem infarction. Recently, however, analysis of our own material showed that cases of vascular disease of the cerebral cortex, particularly of embolic infarction, resulted in recurrent convulsions in about 20 percent of cases, a frequency nearly as high as in traumatic disease of the cerebral cortex. Hypertensive encephalopathy is often attended by convulsions. Venous thrombosis and infarction are a notable cause of focal epilepsy, and the same is true of vascular lesions in infancy and childhood, which may be either arterial or venous in nature. Seizures are also a frequent manifestation of vascular malformations.

CEREBRAL INFECTIONS. All types of cerebral infection may lead to epilepsy. Brain abscess is accompanied by seizures in about 50 percent of cases, and they often continue after the abscess has been drained or removed surgically. The seizures that accompany viral encephalitis, dementia paralytica, and other inflammatory diseases of the brain are related to cortical lesions. Inclusion-body encephalitis and subacute sclerosing encephalitis give rise to arrhythmic myoclonus, which is often combined with progressive dementia. In diseases that do not involve the cerebral cortex, such as encephalitis lethargica, there is little or no disposition to epilepsy.

DEGENERATIVE DISEASES. All types of degenerative diseases, if they affect the cerebral cortex, may be associated with recurrent seizures. Lipid-storage diseases and Jakob-Creutzfeldt disease tend usually to cause myoclonic dementia. Tuberous sclerosis is almost invariably accompanied by seizures. They occur but are infrequent in Alzheimer's disease and Pick's disease. About 3 percent of multiple sclerosis patients have convulsions in some phase of their illness.

CONGENITAL MALDEVELOPMENT OF THE BRAIN. This is frequently associated with epilepsy, which may be part of the syndrome of mental retardation, spastic diplegia, and other disturbances of motor function. The seizures usually develop in the first weeks or months of life. Special types of infantile and childhood seizures are discussed later in Chap. 365.

METABOLIC DISEASES

Conditions that disturb the metabolism of the brain may induce recurrent seizures. With hypoxia of whatever cause the damage to the cerebral cortex is associated with a series of seizures that begin within a few hours and continue intermittently for a variable period of time, usually a few days. Many of the surviving patients are not subject to epilepsy, but a small group develops intention myoclonus. Pyridoxine deficiency, phenylketonuria, and argininosuccinic aciduria are associated with seizures beginning in early life and continuing for the lifetime of the patient. Cerebral edema, resulting from excess ingestion of water or large infusions of glucose and water, may be attended by one or several generalized convulsions followed by headache and mental confusion. Uremia is accompanied by muscular twitching and, occasionally, by one or more terminal convulsions. Low blood calcium due to rickets or hypoparathyroidism often results in both tetany and seizures. Hypoglycemia, as from an overdose of insulin or an insulin-secreting islet cell tumor, often induces seizures, but they invariably follow an initial period of mental confusion, stupor, or coma. The usual history is for the attack to begin several hours after a meal or following a period of fasting. Seizures occur frequently in alcoholic patients and in those who have become addicted to barbiturates during the period of withdrawal.

DRUG INTOXICATION. The classic examples of direct seizure evocation by drugs are camphor, Metrazol, and picrotoxin. Withdrawal from barbiturates and alcohol in addicted individuals also gives rise to generalized convulsions.

APPROACH TO THE CLINICAL PROBLEM OF RECURRENT SEIZURES

A history of recurrent attacks of loss of consciousness or awareness associated with abnormal movements or confusion is usually sufficient to establish a diagnosis of epilepsy. With such patients a very thorough history, a complete physical and neurologic examination, testing of the visual fields, and laboratory studies, including x-ray examination of the skull and an electroencephalogram, should be done. The results of these essential procedures will determine to which of the categories in the above classification the case belongs and whether it should be labeled idiopathic epilepsy.

The history should be particularly searching in regard to epilepsy in the family history and occurrence of head trauma or infections in the past; and careful description of the disease itself, including prodromata, aura, manifestations during the seizure and the postictal period, must be obtained. Seizures in other members of the family favor the diagnosis of idiopathic epilepsy. Signs of pulmonary or ear infection or of congenital heart disease with a right-to-left shunt should suggest, in a patient with recently acquired seizures, the possibility of a brain abscess. The presence of a heart murmur and fever or of atrial fibrillation favor embolism. Head trauma of a serious nature, followed by seizures at an interval of several weeks to 2 years, indicates that an injury may have given rise to convulsions. A regularly recurring aura, especially of a focal nature, may indicate the presence of a localized lesion in the brain. Similarly, a focal convulsive movement at the onset of the seizure probably indicates a localized cerebral lesion. A transient monoplegia or hemiplegia (Todd's paralysis) in the postictal period also has considerable significance in localizing a lesion. In fact, its presence may provide the best clue to a focal brain lesion. A history of other neurologic symptoms such as headache, localized paralysis, or mental changes often indicates the need for special diagnostic studies.

A general physical examination may provide clues to the legion of conditions associated with epilepsy. The presence of protuberances over the skull may suggest an underlying pathologic condition. Vascular nevi over the body, especially over the face and in the retina, may be associated with vascular abnormalities within the skull. Small tumors, often pedunculated, distributed over the body surface bring to mind the diagnosis of von Recklinghausen's disease and, when associated with seizures, may indicate an intracranial glioma or neurofibroma. White spots over the trunk and limbs and sebaceous adenomas of the face point to the diagnosis of tuberous sclerosis. Smallness of an arm or leg points to a congenital defect of brain. Cranial nerve disturbances are also helpful in diagnosis; thus, a sixth-nerve paralysis is often associated with increased intracranial pressure. Localized weakness, differences in reflexes, or the presence of abnormal reflexes, such as Babinski's response, all have potential localizing value.

The question of what laboratory procedures should be done in cases of epilepsy can be answered only on the basis of the clinical findings. With generalized convulsions simple blood chemistries are among the first things to do. The determination of blood glucose helps orient the examiner in instances of hypoglycemia and hyperglycemia; the calcium level provides the main clue to hypocalcemia, the blood urea nitrogen (BUN) to kidney disease, and sodium and potassium levels to multiple metabolic disturbances including dilutional hyponatremia. X-rays of the skull should be taken in all cases. Significant findings related to increased intracranial pressure include erosion of the clinoid processes and, in infants and children, separation of the sutures. Hyperostoses, erosions of the skull, abnormal vascular markings, and intracranial calcifications are other findings of importance that may appear in skull x-rays. Because of the frequency of cerebral metastases from primary carcinoma of the lung, chest films should be made in all patients suspected of having intracranial neoplasm.

Lumbar puncture can be of considerable value in elucidating the causes of epilepsy. If the history, neurologic examination, or skull x-rays show any abnormality, especially if it suggests a focal lesion in the brain, then a lumbar puncture is mandatory. Of special importance are determination of the pressure, cell count, total protein, and serologic tests. Increased pressure points to an expanding intracranial lesion. An abnormal cell count often indicates an infectious process. An elevation in total protein (greater than 100 mg per 100 ml) favors the diagnosis of a tumor. If the pressure is normal, but other symptoms or signs point to a recently acquired, localized brain lesion, an arteriogram or pneumoencephalogram may be needed. If, in addition to localizing signs, the patient shows signs of increased intracranial pressure, whether by papilledema or high cerebrospinal fluid pressure, then a ventriculogram may be preferred to a pneumoencephalogram, although arteriography is now used more frequently than air visualization because of its greater safety. The visualization of the cerebral hemisphere by these procedures may be of particular help to the neurosurgeon in localizing the lesion and in planning a surgical approach to it.

The electroencephalogram, although now routinely employed in the definitive diagnosis of cases with epilepsy, is not absolutely conclusive, since it may be normal in some patients, particularly if the seizures are relatively infrequent, or abnormal in diseases that do not cause epilepsy. The test is of particular value in diagnosing petit mal, for here clinical or subclinical attacks are apt to be frequent enough to register during the electroencephalographic test. Abnormal electrical waves may manifest themselves in other types of epilepsy as well, and the electroencephalogram may be abnormal during the interseizure period, demonstrating either focal or generalized abnormalities of cortical activity. Activation of the electroencephalogram by photic stimulation, drug-induced sleep, or Metrazol injection is now standard procedure in many laboratories.

The type of clinical study in any given case is dictated to some extent by the age of the patient. Up until early adulthood the plan should be outlined as below. Most patients in this age group turn out to have idiopathic epilepsy. With increasing age, the incidence of idiopathic epilepsy becomes less and symptomatic epilepsy increases. Thus the appearance of convulsions for the first time at a period past middle age should be presumptive evidence of brain tumor until every effort has been made to rule it out.

The most frequent causes of recurrent convulsions in different age groups are presented in Table 28-1.

Table 28-1. CAUSES OF RECURRENT CONVULSION IN DIFFERENT AGE GROUPS

Age of onset, yr.	Probable cause
Infancy, 0–2........	Congenital maldevelopment, birth injury; metabolic (hypocalcemia, hypoglycemia), B₆ deficiency, phenylketonuria
Childhood, 2–10......	Birth injury, trauma, infections, thrombosis of cerebral arteries or veins, beginning of idiopathic epilepsy
Adolescence, 10–18...	Idiopathic epilepsy, trauma, congenital defects
Early adulthood, 18–35	Trauma, neoplasm, idiopathic epilepsy, alcoholism, drug addiction
Middle age, 35–60....	Neoplasm, trauma, vascular disease, alcoholism, drug addiction
Late life, over 60.....	Vascular disease, degeneration, tumor

DIFFERENTIAL DIAGNOSIS

The clinical differences between a seizure and a syncopal attack were presented in Chap. 20 and need not be repeated here. It must be emphasized once again that there is no single criterion for distinguishing between them. The author has erred in calling akinetic seizures simple faints and in mistaking cardiac or carotid sinus faints for seizures. Petit mal may be difficult to identify because of the brevity of attacks. One helpful maneuver is to have the patient count for 5 to 10 min. If he is having petit mal, he will blink or stare, pause in counting, or skip one or two numbers. Psychomotor seizures are the most difficult of all to diagnose. These attacks are so variable in character and so likely to induce minor disturbances in conduct rather than obvious interruptions of consciousness that they may be diagnosed as temper tantrums, hysteria, psychopathic behavior, or acute psychosis.

A special problem in diagnosis is offered by states of mental dullness and confusion. Epileptic patients as seen in hospital and office practice usually show no mental deterioration, regardless of the type of seizure. Therefore, the appearance of dementia, confusion, or some other derangement of mental function should suggest the possibility of recurrent subclinical seizures not controlled by medication, drug intoxication, postseizure psychosis, or a brain disease that has caused both dementia and seizures. To distinguish these clinical states may require careful observation, along the lines suggested in Chap. 30, and electroencephalography.

REFERENCES

Lennox, W., and M. Lennox: "Epilepsy," Boston, Little, Brown & Company, 1960.
Penfield, W., and H. Jasper: "Epilepsy and the Functional Anatomy of the Brain," Boston, Little, Brown & Company, 1954.

29 AFFECTIONS OF SPEECH
Raymond D. Adams and Jay P. Mohr

Language or speech functions are of fundamental significance to man, in both his social intercourse and his private intellectual life; and when they are disordered as a consequence of developmental anomaly or disease of the brain, the resultant physiologic loss exceeds all others in gravity—even blindness, deafness, and lameness.

The physician is concerned with all derangements of language function, including those of reading and writing, because they are the source of much unhappiness and disability and are almost invariably manifestations of disease of the brain. Furthermore, language is the means whereby the patient communicates his complaints and his feelings to his physician and, at the same time, the medium for that interpersonal transaction between physician and patient which we call psychotherapy. Thus, any disease process that interferes with speech or the understanding of spoken words touches the very core of the patient-physician relationship. Finally, the clinical study of language disorders serves to illuminate the abstruse relationship between psychologic functions and the anatomy and physiology of the cerebrum. Language mechanisms fall halfway between the well-localized sensorimotor functions and the complex mental functions, such as imagination and thinking, which cannot be localized.

GENERAL CONSIDERATIONS

It has often been remarked that man's commanding position in the world rests on the possession of two faculties: (1) the ability to employ verbal symbols as a "background for his own ideation" and as a means of transmitting his thoughts to others of his kind; and (2) the remarkable facility of his hands. One curious and provocative fact is that the evolution of both speech and manual dexterity occurs in relationship to neurophysiologic pathways located in one cerebral hemisphere. This is a departure from nearly all other localizable neurophysiologic patterns, which are organized according to a bilateral and symmetric plan. The dominance of one cerebral hemisphere, usually the left, emerges with speech and the preference for the right hand, especially in writing; and a lack of development or loss of cerebral dominance as a result of disease disturbs both these traits.

There is abundant evidence that higher animals are able to communicate with each other by vocalization and gestures. However, the content of their communications is their feeling tone at the moment. This *emotional language*, as it is called, was studied by Charles Darwin, who noted that it underwent increasing differentiation in the animal kingdom. Similar instinctual patterns of emotional expression are observed in man. In fact, they are the earliest type of speech to appear (in infancy) and may have been the first to develop in primitive man. Moreover, the language we use to express joy, anger, and fear is retained even after destructive lesions of the dominant cerebral hemisphere; i.e., the neural arrangements that subserve emotional expression are bilateral and symmetric and do not even depend exclusively on the cerebrum. The experiments of Cannon and Bard have amply demonstrated that emotional expression is possible in animals after the removal of both cerebral hemispheres, provided the diencephalon, and particularly the hypothalamus and lower parts of the neuraxis, remain undamaged. In the human infant emotional expression is well developed at a time when the cerebral cortex is still immature.

Propositional, or symbolic, speech differs from emotional speech in several ways. Instead of communicating feeling, it transmits ideas from one person to another and requires in its development the substitution of a series of sounds or marks for objects or concepts. This type of speech is not found in animals nor in the human infant. It is not instinctive but learned and is therefore subject to all the modifying influences of social and cultural environments. However, the learning process becomes possible only after the nervous system has reached a certain degree of maturity. The units of propositional language, i.e., words and phrases, have acquired symbolic value and have become the medium of our thought processes. Facility in symbolic language, which is acquired over a period of 15 to 20 years, depends on both maturation of the nervous system and education.

THE DEVELOPMENT OF LANGUAGE

The acquisition of symbolic language by the infant and child has been observed methodically by a number of eminent scientists, and their findings provide a basis for understanding the various derangements of speech.

First, there is the *babbling* and *lalling stage* during which the infant of a few weeks of age emits a variety of sounds in combinations of vowel and labial or nasoguttural consonants. This predominantly motor speech activity is no doubt stimulated and reinforced by auditory sensations, which become linked to the kinesthetic ones arising from the speech musculature. It is not clear whether the capacity to hear and understand the spoken word precedes or follows the first motor speech. Possibly it varies from one infant to another, but certainly both speaking and auditory perception of words develop very early in life. Soon babbling merges with *echo speech*, in which the infant repeats parrotlike whatever he hears. Thereafter, auditory, visual, and kinesthetic sensations are gradually combined, and a sound comes to stand for or symbolize an object. Nouns are learned first, then verbs and other parts of speech. Single words and groups of words are used meaningfully in thinking and talking. They form propositions, which, according to Hughlings Jackson, are the very essence of speech. By the age of eighteen to twenty-four months the average infant can construct a phrase; in the months and years that follow,

he learns to speak in full sentences. A six-year-old child has a speaking vocabulary of several thousand words and an even larger understanding vocabulary. To learn the name of an object requires the formation of a link between the visual perceptive (association) regions of occipital lobes and the auditory perceptive region in the left temporal lobe, probably by way of the angular gyrus. In order to learn to say a name it is necessary to have a link between the auditory perceptive region (Wernicke) and the center for motor patterns of speech (Broca).

The child is now ready for the next stage, reading. This involves the association of graphic visual symbols with the auditory and kinesthetic images of words that have already been acquired. Usually the written word is learned by associating it with the spoken word rather than the seen object. It is held that the angular gyrus and contiguous parieto-occipital areas are critically involved in the establishment of these cross-modal associations. Writing is learned soon after reading, and word auditory-visual symbols now must become linked to cursive movements of the hand. Only those destined to become literate learn to read and write; and to be a complete master of the art of writing is an attainment of only a few select members of our society.

Language development appears to proceed in an orderly manner, but there are individual variations in the actual time at which each successive stage is reached and, to a limited extent, in the order of the different stages. Maturational delays are frequent. The pattern appears to be set by the neurologic equipment of the individual at any given age. Psychologic factors are of minor importance, at least in the beginning. There is, therefore, good reason why educators have found it unprofitable to teach reading and writing before the sixth year.

Anthropologists have suggested that the individual merely recapitulates the language development of his race. It is supposed that gestures and the utterance of simple meaningful sounds first occurred in primitive man as a differentiation of emotional speech. Gradually these movements and sounds became the conventional signs and verbal symbols of concrete objects, then of the abstract qualities of objects. Signs and spoken language were the first means of human communication; graphic records appeared much later. The American Indian, for instance, never attained a written language. Writing began as pictorial representation, and only much later were alphabets devised. The reading and writing of words and propositions have been relatively recent developments.

The increasing importance of language in contemporary society may be overlooked unless we reflect on the proportion of man's time devoted to purely verbal pursuits. *External speech,* by which we mean the expression of thoughts by spoken and written words and reception of the thoughts of others, is an almost continuous activity when human beings are gathered together; and *internal speech,* or the formation in our minds of unuttered words, is the "coin of mental commerce." It goes on even during a state of preoccupation, when a man is apt to think in words and may, in doing so, subconsciously utter words.

THE ANATOMY OF THE LANGUAGE FUNCTIONS

The conventional teaching is that there are three language areas, situated, in most individuals, in the left cerebral hemisphere (Fig. 31-1). Two are receptive and one executive. The two receptive areas are closely related and embrace what may be referred to as the central language zone. One, subserving auditory language reception, is situated in the posterior part of the first and second temporal convolutions (areas 41 and 42) near the primary auditory receptive area in Heschl's convolutions; the other, subserving visuolexic functions, occupies the angular convolution (area 39) in the inferior parietal lobule adjacent to the primary visual receptive areas. The intervening areas between these auditory and visual language "centers," the inferior temporal region (area 37), and the supramarginal convolution, are also part of this central language zone and are involved in language formulation. The executive area, situated at the posterior end of the third frontal convolution (referred to as Broca's area, or area 44) is for motor aspects of speech. Of dubious significance as a unique "writing center" is the foot of the second frontal convolution above Broca's area. These sensory and motor areas are connected by the arcuate bundle of nerve fibers which passes through the isthmus of the temporal lobe, and other connections may traverse the external capsule of the lenticular nucleus (subcortical white matter of the insula). From Broca's area there are fiber connections with the lower Rolandic cortex which in turn innervates the speech apparatus. These language areas are also connected with the thalamus and to corresponding areas in the minor cerebral hemisphere through the corpus callosum and anterior commissure.

There has been much difference of opinion concerning these cortical areas, and objection has been made to calling them centers, for they do not represent histologically circumscribed structures of constant function and fixed localization. Actually there is relatively little information concerning their anatomy and physiology. A competent neuroanatomist could not distinguish under the microscope some of these cortical speech areas from other parts of the cerebral cortex. Crude electrical stimulation of the parts of the cortex concerned with speech while the patient is alert and talking (during craniotomy under local anesthesia) causes only an arrest of speech. Knowledge of the location of speech functions has come almost exclusively from the study of human beings who have succumbed to focal brain diseases. From the available information it seems almost certain that the whole language mechanism is not divisible into a number of parts, each depending on a certain fixed group of neurones. Instead, speech must be regarded as a sensorimotor process roughly localized in the opercular or peri-Sylvian region of the left cerebral hemisphere, and the more complex elaborations of speech probably depend on the entire cerebrum.

Carl Wernicke, more than any other person, must be credited with the anatomic-psychologic scheme upon which contemporary ideas of *aphasia* rest. Paul Broca, of Paris, had made the fundamental observation that a lesion of the posterior part of the left inferior frontal convolution deprived a man of speech. But Wernicke's original study showed that a lesion in the posterior part of the left superior temporal convolution, near the termination of the acoustic pathway, would result not in loss of speech but in distorted words (paraphasia, i.e., interchange of words of similar sound or meaning, neologisms, and sometimes unintelligible jargon), a failure to comprehend what is said and written, an inability to repeat what is said, and an inability to communicate by writing. The rapid, fluent paraphasic quality of the speech he ascribed to a loss of the internal correction of the activities of the motor speech area of Broca by the receptive language zone. The occurrence of *alexia* with lesions in the auditory language field he explained as a consequence of the fact that one learns to read by associating written symbols with previously learned auditory ones. Similarly, *agraphia* would be expected because one learns to write by linking visual word symbols with kinesthetic ones for hand movement.

In collaboration with his pupils, Wernicke proposed a classification of language disorders, dividing them into three groups according to whether the disorder was (1) of the central receptive or the motor mechanisms of language, (2) of their connections with one another, or (3) of the afferent visual and auditory pathways by which the language mechanism was activated or of the efferent motor pathway by which its executive function was carried out through lower centers. The anatomy of the primary receptive and executive language disorders was said to be *cortical* (localized in the superior temporal and inferior frontal respectively); the anatomy of the lesion which separated the primary receptive zones from frontal motor zones was predicted to be transcortical (perhaps in insula and external capsule); and that which interrupted afferent and efferent pathways was subcortical. The latter were noted to be of two types: (1) motor in the form of *pure word muteness* and (2) sensory in the form of *pure word deafness*. Later Dejerine added a third, (3) *pure word blindness*.

Wernicke and his students established location of the lesions, so they believed, for the cortical and subcortical types of aphasia but those of the transcortical and conduction disorders were inconsistent, being sometimes insular and sometimes in the cortex more posteriorly, i.e., in the posterior Sylvian arc, (the cortex of posterior-superior temporal and inferior parietal lobes).

The verification of Wernicke's scheme by Liepmann, Lichtheim, and other of his pupils required many years of work and the development of systematic clinical and pathologic methods of study. Once the scheme was presented, it came immediately under sharp attack from many quarters. The anatomy of it struck several critics as being too neat, and for the more dynamically oriented workers it gave too little attention to the psychologic aspects of language. Pierre Marie, Henry Head, von Monakow, Arnold Pick, and Kurt Goldstein subsequently offered other ways of subdividing language function, again based on the manner in which speech deteriorated in disease. However, when they sought to correlate clinical and anatomic data, they always came back to an anatomic plan which differed little from that of Wernicke and his colleagues.

Most contemporary students of aphasia, while appreciative of the fundamental importance of Wernicke's contributions, find the division into cortical, subcortical, and transcortical (or conduction) disorders somewhat misleading, for the lesions never respect these anatomic boundaries; and to use these terms, as did Wernicke, to refer to mechanisms that involved predominantly cortical, subcortical, or transcortical organizations of neurones or their connections postulates a kind of physiologic organization, the existence of which is known only by inference. The word *conduction disorder* is especially confusing for it could apply to sensory pathways for the activation of the language mechanism as well as to efferent pathways for the execution of speech and to connections with the medial temporal regions concerned with learning and memory. Furthermore, the idea of subdividing the language mechanism into strictly sensory and motor parts with identifiable anatomic connections with one another can only impress the modern student as a somewhat outdated notion of neurophysiology. Not even the sensorimotor cortex for voluntary hand movements works that way.

Early and recent work on aphasia indicates that human language depends in some way upon the integrity of an anatomic region situated between the primary input zones of the temporal and occipital lobes and the output zone in the inferior frontal lobe of the dominant hemisphere. This places the mechanism in close connection with the cortical sensory association and cross-modal elaboration areas of the superior temporal and inferior parietal lobes, with the corresponding parts of the opposite cerebral hemisphere through the corpus callosum, with medial parts of the temporal lobes (learning-memory mechanisms) and with the diencephalon. The acquisition of language appears to involve, in part, the establishment of specific, item-by-item, cross-modal, verbally-mediated associations. But quite unknown at present is how these verbal relations are organized into a mechanism of extraordinary complexity—one that can be activated (controlled) by a variety of visual and auditory stimuli, that permits variable arrangements of words into an infinite number of sequences with unimaginable speed and efficiency and makes endless combinations of them available for our thinking and problem solving and for communicating our ideas through speech and writing.

From the available clinical and pathologic data it may be concluded that the locus of the anatomic lesion is more significant than the extent of brain damage. Localization of the lesion is in most instances predictable from the clinical symptomatology, but there are variations. For example, patients with lesions of Broca's area (area 44) do not always suffer the same degree of disturbance of speech. This lack of consistency in the anatomy of any given speech disorder has engaged the attention of many students of aphasia, and several different hypotheses have been proposed to explain it. The "classic" one has been that the net effect of any lesion depends not only on locus and extent of lesion but on the degree of cerebral dominance. If cerebral dominance is poorly established, a left-sided lesion has less effect on speech than if dominance is strong. Unfortunately, handedness and cerebral dominance are not recorded in many of the 1,500 cases collected by Henschen from the world's medical literature. Another factor which imparts an element of unpredictability to the anatomy of speech is that no two individuals acquire language in the same way; some depend more on auditory sense, others on visual. Lastly, clinical analyses of speech disorders may fail to identify a biologically meaningful functional deficit. We may then be trying to correlate a phenomenon of secondary importance to the anatomy of the lesion.

CEREBRAL DOMINANCE AND ITS RELATIONSHIP TO SPEECH AND HANDEDNESS

The functional supremacy of one cerebral hemisphere is so crucial to language function that it must be considered in greater detail. There are three ways of determining that the left side of the brain is dominant: (1) the loss of speech when disease occurs in certain parts of the left hemisphere and its preservation in diseases involving the right hemisphere; (2) the greater facility in the use of the right hand, foot, and eye; (3) the arrest of speech immediately after the injection of amobarbital (Amytal Sodium) or some other drug in the left internal carotid artery. Only (2) and (3) are of use in deciding the cerebral dominance of a living and healthy patient. Unfortunately, the Amytal Sodium or Wada test does not reproduce the syndrome of major hemisphere inactivation. There is only mutism followed by a brief period of groping for names. Presumably it gives information about the localization of motor output areas rather than of sensory ones.

Of the general population approximately 90 to 95 percent are right-handed; the remainder prefer the left hand. A person is said to be right-handed if he chooses the right hand for intricate complex acts and is more skillful with it. The preference is more complete in some than others. Most individuals are neither completely right-handed nor completely left-handed but favor one hand for more complicated tasks. Orton refers to this as *intergrading*. The manner in which dextrality and sinistrality are acquired is of interest. Most infants and small children are ambidextrous in their first actions. Writing may be carried out with either hand at first, and "mirror writing" at this early stage is frequent. Between the ages of two and six years one hand and one foot are selected for throwing and kicking a ball, sawing a board, cutting bread, etc. By middle childhood there is usually no doubt as to the dominant side. The reason for hand preference is still controversial. There is strong evidence of a hereditary factor, but the mode of inheritance is uncertain. Learning is also a factor; for many children are shifted at an early age from left to right (shifted sinistrals) because it is a handicap to be left-handed in a right-handed world. Many right-handed persons sight with the right eye, and it has been said that eye preference determines hand preference. Even if true, this still does not account for eye dominance. It is noteworthy that handedness develops simultaneously with language, and the most that can be said at the present is that speech localization and the preference for one eye, one hand, and one foot are all manifestations of some fundamental and inherited tendency not yet defined. Anatomic difference between the dominant and the minor cerebral hemispheres is uncertain except that the occipital horn of the left lateral ventricle is usually larger than the right, and the left sulcus lunatus more prominent. No consistent differences in the electroencephalogram between the two hemispheres have been found.

Left-handedness may result from disease of the left cerebral hemisphere in early life, and this probably accounts for its higher incidence among the feeble-minded and brain-injured. Presumably the neural mechanisms for language then become centered in the right cerebral hemisphere. Handedness and cerebral dominance may fail to develop in some individuals, and this is particularly true in certain families. Developmental defects in speech and reading, stuttering, "mirror writing," and general clumsiness are much more frequent in these families.

Differences in degree of cerebral dominance do unquestionably account for some of the inconsistency in the cerebral localization of speech in different individuals. In studies of groups of left-handed individuals who suffer cerebral derangements of speech it has been noted that approximately 75 percent of them have had lesions in the left cerebral hemisphere. Further, in those aphasias due to the right cerebral lesions, the patient is always left-handed, and the speech disorder tends to be less severe and enduring. The latter may take the form of an expressive disturbance rather than alexia or amnestic aphasia; and visuoconstructive troubles are prominent, as are also faults in calculation and recognition of one's neurologic deficits (anosognosia).

The functional capacities of the minor hemisphere in speech are not fully documented by careful anatomic studies. Always there is some uncertainty as to whether any residual function after lesions of the major hemisphere is due to recovery of parts of its language zones or to the activity solely of the minor hemisphere. Reasonably well established are the following more or less verbal functions of the minor hemisphere: motor responses of mimicry, social anticipation (smiling, handshaking, modesty reactions) and self care (washing and feeding), avoidance behavior to noxious stimuli and capability of training in performances of cross-matching visually presented simple words with pictures.

TYPES OF LANGUAGE DISORDER ENCOUNTERED IN MEDICINE

These can be divided into four categories:

1. Disturbances of speech that occur with diseases affecting the higher nervous integrations, namely, delirium and dementia. Speech is seldom lost in these conditions but is instead merely deranged as part of a general impairment of intellectual functions. These conditions will not be discussed further here (see Chap. 31). *Palilalia* and *echolalia*, in which the patient repeats, parrotlike, the syllables and words which he hears, are special abnormalities usually observed in states of dementia generally with conjoined extrapyramidal signs.

2. The loss or disturbance of speech due to a cerebral lesion that does not deprive a man of his reason or paralyze other motor or sensory functions. This condition has been termed *aphasia;* milder degrees of it have been called *dysphasia.*

3. A defect in articulation with intact mental functions and normal comprehension and memory of words. This is a pure motor disorder of the muscles of articulation and may be due to flaccid or spastic paralysis, rigidity, repetitive spasms (stuttering), or ataxia. The term *anarthria* or *dysarthria* has been applied to some of these conditions.

4. Loss of voice due to a disease of the larynx or its innervation, with resulting *aphonia* or *dysphonia.* Articulation and internal language are unaffected.

In the practice of medicine the most frequent and troublesome disorders of speech are aphasia, stuttering, dysarthria, and aphonia.

Types of Aphasia

Systematic examination will usually make it possible to decide whether the patient has a *global aphasia* (with loss of all or nearly all speech functions; a motor aphasia (*Broca's aphasia*), sometimes called verbal or executive aphasia; *Wernicke's aphasia,* a receptive or sensory aphasia predominantly auditory and visual in type; or *dissociative speech syndromes:* of the central language area from the motor area, of the motor speech area from lower centers, of auditory verbal aphasia (word deafness), of alexia (inability to read), and of amnestic aphasia. Writing is disturbed to some extent in the majority of cases of aphasia and is rarely disturbed alone.

GLOBAL OR TOTAL APHASIA. Global or total aphasia is due to a lesion that destroys a large part of the speech areas of the major cerebral hemisphere. It is an affection of all input and output zones that are concerned with receiving sensory stimuli for speech as well as for expression. Usually it is due to occlusion of the left internal carotid or middle cerebral artery, but it may be caused by a massive hemorrhage (hypertensive or traumatic), an infiltrative tumor, or other lesion. The middle cerebral artery nourishes all the speech areas, and nearly all the aphasic disorders due to vascular occlusion are caused by involvement of this artery or its branches. Left hemispherectomy for glioma or epilepsy has had a similar effect on all speech functions.

Most of the patients with global aphasia are speechless or can say at most a few words; they cannot read or write and can understand only a few simple spoken words and phrases. Related signs include right hemiplegia, hemianesthesia, and homonymous hemianopia. The state of consciousness may vary from full alertness to semicoma. The patient may participate in common gestures of greeting, show modesty and avoidance reactions, and engage in self-help activities. Improvement depends on the nature and extent of the disease and whether or not the right cerebral hemisphere had previously engaged in language formulation and expression. With the passage of time some degree of understanding of spoken speech may be evident and a few words of speech may return. However, if the left hemisphere was strongly dominant, there will usually be little or no recovery, which casts doubt on the popular notion that the right hemisphere can take over speech function.

WERNICKE'S APHASIA. The syndrome has two components. The first is an impairment in phonemic hearing, which reflects the proximity of the lesion to the primary auditory cortex of Heschl's transverse gyri and involvement of auditory association areas, separating them from the angular gyrus. The second is a general impairment of language-dependent behavior, which may reflect the major role the auditory region plays in the regulation of language.

The defect in auditory functions is manifested by an impairment of repetition of spoken words and the matching of two sequences from a series of identical auditory stimuli or rhythms. Repetition is confined to short words or words of which the components are widely separated in phonemic composition. A few simple commands may still be executed but not complex ones. The patient gestures freely, talks volubly, and appears unaware of his deficit. The errors of word formation are in the nature of paraphasia, and take the form of substitution of words or jargon sounds similar in sound to the correct response (literal paraphasia) or the substitution of words of similar meaning for one another (verbal paraphasia). When severely disorganized, the speech may be reduced to an incomprehensible gibberish or jargon.

The general impairment of language-dependent behavior may be more or less disassociated from the deficits in phonemic hearing, and may occasionally appear in more isolated form. Certain neurologists have referred to this as "central aphasia." Although all the sensory and motor apparatus required in the activation and expression of language behavior appears intact, the patient is unable to understand what is said to him, to read aloud or for comprehension, to speak in properly constructed sentences, or to communicate by writing. Vocal speech is marred by paraphasias, as indicated above, and also by impairments in the construction of phrases in spontaneous speech. The patient is unable to name from sight or touch items whose names he can repeat from dictation. He is unable to write from dictation words he can copy from sight or even from touch. The copying performance is slow and laborious and conforms to the exact contours of the model (including the examiner's handwriting style) in a "servile" fashion. He is unable to cross-match words from dictation to sight, yet he can match a word to itself by sight alone and can repeat the word from dictation. Overall, performance is impaired on those tasks which require previous experience to indicate a relationship between two formally dissimilar stimuli (e.g., the sound of the word "cat" and printing the letters of the word "cat"). But preserved are those performances which can be accomplished by indicating or producing a response which is formally identical to that given (e.g., copying from sight the word "cat").

With the passage of time, the impairment in phonemic hearing may improve and with it, the apparent understanding of words. Of the several speech faults, repetition of spoken language, especially of unfamiliar words, is most likely to remain impaired. Extreme variability of performance is frequently striking. When testing is conducted in single steps with pauses between trials, a surprising degree of intact performance may be noted, but any increase in rate and variation of material presented results in failure. A common error is to interpret flaws in verbal production as a primary expressive aphasia, but in actuality, there is no abnormality of the articulatory-phonetic performance as there is in verbal output disorders of purely motor type. This is the reason we prefer to avoid the term *expressive aphasia*, i.e., it includes more than just motor output disorders.

As a rule, the lesion involves the posterior Sylvian region (temporal and parietal) and is usually caused by an embolic occlusion of the lower division of the left middle cerebral artery. Subcortical slit hemorrhage in the temporoparietal region, and involvement of the temporal isthmus and adjacent white matter by tumor, abscess, or extension from putaminal or thalamic hemorrhage may have similar effects.

The posterior Sylvian region, comprising posterior superior temporal, opercular supramarginal, and posterior insular gyri, appears to encompass a variety of language functions, since seemingly minor changes in size and locale of lesion are associated with important changes in syndromes in a spectrum of Wernicke's aphasia, conduction aphasia, pure word deafness, as well as a number of variants of these syndromes. The interesting theoretic problem raised by the consideration of general impairment in language-dependent behavior is whether or not the deficits observed represent disturbance of a unitary language function in the posterior Sylvian region or, instead, a series of sensorimotor activities of which the required anatomic pathways happen to be crowded together in a small region of the brain. In view of the multiple ways in which language deteriorates in disease, the latter hypothesis seems more likely.

MOTOR SPEECH DISORDERS (BROCA'S APHASIA). Although the nature of Broca's aphasia remains somewhat in doubt we have chosen to apply the term, as have others, to a primary deficit in motor speech production. Uncertainty relates always to the degree to which it may be combined with impairment in language-dependent behavior. In our experience there is a wide range of variation in the motor deficit, from the mildest cortical type of dysarthria with entirely intact "inner language" to a complete loss of all means of communication through lingual, phonetic, and manual action. Since the muscles that can no longer be used in speech still function in other acts, the term *motor (kinetic)*, or *ideomotor, apraxia* seems applicable to certain components of the deficit.

In the fully developed syndrome the patient will have lost all power of expressing himself by spoken words. No longer can he speak spontaneously in conversation, read aloud, or repeat words he hears. If any words remain accessible to him, they will be "yes" or "no" and perhaps a few other habitual expressions. One at first suspects the lingual and phonetory apparatus of being paralyzed until it is observed that the patient has no difficulty chewing, swallowing, clearing his throat, licking his lips, and even vocalizing without words. Often the lower part of the face is weak on the opposite (right) side and occasionally the arm and leg as well. The tongue may deviate away from the lesion, i.e., to the right. For a time, despite good preservation of auditory comprehension and ability to read, commands to purse the lips properly, to lick the lips, to blow, smack, and make other purposeful movements are poorly executed, which means that the ideomotor apraxia has extended to other acts. Imitation of the examiner's actions are better performed, and self-initiated actions are normal. The patient may repeat his few remaining words over and over again, as if compelled to do so. The words of well-known songs may be sung, and others are uttered as expletives, when the patient is angered or excited, making the point that he is "speechless" but not "wordless." Usually, the patient recognizes his ineptitude and own mistakes. Failing in attempts to correct them he may exhibit signs of exasperation or despair.

Most patients with Broca's aphasia have as much trouble writing as speaking. Should their right hand be paralyzed, they cannot print with their left one; and if manual mobility is spared, they do not succeed in writing out their replies to questions or in indicating their needs. Writing to dictation is impossible but letters and words can still be copied.

Comprehension of spoken and written language, while normal under many conditions of testing may break down when novel material is rapidly presented, varying with the degree of associated central aphasia.

Broca's aphasia due to vascular lesions (the common ones) usually regresses in time, and as words return, the patient's utterances are noted to be slow, laborious, slurred, and many of the small words (articles, prepositions, conjunctions) are omitted, giving the speech an agrammatic character (*agrammatism*). There is loss also of all the natural accent, word emphasis, and melody of language (*dysprosody*), and the coordination of respiration and speaking are faulty.

The rate of clearing, in fact the natural course of the

neurologic syndrome, varies with the nature of the causative lesion. An embolus in the upper main division (Rolandic) of the middle cerebral artery causes the most abrupt onset and rapid regression (sometimes hours or days). Because of the distribution of this artery there is frequently an associated right-sided faciobrachial paresis and a *left*-sided brachial apraxia. Atherosclerotic thrombosis, tumor, subcortical hypertensive hemorrhage, traumatic hemorrhage, etc., may also declare themselves in this way if they should involve the premotor cortex which lies in the posterior part of the left inferior frontal convolution (area 44 of Broca).

Pure word mutism also causes the patient to be wordless but leaves his inner speech intact. Since this is anatomically more in the nature of a dissociation of the motor cortex for speech from lower centers, we shall describe it with the dissociative syndromes.

DISSOCIATIVE SPEECH SYNDROMES

These are characterized by an impairment in the activation of executive functions of the language mechanism by the interruption of major afferent connections or of major efferent (motor) connections with lower centers, and it also includes separation of the more strictly receptive parts of language from the purely motor ones, i.e., a break in sensorimotor integration. The patient generally appears to be normal except for the specific deficit, sensory or motor, i.e., his behavior with respect to language-dependent tasks and his utilization of words in thinking (inner speech) are normal.

ISOLATION OF BROCA AND WERNICKE AREAS. Here, a lesion (usually hypoxia and ischemia with water-shed infarction) isolates the auditory and motor speech mechanisms separating them from the rest of the brain. The patient exhibits a defect in auditory and visual word comprehension and lacks useful speech. Presumably information from the rest of the brain cannot be transferred to Wernicke's area for conversion into verbal form. Speech is fluent, rapid and paraphrasic. There is dysnomia. Spoken phrases are repeated, parrot-like, unlike the Wernicke aphasic syndrome.

CONDUCTION DISORDER WITH SEPARATION OF CENTRAL LANGUAGE AREA FROM MOTOR SPEECH AREA. Here the principal abnormality consists of paraphasia in self-initiated speech and in repeating what is heard. In contrast, the articulatory-phonetic process is normal and the patient has no difficulty in comprehending what he hears and sees. He is alert and aware of his deficit. One of the best ways of eliciting the defect is to have the patient repeat nonsense syllables. Careful analysis of the disturbance shows that in the formation of words the mistakes are of a type seen in literal paraphasia, that is to say that words of somewhat similar structure (phonemic similarity) but different meaning are interchanged. Often it can be shown that the oral, pharyngeal, lingual musculature is not correctly controlled to produce the word intended, yet there is no element of dysarthria or dysprosody. The disorder becomes more apparent when the rate of presentation of auditory material is increased and as the uttered words become more polysyllabic. Since nouns are the longest words in the sentence, one may gain an inaccurate impression that they are specifically affected.

The lesion in autopsied cases is superficial in the cortex and subcortical white matter and is located in the upper bank of the Sylvian fissure involving the supramarginal gyrus of inferior parietal lobule and occasionally the posterior part of the superior temporal region. It presumably interrupts fiber systems in the insula. The usual cause is an embolus in a branch (ascending parietal or posterior temporal) of the middle cerebral artery. Deeper, larger lesions in position to interrupt the arcuate fasciculus connecting the temporal and frontal lobes are likely to involve other pathways as well, giving rise to a more extensive speech deficit (central aphasia or Wernicke's aphasia and dysnomia). These latter types of aphasia, as they regress, may resolve into conduction aphasia. More anterior insular lesions usually include some degree of Broca's aphasia.

PURE WORD DEAFNESS. This syndrome is characterized by impaired auditory comprehension and inability to repeat what is said or to write to dictation. Inner speech, manifested by facile and correct use of words in thinking and discussing problems, correctly phrased self-initiated utterances, correct writing, reading, and copying are all intact. The patient may declare that he cannot hear, but shouting does not help him, sometimes to his surprise. By audiometric testing no hearing defect is found. Ordinary sounds can be distinguished. Sometimes the patient thinks he has heard a question or statement when he has not; he acts on a combination of visual cues and distorted sounds and then proceeds to give an irrelevant answer. If his listener looks incredulous he reacts by being more insistent. When the patient is able to describe his auditory experience, he says that words are a jumble of noises. Often the syndrome is not pure and elements of paraphasia enter, which helps in distinguishing the condition from true deafness.

In most instances the lesion has been bilateral in the superior temporal gyrus, in position to separate the primary auditory cortex in the transverse gyrus of Heschl from the secondary and tertiary association areas of the superior-posterior part of temporal lobe. The few unilateral lesions have been in the major (dominant) hemisphere. Requirements of smallness and superficiality of lesion in cortex and subcortical white matter are best fulfilled by a small embolic occlusion of a branch of the lower division of the middle cerebral artery. More extensive lesions lead to Wernicke's aphasia.

PURE WORD BLINDNESS. In this state a literate person loses the ability to read, to copy, and often to name colors. He can no longer name or point on dictated command to visual letter stimuli or the words of which they are composed. However, understanding spoken language, repetition, writing to dictation, and conversation are all intact. Often the subject makes no complaint about his difficulty; it is discovered almost by accident. In tests he reads a single letter at a time (this may be seen in otherwise normal patients who have bilateral hemianopia with only central vision remaining) but commonly he utters letter-name responses that seem to have little connection with the presented letters. The response may be corrected and the defect obscured if other visual cues are available, such as the bottle on which the words Coca-Cola appear. Associated with this there may be impaired naming of common colors when presented in isolation, and impaired naming of unseen objects which the subject touches. When the dominant hemisphere is involved, as it usually is in such cases, there may be a right homonymous hemianopia, an amnestic defect (see Chap. 30), and a hemisensory defect on the right due to involvement of the left occipital lobe, the left fornix and its decussation, and the left thalamus, respectively, a combination which nearly always signifies thrombosis or embolism of the left posterior cerebral artery.

The anatomy of the lesions is usually such as to destroy the left visual striate cortex and association areas 18 and 19 as well as the connections of the right visual cortex and association areas to the left angular gyrus. This disconnection usually occurs in the splenium of the corpus callosum. Less often the lesion may be confined to the left occipital lobe and the deep central white matter of the parietal lobe, cutting through the right occipital–left parietal connection. In this case the right homonymous hemianopia may be absent. With purely left cerebral lesions a primary or secondary tumor or, rarely, multifocal leucoencephalopathy or trauma may be the underlying disease. The associated disturbances of color naming are not dependent on a lesion of the corpus callosum. In large lesions of the left parietaloccipital region alexia may be combined with right-left confusion, acalculia, and difficulty in naming of fingers and other parts of the body (Gerstmann's syndrome) (see Chap. 31).

PURE WORD MUTENESS (SUBCORTICAL MOTOR APHASIA). The patient will have lost all capacity to speak, while retaining perfectly the ability to write, to think with words, to understand spoken words, and to read. Although usually paretic, the lips, tongue, pharynx, and larynx show none of the apraxic disturbance seen in Broca's aphasia. With recovery or in milder degrees of the disorder, vocal utterances are dysarthric due to paresis and are extremely slow, with inadequate volume and intonation.

The causative lesion, usually vascular, is located in the motor cortex, separating it from the premotor, or is located beneath both Broca's convolution and the motor cortex, separating them from subcortical motor centers.

AMNESTIC–DYSNOMIC APHASIA. This may be a relatively early or an isolated manifestation of nervous disease. The patient loses the ability to name objects. Partial degrees of it are associated with pauses in speech, groping for a word, the substitution of another word. When shown a series of uncommon objects, the patient may tell of their use instead of giving their names. The difficulty applies not only to objects seen but to the names of things heard or felt, but such tests are more difficult to employ.

Recall of the names for letters, digits, and other printed verbal material is almost invariably preserved. That the deficit is principally one of naming is shown by the fact that the patient makes correct use of the object and is usually able to point to it when asked to do so. As a rule, he will choose the correct name from a series shown him or given to him verbally. There is a tendency among patients to explain failure as one of forgetfulness, which indicates their partial unawareness of the defect.

The causative lesion is usually deep in the temporal lobe, in position, probably, to interrupt connections of sensory speech areas with the hippocampal-parahippocampal regions concerned with learning and memory. Mass lesions, such as a tumor or an otogenic abscess, are the most frequent, and as they enlarge, an upper contralateral quadrantic visual field defect, or Wernicke's aphasia, is produced. Occasionally, dysnomia appears with diseases which occlude the temporal branches of the posterior cerebral artery. Alzheimer's disease and senile dementia may begin or present early a phase in which there is a dysnomic or amnestic type of aphasia. Usually, however, by the time the patient's difficulty is recognized, other disorders of speech have been added, as well as indifference, apathy, and abulia.

APPROACH TO THE CLINICAL PROBLEM OF APHASIA

In investigating a case of aphasia it is first necessary to inquire into the patient's native language, his handedness, and his previous education. Many naturally left-handed children are trained to use their right hand for writing; therefore, in determining this point we must ask which hand is used for throwing a ball, threading a needle, or using a spoon or common tools such as hammer, saw, or bread knife. One should quickly ascertain whether the patient has other signs of a gross cerebral lesion such as hemiplegia, facial weakness, homonymous hemianopia, or cortical sensory loss. When hemiplegia, hemianesthesia, and homonymous hemianopia are present, the aphasic disorder is usually of global type. Such a constellation of signs is but rarely coincident with pure central aphasia, Wernicke's aphasia, or one of the dissociative syndromes. Dyspraxia of limbs and speech musculature, in response to spoken commands or visual mimicry, is generally associated with Broca's aphasia and sometimes central aphasia. Bilateral or unilateral homonymous hemianopia without motor weakness tends often to be linked to pure word blindness (alexia or dyslexia) or to amnestic-dysnomic aphasia. Bilateral hemiplegias are associated not infrequently with pure word muteness. Multiple small embolic vascular lesions, causing a variety of focal cerebral signs, are the lesions most likely to be accompanied by Wernicke's aphasia, alexia, or pure word deafness.

It is important before the beginning of the examination to determine whether the patient is alert and mentally clear or suffering from confusion, because this may interfere with accurate assessment of language. One must also avoid the effects of fatigue as far as possible by making the interview short. Explanation of the purpose of the tests, sympathy, and encouragement are often necessary to assure full cooperation.

Many elaborate examination schemes have been devised for testing the language functions; (see monographs of Weisenberg and McBride, Goldstein, and Schuell); some of them lead to refinements that are of little physiologic or clinical significance. The following procedure will yield sufficient data for diagnosis in most cases.

1. In ordinary conversation does the patient spontaneously utter intelligible words in proper sequence and well-constructed phrases and sentences? The fluency of speech, the extent of vocabulary, the grammatic construction of sentences, the accuracy of word usage, and clarity of enunciation should all be observed and examples incorporated into the record of the interview. Wrong choice of words, misplacement of words or syllables, omission of essential words, and use of disjointed phrases may be slight in degree and take the form of either literal or verbal paraphasia; if severe, they may result in an unintelligible jabbering or jargon. Can the patient repeat or copy what he hears or reads?

2. Can the patient understand what he hears? If he is unable to speak, give him a series of commands of increasing complexity. Ask him to close his eyes, open his mouth, hold up his left hand, place the index finger of the left hand to the right ear, etc. Often the patient will execute the first one or two simple commands correctly and will fail on all others, sometimes repeating the first act over and over (perseveration). Auditory comprehension may be difficult to assess in conversation because of many visual cues that are unwittingly transmitted by the examiner. The most dependable proof of intact repetition is the ability to repeat complex and unusual words and phrases given without gesture and out of context of previous conversation.

3. Can the patient read? Written questions or commands should be present and the responses observed. If motor speech is absent, the patient can be asked to select correct words for objects shown or words spoken by pointing to the corresponding words in a list. Recognition of similarity and dissimilarity between groups of words on the list may be tested by having him point successively to those words designating vegetables, flowers, inanimate objects, etc. If writing is intact, tests of copying or transcribing from print to script or vice versa will indicate whether he can see a word without knowing its meaning.

4. Can the patient write spontaneously? If his right hand is paralyzed, he should be encouraged to try with his left. It must also be determined whether or not he can write from dictation and can copy words or sentences. Transcription from print to script and vice versa should also be tested.

5. If he is able to speak, can he name common objects shown visually, such as a penny, button, pencil, fountain pen, handkerchief, the various parts of a wrist watch, safety pin, key, flashlight, matches? If not, does he recognize the correct name when he hears it? Are gestures appropriate?

Nonfluency distinguishes the anterior or frontal group of aphasias; fluency with failure of comprehension and repetition characterizes the posterior group of aphasias.

Disorders in the Development of Language in Children

A close parallelism exists between the symptoms observed in adults who have suffered a loss in language functions as a result of brain injury and those seen during the development of language skills. This reminds us that there may be faulty development of language and of cerebral dominance. It has been found that a high percentage of these patients have a strong family background of speech disorders and that strong preference for the right or the left hand is not present. Males are affected much more frequently than females (ratios as high as 10:1).

Developmental disorders of language and congenital deafness are far more frequent than aphasia. These include developmental alexia (special reading disability), developmental word deafness, developmental motor aphasia (motor speech delay), and developmental apraxia (abnormal clumsiness of the limbs). The development of language, instead of proceeding in the manner outlined in the early part of this chapter, is arrested or delayed. Disorders of this type are probably due to slowness in the normal processes of maturation rather than an acquired or developmental disease. These conditions are often misunderstood by parents, teachers, and physicians. Sometimes the unfortunate child is judged to be feebleminded or lazy. Another frequent error is to assume the condition is due to psychologic factors, since nervousness, stubbornness, poor sleep, headaches, etc., are frequently associated.

CONGENITAL WORD DEAFNESS. If an individual is born deaf, he can learn to talk only after special training; he is "deaf and dumb." Should deafness develop within the first few years of life, after speech has been acquired, the child gradually loses speech but can be retaught by the lip-reading method. His speech is harsh, poorly modulated, and unpleasant, and he is apt to make many peculiar throat noises of a snorting or grunting kind. Such patients may be bright and alert and also clever at pantomime and gesturing. They are inattentive to household noises and do not appear to understand what is said to them. The deafness can be demonstrated at an early age by careful observation of the child's responses to sounds, but it cannot be accurately tested before the age of three or four years. The psychogalvanic reflex technique for testing reaction to sounds and tests of the labyrinths, which are frequently unresponsive in deaf-mutes, may be helpful. In contrast, the idiot or moron is stupid in all his actions and talks little because he has nothing to say. Developmental word deafness may be difficult to distinguish from true deafness. Usually the parents have noted that the word-deaf child responds to loud noises and music, though obviously this does not assure perfect hearing, particularly for high tones. The word-deaf child

does not understand what is said, and there is delay and distortion of speech. These children are alert, active, and inquisitive and may chatter incessantly. They adopt a language of their own design, and attentive parents come to understand it. This peculiar type of speech is known as *idioglossia*. It is also observed in children who have marked difficulty in the articulation of certain consonants. They learn to lip-read very quickly and are clever at acting out their own ideas.

CONGENITAL WORD BLINDNESS (ALEXIA). In this unusual condition the patient has good eyesight and is able to see the word but not to grasp its meaning. There is no loss of the ability to recognize the meaning of objects, pictures, and diagrams. Usually with assiduous training, the patient, who is otherwise bright and intelligent, can learn to read individual letters and a few simple words. Spelling is impossible. Often the patient cannot write anything of his own composition but can copy skillfully. Lesser degrees of congenital alexia are commoner than the severe forms and pose serious problems in the classroom. Some 10 percent of school children have some degree of this disability. The problem is a complex one, for difficulty in learning to read well is unquestionably influenced by the teaching techniques used in the school. Only a few of the severely handicapped children have a right homonymous hemianopia or a right-sided sensory loss; most of them show no other abnormality. The majority have no other signs. The important genetic study of Hallgren shows that the condition is inherited as an autosomal dominant trait and is unrelated to psychologic factors; speech delay, articulatory abnormalities, and difficulty in reading digits may be associated. Also, there is a statistically higher incidence of left handedness.

ABNORMALITIES OF ARTICULATION AND PHONATION (LISPING, DYSLALIA). A number of odd varieties of deficient articulation may come to the notice of the physician. One is *lisping*, in which the *s* sound is replaced by *th*; e.g., "thister" for "sister." Another condition, called *lallation* or *dyslalia*, a common speech disorder observed in early childhood, is characterized by multiple substitutions or omissions of consonants. In severe forms, speech may be almost unintelligible. These children are unaware that their speech differs from that of other persons and are distressed at not being understood. Milder degrees consist of the failure to pronounce only one or two consonants. For example, there may be imperfect enunciation of the sound *r* so that it sounds like *w*. "Running a race" becomes "wunning a wace." The nature of this disorder is not known. It has been suggested that the development of language in some children is so rapid that there is a partial failure of both perceptive and imitative speech. The patient usually recovers spontaneously from this disorder or responds promptly to speech therapy, which is best carried out at about the age of five years. These abnormalities are more frequent among feebleminded than normal children, and mental defect should always be suspected if numerous consonants are mispronounced and the condition persists beyond the age of twelve or thirteen years. The speech disorder resulting from *cleft palate* is easily recognized. Many of these patients also have a harelip, and the two abnormalities together interfere with suckling and later in life with the enunciation of labial and guttural consonants. The voice has an unpleasant nasality and often, if the defect is severe, there is an audible escape of air through the nose.

STAMMERING AND STUTTERING AND CLUTTERED SPEECH. Stammering and stuttering are difficult to classify. In some respects they belong to the developmental disorders, but they differ from them in being largely centered in articulation. They consist of a spasm of the muscles of articulation when an attempt is made to speak. The spasm may be tonic and result in a complete block of speech, sometimes called *stammering*, or a repetitive spasm that leads to repeated utterance of the first syllable, i.e., a stutter, or the words may come out in rapid clusters, all poorly enunciated. Certain syllables offer greater difficulty than others. The patient falters on an initial consonant or syllable, which he repeats over and over again before he finally succeeds in enunciating the rest of the word, e.g., p-p-paper, b-b-b-boy. The severity of the stutter is increased by excitement, as in speaking before strangers or a group of people. The spasms may overflow into other muscle groups not directly concerned with speech. Males are affected three times as often as females. The time of onset may be when the child first begins to talk, i.e., at two or three years of age, or between the ages of six and eight years. These latter are the two critical periods of language development. Many of these children also have some degree of reading and writing disability. Slowness in developing hand preference or enforced change from left- to right-handedness are noted in many cases. If mild, the condition tends to develop or to be present only during periods of emotional distress; and it usually disappears spontaneously during adolescent or early adult years. If severe, it persists all through life, regardless of treatment, but tends to improve as the patient grows older.

The essential character of stuttering is difficult to define. There is no detectable paralysis or incoordination of speech musculature, which seems to function normally in other commonplace acts and when the patient is alone and relaxed or singing. Stuttering differs from apraxia in that the muscles, when called upon to perform the specific act, go into voluntary spasm; but since the spasm does not occur during other movements in which these muscles are involved, it differs from the intention (tension) spasm of athetosis. It appears to represent a special category of movement disorder and is much like writer's cramp, another motor disorder of unknown etiology.

Everyone who has studied stuttering and stammering has been impressed with the high incidence of similar disabilities in other members of the same family, sometimes going back several generations. This and the preponderance in males suggest a sex-linked characteristic, but the inheritance does not follow a simple pattern.

Many of the patients, probably as a natural result of this impediment to free social intercourse, become increasingly fearful of speaking and have feelings of inferiority after a few years. By the time adolescence and adulthood are reached, emotional factors are so prominent that many physicians have mistaken stuttering for neurosis. Usually there is little or no evidence of any personality deviation before the onset of stuttering, and psychotherapy by competent psychiatrists, though unquestionably helpful in relieving emotional tension and assisting a satisfactory adjustment to the condition, has not significantly modified the underlying defect. Occasionally, stuttering will develop during adult life as a consequence of brain disease.

Emphasis on maturational delay in the language disorders of children is relative. Tumors, vascular lesions of the dominant hemisphere may abolish speech as in the adult, but the effects (especially before the 6th or 7th years) are always transitory.

Disorders of Articulation and Phonation

The third group of speech abnormalities is that of the disorders of articulation. In simple dysarthria there is no abnormality of the cortical centers. The dysarthric patient is able to understand perfectly what he hears, and if literate, he reads and has no difficulty in writing, even though unable to utter a single intelligible word. This is the strict meaning of being inarticulate.

The act of speaking is a highly coordinated sequence of contractions of the larynx, pharynx, palate, tongue, lips, and respiratory musculature. These are innervated by the hypoglossal, vagal, facial, and phrenic nerves. The nuclei of these nerves are controlled through the corticobulbar tracts by both motor cortices. As with all movements, there is also an extrapyramidal influence from the cerebellum and basal ganglions. A current of air is produced by expiration, and the force of it is finely regulated and coordinated with the activity of other muscles engaged in speech. *Phonation*, or the production of vocal sounds, is a function of the larynx. Changes in the size and shape of the glottis and in the length and tension of the vocal cords are effected by the action of the laryngeal muscles. Vibrations are set up and transmitted to the column of air passing over the vocal cords. Sounds thus formed are modified as they pass through the nasopharynx and mouth, which act as resonators. Articulation consists of contractions of the tongue, lips, pharynx, and palate, which interrupt or alter the vocal sounds. Vowels are of laryngeal origin, as are some consonants; but the latter are formed for the most part during articulation. For instance, the consonants *m*, *b*, and *p* are labial, *l* and *t* are lingual and *nk* and *ng* are nasoguttural.

Defective articulation and phonation are best observed by listening to the patient during ordinary conversation or while reading aloud from a newspaper or a book. Test phrases or the rapid repetition of lingual, labial, and guttural consonants may bring out the particular abnormality. Disorders of phonation call for an examination of the apparatus of voice. The movements of the vocal cords should be inspected with the aid of a hand mirror, or, even better, a laryngoscope, and those of the tongue, palate, and pharynx by direct observation.

Defects in articulation may be subdivided into several

types: paralytic dysarthria, spastic and rigid dysarthria, and ataxic dysarthria.

PARETIC DYSARTHRIA. This is due to a neural or bulbar (medullary) paralysis of the articulatory muscles (lower motor neurone paralysis). Bulbar poliomyelitis and "progressive bulbar palsy" are examples of diseases that may produce partial or complete anarthria. In the latter the shriveled tongue lies inert on the floor of the mouth, and the lips are relaxed and tremulous. Saliva constantly collects in the mouth because of dysphagia, and drooling is troublesome. Speech becomes less and less distinct. There is special difficulty in the correct utterance of vibratives, such as *r*; and as the paralysis becomes more complete, lingual and labial consonants are finally not pronounced at all. Lesser degrees of this abnormality are observed in myasthenia gravis. Bilateral paralysis of the palate, which may occur with diphtheria, poliomyelitis, or involvement of the tenth cranial nerve by tumor, produces a disorder of articulation similar to that of the cleft palate. The voice has a nasal quality, since the posterior nares are not closed during phonation, and certain consonants, such as *n, b,* and *k,* are altered. The abnormality is sometimes less pronounced in recumbency and increased when the head is thrown forward. Bilateral paralysis of the lips interferes with enunciation of labial consonants; *p* and *b* are slurred and sound more like *f* and *v*.

SPASTIC AND RIGID DYSARTHRIA. These are more frequent than the paralytic variety. Diseases that involve the corticobulbar tracts, usually vascular disease or motor system disease, result in the syndrome of pseudobulbar palsy. The patient may have had a minor stroke some time in the past affecting the corticobulbar fibers on one side; but since the bulbar muscles are probably represented in both motor cortices, there is no impairment in speech or swallowing from a unilateral lesion. If another stroke occurs involving the other corticobulbar tract and possibly the corticospinal tract at the pontine, midbrain, or capsular level, the patient immediately becomes anarthric or dysarthric and dysphagic. Unlike bulbar paralysis due to lower motor neurone involvement, there is no atrophy or fasciculation of the paralyzed muscles, the jaw jerk is exaggerated, the palatal reflexes are retained, emotional control is poor (pathologic laughter and crying), and sometimes breathing becomes periodic (Cheyne-Stokes). The patient may be anarthric and aphonic for a time, but as he improves, or in mild degrees of the same condition, speech is thick and indistinct, much like that of partial bulbar paralysis.

In paralysis agitans, or postencephalitic Parkinson's syndrome, one observes an extrapyramidal disturbance of articulation. The patient speaks slowly and articulates poorly, slurring over many syllables and trailing off the end of sentences. The voice is low-pitched, monotonous, and lacking inflection. The words are pronounced hastily. In advanced cases speech is almost unintelligible; only whispering may be possible at this stage. It may happen that the patient finds it impossible to talk while walking but can speak if he sits or lies down.

In chorea and myoclonus, speech may also be severely affected, and the defect is distinguished from the speech of pseudobulbar palsy or paralysis agitans by the interruptions of the abnormal movements. Grimacing and other characteristic motor signs must be depended upon for diagnosis. Pyramidal and extrapyramidal disturbances of speech may be combined in generalized cerebral diseases such as general paresis, in which slurred speech is one of the cardinal signs.

In many cases of capsular hemiplegia or partially recovered Broca's aphasia the patient is left with a dysarthria that may be difficult to distinguish from a pure articulatory defect. Careful testing of other language functions, especially writing, may bring out the aphasic quality.

ATAXIC DYSARTHRIA. This is characteristic of acute and chronic cerebellar lesions. It may be observed in multiple sclerosis, Friedreich's ataxia, cerebellar atrophy, and heat stroke. The principal speech abnormality is slowness; imprecise enunciation, monotony, and unnatural separation of the syllables of words (scanning) are other features. Coordination of speech and respiration are poor. There may not be enough breath to utter certain words, and others may be ejaculated explosively. *Scanning dysarthria* is distinctive, but in some cases, especially if there is some possibility of spastic weakness of the tongue from corticobulbar tract involvement, it is impossible to predict the anatomy of disease from analysis of speech alone. Myoclonic jerks involving the speech musculature may be superimposed on cerebellar ataxia in a number of diseases.

Aphonia and Dysphonia

Finally, a few points should be made concerning the fourth group of language disorders, i.e., disturbances of voice. In adolescence and early adult life there may be a persistence of the unstable "change of voice" normally seen in boys soon after puberty. As though by habit, the patient speaks part of the time in a falsetto voice. This can usually be overcome by training.

Paresis of the respiratory movements, as in poliomyelitis and acute infectious polyneuritis, may affect voice because insufficient air is provided for phonation and speech. Also, disturbances in the rhythm of respiration may interfere with the fluency of speech. This is particularly noticeable in so-called "extrapyramidal diseases," and one may note that the patient tries to talk upon inspiration. Reduced volume of speech due to limited excursion of the breathing muscles is another common feature; the patient is unable to speak above a whisper or to shout.

Paresis of both vocal cords causes complete aphonia. There is no voice, and the patient can speak only in whispers. Since the vocal cords normally separate during inspiration, their failure to do so when paralyzed may result in an inspiratory stridor. If one vocal cord is paralyzed, the voice becomes hoarse, low-pitched, and rasping.

Another curious condition about which little is known is *spastic dysphonia.* The authors have seen several cases, middle-aged or elderly men and women, otherwise healthy, who gradually lost the ability to speak quietly and fluently. Any effort to speak resulted in contraction of all the speech musculature so that the patient's voice was strained and phonation was labored. This is apparently a neurologic disorder of undetermined kind. The patients are not neurotic, and psychotherapy has been ineffective. This condition differs from the stridor caused by spasm of the laryngeal muscles in tetany.

Instability or changeableness of voice, a common problem for adolescent boys, may persist into adult life. Its basis is not known. Voice training has been helpful in many patients.

DIAGNOSIS

Speech is such a complex act that it has not been possible to present all its facets. Nothing, for example, has been said here about speech changes during various psychiatric illnesses. This does not mean that the psychiatric syndromes are unimportant, for there is no doubt that hysterical aphonia, the various tics that interrupt the speech of tense individuals, and the altered rate, fluency, and content of speech in the psychoses pose formidable problems.

In diagnosing disorders of speech the physician must attempt in every case to decide first whether the problem is one of aphasia, dysarthria, or dysphonia. The examination procedure outlined above will, if carried out systematically, permit this first and important step to be made.

If the patient is aphasic, it should be determined whether his aphasia is of global, central, Wernicke, or Broca type or whether it is a restricted disorder of motor function, a pure alexia, or word deafness. The differential diagnosis has already been given and also the significance of associated neurologic signs. Identification of the type of aphasia is of localizing value and it may provide an important lead as to the underlying brain disease.

The general physician is frequently called upon to examine children who show some disorder of speech or delay in language development. From the above remarks it will be seen that these disorders fall into several broad categories, of which stuttering, delay in onset of speech, dyslalia, partial or complete deafness, word deafness, cleft palate, lisping, and word blindness are the most frequent. When faced with problems of this type, the physician must ask several questions. *Is the child partially or completely deaf? Does he have a more generalized mental or neuromuscular defect—is he feebleminded or suffering from an infantile hemiplegia or spastic diplegia? Does he stammer, stutter, or show dyslalia?* In attempting to answer these questions, the parents' account of the child's development and his behavior at home is most helpful. Failure to respond to noise of any kind suggests deafness. An interest in sounds and music but not in stories or conversation, together with slow development of understanding and use of speech are indicative of high-tone deafness or word deafness (auditory verbal agnosia). Delayed onset of suckling, head control, sitting, standing, walking, etc., necessitate neurologic examina-

tion; one should look particularly for spastic weakness or rigidity of the limbs and poor motor control of the tongue, as well as mental retardation. The latter can be assessed at an early age by intelligence tests, such as the performance part of the Stanford-Binet test. If the child is otherwise normal, recitation of a nursery rhyme will disclose a stammering, stuttering, lallation of cleft palate speech.

Disturbances of articulation point to involvement of a different set of neural structures, such as the motor cortices, the corticobulbar pathways, the seventh, ninth, and tenth nuclei, the brainstem, and extrapyramidal nuclei and tracts. Often it is necessary to use other neurologic findings to decide which of these are implicated in any given case. The important distinction between the pseudobulbar or supranuclear palsies and the bulbar palsies is grasped only with difficulty by the average student. The information obtained by localizing these two major types of dysarthria is extremely helpful in differential diagnosis.

Dysphonia should lead to an investigation of laryngeal disease either primary or secondary to an abnormality of innervation.

TREATMENT

The sudden loss of speech would be expected to cause great apprehension, but except for almost pure motor defects, most patients show remarkably little concern. It appears that the very lesion that deprives them of speech also causes at least a partial loss of insight into their own disability. This reaches almost a ludicrous extreme in some cases of Wernicke's aphasia, in which the patient becomes indignant when others cannot understand his jargon. Nonetheless, as improvement occurs, many patient do become discouraged. Reassurance and a positive program of speech rehabilitation are the best ways of helping the patient at this stage.

The contemporary methods of training and reeducation in overcoming an aphasic defect have never been critically evaluated. Most aphasic difficulty is due to vascular disease of the brain, and nearly always this is accompanied by some degree of spontaneous improvement in the days, weeks, and months that follow the stroke. Sometimes recovery is complete within hours or days; at times not more than a few words are regained after a year or two of assiduous speech training. Nevertheless, it is the opinion of many experts in the field that speech training is worthwhile.

One must decide for each patient whether speech training is needed and when it should be started. As a rule, therapy is not advisable in the first few days of an aphasic illness, because one does not know how lasting it will be. Also, if the patient suffers a severe global aphasia and can neither speak nor understand spoken and written words, the speech therapist is helpless. Under such circumstances, one does well to wait a few weeks until some one of the language functions has begun to return. Then the physician may begin to encourage and help the patient to use the function to a maximum degree. In milder aphasic disorders the patient may be sent to the speech therapist as soon as the illness has stabilized.

The methods of speech training are specialized, and it is advisable to call in a person who has been trained in this field. However, inasmuch as the benefit is largely psychologic, an interested member of the family or a schoolteacher can be used if a speech therapist is not available in the community.

The language problems of children are serious and demand skillful diagnosis and treatment. Often, excellent results are obtained. Most of the well-organized urban school systems have remedial reading teachers who will take over the problem once it has been evaluated medically. The emotional problems that often accompany the developmental disturbances of language and of cerebral dominance must be dealt with gently and firmly.

The physician should by wise counseling help the patient understand the nature of this problem and try to avoid some of the secondary and emotional problems that the speech disorder creates. Prolonged psychotherapy helps with the emotional problems but has not, in the author's experience, corrected the underlying speech defect. Fortunately, the natural course of mild stuttering is toward improvement during adolescence, and many patients recover spontaneously by adult life. In severe cases a lifelong problem must be faced, and none of the present methods of therapy, including psychoanalysis, has corrected the defect.

There is no special treatment for the dysarthric disturbance of speech.

REFERENCES

Alajouanine, T.: Verbal Realization in Aphasia, Brain, 79: 1–29, 1956.

Brain, R.: Aphasia, Apraxia, Agnosia, chap. 83 in "Neurology, S. A. K. Wilson and N. Bruce (Eds.), 2d ed., vol. 3, Baltimore, The Williams & Wilkins Company, 1955.

Geschwind, N.: Disconnection Syndromes in Animals and Man. Brain, 88:237–294, 585–644, 1965.

Hallgren, B.: Specific Dyslexia. Supp. 65 of Acta Psychiat. Neurol., 1950.

Nielsen, J. M.: "Agnosia, Apraxia, Aphasia: Their Value in Cerebral Localization," 2d ed., New York, Hafner Publishing Company, Inc., 1962.

Orton, S. T.: "Reading, Writing and Speech Problems in Children," New York, W. W. Norton & Company, Inc., 1937.

30 DELIRIUM AND OTHER CONFUSIONAL STATES AND KORSAKOFF'S AMNESTIC SYNDROME

Raymond D. Adams and Maurice Victor

Every physician sooner or later discovers through clinical experience the need for special competence in assessing the mental faculties of his patients. He must be able to observe with detachment and complete objectivity their character, intelligence, mood, memory, judgment, and other attributes of personality in much the same fashion as he observes the nutritional state and the color of the mucous membranes. The systematic examination of these affective and cognitive functions permits him to reach certain conclusions regarding mental status, and these are also of value in understanding the patient and his illness. Without the data obtained from the study of the mental status, errors will be made in evaluating the reliability of the patient's history, in diagnosing the neurologic or psychiatric disease from which he suffers, and in conducting any proposed therapeutic program.

Perhaps the content of this chapter will be more clearly understood if we repeat a few of the introductory remarks of Chap. 17. The main thesis of the neurologic physician is that mental and physical functions of the nervous system are simply two aspects of the same neural process. The mind is no more or less than the self-regulating, goal-seeking activities, the same ones that are manifest in all mammalian life. It is only because of the prodigious complexity of man's brain, his high capacity for memory of past experiences, his imagination, and power of reasoning, his capacity to make conscious choice and to reflect on the working of his own psychic processes that the illusion of separation of mind and body was created. Biologists and psychologists have reached the modern monistic view by placing all protoplasmic activities of the nervous system (growth, development, behavior, and mental function) in a continuum and noting the inherent purposiveness and creativity common to all of them. The physician is persuaded of its truth by his daily experiences with disease, in which every known aberration of behavior, intellect, and personality appear as expressions of diseases of the cerebrum.

In this chapter we are concerned with common disturbances of sensorium and intellection that have not been previously discussed and which stand as cardinal manifestations of certain cerebral diseases. The most frequent of these are confusion, disturbances of memory, and abnormalities of thinking or reasoning.

DEFINITION OF TERMS

The following nomenclature, though tentative, is useful and will be employed throughout this textbook:

Confusion, as stated in Chap. 26, is a term that has two meanings. The commonest refers to a general reduction in alertness, attentiveness, and perception of environmental stimuli, an inability to take notice of, i.e., to register all elements of, a situation within a short period of time. Often there are misinterpretations of stimuli, and hallucinations and drowsiness may be prominent. The other usage designates slowness and inefficiency in thinking, often with failure in subsequent recall. Thus, in the first sense confusion is aligned with disorders of consciousness, attention, and perception, and as was pointed out in Chap. 26, it may represent one stage on the way to coma or emergence therefrom. The term *delirium* is often used to specify a disorder of consciousness, perception, and attention, but it connotes in addition excessive alertness, sleeplessness, and frenzied excitement. Mental activity may be interrupted by the abrupt intrusion of hallucinations, which are frequent. We believe that confusion and delirium represent essentially different types of cerebral disorder. In many textbooks of psychiatry, however, confusion and delirium are grouped together and called toxic-exhaustive psychosis or "organic reaction type," indicating their postulated cause and pathologic basis. Confusion as an impairment of thinking, on the other hand, is related to derangements of intellect, i.e., dementia.

The term *amnesia* means loss of the ability to form memories despite an alert state of mind. It presupposes an ability to grasp the problem, to use language normally, and to maintain adequate motivation. The failure is mainly one of retention, recall, and reproduction, and it should be distinguished from states of drowsiness and confusion, where the learned material seems never to have been adequately assimilated. *Dementia* means loss of reason or, more particularly, a deterioration of intellect. Implied in the word is the idea of a gradual enfeeblement of mental powers in a person who formerly possessed a normal mind. *Amentia*, by contrast, indicates a congenital feeblemindedness.

OBSERVABLE ASPECTS OF BEHAVIOR AND THEIR RELATION TO CONFUSION, DELIRIUM, AMNESIA, AND DEMENTIA

In the strict sense the intellectual, emotional, volitional, and behavioral activities of the human organism are so complex and varied that one may question the possibility of using derangements of them as reliable guides to cerebral disease. Certainly they have not the same reliability and ease of anatomic and physiologic interpretation as sensory and motor paralysis or aphasia. Yet one observes certain of these higher cerebral disturbances recurring with such regularity in certain diseases as to be useful in clinical medicine; and some of them gain in specificity because they are often combined in certain ways to form syndromes, which are essentially what states of confusion, delirium, amnesia, and dementia are. Of course, we do not always know the value of certain elements of these syndromes, i.e., which are of primary or secondary importance.

The components of mentation and behavior that lend themselves to bedside examination are (1) the processes of sensation and perception; (2) the capacity for memorizing; (3) the ability to think, reason, and form logical conclusions; (4) temperament, mood, and emotion; (5) initiative, impulse, and drive; (6) insight. Of these (1), (2), and (3) may be grouped as cognitive, (4) as affective, and (5) as conative or volitional. Insight includes essentially all introspective observations made by the patient concerning his own normal or disordered functioning. Each component of behavior and intellection has its objective side, expressed in the manifest ef-

fects of certain stimulus conditions on the patient and his behavioral responses, and its subjective side, expressed in what the patient says he thinks and feels.

Disturbances of Perception

Perception, i.e., the processes involved in acquiring through the senses a knowledge of the "world about" or of one's own body, involves many things aside from the simple sensory process of being aware of the attributes of a stimulus; it includes the selective focusing and maintaining of attention, elimination of all extraneous stimuli, and recognition of the stimulus by knowing its relationship to personal remembered experience. One must appreciate that the perception of an object undergoes predictable types of derangements in disease. Most often there is a reduction in the number of perceptions in a given unit of time and failure to properly synthesize them and relate them to the ongoing activities of the mind. Or there may be apparent inattentiveness, fluctuations of attention, distractibility (pertinent and irrelevant stimuli now having equal value), inability to persist in an assigned task, and in the reporting and reacting to only a small part of a complex of stimuli. Qualitative changes also appear, mainly in the form of sensory distortions and misinterpretation and misidentification of objects and persons (illusions); and these, at least in part, form the basis of hallucinatory experience in which the patient reports and reacts to stimuli not present in his environment. The loss of ability to perceive simultaneously all elements of a large complex of stimuli is sometimes explained as a "failure of subjective reorganization." Major disturbances in the perceptual sphere, sometimes called "clouding of the sensorium," occur most often in confusional states and deliria, but quantitative deficiency may become evident in the advanced stages of amentia and dementia.

Disturbances of Memory

Memory, i.e., the retention of learned experiences, is involved in all mental activities. It may be arbitrarily subdivided into several parts, namely, (1) registration, which includes all that was mentioned under perception; (2) mnemonic integration and retention; (3) recall; and (4) reproduction. As was stated above, in disturbances of perception and attention there may be a complete failure of learning and memory for the reason that the material to be learned was never assimilated. In Korsakoff's amnestic syndrome newly presented material appears to be temporarily registered but cannot be retained for more than a few minutes, and there is nearly always an associated defect in the recall and reproduction of memories formed before the onset of the illness (retrograde amnesia). Dislocation of events in time and the fabrication of stories, called *confabulation*, constitutes a third feature of the syndrome. Sound retention with failure of recall is at times a normal state; but when it is severe and extends to all events over a given period of time, it is usually due to hysteria or malingering. Proof that the processes of registration and recall are intact under these circumstances comes from hypnosis and suggestion, by means of which the lost items are fully recalled and reproduced. In Korsakoff's amnestic state the patient fails on all tests of learning and recent memory and his behavior accords with his deficiencies of information. Since memory is involved to some extent in all mental processes, it becomes the most testable component of mentation and behavior.

Disturbances of Thinking

Thinking, which is central to so many important intellectual activities, remains one of the most elusive of all mental operations. If by thinking we mean selective ordering of symbols for problem solving and capacity to reason and form sound judgments (the usual definition), obviously the working units of most complex experiences of this type are words and numbers. The activity of substituting word and number symbols for the objects for which they stand (symbolization) is a fundamental part of the process. These symbols are formed into ideas or concepts, and the arrangement of new and remembered ideas into certain orders or relationships, according to the rules of logic, constitute another intricate part of thought, presently beyond the scope of analysis. In a general way one may examine thinking for speed and efficiency, ideational content, coherence and logical relationships of ideas, quantity and quality of associations to a given idea, and propriety of the feeling and behavior engendered by an idea.

Information concerning the thought processes and associative functions is best obtained by analyzing the patient's spontaneous verbal productions and by engaging him in conversation. If he is taciturn or mute, one may then have to depend on his responses to direct questions or upon written material, i.e., letters, etc. One notes the prevailing trends of the patient's thoughts, whether his ideas are reasonable or precise and coherent or vague, circumstantial, tangential, and irrelevant, and whether his thought processes are shallow and completely fragmented. Disorders of thought are frequent in deliria, and in degenerative and other types of cerebral disease. The organization of thought may be disrupted with fragmentation, repetition, and perseveration. This is spoken of as incoherence and marks many confusional delirious states. The patient may be excessively critical, rationalizing, and hairsplitting; this is a type of thinking often manifest in depressive psychoses. Derangements of thinking may also take the form of a virtual flight of ideas. The patient moves nimbly from one idea to another, and his associations are numerous and loosely linked. This is a common feature in hypomanic or manic states. The opposite condition, poverty of ideas (the more frequent condition), is characteristic both of depression, where it is combined with gloomy thoughts, and of dementing diseases, where it is part of a general reduction in all intellectual activity. Thinking may be distorted in such a way that the patient fails to check his ideas against reality. When a false belief is maintained in spite of normally convincing contradictory evidence, the patient is said to have a delusion. Delusion is common to many illnesses, particularly manic-depressive and schizophrenic states. Ideas may seem to have been implanted in the patient's mind by some outside agency such as radio, television, or atomic energy. These reflect the passivity feelings characteristic of manic-depressive and schizophrenic psychoses. Other distortions of logical thought, such as gaps or condensations of logical associations, are typical of schizophrenia, of which they constitute a diagnostic feature.

Disturbances of Emotion, Mood, and Affect

The emotional life of the patient is expressed in a variety of ways, and there are several points to be made about it. In the first place, rather marked individual differences in basic temperament are to be observed in the normal population; some persons are throughout their life cheerful, gregarious, optimistic, and free from worry, whereas others are just the opposite. In fact, the unusually volatile, cyclothymic person is believed to be liable to manic-depressive psychosis and the suspicious, withdrawn, introverted person to schizophrenia and paranoia. Strong, persistent emotional states such as fear and anxiety may occur as reactions to life situations and may be accompanied by derangements of visceral function. If excessive and disproportionate to the stimulus, they have medical significance; they are usually manifestations of an anxiety neurosis or depression. Variations in the degree of responsiveness to emotional stimuli are also frequent and, when excessive and persistent, are important. In depression all stimuli tend to enhance the somber mood of unhappiness. Emotional response that is excessively labile, variable from moment to moment, and poorly controlled or uninhibited is a condition common to many diseases of the cerebrum, particularly those involving the corticopontine and corticobulbar pathways. It may constitute a part of the syndrome of pseudobulbar palsy. All emotional expression may be lacking, as in apathetic states or severe depressions, or the patient may be a victim of every trivial problem in daily life; i.e., he cannot control his worries. Finally, the emotional response may be inappropriate to the stimulus, e.g., a depressing thought is amusing and attended by a smile, as in schizophrenia.

Since there are relatively few overt manifestations of temperament, mood, and other emotional experiences described above, the physician must evaluate these states by the appearance of the patient and by verbalized accounts of his feelings. For these purposes it is convenient to divide emotionality into mood and feeling or affect. By mood is meant the prevailing emotional state of the individual without reference to the stimuli impinging upon him, i.e., his immediate environmental circumstances. It may be pleasant and cheerful or melancholic. The language, e.g., the adjectives used, and the facial expressions, attitudes, postures, and speed of movement most reliably betray the patient's mood.

By contrast, feelings or affects are said to be emotional experiences evoked by environmental stimuli. According to some psychiatrists, feeling is the subjective component and affect, the overt manifestation. Others apply either word to the subjective state. The difference between mood as a prevailing emotional state and feeling and affect as emotional reactions to stimuli may seem rather tenuous, but these distinctions are considered valuable by psychiatrists.

Impulse, that basic biologic urge, driving force, or purpose, by which every organism is directed to reach its full potentialities, appears to be another extremely important and observable but neglected dimension of behavior. Again, one notes wide normal variations from one person to another in strength of impulse to action and thought, and these individual differences are present throughout life. One of the most conspicuous pathologic deviations is an apparent constitutional weakness in impulse in certain neurotic individuals. Moreover, with many types of cerebral disease, particularly those which involve the posterior orbital parts of the frontal lobes, a reduction in impulse is coupled with an indifference or lack of concern about the consequences of actions. In such cases all other measurable aspects of psychic function may be normal. Extreme degrees of lack of impulse, or abulia, take the form of mutism and immobility, called *akinetic mutism.* Psychomotor retardation is a lesser degree of the same state and is also a feature of depression, in which instance mood alternation and extreme fatigability are conjoined, or of cerebral disease.

Lastly, insight, the state of being fully aware of the nature and degree of one's deficits, becomes manifestly impaired or abolished in relation to all types of cerebral disease that cause disorders of behavior. Rarely does the patient with any of the aforementioned states seek advice or help for his illness. Instead, his family usually brings him to the physician. Thus, it appears that the diseases which produce all these abnormalities not only evoke observable changes in behavior but also alter or reduce the capacity of the patient to make accurate introspections of his own psychic function. This fact stands as one of the most incontrovertible proofs that the cerebrum is the organ both of behavior and of all inner psychic experiences; that is to say, behavior and mind are but two inseparable aspects of the function of the nervous system.

COMMON SYNDROMES

This entire group of acute confusional states is characterized principally by clouding of consciousness with prominent disorders of attention and perception that interfere with clarity of thinking and the formation of memories. One syndrome, here called *hyperkinetic delirium,* includes overactivity, sleeplessness, tremulousness, and hallucinations. Convulsions often precede the delirium. In a variant of this syndrome, here called *hypokinetic delirium,* drowsiness, and reduced awareness and responsiveness are the principal abnormalities, and perceptual disorder and degree of activity are less important. A second syndrome is a confusional state in which there

is manifest reduction in alertness, attentiveness, and sensorial registration. A third syndrome consists of a confusional state occurring in a patient with some other cerebral disease. The latter disposes him to the acute psychosis which we have chosen to designate as a *beclouded dementia.* These illnesses tend to develop acutely, to have multiple causes, and to terminate within a relatively short period of time (days to weeks) leaving the patient without residual damage. These two syndromes will be described separately.

Delirium

CLINICAL FEATURES. These are most perfectly depicted in the alcoholic patient. The symptoms usually develop over a period of 2 or 3 days. The first indications of the approaching attack are difficulty in concentrating, restless irritability, tremulousness, insomnia, and poor appetite. One or several generalized convulsions are the initial major symptom in 30 percent of the cases. The patient's rest becomes troubled by unpleasant and terrifying dreams. There may be momentary disorientation or an occasional irrational remark.

These initial symptoms rapidly give way to a clinical picture that, in severe cases, is one of the most colorful and dramatic in medicine. The state of consciousness becomes altered; it is clouded in that the patient is inattentive and unable to perceive all elements of his situation— as though he were in a twilight state. He talks incessantly and incoherently and looks distressed or perplexed; his expression is in keeping with his vague notions of being annoyed or pursued by someone who seeks to injure him. From his manner and from the content of his speech it is evident that he misinterprets the meaning of ordinary objects and sounds around him and has vivid visual, auditory, and tactile hallucinations, often of a most unpleasant type. At first he can be brought momentarily into touch with reality and may in fact answer questions correctly; but almost at once he relapses into his preoccupied, confused state, gives wrong answers, and is unable to think coherently. The clouding of sensorium is revealed by his inability to repeat or reverse series of digits or to do serial additions or subtractions. As a rule he is disoriented. Before long he is unable to shake off his hallucinations even for a second and does not recognize his family or his physician. Tremor and restless movements are usually present and may be violent. The countenance is flushed, and the conjunctivas are injected; the pulse is rapid and soft, and the temperature may be raised. There is much sweating, and the urine is scanty and of high specific gravity.

The symptoms abate, either suddenly or gradually, after 2 or 3 days, although in exceptional cases they may persist for several weeks. The most certain indication of the end of the attack is the occurrence of sound sleep and of lucid intervals of increasing length. Recovery is usually complete.

Delirium is subject to all degrees of variability, not only from patient to patient but in the same patient from day to day and hour to hour. The entire syndrome may be observed in one patient and only one or two symptoms in another. In its mildest form, as so often occurs in febrile diseases, it consists of an occasional wandering of the mind and incoherence of expression interrupted by periods of lucidity. This form, lacking motor and autonomic overactivity, is sometimes referred to as a *quiet delirium* (here, *hypokinetic delirium*) and is difficult to distinguish from other confusional states. The more severe form of active delirium and tremulousness, best exemplified by delirium tremens, is characterized by a great excess of motor activity, severe insomnia, and marked confusion, which may progress to a "muttering stupor" and/or coma, which in about 10 percent of patients ends fatally.

MORBID ANATOMY AND PATHOPHYSIOLOGY. The brains of patients who have died in delirium tremens usually show no pathologic changes of significance. A number of diseases, however, may cause delirium and also give rise to focal lesions in the brain, such as focal embolic encephalitis, viral encephalitis, Wernicke's disease, or trauma. The topography of these lesions is of particular interest. They tend to be localized in certain parts of the brain, particularly in the midbrain and subthalamus and in the temporal lobes, where they involve the reticular activating and limbic systems.

Penfield's studies of the human cortex during surgical exploration clearly indicate the importance of the temporal lobe in producing visual, auditory, and olfactory hallucinations. With subthalamic and midbrain lesions, there may occur visual hallucinations of a pleasurable type accompanied by good insight, namely, the peduncular hallucinosis of Lhermitte.

The electroencephalogram in delirium shows nonfocal slow activity in the 5 to 7 per sec range, a state that rapidly returns to normal as the delirium clears. However, in other cases only activity in the fast beta frequency is seen, and in milder degrees of delirium there is usually no abnormality at all.

An analysis of the several conditions conducive to delirium suggests at least three different physiologic mechanisms. In alcoholism and barbiturate intoxication the clinical manifestations appear after the withdrawal of drugs known to have a strong inhibitory effect on certain areas of the central nervous system. Presumably their release and overactivity are then the basis of delirium. In this respect it is interesting to note that delirium tremens is made up of symptoms which are the antithesis of alcoholic intoxication. In the case of bacterial infections and poisoning by certain drugs, such as atropine and scopolamine, the delirious state probably results from the direct action of the toxin or chemical on these same parts of the brain. Thirdly, destructive lesions such as acute inclusion body encephalitis of the temporal lobes cause delirium by disturbing the function of certain areas.

Psychophysiologic mechanisms have also been postulated. It has long been suggested that some individuals are much more liable to delirium than others. There is much reason to doubt this hypothesis, for it has been shown that all of a group of randomly selected persons would develop delirium if the causative mechanisms were strongly operative. This is to be expected, for any healthy person under certain circumstances may experience phenomena akin to those found in delirium. Thus after repeated auditory and visual stimulation the same impressions may continue to be perceived even though the stimuli are no longer present. Moreover, it has been shown that a healthy individual can be induced to hallucinate by placing him in an environment as free as possible of sensory stimulation. A relation between delirium and dream states has been postulated because in both there is a loss of appreciation of time, a richness of visual imagery, indifference to inconsistencies and "defective reality testing." Moreover, patients may refer to some of these delirious symptoms as a "bad dream," and normal persons may hallucinate in the so-called "hypnagogic state," the short period between sleeping and waking. In general, however, formulations in the field of dynamic psychology seem more reasonably to account for the topical content of delirium than to explain its occurrence. Wolff and Curran, having observed the same content in repeated attacks of delirium due to different causes, concluded that the content depends more on age, sex, intellectual endowment, occupation, personality traits, and past experience of the patient than on the cause or mechanism of the delirium.

The main difficulty in understanding delirium arises from the fact that it has not been possible from clinical studies to ascertain which of the many symptoms have physiologic significance. What is the basis of this altered consciousness, this sensorial alteration, the lack of harmony between actual sensory impressions of the present and memory of those in the past? Obviously, there is something missing from total behavior, something that leaves the patient at the mercy of certain sensory stimuli and unable to attend to others, yet at the same time incapable of discriminating between sense impression and fantasy. There appears to be some lack of inhibition of sensory processes, which may also be the basis of the sleep disturbance (insomnia) and the convulsive tendency.

Acute Confusional State Associated with Reduced Mental Alertness and Responsiveness (Includes Primary Mental Confusion and Hypokinetic Delirium)

CLINICAL FEATURES. Here a conjunction of two syndromes is necessary because at a practical level they may be impossible to distinguish from one another. In the most typical examples all mental functions are reduced to some degree, but alertness, attentiveness, and the ability to grasp all elements of the immediate situation suffer most. In its mildest form the patient may pass for normal, and only failure to recollect and reproduce happenings of the past few hours or days reveals the inadequacy of mental function. The more obviously confused patient spends much of his time in idleness, but what he does do may be inappropriate and annoying to others. Only the more automatic acts and verbal responses are properly performed, but these may permit the examiner to obtain from the patient a number of relevant and accurate replies to questions about age, occupation, and residence. Reactions are slow and indecisive, and it is difficult for the patient to sustain a conversation. He may doze during the interview and is observed to sleep more hours each day than is natural or the same number at more irregular intervals. Responses tend to be rather abrupt, brief, and mechanical. Perceptual difficulties are frequent, and voices, common objects, and the actions of other persons are frequently misinterpreted. Often one cannot discern whether the patient hears voices and sees things that do not exist, i.e., whether he is actively hallucinating, or is merely misinterpreting stimuli in the environment. Inadequate perception and forgetfulness results in a constant state of bewilderment. Failing to recognize his surroundings and having lost all sense of time, he repeats the same question and makes the same remarks over and over again.

As the confusion deepens, conversation becomes more difficult, and at a certain stage the patient no longer notices or responds to much of what is going on around him. Replies to questions may be a single word or a short phrase spoken in a soft tremulous voice or whisper. The patient may be mute. Irritability may or may not be present. It was to this profound impairment of all cognitive functions that Bonhoeffer, a German authority on delirium, gave the name *amentia*. Some patients are extremely suspicious; in fact, a paranoid trend may be the most pronounced and troublesome feature of the illness.

In its most advanced stages confusion gives way to stupor and finally to coma. As the patient improves, he may pass again through the stage of stupor and confusion in the reverse order. All this informs us that at least one category of confusion is but a manifestation of the same disease processes that in their severest form cause coma.

In some instances the mental aberration never exceeds that of confusion with stupor; in others, with more than the usual degree of irritability and restlessness, one cannot fail to notice the striking resemblance to delirium. It is to this latter state that we attach the term *hypokinetic delirium* with all the implications, anatomic and physiologic, described under hyperkinetic delirium. In both there is a clouding of consciousness, impairment of attention, slowness, and disordered perception and association of ideas. The point is that if tremor, vivid hallucinations, vigilant excited attitude, insomnia, and the low convulsive threshold are inconspicuous, the differentiation is nearly impossible. The same diagnostic difficulty arises when a delirium is complicated by an illness that superimposes stupor (e.g., delirium tremens with pneumonia). Actually, typical cases showing one or the other of these two syndromes are easily distinguished. Difficulty in distinguishing these two states is the reason that many writers such as Romano and Engel and Lipowski insist on there being but one disordered mechanism, the manifestations of which they call *delirium*. The present writers would disagree, for they believe several pathogenetic mechanisms of different types and involving different parts of the brain to be included in this category of acute, reversible cerebral disease.

(See Chaps. 118 and 120 for discussions of some of the diseases which cause delirious states.)

MORBID ANATOMY AND PATHOPHYSIOLOGY. All that has been said on this subject in Chap. 26 is applicable to at least one subgroup of the confusional states. In the others no consistent pathologic change has been found. The electroencephalogram is of interest because it is almost invariably abnormal in more severe forms of this syndrome, in contrast to delirium, where the changes are relatively minor. High-voltage slow waves in the 2 to 3 per sec (delta) range or the 5 to 7 per sec (theta) range are the usual finding.

Senile and Other Dementing Brain Diseases Complicated by Medical Diseases (Beclouded Dementia)

Many elderly patients who enter the hospital with medical or surgical illness are mentally confused. Presumably the liability to this state is determined by preexisting brain disease, in this instance senile dementia, which may or may not have been obvious to the family before the onset of the complicating illness. Other cerebral diseases (vascular, neoplastic, demyelinative) may have the same effect of increasing the patient's liability to delirium.

All the clinical features of hypokinetic delirium or confusion described in the previous sections may be present. The severity may vary greatly. The confusion may be reflected only in the patient's inability to relate sequentially the history of his illness, or it may be so severe that he is virtually *non compos mentis*.

Although almost any complicating illness may bring out this confusion, it is particularly frequent with infectious disease, especially in those cases which resist the effects of antibiotic medication; with posttraumatic and postoperative states, notably after concussive brain injuries and removal of cataracts (in which case the confusion is probably related to being temporarily deprived of vision); and with congestive heart failure, chronic respiratory disease, and severe anemia, especially pernicious anemia. Often it is difficult to determine which of several possible factors is responsible for the confusion in this heterogeneous group of illnesses. There may be more than one factor. A cardiac patient with a confusional psychosis may be febrile, have marginally reduced cerebral blood flow, be intoxicated by one or more drugs, or be in electrolyte imbalance. The same is true of postoperative confusional states, where a number of factors such as fever, infection, dehydration, and drug intoxication may be incriminated. The presence of alcoholism may further complicate the matter.

When he recovers from the medical or surgical illness, the patient usually returns to his premorbid state, though his shortcomings, now drawn to the attention of the family and physician, may be more obvious than before.

Coincidental Development of Acute Schizophrenic or Manic-depressive Psychosis during a Medical or Surgical Illness

A certain proportion of psychoses of the schizophrenic or manic-depressive type first become manifest during an acute medical illness or following an operation or parturition. A causal relationship between the two is usually sought but cannot be established. Usually the psychosis began long before but was not recognized. The diagnosis of the psychiatric illness must proceed along the lines suggested in Chaps. 371 and 372. Close observation will usually reveal a clear sensorium and relatively intact memory, which permits differentiation from the acute confusional states.

KORSAKOFF'S AMNESTIC SYNDROMES AND THE RESIDUAL MENTAL STATES FOLLOWING DELIRIUM AND CONFUSION

The majority of patients suffering from the delirious confused states recover completely after a few days or weeks. Afterwards one can detect no evidence of damage to the nervous system. In contrast, in cases of beclouded dementia, as the sensorial disturbance subsides, the patient is left with the same mental weakness that existed before the onset of the confusional state. Sometimes the dementia seems more pronounced afterward, and the family will later remark that the patient's mind failed at the time of the acute illness. However, one has the impression that they merely became aware of the insidiously developing dementia at this time.

There is another group of cases, by no means small or insignificant, in which the acutely delirious or confused patient is left with a severe deficit. The inattentiveness, hallucinations, and sleep disorder disappear. The patient is alert, easily engaged in conversation, and quite proper in his general deportment. Nevertheless, he is incompetent to look after himself. A careful evaluation of his mental status will reveal a severe memory deficit of the type found in Korsakoff's psychosis. The distinguishing feature of this latter illness is not memory loss alone but the disproportionate affection of memory in relation to the patient's alertness and the integrity of other faculties. It is further characterized by the inability to learn new facts and, in its early stages, by confabulation. This state, once fully developed, may be permanent, though often there is some improvement in learning capacity and memory as the months pass. It represents a special type of dementia.

The clinical features of Korsakoff's psychosis are presented in detail in Chap. 363. Although frequently observed in patients who suffer from alcoholism and malnutrition, the same clinical picture may occur with other diseases, such as ruptured saccular aneurysm and subarachnoid hemorrhage, tuberculous meningitis, and tumors in the walls of the third ventricle.

OTHER BEHAVIORAL DISORDERS ASSOCIATED WITH CEREBRAL DISEASE

When one attempts to categorize all the patients with relatively acute or subacute disorders of mentation and behavior under the section headings above, there are still a considerable number that remain difficult to classify. They present themselves as an almost infinite variety of syndromes in which the following abnormalities of function may occur: reduced or increased levels of speech, thought and action; disorientation as to time and place; idleness and lack of interest; loss of spontaneity and sense of humor; muteness and hypokinesia, resistiveness and negativism; hostility, lack of observance of social custom, use of abusive and vulgar language; inexplicable fright, euphoria, and lack of proper concern; complaint of visual distortion, of excess sensitivity to sounds; distortions of smell and taste; inability to find the names of objects, to follow a conversation, to think coherently; sexual indiscretion, lack of modesty, and other signs of disinhibition; seizures; disturbances of sleep. Obviously these many symptoms do not all have the same basic significance and the majority possess only relative localizing value. They may be associated with definite hemiparesis, hemihypesthesia, frank aphasia, or homonymous hemianopia, but even without these lateralizing signs they point to the existence of cerebral disease.

Syndromes comprising these elements may be observed in subacute inclusion body encephalitis, Behcet's meningoencephalitis, adult toxoplasmosis, infectious mononucleosis, acute or subacute demyelinative diseases (acute or subacute recurrent multiple sclerosis), granulomatous and other forms of angiitis, gliomatosis cerebri, carcinomatosis with encephalopathy of multifocal type, multiple tumor metastases, acute and subacute bacterial endocarditis, and thrombopenia with small vessel thrombosis (Moschcowitz's disease). A fuller account of some of these cerebral symptoms will be found in descriptions of these diseases.

Classification of Deliria or Acute Confusional States and Korsakoff's Amnestic Syndrome

The syndrome itself and its main clinical relationships are the only satisfactory basis for classification until such time as the actual cause and pathophysiology are discovered. The tendency in the past to subdivide the syndromes according to their most prominent symptom or degree of severity, e.g., "picking delirium," "microptic delirium," "acute delirious mania," "muttering delirium," has no fundamental value.

I. Hyperkinetic Delirium
   A. In a medical or surgical illness (no focal or lateralizing neurologic signs; cerebrospinal fluid usually clear)
      1. Typhoid fever
      2. Pneumonia
      3. Septicemia, particularly erysipelas and other streptococcal infections

4. Rheumatic fever
5. Thyrotoxicosis and ACTH intoxication (rare)
6. Postoperative and posttraumatic states

B. In neurologic disease that causes focal or lateralizing signs or changes in the cerebrospinal fluid
   1. Vascular, neoplastic, or other diseases, particularly those involving the temporal lobes and upper brainstem
   2. Cerebral contusion and laceration (traumatic delirium)
   3. Acute purulent and tuberculous meningitis
   4. Subarachnoid hemorrhage
   5. Encephalitis due to viral causes and to unknown causes, e.g., infectious mononucleosis

C. The abstinence states (after drug intoxications), exogenous intoxications and postconvulsive states; signs of other medical, surgical, and neurologic illnesses absent or coincidental
   1. Alcoholism (delirium tremens), barbiturates, chlordiazepoxide, glutethimide
   2. Drug intoxications: camphor, caffeine, ergot, bromides, scopolamine, atropine, amphetamine
   3. Postconvulsive delirium

II. Hypokinetic Delirium and Non-Delirious Confusional States Associated with Psychomotor Underactivity
   A. Associated with a medical or surgical disease (no focal lateralizing neurologic signs; cerebrospinal fluid clear)
      1. Metabolic disorders: hepatic stupor, uremia, hypoxia, hypercapnia, hypoglycemia, porphyria
      2. Infective fevers, especially typhoid
      3. Congestive heart failure
      4. Postoperative, posttraumatic, and puerperal psychoses
   B. Associated with drug intoxication (no focal or lateralizing signs; cerebrospinal fluid clear): opiates, barbiturates, bromides, Artane, etc.
   C. Associated with diseases of the nervous system (the focal or lateralizing neurologic signs and cerebrospinal fluid changes of these conditions are commoner than in delirium)
      1. Cerebral vascular disease, tumor, abscess
      2. Subdural hematoma
      3. Meningitis
      4. Encephalitis
      5. Preexisting neurologic disease (e.g., senile dementia) complicated by a medical or surgical disease
   D. Beclouded dementia, i.e., senile brain disease in combination with infective fevers, drug reactions, heart failure, etc.

III. Korsakoff's amnestic syndrome
   A. Deficiency of thiamine
      1. Alcoholic disorders with peculiar dietary habits, gastrointestinal diseases, etc.
   B. Subarachnoid hemorrhage from ruptured aneurysms
   C. Tumors and infective granulomas in walls of the third ventricle
   D. Bilateral post-cerebral artery occlusion
   E. Inclusion-body encephalitis

With reference to the differential diagnosis acute delirious confusional states, one must also have a secure approach because such illnesses are observed almost daily on the medical and surgical wards of a general hospital. Occurring as they do during an infective fever, in the course of another illness such as cardiac failure, or following an injury, operation, or the excessive use of alcohol, they never fail to create grave problems for the physician, the nursing personnel, and the family. The physician often has to diagnose without the advantage of a lucid history, and his program of treatment may constantly be threatened by the patient's agitation, sleeplessness, and uncooperative attitude. The nursing personnel are often sorely taxed by the necessity of providing a satisfactory environment for the convalescence of the patient and, at the same time, maintaining a tranquil atmosphere for the other patients on the ward. And the family is appalled by the sudden specter of insanity and all it entails.

Under such circumstances, it is a great temptation to rid oneself of the clinical problem by transferring the patient to a psychiatric hospital. This, in the author's opinion, is an unwise action, for it may result in the inexpert management of the underlying medical disease and may even jeopardize the patient's life. It is far better for the physician to assume full responsibility for the care of such patients and to familiarize himself with management of this group of nervous disorders.

The first step in diagnosis is to recognize that the patient is confused. This is obvious in most cases, but, as pointed out above, the mildest form of confusion, particularly when some other acute alteration of personality is prominent, may be overlooked. In these mild forms a careful analysis of the patient's thinking as he gives the history of his illness and the details of his personal life will usually reveal an incoherence. Digit span and serial subtraction of 7s from 100 are useful bedside tests of the patient's capacity for sustained mental activity. Memory of recent events is one of the most delicate tests of adequate mental function and may be accomplished by having the patient relate all the details of his entry to the hospital, laboratory tests, etc.

Once it is established that the patient is confused, the differential diagnosis must be made between delirium, simple or primary mental confusion, a beclouded dementia, and Korsakoff's psychosis. This can be done usually by careful attention to the patient's degree of alertness and wakefulness, his capacity to solve new problems, his memory, accuracy of perception, and hallucinations. The presence of Korsakoff's psychosis may not become evident until the patient's general state improves. The distinction between confusional states and dementia is also difficult at times. It has been said that the patient with the acute confusional psychosis has a clouded sensorium, i.e., he is inattentive, and inclined to inaccurate perceptions and hallucinations, whereas the patient with dementia has a clear sensorium. However, it is the authors' impression that many severely demented patients are as beclouded as those with confusional psychoses, and that the two conditions are at times indistinguishable, except for their different time courses. All this suggests that the parts of the nervous system affected may be the same in both conditions. When the physician is faced with this problem, the history of the mode of onset becomes of great value. The confusional psychosis has an acute or subacute onset and is usually reversible, whereas dementia is always chronic and tends to be more or less irreversible.

Once a case has been classified as delirium, primary mental confusion, or Korsakoff's psychosis, it is important to determine its clinical associations. A thorough medical and neurologic examination and often a lumbar puncture should be done. The other medical and neurologic findings are of great value in indicating the underlying disease to be treated, and they also give information concerning prognosis. In the neurologic examination, particular attention should be given to language functions, visual fields and visual-spatial discriminations, cortical sensory functions, and calculation and other test performances that require normal functioning of the temporal, parietal, and occipital lobes. Confusional states are frequent with diseases of these parts of the brain. Moreover, some of the signs of the latter are often mistaken for a confusional psychosis.

Schizophrenia and manic-depressive psychosis can usually be separated from the confusional stress by the presence of a clear sensorium and good memory.

The treatment is directed to eradicating or controlling the underlying disease process.

CARE OF THE DELIRIOUS AND CONFUSED PATIENT

The primary therapeutic effort in treating the delirious and confused patient in a general hospital is to control the underlying medical disease. Delirum seldom lasts more than a few days, and if the patient can be kept on a medical ward, the social stigma that attaches to incarceration in a mental institution is avoided. In the author's experience only a few delirious patients are so agitated and noisy as to annoy others, and should this happen, many general hospitals now have some facilities for isolating the mentally disturbed patient. Delirium of this severity is rare in infectious diseases but is, of course, not infrequent in alcoholism (delirium tremens), drug intoxication, and other medical diseases.

Important objectives are to quiet the patient and protect him against injury. A private nurse, an attendant, or a member of the family should be with the patient at all times, if this can be arranged. Depending on how active and vigorous he is, a locked room, screened windows that cannot be opened by the patient, and a low bed or mattress on the floor should be arranged. It is often better to let the patient walk about the room than to tie him into bed, which may excite or frighten him so that he struggles to the point of complete exhaustion and collapse. If he is less active, the patient can usually be kept in bed by leather wrist restraints, a restraining sheet, or a net thrown over the bed. Unless contraindicated by the primary disease, the patient should be permitted to sit up or walk about the room part of the day.

All drugs that could possibly be responsible for delirium—particularly opiates, barbiturates, bromides, atro-pine, hyoscine, cortisone, adrenocorticotropic hormone (ACTH), and salicylates in large doses—should be discontinued (unless withdrawal effects are believed to underlie the illness). Paraldehyde and chloral hydrate are the only sedatives that can be trusted under these circumstances. Paraldehyde, which is preferred, may be given orally or rectally in doses of 10 to 12 ml. For oral administration, mixing it with fruit juices makes it more palatable, though alcoholic patients will take it in any form and seem to enjoy it. Chlorpromazine, chlordiazep-oxide, and diazepam are often extremely effective if given in full doses, and should be continued until natural sleep is restored. One must be cautious in attempting to suppress agitation completely. To accomplish this may require very large doses of drugs, and vital functions may be dangerously impaired. The purpose of sedation is to assure rest and sleep so that the patient does not exhaust himself. Continuous warm baths or warm packs are also effective in quieting the delirious patient, but very few general hospitals have proper facilities for this valuable method of treatment.

A fluid intake and output chart should be kept, and any fluid and electrolyte deficit should be corrected according to the methods outlined in Chap. 296. The pulse and blood pressure should be recorded at intervals of 2 hr in anticipation of circulatory collapse. Transfusions of whole blood and vasopressor drugs may be lifesaving.

Finally, the physician should be aware of many small therapeutic measures that may allay fear and suspicion and reduce the tendency to hallucinations. The room should be kept well lighted, and if possible, the patient should not be moved from one room to another. Every procedure should be explained in detail, even such simple ones as the taking of blood pressure or temperature. The presence of a member of the family may enable the patient to maintain contact with reality.

It may be some consolation and also a source of professional satisfaction to remember that most delirious patients tend to recover if they are placed in good hygienic surroundings and competently nursed. The family should be reassured on this point. They must also understand that the abnormal behavior and irrational actions of the patient are not wilful but rather are symptomatic of a brain disease.

See also Chapter 31 for care of demented patient.

REFERENCES

Bonhoeffer, K.: Die Psychosen in Gefolge von akuten Infektionen, etc. in "Handbach der Psychiatrie," G. L. Aschaffenburg (Ed.), Spez. Teil 3, pp. 1–60, Leipzig, 1912.

Lipowski, Z. J.: Delirium, Clouding of Consciousness and confusion. J. Nervous Mental Dis., 145:227, 1967.

Romani, J., and G. L. Engel: Physiologic and Psychologic Considerations of Delirium, Med. Clinics N. Am. 28:629, 1944.

Whitty, C. W. M., and O. L. Zangwill (Eds), "Amnesia," London, Butterworth & Co. (Publishers), Ltd., 1966.

Wolff, H. G., and D. Curran: Nature of Delirium and Allied States, Arch. Neurol. Psychiat., 33:1175–1935.

31 DERANGEMENTS OF INTELLECT AND BEHAVIOR INCLUDING DEMENTIA AND OTHER CEREBRAL DEFECT SYNDROMES

Raymond D. Adams and
Maurice Victor

Increasingly, as the number of elderly adults in our population rises, the internist is consulted because an otherwise healthy individual begins to lose his capacity to function effectively as head of a family or as a worker. This may have several significations—indicating the beginning of a brain tumor, the formation of a chronic subdural hematoma, or the development of a chronic drug intoxication, a chronic meningoencephalitis (syphilis), degenerative cerebral disease, a chronic low-pressure hydrocephalus, a degenerative brain disease, or a depressive psychosis. In former times when there was little that could be done about any of these clinical states no great premium was attached to diagnosis. But modern medicine now offers the means of treating several of these conditions and in some instances of restoring the patient to normal health and effectiveness. Early recognition of the underlying pathologic process improves chances of recovery. For this reason and because of the frequency of these problems every practicing physician stands a chance of becoming involved.

The following information will be helpful in understanding the nature of some of these clinical problems.

THE CLINICAL SYNDROME OF DEMENTIA

In current neurologic parlance the term *dementia* usually denotes a clinical state comprised of failing memory and loss of other intellectual functions due to chronic progressive degenerative disease of the brain. It may or may not be associated with signs of disease in one or more of the motor, sensory, or speech areas of the cerebrum. The chronicity of the process is ordinarily emphasized, but the illogic of setting apart any one constellation of cerebral symptoms on the basis of their speed of onset or duration is obvious. We would like to propose that the state of dementia be regarded as a generic syndrome of multiple causation and mechanism, and that a degeneration of neurones is only one of the causes.

The earliest signs of dementia may be so subtle as to escape the notice of even the most discerning physician. Often an observant relative of the patient or an employer is the first to become aware of a certain lack of initiative, irritability, loss of interest, and inability to perform up to the usual standard. Later there is distractibility, inability to think with accustomed clarity, reduced general comprehension, perseveration in speech, action, and thought, and defective memory, especially for recent events. Frequently a change in mood becomes apparent, deviating more often toward depression than elation. The direction of this deviation is said to depend on the previous personality of the patient rather than upon the character of the disease. Excessive lability of mood may also be observed, i.e., an easy fluctuation from laughter to tears on slight provocation. Moral and ethical standards are lost, early in some cases and late in others. Paranoid ideas and delusions may develop. As a rule, the patient has little or no realization of these changes in himself; he lacks insight. As the condition progresses, there is loss of almost all intellectual faculties, with mental retardation and extreme incoherence and irrationality. Mutism, unresponsiveness, dysarthria, aphasia, and sphincteric incontinence may be added to the clinical picture. In a late stage a secondary physical deterioration also takes place. Food intake, which may be increased in the beginning of the illness, is in the end usually limited, with resulting emaciation. Any febrile illness or metabolic upset induces stupor or coma, indicating the precarious state of cerebral compensation. Finally the patient remains in bed most of the time and dies of pneumonia or some other intercurrent infection. This whole process may evolve over a period of months or years, usually the latter.

Many of these alterations of behavior are the direct result of disease of the nervous system; expressed in another way, the symptoms are the primary manifestations of neurologic disease; others are secondary, they are reactions to the catastrophe of losing one's mind. For example, the dement is said to seek solitude to hide his affliction and may thus appear asocial or apathetic. Again, excessive orderliness may be an attempt to compensate for failing memory; apprehension, gloom, or irritability may express general dissatisfaction with a necessarily restricted life. It would appear that even in a state of fairly advanced deterioration, the patient is still capable of reacting to his illness and to the individuals who care for him.

Attempts to relate loss of memory and failing intellectual function to lesions in certain parts of the brain have been eminently unsuccessful. Two types of difficulty have obstructed progress in this field. (1) There is the problem of defining, analyzing, and determining the significance of the so-called "intellectual" functions. (2) The morbid anatomy of these diseases is so diffuse and complex that it cannot be fully localized and quantitated.

In the most careful analyses of the intellectual functions, certain general and certain specific factors have been isolated. The general factors are not localized at the moment to any one area of the brain, whereas the specific ones do have at least a regional localization in the cerebrum. Spearman, Thurstone, and others have been able to single out a number of specific factors such as verbal capacity, ability to appreciate spatial relationships, ability to learn and to reason inductively and deductively, facility in the use of numbers and in numerical calculation, and retentive memory. All these qualities are tested in standard intelligence and achievement tests. Memory correlates poorly with all the other factors and seems to be an independent item. There is an intercorrelation between all the other factors. In other words, a person who performs well in tests of verbal capacity tends to do well on tests of spatial orientation, numerical relationships, learning, and reasoning. Some general factor, ?G factor of Spearman, is being measured by each test and determines in part the level of performance. In addition, there are special aptitudes or factors (S. factors of Spearman) that account for individual superiorities' or (in disease) inferiorities in one or another test.

Morbid Anatomy and Pathologic Physiology of Dementia

In dementia the memory impairment, which is a constant feature, may occur with extensive disease in any part of the cerebrum. Yet it is interesting to note that the function of certain parts of the diencephalon and of the hippocampi may be more fundamental to retentive memory than the rest of the cortex, and as will be pointed out below, it may be certain of the corticothalamic connections that are particularly concerned with this function. Failure in tests of verbal function (the most advanced degree of which is aphasia) is closely associated with disease of the dominant cerebral hemisphere, and particularly the speech areas in the frontal, temporal, and parietal lobes and insula. Loss of capacity for arithmetic, reading, and numerical calculation (acalculia) is related to lesions in the posterior part of the left (dominant) cerebral hemisphere. Impairment in drawing or constructing simple and complex figures with blocks, sticks, picture arrangements, etc., as shown by tests of visual construction is most pronounced in right (nondominant) parietal lobe lesions, as will be pointed out below. Thus, the clinical picture resulting from cerebral disease depends in part on the extent of the lesion, i.e., the amount of cerebral tissue destroyed, and on the specific locality of the lesion.

Dementia is related usually to obvious structural disease of the cerebrum and the diencephalon. Knowledge of the detailed anatomy of the diencephalic nuclei and their connections with one another and with the various parts of the cerebral cortex is so limited that it has thus far been impossible to define either the topography of many of the diseases with which we are concerned or the nature of the lesion. In some diseases, such as Alzheimer's and Pick's presenile or senile dementia, the main process appears to be a degeneration and loss of nerve cells in the association areas, with secondary changes in the cerebral white matter. In others, such as Huntington's chorea, Jakob-Creutzfeldt pseudosclerosis, and the cerebrobasal ganglionic and cerebrocerebellar degenerations, loss of neurones in the cerebral cortex is accompanied by a similar degeneration of neurones in the putamen and caudate nuclei and the cerebellum, respectively. Arteriosclerotic vascular disease results in multiple foci of infarction all through the thalami, basal ganglions, brainstem, and cerebrum and, in the latter, in the motor, sensory, or visual projection areas as well as in the association areas. Severe trauma may cause contusions of cerebral convolutions and degeneration of the central white matter (Strich), which result in protracted stupor, coma, or dementia (rare). Most diseases that produce dementia are quite extensive, and the frontal lobes are affected more often than other parts of the cerebrum.

Other mechanisms than the destruction of brain tissue may operate in some cases. Chronic increased intracranial pressure or chronic hydrocephalus (with large ventricles the pressure may not exceed 180 mm), regardless of cause, is often associated with a general impairment of mental function. There the factor of compression of tracts in the cerebral white matter is the main factor. The compression of one or both cerebral hemispheres by chronic subdural hematomas may cause a widespread disturbance of cortical function. A diffuse inflammatory process is at least in part the basis for dementia in syphilis and in neurotropic virus infections such as "inclusion body encephalitis." Presumably there is loss of neurones and also inflammatory derangement of the function of others. Lastly, several of the toxic and metabolic diseases discussed in Chap. 26 may interfere with nervous function over a long period of time and create a clinical picture similar to, if not identical with, that of dementia. One must suppose that the altered biochemical environment has affected the excitability of the neurones.

(The details of all the diseases which cause dementia will be found in Chaps. 363 and 364.)

Bedside Classification of Dementing Diseases of the Brain

The conventional classification of dementing diseases of the brain is usually according to etiology, if known, or pathology. Another more practical approach, which follows logically from the method by which the whole subject has been presented in this book, is to subdivide the diseases into three categories on the basis of the associated clinical and laboratory signs of medical disease and the accompanying neurologic signs. Once the physician has determined that the patient suffers a dementing illness, he must then decide, from the medical, neurologic, and laboratory data, into which category the case fits. This classification may at first seem somewhat artificial. However, it is likely to be more useful to the student or physician not conversant with the many diseases that cause dementia than a classification based on pathology.

CLASSIFICATION

I. Diseases in which dementia is usually associated with clinical and laboratory signs of other medical disease
   A. Hypothyroidism
   B. Cushing's disease
   C. Nutritional deficiency states such as pellagra, Wernicke's disease and Korsakoff's syndrome, pernicious anemia, and subacute degeneration of spinal cord and brain
   D. Neurosyphilis: general paresis and meningovascular syphilis
   E. Hepatolenticular degeneration
   F. Cerebral arteriosclerosis (coronary disease, pseudobulbar symptoms)
   G. Bromidism

II. Diseases in which dementia is associated with other neurologic signs but not with other obvious medical disease
   A. Invariably associated with other neurologic signs
      1. Huntington's chorea (choreoathetosis)

2. Schilder's disease and related demyelinative diseases (spastic weakness, pseudobulbar palsy, blindness, deafness)
3. Amaurotic family idiocy and other lipid-storage diseases (myoclonic seizures, blindness, spasticity, cerebellar ataxia)
4. Myoclonic epilepsy (diffuse myoclonus, generalized seizures, cerebellar ataxia)
5. Jakob-Creutzfeldt disease (diffuse myoclonus)
6. Cerebrocerebellar degeneration (cerebellar ataxia)
7. Cerebral-basal ganglia degeneration (apraxia-rigidity)
8. Dementia with spastic paraplegia (spastic legs)

B. Often associated with other neurologic signs
1. Cerebral arteriosclerosis
2. Brain tumor
3. Brain trauma, such as cerebral contusion, mid-brain hemorrhage, chronic subdural hematoma

III. Diseases in which dementia is usually the only evidence of neurologic or medical disease
A. Alzheimer's disease and senile dementia
B. Pick's disease
C. Marchiafava-Bignami disease (sometimes with frontal lobe signs)
D. Some cases of brain tumor of frontal lobes and corpus callosum
E. Low-pressure hydrocephalus

Many of these diseases are discussed more fully in other sections of this book. The special features of the dementia that accompanies arteriosclerotic, senile, syphilitic, traumatic, nutritional, and degenerative diseases are discussed in the appropriate chapters.

Differential Diagnosis

The first difficulty in dealing with this class of patients is to make sure of deterioration of intellect and personality change. It may be necessary to examine the patient several times before one is confident of the clinical findings.

There is always a tendency to assume that mental function is normal if patients complain only of nervousness, fatigue, insomnia, or vague somatic symptoms and to label the patients psychoneurotic. *This will be avoided if one keeps in mind that psychoneuroses rarely begin in middle or late adult life.* A practical rule is to assume that all mental illnesses beginning during this period are due either to structural disease of the brain or to depressive psychosis.

A mild dysphasia must not be mistaken for dementia. The aphasic patient appears uncertain of himself, and his speech may be incoherent. Furthermore, he may be anxious and depressed over his ineptitude. Careful attention to the patient's language performance will lead to the correct diagnosis in most instances. Further observation will disclose the fact that the patient's behavior, except for speech, is within normal limits.

The depressed patient presents another type of problem. He may remark that his mental function is poor or that he is forgetful and cannot concentrate. Scrutiny of his remarks will show, however, that he actually remembers all the details of his illness and that no qualitative change in mental ability has taken place. His difficulty is either a lack of energy and interest or an anxiety that prevents the focusing of attention on anything except his own problems. Even during mental tests his performance may be impaired by his emotions, in much the same way as that of the worried student during his examinations. This condition of emotional blocking is called *experiential confusion.* When the patient is calmed by reassurance, his mental function is normal, a proof that intellectual deterioration has not occurred. The hypomanic patient fails in tests of intellectual function because of his restlessness and distractibility. It is helpful to remember that the demented patient rarely has sufficient insight to complain of mental deterioration; and if he admits to poor memory, he seldom realizes the degree of his disability. The physician must never rely on the patient's statements as to the efficiency of mental function and must always evaluate a poor performance on tests in the light of the emotional state and motivation at the time the test is given.

The neurologic syndrome associated with metabolic or endocrine disorders, i.e., ACTH therapy, hyperthyroidism, Cushing's disease, Addison's disease, or the postpartum state may be difficult to diagnose because of the wide variety of clinical pictures that may be shown. As will be stated in Chap. 372, some patients appear to be suffering from a dementia, others from an acute confusional psychosis; or if mood change or negativism predominate, a manic-depressive psychosis or schizophrenia is suggested. In these conditions some degree of clouding of sensorium and impairment of intellectual function can usually be recognized, and these findings alone should be enough to exclude schizophrenia and manic-depressive psychosis. It is well to remember that acute onset of mental symptoms always suggests confusional psychosis or delirium. Inasmuch as many of these conditions are completely reversible, they must be distinguished from dementia.

Once it is decided that the patient suffers from a dementing disease, the next step is to determine by careful physical examination whether there are other neurologic signs or indications of a particular medical disease. This enables the physician to place the case in one of the three categories in the bedside classification. X-rays of skull, electroencephalogram, lumbar puncture and pneumoencephalogram should be carried out in most cases. Usually these procedures necessitate admission to a hospital. The final step is to determine by the total clinical picture which disease within any one category the patient has. Table 372-1 and 2 shows the major points in differential diagnosis.

SPECIAL SYNDROMES CAUSED BY DISEASES OF PARTS OF THE CEREBRUM

Symptoms and signs of disease of one part of the cerebrum may occur singly or in combination with dementia, and they provide important information about the location of a disease process and at times about its nature. This is an appropriate place, therefore, to review briefly the known effects of disease of different parts of the cerebrum. Agnosia, apraxia, and aphasia will be only mentioned, since they are treated more extensively in Chaps. 25, 29, and 357.

FRONTAL LOBES. In Fig. 31-1, it may be seen that the frontal lobes lie anterior to the central, or Rolandic, sulcus and superior to the Sylvian fissure. They consist of several functionally different parts, which are conventionally designated in the neurologic literature by numbers (according to a scheme devised by Brodmann) and by letters (in the scheme of von Economo and Koskinas).

The posterior parts, areas 4 and 6 of Brodmann, are specifically related to motor function. Voluntary movement in man depends on the integrity of these areas, and lesions in them produce spastic paralysis of the contralateral face, arm, and leg. This is discussed in Chap. 21, Motor Paralysis. Lesions limited more or less to the premotor areas (area 6) are accompanied by prominent grasp and sucking reflexes. Lesions in areas 8 and 24 of Brodmann interfere with the mechanism concerned with turning the head and eyes contralaterally. Lesions in areas 44 and 45 of the major hemisphere abolish or reduce verbalization, deglutition, and chewing. Lesions in area 44 of the dominant cerebral hemisphere, usually the left one, have often resulted in loss of verbal expression, the aphasia of Broca. Lesions in the medial limbic or piriform cortex (areas 23 and 24), wherein lie the mechanisms controlling respiration, circulation, and micturition have relatively unclear clinical effects.

The remainder of the frontal lobes (areas 9, 10, 11, 12, and 13 of Brodmann), sometimes called the *prefrontal areas*, have less specific and measurable functions. The following groups of symptoms have been observed in patients with diseases limited to one or both frontal lobes or to the central white matter and anterior part of the corpus callosum by which they are joined.

1. Change of personality, usually expressed as lack of concern over the consequences of any action, which may take the form of a childish excitement (moria of Jastrowitz), an inappropriate joking and punning (*witzelsucht* of Oppenheim), or an instability and superficiality of emotion, or irritability.

2. Slight impairment of intelligence, usually described as lack of concentration, vacillation of attention, inability to carry out planned activity, difficulty in changing from one activity to another, loss of recent memory, or lack of initiative and spontaneity.

3. Motor abnormalities such as decomposition of gait and upright stance, trunk ataxia of Bruns, abnormal postures, reflex grasping or sucking, incontinence of sphincters, and akinetic mutism.

The most pronounced changes have been observed in cases with bilateral disease of frontal lobes, and there has been much doubt as to the effect of a lesion involving only one frontal lobe. Nevertheless, the most careful psychologic tests on patients with lesions of either frontal lobe demonstrate a slight elevation of mood with increased talkativeness and tendency to joke, a lack of tact, inability to adapt to a new situation, and loss of initiative.

Several careful studies of lobotomized patients have

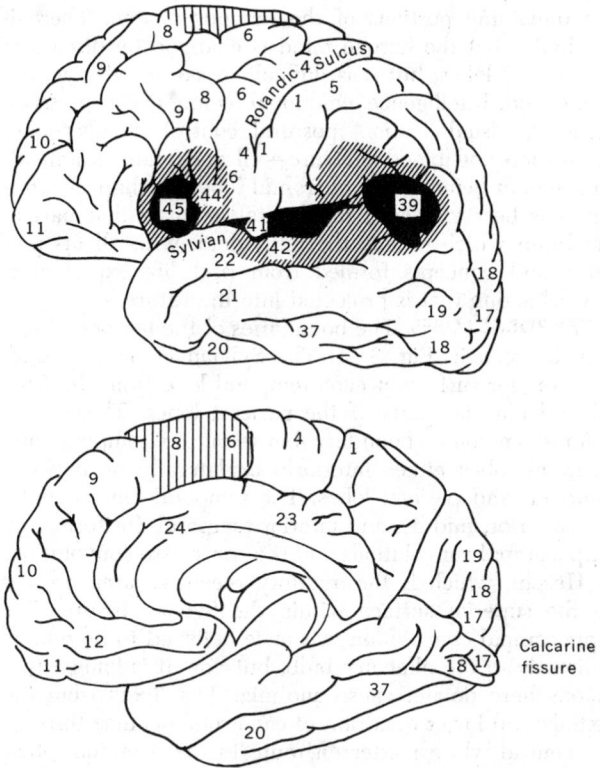

Fig. 31-1. Diagram to show cortical areas, numbered according to the scheme of Brodmann. The speech areas are in black, the three main ones being 39, 41, and 45. The zone marked by vertical stripes in the superior frontal convolution is the secondary motor area which, like Broca's area 45, if stimulated causes vocal arrest. (Redrawn from "Handbuch der Inneren Medizin," Berlin, Springer-Verlag, 1939.)

now been published. Of course, very few of these patients were normal before the operation, so that base-line measurements of mental ability were not always obtainable. However, some patients of normal intellect have received this treatment for severe neurosis or intractable pain. They are said to have shown little or no loss of ability in their performance on intelligence tests, depending on the extent of the procedure; and if worry, fears, compulsions, and suffering from pain were incapacitating, the loss of these traits resulted in test scores actually higher than before the operation. However, careful examination usually will disclose a slight lowering of general intelligence, a decrease in drive or energy, a definite change of personality in the form of shallow emotional life, a lack of tact, and inability to direct and sustain activity toward future goals. Also there is a diminution of traits related to neuroticism, such as suggestibility, rigidity of character, self-criticism, and introversion.

The function of the frontal lobes cannot be determined simply by the study of human beings who have suffered injury or disease of this part of the brain. Symptoms from lesions of a part of the nervous system are not identical with the functions of that part. The symptoms of frontal lobe deficit must depend both on a loss of certain parts of the cerebrum and on the functional activity of the remaining portions of the nervous system. There is no doubt that the human mind is changed by disease of the frontal lobes, but it is difficult to say in what way it is changed. Intelligence, emotional feeling and expression, memory, visual fixation, postural control, regulation of respiration and blood pressure—all are intact in animals and human beings without frontal lobes. Perhaps at present it is best to regard the frontal lobes as that part of the brain which orients the individual, with all his percepts and concepts formed from past life experiences, toward action that is projected into the future.

TEMPORAL LOBES. The boundaries of the temporal lobes may be seen in Fig. 31-1. The Sylvian fissure separates the superior surface of each temporal lobe from the frontal and anterior parts of the parietal lobes. There is no definite anatomic boundary between the temporal and occipital lobes either inferiorly or laterally or between temporal and parietal lobes. The temporal lobe includes the superior, middle, and inferior temporal, fusiform, and hippocampal convolutions and the transverse convolutions of Heschl, which is the auditory receptive area present on the superior surface within the Sylvian fissure. The hippocampal convolution was once believed to be related indirectly to the olfactory bulb, but now it is known that lesions here do not cause anosmia. The fibers from the homolateral lower quadrant of each retina course through the central white matter en route to the occipital lobes, and lesions that interrupt them characteristically produce a contralateral homonymous upper quadrant defect of visual fields. Hearing and labyrinthine function, also localized in the temporal lobes, are bilaterally represented, which accounts for the fact that unless both temporal lobes are affected, there is no demonstrable loss of hearing. Loss of equilibrium has not been observed with temporal lobe lesions. Extensive disease in the superior and middle convolutions of the left temporal lobe in right-handed individuals results in Wernicke's aphasia. This syndrome, discussed in Chap. 29, Affections of Speech, consists of jargon aphasia and inability to read, to write, or to understand the meaning of spoken words. Probably the basic defect in all these is the loss of memory for words.

Between the auditory and olfactory projection areas there is a large expanse of temporal lobe which has no assignable function. This is the temporal association area. Patients with tumors and vascular lesions of this part of the brain have been examined on numerous occasions, but usually the full extent of the disease has not been determined, even by pneumoencephalography, arteriography, or isotopic scanning procedures. Cases of temporal lobectomy for tumor have provided more valuable material, but again it has seldom been possible to be certain that other parts of the brain were not involved. The most careful psychologic studies have shown a difference between cases involving loss of the dominant and the nondominant temporal lobe. With lesions of the dominant side there is impairment in learning verbal material presented aloud; with nondominant lesions there is a similar failure in tests with visually presented material. In addition, about 20 percent of both right and left lobectomy patients have shown a syndrome similar to that described

for the prefrontal parts of the brain; but more significant is the fact that in the other cases little or no defect in personality was exhibited. The study of cases of uncinate epilepsy, with the characteristic dreamy state, olfactory or gustatory hallucinations, and masticatory movements, suggests that all these functions are organized through the temporal lobes. Similarly, stimulation of the posterior parts of the temporal lobes of epileptic patients during surgical procedures has brought to light the interesting fact that complex memories and visual and auditory images, some with strong emotional content, can be aroused in fully conscious human beings. Recent studies of the effect of stimulation of the amygdaloid nucleus, which is in the anterior and medial part of the temporal lobe, have shed additional light on this subject. Symptoms may be evoked not unlike some of those of schizophrenic patients. Complex emotional experiences that have occurred previously may be revived. There are remarkable autonomic effects. Blood pressure rises, pulse increases, respirations are increased in frequency and depth, and the patient looks frightened. These effects have been discussed in Chap. 28, Recurrent Convulsions. Ablation of these nuclei has eliminated uncontrollable rage reactions in psychotic patients. Excision of the hippocampal and adjacent convolutions bilaterally has been carried out recently, with a disastrous loss of ability to learn new experiences or to establish new memories (Korsakoff's psychosis). All this suggests the important role of the temporal lobes in auditory and visual perception and imagery, in learning and memory, and in the emotional life of the individual.

Bilateral ablation of temporal lobes, so far studied only in monkeys, produces an animal that displays a curious tendency to react to every visual stimulus without seeming to recognize it (psychic blindness) and to examine every object in its environment by oral and manual contact. Placidity, with lack of the usual emotional response to stimuli, was another prominent feature.

To summarize, in man the temporal lobe syndromes include the following:

I. Effects of unilateral disease of the dominant temporal lobe
   A. Quadrantic homonymous anopia
   B. Wernicke's aphasia
   C. Impairment in verbal tests of material presented through the auditory sense
   D. Dysnomia or amnestic aphasia
II. Effects of unilateral disease of nondominant temporal lobe
   A. Quadrantic homonymous anopia
   B. Impairment of mental function with inability to judge spatial relationship in some cases
   C. Impairment in nonverbal tests of visually presented material

PARIETAL LOBES. This part of the human nervous system is the subject of one of the most interesting discussions of cerebral function that has occurred in this century: its role in the formation of the body image or body schema.

It has long been known that the postcentral convolution is the terminus of somatic sensory pathways from the opposite half of the body. It has also been learned that destructive lesions here do not abolish cutaneous sensation but instead cause mainly a defect in sensory discrimination with variable impairment of sensation. In other words, pain, touch, and thermal and vibratory sensation are largely retained, whereas stereognosis, sense of position, distinction between single and double contacts (two-point threshold), and the localization of sensory stimuli are lost. There is also the phenomenon of extinction, viz., if both sides of the body are touched simultaneously, only the stimulus on the normal side is perceived. This type of sensory disturbance, sometimes called *cortical sensory defect*, is discussed in Chap. 25, Disorders of Sensation. Later it was noted that extensive lesions deep in the white matter of the parietal lobes produce a contralateral homonymous hemianopia, and lesions in the angular gyrus of the dominant hemisphere result in an inability to read.

More recent investigations have centered about the function of the parietal lobes in perception of position in space and of the relationship of the various parts of the body to one another. Since the time of Babinski it has been known that patients with a large lesion of the minor parietal lobe are often unaware of their hemiplegia and hemianesthesia. Babinski called this condition *anosognosia*. Related psychologic disorders are lack of recognition of the left arm and leg when seen or felt by the other hand, neglect of the left side of the body in dressing, an imperception of external space on the left side, and constructional apraxia, an inability to perform the movements of constructing simple figures. *Agnosia* and *apraxia* are discussed in Chaps. 21 and 25.

Another frequent constellation of symptoms, usually referred to as *Gerstmann's syndrome*, occurs with lesions of the dominant parietal lobe. This consists of inability to write (agraphia), inability to calculate (acalculia), failure to distinguish right from left, and loss of recognition of various parts of the body. An ideomotor apraxia may or may not be conjoined.

The effects of disease of the parietal lobes differ according to whether the dominant (left hemisphere in a right-handed person) or nondominant lobe is involved. These may be tabulated as follows:

I. Effect of unilateral disease of parietal lobe, right or left
   A. Cortical sensory syndrome and sensory extinction (or total hemianesthesia with large acute lesions of white matter)
   B. Mild hemiparesis, unilateral muscular atrophy in children
   C. Homonymous hemianopia or visual inattention, and sometimes neglect of one-half of external space
   D. Abolition of opticokinetic nystagmus to one side
II. Effects of unilateral disease of dominant parietal lobe (left hemisphere in right-handed patients), additional phenomena
   A. Disorders of language (especially alexia)
   B. Gerstmann's syndrome
   C. Bimanual astereognosis (tactile agnosia)
   D. Bilateral apraxia of ideomotor type
III. Effects of unilateral disease of minor parietal lobe (right

hemisphere in right-handed patients), additional phenomena
   A. Anosognosia
   B. Neglect of left side of body
   C. Neglect of visual space to the left of the midline

In all these lesions, if the disease is sufficiently extensive, there may be a reduction in the capacity to think clearly, inattentiveness, and impairment of memory.

It is impossible at this time to present a formula of parietal lobe function in general. It does seem reasonably certain that both the parietal and occipital lobes participate in sensory functions, especially in those which provide consciousness of one's surroundings, of the relationship of objects in the environment to one another, and of the position of the body in space. In this respect, as C. M. Fisher has suggested, the parietal lobe may be regarded as a suprasensory mechanism for transmodal (intersensory) relationships, particularly tactile and visual, which are the basis of our concepts of space.

OCCIPITAL LOBES. The occipital lobes are the terminus of the visual pathways and are essential for visual sensation and perception. Lesions in one occipital lobe result in homonymous defects in the contralateral visual fields. Bilateral lesions cause cortical blindness, a state of blindness without change in optic fundi or pupillary reflexes. If areas 18 and 19 of Brodmann are affected (Fig. 31-1), there is loss of visual recognition, with retention of some degree of visual acuity, a state termed *visual agnosia,* or *mind blindness.* In the classic form of this blindness an individual with intact mental powers is unable to recognize objects, even though by tests of visual acuity and perimetry he appears to see sufficiently well to do so. Psychologists have demonstrated several special types of visual agnosia. In the simultagnosia of Wolpert, the patient, though able to see the individual parts of a picture, is unable to gather the meaning of the whole. Similarly, in prosopagnosia the patient is unable to recognize a human face even though he sees all the individual details of it. Alexia, or inability to read, and visual spatial agnosia, or inability to recognize actual or abstract space, with resulting disorientation, are other special types of agnosia. Often the patient with bilateral lesions of the occipital lobes (cerebral cortical blindness) is unaware of his visual difficulty, i.e., has an agnosia for it. This state is known as *Anton's syndrome.* In *Holmes' syndrome* visual disorientation may be combined with a homonymous hemianopia. Left occipital lobe lesions in combination with a lesion of splenium of corpus callosum causes alexia without agraphia (see Chap. 29).

This whole problem of both visual and tactile agnosia has recently been reexamined. In most of the reported cases tests of primary visual sensation or visual acuity have been inadequate. By controlling the time factor in visual perception and the adaptation time, and by testing the simultaneous perception of multiple points in the visual field, it is possible to show that the visual function is more often impaired than was at first suspected. The division of the visual process into sensation and perception becomes highly artificial.

Visual function is discussed further in Chap. 24.

CORPUS CALLOSUM. A congenital defect or extensive lesion of the corpus callosum disconnects the dominant cerebral hemisphere which controls speech, praxis, and handedness, from the nondominant. The patient speaks, reads, understands spoken words and writes correctly with the right hand. He uses the right hand skillfully. In contrast the left hand is maladroit; and attempts at writing with the left hand result in an aphasic performance. He can read correctly in the right visual field but not in the left. Objects are identified and named by tactile examination with the right hand but not the left. Verbal commands are performed with the right hand but not the left (apraxia). In bifrontal and corpus callosum lesions (tumor, anterior cerebral infarct, Marchiafava-Bignami disease) a corpus callosum syndrome is combined with bilateral grasp reflexes, abulia, and psychomotor impairment.

DIAGNOSIS OF FOCAL CEREBRAL DISEASE. In summarizing the special effects of disease of different parts of the cerebral hemispheres, several points should be made. Extensive lesions in one or both frontal lobes often encroach on motor areas and, in doing so, cause a weakness of muscle groups on the opposite side of the body. This is especially noticeable in the face and is sometimes more pronounced during emotional expression than on voluntary movement. It may affect the arm and leg as well. In some instances the weakness may be rather slight, and a slowness and stiffness of movement with grasp reflex, slightly increased tendon reflexes, and Babinski's sign on the contralateral side are observed. A rather "absent-minded" type of urinary and fecal incontinence is also frequent. Motor aphasia—an inability to speak—indicates involvement of the inferior frontal convolution of the dominant frontal lobe. Anosmia and blindness are neighborhood symptoms, resulting from extension of a lesion on the orbital surfaces of the frontal lobes to the olfactory bulbs and optic nerves.

An upper quadrantic homonymous anopia is the most reliable sign of disease of either the right or left temporal lobes; this localization should always be considered if dementia and this visual disturbance are conjoined. Uncinate or psychic seizures also establish a temporal lobe lesion but do not indicate the laterality. Bizarre disturbances of thinking and affect, often indistinguishable from schizophrenia, may follow temporal lobe seizures. In lesions of the dominant temporal lobe, Wernicke's aphasia is the most characteristic feature.

Cortical sensory deficit is the common neurologic abnormality in disease of either parietal lobe and is often combined with hemiplegia. With left-sided lesions in the inferior parietal lobule there is alexia and a contralateral homonymous hemianopia. Gerstmann's syndrome localizes a lesion in the more posterior parts of the parietal and the lateral occipital lobes of the dominant hemisphere. The curious disturbances of body awareness or body scheme and of parts of the body to the left of the midline are usually found with lesions of the nondominant parietal lobe. Focal seizures arising in the parietal lobe usually consist of a focal or Jacksonian sensory disturbance.

Occipital lesions are distinguished by the almost exclusive affection of visual functions, a circumstance that rarely occurs in pure form with temporal or parietal lesions. The affection may take the form of homonymous hemianopia or of one of the more complex disorders of visual recognition.

In the syndrome of dementia the components of which vary from one disease to another, one may discern the effects of impaired functioning of the several lobes of the brain, and their defects are maximized, always, by bilaterality of lesion and involvement of corpus callosum. Some of these components, such as amnesia, calculation difficulty, reduced verbal function, altered visual spatial relationships, have localizing value even when present in slight degree. In combination they inform the examiner of the diffuse topography of the cortical lesions. Others such as impairment of capacity to think and reason, reduced impulsivity, altered emotionality have little value in localization.

THE APPROACH TO THE CLINICAL PROBLEM OF CONFUSION AND DEMENTIA

The physician presented with a patient suffering from a diffuse or focal cerebral disease must adopt an examination technique designed to expose fully the intellectual defect. Abnormalities of posture, movement, sensation, and reflexes cannot be relied upon for the full demonstration of the neurologic deficit, for it must be remembered that the association areas of the brain may be severely damaged without demonstrable neurologic signs of this type.

Three categories of data are required for the recognition and differential diagnosis of dementing brain disease:

1. A reliable history of illness
2. Findings on mental examination, i.e., so-called "mental status," as well as on the rest of the neurologic examination.
3. Special laboratory procedures, lumbar puncture, x-rays of the skull, electroencephalogram, and sometimes pneumoencephalogram.

The history should always be supplemented by information obtained from a person other than the patient, because through lack of insight he is often unaware of his illness; indeed, he may be ignorant even of his chief complaint. Special inquiry should be made about the patient's general behavior, capacity for work, personal habits, and such faculties as memory and judgment.

This performance of an examination of the mental status must be systematic. At a minimum it should include the following:

I. Insight (patient's replies to questions about his chief symptoms): What is your difficulty? Are you ill? When did your illness begin?
II. Orientation (knowledge of personal identity and present situation):
   Person: What is your name? What is your occupation? Where do you live? Are you married?

Place: What is the name of the place where you are now? How did you get here? What floor is it on? Where is the bathroom? What are you doing now?

Time: What is the date today? What time of day is it? What meals have you had? When was the last holiday?

III. Memory:

Remote: Tell me the names of your children and their birth dates. When were you married? What was your mother's maiden name? What was the name of your first school teacher?

Recent past: Tell me about your recent illness (compare with previous statements). What did you have for breakfast today? What is my name or the nurse's name? When did you see me for the first time. What were the headlines in the newspaper today? Give the patient a simple story orally or written and ask him to retell it after 3 to 5 min.

Retention: Repeat these numbers after me (give series of 3,4,5,6,7,8 digits at speed of 1 per second). Now when I give a series of numbers, repeat them in reverse order.

Visual span: Show the patient a picture of several objects and then ask him to name what he has seen and to note any inaccuracies.

IV. General information: Ask about names of presidents, well-known historic dates, the names of large rivers, of large cities, etc.

V. Capacity for sustained mental activity:

Calculation: Test ability to add, subtract, multiply, and divide. Subtraction of serial 7s from 100 is a good test of calculation as well as of attention.

Abstract thinking: See if the patient can detect similarities and differences between classes of objects, or explain a proverb or a fable.

VI. General behavior: Attitudes, general bearing, stream of thought, attentiveness, mood, manner of dress, etc.

VII. Special tests of localized cerebral functions: grasping, sucking, aphasia battery, praxis with both hands, cortical sensory function, drawing of clock face, map of U.S.A., or Europe, floor plan of house, etc.

In order to enlist the patient's full cooperation, the physician must prepare him for questions of this type. Otherwise, the first reaction will be one of embarrassment or anger because of the implication that his mind is not sound. It should be pointed out to the patient that some individuals are rather forgetful and that it is necessary to ask specific questions in order to form some impression about their degree of nervousness when being examined. Reassurance that these are not tests of intelligence or of sanity is helpful.

A more formal and reliable method of examining the mental capacity of adults is the Wechsler-Bellevue test. This can be given by a psychologist or by the physician if he has carefully read the instructions for administering and scoring the test. The *Mental Examiners' Handbook*, by F. L. Wells and J. Ruesch, published by the Psychological Corporation, is helpful to those not familiar with this type of examination. Tests of retention of verbal material and the recall of a series of learned digits or of visually presented objects are of value in estimating the degree of deterioration. In the Wechsler-Bellevue test the discrepancy between the vocabulary, picture completion, information, and object assembly tests as a group (these correlate well with premorbid intelligence and are relatively insensitive to dementing brain disease) and arithmetic, block design, digit span, and digit-symbol tests provide an index of deterioration.

Although the form of confusion or dementia does not indicate a particular disease, certain combinations of symptoms and neurologic signs are more or less characteristic and may aid in diagnosis. The mode of onset, the clinical course, the associated neurologic signs, and the accessory laboratory data constitute the basis of differential diagnosis. It must be admitted, however, that some of the rarer types of "degenerative" brain disease are at present recognized only by pathologic examination. The correct diagnosis of treatable forms of senile (over sixty years of age) or presenile (forty to sixty years) dementias, such as general paresis, subdural hematoma, brain tumor, bromide or other chronic drug intoxication, normal pressure hydrocephalus, pellagra and related deficiency states, and hypothyroidism, is of greater practical importance than the diagnosis of the untreatable ones.

MANAGEMENT OF THE DEMENTED PATIENT. Dementia is a clinical state of the most serious nature, and usually it is worthwhile to admit the patient to the hospital for a period of observation. The physician then has an opportunity to see him several times in a new and fairly constant hospital environment, and certain special procedures such as x-rays of the skull, lumbar puncture, analysis of blood for drugs, basal metabolic rate, an electroencephalogram, and often a pneumoencephalogram can be carried out at this time. The management of the demented patient in the hospital may be relatively simple if he is quiet and cooperative. If the disorder of mental function is severe, a nurse, attendant, or member of the family must stay with him at all times. Provision must be made for adequate food and fluid intake and control of infection, using the same measures outlined for the delirious patient.

Once it is established that the patient has an untreatable dementing brain disease, a responsible member of the family should be apprised of the medical facts. The patient should be told that he has a nervous condition for which he is to be given rest and treatment. Nothing is accomplished by telling him more. The family should be given the prognosis, if the diagnosis is sufficiently certain for this to be done. If the dementia is slight and circumstances are suitable, the patient may remain at home, continuing activities of which he is capable. He should be spared responsibility and guarded against injury that might result from imprudent action. If he is still at work, plans for occupational retirement should be carried out. In more advanced stages of the disease mental and physical enfeeblement become pronounced and institutional care should be advised. Seizures should be treated symptomatically. Nerve tonics, vitamins, and hormones are of no value in checking the course of the illness or in regenerating decayed tissue. They may, however, offer some support to the patient and family. Sometimes stimulants in the form of dextroamphetamine, caffeine and nicotinic acid cause transitory improvement in mental function. Undesirable restlessness, nocturnal wandering, belligerency or anxiety may be reduced by some of the tranquilizing drugs (see Chap. 121).

Section 4

Alterations in Circulatory and Respiratory Function

32 DYSPNEA
Harry W. Fritts, Jr.

While resting quietly a normal man breathes with effortless ease. His rhythm is leisurely and somewhat irregular; his frequency is usually below 16 breaths per minute; and if he is of average size, his tidal volume is less than 600 ml. To generate this flow of air he expends a very small amount of energy. Indeed, Otis, Fenn, and Rahn have estimated that the calories needed for 24 hr of quiet breathing are fewer than those contained in an ordinary bar of candy. Translated into more precise terms, this indicates that the respiratory muscles of a resting man utilize less than 2 percent of the total energy consumed by the body. It is, therefore, not surprising that quiet breathing is a largely subconscious process.

Even when exercise lifts breathing to the conscious level the normal man does not find the sensation unpleasant. He may complain of breathlessness as he approaches the point of exhaustion, but his discomfort is ameliorated by a feeling of exhilaration or accomplishment. If, however, airflow is artificially impeded, or if ventilatory motion is restricted by strapping his chest and abdomen, awareness of breathing becomes a sensation of distress. Such distress has been characterized by the word *dyspnea*, derived from the Greek roots *dys* (hard) and *pnoe* (breathing). Thus, in its broadest context *dyspnea* denotes an unpleasant awareness of breathing, ranging in intensity from mild discomfort to agony.

Although *dyspnea* has never been a precise term, its current meaning is ambiguous because the word is used in two different ways. On the one hand physicians remark, "The patient complained of dyspnea," while on the other they say, "The patient appeared dyspneic." In the first instance the physician substitutes the noun *dyspnea* for the words used by the patient to describe his symptoms; in the second he employs the adjective *dyspneic* to describe an observed abnormality in the breathing pattern of the patient. Though the choice of definitions is a matter of personal preference, ambiguity can be minimized by using *dyspnea* to denote the overall subject of uncomfortable breathing, by using the words of the patient to describe his symptoms, and by employing precise terms to characterize the breathing pattern, e.g., "a rapid rate with small tidal volumes." This approach has the advantage of separating signs from symptoms, an important distinction because the two are often poorly correlated. Some patients with seemingly normal ventilatory patterns complain bitterly of distress, while others with obviously abnormal frequencies and tidal volumes deny symptoms. As stressed by Gaensler, the patient's account of his discomfort involves many factors, including intelligence, ability to articulate sensations, and threshold for sensory stimuli.

Quantification

Like pain, respiratory discomfort cannot be measured directly, although a number of indices have been devised to predict when discomfort will appear. Three of the most popular have been the Breathing Reserve, the Walking Ventilation, and the Dyspnea Index. All three relate the minute volume of ventilation (MVV) to the maximum breathing capacity (MBC), and all provide information about the fraction of the capacity actually being utilized. For instance the Breathing Reserve, calculated as the difference between the MBC and the MVV, represents the amount of the capacity still available to the person. This amount is customarily expressed as a percentage of the MBC by the following simple formula:

$$\% = \frac{MBC - MVV}{MBC} \times 100$$

Although there is considerable individual variability, most people are asymptomatic when the calculated index is above 70 percent, and most are aware of their breathing when the index is below this level. Accordingly, an average normal man, having an MBC of 150 liters per min, would begin to be breathless only after his MVV exceeded 50 liters per min, a rate of air movement adequate for heavy exercise. In contrast a patient with advanced emphysema, having an MBC of only 50 liters per min, would have discomfort when his MVV reached 15 liters per min, a rate of air movement only slightly greater than that maintained at rest. These calculations shed light on the severe handicap imposed by a disease like emphysema.

Conditions Associated With Respiratory Distress

The foregoing considerations suggest that the relation between the actual ventilation and the maximal capacity to move air is one of the determinants of breathlessness. It therefore follows that stimuli which increase ventilation or disorders which reduce capacity will tend to make discomfort appear. Among stimuli known to be associated with increased ventilation are arterial hypoxemia, arterial hypercapnea, arterial acidemia, muscular exercise, fever, hypermetabolism, systemic hypotension, and an elevated pressure in the great veins and chambers of the right side of the heart. Among disorders known to reduce ventilatory capacity are weakened respiratory muscles, an abnormal chest wall, a low total lung volume, a stiffened lung, and an increased resistance to airflow. All these factors are obvious sources of respiratory discomfort; other influences are less easily understood. For instance, normal man will experience discomfort if he breathes into an apparatus which forces him to maintain a small tidal volume, yet he can obtain relief by taking occasional deep breaths. Also, paralyzing the respiratory muscles with curare can lead to discomfort, even though the alveolar ventilation is adequately maintained by a mechanical respirator.

These observations have led to the view that uncomfortable breathing is related not only to the absolute values of ventilation and capacity, but to a variety of other influences. One is any condition which augments the energy required for a particular level of ventilation. Another is any factor which causes the patient to utilize either a frequency or a tidal volume which is not his normal one.

MECHANISMS OF DYSPNEA

The respiratory center, a complex array of cells in the pons and medulla, is particularly sensitive to changes in carbon dioxide tension and hydrogen ion concentration in the blood and cerebrospinal fluid. The carotid and aortic chemereceptors respond principally to the blood oxygen tension; other receptors in the aortic arch and carotid arteries are sensitive to blood pressure. These peripheral elements transmit impulses centrally through the glossopharyngeal and vagus nerves.

Information about the position and motion of the thorax and lungs travels centrally through several pathways. The intercostal nerves transmit information about the muscles and joints of the chest wall; the phrenic nerves subserve the same function for the muscle of the diaphragm. In addition, the vagi carry impulses from intrapulmonary receptors which signal the state of expansion of the lungs. These impulses, constituting the sensory arm of the Hering-Breuer reflex, provide a means of regulating the respiratory cycle, because inflation tends to limit inspiration and to initiate the expiration of air. Though highly developed in animals, this reflex appears to be relatively weak in normal man.

Despite this detailed knowledge of normal respiration, the precise mechanism producing the sensation of breathlessness remains an enigma. Popular theories have stressed an overloaded respiratory center, fatigue of the respiratory muscles, excessive energy expenditures, and stimulation of intrapulmonary receptors. These re-

ceptors are thought to respond to conditions which increase the stiffness of the lung, and therefore to play a role in the breathlessness occurring in conditions such as pulmonary vascular congestion, pulmonary edema, atelectasis, or diffuse granulomatous disease.

A number of studies have focused attention on the neural circuits regulating the behavior of the respiratory muscles. Campbell has postulated that sensory elements, particularly muscle spindles, play a central role in comparing the tension in the muscle to the degree of stretch. According to him, respiratory discomfort can arise when the tension is inappropriately large for a particular muscle length. Though the exact role of this mechanism has not been determined, there is little doubt that impulses from the respiratory muscles can play an important part in the origin of respiratory discomfort.

Finally, breathlessness often may represent the operation of several mechanisms, rather than the effect of any single one.

DIFFERENTIAL DIAGNOSIS

The separation of an abnormal breathing pattern from respiratory symptoms is an important first step in the approach to the patient. At times, bizarre patterns may be unassociated with distress. One example is the Kussmaul breathing seen in diabetic acidosis. The patient's minute ventilation may be greatly increased, yet he will be unaware of this augmentation. Similarly, many patients with Cheyne-Stokes respiration are oblivious of the change in their breathing pattern. Quite often patients with anemia overventilate, particularly during exercise, but complain chiefly of weakness or tiredness. As a general rule, these diseases produce changes in other organ systems which overshadow the effect on respiration.

Those patients who have breathlessness as a principal symptom usually have one of the following conditions: (1) obstructive disease of the lung, (2) interstitial and alveolar disease of the lung, (3) disease of the chest wall or respiratory muscles, (4) disorders of the heart and circulation, or (5) anxiety neurosis or hysteria. Since each of these conditions is discussed in detail in Part 8, Sec. 3, the ensuing paragraphs stress those points in the evaluation of the patient which will help distinguish one of the conditions from the others.

OBSTRUCTIVE DISEASE OF THE LUNG. (See Chap. 283.) Among the diseases causing acute airway obstruction are asthma, bronchiolitis, and croup. In each, a careful history and a detailed physical examination almost always will establish the diagnosis. In contrast, chronic airway obstruction may be more difficult to recognize, because of the wide variety of signs and symptoms which accompany it. Usually, patients with chronic airway obstruction give a history of shortness of breath for many months. At first breathlessness occurs only with heavy exercise; later with moderate activity; and finally at rest. Characteristically, breathlessness is associated with chronic cough, productive of variable amounts of sputum. Frequent respiratory infections accentuate the cough, quantity of sputum, and breathlessness. The patient may complain of becoming short of breath at night, and he may say that relief comes from bringing up large volumes of secretions. Such a story usually, though not always, permits chronic airway obstruction to be distinguished from the orthopnea or the paroxysmal nocturnal dyspnea that occurs with heart failure. Finally, some patients give a history of wheezing.

The physical examination is especially important; signs of airway obstruction include prolongation of expiration, utilization of the muscles of the neck to lift the anterior part of the upper thorax, retraction of the soft tissues of the thorax during inspiration, and retraction of the lower rib margins as inspiration begins. Often better felt than seen, retraction usually denotes either a low position of the diaphragm or an abnormally low intrapleural pressure, both of which are characteristic of obstructive disease. Other signs include expiratory wheezes and, if the disease is advanced, evidence of right-sided heart failure. Contrary to the popular view, an increased anteroposterior diameter of the chest is one of the less-valuable signs of obstructive lung disease.

Roentgenograms of the chest may be misleading. For instance the leaves of the diaphragm may be low and flat, or they may be at normal levels and rounded. In the latter case their slow rise during a forced expiration will be visible only by fluoroscopy. If the chest is long and narrow, estimating the size of the heart is hazardous, so that even with right ventricular enlargement the transverse cardiac diameter may be normal.

One of the useful bedside tests is to have the patient make a forceful expiration. Prolongation may be plainly evident. If it is not, demonstration that he is unable to blow out a match with his mouth held widely open confirms his failure to achieve a high rate of expiratory flow. When this happens, the MBC will usually be markedly reduced.

Finally, a high hematocrit may reflect chronic arterial hypoxemia and a high venous bicarbonate an elevated tension of carbon dioxide in the blood. Whether or not these changes are present, an analysis of arterial blood is very important.

INTERSTITIAL AND ALVEOLAR DISEASE OF THE LUNG. (See also Chap. 284.) This category embraces a large number of diseases, ranging from acute pneumonia to chronic disorders such as tuberculosis, sarcoid, carcinoma, pneumoconiosis, and idiopathic fibrosis of the lung. The history varies with the etiology, and the signs elicited by physical examination also will depend on the nature and stage of the disease. In almost all these diseases roentgenograms will be abnormal. In the chronic disorders the patient characteristically overventilates at rest and even more while active.

Pulmonary function tests show modest reductions in MBC and vital capacity, and increased stiffness of the lung is often present. Although the oxygen saturation may be low at rest and may fall further with exercise, the carbon dioxide tension is seldom elevated. Indeed, until the late stages of these diseases, the carbon dioxide tension is usually low.

DISEASES OF THE CHEST WALL OR RESPIRATORY MUSCLES. The three most common disorders of the bony thorax causing breathlessness are fractured ribs, kyphoscoliosis, and arthritis of the spine. All interfere with the motion of the thorax and consequently impair ventilation. In each instance the history, physical examination, and standard roentgenograms will permit the diagnosis to be made.

By way of contrast, diagnosing weakness of the respiratory muscles is more difficult. Primary myopathies are uncommon, but almost any debilitating illness, including those associated with prolonged bed rest, can cause the skeletal muscles to atrophy from disuse. When this happens, breathlessness will disappear as the patient regains his general strength.

HEART FAILURE. (See also Chap. 264.) Deciding whether breathlessness originates from disease of the lungs or of the heart often presents a problem. Though a chronic cough usually signifies pulmonary disease, cough as well as wheezing may occur in heart failure. Though breathlessness at night may have a pulmonary origin, acute attacks which awaken the patient and cause him to sit upright are most often caused by heart disease. The important clues, which come from associated symptoms and signs of cardiac dysfunction, include cardiomegaly, hypertension, valvular lesions, or angina. Rales may signify either pulmonary infection or cardiac decompensation, and their diagnostic value is limited. Also, breathlessness of cardiac or pulmonary origin may occur in the absence of rales. In a similar way, the value of roentgenograms is often limited because either pulmonary congestion or pulmonary infection can produce shadows in the lungs.

Tests of pulmonary function usually show some reduction in both the vital capacity and the maximum breathing capacity, and in some instances changes in the mechanical properties of the lungs. Except in the presence of intracardiac shunts, the arterial saturation in nonpulmonary heart disease is almost always above 90 percent, and the carbon dioxide tension is low.

One of the conditions most difficult to distinguish in the differential diagnoses is pulmonary emboli. Right-sided heart failure in the absence of signs of intrinsic lung disease should suggest the possibility of multiple small emboli, but often diagnosis is uncertain without angiography or lung scanning. While the arterial tension of oxygen may be subnormal, the carbon dioxide tension is seldom elevated, an important point of distinction between cor pulmonale secondary to emboli and that caused by obstructive pulmonary disease.

NEUROSIS. Several clues may suggest that breathlessness is associated with psychiatric illness. The most important is the patient's tendency to hyperventilate and occasionally to inspire deeply and expire audibly without relation to exercise. He feels as if he is being smothered, when in fact he is hyperventilating. The breathing pattern is frequently strange, with irregularities in both frequency and tidal volume. At other times the pattern is one of maintained hyperventilation, to the point where the patient complains of tingling in the extremities, or even a sensation of faintness. Watching the patient breathe during sleep is a valuable diagnostic procedure. If the abnormal breathing pattern disappears, psychogenic causes should be suspected. Similarly, observing the patient when he does not know he is being watched is helpful, because the respiratory pattern may be completely different when he is alone.

CONCLUSIONS

The detailed mechanisms of respiratory distress are largely unknown, even though a large number of conditions associated with breathlessness are well characterized. The history, physical examination, roentgenograms, standard laboratory tests, and, where indicated, special tests of respiratory and cardiac function usually will lead to the diagnosis. However, there will remain a group of patients with no measurable abnormalities who appear to have genuine respiratory distress. In these persons careful follow-up during the course of illness will usually reveal concrete signs.

REFERENCES

Campbell, E. J. M.: The Relationship of the Sensation of Breathlessness to the Act of Breathing, pp. 55–63 in "Breathlessness," Oxford, Blackwell Scientific Publications, Ltd., 1966.

Comroe, J.: Some Theories of the Mechanism of Dyspnoea, pp. 1–7 in "Breathlessness," Oxford, Blackwell Scientific Publications, Ltd., 1966.

Cournand, A., D. W. Richards, R. A. Bader, M. E. Bader, and A. P. Fishman: The Oxygen Cost of Breathing, Trans. Assoc. Am. Physicians, 67:162, 1954.

Euler, C. von: The Control of Respiratory Movement, pp. 19–32 in "Breathlessness," Oxford, Blackwell Scientific Publications, Ltd., 1966.

Gaensler, E. A.: "Dyspnea: Diagnostic and Therapeutic Implications," in "Disease a Month," Chicago, The Year Book Medical Publishers, Inc., May, 1961.

——, and G. W. Wright: Evaluation of Respiratory Impairment, Arch. Environ. Health, 12:146, 1966.

Guz, A., M. I. M. Noble, J. G. Widdicombe, D. Trenchard, W. W. Mushin, and A. R. Makey: The Role of Vagal and Glossopharyngeal Afferent Nerves in Respiratory Sensation, Control of Breathing and Arterial Pressure Regulation in Conscious Man, Clin. Sci., 30:161, 1966.

Otis, A. B., W. O. Fenn, and H. Rahn: Mechanics of Breathing, J. Appl. Physiol., 2:592, 1950.

Richards, D. W., Jr.: The Nature of Cardiac and Pulmonary Dyspnea, Circulation, 7:15, 1953.

Sears, T. A.: The Respiratory Motoneurone: Integration at Spinal Segmental Level, pp. 33–45 in "Breathlessness," Oxford, Blackwell Scientific Publications, Ltd., 1966.

Widdicombe, J. G.: Respiratory Reflexes, pp. 585–630 in "Handbook of Physiology," sec. 3, vol. 1, Respiration," American Physiology Society, 1964. Washington, D.C.

Wright, G. W., and B. V. Branscomb: The Origin of the Sensations of Dyspnea, Trans. Clin. & Climatol. Assoc., 66:116, 1954.

33 CYANOSIS, HYPOXIA, AND POLYCYTHEMIA

T. R. Harrison, M. M. Wintrobe,
R. L. Kahler, and E. Braunwald

CYANOSIS

The term *cyanosis* is used to describe the clinical sign of a bluish color of the skin and mucous membranes resulting from an increased amount of reduced hemoglobin, or of hemoglobin derivatives, in the small blood vessels of those areas. Hence it is to be distinguished from *argyria*, in which the deposition of silver salts causes a bluish discoloration of the skin. In the latter condition there is a metallic tint and the blue color persists despite pressure, whereas the truly cyanotic skin becomes pale when sufficient pressure is exerted to express the blood from the vessels.

Cyanosis is usually most marked in the lips, nail beds, ears, and malar eminences. In the last region the line of distinction between true cyanosis and the ruddy color which is commonly seen in robust elderly subjects cannot always be clearly drawn. Furthermore, the "red cyanosis" of polycythemia vera (Chap. 343) must be distinguished from the true cyanosis discussed here. A cherry-colored flush, rather than cyanosis, is caused by carboxyhemoglobin (Chap. 116).

Certain modifying factors influence the degree of cyanosis. These include the thickness of the epidermis, the quality of cutaneous pigment, and the color of the blood plasma, as well as the state of the cutaneous capillaries. The accurate clinical detection of the presence and degree of cyanosis is difficult, as proved by oximetric studies. Some observers can reliably detect central cyanosis when the arterial saturation has fallen to 85 percent; others may not detect it until the saturation has reached 75 percent.

The *fundamental mechanism of cyanosis* consists of an increase in the amount of reduced hemoglobin in the vessels of the skin. This may be brought about either by an increase in the amount of venous blood in the skin as the result of dilatation of the venules and venous ends of the capillaries, or by a decrease in the oxygen saturation in the capillary blood.

As a general rule, cyanosis becomes apparent when the mean capillary concentration of reduced hemoglobin exceeds 5 Gm per 100 ml. It is the absolute rather than the relative amount of reduced hemoglobin which is important in producing cyanosis. Thus, in a patient with severe anemia the relative amount of reduced hemoglobin in the venous blood may be very large when considered in relation to the total hemoglobin. However, since the latter is markedly lowered, the absolute amount of reduced hemoglobin may still be small, and therefore patients with severe anemia and marked arterial desaturation do not display cyanosis. Conversely, the higher the total hemoglobin content, the greater the tendency toward cyanosis; thus, patients with marked polycythemia tend to be cyanotic at higher levels of arterial oxygen saturation than patients with normal hematocrit values. Likewise, local passive congestion, which causes an increase in the total amount of hemoglobin in the vessels in a given area, may cause cyanosis even though the average percentage saturation is not altered.

Cyanosis also is observed when nonfunctional hemoglobin is present in the blood, as little as 1.5 Gm per ml methemoglobin or 0.5 Gm sulfhemoglobin being sufficient to produce cyanosis (Chap. 344).

True cyanosis may be subdivided into two general categories: central and peripheral. In the central type, there is arterial blood unsaturation or an abnormal hemoglobin derivative, and the mucous membranes and skin are both affected. Peripheral cyanosis is generally due to a slowing of blood flow to an area because of vasoconstriction resulting from cold exposure, shock, congestive failure, and peripheral vascular disease; often, in these conditions, the mucous membrane of the oral cavity or those beneath the tongue may be spared. Clinical differentiation between central and peripheral cyanosis may not always be simple, and in conditions such as cardiogenic shock with pulmonary edema there may be a mixture of both types.

Differential Diagnosis

CENTRAL CYANOSIS. Decreased arterial oxygen saturation results from a low oxygen tension in the arterial blood. This may be brought about when there is a corresponding decline in the tension of oxygen in the inspired air without sufficient compensatory alveolar hyperventilation to maintain alveolar oxygen tension. Cyanosis does not occur in a significant degree in an ascent to an altitude of 8,000 ft but is marked in a further ascent to 16,000 ft. The reason for this becomes clear on studying the S shape of the oxygen dissociation

Table 33-1. CAUSES OF CYANOSIS

I. Central cyanosis
   A. Decreased arterial oxygen saturation
      1. Decreased atmospheric pressure—high altitude
      2. Impaired pulmonary function
         a. Alveolar hypoventilation
         b. Uneven relationships between pulmonary ventilation and perfusion
         c. Impaired oxygen diffusion
      3. Anatomic shunts
         a. Certain types of congenital heart disease
         b. Pulmonary arteriovenous fistulas
         c. Multiple small intrapulmonary shunts
   B. Hemoglobin abnormalities
      1. Methemoglobinemia—hereditary, acquired
      2. Sulfhemoglobinemia—acquired
      3. Carboxyhemoglobinemia (not true cyanosis)
   C. Polycythemia (not true cyanosis)
II. Peripheral cyanosis
   A. Reduced cardiac output
   B. Cold exposure
   C. Redistribution of blood flow from extremities
   D. Arterial obstruction
   E. Venous obstruction

curve (Fig. 33-1). At 8,000 ft the tension of oxygen in the inspired air is about 120 mm Hg, the alveolar tension is approximately 80 mm Hg, and the hemoglobin is nearly completely saturated. However, at 16,000 ft the oxygen tensions in atmospheric air and alveolar air are about 85 and 50 mm Hg, respectively, and the oxygen dissociation curve shows that the arterial blood is only about 75 percent saturated. This leaves 25 percent of the hemoglobin in the reduced form, an amount likely to be associated with cyanosis in the absence of anemia.

Impaired pulmonary function, through alveolar hypoventilation, perfusion of unventilated or poorly ventilated areas of lung, or an increase in the barriers to diffusion through which the gas must pass to reach hemoglobin, is common cause of central cyanosis. This may occur acutely, as in extensive pneumonia or in pulmonary edema, or with chronic pulmonary diseases (e.g., emphysema). In the last situation clubbing of the fingers and polycythemia are generally present. However, in many types of chronic pulmonary disease with fibrosis and obliteration of the capillary vascular bed, cyanosis does not occur because there is no significant volume of circulation through unaerated portions.

A less-common, but important, cause of decreased arterial oxygen saturation is shunting of systemic venous blood into the arterial circuit. Certain types of congenital heart disease are associated with cyanosis (Chap. 268). Since blood normally flows from a high- to a low-pressure region, in order for a cardiac defect to result in a right-to-left shunt it must ordinarily be combined with an obstructive lesion distal to the defect or with elevated pulmonary vascular resistance. The commonest congenital cardiac lesion associated with cyanosis is the combination of ventricular septal defect and pulmonary outflow tract obstruction (tetralogy of Fallot). The more severe the obstruction, the greater the degree of right-to-left shunting and resultant cyanosis. The mechanisms for the elevated pulmonary vascular resistance which may produce cyanosis in the presence of intra- and extracardiac communications without pulmonic stenosis are discussed elsewhere (Chap. 268). In patients with patent ductus arteriosus, pulmonary hypertension, and right-to-left shunt, differential cyanosis results; i.e., cyanosis occurs in the lower extremities but not in the upper extremities.

Pulmonary arteriovenous fistulas may be congenital or acquired, solitary or multiple, microscopic or massive. The degree of cyanosis produced by these fistulas depends upon their size and number. They occur with some frequency in hereditary hemorrhagic telangiectasia (Chap. 347). Arterial oxygen unsaturation also occurs in some patients with cirrhosis, although it is uncommon in this condition. A number of factors may explain this observation; pulmonary arteriovenous fistulas or portal vein–pulmonary vein anastomoses have been demonstrated in some patients.

In patients with central cyanosis due to arterial oxygen unsaturation, the severity of cyanosis increases with exercise. With increased extraction of oxygen from the blood by the exercising muscles, the venous blood returning to the right side of the heart is more un-saturated than at rest, and shunting of this blood or its passage into lungs incapable of normal oxygenation intensifies the cyanosis. Also, since the systemic vascular resistance normally decreases with exercise, passage of right ventricular blood into the systemic circuit is made easier by exercise in patients with congenital heart disease and communications between the two sides of the heart.

Arterial blood unsaturation is ascertained by subjecting an arterial blood sample to Van Slyke analysis for de-termining oxygen content and capacity or by directly determining the hemoglobin saturation by oximetric or spectrophotometric techniques. A much more sensitive measurement, especially when the saturation is near normal, is the measurement of arterial blood oxygen tension (P_{O_2}) by means of an oxygen electrode.

Cyanosis is produced by small amounts of circulating methemoglobin and by even smaller amounts of sulfhe-moglobin (Chap. 344). Although they are uncommon causes of cyanosis, these abnormal hemoglobin pigments should be sought by spectroscopic analysis when cy-anosis is not readily explained by malfunction of the circulatory or respiratory systems. Generally, clubbing does not occur with them, but there may be minimal polycythemia.

PERIPHERAL CYANOSIS. Probably the most common cause of peripheral cyanosis is that due to generalized vasoconstriction resulting from exposure to cold air or water. This is clearly a normal response to the stimulus and is transient.

When the cardiac output is low, as in severe con-gestive heart failure or shock, cutaneous vasoconstriction occurs as a compensatory mechanism, so that blood is diverted to more vital areas (kidneys, central nervous system, heart), and intense cyanosis associated with cool extremities may result. Even though the arterial blood may be normally saturated, the reduced volume flow through the skin and the reduced oxygen tension at the venous end of the capillary result in cyanosis.

Acute arterial obstruction to an extremity generally re-sults in pallor and coldness, but there may be associated slight cyanosis. If there is venous obstruction, the ex-tremity is usually congested and markedly cyanotic, and there is true stagnation of blood flow. Stasis of a lesser degree resulting from increased blood viscosity probably contributes to the cyanosis in some patients with poly-cythemia vera.

Certain features are important in arriving at the proper cause of cyanosis.

1. The history, particularly the duration (cyanosis present since birth is usually due to congenital heart disease); possible exposure to drugs or chemicals which may produce abnormal types of hemoglobin.

2. Clinical differentiation of central as opposed to peripheral cyanosis. Objective evidence by physical or radiographic examination of disorders of the respiratory or cardiovascular systems.

3. The presence or absence of clubbing of the fingers. (Clubbing without cyanosis is frequent in patients with

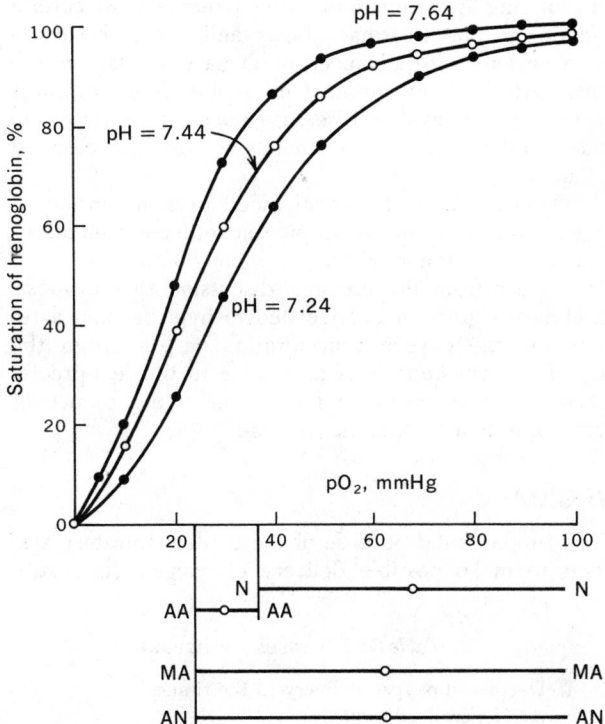

Fig. 33-1. Relationship between oxygen tension and oxygen satu-ration of the hemoglobin of the blood. The heavy line is for blood at pH 7.44. The curves to the right and left are for bloods of pH 7.24 and 7.64, respectively, and indicate quantitatively the magnitude of the Bohr effect for hydrogen ion concentration changes of these magnitudes.

During vigorous muscular effort the increase in acidity of the blood causes the dissociation curve to shift to the right, raises the tissue oxygen tension for any given degree of saturation of the hemoglobin, and thus makes oxygen more available to the muscles. On the other hand, any condition, such as high altitude, which causes respiratory alkalosis moves the dissociation curve to the left. This facilitates oxygen uptake in the lungs by increasing the oxygen saturation at a given level of alveolar oxygen tension.

Beneath the abscissas are plotted the calculated arteriovenous oxygen differences, upon the presumption of the right-heart venous oxygen content normally being 5 vol percent less than the arterial content, and with constant cardiac output in the following states: N = normal person, arterial oxygen content 20 vol percent; AA = same person suffering from arterial hypoxia sufficient to lower the arterial oxygen content to 14.6 vol percent (= 73 per-cent saturation), but with oxygen consumption unaltered; MA = same person with 100 percent increase in oxygen consumption; AN = anemic patient, arterial oxygen content 10 vol percent, with arterial saturation and oxygen consumption same as in normal person. The heavy dots indicate the mean oxygen tension in each instance.

subacute bacterial endocarditis and in association with nonspecific ulcerative colitis, and it may occasionally oc-cur in healthy persons or as an occupational effect.) Slight cyanosis of the lips and cheeks, without clubbing of the fingers, is common in well-compensated patients with mitral stenosis and is probably due to minimal ar-terial hypoxia resulting from fibrotic changes in the lungs secondary to long-standing congestion combined with re-duction of cardiac output. The combination of cyanosis and clubbing is frequent in many patients with certain types of congenital cardiac disease and is seen occasionally in persons with advanced pulmonary disease or pulmonary arteriovenous shunts. On the other hand, cyanosis due to acquired cardiac disease, to acute hypoxia, or to acute disorders of the lungs is not associated with clubbed fingers.

4. Determination of arterial blood oxygen tension or oxygen saturation. Spectroscopic and other examinations of the blood for abnormal types of hemoglobin.

It is clear from the previous discussion that cyanosis is a clinical sign intimately related to hypoxia, i.e., a reduction in the oxygen concentration or tension in the body. The term *hypoxia* is preferable to the less-precise expression *anoxia*, which refers to the total absence of oxygen, a state incompatible with life.

HYPOXIA

The fundamental purpose of the cardiorespiratory system is to make possible delivery of oxygen (and sub-

Table 33-2. CAUSES OF HYPOXIA

I. Decreased oxygen delivery to the tissues
   A. Generalized hypoxia
      1. Arterial hypoxia
         a. Low atmospheric oxygen tension
         b. Diminished oxygenation in the lungs
         c. Systemic venous-to-arterial shunts
      2. Anemic hypoxia
         a. Diminished hemoglobin concentration
         b. Altered hemoglobin
      3. Circulatory hypoxia (ischemia, stagnation)
   B. Specific organ hypoxia
      1. Reflex
      2. Organic
II. Increased oxygen requirements
   A. Thyrotoxicosis
   B. Exercise
III. Improper oxygen utilization

strates) to the cells and to remove carbon dioxide (and other metabolic products) from them. Proper maintenance of this function depends on an intact cardiovascular and respiratory system and a supply of air containing adequate oxygen.

When hypoxia occurs as the result of a decline in oxygen tension in the inspired air, respiration is stimulated, alveolar ventilation increases, and the carbon dioxide tension in the alveoli and in the arterial blood falls. This respiratory alkalosis causes a leftward shift in the oxygen dissociation curve (Fig. 33-1) and enables a given alveolar oxygen tension to cause a greater degree of oxygen uptake by the hemoglobin (Bohr's effect.) Thus, at an alveolar oxygen pressure of 55 mm Hg, a rise in pH from 7.44 to 7.64 will cause the arterial saturation to increase from 80 to nearly 90 percent.

However, when hypoxia results from interference with the passage of air into the lungs or from the perfusion of poorly ventilated alveoli, carbon dioxide tension usually remains normal or even rises; and the oxygen dissociation curve tends to remain unchanged or move to the right. Under these conditions the percentage saturation of the hemoglobin in the arterial blood at a given level of alveolar oxygen tension does not rise and may even fall. Thus arterial hypoxia and cyanosis are likely to be more marked in proportion to the degree of depression of alveolar oxygen tension when such depression results from pulmonary disease than when the depression occurs as the result of a decline in the partial pressure of oxygen in the inspired air.

The respiratory mechanisms may be considerably impaired without the development of a significant degree of arterial hypoxia. This is because the properties of hemoglobin are such that its dissociation curve is practically flat above 100 mm Hg of oxygen tension, and almost flat to about 80 mm Hg. When the tension of oxygen in the alveoli falls below the point at which the slope of the dissociation curve tends to become more nearly vertical, a rapid decline in the amount of oxygen in the arterial blood occurs.

If the flow of blood through the tissues and the oxygen consumption of the tissues remain constant, then the amount of oxygen extracted in the tissues as the blood passes through the capillaries will also remain constant. Therefore, if the oxygen content of arterial blood is reduced, the venous blood emerging from the capillary will have less oxygen by an amount corresponding to the initial abnormal reduction in the arterial blood.

The clinical features of arterial hypoxia depend on how rapidly it develops. Barcroft pointed out that when hypoxia develops rapidly, the picture resembles drunkenness; when it develops slowly, it simulates fatigue. In either case cyanosis is likely to be striking. When the arterial hypoxia is of long duration, clubbing of the fingers usually appears.

Anemic Hypoxia. This includes various states, one of which is associated with anemia and others in which there is a partial conversion to non-oxygen-carrying derivative pigments (Chap. 344). Any decrease in hemoglobin concentration is attended by a corresponding decline in the oxygen-carrying power. Under such conditions the P_{O_2} in the arterial blood remains normal, but the absolute amount of oxygen transported per unit volume of blood is diminished. As the anemic blood passes through the capillaries, and the usual amount of oxygen is removed from it, the P_{O_2} in the venous blood declines to a greater degree than would normally be the case.

Carbon monoxide intoxication (Chap. 116) is accompanied by the equivalent of anemic hypoxia in that the hemoglobin which is combined with the carbon monoxide (carboxyhemoglobin) is unavailable for oxygen transport. But, in addition to this, the presence of carboxyhemoglobin increases the affinity of normal hemoglobin for oxygen at low levels of P_{O_2} (i.e., shifts the lower portion of the dissociation curve of hemoglobin to the left), so that the oxygen can be unloaded only at lower tensions. By such formation of carboxyhemoglobin a given degree of reduction in oxygen-carrying power produces a far greater degree of tissue hypoxia than the equivalent reduction in hemoglobin due to simple anemia.

The P_{O_2} in the venous blood is decreased in both anemic hypoxia and arterial hypoxia. However, the P_{O_2} in the arterial blood is not reduced in anemic hypoxia, and the decrease in mean capillary and in tissue P_{O_2} is less than in arterial hypoxia with similar levels of venous P_{O_2}. Patients with anemia of moderate severity do not exhibit any manifestations of oxygen deficiency while at rest but are likely to display such symptoms on exertion. With severe anemia, symptoms of hypoxia may be present even at rest.

Circulatory Hypoxia. Even though the blood is normal as regards quantity and kind of pigment and is normally saturated with oxygen, and even though the oxygen consumption of the tissues remains normal, reduced P_{O_2} at the venous end of the capillary necessarily occurs if the volume of blood through the tissues (oxygen delivery) is reduced. The clinical pictures which occur when circulatory hypoxia is generalized, as a result of circulatory failure, are discussed in detail in Chap. 264.

Specific Organ Hypoxia. Decreased circulation to a specific organ may be due to organic arterial or venous obstruction or may occur as a reflex phenomenon. The latter may occur when vasoconstriction to, for instance, the limbs, results from an attempt to maintain adequate perfusion to more vital organs, as in severe congestive heart failure. When organic disease of the arteries develops, ischemic hypoxia results, with accompanying pallor. Venous obstruction results in congestion, and the term stagnant hypoxia is applicable.

Increased Oxygen Requirements. Even if oxygen diffusion into arterial blood is unhampered and the hemoglobin is qualitatively and quantitatively normal, the P_{O_2} in venous blood (hence, mean capillary tension) may be reduced if the oxygen consumption of the tissues is elevated without a corresponding increase in volume flow per unit of time. Such a situation may be encountered in febrile states and in thyrotoxicosis. Under such conditions the circulation may be considered deficient relative to the metabolic requirements. Thus, this type of metabolic hypoxia is comparable to circulatory hypoxia, in that in both conditions the volume flow of blood is decreased relative to the needs of the tissues, the difference being that in one case the primary defect is the volume flow of blood and in the other the primary defect is an increased oxygen need by the tissues.

Ordinarily, the clinical picture of patients with hypoxia due to an elevated basal metabolic rate is quite different from that of other types of hypoxia; the skin is warm and flushed, owing to increased cutaneous blood flow which dissipates the excessive heat produced, and cyanosis is absent in these patients.

Exercise is a classic example of increased tissue oxygen requirements. The increased demands are normally met by several mechanisms: (1) by increasing the cardiac output and thus increasing oxygen delivery to the tissues; (2) by preferentially directing the blood to the exercising muscles and away from resting muscles (by changing vascular resistance in various beds, in some areas by direct effects, in others by reflex effects); (3) by increasing oxygen extraction from the delivered blood and widening the arteriovenous oxygen differences. If the capacity of these mechanisms is exceeded, then hypoxia, especially of the exercising muscles, will result.

Improper Oxygen Utilization. The administration of cyanide (Chap. 116) (and several other similarly acting poisons) leads to a paradoxic state in which the tissues are unable to utilize oxygen and the venous blood, in consequence, tends to have a high oxygen tension. This is a type of metabolic disturbance in which the defect is not in the supply of oxygen to the tissues, but in the capacity of the tissues to utilize oxygen. The number of mechanisms transferring electrons to oxygen is limited. It is only by a defect in one or more of these mechanisms, or by failure of preceding oxidations to provide electrons for them, that diminution in oxygen utilization can occur. Thus, cyanide paralyzes the electron-transfer function of cytochrome oxidase so that it cannot pass electrons to oxygen, whereas reduction of tissue temperature slows the rates of metabolic reactions that produce such electrons. Diphtheria toxin is believed to inhibit the synthesis of one of the cytochromes and thus interfere with oxygen consumption and energy production by the cells involved.

Effects of Hypoxia

The symptoms of local oxygen deficiency depend on the tissues affected and are, therefore, protean in nature; they will not be discussed here. When hypoxia is general, all parts of the body may suffer some impairment of function, but those parts which are most sensitive to the effects of hypoxia give rise to symptoms which dominate the clinical picture. The *changes in the central nervous system* are especially important, and here the higher centers are most sensitive. Acute hypoxia, therefore, produces impaired judgment, motor incoordination, and a clinical picture closely resembling that of acute alcoholism. When hypoxia is long-standing, the symptoms consist of fatigue, drowsiness, apathy, inattentiveness, and delayed reaction time, simulating manifestations of severe fatigue. As hypoxia becomes more severe, the centers of the brainstem are affected and death usually results from respiratory failure. The gasping reflex, being a primitive mechanism, persists to the last. Measurements of cerebral blood flow indicate that with reduction of arterial oxygen tension, cerebrovascular resistance decreases and cerebral blood flow increases. This mechanism tends to minimize the cerebral hypoxia. On the other hand, reduction of arterial P_{O_2}, when accompanied by diminution of P_{CO_2}, increases cerebrovascular resistance, and volume flow per unit of time is decreased. It would appear, therefore, that when hypoxia is associated with increased ventilation and hypocapnia, it is enhanced, at least in the higher levels of the central nervous system, by a reduction in volume flow of blood per unit of time. Compared with the brain, the phylogenetically older spinal cord and peripheral nerves are relatively insensitive to hypoxia, and symptoms due to disturbance of these structures usually do not appear. There is evidence that hypoxia causes constriction of pulmonary arteries. This has the advantage of shunting blood away from poorly ventilated areas toward better-ventilated portions of the lung. However, it has the disadvantage of causing increased pulmonary vascular resistance and an increased burden on the right ventricle.

Some of the *metabolic effects of severe acute hypoxia* are well known in regard to the liver and muscles. In these structures the breakdown of the primary foodstuff, carbohydrate, normally proceeds anaerobically (i.e., without oxidation) to the stage of formation of pyruvic acid. The further oxidation of pyruvate requires the availability of oxygen, and when this is deficient, the breakdown is impaired and increasing proportions of pyruvate become reduced to lactic acid, which cannot be further broken down anaerobically (Chap. 75). Hence, there is an increase in the blood lactate, with decrease in bicarbonate and a corresponding acidosis. Since the total energy obtained from foodstuff breakdown is greatly reduced under these circumstances, the amount of energy available for continuing resynthesis of energy-rich phosphate compounds becomes inadequate. As the breakdown of the latter substances is the immediate source of energy driving the myriad of anabolic reactions which take place in tissues, such deficiency of energy-rich phosphate compounds produces a complex disturbance of cellular function. Whether or not the more subtle effects of mild hypoxia upon, for example, the central nervous system are mediated through lesser degrees of such disordered metabolism remains to be demonstrated.

Most of the useful respiratory response to hypoxia originates in special chemosensitive cells in the carotid and aortic bodies, although the respiratory center is also stimulated directly by oxygen lack. The peripheral chemoreceptors are extremely rugged and continue to function after other tissues have been damaged by hypoxemia. The chemoreceptors are stimulated by a reduction in their oxygen supply below their needs either by lowered arterial P_{O_2} or by lowered blood flow to them.

The acute effects of hypoxia on the *reaction of the blood* are complicated, because two different antagonistic influences are at work. If respiration is stimulated by hypoxia, the resulting increase in ventilation, with loss of carbon dioxide, tends to make the blood more alkaline. On the other hand, the diffusion of additional quantities of lactic acid from the tissues into the blood tends to make the blood more acid. In either case the total amount of bicarbonate, and hence the carbon dioxide–combining power, tends to be diminished. With mild hypoxia there is likely to be respiratory alkalosis; severe hypoxia is attended by metabolic acidosis (see Chap. 297).

The heart, although relatively sensitive to hypoxia as compared with most of the structures of the body, is less sensitive than the nervous system. Consequently, in the absence of severe coronary artery disease, serious manifestations of cardiac impairment do not commonly occur when there is generalized hypoxia, and the manifestations arising in the nervous system dominate the picture. It is known that diminished oxygen tension in any tissue re-

sults in local vasodilatation. In generalized hypoxia diffuse vasodilatation results in an elevation of total cardiac output. In patients with preexisting heart disease, particularly coronary artery disease, the combination of hypoxia and the peripheral tissues' requirements for an increase of cardiac output may precipitate congestive heart failure. In prolonged or severe hypoxia hepatic and renal function may also be impaired.

One of the important mechanisms of compensation for prolonged hypoxia is an increase in the amount of hemoglobin in the blood. This is due not to direct stimulation of the bone marrow but to the effect of an erythropoiesis-stimulating factor (erythropoietin). The kidney is the chief site of production or activation of erythropoietin, which then acts upon the stem cells. Assayable levels of erythropietin are increased by hypoxia, and its production has been found to be regulated by the balance between tissue oxygen supply and demand.

POLYCYTHEMIA

The term *polycythemia* signifies an increase above the normal in the number of red corpuscles in the circulating blood. This increase is usually, though not always, accompanied by a corresponding increase in the quantity of hemoglobin and in the volume of packed red corpuscles. The increase may or may not be associated with an increase in the total quantity of red blood cells in the body. It is important to distinguish between *absolute* polycythemia (an increase in the total red corpuscle mass) and *relative* polycythemia, which occurs when, through loss of blood plasma, the concentration of the red corpuscles becomes greater than normal in the circulating blood. This may be the consequence of abnormally lowered fluid intake or of marked loss of body fluids, such as occurs in persistent vomiting, severe diarrhea, copious sweating, or acidosis (Chap. 297). Loss of electrolytes from the extracellular compartment, when not accompanied by corresponding loss of water, leads to a decline of osmolar concentration in the extracellular fluid. The resulting shift of water into the tissue cells may produce relative polycythemia, sometimes of high grade. In certain types of peripheral circulatory failure there is a loss of plasma into the interstitial fluid, again resulting in relative polycythemia. Such a shift takes place largely in the periphery, with the result that the polycythemia may be more marked in capillary blood than in that from central blood vessels.

Because the term *polycythemia* is used loosely to refer to all varieties of increase in the number of red corpuscles, the terms *erythrocytosis* and *erythremia* are preferred in referring to two forms of absolute polycythemia. *Erythrocytosis* denotes absolute polycythemia which occurs in response to some known stimulus; *erythremia* (polycythemia rubra vera) refers to the disease of unknown etiology, which is discussed elsewhere (Chap. 343).

Erythrocytosis develops as a consequence of a variety of factors and represents a physiologic response to conditions of hypoxia. As noted above, sojourn at high altitudes leads to defective saturation of arterial blood with

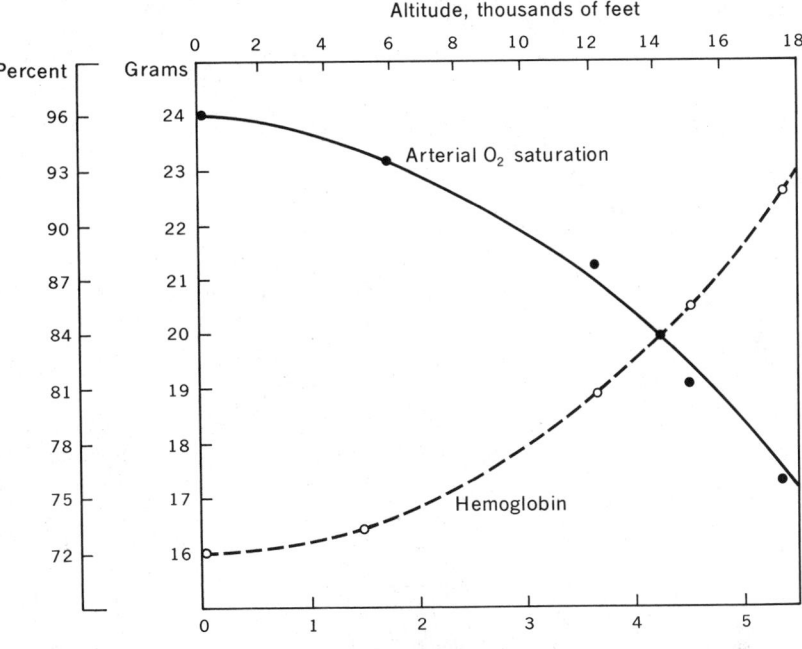

Fig. 33-2. Relationship between mean arterial oxygen saturation (percent) and the mean hemoglobin content (Gm per 100 ml) in healthy male residents at various altitudes. (*Hurtado et al., courtesy, Archives of Internal Medicine.*)

oxygen and stimulates the production of more red corpuscles. There is evidence that oxygen saturation rather than oxygen tension is the more important determinant of the erythropoietic response to chronic hypoxia (Fig. 33-2). Immediately on ascent to a high altitude, symptoms such as fatigue, dizziness, headache, nausea, vomiting, ringing in the ears, and prostration may appear. In most persons adaptation soon occurs, with the development of polycythemia and other compensatory adjustments. However, a disorder may set in insidiously a few years later, or even as long as 20 years after continued residence at high altitudes, leading to the development of a condition known as *chronic mountain sickness* or *seroche (Monge's disease).* Two forms have been described, an emphysematous type in which dyspnea is prominent and bronchitis is common; and an erythremic type in which prominent manifestations are a florid color which turns to cyanosis on mild exertion, mental torpor, fatigue, and headache. Those affected are usually in the fourth to sixth decades. Return to sea level promptly relieves the symptoms. Brisket disease of cattle, a disorder of young calves grazing at high altitudes in Utah and Colorado, which is characterized by pulmonary hypertension and subsquent right-sided heart failure, is not a true counterpart of Monge's disease, since it is not associated with sustained oxygen unsaturation or polycythemia.

Any chronic pulmonary disease which alters ventilation-perfusion relationships or seriously impairs gas diffusion may produce chronic hypoxemia and lead to erythrocytosis. *Emphysema* is the commonest of the chronic pulmonary conditions which is associated with erythrocytosis. Pulmonary arteriovenous fistulas or cavernous hemangioma of the lung may lead to impaired saturation of arterial blood with oxygen, with the conse-

quent development of erythrocytosis and of a clinical picture resembling closely that of certain types of congenital heart disease. The increased blood viscosity secondary to the polycythemia (Fig. 33-3) results in an elevation of pulmonary arterial pressure and, combined with the elevation of pulmonary vascular resistance resulting from hypoxia, the increased viscosity further elevates right ventricular pressure and contributes to the development or intensification of cor pulmonale. Although phlebotomy may be attempted in patients with chronic pulmonary disease with hematocrit values of 50 to 60 percent or more, its value is limited since the diminished blood viscosity is offset by a decrease in oxygen transport.

The mechanical conditions present in very obese individuals may cause primary alveolar hypoventilation and result in arterial unsaturation, erythrocytosis, hypercapnea, and somnolence (Chap. 284). Because certain of these patients resemble the fat, sleepy, red-faced boy of Dickens' *The Pickwick Papers,* the condition has been termed the *Pickwickian syndrome.* This syndrome is observed less commonly in nonobese individuals, and the specific cause is unclear. Decreased sensitivity of the respiratory center to CO_2 may play a role. The increased oxygen cost of breathing found in obese individuals is a contributing factor.

The partial shunting of blood from the pulmonary circuit, such as occurs in congenital heart disease, causes the most striking erythrocytosis resulting from abnormalities in the heart or lungs. Erythrocyte counts as high as 13 million, per cu mm, which are possible only when the red corpuscles are smaller than normal, have been observed in such cases, with volumes of packed red blood cells even as high as 86 ml per 100 ml of blood. As the polycythemia develops, there is a progressive rise in blood viscosity (Fig. 33-3), with the sharpest increase beginning when

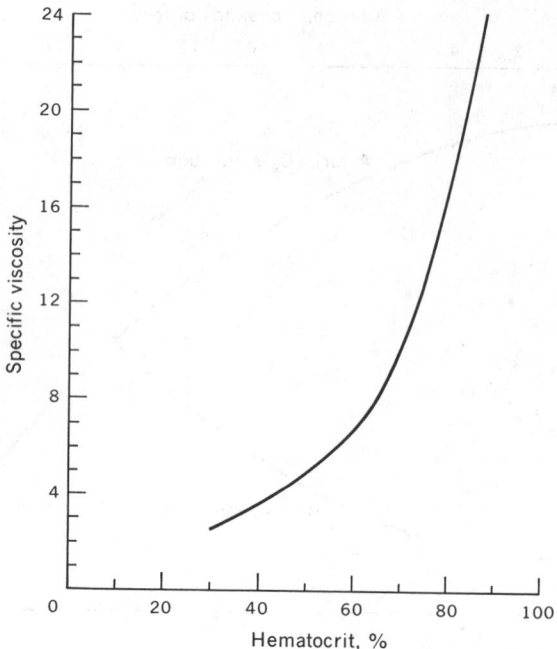

Fig. 33-3. Correlation of hematocrit value with specific viscosity of the blood. (*Rudolph et al.; courtesy, Pediatrics.*)

the volume of packed red blood cells reaches 65 to 70 percent. Cautious phlebotomy is sometimes performed in severely symptomatic patients with extremely high hematocrit levels, but it should not be continued if there is no symptomatic improvement. The commonest defect producing such polycythemia is pulmonary stenosis associated with a right-to-left shunt that allows venous blood to enter the systemic arterial tree without transversing the lungs. Other conditions include transposition of the great arteries, tricuspid atresia, persistent truncus arteriosus, and other less-common anomalies, discussed in Chap. 268. Although erythrocytosis does not usually occur in patients with acquired heart disease, it may occasionally be seen in persons with mitral stenosis.

The excessive use of coal-tar derivatives and other forms of chronic poisoning (Chap. 116), by producing abnormal hemoglobin pigments such as methemoglobin and sulfhemoglobin (Chap. 344), also may cause erythrocytosis. Another chemical agent, cobalt, has produced erythrocytosis in experimental animals, but the mechanism is obscure. Carriers of certain abnormal hemoglobins which have a high oxygen affinity, such as Hb$_{Chesapeake}$ (Chap. 339), are slightly polycythemic.

Erythrocytosis is found in Cushing's syndrome and can be produced by the administration of large amounts of adrenocortical steroids. Especially intriguing are the instances of polycythemia observed in association with various tumors. These have been chiefly of two varieties, *infratentorial* and *renal*. The tumors in the posterior fossa of the skull have usually been vascular (hemangioblastomas). The renal tumors have included hypernephroma, adenoma, and sarcoma. Other tumors that have been associated with polycythemia include *uterine myoma* and

hepatic carcinoma. Polycythemia also has been reported in association with polycystic disease of the kidneys and hydronephrosis. However, only a small proportion (0.3 to 2.6 percent) of the various renal disorders mentioned above have been associated with polycythemia. Plasma erythropoietin levels have been found elevated in a number, though not all, of the cases so studied. Erythropoiesis-stimulating activity has been demonstrated in tumor extracts and in renal cyst fluid, and polycythemia has disappeared after the associated tumor was removed.

The term *stress erythrocytosis* has been applied to the polycythemia seen occasionally in very active, hard-working persons in a state of anxiety, who appear florid but who have none of the characteristic signs of erythremia—no splenomegaly nor leukocytosis with immature cells in the blood. In such individuals the total red blood cell mass is normal and the plasma volume is below normal.

In essence, then, erythrocytosis is known to develop in the presence of:

1. Defective saturation of arterial blood with oxygen, resulting from (*a*) decreased atmospheric pressure and (*b*) impaired pulmonary ventilation

2. Congenital disorders that permit right-to-left shunts

3. Defect in circulating blood pigment

4. Polycythemia produced by the adrenocortical secretions

5. Humoral mechanisms of less well-defined nature which may play a role, as suggested by the cases of polycythemia associated with a variety of tumors, malignant and benign, and with certain renal disorders mentioned above

It is clear, however, that some instances of erythrocytosis cannot be explained by these long-recognized mechanisms.

The differential diagnosis of polycythemia is discussed in the chapter on erythremia (Chap. 343).

REFERENCES

Bakshi, S. P., J. L. Fahey, and L. E. Pierce: Sausage Cyanosis—Acquired Methemoglobeinemic Nitrite Poisoning, New Engl. J. Med., 277:1072, 1967.

Barcroft, J.: "The Respiratory Functions of the Blood," London, Cambridge University Press, 1925.

Burwell, C. S., E. D. Robin, R. D. Whaley, and A. G. Bickelmann: Extreme Obesity Associated with Alveolar Hypoventilation: A Pickwickian Syndrome, Am. J. Med., 21:811, 1956.

Comroe, J. H., Jr.: "Physiology of Respiration," 1st ed., Chicago, The Year Book Medical Publishers, Inc., 1965.

——, R. E. Forster, A. B. Dubois, W. A. Briscoe, and E. Carlsen: "The Lung—Clinical Physiology and Pulmonary Function Tests," 2d ed., Chicago, The Year Book Medical Publishers, Inc., 1962.

Donati, R. M., R. D. Lange, and N. I. Gallagher: Nephrogenic Erythrocytosis, Arch. Intern. Med., 112:960, 1963.

——, J. M. McCarthy, R. D. Lange, and N. I. Gallagher: Erythrocythemia and Neoplastic Tumors, Ann. Intern. Med., 58:47, 1963.

Edwards, M. J., M. J. Novy, C. Waters, and J. Metcalfe:

Improved Oxygen Release: An Adaptation of Mature Red Cells to Hypoxia, J. Clin. Invest., 47:1851, 1968.

Gordon, A. S., G. W. Cooper, and E. D. Zanjani: The Kidney and Erythropoiesis, Seminars Hematol., 4:337, 1967.

Hurtado, A.: Some Clinical Aspects of Life at High Altitudes, Ann. Intern. Med., 53:247, 1960.

Jacobson, L. O., C. W. Gurney, and E. Goldwasser: The Control of Erythropoiesis, pp. 297–327, in "Advances in Internal Medicine," W. Dock and I. Snapper (Eds.), vol. 10, Chicago, The Year Book Medical Publishers, Inc., 1960.

Lundsgaard, C., and D. D. Van Slyke: Cyanosis, Medicine, 2:1, 1923.

Murray, J. F.: Classification of Polycythemic Disorders with Comments on the Diagnostic Value of Arterial Blood Oxygen Analysis, Ann. Intern. Med., 64:892, 1966.

Rudolph, A. M., A. S. Nadas, and W. H. Borges: Hematologic Adjustments to Cyanotic Congenital Heart Disease, Pediatrics, 11:454, 1953.

Weil, J. V., G. Jamieson, D. W. Brown, and R. F. Grover: The Red Cell Mass—Arterial Oxygen Relationship in Normal Man, J. Clin. Invest., 47:1627, 1968.

Wintrobe, M. M.: "Clinical Hematology," 6th ed., Philadelphia, Lea & Febiger, 1967.

34 EDEMA
Louis G. Welt

Edema is defined as an increase in the extravascular component of the extracellular fluid volume. It may be localized or have a generalized distribution depending on the primary lesion. It is recognized by the clinician in its gross generalized form by puffiness of the face (which is most readily apparent in the periorbital areas) and by the persistence of an indentation of the skin following pressure. This is known as *"pitting" edema*. In its more subtle form it may be detected by the fact that the rim of the bell of the stethoscope leaves an indentation on the skin of the chest that lasts a few minutes. One of the first symptoms a patient may note is the ring on a finger fitting more snugly than in the past. Lastly, it should be cautioned that the volume of the interstitial space may increase by several liters before edema is recognized by the patients from the symptoms or by the physician through physical examination. *Ascites* and *hydrothorax* refer to accumulation of excess fluid in the peritoneal and pleural cavities, respectively. *Anasarca*, or "dropsy," refers to gross generalized edema.

PATHOGENESIS

A more detailed discussion of the volume and distribution of body fluids is presented in Chap. 296. About one-third of the total body water is confined to the extracellular space. This compartment, in turn, is composed of the plasma volume and the interstitial space. Under ordinary circumstances the plasma volume represents about 25 percent of the extracellular space, and the remainder is in the interstitium. The forces that regulate the disposition of fluid between these two components of the extracellular compartment are frequently referred to as the *Starling forces*, owing to the masterful description presented by that noted physiologist.

In general terms, two forces tend to promote a movement of fluid from the vascular to the extravascular space, and these forces are the *hydrostatic pressure within the vascular system* and the *colloid osmotic pressure* in the interstitial fluid. In contrast, the factors which promote a movement of fluid into the vascular compartment are the *colloid oncotic pressure* contributed by the plasma proteins, and the *hydrostatic pressure within the interstitial fluid*, referred to as the *tissue tension*. These forces are balanced so that there is a large movement of water and diffusible solutes from the vascular space at the arteriolar end of the microcirculation and back into the vascular compartment at the venous end.[1] In addition, fluid is returned from the interstitial space into the vascular system by way of the lymphatics, and unless these channels are obstructed, lymph flow tends to increase if there is a tendency toward a net movement of fluid from the vascular compartment to the interstitium. In this fashion, all these forces are usually balanced so that a given steady state exists with respect to the size of the two compartments, and yet a large exchange between them is permitted. However, should any one of these factors be altered significantly, one can see how there may be a net movement of fluid from one component of the extracellular space to the other.

An increase in pressure in the vessels of the microcirculation may readily result from an increase in venous pressure due to local obstructive phenomena in the venous drainage, or to congestive heart failure, or to the simple expansion of the vascular volume by the administration of large volumes of fluid at a rate in excess of the ability of the kidneys to excrete these excesses. The colloid oncotic pressure of the plasma may be reduced owing to any of the factors that may induce hypoalbuminemia, such as malnutrition, liver disease, and loss of protein into the urine or into the gastrointestinal tract, or to a severe catabolic state.

Damage to the capillary endothelium increases the permeability of these vessels, which permits the transfer to the interstitial compartment of a fluid containing more protein than usual. Injury to the capillary walls may be the result of chemical, bacterial, thermal, or mechanical agents. Increased capillary permeability may also be a consequence of a hypersensitivity reaction. Lastly, damage to the capillary endothelium is presumably responsible for inflammatory edema, which is easily recognized by the presence of other signs of inflammation—redness, heat, and tenderness.

In any attempts to formulate a hypothesis concerning the pathophysiology involved in edematous states, it is exceedingly important to discriminate between the pri-

---

[1] There is no final resolution of the argument whether the exchange of fluid and solutes occurs between capillary endothelial cells or through the cells themselves.

mary events, which account for the maldistribution of fluid between the two components of the extracellular space, and the predictable secondary consequences, which include the retention of salt and water. There are instances in which an abnormal retention of salt and water may, in fact, be the *primary* disturbance. In these circumstances the edema is a secondary manifestation of the generalized increase in volume of the extracellular fluid. These special instances are usually related to those conditions characterized by an acute reduction in renal function (such as acute tubular necrosis or acute glomerulonephritis) and other disorders characterized by the primary production of excess mineralocorticoid or inappropriate secretion of the antidiuretic hormone.

These latter circumstances aside, one can create a hypothesis which is admittedly at least incomplete but within which one can begin to understand the concatenation of events in a variety of edematous states and perceive many of the features common in the pathophysiology of each. The basic premise is that the primary disorder concerns one or more alterations in the Starling forces such that there is a net movement of fluid from the vascular system into the interstitium or from the arterial compartment of the vascular space into the chambers of the heart or into the venous circulation itself. In either event, a diminished arterial volume may be anticipated to have certain consequences that lead to retention of salt and water. If retention of an increment of salt and water repairs the volume deficit, the stimuli to retain salt and water should be dissipated and a new steady state achieved. If, on the other hand, retention of salt and water does not repair the volume deficit because the increased volume of fluid cannot be sustained in the appropriate component of the vascular bed, the stimuli are not dissipated and the retention of salt and water continues. The sequence of events can be explored in a variety of circumstances.

Obstruction of Venous and Lymphatic Drainage to a Limb

The simplest condition to examine may be the consequences of lymphatic and venous obstruction to a limb. This must increase the hydrostatic pressure in the microcirculation so that more fluid is transferred from the circulation than can be reabsorbed at the venous end; furthermore, the alternate route, the lymphatic channels, are stipulated to be obstructed as well. This event must of necessity cause an increased volume of interstitial fluid in the limb at the expense of the plasma volume. The diminished plasma volume has a variety of consequences:

RENAL HEMODYNAMIC CHANGES. The diminished volume of plasma can be expected to reduce the perfusion of the kidney and decrease the glomerular filtration rate. Since one of the most important influences regulating the excretion of salt (and water) may be the filtered load itself, this would promote the excretion of lesser quantities of salt and smaller volumes of water. Other consequences

of a hemodynamic nature are presumably conditioned by alterations in plasma volume. For reasons that are as yet unclear, it seems quite well established that an influence of "volume" on the rate of excretion of salt functions independently of its filtered load and independently of mineralocorticoid secretion. The nature of this regulatory mechanism is unknown, but a direct correlation occurs between alterations in volume and alterations in the excretion of salt. The phenomenon may be related to the character and distribution of blood flow to the kidney, but there are other alternatives. In any event, a diminished plasma volume can readily diminish the excretion of salt owing to alterations in renal hemodynamic parameters.

HUMORAL FACTORS. Ample evidence reveals that a diminished volume of plasma in some fashion promotes an increased secretion of aldosterone. This is due to an increase in an aldosterone-stimulating agent, which is dependent on the presence of intact kidneys and may well be angiotensin. This, in turn, may be increased in the plasma owing to some influence on the renal circulation related to alterations in flow or pressure, or to the chemical composition of intraluminal fluid that may stimulate the release of renin from the juxtaglomerular apparatus. In turn, the renin reacts with renin substrate to form angiotensin I, and the latter is converted enzymatically to angiotensin II, which stimulates the secretion of aldosterone. Whatever the precise sequence of events, a diminished plasma volume promotes increased secretion of this mineralocorticoid which implements the renal tubular reabsorption of sodium.

The influence of alterations in plasma volume or the excretion of sodium salts was mentioned in relation to possible alterations in renal hemodynamics. There are data that suggest the possibility that the increase in volume of some component(s) of the extracellular space promotes the secretion of a "natriuretic" hormone, also referred to as a *third factor*, or *volume effect*. The unambiguous demonstration of such a hormone, its site(s) of secretion, and its characterization are yet to be presented.

The retention of sodium owing to the hemodynamic and humoral factors alluded to above may, in turn, be accompanied directly by an increased reabsorption of water. If not, then the primary retention of sodium thus dictates some increase in the effective osmolality of body fluids, promotes thirst and the acquisition of water, and promotes the secretion of antidiuretic hormone, which then implements the retention of water.

In the context of the disorder under discussion, the volume of the extracellular fluid (about 140 mM sodium per liter of water) is increased. This increment tends to accumulate in the interstitium of the limb in which venous and lymphatic drainage are obstructed until the tissue tension is great enough to counterbalance the primary alteration in the Starling forces, at which time no further fluid will accumulate in that limb. At this point the additional accumulation of fluid will repair the deficit in plasma volume, and the stimuli to retain more salt and water are dissipated. The net effect is an increase in the volume of interstitial fluid in a local area, and the secondary responses repair the plasma volume deficit incurred by the primary event.

This same sequence may be translated easily to many other edematous states.

Nephrotic Syndrome

The primary alteration in this disorder is a diminished colloid oncotic pressure due to exorbitant loss of protein into the urine. This should promote a net movement of fluid into the interstitium and initiate the sequence of events described above. However, so long as the hypoalbuminemia is severe, the increment of fluid cannot be restrained within the vascular compartment, and hence the stimuli to retain salt and water are not abated.

Cirrhosis

Measurements of blood volume in cirrhosis of the liver are commonly increased when the disorder is accompanied by a fairly large system of dilated venous radicles. Nevertheless, the arterial volume is quite likely diminished in size. If the primary event in the formation of ascites is due to obstruction of the lymphatic drainage of the liver as well as obstruction of the portal venous system, it is likely that the enlarged venous system has promoted a deficit in the arterial component. Once again, the sequence of events already described will come into play, and salt and water will be retained. So long as the venous bed continues to enlarge and the collection of fluid in the peritoneal cavity increases, the deficit in volume of the arterial side of the circulation is not repaired and the stimuli persist to retain salt and water. In addition, considerable data suggest that there are arteriovenous shunts in this disorder. One consequence of these shunts is a reduced renal blood flow despite an increase in cardiac output. In this fashion the alterations due to renal hemodynamic factors are fortified.

Although the diseased liver admittedly may not inactivate aldosterone and antidiuretic hormone in a competent fashion, it is unlikely that this plays a significant role in salt and water retention. Some suggest that this difficulty in inactivation permits the development of higher levels of these humoral agents, which may amplify the responses in terms of salt and water retention. This seems unlikely since, in the first place, a tendency to diminished inactivation of these hormones might be expected to retard their rates of secretion; furthermore, it is apparent that if one provides a mechanism for the loculated ascitic fluid to reach the interstitium of the abdominal wall by the use of a prosthetic device, there is an immediate diuresis of salt and water. This is presumably because if the ascitic fluid reaches the interstitial space elsewhere, it can be reabsorbed into the circulation and this, in turn, will repair the volume deficit and dissipate the stimuli responsible for the retention of salt and water. Unfortunately, these devices are soon obstructed by scar tissue and hence have not been a practical form of

therapy. Nevertheless, this experience emphasizes that deficient inactivation of these hormones by the diseased liver plays no important role in implementing the edematous state.

Congestive Heart Failure

In this disorder it is postulated that the defective systolic emptying of the chambers of the heart promotes an accumulation of blood in the heart and venous circulation at the expense of the arterial volume, and the oft-repeated sequence of events is initiated. In many instances of mild heart failure a small increment of volume may be achieved, which may repair the volume deficit and establish a new steady state. This may result because up to a point an increase in the volume of blood within the chambers of the heart appears to promote a more forceful contraction and may thereby increase the volume ejected in systole. However, if the cardiac disorder is more severe, retention of fluid cannot repair the arterial volume deficit. The increment accumulates in the venous circulation, and the increase in hydrostatic pressure therein promotes the formation of edema in the lungs as well as elsewhere. The pulmonary edema impairs gas exchange and may induce hypoxia, which embarrasses cardiac function still further. The volume of blood within the chambers of the heart becomes ever larger and reaches a point where this increase affects systolic emptying adversely, thus worsening the heart failure.

Cylic Edema

There is a syndrome characterized by periodic episodes of edema without obvious cause. It has been observed most commonly (but not exclusively) in women, and there appears to be some relationship to the menstrual cycle. The fact that most cases are seen in women may be due, in part at least, to the unfortunate cosmetic consequences of facial edema which is more likely to disturb women than men. Another feature of this disorder is fairly constant, large, diurnal alterations in weight so that the patient may weigh several pounds more in the evening than in the morning after having been in the upright posture most of the day.

No one knows whether all these patients represent a single type of disorder with varying degrees of intensity. A large diurnal weight change suggests the possibility that patients may well have increased capillary permeability in general, which is emphasized daily by the upright posture and the consequent increased hydrostatic pressure in the vessels. The episodes of more frankly sustained edema may be the result of a further increase in capillary permeability due to some other influence. If, in fact, it truly occurs more commonly in women and is correlated with the menstrual cycle, there may be some hormonal influence on the permeability of vessels which permits the loss of plasma volume into the interstitial space and the sequence of events secondary to a contraction in plasma volume. An occasional patient has been reported in whom

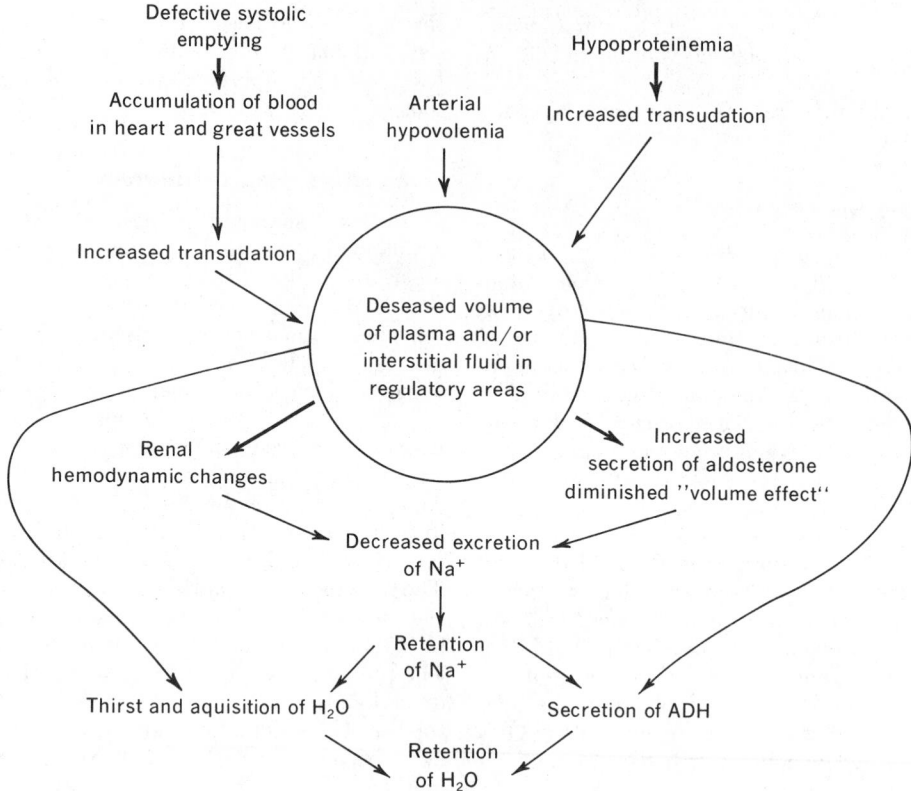

Fig. 34-1. Sequence of events leading to the formation and the retention of salt and water.

the loss of plasma volume was so striking as to induce peripheral vascular collapse; and in one instance, at least, this was so severe as to cause death.

This general formulation is represented graphically in Fig. 34-1. As mentioned earlier, this is certainly incomplete, and the amplification presented in this discussion may well have serious defects of omission and error. Allusion has been made to some of the unknown areas. One more which deserves further comment concerns the precise role of the mineralocorticoid hormone in these problems. Although increased quantities of aldosterone have been demonstrated to be secreted in these various edematous states, it must be emphasized that augmented levels of aldosterone (or other mineralocorticoids) do not always promote the accumulation of edema, as witnessed by the lack of striking fluid retention in most instances of primary aldosteronism. Furthermore, although normal subjects will retain some salt and water under the influence of a potent mineralocorticoid such as deoxycorticosterone acetate or 9-alpha-fluorohydrocortisone, this accumulation appears to be self-terminative despite continued exposure to the steroid and to salt and water. It is probable that the failure of normal subjects to accumulate fluid indefinitely reflects an increase in glomerular filtration rate, other hemodynamic influences, and the effect of the increase in volume which promotes an increased excretion of salt independent of the filtered load of sodium. The role of aldosterone in the accumulation of fluid in these edematous states discussed above may be

more effective because these patients are unable to repair the crucial deficit in volume.

Throughout this discussion it has been assumed that the retention of sodium salts is primary to water retention. This is attested to by (1) the usual failure to accumulate edema if sodium is not available in the diet and (2) the successful use of pharmacologic agents and other measures that promote the excretion of sodium in the urine. In most circumstances the mechanisms responsible for maintaining a normal effective osmolality in the body fluids continue to operate efficiently so that sodium retention promotes thirst and secretion of the antidiuretic hormone, which, in turn, lead to the ingestion and retention of approximately 1 liter of water for each 140 mM sodium retained. Similarly, measures which promote the loss of sodium into the urine are accompanied by antithetical responses leading to the net loss of an equivalent volume of water from the body.

DIFFERENTIAL DIAGNOSIS

Despite numerous inconsistencies encountered in the explanation for the various factors and mechanisms concerned in edema formation, the primary cause can usually be determined. As a rule, localized edema can be readily differentiated from generalized edema. The great majority of patients with noninflammatory generalized edema of significant degree suffer from cardiac, renal, hepatic, or nutritional disorders. Consequently, the differential diagnosis of generalized edema should be directed toward implicating or excluding these several conditions. The considerations listed below should suffice to differentiate the common causes of edema.

Localized Edema

Edema originating from inflammation or hypersensitivity is usually readily identified; allusion has been made to characteristics of this type of edema. Localized edema due to venous or lymphatic obstruction (thrombophlebitis, chronic lymphangitis, resection of regional lymph nodes, filariasis, etc.) may demonstrate in a local area all the characteristics of edema occurring from generalized retention of salt and water. It should be reemphasized that lymph edema is peculiarly intractable because restriction of lymphatic flow results in increased protein concentration in interstitial fluid, a circumstance which severely impedes removal of retained fluid.

Edema of Heart Failure

Evidence of heart disease as manifested by cardiac enlargement, diastolic murmurs, and gallop rhythm plus evidences of cardiac failure, such as dyspnea, basilar rales, diminished vital capacity, prolonged circulation time, venous distension, increased venous pressure, and hepatomegaly, usually provides abundant evidence of the pathogenesis of edema resulting from heart failure.

Edema of the Nephrotic Syndrome

The classic triad—massive proteinuria, hypoproteinemia, and hypercholesterolemia is usually present. This syndrome may occur during the course of a variety of kidney diseases, which include glomerulonephritis, diabetic glomerulosclerosis, amyloid infiltration, renal vein thrombosis, diffuse connective tissue diseases, and hypersensitivity reactions. A history of previous renal disease may or may not be elicited; more commonly, it is not.

Edema of Acute Glomerulonephritis

The edema occurring during the acute phases of glomerulonephritis is characteristically associated with hematuria, proteinuria, and hypertension. Some evidence supports the view that the fluid retention is due to increased capillary permeability; but probably in most instances the edema in this disease results from primary retention of sodium and water by the kidneys owing to acute renal insufficiency and the consequent development of a congested state. However, discrimination between congestive heart failure and a congested state in acute renal insufficiency is often difficult. The congested state differs from congestive heart failure since it is characterized by a normal or increased cardiac output, normal or diminished circulation time, a reduction in the packed cell volume, a normal arteriovenous oxygen difference, and failure to respond to a digitalis preparation. Patients commonly have severe evidence of pulmonary congestion on chest x-ray before cardiac enlargement is significant, and these patients frequently lie supine in bed with no tachypnea. If one cannot discriminate between the congested state and congestive heart failure, use of a cardiac glycoside is more prudent but especial care should be taken to avoid digitalis intoxication.

Edema of Cirrhosis

Ascites plus evidence of hepatic disease (collateral venous channels, hepatomegaly, spider angiomas, and jaundice) characterize edema of hepatic origin. The ascites is frequently extremely refractory to treatment; the lack of therapeutic response can be ascribed to the fact that intraabdominal fluid collects as a result of a combination of obstruction of hepatic lymphatic drainage, portal hypertension, hypoalbuminemia, and relatively high protein content of the ascitic fluid. The latter may be due to escape of a protein-containing fluid through the lymphatic vessels of the liver capsule or through the portal vessels, the lymphatic drainage of which is impeded. Edema may also occur in other parts of the body in patients with cirrhosis as a result of hypoalbuminemia. Furthermore, the sizable accumulation of ascitic fluid may be expected to increase intraabdominal pressure and impede venous return from the lower extremities; hence, it tends to promote accumulation of edema in these limbs as well.

Edema of Nutritional Origin

An inadequate diet over a prolonged period may produce hypoproteinemia and edema. In some instances of extreme malnutrition the degree of transudation appears to be disproportionately great for the degree of serum protein deficit observed. Coexisting beriberi heart disease may augment edema of this origin. In the latter condition, increased cardiac output and blood flow, in addition to those factors usually present in heart failure and capillary dilatation, may further favor edema formation. More striking edema is commonly observed when these famished subjects are provided with an adequate diet. The mechanism is not clear, but the ingestion of more food may increase the quantity of salt taken, which is retained along with water. The edema may be more apparent than under other circumstances, because the subcutaneous tissue is so depleted of fat that modest collections of edema may be more obvious than they would be in an obese subject.

GENERAL DIFFERENTIAL CRITERIA

Aside from the criteria already mentioned, certain other points may help elicit the cause of edema.

The distribution of edema is an important guide to the cause. Thus, edema of one leg or of one or both arms is usually the result of vascular or lymphatic obstruction. Edema resulting from hypoproteinemia characteristically is generalized, but it is especially evident in the eyelids and face and tends to be most pronounced in the morning because of the recumbent posture assumed during the night. Edema associated with heart failure, on the other hand, tends to be more extensive in the legs and to be accentuated in the evening, a feature also determined largely by posture. In the rare types of cardiac disease, such as tricuspid stenosis and constrictive pericarditis, in which orthopnea may be absent and the patient may prefer the recumbent posture, the factor of gravity may be equalized and facial edema observed. Less common causes of facial edema include trichinosis, allergic reactions, and myxedema. Unilateral edema occasionally results from cerebral lesions affecting the vasomotor fibers on one side of the body; paralysis also reduces lymphatic and venous drainage on the affected side.

The color, thickness, and sensitivity of the skin are important. Local tenderness and increase in temperature suggest inflammation. Local cyanosis may signify a venous obstruction. Generalized but usually slight cyanosis commonly indicates congestive heart failure. In individuals who have had repeated episodes of prolonged edema, the skin over the involved area may be thickened, hard, and often red.

The venous pressure is of great importance in evaluating edema. Elevation of this measurement in an isolated part of the body usually reflects venous obstruction. Generalized elevation of venous pressure is almost pathognomonic of congestive heart failure, although it may be present in the congestive state that accompanies acute renal insufficiency. Ordinarily significant increase in venous pressure can be recognized by the level at which cervical veins collapse; in doubtful cases and for accurate recording, the venous pressure should be measured.

Determination of the concentration of serum proteins, and especially of serum albumin, clearly differentiates those patients in whom edema is due entirely or in part to diminished intravascular colloid osmotic pressure. The presence of proteinuria affords useful clues. The complete absence of protein in the urine is evidence against (but does not exclude) either cardiac or renal disease as a cause of edema. In a patient with edema without proteinuria, the presence of a palpable liver constitutes strong evidence that hepatic disease may be the cause of the edema. Slight to moderate proteinuria is the rule in patients with heart failure, whereas persistent massive proteinuria usually reflects the presence of the nephrotic syndrome. Since the liver may be palpable in subjects with heart failure or hepatic disease, the presence of proteinuria in a patient who does not have a palpable liver suggests the possibility of the nephrotic syndrome. Aside from the points mentioned, which bear directly on the question of the type of edema, much valuable information can be obtained from other features of the examination. Some of these are the presence or absence of heart disease, the character of the urinary sediment, the dietary history, and a history of alcoholism.

It should be emphasized that edema may originate from a variety of abnormal states; it is not, therefore, necessarily a consequence of only one of the disorders enumerated above. For example, in a diabetic patient,

edema may be the result of hypoalbuminemia associated with the nephrotic syndrome with intercapillary glomerulosclerosis, increased venous pressure associated with congestive heart failure due to atherosclerotic and hypertensive heart disease, and the anemia consequent to uremia.

SUMMARY

Edema limited to a local area suggests either obstruction or local capillary damage. The obstruction may be lymphatic, venous, or both, and the local capillary damage may be due either to inflammation or to allergy. Significant generalized edema may occur before it can be appreciated clinically. It appears first in tissues that are expansible and may be demonstrable only by pressure against a bony eminence such as the tibia. The presence of generalized edema requires investigation especially for evidence of cardiac, renal, or hepatic disease and occasionally for manifestations of nutritional deficiency.

The primary factors promoting transfer of fluid from the intravascular to the extravascular compartment of the extracellular fluid space are reasonably clear. The secondary factors that induce salt and water retention include a variety of hemodynamic humoral mechanisms, the nature of which, although clarified by recent investigations, can still not be formulated by any single hypothesis with confidence.

REFERENCES

deWardener, H. E., I. H. Mills, W. F. Clapham, and C. J. Hoyter: Studies on the Effluent Mechanism of the Sodium Diuresis Which Follows the Administration of Intravenous Saline in the Dog, Clin. Sci., 21:249, 1961.

Starling, E. H.: The Fluids of the Body, in "The Herter Lectures," New York, W. T. Keener and Co., 1909.

Welt, L. G.: Water Balance in Health and Disease, chap. 6 in "Diseases of Metabolism," 5th ed., G. G. Duncan (Ed.), Philadelphia, W. B. Saunders Company, 1964.

35   PALPITATION
William H. Resnik and Eugene Braunwald

Palpitation is a disagreeable subjective phenomenon which may be defined as an awareness of the beating of the heart. Palpitation is not pathognomonic of any particular group of disorders; even when it occurs as a more or less prominent complaint, the diagnosis of the underlying disease is made largely on the basis of other associated symptoms and data, rather than from an analysis of the palpitation alone. Nevertheless, palpitation is frequently of considerable importance in the minds of patients. The clear association of the symptom with the function of the heart and the fear that it may represent heart disease account for the patient's apprehension about it. Concern is all the more pronounced in patients who know or who have been told that they may have heart disease; to them palpitation may seem to be an omen of impending disaster. Since the resulting anxiety may be associated with increased activity of the autonomic nervous system, with consequent alteration of the cardiac rate and rhythm and the vigor of contraction, the patient's awareness of these changes may then lead to a vicious cycle.

Palpitation may be described by the patient in various terms, such as "pounding," "fluttering," "flopping," and "skipping," and in most cases it will be obvious that the complaint is of a sensation of disturbed heartbeat. Not infrequently, the patient complains of throbbing in the neck or upper part of the abdomen, when under similar circumstances most persons would refer the palpitation to the precordium.

In the various conditions discussed below, palpitation may be the chief source of the patient's discomfort and the outstanding complaint. It must not be inferred, however, that in all these disorders palpitation is always a symptom of great magnitude, even from the patient's standpoint.

The wide variability in the sensitivity to alterations in cardiac activity among different individuals must be appreciated. Some patients seem to be unaware of the most serious tachycardias; others are seriously troubled by an occasional extrasystole.

PATHOGENESIS OF PALPITATION

Under ordinary circumstances the rhythmic heartbeat is imperceptible to the healthy individual of average or placid temperament. Palpitation may be experienced by normal persons who have engaged in strenuous physical effort or have been strongly aroused emotionally. This type of palpitation is physiologic and represents the normal awareness of an overactive heart—i.e., a heart that is beating at a rapid rate and at the same time expelling more than the usual amount of blood with each beat. Since palpitation due to overactivity of the heart may occur also in certain pathologic states, e.g., severe anemia or thyrotoxicosis, it is commonly assumed that it is the overactivity *per se* or the associated increased stroke output that is responsible for the symptom. However, overactivity of the heart is generally associated with several other alterations in cardiac function, including acceleration of heart rate, steeper gradient of development of intraventricular pressure during the period of isometric contraction, and increased intensity of the heart sounds, especially of the first sound.

When palpitation is heavy and regular, it is usually caused by an augmented stroke volume, and it should raise the question of a variety of hyperkinetic circulatory states (anemia, arteriovenous fistula, thyrotoxicosis, and the so-called idiopathic hyperkinetic heart syndrome), aortic or mitral regurgitation, and atrial or ventricular septal defect. But unusual movements of the heart within the thorax are also frequently the mechanism of palpi-

tation. Thus, the ectopic beat and/or the compensatory pause may be appreciated, since both are associated with alterations in cardiac motion.

IMPORTANT CAUSES OF PALPITATION

It is impracticable to enumerate all the circumstances under which palpitation may occur. Hence, only those disorders will be mentioned in which palpitation may be a prominent symptom.

PALPITATION DUE TO DISORDERS OF THE MECHANISM OF THE HEARTBEAT. Extrasystoles. The symptoms are fairly consistent, and in most cases the diagnosis will be suggested by the patient's story. The premature contraction and the post-premature beat are often described as a "flopping" or as if "the heart turns over." The pause following the premature contraction may be felt as an actual cessation of the heartbeat, in contrast with the complete unawareness of pauses of similar duration when the heart beats normally or when atrial fibrillation with a slow ventricular rate occurs. The patient's apprehensions seem to magnify the duration of the interval and sometimes may make him wonder if the heart will ever resume its beat. The first ventricular contraction succeeding the pause may be felt as an unusually vigorous beat and will be described as "pounding" or "thudding." Any one or all of these different symptoms initiated by the premature contraction may be experienced by the patient.

Usually the identification of the extrasystole as the cause of palpitation is a simple matter. When extrasystoles are numerous, clinical differentiation from atrial fibrillation can be made by any procedure that will bring about a definite increase in the ventricular rate; at increasingly rapid heart rates, the extrasystoles usually diminish in frequency and then disappear, whereas the irregularity of atrial fibrillation increases. Heart block, with dropped beats, is the only other common arrhythmia with which the premature contraction is likely to be confused; here, simple auscultation will reveal the absence of the premature beat prior to the pause.

The Ectopic Tachycardias. These conditions, which are considered in some detail in Chap. 265, are other common and medically more important causes of palpitation. Strangely, ventricular tachycardia, one of the most serious arrhythmias, rarely is manifested as palpitation; and this may be related to the abnormal sequence, and hence impaired coordination and vigor, of ventricular contraction.

If the patient is seen between attacks, the diagnosis of ectopic tachycardia and its type will have to depend on the history, but of course the precise diagnosis can be made only when an electrocardiogram and observations on the effect of carotid sinus pressure are made during the episode. The mode of onset and offset gives the most important lead. Determining this mode may prove difficult, for in many cases of rapid heart action, it is not impossible to ascertain with certainty whether there was an actual sudden onset or whether there was a preceding period of anxiety followed by the rapid, but not abrupt, development of sinus tachycardia. It is usually even more difficult to ascertain the exact characteristics of the off-set of the tachycardia.

PALPITATION DEPENDENT ON ORGANIC OR FUNCTIONAL DISTURBANCE ORIGINATING OUTSIDE THE CIRCULATORY SYSTEM. Once again, only the more important and common conditions, particularly those which may not be readily recognized, will be mentioned.

Thyrotoxicosis. In its fully developed form, thyrotoxicosis will usually be evident and offers little difficulty in the way of diagnosis. It is particularly likely to be overlooked in the presence of myocardial failure. The suspicion that thyrotoxicosis is present may be aroused by the detection of any one of its characteristic features, and the diagnosis will be confirmed by the procedures mentioned in Chap. 89.

Anemia. When mild, anemia may cause palpitation during exertion; when severe, it causes palpitation at rest. In some patients the coloring of the skin may not reveal the cause of the symptom, but appropriate studies of the blood will clarify the situation.

Fever. Palpitation may be present in acute infections, particularly in the early stages; but here the symptom is merely an insignificant phenomenon in the midst of other obviously more important ones. Palpitation may be a prominent symptom in an individual suffering from one of the chronic and sometimes more obscure febrile illnesses, such as incipient tuberculosis, chronic brucellosis, subacute bacterial endocarditis, or acute rheumatic fever with carditis and relatively few or no joint manifestations. Carditis in acute rheumatic fever and subacute bacterial endocarditis cannot of course be considered causes of palpitation originating outside the heart. They are considered in this group because the presenting symptoms, including palpitation, are often only those of an infection without localizing symptoms that direct suspicion to the heart. The problem is to determine that the cause of the palpitation is an infectious illness and to carry out the usual procedures to reveal the type of infection.

Hypoglycemia. Palpitation is often a prominent feature of this condition and appears to be related to release of epinephrine. The diagnosis is confirmed by appropriate blood sugar estimations and by prompt relief of all symptoms on the administration of glucose in one form or another (Chap. 96).

Aerophagia. Many patients who complain of "gas" and belching also complain of palpitation, possibly due in some cases to an associated anxiety state. This type of palpitation is readily recognized by the history of relief through eructation.

Tumors of the Adrenal Medulla (Pheochromocytomas). Such tumors may give rise to recurrent attacks, including paroxysms of hypertension and palpitation which are identical to those seen following the injection of epinephrine or norepinephrine. This type of tumor is a rather uncommon cause of palpitation and is mentioned chiefly because cure may be effected by surgical removal (Chap. 93). A similar syndrome may be produced when monoamine oxidase (MAO)-inhibitor drugs are taken concurrently with sympathomimetic drugs, such as ephedrine or amphetamine.

Drugs. The relationship between the development of palpitation and the use of tobacco, coffee, tea, alcohol, epinephrine, ephedrine, aminophylline, atropine, or thyroid extract is obvious.

PALPITATION AS A MANIFESTATION OF THE ANXIETY STATE. Persons who are healthy physically and well adjusted emotionally may have palpitation under certain circumstances. Thus, during or immediately after vigorous physical exertion or during sudden emotional tension, palpitation is common and is usually associated with outspoken tachycardia. Occasionally a healthy person may be conscious of his heartbeat when he is lying on the left side, but this type of palpitation is clearly due to the better transmission of the heart sounds to the ear when he is in that position. Lifting the head from the pillow will bring about a striking diminution or immediate disappearance of the symptom.

In some patients, palpitation may be one of the outstanding manifestations of a transitory episode of acute anxiety which may never recur, i.e., after this one episode or between infrequent bouts of increased nervous tension, the patient may experience no palpitation. In other persons the palpitation may, with other symptoms, represent prolonged anxiety neurosis or anxious depressions or a lifelong disorder indicative of disturbed autonomic function. The latter condition has been called neurocirculatory asthenia (see Chap. 369). Whether these illnesses are simply an expression of a chronic, deep-seated anxiety state superimposed on a normal autonomic nervous system or whether they depend on a constitutional or inherited autonomic instability is not yet entirely clear. At any rate, the clinical significance of this differentiation between the transitory and the enduring forms is that the former is often dissipated by firm reassurance from the physician, whereas the latter is usually resistant even to the most thorough and expert psychiatric care. In the latter case, the patient must be treated with most carefully planned psychologic support and tranquilizing medications. This chronic form of palpitation is known by various names, such as *Da Costa's syndrome, soldier's heart, effort syndrome, irritable heart, neurocirculatory asthenia,* and *functional cardiovascular disease.* Aside from palpitation, the chief symptoms are those of an anxiety state.

Physical examination usually reveals the typical findings of the hyperkinetic syndrome. These include a left parasternal lift, a precordial or apical systolic murmur, a wide pulse pressure, and a rapidly rising pulse. Electrocardiograms may display minor depressions of the S-T junction and inversion of T waves and so occasionally lead to a mistaken diagnosis of coronary disease; this is particularly likely to occur when these findings are associated with complaints by the patients of an aching feeling of substernal tightness, commonly present in emotional stress. The presence of any kind of organic disease is one of the commonest causes of the underlying anxiety which frequently produces this functional syndrome.

The diagnosis of this type of anxiety state depends on

Table 35-1. ITEMS TO BE COVERED IN HISTORY

Does the palpitation occur:	*If so, suspect:*
As isolated "jumps" or "skips"?.....................................	Extrasystoles
In attacks, known to be of abrupt beginning, with a heart rate of 120 beats/min or over, of regular or irregular rhythm?	Paroxysmal rapid heart action
Independent of exercise or excitement adequate to account for the symptom?	Atrial fibrillation, atrial flutter, thyrotoxicosis, anemia, febrile states, hypoglycemia, anxiety state
In attacks developing rapidly though not absolutely abruptly, unrelated to exertion or excitement?......................................	Hemorrhage, hypoglycemia, tumor of the adrenal medulla
In conjunction with the taking of drugs?..........................	Tobacco, coffee, tea, alcohol, epinephrine, ephedrine, aminophylline, atropine, thyroid extract, monoamine oxidase inhibitors
On standing?..	Postural hypotension
In middle-aged women, in conjunction with flushes and sweats?..........	Menopausal syndrome
When the rate is known to be normal and the rhythm regular?..........	Anxiety state

the presence of the findings mentioned above. Even when a patient presents undoubted objective evidence of structural cardiac disease, a superimposed anxiety state should be considered responsible for the symptoms when the clinical picture is that which has been described. Normal values for vital capacity and for circulation time make it extremely improbable that the dyspnea that accompanies this type of palpitation is due to organic cardiac disease. It is noteworthy that an anxiety state, in contrast to heart disease, causes a sighing type of dyspnea. Also pain localized to the region of the apex, lasting for hours or days, and accompanied by hyperesthesia is due usually to an anxiety state, not to structural cardiac disease. Palpitation associated with organic cardiac disease is nearly always accompanied by arrhythmia or by marked tachycardia, whereas the symptom may exist with regular rhythm and with a heart rate of 80 beats per min or less in patients with the anxiety state. Giddiness due to this syndrome can usually be reproduced by hyperventilation (Chap. 20) or by change from the recumbent to the erect posture.

The treatment of the anxiety cardiac syndrome depends on removal of the cause. In many instances a thorough examination of the heart and a statement that it is normal will suffice. Instructions to take more rather than less physical exercise will reinforce these statements. Frequently, the demonstration that the physician can reproduce not only the palpitation but many other symptoms of the anxiety state merely by the subcutaneous injection of 0.5 to 1.0 ml 1:1,000 epinephrine serves to convince the patient that his symptoms are not the result of some mysterious disorder but are rather the effect of a well-understood physiologic mechanism. This is especially true when the initial anxiety has been mainly the result of fear of heart disease. When the anxiety state is a manifestation of chronic anxiety neurosis or depressive psychosis, the symptoms are more likely to persist.

Management of patients with palpitation and the anxiety cardiac syndrome is facilitated by a clear understanding on the physician's part of the mechanisms of the symptoms. The palpitation is probably related to release of epinephrine and to the lower perception threshold. The pain probably arises in the intercostal tissues as a result of the pounding of the heart. The hyperventilation with its ensuing train of symptoms (Chap. 20) is analogous to sighing. It is possible that the entire syndrome is related to decline of the normal inhibitory effect of the cerebral cortex on those hypothalamic centers which normally control the sympathetic system ("cortical-hypothalamic imbalance"). Explanation of these physiologic mechanisms to the patient and reassurance that they are not indicative of serious disease is one of the most important therapeutic steps.

The commonest causes for palpitation have been enumerated and briefly discussed. Because this symptom occurs in such a wide variety of disorders which have no common or closely related underlying disturbance of structure or function, it is impossible to follow closely any predetermined plan of study in elucidating the significance of the symptom. The exact procedure will vary, of course, with the circumstances under which the patient is seen. Table 35-1 summarizes the main points of information that will be ascertained in the history. These questions and others formulated according to circumstances of the individual case will serve to suggest the additional lines of inquiry that may be necessary for analysis and appraisal of palpitation.

One point merits special emphasis. As a rule palpitation produces anxiety and fear out of all proportion to its seriousness. When the cause has been accurately determined and its significance explained to the patient, his concern is often ameliorated and may disappear entirely.

REFERENCES

Cohen, M. E., and P. D. White: Life Stress and Bodily Disease, vol. 29, chap. 56, in "Research Publications of the Association for Research in Nervous & Mental Disease," Baltimore, The Williams & Wilkins Company, 1950.

Kjellberg, S. R., V. Rudhe, and T. Sjöstrand: The Effect of Adrenaline on the Contraction of the Human Heart under Normal Circulatory Conditions, Acta Physiol. Scand., 24:333, 1952.

Siecke, H., and H. E. Essex: Relation of the Difference in Pressure across the Mitral Valve to the Amplitude of the First Heart Sound in Dogs with Atrioventricular Block, Am. J. Physiol., 192:135, 1958.

Wood, P.: "Diseases of the Heart and Circulation," 3d ed., pp. 17 and 18, Philadelphia, J. B. Lippincott Company, 1968.

Yu, P. N., B. J. B. Yim, and C. A. Stanfield: Hyperventilation Syndrome. Changes in the Electrocardiogram, Blood Gases, and Electrolytes during Voluntary Hyperventilation; Possible Mechanisms and Clinical Implications, A.M.A. Arch. Intern. Med., 103:902, 1959.

36 HYPOTENSION AND THE SHOCK SYNDROME

Karl Engelman and Eugene Braunwald

HYPOTENSION

The differential diagnosis of hypotensive states and the development of a rational plan of therapy require understanding of the normal regulation of arterial pressure.

CONTROL OF ARTERIAL PRESSURE. Arterial pressure must be maintained at levels sufficient to permit adequate perfusion of the extensive capillary networks in the systemic vascular bed. The level of pressure in the central arterial bed is in a large measure dependent on two factors—the volume of blood ejected by the left ventricle per unit of time, i.e., the cardiac output, and the resistance to blood flow offered by the vessels in the peripheral vascular bed. The resistance of a blood vessel, in turn, varies inversely as the fourth power of its radius, and at any given level of cardiac output arterial pressure is therefore largely dependent upon the degree of constriction of the smooth muscle in the walls of the arterioles. Though resistance to flow also varies with the viscosity of the fluid and the length of the vessels, alterations in these factors are ordinarily of only secondary importance.

Cardiac output is controlled largely by factors which regulate ventricular end-diastolic volume, the level of myocardial contractility, and heart rate (Chap. 263). The autonomic nervous system plays a major role in the maintenance of arterial pressure by its influences on the cardiac output and on the degree of constriction of the resistance (arterioles) and capacitance (venules and veins) vessels. The afferent limbs of the autonomic reflex arcs regulating arterial pressure arise in stretch receptors in the aortic arch and the carotid sinuses. Impulses are transmitted along afferent fibers in the glossopharyngeal and vagus nerves to extensive central autonomic connections in the medulla. Synapses connect not only the sympathetic and parasympathetic nuclei and efferent arcs, but also the cerebral cortex and hypothalamic nuclei which control hormonal secretion via the pituitary gland.

A rapid reduction of arterial pressure diminishes the stimulation of baroreceptors, which in turn evokes an activation of sympathetic outflow and inhibition of parasympathetic activity. As a result, the vascular smooth muscles in arterioles and veins constrict, while heart rate and myocardial contractility are augmented. In addition, adrenal medullary secretion is increased, as are the output of antidiuretic hormone (ADH), adrenocorticotrophic hormone (ACTH), and aldosterone; all of these effects act to restore the arterial pressure to control levels. Opposite changes occur if arterial pressure is raised acutely. Thus, the operation of the baroreceptor system normally serves to buffer the body from a variety of influences which would otherwise produce marked alterations in arterial pressure.

MEASUREMENT OF ARTERIAL PRESSURE. Arterial pressure is determined clinically with a pneumatic cuff; ordinarily, this indirect method provides slight underestimation of the true arterial pressure. Considerable error may be introduced if proper precautions are not taken in determining blood pressure by this method. The arterial pressure may be significantly underestimated if the air in the cuff is released too rapidly, especially in the presence of bradycardia or an irregular rhythm, or if inadequate inflation of the cuff does not result in complete vascular occlusion. This indirect method is most accurate when, in normal-sized adults, cuffs 12 to 14 cm in width are employed. However, when a cuff of this size is used on children or adults with unusually thin arms, blood pres-

Table 36-1. RANGE OF NORMAL BLOOD PRESSURES

Age, years	Systolic blood pressure, mean ± 2 SD, mmHg		Diastolic blood pressure, mean ± 2 SD, mmHg	
Newborn	80 ± 16*		46 ± 16*	
1......	96 ± 30		66 ± 25	
2......	99 ± 25		64 ± 25	
4......	99 ± 20		65 ± 20	
6......	100 ± 15		56 ± 8	
8......	105 ± 16		57 ± 9	
10......	111 ± 17		58 ± 10	
13......	118 ± 19		60 ± 10	
	Male	Female	Male	Female
20–24....	123 ± 18†	116 ± 18†	76 ± 14†	72 ± 12†
25–29....	125 ± 17	117 ± 15	78 ± 11	74 ± 12
30–34....	126 ± 17	120 ± 18	79 ± 13	75 ± 14
35–39....	127 ± 18	124 ± 19	80 ± 13	78 ± 13
40–44....	129 ± 19	127 ± 23	81 ± 12	80 ± 14
45–49....	130 ± 22	131 ± 25	82 ± 13	82 ± 15
50–54....	135 ± 25	137 ± 27	83 ± 14	84 ± 16
55–59....	138 ± 25	139 ± 28	84 ± 14	84 ± 16
60–64....	142 ± 27	144 ± 29	85 ± 16	85 ± 17

* (Newborn to 13 years). Includes both males and females. From R. J. Haggerty, M. W. Maroney, and A. S. Nadas: Essential Hypertension in Infancy and Childhood, A.M.A. J. Dis. Child., 92:535, 1956.

† (20 to 64 years). From A. M. Master, C. I. Garfield, and M. B. Walters, Normal Blood Pressure and Hypertension, Philadelphia, Lea & Febiger, 1952.

sure may be seriously underestimated, or conversely, it may be overestimated when employed on an arm or thigh greater than 20 cm in girth. Marked vasoconstriction resulting in severely attenuated limb blood flow and/or marked reductions in pulse pressure may also result in serious underestimation of arterial pressure by the auscultatory method. Direct intraarterial recordings may reveal a normal or even an elevated pressure, while the absence of Korotkoff sounds makes the pressure unobtainable by the indirect methods.

THE "NORMAL" BLOOD PRESSURE. The "normal" blood pressure has been difficult to define. Traditional statistical approaches define normality on the basis of values included within two standard deviations of the mean of pressures obtained in a large population of healthy individuals. Analysis of blood pressures obtained from a study of 74,000 presumably healthy, working adults, aged twenty to sixty-four years, revealed that in both sexes the levels of systolic and diastolic pressures rise gradually but progressively with age (Table 36-1). There is little variation in the distribution of pressures at the lower end of the scale over the entire age span, but all curves are skewed to the right for the older subjects. This distribution reflects the increased incidence of hypertension with aging. Chronic hypotension, however, occurs only rarely.

ACUTE HYPOTENSION AND SHOCK

Not commonly, physicians are called upon to treat patients who acutely develop severe hypotension or shock. These two terms are not synonymous; although shock is usually associated with hypotension, a previously hypertensive patient may be in shock despite an arterial pressure within normal limits, and hypotension may occur in the absence of shock. *Shock* may be defined as a state in which there is widespread, serious reduction of tissue perfusion which, if prolonged, leads to generalized impairment of cellular function.

The most common clinical causes of shock are listed in Table 36-2. Since maintenance of arterial pressure is dependent on cardiac output and peripheral vasomotor tone, marked reductions in either of these variables without a compensatory elevation of the other results in systemic hypotension. Reduction of cardiac output due to hypovolemia or acute myocardial infarction is among the most frequently encountered and easily categorized causes of shock. Failure of neurogenic mechanisms resulting in decreased vasoconstrictor impulses is another well-defined category; in many patients, particularly in the late stages of shock, multiple factors play a role in the development of circulatory failure.

Hypovolemia has been studied much more extensively than any other cause of shock; the mechanism of development is usually readily evident and well understood, and therapy, i.e., restoration of blood volume, is both simple and effective if applied before irreversible tissue damage occurs. Whether the primary insult is the external loss of blood, plasma, or water and salt or the internal sequestration of these fluids in a hollow viscus or body cavity, the general effect is similar, i.e., reduced venous return and decreased cardiac output. For purposes of a general discussion of shock, hemorrhagic hypovolemia will be used as the model, but the general physiologic consequences of the various etiologies of reduced tissue perfusion are similar.

Table 36-2. ETIOLOGIC FACTORS IN SHOCK

I. Hypovolemia
  A. External Fluid Losses
    1. Hemorrhage
    2. Gastrointestinal
      a. Vomiting (pyloric stenosis, intestinal obstruction)
      b. Diarrhea
    3. Renal
      a. Diabetes mellitus
      b. Diabetes insipidis
      c. Excessive use of diuretics
    4. Cutaneous
      a. Burns
      b. Exudative lesions
      c. Perspiration and insensible water loss without replacement
  B. Internal sequestration
    1. Fractures
    2. Ascites (peritonitis, pancreatitis, cirrhosis)
    3. Intestinal obstruction
    4. Hemothorax
    5. Hemoperitoneum
II. Cardiogenic
  A. Myocardial infarction
  B. Arrhythmia (paroxysmal tachycardia or fibrillation, severe bradycardia)
III. Obstruction to blood flow
  A. Pulmonary embolus
  B. Tension pneumothorax
  C. Cardiac tamponade
  D. Dissecting aortic aneurysm
  E. Intracardiac (ball-valve thrombus, atrial myxoma)
IV. Neuropathic
  A. Drug induced
    1. Anesthesia
    2. Ganglion-blocking or other antihypertensive drugs
    3. "Ingestion" (barbiturates, glutethimide, phenothiazines)
  B. Spinal cord injury
  C. Orthostatic hypotension (primary autonomic insufficiency, peripheral neuropathies)
V. Other
  A. Infection
    1. Gram-negative septicemia (endotoxin)
    2. Other septicemias
  B. Anaphylaxis
  C. Endocrine failure (Addison's Disease, myxedema)
  D. Anoxia

Depending upon the severity and rate of development of hypovolemia, the shock syndrome may develop abruptly or evolve gradually. If the precipitating factors progress unabated, the endogenous defense mechanisms, while initially competent to maintain adequate circulation, eventually are extended beyond their capacity for compensation. The development of the shock syndrome may be thought to evolve through several stages which merge with one another:

1. The period in which the blood volume deficit is relatively minor and in which the patient may be asymptomatic. In a previously healthy individual compensation for an acute blood loss of as much as 10 percent of the normal blood volume (as with venesection of 500 ml blood from a donor) is achieved acutely by constriction of the arteriolar bed and an augmentation of heart rate and myocardial contractility. Other responses with more gradual effects include the increased secretion of antidiuretic hormone and aldosterone, which results in salt and water retention and the redistribution of fluid into the intravascular compartment. Arterial pressure is maintained and cardiac output is normal, or only slightly reduced, primarily as a consequence of selective reductions of blood flow to the skin, kidney, and muscle beds.

2. With a reduction of blood volume of 15 to 25 percent, cardiac output falls markedly, and despite intense arteriolar constriction in most vascular beds, arterial pressure declines. Generalized venoconstriction occurs, increasing the fraction of the total blood volume in the central circulation and tending to sustain venous return. With this massive reflex adrenergic discharge there is tachycardia, intense cutaneous vasoconstriction, pallor, diaphoresis, piloerection, oliguria, apprehension, and restlessness.

3. Once the patient has achieved this state of maximal mobilization of compensatory mechanisms, small additional losses of blood result in rapid deterioration of the circulation, with life-threatening reductions of cardiac output, blood pressure, and tissue perfusion. The duration of this shock state, the severity of tissue anoxia, and the age and underlying physical state of the patient are of primary importance in determining the ultimate outcome. If tissue perfusion is restored rapidly, recovery may be expected. However, if shock persists, the severe vasoconstriction may itself become a complicating factor and by reducing tissue perfusion even further may initiate a vicious cycle leading to an irreversible state due to widespread cellular injury. Anoxia, hypercapnia, and acidosis result from hypoperfusion of tissues; these metabolic derangements ultimately result in failure of the energy-requiring active transport systems of cell membranes. The integrity of the cells is compromised, and potassium ions, intracellular enzymes, peptides, and other vasoactive compounds are released into the circulation. Of special importance during prolonged profound shock is stasis of the microcirculation of the bowel and breakdown of the mucosal barrier, which leads to the entry of bacteria and bacterial toxins into the bloodstream. Because many of these substances are potent vasodilators, there may be widespread inhibition of vasoconstrictor tone, which depresses arterial pressure despite intense sympathetic activity. Blood flow to the brain and heart is further reduced, and infarction of these vital organs usually leads to death.

Just as cardiac output may fall to dangerous or even fatal levels due to actual fluid losses or sequestration with diminished venous return, cardiac failure or intrathoracic obstruction to blood flow may have a similar effect. Furthermore, even in the presence of a normal blood volume and cardiac function, "vasomotor collapse" due to drug-induced or neuropathic failure of sympathetic vasomotor activity can result in shock due to reduction of peripheral resistance and the pooling of blood in the venous bed. Finally, a complex form of shock may result from infection, especially gram-negative bacteremia with endotoxin release, from anaphylaxis, anoxia, and endocrine disorders which affect myocardial function, fluid and electrolyte balance, vasomotor tone, and general tissue metabolic processes.

Treatment of the patient with shock should be directed toward the rapid restoration of cardiac output and tissue perfusion. General supportive measures must be undertaken immediately, sometimes even before the etiology of the shock state has been identified. Whether shock results from decreased cardiac output due to a primary reduction in intravascular volume or a reduction of "effective blood volume" with pooling of blood in certain vascular beds, the most effective means of restoring adequate circulation is by the rapid infusion of volume-expanding fluids (whole blood, plasma, plasma substitutes, or isotonic electrolyte solutions). However, when shock is secondary to, or is accompanied by, cardiac failure with increased central venous pressure, the infusion of volume-expanding fluids may result in pulmonary edema. Here attention must be directed toward restoring cardiac function with cardiotonic drugs such as the digitalis glycosides and isoproterenol, and an attempt should be made to support arterial pressure at levels sufficient to maintain the coronary perfusion pressure (Chap. 271). Arrhythmias, which may also contribute to the low cardiac output, should be corrected (Chap. 265).

The appearance of the external jugular veins may be helpful in differentiating between shock with high or low central venous pressure. However, a catheter inserted into the superior vena cava is the best means for continuously monitoring venous pressure and is of considerable value in guiding therapy; such a catheter should be inserted in patients with shock whenever possible. Serial measurements of venous pressure, urine flow rate, heart rate, and the clinical and mental state of the patient often provide more important indices of the efficacy of therapy than arterial pressure changes.

There is considerable debate concerning the efficacy of vasocontrictor drugs in shock. In patients with severe peripheral constriction these agents are often ineffective and may actually reduce the already lowered tissue perfusion. However, these drugs are usually helpful in patients with inadequate vasoconstrictor responses. The use of alpha adrenergic blocking agents or massive doses of adrenal glucocorticoids in shock secondary to gram-negative septicemia with endotoxin release is also a matter of considerable controversy and cannot yet be considered a routine procedure.

CHRONIC HYPOTENSION

Although many patients have been treated for chronic "low blood pressure," most of these individuals, with systolic pressures in the range of 90 to 110 mm Hg, are normal and may actually have a greater life expectancy than their cohorts with higher pressures. Patients with true chronic hypotension may complain of lethargy, weakness, easy fatigability, and dizziness or faintness, especially if arterial pressure is lowered further when the erect position is assumed. These symptoms are presumably due to a decrease in perfusion of the brain, heart, skeletal muscle, and other organs.

Although arterial pressure is usually normal or even slightly elevated in patients with congestive heart failure, chronic hypotension occasionally results from severe reductions of the cardiac output, particularly in patients with stenotic valvular lesions and in patients with chronic constrictive pericarditis. The major endocrine causes of chronic hypotension are associated with deficient gluco- and mineralocorticoid secretion and resultant reductions of the intravascular and interstitial fluid volume. Hypotension is usually more pronounced in patients with primary adrenocortical insufficiency than in those with hypopituitarism because secretion of the salt-retaining adrenocortical hormone, aldosterone, is partially preserved in pituitary insufficiency (Chap. 87).

Malnutrition, cachexia, chronic bed rest, and a variety of neurologic disorders may result in chronic hypotension, especially in the standing position. Interference with the neural pathways anywhere between the vasomotor center and the efferent sympathetic nerve endings on the blood vessels or heart may prevent the vasoconstriction and increase in cardiac output which occur as a normal response to a reduction in arterial pressure. Multiple sclerosis, amyotrophic lateral sclerosis, syringomyelia, syphilitic or diabetic tabes dorsalis, peripheral neuropathies, spinal cord section, diabetic neuropathy, extensive lumbodorsal sympathectomy, and the administration of drugs interfering with nerve transmission in the sympathetic nervous system are all associated with orthostatic hypotension. In addition, idiopathic orthostatic hypotension (primary autonomic insufficiency), a rare condition in which there is degeneration of central and/or peripheral autonomic nervous structures, may result in such severe orthostatic hypotension that syncope or seizures occur when the patient arises from recumbency. This condition is progressive and characterized by ascending anhydrosis and loss of hair, decreased BMR, reduced norepinephrine production, deficient secretion of lacrimal and salivary glands, ileus, bladder atony, and absence of tachycardia on standing despite the marked reduction of blood pressure.

Specific therapy is not available for most of the neurologic causes of orthostatic hypotension, and treatment with sympathomimetic drugs has not proved effective over prolonged periods. However, the expansion of extracellular volume, which may be achieved with a high (10 to 20 Gm per day) salt diet and/or the potent synthetic salt-retaining steroid, 9-α-fluorohydrocortisone (0.1 to 0.5 mg per day) may be helpful. Tight, full-length, elastic supportive hose to reduce orthostatic pooling of blood in the legs may also arterial pressure, and in the

most severe cases pressurized aviator suits may be necessary to permit ambulation.

REFERENCES

Beecher, H. K., F. A. Simeone, C. A. Burnett, S. L. Shapiro, E. F. Sullivan, and T. B. Mallory: The Internal State of the Severely Wounded Man on Entry to the Most Forward Hospital. *Surgery* 22:672, 1947.

Master, A. M., C. I. Garfield, and M. B. Walters: Normal Blood Pressure and Hypertension, Philadelphia, Lea and Febiger, 1952.

Weil, M. H., and H. Shubin: Diagnosis and Treatment of Shock, Baltimore, The Williams & Wilkins Company, 1967.

37 ELEVATION OF ARTERIAL PRESSURE

*Karl Engelman and
Eugene Braunwald*

Patients with elevations of arterial pressure are usually asymptomatic, and the blood pressure abnormality often arouses attention only incidentally during military, life insurance, or other periodic physical examination. Because hypertension results in secondary organ damage and a reduced life span, it should be evaluated fully and, when appropriate, treated.

DIAGNOSIS OF HYPERTENSION. Often, however, the first question is whether patients with a moderately elevated routine blood pressure recording are truly hypertensive. It is well established that anxiety, discomfort, physical activity, or other stress can acutely and transiently raise arterial pressure. Most individuals have a higher pressure when initially examined than after several measurements made in the course of a single visit; in order to establish the diagnosis of hypertension it is necessary to document in the course of several examinations that arterial pressure remains elevated. Patients with transient or "labile" hypertension may not require treatment, but should be reexamined periodically, since over the course of time such individuals often develop sustained hypertension.

Systolic hypertension in the presence of a normal or reduced diastolic pressure is rarely considered to be responsible for organ damage, but usually reflects other pathologic processes. It is most commonly seen in elderly patients with decreased compliance of the aortic wall. In patients with severe bradycardia, thyrotoxicosis, severe anemia, fever, aortic valvular insufficiency, arteriovenous shunts or fistulas, and the hyperkinetic heart syndrome, systolic hypertension is due to an elevated stroke volume, often accompanied by a rapid diastolic runoff.

Patients with true systemic hypertension have an increased mean arterial pressure with elevations of both systolic and diastolic pressures. Regardless of the primary etiology, the hemodynamic abnormality in most of these patients is increased vascular resistance, especially at the level of the smaller muscular arteries and arterioles, though a small number of patients may also have an increased cardiac output, particularly in the early stages of the illness. In a small fraction of patients, hypertension is associated with hypervolemia or increased blood viscosity secondary to polycythemia.

ETIOLOGY OF HYPERTENSION

A specific etiology for the increase in peripheral resistance which is responsible for the elevated arterial pressure cannot be defined for at least 90 percent of patients with hypertensive disease. Numerous experimental studies have sought to define the role of a variety of components ultimately responsible for idiopathic, or so-called "essential," hypertension. Evidence for the role played by abnormal psychologic stimuli comes from the finding that chronically stressed animals may become hypertensive, and that sedatives and tranquilizers are helpful in the treatment of many hypertensive patients. Another neurogenic mechanism, the resetting of the sensitivity of the baroreceptors, occurs in hypertensive dogs so that they appear to recognize elevated arterial pressures as normal. The importance of salt intake is suggested by studies showing that rats can be made hypertensive when given excessive dietary salt, and epidemiologic studies have also suggested this as a factor of possible etiologic significance in man; other studies have indicated that increased water and sodium in the walls of arterioles may result in increased peripheral resistance.

It appears that all of the above-mentioned factors play some role in patients with essential hypertension, which might be best regarded as a multifactorial disease related to abnormalities of the regulatory mechanisms normally concerned with the homeostatic control of arterial pressure. Page has described a "mosaic pattern" of how the complex interrelationships of central and sympathetic nervous influences, vascular defects, water and electrolyte metabolism, and cardiac activity can combine to produce the hypertensive state. In addition, hereditary and racial factors seem to play significant roles in the development of hypertension, since this disease is often found in families and is especially prevalent and virulent among certain ethnic groups, such as the American Negro population.

More specific etiologic relationships have been established for a smaller group of patients with systemic hypertension (Table 37-1). Primary renal diseases associated with the development of serious hypertension (as distinguished from renal damage secondary to hypertension) have been recognized for years, although in many cases the exact mechanism of blood pressure elevation is unknown. Hypertension may develop suddenly during the course of acute glomerulonephritis and it is usually a prominent feature in the late stages of renal damage due to chronic glomerulonephritis (Chap. 304) or pyelonephritis (Chap. 303). Polycystic renal disease, renal infarction, or partial occlusion of the renal artery due to congenital or acquired vascular defects are also

Table 37-1. CLASSIFICATION OF ARTERIAL HYPERTENSION

I. Systolic hypertension with wide pulse pressure
   A. Decreased compliance of aorta (arteriosclerosis)
   B. Increased stroke volume or cardiac output
      1. Arteriovenous fistula
      2. Thyrotoxicosis
      3. Hyperkinetic heart disease
      4. Fever
      5. Psychogenic
      6. Aortic valvular insufficiency
      7. Patent ductus arteriosus

II. Systolic and diastolic hypertension (increased peripheral vascular resistance)
   A. Renal
      1. Chronic pyelonephritis
      2. Acute and chronic glomerulonephritis
      3. Polycystic renal disease
      4. Renovascular stenosis or renal infarction
      5. Most other severe renal disease (arteriolar nephrosclerosis, diabetic nephropathy, etc.)
   B. Endocrine
      1. Acromegaly
      2. Adrenocortical hyperfunction
         a. Cushing's disease and syndrome
         b. Primary hyperaldosteronism
         c. Congenital or hereditary adrenogenital syndromes (17-α-hydroxylase and 11-β-hydroxylase defects)
      3. Pheochromocytoma
   C. Neurogenic
      1. Psychogenic
      2. "Diencephalic syndrome"
      3. Familial dysautonomia (Riley-Day)
      4. Poliomyelitis (bulbar)
      5. Polyneuritis (acute porphyria, lead poisoning)
      6. Increased intracranial pressure (acute)
      7. Spinal cord section
   D. Miscellaneous
      1. Coarctation of aorta
      2. Increased intravascular volume (excessive transfusion)
      3. Polyarteritis nodosa
   E. Unknown etiology
      1. Essential hypertension (>90% of all cases of hypertension)
      2. Toxemia of pregnancy
      3. Acute intermittent porphyria

implicated as etiologic factors, the latter having been clearly related to activation of the renin-angiotensin-aldosterone pressor system.

The most clearly defined etiologic relationships in the development of hypertension are found among the endocrine disorders. Adrenocortical hormones have also been implicated in the hypertensive syndromes associated with tumors or hyperplasia of the anterior pituitary (Cushing's Syndrome, primary hyperaldosteronism, Chap. 92), as well as with various congenital or hereditary enzyme defects (hypertensive adrenogenital syndromes). Secretion of excessive qualities of the pressor catecholamines, norepinephrine and epinephrine, associated with pheochromocytomas, i.e., chromaffin cell tumors arising from the adrenal medulla or sympathetic ganglia, are also commonly associated with hypertension (Chap. 93). Patients with acromegaly (Chap. 87) may have hypertension, but the mechanism of their blood pressure elevation is less clear. The presence of these endocrinopathies is usually readily recognizable and distinguishable from essential hypertension by their distinctive clinical and biochemical features.

EFFECTS OF HYPERTENSION

Following an asymptomatic latent period, clinical manifestations which reflect the underlying pathologic sequelae of the hypertensive state usually become apparent. Cardiac, renal, and central nervous system effects due to accelerated vascular damage are most prominent, and if unaltered by therapy, they often ultimately result in symptomatic illness and death.

EFFECTS ON HEART. Cardiac compensation for the excessive work load imposed by increased systemic pressure is at first sustained by the presence of left ventricular hypertrophy. Ultimately, the function of this chamber deteriorates, it dilates, and the symptoms and signs of heart failure appear (Chap. 264). Angina pectoris may also occur due to accelerated coronary arterial disease and/or increased myocardial oxygen requirements as a consequence of the increased myocardial mass which exceeds the capacity of the coronary circulation. On physical examination the heart is enlarged and has prominent left ventricular impulse. The sound of aortic closure is accentuated, and there may be a faint murmur of aortic insufficiency. Presystolic (atrial) gallop sounds appear frequently in hypertensive heart disease and a protodiastolic (ventricular), or summation, gallop rhythm may be present. Electrocardiographic changes of left ventricular hypertrophy are common, while evidence of ischemia or infarction may be observed late in the disease. The majority of deaths due to hypertension result from myocardial infarction or congestive heart failure.

NEUROLOGIC EFFECTS. The neurologic effects of long-standing hypertension can be divided into retinal and central nervous system changes. Because the retina is the only tissue in which the arteries and arterioles can be examined directly, repeated ophthalmoscopic examination provides the opportunity to observe the progress of the vascular effects of hypertension. The Keith-Wagener-Barker classification of the retinal changes in hypertension (Table 37-2) has provided a simple and excellent means for serial evaluation of the hypertensive patient. Table 37-2 includes both the criteria for grouping the retinal findings of hypertension and the secondary arteriolosclerotic changes. Increasing severity of hypertension is associated with focal spasm and progressive general narrowing of the arterioles, as well as the appearance of hemorrhages, exudates and papilledema. These retinal lesions often produce scotomata, blurred vision, and even blindness, especially in the presence of papilledema or hemorrhages of the macular area. Hypertensive lesions may develop acutely, and if therapy results in significant reduction of blood pressure, may show rapid resolution. Rarely, these lesions resolve without therapy. In contrast,

Table 37-2. CLASSIFICATION OF HYPERTENSIVE AND ARTERIOLARSCLEROTIC RETINOPATHY

Degree	Hypertension					Arteriolarsclerosis	
	Arterioles		Hemor-rhages	Exudates	Papilledema	Arteriolar light reflex	AV crossing‡ defects
	General narrowing A/V ratio*	Focal spasm†					
Normal	3/4	1/1	0	0	0	Fine yellow line, red blood column	0
Grade I	1/2	1/1	0	0	0	Broadened yellow line, red blood column	Mild depression of vein
Grade II	1/3	2/3	0	0	0	Broad yellow line, "copper wire," blood column not visible	Depression or humping of vein
Grade III	1/4	1/3	+	+	0	Broad white line, "silver wire," blood column not visible	a) Right-angle deviation, tapering and disappearance of vein under arteriole b) Distal dilatation of vein
Grade IV	Fine, fibrous cords	Obliteration of distal flow	+	+	+	Fibrous cords, blood column not visible	Same as grade III

* This is the ratio of arteriolar/venous diameters.
† This is the ratio of diameters of region of spasm to proximal arteriole.
‡ Arteriolar length and tortuosity increases with severity.

retinal arteriolosclerosis is a degenerative process resulting from endothelial and muscular proliferation, and it accurately reflects similar changes in other organs. Sclerotic changes do not develop as rapidly as hypertensive lesions nor do they regress appreciably with therapy. As a consequence of increased wall thickness and rigidity, sclerotic arterioles distort and compress the veins as they cross within their common fibrous sheath, and the reflected light streak from the arterioles is changed by the increased opacity of the vessel wall.

Central-nervous-system dysfunction also occurs frequently in patients with hypertension. Occipital headaches, most often in the morning, are among the most prominent early symptoms of hypertension. Dizziness, lightheadedness, vertigo, tinnitus, and dimmed vision or syncope may also be observed, but the more serious manifestations are due to vascular occlusion or hemorrhage. With severe long-standing hypertension, patients develop multiple focal or large vascular infarcts or hemorrhages which result in destruction of brain tissue. The focal changes may be manifested as personality or memory deficits, but the larger lesions which produce major strokes are responsible for up to 10 to 15 percent of deaths occurring secondary to hypertension.

RENAL EFFECTS. Vascular damage in hypertension also affects the kidneys. Arteriolosclerotic lesions of the afferent and efferent arterioles and the glomerular capillary tufts are the most common renal vascular lesions and result in decreased glomerular filtration rate and tubular dysfunction. Proteinuria and microscopic hematuria occur due to glomerular lesions, and approximately 10 percent of the deaths secondary to hypertension result from renal failure. Blood loss in hypertension occurs not only from renal lesions, but epistaxis, hemoptysis, and metrorrhagia also occur more frequently in these patients.

MALIGNANT HYPERTENSION. Although these complications of hypertension are serious and are often eventually fatal after many years of the disease, a small fraction, variously estimated as between 1 and 5 percent, of patients with essential hypertension enter an accelerated phase which usually results in rapid death. This "malignant" phase of hypertension is associated with very high levels of arterial pressure and characteristic rapidly progressive necrosis of the walls of small arteries and arterioles with concentric collagenous endothelial thickening leading to diminution or occlusion of the vascular lumen. These lesions of arteriolonecrosis result in massive proteinuria, hematuria and rapidly progressive uremia, grade IV retinopathy with papilledema, and cerebral edema with increased intracranial pressure, mental confusion, and seizures. These manifestations progress rapidly over a period of days to weeks and if therapy is not effective, death occurs from uremia or an intracranial vascular accident.

As a consequence of the pathologic changes secondary to the elevated arterial pressure, treatment of patients with systemic hypertension is directed toward lowering pressure in an attempt to halt or reverse the progressive organ damage. In certain instances specific therapy or cure of the primary etiologic factor can be achieved by repair of a stenotic renal artery lesion or coarctation of the aorta, or by removal or functional suppression of a humor which secretes pressor substances. However, because of the unknown etiology of the hypertension in the majority of patients, therapy is directed primarily toward the major physiologic abnormality, i.e., it is designed to lower systemic vascular resistance. Because the sympathetic nervous system plays such an important role in the maintenance of peripheral resistance, many effective antihypertensive drugs act by interfering with the vasoconstrictor impulses mediated by this system (Chap. 276). Although arterial pressure can be reduced in the majority of patients, hypertension is a chronic disease, and a therapeutic program must usually be maintained for the duration of the patient's life.

REFERENCES

Combined Staff Conference: Recent Advances in Hypertension, Am. J. Med., 39:616, 1965.

Freis, E. D.: Hemodynamics of Hypertension, Physiol. Rev. 40:27, 1960.

Page, I. H., and J. W. McCubbin: The Physiology of Arterial Hypertension, p. 2163, in W. F. Hamilton (Ed.), "Handbook of Physiology," vol. 3, Washington, D.C., The American Physiological Society, 1965.

Scheie, H. G.: Evaluation of Ophthalmoscopic Changes of Hypertension and Arteriolarsclerosis, A.M.A. Arch. Ophthalmol. 49:117, 1953.

38   COUGH AND HEMOPTYSIS
George W. Wright

COUGH

It is estimated that as much as 100 ml secretion is produced daily by the tracheobronchial mucosa. During the night, especially in older persons whose swallowing reflex is less competent, an added amount of secretion trickles into the trachea from the supralaryngeal region The accumulating secretions are moved, in part directly via the ciliary escalator and in part by the cough mechanism, to the pharynx, where the material is then swallowed or expectorated. In some persons, the volume and character of the secretions are such that the entire quantity can be moved by ciliary action alone, but when the secretions are unusually voluminous or difficult to move, the force of coughing is required to maintain clear air passages Under ordinary circumstances cough is considered to be an integral part of the "normal" act of tracheobronchial cleansing.

Cough, with or without the expulsion of secretions, may be a manifestation of disease. In a manner similar to other "clinical manifestations" which are in reality simply altered patterns of normal function, as for example increased frequency of urination or inappropriate breathlessness, sudden changes in cough pattern may be alarming, but gradual changes tend to be ignored by both patient and physician. A more precise delineation of the normal cough and sputum pattern would improve its clinical usefulness. With the increasing awareness that chronic bronchitis in its severe form is one of the common causes of serious morbidity, quantitative and qualitative cough and sputum patterns have been more extensively studied. The pattern indicative of disease has been more sharply defined, but there is still no agreement as to what is "normal." In a population thought to be healthy and having no experience of cigarette smoking, 23 percent admitted to a daily cough with phlegm, swallowed or expectorated, occurring the first thing in the morning only. Thus, a brief period of cough upon arising from sleep would seem acceptable as a normal pattern for clearing the air passages, even if associated with some phlegm. In contrast, cough, with or without phlegm, occurring *throughout* the day should require sufficient medical examination to exclude abnormal causes.

Like sneezing, cough may be a reflex mechanism. It can be invoked or, to some degree, inhibited voluntarily. It is initiated by stimulation of the mucosa or deeper structures in the larynx, trachea, and major bronchi. The nerve pathways involved are the glossopharyngeal and vagus. Direct stimulation of these nerves or their sensory endings in such places as the external ear, neck, and esophagus may also produce cough. Accumulation of mucus on the surface or inflammation, drying, cooling, and chemical stimulation of the mucosa will initiate this reflex, prompting a desire to cough. Changes in the intramural tension of the bronchi by contraction of smooth muscle or effects of gravity invoked by changes in posture may also play a role in initiating the cough reflex.

MECHANISM OF COUGH. The mechanical train of events leading to the expulsive action of a cough is complex. Combined pressure and cinefluorographic studies suggest the following mechanism. After an inspiration, the laryngeal end of the air tubes is firmly closed, and intrathoracic pressure is raised by an expiratory effort. A sudden release of the closed glottis creates a high gradient of pressure between the intrabronchial gas and that in the pharynx. Rates of air flow as high as 600 liters per minute may occur momentarily. It is believed that this high rate of flow moves secretions along the wall of the tubes. At almost the same moment, as the intratracheal pressure rapidly falls, a bronchial transmural pressure gradient is set up because the intrapulmonary air distal to the smaller bronchi is trapped against a higher resistance in the smaller tubes. This momentarily high transmural pressure produces a transient narrowing, if not complete closure, of the lumen of the trachea and major bronchi. These two events, namely narrowing of the lumen and augmented velocity of air flow, push the foreign material toward the oral pharynx in the same manner that a pea is expelled better from a closely fitting tube than from a loosely fitting one. Expulsion of mucus can occur without preliminary closure of the glottis, as for example through a tracheostomy. Cough is, however, not as effective in the tracheotomized person or in one whose respiratory muscles are weakened.

CAUSES OF COUGH. By far the commonest source of bronchial irritation associated with an abnormal cough pattern is that induced by cigarette smoking. Wynder, Lemon, and Mantel, in a study of the epidemiology of persistent cough, demonstrated that 45 percent of their population who smoked from 1 to 10 cigarettes per day and 70 percent of those who smoked more than 21 cigarettes per day had persistent cough. Expectoration of phlegm occurred in 90 percent of those with persistent cough. To what extent cough is directly related to chemical irritation or to hypersecretion has not been determined, but it can be assumed that both play a role. It is apparent from these observations that the use of cough and phlegm as a meaningful early sign of serious underlying lung disease other than chronic bronchitis is of limited value in those who smoke a pack or more of cigarettes daily. Nevertheless, no person with a chronic cough should ever be dismissed lightly as having a "cigarette cough" even though this is often the case.

In most instances of a rather abrupt change in the cough pattern, as for example that associated with the common cold, pneumonia, or pulmonary embolism and infarction, there are other signs and symptoms sufficiently alarming to bring the patient to a physician. Other diseases which begin less abruptly may have as their sole initial symptom an alteration in the cough pattern, and it is in these situations that particular care must be taken to find the cause of a persistently altered cough pattern. Subtle changes in the cough pattern may be due to tuberculosis, fungus infections, tumors, bronchiectasis, sarcoidosis, and many other diseases. Thorough use of roentgenographic and sputum study techniques as well as bronchoscopy must be resorted to under these conditions.

The great importance of cough and sputum as manifestations of chronic bronchitis are discussed in Chap. 283. Cough occurs in emphysema, where the cough mechanism tends to be ineffective and a low-grade chronic bronchitis often develops.

Cough, for the most part not associated with hypersecretion, may occur in diseases of the heart. Pressure of enlarged chambers and vessels on the vagus nerve may play a role in such coughs. Far more common, however, is the peculiar recurring single cough, at times little more than a "clearing of the throat," which is quite characteristic of mild pulmonary edema. In frank pulmonary edema cough is usually more severe.

As a rule, cough has a protective purpose, but it can also be harmful. Distal bronchial secretions tend to be spread peripherally during cough and may spread disease within the lung. Trauma to the tracheobronchial wall or larynx may lead to bleeding or play a role in the development of infection. The muscular effort involved in coughing is relatively great and may aggravate heart failure in patients who have passive congestion of the lungs.

Ribs may be fractured as the result of cough, and this is a not uncommon cause of severe chest pain. Muscle soreness likewise develops in chronic prolonged cough. The pain induced by these two mechanisms often presents a difficulty in differential diagnosis. During a prolonged paroxysm of cough, the persistent high intra-thoracic pressure may so impede venous return that cardiac output falls and cerebral ischemia occurs. This form of "cough" syncope may be associated with fainting and convulsions. It is most common in the elderly with cerebral arteriosclerosis. Such attacks developing in a person operating a mechanical device may lead to disastrous consequences. Cough may also be harmful in a public-health sense because of its potential for spreading infection.

HEMOPTYSIS

Bleeding from the lungs and major air passages is an important and fairly common medical problem. It is, of course, necessary to ascertain that the blood is actually coming from the tracheobronchial tree and not from the gastrointestinal tract or the nasopharynx. Blood which comes from the lungs is usually bright red, frothy in appearance, and mixed with phlegm. That from the stomach tends to be dark red or brown and mixed with food particles. Blood from actively bleeding gums or nasopharynx is virtually always bright red and as a rule is not frothy. In contrast to the retching and vomiting associated with hematemesis and the clearing of the throat or blowing of the nose associated with nasopharyngeal bleeding, the blood which comes from the lung is almost always associated with coughing or with the sensation that something has come into the back of the throat which requires throat clearing. Vomiting often causes coughing and vice versa, but the sequence of these events helps to determine the source of the blood.

In view of the extraordinary vascularity of the lung, it is remarkable that hemoptysis is not more common. It seems likely that some capillary bleeding may occur periodically within the lungs and may never be brought up to the pharynx, but instead be reabsorbed at its point of origin. Pneumonia, chronic passive congestion of the lungs, and pulmonary infarction frequently are associated with frank hemoptysis. However, emphysema, a disease characterized by actual destruction of the most distal pulmonary vascular components, is associated with hemoptysis only infrequently.

CAUSES OF HEMOPTYSIS. The most common causes of hemoptysis are infections, neoplasms, and cardiovascular disorders, but include many other more uncommon causes such as arteriovenous aneurysm, foreign body, parasites, and broncholith. Thoracic trauma, with or without rib fracture, may also produce hemoptysis. Several studies of the etiology of hemoptysis have been made in large groups of patients. The frequency of the various causes differs according to the source, i.e., whether the study is of a population survey, a general hospital, or a surgical clinic. In some groups the cause remains undetermined in as many as 45 percent of cases even after thorough and prolonged search, while in others, only approximately 10 percent of cases is undiagnosed. In general hospitals, hemoptysis is caused by neoplasms in 5 percent, lower respiratory tract infection in 35 percent, tuberculosis in

10 percent, and cardiovascular disease in 10 percent of patients; the remaining 40 percent are undiagnosed. In more limited populations—especially those related to surgical clinics—the proportions are strikingly different, with neoplasm and lower respiratory tract infection accounting for 75 percent of cases and only 7 or 8 percent remaining undiagnosed.

It is not known with certainty whether or not hard coughing alone can lead to hemoptysis. Chronic bronchitis is the cause of most episodes of severe prolonged cough not associated with disorders such as neoplasms or abscess. In view of the altered mucosa in bronchitis, it is not surprising that bleeding or hemoptysis would occur. In some populations chronic bronchitis probably is the underlying etiology of most episodes of mild hemoptysis.

The sputum in bacterial pneumonia nearly always contains blood at some stage in the course of the disease. In the virus pneumonias bleeding is not nearly so common or profuse. In most pneumonias the sputum seldom resembles pure blood but is mixed with mucopurulent material.

In the early stages of pulmonary tuberculosis hemoptysis may be minor but is often persistent. In the more extensive cavitary forms of the disease a large vessel may erode, producing massive or, rarely, even fatal hemorrhage. Because the blood from a tuberculous cavity may be heavily contaminated with organisms, hemoptysis may be associated with an extensive spread of the disease to other parts of the lung via the bronchial system.

It is estimated that hemoptysis occurs on one or more occasion in virtually all patients with bronchiectasis, and in many this is the most frightening aspect of the disease. Chronic inflammation and erosion of the mucosa in the bronchiectatic area presumably causes the bleeding. Hemoptysis is so common and recurrent in bronchiectasis that patients learn to ignore it.

Lung tumors often first manifest their presence by hemoptysis. Bronchial carcinoma should be suspected as the cause of hemoptysis in any patient with a history of smoking a pack or more of cigarettes daily for 20 or more years. At least 50 percent of bronchial neoplasms lead to hemoptysis. With adenoma of the bronchus bleeding may be very profuse.

Pulmonary infarction is one of the commonest causes of hemoptysis occurring in patients hospitalized for reasons other than lung infection. Pulmonary embolism without infarction is less likely to produce hemoptysis. Pulmonary infarction should be suspected as the cause of hemoptysis (1) whenever there is associated pleural pain without clear evidence of pneumonia, (2) in all patients with congestive heart failure, (3) in the postoperative and posttraumatic states, (4) in all bedridden patients, (5) whenever there are signs of phlebothrombosis, and (6) in patients who have transient elevations of serum bilirubin and lactic dehydrogenase with a normal value for serum transaminase.

Pulmonary vascular congestion secondary to heart disease is a common cause of hemoptysis. This is particularly true in mitral stenosis (Chap. 270) but is less common with other causes of congestive failure. Rarely, hemoptysis occurs in patients with systemic arterial hypertension, presumably due to a rupture of a submucosal artery.

Hemoptysis also occurs in the purpuras and leukemias and has been reported in association with anticoagulant therapy. That it does not occur more commonly when clotting is compromised suggests that spontaneous intermittent small-vessel bleeding in the lung parenchyma may in fact be rather uncommon.

REFERENCES

Committee on Etiology of Chronic Bronchitis, Medical Research Council: Definition and Classification of Chronic Bronchitis, Brit. Med. J. (Lancet), 1:775, 1965.

Committee on Therapy, American Thoracic Society: The Management of Hemoptysis, Am. Rev. Resp. Dis., 93:471, 1966.

Loudon, R. G., and L. C. Brown: Cough Frequency in Patients with Respiratory Disease, Am. Rev. Resp. Dis., 96:1137, 1967.

——, and G. B. Shaw: Mechanics of Cough in Normal Subjects and in Patients with Obstructive Respiratory Disease, Am. Rev. Resp. Dis., 96:666, 1967.

Salem, H., and D. M. Aviado: Antitussive Drugs, Am. J. Med. Sci., 247:585, 1964.

Wynder, E. L., F. R. Lemon, and N. Mantel: Epidemiology of Persistent Cough, Am. Rev. Resp. Dis., 91:679, 1965.

Section 5

Alterations in Gastrointestinal Function

39 ORAL MANIFESTATIONS OF DISEASE

Paul Goldhaber

DISTURBANCES OF THE TEETH AND DENTAL TISSUES

DEVELOPMENTAL DISTURBANCES. Since tooth structure, unlike bone, does not undergo physiologic remodeling, developmental disturbances severe enough to cause obvious alterations in the morphologic features or integrity of the teeth provide relatively permanent evidence that a systemic disturbance has acted during that particular phase of tooth development.

The most common type of defect is *enamel hypoplasia,* which results from an aberration in enamel formation due to disturbance of those ameloblasts actively secreting enamel matrix. The defects range from deep pits or grooves extending horizontally around the surface of the crown to defective or completely absent incisal edges or occlusal surfaces. The teeth most frequently affected are the permanent central incisors, cuspids, and first molars, the crowns of which develop during the first year of life. The systemic factors most frequently thought to be involved are serious gastrointestinal disturbances and deficiencies of calcium, phosphorus, or vitamins A and B.

Mottled enamel is a form of hypoplasia due to excessive fluoride ingestion. It consists of white spotting of the enamel or, in more severe forms, of pitting, brownish staining, and brittleness. It should be noted that these effects occur at levels of fluoride significantly higher than that recommended for the artificial fluoridation of drinking water in order to prevent dental caries.

Amelogenesis imperfecta is a hereditary condition in which enamel is absent or is thin, brown, and easily fractured. *Dentinogenesis imperfecta,* also hereditary and usually associated with *osteogenesis imperfecta,* affects the dentin rather than the enamel, giving the teeth a characteristic translucence. Because the union between the dentin and enamel is defective, the latter chips easily, exposing the underlying dentin, which rapidly wears down or fractures.

Congenital syphilis may give rise to characteristic "screwdriver" upper central incisors with notched incisal edges (Hutchinson's incisors) and first molars with rough, pitted occlusal surfaces (mulberry molars).

Complete or partial *anodontia* may occur in *hereditary ectodermal dysplasia,* a syndrome characterized by partial or complete absence of sweat glands, defective or absent sebaceous glands, hair follicles, and other ectodermal structures. When some teeth are present, they are usually cone-shaped.

Intrinsic *staining* of the teeth may be due to a number of factors. Erythroblastosis fetalis may give rise to green, brown, or blue coloration due to the deposition of blood pigment in the enamel and dentin of the developing teeth. In teeth which develop after birth, when hemolysis has ceased, the stain does not develop. A yellow-brown discoloration may be caused by the administration of *tetracycline* to infants or to women in the last trimester of pregnancy In cases of *congenital porphyria,* porphyrins are incorporated in the developing teeth, giving rise to a reddish-brown coloration which fluoresces red in ultraviolet light.

ODONTOGENIC TUMORS. The odontogenic tumors are neoplasms derived primarily from the tissues involved in odontogenesis. The *ameloblastoma*, an example of an ectodermally derived tumor, is the most aggressive tumor in the group and may occur at any age. Most frequently, it occurs in the molar-ramus area, originating as a central lesion of bone which gradually grows and expands the bone. Although the tumor may recur following resection, the prognosis is favorable, since the tumor is slow-growing and rarely, if ever, metastasizes. The *odontomas* are mixed tumors derived from both ectoderm and mesoderm which usually form a slow-growing mass composed of numerous structures having a morphologic resemblance to miniature teeth.

DENTAL CARIES, PULPAL AND PERIAPICAL INFECTION, AND SEQUELAE. Dental caries, the principal cause of tooth loss up to the fourth decade of life, is characterized by a bacteria-induced progressive destruction of the mineral and organic components of the outer enamel and underlying dentin. Numerous long-term public health studies have clearly shown that the artificial fluoridation of drinking water supplies to a level of 1 part per million leads to a 50 to 75 percent reduction in the occurrence of dental caries in permanent teeth of children, presumably due to an alteration of the developing enamel crystals during tooth formation which makes them more resistant to acid dissolution.

If the carious lesion progresses unchecked, there is eventual infection of the dental pulp, giving rise to an *acute pulpitis*. During the early stages of pulpitis moderately severe pain may result from thermal changes, particularly cold drinks. It is noteworthy that toothache in persons flying at high altitudes (aerodontalgia) occasionally occurs in persons having early pulpal inflammation or recently filled teeth. The cause of this phenomenon is not known, but in some instances the pain appears to be related to the sinuses rather than the teeth. As more of the pulp becomes involved because of advanced caries, heat or reclining may stimulate the onset of even more severe and continuous pain. At this stage, damage to the pulp is irreversible, and treatment consists either of extraction or thorough removal of the remaining contents of the pulp chamber and root canals followed by sterilization and filling with an inert material (root canal therapy).

If the pulpitis is not treated, infection may spread beyond the apex of the tooth into the periodontal ligament, giving rise to pain on chewing or percussion. The most common manifestation of periapical disease is the *periapical granuloma*, a localized mass of chronic granulation tissue which slowly expands at the expense of the surrounding alveolar bone. The *chronic periapical granuloma* may present the above symptoms or may be asymptomatic. If allowed to persist untreated the periapical granuloma may give rise to a *periapical cyst* or a *periapical abscess*—all three lesions appearing as radiolucent areas on roentgenograms. The acute periapical abscess may extend into the surrounding bone marrow, resulting in an *osteomyelitis*. More frequently, the abscess perforates the cortical plate and, following the path of least resistance, spreads through various tissue spaces, giving rise to cellulitis and bacteremia, or discharges into

the oral cavity, into the maxillary sinus, or through the skin.

The symptomatology produced by cellulitis depends on which tissue space is affected. For example, *Ludwig's angina* originates from an infected mandibular molar, involves the submaxillary space, and subsequently extends into the sublingual and submental spaces. Clinically, this is manifested by swelling of the floor of the mouth, elevation of the tongue, and difficulty in swallowing and breathing. With continued swelling, there may be edema of the glottis, necessitating an emergency tracheotomy. Spread of the infection to the parapharyngeal spaces may lead to cavernous sinus thrombosis.

PERIODONTAL DISEASE

After the third decade chronic destructive periodontal disease (*periodontitis*) is responsible for the loss of more teeth than dental caries. It begins as a marginal inflammation of the gingivae (gingivitis), which slowly spreads to involve the underlying alveolar bone and periodontal ligament. As the disease progresses, the alveolar bone is resorbed, resulting in loss of periodontal ligament fiber attachment from the tooth to the bone. The separation of the soft tissue from the tooth surface results in "pocket" formation, the inner aspect of which bleeds readily on probing or spontaneously during chewing. Frank pus sometimes exudes from under the gingival margin, accounting for the use of the now outmoded term "pyorrhea." With continued loss of alveolar bone the involved teeth become mobile. As the periodontal pockets deepen, the pocket orifice may become occluded, leading to the formation of a *periodontal abscess*. The prognosis for teeth with advanced bone loss, extreme mobility, and recurrent abscess formation is usually poor or hopeless, and the usual treatment is extraction.

The most important local etiologic factors associated with this disease are thought to be *poor oral hygiene*, resulting in the accumulation of grossly visible adherent masses of bacteria (*bacterial plaque*), calculus (mineralized bacterial plaque), and food impaction. The margins of overextended fillings also play a role as local irritating factors. Occlusal trauma, particularly due to grinding and clenching habits, may be involved. Therapy is aimed at elimination of these factors and the development of a local environment which can be maintained in health by good oral hygiene.

Systemic factors are thought to modify the response of the host to the local factors, but their nature is more obscure. In some instances, however, there are characteristic alterations in the gingiva in response to a number of specific systemic conditions. For example, during *pregnancy* the gingiva may become edematous and friable with a raspberry-like appearance of the interdental papillae. Occasionally, a tumorlike mass may develop in an interdental area (Plate 5-1); this usually regresses following parturition. The use of the anticonvulsant drug *diphenylhydantoin sodium* (Dilantin) frequently results in fibrous hyperplasia of the gingiva which may actually cover the teeth, interfere with mastication, and cause a serious esthetic problem (Plate 5-2). A similar clinical picture, although usually more generalized and extensive, occurs in *idiopathic familial fibromatosis*. The latter condition appears to be hereditary in nature.

A relatively common gingival disease, found predominantly in young adults in college or the armed forces, is *acute necrotizing ulcerative gingivitis* (Vincent's infection; trench mouth) (Plate 5-3). This disease is characterized by tender or painful gingivae, bleeding on pressure, and the pathognomonic sign of papillary or marginal gingival necrosis and ulceration. Clinical evidence suggests that the etiology of this disease has a psychosomatic component. Unlike *acute herpetic gingivostomatitis*, (Plate 5-4), with which this disease is most frequently confused, in patients with acute necrotizing ulcerative gingivitis fever or malaise rarely develop, and patients respond rapidly to penicillin or broad-spectrum antibiotics.

With regard to the *systemic effects of oral disease* it should be noted that both infected periapical lesions and periodontal disease provide potential sources of infection which may spread to other sites. Transient bacteremias have been demonstrated after simple massage of inflamed gingivae, as well as during tooth extraction. The frequent association of tooth extraction with the subsequent occurrence of subacute bacterial endocarditis has led to the prophylactic use of antibiotics in dental patients with a history of rheumatic fever or other evidence of valvular disease.

DISEASES OF THE JAWS

DEVELOPMENTAL DEFECTS. The most serious and common developmental disturbance of the jaws is *cleft palate* (approximately 1 per 1,000 births), which ordinarily presents as a large continuous defect in the midline of the hard and soft palates connecting the nasal and oral cavities and leads to difficulties in eating, drinking, and speech. In mild cases only the soft palate is involved. In more severe cases, the defect may extend anteriorly and follow the line of fusion to the left or right between the premaxilla and the maxilla, producing, in addition, a cleft of the alveolar ridge between the lateral incisor and cuspid, and a cleft lip (*harelip*). A cleft of the lip may occur without a cleft palate. The former is usually repaired surgically before the patient is one month old. Surgery for cleft palate is ordinarily delayed until the patient is about 1½ years old in order to avoid injury to the growth centers in the maxilla. An obturator may be used to close the defect if the cleft is too large.

GENERALIZED SKELETAL DISTURBANCES. There are many systemic bone diseases which may affect the mandible or maxilla. In *Paget's disease* involvement of the jaw occurs relatively late. It is interesting to note that the classic history of the patient needing to buy hats of larger size has its counterpart in the oral cavity, for patients with dentures may need to have them remade periodically because of progressive enlargement of the jaw, usually the maxilla. *Monostotic fibrous dysplasia* of the jaws develops as a painless swelling of the outer plate of bone

leading to malocclusion due to the displacement of the developing tooth germs. The chief complaints of patients with *eosinophilic granuloma, Letterer-Siwe disease*, or *Hand-Schüller-Christian disease* may include sore mouth, tooth mobility, and malodorous breath. When the involved teeth are extracted, the sockets heal with difficulty.

ENDOCRINE DISTURBANCES. The jaws are most severely affected by endocrine diseases which occur during the period of growth and development. In *cretinism* the jaws are small, and eruption and shedding of the primary teeth are delayed. The effects are less severe in *juvenile myxedema*. The oral manifestation of *adult myxedema* is thickening of the lips and tongue. *Hyperthyroidism* in children leads to premature shedding of the deciduous teeth and accelerated eruption of the permanent teeth. In pituitary dwarfs the small jaws cannot accommodate the teeth, giving rise to malocclusion. In *gigantism* the teeth erupt earlier but are widely spaced because of the large size of the mandible and maxilla, which have a normal relationship. In *acromegaly*, accelerated growth of the mandibular condyle leads to a downward and forward elongation of the mandible with resultant prognathism. The tongue enlarges, and often lateral indentations develop from pressure against the teeth. The first sign of *hyperparathyroidism* may be a giant-cell tumor of the jaw, which may appear radiographically as a cystic area in the maxilla or mandible. These cystlike lesions must be differentiated from periapical cysts due to pulpal infection and from fissural cysts, such as median palatine, nasopalatine, and globulomaxillary cysts, which arise from epithelial cells trapped during the fusion of various developing bones. Other radiographic changes, such as loss of lamina dura and alveolar bone resorption, coupled with loosening of teeth are often related to concomitant advanced periodontal disease rather than to hyperaparathyroidism per se (see Chap. 90).

DISEASES OF THE ORAL MUCOSA AND TONGUE

HEMATOLOGIC DISTURBANCES. Oral manifestations are common in both the acute and chronic forms of all types of leukemia, particularly *monocytic leukemia*. They consist of local gingival bleeding, enlargement, and necrosis. Petechiae and ulceration of the oral mucosa may also be evident. Extensive ulcerations of the gingivae, buccal mucosa, lips, soft palate, pharynx, and tonsils may also occur in *agranulocytosis*. In thrombocytopenic states multiple petechiae, ecchymoses, and bleeding gingivae may be observed. The mucous membranes of the oral cavity, including the papillae of the tongue, are atrophic in the *Plummer-Vinson* syndrome (see Chaps. 40, 313). As a result, the tongue is red, smooth, and sore, and there is difficulty in swallowing. Of interest is the finding that the atrophic mucous membranes had a predisposition toward the development of oral carcinoma. The oral symptoms in *pernicious anemia* are similar (see Chap. 337).

VITAMIN DEFICIENCIES. *The oral effects of deficiency of the B group of vitamins* involve the soft tissues primarily, giving rise to reddening and ulceration of the oral

Table 39-1. PIGMENTED LESIONS OF THE ORAL MUCOSA

Condition	Usual location	Clinical features	Course
Black hairy tongue	Dorsum of tongue	Elongation of filiform papillae of tongue, which take on a brown to black coloration.	Long-lasting but may disappear spontaneously.
Heavy metal pigmentation (bismuth, mercury, lead)	Gingival margin	Thin blue-black pigmented line along gingival margin due to prior treatment for syphilis with bismuth or mercury or from accidental absorption of lead.	Long-lasting.
Amalgam tattoo	Gingiva and mucobuccal fold	Small blue-black pigmented areas associated with embedded amalgam particles in soft tissues; these will show up on radiographs as radiopaque particles.	Remains indefinitely.
Fordyce's disease................	Buccal and labial mucosa	Aggregation of numerous, small yellowish spots just beneath mucosal surface; no subjective symptoms.	Remains without apparent change indefinitely.
Addison's disease................	Any area in mouth but mostly on buccal mucosa	Blotches or spots of bluish-black to dark-brown pigmentation occur early in the disease accompanied by diffuse pigmentation of skin; other symptoms of adrenal insufficiency.	Condition controlled by steroid therapy.
Peutz-Jegher syndrome	Any area in mouth	Dark-brown spots on lips, buccal mucosa, and palate with characteristic distribution of pigment around lips, nose, eyes, and on hands; concomitant intestinal polyposis.	Lesions remain indefinitely.
Malignant melanoma	Any area in mouth	The tumor may appear as a raised, painless, brown-black lesion or may be amelanotic; it may be ulcerated and infected.	Early metastasis leads to death.

mucosa and tongue, swelling and burning of the tongue, and fissuring at the corners of the lips (*angular cheilosis*). Severe vitamin C deficiency (*scurvy*) is manifested by petechiae in the oral mucosa; swollen, ulcerated, bleeding gingivae; and loosening of teeth.

PIGMENTATIONS (See Table 39-1). The spread of irregular spots or blotches of brown pigment throughout the oral mucosa, primarily the buccal mucosa, may be the first sign of *Addison's disease*. The pigmentation associated with the *Peutz-Jegher* syndrome is readily differentiated because of its history, characteristic distribution around the lips, eyes, and nostrils, as well as its intraoral distribution. Both *lead poisoning* and *bismuth poisoning* may be manifested by a dark line along the gingival margin, particularly in individuals who have poor oral hygiene. Bismuth poisoning may also demonstrate pigmented patches elsewhere in the oral mucosa.

INFECTIONS. See Tables 39-2 and 39-3 and Chap. 136.

DERMATOLOGIC DISEASES. See Tables 39-2 and 39-3 and Chap. 400.

TONGUE ALTERATIONS. See Table 39-4.

MALODOROUS BREATH. A distinctly unpleasant odor of the breath (halitosis) may emanate from any patient with *infections of the upper respiratory tract,* especially in bronchiectasis and lung abscess. Halitosis may occur with oral sepsis as in *stomatitis, gingivitis,* or extensive *caries.* Some persons who smoke excessively may have halitosis. Occasionally otherwise normal persons will exhibit halitosis without obvious cause. A *fishy odor* of the breath is found in patients with hepatic failure, an *ammoniacal or urinary odor* is found in azotemia, and a *sweet, fruity* odor is typical of diabetic acidosis.

DISEASES OF THE SALIVARY GLANDS

Conditions affecting the salivary glands include mumps parotitis (Chap. 231), Mikulicz's disease (Chap. 386), and Sjögren's syndrome (Chap. 386). Inflammation of the salivary glands (*sialadenitis*) is usually associated with the presence of a salivary stone (*sialolithiasis*) in the duct of one of the major salivary glands. The classic history of pain and swelling of the gland around mealtimes is due to the partial blockage of salivary flow by the stone. Localization of the stone may be accomplished by palpation or by roentgenograms with or without the use of an intraductal injection of radiopaque material (*sialography*).

Xerostomia, or dryness of the mouth, is due to salivary gland dysfunction and may be temporary or permanent. Among the factors which cause temporary dyness are emotional factors (such as fear), infection of the glands, and administration of drugs, such as atropine or antihistamines. Radiation to the area may produce a more permanent xerostomia due to atrophy of the glands. A similar dryness may occur in Sjögren's syndrome.

Table 39-2. VESICULAR, BULLOUS, OR ULCERATIVE LESIONS OF THE ORAL MUCOSA

Condition	Usual location	Clinical features	Course
Viral diseases:			
Acute herpetic gingivostomatitis (herpes simplex)	Lip and oral mucosa	Presence of labial vesicles which rupture and crust, and intraoral vesicles which quickly ulcerate; extremely painful to pressure; acute gingivitis, fever, malaise, foul odor, and cervical lymphadenopathy; occurs primarily in infants and children.	Heals spontaneously in 10–14 days, unless secondarily infected.
Recurrent herpes labialis	Mucocutaneous junction of lip	Eruption of groups of vesicles which may coalesce, then rupture and crust; painful to pressure or spicy foods.	Lasts about 1 week, but condition may be prolonged if secondary infection occurs.
Herpangina (Coxsackie A; also possibly Coxsackie B and ECHO viruses)	Oral mucosa, pharynx, tongue	Sudden onset of fever, sore throat and oropharyngeal vesicles usually in children under 4 years, summer months; diffuse pharyngeal injection and vesicles (1–2 mm), grayish white surrounded by red areola; vesicles enlarge and ulcerate.	Incubation period 2–9 days; fever for 1–4 days; recovery uneventful.
Foot, hand, and mouth disease (Coxsackie A-16)	Oral mucosa, pharynx, palms, and soles	Fever, malaise, headache with oropharyngeal vesicles which become painful, shallow ulcers.	Incubation period 2–18 days; lesions heal spontaneously in 2–4 weeks.
Bacterial or fungous diseases:			
Acute necrotizing ulcerative gingivitis ("trench mouth," Vincent's infection)..........	Gingiva	Painful, bleeding gingiva characterized by necrosis and ulceration of gingival papillae and margins plus lymphadenopathy and foul odor.	Continued destruction of tissue followed by remission, but may recur.
Primary syphilis (chancre)......	Lesion appears where organism enters body; may occur on lips, tongue, or tonsillar area	Small papule develops rapidly into a large, painless ulcer with indurated border; unilateral lymphadenopathy occurs; chancre and lymph nodes contain spirochetes; serologic tests positive by 3d to 4th weeks.	Healing of chancre occurs in 1–2 months, followed by secondary syphilis in 6–8 weeks.
Secondary syphilis	Oral mucosa frequently involved with mucous patches, primarily on palate but also at commissures of mouth	Maculopapular lesions of oral mucosa, about 5–10 mm in diameter with central ulceration covered by grayish membrane; eruptions occur on various mucosal surfaces and skin accompanied by fever, malaise, and sore throat.	Lesions may persist from several weeks to a year.
Tertiary syphilis	Palate and tongue	Gummatous infiltration of palate or tongue followed by ulceration and fibrosis; atrophy of tongue papillae may produce characteristic bald tongue and glossitis.	Gumma may destroy palate, causing complete perforation.
Tuberculosis	Tongue, tonsillar area, soft palate	A solitary, irregular ulcer covered by a persistent exudate; ulcer has an undermined, indurated border.	Lesion may persist.
Histoplasmosis	Any area in mouth, particularly tongue, gingiva, or palate	Numerous small nodules which may ulcerate; hoarseness and dysphagia may occur because of lesions in larynx, usually associated with fever and malaise.	May be fatal.

Table 39-2. VESICULAR, BULLOUS, OR ULCERATIVE LESIONS OF THE ORAL MUCOSA (*continued*)

Condition	Usual location	Clinical features	Course
Dermatologic diseases:			
Mucous membrane pemphigoid..	Primarily mucous membranes of the oral cavity, but may also involve the eyes, urethra, vagina, and rectum	Painful, grayish-white collapsed vesicles or bullae with peripheral erythematous zone; gingival lesions desquamate, leaving ulcerated area.	Protracted course with remissions and exacerbations; involvement of different sites occurs slowly; corticosteroids may control severe cases.
Erythema multiforme..........	Primarily the oral mucosa and skin of hands and feet	Intraoral ruptured bullae surrounded by an inflammatory area; lips may show hemorrhagic crusts; the "iris" or "target" lesion on the skin is pathognomonic; patient may have severe signs of toxicity.	Onset very rapid; condition may last 1–2 weeks; may be fatal.
Pemphigus vulgaris............	Oral mucosa and skin	Ruptured bullae and ulcerated oral areas; mostly in older adults.	With repeated recurrence of bullae toxicity may lead to cachexia, infection and death within 2 years.
Neoplastic diseases:			
Squamous cell carcinoma	Any area in mouth, most commonly on lower lip, tongue, and floor of mouth	Ulcer with elevated, indurated border; failure to heal, pain not prominent; lesions tend to arise in areas of leukoplakia or in smooth or atrophic tongue.	Invades and destroys underlying tissues or may metastasize to regional lymph nodes.
Acute leukemia	Gingiva	Gingival swelling and superficial ulcerations followed by hyperplasia of gingiva with extensive necrosis and hemorrhage; deep ulcers may occur elsewhere on the mucosa complicated by secondary infection.	Fatal.
Lymphosarcoma	Gingiva, palate, tongue, and tonsillar area	Elevated, ulcerated area which may proliferate rapidly, giving the appearance of a traumatic inflammatory lesion; swelling of regional lymph nodes.	Fatal.
Other Conditions:			
Recurrent aphthous stomatitis ..	Any place on oral mucosa	Single or clusters of painful ulcers found anywhere on mucosa with surrounding erythematous border; lesions may be 10–15 mm in diameter.	Lesions heal in 1–2 weeks but may recur monthly or several times a year.
Traumatic ulcers	Any place on oral mucosa; dentures frequently responsible for ulcers in vestibule	Localized, discrete ulcerated lesion with red border; produced by accidental biting of mucosa, penetration by a foreign object, or chronic irritation by a denture.	Lesion usually heals in 7–10 days when irritant is removed, unless secondarily infected.

ORAL CANCER

Oral cancer constitutes more than 5 percent of all human cancers. *Squamous cell carcinoma* is the most common malignant oral tumor, accounting for approximately 90 to 95 percent of all oral malignant tumors. Of interest is the fact that most of these tumors occur on the lips, primarily the lower lip, rather than intraorally (Plate 5-6). About half of the intraoral tumors involve the tongue, primarily the posterior two-thirds and the lateral borders. The major etiologic factor in lip cancer appears to be exposure to intense sunlight. Predisposing factors

for intraoral carcinoma include tobacco (usually in the form of cigar or pipe smoking, or snuff placed in the mucobuccal fold), excessive consumption of alcohol, syphilitic glossitis, and the atrophic mucosa of the Plummer-Vinson syndrome. There is some evidence to suggest that liver disease, particularly cirrhosis, is also important in some types of intraoral carcinoma. Although numerous instances of carcinoma of the tongue adjacent to a sharp tooth or dental appliance have been reported, animal studies with chronic irritation per se, as well as epidemiologic studies, cast doubt on this apparent rela-

Table 39-3. WHITE LESIONS OF ORAL MUCOSA

Condition	Usual location	Clinical features	Course
Pachyderma oris	Any area in mouth	Elevated white lesion due to hyperkeratosis and thickening of the oral epithelium secondary to chronic irritation.	Removal of irritant leads to healing in 2–3 weeks.
Leukoplakia	Any area in mouth	White patch or raised plaque with sharply defined borders; in more severe cases the lesion is indurated and rough, and may be fissured and eroded; pain not present in early lesions.	Carcinoma frequently arises in the more severe type of lesion.
Lichen planus (Plate 5-5)	Any area in mouth but most often on buccal mucosa	Varied appearance of lesion due to arrangement of grayish-white papules which coalesce to make up the pattern; a reticular network is most common; oral lesions may precede skin lesions.	May disappear spontaneously.
Moniliasis (thrush)	Any area in mouth	Creamy white curdlike patches which reveal a raw, bleeding surface when scraped; found in sick infants, debilitated elderly patients, or patients receiving high doses of corticosteroids or broad-spectrum antibiotics.	Responds favorably to antifungal therapy after correction of predisposing causes.
Chemical burns	Any area in mouth	White slough due to necrosis of epithelium and underlying connective tissue caused by contact with agents (e.g., aspirin) applied locally or the use of undiluted sodium perborate or hydrogen peroxide as a mouthwash; removal of slough leaves a raw, painful surface.	Lesion heals in several weeks if not secondarily infected.

tionship. The most common *precancerous lesion* in the oral cavity is *leukoplakia,* which is a whitish patch on the mucosa that histologically shows alterations that include hyperkeratosis, acanthosis, and dyskeratosis. *All chronic ulcerative lesions which fail to heal within 1 to 2 weeks should be considered potentially malignant* and must be biopsied in order to make the definitive diagnosis. It is noteworthy that in their early stages intraoral epidermoid carcinomas are rarely painful, in contrast to similar-appearing inflammatory lesions.

The prognosis for patients with carcinoma of the lip is usually good, since these malignant tumors are noted sooner and apparently metastasize later. On the other hand, patients with carcinoma of the tongue have a poorer prognosis, particularly as the location of the tumor occurs more posteriorly on the tongue. Intraoral carcinomas may spread by direct invasion to the underlying bone. Involvement of nerves, such as the inferior alveolar nerve or mental nerve, may result in numbness or paresthesia of the lower lip on the ipsilateral side. Depending on the site of origin of the intraoral carcinoma, metastases usually spread to the submaxillary or cervical lymph nodes.

NEUROLOGIC DISTURBANCES

A number of neurologic disturbances have a direct effect on oral and paraoral structures. *Trigeminal neu-*

ralgia (tic douloureux) is an example of a syndrome involving the trigeminal nerve. It is characterized by extremely severe, unilateral, lancinating pain of the face occurring spontaneously or set off by pressure on a "trigger zone" on the face. Facial palsy is a unilateral disturbance of the motor branch of the facial nerve due to either trauma, surgical sectioning, or tumor involvement. When it is of acute onset and unknown cause, possibly a localized infection in the nerve, it is called *Bell's palsy.* It may be due to cranial herpes zoster in some instances. The condition is manifested by drooping of the corner of the mouth, inability to close the eye on the same side, and difficulty in speech and eating. In mild cases the symptoms may disappear spontaneously within a month. Alternations in taste sensation in the anterior two-thirds of the tongue due to disturbance of the sensory component of the facial nerve occurs in some cases and indicates a more central location of the lesion in the nerve.

The pain associated with the *glossopharyngeal neuralgia syndrome* is similar in type and intensity to that found in trigeminal neuralgia, being set off by a trigger zone in the pharynx and affecting the posterior region of the tongue, pharynx, soft palate, and ear. Disturbance of the hypoglossal nerve leads to dysfunction of the tongue musculature and atrophy. Bilateral nerve involvement prevents protrusion of the tongue, whereas unilateral involvement leads to deviation of the protruded tongue toward the affected side.

Table 39-4. ALTERATIONS OF THE TONGUE

Type of change	Clinical features
Alterations in size or morphology:	
Macroglossia...............	Enlarged tongue which may be part of a syndrome found in developmental conditions such as Down's syndrome; may be due to tumor (hemangioma or lymphangioma), metabolic disease (such as primary amyloidosis), or endocrine disturbance (such as acromegaly or cretinism).
Fissured ("scrotal") tongue...	Dorsal surface and sides of tongue covered by painless shallow or deep fissures which may collect debris and become irritated.
Median rhomboid glossitis....	Congenital abnormality of tongue with ovoid, denuded area in the median posterior portion of the tongue.
Alterations in color:	
"Geographic" tongue ("wandering rash").	Asymptomatic inflammatory condition of the tongue, with rapid loss and regrowth of filiform papillae, leading to appearance of denuded red patches "wandering" across the surface of the tongue.
Hairy tongue..............	Elongation of filiform papillae of the medial dorsal surface area due to failure of keratin layer of the papillae to desquamate normally; brownish-black coloration may be due to staining by tobacco, food, or chromogenic organisms.
"Strawberry" and "raspberry" tongue.................	Appearance of tongue during scarlet fever due to the hypertrophy of fungiform papillae plus changes in the filiform papillae.
"Bald" tongue.............	Complete atrophy of papillae which may occur in pernicious anemia, severe iron deficiency anemia, pellagra, or syphilis; may be accompanied by painful, burning sensations.

DISTURBANCES OF THE TEMPOROMANDIBULAR JOINT

Pain in the area of the temporomandibular joint frequently causes the patient to seek therapy. It may be due to posterior displacement of the condyle in the fossa leading to displacement of the meniscus and chronic trauma. *Dislocation of the condyle anteriorly* beyond the articular eminence due to sudden stretching or tearing of the capsular ligament may result in a locking of the mandible in an open position. Reduction of the dislocated jaw may be accomplished by a downward and posterior pressure applied bilaterally intraorally to the buccal surfaces of the mandible in the region of the angle of the jaw. Padding of the thumbs is essential to avoid injury due to the sudden closure of the mandible as it snaps back into position. Condylar fracture should be suspected in patients with pain and swelling in the condylar area and a history of recent facial trauma. In *osteoarthritis* the clinical signs and symptoms may be minimal despite extensive changes in the condyle. Temporomandibular joint involvement occurs less frequently in *rheumatoid arthritis*. When affected the joints are swollen and painful, leading to limitation of movement, particularly on arising in the morning. In children the disease may lead to malocclusion. *Ankylosis* of the joint may occur eventually, necessitating a condylectomy.

The myofascial pain syndrome, the most common disorder of the temporomandibular joint, is characterized by facial pain and mandibular dysfunction. The pain is often localized in the ear or jaw and may extend to the neck and shoulder. The mandibular dysfunction is manifested by limitation of movement, particularly an inability to open to the fullest extent. It is thought that such patients are predisposed to the syndrome because of increased musculature tension and hyperexcitable reflexes related to emotional tension. The precipitating factor appears to be the stretching of an abnormal focus of pain which initiates a self-sustaining pain-spasm-pain cycle. Treatment of the pain-dysfunction syndrome involves the use of drugs to relieve the pain, lessen cortical excitability, and relax the muscles. Local anesthetics are used intramuscularly in the region of the trigger zone or as superficial sprays in an attempt to break the pain-spasm-pain cycle.

REFERENCES

Bhaskar, S. N.: "Synopsis of Oral Pathology," St. Louis, The C. V. Mosby Company, 1965.

Gorlin, R. J., and J. J. Pindborg: "Syndromes of the Head and Neck," New York, McGraw-Hill Book Company, 1964.

Jacobson, F. L. (Ed.): Symposium on Oral Diagnosis and Treatment Planning, Dent. Clinics N. Am., 1963.

McCarthy, P., and G. Shklar: "Diseases of the Oral Mucosa," New York, McGraw-Hill Book Company, 1964.

Maccomb, W. S., and G. H. Fletcher: "Cancer of the Head and Neck," Baltimore, The Williams & Wilkins Company, 1967.

Mitchell, D. F. (Ed.): Symposium on Oral Medicine, Dent. Clinics N. Am., 1968.

Shafer, W. G., M. K. Hine, and B. M. Levy: "A Textbook of Oral Pathology," Philadelphia, W. B. Saunders Company, 1966.

40 DYSPHAGIA
Thomas R. Hendrix

Dysphagia, or difficulty in swallowing, is a most reliable symptom and indicates the presence of disease or motor dysfunction. Dysphagia should never be dismissed as an emotional disturbance or be confused with globus hystericus, which is the term used to indicate the sensation of a lump or tightness in the throat independent of swallowing.

The most characteristic manifestation of dysphagia is the sensation of food "sticking" somewhere in its passage to the stomach, usually at the level of the obstructing lesion but sometimes referred to the suprasternal notch, even though the obstruction may be at the lower end of the esophagus. Pain may accompany dysphagia, especially if esophageal spasm is induced by the peristaltic waves attempting to force the bolus through the obstruction. If the pain is mild, it tends to be localized to the site of obstruction; if more severe, it radiates more widely, into the base of the neck, angles of the jaw, arms, epigastrium, or back. Sometimes pain, in a sense, may even cause dysphagia, as when the throat is so sore that swallowing is difficult. For further details regarding these symptoms, see Chap. 313.

Normal swallowing is a complex function dependent upon coordination of voluntary muscular structures of the oropharynx, striated muscles protecting the larynx and respiratory passages, as well as relaxation of the esophageal sphincters and the peristaltic wave itself; hence dysphagia may occur as a consequence of derangement or incoordination of any of the elements of the swallowing act as well as narrowing of the lumen by inflammatory stricture or tumor.

For clinical purposes it is useful to separate dysphagia into that of oropharyngeal or esophageal origin, because symptoms, etiology, and treatment are usually different.

OROPHARYNGEAL DYSPHAGIA. Symptoms associated with dysphagia caused by disorders of oropharyngeal structures include aspiration with swallowing, regurgitation of fluid into the nose, pharyngeal pain with swallowing, and inability of the tongue to move the bolus into the pharynx. Dilatation and atony of pyriform sinuses and pharynx and retention of contrast media in the valleculae are characteristic radiographic findings in patients with pharyngeal dysfunction. In addition, aspiration of contrast medium into the trachea or regurgitation into the nasopharynx and apparent obstruction at the upper esophageal sphincter (cricopharyngeus) may be found.

Neuromuscular disorders are the most common causes of oropharyngeal dysphagia. Examples of these disorders are cerebral vascular accidents which cause pseudobulbar palsy (see Chap. 21) or bulbar palsy, poliomyelitis, motor system disease, diphtheritic polyneuritis, myasthenia gravis, myotonic dystrophies and restricted muscular dystrophies (oculopharyngeal and laryngoesophageal), and dermatomyositis. Ulcerative lesions such as pharyngitis, Vincent's angina, monilia stomatitis, viral infections with herpetic lesions, and retropharyngeal abscess interfere by causing pain and thereby inhibiting the initiation of deglu-

tition. Plummer-Vinson syndrome (Paterson-Kelly syndrome, or sideropenic dysphagia), may also be listed here, since the difficulty in swallowing in this disorder resembles that due to a neuromuscular disorder, although pain may be an additional disturbing feature. Limited pathologic studies have shown both epithelial and muscle atrophy. It is clear that the dysphagia is not due to the characteristic web, or mucosal fold, of the anterior aspect of the cricopharyngeal area, because the web often persists long after the symptoms have been relieved by iron replacement.

Oropharyngeal dysphagia may be caused by narrowing of the lumen of the pharynx or upper esophagus by tumor, granulomatous disease, Zenker's diverticulum, or an enlarged thyroid.

ESOPHAGEAL DYSPHAGIA. Symptoms indicating that the cause of dysphagia is to be found in the esophagus range from retrosternal fullness with swallowing to failure of the bolus to pass through the esophagus associated with pain relieved only by regurgitation of the offending bolus. Barium swallows in patients with dysphagia of esophageal origin show segmental narrowing of the esophageal lumen, failure of peristalsis, or both. Abnormalities of peristalsis may be characterized more precisely by intraluminal manometric studies.

Mechanical narrowing of the esophageal lumen is most frequently caused by carcinoma either of squamous type, arising from the esophagus itself, or adenocarcinoma of the cardia extending up into the esophagus. Rarely, benign tumors may reach sufficient size to cause dysphagia. Inflammatory strictures most commonly result from reflux esophagitis but are also caused by ingestion of corrosive substances, such as lye, or by trauma from foreign bodies or instrumentation. In addition, a lower esophageal ring may produce dysphagia by obstructing the esophageal lumen. Extrinsic pressure from aneurysms, vascular anomalies, mediastinal tumors, or paraesophageal diaphragmatic hernias may compress the esophageal lumen sufficiently to cause dysphagia. Finally, the motility disturbances associated with diffuse esophageal spasm, cardiospasm, and esophageal reflux may be the basis of dysphagia. Although esophageal peristalsis is absent in the majority of patients with scleroderma, dysphagia does not become a prominent symptom until reflux esophagitis has led to an inflammatory stricture.

DIFFERENTIAL DIAGNOSIS. Determination of the basic mechanism responsible for dysphagia is usually a simple matter, but identification of the exact disorder responsible for it may be quite difficult. For example, cancer of the esophagus sometimes presents with a sudden rather than gradual onset, and the x-ray may have a smooth, symmetrical appearance such as is more commonly seen with benign stricture or cardiospasm; even esophagoscopy may be inconclusive, and biopsy may yield deceptive results if the tissue shows only inflammatory reaction and does not include neoplastic cells. Similarly, neuromuscular disorders and disturbances of esophageal motility interfering with swallowing may be difficult to classify.

Certain symptoms associated with dysphagia, however, have diagnostic value. Hiccups, together with difficulty in swallowing, suggest a lesion at the terminal portion of the esophagus, such as carcinoma, achalasia, or hiatal hernia. Dysphagia followed after an interval of some duration by hoarseness usually means extension of a malignant growth beyond the walls of the esophagus and the involvement of a recurrent laryngeal nerve. When the hoarseness comes first and the dysphagia later, the primary lesion is almost always in the larynx. This combination of laryngeal and pharyngeal symptoms may also occur in polymyositis or dermatomyositis or with any disease causing bilateral involvement of vagus nerves or nuclei (poliomyelitis and polyneuritis). In motor system disease, the most common cause of a mixture of bulbar and pseudobulbar palsy, dysphagia is usually combined with dysphonia and dysarthria; the jaw jerk is hyperactive and the tongue atrophic. Dysphagia and unilateral wheezing virtually always indicate a mediastinal mass involving the esophagus and a main or large bronchus. Coughing with each swallow of food or drink means a fistulous communication between the esophagus and the trachea. Coughing occurring sometime after swallowing may be due to regurgitation of food, most common in achalasia and Zenker's diverticulum.

DIAGNOSTIC PROCEDURES. Examination of the mouth and pharynx should disclose those lesions the effect of which is to impede the transfer of food from the mouth to the esophagus, because of either pain or mechanical interference. When lesions of the hypopharynx (e.g., *chronic abscess secondary to tuberculosis of the spine*) or of the larynx (e.g., *tuberculosis* or *carcinoma*) are suspected, examination with a mirror is necessary.

The most important diagnostic technique in the evaluation of dysphagia is a barium swallow. It usually makes it possible to determine whether dysphagia is caused by mechanical obstruction or esophageal motor abnormality. Absence of esophageal peristalsis can best be demonstrated by barium swallows with the patient in Trendelenburg's position. If there is no peristalsis, barium will remain in the esophagus until the patient is tilted upright. Since the muscular action of the pharynx is so rapid, it is useful when studying disorders of the pharynx and upper esophagus to record barium swallows cineradiographically. Projection of the film at slow speed permits detection and analysis of abnormalities of pharyngeal function.

If barium swallow shows a lesion within the esophagus or a narrowing of the lumen, esophagoscopy is the most direct method for establishing the nature of the lesion. In addition to inspecting the lesion, biopsies should be taken to differentiate inflammatory from neoplastic lesions. A malignant stricture is not ruled out with certainty, however, if the biopsy shows only normal tissue or chronic inflammation, because tumors invading the esophagus from the cardia often spread beneath the mucosa and may be missed by a superficial biopsy. In such circumstances repeat biopsies or exfoliative cytology would be necessary. Cytologic studies by experienced personnel are very accurate in the diagnosis of esophageal cancer.

Motor abnormalities of the pharynx and esophagus may be suspected by viewing the movement of a swallowed radiopaque bolus by fluoroscopy, but to characterize these abnormalities definitely the motor response of pharynx and esophagus to swallowing must be studied by recording intraluminal pressure from several points simultaneously. Records are best obtained by use of a train of water-filled, perfused catheters connected to external pressure transducers or strain gages. Examination of manometric records of swallows will demonstrate whether the wave is normally propagated over the length of the esophagus, whether the pressure generated by the peristaltic wave is normal and sufficient to propel the bolus, and, finally, whether sphincter relaxation is complete, of adequate duration, and properly coordinated with the peristaltic wave. Combining manometric with cineradiographic techniques has added greatly to our understanding of pharyngoesophageal function.

REFERENCES

Davenport, H. W.: "Physiology of the Digestive Tract," 2d. ed., Chicago, The Year Book Medical Publishers, Inc., 1966.

Ingelfinger, F. J.: The Physiologic Background of Heartburn, Esophagitis, and Cardiospasm, Arch. Intern. Med., 105: 770, 1960.

Siegel, C. I., and T. R. Hendrix: The Clinical Value of Esophageal Motor Studies, Postgrad. Med., 29:505, 1961.

Stevens, M. B., et al.: Aperistalsis of the Esophagus in Patients with Connective-tissue Disorders and Raynaud's Phenomenon, New Engl. J. Med., 270:1218, 1964.

Winans, C. S., and L. D. Harris: Quantitation of Lower Esophageal Sphincter Competence, Gastroenterology, 52: 773, 1966.

Wynder, E. L., and J. H. Fryer: Etiologic Considerations of Plummer-Vinson (Paterson-Kelly) Syndrome, Ann. Intern. Med., 49:1106, 1958.

41   INDIGESTION

*Kurt J. Isselbacher and
Matthew A. Budd*

"Indigestion" is a term frequently used by patients to describe a multitude of symptoms generally appreciated as distress associated with the intake of food. The term is thus nonspecific and may have a different meaning for the patient and the physician. In approaching the patient with indigestion it is important for the physician first to elicit a good description of this complaint. To some patients indigestion refers to a feeling that digestion has not proceeded naturally. There is a sense of abdominal fullness, pressure, or actual pain. Others may use the term to describe heartburn, belching, distension, or flatulence. These complaints will be considered in this chapter. Discussed elsewhere are the closely related but distinct symptoms of dysphagia, nausea and vomiting, and anorexia (Chaps. 40 and 42).

Indigestion may occur as a result of disease of the gastrointestinal tract or in association with pathologic states in other organ systems. As a result of systematic clinical and laboratory study, a definable pathophysiologic process often can be shown to be responsible for the symptoms in a given case of indigestion. Frequently, however, clear etiologic explanations for the patient's complaints of indigestion are not established. Such cases are often designated as "functional indigestion," with a strong implication that psychosomatic factors underlie the complaints. Although it is clear that psychic factors may lead to symptoms of indigestion, the designation of "functional indigestion" is rarely if ever a satisfactory explanation, serving only to rephrase the patient's symptomatology. A psychogenic cause should not be assumed until organic causes of indigestion have been thoroughly excluded.

After having ascertained the patient's definition of indigestion, it is also important to determine (1) the location and duration of the discomfort, (2) the temporal relation of the symptoms to the ingestion of food, and (3) the possible relation of the symptoms to the ingestion of specific types of food (e.g., fatty foods, milk).

PAIN PATTERNS

True visceral abdominal pain as seen in indigestion is mediated over visceral afferent nerves which accompany the abdominal sympathetic pathways (see Chap. 12). Visceral pain is generally described as dull and aching in nature (with a diffuse midline localization) or as fullness or pressure. The location of the discomfort corresponds generally to the segmental level of the affected organ. Abdominal visceral pain can be produced experimentally by artificially increasing pressure in a hollow viscus. Usually this type of pain is the result of distension or exaggerated muscular contraction of a viscus, and it is noteworthy that inflammation lowers the threshold to such stimuli.

The visceral pain of indigestion should be distinguished from the sharp, lateralized, and localized pain patterns seen in many acute abdominal processes involving the peritoneum. In contrast to true visceral pain, this pain is mediated over cerebrospinal afferent nerves. Again it is of a dull, aching type whether from inflammation of the viscera or of peritoneal surfaces.

In view of the diffuse nature of true visceral abdominal pain, the main clue comes from the segmental level of the viscus; in any given segmental region there is no way of determining which of several viscera are the source of it (Table 41-1). The following rules, already given in Chap. 9, are useful: *Substernal pain* of gastrointestinal origin usually arises from disorders in the esophagus or cardia of the stomach. Because pain in this area is frequently of cardiac origin, heart disease must be considered carefully and excluded. *Epigastric pain* is generally of gastric, duodenal, biliary, or pancreatic origin. As the pathologic process in the biliary tract and pancreas becomes more intense, as, for example, in inflammatory states, the pain lateralizes and localizes, e.g., biliary pain to the right upper quadrant and tip of the right scapula and pancreatic pain to the epigastrium, left upper quadrant, and back. *Periumbilical pain* is generally associated

Table 41-1. DISTRIBUTION OF VISCERAL PAIN AND EXAMPLES OF DISORDERS FREQUENTLY INVOLVING THE SPECIFIC ORGAN

Organ	Location of referred pain	Frequent disorders
Esophagus.........	Substernum, epigastrium	Peptic esophagitis, hiatus hernia stricture, carcinoma
Stomach...........	Epigastrium	Gastritis, peptic ulcer, carcinoma
Duodenum (first and second portion...	Epigastrium	Peptic ulcer
Duodenum (third portion, jejunum and ileum).......	Periumbilical	Regional enteritis, lymphona, gastroenteritis (infectious), intestinal obstruction
Gallbladder........	Epigastrium, right upper quadrant, right side of back	Cholelithiasis, cholecystitis
Pancreas..........	Epigastrium, left side of back	Pancreatitis, pancreatic carcinoma
Liver.............	Right upper quadrant	Passive congestion of liver, hepatitis, cirrhosis
Colon.............	Below umbilicus	Ulcerative colitis, carcinoma, partial obstruction

with small-bowel disease. *Pain below the umbilicus* is often of appendiceal, large-bowel, or pelvic origin.

TEMPORAL RELATIONSHIPS OF PAIN AND INDIGESTION

The establishment of the temporal patterns of a patient's complaints often provides useful diagnostic information. First, it is important to ascertain whether the symptoms are *constant* (continually present over extended periods of time), as may occur, for example, with an infiltrating gastric carcinoma, or *intermittent* as in acute gastritis following an alcoholic binge or in association with the use of certain drugs. Symptoms are occasionally *seasonal;* this can occur in peptic ulcer disease where in some patients symptoms may be more prominent in the spring and autumn.

Another important and often diagnostic feature is the relation of pain or indigestion to ingestion of food. This relationship is especially significant or helpful if symptoms occur either during or minutes after the meal or if they occur several hours (4 or more) after eating. *Early postprandial symptoms* may reflect esophageal disease, because they may be associated with disordered swallowing function. In such instances, the distress or other symptoms of indigestion often are experienced substernally. Early postprandial complaints occur also in gastric disorders such as acute gastritis or carcinoma. *Late post-*

prandial indigestion, i.e., that occurring several hours after eating, may reflect failure of the stomach to empty adequately as in pyloric stenosis or gastric atony. It may also be a symptom of duodenal ulcer, in which case it classically occurs several hours after the meal, when the ulcerated mucosa is exposed to acid secretions of the stomach unbuffered by food. Conversely, the relief of pain following food ingestion is also seen in patients with peptic ulcer and is presumably due to the neutralization of the acid by the ingested food. Late postprandial indigestion also may result from the impaired digestive and absorptive processes, as in pancreatic insufficiency. Pain occurring *nocturnally* and with *recumbency* may be seen in patients with hiatus hernia and carcinoma of the pancreas.

FOOD INTOLERANCE

There are a number of situations in which specific foods or types of foods appear to be related to indigestion. Careful documentation of this relationship is sometimes of great help in arriving at an etiologic diagnosis.

Some foods may be poorly tolerated because of their consistency. For example, patients with esophageal stricture or carcinoma may tolerate liquids well, but the ingestion of solids may be associated with discomfort, especially substernal distress (see Chap. 313). Certain foods may be tolerated poorly because the intestinal tract cannot assimilate them adequately. This may occur following the ingestion of fatty foods in patients with pancreatic or biliary tract disease.

Individuals may lack a specific enzyme required for assimilation of a certain nutrient. As an example, patients may lack or have a deficiency of the mucosal enzyme lactase, which catalyzes the hydrolysis of lactose. When lactase deficiency exists on a congenital or acquired basis (e.g., in sprue, ulcerative colitis) (Chap. 316), the ingestion of milk (where the carbohydrate is lactose) results in distension, flatulence, and diarrhea.

There are a number of other conditions or disorders in which specific foods are poorly tolerated. Foods may be poorly tolerated because they initiate *allergic reactions* or exert a deleterious or *toxic effect* on the intestinal tract of susceptible individuals (e.g., gluten in patients with nontropical sprue). Finally certain substances may lead to systemic effects because of biochemical defects which render them particularly hazardous. Examples of this are galactose intolerance in galactosemia (Chap. 112), and branched-chain amino acid intolerance in maple syrup (urine) disease (Chap. 102).

The above mechanisms do not explain the majority of clinical situations in which indigestion is associated with the eating of specific foods. For example, a history of fatty-food intolerance or an inability to eat cabbage, cucumbers, or spicy foods is commonly obtained from patients with indigestion. However, the mechanisms underlying the production of symptoms in these circumstances is still unclear.

ADDITIONAL SYNDROMES COMMONLY DESCRIBED AS INDIGESTION

GASEOUSNESS, FLATULENCE, AEROPHAGIA. There are a number of common clinical syndromes which may be described by the patient as "indigestion" and which appear to be related to the presence of increased quantities of gas in the intestinal tract. The major portion of intraluminal gas represents swallowed air, with a variable quantity produced within the intestinal lumen itself. A degree of air swallowing, or *aerophagia,* is present in normal individuals and can be observed by the radiologist at fluoroscopy. Under certain circumstances, such as chronic anxiety, poor eating habits, or actual intestinal disease itself, aerophagia may increase in magnitude and lead to symptoms in its own right.

Early postprandial fullness and pressure, relieved by eructation and accompanied by a large amount of air seen on x-ray in the gastric fundus, is often referred to as the *magenblase* (i.e., gastric bubble) *syndrome.* Acute gastric distension by swallowed air can occasionally produce sharp pains which may mimic angina pectoris. This sequence of events may be especially perplexing in older patients with coronary artery disease, because it is well recognized that true angina pectoris may itself be precipitated by the ingestion of a large meal. Fatty meals delay gastric emptying and hence the passage of swallowed air down the intestine. This relationship may explain, in part, the prolonged sense of fullness and eructations experienced by many individuals after a fatty meal.

Swallowed air that is not eructated passes on in the intestinal tract and may either produce diffuse abdominal distension or become trapped in the splenic flexure of the colon. Distension of this segment of the colon produces a sensation of left upper quadrant fullness and pressure with radiation to the left side of the chest. This is known as the *splenic flexure syndrome.* Patients will often describe relief of pain with defecation or with the expulsion of flatus. Diagnosis may be made by demonstrating, on physical examination, a note of increased tympany in the extreme left lateral portion of the upper abdomen or by the visualization of large amounts of air in the splenic flexure of the colon by radiography.

A second major source of intestinal gas is that produced within the lumen by fermentative action of bacteria on carbohydrates and proteins. Increased amounts of intraluminal gas production due to this mechanism have been demonstrated in conditions associated with abnormal bacterial colonization of the small intestine and in patients with carbohydrate malabsorption.

Increased gas production has also been shown to occur following the ingestion of certain foods (e.g., the legumes) which contain significant quantities of nonabsorbable sugars. As in the case of swallowed air, increased amounts of intraluminally produced gas can produce symptoms by causing distension, pain, increased motility (with diarrhea), or flatulence.

HEARTBURN. Heartburn, or pyrosis, is a sensation of warmth or burning located substernally or high in the epigastrium. Experimental studies in human beings have shown that esophageal distension or increased motor activity is associated in most subjects with a feeling of fullness and burning in this area.

Heartburn may occur with organic disease of the intestinal tract and is usually associated with gastroesophageal reflux. This is frequently the case in hiatus hernia. In this setting, heartburn occurs after a large meal or with stooping or bending. Esophageal reflux of acid contents at these times leads to symptoms by either the production of abnormal motor activity or direct mucosal irritation (i.e., esophagitis). Heartburn may also be seen in the absense of a demonstrable anatomic or motor pathologic condition, in which case it is frequently accompanied by aerophagia and for lack of other explanation is often attributed to psychologic factors.

INDIGESTION DUE TO DISEASE OUTSIDE THE INTESTINAL TRACT

A multitude of extraintestinal disease processes may result in indigestion by mechanisms which are poorly understood. Indigestion may be the presenting complaint, for example, in congestive heart failure, uremia, pulmonary tuberculosis, and neoplastic disease. Under these circumstances the symptoms of indigestion may present with no unique features to suggest that they are in fact due to some other systemic disease process.

DIAGNOSTIC APPROACH TO THE PATIENT WITH INDIGESTION

Indigestion represents a challenging and difficult diagnostic problem because of the nonspecific nature of its manifestations. The evaluation of indigestion must include initially a thorough medical work-up, with ultimate confirmation or exclusion of pathophysiologic derangements by the appropriate diagnostic procedures.

A careful history should include an assessment of the patient's general medical health, including the possibility of diseases in extraintestinal organ systems which may produce indigestion. Careful evaluation of psychologic factors is crucial, because they often play an etiologic or contributory role in the patient's problem. Of particular importance is the presence of anxiety, depressive reactions, and hysteria (Chaps. 369 and 370). Evaluation of the patient's intestinal problem must include an assessment of his nutritional status, changes in weight, and appetite.

A clear and detailed description of the specific symptoms should be obtained, particularly the patient's definition of the term "indigestion." The nature of the pain or its frequency and time of occurrence, its relationship to meals, and the special circumstances which lead to its exacerbation or relief should be elicited. Associated intestinal symptoms such as nausea and vomiting, abnormal bowel habits, steatorrhea, diarrhea, and melena should also be sought. Physical examination rarely establishes the specific diagnosis, but it may be useful in detecting disease in other organ systems (for example, congestive heart failure) which can affect intestinal physiology.

X-ray examination of the alimentary tract is crucial to the evaluation of the patient with indigestion. This may involve examination of the esophagus, stomach, small intestine, colon, and biliary tract. Esophagoscopy, gastroscopy or sigmoidoscopy also may be helpful or necessary. Stools should be examined for appearance, occult blood, fat, and muscle fibers. As stated above, careful attempts must be made to exclude nonintestinal disease, especially cardiac disease.

Unfortunately, even after completion of careful diagnostic studies many cases of indigestion will turn out to have no clear explanation. Some of these are psychogenic and may respond to appropriate psychiatric measures. Others represent physiologic derangements which are undetectable by currently available diagnostic methods. Still others represent actual disease processes in early stages which may be diagnosable by conventional methods at a later date. The ultimate evaluation of indigestion requires, therefore, the utmost in sensitivity, diligence, and patience on the part of the examining physician.

REFERENCES

Calloway, D. H.: Respiratory Hydrogen and Methane as Affected by Consumption of Gas Forming Foods, Gastroenterology, 51:383, 1966.

Coghill, N. F.: Dyspepsia, Brit. Med. J., 4:97, 1967.

Jones, C. M.: Digestive Tract Pain, New York, The Macmillan Company, 1938.

Levitt, M. D., and F. J. Ingelfinger: Hydrogen and Methane Production in Man, Ann. N.Y. Acad. Sci., 150:75, 1968.

Pollock, J. H.: "Gaseous Digestive Conditions," Springfield, Ill., Charles C Thomas, Publisher, 1958.

Smith, L. A.: Pattern of Pain in Diagnosis of Upper Abdominal Disorders, J.A.M.A., 156:1568, 1954.

42 ANOREXIA, NAUSEA, AND VOMITING

Kurt J. Isselbacher and Matthew A. Budd

Energy balance in man represents a sensitive coordination and balance between food intake on one hand and work, heat production, and stored energy on the other. Physiologically this balance involves two related phases: a short-term set of mechanisms responsive to the daily changes in energy requirements and long-term mechanisms responsible for the regulation of metabolic reserves and body composition. Energy regulation involves a complex array of neural and chemical stimuli, as yet incompletely understood, which appear to be integrated, at the hypothalamic level, into two centers: a lateral hypothalamic one which initiates feeding and is referred to as the "feeding center" and a medial center resulting in the sensation of satiety and cessation of feeding after a meal has been taken.

Hyperorexia refers to the ingestion of food in excess of metabolic needs and may occur for a variety of neurologic, endocrinologic, and psychologic reasons. *Bulimia* is an extreme form of hyperorexia in which the patient's hunger recurs shortly after eating, resulting in the consumption of frequent large meals throughout the day and night. Such behavior is seen with hypothalamic lesions or in mentally disturbed persons. *Parorexia* describes an appetite for unusual foods and is not strictly concerned with the hunger mechanism. Such behavior may characterize diseases producing metabolic derangements (e.g., Addison's disease) or may be seen in the mentally disturbed.

ANOREXIA

Anorexia, or loss of the desire to eat, is a prominent symptom in a wide variety of intestinal and extraintestinal disorders. It must be clearly differentiated from satiety and from specific food intolerance. Anorexia occurs in many disorders and as a result *by itself is of little specific diagnostic value.* The mechanisms whereby hunger and appetite are modified in various disease states are poorly understood.

Anorexia is commonly seen in diseases of the gastrointestinal tract and liver. For example, it may precede the appearance of jaundice in hepatitis, or it may be a prominent symptom in gastric carcinoma. In the setting of intestinal disease, anorexia should be clearly differentiated from *sitophobia*, or fear of eating because of subsequent or associated discomfort. In such circumstances, appetite may persist, but the ingestion of food is curtailed nonetheless. Sitophobia may be seen, for example, in regional enteritis (especially with partial obstruction) or in patients with gastric ulcer following partial or total gastrectomy.

Anorexia may also be a prominent feature of severe extraintestinal diseases. For example, anorexia may be profound in severe congestive heart failure and contribute significantly to the cachexia in these patients. It may be a major symptom in patients with uremia, pulmonary failure, and various endocrinopathies (e.g., hyperparathyroidism (Addison's disease, and panhypopituitarism). While a frequent accompaniment of organic disease, it is often seen with psychogenic disturbances, such as anxiety or depression.

ANOREXIA NERVOSA

This disease may assume such severe proportions as to be life-threatening. Anorexia nervosa, as the syndrome is called because of present-day attribution to psychogenic factors, is characterized initially by voluntary and marked reduction in the intake of food, leading to malnutrition. Severe caloric restriction in these patients may result in weight loss amounting to as much as 50 percent of the normal body weight and profound deficiencies of essential vitamins and minerals. Death from starvation may result. The disease is seen predominantly in women, although men are also affected occasionally. It generally occurs in early adulthood but can be seen even earlier.

The major clinical feature of anorexia nervosa is profound weight loss in a person with no other signs of demonstrable organic illness. Some patients relate that they experience severe hunger which they consciously curb in the beginning of the illness in order to lose weight. Others complain of a profound loss of appetite. Once anorexia becomes severe, peculiar habits in connection with food may be seen, the main purpose of which is to limit food ingestion which causes distress. Patients may hide or surreptitiously dispose of food; alternatively they may induce emesis or catharsis by a variety of methods. Patients with anorexia nervosa generally demonstrate strength and tolerance for physical activity which is remarkably great in light of their impaired nutritional state. This contrasts with certain endocrine or neoplastic diseases which cause marked weight loss. Only as the degree of malnutrition becomes extreme does weakness become pronounced.

Anorexia nervosa may be a manifestation of a variety of mental disorders and psychiatric diseases. Most often it occurs in adolescents with excessive concern about obesity and physical appearance. These are the most difficult problems of all, and it is to this group that the term anorexia nervosa applies. Occasionally it may be a prominent symptom in hysteria, as a somatic abnormality, and obsessive patients may adhere to ritualistic diets in pursuit of slimness. The severely depressed patient may lose his interest in food, and the psychotic individual may develop delusions about the dangers of eating.

Clinical examination of the patient with anorexia nervosa reveals emaciation, often of extreme degree. There may be signs of vitamin deficiencies as well as caloric undernutrition. The blood pressure, basal metabolic rate, and body temperature may be subnormal. There is neither increased skin pigmentation nor abnormalities in hair distribution; specifically, there is no loss of pubic axillary hair. Mental status surveys usually elicit none of the typical features of hysteria, obsessive-compulsive or phobic neuroses, or depression.

Laboratory tests are of value primarily to aid in the exclusion of systemic diseases which might account for extreme weight loss, such as carcinomatosis, diabetes mellitus, and intestinal malabsorption. However, when the underlying organic disease is subtle and not readily diagnosed by history, physical examination, or laboratory tests, the patient may be prematurely and hence incorrectly labeled as having anorexia nervosa. This is frequently the case in regional enteritis, especially that occurring in childhood and adolescence. It is obviously essential to explore fully all possibilities of underlying organic disease before making a diagnosis of anorexia nervosa.

In the differential diagnosis, anorexia nervosa must be distinguished from panhypopituitarism. There is, however, only a superficial resemblance between these two conditions. While amenorrhea may occur in both diseases, in anorexia nervosa hair distribution, breast tissue, as well as thyroid and adrenal function remain normal until the terminal stages of the disease. In addition, strength and tolerance for exercise are much greater in anorexia nervosa than in panhypopituitarism.

In extreme cases of anorexia nervosa, it may be necessary to give nutriments by nasogastric tube or parenterally in order to sustain life. However, since anorexia nervosa often is accompanied by psychologic conflicts, optimal management includes resolution of the patient's peculiar ideas about food. In some patients a period of anorexia nervosa will terminate spontaneously, even in the absence of psychotherapy. However, in these individuals basic conflicts remain unresolved, and a relapse or other evidence of maladjustment is likely to occur at a later date.

NAUSEA AND VOMITING

Nausea and vomiting may occur independently of one another, but generally they are so closely allied that they can conveniently be considered together. *Nausea* denotes the feeling of the imminent desire to vomit, usually referred to the throat or epigastrium. *Vomiting* refers to the forceful oral expulsion of intestinal contents, while *retching* denotes the labored rhythmic respiratory activity that frequently precedes emesis. Extremely forceful *projectile vomiting* is a special form of vomiting which has significance because it connotes the presence of increased intracranial pressure.

Nausea often precedes or accompanies vomiting. It is usually associated with diminished functional activity of the stomach and alterations of the motility of the duodenum and small intestine. Accompanying severe nausea there is often evidence of altered autonomic (especially parasympathetic) activity: pallor of the skin, increased perspiration, salivation, and the occasional association of hypotension and bradycardia (vasovagal syndrome). Anorexia is also often present.

Following a period of nausea and a brief interval of retching, a sequence of involuntary visceral and somatic motor events occurs resulting in emesis. The stomach plays a relatively passive role in the vomiting process, the major ejection force being provided by the abdominal musculature. With relaxation of the gastric fundus and gastroesophageal sphincter, a sharp increase in intra-abdominal pressure is brought about by forceful contraction of the diaphragm and abdominal wall. This, together with concomitant annular contraction of the gastric pylorus, results in the expulsion of gastric contents into the esophagus. Increased intrathoracic pressure results in the further movement of esophageal contents into the mouth. Reversal of the normal direction of esophageal peristalsis may play a role in this process. Reflex elevation of the soft palate during the vomiting act prevents the entry of the material into the nasopharynx, whereas reflex closure of the glottis and inhibition of respiration helps to prevent pulmonary aspiration.

Repeated emesis may have deleterious effects in a number of different ways. The process of vomiting itself may lead to traumatic rupture or tearing in the region of the cardioesophageal junction resulting in massive hematemesis, the so-called Mallory-Weiss syndrome. Prolonged vomiting may lead to dehydration and the loss of gastric secretions (especially hydrochloric acid) to metabolic alkalosis with hypokalemia. Finally, in states of central nervous system depression (coma, etc.), gastric contents may be aspirated into the lungs with a resulting aspiration pneumonitis.

VOMITING MECHANISM. The act of vomiting is under the control of two functionally distinct medullary centers: the *vomiting center* and the *chemoreceptor trigger zone*. The vomiting center controls and integrates the actual act of emesis. It receives afferent stimuli from the intestinal tract and other parts of the body, from higher cortical centers, especially the labyrinthine apparatus, and from the chemoreceptor trigger zone. The important efferent pathways in vomiting are the phrenic nerves (to the diaphragm), the spinal nerves (to the abdominal musculature), and visceral efferent nerves (to the stomach and esophagus).

The chemoreceptor trigger zone is also located in the medulla but by itself is incapable of mediating the act of vomiting. Activation of this zone results in efferent impulses to the medullary vomiting center, which in turn initiates the act of emesis. The chemoreceptor trigger zone can be activated by many stimuli including drugs such as apomorphine, cardiac glycosides, and ergot alkaloids. Certain of the phenothiazine derivatives appear to antagonize the effects of the above-mentioned drugs on the chemoreceptor trigger zone.

CLINICAL CLASSIFICATION. Nausea and vomiting are common manifestations or organic and functional disorders. The precise mechanisms triggering vomiting in the various clinical states are poorly understood, making classification of mechanisms difficult. The categories mentioned below serve to illustrate some of the many disorders which can be accompanied by nausea and vomiting.

Acute Abdominal Emergencies. Many of the disorders in this category which lead to the "surgical abdomen" are associated with nausea and vomiting. Notably, vomiting may be seen with inflammation of a viscus as in acute appendicitis or acute cholecystitis, obstruction of the intestine, or acute peritonitis (see Chap. 12).

Chronic Indigestion. In many of the disorders falling in this category (see Chap. 41) nausea and vomiting may be prominent. Emesis may be either spontaneous or self-induced and may lead to relief of symptoms, as, for example, in uncomplicated peptic ulcer. Nausea and vomiting may accompany the distension and pain seen in the aerophagic syndromes. Often in patients with chronic indigestion, nausea and vomiting may be provoked by specific foods (e.g., fatty foods) for reasons that are poorly understood.

Acute Infectious Disease. Acute systemic infections with fever, especially in young children, are frequently accompanied by vomiting and often severe diarrhea. The mechanism whereby infections remote from the gastrointestinal tract produce these manifestations is unclear. Viral, bacterial, and parasitic infections of the intestinal tract may be associated with severe nausea and vomiting, often with diarrhea. Severe nausea and vomiting may be prominent in viral hepatitis, even before the appearance of jaundice.

Disorders of the Nervous System. Central nervous system disorders which lead to increased intracranial pressure may be accompanied by vomiting, often projectile. Brain swelling due to inflammation, anorexia, acute hydrocephalus, neoplasms, etc., may thus be complicated by vomiting. Disorders of the labyrinthine apparatus and its central connections which underlie vertigo may be accompanied by vomiting with nausea and retching. Acute labyrinthitis and Ménière's disease are examples of such disturbances. Migraine headaches, tabetic crises, and acute meningitis are additional examples of disorders of the nervous system which can lead to vomiting. In the reactive phase of hypotension with syncope, there may be nausea and vomiting.

Diseases of the Heart. Severe nausea and vomiting may be present in acute myocardial infarction, especially of the posterior wall of the heart. Nausea and vomiting may also be seen in congestive heart failure, perhaps related to congestion of the liver. The possibility that these symptoms may be due to drugs (e.g., opiates or digitalis) should always be borne in mind in patients with cardiac disease.

Metabolic and Endocrine Disorders. Nausea and vomiting commonly accompany several endocrinologic disorders, including diabetic acidosis and adrenal insufficiency, especially adrenal crises. The morning sickness of early pregnancy is another instance of nausea and vomiting possibly related to hormonal changes.

Drugs and Chemicals. The side effects of many drugs and chemicals include nausea and vomiting. In some instances this is due to gastric irritation which stimulates the medullary vomiting center.

Psychogenic Vomiting. This term is applied to the vomiting which may occur as part of any emotional upset on a transitory basis or more persistently as part of a psychic disturbance. Close observation will usually disclose the condition to be one of regurgitation rather than of vomiting, and weight loss may not correspond at all to patients' description of the frequency and severity of vomiting. As discussed earlier in this chapter, anorexia nervosa is an emotional disturbance which may be associated not only with anorexia but also with vomiting. Often patients with emotional disorders and vomiting maintain a relatively normal state of nutrition, because a relatively small amount of the ingested food is vomited.

DIFFERENTIAL DIAGNOSIS. Vomiting should be distinguished from *regurgitation,* which refers to the expulsion of food in the absence of nausea and without the abdominal diaphragmatic muscular contraction which is a part of vomiting. Regurgitation of esophageal contents may occur with esophageal stricture or diverticula. Regurgitation of gastric contents is generally seen with gastroesophageal sphincter incompetence, especially with hiatus hernia or in association with peptic ulcer usually when pylorospasm supervenes.

The temporal relationships of vomiting to eating may be of help diagnostically. Vomiting which occurs predominantly in the morning is often seen early in pregnancy and in uremia. Alcoholic gastritis is commonly accompanied by early morning emesis, the so-called "dry heaves." Vomiting which occurs shortly after eating may suggest pylorospasm or gastritis. On the other hand, vomiting which occurs 4 to 6 hours or longer after eating and involves the elimination of large quantities of undigested food often indicates gastric retention (as in diabetic gastric atony or pyloric obstruction).

The character of the vomitus offers clues to the diagnosis. If the vomitus contains free hydrochloric acid, the obstruction may be due to an ulcer; absence of free hydrochloric is more compatible with gastric malignancy. A feculent or putrid odor reflects the results of bacterial action on the intestinal contents. Such vomiting may be seen with low-intestinal obstruction, peritonitis, or gastrocolic fistula. Bile is commonly present in gastric contents whenever vomiting is prolonged. It has no significance unless constantly present in large quantities, when it may signify an obstructive lesion below the ampulla of Vater. The presence of blood in the gastric contents usually denotes bleeding from the esophagus, stomach, or duodenum.

REFERENCES

Anand, B. K.: Nervous Regulation of Food Intake, Physiol. Rev., 41:677, 1961.

Bliss, E. L., and C. H. H. Branch: "Anorexia Nervosa," New York, Hoeber Medical Division, Harper & Row, Publishers, Incorporated, 1960.

Borison, H. L., and S. C. Wang: Physiology and Pharmacology of Vomiting, Pharmacol. Rev., 5:19, 1953.

Mayer, J.: General Characteristics of the Regulation of Food Intake, chap. I, in "Alimentary Canal," vol. I, Washington, D.C., American Physiological Society, 1967.

43 CONSTIPATION, DIARRHEA, AND DISTURBANCES OF ANORECTAL FUNCTION

Albert I. Mendeloff

NORMAL COLONIC FUNCTION

MOTOR AND ABSORPTIVE FUNCTIONS. When one considers that a north-woods lumberjack may consume several kilograms of foodstuffs per day, furnishing him nearly 6000 Cal, and yet produce a stool which weighs only 100 to 200 Gm, of which nearly three-quarters is water, the efficiency of the gut becomes clearly evident. Just as slight changes in renal function may result in the excretion of abnormal amounts of urine, so relatively minor deviations in the absorption of water, in intestinal tone, in propulsive motility, or in rectal sensitivity may result in dramatic changes in the caliber and consistency of the stools.

On a normal mixed diet the stomach is nearly empty several hours after food is ingested. By the time the head of the food column reaches the ileocecal valve, 99 percent of the carbohydrate, 99 percent of the protein, and 97 percent of the fats have been broken down into absorbable form and entered the portal venules and the lacteals.

When the intestinal bolus reaches the terminal ileum, it proceeds very sluggishly unless the stomach empties; the so-called "gastroileal reflex" causes the ileum to empty into the cecum by a rapid series of small squirts. The ileocecal valve can probably function as a true sphincter, slowing down the entry of ileal contents into the cecum, but it also serves to prevent reflux, at least of gas, from cecum into ileum. The ileal volume reaching the cecum daily is about 600 ml, a slurry thoroughly churned in the right colon by segmental contractions of the haustra. Every now and then a coordinated wave involving a short length of colon pushes the soggy mass along into the next area; reflexes brought on by eating activate an occasional massive contraction; this empties a sizable area of right and transverse colon of its contents, which then are packed into the left colon. Defecatory reflexes originate from the rectal walls, which normally are approximated around a small lumen empty of feces; when sigmoid contraction distends the rectal musculature, the defecatory reflex center in the sacral cord causes an increase in intraabdominal pressure through descent of the diaphragm, closure of the glottis, contraction of the abdominal wall musculature, and tensing of the pelvic floor. The later descent of the pelvic floor and the inhibition of tone of the external anal sphincter complete the skeletal muscular phase of defecation. Central nervous system impulses simultaneously engage sacral parasympathetic nerves to contract the smooth muscle of the pelvic colon. However, if the external sphincter is voluntarily contracted, the sigmoid colon relaxes, and the fecal mass slips back up into the rectosigmoid.

INNERVATION. The colon and rectum are supplied with both sympathetic and parasympathetic nerves carrying both sensory and motor fibers. Sympathetic elements from the lower six thoracic segments travel to the right colon via the superior mesenteric plexus; the left colon receives sympathetic fibers originating in the lumbar segments of the cord gathered into the inferior mesenteric plexus, branches of which follow the inferior mesenteric artery. The rectum receives sympathetic innervation from the hypogastric or presacral nerve. Parasympathetic cholinergic fibers to the right colon are assumed to be part of the vagus, passing through the celiac plexus. The left colon and rectum receive all their parasympathetic innervation via the nervi erigentes, originating in the sacral nerves and joining the sympathetic fibers in the pelvic plexuses, from which some accompany the inferior mesenteric artery. The anus and external anal sphincter are supplied by the inferior hemorrhoidal branch of the internal pudendal nerve and by the perineal branches of the fourth sacral nerves, which nerves also innervate the levatores ani. Sensory nerves from the skin and mucous membrane of the anal canal are plentiful and go to the sacral cord.

The functional significance of the sympathetic supply to the lower bowel is unclear. Careful studies in man following dorsolumbar sympathectomy have failed to reveal any consistent dysfunction of colon or rectum. Attempts to relieve colon pain syndromes by presacral neurectomy have been unavailing. The parasympathetic cholinergic innervation of the colon seems to be of sole importance in the motor and secretory functions of that organ; cholinergic drugs correspondingly activate such functions and result, when large enough dosages are employed, in watery diarrhea, cramps, and pain.

The mechanism of defecation has been previously described, and the important contribution of the abdominal musculature, the levatores ani, and the external anal sphincter noted. The internal anal sphincter, a smooth muscle, relaxes when the rectum is distended and seems to help allow gas to escape without full defecatory movements. Sensory innervation of the anal canal permits the brain to discriminate as to whether rectal contents are liquid, gaseous, or solid.

CONTINENCE AND INCONTINENCE

The defecation reflex depends upon the presence of a neuroreceptor system beginning in the smooth muscle of the upper rectum. When its tension reaches a threshold, this musculature contracts, joining and augmenting an entire complex of abdominal wall contraction, internal anal sphincter relaxation, and opening of the external anal sphincter. The reflex is believed to be further augmented by the anal sensation of feces passing though the anal canal, and perhaps also by associated reflexes like that of micturition. The central representation of defecation lies, in experimental animals, in the medulla near the vomiting center, and it may be transiently disturbed in many vascular insults to the brain. Voluntary inhibition of defecation, described earlier, is mediated through rapid relaxation of the abdominal musculature and the contraction of the external anal sphincter.

This sequence of events can take place in persons whose sacral cord has been destroyed—i.e., all its elements can function in the absence of an intact peripheral nerve supply—but the strength of such a denervated contraction is weak, and evacuation is generally incomplete unless laxation, usually by enema, reenforces the reflex. Cord transection abolishes the cerebral appreciation of the urge to defecate. Thus disease or trauma to the higher spinal cord and the brain can produce in the function of colon and rectum the same range of disturbances of function as occur in the bladder (see Chap. 49). The colon may become hypotonic, the external sphincter ineffective, and the defecatory reflexes dulled; the levatores ani are often weak and the abdominal musculature unable to produce and sustain effective pressure increases.

The inability to appreciate anal sensation, whether due to central disease, peripheral neuritis of sacral nerves, or surgical interruption of anal innervation, as in treatment of hemorrhoids and perirectal abscess, may also weaken the responses and is often particularly troublesome when the stool is semisolid or liquid. The "sensing" of the consistency of rectal contents by anal receptors has been demonstrated only recently; it provides some explanation for the unpleasant fact that many surgical repairs of the anorectal area look anatomically excellent but the patient is incontinent of any fecal material other than a hard dry stool.

Sudden interruption of function of the central nervous system, as by cerebral vascular accident, interferes with this whole defecatory complex at many levels, and usually results in fecal incontinence of some degree. The dysfunction is maximal at the onset of the process and generally returns toward normal over a period of weeks. In most forms of neurologic disease resulting in incontinence, the reflex may be satisfactorily activated by rectal distension, most practically produced by a combination of aperients and enemas, which results in a mass movement in the more proximal bowel, augmenting the reflex evacuation from the rectum. As sensation from the anal area returns, the passage of stool through the anus reenforces the reflex. Since the bowel is filled infrequently, and irrigation techniques are generally effective and not dangerous, fecal incontinence in such patients is usually much less troublesome than is urinary incontinence. Fecal impactions may be prevented by regularly administered enemas, control of diet, use of drugs, and regular exercises for strengthening the voluntary anal muscles.

DISORDERED BOWEL FUNCTION

SYMPTOMS. Exaggerations of the motor components of normal gastrointestinal activity constitute the most important early symptoms of gastrointestinal diseases. In the small intestine rapid propulsive motility may be associated with dyssynergy, the combination giving rise to cramping contractions. Because of the rather imprecise character of man's system for the detection and recognition of the sources of visceral pain, these cramps are usually projected to the midline—if they originate in the duodenum, to the epigastrium; if from the jejunum, to the umbilicus; if from the lower ileum, to the area just below the umbilicus. In the colon, dyssynergic activity is rarely projected to the midline but usually is lateralized along the general course of the offending organ. Since the colon is large, festooning the abdomen, and full of fluid and partially compressible gas, contractions in one or another area of the bowel may force the contents back toward the cecum; a simultaneous dyssynergic contraction anywhere else in the colonic wall may trap gas in the area intervening, distending a relaxed but otherwise innocent portion of the bowel so that discomfort is referred to the distended site, often in the splenic or hepatic flexure. Excessive gas results entirely from air swallowed with food or drink or from such "tics" as sighing or forced belching. Sharp, unpleasant contractions in the left lower quadrant associated with straining at stool and partially relieved by defecation, are called *tenesmus*. A sensation of urgent need to defecate—*rectal urgency*—is an extremely distressing symptom associated with irritability of the rectum. Sharp pain in the anal area is made worse by defecation and is usually associated with an inflammatory response in the skin of the anus—*anal pain*.

After establishing the presence or absence of these deviations, the physician must find out whether or not eating or defecation exacerbates or relieves them, whether the patient tries to mitigate the discomfort by moving about or by lying still, or by holding the abdominal wall immobilized with his hands or against the mattress. Although the general topography of the area of distress may localize findings to large or small intestines, relief by defecation is a feature of disturbance of the left colon, as exacerbation by eating is a feature of malfunction of the small intestine or right colon. Restlessness occurs with colic; peritoneal irritation tends to immobilize the patient. All these disturbances originate as increases in the tone of the bowel wall, and pressure relationships between adjacent segments of intestine determine not only the tension exerted against the wall but also the speed and character of the flow of the fluid contents along the lumen. As increased tension may compress the vessels nourishing the gut wall, so disease or contraction of the nourishing vasculature may deprive the wall of its ability to contract, to absorb, or to secrete. Unabsorbed residue or unduly large volumes of secretions attract more fluid into the lumen, further distending the gut; if large volumes of swallowed air cannot be passed quickly along the small bowel to the cecum, as is usual, the movements of the air-fluid mixture in the small intestine become loud enough to be noticed by the patient; such *borborygmi* are heard normally in the colon. Sudden changes in volume of the abdomen—*distension*—occur when the intraluminal volume of small or large bowel increases, because of paralysis of neuromuscular elements, abnormal handling of gas, or mechanical obstruction behind which muscular contractile activity is greatly increased. Bowel sounds may be absent if the wall is paralyzed, faint if the injury is submaximal, or increased if a viable area is forced to raise its intraluminal pressure in order to drive fluid past an obstructed segment. Sudden changes in pain reference occurring during the course of an illness usually indicate that the peritoneal surfaces have become involved, with more accurate cerebral localization of the underlying disturbance, and perhaps with associated development of spasm or guarding of the overlying musculature.

DIARRHEA AND CONSTIPATION. *Diarrhea* and *constipation* are terms given to alterations in the normal pattern of human defecation habits. There is no standard definition by which patients or physicians may classify strictly the deviation from normal; the range of variation in bowel habits among apparently healthy persons is extraordinarily wide, so that the deviation must, in the last analysis, be compared with each patient's own previous habit pattern rather than with that characterizing the mean, the median, or the mode of the population. Such comparisons involve so many associated functions that it will suffice for the purposes of this discussion to define diarrhea as the frequent passage of unformed stools, and constipation as an undue delay in the evacuation of feces. It is the task of the physician to understand enough of the normal and disturbed physiology of digestion, absorption, and propulsive motility that he may ask pointed questions of the patient which serve to define more precisely the locus, the nature, and, the severity of the disturbance. Since the gastrointestinal tract is a primitive organ upon which all manner of stimuli, from hunger to fear, rage, fever, and fatigue, from grossly infected or chemically toxic ingesta to the most subtly allergenic refined foods, exert effects that disturb function, this task is rarely simple.

ACUTE DIARRHEA. Acute disturbances of bowel function are relatively common and usually manifest themselves as diarrhea. The sudden onset of loose stools in a previously healthy person commonly is due to an active infection, and much less often to the ingestion of preformed toxins, poisonous chemicals or drugs, or to acute radiation sickness. When the patient is first seen, the history will usually point toward the source of the trouble: the eating of a particular meal or food in company with others who have also become similarly ill within 24 hr of eating the suspected food is *prima facie* evidence that a preformed toxin has been ingested; diarrhea developing in a number of patients within 28 to 72 hr after a common meal should make one suspect a salmonella infection. The presence of fever, malaise, muscle aching, and profound epigastric or periumbilical discomfort with severe anorexia suggests an inflammatory disease of the small intestine. The stools are characteristically watery, often accompanied by the explosive passage of gas; there is no rectal urgency or tenesmus and little hypogastric cramping. On physical examination one finds a generally tender abdomen without guarding, and one hears "whooshing" peristaltic sounds. A variant of the syndrome consists only of severe periumbilical pain and vomiting. The hemogram usually is within normal limits. Such an entity is commonly produced by infection with a virus, of which a number of species have been identified. The disease is called *viral gastroenteritis,* runs an acute course for 2 to 3 days, then gradually subsides.

The stool in viral gastroenteritis never contains recognizable exudate—it is singularly free of inflammatory cells, blood, or fibrin. Culture of the stool is usually nonproductive. By contrast, inflammatory diseases of the colon almost always result in leukocytic exudate and fibrin in the feces; stools may give cultures positive for organisms of the genus *Salmonella* or *Shigella* or may on microscopic examination show motile forms and/or cysts of various parasites, the most important of which in the United States is *Endamoeba histolytica.* Colonic infections usually are accompanied by hypogastric cramping, tenesmus, and rectal urgency. The patient may not have true anorexia but may be afraid to eat because eating stimulates the urge to defecate. There is usually fever and leukocytosis.

The physician must remember that an acute diarrhea may be the presenting symptoms of any type of systemic infection or of a hitherto-silent chronic gastrointestinal disease, of which the most well-defined are regional enteritis and ulcerative colitis; the latter may occasionally begin with fulminant dysentery, the former more often presenting as a tender mass in the right lower quadrant with mild diarrhea. Generalized cramping and diarrhea may follow use of a parasympathomimetic drug. Tenesmus, urgency, and left-sided hypogastric tenderness and cramping are classic symptoms of diverticulitis; the stool may contain pus, blood, or both, usually with much mucus. A fecal impaction may make a patient have rectal urgency, ask for a bedpan or visit the toilet often, but expel only a little watery exudate or nothing. Short-circuiting operations on the intestine and stomach usually result in at least mild diarrhea for months after the operation.

Differential diagnosis of these varied entities is made by history, physical examination, gross and microscopic appearance of the stools, appropriate bacteriologic studies, and proctoscopy. It is important to see the excreta put out by the patient, not just to rely on his description or on that of a third party. Toilets are not distinguished for satisfactory lighting nor upset patients for careful observation, and even trained personnel seldom display a curiosity sufficient to overcome the unpleasantness of a stool held close enough for accurate appraisal. Since fluid and electrolyte losses in diarrhea may be so great as to be life-threatening, the patient is given supportive care until studies indicate specific treatment. If no definitive etiologic agent can be identified, barium enema and upper gastrointestinal x-rays should be carried out. Upper gastrointestinal films may be very misleading when the barium meal is fed within the first few days of an acute enteritis or colitis and should be reserved for a time when the whole disease has become more quiescent.

CHRONIC DIARRHEA. A history of bouts of loose stools extending over a period of months or years, usually intermittent in character, calls for painstaking investigation. One particularly wants to know the circumstances of the first such bout—did it follow an acute infection, an operation, an emotional upset of severe degree? The number of days or weeks lost by the patient from his daily occupation on account of the illness, changes in weight and strength, and the appearance of the patient give important leads as to the nature and severity of the underlying disease. By the time the patient sees a physician the presenting symptoms may not be diarrhea but rather those of serious malnutrition, since any long-continued illness of this type may interfere with appetite as well as with the absorptive and digestive functions of the gastrointestinal tract. Associated signs and symptoms may reveal that the diarrhea and malnutrition are due to a generalized disorder which may involve the intestines functionally or structurally—hyperthyroidism, tuberculosis, lymphosarcoma, to name a few. More often, no such disorder will be found, and the physician must consider another, more specifically gastrointestinal disease.

A long history of intermittent diarrhea unaccompanied by fever, weight loss, blood in the stools, or significant loss of working capacity suggests a disturbance of emotional or, less commonly, of allergic origin, and associated symptoms should be elicited (Chaps. 18 and 72). A detailed dietary history is important in such cases, in order to establish the adequacy of the nutrient intake and to allow the patient a chance to ventilate his ideas on the relationship of food and eating to his symptoms. In such disordered functional states, the patient usually has a fairly formed stool on arising in the morning but then has one or two loose stools within the next hour. A similar pattern may occur after the evening meal. The stool caliber is usually small, and there may be mild discomfort, relieved by defecation, in the left lower quadrant of the abdomen. Such a triad of symptoms makes up the diarrheal component of the "irritable colon" syndrome, an extremely common disorder in anxious, nervous people, in which the symptoms result from exaggeration of normal colonic function.

When the history suggests that the diarrheal episodes have been characterized by blood in the stools, or by fever, malaise, anorexia, and weight loss in addition, one suspects a chronic inflammatory process involving either small bowel or colon or both. Regional enteritis may attack any portion of the intestine, producing an encroachment on the lumen and episodes of partial obstruction, ulcerations of the mucous membrane, or local abscesses and fistulas of the abdominal or anal skin, of the bladder, or of other loops of bowel. On proctoscopic examination the rectum is found to be uninvolved, and the stools show little microscopic exudate, although they are often positive for occult blood, gross bleeding being infrequently encountered. Tuberculosis and lymphosarcoma of the intestine can give similar symptoms and may be impossible to differentiate, although usually the roentgenologic appearances are dissimilar. The involvement may be primarily colonic, the most important disease entity being ulcerative colitis, whether idiopathic or due to amebic infestation, venereal lymphogranuloma, or chronic bacillary dysentery. Here the feces show pus cells and red cells when the disease is active, and proctoscopy is usually diagnostic. Stool cultures and examinations for parasites on numerous occasions are important aspects of the medical investigation.

When the patient presents with diarrhea of more than a few months' duration, without fever, blood in the stools, or cramping pain, but with weight loss, weakness, and symptoms of nutritional deficiency diseases (Chaps. 316 and 334), one focuses attention on the small intestine. In children celiac disease and cystic fibrosis of the pancreas are the important disorders to be differentiated; in older patients the same distinction between an absorptive defect and a digestive disorder must still be made in order to distinguish idiopathic steatorrhea from chronic pancreatitis. Whereas the stools in disease of the left colon are loose, often contain exudate on microscopic examination, and weigh less than 200 Gm per 24 hr, the stools associated with malabsorption are bulky, free of exudate, and weigh more than 300 Gm per 24 hr. Such a 24-hr collection, impounded in a collecting vessel, often has a shiny appearance and a foul odor which are almost diagnostic. See Chap. 316 for differential diagnosis of malabsorption.

A history of progressive disease characterized by arthritis, abdominal pain, diarrhea, and weight loss in middle-aged men suggests the diagnosis of Whipple's disease. Lymphosarcomas of low degrees of malignancy may produce malabsorption syndromes by blockage of lymphatic channels from the small bowel; areas of gut with poor motility may become "blind loops" and harbor large numbers of bacteria, which deconjugate bile salts and utilize nutrients needed by the host. The presenting symptoms of such pathologic disturbances may be diarrhea and macrocytic anemia, or watery diarrhea with or without increased fat content. Surgical revisions of the bowel, multiple jejunal diverticulosis, regional enteritis, and mesenteric vascular insufficiency may result in such conditions. Rarer causes of diarrhea are the enormous hypersecretion of gastric juice due to endocrine tumors, and the cramping diarrhea associated with high circulating levels of serotonin (see Chap. 105).

Special techniques are often needed to define clearly all these abnormalities. Duodenal intubation and analysis of digestive juices for pancreatic enzymes is a procedure of considerable importance in ruling out primary disease of the pancreas. Nevertheless, the aid of the skilled radiologist is probably more useful than any test in interpreting all but the earliest manifestations of these syndromes. Pancreatic calcification, fistulas, distortions of the duodenal loop, diffuse granulomatous diseases of the small bowel, diverticula, polyps, ulcerated areas, stenosis, and obstruction—all these can be identified by modern radiologic techniques, which provide in addition baseline data for evaluating the natural history of the disease and response to therapy.

CONSTIPATION. Whereas diarrhea may be a dangerous symptom per se, with its accompaniment of dehydration and loss of cations, constipation of itself is not debilitating, although mild abdominal discomfort and straining at stool are not salutary and tend to increase the severity of preexisting anorectal lesions. The acute onset of severe obstipation in an apparently normal person signifies that something has disturbed the neural, vascular, or muscular integrity of the gut or associated defecatory reflexes and muscles. Such disturbances may result from severe infections, particularly of the central nervous system, from acute mesenteric circulatory catastrophes, from renal colic, from cerebrovascular accidents, from mechanical obstruction of large or small intestine, from painful anal lesions, from certain drugs, or from fecal impaction. Of these, the last is the most embarrassing to overlook, since the puttylike mass filling the rectum makes the patient try to move his bowels and often results in frequent calls for a bedpan or visits to the toilet; such fruitless attempts at defecations may be called diarrhea, and the poor patient may receive antidiarrheal medications! Rapid but complete physical examination including a digital examination of the rectum and proctoscopy is called for in all cases of constipation of acute onset; if no other physical signs to explain the sudden constipation are elicited, a low-pressure barium enema should be given to establish the site of obstruction if present and appropriate measures taken.

A long history of intermittent bouts of constipation, accompanied by abdominal distress relieved by defecation and by passage of hard stools of small caliber, with or without much mucus, is characteristic of the *"irritable colon" syndrome*, one of the most common forms of anxiety met by the physician. The abuse of laxatives over many years is frequently added to the underlying emotional disturbance to aggravate the clinical picture. The symptoms are essentially exaggerations of normal physiologic activity of the colon and in mild degrees have probably been experienced by most healthy people as, for example, the constipation associated with travel. Extensive studies of sigmoid motility in patients with this syndrome have verified the clinical impression that disturbed motor function correlates closely with emotional conflicts. Proctoscopic examination of these patients demonstrates an unremarkable rectum and a rectosigmoid which is often spastic, the lumen smaller than normal, the veins prominent, and the mucus more abundant than usual. The stools are negative for blood, parasites, and pathogenic bacteria; the x-ray examination is usually not abnormal.

Another common form of constipation is also chronic and is not characterized by the triad of symptoms of the irritable colon syndrome. Whether as the result of childhood training or of a perverse understanding of the necessity for bowel movements occurring with chronometric precision, these patients have equated general health with "regularity." This leads to a dependence on laxatives or enemas to hasten the overdue evacuation, so that over the years they lose the sensitivity of the rectal defecatory reflexes. Consequently, they do not have a regular schedule for moving their bowels, which for most normal people is most easily accomplished after breakfast and, if needed, after the heaviest meal of the day; over the years they no longer demonstrate any rhythmicity in defecation, take laxatives whenever they feel "run down," and have stools which may be alternately voluminous and watery or small and hard. Lax abdominal muscles and a pelvic floor weakened by multiple deliveries may contribute to poor defecatory performance. On physical examination these patients often have a palpable colon filled with feces, and on rectal examination feces fill the ampulla, the patient being unaware of this. Such types of rectal insensitivity have been called *atonic constipation, dyschezia,* and *rectal constipation.*

In both the above types of constipation, it is obvious that a thorough analysis by the physician of dietary habits, defecatory habits, use of laxatives, mode of living, and emotional problems must be made before proper therapy can be instituted. At the same time it must be stressed that such patients are not immune to the development of neoplasms of the large bowel, and it is a most difficult task for the physician to decide how often complete studies should be carried out on patients with long-standing, apparently static, complaints. The simplest solution is to do repeated stool examinations for occult blood and digital and proctoscopic examinations, remembering also that in patients who have difficulty with evacuation, anal diseases—fissures, ulcers, and hemorrhoids—are more common than in the general population.

A lifelong history of obstinate constipation may be as-

sociated with the enormous dilatation of the large bowel seen in idiopathic or acquired megacolon. In the former condition, the rectosigmoid is contracted and obstructing, because of its lack of the ganglionic cells necessary to pass on the propulsive waves of the proximal colon; in the latter condition, severe contraction of the voluntary anal sphincter produces enormous dilatation of the rectal ampulla and colon. Radiologic studies are usually very helpful in differentiating these two conditions.

When constipation is of recent onset and progressive, the investigation should be thorough and extremely comprehensive. This is the optimal time to detect a neoplasm of the large bowel. General physical and psychiatric examination may reveal a systemic disorder: hypothyroidism, hyperparathyroidism, tuberculosis, urinary tract disease, congestive heart failure; a major psychosis, profound depression, parkinsonism, or recent cerebrovascular accident may be responsible for progressive constipation. A careful history of drug ingestion may reveal that the patient received ganglionic-blocking agents or opiates prior to onset of symptoms or large amounts of sedation. A marked change in dietary regimen, particularly in combination with sedative drugs, may produce a marked decrease in frequency of bowel movements.

If the digital and proctoscopic findings fail to explain the constipation, a barium enema and upper gastrointestinal x-rays are indicated. Tumors of the gastrointestinal tract comprise nearly half of all cancer, and patients with colonic cancers have a better prognosis for survival after surgical treatment than do those with gastric and esophageal lesions. A high index of suspicion for a neoplastic origin of changes in bowel habits, repeated tests for occult blood in the stools, and careful proctoscopy and x-ray studies will usually justify in salvaged lives the money and time spent.

PROCTALGIA. See Chap. 320.

REFERENCES

Davenport, H. W.: "Physiology of the Digestive Tract," 2d ed., Chicago, The Year Book Medical Publishers, Inc., 1966.

Mendeloff, A. I.: Chronic Diarrhea, Am. J. Dig. Dis., 3:801, 1958.

44 HEMATEMESIS AND MELENA

Kurt J. Isselbacher and Raymond S. Koff

Hematemesis is defined as the vomiting of blood, and melena as the passage of black, tarry stools. These dramatic symptoms of gastrointestinal hemorrhage should not only bring the patient to prompt medical attention but, within certain limits, help define the anatomic site of bleeding. Only rarely will exsanguinating gastrointestinal hemorrhage occur without the appearance of altered or gross blood passed by mouth or rectum. The color of vomited blood will vary from red to black depending upon the duration of contact of the blood with gastric acid in the stomach. Thus if vomiting occurs shortly after the onset of bleeding, the vomitus is likely to be red; if there is delay in vomiting, the appearance will be dark-red, black, or of "coffee grounds" appearance. Since blood entering the gastrointestinal tract below the duodenum rarely reenters the stomach, hematemesis usually indicates that the bleeding is proximal to the jejunum.

Melena may occur independently of, or be associated with, hematemesis. Bleeding of sufficient volume to produce hematemesis usually results in melena. The altered color of the blood results from prolonged contact with gastric juice to produce hematin. In contrast to hematemesis, melena may result from hemorrhage into the jejunum or ileum provided that transit through the bowel is slow. At least 50 to 100 ml blood must rapidly enter the upper gastrointestinal tract to produce a single black, tarry stool. Following a single liter episode of hemorrhage, tarry stools will persist for 1 to 3 days. Subsequently the stools return to normal color, but tests for occult blood may be positive for 3 to 8 days.

The passage of red blood per rectum usually denotes lower intestinal bleeding, i.e., bleeding originating below the duodenum. However, if bleeding is massive and rapid enough, red blood may appear per rectum from an upper intestinal or gastric lesion.

Not all black or red stools are due to blood. Black stools may result from the ingestion of iron, charcoal, or bismuth. Red stools are occasionally seen after ingestion of beets or following intravenous sulfobromophthalein tests. The presence of gastrointestinal bleeding, even if detected only by positive tests for occult blood in the stool or clear aspirate of the gastric contents, indicates potentially serious disease and must be investigated.

The clinical manifestations of gastrointestinal bleeding are dependent upon the extent of hemorrhage, the rate of bleeding, and the presence of associated or coincidental diseases. Unless anemia is present prior to the onset of bleeding, loss of less than 500 ml blood is usually not associated with systemic symptoms. Rapid hemorrhage of greater volume will result in decreased venous return to the heart, decreased cardiac output, reflex vasoconstriction, and increased peripheral resistance. The patient may experience syncope, light-headedness, nausea, sweating, and thirst. He may appear anxious and restless. When blood loss approaches 40 percent of the blood volume, shock with tachycardia and a thready peripheral pulse are usually present. The skin is cold and clammy, and pallor is prominent. Initial hematocrits will not reflect the blood loss accurately until several hours later, when hemodilution has occurred. The platelet count rises, and leukocytosis is found 2 to 5 hr after the onset of bleeding. Occasionally the presence of blood in the intestinal tract is associated with mild fever (100 to 102°F), and the blood urea nitrogen becomes variably elevated 24 to 48 hr after bleeding because of the breakdown of blood proteins to urea by intestinal bacteria.

ETIOLOGY OF UPPER GASTROINTESTINAL BLEEDING

Swallowed blood resulting from epistaxis, hemoptysis, dental extractions, and tonsillectomy may be vomited or result in melena. A careful history and physical examination will exclude these sources.

The three most common causes of upper gastrointestinal hemorrhage are (1) esophageal or gastric varices, (2) peptic ulceration, and (3) erosive gastritis. These three entities encompass 90 to 95 percent of all cases of upper gastrointestinal bleeding in which a definite lesion can be found.

VARICEAL BLEEDING. Bleeding from esophageal or gastric varices is most frequently associated with portal hypertension due to cirrhosis of the liver. Although in the United States alcoholic cirrhosis is by far the most prevalent form of this disease, variceal hemorrhage may occur in other forms of cirrhosis associated with portal hypertension, especially postnecrotic cirrhosis. Portal vein thrombosis may also lead to variceal hemorrhage in the absence of cirrhosis. Bleeding from varices tends to be abrupt and often massive; however, minor bleeding may occur for days from esophageal varices before it is discovered. Upper gastrointestinal bleeding in a patient with cirrhosis suggests a variceal source, but because patients with cirrhosis have a higher incidence of peptic ulceration, bleeding from the latter must be excluded. Furthermore, in the alcoholic patient with cirrhosis who has continued to drink prior to the onset of bleeding, bleeding from gastritis is quite common.

PEPTIC ULCER. Peptic ulcer disease is probably the most common cause of upper gastrointestinal bleeding. The majority of these ulcers are situated in the duodenum. About 20 percent of patients with peptic ulcer will have at least one episode of significant gastrointestinal bleeding. When a patient with known peptic ulcer presents with gastrointestinal hemorrhage, the ulcer is the most probable site of bleeding.

GASTRITIS. Gastritis may be associated with recent heavy alcohol ingestion or with a history of ingestion of salicylates or other drugs. Similarly gastric erosions and ulcerations may occur in "stressful" situations and are not infrequently found in patients with intracranial disease, burns, or recent trauma. Erosive gastritis can rarely be diagnosed by radiologic techniques, and gastroscopy is necessary to confirm this diagnosis.

OTHER LESIONS OF THE UPPER GASTROINTESTINAL TRACT. Less common sources of upper gastrointestinal bleeding originating in the esophagus include esophagitis (with or without hiatus hernia), carcinoma, and peptic ulcer of the esophagus. Lacerations of the mucosa of the distal end of the esophagus associated with severe vomiting (the Mallory-Weiss syndrome) is suggested by a history of nonbloody vomiting followed by hematemesis. While sudden severe hemorrhage is seen in a small number of patients with carcinoma of the stomach, particularly in association with mucosal ulceration, chronic blood loss is a more frequent complication of gastric carcinoma.

Mesenteric venous or arterial occlusion by embolism or thrombosis may produce either occult or overt blood loss.

Lymphoma, polyps, and other tumors of the stomach and proximal small intestine are relatively uncommon lesions and are therefore unusual sources of hemorrhage. The Peutz-Jeghers syndrome of small intestinal polyposis and melanin pigmentation of the lips, mucosa, fingers, and toes may be associated with recurrent melena.

Saccular arteriosclerotic aortic aneurysms may rupture into the upper intestine and are almost invariably fatal. Most commonly rupture occurs into the third portion of the duodenum.

Primary blood dyscrasias including leukemia, thrombocytopenic states, and the hemophilias may result in significant gastrointestinal bleeding. Polycythemia vera, although associated with an increased incidence of peptic ulceration, may also result in gastrointestinal bleeding due to mesenteric or portal vein thrombosis. Periarteritis nodosa, Henoch-Schönlein purpura, and other vasculitides may lead to gastrointestinal blood loss.

Gastrointestinal bleeding, usually mild but occasionally persistent, may accompany amyloidosis, Osler-Rendu-Weber disease, pseudoxanthoma elasticum, Turner's syndrome, single or multiple intestinal hemangiomas, neurofibromatosis, Kaposi's sarcoma, and hemangiectatic hypertrophy. Although the occurrence of hematemesis and melena in uremia is unusual, mild occult intestinal bleeding is quite frequent.

ETIOLOGY OF LOWER GASTROINTESTINAL BLEEDING

ANAL LESIONS. The most common cause of small amounts of bright-red blood on the surface of the stool and on toilet tissue is bleeding from hemorrhoidal veins. Bleeding from internal or external hemorrhoids is frequently precipitated by straining or passage of hard stools. Anal fissures or fistulas likewise first may come to the attention of the patient as a result of rectal bleeding. The presence of an anal pathologic condition *does not preclude other causes and sources of bleeding, such as carcinoma, and these must be sought and excluded.*

RECTUM AND COLONIC DISEASE. Carcinoma of the rectum, rectal polyps, and ulcerative proctitis are the most common bleeding lesions of the rectum. Bleeding from carcinoma in any area of the colon may result in the appearance of gross blood, whether on the stool or mixed with the fecal contents. Bloody diarrhea is often the presenting feature of ulcerative colitis but is uncommon in granulomatous ileocolitis, although occult blood may be present in the stool. Bleeding may accompany bacterial and protozoan diarrhea, especially shigellosis and amebic colitis.

DIVERTICULITIS. Intestinal diverticula may occur in every part of the intestinal tract but are most commonly found in the sigmoid colon. Diverticulosis per se may rarely cause massive gastrointestinal hemorrhage. Bleeding, usually of minimal severity, may originate from these lesions but is more common when inflammation is pres-

ent, i.e., in diverticulitis. Meckel's diverticulum, a congenital anomaly occurring in about 2 percent of the population and located in the ileum usually 20 to 100 cm proximal to the ileocecal valve, is often associated with bleeding. Ectopic gastric mucosa may be present in about 15 percent of these diverticula and may ulcerate with profuse or recurrent rectal hemorrhage, particularly in children and young adults.

APPROACH TO THE PATIENT WITH GASTROINTESTINAL BLEEDING

The approach to the patient with gross bleeding from the gastrointestinal tract is dependent upon the site, extent, and rate of bleeding. In general the patient who presents with hematemesis is more likely to have bled greater amounts and is more likely to exsanguinate than the patient with melena. There is usually a sense of urgency in the immediate diagnosis and treatment of patients with upper gastrointestinal bleeding. When first seen, the patient may be in shock. Before a complete history and physical examination are undertaken, blood must be obtained for typing and cross matching, and an intravenous infusion of saline solution or other plasma expander must be started at once.

HISTORY. A history of epigastric pain relieved by food, milk, or antacids strongly suggests peptic ulcer disease. A history of jaundice and alcoholism suggests chronic liver disease. One must carefully inquire about a recent alcoholic binge or the ingestion of drugs such as aspirin, which may be associated with gastritis or precipitate bleeding from peptic ulcer. Attention must be directed to possible previous episodes of bleeding, vomiting, symptoms of gastrointestinal distress, diarrhea, cramps, weight loss, fever, bleeding from other sites such as the skin and mucous membranes, and a family history of intestinal disease or hemorrhagic diathesis.

PHYSICAL EXAMINATION. Physical examination is directed to excluding a nonintestinal source of blood (i.e., ruling out epistaxis, hemoptysis, pharyngeal lesions). Careful assessment of the skin may reveal the characteristic telangiectasia of Osler-Rendu-Weber disease, the diffuse melanin pigmentation of hemochromatosis, the localized pigmentation of Peutz-Jeghers syndrome, the soft tissue tumors and multiple sebaceous cysts of familial colonic polyposis, or the dermal neurofibromas of neurofibromatosis. The presence of peripheral stigmas of chronic liver disease with hepatosplenomegaly, ascites, and edema suggest the likelihood of portal hypertension and the possibility of bleeding from varices, gastritis, or peptic ulceration. One must look for the presence of abdominal tenderness or masses, determine the frequency and character of the bowel sounds, and look for evidence of malignancy such as a Virchow node or rectal shelf.

LABORATORY STUDIES. Initial studies include the hematocrit, hemoglobin, careful assessment of red cell morphologic features (the finding of hypochromic, microcytic red cells suggests that blood loss is chronic), and white cell count and differential. There should be a platelet count, or platelets should be estimated from the blood smear. Prothrombin time and coagulation studies may be in order to exclude primary or secondary clotting defects. While the initial studies are valuable and essential, it is important that there be *repeated evaluation* of the laboratory data as one follows the clinical course of the bleeding.

DIAGNOSTIC APPROACH

The diagnostic approach (see also Chap. 314 for a more detailed discussion) to the patient with gastrointestinal hemorrhage must necessarily be individualized. It must be emphasized that demonstration of a lesion of the intestinal tract in a patient with gastrointestinal bleeding should be accompanied by evidence that it is *the* bleeding lesion, since more than one potential bleeding lesion may be present. In recent years the number of experienced endoscopists has increased enormously, so that in many medical centers emergency endoscopy and upper gastrointestinal roentgenographic studies can be performed within hours of admission to the hospital. The patient who presents with melena or who has recently experienced hematemesis or is suspected of bleeding from the upper gastrointestinal tract initially should have a stomach tube passed to empty the stomach, to determine whether the bleeding is in the upper gastrointestinal tract and whether the bleeding is continuing.

The next step, provided that blood volume is maintained, will depend on the facilities available. In an increasing number of hospitals esophagoscopy and gastroscopy will be performed immediately thereafter, at the bedside if necessary, followed by emergency upper gastrointestinal roentgenograms. If the patient's condition does not permit these diagnostic measures and bleeding varices or peptic ulcer are strongly suspected, ice water lavage of the stomach may be attempted to slow bleeding, and, in the case of variceal bleeding, intravenous administration of vasopressin may permit hemostasis by reduction of portal venous pressure. Once bleeding is controlled, endoscopy and upper gastrointestinal x-rays are obtained.

If massive bleeding or hematemesis persists, it may be necessary to resort to esophageal tamponade with the Sengstaken-Blakemore tube or some variant of it. Although use of tamponade is extremely hazardous, even under the best of conditions, variceal hemorrhage may be controlled in the majority of patients and the patient's condition stabilized. The initial management of gastrointestinal bleeding may be controlled by the internist, but it is wise to call for the aid of the surgeon, early in the course, because surgical intervention may be necessary if bleeding cannot be controlled.

In the event that bleeding has stopped prior to admission or shortly thereafter and endoscopy and upper gastrointestinal series do not disclose the source of bleeding, one may resort to splenic pulp manometry and splenoportography, especially if varices are suspected. An elevated splenic pulp pressure (>25 to 30 mm Hg) correlates well with hemorrhage from varices. Although splenoportography is generally less useful than the combination of esophagoscopy and barium swallow in demonstrating varices, it provides exceedingly important information on the patency of the portal and splenic veins in the event that surgical decompression of the portal system is contemplated.

If endoscopic and radiologic studies are negative but slow bleeding from the upper intestinal tract persists, a radiopaque string or tape may be passed perorally to aid in localizing the site of bleeding. After the location of the string is checked by fluoroscopy, fluorescein or radioactive-labeled red cells may be injected intravenously; the string is then retrieved and examined for the location of occult blood, fluorescence, or radioactivity. Unfortunately, the string test is subject to a number of methodologic errors and has been (f limited clinical value. Celiac angiography has also been used to localize bleeding from the small intestine, but its overall value remains to be determined.

The most important diagnostic procedure in the evaluation of rectal bleeding is digital rectal examination and proctosigmoidoscopy. Biopsy of lesions may be performed under direct vision through the sigmoidoscope, if necessary. Barium enema examination and air-contrast studies will aid in localizing lesions above the reach of the sigmoidoscope. Obviously bleeding must not be attributed to hemorrhoids or anal fissures unless other lesions are clearly excluded by adequate and repeated examinations. When appropriate, culture of stool specimens and examination of stools for ova and parasites complete the evaluation.

REFERENCES

Brick, I. B., and H. J. Jeghers: Gastrointestinal Hemorrhage, New Engl. J. Med., 253:458, 1955.

Conn, H. O., and J. A. Simpson: Excessive Mortality Associated with Balloon Tamponade of Bleeding Varices, J.A.M.A., 202:587, 1967.

Merigan, T. C., Jr., R. M. Hollister, P. F. Gryska, G. W. B. Starkey, and C. S. Davidson: Gastrointestinal Bleeding with Cirrhosis: A Study of 172 Episodes in 158 Patients, New Engl. J. Med., 263:579, 1960.

Peternel, W. W., A. E. Dagradi, A. I. Rogers, H. M. Nadal, E. B. Perin, and F. C. Jackson: Clinical Investigation of the Portacaval Shunt. III. The Diagnosis of Esophageal Varices, J.A.M.A., 202:1081, 1968.

45 JAUNDICE AND HEPATOMEGALY
Kurt J. Isselbacher

JAUNDICE

Jaundice, or *icterus,* refers to the yellow pigmentation of the skin or scleras by bilirubin. This in turn is a result of elevated levels of bilirubin in the bloodstream. Jaundice may be brought to the attention of the patient or the physician by a darkening of the urine or a yellow discoloration of the skin or sclera; the latter often is the site where clinical icterus may first be detected. Scleral pigmentation is attributed to richness of this tissue in elastin, which has a special affinity for bilirubin. Jaundice must be distinguished from other causes of yellow pigmentation such as carotenemia (see Chaps. 58 and 85), which is due to carotenoid pigments in the bloodstream and is associated with a yellowish discoloration of the skin but not the sclera. Atabrine treatment (see Chap. 241) may produce a yellow color of the skin and urine, but the scleras are usually only minimally discolored, and when pigment is present, it is only seen in the regions of the scleras exposed to light.

Normal serum bilirubin concentrations range from 0.5 to 1.0 mg per 100 ml, and normally most of this is unconjugated (see Fig. 45-1). The precise level at which jaundice becomes clinically evident varies, but usually it can be recognized when the total serum bilirubin exceeds 2 to 2.5 mg per 100 ml. Not infrequently in deep jaundice the skin may take on a greenish hue because of the conversion of bilirubin to biliverdin, an oxidation product of bilirubin. Oxidation occurs more readily with conjugated bilirubin, and hence a greenish hue is seen more frequently in conditions with pronounced conjugated hyperbilirubinemia.

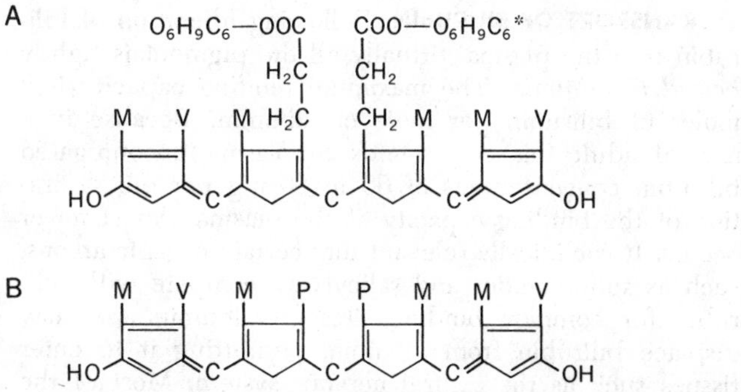

Production and Metabolism of Bilirubin

NORMAL SOURCES OF BILIRUBIN (Fig. 45-2). The majority of the bilirubin is derived from the catabolism of hemoglobin present in senescent red cells. This normally accounts for about 80 to 85 percent of the daily bilirubin production. When a circulating red cell reaches the end of its normal life span of approximately 120 days, it is destroyed in the reticuloendothelial system. In the catabolism of hemoglobin, globin appears to be first dissociated from heme, after which the heme moiety is oxida-

Fig. 45-1. The chemical structures of conjugated (A) and unconjugated (B) bilirubin. Abbreviations: M = methyl, V = vinyl, P = propionic acid. The asterisk (*) refers to glucuronic acid.

tively cleaved and converted to biliverdin by a microsomal heme oxygenase. This enzyme system requires oxygen and a cofactor, reduced nicotinamide adenine dinucleotide phosphate (NADPH). Bilirubin is then formed from biliverdin by another enzyme, biliverdin reductase.

About 15 to 20 percent of the bilirubin is derived from sources other than senescent erythrocytes. One of these is the destruction of maturing erythroid cells in the bone marrow, or so-called "ineffective erythropoiesis" (see Chap. 341). The other is from nonerythroid components, especially in the liver, and involves the turnover of heme and heme proteins (such as cytochrome, myoglobin, and heme-containing enzymes). These two sources of bilirubin are collectively referred to as the *early labeled fraction,* a term which is derived from experiments with labeled glycine and delta-aminolevulinic acid (ALA). Thus when labeled glycine is administered to a normal subject, approximately 15 percent of the label appears in stool stercobilinogen at about 120 days and reflects the bilirubin produced from the normal destruction of senescent red cells.

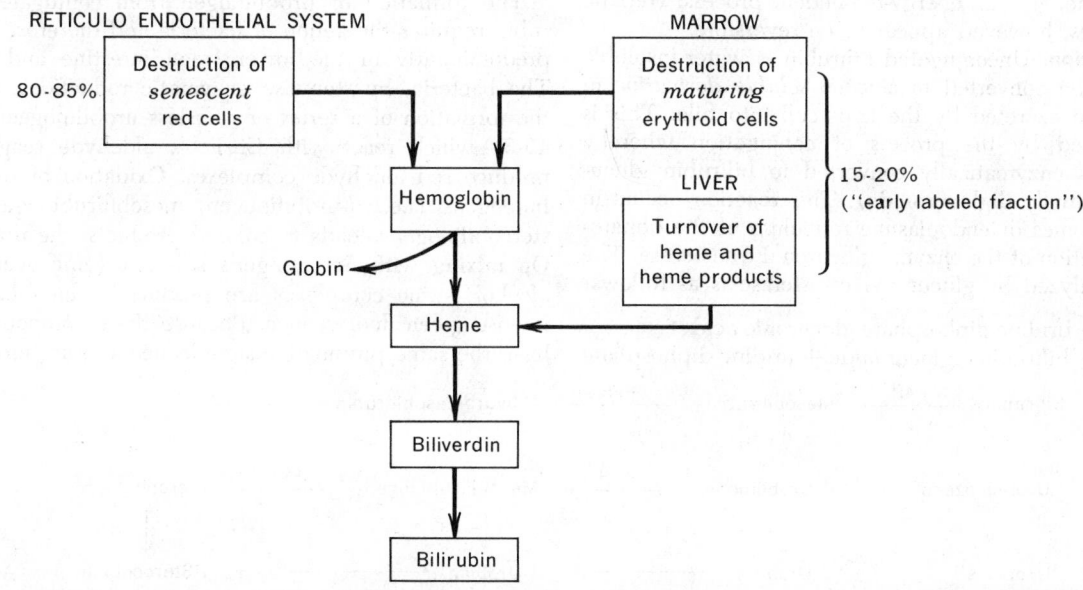

Fig. 45-2. The sources and precursors of plasma bilirubin.

TRANSPORT OF BILIRUBIN. Following liberation of bilirubin into the plasma virtually all the pigment is tightly *bound to albumin*. The maximum binding capacity is 2 moles of bilirubin per mole of albumin. Because in a normal adult this corresponds to plasma unconjugated bilirubin concentrations of 60 to 80 mg per ml, saturation of the binding capacity of the plasma almost never occurs. It is clinically relevant that certain organic anions, such as sulfonamides and salicylates, compete with bilirubin for common binding sites on albumin and may displace bilirubin from albumin, permitting it to enter tissues such as the central nervous system. Most of the evidence for albumin binding has been obtained from studies using unconjugated bilirubin. The conjugated pigment also appears to be bound primarily to albumin, although the binding forces may be different. Some conjugated bilirubin in the plasma is ultrafilterable.

Bilirubin is found in body fluids (cerebrospinal fluid, joint effusions, cysts, etc.) in proportion to the albumin content of the fluids and is absent from true secretions such as tears, saliva, and pancreatic juice. Scar tissue is rarely bilirubin-stained. The appearance of jaundice is also influenced by blood flow and edema. Paralyzed extremities and edematous areas tend to remain uncolored, and "unilateral" jaundice in patients with hemiplegia and edema may be seen if jaundice develops in such patients.

HEPATIC METABOLISM OF BILIRUBIN. The liver occupies a central role in the metabolism of the bile pigments. Three distinct phases are recognized: (1) *hepatic uptake*, (2) *conjugation*, and (3) *excretion* into bile. Of these three steps, excretion appears to be the rate-limiting step and the one most susceptible to impairment when the liver cell is damaged.

Uptake. Unconjugated bilirubin bound to albumin is presented to the liver cell, and upon entry the pigment and albumin became dissociated. Very little is known concerning the mechanism of the uptake phase, particularly whether it is an energy-dependent process. Hepatic uptake does, however, appear to be reversible.

Conjugation. Unconjugated bilirubin is water-insoluble and must be converted to a *water-soluble derivative* in order to be excreted by the liver cell into bile. This is accomplished by the process of conjugation whereby bilirubin is enzymatically converted to bilirubin glucuronide (actually diglucuronide). This reaction occurs in the microsomes or endoplasmic reticulum of the hepatocytes by action of the enzyme glucuronyl transferase. The action catalyzed by glucuronyl transferase is as follows:

Bilirubin + uridine diphosphate glucuronic acid →
      bilirubin diglucuronide + uridine diphosphate

As a result of this enzymatic reaction glucuronic acid is attached to the two carboxyl groups of bilirubin (Fig. 45-1). Glucuronyl transferase is also found in kidney and intestine, but the liver serves as the major site for conjugated bilirubin formation. The hepatic microsomal glucuronyl transferase system also is involved in the formation of glucuronides of other endogenous and exogenous substances (e.g., conjugates of steroids, antibiotics, and salicylates) (see Chap. 323).

The major product of conjugation is bilirubin diglucuronide, sometimes referred to as pigment II. Although some chromatographic evidence has suggested the existence of bilirubin monoglucuride, or pigment I, such a product appears to be a "complex" of unconjugated bilirubin and bilirubin diglucuronide and is perhaps an artifact produced in the course of isolating the pigments. While bilirubin sulfate has also been found in bile, the glucuronide conjugate is the major conjugated bile pigment excreted by the liver cells.

Excretion or Secretion into Bile. In order for bilirubin to be transferred from the liver cell into bile, *the pigment must be in the conjugated form*. Although the overall process is not well understood, the excretion of conjugated bilirubin into bile appears to be an energy-dependent process and the *rate-limiting* step in the hepatic metabolism of bilirubin. When this step is compromised, two consequences occur: (1) decreased excretion of bilirubin into bile and (2) "regurgitation," or reentry of conjugated bilirubin from the liver cells into the bloodstream.

INTESTINAL PHASE OF BILIRUBIN METABOLISM. After its appearance in the intestinal lumen, bilirubin glucuronide may be excreted in the stool or metabolized to urobilinogen and related products. Because of its polarity, conjugated bilirubin is not reabsorbed by the intestinal mucosa, a mechanism which may serve to rid the body of this pigment.

The formation of urobilinogen from conjugated bilirubin requires the action of bacteria and therefore occurs predominantly in the lower small intestine and colon. The bacteria, by stepwise enzymatic reductions, induce the formation of a series of colorless urobilinogens (Fig. 45-3) which react with Ehrlich's aldehyde reagent to produce red aldehyde complexes. Oxidation of the urobilinogens (i.e., *d*-urobilinogen, mesobilirubinogen, and stercobilinogen) leads to colored products, the urobilins. On mixing with Schlesinger's solution (zinc acetate in alcohol), zinc complexes are produced which have an intense green fluorescence. Because these compounds all have the same physiologic significance and are measured

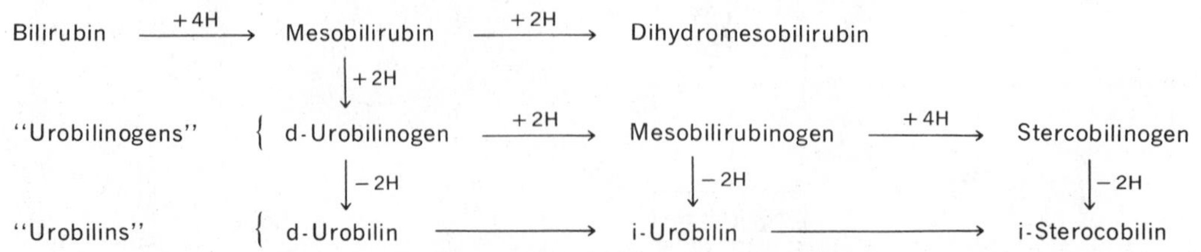

Bilirubin $\xrightarrow{+4H}$ Mesobilirubin $\xrightarrow{+2H}$ Dihydromesobilirubin

$\downarrow +2H$

"Urobilinogens" $\{$ *d*-Urobilinogen $\xrightarrow{+2H}$ Mesobilirubinogen $\xrightarrow{+4H}$ Stercobilinogen

$\downarrow -2H$ $\downarrow -2H$ $\downarrow -2H$

"Urobilins" $\{$ *d*-Urobilin $\longrightarrow$ *i*-Urobilin $\longrightarrow$ *i*-Stercobilin

Fig. 45-3. Chemical steps in the reduction of bilirubin to the urobilinogens and urobilins.

together in most quantitative analyses, they usually are referred to collectively as "urobilinogens" irrespective of their chemical structure or whether they are found in urine, feces, or bile.

In contrast to conjugated bilirubin, urobilinogen is readily reabsorbed from the small intestine into the portal blood and is thus subject to an enterohepatic circulation. Some urobilinogen is reexcreted by the liver into the bile, while the rest is excreted in the urine in an amount usually not exceeding 4 mg daily. When the hepatic excretory mechanism is impaired (e.g., in hepatocellular disease) or the production of bilirubin is greatly increased (e.g., in hemolytic anemia), the urinary urobilinogen may increase significantly.

The normal output of fecal urobilinogen ranges from 50 to 280 mg per day. Under conditions of decreased excretion of conjugated bilirubin into the intestine (e.g., liver disease, bile duct obstruction) or suppression of intestinal flora by antibiotics, fecal output will be diminished. In hemolytic anemia, both urinary and fecal urobilinogen excretion is greatly increased.

In a normal individual with a blood volume of 5 liters and a hemoglobin concentration of 15 mg per 100 ml, the total circulating hemoglobin is 750 Gm. Because approximately 1/120 of the red cells are destroyed daily, 6.3 Gm hemoglobin is released for catabolism. Assuming a quantitative conversion of heme to bilirubin and to urobilinogen, the expected daily output of urobilinogen would be approximately 250 mg plus the additional 15 to 30 mg which would be derived from the other sources described above (i.e., ineffective erythropoiesis, nonhemoglobin heme precursors). Often, however, the amount excreted is considerably less, and it appears likely that there are alternative pathways for hemoglobin degradation that may not involve the formation of bilirubin.

RENAL EXCRETION OF BILIRUBIN. Normally the urine is found to contain no bilirubin by the methods usually employed, although traces may be detectable by sensitive spectrophotometric procedures. In unconjugated hyperbilirubinemia, there is no bilirubinuria, whereas when conjugated hyperbilirubinemia occurs, bilirubin readily appears in the urine. The renal excretion of conjugated bilirubin may serve as a regulatory mechanism and probably accounts for the fact that in complete biliary tract obstruction the serum conjugated bilirubin level usually plateaus between 30 and 40 mg per 100 ml.

Although the renal mechanism for bilirubin excretion is not completely understood, most studies indicate that excretion of conjugated bilirubin occurs by glomerular filtration. The fraction of plasma conjugated bilirubin so filtered appears to be that small fraction which normally is both dialyzable and ultrafilterable. In the urine the dialyzable fraction seems to be associated with a non-albumin plasma constituent of low molecular weight, possibly a peptide. Bile salts enhance the dialyzability of conjugated bilirubin, and it has been suggested that in obstructive jaundice, the elevated plasma bile salts may be responsible for an increased renal excretion of conjugated bilirubin. Unconjugated bilirubin is neither dialyzable nor ultrafilterable, which probably accounts for its failure to be excreted in the urine.

Chemical Tests for Bile Pigments

The most widely employed chemical test for the bile pigments in serum is the van den Bergh reaction. In this reaction the bilirubin pigments are diazotized with sulfanilic acid, with initial conversion of the bilirubin from a tetrapyrrole to dipyrrole. The diazotized dipyrrole molecules are chromogenic and are measured colorimetrically. The van den Bergh reaction can be used to distinguish between unconjugated and conjugated bilirubin because of the different solubility properties of the pigments. When the reaction is carried out in an *aqueous* medium, the water-soluble conjugated bilirubin reacts to give the so-called *direct* van den Bergh reaction. When the reaction is carried out in *methanol*, both conjugated and unconjugated pigments react, giving a measure of the *total* bilirubin level. The total minus the direct-reacting bilirubin give the *indirect* value, which is a measure of the unconjugated bilirubin level.

In the direct van den Bergh reaction, the most accurate measurements are those carried out at 1 min. If the reaction is allowed to proceed longer, a small amount of the unconjugated pigment may begin to react in the aqueous medium. As a result, in a patient with unconjugated hyperbilirubinemia, if the direct reaction is carried out at 30 min, it may give falsely high values and conversely falsely low values for the indirect-reacting bilirubin. This serves to emphasize that the direct and indirect van den Bergh reactions represent *approximations* (not absolute measurements) of the conjugated and unconjugated pigments. A summary of the key differences in the properties and reactions of the bilirubin pigments is presented in Table 45-1.

Table 45-1. COMPARISON OF THE MAJOR DIFFERENCES BETWEEN CONJUGATED AND UNCONJUGATED BILIRUBIN

Properties and reactions	Bilirubin	
	Unconjugated	Conjugated (diglucuronide)
Water solubility............	0	+
Affinity for lipids...........	+	0
Bound to serum albumin....	+++	+
Renal excretion............	0	+
Van den Bergh reaction.....	Indirect (total minus direct)	Direct
Lipid membrane permeability	+	0

The measurement of bilirubin in the urine may be carried out by the Harrison spot test or with Ictotest[1] tablets. The foam test is also a simple and qualitatively valid procedure. When normal urine is vigorously shaken in a test tube, the foam is absolutely white. In a urine

[1] Trademark of Ames Company, Ames, Iowa.

containing bilirubin, the foam will be yellow. This difference may be subtle and may become evident only by comparing a normal urine and one containing bilirubin side by side. Urine urobilinogen may be estimated by the semiquantitative Watson-Schwartz test or the qualitative Diamond test. Fecal measurement must be quantitative to be of value.

Except for concentrated urine, the most common cause of a deep yellow-brown or dark urine is bilirubinuria. However, other mechanisms and diseases associated with a dark urine need to be considered. These include yellow urine due to drugs (e.g., azosulfapyridine); red urine due to porphyria, hemoglobinuria, myoglobinuria, or drugs (e.g., pyridium); and dark-brown or black urine due to homogentisic acid (in ochronosis) or melanin (with melanoma).

Classification of Jaundice

Once the presence of hyperbilirubinemia has been established, the underlying disorder should be approached by considering both (1) the *pathophysiology*

Table 45-2. CLASSIFICATION OF JAUNDICE BASED ON UNDERLYING DERANGEMENT IN BILIRUBIN METABOLISM

I. Predominantly *unconjugated* hyperbilirubinemia
  A. Overproduction
    1. Hemolysis (intra- and extravascular)
    2. Ineffective erythropoiesis
  B. Impaired hepatic uptake
    1. Gilbert's syndrome (constitutional hepatic dysfunction; familial nonhemolytic jaundice)
    2. Posthepatitis hyperbilirubinemia (probably the same as Gilbert's syndrome)
    3. Drugs
  C. Impaired glucuronide conjugation (decreased activity of glucuronyl transferase)
    1. Absence or deficiency (congenital) of transferase (Crigler-Najjar syndrome)
    2. "Immaturity" of transferase (neonatal jaundice)
    3. Deficiency or inhibition of transferase
      a. Inhibition by drugs (e.g., pregnanediol, chloramphenicol)
      b. Hepatocellular disease (e.g., hepatitis, cirrhosis)*
II. Predominantly *conjugated* hyperbilirubinemia
  A. Impaired hepatic excretion (functional or intrahepatic obstruction)
    1. Probable familial or hereditary disorders
      a. Dubin-Johnson, Rotor syndrome
      b. Recurrent (benign) intrahepatic cholestasis
      c. Cholestatic jaundice of pregnancy
    2. Acquired disorders
      a. Hepatitis and cirrhosis
      b. Drug-induced cholestasis
  B. Extrahepatic biliary obstruction (mechanical obstruction, e.g., stones, strictures, tumor of bile duct)

* In hepatitis and cirrhosis, there is usually interference in the three major steps of bilirubin metabolism—uptake, conjugation, excretion. However, excretion appears to be the rate-limiting step and is usually impaired to the greatest extent.

of bilirubin metabolism and (2) the underlying *disease* leading to this deranged metabolism. In many diseases there may be a derangement in *more than one* physiologic parameter of bilirubin metabolism. In any event, it is important first to determine whether the hyperbilirubinemia is predominantly of the *unconjugated* or *conjugated* type. A patient is considered to have predominantly unconjugated hyperbilirubinemia when less than *15 or 20 percent* of the total serum bilirubin is direct-reacting (with the 1-min van den Bergh reaction). A urine determination is important, because *bilirubinuria is found only in conjugated hyperbilirubinemia*.

In Table 45-2, jaundice is classified according to the fundamental derangements in bilirubin metabolism. These consist of (1) overproduction, (2) decreased hepatic uptake, (3) decreased hepatic conjugation, (4) decreased hepatic excretion (due to both intrahepatic and extrahepatic factors). Jaundice may also be described on the basis of the pathogenetic mechanism or disease process leading to deranged bilirubin function, and the terms *hemolytic jaundice, hepatocellular jaundice,* or *obstructive jaundice* are often used. In the past, *retention jaundice* has been used to refer to hemolytic jaundice and *regurgitation jaundice* for cases of hepatocellular or obstructive jaundice.

While these classifications and terms are helpful, in any one patient more than a single derangement or more than one "type" of jaundice may be present. For example, a patient with cirrhosis may have not only impaired liver cell function (and hence hepatocellular jaundice) but also hemolysis. Furthermore, obstructive jaundice may be due either to *mechanical* obstruction of the biliary radicles or to *functional* factors causing impaired hepatic excretion of bilirubin into bile.

In the present chapter a brief description of the major types of jaundice is given. A more detailed discussion of the individual disease entities is found in Chap. 325.

JAUNDICE WITH PREDOMINANTLY UNCONJUGATED BILIRUBIN IN THE SERUM. Overproduction of Bilirubin. When an increased amount of hemoglobin is released from red cells into either the bloodstream or tissues, the net result is an increased production of bilirubin. Hyperbilirubinemia will occur when the liver's capacity to remove the pigment from the circulation is exceeded. In most cases of hemolysis, the total serum bilirubin ranges from 3 to 5 mg per 100 ml. A slight increase in direct-reacting pigment may also be found, but this usually constitutes less than 15 percent of the total serum bilirubin. This finding is probably analogous to the slight elevations of direct-reacting bilirubin which occur when normal subjects are infused with unconjugated bilirubin. Both instances appear to be a reflection of the fact that the rate-limiting step in hepatic bilirubin metabolism is excretion and that when the liver's excretory capacity is exceeded, some reentry of conjugated bilirubin into the bloodstream occurs. For a detailed description of the causes of increased bilirubin production see Chap. 325.

Impaired Hepatic Uptake of Bilirubin. The entry of bilirubin into the liver cell entails a dissociation of the pigment from albumin, but the exact uptake mechanism has not been elucidated. In Gilbert's syndrome and some cases of drug-induced jaundice there may be a derangement in this phase of bilirubin metabolism (see Chap. 325).

Impaired Glucuronide Conjugation. Both acquired and genetic derangements in hepatic glucuronyl transferase occur. In the fetus and at birth, glucuronyl transferase activity is low and appears to account for the *neonatal jaundice* which normally is found between the second and the fifth day of life. There is also a rare congenital disorder associated with a deficiency of glucuronyl transferase, the Crigler-Najjar syndrome, in which marked unconjugated hyperbilirubinemia occurs.

Acquired defects in bilirubin glucuronyl transferase activity may be produced by drugs (i.e., enzyme inhibition) or intrinsic liver disease. However, in most diseases leading to liver cell damage, the excretory capacity of the liver is impaired to a greater extent than is the conjugating capacity. Therefore in most hepatocellular diseases, the hyperbilirubinemia is predominantly of the conjugated type (see Chap. 325).

JAUNDICE WITH PREDOMINANTLY CONJUGATED BILIRUBIN IN THE SERUM. Impaired Excretion of Bilirubin by the Liver. The impaired excretion of bilirubin into the biliary canaliculi, whether due to functional or mechanical factors, results in predominantly conjugated hyperbilirubinemia and bilirubinuria. The presence of *bilirubin in the urine is evidence of conjugated hyperbilirubinemia* and a most important point in the differential diagnosis of jaundice. Such findings are identical to those occurring in complete obstruction of the bile duct, emphasizing that *jaundice due to hepatocellular disease can seldom be differentiated from that due to extrahepatic obstruction solely on the basis of changes in bile pigment metabolism.* Indeed there are often instances when the two conditions are not distinguishable by any biochemical criteria and liver biopsy or laporotomy are needed for the definitive diagnosis.

When there is interference in the excretion of conjugated bilirubin into bile, by what mechanism does this pigment enter the systemic circulation? Several postulates have been proposed for this "reentry": (1) rupture of the bile canaliculi secondary to the necrosis of the hepatic cells that constitute their walls; (2) occlusion of the canaliculi by inspissated bile or their compression by swollen hepatic cells; (3) obstruction of the terminal intrahepatic bile ducts (i.e., cholangioles) by inflammatory cells; (4) altered hepatic cell permeability; and (5) that as a result of impaired excretion, conjugated bilirubin accumulates in the hepatocytes and secondarily diffuses into the plasma. Although some of these postulates are speculative, it is likely that several of these mechanisms occur. For example, occasionally in histologic sections escape of bile through rents in the walls of canaliculi in areas of necrosis is apparent. Also microscopic studies of the liver of rats injected with fluorescent dyes have shown reflux of bile from canaliculi into sinusoids. However, no anatomic damage needs to be in-

voked, because when unconjugated bilirubin is infused into normal subjects at high rates, conjugated hyperbilirubinemia occurs; this is explained most logically by passive diffusion.

Extrahepatic Biliary Obstruction. Complete obstruction of the extrahepatic bile ducts leads to jaundice with predominantly conjugated hyperbilirubinemia, bilirubinuria, and clay-colored stools. Failure of bile to reach the intestine results in virtual disappearance of urobilinogen from the stool and urine. The concentration of bilirubin rises progressively but then usually plateaus at a level of 30 to 40 mg per 100 ml. To some extent this plateau may be explained by a balance between renal excretion and diversion of bilirubin to other metabolites. In hepatocellular jaundice, such a plateau tends not to occur, and bilirubin levels in excess of 50 mg per 100 ml may be found.

Partial obstruction of the extrahepatic bile ducts can also give rise to jaundice but only if the intrabiliary pressure is increased, because the excretion of bilirubin does not diminish until the intraductile pressure approaches the maximal secretory pressure of approximately 250 mm bile. Jaundice may occur at much lower pressures if the obstruction is complicated by infection of the ducts or hepatocellular injury. Therefore, jaundice, bilirubinuria, and clay-colored stools are inconstant findings in partial biliary obstruction, and the amount of urobilinogen in urine and stool varies with the degree of occlusion.

The functional reserve of the liver is so great that *occlusion of the intrahepatic bile ducts* does not give rise to jaundice unless the drainage of bile from a large segment of the parenchyma is interrupted. Either of the two major hepatic ducts or a large number of secondary radicles may be occluded without production of jaundice. In experimental animals the ducts draining at least 75 percent of the parenchyma must be occluded before jaundice appears.

ADDITONAL POINTS OF TERMINOLOGY. In clinical practice, a patient may be described as having *obstructive,* or *cholestatic,* jaundice. By this is meant that clinically, and especially biochemically, there is little to suggest hepatocellular damage and that the main features point to interference with, or obstruction in, the flow of bile. Typically one would expect such a patient to show (1) predominantly conjugated hyperbilirubinemia, (2) minimal biochemical changes of parenchymal liver damage, and (3) a moderate to a marked increase in the serum alkaline phosphatase (usually greater than 15 Bodansky units). As emphasized in Chaps. 323 and 324, an *elevated alkaline phosphatase level* in a patient with jaundice or liver disease in the absence of other disorders such as bone disease is most suggestive of interference with bile secretion or an infiltrative process in the liver. However, often *laboratory tests alone may not permit differentiation of intrahepatic from extrahepatic cholestasis.*

Some clinicians reserve the term obstructive jaundice to those situations where anatomic obstruction can be demonstrated and use the term cholestatic jaundice for cases of parenchymal liver disease in which the obstructive phase is on a functional basis. Nevertheless, because these two entities frequently are indistinguishable by clinical and biochemical criteria, the terms obstructive jaundice and cholestatic jaundice are often used interchangeably.

Hepatocellular disorders in which jaundice associated with an obstructive, or cholestatic, phase occurs include (1) occasional cases of viral hepatitis, (2) drug reactions, especially those due to chlorpromazine and methyltestosterone, (3) some cases of alcoholic hepatitis or alcohol-induced fatty liver, (4) jaundice in the last trimester of pregnancy, (5) most cases of Dubin-Johnson or Rotor syndrome, (6) the disorder of so-called "benign recurrent intrahepatic cholestasis," and (7) certain types of postoperative jaundice. These and other conditions are discussed in Chaps. 325 and 326.

In summary, all forms of conjugated hyperbilirubinemia have by definition an impairment in the excretion of bilirubin into bile. In most cases of parenchymal liver disease, there is a broad derangement in the biochemical tests of liver function. However, when the major detectable alterations of liver function tests include (1) conjugated hyperbilirubinemia and (2) moderate to marked elevation of the serum alkaline phosphatase level, the terms obstructive or cholestatic jaundice may be appropriate. Additional procedures, including operation, are often needed to determine the cause of the cholestasis.

HEPATOMEGALY

In the supine position, the major part of the liver lies beneath the right rib cage. In some normal individuals the liver edge may be palpable 1 to 2 cm below the right costal margin, and a palpable liver edge by itself does not necessarily indicate hepatomegaly. In evaluating liver size by physical examination, two factors other than ability to palpate the liver edge need to be considered, namely, (1) the location of the upper border of liver dullness by percussion and (2) the body habitus.

Normally, the upper edge of liver dullness on the right side in the midclavicular line is at the level of the fifth rib, but in those of asthenic habitus it may be lower. The liver edge normally descends 1 to 3 cm with deep inspiration. In hypersthenic subjects, the liver may extend over to the left abdominal wall, with the lower edge high and not palpable; in hyposthenic subjects with a very acute costal angle the liver may lie in the right half of the abdomen, the edge being palpable by as much as 6 to 8 cm below the right costal margin lateral to the right rectus abdominis muscle. Thus, palpability does not necessarily imply hepatomegaly.

In determining liver enlargement by palpation, one should be certain that the liver is being palpated rather than other right upper quadrant masses such as gallbladder, colonic neoplasm, or fecal material in the colon. Liver enlargement is often confirmed by radiologic studies including hepatic scintiscans, celiac axis angiography, and splenic venography.

In many cases of generalized liver enlargement, the left lobe will be felt in the epigastrium between the xiphoid and umbilicus. The liver should be carefully palpated during deep inspiration to determine whether the edge is tender, regular or irregular, firm or soft, rounded and thickened or sharp. The edge is tender and often rounded with hepatic inflammation as in hepatitis or when the liver is acutely congested as in cardiac decompensation. Pulsation of the liver may be found with tricuspid valvular incompetence. A carcinomatous liver may be rocklike in hardness; the cirrhotic liver is very firm in consistency. The largest livers are often found with carcinoma (primary or metastatic), marked fatty infiltration, congestive cardiac decompensation, Hodgkin's disease, and amyloidosis. Rapid decrease in liver size may occur with improvement of congestive failure or mobilization of fat from the liver.

In a patient with hepatomegaly, auscultation is sometimes helpful. A friction rub may be audible (and palpable) in the right upper quadrant, usually due to a recent biopsy, tumor, or perihepatitis. In portal hypertension a venous hum may be audible between the umbilicus and the xiphoid. An arterial murmur or bruit over the liver may indicate tumor, usually hepatoma.

Table 45-3. CAUSES OF A PALPABLE LIVER AND HEPATOMEGALY

I. Palpable liver without hepatomegaly
   A. Right diaphragm displaced downward (e.g., emphysema, asthma)
   B. Subdiaphragmatic lesion (e.g., abcess)
   C. Aberrant lobe of liver (Riedel's lobe)
   D. Extremely thin or relaxed abdominal muscles
   E. Occasionally present in normal individuals

II. Hepatomegaly
   A. Vascular congestion (e.g., congestive heart failure, hepatic vein thrombosis)
   B. Bile duct obstruction (e.g., lesion in common duct leading to hepatomegaly and subsequently biliary cirrhosis)
   C. Infiltrative disorders
      1. Bone marrow and reticuloendothelial cells
         a. Extramedullary hematopoiesis
         b. Leukemia
         c. Lymphoma
      2. Fat
         a. Fatty liver (e.g., secondary to alcohol or toxins)
         b. Gaucher's disease and some other lipidoses
      3. Carbohydrate (especially glycogen; seen in some patients with diabetes, especially after insulin excess)
      4. Amyloid
      5. Iron (hemochromatosis and hemosiderosis)
      6. Granuloma (tuberculosis, sarcoid)
   D. Inflammatory disorders
      1. Hepatitis—due to drugs or infectious agents
      2. Cirrhosis—except in late stages when prolonged scarring may lead to a *small,* shrunken liver
   E. Tumor—primary or metastatic
   F. Cysts—polycystic disease, congenital hepatic fibrosis

Some of the causes of a palpable liver and hepatomegaly are given in Table 45-3.

REFERENCES

Castell, D. O., K. D. O'Brien, H. Muench, and T. C. Chalmers: Estimation of Liver Size by Percussion in Normal Individuals, Ann. Int. Med., 70:1183, 1969.

Gartner, L. M., and I. M. Arias: Formation, Transport and Excretion of Bilirubin, New Engl. J. Med., 280:1339, 1969.

Lester, R., and R. Schmid: Bilirubin Metabolism, New Engl. J. Med., 270:779, 1964.

Lester, R., and R. F. Troxler: Recent Advances in Bile Pigment Metabolism, Gastroenterology 56:143, 1969.

Sherlock, S.: Jaundice, Chap. 10, in "Diseases of the Liver," 4th ed. Philadelphia, F. A. Davis Company, 1968.

With, T. K.: "Bile Pigments: Chemical, Biological and Clinical Aspects," New York, Academic Press, Inc., 1968.

46 ABDOMINAL SWELLING AND ASCITES

*Kurt J. Isselbacher and
Robert M. Glickman*

Abdominal swelling or distension is a common problem in clinical medicine and may be the initial manifestation of a systemic disease or of otherwise unsuspected abdominal disease. *Subjective* abdominal enlargement, often described as a sensation of fullness or bloating, is usually transient and is often related to a functional gastrointestinal disorder when it is not accompanied by objective physical findings of increased abdominal girth or local swelling. *Obesity* and lumbar lordosis, which may be associated with prominence of the abdomen, may usually be distinguished from true increases in the volume of the peritoneal cavity by history and careful physical examination.

CLINICAL HISTORY. The development of abdominal swelling may be described by the patient as a progressive increase in belt or clothing size, the appearance of abdominal or inguinal hernias, or the development of a localized swelling. Often, considerable abdominal enlargement has gone unnoticed for weeks or months either because of coexistent obesity or because the ascites formation has been insidious, without pain or localizing symptoms. Progressive abdominal distension may be associated with a sensation of "pulling" or "stretching" of the flanks or groins and vague low back pain. Localized *pain* usually results from involvement of an abdominal organ (e.g., a passively congested liver, large spleen, or colonic tumor). Pain is uncommon in cirrhosis with ascites and when it is present, pancreatitis, hepatoma, or peritonitis should be considered. Tense ascites or abdominal tumors may produce increased intraabdominal pressure, resulting in *indigestion* and *heartburn* due to gastroesophageal reflux or *dyspnea, orthopnea,* and *tachypnea* from elevation of the diaphragm. A coexistent pleural effusion, more commonly on the right, presumably due to leakage of ascitic fluid through lymphatic channels in the diaphragm, may also contribute to respiratory embarrassment. The patient with diffuse abdominal swelling should be questioned about increased alcoholic intake, a prior episode of jaundice or hematuria, a change in bowel habits, or a past history of rheumatic heart disease. Such historic information may provide the needed clues to suspect an occult cirrhosis, a colonic tumor with peritoneal seeding, congestive heart failure, or nephrosis.

PHYSICAL EXAMINATION. *Inspection* of the abdomen is an important but often cursorily performed aspect of the abdominal examination. By noting the abdominal contour one may be able to distinguish localized from generalized swelling. The tensely distended abdomen with tightly stretched skin, bulging flanks, and everted umbilicus is characteristic of ascites. A prominent abdominal venous pattern with the direction of flow away from the umbilicus often is a reflection of portal hypertension; the presence of venous collaterals with flow from the lower abdomen toward the umbilicus suggests obstruction of the inferior vena cava; flow downward toward the umbilicus suggests superior vena cava obstruction. "Doming" of the abdomen with visible ridges from underlying bowel loops is usually due to intestinal obstruction or distension. An epigastric mass, with evident peristalsis proceeding from left to right, usually indicates underlying pyloric obstruction. A liver with metastatic deposits may be visible as a nodular right upper quadrant mass moving with respiration.

Auscultation may reveal the high pitched, rushing sounds of early intestinal obstruction or a succussion sound due to increased fluid and gas in a dilated hollow viscus. Careful auscultation over an enlarged liver occasionally reveals the harsh bruit of a vascular tumor, especially a hepatoma, or the leathery friction rub of a surface nodule. A venous hum at the umbilicus may signify portal hypertension and an increased collateral blood flow around the liver. A fluid wave and flank dullness which shifts with change in position of the patient are important signs that indicate the presence of peritoneal fluid. In the obese patient, small amounts of fluid may be difficult to demonstrate; on occasion the fluid may be detected by abdominal percussion with the patient on his hands and knees. Doubt about the presence of peritoneal fluid may be resolved by careful paracentesis with a small gauge (#19 or 20) needle. Careful percussion should serve to distinguish generalized abdominal enlargement from localized swelling due to an enlarged uterus, ovarian cyst, or distended bladder. Percussion can also outline an abnormally small or large liver. Loss of normal liver dullness may result from massive hepatic necrosis; it may also be a clue to free gas in the peritoneal cavity, as from perforation of a hollow viscus.

Palpation is often difficult with massive ascites, and ballottement of overlying fluid may be the only method of palpating the liver or spleen. A slightly enlarged spleen in association with ascites may be the only evidence of an occult cirrhosis. When there is evidence of portal hypertension, the finding of a soft liver suggests that obstruction to portal flow is extrahepatic; the presence of a firm liver suggests cirrhosis as the likely cause of the portal hypertension. A very hard or nodular liver is a clue that the liver is infiltrated with tumor, and when accompanied by ascites, it suggests that the latter is due to peritoneal seeding. A pulsatile liver and ascites may be found in tricuspid insufficiency.

An attempt should be made to determine whether a mass is solid or cystic, smooth or irregular, and whether it moves with respiration. The liver, spleen, and gallbladder should descend with respiration unless they are fixed by adhesions or extension of tumor beyond the organ. A fixed mass not descending with respiration may indicate that it is retroperitoneal. Tenderness, especially if localized, may indicate an inflammatory process such as an abscess; it may also be due to stretching of the visceral peritoneum or tumor necrosis. Rectal and pelvic examinations are mandatory; they may reveal otherwise undetected masses due to tumor or infection.

Radiographic and laboratory examinations are essential for confirming or extending the impressions gained on physical examination. Upright and recumbent films of the abdomen may demonstrate the dilated loops of bowel with fluid levels characteristic of intestinal obstruction or the diffuse abdominal haziness and loss of psoas margins suggestive of ascites. A plain film of the abdomen may reveal the distended colon of otherwise unsuspected ulcerative colitis and give valuable information as to the size of the liver and spleen. An irregular and elevated right diaphragm may be a clue to the presence of a liver abscess or hepatoma. Studies of the gastrointestinal tract with barium or other contrast media are usually necessary in the search for a primary tumor.

ASCITES

In most cases the clinical and laboratory evaluation of the patient with ascites is sufficient to reveal the cause of the fluid accumulation. Often the ascites is a component or complication of cirrhosis, congestive heart failure, nephrosis, or disseminated carcinomatosis. However, even when the cause of ascites seems obvious, it is often important to determine whether another separate or related disease process has supervened. For example, when the compensated cirrhotic with minimal ascites

Table 46-1. ASCITIC FLUID CHARACTERISTICS IN VARIOUS DISEASE STATES

Condition	Gross appearance	Specific gravity	Protein, Gm/100 ml	Cell count		Other tests
				Red blood cells, >10,000/mm³	White blood cells/mm³	
Cirrhosis	Straw colored or bile stained	<1.016(95%)*	<2.5(95%)*	1%	<250(90%)*; predominantly endothelial	
Neoplasm	Straw colored, hemorrhagic, mucinous, or chylous	Variable, >1.016(45%)	>2.5(75%)	20%	>1,000(50%); variable cell types	Cytology, cell block, peritoneal biopsy
Tuberculous peritonitis	Clear, turbid, hemorrhagic, chylous	Variable, >1.016(50%)	>2.5(50%)	7%	>1,000(70%); usually >70% lymphocytes	Peritoneal biopsy, stain and culture for acid fast bacilli
Pyogenic peritonitis	Turbid or purulent	If purulent, >1.016	If purulent, >2.5	Unusual	Predominantly polymorphonuclear leukocytes	+ gram stain, culture
Congestive heart failure	Straw colored	Variable, <1.016(60%)	Variable 1.5–5.3	10%	<1,000(90%); usually mesothelial, mononuclear	
Nephrosis	Straw colored or chylous	<1.016	<2.5(100%)	Unusual	<250; mesothelial, mononuclear	If chylous, ether extraction, Sudan staining
Pancreatitis, pseudocyst	Turbid, hemorrhagic, or chylous	Variable, often >1.016	Variable, often >2.5	Variable, may be bloodstained	Variable	Increased amylase in ascitic fluid and serum

* Since the conditions of fluid examination and patient selection were not identical in each series, the percentage figures (in the parentheses) should be taken as an indication of the order of magnitude rather than the precise incidence of any abnormal finding.
SOURCE: The data in this table are a composite of several large series (Refs. 1–5).

develops progressive ascites that is increasingly difficult to control with sodium restriction or diuretics, the obvious temptation is to attribute the worsening of the clinical picture to progressive liver disease. However, an occult hepatoma, portal vein thrombosis, or even tuberculosis may be responsible for the decompensation. The disappointingly low success of diagnosing tuberculous peritonitis or hepatoma in the patient with cirrhosis and ascites reflects the too-low index of suspicion for the development of such superimposed conditions. Similarly, the patient with congestive heart failure may develop ascites from a disseminated carcinoma with peritoneal seeding. The thorough evaluation of each patient with ascites, even in the presence of an "obvious" cause, will help avoid these errors.

Diagnostic paracentesis (50 to 100 ml) should be part of the routine evaluation of the patient with ascites. The fluid should be examined for its gross appearance, protein content, cell count, and differential, as well as gram and acid-fast stains and culture. Cytologic and cell-block examination may disclose an otherwise unsuspected carcinoma. Table 46-1 illustrates some of the features of ascitic fluid typically found in various disease states. In some disorders, such as cirrhosis, the fluid has the characteristics of a transudate (less than 2.5 Gm protein per 100 ml and a specific gravity less than 1.016); in others, such as peritonitis, the features are those of an exudate. Although there is variability of the ascitic fluid in any given disease state, some features are sufficiently characteristic to suggest certain diagnositic possibilities. For example, bloodstained fluid with more than 2.5 Gm protein per 100 ml is unusual in uncomplicated cirrhosis but consistent with tuberculous peritonitis or neoplasm. Cloudy fluid with a predominance of polymorphonuclear cells and positive gram stain is characteristic of bacterial peritonitis; if the cells are mostly lymphocytes, tuberculosis should be suspected. The complete examination of each fluid is most important for occasionally only *one* finding may be abnormal. For example, if the fluid is a typical transudate but contains more than 250 white blood cells per cu mm, the finding should be recognized as atypical for cirrhosis, nephrosis, or congestive heart failure and should warrant a search for tumor or infection.

Chylous ascites refers to a turbid, milky, or creamy peritoneal fluid due to the presence of thoracic or intestinal lymph. Such a fluid shows Sudan-staining fat globules microscopically, and an increased triglyceride content by chemical examination. A turbid fluid due to leukocytes or tumor cells may be confused with chylous fluid, and it is often helpful to carry out alkalinization and ether extraction of the specimen. Alkali will tend to dissolve cellular proteins and thereby reduce turbidity; ether extraction will lead to clearing if the turbidity of the fluid is due to lipid. Chylous ascites is most often the result of lymphatic obstruction from trauma, tumor, tuberculosis, filariasis (see Chap. 249), or congenital abnormalities. It may also be seen in the nephrotic syndrome.

The etiology of ascites may remain uncertain even after the usual diagnostic procedures have been carried out. Under those circumstances a high proportion of the cases will be due to (1) cirrhosis of the liver, (2) carcinomatosis with peritoneal involvement, (3) tuberculous peritonitis, or (4) hepatoma. In all of these conditions pronounced weight loss, wasting, anorexia, and fever may be found, and hepatomegaly, splenomegaly, and deranged liver function tests may be present. Procedures such as peritoneal biopsy, peritoneoscopy, liver biopsy, splenoportography, or laparotomy may be necessary to provide the diagnosis. Other less common causes of ascites include constrictive pericarditis, hepatic vein obstruction, myxedema and benign tumors of the ovary, particularly fibroma (Meigs's syndrome, with ascites and hydrothorax). The physiologic and metabolic factors involved in the production of ascites are described in Chap. 328.

REFERENCES

Berner, C. et al.: Diagnostic Probabilities in Patients with Conspicuous Ascites, Arch. Intern. Med., 113:687, 1964.

Burack, W. R., and R. M. Hollister: Tuberculous Peritonitis, Am. J. Med., 28:510, 1960.

Hyman, S., F. Villa, and F. Steigmann: Mimetic Aspects of Ascites, J.A.M.A., 183:651, 1963.

Levine, H.: Needle Biopsy of the Peritoneum in Exudative Ascites, Arch. Intern. Med., 120:542, 1967.

Paddock, F. K.: Diagnostic Significance of Serous Fluids in Disease, New Engl. J. Med., 223:1010, 1940.

Rovelstad, R. A. et al.: Helpful Laboratory Procedures in the Differential Diagnosis of Ascites, Proc. Mayo Clin., 34:565, 1959.

Sherlock, S.: Diseases of the Liver and Biliary System, 4th ed., Philadelphia, F. A. Davis Company, 1968.

Section 6

Alterations in Body Weight

47 LOFF OF WEIGHT
47 LOSS OF WEIGHT
George W. Thorn

Weight loss as elicited by history or detected by physical examination constitutes a cardinal manifestation of disease or disordered bodily function, unless an otherwise normal individual has imposed on himself caloric restriction in an effort to reduce.

Under normal circumstances decreased food intake or total starvation initiates a constellation of metabolic changes designed to reduce energy expenditure and heat loss. Chief among these are reduced basal metabolic rate, lowered body temperature, restricted physical activity, and reduced peripheral blood flow (vasoconstriction). By these means the body attempts to maintain the function of vital organs such as the heart, brain, kidneys, liver, and lungs. These mechanisms are seriously impaired when complications such as fever, vomiting, diarrhea, and dehydration supervene.

Anorexia is a frequent accompaniment of chronic as well as acute disease processes. In the absence of specific abnormalities of gastrointestinal function, loss of appetite may be due to toxic products liberated by microorganisms, by breakdown products of tumor tissue, or by retention of metabolic end products as occurs in late-stage renal and hepatic disease. Hypoosmolarity of the body fluid compartment and increased cell water content may give rise to centrally mediated nausea and vomiting through its effect on specific hypothalamic centers. Thus, a patient with malignant hypertension may experience nausea as a consequence of hypertensive cerebrovascular changes in the absence of uremia or, later, as a result of retention of nitrogenous products with progressive renal failure.

In evaluating the implication of weight loss several considerations deserve special attention.

1. Is the patient's history concerning the magnitude and duration of weight loss reliable? Can it be documented by comparison with prior measurements or confirmed by physical examination?

2. Has there been a notable change in appetite or food intake?

3. Has there been evidence of disordered gastrointestinal function with a change in bowel habits?

4. Has there been evidence of polyuria, particularly nocturia?

The determination of the *magnitude of weight loss* is not always easy. Some patients follow changes in weight regularly on bathroom scales or weighing machines, or they have serial physical examinations. Other patients may be quite vague or uninformed regarding actual changes in weight. Questions regarding a change in waist measurement or collar, suit, dress, or shoe size may provide helpful clues. Physical examination should then confirm this, with its opportunity to detect adipose tissue loss and the presence or absence of edema or dehydration. Special consideration should be given to the valuation of overall weight loss in the presence of edema, as the actual tissue loss in such patients will, of course, greatly exceed the apparent decrease in total body weight.

Weight loss with anorexia and decreased food intake occurs in such a diversified range of acute and chronic diseases as not to be particularly helpful in differential diagnosis. The magnitude of weight loss may reflect either the *seriousness* or the *duration* of the underlying disorder. Thought should be given to the diagnosis of psychologic difficulties such as depression and anorexia nervosa, to generalized endocrine and metabolic disorders such as pituitary-adrenal insufficiency and hyperparathyroidism, and to hepatic and renal disease, as well as to chronic infection, neoplasm, and drug intoxication. Weight loss without a significant change in food consumption would suggest hypermetabolic states, such as thyrotoxicosis and anxiety or gastrointestinal hypermotility.

Of course, particular attention will be given in the history to any abnormality in gastrointestinal function as a cause of weight loss. Here again, one is concerned with *decreased food intake* such as might occur in partial intestinal obstruction; *decreased absorption,* which suggests pancreatic or hepatic disease, spruelike syndromes, regional enteritis, or severe food allergies; or *increased loss of food* and *fluids* through vomiting, diarrhea, or draining fistulas. Disorders of gastrointestinal function accompany systemic disorders so frequently that the physician must always maintain a high index of suspicion that what appears to be primarily a disorder of gastrointestinal function may actually reflect deep-seated infection, tumor, or renal, hepatic, cardiac, or pulmonary disease. On the other hand, *specific gastrointestinal disorders* may complicate systemic disease; thus, the patient with nausea, vomiting, and renal azotemia may have an associated peptic ulcer.

The presence of polyuria, and particularly nocturia, in association with anorexia and weight loss suggests diabetes mellitus, diabetes insipidus, chronic renal disease, and disorders giving rise to *hypercalcemia* or *hypokalemia.*

Physicians should encourage patients to weigh regularly and to maintain a lifelong record of changes in body weight, since alterations in weight so frequently mirror abnormalities in bodily function. Loss of weight may be the first indication of serious organic disease or psychologic disorder, the detection and significance of which may be measurably enhanced by carefully recorded changes in body weight.

48   GAIN IN WEIGHT

George W. Thorn

General Considerations

A gradual increase in weight may be secondary to either an accumulation of fluid (edema) or adipose tissue (obesity). However, weight gain in excess of 1 to 2 lb per day will almost invariably indicate excess fluid retention. Excess fluid accumulation or edema (see Chap. 34) should suggest underlying renal, cardiac, or hepatic insufficiency. Hypoalbuminemia usually suggests renal disease, but it may reflect nutritional deficiency or liver disease secondary to small-bowel pathology or inadequate protein intake. Occasionally, primary retention of water with hyponatremia will result from inappropriate antidiuretic hormone secretion. Excess salt intake, licorice, and drugs such as sex hormones, adrenal steroids, diphenylhydantoin, and reserpine may contribute to salt and water retention. The presence of edema and weight gain may mask a significant loss of body tissue. This is best exemplified by the cardiac or hypertensive patient who, following a brisk diuresis, becomes aware for the first time of the extent of body wasting.

Obese patients can retain rather large quantities of extracellular fluid without necessarily exhibiting edema. From a practical point of view, it should be assumed that a markedly obese patient has sequestered a significant volume of extracellular fluid. This can often be demonstrated by administering a diuretic agent; and, of course, this is the approach utilized by many "lose-weight-fast" schemes. Some appreciation of the salt- and water-retaining capacity of obese patients, or of patients with incipient edema, may be obtained by weighing the patient in the morning and again at night. It is not unusual for an obese individual, or a preedematous patient, to gain 4 to 8 lb during the day, particularly if he is up and about.

CYCLIC EDEMA

Idiopathic edema or "periodic swelling" constitutes a physicopsychologic syndrome which uniquely affects adult females. Physiologic mechanisms capable of modifying salt and water metabolism within the body include the antidiuretic hormone (ADH), aldosterone, "third factor," histamine, and the kinins. The intimate relationship between the secretory control of these humoral agents and the central nervous system is well established. Emotional and psychologic factors are readily capable of initiating the release of these agents and, hence, of inducing cyclical retention of fluid and electrolytes. Why the syndrome is limited to the female is still conjectural; however, cyclical retention of fluid and electrolytes occurs physiologically following menstruation and during pregnancy and lactation. Thus, a well-developed pathway is available in the female for psychologic disturbances to manifest themselves pathophysiologically. An understanding of the psychologic and emotional factors is basic to successful therapy. Judicious use of diuretic agents can correct the physiologic abnormalities in most instances; however, the basic symptomatology will not be relieved by diuresis alone. Of particular importance is the avoidance of excessive diuretic therapy with its predilection for inducing potassium and magnesium deficiency, which, in turn, may perpetuate the symptoms of weakness, fatigue, and irritability. The complex nature of this syndrome necessitates astute, thoughtful, and continued medical care.

OBESITY

Obesity occurs when the caloric intake exceeds the energy requirements of the body both for physical activity and for growth. As a result there is an accumulation of fat, which is stored in the adipose tissue. The excessive tissue may be distributed generally over the body, or it may be localized. The factors controlling the location of the fat are not all known, but pituitary, thyroid, and sex hormones play an important role. Obesity is a serious and common disease in those countries in which a combination of generous food supplies and sedentary occupations readily permit the assimilation of more food than is necessary. The excessive deposition of fat is associated with an increased incidence of degenerative diseases such as atherosclerosis, diabetes, and arthritis; indeed, the only common cause of death that does not strike earlier in the obese than in the lean population is suicide! The ill effects of obesity can be prevented and, to some extent, repaired by weight reduction. The treatment of obesity is one of the most serious problems in preventive medicine in the United States today.

Etiology

Under normal circumstances there is a very exact adjustment of food intake to body requirements. Unfortunately, in certain individuals this adjustment is deranged, and intake becomes excessive. The cause of the derangement is not understood, but several important factors are well known.

HYPOTHALAMIC RELATIONSHIPS. It has been known for years that lesions involving the hypothalamus may lead to obesity. Lesions in the ventromedial nucleus of the hypothalamus induce hyperphagia and obesity, whereas lesions in the lateral hypothalamic area lead to a cessation of eating. On the basis of these findings a dual mechanism has been postulated for the regulation of food intake: a "satiety" center in the ventromedial nucleus and a "feeding" center in the lateral hypothalamic area. Studies on gold thioglucose-treated mice have demonstrated fiber connections between these two centers.

Additional experimental studies relate to the theories of "glucostat," "lipostat," and "aminostat" control of food intake. It has been suggested that animals on a free feeding schedule begin to eat when a blood factor falls below a critical level and not because a "hunger" factor increases above a threshold level. Further support of a glucoreceptor is suggested by studies in which phlorhizin, a known inhibitor of glucose uptake in a wide variety of tissues, was tested for a similar effect on hypothalamic glucoreceptors in rats. The infusion of a minute quantity of phlorhizin into the lateral cerebral ventricle resulted in marked hyperphagia and gain in weight, whereas a similar quantity injected intraperitoneally had no demonstrable effect. These data suggest that cerebral glucoreceptors do indeed exist and are involved in the regulation of food intake.

Thus it appears that the basic cause of obesity is a derangement of the appetite-controlling mechanisms, permitting the assimilation of more food than is needed. It has been claimed that certain individuals are more efficient than others in their ability to digest, absorb, and utilize food and therefore that they become obese at lower caloric intakes than might be expected. Extensive balance studies on such patients have never substantiated this explanation; at equivalent levels of physical activity and basal metabolism, there seems to be little variation in the required caloric intake.

DECREASED BASAL METABOLIC RATE AND ACTIVITY. A decrease in basal metabolic rate and activity accompanies hypothyroidism and anterior pituitary deficiency. Some decrease in activity with an increased tendency for obesity occurs with primary gonadal failure—particularly in the female. Advancing age is characteristically attended by a progressive lowering of basal metabolic rate and, of course, in most instances with an appreciable reduction in physical activity. Disorders or diseases which limit ambulation, such as cardiac or pulmonary failure or bone and joint disease, will also predispose to weight gain unless caloric intake is appropriately readjusted.

HYPOTHYROIDISM. Hypothyroidism may be suspected in an individual who has developed intolerance to cold, whose skin has become dry and coarse, and whose reflexes are prolonged (see Chap. 89). Weight gain associated with a more severe degree of hypothyroidism or myxedema may be due to edema, ascites, and pleural effusion. Gordon and his colleagues believe that some obese patients have a specific block in the utilization of fatty acids by peripheral tissues that can be removed by administration of triiodothyronine.

ANTERIOR PITUITARY DEFICIENCY. Anterior pituitary deficiency of a mild degree such as that described by

Sheehan (see Chap. 87) may be accompanied by weight gain. This syndrome is most frequently observed in women after childbirth. Hypopituitarism in males as well as in females may be caused by a chromophobe adenoma or cyst of the pituitary. In such instances, a clue to the disorder may present as a result of local pressure, i.e., headaches or visual disturbances. In all types of mild hypopituitarism, signs of target gland deficiency, i.e., thyroid, adrenal, or gonadal, should be looked for. Gonadal deficiency is characterized by impotence in men and oligomenorrhea or amenorrhea in women. The signs of secondary hypothyroidism do not differ appreciably from those of primary, except that thyroid enlargement is not expected. Secondary adrenal cortical insufficiency is *not* associated with hyperpigmentation and rarely presents as severe mineral (aldosterone) deficiency. Hypoglycemic manifestations are frequently observed.

A decrease in physical activity secondary to a change in occupation, to traumatic injury, to heart disease, or to other incapacitating illnesses will result in increased adiposity if normal caloric intake is maintained. This is of no pathologic significance other than the generally unfavorable effect of obesity on weight-bearing joints.

Increased Caloric Intake

Excessive food intake secondary to *organic* disease occurs most commonly in response to a hypoglycemic stimulus. When hypoglycemic symptoms occur under fasting conditions, hyperinsulinism and pancreatic tumor should be considered. When hypoglycemic manifestations occur 3 to 5 hr after a meal, the paradoxic hypoglycemic response of early diabetes mellitus may be suspected (see Chap. 96). In the latter case it is thought that the prolonged elaboration of insulin represents an inappropriate response to the initial postprandial hyperglycemia. Occasionally, traumatic lesions of the brain, localized encephalitis, and brain tumors appear to modify the satiety centers in the hypothalamus, with resulting stimulation of appetite over and above caloric needs.

FAMILIAL AND CULTURAL EATING HABITS. These are firmly implanted at an early age. In groups in which great emphasis is placed on food, there is a tendency to overeat. Sometimes the cultural pattern equates success with obesity (witness the common caricature of the obese banker) and encourages the ambitious person to achieve a comfortable corpulence. Moreover, when activity patterns change, eating habits may remain constant, so that the man who has previously been physically active may fail to reduce his caloric intake when he suddenly changes to a sedentary occupation. This tendency may be reinforced by the gradual decline of metabolic rate and of muscle activity, which ordinarily accompanies aging.

PSYCHOLOGICAL FACTORS. Certain individuals may have increased appetite for psychologic reasons. Under these circumstances food is used as a substitute for the satisfaction they should obtain from other emotional sources. In this respect, they are similar to alcoholics, who use alcohol as a substitute for such normal sources of satisfaction as their friends, their families, or success in their work.

Psychologists do raise the question, however, whether all individuals describe the changes as "hunger" and eat when the biologic machinery is activated. There is increasing evidence which suggests that major individual differences exist in the extent to which physiologic changes are associated with the desire to eat. Hilde Bruch, a psychoanalyst, has observed that her obese patients literally do not know when they are physiologically hungry. She has suggested that during childhood these individuals were not taught to distinguish between hunger and such states as fear, anger, and anxiety. If this is so, these individuals may be labeling any state of arousal as hunger. That the obese may not know when they are physiologically hungry has been substantiated by Stunkard (1961), who studied the relation of hunger sensation to gastric motility in obese and nonobese individuals. The results indicated that nonobese and obese do not differ in degree of gastric motility and that when the stomach was not contracting, the reports of both groups were similar. However, there was a significant difference between the two groups in the reported coincidence of hunger and gastric motility, i.e., nonobese, 21 percent; obese, 47 percent. Schachter, on the basis of these and many other experiments, suggests that the obese may be relatively insensitive to variations in the correlation of food deprivation but highly sensitive to environmental, food-related cues, and that this may provide one key to understanding the notorious long-run ineffectiveness of virtually all attempts to treat obesity. The use of the anorexigenic drugs such as amphetamine or of bulk-producing nonnutritive substances such as methylcellulose is based on the premise that such agents dampen the intensity of the physiologic symptoms of food deprivation. Probably they do, but these symptoms appear to have little to do with whether or not a fat person eats. Restricted, low-calorie diets should be effective just so long as the obese dieter is able to blind himself to food-relevant cues or so long as he exists in a world barren of such cues.

Therapeutic Considerations

CENTRAL DEPRESSION OF APPETITE. Unfortunately, there is no pharmacologic agent available at this time which acts primarily by depressing the "appetite center." This type of depression is seen regularly in disease states such as hepatitis and uremia and as a toxic manifestation of drugs such as digitalis.

SUBSTANCES WHICH DEPRESS APPETITE BY INDUCING A SENSE OF WELL-BEING. Amphetamine and its derivatives are the prototype of this group of substances. These agents are commonly referred to as "anorexigenic" or "anorectic." There is no evidence to show, however, that their action results from a depression of the appetite center. As a result of stimulation, or a "lift," the patient's drive toward overeating may be significantly modified and as far as he is concerned, the overall effect of the drug is "appetite-depressing." Obviously, drugs which create such a state of euphoria may lead to habituation in certain individuals.

Amphetamine and its derivatives have been shown to depress food intake in man as well as in experimental animals. Patients experience a sense of well-being after the ingestion of these drugs, and it is thought that the reduction in appetite is a consequence of distraction. At least in the hyperphagia which follows frontal lobotomy, no depression of appetite is induced by amphetamine or its congeners.

At present there is a large number of derivatives of amphetamine sulfate (Benzedrine) and closely related compounds available for clinical use, for example, dextroamphetamine sulfate (Dexedrine), levoamphetamine sulfate and phosphate, levoamphetamine alginate (Levonor), methamphetamine hydrochloride (Amphedroxyn, Desoxyephedrine, Desoxyn, Desyphed, Dexoval, Desoxyfed, Drinalfa, Efroxine, Methedrine, Norodin, Semoxydrine, Syndrox), phenylpropanolamine (Propadrine), phenmetrazine (Preludin), phenyl-*tert*-butylamine resin (Ionamin), and diethylpropion (Tenuate and Tepanil).

Although it is unfortunate that manufacturers avoid or disclaim the relationship of many of these substances with amphetamine, the fact is that the structural formulas differ very little (Fig. 48-1). The dextro form of amphetamine differs in its pharmacologic action from the levo form in that the cephalotropic effect is enhanced and the cardiovascular actions are less intense. However, this fact suggests that the dextro form might be expected to cause anxiety, restlessness or sleeplessness at the same dosage level. The action of methamphetamine differs little from dextroamphetamine except in its somewhat enhanced cardiovascular effects. Since phenylpropanolamine may be sold without prescription, it has become a common ingredient of many weight-reducing tablets. Although if given in adequate dosage phenylpropanolamine may reduce appetite, in the usual dosage found in most weight-reducing tablets (25 mg or less) it is no more effective than a placebo. Phenmetrazine, although subjected to intensive study and claimed to be quite different, is a typical congener of amphetamine with the effectiveness of dextroamphetamine. Phenyl-*tert*-butylamine resin is advertised as not being an amphetamine drug, although it clearly belongs to the amphetamine series, as a study of its structural formula indicates (Fig. 48-1).

The usual dosage of amphetamine sulfate (Benzedrine) or dextroamphetamine sulfate (Dexedrine) is 5 mg given 30 to 60 min before meals. It may be necessary in some patients to omit the evening dose because of increased nervousness or sleeplessness. Long-acting preparations which can be given in a single dose of 10 to 15 mg each morning are also useful. These substances may prove helpful for some patients during the early weeks of restricted food intake.

Although serious reactions are rarely encountered with amphetamine and its congeners, the physician

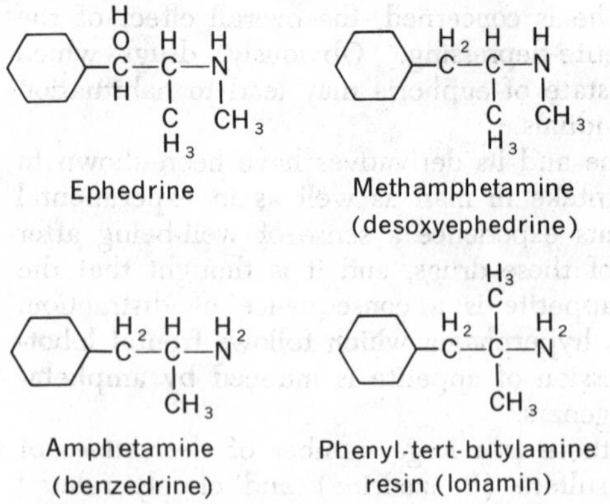

Fig. 48-1. Amphetamine and congeners.

must be alert to the sympathomimetic effect of these agents in causing a rise in blood pressure, increased cardiac rate and work, and the possible development of cardiac arrhythmias. Since tolerance to these drugs develops relatively rapidly, their usefulness is short-lived unless the dosage is increased. The possibility that continued use of amphetamine-like substances such as Menocil may induce pulmonary hypertension has been reported.

BULK PRODUCERS. Repeated attempts have been made to satiate the appetite by means of bulk of low caloric content. Leafy vegetables such as cabbage, spinach, and lettuce are helpful in many patients and constitute an important element in most low-calorie diets. Addition of calorie-free bulk to the diet does not automatically displace calorie-containing food unless specific restrictions are prescribed. Because of the significant reduction in fat content of the diet, patients may experience constipation; for this reason bulk producers such as dioctyl sodium sulfosuccinate (Colace), 50 to 200 mg daily, and agar may be required. However, as suggested earlier, neither appetite depressor nor bulk producer will be particularly effective in a weight-reduction program in an individual who does not normally equate increased gastric contractions with the sensation of hunger or a full intestinal tract with satiety.

METABOLIC STIMULANTS INCLUDING HORMONES. Repeated efforts have been made to discover a nontoxic agent which would maintain a normal metabolic level in the face of weight loss. Dinitrophenol has had the widest use. The consensus today is that its undesirable toxic side reactions make its use unjustified.

In most instances, substances of this type are being employed by physicians or patients in an attempt to induce *weight loss without caloric restriction*. To do this, it is obviously necessary to raise basal metabolic level *above normal*. There is no known substance which can be used safely to increase metabolic level above normal for prolonged periods of time without danger of toxicity.

In the mind of the lay public, "hormones" are the most important cause of obesity and are hopefully considered to be its cure. The well-informed physician recognizes to what a small extent disturbances in hormone secre-

tion are primarily responsible for obesity and how futile most types of hormone therapy are as cures of obesity.

No pituitary preparation now available is useful in weight reduction. Male and female gonadal hormones and adrenal cortical hormones have no place in therapy unless specific deficiency of these hormones exists. Thyroid therapy has received wide application and merits special discussion.

Thyroid therapy is effective substitution therapy in patients with hypothyroidism. Unfortunately, however, the number of patients with hypothyroidism among the obese is relatively small. Thyroid therapy has a definite

Table 48-1. DESIRABLE WEIGHTS FOR MEN AND WOMEN, ACCORDING TO HEIGHT AND FRAME, AGES TWENTY-FIVE AND OVER, WEIGHT IN INDOOR CLOTHING

Height (in shoes)	Small frame	Medium frame	Large frame
Men			
	lb.	lb.	lb.
5 ft. 2 in.	112–120	118–129	126–141
5 ft. 3 in.	115–123	121–133	129–144
5 ft. 4 in.	118–126	124–136	132–148
5 ft. 5 in.	121–129	127–139	135–152
5 ft. 6 in.	124–133	130–143	138–156
5 ft. 7 in.	128–137	134–147	142–161
5 ft. 8 in.	132–141	138–152	147–166
5 ft. 9 in.	136–145	142–156	151–170
5 ft. 10 in.	140–150	146–160	155–174
5 ft. 11 in.	144–154	150–165	159–179
6 ft.	148–158	154–170	164–184
6 ft. 1 in.	152–162	158–175	168–189
6 ft. 2 in.	156–167	162–180	173–194
6 ft. 3 in.	160–171	167–185	178–199
6 ft. 4 in.	164–175	172–190	182–204
Women			
4 ft. 10 in.	92–98	96–107	104–119
4 ft. 11 in.	94–101	98–110	106–122
5 ft.	96–104	101–113	109–125
5 ft. 1 in.	99–107	104–116	112–128
5 ft. 2 in.	102–110	107–119	115–131
5 ft. 3 in.	105–113	110–122	118–134
5 ft. 4 in.	108–116	113–126	121–138
5 ft. 5 in.	111–119	116–130	125–142
5 ft. 6 in.	114–123	120–135	129–146
5 ft. 7 in.	118–127	124–139	133–150
5 ft. 8 in.	122–131	128–143	137–154
5 ft. 9 in.	126–135	132–147	141–158
5 ft. 10 in.	130–140	136–151	145–163
5 ft. 11 in.	134–144	140–155	149–168
6 ft.	138–148	144–159	153–173

and sustained effect on the metabolism of the hypothyroid case. Complete thyroid deficiency may require 0.2 Gm thyroid (USP) daily; 0.1 Gm thyroid (USP) daily should be adequate for milder cases. A given dose of thyroid will produce a predictable rise in basal metabolic rate in a patient with hypothyroidism, and a daily dose of thyroid will maintain the increase in basal metabolic rate indefinitely. It appears that certain patients with obesity can tolerate rather large doses of thyroid without undue symptoms but with sufficient increase in metabolic rate to assist appreciably in their weight-reduction program.

MAINTENANCE OF IDEAL WEIGHT

Patients should understand thoroughly when they undertake a reduction diet that, in all probability, some degree of dietary restriction or discretion will be necessary permanently after ideal weight (Table 48-1) has been attained. The degree of dietary restriction is best attained by establishing the custom of weighing in each morning and adjusting the day's intake of food to the changes in body weight. It may be necessary at this time for the physician to review the comparative caloric content of certain foods which may have been withheld during the diet regimen. It is usually desirable to discuss in detail the calories contained in alcoholic beverages.

Once ideal weight has been attained, a patient should be encouraged to visit his physician every 3 to 6 months for examination and advice. The continued interest of the physician is of paramount importance to the health and happiness of his patient.

REFERENCES

Arees, Edward A., and Jean Mayer: Anatomical Connections between Medial and Lateral Regions of the Hypothalamus Concerned with Food Intake, Science, 157:1574, 1967.

Davis, John, Robert Gallagher, and Robert Ladove: Food Intake Controlled by a Blood Factor, Science, 156:1247, 1967.

Glick, Zvi, and Jean Mayer: Hyperphagia Caused by Cerebral Ventricular Infusion of Phloridzin, Nature, 219:1374, 1968.

Gordon, E. S., E. M. Goldberg, J. J. Brandabur, J. B. Gee, and J. Rankin: Abnormal Energy Metabolism in Obesity, Trans. Assoc. Am. Physicians, 75:118, 1962.

Kekwick, A.: On Adiposity, Brit. Med. J., p. 407, Aug. 6, 1960.

Modell, Walter: Status and Prospect of Drugs for Overeating, J.A.M.A., 173:1131, 1960.

Rose, H. E., and Jean Mayer: Activity, Calorie Intake, Fat Storage, and the Energy Balance of Infants, Pediatrics, 41(1):18, 1968.

Rosenberg, B. A.: A Double-blind Study of Diethylpropion in Obesity, Am. J. Med. Sci., 242:201, 1961.

Schachter, Stanley: Obesity and Eating, Science, 161:751, 1968.

Section 7

Alterations in Genitourinary Function

49 DYSURIA, INCONTINENCE, AND ENURESIS

Bernard Lytton and Franklin H. Epstein

NORMAL MICTURITION

An appreciation of the anatomic and physiologic mechanisms involved in micturition is necessary for a rational approach to the difficult problems of urinary incontinence, enuresis, and other disorders of bladder function.

The bladder muscle, or detrusor, consists of interlacing bundles of muscle that arch around the internal vesicle orifice and continue down into the urethra, where they are interspersed with elastic fibers. The normal tone of these fibers constitutes the internal vesical sphincter. The bladder receives a dual nerve supply from the autonomic system. The sacral parasympathetic, via the pelvic nerves (second, third, and fourth sacral segments), provide the preganglionic fibers to ganglia of the pelvic plexus and bladder wall and these give off postganglionic fibers to the detrusor and posterior urethra. The sympathetic preganglionic fibers (last two dorsal and first two lumbar segments) pass via the lumbar splanchnic nerves to synapse in the paraaortic and pelvic plexuses. The postganglionic fibers supply mainly the blood vessels in the bladder wall and the muscles around the bladder neck. The sympathetic innervation has little influence on bladder function but is probably concerned with closure of the bladder neck at the time of ejaculation; removal of the first lumbar sympathetic ganglion bilaterally is usually followed by infertility due to retrograde ejaculation.

Afferent fibers subserving the sensations of distension and pain pass mainly via the pelvic nerves to the sacral segments of the spinal cord. Some of these fibers are said to pass via the sympathetic nerves, but it is probable that any residual sensation of bladder filling after section of the sacral nerves is due to stretching of the peritoneum overlying the bladder. The internal pudendal nerve supplies motor and sensory fibers from the second, third, and fourth sacral segments to the external sphincter muscle, urethra, and perineal muscles. The action of the detrusor and sphincter muscles is, therefore, both reflex and voluntary.

Micturition is normally a voluntary act. As the bladder fills, a fairly constant low pressure is maintained by the detrusor muscle as it accommodates itself to the increasing volume. When it reaches its capacity, 400 to 500 ml in the normal adult, the stretch receptors transmit impulses via the pelvic afferent nerves, the sacral reflex center, and the fasciculus gracilis to the brain. This initiates the desire to void. Impulses from the brain, which arise in the paracentral lobules, are transmitted via descending fibers just anterior to the corticospinal tracts to the micturition center in the sacral part of the cord and to the pelvic and pudendal nerves to initiate the act of micturition. An initial relaxation of the perineal muscles is followed by detrusor contraction. At this point there is usually tensing of the abdominal muscles and diaphragm, although the resultant rise in abdominal pressure alone cannot initiate voiding normally and is not essential for evacuation. The intravesical pressure rises rapidly to 18 to 43 cm water, the external sphincter relaxes, the bladder neck opens, and voiding occurs with a pressure of 50 to 150 cm. The opening of the bladder neck is the result of active detrusor contraction which widens the bladder neck and shortens the urethra, thus lowering the resistance of the bladder outlet. Closure of the bladder neck occurs with relaxation of the detrusor, which allows a return of the musculature to its normal position, assisted by recoil of the elastic fibers. It is apparent that any interference with detrusor activity or the anatomy of the bladder neck will interfere with the opening mechanism and lead to incomplete emptying or some loss of continence.

DYSURIA

Dysuria denotes difficulty or pain associated with voiding. It may result from a wide variety of pathologic conditions. Frequency, hesitancy, burning, urgency, and strangury (slow, painful emission of urine) are often referred to under the more general term dysuria.

Urgency occurs as a result of trigonal or posterior urethral irritation by inflammation, stones, or tumor. The urge may be so great and so sudden that a patient voids involuntarily.

Frequency of urination in bladder lesions occurs when there is a decreased capacity or when there is pain on distension. In acute inflammatory lesions, edema and loss of elasticity of the bladder wall cause pain or an urge to void when only a small quantity of urine is present in the bladder. Chronic inflammatory lesions such as tuberculosis produce a similar effect and may proceed to permanently diminished capacity from scarring. It can be an early presenting symptom of primary malignant disease of the bladder, due to induration of the bladder wall as a result of tumor invasion and reactionary inflammatory changes.

The majority of conditions producing these symptoms arise in the bladder and urethra. Diseases of other organs and systems may, by invading, compressing, or distorting the lower urinary tract, produce dysuria. Diseases of the nervous system, which involve the nerve supply of the bladder either centrally, as in tabes and multiple sclerosis, or peripherally, as in diabetic neuropathy, produce difficulty in voiding and sometimes pain when secondary infection occurs as a result of residual urine.

The evaluation of a patient with dysuria must include a complete history and physical examination, as well as a complete urologic examination, together with relevant radiologic or laboratory investigations suggested by abnormalities detected during the clinical examination.

Inflammatory lesions in the bladder, prostate, or urethra are the commonest causes of dysuria. These include acute bacterial infections, chronic prostatitis in men, and chronic posterior urethrotrigonitis in women. A great deal may be learned from examination of the external urinary meatus. About 20 percent of children with urinary complaints have a degree of *meatal stenosis*, which may interfere sufficiently with bladder function to result in recurrent infection. Meatal stenosis is often an important etiologic factor in the development and persistence of chronic prostatitis in men and chronic posterior urethritis and trigonitis in women. Unsuspected meatal stenosis of long standing may cause trabeculation of the bladder and other manifestations of obstructive uropathy. Meatotomy results in relief or considerable improvement.

A *urethral caruncle* may present with symptoms of severe discomfort on voiding. This tumor appears as a small cherry-red polyp which may or may not protrude from the posterior lip of the external meatus and which is generally exquisitely tender on palpation. The latter feature helps to distinguish it from the commoner condition of urethral prolapse. Simple excision is the treatment of choice.

Benign overgrowth of the prostate commonly causes frequency, hesitancy, straining, slowing of the stream, and dribbling in older men. Pain is uncommon unless the condition is complicated by infection or vesical calculi.

Frequency and urgency may follow *radiation injury* to the bladder. In the acute phase this may be amenable to treatment with bladder sedatives containing antispasmodics and with small doses of steroids to combat the inflammatory reaction. The persistence of symptoms or bleeding may necessitate surgical intervention. Malignant tumors of the bowel, diverticulitis, regional ileitis, or ulcerative colitis may involve the bladder and cause frequency. Fistula formation results in severe dysuria and pneumaturia.

Chronic interstitial cystitis, a nonspecific chronic inflammatory disease of the bladder wall manifested by small, shallow, stellate hemorrhagic ulcers (Hunner's ulcers), gives rise to a fairly characteristic pattern of dysuria. The patients, generally middle-aged women, complain of persistent frequency and often have severe suprapubic pain, relieved by voiding. There may be an associated terminal hematuria. The urine contains a few white cells and red cells but no bacteria. It may ultimately lead to fibrosis with permanent contraction of the bladder.

Frequency without discomfort on voiding may be associated with a normal bladder capacity and be due to the *polyuria* of diabetes, to conditions causing hypercalcemia or hypokalemia, to the *nocturia* of early congestive heart failure, or to loss of renal parenchyma resulting in the passage of a large volume of poorly concentrated urine. The absence of nocturia in a patient with frequency suggests that it may be of psychogenic origin or due to a polyp or irritative lesion in the posterior urethra that is relieved by recumbency. A patient who complains of recent onset of nocturia should be carefully questioned about diuretic medication.

It should always be remembered that frequency may be due to *paradoxic incontinence* (see below).

Expanding lesions in the pelvis that reduce bladder capacity by external compression are exemplified by pregnancy. Large ovarian cysts and uterine fibroids will have a similar effect. A retroverted gravid uterus or pelvic tumor which becomes impacted may result in stretching and elongation of the urethra and produce difficulty in voiding and finally complete retention.

INCONTINENCE

Paradoxic Incontinence

True incontinence must be distinguished from *paradoxic incontinence,* which accompanies bladder distension caused by mechanical or functional obstruction and is characterized by small, frequent, involuntary "overflow" voidings. In obstruction the increased power of the detrusor suffices to overcome the block, but as soon as a small quantity of urine is voided, the intravesical pressure drops and a large residual remains. Ultimately, the detrusor becomes paralyzed by overdistension, and complete retention ensues. With neurogenic bladders, small voidings occur, sometimes involuntarily, as the pressure of accumulating urine overcomes the resistance at the bladder outlet. With loss of a small amount of urine, pressure falls, and a large residual is left. Often both neurologic and obstructive elements contribute, as in elderly arteriosclerotic patients with prostatic enlargement or in cases of diabetic neuropathy with secondary bladder neck obstruction. The bladder in these patients is flaccid and painless, which may make it difficult to palpate, and the residual urine predisposes to infection. This response of the bladder muscle to obstruction might be compared to that seen in striated and heart muscle under an increased work load.

Congenital Incontinence

Congenital incontinence may be due to a congenital malformation, such as vesical extrophy, epispadias, ectopic ureteral openings in the female, patent urachus, and defects in the spinal cord which occur in association with spina bifida and meningomyelocele. The results of primary reconstructive surgery in cases of extrophy are cosmetically satisfactory, but sphincter control is rarely achieved. Furthermore, most of these children have persistent vesicoureteral reflux, which can lead to progressive renal damage. The majority therefore are still best treated by some form of urinary diversion with excision of the bladder. The results of urethral and bladder neck reconstruction in simple epispadias are better. The management of neurogenic bladder disturbance is principally directed toward the establishment of timed reflex voiding, diminution of residual urine, and control of infection. When there is progressive renal impairment, due to persistent infection and vesicoureteral reflux, urinary diversion is necessary.

Acquired Incontinence

This may occur as a result of disease or injury to the spinal cord, as in tabes, multiple sclerosis, and tumor, or following fractures of the spine. The disruption of the neural mechanism results in complete relaxation of the detrusor and bladder outlet or in ineffective contractions of the detrusor, so there may be overflow incontinence with a flaccid bladder or uncontrollable frequent voidings with a spastic bladder. Cerebral vascular accidents or senility can produce loss of voluntary control of bladder and bowel function.

Parturition can stretch and disrupt the structures of the pelvic floor and perineum to the point that urethral resistance, while sufficient to maintain continence at rest, gives way under stress of straining or coughing, and incontinence ensues. This is probably the result of loss of the urethrovesical angle and urethral shortening. This type of incontinence usually occurs in the erect posture.

Stress incontinence may be aggravated by urgency due to an associated urethrotrigonitis. Relief of the trigonitis will sometimes result in satisfactory control. Treatment is directed toward repair of the pelvic floor, restoration of urethral length, and correction of the urethrovesical angle.

Surgical or radiation injuries can produce vesicovaginal and ureterovaginal fistulas. Incontinence in ureterovaginal fistula occurs with normal voiding, but in vesicovaginal fistula there is generally no normal evacuation of the bladder. The treatment of these fistulas is always surgical. Temporary urinary diversion will enable spontaneous closure to occur in some instances. Excision and reconstruction of a damaged ureter is the treatment of choice, but implantation of the ureter into the bowel or substitution with an ileal segment may be necessary. Nephrectomy is the simplest procedure in the elderly or debilitated patient or when there are serious technical difficulties, provided there is adequate function in the other kidney.

Injury to the sphincter mechanism can occur with pelvic fractures or after prostatic or bladder neck surgery in elderly patients. Gradual improvement may occur for up to a year after injury. Postsurgical incontinence may be controlled with a penile clamp, but this has the disadvantage of producing edema and occasionally ulceration of the penis. A condom catheter may lead to maceration of the penile skin and is often difficult to apply. An indwelling catheter invariably leads to problems of chronic infection. A variety of surgical procedures have been devised to improve control, by using some mechanical means to increase urethral resistance, and are only partially successful. Urinary diversion may become necessary in certain cases.

ENURESIS

Enuresis is generally understood to mean the unintentional voiding of urine, usually at night, when it is synonymously referred to as bedwetting. The term should be restricted to those children in whom there is an absence of any gross urologic abnormality.

Micturition in infancy is governed by a simple spinal reflex. Maturation of the nervous system and development of control over the simple reflexes by the higher centers occurs during the second year of life. By the age of thirty months, most children have voluntary control over rectal and urinary sphincters. The child who persistently wets the bed after the age of three, or who, after a period of control, begins to wet the bed again presents a clinical problem. Enuresis then, may be a delay in the development or a loss of bladder control. It may be affected by physical and psychologic factors. There appears to be no constant single cause.

It is estimated that 15 percent of boys and 10 percent of girls at the age of five are enuretic, but by the age of nine only 5 percent of all children remain bedwetters. The majority of children with simple enuresis are dry by the time they reach puberty. It is more common among children with similarly affected siblings and in children of parents in the lower income groups. This latter finding could be due to the later institution of toilet training.

It is important to distinguish incontinence due to organic urologic disease from enuresis early in the management of these patients. Diabetes mellitus or insipidus may occasionally present with enuresis. Renal disease due to glomerulo- or pyelonephritis or sickle-cell disease producing papillary necrosis may cause bedwetting as a result of the increased volumes of urine passed by these patients. A careful evaluation at the outset should exclude chronic retention with dribbling incontinence due to either bladder neck obstruction or neurologic disease. Patients with organic disease of the bladder are usually incontinent during the day as well as at night, although enuretics may also exhibit this. Those with organic disease often have constant dribbling of urine. Occasionally, however, serious degrees of bladder neck obstruction present with nocturnal enuresis as the only symptom. A congenital decrease in bladder capacity may in part be responsible for enuresis, and is often familial. The enuresis generally ceases as the child gets older and spends less time asleep. Occasionally, a patient with petit mal epilepsy may present with wetting. Urinalysis will reveal any unsuspected infection. Enuresis occurring in retarded

children or in those with serious psychiatric disturbances requires treatment directed to the management of their primary problem.

Contributory factors such as the child's general health, physical environment, and emotional state should be evaluated and the parents encouraged to adopt an understanding rather than a punitive attitude. Correction of minor urologic abnormalities such as meatal stenosis, balanitis, vulvovaginitis, posterior urethritis, and urethral valves will sometimes lead to relief, but this is perhaps attributable only to the dysuria following instrumentation or to the understanding interest shown by the physician. The administration of antiparasympathetic agents to reduce bladder activity, or amphetamines to lighten sleep, have been advocated, but the results are equivocal. Imipramine (Tofranil), a mood-elevating drug whose effect is reinforced by its anticholinergic and stimulant properties, has produced a favorable response in over half the children treated, but may require continuation of treatment for some time. The results of psychotherapy are unconvincing. Considerable success has been claimed for alarm systems which attempt to establish a conditioned reflex. The child is awakened when an electrical circuit is completed by wetting. This method seems to be worth a trial in older children who prove resistant to simpler therapy.

50 OLIGURIA, POLYURIA, AND NOCTURIA

Louis G. Welt

INTRODUCTION

The kidneys provide the main channel for the excretion of water and solutes, and the urine flow and composition is adjusted so as to maintain the internal environment of the body in a remarkably constant steady state. The volume and solute content of the urine in health may vary widely. It is largely dependent on the magnitude and characteristics of the fluid and food ingested and on the quantity of water lost from other routes such as perspiration and insensible water loss. There are many ways in which urine flow can be varied in both health and disease, and it appears essential to review briefly, and in a general fashion, the manner in which urine is formed so that the vicissitudes of life and the impact of disease on urine volume and osmolality may be better understood.

PHYSIOLOGIC CONSIDERATIONS

The final bladder urine represents the net effect of a host of reactions that begin with the formation of an almost protein-free ultrafiltrate of plasma in the glomeruli. The quantity of fluid filtered at the glomeruli per unit of time is the net effect of the difference in the chemical potential of the water of plasma and that of the ultrafiltrate as well as the surface area available for filtration. These factors apply to the filterable solutes as well. The volume of water excreted per unit of time is, then, the difference between the volume filtered and the volume reabsorbed. The quantity of solutes excreted per unit of time is the difference between that which is filtered and that which is reabsorbed or secreted by the renal tubules. Many things remain obscure about these mechanisms, but there is now a general concept around which a description may be presented and from which implications may be drawn with respect to the influence of a variety of circumstances and disease processes. We are indeed indebted to the brilliant micropuncture studies started by Richards and his group in Philadelphia, and continued more recently by Wirz, by Gottschalk and his colleagues, and now by many others.

The water filtered by the glomeruli is reabsorbed at several areas along the nephron by passive diffusion along osmotic gradients, which, in turn, are established by the active transport of solutes. The osmotic gradient is maximized in the medulla and papilla owing to the anatomic arrangement of the loops of Henle and their accompanying blood vessels, which permit the establishment of an ever-increasing osmolality as the papilla is approached. This latter mechanism is referred to as the *countercurrent multiplication system*.

The *initial* step in the reabsorption of water, and the step that represents the largest volume, occurs in the proximal convolution of the nephron. The active transport of solutes, which are primarily sodium, chloride, bicarbonate, and glucose, creates an osmotic gradient so that water follows immediately. In this fashion, approximately two-thirds to three-fourths of the filtered solutes and water are reabsorbed by the end of the proximal tubule. The characteristics of this fluid are altered considerably, not only in volume but in composition. However, it is still iso-osmotic with the parent filtrate.

Another phase in the reabsorption of water occurs in the more distal portions of the nephron, which include the loop of Henle, the distal convolution, and, lastly, the collecting ducts. Although the reabsorption at these levels is smaller in volume than that which occurs in the more proximal segment of the nephron, these latter mechanisms are responsible in one circumstance for the formation of a maximally concentrated urine, and in other circumstances for the formation of a dilute urine. There are, obviously, circumstances wherein the urine osmolality occupies positions intermediate between these polar extremes.

The formation of a *maximally concentrated* urine depends on the presence of antidiuretic hormone, which permits the distal convolution and collecting duct membranes to be completely permeable to water. The micropuncture data reveal that the fluid in the early part of the distal convolution is always hypotonic (whether or not there is maximal antidiuretic hormone activity) to plasma. Furthermore, water is lost between the end of the proximal convolution and the early distal convolution. This clearly implies that solutes have been transported in excess of water, and hence some part of the ascending limb is presumably impermeable to water in the presence or absence of the antidiuretic hormone.

In the presence of antidiuretic hormone activity, the fluid within the distal convolution becomes more concentrated. Where one distal convolution meets with another to form a collecting tubule, the fluid is invariably iso-osmotic (in the rodent) with the parent filtrate. As the fluid courses through the collecting duct (in the presence of antidiuretic hormone activity) and is exposed to a fluid with an ever-increasing osmolality, a passive movement of water causes the fluid within the collecting ducts to remain in osmotic equilibrium with the fluid in the interstitium; thus, it increases in concentration until it exits into the pelvis of the kidney and moves down into the bladder for excretion.

Allusion has been made to the mechanism whereby the fluid in the interstitium is rendered continuously more hyperosmotic from outer medulla to papillary tip. It is dependent upon the anatomic arrangement of the loops of Henle and their blood vessels and is achieved by the transport of sodium salts (in excess of water) from the ascending limb of the loop. This renders the fluid in the interstitium hyperosmotic to the fluid entering the descending limb of the loop of Henle. This difference in osmolality promotes a movement of water from the descending limb fluid; and, in addition, there is entry of solutes into this portion of the limb. The net result is an increase in the osmolality of the fluid in the descending limb. This same process is repeated over and over again, and the fluid in the limb and interstitium becomes more concentrated along its course. When the fluid reaches the ascending portion of the limb and solutes are transported out of the luminal fluid, this fluid and the interstitium become ever less concentrated and are, finally, made hypotonic by the time it reaches the early distal convolution.[1]

In this setting the fluid coursing through the collecting ducts is made more hyperosmotic. Since urea can presumably permeate the collecting ducts largely by passive diffusion, urea moves from the collecting system into the interstitium as water moves along the osmotic gradient. In this fashion, urea contributes significantly to the total solute concentration in the medullary and papillary interstitium and serves to counterbalance the concentration of urea within the collecting ducts.

In man, the maximal concentration of the final urine may be as high as 1,200 to 1,400 mOsm per kg water. This may be considerably higher in rodents, the experimental animals from which the data that permit this formulation have been obtained.

In contrast, in the "complete" absence of antidiuretic hormone, the fluid in the distal convolution is not only

---

[1] The antidiuretic hormone possibly serves to increase the rate of transport of solutes from the ascending limb in addition to its influence on the permeability of the distal tubular and collecting duct permeability.

hypotonic to plasma in the earliest portions but remains so and is excreted as bladder urine with the same or even lower osmolality. Data reveal that salt is transported from the distal convolutions and from the collecting ducts themselves. In the absence of antidiuretic hormone, this aids and abets formation of minimally concentrated urine.

In this fashion, one can visualize the manner in which a highly concentrated or a minimally concentrated urine can be formed. Varying amounts of antidiuretic hormone between none and maximal provide a graded response.

Furthermore, it must be pointed out that even in the two polar situations of maximal antidiuretic hormone activity, or none, the rate of excretion of solutes determines the volume and osmolality of urine. This is to state that a urine may have an osmolality approaching that of the plasma with no antidiuretic hormone activity in the face of a solute diuresis; in contrast, the urine volume may be large and the osmolality may approach that of plasma despite maximal antidiuretic hormone activity in the presence of a solute diuresis. The manner in which a solute diuresis influences the concentration and the volume of urine is not completely clear.

However, within the context of the discussion presented above, it is apparent that a good deal of the water removed from the initial volume of filtrate depends on the active transport of salt and other solutes from the luminal fluid. Even if a constant *percentage* of filtered salt were reabsorbed in the proximal tubule, an increased filtration *rate* would provide a larger volume of fluid to the descending limb of the loop of Henle. Furthermore, to the extent that limitations are placed on the transport of salt from the proximal tubule (owing to the presence in filtrate of a larger concentration of a poorly reabsorbable solute), less water will be reabsorbed. If less salt is transported out of the loop of Henle, or if the flow of fluid through the loop is hastened, the countercurrent multiplier system will operate less efficiently; hence, the maximal osmolality will not be achieved in the interstitium of the medulla and papilla. By the same token, if the reabsorption of solutes is diminished in the distal convolution (e.g., glucose is not reabsorbable at this site), less water will be reabsorbed and a greater volume will reach the collecting duct system. Hence, a large solute excretion will increase the volume and diminish the osmolality of the final urine despite maximal antidiuretic hormone activity.

In contrast, it will be recalled that the efficient transport of solutes prior to, in, and beyond the distal convoluted tubule, coupled with the relative impermeability to water of these latter structures in the absence of antidiuretic hormone, are responsible for the formation of minimally dilute urine. If reabsorption of solutes is less efficient, owing to the filtered load or to the presence of less readily reabsorbable solutes, it is clear that urine osmolality cannot reach minimally dilute levels. As the solute diuresis becomes more intense, urine osmolality will approach that of the plasma.

In summary, a small solute excretion in the absence of antidiuretic hormone would be anticipated to be accompanied by the most dilute urine, and in the presence of antidiuretic hormone, with the most maximally concentrated urine. Varying quantities of antidiuretic hormone will have obvious influences; and the character of the urine anticipated in the presence of maximal antidiuretic hormone activity or none will be modified by the quantity and character of the solute load destined for excretion.

PATHOLOGIC CONSIDERATIONS

Oliguria

DEHYDRATION. There are many causes for oliguria, and the commonest may well be simple dehydration. In the face of a diminished volume of body fluids (especially if the loss has been water in excess of salt to provide an osmotic as well as a volumetric stimulus for the secretion of antidiuretic hormone), one anticipates a diminished filtration rate and a reduced excretion of solutes owing to the influence of a plasma volume deficit on renal hemodynamics. The diminished rate of excretion of solutes accompanied by antidiuretic hormone activity should ensure a small volume of highly concentrated urine.

CONGESTIVE HEART FAILURE. Since the volume of the filtrate plays an important role in the rate of excretion of urine, any circumstance which causes a reduced glomerular filtration rate is likely to be associated with some diminution in the rate of flow of urine. The defective systolic emptying of the heart, which is a characteristic of congestive heart failure, is commonly associated with a reduced flow of blood to the kidney and with a reduced filtration rate. This becomes more and more intense as the failure becomes more profound. Furthermore, in congestive heart failure (see Chap. 34 for more details) the renal excretion of salt is diminished, and the combination is obviously likely to result in a small volume of urine. This may be a striking feature of heart failure.

CIRRHOSIS OF THE LIVER. Cirrhosis is frequently accompanied by diminished renal blood flow and filtration rate (despite a coexistent increase in cardiac output) and by a strikingly low urine flow. In cirrhosis of the liver, as in congestive heart failure, the renal tubular reabsorption of salt is presumably more efficient, and this contributes to a diminished urine volume.

ACUTE RENAL INSUFFICIENCY. A low urine volume is one of the cardinal manifestations of this condition. In acute glomerulonephritis (or disorders with the same basic pathology) this low volume is presumably almost entirely a consequence of the drastic reduction in filtration rate. In acute tubular necrosis there is almost certainly a reduced filtration rate, but other factors as well may contribute to the striking oliguria. It is quite possible that in this latter disorder, the necrotic epithelium represents a nonfunctioning and simply passive membrane. Under these circumstances the intraluminal fluid would be under the same influences with respect to the Starling forces as is the interstitial fluid of the kidney.

It could be anticipated, therefore, that the bulk of the diminished filtrate might be reabsorbed directly into the peritubular vessels, since the tubular walls no longer function as more than a passive diffusion barrier. In other instances the oliguria may be a consequence of nephron obstruction by casts. In many instances, the trivial formation of urine may be a consequence of a combination of these three mechanisms. In renal cortical necrosis, where all elements of the nephron are destroyed, total anuria is common. This may obtain because there is virtually no filtration whatsoever; what little does occur is likely to be subject to the influences suggested above in the context of acute tubular necrosis.

CHRONIC RENAL INSUFFICIENCY. The ability to form a maximally concentrated urine is disturbed early in chronic renal insufficiency. This is accredited to at least two factors. One suggestion is that with a reduced population of nephrons and an elevated concentration of urea the filtration rate and the filtered load of urea per nephron are increased, and in this circumstance there is an osmotic diuresis in those nephrons that contribute to the final urine. In the context of the discussion in the section on physiologic considerations, a framework was provided in an attempt to clarify the influence of the rate of excretion of solutes on the urine concentrating mechanism. Furthermore, if the destruction of renal mass occurs primarily in the medulla (as is so common in pyelonephritis) the nephrons with the longest loops of Henle are more likely to be destroyed. Since these longest loops of Henle set up the highest interstitial osmolality, it is apparent why urine concentrating defects are seen early. Hence, although chronic renal insufficiency may be associated with some polyuria, this is usually not striking. In the patient with end-stage kidney disease, striking reductions in urine flow are frequently observed. This is primarily a consequence of the magnitude of the destruction of renal mass.

OBSTRUCTION OF THE URINARY TRACT. Obstruction of the lower urinary tract, that is, from the bladder to the urethral meatus, is common and is due most frequently to stricture, to compression of the prostatic urethra by an enlarged gland, and, less commonly, to congenital malformations with valve formations that make emptying the bladder difficult. These patients may develop fairly striking acute reductions in urine flow, and this should always be a consideration when a patient is seen with oliguria.

Although it is less common to see oliguria as a consequence of obstruction of the upper urinary tract, it does occur. The reason for its rarity is that there are two kidneys and two ureters, and in order to achieve oliguria from obstruction above the bladder, both ureters must be compromised. However, this does occur in a variety of circumstances which include neoplastic infiltration of the ureters, and bilateral constriction consequent to a retroperitoneal sclerosing inflammatory process. On occasion constrictions may occur at the ureterovesical junctions bilaterally. Hence, although uncommon, bilateral obstruction of the upper urinary tracts may cause oliguria. Uni-

lateral ureteral calculus with ureteral spasm on the opposite side is also possible.

Polyuria

DIABETES INSIPIDUS. This condition results from inability to synthesize and secrete antidiuretic hormone and is the archetype of a disorder accompanied by the excretion of large volumes of dilute urine. In a compilation of several reports, intracranial tumors accounted for 40 percent of the variety of causes for diabetes insipidus, 33 percent were so-called *idiopathic*, and the remainder were scattered among a variety of disorders including trauma. Although not a rare disorder, diabetes insipidus is certainly uncommon. The primary condition from which it must be discriminated is primary polydipsia, which may be due to an intracranial organic lesion but perhaps more often accompanies a basic emotional disorder. These two disorders can be distinguished one from the other in a relatively simple fashion (see Chap. 88).

NEPHROGENIC DIABETES INSIPIDUS. Inability of the renal tubules to respond to antidiuretic hormone of endogenous or exogenous origin characterizes nephrogenic diabetes insipidus. It is a heritable disorder with full expression in males and partial expression in females, which manifests itself quite early in life; these patients are frequently referred to as "water babies." Their management is difficult since they do not respond to any of the available posterior pituitary preparations. However, they do respond to chlorothiazide drugs. The probable manner in which this agent influences the water turnover is by promoting a salt deficit. This, in turn, causes a smaller urine volume. This may be a consequence of a diminished filtration rate but is more likely to be associated with a larger fractional reabsorption of salt, and hence water, in the more proximal portions of the nephron. In this fashion less fluid is delivered to sites where it may escape into the bladder urine.

ACQUIRED RENAL LESIONS. There are acquired renal lesions associated with inability to concentrate the urine maximally.

Potassium depletion is commonly, if not invariably, associated with inability to concentrate the urine appropriately. The nature of the defect is not clear. Although it is at some risk that one translates data from rodents to human beings, information from rats and hamsters does exclude certain possibilities. Micropuncture data obtained by Gottschalk and his colleagues show that the osmolality of fluid in the distal convolution is the same in potassium-depleted rats as in control animals. Hence, there appears to be no lack of osmotic equilibration at this site. Furthermore, more recent data from the same laboratory utilizing normal and potassium-depleted hamsters reveal that there is no osmotic disequilibrium across the collecting duct epithelium. Other data indicate that the interstitial fluid deep in the papilla is not as hyperosmotic in potassium-depleted as in normal animals. The reasons for this are still unclear. Some published data on rats tend to deny the possibility that this is a consequence of a greater flow of fluid through the loop of Henle, since, if anything, the fractional reabsorption of water in the proximal convolution appears to be greater in a state of potassium depletion. Two obvious influences have not yet been evaluated, namely, the rate of medullary blood flow and the rate of active transport of salt in the ascending limb. An increase in medullary blood flow would tend to diminish the hypertonicity of the medullary and papillary interstitium; and a diminished rate of transport of salt across the ascending limb of the loops of Henle would diminish the efficiency of the countercurrent multiplier mechanism. The defect is reversible with potassium repletion.

Hypercalcemia has been known for some time to be accompanied by diminished ability to concentrate the urine maximally. In this instance as well, the precise mechanism is unknown. At this time the available data are somewhat similar to those discussed with respect to potassium depletion. There is no evidence of an osmotic disequilibrium across the collecting ducts and no evidence of an increased flow of fluid through the loop of Henle. The facets that have not been examined in the state of potassium depletion also raise questions about the hypercalcemic state.

Other examples of acquired renal lesions characterized by inability to concentrate the urine are seen frequently in patients with *chronic renal insufficiency*, as alluded to earlier. In addition, some rather striking examples of extreme polyuria have been seen in patients with multiple myeloma, amyloidosis, and, more commonly, after relief of an obstructive uropathy. Marked diuresis is commonly observed in the recovery phase of acute tubular necrosis from a variety of insults. This is frequently referred to as the "diuretic phase" of acute tubular necrosis and may be due in part to the delivery of accumulated fluid but very likely also due in part to renal tubular abnormalities with reference to the reabsorption of solutes and water.

SOLUTE DIURESIS. Large solute diureses, such as are noted in patients with uncontrolled diabetes mellitus and constant glycosuria, are almost always accompanied by large urine flows and complaint of polyuria. Solute diuresis may also occur in patients suffering a "reaction to injury" who are unable to utilize protein but are given large quantities of this foodstuff. In such instances protein is converted to a very large extent to urea and excreted. This increase in solute excretion promotes a large urine flow as described earlier.

Nocturia

The diurnal rhythm that applies to urine flow is such that a larger volume is excreted in the waking 12 hr than during the 12-hr period spent mostly asleep. The precise mechanisms underlying this particular rhythm are not clear, although the evidence suggests a correlation with filtration rate and solute excretion. This rhythm is lost in several circumstances, and in other instances it may appear to have been lost owing to mechanical problems.

The rhythm characterized by a relatively diminished volume of urine at night is frequently disturbed in patients with edema. This may very well be because edema accumulates more during the day owing to activity and the influence of gravity through posture. At night, when the patient is supine, some of the edema may be resorbed into the plasma volume, thereby promoting an alteration in renal hemodynamics that leads to increased excretion of urine.

Nocturia is common in patients with chronic renal insufficiency primarily because they excrete urine at a fairly constant rate, and hence the benefits to sleep of the normal diurnal rhythm are lost. The reasons for this may be similar to those relating to a concentrated urine. In this instance it may be due to a constant osmotic diuresis per nephron.

Partial obstruction of the bladder is often accompanied by nocturia simply because the stimulus to void is so frequently present.

For reasons that are certainly unclear, the patient with untreated adrenal cortical insufficiency loses the normal diurnal rhythm and hence may complain of nocturia.

Lastly, anything that causes dysuria is almost certain to promote nocturia. In this instance, as is the case with obstruction of the bladder, nocturia is characterized by frequent but *small* volumes in contrast to the other cases noted above.

APPROACH TO THE PATIENT

Carefully taken histories usually reveal evidence of disturbances characterized by excretion of small or large volumes of urine, or the presence or absence of nocturia. The associations with disease processes of this type of disturbance have been alluded to, and the questions suggested by these clues are, in a sense, implicit.

The point that bears some emphasis, perhaps, is that wide variations in urine flow exist in health as well as in disease, and a reasonable interpretation can be made only by careful evaluation of the characteristics of the symptom equated with other problems displayed by the patient. The specific evaluation of these disorders is discussed in other sections of this text.

REFERENCES

Gottschalk, C. W.: Osmotic Concentration and Dilution of the Urine, Am. J. Med., 36:670, 1964.

Kleeman, C. R., W. L. Hewitt, and L. B. Guzé: Pyelonephritis, Medicine, 39:3, 1960.

Pitts, R. F.: "Physiology of the Kidney and Body Fluids," Chicago, The Year Book Medical Publishers, Inc., 1963.

Strauss, M. B., and L. G. Welt, "Diseases of the Kidney," Boston, Little, Brown and Company, 1964.

51 HEMATURIA

Bernard Lytton and Franklin H. Epstein

Bleeding from the urinary tract, whether microscopic or gross, is a serious sign. It should be regarded with the same gravity as abnormal bleeding occurring from any other body tract. Hematuria is usually classified as initial, terminal, or total. Total hematuria indicates that the bleeding occurs throughout the urinary stream and suggests that the bleeding originates from either the kidney or the ureter. Initial bleeding is generally associated with lesions in the urethra distal to the bladder neck; terminal bleeding, with lesions in the bladder, usually in the area of the trigone. Severe hemorrhage from the bladder, however, will present as total hematuria. These distinctions as to the type of bleeding are, therefore, only rough indications as to the origin of the bleeding; too much reliance should not be placed on them. About 20 percent of patients who come to the physician with hematuria have it as the only symptom of their urinary tract disease; it is often difficult to persuade these patients to undergo a complete urologic investigation to establish the origin of the bleeding. Ureteral colic is often associated with renal bleeding and is due to the passage of clots.

The finding of an occasional red blood cell in a centrifuged specimen of urine is probably of no significance, since Addis showed that up to 500,000 red cells may normally be excreted in the urine in 12 hr. Vigorous exercise or even intense excitement may increase the numbers of red cells, epithelial cells, and casts in the urinary sediment of normal subjects. Microscopic hematuria may also be increased during certain febrile diseases without implying serious disease of the kidneys. The presence of red blood cell casts is pathologic and further indicates that the source of the bleeding is in the kidneys rather than the lower part of the urinary tract.

Certain dyes and pigments, such as phenolsulfonphthalein, azo dyes, and the indole alkaloids found in beet roots (betanin), may produce red discoloration of the urine which must be distinguished from bleeding. The appearance of the red dye from beet roots occurs only in certain individuals; it is thought to be related to the degree of absorption of the dye from the gastrointestinal tract. Pink or brown discoloration of the urine may occur as a result of hemo- or myoglobinuria. These may be precipitated by cold, exercise, or drug toxicity, especially in susceptible individuals such as those with sickle-cell trait (see Chap. 338).

Diseases of the renal parenchyma, such as glomerulonephritis, malignant hypertension, polycystic kidneys, renal infarction, periarteritis, or poisoning with a nephrotoxic agent, will in most instances be detected by a careful history, physical examination, and the usual laboratory tests. Hematuria may result from a *disorder of blood clotting,* produced by blood dyscrasias, scurvy, or anticoagulant drugs. The increased tendency to bleed in patients on long-term anticoagulant therapy may bring to light another, previously unsuspected, pathologic condition in the urinary tract. *Sickle-cell anemia* or sickle-cell trait may cause bleeding into the urine from disrupted capillaries and microinfarcts in the renal medulla. The aforementioned conditions account for only a small proportion of all patients with hematuria.

Tumors, urinary tract obstructions, calculi, and *infections* account for the bleeding in about 75 percent of patients with hematuria. Tumors alone account for some 20 percent of all cases. It is therefore mandatory in those patients in whom no other cause is found for the bleeding to visualize the upper part of the urinary tract by intravenous pyelography supplemented by retrograde pyelography as indicated and to visualize the bladder and urethra by instrumental examination. Retrograde pyelography may be supplemented by injections of air rather than opaque dye when one is trying to delineate suspected nonopaque calculi or small tumors in the renal collecting system. Doubtful lesions in the kidney may be further investigated by nephrotomography or aortography. The latter is probably best performed by the transfemoral route, which allows selective injections into individual renal vessels to be made if required. Renal tumors generally have greater opacification than the surrounding kidney tissue on tomography, and the aortogram shows the characteristic pooling of the dye in the venous sinusoids that occurs in these tumors and which is a result of the small arteriovenous communications which develop.

On cystoscopy, *acute* and *chronic cystitis,* interstitial cystitis, bladder tumors, and vesical calculi may be readily diagnosed. Bleeding from engorged veins in the prostatic urethra due to benign prostatic hypertrophy is a common source of hematuria. Like prostatitis in men and chronic nonspecific posterior urethritis in women, it should be accepted as the origin of the bleeding only if more serious conditions have been excluded.

Acute cystitis may produce gross hematuria, initially overshadowing all other symptoms. Chronic infections such as *tuberculosis* of the urinary tract or infection with *Schistosoma hematobium* may also have hematuria as their only presenting symptom. Schistosomiasis causes ulceration of the bladder mucosa at the site of deposition of the ova by the adult flukes which inhabit the venules of the bladder and pelvis. It is probably the commonest cause of hematuria in those areas in the Middle East and Africa where it is endemic.

Bleeding associated with the menses should suggest the possibility of *endometriosis* of the urinary tract, provided contamination from the vagina has been excluded.

Trauma to the kidney nearly always manifests itself as hematuria which is often painless and may persist for several days. The incidence of renal injury is increasing because of the increased number of serious automobile accidents. The majority of these cases may be treated conservatively with bed rest and careful observation. Follow-up intravenous pyelography should be carried out, as occasionally the renal injury may produce an anatomic deformity leading to either stone formation or hypertension. A blow on the lower part of the abdomen when the bladder is distended, particularly in children where the bladder is an abdominal organ, may produce a contusion of the bladder, giving rise to painless hematuria.

A group of about 6 to 8 percent of all cases seen have hematuria for which no obvious source can be detected. Further urologic and hematologic investigation 3 to 4 months after the first episode of bleeding will determine the cause in just under half of these. Patients in whom episodes of hematuria persist should have a renal biopsy at a time when they are bleeding. *A focal glomerulitis* has been found to be responsible for the bleeding in many of these cases. The condition appears to have a good prognosis as regards renal function. The severe bleeding which sometimes occurs may be controlled in some instances by the administration of steroids for 2 to 3 months. A small number of cases however, still remain undiagnosed and may have persistent hematuria over a period of many years for which no cause is found.

52 DISTURBANCES OF MENSTRUATION
George W. Thorn

Since normal menstrual cycles depend upon the integrated action of the endocrine and nervous systems, it is to be expected that abnormalities in the menstrual cycle may occur in association with a wide variety of systemic disorders as well as with specific pathologic changes in the reproductive organs. (See Chap. 98 for a discussion of disease of the ovaries and uterus.)

MENARCHE. In temperate climates the menstrual cycle usually begins between the ages of twelve to fifteen, whereas in tropical climates it may appear as early as nine or ten. During the first year or two, the menstrual cycles are likely to be irregular, since many are anovulatory.

Uterine bleeding in the newborn may be noted for 3 to 4 days following delivery and is thought to be due to the sudden decrease in circulating estrogen level which had previously induced endometrial growth in the fetus.

Vaginal bleeding in very young girls should suggest injury from a foreign body introduced into the vagina. Very rarely vaginal bleeding will occur in association with precocious development of breasts due to an ovarian or adrenal tumor.

The delayed onset of menses, beyond the age of sixteen years, suggests *abnormalities* in the development *of the reproductive system,* such as imperforate hymen, uterine hypoplasia, and ovarian agenesis; *endocrine dysfunction,* such as anterior pituitary or thyroid deficiency; or *psychologic disturbances,* which mediate their effect through neurohumoral pathways.

MENSES. Normally periods occur at intervals of 27 to 32 days, and flow lasts an average of 5 days. Approximately 60 to 250 ml blood is lost, with the greatest quantity lost during the first or second day. The volume of menstrual flow can be estimated by the fact that each well-soaked pad will contain approximately 30 to 50 ml blood.

MENOPAUSE. Naturally occurring menopause may be expected by age fifty. Menopause represents the period of change between the years of reproduction and the regression of ovarian function. A gradual reduction in the duration of the menstrual cycle is to be expected at this time. *Irregular bleeding* or *hypermenorrhea* is most often caused by anovulatory cycles, but *neoplasms* should always be suspected. Induced or artificial menopause follows extirpation or irradiation of the ovaries. *Premature menopause* may occur as early as thirty-five without definitive cause; occasionally a familial tendency for this will be noted. However, other causes of amenorrhea such as endocrine abnormalities and emotional factors must be excluded.

ABNORMAL UTERINE BLEEDING. During the reproductive cycle abnormal uterine bleeding should always suggest pregnancy and one of its complications, such as threatened abortion, ectopic pregnancy, or hydatid mole. Having excluded the complications of pregnancy by history, physical examination, and a rapid serologic test, one should consider uterine pathology such as polyps, leiomyomas, and carcinoma of the cervix or body of the uterus. For these a pelvic examination and diagnostic curettage will be required. Ovarian disease, pelvic inflammation, and hormonal abnormalities such as *hypothyroidism* also can induce abnormal uterine bleeding. Systemic disturbances, particularly those associated with anemia, leukemia, abnormalities in blood clotting, and circulatory disturbances such as hypertension should be excluded. The anemia that follows prolonged menstrual bleeding may predispose a patient to further excessive menstruation. In view of the widespread use of hormones, particularly estrogens, progesterone, and contraceptive pills, one should consider the *administration* or *withdrawal* of sex hormonal preparations as potential causes of abnormal uterine bleeding. Finally, disturbed emotional states or serious psychologic difficulties may predispose to abnormal uterine bleeding.

Hypermenorrhea, characterized by excessively long or too profuse menstrual bleeding, may result from delay in the repair of the endometrium and, of course, frequently accompanies anovulatory cyclic bleeding.

Polymenorrhea refers to regular menstrual cycles that occur more frequently than every 23 to 24 days. It is the least common of the menstrual irregularities and tends to occur very early or late in menstrual life. It is due to a shortening of the follicular or luteal phase of the menstrual cycle.

Intermenstrual bleeding refers to the occurrence of irregular bleeding between normally spaced periods. Spontaneous bleeding of this type is more likely to be endometrial in origin in contrast to bleeding of the cervix or vagina.

AMENORRHEA AND OLIGOMENORRHEA. Physiologic amenorrhea precedes the menarche, follows the menopause, and characterizes pregnancy and lactation. *Primary amenorrhea* indicates that menstruation has never occurred, whereas *secondary amenorrhea* refers to cessation of menstruation.

Uterine abnormalities such as agenesis or hypoplasia give rise to primary amenorrhea, whereas destruction of endometrium by irradiation or excessive curettage or removal of the uterus can induce secondary amenorrhea. *Vaginal abnormalities* include such conditions as imperforate hymen. The continued retention of blood may lead to hematometra, hematosalpinx, and eventually hematoperitoneum.

Ovarian agenesis or dysgenesis (Turner's syndrome) is a cause of primary amenorrhea, whereas polycystic disease of the ovary (Stein-Leventhal syndrome), masculinizing tumors of the ovary or adrenal, destruction of ovarian function by irradiation, and hormonal imbalance give rise in most instances to secondary amenorrhea or oligomenorrhea. Hypopituitarism with Simmond's cachexia, Sheehan's syndrome, or the Chiavi-Frommel syndrome will, of course, result in reduced ovarian function and predispose to oligomenorrhea or amenorrhea. With pituitary deficiency, one would expect associated evidence of reduced adrenal and thyroid function (Chap 87). Diabetes mellitus and hyperthyroidism may induce menstrual abnormalities characterized by oligomenorrhea or hypermenorrhea. Malnutrition, obesity, debilitating disease, intoxication, and severe anemia may be associated with oligomenorrhea or amenorrhea as well as with abnormal uterine bleeding. Fear, anxiety, and grief are frequent causes of temporary amenorrhea, and indeed psychologic factors acting on hypothalamic centers constitute one of the most frequent causes of secondary amenorrhea. Amenorrhea is almost an invariable accompaniment of anorexia nervosa.

DYSMENORRHEA. Some form of discomfort normally accompanies ovulatory menstruation in contrast to anovulation bleeding, which is almost never associated with pain. Dysmenorrhea may reflect itself as lower abdominal cramps, backache, headache, and occasionally nausea and vomiting. Of these symptoms, the commonest is abdominal cramps. Many women suffer some discomfort for a few hours on the first day of menstruation, but in the majority of cases this is not incapacitating. Obviously, the degree of pain and discomfort experienced by any individual will depend upon concurrent involvement of the pelvic organs in disease or anatomic abnormalities. The pain threshold of the patient and the effect of emotional and psychologic problems, particularly those related to ignorance or misconception about the significance of the menstrual cycle, are important factors in evaluating the pathogenesis of dysmenorrhea. In *primary spastic* or *intrinsic dysmenorrhea*, there is no evidence of pelvic pathology. It may gradually disappear later in reproductive life, and relief is usually afforded by the birth of a full-term fetus. *Characteristic of secondary dysmenorrhea is the onset of pain after several years of relatively painless periods.* Pain may begin several days before menstrual flow and radiate throughout the entire lower abdomen, into the lower back, and down the legs. It is more constant in nature and not as sharp or cramplike as that noted in the primary type. Secondary dysmenorrhea is usually associated with pelvic pathology such as endometriosis, retroversion of the uterus, pelvic neoplasm, or inflammatory disease such as salpingitis or parametritis. In rare instances intense pain at the time of menstruation may accompany the expulsion of a large mass of shaggy, uterine membrane, i.e., membranous dysmenorrhea. Such events are infrequent and isolated and do not occur with successive periods.

PREMENSTRUAL TENSION. This term is applied to a constellation of symptoms which increase in intensity for 5 to 10 days before menstruation. The most frequent complaints are a sense of abdominal bloating, breast tenderness, headache, irritability, mental depression, and an increase in weight which may be associated with edema of the legs. The abdominal distension and tight feeling may be present without any great increase in weight and ofttimes without gaseous distension of the intestines (Chap. 48). There is no doubt that the wide fluctuation in female sex hormone levels which occurs during the reproductive period, with their important effect on electrolyte and water metabolism as well as upon mood and drive, provide critical "triggering" mechanisms for pathophysiologic changes in peripheral tissues as well as in the central nervous system.

REFERENCES

Behrman, S. J., and J. R. G. Gosling: Fundamentals of Gynecology, chaps. 6–11, New York, Oxford University Press, 1959.

Rogers, J.: Menstrual Disorders, New Engl. J. Med., 270: 194, Jan. 23, 1964.

Thorn, G. W.: Approach to the Patient with Idiopathic Edema or Periodic Swelling, J.A.M.A., 206:333, 1968.

53 DISTURBANCES OF SEXUAL FUNCTION

George W. Thorn

GENERAL CONSIDERATIONS

In men disturbances in sexual function may result from alterations in one or all of three distinct entities.

1. Libido, or the sexual impulse
2. Potentia, or penile erection
3. Ejaculation of semen

In women aberrations of sexual function are more difficult to analyze. Lack or diminution of sexual drive or failure to attain orgasm (frigidity) is much more frequent than in men.

Alterations in Libido

LOSS OF LIBIDO. Loss of libido may occur as a result of either psychologic or somatic factors. It may be complete in the presence of serious organic disease or with advanced age. On the other hand, lost or diminished libido may occur only under particular circumstances or in relation to a particular person, indicating the predominance of psychologic factors. In instances such as these, it is not unusual for a patient to experience nocturnal penile erection and emission of semen. Although loss of libido may accompany serious endocrine disorders such as anterior pituitary deficiency, Addison's disease, or diabetic acidosis or ketosis, it is not likely to be a *primary com-*

plaint of the patient under these circumstances since the impairment in general health and activity is so overwhelming. Under these circumstances, it is more likely that the patient's spouse will have noted or called attention to the difficulty. For practical purposes it is important to bear in mind that the primary complaint of lost or decreased libido in male patients, in the absence of *severe* organic disease or *advanced* age, is almost certainly dependent *upon emotional or psychologic disturbances.*

FRIGIDITY. Inability on the part of women to consummate the sexual act is a distressing complaint of relatively frequent occurrence. The sexual drive of the normal woman is primarily conditioned by psychologic factors, with endrocrine functions in a supporting role. The changes in sexual drive produced by alterations in hormonal level are of relatively little importance in contrast to the role of emotional and psychologic factors. Conditioning from birth or early childhood most often results in a woman's belief that she is frigid. Many experiences in childhood can, later in life, result in incapacity to consummate the sexual act. Such experiences develop a climate of fear, insecurity, and dread concerning the whole subject of sex. Because of these deep-seated emotional conflicts, most patients will require intensive psychotherapy. With an understanding of the real basis of the problem and in conjunction with medical and psychiatric assistance, a small dose of androgenic hormone such as methyl testosterone, 10 mg twice daily, may be given. This may increase sexual drive and more specifically increase the sensitivity of the clitoris. Its continued use, however, may result in menstrual irregularities as well as in hirsutism and acne.

EXCESSIVE LIBIDO. Excessive libido may occur in conjunction with serious neurologic disease such as encephalitis or brain tumor as well as with psychologic and emotional disturbances. *Nymphomania* refers to women who exhibit abnormal behavior that reflects greatly heightened libido.

Alterations in Potentia

IMPOTENCE. Impotence implies the presence of sexual desire in a patient who cannot attain or sustain penile erection. Impotence is rarely of endocrine origin. More frequently it accompanies a neurologic or emotional disorder. In neurologic disorders absence or impairment of parasympathetic nerve activity prevents the development of tumescence of the corpora cavernosa. Impotence is common among patients who suffer disease of the sacral cord segments and their afferent and efferent connections, e.g., cord tumor, tabes, and multiple sclerosis. Approximately one-fourth of male diabetics in the younger age group and about one-half in the fifth decade develop impotence as a consequence of diabetic polyneuritis. Loss of both sexual desire and erection may occur in hypopituitarism, hypothyroidism, and severe eunuchoidism as well as in association with many general debilitating diseases. Patients with trauma to the prostatic urethra and those subjected to perineal operations frequently

have reduced potentia. Malformation of the genitals such as extreme degrees of epispadias, pseudohermaphroditism, growths and edema of the penis, as well as large hernias, hydroceles, and elephantiasis may interfere with sexual function. In the majority of patients, however, impotence is of psychologic origin and fortunately temporary. Fears and phobias which arise about the sexual act, as well as feelings of guilt, may be responsible.

PRIAPISM. True priapism is a state of sustained erection of the penis not accompanied by sexual desire. It is most frequent in the third or fourth decades and is usually accompanied by pain. Two types are recognized: the sustained and the recurrent nocturnal type. Priapism may result from urethral inflammation, from new growth involving the corpora, or from systemic disease such as leukemia or sickle-cell anemia. Diseases of the spinal cord may be accompanied by penile erections, reflexly induced and sustained for long periods of time. The neural apparatus for the control of sexual function is organized through the lower spinal segments, and hence may function effectively even when completely removed from voluntary control by spinal cord lesions. Recurrent, non-sustained, painful priapism is of unknown etiology, although it is often associated with prostatitis. Since it frequently subsides spontaneously, the efficacy of therapy is difficult to document. The administration of amyl nitrite has been noted to cause relaxation during the early phase of priapism. It has also been suggested that an anticoagulant might be effective in minimizing the venous thrombosis which is likely to occur with prolonged priapism. For this, heparin is suggested intravenously in an initial dose of 100 mg, followed by subsequent doses of 50 mg every 6 hr.

Ejaculation

Another type of disturbance consists of *premature ejaculation* of semen, a common complaint in neurotic individuals, though by no means peculiar to them. After lumbar sympathectomy the semen may be ejected into the bladder because of paralysis of the periurethral muscle at the verumontanum.

Dyspareunia

Dyspareunia, or *pain on intercourse,* may be present for a short time at the onset of marriage or sexual intercourse. Pain that continues long after marriage or develops later in life suggests local disease or emotional disturbance. Vaginal and pelvic examination should be made to exclude pelvic inflammatory disease, endometriosis, or tumor. In the absence of demonstrable organic disease, psychologic or emotional factors must be considered. Fear of pregnancy, fear of cancer if contraceptives are used, and tension between husband and wife can prevent enjoyment of intercourse with consequent spasm of vaginal musculature. Explanation of these facts with reassurance by an understanding physician may be followed by appreciable improvement.

Sterility

In the male sterility may result from lack of or impairment of spermatogenesis due to testicular agenesis, hypogenesis, or cryptorchidism; to castration or exposure to roentgen rays or toxic substances; to injury or inflammation; or to endocrine or nutritional disorders. Obstruction of the seminal vesicles and epididymis and pronounced deformity of the penis interfere with the normal passage of the spermatozoa. Infection of the prostate or seminal vesicles may be injurious to the spermatozoa (Chap. 54).

In the female sterility may result from impaired oogenesis as a consequence of deficient ovarian tissue, e.g., ovarian agenesis or hypoplasia, polycystic disease of the ovary with thickened capsule; or as a consequence of the inability of the ovum to become impregnated due to disease of the fallopian tubes, such as infection and endometriosis; or to uterine, cervical, or vaginal abnormalities in structure and function. In addition, debilitating diseases, endocrine abnormalities, and nutritional deficiencies may impair ovulation as well as fertilization and implantation of the ovum.

Infertility

Infertility represents one of the most important and serious disturbances of sexual function. It is estimated that 10 percent of couples in the United States are involuntarily infertile. Of this number it is thought that approximately one-third of cases are due to infertility of the woman, one-third to infertility of the man, and one-third to *decreased fertility* of both partners. Absolute infertility is said to exist when there is complete aspermia or absent or rudimentary ovarian tissue. *Relative infertility* applies to men who have oligospermia, when conception has not taken place. In contrast to other disturbances of sexual function such as impotence, frigidity, and dyspareunia, which are so frequently dependent upon psychologic and emotional factors, sterility and infertility are due primarily to functional and organic disease of the urogenital tract. In most instances the problem of infertility or sterility will be presented by the woman.

The approach to the problem of infertility in both men and women as well as suggestions for corrective therapy are discussed in detail in Chap. 54.

The genesis of *sexual perversions* remains obscure. Endocrine, biochemical, and psychologic studies have failed thus far to clarify either their cause or their mechanism.

REFERENCES

Bell, W. R., and W. R. Pitney: Brief Recordings: Management of Priapism by Therapeutic Defibrination, New Eng. J. of Med., 280:649, 1969.

Calderone, M. S.: "Release from Sexual Tension," New York, Random House, 1960.

Grace, D. A., and C. C. Winter: Priapism: An Appraisal of Management of Twenty-three Patients, J. Urol., 99:301, 1968.

Hamm, F. C., and S. R. Weinberg: "Urology in Medical Practice," 2d ed., Philadelphia, J. B. Lippincott Company, 1962.

Schöffling, K., K. Federlin, H. Ditschuneit, and E. F. Pfeiffer: Disorders of Sexual Function in Male Diabetics, Diabetes, 12:519, 1963.

54 INFERTILITY
Melvin L. Taymor

DEFINITION. Infertility may be defined as the inability to conceive during the course of normal sexual activity. It is generally held that a marriage should not be considered infertile until a year of unprotected coitus has been allowed to pass. However, each couple's problems should be judged individually, and diagnosis and treatment instituted at an earlier or later date as indicated.

ETIOLOGY. The two fundamental concepts to be kept in mind are (1) the multiplicity of etiologic factors and (2) the equal responsibility of male and female partners. To delineate these possible factors working either singly or in concert, one need only review the pathways of conception in male and female and the disorders of these pathways that may ensue.

Deficiency of sperm production in quantity and quality accounts for the majority of the *male's* contribution to the problem of infertility. Sperm production may be adversely affected by congenital influences such as germinal aplasia or cryptorchidism, by hormonal deficiencies of the pituitary or thyroid glands, by infection such as mumps orchitis, and by environmental factors such as nutritional deficiencies, noxious chemicals and drugs, radiation, excess local heat, and altitude. Often the cause is not ascertainable by diagnostic methods available at present. Sperm transport is affected by congenital malformations, surgical trauma, and infections. Impotency, an important factor in many cases, is commonly on a psychologic basis, although local infection or general systemic disorders may play a contributory role.

Defects in the *female* are related to production of ova and interference with their union with spermatozoa. Vaginal causes are organic or functional. Very often these causes are a combination of organic and psychologic factors. The obstruction may be due to an unruptured hymen, or it may be functional due to hypertrophy and contraction of the levator ani muscles. Vaginitis itself is not a serious cause of infertility except in its role as a temporary deterrent to coitus. The cervix is one of the most important areas of obstruction to the passage of sperm. During the few days prior to ovulation the endocervical glands secrete a thin, watery mucus that is beneficial to sperm survival and migration. Infection or estrogen deficiency may decrease the quality of the mucus. Too often the offender is an overly zealous physician who cauterizes the cervix too deeply and destroys the endocervical glands. Uterine abnormalities are not a common cause of infertility. Infertility can be associated with an anomaly such as bicornate, or double, uterus. Uterine fibroids are more likely to result in repeated abortions rather than the failure to conceive. Tubal occlusion is usually secondary to gonorrheal salpingitis. Bacterial salpingitis, secondary to pelvic peritonitis, appendicitis, abortion, or instrumentation, is more likely to result in partial blockage of the fibrated end of the tube. Nongonorrheal infection is also more likely to result in what is called the peritoneal factor. In this condition adhesions may develop between the tube and ovary, or fixation of the ovary may occur. Under these circumstances the chances of union between the sperm and egg are significantly reduced. In addition to infection, the peritoneal factor can be due to endometriosis. Hormonal or endocrine factors are all-important; these may result in deficient corpus luteum function and absence of ovulation.

Immunologic factors may play a significant role in some cases of unexplained infertility.

Finally, emotional factors may play a vital role by interfering with ovulation or initiating tubal spasm or dyspareunia. However, the fact should be stressed that more often than not, the state of infertility with its accompanying diagnostic and therapeutic maneuvers is more likely to produce serious emotional reactions than are primary emotional factors likely to produce infertility.

TREATMENT. The treatment of any defects, minor or major, in both the husband or the wife should be carried out concomitantly so that the total fertility potential of the couple will be raised to an optimum level.

In the *male* with azoospermia, in whom spermatogenesis is normal as shown by testicular biopsy, and in whom a block has been demonstrated, epididymovasostomy can result in return of fertility in 10 to 20 percent of cases. When hormonal studies reveal a deficiency of pituitary gonadotropin, treatment with human chorionic gonadotropin (5,000 units APL intramuscularly twice weekly for 2 to 6 months) is indicated. However, sperm deficiencies not associated with specific pituitary defects will not respond to pituitary or pituitarylike extract. Azoospermia or severe oligospermia will not respond in any significant degree to the administration of hormones, vitamins, thyroid preparations, or diet unless a specific deficiency can be demonstrated. In the present state of knowledge, little can be offered in the vast majority of cases of azoospermia or severe oligospermia.

This degree of pessimism should not be carried over to the infertile male with moderate degree of oligospermia (10 to 30 million per ml) or to the male partner of an infertile couple with only a moderately lowered sperm count (30 to 60 million per ml), particularly if one considers the "couple as a unit" concept of infertility. A modest improvement in the sperm count or motility combined with attention to the factors in the female partner may raise the fertility of the couple above a critical level. Avoidance of excess alcohol and tobacco, sufficient sleep and exercise, an optimum diet, adjustment of local excesses of heat, administration of thyroid preparations in

minor degrees of hypofunction—all these singly or together may prove of definite benefit.

In the *female* specific attention should be directed to the cervical factor by correction of unfavorable coital habits, correction of retroversion of the uterus by a pessary, improvement in quality and quantity of preovulatory mucus by the daily administration of small dosages of estrogen (0.1 mg diethylstilbestrol daily for three or four cycles), by the use of plastic cervical cap, and by the correction of cervicitis by systemic and local antibotics or by cervical cauterization. Cauterization must be conservative lest more harm than good be produced by cervical stenosis or obliteration of mucus secreting glands. When cervical stenosis is found, dilatation under anesthesia is of definite value.

Attempts to overcome tubal occlusion by repeated insufflations, diathermy, and high dosage of estrogen occasionally meet with success. Plastic repair of tubes or cornual implantation is followed by success in only 10 to 20 percent of cases. Surgery for tube-ovarian blockade, due to ovaries fixed by endometriosis, peritubal or periovarian adhesions, but associated with essentially normal tubes, results in a higher percentage of success. Infrequent ovulation accompanied by gross irregularity will respond to thyroid preparations when specifically indicated and to the correction of a specific dietary or vitamin deficiency. Ovulation accompanied by an inadequate luteal phase should be treated with progesterone preparations (Medroxyprogesterone, 2.5 mg daily for 10 days) or injections of human chorionic gonadotropin (HCG, 1,000 units intramuscularly every other day for five doses). Treatment should begin on the fifth or sixth day after the mid-cycle rise in the basal body temperature. Absence of ovulation is rarely corrected by pituitary hormone preparations.

Additional approaches to the medical induction of ovulation, although still experimental and as yet commercially unavailable, show promise for future clinical application. The first is an extract of gonadotropins, high in FSH activity, prepared from the urine of postmenopausal females (HMG). The usual dosage is 150 to 200 FSH units administered intramuscularly daily for 5 to 12 days. When there is evidence of follicular activity, as indicated by increased levels of estrogen in the urine or increasing fern formation in cervical mucus, 8,000 IU of HCG is administered. Each patient responds differently. Overstimulation can result in enlarged cystic ovaries and multiple pregnancies, so each patient should be followed carefully. Polycystic ovaries are most susceptible to massive enlargement and possible rupture.

Clomiphene citrate, a chemical closely related to stilbestrol, also can stimulate ovulation. The mode of action is not completely clarified, but after a 3-to-5-day course of the medication, 100 mg daily, a burst of gonadotropins 3 to 10 days later often stimulates ovulation. It, too, should be used with caution in patients suspected of having polycystic ovaries.

Psychotherapy is of value in improving the coital habits of the couple, in reducing tubal spasm, and in correcting some deficiencies of hormonal nature. Finally, the manner

Table 54-1. TESTS FOR INFERTILITY

I. In the male.
   A. Routine.
      1. Semen analysis. The semen is delivered into a clean glass container by withdrawal or masturbation. The following characteristics are considered normal:
         a. Volume—3 to 5 ml.
         b. Sperm count—above 60 million per ml is unquestionably normal, below 30 million per ml unquestionably indicates reduced fertility. The significance of counts between 30 million and 60 million depends upon the quality of motility and the degree of fertility in the female partner. A highly fertile female would be more susceptible to a count of borderline fertility.
         c. Motility—40 percent or more still actively motile 4 to 5 hr after collection.
         d. Morphology—at least 60 percent of the spermatozoa should be of normal size and shape.
      2. Examination of prostatic smear—excess leukocytes indicate that infection may play a contributory role.
   B. Special tests—for the male with reduced fertility as indicated by semen analysis.
      1. Evaluation of thyroid function by basal metabolic rate, protein-bound iodine, or radioactive iodine uptake.
      2. Testicular biopsy—in most cases this will result in a definitive diagnosis. In only a few cases, however, will it demonstrate a remediable defect.
      3. Urinary gonadotropins—these may be low in pituitary deficiency. Excretion is high in primary gonadal failure.
      4. Sex chromatin determination.
II. In the female.
   A. Routine.
      1. Postcoital test—examination of the cervical mucus for its preovulatory qualities of clarity, spinnbarkeit (ability of the mucus to form a thread 5 to 10 cm in length when stretched between slide and cover slip), ferning (ability of the mucus to form fernlike pattern when dried and examined under low power of microscope), and for the number of viable spermatozoa 8 to 12 hr after coitus.
         a. Good test—more than 20 active spermatozoa per high-power field.
         b. Fair test—5 to 20 spermatozoa per high-power field.
         c. Poor test—less than 5 spermatozoa per high-power field. A poor postcoital test in the presence of good preovulatory mucus suggests a semen deficiency, a deficiency of the coital method, or malposition of the cervix. A poor postcoital test combined with poor mucus in the preovulatory phase and a normal semen analysis indicates a hostile cervix either on an inflammatory or an endocrine basis.

Table 54-1. TESTS FOR INFERTILITY (*Continued*)

      2. The evaluation of tubal patency—initially by insufflation with carbon dioxide (Rubin test) and followed at a later date by hysterosalpingography in those cases which show failure of carbon dioxide to pass or who fail to conceive after an interval of time despite a normal Rubin test.
      3. Evaluation of ovulation and hormonal factors by:
         a. Measurement of basal body temperature, which characteristically shows a sustained rise after ovulation. Studies have shown that actual ovulation may occur as long as 2 days before or 2 days after the beginning of the temperature rise. The value of the temperature chart as an exact indicator of ovulation timing for purposes of timing coitus or insemination treatments can be overestimated.
         b. Endometrial biopsy with the demonstration of secretory changes in the endometrium is valid evidence that ovulation has occurred. The presence of endometrium out of phase with the time of biopsy is evidence of a progestational deficiency.
   B. Special tests should be carried out when indicated.
      1. Evaluation of thyroid function.
      2. Endocrine assays, such as urinary gonadotropin and 17-ketosteroid determination, in cases of anovulation or inadequate luteal function.
      3. Further studies of ovulation timing utilizing vaginal or urinary smears and studies of cervical mucus.
      4. Culdoscopy to detect early endometriosis, pelvic adhesions interfering with tube-ovarian function, or polycystic ovaries.

and attitude of the physician plays a role in the outcome by preventing undue feelings of guilt and depression from gaining the upper hand, and by instilling sufficient hope and fortitude to allow the couple to carry through with the tedious and sometimes painful diagnostic testing and therapeutic maneuvers.

REFERENCES

Gemzell, C. A.: Induction of Ovulation with Human Pituitary Gonadotropins, Fertility Sterility, 13:153, 1962.

Meeker, S. R.: "Human Sterility, Causation, Diagnosis and Treatment: A Practical Manual of Clinical Procedures," Baltimore, The Williams & Wilkins Company, 1933.

Stone, A., and M. E. Ward: Factors Responsible for Pregnancy in 500 Infertility Cases, Fertility Sterility, 7:1, 1956.

Taymor, M. L.: Gonadotropin Therapy, Possible Causes and Prevention of Ovarian Overstimulation, J.A.M.A., 203:362, 1968.

——: Management of Infertility, Springfield, Ill. Charles C Thomas, Publisher, 1969.

Section 8
Alterations in the Integument

55   SKIN LESIONS
Faye D. Arundell and Eugene M. Farber

Examination of the skin should include a detailed history and thorough inspection of the entire surface encompassing the mucous membranes of the mouth and genital region, the hair, and the nails. The patient should be examined undressed, in order to carry out a thorough inspection of the hair, scalp, ears, eyes, mucosae of the nose, mouth, pharynx, teeth, all surfaces of the trunk and extremities, palms, soles, interdigital spaces, and nails. The examination should be performed in unobstructed daylight or artificial daylight illumination. Subtle color changes in the skin may be masked by inadequate artificial lighting. The routine use of a magnifying lens permits the perception of fine details and small lesions.

Orderly notation and description of the lesions are prerequisites to accurate diagnosis and judicious therapy (Chaps. 56 to 60, 400). Four fundamental changes in the skin can be detected by inspection and palpation. These abnormalities, which represent the basic pathologic reactions of skin, are changes in color, mass, fluid content, and texture. Color changes usually result from involvement of the vascular or pigmentary system. Changes in mass caused by cellular proliferation or infiltration result in palpable lesions that may project above the surface of the surrounding normal skin. Free fluid within the epidermis, or between the epidermis and dermis, creates *blisters;* increased free fluid within the dermis results in a solid *mass. Scales,* representing a change in texture of the outermost layers, are caused by defects in the formation or shedding of the horny layer. In any single lesion the changes may occur alone or in combination. The lesion which contains the fewest number of fundamental changes represents the *primary lesion.* The primary lesion should be identified, since its recognition makes it possible to diagnose an eruption. Evolutionary or secondary changes of the primary lesion, their arrangement or configuration, and their distribution on the body surface are additional diagnostic features. Many dermatoses are not accompanied by systemic changes, and their diagnosis is entirely dependent on the analysis of data obtained by observation and palpation of the skin.

PRINCIPAL PRIMARY LESIONS OF DISEASES AFFECTING THE SKIN. Macules.
Macules are small circumscribed changes in color of the skin unaccompanied by any change in mass or fluid content. If there is any palpable elevation or induration present in the colored lesion, it is not a macule. Circumscribed color changes in the skin larger than 1 cm in diameter are referred to as *patches.* Macular changes may be caused by deposition of extrinsic pigment as a consequence of trauma; increase or decrease of the intrinsic skin pigment, melanin, such as freckles and vitiligo; dilatation of cutaneous blood vessels, resulting in erythema; extravasation of erythrocytes to form petechiae or purpuric macules. Firm pressure with a glass slide over the dilated vessels of erythematous macules causes immediate blanching and readily differentiates them from purpuric macules. Erythematous macules are common in drug reactions and in exanthems such as roseola and rubella.

Papules. Papules are small (less than 0.5 cm in diameter) circumscribed increases in mass in the skin produced by tissue proliferation or infiltration. Papules are always palpable and may be accompanied by changes in color and texture. The color, shape, and configuration of papular lesions are characteristic in certain dermatoses. Papules which are violet in color, angular in shape, and have flat tops with adherent scales are the primary lesion of lichen planus. Erythematous papules arranged in rings and semicircles create the characteristic "nickels and dimes" lesions of secondary syphilis.

Papules may extend peripherally or coalesce to form large *plaques.* Erythematous plaques covered by layers of silvery scales are the hallmark of psoriasis (Chap. 400). Firm pebbled plaques occur in *lichen amyloidosis,* a type of amyloidosis confined to the skin.

Nodules. Deep circumscribed lesions that are firmer than the surrounding tissue are termed nodules when they are the result of tissue proliferation or inflammation. Red, hot, firm, tender nodules are present over the shins in erythema nodosum. *Tumors* are circumscribed indurated lesions which are arbitrarily defined as being larger than nodules.

Wheals (hives, urticaria) are a distinctive type of nodule caused by a localized collection of free fluid within the deeper layers of the skin. A hive has a central raised pale nodule surrounded by an erythematous patch, or flare. Wheals may enlarge to form alarmingly large swellings of an extremity or the face (*angioneurotic edema*). Hives, by definition, are transient itchy lesions which involute within hours, though new lesions continue to appear. The commonest causes of such acute urticarial reactions are food allergy, physical allergy, and drug reactions. Chronic urticaria is characterized by transient urticarial lesions that recur for periods longer than 6 weeks. Patients with chronic urticaria require a painstaking history regarding medications, chronic infections, food, environmental, physical, and psychologic factors. Individual urticarial lesions, which are not transient but persist for days or weeks, often form rings or bizarre figures. Persistent figurate urticarial lesions are the only primary lesions present in the chronic erythema group of diseases, such as *erythema annulare centrifugum*. Persistent urticarial lesions also occur as one of the primary lesions in association with blisters and patchy erythema in erythema multiforme (Chap. 400). The diseases characterized by persistent urticarial lesions require a thorough history and investigation for precipitating factors, such as drugs, infection, and neoplastic diseases. Urticarial lesions ordinarily respond to systemic antihistamine therapy. Life-threatening eruptions, such as severe bullous erythema multiforme, require systemic corticosteroid therapy. Under no circumstances should symptomatic therapy, whether antihistamines or corticosteroids, replace a search for and removal of the primary etiologic factor.

Vesicles and bullae. Vesicles are circumscribed small blisters containing free fluid. The free fluid may be located within the epidermis or between the epidermis and dermis. Inflammation of the skin due to chemical irritants, allergens, or physical agents often leads to cellular disintegration and accumulation of free fluid. Vesicles are the prime lesions of acute dermatitis. *Bullae* are vesicles larger than 0.5 cm in diameter. *Pustules* are vesicles containing purulent fluid. It is important for diagnosis to note the following features of the vesicles or bullae: (1) the contents (serous, sanguinous, or purulent fluid); (2) the roof (intact, tough, fragile, or umbilicated); (3) the tension (firm or flaccid); (4) the base (normal skin, erythema, or urticaria); and (5) the relationship of one vesicle to the others (grouped or isolated). These special features, combined with the distribution of the eruption, permit accurate clinical diagnosis of many vesicular diseases. *Herpes simplex* (Chap. 226) is characterized by a single lesion composed of clear or purulent, umbilicated, tough, tense, grouped vesicles on an erythematous base. Multiple lesions, each showing the features of herpes simplex, located in a linear pattern along a nerve root distribution are diagnostic of *herpes zoster* (Chap. 225). Isolated, tense, serous, or serosanguinous bullae on urticarial bases surrounded by concentric rings of normal skin and urticarial rings form the classic "target" or "iris" lesions of erythema multiforme. Isolated pustules surmounting purpuric macules at the tips of the digits represent septic emboli and are cutaneous signs of bacteremia.

SECONDARY LESIONS OF THE SKIN. The secondary lesions of the skin represent sequential or evolutionary changes in primary lesions.

Crusts. Crusts are the dried remains of exudates and may be composed of dried blood, serum, or pus. Crusts are usually situated on oozing erosions or ulcers that can be examined adequately only when the crusts are removed. Linear hemorrhagic crusts mark the sites of excoriations. Honey-colored, clear-yellow crusts are typical of *impetigo*. Impetigo is a superficial bacterial infection of the skin caused by staphylococci and/or beta hemo-

lytic streptococci. Glomerulonephritis is a common accompaniment of impetigo when beta hemolytic streptococci are present in the cutaneous lesions.

Scales. Scales are visible and palpable fragments of the horny outer layer of skin, the stratum corneum. Special features of scales are helpful in diagnosis. Scales may be dry or greasy, lighter or darker than the normal skin, fine or platelike, loose or adherent. Scales may develop on primary lesions, macules, or papules, or on otherwise normal-appearing skin. The greasy yellow scales of seborrheic dermatitis, the silvery piled-up scales of psoriasis, and dark fishlike scales of ichthyosis are diagnostic features of three scaling dermatoses.

Erosions and Ulcers. Erosions are circumscribed superficially denuded areas of skin which usually heal without scarring. Ulcers occur when there is deeper destruction of the cutis and subcutaneous tissues. The etiologic factors concerned in the production of an ulcer may be single or multiple. Although repeated minor trauma is usually the primary cause of leg ulcers in elderly patients, the delayed healing and extension of the ulcer is a consequence of superimposed bacterial infection in individuals with peripheral vascular disease. Table 55-1 lists the conditions which are responsible for ulcers of the lower extremities, including physical agents, infections, vascular diseases, hematologic diseases, neurologic deficits, and neoplasia. The development of squamous cell carcinoma is a recognized risk in chronic ulcers from any cause. The presence of an ulcer demands a thorough investigation to elucidate the underlying causative factor. Biopsy of any ulcer which does not respond to specific therapy for the causative factor is mandatory in order to rule out superimposed neoplastic disease.

Lichenification. Thickening of the skin accompanied by an accentuation of the normal superficial skin markings is termed lichenification. The affected skin is studded with closely set papular elevations separated from each other by delicate furrows. Hyperpigmentation often is present in lichenified areas of skin. Since lichenification is produced by continued irritation of the skin, most commonly from scratching, it is found in many chronic pruritic dermatoses. In localized neurodermatitis (*lichen simplex chronicus*), lichenification and excoriations are the only skin changes to be found. The skin of the antecubital and popliteal fossae classically becomes lichenified in the juvenile and adult types of atopic dermatitis.

Scars. Scars are usually the result of severe dermal injury. In most cases, scars are preceded by ulcers, but dermal diseases, such as discoid lupus erythematosus, cause scars without previous ulceration. It is always dangerous to attempt to make a dermatologic diagnosis from scars alone. Hypertrophy, elevation, and pruritus are common in surgical or traumatic scars. *Keloids* are nodular, firm, generally linear masses of hyperplastic connective tissue which occur in the dermis and subcutaneous tissue after a traumatic injury or burn. The histologic changes in keloids and hypertrophic scars differ only in degree. In keloids the antecedent trauma is often trivial, and constitutional or hereditary factors play a predominant role.

Table 55-1. COMMON ULCERS OF THE
LOWER EXTREMITIES

I. Vascular disorders
   A. Large arteries
      1. Thromboangiitis obliterans
      2. Arteriosclerosis obliterans
      3. Acute arterial occlusion
   B. Small arteries and arterioles
      1. Livedo reticularis
      2. Chronic pernio
      3. Periarteritis nodosa
      4. Hypertensive ischemic leg ulcer
      5. Vasculitis—allergic, rheumatoid
   C. Veins
      1. Chronic venous insufficiency
   D. Arteries and veins
      1. Hemangioma
      2. Arteriovenous fistula
II. Blood dyscrasias
   A. Sickle-cell anemia
   B. Thalassemia
   C. Polycythemia vera
   D. Hereditary spherocytosis
III. Dysproteinemias
   A. Cryoglobulins
   B. Macroglobulins
IV. Infections
   A. Bacterial
      1. Tuberculosis
      2. Syphilis
      3. Chancroid
      4. Granuloma inguinale
      5. Amebiasis cutis
      6. Diphtheria cutis
      7. Pyodermas
      8. Leprosy
      9. Yaws
     10. Leishmaniasis
     11. "Tropical" ulcers
     12. Anthrax
     13. Tularemia
     14. Osteomyelitis
   B. Mycotic
      1. Blastomycosis
      2. Sporotrichosis
      3. Chromoblastomycosis
      4. Coccidioidomycosis
V. Neoplasms
   A. Squamous cell carcinoma
   B. Lymphoma
      1. Mycosis fungoides
      2. Hodgkin's disease
      3. Leukemia cutis
      4. Lymphosarcoma
   C. Melanoma
   D. Sarcoma
      1. Kaposi's sarcoma
      2. Dermatofibrosarcoma
VI. Neuropathic
   A. Trophic ulcers in diabetes, tabes dorsalis, polyneuritis
VII. Drug Reaction
   A. Iododerma
   B. Bromoderma

Table 55-1. COMMON ULCERS OF THE
LOWER EXTREMITIES (*Continued*)

VIII. Traumatic Factors
   A. Factitial
   B. Neurotic excoriations
   C. Insect bites
   D. Radiodermatitis
   E. Decubitus
   F. Physical injury
      1. Trench foot
      2. Immersion foot
      3. Frostbite
      4. Acute pernio
      5. Thermal burns
   G. Chemical burns
X. Miscellaneous
   A. Scleroderma
   B. Lupus erythematosus
   C. Pyoderma gangrenosum
   D. Relapsing febrile nodular nonsuppurative panniculitis

ARRANGEMENT OF LESIONS. Familiarity with the configuration or arrangement of multiple lesions is helpful in establishing a diagnosis of a dermatologic disease. Some dermatoses are characterized by the presence of discrete lesions; other dermatoses are characterized by special relationships or arrangements of multiple lesions in groups, annular or linear patterns, etc.

Grouping. Clusters or close aggregates of multiple vesicles are present in herpes simplex and herpes zoster. A symmetrical eruption of grouped, excoriated vesicles, papules, and scars clustered over the knees, elbows, sacrum, and scapulae occurs in *dermatitis herpetiformis* (Chap. 400).

Annularity. One of the most important configurations seen in the skin is the circle or arc of lesions surrounding normal skin. Annular, papular lesions occur in secondary syphilis, sarcoid, leprosy, discoid lupus erythematosus, and lichen planus. The characteristic lesion of granuloma annulare is a circle of papules or nodules on the extensor surfaces of joints. Evanescent annular erythematous macules occur over the joints in erythema rheumaticum, the cutaneous manifestation of rheumatic fever. Ringworm infections of the glabrous skin (tinea corporis) are characterized by papular, vesicular, scaling, annular lesions which clear centrally and extend peripherally. It is always possible to demonstrate the fungi in scrapings from the lesions of ringworm infections (see below).

Linearity. Linear arrangements of lesions occur in herpes zoster and warty linear epidermal nevi. Localized linear scleroderma may cause deformities by retarding the growth of underlying bones and muscles when it involves the face or extremities of children. Autoinoculation of warts along a scratch results in linear lesions. Similar linear lesions may occur in patients with psoriasis and lichen planus when their skin responds to nonspecific trauma by producing new lesions. Acute vesicular linear lesions aid in differentiating plant dermatitis (poison ivy or oak) from other types of contact dermatitis. Linear distribution of pink, scaling, oval lesions along the cleavage lines of the trunk result in the "Christmas tree" pattern of pityriasis rosea.

Chancriform Complex or Primary Inoculation Pattern. The special configuration of an initial inflammatory papule or ulcerative lesion at the site of inoculation, with the subsequent development of inflammatory nodules in a linear pattern along the lymphatic drainage or with regional adenopathy, is termed the chancriform complex. Primary cutaneous inoculation of bacteria as in syphilis, tuberculosis, and tularemia may follow this pattern (Chap. 155). Sporotrichosis is the commonest naturally occurring deep fungus infection that produces the primary inoculation pattern. Accidental cutaneous inoculation of blastomycosis and coccidiomycosis occurring in laboratory workers also causes a chancriform complex. The recognition of the primary inoculation pattern of reaction is important, since the specific organism can usually be detected in smears or cultures prepared from the primary lesion. Appropriate cultural procedures and biopsies confirm the diagnosis in tuberculosis and the deep mycoses.

DISTRIBUTION OF LESIONS. An important clinical feature of all eruptions is the distribution of lesions over the body. In some dermatoses the distribution is so characteristic of the eruption as to be diagnostic. The lesions may be localized or generalized. Generalized eruptions may be universal and involve the whole cutaneous surface or disseminated and composed of discrete lesions widely scattered over the skin. Disseminated eruptions may be symmetrical or asymmetrical. Areas of the body exposed to specific environmental factors or containing specialized epidermal appendages are the areas of involvement in certain eruptions.

Localized Distribution. In addition to the diseases occurring in linear or chancriform patterns, there are several dermatoses which primarily involve localized areas of the skin surface. Recurrent herpes simplex is characteristically a single lesion which repeatedly involves the same area, most commonly the lips or genitalia. The fixed drug eruption recurs as an acute urticarial or bullous lesion at the same "fixed" site with each exposure to the drug. The fixed site of acute reaction is marked by a hyperpigmented macule that persists between attacks. Certain compounds, such as phenolphthalein in proprietary laxatives, are notoriously associated with fixed drug reactions. Contact allergic dermatitis due to metals in solid objects characteristically causes a localized eruption at the sites of contact, e.g., ear lobes in earring dermatitis and discrete patches on the anterior and posterior thighs in garter dermatitis.

Universal Eruptions. Universal erythema with or without massive scaling is a reaction pattern of the skin. Investigation for the underlying precipitating factor in universal exfoliative erythrodermas is mandatory. Drug reactions, neoplastic diseases, especially the lymphomas, and aggravation of preceding dermatosis, such as psoriasis, may be the cause of universal erythroderma.

Disseminated Symmetrical Eruptions. In several dermatoses the distribution of lesions on one side of the body is an exact mirror image of the other side. Dermatoses due to intrinsic factors, such as drug eruptions, are commonly symmetrical eruptions. Psoriasis is a symmetrical eruption of erythematous silvery scaling plaques involving the elbows, knees, and scalp. Symmetrical, thickened, excoriated plaques of chronic dermatitis involve the antecubital and popliteal fossae in juvenile and adult patients with atopic dermatitis.

Special Areas of Involvement. Dermatoses related to environmental factors involve special areas. Distribution is limited to *exposed areas* in dermatitis where sunlight or air-borne pollens or chemicals play a causative role. Involvement of the face, neck, V-area of the chest, dorsum of the hands and arms, ending abruptly at the sleeve-level, occur in these eruptions. The anatomically shaded areas, the upper eyelids, retroauricular folds, and submental regions, are not involved in photosensitive eruptions, but are involved in air-borne dust dermatitis. *Sebaceous areas,* where sebaceous glands and hair follicles are abundant, are affected by acne, rosacea, and seborrheic dermatitis. In addition to the face, acne involves the neck, shoulders, and upper back and chest, but spares the scalp. Rosacea remains confined to the face, primarily to the flush areas. Seborrheic dermatitis involves the scalp, eyebrows, eyelid margins, sides of the nose, and external auditory canals. The *intertriginous areas, axillae,* inframammary, and anogenital regions, are also common sites of involvement in seborrheic dermatitis, psoriasis, erythrasma, and cutaneous moniliasis. The *pretibial region* is the characteristic site of four dermatoses: erythema nodosum, localized cutaneous myxedema, lichen amyloidosis, and necrobiosis lipoidica diabeticorum. These pretibial eruptions are usually bilateral. Involvement of *mucosal surfaces* is a common and diagnostically helpful feature in diseases which also involve the skin. A lacy white network on the buccal mucosa is pathognomonic of lichen planus. Vesicles and bullae rarely remain intact on mucosal surfaces. Erosions, the sequential lesions of bullae, occur on the tongue, gingiva, buccal, pharyngeal, nasal, and genital mucosa in erythema multiforme and pemphigus vulgaris.

DERMATOLOGIC LABORATORY PROCEDURES. In addition to the laboratory procedures used in general medicine, several special procedures are necessary in establishing or confirming the diagnosis of diseases of the skin.

Wood's Light. A special Wood's filter, which transmits ultraviolet light with wavelengths from 3100 to over 4000 Å, is used in conjunction with a hot quartz or fluorescent light source. Substances that are activated by the wavelengths transmitted through the Wood's filter will fluoresce. The demonstration of fluorescence of a specific color is an important test in porphyria cutanea tarda (Chap. 108), erythrasma, and tinea capitis (ringworm of the scalp hair). The urine in porphyria cutanea tarda fluoresces bright red with the light transmitted through a Wood's filter. Porphyrins produced by cornybacteria cause a distinctive coral-red fluorescence in the involved intertriginous areas in erythrasma (Chap. 400). The teeth are fluorescent in erythropoietic porphyria and in the dental abnormalities in infants caused by tetracyclines. The green-blue fluorescence of infected hairs is a useful screening procedure in epidemic scalp ringworm.

Potassium Hydroxide (KOH) Preparations. The demonstration of hyphae in fungus infections and budding spores in moniliasis is an office procedure which rapidly establishes the diagnosis. The skin is cleansed with alcohol. Scrapings from scaling lesions, tops of vesicles, clippings from nails, or plucked hairs, are placed on a glass slide in a drop of 10% aqueous potassium hydroxide and covered with a cover slip. The KOH preparation is warmed gently over a match or alcohol lamp. Clearing occurs rapidly as the keratin structures dissolve. The fragile hyphae, spores, or budding yeasts are visible in the cleared preparation under "high dry" magnification. A positive KOH preparation is tantamount to a diagnosis. The investigation of all annular scaling or vesicular lesions, all thickened discolored nails, and hairs from

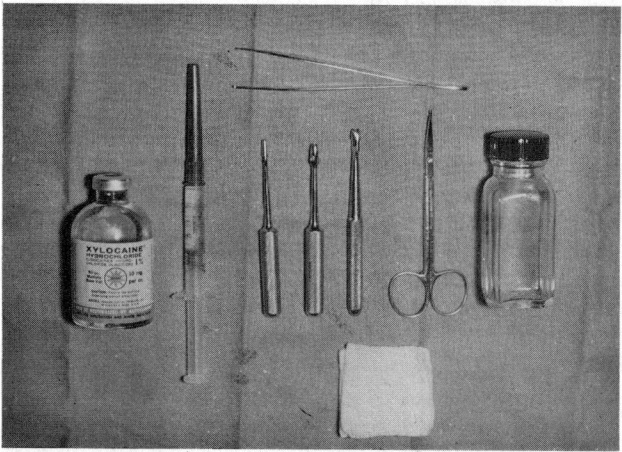

A

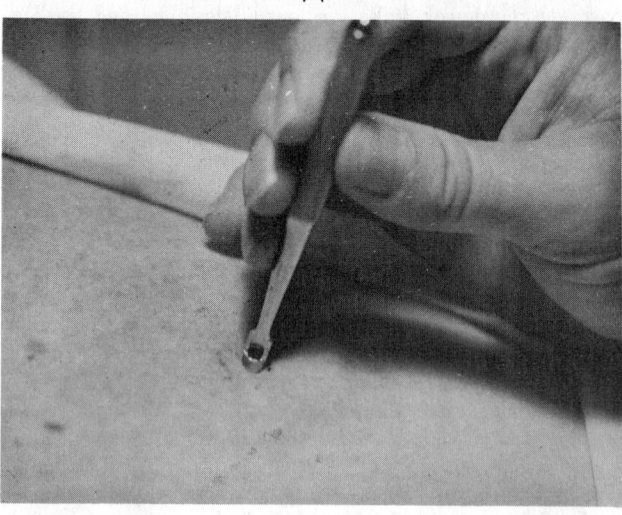

B

Fig. 55-1. *A.* Biopsy of cutaneous lesions requires the following equipment: a local anesthetic, biopsy punches, forceps, and scissors. Biopsy punches are available in graduated sizes from 2 to 6 mm in diameter. *B.* Skin sutures are ordinarily not necessary following punch biopsy. The tissue obtained by biopsy is placed in a formalin fixative.

patchy areas of hair loss, should include a KOH preparation. No dermatitis, nail dystrophy, or localized hair loss should be treated as a fungus infection unless positive KOH preparations have been obtained. The specific fungus or yeast responsible for the positive KOH preparation can be defined by culturing samples of the infected keratin (scales, hairs, nails) on Sabouraud's medium at room temperature. Since it takes approximately 3 weeks of growth to identify fungus cultures, the treatment of superficial fungus infections is ordinarily started on the basis of positive KOH preparations alone.

Cytologic Smears and Imprints. Diagnostic cytologic changes occur in pemphigus, herpes simplex, zoster, and varicella. The roof of the youngest vesicle or bulla is split with a scalpel and reflected. The inner surface of the reflected roof and the denuded floor of the vesicle are scraped gently with a scalpel. The white cellular material is transferred to a glass slide and rapidly air-dried. The slide is placed in Giemsa stain for 1 min, flushed with tap water, and examined microscopically. The giant multinucleated epidermal cells which are the diagnostic cytologic changes of herpes simplex, zoster, and varicella, are not present in vaccinia and variola. Loss of prickles (desmosomes), the basic cellular change in the epidermal cells in pemphigus, is referred to as *acantholysis*. The presence of many acantholytic cells, individual small rounded cells with large nuclei and basophilic peripheral condensations of cytoplasm, in smears from bullae is diagnostic of pemphigus. The definitive diagnosis of the type of pemphigus depends on clinical features and biopsies showing the level of the epidermis at which acantholysis first appears.

Cytologic imprints are prepared by firmly pressing the cut surface of an excised full-thickness piece of skin on a clean glass slide. Inflammatory and neoplastic cells in dermal infiltrates will adhere to the slide and may be stained with any hematologic stain. This procedure is particularly useful in defining the cellular type of lymphomatous lesions of the skin.

Biopsy. Since many cutaneous diseases have specific histologic changes, biopsies are useful in diagnosis. Biopsy is a mandatory procedure in the investigation of lesions suspected of being neoplastic. Tumors of sufficiently small size and suspected malignant melanomas regardless of size should be removed *in toto* by excision biopsy. With other tumors, a 4-mm punch biopsy yields sufficient tissue for histologic diagnosis. Multiple punch biopsies may be required to detect malignant changes in large ulcers. In order to establish the diagnosis in dermatoses, the youngest primary lesion, free from secondary or sequential changes, should be chosen for biopsy. Punch biopsies are particularly useful in the investigation of bullous eruptions; papular scaling eruptions, such as psoriasis and lichen planus; granulomatous diseases, such as tuberculosis, leprosy, and the deep mycoses; purpuric eruptions; and deposition diseases, such as xanthomas and amyloidosis. The characteristic histologic changes in cutaneous lesions aid in establishing the diagnosis in such systemic diseases as sarcoidosis, lupus erythematosus, scleroderma, and dermatomyositis.

Intradermal Tests. The detection of immediate urticarial reactions by scratch or intradermal tests of common pollens, foods, etc. is of limited usefulness in the study of skin diseases. The recognition of the delayed "tuberculin-type" of allergy (Chap. 68) is important dermatologically in the study of both systemic granulomatous and cutaneous granulomatous diseases. The most commonly used intradermal antigens are tuberculin, blastomycin, histoplasmin, and coccidioidin. Less commonly used antigens are mumps, trichophytin, trichenella, Frei antigen of lymphogranuloma venereum, lepromin, and Kveim. Negative reactions to mumps and trichophytin antigen are important in defining anergic states. Kveim antigen is a crude tissue homogenate prepared from lymph nodes or spleens involved with sarcoid. Patients with active sarcoidosis develop pure epithelioid tubercles which are detectable microscopically on skin biopsy of the site where the antigen had been injected intradermally 6 weeks previously.

Patch Tests. The patch test is a useful procedure in the diagnosis of contact allergic dermatitis. The diagnostic patch testing procedure is based on the principle that skin previously sensitized to an antigen will show an eczematous reaction at the site of subsequent applications of that specific antigen (Chap. 68). The suspected substance is applied to the skin and covered by an occlusive cellophane patch held in place by an adhesive plaster. The patch test is removed in 48 hr. A positive patch test, a reproduction of the disease in miniature, consists of erythema, papules, palpable edema, or vesicles. The intelligent use of patch testing depends on careful questioning to detect possible offenders. Known primary irritants such as strong acids, alkalis, soaps, and solvents must be used in only very dilute concentrations for patch testing. Patch tests should not be performed during acute episodes of dermatitis or while the patient is receiving systemic corticosteroid therapy.

PHYSICAL ALLERGY. The production of the disease in miniature by the application of the appropriate stimulus is a useful procedure in the investigation of physical allergies. Cold urticaria is confirmed by the development of an acute urticarial reaction at the site of contact of the skin with an ice cube. A hot bath or exercise induces a generalized eruption of small wheals surrounded by large erythematous flares in generalized cholinergic urticaria. Local heat hypersensitivity is confirmed by eliciting a wheal at the site of local heating of the skin. Photosensitivity testing is a specialized procedure requiring a hot quartz or carbon arc ultraviolet light source. Only small areas of skin should be exposed to light testing in order to avoid generalized or systemic reactions (Chap. 59).

56 ITCHING
Faye D. Arundell and Eugene M. Farber

Pruritus, or itching, is a unique cutaneous symptom that is best described as an unpleasant sensation which provokes the desire to scratch. It is specifically an epidermal sensation which depends on the presence of free unmyelinated nerve endings between the cells of the epidermis. Stimulation of these free nerve endings initiates impulses that travel the same nervous pathways as pain along the lateral spinothalamic tract to the thalamus. Itching evokes the purposive motor response of scratching. Pain, though an allied sensation, evokes reflex withdrawal.

Itching, unlike pain, occurs nowhere but in the skin. Removal of the epidermis abolishes the itching end organ but does not interfere with the perception of pain. Stimuli that will initiate itching are usually of milder degree than those which cause pain. Any mechanical, thermal, or chemical stimulus causing an appropriate degree of injury will induce itching if the epidermis is present. A number of chemicals, released or activated in various ways, appear to function as mediators of pruritus. Extremely low concentrations of proteases, kinins, and histamine cause itching.

Pruritus may be perceived, interpreted, and described by the patient as burning, prickling, stinging, or itching. There is a marked variation in individual itching thresholds. Atopic individuals in general are "itchy people" and have a low itch threshold. Pruritus causes a lowering of the threshold in the affected area, resulting in stimulation of itching by progressively milder stimuli. Scratching, the reflex response to itching, also decreases the itch threshold. A vicious cycle of itching, scratching, and itching may become established in cutaneous regions of lowered thresholds to itch. Vasodilatation lowers the itch threshold and may account for the circadian rhythm of itching, which is usually worse at night. Strong stimuli, such as pain and extremes of temperature, inhibit pruritus. Many severely itching patients learn to substitute pain for itch by pinching the skin adjacent to itching areas or by completely denuding the itchy region. Extremely cold applications give temporary relief which is promptly followed by aggravation of itching.

GENERALIZED PRURITUS

Generalized and persistent pruritus, which is not accompanied by demonstrable skin lesions other than excoriations, is associated with a variety of systemic diseases. Pruritus of sudden onset which is generalized and persistent demands a general medical investigation. The most commonly associated diseases are obstructive jaundice, lymphomas, internal cancers, severe renal insufficiency, and diabetes mellitus. Obstructive hepatic disease causing pruritus is detectable on physical examination, since the patients are invariably jaundiced. Pruritus may be out of proportion to the degree of jaundice, however; severe itching may occur with mild jaundice, and severe jaundice may be unaccompanied by pruritus. The severity of itching correlates better with the accumulation of bile salts than with increased bile pigments. (Chap. 45).

Lymphatic leukemia, Hodgkin's disease, lymphosarcoma, and mycosis fungoides are the lymphomas which cause generalized pruritus. Pruritus in the absence of any primary skin change may be the first manifestation of these diseases. Generalized exfoliative dermatitis, with an aggravation of the pruritus, may develop in the course of any of these lymphomas. The mechanism of the pruritus is unknown, but once specific tumors actually develop in the skin, they no longer itch. Other forms of internal neoplastic disease, such as carcinoma, may also be associated with generalized pruritus. Generalized pruritus in the absence of other systemic diseases always deserves complete study to detect hidden malignancies.

Persistent generalized itching occurs in advanced cases of uremia. Relief of renal failure gives prompt relief of the pruritus. Neither urea nor uric acid is responsible for pruritus, and the chemical mediator of uremic itching is unknown.

Generalized pruritus is usually out of proportion to the severity of diabetes mellitus. In a few diabetics pruritus cannot be explained on any other basis. Most commonly, however, diabetic itching is due to the excessive dryness of the skin rather than to the state of the diabetes. Xerotic skin, which has a decreased water-holding capacity, develops scaling, fine fissures or chapping, and a low itching threshold. Dry heat, cold winds, and frequent bathing aggravate the xerosis. Localized pruritus of the anogenital region of diabetics is usually caused by superficial *Candida albicans* infections.

ITCHY DERMATOLOGIC DISEASES

The cause of pruritus due to dermatologic diseases is evident on inspection of the skin. Since superficial damage causes itching, stimuli of sufficient degrees to cause pruritus usually leave a marker on the skin. Such stimuli may be extrinsic, as in infestations and infections, intrinsic as in immediate urticarial reactions, or a combination of these as in eczematous dermatitis.

INFESTATIONS AND INFECTIONS. Urticarial papules topped by puncta mark the sites of bites. The distribution of the bites depends on the living and feeding habits of the parasite. Flea bites are most common on the lower extremities because fleas are jumping rather than flying insects. The excoriated bites in pediculosis commonly become secondarily infected. The lice and their eggs are usually not found on the skin, since they only feed there, but are present on the hairs or clothing where they reside. A generalized eruption of excoriated papules is present in scabies, but the mite will be found only in burrows in the outer horny layer of the interdigital spaces, flexor surfaces of the wrists, axillary folds, buttocks, areola, and penis.

Pruritus is a common symptom in superficial fungus and yeast infections. Superficial candidiasis is extremely pruritic when it involves the intertriginous areas of the axillae, anogenital, and inframammary regions. The lesions of cutaneous moniliasis are sharply limited, macerated, red patches surrounded by loose epithelial fringes and satellite pustules. Tinea cruris and corporis (ringworm of the groin and body) cause itchy annular lesions with advancing raised scaling or vesicular borders. Potassium hydroxide–treated smears of the scales in moni-

liasis contain budding yeasts, and in tinea they reveal fragile hyphae.

URTICARIA. The pathophysiology of the urticarial reaction is based on the liberation of histamine from mast cells around dermal blood vessels. The liberated histamine increases vascular permeability, and the accumulation of the transudate in the dermis causes visibly raised wheals, "hives." Sufficiently large accumulations compress the subepidermal vascular plexus resulting in a pale or blanched appearance of the wheal. A zone of reflex vasodilation creates an erythematous flare around the wheal. Wheals are transient; each lesion disappears within hours, though new lesions may continue to appear. All of these effects can be induced by injections of histamine intradermally. Amounts of histamine sufficient to cause wheals and flares also cause itching.

The stimuli which result in the release of histamine from mast cells are varied. In clinical medicine the important histamine-releasing stimuli are those which cause physical urticaria and allergic urticaria of the acute and chronic type. Physical stimuli, such as heat, cold, sunlight, and pressure, are causes of urticaria, and this can be confirmed by the reproduction of the lesion with appropriate applications of the stimulus to the skin. Certain drugs, such as morphine and codeine, cause histamine release and urticaria by their direct action on mast cells. Immediate types of allergic reactions are mediated by circulating antibodies which act indirectly through the activation of proteases and esterases to cause histamine release from mast cells. In general, the antigens responsible for these immediate allergic urticarial reactions reach the skin via the systemic circulation after they have been ingested or injected. Food and drug allergies are the commonest causes of acute urticaria. The detection of the underlying factors in chronic recurrent urticaria requires a thorough investigation of drug ingestion, physical factors, infections, parasites, ingested and inhaled allergens, and emotional factors.

ECZEMATOUS DERMATITIS. Itching is the predominant symptom of dermatitis. The hallmarks of acute dermatitis are erythema, vesicles, oozing, and crusting. Scaling and thickening of the skin develop as the dermatitis becomes subacute and chronic. Accentuation of the normal surface markings gives the skin a thick leathery appearance, which is referred to as *lichenification*. The basic histologic change in dermatitis is the accumulation of fluid between the cells of the epidermis. As the amount of fluid increases, disruption of the connections between epidermal cells occurs, and microscopic and macroscopic vesicles and bullae form. The reparative phases, subacute and chronic dermatitis, are marked by an accelerated rate of epidermal cell division and delayed cellular maturation. The number of cell layers in the epidermis increases, resulting in thickening. An imperfect keratin layer forms, and scaling results.

Several types of injury may initiate dermatitis. Physical injury, such as extremes of temperature, radiation, and mechanical trauma, may cause dermatitis. Chemicals, namely acids, alkalis, soaps, and detergents, damage the epidermis and cause dermatitis by their direct primary irritant action. These irritants are responsible for the common hand eczemas of housewives. Allergic mechanisms of the delayed type cause allergic contact dermatitis. Simple chemicals become complete antigens after conjugation with proteins in the skin. Once antibodies have been formed to the protein-chemical conjugate, the skin will react in an eczematous pattern on each subsequent contact between the skin and the chemical. The allergic eczematous reactions are of the delayed type, and 24 or more hours may elapse before detectable changes and itching appear. Contact allergic dermatitis is exemplified by poison ivy dermatitis. Simple chemicals, such as mercury, chrome, and nickel, are common contact antigens responsible for metal (jewelry, garters), leather, and cement dermatitis. More complicated chemicals, such as those in dyes, adhesives, and resins, are important antigens in occupational contact allergic dermatitis (See Chaps. 116 and 117). The most insidious type of contact dermatitis, that caused by antigenic constituents in topical medications, is commonly responsible for prolonging or aggravating dermatitis.

The same factors that initiate dermatitis will aggravate and prolong it. Mechanical damage caused by rubbing and scratching is an important factor. Primary irritation caused by excessive use of soap and water prolongs dermatitis. Excessive dehydration, brittleness, and chapping of the skin are aggravated by overbathing, which further decreases the skin's tolerance to primary irritants. Dryness of the skin aggravated by overbathing is an important factor in the winter, or senile, dermatitis which occurs on the extremities. Stasis in the venous system predisposes to dermatitis of the lower extremities and prolongs any dermatitis in these areas. Sweating tends to aggravate dermatitis, since sweating in the occluded sweat ducts in an area of dermatitis leads to rupture of the ducts and release of irritating sweat into the skin. Vigorous exercise and hot, humid atmospheres will aggravate dermatitis by superimposing *miliaria* ("prickly heat") on the involved areas.

Hereditary or constitutional factors predispose to a common clinical type of dermatitis. *Atopic dermatitis* is an eczematous dermatitis which occurs in individuals who have an inherited tendency to develop asthma and hay fever. The development of atopic dermatitis in these persons is a function of dry, sensitive, itchy skin and does not usually correlate with episodes of allergic rhinitis or asthma. In infants atopic dermatitis is characterized by vesicular crusted eczematous patches on the cheeks and extensor aspects of the extremities. The character and distribution of the eruption change with age. In atopic dermatitis of juveniles and adults the main areas of involvement are thickened, lichenified excoriated plaques of the antecubital and popliteal fossae, face, and neck. At all ages and in all stages atopic dermatitis is an exceedingly itchy eruption, and the patient must be protected from all of the factors which initiate or aggravate pruritus.

Persistent localized patches of chronic dermatitis are prone to develop in patients in whom the itch-scratch cycle has become firmly established. The lichenified patches of *lichen simplex chronicus* are usually single or few in number. They are usually located in areas which the patient can conveniently reach for scratching purposes, namely, the ankles, calves, occiput, vulva, and perianal regions. Underlying factors responsible for initiating or prolonging the itch-scratch cycle should be investigated. Anal and vulvar pruritus may be initiated by seborrheic dermatitis, psoriasis, pinworm infections, moniliasis, reactions to oral antibiotics, diabetes mellitus, and contact dermatitis. Stasis factors, constricting clothing, and superimposed contact dermatitis from topical medications, prolong the itch-scratch cycle.

TREATMENT. Since itching is a symptom, the most effective approach is to detect and eliminate the cause. Removal of the offending parasite, drug, irritant, or antigen in dermatitis or urticaria and institution of appropriate treatment of the underlying systemic disease in cases of generalized pruritus are basic approaches. Ancillary and symptomatic care is directed toward the protection of the skin from all the factors which are known to aggravate and prolong dermatitis. Antihistamines and salicylates are useful oral medications for pruritus. It is inadvisable, however, to prescribe corticosteroids in the absence of a specific diagnosis.

Specific treatment in patients with generalized pruritus is dependent on treating the underlying systemic disease, such as obstructive jaundice, renal failure, diabetes, lymphomas, and malignancies. Such specific approaches offer the only chance for relief of pruritus in these disorders. Cholestyramine therapy, in oral doses of 10 g daily, is helpful in reducing the pruritus accompanying the jaundice of hepatic diseases which are not amenable to surgical relief of the obstruction (Chap. 45).

One application of a thin layer of 1 percent gamma benzene hydrochloride (Kwell) lotion or cream left on the entire skin surface for 24 hr is effective treatment for pediculosis and scabies. Tolnaftate (Tinactin) solution or undecylenic acid (Desenex) ointment applied twice daily to the affected areas is the treatment of choice in tinea pedis, cruris, and corporis. Griseofulvin, the systemic fungistatic agent, is reserved for the treatment of tinea capitis, resistant tinea corporis, and onychomycosis. The average dose of griseofulvin for adults is 1.0 Gm p.o. daily. Better absorption is obtained if the drug is taken at the end of a fatty meal or in the micronized form. Griseofulvin is fungistatic, not fungicidal, and is concentrated in keratin structures such as the hair, nails, and stratum corneum as they are formed. The antibiotic must be taken until the old infected keratin structures are shed and replaced by new keratin containing the drug. Griseofulvin is effective against dermatophytic fungi, but it is not effective against *C. albicans* and the organisms causing tinea versicolor, erythrasma, and the deep mycoses. Nystatin is an effective topical antimonilial agent. It is not absorbed from the gastrointestinal tract and must be applied locally as a lotion, cream, or powder.

Oral antihistamines are effective antipruritic agents and are the mainstay of the symptomatic treatment of urticaria. The specific treatment of the patient with urticaria depends on determining and eliminating the cause, whether it be a drug, food, physical factor, or infection. The most popular antihistamines are diphenhydramine (Benadryl) 50 mg t. i. d., dexachlorpheniramine (Polaramine), 2 mgm t. i. d., and cyproheptadine (Periactin), 4 mg q. i. d. Large doses, up to 600 mg Benadryl daily, are required to suppress severe urticarial drug reactions. Antihistamines may cause drug eruptions when they are administered parenterally. Since they are potent topical sensitizers, they should never be applied to the skin.

Eczematous reactions of the contact type respond to elimination of the offending antigen or irritant. The patient must permanently avoid contact with the antigen in order to remain free of the disease. Patch testing is a valuable investigative procedure in determining the offending antigens in the allergic type of contact dermatitis (Chap. 55).

The therapeutic program for all types of eczematous dermatitis includes symptomatic treatment of pruritus and discomfort and protection of the skin from all factors that aggravate or prolong dermatitis. Oral antihistamines relieve pruritus and prevent aggravation from scratching. Tepid tap water and open compresses relieve oozing, crusting, and vasodilation during the acute vesicular phases of dermatitis. Corticosteroid (0.5 percent hydrocortisone, 0.01 percent fluocinolone acetonide, or 0.025 percent triameinolone acetonide) lotions, creams, and ointments are potent antipruritics when they are applied as a thin layer q. i. d. to the affected areas in the subacute and chronic stages of dermatitis. Avoiding or limiting exposure to bathing and soap prevents aggravation of the dermatitis from excessive dehydration and primary irritation. The addition of bath oils to baths minimizes prolongation of chronic dermatitis. Bed rest and elevation of the legs relieve stasis factors in dermatitis of the lower legs. A uniform environmental temperature, loose clothing, and restriction of physical exercise prevents aggravation of dermatitis from overheating and sweating. The use of compounds which are known potent contact antigens, such as topical anesthetics, topical antihistamines, and certain topical antibiotics, should be minimized.

57 ALOPECIA AND HIRSUTISM

Faye D. Arundell and Eugene M. Farber

The cosmetic and psychologic significance of hair has increased as the biologic need for the protection from cold and trauma that hair provides has decreased. In Western societies, too much facial hair in women, too little scalp hair in men and women, and too much curl in the hair of Negroes are common endocrine and cosmetic concerns. The standards set by society outweigh those that are the physiologic norms determined by genetic and racial factors.

Genetic factors play an important role in determining the quantity, quality, and distribution of hair growth. The diameters of hairs from various body regions are the same in Caucasians and Japanese, but Orientals have scantier growth of beard, axillary, and pubic hair. The incidence of male baldness and female hirsutism is much lower in Japanese. This racial difference in hair growth may be attributable to a decreased sensitivity of the hair follicles to androgens, since there is no difference in the levels of plasma testosterone in Japanese and Caucasians. The ethnic differences in hair growth are striking in Caucasian women. The amount of facial hair and general hair growth which is normal for many women of Mediterranean stock would be grossly abnormal for most Nordics.

Hairs are cylindrical shafts composed of tightly fused hard keratin. The latter is a dead fibrous protein manufactured deep in the dermis. No trauma or treatment applied only to the dead hair can affect the vital proliferating hair follicle. Brushing, combing, shaving, cutting, bleaching, coloring, curling, or straightening may give psychologic and esthetic satisfaction to the individual, but none of these either stimulates or depresses hair growth. The epidermis cannot form new hair follicles after birth.

Hair follicles and sebaceous glands develop from the epidermis as a pilosebaceous unit in the third fetal month. Pilosebaceous units develop in all areas of the skin except the palms and soles. In some areas, such as the axillae and anogenital region, apocrine glands develop in association with the pilosebaceous unit.

The lower end of the hair follicle is expanded into the hair bulb, which lies deep in the dermis. An invagination in the base of the bulb contains a capillary loop in a connective tissue papilla. The papilla is an intrinsic part of the hair follicle that persists through all phases of the hair cycle. A viable dermal papilla is essential for growth of the hair. Melanocytes which furnish pigment for the growing hair are located over the dermal papilla in the bulb. The bulb contains the mitotically active cells of the hair matrix that form the hair. The rapid growth of the matrix pushes toward the surface the differentiating keratinizing cells which make up the hair.

The rate of cellular reproduction in the hair matrix is among the fastest in the body and is equaled only by that of the bone marrow. As many as 30 percent of the cells in the matrix may be in mitosis at any given time. Each scalp terminal hair follicle produces 0.35 mm hair per day. The total production of hair proteins by the approximately 100,000 scalp follicles per day is a phenomenal metabolic task. Metabolic activity of this degree is susceptible to many systemic stresses. Interference with the mitotic activity in the matrix is immediately reflected in disturbances in hair production. Radiation therapy, radiomimetic drugs, antimetabolites, and toxic chemicals, such as thallium, interfere with the cellular reproduction of the hair follicle. Transient interference with protein synthesis results in deformities of the hair shaft, while more prolonged interference causes complete inhibition of hair growth and loss of hair. Increased hair growth occurs with stimuli which increase the temperature or blood flow in the skin. Hair grows faster in summer, in constantly traumatized areas, in skin adjacent to healing bone fractures, and in sympathectomized skin.

Humans have three types of hair: lanugo, vellus, and terminal. *Lanugo* is the prenatal soft, silky, unmedullated, and usually unpigmented hair which normally is replaced by vellus and terminal hairs. In postnatal life, fine, pale, short vellus hairs cover the whole surface of the body except the palms and soles. *Vellus* hairs are almost imperceptible but they persist even in bald scalps, and they are the only hairs present on the glabrous skin. Tactile nerve endings are intimately associated with vellus hair follicles. Specialized tactile sensory end organs are present in the nonhairy areas of the palms, soles, and lips.

Terminal hairs are the coarse, dark, long hairs which develop only in certain areas, such as the scalp, beard, and axillae. The differences in terminal hairs of various regions depend on the growth rate, length of the hair cycle, and physiologic responsiveness. Terminal hairs can be classified into six regional types: (1) scalp, (2) eyebrow and eyelash, (3) beard, (4) axillary, (5) pubic, (6) body. The hairs which make up the secondary sexual characteristics, namely, the beard, axillary, pubic, and body hair, are controlled by androgens in both males and females. The other regional types of hair require no sexual hormone stimulus, although they may be modified by androgens. Androgenic stimulation in genetically predisposed men results in male-pattern baldness. Men who have been castrated before puberty never develop axillary, beard, or pubic hair, and never become bald. Replacement hormonal therapy in eunuchs results in the normal hair growth which comprises secondary sexual characteristics and may result in baldness in the genetically susceptible.

Human hair follicles do not produce hair indefinitely. Each hair follicle's active production of hair is independent of that in neighboring follicles. The activity of each individual follicle is cyclic (Fig. 57-1). A period of mitotic activity and production of hair is followed by a period of involution and rest. The hair in the resting follicle develops a bulbous nonpigmented root, or club, by which it remains attached in the follicle. The resting phase is termed the *telogen* phase and its hair, the club hair. When the follicle becomes active once more, that is, when the *anagen* phase begins, the old club hair is pushed out of the follicle by the newly developing hair beneath it. A certain number of club hairs are shed each day. Approximately 5 to 10 percent of scalp hairs are in the resting phase at any one time, and 20 to 100 club hairs are shed daily. Under normal physiologic circumstances the total population of hair remains constant, since no club hair is shed unless an actively growing hair expels it.

The final length of hair depends on the duration of the growth phase of the cycle in the follicle producing the hair. Follicles in different body regions have active and resting phases of varying lengths. The resting phase of scalp hair must last only a few months, since only 5 to 10 percent of scalp hairs are in the resting phase at any one time. The duration of the growth cycle of hairs on the rest of the body is shorter, probably only 2 to 6 months, and the resting phase of the cycle is of equal duration.

Stimuli which affect the duration of the active part of the hair cycle will obviously have a profound effect on the length of the hair produced and the relative proportions of active and club hairs. A change in the normal proportion of 90 to 95 percent growing hairs and 5 to 10 per-

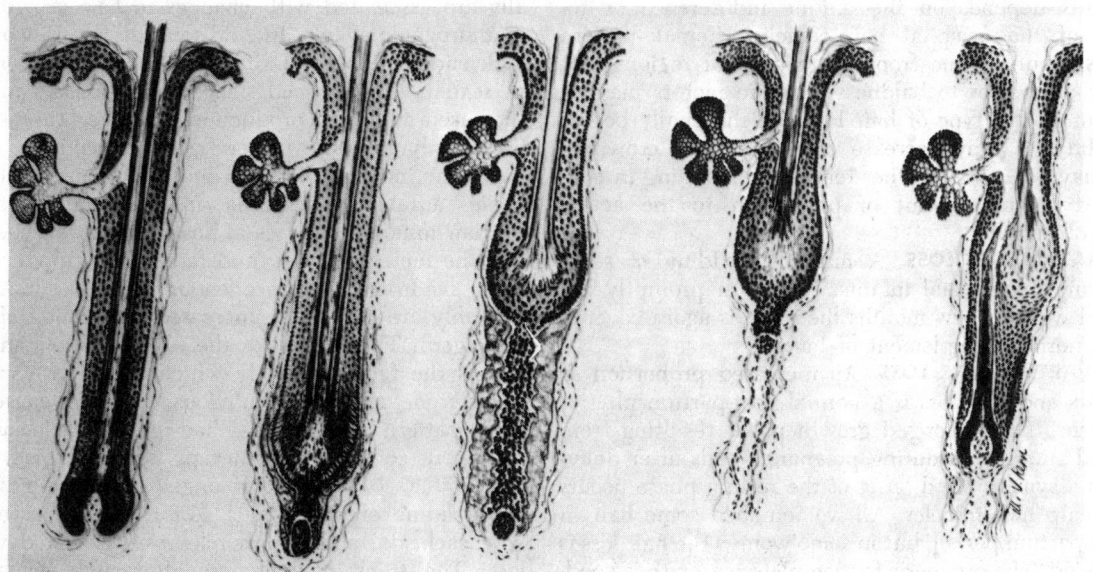

Fig. 57-1. Stages in hair cycle. Progressive changes from a growing (anagen) hair to a resting club hair (telogen)—second from right. In the normal human scalp, some 10 percent of the hairs are in the resting phase. In various types of alopecia, this percentage rises sharply and may be easily determined by the number of hairs which are easily removed by gentle traction. (*D. M. Pillsbury and W. B. Shelley*)

cent resting hairs on the scalp indicates a change in the cycle of hair growth. If the growth period in many follicles is shortened simultaneously, an increased number of club hairs is formed, resulting in a sudden noticeable increase in the hairs shed daily in the succeeding months. Synchronized onset of the resting phase causes the physiologic alopecia seen in newborns and post-partum women. Severe febrile diseases, emotional shock, and debilitating diseases cause a similar synchronized resting phase and hair loss.

ALOPECIA

The psychologic trauma caused by too little hair may be greater than that caused by too much hair. Loss of hair may be the result of physiologic factors or it may be secondary to endocrinologic abnormalities, systemic diseases, cutaneous diseases, infections of the hairs and hair follicles, or physical or chemical trauma.

MALE-PATTERN BALDNESS. A gradual decrease of scalp hair accompanies aging in the human. Male-pattern baldness is inevitable in the presence of androgenic stimuli in men with a genetic predisposition to baldness. The age of onset and the amount of hair lost in men depends on genetic factors. When baldness begins in the late teens, the prognosis is for a significant baldness in the thirties. Some loss over the frontal regions, forming an M-shaped hairline occurs in most men. The loss may progress relentlessly to the parietal regions and vertex, but a marginal fringe of hair in the temporal and occipital regions persists. There is no topical or systemic therapy that will alter the inevitable course of male-pattern baldness. However, the hair follicles from the occipital area maintain their resistance to male-pattern baldness when transplanted into bald areas of the vertex. The success of hair transplants depends on the unique indifference or resistance of the occipital hair follicles. Female-pattern hair loss occurs in the frontal and parietal regions, but it rarely progresses to baldness. Genetic factors may be important in this type of hair loss, which usually begins in middle age. Any decrease of a woman's "crowning glory" may be a threat to her femininity resulting in concern and complaints out of proportion to the actual amount of hair lost.

NEONATAL HAIR LOSS. A marked shedding of scalp hair occurs in neonatal infants. Regrowth promptly begins, and within a few months the scalp is again covered with its normal complement of hairs.

POST-PARTUM HAIR LOSS. An increased proportion of club hairs and hair loss is a normal post-partum physiologic event. The prolonged growth phase resulting from hormonal stimulation during pregnancy ends after delivery, and a synchronized onset of the resting phase occurs in the scalp hair follicles. All women shed some hair in the post-partum period, but in some women the hair loss is pronounced. The prognosis for complete regrowth is good.

ENDOCRINE DISTURBANCES. The effect of individual hormones on the hair growth of various laboratory animals has been the subject of many investigations. In animals growth hormone appears to be responsible for the

increase in hair-shaft diameter, and luteotropin governs the change from infantile to adult pelage. Thyroxine in some species increases both the rate of hair growth and the proportion of hairs in the growing phase of the hair growth cycle. Adrenalectomy also increases the proportion of actively growing hairs, while oophorectomy accelerates the shedding of hairs.

In some types of human hair loss accompanying endocrinologic disturbances, the causes can be deduced from knowledge of the experimental effects of hormones in laboratory animals. However, there are many instances of hair loss associated with endocrine diseases which are unexplained in humans and for which no animal models exist. The hair loss and scanty hair growth in hypopituitarism are compatible with the failure of development or maintenance of adult hair growth in the presence of growth hormone deficiency. The hypopituitary dwarf may be completely hairless, and patients with acquired hypopituitary states and Sheehan's syndrome rapidly lose hair from the axillae, pubis, and at times, the scalp. The importance of the role of growth hormone in human hair growth is confirmed by the increased hair growth and coarse hair of acromegaly.

In congenital cretinism lanugo hair may be retained, and the scalp hair is sparse and dry. In adults, hypothyroidism causes a decrease in the secondary sexual or hormonal hair of the axillae, pubis, and beard, in addition to the characteristic loss of the lateral aspects of the eyebrows. These effects can be related to the retardation of the onset of the growing phase of the hair cycle which follows thyroidectomy in animals. The reason for the growth of long hair on the back, shoulders, arms, and legs of children with hypothyroidism is obscure, as is the hair loss of hyperthyroidism.

Abnormalities of the adrenal glands and ovaries usually are associated with changes in hair growth related to androgenic effects. In Addison's disease in women, the deficiency of adrenal androgens is responsible for the loss of sexual, or hormonal, hair of the axillae and pubis. Increased androgen production in women causes the loss of scalp hair in the pattern of male baldness and produces the increase of facial and body hair which accompanies adrenal hyperplasia and virilizing adrenal and ovarian tumors. The loss of scalp hair in a male pattern and the increased body and facial hair growth of Cushing's syndrome and exogenous ACTH administration probably are caused by increased production of adrenal androgens. The reason for the scalp hair loss and hirsutism of the face and body which occur with exogenous testosterone therapy is obvious, but the cause of the same pattern of abnormal hair growth associated with exogenous corticosteroid therapy is unexplained.

SYSTEMIC DISEASES. Prolonged febrile illnesses, systemic lupus erythematosus (LE), dermatomyositis, severe cachexia, and lymphomas are associated with hair loss. The transient hair loss after high fevers begins within 3 months of the acute illness and is followed by complete regrowth. This type of hair loss was seen more frequently in the preantibiotic era. The alopecia of systemic LE and dermatomyositis may be postfebrile and transient or permanent and associated with cutaneous involvement of the scalp by the disease. A patchy type of moth-eaten alopecia is an uncommon manifestation of secondary syphilis. Permanent hair loss on the extensor surfaces of the fingers is an early sign in systemic scleroderma. Occlusive peripheral vascular diseases are associated with loss of hair from the toes and feet.

PHYSICAL AND CHEMICAL AGENTS. Minor trauma may cause transient alopecia, but any physical damage which is severe enough to destroy the full thickness of the dermis also destroys hair follicles and results in permanent alopecia. The constant traction of certain hair styles causes a marginal alopecia of the frontal and temporal regions. Marginal alopecia occurs in girls and women who constantly wear their hair in braids or "ponytails." A change to a looser hair arrangement usually cures the alopecia. Third degree burns, whether from heat or chemical cauterants, results in permanent alopecia. Ionizing radiation in large doses (1,500r or more) causes permanent hair loss. Fractionated doses of x-rays in lower total doses (400r) result in temporary nonscarring alopecia. Radiomimetic drugs (such as nitrogen mustard), antimetabolites, thallium, heparin, coumarin, and excessive doses of vitamin A produce transient hair loss (Plate 1-2).

CUTANEOUS INFECTIONS. Superficial ringworm infections of the scalp cause patchy alopecia during the stage of active infection but rarely result in scarring and permanent alopecia. Deep pyogenic infections, namely boils and carbuncles, may cause permanent scarred alopecia, but folliculitis rarely does. Leprosy, cutaneous leishmaniasis, severe herpes zoster, and syphilitic gummas are associated with permanent hair loss in the affected area.

CUTANEOUS DISEASES. The permanent alopecia which occurs in lesions of discoid LE (Plate 1-5) localized scleroderma, and sarcoid is only apparent and important when the lesions involve the scalp and eyebrows. Scarring alopecia occurs in the rare dermatologic diseases *lichen planopilaris* and *pseudopelade*. Infants with congenital ectodermal defects characteristically have scanty scalp hair or areas of permanent alopecia. The scalp over nevi, tumors, and cysts may become bald.

TRICHOTILLOMANIA. Compulsive plucking of hairs from the scalp is a habit tic akin to nail-biting. Although the plucked areas may be large, they are never completely bald but contain a stubble of regrowing hairs of varying lengths as yet too short to be pulled.

ALOPECIA AREATA. Alopecia areata is characterized by the sudden development of single or multiple round bald patches of the scalp. The completely bald areas are slightly depressed, but no erythema or gross inflammatory changes are detectable. The patches may enlarge peripherally, and new areas may develop on the scalp, eyebrows, or beard region. Universal loss of all of the scalp and body hair sometimes occurs. The loss of the eyelashes, with the resultant loss of their sun-shading and dust-filtering actions is the only functional problem associated with alopecia areata. The general health is not affected, but the emotional stress caused by the cosmetic defect can be serious.

Although signs of inflammation in the areas of alopecia are grossly lacking, histologic examination reveals an infiltration of inflammatory cells in the papillae of the hair follicles. The cause of alopecia areata is unknown. A family history of the disease is not uncommon. Sudden emotional stress has been reported to precede some cases of alopecia areata, but it is certainly not a common finding. Nail changes, ranging from pitting to complete shedding, may occur. The severity of the nail changes roughly parallels the extent of the disease. The prognosis for spontaneous regrowth is good if the disease begins in adult life and involves only a few areas. If the disease begins in childhood or involves several areas or the whole body, the prognosis for regrowth is poor. Topical applications of corticosteroid creams covered by occlusive plastic dressings and intradermal injections of triamcinolone acetonide into the lesions may stimulate regrowth. Systemic corticosteroid therapy is not justified, since any results are usually transient. Massage, heat, ultraviolet light therapy, dessicated thyroid, and applications of irritants are of no value in the treatment of alopecia areata.

HIRSUTISM

The quantity and distribution of hair is dependent on genetic, racial, and hormonal factors, but the desirable amount of hair depends on cultural factors. The American culture views any hair on women other than on the scalp and pubis as cosmetically undesirable or unfeminine. Hair on the legs and axillae is removed as a matter of course by shaving or chemical depilatories. Hair on the face, breasts, and abdomen represents a threat to the American female's sexual identity for which cosmetic and medical help is commonly sought. Recognition of the psychologic problems created by hirsutism is an essential part of the management of these patients. Sympathetic explanations, reassurance, and cosmetic advice should be given by the physician to the woman whose hirsutism does not have a detectable and correctable endocrinologic basis.

The number of hair follicles in each anatomic region is the same in hirsute women, "normal" women, and men. The complaint of the woman who seeks medical help for hirsutism concerns the development of terminal hairs in regions where only lanugo hairs are usually present. The upper lip, chin, cheeks, chest, and abdomen, that is, the "hormonal" areas of hair growth, are those most commonly involved. Most hirsute women also have increased hair growth on the arms and anterior thighs and increased coarseness of hair. Androgens are known to increase the coarseness of hair and to stimulate the growth of terminal hairs in hormonal areas. A noticeable androgenic effect on hair can occur under three circumstances: (1) an increase in total androgen production, (2) an unusual sensitivity of the target organ (hair follicles) to normal amounts of androgen, (3) a relative preponderance of androgenic effects resulting from a decrease in estrogen. An increase in total androgens is present in virilizing syndromes of adrenal or ovarian origin. End organ insensitivity probably accounts for the decreased hair growth in the Japanese. Conversely, end organ hypersensitivity may account for the so-called "idiopathic" hirsutism of certain Caucasians, such as those of Mediterranean stock. Changes in androgen-estrogen balance may be responsible for the increased growth of facial hair and decrease in scalp hair in postmenopausal women. Hirsutism, once it is established, is relatively refractory to hormonal influences. A castrated man does not rapidly lose an established beard. The removal of a virilizing tumor in a woman stops the further progress of hirsutism but does not result immediately in a noticeable decrease in the established hirsutism.

A complete history and thorough physical examination are prerequisites to the correct diagnosis of the hirsute woman. A careful history of racial origins and family tendency to increased hair growth is important. Familial or genetic hirsutism occurs in 10 percent of Caucasian women. Some facial, abdominal, and chest hair is normal for many women of Mediterranean stock. A heavy growth of scalp hair, coarse hair, a low frontal hairline, and thick eyebrows are common in ethnic hirsutism. Familial hirsutism of this type begins at the menarche and continues to increase into the twenties.

Direct questioning is usually necessary in order to obtain evidence of excess androgen effect on other organs. A change in the voice, increased muscle mass and strength, decrease in breast size, increase in libido, and enlargement of the clitoris are indications of androgen excess. A detailed menstrual history is essential. Delayed onset of menarche, irregular or scanty periods, dysmenorrhea, infertility, or difficulty in conceiving or carrying to

Table 57-1. CAUSES OF HIRSUTISM

I. Localized
   A. Congenital
      1. Hairy nevi
      2. Satyr's tail of spina bifida
      3. Congenital erythropoietic porphyria
   B. Acquired
      1. Occupational—sack carriers
      2. Porphyria cutanea tarda
II. Generalized
   A. Racial, idiopathic, familial
   B. Iatrogenic
      1. Testosterone
      2. ACTH
      3. Corticosteroids
   C. Adrenal Origin
      1. Congenital adrenal hyperplasia
      2. Delayed onset of congenital adrenal hyperplasia
      3. Borderline adrenal dysfunction
      4. Cushing's syndrome
      5. Virilizing adrenal tumors
   D. Ovarian
      1. Virilizing ovarian tumors
         a. Arrhenoblastoma
         b. Adrenal rest tumor
         c. Gynandroblastoma
         d. Hilus or Leydig cell tumor
      2. Polycystic ovary (Stein-Leventhal) syndrome

term may indicate excessive androgen production by the ovary or adrenals.

When an earlier photograph of the patient is available, it is often useful to compare it with the present appearance of the patient. A complete physical examination is in order in all women complaining of hirsutism whether or not ethnic factors are playing a role. The examination should be directed towards determining the degree of hirsutism and detecting signs of virilization or other adrenal or ovarian diseases (Table 57-1). It is not unusual for the hirsute woman to carefully remove excess hair from face before presenting herself for consultation. A cursory inspection of the face and trunk may result in overlooking obvious signs of virilism. The physical manifestations of androgen excess include a husky voice, male body habitus with broad shoulders and slim hips, coarse oily skin, acne, male-pattern baldness of the scalp, enlargement of the thyroid cartilage, hair growth on the chest, atrophy of breasts, male-pattern pubic hair growth, excess hair on the thighs, and enlargement of the clitoris. Palpable enlargement of the ovaries is a sign of polycystic ovaries (Stein-Leventhal syndrome, Chap. 98) or ovarian neoplasms. A plethoric complexion, acne, moon face, central obesity, etc. accompany the hirsutism of Cushing's syndrome (Chap. 92).

Any of these physical findings accompanying hirsutism of even mild degree or even in ethnically predisposed women demands further studies for laboratory evidence of androgen excess. Measurement of total urinary 17-ketosteroids, despite limitations, is a valuable screening test. The delineation of the underlying endocrinologic lesion may require extensive investigation of the physiologic relationships of the pituitary-adrenal-ovarian axis (Chap. 90) with alternate stimulation and suppression of these glands with ACTH, corticosteroids, and human chorionic gonadotrophin.

The problem of excess hair persists even after successful surgical or medical management of the endocrinologic lesion. Hirsutism secondary to the administration of ACTH, corticosteroids, or testosterone may persist for long periods after the medications have been discontinued. Since the expectation is for the hirsuitism present to remain unchanged, explanation and cosmetic advice must be supplied to the patient. Most women have an aversion to shaving the face, although they regularly shave their legs and axillae. Other means of removing or minimizing the excess hair should be discussed. Many excellent bleaches and depilatories, which can be used safely at intervals on the face and are more acceptable to the patient, are available. Electrolysis is the only method of permanently removing excess hairs. In the hands of expert technicians the results of electrolysis are excellent, although the procedure is time-consuming and expensive.

Localized Hirsutism. Localized hirsutism may be congenital or acquired. Congenital localized hirsutism is usually associated with pigmented nevi, which may disfigure large areas of the body. A localized patch of hairs, *Satyr's tail,* may occur in association with spina bifida.

Repeated prolonged trauma to an area may stimulate localized hair growth. This type of hirsutism occurs on the forearms of mentally defective patients who repeatedly bite the affected area, and on the shoulders of men whose occupation entails carrying heavy sacks or other burdens. The hirsutism which develops on exposed areas in porphyria cutanea tarda and erythropoietic porphyria may be related to prolonged trauma from exposure to ultraviolet light.

REFERENCES

Montagna, W. (Ed.): "Aging," New York, Pergamon Press, 1965.

Rogers, G. E.: Structural and Biochemical Features of the Hair Follicle, pp. 179–232 in "The Epidermis," W. Montagna, and W. C. Lobitz, Jr. (Eds.), New York, Pergamon Press, 1964.

Rook, A.: Endocrine Influences on Hair Growth, Brit. Med. J. (Lancet), 1:609, 1965.

Segre, E. J.: Androgens, Virilization and the Hirsute Female, Springfield, Ill., Charles C Thomas, Publisher, 1967.

58 PIGMENTATION

Faye D. Arundell and Eugene M. Farber

The color of normal skin depends primarily on its content of melanin, carotene, and blood. Pathologic changes in skin color result from the deposition of endogenous or exogenous pigmented compounds, such as bile pigments, hemosiderin, homogentisic acid, heavy metals, and tattoo pigments.

MELANIN

The biochemistry of melanin formation, the known mechanisms which influence its synthesis, and the various syndromes associated with decreased or increased amounts of melanin in the skin are discussed in detail in Chap. 109. A normal complement of melanin is the skin's prime protective mechanism against ultraviolet light radiation. Deficiency of melanin, either congenital or acquired, is associated with an increased incidence of photosensitivity and of skin cancer. Inability to form sufficient amounts of melanin in large areas of the skin prevents individuals with albinism and vitiligo from engaging in normal outdoor occupations and activities. The unpigmented patches of vitiligo in the deeply pigmented Africans and Asians are regarded as cosmetic defects and may be social stigmata as well. Excess melanin production associated with systemic diseases, such as Addison's disease and hemachromatosis, is more pronounced in areas of skin which are exposed to sunlight. Long-term treatment of chronic granulocytic leukemia with dimethanesulfonoxybutane (Myleran) causes diffuse hyperpigmentation in some patients.

Genetic factors are of great importance in controlling the function of the melanocytes. The number of melanocytes in the skin is the same in Caucasians and Negroes. Variations in skin color are due to genetically determined differences in the rate at which melanin granules are produced by the melanocytes and transferred to the surrounding epidermal cells. Reflectance spectrophotometry, which gives a quantitative description of skin color, is used in anthropologic studies of melanin pigmentation. The hue of normal skin, which varies from pale tan to black, is a combination of the amounts of melanin in the melanocytes, basal cells, Malpighian cells, and stratum corneum of the epidermis. A normal number of melanocytes is present in albino skin, but the melanocytes do not make pigment because of an inborn error of metabolism (Chap. 101).

Genetic factors also influence the response of melanocytes to a variety of stresses, including local trauma and hormonal, metabolic, and other systemic disturbances. With aging, a varying proportion of melanocytes in hair follicles lose their ability to form melanin. Premature graying of hair is often a familial characteristic. In normal skin an increase in pigmentation occurs after exposure to solar radiation. Individual variations in the amount of tanning developing after sun exposure are influenced by genetic factors. Dark-skinned individuals have very responsive melanocytes. They tan readily and well and have an increased tolerance to sunburn and an increased tendency to develop postinflammatory pigmentary changes in areas of trauma or dermatitis. The incidence of chloasma during oral contraceptive therapy and pregnancy is higher in dark-skinned women.

Unusual ashy, blue-black colors are produced by the presence of melanin outside the epidermis in the deeper layers of the skin. Because of the Tyndall light-scattering phenomenon, these melanin deposits create a gray to blue color in the overlying skin. Mongolian spots and blue nevi owe their unusual blue-black color to the presence of melanin-containing melanocytes in the dermis. Epidermal melanin granules which have been lost into the dermis secondary to epidermal damage may be held within dermal macrophages for prolonged periods of time. This phagocytized melanin gives the previously affected areas of skin a dark brown or ashy color.

PHENOTHIAZINE PIGMENTATION. A peculiar type of bluish-brown hyperpigmentation occurs in a small percentage of patients on long-term, high dosage chlorpromazine therapy. Most cases have occurred in female schizophrenics in mental institutions. The pigmentation occurs only after continuous large doses of 400 to 1,500 mg daily for 2 to 10 years. The pigmentation is blue-gray, violet, or brown and appears on the exposed areas of the face, neck, arms, and hands. Phenothiazines are photosensitizing drugs that bind to melanin in vitro. Drug-induced enhanced reaction to sunlight plays a significant role in the development of phenothiazine pigmentation. The pigment is present as brown granules, both free and within macrophages in the dermis. Melanin pigment is increased in the epidermis, and the dermal pigment is believed to be melanin or a complex of melanin and phenothiazine.

The cutaneous hyperpigmentation caused by phenothiazine drugs may be accompanied by fine stippling of the cornea and anterior capsule of the lens. The eye changes occur equally in males and females who have received large doses of chlorpromazine for prolonged periods of time. The stippling of the cornea and lens, which is visible on slit-lamp examination, and brown discoloration of light-exposed areas of the conjunctiva can occur without the skin pigmentation. Significant visual impairment rarely occurs in patients with phenothiazine eye changes. The skin and eye changes seem to be slowly reversible after the drug is withdrawn.

VARIOUS HEMOGLOBINS. The normal pink shade of skin is attributable to the amount and state of oxygenation of the blood in the skin. The red tint of oxyhemoglobin may be completely masked or almost indiscernible in dark brown or black skins. Cyanosis is due to the presence of reduced hemoglobin in the dermal blood vessels (Chap. 33). Abnormal hemoglobins produce diagnostic changes in the color of skin. Carboxyhemoglobin from carbon monoxide forms a cherry red color. Methemoglobin and sulfhemoglobin, which occur with the ingestion of sulfonamides, sulfones, acetanilid, or phenacetin, create various shades of blue that may mimic the cyanosis of cardiac or pulmonary disease. (Chap. 344).

CAROTENE. The normal yellow tint of skin is caused by carotene in the keratin layer of the epidermis and in the subcutaneous fat. Excessive carotene in the skin (Chap. 84) creates a striking yellow or orange color which is particularly noticeable in the heavily keratinized skin of the palms and soles. Sparing of the scleras is helpful in differentiating this condition from jaundice. The amount of carotene in the skin is increased in excessive dietary intake of yellow vegetables and fruits. Carotenemia is seen in infants, in adults on fad diets, male castrates, panhypopituitarism, myxedema, and diabetes.

JAUNDICE. The intensity of the yellow discoloration of the skin and scleras in jaundice is related to the concentration of bile pigments in the blood. The skin color in jaundice may vary from yellow to greenish-brown.

HEMOSIDERIN. Deposits of hemosiderin in the dermis cause relatively permanent pigmentation of the skin. The color changes created by hemosiderin range from copper to dark brown. Special stains for iron and melanin help to differentiate hemosiderin from melanin in skin biopsies (Chap. 109). Generalized hemosiderin deposits and increased melanin pigmentation occur in hemachromatosis. Localized hemosiderin deposits are common in the skin of the lower extremities in individuals with chronic vascular stasis and capillary fragility.

EXOGENOUS PIGMENTATION. The commonest type of exogenous pigmentation of the skin is the tattoo. The chief danger associated with tattooing is the accidental introduction of infections, such as tuberculosis, infectious hepatitis, and more rarely, syphilis and leprosy. The status symbol of the modern tattoo artist is the sterilizer, which is usually prominently displaced in the parlor. Lo-

cal dermatitis, photosensitivity, or granulomas may be caused by mercury or cadmium in the red areas of tattoos.

Diffuse metallic pigmentation from ingestion or local applications to mucosal surfaces of silver salts (argyria) and parenteral gold salts (chrysiasis) is rare today. The slate color of the pigmentation is usually accentuated in light-exposed areas. The metals can be seen in the dermis in microscopic sections of the affected skin.

A striking yellow pigmentation of the skin occurs with ingestion of quinacrine (Atabrine). During World War II, quinacrine was the most common prophylactic drug used in endemic malarial regions. The yellow pigmentation of the skin gradually disappeared within several months after the drug was discontinued. Absorption of dinitrophenol and tetryl by workers in the explosive industry also causes a marked yellow discoloration of the skin.

REFERENCES

Fox, H. M., and G. Vevers: "The Nature of Animal Colors," London, Sidgwick & Jackson, Ltd., 1960.

Greiner, A. C., and K. Berry: Skin Pigmentation and Corneal and Lens Opacities with Prolonged Chloroquine Therapy, Can. Med. Assoc. J., 90:663, 1964.

Montagna, W., and F. Hu: "The Pigmentary System," vol. 8, "Advances in Biology of Skin," New York, Pergamon Press, 1966.

59 SUNLIGHT AND PHOTOSENSITIVITY REACTIONS

Faye D. Arundell and Eugene M. Farber

Solar radiation is responsible for a number of diverse cutaneous disorders. In order for solar radiation to have an effect on the skin, it must fulfill the following criteria: (1) the radiation must reach the skin surface; (2) the radiation must penetrate the skin; (3) the radiation must be absorbed by some component of the skin; (4) the photon energy of the absorbed radiation must be great enough to initiate a photochemical reaction.

Wavelengths of sunlight shorter than 290 mμ do not reach the earth's surface. The solar radiation which reaches the earth's surface is composed of a continuous spectrum of wavelengths ranging from 290 to 1850 mμ. The shorter wavelengths of solar radiation, namely ultraviolet light (290 to 400 mμ), are responsible for cutaneous disorders. The longer visible and infrared wavelengths (400 to 1850 mμ) are rarely of clinical importance.

SUNBURN. The short "sunburn" wavelengths (290 to 320 mμ) penetrate the epidermis and upper corium. The long-wavelength ultraviolet and visible light penetrate deeply into the dermis and, perhaps, into the subcutaneous tissue. The absorption of long-wavelength ultraviolet light results in an immediate but transient pigmentation due to darkening of preformed melanin. The absorption of sufficient quantities of the sunburn wavelengths in the skin causes photochemical reactions which result in delayed erythema followed by persisting pigmentation. Sunburn erythema appears after a latent period of 6 to 8 hr, increases in intensity, and subsides in 72 to 96 hr. The normal sunburn inflammatory reaction varies from mild erythema to severe painful erythema and bullae. The intensity of the sunburn reaction is inversely proportional to the amount of protective melanin in the skin and directly proportional to the duration of exposure of the skin to solar radiation. Postinflammatory reparative processes are marked by thickening of the epidermis and stratum corneum. The delayed but persistent pigmentation caused by the sunburn spectrum of ultraviolet light is the result of new formation of melanin by melanocytes and upward migration of melanin in the epidermal cells. The new pigmentation begins in 2 days following sun exposure, reaches a maximum at 19 days and subsides over the next 9 months.

CHRONIC ACTINIC CHANGES. Prolonged excessive exposure to sunlight causes persistent leathery thickening of the skin. The collagen and elastin of the dermis degenerate, and the epidermis undergoes such changes as atrophy, hypertrophy, hyperkeratosis, and cellular atypism. These deleterious effects of excessive exposure to sunlight have been equated erroneously with aging. Comparison of the exposed skin of farmers, sailors, and sun worshippers with the protected skin of their trunks reveals that the striking changes are related to solar radiation and not to age. In time, premalignant actinic keratoses and carcinomas are induced in the actinically damaged exposed skin. There is a significant increase in the incidence of basal cell carcinomas and squamous cell carcinomas in individuals living in regions where the sun's radiation is intense. The incidence of skin cancers is greater in Texas than in Minnesota, greater in fair-skinned, freckled individuals than in those with dark complexions, and greater in farmers and ranchers than in office workers. Negroes almost never develop chronic actinic degeneration of the skin, actinic keratoses, or actinic skin cancers. Elderly Negroes look younger than their chronologic age, since their deeply pigmented skin does not undergo the same actinic changes which are commonly considered to be signs of aging in Caucasians.

It is obvious that the skin's main protections against solar radiation are hair and melanin. Actinic degeneration and carcinomas do not occur on the scalp which is shaded by hair but do occur in the exposed areas of the scalp of bald men. The tanning of the skin that results from increased melanin formation affords increased protection against solar radiation. Melanin gives protection by absorbing and scattering light. Greatly increased amounts of ultraviolet light are necessary to produce erythema (sunburn) in tanned skin.

PHOTOSENSITIVITY

Abnormal cutaneous reactions to ultraviolet light are referred to as photosensitivity reactions (Table 59-1).

Table 59-1. SKIN DISEASES RELATED TO SUNLIGHT

I. Phototoxic Eruptions
  A. Endogenous
    1. Congenital erythropoietic porphyria (Chap. 108)
    2. Porphyria cutanea tarda (Chap. 108)
    3. Erythropoietic protoporphyria (Chap. 108)
  B. Exogenous
    1. Drugs—furocoumarins, sulfanilamide, sulfonylurea, chlorpromazine, tetracycline
    2. Chemicals—coal tar, perfumes, chlorophylls, eosin and other dyes
II. Photoallergic Eruptions
  A. Endogenous
    1. Solar urticaria (some types)
  B. Exogenous
    1. Drugs—chlorothiazides, phenothiazines, griseofulvin, promethazine, sulfanilamide
    2. Chemicals—halogenated salicylanilides, bisphenol, para-aminobenzoic acid
III. Idiopathic
    1. Polymorphous light eruptions
    2. Solar urticaria (some cases)
IV. Intrinsic Abnormalities of the Skin
  A. Melanin Deficiency
    1. Albinism
    2. Vitiligo
  B. Idiopathic
    1. Xeroderma pigmentosum
    2. Epidermolysis bullosa
V. Dermatoses Precipitated or Aggravated by Light
    1. Herpes simplex
    2. Lupus erythematosus
    3. Dermatomyositis
    4. Pellagra (Chap. 80)
    5. Hartnup's disease (Chap. 101)
    6. "Photosensitive" psoriasis, lichen planus, seborrheic dermatitis, rosacea, pityriasis rubra pilaris, keratosis follicularis
VI. Excessive Sunlight Exposure
  A. Acute
    1. Sunburn
  B. Chronic
    1. Actinic degeneration of the dermis (farmer's and sailor's skin)
    2. Actinic keratoses
    3. Leukoplakia
    4. Squamous cell carcinoma
    5. Basal cell carcinoma

Photosensitivity is inevitable when the melanocytes of the epidermis are unable to form sufficient amounts of melanin, as in albinism and vitiligo. Photosensitivity in clinical practice most commonly is due to drugs and exogenous chemicals. In the photosensitive porphyrias the photosensitizing agent is an endogenous chemical (Chap. 108). Phototoxic disorders are those in which the basic mechanisms are nonimmunologic, such as porphyria, phototoxic drug eruptions, and phototoxic contact dermatitis. Photoallergic disorders are those photosensitivity reactions in which the basic mechanisms are clearly allergic, such as photoallergic drug reactions, contact photoallergic dermatitis, and some cases of solar urticaria. The pathogenetic mechanisms are unknown in other diseases which may be precipitated or aggravated by light, such as discoid and systemic lupus erythematosus, dermatomyositis, herpes simplex, and pellagra.

The four following groups of chemicals account for the majority of photosensitivity reactions seen in clinical practice:

1. *Sulfonamides,* including the sulfonylurea antidiabetic agents and the chlorothiazide diuretics, are common photoallergic agents.

2. *Phenothiazines,* such as chlorpromazine (Thorazine), promazine (Sparine), and promethazine (Phenergan), are phototoxic agents. Large doses of these drugs for prolonged periods of time may lead to severe hyperpigmentation.

3. *Tetracyclines,* especially demethylchlortetracycline, are phototoxic agents which may also induce shedding of the nails.

4. *Halogenated salicylanilides* and chemically related drugs, such as bisphenol (Bithionol), carbanilides, and hexachlorophene are common photoallergens. These chemicals are present in ever-increasing numbers of commercial antibacterial and deodorant soaps. The incidence of photoallergic dermatitis has shown a remarkable increase, especially in sunny climates, since the introduction of these new soaps in the 1960s.

PHOTOTOXICITY. The phototoxic reaction is similar to an exaggerated sunburn. The erythema begins earlier, and the local reaction is greater in intensity than in normal sunburn. The residual pigmentation is usually more intense and persistent. Phototoxicity can be likened to primary irritant reactions in the skin, since both types of reactions can be provoked in almost all adequately challenged individuals. An adequate challenge for phototoxicity includes two factors: (1) a sufficient amount of the chemical in or on the skin; (2) a concomitant exposure to a sufficient amount of light of the proper wavelength. Phototoxic drugs or chemicals presumably act by absorbing specific wavelengths of light, becoming activated, and passing the extra energy on to a component within the cell with resulting skin damage. The best-known phototoxic systemic drugs are the sulfonilamides, chlorpromazine, sulfonylurea, demethylchlortetracycline, and furocoumarins. Coal tar, perfumes, and furocoumarins are phototoxic agents which are applied topically to the skin. The phototoxicity of coal-tar preparations is used in the Goeckerman treatment for psoriasis, which employs topical applications of crude coal-tar ointment followed by exposure to ultraviolet light. The furocoumarin Tripsoralen (10 mg p.o. daily followed by measured sun exposure) is used to stimulate repigmentation in vitiligo.

PORPHYRIA. The photosensitivity which occurs in some types of porphyria is caused by endogenous phototoxic porphyrins. Severe photosensitivity and scarring occurs in infants and children with congenital erythropoietic porphyria (Chap. 108). In the chronic hepatic type, namely porphyria cutanea tarda, bullae occur on the hands and face following sun exposure and trauma. Urticarial and scarring vesicular lesions (hydroa vacciniforme) develop after sun exposure in erythropoietic protoporphyria. The photensitizing porphyrins are activated by long-wave ultraviolet light; hence, window glass gives these patients no protection.

PHOTOALLERGY. The photoallergic reactions have an immunologic basis which is most commonly a delayed "contact dermatitis" type. Only a small proportion of individuals exposed to the potential photoallergic agent become sensitized. The patient must be specifically sensitized by previous exposure to the chemical. After a latent period of several days, during which sensitization takes place, a delayed abnormal response occurs to specific wavelengths of light. The concentration of the photoallergen necessary to elicit the reaction in a sensitized person is usually much lower than that required for phototoxic reactions. The abnormal response may be urticarial, or papular and vesicular, i.e., a dermatitis. An adequate challenge for photoallergic reactions includes three factors: (1) a sufficient though small quantity of the antigen in or on the skin; (2) the presence of specific antibodies; (3) an exposure to a sufficient amount of the proper wavelengths of light.

Following repeated exposures to the allergen and light, the reaction time becomes shorter, and distant unexposed areas of skin may flare. Two groups of photoallergic patients are seen in clinical practice. The "transient light reactors" are photoallergic individuals in whom the eruption clears promptly when the sensitizing chemical is withdrawn. A small number of photoallergic patients become "persistent light reactors," and for unknown reasons the reaction to light persists for weeks or years after the chemical is withdrawn. Common photoallergic drugs which are administered parenterally include chlorthiazide, chlorpromazine, griseofulvin, and promethazine. Topically applied photoallergic drugs and chemicals include sulfanilamides, promethazine, para-aminobenzoic acid, and the antiseptic agents bisphenol, halogenated salicylanilides, and carbanilides. Photodecomposition products resulting from the action of ultraviolet light have been shown to be the actual sensitizers in the case of sulfanilamide and tribromosalicylanilide.

Clinical Manifestations of Phototoxicity and Photoallergy

The eruption is confined initially to the exposed areas of the face, neck, V-area of the chest, dorsal surfaces of the hands and arms, and the pretibial areas in women. Photoallergic reactions may become generalized, but the disease remains most pronounced in the exposed areas. Local regions which are anatomically shaded in the exposed areas (eyelids, submental regions, etc.) are spared. The primary lesions vary from exaggerated sunburn, bullae, and marked pigmentation in the phototoxic reactions to urticaria and eczematous dermatitis in photoallergic reactions.

Diagnostic tests for photodermatoses are based on the administration of known amounts of light of known wavelengths. There are three basic types of light tests which utilize a hot quartz or carbon arc light source.

1. *MED.* The minimal erythema dose (MED) is

determined by using measured time exposures from a given source of mixed short- and long-wave ultraviolet light. The MED is defined as the shortest exposure causing detectable erythema of the skin at 24 hr. The MED is shorter than normal in phototoxic and photoallergic reactions.

2. *Window-glass Test.* Window glass effectively blocks the short sunburn ultraviolet light wavelengths and provides a convenient method for irradiating the skin with only long wavelengths of ultraviolet light. Normal skin will not develop erythema after exposure to window-glass–filtered ultraviolet light. Prolonged exposures (10 times the MED) will elicit erythema in the phototoxic and photoallergic reactions which are related to long wave ultraviolet light.

3. *Photo Patch Test.* Patch testing with suspected photoallergens followed at 24 hr by exposure of the patch test sites to ultraviolet light is used in the investigation of contact photoallergic reactions. Reproduction of the disease in miniature by this procedure confirms the diagnosis.

The photosensitizer must be identified and eliminated from the patient's environment. These patients may react to light for some period of time after the drug has been withdrawn; therefore, confinement indoors, in darkened rooms and away from windows, may be necessary for several weeks in the more severe reactions. Topical corticosteroid creams give symptomatic relief during the acute stages. Protective clothing and sun-screening lotions or creams, such as red veterinary petrolatum and those containing benzophenones or titanium dioxide, should be used on all exposed skin of the photosensitive patient. The use of these sun-screening agents is necessary throughout the lifetime of patients with actinic degeneration of the skin and idiopathic photosensitive eruptions.

REFERENCES

Baer, R. L., and L. C. Harber: Light Sensitivity in Biologic Systems, Fed. Proc., 24: No. 1, Part III, 14, 15, 1965.

Epstein, S.: Masked Photo Patch Tests. J. Invest. Dermatol., 41:369, 1963.

Urbach, F.: Light Sensitivity, in Dermatologic Allergy: Immunology, Diagnosis, Management, L. H. Criep (Ed.), pp. 501–514, Philadelphia, W. B. Saunders Company, 1967.

60 SWEATING DISORDERS

Faye D. Arundell and Eugene M. Farber

Sweating is one of man's prime thermoregulatory mechanisms. In acclimatized individuals, cooling by evaporation of sweat accounts for 75 to 90 percent of the reduction of body heat. Sweating is a useful mechanism only if the sweat can evaporate and cause cooling of the body surface. The surface of the human body is covered with 3 million separate sweat units, namely, the eccrine sweat glands. The distribution of eccrine sweat glands over the whole body surface is found only in humans and simian primates. In other mammals, eccrine glands are present only in friction surface areas such as the footpads and prehensile tails. The number of sweat glands varies in different body regions of humans; the palms and soles have the greatest number per unit area. In addition to the number of glands, sweating ability depends on the size, output, and responsiveness of the individual glands.

The eccrine sweat gland is an epidermal appendage which develops independently of the pilosebaceous unit. The gland is a simple tubule with a coiled secretory portion located in the depths of the dermis. The duct extends as a straight tubule through the dermis and as a spiral coil through the epidermis to open in a pore on the surface. Two types of cells are present in the secretory portion of the gland: basophilic cells, which secrete mucin; and acidophilic cells, which secrete water and electrolytes.

When the ambient temperature exceeds 31 to 32°C, or 88 to 90°F, there is a sudden onset of visible sweating over the whole body surface. At lower temperatures, periodic insensible sweating occurs in alternate glands. This activity accounts for 10 to 30 percent of the body's total insensible water loss.

The innervation of sweat glands is by cholinergic postganglionic sympathetic fibers, and eccrine glands respond to all cholinergic drugs. Their response is enhanced by anticholinesterases and inhibited by cholinergic blocking agents such as atropine and methantheline bromide (Banthine). The central efferent pathway for sweating runs from the cortex via the hypothalamus, medulla, and lateral horn of the spinal cord to the sympathetic ganglia.

The main stimuli for sweating are psychic for the cortex and thermal for the hypothalamus. Emotion causes immediate, sudden sweating, primarily on the palms and soles but eventually all over the body. Hypothalamic thermoregulatory centers probably are stimulated by warmed blood arriving in the brain from the periphery of the body. Thermoregulatory sweating appears over the whole body surface, but the palms and soles are the last regions to show visible sweating. Axillary eccrine glands respond to both mental and thermal stimulation. In some individuals the axillary glands are as responsive as the palms and soles to mental stimuli. Gustatory sweating, accompanied by blushing, occurs over the lips and nose and may involve the whole face and head. The taste of spicy or acid food causes gustatory sweating in some normal individuals. Excessive gustatory sweating in certain regions (cheek and temple) may follow cervical sympathetic section and injury of the facial nerve (Chap. 355).

Intradermal injection of 0.1 ml of 1:10^5 solution of acetyl-β-methylcholine (Mecholyl) or similar drugs causes sweating by a direct action on the glandular cells. A secondary, more widespread sweating occurring around the site of injection of these agents is the result of the nicotinic effect of these drugs which produce sympathetic axon-reflex sweating. Axonal reflex sweating is also caused by intradermal injections of nicotine and is abolished by infiltration anaesthesia. Intradermal injections of 0.1 ml Mecholyl ($1:10^3$ solution), nicotine sulfate ($1:10^5$ solution), and histamine diphosphate ($1:10^3$ solution) are useful methods for testing the integrity of the peripheral mixed nerves. Absence of the histamine flare indicates degeneration of peripheral sensory neurons. Absence of pilomotor (nicotine) and sweat (nicotine and Mecholyl) reflexes indicates degeneration of peripheral sympathetic neurons. All three axonal reflexes are absent in the lesions of tuberculoid leprosy (Chap. 175). Axonal reflex sweating may explain the local hyperhidrosis seen at the margin of inflammatory dermatoses. Sympathetic denervation is followed by failure of the eccrine glands in the affected area to respond to central thermal stimuli, emotional excitement, or axonal reflexes, but the glands are still able to respond to direct application of heat. This responsiveness to direct stimulation is not abolished by denervation, local anaesthetics, atropinization, or arrest of the circulation.

Eccrine sweat is a clear aqueous solution composed of 99 percent water and 1 percent solids. The normal value of 17 mEq per liter of chlorides in sweat accounts for 80 percent of the osmolality of sweat. The concentration of chlorides in sweat depends on many factors. In mucoviscidosis (cystic fibrosis) the eccrine gland functions at a lower level than normal (Chap. 334). In normal individuals, if the dietary intake of salt is high, the chloride content of the sweat is high. The salt content of sweat is decreased when the dietary intake of water or potassium is unusually high or when the salt intake is low.

The concentration of chlorides increases with time during a single episode of thermal sweating and during increased rates of sweating. With repeated episodes of profuse sweating, the glands begin to function at progressively lower temperatures, the sweat rate increases, and the salt content of the sweat decreases. This acclimatization process results from increased adrenal production of salt-retaining corticosteroids under the stimulus of thermal stress. The three important forms of heat exhaustion which occur in man are (1) heat stroke or hyperpyrexia due to central failure of thermoregulatory centers (Chap. 125); (2) salt-depletion heat exhaustion due to excess loss of salt and water in profuse sweating (Chap. 296); (3) sweat-retention syndrome due to plugging of sweat ducts and pores in hot humid environments.

The *apocrine gland* is a distinct type of epithelial gland which is unrelated anatomically or functionally to the eccrine sweat gland. Apocrine glands are present over the whole body surface in mammals, but they occur only in association with the pilosebaceous apparatus in the axillae, anogenital, and mammary regions of human beings. Specialized apocrine glands are present in the nose, eyelids (Meibomian glands), and external ear canals (where they secrete "ear wax"). The ducts of apocrine glands empty into the upper portion of hair follicles in the axillary, perianal, pubic, and mammary regions. These apocrine glands begin to function at puberty. Under emotional stress and other adrenergic stimuli they secrete a small amount of milky fluid which,

after decomposition by bacteria, creates distinctive regional odors. These odors can be controlled by regular bathing and topical antibacterial agents.

Chronic inflammation of axillary apocrine glands causes acute lesions resembling boils and the persistent draining sinus tracts of hidradenitis suppurativa (Chap. 139).

HYPERHIDROSIS

Thermal sweating performs an essential role in the regulation of body temperature. Emotional sweating, which is most apparent on the palms and soles, may have played an essential role in lubricating the friction surfaces of lower mammals; but in man, it is merely a source of embarassment.

GENERALIZED. The marked sweating during physical exertion, with defervescence, and in hot environments serves a useful function if it can evaporate and cause cooling. Alcohol, hot drinks, and aspirin accentuate any tendency to sweating.

Pain of any type and motion sickness also cause hyperhidrosis. A compensatory increase in the amount and rate of sweating occurs in patients who have undergone sympathectomy for hypertension.

LOCALIZED. Anxiety states are associated in many individuals with excessive outpouring of sweat from the palms, soles, and axillae. Hyperhidrosis of the hands may also occur in otherwise normal individuals. Direct stimulation of the sympathetic nerves causes local hyperhidrosis in inflammatory diseases, such as causalgia, nerve injuries, neuritis, and thrombophlebitis. The immersion foot syndrome is also associated with hyperhidrosis.

Normal amounts of sweating can be controlled with the commercially available antiperspirants containing astringent aluminum salts. Severe axillary hyperhidrosis may require local excision of the skin of the vaults of axillae. The use of systemic anticholinergic agents to control localized hyperhidrosis has been disappointing because uncomfortable side effects of these drugs occur at doses well below those required to stop sweating. Tranquilizers and explanatory reassurance may give some relief.

Diseases or injuries in the region of the parotid gland cause the localized hyperhidrosis which occurs in the auriculotemporal syndrome.

ANHIDROSIS

The confirmation of an inability to sweat depends upon sweat testing during mental or thermal stimulation. The starch-iodine test detects the arrival of sweat at the skin surface. A negative starch-iodine or filter paper test requires special testing procedures to determine whether sweat glands are present but occluded, present but not functioning, or absent. Poral occlusion is confirmed if the previously anhidrotic area sweats after Scotch-tape stripping of the stratum corneum. Sweating after intradermal injections of Mecholyl or nicotine confirms the integrity of the peripheral sympathetic nerves. Failure to sweat in the absence of poral occlusion and the presence of intact sympathetic nerves indicates deep duct occlusion or absence of eccrine glands. A full-thickness biopsy of the skin and subcutaneous fat may be needed to confirm the presence of sweat glands or deep plugging of the sweat duct.

GENERALIZED. Destruction of critical centers of the hypothalamus by tumors, vascular accidents, surgery, or trauma results in complete anhidrosis. Failure of the hypothalamic thermoregulatory centers causes heat stroke. Universal anhidrosis may accompany certain diseases of the peripheral nervous system (Chap. 354). Congenital absence of sweat glands occurs in the syndrome of anhidrotic ectodermal dysplasia. Generalized anhidrosis in which only the face is spared occurs in the *sweat-retention syndrome,* with deep poral occlusion in hot humid climates and in atabrine dermatitis when the sweat ducts are destroyed. Systemic diseases, such as myxedema, Simmonds' disease, and scurvy, may be accompanied by anhidrosis.

The individual with generalized anhidrosis, regardless of cause, is at a special risk during febrile illnesses, physical exertion, or high environmental temperatures. The loss of the evaporative cooling mechanism results in hyperpyrexia, exhaustion, and collapse. A controlled environment with cool temperatures and prevention of exertion and infections is a necessary lifelong pattern in all except the temporary "duct-occlusion" types of anhidrosis.

LOCALIZED. Interruption of the central or peripheral sympathetic nervous systems can result in localized anhidrosis. Syringomyelia, transverse myelitis, multiple sclerosis, tumors of the spinal cord, or interruption of peripheral nerves may cause the condition. Involvement of the peripheral nerves by leprosy, trauma, or other types of neuritis, and involvement of the peripheral sympathetic nerve by leprosy or degeneration secondary to diabetes or gout also cause local anhidrosis. Local anhidrosis due to sweat retention occurs in erythrodermia, psoriasis, atopic dermatitis, stasis dermatitis, and lichen planus. Sweat is still produced in these areas, but since it cannot reach the surface, miliaria and itching result.

REFERENCES

Herxheimer, A.: Excessive Sweating: A Review, Trans. St. Johns Hosp. Dermatol. Soc., 40:20, 1958.

Hurley, H. J., and W. B. Shelley: "The Human Apocrine Sweat Gland in Health and Disease," Springfield, Ill., Charles C Thomas, Publisher, 1960.

Montagna, W., et al. (Eds.): "Eccrine Sweat Gland and Eccrine Sweating," New York, Pergamon Press, 1962.

Shelley, W. B., P. N. Horvath, and D. M. Pillsbury: Anhidrosis: An Etiologic Interpretation, Medicine, 29:195, 1950.

Sulzberger, M. B., and F. Herrmann: "The Clinical Significance of Disturbances in the Delivery of Sweat," Springfield, Ill., Charles C Thomas, Publisher, 1954.

Section 9

Hematologic Alterations

61 PALLOR AND ANEMIA

M. M. Wintrobe and G. R. Lee

PALLOR

The color of the skin depends on many factors, which include the thickness of the epidermis, the quantity and type of pigment contained therein, and the number and degree of patency of the blood vessels, as well as the quantity and nature of the hemoglobin carried within them. Even the nature and fluid content of the subcutaneous tissue are significant factors. It is obvious, therefore, that pallor does not necessarily indicate that anemia is present.

A sallow complexion is present in certain individuals, as it was in their forebears before them, and may exist in the absence of any true anemia; the flush of excitement, on the other hand, or constant exposure to the sun and wind may produce an appearance which masks an underlying anemia. Physicians, at the turn of the present century, spoke of "rosy" chlorotics, as well as of green and pale ones. The number and pattern of distribution of the finer blood vessels vary in different individuals, and in the same person vasoconstriction may produce the appearance of pallor, whereas other factors, such as exercise, for example, may lead to the appearance of a "healthier" color. Certain disorders may affect the skin in such a way that a pallid appearance is produced, even though anemia is absent. These disorders include scleroderma, the various nephrotic states, and myxedema. The last two, however, may be accompanied by actual anemia.

ANEMIA

Definition and Detection

Anemia is most accurately defined as a reduction in the circulating red blood cell mass. However, since direct knowledge of the size of the red blood cell mass is not easily acquired, such a definition is of limited usefulness. It is more practical to define anemia in terms of concentrations per unit volume of blood. In these terms, anemia is a reduction below normal in the volume of packed red blood cells per 100 ml (VPRC), the blood hemoglobin concentration per 100 ml (Hb), and/or the red blood cell count per cubic millimeter (RBC). Under most clinical circumstances, these measurements accurately reflect changes in the red blood cell mass because the total blood volume tends to be kept within relatively narrow limits by a variety of physiologic mechanisms. It is rarely necessary to measure directly the blood volume, but in conditions in which blood volume deviates from normal, such as overhydration, dehydration, fluid retention, or significant blood loss, the usual measures of concentration may be misleading. An increase in the plasma volume may give a false impression of anemia. Of greater importance

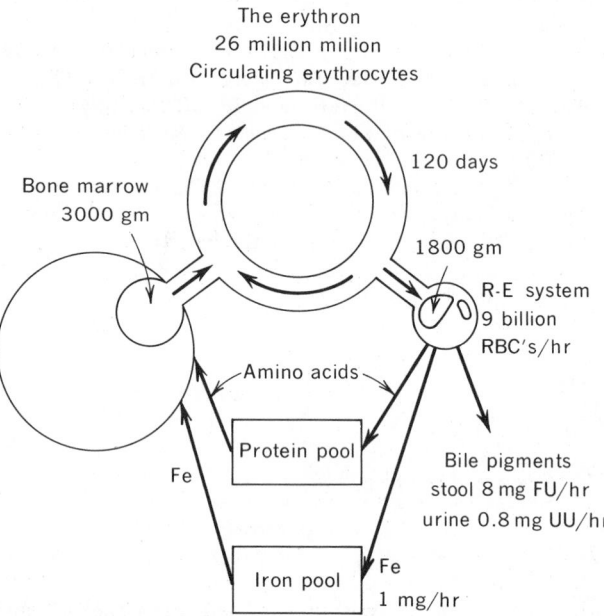

Fig. 61-1. The amount of blood in circulation represents the balance between production and destruction. In a 70-kg man the circulating red corpuscles carry approximately 770 Gm hemoglobin. Since the average life span of the red corpuscles normally is 120 days, the turnover rate per day is the total in the circulation divided by 120. In the average man this comes to approximately 2.16×10^{11} red corpuscles per day, or 9 billion per hour, and 6.4 Gm hemoglobin per day. From this are derived approximately 21 mg iron per day, 250 mg protoporphyrin, and 6.2 Gm globin. The iron and globin are reutilized. Of the protoporphyrin derived from the destroyed red corpuscles, somewhat less than 250 mg appears as fecal urobilinogen, since there are great variations in completeness of evacuation and also because of variations in the extent to which pigments giving this reaction are produced. Under normal conditions, through increased production and transformation of yellow marrow to red, the bone marrow is capable of approximately a seven- or eightfold increase in production capacity. Consequently, other things being equal, anemia will not develop as the result of increased blood destruction until the life span of the red corpuscles has been reduced to less than about 15 to 17 days.

is the fact that an extracellular fluid deficit may mask an underlying anemia.

The VPRC, as measured by the macro hematocrit method, is the simplest and most accurate of the three measures of red blood cell concentration in the blood and is therefore the one most suited for routine use. With relatively little extra effort, this method provides additional information which is extremely useful in the routine survey of a patient, such as the *erythrocyte sedimentation rate*, the *volume of packed white blood cells and platelets*, and the *icterus index*. The VPRC also may be determined by a micro method, and this and the measurement of blood hemoglobin concentration are satisfactory alternatives to the VPRC measured by the macro method when only a small volume of blood is available. Although the red blood cell count was the first available method for detecting anemia, it is rarely used for that purpose at present. When performed by the hemocytometer technique, the determination lacks accuracy; determination by more elaborate instruments, such as the Coulter counter, requires a relatively large initial investment and constant attention to accurate technique and machine maintenance. Consequently, the red blood cell count should be determined only for the purpose of calculating the corpuscular constants (p. 311).

The normal values for red corpuscles for persons at various ages are presented in the Appendix. These data are for persons living at sea level. At higher altitudes, higher values are found, roughly in proportion to the elevation above sea level. In general, the blood of normal persons tends to approach the mean for the sex. Provided the measurements are accurate, a deviation below the mean of more than 10 percent should be looked upon as representing anemia.

Pathologic Physiology

In normal subjects, erythrocytes are produced by the bone marrow and released to the circulation, where they survive approximately 120 days. They are then removed by the reticuloendothelial system, in which the hemoglobin is broken down to bile pigments, iron and globin. It is useful to think of the tissues involved in these processes as if they were one organ, the *erythron*, a concept which is illustrated diagrammatically in Fig. 61-1. It is apparent that the size of the circulating red blood cell mass is related to the rates of production and destruction. In a normal subject, the two rates are equal; therefore, the red blood cell mass remains constant in size, and the subject is said to be in equilibrium. When destruction exceeds production, the red blood cell mass decreases in size and anemia develops. When production exceeds destruction, the red blood cell mass increases.

ERYTHROCYTE PRODUCTION

Considerable evidence has accumulated which indicates that the rate of red blood cell production is under hormonal control. The major source of the hormone erythropoietin is the kidney, and its production appears to be stimulated by hypoxia. Erythropoietin acts to increase the number of immature red blood cell precursors in the bone marrow; the marrow becomes more cellular, fat is replaced by erythroid cells, and formerly inactive or "yellow" marrow becomes active or "red." Under maximum stimulation, the marrow is capable of increasing its production of red blood cells six- to eightfold.

Certain minerals, such as iron, copper, and cobalt, are essential to normal erythropoiesis, and anemia will develop in experimental animals when these are lacking. Certain of the B vitamins also have been shown experimentally to be essential to erythropoiesis, especially vitamin B_{12}, folic acid (pteroylglutamic acid), pyridoxine, ascorbic acid, pantothenic acid, and riboflavin. Nicotinic acid and vitamin E also may be concerned in erythropoiesis.

Since hemoglobin constitutes about 90 percent of the dry weight of the red blood cell, much of red blood cell production is concerned with hemoglobin synthesis. Hemoglobin, a compound of 64,458 mol wt, is made up of a colorless protein (globin) and a prosthetic group known as heme. The globin of adult hemoglobin (hemoglobin A) in man consists of two pairs of polypeptide chains, alpha chains and beta chains, which differ from one another in amino acid sequence. To each of the chains is attached one molecule of heme. Heme, which imparts the red color to the hemoglobin molecule, is a metal complex consisting of an iron atom in the center of a porphyrin structure (Fig. 61-2). The porphyrin has been designated protoporphyrin 9, type III. Like other porphyrin rings, it consists of four pyrrole nuclei connected to one another by methene (=C—) bridges. The iron, which has the capacity of binding oxygen reversibly, is linked to the nitrogen atom in each of the pyrrole groups and also to the imidazole nitrogen of one of the histidines in one of the polypeptide chains of globin.

The structure of heme is identical in all mammals, but the properties of hemoglobin with respect to electrophoretic mobility, solubility, and resistance to denaturation by alkali vary in different species, apparently because of differences in the amino acid composition of globin. In addition, in man a number of different types of hemoglobin, dependent on genetically determined differences in globin structure, have been discovered which in some instances govern the development of hematologic abnormalities and certain clinical manifestations (Chap. 339).

The source materials for the formation of porphyrin are the amino acid glycine and succinyl coenzyme A, which arises from the tricarboxylic acid cycle. In vitro as well as in vivo studies have clarified the steps in the synthetic process (Fig. 61-3). Acetate is transformed into α-ketoglutarate, and this, in the presence of coenzyme A, gives rise to succinyl CoA. This is one of the sites at which pantothenic acid functions in erythropoiesis, since this vitamin is a component of CoA. The vitamin pyridoxine is involved in the next step. The activated form of succinate condenses with a pyridoxal phosphate-glycine-enzyme complex to form delta-aminolevulinic acid

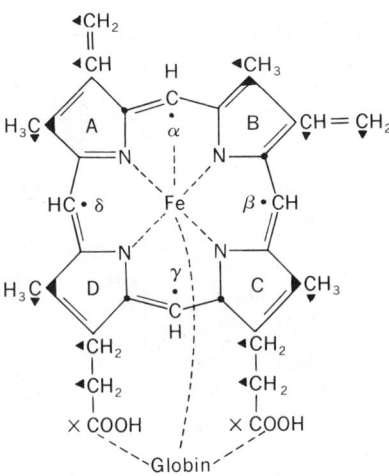

Fig. 61-2. Chemical structure of heme and its manner of union with globin to form hemoglobin. The carbon atoms derived from the alpha carbon of glycine are represented by ●, those supplied from the methyl carbon of acetate by ▼, and those derived from the carboxyl group of acetate by ✕. The unmarked carbons are those derived either from the methyl carbon atom of acetate or from the carboxyl atom.

(Δ-ALA) and carbon dioxide. Two molecules of Δ-ALA condense to form a monopyrrole, porphobilinogen. The subsequent steps leading to the formation of protoporphyrin are shown in the diagram. Ultimately protoporphyrin is converted to hemoglobin in the presence of iron, globin, and an enzyme, heme synthetase. The first and last steps in the heme biosynthetic chain occur in mitochondria; the other steps take place in the cytoplasm.

Globin is synthesized in the cell by a process common to the synthesis of all proteins. This requires messenger RNA, ribosomes, and "activated" amino acids (amino acids which are phosphorylated and attached to specific transfer-RNA molecules). Through a process known as translation, the ribosome travels along the strand of messenger RNA while simultaneously forming amino acids into a polypeptide chain. The specific amino acids selected depend on the sequence of purine and pyrimidine bases in the messenger-RNA molecule, the so-called "genetic code." Messenger RNA is synthesized in the nucleus by a process known as transcription, in the presence of a complementary strand of nuclear DNA (the "gene" or cistrone) and an enzyme, RNA polymerase.

RED BLOOD CELL DESTRUCTION

As noted previously, the normal red blood cell survives about 120 days. Since it contains no nucleus, all the enzymes necessary to maintain this life span must be in the cell when it enters the circulation. The principal factors essential to normal survival are (1) a source of energy, (2) the ability to maintain a stable fluid and electrolyte content, and (3) a system which protects the cell from endogenous and exogenous oxidants.

About 85 to 90 percent of the energy used by red blood cells is derived from the conversion of glucose to lactate by anaerobic glycolysis. The high-energy compound syn-

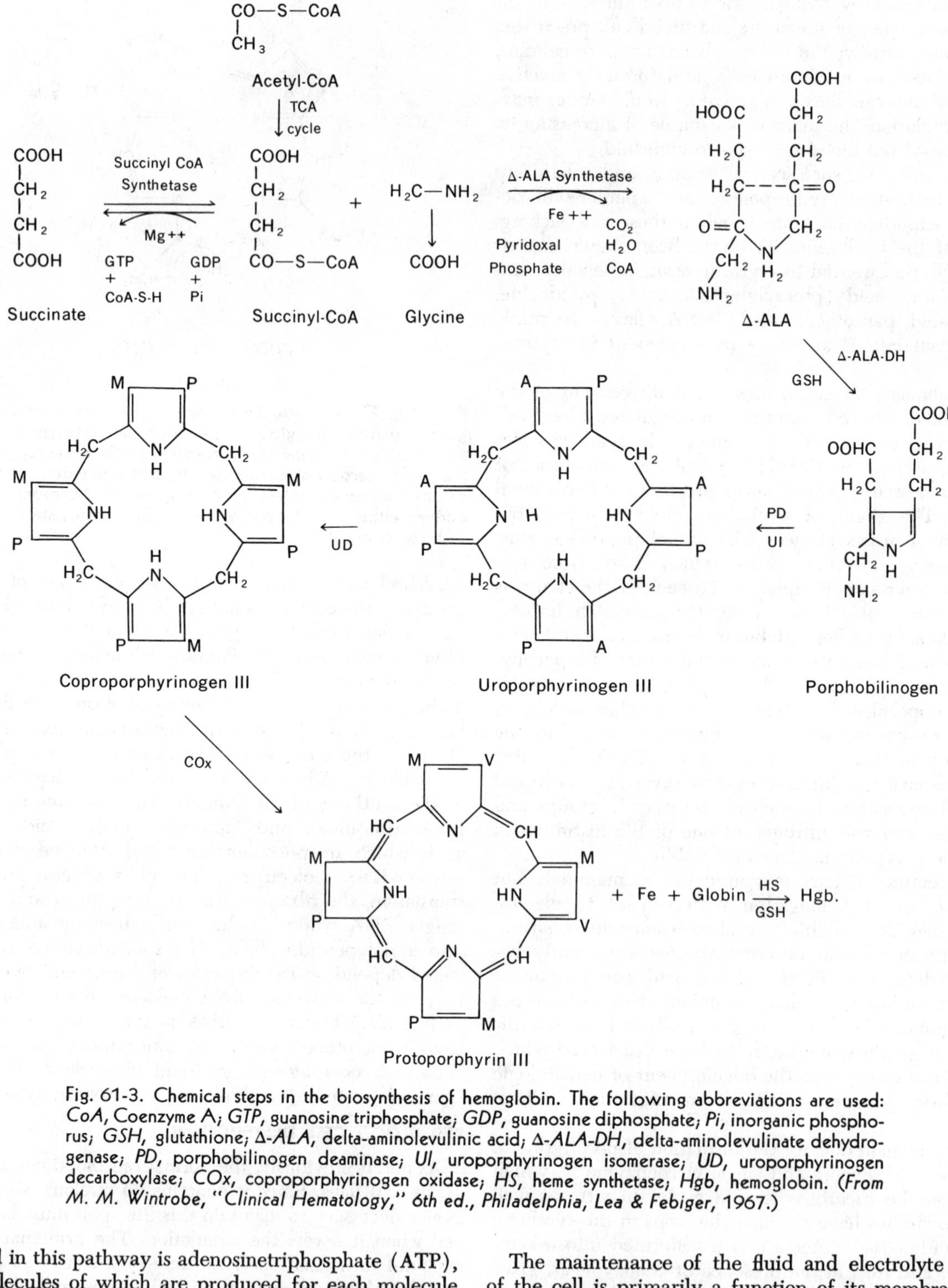

Fig. 61-3. Chemical steps in the biosynthesis of hemoglobin. The following abbreviations are used: CoA, Coenzyme A; GTP, guanosine triphosphate; GDP, guanosine diphosphate; Pi, inorganic phosphorus; GSH, glutathione; Δ-ALA, delta-aminolevulinic acid; Δ-ALA-DH, delta-aminolevulinate dehydrogenase; PD, porphobilinogen deaminase; UI, uroporphyrinogen isomerase; UD, uroporphyrinogen decarboxylase; COx, coproporphyrinogen oxidase; HS, heme synthetase; Hgb, hemoglobin. (From M. M. Wintrobe, "Clinical Hematology," 6th ed., Philadelphia, Lea & Febiger, 1967.)

thesized in this pathway is adenosinetriphosphate (ATP), two molecules of which are produced for each molecule of glucose broken down. The remaining 10 to 15 percent of erythrocyte energy is derived from the hexosemonophosphate shunt. Since no mitochondria are found in mature red blood cells, there is no tricarboxylic acid (Krebs) cycle, and energy from this pathway is not available.

The maintenance of the fluid and electrolyte content of the cell is primarily a function of its membrane. The total volume of the cell must be kept within relatively narrow limits despite an osmotic gradient, and a low sodium and high potassium concentration relative to plasma must be maintained in man. At least three different "pumps" capable of moving sodium out of the cell against an osmotic gradient exist in the erythrocyte membrane. Two of these utilize energy derived from ATP, require the enzyme adenosinetriphosphatase, and are inhibited by cardiac glycosides. They differ from each other in that one requires potassium in the external medium, and the other requires sodium. The third "pump" is inhibited by ethacrynic acid, but not by cardiac glycosides, and requires sodium in the external medium.

The principal components of the system which protect the red blood cell and its contents from oxidation are glutathione, reduced triphosphopyridine nucleotide (TPNH, NADPH), and the enzymes glucose 6-phosphate dehydrogenase, glutathione reductase, and glutathione peroxidase.

At the end of its life span, the red blood cell is removed by components of the reticuloendothelial system, principally the spleen. Within the reticuloendothelial cell, hemoglobin catabolism takes place. Iron and amino acids are extracted and subsequently are reutilized. The porphyrin ring is converted to bile pigments, which are excreted.

In the first step of hemoglobin catabolism, the iron atom is oxidized to the trivalent state, and methemoglobin is formed. Next, the linkage between the heme and the globin is severed, yielding **hematin.** Cleavage of the porphyrin ring is then accomplished by oxidation of the alpha methene bridge, a reaction which requires a ribosomal, mixed-function oxidase enzyme. Products of this reaction are iron, carbon monoxide, and **biliverdin,** a straight chain tetrapyrrole. Most of the liberated iron is transported as "plasma iron" via the transport protein, transferrin, a β_1-globulin, to the bone marrow, where it is used in the synthesis of new hemoglobin. Part of the iron may be retained within the reticuloendothelial cell as ferritin, a ferric iron-protein complex, or as hemosiderin, a ferric hydroxide polymer. The liberated globin is degraded and is returned to the body pool of amino acids. Biliverdin, as discussed earlier, is rapidly reduced to bilirubin, which is then transported from the site of hemoglobin breakdown to the liver via the blood plasma, where it is carried with albumin as a relatively stable protein-pigment complex. On reaching the liver, bilirubin is separated from albumin, conjugated with glucuronic acid, and excreted via the bile ducts in the form of protein-free di- and monoglucuronides.

Under pathologic conditions, free hemoglobin may escape into the circulation. This colors the plasma faint pink to deep red, depending on the concentration. The latter can be measured quantitatively by the benzidine reaction. Hemoglobinemia occurs in severe hemolytic states when there is intravascular hemolysis, as in erythroblastosis fetalis, blackwater fever, and *Clostridium welchii* (*C. perfringens*) sepsis (Chap. 172). Liberated hemoglobin is promptly bound by certain globulins with affinity for hemoglobin, the **haptoglobins,** and is carried to the reticuloendothelial system for breakdown there and conversion to bilirubin. The plasma haptoglobins can usually bind from 100 to 135 mg hemoglobin per 100 ml plasma. When this binding capacity is exceeded, other serum proteins which bind appreciable amounts of hemoglobin and its metabolites include (1) **hemopexin,** a heme-binding β_1-globulin, and (2) albumin which, by union with the ferric complex of protoporphyrin, hematin, forms **methemalbumin.** This compound reacts with benzidine and can be distinguished spectroscopically from other heme and pyrroll pigments. Demonstration of methemalbumin in plasma strongly suggests intravascular hemolysis. This compound may remain in the plasma for many hours or several days.

Hemoglobin liberated in the plasma escapes in the urine. The so-called "renal threshold" for hemoglobin is probably not a true renal barrier, but depends on the capacity of the binding proteins of the plasma and the reabsorptive capacity of the tubules. It is the free, unbound hemoglobin which appears in the urine. Hemoglobin usually appears in the urine if the plasma hemoglobin concentration exceeds the binding capacity of the various binding proteins of the plasma. Hemoglobinuria is then likely to continue until the plasma hemoglobin has fallen to 75 mg per 100 ml. The tubular epithelium of the kidney converts hemoglobin to hemosiderin, and hemosiderin is found regularly in the urine of patients with low concentrations of heme pigments in their plasma. The passage of hemoglobin by the kidney is accompanied and also followed by proteinuria, hemoglobin casts, and precipitates of hemoglobin. The color of urine ranges from pink to deep red with oxyhemoglobin, from purple to black from reduced hemoglobin.

Not all the bile pigment is derived from senescent erythrocytes. Studies of stercobilin excretion following the administration of ^{15}N-labeled glycine indicate that normally at least 10 percent (and in diseases such as pernicious anemia, thalassemia, and congenital porphyria, as much as 30 to 40 percent) is probably derived from heme or porphyrins produced in excess and not utilized in hemoglobin synthesis.

In the intestine, probably through the activity of the bacterial flora, bilirubin is converted to **urobilinogen.** Urobilinogen consists of three colorless chromogens, all of which are characterized by a strong Ehrlich aldehyde reaction, as well as by instability and ease of oxidation to three corresponding orange-yellow pigments which compose the urobilin group. The transition to urobilin can be hastened by mild oxidizing agents, such as iodine, and this is the basis of Schlesinger's qualitative test (alcoholic zinc acetate) for urobilin.

Although some investigators have maintained that the urobilinogens in urine come directly from bilirubin in the plasma, it is more generally held that they are derived from pigments absorbed from the colon into the portal circulation, most of which are returned to the liver and reexcreted in the bile, but a small proportion of which escape into the general circulation and are excreted by the kidney.

The amount of urobilinogen excreted in the urine in 24 hr (UU) by the normal adult is 0 to 3.5 mg, most frequently 0.5 to 1.5 mg. The normal range for fecal urobilinogen (FU), as calculated from a 4-day period of collection, is 40 to 280 mg per day, usually 100 to 200 mg. The expected values are related to the size of the circulating red blood cell mass; thus, lower values are found in young children. Mean values have been found to increase with age. An important qualification should be added. The oral administration of chlortetracycline (Aureomycin) causes a marked decrease in the concentration of fecal urobilinogen. This can be counteracted by the administration of aluminum hydroxide gel. The usefulness and limitations of urine and fecal urobilinogen determinations are discussed in a later chapter (Chap. 338).

Pathogenesis of Anemia

An *etiologic classification* of anemia is given in Table 61-1. The simplest mechanism by which anemia develops is blood loss. Anemia may also develop if red blood cell production is deficient or if red blood cell destruction is excessive. In anemias due to excessive destruction, a rather marked increase in rates of destruction must obtain before anemia occurs, since the normal bone marrow can compensate for a six- to eightfold increase by a like increase in production rates. In some anemias both decreased production and increased destruction play a role.

Anemia due to **blood loss** may be acute or chronic. When the blood loss is acute, the cause of the anemia is usually obvious, although sometimes a large hemorrhage may have occurred under conditions which do not reveal themselves readily. Hemorrhage in the gastrointestinal tract, e.g., from a peptic ulcer, may be dramatic in its symptoms and may be so severe as to cause shock; at other times it may be insidious in character and may occur without the development of pain or of symptoms pointing clearly to the gastrointestinal tract. Hemorrhage into one of the serous cavities may cause puzzling symptoms and signs: profound anemia may develop suddenly and icterus may even appear as the result of absorption of blood from a serous cavity.

Chronic loss of blood occurs most commonly from the pelvic organs in females and from the gastrointestinal tract in the male. A common cause of chronic posthemorrhagic anemia in certain parts of the world is infestation with the hookworm.

It is clear that in man anemia may occur as the result of iron **deficiency**. *Cobalt* deficiency has never been demonstrated in man, but a form of *copper* deficiency associated with hypoproteinemia and microcytic hypochromic anemia has been described in infants. Of the *B vitamins*, anemia due to deficiency has been demonstrated in man only in the case of folic acid and vitamin B_{12}. Deficiency of these substances is characterized by macrocytic anemia and megaloblastic bone marrow. Quite possibly the other B vitamins are available in such amounts, even under the extraordinary circumstances under which man sometimes finds himself, that anemia clearly attributable solely to lack of nicotinic acid, riboflavin, or pantothenic acid has not been demonstrated. Pyridoxine-deficiency anemia has only once been produced experimentally in the human infant, but anemia responding to the administration of pyridoxine has been reported in a number of patients, in whom it may have developed as the consequence of some metabolic defect. More frequently, deficiencies which result in anemia

in man are not due to lack of the substance in the diet but are "*conditioned*" by special circumstances. Thus lack of vitamin B_{12} in pernicious anemia results from an inability to absorb this vitamin because of lack of a gastric "intrinsic factor." Again, in sprue, vitamin B_{12} or folic acid deficiency may develop, presumably as the consequence of inadequate absorption. The same condition is occasionally encountered following extensive resection of the small bowel or in the case of a gastrocolic fistula. Excessive demands in pregnancy and greater needs for growth in childhood and adolescence may "condition" the development of various types of deficiency, and anemia will then ensue (see Table 337-1, p. 1598).

Severe deficiency of *protein* may lead to anemia in man and experimental animals. In the latter, anemia has been shown to be due to reduced production of erythropoietin.

The role of *ascorbic acid* in relation to anemia has not been established clearly; while anemia is seen in scurvy, it has not been shown that this is due directly to lack of vitamin C (see p. 410).

Anemia also results when the **bone marrow fails** for reasons other than the lack of specific nutrients. In these disorders, which are discussed in greater detail in Chap. 341, other bone marrow elements, the granulocytes and platelets, also tend to be reduced in number. Frequently, these "hypoplastic" anemias are due to toxins or drugs. In other instances, the cause of the marrow failure is not clear.

Hemolytic anemias (see Chap. 338) are anemias in which red blood cell destruction has increased to a degree that cannot be compensated for by the bone marrow. These anemias are characterized by certain unique features. Because of the excessive destruction of hemoglobin, there is an increased output of bile pigment. There may be mild to moderate jaundice, because of an increase in the unconjugated or "indirect" serum bilirubin fraction, and urine and fecal urobilinogen output are increased. There also is evidence of increased red blood cell production, the most reliable sign of which is an increase in the reticulocyte count.

Increased red blood cell destruction may result because the cell is *intrinsically defective* or because it is damaged by *extracorpuscular factors*. In a third category are the varieties of hemolytic anemia in which the *intrinsic erythrocytic defect* alone is not sufficient to lead to accelerated hemolysis, the latter occurring only *in the presence of an extraerythrocytic factor*. The various forms of hemolytic anemia are discussed in Chap. 338.

A number of disorders cannot be easily classified among the above three major groups. If red blood cell survival is measured, it is found to be moderately reduced, but not to a degree that would produce anemia. The capacity of the marrow to compensate for this increase in destruction is limited, however, and these two factors together lead to anemia. The extent to which the features of hemolytic anemia are found in these disorders depends on the degree of accelerated blood destruction.

The hemoglobinopathies are included in Table 338-1 among the hemolytic anemias attributable to intrinsic erythrocytic defects because they result from qualitative abnormalities of hemoglobin composition; **the thalassemia syndromes** are included because they are due to quantitative abnormalities of hemoglobin peptide synthesis (Chap. 339). The manifestations of these disorders are variable, however. In some, notably thalassemia major and sickle-cell anemia, there is a marked shortening of red blood cell survival, and it is in such cases that the usual features of hemolysis are present. In others, anemia appears to be due to a combination of reduced red blood cell production and a mild increase in destruction. Still others, including most of the heterozygous conditions, are not accompanied by anemia; in fact, some have been described in which polycythemia occurs as a result of abnormal hemoglobin oxygen binding. Consequently, the hemoglobinopathies and thalassemias may also be classified as disorders with both decreased production and increased destruction of red blood cells, as shown in Table 61-1.

Table 61-1. ETIOLOGIC CLASSIFICATION OF ANEMIA

I. Loss of blood
   A. Acute posthemorrhagic anemia
   B. Chronic posthemorrhagic anemia
II. Deficient red cell production
   A. Deficiency of factors concerned with erythropoiesis
     1. Iron deficiency
     2. Experimentally: copper and cobalt deficiencies
     3. Vitamin B_{12} or folic acid deficiency (pernicious anemia and related megaloblastic anemias)
     4. Experimentally: pyridoxine, riboflavin, pantothenic acid, vitamin E, and protein deficiencies
     5. Posisibly ascorbic acid deficiency
   B. Anemas of bone marrow failure
     1. Hypoplastic and aplastic anemia
     2. Refractory sideoblastic anemia
III. Excessive red blood cell destruction (hemolytic anemias) (see Chap. 338)
   A. Hemolysis principally attributed to intrinsic erythrocytic defects
   B. Hemolysis attributed to an intrinsic erythrocytic defect *plus* an extraerythrocytic factor
   C. Hemolysis principally attributed to extraerythrocytic factors
IV. Disorders with both decreased production and increased destruction of red blood cells
   A. Defective hemoglobin synthesis
     1. Thalassemias
     2. Hemoglobinopathies (sickle-cell anemia and related disorderss)
   B. Anemiae associated with chronic diseases (infection, cancer, rheumatoid arthritis)
   C. Anermia of renal disease
   D. Aemia of liver disease
   E. Annemia of myxedema and other endocrine disorders
   F. Anemias due to bone marrow invasion (myelophthisic anemias)

The **anemia accompanying chronic infection, cancer, and rheumatoid arthritis** (Chap. 340) is unique in that it is associated with a profound disturbance in iron metabolism. This is manifested by a low plasma iron concentration, reduced plasma iron-binding capacity, increased iron stores, and decreased marrow sideroblasts. The defect cannot be altered by iron administration, even if iron is given parenterally in large quantities. An increase in free erythrocyte protoporphyrin and in serum copper occurs at the same time. It is probable that the flow of iron to plasma from reticuloendothelial stores is restricted, but the way in which such a restriction is brought about is unknown. This metabolic defect is overcome and anemia is corrected when the underlying disease, e.g., infection, is treated appropriately.

In the **anemia of renal insufficiency** (Chap. 340), the decrease in red blood cell survival is, in part at least, the consequence of extracorpuscular factors. The nature of these factors has not been defined; there is no evidence of an autoimmune mechanism, nor is there a clear relation with any of the products which are retained in renal insufficiency. Since the kidney is concerned in erythropoietin production, attention has been directed to a possible defect in synthesis of this hormone as an explanation for the decrease in red blood cell production. Plasma erythropoietin levels have been found to be reduced in comparison with comparable degrees of anemia due to other causes. Furthermore, the radioiron marrow transit time, which becomes shortened as erythropoietin stimulates the marrow, is prolonged in renal disease. Unlike the anemia of other chronic disorders, the anemia of renal insufficiency is not characterized by hypoferremia as a constant feature.

Multiple factors are implicated in the pathogenesis of the **anemia of hepatic disease.** Blood loss from esophageal varices may lead to acute or chronic posthemorrhagic anemia. Nutritional folic acid deficiency not uncommonly accompanies cirrhosis in alcoholics. Alcohol itself has been shown to cause reversible depression of red blood cell production. In most cases, however, the cause of the anemia is not clearly defined. The red blood cells are normal or increased in size and tend to be thinner than normal, possibly because of the effect of bile salt retention on membrane lipids. Red blood cell survival is moderately shortened, and red blood cell production is decreased.

The pathogenesis of the anemia observed in **myxedema** is obscure. Defective absorption of vitamin B_{12}, uninfluenced by intrinsic factor, has been demonstrated in some cases. The anemia, which is usually only moderate in degree and is usually normocytic but may be macrocytic, disappears gradually as desiccated thyroid is given, but it seems unlikely that it is attributable directly to deficiency of the hormone. It has been suggested that it is brought about indirectly through the effect of the thyroid on the consumption of oxygen by the tissues. Moderate anemia is encountered in association with adrenocortical insufficiency and in hypopituitarism. The pathogenetic mechanisms are not understood, but in view of what is now known concerning the functions of the hormones secreted by the adrenal glands and the pituitary gland, it is at least plausible that the anemia is the consequence of some metabolic disturbance resulting from deficiency of these hormones.

The pathogenesis of the anemia in **leukemia, malignancy** with metastases to bone marrow (Chap. 340), **myelofibrosis** (Chap. 350), and other similar conditions is as yet obscure. Such anemia has been classified as myelophthisic. The term implies wasting away of the marrow, but it is usually used to refer to encroachment on or replacement of the bone marrow by leukemia or metastases. There is little or no evidence, however, that the erythropoietic tissue is crowded out in these myelophthisic anemias. Measurements of red blood cell production rates have at times yielded normal or increased values. It has been suggested that in some cases erythrophagocytosis contributes to the anemia. A number of studies have shown the "life span" of the red corpuscles to be reduced, and occasionally frank hemolytic anemia develops. It is possible that no single explanation for the anemia associated with these diseases will be found, but it is plausible, at least, that a metabolic fault related to the underlying disease is an important factor.

It should not be overlooked that in any given patient with a chronic ailment accompanied by anemia, more than one factor may play a role. Thus, in any long-standing illness there may be nutritional deficiency because of reduced intake, and sometimes also because of faulty absorption from the gastrointestinal tract. Blood loss may be an added factor. In addition, a metabolic disturbance, such as that which accompanies infection, may play a role as well. In some instances excessive blood destruction complicates the picture still further.

The Signs and Symptoms of Anemia

Anemia should never be thought of as a diagnosis in itself, but rather as a manifestation of an underlying disease process. Thus, the signs and symptoms found in the anemic patient are a mixture of those due to anemia and those due to the underlying disease. Only those symptoms common to all anemias will be discussed below; symptoms more specifically related to the underlying disease are dealt with in the chapters dealing with those entities.

Cardiorespiratory System. Hemoglobin is the vehicle and the cardiovascular system the means of delivery of oxygen to the tissues. When anemia is present, the oxygen-carrying capacity of the blood is reduced. If an equivalent amount of oxygen is to be delivered, blood flow must be increased by means of certain cardiovascular adjustments (Fig. 61-4). Many of the signs and symptoms of anemia reflect these changes in cardiovascular function.

An increased blood flow is accomplished by increases in cardiac stroke volume and heart rate. The patient may be aware of this increased cardiac activity and complain of palpitation. On examination, tachycardia and an increased pulse pressure may be found along with increased pulsations over the precordium and major arteries, and even a capillary pulsation in the fingertips may be detected. The circulation time may be shortened, and there may be a slight rise in right auricular pressure.

Still other signs of the "hyperkinetic syndrome" may be observed (Chap. 264).

The adequacy of the cardiovascular adjustments to anemia depends on the degree of the anemia, the rapidity with which it has developed, and the preexisting status of the cardiovascular system. Symptoms are usually present when the blood hemoglobin concentration is less than 7.5 Gm per 100 ml blood. If anemia has developed so rapidly that there has been little or no time for physiologic adjustment, symptoms are likely to be prominent and to appear comparatively early; on the other hand, if the anemia has been insidious in onset, the adjustment may be so good that the hemoglobin may be as low as 6 Gm per 100 ml, without sufficient functional embarrassment occurring for the patient to be seriously handicapped.

The cardiovascular changes necessarily encroach upon the cardiac reserve; consequently, exercise tolerance is decreased. There may be no symptoms at rest, but signs of oxygen want, such as easy fatigability and dyspnea, develop on exertion. When compensatory adjustments become imperfect or fail, either because of an extreme degree of anemia or because of a previously damaged heart, the clinical picture of cardiac failure ensues. There may be edema, congestion of the neck veins, hepatomegaly, and rales at the bases of the lungs.

Severe anemia may produce a systolic murmur, which is usually most marked at the pulmonic area, but may be heard elsewhere over the precordium, especially at the apex. Very rarely, diastolic murmurs are heard at the base. Over the vessels of the neck a curious humming sound, the *bruit de diable*, may be heard.

Neuromuscular System. Headache, vertigo, faintness, increased sensitivity to cold, tinnitus or roaring in the ears, black spots before the eyes, muscular weakness, and easy fatigability and irritability are common symptoms associated with anemia. Restlessness is an important symptom of rapidly developing anemia. Drowsiness develops in severe anemia. Headache due to anemia may be very severe. Delirium is seldom seen except in pernicious anemia and in the terminal stage of leukemia. Retinal hemorrhage is by no means infrequent.

Alimentary System. Loss of appetite is not unusual as an accompaniment of anemia. Nausea, flatulence, abdominal discomfort, constipation, diarrhea, vomiting, or abnormal appetite may also be found.

Genitourinary System. Menstrual disturbances (most often amenorrhea) in the female, and loss of libido in the male, are frequently encountered in severe anemia. In other instances, excessive menstrual bleeding accompanies anemia. Slight proteinuria and evidence of distinct renal function impairment may be seen in association with anemia.

Epithelial Tissues. The pallor which accompanies anemia has been discussed. The skin itself is an unreliable index of anemia; the mucous membranes (if not inflamed), the nail beds, and the palms of the hands are more dependable. The color of the conjunctiva may be very helpful, but one should not be misled by a coexistent conjunctivitis. The gums are not so useful as would be

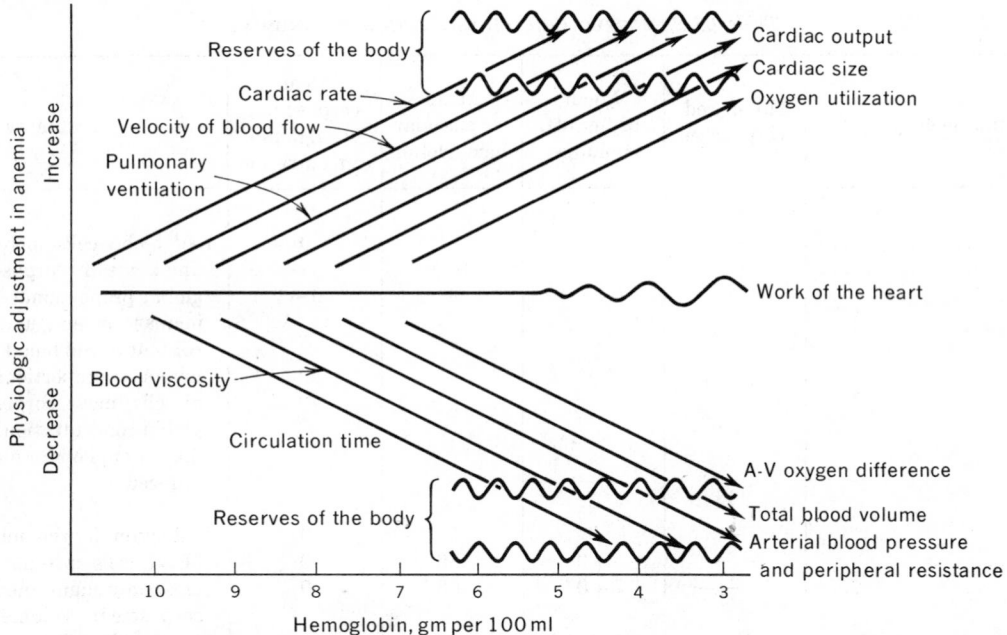

Fig. 61-4. Schematic diagram of physiologic adjustments to anemia. (*From M. M. Wintrobe, Blood,* 1:121, 1946.)

expected, for they may contain pigment or may be inflamed; furthermore, the pressure of the upper lip on the gums may produce some blanching if constriction of vessels results as the lip is retracted. Unless the hand has been held in an awkward position or has been exposed to cold or excessive heat, the nail beds and the palms of the hands will reveal anemia if much exists. In the palms the color of the creases is especially noteworthy, for they retain their red color even after the intervening skin of the palms has become definitely pale; when their color is lost, the hemoglobin may be judged as being below 7 Gm per 100 ml. In addition to pallor, loss of normal skin elasticity and tone, thinning of the hair, and purpura and ecchymoses may develop in the chronic forms of anemia.

The Approach to the Patient with Anemia

Anemia is not a diagnosis in itself, but a manifestation of disease. The challenge to the physician is to diagnose correctly and treat the underlying disease. Failure to appreciate this simple principle may lead to many serious errors in management of the condition. To cite a common example, a patient with anemia secondary to a bleeding cecal carcinoma may be treated with blood transfusions or iron-containing medications or even "hematinic" pills containing a mixture of nutrients and will apparently improve, but the carcinoma will progress to an inoperable stage.

Since literally hundreds of disorders may be associated with anemia, a rational approach to anemia requires that a classification of the causes of anemia be used which forms the basis of a systematic procedure leading to a

diagnosis. Classifications of anemia have been based on etiology (as in Table 61-1), and such an approach may be effective in many cases. However, the necessary information is often difficult to obtain; accurate evaluation of rates of erythrocyte production and destruction often involves rather elaborate, time-consuming, and expensive procedures that needlessly delay proper management. An example is the determination of red blood cell life span. A more practical approach is based on a morphologic classification of anemia. The advantage is that the information necessary to make the classification is quickly obtained at little cost.

The first step in the morphologic classification of a given anemia is to categorize it as belonging in one of three major groups: (1) the macrocytic anemias, (2) the hypochromic and/or microcytic anemias, and (3) the normocytic, normochromic anemias. This is accomplished by the calculation of **corpuscular constants** (erythrocyte indexes) and the careful examination of the stained blood smear.

There are three corpuscular constants, *the mean corpuscular volume* (MCV), the *mean corpuscular hemoglobin concentration* (MCHC), and the *mean corpuscular hemoglobin* (MCH). They are calculated from ratios of the three measures of anemia. Thus,

$$\text{MCV } (\mu^3) = \frac{\text{VPRC}}{\text{RBC}}$$

$$\text{MCHC } (\%) = \frac{\text{Hb}}{\text{VPRC}}$$

$$\text{MCH } (\mu\mu g) = \frac{\text{Hb}}{\text{RBC}}$$

Table 61-2. MORPHOLOGIC CLASSIFICATION OF ANEMIAS

Class and severity	No. of red corpuscles	Mean corpuscular volume	Mean corpuscular hemoglobin	Mean corpuscular hemoglobin concentration	Summary
Macrocytic:					Red blood cells increased in volume; mean corpuscular hemoglobin proportionately increased; increase in size and hemoglobin content of red blood cells roughly inversely proportional to number of cells; mean corpuscular hemoglobin concentration remains normal throughout or may be slightly reduced.
Slight..................	−	+	+	0	
Moderate..............	− −	+ +	+ +	0 −	
Severe.................	− − −	+ + +	+ + +	0 −	
Normocytic:					Reduction in the number of red blood cells without any, or at most only slight, increase in mean corpuscular volume and mean corpuscular hemoglobin; mean corpuscular hemoglobin concentration normal throughout.
Slight..................	−	0	0	0	
Moderate..............	− −	+0	+0	0	
Severe.................	− − −	+0	+0	0	
Hypochromic and/or microcytic:					Reduction in hemoglobin characteristically more marked than reduction in number of cells.
Hypochromic............	−	0	−	−	
Microcytic..............	−	−	−	0	
Hypochromic, microcytic:					
Slight..................	0	−	− −	−	
Moderate..............	−	− −	− − −	− −	
Severe.................	− −	− − −	− − − −	− − −	

+, increase; −, decrease; 0, no change from the normal; 0−, no, or only slight, decrease; +0, slight or no increase. The amount of increase or decrease is indicated by the number of plus or minus signs, respectively.

Normal values for these constants are given in the Appendix. Their use in making a morphologic classification is outlined in Table 61-2.

Since the above determinations are subject to laboratory error, the morphologic impression should always be confirmed by examination of the blood smear. With experience, an accurate assessment of red blood cell size can be made by observing the average red blood cell diameter under the microscope. Hypochromia is seen as an increase in the area of central pallor. It is always wise to compare the observations made on the patient's blood with those made on a normal blood smear, since the magnification and illumination of microscopes vary. Uncommonly, distortions of red blood cell shape may lead to an erroneous impression from examination of the blood smear, especially when cells are unusually flat (leptocytosis), as they are in liver disease, in thalassemia, and after splenectomy. Such cells appear larger and more hypochromic than the corpuscular constants indicate.

The next step in the morphologic approach to anemia varies with the major morphologic category (Table 61-3). Macrocytic anemias are subdivided into two groups, **megaloblastic** and **nonmegaloblastic.** The megaloblastic anemias, of which pernicious anemia is the prototype, result from defective synthesis of nucleic acids, usually because of a deficiency of vitamin B_{12} or folic acid. Certain morphologic features characterize the megaloblastic anemias. The earliest changes are seen in the blood smear and consist of the presence of *oval macrocytes* and *hypersegmented neutrophils.* In the bone marrow, characteristic alterations are seen in nucleated red blood cells; they are larger than normal, and the nuclear chromatin is finer and more particulate. These changes are discussed more fully in Chap. 330, along with a further subclassification of the megaloblastic anemias.

The *nonmegaloblastic* macrocytic anemias make up a heterogeneous group. Macrocytosis is found in patients with markedly increased rates of red blood cell production, because young erythrocytes are somewhat larger than mature erythrocytes; in addition, when demands upon the marrow are great, a "skipped generation" occurs—i.e., the nucleus is prematurely discharged and the red blood cell is released before maturation has progressed fully. Such cells are considerably larger than normal and, since hemoglobin synthesis has not been completed, may be somewhat hypochromic as well. Macrocytosis may also be observed in the anemia accompanying hypothyroidism, liver disease, or aplastic

Table 61-3. MORPHOLOGIC CLASSIFICATION OF ANEMIA

I. Macrocytic anemias (MCV, 94–160 cu μ; MCH, 32–50 $\mu\mu$g; MCHC, 32–36%)
   A. Those related to deficiency of vitamin B_{12} and folic acid (megaloblastic macrocytic anemias)
      1. Pernicious anemia
      2. Sprue and other conditions in which intestinal absorption is impaired
      3. Megaloblastic anemia of infancy
      4. Megaloblastic anemia of pregnancy
      5. Nutritional macrocytic anemias, refractory megaloblastic anemia, etc.
      6. Antimetabolites and increased demands for hematopoietic factors
   B. Where there is intense activity of the bone marrow and in other circumstances (nonmegaloblastic macrocytic anemias)
      1. Reticulocytosis (acute posthemorrhagic anemia, hemolytic anemias, and other conditions usually associated with normocytic anemia)
      2. Some cases of hypothyroidism, liver disease, aplastic anemia
II. Hypochromic, microcytic anemias (MCV, 50–82 cu μ; MCH, 12–27 $\mu\mu$g; MCHC, 24–32%)
   A. Iron deficiency due to
      1. Chronic blood loss
      2. Inadequate intake of iron together with
      3. Faulty absorption (achlorhydria, sprue, etc.) and
      4. Excessive demands for iron (growth, menstruation, pregnancies)
   B. Thalassemia and combinations with abnormal hemoglobinopathies
   C. Anemia of chronic disorders
   D. Sideroblastic (sideroachrestic, hypersideremic) anemias
III. Normocytic anemias (MCV, 82–92 cu μ; MCH, 28–32 $\mu\mu$g; MCHC, 32–36%)
   A. Acute blood loss
   B. Destruction of blood—acute and chronic hemolytic anemias
   C. Anemia of chronic disorders
   D. Anemia due to bone marrow failure
   E. Myelophthisic anemia
   F. Hydremia—not a true anemia

Note: MCV, mean corpuscular volume; MCH, mean corpuscular hemoglobin; MCHC, mean corpuscular hemoglobin concentration.

anemia, but the cause of the macrocytosis in these disorders is not understood.

The **hypochromic** and/or **microcytic anemias** are disorders in which hemoglobin synthesis is deficient. Normal hemoglobin synthesis requires iron, protoporphyrin, and globin, and an abnormality affecting the availability of any of the three may lead to a hypochromic and/or microcytic anemia. By far, the most common cause of this type of anemia is iron deficiency (see Chap. 336). Hypochromia and microcytosis are constant findings in thalassemia and may at times be seen in the hemoglobinopathies (see Chap. 339). The anemia of chronic disorders, such as infection, cancer, and rheumatoid arthritis, is usually normocytic and normochromic, but

at times is hypochromic and occasionally is both hypochromic and microcytic (see Chap. 340). The morphologic changes probably occur because of the disturbance in iron metabolism previously alluded to. Hypochromia and microcytosis are found also in sideroblastic anemias. These are comparatively rare and probably include a variety of entities, some acquired and some inherited. They have in common evidence of excessive iron stores, sometimes producing clinical manifestations of hemochromatosis.

Frequently, a final diagnosis in the hypochromic, microcytic group of anemias can be reached after a careful history and physical examination. Special attention should be given to the dietary history, to evidence of blood loss, and to the possibility of familial transmission. Evaluation of the status of iron metabolism will help to confirm the impression. The principal clinical tools used for evaluating iron metabolism are the serum iron level and iron-binding capacity and the quantitation of iron stores in marrow aspirates stained with the Prussian blue reaction and of iron in nucleated red blood cells (sideroblasts). Results of these procedures are indicated in Table 61-4.

Table 61-4. MEASURES OF IRON METABOLISM IN THE HYPOCHROMIC-MICROCYTIC ANEMIAS

Type of anemia	Serum iron	Serum iron-binding capacity	Marrow iron stores	Marrow sideroblasts
Iron-deficiency....	Decreased	Increased	Absent	Absent
Thalassemia......	Normal or increased	Normal	Normal or increased	Normal or increased
Anemia of chronic disorders	Decreased	Decreased	Usually increased	Decreased
Sideroblastic anemias	Increased	Decreased	Markedly increased	Markedly increased

In evaluating the status of a patient with **normocytic, normochromic** anemia (Table 61-3, III), it is useful to try to draw some preliminary conclusions about the rates of erythrocyte production and destruction. It is rare that measurement of the red blood cell life span with ^{51}chromium is necessary; simpler methods usually provide the necessary information. The most useful, simple method for detecting increased red blood cell production is the reticulocyte count. Increased red blood cell destruction is detected by evaluating bile pigment metabolism by means of serum bilirubin and urinary and fecal urobilinogen determinations. The *anemia of acute blood loss* (Chap. 335) is associated with increased red blood cell production; consequently, the reticulocyte count is usually increased. The *hemolytic anemias* (Chap. 338) are characterized by evidence of both increased production and destruction. In the *anemia of chronic disorders* (Chap. 340), a moderate increase in erythrocyte destruction is accompanied by a modest decrease in production; the changes are subtle, so that the reticulocyte count and measures of hemoglobin catabolism remain within normal limits. The alterations in iron metabolism mentioned above may help to detect the condition. The *anemias due to bone marrow failure* are usually associated with a depressed reticulocyte count; there is no evidence of excessive hemoglobin catabolism, and leukopenia and thrombocytopenia also are present. The *myelophthisic anemias* are characterized by a bizarre blood smear: marked variations in erythrocyte size and shape, nucleated red blood cells, myeloid immaturity, and enlarged, bizarre platelets.

EXAMINATION OF THE BONE MARROW. In some of the above conditions, a final diagnosis is established by study of the bone marrow. This procedure is useful not only in the evaluation of the anemic patient, but also in disorders affecting other formed elements of the blood. There are two basic techniques by which marrow is obtained for study: *aspiration* from the sternum or iliac crest, and *biopsy* of the posterior iliac spine with the Westerman-Jensen needle. Thin smears are prepared from bone marrow aspirates, and such preparations, when stained with Wright's stain, are ideal for the study of fine morphologic details. These smears may also be stained with the Prussian blue reaction in order to assess the amount of iron in reticuloendothelial cells and sideroblasts. Fixed, thick sections of marrow obtained by biopsy are ideal for evaluating the cellularity of the marrow and for detecting fibrosis or granulomatous disorders.

When the patient's condition has been studied thoroughly in the manner indicated above, the number of instances in which examination of the bone marrow will be required is small. In Table 61-5 various types of reaction are listed which may be observed if differential counts on aspirated bone marrow are made. In such preparations, consideration should be given to the following:

Table 61-5. CONDITIONS IN WHICH VARIOUS TYPES OF REACTION MAY BE OBSERVED, AS DEMONSTRATED BY BONE MARROW ASPIRATION

M/E (myeloid/erythroid) ratio increased	*Nonmyeloid cells increased*
Myeloid forms of leukemia	Other forms of leukemia
The majority of infections	Multiple myeloma
Leukemoid reaction	Metastases from carcinoma, etc.
Decrease in nucleated red blood cells	Gaucher's disease, Niemann-Pick disease
	Aplastic anemia (usually relative increase only)
	Infectious mononucleosis

Normoblastic hyperplasia	*Megaloblastic hyperplasia*
Hemorrhagic anemias	Pernicious anemia
Iron-deficiency anemia	Sprue, idiopathic steatorrhea, resection of small intestine (certain cases)
Hemolytic anemias	
Thalassemia	
Cirrhosis of the liver	Tropical macrocytic anemia
Polycythemia vera	Nontropical nutritional macrocytic anemia
Plumbism	
Anemia of chronic renal disease	Macrocytic anemia with Diphyllobothrium infestation
Sideroblastic anemias	Megaloblastic anemia of infancy
	Megaloblastic anemia of pregnancy
	"Refractory megaloblastic" or "achrestic" anemia

1. The myeloid/erythroid (M/E) ratio. By this is meant the proportion of leukocytes of the myeloid series to nucleated red blood cells of all types. A decrease in the M/E ratio (i.e., a greater-than-normal proportion of nucleated red blood cells) may be the result of a decrease in the number of myeloid cells, or it may be the consequence of an increase in erythroid cells. In the latter event, one must differentiate between normoblastic and megaloblastic hyperplasia.

2. The presence of an increased number of cells other than those of the myeloid or erythroid series. These include lymphocytes, plasma cells, reticulum cells, and other forms (myeloma cells, carcinoma cells, Gaucher's cells, etc.).

3. Megakaryocytes. Since these form so small a proportion of the cells of the bone marrow, specific attention should be given them and a number of preparations of marrow should be examined. One should attempt to determine whether they appear to be increased or greatly decreased in number and whether their structure is normal.

4. The absence of marrow elements. In such cases, biopsy may be necessary.

In Table 61-6 are given normal values for the differential nucleated cell count of bone marrow obtained by puncture, and representative findings in a number of conditions are presented. These must be regarded only as examples of findings in typical cases; they do not give the range of variation in disease. The latter obviously depends on the stage of the disease and the presence or absence of modifying factors.

Although in all cases the material obtained by sternal puncture is of interest, bone marrow examination is an essential aid in diagnosis only in a limited number of conditions. These include aleukemic leukemia, multiple myeloma, Gaucher's and Niemann-Pick diseases, and unusual cases of macrocytic anemia. In the last-mentioned condition the demonstration of megaloblasts is very useful, since it suggests vitamin B_{12} or folic acid deficiency. In "aleukemic" leukemia, the bone marrow reveals numerous immature forms, thus dispelling the doubt raised by their absence or scarcity in the blood. In addition to these disorders, in disseminated tuberculosis and histoplasmosis, and in parasitic diseases such as kala-azar, the causative organisms may be discovered in the bone marrow when they cannot be found in any other way. Again, the cells of metastatic lesions may be demonstrated by sternal puncture.

In aplastic anemia it is the negative character of the aspirated marrow material which may be helpful. In cases suspected of being instances of "atypical leukemia," "agnogenic myeloid metaplasia," or "hypersplenism," sternal puncture followed by biopsy may support one of these diagnoses or, instead, may reveal myelosclerosis or myelofibrosis.

Management of Anemia

In the sense that by their administration a specific deficiency is corrected, vitamin B_{12}, folic acid, and iron

Table 61-6. REPRESENTATIVE DIFFERENTIAL COUNTS OF BONE MARROW OBTAINED BY PUNCTURE

Types of cells	Normal[1] average and range	Leukemia, acute[2,3]	Leukemia,[3] chronic myelocytic	Leukemia,[3] chronic lymphocytic	Multiple myeloma[4]	Pernicious anemia	Hemolytic anemias	Iron-deficiency anemia	I.T.P.[7]
Myeloblasts.......	2.0 (0.3–5.0)	*50–95*[5]	4.0	...	0.5	0.8	0.8	0.5	
Promyelocytes.....	5.0 (1.0–8.0)	......	*10.0*	0.8	1.8	2.7	3.0	2.0	1.5
Myelocytes									
Neutrophilic.....	12.0 (5.0–19.0)	......	*26.0*	1.5	1.8	7.7	8.0	9.0	8.0
Eosinophilic.....	1.5 (0.5–3.0)	......	2.0	0.7	...	0.8	2.0	0.8	
Basophilic.......	0.3 (0.0–0.5)	......	0.4	0.2	...	0.3			
Metamyelocytes....	22.0 (13.0–32.0)	......	22.0	8.0	3.3	14.5	18.0	15.0	15.3
Polymorphonuclear									
neutrophils......	20.0 (7.0–30.0)		29.0	8.5	62.0	14.5	9.0	28.0	31.0
Polymorphonuclear									
eosinophils......	2.0 (0.5–4.0)		0.8	1.0	3.5	0.5	0.6	0.2	0.5
Polymorphonuclear									
basophils........	0.2 (0.0–0.7)		0.4	3.0	1.2	0.2	...	...	0.2
Lymphocytes.....	10.0 (3.0–17.0)		1.4	*60.0*	13.0	9.5	10.0	1.0	2.5
Plasma cells.......	0.4 (0.0–2.0)		...	...	*4.3*[4]	0.2	0.4	0.7	0.8
Monocytes........	2.0 (0.5–5.0)		0.2	...	0.2	0.3			
Reticulum cells....	0.2 (0.1–2.0)		1.2	1.5	1.0	2.0	2.6	0.8	
Mitotic figures.....	0		0.2	0.3	...	2.7	1.0		
Abnormal cells.....	0								
Megakaryocytes....	0.4 (0.03–3.0)	......	...	...	...	...	...	...	0.2[6]
Megaloblasts......	0	......	...	...	...	40.0			
Pronormoblasts....	4.0 (1.0–8.0)	......	...	0.2	...	...	5.0	...	4.0
Normoblasts.......	18.0 (7.0–32.0)	......	2.4	14.3	9.0	3.0	*43.0*	40.0	36.0
M/E ratio........	4:1 (3–5:1)	......	40:1	1.5:1	8:1	1:1.5	*1:1*	1.4:1	1.5:1

[1] Adapted from M. M. Wintrobe "Clinical Hematology," 6th ed., Philadelphia, Lea & Febiger, 1967.

[2] The immature forms are listed in the table as myeloblasts merely as a matter of convenience. In acute lymphoblastic leukemia the cells are lymphoblasts, not myeloblasts. Often it is difficult to distinguish the various immature abnormal cells seen in acute leukemia. The essential point is the great preponderance of very young forms.

[3] The bone marrow picture in *aleukemic leukemia* is similar to that of leukemia of the various types, whether or not changes can be demonstrated in the blood.

[4] The characteristic cells in multiple myeloma differ somewhat from typical plasma cells in that the nuclear chromatin is relatively fine and the wheel-spoke arrangement of the chromatin is not present; the cytoplasm is basophilic and bright blue, not blue-green as in the plasma cell. A perinuclear clear zone is unusual.

[5] The most significant changes are shown in *italics*.

[6] Although the number of megakaryocytes may not appear to be increased, in typical idiopathic thrombocytopenic purpura the majority (64 percent in the case cited) have no platelets about them and most of the remainder (32 percent) have very few.

[7] Idiopathic thrombocytopenic purpura.

may be considered to be specific agents for the treatment of certain types of anemia. In macrocytic anemias characterized by megaloblastic bone marrow, of which pernicious anemia is the commonest example, the administration of **vitamin B$_{12}$** corrects the deficiency and the anemia is relieved. In certain rare instances of macrocytic megaloblastic anemia, **folic acid** rather than vitamin B$_{12}$ relieves the anemia. Examples are the megaloblastic anemia of infancy, "refractory megaloblastic" or "achrestic" anemia, many cases of "pernicious anemia of pregnancy," and some cases of sprue. These agents are valueless in anemias other than those in which the bone marrow is megaloblastic.

Likewise **iron** therapy is effective in iron-deficiency anemia and is useless in all other types of anemia. Such therapy is almost always effective by mouth, and only in the rare instances of severe gastrointestinal intolerance and in cases of chronic ulcerative colitis with iron deficiency is it justifiable to give iron parenterally. Under such circumstances, iron-dextran or iron-sorbitol may be given intramuscularly with reasonable safety.

Whether or not desiccated thyroid and ascorbic acid should be classed as specific therapeutic agents, as they are in Table 61-7, is debatable. It is clear that the anemia accompanying hypothyroidism is relieved only by the administration of thyroid, but whether this is the direct consequence of the relief of a deficiency is less certain. The relationship of ascorbic acid therapy to the anemia of scurvy is even less apparent.

Anemias which are neither due to deficiency of iron

Table 61-7. THERAPEUTIC AGENTS FOR ANEMIA

  I. Specific: Vitamin B$_{12}$, folic acid, iron
     Desiccated thyroid (?), ascorbic acid (?)
 II. Nonspecific: Blood transfusions
     Irradiation and chemotherapy (in leukemia, etc.)
     ACTH, adrenocorticosteroids, androgens
     Splenectomy

nor caused by lack of vitamin B$_{12}$ or folic acid are most difficult to manage. Iron or liver therapy, vitamins, or combinations of these, given orally or parenterally, are useless and wasteful of the patient's funds and the physician's time. These anemias cannot, in the present state of our knowledge, be relieved without the elimination of the underlying cause. Thus, the anemia of chronic renal disease is difficult to treat because the renal disease itself is usually so unremittent in character. Likewise, the anemia of chronic infection persists as long as the underlying infection continues. Aplastic anemia in which the bone marrow has been damaged in general carries a very poor prognosis. In some instances the destruction of hematopoietic tissue may not be complete, and in such cases the maintenance of life by transfusion may ultimately be followed by some, or even occasionally by complete, regeneration of bone marrow. The anemia of leukemia is relieved if the leukemic process can be checked by irradiation or chemotherapy. The same is true of the anemia of Hodgkin's disease and other disorders of the lymphoid tissue. In all these conditions the administration of iron, vitamin B$_{12}$, and folic acid or liver is valueless, and the giving of transfusions is but a temporary measure of limited value.

The use of blood transfusions in the treatment of anemia and other hematopoietic disorders is discussed in a separate chapter (Chap. 342).

Adrenocorticosteroids and corticotropin may be very useful in the management of acquired hemolytic anemias, and indirectly, when they affect the leukemic process, they serve to relieve anemia temporarily in acute lymphoblastic leukemia. The corticosteroids and **androgens** also have some value in other instances of anemia, e.g., certain instances of aplastic anemia.

Splenectomy produces permanent relief of the anemia of hereditary spherocytosis and may be valuable in some cases of acquired hemolytic anemia. This is especially true in the more chronic cases and when leukopenia and thrombocytopenia also are present. This operation is also valuable in certain cases characterized by "hypersplenism" (Chap. 350). However, splenectomy should not be undertaken without a thorough diagnostic study and full knowledge of the risks involved—the operative mortality rate, the possibility of postoperative atelectasis or other complications, such as postoperative thrombosis (in association with the marked thrombocytosis which may develop after operation). Finally, one must consider the likelihood of failure to achieve the result desired by this operation.

Details of the management of anemia will be discussed in later chapters in connection with the various types of anemia. In dealing with cases of anemia, the value of a diet containing food factors especially useful in blood regeneration, such as animal protein, the B vitamins, and iron, should not be overlooked. Such a diet offers much more than can be gained from vitamin capsules. The diet should also include all other nutritional essentials, such as ascorbic acid. In addition, the physician should ensure a reasonable balance between rest and activity, and attention should be given to the need for reassurance and the necessity of providing the patient with some understanding of his illness. Palliative measures may also be required for various complaints as they arise.

It should be apparent from what has been said already that adequate management of anemia is impossible without a thorough study of the patient and discovery of the nature and cause of the anemia.

REFERENCES

Gordon, A. S., G. W. Cooper, and E. D. Zanzani: The Kidney and Erythropoiesis, Seminars Hematol., 4:337, 1967.

Lester, R., and R. Schmidt: Bilirubin Metabolism, New Engl. J. Med., 270:779, 1964.

Mauzerall, D.: Normal Porphyrin Metabolism, J. Pediat., 64:5, 1964.

Wintrobe, M. M.: "Clinical Hematology," 6th ed., Philadelphia, Lea & Febiger, 1967.

62 BLEEDING
T. C. Bithell and M. M. Wintrobe

Except for that which occurs during menstruation, spontaneous bleeding is abnormal, and blood loss from even large injuries is usually insignificant. This is a consequence of the efficiency with which vascular integrity is normally maintained and the rapidity with which it is restored following injury. In general, both of these phenomena reflect the function of the hemostatic apparatus. Rapid and voluminous bleeding may develop spontaneously or following trivial trauma, when any of the components involved in hemostasis is lacking.

It must be recognized, however, that the adequacy of the hemostatic apparatus is relative. A ruptured esophageal varix will usually result in serious hemorrhage, while the erosion of blood vessels by a gastric tumor will produce less dramatic but continued bleeding, despite the presence of a normal hemostatic mechanism. Thus, bleeding may result from either a failure of the hemostatic apparatus or from localized pathologic processes which produce vascular erosion or malformation. In either case, this symptom is one of the most serious and significant of the cardinal manifestations of disease.

Localized pathologic processes are by far the most common causes of bleeding; such disorders will be discussed here from a general standpoint only. Although less common, bleeding which results from disorders of hemostasis will be covered in more detail.

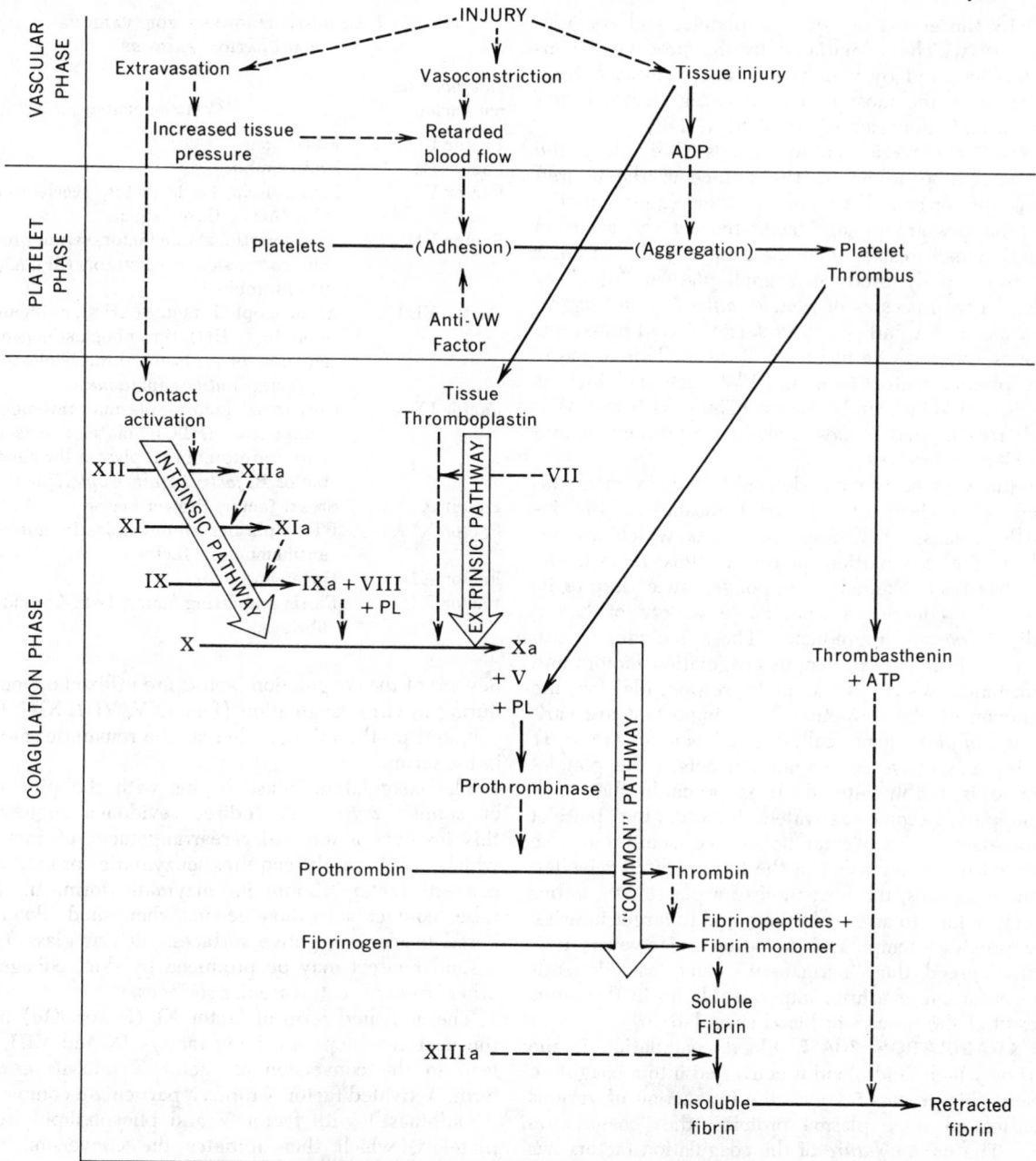

Fig. 62-1. A simplified diagram of the hemostatic process. Subscript *a* denotes the activated forms of the respective factors; PL denotes phospholipid; solid arrows denote transformation; interrupted arrows denote action.

THE PHYSIOLOGY OF HEMOSTASIS

Hemostasis is the process which stops the flow of blood from injured vessels. Completely efficient hemostasis requires normal blood vessels and extravascular tissue, numerically and functionally normal platelets, and a normal coagulation mechanism. A simplified diagram of the hemostatic process is seen in Fig. 62-1, which for descriptive purposes is divided into vascular, platelet, and coagulation "phases."

THE VASCULAR PHASE. The most immediate consequence of injury to small vessels is a reduction of blood flow as a result of vasoconstriction and extravasation of blood. Vasoconstriction tends to markedly reduce blood flow through an injured area. The escape of blood into normal tissue is limited by the extravascular supporting tissue, and the increased tissue pressure which results tends to collapse venules and capillaries which may then rapidly cohere and even become obliterated. These virtually instantaneous phenomena are quickly supplemented by the events of both the platelet and coagulation phases, which are initiated by the process of contact activation, and by various substances released from injured tissues, the most important being tissue *thromboplastins*, and *adenosine diphosphate* (ADP).

THE PLATELET PHASE. Within seconds after injury, the platelets begin to adhere to the surface of the injured vessel (adhesion) and to one another (aggregation). These processes are greatly facilitated by the retarded blood flow which results from the events of the vascular phase, and rapidly produce a small platelet "plug" or thrombus. The processes of *platelet adhesion and aggregation* are complex and poorly understood, and numerous substances appear to be involved. These include a poorly defined plasma factor (the anti-VW factor) which is lacking in von Willebrand's disease (Chap. 346) and ADP derived from injured tissues, including erythrocytes, and the platelets themselves.

Like the vessels, the platelets play both a mechanical and a biochemical role in hemostasis. This involves the release of various substances which are involved in the coagulation phase. In this regard, the platelet has been likened to a sponge, since despite its small size, it contains a remarkable variety of hemostatically important ingredients. These include, in addition to ADP and ATP, various coagulation factors and the substance which is uniquely responsible for the phenomenon of clot retraction. Most important are various *phospholipids* (generically termed *platelet factor 3*) which become active in coagulation before the platelet membrane is visibly altered. It is probable that such phospholipids become activated *in situ*, the platelet membrane serving as a catalytic surface; some may also be released into the plasma in the form of lipid micelles.

In small injuries, the formation of a platelet thrombus alone may suffice to arrest bleeding, and in larger injuries, it may provide "temporary" hemostasis. However, it is generally agreed that "permanent" hemostasis depends on the formation of a firm, impermeable fibrin thrombus as a result of the process of blood coagulation.

THE COAGULATION PHASE. Blood coagulation is the process by which fluid blood is converted into a coagulum or a clot. This process involves the interaction of various poorly defined trace plasma proteins, the "coagulation factors." The *nomenclature* of the coagulation factors has now been standardized by designating each with a Roman numeral (Table 62-1). Factor III originally referred to tissue thromboplastin, factor IV to calcium, and factor VI to the activated form of factor V. These terms are seldom used. The descriptive terms *fibrinogen* and *prothrombin* are generally preferred to the Roman numerals.

The mechanism by which the coagulation factors interact is still uncertain. Evidence suggests that they are proenzymes which are normally inert, but which are transformed into proteolytic enzymes when activated, each sequentially activating the proenzyme next in line (*the "cascade," or "waterfall," hypothesis*). *Calcium* is essential for most steps in the coagulation process, but remarkably little is known concerning its mechanism of action.

Table 62-1. SYNONYMS FOR VARIOUS COAGULATION FACTORS

International nomenclature	Common synonyms
Factor I........	Fibrinogen
Factor II......	Prothrombin
Factor V.......	Proaccelerin, labile factor, accelerator globulin (AcG), thrombogen
Factor VII.....	Proconvertin, stable factor, serum prothrombin conversion accelerator (SPCA), autoprothrombin I
Factor VIII....	Antihemophilic factor (AHF), antihemophilic globulin (AHG), thromboplastinogen, platelet cofactor I, plasma thromboplastic factor A, *facteur antihémophilique* A
Factor IX......	Christmas factor, plasma thromboplastin component (PTC), platelet cofactor II, autoprothrombin II, plasma thromboplastic factor B, *facteur antihémophilique* B
Factor X.......	Stuart factor, Prower factor
Factor XI.....	PTA (plasma thromboplastin antecedent), antihemophilic factor C
Factor XII.....	Hageman factor
Factor XIII....	Fibrin stabilizing factor, Laki-Lorand factor, fibrinase

Several of the coagulation factors are utilized or consumed during in vitro coagulation (factors V, VIII, XIII, fibrinogen, and prothrombin), whereas the remainder are found in the serum.

The coagulation phase begins with the phenomenon of *contact activation*. Indirect evidence suggests that this involves a molecular rearrangement of factor XII, which as a result acquires enzymatic properties and converts factor XI into its enzymatic form. In the test tube, contact activation occurs when shed blood is exposed to electronegative surfaces, such as glass. In vivo, a similar effect may be produced by skin, collagen, and other "foreign" extravascular surfaces.

The activated form of factor XI (factor XIa) initiates the next two steps involving factors IX and VIII, which lead to the conversion of factor X into its enzymatic form. Activated factor X forms a particulate complex (prothrombinase) with factor V and phospholipid from the platelets, which then initiates the conversion of prothrombin into thrombin.

Prothrombinase can be produced by the aforementioned sequence of reactions beginning with contact activation and involving factors XII, XI, IX, and VIII. This is termed the *intrinsic pathway*. The production of prothrombinase by means of this pathway is relatively slow but requires neither tissue thromboplastin nor factor VII. A functionally identical prothrombinase can be produced in a matter of seconds by tissue thromboplastins. This involves a sequence of reactions termed the *extrinsic pathway* which, in addition to factors X and V, requires only factor VII. Consequently this pathway bypasses the steps initiated by contact activation involving factors XII, XI, IX, and VIII. Thus, blood coagulation is initiated by only two processes, i.e., contact activation and tissue thromboplastin; it proceeds initially via two separate pathways, i.e., the tissue-activated extrinsic pathway and the contact-activated intrinsic pathway; later steps leading to the formation of fibrin proceed via a *common pathway,* requiring factors X, V, phospholipid, prothrombin, and fibrinogen.

The final step in the coagulation phase, the *thrombin-fibrinogen reaction,* involves the transformation of fibrinogen into fibrin, which is the physical basis of all blood clots. This occurs in three separate steps; viz., the enzymatic proteolysis of fibrinogen by thrombin which removes four peptides (fibrinopeptides), the formation of a visible but unstable fibrin polymer (soluble fibrin), and finally the formation of a stable fibrin polymer (insoluble fibrin) as the result of the action of factor XIII (fibrin-stabilizing factor). Structurally, fibrin resembles the proteins of muscle and skin and provides an extremely strong and stable framework for the "permanent" hemostatic plug.

CLOT RETRACTION. This is the result of the mechanical shrinkage of fibrin strands within a clot. The platelets supply both the energy (ATP) and the contractile apparatus required for this process (thrombasthenin, a protein which functions like actomyosin of muscle). Despite the teleologic view that clot retraction may constitute a "physiologic" ligature which pulls the edge of a wound together, the hemostatic significance of the process remains uncertain.

PHYSIOLOGIC INHIBITORS OF COAGULATION AND FI-BRINOLYSIS. Mechanisms which maintain the normal fluidity of the blood, restrict the processes of hemostasis to the site of injury, and remove the resulting "debris" when its function has been served, are homeostatically as important as the processes which lead to hemostasis.

The *physiologic inhibitors of coagulation* are poorly understood substances which neutralize the various enzymes produced during blood coagulation and thus prevent the propagation of a thrombus beyond the wound site. They include the antithrombins, the antithromboplastins, inhibitors of prothrombinase, and numerous others. Activated coagulation factors may also be removed from the circulation by cellular mechanisms in the liver and reticuloendothelial system.

Fibrinolysis is usually considered to be the major physiologic means of disposing of fibrin after its hemostatic function has been fulfilled. This process is thus of great importance in wound-healing, and in the recanalization of thrombosed vessels. Fibrinolysis (Fig. 62-2) is accomplished by the leukocytes and by a proteolytic enzyme (plasmin) which, like the coagulation factors, is formed from an inert precursor in the plasma (plasminogen). Various substances activate plasminogen in vitro, including tissue extracts, certain bacterial enzymes, factor XIIa, and thrombin. The mechanism of plasminogen activation in vivo is poorly understood, but fibrinolysis can be initiated by a variety of stimuli, including stress, hypoglycemia, anoxia, and even vigorous exercise. Plasminogen is avidly bound to fibrin (Fig. 62-2, step 1), and when activated (step 2), is present in both a bound form and free in the plasma. The antiplasmins in the plasma rapidly destroy free plasmin but are relatively ineffective against bound plasmin, which is thus free to carry out its physiologic function, fibrinolysis (physiologic proteolysis) (step 3). If plasmin is activated in amounts which exceed the capacity of the antiplasmins, however, other proteins in the plasma, including fibrinogen and most of the coagulation factors, may be destroyed. This abnormal process (pathologic proteolysis) (step 4) may lead to a serious coagulation disorder (Chap. 346).

The process of hemostasis is considerably more complicated than the stepwise reactions illustrated in Fig. 62-1 would suggest, and many of the complexities are of

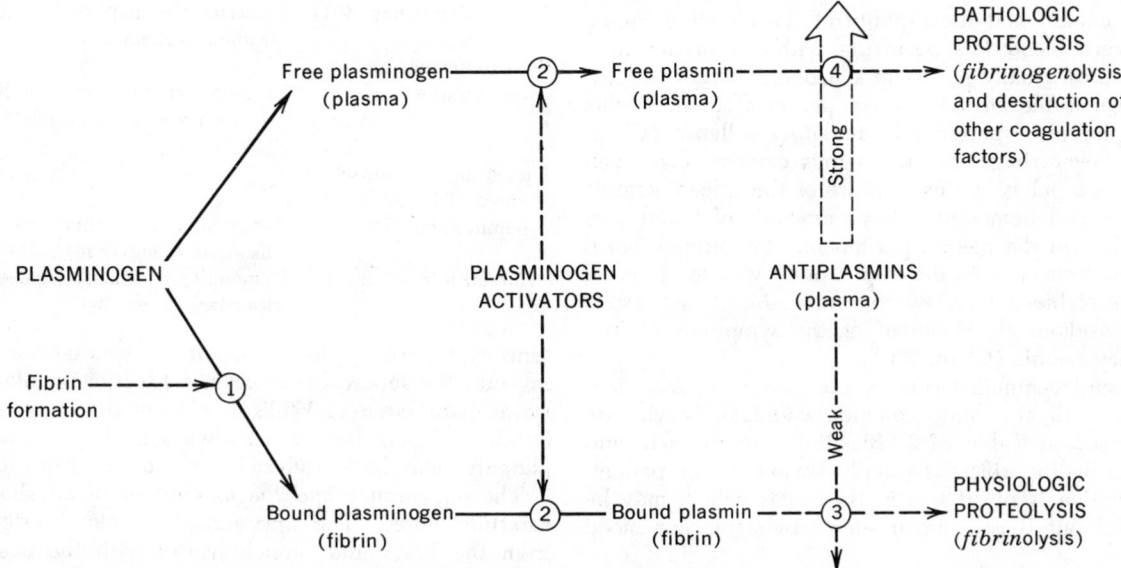

Fig. 62-2. A simplified diagram of the fibrinolytic enzyme system. Plasminogen is synonymous with pro-fibrinolysin; plasmin with fibrinolysin. Solid arrows denote transformation; interrupted arrows denote action.

fundamental homeostatic importance. For example, although the production of thrombin is a relatively slow process at first, when once formed in even trace amounts, this enzyme alters platelets to further their aggregation and also activates factors V and VIII. As a result of such "autocatalytic" feedback mechanisms, the hemostatic process proceeds at an ever-accelerating rate, and once initiated, fibrin formation is virtually instantaneous. This is of great importance in arresting blood loss from a major injury. In this, and in many other respects, the hemostatic apparatus functions in a remarkably interdependent manner. As a result, hemostatic function compatible with life is maintained even when an essential component is completely lacking. The physiologic inhibitors of coagulation and the fibrinolytic enzyme system are also closely integrated with the hemostatic process. For example, fibrin, which provides the basis for the permanent thrombus, also restricts the extent of the thrombus by absorbing large amounts of thrombin. Fibrinolysis may be activated by factor XIIa as a result of the process of contact activation or by thrombin. Thus, the mechanism which activates the process of coagulation also initiates fibrinolysis, and the products of coagulation are themselves potent inhibitors of the process. These relationships are of fundamental importance when homeostasis is threatened by intravascular coagulation.

THE CLINICAL EVALUATION OF BLEEDING

In the evaluation of bleeding, particular attention should be directed to (1) the signs and symptoms of blood loss; (2) the location or source of the bleeding; (3) the appearance and amount of the blood; and (4) certain bleeding manifestations which suggest the presence of a disorder of hemostasis.

The *signs and symptoms* of blood loss per se depend on the amount and the rapidity of the bleeding. Acute and severe blood loss occurring within a matter of a few minutes usually results in syncope, whereas the loss of a comparable amount over a period of hours results in the picture of peripheral circulatory collapse (Chap. 36). In hemorrhage into the serous cavities; e.g., fractures of the pelvis or ribs, rupture of the spleen, ectopic gestation, and hemophilia, large amounts of blood may accumulate in the pleura, peritoneum, or retroperitoneal space, and shock may develop rapidly without external evidence of bleeding. Slow continuous blood loss results in the insidious development of the symptoms of iron deficiency anemia (Chap. 336).

The most common *locations* and *sources of bleeding*, together with the most common causes of each, are summarized in Table 62-2. Bleeding into the skin and from the bodily orifices is usually obvious to the patient. An exception is blood loss in the stools, which may be unnoticed but is a common source of significant blood loss.

Hemorrhage into the confined spaces of the central nervous system rapidly produces definite symptoms and neurologic signs. Intracerebral hemorrhage is a common

Table 62-2. THE CAUSES OF COMMON BLEEDING MANIFESTATIONS

Location or source of bleeding	Most common causes
Gastrointestinal tract (Chap. 44)	Peptic ulcers (Chap. 314), tumors (Chap. 315), gastritis, hiatal hernia, esophageal varices (Chap. 328), colitis, hemorrhoids
Respiratory tract (Chap. 38)	Tumors (Chap. 292), pulmonary emboli (Chap. 285), tuberculosis, mitral stenosis (Chap. 270), bronchiectasis (Chap. 291), other infections
Urinary tract (Chap. 51)	Stones (Chap. 307), glomerulonephritis, infections (Chap. 303), cystitis, tumors (Chap. 310), prostatic hypertrophy
Central nervous sytems (Chap. 26)	Trauma, hypertension, vascular malformations
Vagina (Chap. 52)	Endocrine disorders, tumors, obstetrical complications
Nose and paranasal sinuses	Trauma, hypertension, tumors, polyps, inflammation, perforation of nasal septum, hereditary hemorrhagic telangiectasia (Chap. 347)
Ears	Trauma, basal skull fracture
Serous cavities	Trauma, rupture of spleen, ectopic gestation
Nipples	Fissure, breast tumor
Intraocular (Chap. 401)	Hypertension, nephritis, diabetes, trauma, leukemia
Skin (petechiae and ecchymoses)	Thrombocytopenia or other disorders of blood vessels or platelets (Chap. 345)
Dissecting intramuscular and soft-tissue hematomas	Hemophilia or other coagulation disorders (Chap. 346)
Synovial joints	Hemophilia or other coagulation disorders (Chap. 346)

terminating event in hypertension, and spontaneous bleeding into the subarachnoid space from a congenital aneurysm of the circle of Willis may occur in young persons. Subdural hemorrhage must always be kept in mind in patients who have suffered even trivial head trauma.

The *appearance and the amount of blood* should be carefully noted. The appearance of blood originating from the lungs and bronchi varies with the degree of aeration and the presence or absence of mucus, pus, etc. It is usually bright red and frothy in appearance; e.g., hemoptysis in tuberculosis, but if it originates in areas of consolidation or congestion, it appears dark; e.g., the "rusty" sputum of pneumococcal pneumonia. In most infectious processes, the blood is mixed with pus or mucus and is seldom large in amount. An exception is tuberculosis, where hemoptysis from arteriobronchial fistulas may be alarming. Mitral stenosis may lead to massive pulmonary bleeding when bronchial varicosities rupture (bronchial "apoplexy").

Due to the conversion of red hemoglobin into brown acid hematin by the gastric acid, the appearance of blood from the gastrointestinal tract depends on its site of origin. That originating from the upper gastrointestinal tract, e.g., peptic ulcer, gastritis, resembles coffee grounds if vomited, and if sufficient to discolor the stools, produces a black tarry appearance (melena). In the presence of achlorhydria or when hematemesis is massive, however, the blood may appear red. Blood which originates in the intestinal tract below the ligament of Treitz imparts a bloody red or brown color to the stools (hematochezia) rather than a tarry appearance. In ulcerative colitis, intussuception, volvulus, and mesenteric thrombosis, a bloody mucoid discharge is usually seen. It must be remembered that blood from the nose, sinuses, or lungs may appear in the stools if swallowed, or may be swallowed and then vomited.

Gastrointestinal bleeding from peptic ulcers, Meckel's diverticula, and esophageal varices may be massive, while that which occurs from most polyps, tumors, and infectious processes is seldom so. Esophageal hiatal hernias and hookworm infestation usually produce slow and continued bleeding which is insufficient to change the color of the stools (occult bleeding).

In epistaxis from nasal polyps, various inflammatory processes which produce engorgement of Kiesselbach's plexus, and hypertension, the blood is bright red, and bleeding may be rapid. In epistaxis associated with perforation of the cartilagenous nasal septum, e.g., syphilis, small amounts of blood mixed with mucus are usually seen. Profuse epistaxis is frequently the initial and often the sole symptom in patients with hereditary hemorrhagic telangiectasia.

Small amounts of blood often impart a smoky color to the urine, e.g., glomerulonephritis, whereas in prostatic hypertrophy, renal stones, etc., the urine may appear grossly bloody, and when bleeding is rapid, clots may be passed per urethra. With the exception of renal tuberculosis, infections of the urinary tract, e.g., pyelonephritis, are rarely associated with gross bleeding but commonly produce hematuria which is discovered in the examination of the urine sediment (microscopic hematuria).

Abnormal vaginal bleeding is exceedingly common, and may be manifest as an abnormally heavy menstrual period (hypermenorrhea, menorrhagia), e.g., anovulatory cycle bleeding, or may occur between menses (metrorrhagia), e.g., adenocarcinoma of the uterus. Blood originating from the uterus is usually dark and fluid, but may appear bright red and be mixed with clots if bleeding is rapid, e.g., abruptio placentae. Bleeding from disorders of the cervix, e.g., carcinoma or polyps, is usually intermittent and small in amount.

Clinical Manifestations of Disordered Hemostasis

Although any of the varieties of bleeding summarized in Table 62-2 may be encountered, certain *bleeding manifestations* are more or less *characteristic of the disorders of hemostasis*. For example, bleeding into the synovial joints (hemarthrosis) in the absence of obvious trauma and spontaneous bleeding into the skin are rarely encountered in patients with normal hemostatic function. Moreover, such signs and symptoms fall into two relatively distinct patterns, i.e., those which are most common in disorders of vessels and platelets, and those which are more frequently seen in disorders of coagulation (Table 62-3). *Hemarthrosis* and its sequelae, for

Table 62-3. THE CLINICAL DISTINCTION BETWEEN DISORDERS OF VESSELS AND PLATELETS AND DISORDERS OF BLOOD COAGULATION

Findings	Disorders of coagulation (Chap. 346)	Disorders of platelets and vessels ("purpuric" disorders) (Chap. 345)
Hemarthroses..	Characteristic	Rare
Petechiae......	Rare	Characteristic
Positive family history......	Common	Rare
Sex..........	95% of hereditary forms occur only in males	Relatively more common in females
Traumatic bleeding.....	Onset often delayed; rapid and voluminous	Onset immediate; slow and persistent oozing

example, are almost diagnostic of a severe hereditary coagulation disorder, e.g., hemophilia, and are exceedingly rare in vascular and platelet disorders. Recurrent crops of *petechiae*, on the other hand, are strongly suggestive of an abnormality of the vessels or platelets, e.g., thrombocytopenia, and are rare in the coagulation disorders. Ecchymoses may occur in any disorder of hemostasis, but if they are the result of abnormal blood coagulation, they are large, characteristically dissect deeper structures, and may spread to involve an entire limb.

Profuse and often life-threatening hemorrhage following trivial trauma or surgical procedures is a hallmark of the coagulation disorders, and the onset of bleeding is often delayed for several hours. This phenomenon of *delayed bleeding* is rare in disorders of vessels or platelets, where slow but persistent oozing begins immediately following trauma.

The *sex* of the patient, the *age* when abnormal bleeding was first noted, and the *family history* are of particular importance in evaluating the disorders of hemostasis, since most disorders of vessels and platelets are acquired, whereas most serious coagulation disorders are hereditary, and among these, over 90 percent occur only in males. The absence of a family history of bleeding, however, does not exclude the presence of a hereditary coagulation disorder.

The history remains the best single "screening" test for the presence of a hemorrhagic disorder, and the corollary to this statement is no less true. A history of surgery, major injury, or even multiple tooth extractions without abnormal bleeding is good evidence against the presence of a hereditary coagulation disorder.

THE LABORATORY EVALUATION OF BLEEDING

Laboratory Findings in Acute Bleeding

The acute loss of blood stimulates the hematopoietic system (Chap. 335), resulting in leukocytosis with an increase in immature neutrophils and an elevation of the platelet count (thrombocytosis) and the reticulocyte count (reticulocytosis). Other evidence of accelerated red cell production may be seen in the blood smear (polychromasia and stippling of the erythrocytes), and even nucleated red cells of the normoblastic type may occasionally be found following acute hemorrhage. The erythrocyte sedimentation rate and the indirect reacting serum bilirubin may be increased as a result of bleeding into the tissues. The laboratory findings in anemia are described elsewhere (Chaps. 61, 335, 336). The various procedures which are valuable in the differential diagnosis of the causes of bleeding, other than those concerned with disorders of hemostasis, are considered in the appropriate chapters, as indicated in Table 62-2.

Laboratory Diagnosis of Disorders of Hemostasis

There is no single test which is suitable for the laboratory evaluation of the hemostatic process, but numerous methods of varying complexity and utility are now available for testing the vascular, platelet, and coagulation phases of hemostasis.

TESTS OF THE VASCULAR AND PLATELET PHASES. *The enumeration of the platelets* is considerably more difficult than is the case with erythrocytes or leukocytes. This difficulty is due to the tendency of platelets to aggregate in vitro and the difficulty of visualizing these small highly refractile structures. Among the numerous techniques which have been used, the so-called indirect methods and those hemocytometer methods which employ an ordinary microscope (Rees-Ecker) are very inaccurate and are seldom used. The only satisfactory methods presently available require a phase-contrast microscope (Brecher-Cronkite method) or automated counting equipment, e.g., the Coulter counter. In view of the many variables involved and the relatively large error of even the best methods, the platelet count should always be verified by the examination of a well-prepared peripheral blood smear.

Clot retraction is a specific function of intact platelets.

It is usually deficient in thrombocytopenia and in a rare disorder of platelet function (Glazmann's disease) (Chap. 345). The determination of the presence or absence of clot retraction is seldom necessary in the diagnosis of thrombocytopenia, however, since the platelets can now be enumerated with reasonable accuracy. Qualitative estimates of the extent of clot retraction can be made by incubating one of the samples obtained for the clotting time, where retraction is normally apparent within 2 hr.

Hemostasis in a small superficial wound, such as that produced in measuring *the bleeding time,* depends on the rate at which a stable platelet thrombus is formed and thus measures the efficiency of the vascular and platelet phases. Unfortunately, the bleeding time leaves much to be desired in terms of reproducibility, since no two skin areas are exactly the same and it is impossible to produce a truly standard wound. Despite these intrinsic limitations, the bleeding time is valuable when carefully performed. It is prolonged in the majority of patients with von Willebrand's disease and disorders of platelet function. Although usually prolonged in thrombocytopenia, the bleeding time is seldom of diagnostic importance. Contrary to theory, this test is only inconstantly abnormal in the various disorders attributed to dysfunction of the vessels. The bleeding time is occasionally prolonged in severe coagulation disorders.

In the *tourniquet test,* a "standard" increase in venous and capillary pressure is produced for a short time. Normally, the vessels are unaffected by this procedure, but in the presence of vascular abnormalities or insufficient or abnormal platelets, small capillary hemorrhages (petechiae) may develop. Their number and size is an extremely crude index of the efficiency of the vascular and platelet phases. However, many normal subjects will develop some petechiae and many patients with bleeding due to vascular or platelet disorders will not. The tourniquet test correlates poorly with the platelet count, and although it is usually positive in severe thrombocytopenia, petechiae are usually apparent on physical examination of such patients in any case. The bleeding time, tourniquet test, and platelet count are usually normal in disorders of coagulation.

TESTS OF THE COAGULATION PHASE. Great care must be used in the collection of blood samples for coagulation studies, and foaming and contamination of the specimen with tissue juice, in particular, must be avoided. Because of the innumerable technical variations which are employed in even the simplest tests, only the "normal" range for the particular laboratory and technique utilized is meaningful.

In Fig. 62-1, it can be seen that in addition to the coagulation factors normally present in the plasma, the production of fibrin via the intrinsic pathway requires contact activation, phospholipids from platelets, and calcium. The *partial thromboplastin time (PTT)* is a simple test of this pathway, where contact activation is provided by a glass tube and phospholipid is added in the form of a crude cephalin fraction (platelet substitute, e.g., Thrombofax–Ortho). In the activated PTT, contact activation is further standardized by the addition of various particulate silicates, e.g., Kaolin, Celite. When such a mixture is recalcified, fibrin forms at a normal rate only if the factors involved in the intrinsic pathway (i.e., factors XII, XI, IX, and VIII) as well as those required in the common pathway (i.e., factors X, V, prothrombin, and fibrinogen) are present in normal amounts (Fig. 62-3). Cephalin provides an excess of phospholipid, and the PTT is thus unaffected by the platelets. Since it by-passes the tissue-activated extrinsic pathway, this test is also unaffected by factor VII. The PTT will be prolonged if the level of any of the required factors is below 15 to 20 percent of normal. Since, in severely affected patients coagulation factor levels are as low as 1 or 0 percent, the PTT detects many mildly affected patients. The test is also prolonged by heparin and by inhibitors of any of the essential factors.

The production of fibrin via the extrinsic pathway (Fig. 62-1) requires only tissue thromboplastin and calcium, in addition to the coagulation factors normally present in the plasma. This pathway is measured by the *plasma prothrombin time,* in which plasma is recalcified in the presence of an excess of tissue thromboplastin. Fibrin forms at a normal rate in such a mixture only if the factors involved in the extrinsic pathway (i.e., factor VII) and the common pathway (i.e., factors X, V, prothrombin, and fibrinogen) are present in normal amounts (Fig. 62-3). This test bypasses the intrinsic pathway and the factors concerned there, i.e., factors XII, XI, IX, and VIII. Since tissue thromboplastin contains phospholipids, the prothrombin time is also in-sensitive to platelets. Of the five coagulation factors measured in the prothrombin time, three (i.e., factors VII, X, and prothrombin) are depressed by coumarin-like drugs (Chap. 346). As a result, the prothrombin time is the most widely used test for controlling anticoagulant therapy with such drugs. The prothrombin time is rela-tively more sensitive to deficiencies of factors VII and X than to deficiencies of fibrinogen and prothrombin and is prolonged by inhibitors of any of the essential factors or of tissue thromboplastins and by heparin. The expression of the prothrombin time as a "percentage" of normal is not recommended, since the dilution curves used to arrive at this figure often are misleading.

The *clotting time of whole blood* is the most frequently used and most commonly misinterpreted coagulation test. In theory, it would seem that the rate of fibrin formation in whole blood would provide a measurement of the same coagulation factors as the PTT, as well as the platelets, since the coagulation of blood collected without con-taminating tissue thromboplastins is initiated by contact with glass, bypasses the extrinsic pathway, and depends on the contained platelets as a source of phospholipid. In fact, the coagulation time measures only the time re-quired to form the first traces of thrombin which suffice to produce a visible clot. Even the small amounts of phospholipid which are available in severe thrombocyto-penia are sufficient to produce these requisite traces of thrombin, and consequently, the clotting time is un-affected by the platelet count. For the same reason, the

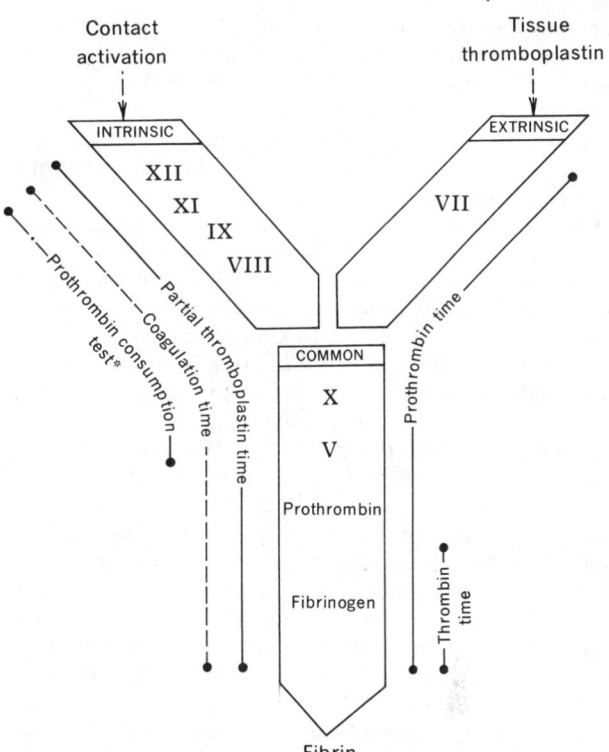

Fig. 62-3. The interpretation of screening tests of blood coagula-tion.
*Platelet phospholipid is also required for normal prothrombin consumption.

clotting time is significantly prolonged only in severe deficiencies of the factors involved in the intrinsic and common pathways (Fig. 62-3) and is usually normal when these factors are present in amounts which exceed 1 percent of normal plasma levels. The clotting time is unaffected by the level of factor VII and remains the most widely used test to control heparin therapy.

Although the clotting time may be normal when only small amounts of prothrombinase are produced, a large amount of unconverted prothrombin will remain; i.e., it will not have been normally utilized or consumed. The qualitative or quantitative measurement of residual pro-thrombin in serum after a standard interval is thus an indirect measurement of the amount of prothrombinase formed and is the essence of the *prothrombin consump-tion test.* This test measures only those factors in the intrinsic pathway required to form prothrombinase, i.e., factors XII, XI, IX, VIII, X, and V (Fig. 62-3). Although more sensitive than the clotting time in that it is abnormal when any of the essential factors are below 2 to 3 percent of normal, the prothrombin consumption test is less sensitive than the PTT and, like the clotting time, fails to detect mildly affected patients. Prothrombin conversion is incomplete and the prothrombin consumption test is abnormal in the presence of thrombocytopenia and qual-itative abnormalities of the platelets.

In the *plasma thrombin time,* preformed thrombin is added to plasma, and the time required to form a clot thus indicates the rate at which the first visible fibrin polymers (soluble fibrin) are formed. The thrombin time is prolonged when the fibrinogen level is low and when the fibrinogen is functionally defective, but is unaffected by the levels of any of the other coagulation factors. It is prolonged by heparin, and by abnormal amounts of antithrombins.

The Fi test is a simple test for hypofibrinogenemia which utilizes latex particles coated with specific antibody to human fibrinogen. When this reagent (Hyland) is mixed with normal blood, visible fibrinogen-latex aggregates are formed which are lacking when the fibrinogen concentration is low. Primarily because it can be quickly performed, this is a valuable test in the diagnosis of the hypofibrinogenemias (Chap. 346).

The *rate of whole blood clot lysis* is a gross measurement of the fibrinolytic enzyme, plasmin. This test requires only the incubation and observation of one of the samples obtained for the clotting time. If fibrinolysis is rapid, the whole blood clot lysis time may be helpful, but otherwise the time required for lysis, which is normally in excess of 72 hr, is usually too long to be of diagnostic help. Relatively simple but more definitive tests, such as the euglobulin lysis time, are available for the study of abnormal fibrinolysis.

All the aforementioned tests of blood coagulation are usually normal in disorders of the vessels or the platelets.

INITIAL LABORATORY STUDY OF THE DISORDERS OF HEMOSTASIS

The definitive diagnosis of the disorders of hemostasis often requires a specially equipped laboratory and relatively elaborate methods. However, the most essential information can usually be obtained from the four simple tests summarized in Table 62-4. The platelet count and the bleeding time together provide the most reliable and reproducible test of the vascular and platelet phases. The PTT measures all of the coagulation factors involved in the intrinsic and common pathways and is generally accepted as the best single screening test for disorders of blood coagulation. This test, and its various modifications, when accurately performed, will be abnormal in over 90 percent of patients with abnormalities of blood coagulation. When supplemented with the plasma prothrombin time, which assesses the extrinsic as well as the common pathway, the abnormality can usually be localized to one of the three pathways and the factors involved therein. In view of their availability, simplicity, and low cost, these four tests are admirably suited to serve as primary screening tests. They should be the first laboratory tests obtained, since they direct further laboratory study, and when interpreted in the light of a careful history, a thorough physical examination, and the laws of probability, they provide a valuable "presumptive" diagnosis, i.e., whether the bleeding is due to a coagulation disorder, to thrombocytopenia, or to a disorder of the vessels or a qualitative disorder of the platelets. Further details concerning the clinical picture, differential diagnosis and treatment of the various hemorrhagic disorders will be found in subsequent sections concerned with the disorders of blood coagulation (Chap. 346) and disorders of vessels and platelets (Chap. 345).

REFERENCES

Biggs, Rosemary, and R. G. MacFarlane: "Human Blood Coagulation," 3d ed., Philadelphia, F. A. Davis Company, 1962.

Cartwright, G. E.: "Diagnostic Laboratory Hematology," 4th ed., New York, Grune & Stratton, Inc., 1968.

Ratnoff, O. D.: "Bleeding Syndromes. A Clinical Manual," Springfield, Ill., Charles C Thomas, 1960.

Williams, W. J.: Biochemical Aspects of Blood Coagulation and Hemostasis, Med. Clinics N. Am., 50:1257, 1966.

Wintrobe, M. M.: "Clinical Hematology," 6th ed., Philadelphia, Lea & Febiger, 1967.

Table 62-4. THE INITIAL LABORATORY EVALUATION OF HEMOSTATIC FUNCTION

Vascular and Platelet Phases		Coagulation Phase		"Presumptive" diagnosis
Platelet count	Bleeding time	Partial thromboplastin time	Prothrombin time	
Reduced	Prolonged	Normal	Normal	Thrombocytopenia (Chap. 345)
Normal or increased	Normal or prolonged	Normal	Normal	Vascular or qualitative platelet disorder (Chap. 345)
Normal	Usually normal	Usually prolonged	Normal or prolonged	Coagulation disorder (Chap. 346)

63 ENLARGEMENT OF LYMPH NODES AND SPLEEN

M. M. Wintrobe and D. R. Boggs

There are some 500 to 600 *lymph nodes* in the body, varying from less than 1 mm to 1 to 2 cm in size. These structures afford mechanical filtration for the lymph stream, removing cellular debris, foreign particles, and bacteria which may have gained access to the lymph from the various structures drained by the lymph channels. In the normal individual very few lymph nodes are palpable, even on careful physical examination. However, the access of disease-producing bacteria and certain viruses sets up an inflammatory reaction in the nodes, and various types of malignant cells can proliferate there. It has been aptly stated that in the exercise of their function the lymph nodes may sacrifice their own integrity for the welfare of the organism as a whole. One may wonder whether they do not mistakenly also nourish neoplastic tissue at their own expense.

These structures are also the site of formation of lymphocytes and of antibodies. Furthermore, in certain diseases, lymph nodes may be the site of formation of erythrocytes, neutrophils, and platelets. This is known as myeloid metaplasia and is a reflection of embryonal hematopoietic potentialities. This reaction also is accompanied by lymph node enlargement.

On physical examination the cervical, supraclavicular, axillary, and inguinal nodes are those most often found to be enlarged. Other lymph nodes which may be found to be enlarged on palpation are the epitroclear, brachial, and very rarely, the popliteal. Enlargement of mediastinal nodes is detected by chest roentgenography. *Lymphangiography* is a technique in which a radiopaque dye is injected into lymphatic channels in the feet. The dye drains into abdominal and even mediastinal lymph node chains, thereby permitting enlarged nodes to be visualized. Roentgenography is the most reliable nonsurgical technique for demonstrating nonpalpable enlargement of abdominal nodes.

CAUSES OF LYMPH NODE ENLARGEMENT

Enlargement of the lymph nodes may be purely local, or it may be widespread. Such enlargement may be accompanied by all the signs of acute inflammation, such as heat, reddening of overlying skin, and tenderness. The nodes may remain discrete or they may fuse with one another as the result of perilymphangitis. Necrosis may even ensue and may be followed by rupture of the nodes and the formation of a sinus. Rapidly enlarging nodes are likely to be tender, but tenderness usually reflects a response to antigen or actual infection within the node. Inflammation of the skin overlying the tender nodes is usually indicative of an infected node. On the other hand, very great enlargement of the lymph nodes may take place in the absence of any signs of inflammation.

Enlarged lymph nodes may be discrete or matted together; they may be extremely hard or only moderately so or they may even be soft or feel cystic. Nontender nodes which feel hard and matted together usually contain metastatic carcinoma or a very aggressive intrinsic neoplasm such as reticulum cell sarcoma. Noninflamed, enlarged lymph nodes usually do not produce serious symptoms unless their enlargement obstructs some vital passageway. Thus, mediastinal lymphadenopathy may be very great and yet produce no symptoms unless the vena cava or bronchi are obstructed.

The chief causes of lymph node enlargement are listed in Table 63-1.

Infection may cause lymph node enlargement as a result of antibody response, granulomatous hyperplasia in response to infection within the node, or because of suppurative infection of the node. Localized infections ordinarily induce lymph node enlargement which is

Table 63-1. CHIEF CAUSES OF LYMPH NODE ENLARGEMENT

I. Antigenic challenge
   A. Infection
      1. Regional lymph node enlargement in the area draining a localized infection
      2. Generalized lymph node enlargement with systemic infection
   B. Allergic reactions such as serum sickness
   C. Diseases associated with "autoimmunity" such as systemic lupus erythematosus
II. Suppurative infections of lymph nodes [e.g., streptococcus, staphylococcus, *Pasteurella tularensis, Treponema pallidum,* virus of lymphogranuloma venereum, *Pasteurella pestis* (plague)]
III. Granuloma formation
   A. Due to infections such as tuberculosis, syphilis, and histoplasmosis.
   B. Diseases of unknown etiology such as sarcoid
IV. Primary lymph node diseases: Hodgkin's disease, lymphosarcoma, reticulum cell sarcoma, etc.
V. Leukemia
VI. Metastases from malignant disease in breast, stomach, etc.
VII. Congenital abnormalities (lymphangiomas)

limited to the regional nodes draining the infected area. If infection is systemic, whether due to steady "seeding" of the bloodstream with bacteria, as in bacterial endocarditis, or due to a systemic virus infection such as infectious mononucleosis, measles, or chicken pox, generalized lymph node enlargement may be present. This, however, is not of the same degree in all parts of the body. In infectious mononucleosis, for example, generalized lymph node enlargement is characteristic, but cervical glandular enlargement is often more striking than that found elsewhere in the body.

Of the *chronic infections,* tuberculosis and syphilis are the commonest causes of lymphadenopathy. In tuberculosis the cervical, mediastinal, or mesenteric glands are most often involved. The enlargement usually is slowly progressive and is easily confused with that caused by Hodgkin's disease. However, tuberculous glands frequently are tender and firm and adhere to one another. Sometimes breakdown of the overlying skin occurs, leading to the production of a stubborn draining sinus. Rarely the lymph node enlargement is acute and rapidly developing, and in such cases the glands may remain discrete and freely movable. In relation to syphilis, mention may be made of the firm, painless swelling in the regional lymph nodes draining the primary lesion; the generalized, firm, shotty, nontender nodes which accompany the secondary stage; and the glandular swelling of various degrees which may accompany the late stages or the congenital form. Other chronic infections in which glandular swelling may be prominent include fungous infections and filariasis.

Serum sickness should not be overlooked as a cause of lymphadenopathy, particularly since it is usually accompanied by fever.

Hodgkin's disease, lymphosarcoma, reticulum cell sarcoma, and giant follicular lymphoma are frequently classed under the single heading of primary lymph node diseases or *"lymphomas"* because, clinically, they are very similar. In these conditions the lymph node enlargement is characteristically localized at first; only as the disease progresses does wider dissemination occur. The node enlargement usually is discrete and firm and ranges greatly in degree. When the adenopathy becomes widespread, nodes may be discovered in locations where the presence of lymphoid tissue may not have been suspected. Such cases of lymph node enlargement are distinguished from those due to leukemia chiefly by the changes in the blood characteristically seen in the latter condition, but also by the asymmetry of the swellings which is often seen in the lymphomas. In leukemia, lymph node enlargement usually is generalized and symmetric, although especially in acute leukemia, adenopathy may be much more prominent in the neck than elsewhere. Tenderness of lymph nodes suggests infection rather than one of the lymphomas, leukemia, or metastatic involvement. However, some degree of tenderness, as well as pain, may be encountered when the glands have enlarged rapidly, especially in Hodgkin's disease. In the last condition, the presence of connective and fibrous tissue in the nodes may cause them to be harder than usual; occasionally they may have the consistency of cartilage.

In *sarcoidosis* the pre- and postauricular lymph nodes, the submaxillary, submental, epitrochlear, and paratracheal glands, are more often affected than in Hodgkin's disease. A history of involvement of the eyes and of the parotid glands (uveoparotid fever) suggests sarcoid, and punched-out areas in the small bones of the hands and feet may be demonstrable by roentgenography (see Chap. 254).

Treatment of convulsive disorders with various *hydantoin or hydantoinlike drugs* may produce a clinical and pathologic syndrome which closely mimics the lymphomas. Lymph node hyperplasia also is encountered in Addison's disease, hyperthyroidism, and hypopituitarism.

Lymph node enlargement due to *metastatic* carcinoma, as a rule, is distinctly localized, and the glandular swelling ordinarily is very hard. Such enlargement may involve nodes which are easily discovered, such as those of the axilla in cases of carcinoma of the breast. Or, the lymphadenopathy may be more often heard about than seen, such as Virchow's sentinel node above the clavicle in cases of carcinoma of the stomach or other abdominal organs. When the adenopathy is present in some region of the body inaccessible to physical examination, it is discoverable only by roentgenography or through the indirect effects of pressure produced by enlargement of the nodes.

Of congenital abnormalities which may lead to lymphoid enlargement, simple or capillary lymphangiomas, cavernous lymphangiomas, and the cystic form (cystic hygroma) may be mentioned.

DIFFERENTIAL DIAGNOSIS OF LYMPH NODE ENLARGEMENT

It should be evident from this discussion that the discovery of the cause of lymph node enlargement requires a thorough examination of the patient.

The location of the glandular enlargement may suggest the site of origin of the disease and may sometimes give some clue to its nature. Acute cervical adenitis should direct attention to the mouth and pharynx, mastoid adenitis to scalp infections, axillary adenitis to the upper extremity and the breast, epitrochlear enlargement to involvement of the ulnar side of the hand or forearm, and inguinal swelling to the lower extremities and genitalia. The examination of the patient must be painstaking, for sometimes secondary glandular enlargement may be much more prominent than the primary cause. Thus, for example, cervical metastases from a nasopharyngeal tumor usually overshadow the primary growth, which is characteristically small and easily overlooked unless a careful nasopharyngoscopic examination is made. The study of the patient should include careful palpation of the sternum for tenderness and of the abdomen for splenic enlargement, as well as examination of the chest for evidence of mediastinal tumor. Rectal and pelvic examination must not be overlooked.

Important laboratory procedures include the serologic test for syphilis; examination of the blood for agglutination reactions; and blood culture and culture of the throat, sputum, and other possible sources which might reveal infection; as well as examination of the blood and sometimes of the bone marrow for morphologic evidences of disease. Skin tests, such as tuberculin, histoplasmin, and coccidiodin, may also need to be performed.

If a disease known to be associated with lymph node enlargement is uncovered by the above studies, it is reasonable to assume that the enlarged nodes are due to this cause. However, if a definitive diagnosis is not made or if doubt exists, a *lymph node biopsy* should be performed. In addition to microscopic examination of the node, culture for bacteria and fungi may be helpful. As a general rule, if more than one area of lymph node enlargement is present, the cervical and supraclavicular areas are better sites for a lymph node biopsy than are the axillary and inguinal areas. Pathologic interpretation of an inguinal node biopsy often proves difficult, presumably because of the frequency with which this area is called upon to respond to the challenge of chronically traumatized feet and legs of man. The surgeon may have difficulty finding axillary nodes unless they are quite enlarged.

In patients with pulmonary lesions of unknown etiology or with a known but apparently localized carcinoma of the lung, scalenus fat pad biopsy may be required (Chap. 292).

THE SPLEEN

A palpable spleen is always a somewhat alarming finding to the physician because of the association of splenomegaly with leukemia and lymphoma. If the spleen is palpable, it is presumed to be enlarged. However, a palpable spleen does not necessarily always imply the presence of disease. Thus, McIntyre and Ebaugh, as a part of a routine physical examination, were able to palpate the spleen in 3 percent of entering college freshmen. Three years later, 30 percent of these students still had a palpable spleen and had no discernible disease.

Structure and Function of the Spleen

The pulp of the spleen is composed of (1) anastomosing strands of lymphoid tissue (white pulp), (2) a reticular network and branching multipolar cells which are placed about blood sinuses and intermingle with the strands of lymphoid tissue (red pulp), and (3) lymphocytes, granulocytes, and erythrocytes. The spleen is a very vascular organ and is capable of changing substantially in size, depending on its content of blood. It is also contractile; its capsule contains a small amount of elastic tissue. The circulation of the spleen is unique. In the lymphatic sheath, capillaries branch at right angles from arterioles. These capillaries rarely contain blood cells but rather appear to "skim" plasma from the arteriole. They serve as afferent lymphatics terminating within the lymphatic sheath. The sinusoidal structure of the red pulp consists of wide sinuses through which blood flow is rapid. These alternate with much narrower sinuses, termed *cords,* in which only a small amount of blood is normally present. The large sinuses and the cords are separated by a basement membrane containing regularly spaced perforations which provide direct communication between the two types of sinuses.

Arterioles terminate in the marginal zone of concentric flattened cells which loosely separates the white and red pulp. Erythrocytes course through the spleen by filtering through these flattened cells and then enter and rapidly traverse the large sinuses. A lesser number of red cells circulate slowly through the smaller sinuses (cords). These cells enter the cords from a few arterioles which terminate in the cords or from the marginal zone or the large sinuses through perforations of the basement membrane. Normally, only a small proportion of the blood, perhaps 20 ml, is present outside the main channel of blood flow.

The spleen, as a lymphoid organ, participates in the cellular events leading to antibody formation. However, splenectomy leads to no detectable defect in antibody production in adults or adolescents. It has been claimed that children who have been splenectomized are more than normally susceptible to infection.

If the spleen is removed, certain characteristic changes in blood cells are observed. Immediately following splenectomy, normoblasts, target cells, and erythrocytes with Howell-Jolly bodies, diffuse basophilia, basophilic stippling, and siderotic granules appear in the blood. Howell-Jolly bodies and target cells are usually demonstrable indefinitely in such patients, but other erythrocyte abnormalities tend to disappear. Neutrophilia and thrombocytosis are present immediately after splenectomy but disappear in a few weeks in most patients. Changes in the blood following splenectomy have been cited as evidence that the spleen exerts an inhibitory action on the bone marrow. Definitive experimental evidence for any humoral influence by the spleen on the bone marrow has not been forthcoming. Insofar as the red cell changes

are concerned, there is experimental evidence to support the view that the spleen normally removes the forms which are not usually seen in the blood. The primary site of destruction of senescent erythrocytes is the spleen.

Approximately one-third of the blood platelets are within the splenic circulation, a much higher figure than that for erythrocytes. There is evidence to suggest that the youngest and presumably most viable platelets are preferentially sequestered by the spleen. When the spleen is enlarged, the proportion of the total body pool of platelets which is in the spleen may increase, resulting in thrombocytopenia. Thrombocytopenia due to accelerated rates of platelet destruction by the spleen occurs when platelets are coated with antibody. There is no evidence that the normal spleen sequesters a significant number of neutrophils, and the mechanism of neutropenia which may develop in association with splenomegaly has not been determined.

During embryonic life the spleen plays an important part in blood formation, and the potentialities of this organ for blood formation persist even in adult life. In certain circumstances, foci of extramedullary blood formation can be found in the spleen; thus, when the functional activity of the bone marrow is impaired, the hematopoietic potentiality of the spleen may become an important asset.

ENLARGEMENT OF THE SPLEEN. This may occur under a great variety of circumstances. The chief ones are listed in Table 63-2.

Of greatest frequency is the enlargement of the spleen which occurs in association with infections. The *"acute splenic tumor"* accompanying various systemic infections such as typhoid fever and septicemia are examples. Like lymph node enlargement, splenic enlargement is frequently encountered in various contagious diseases and is often seen in infectious mononucleosis. Likewise, various subacute infections, notably bacterial endocarditis, are characteristically accompanied by enlargement of the spleen. *Abscess* of the spleen is rare and is usually secondary to pyemia arising from some other site. Frequently multiple and unrecognized, it is unusual for a splenic abscess to achieve prominence and produce local symptoms such as pain, elevation of the left leaf of the diaphragm, or rupture into the peritoneal cavity.

Malaria is, perhaps, the commonest cause of splenic enlargement when the world population is considered. Infection with other parasites which leads to splenic enlargement includes leishmaniasis, trypanosomiasis, and schistosomiasis. In kala-azar the spleen may be huge.

Primary tuberculous splenomegaly is extremely rare, but slight enlargement of the spleen accompanying a widespread tuberculous infection is by no means unusual. Splenomegaly may occur in connection with syphilis, especially congenital syphilis. Enlargement of this organ may also accompany the late stages of syphilis in association with gummas or amyloidosis. Rheumatoid arthritis, brucellosis, and sarcoidosis are other chronic diseases which may be accompanied by splenic enlargement. Splenic enlargement has been observed in about 25 percent of cases of disseminated lupus erythematosus.

Table 63-2. CHIEF CAUSES OF SPLENOMEGALY

I. Inflammatory splenomegaly
    A. "Acute splenic tumor": many acute and subacute infections
        1. Bacterial (typhoid, septicemias, subacute bacterial endocarditis, abscess, etc.)
        2. Viral and miscellaneous (contagious diseases, infectious mononucleosis)
    B. Chronic infections (tuberculosis, syphilis, brucellosis, histoplasmosis, malaria, schistosomiasis, leishmaniasis, trypanosomiasis, etc.)
    C. Miscellaneous diseases (lupus erythematosus, rheumatoid arthritis, sarcoidosis, histiocytosis X, etc.)
II. Congestive splenomegaly (Banti's syndrome)
    A. Cirrhosis of liver
    B. Thrombosis or stenosis, portal or splenic veins
III. Hyperplastic splenomegaly
    A. Hemolytic anemias, congenital and acquired
    B. Thalassemia and certain hemoglobinopathies
    C. Myelofibrosis, myelophthisic anemias
    D. Polycythemia vera
    E. Miscellaneous chronic anemias (pernicious anemia, chronic iron deficiency, "pyridoxine-responsive anemia," etc.)
    F. Thrombocytopenic purpura
    G. Obscure disorders ("big spleen syndrome," "primary splenic neutropenia," and "panhematopenia")
IV. Infiltrative splenomegaly
    A. Gaucher's disease, Niemann-Pick disease
    B. Amyloidosis, hemosiderosis
V. Neoplasms and cysts
    A. True cysts (dermoid, echinococcus, etc.)
    B. False cysts (hemorrhagic, serous, inflammatory, degenerative)
    C. Benign tumors (lymphangioma, hemangioma, etc.)
    D. Leukemia, lymphomas
    E. Malignant tumors (direct invasion or metastatic)

The vascularity of the spleen and its location in the portal bed make this organ liable to swelling as the result of increased venous pressure in that region. Such types of enlargement of the spleen can be classed under the general heading of "congestive splenomegaly" and include the syndromes known as *Banti's disease* and *splenic anemia*, as well as the splenic enlargement which accompanies cirrhosis of the liver and thrombosis of the splenic or portal vein (Chap. 350) and that which may be associated with cardiac failure.

The functions of the spleen in relation to the hematopoietic system result in enlargement of this organ when there is increased blood destruction (acute and chronic hemolytic anemias) or in the presence of chronic anemia of various types such as pernicious anemia, chronic hypochromic anemia, myelophthisic anemia, thalassemia, hemoglobin-C disease, and other hemoglobinopathies. Again, the spleen is enlarged, as a rule, in leukemia. In polycythemia vera splenomegaly is often encountered, and this finding helps to distinguish the primary disorder from secondary forms of polycythemia, where splenic enlargement is rare. The lymphatic hyperplasia which is associated with hyperthyroidism may be accompanied by splenomegaly. The spleen is also enlarged in myelofibrosis, primary splenic neutropenia, and primary splenic panhematopenia (Chap. 350).

Certain rare diseases such as Gaucher's disease and Niemann-Pick disease are characterized by splenic enlargement. In these conditions the swelling of the organ is probably due to the excessive storage of normal and abnormal metabolic products in the cells of the spleen (see Chap. 350).

Like other organs, the spleen may be enlarged as the consequence of the presence of neoplasms of various types. Hodgkin's disease, lymphosarcoma, reticulum cell sarcoma, and giant follicular lymphoma, however, are far commoner causes of splenomegaly than other types of new growth. Carcinoma is the most frequent type of metastatic tumor, but even this is extremely rare. Direct extension from carcinoma of the stomach and hematogenous spread from the stomach, lung, pancreas, and breast and from malignant melanoma may occur. Other tumors that may involve the spleen include lymphangioma, hemangioma and endothelial sarcoma (lymphangiosarcoma), fibrosarcoma, leiomyosarcoma, and myoma. A subcapsular cavernous hemangioma may rupture into the peritoneal cavity and produce acute hemorrhagic shock.

Cysts of the spleen may be of parasitic origin or nonparasitic. Of the latter, those containing serous or hemorrhagic fluid and due to trauma are commonest. They can sometimes be identified roentgenographically because of calcification of the wall. Echinococcus cysts occur more rarely in the spleen than in the liver. "True" cysts are formed from embryonal defects or rests and include dermoids and mesenchymal inclusion cysts.

DIFFERENTIAL DIAGNOSIS OF SPLENOMEGALY

A thorough physical examination, together with the history and the examination of the blood, will serve to differentiate many of the causes of splenomegaly which have been outlined. Sometimes additional procedures may be required, such as blood culture, sternal puncture, a roentgenogram of the chest, serologic tests including thoses for syphilis, liver function tests, and spleen or lymph node biopsy. Since certain of the causes of splenomegaly do not induce diagnostic pathologic changes in the spleen, a splenic aspiration or splenic biopsy will not necessarily yield a diagnosis. In most instances the cause of splenomegaly is not determined by studying the spleen itself but by detecting diseases which are known to be associated with splenomegaly.

The absence of fever is more helpful in differential diagnosis here than is its presence, since most of the conditions which have been mentioned may be accompanied by fever. However, at times, as in malaria and in undulant fever, the characteristic temperature curve is very helpful in making the diagnosis. In the septicemias the splenic enlargement is, as a rule, obviously only a minor feature of the whole clinical picture. The exanthemas are recognized by the respective characteristic changes in the skin. In their absence the skin should be inspected carefully for evidence of the pete-chiae which may accompany acute leukemia, thrombo-cytopenic purpura, or other hematopoietic disorders; the red petechiae occurring in crops together with the larger, slightly nodular and tender Osler nodes so characteristic of subacute bacterial endocarditis; or the spider telangiectases which accompany long-standing liver diseases. The plum-red "cyanosis" of polycythemia vera can hardly be overlooked.

Moderate lymph node enlargement accompanying sple-nomegaly is seen in many infectious diseases as well as in leukemia, but an asymmetric enlargement should arouse suspicion of Hodgkin's disease or lymphosarcoma. Great enlargement of the lymph nodes is seen in the last-named conditions as well as in chronic leukemia, espe-cially in the lymphocytic form. The discovery of icterus suggests hemolytic anemia as a cause or, if there is little or no anemia and the splenic enlargement is only slight, infectious hepatitis. The splenomegaly associated with the Banti syndrome (congestive splenomegaly) and with cir-rhosis of the liver is usually substantial in degree, and jaundice is not the rule under these circumstances. Ma-laria must be kept in mind among the causes of hemo-lytic anemia.

Lesions in the mucous membranes accompanying sple-nic enlargement are seen in measles (Koplik's spots), secondary syphilis (mucous patches), infectious mono-nucleosis (infection of the throat, tonsillar enlargement, sometimes signs of Vincent's angina), and acute leukemia (swollen, thickened gums which may be bleeding or pur-plish in color). In the leukemias, sternal tenderness may be quite pronounced.

The discovery of very great enlargement of the spleen tends to rule out the acute splenic tumor of various sys-temic infections, although sometimes the spleen may ex-tend 4 to 6 cm below the costal margin in septicemia and in subacute bacterial endocarditis. Huge spleens are en-countered in the chronic leukemias, in the Banti syn-drome, in kala-azar, in schistosomiasis, in Gaucher's dis-ease, in Hodgkin's disease and lymphosarcoma, in myelo-fibrosis, and in many instances of chronic hemolytic ane-mia.

Examination of the blood may indicate at once the nature of the disorder, as in malaria, the frank leukemias, or infectious mononucleosis. The discovery of icterus will lead to a reticulocyte count, examination of the stools and urine for the products of blood destruction, an eryth-rocyte fragility test, and other studies (see Chap. 338) to rule out the various hemolytic anemias. The discovery of leukopenia should lead to the consideration of malaria, "aleukemic" leukemia, the Banti syndrome, typhoid fever, histoplasmosis, and leishmaniasis, but it must be kept in mind that the white cell count may sometimes be low also in infectious mononucleosis and in some cases of chronic hemolytic anemia. The demonstration of throm-bocytopenia, as well as prolonged bleeding time, poor clot retraction, and positive tourniquet test, is an important finding, for it suggests acute leukemia. In that condition immature leukocytes will be found in the blood. In the "aleukemic" form, immature cells are absent from the

blood or very scarce, but they are readily demonstrated by sternal puncture. In idiopathic thrombocytopenic pur-pura, the spleen is barely palpable in about 33 percent of cases, but it is never very large. Thrombocytopenia only very rarely accompanies infectious mononucleosis and, while present in other conditions such as pernicious anemia, chronic hypochromic anemia, chronic hemolytic anemias, myelophthisic anemia, the Banti syndrome, Hodgkin's disease, and the related lymph node disorders, it is rarely severe in these diseases.

Sternal puncture may be very helpful if "aleukemic" leukemia, leishmaniasis, or Gaucher's disease is being con-sidered seriously, for the characteristic cells or causative organisms may be demonstrated in this way. Sternal puncture does not often reveal malaria when the parasites have eluded careful study of the blood, but sometimes positive blood cultures for bacteria are obtained by this means when the usual method has failed. Splenic punc-ture is helpful when parasites, storage cells, signs of mye-loid metaplasia, or granulomas are found, but this pro-cedure should not be undertaken when hemorrhagic man-ifestations are present or in the absence of evidence of distinct splenic enlargement.

Various disorders of the spleen are discussed in a later chapter (Chap. 350).

REFERENCES

Jandl, J. H., and R. H. Aster: Increased Splenic Pooling and the Pathogenesis of Hypersplenism, Am. J. Med. Sci. 253:383–398, 1967.

McIntyre, O. R., and F. G. Ebaugh, Jr.: Palpable Spleens in College Freshmen, Ann. Intern. Med. 66:301–306, 1967.

Saltzstein, S. L., and L. V. Ackerman: Lymphadenopathy In-duced by Anticonvulsant Drugs, Cancer, 12:164, 1959.

Wintrobe, M. M.: "Clinical Hematology," 6th ed., Philadel-phia, Lea & Febiger, 1967.

64 ALTERATIONS IN LEUKOCYTES
Dane R. Boggs and M. M. Wintrobe

Unlike the red corpuscles, the leukocytes do not carry out their chief functions in the circulating blood. For them the circulation is mainly a transport system through which they pass from the sites where they are formed to the locations where they are needed. The time that the leukocytes spend in the blood does not reflect their life span, and exact life spans for different types of leukocytes are not known. Their fate, like that of soldiers, probably depends as much on external factors as on the ultimate wearing out of internal metabolic activities.

Little is known about the factors which normally main-tain the leukocyte count and the proportion of different types of leukocytes within a rather narrow range of values, nor is much known about the factors which cause these to change. However, it has been possible

Table 64-1. NORMAL VALUES FOR CONCENTRATION*
OF BLOOD LEUKOCYTES

Cell type	Mean (cells per cu mm)	95% Confidence limits (cells per cu mm)
Neutrophil........	3,650	1,830–7,250
Lymphocyte......	2,500	1,500–4,000
Monocyte........	430	200–950
Eosinophil........	150	0–700
Basophil.........	30	0–150

* Total leukocyte counts from venous blood samples were done in a "Coulter counter," and 200 leukocytes were differentiated on Wright's stained blood smears made on cover glass.

to infer a great deal about the functions of the leukocytes by observing the alterations which are associated with various physiologic states and with different disease entities. In many respects the leukocyte and differential counts serve as mirrors which reflect changes taking place in the body, and thereby, these determinations have proved to be of immense value in differential diagnosis.

The only known function of the leukocytic systems is to defend the body from foreign material by means of phagocytosis and antibody formation. These are interrelated functions; phagocytosis is enhanced by the presence of antibody specific for the substance being phagocytized, and phagocytosis of antigen may be an initiating step in antibody production. Neutrophils, monocytes, eosinophils and basophils are phagocytes, while lymphocytes and plasma cells are concerned with antibody production. Each of these six types of leukocytes probably plays a distinct and unique role in body defense mechanisms, although the role of basophils and eosinophils is unclear.

The concentration in blood of each specific type of

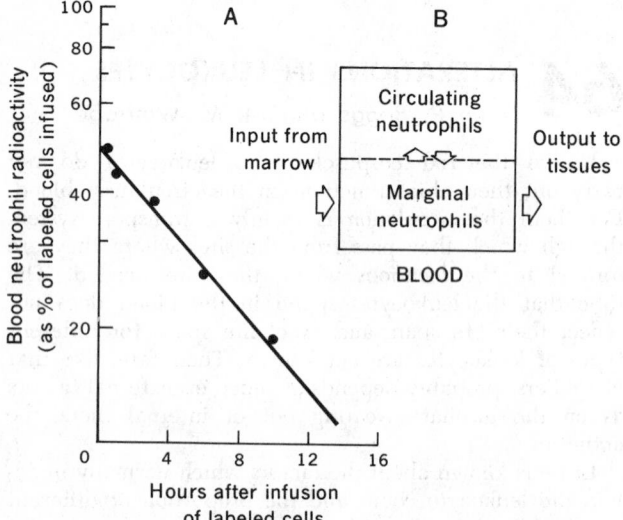

Fig. 64-1. Disappearance of ^{32}DFP-labeled neutrophils in a normal subject (*A*) and a model of blood neutrophil kinetics (*B*).

leukocyte is a much more meaningful value than is total white cell count (total leukocyte concentration). The mean and 95 percent confidence limits of various blood leukocytes as found in 291 prisoners from the Utah State Prison are given in Table 64-1. The number of eosinophils and basophils in the blood is so small that the normal range encompasses zero. Thus, eosinopenia and basopenia cannot be determined from results of routine blood examination.

In this chapter current concepts of the physiology of each of the leukocytic systems will be reviewed, and the diagnostic and clinical significance of changes in the concentration of the various blood leukocytes will be considered.

THE PHAGOCYTIC SYSTEM

Neutrophils

NEUTROPHIL PHYSIOLOGY

During the first half of the last century a number of investigators noted that leukocytes within the confines of blood vessels often are marginated along venule and capillary walls. Modern techniques have made it possible to show that in man approximately one-half of the intravascular neutrophils are marginated and one-half circulate freely (Fig. 64-1*B*). Blood neutrophil concentration, as determined in venous samples, measures the circulating but not the marginal pool.

Neutrophils enter the blood from a storage reservoir in the bone marrow and leave the blood in random fashion after an average intravascular sojourn of 10 hr (Fig. 64-1*A*). They do not return to the blood after leaving it. There are many more neutrophils and neutrophil precursors in the bone marrow than are present in the blood. Bone marrow neutrophils consist of two pools of cells, the mitotic production pool and the postmitotic maturation and storage pool (Fig. 64-2). Morphologic subdivisions within these pools necessarily are somewhat arbitrary. The production pool can be considered as consisting of three compartments of increasing maturity: myeloblasts, promyelocytes, and myelocytes. The postmitotic maturation and storage pool consists of metamyelocytes, "bands" or "juveniles," and segmented neutrophils. Under ordinary circumstances, metamyelocytes are not released to the blood. Bands and segmented neutrophils are readily released to the blood, although segmented neutrophils are released in preference to bands. These cells constitute the storage compartment of bone marrow neutrophils.

From this marrow reserve of neutrophils the rate of cell entry to the blood can be accelerated upon demand before an increase in the rate of cell production occurs. In normal individuals there are enough postmitotic neutrophils to replace those in the blood for approximately 10 days at normal rates of marrow release. Approximately 60 percent of the postmitotic neutrophil pool of normal marrow consists of bands and segmented neutrophils. Thus the effective storage reservoir is approximately 15 times as large as the blood pool (Fig. 64-2).

The fate of neutrophils leaving the blood has not been

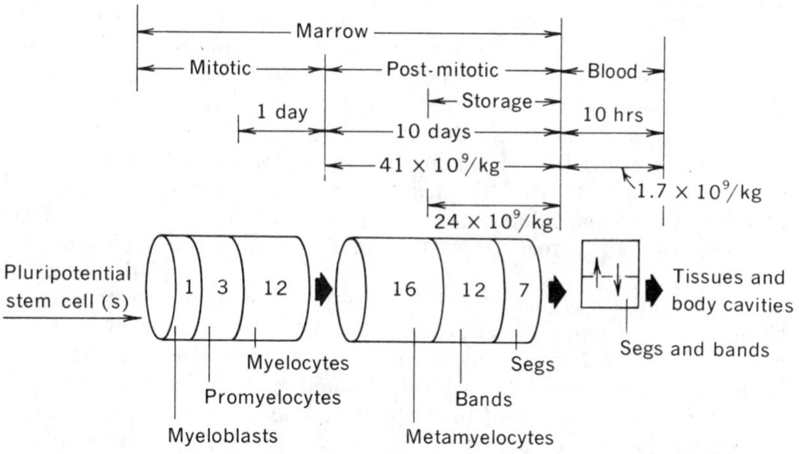

Fig. 64-2. Diagrammatic model of neutrophil kinetics. Neutrophils share with platelets and erythrocytes a common precursor (pluripotential stem cell). The marrow mitotic pool is the site of production. The postmitotic pool consists of cells which continue to mature (metamyelocytes and bands) and a marrow reserve of mature neutrophils. From this, cells enter the blood for a brief sojourn on their way to tissues and body cavities. Only the circulating pool is measured in the traditional leukocyte count of the blood. Data for the size of the system and the transit times through various compartments are based upon studies of neutrophils labeled with radioactive diisopropyl fluorophosphate in normal volunteers from the Utah State Prison. Cell ratios, indicated by the numbers posted on each compartment, are based upon 500 cell differential counts of neutrophils and neutrophil precursors in smears of marrow aspirates from 12 such volunteers.

entirely clarified. In a normal subject, neutrophils appear in bronchial secretions, in urine, and in the lumen of the gut. Whether these sites of egress account for the majority of neutrophils leaving the blood each day or represent but a small proportion of these cells is not known. Following initiation of tissue injury, neutrophils marginate along the walls of the capillaries and venules adjacent to the injured area and by diapedesis traverse the intervening tissue. They enter the area of beginning exudate formation within 1 or 2 hr following the inflammatory stimulus. Diapedesis takes place between endothelial cells of the blood vessel. Neutrophils are delayed for some time at the basement membrane and then move in a seemingly directed fashion through the intervening tissue to enter the exudate. Turnover of neutrophils through an established exudate is almost as rapid as the turnover of neutrophils through the blood.

Neutropenia and neutrophilia may develop by a variety of kinetic mechanisms. Transient changes in blood neutrophil concentration may develop without any change in the rate at which cells enter or leave the blood; rapid shifts of cells between marginal and circulating pools can take place. Since this mechanism does not induce a change in the total number of neutrophils in the confines of the vascular system, it may be designated as producing "pseudoneutrophilia," or "pseudoneutropenia." Strenuous exercise or the administration of epinephrine and perhaps a variety of other stimuli leads to transient demargination of neutrophils with a brief but sometimes striking episode of neutrophilia.

Persistent neutrophilia is usually accompanied by an accelerated rate of entry of new cells from the bone marrow and is of necessity accompanied by increased production. Conversely, in most instances of persistent neutropenia, the storage pool of the bone marrow is exhausted, and usually, production is found to be decreased.

However, changes in egress of neutrophils from the blood can also be the primary cause of changes in blood neutrophil concentration. Administration of pharmacologic doses of hydrocortisone induces neutrophilia, at least in part by reducing the rate of cell loss from the blood. Certain instances of neutropenia, such as those induced by overwhelming infection, by injection of endotoxin, or by administration of antineutrophil antibody, reflect a very marked acceleration in the rate of cell loss from the blood. This acceleration is so great that input from the marrow and increased production cannot keep pace, and neutropenia develops primarily because of accelerated cell loss.

NEUTROPHILIA

An increase in blood neutrophil concentration accompanies most *bacterial infections*. With the exception of a few diseases, such as tuberculosis, brucellosis, and typhoid fever, neutrophilia develops during the inception and persists through the acute phases of bacterial infection. Neutrophilia may be present in some fungal infections, such as actinomycosis; a few viral infections, such as rabies and herpes zoster; and a variety of parasitic and rickettsial infestations. The highest neutrophil levels, often exceeding 30,000 per cu mm, commonly are observed in pneumococcal pneumonia or with localized abscesses. Neutrophilia may not persist as infections become chronic. In some chronic infections, such as bacterial endocarditis and pyelonephritis, neutrophil concentration may be normal.

The presence or absence of neutrophilia is a useful diagnostic sign, and serial determination of neutrophil concentration provides prognostic information during the course of infection. The proportion of blood neutrophils which are not segmented (band/segmented ratio) is of equal or even greater diagnostic and prognostic significance. In the early stages of infection the rate of release of neutrophils from the marrow storage pool to the blood is accelerated in response to demand for phagocytes at the infected site. As the storage pool is reduced, a greater proportion of bands is released, and the band/segmented ratio in the blood increases, leading to a moderate "shift to the left." As the infection is controlled, or as it stabilizes, the demand for neutrophils is reduced or marrow production accelerates to meet continued increased demands. In these circumstances neutrophilia may persist for some time, but as the marrow storage pool is reconstituted, the band/segmented ratio returns toward normal.

On the other hand, if the infection is spreading, the demand for neutrophils may steadily increase and may exceed the ability of the marrow to increase production, so that the storage pool either remains small or may actually become exhausted. In such a patient the shift to the left becomes increasingly more pronounced. Thus the characteristic pattern of early infection is neutrophilia with a modest shift to the left; of healing or well-controlled infection, neutrophilia with little or no cell immaturity; and of severe continuing infection, neutrophilia or even neutropenia with an increasing proportion of bands in the blood.

The magnitude of neutrophilia varies with its cause, being greater as a rule in localized in contrast to systemic infections and in highly virulent infections in otherwise healthy patients as compared with debilitated individuals.

The *transient episodes of neutrophilia* induced by injecting *epinephrine* or by *strenuous exercise* are due to demargination of intravascular neutrophils and are not attended by any change in the band/segmented neutrophil ratio. It is likely that the brief episodes of neutrophilia which are observed in such conditions as *paroxysmal tachycardia, convulsive seizures,* and *delirium tremens* are the result of demargination.

Neutrophilia accompanying many other noninfectious processes probably is produced by accelerating the rate of release of marrow neutrophils, since a modest increase in band/segmented ratio is observed as the neutrophilia develops. This is seen following *acute hemorrhage* and in *acute hemolytic anemia.* The neutrophilia which develops in many diseases can be attributed to the influence of a combination of factors. In some, such as acute *gout, myocardial infarction* or *pulmonary embolism* and *infarction, burns,* and *spider* and *snake bites,* the stimulus for neutrophilia is tissue damage, inflammation, and sterile exudate formation. From what is known about the effects of pharmacologic doses of *hydrocortisone,* described above, it is likely that increased hydrocortisone blood levels, whether resulting from increased production due to stress or decreased degradation, as in hepatic failure, may be, at least in part, responsible for the neutrophilia. Patients with *Cushing's disease* often have mild neutrophilia.

Neutrophilia also is seen in *diabetic acidosis, uremia, eclampsia,* in *Hodgkin's disease,* and sometimes in association with rapidly growing malignant neoplasms. The excessive production of neutrophils, eosinophils, basophils, and platelets, as well as of erythrocytes, so characteristic of *polycythemia vera* may be due to an abnormally functioning pluripotent stem cell compartment.

Unexplained or extreme *neutrophilia* or significant numbers of myelocytes and metamyelocytes and other immature cells in the blood suggests leukemia. The diagnosis of leukemia and its differentiation from "leukemoid reactions" is considered in Chap. 348.

NEUTROPENIA

Neutropenia may be present when the white count (total leukocyte concentration) is decreased, normal, or increased. It should be obvious that the percentage of neutrophils in differential leukocyte counts is relatively meaningless unless it is multiplied by the total leukocyte count to obtain neutrophil concentration.

CLINICAL MANIFESTATIONS. Of itself, neutropenia causes no symptoms unless infection supervenes. However, patients with neutropenia of any cause may suffer from frequent and severe bacterial infections. When neutropenia is related to some disease, the clinical manifestations will be those of the underlying disorder.

The decrease in resistance to infection which attends neutropenia was dramatically exemplified by the syndrome of *agranulocytosis* or *agranulocytic angina,* first recognized in 1922. This disorder is characterized by severe sore throat, marked prostration, and extreme reduction or even complete disappearance of the neutrophils from the blood. Although there may be a prodromal period marked by malaise or moderate fever, the onset is usually acute and fulminating. When first described, agranulocytosis often ended in sepsis and death. It was later recognized that the appearance of this syndrome corresponded with the introduction of certain coal-tar derivatives as therapeutic agents, in particular the antipyretic, aminopyrine (Pyramidon). The course of events was shown to consist of (1) neutropenia; (2) loss of resistance to infection, development of sore throat; and (3) overwhelming sepsis and death. Recognition of the etiologic basis of the syndrome, prohibition of further use of the offending drug, and prompt antibiotic therapy have greatly altered the prognosis.

The symptoms and physical signs directly attributable to neutropenia of any cause are those produced by the infections which attend neutropenia. Infection usually begins in the skin, especially the perineal and axillary areas, the throat, or the lungs, but may be first noted in virtually any area of the body. Initial infections usually are due to common bacteria such as pneumococci, staphylococci, streptococci, and coliform organisms. In patients with recurrent infections, or in patients who receive repetitive courses of antibiotics, more unusual organisms and those resistant to antibiotics, such as *Pseudomonas,* are observed, and infection with fungi, such as *Candida,* becomes more common. With very severe neutropenia infections spread rapidly and bacteremia is common. Patients with a small but significant number of neutrophils in the blood often suffer from chronic, indolent infections which can be contained with proper local and systemic measures but often defy complete cure.

The relationship between the severity of neutropenia and the frequency of infection is far from exact. However, as a general statement, patients with idiopathic neutropenia rarely develop life-threatening infections unless the neutrophil concentration is less than 1,000 per cu mm. In patients with a count of less than 500, this complication is usually observed.

Absolute numbers of monocytes and eosinophils may be increased, and hypergammaglobulinemia is present in some patients with neutropenia. These changes may be due to a physiologic response of other protective systems in compensation for the decreased resistance to infection secondary to the neutropenia or may merely represent the reaction to repeated or chronic infections. Blood lymphocyte concentration is quite variable and may be decreased, normal, or increased.

ETIOLOGY. Neutropenia may exist as an isolated hematologic abnormality or may be associated with anemia and/or thrombocytopenia. All of the causes of aplastic anemia (Chap. 341) are also causes of neutropenia. The major causes of neutropenia can be categorized as (1) drug induced, (2) secondary to known diseases (or syndromes), (3) familial, (4) antibody induced, and (5) idiopathic. Examples of each are given in Table 64-2.

Table 64-2. CAUSES OF NEUTROPENIA

I. Drugs and physical agents (see Table 64-3)
II. Diseases
    A. Infections
      1. Bacterial, e.g., overwhelming infections of any type; also certain other, not necessarily overwhelming infections, e.g., typhoid, paratyphoid, brucella
      2. Viral and rickettsial, e.g., influenza, measles, rubella, hepatitis, Colorado tick fever, psittacosis
    B. Nutritional deficiency, e.g., starvation, selective deficiency of folic acid or vitamin B_{12}
    C. Hematopoietic diseases, e.g., acute leukemia, chronic lymphocytic leukemia, lymphosarcoma, aplastic anemia, paroxysmal nocturnal hemoglobinuria, thymic alymphoplasia, deficient immunoglobulin production
    D. Diseases producing splenomegaly, e.g., congestive splenomegaly, Gaucher's disease, Felty's syndrome
    E. Other diseases, e.g., lupus erythematosus, pancreatic exocrine deficiency
III. Familial chronic neutropenia
IV. Antibody induced neutropenia, e.g., autoantibodies and transplacental antibodies
V. Idiopathic neutropenic syndromes, e.g., cyclic neutropenia, hypoplastic neutropenia, hyperplastic neutropenia

Neutropenia induced by *drugs or by physical agents,* such as x-ray, is probably the most common form of neutropenia (Table 64-3). Drugs which induce neutropenia can be divided into two broad classes, those in which neutropenia can be expected if enough of the drug is given and those in which neutropenia is an unpredictable, "hypersensitivity" reaction. Neutropenia is a common side effect of antitumor therapy, since the alkylating agents, antimetabolies, stathmokinetic agents (those which poison the mitotic spindle, thereby leading to cell death in metaphase), and x-ray (Chap. 348 and 351) all produce neutropenia if given in sufficient dosage. This effect appears to be due to a decrease in neutrophil production, and recovery will usually follow discontinuation of the drug. Certain chemicals, such as benzene, can be added to the above list of agents which produce dose-related neutropenia.

In addition to those listed in Table 64-3, many other drugs have been suspected as a cause of neutropenia. Neutropenia with certain of the above drugs has been accompanied by virtual absence of neutrophil precursors from the bone marrow, while with others mitotic neutrophil precursors have been abundant in marrow aspirates.

Thus it appears that different pathogenetic mechanisms, increased destruction and decreased production, are involved in hypersensitivity reactions.

Certain drugs, notably aminopyrine, appear to destroy mature neutrophils by an immunologic mechanism in sensitized patients. Patients who have recovered from aminopyrine-induced neutropenia become neutropenic again within a few hours following administration of a very small challenging dose of the drug. Blood, withdrawn from such patients 3 hr after a test dose of the drug, induces transient neutropenia when transfused into normal subjects.

Table 64-3. DRUGS AND PHYSICAL AGENTS
PRODUCING NEUTROPENIA

Group I—regularly produce neutropenia if given in sufficient amounts
  Physical agents:
    Radiation with roentgen rays, gamma rays, beta rays, and neutrons.
  Antitumor drugs:
    Alkylating agents (nitrogen mustard, busulfan, chlorambucil, cyclophosphamide, etc.), antimetabolites (methotrexate, 6-mercaptopurine, etc.), stathmokinetics (vinblastine, etc.), antibiotics (daunomycin, etc.).
  Benzene
  Colchicine
Group II—produce leukopenia in "sensitive" persons only
  Analgesics (aminopyrine, dipyrone, phenylbutazone, etc.)
  Phenothiazines (chlorpromazine, promazine, mepazine, etc.)
  Antithyroid drugs (thiouracil, methimazole, etc.)
  Anticonvulsants (trimethadione, phethenylate, etc.)
  Sulfonamides and derivatives [carbutamide, sulfisoxazole (Gantrisin) etc.]
  Antihistamines (Pyribenzamine, etc.)
  Antimicrobial agents (organic arsenicals, chloramphenicol)
  Tranquilizers (meprobamate, etc.)
  Miscellaneous (dinitrophenol, gold salts, etc.)

Neutropenia associated with sensitivity to such drugs as the phenothiazines apparently is due to interference with neutrophil production in the bone marrow rather than to destruction of mature neutrophils. In such cases few or no neutrophil precursors are demonstrable in the bone marrow. The phenothiazine, chlorpromazine, inhibits in vitro nucleic acid synthesis of suspensions of marrow cells.

Many classes of disease are associated with neutropenia (Table 64-2). Mild neutropenia is common in a variety of *viral and protozoal infections* and in infections such as typhoid fever and brucellosis. Neutropenia may also be observed in response to acute, severe, bacterial infections in which neutrophilia is the rule. In the last circumstance neutropenia should be viewed as a very poor prognostic sign for recovery from the infection. In experimental studies of induced pneumococcal pneumonia in dogs, neutropenia developed only in those animals in which the infection was so overwhelming that the marrow reserve of neutrophils was exhausted. If an infected patient runs out of phagocytes, a poor prognosis can be expected. Such patients are not only neutropenic, but very few of their remaining neutrophils are fully mature.

Neutropenia often accompanies *diseases of the hematopoietic system* (Table 64-2). Neutropenia was reported to be the first hematologic change in rare instances of copper deficiency in infants, and mild neutropenia occasionally accompanies severe iron-deficiency anemia. Neutropenia may accompany deficient immunoglobulin production (Chap. 69).

A number of children with pancreatic exocrine insufficiency which is not due to cystic fibrosis also have neutropenia. Since neutropenia is not common in cystic fibrosis, the relationship of the pancreatic dysfunction to the neutropenia is unclear.

Removal of the spleen leads to transient neutrophilia, and in certain diseases the presence of neutropenia seems to be correlated with an *enlarged spleen*. Patients with cirrhosis of the liver often have neutrophilia, but when the spleen is congested and enlarged as a result of increased portal pressure in cirrhosis, neutropenia is more common. Congestive splenomegaly of any cause and splenomegaly due to such diseases as Gaucher's disease may be associated with neutropenia. Neutropenia is rarely observed in rheumatoid arthritis unless the spleen is enlarged (Felty's syndrome). In other diseases, such as systemic lupus erythematosus, the presence of neutropenia correlates poorly with the presence of splenomegaly. The role of the spleen in neutrophil kinetics remains to be clarified, but it is likely that in certain of the above circumstances the spleen traps and destroys an abnormally large number of neutrophils.

Familial neutropenia probably exists in at least two forms: severe neutropenia inherited as an autosomal recessive trait, and a milder form inherited as an autosomal dominant.

Antineutrophil antibodies developing in the absence of such drugs as aminopyrine (autoimmune antineutrophil antibodies) may be responsible for many instances of idiopathic neutropenia, but there is no fully satisfactory in vitro test for detecting their presence. The observation that children born of neutropenic mothers may suffer from transient neutropenia suggests the presence of such antibodies.

Transient neonatal neutropenia also has been observed in children born of multiparous mothers without neutropenia. This suggests that maternal sensitization to fetal neutrophil antigens may occur, resulting in a situation somewhat analogous to erythroblastosis fetalis.

Idiopathic forms of neutropenia are separable into various syndromes, but none of these syndromes is common, and none is very well understood. Neutropenia occurring in regular cycles and sometimes persisting for years has been reported in a number of patients. In some instances the neutropenia has recurred at roughly 3-week intervals. In others the intervals were longer or more irregular. Such cycling of blood levels suggests a disturbance in the regulatory mechanism for neutrophil production. Other examples of chronic idiopathic neutropenia include those with few or no neutrophil precursors (*hypoplastic*) and those with abundant neutrophil precursors in the bone marrow (*hyperplastic neutropenia*).

KINETIC MECHANISM OF NEUTROPENIA. The changes in neutrophil kinetics which can lead to neutropenia are indicated in Fig. 64-3. Blood and/or bone marrow neutrophils can be labeled with radioactive diisopropyl fluorophosphate, and from such in vivo studies the rate of neutrophil production, destruction, blood and marrow transit times, and the sizes of the circulating and marginal pools can be determined. Short-term cultures of bone marrow can be used to study rates of maturation or of proliferation as judged by incorporation of tritiated thymidine into DNA of neutrophil precursors. Neutrophil migration from the blood into induced inflammatory exudates on the skin can be measured. Administration of epinephrine results in demargination of blood neutrophils, and the resultant increase in neutrophil concentration in venous blood samples provides a rough estimate of the size of the marginal pool. Administration of endotoxin, etiocholanolone, or hydrocortisone "flushes" neutrophils from the marrow storage pool into the blood. If the expected increase in blood neutrophil concentration following administration of these drugs does not take place, it is assumed that the patient's storage pool is exhausted.

Either increased cell loss with compensatory increase in production or decreased production can result in exhaustion of the marrow storage pool. In either case, most

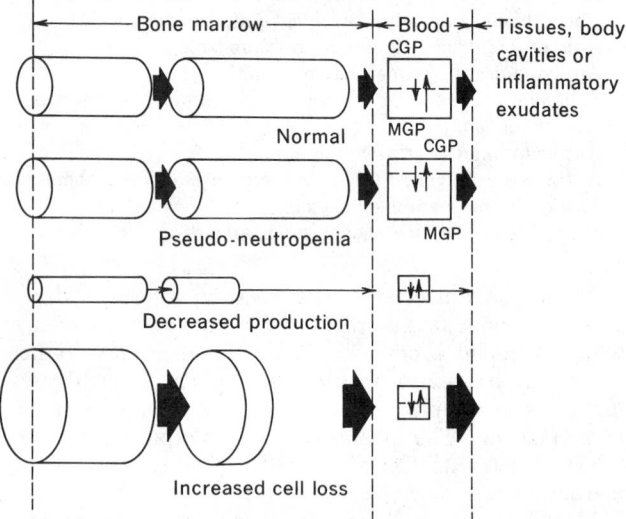

Fig. 64-3. Changes in neutrophil kinetics resulting in neutropenia. The bone marrow is represented as two connected tubes which contain the mitotic and postmitotic compartments, as described in Fig. 64-2. The diameters of the tubes reflect the sizes of the pools, and their length represents their morphologic integrity. The normal neutrophil system is shown at the top of the figure, and three types of change in the system which may lead to neutropenia are illustrated diagrammatically below. In pseudoneutropenia there is a change in the ratio of the circulating (CGP)/marginal (MGP) pools, but the bone marrow is normal. Both when there is decreased production or increased cell loss, the storage compartment of the postmitotic pool is drained, leaving only young metamyelocytes. However, the mitotic pools differ greatly in size in these two neutropenic states.

of the neutrophils in the blood will be "bands." If the bone marrow is examined in these patients, the ratio of mitotic to postmitotic neutrophil precursors is found to be increased. Assuming that the patient is not anemic, the myeloid/erythroid ratio of the bone marrow should distinguish between an increase or a decrease in the size of the marrow mitotic pool of neutrophils. With neutropenia due to increased cell loss, abundant mitotic neutrophil precursors and metamyelocytes should be observed in the bone marrow, producing a pattern which has been termed *maturation arrest*. This is a misnomer because such a pattern probably signifies the reverse of maturation arrest; except in leukemia, it reflects a marrow in which the storage pool is exhausted and from which bands are released to the blood as soon as they are formed.

Careful examination of the blood smear is very useful in interpreting kinetic changes in patients with neutropenia. If the storage pool is exhausted, band form neutrophils are released to the blood as soon as they are formed, and very few will have had time to mature into segmented neutrophils. In this circumstance there will be an increase in the band/segmented cell ratio in the blood. In contrast, if pseudoneutropenia resulting from increased margination of neutrophils along vessel walls is present, the band/segmented cell ratio in blood should be normal.

THERAPY. There is no known method of therapy which will safely and reproducibly accelerate the rate of neutrophil production in a neutropenic patient. Administration of such agents as bacterial endotoxin leads to an accelerated rate of neutrophil production in experimental animals and probably in normal man. However, this acceleration of production appears to be a physiologic response to the acute neutrophil depletion induced by endotoxin. Neutropenic patients would be expected to be under maximal or near maximal stimulation of neutrophil production through normal physiologic mechanisms. Through the years a number of agents have been reported as efficacious in the therapy of neutropenia, but to date none can be considered to be of proven benefit.

If the patient is receiving any drugs or has been exposed to any other agents which might possibly be injurious, further exposure to these drugs and agents should be avoided. Drug-induced neutropenia usually responds to discontinuance of the offending agent, although a few patients die of infection before recovery can occur, and a few others develop chronic neutropenia for reasons which are not clear.

Neutropenia secondary to known diseases such as those listed in Table 64-2 improves or is corrected if general improvement in the disease is brought about.

In a limited proportion of cases of neutropenia, improvement has followed splenectomy, particularly in cases with splenomegaly; for example, in patients with congestive splenomegaly secondary to obstruction in the portal circulation. However, the advisability of the operation must be weighed in the light of the many other problems and complications which may develop. At present there is no means of predicting which patients will respond favorably to splenectomy. Experience with splenectomy in patients who have few neutrophil precursors observable in the bone marrow and who do not have palpable spleens has generally been unfavorable. Only a few of the reported splenectomized cases of idiopathic neutropenia have benefited from the procedure.

Pharmacologic doses of corticosteroids induce neutrophilia in normal human subjects but do so in part by reducing the rate of cell egress from the blood, and such therapy has little or no effect on the rate of neutrophil production. Administration of 40 mg prednisone per day to normal human subjects reduces the number of neutrophils migrating into induced inflammatory exudates to about 10 percent of normal despite doubling of the number of neutrophils in the blood. Even in some patients with neutropenia blood neutrophils may increase with corticosteroid therapy. However, if the mechanism of increase in these patients is the same as it is in normal subjects, the neutrophil increase in the blood is at the expense of neutrophil outflow to the tissues. In that event, steroid therapy would have to be looked upon as dangerous in neutropenic patients.

ALTERATIONS IN NEUTROPHIL MORPHOLOGY AND FUNCTION

MORPHOLOGIC ABNORMALITIES. Microscopically identifiable abnormalities of neutrophils characterize or are associated with a variety of inherited conditions. Most patients, such as those with hereditary hyposegmentation (Pelger-Huët anomaly), hereditary hypersegmentation, or increased, fat-containing azurophilic granulation (Alder's anomaly), do not suffer from frequent infections. It is reasonable to assume that these anomalies do not interfere significantly with neutrophil function. On the other hand, patients who inherit the *Chediak-Higashi syndrome* usually die in childhood of fulminant infection. This anomaly, characterized by the presence of enormous granules (giant lysosomes) in neutrophils and in other leukocytes, is inherited as an autosomal recessive and is associated with partial albinism, hepatosplenomegaly, and development of lymphoid neoplasms. The anomalous leukocytes phagocytize bacteria in an apparently normal fashion. However, the giant lysosomes seem to be functionally defective in killing bacteria, thus reducing the resistance of these patients to infection. Also in the *May-Hegglin anomaly* (cytoplasmic crescent- or spindle-shaped inclusions, dominantly inherited) leukocyte dysfunction at inflammatory sites has been described.

CHRONIC GRANULOMATOUS DISEASE OF CHILDHOOD. Neutrophils of normal morphologic appearance but with decreased ability to kill phagocytized bacteria appear to be responsible for this syndrome. Recurrent infections with bacteria of low virulence develop shortly after birth, and death due to sepsis occurs before adulthood. Chronic lymphadenitis and infected eczematoid dermatitis are usually found in these children. The name of the disease is derived from the granulomas observed in lymph nodes, lungs, liver, spleen, and other viscera. Most patients with the syndrome have been males, and inheritance appears to be sex linked. However, two girls with normal families have been described, and thus, there may be more than one form of disease responsible for this syndrome. Neutrophils from these patients phagocytize bacteria normally, but certain types of bacteria survive for an abnormally long time after being phagocytized. The exact defect in lysosome-phagocytic vacuole interaction in the neutrophils has not been determined.

The environment of the neutrophil may limit its bactericidal capacities. Phagocytosis of bacteria by neutrophils in vitro is inhibited by high concentrations of glucose in the suspending medium. The inhibitory concentrations are within the range of glucose observed in patients with *diabetic acidosis*. The propensity of such patients for developing bacterial infection possibly is explained by inhibition of phagocytosis.

Monocytes

The origin of the monocyte and its relationship to tissue macrophages have been the subject of long-standing controversy. However, recent studies suggest that most exudate macrophages are derived from blood monocytes and that blood monocytes are in turn derived from the bone marrow. Monocyte precursors have not been identified morphologically. Cogent arguments can be raised suggesting their origin from lymphoid or granulocytic systems.

Monocytes migrate into inflammatory exudates at a slower rate and/or in a later phase of inflammation than do neutrophils. Monocyte maturation continues in the inflamed tissue, and the monocyte enlarges, synthesizes enzymes, and assumes the morphologic and chemical characteristics of a macrophage. Macrophages are avid phagocytes and probably play a scavenging role, clearing the exudate of dead neutrophils and other debris in addition to engulfing and killing bacteria.

Macrophages may play some role in the initiation of antibody production under certain circumstances, although there is little to suggest that the monocyte itself is capable of antibody production (Chap. 68). Soluble and particulate antigens are pinocytized and phagocytized by macrophages. Small lymphocytes accumulate around the antigen-bearing macrophage and some form of transfer of antigen or antigen-related material occurs.

Monocytosis is often observed in chronic inflammatory disorders due to infection (tuberculosis, subacute bacterial endocarditis, brucellosis) or other causes, during recovery from infection, in many protozoan (e.g., malaria, trypanosomiasis) and some rickettsial infections (Rocky Mountain spotted fever), in some patients with Hodgkin's disease, and in patients with neutropenia.

Eosinophils

Knowledge concerning the physiology and function of eosinophils is fragmentary. The site of eosinophil production is the bone marrow. If the eosinophilic cells of rodents are the same types of cells as the eosinophils of man, the kinetics of eosinophils probably are similar to those of neutrophils. Eosinophils migrate into induced inflammatory exudates in man, and eosinophil/neutrophil ratios in the exudate approximate those in the blood.

A modest degree of *eosinophilia* (from 600 to 2,000 eosinophils per cu mm) is common in overtly allergic conditions such as seasonal hay fever and asthma, in some skin diseases such as pemphigus, in a variety of parasitic infestations, and in such diseases as periarteritis nodosa. It is also seen in Hodgkin's disease and in Addison's disease. Hereditary eosinophilia, unassociated with overt disease, has been described.

Marked eosinophilia, up to and even exceeding 50,000 eosinophils per cu mm, has been observed in an occasional patient with carcinoma, during acute phases of tissue invasion with parasites such as *Trichina,* and in idiopathic states described as Loeffler's syndrome, tropical eosinophilia, pulmonary infiltration with eosinophilia, and eosinophilic leukemia (Chap. 348).

Eosinophilia usually is present in chronic myelocytic leukemia, myelofibrosis, and polycythemia vera. In these diseases the degree of eosinophilia often parallels the degree of neutrophilia, although in an occasional patient the eosinophilia may be so striking as to overshadow other leukocytic changes. The presence of eosinophilia is useful in distinguishing chronic myelocytic leukemia from leukemoid reactions and polycythemia vera from secondary polycythemia.

During acute bacterial infections eosinophils usually disappear from the blood. Hydrocortisone is known to produce transient eosinopenia.

Basophils

This least common member of the family of normal blood leukocytes is even less well understood than the eosinophil. Whether it is closely related or entirely distinct from tissue mast cells is unclear. However, these two cells are both rich in histamine and may play a role in the allergic response.

Elevated blood basophil concentration is commonly observed in chronic myelocytic leukemia, myelofibrosis, and polycythemia vera. Basophilia is a useful diagnostic sign in distinguishing chronic myelocytic leukemia and polycythemia vera from leukemoid reactions and secondary forms of polycythemia, respectively. A modest increase in basophils may be observed in myxedema, ulcerative colitis, and other chronic inflammatory diseases.

IMMUNOCYTES

Lymphocytes and plasma cells are concerned with the production of antibody rather than with phagocytosis. The exact relationship of plasma cells to lymphocytes is unsettled, but it seems probable that the plasma cell develops directly from the lymphoid system as a specialized cell concerned with the production of circulating antibody.

LYMPHOCYTE KINETICS

Most of the small lymphocytes of the blood, thoracic duct, and lymph nodes constitute a relatively long-lived population, while lymphocytes in the thymus, in the germinal centers of lymph nodes, and in the bone marrow are relatively short-lived. How long the long-lived population may survive without dividing is indicated by studies in patients who have been irradiated. Chromosome defects of a type which induce cell death upon division can be detected for a number of years following therapeutic irradiation. From such studies an estimate of an average intermitotic time of more than a year has been derived.

Lymphocytes do not remain in the blood for this long a period of time but seem to migrate from blood to lymphoid tissue and back to the blood. Vascular exit is through specialized cells in the postcapillary venules of lymph nodes. In the node, recirculating lymphocytes constitute the majority of cells in the cuff surrounding the germinal centers, and from this cuff they migrate into lymph channels and reenter the blood through the thoracic duct or the right lymphatic duct. The number of lymphocytes entering the blood from the thoracic duct is sufficient to replace the total number in the blood several times each day. Such a recirculatory pattern for cells is indicative of very complex cellular kinetics. Any shift or change in the recirculatory pattern at any point in the circuit can induce a profound change in the concentration of lymphocytes in the blood. However, a change in the rate of lymphocyte production may or may not be reflected by a change in blood lymphocyte concentration, and certainly no conclusions can be drawn concerning lymphocyte production from blood levels. The independence of blood lymphocyte levels in relation to events occurring elsewhere in the lymphocyte system is most dramatically illustrated by the pattern of lymphocyte changes which often accompanies hydrocortisone therapy of chronic lymphocytic leukemia. Therapeutic doses of hydrocortisone and its derivatives usually lead to a reduction of the total number of lymphocytes within the body, but for the first few weeks of therapy blood lymphocyte concentration increases.

Injected antigen is delivered to lymph nodes via lymphatics, when it becomes attached to reticular surfaces in the cortex of the node or may be phagocytized by macrophages in the medulla. A new antigen or the product of antigen cellular interaction stimulates conversion of small "uncommitted" lymphocytes to large cells synthesizing DNA. These large blastlike cells may be capable of antibody production or they or their progeny may mature into plasma cells or lymphocytes specialized for antibody production. Immunoglobulins are synthesized by plasma cells as well as by cells which are morphologically similar to the large lymphocyte. Certain studies suggest that most 7s immunoglobin is produced by plasma cells while most 19s immunoglobin is produced by large lymphocytes.

From such cellular proliferation in response to an antigenic challenge, a small lymphocyte eventually emerges. This small lymphocyte is not concerned directly with producing antibody, but carries the capacity ("immunologic memory") to produce a specific antibody. Small lymphocytes of this "committed" compartment may remain dormant for years unless once again exposed to the antigen for which they carry antibody-specific "memory." Faced with a second antigenic challenge, these cells hypertrophy and again develop into or produce antibody-producing cells.

The role of the thymus in the development of the immunocyte system and details concerning the formation of antibody are found in Chap. 68.

The size of the immunocyte system depends, at least in part, upon the degree of antigen exposure. Germ-free animals have fewer lymphocytes than conventional animals but rapidly develop a lymphoid system of normal size when removed from the germ-free environment.

LYMPHOCYTOSIS

The diagnostic significance of lymphocytosis depends in part upon whether the increase is due to normal- or abnormal-appearing lymphocytes. Lymphocytosis due to an increase in normal-appearing small lymphocytes may accompany recovery from acute infections and may be present during *chronic infections,* especially in *tuberculosis* and *syphilis.* In *pertussis* and in a rare syndrome of children and young adults termed **infectious lymphocytosis** very striking increases in the concentration of small lymphocytes may occur. Persistent, unexplained lymphocytosis with normal-appearing small lymphocytes in older patients usually proves to be due to *chronic lymphocytic leukemia* (Chap. 348).

Infectious mononucleosis (Chap. 255) is usually accompanied by lymphocytosis as well as by the appearance of abnormal-appearing lymphocytes in the blood. Known viral diseases, such as *measles,* may be accompanied by lymphocyte changes somewhat similar to those seen in infectious mononucleosis. *Acute lymphoblastic leukemia* (Chap. 348) is characterized by very immature lymphoblasts in the blood, and these cells are easily distinguished from those of infectious mononucleosis by their fine, granular chromatin and prominent nucleoli.

LYMPHOPENIA

Lymphopenia occurs as a relatively nonspecific response to various forms of *stress,* such as *trauma, acute infection,* or *hemorrhage.* Such lymphopenia usually disappears within a few days. Chronic lymphopenia should raise the suspicion of *Hodgkin's disease.*

Plasma Cells

These are but rarely observed in the blood of normal subjects but may appear in small numbers during severe *antigenic challenges,* as in certain *infections* or in *serum sickness.* Large numbers of plasma cells appear in the blood of a few patients with *multiple myeloma* (plasma cell leukemia Chap. 348). Plasma cells constitute less than 1 percent of the nucleated cells of normal bone marrow, but they are not distributed uniformly throughout the marrow, so that the range of normal is quite wide (up to 5 percent in counts of 500 cells from marrow aspirates of normal nonalcoholic inmates of the Utah State Prison). An increased percentage of plasma cells on smears of marrow aspirates should raise the suspicion of multiple myeloma or some other protein-secreting tumor, but may also be observed in such conditions as *liver disease,* during antigenic challenge and in *aplastic anemia. Absence of plasma cells* on smears of marrow aspirates usually is indicative of one of the diseases associated with inadequate production of serum antibody, such as *sex-linked hypogammaglobulinemia* or *chronic lymphocytic leukemia.*

REFERENCES

Boggs, D. R.: The Kinetics of Neutrophilic Leukocytes in Health and in Disease, Seminars in Hematology, 4:359, 1967.

Kauder, E., and A. M. Mauer: Neutropenias of Childhood, J. Pediat., 69:147, 1966.

Wintrobe, M. M.: "Clinical Hematology," 6th ed., Philadelphia, Lea & Febiger, 1967.

65 THE ERYTHROCYTE SEDIMENTATION RATE

M. M. Wintrobe

Measurement of the erythrocyte sedimentation rate (ESR) differs from many other types of laboratory examination because it serves only to indicate a deviation from normal without providing a clue to its cause. Nevertheless, this limitation does not detract from its utility. The procedure has the merit of simplicity and can be classed with the measurement of temperature and pulse rate as an index of disease. The ESR is especially useful as a disease indicator because it may be elevated in the absence of fever.

The blood is a suspension of red corpuscles in plasma. The ESR is a measure of the rate of settling of the red corpuscles, as determined by placing blood, to which an anticoagulant has been added, into a vertical tube and noting the distance the upper level of the column of red corpuscles has fall in a specific period of time, usually an hour. The test is most easily carried out in the "macro" hematocrit (Wintrobe), using blood collected for counts and determination of volume of packed red cells. It is only necessary to allow the tube to stand in a vertical position and to read the level to which the red corpuscles have fallen in an hour. Following this the specimen, after appropriate centrifugation, can be used for measurement of packed red cell volume and for inspection of the plasma (icterus, turbidity) and layers of white cells and platelets. The Westergren method has the advantage of a wider bore and is less likely to give an occasional misleading result, but it entails a special step in the laboratory, rather than being only the first step in a simple screening procedure.

Various technical factors affect the ESR, but if a standard procedure is employed, few will be of great importance. The tube must be placed in a vertical position or the rate of sedimentation will be accelerated. The degree of anemia or polycythemia affects the result, but *correction for this is not entirely satisfactory and is not recommended.* In the presence of severe anemia, the ESR is of limited value.

Normal values for ESR are given in the Appendix. The difference between those for men and for women is largely due to the sex difference in numbers of red corpuscles.

Alterations in ESR depend mainly on the concentration of macromolecules in the plasma, particularly plasma proteins of high molecular weight, such as the α_2 and γ, macroglobulins, and especially fibrinogen. The ESR is more rapid when these macromolecules are present in amounts greater than normal. Under these circumstances, and probably because of changes in the surface charge of the red corpuscles, aggregation of the red corpuscles is increased, and corpuscular aggregates of large volume and relatively small surface area are formed, which causes the ESR to be accelerated.

The only physiologic state in which the ESR is significantly increased is *pregnancy.* The rate gradually increases, beginning about the tenth to twelfth week, and is greater than is attributable to the gradual decrease in volume of packed red cells. It does not return to normal until the third or fourth week post partum. This increase is perhaps a reflection of the tissue changes which take place during delivery and the post-partum period.

The ESR is increased in all acute general infections, but in localized acute inflammatory conditions, variations depend on the nature and severity of the process. Usually the ESR is increased in localized acute suppurations even when the temperature and pulse are normal. In chronic localized inflammation the ESR varies with the extent and nature of the inflammatory process. Uncomplicated new growths are not necessarily associated with rapid sedimentation, even when malignant. When the tumor is very vascular or is undergoing necrosis, the rate may be increased.

The ESR is useful (1) in calling attention to the presence of more or less occult disease; (2) if very rapid, it may be an important clue to collagen vascular disease, notably polymyositis, in a patient with nonspecific complaints, such as headache, muscle aches and pains, and only slight fever; (3) occasionally in differential diagnosis (e.g., pelvic inflammatory disease versus uncomplicated ovarian cyst, psychosomatic versus organic disease), and most important, (4) as a guide to the progress of a disease already recognized (e.g., pulmonary tuberculosis, rheumatic carditis, Hodgkin's disease) when fever or other signs are normal or equivocal. On the other hand, the ESR may be normal when otherwise it might be expected to be accelerated, in patients with multiple myeloma complicated by the presence of cryoglobulin, when there is hypofibrinogenemia, and in circumstances in which rouleau formation does not take place (sickle-cell anemia, hereditary spherocytosis).

Section 10

Other Laboratory Manifestations of Disease

INTRODUCTION

George W. Thorn

There is an increasing interest in the identification of occult disease and in the prevention of ill health, but the acute shortage of physicians compels the recruitment of assistance from "paramedical" personnel and the full exploitation of the potential contributions of improved technology. The basis of good medical practice is, and undoubtedly always will be, a careful history and physical examination. These, in turn, will dictate the specific or appropriate laboratory tests. The automation of quantitative biochemical determinations and the "read-out" potential of computerized data will permit broad scale screening of large segments of our population, and it is important that these technical advances be fully utilized. Physicians, however, will continue to provide the expert consultation needed to plan and evaluate such programs.

In the practice of medicine, it is common for a specific disease process to present initially with nonspecific symptoms, for example, the weakness and increased fatigability of a patient with hypercalcemia secondary to hyperparathyroidism. The classical approach to diagnosis and treatment does not always suggest the appropriate laboratory tests, and the underlying disorder may remain undetected for a long period. It is in this setting that a selected group of biochemical tests may provide an early clue to the correct diagnosis or the presence of an unsuspected "carrier state." This clinical approach is not to be confused with indiscriminate laboratory testing, but accepts the fact that a group of determinations which are known to be frequent harbingers of disease can now be carried out on a single specimen of blood at low cost to the patient. It is also probable that the ready availability of multiple biochemical determinations at relatively low cost will increase the number of individuals who will utilize more regularly scheduled appointments for periodic examinations.

The succeeding chapters describe biochemical analyses and other tests which in the present state of knowledge and technology are feasible for use by physicians in private practice or for public health screening programs.

66 BIOCHEMICAL DETERMINATIONS
George W. Thorn

Serum Electrolytes and Metabolites

With present-day instrumentation, it is possible to determine on a single specimen of blood the concentration of sodium, potassium, calcium, magnesium, chloride, inorganic phosphate, and carbon dioxide–combining power. The possibility of comparing values for several electrolytes on a single specimen is especially useful. For example, an elevated serum sodium value with elevated serum chloride suggests dehydration if serum potassium is normal or elevated; however, if serum sodium is elevated and serum chloride and potassium are low, alkalosis and primary hyperaldosteronism should be considered. Low serum sodium and potassium suggest excessive hydration, serious tissue hypoxia, or excessive diuretic therapy (Thiazide). This last possibility is further strengthened by the finding of elevated serum uric acid and blood glucose levels. If serum calcium level is moderately elevated and serum inorganic phosphorus is low, then primary hyperparathyroidism is almost a certainty— whereas elevated serum calcium with normal or elevated serum phosphate suggests disorders such as breast cancer, multiple myeloma, and sarcoid as possible causes for the hypercalcemia. Tetany and convulsive seizures require determination of blood sugar, serum calcium, and magnesium levels as possible causes.

When screening for diabetes mellitus, blood sugar values should be checked postprandially (2 hr). For detecting disorders associated with hypoglycemia, blood sugar determinations made in the fasting state are more informative. Elevated uric acid with a normal blood-urea-nitrogen suggests gout or other diseases associated with high urate production, e.g., polycythemia, lymphoma, or the effect of x-rays or chemotherapy. Elevated uric acid with elevated blood-urea-nitrogen indicates primary renal disease or severe dehydration.

The level of total serum protein is another very useful determination. An increase in total serum protein with elevated blood-urea-nitrogen and hematocrit suggests dehydration. In the absence of dehydration, elevated total serum protein almost always reflects hyperglobulinemia, whereas lowered total serum protein values usually indicate hypoalbuminemia.

An elevation of serum cholesterol or serum lipids can identify an individual with increased susceptibility to coronary vascular disease, particularly if these abnormalities are associated with an elevated blood glucose.

The most useful and practical screening battery includes the measurement of blood-urea-nitrogen, glucose, serum sodium, potassium, calcium, magnesium, chloride, inorganic phosphate, uric acid, CO_2-combining power, cholesterol and other serum lipids, and total plasma proteins. The time at which blood is taken should be carefully recorded, and stasis should be avoided in obtaining venous samples.

Blood Enzyme Levels

Release of enzymes into the circulation follows injury of any type. In mild or early organic disease, an elevated blood enzyme level may be the sole indicator of underlying pathology. The extent to which the blood enzyme level will reflect the pathologic process depends upon the nature and degree of tissue injury and the capacity of cells to produce enzymes; hence, a diffuse but mild disease may be associated with a significant elevation in blood enzyme level, whereas extensive destruction of cells may be associated with little or no rise. For example, a large increase in plasma alkaline phosphatase level may be observed in the presence of relatively mild intrahepatic cholestasis (Thorazine, methyltestosterone), whereas acute yellow atrophy with widespread total destruction of hepatic parenchymal cells may be accompanied by relatively low levels of alkaline phosphatase, lactic dehydrogenase, and serum glutamic oxalacetic transaminase.

The ability to measure isoenzymes, which are most specific for a particular tissue, will increase appreciably the diagnostic value of blood enzyme levels, particularly since it is possible to observe an increase in the level of a particular isoenzyme without necessarily observing a significant rise in total blood enzyme level.

The capacity to carry out multiple biochemical determinations on a single blood specimen not only is of great value in confirming a clinical impression or detecting an unsuspected disorder or carrier state, but it is also probable that a computer analysis of the different values obtained simultaneously may suggest further possible diagnoses under circumstances in which the magnitude of the deviation of a single biochemical determination is not great enough to be considered abnormal.

67 OTHER SCREENING TESTS
George W. Thorn

Although the following procedures are well recognized as essential components of the complete examination of a patient, their tabulation and a few comments may be found useful. These examinations will provide (1) additional diagnostic potentiality, (2) an initial screen which may suggest more elaborate or definitive examinations, and (3) a point of reference against which changes in the future may be compared and interpreted.

URINALYSIS. Routine examination will include tests for glucose and protein and an examination of the sediment. If the specific gravity is greater than 1.020 and no substances which will elevate it artifactually, such as glucose, large amounts of protein, or organic dyes (an intravenous pyelogram, for example), are present, renal function can be assumed to be normal. On the other hand, a low urine specific gravity is of no clinical significance because in most instances it reflects only greater than average fluid intake. It should be checked with some specific renal function tests such as blood-urea-nitrogen or serum creatinine.

BLOOD EXAMINATION. By collecting 5 ml blood in an anticoagulant which will not alter the size or hemoglobin content of the red corpuscles or injure the leukocytes or platelets (e.g., Sequestrene), together with a few blood smears made directly from the collecting needle, one can determine (1) sedimentation rate, (2) volume of packed red cells, (3) icterus index, (4) volumes of packed white cells and platelets, (5) leukocyte count, (6) platelet count, and (7) differential leukocyte count. The usefulness of these as screening procedures has been discussed in Chap. 61.

STOOL ANALYSIS. Determination of the presence or absence of occult blood is a very important primary screen. In certain parts of the world screening of the stool for parasites is essential.

ELECTROCARDIOGRAM AND CHEST ROENTGENOGRAM. These should be made at the time of the initial examination. In addition to their diagnostic value, they will prove invaluable as a basis for comparison with potential changes in the future.

TIMED VITAL CAPACITY. Timed vital capacity is an essential measurement for the early determination of impaired pulmonary function and for monitoring patients with pulmonary and cardiovascular disease.

TUBERCULIN TEST. The tuberculin test is a valuable determination, particularly in the young or those whose occupation includes a high exposure rate. A negative tuberculin test in a very ill patient requires that other skin tests be carried out to exclude the possibility of anergy.

OCULAR PRESSURE. Since glaucoma is a frequent cause of blindness, measurement of ocular pressure should be carried out routinely on all adult patients.

PAPANICOLAOU EXAMINATION. This should be carried out regularly on the cervical smear of every adult female patient. A similar examination should be made of the sputum, gastric washings, and urine of patients with symptoms suggesting specific organ disease.

SIGMOIDOSCOPY. Although in the asymptomatic patient this procedure will yield a relatively low incidence of serious pathology, it does offer a unique opportunity to detect curable neoplasm in the rectosigmoid region.

It is important from the public health viewpoint as well as that of the individual physician to note that almost all of the procedures included in this and the preceding chapter do not require a physician's participation. A well-trained technician can analyze the urine, stool, and blood specimens as well as the Papanicolaou smears. Ultimately, electrocardiograms and chest roentgenograms will be screened by computer techniques and only those showing significant abnormalities will be referred for professional review and evaluation. Technicians can be trained to administer and evaluate tuberculin tests and vital capacity measurements, as well as to measure ocular pressure. Only sigmoidoscopy, among those procedures outlined above, requires high-level professional skill. Thus, technical advances in instrumentation, coupled with the supervised training of an increased number of paramedical personnel, should permit the physician to devote more time to his individual patient's needs, both physical and emotional.

Nationally, these same developments could facilitate the regular screening of large segments of our population and, hence, increase the possibility of identifying "carrier states" or incipient disease with its exciting remedial possibilities.

Part Four

Disorders Due to Hypersensitivity and Altered Immune Response

68 INTRODUCTION TO CLINICAL IMMUNOLOGY

K. Frank Austen

The immunologic response not only constitutes the principal means of man's defense against pathogenic microorganisms, but also is capable of mediating adverse clinical reactions. Whether an immune response is defined clinically as immunity or hypersensitivity is determined by its effect on the host; the distinction does not necessarily imply different mechanisms of elicitation. The components of the immune system may be considered in terms of the sequential manner in which they contribute to the immune response. The principal features include immunogens, capable of initiating the immune response; cellular processing of immunogenic material; products of the immune response; control mechanisms of the response; and consequences, both beneficial and detrimental, of the immune response. Consideration of the immunologic response in terms of these arbitrary divisions affords a basis for a clinical approach to the diagnosis and management of immune deficiency states and hypersensitivity syndromes.

INITIATION OF THE IMMUNE RESPONSE

A substance must ordinarily be recognized as foreign in order to elicit an immune response. The ability of a substance to evoke such a response is termed *immunogenicity;* the capacity to react specifically with the antibodies induced is termed *antigenicity.* The distinction is useful because many simple substances of less than 1,000 mol wt are not immunogenic unless coupled convalently or by large numbers of ionic bonds to macromolecules but can react with antibodies of appropriate specificity; such simple substances are termed *haptens.*

Deliberate initiation of the immune response is accomplished most reliably by injection of the immunogen. Feeding is not usually effective because being proteins, most immunogens are digested in the gastrointestinal tract. The oral route may, however, be utilized under certain circumstances, such as with attenuated poliomyelitis virus. Natural immunization to environmental substances may occur by such diverse routes as inhalation of plant or tree pollens, ingestion of certain foods or drugs, and skin contact with drugs or natural chemicals such as the catechols of poison ivy plants.

CELLULAR PROCESSING OF IMMUNOGENTIC MATERIALS

After injection, the immunogen is most conspicuous in the macrophages of the reticuloendothelial system, and a variety of observations involving particulate immunogens indicate that ingestion by the macrophage may be an essential step in the immune response. It appears that the macrophage complexes fragments of the immunogen to a unique ribonucleic acid moiety, and that the complexed immunogen is considerably more immunogenic than in the free form. The macrophage ribonucleic acid associated with the immunogenic fragments is distinguished by several criteria, including: (1) low molecular weight, insufficient to contain the base sequence information of messenger RNA; (2) an appreciable representation in the DNA template, as assessed by hybridization techniques, contrasting with the small representation observed with ribosomal RNA; and (3) physicochemical characteristics which do not appear to change as a result of exposing the macrophage to various immunogens, implying a nonspecific carrier function.

Following an immunogenic stimulus the regional lymph nodes (or spleen) become hyperplastic and increase severalfold in weight, and the specific antibody levels in the efferent lymph exceed those in the afferent lymph entering the regional node. Net antibody synthesis by isolated lymph node tissue also has been demonstrated in vitro. The evidence that the plasma cell is particularly active in antibody synthesis includes (1) the prominence of plasma cells as lymphoid tissue becomes hyperplastic in response to an immunogenic stimulus; (2) the approximate relationship between the antibody extractable from such tissue with the plasma cell content; (3) the demonstration by immunofluorescent staining procedures of gamma-globulin in the cytoplasm of plasma cells; and (4) the clinical observations of increased numbers of plasma cells in circumstances of gamma-globulin overproduction and the virtual absence of such cells in heritable disorders of antibody production.

The steps between "activation" of the immunogen by the macrophage and production of specific antibody by the plasma cell are not completely understood but seem to involve the small lymphocyte. In the resting lymph node, plasma cells are rare and about three-fourths of the cells are small lymphocytes while the remainder are large lymphocytes. The population of small lymphocytes is believed to be heterogeneous and is presumed to be capable of several different functions. From their paucity of ribosomes and mitochondria and relatively long generation time of months, certain small lymphocytes seem to be "resting." Directly or, more likely, following processing by the macrophage, the immunogen appears to stimulate these small lymphocytes to differentiate into rapidly dividing, large, ribosome-rich cells termed *immunoblasts*. The immunoblasts are then presumed to differentiate either into plasma cells or back into small lymphocytes which persist as "memory" cells, primed to respond to subsequent encounters with the same or related immunogens. Although the plasma cell is the most active in synthesizing and secreting antibody, both small and large lymphocytes have on occasion been shown to produce antibody.

PRODUCTS OF THE IMMUNE RESPONSE

STRUCTURE OF GAMMA-GLOBULINS. The gamma-globulins are a group of serum proteins with a distinct electrophoretic mobility and the capacity to behave as antibodies. On the basis of different physicochemical and immunochemical properties, these proteins, termed immunoglobulins, have been divided into a number of major classes. The fundamental molecular unit of all classes of immunoglobulins as determined by the employment of reducing and denaturing agents consists of two heavy (H) and two light (L) polypeptide chains linked by interchain disulfide bonds and non-covalent bonds. Disulfide bonds (two or more in man) join the two H chains, and each H chain is linked to its respective L chain by single disulfide bonds. The non-covalent bonds between the polypeptide chains are predominantly hydrophobic bonds. When the enzyme papain is employed, human IgG is split into three fragments; two, termed Fab, are identical and contain the antigen combining sites, and the third, Fc, can be crystallized and is responsible for the unique biologic activities of a class. The Fab fragment consists of an L chain and the N-terminal half of the H chain, termed the Fd fragment, joined by their interchain disulfide bond; the Fc fragment consists of the C terminal portions of the two H chains held by their interchain disulfide bonds. The molecular basis of the specificity of bivalent antibody for antigen resides in the Fab fragments. The combining site is probably constructed predominantly from the Fd fragment of the H chain, while the L chain contributes indirectly by interacting with and stabilizing the neighboring Fd fragment. Differing antibody specificities depend on differing primary amino acid sequences in the region of the combining site; these differences exist in both the H and L chains, which vary in the combining site region but are constant in the C terminal ends of the chains.

For the L chain the constant portion is approximately one-half the chain, whereas in the H chain the invariable portion includes the Fc piece and about one-half of the Fd fragment. It is the antigenic differences in the invariable portion of the H chain which permit division of the human immunoglobulins into five major classes (IgG, IgA, IgM, IgD, and IgE). The constant portion of the L chain allows recognition of two types (kappa and lambda), which occur in combination with all five H chains (gamma, alpha, mu, delta, and epsilon). The molecular formulas for the preponderant immunoglobulin class, IgG, would thus be gamma$_2$ lambda$_2$ ($\gamma_2 \lambda_2$) and gamma$_2$ kappa$_2$ ($\gamma_2 \kappa_2$). IgG is further subdivided into four subclasses, IgG 1 to 4, on the basis of minor intraclass antigenic differences. In addition to the designation of class and subclass by structural differences, there are genetic differences within a class, termed allotypy, expressed by additional discrete structural differences. Genetic control of structural differences in three of the gamma chain subclasses, 1 to 3, has been related to the Gm loci, while allotypic differences in the kappa chain reside in the Inv locus.

PRIMARY IMMUNE RESPONSE. The immune response to the first introduction of an immunogen is termed primary. In a primary response, possibly because of the differential sensitivity of the methodology employed, the IgM antibodies are recognized somewhat earlier than those of the IgG class. The IgM antibodies are observed within the first week of immunization and decline thereafter as the titer of IgG antibodies increases. This relationship and the finding that formation of IgM antibodies requires appreciable levels of immunogen have been interpreted to indicate that IgG antibodies inhibit synthesis of antibodies of the IgM class. Antibodies of the IgA class may be observed following prolonged and rather intensive immunization. The view that IgM antibodies represent a primitive product of the immune response is supported by the predominant synthesis of this antibody class in the newborn and by phylogenic observations. In addition to sequential changes in immunoglobulin class, heterogeneity of the primary response occurs within the IgG class, expressed as an increasing affinity for the antigen. This may be explicable in terms of continued formation of new antibodies capable of interacting with increasing numbers of diverse antigenic determinants on the macromolecular immunogen.

SECONDARY IMMUNE RESPONSE. When the antibody levels have diminished following initial immunogenic exposure, a subsequent encounter will evoke an enhanced response, termed secondary or anamnestic. The anamnestic response requires a lower threshold dose of immunogen for elicitation and is characterized by a shortened lag phase for appearance of detectable product and a higher and more persistent antibody response. Although the quantity of antibody produced per unit time is usually much greater in the secondary response, the doubling time appears to be about the same as in the primary, which is consistent with the participation of more cells rather than an augmentation in the rate of synthesis per cell. The antibodies formed after the secondary stimulus have a much higher affinity for the corresponding antigenic determinant than those appearing after a comparable time during the primary response. The high-affinity antibodies characteristic of the secondary response are of the IgG class.

DETERMINATION OF ANTIBODY SYNTHESIS. Studies by immunofluorescent techniques have demonstrated that individual lymph node cells produce only a single class of heavy and light chains at any one time. Preliminary evidence suggests that L chains are made on small polyribosomes and H chains on large ones; and it is held that half the immunoglobulin molecules, consisting of single L and H chains, are assembled through attachment of free L chains to the polyribosomal-bound H chains, and that the product then is released for assembly into a bivalent immunoglobulin molecule. Although it has been demonstrated that antibody specificity is determined by amino acid sequence, there is no real insight into the molecular basis by which a flexibility sufficient to recognize the vast array of potential immunogens is maintained. Theories of antibody production ranging from instructive, in which the immunogen helps shape the corresponding antibody, to selective, in which the immunogen selectively stimulates a cell or portion of the gene already capable of producing the desired product, continue to be assessed; this theory seems most consistent with the data at hand.

The consequences of the immune response grouped as cellular immunity are of great biologic importance but cannot be presented in physicochemical terms. Accordingly, these cellular phenomena, along with the humoral responses, will be examined in the sections dealing with control mechanisms and the biologic consequences of the immune response.

CONTROL MECHANISMS OF THE IMMUNE RESPONSE

Wide variations usually are observed in the amounts of specific antibody formed in different individuals of the same species in response to a similar immunogenic stimulus. A heritable basis for different responses to certain synthetic immunogens has been well documented in highly inbred strains of guinea pigs and mice. In man there is evidence that the capacity to make antibodies of the IgE class in response to inhaled pollens is associated with an increased incidence of a similar immunoglobulin response to drugs and other environmental antigens.

ROLE OF THE THYMUS. The development of the capacity to respond to an immunogen is dependent on a functioning thymus gland as well as on other lymphoepithelial structures arising embryologically as outpouchings of the gut wall and eventually consisting of lymphocyte populations in close proximity to epithelial cells of endodermal origin. Experimental studies have revealed that neonatal thymectomy interferes with the development of the lymphoid system, profoundly impairs the immunologic capabilities termed "cellular immunity" (such as rejection of foreign-tissue grafts and delayed hypersensitivity), and also under certain circumstances diminishes humoral responses. The manner in which the thymus mediates the development of these aspects of immunologic competence is not entirely clear but may include (1) an environment

in which "stem" cells, possibly of bone marrow origin, differentiate to become immunologically competent before being distributed peripherally to populate node tissue; (2) elaboration of a humoral factor regulating the maturation of peripheral lymphocytes; and (3) the exertion of "censorship," whereby potentially self-reacting clones are eliminated. The consequences of thymectomy are less dramatic in the adult animal, but there is evidence that the thymus continues to provide a mechanism whereby immunologically uncommitted cells acquire the capacity to respond to specific immunogens.

In birds there is an anatomic separation of the central control of the capacity to develop cellular and humoral immunity, the former is regulated by the thymus and the latter by the bursa of Fabricius. In mammals the precise equivalent of the bursa has not been established, but it is assumed to be some portion of the gut-associated lymphoid tissue. The evidence in man for some division of central control resides in the existence of patients with hereditary lesions expressed predominantly as defects in cellular immunity, humoral immunity, or both.

TOLERANCE. The capacity of an individual's immune response to distinguish between his own and foreign macromolecules was termed "horror autotoxicus" by Ehrlich and "self-tolerance" by Burnet. An operational definition of tolerance sufficient to include a variety of terms developed from special experimental circumstances is "a state of specific immunologic nonreactivity to an immunogenic stimulus which would be followed by a recognizable response in a normal animal." Though moderate doses of an immunogen can initiate the immune response, an excessive dose is followed by a state of tolerance or specific nonreactivity to any subsequent dose of the immunogen, although unrelated immunogens, in appropriate dose, are fully active. Tolerance is more easily established in the neonate than in the adult, is maintained by persistence of the immunogen, and can be manifested by impairment of either humoral or cellular immunity. Tolerance to an immunogen has been shown experimentally to be associated with the functional absence of the specifically responding cells or clone. It is held that the excess immunogen destroys the relevant clones as they arise, possibly by bypassing the "activation" step in the macrophage and presenting to the small lymphocyte as free immunogen or as an immune complex in the region of great antigen excess.

AUTOIMMUNITY. The appearance of antibodies in man directed against self represents an autoimmune response. These autoantibodies may reflect a normal response to tissue antigens, which are separated anatomically from the immune system during fetal development and appear later as a consequence of tissue breakdown. Autoantibodies also may arise following abrogation of tolerance in a normal immune system by an exogenous antigen cross-reacting with self or because an abnormal immune system has lost the capacity to distinguish self. Autoantibodies do not necessarily indicate an autoimmune disease. This term must be restricted to situations in which the autoimmune response, humoral or cellular, is responsible for tissue injury.

CONSEQUENCES OF THE IMMUNE RESPONSE: HOST RESISTANCE

The consequences of the immune response are termed *immunity* when beneficial to the host and *hypersensitivity* or *allergy* when detrimental. This is a clinical judgment and does not imply that the basic pathways leading to immunity or hypersensitivity are different.

The constituents of host defense in normal man are both nonimmunologic and immunologic, while those developing as a result of deliberate immunization or overt infection are exclusively immunologic. The nonimmunologic lines of defense include the extrinsic barriers to pathogen penetration, both mechanical and enzymatic, and the intrinsic cellular elements—circulating polymorphonuclear leukocytes and monocytes and fixed mononuclear phagocytic cells. Although these cellular elements are effective in the absence of an immune response, they clearly operate much more effectively in its presence. The so-called *natural antibodies* are present in normal persons who have not been subjected to deliberate immunization or overt infection; these natural antibodies would appear to result from the host's subclinical exposure to the specific pathogen or some cross-reacting pathogen. This makes it possible to consider the role of the immune response in host defense without further reference to a subclinical or overt encounter with the immunogen.

SERUM COMPLEMENT. The humoral immune response participating in host resistance appears to involve a supporting system, known as serum complement; hence it is relevant to examine this system before evaluating the role of the various immunoglobulin classes in host defense. The complement system (C′) consists of distinct serum proteins, numbered 1 through 9, which interact in a well-defined sequence as cytotoxins for target cells and yield a series of by-products representing the essential ingredients of an inflammatory response. When an immune aggregate, or a target cell sensitized by interaction with specific antibody against some cell-surface antigen, interacts with normal serum, the first component of complement (C′1) binds to the complex and is converted from an inactive precursor form to an active enzyme. Complex-bound C′1 then acts on its natural substrates, the fourth and second components of complement, yielding a new cell-bound enzymatic activity consisting of C′4 and the fragment C′2a; the 4,2a unit is termed C′3 convertase. The action of C′3 convertase on C′3 results in the binding of the major portion of the molecule, C′3b, to the complex, leaving the lesser fragment, C′3a or anaphylatoxin, in the fluid phase. The complex, having achieved the 1,4,2a,3b state, can attach to a specific receptor on primate red blood cells or polymorphonuclear leukocytes, a phenomenon known as *immune adherence*, which enhances phagocytosis. The subsequent interaction of the fifth, sixth, and seventh complement components with the complex yields a chemotactic factor for polymorphonuclear leukocytes. The sequential action of the eighth and ninth components to complete the reaction leads to osmotic lysis of the target cell with disruption of the cell membrane by electron microscopy. The system has biologic meaning because it is lethal for some target cells and results in the elaboration of various by-products capable of mediating an inflammatory response. These include *anaphylatoxin*, which produces a local increase in vascular permeability, bringing more antibody and complement to the site of the lesion; the *chemotactic factor*, which attracts polymorphonuclear leukocytes; and a *complex carrying C′3a*, which promotes immune adherence and enhanced phagocytosis. The complement reaction may be beneficial or detrimental to the host, depending entirely on the location of the antigens against which the antibody mediating the reaction is directed.

ANTIBODY. IgG comprises 70 to 80 percent of the serum antibodies of man and is almost exclusively responsible for the antibodies to viruses, toxins, and gram-positive pyogenic bacteria. It is transported across the placenta, while other maternal immunoglobulins mostly are excluded from the fetal circulation. The interaction of IgG with antigen to activate the complement system leads to the development of anaphylatoxin, a release of chemotactic factor, and the capacity of the complex to undergo immune adherence and enhanced phagocytosis; it may be of great importance in controlling man's pyogenic environment.

Between 5 and 10 percent of the total serum antibody is IgM. Antibodies of this class commonly are directed against lipopolysaccharide antigens typified by the somatic O antigens (endotoxins) of gram-negative bacteria. The sensitization of a site on a target cell for subsequent lysis by the nine components of complement can be accomplished either by a single IgM molecule or an IgG doublet. The doublet reduces the efficiency of IgG in mediating cytotoxic reactions, and there is ample evidence that the bactericidal activity of human serum against gram-negative bacteria is mainly dependent on the diverse pool of natural IgM antibodies.

Antibodies of the IgA class comprise about 10 to 20 percent of serum immunoglobulins and are the predominant immunoglobulin in parotid saliva, tears, colostrum, nasal and bronchial secretions, bile, succus entericus, and urine. Secretory IgA has activity against viruses and bacteria, and a specific immune response to experimental virus infection has been demonstrated in the saliva, nasal secretions, and tears of human volunteers. While serum IgA has a sedimentation coefficient of 7S, secretory IgA is principally 11S protein because of an additional structural unit, the T (transport) piece. The T piece probably is responsible for the movement of the molecule into secretions; and it is presumed that such molecules in the external secretions of the respiratory, gastrointestinal, and genitourinary tract contribute to host resistance. The functions in host resistance of the trace immunoglobulins IgD and IgE are unknown.

SPECIFIC CELLULAR IMMUNITY. Specific cellular immunity to intracellular pathogens has been demonstrated experimentally in several models, the most direct of which has involved *Listeria monocytogenes* infection in the mouse. Mice infected with a sublethal dose of this organism developed resistance to a dose 100 times the LD_{50}. Resistance was not associated with the appearance of antibody because agglutination titers were negligible and protection could not be conferred by passive transfer serum; resistance was, however, correlated in time with the development of delayed-type skin hypersensitivity to listeria culture filtrate. Furthermore, monolayer cultures of normal mouse peritoneal macrophages are destroyed readily by innoculation with listeria, while cultures obtained from resistant animals, previously infected with a sublethal challenge, are capable of eliminating the organism. These peritoneal macrophages are demonstrating specific cellular immunity because their activity is not diminished by repeated washing nor enhanced by the addition of normal or immune serum to the culture. Furthermore, these macrophages are capable of destroying intracellular pathogens, other than those used to initiate the immune response such as *Brucella abortus* or *Salmonella typhimurium,* indicating that cellular immunity may be expressed in nonspecific fashion. On the other hand, the induction of cellular immunity is specific because recall can be initiated only by an organism which has previously been used to initiate a primary response. *Induction* of cellular immunity is immunologically specific, while the *expression* by the "activated" macrophage is nonspecific. The association of cellular immunity with the cutaneous reaction of delayed hypersensitivity suggests that the specificity resides in the sensitized lymphocyte, which then "activates" the macrophage to exhibit a nonspecific increased resistance to intracellular pathogens. This is somewhat analogous to humoral immunity, wherein specificity resides with the antibody produced by the plasma cell while the execution involves the nonspecific complement system.

The experimental data considered above imply that a deficiency of IgG would predispose to pyogenic infection, an absence of IgM to infection with gram-negative enteric flora, and a defect in cellular immunity to infection with intracellular pathogens. These generalizations are supported by clinical observations in patients illustrating such heritable or acquired defects (Chap. 69).

CONSEQUENCES OF THE IMMUNE RESPONSE: HYPERSENSITIVITY

The adverse or allergic manifestations of the immune response traditionally have been divided on the basis of their time course following antigen challenge into *immediate, subacute,* and *delayed* hypersensitivity. Clear differences exist in the mechanisms whereby these three broad categories of clinical responses arise; and even differences within a category, such as immediate hypersensitivity, are being appreciated.

IMMEDIATE HYPERSENSITIVITY. Immediate hypersensitivity consists of all the allergic responses that begin within minutes of antigen-antibody interaction and may be divided into *cytotoxic* and *anaphylactic* on the basis of the mediation of the clinical response. In a cytotoxic reaction, such as an acute hemolytic transfusion reaction in man, the critical damage is to the primary target cell

selected because the responsible complement-fixing antibody is directed against some cell-surface antigen. In an anaphylactic reaction, the interaction of antigen with antibody results in the formation and/or release of chemical mediators which act at secondary sites, namely, smooth muscle and vascular tissue.

ANAPHYLAXIS. The chemical mediators of anaphylactic tissue injury known to be specifically formed and/or released from mammalian tissue by antigen-antibody interaction include amines, such as histamine and serotonin, small peptides such as the nonapeptide, bradykinin, and an acidic lipid known as slow-reacting substance of anaphylaxis (SRS-A). Each mediator is capable of causing contraction in a particular group of smooth muscles and of increasing vascular permeability. While the amines, histamine and serotonin, are released from tissue stores, in which they exist in their biologically active form, bradykinin and SRS-A must be formed as well as released as a result of antigen-antibody interaction. SRS-A is the only member of the group without an established chemical structure, but it can be recognized because of a unique combination of chemical and pharmacologic characteristics. This lipid is elaborated in large amounts when lung tissue from individuals with allergic or extrinsic asthma is exposed in vitro to pollen antigen; SRS-A also profoundly constricts the isolated human bronchiole in the presence of specific pharmacologic antagonists of histamine and serotonin.

The anaphylactic reaction may be divided further into cytotropic and aggregate to indicate whether the critical interaction of antigen with antibody leading to release of chemical mediators occurs on a primary target cell, such as a mast cell, or in the fluid phase. The sensitization of human polymorphonuclear leukocytes with antibody of the IgE class for the subsequent antigen-induced release of histamine is an example of a cytotropic reaction. An example of aggregate-induced immediate hypersensitivity is the immune reaction in the fluid phase leading to histamine release via formation of anaphylatoxin. Such a pathway requires IgG and IgM antibodies, which in turn are necessary to activate complement. Not only can the same chemical mediator be released by distinctly different antibody-mediated pathways, but experimental work in the rat has revealed that different chemical mediators of immediate hypersensitivity are released by interaction of the same specific antigen with different homologous immunoglobulins residing on different target cells.

Because an animal or man can respond to an immunogen by making antibodies of several immunoglobulin classes, the clinical picture termed systemic anaphylaxis, which follows a subsequent challenge with specific antigen by a route or dose sufficient to bring about an immediate reaction, represents a composite response to the interaction of antigen with several different immunoglobulins. It is not surprising, therefore, that man exhibits at least three distinct reaction patterns within the anaphylactic syndrome, perhaps reflecting genetic differences in the immune response or variation in the pattern of exposure to the immunogen. Patients may experience respiratory distress due to edema of the hypopharynx and larynx or as a result of intractable bronchospasm. Hypotension then occurs secondary to the hypoxia. Alternatively, a primary vascular collapse without antecedent respiratory difficulty may ensue. It is possible to speculate on the basis of minimal experimental data in man that the pattern of laryngeal edema is mediated by histamine, the intractable bronchospasm by SRS-A, and primary vascular collapse by bradykinin. However, the critical point is that the anaphylactic syndrome has a variable presentation, probably determined by the relative amounts of the different antibodies involved.

ARTHUS REACTION. Subacute hypersensitivity reactions, depending on the deposition of immune complexes, activation of the complement system, and infiltration of polymorphonuclear leukocytes, are termed *Arthus lesions* when produced in the skin and *serum sickness* when they occur systemically. In contrast to the immediate clinical wheal of cutaneous anaphylaxis mediated by the release of chemical mediators, the Arthus lesion is a hemorrhagic reaction which develops over 4 to 10 hr and is associated with a marked polymorphonuclear leukocyte infiltrate of venules with surrounding edema and hemorrhage with or without secondary thrombosis. The reaction is not elicited by precipitating antibodies which do not activate complement and is absent in inborn or acquired complement deficiencies or in acquired leukopenia. The mechanism of the Arthus lesion appears to be as follows: (1) antigen-antibody aggregates are deposited in vessel walls; (2) the complement system is activated, and the chemotactic principle is elaborated; (3) polymorphonuclear leukocytes enter, resulting in (4) enhanced phagocytosis of the aggregates, which, in turn, (5) leads to release of lysosomal enzymes with secondary focal necrosis of the vessel wall.

SERUM SICKNESS. Serum sickness (Chap. 74) may be considered a disseminated form of the Arthus lesion, although the polymorphonuclear leukocytic infiltrate is less striking in the arteritis or glomerulitis of serum sickness than in the classical Arthus lesion. When man or an experimental animal receives a foreign or heterologous protein, the disappearance curve is characterized by three phases: (1) distribution throughout the extracellular compartment; (2) metabolic degradation; and (3) immune elimination due to an immune response with the appearance of specific antibody. The manifestations of serum sickness appear just prior to the onset of the immune elimination phase and are attributed to circulating antigen-antibody complexes formed in the region of antigen excess; these complexes apparently escape the usual clearance mechanisms effective against complexes formed at equivalence or in the zone of antibody excess and are trapped at vascular sites. For example, in experimental glomerular lesion the complexes appearing in association with the complement components are deposited on the epithelial side of the basement membrane. Similarly, immunofluorescent and electronmicrographic techniques have shown deposition of complexes and development of glomerulitis in acute poststreptococcal nephritis and systemic lupus erythematosus in man. However, this is not the only recognized immunologic mechanism of renal disease in man; in Goodpasture's syndrome and certain other instances of nephritis an anti-basement membrane antibody is deposited on the endothelial side of the basement membrane and may produce direct cytotoxic injury.

DELAYED HYPERSENSITIVITY. These reactions are exemplified in the skin by the tuberculin skin test or contact sensitivity and are implicated in the classical allograft rejection reaction of the unmodified recipient. The cutaneous response of erythema and induration is evident within 12 hr and reaches a peak in 24 to 48 hr. Granulocytes about small blood vessels are abundant in 12 hr, but by 24 hr a massive accumulation of mononuclear cells predominates. The delayed hypersensitivity response differs from the cutaneous anaphylactic or Arthus lesion because it is not transferred by serum but requires the transfer of viable lymphocytes in experimental animal models. The lymphocyte plays an essential role because (1) transfer of the delayed reaction can be achieved with thoracic duct cells, (2) the reaction can be suppressed in animals or man treated with an antiserum against the lymphocyte, and (3) the capacity to show contact sensitivity or allograft rejection in heritable or acquired lymphocyte deficiency states is absent. In man, the delayed reaction has been transferred with an extract of peripheral blood cells termed *transfer factor*, which has a molecular weight of less than 10,000. Elicitation of the delayed skin reaction requires a larger portion of the antigen than does interaction with humoral antibody; this phenomenon, referred to as hapten-carrier specificity, means that the specificity for eliciting a delayed response exceeds that of the reaction requiring humoral antibodies. Although this specificity seems to reside in the sensitized lymphocyte, it is only part of the reaction mechanism. Special studies of a skin test site have revealed that the vast majority of the accumulated mononuclear cells are nonsensitive. Studies on the inhibition of macrophage migration in the presence of sensitized lymphocytes and specific antigen have demonstrated an excellent correlation with all aspects of delayed hypersensitivity in vivo and have shown also that the antigen stimulates the lymphocyte to produce a soluble, nondialyzable protein which activates the macrophage. Therefore, the clinical absence of delayed hypersensitivity in acquired diseases such as Hodgkin's disease, sarcoidosis, or measles, may be due not only to defects of the afferent or efferent arcs of the immune response but also to defects in the effector cells.

CONCLUDING COMMENTS

In understanding both heritable and acquired defects in host resistance, it is important to appreciate not only the elements of the immune response contributing specificity, such as the immunoglobulins and the sensitized lymphocyte, but also the role of the nonspecific elements, such as the complement sequence, the polymorphonuclear leukocyte, and the macrophage. These nonspecific elements provide the killing mechanism after a specific immunoglobulin or sensitized lymphocyte has interacted with cell-surface antigens of the pathogen. Defects may occur at any point in the sequential steps in the afferent and efferent arcs of the immune response as well as in the nonspecific humoral and cellular systems which are activated in the final expression of the response. Similarly, in considering hypersensitivity to an exogenous immunogen or an autoantibody, immunochemical and immunopathologic definition of the lesion will assist materially in understanding its mechanism and in arriving at a rational course of therapy, which then may be directed at any point in the afferent and efferent arcs of the immune response or at the nonspecific participants involved in its expression.

REFERENCES

Austen, K. F., and E. L. Becker: "Biochemistry of the Acute Allergic Reactions," Oxford, Blackwell Scientific Publications, Ltd., 1968.

Davis, B. D., R. Dulbecco, H. N. Eisen, H. S. Ginsberg, and W. B. Wood, Jr.: "Microbiology," (see sec. II, Immunology), New York, Hoeber Medical Division, Harper & Row, Publishers, Incorporated, 1967.

David, J. R.: Delayed Hypersensitivity (sec. A, VI), in "Textbook of Immunopathology," P. A. Miescher and H. J. Muller-Eberhard (Eds.), New York, Grune & Stratton, Inc., in press.

Gottlieb, A. A.: The Antigen-RNA Complex of Macrophages, in "Nucleic Acids in Immunology," W. Braun and O. Plescia (Eds.), Berlin, Springer-Verlag, 1968.

Haber, E.: Recovery of Antigenic Specificity after Denaturation and Complete Reduction of Disulfides in a Papain Fragment of Antibody, Proc. Nat. Acad. Sci., 52:1099, 1964.

Janeway, C. A., F. S. Rosen, E. Merler, and C. A. Alper: "The Gamma Globulins," Boston, Little, Brown and Company, 1967.

Mackaness, G. B., and R. V. Blanden: Cellular Immunity, Progr. Allergy, 11:89, 1967.

Muller-Eberhard, H. J.: Chemistry and Reaction Mechanisms of Complement, Advan. Immunol., 8:1, 1968.

Wolstenholme, G. E. W., and R. Porter: "Ciba Foundation Symposium on the Thymus," Boston, Little, Brown and Company, 1966.

69 IMMUNOLOGIC DEFICIENCY DISEASES

(Hypogammaglobulinemia and Related Disorders)

James C. Allen

The greatest benefit of the immune response in man is enhanced resistance to infection. This resistance is impaired in immunologic deficiency states, and repeated or severe infections in patients with immunologic deficiencies bring them to medical attention. The immunologic

defenses in man and animals are divided into two categories: (1) those defense mechanisms mediated by immunoglobulins (antibodies), and (2) those mediated by cells of the lymphocytic series (Chap. 68). Lymphocyte-mediated defense mechanisms are frequently called cellular immunity and are evaluated clinically by delayed hypersensitivity reactions. Immunoglobulins are produced primarily by plasma cells which derive from lymphoid germinal centers and Peyer's patches of the gastrointestinal tract, while the lymphocytes which are of significance in cellular immunity arise from the thymus. Congenital deficiencies in immunoglobulin production usually are associated with poorly developed germinal centers in lymphatic tissue and marked reduction in the usual numbers of plasma cells, while congenital deficiencies in cellular immunity are generally accompanied by lymphopenia and improper development of the thymus. Although the exact significance of each type of immunity in mediating resistance to infection is imperfectly understood, antibodies are of major importance when microbial agents or their products are localized primarily in the bloodstream or extracellular tissues, while cellular immunity may be of greater importance when the microbial agents exist primarily within cells. Exceptions to this generalization probably exist.

Several attempts have been made to categorize the immunologic deficiency diseases, but an entirely satisfactory and logical classification is not available. This apparent confusion exists because the etiology of various deficiency syndromes is not known and the basic defects are not fully defined. In this presentation an attempt is made to organize these disorders according to their immunologic defect: impaired antibody production or impaired cellular immunity.

IMPAIRED ANTIBODY PRODUCTION

The majority of immunoglobulins present at birth are the gamma-G-globulins transferred across the placenta from the maternal circulation. As the neonate catabolizes these proteins, the serum concentration falls to a low of 300 to 500 mg per 100 ml within 4 to 12 weeks. Normally, endogenous production of immunoglobulins gradually increases, the serum level of these proteins rises, and adult levels are attained by the second year. Occasionally, the increases of immunoglobulin synthesis are delayed, and the concentration will fall as low as 75 to 100 mg per 100 ml. In these infants, repeated infection may occur until autogenous production of immunoglobulin reaches satisfactory levels. This syndrome, termed *physiologic hypogammaglobulinemia*, resolves spontaneously.

A sex-linked recessive disease, *familial hypogammaglobulinemia* (*Bruton's*), is characterized by immunoglobulin levels of 50 mg per 100 ml or less. Repeated infections occur usually within the first 2 years of life. *Acquired hypogammaglobulinemia* may occur in either sex and may begin at any age. Generally, immunoglobulin concentrations are somewhat higher than those found in the congenital type, and are between 50 and 150 mg per 100 ml. Impaired antibody production and increased susceptibility to infections may be *secondary* to the replacement of lymphoid tissue by neoplastic or granulomatous disease, as in *chronic lymphocytic leukemia,* or in association with other reticuloendothelial malignancies such as *reticulum cell sarcoma, multiple myeloma,* or *Waldenström's macroglobulinemia.* In addition, *idiopathic* cases of hypogammaglobulinemia occur in which a specific underlying disease cannot be demonstrated; heredity may play a role in these patients. An entity encompassing increased susceptibility to infection associated with hypogammaglobulinemia, thymoma, and absence of eosinophils has been described.

PATHOLOGY. The outstanding pathologic finding in primary and idiopathic forms of hypogammaglobulinemia is the paucity of plasma cells in the bone marrow, lymph nodes, and other tissues. Lymph nodes from patients with congenital hypogammaglobulinemia show ill-defined germinal centers and a thin cortex. Peyer's patches in the gastrointestinal tract are diminished or absent, but the thymus is relatively normal histologically and shows only involution compatible with the patient's age and previous state of health. Pathologic changes associated with the secondary type of hypogammaglobulinemia are those of the underlying disease.

MANIFESTATIONS. The symptoms are a direct consequence of the inability to synthesize protective antibodies in the face of antigenic challenges. There is marked increase in susceptibility to infections, with recurrent and often life-endangering episodes of pneumonia, otitis media, meningitis, sinusitis, septic arthritis, and various infections of the skin. The causative organisms usually are the common pyogenic bacteria, pneumococci, staphylococci, meningococci, and streptococci, but infectious hepatitis, generalized vaccinia, and pneumocystis carinii pneumonia also occur. Approximately one-third of children with congenital sex-linked hypogammaglobulinemia have developed disorders similar to collagen diseases. Recurrent arthritis which is indistinguishable clinically from rheumatoid arthritis is most common, but dermatomyositis, scleroderma, and polyarteritis-like diseases have been reported. Patients with acquired hypogammaglobulinemia also may have recurrent enterocolitis, with marked malabsorption. "Hypersplenism" with leukopenia, thrombocytopenia, and anemia has been described, especially in the idiopathic acquired type of hypogammaglobulinemia. Some studies have shown abnormalities of the immunoglobulins and an increased incidence of collagen vascular disease in relatives of patients with congenital hypogammaglobulinemia.

LABORATORY FINDINGS. The outstanding laboratory finding in these patients is a significant reduction in the concentration of all immunoglobulins which may be demonstrated qualitatively by immunoelectrophoresis or quantitatively by appropriate immunochemical studies. The total immunoglobulin concentration is usually less than 100 mg per 100 ml. Isoagglutinins are lacking or present in low titer, and the expected antibody response to immunization with bacterial antigens is absent. For example, the Dick test is positive, and the Schick test remains positive after immunization with diphtheria toxoid. The demonstration of limited antibody activity does not exclude the diagnosis; small amounts of antibodies to selected antigens are often detectable in serums from these patients. Rarely there is a selective inability to form specific antibodies even though concentration of "normal" immunoglobulins is within the expected range or is only slightly reduced, as in *multiple myeloma* and *Waldenström's macroglobulinemia.* In these instances, specific antibody titers are often low irrespective of the amount of monoclonal immunoglobulin or concentration of the nonmonoclonal immunoglobulins in the patient's serum, and resistance to infection may be impaired. The peripheral blood counts are normal and reflect only intercurrent infections; specifically, chronic lymphopenia is not demonstrable.

IMPAIRED CELLULAR IMMUNITY

Impaired cellular immunity of the familial form classically is associated with imperfect development of the thymus. Two types of *thymic alymphoplasia* without immunoglobulin deficiency have been recognized; they may represent variants of the same disorder. That described by *Nezelof* is associated with normal concentrations of serum immunoglobulins and normal antibody response; in the *dysgammaglobulinemic* form there is an increased concentration of γ_M-globulins with a decrease in the γ_G- and γ_A-globulins. Careful evaluation of antibody production in this disorder is not yet available, but the evidence suggests that no gross deficit exists.

The third and fourth pharyngeal pouches are the embryonic origin of the parathyroid glands and thymus. Failure of these pouches to develop results in congenital absence of the parathyroids and the thymus, leading respectively to hypoparathyroidism and immunologic deficiency. This constellation of defects has been termed the *DiGeorge syndrome.* Cellular immunity is markedly impaired even though lymphopenia may or may not exist. Deliberate immunizations show decreased formation of antibodies, but immunoglobulin levels are normal.

PATHOLOGY. The thymic alymphoplasias are characterized by improper development of the thymus, which is quite small weighing 1 Gm or less at autopsy and is located atypically, often in the area of the thyroid, as a result of improper developmental descent. Histologically, the gland is organized poorly; Hassall's corpuscles and cortical-medullary differentiation are lacking. The primary cell type is epithelial, and the thymus, as well as the spleen, lymph nodes, tonsils, and gastrointestinal lymphoid tissue, has a markedly reduced content of lymphocytes.

MANIFESTATIONS. Increased susceptibility to infections is the hallmark of impairment in cellular immunity. Compared with deficient antibody formation, however, susceptibility to mycotic and viral infections, especially candidiasis, herpes simplex, and cytomegalovirus disease, is more marked. On physical examination, detectable lymphatic tissue (tonsils, peripheral lymph nodes) is diminished markedly, and no thymic shadow is demonstrable radiographically.

LABORATORY FINDINGS. Serum immunoglobulins are grossly normal, although the dysgammaglobulinemic form of thymic alymphoplasia is associated with increased γ_M-globulins and decreased γ_A- and γ_G-globulins in the serum. Antigenic challenge produces a humoral antibody response in these patients. Deficient cellular immunity and deficient delayed hypersensitivity are most easily demonstrated by skin testing with antigens which effectively show this type of immunity, e.g., mumps, trichophyton, histoplasmin, tuberculin (especially PPD—purified protein derivative), Candida, and streptokinase-streptodornase. These patients lack reactivity to the chemical and show delayed or absent rejection of homologous skin grafts. *Lymphopenia* is always present but varies markedly in magnitude, possibly because of differences in expression of the genetic defect. Lymphocyte counts often are less than 2,000 per cu mm; levels as low as 500 per cu mm have been reported.

COMBINED DEFICIENCY OF ANTIBODY PRODUCTION AND CELLULAR IMMUNITY

A combined defect in antibody production and cellular immunity is more common than either alone. Among the most severe of these disorders is *reticular dysgenesis,* a rare disease in which death from infections supervenes shortly after birth. Profound, though poorly studied, immunologic deficits in this disease probably result from failure of a primordial stem cell important to the development of immunologic competence. It is associated with profound leukopenia, lymphopenia, and thymic aplasia.

Two types of thymic alymphoplasia with hypogammaglobulinemia have been described, the autosomal Swiss type and the sex-linked disease, which are both inherited as recessive traits. Aside from the different modes of inheritance, the two diseases are similar and are characterized by hypogammaglobulinemia, impaired antibody response, vestigial thymus glands, and impaired delayed hypersensitivity reactions. Pathologically, sparse plasma cells and diminished lymphatic tissue are characteristic.

Ataxia telangiectasia is a congenital disorder with progressive cerebellar ataxia, cutaneous and conjunctival telangiectasia, and recurrent pulmonary and paranasal sinus infections. It is associated with normal levels of γ_G-γ_M-globulins but very low γ_A-globulins and impaired antibody production. An occasional patient is found to have a greatly elevated concentration of γ_A-globulin. Significant impairment of cellular immunity is also characteristic of this disorder.

The *Wiskott-Aldrich* syndrome is a poorly understood variant of the immunologic deficiency diseases which is characterized by abnormalities of antibody production and cellular immunity. The classical clinical picture is one of eczematoid dermatitis, thrombocytopenia with bleeding diathesis, and increased susceptibility to infections with bacteria, viruses, and fungi. The disease is inherited as a sex-linked recessive trait. The concentra-

tion of γ_M-globulins in the serum is reduced and that of γ_A-globulins may be increased, although there is a selective impairment of antibody response to polysaccharide antigens. Germinal centers and plasma cells are present in normal amount. Lymphopenia is characteristic, but histologically the thymus is within normal limits. Progressive loss of small lymphocytes from lymphatic tissue in males with this disease suggests that it may represent secondary or acquired dysfunction of the immunologic system. A number of patients have developed reticuloendothelial malignancies.

Depression of both antibody production and delayed hypersensitivity reactions may occur in association with the clinical use of *cytotoxic drugs,* either in therapy for malignancy or when these drugs are used as immunosuppressive agents during organ transplantation. In many instances, the occurrence of life-threatening infections is the major limiting factor to the use of these drugs.

DIAGNOSIS OF DISEASES ASSOCIATED WITH THE IMMUNOLOGIC DEFICIENCY STATE

The diagnostic hallmark of this group of diseases is increased susceptibility to infections. When infections occur in association with hypogammaglobulinemia, impaired antibody response, diminished hypersensitivity reactions, lymphopenia, or deficient lymphatic tissue, one of this group of disorders may be involved. It is often difficult to decide with certainty which of the specific syndromes is present, but the age and sex of the patient, the family history, the age at onset, the type of immunologic deficit, the pathologic findings in lymph nodes and bone marrow, and associated findings such as eczema, ataxia with telangiectasia, hypoparathyroidism, or dysgammaglobulinemia are helpful.

TREATMENT

Treatment of these disorders has had limited success. Infections are almost uniformly the presenting problems, and successful management involves accurate microbiologic diagnosis, specific chemotherapeutic or antibiotic treatment, drainage of pus, and general supportive measures. In addition, recognition of the underlying immunologic deficiency state is important. When hypogammaglobulinemia is involved, immediate and chronic replacement therapy with concentrated human γ-globulin is indicated. Fortunately, the half-life of isologous γ-globulin in these patients is generally normal or slightly prolonged. Empirically, resistance to infections in most patients is adequate when the concentration of γ-globulin is about 150 mg per 100 ml. A practical approach is to estimate the amount of γ-globulin which will increase the serum concentration by 100 mg per 100 ml. On the basis of a life of 30 days, monthly administration of 200 mg γ-globulin per kilogram of body weight will maintain this level. Whether therapy is successful should be judged by ensuing resistance to infections, not by the concentration of circulating γ-globulin. Rarely, recurrent infections with the same organism require the use of specific immune γ-globulin. In secondary acquired hypogammaglobulinemia, treatment also is governed by the underlying disease.

Immunologic deficiency states associated with impaired cellular immunity are not amenable to prolonged treatment. Transfer of immunologically competent cells in the form of spleen tissue, bone marrow, or neonatal thymus from normal individuals will restore cellular immunity. Except for one report, however, the use of such transplantation therapy has been followed by a graft-versus-host reaction in which the donor cells reject and destroy the host's tissues.

ABNORMALITIES OF IMMUNE SYSTEMS WITHOUT INCREASED SUSCEPTIBILITY TO INFECTION

That resistance to infection involves many factors is witnessed by the occurrence of immunologic abnormalities without a concomitant increased susceptibility to infections. For example, congenital absence of the γ_A-globulins has been reported in a number of clinically normal individuals. Significant immunoglobulins may be lost in the urine in patients with the *nephrotic syndrome* who usually are not unduly susceptible to infections but who may have an increased incidence of pneumococcal disease.

Intestinal lymphangiectasia is a disease of unknown cause which is characterized by dilated intestinal lymphatics and a protein-losing enteropathy with hypoproteinemia and edema. Serum immunoglobulin concentrations are reduced, but antibody response to immunization is impaired only modestly. Significant lymphopenia (levels to 800 per cu mm is characteristic, and there is profound depression of delayed hypersensitivity reactions, with prolonged homograft survival. Increased susceptibility to infection, however, is not characteristic of this disease. In the nephrotic syndrome and in intestinal lymphangiectasia, the basic mechanisms of antibody formation and cellular immunity are intact. In nephrosis, the detectable defect in immunity is due to loss of immunoglobulins in the urine, while in intestinal lymphangiectasia, both immunoglobulins and lymphocytes are lost in the stool. In both instances, however, there is no significantly increased susceptibility to infections.

Sarcoidosis and *Hodgkin's disease* are classically associated with cutaneous anergy to delayed hypersensitivity reactions. In sarcoidosis, increased susceptibility to infections is unusual, while the occurrence of infection in Hodgkin's disease is dependent on activity of the disease, the type of treatment, and the patient's general condition. Certainly, profound anergy occurs in the course of Hodgkin's disease without clinically apparent increased susceptibility to infection. That passive transfer of delayed hypersensitivity is possible in Hodgkin's disease but not in sarcoidosis suggests different mechanisms for the anergy seen in these instances.

Transient cutaneous anergy may occur during the course of a variety of *acute febrile disorders,* particularly those of viral origin, and in association with *uremia.* Transient anergy to tuberculin may also be demonstrated in association with *miliary or serosal tuberculosis.* In none of these instances has diminution in delayed hypersensitivity reactions paralleled increased susceptibility to infections.

REFERENCES

Cooper, M. D., H. P. Chase, J. T. Lowman, W. Krivit, and R. A. Good: An Immunologic Deficiency Disease Involving the Afferent Limb of Immunity. Wiskott-Aldrich Syndrome: Clinical Studies, Am. J. Med., 4:499, 1968.

Gitlin, D., C. A. Janeway, L. Apt, and J. M. Craig: Agammaglobulinemia, in "Cellular and Humoral Aspects of the Hypersensitive States," H. S. Lawrence (Ed.), New York, Hoeber Medical Division, Harper & Row, Pub., Inc., 1959.

Good, R. A., W. D. Kelly, J. Rotstein, and R. L. Varco: Immunologic Deficiency Diseases, Progr. Allergy, 6:187, 1962.

Hitzig, W., and H. Willi: Hereditary Lymphoplasmocytic Dysgenesis ("Alymphocytosis with Agammaglobulinemia"), Schweiz. Med. Wochschr., 91:1625, 1961.

Hoger, J. R., M. D. Cooper, E. C. Gabrielsen, and R. A. Good: Lymphopenic Forms of Congenital Immunologic Deficiency Diseases, Medicine, 47:201, 1968.

Peterson, R. D. A., W. D. Kelly, and R. A. Good: Ataxia-telangiectasia: Its Association with a Defective Thymus, Immunologic-deficiency Disease, and Malignancy, Lancet, 1:1189, 1964.

Rosen, F. S., S. V. Kevy, E. Merler, C. A. Janeway, and D. Gitlin: Recurrent Bacterial Infections and Dysgammaglobulinemia: Deficiency of 7S Gamma Globulin in the Presence of Elevated 19S Gamma Globulins: Report of 2 Cases, Pediatrics, 28:182, 1961.

Seligmann, M., H. H. Fudenberg, and R. A. Good: A Proposed Classification of Primary Immunologic Deficiencies, Am. J. Med., 45:817, 1968.

Strober, W., R. D. Wochner, P. P. Carbone, and T. A. Waldmann: Intestinal Lymphangiectasia: A Protein-losing Enteropathy with Hypogammaglobulinemia, Lymphocytopenia and Impaired Homograft Rejection, J. Clin. Invest., 46:1643, 1967.

70 IMMUNOGLOBULINS AND SOME OF THEIR DISORDERS

Edward C. Franklin

INTRODUCTION AND CLASSIFICATION

Antibodies with different specificities are known to be dissimilar in their primary structure. Hence, it is not surprising that antibody activity is associated with a heterogeneous group of proteins which are collectively known as the immunoglobulins. Though the bulk of antibody activity resides in the slowly migrating γ-globulin fraction, small amounts of protein related to the immunoglobulins have been identified by serologic tech-

Table 70-1. SOME PROPERTIES OF IMMUNOGLOBULIN

Property	Immunoglobulin class-γ				
	G	A	M	D	E
Molecular weight..........................	145,000	$\pm$160,000	900,000	$\pm$160,000	200,000
Sedimentation coefficient (Svedberg's).........	7	7(9, 11, 13, 15)	19	7	8
Electrophoretic mobility.....................	γ	γ-β	γ-β	γ-β	γ-β
Approx. concentration (mg/100 ml)...........	1,200	200	100	3	0.03
Carbohydrate (%).........................	2.5	10	10	?	10
Valence..................................	2	2(?)	5(?)	?	?
"Paraprotein".............................	G myeloma	A myeloma	Macroglobulin	D myeloma	E myeloma

niques in the β- and the α_2-globulins. In addition to antibodies, the immunoglobulins include a group of structurally related proteins ("paraproteins"), which include myeloma proteins and macroglobulins and are found in several proliferative disorders of plasma cells and lymphocytes. Although these proteins generally appear to be devoid of antibody activity, their structural similarities to classical antibodies have led to their use as models of antibodies. The discovery of antibody activity in some of these paraproteins has raised the possibility that all of them may be antibodies to some as yet undefined antigens.

In spite of the enormous variability among different antibodies, the immunoglobulins show certain properties which permit their grouping into at least five major classes and a limited number of subclasses. Table 70-1 summarizes the relative concentrations and the major physical, chemical, and antigenic features of the five currently recognized classes of immunoglobulins. Though their ultracentrifugal and electrophoretic properties have been of great value in classification, it is their antigenic properties which have been especially useful in clinical practice. In particular, certain unique antigenic determinants which distinguish each class from the others have resulted in the development of class-specific antiserums which are widely used to quantitate and characterize the immunoglobulin fractions in various body fluids by immunoelectrophoretic and immunodiffusion techniques.

Antibodies have been identified in the γ_G-, γ_A-, and γ_M-globulin fractions; the γ_D-fraction has not been shown to possess antibody activity, but its structure suggests that it, too, may contain antibodies. The discovery that reaginic antibodies exist in the hitherto undescribed γ_E-globulin fraction suggests that additional classes of immunoglobulins may be found.

Table 70-1 also lists the paraproteins corresponding to each of the major immunoglobulin classes. When large series of patients with paraproteinemia are studied, the frequency of each paraprotein is closely related to the relative concentration of the corresponding fraction in normal serum. For example, G myeloma proteins occur more frequently than A myeloma proteins, which, in turn, are seen more often than macroglobulins, while D and E myeloma proteins occur only rarely.

The five well-characterized classes of immunoglobulins show striking differences in their distribution in the body and in some of their biologic properties. For example, the γ_G fraction is the only one to cross the placental barrier and thereby provides passive immunity to the newborn infant. During intrauterine life and early infancy, both γ_M and γ_G antibodies are formed by the fetus, while synthesis of γ_A-globulins does not commence until later.

Following an antigenic stimulus later in life, γ_M antibodies generally appear rapidly—the primary response—and production continues only as long as the antigen persists; γ_G antibodies are formed somewhat later, persist for a longer period, and are largely responsible for "immunologic memory," i.e., the ability of the individual to respond more strongly and rapidly to subsequent encounters with the same antigens. However, a clear-cut separation between the properties of these two classes of antibodies is not feasible.

Though all immunoglobulins are widely distributed in the intravascular and, in some instances, the extravascular compartments, the γ_A-globulins are unique in being the major, if not the sole, immunoglobulin fraction in external secretions, such as bronchial and intestinal mucus, saliva, colostrum, and lacrimal fluid, where they provide a first line of defense against bacterial and viral antigens. The γ_A-globulins in these secretions differ from those in the blood in being larger and in containing an extra structural unit with a molecular weight of about 50,000. This unit, known as a "transport piece" or "secretory piece," is synthesized in the epithelial cells of the exocrine glands, and appears to play an important role in the secretion of antibodies into these fluids or possibly in protecting them from proteolysis. The transport piece differs in structure from any of the immunoglobulin subunits, and appears to be under separate genetic control, because it is present in patients with agammaglobulinemia who cannot produce significant amounts of γ-globulins.

STRUCTURAL UNITS OF THE IMMUNOGLOBULINS

The immunoglobulins, like many other complex proteins, are made of multiple polypeptide chains, each of

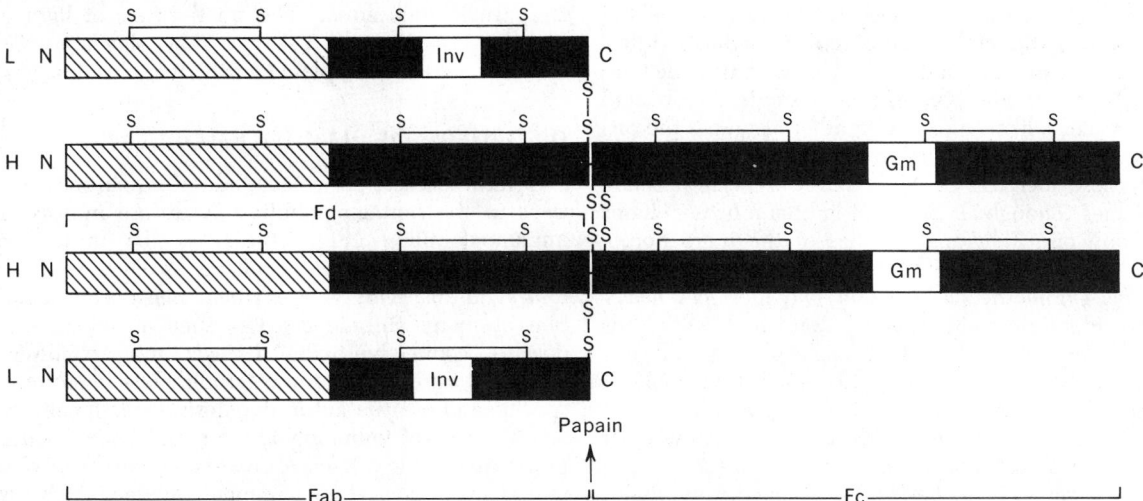

Fig. 70-1. Schematic diagram of γ$_G$-globulin. Heavy chains *H* consist of an Fc fragment, which is the same in all molecules of given subclass, and an Fd fragment, part of which is constant and part of which varies in composition in different myeloma proteins. Similarly, light chains *L* have a constant and a variable half. A light chain and an Fd fragment make up the Fab fragment. S—S = disulfide bond. N and C are N and C terminal ends. *Gm* and *Inv* are genetic factors associated with H and L chains respectively.

which is under separate genetic control. Consequently, similarities in the classes of immunoglobulins may be attributed to the existence of certain structural units found in all of them, while differences among the classes are considered due to structural units unique to each class. In general, each of the immunoglobulins consists of a basic subunit composed of four polypeptide chains held together by disulfide (covalent) and non-covalent bonds (Fig. 70-1). Two of these polypeptide chains have molecular weights of 22,000 and are called light chains. There are two major types, known as κ and λ, which are common to all classes of immunoglobulins. The other two polypeptide chains have molecular weights between 55,000 and 70,000, and are, therefore, called heavy chains. Because the heavy chains are different in each class of immunoglobulin, they are identified by the Greek letter corresponding to the class (γ, α, μ, δ, ε, for the γ$_G$, γ$_A$, γ$_M$, γ$_D$, and γ$_E$ fractions, respectively). The γ$_M$, or macroglobulin, fraction has a molecular weight of about 850,000, compared with 160,000 to 200,000 for the others. It is composed of five such subunits, each of which is probably made of two heavy and two light chains. The disulfide bonds, joining these subunits, can be cleaved readily by sulfhydryl reagents, often with a concomitant loss of antibody activity. This inactivation of antibodies by gentle reduction has been used clinically to identify antibodies in this fraction, but the method appears not to be infallible.

The antigen-binding sites include only a small region of the total molecule and appear to involve both the heavy and light polypeptide chains. They reside in the amino terminal half of the molecule (the Fab fragments) (Fig. 70-1), while many of the other properties generally associated with antibodies reside in the Fc fragment, which constitutes the carboxy terminal end of the heavy chain. Each γ$_G$ molecule, as well as probably all the other 7S immunoglobulins, has two antigen-binding sites. It is not known whether 5 or 10 combining sites exist in the intact γ$_M$-macroglobulin, although it appears likely that 10 sites are potentially available to react with antigens. The elucidation of the amino acid sequence of a number of Bence Jones (light-chain) proteins and parts of several myeloma proteins has demonstrated clearly that both the heavy and light chains contain regions which differ in composition for different proteins. These "variable" regions are located in the amino terminal half of the molecule and, consequently, appear to contribute to the specific conformation required by the antigen-binding sites. Studies of the relatively homogeneous "paraproteins" have extended the knowledge regarding the synthesis and genetic control of the normal immunoglobulins. It has been demonstrated that each class and subclass of heavy and light chains appears to have certain unique structural features in the region of the molecule known as the "constant" region. This region is similar for all molecules belonging to a particular immunoglobulin class and occupies the carboxy terminal half. The synthesis of each of the immunoglobulin chains appears to be under the control of a specific genetic locus. Because of difficulties in the assay system used to define them, not all these loci have been identified. Nevertheless, at least five loci are now known to be involved in the synthesis of the immunoglobulin chains. The constant region of the κ chains is under the control of the Inv locus; the Oz locus may play a similar role for the λ chains. A series of closely linked loci, collectively known as the Gm loci, determine the structure of the different subclasses of γ heavy chains and are known as the γ$_1$, γ$_2$, and γ$_3$ loci. Analogous genetic factors for γ$_4$, α, μ, δ, and ε chains undoubtedly exist but remain to be identified. Multiple alleles exist at each of these loci. In the case of the Inv factors, where studies have progressed furthest, differences between the constant regions of κ chains that are Inv (a+) or Inv (b+) consist of a single amino acid residue. It seems likely also that in other instances the differences between chains under the control of alleles at each of these loci will be limited to only a few amino acid residues. Though all classes of light and heavy chains exist in any one individual, studies of the more homogeneous paraproteins suggest that individual molecules are always symmetric and contain two identical heavy and two identical light chains. Consistent with this finding is the observation that each plasma cell can synthesize only one type of heavy chain and one type of light chain at any one time. Studies with mouse plasma cell tumors in vitro have shown that the synthesis of heavy and light chains occurs on separate polyribosomes, and that, in general, synthesis of light and heavy chains

is approximately equal. The small excess of light chains may be stored in the cell and may play a role in the orderly release of completed antibody molecules.

DISORDERS OF IMMUNOGLOBULINS

Several diseases are associated with quantitative alterations in the immunoglobulins. A diffuse increase in all immunoglobulins (Fig. 70-2B) is the most frequent abnormality and generally reflects an increase in γ-globulin synthesis. This is a common nonspecific manifestation of many chronic diseases such as infections, liver disease, "connective tissue" diseases, and sarcoidosis. This type of diffuse hypergammaglobulinemia is entirely nonspecific and of little aid in diagnosis. Occasionally, one or another class of immunoglobulin may be increased out of proportion to the others. A decrease in one or more of the immunoglobulins (hypogammaglobulinemia) is usually

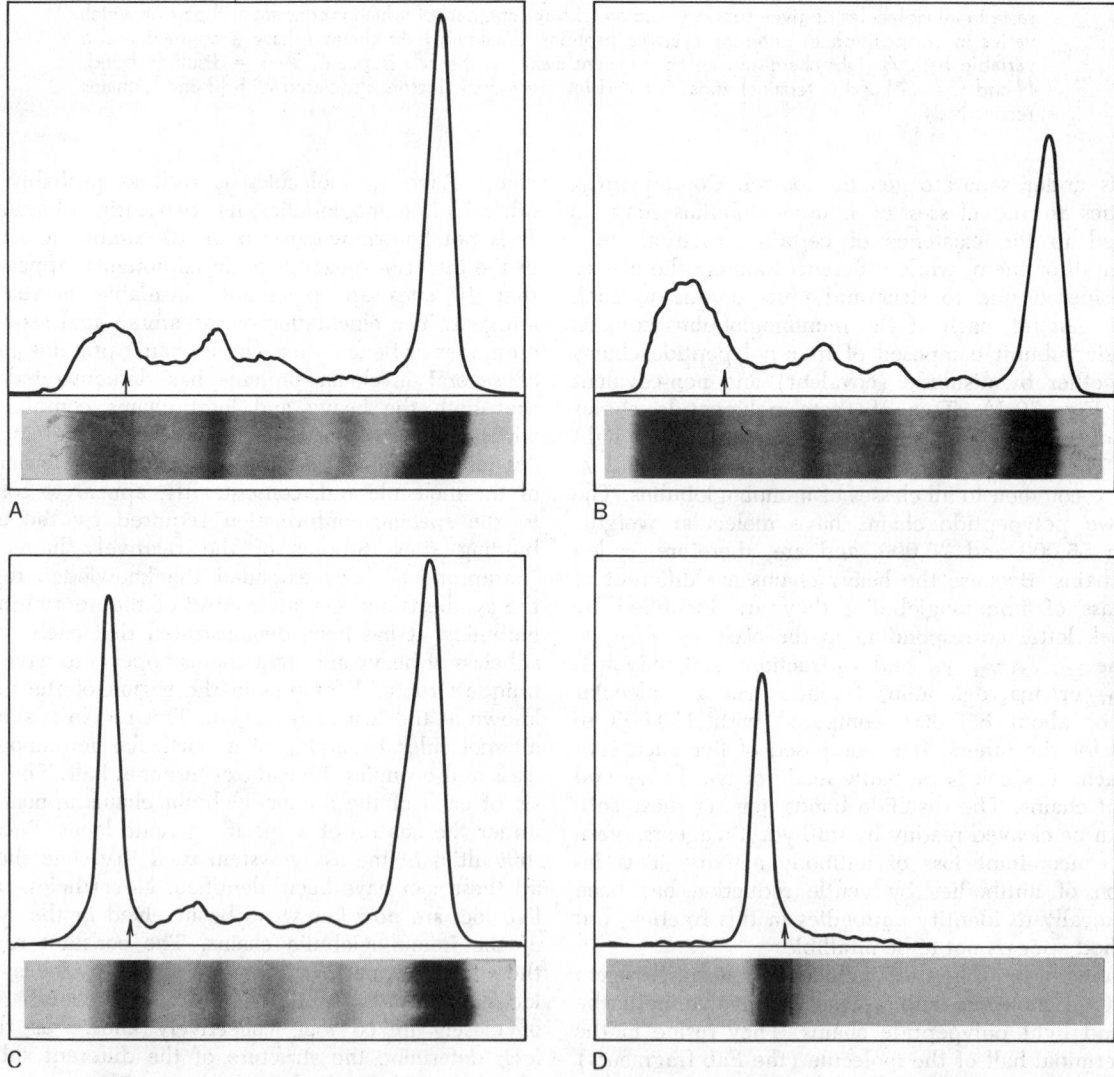

Fig. 70-2. Paper electrophoretic patterns of A. normal serum; B. serum with diffuse hypergammaglobulinemia; C. serum with G myeloma protein ("paraproteinemia"); D. urine with light-chain (Bence Jones) protein.

the result of a decrease in synthesis and is only rarely due to excessive catabolism or loss via the urine or gastro-intestinal tract (Chap. 69). This abnormality is most pronounced in the many types of congenital or acquired agammaglobulinemia or hypogammaglobulinemia. Another type of disorder involves the production of antibodies which react with an antigen present in the host and which have been called "autoantibodies." It seems likely that in many instances, autoantibodies are induced initially by foreign antigens and cross-react with tissue or serum constituents of the host. "Autoantibodies" may be directed against nucleoproteins, autologous or isologous γ-globulin (rheumatoid factors), or against red blood cells, white blood cells, platelets, thyroid antigens, and intrinsic factor. Though "autoantibodies" may be demonstrable in many diseases, their role in the pathogenesis of most of them remains unclear.

A third group of disorders is characterized by the production of immunoglobulin components which appear as homogeneous "spikes" in the electrophoretic pattern of serum or urine (Fig. 70-2C and D). It is not known whether these proteins are abnormal or whether they simply represent a quantitative increase in a normal subfraction. These diseases include a number of neoplastic processes involving plasma cells and lymphocytes, including multiple myeloma, macroglobulinemia, and "heavy-chain" disease. The abnormal proteins range in electrophoretic mobility from the slow γ-globulin to the fast $α_2$-globulin fraction. Precise identification is not possible from the appearance or mobility of the spike on paper electrophoresis and requires immunoelectrophoretic and, in some instances, ultracentrifugal analyses. In about 5 percent of patients with plasma cell dyscrasias, there is no detectable serum or urine abnormality or only a decrease in the γ-globulin level.

The abnormal proteins produced in the so-called dysproteinemias may be viewed best in the light of the normal immunoglobulins and their structural units (Table 70-2). For each normal immunoglobulin there is a

Table 70-2. DISORDERS OF γ-GLOBULIN SYNTHESIS

Heavy and light-chain synthesis	Resultant immunoglobulin disorder
Balanced............	Serum paraprotein (myeloma or macroglobulin)
Light only...........	Urine "L chain" (Bence Jones protein)
Excess light..........	Serum paraprotein and urine "L chain" (Bence Jones protein)
Heavy-chain or fragment only.......	"Heavy-chain" fragment in serum and urine
Excess heavy-chain or fragment*.......	Serum "paraprotein" plus "heavy-chain" fragment in serum and urine

* Not yet observed.

corresponding class of paraprotein. However, the precise nature of the proteins elaborated is determined by the

relative rates of synthesis of the constituent polypeptide chains. For example, in a patient with multiple myeloma or macroglobulinemia, a myeloma protein or macroglobulin is found in the blood if the synthesis of light and heavy chains remains balanced. In certain instances, asynchronous production of heavy and light chains occurs. If only light chains are produced, a homogeneous protein spike, often with the thermal properties of Bence Jones protein, appears in the urine, and no abnormal protein is found in the serum. Bences Jones proteins are defined by their insolubility when heated to 56°C and their resolubilization at 100°C. Since they represent the light polypeptide chains and since many of them fail to demonstrate the characteristic thermal properties, it seems preferable to refer to them as light-chain proteins and to rely on electrophoretic and immunologic methods for their identification. These cases cannot be classified as belonging in any of the major classes of paraproteinemia. If light chains exceed the quantity of heavy chains, both a serum "paraprotein" spike, related to one of the major classes of immunoglobulins, and a light-chain spike are found in the urine. Occasionally, because of the existence of larger polymers or because of decreased catabolism, light chains accumulate in the serum and also can present a spike.

In patients with "heavy-chain disease," a fragment of the heavy chain resembling the Fc fragment is produced and can be identified in both serum and urine (see also Chap. 349). Most of these patients have produced a fragment of the γ chain. However, at least one patient with α heavy-chain disease has been described, and it seems likely that similar disorders of μ, δ, and ε chains will be found. The coexistence of a myeloma protein in the serum and a heavy-chain disease protein in serum and/or urine in patients with asynchronous production of the two types of chain seems conceivable but has not been described.

As judged by a variety of chemical and serologic techniques, these "paraproteins" have significantly greater homogeneity than the normal immunoglobulin fractions. When examined in pure form, they possess only one class of light chain and one subclass of heavy chain, and invariably carry only the genetic markers controlled by one allele at the pertinent locus, even when they occur in an individual who is heterozygous for these factors. In most instances, the proteins produced in these disorders are devoid of antibody activity. However, cold agglutinin and rheumatoid factor activity have been found associated with some macroglobulins, and a few myeloma proteins have shown other antibody activities.

As emphasized in Chap. 349, dealing with the clinical features of the paraproteinemias, the manifestations of macroglobulinemia and multiple myeloma rarely are related to the abnormal proteins, but reflect the existence of a malignant disease. However, in some patients large amounts of the abnormal proteins, the existence of proteins with unusual solubility or antibody properties, and occasionally the marked depression of normal γ-globulins may be responsible directly for certain clinical features, as described below.

Hyperviscosity Syndrome

The presence in serum in high concentrations of a protein, most often a macroglobulin, may cause a marked rise in viscosity, which in turn may interfere with efficient circulation to the brain, digits, kidneys, or eyes. The fundi may show a characteristic appearance, with very dilated venules and many hemorrhages. The hyperviscosity syndrome often results in the sudden onset of confusion, which frequently progresses to severe organic central-nervous-system disturbances. Progressive signs of cardiac and peripheral vascular insufficiency result from the impaired circulation in the small capillaries. The diagnosis may be confirmed by demonstration of increased serum viscosity with an Ostwald viscosimeter. Treatment must be instituted immediately, with repeated plasmaphereses until the viscosity is diminished and symptoms subside. Subsequently, viscosity may be maintained within normal limits by regular plasmaphereses; therapy must be continued indefinitely. Plasmapheresis is particularly successful in patients with macroglobulinemia because these high molecular weight proteins are confined largely to the intravascular space.

Cryoglobulins

Somewhat similar clinical findings may result from the presence of cryoglobulins, which are proteins that precipitate in the cold and redissolve on warming. While cryoglobulins are often detected accidentally in asymptomatic patients, they may on occasion cause peripheral vascular insufficiency and even gangrene after exposure to low temperatures. Cryoglobulins are most often associated with multiple myeloma and macroglobulinemia, but they may occur in systemic lupus erythematosus or other "connective tissue" diseases or even in the absence of any overt illness. About one-third of cryoglobulins are G myeloma proteins, one-third are macroglobulins, and about one-third are mixtures of γ_G- and γ_M-globulins. These mixtures are most often found in patients with one of the "connective tissue" diseases and are associated with purpura and progressive, often fulminant, renal lesions reminiscent of those seen in nephritis caused by antigen-antibody complexes. The precise mechanism for cryoprecipitation is not known, and in general, there is little correlation between symptoms and the amount of cryoglobulins or the temperature at which precipitation occurs. There is evidence that many cryoglobulins may, in fact, be antibodies to γ-globulins.

Cold Agglutinins

Another disorder directly related to an unusual group of abnormal macroglobulins is the hemolytic anemia induced by cold agglutinins (Chap. 338). Though antibodies which cause hemolysis after exposure to the cold may be seen transiently in certain infections, such as infectious mononucleosis or atypical pneumonia, they rarely cause severe hemolysis in any disease other than macroglobulinemia or lymphosarcoma. The cold agglutinins causing hemolysis are generally directed against the I antigen of the red blood cell and usually possess only κ light chains. Unlike antibodies which interact with red blood cells at body temperature, cold agglutinins usually appear free in the circulation because they frequently can be eluted spontaneously from the red blood cells after reacting with certain components of complement.

Bence Jones Proteins

Another abnormality directly related to abnormal proteins is the renal disease seen in patients with Bence Jones proteinuria. The filtration of large amounts of these proteins through the glomeruli exposes the tubules to an enormous reabsorptive load, which may cause degeneration of tubular cells, deposition of proteinaceous inclusions in the cells, and the formation of tubular casts. This is often referred to as "myeloma kidney," and may result in renal failure with uremia or in the appearance of the nephrotic syndrome. Severe dehydration preceding certain diagnostic procedures such as intravenous pyelograms may be sufficient to precipitate acute renal failure in these patients.

Miscellaneous

On rare occasions paraproteins may interact with other substances, such as calcium and some of the clotting factors, or may coat blood platelets and intefere with the normal mechanisms of blood coagulation and hemostasis. There is some evidence that these disorders may be associated with amyloidosis, but it is unlikely that γ-globulins are an integral part of amyloid. Amyloid appears to be a fibrillar protein with several unique properties (Chap. 114).

Hypogammaglobulinemias

The recurrent infections often seen in patients with hypogammaglobulinemias (Chap. 69), are not directly caused by the presence of abnormal proteins but are probably attributable to the decrease in the immune response which is followed by diminished production of immunoglobulins.

SIGNIFICANCE OF PARAPROTEINEMIAS

In rare instances, the paraproteins contribute directly to the pathogenesis of some symptoms. More often they merely provide important clues in the diagnostic classification of these disorders. Evidence in support of the minor role generally played by the paraproteins in the production of clinical symptoms is provided by the ever-increasing number of elderly persons who are found to have a "paraprotein" during a routine study for an unrelated disease, who have no other symptoms, and who cannot be diagnosed as having multiple myeloma or related diseases.

REFERENCES

Cohen, S., and C. Milstein: Structural and Biological Properties of Immunoglobulins, Advan. Immunol., 7:1, 1967.

Fahey, J. L.: Serum Protein Disorders Causing Symptoms in Malignant Neoplastic Diseases, J. Chronic Dis., 16:703, 1963.

———, R. Scoggins, J. P. Utz, and C. Szwed: Infection, Antibody Response and γ-Globulin Components in Multiple Myeloma and Macroglobulinemia, Am. J. Med., 35:698, 1963.

Meltzer, M., and E. C. Franklin: Cryoglobulinemia—A Study of 29 Patients. I. IgG and IgM Cryoglobulins and Factors Affecting Cryoprecipitability, Am. J. Med., 40:828, 1966.

———, ———, K. Elias, R. T. McCluskey, and N. Cooper: Cryoglobulinemia—A Clinical and Laboratory Study. II. Cryoglobulins with Rheumatoid Factor Activity, Am. J. Med., 40:837, 1966.

Osserman, K., and K. Takatsuki: Plasma Cell Myeloma—γ-Globulin Synthesis and Structure—A Review of Biochemical and Clinical Data with the Description of a Newly Recognized and Related Syndrome Hγ₂ Chain (Franklin's) Disease, Medicine, 42:357, 1963.

Solomon, A., and J. L. Fahey: Bence Jones Proteinemia, Am. J. Med., 37:206, 1964.

71 TRANSPLANTATION

John P. Merrill

Transplantation of the human kidney is now a justified procedure for the treatment of advanced chronic renal failure. An analysis of more than 2,000 cases performed as of July, 1968, shows a 2-year survival rate of 80 percent for transplants between siblings done since January, 1966. For a similar period, 2-year survival rates for parent-to-child transplants are 60 percent and those for cadaver kidneys, 40 percent. The data show a striking improvement in results since the first successful kidney transplant in 1954, and further improvement can be expected. The results compare favorably with such accepted procedures as open heart surgery for acquired valvular heart disease. Human liver, pancreas, bone marrow, heart, and endocrine glands also have been transplanted but with less success. Even for these tissues, however, the problem does not appear insurmountable.

IMMUNOLOGIC CONSIDERATIONS

Necessary to the understanding of transplantation immunity are the following terms: *autograft*—the transplantation of tissue from one part of an individual to another part of that same individual; *isograft*—the transplantation of tissues between two individuals of the same inbred strains. Because in these cases the antigens of the donor and recipient are identical, no *histocompatibility* difference exists and no immune response to the graft occurs. A case in point in man is transplantation between identical twins. In an *allograft*, i.e., a graft of tissues between two individuals of the same species, histocompatibility differences may be strong or weak, depending on the individual and the species. A *xenograft* is a graft between individuals of two different species. The term "heterograft" is still used synonomously with xenograft.

Most of the knowledge of the biology of human tissue transplantation stems from experimental work in animals. Though species differences do exist, a justifiable analogy to data from animal experiments may be made and can be summarized by the following generalizations. The rejection of an allograft in man is due to an immune response in the recipient against an antigen present on the tissues of the donor and absent in the host. In man, it is probable that the three major antigenic mosaics of the human histocompatibility system (HU-1) are strong antigens. These antigens not only are detectable by serologic techniques but also may, by virtue of their presence or absence in the donor and recipient pair, modify the course of transplants and the amount of immunosuppressive therapy necessary. In experimental animals, by long and careful inbreeding it is possible to control histocompatibility, and the immune response between animals of different histocompatibility can be delineated by carefully controlled experiments involving grafting in a large number of lower mammals. For obvious reasons this is not true for man. However, it is possible in man to transplant skin, to inject peripheral leukocytes and platelets, to study the reactions of peripheral leukocytes from various individuals to a single anti-human leukocyte serum, and to correlate this information with the results in kidney transplantation.

HOST VERSUS GRAFT REACTION. If a piece of skin is transplanted from *A* to *B*, ingrowth of capillaries from the host into the graft occurs and the graft becomes vascularized in a normal fashion for 3 or 4 days. During this time it is probable that antigens of the graft reach the host by way of both the lymphatics and the bloodstream. The graft antigens appear to consist of lipoprotein complexes. The recipient becomes sensitized to the antigens released by the graft in the following fashion: Fig. 71-1 (1) Antigen from the graft reaches the regional lymph nodes by the afferent lymphatic vessels and reacts with a macrophage. Here the antigen acquires an RNA component, which is then transfered to an unsensitized or "uncommitted" lymphocyte. This small lymphocyte enlarges into a large pyroninophilic cell (lymphoblast), which divides repeatedly, giving rise to many sensitized lymphocytes, i.e., lymphocytes containing antibody directed against the graft. These cells then reach the vasculature of the graft, causing damage to its vascular endothelium, and eventually pass through the wall of the vessels where they infiltrate the interstitium of the graft. (2) It is possible that this process also takes place outside the lymph nodes, including the kidneys and other directly vascularized grafts, where lymphocytes or macrophages come in direct contact with antigens of the graft. Once these sensitized cells reach lymphatic tissue anywhere in the body, they may stimulate the process described above. It is probable also that cell-free or soluble antibody in the form of gamma-globulin (IgG)

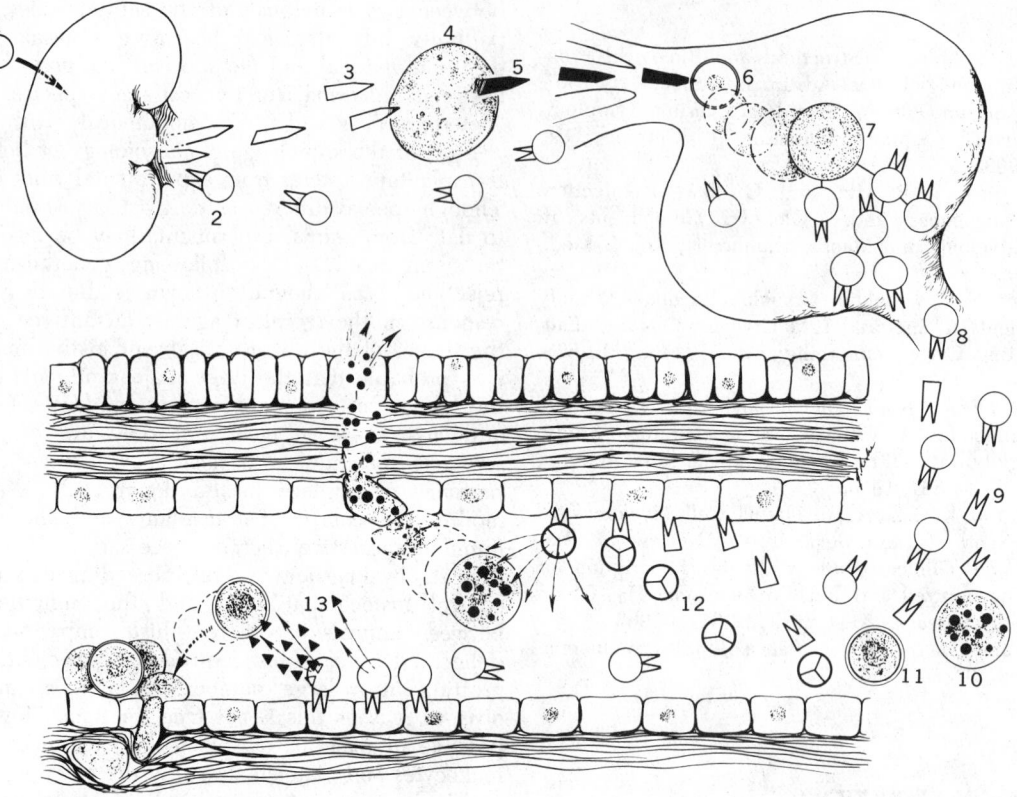

Fig. 71-1. (1) Unsensitized lymphocyte (2) Lymphocyte sensitized by passage through kidney (3) Antigen released from kidney (4) Macrophage (5) Processed antigens (6) Lymphocyte (7) Lymphoblast (8) Sensitized lymphocyte (9) Antibody globulin (10) PMN leukocyte (11) Macrophage (12) Complement (13) MIF factor.

There are two current concepts of the mode of sensitization of a recipient to a transplanted kidney. In the first, antigens of the kidney (3) may be engulfed by the macrophage system (4) of the recipient and the processed antigen (5) induces transformation of some of the lymph node lymphocytes (6) into lymphoblasts. Alternatively, circulating lymphocytes (1) may become sensitized directly as they pass through the kidney (2). Either way, the result is production of lymphocytes (8) particularly sensitized to the graft. When these cells arrive at the vasculature of the graft along with antibody globulin (9), which is also produced by the lymph nodes, they attach to antigenic binding sites on the wall of the vessel. Complement is bound at the antibody sites and the complement (12) sequence is initiated. As a result of this initiation, the polymorphonuclear (PMN) chemotactic factor is released and PMN's (10) are attracted to the graft where the release of lysosomal enzymes from the leukocytes may result in damage to the vascular wall. Similarly the interaction of sensitized lymphocytes and antigens at the graft site releases macrophage migration inhibitory factor (MIF) (13) which causes the accumulation of cells (11) at the graft site. Some mononuclear cells migrate through the vessel wall and are seen as perivascular accumulations. Intravascular accumulation results in slowing of flow, stasis, and graft ischemia. Not shown here are platelet deposition and small thrombi, which may accompany this reaction.

may react directly with the vascular endothelium of the graft. When this occurs, the cellular reaction is secondary. An example in man is the accelerated rejection that occurs when an individual (B) who has been sensitized by a previous skin graft from A receives a second skin graft; if the second graft is placed a certain length of time following the initial transplant, it may be rejected in an "accelerated fashion." Under these circumstances the second graft never becomes vascularized. Small-vessel thrombosis occurs with rapidity. No lymphocytes are seen at the site of the rejected graft, and the polymorphonuclear leukocytes that appear seem to be due to a response to necrosis rather than to an immune reaction. Alternatively, it is possible that sensitized lymphocytes

reach the vascular endothelium but are destroyed upon contact with it, liberating proteolytic enzymes which cause further endothelial destruction and injury. Finally, both mechanisms may be operative in previously sensitized individuals. Soluble antigens from the graft encounter a sensitized lymphocyte at the vessel wall. The antigen combines with the cell-bound antibody, and a protein factor is released which interferes with the migration of monocytes by making them adhere to the vessel wall and injure its endothelial lining. The monocytes activated by this migration-inhibitory factor (MIF) are transformed into macrophages which force themselves through the endothelium of the vessel wall, releasing lysosomal hydrolases which attack both the vessel wall and the parenchymal elements. Many similarities between the rejection of transplanted tissue and the so-called delayed hypersensitivity reaction have been noted, and graft rejection is thought to be a manifestation of delayed hypersensitivity.

IMMUNOSUPPRESSIVE TREATMENT

When histocompatibility differences exist between donor and recipient, it is necessary to modify or suppress the immune response in order to enable the recipient to "tolerate" a graft. Immunosuppressive therapy in general suppresses all immune responses, including those to bacteria, fungi, and even malignant tumors. Agents used in man to suppress the immune response are the following:

TOTAL-BODY IRRADIATION. Lethal doses of x-irradiation in animals destroy the lymphopoietic system and the ability to reject a tissue graft. However, because irradiation also destroys the bone marrow, it is necessary to transplant bone marrow in order to enable the animal to survive. Attempts to utilize this technique in man generally have been unsuccessful, but one patient at least has done well.

DRUGS. *Azathioprine* (Imuran), an analogue of 6-mercaptopurine, is the keystone of immunosuppressive therapy in man. This agent inhibits synthesis of deoxyribonucleic acid (DNA) or ribonucleic acid (RNA) or both. Because cell division and proliferation result as part of the immune response to antigenic stimulation, suppression may be mediated by the inhibition of mitosis of immunologically competent lymphoid cells interfering with synthesis of DNA. Alternatively, inhibition may occur by blocking the synthesis of ribonucleic acids (possibly messenger RNA) which is thought to play an important role in the processing of antigens prior to lymphoid stimulation. Therapy with azathioprine is generally instituted 2 to 10 days prior to transplantation of the kidney and is continued as long as the allograft functions. Because the drug is excreted by glomerular filtration, the dose must be varied according to the functional status of the kidney. Bone marrow depression may occur as a result of excess dosage of azathioprine, as may jaundice, anemia, and alopecia. *Actinomycin C* formerly was employed in the treatment of rejection crises but because of its toxicity is used infrequently.

The *corticosteroids,* usually in the form of prednisone, are important adjuncts to immunosuppressive therapy. Of all the agents employed, the effect of prednisone is easiest to assess, and in large doses it is unquestionably the most effective agent for the reversal of rejection. In general, 150 to 200 mg prednisone is given immediately prior to or at the time of transplantation, and the dosage is reduced to maintenance levels, over a period of 2 weeks. The well-known side effects of the corticosteroids, particularly impairment of wound healing and predisposition to infection, make it desirable to taper the dose as rapidly as possible in the immediate postoperative period. Prednisone should be used in large doses (200 to 500 mg) immediately upon detection of beginning rejection. When the drug is effective, the results are usually apparent within 24 to 48 hr, and the dose then may be reduced again. Although most patients whose renal function is stable after 6 months or a year do not require large doses of prednisone, maintenance doses of 20 mg per day are the rule.

THORACIC DUCT FISTULA. Lymphocyte depletion by cannulation and drainage of the thoracic duct appears to lessen the number of rejection crises in the early post-transplant period in man.

EXTRACORPOREAL IRRADIATION. Irradiation of blood as it passes through an extracorporeal source connected to the patient by the arteriovenous cannula usually utilized for dialysis with the artificial kidney, has resulted in lymphocyte depletion and is an adjunct to other forms of immunosuppressive therapy but not a substitute for them. It is particularly useful in maintaining immunosuppression when toxicity of other agents requires their temporary discontinuance.

ANTILYMPHOCYTE SERUM. When serums from animals made immune to host lymphocytes are injected into the recipient, they destroy lymphoid cells and suppress the immune response to tissue grafts. Antilymphocyte serum is unquestionably effective in prolonging grafts in experimental animals, but its efficacy in human beings is somewhat less clear. In practice, peripheral human lymphocytes or lymphocytes from cadaver spleens or thoracic duct fistulas are injected into horses to produce antilymphocyte serums, from which the specific globulin is then separated. The globulin is injected intramuscularly into patients 5 days to a week prior to transplantation, and injections are continued for 2 to 3 weeks thereafter. Pain and swelling occur at the site of injection, and occasional anaphylaxis has been reported. No deaths attributable to the use of horse serum have occurred. When an effective preparation of antilymphocyte globulin is used, delayed-type hypersensitivity skin tests disappear in the recipient. There is suggestive but not conclusive evidence that the mortality rate of patients treated in this fashion is decreased and that when antilymphocyte serum is used, smaller doses of azathioprine and steroids will prevent rejection. Although antilymphocyte serum should be used with extreme caution in man, it seems probable that further exploration of this preparation may yield an effective agent which can be used with relatively little hazard of serum sickness or nephrotoxic nephritis.

Other techniques of immunosuppression, including thymectomy, splenectomy, and local irradiation of the kidney, have not influenced the course of human kidney transplants favorably.

COMPLICATIONS OF RENAL TRANSPLANTATION

The complications of human renal transplantation often result from the use of *immunosuppressive therapy.* Wound infection with gram-negative organisms is common, as is breakdown of wounds, particularly the ureteral anastomosis. Pulmonary infections with a variety of unusual organisms, including *Candida* (Chap. 190), *Aspergillus* (Chap. 193), *Nocardia* (Chap. 192), *Pneumocystis*

(Chap. 245), and cytomegalovirus (Chap. 232), also occur. Their relationship to a general defect in immunologic integrity is clear. The complications of *corticosteroid* therapy are well known and include gastrointestinal bleeding, hemorrhagic pancreatitis, and impairment of wound healing. Leukopenia, anemia, and jaundice occur as a result of azathioprine administration.

Even identical twins who do not require immunosuppressive therapy develop complications. In 18 sets of identical twins, whose original disease was glomerulonephritis, 11 developed a similar histologic lesion in the transplanted kidney. The glomerular lesion is not, however, limited to the isograft, nor is it necessarily a question of "catching" the disease in the transplant because of continuing antiglomerular activity. A number of patients with true allografts treated with immunosuppressive therapy have developed typical glomerular lesions over a period of years. One patient who received a successful allograft from his mother developed a classical nephrotic syndrome with glomerulonephritis 2½ years after transplantation. Because the reason for transplantation initially was the accidental removal of a single normal ectopic kidney, the development of glomerulonephritis in the transplant cannot be attributed to "continuing activity."

Another long-term complication of renal allografting has been the development of *nephrosclerosis* with proliferation of the vascular intima of renal vessels, intimal fibrosis, and marked decrease in the lumen of the vessels. The result is renal ischemia, hypertension, widespread tubular atrophy, interstitial fibrosis, and glomerular atrophy with eventual renal failure. Both the long-term vascular lesions and the glomerular lesions are probably the result of subclinical episodes of rejection with damage to capillary and vascular endothelium and resultant healing with fibrosis and sclerosis.

Sensitization of the human recipient to subsequent skin grafts from any donor may occur following the intradermal injection of donor leukocytes, and uremic recipients, particularly when maintained for long periods on hemodialysis, require repeated transfusions and thus have repeated exposure to formed elements in the blood which are capable of sensitizing the recipient to subsequent tissue grafts. Rapid rejection of a first kidney allograft has been documented in a number of patients who presumably have been sensitized by platelets or leukocytes in transfusions administered prior to operation. Antibodies to human leukocytes have been demonstrated in the serum of these patients and are associated in a significant number of instances with a rapid rejection of the renal transplant.

Tumor cells have been transplanted inadvertently with kidneys taken from cadaver donors dying from bronchogenic carcinoma and other malignancies. The immunosuppressive therapy which allows the kidney to be tolerated in the recipients also apparently permits survival and propagation of the malignant tumor. With cessation of immunosuppressive therapy both the renal allograft and the tumor are destroyed.

TISSUE TYPING

In the experimental animal the duration of allograft survival depends on the "strength" of the difference in histocompatibility between the donor and the recipient. A number of techniques for "typing" tissue have been developed. Of these, the most important are (1) serotyping of leukocytes and (2) use of mixed lymphocyte cultures. In serotyping, serums obtained from patients who have been immunized inadvertently to human leukocytes (either multiparous women or patients who have received repeated transfusions) are evaluated with respect to their ability to agglutinate leukocytes and to elicit a cytotoxic effect. In the performance of both tests, donor and recipient cells are tested against a single antiserum; as many different antiserums as feasible are used. If agglutination or cytotoxicity is detected for both sets of cells, antigenic configurations are said to be similar; the same holds true if neither is affected. If one set of cells is affected and the other is not, a difference is assumed to be present. Serial dilutions of serum may sharpen differences in agglutination or cytotoxicity. By cross absorption of antiserums it is theoretically possible to obtain monospecific antiserums capable of recognizing a single leukocyte antigen. Five of these antigen groups have been characterized and predict important histocompatibility antigens in man. In general, there has been a good correlation between close histocompatibility and transplant survival. Predictably, the correlation has been better between siblings and parent-child combinations than with cadaver kidneys, probably because not all antigens recognized by these techniques are related to true histocompatibility. The *mixed lymphocyte culture technique* involves culturing peripheral blood lymphocytes from donor and recipient. When these cells are stimulated, they are transformed into large basophilic blastlike cells, presumably an indication of antibody synthesis which can be quantitated either by a number of morphologic changes or by the uptake of tritiated thymidine or iodouridine. Stimulation to form antibody will be greater when histocompatibility difference between donor and recipient is marked. Inhibition of the immunologic potential of cells at a certain point in their inactivation by mitromycin interferes with the ability of cells to react, but these cells still can be stimulated, making it possible to predict how strongly a potential recipient may be stimulated by donor cells. These techniques in selecting donor recipient pairs are promising and may lead to a rational decrease in the dose of toxic immunosuppressive therapy which must be utilized to prevent rejection.

SELECTION OF RECIPIENTS FOR KIDNEY TRANSPLANTATION

Table 71-1 lists practical considerations in the selection of a recipient for a human renal allograft. Such a procedure should be undertaken only when conservative treatment has failed, when there are no reversible ele-

Table 71-1. CONTRAINDICATIONS TO HUMAN KIDNEY
TRANSPLANTATION

1. Absolute contraindications:
   a. Reversible renal involvement
   b. Ability of conservative measures to maintain useful life
   c. Major extrarenal complications (cerebrovascular or coronary disease; neoplasia)
   d. Active infection
   e. Active glomerulonephritis
   f. Previous sensitization to human tissue
2. Relative contraindications:
   a. Age
   b. Presence of vesical or urethral abnormalities
   c. Iliofemoral occlusive disease
   d. Diabetes mellitus
   e. Inactive lupus erythematosus
   f. Psychiatric problems

ments in the patient's renal failure, and when he is too sick to be maintained comfortably with the usual methods of treatment. However, the considerable success with kidneys transplanted from blood relatives, reports of success with second or third kidney transplants, and the ability to maintain patients who have had transplant failures on hemodialysis justify consideration of kidney transplantation before the patient is critically ill and possibly even before it is obvious that hemodialysis is the only other course. The recipient should be free of life-threatening extrarenal complications such as cancer, severe coronary artery disease, and cerebrovascular disease. Provided that diffuse vascular involvement is not present, diabetes itself is not a contraindication. Although age may be a limiting factor, the "physiologic" age rather than the chronologic age contraindicates transplantation. A cadaver transplant into an eighty-two-year-old patient is on record, and adult renal allografts have been transplanted into recipients as young as three. Although abnormalities of the bladder and urethra present additional hazards, successful renal allografts have been placed in individuals with these abnormalities by prior construction of an artificial bladder (i.e., ileal conduit) into which the donor ureter is placed. The demonstration of "preformed antibodies" in the potential recipient prior to transplantation is a contraindication when it can be shown that these antibodies react specifically to donor cells.

DONOR SELECTION

Donor sources are cadavers or volunteer blood-related living donors. Living volunteer donors should be found completely normal on physical examination and should be of the same major ABO blood group, because there is good evidence that crossing major blood group barriers prejudices survival of the allograft. It is, however, possible to transplant a kidney of a type O donor into an A or B recipient. Selective renal arteriography should be performed on volunteer donors to rule out the presence of multiple or abnormal renal arteries, because the sur-

gical procedure is inordinately difficult and the ischemic time of the normal kidney prohibitively long when vascular abnormalities exist. Cadaver donors should be free of malignant neoplastic disease because of possible transmission of cancer to the recipient. Tissue typing of donor and prospective recipient and direct crossmatching are mandatory.

CLINICAL COURSE OF THE RECIPIENT

Usually, but not invariably, bilateral nephrectomies are performed prior to transplantation, and the recipient is maintained on intermittent hemodialysis. Removal of the patient's own diseased kidneys obviates a source of infection in the postoperative period and facilitates the diagnosis of rejection of the allograft, because variations in renal function and urine sediment are then related only to changes in the allograft.

Psychologic complications following transplantation are common. Depression and anxiety may reflect both the difficult and stressful postoperative course and the anxiety and uncertainty of the physician.

THE REJECTION CRISIS. Early diagnosis of rejection is imperative because prompt institution of vigorous therapy may reverse renal function and prevent irreversible damage due to fibrosis. Clinical evidence of rejection is characterized by fever, swelling, and tenderness over the allograft, and by oliguria. In patients whose renal function is good initially, oliguria may be accompanied by decreased urinary sodium concentration and increased urine osmolarity. These changes may not be present in more chronic stages of rejection or when renal function is impaired at the onset of rejection. A transplanted cadaver kidney more often than not undergoes a period of anuria which may last as long as 3 months without prejudicing the eventual function of the graft. In this instance, the reversible lesion is presumably due to ischemia, and the diagnosis of rejection becomes more difficult. Renal arteriography and radioactive Hippuran renograms may be useful in ascertaining changes in the renal vasculature and in renal blood flow even in the absence of urine flow. When renal function has been good initially, a rise in the blood urea nitrogen level and a decrease in the creatinine clearance may herald the onset of rejection. The creatinine clearance is perhaps more reliable, because fever and the administration of prednisone may influence the concentration of blood urea nitrogen without necessarily reflecting a decrease in urea clearance. Increase in the 24-hr excretion of urinary lysozyme has been helpful. Increase in proteinuria may reflect rejection, but when it occurs later in the course of the postoperative period, predominant glomerular disease may be present. Hypertension is also a concomitant of rejection. When hypertension responds to prednisone, it is likely that rejection has been responsible for the elevation of blood pressure, because other forms of hypertension usually do not improve with corticosteroid therapy. The measurement of the intrarenal distribution of blood by the xenon washout technique has been valuable in assessing rejection both in man and in experimental animals. It is possible at operation to leave in the renal artery a small polyvinyl catheter through which these studies may be done repeatedly.

TRANSPLANTATION OF OTHER VISCERAL ORGANS

Organs other than the kidney which have a potential for clinical transplantation are the liver and heart. Two possible indications for *liver transplantation* are chronic hepatic failure and malignancy which is localized to the liver. Two techniques for liver transplantation have been utilized in man: (1) *Orthotopic*—the recipient's own liver is removed and the transplant is substituted for it in the anatomic position. (2) *Auxiliary*—the recipient's liver is left in place and the allograft is placed in the right paravertebral gutter. The donor's vena cava then is interposed in the recipient terminal inferior vena cava, and the hepatic artery is anastomosed to the right common iliac artery. Finally, the end of the allograft portal vein is anastomosed to the recipient's superior mesenteric vein.

Immunosuppressive regimens are similar to those in kidney transplantation. There is some suggestion that the use of antilymphocyte globulin is more effective in liver allografting. Obviously, the donor source must be a cadaver. Complications of liver transplantation have been strikingly different from those encountered with renal allografts. In many instances an initial hemorrhagic diathesis with fibrinolysis ocurs. This is followed by a phase of hypercoagulability in the successfully transplanted recipient, which in one instance resulted in fatal pulmonary emboli. Infections also seem to present a greater problem than with renal allografts. These complications are not insurmountable, and although no patient with a liver transplant has survived for more than 1 year, the prospects for the future are promising.

Transplantation of the heart has been accomplished successfully in man in a number of instances. Early results suggest that it is comparable to transplantation of the kidney and that results certainly will improve. Indications for cardiac transplantation are myocardial insufficiency, usually due to severe coronary artery disease and myocardial fibrosis, and failure to respond to the most rigorous medical measures. The donor must be a cadaver and is usually an individual whose death has resulted from trauma or suicide. The question of the ethics and morals raised by the removal of a heart capable of sustaining life in another individual has been discussed by many medical and lay authors. It seems eminently reasonable that if "death" of the brain has occurred, as evidenced by lack of electrical activity in the electroencephalogram over a period of 24 to 36 hr, dilated pupils, failure of spontaneous respiration, and lack of peripheral reflexes, the ability to maintain respiration or cardiac output by artificial methods is academic. Nevertheless, the decision as to when to discontinue these efforts should be made independently by the physician caring for the prospective donor in consultation with one or two colleagues. The question of whether or not the heart is to be used for transplantation should not affect this decision. Once the decision has been made, the donor can be maintained until the recipient is prepared for operation.

Human *spleen* and *pancreas* have been transplanted with limited success. If it could be shown that normal spleen can produce a useful amount of antihemophilic globulin, transplantation of that organ to some patients with hemophilia would provide a distinct advantage over standard substitution therapy. Transplantation of lymphoid tissue (including spleen) for total agammaglobulinemia has resulted in temporary improvement, but eventually the transplanted lymphoid tissue rejects the host (graft versus host reaction). Temporary success in transplanting pancreas in diabetics also has been reported, but substitution therapy seems more feasible.

Various other *endocrines*, including parathyroid, adrenal, and thyroid, have all been transplanted, with only temporary success. A large percentage of *corneal grafts* survive as allografts in man, primarily because the cornea is not vascularized, which excludes immunologically competent cells. Grafts of bone and blood vessels do not survive as living allografts but act as a "scaffolding" over which host tissue may grow.

Transplantation of allogenic marrow in man is of particular interest because when allogenic marrow is transplanted successfully following irradiation, the marrow recipient "tolerates" skin grafts from animals isologous with the marrow donor.

The obvious application of marrow transplantation to patients with leukemia and aplastic anemia has resulted in a number of attempts at human marrow transplantation. When identical twin donors have been used, the results have been uniformly promising. For example, marrow transplants were carried out in four patients with leukemia following lethal total-body irradiation. In every instance the transplant was successful and the patient died later of recurrent leukemia. Also using identical twin donors, successful marrow transplants have been performed in at least four patients with acute bone marrow failure and in one patient following accidental lethal whole-body irradiation. In these cases the transplants were successful and appear to have been lifesaving. A complication of marrow transplantation is a reaction of the grafted cells against the host whose immunosuppressive potential has been ablated by irradiation or nitrogen mustard. This reaction is characterized by fever, anorexia, diarrhea, dermatitis, and alopecia and is similar to that demonstrated in animals who have been treated in this fashion. Encouraging results in preventing the "graft versus host reaction" by the early administration of Amethopterin and cyclophosphamide have been reported.

ORGAN PRESERVATION

If it were possible to remove cadaver organs and to store them for a period of days or longer under conditions permitting their successful replantation, one of the difficult problems in organ procurement would be solved. Bone marrow is the only organ that can be stored easily for prolonged periods. The hope of kidney, heart, or liver banks in which suitably typed organs could be stored for subsequent transplantation to a suitable recipient is still a long way from reality. The most effective technique for preservation is hyperbaric, hypothermic perfusion, but organs treated in this fashion must be transplanted within 24 to 36 hr.

XENOGRAFTS

Kidneys, lungs, and hearts have been transplanted to human beings from various primates, including chimpanzees and baboons. Although one chimpanzee kidney graft functioned well for more than 7 months, clinical efforts in this area have been abandoned. It seems quite possible, however, that continuing efforts to find other species whose tissues may be more compatible to man's (e.g., the pig) may result eventually in a source of organs which might eliminate many of the present problems. In fact, it might be possible to breed pigs for histocompatibility with man in the same fashion that mice were bred to produce purebred lines with predictable tissue antigenicity.

REFERENCES

Amos, B.: Immunologic Factors in Organ Transplantation, Am. J. Med., 44:767, 1968.

Merrill, J. P.: Human Tissue Transplantation, in F. J. Dixon and H. G. Kunkel (Eds.), Advan. Immunol., 7:276, 1968.

Rapaport, F. T., and J. Dausset: "Human Transplantation," New York, Grune & Stratton, Inc., 1968.

Russell, P. S.: Kidney Transplantation, Am. J. Med., 44:776, 1968.

Starzl, T. E.: "Experience in Renal Transplantation," Philadelphia, W. B. Saunders Company, 1964.

72 ASTHMA, HAY FEVER, AND OTHER MANIFESTATIONS OF ALLERGY

Philip S. Norman

ASTHMA

DEFINITION. Asthma is characterized by paroxysms of expiratory dyspnea and wheezing, overinflation of the lungs, cough, and rhonchi. The onset of paroxysms may be sudden or insidious; their duration may be brief or they may last weeks. Symptoms are due to generalized bronchial airway obstruction, which occurs as a result of contraction of bronchial smooth muscle, hypertrophy of the bronchial wall, edema of the bronchial mucosa, and accumulation of secretions in the bronchial lumens.

MANIFESTATIONS AND PATHOPHYSIOLOGY. In asthma, it is probable that bronchospasm, mucosal edema, and bronchial secretions are the principal mechanisms producing airway obstruction, which is localized primarily in the small bronchioles. Normally, the bronchial lumens enlarge upon inspiration and narrow upon expiration. Dyspnea, therefore, is most pronounced, and wheezing and rhonchi are audible, during expiration. The expiratory phase of respiration is prolonged, and inspiration characteristically is not as difficult as expiration. Expiratory dyspnea requires the use of accessory muscles to deflate the lung, increasing the intrathoracic pressure. During inspiration, on the other hand, the negative intrathoracic pressure is accompanied by retraction of the intercostal, suprasternal, and supraclavicular spaces. The expiratory airway obstruction leads to hyperinflation or reversible emphysema of the lungs.

Asthma characteristically occurs in attacks of variable duration; between attacks pulmonary function is normal or nearly normal and patients are relatively free of symptoms. Such spasmodic asthma is more frequent at night, and attacks usually last several minutes to several hours. Occasionally spasms last several days, and some asthmatic patients maintain an almost continuous state of airway obstruction nearly every day.

The precise mechanism of dyspnea in asthma is not known, but it probably results from a combination of conscious recognition of obstruction to breathing, hyperinflation, changes in intrapleural pressure, and increased work. Wheezing, dyspnea, and cough are worse with effort, are exaggerated by anxiety, and tend to be most severe at night. During a paroxysm, the patient is usually most comfortable while sitting with the trunk forward and the arms elevated to rest at shoulder level. Elevation of the diaphragm while the patient is recumbent reduces the respiratory reserve. The sitting posture reduces intraabdominal pressure and allows the viscera to move downward and forward.

The physical properties of the bronchial secretions undoubtedly influence the manifestations of asthma, but very little is known of the changes that may occur in sputum viscosity, elasticity, and stickiness. The ease with which sputum can be evacuated from the bronchi, however, obviously is an important factor in the severity of airway obstruction. Cough frequently becomes more severe during recovery from an asthmatic attack, when sputum seems more liquid and is raised in larger quantities. Syncope may occur when prolonged periods of increased intrathoracic pressure associated with paroxysms of coughing interfere with venous return to the heart. The sputum usually is white and mucoid and contains no blood or pus. Microscopic examination often shows eosinophils and Charcot-Leyden crystals. In addition, as an asthmatic attack subsides, mucous casts of the bronchi or bronchioles may be seen in the sputum (Curschmann's spirals). Purulent sputum indicates bronchial or pulmonary infection.

There is no fever unless asthma is caused by or associated with infection. After a prolonged attack the patient may complain of soreness in the chest or abdomen as well as tiredness, but otherwise there are no systemic manifestations of the disease.

During a mild attack the sensation of obstruction to breathing may lead the patient to overcompensate by hyperpnea and there will be a reduction in blood CO_2 tension. If airway obstruction becomes more severe, there may be a fall in oxygen tension with cyanosis and a rise in CO_2 tension due to ventilatory failure. Such rises in P_{CO_2} are often uncompensated and are accompanied by a low plasma bicarbonate concentration. There is also an altered ventilation/perfusion ratio in asthma which arises from regional defects in ventilation due to bronchial plugging. These ventilation defects may reflexly cause transient regional reduction in blood flow, which can be detected during asthmatic attacks by pulmonary scanning techniques.

When an asthmatic episode is prolonged for many hours or days and is resistant to therapy, it is defined as *status asthmaticus*. The chest is greatly distended, the patient works desperately to move air through the obstructed airways, using the accessory muscles of respiration, and breath sounds and wheezes may become very faint because movement of air is poor. Cough is virtually impossible, and the patient is often volume-depleted and extremely fatigued. If status does not resolve, the chest becomes almost silent and severe respiratory acidosis ensues. Death from respiratory arrest is possible, and vigorous emergency treatment is necessary.

Asthmatic episodes may be complicated by *atelectasis* due to mucoid plugging of bronchi with subsequent extraction of gases from the unventilated portion of the lung. *Pneumonia* may supervene in poorly ventilated or atelectatic portions of lung. *Spontaneous pneumothorax* and *mediastinal emphysema* are rare complications of an asthmatic attack. Ordinarily, asthma does not affect cardiac function unless the attack is protracted or is accompanied by irreversible emphysema. Under these circumstances, cor pulmonale may develop.

ETIOLOGY. Asthma begins before age ten in about one-half of cases and before age thirty in another third, but it may begin *de novo* even in old age. Before age ten, asthma is twice as frequent in boys, but by age thirty the incidence is equal in men and women. Asthma is present in members of the immediate family of about one-third of patients.

In most asthmatics four main factors are thought to interact to a variable degree in producing attacks: (1) allergy to external inhaled allergens; (2) respiratory infections; (3) psychophysiologic reactions to life stress; and (4) air pollution. Although asthma is regarded as an allergic disease, hypersensitivity is found to be the predominant cause in only about one-third of cases and a contributing factor in perhaps another third.

Hay fever and urticaria sometimes precede development of asthma, or occur simultaneously, suggesting that asthma is attributable to inhaled or ingested antigens in an individual with reaginic or atopic allergy. This type of asthma is observed most commonly in young persons and usually is seasonal. The same inhaled pollens, molds, dusts, danders, etc., described further on in this chapter under Allergic Rhinitis (Hay Fever) are implicated in allergic asthma. The relationship to seasonal exposure, positive skin tests, and family history of allergy are the same as in hay fever. Nonseasonal asthma may also be due to allergy to dust, feathers, animal danders, foods, or drugs.

A syndrome of chronic sinusitis, nasal polyps, poorly remitting asthma, and unusual sensitivity to aspirin has been observed in some adults. These individuals have onset of symptoms as adults and may have rapidly developing life-threatening paroxysms of bronchospasm after a single aspirin tablet.

Respiratory infections appear to be the predominant etiologic factor in about 40 percent of cases and are most common in the very young, the elderly, and those with the most serious disease. Initially these infections may appear to be no more than a common cold, but they may set off a train of asthmatic symptoms lasting days or weeks. There has been no systematic attempt to isolate and identify the specific bacteria or viruses which initiate these infections; presumably the same organisms implicated in respiratory infections in normal individuals are involved.

Allergic bronchopulmonary aspergillosis is a specific infection occurring in asthmatic patients in whom endobronchial growth of *Aspergillus fumigatus* is accompanied by prolonged asthma, expectoration of small brown "plugs" of mycelia, transient pulmonary infiltrates, and eosinophils in the sputum and blood. The diagnosis may be suspected from the character of the pulmonary infiltrates and the appearance of the sputum and is established by demonstration of mycelia on microscopic examination of the sputum and positive cultures for *A. fumigatus*. These infections have been recognized repeatedly in Great Britain but appear to be rare in the United States. They respond to the usual measures for asthma but may recur.

In about a third of patients, emotional strain and specific stressful life situations appear to be important factors in initiating asthmatic episodes. It would be presumptuous to identify a specific kind of psychologic stress as generating asthma or to describe an "asthmatic personality." Nevertheless, many asthmatic episodes occur when there are no detectable external factors except psychologic stress.

"Tokyo-Yokohama asthma" or *"New Orleans asthma"* refers to a greatly increased rate of asthmatic attacks which have appeared at times of heavy air pollution in highly industrialized urban areas in individuals not otherwise troubled with asthma. The relationship to industrial air pollution is suggestive but not proved. Nevertheless, several surveys in large cities have indicated that emergency room visits by patients with known asthma are much more frequent on days of increased air pollution. The specific pollutants acting as irritants in these situations are unknown.

The etiologic factors which have been incriminated in asthmatic episodes may be acting in individuals with an underlying physiologic defect which predisposes them to bronchospasm. For example, asthmatic patients will react with a greater degree of bronchospasm for a longer period to drugs such as acetylcholine, mecholyl, histamine, serotonin, or cholinesterase inhibitors than normal, and are also unusually sensitive to nonspecific irritants such as dusts, cooking odors, and gaseous air pollutants. They will respond to vigorous exercise with bronchospasm and react more vigorously to the above-mentioned stimuli after treatment with β-adrenergic blocking agents such as propranolol. Therefore, these drugs are contraindicated in asthmatic patients. If there is an acquired or innate physiologic defect in some or all asthmatic patients, its nature is unknown.

DIAGNOSIS. Certain specific causes of local or generalized airway obstruction must be considered when a patient comes initially to the physician with asthma. Generally, wheezing and rhonchi are heard throughout the chest; localized wheezing indicates endobronchial disease, such as foreign body aspiration, neoplasm, or stenosis. The symptoms of airway obstruction in localized endobronchial disease are at times spasmodic and may mimic asthma closely. "Cardiac asthma" or wheezing occurring during cardiac failure or pulmonary edema usually can be differentiated from paroxysmal asthma by the presence of moist rales, blood-tinged sputum, and other signs of heart failure (Chap. 264). Asthma occasionally is a presenting manifestation of polyarteritis nodosa (Chap. 391). Reactions to drugs, particularly aspirin, are an occasional cause of severe asthma. Loeffler's allergic pneumonitis, caused by parasitic infestation of the lungs, is often accompanied by asthma.

Poisoning with cholinergic drugs or insecticides may induce bronchoconstriction and expiratory dyspnea that can be specifically relieved with atropine (Chap. 116). Carcinoid tumors which elaborate serotonin may be associated with asthma (Chap. 105). Sometimes, cerebral trauma may result in asthmatic symptoms.

Chemical pneumonias such as silo-filler's disease (Chap. 289) may be accompanied by difficult breathing resembling asthma. On the other hand, allergic interstitial pneumonitis, which is a hypersensitivity reaction to inhaled organic dusts, usually is not accompanied by bronchospasm.

LABORATORY FINDINGS. Skin tests used for the diagnosis of allergic asthma are no different from those used for the diagnosis of hay fever (see below). There are no specific laboratory tests that define the allergic etiology, but finding an increased number of eosinophils in sputum and blood occasionally will suggest an allergic cause of asthma. Measurements of pulmonary function will demonstrate increased airway resistance and hyperinflation which are almost completely reversible between attacks. Frequent measurements of arterial P_{O_2} and P_{CO_2} may be crucial in assessing the severity of status asthmaticus and the response to therapy.

THERAPY. Specific Treatment. As is the case in hay fever, elimination of the offending antigen from the patient's environment is the most successful means of preventing and treating allergic asthma. Mechanical obstruction of the tracheobronchial tree should be corrected, and infection of the sinuses should be treated.

Specific desensitization or hyposensitization of the pa-

tient with asthma due to inhaled antigens is performed as in hay fever but may be less effective, and improvement usually does not persist when desensitization is discontinued.

The frequent occurrence of bronchial infection in adults with nonseasonal or chronic asthma necessitates special consideration. The pneumococcus and *Hemophilus influenzae* are the microorganisms most often isolated from the bronchi and sputum of patients with asthma and chronic bronchitis, and exacerbations of cough and dyspnea may be associated with an increase in the number of these bacteria. These patients may be treated with tetracycline, 0.5 to 1.0 Gm per day, or ampicillin, 1.0 Gm per day, continuously during the winter months or at the earliest sign that symptoms are increasing. This approach may lead to a significant decrease in the severity and frequency of exacerbations.

Nonspecific Treatment. Treatment of acute asthma is most effective when begun soon after onset of the paroxysm. Mild attacks may be readily relieved by inhalation of 50 to 150 μg of nebulized isoproterenol. A variety of commercial products which furnish a measured dose of isoproterenol with inert freon as a propellant are available. The smallest amount consistent with relief should be employed, and administration should not be repeated more often than every 3 hr. With a rapidly developing severe paroxysm, 0.3 to 1.0 ml of 1:1,000 epinephrine should be injected subcutaneously; this dose may be repeated as needed but no more often than every 30 min. Both isoproterenol and epinephrine may become ineffective after repeated use in a prolonged asthmatic attack. There are reports that a single inhalation of isoproterenol may have caused paradoxic bronchospasm (following an initial transient decrease in airway resistance) in a few patients who had used the drug excessively for unremitting asthma over several days. Some asthmatic deaths may be associated with overuse of isoproterenol, as its effectiveness in relieving bronchospasm becomes progressively less.

Early in attacks, a sedative such as amobarbital, 50 or 100 mg, may be desirable to allay agitation and relieve anxiety. As the attack becomes more severe and prolonged, sedatives become less desirable because the patient needs every faculty for the work of breathing. Respiratory arrest has been reported in severely asthmatic patients shortly after injections of sedative or tranquilizing drugs. Drugs which depress respiration such as morphine have been the apparent cause of sudden death and should never be used during asthmatic episodes.

Aminophylline is an active bronchodilator and may be used with, or in preference to, epinephrine. It may be given intravenously or rectally; a dose of 0.5 Gm is usually required for adequate bronchodilatation. It is ordinarily not possible to give this dose orally without gastric irritation. Intravenous aminophylline must be given slowly, and it is desirable to dilute 0.5 Gm in 50 ml of 5 percent glucose and to administer it in a drip over a 20-min period. Hydration to prevent inspissation of mucus is important, and it is often convenient to follow intravenous medication with a liter or more of 5 percent glucose.

When epinephrine and aminophylline are poorly effective in relieving bronchospasm or there is prompt recurrence, administration of corticosteroids is necessary. Daily doses will range between 15 and 80 mg prednisone, and a favorable response cannot be expected for several hours. Considerable foresight is required to select those patients who will require steroids for adequate control, because the physical signs of asthma are often misleading. Early determination of arterial P_{O_2} and P_{CO_2} often will help to recognize those patients who are on the verge of ventilatory failure and who will require prompt and vigorous therapy. Increasing carbon dioxide tension despite treatment is a grave prognostic sign and may mean that tracheostomy and mechanical ventilation will be necessary to prevent death.

When steroids are required, 100 to 300 mg hydrocortisone may be given intravenously, although this route probably is no more effective than the oral route. Once initiated, steroids should be continued to maintain improvement, and then tapered as rapidly as is consistent with continued control of asthma.

Continuous administration of adrenal steroids to patients with chronic asthma or asthmatic bronchitis has been effective and safe in preventing paroxysms. The dose required is usually less than 20 mg prednisone or its equivalent per day. This regimen has been continued for several years in many patients without serious side effects or complications. In fact, patients with severe asthma accompanying infections often have fewer episodes of infection while receiving adrenal steroids continuously.

Prophylactic management of asthmatic patients involves the use of drugs to abort paroxysms. Oral ephedrine, 25 to 50 mg, and phenobarbital, 30 to 60 mg, may be given three or four times a day when the patient is most likely to develop asthma. Recommended doses of oral theophylline or aminophylline preparations contain too little drug to be effective, and effective doses usually cause gastric irritation. Smoking is undesirable in asthmatics, as are obesity, excessive exertion, fatigue, and dietary indiscretion.

ALLERGIC RHINITIS (Hay Fever)

DEFINITION. Allergic rhinitis is characterized by sneezing, rhinorrhea, swelling of the nasal mucosa, itching of the eyes, and lacrimation. Hay fever is the common term for allergic rhinitis due to seasonal spread of pollens in the air, but the disease is not necessarily seasonal and may result from exposure to antigens other than pollen. *Vasomotor rhinitis* designates those diseases without allergic or infectious etiology which resemble hay fever.

ETIOLOGY. Plants that spread large amounts of airborne pollen are common sources of antigens responsible for hay fever, but those pollinated by insects, including most flowering plants such as roses and goldenrod, are not. Ragweed pollen is the principal offender

in the United States. It is prevalent in the central, eastern, and southeastern part of the country, but virtually absent west of the Rocky Mountains. Ordinarily ragweed pollinates between early August and late October, the most likely season for hay fever.

In the northern half of the United States, grasses pollinate from May to July, while in the South grass may pollinate throughout the year. Although the time of year when trees pollinate may vary, they ordinarily do so in early spring, and earlier in the South than in the North. Some widespread airborne pollens are nonallergenic; pine pollen, for instance, almost never causes hay fever. Certain widespread molds, found most frequently on decaying vegetation, which also propagate by means of airborne spores, appear in definite seasons. *Hormodendrum* has a peak incidence in July and *Alternaria* in October; both may cause seasonal allergic rhinitis.

Most pollen particles are about 25 to 40 μ in diameter and settle promptly from the air. The settling properties of pollen are used for crude estimations of the "pollen count" in the air by collecting and enumerating particles on a greased glass slide. There is an approximate but regular correlation between the pollen count and the frequency and severity of hay fever in the exposed population. Pollen particles from plants, grasses, or trees of varying types can be differentiated by microscopic examination, permitting precise definition of the airborne pollens responsible for hay fever.

Pollen particles are relatively large and, when inhaled, will impinge on and be deposited within the nose. Very few particles would be expected to reach the terminal bronchioles. House dust, fungus spores, animal danders, feathers, broken insect parts, facial powders, vegetable dusts, insecticides, and food particles disseminated during cooking also have been incriminated as causes of hay fever; the etiologic relationship between ingested food and respiratory allergy has been difficult to document.

PATHOGENESIS. When pollens and mold spores land on the nasal mucosa, their carbohydrate coat is digested by the lysozyme of respiratory mucus, which releases the protein contents. Careful analysis reveals that the grains of ragweed and grass pollens contain several specific proteins, referred to as *allergens,* which account for the sensitizing potential of the pollen. The allergens are of relatively low molecular weight (10,000 to 40,000) and consist of 1 percent or less of the extractable solids of the pollen. The biologic potency of these allergens is such that intradermal injection of 1 $\mu\mu$ will cause a wheal and erythema reaction when injected intradermally in a sensitive patient. Other pollen, mold, and dander allergens are less well characterized but appear to have similar properties. Presumably, it is the unusual ability of allergic individuals to become sensitized following release of these allergens in the respiratory tract that leads to allergic disease.

The sensitivity in hay fever is not confined to the mucous membranes but is general and is exemplified by the ability of the entire skin to react. Furthermore, the granulocytic leukocytes in vitro will respond to the addition of pollen extract by secreting histamine into the surrounding medium. This process requires living metabolizing cells and is independent of the presence of complement. These reactions are conferred by the fixation to cells of "reaginic" antibodies, a special type of antibodies which are usually of the IgE class, which have a particular affinity for cells, and which are usually detected by the Prausnitz-Küstner test (see below). Allergen-induced release of histamine from mucosal tissue mast cells sensitized by reaginic antibody probably accounts for the major manifestations of respiratory allergies. The ability to synthesize reagins is not confined to allergic individuals; nearly everyone will develop wheal and erythema skin reactivity to repeated intradermal injections of antigens such as ascaris extract and bovine ribonuclease. Allergic individuals, however, are likely to develop such reactions to antigens instilled into the nose, while normal individuals rarely do. The nature of the defect responsible for this phenomenon is unknown, but it is probably hereditary, because there is a strong tendency for allergic disease to run in families. The mode of inheritance has not been determined, but when both parents have "atopic" disease, the allergy in the offspring is apt to be unusually severe. In all, from 5 to 15 percent of individuals are atopic—i.e., they are capable of developing allergy to inhaled antigens.

The nasal mucosa of patients with hay fever or allergic rhinitis also appears to be more susceptible to the effects of irritants than is the nasal mucosa of normal persons. Furthermore, studies in volunteers indicate that persons with allergic rhinitis are more susceptible to infection by respiratory viruses than are normal persons. This enhanced reactivity of the nasal mucosa to a variety of stimuli also may explain the effects of emotional disturbances in exaggerating and possibly initiating symptoms of rhinitis in the allergic individual.

MANIFESTATIONS. Pruritus about the eyes, nose, throat, and mouth, nasal discharge, sneezing, and lacrimation are the characteristic features of hay fever or allergic rhinitis. Particularly troublesome to the patient is mucosal swelling with occlusion of the airway, making breathing difficult and often causing insomnia. Symptoms vary in severity from day to day.

Occlusion of the nasal passages by swelling of the turbinates and mucous membranes may result in obstruction of the sinus ostiums or the eustachian tube, and infection of the sinuses and middle ear is a relatively common complication of perennial allergic rhinitis but is uncommon in seasonal hay fever. In addition, infection of the sinuses or nose in patients with allergic rhinitis results in formation of nasal polyps. These polyps further obstruct the nasal passages, increase symptoms, and exaggerate infection.

Many persons with hay fever or allergic rhinitis subsequently develop asthma. Retrobulbar neuritis, laryngeal edema with hoarseness, angioedema, urticaria, and other allergic illnesses occasionally accompany allergic rhinitis.

DIAGNOSIS. Symptoms of allergic rhinitis or hay fever occur in situations where allergy cannot be incriminated. For example, sneezing, watery nasal discharge, and lacrimation may develop upon exposure to an atmosphere heavily contaminated with smoke, dust, or other irritants. Similarly, these symptoms often herald the onset of a viral upper respiratory tract infection. The symptoms of hay fever are attributable to nonsuppurative inflammation of the nasal mucosa, and any situation resulting in inflammation of the nose can produce an illness which is indistinguishable from allergic rhinitis. Ingestion of alcoholic beverages and emotional stimuli may also produce hyperemia of the nasal mucous membranes, exaggerating the symptoms of allergic rhinitis. Polycythemia vera may occasionally be recognized initially because of nasal and conjunctival hyperemia, resulting in symptoms resembling those of hay fever. Certain drugs, particularly rauwolfia derivatives, may have similar effects.

The pale and edematous appearance of the nasal mucosa helps to distinguish allergic rhinitis or hay fever. The conjunctivas and the skin about the eyes, nose, and occasionally the mouth are reddened. In addition, nasal polyps are characteristic of allergic nasal disease, although infection in the nose or sinuses may also be present. Microscopic examination of nasal secretions shows many eosinophils.

Of great importance in the diagnosis of hay fever is its seasonal occurrence, which coincides with pollination of weeds, grasses, or trees. Allergic rhinitis due to local contamination of the patient's environment is diagnosed by carefully correlating the patient's symptoms with exposure to potential allergens at home, at work, and at play. The continuous character of perennial allergic rhinitis makes an allergic etiology less readily recognizable. Examination of nasal secretions for eosinophils, however, is often helpful. Blood eosinophilia also is found occasionally in patients with allergic rhinitis.

Skin Tests. Approximately 25 percent of the normal population will develop wheal and erythema skin reactions following intracutaneous inoculation of common airborne antigens. Not all persons with positive skin reactions, however, have allergic rhinitis. The allergic patient commonly has positive skin reactions to many antigens when from the history only one or two are incriminated as the cause of symptoms. Skin tests with allergenic antigens, therefore, are of more value in detecting an allergic propensity than in detecting the specific antigen responsible for the patient's symptoms. Only careful correlation of the skin reactivity with the environmental circumstances will delineate the responsible antigen.

Tests are performed with crude aqueous extracts of pollen, dust, foods, animal dander, insects, and other substances. These extracts are commercially available, but their potency varies considerably. No method of standardization is very reliable, because the extracts are crude and the measurement of specific antigen has not been possible.

Skin tests are done by applying a drop of antigen to a skin scratch or by intradermal inoculation of 0.01 to 0.02 ml. In the beginning, very dilute extract should be used. The concentration may be increased gradually until there is certainty that the patient has a negative reaction. Ordinarily, it is unwise to test a patient repeatedly on the same day or to test with many extracts at one time. Positive reactions appear within 15 to 20 min and are characterized by wheal and erythema formation and local pruritus. If large doses of extract are given, symptoms of hay fever or even a generalized reaction may be produced. Extracts of foods are available for skin testing, but their use should be limited because it is preferable to diagnose allergy to foods by history and by elimination diets. Identification of bacteria in the respiratory tract which are potentially responsible for infection is more valuable than skin testing with bacterial extracts.

When it is undesirable to perform skin tests in young children or in persons with generalized skin disease, passive transfer of the patient's serum to normal recipients may be performed (Prausnitz-Küstner, or P-K test). Ordinarily, 0.05 to 0.1 ml of the patient's serum is injected intradermally into the recipient, and 24 hr later normal skin and sites injected with serum are tested with the antigenic extracts.

Epinephrine and ephedrine greatly reduce the wheal and erythema response to intradermally injected antigen, as do large doses of antihistamines; these drugs should not be administered before skin testing. Adrenocortical steroids have little effect on these reactions.

THERAPY. Specific Treatment. Elimination of the offending antigen from the patient's environment is the most effective means of controlling allergic disease. This is not always easy, even when the antigen is known. If it is determined that dander from dogs or cats is responsible, for example, then animals should be avoided. When feathers are found to be responsible for allergic symptoms, a feather pillow should be replaced by one of foam rubber. Air filtration is often useful in controlling symptoms due to airborne pollens, but occasionally it may be necessary to advise the patient to live in a pollen-free area during the hay fever season. Mechanical obstruction of the nasal airway, which may aggravate the symptoms of rhinitis, should be corrected, and infection should be treated with an antibacterial drug capable of eradicating the specific microorganism. Alleviation of emotional disturbances by the use of drugs, correction of the environment, or psychiatric guidance occasionally will alleviate the symptoms of allergy.

Desensitization, hyposensitization, or immunization with the antigens recognized as specifically responsible for allergic respiratory disease may be effective. Controlled studies of desensitization in patients with hay fever due to ragweed pollen have shown that approximately 80 percent of patients are partially relieved of their symptoms, while only 25 percent of patients given a placebo improved. Improvement appears to be related to two factors: the development of normal circulating IgG antibodies ("blocking" antibodies) which can combine with the antigen and block its ability to trigger cellular histamine release, and an actual reduction (sometimes complete abolition) of the cellular sensitivity which confers the allergic reaction. The reasons for the reduction in cellular sensitivity are not clear, because the patient continues to have circulating reaginic antibody, although in reduced titer.

Treatment by desensitization may be perennial, coseasonal, or preseasonal. Continued therapy throughout the year probably is preferable to intermittent treatment, but the dose of antigen in some patients must be reduced considerably during the season of the year when symptoms are expected to occur. The beneficial effects of desensitization persist for some months after treatment is discontinued, but the allergic symptoms tend to recur eventually.

Bacterial vaccines have been employed in desensitizing patients with allergic rhinitis. Because of the lack of evidence for bacterial hypersensitivity as a cause of allergic respiratory disease and the lack of data that such treatment is effective, it cannot be recommended.

Nonspecific Treatment. Many patients can be relieved of their complaints with symptomatic therapy. The severity, recurrence, and refractoriness to symptomatic treatment will determine whether or not specific desensitization should be attempted. Antihistamines, such as tripellenamine, 50 mg; diphenhydramine, 50 mg; chlorpheniramine, 4 mg; and many others, often are effective in controlling hay fever. Their repeated use frequently is associated with gradually decreasing effectiveness, but when one drug fails, another may be effective. In addition they may produce drowsiness and reduce physical and mental dexterity.

Oral adrenocortical steroids are extraordinarily effective in relieving the symptoms of most patients with allergic respiratory disease and were it not for their side effects, could be generally recommended as the drugs of choice in hay fever. Nevertheless, they can be used to manage acute symptoms, and in some patients small daily doses will suppress symptoms completely during an entire season. Hydrocortisone, 25 to 100 mg, prednisone 5 to 20 mg, and methylprednisolone, 4 to 12 mg each day, are all usually quite effective. Adrenal steroids can cause a remarkable disappearance of nasal polyps when used in patients with perennial rhinitis. The benefit derived from adrenal steroids always must be balanced against the potential side effects of these potent drugs.

Small doses of the water-soluble steroid dexamethasone sprayed into the nose three or four times a day effectively suppress the symptoms of all but the severest hay fever without danger of systemic side effects. The effect of the steroid is local and cannot be duplicated by the same dose given orally. As further experience accumulates, intranasal dexamethasone may become accepted as the treatment of choice in allergic rhinitis. Shrinkage of polyps also can be achieved by this treatment.

A variety of agents are available for shrinking the nasal mucous membrane to relieve obstruction of the nasal airways. Aqueous phenylephrine (0.25 or 0.5 percent) is an effective nasal decongestant that is useful in patients who are very uncomfortable from hay fever or allergic rhinitis until other remedies can correct the underlying disease. Repeated use of the drug, however, may cause reactive hyperemia of the nasal mucosa, further exaggerating the symptoms of rhinitis. Orally administered ephedrine, 25 mg, or pseudoephedrine, 60 mg, may also be used to shrink nasal mucous membranes, but they have limited effectiveness. Atropine-like drugs may help to dry up excessive nasal secretions, if there is no concomitant asthma.

ALLERGIC SKIN DISEASE

There are many dermatologic manifestations of allergy, including contact dermatitis, urticaria, angioedema, erythematous rashes, and eczema. These are roughly divisible into those related to "delayed" and "immediate" hypersensitivity. Urticaria and angioedema usually are manifestations of immediate hypersensitivity, while contact dermatitis and many instances of eczematous dermatitis are attributable to delayed hypersensitivity. At times an antigen may induce and elicit both immediate and delayed hypersensitivity reactions, resulting in both urticaria and eczema.

Urticaria, angioedema, contact dermatitis, and erythematous rashes are the principal forms of allergy in which the skin is the major target organ. Many other rashes are attributed to systemic allergic disease, including erythema nodosum, erythema multiforme, exfoliation, bullae, purpura, "fixed" drug eruptions, and photosensitivity. Certain supposed immunologic diseases such as systemic lupus erythematosus, dermatomyositis, rheumatic fever, and scleroderma also are characterized by "allergic" skin lesions.

CONTACT DERMATITIS. See Chap. 400.

URTICARIA. Urticaria (hives) is characterized by white or red evanescent wheals, papules, or macules that are surrounded by erythema and are pruritic. They may be generalized, but they commonly appear in areas of skin covered by clothing. Urticaria also may involve mucous membranes such as the stomach and mouth and frequently is accompanied by eosinophilia. It often occurs in serum sickness (Chap. 74) or in combination with hay fever and allergic asthma. Emotional tension, increased heat, and physical exercise may exaggerate urticaria. Urticaria can be induced by histamine and acetylcholine, and good evidence indicates that liberation of histamine during an allergic reaction is responsible for hives. Urticaria may occur from ingestion, inhalation, injection, or contact with the offending antigen. Foods and drugs frequently are responsible, but hives also have been related to a great variety of inhalants and contactants, such as pollen, dander, dust, feathers, and wool. As in other allergic diseases, the responsible antigen may be detected by careful history, skin test, or elimination diets.

If a specific cause of urticaria is found, it should be corrected or the antigen eliminated from the environment. Acute symptoms usually respond to antihistamines, but adrenal steroids may be needed. Epinephrine, 0.2 to 0.5 ml of 1:1,000 aqueous solution intramuscularly, provides prompt but transient relief. Chronic, idiopathic urticaria is often refractory to treatment, and many of these patients require psychiatric assistance. Prolonged use of adrenal steroids in chronic urticaria is inadvisable.

When first seen, subacute lupus erythematosus occasionally resembles recurrent urticaria.

Angioedema is characterized by edema of the eyelids, lips, external genitalia, and the mucous membranes of the mouth, tongue, or gastrointestinal tract. The swelling may be localized to one area or may be diffuse, and commonly is acompanied by urticaria elsewhere. When the respiratory tract is involved, the patient may have laryngeal edema with hoarseness, stridor, and cyanosis, and rarely death may ensue. Generally, angioedema is attributed to food allergy; shellfish very commonly are incriminated. In addition, the reaction may occur from the many antigens responsible for urticaria. The treatment of angioedema is the same as for urticaria. If respiratory tract obstruction occurs, tracheostomy may prove lifesaving.

A rare form of angioedema is inherited as an autosomal dominant trait and begins in childhood. Nonpruritic angioedematous swellings in the skin characteristically are acompanied by angioedema of the gut, which may result in abdominal pain and lead to unnecessary laparotomy. The diagnosis is made by demonstrating a specific deficiency of a serum protein that inhibits the first component of complement and the proteolytic enzyme kallikrein. There is no specific treatment.

REFERENCES

ALLERGIC RHINITIS

Lowell, F. C., and W. Franklin: A "Double-blind" Study of Treatment with Aqueous Allergenic Extracts in Cases of Allergic Rhinitis, J. Allergy, 34:165, 1963.

Norman, P. S.: Treatment of Allergic Rhinitis, Johns Hopkins Med. J., 121:49, 1967.

Samter, M., and H. L. Alexander: "Immunological Diseases," Boston, Little, Brown and Company, 1965.

ALLERGIC SKIN DISEASE

Waughan, W. T., and J. H. Black: "Practice of Allergy," St. Louis, The C. V. Mosby Company, 1954.

ASTHMA

Bates, D. V., and R. U. Christie: "Respiratory Function in Disease," Philadelphia, W. B. Saunders Company, 1965.

Gay, L. N.: The Pathology of Asthma, Clinics, 5:347, 1946.

Williams, D. A., E. Lewis-Fanning, L. Rees, J. Jacobs, and A. Thomas: Assessment of the Relative Importance of the Allergic, Infective and Psychologic Factors in Asthma, Acta Allergol, 12:376, 1958.

73 REACTIONS TO DRUGS
Leighton E. Cluff

The incidence of adverse reactions to drugs has paralleled the growing use of pharmaceuticals, and with continued introduction of new drugs, this problem has become even more serious.

DEFINITION. Classification of drug reactions is not easy, but undesired responses to therapeutic agents have certain specific features that facilitate categorization. Nearly any drug can elicit pharmacologic effects other than those for which it is usually administered, and when these appear, they are referred to as *side effects*. Some patients show unusual susceptibility to the pharmacologic actions of a drug and are said to have an *idiosyncrasy*. Reactions not explained by the pharmacologic properties of a drug, and therefore indicative of altered reactivity of the patient, are termed *allergic*. Pharmacologic effects, as a rule, are intensified by increasing dosage or cumulative action (*toxic effects*), and readministration is not associated with increased reactivity of the patient. For example, nausea, hyperpnea, and tinnitus in a person given aspirin are side effects, and reduction in dosage will usually alleviate the situation. The occasional patient who displays these symptoms after taking a small amount of aspirin has an idiosyncrasy to the drug. However, if ingestion of aspirin is followed by bronchial asthma or urticaria, reactions not explainable by the pharmacologic action of the drug, the patient is allergic to it. This type of reaction is likely to be associated with symptoms commonly ascribed to hypersensitivity (rash, asthma, pruritus, arthritis, fever, leukopenia, etc.), frequently recurs promptly on readministration of the drug, and is not closely dependent on dosage or cumulative action.

The clinical importance of differentiating side effects, idiosyncrasy, and allergy relates to the hazard of readministration of a drug or to its probable safety in lower dosage.

ETIOLOGY. Allergy to drugs is attributed to immunologic mechanisms and may be manifested by immediate or delayed hypersensitivity. Most pharmacologic agents, however, are incapable of initiating an immunologic response by themselves, and the actual antigen is a conjugate of the drug or its derivatives with autologous proteins. Under such circumstances, the drug acts as a *hapten,* is nonantigenic by itself, but confers antigenic specificity to the protein, which is able to combine with the antibody or react with cells of the sensitized person. Many drugs are bound by body proteins, and there is experimental evidence that the ability of chemical compounds to elicit allergic contact dermatitis can be correlated with their affinity for sulfhydryl-containing proteins of skin. Practically all drugs bind to serum protein, particularly albumin, after absorption, but there is little to suggest that these protein-drug conjugates are important in drug allergy. Other tissue proteins also may bind drugs, but those specifically responsible for rendering a chemical antigenic are not known. The firmness of the combination of a drug or chemical to protein is a determinant of the antigenicity of the complex. Furthermore, the administered drug may be less important in inducing an immunologic response than its degradation products. For example, penicillenic acid and penicilloic acid, degradation products of penicillin, are believed to be responsible for most instances of penicillin allergy. Identification of penicilloyl derivatives in penicillin allergy was predicated upon the knowledge that they could conjugate firmly to proteins.

Serum antibody has been demonstrated in some persons with drug allergy involving cellular elements of blood, as in agranulocytosis, hemolytic anemia, and thrombocytopenia. In other types of drug hypersensitivity, however, precipitation, hemagglutination, or complement fixation tests with a patient's serum may be negative, and direct intradermal or passive transfer tests of the Prausnitz-Küstner type are often unrevealing. In addition, demonstration of agglutination by serum of erythrocytes sensitized with a drug such as penicillin may fail to differentiate the allergic from the nonallergic individual. These results however, are more indicative of the inadequacy of present methods of testing than an argument against an immunologic basis for hypersensitivity to drugs. Demonstration of penicilloyl derivatives associated with penicillin hypersensitivity has provided an important diagnostic test for penicillin allergy. A significant proportion of persons who have penicillin allergy will have a positive wheal and flare skin test to penicilloyl conjugated to a polylysine carrier. Moreover, a positive skin test to minor determinants (which is usually elicited by penicillin G) reflects individuals with the greatest propensity to develop serious systemic anaphylaxis. Though these skin tests indicate that some progress has been made in detecting drug reactions, particularly those to penicillin, the lack of effective testing methods is a great handicap to clinical investigation of these reactions.

Most types of allergic reactions to drugs are nonfamilial; however, anaphylaxis may occur more commonly in persons with other allergic disease, such as hay fever, asthma, or urticaria. Certain diseases seem to predispose to the development of drug allergy. For example, patients with inflammatory or necrotizing gastrointestinal lesions appear to be particularly susceptible to orally administered drugs. Furthermore, the patient acquiring a reaction to one drug often develops allergic reactions to other drugs, but manifestations may differ.

The likelihood of a patient developing an adverse reaction to a drug is directly related to the number of different medications administered. Approximately 5 percent of hospitalized individuals receiving fewer than six different drugs will experience a drug-induced illness. Over 40 percent of hospitalized patients receiving more than 16 different drugs will have an adverse reaction. In part this is attributed to an additive effect, but pharmacologic interactions or incompatibilities also account for the increased rate of adverse reactions when many drugs are given.

Five percent of patients admitted to a hospital have a drug-induced illness; they are three times more likely to acquire another drug-induced illness during hospitalization than patients admitted without an adverse drug reaction. Similarly, a prior history of untoward drug effects is associated with predisposition to subsequent drug-induced illness. In part, this predisposition may be due to genetic differences between patients, exemplified by the susceptibility of individuals with glucose-6 phosphate dehydrogenase deficiency to hemolytic anemia following administration of primaquine and nitrofurans.

Renal and liver dysfunction obviously influences drug metabolism and excretion, and may affect the frequency of adverse reactions to certain drugs. The dosage of many drugs, particularly antibiotics, should be adjusted in the presence of renal and hepatic disease.

Sedatives and tranquilizers most often are incriminated as causes of adverse drug reactions in hospitalized patients. The antibiotics, digitalis, and diuretics are next in importance. Penicillin is the drug most frequently incriminated as a cause of drug allergy, particularly anaphylaxis.

EPIDEMIOLOGY. The incidence of adverse reactions to drugs is not known accurately because there have been few efforts to relate the number of adverse reactions observed to the patients at risk who are taking the drug. From the information available, it appears that most adverse reactions to drugs are not serious and that reactions vary in frequency among drugs. Women are more likely to show adverse reactions to drugs than men. With a few exceptions, exemplified by adverse drug reactions related to genetically abnormal erythrocytes, race and age in adults do not affect the incidence of reaction to drugs. Most reactions develop within 7 to 10 days of drug administration. There appears to be an increased likelihood of adverse drug reaction when multiple drugs are taken by the same patient.

MANIFESTATIONS. Adverse effects of drugs attributed to their pharmacologic action are drug-specific. Allergic reactions, however, are often the same irrespective of the incriminated drug. Some presumed allergic reactions, however, are more common with certain drugs than with others.

The commonest manifestations of allergy to drugs are no different from hypersensitivity reactions of other types and include rashes, asthma, and the symptoms of serum sickness. These are easily recognized clinically as allergic in origin. Other features of drug allergy are less easily characterized. The tabulation in Table 73-1 of common drugs and reactions they may elicit includes some effects that may not be allergic at all.

Skin. Morbilliform, urticarial, and maculopapular rashes are probably the most common skin reactions, but many others are observed, including vesicular, bullous, exfoliative, eczematous, and purpuric eruptions. Pruritus is frequent. Although the type of skin lesion usually will not help identify the causative drug, certain skin reactions are relatively specific. Erythema multiforme or nodosum is seen in allergy to Dilantin, bromides, iodides, trimethadione, and sulfonamides. "Fixed" drug eruptions are most frequently due to aminopyrine, phenolphthalein, or atabrine. Photosensitization during drug therapy occurs characteristically with chlorpromazine, phenothiazine, sulfonamides, and tetracycline derivatives.

Fever. Fever may be an isolated manifestation of drug allergy, and most pharmaceuticals in common use can produce a febrile reaction, including most antibiotics and chemotherapeutic agents. However, the tetracycline derivatives are uncommon causes of drug fever, and digitalis has rarely, if ever, been incriminated as the cause of a pyrogenic reaction. Elevation of temperature may appear abruptly after treatment begins, or it may develop in a stepwise fashion during or after the second week of drug administration. Drug fever is often associated with chills and constitutional symptoms and may be accompanied by leukocytosis. Discontinuing therapy usually results in defervescence within a short period, although several days may be required for return of temperature to normal.

Blood. Changes in the formed elements of the blood are common during drug allergy and may have no specificity. Some drugs have been found to have limited or no effects on the blood, while others produce specific abnormalities. For example, penicillin has not been incriminated as a cause of serious hematologic abnormalities. In therapeutic doses, acetanilid is probably not a cause of anemia, agranulocytosis, thrombocytopenia, or aplastic anemia; in high dosage, however, it may produce leukocytosis, methemoglobinemia, and acute hemolysis. *Methemoglobinemia* also occurs with antipyrine, nitrites, sulfonamides, primaquine, and pamaquine, but this reaction is probably not allergic in origin. Barbiturates, salicylates, and para-aminosalicylic acid rarely, if ever, produce agranulocytosis. *Eosinophilia* may accompany allergic reactions of many types, but it occurs with such frequency as an isolated finding during therapy with streptomycin or nirvanol that it has no significance. *Lymphocytosis* is common in patients receiving Dilantin and nirvanol, and polymorphonuclear leukocytosis may be found in individuals taking Dilantin or atropine. Studies of the erythrocyte abnormality responsible for the *acute hemolytic anemia* induced by primaquine, sulfonamides, and nitrofurans in certain individuals indicate that what was thought to be drug allergy is actually a genetically determined enzyme deficiency. Jaundice due to pharmaceutical agents is discussed elsewhere (Chap. 327).

Nervous System. A variety of neurologic manifestations may appear during drug therapy, but in the majority of instances there is little evidence to incriminate allergy as a cause. The commonest reaction is delirium, seen particularly with digitalis, atropine, thiocyanates, and sedatives. Other drugs that produce adverse effects on the nervous system (ranging from paresthesias and peripheral neuritis to deafness) are streptomycin, hydralazine, chlorpromazine, Diamox, isoniazid, polymyxin, neomycin, and kanamycin.

Others. Nausea, vomiting, and diarrhea are exceedingly common drug reactions. In addition, *abdominal pain* in the absence of other symptoms may be produced by quinidine, chlorpromazine, and primaquine. *Albuminuria* and *cylindruria* occur particularly with heavy metals, bacitracin, polymyxin, and colimycin. Dilantin, chloral hydrate, sulfonamides, trimethadione, Phenurone, colchicin, thiocyanate, and amphotericin B occasionally produce renal dysfunction, probably because of their direct toxic action. Amphotericin B may produce tubular necrosis and renal calcification, but this is only occasionally associated with significant evidence of renal insufficiency and nitrogen retention. Hypersensitivity to sulfonamides has resulted in acute hemorrhagic nephritis.

Histologic lesions indistinguishable from those of *polyarteritis nodosa* have been found in the tissues of patients who have experienced allergic reactions to iodides, Dilantin, sulfonamides, and penicillin. Manifestations of

Table 73-1. ADVERSE REACTIONS TO DRUGS

Drug	Gastrointestinal				Cutaneous							Hematologic (Marrow failure)							Metabolic			Neurologic				Ear and eye		Allergic			Cardiorenal			Collagen-vascular syndromes	Fetal and neonatal effects
	Nausea-vomiting	Diarrhea	GI bleeding	Jaundice	Dermatitis	Acneiform eruption	Erythema multiforme	Urticaria	Purpura	Fixed eruption	Photosensitization	Red blood cells	White blood cells	Platelets	Hemolysis	Leukocytosis	Eosinophilia	Hypoprothrombinemia	Hypokalemia	Hyperuricemia	Hyperglycemia	Delirium	Convulsions	Peripheral neuropathy	Extrapyramidal syndrome	C$_8$ nerve damage	Ocular damage	Anaphylaxis	Fever	"Serum sickness"	Arrhythmia	Hypotension	Renal disorder		
Acetazolamide					+						+	+	+	+					+					+					+				+		
Acetophenetidin					+			+	+	+		+	+	+	+	+													+				+		
Alkylating agents	+	+	+	+	+			+			+	+	+	+						+									+				+		+
Aminopyrine					+			+		+			+		+														+		+				
Aminosalicylic acid	+	+	+	+	+								+	+	+	+	+	+											+	+	+				
Amphotericin B	+	+										+												+					+				+		
Anabolic steroids	+			+		+																													+
Antihistamines	+				+			+				+	+	+														+	+	+		+			
Antimetabolites	+	+	+	+					+			+	+	+						+									+						+
Barbiturates					+		+	+	+	+		+										+							+	+					
Belladonna alkaloids					+											+						+							+						
Benzothiadiazines	+		+	+	+						+		+	+					+	+	+												+		+
Bromides	+					+	+	+														+							+				+		
Chloral hydrate	+				+			+	+																								+		
Chloramphenicol	+		+	+	+			+				+	+	+																					+
Chlordiazepoxide					+											+	+					+			+				+		+				
Chloroquine	+	+			+						+					+											+								
Chlorpropamide	+			+				+				+	+	+																					
Cocaine (derivatives)	+				+																	+	+					+	+						
Codeine	+				+			+																											
Colchicine	+	+										+	+	+										+					+				+	+	
Colistin and polymyxin					+																			+					+				+		
Corticosteroids			+			+										+			+		+	+						+							+
Coumarin derivatives	+	+	+		+													+																	+
Diethylstilbestrol	+				+											+																			
Digitalis	+	+			+		+	+								+	+											+	+						
Dimercaprol (BAL)	+				+			+				+			+														+		+				
Ergot alkaloids	+																												+						
Erythromycin	+	+		+				+																					+						
Ethynyl estradiol	+			+	+						+																								
Gold		+	+	+	+		+	+	+	+		+	+	+															+	+			+	+	
Griseofulvin	+	+			+			+														+				+							+		
Guanethidine		+			+																										+	+	+		
Heparin				+										+														+			+	+			
Hydantoin derivatives			+	+	+	+		+				+	+	+	+	+	+							+					+	+				+	+
Hydralazine	+	+	+		+		+					+	+	+										+					+	+	+			+	
Imipramine and amitriptyline				+	+							+											+		+						+	+			
Insulin					+																							+		+					
Iodides	+	+			+	+	+	+	+	+		+	+				+											+	+	+				+	+
Isoniazid	+			+	+			+	+				+				+					+	+	+					+						
Kanamycin and neomycin	+																+									+									
Meperidine	+							+																					+			+			+
Meprobamate					+							+	+	+															+						

Table 73-1. ADVERSE REACTIONS TO DRUGS (*Continued*)

Drug	Gastro-intestinal				Cutaneous							Hematologic (Marrow failure)							Metabolic			Neurologic				Ear and eye		Allergic			Cardiorenal				
	Nausea-vomiting	Diarrhea	GI bleeding	Jaundice	Dermatitis	Acneiform eruption	Erythema multiforme	Urticaria	Purpura	Fixed eruption	Photosensitization	Red blood cells	White blood cells	Platelets	Hemolysis	Leukocytosis	Eosinophilia	Hypoprothrombinemia	Hypokalemia	Hyperuricemia	Hyperglycemia	Delirium	Convulsions	Peripheral neuropathy	Extrapyramidal syndrome	C8 nerve damage	Ocular damage	Anaphylaxis	Fever	"Serum sickness"	Arrhythmia	Hypotension	Renal disorder	Collagen-vascular syndromes	Fetal and neonatal effects
Mercurials	+				+		+	+		+			+						+									+	+	+			+		
Methyldopa		+		+	+							+	+																				+	+	
Methimazole				+	+			+					+				+												+						
Methylphenidate	+																						+								+	+			
Methyltestosterone				+		+																													+
Morphine	+			+				+													+														+
M.A.O. inhibitors				+	+								+									+	+										+		
Nitrofurantoin	+				+			+							+	+								+				+	+						
Novobiocin	+	+		+	+																								+						+
Penicillins					+		+	+	+								+											+	+	+				+	
Phenformin	+	+																																	
Phenindiones	+	+	+	+	+								+				+	+											+	+					
Phenolphthalein		+			+		+	+		+									+										+	+					
Phenothiazines	+			+	+		+	+		+	+		+			+	+						+		+		+		+		+	+			+
Phenylbutazone		+	+	+	+			+				+	+	+															+	+			+	+	
Primaquine	+	+		+									+		+	+							+				+								
Probenecid	+			+	+										+													+	+						
Procaine amide	+	+			+			+			+		+											+				+	+	+	+	+		+	
Progesterone	+																																		+
Propoxyphene	+				+																														
Propylthiouracil				+	+								+				+												+	+				+	+
Quinidine/quinine	+	+			+			+	+	+			+	+	+		+						+			+		+	+		+	+			+
Rauwolfia	+	+	+		+																				+							+			+
Salicylates	+		+		+		+	+	+							+	+			+		+				+		+	+	+		+	+		+
Spironolactones					+																	+									+	+			
Streptomycin	+	+			+			+				+	+	+			+						+			+	+	+	+						+
Sulfonamides				+	+		+	+	+	+	+	+	+	+	+		+							+				+	+	+			+	+	+
Sympathetic amines					+																+	+	+	+							+				
Tetracyclines	+	+		+	+					+																			+				+		+
Tolbutamide	+	+	+				+	+			+	+	+	+																			+		
Trimethadione		+		+	+		+					+	+	+																			+	+	
Vancomycin					+																					+		+					+	+	
Xanthine derivatives	+		+		+					+													+								+	+			

systemic lupus erythematosus have appeared during therapy with gold, hydralazine, and a few other drugs. The manifestations of lupus associated with drug reactions usually have been reversible following discontinuation of the drug (Chap. 392).

Anaphylaxis may follow the parenteral administration of a variety of drugs, but the agent incriminated most often is penicillin. The risk of any particular patient's developing anaphylaxis to penicillin is very small, but because a large number of patients (20 to 30 percent in general hospitals) receive the drug, this reaction may be observed relatively frequently. Radiopaque iodinated dyes, particularly those used for intravenous pyelography, and Bromsulphalein are two other common diagnostic agents which have been incriminated in anaphylaxis.

TREATMENT AND PROPHYLAXIS. Allergic reactions to drugs usually subside promptly when the agent is discontinued. For reasons that are not understood, however, the reaction occasionally persists for prolonged periods despite withdrawal of the drug. Recurrent urticaria for many months after a penicillin reaction is a common example.

The management of serum sickness is described in Chap. 74. In the event of persistent or severe manifestations of drug allergy, the use of adrenocortical steroids is indicated. Adrenal steriods, antihistamines, and epinephrine are usually ineffective in alleviating reactions due to idiosyncrasy or side effects of a drug. Reactions of this type are best managed by withdrawing the offending drug and administering other drugs with appropriate pharmacologic actions, e.g., sedatives for excitability, stimulants for depression, etc.

Although it is usually not possible to predict the occurrence of drug allergy in a patient, the fact that hypersensitivity to drugs may be commoner in individuals with other allergic reactions makes it reasonable to inquire about this before beginning treatment with any agent. A specific history of hypersensitivity to a given drug contraindicates its readministration unless the clinical situation is serious. When confronted with such a situation, the procedure of choice is to look for an alternative agent which is just as efficacious. For example, vancomycin may be used as effectively as a penicillin in staphylococcal endocarditis. In a number of instances when it has been judged necessary to prescribe a drug to which a patient is known to be allergic, the concomitant administration of adrenal steroids has completely suppressed the manifestations of hypersensitivity. The third alternative, namely "desensitizing the patient" by administering progressively increasing dosages of a drug such as penicillin, should be used only as a last resort. Though desensitization is often successful, there are occasional examples of an individual who was believed to have been "desensitized" and who experienced a fatal anaphylactic reaction upon receiving a large systemic dose of the drug in question.

Although it is said that sensitivity to a drug will subside if its administration is continued, this is not a regular occurrence and should not be accepted as a basis for further therapy with the incriminated agent.

The U.S. Food and Drug Administration and the Council on Drugs of the American Medical Association are accumulating information on adverse drug reactions. They solicit the cooperation of all physicians in reporting reactions to them.

REFERENCES

Alexander, H. L.: "Reactions to Drug Therapy," Philadelphia, W. B. Saunders Company, 1956.

Carr, E. A., Jr.: Drug Allergy, Pharmacol. Rev., 6:365, 1954.

Cluff, L. E., and J. E. Johnson: Drug Fever, Progr. Allergy, 8:149, 1964.

Eisen, H. N.: Hypersensitivity to Simple Chemicals, in "Cellular and Humoral Aspects of Hypersensitivity," New York, Hoeber Medical Division, Harper & Row, Publishers, Incorporated, 1959.

Landsteiner, K.: "The Specificity of Serological Reactions," Cambridge, Mass., Harvard University Press, 1945.

Seidl, Larry G., G. F. Thornton, J. W. Smith, and L. E. Cluff: Studies on the Epidemiology of Adverse Drug Reactions: III. Reactions in Patients on a General Medical Service, Bull. Johns Hopkins Hosp., 119:299, 1966.

Smith, J. W., L. G. Seidl, and L. E. Cluff: Studies on the Epidemiology of Adverse Drug Reactions: V. Clinical Factors Influencing Susceptibility, Ann. Intern. Med., 65:629, 1966.

74 SERUM SICKNESS AND RELATED DISORDERS

Leighton E. Cluff

DEFINITION. Serum sickness is a systemic illness which occurs in individuals allergic to foreign serum or serum protein. An identical illness may also develop from allergic reactions to drugs. The reaction is characterized by fever, skin eruptions, lymphadenopathy, and arthralgia.

ETIOLOGY AND PATHOGENESIS. Serum sickness was first recognized when the use of immune horse serum for prophylaxis and therapy of diphtheria became widespread. With advances in chemotherapy, foreign serum is employed less and less frequently, and its use is now limited for the most part to diphtheria, tetanus, gas gangrene, botulism, envenenation by reptiles, and rabies. The increasing availability of human immune globulin for treatment and active immunization in many diseases has decreased significantly the importance of allergic reactions to foreign serum. For reasons not entirely clear, transfusion of blood is occasionally followed by serum sickness. Though whole foreign serum is more likely to elicit a reaction, purified fractions are also capable of producing illness. The incidence and severity of serum sickness increase with dosage of the antigen.

Serum sickness is an immunologic reaction dependent on antigen and serum antibody. Following an initial injection of foreign serum, serum fraction, or some drugs, antibody will develop within 7 to 10 days. The reaction leading to illness occurs while the antibody is appearing in the serum and antigen is present in excess of available antibody. Circulating antigen-antibody complexes may be found in the blood. As the reaction develops, serum complement declines. An individual previously exposed to an antigen and possessing specific serum antibody may develop an immediate reaction with anaphylactic shock upon subsequent exposure to the antigen. The previously exposed person who possesses no specific serum antibody may have an accelerated reaction after a second exposure to the antigen, because the booster or anamnestic response results in rapid reappearance of antibody. Depending on the degree of prior sensitization and the level of serum antibody, a severe reaction may occur within minutes or hours.

Apparent relapses or recurrences of serum sickness are not unusual. Serum is not a single antigenic substance, and such a course results from a series of reactions to different antigenic components of the injected material.

The mode of injury to tissue, the release of histamine, serotonin, acetylcholine, etc., by antigen-antibody union are discussed in Chap. 68. The elicitation of illness by nonprotein drugs involves immunologic mechanisms also. These are discussed in Chap. 73.

PATHOLOGY. Serum sickness is rarely fatal. However, examination of tissues of patients dying of other causes during or shortly after an episode of serum sickness often shows lesions indistinguishable from those of periarteritis nodosa. Similar lesions are readily produced in rabbits by injection of foreign protein. The finding of vasculitis in allergic reactions is one of the several factors that have led to the idea that hypersensitivity may be important in the causation of periarteritis nodosa, rheumatic fever, systemic lupus erythematosus, and other diseases characterized by vascular damage.

MANIFESTATIONS. After an incubation period of 4 to 10 days (it may be much shorter in sensitized persons or as long as 21 days in others), there is the onset of *pruritus*, followed shortly by *rash*. The rash may take the form of erythematous, morbilliform, or petechial eruption, but by far the commonest pattern is urticaria. Often, the skin lesions appear at the local site of injection of the serum several hours before the rash becomes generalized. *Lymphadenopathy*, most prominent in the area draining the injection site, is usual, as is *edema* of the face, lips, eyelids, or, rarely, the glottis. Most patients with serum sickness have fever which is often accompanied by arthralgia and at times by arthritis, with effusion into one of the large joints. The joint manifestations may be, in fact, the overshadowing feature of serum sickness. Other symptoms include headache, nausea, vomiting, abdominal pain, diarrhea, cardiac arrhythmias, and pericarditis.

The most disabling complications of serum sickness are neurologic disorders, which occur in a minority of cases. Unilateral mononeuritis which involves the shoulder girdle or arm and is characterized by weakness and sensory deficit, may appear. Isolated facial palsy occurs, and occasionally, there may be extensive polyneuritis or meningoencephalitis.

LABORATORY FINDINGS. There is usually a mild peripheral neutrophilic leukocytosis, and the bone marrow shows an increase in number of plasma cells. Eosinophilia is not a feature of classical serum sickness, but it occasionally accompanies the drug-induced syndrome. The urine may contain protein, casts, and erythrocytes. Electrocardiograms sometimes show transient conduction defects. Slight pleocytosis in the cerebrospinal fluid is frequent even in the absence of demonstrable neurologic dysfunction.

COURSE. Serum sickness is a benign, self-limited disease which subsides within 1 to 3 weeks. In patients with neuropathy, residual weakness may require several weeks to abate, but complete restoration of function is the rule. Rare deaths from edema of the glottis are recorded, but a fatal outcome is more often a result of the intercurrent disease.

TREATMENT. Urticaria usually responds to small doses of epinephrine and can be controlled with ephedrine and antihistaminics. Joint pains are usually relieved promptly by aspirin or other salicylates.

For severely ill and uncomfortable patients, adrenal steroids offer prompt relief, and the great efficacy of these compounds has led to their increasing use for symptomatic treatment. They need to be given for only 4 to 7 days in most patients.

Tracheostomy or tracheal intubation is needed at times for sudden respiratory obstruction by edema, and equipment for these procedures should be at hand during the early stages of the disease. Adrenal steroids relieve incipient respiratory obstruction promptly.

In patients who have developed serum sickness as a result of administration of tetanus or diphtheria horse antiserum, active immunization with toxoid should be initiated before the patient is released from medical care. Once a foreign serum has produced serum sickness it should never be given again.

ANAPHYLAXIS. Occasional patients given an injection of serum, of skin-test antigen, or a drug will become profoundly ill and may collapse and die within minutes. Asthmatic wheezing, cyanosis, and severe pruritus involving the hands often occur at the onset of illness. This reaction is the human counterpart of anaphylactic shock in lower animals. Because it rarely occurs in individuals who give no history of hypersensitivity and because fatalities have followed the injection of tiny amounts of serum for the purpose of determining a patient's state of sensitization, prevention is very difficult. Perhaps the most important step in reducing the incidence of anaphylaxis is to follow the dictum that no serum product or drug should be given to any patient without clear indications. Although most severe reactions occur after parenteral administration of the antigen or drug, fatalities have been reported after oral ingestion.

Treatment consists of the intravenous or intracardiac administration of epinephrine and vigorous support of respiration and circulation. Adrenal steroids may be given parenterally but are of little or no value in treating this acute situation. When the injection site permits, a tourniquet may be applied to slow absorption of the antigen.

ARTHUS REACTION. When experimental animals are sensitized to foreign serum or other proteins, reinjection of antigen into the skin often elicits transient erythema and edema, similar to a "positive" skin test in man. If animals are highly sensitive or if the dose of antigen is large, the skin lesion may progress to hemorrhage and necrosis, with eventual ulceration and scarring. This irreversible tissue damage after local application of antigen in a sensitive animal is the classic Arthus phenomenon. Rarely, a similar type of hemorrhagic necrosis occurs at sites of injection of serum or drugs in man. These Arthus-like reactions are unusual, however, and are far outnumbered by inflammatory reactions at injection sites attributable to the intrinsic irritating properties of a drug, to hemorrhage in patients with hemophilia, thrombocytopenia, or drug-induced coagulation defects, or to secondary bacterial infection. Until these disorders have been ruled out, an Arthus reaction should not be invoked as the cause of tissue damage in man.

SHWARTZMAN REACTION. Appropriately timed intradermal injections of bacterial endotoxins or endotoxins in combination with various other substances can elicit in rabbit skin a hemorrhagic necrosis that resembles the Arthus reaction. The mechanism of the reaction is not clear, but it may have a pathogenesis similar to that of immunologic reactions. Numerous attempts have been made to demonstrate the importance of this reaction in the pathogenesis of human disease, including peptic ulcer, acute pancreatitis, and focal reactions in tuberculosis, but it remains, for the most part, a dramatic laboratory phenomenon. The confluent purpura and the adrenocortical hemorrhage of meningococcemia may be the human counterpart of a Schwartzman reaction (Chap. 142).

REFERENCES

Austen, K. F.: Systemic Anaphylaxis in Man, J.A.M.A., 192: 116, 1963.

Dixon, F. J., J. J. Vazquez, W. O. Weigle, and C. G. Cochrane: Pathogenesis of Serum Sickness, A.M.A. Arch. Pathol., 65:18, 1958.

Kojis, F. G.: Serum Sickness and Anaphylaxis, Am. J. Dis. Child., 64:93, 313, 1942.

Longcope, W. T.: Serum Sickness and Analogous Reactions from Certain Drugs, Particularly the Sulfonamides, Medicine, 22:251, 1943.

v. Pirquet, C., and B. Schick: "Serum Sickness," Baltimore, The Williams & Wilkins Company, 1951.

Part Five
Nutritional, Hormonal, and Metabolic Disorders

Section 1
Basic Considerations

INTRODUCTION

Nutrition, the science of food, is concerned with types and amounts of foodstuffs with respect to their basic components (minerals, amino acids, lipids, carbohydrates, or vitamins) and the ways they are carried through the processes of digestion, absorption, transport utilization, and excretion. It is a widely held view among the laity that all health is somehow attributable to poor food habits, and patients will expect physicians to be attentive to this possibility and to give knowledgeable advice.

The term *nutrition,* however, does not confine one necessarily to a consideration of dietary or exogenous materials. Even though the diet may contain all of the 40-odd essential nutrients, a variety of causes may precipitate conditioned deficiency states which will prevent the fulfillment of all the nutritional requirements of the cells and tissues of the body. In nations in which technology, education, social security, medical services, food, clothing, housing, and many other socioeconomic factors are highly developed and food of all types is abundant, disorders of nutrition generally are due to factors which interfere with assimilation or absorption of nutrients, produce excess loss, or cause excess elimination of an adequate intake. Psychic factors, such as those which play an important role in anorexia nervosa or food fads, also are important considerations.

In less favored societies ("developing nations") reduced intake of calories and essential nutrients is likely to be the most important cause of nutritional deficiency—the result of poverty, insufficient education, and cultural and religious practices. In such countries the classical nutritional diseases are seen.

Nutritional lack finds expression in various ways, and the physician must recognize and understand its effects. He must bear in mind that malnutrition will often complicate an illness and may aggravate it. On the other hand, good nutrition can facilitate the management of disease, and thus, food habits and diet therapy become inextricably a part of diagnosis and therapeutics.

In medical centers the availability of dieticians, specialized dietary services, and a large variety of laboratory facilities has eased the application of nutrition science for physicians early in their careers. A hidden danger is that such readily available assistance leaves them relatively unprepared for their possible subsequent isolation from such facilities. This section reviews the essential elements of nutrition and metabolism and discusses the application of the principles of nutrition science to diagnosis and management. The classical deficiency states are described, but the emphasis is upon the more relevant matter of relating nutritional disturbances to the prevention and management of other illnesses.

75 INTERMEDIARY METABOLISM OF PROTEIN, FAT, AND CARBOHYDRATE

George F. Cahill, Jr.

Life may be defined as a system of matter having heritability and mutability; as such, it requires continued or intermittent capture of both energy and matter. The processes maintaining life in the cell may be divided accordingly: the transformation of captured energy into forms useful to and usable by cells, and the transformation of matter (molecules) to make more available their energy content or to use the matter to replace the machinery of the cell or to synthesize new machinery for growth or reproduction. Disturbances in transformation of energy or molecules may become manifest as disease processes, though our knowledge of the precise metabolic events in most cases is as yet fragmentary.

These functions of the cell are carried out in specialized subcellular compartments: maintenance and renewal of cell structure is governed by information contained in nuclear deoxyribonucleic acid (DNA); energy transformations are performed mainly by mitochondria; and synthetic and degradative processes are accomplished in microsomes and in the surrounding soluble fluid or cytoplasm.

ENZYMES

The functioning unit of the cell which catalyzes all the molecular changes is a protein molecule, an *enzyme*. A biochemist's view has been summarized: "Except for those rare phenomena in biology which are purely physical, the 'aliveness' of cells is basically the summation of enzymatic catalysis and its regulation" (Anfinsen). Enzyme function is localized to a small portion of the usually large polypeptide sequence, the active site E. This site binds the substrate molecule S transiently during the act of catalysis to form the enzyme-substrate complex ES, which then dissociates to liberate free enzyme and product P. The process of catalysis by the enzyme can be formulated as a set of rates maintaining a chemical equilibrium:

$$E + S \underset{k_{-1}}{\overset{k_1}{\rightleftharpoons}} ES \overset{k_2}{\rightarrow} P + E \qquad (1)$$

The velocities are expressed by the constants k_1, k_{-1}, and k_2 and are properties of the enzyme molecule arising from its three-dimensional structure and from the arrangement of its active sites. The overall chemical equilibrium $S \rightleftharpoons P$, which in the absence of the catalytic enzyme might be reached only after a prolonged period of time, is accelerated by the enzyme, which, by forming complexes as in Eq. (1), imparts much higher velocities to some of the individual steps of the reaction. An interrelationship between these velocity constants can be expressed through a constant that depends on the features of the enzyme and the conditions of the reaction:

$$K_m = \frac{k_{-1} + k_2}{k_1} \qquad (2)$$

K_m is the Michaelis constant. When k_2 is small compared with k_{-1}, K_m is also the measure of the affinity of the active site for the substrate, the dissociation constant of the enzyme-substrate complex; K_m can also be thought of as the concentration of substrate that half-saturates the active enzyme sites. These concepts are of increasing importance in understanding normal and disease mechanisms, since controls can be exerted on enzymes which catalyze "rate-limiting" steps in a sequence of reactions

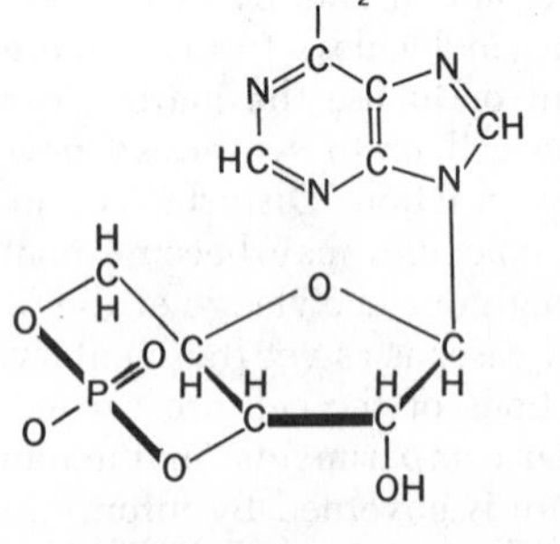

Adenosine-3',5'-Monophosphate
(Cyclic-3', 5'-AMP)

Fig. 75-1. The structure of cyclic-3',5'-adenosinemonophosphate (cyclic-3',5'-AMP or cyclic adenylate). It is produced in the cell from adenosinetriphosphate (see Fig. 75-2).

or on enzymes at points in the pathways of intermediary metabolism (or of energy transfer) which are "switching stations," where more than one path is possible. The mechanism of control at these points may be a chemical reaction between the controlling agents and the effector molecule, and is governed by the properties of the enzyme and agent and their interactions, much the same way as the reactions shown in Eq. (1).

CONTROL MECHANISMS

The state of simple chemical equilibrium is probably seldom attained in reactions in the living cell. Since the product is usually being removed by another process, the reaction, although potentially bidirectional, usually carries substrate in only one direction. In certain cases, the nature of the reaction catalyzed by the enzyme is so heavily favored in one direction, because of loss of free energy in the reaction (exergonic), that the enzyme catalyzes a reaction which is essentially unidirectional. Wherever this occurs, there appears to be an important site of overall metabolic control, as by a hormone or some other regulatory process, which by changing the activity or quantity of the enzyme is able to alter profoundly the rate of the reaction and therefore the flow of substrate over this and subsequent reactions.

Knowledge of enzymes has so far been of medical value in two areas: the empiric use of enzyme activity measurements as diagnostic aids and the recognition that certain genetically transmitted diseases or disease traits are the result of a single discrete biochemical lesion, due to a defect either in the synthesis or in the action of an enzyme. The usefulness of diagnostic enzymology is being increased by observations that *isozymes*, enzymes catalyzing the same reaction but possessing different structural or functional (e.g., K_m) properties, can be identified in body fluids as originating in a specific organ or tissue. The catalytic nature of enzymes (some enzymes handle the alteration of more than 5 million substrate molecules per min per molecule of enzyme) makes them key control points for the regulation of metabolic flux by hormones, vitamins, trace metals, pharmacologic agents and toxins, and specific metabolites which can bind to an enzyme and either alter the three-dimensional conformation of the enzyme (allosteric transitions) or compete with the substrate and cause inhibition.

Other control mechanisms include (1) changes in the state of polymerization of enzyme molecule structure, e.g., the transformation of inactive phosphorylase dimers into the active tetramer under the indirect influence of a unique molecule, cyclic-3',5'-adenosinemonophosphate (Fig. 75-1); (2) the availability of oxidized or reduced coenzymes; (3) actions on membrane permeability. There is also evidence that hormones act on membranes that enclose and partition the interiors of cells to control the transport of substrates or cofactors from one compartment to another. With the discovery that the membrane of the mitochondrion, for instance, contains oriented enzymes, this distinction may lose some of its sharpness. Nevertheless, the phenomena of diffusion, active membrane transport, and pinocytosis (an action engulfing external particles or molecules, in which part of the membrane forms a shell around the object of transport) have been shown to be affected by hormone action. (4) The amount of an enzyme present in the cell also controls the catalytic action exerted. Enzymes are made via the usual routes of synthesis of proteins, but there are more specific influences on enzyme synthesis than those governing the general production of proteins. In primitive unicellular organisms, where the supply of substrates can be controlled, production of an enzyme can be induced *de novo* by supplying a new substrate. The role of enzyme induction in mammals is not so clear, although some examples of adaptation of tissues to metabolize certain compounds more rapidly have been reported. When an enzyme contains a special organic or inorganic prosthetic group that is not synthesized via the ordinary metabolic routes, interference with the supply of the prosthetic group may decrease the amount of active enzyme synthesized; conditioned or dietary deficiencies of vitamins and inorganic elements may also cause such defects.

Energy Transformation

The energy that allows living protoplasm in heterotrophic cells to maintain its structure and growth and therefore its function against the demands of the less-organized environment is derived from the potential energy inherent in the chemical bonds of large, moderately complex organic molecules—biologic fuels. This energy is transformed by various catalytic mechanisms partly into heat, which in homotherms maintains a constant body temperature higher than that of the environment, facilitating enzyme catalyses. In autotrophic cells, energy for useful work is derived not from organic molecules, but from sunlight, which is used to fix carbon dioxide from the air and to synthesize carbohydrate; this is the ultimate source of the substrates needed by heterotrophic cells to survive.

High-energy Bonds

The carrier molecule for the free energy derived from foodstuffs (or from sunlight) is adenosinetriphosphate (ATP) (Fig. 75-2). In the cells, the terminal phosphate groups are transferred to "activate" other molecules; the free energy of the ATP molecule is conserved in part in this transfer so that the activated acceptor molecule can thereafter participate in energy-requiring processes such as muscle contraction or syntheses. The high-energy bond of ATP is the pyrophosphate linkage of its terminal phosphate groups ($\sim$P), and the free energy content of each $\sim$P is about 8 kcal per mole. This may be thought of as the energy evolved when the phosphate ester linkage is simply hydrolyzed in solution. Ordinary "energy-poor" phosphate ester linkages have a free energy content of approximately 2 kcal per mole. The high energy is apparently imparted to the bond by the other resonant chemical bonds immediately adjacent to the phosphate group: it is as if they supplied negative charges like the

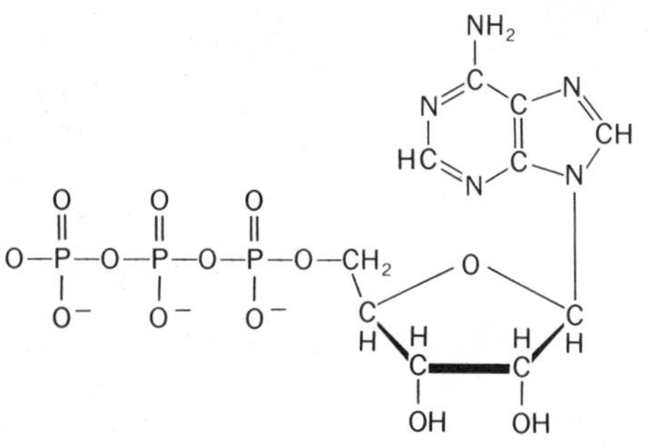

Adenosine-5'-Triphosphate (ATP)

Fig. 75-2. The structure of adenosinetriphosphate. Energy is stored in the two terminal high-energy phosphate bonds (denoted in the text as $\sim$P) and is released or transferred to support reactions requiring energy (endergonic).

negative poles of a magnet, kept together only by the phosphate bond; when hydrolysis or transfer occurs, this highly "stressed" bond releases or transfers its potential energy content.

High-energy bonds are not found solely in ATP, although it is probably the principal source of these bonds in the cell. In mammalian muscle, the main storage form of high energy is in the phosphoamide bond of creatine phosphate (in lower animals, in arginine phosphate). Other forms are the phosphoenols like phosphoenolpyruvate and acetyl phosphate; pyrophosphate and polypyrophosphate; thioesters like acetyl coenzyme A; and sulfonium compounds like S-adenosylmethionine, which activate methyl groups for the synthesis of choline, creatine, N-methylnicotinamide (for coenzyme I or DPN+),[1] and norepinephrine.

There are two major pathways by which high-energy bonds in ATP are generated. (1) *Intra*molecular H transfer (hydrogen atom transfer), which is performed by single or complex soluble enzymes in the cytoplasm or in the free fluid inside mitochondria. (2) *Inter*molecular H transfer, which is performed by solid-state, insoluble complexes of oriented enzymes in mitochondrial membranes. Mitochondria transduce energy in heterotrophic cells, transforming substrate energy to ATP bonds through the use of over 90 percent of the O_2 consumed by the cell.

In mitochondria, the enzymes, starting with that one specific for the substrate being utilized, transfer H atoms or electrons stepwise to each other (diphosphopyridine nucleotide, flavins, cytochromes) in the membrane portion, and at the same time esterify inorganic phosphate to make an (as yet hypothetic) high-energy intermediate compound, X $\sim$P (Fig. 75-3). In the presence of adenosinediphosphate (ADP) the high-energy phosphate is transferred from the intermediate compound on the mito-

[1] Diphosphopyridine nucleotide (DPN+) and reduced diphosphopyridine nucleotide (DPNH) have been renamed nicotinamide adenine dinucleotide (NAD+ and NADH), and the respective triphosphopyridine nucleotide compounds TPN+ and TPNH have been renamed nicotinamide adenine dinucleotide phosphate (NADP+ and NADPH).

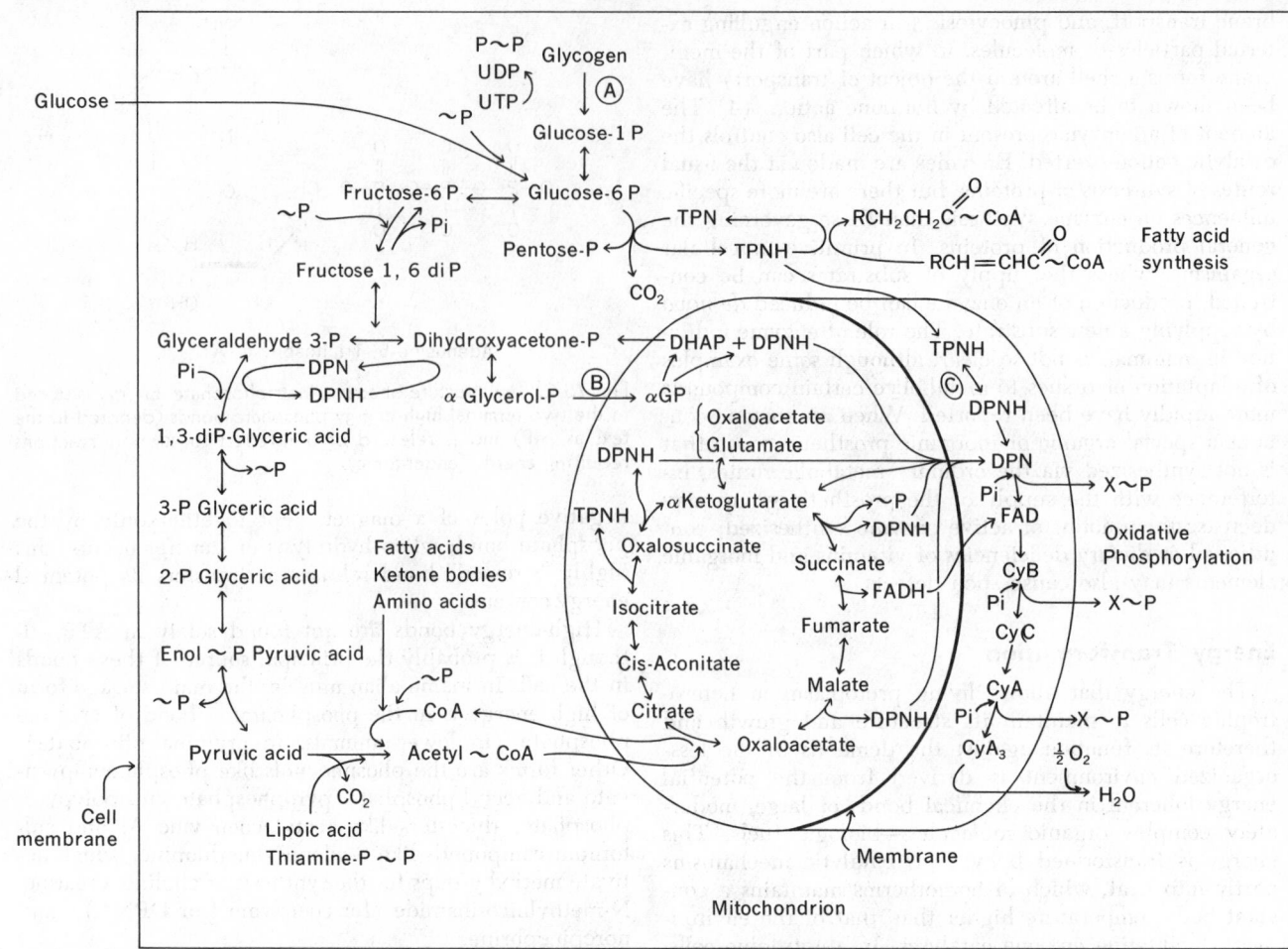

Fig. 75-3. A general scheme of energy and molecular transformations in compartments of the cell. Glucose is transported across the cell membrane, phosphorylated through use of a high-energy phosphate bond ($\sim$P), and then transformed either to store its energy content (upward, glycogenesis) or to release its energy content (downward) via (1) breakdown of glycogen by phosphorylase (A); (2) oxidation through the glycolytic cycle to form acetyl CoA; (3) hydrogen transfer (B) to enter the mitochondrial apparatus; (4) oxidation through the pentose pathway. Energy is transformed into useful form via the consumption of O_2 in mitochondrial membranes, with concomitant esterification of inorganic phosphate (P_i) to form a (hypothetic) high-energy phosphate intermediate compound ($X \sim P$), which can be used to synthesize ATP (see Fig. 75-2); this mitochondrial process is oxidative phosphorylation. The mitochondrial matrix contains enzymes catalyzing the Krebs (tricarboxylic acid) cycle, transforming the energy released from acetyl CoA produced from glucose, amino acids, ketone bodies, or fatty acids. Further details are discussed in the text.

chondrion to make ATP; three ATP molecules are produced for each atom of oxygen used in oxidizing most substrates. This process is *oxidative phosphorylation*. The mitochondrial apparatus, besides transforming energy, also contains its own control mechanism for respiration. When the high-energy intermediate remains *in situ*, i.e., when no ADP is present to accept the high-energy bond from $X \sim P$, oxidation proceeds at a relatively slow rate; when acceptor ADP is added, the oxidative rate increases up to tenfold or more as substrate is consumed. The demand for useful energy thus controls the generation of useful energy, a mechanism of *respiratory control*. Living cells, surprisingly perhaps, respire at the lower rate and so are in a state of controlled respiration. The oxygen con-

sumption of man, measured as the BMR, is predominantly due to this basal mitochondrial oxygen utilization. The coupling between oxidation and phosphorylation in the normal cell may be compared to the clutch of a car, which engages and harnesses the consumption of fuel and oxygen to rotating the wheels; the phosphate-acceptor function of ADP is like releasing a set brake and advancing the throttle.

The transformation of energy by oxidative phosphorylation in mitochondria can be inhibited by chemical agents in vitro and in vivo. Dinitrophenol and salicylates act this way, reducing phosphorylation but allowing oxidation to continue. Indeed, when this "uncoupling" of phosphorylation occurs, the rate of oxidation increases severalfold, as if the clutch of the car had been disengaged while the throttle was still advanced, allowing the motor to run faster and overheat without doing useful work. This accounts for the toxic actions of dinitrophenol and salicylates, which raise the BMR and eventually the body temperature; toxic amounts of thyroid hormone induce a similar change.

INTERMEDIARY METABOLISM

Mitochondrial Oxidation

Mitochondria can oxidize a number of substrates as fuel for generation of high-energy bonds, through the presence of enzymes specific for the substrate; the H atoms so obtained all traverse the common mitochondrial membrance pathway of electron transport and H transport to produce useful energy. The following metabolic fuels or molecules derived from them can be oxidized by mitochondria to serve as the important sources of energy (Fig. 75-3): (1) glucose, (2) amino acids, (3) ketone bodies, and (4) fatty acids. As detailed below, the proportion and amount utilized of each of these is under physiologic and biochemical control. Products of the metabolism of glucose and amino acids (after transamination) enter the Krebs cycle in the soluble matrix of the mitochondrion mainly as acetyl CoA, an activated thioester of acetate and coenzyme A, which contains the vitamin pantothenic acid. The esterification proceeds from energy derived from ATP. Fatty acids and ketone bodies are also oxidized by mitochondria as CoA esters. Studies suggest that the fatty acid molecules enter mitochondria combined with carnitine, a known growth factor. There is a complex mitochondrial fatty acid oxidation cycle, whereby fatty acids are activated using CoA and ATP. Dehydrogenation is accomplished by flavoproteins which contain the vitamin riboflavin and the metals Cu or Fe. The unsaturated fatty acid is then hydrated, dehydrogenated (using DPN^+, containing the vitamin nicotinamide); and split by a molecule of CoA, liberating acetyl CoA to enter the Krebs cycle and generate ATP). From this process there remains a fatty acid two carbons shorter than the original, which in turn re-enters the fatty acid cycle to repeat the above sequence. In the cycle, the reducing equivalents obtained from the two dehydrogenation steps may also enter the electron-transport chain to generate high-energy bonds.

Glucose Metabolism

Mitochondrial generation of ATP is not the only source of utilizable energy in the cell, though it accounts for more than 90 percent. Anaerobic glycolysis in the cytoplasm also produces via intramolecular H-atom transfers two ATP molecules per molecule of glucose oxidized, as indicated in Fig. 75-3. The efficiency of energy transformation, the amount of useful energy obtained per unit of fuel burned, is much lower in glycolysis than in mitochondrial oxidative phosphorylation; in other words, glycolysis is a relatively inefficient means of supplying large amounts of energy.

In the utilization of glucose by a cell, it is first phosphorylated to glucose 6-phosphate by the enzyme hexokinase. Adenosinetriphosphate is utilized in the process, yielding ADP and glucose 6-phosphate. Thus a high-energy phosphate bond is transferred to form a low-energy bond with loss of heat, which makes the reaction essentially unidirectional and therefore a potential site of metabolic control. Glucose 6-phosphate occupies a strategic position with reference to several biochemical pathways (see further on).

GLYCOLYSIS. This sequence of reactions is the most important route of glucose 6-phosphate metabolism. The first step is the conversion of glucose 6-phosphate to fructose 6-phosphate by phosphoglucose isomerase. Then another high-energy phosphate is added from ATP by phosphofructokinase to form fructose 1,6-diphosphate. This is another exergonic or unidirectional step, and it has been suggested that this step controls the entire glycolytic pathway. Phosphofructokinase action is opposed by another enzyme, fructose 1,6-diphosphatase, which converts fructose 1,6-diphosphate back to fructose 6-phosphate. This latter enzyme, as expected, is located in tissues which *produce* glucose, and therefore is found in liver; there its activity is increased by any one of a numerous group of metabolic stimuli which accelerate gluconeogenesis, e.g., glucocorticoids. Conversely, fructose 1,6-diphosphatase is essentially lacking in tissues such as muscle, adipose tissue, or brain, where the only route of glucose metabolism is via glycolysis to pyruvate and lactate and then via acetate and the Krebs cycle to CO_2, in the presence of oxygen.

After formation of fructose 1,6-diphosphate, the hexose unit is split into two interconvertible 3-carbon phosphorylated sugars. One of these, glyceraldehyde 3-phosphate, is dehydrogenated and phosphorylated to form DPNH $(NADH)$[1] and 1,3-diphosphoglyceric acid, which through a series of reactions yields pyruvate and two high-energy phosphate bonds. Thus the overall reaction is:

$$Glucose + 2 \sim P + 2\ Pi + 2\ DPN^+ \rightarrow 2\ pyruvate$$
$$+ 4 \sim P + 2\ DPNH + 2\ H^+$$

If oxygen is lacking and the DPNH cannot be oxidized to DPN^+, its hydrogen atom can be disposed of in the conversion of pyruvate to lactate, and thereby DPN^+ is replenished for further glycolysis. Thus the overall reaction is:

$$Glucose + 2 \sim P \rightarrow 2\ lactate + 4 \sim P$$
or $$Glucose \rightarrow 2\ lactate + 2 \sim P \qquad (3)$$

This sequence, termed *anaerobic glycolysis* since it can occur in the absence of oxygen, can provide a small but, in an emergency, significant and necessary amount of energy. *Anaerobic glycolysis is limited, however, by the accumulation of lactic acid which eventually lowers the pH to a degree not compatible with cellular function.*

GLYCOGENESIS. Glucose 6-phosphate can alternatively be converted to glycogen by first being altered to glucose 1-phosphate by phosphoglucomutase. The glucose 1-phosphate is condensed with uridine triphosphate (UTP) to form uridine diphosphoglucose (UDGP) and pyrophosphate, which in turn is hydrolyzed to free inorganic phosphate. Thus two high-energy phosphate bonds are utilized, an exergonic reaction. As expected, the activity of this system is a site of metabolic control, being increased in muscle by insulin, and possibly also in liver. The UDP-glucose is then condensed with one of the many outer chains of an already existing glycogen molecule to form one more glucose unit attached by a 1,4 link. The glycogen chain can be modified by the "branching" enzyme to form another chain. In the opposite direction, glycogen is broken down to glucose 1-phosphate by another enzyme, phosphorylase (Fig. 75-3,A). This also is an exergonic process and essentially unidirectional. Phosphorylase activity is increased by different hormones in different tissues, e.g., epinephrine and glucagon in liver, epinephrine in muscle, norepinephrine and epinephrine in adipose tissue, and probably others. The precise activations of phosphorylase are different in various tissues, i.e., in muscle a condensation of two proteins takes place, in liver a phosphate is joined to the inactive enzyme. In all tissues, cyclic-3′,5′-adenosinemonophosphate (Fig. 75-1) appears to be the intermediate effector molecule between the stimulator and the activation of phosphorylase. The end result is glycogenolysis and presentation of extra fuel for glycolysis in whatever tissue is activated. These reactions are discussed in further detail in Chap. 111.

DIRECT OXIDATIVE PATHWAY. In several tissues (adipose, liver, adrenal, mammary) reduced TPN^+ (TPNH or NADPH) is required to provide the hydrogen and electrons for synthesis of lipid. Thus a certain proportion of glucose 6-phosphate and TPN^+ is oxidized by glucose 6-phosphate dehydrogenase to TPNH and 6-phosphogluconic acid, and the last in turn to a compound which loses carbon-1 as CO_2 and produces another TPNH and a pentose phosphate, ribulose 5-phosphate. Through a complicated series of reactions, the pentose phosphates return to the main glycolytic sequence as fructose 6-phosphate or triose phosphate.

GLUCOSE 6-PHOSPHATASE. This enzyme comprises yet another pathway of glucose 6-phosphate metabolism and is located only in those tissues capable of producing glucose: liver and kidney, and also placenta. In the liver, it is the final common pathway for glucose production, and opposes the activity of the glucose-phosphorylating system. The activity of glucose 6-phosphatase in liver is increased in states associated with increased glucose production (diabetes, excess adrenal glucocorticoids) and is decreased in those associated with increased insulin or carbohydrate intake. Again there are two "unidirectional" enzymes at an important site of metabolic control, the production or uptake of glucose by liver. The role of the enzyme in kidney is apparently different and may be related to the process of reabsorption of metabolic intermediates which are converted to glucose 6-phosphate and then released into the bloodstream. It is clearly not related to the renal tubular reabsorption of

glucose, since this process does not involve phosphorylation or dephosphorylation.

GLUCURONIC ACID PATHWAY. An alternative route of glucose 6-phosphate metabolism is the oxidation of carbon-6 of glucose, the glucose having been condensed with UTP to form uridinediphosphate glucose, similar to its route to glycogen. The glucuronic acid thus formed may become a moiety in many of the complex carbohydrates which serve as structural units (glycoproteins) or may be used to conjugate and detoxify endogenous and exogenous compounds prior to their elimination from the body. As part of this pathway, carbon-6 of UDPG can be cleaved to form CO_2 and a 5-carbon sugar which, through a series of reactions, enters the glycolytic pathway. One of the intermediates in this sequence, 1-xylulose, may accumulate and be excreted in the urine in the benign disease, essential pentosuria, which is due to lack of the enzyme which catalyzes the subsequent step in the sequence (Chap. 95).

Acetate and Pyruvate Metabolism

Just as glucose 6-phosphate occupies a position at the crossroads of many metabolic reactions, so do acetate and its closely related products. Pyruvate, the terminus of the previously mentioned pathways, to be further metabolized, must be decarboxylated in the presence of DPN^+ and coenzyme A (thiamine or vitamin B_1 and lipoic acid are essential cofactors) to form CO_2 and acetyl CoA (see Chap. 81). Free acetate itself is of only minor importance in nonruminants as a metabolic fuel. It is the acetyl CoA, therefore, which can enter the subsequent metabolic routes.

In the process of fatty acid synthesis, the acetyl CoA accepts CO_2 to form malonyl CoA and through a series of reactions involving condensations and reductions [TPNH derived from glucose oxidation via the direct oxidative pathway or via transhydrogenation from DPNH (Fig. 75-3C) is the reducing agent] a 16-carbon, saturated, long-chain fatty acid, palmitic acid, is formed; this can then be extended or unsaturated by other enzyme systems. This sequence takes place primarily in adipose tissue but also in liver and to a lesser extent in other tissues. Another route open to acetyl CoA is the formation of ketone bodies, a reaction which occurs exclusively in liver. There is some question as to whether ketones are formed by direct condensation of two acetyl CoA's or via an intermediate comprised of three acetyl CoA's, namely, β-hydroxy-β-methylglutaryl CoA. A third route for acetyl CoA metabolism, via β-hydroxy-β-methylglutaryl CoA, is in the formation of the steroid nucleus and the various compounds derived from it by further metabolic changes, such as cholesterol, steroid hormones, and bile salts. The fourth and perhaps most important route is the condensation of acetyl CoA with oxaloacetate to form citrate, the first step in the sequence of intramitochondrial reactions involving the Krebs or citric or tricarboxylic acid cycle, as previously described.

Another pathway of pyruvate metabolism is the direct

condensation with CO_2 to form oxaloacetate. This sequence is unique in liver and is catalyzed by an enzyme, pyruvic carboxylase. In fasting, or in diabetes mellitus in which fat breakdown to acetyl CoA occurs at a rapid rate, the high level of acetyl CoA accelerates this reaction. Normally oxaloacetate would accept the acetyl CoA to form citrate for oxidation via the citric acid cycle, but this reaction is apparently blocked under fasting conditions or diabetes, and under these conditions the oxaloacetate is phosphorylated and decarboxylated to form phosphoenolpyruvate by another enzyme unique to liver, phosphoenolpyruvate carboxykinase. By this sequence, pyruvate is converted to phosphoenolpyruvate and then to glucose, a reaction which cannot proceed directly in this direction because of the energy differential.

Hydrogen Shuttles

H atoms (reducing equivalents) can be shunted between different metabolic or structural compartments or pathways which eventually generate ATP. Thus, H atoms can be transferred from the low-efficiency glycolytic-cytoplasmic pathway to the high-efficiency mitochondrial apparatus, increasing the generation of ATP. Any metabolite that is reduced in the cytoplasm to a product which is a substrate for an intramitochondrial oxidation can act as an H carrier. One such system is the α-glycerophosphate-dihydroxyacetone shuttle:

α-Glycerophosphate $+$ DPN$^+$ $\rightleftharpoons$
$\qquad$ dihydroxyacetone phosphate $+$ DPNH $+$ H$^+$ (4)

A soluble cytoplasmic α-glycerophosphate dehydrogenase uses DPN$^+$ to oxidize α-glycerophosphate (αGP) to dihydroxyacetone phosphate (DHAP) (both produced by the glycolytic cycle) and DPNH. DPNH cannot apparently enter mitochondria to act as a carrier of H equivalents from the cytoplasm, but α-glycerophosphate can (Fig. 75-3B). Then a distinctly different α-glycerophosphate dehydrogenase within mitochondria oxidizes αGP to DHAP, producing intramitochondrial DPNH, which in turn generates mitochondrial ATP. The DHAP then diffuses into cytoplasm to reenter the shuttle cycle. In rats, thyroid hormone rapidly produces a marked increase in the activity of only the mitochondrial dehydrogenase, making possible increased H-shuttle activity, which in turn increases metabolic ATP generation. A similar H shuttle exists between the fatty acid synthetic cycle and mitochondria, consisting of two β-hydroxybutyric acid dehydrogenases, DPN$^+$, β-hydroxybutyric acid, and acetoacetate.

A different sort of H shuttle can transfer H atoms between the two coenzymes for dehydrogenation, DPN$^+$ and TPN$^+$ (Fig. 75-3C). This is of importance in that H atoms carried into the mitochondrial electron-transport system by DPNH generate ATP; H atoms carried into extramitochondrial oxidizing systems by TPNH generate no high-energy phosphate bonds but are available for the reductive steps of fatty acid and other syntheses.

These transhydrogenations between DPN$^+$ and TPN$^+$ are thus a switching point where reducing equivalents generate useful energy, are used in syntheses directly, or are dispelled as heat. A specific transhydrogenase enzyme is found in mitochondrial membranes, and there are probably many additional de facto transhydrogenases. Any enzyme that has a coenzyme specificity broad enough so that it can react with both DPN$^+$ and TPN$^+$, e.g., glutamic dehydrogenase in mitochondria or steroid dehydrogenase in microsomes, can act as a molecular H shuttle.

Uses of ATP

A detailed listing of specific reactions into which ATP enters may be found in standard biochemical texts. A selected few are of illustrative interest. Studies indicate that the mitochondrion, a self-sufficient apparatus in many ways, transforms energy, and also has a capacity to maintain high internal electrolyte concentrations when it is functioning in its energy-producing role. Mitochondria can accumulate K$^+$, Ca^{++}, Mg^{++}, Mn^{++}, and phosphate ions while oxidizing and phosphorylating, but not when phosphorylation is uncoupled. The purpose of the accumulation is as yet obscure, for Ca^{++} ions, for instance, are themselves uncoupling agents. However, demonstrations that parathyroid hormone is capable of affecting phosphate and Ca^{++} exchanges in mitochondria in vitro are of obvious importance in understanding the mechanism of action of the hormone. The contribution of the osmotic work done by mitochondria toward that of the whole cell is not yet clear.

A major role of ATP in the body is to serve as the ultimate energy source for muscle contraction. The detail of the molecular events concerned with this physical process is still a matter for investigation, but ATP is necessary for the relaxation phenomenon, whereby the contracted actomyosin fibrils resume their more elongated form, primed for the next contraction. Indeed, so definite is the association between the use of ATP and muscle contraction that the actomyosin molecule is called an "ATPase." The dependence of muscle contraction on ATP is reflected in the demands of the myocardium, for instance, for a continued supply of utilizable energy derived from oxidation. The myocardium is supplied with large intricate mitochondria, and interference with the supply of oxygen by a decrease in blood flow produces noncontracting myocardial areas with differences in electric potential (see Chap. 260). Such changes probably increase cellular permeability so that enzymes (e.g., lactic dehydrogenase and the transaminases from cytoplasm, and intramitochondrial enzymes such as malic dehydrogenase) leak into the circulation to provide biochemical diagnostic criteria of impaired myocardial function. Biochemical lesions of the myocardium that interfere with the generation of ATP occur in anemia, thyrotoxicosis, and beriberi, and result in a myocardial contractile defect which is not susceptible to the beneficial action of digitalis, ordinarily so effective when the contractile mechanism itself operates at a disadvantage but has an adequate energy supply. Defects in energy transformation in *skeletal* muscle appear to be present in at least two diseases, as demonstrated by functional and structural changes in muscle mitochondria in patients with thyrotoxicosis, and in a reported case of hypermetabolism in a euthyroid woman.

Another significant use of ATP is the generation of heat to maintain body temperature. In the synthesis of ATP by oxidative phosphorylation, for example, only 60 percent of the energy liberated from oxidation of its substrates is transformed by the mitochondrion to phosphate bond energy. An appreciable portion of the liberated energy is evolved as heat, which assists in maintaining body temperature. When the external environment increases the need for heat production, the body responds with an increased rate of oxygen consumption. Fat depots may function actively in controlling body temperature, not only as an insulator but possibly by increased heat production. The free fatty acids liberated under hormonal control from adipose tissue are reesterified and reincorporated through a burst of O_2 consumption and ATP utilization, and heat is generated concomitantly. The major toxic symptom of agents that uncouple oxidative phosphorylation is hyperthermia, seen with salicylates and dinitrophenol, and in thyroid crisis.

The syntheses of the polymeric compounds that store energy in the body require ATP, e.g., the condensation of glucose 1-phosphate to form glycogen, of acetyl CoA to form fatty acids, of soluble RNA–amino acid complexes to form polypeptides and proteins, and of nucleosides to form nucleotides.

ENERGY TRANSFORMATION

To survive, a species must possess mechanisms whereby it can deposit and store fuel during periods of availability, and be able to mobilize this fuel at times of increased need, in addition to storing and mobilizing fuel for the necessary chemical reactions required to maintain the integrity of its structure.

The human body contains numerous organic compounds with energy potential: lipids, carbohydrates, proteins, and nucleic acids. The lipids are by far the most quantitatively important form of storage of fuel, in addition to providing other functions such as insulation of the body as a whole or as essential components in the structure of cell walls, myelin, and other membranes. Carbohydrates serve as a lesser form of fuel storage except for the nervous system. Protein serves as the structural basis for all enzymes, as well as for contracting elements such as muscle or supporting structures such as collagen, and as a fuel, as a precursor for carbohydrate in the process of gluconeogenesis. Nucleic acids form fundamental components in the hereditary and synthetic mechanisms and, fortunately, are not available as fuels. The body can be divided into four main metabolic compartments, adipose tissue, nervous tissue, muscle, and liver.

Adipose Tissue

Adipose tissue is composed of between 60 and 90 percent triglyceride and thus contains 6 to 8 kcal per Gm tissue. A normal 70-kg male may have 10 kg adipose tissue and thereby a potential fuel reserve of approximately 75,000 kcal, which theoretically could support life for well over 2 months. In obesity, 100 kg of adipose tissue may be present—an entire year's supply!

Adipose tissue metabolism (Fig. 75-4) is controlled by many factors, which may be grouped into two general classes, anabolic and catabolic. A rise in blood glucose level following ingestion of carbohydrate stimulates insulin production; insulin directly increases glucose uptake into adipose tissue, where, in the process of lipogenesis, it is metabolized via acetate into fatty acids, which are then esterified with glycerol to form triglycerides. Thus the individual has converted a less efficient fuel on a weight basis (carbohydrate) to a more efficient form of energy storage (lipid). Some of the ingested glucose may be converted to glycogen in liver, muscle, and adipose tissue. These carbohydrate stores serve two ancillary purposes: (1) as a temporary storage site during ingestion of large amounts of carbohydrate until the lipogenetic process can store the energy as fat; (2) as an emergency store of quickly available glucose for anaerobic glycolysis during periods of stress. The increased economy of storage of energy as lipid far surpasses that as carbohydrate, since triglyceride is deposited in an extraaqueous phase, whereas glycogen is stored with water and electrolytes; 1 Gm glycogen-containing tissue yields only 1 to 1½ kcal and it is therefore one-fourth to one-sixth as efficient for storage of energy as an equivalent unit of lipid-containing tissue.

Insulin appears to exert other effects on adipose tissue. Following a fatty meal, triglycerides enter the bloodstream as particulate aggregates—chylomicrons—via the thoracic duct. They may then enter the liver and be chemically remodified and released into the circulation or they may be directly incorporated into adipose tissue where they are hydrolyzed into free fatty acids and reesterified into triglyceride. These many rearrangements of the originally ingested fat may be the animal's mechanism to ensure that the fat which it stores in its adipose tissue contains the correct number and types of fatty acids. Insulin in the fed individual apparently plays an important role in the uptake of circulating triglycerides into adipose tissue, in addition to its role in promoting lipogenesis from glucose.

Fuel stored as adipose tissue triglyceride is released in only one form, free fatty acids. Adipose tissue free fatty acid concentration is in equilibrium with the fatty acid bound to albumin in the circulation; thus, a rise in adipose tissue free fatty acids induces a release of these into the circulation. The level of free acids in adipose tissue is controlled by several factors. Insulin decreases this level by providing increased glucose uptake, which supplies increased glycerol acceptor for esterification of fatty acids in the cell. Insulin also inhibits the breakdown of triglyceride into free fatty acid.

ADIPOSE TISSUE

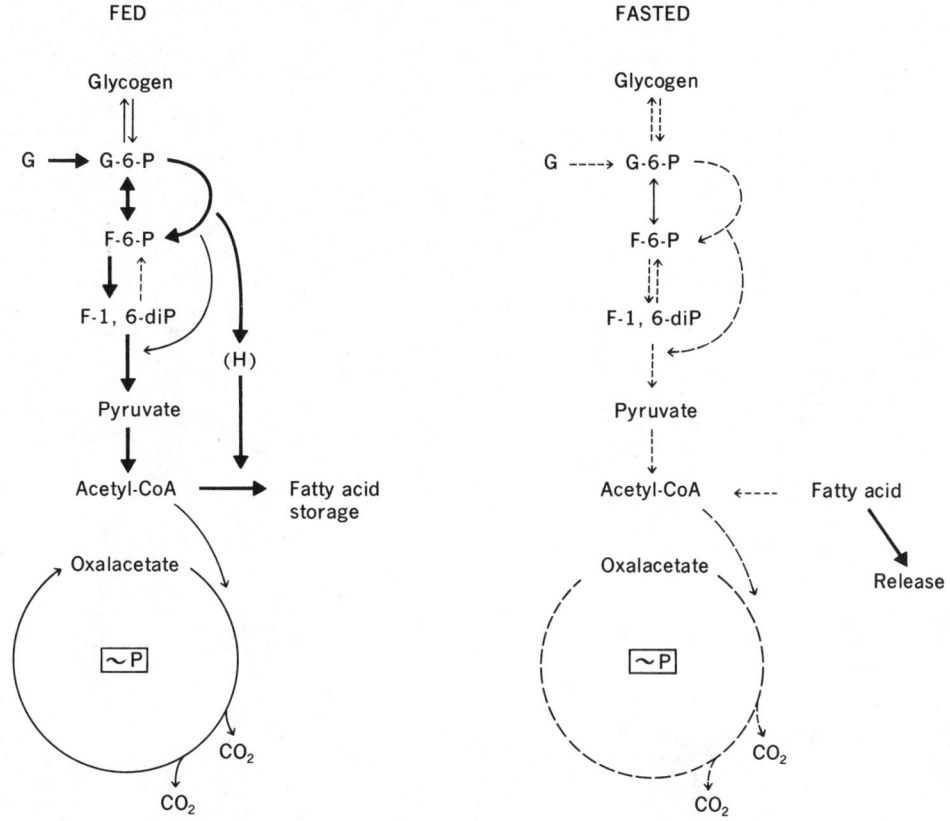

Fig. 75-4. Comparison of flow of substrate across metabolic pathways in adipose tissue in the fed and fasted state. In the former, glucose (G) is metabolized to acetyl CoA, which is then resynthesized to fat and stored. During fasting, glucose metabolism is limited and fatty acids are released for fuel for the remainder of the body.

Conversely, lack of insulin, as in fasting, increases adipose tissue free fatty acid by a reversal of these processes and thereby augments fatty acid release. Among other substances which increase fatty acid production by adipose tissue are norepinephrine, epinephrine, and growth, thyroid, and adrenal hormones. The action of epinephrine on free fatty acid mobilization depends on the thyroid status, being increased in hyperthyroidism and decreased or absent in hypothyroidism.

Nervous Tissue

Nervous tissues require glucose as fuel at all times (Fig. 75-5). This glucose utilization is independent of insulin, or of glucose concentration (as long as it is adequate), or of the state of nervous activity. Only in severe metabolic derangements producing coma is there a significant decrease in the use of glucose (except for a gradual slight decrease with age).

During prolonged starvation, however, and probably in individuals who have been on a very high fat (ketogenic) diet, the brain may decrease its glucose utilization without loss of function because of its capacity to

adapt to utilization of acetoacetate and β-hydroxybutyrate.

In nervous tissue glucose is totally glycolyzed and then oxidized to CO_2 by the tricarboxylic acid cycle. Thus glucose and oxygen must always be available; if their supply is interrupted, brain function ceases immediately.

Muscle

Muscle tissue is versatile in that it can utilize several different fuels to support activity (Fig. 75-5). Glucose is readily removed by muscle from the circulating fluids under the stimulus of insulin, although increased muscular activity or anoxia can also increase glucose uptake. The glucose in muscle is readily glycolyzed to lactic acid and, if there is adequate oxygen, to CO_2 and water. The glucose may also be stored to be used as emergency fuel for glycolysis when oxygen is unavailable or relatively inadequate.

Muscle mitochondria also readily utilize fat as fuel. The fat can come from several sources, from circulating particulate fat (triglyceride) derived from the diet or

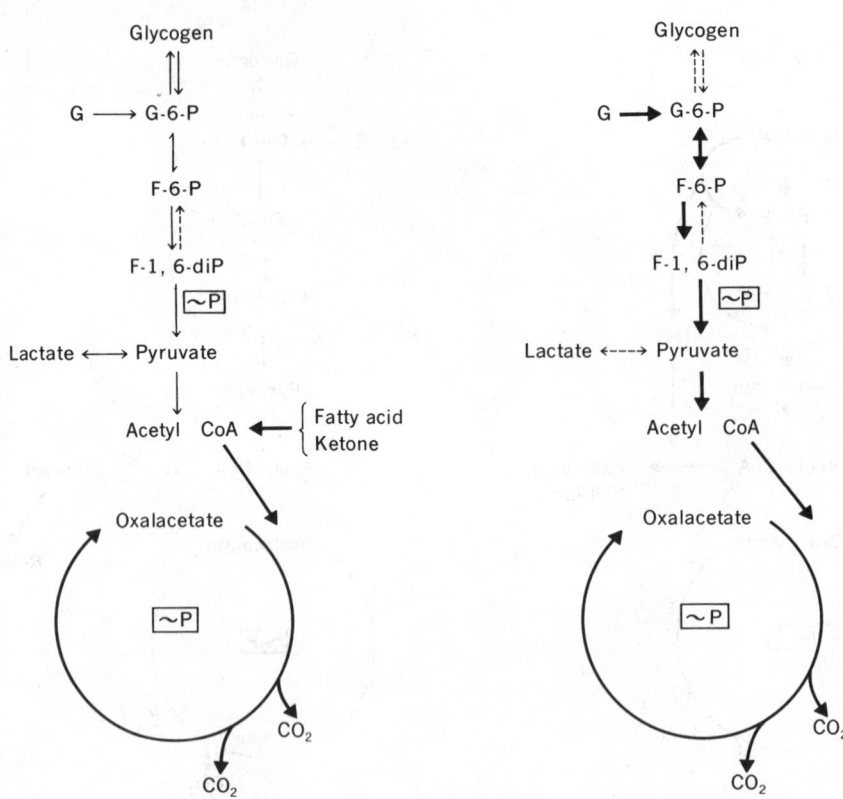

MUSCLE   NERVOUS TISSUE

Fig. 75-5. Muscle tissue utilizes predominantly fatty acid or ketone as a source of fuel, but it is also able to derive limited amounts of energy ($\sim$P) from the conversion of glucose to lactate (anaerobic glycolysis). Nervous tissue is able to utilize only glucose as its metabolic fuel, and requires a constant supply of oxygen for total combustion of the glucose to CO_2 in order to derive energy for adequate function.

secondarily from the liver, from free fatty acids circulating in the blood, having been released from adipose tissue, or from a third source, fat stored directly in the muscle itself. Whatever the origin, the fatty acid is oxidized completely to CO_2 and water, and it is fat which serves as the major contributor of energy to muscle metabolism.

A third type of fuel for muscle is derived from the liver as a product of the incomplete combustion of fatty acids, namely, acetoacetic and β-hydroxybutyric acids, which, with acetone, form the *ketone bodies*. These two acids are also completely metabolized to CO_2 and water in muscle and in certain circumstances can provide a major share of muscle fuel.

By mechanisms not yet clarified, muscle selectively metabolizes ketone bodies, then fatty acids, and, as a last resort, glucose. If ketones are unavailable and free fatty acid concentration is low, as after carbohydrate or insulin administration, muscle will then readily metabolize glucose. Conversely, if ketone or fatty acid concentrations are high, glucose metabolism is minimized, even in the presence of insulin and the glucose which is taken into the tissue is converted to and stored as glycogen. One major role of muscle is to serve as a storehouse

for amino acids. It is now accepted that a primary site of insulin action is to stimulate the incorporation of circulating amino acids into muscle protein. This action is biochemically distinct from the effect on glucose. If insulin is lacking, this process is decreased or even reversed, and amino acids are mobilized. Adrenocortical hormones oppose the insulin effect. In fasting, amino acids are mobilized from muscle, and during feeding, when insulin increases, amino acids are incorporated into muscle protein. Removal of both insulin and adrenal hormones achieves a new balance, but one without flexibility in either direction.

Liver

Of the four groups of tissues playing a major role in body fuel economy, liver (Fig. 75-6) serves as the director of traffic and, as such, is more complicated than adipose, nervous, and muscle tissues. During fasting, it must provide glucose for those tissues requiring glucose for survival (mainly the brain), and during times of carbohydrate ingestion, it stops producing glucose and, instead, removes glucose and stores it as glycogen, transiently if the glycogen reserve is already adequate, or more permanently if the glycogen reserve has been previously depleted by prolonged fasting or other stress.

Unlike peripheral cells, the liver cell is freely permeable to glucose, and the concentration of glucose in the blood is approximated by the concentration in the liver cell, being slightly greater if glucose is being produced by the liver and slightly less if glucose is being removed. The net flow of glucose inside the liver cell into and out of the metabolically activated pool of glucose, glucose 6-phosphate, is a function of two enzymes unique to liver, glucokinase and glucose 6-phosphatase. The activity of the former of these is increased by insulin or carbohydrate feeding, and that of the latter by fasting, insulin insufficiency, or adrenal steroids. Thus the activities of these two opposing systems direct the net flow of glucose into and out of the liver, and are a control over the concentration of glucose in the circulating fluids.

Liver is also unique in possessing other enzymes which are located at metabolic control sites in the sequence of reactions between amino acids and glucose and which increase in activity during times of increased gluconeogenesis, as associated with fasting, diabetes, or adrenal steroid administration, and are decreased by carbohydrate feeding or insulin administration.

During fasting, liver must provide glucose for fuel for those tissues requiring glucose, primarily brain, but also spinal cord, peripheral nerve, leukocytes, erythrocytes, renal medulla, and probably others. This it does by synthesizing new glucose (gluconeogenesis) from glycogenic amino acids released into the circulation from muscle, and, to a lesser extent, from lactate or pyruvate returning to the liver from peripheral tissues, as well as from glycerol arising from lipolysis in adipose tissue. Normally liver contains only 70 to 80 Gm glycogen, less than one-half a day's supply of carbohydrate, should gluconeogenesis not be stimulated to provide the glucose needed by the organism. The liver in a fasting normal man produces approximately 180 Gm glucose daily, of which approximately 144 Gm is oxidized to CO_2 and water and 36 Gm is returned as lactate and pyruvate. To accomplish this, about 75 Gm muscle protein is metabolized to amino acids, which are removed by the liver as precursors for the bulk of the glucose which has to be synthesized. Although net conversion of fat into carbohydrate has not been shown in mammalian tissues, 128 Gm glucose (glycerol from adipose tissue mobilization of triglyceride provides about 16 Gm) cannot be synthesized from 75 Gm protein; many explanations for this process have been offered, such as utilization of fat or ketones or utilization of a small amount of the stored glycogen for a brief period of time.

The liver in the normal fed individual uses as its source of fuel mainly amino acid. During fasting, the amino acid which is presented to the liver is diverted, for

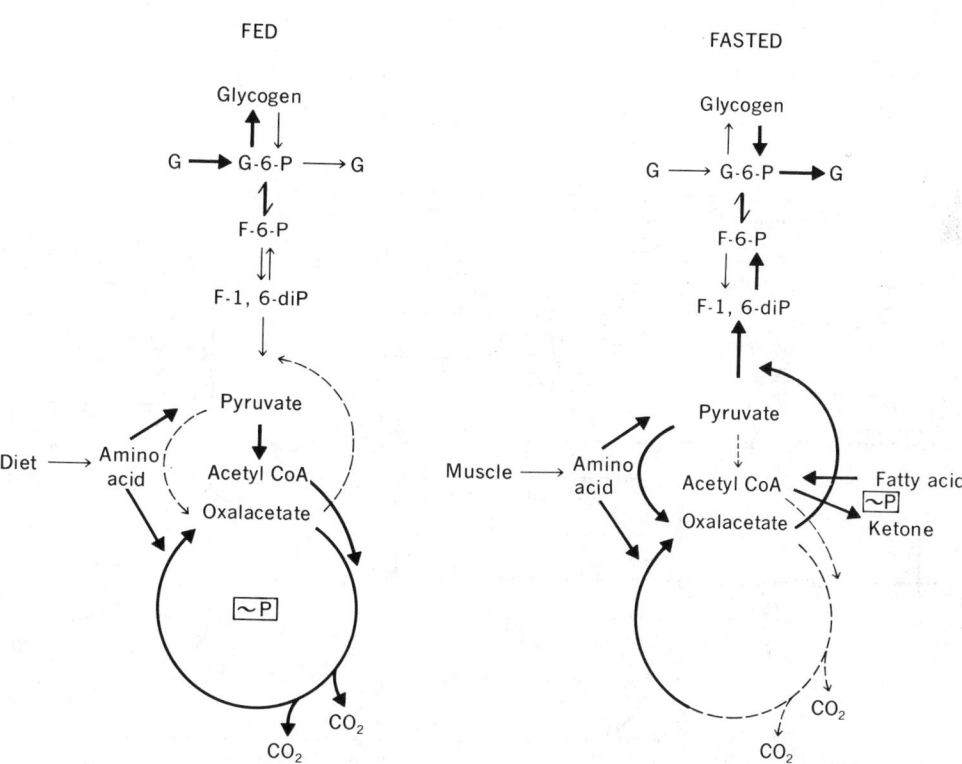

Fig. 75-6. As described in the text, the liver in the fed animal stores glucose as glycogen and derives its own energy from amino acid metabolism. During fasting, its energy (~P) is derived from the conversion of fatty acids to ketone, and amino acids are diverted into glucose synthesis.

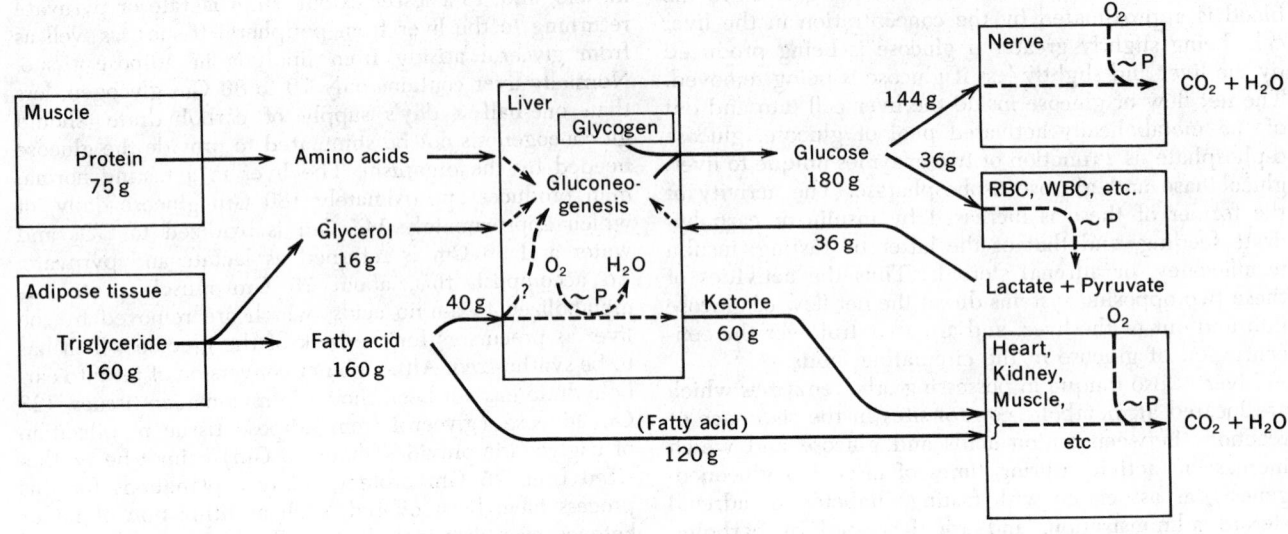

FASTING MAN

ORIGIN OF FUEL

FUEL CONSUMPTION

Muscle — Protein 75 g → Amino acids → Liver

Glycogen

Gluconeogenesis

Adipose tissue — Triglyceride 160 g → Fatty acid 160 g

Glycerol 16 g

O_2 ? ~P H_2O

Glucose 180 g

Ketone 60 g

(Fatty acid) 120 g

Nerve O_2 ~P → $CO_2 + H_2O$ 144 g

RBC, WBC, etc. ~P 36 g

Lactate + Pyruvate 36 g

Heart, Kidney, Muscle, etc O_2 ~P → $CO_2 + H_2O$

40 g

Fig. 75-7. Quantitative estimation of the flow of metabolic fuels by a normal fasted man for a period of 24 hr, utilizing 1800 kcal.

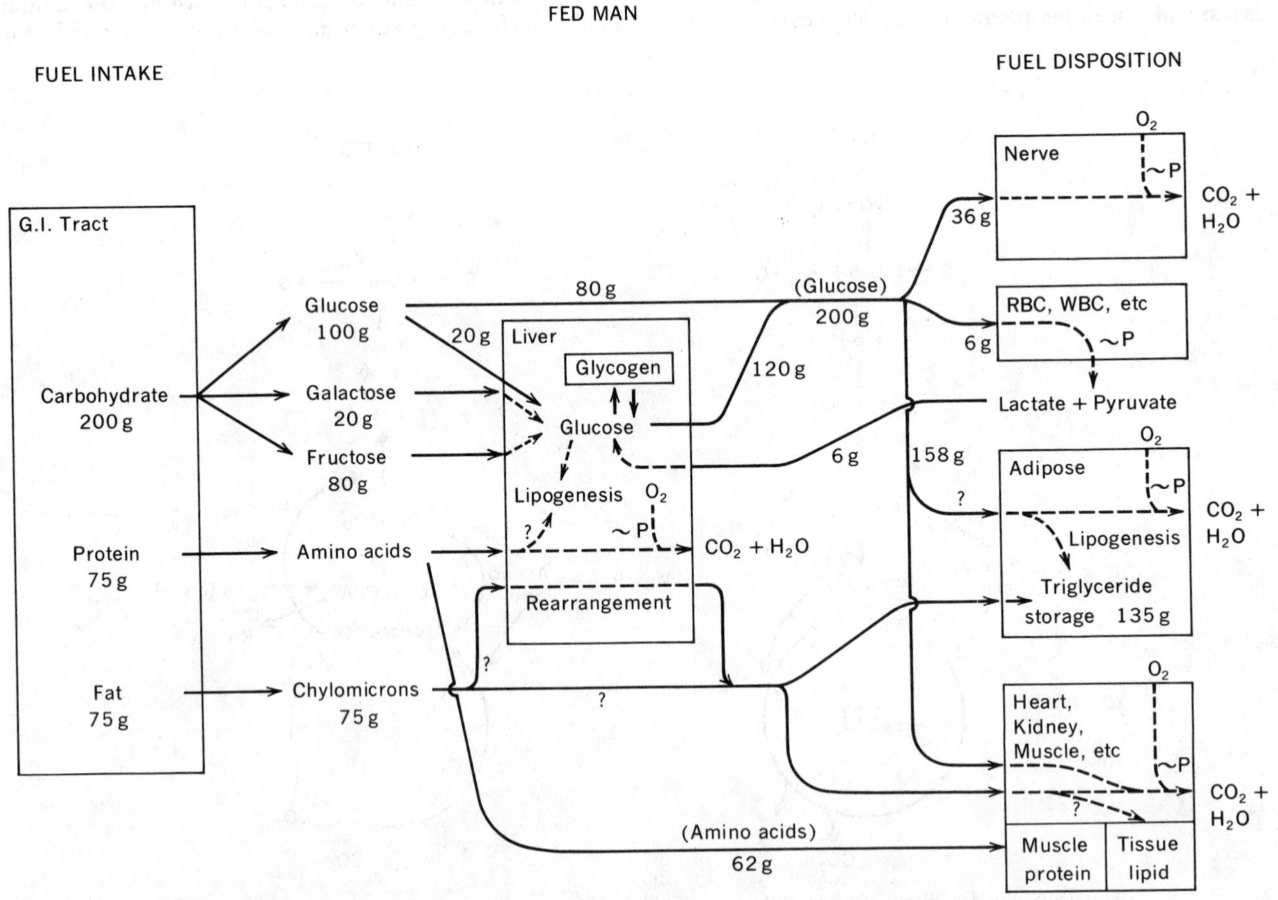

FED MAN

FUEL INTAKE

FUEL DISPOSITION

G.I. Tract

Carbohydrate 200 g → Glucose 100 g / Galactose 20 g / Fructose 80 g

Protein 75 g → Amino acids

Fat 75 g → Chylomicrons 75 g

Liver

Glycogen

Glucose

Lipogenesis O_2 ? ~P → $CO_2 + H_2O$

Rearrangement

80 g   (Glucose) 200 g

20 g

120 g

6 g

?

?

?

Nerve O_2 ~P → $CO_2 + H_2O$ 36 g

RBC, WBC, etc 6 g ~P

Lactate + Pyruvate

Adipose O_2 ~P → $CO_2 + H_2O$ Lipogenesis

Triglyceride storage 135 g

158 g

?

Heart, Kidney, Muscle, etc O_2 ~P → $CO_2 + H_2O$

(Amino acids) 62 g

Muscle protein | Tissue lipid

?

Fig. 75-8. Quantitative estimation of the flow of metabolic fuel of a man eating a theoretic meal containing 200 Gm carbohydrate (100 Gm as glucose, 20 Gm galactose, and 80 Gm fructose), 75 Gm protein, and 75 Gm fat and disposing of the meal in peripheral depots in 4 hr.

economical reasons, into glucose synthesis, and the liver now uses for its own energy needs the partial oxidation of fatty acids to ketone bodies, from which one-third of the total potential energy of the fatty acid is derived. Thus the process of gluconeogenesis, amino acid metabolism (and therefore urea production), and the production of ketone bodies are intimately related.

When the animal is fed, liver metabolism is grossly altered through a number of complicated mechanisms. Gluconeogenesis ceases, those amino acids which enter the liver are metabolized, providing the needed energy for the liver's own metabolic processes, and ketone production ceases. The level of free fatty acids in the circulation falls, since their release from adipose tissue is inhibited. The liver, however, continues to remove about one-fourth of the total turnover of free fatty acids, but now, since its own energy is adequately provided by amino acid oxidation via its citric acid cycle, esterifies these free fatty acids and returns them to the periphery instead of converting them to ketone bodies. In other words, during fasting, amino acid carbon is diverted into gluconeogenesis, the liver citric acid cycle is inoperative, and the liver's energy is derived from ketogenesis. During feeding, the citric acid cycle predominates, amino acids are deaminated, and their products are oxidized via the cycle, and ketone production essentially ceases.

Total Organism

Figures 75-7 and 75-8 summarize the two metabolic phases of fasting and feeding in a normal man at rest. The basal metabolic expenditure, that amount of fuel as determined by the oxygen consumed to burn it, is a function of body surface, age, and sex and is remarkably constant in a single person and, more important, between persons of similar age, size, and sex. The basal metabolic rate (BMR) is expressed as a percentage variation of the mean oxygen consumption obtained from a normal population of similar sex and surface area, or substituting for surface area, height and weight, from which surface area is derived. The appetite mechanism in a normal individual appears to be exquisitely set so as to maintain the body at constant weight and to be able to compensate for the increased fuel consumption during muscular work. Thus the weight normally varies little from year to year. For example, if an additional 100 kcal, i.e., one slice of bread, were to be stored daily as adipose tissue, at the end of the year there would have been over a 10-lb weight gain. The sensitivity of the appetite mechanism and, obviously, of the capacity to expend the calories beyond those required to maintain basal metabolism, and the equality between these two processes in the normal individual are overtly disturbed

SEVERE DIABETES

ORIGIN OF FUEL   FUEL CONSUMPTION

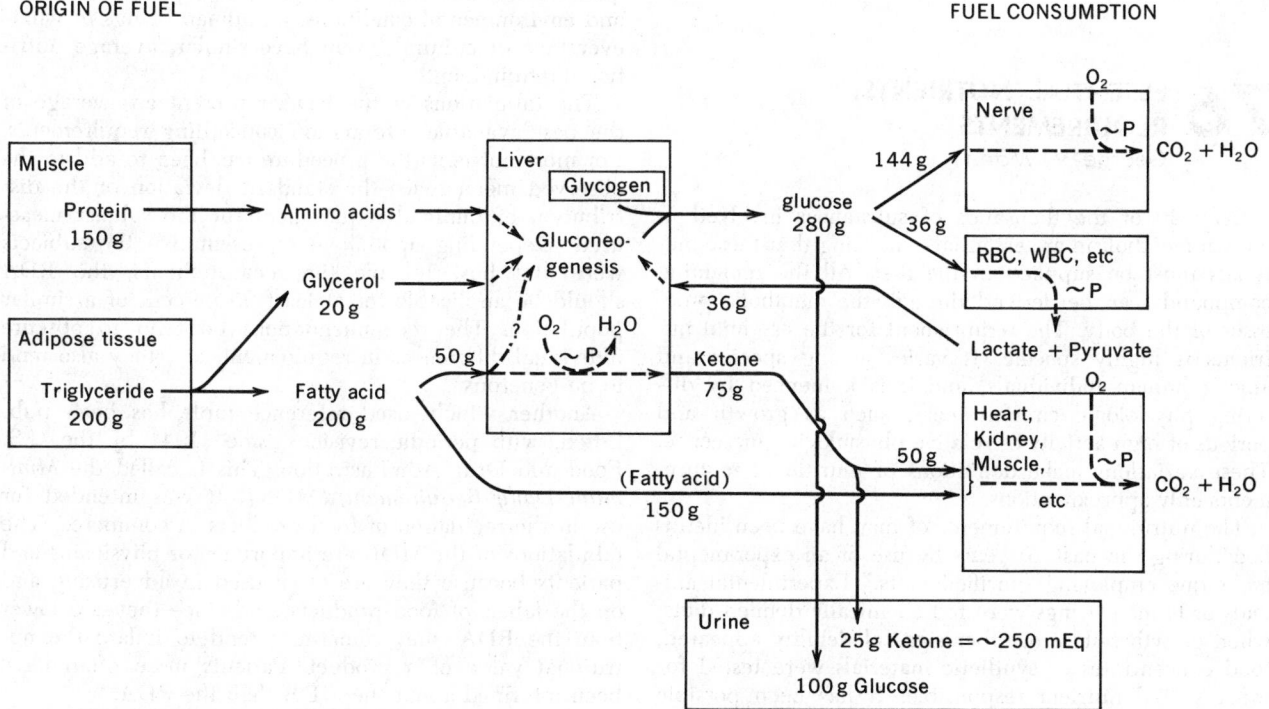

Fig. 75-9. Quantitative estimation of the flow of metabolic fuel for a period of 24 hr in a subject with diabetes mellitus; the subject was losing 25 Gm ketone and 100 Gm glucose in the urine. This glucose is in addition to that amount lost in the urine if the subject were eating and spilling the ingested carbohydrate. Thus a net negative carbohydrate balance of this degree is the causative factor which necessitates increased gluconeogenesis and the resultant ketosis. Net energy loss is 2400 kcal.

in states of abnormal energy storage such as anorexia nervosa, or its antithesis, obesity (discussed further in Chaps. 42 and 48).

Diabetes Mellitus

The metabolic changes of the normal fasted man may be extrapolated into those of the subject with diabetes, who loses glucose in the urine because of hyperglycemia (Fig. 75-9). Thus, muscle protein is mobilized at a faster rate to supply precursors for the accelerated gluconeogenesis. Fatty acids are released more rapidly from adipose tissue, and concomitantly ketones are produced more rapidly by the liver, and these also are spilled in the urine; being relatively strong acids, their loss is associated with sodium and potassium loss, thereby producing a metabolic acidosis. The entire sequence progresses (as described in Chap. 94) until reversed by the administration of insulin.

REFERENCES

Anfinsen, C.: "The Molecular Basis of Evolution," New York, John Wiley & Sons, Inc., 1959.

Lehninger, A. L.: "The Mitochondrion," New York, W. A. Benjamin, Inc., 1964.

Stanbury, J. B., J. B. Wyngaarden, and D. C. Fredrickson: "The Metabolic Basis of Inherited Disease," 2d ed., McGraw-Hill Book Company, New York, 1966.

76 ESSENTIAL NUTRIENTS: REQUIREMENTS
George V. Mann

Only 40 of the thousands of substances involved in human metabolism are essential—meaning that these materials must be supplied in the diet. All the remaining compounds can be derived through the metabolic processes of the body. The requirement for the essential nutrients is highly specific. It varies among species and among human individuals, and it is influenced by differing physiologic circumstances, such as growth and periods of high activity or relative physiologic quiescence. These variations make definitions of nutritional requirements only approximations.

The nutritional requirements of man have been identified during the past 70 years by use of an experimental technique employing "purified diets." Experimental animals or human beings were fed chemically defined diets; when growth failure or other signs of debility appeared, food concentrates or synthetic materials were tested for the essential nutrient responsible. It has been possible by this method to produce in animals disorders which mimic human disease and to isolate the essential organic factors (vitamins). The vitamins were first named alphabetically and were then, when they were identified, given chemical names. Systematic studies with purified diets

were begun about 1900 by F. G. Hopkins and E. V. McCollum and were extended by H. C. Sherman, H. Steenbock, the Mellanbys, C. Elvejhem, and many others. This immensely useful work has been reviewed by McCollum, a pioneer in the field who died in 1967.

The major nutrients, fat, protein, and carbohydrate, were first defined, and then certain of the bulkier minerals which are indispensable for growth and health were identified. The vitamins, the essential amino acids, and the essential trace elements were recognized later. Estimates of daily requirements have been summarized and published since 1943 by the Food and Nutrition Board of the National Research Council of the United States. These recommendations are intended to serve as standards of reference rather than final judgments. They are sometimes misinterpreted because of failure to note that the *Recommended Dietary Allowance* (RDA) includes a generous margin of safety above the current estimates of minimal daily requirements. It does not follow that all persons taking less than the RDA are malnourished. The RDA attempts to set a goal which will ensure good nutrition in healthy individuals under current living conditions in the United States.

Other official agencies have published similar recommendations for nutrient intake which are more applicable to their particular needs or national situations. The differences among these recommendations do not imply that various racial and ethnic groups have different nutritional requirements. While there are differences of requirement due to variations in body size, physical activity, and environmental conditions, all human beings of whatever race or cultural group have similar, average nutritional requirements.

The tabulations in the RDA represent an average of the best available information concerning requirements. For most nutrients the procedure has been to add to the observed mean twice the standard deviation of the distribution of minimal requirement for the subject measured. Depending upon how representative the subjects were and how reliable the measurements, the RDA should be applicable for at least 95 percent of a similar population. The recommendations do tend to obscure individual differences in requirement, and they also tend to be generous.

Another widely used reference table has been published, with periodic revisions, since 1941 by the U.S. Food and Drug Administration. This is called the *Minimum Daily Requirement* (MDR). It was intended for use in the regulation of food products in commerce. The tabulations of the MDR are important for physicians and patients because they are often used in advertising and on the labels of food products, and since they are lower than the RDA, they sometimes tend to inflate the nutritional value of a product. Patients more often have been informed about the MDR than the RDA.

The 40 essential elements and compounds necessary in the human diet are listed in Table 76-2. The essentiality of a nutrient is determined by species, by individual constitution, and by the metabolic circumstances.

Ascorbic acid is necessary for primates and a few ro-

Table 76-1. RECOMMENDED DAILY DIETARY ALLOWANCES, FOOD AND NUTRITION BOARD,
NATIONAL ACADEMY OF SCIENCES, NATIONAL RESEARCH COUNCIL

	Age,[1] years	Weight kg	Height cm	Kcal[2]	Protein, Gm	Fat soluble vitamins			Water soluble vitamins							Minerals				
						A[5] IU	D, IU	E, IU	Ascorbic acid, mg	Folic acid, mg	Nicotinic acid,[3] mg.Eq.	Riboflavin, mg	Thiamine, mg	Vitamin B$_6$, mg	Vitamin B$_{12}$ μgm	Ca, Gm	P, Gm	I$_2$, μg	Fe, mg	Mg, mg
Infants[4].......	0–1	4–9	55–72	kg × 120	kg × 2	1500	400	5	35	0.05	6	0.4	0.3	0.3	1.5	0.6	0.5	40	10	100
Children......	1–10	12–28	81–131	1100–2200	25–40	2500	400	10	40	0.2	10	1.0	0.7	1.0	4	0.8	0.8	80	10	200
Adolescent																				
Male.......	10–18	35–59	140–170	2500–3000	45–60	5000	400	20	50	0.4	18	1.4	1.2	1.8	5	1.4	1.4	135	18	350
Female.....	10–18	35–54	142–160	2250–2300	50–55	5000	400	20	50	0.4	15	1.4	0.9	1.8	5	1.3	1.3	115	18	350
Adult[6]																				
Male.....	18 up	67–70	175 up	2800	60 up	5000	....	30	60	0.4	17	1.7	1.0	2.0	5	0.8	0.8	130	10	350
Female.....	18 up	58 up	163 up	2000	55 up	5000	....	25	55	0.4	12	1.7	0.8	2.0	5	0.8	0.8	100	18	300
Pregnant......	....	....	....	+200	65	6000	400	30	60	0.8	15	1.8	1.0	2.5	8	+0.4	+0.4	125	18	450
Lactating.....	....	....	....	+1000	75	8000	400	30	60	0.5	20	2.0	1.2	2.5	6	+0.5	+0.5	150	18	450

[1] The age ranges are more abridged here than in the original table.
[2] Calorie adjustment must be made for size and expenditure.
[3] Nicotinic acid equivalents include preformed nicotinic acid and tryptophane, 60 mg.Eq. to 1 mg nicotinic acid.
[4] Allowances for calcium, thiamine, riboflavin, and nicotinic acid are proportional to calorie requirement.
[5] Assuming one-fifth from preformed vitamin A and four-fifth from beta-carotene.
[6] These allowances will include a range of individual requirements for individuals living in the United States under usual environmental conditions. They can be achieved with a variety of common foods which will also supply other nutrients for which human requirements are uncertain.

SOURCE: This table is adapted from the more detailed table of the "Recommended Dietary Allowances" of the National Research Council, Food and Nutrition Board, 7th ed. Publication 1694 Price $1, NAS Printing and Publications Office, 2101 Constitution Ave. N.W., Washington, D.C. 20418.

dents and birds because they lack the enzyme necessary for one step in the formation of ascorbic acid from glucose. The essential amino acids illustrate the relativity of the term *essential*. Arginine and histidine are essential for growing children but not for human adults. Glycine and L-cystine are essential for chickens during periods of feather growth but not at other times.

DIET MIXTURES. The energy for growth, metabolism, and physical activity is supplied by the major foodstuffs, fat, carbohydrate, and protein. In the United States ap-

Table 76-2. ESSENTIAL NUTRIENTS FOR
HUMAN BEINGS

Elements	Major	Ca, P, Na, Cl, K, Mg
	Minor	Fe, I, Mn, Mb, Co, Zn, Cu
	Uncertain	Se, Cr, Fl
Vitamins	Water soluble	Thiamine, riboflavin, pyridoxine, niacin, folacin, pantothenic acid, cobalamine, biotin, ascorbic acid
	Fat soluble	Vitamin A-carotene, D, E, K essential fatty acids (linoleic, arachidonic)
Nitrogenous	Essential amino acids	Lysine, threonine, leucine, isoleucine, methionine, tryptophane, valine, phenylalanine (for children, arginine and histidine)
	Nonessential nitrogen	

Notes—Carbon and oxygen are essential. Choline is not considered a vitamin. When optimal amounts of cobalamine, serine, and methionine are available, choline is synthesized from them.

proximately 15 percent of the calories of this fuel mixture is derived from protein, 40 percent from fat, and 45 percent from carbohydrate. These proportions are strongly influenced by cultural and socioeconomic conditions. The proportion of fat and protein in the diet mixture has tended to increase since 1900 in the United States as the proportion of carbohydrates, especially the complex polysaccharides from foods such as potatoes and cereal flours, has decreased.

The human organism has an astonishing versatility in adapting to different food mixtures. Thus, the hunters and pastoralists of the world exist in good nutritional health on meat or milk diets which contain less than 50 Gm carbohydrate daily, whereas agriculturists and vegetarians maintain good health on diets with only 30 to 40 Gm protein and 25 Gm or less fat daily. It is important to recognize that dietary adequacy can be obtained with widely different fuel mixtures (Fig. 76-1).

CALORIES. The recommended dietary allowances include energy allotments according to age, size, sex, and activity. These recommendations are more useful for economic planners than for physicians because of the wide variation of individual calorie requirement. It has been useful to define a reference man who is twenty-two years old and weighs 70 kg and a reference woman age twenty-two and weighing 58 kg. Resting metabolism is related to size as body weight in $kg^{0.72}$. This energy requirement declines with age at the rate of about 2 percent per decade after age twenty. Energy costs are also increased by deviations from ambient temperature below 14°C and above 30°C.

Pregnancy requires the accumulation of about 55,000 Cal, an average of 200 Cal per day. The production of 850 ml milk per day requires about 1000 Cal. The re-

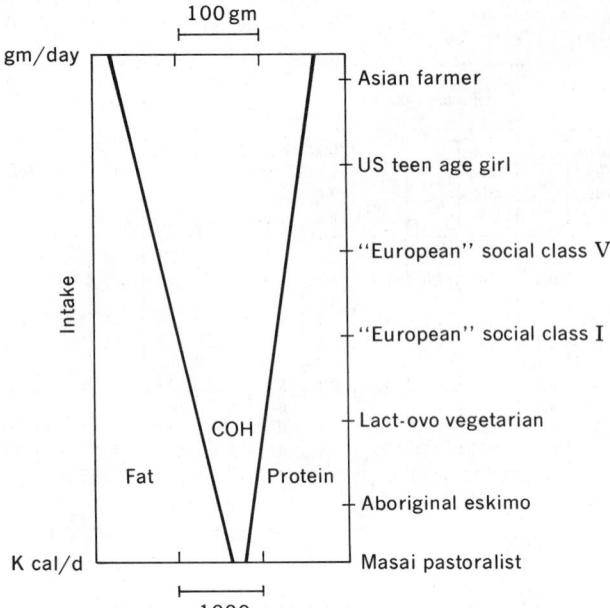

Fig. 76-1. The range of dietary mixtures compatible with good nutrition encountered in various groups of individuals. Social classes I to V are those designated by the Registrar General of the United Kingdom in accordance with socioeconomic status. Class I refers to professional persons, and Class V to unskilled laborers.

maining energy cost for adult persons is attributable to physical activity, and this is almost always the critical determinant of the amount of adipose tissue. The preoccupation with appetite as the cause and with restriction of food in the treatment of obesity to the neglect of expenditure rates has been a major error of nutritional science (See Chap. 48). The cost of maximal physical activity for man can be increased by exertion to twenty times the resting level of 65 Cal per hr. Cultural attitudes and technical developments have largely abolished such high and protracted levels of energy expenditure in the Western world, and the consequences are increasing obesity and health problems of many kinds.

The energy cost of fever is discussed in Chap. 16.

CARBOHYDRATE. With the exception of ascorbic acid there are no particular carbohydrates known to be essential in the human diet. Despite statements to the contrary, there are no persuasive reasons to believe that refined carbohydrates in the diet are damaging or predispose to disease. There is evidence that the ability of some individuals to metabolize lactose is progressively impaired with age, probably through a loss of intestinal lactase. The increasing evidence of intolerance to milk in older persons is explained on this basis. The amount of carbohydrate in the diet has a distinct but transitory influence on the plasma level of triglycerides.

FAT. The dietary fat furnishes 9 Cal per Gm, while protein and carbohydrate supply only 4 Cal per Gm. Fats add palatability to food. The fat content of the diet in the United States has steadily increased over the last 50 years, more in the content of polyunsaturated vegetable

fatty acids than in saturated animal fat. It has not been established that the kind of dietary fat is a factor in the development of disease, although it is widely assumed, on the basis of circumstantial evidence, that saturated animal fat contributes to hypercholesteremia and atherosclerosis (see Chap. 275).

Two unsaturated fatty acids, linoleic and arachidonic, have been shown to be essential nutrients for experimental animals and for children, but essential fatty acid deficiency is unknown in human adults. Diets low in fat have an additional significance because dietary fat is the vehicle for absorption of other fat-soluble nutrients, especially vitamin A and carotenes. Fatty acids with 8 to 12 carbons are absorbed directly into the portal system. Mixtures of triglyceride made with these "medium chain" fatty acids are useful because they are better absorbed than the long-chain fatty acids more prevalent in natural foodstuffs. They are useful in the management of intestinal malabsorption (Chap. 316).

PROTEIN. Protein is a dietary essential because of its component amino acids. Food proteins contain various combinations of the 20 natural amino acids, of which 10 have been shown to be essential for human beings. Arginine and histidine are essential only for growing children.

The amino acids recovered from the hydrolysis of dietary protein are either used for the synthesis of body protein or they are catabolized for energy. The energy requirements of the body take priority so that catabolism can supersede anabolism, thus accounting for the interdependence of amino acid requirement and energy supply. As described in Chap. 79, there is a spectrum of protein-calorie malnutrition ranging from protein deficiency with sufficient calories to a dietary energy deficiency which is not relieved even by high quality protein in the diet.

Genetic determinants govern the formation of proteins. The body protein can only be formed or replaced with the amino acid mixture appropriate for the protein being synthesized, and all the constituent amino acids must be present simultaneously. Lacking one or more of the amino acids, the body cannot make proteins, since it cannot make incomplete ones, and it has a limited ability to conserve an incomplete mixture until the missing amino acids can be obtained. The 10 to 12 nonessential amino acids are part of this mixture and differ in the capability of the body to synthesize them from simpler available substrates. The actual essential chemical substances are not the amino acids themselves but the alpha-keto acids which are readily aminated to furnish amino acids. This fact is important in the search for a nutritionally adequate dietary mixture which will minimize the urinary nitrogen in patients with uremia. Thus, in addition to the nutritional requirement for each of the essential amino acids there is a need for nitrogen which can be used for aminating the nonessential alpha-keto acids as they are synthesized.

Deficiencies of essential amino acids in human beings result in no specific signs or symptoms. The requirements for the essential amino acids have been established by measurement of nitrogen balance. Balance is a statement of the net economy of a substance, positive during retention, negative during loss. The major nitrogen loss from the body is in the urine, and this amount is highly dependent upon protein intake. Urea nitrogen tends to predominate in the urine with high protein diets and become negligible on protein-free diets. The fecal nitrogen is relatively constant, averaging about 1 Gm per day in adults. With sweat and desquamation a small loss of nitrogen occurs through the skin.

The *nutritional quality of a dietary protein* can be determined in several ways. The most useful experimental method has been the measurement of *biological value*, which is the percent nitrogen absorbed from a given protein which is retained in the body. For identifying the essential amino acids and measuring the minimum daily requirement of each in man, determination of the minimal protein level necessary to maintain nitrogen balance has been more useful. The measurements must be precise, the observational periods long, and the environmental conditions carefully controlled. These technical requirements make the method tedious and costly, and it has not been applied to large numbers of subjects. A third method for evaluating nitrogen requirement is to sum up nitrogen losses through the urine, the feces, and the skin while the test subject is fed a protein-free diet. When allowances are made for growth, the requirement is the sum of all these channels. Because the nitrogen content of protein is about 16 percent, the sum of the excreted nitrogen × 6.25 (100/16) equals the daily protein requirement in grams.

If minimal total body nitrogen loss in adults and children is 3.2 mg per basal Cal energy exchange, then the daily maintenance requirement is 20 mg (3.2 × 6.25) of protein per basal Cal. Assuming the basal energy requirement for the reference man is 1750 Cal, then (1750 × 20)/1000 gives a minimal requirement of 35 Gm of an ideal protein daily. However, because the coefficient of variation among individuals for protein required per basal Cal is about 15 percent, twice this, or 30 percent of 35 Gm, is added, giving a daily requirement of the ideal protein of 45 Gm. This is the generous margin of the estimate. On the average, dietary proteins are only about 70 percent utilized because of limitations of absorption and retention. Consequently 45 × 100/70 equals 65 Gm daily as the requirement for ordinary protein. This amounts to 0.93 Gm protein per kg of body weight for the reference man and is the basis for the commonly used estimate of requirement (1 Gm protein per kg body weight per day). Growing children and pregnant or lactating women are given additional allowances for growth and secretion of protein.

The quality of dietary protein is critically important. Proteins which are low in one or more of the essential amino acids must be taken in large amounts in order to furnish the amino acid mixture necessary for synthesis of body protein. This relationship has additional nutritional significance. Two or more proteins, each deficient in different essential amino acids, can complement one another when eaten together. Between them they may furnish a high-grade protein. This is one reason for advising people to eat a variety of foods to ensure a sound diet. It is also the basis for the search for indigenous food proteins in areas of the world where protein malnutrition is prevalent in order to find a combination of native proteins which will yield an adequate mixture of high biological value. This usually is a more economical and feasible solution than importing a complete protein or introducing entirely new foods.

Generally, the available amino acid pattern of plant proteins is less like that of human tissues than proteins from animal sources. Whole egg protein has a high biologic value and is often used as a reference standard. However, since animal proteins require that time, labor, plant proteins, and other foodstuffs be used to feed livestock for their production, a long-term goal has been to find ways in agriculture, food technology, and cookery to make mixtures of complementary plant proteins which will be as nutritious as the animal proteins which approximate the composition of human proteins.

It is possible in animals to produce imbalances of amino acid intake which lead to growth failure, but this has not been shown to be important in man. There is no known dietary requirement for any whole protein or polypeptide. There is probably some upper limit of dietary nitrogen intake, although this must be very high. Some pastoralists are well nourished on a diet of milk and meat which entails a daily protein intake of 300 Gm and an equal amount of fat.

ESSENTIAL ELEMENTS. In addition to the elements which are furnished as components of the major foodstuffs (O, H, N, S, C), there are 16 others which are known or suspected to be essential. These are shown in Table 76-2.

CALCIUM AND PHOSPHORUS. Calcium and phosphorus are particularly important during growth. They are especially abundant in bone and are also essential ionic components of soft tissues. There is accumulating evidence that the mass of bone mineral accumulated in young adult life is steadily depleted thereafter and that the appearance of subsequent disorders involving demineralization may be a function of this starting mass.

Calcium is not absorbed efficiently from the intestine. Vitamin D is required for this process. Circumstances which produce malabsorption as well as dietary phytates, oxalates, and excessive phosphate may compromise absorption of calcium. The obligatory loss of calcium in the urine of an adult is about 175 mg per day, while the fecal loss of endogenous calcium is 125 mg daily. An additional 10 to 20 mg is lost each day through the skin, making the total loss about 300 mg daily. Only about 40 percent of the dietary calcium is absorbed, so that an allowance of 800 mg per day in the food is necessary to replace this loss. Nevertheless, it has been shown that many individuals can, by adaptive processes, come into balance on as little as 300 mg daily intake. It is not established that a long-continued intake which is low or marginal in calcium is a cause of osteoporosis (Chap. 381). During growth, pregnancy, and lactation, additional allowances of 100 to 600 mg daily are recommended.

SODIUM AND CHLORIDE. While sodium and chloride are essential ions, they often are consumed in great excess. The best estimate of the usual adult intake in the United States is between 6,000 and 18,000 mg sodium chloride daily. This is in contrast to an estimated sodium chloride requirement of 800 to 1,000 mg daily. That this excess intake contributes to ill health is not clear. The intake of sodium chloride in the United States has tended to decline as other methods for preserving food have been developed. A drive for eating salt occurs in animals which subsist on a vegetarian diet low in sodium and high in potassium. Carnivores have no craving for salt because they obtain sufficient sodium from the meat they eat. The ratio of K to Na intake of herbivores is 20, as compared with 5 for most carnivores and 1.0 for human beings in the Western world.

Only severe and prolonged heat exposure requires supplementary salt, since dietary intake usually is high, and because of the efficient adaptation reaction mediated by aldosterone secretion (Chap. 92) which diminishes the sodium in sweat and urine after heat exposure. Disorders of sodium homeostasis occur where the adaptation is overwhelmed or, as in mucoviscidosis (Chap. 334), when full adaptation cannot be achieved. The availability of potent saluretic drugs has diminished but not abolished the need for salt-restricted diets (see Chap. 264). Sodium depletion is generally the consequence of a restricted intake and urinary wastage caused by either a saluretic agent or renal disease (see Chap. 300).

POTASSIUM. The principal intracellular cation is potassium. Appreciation of the clinical significance of potassium was delayed because the plasma concentration of potassium is not a sensitive index of changes in intracellular concentration. Disorders attributable to hyper- or hypokalemia are described in Chaps. 92, 264, and 300.

There are no recommended dietary allowances for sodium, potassium, or chloride because they are widely distributed in food, and disorders are more commonly the result of excessive losses or retention than of dietary deficiency.

IRON. Iron is an indispensable element which is often taken in marginal or low amounts in human diets. Iron deficiency will be discussed in Chap. 336. Iron toxicity can occur (Chap. 107), especially when iron intake is high in the face of a low protein diet. Since only 10 percent of dietary iron is absorbed and absorption varies with the source of iron, the RDA ranges from 12 to 18 mg per day for men, pregnant women, and growing children. The three physiologic conditions which require particular attention to iron intake are infancy and adolescence, when growth is rapid; menstruation, which causes a loss of an average of 15 mg of iron during each cycle; and pregnancy, when maternal iron-bearing tissues are enlarging and the fetus is accumulating iron as well.

MAGNESIUM. Magnesium is a cofactor for many body enzymes. Adult tissues contain about 20 to 25 Gm magnesium, about half of which is in bone. The RDA is 350 mg per day for men and 300 mg per day for women. This is readily obtained in ordinary diets. The average American diet contains about 120 mg of magnesium per 1000 Cal.

Experiments with a small group of human subjects fed a diet deficient in magnesium but adequate in other respects produced a nonspecific spectrum of neurologic, muscular, and gastrointestinal manifestations which seemed related to a marked decrease in serum calcium and potassium levels. It appeared in these studies that magnesium is well conserved by both the kidney and the bowel when the supply is limited, but it is poorly stored so that a regular intake is necessary to avoid deficiency. The manifestations of magnesium depletion are described in Chap. 85.

HALOGENS. The daily requirement of *iodine* is 50 to 70 μg. It is an essential part of the thyroid hormones. Its metabolism is discussed in Chap. 89. An efficient way to assure this intake, especially in areas with soil depleted of iodine, is by the use of iodized salt. In the United States such salt is offered optionally with 100 ppm of iodide. Since 1920, this practice has dramatically reduced the prevalence of goiter. Some nations by mandate require iodinization of salt.

While *fluoride* is not known to be essential, its administration during the formative years of life at a rate of about 1 ppm in drinking water will approximately halve the rate of dental caries. An excess of fluoride, above 3 to 5 ppm in water, leads to cosmetic disfigurement of teeth, and larger excesses cause osteopetrosis and ossification of ligaments. It has been proposed that a fluoride intake of 1 to 5 ppm may diminish the prevalence of osteoporosis in adult life. The fluoride ion is thought to change the crystalline structure of apatite in bone by replacing an hydroxyl ion. This action in bone may resemble its effect on teeth.

COPPER. Copper is known to be essential in man, but deficiency is thought to be very rare. An adult man's tissues contain 75 to 150 mg copper. The concentration is highest in the liver at birth. Most of the serum copper is bound to the protein ceruloplasmin. Copper intoxication is well known in Wilson's disease (Chap. 110). A daily intake of 2 mg copper maintains balance and is easily obtained even in relatively poor diets. Deficiency is usually associated with an iron deficiency or with major malabsorptive disorders.

TRACE ELEMENTS. The trace or microelements include chromium, cobalt, manganese, molybdenum, selenium, and zinc.

Chromium may influence carbohydrate metabolism, since chromium-deficient rats show abnormal glucose tolerance. *Cobalt* appears to function in man only as a component of vitamin B_{12}. *Manganese* is a component of several enzyme systems and is also found in bone, but deficiency of this element in man has not been recognized. *Molybdenum* is essential for experimental animals, but a deficiency in man is unknown. *Selenium* has been shown to have functions like those of vitamin E, and clear-cut deficiency has been produced in animals. Selenium intoxication is also well known in animals raised in areas with a high selenium content in the soil and vegetation.

Zinc deficiency has been demonstrated in animals, but

the existence of definite human deficiency is still uncertain. In patients with cirrhosis, low levels of plasma zinc and high urinary levels have been reported, but the relation of these changes to the disease is not established.

The vitamins are discussed in the chapters which follow.

REFERENCES

DuBois, E. F.: "Basal Metabolism in Health and Disease,"

pp. 410–442, chap. 18, Philadelphia, Lea & Febiger, 1936.

Holt, P. R.: Medium Chain Triglycerides. A Useful Adjunct in Nutritional Therapy, Gastroenterology, 53:961, 1967.

McCollum, E. V.: "A History of Nutrition," Boston, Houghton Mifflin Company, 1964.

Shils, M. E.: Experimental Human Magnesium Depletion, Medicine, 48:61, 1969.

Underwood, E. J.: "Trace Elements in Human and Animal Nutrition," 2nd ed., New York, Academic Press Inc., 1962.

Section 2

Nutritional Deficiency States

77 NUTRITIONAL DEFICIENCY STATES

George V. Mann

Malnutrition in Western developed countries has two aspects, overnutrition and undernutrition. Sporadic instances of scurvy and rickets in United States children usually result from some combination of misinformation or ignorance and are not indicative of widespread deficiency. Lamentations about the nutrition of teenagers are often heard, but these are more often based on the misapplication of generous dietary allowances rather than on the documentation of physical or chemical signs of nutritional deficiency.

THE PATHOGENESIS OF NUTRITIONAL DISEASE. Human beings cannot select an adequate diet from a variety of foods by instinctive reliance upon taste or the other senses, but require nutrition education. Moreover, poor food habits are very difficult to change. Margaret Mead has observed that one can change religion more easily than food habits.

Dietary deficiencies result from two kinds of changes. Thus the food supply may change as with the introduction of maize into Europe, which led to pellagra, or the change to polished rice in the Orient, which led to endemic beriberi. Another cause of dietary deficiency is a shift from a wide to a narrow assortment of food choices. When a varied diet gives way to alcohol, when meat is replaced by crackers and tea, when fresh vegetables are replaced by a few canned foods, or when civilization and northerly migration bring smoke and clothing which prevent the exposure of the skin to sun, then nutritional deficiencies may occur.

Seven principles should be kept in mind in relation to the causes and management of nutritional disease.

1. Animals, including man, adapt to the available food. This adaptation occurs for many nutrients, but that for protein is better understood. When the protein supply is low, the organism becomes more efficient in nitrogen utilization and it can come into nitrogen balance on as little as 20 to 30 Gm protein per day.

2. Culture determines food behavior. A child learns the way his culture has dealt with food and he follows this through life. The most important teacher of nutrition is the mother. Elementary schools offer an important opportunity to correct or modify food habits.

3. Food deprivation alters behavior. This is a conspicuous effect, especially during periods of calorie deprivation. Starvation causes profound deterioration of personality, whether caused by cancer, famine, or the faddist treatment of obesity.

4. Foods complement one another in their nutrient content. Two proteins, each incomplete in content of essential amino acids, may when taken together, serve as a complete protein. The incidence of nutritional deficiency increases when the diet has been restricted in variety.

5. Nutrient deficiencies are generally multiple because a diet of natural foods rarely will be low in only one essential nutrient. This is important in therapy for treatment with a single nutrient will often aggravate coexistent deficiencies of other nutrients.

6. The nutrient requirements of human beings are known. While this may seem an overconfident statement, it is a reasonable assumption. There is no foundation for the faddists' argument which advocates bizarre foods for managing ill health because it is contended that "unknown essential nutrients" are supplied by these crude or unprocessed foods.

7. Frank deficiency disease appearing in a few individuals usually is indicative of subclinical or occult disease in others of the same family or social group.

The patterns of nutritional disease can be seen in two quite different social circumstances (Figs. 77-1 and

77-2). In the technically developed countries and among affluent classes, and even in underdeveloped areas, the pattern is one of "malnutrition amid plenty." Despite abundance of food, misguided or misinformed choices and consumption of highly refined and processed foods can result in dietary imbalance and nutritional deficiency. In the underdeveloped areas of the world and among the poor and underprivileged classes of all countries, the problems of too little food and too little choice are compounded by lack of judgment in the selection of food or its optimal preparation. The stress of parasitic infestation and infection often aggravates the already marginal intakes of energy and nutrients in these groups. There is no doubt that nutritional deficiency may be precipitated by other diseases, but it is not well established that malnutrition predisposes to other diseases. The morbidity and mortality from infectious disease is higher in malnourished populations than in the well nourished, but it has been difficult to show that malnutrition increases the incidence of infections.

FACTORS LEADING TO THE DEVELOPMENT OF DEFICIENCY STATES. These are six in number.

1. A low dietary intake of essential nutrients. This may be a result of poverty, ignorance, social isolation, or food faddism or the result of other behavioral abnormalities.

2. Low intakes may be caused by a disorder of the oral or pharyngeal cavities which impairs food intake.

3. Deficiency states may be the consequence of malabsorption. They will often be seen as a complication of sprue or of other malabsorption syndromes (Chap. 316).

4. Deficiency states may result from poor utilization of a nutrient of which intake is adequate. For example, the utilization of carotene, the provitamin A, is poor in the presence of hypothyroidism, and carotene is poorly absorbed if the diet is exceptionally low in fat. Vitamin K is poorly absorbed in the absence of bile in the intestinal tract, and the synthesis of prothrombin is often impaired in the presence of advanced liver disease.

5. Nutrient wastage may account for malnutrition, as

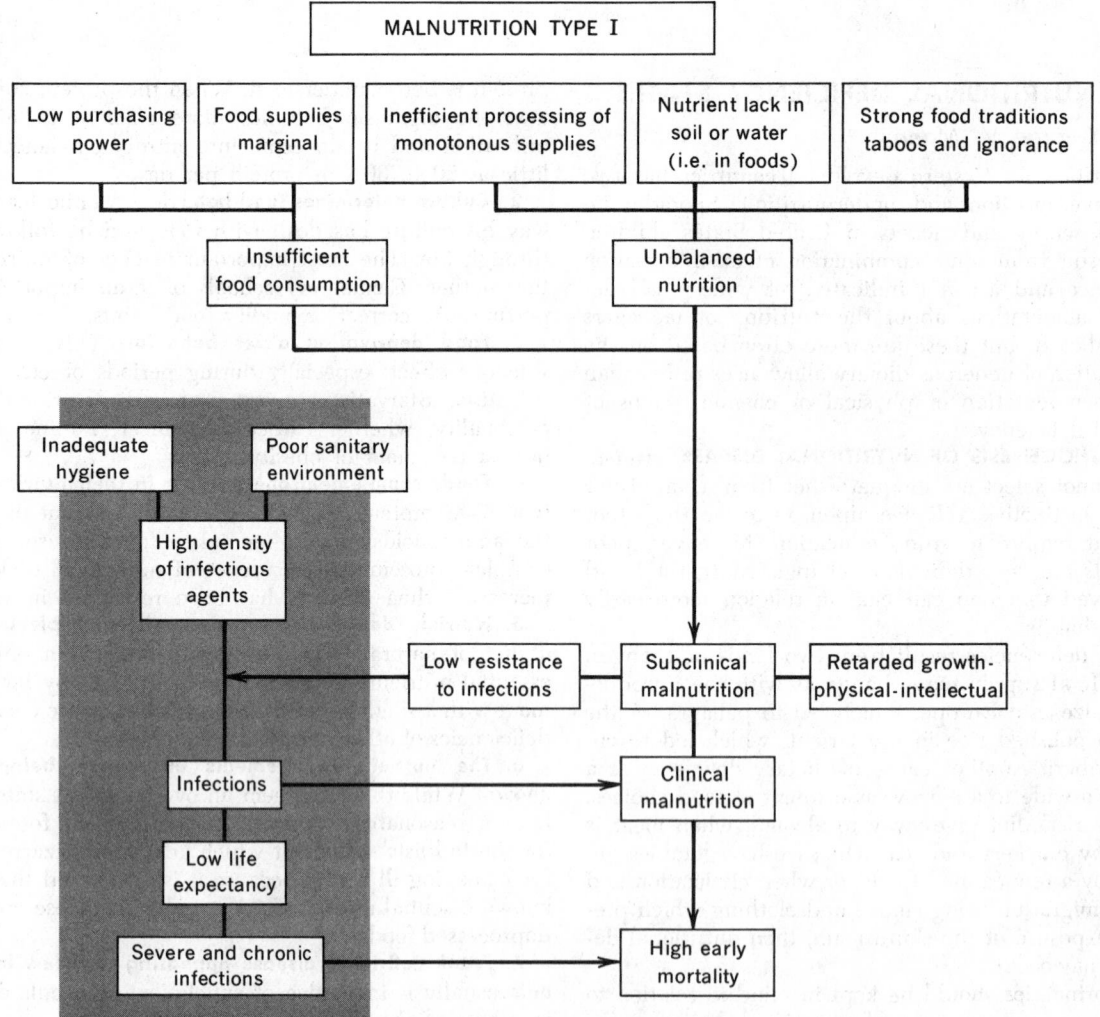

Fig. 77-1. The pattern of malnutrition in underdeveloped cultures.

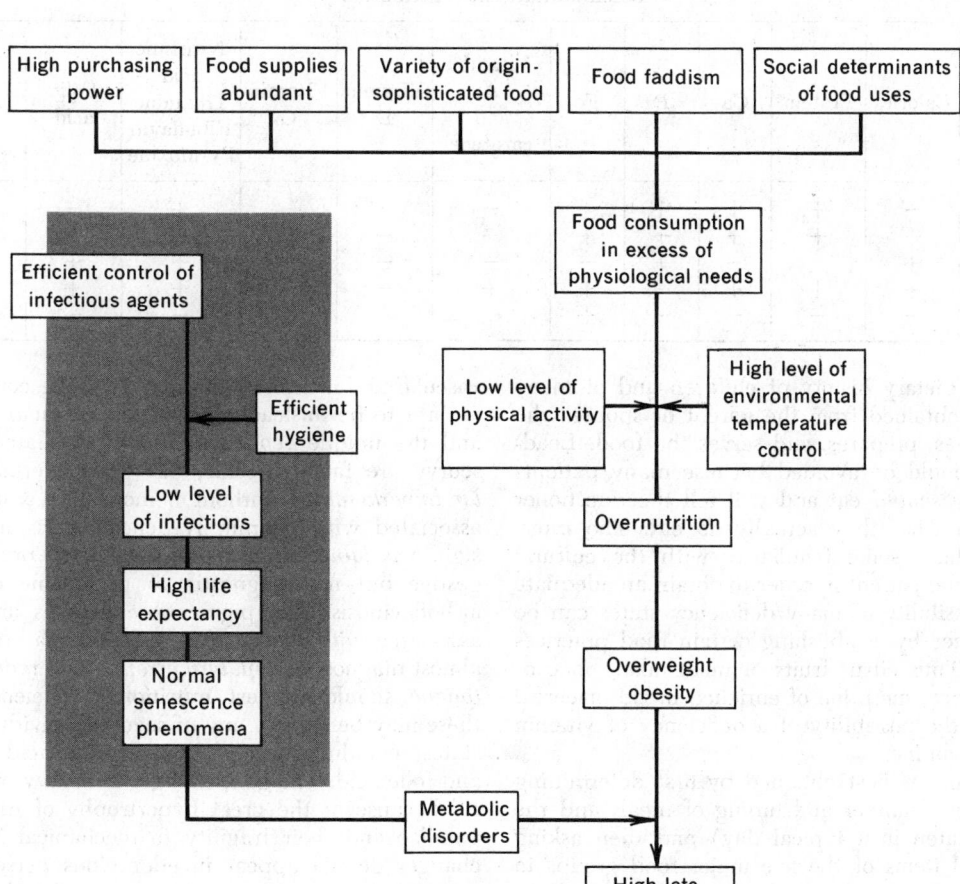

Fig. 77-2. The pattern of malnutrition in technically advanced cultures.

in the aminoacidurias or phosphaturias associated with renal tubular disease.

6. The utilization of a nutrient may be impaired even though intake is adequate, as when goitrogens impair iodine utilization. Substances with antivitamin activity are well known in experimental nutrition. Certain drugs impair the utilization of pyridoxine (Chap. 336).

REFERENCES

Behar, M., F. Viteri, R. Bressani, G. Arroyave, R. L. Squibb, and N. S. Scrimshaw: Principles of Treatment and Prevention of Severe Protein Malnutrition in Children (Kwashiorkor), Ann. N.Y. Acad. Sci., 69:854, 1959.

Mitchell, H. H.: Nutritional Adaptation, chap. 6 in "Nutrition," vol. 2, "Vitamins, Nutrient Requirements and Food Selection," G. H. Beaton, and E. W. McHenry (Eds.), New York, Academic Press Inc., 1964.

Scrimshaw, N. S., C. E. Taylor, and J. E. Gordon: Interactions of Nutrition and Infection, World Health Organ. Monogr., 1965.

78 EVALUATION OF NUTRITIONAL STATUS
George V. Mann

The diagnosis of malnutrition depends on the diet history, the recognition of distinctive physical signs, the demonstration of biochemical abnormalities, and the response to therapeutic trials.

DIET HISTORY. Of the several ways of measuring dietary intake, only the dietary history is likely to be applicable for physicians. In dietary surveys measurements of food intake often are made in the home by a household food inventory method. Dietitians may use the patient's 3- or 7-day food diary, and economists rely on evidence from commodity balance sheets and food available for consumption.

Obtaining a dietary history is simplest when food choice and variety have been limited. The inquiry must determine food habits over a period of weeks and months rather than a few days because the long-term intake is

Table 78-1. A SYNOPSIS OF U.S. BASIC FOOD GROUPS AND THEIR NUTRIENT CONTRIBUTION

Food group	Essential nutrient contribution											
	Calories	Protein	Ca	P	Fe	Vitamin A and carotene	Vitamin D	Vitamin C	Nicotinic acid Thiamine Riboflavin Pyridoxine	Folic acid	B$_{12}$	Vitamin E
Dairy	−	+	+	+	−	−	+	−	+	−	+	−
Meat	+	+	+	+	+	−	−	−	+	−	+	+
Cereal and bread	+	−	−	+	−	−	−	−	+	+	−	+
Vegetables	+	+	+	−	+	+	−	−	+	+	−	−
Fruit	−	−	−	−	+	+	−	+	−	−	−	−

important. The dietary history of children and of many adults must be obtained from the parent or spouse who actually purchases, prepares, and serves the food. Leading questions should be avoided because many patients know what they *should* eat and will tell the questioner this rather than what they actually *do* eat. The interviewer should have some familiarity with the cultural environment of the patient in order to obtain an adequate history. The possibility of many deficiency states can be eliminated at once by establishing certain food practices of the patient. Thus citrus fruits or meat taken once or twice a week or consumption of enriched bread or cereal daily eliminate the possibility of a deficiency of vitamin C, protein, or thiamine.

The diet history is best obtained by first determining the meal pattern (number and timing of meals and the kinds of food eaten in a typical day) and then asking about individual items of the five major food groups in Table 78-1. This type of cross-check will bring to light inconsistencies that should be explored. The physician's needs are met by ruling out possibilities rather than by aiming for quantification of intake of nutrients.

PHYSICAL SIGNS. The diagnostic specificity of the physical signs of nutritional disease, such as cheilosis, perleche, nasolabial seborrhea, follicular hyperkeratosis, conjunctival injection, dry hair, swollen gums, and even bowed extremities or bossed skulls, as evidence of past or present nutritional disease has been exaggerated.

The posture and muscle tone and the patient's attitude may be helpful in the appraisal of malnutrition, but these signs are not specific. The amount of subcutaneous fat can be useful in appraising calorie deficiency and can be quantitated with standard calipers. By using the principles of isotopic dilution, it is possible to calculate the size of the body compartments, and body composition can be measured, but such measurements are not practical for physicians. Body fat can also be derived from measurements of body density, but inspection and palpation of subcutaneous fat will serve almost as well.

There are a few changes in mucous membranes and the skin and hair which are useful because they are fairly specific for nutritional deficiency. *Bitot's spot* (Chap. 84) generally indicates deficiency of vitamin A. Other vascular and membranous changes in the conjunctival sac are apt to be misleading. The *perifollicular hemorrhages* and the unique *"corkscrew" hair* associated with adult scurvy are fairly specific, but phrynoderma, or *follicular hyperkeratosis* without hemorrhage, which has been associated with vitamin A deficiency, is not a specific sign. *Nasolabial seborrhea* and *scrotal dermatitis* are suggestive but not diagnostic of pyridoxine deficiency or ariboflavinosis. The pigmentary changes and dermatitis associated with kwashiorkor and pellagra are typical and almost diagnostic. *Papillary atrophy and reddening of the tongue* should suggest nutritional deficiency, although these may be seen in any of several individual deficiency states, including those of iron, nicotinic acid, vitamin B$_{12}$, and folic acid. The *gum changes* in scurvy often are typical because of the great hypertrophy of the interdental papillae and their fragility to mechanical injury. These changes do not appear in edentulous persons. Enlargement of the salivary glands is seen in malnutrition, but it is not a specific sign.

Neuropathy is a feature of many deficiency states, including those of thiamine, pyridoxine, cobalamine, and nicotinic acid. Thiamine deficiency is associated with peripheral weakness, wasting, and paresthesia, as well as Wernicke's ophthalmoplegia and psychosis. Pyridoxine deficiency often leads to convulsions in infants and in experimental animals to lesions of sensory neurons. Deficiency of cobalamine may cause subacute degeneration of the spinal cord. Psychosis is a common complication of pellagra (Chap. 363).

The *radiologic signs* of rickets, osteomalacia, and juvenile scurvy often are decisive in the acute stages of the disorder. The intestinal mucosal pattern formerly described as a *deficiency pattern* is misnamed. Although the changes are often seen in sprue as a result of atrophy of the villi and changes in the mucous secretions, they do not reflect any specific vitamin deficiency.

There are no typical electrocardiographic signs of vitamin deficiency, but the changes in the ECG during hyper- and hypokalemia are typical. These are described in Chap. 265.

BIOCHEMICAL TESTS. The many biochemical tests for assessing nutritional status are summarized in Table 78-2.

Table 78-2. BIOCHEMICAL AIDS IN DIAGNOSING NUTRITIONAL DEFICIENCY

Nutrient	Test	Level suggesting nutritional disorder	Normal range
Protein..................	Plasma total protein	< 6.0 Gm%	6.5–8.0 Gm%
	Serum albumin	< 3.5 Gm%	4.0–5.2 Gm%
	Plasma Essential amino acid/ Total amino acid	< 0.3	0.3–0.5
Vitamin A and carotene...	Plasma vitamin A	< 20 μg%	50–100 μg%
	Plasma carotenoids	< 30 μg%	100–200 μg%
	Response to 200,000 IU Vitamin A	Plasma level increases × 2	< × 1
Vitamin D..............	Serum Ca	< 35 mEq/L	4.5–6 mEq/L
	Serum P	< 0.8 mEq/L	1.0–1.5 mEq/L
	Serum alkaline phosphatase	> 15 units—adults	5–13 K-A units
		> 20 units—children	10–20 K-A units
Vitamin C..............	Whole blood	< 0.20 mg%	0.4–1.0 mg%
	Buffy coat	< 10 mg%	25–40 mg%
Thiamine...............	Blood lactate	> 15 mg%	9–15 mg%
	Plasma pyruvate	> 2.0 mg%	0.8–2.0 mg%
	Transketolase (TK) RBC	< 850 μg hexose/ml/hr.	900–1500 μg hexose/ml
	Thiamine pyrophosphate effect on TK	> 15%	< 15%
	Urinary thiamine	< 50 μg/Gm creatinine	100–500 mg/Gm creatinine
Riboflavin..............	Plasma flavin adenine dinucleotide	< 1.5 μg	2–3 μg%
	Urinary riboflavin	< 50 μg/gm creatinine	100–500 μg/Gm creatinine
Pyridoxine..............	Urinary xanthurenic acid after 10 Gm *dl*-tryptophane	> 50 mgm/24 hr	trace
Vitamin B$_{12}$.............	Plasma B$_{12}$ level (*Euglena gracilis* in serum)	< 100 $\mu\mu$g/ml	200–900 $\mu\mu$g/ml
	Schilling test	< 8% ^{60}Co B$_{12}$	> 8% nucleide following 1 mg B$_{12}$ IM
Pantothenic acid..........	Serum	< 50 mμ Gm/ml	100 mμ Gm/ml
Folic acid...............	Serum level (*L. casei*)	< 5 mμg/ml	5–20 mμg/ml serum
	Formimino glutamic acid (Figlu) after 20 Gm 1-histidine HCl p.o.	> 75 mg/12 hr in urine	0–55 mg/12 hr
Iron....................	Serum iron	< 60 μg/100 ml	60–190 μg%
	Serum iron-binding capacity	> 400 μg	250–400 μg%
Magnesium..............	Serum	< 1.5 mEq/L	1.5–3.0 mEq/L
Copper..................	Serum	< 85 μg%	114 μg%
Zinc....................	Plasma	< 80 μg%	120 μg%
Vitamin K..............	Plasma Prothrombin Time	> 20 sec	10–15 sec
Tocopherol..............	Plasma	< 0.4 mg%	0.5–2.0 mg%
Sodium.................	Serum	< 132 mEq/L	132–142 mEq/L
Potassium..............	Serum	< 3.5 mEq/L	3.5–5.0 mEq/L

Sampling for these tests must be done promptly, before the hospital diet or dietary suggestions alter the findings and confuse the diagnosis.

A practical strategy in nutritional diagnosis is to use the dietary history to establish the possibility of nutritional deficiency, to use the results of physical examination and appropriate laboratory tests to establish a tentative diagnosis, and to employ the therapeutic trial to confirm it.

THERAPEUTIC TRIALS. The urgency of circumstances, coupled with unavailability or delays in obtaining biochemical tests, sometimes forces the immediate application of a therapeutic trial as a diagnostic measure. In following this course, three precautions should be observed: (1) If therapy includes multiple nutrients, the patient's recovery may not be attributable to a single cause, and if such information is lacking, the disorder may recur because of failure to correct the cause. (2) The ease with which the deficiency is treated and with which recovery occurs may prevent adequate explanation or nutrition education and invite recurrences. (3) There are certain definite hazards associated with nutrient therapy because both vitamins A and D are toxic in excessive dosages. Vitamin A given in amounts over 25,000 units per day will in time produce anorexia, irritability, decalcification of bone, headache, and loss of hair. For vitamin D the margin between requirement and toxicity is lower. Doses of over 2,000 international units (IU) per day are potentially dangerous and may cause hypercalcemia. The vitamin D intake should not exceed 400

IU per day. Another hazard in vitamin therapy is the danger of administering folacin to a person with vitamin B_{12} deficiency. This will lead to relief of anemia, but neurologic lesions of vitamin B_{12} deficiency will persist and may progress to irreversible stages before B_{12} deficiency is recognized (Chap. 337).

Vitamin Supplements. Multivitamin preparations are readily available without prescription and are aggressively promoted. They often are used wastefully. A physician may be tempted to prescribe them because they are thought to be harmless or because he looks upon this as a simple way to protect patients against the small chance of developing a deficiency state. This practice is undesirable on three counts: it is wasteful; the use of unnecessary medication is to be deplored; and such use of vitamins lulls many patients and a few doctors into neglecting needed diagnostic studies.

With the exception of occasional pregnant or lactating women, well people do not need supplemental vitamins in their diets.

The Council on Nutrition of the American Medical Association has published suggestions for composition of therapeutic vitamin mixtures. Multiple vitamin mixtures should contain only those nutrients known to be essential for man. Supplements should not include such natural mixtures as liver, yeast, or wheat germ. The available multivitamin preparations fall into three general categories according to the amount of nutrients supplied. The first class should supply about one-half of the RDA and is indicated as a supplement in the prophylaxis of nutritional deficiencies for persons with minor disturbances of dietary intake or with unusually large temporary requirements. The second class should contain about 1½ times the recommended dietary allowance and is intended as a therapeutic supplement for proven or suspected deficiency states. The third type of multivitamin supplement should contain from three to five times the RDA and is recommended for use in disorders of absorption, retention, or excessive vitamin losses. This type should not be used as a dietary supplement for protracted periods. The levels of individual nutrients in the mixtures should be proportionate multiples of the recommended dietary allowances.

There is no justification for the widespread marketing of multivitamins to families for their purported value in preventing colds or infections. This effect cannot be documented. The tendency among food merchants to increase the vitamin content of breakfast cereals to therapeutic levels is an insidious marketing device that cannot be justified.

Cereal Enrichment. During World War II a program of enrichment of certain basic cereal foods was begun in the United States, and it has since been continued. Because one-half or more of the food energy supply of the majority of human beings comes from carbohydrate, the National Research Council recommended the enrichment of white flour and bread. It is estimated that about 90 percent of all white breads presently sold in the United States are enriched. The significant addition of nutrients to the composition of those products is indicated in Table

Table 78-3. NUTRIENT LEVELS IN FLOUR,
UNITED STATES
(in mg/lb)

	Thiamine	Riboflavin	Nicotinic acid	Iron
Whole wheat flour..	2.49	0.54	19.7	15.0
White flour........	0.28	0.21	4.1	3.6
Enriched white flour	2.00	1.20	16.0	13.0

78-3. Five southern states also require that corn meal and grits be enriched. South Carolina requires that rice be enriched.

The most dramatic demonstration of enrichment as a means of preventing nutritional disease is the Philippine experiment with enriched rice. The project demonstrated in Bataan that enrichment of rice with thiamine and riboflavin was feasible, economically desirable, acceptable, and a highly efficient way of preventing sickness and death from beriberi.

In addition to these required enrichments, a number of other common foods in the United States are permitted to contain nutrient additives. An early additive was milk powder to bread, which significantly increased its protein and vitamin content. With the development and patenting of the process for obtaining vitamin D_2 by irradiating ergosterol, whole milk was allowed to be enriched to a level of 400 IU per quart, and represents an important source of vitamin D for children.

REFERENCES

Pearson, W. N.: "Assessment of Nutritional Status: Biochemical Methods," chap. 7 in "Nutrition, A Comprehensive Treatise," vol. 3, G. H. Beaton, and E. W. McHenry (Eds.), New York, Academic Press Inc., 1967.

Quiogue, E. S.: The Rice Enrichment Project in Bataan, Philippines, Am. J. Public Health, 42:1086, 1952.

White, P. L.: Vitamin Preparations as Dietary Supplements and as Therapeutic Agents, J.A.M.A., 169:41, 1959.

Young, C. M., and M. F. Trulson: Methodology for Dietary Studies in Epidemiological Surveys. II. Strengths and Weaknesses of Existing Methods, Am. J. Public Health, 50:803, 1960.

79 STARVATION AND PROTEIN MALNUTRITION

George V. Mann

STARVATION. Starvation emphasizes the importance of the principle of adaptation in nutrition. As people starve, their physiologic processes change in ways to conserve energy. Their surfaces become smaller and cooler, their pulses slower, and their spontaneous activity lessens. Secondary sexual characteristics disappear and personality is altered as all interests become preoccupied with food.

The changes consequent to starvation are the same whether in sick patients or in starving populations. They have been recorded systematically in two scientific studies, Benedict's experiment in 1919 and that of Keys in 1950.

The compositional changes in simple starvation are largest for body fat because fat comprises the main energy reserve. The stores of energy available to a well-nourished man of average composition are summarized in Table 79-1. It is significant that such a man, with the usual

Table 79-1. ENERGY STORES IN A "STANDARD" MAN

Component	Cal/g, kcal	Total weight, Gm	Caloric equivalent	Available as energy
Protein.......	4	11,000	44,000	8,000
Fat..........	9	9,000	81,000	72,000
Carbohydrate.	4	500	2,000	800
Water........	...	45,000		
Mineral......	...	4,500		
Total......	...	...	...	81,000*

* 81,000/1,200 = 67 days

adaptation to starvation, might reduce his daily resting metabolism from 1750 to 1200 Cal or less. With these stores he would be predicted to survive about 67 days, when he would have exhausted his fuel supply. In fact, this is about the survival time of adult men during famines. Women, starting with more body fat, have typically survived longer than men. Chassat's Rule is that recovery from starvation is doubtful after half the normal weight has been lost.

Starvation often is associated with fluid retention, the *hunger edema* which still is unexplained. It is probably due in part to the hypoproteinemia consequent to the profound negative nitrogen balance, this leading to alterations in the osmotic concentrations of the body, especially in the renal interstitial tissues, which in turn result in impaired excretion of water and salt. The edema may also reflect some alteration in the functions of adrenal corticoid hormones with starvation.

Contrary to previous belief, rehabilitation can be achieved with an abundance of almost any balanced diet. Starvation and episodes of malnutrition, especially in the young, have been shown to impair physical and intellectual growth in experimental animals. Whether periods of malnutrition may produce permanent intellectual damage, analogous to the arrests and opacities seen in bone by x-ray after these nutritional disorders, is presently unknown. If this were true, it might contribute to the backwardness of human beings in the so-called "underdeveloped areas" at home and abroad.

Clinical Changes. The changes occurring with starvation are most clearly seen in anorexia nervosa where the usual sociologic and physical disturbances of famine are not present. Anorexia nervosa is discussed in Chap. 42. The increased pigmentation of a starving person is prob-

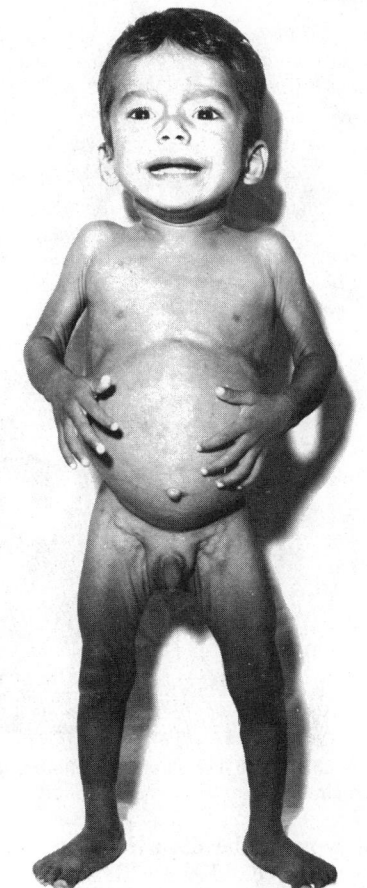

Fig. 79-1. An example of marasmus. (*Photograph courtesy of Nevin S. Scrimshaw*)

ably due to closer juxtaposition of melanocytes in the skin. The prevalence of infection in famine probably is due to the usual deterioration of housing facilities and public health barriers to infection rather than to a decline of individual resistance.

The current fad of using total starvation in the treatment of obesity requires the reminder that these starving patients do not develop deficiencies of the micronutrients and do not require supplementary vitamins.

MARASMUS AND KWASHIORKOR. *Marasmus* is the term applied to a child with exhaustion of protein and energy stores (Fig. 79-1). It is the end stage of both protein and calorie insufficiency. *Kwashiorkor* is primarily a protein deficiency. It was first identified, described, and recorded by Dr. Cicely Williams in Ghana in 1931. The name is that used by the Ga people, to whom the disorder was well known. Kwashiorkor is protein deficiency occurring in the presence of sufficient energy intake. The child is edematous, although its muscles are wasted. It is apathetic and often anorexic, and may present a characteristic dermatosis (Fig. 79-2). The hair often is depigmented, assuming a reddish hue with thinning and straightening of the kinky texture normal in Negro children. There are profound deficiencies of intestinal enzymes. The liver is fatty and enlarged, and persistent

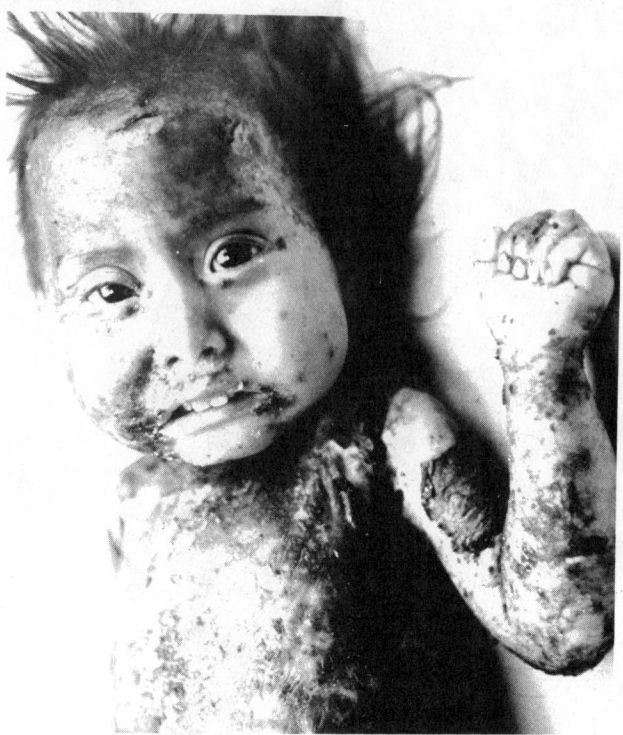

Fig. 79-2. A child with kwashiorkor. (*Photograph supplied by Nevin S. Scrimshaw*)

diarrhea is typical. The disorder often is precipitated by an infection in a child weaned from breast milk to a pablum of cassava meal in water which, although supplying energy, is disastrously low in protein. Initially this disorder was confused with adult pellagra. Since World War II, it has been clearly established as a major cause of death and disability in children throughout the world.

The term *protein-calorie malnutrition* has been widely used to designate collectively the spectrum ranging from pure protein deficiency to total energy deficiency. The hungry, emaciated, marasmic child can usually be distinguished from the sullen, anorexic, edematous child with a dramatic dermatosis. There are, however, all shades of intermingling of these classical extremes of marasmus and kwashiorkor. The relationship of calorie and protein de-

ficiency to this terminal state is shown graphically in Fig. 79-3. Marasmus and kwashiorkor are not always separable as the diagram suggests. These children waste away without the typical physical signs of any particular nutrient deficiency, although vitamin A deficiency is a common complication and many other stores of nutrients are depleted. Kwashiorkor represents one end of this spectrum, marasmus the other.

There is no efficient biochemical indicator of protein-calorie malnutrition. The serum albumin will generally be reduced. Levels of 3.50 to 2.75 Gm per 100 ml indicate a probable protein deficiency, and levels below 2.75 Gm per 100 ml are highly probable indicators. In time the plasma total protein becomes reduced although the tendency to hyperglobulinemia in persons who live in underdeveloped areas tends to obscure this sign. The ratio of essential to nonessential amino acids in plasma will decline, but this has not been a dependable sign.

Extracellular fluids tend to increase until frank edema develops. The diagnosis largely depends upon the dietary history and the clinical appearance. The skin and hair changes in children with kwashiorkor are often dramatic, while in adults such skin changes are rarely seen, although apathy, wasting, and great weakness are found. Even though some intestinal enzymes may be depleted, the disorder responds to hydration and refeeding with an abundance of protein of high biologic value. Because of the frequency with which infection is seen as the immediate precipitating cause, broad-spectrum antibiotics are used immediately, along with therapeutic levels of vitamins. Even with optimum treatment the death rate in children remains high. Malnourished children tend to have repeated bouts of malnutrition unless the mother can be made to understand the relationship between the poor diet and the illness.

Trauma. The metabolic response to trauma is characteristic and predictable (Chap. 92). Even in well-nourished persons the stress of injury, infection, or surgery will induce a sequence of catabolism that entails loss of body fat, nitrogen, potassium, magnesium, sulfur, and calcium and retention of water and sodium. The reactions appear to be mediated hormonally. It is not established that any amount of forced feeding will abolish this sequence. The metabolic wasting that occurs with a combination of starvation and infection has been termed *sep-*

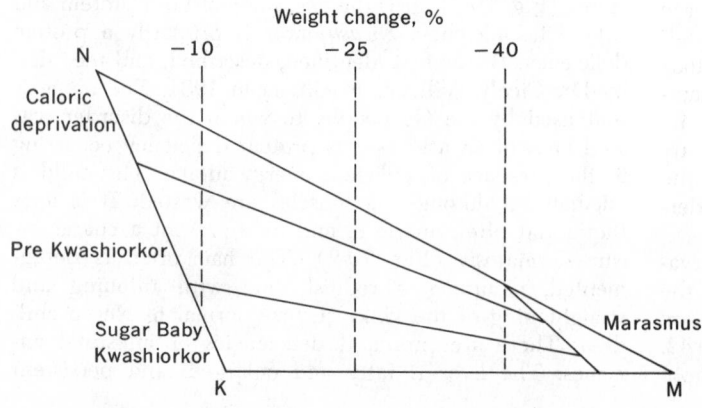

Fig. 79-3. The relationship of marasmus (*M*) and kwashiorkor (*K*). The energy depletion is indicated along the abscissa, the extent of protein depletion, along the ordinate. The classical example of kwashiorkor, the sugar baby fed a pablum of starch, will show but little weight loss because his energy stores are preserved. The child with marasmus is greatly underweight and protein depleted. Infection may move a child rapidly toward *K* and *M*. (*Adapted from Scrimshaw and Behar*)

tic starvation. Intracellular water diminishes, but the total body water increases. The wasting may reach a rate of 1.5 kg tissue daily. As minimal trauma as a venesection of 500 ml produces similar but lesser changes. The wasting disorder called *cardiac cachexia* is seen in patients with chronic heart failure (Chap. 264).

Ethanol. The role of ethanol in causing or contributing to nutritional disease is exceedingly important. Ethanol yields about 7 Cal per Gm and is often an important source of calories in the diet. There is a tendency for light drinkers to become obese because they seem not to compensate for this increased caloric intake. Heavy drinkers tend to decrease their intake of foods as their intake of alcohol increases and to lose weight. It has been widely supposed that the malnutrition associated with alcoholism is a consequence of replacement of food by alcohol, but this is not true. The pathologic effects of ethanol are discussed in Chaps. 118 and 328. Ethanol is toxic to many tissues.

REFERENCES

Brock, J. F.: Dietary Protein Deficiency, Ann. Intern. Med., 65:877, 1966.

Keys, A., et al.: "The Biology of Human Starvation," vol. 1, chap. 1, the University of Minnesota Press, 1950.

Lieber, C. S.: Metabolic Derangement Induced by Alcohol, Ann. Rev. Med., 18:35, 1967.

Moore, F. D., et al.: "The Body Cell Mass and its Supporting Environment—Body Composition in Health and Disease," Philadelphia, W. B. Saunders Company, 1963.

Scrimshaw, N. S., and M. Behar: Malnutrition in Underdeveloped Countries, New Engl. J. Med., 272:137, 1965.

Terris, M.: Epidemiology of Cirrhosis of the Liver: National Mortality Data, Amer. J. Public Health, 57:2076, 1967.

80   PELLAGRA

*Richard H. Follis, Jr. and
George V. Mann*

HISTORY. During the eighteenth century, a new disease began to appear with increasing frequency in northern Spain and Italy. First called *mal de la rosa* by Casal (from the erythematous skin lesions), the malady soon came to be known as *pelle agro* (skin, rough), from which the present-day name, *pellagra*, is derived. Casal described the prominent features: "a horrible crust" involving the skin, particularly of the hands and neck; "painful burning of the mouth"; "perpetual shaking of the body"; and "mania." He noted the prominence of maize in the diet of the people whom he had studied. During the nineteenth century, the principal focus of the disease was northern Italy, where in some areas as many as 5 percent of the population in a given area might be affected. A number of explanations were advanced for the cause: that maize acquired toxic properties as a result of infestation with molds or fungi; that a material present

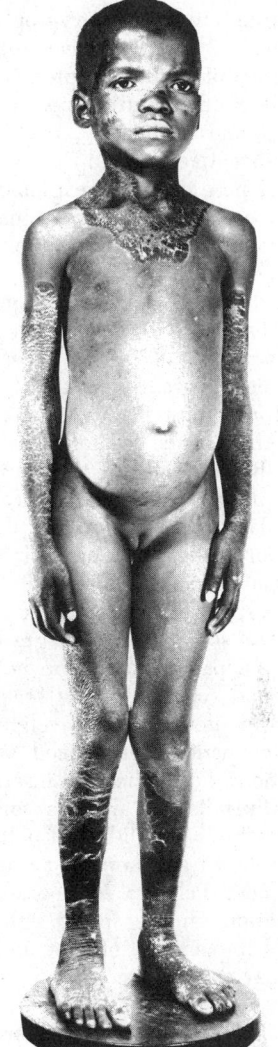

Fig. 80-1. Pellagra in a young girl. (*Photograph courtesy of Dr. J. G. Prinsloo and the American Journal of Clinical Nutrition*)

in the grain was transformed into a poisonous substance in the intestinal tract of man; that maize contained some chemical that sensitized the skin to the photodynamic action of sunlight; that some specific microorganism was present; or that a diet predominantly of maize was a poor source of nourishment.

Pellagra began to appear in epidemic proportions in the southern United States in the early 1900s. Joseph Goldberger, of the U.S. Public Health Service, soon showed in classic studies that diet alone could cure, prevent, or cause the disease. He demonstrated the importance of protein in the diet and for a time he favored the idea that lack of specific amino acids was the cause. His interest then shifted to the curative effects of yeast and to the identification of an antipellagra vitamin. In 1937, Elvehjem and his coworkers showed that nicotinic acid would cure black tongue, a pellagra-like disease, in dogs. Shortly thereafter nicotinic acid proved effective in the therapy of clinical pellagra. When it was found that the essential amino acid, tryptophan, is a precursor of nicotinic acid, it became clear that pellagra results from a deficiency of dietary tryptophan and/or nicotinic acid; deficiency of other nutrients, such as riboflavin, thiamine, folic acid, and vitamin B_{12}, may complicate the disease. The persistent relationship of dietary maize to the development of pellagra is not explained. Pellagra is rare in populations consuming other grains with even lower content of nicotinic acid and tryptophan than maize. It has not been possible to demonstrate the significance of substances binding nicotinic acid in maize, which may interfere with its utilization.

PREVALENCE. After 1940, the prevalence of endemic pellagra diminished greatly in the United States. The disease is still important in Yugoslavia, Rumania, Egypt, India, South Africa, and Yucatan. Cases of sporadic pellagra are rarely observed in the United States; when encountered, they often accompany chronic disease states, particularly those affecting the gastrointestinal tract. In addition, pellagra occurs in individuals who consume large quantities of alcohol and whose diets are restricted with respect to a number of essential nutrients.

CLINICAL FINDINGS. Before pellagra becomes clinically manifest and the patient seeks the help of a physician, certain prodromal symptoms may be present. These include loss of appetite leading to weight loss, indigestion, diarrhea or constipation, generalized weakness, lassitude, burning sensations, headache, and insomnia. These symptoms are usually followed after varying periods of time by the manifestations of full-blown pellagra, which affect the skin, alimentary tract, nervous system, and to a lesser extent, the blood. Pellagra is a seasonal disease with acute exacerbations in the spring, when a combination of the winter's impairment of diet and a new exposure to sun and heavier work seem to precipitate the acute episodes.

The *skin lesions* may begin as an erythema that looks very much like sunburn. Burning or itching may be intense. The initial changes may be followed by the formation of vesicles or by peeling. The erythematous skin may assume a dirty-brown color and then becomes rough and scaly. This stage, which may not necessarily be preceded by erythema, may remain for prolonged periods. Characteristically, the skin lesions are symmetric and tend to be localized over exposed areas: backs of hands in adults and backs of feet in children, on the face, neck, elbows, and knees. In addition, the scrotum, vulva, and perianal region may be involved. Unilateral dermatitis is usually associated with local pressure, trauma, heat, or sunlight. The evolution of the lesions may differ; erythema of the hands may appear while hyperkeratosis of the legs is already present. Seborrhea about the nose with comedo formation may be conspicuous in some patients.

Sore mouth is a common complaint. Changes in the tongue are conspicuous, and glossitis is thought by some to be a more sensitive gauge of the disease than skin lesions. The tip and margins of the tongue become hyperemic, a change that may spread to involve the entire surface so that the structure acquires a beef-red appearance. Small ulcers sometimes appear. Inflammatory lesions may be found in the mucous membrane of the mouth. Secondary infection is common, particularly with fusospirochetal organisms. In advanced stages of the disease, the tongue may be pale with complete atrophy of the papillae. Angular lesions, i.e., gray macerated or ulcerated areas at the corners of the mouth, are frequently present. Pain on swallowing is common. Anorexia, accompanied by epigastric discomfort, is a frequent complaint. *Diarrhea* has always been a prominent part of the pellagra syndrome. Stools are small, frequent, and watery, quite different from those in sprue. The liver ordinarily is not enlarged.

Neurologic signs rarely appear at the beginning of the disease but are common when skin or alimentary manifestations are prominent. Subjectively, the patient may complain of vertigo, weakness, headache, paresthesia, anesthesia, and general aches. Severe pain of the hands and feet may be present. Objectively, tendon reflexes are abnormal, usually diminished. Coarse tremors of the tongue, head, or extremities may be noted on examination. Muscular spasms are sometimes prominent. Mental disturbances have always been a feature of endemic pellagra; they include general "nervousness," confusion, depression, insomnia, apathy, and delirium. The picture is a varied one.

The above clinical manifestations account for the old description of pellagra as the disease of the four D's: "dementia, diarrhea, dermatitis, and death."

LABORATORY FINDINGS. Chemical examinations of the blood are of little help in pellagra. Occasionally hypoproteinemia, with low serum albumin values, is found. Gastric analysis reveals achlorhydria in about one-half the cases. On examination, the stools may show the presence of hookworm ova or other parasites in areas where infestations are prevalent. The content of N-methyl nicotinamide in the urine is helpful in assessing tryptophan-nicotinic acid nutriture in population groups, but this determination is of little help in the individual case. The urinary excretion of riboflavin may be decreased in pellagra.

Anemia is present in approximately one-half the cases of pellagra, but in only about one-quarter is it of any consequence. The anemia is not particularly specific.

PATHOLOGY. The earliest skin lesions show dilatation of the superficial blood vessels and proliferation of their endothelial cells. The superficial connective tissue elements of the corium assume a spongy appearance. The epidermis, which may already show hyperkeratosis, separates from the corium with the formation of a vesicle. There may be increased pigmentation of the superficial hyperkeratotic layer with decrease in pigment cells in the basal region. Chronic lesions merely show hyperkeratosis. The epithelium of the tongue is atrophic, with loss of papillae; a subacute inflammatory reaction may be present. The esophagus is commonly the site of acute inflammation with loss of epithelium. Alterations in the remainder of the intestinal tract are not particularly noteworthy, save in the colon. Here small ulcers may be present with abscess formation in the submucosa. Cystic dilatations of the mucous glands are prominent. The liver may contain excessive fat, which is usually periportal in distribution. The lining of the vagina frequently is acutely inflamed with superficial ulceration. The neurologic changes are variable and consist of atrophy of cerebral neurones, degeneration of peripheral nerves, nerve roots, and tracts in the spinal cord. Bone marrow, if abnormal, may show a megaloblastic response or erythroblastic hyperplasia.

Pathogenesis. When man subsists on a diet of which the main staple is maize and in which there is little other protein, pellagra is likely to ensue. Maize is nutritionally inferior to other foods in a number of ways, particularly when modern milling procedures are employed. Its protein is low in quantity and, more important, in quality because it is low in two essential amino acids. Maize protein contains only a trace of tryptophan and low levels of lysine. Although maize contains appreciable quantities of nicotinic acid when assayed chemically, much of this vitamin is unavailable, since it cannot be assimilated from maize in the intestinal tract. Nicotinic acid is found in high concentrations in liver, yeast, red muscle meats, fish, and wheat germ. Vegetables and cereals contain much less. Coffee is a significant source of nicotinic acid.

In India, in contrast to many other countries, the use of millet and sorghum (jowar) in the diet, rather than maize, has been associated with the development of pellagra.

Meat protein, dairy products, and eggs are generally limited or entirely lacking in the pellagrin's diet. Furthermore, diets that have been associated with pellagra have been deficient not only in protein, but also in available nicotinic acid, riboflavin, thiamine, and vitamin B_{12}.

The multiple nutrient deficiency aspects of pellagra have been recognized for some time, and they cause one to ask: What is the definition of pellagra? Some workers would be restrictive and define the disease as pure tryptophan–nicotinic acid deficiency. The argument is that since the cardinal symptoms respond to nicotinic acid, pellagra should be regarded as a deficiency of this vitamin. Since, however, some of the classic symptoms and signs are alleviated not by nicotinic acid therapy but by other nutrients, it may be preferable to define pellagra as a multiple deficiency syndrome produced principally by deficiencies of tryptophan–nicotinic acid, riboflavin, and thiamine, and occasionally by folic acid, vitamin B_{12}, and possibly pyridoxine.

It is generally agreed that exposure of the skin to ultraviolet radiation may precipitate the appearance of dermal lesions or may increase the severity of those already present. In addition, the exposure of pellagrous subjects to sunlight may lead to effects in areas other than the skin; for instance, glossitis may be induced, nausea and vomiting may occur, or diarrhea may appear. The effect of sunlight helps to explain the seasonal variations in the prevalence of pellagra in the north temperate zones.

Individuals of different age groups are not equally affected by the disease. The greatest prevalence is in females, aged twenty to forty-five, i.e., the childbearing,

lactating group. The next most common prevalence is usually found in children aged nine to fifteen years, but this statement must be qualified since these data come from Goldberger's studies in the southern United States at a time when child labor was extensive.

Sporadic cases of pellagra, not associated with a maize diet, are important, for today they comprise in the United States the commonest group of pellagrins. "Secondary" or "conditioned" pellagra may develop in persons who have some other disease. Disturbances of the gastrointestinal tract are the most common cause, e.g., gastric ulcer or carcinoma and various disturbances of the large and small intestine, particularly those which lead to diarrhea. The second most important group are the chronic alcoholics, although it is more usual for the chronic alcoholic to develop symptoms of thiamine deficiency. Polyneuritis, as well as the skin and other signs characteristic of pellagra, may be observed in the same individual.

DIAGNOSIS. Signs in endemic pellagra often are diagnostic. The dietary history is especially important. The diagnosis of incipient pellagra or the recognition of cases without skin manifestations ("pellagra sine pellagra") is more difficult. Here it may be necessary to evaluate the response to therapy with nicotinic acid and other nutrients. The estimation of N^1-methylnicotinamide concentration in the urine may be of help. The possibility of overt or subclinical pellagra should be considered in every person with a compatible diet history who suffers from gastrointestinal disease, particularly those conditions which lead to the malabsorption syndrome (Chap. 316). So, too, with any chronic alcoholic, the question of adequate nutrition with respect to nicotinic acid and other vitamins must always be considered.

Three forms of disorder with pellagra-like skin lesions, though uncommon, are worthy of mention. The first is an hereditary affliction called *Hartnup's disease* (Chap. 96). This syndrome consists of a pellagra-like skin rash following exposure to sunlight, intermittent cerebellar ataxia, renal aminoaciduria, and the excretion of large amounts of indole-3-acetic acid and indican in the urine. Increased quantities of protoporphyrin are found in the stool. Other manifestations of pellagra, such as glossitis, stomatitis, or gastrointestinal symptoms, are not present. The skin lesions respond to nicotinic acid therapy, suggesting that the metabolic disorder results from diversion of tryptophane from its normal route of degradation to pyrrole metabolites.

A second form of pellagra-like disease has been reported in patients receiving isoniazid, the *tuberculostatic* drug which is also a vitamin B_6 antagonist. In such patients peripheral neuritis and pellagra-like skin lesions appear and may not regress even when the drug is discontinued. Treatment with nicotinic acid often is efficacious in curing the skin lesions. Pyridoxine or B-complex preparations will usually relieve the neurologic manifestations.

The third disturbance in which pellagra-like skin lesions have been observed is associated with malignant carcinoid tumors (*malignant argentaffinomas*). These tumors produce such large amounts of 5-hydroxytryptamine (serotonin) from tryptophan that a conditioned form of tryptophan deficiency results. In addition to skin lesions, the patients may exhibit other characteristics of pellagra: mental confusion, diarrhea, and glossitis.

TREATMENT. Severely ill pellagrins, particularly those with diarrhea and dementia, should be treated as emergencies. Water and electrolyte deficits must be corrected immediately. Intravenous administration of nicotinic acid or nicotinamide in doses of 100 mg two or three times a day is recommended. These amounts can be added to physiologic salt solution containing 5% glucose. Nicotinamide is free from the unpleasant vasomotor effects of nicotinic acid. Other nutrients, particularly riboflavin, also are necessary. A practical, economical form of therapy is the administration of ½ to 1 oz debittered brewer's yeast in tomato juice three times a day. A high (3000 to 4000) calorie, high protein diet is desirable. Frequent feedings are advocated at first. Stomatitis, diarrhea or constipation, and oozing or ulcerated lesions of the skin will necessitate symptomatic medication.

PROGNOSIS. Until the advent of yeast and vitamin therapy, the prognosis of pellagra was grave, but now the prognosis is excellent. The glossitis begins to decrease in 24 hr; the papillae of the tongue will begin to regenerate by the end of the first week. Lesions of the lips begin to heal in 2 to 3 days. Gastrointestinal symptoms improve in 24 to 48 hr, and diarrhea will usually have ceased by the end of the first week. Demented patients usually become rational after 3 or 4 days, unless, of course, damage to the brain is irreversible. Polyneuritis, if present, may take some time to improve.

REFERENCES

Bean, W. B., T. D. Spies, and M. A. Blankenhorn: Secondary Pellagra, Medicine, 23:1, 1944.

FAO Nutritional Stuidies, "Maize and Maize Diets," no. 9, Rome, 1953.

Gillman, J., and T. Gillman: "Perspectives in Human Malnutrition: A Contribution to the Biology of Disease from a Clinical and Pathological Study of Chronic Malnutrition and Pellagra in the African," New York, Grune and Stratton, Inc., 1951.

Goldsmith, G. A., H. P. Sarett, V. D. Register, and J. Gibbens: Studies of Niacin Requirement in Man: I. Experimental Pellagra in Subjects on Corn Diets Low in Niacin and Tryptophan, J. Clin. Invest., 31:533, 1952.

Sydenstricker, V. P.: The History of Pellagra, Its Recognition As a Disorder of Nutrition and Its Conquest, Am. J. Clin. Nutrition, 6:409, 1958.

Terris, M. (Ed.): "Goldberger on Pellagra," Baton Rouge, La., Louisiana State University Press, 1964.

81 BERIBERI

Richard H. Follis, Jr. and George V. Mann

HISTORY. During the seventeenth, eighteenth, and nineteenth centuries, as a result of the increasing contacts of European physicians with the Far East, a disease peculiar to that area became known to Western physicians. The principal characteristics of this disease, oriental beriberi, as described by a nineteenth-century physician, were "a feeling of numbness, sense of weight and weakness" in the legs, "edema of the feet," "unsteady and tottering walk" with "almost total palsy," "rigidity and various affections of the nerves," "oppression and weight in the precordium," and, occasionally, "sudden death." The disease was endemic throughout South China, Southeast Asia, the Philippines, the East Indies, and parts of India.

Studies soon revealed the close relationship of rice in the diet to the disease. Beriberi was eradicated from the Japanese Navy by Takaki, who added meat, vegetables, and condensed milk to the rice diet of the common sailor. In Batavia (now Djakarta), Eijkman observed a beriberi-like disease in fowl fed polished rice; the birds could be cured with unpolished grain. In Malaya, differences were noted in the prevalence of beriberi among persons who consumed parboiled rice and those who were accustomed to eat highly polished grain. By 1912, the therapeutic effectiveness of rice polishings had been demonstrated, particularly in patients with acute cardiac manifestations of beriberi. This led E. B. Vedder, a U.S. Army physician, to recommend to R. R. Williams, a chemist then working in Manila, that the protective substance be isolated. As a result, 20 years later Williams and his coworkers announced the chemical structure and synthesis of the active principle, thiamine. The metabolic role of thiamine was demonstrated at once.

PREVALENCE. Today the prevalence of clinical beriberi in the Far East is much reduced. One may encounter occasional cases of the disease, particularly in infants and pregnant or lactating women. Thiamine deficiency in the United States is most often seen in alcoholics. The presence of thiamine in enriched flour and white bread has no doubt diminished the prevalence of this disorder. The dramatically successful rice enrichment program in the Philippines has been discussed (Chap. 78). The desirability of enriching wines, beers, and whiskeys with thiamine has been considered but thought to be an undesirable endorsement.

CLINICAL FINDINGS. Three main types of beriberi have been recognized in the Orient: a chronic form in which neurologic involvement is prominent, an acute form with heart failure, and a less acute state in which edema is the most characteristic manifestation. The onset of the chronic neurologic form is insidious. Over the course of days or weeks, the patient comes to be easily fatigued and experiences heavy feelings in the legs, together with stiffness and aching in the muscles. In time the muscles become weaker, acutely painful, and then atrophic. The extensors of the foot usually are first affected, then the muscles of the calf and thigh. Pain followed by atrophy soon occurs in the muscles of the arms; the muscles of the trunk may be affected later. Associated with these signs and symptoms are foot drop and wrist drop, together with loss of reflexes at the ankle and knee. Paresthesias and anesthesias may be demonstrated, particularly over the lower extremities. Circumoral anesthesia may be present. Aphonia is sometimes a symptom. Walking becomes difficult, and the patient can only shuffle about with a cane or is forced to hold on to objects about him to keep from falling. Evidences of neurologic involvement may fluctuate. In time, however, the patient becomes completely bedridden. Involvement of the cerebrum is absent.

All the while, weight loss will have been progressing, and anorexia usually is persistent. Diarrhea may be more or less continuous. Evidences of cardiac involvement may accompany these neurologic disturbances or may appear suddenly in the absence of any evidence of involvement of the nervous system. The cardiac manifestations consist of palpitation, precordial pain, and dyspnea which may come on in paroxysms without warning. The heart is found to be enlarged and tachycardia is present. Prominent venous pulsations are noted in the neck. Edema usually is present. The blood pressure is not elevated, but the pulse pressure is increased and venous pressure is elevated. Death may result suddenly, with or without exertion.

Beriberi in infants has been and continues to be a health problem in the Far East. In babies the clinical classifications are the aphonic, in which the child loses his voice; the cardiologic, a sudden episode of cyanosis and cardiac arrest leading to death; and the pseudomeningitic with the manifestations of meningitis. These babies are typically born of mothers with low dietary intakes of thiamine and consequently low levels in their milk. The baby seems to flourish until quite suddenly it is stricken, usually at three to six months of age. The disorder is prevented by giving the mother thiamine and treated by the administration of thiamine to the infant. This will often bring a dramatic cure in a matter of hours.

In the mid-1930s, observers in large urban clinics in the Occident began to recognize instances of cardiac and neurologic disease occurring predominantly in alcoholics. In some areas the prevalence of these forms of *Occidental beriberi*, as these entities came to be called, was high. The clinical aspects of this form of heart disease are described in Chap. 264.

The symptoms and signs relative to neurologic involvement in alcoholics have the characteristics of a progressive polyneuritis with sensory and motor defects (Chaps. 118 and 363). Almost invariably there is a history of excessive consumption of alcohol and poor dietary intake. In addition, such patients frequently exhibit manifestations of delirium tremens, Korsakoff's syndrome, or Wernicke's disease. To such examples of neurologic involvement in poorly nourished, chronic alcoholics have been added other syndromes in recent years, such as amblyopia, central pontine myelinolysis, and corticocerebellar degeneration. None of these changes, including Wernicke's disease, has been described in beriberi occurring in Oriental peoples.

Thiamine is involved in a number of key reactions in glycolysis. Consequently, disturbances of lactate metabolism and of pentose phosphate shunt reactions would be expected to reflect alterations of these functions. However, the significance of elevated plasma levels of lactate and pyruvate in the diagnosis of thiamine deficiency is limited by the sensitivity of these to other factors, particularly physical exercise or the hypoxia associated with congestive failure. More useful is the measurement of the transketolase content of red blood cells. This enzyme functions in the pentose phosphate shunt and requires thiamine as a cofactor. Thus it is sensitive to deficiency states. The test is combined with an assessment of the effect of thiamine pyrophosphate added to the in vitro system, the so-called "TPP Effect." This amounts to an in vitro therapeutic trial. It is proving to be a most useful diagnostic procedure.

PATHOLOGY. From the above account of the clinical manifestations of beriberi, anatomic alterations might be expected in the nervous tissues and heart. Post-mortem examinations performed on patients dying with neurologic manifestations of beriberi at the turn of the century in the Orient revealed myelin degeneration of the peripheral nerves, with loss of axoplasm. Lesions in the brain and spinal cord have not been reported from the Orient. Among the sporadic cases designated as neurologic beriberi encountered in the Occident, usually among alcoholics, lesions of peripheral nerves have also been described. More prominent, however, are changes in the brain. Alterations characteristic of Wernicke's disease— bilateral hemorrhagic necrotic foci in the mammillary bodies, the hypothalamic nuclei, and midline structures —are found. Damage to the optic nerve and lesions in the spinal cord have been reported.

The heart is usually described as enlarged, but this increase in size is usually due to dilatation, although hypertrophy of the right ventricle has sometimes been noted. The myocardial fibers do not exhibit necrosis, although swelling and vacuolization may be prominent. No cellular infiltration is present.

PATHOGENESIS. Rice is the principal foodstuff of onehalf or more of the inhabitants of the world. The introduction of power milling machinery at the end of the nineteenth century led to a great increase in beriberi in the Far East. When rice is highly milled, most of its vitamin content, such as thiamine, riboflavin, nicotinic acid, pantothenic acid, and pyridoxine, is removed. Lipids and minerals, such as calcium, iron, and iodine, which are present in the outer portions of the grain, are lost as well. Rice is milled to preserve its storage quality and, as with highly milled flour in the Western world, the refined product has come to be preferred by consumers. The protein content of rice is low, though its quality is good.

Although the rice eater's diet is deficient in a number of nutrients, the principal manifestations of beriberi— the derangements in cardiac and neurologic function— appear to be related to thiamine deficiency. The therapeutic response of the patient with cardiac beriberi, whether infant or adult, to thiamine is good evidence for this relationship. The development of anatomic lesions in the heart of experimental animals deprived of thiamine is further proof for the relation of this vitamin to the integrity of the myocardium. Thiamine is involved in several enzymatic transformations involving pyruvate, alpha-ketoglutarate and in the transketolase reaction mentioned above. The explanation for the edema probably is two-fold; heart failure and protein malnutrition.

The precise relationship of thiamine to maintenance of the integrity of the peripheral nervous system is uncertain. The predilection of the nervous system for injury in thiamine deficiency suggests that the vitamin is especially crucial for those tissues which depend upon carbohydrate metabolism exclusively for their energy sources. The clinical response to thiamine usually is not rapid, though this can be explained on the basis that damage has been severe enough to have caused structural loss. Hence, regeneration is necessary if function is to be restored. Lesions of the peripheral nerves have been difficult to produce in experimental animals. In contrast, the manifestations of Wernicke's disease may clear up in a few hours after thiamine administration, and lesions similar to those observed in Wernicke's disease have been demonstrated in the brains of thiamine-deficient animals. The enigma of the absence of Wernicke's disease in the Orient (except among Western prisoners of war) remains.

DIAGNOSIS. In the Orient, the symptoms are characteristic enough. Certain simple tests are helpful: pain when the calf muscles are squeezed, anesthesia to pinprick over the anterior surface of the tibia, loss of patellar reflex, and inability to rise from the squatting position. The presence of pitting edema and manifestations of cardiac involvement help with the diagnosis when they are present.

The diagnosis of the occasional case in the Occident is more difficult. Here the dietary history, particularly if alcoholism has been present, is important. Evidence of neurologic involvement usually is the most prominent symptom.

TREATMENT. When there is cardiac involvement in infants or adults, beriberi becomes a medical emergency. The immediate administration of thiamine is important. Intravenous administration of 10 to 20 mg thiamine, two or three times a day, is recommended. Doses of thiamine, 3 to 5 mg orally two or three times a day, should be adequate for the ordinary patient. A balanced diet is important in prevention.

PROGNOSIS. The response of infants and adults with cardiac beriberi in the Orient is one of the most dramatic in medicine. Cardiac symptoms improve rapidly. Diuresis begins within the first 12 hr. In the Occident such dramatic responses are not seen as often. When neurologic involvement is present, response to therapy is much more gradual. However, as mentioned above, the ophthalmoplegia, ataxia, and nystagmus of Wernicke's disease respond to thiamine, as do mental symptoms such as apathy and drowsiness. Amentia responds less rapidly.

REFERENCES

Brin, M.: Erythrocyte Transketolase in Early Thiamine Deficiency, Ann. N.Y. Acad. Sci., 98:528, 1962.

Kinney, T. D., and R. H. Follis, Jr. (Eds.): Nutritional Disease: Beriberi, Fed. Proc., 17: Supp. 2, 3, 1958.
Vedder, E. B., "Beriberi," New York, William Wood & Company, 1913.
Victor M., and R. D. Adams: On the Etiology of the Alcoholic Neurological Diseases, Am. J. Clin. Nutrition, 9:379, 1961.
Williams, R. R.: "Toward the Conquest of Beriberi," Cambridge, Mass., Harvard University Press, 1961.

82 SCURVY
Richard H. Follis, Jr. and George V. Mann

HISTORY. Although accounts of a disease which might be construed as scurvy are found in ancient writings, the first clear-cut descriptions appear in records of the Crusades. When the long sea voyages of discovery began toward the end of the fifteenth century, scurvy became commonplace and soon ranked first among causes of disability and mortality in sailors. Scurvy on land appeared among military and civilian population groups as a result of the many European wars which led to troop movements and civilian displacement.

In 1747 James Lind, a British naval surgeon, in a model experiment, studied the effects of several types of treatment, including one composed of "two oranges and one lemon given every day" on sailors with typical signs of scurvy: "putrid gums, the spots and lassitude, with weakness of their knees." The curative efficacy of these citrus fruits was clear.

Infantile scurvy began to receive attention after 1883, when Barlow described the syndrome as it is recognized today: the swollen, tense, exquisitely painful, flexed lower extremities; crepitus at the ends of the shafts of the bones; swollen, bleeding gums; and subcutaneous hemorrhages. With increasing use of breast milk substitutes, scurvy became common in the urban areas of Europe and the United States at the turn of the century.

A disease of the growing bones of guinea pigs, quite like that seen in children, was produced by dietary means in 1907. Investigators then had a way to assay antiscorbutic materials, and 25 years later, C. G. King and his associates isolated from lemon juice a biologically active, crystalline material. This compound was later synthesized and shown to be ascorbic acid.

PREVALENCE. In previous times scurvy in adults tended to occur in epidemic-like outbreaks. Scurvy now is seen in isolated individuals, usually lonely men whose diet is grossly unbalanced and devoid of sources of ascorbic acid (*bachelor scurvy*). Each year in urban clinics in the United States and Europe such examples of adult scurvy are encountered. Occasional cases of scurvy continue to appear in pediatric clinics, usually a result of maternal error or ignorance.

CLINICAL FINDINGS. There are three principal manifestations of scurvy in the adult: swollen gums with loss of teeth, skin lesions, and pain and weakness in the lower extremities. The clinical course of the disease is understood as a result of studies on volunteers in whom ascorbic acid deficiency was deliberately produced. The first change, which was observed after approximately 140 days, was prominence of the hair follicles, usually those over the back and thighs. This prominence is due to plugging of the lumens with an excessive amount of keratin, which leads to an impediment to hair growth so that the hair becomes coiled upon itself within the follicle. The epithelium surrounding each follicle becomes hyperemic, and blood cells extravasate into the tissues. These disappear leaving deposits of pigment, so that the perifollicular area becomes discolored. Large confluent ecchymoses appear over the seat in a saddle pattern. Petechiae tend to appear on the dorsal surfaces with application of a tourniquet. Lesions in the mouth appear after approximately 200 days of deprivation. Reddening and swelling of the interdental papillae occur first, soon followed by hemorrhage. The time of appearance and degree of severity of the gum changes are related to the state of oral hygiene. Pain and weakness in the extremities have been prominent in experimental studies. Old scars become tender and livid, and new injuries heal slowly.

The clinical picture in children is very different from that observed in adults. The peak incidence is 8 months; few cases are seen after the first year. The most prominent sign on physical examination is tenderness of the lower extremities, which are also usually somewhat swollen. The legs are characteristically partially flexed and guarded. Involvement of the upper extremities is less common. The extremities are obviously painful; the child screams when approached. The costochondral junctions may be enlarged. Crepitus of the epiphyseal areas of the ankles and wrists may be felt. The gums are swollen and hemorrhagic when teeth are present, but show little change before teeth erupt. Subcutaneous hemorrhages may be observed; these tend to be in the form of ecchymoses, not the pinpoint hemorrhages seen about the follicles in the adult. Follicular lesions are uncommon in children. Hemorrhages occur elsewhere: suborbital with proptosis, epistaxis, hematuria, or signs of subdural bleeding.

LABORATORY FINDINGS. The concentration of ascorbic acid may be determined in samples of plasma or in the buffy coat layer. Zero levels may be present in the plasma of adults for months before tissue stores are depleted. The plasma level mirrors the recent intake of ascorbic acid. Even if minimal or zero concentrations of ascorbic acid are present in plasma, the clinical syndrome will likely not be present. When adults subsist on an intake of 10 mg ascorbic acid per day, the concentrations of the vitamin in the buffy coat average about 2 mg per 100 ml. In such instances no clinical evidence of scurvy is present. On a vitamin C-deficient diet, the ascorbic acid concentration in the buffy coat falls to 1 mg or less after 4 to 6 months. At these values clinical scurvy may become manifest.

Saturation or load tests may be of some help in evalu-

ating ascorbic acid nutriture. When adequate amounts of the vitamin are being ingested, the urinary output will be about 25 to 75 mg per 100 ml. Urinary output will be virtually zero when the body stores are depleted. If 200 mg ascorbic acid is administered each day and urinary excretion of the vitamin is small during the first 3 or 4 days, this indicates that the stores are reduced.

PATHOLOGY. In adults studied at autopsy, the most conspicuous finding is the presence of generalized hemorrhage. The perifollicular lesions and ecchymoses noted clinically are conspicuous. In addition, extravasations of blood are found in the pericardial or pleural cavities, walls of the intestinal tract, bladder, and renal pelves. In young adults separation of the epiphyses or costochondral junctions may be present, as well as subperiosteal hemorrhage.

In children the most characteristic changes at autopsy are in the skeleton. The periosteum has separated or may be easily stripped from the shaft of a bone; the costal or epiphyseal cartilages have separated from the shaft of the rib or a long bone. Microscopic examination at the cartilage-shaft junction shows a dense "lattice" of spicules of calcified cartilaginous matrix, many of which have fractured. Little bone has formed on this lattice, which furthermore, has not been destroyed. In less advanced cases, fractures occur only at the edges or corners of the bone. Hemorrhage may be observed in the marrow or beneath the periosteum. As a result of decreased osteoid formation, the cortex and trabeculae of the shaft are reduced in thickness. Aside from hemorrhages elsewhere—subdural, subpleural, and subcutaneous—little else is found that is specific for scurvy. Rickets frequently coexists in such children.

PATHOGENESIS. Scurvy represents the reaction of particular hosts, such as man, other primates, and the guinea pig, to a lack of ascorbic acid in the diet. Most mammalian species can synthesize the vitamin. Ascorbic acid is found in high concentrations in citrus and other fruits, leafy vegetables, tubers, most grasses, and sprouting plants. The vitamin content of human milk varies, since the mother is dependent on dietary sources. Milk from a well-nourished woman contains 5 to 7 mg per 100 ml. Fresh cow's milk contains 1.0 to 2.6 mg per 100 ml; however, storage and sterilizing reduces this to virtually zero in dairy milk. Scurvy is virtually unheard of in breast-fed infants unless the mother is deficient. On the other hand, the use of sterilized infant formulas prepared from cow's milk or proprietary foods may be expected to produce scurvy in infants if the diet is not supplemented with a source of ascorbic acid.

Scurvy is, broadly speaking, a genetic disease in that the tissues of these species appear to have lost their ability to synthesize ascorbic acid. The chemical steps in the formation of the vitamin are well known:

a. D-glucuronate + TPNH + H^+ → L-gulonate + TPN^+

b. L-gulonate + DPN^+ → L-gulonolactone + DPN^+ + H^+

c. L-gulonolactone → L-ascorbate + H_2O

Liver and kidney tissues of all mammalian species so far studied can carry out reactions *a* and *b*. Only liver cells can form L-ascorbate via reaction *c*, but the hepatic tissues of man, other primates, and guinea pigs cannot carry this out.

The basic structural disturbance in scurvy is the failure of various types of connective tissue cells to form their respective collagenous matrices. Fibroblasts are unable to elaborate collagen; osteoblasts and odontoblasts do not synthesize osteoid and dentine. The lack of formation of these matrices explains the failure of wounds to heal, the changes in the growing bone of infants and children, and the alterations in the teeth of experimental animals. What is the underlying biochemical lesion? Collagen is characterized chemically by large amounts of glycine, proline, and hydroxyproline. The presence of the latter, a hydroxy-amino acid, and of hydroxylysine make collagen unique, since these amino acids are not found in other proteins. Hydroxyproline is not synthesized in the absence of ascorbic acid. This is most important when it is recalled that exogenous hydroxyproline is normally not incorporated into collagen. All the hydroxyproline in the basic

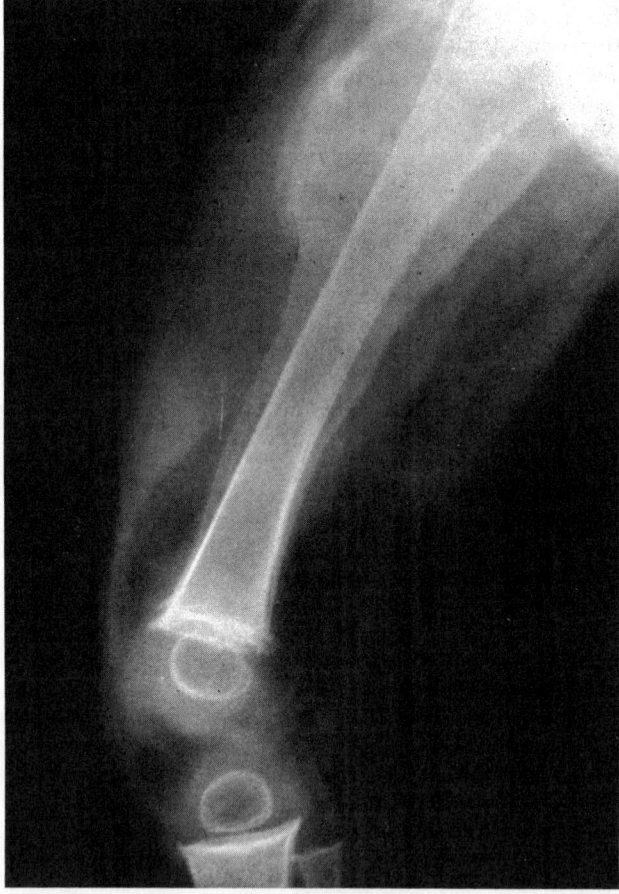

Fig. 82-1. The film shows four characteristic changes of scurvy. A large subperiosteal hemorrhage is being calcified. The epiphyseal margin shows a translucent line medially, the "corner sign" of Park. The epiphyseal plates are dense, and the bone shaft shows a ground-glass appearance with lack of trabecular detail. (*Photograph courtesy, Dr. Henry Burko, Vanderbilt University*)

collagen molecule is derived from the hydroxylation of proline in vivo. The point in collagen synthesis at which hydroxylation of proline takes place is not clear at this time. In ascorbic acid–deficient organisms, the connective tissue cells can proliferate. However, their microscopic appearance implies their functional impotency. Their cytoplasm is scanty, and virtually no stainable RNA is present. What this means in terms of altered synthetic mechanisms is obscure at this time.

The role of ascorbic acid in the integrity of blood vessels is not clear. The characteristic perifollicular hemorrhages indicate a defect in the vascular wall. Under the biomicroscope, capillary dilatation may be observed. Since the integrity of collagen is affected as a result of ascorbic acid deficiency, it is possible that the blood vessels may lose the support provided by these fibers and, hence, become more liable to the effects of minor trauma.

Certain other metabolic defects may be observed as a result of ascorbic acid deficiency, though these are not usually considered part of the scurvy syndrome. One of the most interesting aspects of ascorbic acid function is its nonspecific relation to metabolism of the aromatic amino acids, phenylalanine and tyrosine. Premature infants deficient in ascorbic acid excrete relatively large amounts of parahydroxyphenyllactic acid and para-hydroxyphenylpyruvic acid in the urine when excess phenylalanine and tyrosine are administered. The defect appears to be an inability to metabolize the tyrosine. Ascorbic acid is implicated in the secretion of the aqueous humor. The vitamin also plays a role in the metabolism of folic acid, i.e., in the transformation of this material to folacin (citrovorum factor). Occasionally, scurvy is associated with a macrocytic anemia which responds to citrovorum factor.

DIAGNOSIS. The clinical features of full-blown scurvy in adults or infants are characteristic. A most important point to emphasize is the feeding history in infants. If an infant four to six months or older has been bottle-fed with boiled milk or milk substitutes from birth or shortly after and has received no supplemental ascorbic acid, the possibility of scurvy should be considered. The feeding history of adults is likewise important because the disease often is observed in individuals subsisting on diets obviously low in ascorbic acid content. The history relative to vitamin C intake is easy to obtain.

X-ray examination in the adult is not of particular help in diagnosing scurvy, except that one may see alterations in the lamina dura of the jaws. In infants, x-ray examination of the skeleton may be helpful. At the junction between the epiphyseal cartilage and shaft of the long bones, there may be a zone of increased density, which represents the area of excess spicules of calcified cartilaginous matrix, some of which may have fractured (Fig. 82-1). There may also be defects, i.e., areas of rarefaction, at the "corners" of the bones, and these result from fractures at the periphery of the junction between cartilage and shaft. The formation of spurs or projections of the periosteum about the margins of the cartilage also are characteristic. In addition, the bone film will show a "ground glass" appearance, which reflects the decrease in density due to diminished width of the cortices and size of the medullary trabeculae.

TREATMENT. In infants the administration of fresh orange juice in single or multiple doses per day is advised. This may be sweetened with sugar. If orange juice is refused, twice the amount of tomato juice is the next choice. Synthetic ascorbic acid may be employed orally, 100 to 300 mg per day. There is little need for parenteral therapy. In view of the changes that have taken place in the skeleton, children in whom the disease is in the stage of healing should be handled as little and as gently as possible. It is not necessary to manipulate any bony deformities, nor should splints or casts be applied.

Treatment in adults involves administration of orange juice or ascorbic acid in divided doses up to 500 mg per day. A diet rich in vitamin C should be initiated and continued in both children and adults.

PROGNOSIS. Under therapy gum lesions, if present in infants and in adults, begin to regress in 2 to 3 days. Periosteal shadows, resulting from new bone formation, begin to appear in the long bones of infants after approximately a week. Hemorrhages in the skin usually disappear in 2 to 3 weeks.

REFERENCES

Barlow, T.: On Cases Described as "Acute Rickets" Which Are Probably a Combination of Scurvy and Rickets, the Scurvy Being an Essential and the Rickets a Variable Element, Med. Chir. Trans., 66:159, 1883.

Gould, B. S.: Collagen Formation and Fibrogenesis with Special Reference to the Role of Ascorbic Acid, Int. Rev. Cytol., 15:301, 1963.

Hess, A. F.: "Scurvy, Past and Present," Philadelphia, J. B. Lippincott Company, 1920.

Medical Research Council: Vitamin C Requirements of Human Adults, Spec. Rep. Ser., no. 280, London, 1953.

Park, E. A., H. G. Guild, D. Jackson, and M. Bond: The Recognition of Scurvy with Special Reference to the Early X-ray Changes, Arch. Dis. Child., 10:265, 1935.

83 VITAMIN D DEFICIENCY AND HYPERVITAMINOSIS D

George Nichols, Jr.

VITAMIN D DEFICIENCY

INTRODUCTION. Deficiency of vitamin D, whether the result of dietary inadequacy, lack of exposure to sunlight, failure of absorption, or defective metabolism and utilization, results in either rickets or osteomalacia—conditions which differ from each other only because of the presence or absence of active bone growth. Thus rickets begins in childhood, although its manifestations may persist throughout life, while osteomalacia begins after skeletal growth has been completed.

HISTORY. These diseases have been known since an-

tiquity, with references to soft, waxy bones being found in Plato's writings. The prevalence of these diseases seems to have increased when people began living in cities, presumably because of dietary lack or inadequate exposure to ultraviolet light rather than poverty; even Charles I of England and his second daughter were severely afflicted with rickets. The first complete description of the disease is usually attributed to Glisson, in whose book, published in 1650, the well-known physical signs, "swellings and knotty excrescences about some of the joynts," "tumors in the tops of the ribs where they are conjoyned with gristles in the breast," "breasts of a hen or capon," and "crooked bones" are described. However, an equally careful description was published 5 years earlier by Whistler, then a medical student at Leiden.

The true nature and origins of these diseases were not understood until Mellanby produced, by dietary means, a ricketslike condition in dogs which could be prevented by an antirachitic vitamin found in certain fats and oils. Between 1918 and 1927 the pathogenesis of rickets was virtually completely elucidated: The disease was induced and studied histologically in experimental animals; the importance of the concentrations of calcium and phosphorus relative to one another was demonstrated; the antirachitic vitamin was proved to be a specific compound, vitamin D, which by 1927 had been chemically identified; the role of ultraviolet radiation in activating a provitamin in foods and in the skin was demonstrated; deranged concentrations of calcium and phosphorus in the serum of rachitic children were described and found to return to normal after therapy with vitamin D; healing processes in the bones were followed roentgenographically and histologically; and calcification of rachitic cartilage *in vitro* was produced by suitable concentrations of calcium and phosphorus in the incubation medium.

PREVALENCE. Vitamin D enrichment of animal and human food has effectively prevented rickets so that the disease in its florid forms has become a rarity in technically advanced countries. Rickets was found only in 1 in 2,800 North American pediatric admissions in 1962. However, rickets has persisted in North Africa and other underdeveloped areas, and the disease is still seen in urban areas in the United Kingdom, where migratory populations from the West Indies and Pakistan, especially, have come from a sunny to a clouded climate and have not taken advantage of the preventive measures.

While the most common type of rickets continues to be that due to vitamin D deficiency, abnormalities of calcium and phosphorus metabolism are beginning to be recognized more and more frequently as causes of so-called "endogenous," or "conditioned," rickets.

Osteomalacia is now uncommon in both developed and developing countries. In the past, however, famine accompanying war gave rise to many cases of osteomalacia, particularly in women. In North China, osteomalacia has been common as a result of low calcium intake, insufficient sunlight, and many pregnancies. A similar situation has been described in Moslem women in *purdah*. Virtually all instances of osteomalacia encountered in the

Western World now are due to some conditioning factor related to abnormal vitamin D or calcium and phosphorus metabolism, such as poor absorption, excessive intestinal loss, disordered metabolic turnover, or increased renal excretion.

CLINICAL FINDINGS. Uncomplicated Rickets. The cardinal signs of *uncomplicated rickets* are muscular hypotonia and skeletal deformities. The pattern of the skeletal deformities is influenced largely by the age at which the disease becomes manifest. If it begins when the infant is recumbent, the effects of pressure due to gravity tend to produce flattening of the skull, thorax, and pelvic girdle. If the child has been able to sit up, kyphosis or deformity of the forearms and anterior bowing of the lower legs are found if the extremities have been crossed or if the feet hang over the edge of a chair. When the child can walk, further vertebral and pelvic deformity may ensue, as well as curvatures of the lower extremities such as bow legs, knock-knees, and even fractures.

Among the first physical signs of rickets to appear in the infant are softened areas in the skull, *craniotabes*. The bone may be readily depressed because of lack of rigidity, resulting from decreased deposition of inorganic materials. Craniotabes is not a specific sign of rickets, however, and may be observed in other diseases such as osteogenesis imperfecta and hydrocephalus. There may also be thickening and/or bossing of the cranial bones, particularly the parietal or frontal structures. Costochondral swellings, or beadings (*rachitic rosary*),

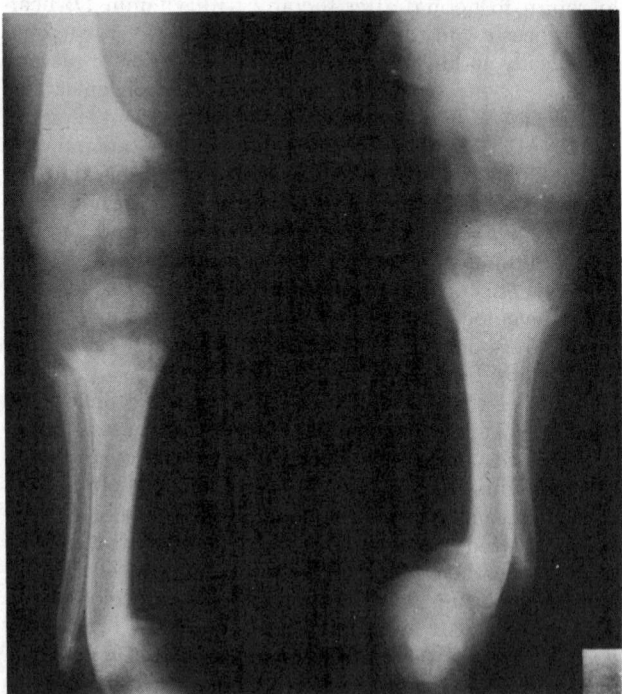

Fig. 83-1. The x-ray changes of the long bones in juvenile rickets. The shaft of the tibia is deformed; the metaphysis is widened, irregular, cupped, and translucent. (*Photo courtesy, Dr. Henry Burko, Vanderbilt University.*)

are among the cardinal signs of rickets, but similar changes may be observed in scurvy. With the development of the rachitic rosary, the lateral configuration of the thorax becomes flattened, and the sternum is pushed forward to form the so-called "*pigeon breast.*" The ribs are deformed by inward stress at the points of attachment of the diaphragm and form "*Harrison's grooves.*" These deformities reduce the volume of the thorax sometimes to such a degree that ventilation may be seriously impaired. Kyphosis of the lower thoracic and upper lumbar spine is found if the child has begun to sit up but disappears if the infant is suspended. Bilateral swellings of the ankles, and particularly the wrists, are characteristic. The shafts of the long bones may be thickened. Greenstick fractures may occur. Curvatures, either outward (bowlegs, *genu varum*) or inward (knock-knees, *genu valgum*) are prominent, and bending of the lower leg may lead to anterior curvature. Twisting of the metaphysis may result in *coxa vara*.

Primary dentition is delayed, and the order of tooth eruption may be abnormal. The enamel of the permanent teeth may show pits or grooves. In severe cases enamel may be virtually absent.

Hypocalcemic tetany can occur in rickets, usually appearing near the onset of the disease and sometimes in the healing stage. The lowered serum calcium concentration may on occasion be sufficient to lead to laryngeal spasm, convulsions, and death.

Both growth and weight gain generally are normal in uncomplicated rickets. There is, however, an extreme form of this disorder known as *dystrophic rickets,* or *osteomalacic rickets,* which apparently also is due to vitamin D deficiency. Here the muscular hypotonia and bony deformities are extreme, growth and weight gain cease, and multiple fractures as well as severe anemia and hepatosplenomegaly can occur. Whether other nutritional deficiencies besides vitamin D are involved in this condition is not clear, but like the more common form of rickets, dystrophic rickets responds dramatically (if more slowly) to treatment with vitamin D.

Osteomalacia. The clinical aspects of *osteomalacia* in adults are not as dramatic as those seen in the growing child. Weakness and/or vague aches and pains in various parts of the skeleton, back, pelvis, ribs, and extremities usually are the earliest signs. When skeletal pain is present, it tends to be generalized and persistent in contrast to the episodic "lumbago" of osteoporosis. As the disease progresses, weakness becomes sufficiently severe to confine the patient to bed, and spontaneous fractures or collapse of vertebras can occur. Tetany may be encountered, and, if the disease has been present for a long time, curvatures of the extremities may be present. Bone pain on pressure may also be present. As noted, osteomalacia due solely to dietary deficiency is rare, so that the presence of conditions such as intestinal malabsorption or certain renal or other abnormalities which create an increased demand for vitamin D should be suspected, and vice-versa.

LABORATORY FINDINGS. The serum calcium concentration in rickets generally is normal or at the lower limit of normal, while serum phosphorus values are reduced from the normal childhood level of 5 to 6 mg to 2 to 4 mg per 100 ml. In some individuals, serum calcium and not phosphorus may be reduced. In premature babies both calcium and phosphorus concentration may be lower than normal. Adults with vitamin D–deficient osteomalacia show similar changes, with serum calcium values being normal, while serum phosphorus concentration usually is somewhat reduced below the normal level of 3 to 4 mg per 100 ml. Serum alkaline phosphatase activity generally is elevated in both disorders, although normal values are occasionally encountered in mild cases. Other abnormalities include mild metabolic acidosis, amino aciduria, glycosuria, and increased excretion of hydroxyproline in the urine. Reductions in plasma and urinary citrate values together with increased fecal excretion of calcium and phosphate may be observed.

RADIOLOGY. The radiologic signs of rickets reflect the inadequate mineralization and overproduction of osteoid which are the hallmarks of the skeletal pathology in this disease. Thus, in the growing child, the metaphyses of the long bones are wide, their upper surfaces tend to be cupped, and the span of the growth cartilage is markedly widened. The epiphyses are small and irregular and the trabeculae are indistinct. Thinning of the cortex, bowing, fractures (especially of the greenstick type), and other deformities are present (Fig. 83-1).

In osteomalacia, the epiphyseal changes are not seen because the disease develops after they have closed. Therefore, thinning of the cortex of the long bones; deformities, including marked bowing, especially of the weight-bearing bones of the lower extremities; fractures, and pseudofractures are the distinguishing features. "Pseudofractures," or *Looser's zones*, are characteristic bands of decalcification which are perpendicular or oblique to the surface of the bone. They are considered pathognomonic of osteomalacia but are seen in rickets as well. While usually straight, they may zigzag. On either side of the band, a denser shadow of callus often helps make the band more obvious. Looser's zones tend to be symmetrical, and their distribution is fairly constant: the neck of the humerus and femur, the pubic rami, the ribs, and especially the axillary borders of the scapulae. In addition, subperiosteal erosions, similar to those found in hyperparathyroidism, have been reported to occur in as many as 50 percent of cases.

Although the reversal of radiologic changes with treatment is relatively slow in osteomalacia, reversal begins quite promptly in rickets, the first change being the appearance of a dense band of calcification midway between the epiphysis and metaphysis. This becomes quite distinct between the eighth and thirteenth day following the onset of vitamin D therapy. Mineralization begins in this area and ultimately spreads to involve the entire uncalcified metaphyseal area. After several months, complete healing may be found; alternatively, the cortical bone in the concavity of bowed bones may remain thickened, resulting in some narrowing of the normal marrow cavity. Islands of cartilage which fail to calcify adequately occasionally are trapped in the diaphysis and

appear as translucent defects in otherwise healthy tissue.

The radiologic changes found in rickets and osteomalacia generally are quite easy to distinguish from other conditions, although in the absence of pseudofractures, osteomalacia may not be easily differentiated from osteoporosis by radiologic criteria alone. Biopsy will show a striking excess of osteoid in osteomalacia which is not found in osteoporosis, thus establishing the diagnosis in doubtful cases.

PATHOLOGY. The distinguishing features of the skeletal changes in both rickets and osteomalacia are defective mineralization and a relative overabundance of new uncalcified bone matrix or osteoid. The relative undermineralization of the skeleton is manifested *chemically* by a reduction in the mineral ash content of the dried bone solids from more than 60 to less than 50 percent. In addition to excess osteoid there is a greater than normal number of osteoblasts. Widened osteoid seams are noted in the cortical bone in areas which have been remodeled recently. The trabeculae have prominent borders of osteoid. In some patients, evidence of excessive destruction of the bone formed before the disease began or of newly produced osteoid may be observed; the number of osteoclasts may be increased as well as osteoblasts. In addition, in the growth cartilage defective calcification along the columns of hypertrophic cells is found.

In rickets, the degree of involvement of the different parts of the skeleton is related to the rate of growth of the different bones. Because the anterior ends of middle ribs grow fastest, the disease is most marked there. For the same reason, the epiphyses about the knee, shoulder, and wrist show more change than the opposite ends of these bones. Since osteomalacia is rickets in adults in whom epiphyseal growth has ceased, the conspicuous change is found only in the bone biopsy, where the osteoid seams noted above are seen.

As healing of rickets occurs, inorganic material appears in the matrix about the most recently matured hypertrophic cartilage cells (Muller's line). Calcification of the oldest osteoid seems to occur first in membranous bones. Healing of osteomalacia is indicated by disappearance of the osteoid borders and ultimately of the osteoid seams in the dense cortical bone.

In cases of classic vitamin D–deficiency rickets, little that is specific besides bone lesions is to be found at autopsy. A fairly constant finding in cases of long-standing rickets and osteomalacia is enlargement and increased cellularity of the parathyroid glands. However, when rickets or osteomalacia is secondary to malabsorption or renal disease, pathologic changes in the gastrointestinal tract, including obstruction of the bile or pancreatic ducts may be present. The kidney may show abnormalities in the structure of the nephron; such as the shortening of the renal tubules which has been reported in cases of phosphate diabetes with aminoaciduria. In addition, chronic renal disease in the form of chronic glomerulonephritis, interstitial, or pyelonephritis may be present.

PATHOGENESIS. Rickets may be defined as a disease of the developing skeleton characterized by defective mineralization of the organic matrices of the cartilage and bone. Because osteomalacia is rickets in adults in whom cartilagenous growth has ceased, it may be defined as the skeletal disease in adults which is characterized by defective mineralization of the bone matrix.

Several lines of evidence indicate that both rickets and osteomalacia are due to lack of vitamin D specifically and not just to a decreased calcium-phosphorus ion concentration product in the body fluids as was once thought. In brief, experimental rickets characterized by increased osteoid and decreased mineralization can be produced in animals by vitamin D–deficiency alone and occurs regardless of the levels of calcium and phosphate which are fed. Indeed, calcium deficiency alone inhibits bone growth (and has been cited as a cause of osteoporosis), but the osteoid which is laid down is normally calcified and excessively wide osteoid seams are never seen. It is important to note that *phosphate deficiency* (with or without lowered serum phosphate concentrations) and ingestion of a number of foreign ions, notably strontium, beryllium, and fluoride, can produce bone disease with many of the outward features of rickets and osteomalacia. These differ in several important respects, however, from the condition produced by vitamin D deficiency; parathyroid enlargement is absent, serum calcium concentrations are almost invariably normal, and vitamin D is not curative.

Vitamin D is a sterol derivative formed in nature by the irradiation of ergosterol or 7-dehydrocholesterol, with ultraviolet light of a wave length between 250 and 312 mμ. This opens the B ring to produce either ergocalciferol (vitamin D_2) when ergosterol from plant sources is irradiated, or cholicalciferol (vitamin D_3) when 7-dehydrocholesterol, the precursor found in normal human skin, is exposed. The sterol derivative, AT-10 has vitamin D activity but offers no advantage over vitamin D_2 and is more expensive.

The international unit of vitamin D activity is defined as the amount that is equal in potency to 1 mg of the international standard of the irradiated ergosterol. This is equivalent to 0.025 μg of pure crystalline calciferol (40,000 units = 1 mg of calciferol). Thus two related substances with vitamin D activity are available to the organism: Vitamin D_2 is less effective biologically in birds and at least some of the New World primates, but the two forms appear to be equally effective in human beings.

Vitamin D occurs only in very small amounts in common foods such as cereals, vegetables, and fruit. Liver, butterfat, and egg yolk contain small amounts (8 to 20 units per 100 grams). Human and cow's milk also are poor sources, but most marine fish contain appreciable amounts and liver oils are particularly high in vitamin D content. Cod-liver oil contains 8,500 units; halibut, 60,000; and the oil from the liver of the blue-fin tuna, some 4,000,000 units per 100 ml. In many countries, including the United States, dietary sources, usually milk, margarine, or butter are fortified with additional vitamin D. The required level in this country is 400 international units per quart of milk.

The high fat solubility of vitamin D and its insolubility in water explain the failure of dietary sources to provide adequate amounts of the vitamin under a variety of pathological conditions; an example is steatorrhea due to intestinal malabsorption, blockade of the bile ducts, or pancreatic disease. Occasionally rickets or osteomalacia occurs in individuals ingesting excessive amounts of mineral oil. Similarly, the need for exposure to sunlight explains the geographical prevalence of these disorders in northern countries and the particular susceptibility of Negroes to these diseases, because the pigment in their skins tends to absorb much of the ultraviolet radiation before it can reach the Malpighian layer where the vitamin D precursor is found.

The absorption of dietary vitamin D from the gastrointestinal tract has been studied with isotopically labeled materials. Vitamin D is absorbed with the chylomicrons and very low density lipoproteins into the lymph. Thus the presence of fat and bile salts in the gastrointestinal tract is of great importance to normal absorption of vitamin D. The vitamin is transported via the circulation to the liver, where it is converted to the metabolically active form, 25-hydroxycholecalciferol. From there it is distributed to its target organs, gut, skeletal tissue, and kidney. The highest concentrations per cell are found in the intestine and skeleton.

The presence of vitamin D is apparently of critical importance to the absorption of calcium by the intestinal mucosa. This action seems to be particularly important in the upper part of the small intestine, the major site of active transport. The exact biochemical mechanism involved in this action has yet to be identified. However, DeLuca and Avioli, while searching for an explanation of the delay in the onset of vitamin D action following its administration, were able to demonstrate metabolic conversion of the vitamin to a biologically active form during this interval. Other work in which binding of the metabolically active derivative of vitamin D (25-hydroxycolicalciferol) to the nuclear membrane in the cells of target tissues (bone and gut) and the induction of RNA synthesis in these tissues under its influence, suggest that the primary action of the metabolic derivative is upon the synthesis of messenger RNA and thereby, perhaps, the synthesis of a specific calcium-binding protein.

For many years, it was thought that the sole action of vitamin D was on the intestine, but it is now clear that it acts on the skeleton as well, in two ways. First, without vitamin D normal calcification of the osteoid laid down during remodeling does not occur in vitro or in vivo, regardless of the calcium and phosphate concentration. Some vitamin D also seems to be required for the calcium-mobilizing action of parathyroid hormone on the skeleton. In addition, *large* doses of vitamin D appear to mimic the action of parathyroid hormone because they cause mobilization of mineral from the skeleton, resulting in increases in serum calcium concentration and urinary calcium excretion, both to abnormally high levels.

Less information is available concerning the action of vitamin D on the kidney. Both increases and decreases in tubular absorption of calcium have been reported, although the most recent and well-controlled studies suggest that calcium reabsorption in the proximal tubule is probably increased as a result of the action of the vitamin. On the other hand, it is clear that phosphate excretion may be increased by vitamin D just as it is by parathyroid hormone.

Vitamin D–deficient Rickets and Osteomalacia. With these facts in mind, the mechanism of the development of rickets and osteomalacia secondary to a deficient supply of vitamin D can be understood. Calcium absorption from the gut is decreased, and its excretion in the feces is increased by taking with it larger amounts of phosphate. Decreased mineralization of the growing cartilage of bone occurs partly because the availability of calcium is inadequate, but more importantly, because the mechanism for calcium deposition in the plate is somehow blocked. Failure of adequate intestinal absorption of calcium together with deficient resorption of bone tends to lower the serum calcium, and this in turn stimulates the parathyroid gland to excessive secretion. While the parathyroid hyperactivity maintains the serum calcium at normal concentration, it is also accompanied by decreased concentration of serum phosphate because of increased urinary excretion of that ion. This secondary hyperthyroidism is probably responsible for the interesting effects of feeding phosphate to rachitic children. Ingestion of 100 mg per kg of this ion is without effect in normal children but often sharply lowers the calcium concentration in the serum of rachitic children, sometimes to tetanic levels. Indeed an acute illness which causes tissue lysis with release of tissue phosphate into the circulation may produce hypocalcemic tetany in rachitic children. The mechanism for the developement of osteomalacia is presumably identical to that described for rickets.

"Conditioned" or Secondary Rickets and Osteomalacia. Because diets in the United States are quite adequate in vitamin D, the presence of rickets or osteomalacia should call attention to the possibility that the disease is secondary to some other disorder. If calcium intake is relatively low and there is an inadequate supply of sunlight, multiple pregnancies may lead to vitamin D and calcium deficiency and the early appearance of osteomalacia, presumably related to losses of vitamin D, calcium, and phosphorus with lactation. Other factors such as the pH of the intestinal contents, the presence of certain insoluble compounds, such as phytic acid from cereals, which bind calcium, or the presence of excessive nonmetabolized or absorbed lipids in the diet (for example, mineral oil) may restrict the absorption of vitamin D and/or calcium and produce rickets or osteomalacia.

Either glomerular or tubular *renal disease* may be accompanied by clinical rickets in children and by evidence of osteomalacia in adults. Hypocalcemia and hyperphosphatemia are commonly found. While hyperphosphatemia can be partially reduced by feeding the patient compounds which bind phosphate in the gastrointestinal tract, thus controlling absorption of phosphate, the hypocalcemia of renal disease is notoriously resistant to the usual therapeutic doses of vitamin D (*vitamin D resistance*). In patients with chronic renal disease the plasma concentration of the metabolically active derivative of vitamin D is decreased because of accelerated destruction or loss and increased turnover. Furthermore, serum calcium concentrations are not restored to normal by secondarily increased parathyroid function because of a lack of the amounts of metabolically active derivative of vitamin D required for the normal functioning of the skeletal cellular mechanisms responsible for maintaining serum ionized calcium concentrations at their normal level (Chap. 379).

At the renal tubular level, disturbances of renal hydrogen ion excretion (renal tubular acidosis) may lead to excessive losses of calcium through the kidneys with secondary nephrocalcinosis and hypocalcemia, in addition to metabolic acidosis. Although the mechanism of this syndrome is not clear at the present time, it is generally thought to result from the excretion of acid metabolites in association with sodium, potassium, calcium, and other "fixed" cations.

Phosphate Deficiency. Although a lack of dietary phosphorus probably is sufficiently rare as to have no clinical significance in normal man, failure to absorb adequate phosphate from the gastrointestinal tract, with or without excessive urinary losses, may lead to a condition which strongly resembles rickets or osteomalacia with respect to its biochemical alterations and the microscopic appearance of the skeletal tissues, though the mechanisms which underlie its appearance are still unclear. Like renal tubular acidosis, this condition appears most commonly to result from defects in renal tubular function. These may involve phosphate reabsorption only (*phosphate diabetes*) or be multiple, involving in addition to phosphate, glucose and amino acids (*Fanconi's syndrome*). The most striking features of these conditions are the abnormal amounts of phosphate and the other materials in the urine and the resistance of the conditions to the therapeutic effects of usually curative doses of vitamin D.

Hypophosphatasia. This condition is another, probably genetically determined disorder which leads to defective mineralization of skeletal tissues. It is easily identified by the low levels of alkaline phosphatase activity which are found in the plasma together with the excessive excretion of phosphoethanolamine in the urine.

A list of the various conditions which may underlie or appear in conjunction with rickets and osteomalacia with or without associated secondary hyperparathyroidism is given in Table 83-1.

DIAGNOSIS. The diagnosis of both rickets and osteomalacia must be made on clinical grounds because a suitably sensitive, convenient assay for vitamin D activity in the circulating fluids still is not available. However, the diagnosis is generally not difficult and can be made on the basis of history, the presence of characteristic clinical and radiologic features, and the concentration of serum calcium, phosphorus, and alkaline phosphatase activity. The presence of widened osteoid seams on histologic examination of samples of bone obtained at biopsy provides important confirmatory evidence. Finally, a prompt therapeutic response to orally or paren-

Table 83-1. THE PATHOGENESIS OF RICKETS
AND OSTEOMALACIA

I. Vitamin D deficiency
  A. Defective endogenous formation in skin
  B. Exogenous dietary deficiency
  C. Decreased absorption
    1. Malabsorption syndromes
    2. Absence of bile or pancreatic juice
II. Phosphorus deficiency
  A. Dietary deficiency
  B. Formation of insoluble complexes
  C. Malabsorption syndromes
  D. Phosphate diabetes (vitamin D–resistant rickets)
  E. Fanconi syndrome
    1. With glycosuria
    2. With glycosuria and aminoaciduria
    3. With cystinosis
    4. With glycinuria
    5. Associated with heavy-metal toxicity
    6. Associated with Wilson's disease
    7. Associated with multiple myeloma
    8. Associated with neurofibromatosis
    9. Lowe's syndrome
III. Miscellaneous
  A. Hypophosphatasia
IV. Contributing causes
  A. Calcium deficiency
    1. Dietary deficiency
    2. Poor absorption (vitamin D deficiency)
    3. Insoluble complex formation
    4. Increased pH of intestinal contents
    5. Steatorrhea and malabsorption syndromes
    6. Idiopathic hypercalcuria
    7. Chronic renal disease
    8. Renal tubular acidosis
    9. Pregnancy and lactation
    10. Excessive sweating

terally administered vitamin D can serve to confirm the diagnosis, especially in vitamin D–deficiency rickets.

TREATMENT. Simple rickets requires less than 5 mg vitamin D by mouth given in doses of 0.05 to 0.1 mg (2,000 to 4,000 units) each day for 6 to 12 weeks. Even smaller doses may be quite adequate; larger doses may be detrimental (see below) and are required only in specific instances where a therapeutic response is not obtained due to relative resistance to vitamin D. However, if rickets is complicated by tetany, large doses of vitamin D as well as intravenous infusion of calcium chloride or calcium gluconate may be required in the early stages of treatment.

The addition of calcium to the therapeutic regimen usually is desirable, partly to provide the calcium needed for mineralization of previously uncalcified osteoid, partly to avoid the complication of hypocalcemia, which occurs not infrequently in the early days of treatment. Because the normal human diet contains excessive amounts of phosphate, the particular calcium salt employed probably is of relatively little significance; many prefer to use calcium phosphate salts ($CaHPO_4$) with the thought that both calcium and phosphate will be provided in this way in adequate amounts.

Prevention of rickets can be achieved by feeding as little as 400 units vitamin D daily to infants until the age of two years and by also giving this amount until full growth is achieved if sunshine is absent during the winter months. The absolute amount required varies considerably from individual to individual and with the circumstances of living, especially the amount of exposure to ultraviolet radiation and sunshine. Premature infants probably have no store of vitamin D at birth and require larger amounts (2,000 to 3,000 units daily for the first 2 or 3 months of life), and darkskinned people, who are relatively insensitive to ultraviolet radiation and hence have lower rates of endogenous vitamin D production, also may require larger amounts.

In cases of Vitamin D resistance, the use of 25-hydroxycholecalciferol may be effective.

HYPERVITAMINOSIS D

INTRODUCTION. Vitamin D, like vitamin A, can cause toxic manifestations if administered in excessive amounts. The dangers of excessive dosage came to light soon after the crystalline form of the vitamin became available and began to be used, often in huge doses, in the unsuccessful treatment of such varied conditions as rheumatoid arthritis, psoriasis, and tuberculosis of the skin. Recognition of the syndrome of hypervitaminosis D in the late 1940s led to a marked reduction in the number of cases. Now, the condition is relatively rare, occurring only through inadvertent excessive intake, as in the "idiopathic" hypercalcemia of infants which proved to be secondary to excessive fortification of cow's milk with vitamin D. Vitamin D intoxication also has occurred in the course of treatment of vitamin D–resistant rickets, renal osteodystrophy, and hypoparathyroidism.

The exact amount of the vitamin needed to cause intoxication varies from patient to patient as well as with age, renal function, and calcium intake, but as little as 50,000 units per day has been reported to be toxic in some patients.

CLINICAL FEATURES. The signs and symptoms of vitamin D intoxication are largely those of hypercalcemia and include weakness, lethargy, anorexia, nausea and vomiting, weight loss, polyuria and polydipsia, irritability, mental depression, and calcific keratitis (band keratitis). Albuminuria and casts are often present, and the signs and symptoms of renal stones or uremia, secondary to nephrocalcinosis, may ultimately appear. Diarrhea with cramping abdominal pain and acute pancreatitis also can occur. Hypertension, secondary to renal damage, is a frequent late complication.

LABORATORY FINDINGS. Elevations of serum calcium, which may be marked, and phosphorus concentrations, with depression of serum alkaline phosphatase activity, are found. In addition, alkalosis with decreased serum potassium concentration is frequent. Increased urine calcium excretion is present in the early phases of the disease, but calcium excretion may fall to normal or low levels as renal failure secondary to nephrocalcinosis develops. Despite increased calcium absorption from the gut, the total body balance of calcium is negative.

RADIOLOGY. In advanced cases of vitamin D intoxication, especially in children, increased density of the metaphysis of the long bones may occur in association with decreased density in the shafts. Lines, not unlike those seen in lead poisoning, have been reported in the metaphyseal region and correspond to the time of peak vitamin D ingestion.

Much more striking when it is present is soft-tissue metastatic calcification. Although the diffuse calcium deposits in the kidney usually are not easy to see, calcification in the media of the larger vessels, deposits of calcium adjacent to joints, and renal stones may be very prominent.

PATHOLOGY. Significant pathologic changes are found in kidneys, arteries, and bones. In the kidneys, deposits of calcium are found first in the tubular basement membranes, especially near the corticomedullary junction, and gradually extend to involve the tubular cells and even the membrane of Bowman's capsule. Hyaline and calcium-containing casts also are found in the tubules. Inflammatory changes and fibrosis develop in later stages.

Surprisingly, the bony trabeculae show increased osteoid borders reminiscent of rickets. However, other features of bone histology are generally normal in man, although changes strongly resembling those of hyperparathyroidism have been induced in animals with vitamin D.

In addition to these changes, deposits of calcium may be found in the skin, heart, pancreas, stomach, lung, thyroid, and other tissues.

PATHOGENESIS. The precise roles played in the development of this syndrome by the various vitamin D–sensitive mechanisms are not yet clear. While increased calcium absorption from the gut doubtless plays some role, excess mobilization of calcium and phosphorus from skeletal stores accounts for most of the elevation of serum calcium.

TREATMENT. The treatment of this disorder clearly is to stop excessive intake of vitamin D. This usually is sufficient to reverse the process. However, dehydration and electrolyte imbalance secondary to disturbed renal function may demand attention. Details concerning treatment of the acute hypercalcemic syndrome will be found in Chap. 90.

PROGNOSIS. Generally, the prognosis is favorable if the condition is recognized early and vitamin D is withdrawn. The serum calcium falls to normal over a period of days. Gradually the skeleton becomes normal, metastatic calcification disappears, and normal renal function returns. However, in young children or in adults in whom the process has advanced to renal fibrosis and hypertension, the prognosis may be grave.

REFERENCES

Avioli, L., Birge, S., Lee, S. W., and Slatopolsky, E.: The Metabolic Fate of Vitamin D_3-^{3}H in Chronic Renal Failure, *J. Clin. Invest.*, 47:10, 1968.

Blunt, J. W., De Luca, H. F., and Schnoes, H. K.: 25-Hydroxycholecalciferol. A Biologically Active Metabolite of Vitamin D_3, Biochemistry, 7:10, 1968.

Fourman, P., and Royer, P.: "Calcium Metabolism and the Bone," Philadelphia, F. A. Davis Company, 1968.

Loomis, W. F.: Skin-pigment Regulation of Vitamin D Biosynthesis in Man, *Science*, 157:3788, 1967.

Wasserman, R. H.: "Transport Proteins from Animals, Proceedings of the Symposium on Membrane Proteins, New York Heart Association, New York, Nov., 1968.

84 VITAMIN A DEFICIENCY, XEROPHTHALMIA, NIGHT BLINDNESS AND HYPERVITAMINOSIS A

Richard H. Follis, Jr. and George V. Mann

HISTORY. Inability to see in subdued light, called *night blindness*, and dryness, haziness, and spontaneous necrosis of the cornea are abnormalities which have been recognized for many years. Over a century ago, Bitot called attention to the simultaneous occurrence of night blindness and lesions of the conjunctiva. By the turn of the century, Mori had suggested that ocular lesions in Japanese children might be related to a lack of fat in the diet. Soon a fat-soluble material (later to be called vitamin A) was shown to enhance the growth of rats and prevent the development of ocular lesions that histologically resembled those which had been observed in man. During the second decade of this century, investigators in Denmark clearly established the relationship of vitamin A to xerophthalmia in children. In 1930 carotene was demonstrated to be provitamin A. Vitamin A was chemically identified in 1931 and synthesized in 1936.

PREVALENCE. Today the areas of greatest prevalence of endemic vitamin A deficiency are found in Indonesia, particularly Java and parts of Sumatra; India; the Near East; and North Africa. Isolated instances of conditioned vitamin A deficiency have been described in Europe and the United States.

Vitamin A deficiency is the first cause of blindness in the world, and yet this occurs mostly in tropical areas where the carotenes which would prevent it are plentiful. The real need is for nutrition education.

CLINICAL FINDINGS. The term *xerophthalmia* is used here in an inclusive sense to refer to certain anatomic abnormalities of the eye resulting from vitamin A deficiency. The lesions usually exhibit a definite sequence of stages in development. The initial change, which is called xerosis (*xerosis epithelialis conjunctivae*), consists of dryness and opacity of the bulbar conjunctiva. Secretion of tears is decreased. At the lateral margin of the cornea, a triangular-shaped accumulation of sticky secretion may appear. This is the Bitot spot, which resembles a plaque or pseudomembrane filled with bubbles (Fig. 84-1). As the photograph indicates, the lesion has the appearance of a fleck of meringue. This material is difficult to scrape off. Fine pigmentation may also be present throughout the conjunctiva. These alterations are either accompanied or soon followed by haziness and dryness of the cornea (*xerosis corneae*). The tarsal glands along the eyelid frequently are enlarged. Photophobia may be marked. The most serious consequence is the appearance of small epithelial erosions on the cornea. These soon become infected and enlarged. If this ulceration continues, destruction of the cornea (*keratomalacia*) occurs, a process that may be extremely rapid. Thus a child with conjunctivitis and photophobia may open his eyes one morning to reveal the lens extruded, the bulb collapsed, and vision irrevocably lost (Fig. 84-2). Short of this, the cornea may heal but with a scar that greatly limits vision.

As already noted, visual acuity in subdued light is reduced as a result of vitamin A deficiency. This disturbance is called night blindness. Two other terms, *nyctalopia* and *hemeralopia*, have been used to refer to this condition. Nyctalopia means an inability to see in subdued light. Hemeralopia refers to a decrease in vision that follows exposure to bright light. Defective ability to see in subdued light may be established by certain tests; however, these are difficult to perform under routine conditions and are particularly unsuited for children. An instrument, the electroretinogram, has been developed for objective testing in research.

The nonocular manifestations of vitamin A deficiency are not conspicuous and are usually obscured by signs of general malnutrition or the presence of some conditioning disturbance, such as obstruction of the pancreatic or biliary ducts, which may lead to poor absorption of the vitamin. Tracheitis, bronchitis, and pneumonia are the commonest clinical manifestations.

LABORATORY FINDINGS. Vitamin A nutriture may be assessed by determining the carotene and/or vitamin A content of blood serum. Values are expressed in International Units (IU) or micrograms per 100 ml. One IU is equivalent to 0.3 μg vitamin A or 0.6 μg β-carotene. Vitamin A concentration is decisive; carotene values may be misleading, since other pigments may be present.

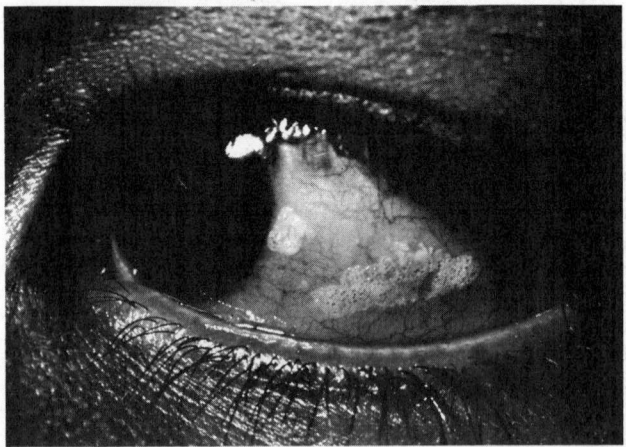

Fig. 84-1. Bitot's spots showing the characteristic meringue texture. (*Photograph courtesy of Professor D. S. McLaren and the American Journal of Clinical Nutrition*)

Serum values for carotene and vitamin A are usually considered to be normal if over 40 and 20 μg per 100 ml, respectively. When values for carotene and vitamin A fall below 20 and 10 μg per 100 ml, respectively, the deficient state is probably present. Valuable information on vitamin A nutriture among population groups has been obtained from analyses of liver tissue. For instance, among well-nourished groups in Great Britain, values averaging 450 IU per Gm have been obtained. In contrast, data derived from Chinese subjects indicate much lower levels, averaging 79 IU per Gm.

PATHOLOGY. The tissues chiefly affected are epithelial in nature, principally those which ordinarily are not keratinized. These include the lining epithelium of the upper and lower respiratory passages, genitourinary tract, eye and paraocular glands, salivary glands, accessory glands of the tongue and buccal cavity, and pancreas. The fundamental change is metaplasia of the normal nonkeratinized lining cells into a keratinizing type of epithelium. The cornea becomes dry, wrinkled, and hazy due to intrinsic changes as well as to lack of tears as a result of obstruction of the ducts. The ciliated epithelium of the respiratory tract is replaced by a keratinizing lining so that the important mechanical effects of the cilia are lost. The basal cells in all areas retain, however, their potentiality for reverting to normal if their supply of vitamin A is restored.

At autopsy other changes may be found that are responsible for conditioned vitamin A deficiency. For instance, obstruction to the biliary tract or pancreatic duct may interfere with fat absorption. Liver disease may have interfered with storage.

PATHOGENESIS. At least two forms of vitamin A alcohol are known (A_1 and A_2), together with acid and aldehyde derivatives. The vitamins A are intimately related to provitamins, the carotenes, and certain other pigmented compounds. A part of ingested carotene is absorbed by the cells of the intestinal mucosa and transformed into vitamin A. Bile is important in this process. Vitamin A is usually present in ester form in foods; it is hydrolyzed in the intestinal tract and absorbed as the alcohol (*retinol*). Within the cells of the intestinal mucosa, vitamin A is esterified, usually with palmitic acid, and transported via the thoracic duct as the ester to the liver, where it is stored. As needed, vitamin A ester is hydrolyzed to the alcohol and transported, attached to plasma protein, to the tissues. Vitamin A aldehyde (*retinal* or *retinene*) is found in the retina and is important in the visual process. The interrelations between alcohol, acid, and ester forms of vitamin A have been greatly clarified. It is possible that vitamin A acid (*retinoic acid*) may be the "active form." The alcohol (retinol) is converted to aldehyde (retinal or retinene). The latter may be converted to the acid by an enzyme in the liver. The reverse reaction, i.e., acid to alcohol or aldehyde, does not appear possible. The acid is more effective for growth in experimental animals than is the aldehyde. The acid is not active in the visual process.

The greatest concentration of vitamin A in man is found in the liver. Concentrations are also appreciable in kidneys, adrenals, lungs, and the retina. Fat depots contain a small amount of the vitamin.

Vitamin A deficiency may result from an insufficiency of this vitamin or its precursors in the diet or because of some process which interferes with absorption from the intestinal tract, transport, or storage in the liver. Obstruction of the biliary tract or pancreatic ducts in children or adults may lead to diminished absorption of vitamin A. Diarrhea and the various types of malabsorption syndromes are accompanied by vitamin A malnutrition. Of particular importance is the interrelation of vitamin A and protein nutrition, since vitamin A alcohol appears to be transported by plasma albumin. Transport to and mobilization from the liver may be impaired as a result of protein malnutrition.

The intricate reactions whereby vitamin A enters into the visual process may be briefly summarized. Vitamin A aldehyde (retinal or retinene) is found in the retina bound to a protein called *opsin.* Together these form the compound *rhodopsin,* the red pigment of the retinal rods. Under the influence of light, *rhodopsin* breaks down into its two components, thereby initiating a nerve impulse. The mechanism of this reaction was worked out by the Nobel Prize-winning studies of George Wald and his associates.

How vitamin A maintains the integrity of epithelial structures remains a mystery. Vitamin A appears to be implicated in the metabolism of intracellular structures, the lysosomes, in mucopolysaccharide metabolism, and in steroid hormone formation. While the integrity of specialized epithelial structures does require vitamin A, it has not been shown that high intakes of vitamin A will prevent infections. The old remark that carrots are good for vision applies only to persons with vitamin A deficiency and nyctalopia.

DIAGNOSIS. McLaren observed that the eye changes and biochemical findings in vitamin A deficiency often are poorly correlated. The diagnosis and treatment must not wait for all the confirmatory information. A dietary history suggesting a low carotene intake, and especially if the diet is also low in fat and thus one which causes poor absorption of carotene, should be suggestive. Protein deficiency appears to aggravate vitamin A deficiency by impairing transport of the vitamin in vivo. Sprue and diarrheal states will also predispose to vitamin A deficiency.

Measurements of plasma carotene may be misleading because of the presence of other carotenes which are poor provitamins. Vitamin A levels below 20 μg per 100 ml signalize the need for immediate therapy. Distinctive eye changes demand therapy even without laboratory confirmation.

THERAPY. Oral administration of 500,000 IU vitamin A daily as the palmitate or acetate for 3 or more days is recommended. In addition, it may be well to administer similar-sized doses intramuscularly. The diets of children with vitamin A deficiency are usually also lacking in other nutrients and hence should be improved, particularly with respect to protein.

PROGNOSIS. The outcome as far as sight is concerned

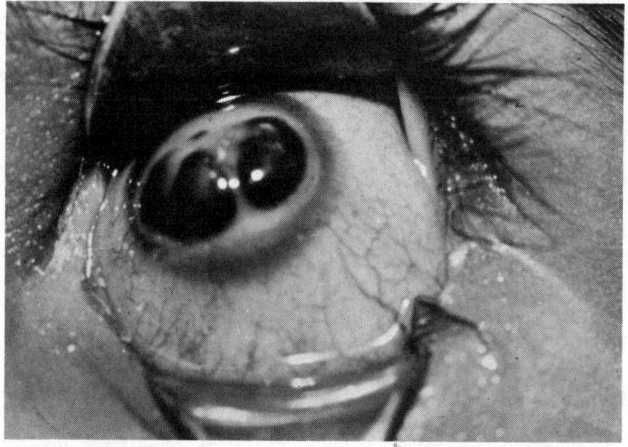

Fig. 84-2. The destruction of the eye by colliquative necrosis of the cornea. The lens is about to drop out. (*Photograph courtesy of Professor D. S. McLaren*)

will depend on the degree of involvement of the ocular structures before therapy is instituted. If only clouding of the cornea has occurred, prognosis is excellent. However, if perforation and infection of the anterior chamber have taken place, restoration of sight is virtually unknown.

Hypervitaminosis A

The ingestion of large amounts of vitamin A, in doses ranging from 75,000 to 500,000 IU daily to infants or adults, results in a variety of signs and symptoms that sometimes may be extremely confusing, particularly if a history of ingestion has not been elicited. Ignorance is usually the reason for taking excessive amounts of vitamin A.

In infants, the effects of acute toxicity are drowsiness, vomiting, and bulging of the fontanels as a result of increased intracranial pressure. More chronic evidences of toxicity include failure to gain weight, alopecia, coarseness of hair texture, hepatomegaly, and evidences of bone pain. X-ray examination of the skeleton reveals characteristic areas of periosteal new bone formation, particularly prominent in the shafts of the long bones.

In adults, headache, blurred vision or diplopia, nausea, and vomiting all may be present. Bone pain and osseous changes similar to those occurring in children may be observed. In addition, calcification of ligaments and tendons may be seen on x-ray examination. Peeling of the skin, neuritis, fissures and sores at the corners of the mouth, coarsening of the skin, alopecia, and localized areas of hyperpigmentation of the epidermis are common. As might be expected, the level of vitamin A in the serum is elevated; values as high as 2,000 μg per 100 ml have been reported. Fortunately, the prognosis is good when vitamin A ingestion halts.

Mention should be made of *carotenemia,* because it may be confused with jaundice. When large amounts of carotene-containing foods are ingested, the blood plasma may contain a high enough concentration of pigment to impart a yellowish color to the skin (especially the palms of the hands and the nasolabial folds) but not the conjunctivas.

REFERENCES

Dowling, J. E. and G. Wald: Vitamin A Deficiency and Night Blindness, Proc. Nat. Acad. Sci., 44:648, 1958.

McLaren, D. S.: "Malnutrition and the Eye," New York, Academic Press, Inc., 1963.

Medical Research Council: Vitamin A Requirements of Human Adults, Special Report Series no. 264, 1949.

Moore, T.: "Vitamin A," New York, Elsevier Publishing Company, 1957.

Oomen, H. A. P. C.: An Outline of Xerophthalmia, Int. Rev. Trop. Med., 1:131, 1961.

85 OTHER DEFICIENCY STATES
George V. Mann

There are a number of nutritional deficiencies other than those discussed already which often appear as complications of other diseases or of therapy. These will be considered in the present chapter.

SODIUM DEPLETION. Although the usual intake of sodium chloride is five to ten times the daily requirement, there are a few disorders in which excessive losses of sodium produce depletion of body stores. The excessive losses in Addison's disease result from failure of the hormone-conditioned retrieval of sodium in the kidney (Chap. 92).

Diarrhea, especially when coupled with fever and salt loss from excessive sweating, may produce salt depletion. This is most often seen in children and may be aggravated by excessive replacement of fluids without adequate attention to serum sodium levels. Thus hyponatremia may reflect either depletion of sodium or excessive dilution of the serum.

Some stages of chronic nephritis are associated with excessive urinary loss of sodium. This may be complicated by low sodium diets and the use of diuretic agents. Diagnosis and management are discussed in Chap. 301.

The normal organism has a remarkable ability to adapt to sodium deprivation so that either low-salt diets, as used in the treatment of hypertension, saluretic agents or heat exposure lead to a hormonal response which conserves sodium. This reaction cannot be efficient in the presence of congenitally absent or diseased sweat glands, as in mucoviscidosis or in renal or adrenal disease. The signs of hyponatremia are weakness, apathy, confusion, nausea, muscle cramps, and azotemia. The diagnosis depends upon the presence of clinical manifestations of dehydration and appropriate biochemical measurements.

POTASSIUM DEPLETION. The potassium of the body is predominantly intracellular so that serum measurements are poor criteria for the level of body stores. Hypokalemia may be associated with nausea, weakness, and confusional states in addition to paralytic ileus and cardiac irregularities, such as flattening of T waves and prolongation of the Q-S intervals in the ECG. A common cause of hypokalemia is the use of diuretic agents which cause the kidney to lose potassium as well as sodium. Potassium losses also can be great from the gastrointestinal tract and during metabolic acidosis, during starvation, or in any wasting disorder. Excessive adrenal steroids induce potassium loss. Potassium deficiency leads to necrosis of muscle fibers and vacuolization of renal epithelium. In familial periodic paralysis the potassium disturbance is associated with a shift of the ion among body compartments rather than loss in the urine.

Potassium is rich in plant foods. The requirement for potassium is influenced by the sodium intake because the sodium/potassium ratio appears to be critical. Repletion of potassium losses involves two possible hazards. Excessive parenteral potassium may cause cardiac irregularities and standstill if the plasma level is raised too rapidly. Oral preparations of potassium, especially enteric coated pills, have been a cause of intestinal ulceration, bleeding, and stenosis. The proper management of potassium deficiency is prevention by ensuring an adequate intake of potassium-rich foods, especially when potassium-wasting drugs are given. Readily available foods such as bananas, orange juice, tomato juice, or meat broth are good sources of potassium for this purpose. Repletion of stores may require parenteral administration but this should be carried out very cautiously in the presence of oliguria or anuria and serum levels should be checked at frequent intervals (see Chaps. 296 and 297).

MAGNESIUM DEPLETION. Magnesium deficiency in man is well known as a complication of alcoholism and of intestinal malabsorption. It occurs occasionally as a complication of diabetes mellitus, of kwashiorkor in children, and of disturbances in parathyroid and adrenal function. Magnesium is predominantly an intracellular cation. The serum contains only 2 mEq per liter, but there is a total of 25 Gm in the body of which about half is in the skeleton (Chap. 76). Like deficiencies of sodium and potassium, magnesium depletion may occur from deficient intake, poor absorption, and increased renal excretion. A syndrome characterized by vertigo, weakness, distension, positive Chvostek sign, and convulsive seizures with or without tetany has been ascribed to a decrease in serum concentration of magnesium (Chap. 21). The deficiency signs respond quickly to magnesium therapy but not to calcium. The typical symptoms of Tetany may even be aggravated by calcium in such cases.

RIBOFLAVIN DEFICIENCY. It is something of a paradox that riboflavin deficiency has not produced more profound or characteristic signs because flavoproteins play a central role in many metabolic processes. In young experimental animals, riboflavin deficiency causes cessation of growth and extensive skin changes. In adult animals fatty changes in the liver and sudden death may occur. Dietary deficiency has been produced in a number of human trials and has been shown to cause only mild angular lesions of the lips (cheilosis) and a scrotal, seborrheic dermatitis. Riboflavin deficiency also has been produced by feeding human subjects the riboflavin antagonist galactoflavin. This procedure caused an anemia, a change not seen in dietary riboflavin deficiency. The level of flavine-adenine-dinucleotides in the plasma in riboflavin deficiency is a good index of deficiency, but this measurement is not widely available. Diagnosis depends upon the dietary history, the suggestive skin signs and a therapeutic trial.

PYRIDOXINE DEFICIENCY. Vitamin B_6 denotes a group of three compounds, pyridoxine, pyridoxal, and pyridoxamine. The first is found in plant foods and the last two are found in animal products. All are unstable to heat and light, but they are so widely distributed that simple dietary deficiency is very unusual in man. In experimental animals a deficiency of vitamin B_6 causes cachexia and scaling of the skin, as well as a profound, microcytic hypochromic anemia. Convulsive seizures may be seen, and sensory neurone degeneration develops. In babies fed diets deficient in vitamin B_6 convulsive seizures occurred. The diagnosis of deficiency can be substantiated by the disappearance from the urine of the metabolite 4-pyridoxic acid or by measuring the amount of xanthurenic acid in the urine before and after administering l-tryptophan. In pyridoxine deficiency, the conversion of this amino acid to nicotinic acid is impaired, and xanthurenic acid excretion is increased.

A number of drugs interfere with vitamin B_6 utilization. Isoniazid and hydralazine form inactive derivatives and increase the pyridoxine requirements. Polyneuritis may appear as a complication of therapy with these agents and can be relieved by supplying large amounts of the coenzyme.

Certain microcytic anemias have been found to be partially responsive to pyridoxine therapy (Chap. 336). Convulsive seizures have been described in infants receiving normal diets which could be relieved by administration of pyridoxine. Such observations have lead to the concept of *pyridoxine dependency* arising from a genetically determined requirement for unusually large amounts of pyridoxine. Such dependency may represent an example of a metabolic "in-born error" caused by a deficiency of the coenzyme pyridoxine, which contrasts with the metabolic error caused by deficiency of the protein apoenzyme in phenylketonuria. The latter can only be managed by dietary reduction of the enzyme substrate phenylalanine in order to minimize accumulation of an injurious metabolite (Chap. 102).

PANTOTHENIC ACID DEFICIENCY. This deficiency is well known in experimental animals and has been produced in mild form in human beings by feeding a pantothenate antagonist. The vitamin is widely available in foods. A natural deficiency has not been described in man, but pantothenic acid deficiency may contribute to multiple deficiency states observed with grossly defective diets or with severe malabsorption. A daily intake of 5 to 10 mg is considered adequate. The American diet supplies an average of 10 to 15 mg daily.

BIOTIN DEFICIENCY. This deficiency occurs only when the diet contains large amounts of a protein called *avidin* which binds biotin and prevents absorption from the intestine. Avidin occurs especially in raw egg white. It is inactivated by heating. An experimental deficiency of biotin in human beings causes a dermatitis, malaise, anxiety, hyperesthesia, and nonspecific ECG changes. The vitamin is widespread in animal food products. Deficiency in man must be very rare.

VITAMIN E DEFICIENCY. There is a widespread misconception that vitamin E facilitates reproductive function. While it is true that a deficiency of alphatocopherol in rats and certain other species has led to resorption of fetuses, it does not follow that vitamin E will augment lagging reproductive activity in man. A number of isomeric tocopherols, which are abundant in vegetable oil, have vitamin E activity. Deficiency of these materials typically causes muscular degeneration and creatinuria in several species. Because storage capacity for the vitamin is large, experimental deficiency develops slowly and requires 400 to 600 days in Rhesus monkeys. In these animals the red blood cells became fragile and an anemia developed. Anemia responding to tocopherol has also been reported in malnourished infants. It appears that the requirement for vitamin E is determined in part by the amount of polyunsaturated fatty acid in the diet. Diets rich in polyunsaturated fat may increase the requirement for alphatocopherol, but the two substances generally occur in the same food sources, so that in practice, these diets should not require supplementation with vitamin E.

FOLIC ACID DEFICIENCY. *Folic acid* or *folacin* refers to a group of substances widely distributed in both vegetable and animal foods. It exists in several forms, either free or conjugated, with one or more molecules of glutamic acid. The vitamin acts with vitamin B_{12} in the transfer of single carbon units which are essential for hematopoiesis and mucosal proliferation. The pathogenesis and clinical manifestations of folic acid deficiency are discussed in Chap. 337. Megaloblastic anemia due to folate deficiency has been more commonly recognized than previously as biochemical techniques for assays of blood folate (Chap. 78) have improved. In the United Kingdom the ratio of anemia caused by folate deficiency to pernicious anemia is about 1:1.25. The deficiency tends to be commoner in the aged, in pregnancy, and in persons with malabsorptive disorders. Lacking biochemical confirmation, the diagnosis is confirmed by a therapeutic trial by following the reticulocyte response after treatment with folate (Chap. 337). Occasionally a response to folic acid will be seen in the anemia of scurvy, and sometimes folate deficiency will respond incompletely to vitamin B_{12} therapy. These must represent multiple deficiency states.

An average United States diet supplies 150 to 200 μg of folic acid daily. While the minimal requirement may be only 50 μg per day, some of the dietary supply is lost in food preparation, and the efficiency of absorption is variable. The recommended dietary allowance (RDA) is 400 μg per day, and this should be doubled in pregnancy.

The sale of vitamin preparations containing more than

100 μg folic acid in the daily dose is now prohibited by federal regulations which are aimed at preventing inadvertent treatment of pernicious anemia while the neurologic manifestations progress. This amount of folate will supply the daily requirement for a normal adult.

VITAMIN K DEFICIENCY. The family of substances with vitamin K activity occurs in plants (phylloquinones) and in bacteria. They are essential for blood clotting because they are needed for the production of prothrombin and several other clotting factors (Chap. 62). Vitamin K deficiency may occur in the newborn before the intestinal flora and the diet begin to supply the vitamin (Chap. 346). This is prevented by prepartum treatment of the mother with the vitamin, thus assuring the infant a normal clotting mechanism during birth trauma. The natural vitamin derived from plants is called vitamin K_1 (phylloquinone) and that derived from bacteria, K_2 (farnoquinone). A commonly used therapeutic agent is menadione, or vitamin K_3, which is the synthetic compound 2-methyl 1,4 napthoquinine. The dosage given premature infants should be no more than 1 to 2 mg per day or kernicterus may develop. Because vitamin K_1 does not show this toxicity for premature infants, the present regulations prohibit the inclusion of menadione in over-the-counter vitamin supplements available to expectant mothers. Water-miscible forms of vitamin K are available for parenteral use especially to reverse the hypoprothrombinemia and bleeding caused by excessive therapy with anticoagulants.

Because the supply of vitamin K is derived from the intestinal flora as well as the diet, treatment with antimicrobials by depressing intestinal flora may diminish the vitamin supply and lead to hypoprothrombinemia. This is particularly likely to occur when there is concomitant administration of anticoagulants. Vitamin K deficiency rarely occurs from simple lack in the diet. No recommended dietary allowance has been established.

REFERENCES

Folic Acid and Pregnancy, Nutr. Rev., 25:325, 1967; 26:5, 1968.

Fomon, S. J., et al.: Vitamin K Compounds and the Water Soluble Analogues, Pediatrics, 28:501, 1961.

Horwitt, M. K.: Nutritional Requirements of Man with Special Reference to Riboflavin, Am. J. Clin. Nutr., 18:458, 1966.

Mason, K. E., et al.: Symposium—Hematological Aspects of Vitamin E, Am. J. Clin. Nutr., 21:1, 1968.

Raskin, N. H., and R. A. Fishman: Pyridoxine Deficiency Due to Hydralazine, New Engl. J. Med., 273:1182, 1965.

Wacker, W. E. C.: Magnesium Metabolism, J. Am. Diet. Ass., 44:362, 1964.

Section 3

Hormonal Disorders

86 GENERAL CONSIDERATIONS AND MAJOR SYNDROMES

George W. Thorn

INTRODUCTION

Isolation, purification, identification, and synthesis of new hormones continue at a rapid rate, and it is reasonable to assume that within the near future those few remaining unidentified principles will also succumb to the technical advances of chemistry and biophysics. Noteworthy among recorded achievements are the determination of the structure and amino acid sequence of adrenocorticotropin, melanocyte-stimulating hormone, and insulin; the synthesis of posterior pituitary hormone and a host of adrenal and gonadal steroid hormones; and the isolation of several new thyroid substances as well as the isolation, identification, and synthesis of glucagon and calcitonin.

Coupled with these chemical advances is a rapidly expanding body of knowledge concerning the regulation of hormonal secretion and the precise locus of hormonal action. Although this latter field has barely been opened, the effect of insulin on permeability to certain sugars, the mechanism whereby estrogens provide energy for the growth of their target organs, and the physical modification of mitochondrial particles by thyroxin illustrate the type of information rapidly becoming available.

It is now generally agreed that hormones do not initiate new events in the complicated biochemistry of metabolic processes, but rather produce their effects by regulating enzymatic and other chemical reactions already present. In view of the relatively large number of hormones, their diverse chemical structures, and their multiple sites of action, it can be assumed that scarcely a single important metabolic event can escape the effect of their primary or secondary action. From this one may conclude that a true understanding of any disease process or physiologic disorder must encompass an appreciation of the possible etiologic role of hormones and the factors regulating their synthesis, release, and degradation. In this regard, one can point to such widely diverse actions as the effect of catechol amines (adrenal medulla) on brain metabolism and psychologic behavior; the effect of adrenal steroids on the inflammatory reaction associated with infection, trauma, surgery, or burns; the effect of insulin on adipose tissue metabolism; and the importance of growth hormone on the fabrication of body proteins.

MECHANISMS OF ENDOCRINOPATHIES

Characteristically, endocrine abnormalities arise as a consequence of increased or decreased hormone secretion. In the majority of patients, the clinical manifestations derive from an excess of or deficiency of the *normally* secreted hormone. However, in certain syndromes, such as some cases of adrenal virilism, the endocrinopathy may result from secretion of an abnormal hormone. In addition, hormonal disorders may result from aberrations in the metabolism or degradation of hormones. For example, a deficiency of plasma proteins may decrease the quantity of hormone-carrying protein in the blood and hence modify significantly the balance between "free" and "bound" thyroid hormone; liver disease may alter the conjugation or degradation of steroid hormones, giving rise to abnormal blood and tissue hormone levels. In such types of abnormalities, however, serious endocrine disorders will result only if the "servo-regulating" mechanism, or feedback response, fails to stimulate the appropriate reaction in the trophic gland. Endocrine abnormalities may also develop when local tissues are unable to respond to a normal hormonal level. For example, localized myxedema over the tibia may occur in the presence of thyrotoxicosis or euthyroidism; in cases of pseudohypoparathyroidism, the abnormalities observed in hypoparathyroidism occur despite the presence of normal parathyroid glands. In some endocrinopathies, heightened tissue susceptibility to hormone action is the determining factor in the genesis of the syndrome, for example, hirsutism in young women with a minimal abnormality in androgenic steroid secretion, or extreme degrees of hyperpigmentation observed in patients with early adrenal insufficiency and increased melanin pigmentation on a racial basis.

Hormonal secretions in general show wide fluctuations throughout the 24-hr period, periods of high activity often alternating with those of reduced secretion; for example, in the early morning the level of adrenal cortical secretory activity is high. Evidence is accumulating that endocrinopathy may result from a loss of cyclic diurnal pattern due to a more or less constant hormonal elaboration throughout the day and night, resulting in only a slight increase, if any, in total secretion. Two important considerations have been derived from these observations: (1) Interpretation of single determinations of hormone content—of blood, tissues, or urine—reflecting instantaneous or relatively short collection periods may be unreliable; for final evaluation, repeated determinations, longer collection periods, or isotopic "turnover" studies may be required. (2) Clinical application of the cyclic method of hormone administration has been quite successful in minimizing undesirable hormone side effects

while maintaining control of the underlying disease process.

DIAGNOSTIC APPROACH TO ENDOCRINE ABNORMALITIES

The suspicion that an endocrine abnormality may play a role in a patient's illness will often derive initially from the gross physical appearance of the patient, as in myxedema, hyperthyroidism, pituitary dwarfism or gigantism, acromegaly, hypogonadism, carotenemia (diabetes mellitus or hypothyroidism), Addison's disease, Cushing's syndrome, and the adrenogenital syndrome. Although a careful history and physical examination will in most instances provide presumptive evidence of an underlying endocrine disorder, the definitive diagnosis will almost invariably depend upon the values obtained from laboratory examinations. Here, accuracy in diagnosis depends upon the specificity of the laboratory test, its precision and its reproducibility, the care and understanding with which specimens are collected, and the reliability of the laboratory that carries out the procedures. In the past, endocrine abnormalities were established for the most part on the basis of nonspecific laboratory examinations such as the basal metabolic rate; roentgenograms; glucose tolerance test; and blood sugar, calcium, sodium, and potassium determinations. Today, tests of endocrine dysfunction are employing more and more frequently measurement of the specific hormones under consideration, for example, protein-bound iodine level, blood and urinary steroid values, urinary gonadotropins, and blood ACTH or insulin levels. It is essential for the practicing physician to realize, however, that a single determination of a specific hormone (in blood, urine, or tissue) does not necessarily establish or exclude an endocrine abnormality. The addition of hormonal "turnover" or "secretory" measurements by means of isotopic techniques represents a great step forward. The use of stressful situations or specific substances such as ACTH (adrenocorticotropin) for the adrenal, thyroid-stimulating hormone (TSH) for the thyroid, and glucose for the detection of early diabetes permits one to test the functional reserve of these endocrine systems and thereby facilitates the diagnosis of potential endocrine deficiency at a time when prophylactic measures may prove effective. In the succeeding chapters, particular attention will be devoted to indicating the usefulness and limitations of diagnostic methods and the degree of specificity attached to the procedure. Because of its great practical importance, the source of common errors related to these determinations will also be emphasized.

ENDOCRINE SYNDROMES

Although secretions of the endocrine glands govern widespread metabolic activities throughout the body, from the viewpoint of the internist, major endocrine disorders present over and over again as a limited number of syndromes. These will be reviewed briefly in relation to the cardinal manifestations of disease.

WEAKNESS AND INCREASED FATIGABILITY (see also Chap. 19). These are without doubt the most frequent presenting symptoms of adult patients seeking assistance from the internist or general practitioner. Although in the majority of instances these complaints derive primarily from emotional or psychologic disturbances, underlying organic disease must always be considered. When endocrine abnormalities are suspected, one should inquire first whether the symptoms have been accompanied by *weight loss*—if so, adrenal cortical insufficiency, hyperthyroidism, and diabetes mellitus should be considered. Adrenal cortical insufficiency, if present, should be accompanied by some increase in pigmentation, hypotension, gastrointestinal disturbances, and perhaps salt craving. Hyperthyroidism would be suggested by goiter, eye changes, tremor, intolerance for heat, etc., and diabetes mellitus by polyuria and polydipsia.

Without weight loss, but with symptoms of weakness and fatigability, one would consider hypothyroidism, hypopituitarism, hyperparathyroidism, and hyperaldosteronism. The first of these is characteristically associated with delayed reflexes, intolerance to cold, dry skin, and carotenemia. Hypopituitarism is suggested by oligomenorrhea or amenorrhea in the female, impotence in the male, decreased tolerance to cold, hypoglycemic episodes, and hypotension. Hyperparathyroidism is suggested by the association of bone pain, renal calculi, and polyuria. Hyperaldosteronism might be accompanied by significant hypertension, demonstrable muscular weakness, polyuria, and electrocardiographic changes that suggest potassium depletion.

MENSTRUAL IRREGULARITIES (see also Chap 98). In addition to pregnancy and local disease of the uterus, menstrual irregularities are associated with four major endocrine disturbances: (1) *primary ovarian failure*, prior to natural menopause and characterized by hot flashes, gain in weight, increased emotional instability, and elevated urinary values of follicle-stimulating hormone; (2) *secondary ovarian failure*, associated with reduced or absent urinary gonadotropins and evidence of other target gland deficiencies, i.e., thyroid and adrenal; (3) *hypothyroidism*, in which menorrhagia as well as oligomenorrhea frequently occur; (4) *adrenogenital syndrome*, in which oligomenorrhea or amenorrhea is seen in combination with increased muscular development, hirsutism, and other signs of masculinization.

HIRSUTISM (see also Chap 57). Increased body hair in females and decreased scalp hair in both sexes is a frequent disorder for which patients seek medical attention. Unfortunately, to date, most female patients with increased hair do not have a demonstrable excess of adrenal or ovarian androgens. Increased androgenic secretion should be considered when *hirsutism* is associated with menstrual irregularities and amenorrhea, or with other evidence of virilism, i.e., increased muscular development and increased size of clitoris.

Although loss of scalp hair and baldness is almost never due to a specific endocrinopathy, a receding hair line in female patients associated with *increased* body hair should always suggest excessive androgenic hormone secretion of adrenal or gonadal origin. Thinning of the hair is frequent in patients with Cushing's syndrome, hypothyroidism, or hypopituitarism. It is rare, however, to observe disturbances in hair growth as a manifestation of serious endocrine abnormality in the absence of rather well-defined signs and symptoms of adrenal, pituitary, or gonadal dysfunction.

IMPOTENCE AND DECREASED LIBIDO (see also Chap. 53). Although these cardinal manifestations of functional disorder are a frequent basis for medical consultation, they are rarely due primarily to endocrinopathies. In addition to primary disease of the generative organs, however, *anterior pituitary deficiency*, especially associated with chromophobe adenomas, should be considered. Evidence of local tumor (changes in vision, headache, etc.) and associated target gland deficiencies (adrenal, thyroid, and gonadal) should be sought. Patients with diabetes mellitus will often exhibit both impotence and decreased libido, but in most instances this occurs after the disease has been present for some time.

OBESITY (see also Chap. 48). Obesity suggests the possibility of an underlying endocrine disturbance, which in practice rarely is causative. However, two serious disorders must be considered in patients with marked, generalized obesity. The first is diabetes mellitus, and this should be investigated with a postprandial glucose determination and a glucose tolerance test, if fasting blood glucose levels are within the normal range and if sugar is not present in the urine. The second serious disorder is insulinoma. Hunger, increased appetite, and weight gain are characteristic of patients with insulinoma as well as those with "reactive" hypoglycemia. The former experience greatest hunger and symptomatology after prolonged fast, the latter shortly after eating, particularly a meal of high carbohydrate content. In both instances appetite and food intake are stimulated by absolute or relative hypoglycemia, and the vicious cycle is continued.

Hypothyroidism and mild hypopituitarism may be associated with moderate obesity. The final diagnosis of the former will require laboratory tests of thyroid function; the latter requires tests for the adequacy of target gland function.

Gross obesity in Cushing's syndrome is rare—what is more common is loss of adipose tissue in the extremities with an increase in abdominal fat pad, straie, and "buffalo hump."

There is no doubt that castration or ovarian failure predispose to obesity. This is not only well-established in man but of practical significance to poultry and cattle raisers. However, in young women there often occurs a reversal of this cycle; namely, rapid weight gain secondary to excess food intake, stress, and anxieties, which may be *followed* by oligomenorrhea or amenorrhea. Whether the weight gain itself is of primary importance in the genesis of the ovarian dysfunction, or whether weight gain and altered gonadal function are both secondary to changes in the hypothalamic centers is not known. However, it is well established that with improvement in emotional status and with weight loss, normal ovulation and menstruation will often ensue. In contrast, primary ovarian failure from organic disease is usually attended by hot flushes and other evidence of vasomotor instability as well as by elevated urinary gonadotropin levels.

HYPERTENSION (see also Chaps. 92, 93, and 276). Hypertension is another frequent disorder encountered in medical practice that should suggest an underlying endocrine abnormality. The hypertensive patient with minimal abnormalities in urinary constituents but with polyuria and nocturia suggests hypokalemia (hyper-aldosteronism) or hypercalcemia (hyperparathyroidism). Clinically the hypokalemic patient with *hyperaldosteronism* rarely presents with the malignant form of hypertension and characteristically exhibits neuromuscular weakness. The electrocardiogram will often reveal changes consistent with potassium depletion, whereas serum sodium concentration is usually *elevated*. The problem is to exclude hypokalemia induced by diuretic administration, especially the thiazides, and the ensuing secondary hyperaldosteronism.

The patient with hypertension, polyuria, and hypercalcemia associated with *hyperparathyroidism* will frequently give a history of urinary calculi or bone pain. He may also present the stigmas of psychoneurosis as a consequence of sustained hypercalcemia. Band keratopathy is rare except with long-continued elevated serum calcium level. A palpable tumor in the neck, unfortunately, is usually a thyroid nodule.

Two characteristic findings in patients with hypertension secondary to *pheochromocytoma* are the cyclic nature of hypertension in the classic syndrome and the absence of obesity. Unfortunately, most tumors secrete predominantly norepinephrine; hence, the textbook picture of tachycardia, nervousness, sweating, and glucosuria is infrequent. Catechol amine excretion may be within normal values between episodes.

Hypertension and moderate obesity, particularly of the truncal type, suggest the possibility of underlying *Cushing's syndrome*. This possibility is greatly increased if diabetes mellitus, easy bruisability, and pink abdominal striae are present. Every hypersensitive patient with diabetes mellitus should be screened for adrenal overactivity. The simplest test is a direct eosinophil count. With a count of more than 100 per cu mm, Cushing's syndrome can be reasonably excluded; with a value under 50, definitive tests should be carried out.

Hypertension as an early manifestation of diabetes mellitus is uncommon. However, since hypertensive-vascular disease is such a frequent complication of diabetes mellitus, hypertensive patients—especially those who are obese—should have postprandial blood glucose determinations evaluated and glucose tolerance tested.

Hypertension as a manifestation of *adrenogenital syndrome* should be considered in young subjects with associated evidence of virilism.

ABNORMALITIES IN GROWTH (see also Chaps. 87 and 89). Abnormalities in growth, particularly in children, are associated with *hypothyrodism* and *cretinism*. The latter must be detected within the first few weeks after birth if serious damage to the central nervous system is to be prevented. All babies with *persistent* umbilical hernia should be screened for possible *hypothyroidism*. Untreated diabetes mellitus will result in retarded growth as will excess cortisol and androgen secretion. Long-standing renal disease will impair skeletal growth and mimic an endocrinopathy because of the frequent co-existence of secondary hyperparathyroidism.

Closely related to abnormalities in growth among adolescent boys is the problem of undescended testes. A conservative approach is urged, and the reader is referred to Chap. 97 for details as to the management of this important problem.

Other cardinal signs that should call attention to possible endocrine abnormalities include the following:

1. Changes in the skin (see also Chaps. 58–60). Dryness in hypothyroidism and Addison's disease; thin, atrophic skin with "wrinkles" in pituitary and gonadal failure; easy bruisability in Cushing's syndrome; moist, fine, warm skin in hyperthyroidism; coarse, reduplicated skin in acromegaly; hyperpigmentation in Addison's disease.

2. Arthropathies are not infrequent in acromegaly, gigantism, myxedema, and primary gonadal failure.

3. Tetany and convulsive seizures (see Chap. 28) may indicate hypoglycemia (insulinoma, reactive hypoglycemia, Addison's disease, hypopituitarism), hypocalcemia (hypoparathyroidism), or hypokalemia (hyperaldosteronism, Cushing's syndrome).

4. The presence of edema (see Chap. 34) should suggest hypothyroidism or myxedema as well as secondary hyperaldosteronism and Cushing's syndrome.

5. Psychologic abnormalities (see Chap. 18) are frequently observed in Addison's disease and Cushing's syndrome as well as in hypopituitarism, hypothyroidism, hyperthyroidism, hyperparathyroidism, and acromegaly.

IATROGENIC ENDOCRINOPATHIES

With the general use of the corticosteroids, thyroid, and the sex hormones as nonspecific therapeutic agents, new and difficult problems present themselves to the internist and endocrinologist. One may be faced on the one hand with iatrogenic Cushing's syndrome, hyperthyroidism, or virilism—or severe adrenal insufficiency or hypothyroidism if hormone therapy is discontinued rapidly or completely. Special problems relating to these phenomena will, because of their seriousness, be discussed at length in relation to each of the specific hormones so implicated. The use of hormones as nonspecific therapeutic agents, while offering great promise in many serious and often fatal diseases, is fraught with difficulties and requires, in addition to a thorough knowledge of the endocrine preparations a comprehension of their physiologic and pharmacologic effects, the exercise of sound judgment on the part of the physician, and complete cooperation on the part of the patient. Without these the end result accompanying endocrine pharmacotherapeutics may be more disabling than the untreated cause of the primary disease.

87 DISEASES OF THE ANTERIOR LOBE OF THE PITUITARY GLAND

Don H. Nelson and George W. Thorn

The pituitary gland lies at the base of the brain in a bony cavity, the sella turcica, within the sphenoid bone. The normal gland measures $10 \times 13 \times 6$ mm and weighs approximately 0.6 Gm. Anatomically it is divided into the anterior lobe, which constitutes three-quarters of the weight of the gland, a rudimentary intermediate lobe, and a posterior or neural lobe. The classic histology of the anterior lobe divides the cells into three types, depending on the presence and staining characteristics of the intracellular granules. These are the chromophobes, which are agranular, the eosinophils and the basophils, in the proportions of approximately 52, 37, and 11 percent, respectively. More detailed studies suggest that some of the agranular cells may contain fine acidophilic and basophilic granules; hence the term "amphophils."

The anterior lobe secretes a variety of peptide hormones, of which six are clearly defined. Growth hormone (HGH) has a generalized somatic effect on growth; adrenocorticotropin (ACTH) stimulates the secretory activity of the adrenal cortex; thyroid-stimulating hormone (thyrotropin, TSH) stimulates the formation and release of thyroid hormones; follicle-stimulating hormone (FSH) stimulates growth of the graafian follicle and estrogen secretion in the female and spermatogenesis in the male; luteinizing hormone (LH) initiates ovulation and luteinization of the mature follicle in the female; in the male, this hormone is the testicular interstitial cell-stimulating hormone (ICSH), responsible for male hormone secretion. Prolactin or lactogenic hormone (LtH) is responsible for secretion of milk by the properly developed mammary gland. Although production of the melanocyte-stimulating hormone (MSH) is classically ascribed to the intermediate lobe, this hormone may also be a secretion of the anterior lobe.

According to classic concepts, the chromophobe cells are considered to be nonsecretory, the eosinophilic cells responsible for secretion of GH, LH, and LtH, and the basophilic cells producing ACTH, TSH, and FSH. Such a simple classification, however, does not now seem probable; some pituitary tumors associated with Cushing's syndrome have been found to be composed of chromophobe as well as eosinophilic cells, although the largest number are small basophilic tumors. Similarly, eosinophilic tumors are most often associated with increased growth hormone production, but tumors of other cell types may occasionally be responsible.

PITUITARY TUMORS

Pituitary tumors account for approximately 10 percent of all intracranial tumors. By far the commonest pituitary tumor is the *Chromophobe adenoma,* which is usually nonsecretory in nature. Active pituitary tumors usually secrete only one pituitary hormone in excess.

Tumors secreting GH, ACTH, MSH, TSH, and LtH have all been described, although the last three types of tumor are very rare. FSH- or LH-secreting tumors are notable by their absence.

In addition to producing the *signs and symptoms* of hormone excess, discussed in later sections on the specific hormones, these tumors may compress and destroy normal pituitary tissue within the sella turcica and produce hormonal deficiency states, or they may extend out of the sella turcica to compress the optic nerves, hypothalamus, and other nervous structures in the vicinity. Pressure on the optic chiasma most often involves the decussating nerve fibers supplying the nasal retinal fields and leads to loss of the temporal fields of vision and classical bitemporal hemianopsia. Further extension of the tumor may involve one or both optic nerves and result in loss of visual acuity and even in complete blindness. These tumors may also compress the hypothalamus and result in disturbances in sleep, temperature control, appetite, and autonomic nervous functions. Curiously, these tumors are not known to damage the supraopticohypophyseal tract to a degree to cause diabetes insipidus. Involvement of the third, fourth, and sixth cranial nerves is rare but may occur. Headache is a frequent complaint in patients with this condition and has no well-defined pattern.

Clinical evaluation of these patients should include roentgenograms of the skull and visual fields, ophthalmoscopic examination, spinal fluid examination (particularly for increased protein content), and pneumoencephalography, especially in patients with severe optic nerve compression, increased intracranial pressure, or signs of hypothalamic and brain involvement. Carotid angiography may also be useful in delineating any extension of a tumor out of the sella.

Therapy of pituitary tumors generally involves a choice between pituitary irradiation or surgery. Postponement of specific treatment is justifiable in occasional patients with small, localized chromophobe adenomas, in which case specific hormonal replacement therapy should be initiated and the patient carefully observed for signs of tumor growth and extension. Surgical resection of tumor tissue is indicated when there is rapid deterioration of vision, ventricular obstruction, or significant brain compression. Although surgery provides the greatest opportunity for arrest of tumor growth, there is a calculated morbidity and mortality, particularly with the large tumors extending outside the sella turcica.

Radiotherapy in tissue doses of 3,500 to 4,500 r is often associated with regression of the tumor and relief of local signs and symptoms. In these doses, normal pituitary tissue and surrounding nervous structures are unharmed. Some tumors recur and may require further x-ray therapy, or surgery. Further experience with such experimental techniques as cryohypophysectomy, high-voltage and proton-beam irradiation, and radioactive implantations offers hope for better methods of treating these tumors.

Hemorrhage into a tumor, so-called "pituitary apoplexy," may result in an acute catastrophe accompanied by severe headache, blindness, hypotension or shock, fever, and signs of meningeal irritation or brain involvement. Emergency treatment is required, which may include surgical aspiration of the sella turcica, use of adrenal-steroids, and other supportive measures. Pituitary apoplexy may occur spontaneously and is occasionally observed following irradiation.

The craniopharyngioma, which is usually suprasellar in position, is the most common type of tumor involving the pituitary gland in childhood and thus the most common cause of prepuberal hypopituitarism. The tumor represents a secretory vestige of Rathke's pouch cut off from its origin in the roof of the pharynx and carried cephalad by the migrating pituitary anlage. The viscous, cholesterol-containing fluid of such suprasellar cysts is prone to calcification, which provides a useful diagnostic sign on x-ray examination. Although these tumors are more frequent in the younger age group, occasionally they are slow-growing and may not be clinically apparent until adult life. These patients often mature normally and come to the physician with an adult form of hypopituitarism. These tumors usually require surgical intervention. *Other tumors* which may involve the pituitary or the suprasellar area include meningiomas, epidermoid or dermoid tumors, primary or metastatic carcinomas, and granulomatous disorders such as sarcoidosis, gummas, tuberculomas, and Hand-Schüller-Christian disease.

GROWTH HORMONE

Growth hormone, unlike the other anterior pituitary hormones, does not have a specific "target organ" but has a generalized effect on all tissues and organs. This hormone has a molecular weight of 22,000, although there is some indication that an "active core" may be considerably smaller. Though once thought to be solely concerned with growth in the early years of life, growth hormone has been found to exert significant physiologic functions throughout life. It has been shown to facilitate amino acid transport and incorporation into protein, to mobilize free fatty acids from peripheral fat stores, and to reduce lipid synthesis. Growth hormone also causes renal retention and body storage of calcium, phosphorus, sodium, potassium, and nitrogen as part of its generalized anabolic action. It has an anti-insulin or diabetogenic action and, in large doses, can produce glucosuria, impaired glucose tolerance, and insulin resistance. Growth hormone is responsible for the elevated level of serum inorganic phosphorus and alkaline phosphatase observed in growing children.

Growth hormone is species-specific, and only primate growth hormone has been found to have significant physiologic effects in man and to be capable of stimulating growth in pituitary dwarfs.

Concentration of plasma growth hormone can now be determined with immunologic techniques, and elevated levels have been found in most patients with acromegaly. Significantly, growth hormone levels have been shown to increase following exercise, prolonged fast, and during hypoglycemia, which suggests a dynamic physiologic role for this hormone throughout life, in addition to its growth-promoting effects in childhood.

Other substances which may produce an increase in plasma growth hormone are arginine, vasopressin, pyrogens, and estrogens. The latter, due to their widespread use in contraceptive preparations, may give falsely high growth hormone values in patients suspected of having acromegaly.

Growth Hormone Secreting Tumors

Marie, in 1886, first described the classical clinical manifestations of acromegaly. One year later, Minkowski reported a case with a pituitary tumor, and Benda subsequently showed that such tumors were eosinophilic in nature. In 1895, Brissaud and Meige suggested an association between gigantism and acromegaly, and Hutchinson subsequently reported the pathologic findings in three cases of gigantism associated with pituitary tumors. Acromegaly and gigantism are now recognized as identical disturbances of growth hormone secretion, differing only in the age of onset of the disorder.

GIGANTISM

Prior to puberty, excess growth hormone secretion results in a generalized overgrowth of the skeleton and soft tissues. Early in the course of the disorder, these patients are usually physically strong and alert. Later in the disease, however, pituitary insufficiency may develop, with its associated weakness and easy fatigability. Hypogonadism of the pituitary type develops during the course of the disease.

The underlying lesion is generally an *eosinophilic or mixed cell adenoma of the anterior lobe* which is usually visible radiologically. The condition, although rare, presents no difficulty in diagnosis and needs only to be differentiated clinically from the tall stature of primary gonadal failure. Persons with the latter condition exhibit the characteristic eunuchoid habitus and associated gonadal failure and, unlike the patient with gigantism, have increased titers of urinary follicle stimulating hormone characteristic of primary hypogonadism. Treatment of pituitary gigantism is similar to that for acromegaly.

ACROMEGALY

In adults, the same type of pituitary tumor producing excess growth hormone results in the clinical picture of acromegaly. The disease is usually first manifested by changes in facial features and overgrowth of the head, hands, and feet which may necessitate an increase in hat, glove, or shoe size (Fig. 87-1). In other instances, headache or visual disturbances from local effects of the expanding pituitary tumor may be the first indications of the disorder.

The fully developed syndrome is easily recognized, but in the earlier stages, comparison of serial photographs over a span of years may be extremely helpful in documenting a gradual and progressive change in features.

The hands and feet are broad and greatly enlarged, the ends of the digits are square, and prognathism may be so marked as to interfere with mastication (Fig. 87-2). Arthritic manifestations are not unusual, and widespread osteoarthritic-like changes in the bones and joints are often demonstrable. Patients with acromegaly are particularly subject to psychologic disturbances and almost always exhibit considerable emotional instability.

Among the associated endocrine disturbances, enlargement of the thyroid and an increased basal metabolic rate are frequently found. Hyperthyroidism, however, occurs in only a small percentage of cases. Although frank diabetes mellitus is present in only 10 to 15 percent of these patients, glucose tolerance is impaired in the majority of patients during the active phase of the disease. Diabetes mellitus, when present, is typically mild but may be relatively resistant to insulin therapy. Libido may be increased at the onset but is lost subsequently, and gonadal atrophy may occur late in the disease. The course of the disease is usually one of benign chronicity, but fatal termination may occur as a result of cardiac failure, diabetic acidosis, local complications of the tumor, or unrecognized hypopituitarism.

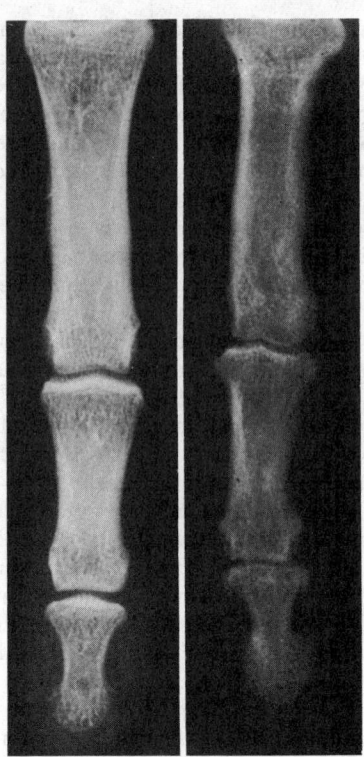

Fig. 87-2. Characteristic tufting or "arrowhead" appearance of the terminal phalanx in acromegaly (right). Normal phalanx for comparison (left). Note also the thickness of the acromegalic finger.

Diagnosis

Diagnosis is made by the typical changes in body configuration, possible demonstration of a pituitary tumor by x-ray or visual field defects, and most importantly, by an elevated basal plasma growth hormone level which does not decrease during a standard glucose tolerance test. Because the skeletal changes are permanent, it is important in the treated as well as the untreated case to determine whether there is continual hypersecretion of growth hormone, or whether a deficiency of growth hormone and perhaps of other hormones has resulted from pituitary destruction from pressure, hemorrhage, or earlier x-ray therapy. Activity of the process is implied by continued skeletal and soft-tissue growth, by the presence of diabetes mellitus or a significantly impaired glucose tolerance test, by elevated levels of serum inorganic phosphorus and alkaline phosphatase, and by increased excretion of hydroxyproline in the urine. The basal plasma growth hormone determination is usually necessary for final determination of activity. Patients with active acromegaly may show a hyperactive increase in urinary 17-ketosteroid excretion following intravenous ACTH while 17-hydroxysteroid excretion is normal.

There is one familial condition without evidence of increased growth hormone, the Touraine-Solenti-Golé syndrome, in which afflicted individuals present acromegalic features. Particularly suggestive of acromegaly

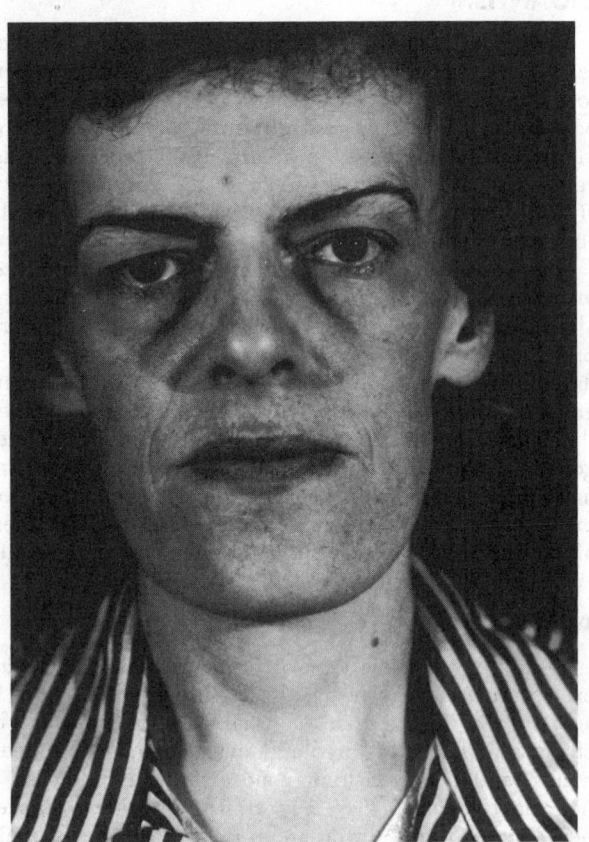

Fig. 87-1. A forty-four-year-old woman with arrested acromegaly. Onset of the disease occurred when patient was twenty-four years of age, when enlargement of the sella turcica was demonstrated. Following x-ray therapy of the pituitary no further progression of the disease has been observed.

in this condition are the skin changes; thus its common designation, pachydermoperiostitis (idiopathic hypertrophic osteoarthropathy). Although the fingers are often clubbed, the periosteal thickening of the bones is not what one would expect to see in acromegaly. The amount of growth hormone is of course not increased.

TREATMENT. Eosinophilic adenomas may respond to irradiation, but in general this form of therapy is not presently considered to be so effective as an ablative procedure of the pituitary gland. The presence of hypopituitarism must be suspected and the appropriate substitution therapy instituted (adrenal, thyroid, and gonadal hormones), particularly if surgery is contemplated. Because of the permanent disfigurement which acromegaly produces, the progress of the disease must be watched closely, particularly in women, and earlier surgical intervention should be considered in an attempt to minimize the cosmetic complications. Although successful therapy will not reverse the bony changes, the decrease in hypertrophy of the skin and subcutaneous tissues may produce an important improvement in appearance.

ADRENOCORTICOTROPIN (ACTH)

This hormone is a polypeptide composed of 39 amino acids with a molecular weight of approximately 4,500. The primary structure has been elucidated, and small quantities have been synthesized (Fig. 87-3).

The principal physiologic effect of this hormone is to stimulate the secretion of hydrocortisone from the adrenal cortex. Under the stimulus of ACTH, the adrenal gland also secretes corticosterone, aldosterone, estrogens, and certain so-called "adrenal androgens." In the case of aldosterone, ACTH is not the chief controlling factor regulating its secretion. As part of its adrenal stimulating

effect, ACTH promotes an increase in adrenal blood flow and hypertrophy of the gland. Certain extra-adrenal actions of ACTH of obscure physiologic significance include a lipid-mobilizing effect and a hypoglycemic action. ACTH has intrinsic melanocyte-stimulating activity because of similarities between its N-terminal amino acid sequence and the structure of MSH (Fig. 87-3).

Secretion of ACTH is regulated by the concentration of hydrocortisone in plasma and by various parts of the brain, particularly the anterior median eminence of the hypothalamus. Nerve cells in this area are thought to produce one or more peptide neurohormones, termed corticotropin-releasing factors (CRF), which are released into the pituitary portal circulation and stimulate the secretion of ACTH by the anterior pituitary cells. Higher centers of the brain may act to stimulate or inhibit ACTH secretion.

Central-nervous-system activity maintains a diurnal rhythm of ACTH secretion, which results in highest levels in early morning and lowest levels at night. There is a considerable increase in plasma ACTH concentration in adrenal insufficiency because of loss of the normal reciprocal relationship between plasma hydrocortisone concentration and ACTH secretion. Substantial increases in ACTH secretion occur during stress irrespective of the plasma steroid level. Prolonged administration of corticosteroids depresses the secretion of ACTH and results in adrenal atrophy indistinguishable from that observed in spontaneous hypopituitarism.

CUSHING'S DISEASE

(Also see Chap. 92.) In 1932, Cushing described the clinical disorder of pituitary basophilism associated with adrenocortical hyperplasia. This concept led to consid-

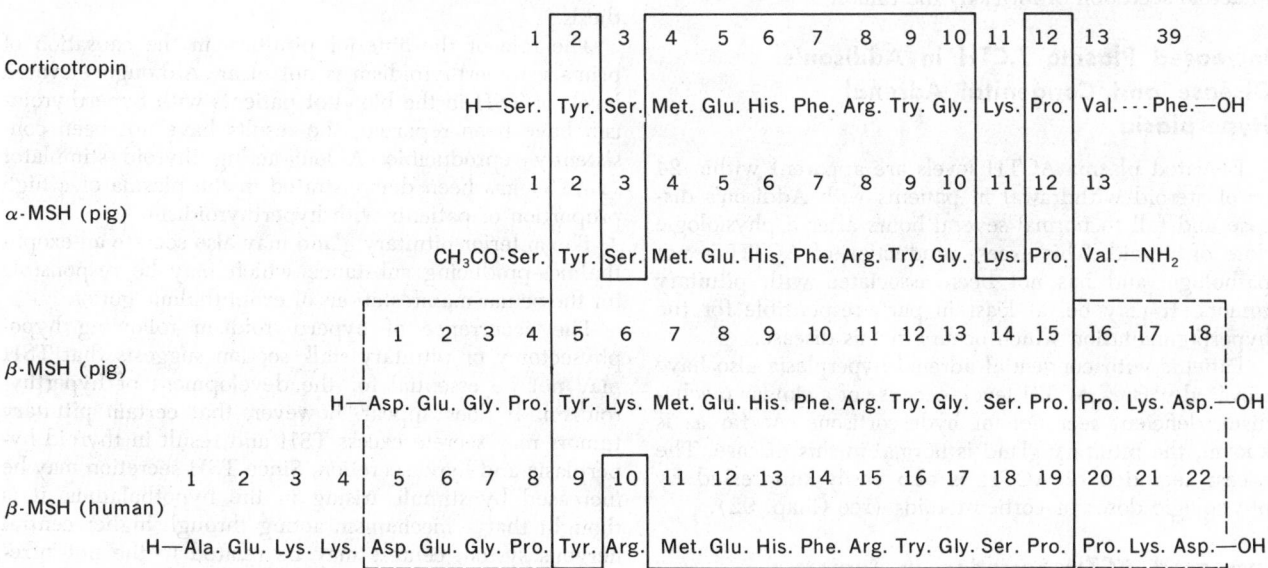

Fig. 87-3. Amino acid sequences of corticotropin and melanocyte-stimulating hormones. (Modified from I. Harris.)

erable controversy and a voluminous literature on the presence and significance of basophilic adenomas in patients with adrenocortical hyperfunction.

Relatively few patients with adrenocortical hyperfunction first come to the physician with definite enlargement of the pituitary gland; however, the incidence of pituitary tumor is significantly increased in those patients subjected to total adrenalectomy. Since bilateral total adrenalectomy has only been widely practiced for little more than a decade, it is possible that more patients will develop clinically evident pituitary tumors in due time. Curiously, most of the postadrenalectomy pituitary tumors have proved to be chromophobe adenomas Eosinophilic and mixed-type tumors have also been found in Cushing's disease, but the largest number are associated with small basophilic tumors or hyalinization of the basophils.

Biologic tests for the measurement of ACTH in plasma, and more recently immunoassay techniques, may be of value in establishing the cause of adrenocortical hyperfunction. The finding of an elevated plasma ACTH level suggests a pituitary origin, but such an elevation may also be found in patients who have nonendocrine carcinomas that also secrete ACTH-like substances. In a series that we have undertaken, an elevated plasma ACTH level was found more often in those patients with a nonendocrine tumor, e.g., in the lung or pancreas, than in patients with Cushing's syndrome and adrenal hyperplasia. In an adrenalectomized patient with Cushing's disease, an abnormal elevation in ACTH, exceeding the level observed in Addison's disease or in patients adrennalectomized for other diseases, is highly suggestive of an ACTH-secreting pituitary tumor. These patients often show intense pigmentation of the skin which may be due to the MSH-like activity of ACTH referred to above or to actual secretion of MSH by the tumor.

Increased Plasma ACTH in Addison's Disease and Congenital Adrenal Hyperplasia

Elevated plasma ACTH levels are apparent within 24 hr of steroid withdrawal in patients with Addison's disease and fall to normal several hours after a physiologic dose of steroid. This excess production of ACTH is not pathologic and has not been associated with pituitary tumors. It may be, at least in part, responsible for the hyperpigmentation which occurs in this disease.

Patients with congenital adrenal hyperplasia also have elevated plasma ACTH level, because of a similar mechanism, deficient secretion of hydrocortisone. As far as is known, the pituitary gland is normal in this disease. The excess secretion of ACTH is also easily suppressed by physiologic doses of corticosteroids (see Chap. 92).

Increased ACTH Secretion in Tumors of Nonendocrine Origin

A number of patients with Cushing's syndrome secondary to the release of ACTH-like substances from non-

endocrine neoplasms has been reported. Carcinoma of the lung is the most frequent type of tumor associated with this syndrome. Of particular interest has been the association of Cushing's syndrome with benign bronchial adenomas as well as malignant tumors. In a few cases the substance produced by the tumor has been shown to be, in all probability, ACTH. It is possible that neoplastic tumors could also secrete an ACTH-releasing factor which would in turn stimulate the secretion or release of ACTH. The latter could be detected biologically by its effectiveness in the presence of an intact pituitary-adrenal system and its ineffectiveness in the absence of the anterior pituitary gland. To date, there is no evidence that these nonendocrine neoplasms secrete adrenal steroids; hence, removal of both adrenals should result in a cure of the Cushing's syndrome in circumstances which prevent the complete removal of the primary neoplasm.

THYROTROPIN (TSH)

(See Chap. 89). Thyrotropin is a glycoprotein of approximately 26,000 molecular weight. It stimulates the uptake of iodide by the thyroid gland and the synthesis and release of thyroid hormones. Continued stimulation results in hypertrophy of the gland and an increase in the vasculature. Thyrotropin deficiency results in glandular atrophy and depressed thyroid function. The administration of thyroid hormone depresses the secretion of thyrotropin and produces similar changes in thyroid function. There is good evidence that the ventral medial nuclei and paraventricular nuclei of the hypothalamus are involved in the control of TSH secretion, and that destruction of these areas depresses thyroid hormone synthesis.

The role of the anterior pituitary in the causation of primary hyperthyroidism is not clear. Although elevated levels of TSH in the blood of patients with hyperthyroidism have been reported, the results have not been consistently reproducible. A long-acting thyroid stimulator (LATS) has been demonstrated in the plasma of a high proportion of patients with hyperthyroidism.

The anterior pituitary gland may also secrete an exophthalmos-producing substance which may be responsible for the ocular manifestations of exophthalmic goiter.

The occurrence of hyperthyroidism following hypophysectomy or pituitary stalk section suggests that TSH may not be essential for the development of hyperthyroidism. It does appear, however, that certain pituitary tumors may secrete excess TSH and result in thyroid hyperplasia and hypersecretion. Since TSH secretion may be increased by stimuli arising in the hypothalamus, it is thought that a mechanism acting through higher central nervous system centers may be related to the not-infrequent development of thyrotoxicosis following major emotional or psychic trauma. It is also probable that increased TSH secretion is involved in the hyperthyroidism associated with acromegaly.

GONADOTROPINS

(See Chap. 98). The gonadotropins, FSH and LH, are large protein hormones of approximately 30,000 molecular weight. These hormones regulate the development, reproductive functions, and hormonal secretions of the ovary and testicle. Prolactin (LtH) is also classed as a gonadotropin; however, its primary action is on the mammary gland and though it may be luteotrophic (i.e., sustaining the function of the corpus luteum) in lower animal species, this action has not been shown to be of physiologic significance in man.

The secretion of gonadotropins is influenced by the rate of sex hormone production and by certain areas of the hypothalamus. Castration increases and estrogens decrease the secretion of FSH, probably by modifying the hypothalamic centers which control FSH secretion by the anterior pituitary. The secretion of LH is also increased by castration but is less sensitive to inhibition by estrogens. Progesterone depresses LH secretion in some species. Testosterone is a poor inhibitor of FSH secretion but does block the secretion of LH.

Secretion of LH has been clearly shown to be regulated by the posterior hypothalamus. This area is also important in prolactin secretion, probably by producing a hormone that inhibits the production and release of LtH by the anterior pituitary. Lesions in this area block LH secretion and result in enhanced secretion of prolactin and pathologic lactation.

Gonadotropins are not found in the urine until puberty. Thereafter, they are present in significant quantities throughout life, with peaks of excretion appearing at the time of ovulation and greatly increased levels occurring after the menopause or following castration. Although relatively crude, the bioassay for urinary gonadotropins (FSH assay) is the most widely used direct assay of a pituitary hormone in general use. The assay is not specific for FSH, since even small quantities of LH appear to be necessary for the biologic action of FSH. Low urinary FSH levels are occasionally found in normal individuals, and several determinations are necessary for accurate clinical evaluation. Increasing availability of radioimmunassay of these and other pituitary hormones makes diagnosis of gonadotropin abnormalities much more reliable.

Chorionic gonadotropin (HCG) is derived from the placenta and appears in the urine in large quantities during pregnancy. Preparations from human pregnancy urine are available for clinical use. This hormone has predominantly an LH action and is used clinically to stimulate Leydig cell function and ovulation (Chap. 98).

Sexual Precocity

No definite pituitary disorders are associated with increased secretion of LH or FSH. There are cases of isosexual precocity, often familial, in which premature but normal sexual development occurs, probably on the basis of early maturation of central nervous system centers regulating gonadotropin formation and release. Lesions of the hypothalamus or pineal gland also may result in premature secretion of gonadotropic hormones and precocious puberty (Chap. 100).

Galactorrhea

Abnormal lactation is sometimes observed in patients with acromegaly or chromophobe adenomas and also may occur after pituitary stalk section. A condition associated with persistent post-partum lactation and amenorrhea is referred to as the Chiari-Frommel syndrome. The galactorrhea in these disorders is most likely the result of excess prolactin secretion. If a pituitary tumor is found, it should be treated. In the absence of evidence of a tumor, galactorrhea may be suppressed by estrogen administration.

PANHYPOPITUITARISM

PREPUBERAL. Prepuberal panhypopituitarism, which was first described in 1871 by Lorrain, is a rare condition usually associated with suprasellar cyst or craniopharyngioma. The disease is characterized by dwarfism and subnormal sexual development but normal mentality. The impairment of growth is symmetric and the body proportions are normal. As in other cases of hypopituitarism, the skin often has a pale yellowish appearance and increased wrinkling. Sexual maturation is delayed, and in rare cases there may be obesity from hypothalamic involvement. Diabetes insipidus is not an infrequent accompaniment.

If the tumor is of sufficient size to affect the optic chiasma, there may be bitemporal hemianopsia or complete blindness. X-ray studies reveal delayed fusion of the epiphyses, supresellar calcification, and, often, destruction of the sella turcica. The condition must be distinguished from genetic dwarfism and from hypothyroidism. Children with a familial type of dwarfism have isolated deficiency of growth hormone secretion but normal production of other pituitary hormones and development of epiphyses consistent with chronologic age. Hypothyroid children have subnormal mentality, infantile body proportions, dwarfism, and the characteristic epiphyseal dysgenesis.

Treatment with cortisone, thyroid, and sex hormones, described in more detail in the next section, should be instituted, with dosage adjusted for body size and age. Although limited by the availability of material, human or monkey growth hormone in doses of 1 to 3 mg weekly has had considerable success in producing growth in these patients. Because of the psychologic and sociologic importance of reaching normal stature, every attempt should be made to obtain such therapy for these patients if the epiphyses have not closed. Growth hormone from nonprimate sources has had no effect on growth in human beings.

POSTPUBERAL PANHYPOPITUITARISM. The common causes for panhypopituitarism in the adult include chromophobe adenoma, post-partum pituitary necrosis, craniopharyngiomas, and the end stages of acromegaly. Less common lesions include gliomas, basilar meningitis, head injuries associated with hemorrhage into the pituitary or the suprasellar region, and granulomatous disorders such as sarcoidosis and Hand-Schüller-Christian disease.

Post-partum pituitary necrosis (Sheehan's syndrome) is due to extensive thrombosis of the pituitary circulation during delivery, usually associated with uterine hemorrhage but occasionally developing after a bout of hypotension without blood loss. Characteristically, these patients fail to lactate in the puerperium and do not have a recurrence of menstrual function. The association of these signs should always suggest this diagnosis. There follows the insidious onset of a host of vague symptoms, including asthenia, lethargy, loss of libido, loss of axillary and pubic hair, and cold intolerance (Fig. 87-4). Some patients appear quite healthy and often are classified as psychoneurotic until the true diagnosis is revealed. Others gradually lapse into a far-advanced state of anterior pituitary insufficiency involving gonadal, thyroid, and adrenal function in approximately that order of development. Physical signs consist of bradycardia, hypotension, loss of axillary, pubic, and scalp hair, premature wrinkling and pallor of the skin, which is fine and atrophic, and a general loss of secondary sex characteristics, with atrophy of the breasts and genitalia.

Irrespective of the cause of panhypopituitarism, the secondary effects on the endocrine glands are similar. There is marked atrophy of the thyroid, adrenals, and gonads. Interference with growth occurs if the lesion appears prior to epiphyseal closure. The pituitary gland has a large reserve, and substantial amounts of pituitary tissue must be damaged before significant hormone deficiency develops. Not all patients develop hypofunction of all three target glands; isolated gonadal failure is relatively common, or gonadal failure may be associated with either thyroid or adrenal insufficiency. Isolated growth hormone deficiency, TSH or ACTH deficiency may also be seen although the latter is quite rare.

LABORATORY FINDINGS. Laboratory findings reflect decreased function of the target endocrine glands. Thus, the serum protein-bound iodine and thyroidal radioiodine uptake are low, and there is a decrease in the basal metabolic rate. The level of serum cholesterol, unlike that in primary myxedema, is rarely elevated, despite lowered thyroid function. Levels of urinary 17-ketosteroids, 17-hydroxycorticosteroids, and 17-ketogenic steroids are depressed, and urinary gonadotropins are subnormal or absent. Blood levels of ACTH and growth hormone are depressed. A normochromic anemia is often present, and there may be leukopenia and relative lymphocytosis in the presence of adrenal insufficiency. Fasting hypoglycemia is rarely found but may occasionally be severe enough to produce coma. The serum sodium concentration is usually normal, but hyponatremia may occur during periods of stress. The serum potassium level and BUN are usually normal, in contrast to increases seen in the patient with Addisonian crisis.

DIAGNOSIS. The diagnosis of hypopituitarism is generally not difficult to establish once it is suspected, but because of the insidious onset and the variable signs and symptoms, the disorder may escape detection for many years. These patients often come to the physician with acute medical emergencies associated with infection or trauma and fail to respond normally to the usual therapeutic measures. In such instances, clinical evidence of gonadal, thyroid, or adrenal insufficiency should be sought; if present, it will quickly suggest the diagnosis.

Patients with pituitary myxedema must be differentiated from those with primary thyroidal failure. Patients with the pituitary form often do not appear to be so myxedematous as those with primary hypothyroidism. An enlarged thyroid gland is indicative of primary hypothyroidism, since the thyroid is atrophic in hypopituitarism. In the absence of clear evidence of a primary thyroid disorder such as might result from radioiodine therapy, thyroidectomy, or thyroiditis, pituitary insufficiency should be ruled out in every patient with hypothyroidism. The response to TSH is helpful in differentiating primary from pituitary hypothyroidism. In contrast to the lack of response to TSH in the patient with primary hypothyroidism, a marked increase in the protein-bound iodine and the radio-iodine uptake will be produced in the patient with the pituitary type of hypothyroidism by the administration of 10 units of TSH intramuscularly daily for 2 days. Some patients with pituitary myxedema may not respond to TSH, probably because of advanced thyroidal atrophy.

The patient with adrenal failure secondary to pituitary disease will usually show an increase in the 24-hr urinary excretion of 17-ketosteroids, 17-hydroxycorticosteroids, and 17-ketogenic steroids with administration of ACTH. These patients often do not respond to a single day's infusion of ACTH, but administration of 40 units intravenously over an 8-hr period on three or four successive days characteristically will reveal a step-wise increase in steroid excretion by the third or fourth day of administration. Hypopituitary patients secrete near-normal quantities of aldosterone and thus are usually in sodium balance. Hyponatremia, when it does occur, however, may be due to sodium depletion as well as to extracellu-

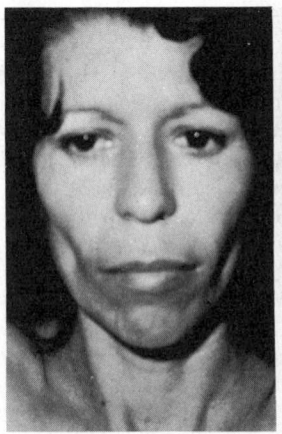
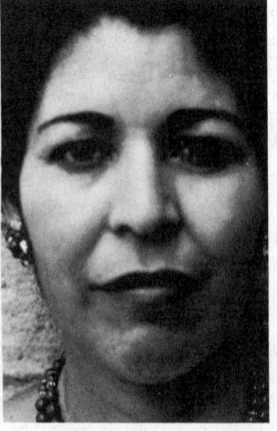

Fig. 87-4. Photographs of a forty-year-old woman when first seen for hypopituitarism (Simmond's disease) and after 6 months' therapy.

lar dilution. The hyponatremia seen secondary to hypopituitarism is easily corrected by the intravenous administration of cortisol in contrast to hyponatremia secondary to the inappropriate secretion of antidiuretic hormone.

Measurement of urinary steroids following the administration of 2-methyl-1,2 bis-(3-pyridyl)-1-propane [SU 4885 (Metopirone)] provides a particularly useful index of the ability of the pituitary gland to increase ACTH secretion. This compound inhibits the 11-hydroxylation of the steroid molecule in the adrenal gland and leads to decreased secretion of 17-hydroxycorticosterone (hydrocortisone) and increased secretion of 17-hydroxy-11-deoxycorticosterone (substance S). The hydrocortisone deficiency results in increased ACTH secretion from the anterior pituitary gland, a marked increase in the adrenal secretion of substance S, and a resultant increase in the urinary excretion of 17-hydroxycorticosteroids and 17-ketogenic steroids. Patients with normal pituitary-adrenal function will show an increase in these urinary steroids with this drug, but patients with either primary or secondary adrenal insufficiency will fail to demonstrate such an increase in urinary 17-hydroxycorticosteroids (Fig. 87-5). This test is of particular value in assessing pituitary ACTH reserve in patients who have normal or only slightly depressed basal urinary steroid levels. It is a hazardous test in patients with obvious deficiency in adrenal steroid secretion and can induce adrenal crisis in patients with primary adrenal insufficiency or those with adrenal atrophy secondary to deficient ACTH production. For this reason the test is best performed on hospitalized patients. If adrenal insufficiency occurs, it can be relieved quickly by IV cortisol.

Hypogonadism secondary to pituitary disease is characterized by decreased or absent urinary gonadotropins, in contrast to the increased titers found in primary gonadal failure. The prolonged amenorrhea observed in many patients with chronic illness and especially in those with anorexia nervosa is often confused with that due to panhypopituitarism. Urinary gonadotropin concentration may be low in these patients, but adrenal and thyroid function is usually normal. Thus, detailed study of each target gland will often be necessary to establish or rule out pituitary insufficiency in patients with obscure hypogonadism, hypothyroidism, or hypoadrenalism.

Other physiologic tests which have been employed in the past in establishing a diagnosis of hypopituitarism, such as the insulin tolerance test and the water test are less specific and may be life-threatening if not carried out under close supervision.

Patients with pituitary-adrenal insufficiency excrete administered water at a depressed rate, similar to the rate of excretion in patients with primary adrenal failure; however, this test may be falsely positive in the presence of renal, hepatic, or cardiac disease. These patients may develop water intoxication during the test and should be carefully observed for this complication and treated with I.V. cortisol if required.

TREATMENT. The use of pituitary hormones would be true replacement therapy for panhypopituitarism. However TSH and ACTH must be given daily by intramus-

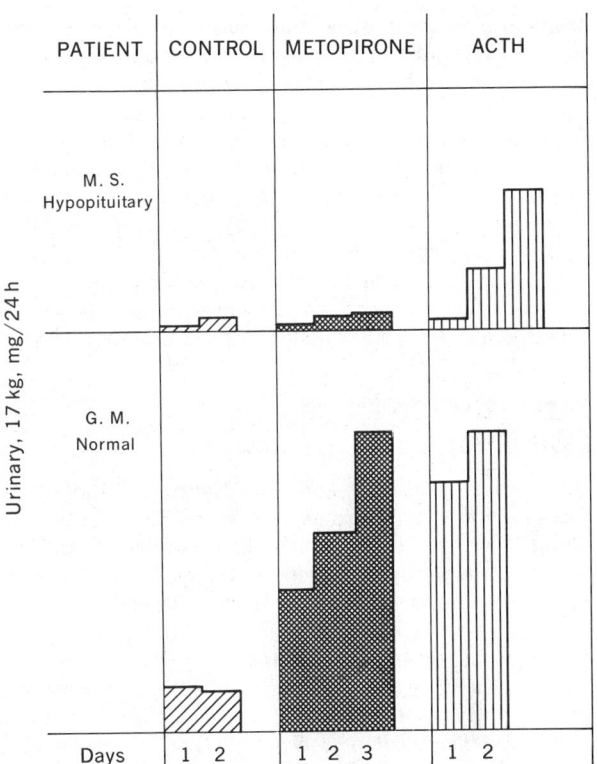

Fig. 87-5. Response of urinary 17-ketogenic steroids in a hypopituitary patient (M.S.) and a normal subject (G.M.) to Metopirone (750 mg every 6 hr for 48 hr) and ACTH (40 units intravenously over 8 hr on two or three successive days). Note the lack of response to Metopirone and delayed response to ACTH in the hypopituitary patient.

cular injection, and pituitary gonadotropins cannot be used successfully for any prolonged period because of the tendency to antibody formation. In practice, excellent results are obtained by oral replacement therapy with the target gland hormones. Thyroxin should be given at first in a dose of 0.05 mg a day, with the amount gradually increased over a period of several weeks to a total daily dose of 0.2 to 0.3 mg. Cortisone acetate should be initiated at a level of 5 to 10 mg per day and increased to 15 to 30 mg as needed. Since the administration of thyroid hormone alone in a patient with associated pituitary-adrenal insufficiency may precipitate a serious adrenal crisis, it is important to initiate cortisone therapy prior to or at least simultaneously with thyroxin therapy in these patients. Salt-retaining hormone therapy is generally not needed, but if required, can be achieved with the oral administration of 0.05 to 0.1 mg fluorohydrocortisone daily.

A long-acting testosterone preparation should be given intramuscularly in doses of 100 to 200 mg every 2 to 4 weeks to male patients; proportionately smaller doses are often beneficial in female patients. In the female patient, estrogens may be given daily by mouth or at intervals of 2 to 4 weeks by injection. If desired, cyclic therapy with estrogens and progesterone may be given to induce artificial menstrual function.

It should be emphasized that hormonal therapy is intended only to provide normal replacement of physiologic levels for proper body function. Although the harmful effects of large-dose corticosteroid administration may not be observed with this schedule, psychic disturbances of various kinds are occasionally noted in patients suddenly exposed to full replacement therapy after a long period of adrenal or thyroid hormone deficiency. Another problem often noted is that of excessive appetite in some patients receiving even small doses of cortisone. In this instance, it may be necessary to institute a restrictive diet or to decrease cortisone dosage to bare minimum levels.

OTHER SYNDROMES OF POSSIBLE PITUITARY ORIGIN

Froehlich's syndrome and the Laurence-Moon-Biedl syndrome are two disorders associated with failure of gonadal development in which disturbances in anterior pituitary gonadotropin secretion are postulated. However, no consistent lesions have been observed in the anterior pituitary; and it is thought that the primary disturbance is in the hypothalamus.

Froehlich's syndrome is associated with adiposity and sexual infantilism. In addition to truncal obesity, there are underdevelopment of the gonads and an absence of the secondary sex characteristics. The condition may be associated with mental retardation, visual disturbances, diabetes insipidus, and impaired skeletal growth. It is important to differentiate between cases of Froehlich's habitus (obesity and apparently delayed genital development) and true Froehlich's syndrome. The former condition is often observed in normal prepuberal boys who may have normal sex organs hidden in the adipose tissue. With the onset of puberty, these boys develop normally and often lose their adiposity and assume normal adolescent body proportions. Froehlich's syndrome may be associated with tumors or other disorders of the hypothalamic-pituitary area. The obesity may be caused by damage to hypothalamic centers regulating appetite.

The Laurence-Moon-Biedl syndrome is a hereditary disease characterized by adiposity, genital atrophy, mental retardation, skull deformities, retinitis pigmentosa, and associated congenital malformations such as polydactyly and syndactyly. Fewer than 100 cases have been reported, and there is no evidence of pituitary lesions in these patients. The adiposity and genital atrophy are assumed to be caused by hypothalamic-pituitary dysfunction.

INTERMEDIATE LOBE OF THE PITUITARY GLAND

The intermediate lobe of the pituitary gland is the probable site of production of melanocyte-stimulating hormone (MSH). Two types of MSH have been identified. Alpha-MSH is a polypeptide composed of the same 13 amino acids found in the N-terminal position of ACTH (Fig. 87-3). Human β-MSH contains 22 amino acids and is closely related structurally to α-MSH as well as to ACTH. Because of the common N-terminal sequence, ACTH preparations have intrinsic melanocyte-stimulating effects; however, pure MSH does not stimulate adrenal cortical secretion. It is of interest that cortisone administration may suppress MSH as well as ACTH secretion from the pituitary gland.

There have been descriptions of MSH-secreting tumors of the pituitary gland. These rare tumors are associated with a generalized increase in pigmentation similar to that observed in patients with pituitary tumors following adrenalectomy for Cushing's syndrome. The hyperpigmentation observed in patients with Addison's disease may be due to increased production of MSH as well as ACTH. Increased MSH secretion may also be responsible for the hyperpigmentation observed in some cases of hyperthyroidism, biliary cirrhosis, sprue, and other chronic diseases. Conversely, it is probable that the decreased pigmentation often apparent in patients with panhypopituitarism is due to decreased production of MSH.

REFERENCES

Antoniades, H. N.: "Hormones in Human Plasma," Boston, Little, Brown and Company. 1960.

Brasel, J. A., J. C. Wright, L. Wilkins, and R. M. Blizzard: An Evaluation of Seventy-five Patients with Hypopituitarism Beginning in Childhood, Am. J. Med., 38: 484, 1965.

Harris, G. W., and B. T. Donovan: "The Pituitary Gland," London, Butterworths, 1966.

Lerner, A. B.: Hormonal Control of Pigmentation, Ann. Rev. Med., 11:187, 1960.

Liddle, G. W., D. Island, and C. K. Meader: Normal and Abnormal Regulation of Corticotropin Secretion in Man, Recent Progr. Hormone Res., 13:125, 1962.

Nelson, D. H., J. W. Meakin, and G. W. Thorn: ACTH-producing Pituitary Tumors Following Adrenalectomy for Cushing's Syndrome, Ann. Intern. Med., 52:560, 1960.

Odell, W. D., G. T. Ross, and P. L. Rayford: Radioimmunassay for Human Luteinizing Hormone, Metabolism, 15: 287, 1966.

Poppen, J. L.: Changing Concepts in the Treatment of Pituitary Adenomas, Bull. N.Y. Acad. Med., 39:21, 1963.

Purnell, D. C., R. V. Randall, and E. H. Rynearson: Postpartum Pituitary Insufficiency (Sheehan's Syndrome): Review of Eighteen Cases, Proc. Staff Meetings Mayo Clin., 39:321, 1964.

Rabkin, M. T., and A. G. Frantz: Hypopituitarism: A Study of Growth Hormone and Other Endocrine Functions, Ann. Intern. Med., 64:1197, 1966.

Rimoin, D. L., T. J. Merimee, and V. A. McKusick: Growth Hormone Deficiency in Man: An Isolated, Recessively Inherited Defect, Science, 152:1635, 1966.

Roth, J., S. M. Glick, P. Cuatrecasas, and C. S. Hollander: Acromegaly and Other Disorders of Growth Hormone Secretion, Ann. Intern. Med., 66:760, 1967.

Utiger, R. D.: Radioimmunassay of Human Plasma Thyrotropin, J. Clin. Invest., 44:1277, 1965.

88   DISEASES OF THE NEUROHYPOPHYSIS

Joseph F. Dingman and
George W. Thorn

Oliver and Schaefer in 1894 demonstrated a pressor effect of pituitary extracts, and in 1897 Howell showed that the pressor principle resided in the posterior lobe. The oxytocic action of posterior pituitary extracts was described by Dale in 1909 and the antidiuretic action by von den Velden in 1913. Fisher, Ingram, and Ranson in 1938 demonstrated a functional relationship between certain hypothalamic nuclei and the posterior pituitary. The studies of Scharrer and Scharrer since 1928 concerning the secretory activity of nerve cells (neurosecretion), the demonstration by Bargmann in 1949 of secretory granules in the neurones of the supraoptic and paraventricular nuclei of the hypothalamus, and the successful synthesis of oxytocin and vasopressin by du Vigneaud and coworkers represent important advances in current understanding of the endocrine functions of the neurohypophysis.

General Considerations

The principal effects of posterior pituitary extracts are to enhance the reabsorption of water by the renal tubules (antidiuretic effect); stimulate uterine contraction (oxytocic effect); promote the secretion of milk from the lactating breast (milk-ejecting effect); and, only in anesthetized mammals, produce a rise in blood pressure (vasopressor effect). The neurohypophyseal hormones are vasopressin (antidiuretic hormone, ADH) and oxytocin. The former is predominantly responsible for pressor and antidiuretic actions, whereas the latter is most potent in uterine stimulation and milk ejection. The neuroendocrine unit responsible for production and secretion of these hormones has been designated the neurohypophysis (Fig. 88-1) which includes the neurones of the supraoptic and paraventricular nuclei of the anterior hypothalamus, the axons that form the supraopticohypophyseal tract, and the posterior lobe of the pituitary body, the pars nervosa, in which the axone endings terminate.

Classic concepts of the endocrine function of the neurohypophysis ascribed the role of hormone production to parenchymatous secretory cells in the posterior lobe; however, an impressive body of evidence has been accumulated to show that vasopressin is actually secreted by the neurones of the supraoptic nuclei and oxytocin by the paraventricular nuclei. Gomori's chrome hematoxylin stain for the beta cells of the pancreatic islets demonstrated the presence of secretory granules within the cytoplasm of these neurones. These granules migrate along the axons and accumulate in the perivascular axone endplates in the posterior pituitary. The bulk of neurohypophyseal hormone is contained in the posterior lobe and only a small fraction of total activity is found in the tuber cinereum, stalk, and hypothalamic nuclei. The posterior pituitary then serves mainly as a reservoir of hormone readily available for rapid release into the systemic circulation.

Removal of the posterior lobe will lead to hormonal deficiency only if most of the axons of the hypothalamohypophyseal tract are severed and retrograde degeneration of the hypothalamic neurones occurs. With severance of the stalk close to the posterior pituitary body, short axons terminating at a higher level may escape injury and the remaining viable neurosecretory cells apparently

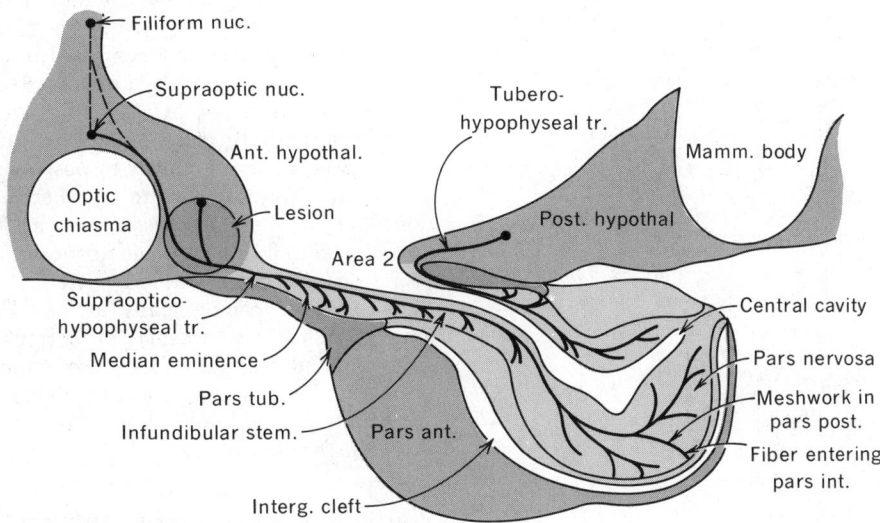

Fig. 88-1. Diagram of a midsagittal section through the hypothalamus and hypophysis. The broken lines indicate proposed filiform-supraoptic connections and the tractus paraventricularis. The gray circle indicates the position of a typical lesion designed to produce diabetes insipidus. (*Fisher, Ingram, and Ranson: "Diabetes Insipidus and the Neuro-Hormonal Control of Water Balance," Fig. 2, Ann Arbor, Mich., J. W. Edwards, Publisher. Incorporated, 1938.*)

can maintain secretion and release of hormones, probably into the vessels of the stalk and the hypothalamus.

The physiologic significance of the peculiar anatomic location of this neurosecretory organ, in which hypothalamic neurones extend their processes over relatively great distances into the posterior pituitary, is obscure. Such an arrangement may have been necessary, teleologically, in order to provide a ready route for hormone release into the systemic circulation through the highly vascularized posterior pituitary. In addition, posterior lobe extracts contain one or more hypothalamic neurohormones, which regulate the release of ACTH from the anterior pituitary (corticotropin-releasing factor, CRF), and oxytocin may play a role in regulating the secretion of prolactin (lactogenic hormone). Thus, the neurohypophysis may provide an important link between the central nervous system and the secretion of anterior pituitary tropic hormones which so profoundly influence the body economy.

In view of this evidence, consideration of the posterior pituitary as an endocrine gland warrants revision, and reference should be made to the neurohypophysis when discussing this endocrine system. However, the terms posterior pituitary gland and posterior lobe hormone are still in common usage at the present time.

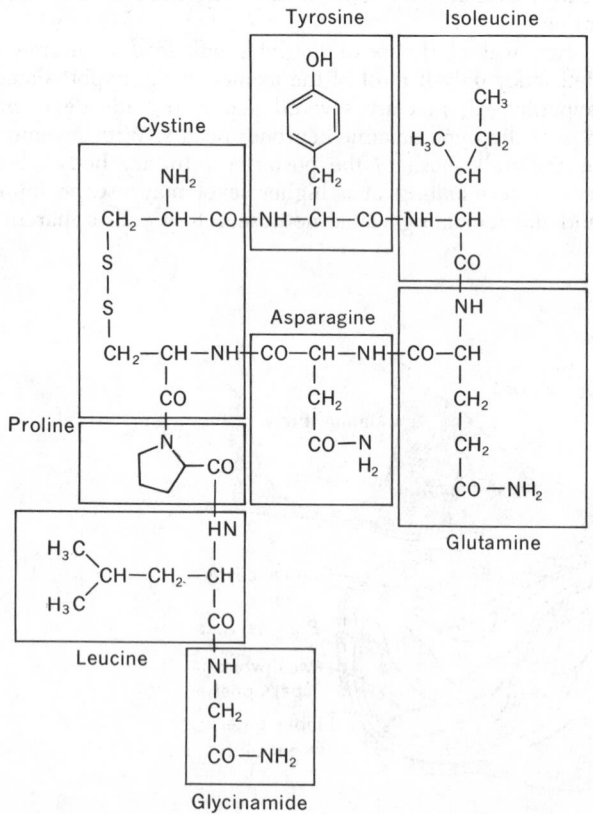

Fig. 88-2. Oxytocin. (B. Berde: "Recent Progress in Oxytocin Research," Fig. 1, Springfield, Ill., Charles C Thomas, Publisher, 1959.)

Nature of Neurohypophyseal Hormones

Extracts of the neurohypophysis are assayed biologically with reference to oxytocic, vasopressor, and antidiuretic activities. One international USP or BP unit is defined as the activity of 0.5 mg of an international standard bovine posterior pituitary powder. In crude extracts of the posterior lobe the biologic activity appears to reside in a homogeneous protein or polypeptide fraction having a molecular weight of the order of 30,000 and an isoelectric point of pH 4.8. Such fractions show approximately equal vasopressor and oxytocic activities in terms of the reference powder, of the order of 16.6 IU per milligram. It has not been conclusively established whether this protein represents the natural secretion of the neurohypophysis or whether vasopressin and oxytocin loosely bound to the protein by electrostatic forces are released in a free form into the circulation.

Using modern technics of ion exchange chromatography and countercurrent distribution, highly purified preparations of *vasopressin* (600 IU per milligram) and oxytocin (500 IU per milligram) have been obtained from posterior lobe extracts. Both vasopressin and oxytocin contain eight amino acids and 3 moles of ammonia. The peptide structure of each hormone has been determined, and both hormones have been successfully synthesized by de Vigneaud and his coworkers, representing a milestone in peptide chemistry and hormone research. Both hormones are composed of five amino acids arranged in the form of a ring closed by the disulfide linkage of cystine, with a side chain of three amino acids. Oxytocin contains cystine, tyrosine, isoleucine, glutamine, and asparagine in the ring, with proline, leucine, and glycinamide in the side chain (Fig. 88-2). Vasopressin differs from oxytocin by only two amino acids. Phenylalanine replaces isoleucine in the ring, and leucine in the side chain is replaced by arginine (human, beef vasopressin, Fig. 88-3) or lysine (hog vasopressin). The molecular weight of oxytocin is 1,007 and of arginine vasopressin, 1,084. Both are ampholytes, oxytocin having an isolectric point of pH 7.7, and arginine vasopressin being considerably more basic, with an IP of pH 10.9.

Oxytocin has been shown to possess slight but definite pressor and antidiuretic effects, whereas vasopressin contains not only equal pressor and antidiuretic activities but also significant intrinsic oxytocic and milk-ejecting properties. Partially purified posterior pituitary preparations available commercially include Pitocin (oxytocin) and Pitressin (vasopressin), each fraction being slightly contaminated by the other in pharmaceutical preparations. Synthetic oxytocin (Syntocinon) is now available, and synthetic lysine vasopressin should soon become available for clinical use.

Physiology of Neurohypophyseal Secretion

Secretion of vasopressin is regulated by the total solute concentration or osmolality of plasma (osmoregulation),

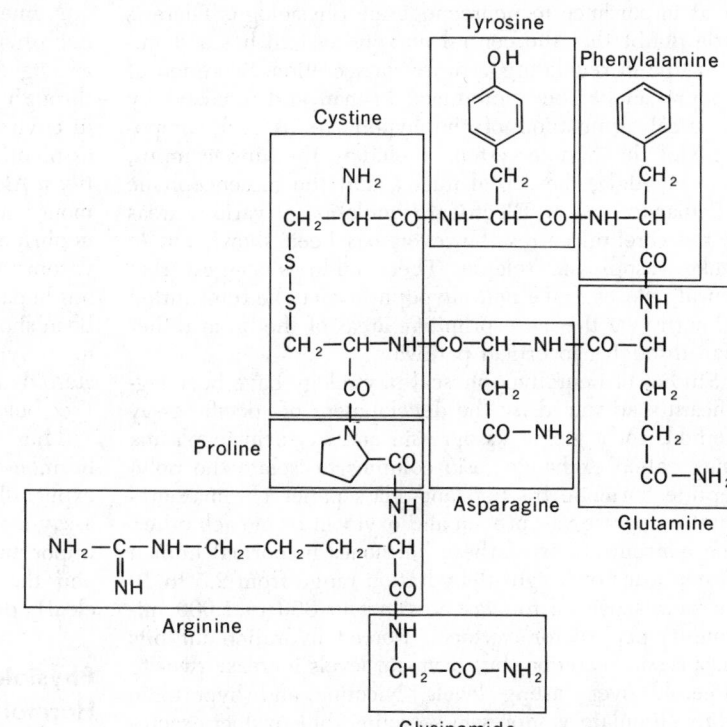

Fig. 88-3. Vasopressin. (*B. Berde: "Recent Progress in Oxytocin Research," Fig. 2, Springfield, Ill., Charles C Thomas, Publisher, 1959.*)

the intravascular or extracellular fluid volume (volume regulation), and by central nervous system activity (neural regulation). Secretion of oxytocin has been demonstrated during labor and milk release, consistent with the known uterotonic and milk-ejecting actions of the hormone. (Other factors regulating oxytocin secretion will be discussed below).

The osmoregulatory mechanism controlling vasopressin release is exquisitely sensitive to slight changes in plasma osmolality. Dilution of the plasma solutes by administration of water inhibits the secretion of vasopressin, and rapid excretion of water by the kidneys ensues; secretion is restored when plasma osmolality returns to normal. An increase in plasma osmolality resulting from a deficit of water or a relative increase in the ratio of extracellular to intracellular solutes stimulates the secretion of vasopressin and maximum conservation of water by the kidneys. This mechanism is probably the first line of defense in day-to-day preservation of water balance and is mediated principally by changes in the concentration of sodium in the extracellular fluid.

A poorly understood auxiliary mechanism regulating vasopressin secretion, which may be more important than plasma osmolality, especially in pathologic conditions, is the influence of the volume of the body fluids on neurohypophyseal function. Various procedures which reduce effective blood volume such as quiet standing, venous congestion, and hemorrhage are known to stimulate vasopressin secretion. The acute release of vasopressin with graded hemorrhage in the dog can be effectively blocked by severance of the vagi and maintenance of carotid sinus perfusion pressure. Thus, it appears that a contrac-

tion of blood volume activates afferent neural pathways to the neurohypophysis which arise in the carotid and aortic baroreceptors and the stretch receptors in the wall of the left atrium.

Of the two vascular modalities, osmolality and volume, the former apparently operates effectively in most normal situations by retaining or releasing body water to suit the needs of the body. However, in pathologic conditions characterized by a decrease in intravascular or extracellular fluid volume or in cardiac output, volume regulation supersedes osmoregulation. In this situation, vasopressin secretion may persist despite the simultaneous occurrence of hypotonicity. A primary decrease in osmolality, such as that seen in the hyponatremia of Addison's disease, salt-losing nephritis, or long-standing congestive heart failure, would severely deplete body water if osmolality were the only factor governing vasopressin secretion. A regulator of secretion sensitive to the volume of the body water or the fullness of the vascular compartment or both would protect against desiccation and vascular collapse in these situations, the body giving up an optimal osmotic state for the vital requirements of the tissues for water. This antidiuretic mechanism, although protective in nature, may lead to serious complications, particularly in disorders already characterized by fluid retention and edema, since persistent water retention in salt-restricted subjects may lead to severe hyponatremia, water intoxication, and further compromise of circulation and renal function (Chap. 296).

Since neurohypophyseal hormones represent secretions of the central nervous system, studies of the central neural control of the neurohypophysis have assumed great importance in neuroendocrine physiology. There is little doubt that the central nervous system has a dominant role in regulating vasopressin secretion. Secretion of vasopressin has been produced in man and monkeys by electrical stimulation of the hypothalamus and components of the "limbic system" including the hippocampus, the amygdala, the septal nuclei, and the mesencephalic reticular formation. Electrical stimulation of various areas of the cerebral cortex, however, has been shown not to evoke vasopressin release. These findings suggest that neural reflexes to the neurohypophysis may be transmitted primarily via the more primitive areas of the brain rather than through neocortical pathways.

Studies of neurohypophyseal physiology have been significantly advanced by the development of specific assay methods for arginine vasopressin and oxytocin in plasma using cation exchange resin columns to isolate the polypeptide hormone fraction and glass paper chromatography to separate vasopressin and oxytocin from each other. The concentrations of these hormones in normal human plasma after overnight dehydration range from 2.5 to 10 microunits per ml for vasopressin and 300 to 1,000 microunits per ml for oxytocin. Forced hydration inhibits vasopressin secretion, but oxytocin levels increase two- to threefold over fasting levels. Nicotine and hypertonic saline stimulate vasopressin secretion, but oxytocin secretion is acutely inhibited in most subjects. Specific increases in oxytocin secretion accompanied by an abrupt cessation of vasopressin secretion have been observed both during active labor as well as during breast feeding.

The release of vasopressin with increased plasma osmolality and contracting blood volume and its inhibition with plasma dilution are consistent with this hormone's physiologic role in water metabolism. The release of oxytocin during labor and breast feeding is also representative of specific physiologic responses. However, the inhibition of oxytocin secretion during vasopressin release and the converse response during active oxytocin secretion suggest a reciprocal relation in neurohypophyseal hormone secretion which may have important but still undefined implications in health and disease. Of obscure physiologic significance are the findings of measurable oxytocin levels in mildly dehydrated subjects of both sexes and the increase in oxytocin secretion observed with hypotonic expansion of the body fluid volume.

Normal to elevated plasma oxytocin levels have been found in most patients with spontaneous diabetes insipidus, and oxytocin deficiency has been observed only in patients subjected to hypophysectomy or pituitary stalk section. These findings corroborate the experimental evidence for separate sites of secretion of vasopressin and oxytocin by the supraoptic and paraventricular nuclei respectively. Lesions of the median eminence or anterior hypothalamus which interrupt the supraoptico-hypophyseal tract apparently spare certain paraventricular axons which enter the stalk from more lateral and caudal areas of the hypothalamus. Severance of the pituitary stalk would be expected to interrupt all nerve tracts to the posterior pituitary and thus lead to combined vasopressin and oxytocin deficiency.

Numerous centrally acting substances stimulate the neurohypophysis. These include emotional stresses such as fright, noise, and pain; fainting, which may also act through volume regulators; coitus, suckling, and changes in environmental temperature; and numerous drugs such as nicotine, acetylcholine, and many hypnotics and sedatives. Alcohol inhibits ADH secretion. Of the various hormones and endogenous substances, small doses of epinephrine inhibit and large doses stimulate the release of vasopressin, at least in animals. Ferritin, the iron-containing hepatic vasodepressor substance, and bradykinin have been shown to be antidiuretic by virtue of stimulating the neurohypophysis, and the hydrocortisone-like adrenal steroids have been shown to inhibit vasopressin secretion (see below).

Thus it is readily apparent that the neurohypophyseal hormones are secreted under diverse and seemingly inexplicable situations. With the availability of specific assay methods for these hormones in human plasma, their importance in the body economy and in the pathogenesis and the complications of disease should soon be more clearly defined.

Physiologic Actions of Neurohypophyseal Hormones

VASOPRESSIN (ADH). The pressor and antidiuretic activities of vasopressin are properties of a single molecule. The antidiuretic action is of profound importance in regulating water balance. The current hypothesis as to the mechanism of action of vasopressin on water reabsorption by the kidney, based on experiments with various biologic membranes, such as frog skin and toad bladder, is that it renders the cells of the distal portions of the nephron permeable to water, permitting passive diffusion of tubular water along an osmotic gradient across the cell and into the peritubular vessels. The antidiuretic action of vasopressin is best demonstrated during water diuresis; *this effect represents the true physiologic role of the hormone on water metabolism, which is to prevent the bulk of the filtered water entering the distal tubular segment from escaping into the urine.* The effect of vasopressin during hypertonic urine flow is extremely variable and limited by the maximum rate of water reabsorption which the concentrating mechanism of the collecting tubules can achieve.

An interesting aspect of the studies of the action of vasopressin on biologic membranes has been the demonstration that this hormone has a pronounced effect on transport of sodium as well as water across cell boundaries. The effect of vasopressin on sodium excretion by the kidney is, however, extremely variable and depends upon experimental conditions. It is probable that vasopressin does not have a direct effect on sodium excretion and that any observed change in sodium balance is secondary to the modifying influence of this hormone on the total volume and distribution of body water.

Vasopressin has been shown to exert a pressor effect in persons with postural hypotension, and large intravenous doses may also produce transient increases in blood pressure even in normal man. The significance of this observation in relationship to blood pressure regulation in normal persons is unknown. Generally, posterior lobe preparations used therapeutically in man have no consistent effect on blood pressure, probably because of compensatory adjustments elsewhere in the circulation.

Lysine vasopressin has also proved to be of value as a means of assessing adrenocorticotropin secretion by the anterior pituitary. Although other corticotropin-releasing factors (CRF) differing from vasopressin have been extracted from the hypothalamus and posterior lobe, vasopressin itself has been shown to be a potent CRF. In clinical investigation, large intramuscular doses of 5 to 10 units are required to produce measurable increments in plasma steroid levels; however, intravenous doses as low as 50 to 80 microunits have been shown to produce significant increments in ACTH secretion in the rat. Since these vasopressin levels fall well within the physiologic range of stressed animals, it is possible that vasopressin may serve a physiologic role as an ACTH-releasing neurohormone in addition to its direct peripheral actions.

OXYTOCIN. Recent studies with purified and synthetic oxytocin have significantly advanced understanding of the role of this hormone in uterine function and milk secretion. Oxytocin has been shown to be the hormonal substance of posterior lobe extracts responsible for release of milk from the lactating breast, as little as 0.5 units, or 1 μg, synthetic hormone producing a copious flow of milk within 30 sec of intravenous injection. Synthetic oxytocin has also been used successfully to initiate labor, and as previously mentioned, there is some evidence that oxytocin stimulates or sustains the secretion of prolactin by the anterior pituitary. Oxytocin, therefore, appears to play a very important and fundamental role in reproduction. Vasopressin also possesses oxytocic and milk-ejecting properties but is much less potent than oxytocin in this regard.

Other effects of oxytocin that warrant consideration include its marked but evanescent vasodepressor action demonstrable both in human beings and experimental animals and its effect on water excretion and renal function. In appropriate experimental situations, oxytocin has been shown to antagonize the antidiuretic action of vasopressin and to increase renal plasma flow and sodium excretion. The latter effect is currently attributable to an action of the hormone on the brain, which is abolished by hypophysectomy or the induction of diabetes insipidus. The demonstration that some of the actions of oxytocin are directly opposed to those of vasopressin implies a physiologic system for regulation of the volume and composition of the body fluids as well as the arterial pressure under the control of the central nervous system and the hypothalamus, which, although obscure at this time, may prove to be of clinical significance in the future.

Adrenocortical-neurohypophyseal Relationships

Patients with primary and secondary adrenocortical insufficiency characteristically show increased body water, hyponatremia and an inability to excrete a water load. These patients have been shown to have in the fasting state abnormally elevated plasma vasopressin levels which remain above the normal range despite forced hydration and further dilution of the plasma solutes. Curiously, plasma oxytocin is immeasurable both in the fasting and overhydrated state. Administration of hydrocortisonelike steroids to dehydrated patients is accompanied by a fall in plasma vasopressin and an increase in oxytocin levels into the range of fasting normal subjects. Water administration in the steroid-treated patient is accompanied by a normal osmoreceptor response to hemodilution with a fall in plasma vasopressin to zero and an increase in oxytocin levels to those observed in hydrated normal subjects. The inhibition of vasopressin secretion is accompanied by a normal water diuresis. Thus, it is apparent that the abnormal water metabolism of adrenocortical insufficiency is related to increased and sustained vasopressin secretion despite hypotonicity of the body fluids. Glucocorticoids restore normal water metabolism in this disease by a direct inhibitory action on vasopressin secretion and restoration of a normal osmoreceptor response to induced expansion of the body water. The observed changes in oxytocin secretion in untreated and steroid-treated patients suggest that the adrenal cortex influences oxytocin release either directly or indirectly through its effect on vasopressin secretion.

Hydrocortisone induces a transient water diuresis within the first few hours of administration even in subjects with normal adrenocortical function, an effect which is probably due to an acute decrease in vasopressin secretion. The resulting loss of body water would lead to relative hypertonicity of the body fluids and reactivation of vasopressin release via osmoregulatory pathways, even though blockade of neural pathways for ADH secretion may persist. The physiologic significance of this effect of hydrocortisone on the secretion of a hormone of prime importance in regulating water metabolism has not been delineated, but it may represent a hormonal mechanism for independently regulating the body content of sodium and water, which may be of fundamental importance in clinical disorders of sodium and water metabolism.

The adrenal steroids have not been shown to modify the antidiuretic effect of vasopressin in man. Thus, it has been shown that the diuretic effect of adrenal steroids is mediated not through a direct effect on the renal tubular reabsorption of water but by an indirect pathway involving inhibition of vasopressin secretion and a decrease in antidiuretic hormone action on the kidney.

In patients with partial neurohypophyseal insufficiency, a more complete state of diabetes insipidus can be induced with hydrocortisone administration, and a greater loss of solute-free water from the kidney occurs. Patients with a complete absence of vasopressin secretion do not have a true water diuresis with adrenal hormone administration. Since these hormones, at times, increase solute excretion by the kidney, there may be a concomitant increase in water excretion because of an inability of the kidney, in the absence of vasopressin, to increase solute concentration of the urine.

Adrenal steroids affect water metabolism in several other ways. Prolonged steroid therapy may occasionally result in extensive potassium depletion and the development of kaliopenic nephropathy associated with isosthenuria and a two- to threefold increase in urine flow. Very rarely, adrenal steroids may produce a striking polydipsic syndrome with urine volumes as high as 15 to 20 liters per 24 hr. Steroid effects on thirst-regulating centers in the anterior hypothalamus or other parts of the brain may be implicated in this disorder.

The adrenal steroids thus appear to influence water metabolism in man (1) by inhibiting the central neural control of vasopressin secretion and decreasing vasopressin action on the kidney; (2) by increasing solute excretion and the obligatory excretion of water in patients with vasopressin deficiency; (3) by producing the sensation of thirst, possibly by an effect on hypothalamic and other central nervous system thirst centers; (4) by producing potassium deficiency and kaliopenic nephropathy.

Vasopressin Deficiency— Diabetes Insipidus

Diabetes insipidus is a chronic symptom complex characterized by the passage of large quantities of pale, dilute urine, with secondary polydipsia. It results from a defect in the chain of events by which vasopressin is released from the neurohypophysis and acts on the cells of the renal tubules. The classic anatomic and physiologic studies of Fisher, Ingram, and Ranson, revealed that the disease may be caused by interference with the functional integrity of the neurohormonal unit comprising the supraoptic and paraventricular nuclei of the hypothalamus, the supraoptico hypophyseal tract, and the posterior lobe of the hypophysis. The full-blown disease occurs only when the tract is interrupted close enough to the hypothalamus to cause degeneration of at least 85 percent of the supraoptic and paraventricular neurones. There is also a relatively rare disorder, nephrogenic diabetes insipidus, which is mostly familial. This disorder may be due to a hereditary refractoriness of the renal tubules to vasopressin, and it is presumed that there is no neurohypophyseal disease in this group.

The incidence of classic diabetes insipidus following hypophysectomy may be significantly diminished if damage to the supraoptic neurones is minimized by careful severance of the pituitary stalk as close to the pituitary gland as possible. The polyuria of hypophysectomized human beings has been shown to vary with the magnitude of vasopressin deficiency. Patients who lack this secretion demonstrate persistent polyuria despite withdrawal of adrenocortical replacement therapy. These observations illustrate the important role of vasopressin indetermining the rate of water excretion and corroborate the concept that the diuretic effect of adrenal steroids is mediated indirectly through an effect on vasopressin secretion. The adrenal steroids may increase urine volume in such patients, however, by increasing solute excretion.

The thyrotropic and growth hormones of the anterior pituitary are necessary to maintain polyuria, probably by influencing the nutritional state and solute turnover as well as by sustaining renal function. A peripheral antagonism of vasopressin by thyroid hormone has been demonstrated, but this effect may not be a direct one.

INCIDENCE. Diabetes insipidus is a rare disease, with a slightly greater incidence in youth and in males. In 1924 Rowntree reported 10 and 16 cases, respectively, in two series of 100,000 admissions to the Mayo Clinic. With the advent of hypophysectomy in recent years for the treatment of far-advanced breast carcinoma and other serious disorders, the disease is becoming much more prevalent in the general hospital population.

ETIOLOGY. As shown by Fink's pathologic studies in 107 cases, the great majority of instances of this disease are due to anatomic lesions involving the hypothalamic-hypophyseal system and, hence, presumably interfering with vasopressin production. In clinical practice, it will often be impossible to elicit any other evidence of such a lesion; while the label *idiopathic* may be justifiable for such cases antemortem, the finding of an anatomic lesion at autopsy generally may be predicted.

PATHOLOGY. The primary pathologic processes associated most frequently with the syndrome have been tumors of the diencephalopituitary region, basilar meningitis, sarcoidosis, and the histiocytic disorders. Transitory and occasionally permanent polyuria may follow severe head injuries. Pathologic changes consist of those due to the primary disorder, such as tumor, brain injury, and inflammation, and secondary changes in the urogenital tract, such as dilatation and hypertrophy of the bladder with megaloureter.

CLINICAL PICTURE. The chief symptoms of diabetes insipidus are polyuria and polydipsia. The loss of large amounts of pale, dilute urine, occasionally as much as 15 to 29 liters per day, results in dehydration and, consequently, in such related symptoms and signs as dry skin, constipation, and an intense, almost insatiable thirst. Water deprivation to the limit of tolerance does not prevent polyuria, nor does it lead to a significant increase in urine concentration. Thus, in this disease, polydipsia is secondary to polyuria, in contrast to patients with psychogenic polydipsia, who pass large quantities of urine as an aftermath of a large fluid intake. In patients with diabetes insipidus, no consistent physical or chemical changes are noted other than those of dehydration. However, there may be symptoms referable to the localized disease process causing the syndrome.

The role of trauma in the production of diabetes insipidus deserves special comment, since the polyuria that sometimes follows head injury is not infrequently transient, as contrasted with the chronicity of most other forms of the disease. A similar syndrome may develop subsequent to cerebrovascular accidents or intracranial surgery, and in association with other forms of cerebral disease. When the full-blown syndrome develops under these conditions, serious dehydration may occur before the diagnosis is suspected, particularly in the incontinent patient or in the patient with clouded sensorium who is unable to request or partake of an adequate volume of fluids. The dehydration, which is due principally to water loss, may be accentuated by the administration of isotonic saline or solutions containing large amounts of protein. Such large solute loads will aggravate the renal loss of water in these patients because of an inability of the kidney to increase the solute concentration of the urine in the absence of vasopressin.

DIAGNOSIS. The symptoms plus the large urine volume, with specific gravity below 1.010 and urinary osmolality less than that of plasma, unassociated with a history or other findings of diabetes mellitus or of chronic renal disease, will quickly suggest diabetes insipidus. Since this diagnosis commits the patient to sustained replacement therapy for an indefinite period, it is not to be made lightly, and the clinical impression should be supported by careful studies made under hospital conditions. All cases of diabetes insipidus, moreover, should be studied carefully for active intracranial lesions, which should be presumed to be present until proved otherwise. Thus, examination should include, in addition to the differential tests of water excretion outlined below, a study of the spinal fluid, roentgenograms of the skull and chest (metastatic disease), electroencephalogram, serologic test (syphilis), the serum protein level, sternal marrow aspiration (multiple myeloma), and visual fields.

DIFFERENTIAL DIAGNOSIS. The syndrome must be differentiated from psychogenic polydipsia, chronic nephritis, and diabetes mellitus as well as from the polydipsia and polyuria so characteristically associated with the hypochloremic alkalotic syndrome and the hypercalcemia of hyperparathyroidism and vitamin D intoxication. Chronic nephritis may be excluded by the absence of protein or formed elements in the urine, a normal blood urea nitrogen level, and normal kidney function tests. Often the most difficult differential diagnosis is that between diabetes insipidus and psychogenic polydipsia. Other procedures helpful in making a differential diagnosis are the following:

1. Dehydration for 8 to 12 hr should be performed cautiously during the day, with close observation of the patient for signs of vasomotor collapse, which can occur with sudden severe dehydration. An inability to increase the specific gravity and osmolality of the urine to hypertonic levels is characteristic of diabetes insipidus and serves to differentiate this syndrome from psychogenic polydipsia but not from chronic nephritis. Great care must be taken in suspected psychogenic cases to be certain that the patient does not have access to water or other fluids.

2. Alleviation of symptoms will follow repeated small doses of aqueous vasopressin, i.e., 5.0 units intramuscularly every 3 to 4 hr. This differentiates diabetes insipidus from chronic nephritis but not from psychogenic polydipsia. The possibility of vasopressin-resistant diabetes insipidus must always be kept in mind, since 5 to 15 percent of cases of diabetes insipidus fall into this category.

3. Secretory function should be tested. Since the secretion of vasopressin can be initiated by either neurogenic or osmotic stimuli, both the hypothalamic neurones and the osmoregulators must be stimulated in turn for the integrity of this neurohormonal unit to be properly evaluated. In addition, the adequacy of renal tubular responsiveness to vasopressin must also be measured to understand fully the nature of the polyuria. The functional integrity of the neurohypophyseal-renal system may be evaluated within a few hours by serial intravenous injections of nicotine, hypertonic saline solution, and vasopressin under constant water-loading conditions. Acute changes in urinary osmolality and free water clearance (C_{H_2O}) during water diuresis reflect the action of vasopressin on the renal tubular reabsorption of water and may be regarded as a useful index of the secretory capacity of the neurohypophysis.[1]

Technique for Studying Neurohypophyseal Function. The patient is hydrated with 20 ml water per kg body weight over 30 to 60 min. Preliminary dehydration is unnecessary and may be dangerous. Urine is collected at 15- to 30-min intervals by spontaneous voiding if at all possible or else through an indwelling catheter. In the latter case, it is worthwhile to administer 0.5 Gm tetracycline by mouth several hours before catheterization to prevent urinary tract infection. A constant state of hydration is maintained by oral or intravenous administration of a volume of fluid equal to that excreted during the preceding collection period. When a sustained high rate of urine flow is reached (over 5 ml per min), 1.0 mg nicotine in solution is injected intravenously over a period of 0.5 to 2 min. The dose of nicotine is gradually increased by 0.5 to 1.0 mg at intervals of 30 min until a clear-cut antidiuretic response ensues or symptoms of nicotine intoxication (i.e., vertigo, nausea, vomiting) preclude further administration. As an alternative, the subject can smoke one to three cigarettes rapidly and with deep inhalation.

The normal antidiuretic response to nicotine, which occurs within 15 to 30 min after injection, is a decrease in urine flow and free water clearance, accompanied by an increase in urinary creatinine, chloride, and total solute concentrations (Fig. 88-4). Patients with diabetes in-

---

[1] The urine volume, V, is equal to the algebraic sum of the osmolal clearance, C_{osm}, and the free water clearance, C_{H_2O}.

$$V = C_{osm} + C_{H_2O}$$
$$C_{osm} = V \frac{\text{total solute conc. urine}}{\text{total solute conc. plasma}}$$

C_{osm} represents the volume of water required to contain the urinary solutes in a solution isosmotic with plasma. C_{H_2O} represents the net excess or deficit of water beyond the osmolal clearance; it will be positive during a water diuresis and negative when urine is concentrated by the abstraction of solute-free water, as in antidiuresis. C_{H_2O} usually parallels urine flow during water diuresis studies, since osmolal clearance remains relatively constant. This index is particularly useful in determining the changes in water excretion occurring during the solute diuresis usually observed with hypertonic saline administration. Not infrequently, a large increase in C_{osm} may mask a concomitant decrease in C_{H_2O}. In this instance, urinary flow may fall only slightly or may actually increase, even though an increase in water reabsorption may be under way under the influence of released vasopressin.

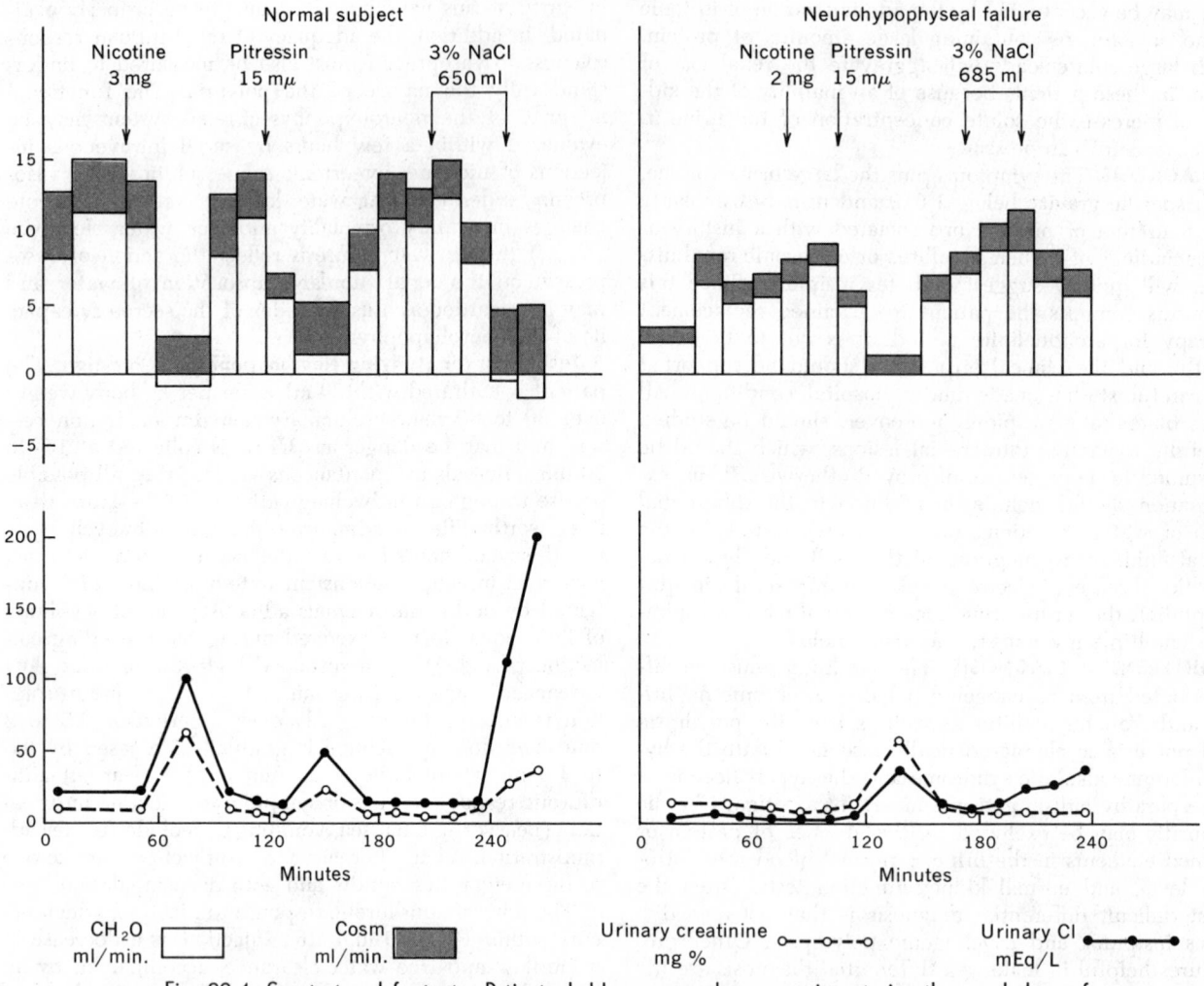

Fig. 88-4. See text and footnote. Patient, J. H., a nonsmoker, was given twice the usual dose of nicotine.

sipidus usually do not show a fall in water excretion with normal doses of nicotine; however, some may have a minimal antidiuretic response with much larger amounts (5 to 6 mg nicotine base), which may be due to residual neurohypophyseal activity or transient hemodynamic effects on the kidney. When urine flow returns to control levels, 15 to 25 milliunits aqueous vasopressin is injected intravenously. The response to vasopressin differentiates renal disease from true diabetes insipidus.

The administration of water is discontinued with the vasopressin injection to decrease the volume of retained water in preparation for the intravenous administration of hypertonic saline solution, since excessive hydration may abolish the osmotic response by diluting the hypertonic saline as it enters the circulation. When the antidiuresis to vasopressin is completed, 3 percent saline (10 ml per kilogram) is infused rapidly over 30 to 45 min. In normal persons a marked antidiuretic response will occur during the infusion or within the following 60 min. In patients with diabetes insipidus, this antidiuresis does

not occur and a rise in free water clearance is frequently observed due to the associated solute diuresis (Fig. 88-4). Patients with psychogenic polydipsia demonstrate normal antidiuresis to the hypertonic saline infusion, but, curiously, many do not respond normally to nicotine, suggesting some derangement in hypothalamic function and neural regulation of vasopressin release in this disorder.

The response to nicotine, to hypertonic saline solution, and to vasopressin may be used to differentiate the locus of the functional disturbance responsible for the polyuria, i.e., hypothalamus, osmoregulators, and renal tubules. Patients with vasopressin-deficient diabetes insipidus classically do not respond to hypertonic saline. However, certain patients with diabetes insipidus apparently have secreting neurohypophyseal tissue that responds to normal doses of nicotine but not to hypertonic saline solution. Post-mortem studies on one such patient with metastatic breast carcinoma demonstrated an abundance of secretory granules within the neurones of the intact supraoptic nuclei, but the posterior pituitary and stalk were devoid of neurosecretion and completely destroyed by tumor. This phenomenon suggests that isolated posterior pituitary damage may lead to a selective failure of the osmoregulatory control of vasopressin secretion and a clinical syndrome of vasopressin-deficient diabetes insipidus despite the presence of functioning neurohypophyseal tissue.

TREATMENT. Treatment of diabetes insipidus may be divided into two phases: (1) correction of the underlying intracranial difficulty, if present; (2) replacement therapy with vasopressin, which usually must be continued throughout life.

Pitressin is a partially purified vasopressin fraction obtained from animal posterior lobes supplied as an aqueous solution in 0.5- and 1-ml ampuls with a strength of 20 IU pressor activity per milliliter. The quantity of Pitressin required to ameliorate polyuria is very small (0.1 to 0.2 ml), but the evanescent action of the aqueous preparation necessitates repeated injections at 3- to 4-hr intervals, making this form of treatment impractical for prolonged periods. Synthetic lysine vasopressin solution for parenteral use is comparable in action to aqueous Pitressin.

Nasal insufflations of dried posterior pituitary powder (supplied in 5- and 30-Gm bottles) every 3 to 6 hr accomplish the same purpose and are more easily administered, but most patients develop a chronic rhinopharyngitis and even gastritis from swallowed powder. Systemic allergic reactions are rare but have been observed.

A synthetic *lysine vasopressin* solution containing 50 pressor units per milliliter in 5-ml plastic spray vials is available for intranasal use as a spray or as drops. Its activity is as rapid and as prolonged as posterior lobe powder, but this preparation has the decided advantage of eliminating the local or systemic allergic reactions to the foreign protein in posterior pituitary preparations of animal origin. This material currently is the treatment of choice for ambulatory patients.

Pitressin tannate in oil is supplied in 1-ml ampuls with a strength of 5 IU per milliliter. This preparation provides relatively prolonged hormonal action; a single injection is usually effective for 24 to 72 hr. A test dose of 0.3 to 0.5 ml (1.5 to 2.5 IU) should be given initially to determine the effectiveness of treatment and to guard against the serious, but fortunately rare, occurrence of excess fluid retention and water intoxication in particularly sensitive individuals. For practical purposes chronic treatment with 1.0-ml doses of hormone should be tried and the frequency of injection gauged by the recurrence of polyuria. Most patients will retain 1 to 2 kg water following an injection, and the dissipation of effective hormone levels will be attended with a sudden polyuria and loss of body weight before onset of polydipsia. In general, injections should be timed to coincide with the onset of polyuria in order to prevent marked fluctuations in body water content and fluid compartmental shifts. Abnormal fluid retention may be mitigated by instructing the patient to guard against excessive fluid ingestion after treatment. The hormone is preferably given in the evening to ensure a restful night. *It is very important to instruct the patient to warm the vial and to shake it thoroughly, since the active material has a tendency to precipitate out in the vial.* This is the commonest cause of so-called "vasopressin resistance."

Occasionally, patients with vasopressin-sensitive diabetes insipidus may develop resistance to the action of the hormone, in some cases accompanied by allergy either to the hormone or to the oily menstruum. Allergy to the latter may be easily corrected by use of a different medium, and hormone allergy may be overcome by desensitization. Vasopressin resistance is also observed in patients with hypokalemia and hypercalcemia or hypercalciuria, either of which blocks the full action of ADH on the renal tubules. Serum and urinary calcium and potassium measurements should be made in all patients with vasopressin-resistant polyuria and appropriate investigations and treatment carried out.

Both *chlorothiazide* and *hydrochlorothiazide* have been shown to increase free water reabsorption in diabetes insipidus. These drugs, however, will decrease urine flow by no more than about 30 to 50 percent, and most patients usually will continue to require vasopressin therapy as well to prevent abnormally large urine volumes. The thiazide derivatives may have their greatest usefulness in lessening polyuria in the rare form of vasopressin-resistant diabetes insipidus. The average daily dose of chlorothiazide is 0.5 to 1.0 Gm and of hydrochlorothiazide, 0.05 to 0.1 Gm given in divided doses. Since the thiazides may produce potassium depletion, which can impair the concentrating ability of the kidney, it is worthwhile to administer 1.0 to 2.0 Gm KCl syrup by mouth with each dose of thiazide drug. Simultaneous administration of spironolactone (Aldactone[R]) with the thiazide may prevent hypokalemia by blocking the aldosterone-mediated NaK exchange in the distal renal tubule.

Chlorpropamide in doses of 250 to 500 mg per day is also effective antidiuretic therapy in some patients. The value of this drug is that the volume depletion and hypokalemia from thiazides can be avoided. The possible development of hypoglycemia from chlorpropamide should be investigated and corrected by decreasing the dose or discontinuing therapy if necessary. The mechanism of action of this drug on renal water reabsorption has not been clarified.

The prognosis of diabetes insipidus is determined by the outcome of the primary disease process. With regular treatment, patients with isolated neurohypophyseal atrophy can lead normal lives.

Excess of Antidiuretic Hormone

Abnormally elevated levels of antidiuretic substances in blood and urine have been reported in a variety of disease states associated with edema or defects in water diuresis, including cardiac failure, cirrhosis with ascites, nephrosis, and Addison's disease. While the hypothesis that excessive antidiuretic activity may be responsible for the water retention observed in edematous patients is quite attractive, proof has not been clearly established.

It is generally agreed that patients with these disorders do not show excessive sensitivity to or delayed inactivation of administered vasopressin. Some studies with nicotine stimulation of endogenous vasopressin secretion in patients with edema have yielded normal results, but some patients whose disease is associated with severe hyponatremia have shown enhanced neurohypophyseal response to nicotine and other stimuli. Many of the studies that minimize a role of vasopressin in edema formation are based upon data observed in patients in equilibrium with their fluid retention who can excrete water loads, albeit at a somewhat depressed rate. It is obvious that vasopressin release mechanisms should be evaluated during the active phase of edema formation, but studies have been hampered by the fact that such patients frequently cannot excrete administered water, which automatically vitiates the only reliable biologic end point of vasopressin action, i.e., antidiuresis. Further advances in this field will depend upon the application of precise and reliable methods for measuring vasopressin levels in the plasma.

The level of vasopressin in the body fluids need not necessarily be increased to account for water retention, since even physiologic amounts effectively halt a water diuresis. The abnormality in water metabolism may be primarily related to a *persistence* of vasopressin secretion despite the presence of excess body water or hypotonicity, both of which normally should induce water diuresis. It appears that the distribution rather than the total quantity of body water may determine the secretory activity of the neurohypophysis, and more extensive studies of the precedence of volume versus osmolal regulation of vasopressin secretion should shed more light on the nature of fluid retention in these disorders.

Inappropriate ADH Syndrome

The above discussion is particularly pertinent in understanding the nature of the antidiuretic factors responsible for the *inappropriate ADH syndrome*, described in patients with oat cell carcinoma of the lung, acute intermittent porphyria, various central nervous system disorders, etc. Antidiuretic assays of whole plasma and urine purport to show increased ADH levels in several patients. The situation is made more complex by the finding of antidiuretic activity in extracts of primary and metastatic tumor tissues. These antidiuretic substances have not been confirmed as ADH, however; the bioassay methods employed are not specific for vasopressin and may be interfered with by vasoactive peptides other than ADH in the biologic extracts or by a nonspecific release of ADH by the assay animal following injection of noxious substances or heterologous tissue extracts. The fact that the characteristic syndrome is also observed in nontumorous conditions suggests that abnormalities in neurohypophyseal secretion of vasopressin may well prove to be the common denominator in these diverse clinical disorders. Proof of vasopressin synthesis by these nonendocrine tumors must await results of tissue culture of tumor cells or specific radioimmunologic or ultramicrochemical measurements of arginine vasopressin in the tumors.

The interrelationships between neurohypophyseal secretion and the adrenal secretion of aldosterone are not well defined. Patients with aldosterone-secreting tumors do not usually develop edema, and normal subjects treated with aldosterone have been shown to escape readily from sodium and water retention. Furthermore, patients with diabetes insipidus will retain sodium with aldosterone therapy but will not retain isosmotic quantities of water unless they receive vasopressin simultaneously.

Aldosterone secretion may be inhibited by expansion of body fluids despite the presence of hyponatremia. In this respect, the regulation of aldosterone secretion resembles that for vasopressin secretion, the influence of fluid volume having precedence over osmolal concentration. It is probable that there is an intimate physiologic interrelation between aldosterone, which governs sodium metabolism, and vasopressin, which regulates water metabolism. Both vasopressin and aldosterone are probably necessary for the isosmotic retention of fluid, and persistent secretion of both hormones could be responsible for the development of edema in patients with fundamental derangements in circulation.

REFERENCES

Ahmed, A. B. J., B. C. George, C. Gonzalez-Auvert, and J. F. Dingman: Increased Plasma Arginine Vasopressin in Clinical Adrenocortical Insufficiency and Its Inhibition by Glucosteroids, J. Clin. Invest., 46:111, 1967.

Bartter, F. C., and W. B. Schwartz: The Syndrome of Inappropriate Secretion of Antidiuretic Hormone, Am. J. Med., 42:790, 1967.

Dingman, J. F., and J. Hauger-Klevene: Treatment of Diabetes Insipidus: Synthetic Lysine Vasopressin Nasal Solution, J. Clin. Endocrinol. Metab., 24:550, 1964.

du Vigneaud, V.: Trail of Sulfur Research: From Insulin to Oxytocin, Science, 123:967, 1956.

Symposium on Antidiuretic Hormones, Am. J. Med., 42:651, 1967.

Verney, E. B.: Absorption and Excretion of Water: Antidiuretic Hormone, Lancet, II:739, 1946.

89 DISEASES OF THE THYROID
Herbert A. Selenkow and
Sidney H. Ingbar

Diseases of the thyroid gland are manifested by increases in gland size (goiter, neoplasm), alterations in hormonal secretion, or both. Changes in gland size and weight (normally 15 to 35 Gm) are associated with toxic or nontoxic goiter, adenomas, thyroiditis, or malignancies. Symptoms may arise from local compression in the neck and superior mediastinum, from disturbances in hormonogenesis resulting in hypothyroidism or hyperthyroidism, or from malignancy. Alterations in thyroid hormone secretion produce a wide variety of anatomic, physiologic, and metabolic effects, characteristic of which are increased oxygen consumption (hypermetabolism) from excessive secretion and decreased oxygen consumption (hypometabolism) from thyroid insufficiency.

In 1891, Murray, an English physician, administered thyroid substances to a myxedematous patient, who subsequently improved remarkably. The material employed was a glycerin extract obtained from sheep thyroids. Magnus-Levy, in 1895, observed that administration of thyroid extract to patients with hypothyroidism was followed by an increase in basal metabolic rate. In 1896, Baumann obtained an acid hydrolyzate of thyroid tissue in powder form that contained 10 percent iodine, thus establishing the high iodine content of this hormone. Oswald, 8 years later, prepared iodothyroglobulin, which indicated that thyroid hormone was a protein substance. *Thyroxin* was first isolated by Kendall in 1915 and subsequently synthesized by Harington and Barger in 1927. The potent homologue of thyroxin, 3,5,3'-triiodothyronine, was isolated chromatographically from plasma and thyroid tissue and identified simultaneously in 1952 by Gross and Pitt-Rivers and by Roche, Lissitsky, and Michel.

ANATOMY AND EMBRYOLOGY

The human thyroid originates embryologically from an invagination of the pharyngeal epithelium with some cellular contributions from the lateral pharyngeal pouches. Progressive descent of the midline thyroid anlage gives rise to the thyroglossal duct, which extends from the foramen cecum at the base of the tongue to the isthmus of the thyroid. Remnants of tissue may persist along the course of this tract as "lingual thyroid," as thyroglossal cysts and nodules, or as a structure contiguous with the thyroid isthmus, called the *pyramidal lobe*. The cephalad portion of the pyramidal lobe in adults is usually a vestigial structure consisting of a thin fibrous cord. The remnant close to the thyroid isthmus may contain significant amounts of thyroid tissue that can be identified by careful palpation as the pyramidal lobe. This lobe usually extends from the thyroid cartilage to the thyroid isthmus and is more commonly located to the left than to the right of the midline. Hypertrophy of this lobe is found in disorders of diffuse thyroid enlargement such as hyperthyroidism, diffuse hyperplasia of adolescence or pregnancy, and in lymphoid thyroiditis. Ectopic thyroid tissue may occur rarely in the trachea or esophagus.

The human fetal thyroid becomes detectably functional around 14 to 16 weeks and during the latter part of gestation develops the capacity to synthesize and secrete thyroid hormones. The extent to which fetal requirements for thyroid hormones are met by secretion from the maternal or fetal thyroid is not clear. The thyroid gland enlarges progressively during fetal development and neonatal life and reaches the adult size of about 20 to 25 Gm. The precise weight of the "normal" adult thyroid gland varies considerably with geographic, genetic, and environmental factors.

BIOCHEMICAL PHYSIOLOGY

The hormonal activity of the thyroid gland is controlled mainly by the thyrotropic or thyroid-stimulating hormone (TSH) of the anterior pituitary gland (see Chap. 87). Release of TSH from the pituitary is regulated, at least in part, by hypothalamic centers and generally depends upon the quantity of thyroid hormones available to the tissues. A reduction in the availability of thyroid hormones stimulates TSH output, which, in turn, tends to increase the secretion and size of the thyroid gland. Conversely, in normal persons, an excess of available thyroid hormones tends to depress secretion of TSH and so, in turn, to reduce thyroid activity and size. Certain chemical compounds, as well as congenital or acquired enzymatic defects within the thyroid, reduce hormonal secretion leading to increased TSH secretion and goiter formation (goitrogenesis). Conversely, thyroid hormones inhibit secretion of TSH and thus act as antigoitrogenic agents.

Pathways of iodine metabolism are schematically represented in Fig. 89-1. Approximately 100 to 200 μg dietary iodide is absorbed daily via the gastrointestinal tract, and a similar amount is excreted in the urine. Circulating inorganic iodide is usually present in serum in minute amounts of the order of 0.5 μg per 100 ml. This ionic iodide is available to the thyroid, kidneys, and exocrine glands. That portion not concentrated by the thyroid is rapidly cleared by the kidneys. Iodide extracted by the exocrine glands is recirculated via intestinal resorption. The intrathyroidal processes leading to synthesis and secretion of thyroid hormones may be divided into four sequential stages (Fig. 89-2). Iodine in the plasma is available to the thyroid gland for hormonal synthesis only as inorganic iodide. This is derived from two major sources, the peripheral degradation and deiodination of hormonal as well as nonhormonal iodinated compounds and, more importantly, the diet. In most areas of the world the dietary intake of iodine is sufficiently low so that the concentration of iodide in plasma is well below 1 μg per 100 ml. The first step in hormonal biosynthesis is active transport of iodide from plasma at a rate exceeding efflux from the gland, with the result that a concentration gradient for iodide is maintained. Thyroid/serum gradients may vary from 10 to 500, or more, under varying physiologic conditions. The activity of the iodide transport or trapping mechanism is increased directly by TSH or indirectly via low thyroidal iodine stores. Next, through a reaction apparently mediated by an intrathyroidal peroxidase, iodide is oxidized to a higher valence form, possibly iodine or hypoiodite. This highly reactive form of iodine exists only momentarily, as it combines rapidly with tyrosyl groups in thyroid proteins (organification) to form monoiodotyrosine (MIT) and diiodotyrosine (DIT). These iodotyrosines then undergo oxidative condensation (coupling), possibly again through the mediation of a thyroidal peroxidase, to yield a variety of iodothyronines, including thyroxin (T4) and 3,5,3"-triiodothyronine (T3). The latter compound (hereafter referred to as triiodothyronine) and thyroxin are the major hormonally active products secreted by the thyroid gland. These, as well as the other iodinated amino acids, are formed within the thyroglobulin molecule and stored as such in the thyroid follicle. Under physiologic condi-

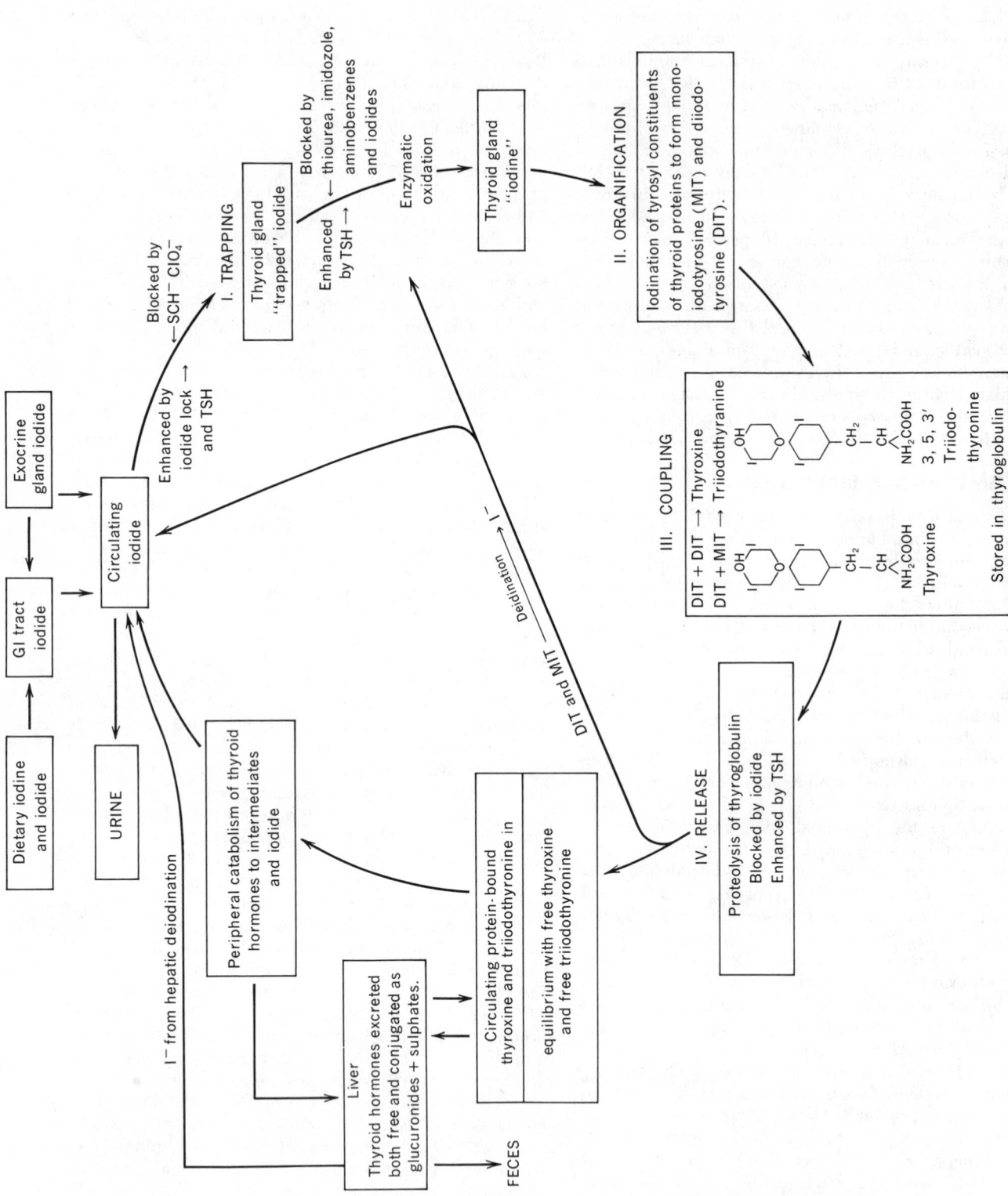

Fig. 89-1. Simplified schematic representation of pathways of iodine metabolism.

446

I. TRAPPING

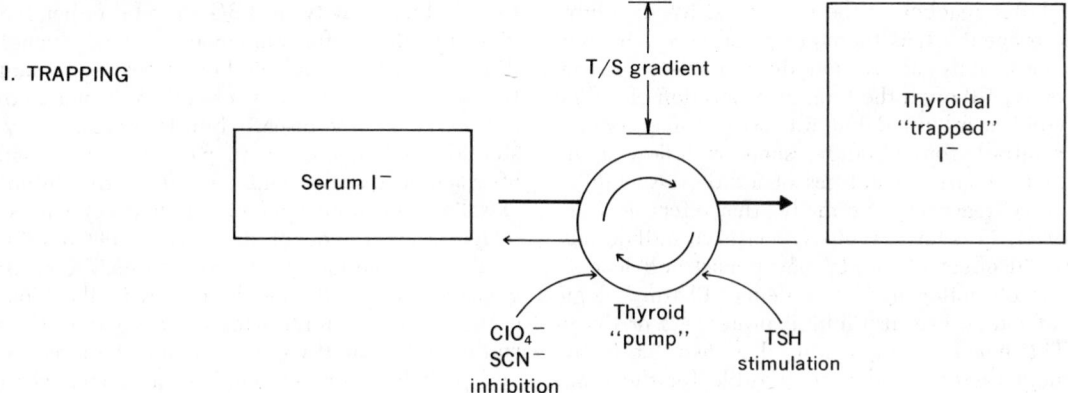

II. ORGANIFICATION

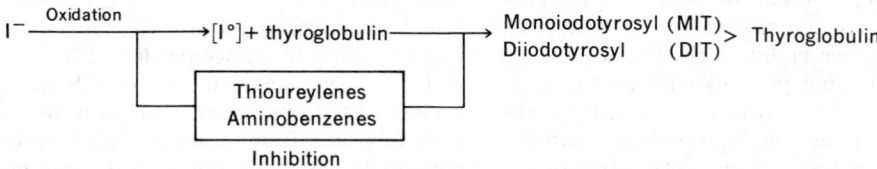

III. COUPLING

$$2 \text{ DIT} \longrightarrow \text{Thyroxinyl} \quad (T4)$$
$$1 \text{ MIT} + 1 \text{ DIT} \longrightarrow \text{Triiodothyroninyl (T3)} \Big\rangle \text{Thyroglobulin}$$

IV. RELEASE

$$\text{T4-T3-MIT-DIT-Thyroglobulin} \xrightarrow[\text{thyrotopin activated}]{\text{Enzymatic hydrolysis}} \begin{array}{l} \nearrow \text{T4} + \text{T3 (plasma)} \\ \searrow \text{MIT} + \text{DIT (thyroid)} \end{array}$$

$$\text{MIT} + \text{DIT (Thyroid)} \xrightarrow[\text{deiodinase}]{\text{Tyrosine}} \text{Tyrosine} + I^- \text{(recycled)}$$

Fig. 89-2. *Sequential stages of intrathyroidal synthesis and secretion of thyroid hormones.*

tions, thyroglobulin does not enter the circulation. Secretion of hormonally active materials requires hydrolysis of thyroglobulin (release), which is effected by thyroidal proteases and peptidases. The thyroid hormones released by proteolysis of thyroglobulin are free to enter the bloodstream, whereas MIT and DIT are prevented from entering the circulation by action of an iodotyrosine deiodinase, which removes their iodide. This iodide is in part reutilized for synthesis of hormone and in part lost from the thyroid gland into the circulation.

The foregoing reactions are subject to inhibition by a variety of chemical compounds. Such agents are generally termed *goitrogens,* since, by virtue of their ability to inhibit hormonal synthesis, they induce goiter formation. Certain inorganic anions, notably perchlorate and thiocyanate, inhibit the iodide transport mechanism and thus either prevent thyroid cells from concentrating iodide or cause release at thyroidal iodide into the circulation. The goiter and hypothyroidism that follow chronic depletion of intrathyroidal iodide, such as these agents induce, can be prevented or relieved by doses of iodide sufficiently large to enable adequate quantities to enter the gland by simple diffusion. The commonly employed antithyroid agents, such as the derivatives of thiourea and mercaptoimidazole, exert more complex actions upon pathways of hormonal biosynthesis. These agents, as well as certain aniline derivatives, inhibit the initial oxidation (organic binding) of iodide, decrease the proportion of DIT relative to MIT, and block coupling of iodotyrosines to form the hormonally active iodothyronines. The latter reaction is the most sensitive to inhibition by these agents. It is therefore possible for the synthesis of hormonally active iodothyronines to be decreased greatly, although the total incorporation of iodine by the thyroid is inhibited but little. Excessive concentrations of intrathyroidal iodide, such as follow acute administration of large quantities of iodide, also inhibit these oxidative reactions. Normally, this effect is transient; however, in a few peculiarly sensitive individuals, the antithyroid effect of iodide may persist and lead to development of goiter and myxedema. Pharmacologic quantities of iodide can also inhibit proteolysis of thyroglobulin. This effect is most readily demonstrable in hyperfunctioning thyroids and is responsible for the rapid ameliorative action of iodides in thyrotoxicosis.

In the bloodstream, T4 and T3 are almost entirely bound to plasma proteins. Electrophoretic analyses indicate that T4 is bound primarily to an interalpha-globulin termed *thyroxin-binding globulin*, or TBG, to a prealbumin, *thyroxin-binding prealbumin,* or TBPA, and to albumin in decreasing order of intensity. The interaction between T4 and its binding proteins conforms to a reversible binding equilibrium in which the majority of the hormone is bound and a very small proportion (normally less than 0.1 percent) is free. Since only the free or unbound hormone is available to tissues, the metabolic state of the patient will correlate more closely with the concentration of free hormone than with the total concentration of hormone. Furthermore, homeostatic regulation of thyroid function will be directed toward maintenance of a normal concentration of free rather than total hormone. Disturbances of the thyroid hormone–plasma protein interaction are of two general types (see Table 89-2). In the first, the thyroid-pituitary axis is intrinsically normal, and the homeostatic control of thyroid secretion is intact. Under these circumstances, disordered binding interactions result from primary alterations in the concentration or avidity of the thyroxin-binding proteins. For example, an increase in binding activity will lower the concentration of free hormones and thus diminish the quantity of hormones available to tissues. Total hormonal concentration in serum will then increase until the *concentration* of free hormones is restored to normal, but at this time, the proportion of hormones which is free will be decreased. The increase in total hormonal concentration counterbalances the decrease in the proportion which is free, with the result that the concentration of free hormones is normal and the metabolic state of the patient is unchanged. Converse changes occur when the binding of T4 by plasma proteins declines. The binding activity of TBG is increased in serum of normal pregnancy, during administration of estrogens, in patients with estrogen-secreting tumors, and in some patients with acute idiopathic porphyria. Binding activity of TBG is decreased in serum of patients given androgenic steroids, some anabolic drugs, or large doses of glucocorticoids; in nephrosis (where substantial quantities of TBG are lost in the urine); and in patients receiving hydantoins that are competitive inhibitors of T4-binding by TBG. Rarely,

the binding activity of TBG may be either increased or virtually absent for unknown reasons. Such idiopathic disorders of hormonal binding appear to be familial. The thyroxin-binding activity of TBPA is not known to be enhanced in any disease but is increased by anabolic steroids. It is decreased in patients with a wide variety of systemic diseases and by competitive inhibitors such as salicylates, dinitrophenol, or their congeners.

The second type of disturbance of thyroid hormone binding interaction results from primary alterations in the concentration of thyroid hormones in the blood such as occur in hypothyroidism or thyrotoxicosis. Here, homeostatic control of thyroid hormone secretion is disrupted and pathologic factors regulate hormonal secretion independent of the thyroid-pituitary axis. Under these circumstances, the activity of the thyroxin-binding proteins is changed little, if at all, and the concentration of free hormones will vary directly with the total concentration. Since such changes in circulating hormone usually result from intrinsic thyroidal disease, homeostatic mechanisms cannot restore the concentration of free hormones to normal. Primary changes in thyroidal function are therefore associated with persistent changes in the concentration of both total and free hormone, and therefore, with alterations in the anabolic status of the patient. In these disorders, the relative change on the *concentration* of free hormones is greater than the change in total hormones, with the result that the proportion of free hormones varies *pari passu* with the total hormonal concentration.

Because the free thyroid hormones in blood represent only a very small proportion of the total, even in abnormal states, the concentration of protein-bound hormone will closely reflect the total concentration of thyroid hormones in the blood. This is generally measured as the protein-bound iodine (PBI) or the serum thyroxin (serum T4). Direct measurement of the proportion of free thyroid hormones can be accomplished by dialysis techniques. The mathematical product of this value and the serum PBI or T4 will indicate the concentration of free T4. Dialysis methods for determining free T4 are technically difficult; however, a reflection of the proportion of free hormones can be obtained from one of the several in vitro triiodothyronine "uptake" methods such as the Resin sponge ^{131}I-triiodothyronine uptake test (Resin-T3, Triosorb). In a manner analogous to calculation of the absolute concentration of free T4, the product of the Resin-T3 and the PBI (or serum T4) yields the *free thyroxin index*. This value is proportional to the free T4 concentration and, like the free T4, by dialysis varies with the metabolic state of the patient.

Triiodothyronine is not bound by TBPA and is bound by TBG only weakly. As a consequence, the unbound proportion of T3 is normally eight to ten times greater than T4. T3 is, therefore, removed from the blood much more rapidly than T4, which accounts for its failure to contribute materially to the total hormonal iodine concentration in the blood and possibly for its more rapid onset and offset of action. Its binding characteristics, however, do not account fully for the fact that it has a three-to fourfold greater metabolic potency than thyroxin when administered orally.

In the normal individual, the metabolic state reflects a summation of the action of T4, which contributes substantially to PBI, and of T3, which does not. Therefore, when exogenous hormones are employed to treat hypothyroidism or to suppress endogenous thyroid function, a normal metabolic state will be associated with a slightly elevated PBI if T4 is used and with a subnormal PBI if T3 is employed. Under physiologic circumstances, normal levels of free thyroxin in serum are maintained via an intact thyroid-pituitary axis through a negative feedback (servo) relationship with TSH. However, under pathologic circumstances, such as in the thyrotoxicosis of Graves' disease or autonomous thyroid tumors, pituitary thyrotropin is inhibited fully by the elevated serum levels of free T4 and the excessive thyroidal hormone secretion results from stimulatory factors which are not suppressed by even high levels of free T4. In Graves' disease, the persistently excessive thyroid secretion appears to be mediated via a circulating immunoglobulin with prolonged TSH-like properties known as LATS (long-acting thyroid stimulator). Thyrotoxicosis also results from excessive secretion of autonomous thyroid tumors (as in single or multiple hyperfunctioning nodules) and, rarely, from multiple metastases of thyroid cancer. Thyroidal independence of pituitary thyrotropic activity in patients with thyrotoxicosis forms the basis for the thyroid suppression test. A separate serum factor has been postulated to be etiologically responsible for the ophthalmopathy associated with Graves' disease, but to date this has not been identified or characterized with certainty.

DIAGNOSTIC LABORATORY TESTS

Availability of a variety of useful laboratory tests makes possible accurate evaluation of thyroid hormone economy under diverse clinical circumstances (Table 89-1). For simplicity, such tests may be divided into two major categories: the first, *thyroid indices,* includes those which measure some aspect of thyroid hormone metabolism involving iodine, such as hormonal synthesis, secretion, or plasma concentration. The second category, *metabolic indices,* includes those tests which measure some metabolic action of thyroid hormones on cellular metabolism. Unfortunately, the latter are to a large extent influenced by a variety of nonthyroidal factors and therefore tend to be less specific.

The *basal metabolic rate* (BMR) measures oxygen consumption in the basal state and is expressed as a percentage of values found in normal individuals of the same age, sex, and body surface area. Nonthyroidal disorders that alter oxygen consumption must be excluded if this test is to be of diagnostic value. Febrile illnesses, leukemia, neoplasms, hypertension, congestive heart failure, aortic stenosis, diabetes, pheochromocytoma, chronic pulmonary insufficiency, polycythemia, or perforated eardrums may be associated with an increased BMR. The BMR is most helpful in following changes in oxygen con-

sumption in the same individual during therapy. Similarly, the serum cholesterol, creatine tolerance tests, photomotogram, and electrocardiogram are of ancillary but limited diagnostic value because of their nonspecificity.

The *serum protein–bound iodine* (PBI) usually reflects the concentration of circulating thyroid hormones and represents an excellent diagnostic laboratory test for estimating thyroid function in the absence of interfering substances. Under abnormal circumstances, the PBI may include iodinated materials of either endogenous or exogenous origin. These may be either iodinated proteins, as in lymphoid thyroiditis, or iodinated organic compounds, such as radiopaque contrast drugs, which bind to plasma proteins (usually albumin). The iodinated proteins can be separated physically from the thyroid hormones by a butanol extraction procedure (BEI). On the other hand, most organic iodinated compounds are also extracted by butanol and therefore measured by the BEI. Thyroid hormones can be distinguished from iodinated proteins and most organic iodinated compounds by column chromatographic techniques, particularly when the latter are not present in high concentration.

Serum Thyroxin (serum T4) can be assayed directly by a method which depends upon the ability of thyroxin (T4) extracted from serum to displace radioactive T4 from a protein mixture containing TBG (binding displacement analysis). This test requires no chemical determination of iodine and is therefore not influenced by iodinated contaminants or heavy metals such as mercury. Furthermore, the high specificity of TBG for T4 renders this test independent of endogenous iodinated substances other than T4. In view of this remarkable specificity, the serum T4 test is more widely applicable for most clinical situations than the PBI or BEI. The designation serum T4 will be used hereinafter for the measurement obtained by this method.

Serum "free" thyroxin (free T4) is an important constituent of the metabolically active T4 pool. The small fraction of the total serum T4 which circulates free can be measured directly by dialysis techniques using radioactive T4 added to serum samples. The product of free T4 *fraction* and the total serum T4 gives the *concentration* of free T4. According to current concepts, the free T4 concentration relates directly to the patient's metabolic status and to regulation of thyroid gland secretion via pituitary thyrotropin in most circumstances.

The *Resin-Triiodothyronine uptake* (Resin-T3) is used commonly as a diagnostic test of thyroid function. This in vitro test depends upon competitive binding for radioactive T3 between serum TBG and a resin. If the thyroid hormone binding sites on TBG are saturated with endogenous T3 and T4 or are not available for binding, the radioactive T3 added to the system will be bound preferentially by the resin and Resin-T3 "uptake" will be high, as in thyrotoxicosis or congenital TBG deficiency. The converse occurs when the TBG binding sites are undersaturated or available in excessive amounts as in myxedema or pregnancy. The Resin-T3 uptake is directly proportional to the fraction of free T4 in serum and inversely

Table 89-1. COMPARATIVE VALUES COMMONLY OBTAINED FOR TESTS OF
THYROID FUNCTION IN VARIOUS CLINICAL SITUATIONS

Diagnostic and Clinical Status	24-hr ^{131}I uptake, %	Serum PBI,* µg/100 ml	Serum T4† µg/100 ml	BMR, % normal standard	Resin T3‡ uptake, % normal control
Euthyroidism:					
Normal values	15–50	4–8	4–11	−15–+15	85–115
Pregnancy	Normal/high	High	High	+20–+25	Low
Iodide deficiency	High	Normal/low	Normal/low	Normal/low	Normal/low
Iodide therapy, 3.0 mg/day	Low	High	Normal	Normal	Normal
Thyroid, USP, >120 mg/day	Low	Normal/high	Normal/high	Normal/high	Normal/high
L-thyroxin, >0.4 mg/day	Low	Normal/high	Normal/high	Normal/high	Normal/high
L-triiodothyronine, >0.1 mg/day	Low	Low	Low	Normal/high	Normal/high
Congestive heart failure	Variable	Normal/low	Normal/low	Variable	Normal/high
Hyperthyroidism:					
Untreated	50–100	7–20	11–20	High	115–160
Pregnancy	High	High	High	High	Normal/high
Iodide therapy, >2.0 mg/day	Low	>20	5–15	High/normal	High/normal
Thyroid, USP, >120 mg/day§	>20	High	High	High	High
L-Thyroxin, 0.4 mg/day§	>20	High	High	High	High
L-Triiodothyronine, 0.1 mg/day§	>20	High	High	High	High
Antithyroid drug therapy (euthyroid)	Variable	Normal	Normal	Normal	Normal
Thyroiditis (acute):	Low	Normal/high	Normal/high	Normal/high	Normal/high
Myxedema (primary):					
Untreated	0–15	0–4	0–4	−20–−50	Low‡
Thyroid USP, 120 mg/day (euthyroid)	Low	Normal¶	Normal¶	Normal	Normal
L-Thyroxin, 0.4 mg/day-euthyroid	Low	Normal/high	Normal/high	Normal	Normal/high
L-Triiodothyronine, 0.1 mg/day (euthyroid)	Low	Low	Low	Normal	Normal

* The presence in serum of trace quantities of mercurial salts will render values for the PBI and BEI factitiously low by the usual methods. Normal values for the serum butanol–extractable iodine (BEI) and the serum T4 by column are 3.2 to 6.5 µg%.

† Serum T4 designates values obtained by the binding displacement method of Murphy and Pattee (J. Clin. Endoc. 26: 247, 1966).

‡ The Resin-T3 values listed here are for the resin sponge method (Triosorb, Abbott) expressed as a percent of a standard control serum. This test is also expressed as an absolute percent uptake with normal values ranging from 25 to 35 percent (See JAMA 202: 135, 1967). The Resin-T3 test is not generally diagnostic of hypothyroidism because of excessive overlap of values in the low normal range with those in hypothyroidism.

§ Suppression test (see text).

¶ The PBI and serum T4 values may be lower than normal in patients receiving some lots of desiccated thyroid, USP, or thyroglobulin (Proloid).

proportional to the available TBG binding sites. It is more readily performed than the direct measurement of the fraction of free T4 by dialysis and serves as a useful indirect measure thereof. Unfortunately, this test depends upon the integrity of the thyroxin-binding proteins and is thus influenced by factors which modify the quantity or binding affinity of these proteins. Common among these are wasting diseases, hepatitis, acidosis, pulmonary insufficiency, renal diseases, and supraventricular tachycardias. A "free T4 index" can be derived from the mathematical product of the concentration of serum T4 (or PBI) and the Resin-T3 uptake (see Table 89-2) in a manner analogous to calculating the actual concentration of free T4 in serum.

The *thyroidal* (^{131}I) *uptake* indicates the *proportion* of ingested iodide accumulated by the thyroid gland. A normal value suggests a physiologic rate of hormone syn-

thesis if it is assumed that the total quantity of iodide being metabolized is normal and that the iodide, once accumulated by the thyroid, is incorporated into active hormonal products. When body iodide stores are expanded, the ^{131}I uptake will almost invariably decrease, although the patient remains metabolically normal. The converse will occur in iodide deficiency.

The *thyroid suppression test* has come into wide clinical usage. This test reflects the integrity of the pituitary-thyroid mechanisms that maintain homeostasis, as described in an earlier section. It is based on the fact that when normal homeostatic mechanisms are disrupted, exogenous thyroid hormone will not suppress the patient's thyroid function. Abnormal tests are therefore found in patients with thyrotoxicosis resulting from hormonal overproduction, whatever its cause. In addition, abnormal tests reflect the physiologic disturbance which, in Graves'

Table 89-2. CLASSIFICATION OF THE VARIETIES OF
DISORDERED THYROID HORMONE-PLASMA
PROTEIN INTERACTIONS

Clinical condition	Total T4 (serum T4 or PBI)	Proportion free T4 (Resin-T3)	Concentration free T4 (free T4 index)
1. Primary Abnormality in Thyroid Binding Proteins			
a. Increased Binding	↑	↓	N
b. Decreased Binding	↓	↑	N
2. Primary Disorder of Thyroid Function			
a. Myxedema	↓	↓	↓
b. Thyrotoxicosis	↑	↑	↑

disease, may exist in the absence of thyrotoxicosis. Examples occur in some patients whose hyperthyroidism has been treated and in some exhibiting solely the ophthalmic manifestations of Graves' disease (hyperophthalmic Graves' disease).

The test is usually performed using a standard dose of liothyronine (sodium L-triiodothyronine). After an initial radioactive iodine uptake (usually at 24 hr), the patient is given a course of liothyronine, 100 μg daily. On the seventh day of liothyronine administration, the radioactive iodine uptake is repeated. If, after appropriate correction for residual radioactivity, the 24-hr radioactive iodine uptake is less than 20 percent, thyrotropin suppression is presumed. Values above 20 percent in 24 hr indicate a disturbance of homeostatic control such as in Graves' disease or autonomous thyroid tumors. Since technical factors vary, the test should be standardized for each laboratory. Desiccated thyroid or sodium L-thyroxin in calorigenically equivalent doses can also be used. It is generally inadvisable to undertake this test in patients over the age of fifty or in those with potential or actual cardiac or vascular disease, since the excessive metabolic activity induced by thyroid hormone stimulation may induce atrial fibrillation, cardiac failure, or vascular accidents. The thyroid suppression test is particularly helpful in the differential diagnosis of various forms of goiter in young adults. It is also useful in evaluating whether the homeostatic disturbance persists in thyrotoxic patients who have been treated.

The *thyrotropin stimulation test* (TSH test) is useful to distinguish primary thyroidal failure, either complete or partial (decreased thyroid reserve) from thyroid hypofunction caused by inadequate TSH stimulation. The latter may result from either intrinsic pituitary disease or from pituitary suppression by exogenous hormone. An increase in radioactive iodine uptake of 10 to 15 percent or more or a rise in serum PBI of more than 1.5 to 2.0 μg per 100 ml indicates that the thyroid gland can respond to exogenous TSH stimulation. The usual dosage of thyrotropin, USP (Thytropar, Armour) is 5 or 10 units given as a single intramuscular injection to determine primary thyroid insufficiency or diminished thyroid reserve. In pituitary failure, this dosage may be insufficient due to thyroidal refractoriness, and doses of 15 to 30 units can be given over a 24 to 48 hr period, 5 to 10 units each 12 to 24 hr. The second uptake test or PBI is obtained 24 hr after the last dose of TSH. Absence of a measurable response to TSH may be caused by several factors but is most commonly the result of primary thyroid failure.

Immunoreactive thyrotropin (TSH) can be measured in serum directly by radioimmunoassay. Although this assay has been of assistance in confirming pathophysiologic concepts of thyroid-pituitary interaction, it is not available generally for clinical testing.

Values for the 24-hr thyroidal radioactive iodine uptake, serum PBI, and serum T4 as well as the in vitro resin-triiodothyronine uptake test are listed in Table 89-1 for common clinical situations. Despite the specificity of these tests, numerous factors may alter their absolute value and yield a result inconsistent either with other results or with the clinical condition of the patient. Modification of test results by extraneous factors most commonly follows administration of iodine, in either organic or inorganic form. Here, high values for tests measuring serum iodine levels and low thyroidal uptakes of ^{131}I are seen. Under such circumstances, the tests of serum T4 and hormonal binding (RBC-T3 and Resin-T3 are useful, since they are not influenced by nonhormonal iodinated compounds. The presence of mercury in serum will produce factitiously low values for PBI and BEI but will not alter the serum T4 or binding tests. On the other hand, systemic disorders and drugs that alter protein binding also affect the values for the RBC-T3 and Resin-T3 tests. Liver disease, cachexia, pulmonary insufficiency, acidosis, androgens, anticoagulants, and anticonvulsants produce increases in the RBC-T3 or Resin-T3 uptake test. Contrariwise, estrogens and pregnancy reduce these uptake tests. Under these circumstances, the values reported differ from the patient's clinical status. When there is some apparent contradiction in the values for different tests, the explanation can usually be found by a careful history of drug ingestion and by a physiologic interpretation of the observed facts.

SIMPLE (NONTOXIC) GOITER

There is considerable confusion concerning the descriptive terms *endemic* and *sporadic goiter*. Endemic implies an etiologic factor or factors common to a particular geographic region. The term has been defined as the presence of generalized or localized thyroid enlargement in over 10 percent of the population. The connotation of sporadic is that goiter arises in nonendemic areas as a result of a stimulus that does not affect the population generally. Since these terms fail to define or distinguish the causes of such goiters and since thyroid enlargement of diverse etiology may exist in both endemic and nonendemic regions, it seems prudent to employ a general term such as *simple* or *nontoxic goiter*. This all-inclusive category can be further subdivided into specific etiologic groups as defined by objective procedures. Simple or nontoxic goiter may be defined as any enlargement of the thyroid gland that does not result from an inflammatory or neoplastic process and does not lead to thyrotoxicosis or myxedema.

HISTORY. Goitrous enlargement of the thyroid gland has been recognized since antiquity by many cultures in diverse parts of the world. Its existence has been documented in historic accounts dating back to the fifteenth century B.C. and has been incorporated into the art, literature, and folklore of many cultures. By the nineteenth century, goiter became recognized medically as a common entity in many geographic areas, particularly in mountainous regions such as the Pyrenees, Alps, Carpathians, Himalayas, Sierras, and Andes. Cretinism was described in many goitrous regions of the world and, in the Americas, was noted in pre-Columbian art forms.

Iodine was discovered in the residue of burned seaweed by Courtois in 1812 and identified as a new element by Gay-Lussac. It has been used empirically for therapy of goiter since ancient times. In 1896, iodine was found to be a normal constituent of the thyroid gland by Baumann, but it was not until 1915 that Kendall isolated L-thyroxin. The chemical structure of this hormone was determined and proved by chemical synthesis in 1927 by Harington and Barger. A second hormonal constituent of the thyroid gland, L-triiodothyronine, was isolated and identified in 1952 by Roche, Lissitsky, and Michel in France and by Gross and Pitt-Rivers in England. Coindet in 1820 first described in scientific fashion the results of iodide therapy before the Swiss Society of Natural Sciences. However, because of complications of overdosage and the poor comprehension of thyroid disease prevalent at that time, iodine therapy failed acceptance by most physicians for the next century. The important relationship of iodine deficiency to goiter was renewed through the devoted labors of Marine who in 1905 began a systematic investigation of this association. His research reached a peak of excellence in 1917 when Marine and Kimball initiated the now classic controlled study of elementary school children in Akron, Ohio and concluded several years later that iodide deficiency was a major cause of goiter and that such goiters could be prevented by supplementation of dietary iodine. Despite this remarkable discovery, most nations have yet to pass adequate legislation to guarantee this important dietary mineral to all people. It was estimated by the World Health Organization in 1960 that approximately 200 million people were goitrous. The incidence varies with the prevalence of dietary iodine and has tended to decrease with the introduction of iodine as a public health measure. It is, however, still a major public health problem even in highly industrialized countries, despite a concerted, albeit inadequate, effort to reduce the high incidence of goiter by dietary measures.

ETIOLOGY. Although the causes of simple goiter are manifold, their clinical manifestations reflect the operation of a common pathophysiologic mechanism. Simple goiter results when one or more factors impair the capacity of the thyroid, in the basal state, to secrete sufficient quantities of physiologically active hormones to meet the needs of peripheral tissues. Under these conditions, secretion of TSH is enhanced, and this stimulates both glandular growth and the activity of all intrathyroidal reactions involved in synthesis and secretion of thyroid hormone. Such compensatory increases in functioning thyroidal mass and stimulation of cellular activity are sufficient to overcome mild or moderate impairments of hormonal synthesis, and the patient remains metabolically normal although goitrous. When, however, impairment of hormonal synthesis is severe, compensatory responses are inadequate and the patient is both goitrous and more or less severely hypothyroid. Thus, the entity of simple goiter cannot be separated clearly, in the pathogenetic sense, from goitrous hypothyroidism. Specific causes of simple goiter are included in Table 89-3 and may exist with or without hypothyroidism.

PATHOLOGY. The histopathology of the thyroid in simple goiter will vary with the severity of the etiologic factor and the stage of the disorder at which the examination is made. In its initial stages, the gland will reveal a uniform hypertrophy, hyperplasia, and hypervascularity. As the disorder persists or undergoes repeated exacerbations and remissions, uniformity of thyroidal architecture is usually lost. Occasionally, the greater part of the gland may display a reasonably uniform degree of involution or hyperinvolution with colloid accumulation. More often such areas are interspersed with patchy areas of focal hyperplasia. Fibrosis may demarcate a variable number of nodules, which may be hyperplastic or involuted; these may resemble, but do not really represent, true neoplasms (adenomas). Areas of hemorrhage and calcification may be present.

CLINICAL PICTURE. In simple goiter, the clinical manifestations arise solely from enlargement of the thyroid, since the metabolic state of the patient is normal. In goitrous hypothyroidism, symptoms caused by thyromegaly are similarly present but are accompanied by signs and symptoms of hormonal insufficiency. Mechanical sequelae include compression and displacement of the trachea or esophagus, occasionally with obstructive symptoms if the goiter becomes sufficiently large. Superior mediastinal obstruction may occur with large intrathoracic goiters. Signs of compression can be induced in the case of large cervical goiters when the patient's arms are raised above the head (Pemberton's sign); suffusion of the face, giddiness, or syncope may result from this maneuver. Compression of the recurrent laryngeal nerve leading to hoarseness is rare in simple goiter and suggests neoplasm. Sudden hemorrhage into a nodule may lead to an acute, painful swelling in the neck and may produce or enhance compressive symptoms. Hyperthyroidism not uncommonly supervenes in long-standing multinodular goiter (toxic multinodular goiter). It is not known whether this represents the superimposition of Graves' disease upon a chronic nontoxic goiter or a separate disease entity.

In geographic regions where iodine deficiency is severe,

acquired goitrous enlargement may also be associated with varying degrees of hypothyroidism. Cretinism, both goitrous and nongoitrous, occurs with increased frequency in the children of goitrous parents, and contributes a significant sector of the socially dependent population in many countries where goiter is common. The association of deaf-mutism, goiter, and varying degrees of mental retardation has been termed *Pendred's syndrome*.

DIAGNOSIS. The *diagnosis* of simple goiter can often be suspected on clinical grounds. However, other goitrous conditions such as forms of chronic thyroiditis, drug or iodide goiter, or primary thyroid neoplasms, cannot always be excluded by the consistency, size, or symmetry of the enlargement. A careful history is important to determine the prevalence of thyroidal pain and tenderness, drug ingestion, rapid changes in size, or hoarseness. High titers of circulating thyroglobulin antibodies suggest but do not necessarily indicate lymphoid thyroiditis (Hashimoto's struma). At times, needle biopsy of the thyroid is indicated to confirm or exclude the diagnosis of thyroiditis, but it should not be used if thyroid cancer is suspected. Laboratory tests of thyroid function in the inhabitants of countries where goiter is highly endemic (greater than 10 percent of the population) may vary considerably. An elevated thyroidal uptake of radioactive iodine often accompanies low levels of inorganic serum and urinary iodide. Serum T4 (and PBI) levels are usually in the low normal range or may be moderately reduced if hypothyroidism coexists.

TREATMENT. The object of treatment is to remove the stimulus of thyroidal hyperplasia, either by relieving external encumbrances to hormone formation or by providing sufficient quantities of exogenous hormone to inhibit TSH and thereby put the thyroid gland almost completely at rest. In disorders characterized by decreased thyroidal iodide stores, such as iodine deficiency or impairment of the thyroidal iodide–concentrating mechanism, small doses of iodide may prove effective. Occasionally, a known extrinsic goitrogen can be withdrawn. Most commonly, however, no specific etiologic factor can be detected, and *suppressive thyroid therapy* is required. For this purpose, desiccated thyroid in dosage usually ranging from 120 to 180 mg is the agent of choice. Purified hormones such as the sodium salts of thyroxin or triiodothyronine are equally effective metabolically but may render it difficult to assess overdosage through measurement of the PBI. Suppression of endogenous thyroid function is most readily assessed by serial measurements of the 24-hr thyroidal uptake of ^{131}I. Partial suppression is indicated when ^{131}I uptake is reduced below control values and complete suppression when the 24-hr uptake falls below 10 percent. In multinodular, nontoxic goiter, lack of complete suppression usually indicates the presence of autonomously functioning foci, demonstrable by scanning techniques. Radioactive iodine uptake studies can be obtained at appropriate intervals and the dose of exogenous hormone gradually adjusted as needed to achieve maximum suppression. Occasionally, physiologic replacement doses of exogenous hormones will induce mild but usually transient symptoms of thyrotoxicity. In such patients, more prolonged intervals between dosage changes will usually permit achievement of full thyroid suppression without inducing symptoms of toxicity.

Reported results of therapy vary widely. There is general agreement that the early diffuse, hyperplastic goiter responds well, with regression or disappearance in 3 to 6 months. In the authors' experience, the later, nodular stage responds less favorably, and significant reduction in gland size is achieved in approximately half the cases. Internodular tissue regresses more often than do nodules themselves. The latter may therefore become more prominent during treatment. After maximum regression of the goiter, suppressive medication may be maintained for prolonged periods, reduced to minimal levels, or at times withdrawn. In an unpredictable manner, goiter will in some cases remain relieved while in others it will recur. In the latter instances, suppressive therapy should be reinstituted and should be continued indefinitely. When treatment is initiated in patients of childbearing age, it should probably be continued through the menopause.

Surgical therapy of simple goiter is physiologically unsound, but it may occasionally be necessary to relieve obstructive symptoms, especially those which persist after a conscientious trial of medical therapy. Surgical exploration of nodular goiter may be indicated in some individuals when evidence suggests carcinoma. However, the suggestion that subtotal resection of multinodular, nontoxic goiter affords effective prophylaxis against the development of thyroidal carcinoma is unsound. If for some reason subtotal thyroidectomy has been performed, use of physiologic replacement doses of desiccated thyroid, 120 to 180 mg daily, is recommended to inhibit regenerative hyperplasia and further goitrogenesis.

HYPOTHYROIDISM

HISTORY. The concept that sporadic cretinism is caused by absence of the thyroid gland was first expressed by Dr. C. H. Fagge at Guy's Hospital in 1871. In 1874, Gull described adult myxedema, stating that it resembled cretinism but occurred in adult life. The term *myxedema*, or *mucous edema*, has been credited to Ord (1878). During the subsequent 4 to 5 years, the Reverdin brothers, of Geneva, and Kocher, of Berne, observed that following thyroidectomy for goiter there appeared what they termed *postoperative myxedema* or *cachexia strumipriva*. The striking effects of thyroid replacement therapy in myxedematous patients were described in 1891 by Murray, who was the first to administer a glycerin extract of animal thyroid. The next year, Mackenzie and Fox noted independently that animal thyroid was equally effective by mouth, and for over 75 years this natural hormone has been used extensively. Standardization of desiccated thyroid was introduced into the U.S. Pharmocopoeia in 1915 and persists to the current edition. Synthetic L-thyroxin was reintroduced into therapy around 1953 after a commercially feasible synthesis was devised by Hems and his associates. Use of L-triiodothyronine (liothyronine) followed shortly thereafter.

INCIDENCE. Cretinism is rare. The incidence of myxedema (juvenile and adult) is estimated to be 1 in every 1,500 hospital admissions. Adult myxedema occurs about five times as frequently in women as in men and most frequently between the ages of thirty and sixty years.

ETIOLOGY. Hypothyroidism may be either primary (thyroid gland failure) or secondary (anterior pituitary failure) (Table 89-3). Primary hypothyroidism dating

Table 89-3. CLASSIFICATION OF HYPOTHYROIDISM

I. Primary (sporadic and endemic)
  A. Nongoitrous
    1. Idiopathic
    2. Postablative (surgery, radiation)
    3. Postinflammatory
  B. Goitrous
    1. Congenital and hereditary defects
      a. Trapping
      b. Organification
      c. Coupling
      d. Dehalogenation
      e. Release
      f. Maternal-induced (iodide, antithyroid compounds)
    2. Acquired
      a. Iodides (excess or lack)
      b. Drugs (thiocyanates, PASA, butazolidine, cobalt)
      c. Natural goitrogens (food, milk)
      d. Thyroiditis (Hashimoto's)
II. Secondary
  A. Pituitary failure
  B. Transport abnormalities
  C. Utilization defects (hypothetic)

from birth results in a clinical picture characteristic of cretinism. Two varieties of cretinism can be distinguished, athyreotic and goitrous. In areas of endemic goiter, cretinism is common and is usually, but not invariably, goitrous. The sporadic cretinism of nonendemic areas is usually athyreotic but may be goitrous. In the latter patients, hereditary disorders of thyroid hormone biogenesis can usually be identified. Deaf-mutism is a common accompaniment of cretinism and, when associated with goiter, has been termed *Pendred's syndrome.*

The occurrence of primary thyroid deficiency later in life gives rise to the syndromes of juvenile and adult myxedema. Under these circumstances, inadequate production of thyroid hormones results from destruction of the thyroid gland by disease, atrophy, or ablative procedures (thyroidectomy, radioactive iodine therapy, or external radiation). Secondary hypothyroidism results from a deficiency of pituitary TSH and may occur at any age as a consequence of anterior pituitary failure (Chap. 87).

A classification of the more important pathophysiologic etiologies of hypothyroidism is presented in Table 89-3.

The most frequent cause of spontaneous hypothyroidism is idiopathic atrophy of the thyroid gland. In children, this may result from developmental abnormalities. In adults, such atrophy may represent the final stage of an autoimmune response to thyroglobulin or other thyroid antigens and may therefore be related to one form of chronic thyroiditis, struma lymphomatosa (Hashimoto's struma). Circulating thyroid antibodies may be detected in a majority of patients with spontaneous hypothyroidism (see under Thyroiditis). Postthyroidectomy and postradiation hypothyroidism occur more frequently than the spontaneous varieties, and radioactive iodine therapy of hyperthyroidism is currently the most common cause of hypothyroidism. Occasionally, in patients who have undergone thyroid ablative procedures or have experienced chronic thyroid inflammation, thyroid function is not completely abolished but is insufficient to meet peripheral hormonal needs. Such patients, who may have mild symptoms of hypothyroidism, can be distinguished by their failure to respond to TSH and have been described as having decreased thyroid reserve.

CLINICAL PICTURE. The general appearance of children with hypothyroidism varies considerably, depending on the age at which the deficiency begins and the promptness of replacement therapy. Signs and symptoms of cretinism may be clinically evident at birth, or more commonly, within the first several neonatal months, depending upon the completeness of thyroid failure. These children are dwarfed, stocky, and somewhat overweight, with a broad flat nose, eyes set apart because of failure of nasoorbital development, coarse features with thick lips, protruding tongue, pale mottled skin, poor muscular tone and intestinal activity, spadelike stubby hands with x-ray evidence of retarded bone age and epiphyseal dysgenesis, delayed eruption of teeth, and malocclusion resulting from macroglossia. *In infancy, the characteristic facies, the hoarse cry, the large tongue, the "potbelly" and the presence of an umbilical hernia should call attention to the diagnosis of severe degrees of thyroid deficiency. Diagnosis and treatment at the earliest possible date in infancy are important,* since the extent of mental retardation may be related to the age at which treatment is instituted. Good results are obtained only when the diagnosis is established early and adequate therapy is instituted at once. If therapy is delayed, most of the clinical features of cretinism may still be reversed but some degree of mental retardation usually persists.

The adult and older child with myxedema have a typical facies, characterized by a dull, uninterested expression and puffy eyelids, often with alopecia of the outer third of the eyebrows. The skin of the face exhibits creamy pallor, and occasionally there is palmar yellowing. The changes in coloring result from anemia combined with carotenemia. The skin elsewhere on the body is dry and rough. The subcutaneous tissue is indurated and doughy because of interstitial fluid of high protein content. The hair is brittle and dry. There is swelling of the tongue and larynx and a halting, slurred, hoarse speech with slowing of physical and, seemingly, of mental activity. Anemia, constipation, and increased sensitivity to cold are present as well as increased capillary fragility, as evidenced by susceptibility to bruising. Women with myxedema during the active ovarian cycle usually note prolonged or excessive menstrual bleeding. Some patients with hypothroidism complain of constant rhinorrhea, coryza, or deafness. There may also be arthralgia, symptoms indistinguishable from those of peripheral neuropathy, signs and symptoms of cerebellar disturbance, muscular weakness, or myotonia.

The cardiac silhouette is usually larger than normal, partially because of dilation but mostly from pericardial effusion, which is commonly present. Rarely, the cardiac silhouette may be small; if so, pituitary myxedema should be considered. Thyroid tissue is rarely palpable except in presence of chronic thyroiditis, endemic goiter, goitrogen ingestion, or goitrous cretinism. Skeletal growth is usually normal in the adult patient with myxedema, but in children or adolescents both growth and skeletal maturation are usually retarded significantly. The relaxation time of the deep tendon reflexes is characteristically slowed in patients with myxedema. Severe ileus with a picture of megacolon is also seen. Rarely, psychoses (myxedema madness) may dominate the clinical picture in patients with myxedema. Untreated patients with profound degrees of myxedema may exhibit hypothermic coma (myxedema coma), a serious and usually fatal complication. Some features of myxedema coma are related to respiratory depression and consequent CO_2 narcosis. Occasional hyponatremia, not responsive to glucocorticoids, is present and may represent a form of refractive dilutional hyponatremia. Hydrothorax, ascites, and pericardial effusions of high protein content are not uncommon.

DIAGNOSIS. Laboratory examinations in primary thyroid atrophy usually reveal a low basal metabolic rate, elevated serum cholesterol level, low plasma protein-bound iodine or serum T4, low resin T3 uptake of labeled triiodothyronine, and decreased radioiodine uptake in the thyroid. Extraneous factors that may modify the plasma PBI level or the radioiodine uptake of the gland are enumerated in Table 89-2. In some varieties of goitrous hypothyroidism, the thyroid uptake of radioactive iodine may be increased. In those in whom ^{131}I remains unbound, it may be discharged from the gland after administration of potassium thiocyanate or perchlorate.

It is noteworthy that the spinal fluid protein concentration may be elevated in patients with profound myxedema. There may be a significant normocytic or slightly macrocytic anemia as well as gastric achlorhydria. When losses of iron are excessive, such as may occur with menorrhagia, a picture of hypochromic anemia may predominate. The electrocardiograph may reveal a marked decrease in voltage with flattened or inverted T waves. Serum enzyme levels are often increased in myxedema, the lactic dehydrogenase (LDH) usually being elevated to a greater extent than the creative phosphokinase (CPK) or glutamic oxaloacetic transaminase (SGOT). These findings may be confusing when myocardial infarction is suspected as a complication in myxedema, particularly since this elevation results principally from the cardiac isoenzymes of LDH. Serum uric acid may also be elevated in myxedema.

The signs and symptoms of mild or moderate hypothyroidism are less striking. The symptoms are similar to those in frank myxedema but are less severe. Such symptoms are, however, readily confused with those of many other organic or psychogenic disturbances. Even the BMR may be low for reasons other than the presence of thyroid disease. It is important, therefore, to establish the diagnosis of true, mild hypothyroidism on the basis of objective criteria. Such criteria may be met either by the finding of subnormal values for serum T4, PBI, Resin T3 uptake, and the thyroidal ^{131}I uptake or, in the presence of marginal values for these tests, by their failure to increase after TSH.

Hypothyroidism secondary to anterior pituitary deficiency may present a picture indistinguishable from that of primary myxedema. However, the accumulation of subcutaneous fluid (myxedema fluid) is usually not so pronounced in patients with pituitary myxedema as in those with primary myxedema. Careful investigation will usually reveal associated gonadal and adrenocortical deficiency out of proportion to that seen in primary myxedema. In general, the serum cholesterol level is within, or close to, normal limits in patients with hypothyroidism secondary to anterior pituitary failure, whereas it is usually elevated in primary myxedema. Patients with primary myxedema respond readily and satisfactorily to thyroid replacement therapy. In contrast, administration of this hormone to patients with pituitary myxedema is usually less effective and may precipitate adrenal crisis. The administration of TSH to patients with pituitary hypothyroidism is usually followed in 24 hr by a rise in the thyroidal uptake of radioactive iodine and in serum protein–bound iodine or serum T4.

DIFFERENTIAL DIAGNOSIS. Little difficulty will be experienced in diagnosing classic cretinism or juvenile and adult myxedema. Occasionally, a mongoloid infant may be confused with a cretin. However, the characteristic mongoloid eyes, hyperextensibility of the finger joints, and normal skin and hair texture distinguish the mongoloid imbecile from the hypothyroid cretin. Chronic nephritis and especially nephrosis may simulate myxedema. This is particularly true of the chronic uremic patient with retarded mental acuity and characteristic facial expression. In nephrosis, the basal metabolic rate is usually below normal as is the level of the serum PBI, or serum T4. Since the nephrotic patient may also exhibit anemia, hypercholesterolemia, and anasarca (simulating myxedema fluid), the differential diagnosis may be confusing. However, the uptake of radioactive iodine is usually normal in nephrotic patients, the low level of serum PBI or serum T4 being caused by a decrease in throxin- binding proteins in the blood, resulting from proteinuria. The hyperactive deep tendon reflexes of the uremic patient, as contrasted with the slowed relaxation phase of the reflexes in patients with myxedema, may aid in distinguishing the two conditions. Not infrequently hypothyroid patients exhibit anemia and clinically resemble patients with pernicious anemia. Though usually separate, myxedema and pernicious anemia may coexist; recent evidence suggests that they may share related immunologic abnormalities.

Patients with secondary hypothyroidism, because of attendant adrenocortical failure, must be distinguished carefully from patients with primary myxedema. Urinary 17-ketosteroid and 17-hydroxycorticoid excretion may be reduced in both conditions, and the response to the 2-day ACTH test may occasionally be misleading in differentiating these conditions (see Chap. 87). The finding of elevated levels of urinary FSH, a normal water-loading test, and a good response to metyrapone (SU-4885) helps distinguish primary myxedema from anterior pituitary failure. In addition, the rise in serum immunocreative growth hormone (HGH) in response to insulin-induced hypoglycemia or arginine infusion is characteristically absent in panhypopituitarism, but present in primary myxedema. Although the patient with Addison's disease is frequently hypometabolic, absence of excessive pigmentation, a normal water-loading response, and low values for PBI, serum T4, and radioactive iodine uptake help distinguish myxedema from Addison's disease.

Table 89-4. APPROXIMATE EQUIVALENT DOSES OF VARIOUS THYROID PREPARATIONS

Preparation	Average daily oral maintenance dose, mg*	Serum PBI†
Thyroid, USP.........	120–180	Normal
L-Thyroxin (T4).......	0.3–0.4	Slightly elevated
L-Triiodothyronine (T3).............	0.075–0.125	Depressed
L-T4+L-T3........... (Liotrix)	L-T4:0.20–L-T4:0.180 L-T3:0.030–L-T3:0.045	Normal

* Infants and children require proportionally larger doses of thyroid preparations than adults.

† Serum levels of PBI vary according to preparation used and may not be a direct measure of thyroid hormone effect (see text).

TREATMENT. Desiccated thyroid (thyroid, USP) is the most commonly used preparation and is usually administered in 30-, 60-, 120-, or 180-mg tablets. Its major disadvantage is inadequate standardization of hormonal content. Sodium L-thyroxin is available as 0.05-, 0.1-, 0.2- and 0.3-mg tablets (Synthroid, Flint), and sodium L-triiodothyronine is marketed in 0.005-, 0.025-, and 0.050-mg tablets (Cytomel). A new combination containing synthetic sodium L-thyroxine and sodium L-triiodothyronine in a ratio of 4:1 by weight (Euthroid) has been introduced to obviate some of the problems inherent in the standardization of thyroid, USP. Serum T4, PBI, and resin T3 uptake tests in patients receiving this synthetic

thyroid combination are usually representative of their metabolic status. The average daily maintenance dosages of these preparations are listed in Table 89-4. Some commercially available lots of UTP thyroid, as well as some lots of a thyroglobulin preparation (Proloid) give levels of PBI lower than anticipated by the patient's metabolic status. This is presumably a result of increased ratio of triiodothyronine to thyroxin in these preparations.

In all instances, except perhaps in myxedema coma, it is desirable to institute therapy with relatively small doses of a thyroid substance, since sudden changes in metabolic level may induce undesirable psychologic or cardiovascular disturbances, especially in elderly patients. The occurrence of angina pectoris or congestive heart failure during therapy for myxedema is an indication to proceed with caution, since rapid changes in metabolic rate may precipitate as well as increase the severity of these conditions. In adults, one may begin with a dose of 15 mg USP thyroid or less per day, gradually increasing the dosage at weekly or biweekly intervals. In patients over forty or fifty years of age, thyroid therapy should be given cautiously with longer intervals between increments in dosage. The usual daily dose of desiccated thyroid necessary to maintain an athyreotic patient in euthyroidism is 90 to 180 mg. In the presence of any evidence of cardiovascular disease, the total dosage should not exceed 30 to 60 mg daily until the patient has been followed for several weeks at this level. The maximum effect from a given dosage level will not be obtained for at least 7 to 10 days, and thyroid hormone action will persist for several weeks after the last dose. It is not necessary to give desiccated thyroid more than once daily. Because of its relatively more rapid onset and shorter duration of action, triiodothyronine may be given in divided doses.

In many patients, generalized muscular aching follows initiation of therapy regardless of the dosage of thyroid hormone, and occasionally coryza is noted. It is essential in patients with cretinism or juvenile myxedema to maintain therapy at close to toxic levels in order to ensure the desired growth response. The requirement for optimum bone growth appears to be higher than that usually needed for satisfactory maintenance of the overall clinical status. Children need somewhat more thyroid in proportion to their size than do adults. Dosage usually must be adjusted according to clinical evaluation of the effects obtained, at the same time avoiding symptoms of overdosage such as tachycardia, irritability, continuous weight loss, diarrhea, or sweating. In panhypopituitarism, thyroid hormone therapy should *not* be instituted until after adrenocortical replacement therapy has been initiated. The initial dose of desiccated thyroid should be small and increased gradually by 15-mg increments at 3-week intervals.

It should be noted that patients with untreated myxedema, like patients with Addison's disease, are extremely sensitive to the pharmacologic actions of many drugs such as narcotics, barbiturates, and tranquilizers as well as to most stressful situations such as operations. Patients with myxedema coma should be treated with parenteral triiodothyronine, adrenocortical steriods, artificial respiration (if CO_2 narcosis exists), and correction of any electrolyte disturbances.

HYPERTHYROIDISM

The terms *hyperthyroidism* and *thyrotoxicosis* usually denote the complex of physiologic and biochemical disturbances that result when the tissues are exposed to excessive quantities of thyroid hormones. This occurs most commonly in association with diffuse hyperplasia of the thyroid gland often accompanied by specific ophthalmic abnormalities and is usually designated *Graves' disease*. It is also termed *Parry's* or *Basedow's disease*. It should be recognized, however, that hyperthyroidism may result from overproduction of thyroid hormone by a hyperfunctioning adenoma, multinodular goiter (Plummer's disease), or ectopic thyroid tissue. The peripheral features of hyperthyroidism also result when thyroid medication is taken in excess (thyrotoxicosis factitia). The following discussion will deal mainly with Graves' disease. In addition, features of other disorders that may produce hyperthyroidism will be discussed.

HISTORY. In 1786, Dr. Caleb Parry described a disease characterized by thyroid enlargement, dilatation of the heart, palpitation, exophthalmos, and nervous as well as menstrual symptoms. Graves and Basedow, between the years 1835 and 1843, published treatises independently on the syndrome that now bears their names. That hyperthyroidism was the fundamental disorder in Graves' disease was formulated by Möbius in Germany in 1887. The use of iodine in the treatment of thyrotoxicosis was popularized by Plummer. Recent advances in the medical therapy of hyperthyroidism include the introduction in 1942 of antithyroid substances such as derivatives of thiourea and imidazole. Radioactive iodine, introduced in 1942, now occupies a prominent position as a therapeutic agent in the treatment of thyrotoxicosis.

INCIDENCE. Graves' disease is a relatively common disorder which may occur at any age but occurs especially in the third and fourth decades. The disease is much more frequent in women than in men. In nongoitrous areas the ratio of predominance in females may be as high as 8:1. In endemic goitrous areas the ratio is lower. Hyperthyroidism is comparatively rare in children. When it occurs, there is usually a diffuse goiter free of nodules.

ETIOLOGY. Basic to Graves' disease is a derangement of those homeostatic mechanisms that normally adjust thyroid hormone secretion to meet the physiologic needs of the peripheral tissues. In the past, it was suggested that this homeostatic disruption resulted from either overproduction of TSH by the pituitary or development of autonomous hyperfunction within the thyroid itself. The weight of evidence now indicates, however, that neither is the case. Rather, thyroidal hyperfunction in Graves' disease appears to result from the action of an hormonotropic serum globulin called the "long-acting thyroid stimulator" (LATS). Under appropriate bioassay conditions, LATS is demonstrable in the serum of approximately 90 percent of thyrotoxic patients with Graves'

disease. Its designation as LATS derives from the fact that in the test system its action is more prolonged than that of TSH. The initial action of LATS on thyroidal iodine metabolism is to stimulate hormonal release, but it is also capable of increasing ^{131}I uptake and inducing thyroidal hyperplasia. Like thyrotropin, it stimulates several aspects of thyroid intermediate metabolism. It has not been possible, by means of available fractionation techniques, to separate LATS from other 7S gamma-globulins of plasma. Furthermore, the action of LATS on the thyroid is inhibited by antibodies to normal human 7S gamma-globulin, but not antibodies to TSH. Although the nature of the putative antigen is unknown, these findings suggest that LATS is itself an antibody to some cytologic component of the thyroid. If so, Graves' disease should be included among those disorders associated with, if not necessarily caused by, autoimmune phenomena. Titers of LATS in the patient's serum do not correlate completely with the presence or absence of thyrotoxicosis or with its degree of severity. Indeed, some authorities believe that titers of LATS correlate best with the presence and severity of ophthalmopathy or pretibial myxedema. Hence, it is likely that factors other than LATS also serve to condition the state of thyroid function in Graves' disease.

PATHOLOGY. In Graves' disease the thyroid gland is diffusely enlarged bilaterally, soft, and vascular. The essential pathology is that of parenchymatous hypertrophy and hyperplasia, characterized by increased height of the epithelium and redundancy of the follicular wall, giving the picture of papillary infoldings and cytologic evidence of increased activity. Such hyperplasia is usually accompanied by lymphocytic infiltration. In hyperthyroidism associated with nodular goiters (Plummer's disease), the major part of the thyroid tissue shows colloid involutional changes with hyperplastic paranodular areas that exhibit the functional changes responsible for the hyperthyroidism. This type of gland is thought to represent the end stage of an involuted nodular goiter and is erroneously termed *toxic adenoma*. True thyroid tumors (adenomas) that produce hyperfunction occur only rarely; in these, the paranodular tissue is inactive. Following iodine medication, there is colloid storage, which sometimes causes enlargement and increased firmness of the gland. Graves' disease is associated with generalized lymphoid hyperplasia and infiltration. Thyrotoxicosis may lead to degeneration of skeletal muscle fibers, enlargement of the heart, fatty infiltration or diffuse fibrosis of the liver, decalcification of the skeleton, and loss of body tissue (including fat deposits, osteoid, and muscle).

CLINICAL PICTURE. Common manifestations of Graves' disease include exophthalmos, goiter, fine tremor (especially of the extended fingers and tongue), increased nervousness as well as emotional instability, excessive sweating and heat intolerance, palpitations, and hyperkinesis. Loss of weight and of strength usually exist, often despite increased appetite. Hyperdefecation and occasionally anorexia, nausea, and vomiting may occur. Dyspnea, paroxysmal arrhythmias, and in individuals over the age of forty, cardiac failure occur not infrequently.

Oligomenorrhea and amenorrhea are commoner than menorrhagia. In general, nervous symptoms dominate the clinical picture in younger individuals, whereas cardiovascular and neuromusuclar symptoms predominate in older subjects.

The skin is warm and moist with a velvety texture, and palmar erythema is often found. The hair is fine and silky. Occasionally, increased loss of hair from the temporal aspects of the scalp may be noted. Excessive melanin pigmentation is not uncommon. Ocular signs include a characteristic stare with widened palpebral fissures, blinking, lid lag, failure of convergence, and failure to wrinkle the brow on upward gaze. These signs are thought to result from sympathetic overstimulation and usually subside when the thyrotoxicosis is corrected. The *infiltrative ophthalmopathy* characteristic of Graves' disease will be discussed in a later section.

The diffuse toxic goiter may be asymmetric and lobular. A bruit heard best directly over the gland is not found invariably. When heard, it usually signifies that the patient is thyrotoxic, but may also rarely be present in association with other disorders in which the thyroid is markedly hyperplastic. Venous hums and carotid souffles should be distinguished from true thyroid bruits. A hyperplastic pyramidal lobe of the thyroid may often be palpable if carefully sought.

Cardiovascular findings include a wide pulse pressure, sinus tachycardia, atrial arrhythmias (especially atrial fibrillation), systolic murmurs, increased intensity of the apical first sound, cardiac enlargement, and at times, overt heart failure. A to-and-fro, high-pitched sound may be audible in the pulmonic area and may simulate a pericardial friction rub (Means-Lerman scratch).

DIAGNOSIS. When severe, Graves' disease (as well as other thyrotoxic disorders) is so striking that the diagnosis presents little difficulty. Goiter, eye signs, loss of weight despite good appetite, tachycardia, sweating, psychic instability, tremor, increased basal metabolic rate, high serum PBI and T4 increased resin uptake of radioactive triiodothyronine, and a rapid, increased thyroidal uptake of radioiodine all serve to establish the diagnosis (Table 89-2).

In a few patients the clinical picture may be one of apathy rather than of hyperactivity, and the basal metabolic rate elevation may be relatively slight. In such instances the clinical detection of underlying thyrotoxicosis is difficult, but the thyroidal uptake or radioactive iodine and the serum PBI levels are usually diagnostic. A barium swallow may be helpful in demonstrating displacement of the esophagus or trachea by substernal enlargement of the thyroid. All patients with unexplained cardiac failure or irregularities in rhythm, especially atrial fibrillation, should be surveyed carefully for underlying thyrotoxicosis. In patients with preexisting cardiac disease, even mild thyrotoxicosis may induce severe disability. The circulation time may be rapid or normal in the presence of an elevated venous pressure, and the response to digitalis is usually poor.

Although eye signs are important, it should be recognized that infiltrative ophthalmopathy may occur antecedent to or in the absence of thyrotoxicosis. Prominent eyes and wide palpebral fissures without infiltrative ophthalmopathy occur normally in some individuals. Proptosis and occasionally mild degrees of conjunctival hyperemia are seen in advanced uremia, Cushing's syndrome, cirrhosis of the liver, and malignant hypertension; in such instances, thyroid function is normal and the ophthalmopathy is not of thyroidal origin.

DIFFERENTIAL DIAGNOSIS. Signs and symptoms in a number of nonthyroidal disorders may simulate certain aspects of the thyrotoxic syndrome. *Anxiety* is a prominent feature of hyperthyroidism, and there is thus some overlap in the symptomatology of this disorder with pure anxiety states of emotional origin. Such symptoms as tachycardia, tremulousness, irritability, weakness, and fatigue are common to the anxiety of both disorders. In anxiety of emotional origin, however, the peripheral manifestations of excessive thyroid hormones are absent; thus, the skin of the extremities is usually cold and clammy rather than warm and moist. *Weight loss,* when present in emotional anxiety, is characteristically accompanied by anorexia, whereas in hyperthyroidism it is generally but not invariably accompanied by excessive appetite. Hyperthyroidism can occasionally be confused with such disorders as metastatic carcinoma, cirrhosis of the liver, hyperparathyroidism, sprue, and neuromyopathies such as *myasthenia gravis* and *periodic paralysis*. These conditions may be mimicked by hyperthyroidism or, rarely, may coexist with it. Sympathetic activity of thyrotoxicosis may result in an overlap of signs and symptoms with those of *pheochromocytoma*, including heat intolerance, excessive perspiration, tachycardia with palpitations, and a hypermetabolic state, which may often be severe. In all the above disorders, as well as other conditions considered in the differential diagnosis of hyperthyroidism, careful evaluation of one or more of the specific laboratory procedures previously described will usually distinguish hyperthyroidism from the others.

Hyperthyroidism is a disorder of so many diverse clinical manifestations that it may masquerade as one of many seemingly unrelated disorders. Signs and symptoms directing the physician's attention to gastrointestinal, cardiovascular, or neuromuscular diseases are not infrequent, particularly in older individuals. This differential diagnosis is extremely important in patients with heart disease in whom thyrotoxicosis must be considered in the etiology of atrial fibrillation and congestive heart failure. Subacute bacterial endocarditis, myocarditis, pericarditis, acute rheumatic fever, and coronary heart disease may be mimicked by uncomplicated hyperthyroidism.

TREATMENT. Graves' disease is a disorder often characterized by cyclic phases of exacerbation and remission. Occasionally, patients with forms of the disease may recover spontaneously. This characteristic of Graves' disease has important implications in the choice of and response to therapy.

There are two major approaches to the treatment of hyperthyroidism; both are directed to limiting the quantity of thyroid hormones the gland can produce. The first major therapeutic category, the use of antithyroid agents, interposes a chemical blockade to hormone synthesis, the effect of which is operative only as long as the drug is administered or until a spontaneous remission occurs. Thus, the agents can control successfully a single phase of active thyrotoxicity but probably will not prevent exacerbation at some subsequent period. The second major approach is ablation of thyroid tissue, thereby limiting hormone production. This may be achieved either surgically or by means of radioactive iodine. Since these procedures induce permanent anatomic alterations of the thyroid, they can control the individual active phase and are more likely to prevent recurrence of thyrotoxicity during a later exacerbation. On the other hand, the permanency of the effects of surgery or radiation makes these modes of therapy capable of leading to hypothyroidism, either shortly after treatment or with the passage of years.

Each major mode of therapy has advantages and disadvantages, indications and contraindications. The latter are more often relative than absolute. In general, a trial of long-term antithyroid therapy is desirable in children, adolescents, young adults, and pregnant women, but it may also be employed in older patients. Indications for ablative procedures include relapse or recurrence following drug therapy, a large goiter, drug toxicity, and failure of the patient to follow a medical regimen or to return for periodic examinations. Subtotal thyroidectomy is usually elected for patients under the age of forty in whom ablative therapy is required. With older patients, radioactive iodine is clearly the ablative procedure of choice, as it is for patients who have had previous thyroid surgery or those in whom serious systematic disease contraindicates elective surgery.

In those patients selected for *long-term antithyroid therapy,* satisfactory control can almost always be achieved if a sufficient dosage of the drug is administered. Most patients can be managed successfully by propylthiouracil, 100 mg every 8 hr. Methimazole is at least as effective as propylthiouracil when administered in one-tenth the dosage. Once euthyroidism is achieved, the initial daily dosage may be reduced to the smallest doses that control the thyrotoxicosis fully. In many clinics, however, the initial dose is continued and is supplemented with 120 to 180 mg USP thyroid or its equivalent in synthetic thyroid preparations. By this latter regimen, hypothyroidism resulting from overdosage of antithyroid drugs can be prevented. This is especially important in pregnant patients. Furthermore, the undesirable consequences of hypothyroidism, such as enhancement of oculopathy and enlargement of the goiter, may thereby be forestalled. The precise duration of therapy is difficult to predict in the individual patient and may be a function of the spontaneous course of the disease itself. If this is the case, the longer the course of therapy, the more likely it is that the patient will remain well when the drug is discontinued. In general, however, an 18- to 24-month course is usually employed. A normal suppressive response to exogenous thyroid hormone when the antithyroid compound

is discontinued indicates that the patient is likely to remain well for some time. Following a regimen of this type, approximately 50 percent of patients will remain well for a prolonged period or indefinitely.

The *treatment of hyperthyroidism during pregnancy* is a subject of disagreement. Most physicians agree that antithyroid therapy is preferable to subtotal thyroidectomy, and this is particularly true during the first and third trimesters. The major disadvantage of antithyroid therapy is the possibility of inducing goiter and hypothyroidism in the fetus, since antithyroid agents readily traverse the placenta. Maintenance of a metabolic state in the mother consistent with the pregnant state greatly decreases the likelihood that fetal hypothyroidism will ensue. Antithyroid therapy should therefore be adjusted to permit maintenance of a serum protein–bound iodine of between 7 and 11 μg per 100 ml throughout pregnancy with a resin-T3 level below 85 percent and a basal metabolic rate of $+25$ to $+30$ percent during the last half or trimester. This can be achieved by careful regulation of dosage, but some authorities regularly supplement the antithyroid regimen with replacement doses of thyroid hormone. The latter program is highly successful, provided that a false sense of assurance does not lead to administration of excessive doses of antithyroid agent or neglect of frequent observation of the patient.

Leukopenia is the principal undesirable side effect of antithyroid drugs. Mild transient leukopenia may occur in approximately 10 percent of patients treated and is not necessarily an indication for discontinuing therapy. When the absolute number of polymorphonuclear leukocytes reaches 1,500 or less, antithyroid medication should be discontinued. Allergic rashes and drug sensitivity develop in a small percentage of patients. These may disappear with antihistamine therapy at the same or reduced dosage of antithyroid agent, but it is probably preferable, when sensitivity reactions occur, to change to another drug. On rare occasions (in less than 0.2 percent), agranulocytosis may occur. This may be sudden in onset.

Iodides inhibit the release of thyroid hormones from the thyrotoxic gland, and their ameliorative effects occur more rapidly than those of antithyroid compounds. However, response to iodides is often incomplete and transient. Furthermore, by expanding the thyroidal stores of hormones, iodides may prolong greatly the latency of response to subsequently instituted antithyroid therapy. Therefore, in the medical therapy of hyperthyroidism, iodides are mainly useful as an adjunct to other therapeutic measures in those cases in which rapid control of thyrotoxicosis is mandatory. Only rarely will contraindication to other forms of therapy dictate the use of iododes alone.

Radioactive iodine (^{131}I) affords a relatively simple, effective and economical means of treating thyrotoxicosis. Its major advantage is that it can produce the ablative effects of surgery without the immediate operative and postoperative complications. The principal disadvantage of ^{131}I therapy, in the dosage which has usually been employed, is its tendency to produce hypothyroidism with a frequency that increases progressively with time. As many as 30 to 70 percent of patients may develop this complication by 10 years after treatment. Although hypothyroidism is readily treated, once diagnosed, the insidious onset of the disorder may obscure the diagnosis until serious complications of hypothyroidism have developed. Hence, some recommend that all patients be treated with large doses of ^{131}I to ensure relief of thyrotoxicosis and then be placed on permanent physiologic replacement doses of thyroid hormone.

To date, studies have provided no evidence of a significant carcinogenic or leukemogenic effect of radioiodine in those doses commonly used in treating hyperthyroidism. Nevertheless, many physicians prefer to reserve radioiodine therapy for patients over forty years of age, thinking that it is currently not justifiable to administer an agent of undetermined radiation potentialities to younger persons, particularly those of childbearing potential. Patients with recurrent thyrotoxicosis following surgery, those who refuse surgery, or those who have complicating illnesses contraindicating surgery are excellent candidates for radioiodine therapy. The usual therapeutic dose for diffusely enlarged thyroid glands ranges between 120 to 140 μc per estimated Gm thyroid tissue (approximately 4 to 8 mc total dose). Nodular goiters may require somewhat larger doses, usually 8 to 12 mc. Repeated doses are sometimes required, and these may be given at intervals of 3 to 6 months until euthyroidism is achieved.

The foregoing doses are those which have been used commonly and are intended to produce relief of thyrotoxicosis within a few months of treatment. Smaller doses (approximately half as much ^{131}I) may not induce delayed hypothyroidism as frequently, but are also less likely to relieve thyrotoxicosis within a relatively short period. Antithyroid agents can be employed, however, to maintain metabolic control while the effect of the ^{131}I is taking hold.

Radiation thyroiditis from radioiodine may contraindicate its use in patients with large substernal goiters likely to induce respiratory embarrassment upon swelling. Patients exhibiting severe hyperthyroidism, heart failure, or progressive ophthalmopathy may first be rendered euthyroid by the use of methimazole or prophylthiouracil; by discontinuing antithyroid treatment for 2 or 3 days, or longer, and then administering radioactive iodine, a good therapeutic response may be obtained and the potential complication of radiation thyroiditis avoided.

Before radioactive iodine was introduced, subtotal thyroidectomy was the classic form of ablative therapy and it is still widely employed in younger patients in whom antithyroid therapy is unsuccessful. Although precise preoperative programs differ, several general principles should be emphasized. Patients should first be rendered fully euthyroid by means of antithyroid agents. Only then should iodides (5 to 10 drops Lugol's solution three times a day for approximately 2 weeks) be administered concomitantly to effect an involutional response in the gland. Antithyroid drugs should not be discontinued merely because treatment with iodides is instituted.

Hazards of *subtotal thyroidectomy* include immediate operative complications such as anesthetic accidents, hemorrhage sometimes leading to respiratory obstruction, and hypoparathyroidism. As time progresses, wound infection, cord paralysis, and hypothyroidism may occur. In experienced hands, surgery is an effective and relatively safe mode of therapy. Postoperative recurrences are quite uncommon. However, carefully conducted follow-up studies reveal that hypothyroidism follows surgery more frequently than previously suspected, although not as commonly as following ^{131}I.

Thyrotoxic Crisis

The clinical picture of thyrotoxic crisis or storm is that of a fulminating increase in all the signs and symptoms of thyrotoxicosis. In the past, this disturbance was most often observed postoperatively in patients poorly prepared for surgery. However, with the preoperative use of antithyroid drugs and iodide and with appropriate measures directed to control of metabolic factors, weight, and nutritional status, postoperative thyrotoxic crisis should not occur. At present, so-called "medical storm" is more common and occurs in untreated or inadequately treated patients. It is precipitated by surgical emergency or complicating medical illness, usually sepsis. The syndrome is characterized by extreme irritability, delirium or coma, hyperpyrexia to 106°F or more, tachycardia, restlessness, hypotension, vomiting, and diarrhea. Rarely, the clinical picture may be more subtle, with apathy, severe prostration, and coma with only slight elevation of temperature. Such postoperative complications as sepsis, septicemia, hemorrhage, and transfusion or drug reactions may mimic thyrotoxic crisis. It is thought that in certain patients thyrotoxic crisis is associated with or precipitated by adrenocortical insufficiency. The possibility of this complication gains support from evidence indicating increased adrenocortical hormone requirements in thyrotoxicosis and from evidence indicating reduced adrenocortical reserves in this disorder.

TREATMENT. Treatment of thyroid crisis should include the intravenous administration of large quantities of hypertonic glucose, hydrocortisone, and iodide; the intramuscular administration of B-complex vitamins, particularly thiamine, and where indicated, reserpine, guanethidine, or propranolol. Large doses of antithyroid drugs should be continued or instituted. The patient should be placed in a cooled, humidified oxygen tent and the hyperpyrexia treated as indicated. Full digitalization should be employed only in the presence of cardiac failure. If shock exists, intravenous pressor agents may be employed with extreme caution since patients with hyperthyroidism are particularly sensitive to pressor amines.

Ophthalmopathy

The clinical signs associated with the ophthalmopathy of Graves' disease may be divided into two components: the spastic and the mechanical. The former includes the stare, lid lag, and lid retraction that accompany thyrotoxicosis and account for the "frightened" facies and classic eye signs previously described. These findings need not be associated with actual proptosis and usually return to normal after appropriate correction of thyrotoxicosis. The mechanical component includes proptosis of varying degrees with ophthalmoplegia and congestive oculopathy characterized by chemosis, conjunctivitis, marked periorbital swelling, and the resultant complications of corneal ulceration, optic neuritis, and optic atrophy. These changes are associated with and may result from an increase in retrobulbar volume and pressure produced by accumulation of fat, water, and inflammatory cells in the retroorbital connective tissue and ocular musculature. When exophthalmos progresses rapidly and becomes the major concern in Graves' disease, it is usually referred to as *progressive* and, if severe, *malignant* exophthalmos. The term *exophthalmic ophthalmoplegia* refers to the ocular muscle weakness that so commonly accompanies this disorder and results in strabismus with varying degrees of diplopia. Exophthalmos may be unilateral early in the course of the disorder but usually progresses to symmetric involvement. It must be differentiated from retrobulbar tumors of various types as well as from a rare granulomatous disorder, *pseudotumor oculi*. Exophthalmos can be familial, is more common in some ethnic groups, and is seen in other endocrine disorders such as Cushing's syndrome and acromegaly, as well as in uremia, malignant hypertension, severe aortic stenosis, and superior mediastinal obstruction. Where doubt as to the cause of exophthalmos exists, an abnormal thyroid suppression test affords strong presumptive evidence that the oculopathy takes its origin in Graves' disease.

It is probable that the ophthalmopathy of Graves' disease results from some factor or factors of the anterior pituitary gland or the hypothalamus, although the genesis of this disorder is not known definitely. The exophthalmos may stabilize or decrease after treatment of hyperthyroidism but usually follows a course independent of the metabolic response to therapy. Rapid progression of exophthalmos with marked chemosis and edema is generally a grave prognostic sign and should serve as a warning that progressive eye changes may be anticipated. In treating this type of exophthalmos it is important to bring the thyrotoxicosis under control gradually and to prevent the development of hypothyroidism. Subtotal thyroidectomy or radioactive iodine therapy early in the course of this disease may enhance the progression of exophthalmos. Although there appears to be little difference in the incidence of progressive eye changes following the various forms of therapy of hyperthyroidism, antithyroid drug therapy seems to be the least provocative of severe or malignant exophthalmos. The long-continued administration of thyroid to forestall hypothyroidism may favor the regression of exophthalmic changes.

In mild forms of the disorder, considerable benefit may be derived from simple measures, such as elevating the head of the bed at night, administration of mercurial or thiazide diuretics or spironolactone to reduce edema, and provision of tinted glasses for protection from wind and foreign bodies. A 1% solution of methylcellulose or plastic shields may help to prevent corneal drying in patients unable to appose the lids during sleep. In more severe cases, as evidenced by progressive exophthalmos, increasing chemosis, ophthalmoplegia, or loss of vision, large doses of prednisone (120 to 140 mg daily) may be administered. Following improvement, the dosage is reduced to the lowest effective level. Prolonged administration is usually not feasible because of undesirable glucocorticoid side effects. In cases that appear to progress despite these measures, orbital decompression, if performed sufficiently early, will at times halt progression of the disease and preserve vision.

Localized or Pretibial Myxedema

Localized myxedema, a circumscribed deposition of mucinous material in the deeper layers of the skin over the lower portion of the legs or dorsa of the feet, occurs in patients with past or present Graves' disease and is not a manifestation of hypothyroidism. The affected area of skin may be pruritic with increased pigmentation, hirsutism, and a *peau d'orange* appearance that is sharply delineated from the normal skin. The clinical course resembles that of exophthalmos, with which it is associated frequently. It may also be associated with clubbing of the fingers. About half the cases occur during the active stage of thyrotoxicosis, and in the remainder the lesions develop after treatment. The activity of the disorder is usually self-limited. No form of therapy is entirely satisfactory, although the local injection of hyaluronidase or hydrocortisone has been beneficial transiently in some cases.

Thyrotoxic Heart Disease

The cardiac manifestations of hyperthyroidism have been described, Many elderly patients may exhibit obvious cardiac disease but without the usual clinical appearance of hyperthyroidism. These thyrocardiac patients have been called *apathetic* or *masked*. Occasionally they represent difficult diagnostic problems, but if one maintains a constant awareness of thyrotoxicosis in patients with heart disease, the correct diagnosis is almost always suspected. In these patients hyperthyroidism is usually associated with a toxic multinodular goiter. Although the basal metabolic rate may not be grossly abnormal, the PBI (in the absence of antecedent mercurial therapy) or the serum T4 and the radioactive iodine uptake of the thyroid are usually diagnostic.

In patients with cardiac decompensation and thyrotoxicosis, the cardiac output is frequently above normal, with a rapid or normal circulation time in spite of an elevated venous pressure. This condition is one of several examples of so-called "high-output failure." Even though elevated, the cardiac output is unable to satisfy the high metabolic requirements of the body, and thus heart failure occurs. It is probably wise to obtain such thyroid studies as the PBI or serum T4 and the radioactive iodine uptake in all patients with atrial fibrillation or congestive heart failure of undetermined etiology, since the finding of thyrotoxicosis affords a remediable form of cardiac disease.

Evidence suggests that the production of hypothyroidism and, consequently, hypometabolism is beneficial in appropriately selected *euthyroid* patients with congestive heart failure from any cause or in those with angina pectoris or intractable supraventricular tachycardia. Hypothyroidism may be produced readily by the administration of radioactive iodine.

Thyrotoxic Myopathy

Weakness, impairment of muscular function, and wasting of varying severity often accompany thyrotoxicosis and may suggest the presence of a primary muscular disorder. In certain patients, severe myopathy may be the dominant feature of thyrotoxicosis. Creatinuria is present under these circumstances, as it is in nonthyrotoxic myopathies. Myasthenia gravis and periodic paralysis occur more commonly with, or may be exacerbated by, thyrotoxicosis. A moderately beneficial response to prostigmine and related drugs may occur in thyrotoxicosis and does not of itself indicate the presence of myasthenia gravis (see Chap. 377).

Thyrotoxic Bone Disease

Skeletal demineralization is a not uncommon manifestation of thyrotoxicosis and is associated with hypercalcuria and hyperphosphaturia even when loss of bone salts is not demonstrable radiologically. Serum calcium, phosphorus, and alkaline phosphatase levels are usually normal. In some patients, however, serum calcium and alkaline phosphatase may be elevated. The latter findings may be purely a manifestation of uncomplicated thyrotoxicosis rather than associated hyperparathyroidism, but at times the two diseases coexist. Clinically, significant degrees of skeletal demineralization are rarely seen except in elderly patients in whom thyrotoxicosis may accentuate the effects of preexisting osteoporosis (see Chap. 380).

THYROID NEOPLASMS

Adenomas

True adenomas, as contrasted with localized adenomatous areas, are encapsulated and usually compress contiguous thyroid tissue. Such adenomas are generally present in the thyroid gland but may also occur ectopically. They vary greatly in size and histologic characteristics. Adenomas are often classified into three major types: papillary, follicular, and Hürthle cell. The follicular adenomas can be subdivided according to the size of the follicle into colloid or macrofollicular, fetal or microfollicular, and embryonal varieties. There is considerable variation in physiologic differentiation as judged by their ability to concentrate radioiodine. Generally, the more highly differentiated adenomas (follicular) are most likely to mimic the function of normal thyroid tissue. Function-

ing adenomas are usually independent of TSH stimulation and may produce sufficient thyroid hormone to suppress completely the activity of the remainder of the thyroid gland. Ultimately, production of hormone by the adenoma may be sufficient to produce thyrotoxicosis (toxic adenoma). Such lesions can be distinguished by isotopic scanning procedures, which reveal localization of

Table 89-5. CLASSIFICATION OF THYROID TUMORS

I. Tumors of low malignancy
   A. Adenomas with blood vessel invasion
   B. "Histologic carcinoma" (small tumors found incidentally at operation; without symptoms, recurrence, or metastases)
   C. Papillary adenocarcinoma (occurs in young age group; lymphangioinvasive)
II. Tumors of moderate malignancy
   A. Nonpapillary, solid, or alveolar, adenocarcinoma (occurs in older age group; hemangioinvasive; histologically the metastases may appear benign—"benign metastasizing struma")
   B. Hürthle cell adenocarcinoma (occurs in middle age group; usually locally invasive, occasional skeletal or pulmonary metastases)
   C. Medullary carcinoma with amyloid stroma (usually occurs after the age of 50, usually metastasizes via both lymphatics and bloodstream, may be familial and associated with other endocrine and mesodermal disorders)
III. Tumors of high malignancy (rare)
   A. Small-cell carcinoma (simplex)
   B. Giant-cell carcinoma
   C. Epidermoid carcinoma
   D. Fibrosarcoma
   E. Lymphoma

radioiodine solely in the area of the adenoma ("hot nodule"). In such instances, function in the suppressed portion of the thyroid can be restored by exogenous TSH, and this can be demonstrated by isotopic scanning. Following excision of a "hot" nodule, endogenous TSH usually restores function in the previously suppressed tissue. This uncommon disorder should not be confused with Graves' disease. When the toxic adenoma is ablated by surgery or radioiodine, the remainder of the thyroid tissue almost always resumes entirely normal function. The incidence of adenomas varies considerably and is usually increased in areas of endemic goiter. The etiology of true encapsulated adenomas is unknown and doubtless differs from that of adenomatous goiter. As in other organs, the role of benign adenomas as forerunners of carcinoma is uncertain.

Ectopic thyroid tissue, both encapsulated and nonencapsulated, can occur along the thyroglossal tract from the base of the tongue to the diaphragm. Lingual goiters, thyroglossal duct cysts, pyramidal lobe adenomas, and both esophageal and tracheal rests have been described. Ectopic thyroid tissue in the ovary (struma ovarii) may produce thyroid hormone and has been alleged to cause thyrotoxicosis. Isotopic scanning techniques can be helpful in diagnosing ectopic thyroid tissue if it is sufficiently differentiated to concentrate radioiodine.

Carcinoma

Cancers of the thyroid gland are pathologically pleomorphic and seldom of a pure type. Definitive pathologic classification is difficult, and the degree of malignancy as determined histologically is not necessarily consistent with the clinical course of the disease. A modification of Warren's classification is given in Table 89-5.

From a clinical point of view, primary thyroid carcinomas are of four major types: (1) A small number are highly anaplastic and histologically undifferentiated. These are often quite malignant and for the most part not amenable to surgical or radiation therapy. (2) A similarly uncommon type is the follicular carcinoma, whose structure so closely mimics that of normal thyroid tissue that it has been termed *benign metastasizing thyroid carcinoma*. This variety has a predilection for metastases to bone and is often first discovered radiologically or when a metastatic lesion is biopsied. (3) Medullary or solid carcinoma with amyloid stroma is the most distinctive type of malignant thyroid neoplasm. It occurs after the age of fifty and metastasizes via both lymphatic and blood vessel invasion. The disease is sometimes familial and may be associated with pheochromocytoma, intestinal polyps, or fibromata. An unusual association with Cushing's syndrome and a syndrome similar to that produced by carcinoid tumors has been reported. Convincing evidence that amyloid tumors may secrete thyrocalcitonin, sometimes in huge quantities, has been presented and some patients develop severe hypocalcemia. (4) The largest number of thyroid cancers present with varying degrees of differentiation. The most common of these is papillary adenocarcinoma, which is generally of low virulence, metastasizes to regional lymph nodes, and is the most amenable to therapy.

DIAGNOSIS AND MANAGEMENT. The diagnosis and management of malignancies of the thyroid gland present several problems, each of which must be taken in proper perspective. In the past, statistical analyses of the incidence of thyroid cancer in surgical specimens led to a concept upon which was based the rationale for surgical removal of thyroid nodules in the prophylaxis or therapy of thyroid cancer. This concept proposes that goiters be removed surgically to prevent cancer and is predicated upon the finding of a high incidence of cancer in surgical specimens of goiters containing either a single nodule or multiple nodules. Recent reappraisal of this concept has shown that, although the incidence of thyroid cancer in surgical specimens appears to be increasing, the actual incidence of thyroid cancer in the general population is quite low, somewhere in the range of 2.5 cases per 100,000 population per year. This is in contrast to the high incidence of nodular goiter in the population. The death rate from thyroid cancer is quite low, probably less than 0.6 per 100,000 population per year. The low death rate from this disease has suggested that the high

incidence of carcinoma in surgical specimens results from effective selection of high-risk patients and that the pathologic criteria of thyroid malignancy may not truly reflect the natural history of this lesion.

Signs and symptoms most suggestive of more virulent varieties of thyroid cancer are rapid and progressive growth (not to be confused with overnight enlargement of a nodule, which is usually the result of hemorrhage or infarction), hoarseness caused by recurrent laryngeal nerve paralysis, presence of lymph node enlargement in the neck or supraclavicular area, or fixation of the thyroid gland to contiguous structures. Papillary and follicular adenocarcinoma of the thyroid are often clinically indolent. Thyroid nodules or lymph nodes harboring these varieties of thyroid cancer may not show clinical evidence of growth over periods of years. Follicular carcinoma of the thyroid is frequently diagnosed for the first time by the finding of skeletal or pulmonary metastases on routine x-ray. Hyperthyroidism or hypothyroidism is rarely associated with thyroid cancer. Needle biopsy of the thyroid is considered by some physicians to be contraindicated in the diagnosis of thyroid malignancy because of the tendency of these neoplasms to "seed" in the incised area.

The relative degree of functional differentiation can be determined by use of the scintigram obtained after administration of radioactive iodine. The degree of ^{131}I uptake in the nodule can thus be determined and compared to that present in the normal tissue. In this manner, thyroid nodules may be divided arbitrarily into "hot" or "cold," depending upon whether or not they take up more or less ^{131}I than the normal portions of the gland. Generally speaking, the "cold" nodules have a greater likelihood of being malignant. However, it must be remembered that many benign nodules and cysts are likewise "cold" and that this test should not be used as the sole determinant of malignancy or operability. There appears to be an etiologic relationship between radiation therapy directed to the head and neck regions of children and young adults and the later development of thyroid cancer.

Conservative treatment of most thyroid malignancies is a growing trend in the approach to this problem. Such conservatism stems from several factors. First, thyroid cancer of a high degree of malignancy usually progresses so rapidly that it is frequently beyond any form of treatment at the time diagnosis is established. Second, nodular goiter is common, while carcinoma of the thyroid is rare; hence, indiscriminate operation on all nodular goiters in the hope of uncovering the occasional malignancy may result in a greater morbidity and mortality than would be produced by the carcinoma if left untreated. However, as indicated above, a presumptive diagnosis of carcinoma in the thyroid can usually be made with a reasonable degree of accuracy on the basis of the criteria previously mentioned. Therefore, it should be possible to select a group of high-risk patients in whom surgery may be indicated. When such a high-risk patient is young, most authorities agree that surgery should be performed. There is less agreement as to the benefits of surgery when similar lesions are detected in older patients. When, at surgery, a carcinoma is found, excision with a generous portion of surrounding normal tissue is recommended. Removal of lymph nodes in which cancer is obviously present is justified. In addition, selected nodes from areas of drainage should be removed to provide information concerning the extent and localization of distant metastases. Radical neck dissections do not appear to be justified at this time.

Although ablation of thyroid carcinoma with large therapeutic doses of radioactive iodine is theoretically possible and has been used occasionally, instances are rare in which the primary or metastatic lesions concentrate sufficient radioiodine to make this possible. External radiation may be helpful especially when metastases are localized to a single accessible area.

The use of suppressive doses of exogenous thyroid hormone to inhibit tumor growth is being evaluated further. Because of the virtual absence of serious side effects from such medication (120 to 240 mg USP thyroid daily), all patients with thyroid cancer, regardless of whether or not surgery has been undertaken, should be treated with thyroid suppression.

THYROIDITIS

Thyroiditis is a comparatively rare disease. It may be specific (suppurative or nonsuppurative), nonspecific (acute or subacute), or chronic (Hashimoto's or Riedel's struma).

Specific Thyroiditis

This condition may be caused by almost any known pathogenic organism, pyogenic or nonpyogenic, and is relatively rare compared to the nonspecific varieties. It may occur after infection of the mouth, pharynx, upper respiratory tract, or cervical lymph nodes. Very rarely tuberculosis, actinomycosis, syphilis, or infection with pyogenic organisms may result in single or multiple abscesses. Classically, redness, swelling, and tenderness of the skin over the thyroid occur together with fever and other systemic signs of infection. Treatment consists, for the most part, of specific antibiotic or chemotherapeutic agents along with surgical drainage where indicated.

Nonspecific Thyroiditis

This variety of thyroiditis is of unknown etiology, is probably not an autoimmune disorder, and may be viral in origin. It is usually self-limited, with repetitive episodes of progressively less severity. It is seen predominantly in middle-aged women and rarely progresses to hypothyroidism. The most common form of acute or subacute thyroiditis is associated histologically with giant-cell formation (de Quervain's thyroiditis). The onset of symptoms may be dramatic and often seems to follow an upper respiratory tract infection. There is usually progressive swelling and tenderness in the thyroid gland, with radiation of pain to the ears or jaw, associated with systemic manifestations of fever, nervousness, myalgia, and headache. Laboratory investigation often shows an elevated sedimentation rate, a normal or low leukocyte count, and a slightly increased PBI and BMR. The thyroidal ^{131}I uptake is characteristically depressed but may at times be normal. Each lobe of the thyroid can be affected separately, but the entire gland is involved as the disease progresses. A needle biopsy is helpful if the diagnosis is not clear and may be necessary to differentiate thyroiditis from hemorrhage or from a suppurative process.

Therapy should be conservative, since complete spontaneous recovery is the general rule. Hypothyroidism only rarely results from this inflammatory process. Rest, fluids, and aspirin often suffice. When symptoms are severe, a short course of steroid therapy (50 mg cortisone or its equivalent every 6 hr) usually will relieve them, but they often return upon withdrawal of the steroid. X-ray therapy in doses of 300 to 400 r has been reported to be efficacious in this disorder.

Chronic Thyroiditis

Two varieties of chronic thyroiditis of undertermined etiology may be diagnosed histologically: *Hashimoto's struma* (struma lymphomatosa, lymphadenoid goiter) and *Riedel's struma*. Struma lymphomatosa, by far the more common of the two, occurs predominantly in middle-aged women. It is characterized by a firm, rubbery, lobular swelling of the thyroid, simulating multinodular goiter. The serum of patients with this disorder may contain increased amounts of gamma-globulin, and the thymol turbidity and cephalin flocculation tests may be abnormal.

In the early stages of this disorder, the patients are metabolically normal, and thyroid function studies are either normal or may reveal a slightly elevated ^{131}I uptake. Occasionally there are abnormal, noncalorigenic, iodinated proteins in the blood. As a result, the PBI may be inordinately high compared to the metabolic state of the patient and to the serum T4 concentration. Such dissociation between the PBI and the serum T4, although occasionally seen in other nontoxic goiters, most commonly occurs in Hashimoto's disease. Ultimately, hypothyroidism results from replacement of the functional thyroid structures by lymphoid or fibrous tissue. At this time, the serum protein–bound iodine and the 24-hr radioactive iodine uptake are usually low, and there is often no response in these indices to TSH administration.

Of particular interest in this disorder is the detection of circulating autoantibodies to thyroglobulin as well as to cellular antigens. A variety of antibodies has been described, certain of which may be measured by gel diffusion or fluorescent antibody techniques or by the tanned erythrocyte hemagglutination assay. It has been postulated that Hashimoto's struma is an example of an autoimmune disease in which the damaging effects of the antigen-antibody combination in the thyroid gland lead to destruction of functional thyroid tissue. Proof of this is lacking, however. Detection of circulating antibodies to thyroglobulin is not specifically diagnostic of Hashimoto's struma, however, since they may be found in other thyroidal disorders.

Diagnosis of Hashimoto's struma is suspected on clinical grounds when nodular goiter is present with hypothyroidism. Definitive diagnosis depends upon histologic confirmation, which may be obtained by needle biopsy, and by the presence of high titers of thyroglobulin antibody. Treatment consists of replacement doses of 120 to 180 mg USP thyroid daily to correct or avoid hypothyroidism and, in some patients, to reduce the size of the goiter. When Hashimoto's disease is first diagnosed following subtotal thyroidectomy, it is particularly important to institute thyroid substitution therapy to avoid the unusually common postoperative consequences of hypothyroidism.

Riedel's struma produces a firm, ligneous swelling of the thyroid, which may involve surrounding neck structures. This disorder is exceptionally rare and must be differentiated from thyroid neoplasia.

REFERENCES

Forester, C. F.: Coma in Myxedema: Report of a Case and Review of the World Literature, A.M.A. Arch. Intern. Med., 111:734, 1963.

Hazard, J. B.: Thyroiditis: A Review, Am. J. Clin. Pathol., 25:289, 399, 1955.

Ingbar, S. H., and N. Freinkel: Hypothyroidism, Disease-a-Month, September, 1958.

——: Physiological Considerations in Treatment of Diffuse Toxic Goiter, A.M.A. Arch. Intern. Med., 107:932, 1961.

—— and K. A. Woeber: The Thyroid Gland, chap. 4 in "Textbook of Endocrinology," R. H. Williams (Ed.), Philadelphia, W. B. Saunders Company, 1968.

Lindsay, S.: "Carcinoma of the Thyroid Gland," Springfield, Ill., Charles C Thomas, Publisher, 1960.

McGill, D. A., and S. P. Asper, Jr.: Endocrine Exophthalmos. A Review and a Report on Autoantibody Studies, New Engl. J. Med., 267:133, 188, 1962.

Means, J. H., L. J. DeGroot, and J. B. Stanbury (Eds.): "The Thyroid and Its Diseases," 3d ed., New York, McGraw-Hill Book Company, 1963.

Pitt-Rivers, R. (Ed.): "Advances in Thyroid Research," London, Pergamon Press, 1961.

—— and W. R. Trotter (Eds.): "The Thyroid Gland," vols. 1 and 2, London, Butterworth & Co., Publishers, Ltd., 1964.

Selenkow, H. A., and C. S. Hollander: Physiologic, Pharmacologic and Therapeutic Considerations in Surgery for Hyperthyroidism, Anesthesiology, 24:425, 1963.

Veith, F. J., J. R. Brooks, W. P. Grigsby, and H. A. Selenkow: The Nodular Thyroid Gland and Cancer: A Practical Approach to the Problem, New Engl. J. Med., 270:431, 1964.

Werner, S. C. (Ed.): "The Thyroid," New York, Harper & Row Publishers, Inc., 1962.

90 DISEASES OF THE PARATHYROID GLANDS

*Daniel S. Bernstein
and George W. Thorn*

The parathyroid glands were first recognized as separate structures and described by Sandstrom in 1880. Shortly thereafter Gley (1881) and others performed extirpation experiments demonstrating that tetany ceased with the intravenous injection of calcium. Further proof of the endocrine nature of these glands followed from the preparation of parathyroid extracts by Collip in Canada, and by Hanson and Berman in the United States, and from the demonstration that these extracts could induce elevation of plasma calcium level.

ANATOMY

The parathyroid glands originate from the posterior halves of the third and fourth pairs of pharyngeal pouches. Therefore, like the thyroid, the parathyroids are entodermal in origin. In man the parathyroids are reddish- or yellowish-brown and are flattened, ovate, or pyriform bodies located on the posterior surfaces of the lateral lobes of the thyroid. There are normally 4 glands. The number may vary from 2 to 10, and their location is extremely variable. They have been found within the thyroid gland, in the mediastinum, and in scattered regions of the neck. The average size of a human parathyroid gland is $5 \times 3 \times 3$ mm, and the combined weight of 4 glands averages about 120 mg.

In the adult, the parathyroid gland contains chief cells and oxyphil cells. The chief cells are more numerous and are the source of the parathyroid hormone. These cells are 6 to 8 μ in diameter and contain glycogen. The oxyphil cells appear in the human gland at about the tenth year of life. They contain no glycogen, and their nuclei are somewhat pycnotic. They may represent a more mature or inactive chief cell. Another cell, the large water-clear cell (*wasserhelle* cell) derived from the chief cell, is the commonest cell type observed in hypertrophy and hyperplasia of the parathyroids.

EFFECTS OF PARATHYROID HORMONE

The function of parathyroid hormone is to maintain a normal level of plasma calcium. In the normal human being, the hormone performs this action so well that the plasma calcium varies only slightly from time to time even though the entry and egress of calcium to and from the body may vary widely. This regulation is mediated by an effect on the skeleton, the largest reservoir of calcium in the body. The significance of the phosphaturic effect of parathyroid hormone is unknown, although it may be a factor in stabilizing the plasma calcium.

Bone

Parathyroid hormone causes dissolution of the relatively stable fraction of bone mineral as well as the bone matrix, releasing calcium, phosphate, magnesium, and hydroxyproline to the extracellular fluid. The precise mechanism is unknown, but it has been shown that the major portion of bone mineral and matrix resorption is normally a function of the osteocyte (and, to a smaller extent, of the osteoclast), which under abnormal situations such as hyperparathyroidism, becomes the predominant cell causing bone resorption. Thus, the mobilization of bone mineral is a product of bone cellular metabolism, perhaps because of changes in bone mineral solubility produced by metabolic organic end products or by release of lysosomal enzymes stored intracellularly and released at appropriate times secondary to hormonal influences or other substances which labilize lysosomal membranes.

There is little doubt now that the action of parathyroid hormone on bone is a direct one. Bone tissue culture implants can be seen actively to resorb bone after minute amounts of parathyroid hormone are added. Parathyroid glands transplanted directly to bone cause local resorption around the area of transplantation. Histologically, the end product of parathyroid hormonal activity is a cystic space in the bone filled with fibrous tissue, i.e., osteitis fibrosa cystica. Any theory explaining the action of parathyroid hormone on bone must account for this pathologic picture.

Urinary Inorganic Phosphate

Since the advent of a more purified parathyroid preparation, arguments over the major site of the phosphaturic action of the hormone have been, for the most part, resolved. It is apparent that the hormone inhibits the well-documented process of renal tubular reabsorption of phosphate. There is, however, a small group who maintain that the hormone causes an increase in tubular secretion of phosphate, although the evidence for this process of tubular secretion of phosphate is scanty. The site in the kidney for tubular phosphate absorption is the proximal tubule, and the hormone exerts its effect on this function with little, if any, action on glomerular filtration rate.

Urinary Calcium

Renal handling of calcium is a complex process complicated by an interrelationship with sodium excretion. Calcium is probably actively resorbed from the distal tubule, although there may be some passive diffusion of calcium in the proximal tubule. In human beings with hypocalcemia, it appears that the TR Ca^{++} (TR = tubular reabsorption, Ca = calcium) is decreased. When parathyroid hormone is given, the TR Ca^{++} increases somewhat, although the evidence for this has not been sufficiently documented as yet. It would fit the scheme that parathyroid hormone tends to maintain the plasma Ca^{++} level within narrow limits. Excessive calcium loads presented to the kidney cause increased excretion of sodium, and vice versa, although mechanisms are not well understood. One may conclude that the majority of

investigators now feel that parathyroid hormone effects an increase in the renal tubular reabsorption of calcium, although additional evidence is needed to substantiate this hypothesis.

Gastrointestinal Absorption and Secretion

The effect of parathyroid hormone on the intestinal transport of calcium is probably to increase the amount of calcium absorbed against the mucosal-serosal gradient. The experimental evidence for this effect is disputed, and, even if substantiated, probably is of such small magnitude as to be relatively insignificant in affecting the overall calcium balance.

Lactation

It has been postulated that parathyroid hormone controls the amount of calcium in breast milk in animals, although there are no data regarding this point in human beings. Experimentally, parathyroidectomy in a lactating animal increases the calcium content of breast milk, and parenterally administered parathyroid extract given to such animals will restore the calcium content by reducing the amount of calcium secreted by the tubular epithelium of the breast. Therefore, parathyroid hormone may act to conserve blood calcium not only by its action on bone, kidney, and gut, but also on another portal of egress of calcium, the breast.

Lens

It has long been recognized that the incidence of cataracts is high in untreated hypoparathyroidism. Some experimental evidence suggests that the lens calcium is increased in hypoparathyroidism at a time when extracellular fluid calcium is reduced. Incubation of the lens in vitro with parathyroid hormone can reduce the lens calcium.

In summary, parathyroid hormone has an effect on any organ system involved in the handling of calcium. This action, at any specific site, is designed to maintain a constant level of plasma calcium. The exact manner by which the parathyroid hormone exerts its effects on single organ systems remains an enigma, however, and a fertile field of future research.

CHEMISTRY OF PARATHYROID HORMONE

In recent years major progress has been made in purifying parathyroid hormone. The purest preparation has been made by phenol extraction of bovine parathyroid glands and subsequent purification by gel filtration. Various estimates of the molecular weight range from 8,400 to 9,400. All the common amino acids, with the exception of cystine, 17 in number, are represented. Methionine accounts for the sulfur content of the polypeptide. The absence of cystine and the isolation of a single N-terminal amino acid, alanine, support the conclusion that the hormone is a single-chain polypeptide. Parathyroid extracts can be reversibly inactivated by oxidation (as by hydrogen peroxide) and the biologic activity restored or increased above preinactivation values by reducing agents (mercaptoethanol; cysteine). Other agents, such as heparin, oil, and gelatin, appear to stabilize the activity of the hormone. The active, purified hormone contains both calcium-mobilizing and renal-tubular-phosphate–blocking properties. Parathyroid extract is available commercially. Parathyroid extract, USP, is standardized by biologic assay so that 1 ml contains 100 to 120 USP units. The USP unit is defined as $\frac{1}{100}$ of the amount required to raise the plasma calcium level of a normal male dog weighing 10 to 12 kg by 1.0 mg per 100 ml within 16 to 18 hr after a single subcutaneous injection.

REGULATION OF PARATHYROID ACTIVITY

The parathyroid glands do not appear to be under direct control of a tropic hormone elaborated by the anterior pituitary, nor is there evidence of nervous control of their secretory activity. However, a number of observations point to an indirect relationship to other endocrine organs. Parathyroid hyperplasia has been reported in cases of acromegaly, Cushing's syndrome, Addison's disease, and pancreatic islet cell adenomas. Experimentally, hypophysectomy in animals causes some involution of the parathyroids, whereas growth hormone, adrenocorticotropin, crude anterior pituitary extracts, and adrenal steroids cause hyperplasia. It is possible that these changes are secondary to the alteration in serum mineral levels mediated by the pituitary, thyroid, adrenal, gonadal, and islet cell hormones. A number of cases of multiple tumors involving the anterior pituitary, pancreatic islet tissue, and the parathyroids have been reported. Since tumors of these glands are quite rare, their association can scarcely be explained as a matter of chance. Also the familial occurrence of multiple tumors of this type has been noted. Although unexplained, the association of these tumors is of clinical importance.

The parathyroid glands alter their production of hormone in response to change in the **plasma level of ionized calcium.** It is generally agreed that hormone production is stimulated by hypocalcemia and decreased by hypercalcemia. Hyperplasia of the parathyroids is found in those conditions in which there is a tendency toward a low plasma calcium level, namely, rickets (or osteomalacia), calcium deprivation, and renal insufficiency with acidosis. There is conflicting evidence concerning an increase in parathyroid hormone production in patients with hyperphosphatemia in the absence of hypocalcemia.

With the application of newer methods of radioimmunoassay techniques, it has been shown that there is probably not a normal circadian rhythm to parathyroid synthesis or release. As measured by radioimmunoassay, parathyroid hormone levels in man respond proportionally to changes in plasma calcium concentration as produced

by EDTA (ethylenediaminetetraacetic acid). Extraordinarily high plasma levels of parathyroid hormone occur in hypocalcemia associated with chronic renal disease. Concentrations of parathyroid hormone in cases of parathyroid adenoma show considerable variation, with an appreciable proportion of such patients showing a normal plasma parathyroid hormone concentration. However, such a finding in the presence of hypercalcemia, which ordinarily would decrease plasma immunoreactive parathyroid hormone levels, suggests an autonomously functioning nonsuppressible gland. In patients with azotemic renal disease and hypocalcemia the values are uniformly higher than in primary hyperparathyroidism. These findings only point out the difficulty in deciding whether a patient with severe renal impairment and a high normal plasma calcium level in the presence of elevated serum phosphate has a primary parathyroid adenoma and secondary renal disease or primary renal disease and secondary or autonomous parathyroid hyperplasia ("tertiary hyperparathyroidism"). Since the consequences of "tertiary hyperparathyroidism" are extensive osteitis fibrosa cystica and metastatic soft-tissue calcification, subtotal (seven-eighths) parathyroidectomy may be justified, especially if future renal homotransplantation is contemplated. Although measurements of plasma parathyroid hormone have added a new tool aiding in the diagnosis of hyperparathyroidism, it may be seen from the above discussion that changes in the plasma calcium, phosphate, and alkaline phosphatase levels are still reliable and important indicators of parathyroid function.

HYPOPARATHYROIDISM
History

One of the causes of tetany is total or extensive parathyroidectomy. Tetany received its name from Corvisart in 1852. MacCallum and Voegtlin in 1908 showed that the mechanism of this type of tetany was dependent upon hypocalcemia. The Swiss surgeons Reverdin and Kocher in 1882 described postoperative tetany after a complete thyroidectomy for goiter without realizing that the condition was due to parathyroid deficiency.

Etiology and Pathology

Primary parathyroid deficiency is extremely rare, usually occurring in patients under the age of sixteen, but often persisting throughout adult life. In most instances, clinical evidence of parathyroid deficiency is secondary to thyroidectomy. During the past decade increased knowledge and experience in surgical techniques have decreased the incidence of permanent parathyroid deficiency secondary to thyroidectomy. Transient deficiency is not unusual and is attributed to trauma, edema, hemorrhage, and temporary interference with the blood supply to the remaining parathyroid glands. There have been no documented cases of hypoparathyroidism secondary to the administration of radioactive iodine in the treatment of thyrotoxicosis.

Pathologic Physiology

There is a pronounced disturbance of calcium and phosphate metabolism as reflected by plasma calcium levels as low as 2.5 mEq per liter (5 mg per 100 ml) and plasma inorganic phosphate levels as high as 3 to 4 mM per liter (9.3 to 12.4 mg per 100 ml). The decrease in calcium facilitates the transmission of impulses across the myoneural junction, which is responsible for much of the clinical picture.

Clinical Picture

The most striking symptom is an increased neuromuscular excitability resulting from a decrease in the plasma ionized calcium. The presenting complaint in most (70 percent) of these patients is tetany or tetanic equivalents. Tetany is manifested by carpopedal spasm in which the stiff, hollowed hand with rigid fingers is flexed at the metacarpal-phalangeal, wrist, and elbow joints and the legs and feet are extended. The tetanic equivalents include tonic and clonic convulsions, laryngeal stridor (spasm) which may be fatal, paresthesias, numbness, muscle cramps, dysphagia, dysarthria, muscular palsies, and cardiac irregularities. Spasm may involve the smooth muscle of the eye, gastrointestinal tract, bladder, and blood vessels. About 40 percent of these patients are seen because of epileptic seizures. The electroencephalographic findings in these patients suggest that occasionally underlying factors unrelated to plasma calcium levels play an important part in lowering the threshold for convulsive seizures. Mental changes are frequent and include anxiety, depression, increased irritability, and psychoses. Acute symptoms may be precipitated by infection, undue fatigue, menstruation, and emotional upsets and by an increase in the phosphate content of the diet. In some cases, the symptoms may be quite mild, varied, and even vague. Patients have manifested fatigue, muscular weakness, palpitations, numbness and tingling of the extremities, and other signs of latent tetany for as long as 30 years before a diagnosis of chronic hypoparathyroidism was established.

On examination, increased neuromuscular excitability may be demonstrated by contraction of the facial muscles in response to a light tap over the facial nerve in front of the ear (Chvostek's sign). This test is almost always positive in untreated hypoparathyroidism; however, it does occur occasionally in normal individuals. Dorsal flexion and abduction of the foot may be elicited by tapping the lateral surface of the fibula just below its head (peroneal sign). If the circulation to the arm is occluded by inflation of a blood pressure cuff above the level of systolic pressure, the hand may assume the typical position seen in carpopedal spasm within 3 min (Trousseau's sign). This sign is sometimes negative in marked hypoparathyroidism. Extensive tropic changes of the ectoderm may be seen. The hair is likely to be sparse, prematurely gray, and is occasionally absent in the axillary and pubic regions. Generalized or patchy erythema may be found. The skin is rough, dry, and scaling, and

there may be papules, vesicles, or bullae. A number of skin diseases have been described in association with hypoparathyroidism, including moniliasis of the skin, nails, tongue, and mouth. However, no etiologic relationship has been established. The nails are deformed and brittle, showing transverse ridging. In children one finds evidence of faulty dentition, including pitting and ridging of the enamel. Cataracts are frequently present, their extent being related to the duration and severity of the hypocalcemia. Early lens changes, not apparent on ophthalmoscopic examination, can usually be found with the aid of a slit lamp. Papilledema has been observed. The electrocardiogram usually shows a prolongation of the Q-T interval. The density of the bone may appear normal or increased. Abnormalities of dentition, such as deformed or absent roots, may be helpful in determining the age of onset of the disease. The pronounced disturbance of calcium and phosphate metabolism is reflected by lowered plasma calcium and elevated plasma inorganic phosphate levels. The alkaline phosphatase is normal or low. Hypocalciuria may be present, as shown by a negative Sulkowitch test (see p. 470). The spinal fluid may be under increased pressure without other abnormalities. When this occurs in the presence of papilledema, the diagnosis of a brain tumor may be made incorrectly. In primary hypoparathyroidism, bilateral symmetric calcification of the basal ganglions is commonly seen on the skull film. Other areas, such as the cerebellum and choroid plexus, are occasionally calcified.

Differential Diagnosis

The principal causes of tetany are hypocalcemia and alkalosis. Of the nonparathyroid causes of hypocalcemia, rickets, osteomalacia, steatorrhea, and renal insufficiency are the most common. Recently, there has been described a new syndrome of "decreased tissue calcium with tetany." This condition is manifested by severe tetany with normal plasma levels of calcium, magnesium, potassium, and carbon dioxide content. It has been demonstrated by radioactive calcium studies that the tissue calcium pool is lower than normal and that treatment with vitamin D will tend to bring the level of calcium in this pool toward normal. Extreme caution must be employed since the difference between the therapeutic and toxic dose of vitamin D is narrow.

In rickets, osteomalacia, and steatorrhea, a low value for plasma calcium is almost invariably associated with a normal or low value for plasma phosphate. In late-stage renal insufficiency with hypocalcemic tetany, the elevation in plasma phosphate level is disproportionately higher than that which occurs with a given level of hypocalcemia in parathyroid tetany. Nitrogen retention, as evidenced by an elevated blood urea nitrogen or nonprotein nitrogen, is early always present and differentiates the two conditions. A lowered plasma magnesium can also produce tetany. Magnesium salts have been used to eliminate hypocalcemic tetany. Furthermore, the level of plasma potassium plays an important part in the clinical manifestation of hypocalcemic tetany. The relationship of these three ions in the serum as regards tetany can be formulated as follows: calcium × magnesium/potassium. This is especially important in the treatment of renal failure, in which all three of these ions are drastically altered.

In addition to general renal insufficiency, two specific tubular lesions are to be considered. The first is a failure of reabsorption of certain amino acids (Fanconi syndrome, Chap. 103) in which there is increased excretion of phosphate and low-phosphate rickets, and the second is a rare selective failure of calcium reabsorption accompanied by metabolic acidosis and often by renal calcinosis.

Alkalosis causes tetany with no demonstrable change in the concentration of calcium in the plasma. It may be due to hyperventilation, to prolonged vomiting of acid gastric contents, or to excessive alkali ingestion. With hyperventilation, the carbon dioxide *content* of the plasma is reduced; whereas with vomiting, and alkali ingestion, the carbon dioxide–combining power of the plasma may be increased greatly (see Chap. 297). Alkalotic tetany occurs most frequently in association with acute infection, particularly in children.

Treatment

The object of treatment is to increase and maintain the plasma calcium at an approximately normal level.

MANAGEMENT OF ACUTE HYPOPARATHYROIDISM. Immediate correction of hypocalcemia may be accomplished by intravenous injections of calcium gluconate (10 ml of a 10 percent solution) or calcium chloride (10 ml of a 5 percent solution or an intravenous drip of 500 ml of 0.2 percent solution over a 1-hr period) (see Table 90-1). The effect is transitory, lasting only a few hours, and additional calcium may have to be administered. Caution should be exercised with patients on digitalis, since rapid infusion of calcium may cause cardiac arrest. Parathyroid extract injection may be instituted along with the infusion of calcium and will give more prolonged action (12 to 24 hr). Parathyroid extract is available in injectable form containing 80 to 120 USP units per milliliter. From

100 to 200 units should be administered intravenously. Administration should proceed slowly initially since anaphylactoid reaction may occur and necessitate discontinuance. From 25 to 50 units of parathyroid extract may be given every 6 to 12 hr during the acute phase of hypoparathyroidism.

Dihydrotachysterol should be administered in doses of 1 to 3 ml (1.25 to 3.75 mg) one to three times daily by mouth until calcium appears in the urine, as indicated by the Sulkowitch test. The dose is then adjusted to maintain a normal serum calcium level. Treatment may be continued with this preparation or with a cheaper but just as adequate preparation of calciferol (vitamin D_2). Supplementary calcium preparations should be given orally as soon as possible. Calcium chloride is most effective, since it forms an acid solution which favors calcium absorption and also contains a higher percentage of available calcium. It may be administered in doses of 10 ml of a 30 percent solution, well diluted, three times a day after meals (see Table 90-1). A licorice syrup medium will conceal the taste of calcium chloride solution.

MANAGEMENT OF CHRONIC HYPOPARATHYROIDISM. The objective of therapy in chronic hypoparathyroidism is to reduce the plasma phosphate and raise the plasma calcium levels. This is best accomplished by a combination of dietary and drug therapy. The diet should include as much calcium as can be tolerated, but there is nothing to be gained by reducing the amounts of phosphate in the diet unless it is eaten in excess. From 4 to 8 Gm of the various calcium salts shown in Table 90-1 should be given.

Parathyroid hormone is rarely used except in critical situations since it must be given daily and may be associated with local reactions. There is no evidence that antibodies will develop to chronically administered parathyroid hormone. It is almost always advantageous to administer vitamin D_2 (calciferol) in ranges of 50,000 to 150,000 units daily, in order to enhance plasma calcium levels. Dihydrotachysterol, a synthetic derivative of ergosterol, may also be used, but while its action is sim-

Table 90-1. CALCIUM-REGULATING COMPOUNDS

Type	Route of administration	Dosage	Effect on plasma calcium
Calcium gluconate (USP).....	Intravenous Intramuscular Oral	5 to 20 ml of 10% aqueous solution (IV) 10 ml of 5% solution (1 to 2 times daily IM) 10 to 25 Gm daily	Immediate but of only short duration
Calcium chloride (USP).......	Intravenous Oral	55 ml of 0.2% over 1 hr (IV) or 10 ml of 5% aqueous solution slowly (IV) 10 ml of 30% aqueous (2 to 3 times daily)	Immediate but of only short duration
Calcium lactate.............	Oral	10 to 15 Gm daily (as a clear solution)	Immediate but of only short duration
Dihydrotachysterol (AT 10)...	Oral	3 to 4 ml (1.25 mg per ml) daily initially; 1 ml (3 to 5 times weekly) as maintenance	Delayed, with a maximum in 48–96 hr. Prolonged effect
Calciferol (vitamin D_2).......	Oral	50,000 to 200,000 units daily (1.25 to 5 mg)	Delayed. Prolonged effect
Parathyroid.................	Subcutaneous or intramuscular	100 to 200 units in severe tetany and then 25 to 50 units every 6 to 12 hr. Not recommended maintenance	Moderately rapid, with maximum in 8 to 18 hr

ilar to that of vitamin D_2 in all respects, it is much more expensive and rarely must be resorted to in favor of vitamin D_2. When vitamin D_2 or AT 10 (dihydrotachysterol) is used in therapy, the plasma calcium should be determined at frequent intervals, because persistent hypercalcemia and hypercalcuria may lead to deleterious effects. Since vitamin D_2 or AT 10 will cause an increase in the urine calcium before affecting a rise in blood calcium levels, it is important to check the urine level of calcium often as well as the plasma calcium, either by total 24-hr calcium excretion or by the Sulkowitch test. The Sulkowitch solution has the following composition:

Oxalic acid	2.5 Gm
Ammonium oxalate	2.5 Gm
Glacial acetic acid	5.0 ml
Distilled water q.s. ad	150.0 ml

The test is performed by adding 5 ml of the reagent to 5 ml urine in a test tube and noting the speed of appearance and the density of the precipitate. The result is graded 0, 1, 2, 3, or 4+. Routine use of the test for a short time enables one to become familiar with a normal response. The calcium intake (e.g., quantity of milk) as well as marked concentration or dilution of the urine should be taken into account. A negative test after a week on a diet free of milk and cheese suggests hypocalcemia —less than 3.5 mEq per liter (7.0 mg per 100 ml)—and a 3 to 4+ test suggests hypercalcemia—more than 5.2 mEq per liter (10.4 mg per 100 ml). Although this test can be run by the patient, it is important to check plasma levels from time to time. A 2+ Sulkowitch reaction is the most desirable.

An adjunctive mode of therapy is the use of probenecid (Benemid) by mouth in doses ranging from 0.5 to 1.5 Gm (daily). This agent is most useful in treating the tetany seen directly after inadvertent surgical removal of the parathyroids but is of little help in the chronic treatment of hypoparathyroidism. Rarely can Benemid be used alone. It acts on the kidney, blocking the reabsorption of phosphate by the renal tubule in a similar manner to the way it blocks the tubular reabsorption of uric acid. If epilepsy is evident, Dilantin or other antiepileptic drugs should be employed.

PSEUDOHYPOPARATHYROIDISM

The first description of this rare condition was given by Albright and his coworkers in 1942. This disease presents the same clinical and chemical features as hypoparathyroidism, except that these patients have round faces and short, thick figures. Subcutaneous centers of ossification are seen. There is a characteristic shortening of some of the metacarpal and metatarsal bones as a result of early epiphyseal closure, so that a dimple rather than a knuckle shows upon clenching of the fist. Most of the patients show some degree of mental deficiency. Not all these characteristics are necessarily present; any one

or a combination of them may be found. The apparent parathyroid deficiency in these patients appears to be due to a lack of end organ response. This is supported by the failure to respond to parathyroid extract, the finding of normal or hyperplastic glands where biopsy specimens have been obtained, and the failure to demonstrate antibodies to parathyroid hormone in the serum of patients in whom studies were done. The failure of these patients to respond to parathyroid extract need not be complete, and there are patients who have almost normal response to injected hormone. The finding of a 100-fold increase in thyrocalcitonin in the thyroid of one such pseudohypoparathyroid patient may provide an important clue in the pathogenesis of this disease.

It was suggested that the abnormalities seen in pseudopseudohypoparathyroidism and which are also found in pseudohypoparathyroidism are probably due to separate genetic factors, which may penetrate independently. Subsequent reports support this concept. Albright and his group have reported a case of a young woman with a rounded face, thickset figure, characteristic smile, shortened fingers and toes, and subcutaneous calcium deposits. However, the plasma calcium and phosphate levels were normal, and the Chvostek and Trousseau signs were absent.

Diagnosis

Because of the frequent history of convulsions, the condition may be incorrectly labeled epilepsy. The symptoms, chemical findings, and physical signs are those of hypoparathyroidism. The relative resistance to parathyroid extract as measured by failure to produce a phosphate diuresis (Ellsworth-Howard test) serves to distinguish it from hypoparathyroidism.

THE ELLSWORTH–HOWARD TEST. The test is performed as follows: The patient, in the fasting state, is given 2 ml (200 units) of parathyroid extract intravenously, and the urinary phosphate content is determined hourly for 3 hr prior to, and for 3 to 5 hr following, the injection. Occasional anaphylactoid reactions to the extract make slow and careful administration necessary. Parathyroid extracts are assayed by their effect on the plasma calcium level, and recent preparations have not been so effective in producing an increased phosphate excretion as those previously available. It is best to compare the response of the patient to that of a normal control given the same amount of hormone. The degree of phosphate diuresis induced by parathyroid hormone is dependent upon both the level of endogenous parathyroid secretion and the responsiveness of the phosphorus-reabsorbing mechanism of the renal tubules. Following the injection of a standard amount of parathyroid extract, there is a five- to sixfold increase in urine phosphate in normal persons, a tenfold or greater increase in patients with hypoparathyroidism, and at the most a twofold increase in patients with pseudohypoparathyroidism (parathyroid hormone resistance). Patients with hyperparathyroidism show a variable response to the extract.

Treatment

The therapy is the same as that outlined under chronic hypoparathyroidism.

PRIMARY HYPERPARATHYROIDISM

History

Generalized osteitis fibrosa cystica, a generalized disease of bones, was described in 1891 by von Recklinghausen. Askanazy associated this condition with a parathyroid tumor in 1904, and in 1925 Mandl removed a parathyroid adenoma from a patient suffering from this disease and noted a remarkable improvement. The occurrence of hyperparathyroidism without bone disease was pointed out by Albright in 1934. The clinical and metabolic studies subsequently carried out by Albright, Bauer, Aub, and Cope are classic.

Incidence

The exact incidence of the disease is unknown, but thanks to the work of Albright and his colleagues there has been a deliberate search for the disease, with a consequent increase in the frequency of diagnosis. The disease occurs most often in middle life, and about 70 percent of the patients reported are women. It has been shown that hyperparathyroidism can exist without evident disease of bone and that skeletal involvement represents a relatively late development. Involvement of the urinary tract is much more common than bone disease in the United States, presumably because of the high calcium intake, and in several series of cases more than 5 percent of all kidney stones have been associated with hyperfunction of these glands. Many cases of hyperparathyroidism in the United States are "masked" by insignificant or atypical alterations in plasma calcium and phosphate levels resulting from a high phosphate intake.

Etiology

Hypersecretion of the parathyroid glands may be caused by adenoma, hyperplasia, or carcinoma. The most common cause of primary hyperparathyroidism is an adenoma (90 percent of cases), hyperplasia is rather infrequent, and carcinoma is rare.

Pathology

Adenomas are usually limited to one gland. Norris collected from the literature 322 cases of parathyroid adenoma, with only 20 cases (6.2 percent) having multiple tumors. The pathologic overactivity of these tumors is not closely associated with their size. The adenomas are encapsulated, soft, orange-brown masses embedded in fat. They are occasionally lobular. The appearance, grossly, differs from that of the hyperplastic gland, which is irregular in shape and a darker, mahogany brown in color. The adenoma usually involves the entire gland but may involve only part of it. Adenomas are found in all the locations of the normal parathyroid glands. In one large series, 75 percent were found in the mediastinum. All cell types may be present, forming cords, glands, and solid masses. Cyst formation is common.

In primary diffuse hypertrophy and hyperplasia all the glands are involved but not necessarily to the same extent. The glands show a uniformity of structure, with a predominance of very large *wasserhelle* cells and a tendency to gland formation. There is a good correlation of size to the degree of overactivity.

Carcinoma of the parathyroid gland is extremely rare, accounting for 1 percent of functioning parathyroid tumors. They are generally larger than adenomas and in most cases have been clinically palpable. All these tumors have been associated with severe hyperparathyroidism with bone disease. They are generally slow-growing, tending to recur locally when excised, and are very resistant to x-ray therapy. Metastases to the regional lymph nodes, lungs, and liver may occur. Evidence indicates that carcinoma may develop from an adenoma.

The skeletal lesions observed in conjunction with long-standing hyperparathyroidism are discussed in Chap. 380, Osteoporosis. Degenerative changes occur in the renal tubular epithelium, heart muscle, and gastric mucosa and are often followed by calcification. About 80 percent of the cases show some evidence of renal damage such as nephrolithiasis, pyelonephritis, and calcium deposits in and around the tubules.

Mineral Levels

Characteristically, the plasma calcium is elevated and may attain values as high as 10 mEq per liter (20 mg per 100 ml). The plasma inorganic phosphate level is reduced below 1 mm per liter (3.1 mg per 100 ml) unless renal damage has resulted in secondary phosphate retention. In the presence of a high phosphate intake, many patients with hyperparathyroidism have plasma phosphate levels which fall within normal limits, with minimal elevation in plasma calcium levels. The excretion of calcium and phosphate in the urine is increased. With extensive bone involvement, the alkaline phosphatase may reach levels as high as 20 to 30 Bodansky units.

Clinical Picture

The earliest symptoms rarely lead to a diagnosis. They may be recognized in retrospect as an accompaniment of hypercalcemia. The symptoms include muscular weakness, anorexia, nausea, and constipation. Polyuria and polydipsia accompany the excessive calcium, phosphate, sodium, and potassium excretion as well as the renal lesions, which cause a loss of the ability of the kidney to concentrate urine even before structural changes have occurred. Often the first indication of hyperparathyroidism is renal colic or a spontaneous fracture. Deafness, paresthesias, and bone pain have been observed, and weight loss may be marked. On examination one may find hypotonia, muscular weakness, calcific keratitis (band keratitis), skeletal deformities, fractures, and tumor masses, especially in the jaw (epulis). When bone disease is present, x-ray studies may show a generalized decrease in bone density, cysts, tumors, fractures, and deformities, which are most marked in the hands, long bones, vertebras, pelvis, skull, and jaw. Bone marrow depression is common, with anemia, leukopenia, and occasionally thrombocytopenia. Peptic ulcer occurs in many patients with this disorder.

Diagnosis

Classic cases of chemical hyperparathyroidism with von Recklinghausen's disease (osteitis fibrosa generalisata or osteitis fibrosa cystica) are diagnosed easily from the clinical picture and the chemical findings of hypercalcemia, hypophosphatemia, hypercalcuria, and an increased plasma alkaline phosphatase (Table 90-2). It is important to carry out simultaneous calcium and total protein determinations, as marked hypoproteinemia (with accompanying decrease in calcium proteinate) may mask an increase in diffusible ionized calcium, the fraction of importance in this disease. It is also important to obtain plasma calcium levels on several occasions, particularly if the first determination is not elevated. The ion activity of calcium can be accurately and rapidly measured by the use of a special calcium ion activity electrode. Usually the calcium ion activity is about 48 to 50 percent of the total calcium, with 49 percent bound to protein and 2 to 3 percent bound to complexes such as citrate and phosphate. Bone lesions may be absent or minimal when calcium and protein intake have been high or when the disease is relatively mild or of short duration. In such cases the plasma alkaline phosphatase level may not be elevated. The diagnosis of hyperparathyroidism should be carefully ruled out in all patients with renal stones. Lithiasis often occurs in mild cases in which no other symptoms are present and plasma mineral levels show minimal changes.

Although hypercalcuria occurs in the absence of hyperparathyroidism, particularly in patients with nephrolithiasis, it is helpful in establishing the diagnosis from other causes. If after 7 to 14 days on a diet of 200 mg calcium the patient excretes more than 200 mg calcium in the urine in 24 hr, hypercalcuria is present. In the presence of avitaminosis D or renal insufficiency, hypercalcuria may not be found in hyperparathyroidism. An approximation of the urinary calcium concentration may be made with the Sulkowitch test.

The early diagnosis of hyperparathyroidism in the absence of renal and skeletal lesions may be extremely difficult, and several procedures have been devised to facilitate diagnosis.

INTRAVENOUS CALCIUM TEST. When a calcium load is administered intravenously, the normal individual responds with a rise in the plasma phosphate level and a fall in the urinary phosphate excretion. This is due to the fact that calcium will "shut off" the parathyroids if the plasma level is high enough. Theoretically, patients with hyperparathyroidism should not show the decrease in urinary excretion of phosphate, but the results are often inconclusive. Patients with hypoparathyroidism show a

Table 90-2. SUMMARY OF CHEMICAL FEATURES OF DISEASES WITH DISTURBED PLASMA CALCIUM AND PHOSPHATE

Disease	Serum			Urine		Feces*	
	Calcium	Phosphate	Alkaline phosphatase	Calcium	Phosphate	Calcium	Phosphate
Hyperparathyroidism.......	Increased	Decreased	Normal or increased	Increased	Increased	Normal	Normal
Paget's disease............	Normal	Normal	Increased	Normal	Normal	Normal	Normal
Hypoparathyroidism........	Decreased	Increased	Normal	Decreased	Decreased	Normal	Normal
Renal insufficiency.........	Decreased	Increased	Normal or increased	Decreased	Decreased	Normal	Increased
Osteomalacia..............	Decreased or normal	Decreased	Increased	Decreased	Decreased	Normal or increased	Decreased
Senile osteoporosis	Normal	Normal	Normal	Normal	Normal	Normal	Normal
Multiple myeloma..........	Normal to increased	Normal	Normal	Normal to increased	Normal to decreased	Normal	Normal
Milk-alkali syndrome.......	Increased	Normal to increased	Normal	Normal to decreased	Normal to decreased		
Vitamin D intoxication	Increased	Increased	Normal	Increased	Decreased	Decreased	Decreased
Metastatic carcinoma.......	Normal to increased	Normal	Normal to increased	Increased	Normal		
Sarcoidosis...............	Increased	Normal to increased	Normal to increased	Increased	Decreased	Decreased	Decreased
Hyperventilation (alkalosis)	Normal	Normal	Normal	Normal	Normal		

* On low-calcium diet.

marked phosphate diuresis, and this test is probably most useful in diagnosing true hypoparathyroidism.

TUBULAR REABSORPTION OF PHOSPHATE. Parathyroid hormone decreases the tubular reabsorption of phosphate in the renal tubules, and it has been found that patients with hyperparathyroidism have a tubular reabsorption of phosphate which is distinctly lower than normal. This can be best demonstrated by giving these patients an oral phosphate load (1 mM phosphate per kg body weight, made up of buffered mono- and dibasic sodium phosphate at pH 7.4), following which the tubular maximal transport of phosphate can be calculated (expressed as tubular reabsorption of phosphate in micromoles per 100 ml glomerular filtration rate per minute). Normal values range from 110 to 150. It can be shown that when there is a normal inulin clearance, this type of determination is valid and is further evidence for the tubular blocking action for phosphate by parathyroid hormone.

CORTISONE TEST. The action of cortisone on the normal subject is to decrease the absorption of calcium from the gastrointestinal tract and to increase the urinary output of calcium. In those patients with sarcoidosis and hypercalcemia, multiple myeloma, vitamin D intoxication, infantile hypercalcemia with failure to thrive, and metastatic carcinoma with hypercalcemia, cortisone acetate (150 mg per day in divided doses for 10 days, or its equivalent) has been shown to lower the plasma calcium within a matter of a few days to 2 weeks. When the diagnosis of hyperparathyroidism is uncertain, this test can often help make the correct diagnosis, since cortisone in most instances does not affect the hypercalcemia due to a parathyroid adenoma.

Differential Diagnosis

Careful observation may be required to differentiate less-typical cases from the following skeletal disorders.

OSTEOPOROSIS. This disease is characterized by a relative increase in bone resorption over bone formation, leading to an eventual decrease in bone mass and a negative calcium balance. It may arise from various hormonal disturbances such as hyperparathyroidism, hyperthyroidism, hyperadrenocorticism, and acromegaly, but it is considered most often to be of an idiopathic variety. Osteoporosis is frequently seen in women after the menopause and involves the spine and pelvis, very rarely the skull. Plasma calcium, phosphate and alkaline phosphatase levels, and the percentage of phosphate reabsorption by the renal tubules are generally within normal limits.

The negative calcium balance may be affected favorably by the administration of estrogens, fluoride, vitamin D in small amounts, calcium suplements, and phosphate administration.

OSTEOMALACIA. This implies failure to mineralize an otherwise normal matrix, seen especially in steatorrhea, vitamin D deficiency, and primary renal acidosis. Both plasma calcium and phosphate levels are decreased, while that of plasma alkaline phosphatase is increased. The urinary calcium excretion is decreased in the first two disorders and increased in the last.

MULTIPLE MYELOMA. This condition may show sharp demarcation of bone lesions by x-ray, with increased plasma and urine calcium, possible stones, a variable phosphate level, increased globulin, Bence-Jones protein (50 percent), and plasma cells in the bone marrow. Even though massive bone disease may be seen by x-ray, the alkaline phosphatase usually remains within normal limits.

METASTATIC MALIGNANCIES. These may present a variable roentgenogram, depending on whether the origin of the primary tumor is the breast, prostate, kidney, bronchus, or thyroid. Plasma calcium and alkaline phosphatase may be increased. An increase in the prostatic fraction of the total acid phosphatase is presumptive evidence for carcinoma of the prostate. The acid phosphatase level may be elevated in other types of metastatic cancer to bone.

RENAL OSTEITIS FIBROSA. In this condition there exists a history of onset of renal difficulties prior to skeletal changes. However, this differentiation is often extraordinarily difficult to ascertain. It should be stated that if an elevated plasma calcium level is found with severe long-standing renal disease, this is most likely due to primary hyperparathyroidism.

SARCOIDOSIS. It once was believed that the bone lesions seen as punched-out lesions in the hands and feet were responsible for the cases of hypercalcemia in association with sarcoid, but this has been shown not to be the case. Indeed, the association of hypercalcemia in sarcoidosis is rarely seen in those cases where the bones are involved. There is little doubt at present that the hypercalcemia is secondary to an increased sensitivity to vitamin D and that moderate exposure to bright sunlight is enough to induce hypercalcemia in the 20 to 30 percent of those afflicted with sarcoid who have this sensitivity. The hypercalcemia responds rapidly to cortisone administration and serves to distinguish this disease from hyperparathyroidism in most instances. An increased globulin, pulmonary fibrosis, splenomegaly, hepatomegaly, and a positive Kveim test help to establish the diagnosis.

OTHER SKELETAL DISEASES. Gaucher's disease, Niemann-Pick disease, Hand-Schüller-Christian syndrome, Hodgkin's disease, osteogenesis imperfecta, osteomyelitis, xanthomatosis, chronic radium poisoning, polycythemia vera, erythroblastosis, etc., may have to be considered in the different diagnosis. A more complete discussion of these individual skeletal disorders is given in Part VIII, Sec. 12, Disorders of Bone.

HYPERCALCEMIA ASSOCIATED WITH RENAL INSUFFICIENCY AND PROLONGED MILK OR ALKALI INGESTION. Burnett and his coworkers (1949) described a syndrome with many features common to primary hyperparathyroidism and secondary renal damage. The characteristic features in patients with this syndrome were a history of prolonged and excessive intake of milk and absorbable alkali, hypercalcemia without hypercalcuria or hypophosphatemia, marked renal insufficiency, calcinosis, and mild alkalosis. The differentiation of this syndrome from primary hyperparathyroidism may be very difficult because of the high incidence of ulcer symptoms in hyperparathyroidism. Treatment consists of a low-milk, low-alkali diet and a high fluid intake. The azotemia and hypercalcemia may diminish and the chemical imbalance may be restored to normal, but residual renal damage may persist.

VITAMIN D INTOXICATION. Excessive vitamin D administration induces a clinical and pathologic picture similar to that of hyperparathyroidism. The symptoms of intoxication are those secondary to hypercalcemia and hypercalcuria already described. Recovery depends on prompt diagnosis and on the severity of the toxicity. Cortisone is the treatment of choice, as well as complete elimination of all sources of vitamin D, in moderate to severe cases of poisoning. The dosage of cortisone should range from 75 to 150 mg per day and should be maintained at this level until a normal plasma calcium is attained. The severe manifestations of the hypercalcemia will recede in a week to 10 days under such treatment, but other minor side effects, such as lassitude, weakness, and loss of appetite, may linger weeks or months before disappearing.

HYPERCALCEMIA IN CARCINOMA WITHOUT METASTASES. Recently there have been numerous instances in which a picture resembling hyperparathyroidism was abolished by removing a cancer locally. These cases were not associated with any demonstrable bony metastases. The cause of the hypercalcemia is not evident, although it has been presumed that these tumors have secreted a substance with plasma calcium–raising properties. The cortisone test is often a useful tool in differentiating this cause of hypercalcemia from hyperparathyroidism.

IMMOBILIZATION. Any patient with diffuse skeletal disease or chronic disease, if immobilized, may develop hypercalcemia and hypercalcuria, unless appropriate measures to prevent its occurrence are taken. No patient with Paget's disease should be put to bed for any long interval, since such a patient is especially likely to develop hypercalcuria.

IDIOPATHIC HYPERCALCEMIA OF INFANCY WITH FAILURE TO THRIVE. This is a new syndrome first described in Great Britain by Lightwood and his associates. These infants often have mental retardation, elfin facies, elevated cholesterol levels in the plasma, and hypercalcemia with all its secondary effects on the kidney and elsewhere. They will respond to cortisone or a diet devoid of vitamin D and calcium. It has been postulated that these children have an abnormal sensitivity to vitamin D similar to that found in sarcoidosis.

IDIOPATHIC HYPERCALCURIA. A large group of patients in whom renal calculi occur characteristically have hypercalcuria, low plasma phosphate, and normal plasma calcium. They may or may not have a lowered tubular reabsorptive rate for phosphate. Bone lesions and elevation of the alkaline phosphatase level are absent. Though the etiology of this syndrome is not clear at the present time, it is possible that these patients have a variant of hyperparathyroidism, and their condition should be followed carefully. Should they develop hypercalcemia at any time in their clinical course, neck exploration for an adenoma should be considered seriously.

OTHER CAUSES OF HYPERCALCEMIA. Thyrotoxicosis has been described in association with hypercalcemia, although this is a rare phenomenon.

Treatment

Once the diagnosis of primary hyperparathyroidism is established, fluids should be forced, intake of calcium restricted, and surgical consultation obtained with a view toward neck exploration. Difficulty in locating the offending gland or glands because of inconstant anatomic positions, and because the noninvolved glands show compensatory atrophy, may necessitate not only extensive but also repeated surgical exploration. Careful x-ray studies of the neck, including the esophagus and the mediastinum, may be helpful in locating the tumor before exploration, but they are often misleading. Removal of an adenoma or removal of all except a portion of one gland in case of hypertrophy and hyperplasia may be expected to cure the condition. When plasma alkaline phosphatase level is markedly elevated, large quantities of calcium may be required postoperatively to prevent recurrent tetany, since the bone will avidly remove calcium from the plasma in order to recalcify the bone lesions. The treatment of postoperative tetany is similar to that described in the treatment of hypoparathyroidism except that more vigorous treatment may have to be continued for some time to control the acute manifestations. A diet high in calcium and phosphate should be given postoperatively, but there is no need for increased doses of vitamin D over the normal intake unless there is a problem of chronic tetany. Under normal circumstances great improvement may be noted in the skeletal lesions as well as the renal function.

ACUTE HYPERCALCEMIC SYNDROME

Hypercalcemia caused by acute parathyroid intoxication or nonendocrine tumor constitutes an acute medical emergency. Acute parathyroid intoxication, with marked elevation of the plasma calcium level, occurs occasionally as a complication of hyperparathyroidism. It is characterized by weakness, lethargy, intractable nausea and vomiting, coma, and sudden death. The oral, rectal, or intravenous administration of phosphate is probably the most effective medical therapy for the treatment of hypercalcemia. A solution containing NaH_2PO_4 and Na_2HPO_4 (Fleet's Phospho-Soda), each 5 ml containing 3.3 Gm sodium phosphate, may be given orally. The usual dose is 10 to 20 ml (diluted with water or juice) daily, and the maintenance dose depends on the level of plasma calcium. The hypocalcemic effect of phosphate is apparent usually in 12 to 24 hr. If the patient is anorectic or comatose, a Fleet's Phospho-Soda enema may be used, since phosphate is readily absorbed through the sigmoid colon. One to three enemas daily may be used until the patient is able to swallow liquids. Intravenously, one may administer 500 ml of 0.1 M phosphate (0.08 mole Na_2HPO_4 plus 0.02 mole KH_2PO_4 per liter) over a 4- to 8-hr period, followed, if necessary, by an additional 500 ml INPHOS (Davies, Rose-Hoyt), a commercial preparation, available for intravenous use. One should be extremely cautious when using intravenous phosphate in azotemic patients, since profound hypocalcemia with tetany and convulsions has been reported. Great care should be taken as well to prevent infiltration of the phosphate infusion, since this will lead to subcutaneous calcification at the site of infiltration. It should be pointed out that early operation is indicated, because phosphate administration is not indicated as permanent treatment for hypercalcemia.

SECONDARY HYPERPARATHYROIDISM
History

Enlargement of the parathyroid glands secondary to another disease process in the body was first noted in 1905 by MacCallum in a case of nephritis. One year later, Erdheim noted similar findings in rickets, and since that time the syndrome of secondary hyperfunction of the parathyroids has been recognized.

Incidence

As a complication of advanced renal disease, hyperfunction of the parathyroids is relatively common. In 1933 Pappenheimer and Wilens reported that in a series of 21 cases of nephritis the mean parathyroid weight was 50 percent greater than in a control group.

Etiology

The most common cause of this condition is chronic, long-standing renal disease, as in glomerulonephritis and pyelonephritis. The term *renal rickets* does not apply to cases of secondary hyperparathyroidism and should be reserved for those cases seen most often in children in whom true rickets is secondary to prolonged and chronic renal disease and the supervening acidosis. Both secondary hyperparathyroidism and rickets have been described in the same patient as a complication of chronic renal disease. Reports of secondary hyperparathyroidism have been noted in a variety of diseases, such as osteogenesis imperfecta, Paget's disease, multiple myeloma, carcinoma with bone metastases and pituitary basophilism.

Pathology

The parathyroid glands are enlarged diffusely and are hyperplastic. No single adenomas are visible. The cells are normal in size and easily differentiated from those seen in primary hyperparathyroidism. The former are principally chief cells with some increase in oxyphil cells, as opposed to the huge, water-clear cells of primary hyperparathyroidism due to hypertrophy and hyperplasia. The bone lesions are entirely similar to those seen in primary hyperparathyroidism, namely, generalized decalcification and bone cysts, with or without outright fracture.

Pathologic Physiology

It is unclear at the present time what the precise mechanisms for the development of parathyroid hyperplasia are in renal disease. It was believed that long-standing phosphate retention was the *sine qua non* for the development of the syndrome. The metabolic acidosis which invariably accompanies chronic renal disease leads to a negative calcium balance, since bone mineral constitutes in effect an important homeostatic mechanism for the neutralization of fixed acid, and an effective, although costly, device for the defense against progressive acidosis in patients whose kidneys have lost their capacity to regulate the acid balance of the body. Whether or not acidosis affects the skeleton by modifying the physiologic actions of vitamin D, parathyroid hormone, or thyrocalcitonin has not, as yet, been determined. Correction of the acidosis by alkali administration, vitamin D, or renal homotransplantation has led to variable degrees of bone repair.

Clinical Picture

The symptoms are usually those of the primary disease process before any evidence of hyperparathyroidism is noted. Classic glomerulonephritis or pyelonephritis, uremia, and evidence of renal insufficiency dominate the clinical picture. In children, dwarfism and pathologic fractures may be the presenting complaints.

Diagnosis

The chemical findings of normal or low-normal plasma calcium with hyperphosphatemia and high alkaline phosphatase, with the classic skeletal roentgenograms of bone cysts and generalized demineralization, lead to the diagnosis of parathyroid hyperfunction with renal disease. The history of early renal disease is often the only differential diagnostic point, since the primary cases are often complicated late in the disease by renal failure secondary to long-standing hyperparathyroidism. An elevated plasma calcium level in the presence of uremia indicates autonomous parathyroid hyperfunction due either to a primary adenoma or to "tertiary" parathyroid hyperplasia.

Treatment

Of greatest importance is a correct diagnosis. Once this is established, all therapy is directed at the primary disease, and an attempt is made to correct the acidosis by the administration of alkaline salts, such as bicarbonate or citrate. Attempts to elevate the plasma calcium level by large amounts of vitamin D (calciferol, in doses of 50,000 to 150,000 units per day, or the equivalent in vitamin D_3 or dihydrotachysterol) are often indicated when the plasma calcium is reduced in order to suppress excessive parathyroid hormone secretion. However, this type of therapy is extremely dangerous and must be carefully regulated, since the difference between therapeutic and toxic doses of vitamin D is quite narrow. Certain patients with chronic renal disease and severe secondary hyperparathyroidism have had subtotal parathyroidectomy followed by vitamin D therapy. Though the bone disease is strikingly cured by such means, the basic renal disorder is unaltered and the patients have ultimately died of uremia.

NONFUNCTIONING TUMORS OF THE PARATHYROID GLANDS

Nonfunctioning carcinoma of the parathyroids has been reported, but these cases have not been generally accepted, because of the difficulty in establishing the origin of the tumor. Other nonfunctioning tumors include oxyphil adenomas which may be burned-out primary adenomas), metastatic carcinoma, and cysts. Microscopic cysts are common in hyperplastic and adenomatous glands, whereas gross cysts are quite rare. Symptoms, when present, are due to pressure on local structures, including the recurrent laryngeal nerve. Most tumors have been found in the lower glands.

REFERENCES

Baker, W. H.: Abnormalities in Calcium Metabolism in Malignancy: Effects of Hormone Therapy, Am. J. Med., 21:714, 1956.

Bernstein, D. S., and C. D. Guri: Hyperparathyroidism and Hypoparathyroidism: Preoperative and Postoperative Care, Anesthesiology, 24:448, 1963.

Bogdonoff, M. D., A. H. Woods, J. E. White, and F. L. Engel: Hyperparathyroidism, Am. J. Med., 21:583, 1956.

Bourne, G. H.: "The Biochemistry and Physiology of Bone," New York, Academic Press, Inc., 1956.

Bronsky, D., D. S. Kushner, A. Dubin, and I. Snapper: Idiopathic Hypoparathyroidism and Pseudohypoparathyroidism, Medicine, 37:317, 1958.

Chambers, E. L., G. S. Gordan, L. Goldman, and E. C. Reifenstein, Jr.: Tests for Hyperparathyroidism: Tubular Reabsorption of Phosphate, Phosphate Deprivation, and Calcium Infusion, J. Clin. Endocrinol. & Metab., 16:1507, 1956.

Goldsmith, R. S., and S. H. Ingbar: Inorganic Phosphate Treatment of Hypercalcemia of Diverse Etiologies, New Eng. J. Med., 274:1, 1966.

Heaney, R. P., and G. O. Whedon: Radiocalcium Studies of Bone Formation Rate in Human Metabolic Bone Disease, J. Clin. Endocrinol. & Metab., 18:1246, 1958.

Munson, P. L., P. F. Hirsch, and A. H. Tashjian: Parathyroid Gland, Ann. Rev. Physiol., 25:325, 1963.

Rasmussen, H.: Purification of Parathyroid Polypeptides, J. Biol. Chem., 235:3442, 1960.

Underdahl, L., L. B. Woolner, and B. M. Black: Multiple Endocrine Adenomas: Eight Cases Involving Parathyroids, Pituitary, and Pancreatic Islets, J. Clin. Endocrinol. & Metab., 13:20, 1953.

91 CALCITONIN

Daniel S. Bernstein and Menelaos A. Aliapoulios

Historical Development

That precise regulation of plasma calcium is mediated by parathyroid hormone acting on bone, intestine, and kidneys has been recognized over the past 40 years. In 1961, this classic concept was challenged as a result of the demonstration of a second substance involved in calcium homeostasis by Copp and his coworkers, who showed that perfusion of the thyroparathyroid glands with a hypercalcemic solution produced a rapid fall in plasma calcium level. In 1963, Hirsch and colleagues demonstrated a fall in plasma calcium and phosphate in rats given a crude extract of hog thyroid. They appropriately named this new hormone *thyrocalcitonin*. The presence of the new hormone originating in the thyroid gland was established in other species as well as in man.

Anatomy and Physiology

Initially it was thought that thyrocalcitonin originated in the epithelial cells of the thyroid gland. It is now known that thyrocalcitonin is derived from the ultimobranchial bodies which fuse with the thyroid in mammals. These bodies, whose function hitherto was obscure, remain as separate structures in birds, fish, reptiles, and amphibians. They develop from the ventral part of the pharyngeal entoderm immediately behind the last pair of gill pouches. Their cells have a particular microscopic appearance, which is now recognized to be similar to that of the thyroid "C" cells. These "C" cells were identified long ago as differing from the thyroid follicular cells and now have been shown to be the site of production of thyrocalcitonin. Stimulation of the thyroid by TSH produces no increase of thyrocalcitonin, and propylthiouracil administration induces no decrease in the secretion of this substance. The term *thyrocalcitonin* can now be discarded because this hormone is derived from ultimobranchial tissue which is not necessarily confined to the thyroid.

Chemical Structure

The chemical structure of calcitonin (porcine) was determined independently by three groups of investigators. Following this, the total synthesis of the hormone was accomplished. Calcitonin is a 32-chain polypeptide with a disulfide bridge and a molecular weight of approximately 3,600. The amino acid composition is unique in the absence of isoleucine and in the high content of glycine, proline, and serine. Calcitonin is highly potent, and its biologic activity is demonstrable in microgram quantities.

Physiologic Action

It has been established that calcitonin, when injected into various test animals as well as humans, induces a rapid fall in plasma calcium, with ionized calcium and phosphate levels rarely lasting longer than 3 to 4 hr. It has been shown that the fall in plasma calcium and phosphate levels following injection of calcitonin is not dependent upon the presence of the parathyroid gland. Calcitonin has no significant effect on calcium transport across the duodenum, and nephrectomy does not alter its hypocalcemic effect. Investigators, using varied experimental models, have shown that calcitonin has a direct inhibiting effect on bone resorption which is proportional to the concentration of calcitonin employed. With decreased bone resorption, there is an associated decrease in the excretion of urinary hydroxyproline. In long-term use, calcitonin has been shown to increase trabecular bone formation in parathyroidectomized rats. The extent to which calcitonin can inhibit bone resorption is probably dependent upon the existing rate of bone resorption, a greater response being evoked in the presence of increased bone resorption. Calcitonin also produces a decrease in the urinary excretion of calcium, magnesium, and hydroxyproline, whereas the effect on renal phosphate excretion has not been clearly elucidated.

Clinical Significance

Human thyroid tissue has been shown to contain significant amounts of calcitonin. The presence of calcitonin in the plasma of two normal persons at rest has been detected by rat bioassay and by radioimmunoassay. This implies that the hormone has a physiologic role other than combating periodic hypercalcemia. Furthermore, the concentration of calcitonin is increased in response to an infusion of calcium. In two cases of pseudohypoparathyroidism, calcitonin concentration 100 times greater than normal was found and deserves attention as a possible factor responsible for the alteration in calcium metabolism observed in this syndrome. In cases of thyroid goiter, adenoma, and hyperplasia, calcitonin is absent or found in decreased amounts. In hyperparathyroidism, there is decreased calcitonin in the thyroid gland.

Several patients have been described with medullary carcinoma of the thyroid and an excess of hypocalcemic activity in the blood or tumor. A variety of laboratory techniques as well as radioimmunoassay of serum in one instance confirmed that the active substance was calcitonin. Only one patient was noted to have hypocalcemia and hypophosphatemia, and none was reported to have dense bones on x-ray examination. It now appears certain that medullary carcinoma results from malignant proliferation of thyroid "C" cells. No other syndrome in man has been formally proved to result from abnormal production of calcitonin, but studies in cows with hypocalcemia and hypophosphatemia at parturition showed that excess release of calcitonin might be responsible for this condition.

The practical importance and the possible clinical application of this new hormone are speculative at present. There may be pathogenetic significance in the elevated levels of calcitonin found in pseudohypoparathyroidism and in medullary carcinoma of the thyroid. The direct effect of calcitonin in decreasing bone resorption could be of benefit to patients with osteoporosis, hypercalcemia of diverse etiology, bone fractures, Paget's disease, and other demineralizing bone disorders accompanied by excessive bone resorption. Calcitonin administration has produced a temporary fall in plasma calcium level in a patient with hypercalcemia due to metastatic carcinoma.

In a patient with hypercalcemia associated with a malignant parathyroid tumor, calcitonin administration for periods of approximately 2 to 3 weeks on two occasions resulted in a decrease in serum calcium level and a reduction in urinary calcium excretion.

REFERENCES

Aliapoulios, M. A., D. S. Bernstein, and M. C. Balodimos: Thyrocalcitonin: Its Role in Calcium Homeostasis, Arch. Intern. Med., 123:88, 1969.

——, and P. L. Munson: Thyrocalcitonin, Surg. Forum, 16:55, 1965.

Dambacher, M. A., J. Guncaga, T. Lauffenburger, and H. G. Haas: Human Calcitonin, Germ. Med. Mth., 14:356, 1969.

Foster, G. V.: Calcitonin (Thyrocalcitonin), New Engl. J. Med., 279:349, 1968.

Galante, L., T. V. Gudmundsson, E. W. Matthews, E. D. Williams, A. Tse, N. J. Y. Woodhouse, and I. MacIntyre: Thymic and Parathyroid Origin of Calcitonin in Man, Lancet, p. 537, September 7, 1968.

Hirsch, P. F., and P. L. Munson: Thyrocalcitonin, Physiol. Rev., 49:548, 1969.

Pechet, M. M.: Symposium on Thyrocalcitonin, Am. J. Med., 43:645, 1967.

92 DISEASES OF THE ADRENAL CORTEX

David P. Lauler, Gordon H. Williams, and George W. Thorn

INTRODUCTION

Thomas Addison's description in 1849 of a clinical syndrome resulting from destruction of the adrenal glands first attracted attention to these organs. Seven years later Brown-Séquard demonstrated that removal of both adrenals from experimental animals caused death soon after operation, whereas control animals subjected to a sham operation survived. Subsequent investigations established that the life-maintaining hormone was elaborated by cells in the cortex, since destruction of all medullary tissue was not accompanied by the classic signs and symptoms of adrenal insufficiency noted after complete removal of the glands.

Between 1927 and 1930, Hartman and his associates, Rogoff and Stewart, and Pfiffner and Swingle all independently described methods for preparing potent adrenocortical extracts. During the following decade, crystalline steroid substances were isolated from these extracts by Kendall, by Grollman, and by Reichstein. In 1937, Steiger and Reichstein synthesized the first natural corticosteroid, 11-deoxycorticosterone, a year before it was identified in adrenal extracts. From 1940 to 1950, the synthesis of several 11-oxygenated compounds was achieved, including cortisone and hydrocortisone. The contributions of Sarett and his collaborators, Reichstein et al., and Kendall and his coworkers were outstanding in this regard. In 1954 aldosterone, the principal salt-retaining hormone of the adrenal, was identified by Simpson and Tait in collaboration with the Swiss group under Reichstein.

Since 1954, a number of remarkable advances have occurred. ACTH has been isolated, its amino acid sequence determined, and the complete molecule synthesized. A number of substances which interfere with the action of adrenal steroids have also been synthesized. For example, amphenone and 2-methyl-1,2-bis-(3-pyridyl)-1-propanone (metyrapone) interfere with the synthesis of hydrocortisone. Spironolactone and 2,4,7-tri-amino-6-phenylpteridine (triamterene) block the physiologic effects of aldosterone. Among the most significant advancements have been the refinements in the ease and accuracy with which steroids and their metabolic products may be measured, e.g., by double isotope derivative, competitive protein-binding radioassay, and radioimmunoassay techniques.

BIOCHEMISTRY AND PHYSIOLOGY

Steroid Nomenclature

The adrenal steroids contain as their basic structure a cyclopentanoperhydrophenanthrane nucleus consisting of three 6-carbon hexane rings and a single 5-carbon pentane ring (D). The carbon atoms are numbered in a predetermined sequence beginning with ring A (Fig. 92-1). The Greek letter Δ indicates a double bond, as does the suffix -ene. The position of a substituent below or above the plane of the steroid molecule is indicated by the letters α and β respectively. The α-substituent is drawn with a broken line (− −OH), and the β-substituent is drawn with a solid line (—OH). The C_{19} steroids are those which have substituent methyl groups at positions C-18 and C-19. C_{19} steroids that also have a ketone group at C-17 are termed *17-ketosteroids*. These C_{19} steroids have predominant androgenic activity. The C_{21} steroids are those which have a 2-carbon side chain (C-20 and C-21) attached at position 17 of the D ring and, in addition, have substituent methyl groups at C-18 and C-19. C_{21} steroids that also possess a hydroxyl group at position 17 are termed *17-hydroxycorticosteroids* or *17-hydroxycorticoids*. The C_{21} steroids may have either predominant glucocorticoid or mineralocorticoid properties. *Glucocorticoid* signifies a C_{21} steroid with predominant action on intermediary metabolism, and *mineralocorticoid* indicates a C_{21} steroid with predominant action on the metabolism of the body minerals, sodium and potassium.

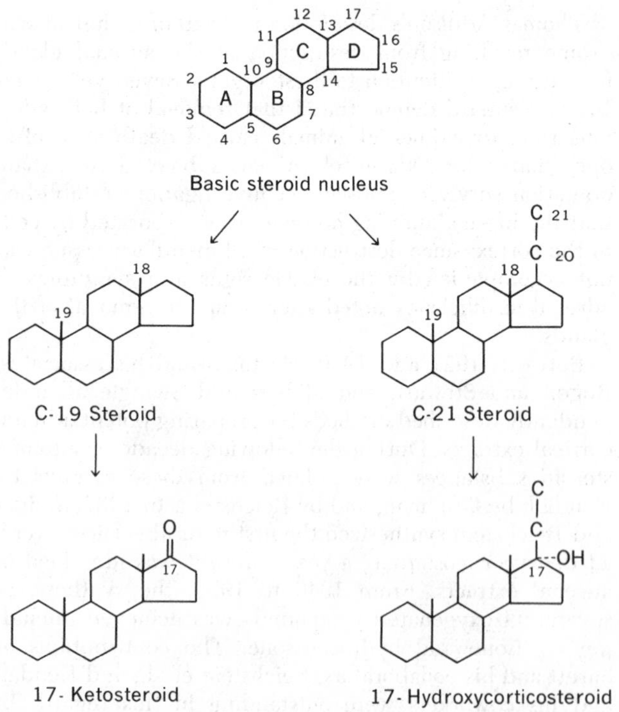

Biosynthesis of Adrenal Steroids

Cholesterol, derived from the diet and from endogenous synthesis via acetate, is the principal starting compound in steroidogenesis. The three major adrenal biosynthetic pathways lead to the production of glucocorticoids (cortisol), mineralocorticoids (aldosterone), and adrenal androgens (dehydroepiandrosterone) (Fig. 92-2).

GLUCOCORTICOID PATHWAY. $\Delta5$-Pregnenolone is formed after cleavage of the side chain of cholesterol. $\Delta5$-Pregnenolone is converted to progesterone by the action of the enzymes 3β-hydroxydehydrogenase and $\Delta5,\Delta4$-isomerase. These enzymes transform the 3β-hydroxy group of $\Delta5$-pregnenolone to a C-3-ketonic group and transform the double bond between C-5:C-6 of $\Delta5$-pregnenolone to position C-4:C-5 of progesterone. A series of hydroxylations mediated by specific hydroxylating enzymes then occurs in sequential fashion at C-17, then at C-21, and finally at C-11. With the introduction of a hydroxyl group at position C-17 of progesterone by the enzyme C-17 hydroxylase, 17α-hydroxyprogesterone is formed, which in turn has a hydroxyl group introduced at C-21 by the enzyme C-21 hydroxylase, producing 11-deoxycortisol (Compound S), the major precursor of cortisol. Finally, a third hydroxyl group is introduced at the C-11 position of 11-deoxycortisol by the enzyme C-11 hydroxylase, to produce cortisol (Compound F, hydrocortisone), the major glucocorticoid. The chemical name for cortisol is 11β,17α,21-trihydroxy-4-pregnene-3,20-dione.

MINERALOCORTICOID PATHWAY. Progesterone, after transformation from $\Delta5$-pregnenolone, is hydroxylated at the C-21 position to form 11-deoxycorticosterone. This C-21 hydroxylase, rather than being identical to the enzyme used to form 11-deoxycortisol, may be an isoenzyme of it; 11-deoxycorticosterone is then hydroxylated at the 11 position to form corticosterone, compound B. A hydroxyl group is then introduced at the 18 position to form 18-hydroxycorticosterone, the immediate precursor of aldosterone. With conversion of the hydroxyl group at C-18 to an aldehyde group, the major mineralocorticoid, *aldosterone*, is formed. The 18-aldehyde group exists free

Basic steroid nucleus

C-19 Steroid

C-21 Steroid

17- Ketosteroid

17- Hydroxycorticosteroid

Fig. 92-1. Basic steroid structure and nomenclature.

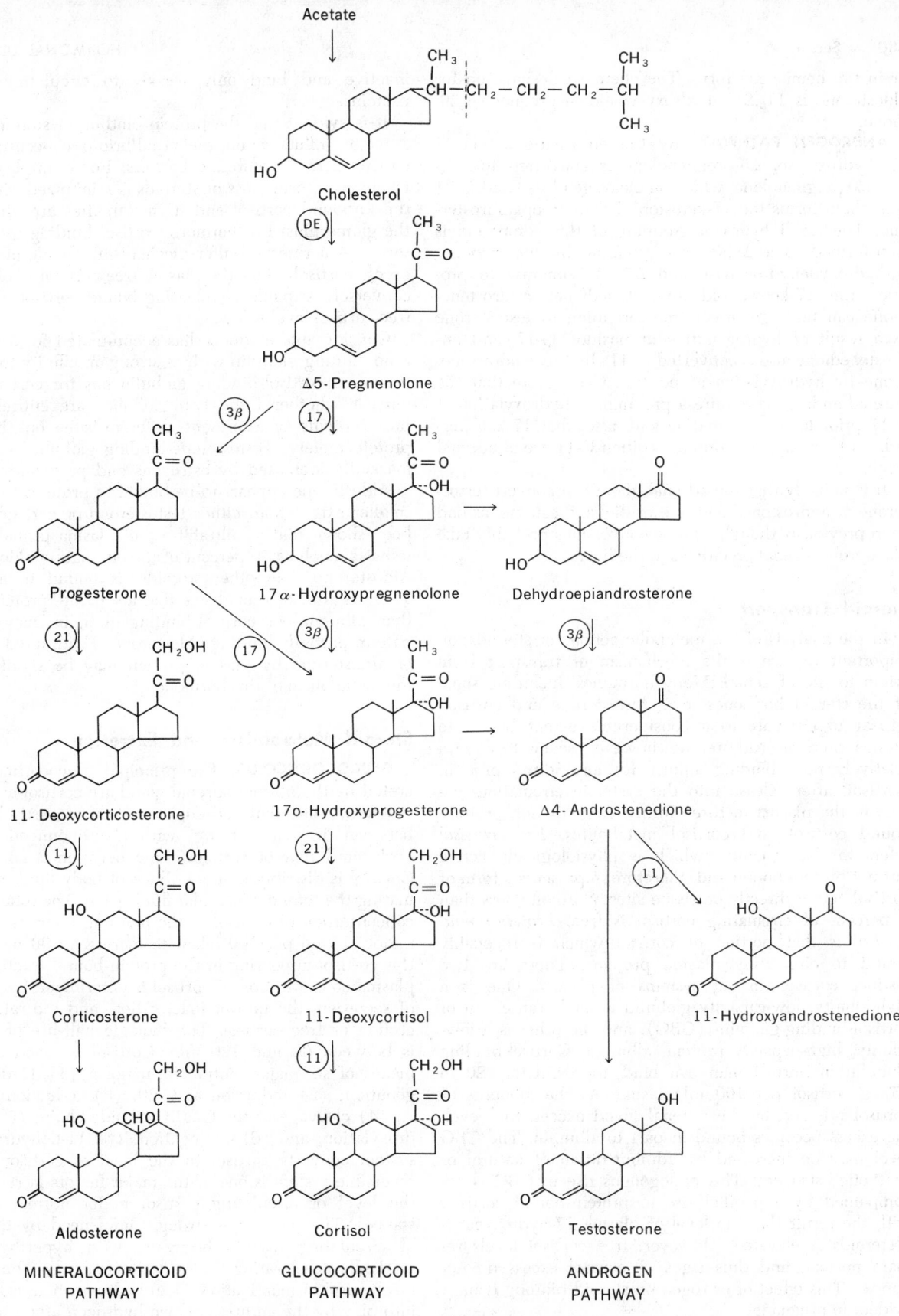

Fig. 92-2. Biosynthetic pathways for adrenal steroid production. Major pathways to mineralocorticoids, glucocorticoids, and androgens. Circled letters and numbers denote specific enzymes: *DE* = debranching enzyme; 3β = 3β-ol-dehydrogenase with Δ4–Δ5 isomerase; 11 = C-11 hydroxylase; 17 = C-17 hydroxylase; 21 = C-21 hydroxylase.

or in the hemiacetal form. The chemical designation for aldosterone is $11_\beta,21$-dihydroxy-18-aldo-4-pregnene-3,20-dione.

ANDROGEN PATHWAY. By the enzymatic action of 17_α-hydroxylase, $\Delta5$-pregnenolone is converted to 17_α-hydroxypregnenolone, which on cleavage of its C-20:C-21 side chain forms the 17-ketosteroid dehydroepiandrosterone. The $\Delta5,-3$ hydroxyl grouping of this compound is transformed to a $\Delta4,-3$ oxo- grouping by the enzymes 3_β-hydroxydehydrogenase and $\Delta5,\Delta4$ isomerase to produce the 17-ketosteroid androstenedione. Androstenedione can undergo direct transformation to testosterone as a result of hydrogenation at position C-17, and androstenedione also is converted to 11_β-hydroxyandrostenedione by hydroxylation at position C-11. Note that the adrenal androgens require a preliminary hydroxylation at C-17 prior to their formation and, also, that 17-ketosteroids with an oxygen group at position C-11 are of adrenal origin.

It is unlikely that the adrenal gland can convert testosterone or androstenedione to estradiol and estrone, as had been previously thought. These conversions probably take place from adrenal precursors in the liver.

Steroid Transport

In the analysis of the metabolic actions of steroids, an important feature is the mechanism of transport from origin to site of action. Many hormones, including some of the steroid hormones, e.g., testosterone and cortisol, appear to circulate to a considerable extent bound to plasma proteins. Aldosterone, however, seems to have a relatively poor binding affinity for any serum protein. Cortisol, after release into the systemic circulation, occurs in the plasma in three forms: free cortisol, protein-bound cortisol, and cortisol metabolites. *Free cortisol* refers to that quantity which is physiologically active but not protein bound and, therefore, represents a form of cortisol acting directly on tissue sites. Normally, less than 5 percent of circulating cortisol is free. *Protein-bound cortisol* is that portion of cortisol which is reversibly bound to circulating plasma proteins. There are two distinct cortisol-binding systems of plasma. One is a high-affinity, low-capacity globulin termed transcortin or cortisol-binding-globulin (CBG), and the other is a low-affinity, high-capacity protein, albumin. Cortisol-binding globulin in normal man can bind approximately 20 to 25 μg cortisol per 100 ml plasma. As the amounts of cortisol released by the adrenal gland exceed this level, the excess becomes bound in part to albumin. The CBG level may be increased by administration of natural or synthetic estrogens. This endogenous rise in CBG is accompanied by a parallel rise in protein-bound cortisol, with the result that the level of plasma 17-hydroxycorticosteroids is elevated. However, free cortisol levels remain normal, and thus signs of cortisol excess do not appear. This effect of estrogen on steroid binding is most evident in pregnancy.

Cortisol metabolites such as tetrahydrocortisol also circulate in the plasma. These metabolites are biologically inactive and bind only weakly to circulating plasma proteins.

It is evident that the protein binding of steroids exerts a major influence on the equilibrium concentration of cortisol across membrane barriers. For example, by this mechanism, urine loss of steroids is minimized, since only the unbound cortisol and its metabolites are filtrable at the glomerulus. Furthermore, cortisol binding to proteins serves as a reserve buffer mechanism capable of binding excess cortisol when the plasma free cortisol is high, and conversely, capable of releasing bound cortisol when the free cortisol level is low.

Considerable evidence has accumulated for a testosterone-binding globulin with as strong an affinity for testosterone as cortisol-binding globulin has for cortisol. It is unclear whether these two globulins are entirely separate proteins or represent different sites on the same protein moiety. Testosterone-binding globulin is likewise markedly increased by estrogens and pregnancy.

Aldosterone appears to be bound to proteins to a much smaller extent than either testosterone or cortisol. It has been shown that an ultrafiltrate of plasma probably contains as much as 50 percent of the circulating aldosterone. Aldosterone, like other steroids, is bound to albumin. There is also some evidence that a separate protein, other than albumin- or cortisol-binding globulin, may participate in partially binding aldosterone. The limited binding of aldosterone by plasma protein may be significant in the metabolism of this hormone.

Steroid Metabolism and Excretion

GLUCOCORTICOIDS. The principal glucocorticoids secreted by the normal adrenal gland are cortisol and corticosterone. The daily adrenal secretion of cortisol ranges between 15 and 30 mg, with a pronounced diurnal cycle, and that of corticosterone between 2 and 4 mg. Cortisol is distributed in a volume of body fluids approximating the total extracellular fluid space. The total plasma concentration of cortisol in the morning hours is approximately 15 μg per 100 ml, with more than 90 percent of this cortisol appearing in the protein-bound fraction. The plasma concentration of cortisol is determined by the rate of secretion, the rate of inactivation, and the rate of excretion of free cortisol. The biologic half-life of cortisol is between 60 and 120 min. Cortisol is inactivated by means of six major biotransformations: (1) 11-dehydrogenation; (2) reduction at C-20; (3) reduction of ring A; (4) cleavage of the C-20:C-21 side chain; (5) 6_β-hydroxylation; and (6) conjugation. The 11-dehydrogenase system converts cortisol to the inactive cortisone. This reversible system is one of the major factors in regulating the level of circulating cortisol under normal circumstances. The enzyme is strongly influenced by the level of circulating thyroid hormone, with hyperthyroidism markedly accelerating the oxidative reaction. The second mechanism of inactivation, C-20 hydroxylation, is brought into play by the addition of two hydrogen atoms at C-20. Further reduction elsewhere in the molecule is possible, and the products are the cortols and the cortolones. The third mechanism is the reduction of ring A. The initial saturation of the C-4:C-5 double bond in ring A by the introduction of two hydrogen ions produces *dihydrocortisol* (Fig. 92-3). Next the C-3 ketonic group of dihydrocortisol is reduced by further addition of two hydrogen atoms to form *tetrahydrocortisol* (THF). Furthermore, cortisone may go through a similar reduction process to produce tetrahydrocortisone (THE). From 5 to 10 percent of the secreted cortisol is metabolized in the liver by cleavage of the C-20:C-21 side chain to form

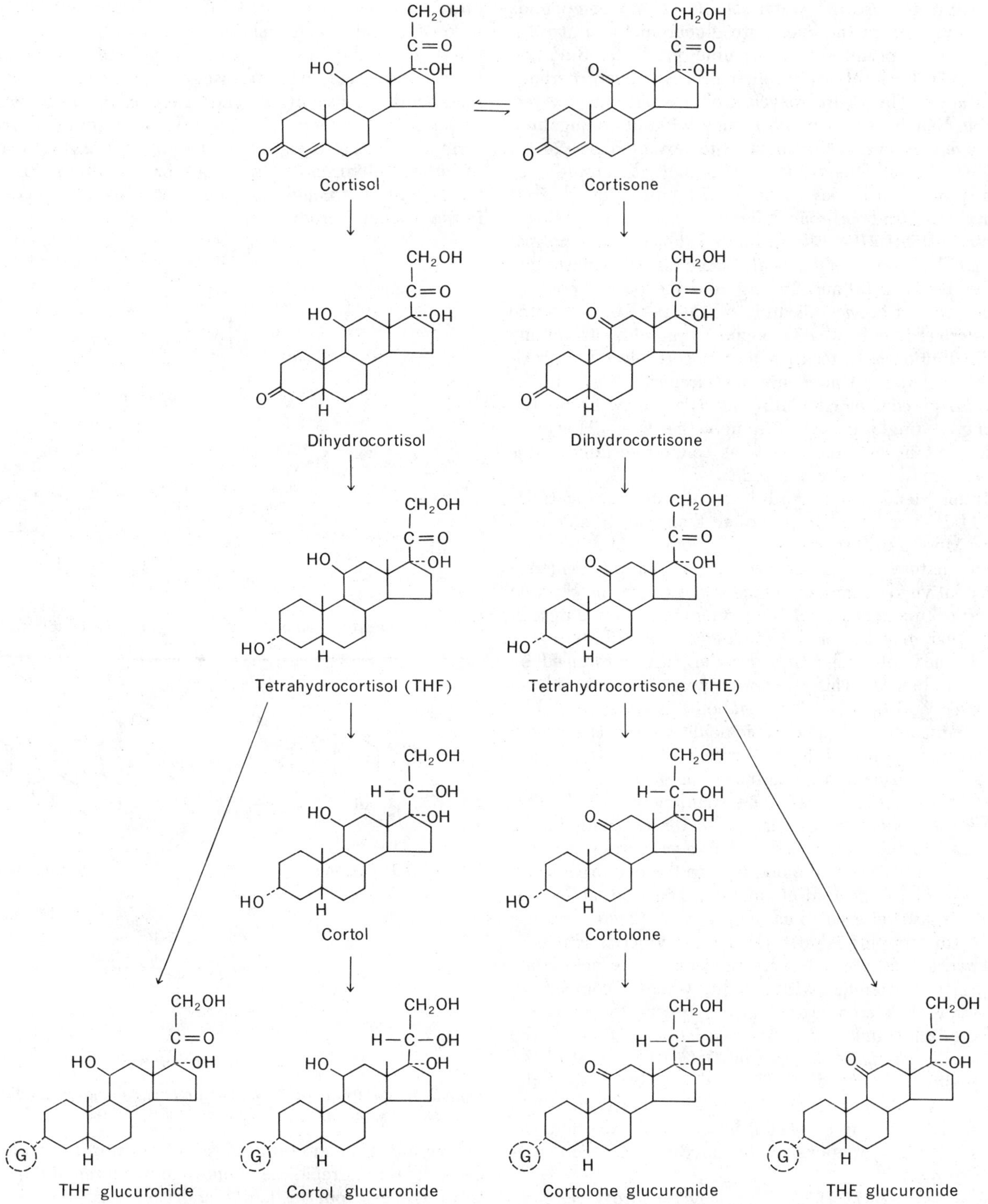

Fig. 92-3. Metabolism of cortisol to tetrahydrocortisol, tetrahydrocortisone, cortol, and cortolone. Conjugation occurs with glucuronic acid at C-3 position. Note interconversion of cortisol and cortisone.

the corresponding 11-oxyketosteroid. Finally, in normal man, 6β-hydroxylation of cortisol represents a relatively minor metabolic transformation. However, under certain circumstances, in infancy and toxemia of pregnancy and with certain drugs, the formation of this product becomes important. The first four transformations produce compounds which are not water-soluble. These compounds are conjugated in the liver with glucuronic acid at position C-3 to produce water-soluble products. Sulfation appears to be a relatively minor process, except perhaps in infancy. The 6β-hydroxycortisol is sufficiently water-soluble that it can clear the kidney without conjugation. The average amounts of metabolites excreted per 24 hr. are as follows: free cortisol, 0.05 mg; glucuronides of cortols and cortolones, 3 mg; 17-ketosteroids derived from cortisol and cortisone, 1.5 mg.

MINERALOCORTICOIDS. In normal subjects on a normal salt intake, the average daily secretion of aldosterone ranges between 50 and 250 μg, and the plasma concentration ranges between 5 and 15 mμg per 100 ml. Since aldosterone is only weakly bound to proteins, its volume of distribution is larger than that of cortisol and approximates 35 liters. Under normal circumstances, greater than 75 percent of circulating aldosterone is inactivated during a single passage through the liver. However, under certain conditions, such as congestive failure, this percentage is markedly reduced.

Under steady-state conditions, aldosterone exists as the 11-18-hemiacetal form rather than the 18-aldehyde form. Most transformations of this compound are reductive in nature. There has been no substantial evidence of oxidative reactions involving aldosterone, in contrast to cortisol metabolism. Of the numerous reductive metabolites that may be formed, 50 percent of aldosterone is transformed into the tetrahydro derivative produced by ring A reduction. This reaction appears to occur only in the liver, and because this metabolite is water-insoluble, it is conjugated with glucuronic acid before it is excreted in the urine. From 7 to 15 percent of aldosterone appears in the urine as a glucuronide conjugate, from which free aldosterone is released on standing at pH 1. This *acid-labile conjugate* appears to be formed both in the liver and in the kidney. The relative proportions appear to be related to relative blood flow to the two organs and the state of the general circulation. The acid-labile conjugate is also referred to as the *3-oxo conjugate*, because the 3-oxo grouping is not irreversibly reduced, as it is in tetrahydroaldosterone. Ninety percent of the acid-labile conjugate is excreted within 6 hr, whereas comparable tetrahydroaldosterone excretion requires 24 to 36 hr. For average salt intake, the 24-hr urine excretion of the acid-labile conjugate ranges from 1 to 10 μg, that of the tetrahydro derivative from 25 to 35 μg, and that of the nonconjugated, nonreduced free aldosterone from 0.2 to 0.6 μg. Aldosterone excretion, like cortisol excretion, exhibits diurnal variations, with daytime excretion predominating.

ADRENAL ANDROGENS. The major androgenic compound secreted by the adrenal gland is dehydroepiandrosterone (DHEA) and its C-3 sulfuric acid ester.

From 15 to 30 mg of these compounds is secreted daily. Much smaller amounts of Δ4-androstenedione and 11β-hydroxyandrostenedione and testosterone are secreted. The major fraction of dehydroepiandrosterone is found in the urine as the sulfate. However, only a small portion of the secreted compound reaches this stage without other metabolic alterations. The first step, which is irreversible, is the conversion to Δ4-androstenedione (Fig. 92-4). This compound is then interconvertible with testosterone and shares with testosterone a common group of metabolites, consisting of androsterone, epiandrosterone, and etiocholanolone. The second major route of transformation is the formation of the 16α-hydroxyl derivative of either dehydroepiandrosterone or its sulfate. In pregnancy, this compound performs a vital role as a precursor in the placental production of estriol.

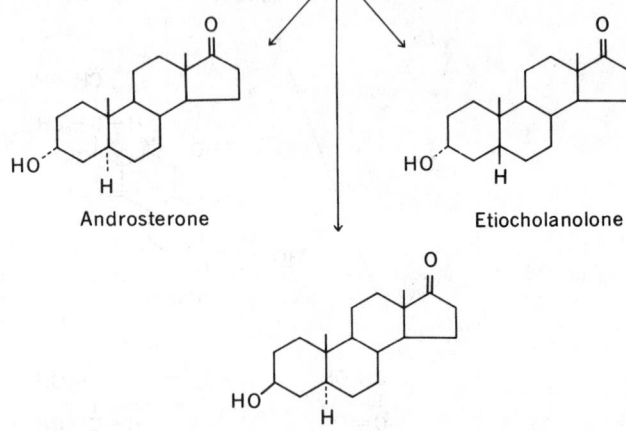

Fig. 92-4. Metabolism of adrenal androgens. Δ4-androstenedione and testosterone contribute to the same metabolites.

Two-thirds of the urine 17-ketosteroids in the male are derived from adrenal metabolites, and the remaining one-third comes from testicular androgens. In the female, almost all urine 17-ketosteroids are derived from the adrenal gland. It is improbable that estrogens are synthesized by the adrenal gland. There has been no substantial proof of aromatic enzymes being present in adrenal tissue. The increased estrogens in ovariectomized patients and in feminizing adrenal tumors are probably secondary to the action of liver enzymes on androgenic precursors secreted by the adrenal glands.

ACTH Physiology

The adrenocorticotropin hormone (ACTH) (see Chap. 87) is an unbranched long-chain polypeptide containing 39 amino acids. It is stored in and released from the anterior pituitary gland, where histologically it appears to be localized to basophil cells. Only 50 units, or roughly 0.25 mg, of the active peptide are stored in the anterior pituitary. Much of the potential for producing the corticotropic actions of ACTH is present in smaller polypeptide fragments. It appears that the significant structure necessary for high adrenocorticotropin activity is the unusual sequence of basic amino acid lys-lys-arg-arg occurring in the 15 to 18 position. The biologic half-life of ACTH is less than 10 min. The release of ACTH from the anterior pituitary gland is governed by a "corticotropin-releasing center" in the median eminence of the hypothalamus, which upon stimulation releases a chemical mediator (corticotropin-releasing factor, CRF) that travels via the pituitary-stalk portal bloodstream to the anterior pituitary gland, where it effects the release of stored ACTH (Fig. 92-5). CRF is thought to be a short-chain polypeptide whose release is facilitated by a large number of nervous stimuli, including those arising from higher centers. The principal regulator of CRF release is the plasma free cortisol level, which by a negative feedback mechanism causes increased release of CRF when plasma cortisol level is low and a decreased release of CRF when plasma cortisol concentration is elevated. This servomechanism establishes the primacy of blood cortisol concentration and serves to buffer deviations in blood cortisol levels from a supposed optimal level. It also appears that cortisol feeds back directly on the pituitary gland and higher brain centers, and perhaps even on the adrenal cortex as well.

Besides its major action in stimulating the biogenesis and release of steroid hormones by the adrenal gland, ACTH can stimulate melanocytes of amphibians and can increase adipokinetic activity in a number of species. Both these extraadrenal actions have been verified with synthetic ACTH molecules.

The action of ACTH on the adrenal gland itself is rapid; within minutes of its release, there is an increased concentration of steroids in the adrenal venous blood. It produces a number of biochemical changes: (1) an increase in adrenal weight; (2) a decrease in amount of adrenal lipids, cholesterol, and ascorbic acid; (3) an increase in protein synthesis and oxidative phosphorylation; and (4) an accelerated rate of glycolysis. The molecular basis of ACTH action has not been elucidated. Some investigators suggest that ACTH accelerates the production of Δ5,pregnenolone from cholesterol in a rate-limiting manner; others have suggested that ACTH acts by

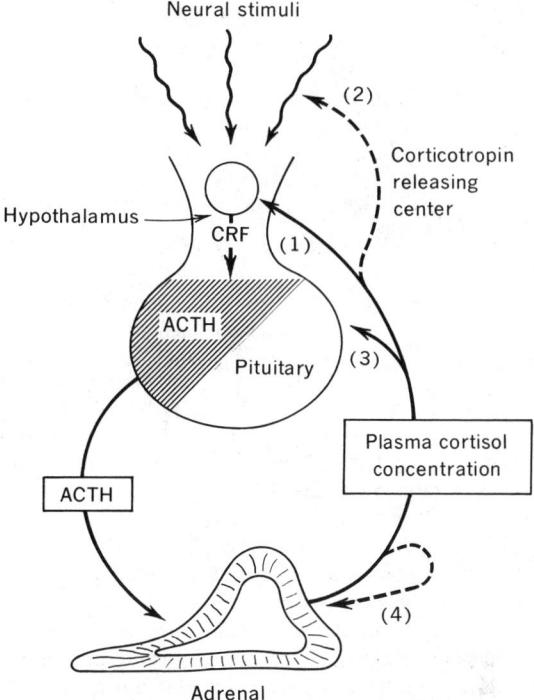

Fig. 92-5. Hypothalamic-pituitary-adrenal axis. *CRF* = corticotropin-releasing factor. (1) Dominant feedback control on the hypothalamus; (2) possible feedback of plasma cortisol on higher nerve centers; (3) feedback on the pituitary gland; and (4) possible direct feedback on the adrenal gland itself.

increasing the formation and availability of adenosine-3′,5′-monophosphate in the adrenal gland, which would lead to an increase in the synthesis of reduced coenzymes needed for steroid biosynthesis. Evidence has been obtained which suggests that activation of protein biosynthesis is an important if not an essential part of the action of ACTH and possibly of other tropic hormones. ACTH apparently increases protein biosynthesis either by stimulation of messenger ribonucleic acid or by enzyme activation.

Renin-Angiotensin Physiology (See Chap. 276)

Renin is a proteolytic enzyme with an approximate molecular weight of 35,000 to 40,000. It has been semipurified. It is produced and stored in the granules of the juxtaglomerular cells surrounding the afferent arterioles of the cortical glomeruli. The juxtaglomerular apparatus consist of both the juxtaglomerular cells and the cells of the macula densa. The latter area also contains some renin. Renin acts on the basic substrate angiotensinogen (a circulating alpha$_2$-globulin) made in the liver, to form the decapeptide angiotensin-I. Various inhibitors of intrarenal renin formation are believed to exist (Fig. 92-6). Angiotensin-I is then enzymatically converted by converting enzyme to the octapeptide angiotensin-II by the splitting off of the two C-terminal amino acids. Angiotensin-II is the most potent pressor compound (on a milli-

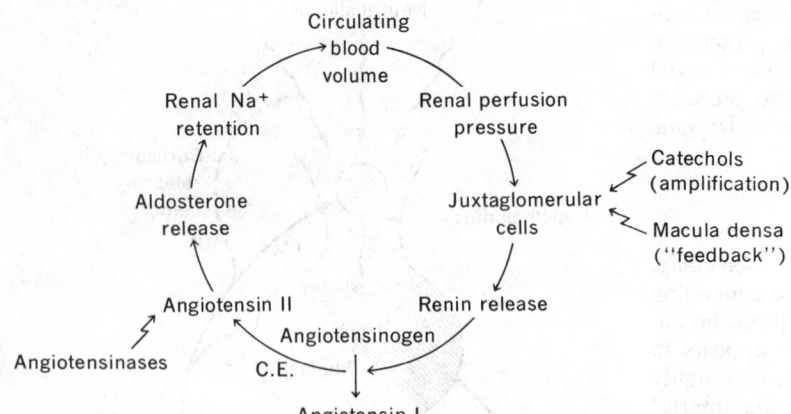

Fig. 92-6. Renin-angiotensin-aldosterone volume regulation in normal man.

gram-for-milligram basis) made in the body, and it exerts this pressor action by a direct effect on arteriolar smooth muscle. In addition, angiotensin-II is the most potent direct stimulus to the production of aldosterone by the zona glomerulosa of the adrenal cortex. Various peptidases, collectively termed "angiotensinases," in organ tissue, vessel walls, and circulating plasma are responsible for the ultimate biochemical degradation of circulating angiotensin-II. Angiotensin-II may also play a role in modifying the renal tubular transport of sodium. Such a direct tubular effect, independent of its effect on renal hemodynamics, remains controversial.

Renin release is controlled both by extrarenal and intrarenal mechanisms. The extrarenal mechanism is capable of overiding the intrarenal mechanism, although in many situations they act synergistically in series. The common denominator for the release of renin by the *extrarenal* mechanism is that of volume depletion. Volume depletion may be induced (by hemorrhage, ganglionic blockade, diuretic administration, salt restriction) or may exist on a chronic basis, as in certain disorders associated with edema.

The juxtaglomerular cells, which are specialized myoepithelial cells cuffing the afferent arterioles, act as miniature pressure *transducers*, sensing renal perfusion pressure and corresponding changes in afferent arteriolar perfusion pressures. The changes in pressure are perceived as distortions in the existing stretch on the arteriolar walls. For example, under conditions of a reduction in circulating blood volume, there will be a corresponding reduction in renal perfusion pressure and, therefore, in afferent arteriolar pressure. This will be perceived by the juxtaglomerular cells as a decreased stretch exerted on the afferent arteriolar walls. The juxtaglomerular cells will then release increasing quantities of renin within the kidney circulation, leading to the formation of angiotensin-II. Angiotensin-II leaves the kidney both by a renal lymphatic and a renal venous outflow. It directly stimulates the adrenal cortex to release increasing quantities of aldosterone. (At higher levels, angiotensin may have a direct pressor effect.) Increasing plasma levels of aldosterone lead to increasing renal sodium retention and thus result in expansion of extracellular fluid volume, which, as it is completed, dampens the initiating signal for renin release. Within this context, the renin-angiotensin-aldosterone system is subserving volume control by appropriate modifications of renal tubular sodium transport. Circulating catecholamines, and perhaps the renal sympathetic nerves, are capable of amplifying the response of the juxtaglomerular cells to changes in perfusion pressure. The renal nerves per se are not a prerequisite for such an amplification, however, since the denervated kidney can successfully adapt to salt restriction.

An *intrarenal* control mechanism for renin release has been postulated. Such a theory centers on the macula densa cells. These are a group of special-staining distal convoluted tubular epithelial cells found in direct apposition to the juxtaglomerular cells. It has been suggested that they may function as chemoreceptors, monitoring the sodium load presented to the distal tubule, and that such formation, while it is being monitored, is directly fed back to the juxtaglomerular cells where appropriate modifications in renin release may take place. Such an intrarenal renin-release mechanism is said to be capable of operating independently of changes in renal perfusion pressure. Under conditions of increased delivery of filtered sodium to the macula densa, such feedback may occur to the juxtaglomerular apparatus, resulting in a release of increasing quantities of angiotensin, which could then be capable of decreasing glomerular filtration rate, thereby reducing the filtered load of sodium (hypothesis of Thurau). The evidence for the hypothesis is conflicting.

The pressor response to infused or circulating angiotensin is conditioned by at least two factors: (1) it is inversely related to the circulating levels of angiotensin; (2) it is modified by the concentration of plasma sodium. Pressor response is dampened by a decrease in plasma sodium concentration.

Glucocorticoid Physiology

The division of adrenal steroids into glucocorticoids and mineralocorticoids is somewhat arbitrary in that most glucocorticoids have some mineralocorticoid-like properties, and vice versa. The descriptive term *glucocorticoid* is applied to those adrenal steroids having a predominant action on intermediary metabolism. The principal glucocorticoid is cortisol (hydrocortisone). The actions of the glucocorticoids on intermediary metabolism include the regulation of protein, carbohydrate, lipid, and nucleic acid metabolism. Their actions appear mainly to be catabolic in effect, with an increased protein breakdown and nitrogen excretion. Glucocorticoids also increase hepatic glycogen content by increasing hepatic glucose synthesis. This is brought about by increasing the quantity of intermediary metabolites, especially those derived from glycogenic amino acids. Hepatic trapping and deamination of amino acids derived from peripheral supporting structures, such as bone, skin, muscle, and connective tissue, appears to be essential to the process. The increased mobilization of protein results in increased plasma amino acid levels and increased urinary nitrogen excretion. Glucocorticoids are capable of directly increasing the level of specific hepatic enzymes, such as tryptophan pyrrolase and tyrosine-α-ketoglutarate transaminase. The elevated levels of these hepatic enzymes can influence the balance of serum amino acids, which in turn can be responsible for diminished protein metabolism and subsequent cytolysis of lymphoid tissues and muscle. Cortisol enhances the release of free fatty acids from adipose tissue during fasting or adrenergic stimulation. The action of cortisol on structural protein and adipose tissue varies considerably in different parts of the body. For example, depletion of protein matrix of the vertebral column may be striking, whereas long-bone structure may be affected only minimally; peripheral adipose tissue may diminish, whereas abdominal and interscapular fat may accumulate. Cortisol has a major effect on body water in both its distribution and its excretion. It subserves the extracellular fluid volume by a retarding action on the inward migration of water into cells. It affects renal water excretion in a dual manner, by increasing the rate of glomerular filtration and by a direct action on the renal tubule, both of which summate to increase solute-free water clearance. Glucocorticoids, in general, will increase renal tubular sodium reabsorption and cause an increased urine potassium excretion. Cortisol is also necessary for normal vascular reactivity, ensuring the response of vascular smooth muscle to circulating vasoconstrictor factors. The glucocorticoids have significant anti-inflammatory effects, producing lysis of lymphoid tissues and diminishing circulating eosinophils. Some of these actions may be due to the ability of the glucocorticoids to stabilize lysosomal membranes. In this way, cortisol can suppress the release of acid hydrolases which are stored within the lysosomes. The integrity of personality is enhanced by cortisol, and emotional disorders are common with either excesses or deficits of cortisol. Lastly, cortisol is the major determinant of pituitary ACTH release by its direct effect on the hypothalamic corticotropin-releasing center.

Mineralocorticoid Physiology

Three major mineralocorticoids are produced by the human adrenal cortex: 11-deoxycorticosterone (DOC), corticosterone, and aldosterone. DOC and corticosterone are the immediate precursors in the biosynthetic pathway for aldosterone, and the production of DOC and corticos-

terone is governed by ACTH levels. Production rates for these hormones on a normal sodium intake are DOC, 50 to 250 μg per day; corticosterone, 900 to 4,500 μg per day; and aldosterone, 50 to 250 μg per day. The effects of these various mineralocorticoids on sodium and potassium metabolism are indistinguishable, but the potency of aldosterone is much greater than that of the other compounds. For this reason, aldosterone is considered the principal mineralocorticoid.

Aldosterone has two important physiologic functions: (1) it is the prime regulator of extracellular fluid volume, and (2) it is a major determinant of potassium metabolism. It regulates volume through a direct effect on the renal tubular transport of sodium. Aldosterone acts predominantly at the site of the distal convoluted tubule, where it accelerates the exchange of tubular sodium ions for secreted potassium and/or hydrogen ions. Aldosterone increases the efficiency of this distal tubular sodium-potassium exchange site. The reabsorbed sodium ions are then transported out of the tubular epithelial cells into the interstitial fluid volume of the kidney and from there into the renal capillary circulation. Since sodium ions are the prime determinant of extracellular fluid volume, aldosterone, through its regulation of renal sodium transport, may be said to be the prime regulator of extracellular fluid volume. Water will passively follow the aldosterone-mediated transported sodium. In effect, through the agency of aldosterone, extracellular fluid can be expanded by a mechanism analogous to an endogenous infusion of normal saline solution.

Aldosterone, under conditions of extracellular fluid volume depletion, also markedly influences the iso-osmotic reabsorption of proximal tubular sodium. Contrariwise, expansion of extracellular fluid volume, with the associated suppression of aldosterone release, will be characterized by a decrease in the percentage of the filtered sodium load reabsorbed by the proximal tubules. A definitive action of aldosterone on the transport of sodium in the ascending limb of Henle has not been clearly documented.

Aldosterone also acts directly on the epithelium of the salivary ducts and sweat glands and on the mucosal cells of the gastrointestinal tract to cause direct reabsorption of sodium in exchange for potassium ions. A direct cellular action, as on muscle cells, of aldosterone has been difficult to prove. It has been reported that in the absence of aldosterone, sodium tends to leave the extracellular fluid base by migrating into cells, onto tendon and bone surfaces, and increasing sodium wasting by the kidneys will occur. The d-isomer of aldosterone is the biologically active form.

There are three well-identified *control mechanisms* for aldosterone release, and in all probability several as yet undiscovered control systems also exist. The recognized control systems are renin-angiotensin system, potassium, and ACTH. The renin-angiotensin system is the major system for control of extracellular fluid volume, via regulation of aldosterone secretion. In effect, the renin-angiotensin system attempts to maintain circulating blood volume constant by causing increasing aldosterone-induced sodium retention during periods registered as volume deficiencies, and by decreasing aldosterone-dependent sodium retention under conditions in which volume is registered as being ample. In clinical medicine, volume deficits are much more common than volume excesses. Such deficits are repaired by stimulation of the renin-angiotensin-aldosterone system and its consequent effect on the renal retention of sodium and water. Volume regulation in the absence of the renin-angiotensin system (renoprival man) is extremely difficult and is characterized by marked oscillations of blood pressure. Such information documents that the renin-angiotensin system is the major control system for aldosterone-mediated volume regulation.

Potassium ions can regulate aldosterone secretion independently of the renin-angiotensin system. If a solution of potassium ions is injected into the adrenal artery, immediate increase in adrenal venous aldosterone levels can be documented. It appears that potassium has a direct stimulatory effect on adrenocortical production of aldosterone, presumably via a transmembrane effect. Adrenocortical cells act as if they monitor the flux of potassium across their membranes, and under conditions of increased flux to the cell, there is an increase in aldosterone production and release; contrariwise, under conditions of decreased potassium influx, there is a decrease in aldosterone release. This potassium-mediated control system for aldosterone release operates in parallel with the renin-angiotensin system and can be of comparable potency. When the renin-angiotensin system may be impaired, as in acute and chronic renal failure, this potassium-aldosterone control system assumes even greater importance.

Potassium stimulation of aldosterone release may be a protective mechanism against potassium intoxication. When the human organism receives an acute load of potassium, aldosterone release will be stimulated, and the released aldosterone, by accelerating the potassium-sodium distal tubular exchange, will result in increased urinary loss of potassium, thus minimizing the increase in plasma potassium concentration. Under conditions of potassium depletion and hypokalemia, there is a marked diminution in aldosterone production and release. Adrenal responsiveness to potassium stimulation can be potentiated by activation of the renin-angiotensin system through sodium restriction.

ACTH plays a permissive role in aldosterone release. Hypophysectomized patients, or patients with pituitary insufficiency, have a suboptimal aldosterone response to sodium restriction. In normal persons, with ACTH administration, there is an acute rise in aldosterone secretion to levels three to four times above the base line. However, with the continued administration of ACTH, aldosterone production rates return to control levels, providing suggestive evidence that ACTH is not an important control mechanism in day-to-day physiologic conditions. Such a control mechanism would assume importance, however, under conditions of acute stress, burns, hemorrhage, etc. More recently, it has been suggested that there may exist pituitary factors other than ACTH which are necessary for a maximal adrenal aldosterone response. When normal individuals are given a long-term course of aldosterone (or a comparable mineralocorticoid, such as parenteral DOC), an initial period of sodium retention is followed by a natriuresis, and sodium balance is reestablished. As a result, clinical edema formation does not develop. Thus, with continuous administration of the potent sodium-retaining hormone aldosterone, patients reachieve sodium homeostasis and do not continue to exhibit sodium retention. This phenomenon is referred to as the "escape phenomenon," signifying an "escape" by the renal tubules from the sodium-retaining action of chronically administered aldosterone. The mechanism responsible for the escape phenomenon has remained elusive. It does appear to be dependent on normal renal hemodynamics, and it has been suggested that an as-yet-unidentified natriuretic principle may be involved. Such an "escape" phenomenon is also exhibited by patients with essential hypertension (primary aldosteronism) but is characteristically absent in patients with edema disorders.

Androgen Physiology

The principal adrenal androgens in terms of quantitative secretion are dehydroepiandrosterone (DHEA), androstenedione, and 11-hydroxyandrostenedione. Of these, androstenedione is the major androgen, five times more active than DHEA. Testosterone, which is interconvertible with androstenedione peripherally and which has been isolated from the adrenal gland, exhibits an additional fivefold increase in androgenic potency when compared to androstenedione, pointing up that DHEA, androstenedione, and 11-hydroxyandrostenedione are biologically weak androgens. The release of adrenal androgens is stimulated by ACTH and not by gonadotropins. With ACTH stimulation urine 17-ketosteroids increase but to a much lesser extent than do urine 17-hydroxycorticoids. Part of this increment in 17-ketosteroid excretion is due to the metabolism of the increasing 17-hydroxycorticoids by the mechanism of C-20:C-21 side chain cleavage, producing 11-oxy-17-ketosteroids. Adrenal androgens are suppressed by exogenous glucocorticoid administration, as judged by decrements in urine 17-ketosteroid excretion. Additional specific control mechanisms for adrenal androgen release may exist independently of the ACTH system.

The major effects of these androgenic hormones are on protein metabolism and on secondary sexual characteristics. Androgens increase the synthesis of protein from amino acids, and this anabolic action leads to increased muscle mass and strength. Linear growth is accelerated by androgens prior to epiphyseal closure, which is hastened by androgen excess. The secondary sexual characteristics are affected through inhibition of the female characteristics (defeminization) and accentuation of the male characteristics (masculinization). These are seen clinically as hirsutism and virilization in the female with amenorrhea, atrophy of breasts and uterus, enlargement of the clitoris, deepening of the voice, acne, increased muscle mass, increased heterosexual drive, and receding hairline. In the male there are increased body and sexual hair and enlargement of the sexual organs.

The bioassay of androgens has been largely replaced by more specific analytic techniques, such as double isotope derivative analysis using S-35 thiosemicarbazide, electron capture gas-liquid chromatography, and competitive protein-binding radioassay. The first two techniques require a great deal of biochemical and electronic sophistication in order to achieve reliable results. However, the competitive protein-binding method requires fewer technical skills and, therefore, may become the more practical way of determining adrenal androgen levels.

LABORATORY EVALUATION OF ADRENOCORTICAL FUNCTION
Blood Levels

ACTH. Before 1964, blood ACTH levels were determined by bioassay preparations. However, since then it has been possible in a number of laboratories to determine ACTH by radioimmunoassay. Problems of specificity and sensitivity have limited the general application of this technique. Plasma ACTH levels show a diurnal cycle, with lower blood levels detected in late afternoon and early evening. In normal man, the morning ACTH concentration is between 0 and 10 mμg per ml.

ANGIOTENSIN–RENIN. Chemical measurements of plasma angiotensin levels have been attempted, but because of problems of extraction and precise chemical identity, such methods have been largely abandoned. Radioimmune assays for angiotensin are being developed by the production of antibodies to the octapeptide angiotensin-II by linkage to a larger molecule, such as albumin or poly-1-lysine. By such methods, values for normal subjects on a low salt diet have been found to be supine, 40 $\mu\mu$g per ml; upright, 60 $\mu\mu$g per ml.

Measurements of the enzyme renin are made by several laboratories utilizing a purified renin substrate. The majority of clinical determinations of the renin-angiotensin system, however, involve measurements of peripheral "plasma renin activity" (PRA) in which the renin activity is gauged by the generation of angiotensin during a standardized incubation period. This method depends on the presence of sufficient angiotensinogen in the patient's plasma as substrate. The generated angiotensin then is measured in a standardized rat pressor bioassay. Plasma renin activity levels will depend on dietary intake of the patient and whether or not the patient is ambulatory. Values for resting supine patients on a normal salt intake range between 100 to 300 (angiotensin produced, mμg/ml/4 hr).

CORTISOL. Blood levels of cortisol can be measured in a number of ways; the most sensitive of these is the double isotope derivative technique. However, the level of plasma cortisol determined by competitive protein-binding radioassay also appears to be reliable. A less-sensitive and specific method is measuring Porter-Silber chromogens in the blood by a fluorimetric technique. The morning plasma levels of 17-hydroxycorticoids range between 10 and 20 μg per 100 ml. These blood levels exhibit a marked diurnal pattern, with highest values between 6 and 8 A.M. and the lowest value at 10 P.M. to 12 midnight.

ALDOSTERONE. Because of the minute quantities of plasma aldosterone present, it has been difficult to determine it directly. Only a few laboratories, utilizing double isotope dilution techniques, can measure peripheral plasma levels. On normal salt intake, the values range from 5 to 15 mμg per 100 ml.

ANDROGENS. Testosterone in plasma has been measured by isotopic and competitive protein-binding means; the range for nonhirsute females is 30 to 100 and for males 400 to 1,000 mμg per 100 ml.

Urine Levels

The principal determinations are of urine 17-hydroxycorticoids, 17-ketosteroids, 17-ketogenic steroids, free cortisol, and aldosterone. The urine 17-hydroxycorticoids are determined as Porter-Silber chromogens, i.e., these steroids react with the reagent phenylhydrazine to produce a characteristic color. This reaction is specific for steroids with a "dihydroxy acetone" C-17 side chain, i.e., with hydroxyl groups on C-17 and C-21 and a ketone group on C-20 (Fig. 92-7). Therefore, this determination will include cortisol, cortisone, tetrahydrocortisol, tetrahydrocortisone, and 11-dexoycortisol but not cortols, cortolones, and pregnanetriol. Normal values for 24 hr range from 1 to 10 mg per day, with daytime (7 A.M. to 7 P.M.) excretion exceeding night values (7 P.M. to 7 A.M.). It is of extreme importance that the completeness of any and all urine steroid collections be checked by urine creatinine determinations.

The urine 17-ketosteroids are those containing a ketone group at C-17; two-thirds of these originate from the adrenal gland and the remainder from the testes. Their measurement depends on the Zimmerman reaction, whereby color is produced when 17-ketosteroids are condensed with *m*-dinitrobenzene. This reaction is specific for steroids with a ketone substituent with an adjacent unsubstituted carbon atom. The major urine 17-ketosteroids are dehydroepiandrosterone, epiandrosterone, androsterone, etiocholanolone, 11-oxoetiocholanolone, 11-hydroxyetiocholanolone, and 11-hydroxyandrosterone (Fig. 92-8). Normal values for males range between 7 and 25 mg per day and for females between 5 and 15 mg per day. The diurnal pattern for 17-ketosteroid excretion is definite but less accentuated than that for 17-hydroxysteroids. Urine 17-ketosteroid values are highest in young adults and decline with age.

The total urine 17-ketosteroids may be subdivided into those having either an oxygen or hydroxyl substituent at position C-11 (11-oxy-17-ketosteroids) and those having no such groups (11-deoxy-17-ketosteroids). The *11-oxy-17-ketosteroids* include 11-oxoetiocholanolone, 11-hydroxyetiocholanolone, and 11-hydroxyandrosterone. These

11-oxy-17-ketosteroids are uniquely derived from the adrenal gland, since other tissues do not possess the enzymes for active C-11 hydroxylation, whereas the 11-deoxy-17-ketosteroids may arise from adrenal, testicular, and ovarian tissue.

Ketogenic steroids is a descriptive term for those C-21 hydroxycorticoids potentially capable of transformation into 17-ketosteroids in vitro. After the excreted 17-ketosteroids are reduced to noninterfering compounds, the side chains of C-21 hydroxycorticosteroids are oxidized to 17-ketonic groups, which then can be measured by the Zimmermann reaction as 17-ketosteroids. The Norymberski technique for ketogenic steroid analysis is specific for compounds containing the following groups:

17-HYDROXY-CORTICOIDS (Porter-Silber chromogens)

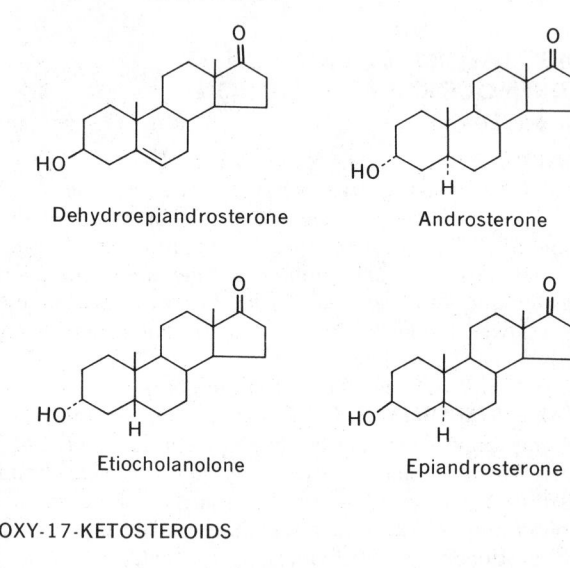

e.g. cortisol

17-KETO-STEROIDS (Zimmerman reaction)

e.g. etiocholanolone

17-KETOGENIC-STEROIDS (Norymberski technique)

e.g. porter-silber
chromogens

e.g. cortols
cortolones

e.g. pregnanetriol

Fig. 92-7. Key reactive groups (enclosed by dashed circle) in urine steroid determinations.

17,21-dihydroxy-20-keto; 17,20,21-trihydroxy-; and 17,20-dihydroxy-21-deoxy-. It may be seen that the first of these groupings represents those compounds capable of reacting as *Porter-Silber chromogens;* the second, or trihydroxy, grouping would include the cortols and the cortolones; and the third, or 21-deoxy, grouping would include pregnanetriol. Thus, urine 17-ketogenic steroid determination includes all steroids determined as 17-hydroxysteroids by the Porter-Silber method and, in addition, includes the cortols, cortolones, and pregnanetriol. The normal range for urine **17-ketogenic steroids** is 5 to 20 mg per day.

11-DEOXY-17-KETOSTEROIDS

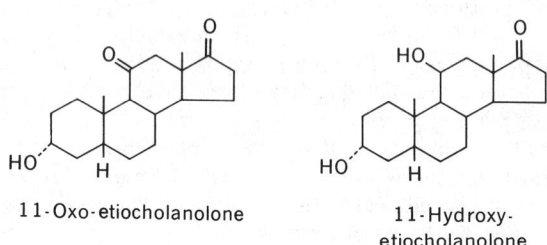

Dehydroepiandrosterone   Androsterone

Etiocholanolone   Epiandrosterone

11-OXY-17-KETOSTEROIDS

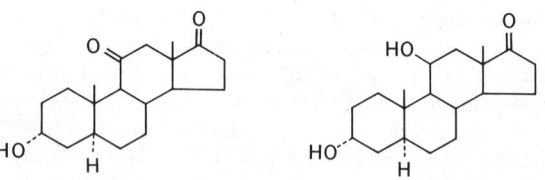

11-Oxo-etiocholanolone   11-Hydroxy-
                                etiocholanolone

11-Oxo-androsterone   11-Hydroxy-androsterone

Fig. 92-8. Principal urine 17-ketosteroids, 11-oxy-17-ketosteroids derived from the adrenal glands.

The determination of either urine free cortisol or aldosterone excretion is more difficult, usually requiring double isotope derivative techniques. Urinary free cortisol may also be determined by partition chromatography or competitive protein-binding radioassay. Normal subjects excrete less than 100 μg per day.

Aldosterone excretion rate is tested by determining the excretion of a major metabolite, usually the acid-labile conjugate. A carefully timed urine collection is a prerequisite for all excretory determinations. Normal values for the 24-hr aldosterone excretion rate range between 2 and 10 μg.

Steroid Secretion Rates

The basic assumption in the interpretation of urine steroid values is that excreted adrenal steroid metabolites (17-hydroxycorticoids, 17-ketogenic steroids) accurately reflect adrenal secretory rates of that steroid (cortisol). Measurement of the actual adrenal secretory rate of a given steroid would, of course, be preferable, and such methods are finding increasing clinical application. The adrenal secretory rate is calculated by the dilution that an administered radioactive steroid undergoes as a consequence of the admixture of endogenously secreted nonradioactive steroid hormone with the exogenous radioactive steroid. In practice, a major metabolite of the steroid is isolated and purified by chromatography; from a determination of its specific activity (counts per minute per microgram of steroid) and knowledge of the specific activity of the administered steroid one may calculate by the dilution principle the actual amount of the steroid secreted by the adrenal gland during the period of urine collection (usually 24 hr). Such secretory rate determinations have been standardized for cortisol and aldosterone. The average daily cortisol secretory rate determined by such methods is 8 to 30 mg per day, and the average aldosterone secretory rate 50 to 250 μg per day on a normal sodium intake.

The determination of secretion rates of the adrenal androgens is complicated by two facts: most androgens are derived from two different sources (adrenals and gonads), and they are readily interconvertible after secretion. Because of this, classic secretory techniques are probably not applicable. Instead, androgen production rates are usually determined by the use of metabolic clearance rates and plasma concentrations of the particular steroid. Because these methods are more cumbersome, less information has been obtained about androgen metabolism.

Stimulation Tests

Stimulation tests are useful in documenting the existence of a hormonal deficiency state. A standardized and specific stimulus for the production and release of a given hormone is applied, and the quantity of the released hormone is then measured.

GLUCOCORTICOID STIMULATION TESTS. Within minutes after initiating an infusion of ACTH, increased cortisol levels are noted in adrenal venous blood. This responsiveness of the adrenal gland to ACTH is utilized as an index of the "functional reserve" of the gland to produce cortisol. Under maximal ACTH stimulation the cortisol secretion increases tenfold to 300 mg per day. Such maximal stimulation is obtainable only with prolonged ACTH infusions. For clinical purposes, the functional adrenal reserve for cortisol production is standardized with a shorter infusion time (8 hr). The standard intravenous ACTH test is performed by administering 40 units of aqueous ACTH in 500 ml normal saline solution intravenously over an exact 8-hr interval (from 8 A.M. to 4 P.M.) on two successive days and collecting the complete 24-hr urine output for analysis of creatinine, 17-hydroxycorticoids (or 17-ketogenic steroids), and 17-ketosteroids. The patient may be ambulatory during this period. With such a method of testing, an average increment of 15 mg (range, 5 to 25) has been noted in urine 17-hydroxysteroids on the first day of testing and an average increment of 25 mg (range, 15 to 35) on the second infusion day, by one commonly used method. Much smaller rises in urine 17-ketosteroid excretion are noted, with average increments of 4 to 8 mg per day on the first and second day of testing, respectively. In the performance of the test the duration of the infusion must be strictly adhered to. Screening tests utilizing the intramuscular injection of ACTH (40 to 80 units twice daily) have been employed and offer the occasional advantage of ease of performance, but they have a more serious disadvantage in that the responses often vary because of irregular absorption of the ACTH from the injection site.

Occasionally it is necessary to prolong the ACTH infusion in order to separate primary from secondary tion, diuretic administration, or venesection. The simplest adrenal insufficiency. This can be accomplished by using an 8-hr infusion on four or five consecutive days or by a continuous 48-hr infusion. The 48-hr infusion is given as 80 units of ACTH in 1,000 ml 5 percent dextrose in water or dextrose in normal saline every 24 hr for two consecutive days. Fluid retention due to the contamination of most commercial preparations of ACTH with ADH is a problem in some patients.

MINERALOCORTICOID STIMULATION TESTS. Standardized aldosterone stimulation tests have been devised utilizing a protocol of programmed volume depletion. Volume depletion may be engendered by sodium restriction, diuretic administration, or venesection. The simplest stimulation test involves the modality of sodium restriction. The patient is placed on a constant diet containing 200 mEq sodium and 100 mEq potassium, with defined physical activity. After a 5-day equilibration period on this diet, dietary sodium intake is abruptly lowered to 10 mEq per day and held constant. The diet-physical activity program is left unchanged. After 3 to 5 days of such sodium deprivation, aldosterone secretion rates (or excretion rates) should exhibit a two- to threefold increase.

Stimulation tests may also be carried out by the **administration of a potent diuretic,** such as ethacrynic acid or furosemide, with measurements of aldosterone secretion being made on the day preceding, the day of, and the day after diuretic administration. The diuretic is administered throughout a 24-hr period in doses sufficient to cause an increase in urine output (over control) of

1,500 ml and/or a weight loss of 3 lb in 24 hr. The test may be carried out while the patient has a high or low sodium intake. Again, a two-to threefold rise in aldosterone production should be observed. The difficulty with this testing procedure is that the diuretic will induce variable losses of potassium, which will tend to dampen the hypersecretion of aldosterone that otherwise would have occurred for a corresponding degree of volume depletion.

Hemorrhage, either functional or induced, may also be used as an aldosterone-stimulating test. As measurements of plasma aldosterone become available, this may become the preferred method of stimulating the aldosterone system via the renin-angiotensin mechanism. Functional hemorrhage may be tested by making measurements of plasma aldosterone before and after 4 to 5 hr of ambulation. There is a minimum of three- to sixfold rise in plasma aldosterone levels under such conditions, which is presumably a response to transthoracic volume depletion which occurs with assumption of the upright position. Aldosterone secretion or excretion rates can be made on the day before and the day of acute venesection, with withdrawal of 400 to 600 ml of venous blood over a period of 30 to 40 min. The normal response is a twofold rise in aldosterone secretion/excretion.

Because of adverse effects on the coronary circulation, angiotensin infusions have not found favor as a means of performing tests of adrenal aldosterone responsiveness.

Suppression Tests

Suppression tests are used to document hypersecretion of adrenocortical hormones and are based on the demonstration of a decrease in the target hormone following standardized suppression of its tropic hormone. Thus, suppression testing for cortisol hypersecretion would involve suppression of ACTH release, with the documentation of an appropriately normal decrease in cortisol production, while suppression testing of aldosterone would involve demonstration of a decrease in aldosterone secondary to suppression of the renin-angiotensin system.

GLUCOCORTICOID SUPPRESSION TESTS. The hypothalamic-pituitary ACTH release mechanism is sensitive to the circulating blood level of glucocorticoids. When such blood levels are increased in the normal individual, the corticotropin-releasing center decreases its production of the corticotropin-releasing factor (CRF), and consequently less ACTH is released from the anterior pituitary; secondarily, less steroid will be produced by the adrenal gland. The integrity of this feedback mechanism can be tested clinically by giving a potent glucocorticoid and judging suppression of the corticotropin-releasing center by analysis of urine steroid excretory values. A potent glucocorticoid such as dexamethasone is utilized in order that the administered compound may be given in such small amounts that it will not contribute significantly to the steroids to be analyzed.

One or more of three standard tests are usually employed. The simplest is the overnight dexamethasone suppression test. This involves the measurement of plasma corticoid levels at 8 A.M. and/or the urine 17-hydroxycorticoid and creatinine excretion between 7 A.M. and 12 noon following the oral administration of 1 mg dexamethasone the previous midnight. The 8 A.M. value for plasma corticoids in normal subjects should be less than 10 μg per 100 ml, and the ratio of urine Porter-Silber chromogens per milligram of creatinine in the 5-hr urine specimen should be less than 0.004.

The usual method of testing adrenal suppressibility is to administer 0.5 mg dexamethasone every 6 hr for two successive days while collecting urine over a 24-hr period for determination of creatinine, 17-hydroxysteroids, and 17-ketosteroids. In patients with a normal hypothalamic-pituitary ACTH release mechanism, a fall in the urine 17-hydroxycorticoids to less than 3 mg a day on the second day of dexamethasone administration is seen.

An intravenous dexamethasone suppression test is used less often. One milligram of dexamethasone is administered intravenously per hour for a total of 3 hr, and blood is collected for plasma glucocorticoid determinations. A 50 percent fall in plasma cortisol at the end of 3 hr of infusion is normally expected. Normal response to any of the suppression tests implies that the ACTH control of the adrenal glands is physiologically normal. However, an isolated abnormal result, particularly when the overnight suppression test is being used, does not in itself imply pituitary and/or adrenal disease.

MINERALOCORTICOID SUPPRESSION TESTS. Mineralocorticoid suppression testing procedures have been devised using saline infusions, oral salt loading, or DOCA administration as the means for expansion of the extracellular fluid volume. With expansion of extracellular fluid volume, there will be a decrease in renal renin release, a decrease in circulating plasma renin activity, and a decrease in aldosterone secretion and/or excretion. This would be the appropriate "normal" response. Varied tests differ in the rate at which extracellular fluid volume is expanded. The "normal saline suppression test" involves the intravenous administration of 2 liters of normal saline solution over a 4-hr period from 9 A.M. until 1 P.M. on two consecutive days. Aldosterone secretion or excretion rate is measured the day before and on the second day of saline loading. The patient previously has been permitted to come into equilibration on a 10 mEq sodium/100 mEq potassium constant diet. Normal response of suppression of aldosterone secretion by this maneuver is to a value of less than 200 μg per day. The "oral salt-loading suppression test" is conveniently caried out by abruptly increasing the patient's sodium intake from a constant level of 10 mEq per day to 200 mEq per day for a period of 3 to 5 days, with measurements of aldosterone secretion on the fourth or fifth day, at which time a 24-hr secretion rate should be less than 200 μg per day. Potassium intake is held constant throughout the test, since potassium will cause aldosterone secretion to vary independently of the renin-angiotensin system. The "DOCA suppression test" is carried out by placing the patient on a normal (100 mEq) or high (200 mEq) sodium intake. After the patient is in sodium balance, deoxycorticosterone acetate is administered intramuscularly

(10 mg every 12 hr) for a period of 3 to 5 days. Normal subjects on a sodium intake of 100 mEq daily demonstrate a 70 percent decrease in aldosterone excretion rate, when compared with control levels, which means that the aldosterone excretory value should be less than 5 μg per day.

Test of Pituitary Responsiveness

A number of stimuli, such as insulin hypoglycemia, arginine vasopressin, and pyrogen, will cause release of ACTH from the pituitary by an action on higher nerve centers, the hypothalamus, or the pituitary gland itself. By measuring plasma ACTH, or urine or blood glucocorticoids, the status of pituitary ACTH can be evaluated.

Metyrapone [SU4885 (Metopirone)] is a drug that selectively inhibits the enzyme action of 11-beta-hydroxylase in the adrenal gland. As a result, the conversion of 11-deoxycortisol (Compound S) to cortisol is interfered with and increased amounts of 11-deoxycortisol accumulate while blood levels of cortisol decrease (Fig. 92-2). Since 11-deoxycortisol is a weak suppressor of the hypothalamic-pituitary axis, the anterior pituitary responds to the declining cortisol blood levels by releasing larger quantities of ACTH in an attempt to stimulate the adrenal gland to release additional cortisol, which attempt, however, is thwarted by the metyrapone-induced enzymatic blockade. The metabolites of 11-deoxycortisol are excreted in increasing amounts in the urine, where they are measured as 17-hydroxycorticoids. *Note that the adrenal glands must be capable of being stimulated by ACTH, since assessment of the response depends on adrenal steroid production.*

The metyrapone response has been standardized for clinical evaluation of the reserve capacity of the anterior pituitary gland to release ACTH. Every 4 hr over a 48-hr period 750 mg metyrapone is administered orally, and daily urine collections for 17-hydroxycorticosteroids are obtained the day before testing, the 2 days of testing, and the day after the last dose of metyrapone. The peak response of increased urine 17-hydroxysteroid excretion may be seen on the day after completion of metyrapone administration, and normal individuals will respond with at least a doubling of their basal 17-hydroxysteroid excretion.

Tests for Renin Responsiveness

Attempts have been made to standardize measurement of renin responsiveness by the acute induction of volume depletion and/or hypotension. Acute hypotension, induced either by diazoxide or by hydralazine, has been tried, but the results have been variable. Standardization has been improved by controlled volume depletion, induced by diuretics or by the assumption of the upright position. Diuretic-induced volume depletion is limited by patient-to-patient variability to the same dose of diuretic.

The most widely accepted test, suggested by Conn, is based on postural augmentation of plasma renin activity. This test involves determination of plasma renin activity in the supine patient before and immediately following 4 hr of ambulation. The normal response is a two- to threefold rise in plasma renin activity. In normal persons, a diurnal rhythm for plasma renin activity is characterized by peak values occurring between 10 A.M. and 12 noon, with decreases in activity in the afternoon.

HYPERFUNCTION OF THE ADRENAL CORTEX

Distinct clinical syndromes are produced when excess amounts of the principal adrenocortical hormones are secreted. Thus, excess production of the principal glucocorticoid cortisol is associated with Cushing's syndrome; excess production of the principal mineralocorticoid aldosterone with clinical and chemical signs of aldosteronism; excess production of adrenal androgens with adrenal virilism. As would be expected, these syndromes do not always occur in the "pure" form but may have overlapping features.

Cushing's Syndrome

From an analysis of the clinical and pathologic findings in a series of 12 patients, Harvey Cushing, in 1932, established a syndrome characterized by truncal obesity, hypertension, fatigability and weakness, amenorrhea, hirsutism, purplish abdominal striae, edema, glucosuria, and osteoporosis. As knowledge of this syndrome increased and as clinical tests of adrenocortical function became standardized and readily available, the diagnosis of Cushing's syndrome has been broadened into the following classification:

CAUSES OF CUSHING'S SYNDROME

   I. *Adrenal hyperplasia*, 70 percent of cases
     A. Secondary to hypothalamic dysfunction
     B. Secondary to ACTH-producing tumors
       1. Pituitary tumors
       2. Nonendocrine tumors (bronchogenic carcinoma)
  II. *Adrenal adenoma*, 15 percent of cases
 III. *Adrenal carcinoma*, 10 percent of cases
 IV. *Exogenous*, iatrogenic
     A. Prolonged use of glucocorticoids
     B. Prolonged use of ACTH

It is apparent that, regardless of etiology, all cases of Cushing's syndrome are due to increased production of cortisol by the adrenal gland. The majority of cases are due to *bilateral adrenal hyperplasia*, in which the adrenal gland weight usually exceeds the normal combined total weight of 10 Gm. Harvey Cushing originally postulated that the adrenal hyperplasia in these patients was attributable to the presence of pituitary basophilic adenomas. However, many cases are found without basophilic adenomas. Some are due to ACTH-producing chromophobe adenomas, but these cases represent a small fraction of the total. In the remaining cases attention has focused also on the elaboration of increased amounts of ACTH in the absence of pituitary tumors, possibly as a result of hypothalamic dysfunction, whereby the cortico-tropin-releasing center is reset to respond to a higher level of circulating cortisol. Proof of such a theory may now be possible with the availability of sensitive methods for determining plasma ACTH. Such cases of Cushing's syndrome due to adrenal hyperplasia, presumably due to excessive ACTH stimulation, always affect both adrenal glands.

In some 15 percent of cases of Cushing's syndrome, unilateral *adrenal adenomas* are found. On occasion they may occur bilaterally. These adenomas may or may not function in autonomous manner; i.e., they may or may not be independent of ACTH stimulation and control. In addition, approximately 10 percent of cases of Cushing's syndrome are associated with *adrenal carcinomas,* most often unilateral and most often functioning autonomously. In those cases of Cushing's syndrome due to unilateral adrenal adenomas or carcinomas functioning independently of ACTH, atrophy of the contralateral gland is often found, attributable to suppression of ACTH release by the high levels of cortisol secreted by the tumors. A small number of patients with Cushing's syndrome are found to have *adrenal rest tumors,* i.e., aberrant adrenocortical tissue occurring outside the adrenal gland. These embryologic remnants may be in the perirenal area, ovaries, or testes and exhibit histologic features of hyperplastic or adenomatous changes.

Nonendocrine tumors secreting polypeptide fractions that have an ACTH-like action are also occasionally responsible for Cushing's syndrome secondary to bilateral adrenal hyperplasia. The major association of a nonendocrine tumor has been with primitive "oat-cell" carcinomas of the lung. Hypokalemic alkalosis is often prominent in such cases, whereas many of the distinctive physical findings usually associated with Cushing's syndrome may be absent.

INCIDENCE. As steroid analyses have become more available, increasing numbers of patients with Cushing's syndrome are being detected among persons undergoing evaluation for such diverse entities as diabetes mellitus, hypertension, obesity, and osteoporosis. Many of these patients exhibit mild degrees of adrenal hyperfunction. The incidence of Cushing's syndrome in the female is three times that in the male. The most frequent age of onset is the third or fourth decade.

CLINICAL SIGNS AND SYMPTOMS. The frequency of clinical findings is listed in Table 92-1. Knowledge of

Table 92-1. INCIDENCE OF SIGNS AND SYMPTOMS IN 35 CASES OF CUSHING'S SYNDROME, PERCENT

Typical habitus	97	Amenorrhea	77
Increased body weight	94	Cutaneous striae	67
Fatigability and weakness	87	Personality changes	66
		Ecchymoses	65
Hypertension (above 150/90)	82	Edema	62
		Polyuria, polydipsia	23
Hirsutism	80	Hypertrophy of clitoris	19

the physiologic effects of glucocorticoids shows that many of the signs and symptoms logically follow. As a result of mobilization of peripheral supportive tissue, there are muscle weakness and fatigability, osteoporosis, and cutaneous striae. The latter involve a weakening and rupture of collagenous fibers in the dermis, so that the heavily vascularized subcutaneous tissues are exposed. Likewise, because of the loss of perivascular supporting tissue, there is easy bruisability, and ecchymoses often appear at sites of mild trauma. The osteoporosis may be so severe that collapse of vertebral bodies and pathologic fractures of other bones are frequently encountered. As a result of increased hepatic gluconeogenesis from these mobilized precursors, there may be frank diabetes with polydipsia and polyuria. More frequently, with the presence of an adequate reserve of insulin, there is deposition of this excess glucose in fat depots. This is observed most notably in the upper part of the face, the classic "moon" facies; in the interscapular area, the "buffalo" hump; and in the mesenteric bed, where it produces the classic "truncal" obesity (Fig. 92-9). Rarely, there may be episternal fatty tumors and mediastinal widening secondary to fat accumulation. The reason for this peculiar distribution of lipid is not known. The face also appears plethoric, even in the absence of any increase in red blood cell concentration. Hypertension is most always present, and frequently there are profound emotional changes, ranging from irritability or emotional lability to severe depression, confusion, or even frank psychosis. Acne and hirsutism are frequent in female patients, hirsutism often appearing as a fine "downy" coat over the face, forehead, and upper part of the trunk. Likewise in women patients, oligomenorrhea or amenorrhea is a frequent disturbance.

LABORATORY FINDINGS. With rare exceptions, plasma and urinary 17-hydroxycorticoid levels are elevated. Cir-

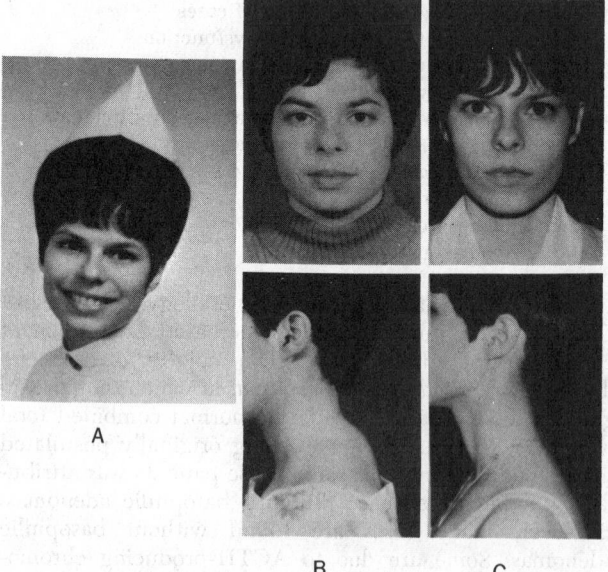

Fig. 92-9. A twenty-year-old female with Cushing's syndrome due to a right adrenal cortical adenoma: *A,* 2 years prior to surgery, age eighteen; *B,* 1 month prior to surgery, age twenty; and *C,* 1 year after surgery, age twenty-one.

culating eosinophils are below 100 cells per cu mm in 90 percent of cases, and patients characteristically show a mild neutrophilic leukocytosis. In spite of markedly plethoric facies, the hematocrit is usually within the normal range, but occasionally erythemia with higher hematocrits is encountered, particularly when the syndrome is associated with excessive production of 17-ketosteroids. Serum sodium concentration is usually normal; however, with marked excess secretion of cortisol, there may be hypokalemia, hypochloremia, and metabolic alkalosis. More than three-fourths of patients exhibit intermittent glucosuria, and nearly all have a decreased rate of disappearance of infused glucose from the circulation. Some patients may have frank diabetes, necessitating insulin therapy. X-ray studies usually reveal generalized osteoporosis, most marked in the spine and pelvis, but also frequently found in the skull, with disappearance of the lamina dura, and fractures are often seen in the ribs and vertebras. Intravenous pyelography and laminograms with or without retroperitoneal insufflation may demonstrate adrenal enlargement, particularly when an adenoma or carcinoma is the pathologic cause of the disease. More sophisticated x-ray techniques, such as selective adrenal arteriography or venography, may make the localization and diagnosis more specific. However, in many cases, these sophisticated procedures are probably not necessary, particularly since they are not without risk. The increased friability of the adrenal veins in Cushing's syndrome makes venography particularly hazardous.

DIAGNOSIS. The diagnosis of Cushing's syndrome depends on the direct or indirect demonstration of increased cortisol production in the absence of stress. Once this is established, further testing is carried out to determine whether or not the excess cortisol is being produced in an autonomous manner, since such knowledge will permit a more specific etiologic diagnosis.

For initial screening purposes, 24-hr urine 17-hydroxy- and 17-ketosteroid determinations are carried out, since values in excess of 10 mg per day for urine 17-hydroxy-steroids (Porter-Silber) justifies further evaluation (Ta-

Table 92-2. LABORATORY EVALUATION AND TESTING OF ADRENOCORTICAL FUNCTION IN NORMAL SUBJECTS AND IN PATIENTS WITH CUSHING'S SYNDROME*

Normal values	Plasma ACTH	Plasma cortisol	Cortisol secretory rate	Urine values	Control base line	Days of ACTH stimulation		Days of dexamethasone suppression, mg q 6h			
								0.5		2.0	
						1	2	1	2	1	2
	N	N	N	17-OH : 1–10		18–40	25–50	1–6	0–3	0–3	0–3
	N	N	N	17-KS : 5–25		15–30	20–40	6–18	5–15	4–12	4–8

Cushing's syndrome:

Hyperplasia...............	N–I ↗	I ↑	I	17-OH :	15 ↑	50	↑ 90	12	10	8	5 ↓
				17-KS :	20 ∿	50	90	18	15	12	10
Adenoma:											
Complete autonomy........	D ↓	I ↗	I	17-OH :	30 ↑	30	30	30	30	30	30
Incomplete				17-KS :	12 ∿	14	18 ↗	12	10	8	6
autonomy..............	N–D ↓	I ↗	I	17-OH :	15 ↑	50	90 ↗	15	15	12	10
				17-KS :	12 ∿	14	16	12	10	10	10 ✓
Carcinoma:											
Adrenal..................	D ↓	I ↑	I	17-OH :	50 ↑	50	50 ○	50	50	50	50
				17-KS :	60 ↗	60	60	60	60	60	60 ○
Extraadrenal	I ↑	I ↗	I	17-OH :	30 ↗	65	80 ○	30	30	30	30
(ACTH-producing tumor)				17-KS :	25 ↗	55	70	25	25	25	25 ○
Exogenous steroids	D ↓	D ↓	D	17-OH :	1 ↓	1	2	1	1	1	1
(iatrogenic)				17-KS :	4 ↓	5	6	5	4	4	4 ○

* Clinical status charted vertically and *representative* values for steroid tests charted horizontally. 17-OH, 17-KS refer to 24-hr urine 17-hydroxycorticosteroid and 17-ketosteroid excretion. 17-KS base-line excretion higher in males than in females. All laboratory values given in milligrams per day. Urine ketogenic steroid values will be approximately twofold greater than those listed for urine 17-OH (except in adrenogenital syndrome). See text for normal blood steroid values. Note that only in the iatrogenic form of Cushing's syndrome are both the plasma ACTH and plasma cortisol levels decreased. ACTH stimulation causes brisk rise in *both* 17-OH and 17-KS in hyperplasia; disproportionate rise in 17-OH in adenoma; and no change in steroid excretion in adrenal carcinoma. Dexamethasone suppression is usually incomplete at the 2-mg daily dosage level in hyperplasia but complete with 8-mg dosage; incomplete at both 2- and 8-mg daily dosage in both adenomas and carcinomas with complete autonomy; incomplete in Cushing's syndrome secondary to extraadrenal ACTH-producing tumors. Abbreviations: N = normal; I = increased; D = decreased.

ble 92-2). An ancillary screening procedure is to determine the diurnal excretion pattern for urine 17-hydroxysteroids by collecting urine between 7 A.M. and 7 P.M. and 7 P.M. to 7 A.M. The patient with Cushing's syndrome will generally excrete an equivalent or greater amount of the 17-hydroxysteroids in the night collection, in contrast to most normal subjects. Creatinine determinations are of critical importance to demonstrate the accuracy and adequacy of the collection procedure. An adult female excretes approximately 1,000 mg creatinine daily, with about 50 to 60 percent found in the daytime collection; an adult male excretes approximately 1,800 mg daily. Day-to-day variation in creatinine excretion by a patient should not exceed 20 percent. If it is demonstrated that the diurnal cycle for steroid excretion is "reversed," i.e., night urine 17-hydroxysteroids are almost equal to or greater than daytime excretion, one then knows that excessive cortisol is being released continuously "around the clock." These urine steroid determinations, which reflect the metabolites of cortisol, are indirect but adequate proof of excessive cortisol production. A direct method is available utilizing radioisotopic cortisol to determine the actual cortisol secretory rate, which in cases of Cushing's syndrome is in excess of 30 mg per day. Another method of direct confirmation of excess cortisol is the determination of the free cortisol in the urine, which reflects the active free cortisol in the blood. Normal persons excrete less than 100 μg daily of free cortisol, whereas patients with Cushing's syndrome may excrete up to ten times this amount. The sensitivity of this urine free cortisol test resides in the fact that only free cortisol of the plasma is freely filtrable at the glomerulus, and thus increments in the plasma level of this biologically active form are magnified in terms of urine excretory values.

Owing to a marked diurnal variability plasma 17-hydroxycorticoid determinations are not meaningful when performed in isolated fashion, but demonstration that the expected normal fall in late afternoon blood levels does not occur is increasingly used as a diagnostic measure. Normally, the plasma level declines by half or more; if such a decrease is not noted, one assumes that continuous hypersecretion of cortisol is occurring.

An additional screening procedure involves the use of the rapid dexamethasone suppression test.

Specific diagnosis of the type of lesion causing Cushing's syndrome can usually be made by the combined use of ACTH-stimulation and dexamethasone-suppression tests. Adrenal hyperplasia, whether caused by hypothalamic dysfunction or by an ACTH-producing tumor, is characterized by hyperreactivity to exogenous ACTH. The continuous stimulation of the hyperplastic glands by endogenous ACTH appears to "prime" the adrenals to this hyperactive response to exogenous ACTH testing. This hyperactive response is evidenced in the parallel rise of both urine 17-hydroxy- and urine 17-ketosteroids. Whereas adrenal cortisol production is suppressed in normal subjects given dexamethasone 0.5 mg every 6 hr for 48 hr, no suppression occurs in patients with bilateral adrenal hyperplasia given this dosage. Suppression of cortisol production in normal subjects is judged by a decrease in urine 17-hydroxysteroids to less than 3 mg per day, demonstrating that the hypothalamic-pituitary axis is appropriately responsive to increases in blood glucocorticoid levels, with a resultant decline in ACTH release. Lack of suppression in patients with adrenal hyperplasia given 2 mg daily of dexamethasone suggests that their hypothalamic-pituitary axis is "reset" to a higher blood level of glucocorticoids. On higher doses of dexamethasone (2 mg every 6 hr) suppression of urine 17-hydroxysteroid levels to values less than half the base-line levels can be demonstrated, consistent with the view that the hypothalamic-pituitary axis in these patients is reset upward and is responsive only to higher blood levels of glucocorticoids, at which point an appropriate decline in ACTH release does occur. The finding of a normal plasma ACTH level in these patients is an abnormal sign, since with the elevated blood cortisol levels one would expect a decreased blood ACTH level. On metyrapone testing, patients with adrenal hyperplasia due to hypothalmic dysfunction will again demonstrate a hyperactive response. In patients with adrenal hyperplasia secondary to an *ACTH-producing tumor,* such as an oat-cell bronchogenic carcinoma, no suppression will occur after dexamethasone administration and an abnormally depressed metyrapone test results, since the ACTH production by the tumor functions in an autonomous manner.

In patients with Cushing's syndrome secondary to an *adrenal adenoma,* hyperreactivity to exogenous ACTH testing may or may not occur, depending on whether the adenoma is functioning in an autonomous manner; if it is, it will be found ACTH-insensitive and thus fail to demonstrate a brisk rise in urine 17-hydroxycorticoids on ACTH stimulation. The diagnosis of adrenal adenoma is suggested by the disproportionate elevation in base-line urine 17-hydroxycorticoids with only a modest rise in 17-ketosteroids. Those adenomas which function autonomously fail to suppress after administration of dexamethasone at either the 2- or 8-mg daily dosage schedule, whereas the ACTH-sensitive adenomas most often fail to suppress with the lower, 2-mg daily dosage but may demonstrate suppression at the higher, 8-mg daily dosage. The variability of dexamethasone suppression testing is greater at the higher dose levels, and the distinction between adenomas and carcinomas is as a result less decisive. Another entity in the differential diagnosis is multinodular ("adenomatous") adrenal hyperplasia, which is an uncommon condition characteristically having features of both hyperplasia and of adenomas. Response to ACTH stimulation is abnormally brisk, but patients with multinodular adrenal hyperplasia most often do not show suppression after dexamethasone. Bilateral enlargement of the adrenals may be noted in such patients on the roentgenogram, and some patients excrete high levels of 3β-hydroxy-Δ5-steroids. Such patients usually do not show suppression with the standard doses of dexamethasone. However, with large doses, such as 4 to 8 mg every 6 hr, suppression often occurs.

Metyrapone testing is useful in differentiating adrenal tumors (adenoma or carcinoma) from adrenal hyperplasia, since the adrenal tumors by their autonomy suppress the ACTH-releasing capacity of the pituitary, with the result that on metyrapone challenge testing the pituitary fails to release ACTH in an appropriate manner and the usual rise in urine 17-hydroxycorticoids fails to occur. This finding of impaired response to metyrapone challenge separates adrenal tumors from adrenal hyperplasia, in which normal or hyperactive responses occur.

The diagnosis of *adrenal carcinoma* as a cause of Cushing's syndrome is suggested by markedly elevated baseline values of *both* urine 17-hydroxycorticoids and urine 17-ketosteroids. Adrenal carcinoma is usually resistant to both ACTH stimulation and dexamethasone suppression because of the autonomy of the tumor tissue itself and because of extreme atrophy of the normal remaining adrenal tissue. Virilization is often present. Functioning adrenal carcinomas that produce Cushing's syndrome are most often associated with elevated urine excretory values for the metabolites of the intermediates of steroid biosynthesis (such as tetrahydro-11-deoxycortisol) in addition to the cortisol metabolites, suggesting inefficient conversion of the intermediates to the final product. This is in contrast to Cushing's syndrome associated with adrenocortical hyperplasia, where the elevation of urine steroids is largely accounted for by cortisol metabolites.

Cushing's syndrome is being reported with increasing frequency in association with *nonendocrine tumors* producing an ACTH-like material in an autonomous manner, with the resultant development of adrenal hyperplasia. Approximately half these cases have been associated with the primitive small-cell type of bronchogenic carcinoma, and the remainder have been reported chiefly with tumors of thymus, pancreas, ovary, or thyroid. The onset of Cushing's syndrome is distinctively sudden in these patients, and this partly accounts for their failure to exhibit all the classic physical findings of the syndrome. Extracts of some of these nonendocrine tumors have produced a compound that is biologically, physiochemically, and immunologically similar to pituitary ACTH. Since such tumors often produce large amounts of this ACTH-like material, base-line urine steroid values are usually markedly elevated, and increased skin pigmentation is almost always present. These changes may be due to a MSH- or CRF-like material produced by the tumor. Hypokalemic alkalosis is much more common in these patients than in patients with Cushing's syndrome due to other causes. Edema and hypertension are also seen with greater frequency in these patients. On being tested, these patients will demonstrate a hyperactive response to ACTH stimulation but no suppression with dexamethasone and no increment in urine 17-hydroxycorticoid excretion after metyrapone administration. Plasma ACTH levels are most often markedly elevated in these patients, a helpful diagnostic finding, since plasma ACTH levels in other categories of Cushing's syndrome are at most modestly elevated.

Hyperpigmentation in patients with Cushing's syndrome always points to an extraadrenal tumor, either in an extracranial location, as discussed in the previous paragraph, or within the cranium. In the first 100 cases reported of Cushing's syndrome associated with pituitary tumors the majority had associated basophilic adenomas; chromophobe adenomas were in a distinct minority. Since this original series, chromophobe adenomas and carcinomas are being reported in much greater frequency than are basophilic adenomas. Basophilic adenomas do not cause enlargement of the sella turcica, whereas chromophobe tumors are the commonest cause of ballooning of the sella. The chief complaint of patients with chromophobe tumors is decreasing visual acuity, often with blurred vision and always with headaches. The chromophobe adenomas are asymmetric in growth, and as they progress upward, pressure on the optic nerve tracts results in visual field defects in most patients, with earliest losses occurring in the superior temporal quadrants; later a full bitemporal hemianopsia results. Headaches would appear to be caused by traction on surrounding dural structures or on the diaphragma sella. This association of pituitary tumors with Cushing's syndrome has generated interest as to whether all cases of adrenal hyperplasia may be caused by extraadrenal tumors and has led further to the speculation that chronic hypothalamic dysfunction may lead to the development of anterior pituitary tumors. A limitation to such interpretation has been the finding that approximately one-tenth of patients undergoing bilateral adrenalectomy for Cushing's syndrome have developed enlarged sella turcica and pituitary tumors, clinically evident only *after* the surgery, strongly suggesting that the loss of adrenal tissue, and consequent loss of the usual negative cortisol feedback on ACTH release, may be instrumental in the genesis of such tumors. Since intrasellar tumors may be present at an early stage in many patients *without* sellar enlargement, a decisive opinion as to their role in the genesis of Cushing's syndrome, or in the sequelae of its surgical therapy, must be withheld for further investigation. Clinically, all patients suspected of having Cushing's syndrome must be carefully examined for visual field defects and enlargement of the sella turcica; if defects are found, further diagnostic procedures may be warranted, such as sellar tomography, pneumoencephalography, and angiography.

DIFFERENTIAL DIAGNOSIS. Patients with exogenous obesity, hypertension, and diabetes mellitus, occurring singly or in combination, present major problems in diagnosis. Extreme *obesity* is uncommon in Cushing's syndrome; furthermore, with exogenous obesity, the adiposity is generalized, not truncal. On adrenocortical testing, abnormalities, if noted in patients with exogenous obesity, are never extensive but only modest. Basal urine steroid excretion levels in obese patients are either normal or slightly elevated, a finding similar to their cortisol secretory values. Some patients demonstrate an increased percentage of conversion of secreted cortisol into excreted metabolites. Blood cortisol levels are normal, and, of greater importance, a normal diurnal pattern in blood and urine levels is seen. On ACTH stimulation some of the patients will demonstrate a brisk response; however, in most cases this response is suppressed easily with dexamethasone. It would appear that exogenous obesity may *cause* alterations in the secretion and metabolism of steroids, pointing up the secondary nature of altered steroid testing patterns sometimes encountered. These patients are best treated by a concerted weight reduction program with periodic retesting of adrenal function.

Patients with *hepatic disease*, notably cirrhosis, often with obesity, may exhibit some of the manifestations of Cushing's syndrome. The reason for this resides in their impaired ability to inactivate circulated steroids, owing to decreased hepatic blood flow, with the result that blood levels may increase but secretory rates generally are found in the normal range. The defect is in inactivation of steroids, not in excessive secretion, so that therapy is initiated only for the underlying hepatic disease.

Iatrogenic Cushing's syndrome, induced by the administration of either glucocorticoids or ACTH, is indistinguishable by physical findings from the endogenous forms of adrenocortical hyperfunction. On occasion one may wish to rule out an underlying endogenous form of Cushing's syndrome that may be clinically magnified by exogenous therapy. This is accomplished by changing the patient's therapy to 1.0 mg dexamethasone daily while collecting base-line and diurnal split urine output for corticosteroid analysis. Patients with a pure exogenous form of Cushing's syndrome due to prolonged suppression of their hypothalamic-pituitary axis by administered steroid will demonstrate low base-line steroid excretion, predominantly in the daytime, a finding in distinct contrast to that in patients with endogenous Cushing's syndrome. Patients receiving long-term ACTH therapy, in addition to the features of Cushing's syndrome, may also have melanodermia. The production of iatrogenic Cushing's syndrome is related both to the total steroid dose and to the duration of therapy. Also, patients on afternoon and evening doses of steroid develop Cushing's syndrome more readily and on smaller daily steroid doses than do patients on a steroid program limited to morning doses only. In addition, there appears to be a marked interpatient difference in the enzymatic disposition of administered steroid. Several cases have been reported in which a spontaneous remission of Cushing's syndrome occurred; some have been characterized by intermittent abnormalities in adrenal testing. It is difficult to know whether such abnormalities are functional in nature or true pathophysiologic processes.

THERAPY. When an adenoma or carcinoma is suspected, adrenal exploration is performed, with excision of the tumor. Since cortisol production by the tumor generally causes atrophy of the contralateral gland, if an atrophied gland is noted on the initial side of exploration, the tumor must be on the opposite side. Because of this probable atrophy of the contralateral adrenal, the patient is prepared and treated pre- and postoperatively for total adrenalectomy even when a unilateral lesion is suspected, the routine being similar to that for an Addisonian patient undergoing elective surgery (Table 92-3).

The possibility of chemically inhibiting adrenocortical hyperfunction due to carcinoma is under active investigation. The principal antitumor drug under evaluation is *o,p'*-DDD [2,2-bis-(2-chlorophenyl,4-chlorophenyl)-1,1-dichloroethane], an isomer of the insecticide DDT. *o,p'*-DDD originally was demonstrated to induce adrenal atrophy of the "cytotoxic type" in experimental animals. This drug suppresses cortisol production and decreases plasma and urine steroid levels. It also suppresses peripheral enzyme systems responsible for steroid transformations. Daily dosage of *o,p'*-DDD has ranged from 2 to 12 Gm. Its cytotoxic action appears specific for adrenal glandular tissue, but histologic hepatic abnormalities have

Table 92-3. STEROID THERAPY SCHEDULE FOR PATIENTS WITH CUSHING'S SYNDROME UNDERGOING ADRENALECTOMY*

	Steroid							
	Cortisone acetate (intramuscularly)		Cortisone acetate (orally)				Fluorohydrocortisone (orally)	Hydrocortisone infusion
	7 A.M.	7 P.M.	8 A.M.	12 M.	4 P.M.	8 P.M.	8 A.M.	Continuous
Day before operation.........	...	100						
Day of operation............	100	50	...	...	...	...	...	300
Postoperative day 1..........	50	50	...	...	...	...	...	200
" 2..........	50	50	...	...	...	...	...	150
" 3..........	50	50	...	...	...	...	...	100
" 4..........	50	25	25	25	25	25	...	
" 5..........	50	...	25	25	25	25	0.1	
" 6..........	...	...	50	25	25	25	0.2	
" 7..........	...	...	25	25	25	25	0.2	
" 8..........	...	...	25	12.5	25	12.5	0.2	
" 9–14.......	...	...	25	12.5	25	...	0.1	
" 15–21......	...	...	25	12.5	12.5	...	0.1	
" 22–........	...	...	25	...	12.5	...	0.1	

* Both intravenous and intramuscular routes are utilized to minimize hazards of infusion infiltration. All steroid doses are in milligrams.

been reported. Almost all patients experience side effects of anorexia, diarrhea, or vomiting, and patients on long-term therapy must be observed closely for signs of adrenal insufficiency. For this reason patients may be placed on long-term glucocorticoid replacement therapy. In some patients dramatic regression of both tumor and metastases may occur, but long-term survival remains discouragingly limited. Predictability of expected response is poor. Investigation of this drug, however, has expanded the search for a more perfect chemical inhibitor of hyperactive adrenal tissue. For example, aminoglutethamide appears to inhibit steroid synthesis at a step between the conversion of cholesterol to pregnanelone. Because of this, it has been used in the treatment of Cushing's syndrome. However, it also may induce hypothyroidism and has moderate to severe side effects, severely limiting its usefulness. Another compound is DL-2-(p-aminophenyl)-2-phenylethylamine. At present, there has been little clinical experience with this compound, but it seems to exert its effect by blocking 11_β-hydroxylation thereby offering promise as an effective inhibitor of adrenal biosynthesis.

In patients with a severe form of Cushing's syndrome due to adrenal hyperplasia, with features of hypertension, overt diabetes, psychosis, and osteoporosis with pathologic fractures and in the absence of an enlarged sella turcica, a complete total bilateral adrenalectomy is preferred. Since, as mentioned earlier, one-tenth of these patients develop pituitary tumors after surgery, pituitary irradiation is also indicated in any patient who develops increased pigmentation or in whom the sella turcica size increases postoperatively. In patients past the reproductive years, pituitary irradiation may be carried out prophylactically in conjunction with complete adrenalectomy. It cannot be stressed too strongly that the status of all patients with bilateral adrenalectomy must be followed diligently with periodic reexaminations for evidence of increasing sellar size or pigmentary changes.

If patients with adrenal hyperplasia are noted to have signs of pituitary tumor (melanodermia, increased sellar size, visual field defects), specific therapy directed at the pituitary gland must be undertaken. In general, the type of therapy is either surgery or some form of radiation. Complications of surgical therapy include cerebrospinal fluid rhinorrhea, optic nerve and posterior pituitary injury, as well as removal of all tropic hormones. The morbidity and mortality rates are greater than with radiotherapy, and therefore surgery is often reserved for those cases not amenable to treatment with radiation. There are three major methods of directing radiotherapy at the pituitary gland. (1) The classical approach is the use of conventional external radiation at a dose of 3,000 to 5,000 r delivered over several weeks. The total dosage is limited by possible damage to surrounding neural structures and by the loss of additional pituitary tropic function. Treatment has been successful in fewer than one-third of the patients with Cushing's syndrome who were treated solely by this method. (2) The second method is internal pituitary irradiation by the stereotactic implantation of ^{90}yttrium pellets in the pituitary via the transnasosphenoid route. Possible limitation of this form of

therapy may be found once long-term evaluation on the effects of the radiation on perisellar structures (such as the internal carotid artery) has been made. (3) The most recent development has been the use of the alpha particle or proton beam as a source of external radiation. By this method as much as 12,000 r can be directed at the pituitary gland without evident damage to surrounding structures. This is because the beam can be focused more sharply than the more commonly used gamma radiation and because multiple portals of entry can be used. Even with this therapy there is a significant incidence of ocular motor palsies. This form of therapy holds great promise because of its ease of application, insignificant mortality rate, and low morbidity rate. However, final evaluation awaits long-term follow-up studies on treated subjects.

In patients with milder forms of adrenal hyperplasia without serious steroid-induced complications, several methods of approach are available, such as unilateral adrenalectomy with or without pituitary irradiation, or external or internal pituitary irradiation. Unilateral adrenalectomy without pituitary irradiation must be reserved for those patients with the mildest forms of adrenal hyperplasia.

If Cushing's syndrome redevelops after bilateral adrenalectomy, excessive stimulation of a remnant of adrenocortical tissue must be occurring. In very rare instances an embryologic extraadrenal remnant may be stimulated to produce excess cortisol. Surgical exploration has not been rewarding because of the difficulty in identifying small adrenocortical remnants. What is needed is an isotopic detection method whereby radioactive incorporation into the aberrant tissue can be monitored, and thus identification secured, at the operative field.

Aldosteronism

Aldosteronism is a syndrome associated with hypersecretion of the major adrenal mineralocorticoid aldosterone. *Primary* aldosteronism signifies that the stimulus for the excessive aldosterone production resides within the adrenal gland, whereas in *secondary* aldosteronism the stimulus is of extraadrenal origin.

PRIMARY ALDOSTERONISM

The constellation of signs and symptoms of excessive inappropriate aldosterone production was first summarized by Conn in 1956. The disease results from an aldosterone-producing adrenal adenoma (Conn's syndrome) or, in some cases, an adrenal carcinoma; cases have occurred with adrenal hyperplasia, and in rare instances the disease has occurred in the absence of pathologic changes in the adrenal gland as judged by light microscopy.

The majority of cases (75 percent) involve a unilateral adrenal adenoma, usually small and occurring with equal frequency on either side. It is twice as common in women as in men, presenting between the ages of thirty and fifty.

INCIDENCE. Primary aldosteronism is an uncommon disease. An estimated 400 cases have been reported worldwide in the first 10 years after its description. The incidence in unselected hypertensive patients is less than 0.5 percent. Because of special diagnostic procedures involved, diagnosis has been largely restricted to symptomatic patients. With greater availability of these procedures an increased incidence may be seen.

SIGNS AND SYMPTOMS. The continual hypersecretion of aldosterone increases the renal distal tubular exchange of intratubular sodium for secreted potassium and hydrogen ions, with progressive depletion of body potassium and development of hypokalemia. Almost all patients have diastolic hypertension, usually not of marked severity, and complain of headaches. The hypertension is related in some unknown manner to the increased sodium reabsorption. *Potassium depletion* is responsible for the major complaints of muscle weakness and fatigue and is related to the effect of intra- and extracellular potassium ion depletion on muscle membrane. The muscle weakness is most striking in the legs and may progress to transient paralysis. Muscles innervated by cranial nerves are usually spared. Most patients have nocturnal polyuria due to a vasopressin-insensitive, potassium-depletion-induced nephropathy. The polyuria results from impairment of concentrating ability and is often associated with polydipsia. These patients may have electrocardiographic and roentgenographic signs of left ventricular enlargement secondary to their hypertension, and hypertensive retinopathy is often seen but papilledema is absent. Electrocardiographic signs of potassium depletion such as prominent U waves are often present. In the absence of associated congestive heart failure, mental disease, or preexisting abnormalities (such as thrombophlebitis), edema is characteristically absent in these patients.

In cases of long duration, potassium-depletion nephropathy becomes manifest, with azotemia, often with superimposed bacilluria, and in some instances with congestive heart failure and edema.

LABORATORY FINDINGS. Laboratory findings are dependent on both the duration and the severity of the potassium depletion. On examination of the urine, negative to trace amounts of protein are found, sometimes with superimposed pyuria and bacilluria, presumably because of the predilection of potassium-depleted kidneys for infection. Urine specific gravity is low (less than 1.015), and an overnight concentration test with simultaneous vasopressin administration reveals impaired ability to concentrate the urine. Urine pH is often neutral to alkaline, because of excessive secretion of ammonium and bicarbonate ions; potassium depletion may lower the maximal tubular transfer rate for bicarbonate. Urine 17-hydroxycorticosteroid and 17-ketosteroid excretion levels are always within the normal range in patients with aldosteronomas but may occasionally be elevated in those rare instances of primary aldosteronism due to adrenal carcinoma. Mild azotemia is an inconstant finding.

Serial blood sampling usually reveals *hypokalemia* and hypernatremia. Serial blood sampling is stressed. The hypokalemia may be severe (less than 3.0 mEq potassium per liter) and reflects significant body potassium depletion, usually in excess of 300 mEq. *Hypernatremia* is due to both sodium retention and a concomitant water loss from polyuria. The serum bicarbonate level may be elevated as a result of hydrogen ion loss into the urine and migration into potassium-depleted cells, with alkalosis then developing. The alkalosis is perpetuated with potassium deficiency, since such deficiency increases the capacity of the proximal convoluted tubule to reabsorb filtered bicarbonate. This alkalosis predisposes to signs and symptoms of tetany. If hypokalemia is severe, serum magnesium levels will be reduced. In the absence of azotemia, serum uric acid concentration is normal.

Salivary sodium potassium ratios are reduced in the majority of cases, as is thermal sweat sodium concentration.

Total body sodium content is increased but not to the degree seen in edematous states. Total exchangeable sodium is moderately elevated, and total exchangeable body potassium is usually, but not invariably, reduced. The volume of extracellular fluid is expanded in most cases, with expansion of plasma volume in many. The expanded extracellular fluid volume is thought to be responsible for the reversed diurnal excretory pattern for salt and water that many of these patients exhibit, with predominant salt and water excretion occurring during the night. Polyuria contributes to the nocturia.

DIAGNOSIS OF PRIMARY ALDOSTERONISM. The major criteria which permit the clinician to derive an unequivocal diagnosis of primary aldosteronism are (1) diastolic hypertension without edema; (2) hypersecretion of aldosterone which fails to be suppressed appropriately during volume expansion (salt loading); (3) hyposecretion of renin (as judged by low plasma renin activity levels) which fails to increase appropriately during volume depletion (upright posture); (4) hypokalemia and/or inappropriate urine potassium loss.

Diastolic hypertension is a prerequisite for the diagnosis of primary aldosteronism, even though transient periods of relative normotension may be observed during long-term evaluation. Diastolic hypertension exhibited by patients with primary aldosteronism does not differ from the labile variety of essential hypertension. Blood pressure readings characteristically become reduced after hospitalization, but moderate to severe rises may occur in hospital and are often related to emotional situations. Accelerated (sustained) diastolic hypertension is uncommon but has been reported.

Patients with primary aldosteronism characteristically *do not have edema,* since they are exhibiting a perpetuated "escape" phenomenon. Since they are in a chronic state of escape from the sodium-retaining aspects of mineralocorticoids, they characteristically excrete an administered salt load with a greater rapidity than do normotensive subjects, a characteristic which is shared by patients having essential hypertension. Only a limited sodium retention occurs when patients with primary aldosteronism are given sodium-retaining hormones parenterally. Rarely in patients with associated potassium-depletion nephropathy and azotemia, pretibial edema may be present.

Since hypersecretion of aldosterone may occur either in primary or in secondary aldosteronism, documentation of this parameter alone is not sufficient to arrive at a diagnosis of primary aldosteronism. It must be further documented that this hypersecretion of aldosterone *fails to be suppressed* normally during volume expansion of a sufficient degree to suppress the renin-angiotensin system. It is to be noted that the autonomy exhibited by aldosterone tumors in these patients refers only to their resistance to suppression of hypersecretion during volume expansion; such tumors can and do respond either in normal or supernormal fashion to the stimuli of potassium loading or ACTH infusion. Patients with primary aldosteronism do not respond to volume expansion since their renin-angiotensin system is already suppressed. Appropriate suppression testing may be carried out by saline loading, oral salt loading, or DOCA administration (see Mineralocorticoid Suppression Tests, earlier in this chapter). The autonomy of these tumors to volume expansion is not necessarily complete; many patients with primary aldosteronism will demonstrate some decrease of hypersecretion of aldosterone during volume expansion maneuvers, but such decreases are significantly less than the expected normal response.

The finding of a *low plasma renin activity level* which fails to respond appropriately to volume depletion, in conjunction with documentation of hypersecretion of aldosterone, constitutes the unique biochemical finding for a diagnosis of primary aldosteronism (see Fig. 92-10). Since some patients with essential hypertension, for reasons not known, have low plasma renin levels, it is essential to demonstrate that these low levels in patients with suspected primary aldosteronism fail to respond appropriately to volume depletion (see pp. 485 to 486). (This finding is comparable to the situation of long-term pituitary ACTH suppression resulting from hypersecretion of cortisol.)

A major criterion for the diagnosis of primary aldosteronism is the demonstration of *hypokalemia* associated with an inappropriately high urine potassium excretion. Judgments as to the significance of a given degree of hypokalemia for a given rate of urine potassium excretion must take into account the patient's potassium and sodium intake. Patients with hypokalemia secondary to diuretics, laxatives, etc., will generally have a 24-hr urine potassium excretion of less than 40 mEq per day, and often the value is markedly less than this. Most patients with primary aldosteronism, on the other hand, with a potassium intake of 100 mEq per day always have a 24-hr urine potassium excretion of greater than 40 mEq per day. Since potassium excretion can be modified by manipulations in sodium intake, this latter factor must be taken into consideration. During periods of high sodium intake, delivery of sodium ions to the distal tubular sodium-potassium exchange site will be increased, resulting in a rise in potassium excretion over control values. Contrariwise, potassium excretion can be minimized for any degree of hypokalemia by restriction of sodium intake, which limits the amount of sodium reaching the

Primary aldosteronism

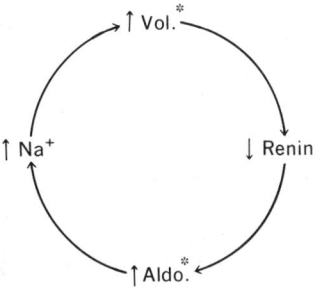

Secondary aldosteronism

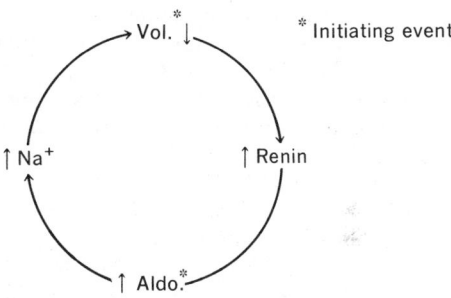

Fig. 92-10. Responses of the renin-aldosterone volume control loop in primary versus secondary aldosteronism.

distal tubular exchange site. Patients with primary aldosteronism will always exhibit inappropriate urine potassium losses during either saline or oral salt loading procedures.

Precise localization of aldosterone-producing adenomas may be determined preoperatively in many cases by the technique of percutaneous transfemoral bilateral adrenal vein catheterization with simultaneous adrenal arteriography and venography. Such a technique permits radiologic localization, and, in addition, the adrenal vein sampling may demonstrate a two- to threefold increase in plasma aldosterone concentration on the involved side compared with the uninvolved side.

DIFFERENTIAL DIAGNOSIS. All patients with *accelerated hypertension* and hypokalemia must be evaluated for unilateral renal disease. If such a diagnosis is confirmed, an additional diagnosis of primary aldosteronism is unlikely, although in rare instances both have been recorded to occur simultaneously. A useful maneuver in distinguishing between secondary aldosteronism due to accelerated hypertension and primary aldosteronism is to monitor serum potassium levels and aldosterone secretion (or excretory rates) prior to and following therapeutic correction of the hypertension. In patients with accelerated hypertension and secondary aldosteronism, the aldosteronism will subside with successful antihypertensive therapy, i.e., aldosterone parameters will return to normal and the hypokalemia and/or alkalosis will disappear. In distinct contrast, patients with primary aldosteronism in

Table 92-4. CHARACTERISTICS OF VARIOUS HYPERMINERALOCORTICOID STATES

Disorder	Blood pressure	Edema	Serum Na+	Serum K+	Plasma renin activity	Aldosterone
Primary aldosteronism	↑	0	↑,N	↓	↓↓	↑
Secondary aldosteronism:						
Accelerated hypertension	↑↑	0	↓,N	↓	↑↑	↑↑
Edema disorders	N,↓	+	↓,N	N,↓	↑	↑
DOC tumor	↑	0	↑,N	↓	↓↓	↓,N
Licorice ingestion	↑	0	↑,N	↓	↓	↓,N
Cushing's syndrome	↑	0,+	N,↑	↓,N	N,↓	N,↓
Bartter's syndrome	N,↓	0	N,↓	↓	↑↑↑	↑↑

whom successful blood pressure reduction is undertaken will continue to exhibit hypokalemic alkalosis with hypersecretion of aldosterone. An additional maneuver is sometimes useful. This is based on the observation of Melby that the majority of patients with primary aldosteronism become normotensive when treated with the aldosterone antagonist, spironolactone (Aldactone A), when given in a dose of 50 mg every 6 to 8 hr daily over a period of 2 to 5 weeks, whereas a minority of patients with essential hypertension become normotensive. Such therapy in patients with accelerated hypertension and secondary aldosteronism often will correct the electrolyte abnormalities, but hypertension will persist. It is of interest that patients with primary aldosteronism have been successfully managed medically for as long as 6 years through the chronic use of spironolactone therapy.

Primary aldosteronism must also be distinguished from other *hypermineralocorticoid states.* In a few instances, hypertensive patients with hypokalemic alkalosis have been found to have DOC-secreting adenomas. Such patients will have reduced plasma renin activity levels, but **aldosterone measurements will be either normal or reduced,** suggesting the diagnosis of mineralocorticoid excess due to a hormone other than aldosterone (see Table 92-4).

Licorice ingestion produces a syndrome mimicking primary aldosteronism. Licorice contains a sodium-retaining principle, glycyrrhizinic acid, which causes sodium retention, expansion of the extracellular fluid volume, hypertension, depressed plasma renin levels, and suppressed aldosterone levels. The diagnosis is excluded by a careful history.

Hypokalemic alkalosis is a prominent feature of *Bartter's syndrome* (juxtaglomerular hyperplasia). Patients with this disorder are easily distinguished by the finding of normotension and moderate to marked increases in plasma renin levels.

Base-line measurements of plasma renin activity and aldosterone secretion/excretion rate are not sufficient for a diagnosis of primary aldosteronism, since a small segment of the hypertensive population has been documented to have low-level plasma renin activity for undetermined reasons. Such patients may demonstrate an appropriate response in terms of plasma renin levels to volume depletion but display a subnormal rise in aldosterone secretion. Data are not available as to the response of this group of patients to the maneuver of volume expansion. It should also be pointed out that autonomous hypersecretion of aldosterone *without* demonstration of a low plasma renin level is not of sufficient accuracy to permit the diagnosis of primary aldosteronism, since it may occur in either secondary or "tertiary" aldosteronism.

SECONDARY ALDOSTERONISM

Secondary aldosteronism refers to an appropriately increased production of aldosterone by the adrenal gland in response to stimuli originating outside the gland. The adrenal production rates of aldosterone are often higher in patients with secondary aldosteronism than in those with primary aldosteronism. Most patients with secondary aldosteronism exhibit this syndrome either as an associated feature of the accelerated phase of hypertension (regardless of the primary disease) or on the basis of an underlying edema disorder.

The majority of patients in the *accelerated phase* of hypertensive disease exhibit a secondary aldosteronism characterized by hypokalemic alkalosis, absence of edema, moderate to severe increases in plasma renin levels, and moderate to marked increases in aldosterone secretion/excretion rates. It has been postulated that the profound renal vasoconstriction which may be present in such patients is responsible for the excessive release of renin and hence initiates the state of secondary aldosteronism. Such a suggestion is supported by the observation that therapeutic correction of the hypertension results in the disappearance of the hyperaldosteronism.

Secondary aldosteronism is present in most *edema* disorders. Edema may be said to be the cardinal finding on physical examination for the presence of secondary aldosteronism. Hypersecretion of aldosterone in such clinical states correlates best with the phases of rapid accumulation of edema fluid. During phases of stable body weight, aldosterone measurements are often reported to be within the normal range. Patients with secondary aldosteronism due to edema disorders differ qualitatively from normal subjects and from patients with primary aldosteronism, in that they fail to exhibit a normal "escape" pattern in response to the chronic administration of DOC. These patients are exquisitely sensitive to the sodium-retaining properties of the mineralocorticoids and will exhibit a profound decrease in urine sodium excretion, often to barely detectable levels. They retain excess salt and water, but this retained fluid is ineffective in terms of reexpanding what is registered by the renin-angiotensin system as a deficient circulating blood volume. Instead, the excess salt and water that are retained accumulate in increasing quantities as edema fluid. Diuretic therapy often exaggerates the features of secondary aldosteronism via the mechanism of acute volume depletion; when this happens hypokalemia and on occasion alkalosis become prominent features.

Increased aldosterone secretion rates have been amply documented in patients who form edema as a result of either cirrhosis or the nephrotic syndrome. In congestive heart failure, however, elevated aldosterone secretion is a variable finding. The stimulus for aldosterone release in these clinical conditions appears to be *arterial hypovolemia*. Arterial blood volume may be depleted in cirrhosis as a result of decreased hepatic protein synthesis and protein loss into ascitic fluid; likewise, urine protein losses in the nephrotic syndrome may lead to arterial hypovolemia. Despite venous congestion, arterial hypovolemia may occur in congestive heart failure as a result of a failing cardiac output. The finding of normal aldosterone secretory rates in some patients with congestive heart failure requires explanation. It has been shown that approximately 95 percent of the circulating blood aldosterone is removed from the plasma and metabolized or extracted by the liver during a single passage. The rate of removal of aldosterone from plasma is termed its *metabolic clearance rate*, and since aldosterone is almost exclusively "cleared" by the liver, hepatic blood flow will approximate the aldosterone clearance rate. Since the blood level of circulating aldosterone is presumed to be the critical factor in its biologic activity, it is to be appreciated that the blood level will be determined by both the aldosterone secretion rate and the rate of hepatic inactivation. Thus, in clinical states characterized by reduced hepatic blood flow, such as congestive heart failure, an increased blood circulating aldosterone level can occur and result in sodium retention, even though the secretion rate of the hormone is within the normal range. Some of the patients currently being reported as having primary aldosteronism due to bilateral adrenocortical hyperplasia may in the future be classified as having secondary aldosteronism. Such a possibility would have to await the demonstration of an extraadrenal stimulus to aldosterone production other than ACTH and angiotensin. It is postulated that if such patients were to have secondary aldosteronism, they would have hypersecretion of aldosterone because of this unidentified stimulus. The excess aldosterone would then suppress plasma renin activity to a low level, thus mimicking primary aldosteronism.

"TERTIARY" ALDOSTERONISM

An increasing number of patients are being reported who do not fulfill precise criteria for either primary or secondary aldosteronism. This is analogous to the clinical evolution of our concepts of parathyroid disease, and one may predict that some of these patients will in time be classified as having "tertiary" aldosteronism. Such a diagnosis implies that in the initial phase of their disease, hyperaldosteronism occurs as an appropriate response to an extraadrenal stimulus but that at a later stage, hypersecretion of aldosterone becomes independent of the initiating stimulus. For example, a patient has been observed who had profound hypovolemia due to abnormal capillary permeability; after a decade of diuretic therapy he was found to have an aldosteronoma.

Adrenal Virilism

The adrenal virilizing syndromes result from excessive productions of adrenal androgens, such as dehydroepiandrosterone and Δ4-androstenedione which are converted to testosterone, the elevated testosterone levels account for most of the virilization. As in other states of adrenocortical hyperfunction, the syndrome may result from hyperplasia, adenoma, or carcinoma. It also may arise in a congenital form, termed *adrenogenital hyperplasia,* due to enzymatic deficits. The adrenal virilizing syndromes may be associated with secretions of greater or smaller amounts of other adrenal hormones and may, therefore, present as a "pure" syndrome of virilization or a "mixed" syndrome associated with excessive production of glucocorticoid and some of the characteristics of Cushing's syndrome. In *congenital* adrenal hyperplasia the virilizing syndrome may be associated with either excessive or decreased secretion of mineralocorticoid or decreased production of glucocorticoid.

The enzymatic composition of the adrenal as determined by heredity (and perhaps other factors as well) determines the relative rate of synthesis of hormones with glucocorticoid activity and of hormones with androgenic activity.

Since in man hydrocortisone is the principal adrenal steroid regulating ACTH elaboration, and since ACTH stimulates both hydrocortisone and adrenal androgen production, it stands to reason that an enzymatic interference with hydrocortisone synthesis may result in the enhanced secretion of adrenal androgens. In severe congenital virilizing hyperplasia, the adrenal output of hydrocortisone may be so compromised as to cause clinical evidence of glucocorticoid deficiency despite anatomic adrenal hyperplasia. Conversely, a high hydrocortisone output as the result of primary adrenal pathology (adenoma) may inhibit ACTH secretion and thus result in a low adrenal androgen output.

INCIDENCE. Congenital bilateral adrenocortical hyperplasia is by far the most common adrenal disorder of infancy and childhood. It has also been described later in life, predominantly in women. Its appearance in postpuberal men would obviously not be as clinically apparent; nevertheless, it has been reported. In its various forms, adrenogenital hyperplasia is thought to be related to a defective autosomal recessive gene. The most common form of significant "noncongenital" adrenal virilization is that seen with bilateral adrenocortical hyperplasia and is most frequently associated with various degrees of excessive production of glucocorticoid hormone and the clinical signs and symptoms of Cushing's syndrome.

CLINICAL SIGNS AND SYMPTOMS. In the adult female, regardless of etiology, the clinical signs and symptoms are those anticipated from excessive androgen production. These include hirsutism, acne, increased sebum production, temporal baldness, deepening of voice, increased muscle mass and strength, decreased breast size, atrophy of the uterus, amenorrhea, enlargement of the clitoris, increased heterosexual drive, and development of a male habitus. The clinical distinction between excessive hair growth (hirsutism) and virilization is useful. Virilization signifies that multiple signs of androgen excess are present in addition to hirsutism, and one of the more easily recognized of these signs is hypertrophy of the clitoris. Hirsutism in the absence of other signs of virilization is uncommon in these patients. The virilizing syndromes are difficult to document in the adult male, for obvious reasons.

The congenital form of adrenal hyperplasia is secondary to a defect in steroid enzymatic activity. To date, defects have been described in the C-21, C-18, C-17, and C-11 hydroxylase enzymes, as well as in the 3β-ol-dehydrogenase enzyme. Most of these defects produce virilization. However, the C-17 hydroxylase defect may actually produce sexual immaturity. These enzymatic deficits may occur singularly or in combination. Adrenal virilization at birth is almost always due to congenital adrenal hyperplasia; however, the disease may not become apparent until many years later, and sometimes only in adult life. In the most common form of congenital adrenal hyperplasia, that due to impairment of *C-21 hydroxylation,* there will be reduced conversion of 17-hydroxyprogesterone to 11-deoxycortisol and thus reduced formation of cortisol from 11-deoxycortisol (Fig. 92-2). In addition to cortisol deficiency, there may or may not be an associated reduction in aldosterone secretion as a result of impaired C-21 hydroxylation of progesterone to 11-deoxycorticosterone, a precursor of aldosterone. Thus, with congenital adrenal hyperplasia secondary to C-21 hydroxylase deficiency, adrenal insufficiency will be present with or without an associated salt-losing tendency due to aldosterone deficiency. It is probable that the C-21 hydroxylase enzymes, rather than being identical, are isoenzymes.

Therefore, the difference between the salt-losing variety and the non-salt-losing variety resides in whether the genetic abnormality involves one or both of these isoenzymes. As a result of the C-21 hydroxylase deficit, precursor products accumulate and are shunted into alternate pathways of metabolism, chiefly the androgen pathway, accounting for the production of excessive androgens. The accumulation of progesterone may also exaggerate any salt-losing tendency, since progesterone has an antialdosterone effect on renal tubular salt conservation. Since a cortisol deficiency exists, the adrenal glands become hyperplastic because of excessive ACTH stimulation.

With a *C-11 hydroxylase* deficiency a "hypertensive" variant of congenital adrenal hyperplasia develops with cortisol deficiency, since there is impaired conversion of 11-deoxycortisol to cortisol. Hypertension occurs because of the impaired conversion of 11-deoxycorticosterone to corticosterone, resulting in the accumulation of 11-deoxycorticosterone, a potent mineralocorticoid. Increased shunting again occurs into the androgen pathway.

Recently, two new enzymatic defects have been reported. One is a pure C-17 hydroxylase deficiency. The other is a combined C-17 hydroxylase and C-18 hydroxylase deficiency. In those patients with a C-17 hydroxylase deficiency alone, there is increased production of progesterone and its metabolite pregnanediol, with decreased production of cortisol and shunting into the mineralocorticoid pathway. This leads to the characteristic clinical picture of excess aldosterone secretion with low plasma renin activity. The effects of an increased aldosterone secretion are also noted, in that hypertension and hypokalemia are frequent. Because C-17 hydroxylation is also necessary for androgen formation, virilization has not been described with this defect. C-17 hydroxylation is also important in gonadal biosynthesis, and defects in gonadal biosynthetic pathways have been described. With the combination of C-17 and C-18 hydroxylase deficiency, a similar clinical picture is seen except that there is a decrease in aldosterone synthesis. Most, if not all, of these patients with combined deficiencies have gonadal enzymatic abnormalities and an exaggerated salt-losing tendency because of the accumulation of progesterone behind the block (Table 92-5).

Table 92-5. URINE EXCRETORY PRODUCTS IN CONGENITAL ADRENAL HYPERPLASIA

	17-KS	17-OH	THS	Pregnanetriol	Pregnanediol	THDOC	THB	Aldosterone
C-21 hydroxylase deficiency:								
Salt-losing.................	I	N–D	N–D	I	I	D	D	D
Non-salt-losing............	I	N–D	N–D	I	N–I	N–I	N–I	N–I
C-11 hydroxylase deficiency....	I	I	I	I	N–I	I	D	D
C-17 hydroxylase deficiency....	N–D	N–D	N–D	N–D	I	I	I	I
C-17 and C-18 hydroxylase deficiency..................	N–D	N–D	N–D	N–D	I	I	I	D
3β-ol-Dehydrogenase deficiency.	I	N–D	N–D	N–D	N–D	N–D	N–D	N–D

Note: THS, tetrahydro 11-deoxycortisol; THDOC, tetrahydro 11-deoxycorticosterone; THB, tetrahydrocorticosterone; I, increased; N, normal; D, decreased.

With *3β-ol-dehydrogenase* deficiency, there is impaired conversion of pregnenolone to progesterone, with the result that pathways to both cortisol and aldosterone are "blocked," with shunting then occurring into the adrenal androgen pathway via 17α-hydroxypregnenolone to dehydroepiandrosterone.

Clinically adrenal virilism due to congenital adrenal hyperplasia manifests itself as *pseudohermaphroditism* of females and *premature virilization* of males. The age of onset of virilization is most probably prenatal, after the fifth month of embryonic development. At birth there may be macrogenitosomia in the male infant and enlargement of the clitoris, partial or complete fusion of the labia, and sometimes a urogenital sinus in the female. If the labial fusion is nearly complete, the female infant will have external genitalia resembling a penis with hypospadias, changes consistent with female pseudohermaphroditism. Chromosomal sex can be determined by skin biopsy or examination of oral mucosal smears. Those infants with a salt-losing tendency often crave salt, and episodes of acute adrenal insufficiency are common. This salt-losing variant of congenital adrenal hyperplasia is often associated with vomiting, diarrhea, and hypotension. Hypertension is, of course, a key feature of the hypertensive variant of congenital adrenal hyperplasia, and its severity may dominate the clinical picture. In the *postnatal period* from infancy through adolescence, congenital adrenal hyperplasia will be associated with virilization in the female and isosexual precocity in the male. The excessive androgens produced will result in accelerated growth before fusion of epiphyses occurs, with skeletal growth exceeding the chronologic age. With epiphyseal closure, which is hastened by excessive androgens, growth stops but truncal development continues, giving the characteristic appearance of a child of short stature with a well-developed trunk. Incomplete variants of congenital adrenal hyperplasia sometimes occur in adult life, with virilization occurring in the female. It is not apparent why the adrenogenital syndrome should be dormant until adult life. One possibility may be that only a partial deficiency of an enzyme system such as C-11 hydroxylase was inherited and that the production of androgens in adult life may further inhibit the action of this enzyme, with consequent overproduction of adrenal androgens.

DIAGNOSIS. The diagnosis of adrenal virilism due to *congenital adrenal hyperplasia* should be considered in all infants exhibiting "failure to thrive," particularly those having episodes of acute adrenal insufficiency or having sustained hypertension. The diagnosis is further suggested by the finding of hypertrophy of the clitoris, fused labia, or urogenital sinus in the female and isosexual precocity in the male infant. In infants and children with a *C-21 hydroxylation block*, increased urine 17-ketosteroid excretion is typically associated with an increase in the excretion of pregnanetriol, which is a metabolite of 17α-hydroxyprogesterone. These children will show low urine 17-hydroxycorticoid excretion levels and elevated levels of plasma ACTH. Ketogenic steroid excretion will be elevated, since the depressed 17-hydroxycorticoid excretion is more than offset by increments in pregnanetriol excretion, which metabolite is included in the analysis. On testing with ACTH, the altered metabolic pathways

Table 92-6. LABORATORY EVALUATIONS AND TESTING OF ADRENOCORTICAL FUNCTION IN THEORETICAL CASES OF ADRENAL VIRILIZING SYNDROMES*

Syndromes	Plasma ACTH	Plasma cortisol	Cortisol secretory rate	Urine values	Control base line	Days of ACTH stimulation		Days of dexamethasone suppression, mg q 6h			
								0.5		2.0	
						1	2	1	2	1	2
Benign androgenic hyperplasia...............	N†	N	N	17-OH :	7	20	35	4	2	1	1
				17-KS :	17	35	50	10	5	4	3
Virilizing carcinoma..........	N–D‡	N–I	N–I§	17-OH :	12	24	35	10	5	4	4
				17-KS :	150	150	150	150	150	150	150
Virilizing adenoma...........	N	N	N	17-OH :	8	17	30	6	4	3	3
				17-KS :	150	160	170	150	140	130	120
Congenital adrenal hyperplasia...............	I	D	D	17-OH :	3	12	20	3	4	5	5
				17-KS :	40	60	90	25	20	15	10

* Clinical status charted vertically and representative values for steroid tests charted horizontally. 17-OH, 17-KS refer to 24-hr urine 17-hydroxycorticosteroid and 17-ketosteroid excretion. All laboratory values given in milligrams per day. Base-line urine 17-KS are either at upper limits of normal or slightly elevated in benign androgenic hyperplasia, whereas they are markedly elevated with virilizing carcinoma or adenoma. With ACTH stimulation, in benign androgenic hyperplasia, there is disproportionate rise in 17-KS; in virilizing tumors, there is no increment in 17-KS; in congenital adrenal hyperplasia, there is a rise in 17-KS (unless base-line 17-KS are very high). With dexamethasone suppression, in benign androgenic hyperplasia, there is complete suppression; in virilizing tumors, no suppression; in congenital adrenal hyperplasia, complete suppression.

† N, normal.

‡ D, decreased.

§ I, increased.

are exaggerated, with sharp rises occurring in 17-keto-steroid excretion and little or no rise in 17-hydroxycorticoid excretion (Table 92-6).

The diagnosis of a *salt-losing form* of congenital adrenal hyperplasia due to defects in both C-21 hydroxylase enzymes is suggested by episodes of acute adrenal insufficiency with hyponatremia, hyperkalemia, dehydration, and vomiting. These infants and children often "crave" salt and exhibit laboratory signs of concomitant deficits in both cortisol and aldosterone secretion.

With the *hypertensive form* of congenital adrenal hyperplasia due to impaired C-11 hydroxylation, the precursor 11-deoxycortisol will accumulate. As a result, both urine 17-keto- and 17-hydroxycorticoid excretion may be elevated, since 11-deoxycortisol would be included in the analysis of Porter-Silber chromogens. The diagnosis is secured by demonstrating increased amounts of tetrahydro-11-deoxycortisol in the urine with decreased amounts of tetrahydro metabolites of cortisol.

The finding of very high levels of urine dehydroepiandrosterone with low levels of pregnanetriol and of cortisol metabolites is characteristic of patients with congenital adrenal hyperplasia due to 3_β-ol-dehydrogenase deficiency. These patients also exhibit marked salt wasting.

The C-17 hydroxylase deficiency results in low levels of all cortisol precursors up to progesterone and its metabolite, pregnanediol, which are increased. Also, there is increased excretion of aldosterone and corticosterone. Patients with the combined C-17 and C-18 hydroxylase deficiencies have a similar excretion pattern except that corticosterone excretion is elevated while aldosterone secretion is decreased (see Table 92-5).

The adrenal virilizing syndrome in adults is most often due to noncongenital causes, namely, adrenal hyperplasia or tumor. *Benign androgenic adrenal hyperplasia* refers to those patients with hirsutism with normal or slightly elevated urine 17-ketosteroids and normal 17-hydroxycorticosteroids (Table 92-7). With ACTH stimulation there is a brisk rise in the urine 17-ketosteroids when compared to the 17-hydroxysteroids. Base-line 17 ketosteroids are easily suppressed on 2 mg daily of dexamethasone. An estimated one-third of patients with the polycystic ovarian syndrome and one-third of females with idiopathic hirsutism have findings consistent with benign androgenic adrenal hyperplasia. In adrenocortical hyperfunction of Cushing's syndrome, both urine 17-ketosteroid

Table 92-7. CAUSES OF HIRSUTISM IN FEMALES

1. Idiopathic
2. Familial
3. Ovarian
   a. Polycystic ovaries
   b. Tumor: arrhenoblastoma, hilus cell, adrenal rest
4. Adrenal
   a. Benign androgenic hyperplasia
   b. Congenital adrenal hyperplasia
   c. Virilizing carcinoma
   d. Virilizing adenoma
   e. Noncongenital adrenal hyperplasia (Cushing's)

and 17-hydroxysteroid base-line values will be elevated, the latter separating Cushing's syndrome from benign androgenic hyperplasia.

Adrenal adenomas and *carcinomas* may also cause a pure or mixed virilizing syndrome. Since adrenal androgens are weak androgens compared with gonadal androgens, adrenal virilization is characterized by large increments in urine 17-ketosteroids, often with less impressive clinical signs of virilism. Virilizing adrenal cortical adenomas are rare. They produce very high levels of urine 17-ketosteroids, often greater than 200 mg per day, and are associated with no rise or only a slight rise in urine 17-hydroxysteroids. They may or may not be sensitive to ACTH stimulation and likewise may or may not be sensitive to dexamethasone suppression. *Virilizing adrenal carcinomas* are the most common adrenal tumor causing virilization. They are also associated with very high urine 17-ketosteroid excretion and may have normal 17-hydroxycorticoid excretion or a moderate rise in 17-hydroxysteroid excretion. They characteristically show no increase in steroid excretion upon stimulation with ACTH and also characteristically fail to be suppressed with dexamethasone administration. These tumors are often associated with marked virilization of sudden onset. The very high ketosteroid excretion of both virilizing adenomas and carcinomas is made up in large part of the weak androgen dehydroepiandrosterone, which has approximately 5 percent of the androgenicity of testosterone. The clinical differentiation between virilizing adrenal adenoma and carcinoma is tenuous and cannot be made with certainty preoperatively.

DIFFERENTIAL DIAGNOSIS. The chief consideration in the differential diagnosis of adrenal virilization is virilization due to ovarian causes (Table 92-6). The low to slightly elevated urine 17-ketosteroid values associated with "idiopathic" hirsutism are in sharp contrast to the very high values with adrenal virilization. The hirsutism associated with polycystic ovaries is associated with other signs of virilization in 10 to 15 percent of patients. The association of amenorrhea with bilaterally large ovaries suggests polycystic ovaries, although some polycystic ovaries are of normal size. Urine 17-ketosteroid excretion in polycystic ovarian syndrome is either normal or slightly increased and characteristically fails to exhibit normal suppression with dexamethasone administration. In some of these patients a modest rise in urine 17-ketosteroids is shown on ACTH administration and purified FSH preparations cause a rise in the 11-deoxy-17-ketosteroid fraction with no or little change in the urine 11-oxy-17-ketosteroids. Hirsutism in these patients is thought to be due to defective ovarian aromatization whereby the androgen precursors, $\Delta 4$-androstenedione and testosterone, are not completely aromatized to the estrogens, estrone and estradiol, with the result that the blood level of the androgens will increase.

The most common *ovarian tumor* causing virilization is the arrhenoblastoma, but other ovarian tumors such as adrenal rest tumor, granulosa cell tumor, hilar cell tumors, and Brenner tumors have been associated with virilization. These masculinizing ovarian tumors may secrete testosterone as the major androgen, and the secretion of a few milligrams of testosterone, in view of its high androgenicity, can cause overt hirsutism. As a result, urine 17-ketosteroids are within the normal range in half these patients, and moderate elevations occur in the remainder. Urine base-line 17-ketosteroid excretion in excess of 40 mg per day is rare, with the exception of adrenal rest tumors. Urine 17-hydroxycorticoid excretion is normal. These ovarian tumors characteristically fail to be suppressed with dexamethasone; with the exception of adrenal rest tumors, they are largely independent of ACTH stimulation. Adrenal virilization due to *adrenal tumor* is characterized by high urine 17-ketosteroid excretion representing metabolites of weak adrenal androgens (such as dehydroepiandrosterone), whereas virilization due to ovarian tumors is characterized by normal or moderate elevation of urine 17-ketosteroids, since the ovaries are secreting the extremely potent androgen, testosterone. The principal difference between biosynthesis of androgens by the ovaries and by the adrenals is that tropic control is exerted principally by gonadotropins in the former and by ACTH in the latter case.

Direct inspection of the ovaries by culdoscopy is a valuable means of differentiating between ovarian and adrenal causes of hirsutism. Polycystic ovaries have a characteristic "oyster" appearance, and varying degrees of bilateral enlargement may be seen. Unilateral ovarian enlargement suggests ovarian tumor. If on culdoscopic examination "normal" ovaries are found, this, of course, strengthens the probability of an adrenal etiology for virilization. Suprarenal and ovarian tomography, with or without contrast studies, is helpful in delineating this problem.

With the finding of isosexual precocity in young boys, in addition to congenital adrenal hyperplasia, one must consider the possibility of hyperplasia of adrenal rest tissue occurring in the epididymis or testes. These *testicular adrenal rests* secrete high quantities of ketosteroids and operate under ACTH control. The aberrant adrenal rest tissue usually causes bilateral testicular enlargement, in contrast to the unilateral testicular enlargement with contralateral atrophy usually seen with true interstitial cell tumors. Further differentiation from interstitial testicular cell tumors is afforded by the insensitivity of the latter to ACTH stimulation.

TREATMENT. Treatment of adrenal virilism is dictated by the type of lesion suspected. The patients with *congenital adrenal hyperplasia* have the fundamental defect of cortisol deficiency with resultant excessive ACTH stimulation producing hyperplasia of the adrenal glands and causing additional "shunting" into the adrenal androgen pathway. Therapy in these patients consists of daily glucocorticoid (dexamethasone, prednisone, cortisone, etc.) administration to suppress pituitary ACTH secretion. In children, this not only suppresses urinary ketosteroid excretion but also ends virilization and the associated problems of hyperandrogenicity. The dosage schedule is governed by repetitive analysis of the urine 17-ketosteroids and by skeletal growth and maturation. Those children born with abnormalities of external genitalia may require surgical correction of labial fusion, urogenital sinus, etc. Response of these children to steroid therapy is gratifying in that normal growth and development occur and the menarche and onset of spermatogenesis occur at the appropriate age. Many females with this disorder have married and borne children. Steroid therapy is indicated throughout the life span of these patients.

Some infants and children with the associated defect of salt wasting require vigorous correction of salt deficits in conjunction with small doses of a potent mineral corticoid such as 9_α-fluorohydrocortisone.

In patients with adrenal virilization due to adrenal tumors, prompt surgical intervention with complete excision of the tumor is, of course, indicated. One cannot postpone surgical intervention in patients suspected of having virilizing adrenal adenomas, since such adenomas are practically indistinguishable from adrenal carcinomas, both clinically and biochemically. Preoperative localization of adrenal tumors is attempted with renal tomography or selective adrenal angiography. Since "pure" virilizing adrenal tumors do *not* cause contralateral adrenal atrophy, thorough inspection and exploration of both suprarenal areas is mandatory. If metastases have occurred, one may consider the use of antitumor drugs such as o,p'-DDD with or without local irradiation. o,p'-DDD in some patients has been associated with striking regression in peripheral metastases paralleled by a decrease in urine 17-ketosteroid and 17-hydroxycorticoid excretion; however, long-term survival is rare. In some patients given a trial of o,p'-DDD, regression of metastases is not seen but a fall in urine 17-hydroxycorticoids occurs. The explanation resides in the fact that o,p'-DDD can alter the extraadrenal metabolism of cortisol so as to decrease the metabolism and excretion of the usual metabolite, tetrahydrocortisol, causing the decrease in Porter-Silber chromogens; yet at the same time, there is increased conversion to and excretion of 6_β-hydroxycortisol, a steroid not included routinely as a Porter-Silber chromogen because of its poor solubility in the preliminary extracting solvent (dichloromethane).

Adrenal Feminization

Adrenal feminization is an exceedingly rare entity and, when present, is almost always due to adrenal tumor. These adrenal tumors will cause feminization in the male, with development of gynecomastia (often with breast tenderness), change in body habitus, testicular atrophy, feminizing hair changes, and loss of libido. They may occur in "pure" form, i.e., with normal levels of urine 17-ketosteroids, or in "mixed" form, with feminization despite high 17-ketosteroid excretion. They are always associated in the male with increased excretion of estrogen metabolites, such as estrone and estradiol. These adrenal tumors secrete increased amounts of androstenedione, which undergoes conversion, either in the adrenal or peripherally in the liver, into the estrogens, estrone and estradiol. Some patients have had elevated urine values for pregnanetriol, suggesting that 11_β-hydroxylation may be impaired.

The majority of adrenal tumors causing feminization are carcinomas. They are most common in the age group twenty-five to forty-five. These tumors are almost always unilateral and occur with equal frequency on either side. In rare instances they have occurred in an extraadrenal locus such as the testis. The feminizing adrenal carcinomas are large tumors (weighing several hundred grams) and often are easily palpable on physical examination, whereas feminizing adrenal adenomas are characteristically small tumors. Metastases occur most often to the liver and lungs. Feminizing adrenal tumors do not cause contralateral adrenal atrophy, which makes bilateral exploration mandatory if the initial adrenal explored is normal. Almost all cases of feminizing adrenal carcinoma are evident on suprarenal tomography studies. Patients with feminizing adrenal tumors usually have normal to moderately elevated 17-ketosteroid excretion levels. If the urine 17-ketosteroid excretion is greater than 100 mg per day, the diagnosis of a feminizing adrenal carcinoma is almost certain. Urine 17-hydroxycorticoid excretion is usually within the normal range or slightly elevated. Associated Cushing's syndrome is rare. ACTH stimulation causes little change in 17-ketosteroid excretion. The chemical determination of urine estrogen titers always demonstrates an elevated value. The elevated urine estrogen excretion level is principally due to increased estriol and also to increments in estradiol and estrone. Since the estrogens produced by adrenal feminizing tumors are conversion products from androgen precursors, the amount of estrogens elaborated will depend both on the amount of androgen precursors formed and on the efficiency of the androgen-to-estrogen conversion process.

Radiotherapy has not been helpful in treatment. Despite operative intervention, most patients with adrenal feminizing carcinoma die within 3 years of diagnosis. With successful operative removal of feminizing tumors, the urine estrogen titer falls; a failure of the titer to fall or a recurrence of elevated urine titers indicates functioning tumor tissue.

The diagnosis of adrenal feminization in the male is strongly suggested by the onset of gynecomastia associated with a flank mass. The additional finding of increased urine estrogen titers confirms the diagnosis. Gynecomastia may also be seen with *testicular tumors* (chorioepithelioma, Sertoli cell, seminoma, interstitial cell tumor) because of increased production by the tumors of chorionic gonadotropin, with an associated elaboration of estrogens by the testes. Adrenal feminization in the female is more difficult to detect, but it has been reported.

HYPOFUNCTION OF ADRENAL CORTEX

Adrenocortical hypofunction includes all conditions in which the secretion of adrenal steroid hormones falls below the requirements of the body. Various types of adrenal insufficiency are encountered and may be divided into two general categories: (1) those associated with primary inability of the adrenal to elaborate sufficient quantities of hormone and (2) those associated with a secondary failure due to a primary failure in the elaboration of ACTH (Table 92-8).

Table 92-8. CLASSIFICATION OF CAUSES OF ADRENAL INSUFFICIENCY

I. Primary adrenal insufficiency
   A. Anatomic destruction of gland (chronic and acute)
     1. Infection
     2. Invasion: metastatic, fungal, etc.
     3. Hemorrhage
     4. "Idiopathic" atrophy, autoimmune
     5. Surgical removal
   B. Metabolic failure in hormone production
     1. Virilizing hyperplasia, congenital (certain types)
     2. Enzyme inhibitors
       a. Specific: metyrapone
       b. Nonspecific: amphenone
     3. Cytotoxic agents: *o,p'*-DDD, aminoglutethamide
II. Secondary adrenal insufficiency
   A. Hypopituitarism due to pituitary disease
   B. Suppression of hypothalamic-pituitary axis
     1. Exogenous steroid
     2. Endogenous steroid from tumors after tumor removal
     3. Pharmacologic agents

Chronic Adrenocortical Deficiency

This disorder is also called Addison's disease or chronic glucocorticoid deficiency. Addison's classic description in 1855, namely, "general languor and debility, remarkable feebleness of the heart's action, irritability of the stomach, and a peculiar change of the color of the skin," summarizes the dominant clinical features of the disease. Advanced cases usually cause little difficulty in diagnosis, but recognition of the disease in its earlier phases may present a real challenge. The disease, when unrecognized and untreated, carries an almost uniformly poor and frequently fatal prognosis. Early diagnosis is important, since present-day therapy may provide complete correction of the metabolic derangement.

INCIDENCE. Primary adrenocortical insufficiency is relatively rare. It may occur at any age in life and affects both sexes with equal frequency. Because of increasing therapeutic use of exogenous steroids, secondary adrenal insufficiency is seen with increasing frequency.

CLINICAL SIGNS AND SYMPTOMS. Adrenocortical insufficiency is most frequently characterized by an insidious onset with slowly progressive fatigability, weakness, anorexia, nausea and vomiting, weight loss, cutaneous and mucosal pigmentation, hypotension, and occasionally hypoglycemia. These signs and symptoms compose the classic syndrome of Addison's disease; however, the spectrum may vary, depending on the duration and degree of adrenal hypofunction, from a complaint of mild chronic fatigue to the fulminating shock associated with acute massive destruction of the glands in the type of syndrome described by Waterhouse and Friderichsen. Table 92-9 lists the incidence of symptoms and signs noted in cases of Addison's disease.

Table 92-9. INCIDENCE OF SYMPTOMS AND SIGNS IN 125 CASES OF ADDISON'S DISEASE, PERCENT

Weakness	99	Hypotension (below	
Pigmentation of skin	98	110/70)	87
Pigmentation of mucous		Abdominal pain	34
membranes	82	Salt craving	22
Weight loss	97	Diarrhea	20
Anorexia, nausea, and		Constipation	19
vomiting	90	Syncope	16
		Vitiligo	9

Asthenia is the cardinal symptom of Addison's disease. Early it may be sporadic, usually most evident at times of stress; as adrenal function becomes more impaired, the weakness progresses until the patient is continuously fatigued, necessitating bed rest. Even the voice may fail, so that speech finally becomes listless and indistinct.

Pigmentation is the most striking sign of the disease. It commonly appears as a diffuse brown, tan, or bronze darkening of both exposed and unexposed points such as elbows or creases of the hand and in areas normally pigmented such as the areolas about the nipples. In many patients, bluish-black patches appear on the mucous membranes. Some patients develop dark freckles, and occasionally irregular areas of vitiligo may appear paradoxically. As an early sign, patients may notice an unusually persistent tanning following exposure to the sun.

Arterial hypotension is also extremely frequent, and in severe cases blood pressures may be in the range of 80/50 or less. Postural accentuation is common, and syncope may occur.

Abnormalities of gastrointestinal function are not only extremely frequent but often are the presenting complaint. Symptoms may vary from mild anorexia with weight loss to fulminating nausea, vomiting, diarrhea, and various types of ill-defined abdominal pain, which at times may be so severe as to be confused with an acute condition of the abdomen requiring surgery. Rarely a Landry's type of ascending paralysis with flaccid quadriplegia and mixed sensory defects accompanied by ascending muscular weakness has been noted in conjunction with a high serum potassium level. In these instances, the electrocardiogram may reflect the hyperkalemia. In addition, patients with adrenal insufficiency frequently have marked personality changes, usually in the form of excessive irritability and restlessness. Enhancement of the sensory modalities of taste, olfaction, and hearing is often present and is reversible with therapy.

LABORATORY FINDINGS. In the milder forms, sometimes called *partial* or *incomplete* Addison's disease, there may be no demonstrable abnormalities in any of the parameters measured in the routine laboratory, and even plasma and urinary steroid determinations may indicate values relatively low yet within normal range. However, definitive studies of adrenal stimulation with ACTH show abnormalities even in this stage of the disease. In the more advanced stages, levels of serum sodium, chloride, and bicarbonate are reduced while serum potassium is elevated. The hyponatremia is due to extravascular loss of sodium both into the urine (due to aldosterone defi-

ciency) and from the vascular compartment into tendon, cartilage, and bone. This extravascular sodium loss depletes extracellular fluid volume and accentuates hypotension. Elevated plasma levels of vasopressin and angiotensin have been reported, and these may be contributing factors to hyponatremia through impairment of free-water clearance. The hyperkalemia is due to a combination of factors including aldosterone deficiency, impaired glomerular filtration rate, and acidosis. These patients may show marked reduction in heart size, and in about one-quarter of the patients suprarenal calcification is seen but is unfortunately not pathognomonic. The electrocardiogram may show nonspecific changes and the electroencephalogram a striking reduction and slowing of the predominant activity. The basal metabolic rate may be low, but other thyroid indexes are usually normal. There may be a normocytic anemia, a relative lymphocytosis, and usually a moderate eosinophilia.

DIAGNOSIS. The diagnosis of adrenal insufficiency requires demonstration either directly or indirectly of decreased cortisol production by the adrenal in the basal state (*complete* adrenal insufficiency) or the unmasking of decreased cortisol production only in the stimulated state (*incomplete* adrenal insufficiency) (Table 92-10).

In all cases of *complete* adrenal insufficiency the cortosol secretory rate is markedly decreased, and this may be ascertained indirectly by the finding of low to absent 24-hr urine 17-hydroxycorticoids and urine 17-ketosteroids. Because of the contribution of the male gonads to urine 17-ketosteroids, basal excretory values in complete adrenal insufficiency will be higher for males than females. With incomplete adrenal insufficiency, urine steroid excretion values overlap into the normal range; because of this, a diagnosis of adrenal insufficiency cannot be made solely on the values of basal urine steroid determinations. Plasma cortisol values are from zero to the lower range of normal. Aldosterone secretion is very low judged by isotopic secretory rate determinations, as are aldosterone excretory values. In patients with primary adrenal insufficiency, plasma ACTH levels are elevated because of loss of the usual cortisol-hypothalamic feedback relationship, whereas in secondary adrenal insufficiency plasma ACTH values are low, a finding consistent with the absence of increased pigmentation in patients having the latter condition.

The specific and definitive diagnosis of adrenal insufficiency can be made only with the ACTH stimulation test to assay the adrenal reserve capacity for steroid production. In addition, ACTH testing is helpful in establishing whether adrenal insufficiency is primary or secondary. In patients undergoing ACTH testing as a diagnostic method for adrenal insufficiency, saline solution should be utilized as the diluent for the ACTH to be infused, since on occasion patients may experience an acute febrile episode when glucose is used. An additional advantage of using saline diluent is that a clinical estimate of adrenal responsiveness may be made by the presence or absence of weight gain during the infusion period, weight gain commonly occurring when adrenocortical function is intact. The potential dangers of ACTH testing in patients

Table 92-10. LABORATORY EVALUATION AND TESTING OF ADRENOCORTICAL FUNCTION IN ADRENAL INSUFFICIENCY*

	Plasma ACTH	Plasma cortisol	Cortisol secretory rate	Urine values	Control base line	Days of ACTH stimulation			
						1	2	3	4
Primary:									
Complete..................	I†	D‡	D	17-OH : 0–2	0–2	0–2	0–2	0–2	0–2
				17-KS : 3–6	3–6	3–6	3–6	3–6	3–6
Incomplete...............	I	D	D	17-OH : 1–4	5–10	6–12	5–10	5–10	5–10
				17-KS : 5–7	7–10	8–12	7–10	7–10	7–10
Secondary:									
Complete..................	D	D	D	17-OH : 0–2	2–6	5–10	7–14	10–20	
				17-KS : 0–6	4–8	5–8	6–10	8–15	
Incomplete...............	D	D	D	17-OH : 1–4	5–10	7–14	10–20	20–30	
				17-KS : 5–7	5–8	6–10	8–15	15–20	

* Clinical status charted vertically, and representative values for steroid tests charted horizontally. 17-OH, 17-KS refer to 24-hr urine 17-hydroxycorticosteroid and 17-ketosteroid excretion. All laboratory values given in milligrams per day. Note that plasma ACTH values are increased in primary forms and decreased in secondary forms. Note also that differentiation between primary and secondary forms on ACTH stimulation testing becomes greatest on day 3 and day 4 of stimulation.

† I, increased.

‡ D, decreased.

with limited adrenal reserves may be minimized by the prior **administration of 1 mg of a potent steroid such as dexamethasone.** The excretory products of 1 mg of this compound will not add appreciably to the amount of 17-hydroxycorticoids measured in the urine and therefore will not interfere with the test. For testing purposes, 40 units of ACTH is infused in the standard manner for 4 to 5 successive days, with daily urine collections tested for creatinine, 17-hydroxycorticoid, and 17-ketosteroid levels. Alternatively, a continuous 48-hr ACTH infusion may be used by giving 40 units of ACTH in 500 ml of 5 percent dextrose in normal saline solution every 12 hr for four consecutive 12-hr periods. In patients with complete primary adrenal insufficiency, ACTH stimulation by either method will cause a rise in steroid excretion of less than 2 mg per day.

In *incomplete* adrenal insufficiency, ACTH testing carried out by either method will result in subnormal increments in urinary 17-hydroxycorticoids. A variant of this response is sometimes seen in which small increments in steroid excretion occur on the first 3 days of the 5-day infusion test, while on the last 2 days, there is an actual decline in the level of steroids. Alternately, the last 12 hr of the continuous 48-hr infusion will show a decline in 17-hydroxycorticoid excretion. These results suggest that the limited adrenal tissue has been maximally stimulated and has insufficient steroid reserve capacity. In patients with adrenal insufficiency secondary to *anterior pituitary hypofunction*, a "staircase" response in steroid excretion is seen on successive days of ACTH stimulation, signifying that the adrenal can respond to exogenous ACTH and that the deficit must reside in the failure to produce and/or release endogenous ACTH.

Patients receiving long-term steroid therapy, despite physical findings of Cushing's syndrome, develop adrenal insufficiency both because of prolonged suppression of the hypothalamic corticotropin-releasing center and because of actual adrenal atrophy. Adrenal atrophy results from the loss of endogenous ACTH stimulation, which stimulus is prerequisite for maintaining normal adrenal size. Thus, these patients acquire two deficits, a loss of adrenal responsiveness to ACTH and a failure of pituitary ACTH release. These patients are characterized by low blood cortisol and ACTH levels, low base-line steroid excretion, and abnormal ACTH and metyrapone test results. On testing these patients with ACTH, one looks for the "staircase" response, with successive daily increments in steroid excretion; however, *prolonged ACTH testing* may be needed to elicit such a response. The urine steroid pattern, when adrenal reactivation does occur, often reveals increments in 17-hydroxycorticoids without parallel increments in 17-ketosteroids. Practically all patients with steroid-induced adrenal insufficiency will eventually respond to ACTH testing, but individual response time is most variable, ranging from days to months. Once such patients are shown to have reacquired adrenal sensitivity to exogenous ACTH, their ability to release endogenous pituitary ACTH must be determined. The standard metyrapone test is utilized for this purpose. For a valid metyrapone test, it must be previously documented that the patient's adrenal glands are sensitive to ACTH, since the metyrapone test response depends on adrenal responsiveness to released ACTH. For this reason the test is *contraindicated* in patients with suspected or proved adrenal insufficiency. In patients with steroid-induced adrenal insufficiency, abnormal (low) metyrapone tests usually continue for several months after the adrenal glands have regained responsiveness to ACTH. In interpreting the metyrapone test it is useful to consider it as an endogenous ACTH stimulation test and compare the peak urine 17-hydroxycorticoid excretion with the maximal values previously obtained with exogenous ACTH stimulation.

Plasma ACTH levels help distinguish between primary

and secondary adrenal insufficiency, since they are elevated in the former and decreased to absent in the latter.

Indirect tests of adrenocortical function include (1) a delay in water excretion following an acute water load; (2) defective renal conservation of sodium when a low sodium, high potassium diet is imposed; (3) a tendency toward hypoglycemia during fasting and hypoglycemic unresponsiveness following the intravenous administration of insulin. Since ACTH is available for direct evaluation of adrenocortical function, these procedures are *rarely* indicated; furthermore, in a patient with adrenocortical insufficiency, water intoxication, sodium deprivation, or hypoglycemia may all be life-threatening situations.

DIFFERENTIAL DIAGNOSIS. Since weakness and fatigue are such common complaints, clinical diagnosis of early adrenocortical insufficiency is frequently difficult (Table 92-9). However, mild gastrointestinal distress with weight loss, anorexia, and a suggestion of increased pigmentation make mandatory ACTH stimulation testing to rule out adrenal insufficiency, particularly before steroid treatment is begun. Weight loss is useful in evaluating the significance of weakness and malaise. Racial pigmentation in Negroes, Orientals, Indians, Spanish Americans, and Latins and hyperpigmentation in other diseases represent a major problem. These diseases include hemochromatosis, acanthosis nigricans, porphyria, thyrotoxicosis, polyostotic fibrous dysplasia, chronic metal poisoning (bismuth, lead, arsenic, silver), chronic malnutrition (starvation, anorexia nervosa, sprue syndrome, pellagra), progressive malignancy, chronic anemia, salt-losing nephritis with hypotension, renal tubular acidosis, scleroderma, excess nicotinic acid, and hepatic cirrhosis. In most cases, differentiation from Addison's disease is not difficult, but when doubt exists, ACTH administration ordinarily provides clear-cut differentiation.

ETIOLOGY AND PATHOGENESIS. Addison's disease results from progressive adrenocortical destruction, which must involve more than 75 percent of the glands before clinical signs of adrenal insufficiency appear. The adrenal is a frequent site for chronic infectious diseases of the granulomatous variety, predominately tuberculosis but also including fungal infections such as histoplasmosis, coccidioidomycosis, and cryptococcosis. In previous years, tuberculosis was found at postmortem examination in 70 to 90 percent of cases; however, the most frequent finding at present is *idiopathic* atrophy, and it has been suggested that an autoimmune mechanism may be responsible for this process. Rarely, other lesions are encountered, such as bilateral tumor metastases, amyloidosis, or sarcoidosis.

The possibility that some patients may have primary adrenal insufficiency on an *autoimmune basis* has been strengthened by the finding that one-half of patients with Addison's disease have circulating adrenal antibodies, tested by the indirect Coons method. These antibodies appear species-specific but lack organ specificity. Certain of these patients also have additional circulating antibodies to thyroid or parathyroid tissue, a finding of inter-

est because of the increased incidence of hypothyroidism and hypoparathyroidism in Addison's disease.

ADDISON'S DISEASE ASSOCIATED WITH OTHER ENDOCRINE DYSFUNCTIONS. In 1926, Schmidt described two patients with nontuberculous Addison's disease and chronic lymphocytic thyroiditis. Subsequent reports have documented association of thyroid insufficiency and Addison's disease, and the possibility of a common autoimmune process has been raised as the etiologic factor responsible for *Schmidt's syndrome*. More than 20 patients have been described with concomitant parathyroid and adrenal insufficiency. In most of these patients, autoantibodies have been discovered, raising the possibility that these two diseases may be related to a common event. Diabetes mellitus has now been reported as being associated with Addison's disease in more than 100 cases. Again, what role genetic predisposition and/or autoimmunity may play in the occurrence of these two diseases in the same individual is unknown. Rarely, the combination of Addison's disease, myxedema, and diabetes mellitus has been described. Between 3 and 4 percent of patients with Addison's disease have coexistent hyperthyroidism. The presence of both disorders in the same individual poses a difficult diagnostic problem, since many of the clinical manifestations are similar. Furthermore, the hyperthyroid state may change a subclinical insufficiency to complete adrenal insufficiency, because of the effect, mentioned above, of thyroid hormone on cortisol metabolism.

Further study of patients with combined endocrine dysfunction may prove valuable in revealing the cause of spontaneous adrenal destruction.

TREATMENT. All patients with Addison's disease should receive specific hormone replacement therapy. Like diabetics, these patients require careful and persistent education in regard to their disease. Since the adrenal gland elaborates three general classes of hormone, of which two, glucocorticoids and mineralocorticoids, are of primary clinical importance, replacement therapy should correct both deficiencies. Cortisone (or hydrocortisone) is the mainstay of treatment; however, its mineralocorticoid effect, when it is given in sufficient dosage to replace the endogenous hydrocortisone deficiency, is inadequate for complete electrolyte balance; therefore, the patient usually requires other supplementary hormone. Cortisone dosage varies from 12.5 to 50 mg daily, with the majority of patients taking 25 to 37.5 mg in divided doses. Because of its direct local effect on gastric mucosa, patients are advised to take their cortisone with meals or, if this is impractical, with milk or an antacid preparation. In addition, the larger proportion of the dose (25 mg) is taken in the morning and the remainder (12.5 mg) in the late afternoon, to simulate somewhat the normal diurnal adrenal rhythm. Some patients may exhibit insomnia, irritability, mental excitement, and even frank psychosis soon after initiation of therapy; in these the dosage should obviously be reduced. Other indications for maintaining the patient on smaller amounts are hypertension, diabetes, or active tuberculosis.

Since, as mentioned earlier, this amount of cortisone or

hydrocortisone fails to replace the mineralocorticoid component of the adrenal gland, supplementary hormone is usually needed. The simplest means is daily oral administration of 0.1 to 0.2 mg of 9_α-fluorohydrocortisone. If parenteral administration is indicated, 2.0 to 5.0 mg deoxycorticosterone acetate in oil may be given every day intramuscularly. An alternative method of therapy is an injection of 25 to 50 mg deoxycorticosterone trimethylacetate in oil intramuscularly every 3 to 4 weeks, but as with the previous use of subcutaneous implantation of pellets of deoxycorticosterone which lasted for 8 to 10 months, most patients prefer the simplicity of daily oral administration of the 9_α-fluorohydrocortisone.

Complications of cortisone therapy, with the exception of peptic disease, particularly ulcer or gastritis, are *extremely rare* in the dosage used in the treatment of Addison's disease. However, overtreatment with deoxycorticosterone preparations or 9_α-fluorohydrocortisone is more frequent and may present as edema, hypertension, cardiac enlargement, or even congestive failure due to sodium retention. Overtreatment may also present as weakness, progressing to total paralysis, due to hypokalemia. In the management of patients with Addison's disease, regular measurements of body weight, serum potassium, heart size, and blood pressure, and serial electrocardiograms are useful.

All patients with adrenal insufficiency, including bilaterally adrenalectomized patients, should carry medical identification, should be educated and instructed in the parenteral self-administration of steroids, and should be registered with a national medical alerting system.

SPECIAL THERAPEUTIC PROBLEMS. During periods of intercurrent illness, the dose of cortisone or hydrocortisone should be increased to levels of 75 to 150 mg per day. When oral administration is not possible, parenteral routes should be employed. Likewise, before surgery or dental extractions, excess steroid should be administered. For a representative program of steroid therapy for an Addisonian patient or an adrenalectomized patient undergoing a major operation, see Table 92-11. The patients should all be advised of these facts and should carry an identification card bearing detailed instructions for the administration of steroid in case of acute illness or injury. Patients should also be advised to increase the dose of 9_α-fluorohydrocortisone and add excess salt to their otherwise normal diet during periods of excessive exercise with sweating, during extremely hot weather, or during periods of gastrointestinal upsets. In spite of animal studies demonstrating an increased susceptibility to tubercular spread associated with excess steroid administration, patients with Addison's disease and tuberculosis may be maintained safely on 12.5 to 25 mg cortisone daily.

COURSE AND PROGNOSIS. Untreated Addison's disease characteristically runs a chronic and relentless course. In some patients, its advance is relatively slow, but in all patients the condition may rapidly deteriorate into adrenal crisis. With treatment, the prognosis of the disease is extremely favorable. In fact, some of the degenerative vascular problems such as hypertension or congestive failure are more easily handled in an Addisonian patient than in one with intact adrenal glands.

Acute Adrenocortical Insufficiency

Acute adrenocortical insufficiency may result from several processes. One of these, usually termed *adrenal crisis,* is a rapid and overwhelming intensification of chronic adrenal insufficiency. Another process involves an acute hemorrhagic destruction of both adrenal glands, usually associated with an overwhelming septicemia. Adrenal hemorrhage due to excessive anticoagulants is being seen with increasing frequency. A third, and probably the most

Table 92-11. STEROID THERAPY SCHEDULE FOR ADDISONIAN PATIENT UNDERGOING A MAJOR OPERATION*

	Cortisone acetate (intramuscularly)		Cortisone acetate (orally)				Fluorohydro-cortisone (orally)	Hydro-cortisone infusion
	7 A.M.	7 P.M.	8 A.M.	12 M.	4 P.M.	8 P.M.	8 A.M.	Continuous
Routine daily medication.....	...	...	25	...	12.5	...	0.1	
Day before operation........	...	50	25	...	12.5	...	0.1	
Day of operation............	100	50	...	...	...	...	...	200
Postoperative day 1..........	50	50	...	...	...	...	...	100–150
" 2..........	50	50	...	...	...	...	...	50–100
" 3..........	50	50	25	...	...	25	...	
" 4..........	50	...	25	25	25	...	0.1	
" 5..........	...	...	25	25	25	25	0.1	
" 6..........	...	...	25	25	25	...	0.2	
" 7..........	...	...	25	12.5	25	...	0.2	
" 8..........	...	...	25	12.5	25	...	0.2	
" 9–13.......	...	...	25	12.5	12.5	...	0.1	
" 14........	...	...	25	12.5	...	...	0.1	

* All steroid doses are given in milligrams.

frequent, cause of acute insufficiency results from the rapid withdrawal of steroids from patients with adrenal atrophy secondary to chronic steroid administration.

Adrenal Crisis

The long-term survival of patients with Addison's disease largely depends upon prevention and treatment of adrenal crisis. Consequently, the occurrence of infection, trauma (including surgery), gastrointestinal upsets, or other forms of stress requires an immediate increase in hormone. In previously untreated patients, preexisting symptoms are intensified. Nausea, vomiting, and abdominal pain may become intractable. Fever is frequently severe but may be absent. Lethargy deepens into somnolence, and the blood pressure and pulse fail as hypovolemic vascular shock ensues. In contrast, patients previously maintained on hormone therapy may not exhibit severe dehydration or hypotension until preterminally, at which time there is an extremely rapid decline.

Treatment is primarily directed toward the rapid elevation of circulating adrenocortical hormone, in addition to the replacement of the sodium and water deficit. Hence, an intravenous infusion of 1,000 ml 5 percent glucose in normal saline solution containing 100 to 200 mg of any of several soluble hydrocortisone preparations is begun rapidly, with the first 250 ml infused in the first ½ to 1 hr and the remainder over the ensuing 4 to 8 hr. If the condition is extreme, immediate intravenous infusion of 100 mg hydrocortisone in the first few minutes is suggested, followed by a rapid infusion as described above. Epinephrine, 0.2 mg intravenously, may also be indicated. In any case, it is also advisable to administer 100 mg cortisone acetate intramuscularly in case the infusion becomes infiltrated or inadvertently stopped. If the crisis was preceded by prolonged nausea, vomiting, and dehydration, several liters of saline replacement is indicated. With large doses of steroid, as, for example, 200 mg cortisone or hydrocortisone, the patient receives a maximal mineralocorticoid effect, and supplementary deoxycorticosterone is superfluous. After the initial infusion, depending on the patient's condition, a second similar infusion may be given; if there has been marked improvement, the patient may be offered oral fluids and be given 50 mg cortisone acetate intramuscularly every 12 hr until gastrointestinal absorption is guaranteed, at which time the steroid can be given orally. Steroid dosage is then tapered over the next few days to maintenance levels, with reinstitution of supplementary mineralocorticoid if needed.

Adrenal Hemorrhage

Adrenal hemorrhage (adrenal apoplexy) is usually associated with overwhelming septicemia (Waterhouse-Friderichsen syndrome); however, it may also occur in the absence of sepsis. Occasionally, massive bilateral adrenal hemorrhage results from birth trauma. The infant may either be stillborn or die soon after birth of shock and hyperpyrexia. Adrenal hemorrhage also occurs in patients with advanced hypertension and arteriosclerosis, during pregnancy, following idiopathic adrenal vein thrombosis, during convulsions in epilepsy or during electroconvulsive therapy, with excessive anticoagulant therapy, and after trauma or surgery. Pain in the flank and epigastrium is frequent, and if the hemorrhagic process ruptures into the abdomen, signs of peritoneal inflammation are present.

The adrenal hemorrhage associated with septicemia is most frequent with meningococcemia but is also seen with overwhelming infections due to pneumococcus, staphylococcus, or *Hemophilus influenzae*. The onset is often explosive, with a shaking chill, violent headache, vertigo, vomiting, and prostration. A petechial rash appears on the skin and mucous membranes and progresses rapidly to a confluent, extensive purpura. Large areas of skin may become grossly hemorrhagic. Body temperature may be subnormal but is usually markedly elevated. Circulatory collapse rapidly ensues, and death may occur within 6 to 48 hr. Specific diagnosis requires immediate identification of the organism. Frequently, the septicemia is so massive that organisms may be seen in peripheral blood smears or petechial scrapings. Time is not sufficient for determination of adrenal function; however, a plasma sample for later determination of 17-hydroxysteroid level may be of academic interest.

Treatment must be immediate and intensive. Control of the infection by vigorous administration of parenteral, preferably intravenous, antibiotics is indicated in addition to the steroid schedule delineated for adrenal crisis. Intravenous norepinephrine (4 to 8 mg per liter) may also be required to maintain vascular tone. Since shock may also be associated with massive septicemia without adrenal hemorrhage, one is never completely certain whether adrenal insufficiency is contributing to the patient's decompensation; however, the authors think that because of the increasing frequency of survival of patients treated with steroid, some degree of adrenal insufficiency, whether relative or absolute, is present and that steroid treatment is therefore indicated in all patients in whom fulminating septicemia is associated with shock.

Adrenal Insufficiency Due to Metabolic Failure in Hormone Production

This group of patients includes those with congenital adrenal hyperplasia and those receiving one of several pharmacologic agents which are capable of inhibiting hormone synthesis in the gland. These include Amphenone, which appears to inhibit synthesis of all hormones early in the sequence of reactions from cholesterol and concomitantly results in hypertrophy of the gland; and various derivatives of diphenyl dichloroethane, of which the o,p-dichloro-derivative is the most active [o,p'-DDD (Perthane)] and causes atrophy and even necrosis of adrenocortical tissue. Three other compounds specifically block an enzymatic step in the formation of cortisol: 2-methyl-1,2-bis-(3-pyridyl)-1-propanone (metyrapone, SU-4885) and p-aminophenyl-2-phenylethylamine selectively inhibit 11-hydroxylation of the steroid nucleus, and aminoglutethamide appears to block the conversion of cholesterol to pregnanelone. Furthermore, thyroid hormone, increases the conversion of cortisol to the biologically inactive cortisone and thereby can produce a state of relative adrenal insufficiency.

Hypoaldosteronism

Patients with *isolated* aldosterone deficiency are rare. Such a deficiency accompanied by normal cortisol production has been reported as a congenital biosynthetic defect; postoperatively following removal of aldosteronoma; during protracted heparin or heparinoid administration; in pretectal disease of the nervous system; in severe postural hypotension; and in association with complete heart block.

In severe cases urine sodium wastage is present on a normal salt intake, whereas in milder forms excessive urine sodium losses occur only during salt restriction. The patients always develop hyponatremia and hyperkalemia, the latter often to a severe degree.

A biosynthetic defect has been noted in some patients who are unable to transform the angular C-18 methyl group of corticosterone to the C-18 aldehyde grouping of aldosterone. This C-18 transformation requires first the formation of 18-hydroxycorticosterone from corticosterone, and then, secondly, dehydrogenation of the C-18 hydroxyl group to form the characteristic C-18 aldehyde group of aldosterone. These patients will manifest low to absent aldosterone secretion and excretion in association with elevated secretion and excretion values for corticosterone and 18-hydroxycorticosterone.

The feature common to all patients with hypoaldosteronism has been their inability to *increase* aldosterone secretion appropriately during severe salt restriction. An additional feature has been the reversal of the signs of salt wasting, hyponatremia and hyperkalemia, with the administration of potent mineralocorticoids. For practical purposes the oral administration of 9_α-fluorohydrocortisone in a dose of 0.1 to 0.3 mg daily restores electrolyte balance.

NONSPECIFIC USE OF ACTH AND ADRENAL STEROIDS IN CLINICAL PRACTICE

The widespread application of ACTH and adrenal steroid therapy in many branches of medicine and surgery emphasizes the need for a thorough understanding of the metabolic effects of these agents if clinical use is to be most effective and if undesirable side reactions are to be minimized. Before instituting adrenal hormone therapy, a physician should weigh carefully the gains that can reasonably be expected versus the potentially undesirable metabolic actions of the particular hormone. Accurate appraisal will require familiarity with the reports of others in similar instances, a critical evaluation of the statistical significance of such reports, as well as a clear understanding of the chemical, physiologic, and psychologic changes

Table 92-12. ADRENAL PREPARATIONS

Commonly used name	Other names	Estimated potencies*	
		Glucocorticoid	Mineralocorticoid
Hydrocortisone......................	Cortisol, hydrocortone Compound F, 17-hydroxycorticosterone PREGN-4-ene-11$_\beta$,17$_\alpha$,21-triol-3,20-dione	1	1
Cortisone...........................	Cortone, compound E 11-Dehydro-17-hydroxycorticosterone PREGN-4-ene-17$_\alpha$,21-diol-3,11,20-trione	0.8	0.8
DOC...............................	Percorten, cortexone, 11-deoxycorticosterone PREGN-4-ene-21-ol-3,20-dione	0	15
Aldosterone........................	Electrocortin PREGN-4-ene-11$_\beta$, 21-diol-18-ol-3,20-dione	0.3	400
Prednisolone........................	Meticortelone, Δ1-hydrocortisone PREGN-1,4-diene-11$_\beta$,17$_\alpha$,21-triol-3,20-dione	4	0.25
Prednisone.........................	Meticorten,Δ1-cortisone PREGN-1,4-diene-17$_\alpha$,21-diol-3,11,20-trione	4	0.25
Methyl prednisolone.................	Medrol, 6-methyl-Δ1-hydrocortisone	5	±
Triamcinolone......................	Aristocort, Kenacort 16$_\alpha$-Hydroxy-9$_\alpha$-fluoro-Δ1-hydrocortisone	5	±
Dexamethasone.....................	Decadron, Hexadrol 16$_\alpha$-Methyl-9$_\alpha$-fluoro-Δ1-hydrocortisone	30–40	±
Fluorohydrocortisone................	Florinef, Fluoro-F 9$_\alpha$-Fluorohydrocortisone	10	300

* Relative milligram comparisons to cortisol, setting the glucocorticoid and mineralocorticoid properties of cortisol as 1. Sodium retention insignificant in usual doses employed of methyl prednisolone, triamcinolone, and dexamethasone.

Table 92-13. CONSIDERATIONS PRIOR TO THE USE
OF CORTICOSTEROIDS AS PHARMACOLOGIC AGENTS

1. How serious is the underlying disorder?
2. How long will therapy be required?
3. What is the anticipated effective dose range?
    a. To ameliorate symptoms?
    b. To suppress effectively the signs and symptoms of the disorder?
4. Is the patient predisposed to any of the known hazards of steroid therapy by virtue of having:
    a. Hypertension or cardiovascular disease?
    b. Peptic ulcer, gastritis, or esophagitis?
    c. Osteoporosis?
    d. Diabetes mellitus?
    e. Tuberculosis or other infections?
    f. Psychologic difficulties?
5. Which adrenal preparation is preferable?
    a. Choice of steroid preparation?
    b. ACTH versus steroids?
    c. Steroids by mouth versus steroids by injection?
6. Alternate day therapy.
7. Supplementary adjuvants employed to minimize metabolic disabilities.
8. A schedule for withdrawing corticosteroids.
9. Summary.

that hormone preparations of this type are known to induce (Table 92-12).

Perhaps an approach to the problem presented by a particular patient may be facilitated by reviewing the specific considerations outlined in Table 92-13.

How Serious Is the Underlying Disorder?

The use of any nonspecific or "symptomatic" pharmacologic agent must be weighed against the seriousness of the underlying disorder. Each pharmacologic agent has a "price tag," which must be evaluated carefully before a therapeutic program is begun. With the antibiotic agents this price tag may consist of the possibility of inducing drug-sensitivity reactions or the development of antibiotic-resistant strains of pathogenic organisms; with the agents employed for hypertensive cardiovascular disease the price tag may consist of disturbing side effects referable to the autonomic nervous system. With the corticosteroids, effective therapy may be purchased at the risk of inducing undesirable side reactions such as peptic ulceration, osteoporosis, or psychologic abnormalities. Clearly, in a patient whose life is threatened by unexplained shock or in whom other measures have failed to modify the course of disseminated lupus erythematosus, the physician need not hesitate to employ massive steroid therapy. On the other hand, one should exercise restraint in administering suppressive steroid therapy to a patient with early rheumatoid arthritis who as yet has not received the possible benefits of physiotherapy and a well-organized program of general medical care.

How Long Will Therapy Be Required?

The problems which arise in connection with evaluating the seriousness of the underlying disorder naturally involve the expected or anticipated duration of therapy. Thus the use of intravenous hydrocortisone for 24 to 48 hr in the treatment of severe status asthmaticus or acute serum sickness or a drug reaction does not present the same problem as the treatment of chronic, lifelong asthma or psoriasis. In general, contraindications to steroids for severe, short-lived disorders will be few, whereas in suppressive therapy for chronic, persistent disorders one must envisage the serious problem presented by Cushing's syndrome, which results from prolonged ingestion of exogenous glucocorticoid.

What Is the Anticipated Effective Dose Range?

Hormone therapy may be employed in a relatively low dosage schedule calculated to achieve clinical improvement but not necessarily complete suppression of all signs and symptoms of the disorder. In the former case, 50 to 75 mg cortisone or hydrocortisone (or the equivalent amount of one of its derivatives) may be adequate to attain worthwhile clinical improvement, whereas 150 to 300 mg cortisone or hydrocortisone may be needed to suppress all evidences of activity of the disease. At the 50- to 75-mg dosage of cortisone or hydrocortisone, it might be feasible to embark on long-term therapy with minimal risk of serious complications resembling Cushing's syndrome, whereas at the 150-mg dosage level, relief of one disease may be attained only at the risk of inducing another (Cushing's syndrome). In general, doses of hydrocortisone or cortisone of 75 mg or less may be tolerated by most patients for prolonged periods of time with a minimum of underlying metabolic disabilities, whereas doses of cortisone or hydrocortisone of 100 mg or more will usually be associated with progressive metabolic aberrations. Dosage of cortisone or hydrocortisone in the range of 25 to 50 mg daily can, in all probability, be tolerated by most patients for life.

Is the Patient Predisposed to Any of the Known Hazards of Steroid Therapy by Virtue of Having Any of the Following Conditions?

HYPERTENSION OR CARDIOVASCULAR DISEASE. In general, the sodium-retaining propensity of most adrenal steroid preparations requires that caution be used when they are given to patients with preexisting hypertension or cardiovascular or renal disease. The availability of preparations in which sodium-retaining activity is minimal (triamcinolone and dexamethasone), restriction of dietary sodium intake, and the use of resins, diuretic agents, and particularly supplementary potassium salts will permit the safe use of steroid therapy where important indications exist. Of course, in congestive failure or pericardial effusion associated with acute rheumatic activity or in patients with nephrotic edema, steroid hormone preparations may act as effective diuretic agents.

For all patients in whom prolonged steroid therapy is contemplated cardiovascular-renal status should be carefully evaluated, with a chest film for *heart size* and an electrocardiogram included.

PEPTIC ULCER, GASTRIC HYPERSECRETION, OR ESOPHAGITIS. Patients with a history of gastric hypersecretion or peptic ulcer are likely to experience aggravation of their symptoms while receiving adrenal hormone therapy. It is not known for certain whether aggravation of peptic ulceration and complicating gastrointestinal hemorrhage reflect the increased gastric secretory activity so frequently associated with adrenal hormone therapy or whether the nitrogen-depleting effect of these hormones accelerates the process of ulceration and perforation. Antacid therapy and an ulcer diet are useful precautions in susceptible patients. *The development of anemia in a patient on ACTH or cortisone therapy should immediately suggest gastrointestinal bleeding,* and patients should be cautioned to note black or tarry stools. A clear-cut history of peptic ulcer is a contraindication to ACTH and cortisone therapy unless extreme precautions are taken.

OSTEOPOROSIS. All patients on prolonged cortisone-like steroid therapy are likely to develop some degree of osteoporosis. Obviously a considerable change in bone structure must occur before it is radiologically demonstrable. For this reason patients should have standard films of the spine and pelvis in order to establish the status of the bony framework before therapy and for comparative purposes later. Postmenopausal women and men and women of advanced age will be predisposed to the earlier development of serious changes of this type. The skin also participates in the depletion of body protein, becoming thin and atrophic and easily bruisable. It is possible that ACTH may cause less osteoporosis for a given level of steroid therapy because of a concomitant increase in adrenal androgen secretion. This possible advantage of ACTH over crystalline steroids is offset by the difficulty with which an exact pharmacologic dosage of endogenous steroid is maintained with the tropic hormone. Since corticosteroids, in general, exert an anti-vitamin-D-like action, all patients on adrenal steroids should receive a generous supplement of vitamin D, i.e., 1,500 IU daily. Supplementary calcium therapy in the form of calcium lactate, 1 Gm three times daily, and estrogen and androgen therapy should be considered in those patients known to be susceptible to the catabolic action of adrenal steroids. Sodium fluoride therapy (3 mg daily) may also be beneficial. Of course, any degree of osteoporosis a priori would constitute evidence against the desirability of prolonged high-dosage adrenal hormone therapy.

DIABETES MELLITUS. Prolonged ACTH or cortisone-like steroid therapy may unmask latent diabetes mellitus and aggravate preexisting disease. For this reason a careful history is important to exclude familial incidence of diabetes, as well as an examination of the blood and urine for excess glucose levels. It is more valuable to carry out these examinations following a test load of carbohydrate. A convenient method consists in measuring blood and urinary glucose 2 to 3 hr after the ingestion of a breakfast containing approximately 100 Gm carbohydrate (see Chap. 94). Obviously the presence of frank diabetes mellitus or the demonstration of impaired glucose tolerance will affect the physician's decision to institute adrenal hormone therapy. However, if such therapy appears necessary or desirable in the presence of latent diabetes, the judicious use of supplementary insulin should be seriously considered. The insulin requirement of known diabetics will usually need to be increased with ACTH or cortisone-like therapy except in those rare instances in which the diabetic patient is suffering from some degree of insulin-protein reaction in which the anti-inflammatory or antiallergic effect of cortisone enhances the metabolic effectiveness of the insulin sufficiently to balance off the diabetogenic action of the former.

TUBERCULOSIS OR OTHER INFECTIONS. Before prolonged steroid therapy is seriously considered, it is imperative to exclude tuberculosis and other infections. Continued steroid therapy, without a specific antibiotic agent, can lead to serious spread of infection. A chest film is essential before prolonged steroid therapy is begun, and the desirability of cultures from the nose and throat and of the urine and feces, if symptoms point to any disturbances, is evident.

PSYCHOLOGIC DIFFICULTIES. From time to time steroid therapy may be complicated by severe psychologic disturbances, and, of course, less-severe abnormalities are relatively frequent. In general, serious psychlgic disturbances are more closely related to the patient's personality structure than to the actual dose of hormone, although, as might be anticipated, larger doses of hormone will be associated with more frequent serious reactions. At present there is no reliable method of determining beforehand a patient's psychologic reaction to steroid therapy. Patients with known psychologic difficulties undoubtedly experience more frequent and more severe disturbances. Further difficulty arises because previous tolerance of steroids does not necessarily ensure immunity from subsequent courses of therapy, and untoward psychologic reactions on one occasion do not invariably mean that the patient will respond unfavorably to a second course of treatment. This is one area in which the physician must follow his patient carefully during the early period of steroid therapy and one in which he must take a responsible member of the patients' family into his confidence.

Consideration of the foregoing conditions will produce important data on which the physician's ultimate decision for or against hormone therapy will rest.

Which Adrenal Preparation Is Preferable?

CHOICE OF STEROID PREPARATION. Four considerations need to be taken into account in deciding which steroid preparation to use. The first of these is the biologic half-life of the particular compound. The rationale behind every-other-day therapy is to decrease the metabolic effects of the steroids for a significant amount of time over the 2-day period, yet at the same time to produce pharmacologic suppression of sufficient duration to maintain the disease in remission. Too long a half-life would defeat the first purpose, and too short a half-life would defeat the second. In general, the more potent the steroid, the longer its biologic half-life tends to be. The second consideration is whether the mineralocorticoid effects of the steroid are important. The newer synthetic steroids have much less mineralocorticoid effect relative to their glucocorticoid effect than cortisol or cortisone (Table 92-12). This may be an important consideration in certain disease states. Thirdly, cortisone and prednisone, in contrast to the other glucocorticoids, have to be converted into their biologically active equivalents before any anti-inflammatory effects can occur. Finally, the cost of the medication needs to be considered seriously, particularly if chronic administration is to be undertaken. Per tablet, prednisone is the least expensive of all adrenal steroids. However, the physician should be aware that there are probably a number of steroid preparations whose formulation is inferior, so that they result in less than the optimum therapeutic effect.

ACTH VERSUS STEROIDS? In most cases, the only decision of major consequence is whether to use ACTH rather than one of the adrenal steroid preparations. In general, adrenal steroid therapy is effective by mouth and can be regulated more accurately than ACTH therapy. The latter will fluctuate considerably in the amount of steroid produced from day to day, depending on the rate and extent of absorption of ACTH and on the state of the adrenal cortex. ACTH therapy does stimulate the secretion of adrenal androgens as well as hydroxysteroids. The former may have advantages in certain diseases, such as dermatomyositis, in which the adrenal androgens may prove helpful in maintaining the muscle mass while the inflammatory reaction is being suppressed by the 17-hydroxycorticosteroids. Combined androgen and corticoid therapy may, of course, attain the same objective. Sodium retention with ACTH has often been more marked than with cortisone or, particularly, with prednisone therapy.

There is little support for the belief that ACTH stimulates the production of naturally useful steroids qualitatively different from those available commercially. The use of ACTH, of course, presupposes a normally responsive adrenal cortex, an assumption that cannot always be verified in serious or prolonged disorders. Both ACTH and steroid administration induce pituitary inhibition. In addition, steroid therapy also induces adrenal suppression. For practical purposes ACTH is used to initiate a therapeutic response and to activate the adrenal cortex before steroid therapy is discontinued. It has, of course, a very important use in the diagnostic approach to disorders of adrenal function.

STEROIDS BY MOUTH VERSUS STEROIDS BY INJECTION. In acute emergencies such as brain tumor, allergic reactions, and shock, steroids will be administered intravenously in large doses, i.e., 300 to 500 mg hydrocortisone or 10 to 20 mg dexamethasone in 24 hr. For patients on long-term steroid therapy who develop gastrointestinal bleeding or symptoms of peptic ulcer, it may prove helpful in addition to the usual medical measures, to administer the daily steroid requirement *intramuscu-*

larly. This reduces the concentration of steroid reaching the gastrointestinal tract, without impairing the systemic effect.

"Alternate-Day" Therapy

It has been shown that twice the daily maintenance dose, given every other day, may minimize pituitary and adrenal atrophy as well as reduce the degree of Cushingoid changes. Such a schedule is well worth considering for any patient destined to receive corticosteroids for prolonged periods.

Supplementary Adjuvants Employed to Minimize Metabolic Disabilities

Since the continued use of ACTH or adrenal steroids induces a hypokalemic, hypochloremic metabolic alkalosis, supplementary potassium therapy should be given daily to patients receiving these hormone preparations. Potassium may be given as an elixir of potassium chloride, 2 to 3 tsp three times daily with meals (4 mEq potassium per tsp). Potassium chloride has a great theoretical and practical advantage over "mixed" potassium salts, particularly those containing potassium bicarbonate or citrate. Renal insufficiency is the primary complication in which supplementary potassium medication must be monitored carefully.

Antacid therapy and an ulcer-type diet *should be instituted* for all patients on steroid or ACTH therapy who give evidence of past or present increased gastric acidity, peptic ulceration, or upper gastrointestinal bleeding.

In patients who will require long-term ACTH or steroid therapy, the attending physician should make repeated efforts to ascertain whether the major manifestations of the underlying disorder cannot be held in satisfactory abeyance with a reduced hormone dosage. The ultimate development of Cushing's syndrome and its serious complications may prove more disastrous 3 to 5 years hence than the disease for which steroids were initially prescribed. Therefore *any* reduction in hormone dosage, however small, may be important in postponing the day of reckoning.

It is often possible to effect a considerable reduction in steroid maintenance dosage, if very small decrements are made, such as 5 percent per month. *Percentage* reduction should always be employed, as a reduction of 5 mg prednisone per day from a level of 100 mg to 95 mg is quite different from a reduction from 30 to 25 mg. It is also important for both patient and physician to appreciate that steroid therapy in general creates some degree of "euphoria" and hence a tendency to addiction. Thus a reduction in steroid dosage will initially be accompanied by a decrease in "energy" or sense of well-being. This may reduce the patient's threshold for tolerating the symptoms of his underlying disease without necessarily representing a true exacerbation. With a very small percentage decrease in dosage and with reassurance by the physician and understanding on the part of the patient, it is remarkable what can be accomplished in reducing the steroid level over a prolonged period. Patients are extremely grateful for any help that they can be given in this direction, when the long-range threat of steroid-induced complications is carefully explained.

When carrying out a slow, gradual reduction in steroid dosage, it must be realized that a sudden exacerbation of the underlying process may occur in conjunction with an acute infection or unusual stress. Under these circumstances the steroid dosage must be increased immediately, but it can usually be reduced promptly to the former dosage level once the precipitating factor is alleviated.

A Proposed Schedule for Attempting Withdrawal of ACTH or Corticosteroids Following Their Long–term Use as Pharmacologic Agents

Corticosteroid therapy induces both pituitary and adrenal suppression, whereas ACTH therapy affects only the former. For practical purposes it should be assumed that the majority of patients on prolonged steroid therapy will ultimately regain sufficient pituitary-adrenal activity to meet everyday needs. Regardless of how far in the past prolonged steroid therapy was given, in case of emergencies such as surgery, injuries, and severe infections, *supplementary cortisol or cortisone should always be employed*. It will also be apparent that regardless of the stepwise manner in which complete withdrawal of steroids is accomplished, there must always be a period of relative hypoadrenalism before endogenous ACTH-adrenal activity is restored. This is a point that must be seriously considered in patients with systemic lupus or widespread skin diseases, in which temporary hypoadrenalism may precipitate a serious or life-threatening exacerbation and hence is contraindicated. In such patients, Addisonian maintenance therapy for the long term may be indicated. For those patients, however, in whom it would appear advantageous to withdraw steroid therapy, the following schedule is suggested. *Steroid medication should not be withdrawn* until a patient's daily requirement is less than 50 mg hydrocortisone, 10 mg prednisone, or 1 to 1.5 mg dexamethasone.

The patient's steroid is changed to dexamethasone in a dosage equivalent to that of the steroid being employed, i.e., 1 mg dexamethasone for each 25 to 30 mg hydrocortisone; 1 mg dexamethasone for each 5 to 8 mg prednisone.

After 3 to 5 days on dexamethasone alone, base-line 24-hr urinary hydroxysteroid levels are determined (dexamethasone at this dosage level does not add appreciably to urinary steroid values).

While dexamethasone therapy is continued, ACTH is added in relatively large doses, i.e., 40 units intravenously over 8 hr daily for 3 to 5 successive days, or 80 units given in a continuous 24-hr infusion for 2 days or 80 units intramuscularly twice daily until urinary hydroxysteroids have attained a value at least three times the normal base line.

With evidence of adequate adrenocortical response, the maintenance dose of dexamethasone should be appropriately reduced and discontinued.

During this entire period the patient remains vulnerable to undue stress and must be protected on such occasions by administration of ACTH or an appropriate dose of glucocorticoid.

When a patient being maintained on dexamethasone and receiving ACTH in the larger dose as outlined above, fails to display a brisk adrenal response, he must be returned to a maintenance dose of steroid. ACTH can then be given intramuscularly two to three times weekly in a dose of 80 units in addition to the maintenance dose of steroid, and at a later date (4 to 6 weeks) the original schedule may be tried again. Failure to observe a satisfactory adrenal response on the second occasion implies, for practical purposes, permanent primary adrenocortical insufficiency, and the patient should be treated as for Addison's disease.

Summary

Several general facts should be considered in the management of patients receiving prolonged steroid therapy.

1. There is real danger of inducing acute adrenal failure if steroid therapy is suddenly withdrawn. Furthermore, adrenal reserve may be inadequate for a *prolonged* period after steroid therapy ends. Under these circumstances, patients must be warned about the additional risk of acute stress reactions such as injuries, operations, and infections. Both the patient and his doctor should be aware of this problem, and supplementary corticoid therapy should be readily available at all times.

2. Patients being maintained on a constant dose of steroid over a prolonged period should be protected by an increase in hormone therapy during a period of surgery or endocrine stress. It may be necessary to increase the basic dose of glucocorticoid by the equivalent of 100 mg cortisone per day.

3. When steroids such as prednisone, which usually do not invoke appreciable sodium retention or edema, are being used, one must be on the alert for more subtle evidence of overdosage during a prolonged therapeutic program. Special attention should be given to disturbance in the gastrointestinal tract, as indicated by the appearance of digestive symptoms or occult blood in the stool. Signs suggestive of bone pain due to the development of underlying osteoporosis should be carefully watched for.

4. All patients receiving prolonged steroid therapy should have periodic checks, which should include body weight, blood pressure, urine sugar, and appraisal of the cardiovascular, digestive, and skeletal systems. The possibility of the development of posterior subcapsular cataracts must be considered.

Adrenal hormone therapy constitutes a potent pharmacologic agent in the armamentarium of every practicing physician. As with all potent medicaments, a physician's responsibility must include an adequate knowledge of the pharmacologic actions of these agents as well as of the indications and contraindications for their use.

REACTION TO INJURY AND STRESS

A febrile response, leukocytic changes, and alterations in the erythrocyte sedimentation rate are well recognized indexes of injury and the body's reaction to it. It is now recognized, however, that the reaction to injury involves a series of integrated responses which affect the whole organism. Changes in the circulation are accompanied by important psychologic and neuromuscular alterations. These are mediated via a group of chemical and metabolic reactions initiated by neurohormonal mediators and chemical substances—the latter derived from injured tissue. These reactions involve the pituitary and adrenal gland secretions, as well as the liver, kidney, and hematopoietic tissues. Alterations in protein, carbohydrate, and fat metabolism occur, as well as significant changes in electrolyte concentration and distribution. In addition, immunologic changes accompany the general reaction to stress and represent important defense mechanisms for the organism (see Chap. 68).

Selye has applied the descriptive title of "the alarm reaction" to the series of events which may be initiated by such varied stresses as emotional disturbances, infection, hemorrhage, trauma, or undue exposure to heat and cold. Injury such as occurs with full-thickness burns gives rise to the most intense pattern of reaction.

In the original hypothesis, it was assumed that the increased liberation of adrenal hormones, both medullary and cortical, was largely responsible for initiating the widespread metabolic changes characteristic of this syndrome. Indeed, by the use of highly purified ACTH preparations or synthetic adrenal steroids, it has been possible to reproduce many of the changes characteristic of this general response. Thus, increased excretion of nitrogen, potassium, and phosphorus, retention of sodium chloride and water, reduction in circulating eosinophils and lymphocytes, increase in polymorphonuclear leukocytes, elevation of blood sugar level with decreased glucose tolerance, changes in important plasma constituents such as cholesterol and globulin, and alterations in gastrointestinal secretions, as well as fundamental changes in psychologic behavior and neuromuscular function, have all been observed in patients and in normal persons given large quantities of ACTH or cortisol. Although widespread effects of this type can be induced by stimulating the intact adrenal gland of man with purified ACTH preparations or by the administration of the appropriate adrenal steroids, there is evidence that mechanisms other than those related to activation of the pituitary-adrenal axis are capable of inducing similar metabolic and chemical changes. In fact, only in severe stress or tissue injury is a measurable increase in blood or urine adrenal steroid level demonstrable. Thus, it appears more correct to interpret the total response of the organism to stress as representing the effects of pituitary–adrenal cortical stimulation acting in combination with a variety of other metabolic and immunologic alterations.

REFERENCES

Addison, T.: "On the Constitutional and Local Effects of Disease of the Suprarenal Capsules," London, S. Highley, 1855.

Afifi, A. K., R. A. Bergman, and J. C. Harvey: Steroid Myopathy. Clinical, Histologic, and Cytologic Observations, Johns Hopkins Med. J., 123:158, 1968.

Beisel, W. R., V. C. DiRaimonde, and P. H. Forsham: Cortisol Transport and Disappearance, Ann. Intern. Med., 60:641, 1964.

Berson, S. A., and R. S. Yalow: Radioimmunoassay of ACTH in Plasma, J. Clin. Invest., 47:2725, 1968.

Biglieri, E. G., M. A. Herron, and N. Brust: 17-Hydroxylation Deficiency in Man, J. Clin. Invest., 45:1946, 1966.

Blizzard, R. M., R. W. Chandler, M. A. Kyle, and W. Hung: Adrenal Antibodies in Addison's Disease, Lancet, II:901, 1962.

Conn, J. W., and L. H. Louis: Primary Aldosteronism, A New Clinical Entity, Ann. Intern. Med., 44:1, 1956.

Cushing, H.: The Basophil Adenomas of the Pituitary Body and Their Clinical Manifestations (Pituitary Basophilism), Bull. Johns Hopkins Hosp., 50:137, 1932.

Dexter, R. N., L. M. Fishman, R. L. Ney, and G. W. Liddle: Inhibition of Adrenocortical Steroid Synthesis by Amino Glutethamide: Studies of Mechanisms of Action, J. Clin. Endocrinol. & Metab., 27:473, 1967.

Graber, A., R. L. Ney, W. E. Nicholson, D. P. Island, and G. W. Liddle: Natural History of Pituitary Adrenal Recovery Following Long-term Suppression with Corticosteroids, Trans. Assoc. Am. Physicians, 77:296, 1964.

Hellman, L., H. L. Bradlow, B. Zumoff, and T. F. Gallagher: The Influence of Thyroid Hormone on Hydrocortisone Production and Metabolism, J. Clin. Endocrinol. & Metab., 21:1231, 1961.

Herrera, M. G., G. F. Cahill, Jr., and G. W. Thorn: Cushing's Syndrome: Diagnosis and Treatment, Am. J. Surg., 107:144, 1964.

Hutter, A. M., Jr., and D. E. Kayhoe: Adrenocortical Carcinoma: Clinical Features in 138 Patients, Am. J. Med., 41:572, 1966.

Lauler, D. P.: Preoperative Diagnosis of Primary Aldosteronism, Am. J. Med., 41:855, 1966.

Luetscher, J.: Primary Aldosteronism: Observations in Six Cases and Review of Diagnostic Procedures, Medicine, 43:137, 1964.

Maeda, R., M. Okamoto, L. C. Wegienka, and P. H. Forsham: A Clinically Useful Method for Plasma Testosterone Determination, Steroids, 13:83, 1969.

Murphy, B. E.: Some Studies of the Protein Binding of Steroids and Their Application to the Routine Micro and Ultramicro Measurements of Various Steroids in Body Fluids by Competitive Protein Binding Radioassay, J. Clin. Endocrinol. & Metab., 27:973, 1967.

Paris, J.: On the Diagnosis of Addison's Disease and Cushing's Syndrome by Laboratory Methods, Mayo Clinic Proc., 39:26, 1964.

Ross, E. J.: Aldosterone and Its Antagonists, Clin. Pharm. & Therap., 6:65, 1965.

Thorn, G. W.: Clinical Considerations in the Use of Corticosteroids, New England. J. Med., 274:775, 1966.

93 PHEOCHROMOCYTOMA

Roger B. Hickler and George W. Thorn

The first pheochromocytoma was described by Frankel in 1886, with the term subsequently given by Pick to describe tumors which are selectively colored by chromium salts. The syndrome of paroxysmal hypertension due to this tumor was first clearly described by Labbe, Tinel, and Coumier in 1922. In 1926 Roux and in 1927 Mayo performed the first successful surgical removals of the tumor. In 1936 Beer, King and Prinzmetal determined that the characteristic paroxysmal rise in blood pressure was associated with the release of hormone from the tumor into the blood. *Persistent* hypertension was first attributed to the tumor in the same year by Kremer.

INCIDENCE. It is estimated that over 1,000 cases of pheochromocytoma have been identified, the incidence rising with improved diagnostic techniques. Anatomic statistics from the Mayo Clinic showed 15 of these tumors in 15,984 autopsies, an overall incidence of 0.1 percent. Smithwick estimated the incidence in a hypertensive population explored for sympathectomy to be 0.5 percent.

ANATOMY. Embryologically two cell types differentiate from a common stem cell, the sympathogonia of the primitive neuroectoderm, to form the adrenal medulla: the chromaffinoblast and the neuroblast, which mature into the chromaffin cell and sympathetic ganglion cell, respectively. These medullary cells are richly supplied with preganglionic fibers from the splanchnic nerves.

The chromaffin cell is so named because of its capacity to show brown intracytoplasmic granules on treatment with chromium salts, a result of oxidation and polymerization of the catecholamine stored in the granules. Chromaffin cells are found in widely dispersed sites at birth: the adrenal medulla, the paraganglia (along the retropleural and retroperitoneal sympathetic chains), the organs of Zuckerkandl (paired structures lying anterior to the bifurcation of the abdominal aorta), chemoreceptor areas ("glomic tissue" at the carotid bifurcation, along the aortic arch, and at the jugular bulb), and the human dermis. Many of the extraadrenal sites undergo progressive involution until puberty, but remnants account for the extraadrenal occurrences of pheochromocytomas, reported in all of the areas cited with the exception of the skin.

PATHOLOGY. Over 50 percent of pheochromocytomas occur in the region of the adrenals, sometimes bilaterally, and over 90 percent lie between the diaphragm and pelvic floor. As indicated by metastases, 6 percent are malignant and 7 percent occur simultaneously in more than one focus. Metastases may be functional and have occurred in liver, lungs, and central skeleton, as well as paraaortic lymph glands. The tumor weight may vary from a gram to several thousand grams (averaging about 100 Gm) and correlates poorly with the severity of the symptomatology. The tumors are round, frequently lobulated, and highly vascular. They may show hemorrhagic and necrotic areas with cystic degeneration, particularly large tumors. On section they appear brown or gray. Histologically they resemble the adrenal medulla; the nuclei are often multiple, cytoplasmic vacuolization is common, and dark staining with chromium salts is characteristic. Benign tumors may invade the capsule and are difficult if not impossible to distinguish from malignant forms on purely histologic grounds.

PHYSIOLOGY. The chromaffin cells of the adrenal medulla synthesize, store, and secrete epinephrine and norepinephrine. The biosynthesis of these hormones proceeds as follows: conversion of phenylalanine to tyrosine; oxidation of tyrosine to dopa (3,4-dihydroxyphenylalanine); decarboxylation of dopa to dopamine (3,4-dihydroxyphenylethylamine); and oxidation of dopamine to norepinephrine; epinephrine is formed by methylation of norepinephrine (Fig. 93-1). Epinephrine is the major hormone of the adrenal medulla, constituting 80 percent of its stored content of catecholamine; the major source of norepinephrine is the postganglionic sympathetic neurone, where it acts as the neurotransmitter.

The catecholamines are stored in cytoplasmic granules in the medullary chromaffin cells, which also contain a high content of adenosine triphosphate (ATP). It has been suggested that hydrolysis of adenosine triphosphate in the granules by an adenosine triphosphatase disrupts the granules and permits release of the hormone, which is normally released by cholinergic preganglionic sympathetic nerve impulses. A number of agents can directly stimulate chromaffin cells or the adrenergic neurones to release catecholamines, including acetylcholine, nicotine, histamine, 5-hydroxytryptamine, tyramine, and reserpine. A number of physiologic stimuli cause an increase in the release of both epinephrine and norepinephrine such as severe muscular work, asphyxia and hypoxia, and hemorrhagic hypotension. Insulin hypoglycemia causes a selective release of epinephrine alone, favoring the concept of separate cells for the synthesis and separate control of the release of adrenomedullary epinephrine and norepinephrine.

The physiologic effects of the adrenomedullary hormones may be characterized as preparing the organism to meet an emergency situation. Both epinephrine and norepinephrine have a direct inotropic and chronotropic effect on the heart. However, the purely vasoconstrictor effect of norepinephrine results in diastolic and systolic hypertension, producing reflex slowing of the heart, so that cardiac output is generally unchanged or reduced. The net peripheral vasodilator effect of physiologic doses of epinephrine (due primarily to vasodilatation of resistance vessels of skeletal muscle) permits a rise in cardiac output, with widening of pulse pressure through a rise in systolic pressure; diastolic pressure may fall slightly. Cutaneous and renal vasoconstriction is common

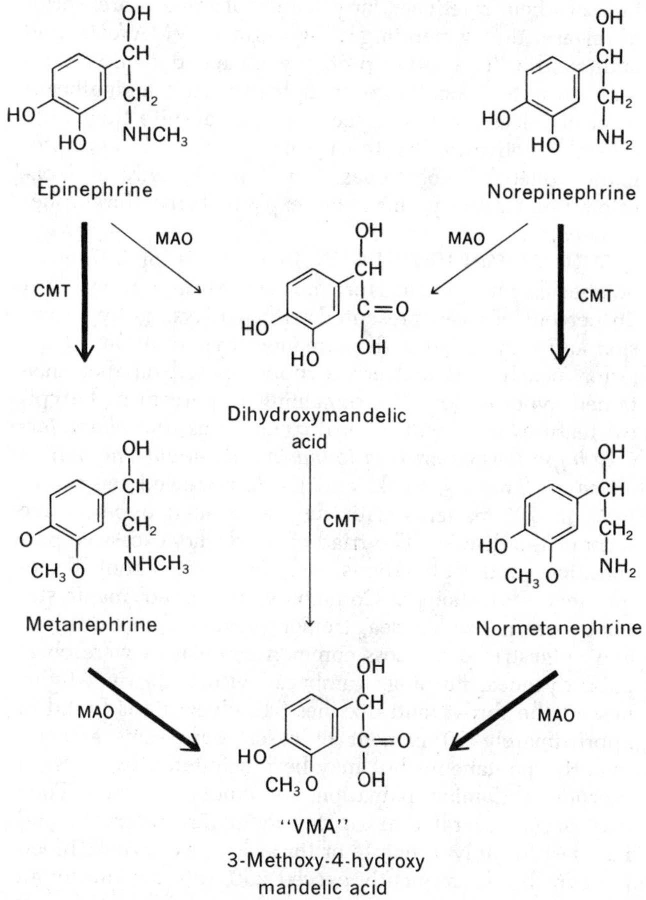

Fig. 93-1. The degradation of epinephrine and norepinephrine by catechol-O-methyl transferase (CMT) and monamine oxidase (MAO). All the above compounds appear in the urine in the free form or conjugated to glucuronide or sulfate. The heavier arrows indicate the major pathways. 3-Methoxy-4-hydroxy-mandelic acid is also designated as vanil mandelic acid (VMA).

to both hormones. Both increase the rate and depth of respiration and stimulate the release into plasma of non-esterified fatty acids from neutral fat depots. Other metabolic effects characteristic of epinephrine and, to a lesser extent, of norepinephrine, include increased formation of active phosphorylase in liver and skeletal muscle, resulting in accelerated hepatic glycogenolysis and release of lactic acid from muscle. These effects lead to hyperglycemia, increased oxygen consumption, and a high respiratory quotient.

CATECHOLAMINE METABOLISM. Figure 93-1 shows the major paths of metabolism of norepinephrine derived from sympathetic nerve endings, and of norepinephrine and epinephrine derived from the adrenal medulla. Most of the norepinephrine which is synthesized is converted *in situ* to metabolically inactive dihydroxymandelic acid by the action of intraneuronal monamine oxidase (MAO) before it can exert any biologic effect. This is discharged into the circulation and may be further metabolized by the enzyme catechol O-methyl transferase (COMT), present in high concentration in liver and kidney, to 3-methoxy, 4-hydroxy mandelic acid (vanil mandelic acid or VMA). Of the catecholamine which is released "intact," a small fraction interacts with receptor sites. The rest is either recovered and again bound in the storage granules, or carried in the circulation and rapidly converted by catechol O-methyl transferase to inactive

methoxy derivatives: norepinephrine to normetanephrine and epinephrine to metanephrine (collectively referred to as *metanephrines*). A portion of the metanephrines so formed may, in turn, be oxidized by monamine oxidase, present in most tissues, to vanil mandelic acid. Bilateral adrenalectomy results in only a minor depression of urinary catecholamines, since 80 percent is normally norepinephrine, largely derived from sympathetic nerve endings. The high activity of these two enzyme systems (MAO and COMT) is indicated by the fact that, by weight, the daily urinary content of the metanephrines (after hydrolyzing the major conjugated fraction free of its glucuronide or sulfate) is approximately seven times, and of VMA approximately thirty times that of the total catecholamines. Half of the catecholamine is in the "free" form and half as glucuronide or sulfate conjugates.

Crout and Sjoerdsma have defined the abnormal turnover and metabolism of catecholamines in patients with pheochromocytoma. Individual tumors vary widely in rates of production and turnover of catecholamines. Small tumors tend to release in active form (and rapidly replace) a comparatively high proportion of their relatively small total content of stored catecholamines. This relates to a low rate of oxidation by the tumor of stored catecholamines to inactive metabolites, as judged by a comparatively low urinary VMA catecholamine ratio. By contrast, large tumors tend to metabolize a considerable portion of their relatively large catecholamine stores prior to release, thus generating a high urinary VMA/catecholamine ratio. The latter probably escape detection until they grow to a size large enough to permit a significant level of release of free catecholamines despite their high rate of inactivation by the tumor. Reports of "asymptomatic" pheochromocytomas, found incidentally at laparotomy or autopsy, may be explained by these phenomena.

CLINICAL MANIFESTATIONS. In a review of 507 cases of pheochromocytoma, Hermann and Mornex report that 26 percent of cases presented with paroxysmal hypertension and 60 percent with permanent hypertension; of the latter, nearly half had crises superimposed on their sustained hypertension. The remaining 14 percent had atypical features or absent clinical signs. Thus, *the characteristic hypertensive crisis is found in only about one-half of all cases.* Thomas, Rook, and Kvale reviewed the symptoms in 100 patients with the paroxysmal hypertensive form of the disease. The triad of headache, excessive perspiration, and palpitations was found in about three-quarters of instances. Commonly associated manifestations were pallor, nausea, tremor, weakness, nervousness, and epigastric pain. Less common complaints were chest pain, dyspnea, flushing, numbness, visual blurring, tightness of the throat, and dizziness. Bradycardia is found in approximately 20 percent of cases. Paroxysms are frequently spontaneous but may be precipitated by physical exertion, abdominal palpation, and emotional upset. They may occur several times a day or at rare intervals, and may last for only a minute or for as long as a week. Blood pressure levels frequently exceed 250/150 mm during an attack in association with the paroxysmal release of catecholamine, as shown in Fig. 93-2. Shock and renal failure may attend or follow a paroxysmal attack. During a paroxysm death may occur from pulmonary edema, ventricular fibrillation, or cerebral hemorrhage.

Cases of *persistently* secreting tumors may be difficult

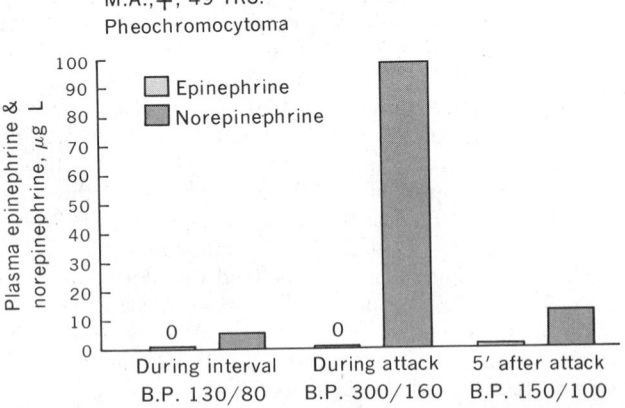

M.A., ♀, 49 YRS.
Pheochromocytoma

Fig. 93-2. The plasma epinephrine and norepinephrine levels before, during, and after a spontaneous paroxysm. The change in levels illustrates the intermittent secretory activity shown by some tumors and underlines the importance of obtaining samples for diagnostic purposes at the height of a spontaneous or induced attack.

to distinguish from cases of essential hypertension, but hyperglycemia and hypermetabolism (elevated BMR) are found in approximately 50 percent of patients with these tumors. Progressive weight loss and the demonstration of postural hypotension are further suggestive clinical evidence of sustained catecholamine secretion by a tumor. Frank retinopathy (grade 3 to 4 funduscopic changes) is found in more than half of these patients, an appreciably higher incidence than is found in the purely paroxysmal variety. This underscores the gravity of this form of hypertension and the importance of early clinical detection.

Special Features. Several unique aspects of the disease deserve emphasis. The tumor may first appear in early childhood or old age, but the average age of onset is during the fourth decade. In childhood pheochromocytoma the hypertension is almost always of the sustained variety, and the tumor tends to be bilateral and show a higher incidence of malignancy than in the adult. Distinct genetic factors are implicated in some instances by the prevalence of the tumor in certain families, sometimes in association with other congenital disorders of the neuroectoderm such as neurofibromatosis and central nervous system hemangioblastoma. A number of reports deal with the familial coincidence of pheochromocytoma and thyroid cancer, which is usually the medullary or solid type with amyloid production. This complex also has been coupled with parathyroid tumors as in the form of "multiple endocrine neoplasia" (Chap. 87).

Chromaffin-positive norepinephrine-secreting tumors of the glomic tissue of the carotid body and jugular bulb have been reported. These may represent further examples of the relationship between dysplasia of the neuroectoderm and the paroxysmal syndrome. There is an isolated case report of unilateral adrenal medullary hyperplasia in which removal of the hyperplastic gland resulted in complete amelioration of the signs and symptoms of excessive catecholamine secretion.

True polycythemia has been reported in association with the tumor, with return of the red cell mass to normal after successful surgery. Pheochromocytoma of the bladder wall produces a unique syndrome of paroxysmal symptoms, particularly throbbing headache, on micturition. While the majority of pheochromocytomas produce more norepinephrine than epinephrine (in contradistinction to the normal adrenal medulla), a few have been reported which are predominantly epinephrine secretors. These tend to be of the paroxysmal type and to produce hypotension and shock during a paroxysm, perhaps due to the vasodilating effect of the beta-adrenergic stimulation on the peripheral vasculature. The frequency of a diabetic tendency increases as the proportion of the epinephrine to the total catecholamine content of the tumor increases, perhaps because of the greater glycogenolytic activity of epinephrine. However, impaired carbohydrate tolerance has been found in pure norepinephrine secretors, and recent evidence indicates that the associated excessive alpha-adrenergic stimulation will inhibit insulin release to account for the impairment.

Over 50 percent of patients dying with a pheochromocytoma have an active myocarditis at autopsy. In the majority of these instances there was prior clinical evidence of left ventricular failure. In all probability this is a direct, "toxic" effect of the high levels of catecholamines on the myocardium.

Finally, a hypertensive response to smoking, to anesthesia, or to therapy with ganglionic blocking agents and guanethidine should raise the strong suspicion of a pheochromocytoma.

DIAGNOSIS. The clinical picture of essential hypertension with marked vasomotor lability strongly suggests pheochromocytoma, but pheochromocytoma with sustained hypertension in the absence of paroxysms may be indistinguishable from essential hypertension. Thus, routine laboratory screening of all patients with significant hypertension is desirable for this potentially curable form of hypertension.

Urinary Assay for Catecholamines and Their Methoxy Derivatives. Modern chemical methods for the determination of 24-hr urinary catecholamines and their methoxy derivatives have largely replaced the older pharmacologic tests in routine screening because of their safety and greater accuracy. Current chemical methods for determining urinary free catecholamines involve modifications of the trihydroxyindole (THI) method of Lund. The urinary-free catecholamines are adsorbed on an alumina or resin column, eluted with acid, oxidized to form "chromes," which, in turn, are tautomerized in alkali to form strongly fluorescent trihydroxyindoles. Free epinephrine and norepinephrine may be measured separately from fluorometric readings at different wave lengths. After acid hydrolysis to free the conjugated fractions, metanephrine (MN) and normetanephrine (NMN) may be isolated on resin and converted to trihydroxyindoles for fluorometric assay or oxidized to vanillin and read photometrically. VMA is measured by isolation and oxidation to vanillin, which may be read photometrically directly or after color development with added indole.

With these techniques Sjoerdsma and associates determined, simultaneously, the 24-hr urinary free catecholamines, metanephrines, and vanil mandelic acid on 64 patients with proven pheochromocytoma. The results are shown in Fig. 93-3 and indicate that the values obtained for all three assays were above the upper limit of normal in all but a few instances, giving an overall diagnostic reliability in the range of 90 percent. The upper limits of normal are (1) free catecholamines (epinephrine plus norepinephrine), 100 μg; (2) metanephrine plus normetanephrine, 1.3 mg; (3) VMA, 6.5 mg. Therapy with alpha-methyl dopa will produce false elevations in the free catecholamines and, potentially, in the metanephrines. Dietary sources of p-hydroxy-mandelic acid such as bananas produce false positives in the VMA determination. In general, *it is important to discontinue sympathomimetic agents and monamine oxidase inhibitors when performing these assays.* The relative diagnostic merits of the three different indices is debated, and it is probable that any one of them, carefully done, will serve equally well.

Pharmacologic Tests for Pheochromocytoma. In the absence of facilities for these chemical determinations, re-liance may be placed on the various intravenous pharmacologic tests. Along with the phentolamine (Regitine[R]) test, which produces a precipitous fall in blood pressure in pheochromocytomas, there are now in use three "provocative" tests: the older histamine and the newer tyramine and glucagon tests. Unfortunately, deaths have occurred after both phentolamine and histamine in pheochromocytomas, and the pharmacologic approach probably fails to detect as many as 25 percent of cases. The matter is further complicated by the prevalence of false positives with these agents. The intravenous tyramine test has the advantage over histamine and glucagon of causing a milder rise in blood pressure in the presence of a pheochromocytoma, but, by the same token, the end point of a positive reaction is less succinct. It is strongly contraindicated in any patient receiving amine oxidase inhibitor therapy, where the administration of tyramine may precipitate a hypertensive crisis. Histamine and probably glucagon should not be used if the control pressure is 170/110 mm or above, and phentolamine should be ready for immediate administration in the advent of a precipitous rise in blood pressure when these tests are performed. With pressures in the range of 170/110 mm or above, the tyramine and phentolamine tests are the ones of choice.

In a small percentage of patients, particularly during a normotensive period in those with intermittently secreting tumors, 24-hr urinary assay for catecholamines (or derivatives thereof) may not be clearly elevated into a diagnostic range. If suspicion is still strong on clinical grounds, the tumor may be provoked to secrete with 0.01 to 0.025 mg histamine base, given intravenously. This should be followed by the rapid injection of 5 mg phentolamine intravenously, should an alarming rise in blood pressure ensue. Blood may be drawn during the control period and at intervals of 2 min in the immediate posthistamine period for plasma assay for catecholamines, or a timed urine specimen (after prior emptying of the bladder) may be collected for a period of 6 hr for analysis for catecholamines or methoxy derivatives which may be expressed as amount excreted per milligram of creatinine.

The upper limit of normal for plasma epinephrine and norepinephrine varies with the method employed (trihydroxyindole or ethylenediamine condensation) and must be established in a given laboratory to determine a diagnostic rise following histamine administration. The upper limit of normal for urinary catecholamines (epinephrine plus norepinephrine) is 0.05 μg per mg creatinine; for metanephrine plus normetanephrine, it is 2.1 μg per mg creatinine; for VMA, it is 9.5 μg per mg creatinine. Levels above these following histamine administration are diagnostic. If a spontaneous attack should occur while a patient is under observation, blood and urinary determinations should be made immediately (Fig. 93-2). The plasma ethylenediamine condensation method for plasma catecholamines is invalid in the presence of uremia.

Localization of Tumor. While rarely palpable, a tumor mass may be detected on a plain film of the abdomen. Traditional and more specialized techniques for tumor localization have been tomography of the suprarenal areas

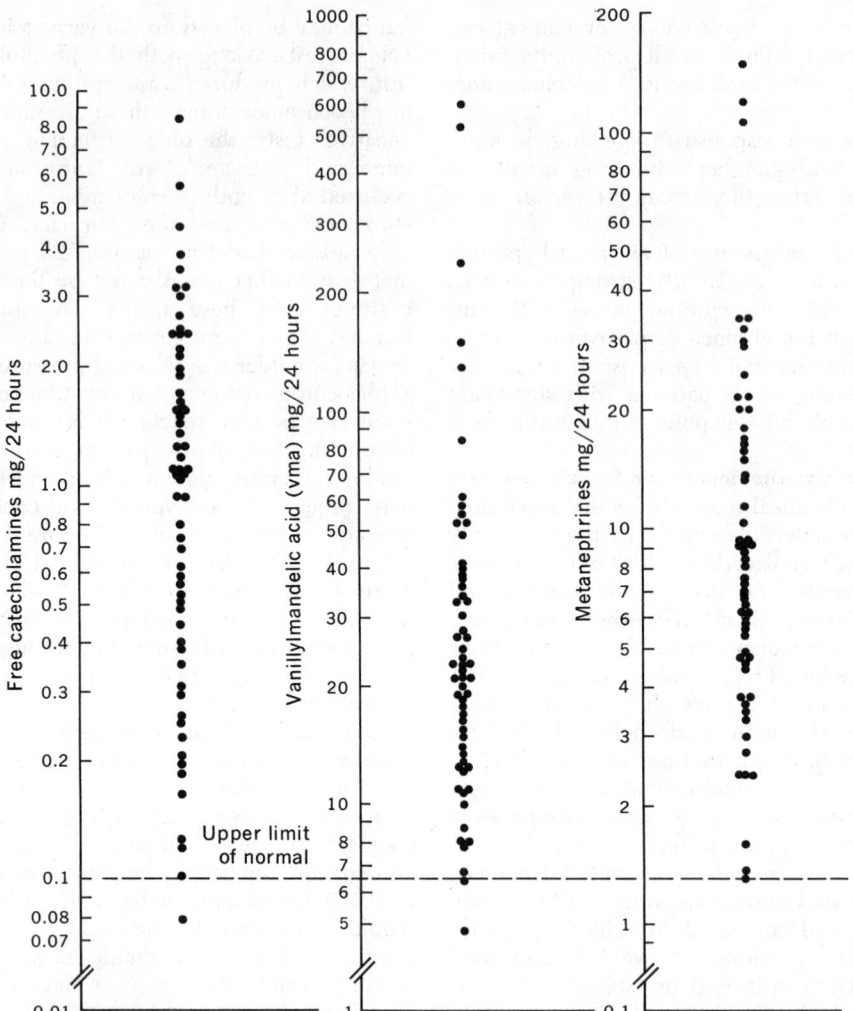

Fig. 93-3. Urinary excretion of catecholamines and metabolites in 64 patients with proved pheochromocytoma. (By permission of The Annals of Internal Medicine 65: 1966, Fig. 2, p. 1306. Sjoerdsma, A., Engelman, K., Waldmann, T. A., Cooperman, L. H., and Hammond, W. G., Combined Clinical Staff Conference at the National Institutes of Health. Pheochromocytoma: Current Concepts of Diagnosis and Treatment.)

during an intravenous pyelogram, and abdominal filming following the contrast afforded by presacral carbon dioxide insufflation. More recently, the advent of selective renal and adrenal angiography has afforded superb information in this regard; in some hands, these newer radiologic procedures are proving to be the ones of choice. The hazards attending these contrast techniques (including the potential for direct tumor stimulation) are apparent, and phentolamine should be ready for immediate administration during their performance. The analysis of catecholamines in plasma obtained by catheter at different levels in the venous system under fluoroscopic control has also been useful. Thoracic tumors, while rare, may be seen on a plain chest film.

Crout and Sjoerdsma report that the separate determination of urinary epinephrine and norepinephrine is of predictive value in tumor localization. If there is a significant elevation of epinephrine as well as norepinephrine

(42 percent of all cases), the tumor may be expected to lie in or adjacent to one of the adrenal glands or, rarely, in the organs of Zuckerkandl. If the urine contains elevated norepinephrine alone (58 percent of all cases), the tumor, of course, may still be found in one of the adrenal areas. Less than 10 percent of tumors are extra-abdominal, and these will generally show only an elevation of urinary norepinephrine and probably reflect a deficiency of N-methylating enzyme, present in the normal adrenal medulla and necessary for the conversion of norepinephrine into epinephrine.

DIFFERENTIAL DIAGNOSIS. Incorrect diagnoses in the presence of a pheochromocytoma have included diabetes mellitus, thyrotoxicosis, anxiety neurosis, "vascular" headache, epilepsy, and hypertensive crises due to lead poisoning and porphyria.

Patients with "nonchromaffin" sympathetic tumors, i.e., ganglioneuromas and, particularly, neuroblastomas have shown elevated levels of norepinephrine in the urine as well as increased excretion of its precursors (dopa and dopamine) and of its methoxy metabolites (metanephrines and VMA). Since some of these patients have associated hypertension, these tumors are to be distinguished from true "chromaffinomas." Another condition in which hypertension may be associated with markedly elevated urinary catecholamine excretion in the absence of a pheochromocytoma is Guillain-Barre syndrome, which perhaps results from a pathologic alteration in the sympathetic nervous system.

TREATMENT. In patients in whom surgical resection of the tumor cannot be performed, as with functioning metastases, the regular oral administration of the alpha-adrenergic blocking agent phenoxybenzamine (Dibenzyline^R) has been reported to have controlled most of the disturbing signs and symptoms for a period of many months. This approach has also been recommended routinely for a period of several weeks in order to get patients into an optimum condition in preparation for surgery, as in the presence of malignant hypertension with congestive heart failure. The use of beta-adrenergic blockers, such as propranolol, may also be useful in protecting against beta-adrenergic mediated cardiac arrhythmias from high circulating levels of catecholamines. The use of inhibitors of catecholamine synthesis is another approach to the pharmacologic treatment and preoperative control of patients with pheochromocytoma; preliminary reports of the use of alpha-methyl-para-tyrosine in this regard are very encouraging.

Surgical removal of the tumor is the treatment of choice for this potentially lethal disease. Since over 90 percent of all such tumors are located in the abdomen, a careful abdominal exploration through a generous transverse upper abdominal incision may be undertaken, even without the certain exclusion of a rare extraabdominal site. To avoid extremes of hypertension during induction of anesthesia and surgical manipulation, an intravenous drip of phentolamine should be ready at all times. To avoid extremes of hypotension on clamping the blood supply of the tumor and following its removal, an intravenous drip of norepinephrine or other pressor amine should also be prepared in advance. *Administration of whole blood or plasma on removal of the tumor may be of paramount importance in preventing postoperative shock,* since the sudden relief of the prolonged vasoconstriction attending the disease produces a state of disparity between the vascular capacity and effective blood volume.

REFERENCES

Crout, J. R., and A. Sjoerdsma: Turnover and Metabolism of Catecholamines in Patients with Pheochromocytoma, J. Clin. Invest., 43:94, 1964.

Hermann, H., and R. Mornex: Human Tumours Secreting Catecholamines: Clinical and Physiopathological Study of the Pheochromocytomas, Oxford, Pergamon Press, 1964.

Mitchell, P. L., and E. Meilman: The Mechanism of Hypertension in the Guillain-Barre Syndrome, Am. J. Med., 42:986, 1967.

Page, L. B., and R. B. Copeland: Pheochromocytoma, Disease-a-Month, January, 1968.

Sjoerdsma, A., K. Engelman, T. A. Waldmann, L. H. Cooperman, and W. G. Hammond: Combined Clinical Staff Conference at the National Institutes of Health. Pheochromocytoma: Current Concepts of Diagnosis and Treatment, Ann. Intern. Med., 65:1302, 1966.

Sheps, S. G., and F. T. Maher: Histamine and Glucagon Tests in Diagnosis of Pheochromocytoma, J.A.M.A., 205:895, 1968.

Steiner, A. L., A. D. Goodman, and S. R. Powers: Study of a Kindred with Pheochromocytoma, Medullary Thyroid Carcinoma, Hyperparathyroidism and Cushing's Disease: Multiple Endocrine Neoplasia, Type 2, Medicine, 47:371, 1968.

Thomas, J. E., E. D. Rooke, and W. F. Kvale: The Neurologist's Experience with Pheochromocytoma: A Review of 100 Cases, J.A.M.A., 197:754, 1966.

Wurtman, R. J.: Catecholamines, New England Journal of Medicine Medical Progress Series, Boston, Little, Brown and Company, 1966.

94 DIABETES MELLITUS
Jurgen Steinke and George W. Thorn

Knowledge of diabetes is important because of its high prevalence, it has been estimated that there are 200 million diabetics in the world, and because the treated diabetic individual has the potential for a nearly normal life-span. Diabetes has metabolic and vascular components, which are both probably interrelated. The metabolic syndrome is characterized by an inappropriate elevation of blood glucose, associated with alterations in lipid and protein metabolism for which a relative or absolute lack of insulin is responsible. The vascular syndrome consists of accelerated nonspecific atherosclerosis and a more specific microangiopathy particularly affecting the eye and kidney.

HISTORY

Diabetes has been recognized from antiquity. Chinese medical writings mentioned a syndrome of polyphagia, polydipsia, and polyuria. Aretaeus (*ca.* A.D. 70) described the disease and gave it its name, meaning in Greek "to run through."

The study of the chemistry of diabetic urine was initiated by Paracelsus in the sixteenth century; however, he mistook the residue of the boiled urine for salt instead of sugar. Some 100 years later, Thomas Willis described the sweetness of the diabetic urine, "as if imbued with honey or sugar," which Dobson proved to be sugar. This led to a rational dietary approach, introduced by Rollo 29 years later. Morton (1686) noted the hereditary character of diabetes. In 1859, Claude Bernard demonstrated the increased glucose content of diabetic blood and recognized hyperglycemia as the cardinal sign of the disease. In 1869, Langerhans, still a medical student, described the islet cell formation in the pancreas, which now bears his name. Kussmaul characterized the air hunger and labored breathing of the patient in diabetic coma in 1874. The careful work by clinicians such as Bouchardat, Naunyn, von Noorden, Allen, and Joslin led to a significant therapeutic success with diet. Von Mering and Minkowski carried out their studies in 1889, demonstrating that dogs could be made diabetic by pancreatectomy. However, it took more than 30 years before Banting and Best were able to prepare an extract from dog pancreas capable of reducing an elevated blood glucose level. In 1939, the first long-acting insulin was introduced by Hagedorn. The chemical structure of ox insulin was established by Sanger in 1953; Nicol and Smith described the chemical structure of human insulin in 1960. The basic unit contains two polypeptide chains united by disulfide bridges. In 1964, Katsoyannis in the United States and Zahn in Germany completed the synthesis of both the A and B chains of insulin and were able to combine both chains into biologically active material. In 1967 Steiner described a large "proinsulin" molecule which is converted by enzymatic cleavage into the smaller biologically active insulin.

The accidental discovery of the hypoglycemic action of carbutamide by Franke and Fuchs in Germany, in 1955, and the earlier experimental work of Loubatieres in France initiated the use of oral hypoglycemic agents.

PREVALENCE

Diabetes mellitus is a disease of worldwide distribution. If it is more frequent in some countries than in others, it will have to be established when diagnostic criteria are agreed upon and uniformly controlled detection drives are executed. In the United States there are approximately 4 million persons with diabetes, close to 2 percent of the total population. Diabetes is more frequent in older people. The United States Public Health Service estimates that there are 2 diabetics for every 1,000 people up to age twenty-four, 10 between the ages of twenty-five and forty-four, 33 in the age group forty-five to fifty-four, 56 between ages fifty-five and sixty-four, and 69 per 1,000 between sixty-five and seventy-four years of age. Unless a cure or some preventive measure is found for diabetes, this number will continue to increase for the following reasons: (1) the population grows and becomes older; (2) the life expectancy of the treated diabetic is close to normal, or is at least two-thirds that of the general population at a given age; (3) since more diabetics live long enough to have children, an increasing number of children will inherit the diabetic gene; and (4) obesity, which appears to precipitate diabetes among those predisposed to it, is also on the rise, thus allowing more potential diabetics to emerge.

The undiagnosed adult diabetic presents a major challenge to the practicing physician. Not infrequently diabetic symptoms are minimal, and the patient does not seek medical advice. In the United States, approximately 50 percent of the 4 million diabetics are unidentified. Because early treatment prolongs life, these undiagnosed diabetics must be found. As it is not feasible to test the entire population, it is advisable to concentrate on those individuals with predisposition for the disease. They are (1) relatives of known diabetics, among whom diabetes is 2½ times more frequent than in the general population; (2) obese persons, since 85 percent of diabetic patients are, or were at one time, overweight; (3) persons in the older age groups, as four out of five diabetics are over forty-five; and (4) mothers delivered of large babies, since the birth of a large infant may be an indication of maternal prediabetes.

Apart from these high-risk groups, routine testing for diabetes should be performed whenever a new patient visits a physician's office or is admitted to a hospital. Furthermore, it would be desirable to include testing for diabetes in preemployment examinations and to retest employees at yearly intervals.

INHERITANCE

It is well-established that diabetes mellitus is inherited; the *mode* of inheritance is still under discussion.

The acceptance of heredity for diabetes is based on the greater frequency of diabetes among blood relatives of known diabetics. The pattern of inheritance is characterized by (1) a more frequent occurrence in the mates of identical than of nonidentical twins; (2) the equilateral transmission of the trait by either affected parent; and (3) the susceptibility of both sexes. However, genetic study is complicated by the fact that susceptibility to diabetes is inherited, but the disease itself may not become apparent clinically for years. Genetic studies are based on occurrence of clinical diabetes (phenotype), not on presence of the genetic predisposition (genotype), for the latter cannot be detected at the present time. It is possible that the diabetic trait may be dominant and the manifest diabetic disease recessive. There is further confusion because diabetes is a syndrome; for example, chronic pancreatitis may be associated with hyperglycemia indistinguishable from that observed in genetic diabetes. This could lead to false designation of an individual as affected with genetic diabetes. Diabetes has a variable age of onset (youth onset and maturity onset), each with a characteristic clinical pattern. This has led, on the one hand, to the hypothesis of multifactorial inheritance and to the hypothesis that the mode of inheritance in juvenile diabetes is homozygous, whereas the hereditary factor in maturity onset diabetes is heterozygous. On the other hand, Steinberg has reviewed all available genetic data and expressed the belief that diabetic inheritance is consistent with homozygosity for a recessive gene at a single locus, with variable penetrance.

CLASSIFICATION

It is helpful to classify the diabetic patient not only according to the type of his diabetes but also according to his present stage of carbohydrate decompensation.

The latter implies that progression or regression from one stage to the next occurs and may be very rapid, may proceed slowly, or may never take place. The following *stages* of diabetes are almost universally accepted: (1) Overt or clinical diabetes: this is frank diabetes either of the ketosis-prone (juvenile) or ketosis-resistant (adult) type. Fasting and random blood glucoses are definitely elevated, symptoms related to hyperglycemia and glycosuria can usually be elicited. (2) Chemical or asymptomatic diabetes: the fasting blood glucose level is usually normal, but the postprandial level is frequently elevated. An oral or intravenous glucose tolerance test performed in the absence of stress is clearly abnormal. There are no diabetic symptoms. If observed in children, this stage is usually of short duration, as they progress rapidly to overt diabetes; in adults it may be present for years, and some patients never progress beyond it. Despite this, diabetic angiopathy may be present. (3) Latent or stress diabetes: present in a person who at the *present* time has a normal glucose tolerance but who is known to have been a diabetic at some *previous* time, i.e., during pregnancy (gestational diabetes), during infection, when obese, or when under stress, such as cerebrovascular accident, myocardial infarction, extensive burns, or endocrinopathies. Patients with such temporary carbohydrate intolerance should be watched closely, particularly when there is a family history of diabetes. (4) Prediabetes: this is a conceptual term, a retrospective diagnosis, applied to the period of time preceding any glucose intolerance. By definition it cannot be diagnosed with certainty in the current state of our knowledge except in the nondiabetic identical twin of a diabetic patient and possibly in the offspring of two diabetic parents.

As to the *types* of diabetes, the following etiologic classification can be applied:

1. *Genetic (hereditary, idiopathic, primary, essential) diabetes,* subdivided according to the age of onset into juvenile and adult diabetes.

2. *Pancreatic diabetes,* where the carbohydrate intolerance can be attributed directly to destruction of the pancreatic islets by chronic inflammation, carcinoma, hemochromatosis, or surgical removal.

3. *Endocrine diabetes,* when the diabetes is associated with endocrinopathies such as hyperpituitarism (acromegaly, basophilism), hyperthyroidism, hyperadrenalism (Cushing's syndrome, primary aldosteronism), pheochromocytoma, and pancreatic islet cell tumor of the A-cell type. Under this category can also be included the gestational diabetes and the various forms of stress diabetes listed above.

4. *Iatrogenic diabetes,* when precipitated by administration of corticosteroids, certain diuretics of the benzothiadiazine type and possibly also by estrogen-progesterone combinations.

PATHOLOGY

Pancreas

With the use of special stains with the light microscope and with the availability of the electron microscope, it now appears very likely that almost all diabetic patients exhibit a correlation between severity of their diabetes, on the one hand, and reduced total mass of beta cells and degree of beta cell degranulation, on the other. These two factors correlate with the amount of extractable pancreatic insulin. Generally speaking, after several years of established clinical diabetes, the patients with youth-onset diabetes shows essentially no extractable pancreatic insulin, whereas the pancreas of the adult-onset diabetic still contains some insulin, approximately half that found in control pancreases. Patients with maturity-onset diabetes studied at autopsy reveal a significant incidence of hyalinization of pancreatic islets. It has been suggested that this material is related to amyloid (Lacy).

Of special interest is the finding that some juvenile diabetics who come to autopsy shortly after clinical onset of diabetes show large islets of Langerhans. This would support the concept that the *initial* lesions is not necessarily decreased insulin production by the pancreas.

There is also the admittedly rare patient with recent onset of diabetes whose pancreatic islets indicate lymphocytic infiltration (insulitis), a lesion again found only in young diabetics. This raises the possibility of an infection or autoimmune mechanism.

Blood Vessels

Atherosclerosis in the diabetic patient is not different from that commonly observed, but it is equally present in both sexes and occurs earlier in life. Coronary artery disease is a frequent cause of death, and cerebrovascular accidents are significantly more common. In addition, these patients usually have small-vessel disease, or microangiopathy, of which the initial lesion is a thickened basement membrane.

Retina

Microaneurysms, small hemorrhages, and exudates are frequently seen in patients with long-standing diabetes. Frequently, there is also a striking dilatation of venules. Hemorrhage into the vitreous may be the cause of sudden loss of vision. Proliferative retinopathy is found frequently in juvenile diabetes of long duration. There is formation of new blood vessels around the optic disc. If, in response to hemorrhage into the vitreous, scar tissue forms, it may upon retracting produce retinal detachment. In proliferative retinopathy, a secondary hemorrhagic glaucoma is often the final step leading to total blindness. At the present time, in the United States, diabetic retinopathy is the third most frequent cause of blindness, after cataracts and glaucoma.

A better understanding of the mechanism of early vascular changes has been made possible by the introduction of the in vitro trypsin digestion of the flattened retina. Cogan and Kuwabara describe two types of vascular cells, the endothelial and the mural cell. In diabetics, there is a specific loss of mural cells, resulting in loss of tone with formation of microaneurysms and some diffuse distension with consequent ischemia of adjacent areas. This theory is supported by in vivo findings employing fluorescein, injected intravenously in the general circulation, followed by serial photographs of the fundus. In diabetics, there is not only delayed emptying but also leakage of the dye from blood vessels in areas where exudates and hemorrhages are occurring.

Kidney

Specimens for histologic study can be obtained by open or percutaneous biopsy or, of course, at autopsy. The specific diabetic lesion is the nodular glomerulosclerosis described by Kimmelstiel and Wilson. The lesions consist of PAS-positive material, believed to accumulate first in the mesangial region. With time, nodules form. In addition, the basement membrane of the glomerular loops becomes diffusely or focally thickened, and furthermore, the effects of arterial and arteriolar sclerosis become manifest. Pyelonephritis, a frequent complication, is a local manifestation of the generalized increased susceptibility to infection. The combination of these lesions constitutes diabetic nephropathy and manifests itself clinically with proteinuria, edema, and hypertension.

Link Between Metabolic and Vascular Changes

Some of the pathologic changes observed in diabetic patients are obviously secondary to hyperglycemia, such as deposition of glycogen in the renal epithelium, especially in the proximal convoluted tubule and the loop of Henle, where it is directly correlated to the glucose concentration in the urine. Hyperglycemia also results in deposition of glycogen in non-insulin-dependent organs, such as skin, heart muscle, iris, and ciliary bodies of the eye. The liver of the diabetic patient, except in the terminal stages, contains normal amounts of glycogen; however, the distribution may be abnormal within the nuclei of the hepatic parenchymal cells. Occasionally the liver is enlarged and infiltrated with fat, mainly in untreated or poorly treated diabetics.

The relationship between derangement of intermediary metabolism and microangiopathy has not been clarified and is the subject of controversy. Except for the patient with mild diabetes, perfect control is almost impossible to achieve in the immediate postprandial state, and therefore, most patients present varying shades of insufficient control.

Biochemically it is possible that excessive synthesis of mucopolysaccharides from glucose, via an insulin-dependent pathway, leads to derangement of the basement membrane, with secondary infiltration by materials from the bloodstream. It has been questioned whether such a derangement is necessarily the consequence of an abnormal glucose metabolism or if both the level of blood glucose and the state of the basement membrane could be influenced by a third factor. On the other hand, it is now well documented that all the complications of genetic diabetes can occur in secondary forms of diabetes in man

and furthermore that they can be reproduced in animals with experimental diabetes (Bloodworth).

Pathophysiology

In all likelihood the diabetic syndrome develops as a consequence of an imbalance between insulin production and release, on the one hand, and hormonal or tissue factors modifying the insulin requirement, on the other.

Insulin is absolutely lacking in those forms of secondary diabetes where destruction or removal of the pancreas has taken place. Similarly overt growth-onset diabetes is characterized by insulin deficiency. There is essentially no extractable pancreatic insulin, no response to oral hypoglycemic agents of the sulfonylurea type, a marked tendency to ketoacidosis, and therefore dependence on exogenous insulin for survival. It is assumed that diabetes in the child begins when the pancreatic production of insulin declines. However, this is not always irreversible, as at least one-third of all juvenile diabetics will develop a phase of remission, usually within 3 months after the acute onset of the disease. If present, the remission may last from several days to several months; it rarely exceeds 1 year. Often during such a remission no insulin treatment is necessary, and a glucose tolerance test may be normal. Nevertheless, after this remission the juvenile diabetic progresses rapidly to a state of total insulin deficiency.

The patient with adult-onset diabetes develops his disease considerably more slowly. At the early stage no symptoms may be present, and diagnosis is suspected by discovery of elevated blood glucose levels 1 or 2 hr postprandially. Measurement of serum insulin may indicate close to normal fasting levels; however, the insulin response to administered glucose is abnormal in that it occurs late. This is responsible for the elevated blood glucose 1 to 2 hr postprandially. As insulin release increases with the rising blood glucose, the blood glucose declines; with excess insulin, the blood glucose may fall precipitously, provoking the symptoms of reactive hypoglycemia between the *third and fifth hour* postprandially. As the disease progresses further, the insulin release becomes less pronounced, the episodes of reactive hypoglycemia tend to disappear; finally the amount of circulating insulin is insufficient to return the blood glucose to normal levels between meals. In maturity-onset diabetes the pancreatic insulin reserve is decreased, but rarely totally absent. Thus the occurrence of diabetic ketoacidosis is uncommon.

Although in many patients the contrast between growth-onset and maturity-onset is initially at least quite sharp, there are crossovers between these two types and the above comments must be considered only as generalizations.

Regardless of the type of diabetes, by definition, the cardinal sign is hyperglycemia, frequently associated with glycosuria. The hyperglycemia has two components: hepatic overproduction and peripheral underutilization. The source of the glucose released from the liver is dietary carbohydrate, liver glycogen, and gluconeogenesis from protein. Underutilization of glucose in the peripheral tissue takes place mainly in adipose tissue and muscle, both of which are insulin-sensitive, and is attributed to a lack of circulating insulin. Impaired glucose uptake by muscle leads to loss of muscle glycogen and release of amino acids for gluconeogenesis. Impaired glucose uptake by adipose tissue causes impaired triglyceride synthesis. In addition, with lack of insulin, there is release of free fatty acids from adipose tissue into the bloodstream. In the liver, the fatty acids are metabolized to ketone bodies. Although they can be utilized by certain tissues, they are formed in excess in the diabetic person. They accumulate in the blood and lead to ketonuria. As they are strong acids, it is necessary for the kidney to excrete a fixed base with them, leading to both sodium and potassium loss. Therefore, the diabetic organism loses glucose, water, ketone bodies, and base. This will result in dehydration, ketoacidosis, and weight loss, and in extreme cases, may proceed to diabetic coma and death.

The exact mechanism by which insulin acts remains unknown. However, it is well established that tissues vary widely in sensitivity and responsiveness to insulin. For example, in muscle and adipose tissue, insulin probably acts on cell membrane permeability and so facilitates the entry of glucose into the cell. On the other hand, liver cells exhibit no demonstrable permeability barrier to glucose. The insulin effect on liver appears to be on the phosphorylating mechanism. It has recently been suggested that the liver contains two enzymes for phosphorylation of glucose: hexokinase and glucokinase. Hexokinase is insulin-*independent,* and glucokinase is insulin-*dependent.* In addition, insulin affects glycogen synthesis. The effect of insulin on fatty acids has been mentioned above. It is noteworthy that this antilipolytic action requires a lower level of insulin than that for glucose uptake. Therefore an absolute deficiency of circulating insulin as in juvenile diabetes will lead to hyperglycemia and marked lipolysis with resultant ketosis, whereas only a decrease of circulating insulin such as in adult-onset diabetes will lead to hyperglycemia without ketosis.

In diabetes the primary inherited defect responsible for the failing insulin production remains unknown. The recent discovery of proinsulin may be a step forward. Proinsulin is a larger molecule than insulin (molecular weight 9000, versus 6000) because of some 30 additional amino acids, but it exhibits considerably less biological activity. Controversy exists whether proinsulin is an inactive storage form or a precursor of insulin. It is transformed into insulin by cleavage of the intermediate chain.

It is conceivable that in some diabetic patients there is a failure to activate proinsulin. As large quantities of proinsulin would be required to meet the body's insulin demand, this failure could eventually lead to pancreatic exhaustion and thus to frank diabetes.

PRECIPITATION OF DIABETES BY EXTRAPANCREATIC FACTORS

Obesity is frequently associated with diabetes, though it should not be inferred that all obese individuals are potential diabetics. Biopsy studies have shown that adult onset obesity is associated with hypertrophy of adipose cells and that the larger the cell, the less responsive to insulin it becomes. As less glucose can be disposed of, the resulting hyperglycemia will lead to hyperinsulinemia. In patients genetically predetermined, this may lead to pancreatic exhaustion or at least to a relative insulin deficiency.

Pregnancy also exerts a definite diabetogenic action in women so predisposed. Initially, diabetes may become apparent only during pregnancy and disappear following delivery; rarely it remains; frequently, years or decades later, permanent diabetes develops. There is evidence that hormonal factors, such as placental lactogen and marked destruction of endogenous insulin by the placenta, may play a role in precipitating diabetes. It is speculated that the higher frequency of diabetes in adult females may be due to pregnancies and obesity.

Recently, the diabetogenic action of certain *diuretics* of the benzothiadiazine type has been noted. There is evidence that these drugs mediate such mechanism by inhibiting pancreatic insulin release. This effect is reversible, contrary to the damage produced by the administration of alloxan. Growth hormone is diabetogenic by decreasing peripheral glucose utilization and by increasing release of free fatty acids. Excess epinephrine causes increased hepatic glycogenolysis and, in addition, exhibits pancreatic insulin release. The steroids act by increasing hepatic gluconeogenesis and decreasing glucose uptake by adipose tissue. Thyroxin increases hunger and food intake and generally heightens the level of metabolic activity. Infection of any sort will impair glucose tolerance and may unmask the tendency to diabetes. The diabetogenic mechanism of infection is probably nonspecific and consists of elevated levels of corticosteroids, fever that increases the general metabolic load, and possibly catecholamine release, all of which decrease the effectiveness of circulating insulin. In rare instances inflammation of the pancreatic islets takes place.

DIAGNOSIS

The diagnosis of diabetes mellitus is frequently suggested by a history of polydipsia, polyuria, and polyphagia, associated with weight loss. A clinical suspicion of diabetes is confirmed by finding glucose in the urine *and* by detecting an abnormally elevated blood glucose. If hyperglycemia is associated with glycosuria *and* with ketonuria, the diagnosis of diabetes mellitus is certain.

In the patient without any obvious symptoms suggestive of diabetes, the following procedures are recommended as screening tests for diabetes. By far, the simplest tests is to obtain a urine specimen 1 to 2 hr after a heavy carbohydrate meal. However, in older persons with an elevated renal threshold, the blood glucose may be elevated without being associated with glycosuria; furthermore, the finding of urinary sugar alone is not diagnostic of diabetes. Therefore, determination of blood glucose not only is preferable as a screening procedure but is mandatory to establish the diagnosis of diabetes. Unfortunately much confusion exists as to what represents an abnormal blood glucose value. Whereas there is general agreement that a 1-hr postprandial blood glucose of 200 mg per 100 ml or higher indicates diabetes, there is considerable discussion if abnormality starts above a value of 160, 170, or 180 mg per 100 ml. It has become apparent that clinical information and follow-up studies as well as the methodology of the blood glucose determination have to be taken into account. In general terms it can be stated that upper limits of normalcy increase with age and during pregnancy. As to methodology, the physician needs to know (1) if capillary or venous blood was used (the capillary blood glucose will be higher); (2) if the blood glucose was determined on whole blood or plasma (plasma or serum will render higher values than whole blood; on the other hand, severe anemia will give falsely elevated values with whole blood); (3) which particular technique for measuring blood glucose was employed. A rather less specific method such as Folin-Wu will give the highest values as it measures in addition to glucose also fructose, lactate, pyruvate, etc. The glucose oxidase method will reflect the "true" glucose content and therefore yield the lowest value. The autoanalyzer employs the ferricyanide method which is slightly higher than the glucose oxidase technique. It is apparent that the possible variations are many, therefore the best advice is to be familiar with the methods and normal range in a given hospital. When blood glucose values are reported to outlying institutions or life insurance companies, the type of blood and the technique employed should be noted.

Fasting and Postprandial Blood Glucose

The normal range for fasting blood glucose as measured by the autoanalyzer is between 70 and 110 mg per 100 ml whole blood. An elevated fasting blood sugar is highly suggestive of diabetes; on the other hand, diabetes can never be ruled out by presence of a normal fasting blood sugar. Therefore, it is advisable to obtain a blood sugar determination 1 or 2 hr after a meal which has

Table 94-1. 100-GM CARBOHYDRATE BREAKFAST

Food	Quantity	Carbohydrate, Gm
Orange juice............	8 oz	24
Cooked cereal..........	4 oz ⎫	
or	⎬	16
Dry cereal.............	1 oz ⎭	
Bread.................	2 slices	32
Egg..................	1	
Butter................	2 pats	
Milk..................	6 oz	9
Cream................	3 oz	4
Sugar.................	3 tsp	15
Coffee or tea...........	ad lib.	
		100

contained approximately 100 Gm carbohydrate, as indicated in Table 94-1, or a regular breakfast to which 50 Gm glucose have been added. A 1-hr value of 170 mg per 100 ml or higher is highly suspicious of diabetes, as is a 2-hr value above 120 mg per 100 ml. If the level is borderline, or especially if one wishes definitely to rule out diabetes, then a formal 3-hr glucose tolerance test is indicated.

Oral Glucose Tolerance Test

Following a fasting blood glucose determination, 100 Gm glucose (available commercially in solution) is given and the blood glucose measured at ½ hr, 1 hr, 2 hr, and 3 hr; the urine is examined for the presence of sugar. The following are considered upper normal values obtained with venous blood as measured by the autoanalyzer method: Fasting, 110 mg per 100 ml; ½ hr (or peak value), 170 mg; 1 hr, 170 mg; 2 hr, 120 mg; and 3 hr, 110 mg per 100 ml. There should be no glucose in the urine at any time. The result of the glucose tolerance test in an apparently healthy subject is influenced by at least three factors: diet, physical activity, and age. It is mandatory that the patient be on a preparatory diet containing 250 to 300 Gm carbohydrate for 3 days before testing; otherwise a decreased carbohydrate tolerance can be observed, known as *starvation diabetes*. Physical inactivity also decreases carbohydrate tolerance, and therefore prolonged bed rest may give false-positive results. Finally, age exerts an effect on glucose tolerance. Although standards are not available for individuals of different decades, especially over the age of fifty, Fajans suggests that between the ages of fifty and fifty-nine the 2-hr level can be considered normal up to 130; between the ages of sixty and sixty-nine, up to 140; between the ages of seventy and seventy-nine, up to 150; and above age eighty, above 160 mg per 100 ml. Additional factors known to affect glucose tolerance are fever, infection, endocrinopathies, liver disease, myocardial infarction, cerebrovascular accident, and certain medications such as diuretics of the benzothiodiazine type.

Intravenous Glucose Tolerance Test

As intestinal absorption of glucose may interfere with a glucose tolerance test, it is occasionally desirable to perform an intravenous glucose tolerance test. This is especially indicated if there is a history of gastrointestinal surgery. Accelerated intestinal absorption of glucose, as in the "dumping syndrome" may result in a diabetic-type oral glucose tolerance curve; however, the intravenous glucose tolerance may be well within normal limits.

The dose of glucose is 0.5 Gm per kg body weight as a 25 percent solution. It is administered intravenously within 2 to 4 min, and blood is collected every 10 min for 1 hr. Under these conditions, the rate of blood glucose decreases in an exponential manner, and the glucose disappearance can be calculated. Disappearance rate = $70/t\frac{1}{2}$, where $t\frac{1}{2}$ = number of minutes it takes for the blood glucose to fall 50 percent. In normal individuals it usually exceeds 1.5 percent of the administered dose per minute, and values below 1 percent are clearly diabetic.

If glucose tolerance tests are performed routinely in a large hospital population, many patients afflicted with chronic diseases like rheumatoid arthritis, cancer, or amyotrophic lateral sclerosis may exhibit impaired glucose tolerance curve without any clinical evidence of diabetes. Because many of these patients with "chemical diabetes" will not progress to a state of overt clinical diabetes, one has to be careful not to overdiagnose diabetes.

Cortisone Glucose Tolerance Tests

Fajans and Conn have proposed performing the oral glucose tolerance test after priming with cortisone in an attempt to establish the diagnosis of chemical diabetes at a time when the conventional oral glucose tolerance test is still within normal limits. The technique consists of administering 50 mg cortisone acetate 8 and 2 hr before the glucose tolerance test. The cortisone glucose tolerance test may detect carbohydrate intolerance earlier than the standard oral glucose tolerance test.

DIFFERENTIAL DIAGNOSIS OF GLYCOSURIA (See Chap. 95)

The presence of glucose in the urine should be considered to indicate diabetes until an alternate diagnosis can be definitely established. Glycosuria may indicate a low renal threshold, which is present in pregnancy, in patients with chronic renal disease, and in patients with idiopathic renal glycosuria. In the latter, glucose is present in most urine specimens, including a second voided specimen after an overnight fast, but the glucose tolerance test is normal. The transient glycosuria that occurs occasionally in apparently healthy persons under conditions of stress or infection or following ingestion of a high carbohydrate meal is usually associated with an abnormal glucose tolerance test and, therefore, indicates chemical diabetes.

CLINICAL PICTURE

Growth-onset Type

The growth-onset type of diabetes if characterized by a rapid onset with symptoms, such as polydipsia, polyuria, polyphagia, loss of weight and strength, marked irritability, and in children frequently, recurrence of bedwetting. The diabetes is apt to be of the unstable or brittle type, being quite sensitive to the administration of exogenous insulin and easily influenced by physical activity. The patient is prone to ketoacidosis. For adequate treatment, diet and insulin therapy are mandatory. Since the introduction of insulin therapy, diabetic ketoacidosis has been markedly reduced as a major cause of death; the primary causes of death in diabetic patients are now cardiovascular and renal. Diagnosis of diabetes in the growth-onset-type patient is usually not difficult. However, occasional children and adolescents have asymptomatic diabetes demonstrable only by glucose tolerance test. In these patients the disease appears to progress very slowly.

Maturity-onset Type

The maturity-onset diabetic patient has a less stormy beginning, frequently symptoms are minimum or absent. The chief complaint may be moderate weight loss or occasionally, weight gain. There may be some nocturia. A female patient might consult her gynecologist because of vulvar pruritis. Frequently, however, the patient seeks medical attention because of vascular complications. As a consequence of blurred or decreased vision, the patient may see an ophthalmologist first, who may diagnose diabetic retinopathy. Fatigue and anemia may be caused by fairly advanced diabetic nephropathy. Diabetic neuropathy may present as paresthesias, loss of sensation, impotence, nocturnal diarrhea, postural hypotension, or neurogenic bladder. Not infrequently, the patient presents with an ulcer or gangrene of his toes or heel and on examination has a pulseless or painless foot. Thus the patient with maturity-onset diabetes usually does not present with the dramatic, acute metabolic syndrome observed in the juvenile patient but rather with a chronic vascular syndrome. It is therefore important to suspect diabetes as an underlying disease under a wide variety of circumstances.

TREATMENT

The aims of managing diabetes are (1) correction of the underlying metabolic abnormalities by diet, oral hypoglycemic agents, or insulin; (2) attainment and maintenance of ideal body weight; and (3) prevention, or at least delay, of complications commonly associated with the disease.

Successful therapy will depend upon the thoroughness with which the physician understands the particular problems in each individual case, upon how well the patient has been instructed, and upon how conscientious the patient is about following instructions.

On initiating treatment of a patient with diabetes, it is essential to be certain that there is no active focus of infection, as it will aggravate the diabetic state. Infection of the urinary tract should be looked for particularly, and a chest x-ray is imperative. It is also advisable to obtain careful baseline evaluations of the state of the cardiovascular, nervous, and renal systems and of the eye grounds to serve as subsequent points of reference.

Diet

Dietary treatment of diabetes still constitutes the basis for management. The principal considerations in designing diabetic diets are (1) the basic nutritional requirements of a patient with diabetes are the same as those of a nondiabetic patient; (2) the diet should be varied and palatable.

THE BASIC CALORIC REQUIREMENT. This is dictated by the desirable, or ideal, weight, the age, and the occupation of the patient. If he is obese, the diet will be restricted in calories; if the patient is undernourished, the diet initially will exceed the basic caloric requirement. The desired weight is calculated from the height, taking frame size into consideration. For an approximate calculation of the basic caloric requirement, the ideal weight is multiplied by 10. Example: A patient's ideal weight is 180 lb, his total caloric requirement will be 1800 Cal. Additional calories should be allowed according to the patient's occupation and activities. Calories may be reduced for patients over fifty years of age who are less active.

PARTITION OF CALORIES. The average American diet consists of carbohydrate, 40 to 45 percent; protein, 15 to 20 percent; and fat, 35 to 40 percent. The diabetic diet can approximate this distribution. The caloric value of carbohydrate and protein is approximately 4 Cal per Gm and of fat, 9 Cal per Gm.

CARBOHYDRATE. To prevent acetonuria, a minimum of 1 Gm per lb body weight is necessary, or in the example of the patient weighing 180 lb, 180 Gm. This minimum requirement should be increased if indicated by occupation or during the growth period in children. It is obvious that regulation of diabetes will be simpler with a greater number of feedings involving smaller quantities of carbohydrate than with three large meals. In particular, diabetic patients receiving insulin or oral hypoglycemic agents should receive a midafternoon and bedtime snack in order to minimize fluctuation of the blood glucose.

PROTEIN. A *minimum* of 0.5 Gm per lb body weight is indicated. This is increased during pregnancy and during childhood and decreased only in the presence of azotemia.

FAT. It can be metabolized without the direct influence of insulin. However, dietary fat, particularly of animal origin, together with other factors such as decreased physical activity, seems to play an important role in the pathogenesis of atherosclerosis; therefore, fat intake should be kept to a minimum. The amount prescribed is calculated by subtracting calories allowed for carbohydrate and protein from the total caloric requirement.

Example: Total Calories based on an ideal weight of 180 lb are 1800. Assigned for carbohydrate $180 \times 4 = 720$, for protein $90 \times 4 = 360$ Cal, there remain $(1800 - 720 - 360) = 720$ Cal. These are given as fat, or $720/9 = 80$ Gm fat. The final diet then consists of carbohydrate 180 Gm, protein 90 Gm, and fat 80 Gm. It is probably advisable to reduce the total amount of cholesterol and to supply some of the fat as unsaturated fatty acids.

The American Diabetes Association and the American Dietetic Association have published a booklet on meal planning with exchange lists. In it all the available foods are divided into six types. Foods cannot be switched between the lists but can be interchanged within each list. Food is subdivided into (1) milk exchanges; (2) (*a*) essentially unlimited vegetables, (*b*) somewhat limited vegetables; (3) fruits; (4) bread exchanges which include apart from bread also cereal, rice, spaghetti, potato, etc.; (5) meat exchanges which include meat, cold cuts, egg, fish, cheese; and (6) fat exchanges. In Tables 94-2 and 3 these exchange lists are presented in more detail. Food can be weighed or measured with a standard 8-oz measuring cup, teaspoon, and a tablespoon.

Oral Hypoglycemic Agents

These have a definite place in the treatment of maturity-onset diabetes, provided it is of the nonketotic type and that dietary treatment alone is unsuccessful in achieving adequate control. Patients falling into this category constitute approximately two-thirds of all maturity-onset diabetics. It should be emphasized that none of the oral hypoglycemic agents is insulin, nor can they replace it in conditions such as diabetic ketoacidosis. The agents presently in use are of two types: the sulfonylureas and the biguanides.

SULFONYLUREAS. The sulfonylureas available by prescription are tolbutamide (Orinase), acetohexamide (Dymelor), chlorpropamide (Diabinase), and tolazamide (Tolinase). Although there is some evidence that they directly decrease hepatic glucose output, they act primarily by enhancing the secretion of endogenous insulin. Thus, to be effective, at least residual function of the beta

Table 94-2. FOOD EXCHANGES

LIST 1. MILK[1]
Calories 170, Carbohydrate 12 Gm, protein 8 Gm, fat 10 Gm per serving.

Food	Approximate measure 1 exchange	Weight, Gm
Milk, plain...............	1 cup (8 oz)	240
Milk, evaporated.........	½ cup	120
Milk, powder, skim[2]......	⅓ cup (5⅓ tbsp level)	48
Milk, powder, whole......	½ cup (8 tbsp level)	35
Buttermilk[2].............	1 cup	240
Milk, skim[2].............	1 cup	240

LIST 2. VEGETABLES
One or more fat exchanges from the diet allowance may be used to season the vegetables.
Carbohydrate 7 Gm, protein 2 Gm, fat negligible
One exchange equals ½ cup.

Beets	Peas, green	Squash, winter
Carrots	Pumpkin	Turnip
Onions	Rutabagas	

[1] Modified from Meal Planning with Exchange Lists. Obtainable from the American Diabetes Association, Inc., New York, N.Y.

[2] Add 10 Gm fat (2 fat exchanges). Most commercial buttermilk is skimmed. Check local supplies.

All other vegetables, except those listed under Bread Exchanges, contain negligible carbohydrate, protein, and fat. They may be used as desired.

Table 94-2. FOOD EXCHANGES (*Continued*)

LIST 3. FRUITS

Fresh, cooked, canned, or frozen *unsweetened*. Carbohydrate 10 Gm per exchange; protein and fat negligible.

Fruit	Approximate measure 1 exchange	Weight, Gm
Apple, 1 small...........	2″ diameter	80
Applesauce..............	½ cup	100
Apricots, dry...........	4 halves	20
Apricots, fresh..........	2 medium	100
Banana.................	½ small	50
Berries (blackberries, raspberries, and strawberries)..........	1 cup	150
Blueberries.............	⅔ cup	100
Cantaloupe.............	½ (6″ diameter)	200
Cherries................	10 large or 15 small	75
Dates.................	2	15
Figs, dried.............	1 small	15
Figs, fresh.............	2 large	50
Grapefruit.............	½ small	125
Grapefruit.............	½ cup	100
Grapes................	12	75
Grape juice............	¼ cup	60
Honeydew melon........	⅛ (7″ diameter)	150
Mango.................	½ small	70
Nectarines.............	1 medium	100
Orange................	1 small	100
Orange juice...........	½ cup	100
Papaya................	⅓ medium	100
Peach.................	1 medium	100
Pear..................	1 small	100
Pineapple.............	½ cup, cubed	80
Pineapple juice.........	⅓ cup	80
Plums.................	2 medium	100
Prunes, dried...........	2 medium	25
Raisins................	2 tbsp level	15
Tangerine.............	1 large	100
Watermelon............	1 cup diced 1 slice 3″ × 1½″	175

LIST 4. BREAD EXCHANGES

Carbohydrate 15 Gm, protein 2 Gm, fat negligible.

Food	Approximate measure 1 exchange	Weight, Gm
Bread, baker's..........	1 slice	25
Biscuit, roll.............	2″ diameter	35
Muffin.................	2″ diameter	35
Cornbread.............	1½″ cube	35
Cereals, cooked.........	½ cup, cooked	100
Cereals, dry (flakes, puffed, and shredded varieties)............	¾ cup, scant	20
Rice, macaroni, noodles, spaghetti............	½ cup, cooked	100
Crackers:		
Graham..............	2 (2½ × 2¾″)	20
Oyster..............	20 (½ cup)	20
Saltines.............	5 (2″ square)	20
Soda................	3 (2½ × 2½″)	20
Round, thin varieties...	6–8 (½″ diameter)	20
Vegetables:		
Beans, peas, dried (cooked) Includes limas, navy, kidney beans, black-eyed peas, cowpeas, split peas, etc............	½ cup, scant	100
Corn.................	⅓ cup or ½ ear	80
Parsnips..............	½ cup	125
Potatoes:		
White, baked.......	2″ diameter	100
White, boiled, mashed...........	½ cup	100
Sweet or yam.......	¼ cup	50
Ice cream, vanilla[3].......	⅛ qt	70
Sponge cake, no icing.....	1½″ cube	25

[3] Omit 2 fat exchanges.

cells is necessary. They are indicated in the maturity-onset diabetic patient in whom diet alone has failed, acetonuria has not been demonstrated, and there is no history of diabetic ketoacidosis. Such a patient can be started on sulfonylureas without the prior use of insulin, or he can be transferred from insulin to sulfonylureas. The chance of therapeutic success with these agents is better when clinical diabetes has been present for a relatively short period of time, if the patient is over the age of forty, and if he or she is overweight. A large initial loading dose is now not considered necessary for the sulfonylureas. In general, side effects are rare; and except for chlorpropamide in high doses, these agents have a good record, especially with respect to hepatic function. Alcohol intolerance has been observed under treatment with sulfonylureas. Occasionally, in elderly undernourished patients, severe hypoglycemia may follow their ad-

ministration. Apart from this, prolonged hypoglycemia is frequently observed when a sulfonylurea is administered to a patient with uremia, as renal excretion of the drug will be delayed. This is the case particularly with chlorpropamide and acetohexamide, as the former is not metabolized to any significant extent and the latter is transformed by the liver to hydroxyhexamide, which also exhibits a potent hypoglycemia property. In both instances, elevated blood levels of the respective drug will lead to severe and protracted hypoglycemia. If this occurs, prolonged and intensive treatment with intravenous glucose (i.e., 200 Gm within 24 hr) and close medical supervision for at least 48 to 72 hr is mandatory.

Between 20 to 30 percent of diabetic patients initially considered to be good candidates for treatment with sulfonylurea will fail to respond after several months or years. This secondary failure can often be attributed to

Table 94-2. FOOD EXCHANGES (*Continued*)

LIST 5. MEAT EXCHANGES
Carbohydrate negligible, protein 7 Gm, fat 5 Gm per serving.
All items expressed in cooked weight.

Food	Approximate measure 1 exchange	Weight, Gm
Meat: Beef, fowl, lamb, veal (medium fat), liver, pork, ham (lean).......	1 oz	30
Cold cuts: Salami, minced ham, bologna, cervelat, liver sausage, luncheon loaf.................	1 slice 4½″ diam. × ⅛″	45
Frankfurters (8 to 9 per lb)	1	50
Fish:		
Cod, haddock, halibut, herring, etc..........	1 oz	30
Salmon, tuna, crab-meat, lobster.......	¼ cup	30
Shrimp, clams, oysters (medium)..........	5	45
Sardines...............	3 medium	30
Cheese:		
Cheddar type..........	1 oz	30
Cottage...............	3 tbsp level	45
Peanut butter[4]..........	2 tbsp scant	30
Egg...................	1	50

[4] Limit to one serving per day unless adjustment is made to balance carbohydrate content.

LIST 6. FAT EXCHANGES
Carbohydrate and protein negligible, fat 5 Gm per serving. Fat exchanges utilized in cooking should be accounted for.

Food	Approximate measure 1 exchange	Weight, Gm
Avocado................	⅛ (4″ diam.)	24
Butter or margarine......	1 tsp level	5
Bacon, crisp.............	1 slice	10
Cream, light, sweet, or sour—20%.......	2 tbsp level	30
Cream, heavy—40%......	1 tbsp level	15
Cream cheese...........	1 tbsp level	15
French dressing.........	1 tbsp level	15
Mayonnaise.............	1 tsp level	5
Nuts...................	6 small	10
Oil or cooking fat........	1 tsp level	5
Olives.................	5 small	50

poor adherence to a prescribed diet, the presence of infection, or the gradual progression of the diabetes to a more insulin-deficient state. Sometimes, a secondary failure is due to destruction of the pancreatic islets by carcinoma or hemochromatosis.

Table 94-3. EXAMPLE OF AN 1800 CALORIE DIABETIC DIET ORDER
(CARBOHYDRATE 181 GM, PROTEIN 90 GM, FAT 80 GM)

Exchange	Break-fast	Lunch	Snack	Supper	Snack
Milk.............	½	1	—		½
Bread............	2	2	1	2	1
Meat............	1	2	1	3	1
Fat.............	1	1	—	2	—
Fruit............	1	1		1	—
Vegetable........	—	1	—	1	
Partition in Gm:					
Carbohydrate......	46	52	15	47	21
Protein...........	15	26	9	27	13
Fat.............	15	25	5	25	10

TOLBUTAMIDE. This is the most widely used oral hypoglycemic agent. Each tablet contains 500 mg. The biologic half-life is approximately 6 hr. It is administered before breakfast *and* before supper, the total daily dose ranging from 1 to 3 Gm. The excretory product in the urine may give a false positive test for albumin, since it is precipitated by acidifying the urine.

ACETOHEXAMIDE. Tablets are available in strengths of 250 and 500 mg. Its half-life is longer and, therefore, a *single* dose may be effective. Recently, a moderate uricosuric property has been attributed to acetohexamide, which would make it a useful drug in subjects with co-existing diabetes and gout.

CHLORPROPAMIDE. Tablets are available containing 100 or 250 mg. The biologic half-life is approximately 36 hr, and daily administration may result in a cumulative effect. The recommended daily dose is 100 to 250 mg before breakfast; it should not exceed 500 mg. Because of its long action, a bedtime snack containing carbohydrate, protein, and fat, e.g., milk with crackers, is advisable. As it has a slightly greater toxic effect on the liver than has tolbutamide or acetohexamide, and since its long half-life may occasionally result in hypoglycemia

Table 94-4. ORAL HYPOGLYCEMIC AGENTS

Generic name	Available form	Average dose	Duration of action
Tolbutamide	500 mg	500–1,000 mg b.i.d.	6–12 hr
Acetohexamide	250 mg 500 mg	250–1,000 mg A.M.	12–24 hr
Tolazamide	100 mg 250 mg	100–500 mg A.M.	16–24 hr
Chlorpropamide	100 mg 250 mg	100–500 mg A.M.	24–36 hr
Phenformin	25 mg tablet 50 mg capsule	25 mg b.i.d. 50 mg b.i.d.	4–6 hr 8–12 hr

in the early morning, it is advisable to keep the daily dose as low as possible.

TOLAZAMIDE. This is available in 100 and 250 mg tablets with a half-life of approximately 12 hr. It is administered in a single or divided dose, not exceeding 500 mg per day.

Biguanides

PHENFORMIN. Of the biguanides, *phenformin,* a phenethyl biguanide (DBI), is commercially available as a 25-mg tablet with a biologic half-life of 3 to 4 hr and as a 50-mg time-disintegration capsule of longer half-life. The mechanism of action differs fundamentally from that of the sulfonylureas in that it can correct hyperglycemia in the pancreatectomized animal and the hypoglycemic effect cannot be produced in nondiabetic-fed subjects. The mechanism of action is still poorly understood, but it appears that phenformin influences the anaerobic pathway of glucose and inhibits hepatic gluconeogenesis. As phenformin makes a diabetic patient occasionally more sensitive to exogenous insulin, it has been suggested that phenformin inhibits an insulin antagonist. The use of phenformin as the only antidiabetic agent is limited because the effective dose is frequently associated with gastrointestinal side effects such as anorexia, nausea, vomiting, and diarrhea. Furthermore, phenformin may contribute to excess lactic acid; it should not be used in those circumstances in which marked tissue hypoxia might be expected to occur, i.e., myocardial infarction, hypotension, low arterial blood oxygen saturation, etc. Fatalities have been reported in which severe lactic acidosis apparently facilitated by the administration of phenformin constituted an important contributory effect. The indications for its use are (1) the very rare diabetic patient of maturity onset who is allergic to the sulfonylureas (the daily recommended dose of phenformin ranges from 50 to 200 mg, to be given either as tablets t.i.d. or as capsules b.i.d.); (2) in combination with sulfonylurea in the elderly patient who fails to respond to a maximum dose of a sulfonylurea; (3) in the brittle diabetic on insulin with frequent hypoglycemic reactions, in whom the addition of phenformin might result in reduction of the insulin requirement and thus facilitate control. Unfortunately, the use of phenformin in this type of patient is often disappointing; (4) in the obese overeating non-insulin-dependent diabetic in whom the sulfonylureas have failed.

The adult-onset diabetic patient can often be controlled by diet alone, and he should be given an adequate trial for several weeks, unless dictated otherwise by clinical circumstances such as acute infection. The multitude of oral agents available, each with somewhat different dosages and durations of actions, make it difficult to master them all; therefore, it is recommended to become familiar with a short-acting drug such as tolbutamide and a longer acting, more powerful agent such as chlorpropamide. A summary of all the available agents is given in Table 94-4. In general, the safety record of the sulfonylureas has been good, however potentiation of their actions by other drugs such as Gantrisin, Butazolidin, and Dicumarol have been reported; therefore, the physician should be aware of such possibilities.

Insulin

The use of insulin is clearly indicated in the youth-onset diabetic and in those patients with maturity-onset diabetes in whom diet and oral hypoglycemic agents have proved inadequate to maintain satisfactory levels of blood glucose in both the fasting and the postprandial state. Furthermore, the use of insulin is mandatory in diabetic ketoacidosis.

TYPES OF INSULIN. In the United States the animal sources for insulin are beef and pork. As human insulin has a structure similar to that of pork, the use of pure pork insulin rather than a beef-pork mixture may be preferred. Apart from the species difference, seven types of insulin are commercially available. They can be divided into insulins of fast, intermediate, and long action. Their properties are summarized in Table 94-5.

Each of the insulins is available in two different strengths, namely, 40 or 80 units per milliliter. The choice between the two is governed according to the amount of insulin required by the patient. If only a small amount is necessary, for example, 16 units, the use of U 40 will allow a more accurate dosage; if a larger amount is required, U 80 has the advantage of a smaller volume.

CHOICE OF INSULIN. (1) Crystalline insulin is best for emergencies, such as the treatment of diabetic ketoacidosis or the achievement of fast control in the patient with

Table 94-5. INSULIN ACTION CURVES

Action	Insulin	Modifier	Duration of action, hr	Maximum effect, hrs postinjection
Fast.....................	Crystalline zinc (regular)	None	6	2–3
	Semi-Lente	Zinc	12	3–6
Intermediate..............	Globin	Globin	18	6–8
	NPH	Protamine	24	8–10
	Lente	Zinc	24	8–10
Long....................	Ultralente	Zinc	36	12–20
	Protamine zinc	Protamine	36	12–20

marked hyperglycemia; it is also employed for daily use in combination with an intermediate insulin to bring on earlier action. (2) Intermediate insulins in a single dose injected before breakfast will control the majority of diabetics. The dosage will be gauged by the prelunch, midafternoon, and fasting blood sugar values. The midafternoon blood glucose corresponds to the peak of insulin action and will dictate the maximum morning dose. It is advisable that all patients receiving an intermediate insulin be given a midafternoon snack. If the midafternoon blood glucose level is between 80 and 120 mg per 100 ml, and the prelunch value is still unduly elevated, the addition of a small amount of crystalline insulin at breakfast time is indicated. It can be mixed with NPH or lente in the same syringe. Almost all maturity-onset diabetics can be adequately controlled by intermediate insulins alone or in combination with crystalline insulin administered before breakfast.

The patient with youth-onset diabetes often develops nocturnal hyperglycemia and, consequently, will exhibit a high fasting blood glucose associated with glycosuria. Further increase in the morning dose of intermediate insulin will often lead to hypoglycemia in the midafternoon. To reduce the fasting blood glucose to normal levels, a long-acting insulin can be tried, but often a second small dose of the intermediate insulin before supper or at bedtime is preferable. The latter regime is eminently satisfactory in the 24-hr control of the juvenile diabetic, and usually patients do not complain about the second injection because they feel so much better. Very rarely, sugar is spilled at bedtime but none before supper. Then the addition of a small amount of crystalline insulin to the evening dose of NPH is indicated, and both are given before supper. As a general rule, it can be stated that whenever insulin is given in the evening in addition to the morning dose, the latter should be reduced. (3) The use of long-acting insulin with the hope of establishing control with a single morning injection, in general, has been disappointing.

INITIATION OF INSULIN THERAPY. If the patient has massive glycosuria and elevated blood glucose, insulin therapy is begun immediately with crystalline insulin. The following schedule is recommended: 20 units for a 4+, 15 units for a 3+, and 10 units for a 2+ urine test. Once the acute syndrome is under reasonable control, or if the metabolic derangement is less dramatic, a longer acting insulin can be started. It is best to start with 10 or 20 units of NPH or lente and increase this by 5 units per day, as indicated by urine tests and blood glucose levels. Most diabetic patients will require between 30 and 50 units of insulin daily.

COMPLICATIONS OF INSULIN THERAPY. Insulin Reactions. These are commonly caused by excess insulin dosage, delayed food intake, or unusual physical activity. Very rarely, an increased sensitivity to insulin is due to early adrenal or pituitary hypofunction and, even more exceptionally, to development of a functioning islet cell tumor. Occasional insulin reactions are almost unavoidable, especially in the juvenile insulin-sensitive diabetic, but they are harmless if recognized and treated early. To

reduce them to a minimum, it is essential that the patient knows how to test his urine for glucose and, provided he does not have an elevated renal threshold for glucose, how to reduce his insulin dose when his urine tests indicate absence of glucose for several days. The patient also has to be instructed to eat his meals on time and, when unusual physical activity is anticipated, either to reduce his morning insulin dose or to ingest extra calories to compensate for the blood-sugar-lowering effect of exercise.

The signs and symptoms of an insulin reaction vary with the type of insulin used. *Crystalline insulin produces a characteristic reaction* of rapid onset consisting of hunger, a peculiar abdominal sensation, sweating, palpitation, tremor, tachycardia, weakness, irritability, and pallor. Patients usually recognize these symptoms early, and they are relieved within minutes by ingestion of carbohydrate: sugar, orange juice, candy, etc. To prevent any awkward situation, every diabetic patient on insulin should carry several lumps of sugar with him at all times. As a patient in insulin reaction may act as though he were intoxicated, *it is further recommended that all diabetics carry a card identifying them as such.* This is especially important in patients with a long history of diabetes. Due to neuropathy, sympathetic nervous system signs may gradually be lost, and thus the patient lacks indications of impending reaction and may exhibit only impairment of cerebral functions. *The intermediate and long-acting insulins produce a more gradual decline in blood glucose* with consequently less release of epinephrine; symptoms are produced by deficient glucose metabolism of the higher nervous centers. They consist of headache, blurred or double vision, fine tremor, uncontrollable yawning, hypothermia, mental confusion, incoordination, and eventually, unconsciousness. In elderly persons an insulin reaction may mimic a cerebrovascular accident. Treatment is administration of glucose by mouth or by vein. In severe and prolonged insulin reactions it is advisable to administer a glucocorticoid to produce maximum stimulation of gluconeogenesis. Relatives of diabetic patients prone to severe insulin reactions, and especially parents of diabetic children, should be instructed in the use of glucagon. It can be injected subcutaneously, just as insulin, and will lead to a transient rise in blood glucose that is long enough to wake the patient up and enable him to receive some carbohydrate by mouth.

Recurrent hypoglycemic attacks, with their attendant anxiety, headache, loss of concentration power, etc., constitute a nuisance to the diabetic patient, but only *severe and prolonged* attacks of hypoglycemia will lead to intellectual deterioration as a result of irreversible damage to cortical neurones.

An insulin reaction initiates a counterregulatory mechanism characterized by release of epinephrine, adrenal corticosteroids, and growth hormone. This will result in a rebound hyperglycemia, for "hypoglycemia begets hyperglycemia." Knowledge of this physiologic defense mechanism will prevent the physician from administering extra insulin to combat this hyperglycemia. If the insulin reaction is due to excess insulin, the patient will benefit from a reduced insulin dosage.

Reactions at the Site of Insulin Injection

Such reactions are not uncommon at the beginning of treatment. They are characterized by redness, swelling, pain, and nodule formation. As they usually disappear within a few days or weeks, the patient can be reassured, and no treatment is indicated. If the local reaction persists, it can be improved by changing to an insulin of the lente type, which does not contain protamine. Skin infections at the site of injection are extremely rare.

Insulin Lipodystrophy

This reaction is characterized by either hypertrophy or atrophy of the subcutaneous adipose tissue at the site of insulin injection. This is frequent and affects children and females more than males. If the patient is bothered by the esthetic aspect of this complication, injection of insulin into other sites is recommended until the lesion improves; then the atrophic area may again be used in the hope of inducing lipogenesis.

Insulin Resistance

Almost all diabetic patients treated with insulin for several months will develop circulating antibodies to insulin. However, only a few (approximately 1 in 1,000 insulin-treated diabetics) will develop insulin resistance. By definition it is present if the daily insulin requirement in the absence of ketoacidosis exceeds 200 units. Patients with insulin resistance may require several thousand units daily. When insulin resistance is associated with hemochromatosis, severe infections, Cushing's syndrome, acromegaly, or hyperthyroidism, it is secondary. Frequently, no obvious cause can be detected. Examination of serum will demonstrate the presence of large quantities of antibodies to insulin and an increased insulin-binding capacity. In such patients a trial with pure pork insulin is always justified, and very often a sizable reduction in insulin requirement can be achieved. If such a simple measure fails, the use of steroids is indicated, for their anti-insulin effect is outweighed by their antiallergic effect. Rarely the sulfonylureas are helpful. The natural course of idiopathic insulin resistance is characterized by spontaneous remission within several weeks or months. Frequently, the resistance breaks abruptly and the patient exhibits episodes of severe hypoglycemia as the antibody-bound insulin is released and becomes suddenly available.

COMPLICATIONS OF DIABETES

Diabetic Ketoacidosis and Coma

Lack of insulin is the cause of diabetic ketoacidosis. The patient may be (1) an undiagnosed diabetic, (2) a known diabetic who fails to increase his insulin dose despite poor urine tests, or (3) a known diabetic who suffers from nausea and vomiting and, as he does not eat, reasons that he does not need his daily insulin. Omission of insulin probably constitutes the single largest cause of diabetic acidosis.

DIAGNOSIS. Among clinical signs and symptoms, vomiting is present in approximately two-thirds of patients with acidosis. Abdominal pain and tenderness may be related to nausea and vomiting or sodium depletion and may be so severe as to mimic an abdominal emergency ("pseudoappendicitis" of diabetic acidosis). Air hunger and heavy labored breathing as described by Kussmaul are expressions of the acidosis and correlate with the reduction in serum CO_2. There is dehydration as evidenced by soft eyeballs, dry skin, poor urinary output, and hypotension. Laboratory findings include the following: the urine usually contains massive amounts of glucose and acetone; frequently there is also transient albuminuria. The diagnosis of diabetic ketoacidosis is made, however, by finding hyperglycemia, ketonemia, and reduction of serum CO_2 content. The acidosis is metabolic and is caused by accumulation of ketone bodies associated with loss of sodium and potassium. The azotemia is due partly to dehydration and partly to tissue protein breakdown. Serum lipids are generally increased. The rise in hematocrit indicates dehydration; usually there is leukocytosis.

DIFFERENTIAL DIAGNOSIS. On clinical grounds alone it is sometimes difficult to distinguish between diabetic acidosis and an insulin reaction. If any doubt exists, blood should be drawn for laboratory tests and 50 ml of 50 percent glucose injected intravenously. If the coma is due to insulin reaction, the patient will wake up immediately; if he is in diabetic coma, no harm has been done. Among diagnoses to be considered are salicylate poisoning; lactic acidosis; hyperglycemic, hyperosmolaric, nonketotic coma; or far-advanced renal failure—all conditions which can occur in a diabetic patient.

TREATMENT. This will vary greatly from patient to patient; however, the general principles are as follows: (1) through a large needle blood is withdrawn for laboratory tests (blood glucose, BUN, Na, K, Cl, CO_2 Hct, plasma acetone), and the vein is kept open with an infusion of normal saline. The rationale for this rests on the observation that patients in diabetic coma may decompensate very rapidly, and precious time will be lost in finding a vein and performing a venous cutdown. (2) Crystalline insulin is administered both subcutaneously and intravenously. The average dosage of insulin required for patients in diabetic coma is 200 units, 100 units intravenously and 100 units subcutaneously. The dosage, of course, will vary from patient to patient and may have to be larger for an obese diabetic and less in a frail, elderly diabetic. If the patient has been in diabetic coma previously and required 300 units to respond, chances are he may require a similar dose again. Severe acidosis necessitates reevaluation of blood glucose, serum CO_2, and serum acetone levels every 2 hr; if less severe, every 4 hr will suffice. If the blood glucose level remains above 500 mg per 100 ml and serum acetone is positive at 1:4 dilution, another 100 units of insulin should be given. If the patient does not respond at all or if he deteriorates, successive doses are increased rapidly and given at hourly intervals. An occasional patient may require 5,000 or 10,000 units within the first 24 hr of treatment. If, on the other hand, at the fourth hour the level of blood glucose has decreased but remains above 400 mg per 100 ml, administration of another 50 units of insulin is indicated. (3) All patients in diabetic acidosis are severely dehydrated and depleted of sodium and potassium. They will require a large amount of fluid, usually a total of 4 to 8 liters during the first 24 hr. Many electrolyte formulas have been proposed for adequate replacement, and though their value is not doubted, it is important to start fluid therapy *immediately*, which is best done with the universally available normal (0.9 percent) saline solution. Once treatment is under way and the laboratory has reported values for blood glucose, serum CO_2, and electrolytes, finer adjustments can be made. The addition of bicarbonate is certainly indicated if the acidosis is severe (CO_2-combining capacity less than 10). It may also counteract the inhibitory effect a lowered pH has on insulin activity and therefore restore the patient's sensitivity to insulin. Once the blood glucose approaches 200 mg per 100 ml, the intravenous fluid should be changed to 5% glucose in saline in order to avoid hypoglycemia. Usually there is also a deficiency of potassium, and this should be replaced, starting at the second or third hour, at a rate not exceeding 20 mEq per hour; rarely more than 80 mEq is needed during the initial 24 hr of treatment. The need for and administration of potassium can be monitored with an electrocardiograph. Signs of hypokalemia are flattening or inversion of T waves and prolongation of the Q-T intervals. (4) There are useful accessory procedures in treatment of diabetic acidosis. If the patient is unconscious, gastric lavage should be performed to prevent aspiration pneumonia. If the patient is in obvious circulatory collapse, blood, plasma, or a plasma volume expander should be given. Finally, the precipitating cause for the development of diabetic acidosis has to be established for each patient before specific treatment can be initiated. (5) The acute phase of diabetic acidosis is considered ended once the patient is completely responsive, the blood glucose is below 200 mg per 100 ml, the undiluted serum shows no evidence for acetone, serum CO_2 is normal, and the urine shows minimal glycosuria and not more than 1+ acetone. Now is the time to start the patient on intermediate insulin in a small dose to prevent a relapse into ketosis and also, if needed, to give crystalline insulin in amounts dictated by urine sugar levels. A soft diet should be started. It is essential to begin with frequent small feedings. Intravenous fluid administration may be discontinued as soon as the patient is able to retain liquids by mouth. The overall mortality of patients with diabetic acidosis is approximately 5 percent. A very rare but serious complication of diabetic ketoacidosis is facial mucormycosis, see Chap. 191.

Hyperglycemic Nonketotic Coma

This entity is characterized by extreme elevation of blood glucose (values of 1,000 mg per 100 ml or higher are not rare; "syrupy" blood), and absence of ketonemia or acetonuria. The marked hyperglycemia and the associated hypernatremia secondary to water loss lead to an increase in extracellular fluid osmolarity with consequent intracellular dehydration, the effect of which on the central nervous system accounts for the neurologic symptoms and coma. Serum osmolarity can be estimated by multiplying the Na concentration times 2 and adding 5.5 for each 100 mg of glucose (molecular weight of glucose is 180, therefore $100/18 = 5.5$). Normal values range between 290 and 310 mOsm per liter. A patient with values of Na of 160 mEq per liter and of blood glucose of 1,000 mg per 100 ml exhibits an approximate serum osmolarity of $320 + 55 = 375$ mOsm per liter. The highest level recorded is 458 mOsm per liter.

It is observed usually in the middle-aged or older person, frequently associated with corticosteroid therapy or peritoneal dialysis and may be the first indication of diabetes. Awareness of this syndrome is important, as a comatose patient seen for the first time may be misdiagnosed, as he will show massive glycosuria but no acetone, and therefore it is reasoned that the cause for his coma is not diabetic ketoacidosis and no antidiabetic treatment is initiated. Thus valuable time may be lost. Treatment consists of intravenous fluid, preferably hypotonic saline and insulin. Some patients are markedly sensitive to insulin, and 25 to 50 units may suffice, whereas others may require 200 or more units. According to the literature the mortality of this diabetic complication approximates 50 percent; however, in our personal experience with eight patients only one patient died. After recovery not all patients will require insulin. Some can be carried with oral agents or diet alone.

Diabetic Retinopathy

This can be detected in varying degrees in more than 90 percent of diabetic patients after 20 years of clinical diabetes.

The earliest recognizable lesions on fundoscopy are dilatation of veins and "microaneurysms" which actually consist of small punctate hemorrhages. Unless they occur within the macula, the vision will not be impaired. Other relatively early lesions are waxy exudates. This stage of the retinopathy can remain stationary for many years. It is the long-term juvenile diabetic who may progress to a more malignant stage, that of neovascularization and proliferative retinopathy. The new blood vessels usually emanate from the disk and grow toward the vitreous. If a preretinal hemorrhage occurs, organization takes place with formation of fibrous and collagenous tissue. Shrinkage of the scar tissue will produce retinal detachment (Fig. 94-1 and color plate). Advanced diabetic retinopathy is frequently associated with retinal lesions caused by atherosclerosis, arterial hypertension, and renal insufficiency.

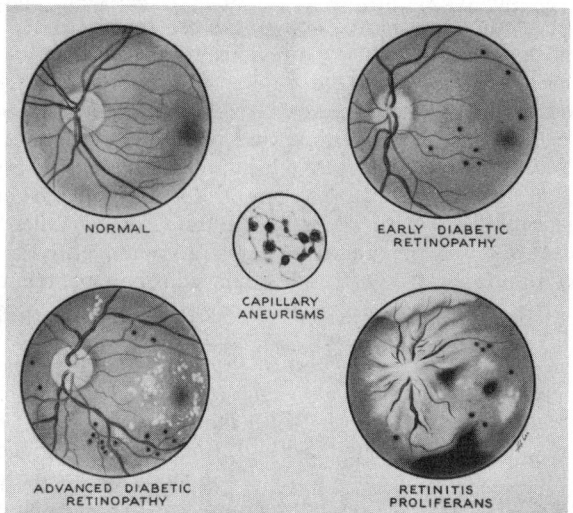

Fig. 94-1. Note the early dilatation of the venules and the punctate hemorrhages *in early diabetic retinopathy* actually representing capillary aneurysms surrounded by hemorrhages, as shown in a microscopic preparation of the retina (*center*). In *advanced diabetic retinopathy*, note in addition the typical hard, waxy exudates. In *retinitis proliferans* is seen the spread of connective tissue, revealed as a white material emanating from the optic disk, together with endovascularization in the form of small irregular vessels. Note the detachment of the retina at the top of the figure, and the larger hemorrhages.

The appearance of retinopathy is fundamentally related to duration of diabetes; one of the reasons for strict chemical control of the metabolic component of diabetes is the possibility of delaying its onset and if possible, making it less severe. If incapacitating retinopathy is present, pituitary ablation should be considered, either by stalk section, total hypophysectomy, or irradiation. Poor vision in one eye and rapidly progressing retinopathy in the other eye constitute the major indication. However, the patient needs to be carefully selected as to emotional stability, long-term willingness to cooperate, and relative freedom from coronary artery disease or nephropathy. As hypoglycemia presents a major hazard after pituitary intervention, the patient should preferably not be living alone. After ablation of the pituitary, preliminary results indicate that two-thirds of patients have stabilized or improved their vision. The factor responsible for improvement has not been identified. Whereas pituitary manipulation represents a last effort to salvage vision, and is associated with the iatrogenic induction of thyroid, adrenal, and gonadal deficiency, newer forms of treatment are directed towards the affected eyes themselves. They are photocoagulation, introduced by Meyer-Schwickerath, and laser beam treatment of the retina. Preliminary results indicate that these procedures may be applied to *early* retinal lesions, and the results obtained are encouraging.

Diabetic Nephropathy

(See Chap. 311 for discussion.)

Diabetic Neuropathy

This is a common, distressing, and therapeutically unsatisfactory complication of diabetes at any stage. Although it most frequently involves peripheral nerves, it may involve any portion of the nervous system and, thus, has an almost unlimited range of manifestations (Table 94-6). The peripheral neuropathy is characterized by a

Table 94-6. DIABETIC NEUROPATHIES

Peripheral:
    Sensory: loss of vibratory sense, paresthesias, pain, loss of pain
    Neuromuscular: weakness, paralysis, absent tendon reflexes, diabetic amytrophy (thighs), extraocular muscle palsies
Autonomic:
    Eye: pupillary changes
    Gastrointestinal: delayed gastric emptying, gallbladder dysfunction, nocturnal diarrhea
    Genitourinary: sexual impotence, atonic urinary bladder, retrograde ejaculation
    Vascular: orthostatic hypotension
    Bones and joints: neuropathic joint (Charcot)
    Skin: neurogenic ulcer, absent sweating, dependent edema

nonsegmental distribution. An interesting differential diagnosis is presented by the patient with severe headache and ocular palsy. If an intracranial aneurysm can be ruled out by angiogram, diabetic neuropathy may be the underlying cause. The neuropathy may be primarily metabolic, which is potentially reversible, or primarily vascular, which is less amenable to treatment.

Treatment of diabetic neuropathy consists of careful control of the diabetes; however, it is not specific, and weeks or months may pass before improvement takes place. If the neuropathy is associated with hyperlipemia, a trial with Clofibrate, 2 Gm daily, is justified.

Gangrene of the Feet

This is a serious and frequent complication of diabetes, especially in the older age group. It may be due to vascular lesions ("pulseless" foot) or to neuropathy ("painless" foot), usually with a superimposed infection or injury. Gangrene may also be associated with small vessel disease in which pedal pulses are not decreased. Arterial insufficiency is diagnosed by a history of claudication and by finding, on examination, weak or absent pedal pulses, blanching of the foot when raised above a 45° angle, and delayed venous filling when the foot is dependent. An arteriogram is indicated. Amputation is the treatment; hence, prevention, or at least delay of onset, of gangrene is of paramount importance. Simple rules for prevention include (1) washing the feet with warm but never *hot* water each evening; (2) applying lanolin two or three times weekly if the skin is dry; (3) inserting lamb's wool between overlapping toes; (4) avoiding injuries to feet (the patient should never go barefoot); (5) not cutting toenails if vision is poor; (6) treating of corns and calluses by a qualified podiatrist or surgeon.

SURGERY AND DIABETES MELLITUS

Diabetic patients may be affected by any surgical disease, but there are certain conditions, such as gangrene of the foot and cholelithiasis, to which they are more prone than the average person. There is also a strong association between cancer of the pancreas and diabetes. In addition, surgical problems may be unrelated to diabetes, such as repair of a hernia. As diabetes is a relatively common condition, from time to time every surgeon and anesthesist will be confronted with a diabetic patient.

The present surgical mortality in diabetics is approximately that of the general population. The surgical risk is increased in diabetics in the presence of poor regulation, obesity, arteriosclerosis, and cardiovascular-renal disease. However, even for the uncomplicated diabetic patient, operation and anesthesia constitute an additional metabolic stress, which will accentuate the predisposition to hyperglycemia and ketosis. Nevertheless, diabetes constitutes no contraindication to surgery; and if the case is an emergency, only a few hours are generally needed to evaluate and prepare such a patient for operation.

On admission for elective or emergency surgery, the patient with diabetes presents in either of two ways: either he is a known diabetic under treatment with varying degree of metabolic control, or the diagnosis of diabetes is suggested by routine preoperative testing. If the scheduled surgery is elective in nature and the diabetes requires further regulation, surgery should be postponed until glycosuria is minimal, acetonuria absent, and preprandial blood glucose close to normal. If, on the other hand, surgery is urgent and there is marked hyperglycemia and ketosis, vigorous treatment is started immediately with intravenous fluid and insulin. The majority of diabetic patients will not present in this dramatic way; most of them are under reasonable metabolic control. Their management during surgery will vary according to the severity of their condition. As a general principle, one should aim to prevent acetonuria and excessive protein breakdown by providing an adequate carbohydrate intake. This is done on the day of surgery by replacing the oral feedings with intravenous 5% or 10% glucose in water or saline, the volume being dictated by the cardiac state and fear of overhydration. Usually, 1,000 to 1,500 ml of 5% glucose in saline is sufficient. By history and laboratory evaluation three types of diabetes are encountered: (1) mild diabetes, treated with diet alone; only close surveillance with frequent urine testing and daily blood glucose is required. (2) Patients on oral agents, such as tolbutamide, acetohexamide, tolazamide, chlorpropamide; or phenformin. As oral intake is usually impossible on the day of surgery, these patients are best changed to a small amount of intermediate-acting (lente or NPH) insulin, for example, 10 to 20 units. Once oral feedings are resumed in the postoperative period, insulin is discontinued and the respective tablets restarted at the former dose. (3) Patients previously on insulin and well controlled receive on the day of surgery two-thirds of their usual *total* dose, preferably divided into a preoperative and postoperative dose, and omitting crystalline insulin. Example: Preoperative insulin dose = 10 units crystalline insulin, 35 units NPH, total dose 45 units. Therefore, on the day of surgery, one-third, or 15 units, of NPH is given preoperatively, and 15 units of NPH is given postoperatively. It is customary in some centers not to give any preoperative insulin, presumably due to fear of hypoglycemia, and only to administer crystalline insulin according to urine test in the postoperative period. In our experience, hypoglycemia occurs rarely if the preoperative insulin is only NPH or lente, provided the total dose is reduced by one-third and, furthermore, if glucose is administered intravenously throughout the operative period. The benefits of this regimen are that the patient does not escape into severe hyperglycemia or ketosis with resultant electrolyte imbalance during surgery or the immediate postoperative period.

PREGNANCY AND DIABETES MELLITUS

The problem of management during pregnancy has assumed increasing importance, as young diabetic patients now survive longer and are thus capable of procreation. Infertility in female diabetic patients, common before insulin therapy, is rarely seen with good control of the diabetes. The problems engendered by pregnancy in diabetics concern maternal survival, fetal salvage, and prevention of diabetes in the offspring.

Today pregnancy carries but slightly added risk to the well-managed diabetic mother; the maternal survival is 99.7 percent (White). In contrast, fetal mortality is still high. Stillbirths among diabetics are six times as common as among nondiabetics. Fetal salvage will depend on the duration of the mother's disease and presence or absence of vascular lesions such as nephropathy.

Diagnosis

In patients not previously known as diabetic, pregnancy may induce a temporary state of diabetes. The diagnosis may offer some difficulty, since with the lowered renal threshold of pregnancy, glycosuria is not uncommon even among nondiabetic pregnant women. If urinary glucose is found during pregnancy and there is, in addition, a history of frequent miscarriages, of babies with a birth weight exceeding 9 lb, or a family history of diabetes, diabetes should be suspected. The diagnosis can be firmly established only by the presence of abnormal blood glucose levels, whether fasting or postprandial. If they are borderline, performance of a glucose tolerance test is definitely indicated.

Treatment

The best results are obtained by close cooperation between the patient, the internist, and the obstetrician. The treatment of pregnant diabetic patients entails the same general health measures as those recommended for nondiabetic pregnant women. It is desirable to maintain a high intake of protein (i.e., at least 2 Gm per kg body weight per day) with a total caloric intake of 30 Cal per kg body weight and an adequate intake of calcium and iron. To prevent edema and minimize hydramnios, a low-salt diet is indicated, and the liberal use of diuretics is advisable. In most women, diabetes is regulated throughout pregnancy with insulin. Because of the lowered renal threshold for glucose one should not attempt to keep the urine sugar-free. It is admittedly often difficult to avoid excessive weight gain, but at least 200 Gm carbohydrate must be utilized to prevent ketosis.

Care of a diabetic patient through the first trimester may be difficult because of nausea and vomiting. If antiemetic drugs fail to control nausea and vomiting and frequent small feedings are not well tolerated, intravenous glucose must be administered. In the last trimester the insulin requirement usually increases concurrently with a rise in adrenal cortical activity, the presence of hormonal anti-insulin factors of placental origin, and placental destruction of insulin. It is of utmost importance to detect preeclamptic toxemia and hydramnios, since treatment will reduce fetal mortality. Timing of delivery is also important. The more advanced the diabetic state of the mother, the earlier the delivery should be attempted. Patients with only chemical diabetes can be delivered at term, patients with vascular complications should be delivered at the thirty-sixth week. The child may be delivered vaginally or by section. Early delivery has the advantage of removing the infant before it becomes too large and before placental circulation is impaired. The latter may be either the cause or the effect of the tendency to toxemia. A sudden decrease of insulin requirement to prepregnancy level usually follows delivery; therefore, it is advisable to omit the insulin dose on the day of delivery and to administer glucose intravenously.

CARE OF THE NEWBORN

Special attention has to be paid to the predisposition of newborn infants of diabetic mothers to develop the respiratory distress syndrome (hyaline membrane disease) and hypoglycemia.

The incidence of diabetes later in life in a child delivered of a diabetic mother is 22 percent and thus not essentially different from that of the general population with either a diabetic mother or a diabetic father.

REFERENCES

Bressler, R.: Investigative Issues in Diabetes Mellitus, Arch. Int. Med., 123:219, 1969.

Butterfield, W. J. H., and W. Van Westering: Tolbutamide after Ten Years, Excerpta Med., 1967.

Clarke, B. F., and Duncan, L. J. P.: Comparison of Chlorpropamide and Metformin Treatment of Weight and Blood Glucose Response of Uncontrolled Obese Diabetics, Lancet, I:123, 1968.

Duncan, L. J. P.: Diabetes Mellitus, Edinburgh, University Press, 1966.

Goldberg, M. F., and S. L. Fine: Symposium on the Treatment of Diabetic Retinopathy, Public Health Service Publication No. 1890, 1969.

Grodsky, G. M., and P. H. Forsham: Insulin and the Pancreas, Ann. Rev. Physiol., 28:347, 1966.

Halmos, P. B., J. K. Nelson, and R. C. Lowry: Hyperosmolar Non-ketoacidotic Coma in Diabetes, Lancet, I:675, 1966.

Hirsch, J., and P. W. Han: Cellularity of Adipose Tissue: Effects of Growth, Starvation, and Obesity, J. Lipid. Res., 10:77, 1969.

Lacy, P. E.: The Pancreatic Beta Cell, Structure and Function, New Engl. J. Med., 276:187, 1967.

Special Report: Classification of Genetic Diabetes Mellitus, Diabetes, 16:540, 1967.

Steiner, D. F., D. Cunningham, L. Spigelman, and B. Aten: Insulin Biosynthesis, Evidence for a Precursor, Science, 157:697, 1967.

U.S. Department of Health, Education, and Welfare: "Diabetes Source Book," No. 1168, May, 1964.

Warren, S., P. M. LeCompte, and M. A. Legg, "The Pathology of Diabetes Mellitus," 5th ed., Philadelphia, Lea & Febiger, 1966.

White, P. (ed.): "Diabetes," Med. Clinics N. Am., 49:4, 1965.

95 NONDIABETIC MELITURIA
Alexander Marble

DEFINITION. Nondiabetic melituria includes a variety of conditions in which, apart from diabetes mellitus, sugar appears in the urine in amounts large enough to yield positive tests by methods in common clinical use. It is, therefore, not a precisely defined entity. Certain of the conditions appear to be inborn errors of metabolism, and most, though not all, are asymptomatic anomalies with no apparent influence on longevity.

CLASSIFICATION. The nondiabetic meliturias may be classified by whether or not the sugar found in the urine is glucose, as shown in Table 95-1.

GLUCOSURIC MELITURIA

PHYSIOLOGY. Normally, the concentration of glucose in the glomerular filtrate is the same as that in the plasma water. Glucose is reabsorbed in the proximal convoluted tubules, chiefly in their proximal portions. Since the passage of glucose through the tubular mucosa takes place against an ever-increasing gradient, the reabsorption involves an active transport process requiring energy. As the concentration of glucose in the plasma increases, the amount of glucose absorbed by the tubules reaches a

Table 95-1. TYPES OF NONDIABETIC MELITURIA

I. Glucosuric melituria
   A. Renal glucosuria
      1. Hereditary
         a. "True" renal glucosuria with glucosuria invariably
            present even during fasting
         b. Associated with other renal tubular defects, as in
            the Fanconi syndrome
      2. Nonhereditary
         a. Pregnancy
         b. Nephropathy, with damage to proximal tubules
   B. Transient glucosuria in diverse conditions in which there
      is temporary hyperglycemia considered not to be due to
      diabetes
II. Nonglucosuric melituria
   A. Pentosuria
   B. Fructosuria
      1. Essential fructosuria
      2. Hereditary fructose intolerance
   C. Lactosuria
   D. Galactosuria
   E. Mannoheptulosuria
   F. Other conditions

transfer maximum (Tm_G), which in the normal adult is about 300 to 350 mg per minute. When the arterial blood glucose exceeds a certain level (usually about 150 to 180 mg per 100 ml) and the amount of glucose presented to the tubules for reabsorption is greater than the Tm_G, glucose appears in the urine. However, this concentration of blood glucose, often called the *renal threshold,* is not rigidly fixed and is not the sole factor concerned. Changes in the glomerular filtration rate alter the total quantity of glucose reaching the proximal tubules per unit of time and variations in the activity of tubules of individual nephrons influence the composite effect.

RENAL GLUCOSURIA. "True" renal glucosuria with glucose in the urine constantly and persistently even during the fasting state (with blood glucose levels below 100 mg per 100 ml) is a rare condition. Among approximately 50,000 patients with melituria, this type and degree of renal glucosuria was recognized in only 85 cases. However, if the designation of renal glucosuria is made more loosely so as to include situations in which the renal threshold is lower than average but not below 100 mg per 100 ml, the number of cases may be large. Whether or not there is any basic difference in the situations responsible for these varying degrees of lowering of the renal threshold, and whether or not one is justified in considering "true" renal glucosuria an entity, cannot be answered with the information available. Indeed, the cause and nature of the tubular abnormality in renal glucosuria remain obscure. Renal biopsy studies, admittedly few in number and limited in scope, have failed to demonstrate any specific anatomic or enzymatic defect.

Renal glucosuria is a condition set apart from diabetes mellitus. Glucosuria is invariably present, and the blood glucose is unquestionably normal both on random sampling and during an oral glucose tolerance test. Measures designed to evaluate carbohydrate utilization yield normal results, and ketosis develops during starvation rather than after dietary excesses. Symptoms characteristic of diabetes are lacking, and without treatment the condition is not progressive.

Renal glucosuria has been thought to be inherited as a dominant trait. However, the results of certain family surveys suggest that it is transmitted as a single autosomal gene which, in its homozygous expression, is manifested by persistent, gross glucosuria and in its heterozygous expression by slight or no glucosuria. Although, as stated above, it appears to be unrelated to diabetes mellitus, diabetes seems to occur in the families of persons with renal glucosuria with a frequency greater than expected. There is no evidence that diabetes develops later among persons with "true" renal glucosuria to a greater extent than would be expected in the general population. Care must be taken at the time of original study to exclude those persons in whom glucose tolerance tests yielded borderline results. It is important that persons thought to have renal glucosuria be observed closely, particularly for the first few years in order to establish with reasonable certainty the diagnosis of a benign condition.

Decreased capacity of the renal tubules to reabsorb glucose may be part of a more extensive disturbance of tubular function, as in the *Fanconi syndrome,* which is characterized also by defective reabsorption of amino acids, phosphate, and bicarbonate (see Chap. 103 and 104).

Temporary renal glucosuria occurs frequently in *pregnancy,* particularly during the latter half. The mechanism is poorly understood. The chief responsibility of the physician is to make sure that the condition is benign glucosuria and not diabetes mellitus, which may well have its onset or be recognized first during pregnancy. "Screening" tests should be made by determining the level of blood glucose at 1 hr after 50 Gm glucose, after a meal liberal in carbohydrate, or after the intravenous administration of glucose (see Chap. 94).

Glucosuria of varying degree and duration may also occur in nephropathies in which there is tubular damage and impaired absorption of glucose. These include certain nephritides and particularly nephrosis resulting from the administration of chemical agents such as heavy metals and (in animals) phlorhizin.

Patients with diabetes mellitus may also have a renal threshold lower than normal. When insulin is used in treatment, the dosage must be chosen carefully with special attention to the blood glucose. Parallel studies of blood and urine glucose will furnish a practical guide as to what degree of glucosuria must be allowed to prevent episodes of hypoglycemia.

TRANSIENT GLUCOSURIA IN DIVERSE CONDITIONS. Glucose may appear in the urine transiently and intermittently in a wide variety of conditions, including disorders of the pituitary (acromegaly, pituitary basophilism), adrenals (Cushing's syndrome, pheochromocytoma), and thyroid (hyperthyroidism); stimulation of intracranial nerve centers as with brain tumors, cerebral hemorrhage, and injuries of the skull; infections, toxemias, anesthesia, and asphyxia; administration of carbohydrate following starvation ("hunger glucosuria"); following subtotal gastrectomy; acute myocardial infarction; and malignant disease. In most of these conditions hyperglycemia is present temporarily and affords a satisfactory explanation for the glucosuria. However, recent studies and experience suggest that often diabetes mellitus is actually present in early or latent form and has been brought to the level of clinical recognition by the stressful situation. Accordingly, patients with temporary hyperglycemia and glucosuria require careful observation and periodic examinations for years so that if overt diabetes should develop, it may be recognized early. Such individuals should be encouraged to keep the body weight throughout life at a level appropriate for age, height, and body build.

NONGLUCOSURIC MELITURIA

In patients with persistent normoglycemic melituria it is important to ascertain the type of sugar excreted. In most instances the reducing substance will be found to be glucose, but in a number of cases sufficiently large to make special study definitely worthwhile, the sugar is not glucose but pentose, fructose, or some other sugar less commonly encountered. These sugars bear no relation to diabetes mellitus, and their recognition has practical importance as regards eligibility for employment, life insurance, etc., since for the most part these conditions are benign. A systematic study includes the following procedures:

1. Benedict's test, or a modification (Clinitest). This is positive for all sugars found in the urine. The ketoses, particularly fructose, the pentoses, and mannoheptulose, reduce Benedict's solution after a few hours at room temperature (i.e., without heating) and within 10 min at 50 to 60°C.

2. Glucose oxidase test (specific for glucose). Paper strips (Tes-tape and Clinistix) are available for quick testing.

3. Bial (orcinol hydrochloride) reaction. It is positive for pentose.

4. Seliwaroff (resorcinol hydrochloride) reaction. It is positive for fructose.

5. Paper chromatography to confirm the identity of the sugar.

6. Formation of characteristic osazone crystals with phenylhydrazine or (in the case of fructose) methylphenylhydrazine. This may be carried a step further by determination of the melting point of the crystals (glucosazone, 205°C; pentosazone, 157 to 160°C).

7. Fermentation with baker's yeast. Glucose and fructose are always, galactose usually, lactose occasionally, and pentose and mannoheptulose never fermented.

PENTOSURIA. Essential pentosuria is a benign condition inherited as an autosomal recessive trait. Its rarity is indicated by the fact that among 50,000 patients with melituria, only 11 cases of essential pentosuria were recognized. It is characterized by the constant presence in the urine of pentose 1-xylulose in small amounts varying from 1 to 4 Gm daily. With Benedict's method one usually obtains a constant green test. Most reported cases have been in Jews, although some have been in Lebanese families. Although pentosuria was thought formerly to occur predominately in males, recent studies suggest that the sex distribution may be more nearly equal. Most of the families of pentosurics in the New York City area studied by Lasker came originally from geographic foci of relatively limited extent, largely Poland and Germany. The condition is harmless, asymptomatic, and unrelated to diabetes. It requires no treatment

The enzymatic defect concerned in pentosuria appears to be related to the metabolism of glucuronic acid. Normally, uronic acids are converted to a pentose(1-xylulose), then to a sugar alcohol (xylitol), and finally through a series of steps to hexose. In individuals with pentosuria the enzyme responsible for the conversion of 1-xylulose to xylitol apparently is deficient. As a result, 1-xylulose accumulates and is excreted in the urine.

FRUCTOSURIA. Essential Fructosuria. Like pentosuria, this is a benign, asymptomatic anomaly of metabolism, probably inherited as an autosomal recessive trait. All reported cases have been in Jews. Fructosuria appears in males and females with about equal frequency. Fructosuria is rarer than pentosuria. Among 50,000 persons seen with melituria, only 4 cases of fructosuria, 2 in males and 2 in females, were recognized. Two of the patients were brother and sister.

Following the ingestion of fructose by persons with essential fructosuria, the concentration of that sugar in the blood reaches higher levels and remains high longer than in the normal individual. As a consequence, some 10 to 20 percent of the amount administered is excreted in the urine. Furthermore, the rise of the respiratory quotient is less than normal and the blood lactic and pyruvic acid concentrations remain unchanged. Available evidence strongly suggests that the faulty metabolism is due to a primary deficiency of hepatic fructokinase, an enzyme that catalyzes the conversion of fructose to fructose 1-phosphate.

Hereditary Fructose Intolerance. Hereditary fructose intolerance is an uncommon error of metabolism characterized by symptomatic hypoglycemia and vomiting after the ingestion of fructose. In this condition, thought to be inherited as an autosomal recessive trait, the primary defect is a deficiency of fructose 1-phosphate aldolase in the liver. The accumulation of fructose 1-phosphate supposedly inhibits fructose phosphorylation by fructokinase and this results in fructosemia and fructosuria. The mechanism for the secondary hypoglycemia is not clear. Indirect evidence favors inhibition of glucose production or release by the liver by fructose 1-phosphate, although the details of this action have not been clarified.

Treatment consists of elimination of fructose-containing foods from the diet. The outlook is excellent if the condition is recognized early in infancy and appropriate steps taken. If fructose is not avoided, long-term effects may include liver damage, renal impairment, and finally, cachexia and death.

LACTOSURIA. Lactose appears in the urine toward the end of pregnancy and during lactation. It may be considered as a physiologic event and need cause no concern. However, particularly during pregnancy, the finding of sugar in the urine should prompt the determination of the blood glucose at 1 hr after 50 Gm glucose or a meal liberal in carbohydrate in order to detect diabetes if present. Lactose gives a positive test with Benedict's solution. It is best identified by paper chromatography.

GALACTOSURIA. (See Chap. 112).

MANNOHEPTULOSURIA. Mannoheptulose appears in the urine of certain persons in small amounts after the eating of avocado. It is of no importance clinically.

OTHER MELITURIAS. Maltosuria has been reported rarely but has not been shown to be of clinical significance. Sucrose is promptly excreted in the urine following its administration intravenously, since under these conditions there is no provision in the body for hydrolyzing it to simpler sugars. Alimentary sucrosuria of slight degree may occur in normal individuals following a loading dose of cane sugar. Endogenous sucrosuria, difficult to explain, has been noted rarely and then only in association with disease of the pancreas. In reported cases the specific gravity of the urine reached values as high as 1.070. One must be on guard for cases of deception in which patients add cane sugar to urine brought for examination, not realizing that sucrose will not reduce Benedict's solution. An unusually high specific gravity of the urine leads one to think of the possibility of sucrose in the urine.

REFERENCES

Freeman, J. A., and K. E. Roberts: A Fine Structural Study of Renal Glycosuria, Exper. Mol. Pathol., 2:83, 1963.

Froesch, E. R., H. P. Wolf, H. Baitsch, A. Prader, and A. Labhart: Hereditary Fructose Intolerance. An Inborn Defect of Hepatic Fructose 1-phosphate Splitting Aldolase, Am. J. Med., 34:151, 1963.

Khachadurian, A. K., and L. A. Khachadurian: The Inheritance of Renal Glycosuria, Am. J. Human Gen., 16:189, 1964.

Marble, A.: Nondiabetic Melituria, pp. 717–738 in E. P. Joslin, H. F. Root, P. White, and A. Marble: "The Treatment of Diabetes Mellitus," 10th ed., Philadelphia, Lea & Febiger, 1959.

Stanbury, J. B., J. B. Wyngaarden, and D. S. Fredrickson: "The Metabolic Basis of Inherited Disease," 2d ed., New York, McGraw-Hill Book Company, 1966; see chapts. on Pentosuria by H. H. Hiatt, p. 109; Fructosuria by E. R. Froesch, p. 124; and Renal Glycosuria by S. M. Krane, p. 1221.

96 HYPERINSULINISM, HYPOGLYCEMIA, AND GLUCAGON SECRETION

*Stefan S. Fajans and
George W. Thorn*

INTRODUCTION

The maintenance of a constant blood glucose level is an essential part of homeostasis. The blood glucose level at any given time reflects the balance of two groups of physiologic processes: (1) those which add glucose to the blood, namely, (*a*) mobilization of glucose from glycogen stores, (*b*) formation of carbohydrate from nonglucose sources (gluconeogenesis), and (*c*) absorption of ingested carbohydrate; and (2) those which remove glucose from the blood, namely, utilization of glucose by liver, adipose tissue, muscle, brain, and other tissues.

CLASSIFICATION. Hypoglycemia may be produced by a variety of factors. In some the mechanism is poorly understood. Hence, a complete classification based on pathologic physiology is difficult. Nevertheless, the common causes of spontaneous hypoglycemia can be grouped as listed in Table 96-1. From the clinical view, patients with

Table 96-1. ETIOLOGIC CLASSIFICATION OF SPONTANEOUS HYPOGLYCEMIA

I. Organic hypoglycemia*
  A. Pancreatic islet cell tumor, functioning
  B. Nonpancreatic tumors associated with hypoglycemia
  C. Anterior pituitary hypofunction
  D. Adrenocortical hypofunction
  E. Acquired extensive liver disease
II. Hypoglycemia due to specific hepatic enzyme defect
  A. Glycogen storage diseases*
  B. Hereditary fructose intolerance
  C. Galactosemia
  D. Familial fructose and galactose intolerance
III. Functional hypoglycemia
  A. Reactive functional
  B. Reactive secondary to mild diabetes
  C. Alimentary hyperinsulinism
  D. Transient postnatal hypoglycemia in infant of diabetic mother*
  E. Transient hypoglycemia in the newborn of low birth weight*
  F. "Idiopathic hypoglycemia" of infancy and childhood*
  G. Alcohol and poor nutrition*
IV. Exogenous hypoglycemia*
  A. Iatrogenic ⎫ insulin or sulfonylurea compounds
  B. Factitious ⎭

*Fasting hypoglycemia.

hypoglycemia can be divided into two groups, according to the usual relationship of hypoglycemia to the fasting or postprandial state. Regardless of etiology, the conditions listed in Table 96-1 interfere with the homeostatic mechanism, which regulates the blood glucose level. Such interference may take place at different levels, even if the underlying cause of hypoglycemia is a single one. For example, in patients with functioning islet cell tumors, hypoglycemia is the result not only of increased glucose uptake in insulin-sensitive tissues and decreased hepatic glucose output but also of decreased inflow to the liver of substrates needed for gluconeogenesis. For example, the mobilization of amino acids from muscle is reduced.

CLINICAL PICTURE. The clinical symptoms and signs of hypoglycemia are the same regardless of the underlying cause. The symptoms which occur in any given patient vary with the degree and the rate of decline of blood glucose levels and with the variable and individual susceptibility of the underlying state of the central and autonomic nervous systems. Symptoms associated with a rapid decline in blood glucose levels are due in part to activation of the autonomic nervous system and the ensuing release of epinephrine. These symptoms are sweating, shakiness, trembling, tachycardia, anxiety, nervousness, weakness, fatigue, hunger, nausea, and vomiting. Other symptoms of hypoglycemia result from decreased uptake of glucose and decreased utilization of oxygen by the brain and usually occur when the decline in blood glucose levels is slow and/or when hypoglycemia is severe or prolonged. These symptoms are headache, visual disturbances, lethargy, yawning, faintness, restlessness, and difficulty with speech and thinking. Other manifestations may be agitation, mental confusion, somnolence, stupor, prolonged sleep, loss of consciousness, coma, and hypothermia. Twitching, convulsions, "epilepsy," and bizarre neurologic signs, motor as well as sensory in nature, may occur. Prominent signs observed in patients with alcohol-induced hypoglycemia are hypothermia, conjugate deviation of eyes, extensor rigidity of extremities, positive Babinski signs, and trismus. Repeated hypoglycemic episodes may lead to loss of intellectual ability and personality changes characterized by outbursts of temper or queer, bizarre, and psychotic behavior. Extensive and permanent mental or neurologic damage may result from frequent and prolonged episodes of hypoglycemia.

FUNCTIONING ISLET CELL TUMORS
Pathology

Approximately 90 percent of functioning islet cell tumors are benign adenomas; approximately 10 percent are definitely malignant with identified metastases. Hyperplasia of the islet cells has not been proved to occur in adults. Functioning islet cell tumors may be diagnosed at any age, with a majority of cases occurring between thirty and sixty years. Benign islet cell adenomas vary in size from 0.14 to 15 cm in diameter, but the majority are between 0.5 and 3.0 cm. They are usually encapsulated, firmer than the normal pancreas, highly vascular, purplish and occasionally whitish in color, and they present an irregular surface. They are found to be equally distributed throughout the head, body, and tail of the pancreas. Benign adenomas of islet cell tissue rarely occur outside the pancreas. Multiple adenomas are found in approximately 5 to 10 percent of cases. Multiple adenomas of islet cells may be associated with adenomas of the pituitary, parathyroids, and other endocrine glands and with peptic ulceration. In recent years it has been emphasized that this association frequently has a familial basis. A family history of diabetes has been found also in 25 to 30 percent of patients with functioning islet cell tumors.

Clinical Picture

Symptoms of hypoglycemia due to islet cell adenoma may develop insidiously, with periodic hypoglycemic attacks becoming more frequent and more severe. Fasting and exercise precipitate attacks. Attacks usually occur in the early morning hours, during the longest daily fasting period, or they may occur in late afternoon, especially if the noon meal is missed. Symptoms may also occur 2 to 5 hr after meals. Symptoms and signs secondary to decreased cerebral oxygen utilization usually predominate over symptoms secondary to hyperepinephrinemia. The pattern of symptoms is usually repetitive in the same patient, but it may differ from patient to patient. Many patients learn to avert symptoms by taking frequent feedings, including a feeding at 2:00 or 3:00 A.M. Obesity may thereby result. Chronic hypoglycemia may not only produce profound personality changes but may result also in damage to anterior horn cells of the spinal cord, with progressive muscular atrophy.

Diagnosis

A typical symptomatic attack with demonstrated hypoglycemia and relief of symptoms and signs by administration of glucose constitute the diagnostic criteria outlined by Whipple. This *triad of Whipple* is not specific for patients with functioning tumors of the pancreas, as it may occur in patients with other types of hypoglycemia. The level of the overnight fasting blood glucose is usually below normal. More prolonged fasting is the most helpful diagnostic procedure and will cause a fall in blood sugar below 30 to 35 mg per 100 ml (true blood glucose method). In the majority of cases, a typical attack with associated hypoglycemia can be induced within the first 24 hr of fasting. If hypoglycemia and typical symptoms are not induced, fasting should be prolonged for up to 72 hr, at which time the patient should be exercised vigorously. In patients with insulinomas, or other types of fasting hypoglycemia, exercise produces a further fall in blood sugar levels, but it produces a rise in blood glucose in patients with functional hypoglycemia.

Assays of serum insulin (Chap. 94) performed in conjunction with fasting blood glucose levels may be valuable in diagnosing insulinoma. Elevated fasting levels of serum insulin in peripheral blood are found in only two-thirds of patients with functioning islet cell tumors. Thus, diagnosis of insulinoma is strengthened by an elevated fasting insulin level, but a "normal" level does not rule out this diagnosis. When fasting insulin levels are measured daily for several days in the same patient, an elevated level can frequently be found in at least one specimen. A serum insulin level in the "normal range" associated with a fasting blood sugar level in the hypoglycemic range is also significant. In addition, when the overnight fast is prolonged for 4 hr or more in patients with fasting blood sugar levels in the borderline range, the blood glucose level may fall into the hypoglycemic range, while the level of serum insulin remains constant or rises, indicating an abnormal glucose-insulin homeostatic relationship. This is good evidence for the presence of an autonomous insulin-producing tumor. An elevated fasting level of plasma insulin after an overnight fast is not specific for insulinoma as it is also seen in obese patients and has been reported in patients with galacto-semia and familial fructose and galactose intolerance.

The intravenous tolbutamide test is valuable in the differential diagnosis of spontaneous hypoglycemia. After blood for a fasting blood glucose determination is obtained, 1 Gm sodium tolbutamide dissolved in 20 ml distilled water is injected intravenously over 2 min. Subsequently blood levels of glucose are determined every 15 min for the first hour and every 30 min during the second and third hours of the test. If plasma levels of insulin can be obtained during the test (see below), blood samples for insulin assay should be obtained every 5 min during the first 15 min after administration of tolbutamide. The greatest usefulness of the test is in obtaining evidence against a diagnosis of insulinoma in patients suspected of having functional hypoglycemia but whose history is unusual or in whom fasting blood glucose levels are in the lower range of normal. In such patients a normal 3-hr intravenous tolbutamide test (return of blood glucose to 70 percent or more of fasting blood sugar level) may obviate hospitalization and determination of blood glucose during prolonged fasting. In patients suspected of harboring insulinoma the test can be used for confirmation, but it should be carefully performed with the patient in the hospital. Tolbutamide-induced hypoglycemia persisted for 3 hr in 50 of 55 patients subsequently proved to have insulinomas. In these 55 patients fasting blood sugar levels were 50 mg per 100 ml or above. The lower the fasting blood sugar, the more frequently will the test have to be terminated early because of severe neurologic symptoms. False positive responses can occur in association with severe liver disease, alcoholic hypoglycemia, idiopathic hypoglycemia of infancy, severe undernutrition, and azotemia. They also may occur in some patients with nonpancreatic tumors and associated hypoglycemia, particularly in those patients in whom blood sugar levels decrease rapidly on fasting. In contrast, no false positive responses have occurred in patients with functional hypoglycemia, diabetes mellitus with reactive hypoglycemia, or patients without spontaneous hypoglycemia. Obviously the test is of little help if the fasting blood glucose level is very low.

Assays of blood insulin in conjunction with the intravenous tolbutamide test increase the value of the test. The finding of excessive increases in plasma insulin levels (above 190 μU per ml) within the first 15 min after intravenous administration of tolbutamide and/or prolonged elevation of plasma insulin thereafter (1) increases the specificity of this test in patients with insulinoma; (2) increases the usefulness of the test in patients with low fasting blood sugar levels, since it allows termination of the test when necessary; and (3) may differentiate insulinoma patients from patients with false positive blood glucose responses. Approximately 80 percent of patients with islet cell tumors exhibit an abnormal insulin response to intravenously administered tolbutamide. However, an increase in levels of insulin in the high normal range after intravenous tolbutamide does not rule out the existence of an insulinoma.

Sensitivity to leucine may be useful diagnostically. In adult patients a large decrease in blood glucose (over 25 mg per 100 ml) and a large increase in plasma insulin (over 30 μU per ml) after administration of leucine strongly suggest diagnosis of an insulinoma. Approximately 70 percent of patients with functioning islet cell tumors exhibit an exaggerated response to leucine. In childhood, sensitivity to leucine does not differentiate between idiopathic hypoglycemia and insulinoma. Severe leucine-induced hyperinsulinemia and hypoglycemia will also be obtained in factitious hypoglycemia due to surreptitious administration of sulfonylureas, since profound sensitivity to leucine-hypoglycemia can be produced in normal subjects by pretreatment with such compounds. A negative response to leucine does not rule out the existence of an insulinoma.

An exaggerated increase in serum levels of insulin over 160μU per ml after the intravenous administration of 1 mg of glucagon is observed in 50 to 75 percent of patients with proven islet cell tumors. When this occurs, the hyperglycemic effect of glucagon may be subnormal and followed by a profound fall in blood glucose.

In patients with suspected islet cell tumors all three provocative tests should be employed, since an abnormal response may be obtained with one but not another of these tests. Obese patients have an exaggerated rise in plasma insulin with any of these stimuli to insulin secretion, but the hyperinsulinemia is not accompanied by abnormal secondary hypoglycemia.

The oral glucose tolerance test (Chap. 94) may give a relatively flat curve with rapid return of the blood glucose into the hypoglycemic range due to excessive insulin release from the tumor in response to a rising concentration of blood glucose. Occasionally a high plateau curve may be found due to factors counterregulatory to chronic hypoglycemia and normal or subnormal release of insulin from the tumor in response to a rising blood glucose level. The intravenous glucose tolerance test with calculation of an index of glucose utilization is also of limited usefulness, as variable results are obtained in patients with functioning islet cell tumors.

TREATMENT. When the diagnosis of functioning islet cell tumor is made, relief of hypoglycemia by early surgery is indicated to prevent any further damage to the central nervous system and to prevent obesity, which makes surgical management more difficult. Identification of the tumor at the time of surgery may present a problem, particularly in the case of a relatively small tumor not located on the anterior surface of the pancreas. Selective pancreatic arteriography has made it possible to localize some of these tumors preoperatively. It was successful in locating a tumor radiographically in 5 of 11 patients with proven islet cell tumors. Of these five tumors three were located in the head of the pancreas and could not be palpated by the surgeon at the time of laporatomy.

Glucocorticoids have been used as an adjunct in the preoperative preparation of patients with insulinomas or in patients with persistent hypoglycemia following unsuccessful surgery. Cortisone, 100 to 200 mg per day, may be required preoperatively, but of course, continued administration at this level will lead to increased obesity and signs of Cushing's syndrome.

The benzothiadiazine compound, diazoxide, particularly when used in conjunction with one of the diuretic thiazides, such as trichlormethiazide, has been useful to elevate blood levels of glucose into the normoglycemic or hyperglycemic range prior to operation. Diazoxide causes increases in blood glucose by decreasing the secretion of insulin. In addition, diazoxide and the diuretic thiazides elevate blood glucose by one or more extrapancreatic mechanisms. Effective dosage ranges between 150 and 450 mg for Diazoxide and 2 and 3 mg for trichlormethiazide. The drugs should be discontinued 2 days before surgery.

The surgical approach to insulinomas may be complicated by difficulty in identifying the tumor, by difficulty encountered in "shelling out" completely all tumor tissue, and by the fact that multiple tumors are not at all uncommon. In the absence of a definite insulinoma, resection of first the tail and then the body of the pancreas is justified, as a significant proportion of tumors are located in these areas. After excision of the adenoma or subtotal pancreatectomy to find the adenoma, the patient is usually cured except in cases of multiple tumors or unlocated tumors in the head of the pancreas. Difficulty in shelling out the complete tumor is undoubtedly a significant factor in tumor recurrence. In approximately 20 percent of cases diagnosed histologically as carcinoma, follow-up observations have failed to reveal a recurrence of symptoms or tumor for several years.

Patients with nonresectable metastatic islet cell tumors present a management problem, as their hypoglycemia may be so severe as to respond only poorly to oral and even intravenous glucose administration. Since diazoxide is a potent and consistent inhibitor of pancreatic insulin release, it has proved to be an effective agent for the alleviation of symptomatic and biochemical hypoglycemia in many of these patients. To counteract the sodium-retaining effect of diazoxide administered in a dose of 600 to 1000 mg per day, a naturetic thiazide, such as trichlormethiazide, should be used in a dose of 2 to 3 mg per day.

In patients with metastatic islet cell carcinoma who do not respond to the hyperglycemic effect of diazoxide, the use of streptozotocin may be indicated. Streptozotocin, an antibiotic and an experimental antitumor agent, is a highly effective cytotoxic agent for pancreatic beta cells. Although not devoid of renal and hepatic toxicity, it has considerably greater specificity for normal or abnormal beta cells than is true for alloxan. Two patients with metastatic islet cell cacinoma who were teated with streptozotocin have had complete relief from hypoglycemia and regression of tumor mass.

The use of glucocorticoids and injections of glucagon may also be valuable.

NONPANCREATIC TUMORS ASSOCIATED WITH HYPOGLYCEMIA

Severe hypoglycemia has been reported in more than 100 patients harboring nonpancreatic tumors of meso-thelial, epithelial, or endothelial origin. Most of these tumors are mesothelial in type and are classified as fibromas, sarcomas, or fibrosarcomas. They are usually situated in the thorax, the retroperitoneal space, or the pelvis. They may be attached to the diaphragm or found within the liver. Other cases of nonpancreatic tumors associated with severe hypoglycemia include 28 patients with primary hepatic carcinoma, 14 patients with carcinoma of the adrenal cortex, 5 patients with gastrointestinal carcinomas, 2 patients with pseudomyxoma peritonei, 2 patients with bronchogenic carcinoma, and 1 with a bronchial carcinoid tumor. The common clinical characteristics of these tumors, particularly of the fibrosarcomas, are their slow growth and their massive size (up to 9 kg). Hypoglycemia disappears after resection or occasionally after irradiation of the tumor. Many theories have been advanced to explain the mechanism by which these tumors cause hypoglycemia, but none of these is applicable to all patients. A block in hepatic glucose output, excessive glucose consumption by tumor tissue with a high rate of anaerobic glycolysis, and inhibition of lipolysis have been reported in some of these patients. In the majority of patients immunoreactive insulin and insulinlike activity in serum or extract or tumor tissue have been normal or subnormal. High levels of serum insulin have been reported in one patient with severe hypoglycemia due to a large fibrosarcoma and in another patient with a bronchial carcinoid tumor with metastases. Only rarely have tumor extracts contained immunologically recognizable insulin. Twelve reports indicate that extracts of tumors from some of these patients contain an insulinlike substance stimulatory in either isolated rat diaphragm or epididymal fat pad systems. It is possible that some of these tumors synthesize a polypeptide closely related to insulin, but which in the majority of instances is not recognized immunologically as insulin.

OTHER CAUSES FOR FASTING HYPOGLYCEMIA

Although it is infrequent, fasting hypoglycemia may occur in patients with hypofunction of the anterior pituitary (Chap. 87) or hypofunction of the adrenal cortex (Chap. 92). Usually, other stigmas of these disorders enable one to make a diagnosis. In infants and children hypoglycemia due to isolated growth hormone deficiency has been reported.

Alcohol ingestion superimposed upon an inadequate dietary intake can precipitate acute hypoglycemia. Blood glucose levels as low as 10 or 20 mg per 100 ml have been observed. Inhibition of gluconeogenesis is primarily responsible for hypoglycemia in conjunction with depletion of liver glycogen stores.

Occasionally, diffuse hepatic disease (Chap. 323) may be associated with hypoglycemia. Very seldom, fasting hypoglycemia can be traced to a glycogen-storage disease (Chap. 111) or to galactosemia (Chap. 112).

In children the most common type of fasting hypoglycemia is that classified as *idiopathic hypoglycemia of infancy and childhood*. This entity is probably heterogeneous. Fasting hypoglycemia may begin in early postnatal life or in the first 2 years of life. The hypoglycemia may be mild and intermittent or more persistent and severe. Usually by seven to nine years of age these children "outgrow" the occurrence of hypoglycemia. Differentiation from functioning islet cell tumor is most difficult, although the occurrence of insulinoma is rare in this age group.

POSTPRANDIAL HYPOGLYCEMIA
Reaction Functional Hypoglycemia

Reactive functional hypoglycemia occurs almost uniformly in patients with emotional problems. It has been thought to be due to excessive secretion of insulin in response to a normal rise of blood glucose following meals. This is not a consistent finding. The diagnosis is suspected by a history of hypoglycemic symptoms occurring 2 to 4 hr after ingestion of a meal rich in carbohydrates, and it is confirmed by an oral glucose tolerance test extended for 4 or 5 hr, blood samples being obtained at half-hour intervals. It is not unusual in such patients to find blood glucose levels of 30 or 40 mg per 100 ml between the second and fourth hour of the test.

However, the usual symptoms produced by reactive hypoglycemia are transitory and often subside spontaneously in 15 to 30 min. Weakness, hunger, inward trembling, sweating, and tachycardia are the most common symptoms in these patients. Loss of consciousness or convulsions do not occur, and the severity of symptoms is not progressive. In patients with functional hypoglycemia attacks are more frequent when emotional stress and anxiety are greater. A 72-hr fast is well tolerated, and the concentration of blood glucose rarely drops below 45 mg per 100 ml. The intravenous tolbutamide test is normal. A family history for diabetes mellitus is usually absent.

In some patients with advanced cerebrovascular disease, reactive functional hypoglycemia may be the trigger which initiates a cerebral ischemic episode and its subsequent potential chain of events. Similarly, in patients with a hypersensitive carotid sinus or with postural hypotension, the same procedures that do not induce the vascular response at other times may do so during an episode of reactive hypoglycemia. Likewise, there are a number of patients with ectopic tachycardias of various types in which an episode of reactive hypoglycemia is either the sole "trigger" initiating the attacks, which is quite rare, or one of several "triggers," which is quite common. Episodes of reactive hypoglycemia may precipitate attacks of angina as well as bouts of acute pulmonary edema in predisposed cardiac patients. For this small but important group of patients serious cerebral and cardiovascular complications may be minimized by *recognizing* the possible role that reactive functional hypoglycemia may play as an initiating factor.

TREATMENT. The distressing symptoms experienced by patients with functional hypoglycemia may be prevented by a diet low in carbohydrate and high in protein, with adequate fat to maintain caloric requirements. The diet is divided into three to six feedings, with protein and carbohydrate proportions divided equally among the meals. In patients with a history suggestive of reactive hypoglycemia but in whom the diagnosis cannot be substantiated by a glucose tolerance test, diet therapy may be tried. An important approach is to improve the psychologic and emotional status of the patient with functional hypoglycemia. In this regard the use of sedatives such as Phenobarbital, 30 mg at 10:00 A.M., 3:00 P.M.; and bedtime, as well as tranquillizers such as Librium, 10 mg two to three times daily, may prove useful. The prognosis is good, as usually it is a self-limiting disease within a few months or years.

Reactive Hypoglycemia Secondary to Mild Diabetes

This condition has to be distinguished from reactive functional hypoglycemia, for both the underlying mechanism and the prognosis are different. Whereas in patients with reactive functional hypoglycemia the pancreatic insulin release is thought to be excessive but well-timed in response to the rising postprandial blood glucose, in patients with mild diabetes the insulin release is delayed. It is not until the blood glucose rises to frank diabetic levels that insulin is secreted in excess. Measurements of serum insulin during glucose tolerance tests in such patients have demonstrated that relatively large amounts of insulin are released, albeit late; the blood glucose then decreases from diabetic to normal levels and further to hypoglycemic levels. This type of hypoglycemic response is most likely to occur between the third and the fifth hours. It is apparent that these patients have only mild diabetes, as endogenous insulin is available and their fasting blood glucose is within normal limits. Their carbohydrate intolerance can only be detected by a postprandial blood glucose determination or an oral glucose tolerance test. Frequently there is a family history of diabetes mellitus.

Treatment consists of a diabetic diet with frequent feedings. Weight reduction in the obese patient may normalize glucose tolerance, with disappearance of reactive hypoglycemia. Contrary to the relatively benign prognosis of reactive functional hypoglycemia, the disorder is not self-limiting and such patients may eventually progress to a more advanced state of insulin deficiency and the clinical syndrome of diabetes mellitus (Chap. 94).

Alimentary Hypoglycemia

In patients with gastroenterostomy or subtotal gastrectomy, hypoglycemia is due to excessive insulin release in response to excessive postprandial hyperglycemia (alimentary hyperinsulinism). The diagnosis is made by history of abdominal surgery, an *abnormal oral glucose tolerance test* with elevation of the peak blood glucose level, but a *normal intravenous glucose tolerance test*.

Other Causes of Postprandial Hypoglycemia

Leucine sensitivity in the adult is extremely rare. Approximately 70 percent of patients with functioning islet cell tumors and 30 percent of patients with idiopathic hypoglycemia of infancy and childhood may be sensitive to leucine. Recently, hypoglycemia following the ingestion of fructose has also been described, due to an inborn error of metabolism in which there is a deficiency of the enzyme hepatic fructose 1-phosphate aldolase. It is very infrequent.

EXOGENOUS HYPOGLYCEMIA

The possibility of factitious hyperinsulinism as a result of surreptitious administration of insulin or sulfonylureas should always be considered, particularly in nurses, other medical personnel, and relatives of diabetic patients. If self-administration of insulin is suspected, presence of *insulin antibody in serum* from such patients may point to the proper diagnosis, provided there is no history of previous insulin administration.

In the case of ingestion of tolbutamide (Orinase) in large amounts, acidification of the urine will disclose a white precipitate which is a crystallization of the carboxylated excretion product of tolbutamide.

REGULATION OF GLUCAGON SECRETION AND EFFECTS OF GLUCAGON
Source and Characteristics

Glucagon is a polypeptide hormone secreted by the alpha cells of the islets of Langerhans. The hormone is made up of 29 amino acids in a straight chain and has a molecular weight of 3485. With a sensitive radioimmunoassay employing an antiserum specific for glucagon, its concentration can be assayed in pancreatic tissue and in blood. From different portions of the gastrointestinal mucosa (stomach, but particularly small intestine) extracts have been prepared which have immunological characteristics similar to but not identical with pancreatic glucagon. This immunoreactive material, called "gut glucagon," "entero-glucagon," or "glucagon-like immunoreactive material," has been found to be separable into two fractions, one of molecular weight of approximately 7000 and the other with a molecular weight of 3500. The former differs from glucagon in biologic activity (see following). The plasma concentrations of pancreatic glucagon in peripheral blood is approximately 100 pg per ml in the basal state.

Factors Influencing Secretion of Glucagon

Unger and associates have demonstrated that insulin-induced hypoglycemia is followed by increases in the concentration of glucagon in pancreatic and peripheral blood. Starvation is another stimulus to increased secretion of glucagon. On the other hand, hyperglycemia due to orally or intravenously administered glucose causes suppression of glucagon secretion. The ingestion of protein meals or the intravenous or oral administration of certain amino acids (arginine) are other potent stimuli to the secretion of pancreatic glucagon. Administration of pancreozymin, a gastrointestinal hormone released after protein ingestion, has also been found to increase plasma levels of glucagon and to augment the effect of amino acids on glucagon secretion.

The oral but not the intravenous administration of glucose is followed by a significant increase in immunoreactive glucagon in peripheral blood which is due to release of "gut-glucagon."

Metabolic Effects of Glucagon

Glucagon exhibits a marked effect on carbohydrate, protein, and lipid metabolism in vivo and in vitro. Glucagon stimulates hepatic glycogenolysis by increasing cyclic 3', 5' adenosine monophosphate (AMP) which leads to increased phosphorylase activity. Increased glycogenolysis and inhibition by glucagon of hepatic glycogen synthetase (also via cyclic AMP) cause hyperglycemia. Glucagon stimulates gluconeogenesis by promoting the hepatic uptake of amino acids,. It inhibits the incorporation of amino acids into liver protein and increases excretion of nitrogen. Glucagon, by activating the adenyl cyclase systems, also promotes lipolysis in liver and adipose tissues. The resulting increased hepatic concentration and oxidation of free fatty acids stimulate hepatic gluconeogenesis and ketogenesis.

In addition to these effects of glucagon on hepatic and adipose tissues, glucagon has a direct effect on stimulating increased release of insulin from the pancreatic beta cells independent of the increases in blood glucose. Glucagon's effect on pancreatic beta cells may also be mediated by activation of the adenyl cyclase system. "Gut glucagon" of molecular weight 7000 also increases the secretion of insulin but does not have the hepatic effects of pancreatic glucagon.

Other extrahepatic effects of glucagon are a positive inotropic effect upon cardiac muscle, a stimulation of adrenal medullary secretion, and a slight lowering of serum levels of calcium and phosphate.

Physiologic Role of Glucagon

The extreme sensitivity of hepatic and adipose tissues to glucagon and the fact that increased secretion of glucagon is stimulated by fasting and hypoglycemia suggest that glucagon is released in order to provide for increased distribution of energy substrates during periods of glucose need. Glycogenolysis and gluconeogenesis will lead to increased levels of blood glucose, and increased lipolysis will furnish free fatty acids for energy and will stimulate gluconeogenesis. In contrast to the effects of fasting and hypoglycemia, rapid increases in blood glucose inhibit the secretion of glucagon. In birds the removal of the pancreas, rich in alpha cells and glucagon, is followed by the development of severe hypoglycemia. This hypoglycemia can be alleviated by the injection of glucagon. Amino acid–induced glucagon release after protein feeding may be an important factor in preventing hypoglycemia which might otherwise occur during amino acid–induced insulin release.

Whether or not pancreatic glucagon plays a physiologic

role in mediating increased release of insulin is still to be demonstrated. It is possible, although not established, that release of "gut glucagon" after ingestion of carbohydrate is one of the mediators of insulin secretion when glucose is ingested.

Abnormalities of Glucagon Secretion

McGavran and his associates have reported a patient with a malignant tumor of the alpha cells of the pancreas who also had diabetes. There was an increase in concentration of glucagon in tumor tissue and plasma. Removal of part of the tumor resulted in decreased concentration of plasma levels of glucagon and in amelioration of the hyperglycemia. At the present time there is no evidence that abnormalities of glucagon secretion play a role in diabetes of genetic origin. Some patients with familial multiple endocrine adenomatosis have been described to have elevated levels of plasma glucagon in addition to evidence of hyperinsulinism, hyperparathyroidism, and other hormonal hypersecretion. A syndrome caused by decreased secretion of glucagon has not been described as yet. However, it can be anticipated that a hypoglycemic state due to glucagon deficiency will eventually be documented. Some infants and children with so-called "idiopathic hypoglycemia" may be found to be deficient of glucagon. Decreased plasma levels of glucagon and decreased glucagon reserve have been reported in some patients with severe chronic pancreatitis and associated diabetes. The plasma glucagon response to intravenously administered arginine should prove to be a valuable test for pancreatic glucagon reserve.

Clinical Usefulness of Glucagon Administration

In the presence of normal glycogen stores glucagon produces a hyperglycemic effect when given subcutaneously, intramuscularly, or intravenously. The acute administration of glucagon has been used clinically most frequently in the treatment of severe insulin-induced hypoglycemia of labile diabetics when oral or intravenous administration of glucose is not possible. More prolonged administration of a repository form of glucagon (zinc glucagon) has been of some help in the treatment of some patients with inoperable pancreatic islet cell tumors. Recently, large amounts of glucagon have been administered to selected patients with severe heart failure and cardiogenic shock. A beneficial effect has been obtained in some patients due to the positive inotropic effect exerted by glucagon.

Glucagon Tests

Several types of glucagon tests have been employed. One test takes advantage of the glycogenolytic properties of glucagon as a means for assessing adequacy of hepatic glycogen stores and the competency of enzymes in producing glycogenolysis. One milligram of glucagon is injected intravenously over 4 min and blood specimens are obtained at 0, 20, 30, 45, 60, 90, and 120 min. In healthy subjects the blood sugar level rises from 30 to 90 mg per 100 ml 20 to 30 min after injection of glucagon. In patients with cirrhosis or glycogen storage disease there is a subnormal or no rise in blood sugar.

Another glucagon test takes advantage of the insulin-releasing property of glucagon. In patients with functioning pancreatic islet cell tumors, injection of 1 mg glucagon may be followed by excessive increases in plasma insulin. Blood samples are obtained at −15 min and 0 time, and again 3, 5, 10, 15, 30, 45, 60, 90, 120, 150, and 180 min after injection of glucagon. Excessive increases in plasma insulin (over 160 microunits per ml) may occur during the first few minutes after injection of glucagon in 50 percent or more of patients with insulin secreting tumors. This may be associated with a subnormal rise in blood glucose but may be followed by excessive secondary decreases in blood glucose. The test may have to be interrupted if severe hypoglycemic symptoms develop. Such patients should be treated with intravenous glucose.

Intravenous administration of 0.5 to 1.0 mg of glucagon has also been used as a provocative test in patients suspected of harboring pheochromocytoma. In patients with pheochromocytoma glucagon evokes release of excessive quantities of pressor amines, resulting in a hypertensive paroxysm.

REFERENCES

Black, J.: Diazoxide and the Treatment of Hypoglycemia, Ann. N. Y. Acad. Sci., 150:194, 1968.

Conn, J. W., and H. S. Seltzer: Spontaneous Hypoglycemia, Am. J. Med., 19:460, 1955.

Dormandy, T. L., and R. J. Porter: Familial Fructose and Galactose Intolerance, Lancet, 1:1189, 1961.

Fajans, S. S., J. C. Floyd, Jr., R. F. Knopf, J. Rull, E. M. Guntsche, and J. W. Conn: Benzothiadiazine Suppression of Insulin Release from Normal and Abnormal Islet Tissue in Man, J. Clin. Invest., 45:481, 1966.

Field, J. B., H. Keen, P. Johnson, and B. Herring: Insulin-like Activity of Nonpancreatic Tumors Associated with Hypoglycemia, J. Clin. Endocrinol. & Metab., 23:1229, 1963.

Floyd, J. C., Jr., S. S. Fajans, R. F. Knopf, and J. W. Conn: Plasma Insulin in Organic Hyperinsulinism: Comparative Effects of Tolbutamide, Leucine and Glucose, J. Clin. Endocrinol. & Metab., 24:747, 1964.

Freinkel, N., D. L. Singer, R. A. Arky, S. J. Bleicher, J. B. Anderson, and C. K. Silbert: Alcohol Hypoglycemia: I. Carbohydrate Metabolism of Patients with Clinical Alcohol Hypoglycemia and the Experimental Reproduction of the Syndrome with Pure Ethanol, J. Clin. Invest., 42:1112, 1963.

Froesch, E. R., H. P. Wolf, H. Baitsch, A. Prader, and A. Labhart: Hereditary Fructose Intolerance: An Inborn Defect of Hepatic Fructose-1-Phosphate Splitting Aldolase, Am. J. Med., 34:151, 1963.

Graber, A. L., D. Porte, Jr., and R. H. Williams: Clinical Use of Diazoxide and Mechanism for Its Hyperglycemic Effects, Diabetes, 15:143, 1966.

Lawrence, A. M.: Glucagon Provocative Test for Pheochromocytoma, Ann. Int. Med., 66:1091, 1967.

McGavran, M. H., R. H. Unger, L. Recant, H. C. Polk, C. H. Kilo, and M. E. Levin: Glucagonoma: The Identification of A Glucagon-Secreting-Alpha-Cell Carcinoma of the Pancreas, New Eng. J. Med., 274:1408, 1966.

Murray-Lyon, I. M., A. L. Eddleston, R. Williams, M. Brown, B. M. Hogbin, A. Bennett, J. C. Edwards, and K. W. Taylor: Treatment of Multiple-Hormone-Producing Malignant Islet-Cell Tumour with Streptozotocin, Lancet, 2:895, 1968.

Ohneda, A., E. Aguilar-Parada, A. M. Eisentraut, and R. H. Unger: Characterization of Response of Circulating Glucagon to Intraduodenal and Intravenous Administration of Amino Acid, J. Clin. Invest., 47:2305, 1968.

Ohneda, A., E. Aguilar-Parada, A. M. Eisentraut, and R. H. Unger: Control of Pancreatic Glucagon Secretion by Glucose, Diabetes, 18:1, 1969.

Pek, S., S. S. Fajans, J. C. Floyd, Jr., R. F. Knopf, and J. W. Conn: Effects upon Plasma Glucagon of Infused and Ingested Amino Acids and of Protein Meals in Man, Diabetes, 18:328, 1969.

Samols, E., and V. Marks: Insulin Assay in Insulinomas, Brit. Med. J., 1:507, 1963.

Samols, E., G. Marri, and V. Marks: Promotion of Insulin Secretion by Glucagon, Lancet, 2:415, 1965.

Shames, J. M., N. R. Dhurandhar, and W. G. Blackard: Insulin-Secreting Bronchial Carcinoid Tumor with Widespread Metastases, Am. J. Med., 44:632, 1968.

Unger, R. H., A. M. Eisentraut, and L. L. Madison: The Effects of Total Starvation Upon the Levels of Circulating Glucagon and Insulin in Man, J. Clin. Invest., 42:1031, 1963.

Unger, R. H., A. Ohneda, I. Valverde, A. M. Eisentraut, and J. Exton: Characterization of Response of Circulating Glucagon-Like Immunoreactivity to Intraduodenal and Intravenous Administration of Glucose, J. Clin. Invest., 47:48, 1968.

97 DISEASES OF THE TESTES

John F. Crigler, Jr., Eugenia Rosemberg, and George W. Thorn

History

Androgen deficiency resulting from loss of testicular tissue was undoubtedly recognized by prehistoric man, as was the associated sterility; indeed, testicular tissue was recommended for impotence over 30 centuries ago. This dual function of the testes, as both the site of spermatogenesis and the primary site of male hormone production, was clearly defined in the middle of the nineteenth century when Berthold returned to the capon the characteristics, both physical and behavioral, of the cockerel by testicular grafts, and when his contemporaries, the anatomists von Kolliker, Leydig, Sertoli, and Schweigger-Seidel, defined the morphology of the gland. They recognized the spermatogonia, spermatids, the Sertoli (or sustentacular) cells, and cells located interstitially between the tubules (the Leydig or interstitial cells).

The tropic role played by the anterior pituitary gland in the development and maintenance of testicular function was demonstrated by Smith and Engle in 1927, and several years later Butenandt isolated androsterone from male urine. By 1935, testosterone had been synthesized from cholesterol and isolated in crystalline form from bull testes. In addition, it was conclusively shown to be the most significant natural androgenic material.

Embryologists had debated for many years the relative importance of sex chromosomal pattern, hormones or "determiners" secreted by the embryonic gonads, and maternal hormones on sex differentiation. In 1917, Lillie described the role of sex hormones in the development of freemartins. Wiesner proposed in 1935 that there is an autonomous tendency which results in female development unless opposed by male hormone. However, it was not until the late 1940s and early 1950s that Alfred Jost (1947) and other experimental embryologists clearly demonstrated that secretions of the fetal testes are necessary for development of male genital ducts and external genitals and that female development occurs in the absence of gonads. About the same time, Barr and Bertram (1949) described sex chromatin masses at the periphery of the nucleus in resting ganglion cells of female cats, a distinguishing characteristic of the female sex subsequently shown to be present in the peripheral cells of most mammalian species. The application of this simple cytologic means of assessing the number of X chromosomes and, more recently, of more sophisticated cytogenetic techniques, to the study of patients with sexual abnormalities has added to our advances in the fields of embryology and cytogenetics, which have been of great importance in elucidating the pathophysiology of testicular disorders.

Development

EMBRYOGENIC. In the fourth to sixth weeks of fetal development, the primitive genital ridge differentiates into cortical and medullary components capable of becoming either a testis or an ovary. If the primordial germ cells which migrate from the dorsal endoderm of the yolk sac to the urogenital ridge have a Y chromosome, the primary sex cords of the medulla undergo proliferation to form seminiferous tubules, which subsequently link up with convoluted tubules of mesonephric origin (rete testis and epididymis) and channel into the Wolffian duct. Ingrowths of coelomic epithelium carry germ cells to the seminiferous tubules. The cortex of the primitive gonad becomes isolated by the tunica albuginea and involutes. Interstitial cells of Leydig are abundant by the age of eight weeks and secrete fetal masculinizing hormones necessary for development of Wolffian duct structures (vas deferens, seminal vesicles), involution of the Müllerian system (appendix testis), and enlargement of the genital tubercle and fusion of the urethral and labioscrotal folds to form male external genitalia. If the primordial germ cells have two X chromosomes, the medullary component of the primitive gonad involutes and the cortical component proliferates and persists as the future ovary. In the absence of masculinizing factors of the interstitial cells of the fetal testis, development presumably evoked by the presence of a Y chromosome, normal female development of genital ducts and external genitalia takes place, with the formation of the fallopian tubes, uterus and upper vagina from the Müllerian ducts, regression of the Wolffian system, and persistence of the small genital tubercle and unfused urethral and labioscrotal folds.

POSTNATAL. Shorty after birth the testes measure 1.5 to 2.0 cm in length and 0.7 to 1.0 cm in width and weigh approximately 0.5 Gm each. The interstitial cells, active during uterine life as a result of chorionic gonadotropin, undergo differentiation and remain quiescent or semiquiescent until puberty. Studies using sufficiently sensitive techniques, however, demonstrate measurable levels of both gonadotropic and sex steroid hormones at all ages. It is recognized, also, that hypogonadal children show an earlier rise of gonadotropins than normal children, indicating a restraining influence of the prepuberal gonad upon the gonadotropic activity of the pituitary. At birth, 10 percent of male infants have incompletely descended testes, but after the first year, this figure drops to 2 to 3 percent. Late prepuberal descent further decreases the number, so that only 0.3 to 0.4 percent of males have either unilateral or bilateral undescended testes, postpuberally, unilateral undescended testes being four to five times more frequent.

During adolescence, each testis increases in size, as a result chiefly of changes in the seminiferous tubules under the stimulation of pituitary follicle–stimulating hormone (FSH) and androgens produced locally by developing interstitial cells. The fully developed testis measures 3.5 to 5.5 cm in length and 2.1 to 3.2 cm in width, and weighs 15 to 20 Gm each. Interstitial cell–stimulating hormone (ICSH) induces interstitial cell differentiation, with the production of male sex hormones, genital enlargement, and the development of secondary sexual characteristics. Normal function, including demonstrated fertility, has been noted when testes were less than half the mean size.

ABERRATIONS IN EMBRYONIC DEVELOPMENT. It is currently postulated that sex-determining genes on the X and Y chromosomes are responsible, through their effects on cellular function of the primitive cortex or medulla, for gonadal differentiation of these tissues into either a testis or an ovary. Embryologic studies have indicated that normally functioning fetal testes are required for male differentiation of genital ducts and external genitalia. The fetal testis appears to produce, at least, two types of substances: (1) a "duct-organizing substance," which stimulates development of the Wolffian system and involution of the Müllerian duct; and (2) an androgen, which may play a role in Wolffian duct development but is required for masculinization of the external genitalia. The correlation between chromosomal patterns, gonadal differentiation, and subsequent genital development in human beings has been quite consistent. Some cases, however, remain unexplained by the above stated concepts, although they do not disprove the hypothesis, since current techniques do not detect all chromosomal anomalies (mosaicism, interchange of sex-determining factors between X and Y chromosomes, etc.) or measure directly fetal gonadal function.

If gonadal tissue does not develop (gonadal dysgenesis, genotypic XO, X isochromosome X, X deleted X, etc.) or interstitial cells are nonfunctioning before differentiation of genital ducts in a genotypic male (XY), **both internal and external genitalia are entirely female.** Partial failure in testicular development or in the elaboration of fetal masculinizing hormones (genotypic XY or mosaics having a cell line with a Y chromosome) results in ambiguous internal and external genital development, the type of abnormality reflecting the age of onset and degree of fetal gonadal dysfunction. Patients with abnormal fetal testes, therefore, may have genital development ranging from almost complete feminization through incomplete fusion of the urethral and labioscrotal folds with some enlargement of the genital tubercle and various degrees of development of the Müllerian ducts to mild degrees of hypospadias. In addition, if testicular tissue exists unilaterally (true hermaphrodite, mixed gonadal dysgenesis), male development of genital ducts occurs on the side of the testes and Müllerian duct structures develop on the side with the ovary or missing gonad. These findings are consistent with observations in other animal species which demonstrate a local effect by diffusion of fetal masculinizing hormones (Chap. 4).

Some genotypic males (XY) who have histologically normal-appearing testes before puberty show total **feminization of external genitalia although internal genitals are masculinized** (syndrome of testicular feminization). This abnormality is inherited as either a sex-limited recessive or a sex-limited autosomal dominant mutant gene, as half of the genotypic males are affected. The lack of masculinization of external genitals (but not of internal genitalia), the absence of sexual hair (present in approximately one-third of the patients), and the occurrence of feminization at adolescence with normal plasma and urine testosterone concentrations indicate an abnormality in the response of tissues to androgens. Decreased reduction of testosterone to 17β-hydroxyandrostane urinary metabolites and activity of the Δ^4-5α-reductase of skin, which catalyzes the transformation of testosterone to 17β-hydroxy-5α-androstan-3-one (dihydrotestosterone), a metabolite with biological activity comparable to testosterone, has been demonstrated in these patients. Intramuscular administration of dihydrotestosterone to a patient with testicular feminization, however, failed to produce the changes in urinary nitrogen, phosphorus, and citric acid excretion observed in a control individual. Nevertheless, these new biochemical observations are consistent with the hypothesis that the basic defect is an inability of end-organ tissues to metabolize testosterone in a normal manner. Feminization of the external genitals of these patients may be so complete that the abnormality is only discovered later in life when primary amenorrhea, the absence of sexual hair, or the appearance of inguinal masses make the diagnosis apparent. Surgical exploration of these patients reveals the presence of vas deferens, epididymis, and testes, the latter showing variation in histologic findings with age and the completeness of the defect. After adolescence, tubular adenomas and hyperplasia of Leydig cells (often adenomatous) are common.

Finally, **masculinization** of **external genital development** of a **genotypic female** fetus (XX) may be induced by excess fetal adrenal androgens (patients with congenital adrenal hyperplasia) or by excess androgens produced or taken (usually synthetic progestational steroid hormones) by the mother during pregnancy. Defects induced by these extragonadal androgens are limited to the external genitalia (hypertrophy of the genital tubercle with various degrees of fusion of the urogenital and labioscrotal folds), so that if the condition is recognized, an appropriate sex assignment can be made and the genital abnormality surgically corrected.

Physiology

The role of fetal testicular function on genital development has been described above. The precise interrelationships of hypothalamic-pituitary and testicular functions (Fig. 97-1) at adolescence and in adult life are not completely defined. The hormone elaborated by the anterior pituitary gland that appears to induce development and then functional maintenance of the testicular interstitial (Leydig) cells has been appropriately labeled interstitial cell–stimulating hormone (ICSH) and reportedly is identical to luteinizing hormone (LH) in the female. Pituitary FSH stimulates development of the seminiferous tubules. At the moment, the role of ICSH and testosterone in seminiferous tubular development and spermatogenesis is not well defined. It is generally accepted that the Leydig cell is the principal site of synthesis of steroid hormones (testosterone, estrogens, and others). The probable role of ICSH and the Leydig cell in hormonal production in human beings is illustrated by observations on so-called "fertile eunuchs," patients who show spermatogenesis but lack masculine secondary changes and in whom testicular biopsies show an absence of Leydig cells.

FSH and *ICSH* have been measured by specific bioassays and radioimmunoassays in the urine and serum of prepuberal children. It has been suggested that sexual maturity is accompanied by a marked increase in the excretion of LH, with a relatively smaller increase in FSH. Though these changes in gonadotropins at adoescence have been demonstrated, the factors, probably neural, initiating pubery are still unknown. Nevertheless, production of androgenic hormones by the testes at puberty effects the numerous somatic changes noted in the adolescent male. These include enlargement and increased pigmentation of the external genitalia, hypertrophy of the larynx with lowering of the voice, a generalized increase of amount of hair to hirsutism with growth of a beard and a typical masculine pelvic escutcheon and forehead hair line, enlargement of the prostate and seminal vesicles,

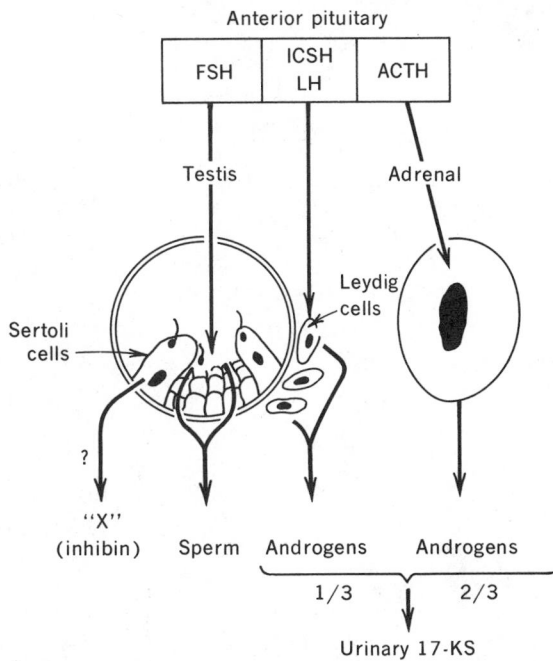

Fig. 97-1. Scheme showing anterior pituitary–testis relationship.

and an overall increase in muscular development. Metabolic balance studies demonstrate retention of electrolytes, nitrogen, and phosphorus; and radiologic examination shows acceleration of osseous development with subsequent epiphyseal fusion.

The testes of the normal, young male secrete between 4 and 8 mg testosterone daily and, approximately 40 μg of estradiol, another 20 to 25 μg of estradiol being formed from testosterone and androstenedione in other tissues. Approximately half the testosterone appears in the urine as measurable 17-ketosteroids, primarily androsterone and etiocholanolone (Fig. 97-2). The total 17-ketosteroid daily excretion for males, which includes the steroid derivatives from the testes and adrenal cortex, is 8 to 18 mg, of which approximately 4 mg is derived from the testes and the remainder from the adrenals. Plasma testosterone concentrations in young adult males vary from 0.4 to 1.0 μg per 100 ml (mean 0.7 μg per 100 ml), whereas normal females of similar age have plasma concentrations between 0.02 and 0.07 μg per 100 ml. Recent studies of testosterone production rates in normal men aged sixty-six to eighty-six years suggest that with advancing years, there may be a significant fall in testosterone secretion. It is well known that urinary 17-ketosteroid excretion diminishes with increasing age. It seems unlikely, however, that a sudden cessation in gonadal function analogous to the process in the female ever occurs in the male.

TESTICULAR DISORDERS

The principal abnormalities of testicular function, listed according to their effect on both interstitial and seminiferous tubular activity, are summarized in Table 97-1.

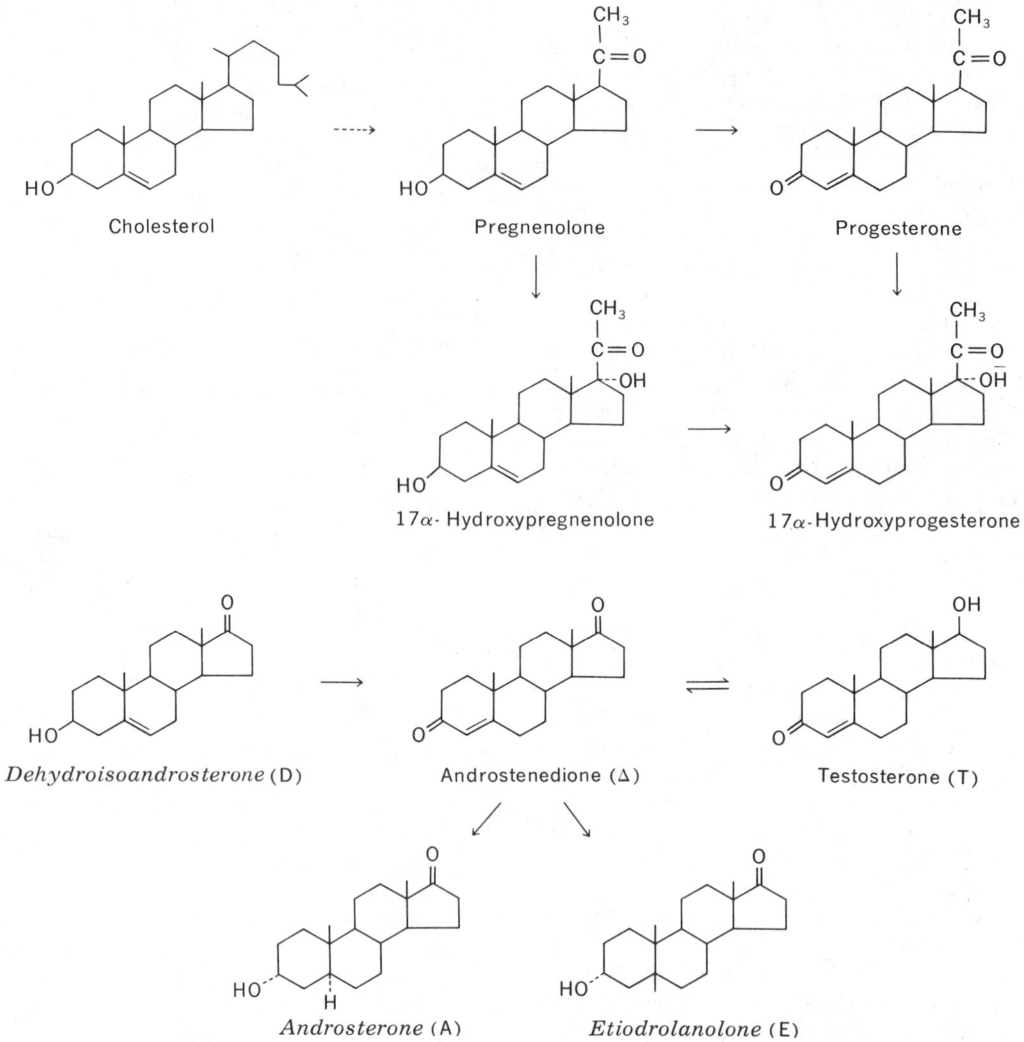

Fig. 97-2. Synthesis and metabolism of androgens. The broken line between cholesterol and pregnenolone signifies a series of reactions, all of which, including the conversion to 17α-hydroxyprogesterone to Δ4-androstenedione (Δ) and to testosterone (T), occur in the testis. More recently there is evidence that dehydroisoandrosterone (D), principally secreted by the adrenal, is also normally synthesized by gonadal tissue. In addition, it is now well recognized that D, Δ, and T are peripherally interconvertible, as shown by the arrows. Further metabolism of these compounds to the principal urinary metabolites (italicized in the diagram) occurs mainly in liver, where they are also conjugated to excretion as glucuronides or sulfates.

Hypogonadism

The clinical term *hypogonadism* as most often used refers to failure in interstitial cell function which results in decreased or absent production of male sex hormones. Seminiferous tubular failure, however, often is associated and, indeed, may occur without significant changes in testicular hormonal production (Sertoli-cell-only syndrome and postpuberal abnormalities). Both testicular functions may be decreased either primarily by a developmental or destructive lesion of the testes or secondarily by failure in production of pituitary gonadotropins.

PREPUBERAL HYPOGONADISM. The clinical picture of hypogonadism is directly related to the time of development of androgen deficiency. Prepuberal deficiency results in varying degrees of failure to develop the expected secondary sexual characteristics associated with maturity. Total lack of androgen production by the testes is associated with persistent infantile structure, a high voice, partial or total lack of facial, axillary, and pubic hair, infantile genitalia, and a barely palpable prostate. Because of lack of osseous maturation, epiphyseal closure is delayed, resulting eventually in a tall "eunuchoid" habitus with long arms and legs and a span 2 in. greater than height. Gynecomastia, wide hips, and girdle obesity may also be present. The skin is pale and delicate and may show early wrinkling. Acne and seborrhea are absent.

Prepuberal hypogonadism remains inapparent (unless there are gross anomalies of the testes, which may signal

Table 97-1. ABNORMALITIES OF TESTICULAR FUNCTION

I. Hypogonadism (decreased androgen production and/or spermatogenesis).
  A. Primary (increased urinary gonadotropins).
    1. Developmental abnormalities.
      a. Klinefelter's syndrome (seminiferous tubule dysgenesis). Classic form—eunuchoidism, gynecomastia, mental retardation, and small firm testes. Buccal smear—chromatin-positive. Leukocyte karyotype usually XXY or XXYY but may have other poly X and Y chromosomal constitution and mosaicism with combination of many cell lines.
      b. Reifenstein's syndrome (male pseudohermaphroditism). Hereditary testicular disorder with hypospadias, varying degrees of gynecomastia and eunuchoidism, and postpuberal seminiferous tubular atrophy. No chromosomal abnormality.
      c. Male Turner's syndrome. Somatic anomalies of phenotypic female Turner's syndrome. Leukocyte karyotype usually XY, although occasionally show abnormal chromosomes or mosaicism. Variable testicular histology and function.
      d. Sertoli-cell-only syndrome (germinal aplasia). Normal development. Infertility. No chromosomal abnormality. Etiology unknown.
      e. Anorchia. Cryptorchid with no somatic anomalies. No chromosomal abnormality. Etiology unknown.
    2. Postpuberal abnormalities.
      a. Seminiferous tubule failure.
        1. Orchitis (mumps, tuberculosis, leprosy, gonorrheal infection, brucellosis, syphilis, etc.), hyperpyrexia, irradiation, trauma, neoplasm, or surgical castration.
        2. Congenital disorders—myotonia dystrophica, cystic fibrosis, Laurence-Moon-Biedl syndrome.
        3. Idiopathic.
      b. Leydig cell failure (male climacteric).
  B. Secondary (decreased urinary gonadotropins).
    1. Isolated gonadotropin deficiency. Often associated with congenital anomalies including anosmia or hyposmia, harelip, cleft palate, etc. May be inherited as a sex-linked recessive or sex-limited autosomal dominant.
    2. Isolated ICSH deficiency (fertile eunuch).
    3. Multiple pituitary deficiencies (panhypopituitarism).
      a. Idiopathic prepuberal.
      b. Secondary to neurophyophyseal lesions—neoplasm (chromophobe, astrocytoma, hamartoma, teratoma), cyst (craniopharyngioma) or granulomatous process (sarcoid, etc.).
      c. Congenital disorders—Laurence-Moon-Biedl syndrome.
II. Hypergonadism (excess androgen production).
  A. Primary (functioning interstitial cell tumor).
  B. Secondary (measurable urinary gonadotropins).
    1. Familial.
    2. Tumor in region of third ventricle (pinealoma, astrocytoma, hamartoma, teratoma, and craniopharyngioma).

pathologic changes at an earlier age) until the expected time of puberty. A total absence of any of the usual changes of adolescence at approximately age fourteen or fifteen suggests that interstitial cell function may be abnormal. However, as in other developmental states, there is a wide range of normal variation, so that puberal changes may not be noticeable in some normal boys until the sixteenth or seventeenth year, when genital and secondary sexual changes may begin to be apparent. This delay in adolescent development causes much concern to patient, family, and physician, and not infrequently some form of hormonal therapy is given, followed by somatic changes that undoubtedly would have occurred without treatment.

POSTPUBERAL HYPOGONADISM. Postpuberal hypogonadal changes decrease or are minimized when the hypogonadal state develops late in adult life; thus castration of elderly men may cause none of the alterations seen in younger individuals. In young males, there are usually diminished beard growth and thinning axillary and other body hair. The skin becomes smoother, the prostate atrophies to the point of being barely palpable, and sexual desire and performance wane. The genitalia lose pigmentation and may decrease somewhat in size. The voice does not change, but gynecomastia may appear. In older men none of these changes may be noted; beard and body hair growth usually persist, and there may be no noticeable change in libido or sexual function.

PRIMARY HYPOGONADISM. The causes of primary hypogonadism in males are listed in Table 97-1. The testicular abnormality may be present at birth as either a genetic or an embryologic defect, or it may occur at any time later in life as a result of either testicular infections (such as mumps, tuberculosis, brucellosis, leprosy, syphillis) or following trauma, irradiation, neoplasm, or castration, either surgical or accidental. Beginning in early adolescence, even before the appearance of the obvious physical characteristics of hypogonadism, the patient may have increased serum concentrations of pituitary gonadotropin hormones (measured by radioimmunoassay) and may excrete excessive quantities in the urine. The immature mouse uterine weight assay, which measures both ICSH and FSH, is used most frequently for determination of total urinary gonadotropin content. In addition, because of lack of testosterone synthesis, plasma testosterone concentrations as well as urinary 17-ketosteroid excretion of adult patients are significantly decreased. It should be stated here with emphasis, however, that the patient's own tissues clinically observed frequently provide the most significant assay of androgen production. The following syndrome is an example of primary hypogonadism.

KLINEFELTER'S SYNDROME (Semniferous Tubule Dysgenesis). Klinefelter, Reifenstein, and Albright described in 1942 a clinical syndrome of hypogonadism that includes gynecomastia, eunuchoidism, elevated level of urinary gonadotropins, and decreased testicular size associated with hyalinization of the tubules. Barr demonstrated that many of these patients were *chromatin-positive*, exhibiting nuclei similar to those seen in females (see Chap. 4). Culture of marrow cells and leukocytes in vitro in the presence of colchicine has permitted direct

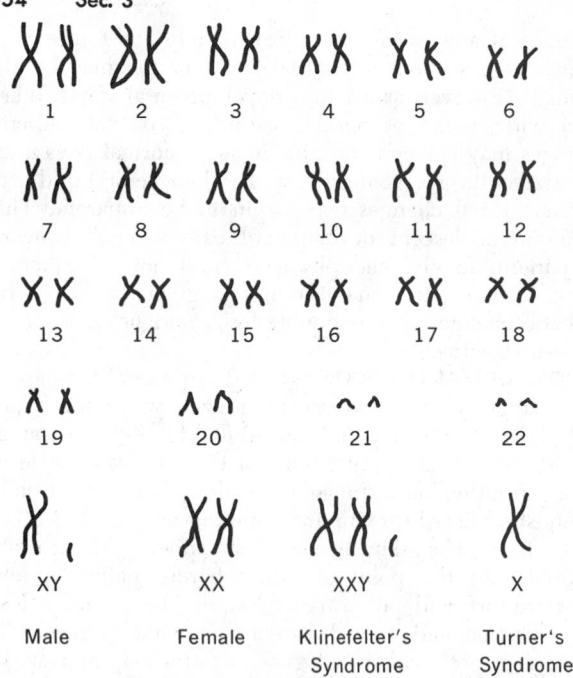

Fig. 97-3. Schematic drawing of 22 pairs of autosomes and sex chromosomes, including two aberrant forms of sex chromosomes as seen in patients with Klinefelter's or Turner's syndrome.

chromosomal counting and classification (see Fig. 97-3); and indeed, many patients with the triad described by Klinefelter et al. have been shown to possess an extra sex chromosome, resulting in a karyotypic classification of 22 autosomes plus 2 X chromosomes and 1 Y chromosome (See Chap. 4). Thus, they have 47 instead of 46 chromosomes, and it is therefore not surprising that many of these patients also have various degrees of mental deficiency. A clue to the diagnosis of this disorder often lies in the behavior and personality of the Klinefelter patient. Talkativeness with little substance to the content is an outstanding behavioral trait. Klinefelter's syndrome in some patients who lack the classical chemical findings of gynecomastia, eunuchoidism, and small testes may be discovered only when they appear in an infertility clinic. In addition, Klinefelter's syndrome is not infrequently discovered when the patient seeks medical care for chronic pulmonary disease, obesity, diabetes mellitus, varicose veins, and thrombophlebitis, disorders which appear to be more prevalent in these individuals; thus, the spectrum of Klinefelter's syndrome is broad, including obviously feminized males on one end and, on the other end, normally virilized men with only abnormal microscopic testicular anatomy but often with the associated diseases listed above.

SECONDARY HYPOGONADISM. Secondary hypogonadism results from failure of pituitary elaboration of the necessary tropic hormones, specifically ICSH and FSH (Table 97-1, I-B). Isolated deficiencies of gonadotropic hormones without demonstrable loss of other pituitary hormones have been described in males in association with anosmia or hyposmia by Kallman. The condition is inherited either as a sex-linked recessive defect or as a sex-

limited autosomal dominant one. Very rarely, an isolated ICSH deficiency occurs. In most cases, however, there is an associated loss of other pituitary tropic hormones, resulting in growth failure before adolescence and in decreased thyroid, adrenal, and gonadal function at all ages. When there is a progressive loss of hypothalamic-pituitary function because of a neoplasm (chromophobe, astrocytoma, hamartoma, teratoma), cyst (craniopharyngioma), or granulomatous process (sarcoid), a decrease of gonadotropins is often the first deficiency observed, and the patient, therefore, may appear in the clinic with isolated hypogonadism. Prepuberal hypopituitarism is usually recognized because of the dwarfism that results from growth hormone deficiency. Occasionally, however, testes of preadolescent boys with other evidences of pituitary dysfunction are significantly small. Froehlich in 1901 described such an obese hypogonadal boy with signs of a tumor in the hypothalamic area. Since then, Froelich's name has been inappropriately applied to the condition of a large group of overweight boys with slightly retarded maturation but with normal linear growth and no demonstrated hypothalamic lesion; in such cases the delay in maturation is without any real clinical significance. Patients with the Laurence-Moon-Biedl syndrome have been described with both primary (germinal aplasia) and secondary (hypogonadotropic) hypogonadism.

The absence of serum and urinary gonadotropins after the age of adolescence in patients with diminished gonadal function is diagnostic of secondary hypogonadism. Studies of growth, thyroid, adrenal, and antidiuretic hormones may reveal clinically unsuspected deficiencies. Skull roentgenogram may also show intracranial calcification, enlargement of the sella turcica, or erosion of the clinoid processes, and visual field examination may demonstrate early involvement of the optic nerves.

TREATMENT OF HYPOGONADISM. Patients with primary hypogonadism (increased urinary gonadotropins) require testosterone replacement therapy. Preparations commonly used are listed in Table 97-2. The usual method of ther-

Table 97-2. HORMONAL THERAPY FOR HYPOGONADISM

Preparations	Route and Dosage
Methyltestosterone (linguets)	Sublingual 5–10 mg, 4 times daily.
Testosterone propionate	Intramuscular 25–50 mg, 3 times weekly.
Testosterone enanthate Testosterone cyclopentyl-propionate Testosterone phenylacetate	Intramuscular 100–200 mg every 1–2 weeks for maximum effect, 200 mg every 3–5 weeks for maintenance.
Human chorionic gonadotropin	Intramuscular 1,000–4,000 IU 3 times weekly for 6 to 9 months. Repeated courses as required.

apy is to start with relatively small doses of the long-acting depot preparations of testosterone, giving either 50 mg every 2 weeks or 150 mg every 3 to 4 weeks. The dosage subsequently (after epiphyseal fusion in adolescent boys) is increased to 200 mg every 2 weeks to obtain full androgen effect, including deepening of the voice and increased facial hair. Final adult maintenance requirements are usually satisfied by 200 mg of the depot preparations every 3 to 5 weeks. Excessive acne formation, edema from retention of sodium, and undesirable personality changes all indicate overtreatment, and the dosage should be diminished appropriately.

In patients with secondary hypogonadism, a trial on human chorionic gonadotropin (HCG) may be indicated. Usually 6 to 9 months of 1,000 to 4,000 IU of HCG are given as a single course. If regression to a hypogonadal state occurs when HCG is discontinued, either a second course of HCG may be given or testosterone therapy as outlined above may be begun. In the past, long-term therapy with HCG has not proved practical. A gonadotropin preparation rich in FSH has been obtained from human menopausal urine. Experience with this preparation in gonadotropin-deficient postpuberal males indicates that it can restore spermatogenesis to normal. The prepuberal testes seem to require stimulation with HCG before spermatogenesis can be induced by administration of the human menopausal gonadotropin preparation.

Hypergonadism

The production of excessive quantities of androgenic hormones in the adult male results in little, if any, morphologic or functional change. However, in the child, the somatic changes associated with puberty may be induced at an early age and therefore become clinically apparent (precocious puberty). The causes of hypergonadism and isosexual precocity in the male are listed in Table 97-1. Hypergonadism may be due to excessive androgen production from a functioning testicular tumor, the Leydig, or interstitial, cell carcinoma. Children with these tumors show all the changes associated with puberty, such as increased hair growth and phallic enlargement, and usually have a palpable testicular tumor. However, the presence of the tumor may be difficult to determine if the testes are undescended, or if the tumor is extremely active in producing hormone but is very small. Plasma testosterone concentrations are increased. Urinary 17-ketosteroids, however, may be normal or only slightly increased, because of the marked potency of testosterone. Urinary pituitary gonadotropins are usually absent. Hypergonadism may also result from an early onset of puberty due to altered hypothalamic-pituitary function. The sequence of development is similar to that observed in adolescence, with enlargement of genitalia, appearance of pubic and axillary hair, deepening of the voice, and appearance of acne and seborrhea occurring in that order and beginning at two to three years of age or earlier. The testes are large for the patient's chronologic age but are in accord with the size expected for the degree of maturity exhibited by the remainder of his somatic development. Gonadotropins may be present in the urine but are not invariably measurable by routine assay procedures. In the early stages, the level of 17-ketosteroids may not be significantly elevated for the patient's chronologic age (in contrast to virilism produced by adrenal abnormalities), but

subsequently it rises to a degree appropriate for his developmental age. Isosexual precosity of this type in males, although uncommon, is often familial, in contrast to the more frequently occurring true precocity in females, from whom a family history of early puberty is seldom obtained. When true precosity occurs in males without a family history, it is almost always associated with space-occupying lesions in the region of the third ventricle (pinealoma, astrocytoma, hamartoma, and rarely a craniopharyngioma). The continued production of androgens excessive for their age in these patients results in accelerated growth during childhood, followed by early closure of the epiphyses, ending in an adult who frequently is smaller than his contemporaries.

Isosexual precosity in the male may also result from excessive quantities of adrenal androgens. The pattern of accelerated growth and development is similar to that produced by testicular hormones. The testes remain, however, infantile and atrophic; and gonadotropins are invariably absent. The diagnosis is made on the basis of markedly elevated level of urinary 17-ketosteroids. For further discussion, see Chap. 92.

NEOPLASMS OF THE TESTES

Neoplasms of the testes are relatively uncommon. It is generally believed that they occur more often in the cryptorchid testis (1 in 2,000) than in the normal testis (1 in 100,000). They may be classified as follows, in their relative order of frequency:

1. Seminoma (germinoma)
2. Teratocarcinoma
3. Embryonal carcinoma
   a. Chorioepithelioma
4. Teratoma
5. Interstitial cell tumor
6. Fibroma, lipoma, adrenoma, myxoma
7. Unclassified varieties

In addition, lymphoma, plasmacytoma, leukemia, and carcinoma of other tissues occasionally produce secondary tumors in the testes. The incidence of teratocarcinoma is roughly constant throughout life, whereas the incidence of seminoma tends to rise with age. One-year survival is rare for patients with embryonal carcinomas and chorioepitheliomas, not uncommon for those with teratocarcinomas and teratomas, and the rule for those with seminomas.

Endocrine changes (such as gynecomastia and increased secretion of gonadotropins, giving a positive Aschheim-Zondek test result) are occasionally seen with chorioepitheliomas, as well as with embryonal carcinomas and teratocarcinomas. The endocrine effects of interstitial cell tumors have been discussed.

Diagnosis

The diagnosis is made by palpating a mass, usually firm, smooth, and painless. Neoplasms must be distinguished from the changes induced by tuberculosis or gonorrheal epididymitis, from syphilis (usually accompanied by a positive serologic test and a response to specific therapy), and from the various fluid-containing cysts (hydrocele, spermatocele), which may be transilluminated. The diagnosis may be aided also by increased urinary excretion of 17-ketosteroids, estrogens, or gonadotropins; the latter give a positive Aschheim-Zondek test. Rarely, tumor cells may be identified in the semen.

Treatment

Surgical removal is always indicated in any tumor of the testes and will usually effect a cure in the benign varieties. If the tumor is malignant, a radical operation, followed by irradiation, should be employed. X-ray therapy has been shown to effect a cure in the majority of cases of seminoma. Results of therapy may be followed by repeated determinations of the 17-ketosteroids or estrogens or by the Aschheim-Zondek test, if it was originally positive. Certain testicular tumors, particularly the chorioepitheliomas, have been shown to be exquisitely sensitive to certain antimetabolic agents such as 4-amino-N^{10}-methylpteroylgutamic acid (Methotrexate).

DISEASES OF THE PROSTATE

Benign Prostatic Hypertrophy

This pathophysiologic disorder, which affects a high proportion of elderly men, is a significant cause of dysuria and incontinence (see Chap. 49) and urinary tract obstruction (see Chap. 302). It has been also considered a potentially precancerous lesion. Hormonally, the prostate is significant as a clinical indicator of androgen secretion, since appreciable reduction in prostatic size accompanies either primary or secondary hypogonadism as well as those disorders of liver function characterized by excessive estrogen activity.

Carcinoma of the Prostate

Adenocarcinoma of the prostate is one of the most common tumors of men. It is rare before the age of forty; the incidence rises rapidly with advancing age, with the condition occurring microscopically in 10 to 15 percent of men in the fifth decade and in as many as 40 percent of those in the eighth decade. However, only one-fourth of these cases may become clinically apparent before death. Three-fourths of these tumors arise in the posterior lobe. The majority are easily palpable; hence, frequent routine rectal examinations are indicated to demonstrate early, operable tumors. Although the whole gland need not be enlarged, the presence of stony, hard, indurated nodules or masses strongly suggests an adenocarcinoma. Frequently, there may be an elevation in the "prostatic" fraction of serum acid phosphatase while the tumor is still located within the prostatic capsule, and elevation of this enzyme may serve to differentiate a benign hypertropic nodule from a malignancy. Once the tumor has spread locally from the gland, particularly after it has

metastasized, total serum acid and alkaline phosphatase levels may be greatly elevated.

Therapy consists of radical prostatectomy; irradiation by x-ray, radium, or radioactive isotopes (colloidal gold); and estrogen hormonal treatment (especially when metastatic disease develops). Androgens are decreased by orchidectomy and by adrenalectomy or adrenocortical suppression following dexamethasone administration (1 to 2 mg given orally in divided doses); estrogen levels are increased by administering diethylstilbestrol, 10 to 15 mg daily, or the equivalent dosage of other estrogenic products.

REFERENCES

Albert, A.: Bioassay and Radioimmunoassay of Human Gonadotropins, J. Clin. Endocrinol. & Metab., 28:1683, 1968.

Albert, A., L. O. Underdahl, L. F. Greene, and N. Lorenz: Male Hypogonadism: I, II, III, IV, V, VI, VII, Proc. Staff Meet. Mayo Clinic, 28:409, 557, 698, 1953; 29:131, 317, 368, 1954; 30:31, 1955.

Dorfman, R. I., and R. A. Shipley: "Androgens–Biochemistry, Physiology and Clinical Significance," New York, John Wiley & Sons, Inc., 1956.

Federman, D. D.: "Abnormal Sexual Development. A Genetic and Endocrine Approach to Differential Diagnosis," Philadelphia, W. B. Saunders Company, 1967.

Howard, R. P., R. C. Sniffen, F. A. Simmons, and F. Albright: Testicular Deficiency: A Clinical and Pathological Study, J. Clin. Endocrinol., 10:121, 1950.

Klinefelter, H., E. Reifenstein, Jr., and F. Albright: Klinefelter Syndrome Characterized by Gynecomastia, Aspermatogenesis without A-Leydigism, and Increased Excretion of Follicle-stimulating Hormone, J. Clin. Endocrinol., 2:615, 1942.

McCullagh, E. P., J. C. Beck, and C. A. Schaffenburg: A Syndrome of Eunuchoidism with Spermatogenesis; Normal Urinary FSH and Low or Normal ICSH ("Fertile Eunuchs"), J. Clin. Endocrinol. & Metab., 13:489, 1953.

Patton, J. F., D. N. Seitzman, and R. A. Zone: Diagnosis and Treatment of Testicular Tumors, Am. J. Surg., 99:525, 1960.

Paulsen, C. A.: The Testes, p. 405 in "Textbook of Endocrinology," R. H. Williams (Ed.), Philadelphia, W. B. Saunders Company, 1968.

Strickland, A. L., and F. S. French: Absence of Response to Dihydrotestosterone in the Syndrome of Testicular Feminization, J. Clin. Endocrinol., 29:1284, 1969.

98 DISEASES OF THE OVARY
Janet W. McArthur

HISTORY

The ovulatory function of the ovaries was first described by a Dutch physician, Reinier de Graaf, in 1673. He recognized small fluid blisters, now known as *graafian follicles*, which had succeeded in reaching the surface of the ovaries before ovulation. The hormonal function of the ovaries was first demonstrated in 1896, by the German biologist, Knauer, who showed that ovarian grafts in the dog would prevent the uterine atrophy that follows castration. It was next observed, by Marshall and Jolly, that the ovarian secretion which produced estrus differed from that which was formed by the corpus luteum. The presence of estrogens in the follicles was proved by R. T. Frank, and their occurrence in urine was established by Allen and Doisy, who demonstrated the effectiveness of potent urinary extracts in producing estrus in the vaginal mucosa of rodents. This relatively simple biologic assay method became of incomparable help in the isolation and synthesis of estrogenic compounds. In 1929, Butenandt and Doisy and associates isolated estrone in a crystalline form from the urine of pregnant women. In 1930, estriol was identified by Browne in human placentas, and in 1936, MacCorquodale obtained estradiol, the most potent natural estrogen, from ovarian follicular fluid. The progestational activity of the corpus luteum hormone was first demonstrated by Corner and Allen in 1929. Five years later progesterone was isolated and identified simultaneously and independently by Butenandt, Allen, Slotta, and Hartmann.

INTRODUCTION

The ovary is a specialized organ of reproduction which serves (1) as an exocrine gland which liberates gametes for fertilization, and (2) as a complex of endocrine glands which secretes hormones responsible for (a) the growth and cyclic function of the reproductive tract, and (b) a variety of metabolic effects in nongenital tissues. During mature reproductive life a new endocrine gland, the follicle, is activated each month. After ovulation the follicle undergoes transformation into a second gland of internal secretion, the corpus luteum. To the extent that the formation of the corpus luteum requires the prior existence of a follicle, the two structures are interdependent. Nevertheless, differences of fundamental significance obtain between their secretory products. Both structures are embedded in an interstitium, or stroma, which constitutes a third endocrine gland.

A major difference between the ovary and the testis is that the former is endowed with a finite stock of germ cells, whereas the latter proliferates gametes continuously. The number of ova reaches a maximum 5 months before birth. Thereafter the number declines, mainly as the result of atresia, until by the end of the fifth decade the original complement of germ cells is exhausted. An inexorable, though less-rapid, decline in follicular hormone secretion begins in the fifth decade. In addition, the secretion of luteal hormones becomes more and more erratic as the incidence of anovulatory cycles increases. By old age, only the ovarian stroma retains any semblance of functioning tissue.

DEVELOPMENT

The formation of the gonads begins at a very early stage, when the embryo has attained a crown-rump length of 5 mm (twenty-one to twenty-eight days of age). The genetic sex of the conceptus is identifiable even earlier, at the age of fifteen days, by the presence of nuclear sex chromatin in the female. During the seventh week, the ovarian destiny of the "indifferent gonad" can be inferred histologically by the absence of the epithelial cords which characterize the developing testis.

Four major phases in the development of the ovary are recognized: (1) migration of primordial germ cells from their site of origin in the endoderm of the primitive gut to bilateral thickenings (the "germinal ridges") of the coelomic epithelium ventral to the developing mesonephros, (2) proliferation of the germinal and nongerminal cells in the genital ridges, (3) division of the gonads into a peripheral cortex and a central medulla, and (4) sex differentiation, consisting of proliferation of the cortex and involution of the medulla in the female, and the reverse process in the male. A complex sex-determining mechanism, the details of which are obscure, is responsible for the conversion of the "indifferent gonad" into an ovary or testis. The cortical germ cells (oogonia) increase rapidly in number as a result of mitotic division, whereupon they enter the meiotic prophase, to become, by definition, oocytes. Each is soon invested by a single layer of smaller supporting cells to form the primordial follicles. In this resting phase the oocytes remain throughout childhood and adult life until either preovulatory maturation or pseudomaturation with atresia occurs. The oocytes appear to exert an inductive influence upon the surrounding granulosa cells, since follicles fail to develop in ovaries which lack oocytes, and oocyte atresia is followed by granulosal degeneration.

COMPARTMENTS

The complexity of the tasks devolving upon the ovary is reflected in the heterogeneity of its structure. Throughout active reproductive life, morphologic and biochemical events are occurring simultaneously in the follicular, luteal, and interstitial compartments. Anatomic specialization in the ovary is paralleled by a degree of biochemical specialization. Thus, although in vitro studies reveal that upon incubation with acetate, each of the compartments is capable of synthesizing all the major categories of gonadal steroids, in vivo there is a preferential formation of estrogen by the follicle, of progestogens by the corpus luteum, and of androgens by the stroma.

Follicle

Follicular growth comprises two phases. During the first, the oocyte enlarges rapidly to virtually adult dimensions while the investing cortical cells (the membrana granulosa), which convert the germ cell into a primordial follicle, grow very slowly. During the second phase, further growth of the oocyte is minimal but the follicle enlarges rapidly and develops an antrum, which fills with fluid secreted by the granulosa cells. The antrum first appears when the follicle attains a diameter two or three times that of the contained oocyte. Once a follicle has acquired an antrum it becomes, by definition, a graafian follicle.

Maturation falls short of completion in all but that minute proportion of graafian follicles destined to ovulate. Periodically, in response to gonadotropin stimulation (see below), the elected follicle exhibits an intense preovulatory growth spurt, accompanied by increasing antral distension, the loosening of the cumulus oophorus (those granulosa cells which hold the egg in suspension), and the hypertrophy and hyperemia of the theca interna. As the follicle enlarges, its wall thins and presently ruptures, releasing the ovum into the peritoneal cavity. A complex of satellite follicles enlarges concomitantly, but to a lesser extent; and after ovulation they undergo rapid atresia.

Growth of the follicle is paralleled by biochemical processes resulting in the secretion of estrogen and, during the immediately preovulatory phase, of small amounts of progesterone. At the peak of follicular activity, the secretion rate of estradiol varies from 0.2 to 0.5 mg per 24 hr. The prime locus of estrogen synthesis has not been directly identified but is believed to be the theca interna.

Corpus Luteum

Following ovulation the ruptured follicle is converted into a corpus luteum, which likewise has a limited anatomic and biochemical life span. This is divisible into stages of proliferation and hyperemia, vascularization, maturity, and retrogression. The secretion of estrogen is continued and is supplemented by the secretion of progesterone. Biosynthetic activity increases steadily and becomes maximal on days 21 to 22 of the menstrual cycle, when implantation of the fertilized ovum occurs. Estimates of the progesterone secretion rate, though discrepant, agree qualitatively in that they reveal a phenomenal increase in the biosynthetic capacity of the transformed follicle, to the vicinity of 20 to 40 mg progesterone per day.

How the follicular-to-luteal change in the pattern of hormone synthesis is effected is the subject of much speculation. One view is embodied in the so-called "two-cell" theory. This postulates that the cells of the theca interna are endowed with the full enzyme complement required for the synthesis of estradiol-17β, whereas the cells of the granulosa possess little or no 17-desmolase activity and only weak 17-hydroxylase activity. During the follicular phase, the well-vascularized theca internal cells synthesize estrogens, which have ready access either to the follicular fluid or the systemic circulation, whereas the granulosa cells, lacking a blood supply, are presumably deprived of the nutrients required for hormone synthesis. After ovulation, the granulosa cells become richly vascularized, undergo enlargement, and form the corpus luteum. However, in consequence of their enzymic endowment, they are ill equipped to synthesize estrogen in quantity and secrete mainly progesterone.

In the event that conception occurs, the trophoblast of the implanted ovum secretes a complex of proteins known collectively as "human chorionic gonadotropin" (HCG) into the maternal circulation. By a luteotropic action, HCG then prolongs the life of the corpus luteum until the placenta gains secretory competency. If conception fails to occur, the corpus luteum undergoes rapid regression and over the course of 7 to 10 months is replaced by a hyaline remnant, the corpus albicans.

Interstitium

The interstitium, or stroma, acts as a supporting matrix for the follicles, corpora lutea, and corpora albicantia, and, in addition, it secretes steroids. Qualitative and quantitative changes in its structure occur in association with various reproductive processes. During pregnancy there is increasing luteinization of the stroma, and during the postmenopausal years stromal proliferation and luteinization are frequent. In extreme old age, the stroma tends to lose its stimulated appearance. The higher grades of stromal luteinization are sometimes associated with clinical indications of androgen hypersecretion.

The hilus may come eventually to be regarded as a fourth ovarian compartment, but at present it is generally treated as a specialized portion of the interstitium. It contains elements resembling testicular Leydig cells, which occur in nests, the size of which varies at different ages. Hyperplasia of these cells may occur during pregnancy, and the larger hilus cell complexes are more frequent in elderly women.

Androstenedione and dehydroepiandrosterone can be extracted from normal ovarian stroma, the highest concentrations being found in the hilus.

PHYSIOLOGIC CONTROL OF THE OVARY

The **follicles of the ovary** can develop to the antrum stage in the absence of pituitary function. However, maturation of the follicles and the sequential changes which characterize the normal menstrual cycle are contingent upon the release of the gonadotropins from the anterior lobe of the pituitary. The pituitary, in turn, is subject to the control of the hypothalamus. When stimulated by pituitary follicle–stimulating hormone (FSH) the follicles acquire an investment of multiple layers of granulosa cells, and they secrete estrogen in response to the joint action of FSH and luteinizing hormone (LH). Preovulatory growth of the follicle, ovulation, and transformation of the spent follicle into a corpus luteum are effected by LH, possibly in conjunction with FSH. Once formed, the human **corpus luteum** requires no additional gonadotropin support in order to secrete estrogen and progesterone. The in vitro synthesis of steroids by the stroma is increased by LH and human chorionic gonadotropin, (HCG), which, in the female as in the male, appear to be interstitial cell–stimulating hormones.

The central nervous system controls the synthesis and release of FSH and LH by the pituitary via two mechanisms. The first is a system which is localized in the ventromedial arcuate nuclear region of the hypothalamus. By discharging tonic quantities of the so-called FSH- and LH-releasing factors into the hypophyseal-portal circulation, this system assures the basal secretion of gonadotropin in quantities sufficient to maintain estrogen production. However, the ovulatory surge of gonadotropin cannot be independently initiated at this level. The second system comprises sex steroid–sensitive (and perhaps gonadotropin-sensitive) neural elements which are located mainly in the preoptic region of the anterior hypothalamus, the thalamohypothalamic border region, and the limbic system. Afferent pathways from the external environment also converge upon this region of the hypothalamus, which integrates all the relevant information. Under proper hormonal and environmental conditions, the preoptic region activates the more terminal infundibular region and evokes an ovulatory discharge of gonadotropins from the pituitary (Fig. 98-1).

HORMONES OF THE OVARY

The ovary secretes a water-soluble nonsteroid hormone or hormone complex known as relaxin and three types of steroid hormones: estrogens, progestogens, and androgens.

Nonsteroid (Relaxin)

Relaxin has not been isolated as a chemical entity, but its activity is associated with a water-soluble polypeptide structure. In conjunction with estrogens and progestogens, it facilitates parturition in certain mammals by loosening the symphysis pubis and sacroiliac joints. Relaxin has also been reported to soften the cervix, increase the uterine content of glycogen, nitrogen, and water, decrease the tone and motility of the uterus, increase uterine responsiveness to oxytocin, and promote lobuloalveolar growth of the mammary gland. In human pregnancy, blood relaxin values reach a maximum during the thirty-sixth week and remain high until delivery, whereupon a precipitous fall occurs. The cellular source in the ovary is unknown, and since the hormone can apparently be formed in other organs of the reproductive tract, its specificity as an ovarian secretion is in doubt.

Steroids

The ovarian steroids are synthesized from acetate via cholesterol and pregnenolone by essentially the same pathways as exist in other steroid-producing organs, the testis, adrenal cortex, and placenta.

ESTROGENS. The term *estrogen* refers strictly to substances capable of inducing estrus, or sexual receptivity, in female mammals. However, it has been extended to include compounds which produce certain uterine changes and to the steroid metabolites of true estrogens, whether or not these possess biologic activity. In the nonpregnant female, the ovary is the principal site of estrogen formation; during pregnancy, placental estrogen formation gradually increases until, by the third trimester, it may exceed ovarian production by a thousand fold.

Estradiol-17$_\beta$ is believed to be the primary secretory product of the human ovary, and to be interconvertible

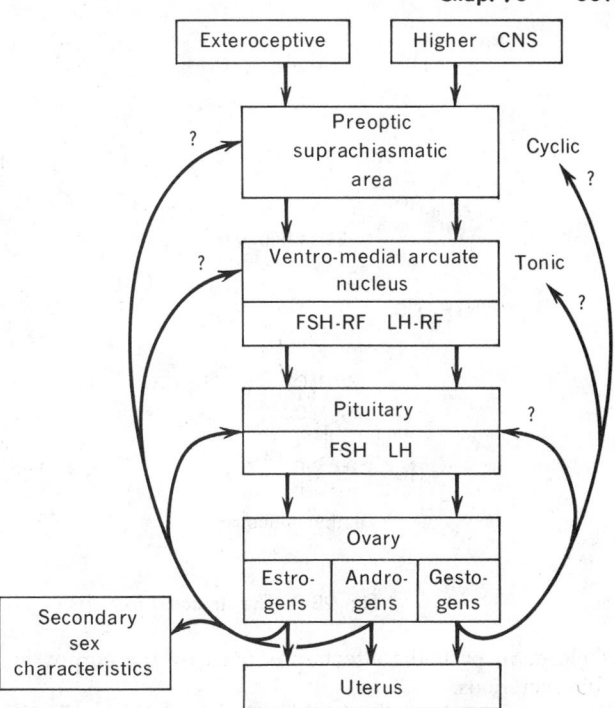

Fig. 98-1. The central nervous system–pituitary–ovarian–uterine chain. (*Adapted from R. Hertz, W. D. Odell, and G. T. Ross, Ann. Int. Med., 65:800, 1966.*)

with estrone by dehydrogenases which are present in the ovary and in many other tissues. Estrone and estradiol are, in turn, irreversibly converted to estriol, an estrogen of human urine that is quantitatively important, especially during pregnancy. Additional estrogenic metabolites of low biologic activity have been isolated in great number from human tissues and from the urine of pregnant and nonpregnant women.

The natural estrogens are all 18- or 19-carbon steroids which are characterized by the aromatic nature of ring A, the oxygen substituent at C-17, and the phenolic hydoxyl group at C-3. Many nonsteroidal estrogens have been synthesized for clinical use; they produce biologic effects resembling those of the natural estrogens. Representative examples from both the natural and synthetic categories are depicted in Fig. 98-2.

The liver is the principal site of the interconversion of estradiol and estrone, and is largely responsible for the inactivation of estrogen in the body. Protein-bound estrogen is abstracted from the plasma and excreted into the bile, from which it returns to the liver via the enterohepatic circulation. Degradation of estrogen is accomplished by (1) conversion to relatively inactive estrogenic compounds, (2) conjugation with glucuronic and sulfuric acids for excretion in the urine as water-soluble complexes, and (3) oxidation to unknown nonestrogenic substances.

PROGESTERONES. The term *progestogen* refers to substances which serve to prepare the uterus for the reception and development of the fertilized ovum. It has been extended to include compounds capable of duplicating, in

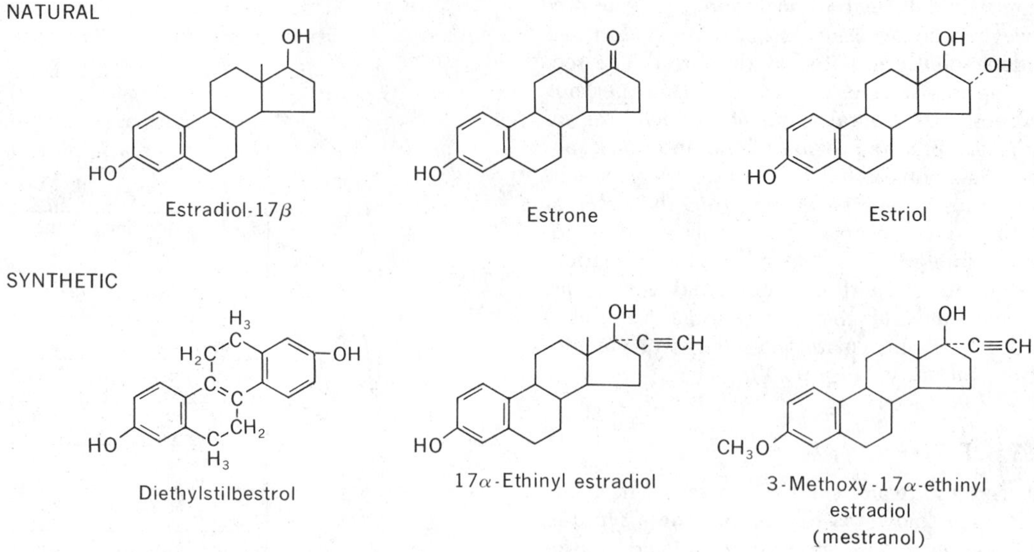

NATURAL

Estradiol-17β   Estrone   Estriol

SYNTHETIC

Diethylstilbestrol   17α-Ethinyl estradiol   3-Methoxy-17α-ethinyl estradiol (mestranol)

Fig. 98-2. The structural formulas of some important estrogens, natural and synthetic.

whole or in part, the effects produced by the corpus luteum secretions.

Progesterone is synthesized by all the steroid-producing glands. When secreted by the corpus luteum and placenta it exerts powerful physiologic effects in its own right; in addition, it is thought to serve as the key intermediate from which the androgens, estrogens, and corticosteroids are ultimately derived.

The ovarian progestogens consist of progesterone, the most important and abundant compound, and at least two other steroids: 20_β- and 20_β-dihydroprogesterone. Both of these partially reduced compounds have been detected in human follicular fluid and in the corpus luteum and placenta, the 20_α isomer in higher concentration than the

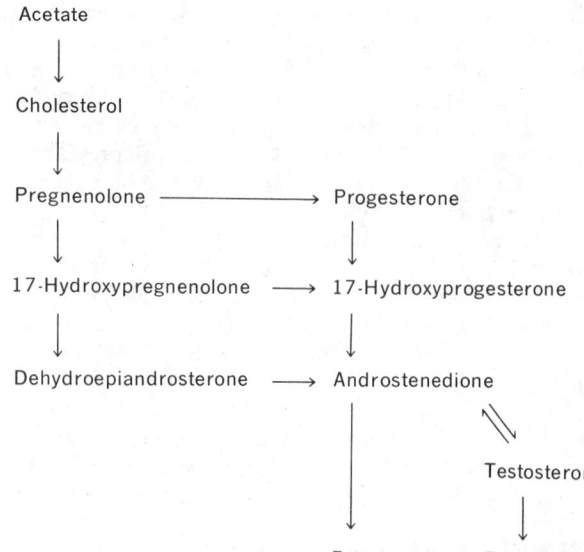

Fig. 98-3. Biosynthetic pathways for the synthesis of ovarian estrogens in the human female. (*Adapted from O. W. Smith and K. J. Ryan, Am. J. Obstet. & Gynecol., 84:141, 1962.*)

20_β. The basic molecule consists of 21 carbon atoms, two of which are contained in the side chain at C-17. These compounds are secreted by the follicle just prior to ovulation and are produced in much larger amounts by the corpus luteum. The quantity of progesterone which can be isolated from the corpus luteum is small compared with the amounts of progesterone secreted during the luteal phase of the cycle, indicating that progesterone is secreted almost as rapidly as it is produced.

A number of progestational steroids which mimic various facets of natural progesterone action have been synthesized. Many exhibit androgenic or estrogenic as well as progestational properties and, in these qualitative differences from the natural hormone, differ materially from the synthetic estrogen compounds. The short half-life of progesterone and the large doses consequently required to elicit biologic effects have prompted efforts to alter the progesterone molecule so as to increase its potency. Two groups of progestogens far surpassing the natural hormone in oral activity have been synthesized: (1) derivatives of testosterone (ethisterone) and of 19-nortestosterone (e.g., norethynodrel and norethindrone), the latter exhibiting the marked enhancement of oral potency which results from the removal of the angle-methyl group (C_{19}) attached to C_{10}, and (2) compounds derived from 17-hydroxyprogesterone [e.g., medroxyprogesterone (Provera), chlormadinone]. Esterification of 17_α-hydroxyprogesterone by caproic or other long-chain fatty acids yields long-acting preparations useful for parenteral administration.

The structural formulas of some representative synthetic progestational steroids are shown in Fig. 98-4, together with allied natural compounds.

The liver is largely responsible for the inactivation of progesterone, which it first reduces to pregnanediol and then conjugates with glucuronic acid for excretion in the urine. These processes are aided by an enterohepatic circulation which differs from that of the estrogens in that approximately 30 percent of progesterone or its metabolites are lost in the feces, whereas the estrogens are almost completely absorbed from the intestine. Some 10 to 15 percent of exogenously administered progesterone can be accounted for by urinary pregnanediol, and a small additional percentage by several isomers and closely related pregnane derivatives. The major degradation products of progesterone are unknown.

ANDROGENS. That the ovary possesses the biochemical potential for androgen production has long been evident from physiologic and clinical observations. In vitro incubations reveal, moreover, that testosterone is a product of the stroma and of no other ovarian compartment. However, in vivo studies are bringing to light an exceedingly complex situation.

Although **testosterone** is present in measurable amounts

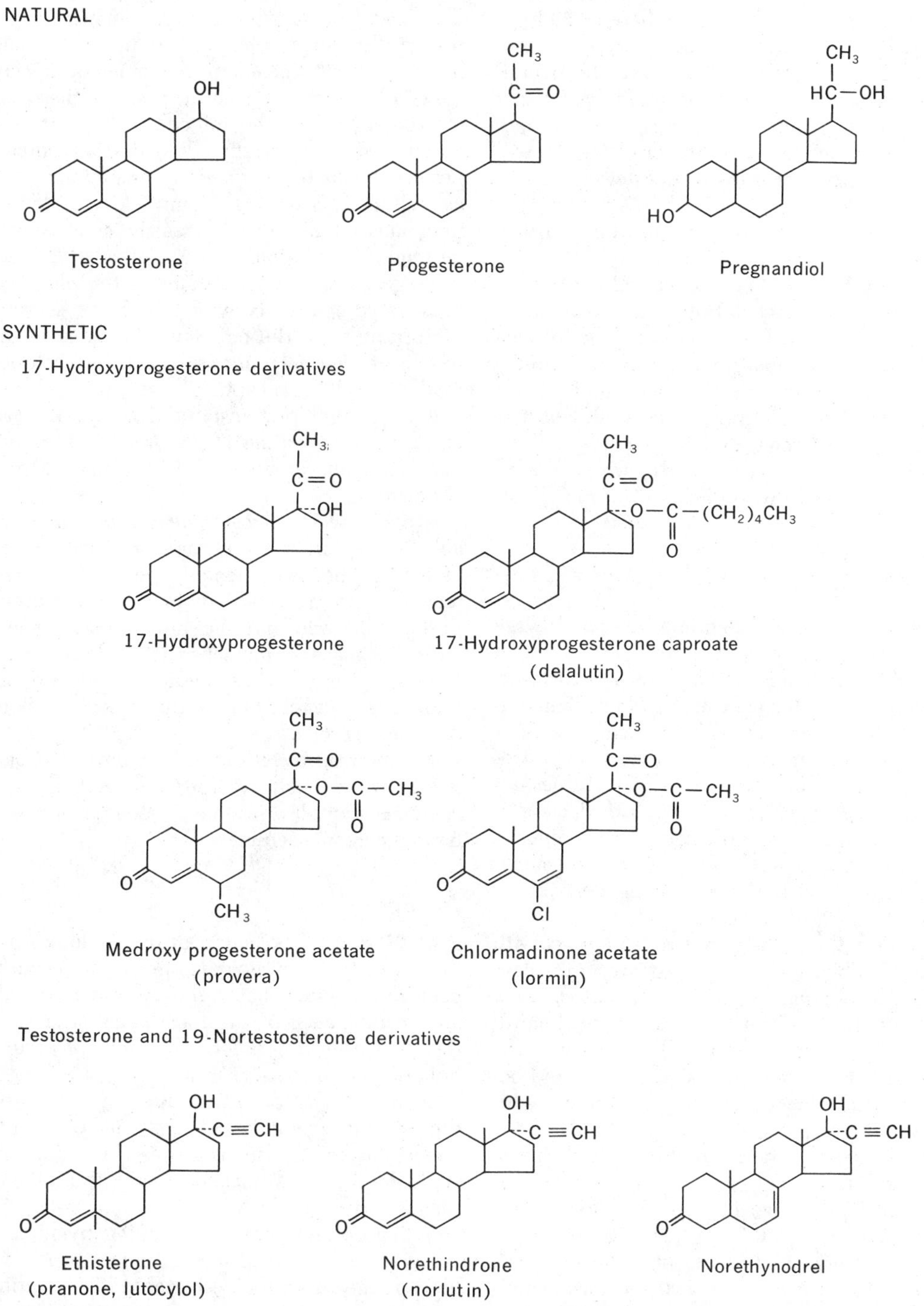

Fig. 98-4. The structural formulas of some important progestogens and allied compounds.

in the circulation of the human female, the ovarian contribution, as measured in the venous effluent, is negligible. It would appear that such androgen precursors as androstenedione and dehydroepiandrosterone, which are secreted to a small extent by the ovaries and to a greater extent by the adrenal cortex, are converted to active androgens in the peripheral tissues. According to one view, the function of androstenedione and dehydroepiandrosterone may be to serve as prehormones (endocrine secretions which possess little or no inherent biologic activity but which, after peripheral conversion to more active compounds, contribute significantly to the overall biologic effect). Peripheral conversion could be by any tissues, including those of the target organs. This arrangement would enable effective concentrations of an active product (e.g., testosterone or dihydrotestosterone) to be achieved locally in regions such as the clitoris without the high circulating levels of androgen which would virilize a female subject.

Androstenedione is thought to be converted in the liver to testosterone and to undergo intrahepatic conjugation with glucuronic acid without mixing with the plasma testosterone. Thus, testosterone glucosiduronate is not a unique metabolite of testosterone. A proportion of plasma testosterone is reduced by the liver to the weakly androgenic compound, androsterone, and its inactive isomer, 5_β-androsterone, and these compounds are rendered water-soluble by conjugation with glucuronic and sulfuric acid.

Levels in Body Fluids

ESTROGENS. Colorimetric and fluorimetric methods are available for measurement of the natural estrogens in urine. During the menstrual cycle, two peaks of estrogen excretion are generally noted, one in midcycle immediately prior to ovulation, and the other during the midluteal phase. During the midcycle peak, the "total" estrogen excretion (estradiol plus estrone and estriol) does not normally exceed 100 μg per 24 hr. In the fifth decade of life, the urinary estrogen levels of women commence a steady decline. The urinary estrogen level of postmenopausal women is low and is thought to be derived, in large part, from the adrenal cortex.

Urinary levels of endogenous estrogen in patients with liver disease are variable, with only a proportion displaying the increased levels that might be anticipated.

Urinary estrogen determinations are sometimes helpful in detecting granulosa cell or theca cell tumors in postmenopausal women. The adrenogenital syndrome and occasional adrenocortical tumors are also associated with elevated levels of urinary estrogen.

Levels of "free" estrone and estradiol have been measured throughout the menstrual cycle by fluorimetric and isotopic techniques. The range of normal concentration of both compounds is 0.01 to 0.03 μg per 100 ml plasma during the follicular and luteal phases of the cycle, with increases in the levels to 0.1 μg per 100 ml during midcycle.

PROGESTOGENS. *Pregnanediol,* the most important reduction product of progesterone, is excreted in the urine as the glucosiduronate and is measurable by gravimetric, colorimetric, and gas chromatographic techniques. Although pregnanediol is not a unique metabolite of progesterone, there is a rough correlation between the rate of pregnanediol excretion and the rate of progesterone secretion. Low and relatively constant levels of urinary pregnanediol (in the vicinity of 1 mg per 24 hr) are detected during the follicular phase of the cycle; higher levels, with a range of 2 to 8 mg per 24 hr, are found during the luteal phase. The urine of children, adult males, and postmenopausal women also contains pregnanediol in low concentrations; in these subjects and in women during the follicular phase of the cycle, the adrenal cortex is presumed to be the source. Since progesterone can be secreted by a luteinized theca interna as well as by a corpus luteum, elevated levels of urinary pregnanediol do not necessarily connote the prior occurrence of ovulation.

Progesterone concentrations in the plasma are low because of the rapidity with which the secreted hormone disappears from the circulation. Plasma levels are measurable in nonpregnant subjects by isotope derivative methods, electron-capture gas-liquid chromatography, and competitive protein-binding assays. In normal women, follicular phase values of the order of 0.05 μg per 100 ml and luteal phase values of 1.5 μg per 100 ml have been obtained.

ANDROGENS. Testosterone glucosiduronate is measurable in the urine by isotopic and gas chromatographic methods. The levels tend to be several times higher in men than in women, and in the latter they are higher during midcycle and the luteal phase than during the follicular phase of the menstrual cycle.

Testosterone, androstenedione, and dehydroepiandrosterone are measurable in the blood by double isotope dilution methods.

For the reasons set out earlier, these androgen measurements are difficult to interpret, and until various biochemical complexities have been resolved they are of limited clinical usefulness.

Actions

ESTROGENS. The name estrogen does scant justice to the diversity of physiologic effects produced by the estrogenic hormones. Their primary role is the development and maintenance of the female sex organs, and perhaps their most general effect is to promote tissue growth. At puberty the tubes, uterus, and vagina enlarge in response to increased estrogen stimulation, and the appearance of the external genitalia changes in consequence of fat deposition in the mons pubis and labia majora. The vaginal epithelium thickens during the follicular phase of the menstrual cycle, with shedding of large numbers of cornified epithelial cells containing pyknotic nuclei. The cervix is stimulated to secrete mucus of low viscosity and high permeability to spermatozoa. The uterine and tubal mocosa and their vasculature proliferate, and their musculature becomes contractile.

The estrogens exert direct effects on the ovary as well as indirect effects via the hypothalamic-pituitary system. Small amounts of estrogen promote the growth of vesicular follicles and increase their responsiveness to FSH. Puberal estrogen secretion causes the breasts to enlarge because of increased fat deposition, development of the supporting stroma, and ductal growth. The increased melanin pigmentation of the nipples and perineum is due, at least in part, to estrogen. There is a widespread deposition of fat in the subcutaneous tissues, particularly in the buttocks and thighs, leading to the characteristic rounding of the female figure.

The estrogens stimulate cell division in the deeper layers of the skin and gingivae, and in the mucosae of the oral cavity, nose, and urethra, causing a more rapid replacement of the outer cornified layers. Bone metabolism is significantly affected with increased osteoblastic activity, a positive calcium and phosphorus balance, widening of the pelvic outlet, and accelerated epiphyseal closure. The composition of the circulating lipids is altered, with a fall in total cholesterol and an increase in the α-lipoprotein fraction over the β fraction. Estrogens increase the levels of serum thyroxine-binding globulin, corticosteroid-binding globulin, ceruloplasmin, total copper, prothrombin, and AC-globulin. Antithrombin activity is decreased by estrogens.

PROGESTOGENS. Although secreted in far greater amounts than estrogen, progesterone exerts only negligible effects on the general body economy. It produces few specific changes when present alone, acting ordinarily in conjunction with estrogen. Progesterone tends to encourage tissue differentiation, rather than growth. Its most important function is to induce secretory changes in the lining of the tubes and uterus, the endometrium being thereby adapted for the implantation of the fertilized ovum. The viscosity of the cervical mucus is increased during the postovulatory phase, rendering it impermeable to spermatozoa, and ferning disappears. Tubal and uterine contractility are altered to favor transport of the fertilized ovum and to prevent its expulsion from the uterus. Lobuloalveolar proliferation of the breast is stimulated. Progesterone exerts a thermogenic action, the basal body temperature increasing by approximately 1° in midcycle and remaining elevated during the luteal phase. A slightly negative nitrogen balance is induced by progesterone, and by antagonism to aldosterone, a negative balance of sodium, chloride, and water is favored. Progesterone acts as a mild respiratory stimulant, increasing minute ventilation while decreasing alveolar and arterial CO_2 tension and the respiratory quotient.

ANDROGENS. The physiologic role of the androgens in the human female has not been clearly delineated. However, it is probable that they act to promote a positive nitrogen balance and to increase libido and muscular strength. Experimental evidence suggests that by local action within the ovary small amounts of androgen hasten antrum formation by separating the granulosa cells; larger amounts cause destruction of ova and granulosa cell atrophy. It may be that atresia of those follicles not destined to ovulate is promoted by androgens. In excess, these compounds may blight the follicles of the ovary in the Stein-Leventhal syndrome, contributing to its polycystic structure.

ENDOCRINE DISORDERS OF THE OVARY

Diseases of the ovary may be classified as endocrine and nonendocrine, depending on the presence or absence of disturbances in hormonal secretion. Endocrine diseases of the ovary, because of the prominence of their systemic manifestations, are of concern to the internist as well as the gynecologist and will be considered here. Nonendocrine diseases, which comprise such entities as endometriosis, infections, and nonfunctioning tumors of the ovary, tend to produce localized effects and will not be treated in this chapter. The endocrine disorders of the ovary may be classified as (1) hypo-hyper-, or dysfunctional, (2) primarily ovarian in origin or secondary to disturbances elsewhere, and (3) congenital or acquired. Some disorders, particularly those secondary to disturbances of hypothalamic or pituitary secretion, are general in that they affect follicular, luteal, and interstitial function. Others are compartmental in that they involve only one or two of the major subunits of the ovary (Table 98-1). Methodologic difficulties are responsible for the

Table 98-1. A CLASSIFICATION OF THE ENDOCRINE DISORDERS OF THE OVARY

I. Ovarian hypofunction
  A. Primary
    1. General
    2. Gonadal dysgenesis (Turner's syndrome)
    3. Menopause
  B. Secondary
    1. General
      a. Hypothalamic disorders
      b. Hypopituitarism
      c. Constitutional and metabolic disturbances
    2. Compartmental
      a. Anovulatory bleeding
      b. Inadequate luteal phase
II. Ovarian hyperfunction
  A. Primary
    1. Feminizing tumors
    2. Masculinizing tumors
  B. Secondary
    1. General: true precocious puberty
    2. Compartmental
      a. Persistent follicle cyst
      b. Corpus luteum cyst
      c. Stein-Leventhal syndrome and hyperthecosis
III. Ovarian dysfunction
  A. Choriocarcinoma
  B. Struma ovarii
  C. Carcinoid

meager documentation of many ovarian syndromes. However, as these are overcome, a rational biochemical schema for classification is emerging.

Because of the specialized role of the ovary as an **organ of reproduction,** its disturbances tend to give rise to more restricted symptoms than do those of many other endocrine organs. Unless the influence of a feminizing tumor, for example, is projected against the barren sexual background of childhood or the postmenopausal years, the manifestations may be so inconspicuous as to escape notice. Disorders heralded by infrequent menstruation, staining, or the disappearance of cramps may be trivial in systemic terms and yet have profound reproductive consequences. This is attributable to the fact that except during periods of temporary dissociation, such as adolescence and lactation, the exocrine and endocrine activities of the ovary are firmly integrated. Any deficiency in either results in impaired reproductive function.

OVARIAN HYPOFUNCTION

Although the suspension of established ovarian function is readily recognizable as pathologic, it may be less easy to determine whether delayed sexual maturation in a child reflects hypofunction of clinical significance. The menarche presently occurs at a mean age of 13.5 ± 5 years; since its timing is significantly influenced by genetic factors, the family history as regards menarcheal age should be investigated. The menarche is ordinarily preceded by breast development, a spurt in skeletal growth, and the appearance of pubic hair (axillary hair tends to appear almost simultaneously with the menarche). The presence of any of the secondary sex characters, or of superficial cells in the vaginal smear or urinary sediment, constitutes presumptive evidence of incipient ovarian activation.

Gonadal Dysgenesis (Turner's Syndrome)

Upon gaining the germinal ridges, the primordial germ cells may, for obscure reasons, degenerate without undergoing transformation into primordial follicles. A "streak gonad," incapable not only of ovulation but of estrogen secretion, is thereby formed. In rare instances, the medullary stroma and hilus cells of such gonads secrete sufficient androgen to induce mild virilization.

In patients with this genetic disorder, the breasts fail to develop, sex hair growth is sparse, and the titers of FSH and LH early rise to menopausal levels. Although amenorrhea is the rule, the germ cell endowment is occasionally sufficient to permit menstruation for a few years, and one well-documented instance of pregnancy has been reported. The key genetic defect is an abnormality of the second X chromosome in some or all of the cells of the patient. Approximately one-half of the patients have a 45-X chromosome constitution, one-third have mosaicism (most frequently 45-X-46-XX), and a small proportion have a structural defect of the 1-X chromosome with the loss of a proportion of its genetic material. The presence of other congenital anomalies such as short stature, webbing of the neck, short metacarpals, and coarctation of the aorta often suggests the diagnosis during the prepuberal years.

Cyclic replacement therapy is indicated to prevent osteoporosis, premature aging of the skin, and other consequences of estrogen deficiency. Diethylstilbestrol 0.5 to 2.0 mg, or the equivalent dosage of other estrogenic preparations, should be given daily during the first 3 weeks of each month. Once withdrawal bleeding has begun to occur, medroxyprogesterone acetate 5 to 10 mg, or the equivalent dosage of other progestational agents, should be added during the last 5 to 10 days of each course to effect secretory differentiation of the endometrium, thereby preventing cumulative hyperplasia and functional bleeding. "Sequential" antiovulatory preparations are a convenient form of therapy.

Menopause

The menopause, or final cessation of menses, occurs at a mean age of approximately forty-eight years and is frequently delayed until the early fifties. Termination of menstrual function before the age of forty may be considered premature. A small proportion of patients experiencing a precocious menopause have sex chromosomal mosaicism. Additional patients exhibit an unusual propensity to autoimmune disease, which may conceivably affect the ovaries. In the majority of instances, no explanation is available. The cause of the normally timed climacteric is also somewhat obscure. It appears to reflect an unduly rapid depletion of the oocytes, with the loss of their inductive effect upon the granulosa and theca cells. With a diminution of the steroid feedback influence upon the hypothalamus, the gonadotropin titer rises and the release of FSH and LH is no longer coordinated. Eventually, the stroma remains as the only functioning compartment.

The menopause is usually heralded by a period of menstrual irregularity. Amenorrhea tends to alternate with scanty periods or with bleeding which may be disconcertingly profuse. Hot flashes, the classic symptom of the climacteric, may begin at an early stage but tend to become more frequent after the periods have entirely ceased. They occur in approximately 85 percent of menopausal women and are brief in duration, lasting only a few minutes. The sensation of warmth is confined to the chest, neck, and face and may be accompanied by diffuse or patchy flushing of the skin and sweating. Hot flashes occur most frequently when heat production is increased (e.g., after meals or emotional stress) or when the dissipation of heat is impaired by bedclothes or by high ambient temperatures and humidity. Fatigue, arthralgias, insomnia, and emotional instability are common complaints in middle life; whether they are integral components of the climacteric or are only temporally related is in dispute. The rate at which involution of the ovary takes place affects the severity of menopausal symptoms. In women experiencing a sudden (not necessarily surgical) loss of ovarian function, hot flashes are likely to be severe and dyspareunia due to atrophy of the vagina may be troublesome. In women experiencing a gradual decline of ovarian activity, amenorrhea may be the sole symptom.

Treatment of the menopause comprises (1) the exclusion of organic causes of any associated menorrhagia, (2) explanation of the physiologic changes wrought by the climacteric, ventilation of the patient's anxieties, and reassurance, and (3) hormonal replacement. Estrogen therapy not only suppresses hot flashes, diminishes arthralgia, and relieves dyspareunia but also helps to prevent osteoporosis and may delay the onset of coronary arteriosclerotic heart disease. Sex steroid treatment should be administered indefinitely, as described in the section on gonadal dysgenesis. After a number of years, withdrawal bleeding will no longer occur and the progestational component can be omitted. Mild sedatives, such as phenobarbital 15 mg several times daily, are helpful in diminishing tension. Regular periodic examinations of the breasts and pelvis are essential, as are vaginal smears. The latter serve as a screening test for malignancy, particularly of the cervix. Smears are less reliable for the detection of carcinoma of the endometrium and, in the event of bleeding which is abnormal in timing or quantity, should be supplemented with endometrial biopsy and curettage. The maturation index obtainable from vaginal smears is useful for regulating estrogen dosage. If estrogen is given in amounts sufficient to maintain the superficial cells at a level of 10 percent, dyspareunia can be prevented.

Hypothalamic Disorders

Ovarian hypofunction associated with congenital disorders affecting the hypothalamus, such as the **Laurence-Moon-Biedl syndrome,** has been described elsewhere (see Chap. 87).

Destructive lesions of the hypothalamus, such as those resulting from the expansion of tumors and cysts, may induce ovarian hypofunction. The **Frommel-Chiari syndrome** of continued lactation and genital atrophy following childbirth appears to be due to a lesion which somehow impairs the secretion of the prolactin-inhibiting factor and that of the FSH- and LH-releasing factors. In a high proportion of such patients, ovulation can be induced by treatment with clomiphene citrate (Clomid) in 5-day courses at a dosage of 50 to 100 mg per day (Fig. 98-5). This agent, a congener of the synthetic estrogen trichloranisene, evokes the release of FSH and LH from the pituitary.

Emotional strain which alters the afferent neural input to the hypothalamic centers controlling the secretion of the FSH- and LH-releasing factors is perhaps the commonest cause of amenorrhea, apart from pregnancy. The vulnerability of girls in the ten- to twenty-year age group to such stresses as attending school away from home has given rise to the term "boarding school amenorrhea." In older women the menstrual cycle is more resistant to disturbance, and either exceptional stress or frank emotional illness, such as depression, is required to suspend ovarian function. Treatment with Clomid will sometimes bring about ovulation, but in severe cases, psychotherapy may be needed to restore normal cyclicity.

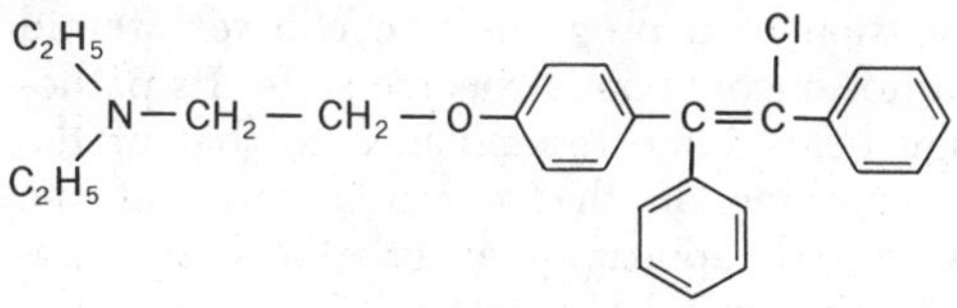

Fig. 98-5. The structural formula of Clomid.

Hypopituitarism

In early life, the commonest pituitary cause of sexual infantilism is a **craniopharyngioma;** in adult life, **chromophobe** or **eosinophil adenomas of the pituitary** and **necrosis resulting from postpartum hemorrhage (Sheehan's syndrome)** are the most frequent pituitary lesions resulting in ovarian insufficiency (Chap. 87). **Granulomatous diseases** (Hand-Schüller-Christian syndrome, sarcoid) and metastatic tumors or neoplasms arising in surrounding structures (meningioma) may diminish pituitary function at any age.

Headache, visual disturbances, or impaired growth suggest the possibility of a pituitary disorder in prepuberal girls, although failure of the menses to begin (primary amenorrhea) may be the sole manifestation. In adults, the cessation of menses previously present (secondary amenorrhea) and the coupling of lactation with amenorrhea should suggest the possibility of a chromophobe or acidophil tumor of the pituitary. X-ray visualization of the sella turcica is an essential component of the investigation of all patients with obscure amenorrheas. Sequential treatment with preparations of human menopausal urinary gonadotropin (as a source of FSH) and of human chorionic gonadotropin (as a source of LH-like activity) has, in occasional cases, resulted in ovulation.

Constitutional and Metabolic Disturbances

Severe constitutional illnesses such as **congenital heart disease, chronic renal disease,** or **rheumatoid arthritis** may delay the menarche and, in adult life, may cause amenorrhea and sterility. Injudicious dieting with too-rapid weight loss, anorexia nervosa, poorly controlled diabetes mellitus, and hyperthyroidism may also impair reproductive function. The point of impact of these different disorders upon the hypothalamic-pituitary-ovarian chain is poorly defined. A recovery of ovarian function generally follows successful treatment of the primary condition.

The **adrenogenital syndrome** (Chap. 92), a severe metabolic disorder commonly due to adrenocortical hyperplasia, is associated with pseudohermaphroditism and sexual infantilism. The adrenal cortex secretes estrogens as well as the "adrenal androgens" in greatly increased amounts, and the former, in particular, impair the hypothalamic control of FSH and LH release. Suppression of adrenal estrogen secretion by the administration of corticosteroids is speedily followed by sexual maturation and menstruation.

"Postcontraceptive amenorrhea" (i.e., that ensuing

upon the suspension of a program of cyclic sex steroid treatment) is a not uncommon iatrogenic state. Its pathologic physiology bears some resemblance to that of the adrenogenital syndrome, in that elevated levels of the circulating sex steroids appear to disturb the hypothalamic regulation of FSH and LH secretion. Omission of the contraceptive preparation is generally followed promptly by a return of menstrual function (i.e., within a period of a year or less). In some instances prolonged amenorrhea can be aborted by the administration of Clomid.

Anovulatory (Functional) Bleeding

Puberty and the premenopausal years are epochs during which the sluggish waxing and waning of the ovarian follicles, with an abnormally prolonged secretion of estrogen and an absence of ovulation, are particularly likely to occur. A teetering level of circulating estrogen results and is likely to be accompanied by painless menorrhagia (excessive menstrual bleeding), metrorrhagia (intermenstrual bleeding), or both, interspersed with long periods of amenorrhea. Anovulatory (functional) uterine bleeding, or "metropathia hemorrhagica," is so common at the two extremes of reproductive life as to be virtually physiologic. During the postmenarcheal and adult years, the condition is traceable to an absence of the midcycle LH surge with abnormally low levels of estrogen in the circulation and an absence of progesterone.

On rare occasions, a persistent follicle cyst is large enough to be outlined on bimanual examination. However, the diagnosis must ordinarily be made by exclusion. The disorders requiring differentiation vary according to the age of the patient (Table 98.2).

Table 98.2. SOME IMPORTANT CAUSES OF VAGINAL BLEEDING DURING DIFFERENT EPOCHS OF REPRODUCTIVE LIFE

1. Adolescence
   a. Functional uterine bleeding
   b. Blood dyscrasias
2. Maturity
   a. Complications of pregnancy
   b. Benign tumors (fibromyomas of the uterus, polyps of the endometrium and cervix)
   c. Malignant tumors of the cervix and corpus of the uterus
   d. Pelvic inflammatory disease
3. Premenopause
   a. Functional uterine bleeding
   b. Benign and malignant tumors of the uterus
4. Senescence
   a. Estrogen treatment
   b. Senile vaginitis
   c. Malignant tumors of the uterus
   d. Feminizing tumors of the ovary

Functional uterine bleeding is rarely fatal, but anemia is frequent and requires replacement treatment with iron. In younger patients, the oral progestational agents, fortified with estrogen, are exceedingly effective hemostatic agents. Doses of, for example, 5 to 30 mg daily of norethynodrel with mestranol (Enovid) may be given for a period of 3 weeks and then withdrawn to permit a "medical curettage." When the bleeding has been checked and the hemoglobin level restored, normal ovulatory menstrual function may resume spontaneously. If this does not occur, intermittent treatment with Clomid may establish a normal feedback mechanism, with cyclic release of the gonadotropic hormones. In older patients, pelvic examination under anesthesia and curettage are required to exclude organic lesions.

Inadequate Luteal Phase

A clinically inconspicuous syndrome characterized by somewhat abbreviated menstrual cycles, infertility, and tendency to abortion is the so-called "inadequate luteal phase." In this disorder, the secretory activity of the corpus luteum is deficient and its term of activity is abbreviated.

A short luteal phase is physiologic (1) in the later phases of the postmenarcheal period, when it is an important cause of "adolescent sterility" (anovulation is the proximate cause of infertility during the immediately postmenarcheal years), and (2) in the puerperium, when menstrual periodicity is gradually being regained. At other times it is pathologic.

The diagnosis may be suspected from the character of the basal body temperature pattern, which is characterized by a slow rise to the luteal level and abbreviation of the luteal plateau. Confirmatory evidence may be obtained by histologic dating of appropriately timed endometrial biopsies. In some patients, the LH-like action of chorionic gonadotropin administered during the postovulatory phase has resulted in the formation of a mature endometrium which can support a conceptus. It would thus appear that in certain instances, at least, the disorder reflects the midcycle release of LH in amounts insufficient to form a corpus luteum capable of normal secretory activity.

OVARIAN HYPERFUNCTION

Ovarian hyperfunction may be relative or absolute. Thus, the elaboration of estrogen in amounts which are supraphysiologic for the reproductive age of the subject constitutes hyperfunction, even though the quantity secreted is less than that characteristic of mature reproductive life.

Feminizing Tumors

Granulosa and theca cell tumors and, on occasion, certain other ovarian neoplasms may secrete estrogen. The stromal elements of tumors in the latter category (e.g., cystadenofibroma and primary adenocarcinoma of the ovary) may resemble those of the thecoma or may contain elements resembling theca-lutein or stroma-lutein cells. The histogenesis of these tumors is uncertain. However, it would appear that granulosa and theca cell tumors arise from the stroma or its follicular wall derivatives and recapitulate the elements of the follicular wall. Approximately 5 percent of the reported granulosa cell tumors arise before puberty, 55 percent during the period of reproductive life, and 40 percent after the menopause. Theca cell tumors tend to occur in a slightly older age group.

The **symptoms** depend on the age of the patient. Precocious pseudopuberty and intermittent uterine bleeding result from the function of such tumors during the premenarcheal years; irregular uterine bleeding, frequently alternating with periods of amenorrhea, is common during active reproductive life; bleeding is the characteristic manifestation of these tumors during the postmenopausal years.

Granulosa cell tumors comprise approximately 10 percent of all primary ovarian carcinomas and are the most common hormone-secreting tumors of the ovary. From 10 to 15 percent of granulosa cell tumors exhibit a low degree of malignancy, in contradistinction to theca cell tumors, which are rarely, if ever, malignant. Both are almost invariably unilateral and tend at times to produce ascites. The Meigs syndrome of ascites and hydrothorax has been observed, especially with the theca cell tumor. Endometrial hyperplasia is a frequent concomitant, and the incidence of uterine leiomyoma, adenomyosis, and adenocarcinoma is increased.

The **diagnosis** is sometimes suggested by an unexpectedly high proportion of superficial cells in the vaginal smear. Urinary estrogen levels tend to be somewhat increased, and gonadotropin levels are occasionally depressed for age. Surgical removal is the treatment of choice.

Masculinizing Tumors

The **arrhenoblastoma** and the **hilus cell tumor of the ovary** are rare androgen-secreting lesions, the histogenesis of which is uncertain. The majority of arrhenoblastomas tend to occur in comparatively young women, while the hilus cell tumor is characteristically a neoplasm of the late reproductive or postmenopausal years. Both are ordinarily unilateral and benign. The clinical course is one of defeminization followed by masculinization. The 17-ketosteroid excretion tends to be normal or only slightly increased and to be refractory to dexamethasone suppression. Plasma testosterone levels are often elevated. The treatment is surgical.

The so-called "**lipoid cell tumor**" **of the ovary** is a lesion with an uncertain histogenesis, although in certain instances it appears to arise from the ovarian stroma. The large rounded polyhedral cells of which the tumor consists lack the pathognomonic crystalloids of Reinke but are otherwise identical with Leydig cells. The syndrome of masculinization resulting from the secretion of this tumor may be clinically indistinguishable from that produced by the arrhenoblastoma. The 17-ketosteroid excretion may assist in the differentiation in that it is generally elevated, sometimes to a marked degree. Both premenarcheal and postmenopausal cases have been re-

ported, but twice as many tumors have occurred in premenopausal as in postmenopausal women.

True Precocious Puberty

Sexual precocity associated with pituitary activation of graafian follicles is generally idiopathic or "constitutional" in origin. Constitutional precocity is presumed to be due to preternaturally early maturation of the hypothalamus, which escapes from the inhibition exerted by the small but physiologically significant amounts of estrogen secreted by the infantile ovary. Gonadotropin secretion can be materially reduced, with regression of the secondary sexual characteristics and protection from the hazard of pregnancy, by intramuscular injections of medroxyprogesterone acetate. The dosage is easily monitored by periodic determinations of the maturation index, either from vaginal smears or from the sediment of freshly voided urine.

Sexual precocity is a cardinal feature of **Albright's syndrome** of **polyostotic fibrous dysplasia** (Chap. 384). There is no clear indication of the pathogenesis, and a genetic basis for the precocity has been postulated. In rare instances, the ovary is activated prematurely by gonadotropic hormones released in consequence of hypothalamic stimulation by cysts or tumors, and by postencephalitic or postmeningitic lesions.

An unusual form of precocity is that associated with **hypothyroidism**, which increases ovarian sensitivity to endogenous gonadotropins. The precocity can be reversed by the administration of desiccated thyroid in doses sufficient to provide physiologic replacement. These observations contrast with the effects of hypothyroidism on adult women, who commonly experience a failure of ovulation, with a tendency to functional bleeding.

Persistent Follicle Cysts

Follicle cysts which persist during the climacteric tend to differ from those of puberty and the reproductive years in that, because of the hypersecretion of FSH and LH, they are likely to secrete estrogen in amounts which exceed those which are physiologic during mature reproductive life. Massive estrogen treatment designed to inhibit the gonadotropic support of a palpable mass presumed to be a cystic follicle is warranted and is sometimes successful. However, because of the impossibility of distinguishing benign cysts from malignant tumors by palpation, the length of such trials should be carefully limited.

Corpus Luteum Cysts

The classic instance of physiologic luteal hyperfunction is the first trimester of pregnancy. In response to stimulation by chorionic gonadotropin, the corpus luteum of pregnancy secretes estrogen and, to a lesser extent, progesterone in amounts which exceed those characteristic of the luteal phase of the menstrual cycle.

A biochemically similar, but pathologic, state results from the formation of corpus luteum cysts. These may arise spontaneously or iatrogenically as a result of the **administration of Clomid.** Those occurring in Clomid-treated patients may be multiple, giving rise to a several-fold enlargement of the ovary; those occurring spontaneously tend to be single, seldom exceeding a walnut in size.

The presenting complaint of patients with spontaneous cysts is often that of **sudden amenorrhea.** Such cases are frequently mistaken for ectopic pregnancy because of the adnexal enlargement, hyperemia of the vagina and cervix, and the swelling and tenderness of the breasts. The cysts are sensitive to touch, with fragile walls which are likely to rupture. The suspicion of ectopic pregnancy is therefore likely to be compounded by the occurrence of acute abdominal pain. So difficult is the clinical diagnosis that many patients are, in fact, operated upon to exclude the possibility of ectopic pregnancy.

The cysts resulting from Clomid treatment may enlarge with sufficient rapidity to induce lower abdominal discomfort. They are less fragile than the spontaneous variety and ordinarily regress spontaneously after the drug is discontinued.

Stein-Leventhal Syndrome and Hyperthecosis of the Ovary

These uncommon but important conditions reflect hypersecretion of androgens by the ovarian stroma and perhaps by the hyperplastic and lutenized theca interna enveloping the subcapsular cysts and atretic follicles. **Plasma levels of androstenedione** and **dehydroepiandosterone,** which may be converted peripherally to **testosterone,** are elevated, as, on occasion, are plasma levels of testosterone itself. The history is one of **irregular menstrual cycles,** generally experienced from puberty onward, and sometimes interspersed with long periods of amenorrhea and abnormal bleeding. Perhaps in consequence of erratic bursts of LH secretion (with an absence of the normal midcycle surge), the ovaries become polycystic, and, since ovulation occurs only rarely, there is associated sterility. Over a period of time the patients tend to develop hirsutism and, in occasional cases, frank virilism.

If the stroma contains nests of lipid-laden lutein cells, the term **hyperthecosis** is applied. Whether the Stein-Leventhal syndrome and hyperthecosis represent a pathologic continuum or distinct entities is uncertain. Hyperthecosis generally evolves in a manner similar to that described for the Stein-Leventhal syndrome. Occasionally, however, there is an abrupt onset in older women (sometimes after pregnancy), and there may be associated hypertension and impaired glucose tolerance.

There is much to suggest that an abnormal hypothalamic-ovarian feedback mechanism is responsible for the disorder. Prior to the introduction of Clomid treatment, **wedge resection of a substantial amount of ovarian tissue** was the treatment of choice for the induction of ovulation. It is still of value in those patients who prove to be refractory to Clomid. Because of the characteristic hyperresponsiveness of the polycystic ovary, **Clomid is best administered initially** in a dose of 25 to 50 mg daily for 3 to 5 days, which is somewhat lower than that ordinarily effective in patients with persistent anovulation due to other causes. Neither Clomid treatment nor wedge resection ameliorates the hirsutism, except in rare instances.

In a proportion of patients with menstrual irregularities, hirsutism and a high normal or slightly elevated 17-ketosteroid excretion, differentiation of mild adrenocortical hyperplasia from the Stein-Leventhal syndrome may be difficult (Chap. 92). Patients with this complex of findings should be given the benefit of a suppression test with small doses of a glucocorticoid, such as prednisone 2.5 mg three times a day.

OVARIAN DYSFUNCTION

In rare instances, bizarre dysfunction results from the presence of **ovarian teratomas. Choriocarcinoma,** a highly malignant tumor which secretes chorionic gonadotropin, may arise in the ovary of a prepuberal girl and induce sexual precocity. **Struma ovarii,** which is generally a benign neoplasm, may secrete thyroid hormone at any age. Occasionally, the rate of secretion is so rapid as to induce thyrotoxicosis. **Carcinoid tumors** are sometimes found in dermoid cysts containing intestinal or bronchial epithelium. They may induce the characteristic "carcinoid flush," together with cyanosis and diarrhea, and may, in rare instances, exhibit metastatic spread.

REFERENCES

Baird, D., R. Horton, C. Longcope, and J. F. Tait: Steroid Prehormones, Perspect. Biol. Med., 11:384, 1968.

Grady, H. G., and D. E. Smith (Eds.): "The Ovary," Baltimore, The Williams & Wilkins Company, 1963.

Morris, J. M., and R. E. Scully: "Endocrine Pathology of the Ovary," St. Louis, The C. V. Mosby Company, 1958.

Richardson, G. S.: "Ovarian Physiology," Boston, Little, Brown & Company, 1967.

Rogers, J.: "Endocrine and Metabolic Aspects of Gynecology," Philadelphia, W. B. Saunders Company, 1963.

Savard, K., J. M. Marsh, and B. F. Rice: Gonadotropins and Ovarian Steroidogenesis, Recent Progr. Hormone Res. 21:285, 1965.

Zuckerman, S. (Ed.): "The Ovary," vols. I and II, New York, Academic Press, Inc., 1962.

99 DISEASES OF THE BREAST
Kendall Emerson, Jr.

History

The earliest description of cancer of the breast, and probably of cancer in any form, is credited to the Egyptian physician Imhotep in 3000 B.C. and is recorded in the Edwin Smith Surgical Papyrus under Case number 39, "Bulging Tumor of the Breast." The gross anatomy of the lactating breast must have been familiar to the author of the Song of Solomon in the year 1014 B.C., who likened it to "a cluster of grapes." Aside from its obvious function of lactation, however, little was known about the mammary gland, and interest in it throughout the ages has been more esthetic and symbolic than scientific until the studies of Sir Astley Cooper in 1845 provided us with an adequate morphologic description of this organ and the first suggestion of its possible relationship to menstrual dysfunction. In the latter half of the nineteenth century the German investigators discovered that normal breast development in animals depended upon intact ovarian function, and in 1896 Sir George Beatson first demonstrated the inhibition of the growth of mammary cancer by oophorectomy in human beings. The role of the corpus luteum and pituitary in the development of the breasts has been brought to light during the present century by the works of L. Loeb, Gardner, Riddle, Corner, Turner, and many others.

Congenital Anomalies

The occurrence of aberrant breast tissue (polymastia) and supernumerary nipples (polythelia) situated along the so-called "milk line" extending from the midclavicle to the inguinal ligament has been noted in art and legend since recorded time. One wonders if these anomalies may not have been more common when man was closer in evolution to his multiparous animal forebears, since the number of breasts allotted to each member of the animal kingdom is in proportion to the average size of its litter. Absence of one or both breasts (amastia) occurs very rarely but was recorded long ago by the aforementioned author of the Song of Solomon.

Endocrine Relationships

The most comprehensive recent studies of the endocrine factors determining the growth and function of the mammary glands are those of Lyons in rats, which are very briefly summarized here because they seem to support most of the observations in human beings. The development of the normal nonlactating breast is directly dependent upon the synergistic action of three major hormones: estrogens, pituitary growth hormone, and adrenal cortical steroids. Growth hormone alone will cause some growth of mammary ducts, whereas estrogens and adrenal hormones have no effect by themselves. Prolactin (luteotropic hormone, LTH) and progesterone are essential for the functional development of the alveolar lobules and the secretion of milk, whereas in the adult gland estrogens inhibit lactation by suppression of LTH activity. Prolactin with adrenal steroids can induce lactation in the absence of progesterone. Persistent lactation may occur in association with hyperplasia or with prolactin-producing tumors of the pituitary with acromegaly or without (Argonez-del Castillo and Forbes-Albright syndromes); following pregnancy by chronic stimulation of the nipple or in association with amenorrhea, low urinary FSH, and hypothyroidism (Chiari-Frommel syndrome); and occasionally during the administration of certain drugs such as the phenothiazines, methyl DOPA, and reserpine.

The hormones of greatest clinical importance in relation to the breast in man are the estrogens. Engorgement of the breasts may be seen as a transient phenomenon in newborn infants due to the high level of circulating estrogens of placental origin. The normal development of the female breast at puberty, which is sometimes accompanied by intermittent tenderness and edema, results from the rising levels of circulating estrogens secreted by the maturing ovarian follicles just prior to the menarche. Precocious breast development may occur as a result of inherited or constitutional factors; of abnormal pituitary, ovarian, or adrenal activity associated with functional tumors or hyperplasia of these organs; or of locally irritating lesions such as tumors of the pineal or fourth ventricle, fibrous dysplasia of the bones of the base of the skull, as occurs in Albrights' disease (polyostotic fibrous dysplasia), or rarely following viral encephalitis.

Gynecomastia

Gynecomastia occurs physiologically in normal males at puberty and may persist through adolescence. (In some animals such as the bat, the function of lactation is retained by the male who may assist his partner in suckling their young.) This breast enlargement usually subsides spontaneously, but if it presents a sufficiently serious psychologic problem simple mastectomy with preservation of the nipples is justified since any hormonal treatment is ineffective. Gynecomastia should always raise the suspicion of seminiferous tubule dysgenesis with fibrosis, a variant of Klinefelter's syndrome, in which there is usually an elevated urinary excretion of follicle-stimulating hormone and a female pattern of sex chromatin (see Chap. 97).

Marked degrees of breast development in adolescent males or the onset of gynecomastia in later life may indicate the presence of an estrogen-secreting tumor of the adrenal. These tumors are usually associated with an elevation of the urinary 17-ketosteroids, the excretion of which is not further stimulated by ACTH or suppressed by adrenal steroids. Every effort should be made to locate such tumors by radiographic means and to remove them surgically because, though rare, a high percentage, if not all, are malignant.

Choriogenic tumors and, more rarely, interstitial cell and granulosa cell tumors of the testes, may produce gynecomastia. This condition is also seen in males with cirrhosis of the liver and in states of severe malnutrition, presumably in both instances due to failure of inactivation of circulating estrogens. It regularly follows iatrogenic administration of estrogenic compounds in the treatment of carcinoma of the prostate and even occasionally occurs during testosterone therapy in eunuchoidism. Transient gynecomastia occurs as a normal physiologic phenomenon in elderly men and may be associated with the administration of common therapeutic agents having a basic steroid structure such as digitalis and spironolactone.

Infections of the Breast

Acute pyogenic infections of the breast are largely confined to the first 2 months of lactation and usually involve the staphylococcus, less often a beta streptococcus. They should be prevented by proper hygiene and treated with appropriate antibiotics. Very rarely an acute mastitis may occur during the course of paratyphoid or typhoid fever, brucellosis, or mumps, unassociated with lactation.

Chronic tuberculous mastitis is a rarity today. It usually results from the extension of tuberculosis of the underlying bone into the breast tissue and should be suspected from the presence of multiple sinus tracts and the finding of active tuberculosis elsewhere.

Inflammatory Lesions

Mammary duct ectasia (Haagensen) is a benign condition usually seen in elderly women with atrophic breasts wherein the mammary ducts in or just beneath the nipple become dilated and filled with cellular debris and lipid-containing material. Intermittent pain and local inflammatory changes may be present, and because a discharge, at times bloody, and retraction of the nipple may occur, this condition must be differentiated from carcinoma. Excision of the nipple is usually indicated.

Fat necrosis is a common occurrence following trauma, which may be so slight as not to have been noticed. It presents as a painful lump usually associated with some ecchymosis and may be followed by local atrophy and dimpling of the skin, at which stage biopsy must be performed to distinguish it from carcinoma.

Thrombosis of the thoracoepigastric veins and sclerosing subcutaneous phlebitis (Mondor's disease) occur after trauma or for no apparent reason and are manifest by the appearance of long cordlike structures, initially tender, in the outer half of the breast, frequently extending up into the axilla or down toward the epigastrium. They may persist up to a year, but no treatment is indicated.

Sarcoid may very rarely involve the skin of the chest. Eosinophilic granuloma may occur in the submammary folds.

It must not be forgotten that carcinoma of the breast may rarely present as a subacute red, warm, indurated mass, resembling a bacterial cellulitis, the so-called "inflammatory carcinoma." This lesion may be suspected when the skin over it presents the characteristic *peau d'orange* appearance.

Fibrocystic Disease

With each menstrual cycle there is a recurring biphasic stimulation first of proliferation of breast tissue by estrogens, then of alveolar secretory activity by progesterone, followed by a period of involution. In most women these changes are of such slight degree as to cause few if any clinical symptoms. Not infrequently, however, well-marked inflammatory changes may occur preceding each menses, with tenderness, engorgement, and increasing nodularity of the breasts. This is more often seen in nulliparous women and may subside after childbearing and lactation. Methyl testosterone, 5 mg daily for 7 to 10 days before each menstrual period, will often provide relief.

In the later years of reproductive life the continued recurrent stimulation and involution of the breasts in the course of each menstrual cycle may result in diffuse and nodular fibrosis and the formation of cysts of varying sizes, so-called "chronic cystic mastitis." This condition can simulate carcinoma but is usually distinguishable by the fact that it is intermittently painful and may subside to some extent following menstruation. Nevertheless, carcinoma may coexist and be masked by the diffuse nodularity of the cystic disease. Moreover, the incidence of mammary carcinoma is greater in patients with fibrocystic disease of the breasts, and it is unwise to delay biopsy of suspicious areas in the hope that they may subside by the end of the next menstrual cycle. In severe cases simple mastectomy is fully justified.

Tumors of the Breast

Benign fibroadenomas of the breast may occur at any age but are more common in women under the age of thirty. They may be distinguished from carcinomas by their mobility and well-defined margins, but biopsy is nonetheless imperative.

Benign intraductal papillomas may occur and cause a bloody discharge from the nipple. They are usually small and difficult to feel but may be located by noting that area of the breast on which pressure causes the bleeding. Excision is always advisable.

Sarcomas of all types make up less than 3 percent of all breast tumors. Fibrosarcomas are the most frequent; lymphosarcomas occasionally originate in the breast. Liposarcomas and hemangiosarcomas have been reported rarely. Cystosarcoma phyllodes is a curious, very large, relatively rapidly appearing tumor arising usually from a preexisting fibroadenoma. It presents as a tender, warm, cystic mass often replacing the whole breast. The skin over it is thinned, and the superficial veins are dilated. The tumor consists of fibrous cords covered with epithelium arising from the duct system. The cords are separated by cystic areas which become filled with leaflike (phyllodes) projections of epithelial tissue. Although these tumors are usually benign, blood-borne metastases have been reported and surgical removal of the tumor is always indicated.

CARCINOMA OF THE BREAST

In western civilization carcinoma of the breast is the most frequent malignant tumor to which the human female is subject and accounts for a greater number of deaths than any other single form of cancer in women. It occurs with increasing frequency from the age of twenty up to the menopause, when its incidence levels off until a second rise in frequency occurs after the age of sixty-five. For reasons as yet not entirely clear, breast cancer is very much less common in Japan and other oriental countries.

ETIOLOGY. In common with most forms of malignant disease, the etiology of breast cancer is not known. A few factors affecting its incidence are, however, reasonably well established. The very strong hereditary influence seen in mice can be carried over, though in a much smaller degree, to human beings. A two- to sevenfold increase in the familial incidence of the disease is reported.

The role of the estrogenic hormones in the genesis of breast cancer in human beings is still controversial. The incidence of mammary cancer appears to be directly related to the duration of the period of ovarian activity. It is more common in childless women with a late menopause and less frequent in women with multiple pregnancies and a history of prolonged nursing during which ovarian estrogen production is suppressed. The view most widely accepted at the present time is that estrogens do not initiate the cancer but may, nevertheless, hasten its development in genetically susceptible individuals. The prolonged use of these hormones, especially at or beyond the menopause in patients with a family history of cancer, should be discouraged.

Recent observations on the epidemiology of breast cancer suggest that environmental influences may play a role. The disease is more common in Japanese women living in the United States than in Japan, in the women of Denmark than in their Scandinavian sisters in Finland, and in fat women than in thin. Wynder has gone so far as to speculate that one common variable, the quantity of saturated fat in the diet, might affect the growth of mammary cancer directly by providing precursors for the synthesis and/or a vehicle for the storage of the fat-soluble estrogens. Of particular interest is the high incidence of both breast cancer and polycystic ovaries among the Parsis in Bombay, more than twice that of the general population in India. This ancient religious sect comprises a closely interrelated and affluent community having access to a relatively rich diet, thus combining both genetic and environmental factors which might favor the growth of mammary cancer.

PATHOLOGY. The primary site is usually in the ducts, less often in the alveoli. Multicentric origins are a frequent occurrence, and all gradations of differentiation may be observed. It is common to see a marked proliferation of dense connective tissue surrounding groups of malignant cells, whether primary or metastatic, the so-called "scirrhous carcinoma." Unfortunately all degrees of differentiation may be found in different portions of the same tumor and little prognostic value can be attached to the histologic appearance of any one area of such a malignancy.

Mammary carcinoma is prone to metastasize relatively early to the regional lymph nodes—axillary and supraclavicular if the primary site is in the outer half of the breast, the internal mammary chain if the disease arises in the inner quadrants of breast tissue. From thence spread occurs primarily to bone, lungs, liver, skin, and subcutaneous tissues generally, less frequently to the brain. Blood-borne metastases may occur even before lymphatic spread is clinically evident. It is interesting that there is a predilection for metastases to occur in the ovaries, adrenals, and pituitary—areas rich in the hormones stimulating the growth of this type of epithelial cell.

DIAGNOSIS. The diagnosis of breast cancer is facilitated by the fact that it is possible to palpate directly this type of neoplasm, a procedure which should be done gently because of the possibility of spreading the disease. Unfortunately, the diffuse nodularity of the adult female breast makes it difficult to detect early lesions. As a rule the physician must depend on such evidence as hardness, fixation to underlying structures, or dimpling of the overlying skin to distinguish a malignant mass from a benign nodule of breast tissue, and by the time these distinguishing signs have become apparent the cancer has all too often metastasized. Direct exposure of the breasts to irradiation with low-voltage x-rays in order to bring out contrasts in soft tissue densities, so-called "mammography," has been of great value in screening for breast cancer and in eliciting small lesions in large, fatty breasts. When secretions are obtainable from the nipple, cytologic examination may be helpful. The majority of patients with breast cancer suggest the diagnosis themselves because of their ready detection of abnormal lumps or masses during self-examination. Although the procedure of periodic self-examination of the breast may be decried as tending to encourage neuroticism and cancerphobia, it is the only practical way by which we can succeed in reducing the death rate from cancer of the breast until a final cure for cancer has been found.

TREATMENT. Total *surgical excision* provides the only permanent cure for carcinoma of the breast, and x-ray therapy the best palliation for localized disease. The technical details of the surgical and radiologic treatment of breast cancer are beyond the scope of this chapter, as is the controversy over radical versus simple mastectomy with extensive local irradiation, as advocated by McWhirter and others. Because of the susceptibility of breast cancer to changes in its endocrine environment, however, every physician should be cognizant of the remarkable palliative effect which can be achieved in inoperable mammary cancer by intelligent hormonal manipulations.

The two most important factors governing the prognosis of disseminated breast cancer and the success of its treatment or palliation are first, the age of the patient and second, the length of the free interval between the discovery of the primary tumor and the appearance of metastases. In common with neoplasia in general the younger the age at which it occurs, the more rapid and malignant is its growth. The only exceptions to this rule are the rare cases of juvenile breast cancer reported in patients from three to fifteen years of age, which appear to have a more benign course. The length of the free interval is a rough measure of the balance between the biologic activity, or turnover rate, of tumor cells and the poorly understood factors of host resistance.

The rationale of the *endocrine treatment of breast*

cancer is predicated on the assumption that in the total population of malignant cells some portion retain their metabolic dependency for growth upon estrogens for variable lengths of time before ultimately becoming autonomous. The first aim of therapy, therefore, is to remove all sources of estrogen from the afflicted subject. There is increasing evidence, but not universal agreement, that prophylactic oophorectomy and prednisone suppression of adrenal estrogen precursors at the time of initial mastectomy may significantly prolong the free interval, if not the total survival time of those patients with metastases ostensibly confined to axillary lymph nodes. Surgical or adequate x-ray castration will induce subjective and/or objective remissions in approximately 40 percent of patients with demonstrable metastases up to 10 years or even longer after the menopause, the incidence of favorable responses tending to vary directly with age.

A very high incidence of ovarian stromal hyperplasia, which is considered to be evidence of persistence of estrogen synthesis beyond the period of ovulation, has been observed among postmenopausal patients with mammary cancer. Such estrogen activity may be most easily detected by demonstrating the presence of more than 10 percent of cornified cells in the vaginal smear stained by the Papanicolaou method. When this activity is present, oophorectomy is indicated and may produce dramatic remissions even in patients over the age of seventy years.

With cessation of ovarian activity the adrenal cortex takes over the function of supplying precursors for estrogen production, and *bilateral adrenalectomy* will then bring about a further remission in approximately 50 percent of subjects. The remissions following these procedures may last anywhere from 6 months to 5 years or longer. Although no statistics are currently available, some investigators believe that oophorectomy and adrenalectomy carried out simultaneously will bring about a more prolonged remission in a larger percentage of patients than when adrenalectomy is deferred until the remission following oophorectomy is ended or fails to occur. In particular, when the metastatic disease is far advanced, the condition of the patient may preclude the performance of a second operation.

Surgical hypophysectomy, or pituitary stalk section, induces a functional ovarian and adrenal ablation and results in a remission rate equal to but no greater than the surgical extirpation of these target organs. The technical problems involved in total removal of the hypophysis and the degree of morbidity rising therefrom have tended to discourage this procedure. Pituitary ablation by roentgen or nuclear bombardment is too gradual to be of value in retarding the progress of a rapidly growing neoplasm.

Functional suppression of estrogen production by the ovaries may be achieved by the administration of depot progesterone, 200 mg intramuscularly, at monthly intervals, and simultaneously, the production of adrenal estrogen precursors can be inhibited by prednisone, 5 mg at 8-hr intervals daily. Such measures may be successful in retarding mammary cancer growth when surgical procedures are unavailable or unwarranted, but they are less certain and suppression is rarely as complete.

As yet, no reliable means has been found to select beforehand those individuals who will respond favorably to endocrine ablative procedures. A marked stimulation of tumor growth by estrogen administration usually implies a favorable response to oophorectomy, and similarly, a suppression of growth by prednisone indicates that adrenalectomy will have a good effect. The converse is not always true, however, and even lack of response to oophorectomy does not necessarily preclude a favorable response to subsequent adrenalectomy. Bullbrook and associates have presented statistical evidence indicating that in women under sixty-five who excrete a low ratio of androgens (11-deoxy-17-ketosteroids) to 17-hydroxy-corticosteroids in their urine, breast cancer has a poorer prognosis in terms of recurrence rate, 3-year survival, and response to adrenalectomy than in women of similar age with a higher androgen excretion rate. Moore and coworkers have noted a tendency for patients who respond favorably to adrenalectomy to show a greater rise in the urinary excretion of 17-keto- and 11-17-hydroxy-steroids following ACTH stimulation than those who fail to respond. Statistical discriminants based on data derived from such urinary hormone measurements have been advocated for the preselection of patients for adrenalectomy, but have not yet found general applicability. The length of the free interval is still a much more reliable predictor of response. As a rule of thumb, a free interval of less than 12 months indicates a poor prognosis.

Developments in *cancer chemotherapy,* however, have changed strikingly these predictions. The combination of ovarian and adrenal extirpation followed immediately by 5-Fluoro-uracil (5-FU), 15 mg per kg body weight given as a daily intravenous infusion over 4 to 6 hr for 5 to 7 days has sharply increased the remission rate and extended it to include many patients with a free interval less than 12 months. The 5-FU is well tolerated on this dosage schedule and should be continued as a single weekly intravenous injection as long as the remission lasts, provided no evidence of bone marrow suppression intervenes. Many patients too sick for surgical procedures may show striking improvement for 1 to 2 years following combined administration of prednisone 20 to 40 mg daily and 5-FU in the aforementioned dosage schedule. Undoubtedly other chemotherapeutic agents will be found which are equally or more effective but, hitherto, no agent has been shown to be effective in more than 20 percent of patients unless combined with simultaneous manipulation of the endocrine environment of the cancer cell.

In older patients, 15 years or more past the menopause, *large doses of estrogens* may provide remarkable palliation, and this is the treatment of choice. This paradoxic effect of estrogens, first clearly described by Nathanson, has never been fully explained.

The place of *androgens and estrogens* in the treatment of metastatic breast cancer has been well defined by the recent report of the American Medical Association's

Council on Drugs, based on a 10-year nationwide co-operative study. In summary, androgens produced objective remissions in approximately 20 percent of patients both before and after the menopause. Estrogens, which should not be used before the menopause, will induce remissions in about 36 percent of patients during the first 8 postmenopausal years and in more than 38 percent in later years. Estrogens have a greater relative effect on soft tissue and visceral metastases than on bone but equal or exceed the effect of androgens on all types of tissue. It should be emphasized that estrogens must be employed in large doses to achieve these results, such as stilbestrol, 15 mg, or ethinyl estradiol, 3 mg daily. Smaller amounts may adversely affect the tumor. Nausea and vomiting may occur at the onset of treatment but can be controlled by antiemetic agents and will disappear in time. Uterine bleeding may be troublesome but can usually be controlled by the cyclic administration of progesterone or methyl testosterone.

The optimum dose of *androgens* has been found to be equivalent to 100 mg of testosterone propionate given intramuscularly three times weekly. Recent experience indicates that the newer anabolic androgens such as fluoxymestrone in oral doses of 20 mg daily may be equally effective with much less tendency to produce the undesirable masculinizing side effects of testosterone.

All patients, but especially those within the first 8 postmenopausal years, should be observed carefully during the first few days and weeks of treatment because both androgens and estrogens may cause an exacerbation of their disease, estrogens by a direct stimulating effect and androgens presumably by being converted in small but effective amounts to estrogens. One of the most serious complications produced by administration of these hormones in patients who exhibit extensive skeletal metastases is calcium intoxication. This is presumed to result from the sudden stimulation of growth of the bony metastases by the hormone, with correspondingly rapid destruction of bone and flooding of the circulation with calcium. There is a marked increase in urine calcium excretion, and the serum calcium level may rise to as high as 15 to 20 mg per 100 ml, and drowsiness, coma, convulsions, and death from renal failure may ensue. It is important to distinguish this condition from cerebral or liver metastases or the terminal effects of widespread cancer because it can be reversed by forcing fluids, withdrawal of the offending hormone, and administration of large amounts of hydrocortisone, 200 mg daily by slow intravenous drip or in divided oral doses daily, until symptoms subside. The administration of neutral phosphate salts, in doses equivalent to 1.5 Gm phosphorus daily, may be of great value presumably by redirecting the flow of calcium away from the kidneys back into bone.

Hypercalcemia may, of course, occur spontaneously in far advanced autonomously growing malignancy with widespread skeletal metastases but can still usually be controlled with the above measures plus the addition of a chemotherapeutic agent. Occasionally hypercalcemia may be found in the absence of demonstrable bony involvement. It has also been reported that a "calcium-mobilizing" steroid may be elaborated by breast tumors.

Carcinoma occurs in the *male breast* at least one hundred times less frequently than in the female. Otherwise it behaves in exactly the same manner. The treatment is the same except that orchiectomy replaces oophorectomy. Prednisone and hypophysectomy have both been shown to induce remissions when the primary disease has metastasized, and progestational compounds may be of value.

REFERENCES

Barnes, A. B.: "Current Concepts: Diagnosis and Treatment of Abnormal Breast Secretions," New Engl. J. Med., 275: 1184, 1966.

Bulbrook, R. D., J. L. Hayward, and B. S. Thomas: "The Relation between the Urinary 17-Hydroxy Corticosteroids and 11-Deoxy-17-Oxysteroids and the Fate of Patients after Mastectomy," Lancet, 1:945, 1964.

Haagensen, C. D.: "Diseases of the Breast," Philadelphia, W. B. Saunders Company, 1956.

Lyons, W. R., C. H. Li, and R. E. Johnson: "Hormonal Control of Mammary Growth and Lactation," Recent Prog. Hormone Res., 14:219, 1958.

Moore, F. D., S. I. Woodrow, M. A. Aliapoulios, and R. E. Wilson: "Carcinoma of the Breast, A Decade of New Results with Old Concepts," New Engl. J. Med., 277:293, 343, 411, 460, 1967.

Wynder, E. L., L. Hyams, and T. Shigematsu: "Correlation of International Cancer Death Rates, An Epidemiological Exercise," Cancer, 20:113, 1967.

100 DISEASES OF THE PINEAL GLAND

Richard J. Wurtman

INTRODUCTION

The past decade has witnessed a great increase in knowledge about the pineal gland. Only a short time ago it was widely believed that this organ was vestigial in mammals, that the pineal had once been a photoreceptor (the "third eye") in amphibians, but with evolution had lost even this function and bore the stigma of calcification. Since the discovery of melatonin in 1958, compelling evidence has accumulated that the mammalian pineal is not a vestige but an important component of a neuro-endocrine control system. This organ has been shown to function as a neuroendocrine transducer: it receives a cyclic input of sympathetic nervous "information" which is generated by retinal effects of environmental lighting. In response to this input, the pineal secretes a hormone, melatonin, into the bloodstream, much as the adrenal medulla releases epinephrine in response to cholinergic nervous stimulation. The synthesis and secretion of melatonin vary with a 24 hr periodicity, thereby providing the body with a circulating "clock" apparatus. Largely because of technical difficulties, few attempts have been made to exploit this new knowledge of pineal function in clinical medicine. Hence, the principal circumstance which forces the clinician to think about the pineal continues to be the rare case of a disorder with evidence of a pineal neoplasm. It can be anticipated that as information about pineal physiology increases, more situations will suggest themselves in which pineal malfunction might be a factor in causing a disease.

ANATOMY AND BIOCHEMISTRY OF THE PINEAL

The human pineal gland is a flattened, conical organ which lies beneath the posterior border of the corpus callosum and between the superior colliculi. It originates embryologically as an evagination of the ependyma which lines the roof of the third ventricle, and remains connected to this region by the pineal stalk. The adult gland weighs about 120 mg; its dimensions are 5 to 9 mm in length, 3 to 6 mm in width, and 3 to 5 mm in thickness. Most of the pineal is enveloped by pia mater, from which blood vessels, unmyelinated nerve fibers, and septums of connective tissue penetrate the gland, thereby dividing it into lobules. The pineal glandular or parenchymal cells on the periphery of the lobule are elongated; those in the central zone are ovoid. They contain numerous granular bodies (which might represent a stored secretion), and give rise to processes that terminate adjacent to the capillary endothelium.

For many years it was assumed that the pineal gland was innervated by fibers which originated in the epithalamus, most likely in the habenula or posterior commissure. The pineal was known to share a common embryonic origin with these structures, and tracts were demonstrable in lower vertebrates (e.g., the frog) that ran from pineal photoreceptors to the epithalamus. Moreover, nerve bundles from the brain clearly could be shown to enter the pineal stalk in most mammals. In 1960, however, Kappers made the important discovery that the primary innervation of the mammalian pineal originates not within the brain but rather from sympathetic cell bodies in the superior cervical ganglions. Subsequent studies using the electron microscope revealed that the sympathetic nerve endings terminate directly on pineal parenchymal cells in an anatomic relationship that resembles the synapse. The sympathetic innervation of pineal glandular cells appears to be a new evolutionary adaptation. Such a parenchymal innervation may be unique in the body, and itself invalidates the vestige theory of pineal function.

In 1917, McCord and Allen showed that the pineal gland of the cow contained a factor which caused amphibian skin to blanch. When pineal homogenates were fed to tadpoles, the melanin granules within dermal melanophores aggregated around the cell nuclei, thereby lightening the skin. (This effect is opposite to that produced by the melanocyte-stimulating hormone, MSH, which is secreted by the pars intermedia of the pituitary gland.) Four decades later, Lerner and his colleagues identified this pineal factor as melatonin (5-methoxy-N-acetyltryptamine) (Fig. 100-1). Melatonin appears to have no effect on the melanocytes which are responsible for normal skin pigmentation in human beings.

Melatonin was shown to be a derivative of serotonin (Fig. 100-1), a widely distributed indole stored in very large quantities in mammalian pineals. It differs from all indoles previously identified in mammals in that it contains a methoxy- group. The enzyme which catalyzes this methoxylation reaction (hydroxyindole-O-methyl transferase, HIOMT) was shown to be highly localized

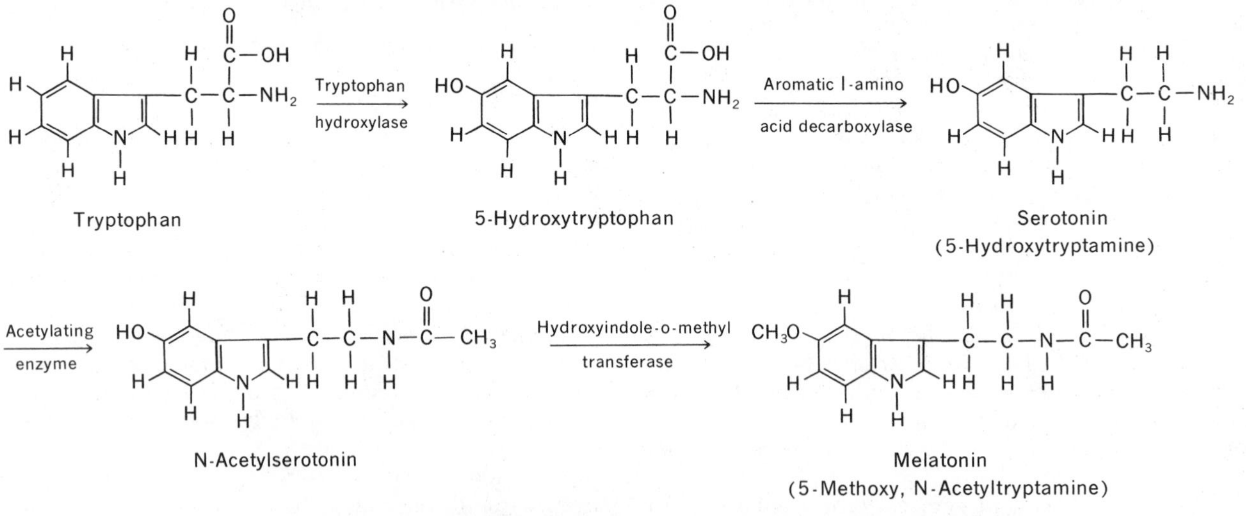

Fig. 100-1. Synthesis of melatonin in the pineal gland. The pineal takes up tryptophan from the circulation; the amino acid is hydroxylated to form 5-hydroxytryptophan; this is then converted to the amine serotonin (5-hydroxytryptamine) by the enzyme aromatic L-amino acid decarboxylase. Most of the serotonin formed in the pineal and elsewhere is destroyed by oxidative deamination, forming 5-hydroxyindole acetic acid. However, the pineal has the unique capacity to acetylate serotonin and to O-methylate the product to form the hormone melatonin.

within the pineal gland in mammals. All pineals contain this enzyme, and no other mammalian tissues appear capable of making melatonin. (The enzyme is not as highly localized in lower vertebrates; it is present in the eye and brain of the frog, in which species melatonin may function as a neurotransmitter.) The extreme localization of HIOMT has recently been used as a "marker" to differentiate true pinealomas from pineal tumors of glial or other origin.

PHYSIOLOGY OF THE MAMMALIAN PINEAL

Environmental lighting conditions exert several important effects on the mammalian neuroendocrine apparatus. Light acts as an "inducer" that modifies the rate of sexual maturation; girls who have been deprived of light perception from birth may show early pubescence. The sequence of day and night also acts to generate certain 24-hr biologic rhythms, or to synchronize similar rhythms which are produced by signals arising from within the body. There is evidence that one function of the mammalian pineal might be to mediate some of these endocrine effects of light. When rats are placed in continuous light for 2 or 3 days, a significant reduction in pineal weight occurs, accompanied by a marked decrease in the ability of the pineal to make melatonin. Continuous darkness has opposite effects. The effects produced by artificial lighting environments appear simply to be an exaggeration of the changes in pineal metabolism accompanying the normal cycle of day and night. This effect of light on the pineal is indirect and is initiated by the retinal response to light. The "information" about light travels to the pineal by a route which involves (1) the inferior accessory optic tract, (2) centers in the brain and spinal cord that regulate the sympathetic nervous system, and (3) the sympathetic nerves to the pineal which originate in the superior cervical ganglions. The diurnal variation in pineal melatonin secretion provides the body with a circulating "clock" which is under the direct control of the lighting environment.

Less is known about which organs take cues from the pineal "clock" than about the mechanism responsible for its rhythmic changes. It seems likely that melatonin exerts physiologic inhibitory effects on gonadal and thyroid function and also modifies behavior and electroencephalographic activity. For example, when rats are treated with small doses of the indole, the uptake of radioactive iodine by the thyroid is depressed, ovarian growth is inhibited, and the cyclicity of ovulation is disturbed. Circulating melatonin releases MSH from the rat pituitary and inhibits the spontaneous and serotonin-induced contractility of bronchial and gastrointestinal smooth muscle. It is possible that all the endocrine effects of melatonin operate via a common mechanism which involves an action on the brain. When tiny amounts of melatonin are implanted in the median eminence of the hypothalamus or the midbrain reticular formation, the increase in pituitary luteinizing hormone (LH) content which normally follows castration is blocked.

It had been suggested that the mammalian pineal secretes a hormone, "adrenoglomerulotropin," which acts on the adrenal cortex to stimulate the release of aldosterone. This hormone was tentatively identified as 1,methyl-6-methoxy1,2,3,4-tetrahydro-2-carboline; however, subsequent studies failed to demonstrate that the pineal is capable of synthesizing this compound, or that its administration invariably produces a rise in aldosterone secretion. 5-Methoxytryptophol, another indole closely related to melatonin, has been identified in rat and bovine pineals, and may exert effects on gonad function similar to those of melatonin.

PINEAL PATHOLOGY

Two pineal lesions have been of interest to the clinician: pineal calcification, which is a universal autopsy finding, and pineal tumors, which are best known for their endocrine sequelae. In rare instances, pineal glands have also contained cancer metastases, gummas, tuberculous granulomas, or isolated segments of skeletal muscle.

Pineal calcification often first becomes visible on skull roentgenograms around the time of puberty, and it has been suggested that the gland degenerates at this time of life, and then becomes calcified. However, recent studies have not supported this hypothesis. If pineals are examined by appropriate microscopic techniques, evidence of calcification often is seen in patients who died long before the age of puberty. A ground substance believed to serve as the matrix for calcification was seen in 8 of 28 pineals taken from children under one year of age. Moreover, studies of pineal function have failed to show any differences between heavily calcified glands taken from aged subjects and pineals from young subjects with no gross evidence of calcification. The functional significance of pineal calcification remains entirely unexplained. The chemical identity of the calcified material appears to be hydroxyapatite; crystals of this compound taken from human pineals are similar to those prepared from bone or tooth.

Pineal tumors may be divided into several distinct categories by their microscopic appearance. Somewhat more than half of all pineal tumors may be classified as true pinealomas. These tumors contain clusters of two distinct types of cells: large, spheroidal, epithelial cells, and small, dark-staining cells with little cytoplasm and an ultrastructure indistinguishable from that of the lymphocyte. About 10 to 15 percent of all reported pineal tumors have been teratomas; these may contain mucus-secreting columnar epithelial cells, adenocarcinoma tissue, and areas resembling thyroid, muscle, cartilage, bone, and nerve. Like other midline teratomas, they are often malignant. The remainder of pineal tumors have been of vascular or glial origin.

Several theories have been propounded to explain the existence of two distinct cell types in the classical parenchymal pinealoma. Globus and Silbert suggested that the pinealoma arises from an embryonic rest and that consequently its appearance is similar to that of the normal gland during one phase of its prenatal development. Late in prenatal life the human pineal contains two types of cells arranged in a mosaic pattern which superficially resembles that seen in true pinealomas. Pineal embryonic rests without evidence of neoplastic degeneration have, in fact, been observed in normal brains. Russell held that the two-cell types are actually a single cell, and that most tumor specimens classified as parenchymal pinealomas are really only segments of pineal teratomas. Marshall and Dayan have proposed that the presence of cells resembling lymphocytes in pinealomas (and in seminomas, dysgerminomas, and certain mediastinal tumors) results from an immune reaction on the part of the host: all four tumors may release unidentified antigens, and the immunologic responses to these antigens may serve to retard tumor growth. Few data are available on the general immunologic status of patients who have pinealomas.

Confirmation of pineal origin of the large pinealoma cells has been hampered by the lack of a specific pineal function which could be measured in these cells (such as the uptake of 131 iodine by thyroidal cells in follicular adenomas). However, recent studies suggest that assays for the melatonin-forming enzyme (HIOMT) may provide such a "marker." Two pineal tumors containing this enzyme have been described; one was a metastasis from a parenchymal pinealoma, and the other, a specimen from an ectopic pinealoma. Both tumors had the characteristic histologic appearance of the parenchymal pinealoma.

The natural history of a pineal tumor is related to its size and its histologic appearance. Tumors which originate within the pineal gland usually become clinically manifest because of symptoms which arise from their location (e.g., internal hydrocephalus, elevated cerebrospinal fluid pressure, and oculomotor signs such as paralysis of upward gaze, or Parinaud's syndrome); less frequently, the patient's family initially seeks medical attention because of the development of precocious puberty. About one-third of all boys below the normal age of sexual maturation who have pineal tumors develop precocious puberty. This neoplasm accounts for about 10 to 15 percent of all precocious sexual development in males. For unexplained reasons, pineal tumors are much less common among girls and are not associated with precocious menarche. Some investigators have suggested that the precocious sexual development in pinealoma patients is a nonspecific consequence of the pressure that these tumors exert on surrounding brain tissue. Kitay and others have summarized the evidence against this "pressure hypothesis": (1) Pineal tumors may produce precocious puberty, no gonadal signs, or even delayed pubescence. The endocrine effects of a particular tumor appear to be unrelated to its size. (2) Most cases of precocious puberty develop in patients with nonparenchymal tumors (frequently teratomas). An occasional parenchymal tumor leads to gonadal enlargement, but more commonly these neoplasms are associated with delayed pubescence or with

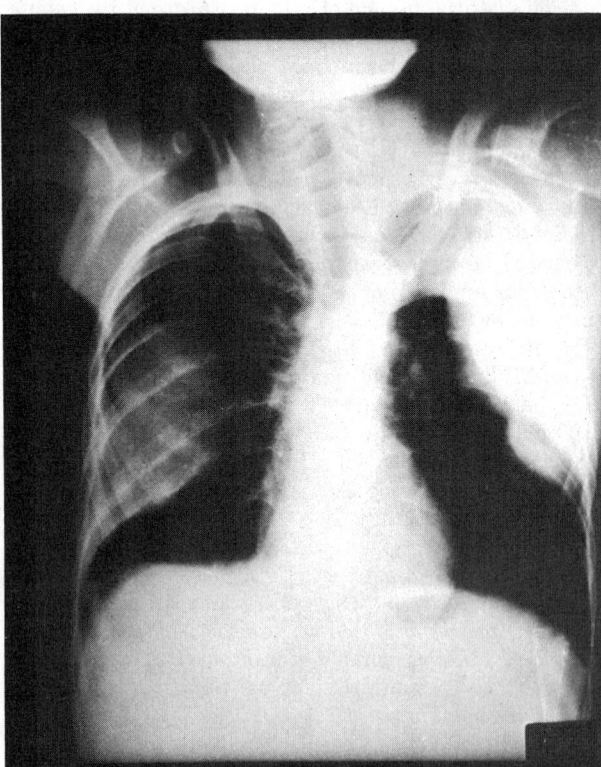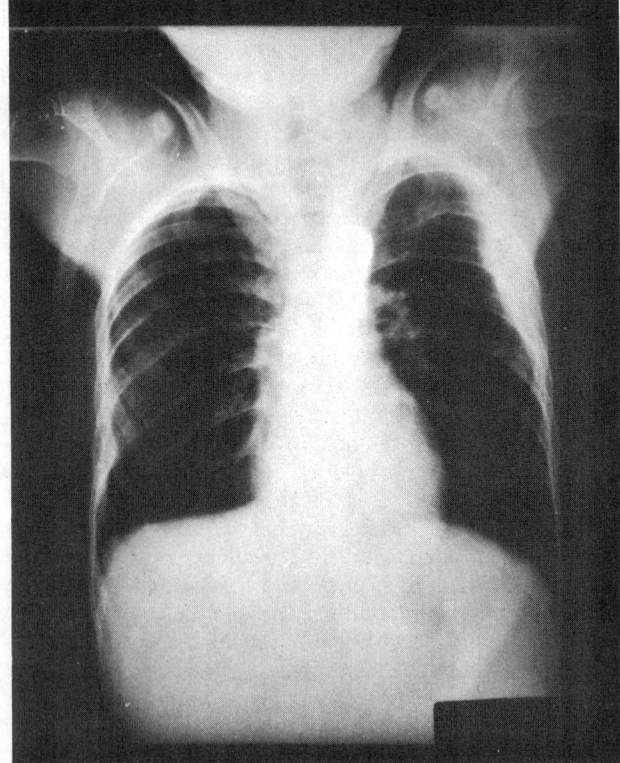

Fig. 100-2. Metastases of parenchymal pinealoma to lung, and response to chemotherapy. Roentgenogram at right was taken 3 weeks after patient received methotrexate, cytoxan, and actinomycin D. (*Photograph courtesy of Dr. Rudolf Toch, Massachusetts General Hospital, Boston.*)

secondary gonadal failure. (3) Gonadal abnormalities have been observed in a large number of pinealoma patients whose tumors had neither produced signs of a chronic elevation in cerebrospinal fluid pressure nor invaded other brain areas. The demonstration that a pineal hormone, melatonin, influences normal sexual maturation in rats supports the hypothesis that precocious puberty develops in pinealoma patients because the damaged pineal fails to release an inhibitory hormone. It has not been possible to test this hypothesis directly, because no assay is available which can be used to measure the level of melatonin or its metabolic products in blood or urine. It is noteworthy, perhaps, that both patients described above whose tumors contained melatonin-forming activity showed evidence of depressed sexual function.

Parenchymal pinealomas frequently show a good, if temporary, clinical remission following irradiation. Patients generally receive 3,000 to 5,000 rads; radiation is administered over a wide portal because pinealomas not infrequently metastasize throughout the ventricles and the subdural space. Japanese surgeons have reported encouraging results following the surgical extirpation of pinealomas; however, this method is complicated by the relative inaccessibility of the pineal, and consequently is used rarely in the United States. A patient with metastatic parenchymal pinealoma has been repeatedly treated during an 8-year period with x-ray and chemotherapeutic agents; each time an objective decrease in tumor mass occurred (Fig. 100-2).

A small number of tumors with the histologic appearance of pinealomas originate elsewhere in the brain at some distance from the normal pineal gland. These "ectopic pinealomas" generally arise in the hypothalamus in the region of the infundibulum. Hence, patients usually present a picture similar to that seen with craniopharyngioma with a clinical triad of bitemporal hemianopsia, hypopituitarism, and diabetes insipidus. Most ectopic pinealomas show a good clinical response to irradiation.

REFERENCES

Kappers, J. A.: Survey of the Innervation of the Epiphysis Cerebri and the Accessory Pineal Organs of Vertebrates, Progr. Brain Res., 10:87, 1965.

Kelly, D. E.: Pineal Organs: Photoreception, Secretion, and Development, Am. Sci., 50:597, 1962.

Kitay, J. I., and M. D. Altschule: "The Pineal Gland: A Review of the Physiologic Literature," Cambridge, Mass., Harvard University Press, 1954.

Ramsey, H. J.: Ultrastructure of a Pineal Tumor, Cancer, 18:1014, 1965.

Scharenberg, K., and L. Liss: The Histologic Structure of the Human Pineal Body, Progr. Brain Res., 10:193, 1965.

Wurtman, R. J.: The Pineal Gland, p. 117 in "Endocrine Pathology," J. M. B. Bloodworth (Ed.), Baltimore, The Williams & Wilkins Company, 1968.

——: Effects of Light and Visual Stimuli on Endocrine Function, p. 20 in "Neuroendocrinology," vol. 2, L. Martini and W. F. Ganong (Eds.), New York, Academic Press, Inc., 1967.

Section 4

Errors of Metabolism

101 INTRODUCTION

Lloyd H. Smith, Jr.

Few diseases are either wholly genetic or environmental in their pathogenesis. The degree to which "environment" (microbiologic, physical, psychologic, chemical) is injurious depends on the genetic legacy of the host. This may represent a specific genetic defect phenotypically expressed as altered structure and function or inappropriate amount of a given protein, a group of disorders still often designated by Garrod's term as "inborn errors of metabolism." Perhaps more often the genetic propensity toward disease represents polymeric gene action, the summation of a number of genic expressions which can now be described only by statistical approaches. A number of factors have contributed to recent interest in genetic diseases: (1) With improved control of environment, disease is increasingly endogenous rather than exogenous. (2) Advances in molecular biology have elucidated the mechanisms of transmission and expression of genetic information, allowing the definition of certain diseases with increased precision. (3) Although genetic diseases cannot be cured in the host, knowledge of the resulting biochemical derangements often allows rational means of treatment to be devised.

In this section major attention will be directed to individual genetic diseases rather than to broader topics in population genetics or molecular biology. It is not clear just how many inborn errors of metabolism there are. By the use of current estimates of the number of different kinds of proteins in the body, the average number of amino acids per protein, and the possibility that at a given point any one of 20 amino acids might be substituted, it may be estimated that the possibilities for variation in structural genes alone are $>10^{10}$. Many factors reduce the number of diseases which are recognized.

Certain variations are trivial, lead to no biologic disadvantage, and merely constitute the chemical basis of individuality. Other defects are intrinsically lethal and contribute to the high incidence of spontaneous abortions. Variations may occur not only among diseases but also within diseases, depending on the site of alteration in the protein and the degree of resulting dysfunction. More than 50 types of abnormal hemoglobins have been described. It may well be, by analogy, that there are more than 50 types of galactosemia or phenylketonuria. Individual genetic diseases vary widely in frequency, from diabetes mellitus (3 to 5 percent of the population) to sulfituria (a single case description). The variables in frequency—mutation rate and the balance of biologic advantage and disadvantage—are now the subject of considerable interest in human genetics.

The usual **inborn error** of **metabolism** results from the absence or severe reduction in catalytic activity of an enzyme, whether the protein is physically missing or is present but altered in a fashion which impairs its function. In microorganisms genetic disorders of too much enzyme activity occur. The recent description of increased activity of Δ-aminolevulinic acid synthetase in acute intermittent porphyria suggests that this type of activity may also occur in human disease. In the latter case, however, the process may be a biochemical epiphenomenon rather than the basic defect productive of the neurologic complications. **Genetic disorders** usually produce disease by the **accumulation** of the **substate** of the **enzyme and/or some** of its **by-products** or by **absence or reduced availability** of the **product of the reaction** normally catalyzed by the defective enzyme. This concept is illustrated simply in diagrammatic form first introduced by Charles Dent:

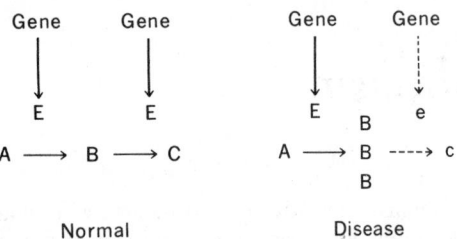

Normal   Disease

The accumulation of substrate B is the most frequently encountered abnormality productive of disease. This may be related to the fact that most genetic disorders so far discovered have dealt with degradative pathways of metabolism. Some examples of substrate (and substrate by-product) toxicity are described in greater detail in subsequent chapters: phenylalanine and its by-products in phenylketonuria, galactose 1-phosphate in galactosemia, oxalate in primary hyperoxaluria, homogentisic acid and its pigment polymer in alcaptonuria. Such defects may result in storage diseases such as the lipidoses, cystinosis, glycogen storage diseases, etc. The accumulated precursor may inhibit other metabolic pathways or interfere with amino acid transport into cells. Often the biochemical mechanism of injury is obscure.

Genetic disorders may lead to disease because of **absence** or **reduced availability** of **the product** rather than through accumulation of the precursor. Most of the recognized examples lie in defects in plasma protein synthesis or in the sequence of hormone synthesis, described elsewhere in this book. For example, deficiency of circulating thyroxine and triiodothyronine is the major defect in the various specific genetic forms of familial cretinism (Chap. 89), producing damage to the developing central nervous system, delayed maturation of the skeleton, hypometabolism, and failure of inhibition of TSH (thyroid-stimulating hormone) release, with resulting goiter. Similarly, deficiency of hydrocortisone in congenital adrenal virilism (Chap. 92) is the ultimate cause of adrenocortical hyperplasia (via ACTH) and of the excessive synthesis of steroidal precursors into adrenal androgens. A large number of genetic disorders of the synthesis of circulating proteins which participate in hemostasis have been described. In fact these proteins have been largely discovered in the study of patients with a hemorrhagic diathesis. The ultimate deficiency common to these disorders is that of appropriate formation of cross-linked fibrin polymer. The multiple types of genetic blocks in glycolysis associated with chronic nonshperocytic hemolytic anemia probably share a common deficiency of erythrocytic ATP (adenosinetriphosphate). The defect in albinism is absence of melanin; and a major defect in the von Gierke form of glycogen storage disease is deficiency of circulating glucose secondary to loss of glucose 1-phosphatase activity. In hereditary orotic aciduria, uridine becomes an essential metabolite. In a sense these disorders represent analogs of auxotrophism in bacteria.

A number of *genetic diseases* have now been described in which there is a **defect** in **the active transport of metabolites across membranes,** as summarized in Chap. 104. Occasionally the physical properties of the abnormal protein may constitute the mechanism of disease, as in the propensity toward stacking and tactoid formation in sickle-cell anemia and the heritable disorders of connective tissue. Pharmacogenetics refers to inherited alterations in drug metabolism, sensitivity of response, and toxicity. As an example, pseudocholinesterase deficiency is innocuous except during the use of certain muscle relaxants in anesthesia, when prolonged paralysis may result. Immunogenetics refers not only to immunologic markers in gamma-globulins but also to the inherited basis of antigenic (chemical) individuality. It is apparent that genetic alterations may be productive of disease through a variety of mechanisms, both subtle and direct.

Genetic diseases cannot be cured in the host. Knowledge of the mechanism of disease, however, often allows effective palliative measures to be instituted. Many of these are illustrated in the discussion of specific diseases in the chapters of this section. The approaches which have been used may be summarized briefly:

1. *Replace the enzyme.* This could be done phenotypically or, in theory, genotypically. The latter would clearly be preferable if genotypic replacement, augmen-

tation, or repair becomes feasible in multicellular organisms. Replacement now is largely limited to extracellular proteins such as coagulation factors, gamma-globulins, or hormones, of transient value only. Homotransplantation raises the possibility of localized extirpation and "cure" of genetic disease. The cystinuric kidney has been replaced. Drugs may alter the expression of genetic information. Phenobarbital has been used successfully to cause marked proliferation of the smooth-surfaced membranes of the endoplasmic reticulum in liver cells and thereby enhance pathways of bilirubin metabolism in certain cases of congenital hyperbilirubinemia.

2. *Reduce the accumulation of substrate.* This is usually carried out by dietary therapy, such as galactose-free diets in galactosemia or phenylalanine-restricted diets in phenylketonuria. The accumulation may be that of a by-product, such as uric acid or oxalate. In these cases new approaches to drug management are being pursued to inhibit the by-product formation or increase its excretion.

3. *Supply the product.* At the present time this approach is rarely employed except in endocrine replacement therapy, e.g., administration of a glucocorticoid in congenital adrenal hyperplasia or of thyroxin in the various forms of familial cretinism. The requirement for uridine in hereditary orotic aciduria is an exception, since this is replacement of an intermediate on a specific biosynthetic pathway.

4. *Miscellaneous.* A number of miscellaneous approaches have been successfully employed to compensate for errors of metabolism. Phlebotomy removes the excess iron of hemochromatosis, and D-penicillamine removes the excess copper of Wilson's disease. D-penicillamine forms a more soluble mixed disulfide of cystine in cystinuria. Chlorothiazide reduces the diuresis of vasopressin-resistant diabetes insipidus. Other examples could be cited. In summary, the treatment of genetic diseases is a challenging and often rewarding category of therapeutics.

Garrod wrote in 1908, "The existence of chemical individuality follows of necessity from chemical specificity, but we should expect the differences between individuals to be still more subtle and difficult of detection." The molecular biology of genetic transmission and expression is perhaps the most important area of scientific advance in the past two decades. Application of these advances in man has elucidated a large number of genetic errors of metabolism, some of which are described in specific detail in the following chapters.

REFERENCES

Harris, H.: "Garrod's Inborn Errors of Metabolism," New York, Oxford University Press, 1963.

Stanbury, J. B., J. B. Wyngaarden, and D. S. Fredrickson (Eds.): "The Metabolic Basis of Inherited Diseases," 2d ed., New York, McGraw-Hill Book Company, 1966.

Crow, J. F., and J. V. Neel (Eds.): "Proceedings of the Third International Congress of Human Genetics," Baltimore, The Johns Hopkins Press, 1967.

102 ERRORS OF METABOLISM ASSOCIATED WITH MENTAL DEFICIENCY

Lloyd H. Smith, Jr.

The biochemistry of cerebral function is not well understood, but is now the subject of extensive investigation. The brain shares with other specialized tissues many common pathways of biosynthesis and catabolism of cell constituents and of energy metabolism. Some biochemical reactions are found uniquely in nervous tissue; and some of its common pathways are catalyzed by isozymes under separate genetic control. Inherited metabolic disorders which affect cerebral function may be considered to be in two general categories: those with abnormal genetic expression in the brain itself (in the synthesis or control of synthesis of proteins) and those in which a metabolic abnormality elsewhere in the body indirectly affects cerebral function (accumulation of a toxic product, deficiency of required metabolite). It is not always possible to distinguish clearly between these categories. No attempt will be made to present all the genetic disorders which could be considered in the classification of this chapter. Phenylketonuria, homocystinuria, and maple syrup urine disease will be reviewed. Some of the other disorders have been summarized in Table 102-1, with reference to review articles. Since almost any disorder which affects general health may influence cerebral function, the selection of disorders included has been an arbitrary one. As an example, chromosomal disorders associated with mental deficiency, such as mongolism, have been excluded. The reader should refer to Chap. 363 for discussion of other metabolic diseases and to Chap. 31 and 365 for a more complete account of the neurologic effects thereof.

PHENYLKETONURIA

Definition

Phenylketonuria, first described by Folling in 1934, is a metabolic disorder secondary to an inherited deficiency of phenylalanine hydroxylase. This results in the accumulation of phenylalanine and some of its metabolites (notably phenylpyruvate, phenyllactate, phenylacetate and O-hydroxyphenylacetate) and a syndrome of mental deficiency. Other neurologic deficits, epileptic seizures, and reduced pigmentation may also occur.

Genetics and Pathogenesis

Phenylketonuria is transmitted as an autosomal recessive trait, occurring in its clinical (homozygous) form with a frequency of about 1 in 10,000 to 15,000 births in the United States. About 0.7 percent of the inmates in institutions for the mentally defective are patients with homozygous phenylketonuria. Heterozygotes (at least 1 percent of the population) usually exhibit slightly elevated fasting levels of plasma phenylalanine and reduced rates of plasma clearance of phenylalanine after its oral

Table 102-1. ERRORS OF METABOLISM ASSOCIATED WITH MENTAL DEFICIENCY

Disease	Enzyme deficiency	Signs and symptoms	Laboratory abnormalities	Transmission	References
Phenylketonuria	Phenylalanine hydroxylase	Severe mental deficiency, tremors, seizures, muscular hypertonicity, hyperkinesis, reduced pigmentation	Plasma phenylalanine elevated, phenylalanine, phenylpyruvate, phenyllactate, phenylacetate, and O-hydroxy phenylacetate, elevated in urine	Autosomal recessive	W. E. Knox, in J. B. Stanbury et al. (Eds.), "The Metabolic Basis of Inherited Disease," 2d ed., New York, McGraw-Hill, 1966.
Homocystinuria	Cystathionine synthetase	Mild mental deficiency (sometimes absent), ectopia lentis, osteoporosis, thromboembolic complications, skeletal deformities resembling Marfan syndrome	Elevated plasma and urine methionine and homocystine	Autosomal recessive	R. N. Schimke, et al., in W. L. Nyhan (Ed.), "Amino Acid Metabolism and Genetic Variation, New York, McGraw-Hill, 1967.
Maple syrup urine disease (branched chain ketoaciduria)	Oxidases of α-ketoisocaproic acid, α-ketoisovaleric acid, α-keto-β-methylvaleric acid	Progressive deterioration of central nervous system function usually beginning shortly after birth and leading to early death; sweet, maple syruplike odor to urine and sweat	Elevated levels of leucine, isoleucine, valine, and their corresponding keto acids in blood and urine	Autosomal recessive	J. Dancis and M. Levitz, in J. B. Stanbury, et al. (Eds.), "The Metabolic Basis of Inherited Disease," 2d ed, New York, McGraw-Hill, 1966.
Galactosemia	Galactose 1-phosphate uridyl transferase	Vomiting, diarrhea, failure of growth and development, hepatosplenomegaly, cataracts, mental retardation; improvement on omission of milk	Blood galactose elevated, abnormal galactose tolerance test; galactose, amino acids, and protein in urine; enzyme defect demonstrable in RBCs	Autosomal recessive	K. J. Isselbacher, in J. B. Stanbury et al. (Eds.), "The Metabolic Basis of Inherited Disease," 2d ed., New York, McGraw-Hill, 1966.
Cystathioninuria	Cystathionine cleavage enzyme (binding site for pyridoxal phosphate)	Mental deficiency may or may not be present; no other specific clinical picture has emerged	Excessive excretion of cystathionine in urine	Not established; probably autosomal recessive	G. W. Frimpter et al., New Eng. J. Med., 268:333, 1963; T. L. Perry et al., New Engl. J. Med., 278:590, 1968.
Argininosuccinic aciduria	Argininosuccinase	Severe mental retardation, ataxia, seizures, hepatic dysfunction, abnormally friable hair	Elevated plasma and CSF argininosuccinate, citrulline, and sometimes ammonia; argininosuccinate in urine	Autosomal recessive	H. W. Moser et al., Am. J. Med., 42:9, 1967.

Disease	Enzyme Defect	Clinical Features	Biochemical Findings	Genetics	Reference
Hyperlysinemia	Not established. Probably block in saccharopine synthesis.	Mental and physical retardation, impaired sexual development, lax ligaments, occasional convulsions	Hyperlysinemia and hyperlysinuria; one patient had hyperammonemia; ornithine, arginine, and cysteine may be increased in urine because of renal tubular competition	Not established; probably autosomal recessive	H. Ghodimi et al., New Engl. J. Med., 273:723, 1965.
Gaucher's disease (cerebroside lipoidosis)	Glucocerebrosidase	Infantile or cerebral form: hyperextension of head, hypertonicity, strabismus, apathy, seizures, mental retardation, hepatosplenomegaly	Gaucher cells in marrow, high levels of serum acid phosphatase	Probably autosomal recessive	D. S. Fredrickson, in J. B. Stanbury et al. (Eds.), "The Metabolic Basis of Inherited Disease," 2d ed., New York, McGraw-Hill, 1966.
Hyper-β-alaninemia	Not established, probably β-alanine: α-ketoglutarate transaminase	Lethargy, somnolence, hypotonicity, seizures, early death in single described case	β-alanine elevated in plasma; β-alanine, taurine, β-aminoisobutyric acid and γ-aminobutyric acid elevated in urine	Not established	C. R. Scriver et al., New Engl. J. Med., 274:635, 1966.
Methylmalonic aciduria	Probably methylmalonyl CoA isomerase	Developmental retardation, severe metabolic acidosis	Large amounts of methylmalonic acid in urine, long chain ketonuria, intermittent hyperglycinemia	Not established	V. G. Oberholzer et al., Arch. Dis. Child., 42:492, 1967; L. E. Rosenberg et al., New Engl. J. Med., 278:1319, 1968.
Sulfituria	Sulfite oxidase	Severe neurologic abnormalities at birth, deteriorating to an almost decorticate state; ectopia lentis in single described case	Excessive urinary excretion of sulfite, thiosulfate, and S-sulfo-L-cysteine; reduced urine sulfate	Not established	L. Laster et al., J. Clin. Invest, 46:1082, 1967.
Hyperglycinemia (ketotic variant)	Not established	Developmental retardation, periodic ketosis, with vomiting, neutropenia, thrombocytopenia, lethargy, coma, seizures, osteoporosis	Glycine elevated in plasma and urine; alanine, serine, leucine, isoleucine, and valine variably elevated in plasma	Not established; probably autosomal recessive	W. L. Nyhan et al., in W. L. Nyhan (Ed.), "Amino Acid Metabolism and Genetic Variation," New York, McGraw-Hill, 1967.
Hyperglycinemia (nonketotic variant)	Not established; possibly glycine oxidase	Developmental retardation, spastic paraplegia, opisthotonos, seizures	Glycine elevated in plasma and urine; urine oxalate lowered	Not established	T. Gerritsen et al., Pediatrics, 36:882, 1965.

Table 102-1. ERRORS OF METABOLISM ASSOCIATED WITH MENTAL DEFICIENCY (*Continued*)

Disease	Enzyme deficiency	Signs and symptoms	Laboratory abnormalities	Transmission	References
Lowe's syndrome (oculo–cerebrorenal syndrome)	Not established	Mental and somatic retardation, cataracts, buphthalmos, corneal clouding, epicanthal folds, typical or atypical Fanconi syndrome, sometimes with rickets	Generalized aminoaciduria (except for valine, leucine, and isoleucine), phosphaturia, and tubular acidosis	X-linked recessive	E. J. Sehoen and G. Young, Am. J. Med., 27:781, 1959.
Hypervalinemia	Valine–α-ketoglutarate transaminase	Mental and somatic retardation, nystagmus, hypotonicity, unresponsiveness, vomiting	Valine elevated in plasma and urine	Presumed autosomal recessive	J. Dancis et al, Pediatrics, 39:813, 1967.
Hydroxyprolinemia	Hydroxyproline oxidase	Severe mental retardation; single case	Free L-hydroxyproline elevated in plasma and urine; bound hydroxyproline normal	Not established	M. L. Efron et al., New Engl. J. Med., 272:1299, 1965.
Niemann-Pick disease (sphingomyelin lipoidosis)	Sphingomyelinase	Physical and mental retardation, cherry-red spots in eyes, massive hepatosplenomegaly, foam cells in marrow, early death	Foam cells in marrow; sphingomyelin storage	Probably autosomal recessive	D. S. Fredrickson, in J. B. Stanbury et al. (Eds.), "The Metabolic Basis of Inherited Disease," 2d ed., New York, McGraw-Hill, 1966.
Tay-Sachs disease (ganglioside lipoidosis)	Not established	Progressive retardation, paralysis, dementia, blindness beginning by age 4–6 months, and progressing to death by age 4 years	Accumulation of a monosialoganglioside in ganglion and glial cells of the CNS	Autosomal recessive	D. S. Fredrickson and E. G. Trams, in J. B. Stanbury et al. (Eds.), "The Metabolic Basis of Inherited Disease," 2d ed., New York, McGraw-Hill, 1966.
Metachromatic leukodystrophy (sulfatide lipoidosis)	Cerebroside sulfatase	Progressive generalized neurologic deterioration, beginning about age 12–18 months and leading to death in a few years in the typical late infantile form	Metachromatic granules of sulfatides in white matter; excess sulfatide excreted in the urine	Probably autosomal recessive	H. W. Moser and M. Lees, in J. B. Stanbury et al. (Eds.), "The Metabolic Basis of Inherited Disease," 2d ed., New York, McGraw-Hill, 1966.
Lesch–Nyhan syndrome	Hypoxanthine guanine phosphoribosyltransferase	Mental deficiency, choreoathetosis, self-mutilation, gout	Severe hyperuricemia with hyperuricosuria	X-linked recessive	M. Lesch and W. L. Nyhan, Am. J. Med., 36:561, 1964; W. N. Kelley et al, Proc. Nat. Acad. Sci, 57:1735, 1967.

Histidinemia	Histidase (histidine α-deaminase)	Variable mental retardation	Increased histidine in blood and urine; increased excretion of imidazole pyruvate, imidazolelactate, and imidazoleacetate; low plasma glutamate; high blood and urine alanine	Autosomal recessive	H. Ghadimi and R. Zischka, in W. L. Nyhan (Ed.), "Amino Acid Metabolism and Genetic Variation," New York, McGraw-Hill, 1967.
Citrullinemia	Argininosuccinic acid synthetase	Mental retardation, nausea, vomiting, tremors, hypotonicity, intermittent hyperammonemia	Citrulline elevated in blood and urine; blood NH_3 elevated postprandially; urea normal	Not established; probably autosomal recessive	W. C. McMurray et al., Pediatrics, 32:347, 1963.
Hyperammonemia	Ornithine transcarbamylase and carbamyl phosphate synthetase	Chronic ammonia intoxication with mental retardation, lethargy, stupor, usually early death	High blood and CSF ammonia; mild general aminoaciduria; glutamine elevated in CSF	Not established	B. Levin, Am. J. Dis. Child., 113:142, 1967; A. Russel et al., Lancet, 2:699, 1962.
Isovaleric acidemia	Probably isovaleryl-CoA dehydrogenase	Mild psychomotor retardation, intention tremor, attacks of acidosis, stupor, and coma; "sweaty-foot smell" of breath	Elevated plasma isovaleric acid	Not established; probably autosomal recessive	M. A. Budd et al., New Engl. J. Med., 277:321, 1967.
Carnosinemia	Probably carnosinase	Mental deterioration in early life, somnolence, seizures, flaccid muscles, myoclonic jerks	Excessive plasma and urine carnosine, increased homocarnosine in CSF	Not established; probably autosomal recessive	T. L. Perry et al., New Engl. J. Med., 277:1219, 1967.

administration. Although some studies have suggested an increased incidence of mental deficiency or psychiatric disturbances in families of patients with phenylketonuria, the heterozygous state has not been demonstrated to be injurious.

Phenylalanine is normally hydroxylated in the para position to form tyrosine, involving a complex biochemical reaction catalyzed by phenylalanine hydroxylase. This enzyme is restricted to liver, where it exhibits increasing activity in the first few weeks after birth. Active enzyme fails to appear in the phenylketonuric infant. This results in accumulation of dietary phenylalanine in the plasma and presumably in cells, with secondary diversion (by transamination) into phenylpyruvate, phenyllactate, phenylacetate, and O-hydroxyphenylacetate, all four of these phenyl acids being excreted together with phenylalanine in the urine. Phenylalanine is a competitive inhibitor of tyrosinase on the pathway of melanin synthesis, which explains the decreased pigmentation of hair, eyes, and skin. High levels of phenylalanine in body fluids inhibit transport of amino acids into cells. The resulting deprivation of essential amino acids in the developing brain may be the immediate cause of cerebral damage, although this has not been established. Other explanations relate to altered patterns of synthesis of pharmacodynamic amines (serotonin, norepinephrine, phenylethylamine, etc.).

Clinical Presentation and Diagnosis

Retardation of mental development, usually of severe degree, is the major manifestation of phenylketonuria. Since the mental defect is stationary and not progressive in older children or adults, the brain injury appears to be limited to a particularly sensitive stage in brain development. Other neurologic abnormalities sometimes found are tremors, seizures, muscular hypertonicity, hyperkinesis, and EEG abnormalities. As noted, there tends to be reduced pigmentation of skin, hair, and eyes. Eczema has been commonly described.

Early diagnosis is essential for successful treatment since the neurologic abnormalities, once established, are largely irreversible. Diagnosis before one month of age requires the demonstration of grossly elevated levels of plasma phenylalanine. The excretion of the associated metabolites may not be remarkable at this time. Testing by screening for phenylketonuria of all newborn infants and of all infants of thirty days and under when admitted to another hospital is now mandatory in 37 states. This routine blood testing can be carried out quite simply using the bacterial inhibition assay (Guthrie) or a fluorometric procedure. Positive tests must be carefully followed up with quantitative measurements of plasma phenylalanine and study of urinary metabolites to differentiate the disease from transient hyperphenylalaninemia related to prematurity, tyrosinemia, or heterozygosity. This is important because restrictive diets may be injurious in patients other than those with phenylketonuria. The ferric chloride test, a transient blue or olive-green color appearing on the addition of a few drops of 5%

$FeCl_3$ to 5 ml urine, is still useful for screening older children or adults and is usually positive in infants.

Treatment

The biochemical abnormalities can be corrected by preventing the accumulation of phenylalanine. This is done by a special diet in which protein is replaced by an amino acid mixture low in phenylalanine (Ketonil, Lofenolac). Supplementary foods are given to supply only the amount of L-phenylalanine needed for body growth. The program should attempt to maintain normal weight gain and near normal plasma phenylalanine levels and should be continued until the child is at least four years of age. The results of dietary treatment are still being assessed. Normal development has been obtained in some patients treated from early infancy. Little permanent improvement can be achieved by treatment begun later, the main effect being that of prevention of further intellectual deterioration.

HOMOCYSTINURIA

Definition

Homocystinuria is a genetic disease resulting from absence of cystathionine synthetase, an enzyme which catalyzes an important step in the transsulfuration pathway converting methionine to cysteine. It is characterized clinically by ectopia lentis, osteoporosis, thromboembolic phenomena, and mental retardation, and chemically by excessive urinary excretion of homocystine. It was described initially in 1962, and approximately 100 cases have been reported.

Genetics and Pathogenesis

Homocystinuria is transmitted as an autosomal recessive trait. Heterozygotes have no stigmata of the disease and have no detectable plasma homocystine and no elevation of plasma methionine. They sometimes exhibit delayed plasma clearance of methionine loads given orally or intravenously. Assays of liver biopsy material from parents of homocystinurics (presumed heterozygotes) have revealed cystathionine synthetase activities intermediate between those of patients and controls. Homozygotes exhibit virtual absence of this enzyme activity in liver and brain.

In the absence of cystathionine synthetase, homocystine and methionine accumulate and cysteine (or cystine) becomes an essential amino acid. There is no clear information about how these chemical derangements result in the diverse structural and functional manifestations of the disease. It has been suggested that the ability of homocystine to form mixed disulfides may inactivate critical sulfhydryl groups of enzymes or impair disulfide cross linkages in structural proteins. No role of cysteine deficiency has been established. Current studies are directed to other sulfur-containing metabolites in urine, such as the recent demonstration of 5-amino-4-imidazole-carboxamide-5'-S-homocysteinyl-riboside.

Clinical Presentation and Diagnosis

Patients with homocystinuria often exhibit a superficial resemblance to the Marfan syndrome (Chap. 395). Some of the skeletal and connective tissue abnormalities which have been described are ectopia lentis, severe juvenile osteoporosis, kyphosis, scoliosis, genu valgum, deformities of the sternum such as pectus excavatum and pectus carinatum, abnormalities of the palate, and arachnodactyly. Mental deficiency is common, but may be absent; when present, it is not usually as severe as that of phenylketonuria. Recurrent arterial and venous thromboses may complicate the course and lead to early death from pulmonary embolism or coronary or carotid occlusion. Patients with homocystinuria tend to resemble one another with their skeletal deformities, light-colored hair, and coarse skin with malar flush and livido reticularis. Diagnosis is established by finding homocystine in the urine using paper or ion exchange column chromatography. As a disulfide, homocystine will also give a positive nitroprusside reaction in urine, but must then be differentiated from cysteine by chromatographic techniques. Plasma methionine is also elevated.

Treatment

In the absence of clear evidence of the mechanism by which loss of cystathionine synthetase activity is injurious, therapy has been attempted with low methionine, cystine-supplemented diets. Early reported results have been encouraging but difficult to evaluate in view of the variability of the clinical course. Some patients have been maintained on coumadin anticoagulation.

MAPLE SYRUP URINE DISEASE
(Branched Chain Ketoaciduria)

Definition

Maple syrup urine disease, so named because of the characteristic odor of the urine and sweat of affected patients, is a rare genetic disorder of the metabolism of branched chain amino acids and their corresponding keto acids. It is associated with severe neurologic damage and mental retardation occurring in the early neonatal period, usually leading to early death. A few atypical milder cases have been described in older children. Approximately 25 to 30 cases have been reported since its initial description in 1954.

Genetics and Pathogenesis

Leucine, isoleucine, and valine are normally metabolized to their corresponding ketoacids (α-ketoisocaproic acid, α-keto-β-methylvaleric acid, and α-ketoisovaleric acid, respectively). These keto acids then undergo oxidative decarboxylation in complex reactions comparable to those catalyzed by pyruvate and α-ketoglutarate oxidases, each keto acid having a specific oxidase. In maple syrup urine disease the activities of all three keto acid oxidases are markedly reduced or virtually absent in brain, kidney, liver, and peripheral leukocytes. The loss of activity of three analogous but distinct enzymes suggests that this disease is caused by the mutation of an operator gene (if this hypothesis is applicable to mammalian genetics) or of a gene controlling a common enzyme subunit. The disease is transmitted as an autosomal mendelian recessive trait. Presumed heterozygotes have reduced activities of the keto acids oxidases in their leukocytes, but otherwise exhibit no clinical or chemical stigmata of the disease. The metabolic block in these parallel degradative pathways leads to the accumulation of three branched chain keto acids and the corresponding amino acids in blood and their excessive excretion in urine. The mechanism of neurologic damage has not been established, although several hypotheses have been advanced. The keto acid derivatives of leucine and valine inhibit the activity of L-glutamic dehydrogenase in brain homogenates. Another suggestion relates to the inhibition of transfer of other essential amino acids into the central nervous system in the presence of elevated plasma levels of the branched chain amino acids.

Clinical Presentation and Diagnosis

Infants with maple syrup urine disease are normal at birth but begin within a few days to exhibit progressive deterioration with lethargy, poor feeding, diminished awareness, hypertonicity alternating with flaccidity, and convulsions. The characteristic urine odor from which the name derives is present. Death generally occurs within the first few weeks of life from severe neurologic damage with respiratory disturbances. If death is delayed, mental retardation becomes apparent. The diagnosis is usually first suggested from the odor of the urine, described as sweet, caramel-like, or like maple syrup. The urine gives a positive ferric chloride test and dinitrophenylhydrazine reaction for keto acids. The diagnosis is best established by ion exchange column chromatography of plasma to demonstrate elevated levels of leucine, isoleucine, and valine. Methods for demonstrating the enzyme defect in circulating leukocytes have been described.

Treatment

The treatment of maple syrup urine disease, like that of phenylketonuria, is based on the use of a diet restricted in the corresponding amino acids beginning early in life before the onset of permanent neurologic damage. In practice this has been very difficult because of the necessity to balance three different amino acids, the ubiquitous distribution of the branched chained amino acids in foods, and the large number of plasma chromatographic analyses required. A few encouraging results have been reported using strict dietary therapy. It is not clear whether such treatment can be omitted in later life.

REFERENCES

Auerbach, V. H., A. M. DiGeorge, and G. G. Carpenter: Phenylalaninemia, p. 5 in W. L. Nyhan (Ed.), "Amino Acid Metabolism and Genetic Variation," New York, McGraw-Hill Book Company, 1967.

Carson, N. A. J., D. C. Cusworth, C. E. Dent, C. M. B. Field, D. W. Neill, and R. G. Westall: Homocystinuria: A New Inborn Error of Metabolism Associated with Mental Deficiency, Arch. Dis. Child., 38:425, 1963.

Dancis, J., and M. Levitz: Maple Syrup Urine Disease (Branched Chain Ketonuria), p. 353 in J. B. Stanbury, J. B. Wyngaarden, and D. S. Fredrickson (Eds.), "The Metabolic Basis of Inherited Disease," 2d ed., New York, McGraw-Hill Book Company, 1966.

Jervis, G. A.: Phenylketonuria, p. 5 in W. L. Nyhan (Ed.), "Amino Acid Metabolism and Genetic Variation," New York, McGraw-Hill Book Company, 1967.

Knox, W. E.: Phenylketonuria, p. 258 in J. B. Stanbury, J. B. Wyngaarden, and D. S. Fredrickson (Eds.), "The Metabolic Basis of Inherited Disease," 2d ed., New York, McGraw-Hill Book Company, 1966.

Menkes, J. H.: The Pathogenesis of Mental Retardation in Phenylketonuria and Other Inborn Errors of Amino Acid Metabolism, Pediatrics, 39:297, 1967.

———, P. L. Hurst, and J. M. Craig: A New Syndrome: Progressive Familial Cerebral Dysfunction with an Unusual Urinary Substance, Pediatrics, 14:462, 1954.

Mudd, S. H., J. D. Finkelstein, F. Irreverre, and L. Laster: Homocystinuria: An Enzymatic Defect, Science, 143:1443, 1964.

Schimke, R. N., V. A. McKusick, and R. G. Weilbaecher: Homocystinuria, p. 297 in W. L. Nyhan (Ed.), "Amino Acid Metabolism and Genetic Variation," New York, McGraw-Hill Book Company, 1967.

Snyderman, S. E.: Maple Syrup Urine Disease, p. 171 in W. L. Nyhan (Ed.), "Amino Acid Metabolism and Genetic Variation," New York, McGraw-Hill Book Company, 1967.

103 STORAGE DISEASES. ALCAPTONURIA AND OCHRONOSIS, PRIMARY HYPEROXALURIA WITH OXALOSIS, AND CYSTINE STORAGE DISEASE

Lloyd H. Smith, Jr.

A number of genetic diseases are characterized by excessive storage of metabolites in the host. Most often these represent blocks in degradative pathways. Examples may be cited in the glycogen storage disease (Chap. 111), the lipidoses (Gaucher's disease, Fabry's disease, Niemann-Pick disease, Tay-Sachs disease, Tangier disease, metachromatic leukodystrophy) (Chap. 113), certain amino acid degradative diseases (primary hyperoxaluria with oxalosis, alcaptonuria with ochronosis, possibly cystine storage disease), and possibly in some disorders of connective tissues (Hurler's syndrome) (Chap. 399). In addition excessive retention of dietary minerals may occur, as in hemochromatosis (Chap. 107) and Wilson's disease (Chap. 110). Tophaceous gout represents a special case, with excessive production and/or renal retention of a metabolic end product, uric acid (Chap. 106). Most of the above disorders have been described elsewhere in this book. This chapter will be concerned only with certain storage diseases of amino acid metabolism.

ALCAPTONURIA AND OCHRONOSIS

Definition

Alcaptonuria, one of the original inborn errors of metabolism studied by Garrod, is a rare disorder in the degradative pathway of phenylalanine and tyrosine metabolism. The genetic defect in the activity of the enzyme homogentisic acid oxidase leads to the accumulation and excessive urinary excretion of homogentisic acid. There is an associated deposition of dark pigment in connective tissues (ochronosis) and a particular form of degenerative arthritis. Over 600 cases have been reported.

Genetics and Pathogenesis

Homogentisic acid, a normal intermediate in the metabolism of phenylalanine and tyrosine, is oxidized with opening of the phenyl ring to form maleylacetoacetic acid. The enzyme homogentisic acid oxidase, which catalyzes this step, has been found to be missing in activity in liver and kidney from patients with alcaptonuria. The disease seems to be transmitted as an autosomal mendelian trait, with a frequency of about one in 200,000 births. No biochemical method for detection of presumed heterozygotes has been devised, nor do they exhibit any of the clinical features of the disease. The renal excretion of excessive homogentisic acid (3 to 7 Gm per day) fully accounts for the reducing properties of urine, gentisic acid being the only other metabolite excreted in excess. At neutral pH or above, homogentisic acid is rapidly oxidized to a brown or black polymer, with darkening of the urine on standing and with staining of wet diapers or linen. The slower accumulation in the body of a similar polymer bound to cartilage and other connective tissues is presumably the origin of ochronosis. Recently an enzyme has been described in skin and cartilage which oxidizes homogentisic acid to a melanin-like polymer. The mechanism by which this oxidation produces cartilagenous degeneration and arthritis is not clear.

Clinical Presentation and Diagnosis

Alcaptonuria is a benign disorder until middle life, when degenerative joint changes begin in the majority of cases. Prior to this time the darkening of urine is often unnoticed, although a positive but atypical Benedict's test for urine glucose may call it to one's attention. The increasing use of the glucose oxidase test will diminish this method of discovery. With the onset of arthritis, the large joints and the spine are affected with pain and stiffness, interspersed with periods of acute inflammation, which may resemble rheumatoid arthritis. Limitation of motion of the joints and ankylosis of the lumbosacral spine often occur later in the course. The roentgenogram of the spine is often almost pathognomonic, with degeneration and dense calcification of the intervertebral disks and resulting narrowing of the spaces. Ochronotic pigmentation may often be seen in the transmitted blueness of cartilages of the ear, nose, and costochondral junctions, and in brown areas in the sclerae, most frequently located at the insertions of the lateral rectus muscles. A high incidence of degenerative cardiovascular disease has been described in older ochronotic patients, but a cause-and-effect relationship has not been firmly established. The diagnosis is usually made from the triad of *arthritis, ochronotic pigmentation,* and *urine which darkens* on the addition of strong alkali. As noted, the urine reduces alkaline copper solutions, but since it turns black in the process, the erroneous diagnosis of glucosuria can be avoided. Homogentisic aciduria can be further identified by the ability of the urine to blacken undeveloped photographic film exposed to light. It may be conclusively demonstrated by chemical tests, chromatographic characteristics, or a specific enzymatic assay. Reversible acquired ochronosis has been described in the past after the prolonged use of carbolic acid dressings for cutaneous ulcers.

Treatment

Alcaptonuria carries with it no metabolic disadvantage other than the deposition of polymerized pigment in connective tissues and the associated degenerative changes. Ascorbic acid, as a strong reducing agent, will impede the oxidation and polymerization of homogentisic acid in vitro. Its use in large doses has been suggested as a possible means of preventing pigment formation and deposition in ochronotics, but its efficacy has not been demonstrated. The long and relatively benign course of the illness discourages attempts at rigid control of phenylalanine or tyrosine in the diet. Symptomatic treatment is similar to that of osteoarthritis (Chap. 387).

PRIMARY HYPEROXALURIA AND OXALOSIS

Definition

Primary hyperoxaluria is a genetic disorder characterized biochemically by continued excessive urinary excretion of oxalic acid and clinically by calcium oxalate nephrolithiasis and nephrocalcinosis. At postmortem examination calcium oxalate is usually found to be widely deposited in the tissues, a condition called oxalosis. In its typical form primary hyperoxaluria generally leads to uremia and early death. A few milder cases have been described in adult life with recurrent calcium oxalate kidney stones.

Genetics and Pathogenesis

Primary hyperoxaluria has been shown to represent two distinct genetic disorders, associated with glycolic aciduria and L-glyceric aciduria, respectively. They are described here together, since both diseases have similar levels of urinary oxalate and are indistinguishable clinically. The excessive synthesis of oxalate results from a block in an alternate route of metabolism of its precursor, glyoxylic acid. In glycolic aciduria the activity of the enzyme α-ketoglutarate:glyoxylate carboligase, which catalyzes the synthesis of α-hydroxy-β-keto adipic acid, has been found to be markedly reduced in liver, spleen, and kidney preparations. The resulting expansion of the glyoxylate pool behind the site of the metabolic block leads to its excessive oxidation to oxalic acid and reduction to glycolic acid. All three of these 2-carbon acids are excreted in increased amounts in the urine. The disease seems most likely to be transmitted as an autosomal Mendelian recessive trait, but no means of detecting presumed heterozygotes has been found. In L-glyceric aciduria there is absent activity of D-glyceric dehydrogenase (demonstrated in leukocytes), an enzyme which catalyzes the reduction of hydroxypyruvic acid in the catabolic pathway of serine metabolism. The accumulated hydroxypyruvate is reduced by lactic dehydrogenase to the unnatural L isomer of glyceric acid, which is excreted in the urine. D-Glyceric dehydrogenase appears to be the same enzyme as glyoxylate reductase which is an explanation for the accompanying excessive synthesis and excretion of oxalic acid. L-Glyceric aciduria is transmitted as an autosomal recessive trait and partial reductions in D-glyceric dehydrogenase activity are found in heterozygotes. The pathogenesis of stone formation, nephrocalcinosis, and oxalosis seems to relate directly to the insolubility of calcium oxalate. The disease can be simulated in animals, and in man, by pyridoxine deficiency, which presumably inhibits the transamination of glyoxylate to glycine. Glycolic acid and L-glyceric acid have no known toxic effects.

Clinical Presentation and Diagnosis

Primary hyperoxaluria usually presents in childhood with recurrent kidney stones, with or without radiographically demonstrable nephrocalcinosis (Chap. 307). Rarely renal failure secondary to nephrocalcinosis may be the initial finding. The course of the childhood form of the disease is usually that of progressive renal failure leading to death from uremia. In adults kidney stones are frequent and occasionally mild nephrocalcinosis is found, but renal function is usually well preserved. The diagnosis is established by demonstrating excessive excretion of oxalic acid in the absence of pyridoxine deficiency. The normal child or adult excretes less than 60 mg oxalic acid/1.73m²/24 hr. Patients with primary hyperoxaluria usually excrete at least two or three times that amount. The differential diagnosis of the glycolic aciduria (most frequent) and L-glyceric aciduria subvariants depends on specific measurements of those metabolites in urine.

Treatment

There is no specific treatment for primary hyperoxaluria at this time. Large doses of pyridoxine (100 mg per day) may reduce urine oxalate, but the effect is not striking. Measures which may reduce the risk of stone formation are of use, such as forcing fluids, the use of a high phosphate regimen, and oral magnesium oxide (Chap. 307). Because of the seriousness of the disorder, attempts are being made to develop an inhibitor of oxalate synthesis, comparable to the use of allopurinol in gout.

CYSTINOSIS AND FANCONI'S SYNDROME

Definition

Cystine storage disease, or cystinosis (Lignac-de Toni-Fanconi syndrome), is a rare genetic disorder, usually found in childhood in association with Fanconi's syndrome. Rarely, ocular and systemic cystine storage occurs in an adult form in the absence of renal disease. Fanconi's syndrome is a descriptive phrase for a group of physiologic abnormalities which occur with proximal renal tubular dysfunction, notably glucosuria, generalized aminoaciduria, phosphaturia, and renal tubular acidosis. Cystinosis is only one of many diseases which may be associated with Fanconi's syndrome, a classification of which is given in Table 103-1.

Table 103-1. CLASSIFICATIONS OF FANCONI'S SYNDROME

I. Idiopathic
   A. Sporadic
   B. Familial
II. As part of a genetic disease
   A. Cystinosis
   B. Wilson's disease
   C. Tyrosinemia
   D. Lowe's syndrome
   E. Hereditary fructose intolerance (with fructose)
III. Medullary cystic disease
IV. Acquired
   A. Abnormality of protein metabolism
      1. Nephrotic syndrome
      2. Multiple myeloma
      3. Sjögren's syndrome
      4. Amyloidosis
   B. Drugs
      1. Outdated tetracycline
      2. 6-Mercaptopurine
      3. Isophthalanilide
   C. Heavy metals
      1. Mercury
      2. Uranium
      3. Cadmium
   D. Malignancy
V. Experimental (animals)
   A. Maleic acid
   B. Malonic acid

SOURCE: After R. C. Morris, Jr., The Clinical Spectrum of Fanconi's Syndrome, Calif. Med., 108:225, 1968.

Genetics and Pathogenesis

The metabolic defect resulting in cystine storage has not yet been discovered. A number of enzymes in cystine metabolism have been assayed without finding any consistent abnormality, and earlier claims of reduced levels of blood cystine reductase have not been confirmed. Marked increases in cystine have been found in circulating leukocytes and in fibroblasts grown in tissue culture from patients with cystinosis. The free cystine is compartmentalized within the "granular" fraction of the cell. The disease seems to be transmitted as an autosomal recessive trait, with heterozygotes demonstrating intermediate levels of intracellular cystine. Plasma cystine levels are usually normal or slightly elevated only. The biochemical link between cystine storage and proximal renal tubular dysfunction is obscure in the childhood form of the disease and missing in adults. Cystine has the ability to form mixed disulfides with sulfhydryl groups. It has been suggested that the injurious effect of cystine storage may result from inhibition of sulfhydryl-containing enzymes by the formation of half-cystine residues on the proteins.

As outlined in Table 103-1, Fanconi's syndrome may be of diverse origins, both inherited and acquired. It represents a nonspecific pattern of failure of proximal renal tubular absorptive function, varying greatly in the degree of severity and the spectrum of functions impaired. The individual disease processes will not be discussed here. In idiopathic Fanconi's syndrome and that associated with cystinosis, microdissection studies have demonstrated a consistent structural change in the proximal tubule, the so-called "swan neck deformity." The proximal tubule is shortened and exhibits atrophy with flattened epithelium in the region adjacent to a normal-appearing glomerulus.

Clinical Presentation and Diagnosis

Cystine storage disease with Fanconi's syndrome is a serious disorder which usually leads to death from uremia by the age of ten. Failure to thrive and severe resistant rickets with stunting of growth develop in the first few months of life. Rickets results from several derangements: (1) failure of tubular reabsorption of phosphate with hypophosphatemia, (2) proximal renal tubular acidosis with bicarbonate wastage and chronic systemic acidosis, (3) hypercalcuria secondary to acidosis, and (4) the inhibition of osteoid calcification (vitamin D resistance) produced by azotemia. A more complete description of rickets and osteomalacia is presented elsewhere in this book (Chap. 83). Secondary hyperparathyroidism is a frequent complication. Glucosuria may be scanty and intermittent or profuse and constant at a normal blood glucose level; it is sometimes sufficient to produce ketosis and contribute to further exacerbation of acidosis. Excessive urinary loss of potassium associated with renal tubular acidosis may lead to hypokalemia with muscle weakness or paralysis. Potassium depletion may produce "clear-cell nephropathy" with further deterioration of renal tubular function, especially a renal tubular concentration defect productive of polyuria. Generalized aminoaciduria occurs, with a nonspecific pattern. Although cystine is usually excreted in excess, the urinary concentration is not sufficient to lead to cystine kidney stones. Hypouricemia may result from failure of reabsorption of uric acid.

It has been recently found that patients with Fanconi's syndrome excrete lysozyme in the urine as well. Pyelonephritis is frequent and may contribute, along with interstitial fibrosis, to the onset of renal failure. The idiopathic Fanconi's syndrome may occur in an identical clinical and pathologic combination except for the absence of cystine storage. Individual patients may exhibit some but not all of the proximal tubular defects. The clinical presentation may be dominated by other manifestations of the primary disease productive of Fanconi's syndrome (Table 103-1). Rarely, cystinosis may occur in the adult in the absence of renal dysfunction (Cogan's syndrome). Crystalline rods or plates of cystine are found in the cornea and conjunctiva as the only manifestation of adult cystinosis. Similar ocular cystinosis occurs in the infantile form of cystinosis.

The diagnosis of Fanconi's syndrome depends on the demonstration of the characteristic pattern of proximal renal tubular defects, of which the most important are phosphaturia, generalized aminoaciduria, glucosuria, and renal tubular acidosis of the proximal (bicarbonate flooding) type. All these defects may be found individually or in various combinations, and may even vary with time in a given patient. It is therefore most useful to describe the actual physiologic derangements rather than to take refuge in the eponym. Cystinosis as cystine crystals may be demonstrated by slit-lamp examination of the eye, or may be found in bone marrow or circulating leukocytes. Cystinotic leukocytes have very high levels of cystine by chemical analysis, even in the absence of demonstrable crystals.

Treatment

Treatment would logically be directed toward the disease resulting in Fanconi's syndrome and toward replacement therapy to compensate for renal dysfunction. Some of the diseases listed in Table 103-1 can be treated (Wilson's disease, hereditary fructose intolerance, etc.); others cannot. In the absence of specific information about its biochemical defect, attempts to treat cystinosis have generally been unrewarding. The use of D-penicillamine or dimercaptopropanol has been advocated in an attempt to regenerate active sulfhydryl groups on enzymes (see Wilson's disease, Chap. 110). Further information will be required to evaluate the hypothesis on which this form of treatment is based, as well as its efficacy. Cystine is synthesized from the essential amino acid methionine, so that specific dietary treatment has not been vigorously pursued. Treatment of the secondary physiologic derangements has been more successful and has been directed toward replacement of calcium, phosphate, sodium, and potassium to reverse chronic acidosis, rickets (osteomalacia in the adult), and hypokalemia. Large amounts of vitamin D are required (usually 50,000 to 400,000 IU daily) to promote normal calcification of bone. It has been reported that vitamin D may improve certain parameters of tubular function as well, reducing aminoaciduria, glucosuria, and bicarbonate wasting. Shohl's solution (98 Gm sodium citrate and 140 Gm citric acid per liter) is a suitable source of buffer base for chronic treatment of acidosis. Chronic potassium supplementation is not usually required after its initial repletion and the correction of acidosis. Improved healing of rickets may occur with supplemental phosphate if phosphaturia is severe. Despite considerable symptomatic improvement and healing of rickets, progressive renal damage in cystinosis leads to early death from uremia. Adult cystinosis is a benign disorder which does not require treatment. The treatment of adult Fanconi's syndrome is similar to that described for the infantile form, but the prognosis is much better (for detailed therapy see Chap. 104, pp. 592 to 593).

REFERENCES

Cogan, D. G., T. Kuwabara, and C. S. Hurlbut, Jr.: Further Observations on Cystinosis in the Adult, J.A.M.A., 160: 1725, 1958.

Hockaday, T. D. R., J. E. Clayton, E. W. Frederick, and L. H. Smith, Jr.: Primary Hyperoxaluria, Medicine, 43:315, 1964.

La Du, B. N.: Alcaptonuria, p. 303 in "The Metabolic Basis of Inherited Disease," 2d ed., J. B. Stanbury, J. B. Wyngaarden, and D. S. Fredrickson (Eds.), New York, McGraw-Hill Book Company, 1966.

Leaf, A.: The Syndrome of Osteomalacia, Renal Glycosuria, Aminoaciduria, and Increased Phosphorus Clearance (the Fanconi Syndrome), p. 1205 in "The Metabolic Basis of Inherited Disease," 2d ed., J. B. Stanbury, J. B. Wyngaarden, and D. S. Fredrickson (Eds.), New York, McGraw-Hill Book Company, 1966.

Morris, R. C., Jr.: The Clinical Spectrum of Fanconi's Syndrome, Calif. Med., 108:225, 1968.

O'Brien, W. M., B. N. La Du, and J. J. Bunim: Biochemical, Pathologic, and Clinical Aspects of Alcaptonuria, Ochronosis, and Ochronotic Arthropathy, Am. J. Med., 34:813, 1963.

Schneider, J. A., F. M. Rosenbloom, K. H. Bradley, and J. E. Seegmiller: Increased Free-cystine Content of Fibroblasts Cultured from Patients with Cystinosis, Biochem. Biophys. Res. Commun., 29:527, 1967.

Williams, H. E., and L. H. Smith, Jr.: L-Glyceric Aciduria: New Genetic Variant of Primary Hyperoxaluria, New Engl. J. Med., 278:233, 1968.

—— and ——: Disorders of Oxalate Metabolism, Am. J. Med., 45:715, 1968.

Wyngaarden, J. B., and T. D. Elder: Primary Hyperoxaluria and Oxalosis, p. 189 in "The Metabolic Basis of Inherited Disease," 2d ed., J. B. Stanbury, J. B. Wyngaarden, and D. S. Fredrickson (Eds.), New York, McGraw-Hill Book Company, 1966.

104 ERRORS IN MEMBRANE TRANSPORT

Lloyd H. Smith, Jr.

The transfer of metabolites across cell membranes is usually an active energy-requiring process of considerable specificity. The enzymology of these processes and the required structural characteristics of cell membranes are poorly understood, although this now represents an important area of biochemical and biophysical investigation. A number of diseases in man are best described as genetic defects in active transport of specific substances across epithelial cell membranes. In none of them has a specific enzymatic or structural defect been identified, other than in the description of the functional derangement. It is possible that defects may occur in the active transport of metabolites among the specific compartments or organelles within cells.

Some of the genetic diseases which might be classified as errors in membrane transport are cystinuria; Hartnup disease; hereditary renal tubular acidosis; renal glycosuria, familial renal gout; vasopressin—resistant diabetes insipidus; congenital hemolytic anemia with high sodium, low potassium in the red cells; familial goiter with iodide transport defect; methionine malabsorption syndrome; isolated tryptophan malabsorption (blue diaper syndrome); glucose and galactose malabsorption disease; congenital alkalosis with diarrhea (chloridorrhea); and hereditary intestinal malabsorption of vitamin B_{12}. Hemochromatosis might qualify in this category as an error of excessive transport of iron. There are data which suggest that vitamin D–resistant rickets ("phosphate diabetes") represents a defect in vitamin D metabolism rather than a primary transport defect. Similarly cystinosis with the Fanconi syndrome seems to represent a disorder in cystine metabolism rather than a primary renal tubular defect. This section will be limited to brief presentations of cystinuria, Hartnup disease, renal glycosuria, and hereditary renal tubular acidosis.

CYSTINURIA

Definition

Cystinuria is a genetic disorder (or group of closely related disorders) characterized by continued excessive excretion of the dibasic amino acids cystine, lysine, arginine, and ornithine. This results from a transport defect for these amino acids in the renal tubule. Similar transport defects occur in the intestinal mucosa. The sole clinical manifestations are those of recurrent cystine kidney stones and their sequelae. Patients tend to be of short stature, which has been attributed, without supporting evidence, to lysine deficiency.

Genetics and Pathogenesis

Cystinuria has been known to be a familial disease for almost a century. It was one of the four original "inborn errors of metabolism" studied by Sir Archibald Garrod, who demonstrated its transmission in a pattern consistent with autosomal recessive inheritance. Further advances awaited the application of modern methods of amino acid analysis and the study of transport in kidney and in gut mucosal biopsies in vitro. In approximately two-thirds of the families (parents and children) the presumed heterozygotes of affected patients, have normal levels of urinary dibasic amino acid excretion. In the remaining families heterozygotes excrete increased amounts of cystine and lysine. At least one additional phenotype can be identified on the basis of intestinal transport studies. Several families have been studied with different genetic types in conjugal heterozygotes of cystinuria. The resulting patterns of double heterozygote defects have been interpreted as evidence for multiple allelic mutations. The incidence of homozygous cystinuria is approximately 1:20,000.

For many years cystinuria was attributed to a defect in cystine metabolism and was often confused with cystine storage disease (cystinosis). Dent and Rose first demonstrated by clearance techniques that impaired renal tubular reabsorption of the specific amino acids cystine, lysine, and arginine was the explanation of aminoaciduria. Subsequent studies indicated similar defects in tubular reabsorption of ornithine and more recently homocysteine, the mixed disulfide of cysteine. Clearance of cystine may significantly exceed glomerular filtration rate, indicating net tubular secretion of this amino acid. Plasma levels of the four amino acids are reduced. A common mechanism in the kidney has been confirmed by competition of the amino acids for transport during infusion in vitro and in part in tissue slice preparations of kidney in vitro. It has not been possible to demonstrate a defect in cystine transport in vitro in renal biopsies from patients with cystinuria.

The transport defect for dibasic amino acids in cystinuria is also found in the gut. This was first demonstrated by oral tolerance tests. It has been clearly confirmed in studies of active transport in jejunal mucosal biopsy specimens in vitro. With impaired absorption, lysine and ornithine are decarboxylated by intestinal bacteria to cadaverine and putrescine, respectively. These diamines are partially metabolized to pyrrolidine and piperidine, and all these compounds are excreted in increased amounts in cystinuric urine. No impairment of amino acid transport has been found in tissues other than the renal tubules and the gut mucosa in cystinuria.

Normal urinary excretion of cystine varies with size and diet, but has an upper normal range of about 18 mg per Gm creatinine. In homozygous cystinuria cystine excretion usually varies between 0.4 to 1.0 Gm per day, although values as high as 3.0 Gm per day have been found. The solubility of cystine in urine is approximately 350 to 400 mg per liter. Supersaturation and crystallization readily occur, particularly during nocturnal concentration of the urine. The accretion of such crystals as stones, with the resulting complications of obstruction and infection, is the direct cause of disability in cystinuria.

Diagnosis

The clinical manifestations of cystine kidney stones are indistinguishable from those of other kidney stones: flank pain, colic, hematuria, obstructive uropathy, infection. Cystine stones are as densely radiopaque as calcium-containing kidney stones. In overall incidence they constitute approximately 1 to 2 percent of all kidney stones. It is important to establish the composition of kidney stones in order to institute rational programs of stone prophylaxis (Chap. 307).

The most direct diagnostic procedure is that of stone analysis because cystine stones occur only in the genetic disorder cystinuria. The appearance of cystine crystals in the sediment of concentrated, acidified (addition of glacial acetic acid to pH 4.5), chilled urine specimens usually indicates a cystine concentration of greater than 200 to 250 mg per liter. The crystals are hexagonal plates resembling the formula of a benzene ring. The nitroprusside test for cystine is a nonspecific reaction for sulfhydryl groups after reduction of disulfides by sodium cyanide. It can be made semiquantitative for cystine in the absence of other sulfhydryl compounds.

The specific aminoaciduria of cystine, lysine, arginine, and ornithine can be directly demonstrated by paper or ion exchange column chromatography of urine. This pattern is diagnostic of genetic cystinuria. The urinary amino acid pattern of cystinuria may sometimes be found in the rare disorder of familial pancreatitis.

Treatment

As a genetic disease cystinuria cannot be "cured" in the host (except by renal homotransplantation). In order to prevent formation and growth of stones, attempts are made to reduce the concentration of cystine in urine and to increase the solubility of cystine at a given urine concentration. Urinary excretion of cystine can sometimes be minimized by a diet low in methionine, the most important cystine precursor. Of greater practicality, cystine concentration can be reduced by increasing urine volume by forcing fluids, especially at night. Some increase in cystine solubility is obtained by alkalinizing the urine, but the solubility curve rises steeply only at pHs higher than 7.2.

A promising new approach is that of forming mixed disulfides of cysteine with other sulfhydryl compounds with enhancement of solubility. The use of D-penicillamine (1.0 to 2.0 Gm daily) leads to the excretion of a soluble cysteine-penicillamine disulfide (solubility fifty times greater than cystine) with reduction of cystine excretion below saturation concentrations. The toxicity of D-penicillamine has stimulated current attempts to find more suitable compounds with similar properties.

HARTNUP DISEASE

Hartnup disease (also called H disease) is a genetic disorder of the transport of a group of monoamino-monocarboxylic acids which share a common transport mechanism in the renal tubule and in the gut mucosa. The disease, so far described in about 25 patients, seems to be the homozygous manifestation of an autosomal recessive trait; the heterozygous state is not detectable by current techniques. Hartnup disease is characterized by massive aminoaciduria of alanine, serine, threonine, asparagin, glutamine, valine, leucine, isoleucine, phenylalanine, tyrosine, tryptophan, histidine, and citrulline. In contrast to cystinuria, the associated gut defect is more

important in producing the symptoms of the disease—intermittent pellagra-like rash appearing after exposure to sunlight, attacks of cerebellar ataxia often accompanying the skin manifestations, and psychiatric changes varying from emotional instability to dementia. Impaired absorption allows for bacterial degradation of amino acids which may (1) lead to nicotinamide deficiency from loss of precursor tryptophan, thereby producing pellagra, and (2) allow for the production and absorption of toxic metabolic products injurious to the central nervous system. The specific amino acid metabolites responsible for the signs and symptoms of cerebral and cerebellar dysfunction have not been identified. The diagnosis can be established by the pattern of urinary amino acids, measured by paper or ion exchange chromatography. Most patients respond well to maintenance treatment with oral nicotinamide (50 to 200 mg per day). A high protein diet is also recommended to counter the amino acid loss in the gut and in the urine.

RENAL GLYOSURIA

Definition

Renal glycosuria is a genetic disorder in which glucose is excreted in the urine at normal concentrations of blood glucose. In order to avoid confusion with other conditions associated with melituria, Marble's strict criteria should be followed (Chap. 95): (1) glycosuria occurs in the absence of hyperglycemia; (2) all specimens of urine should contain glucose with relatively little fluctuation in glycosuria related to diet; (3) the oral glucose tolerance test is normal (sometimes slightly flat); (4) the reducing substance is specifically identified as glucose, ruling out other meliturias such as pentosuria, fructosuria, galactosuria, sucrosuria, maltosuria, mannoheptulosuria; (5) the storage and utilization of carbohydrates are normal. By these criteria, including the absence of other disorders of proximal renal tubular function, renal glycosuria can be identified as a rare (94 cases in 50,000 cases of melituria at the Joslin Clinic) isolated transport defect. Use of the more liberal criteria proposed by Lawrence, i.e., glycosuria which occurs with a normal glucose tolerance test, will detect many more abnormalities.

Genetics and Pathogenesis

Current information is most consistent with the transmission of renal glycosuria as a mendelian dominant characteristic, although the suggestion has been made that the defect may be expressed in heterozygotes with homozygotes representing severer forms of the disease. Diabetes mellitus is frequently found in the families of patients with renal glycosuria; whether renal glycosuria defined by the strict Marble criteria is a precursor of diabetes is disputed. Many patients with renal glycosuria by the Lawrence criteria will develop clinical diabetes mellitus within a few years of diagnosis.

No consistent structural alteration has been demonstrated in the renal tubule by light or electron microscopy. Most studies of the renal defect have been carried out by classical clearance techniques. Plasma glucose is completely filterable in the glomerulus and is reabsorbed by an active process in the proximal tubule. The biochemical basis of active reabsorption of glucose has not been demonstrated; specifically, no intermediary product has been found. Reabsorption exhibits saturation kinetics with a transfer maximum (TM) of about 250 to 325 mg glucose per min in the normal adult. Clearance studies in renal glycosuria have failed to yield a consistent pattern. In some patients a low TM for glucose has been found; in others the TM has been normal but there has been an increased splay in the curve describing the relationship of glucose reabsorbed to that filtered. Renal glycosuria could result from any one of the following defects: decrease in the anatomic mass of the proximal tubule in relation to its glomerulus (glomerulotubular imbalance), abnormal distribution of the transport system relative to glomerular filtration whether on a functional or anatomic basis, an abnormality in the presumed enzymatic step or steps (permeability, hypothetical membrane carrier, energy-yielding reactions) which constitute the active transport process. It is likely that there may be different genetic and pathogenetic forms of the disease.

Diagnosis and Clinical Implications

The criteria for diagnosis have been included in the definition. It is important to identify the reducing substance as glucose (by glucose oxidase, for example) and also to rule out other primary or secondary renal tubular defects (aminoaciduria, phosphaturia, renal tubular acidosis, etc.) The recently described disorder of glucose and galactose malabsorption is characterized by impaired intestinal absorption of these monosaccharides and renal glycosuria. The prognosis of renal glycosuria appears to be excellent except insofar as it may herald subsequent clinical diabetes. No treatment is required.

RENAL TUBULAR ACIDOSIS

Definition

Renal tubular acidosis (RTA) is a clinical disorder characterized by inability of the kidney to excrete an appropriately acid urine. This results in a persistent metabolic acidosis with hyperchloremia, and may be complicated by potassium depletion and/or hypercalcuria. RTA may occur as an isolated tubular defect or as one component of more extensive tubular dysfunction (such as in the De Toni-Fanconi syndrome). It has been described in association with glycogenosis, cystinosis, galactosemia, Wilson's disease, Lowe's syndrome, hereditary fructose intolerance, thyrotoxicosis, cadmium poisoning, and in a variety of disorders associated with hypergammaglobulinemia. The syndrome of RTA may be closely simulated by the chronic administration of potent carbonic anhydrase inhibitors. Its extracellular fluid pattern of hyperchloremic acidosis may be found following bilateral ureterosigmoid transplantations, during the in-gestion of large amounts of ammonium chloride, or in some patients with chronic pyelonephritis.

Genetics and Pathogenesis

Although often secondary to other metabolic disorders, RTA may occur with otherwise normal or nearly normal renal function and in the absence of associated diseases. Some of these cases have appeared to be sporadic; others have exhibited definite familial aggregation. The pattern of inheritance, including transmission in three successive generations, is consistent with a mendelian dominant trait. It seems unlikely that the transient infantile form of RTA, with a negative family history, represents the same disorder.

A complete discussion of the pathogenesis of RTA would demand a full treatment of the role of the kidney in the defense of acid-base balance. In brief, the kidney serves this homeostatic function in several closely related ways: by excretion of certain anionic products of metabolism (phosphate, sulfate), by conservation of filtered bicarbonate, by tubular secretion of hydrogen ions in exchange for sodium, and by tubular synthesis and excretion of ammonia. In RTA phosphate and sulfate excretions are not impaired in the absence of secondary renal failure. Normally the filtered bicarbonate is reclaimed in the proximal renal tubule by hydrogen ion secretion, and the TM for bicarbonate reabsorption is normal. The excretion of ammonia is often reduced, but only in proportion to the reduced urine acidity. The most plausible mechanism for RTA is that of inability of the distal renal tubule to develop a steep H+ gradient between extracellular fluid and tubular urine. This transport defect or "gradient defect" for H+ in the distal tubule results in reduced urine titratable acidity and ammonia, increased urinary loss of sodium and potassium (due to increased tubular exchange of potassium in lieu of H+ for sodium), and systemic acidosis. Sustained acidosis results in mobilization of calcium from bone and hypercalcuria. A few patients have been described with "proximal RTA," i.e., a partial failure of bicarbonate reabsorption with flooding of the normal distal tubular acidification mechanism.

Diagnosis and Clinical Implications

The diagnosis of RTA depends upon demonstration of impaired acidification of the urine in the face of systemic acidosis and in the absence of uremia. In mild cases this may require a further acid challenge (0.1 Gm ammonium chloride per kg body weight). The serum chloride is usually elevated commensurate with the reduction in serum bicarbonate. Other disorders noted above which may lead to secondary impairment of renal tubular acidification must be excluded. The most important complications of RTA are potassium depletion (weakness, paralysis, secondary renal tubular dysfunction), hypercalcuria (nephrocalcinosis, nephrolithiasis, osteomalacia, or rickets), pyelonephritis, and renal failure secondary to these factors.

Treatment

Acidosis, hypercalcuria, and potassium wasting are usually corrected by the oral administration of 1.0 to 1.5 mEq/kg/day of sodium bicarbonate, given in three divided doses. Alkali replacement may be better tolerated as Shohl's solution (140 Gm citric acid and 98 Gm hydrated crystals of sodium citrate per liter), given in a dosage of 50 to 100 ml per day in divided doses. The amount of alkali given should be sufficient to return the serum bicarbonate and pH to a normal range. Supplementary potassium and/or calcium and vitamin D may be required temporarily until body stores of these minerals have been repleted.

REFERENCES

Barron, D. N., C. E. Dent, H. Harris, E. W. Hart, and J. B. Jepson: Hereditary Pellagra-like Skin Rash with Temporary Cerebellar Ataxia, Constant Renal Amino-Aciduria and Other Bizarre Biochemical Features, Lancet, 2:421, 1956.

Bartter, F. C., M. Lotz, S. Thier, L. E. Rosenberg, and J. T. Potts: Cystinuria, Combined Clinical Staff Conference at the National Institutes of Health, Ann. Intern. Med., 62: 796, 1965.

Crawhall, J. C., and R. W. E. Watts: Cystinuria, Am. J. Med., 45:736, 1968.

Gill, J. R., Jr., N. H. Bell, and F. C. Bartter: Impaired Conservation of Sodium and Potassium in Renal Tubular Acidosis and Its Correction by Buffer Anions, Clin. Sci., 33:577, 1967.

Jepson, J. B.: Hartnup Disease, p. 1283 in J. B. Stanbury, J. B. Wyngaarden, and D. S. Fredrickson (Eds.), "The Metabolic Basis of Inherited Disease," 2d ed., New York, McGraw-Hill Book Company, 1966.

Krane, S. M.: Renal Glycosuria, p. 1221 in J. B. Stanbury, J. B. Wyngaarden, and D. S. Fredrickson (Eds.), "The Metabolic Basis of Inherited Disease," 2d ed., New York, McGraw-Hill Book Company, 1966.

Lawrence, R. D.: Symptomless Glycosurias: Differentiation by Sugar Tolerance Tests, Med. Clin. N. Am., 31:289, 1947.

Marble, A.: Non-Diabetic Melituria, in E. P. Joslin, H. F. Root, P. White, and A. Marble (Eds.), "The Treatment of Diabetes Mellitus," Philadelphia, Lea & Febiger, 1959.

Milne, M. D., A. M. Asatoor, K. D. G. Edwards, and L. W. Loughridge: The Intestinal Absorption Defect in Cystinuria, Gut, 2:323, 1961.

Morris, R. C., Jr.: Renal Tubular Acidosis: Mechanisms, Classification and Implications; New Engl. J. Med., 281: 1405, 1969.

Relman, A. S.: Renal Acidosis and Renal Excretion of Acid in Health and Disease, Advances Intern. Med., 12:295, 1964.

Seldin, D. W., and J. D. Wilson: Renal Tubular Acidosis, p. 1230 in J. B. Stanbury, J. B. Wyngaarden, and D. S. Fredrickson (Eds.): "The Metabolic Basis of Inherited Disease," 2d ed., New York, McGraw-Hill Book Company, 1966.

105 THE CARCINOID SYNDROME
John A. Oates

The association of carcinoid tumors with cutaneous flushes, telangiectasia, diarrhea, cardiac valvular lesions, and bronchial constriction eluded recognition until 1953. Once this connection was established by Thorson, Biörk, Björkman, and Waldenström, and independently by Isler and Hedinger, it was clear that the syndrome was mediated by release of one or more biologically active agents by the tumor. Serotonin was the first such agent to be discovered, and overproduction of this amine is the most consistent biochemical indicator of the carcinoid syndrome. Serotonin, however, is not the sole mediator of the clinical syndrome. These tumors vary in their metabolism of indoles and may elaborate chemically unrelated agents such as bradykinin, histamine, and adrenocorticotropic hormone (ACTH). Furthermore, there is evidence suggesting that an additional unidentified substance participates in the production of flushing. Within the broad classification of carcinoid tumors there is great diversity in the production of biologically active substances and in the mechanisms for their storage and release. Accordingly, there is a varied spectrum of clinical manifestations.

Pathologic Anatomy of the Tumor

Carcinoid tumors are slowly growing neoplasms of enterochromaffin cells. The metastatic tumors associated with carcinoid syndrome usually arise from small primary tumors in the ileum. The syndrome is also produced by neoplasms arising from the remainder of the small intestine, from organs derived from the embryonic foregut (e.g., bronchus, stomach, pancreas, and thyroid), and from ovarian or testicular teratomas.

Carcinoid tumors have an unusual proclivity for metastasis to the liver and may involve this organ extensively with minimal metastatic disease elsewhere. Extrahepatic metastases occur in bone, where they are often osteoblastic, and in lung, pancreas, spleen, ovaries, adrenals, and other organs.

Primary carcinoid tumors of the appendix neither metastasize nor produce carcinoid syndrome. Those from the large bowel may metastasize but do not exhibit an endocrine function.

The usual carcinoid tumor arising from the ileum has the classical histologic pattern of dense nests of cells with uniform size and nuclear appearance. Histochemically, they typically exhibit an argentaffin reaction in which the cells convert a silver salt to metallic silver. A positive argentaffin reaction is not required for the diagnosis, however, and carcinoid tumors arising from organs of the embryonic foregut do not usually contain many argentaffin cells. Tumors from these organs also have a broad histologic spectrum, which in the lung ranges from typical bronchial carcinoid to a form indistinguishable from oat cell carcinoma.

Clinical Features

Unlike most metastatic neoplasms, carcinoid tumors have an unusually slow rate of growth; most patients survive for 5 to 10 years after the disease is recognized. For much of the duration of the illness, morbidity may result largely from the endocrine function of the tumor. Death results from hepatic or cardiac failure and from complications associated with tumor growth.

VASOMOTOR PAROXYSMS. The most common clinical feature is cutaneous flushing. The typical flush is erythematous and involves the head and neck (blush area). Some patients exhibit vivid color changes from red to violaceous to pallor during its course. Prolonged flushing attacks may be associated with lacrimation and periorbital edema. The systemic effects of the flush are variable. It may be accompanied by tachycardia, and the blood pressure usually falls or does not change. A rise in

blood pressure during flushing is rare, and carcinoid syndrome is not a cause of sustained hypertension.

Flushing may be provoked by excitement, exertion, eating, ethanol, and epinephrine.

TELANGIECTASIA. In addition to paroxysms of cutaneous vasodilation, some patients also develop purple telangiectasia, primarily on the face and neck and most marked in the malar area.

GASTROINTESTINAL SYMPTOMS. Intestinal hypermotility with borborygmi, cramping, and explosive diarrhea may accompany the episodic flushes. Chronic hypermotility with diarrhea is more common. When this is severe, malabsorption can occur.

CARDIAC MANIFESTATIONS. There is a unique deposition of fibrous tissue on the endocardium of the valvular cusps and cardiac chambers. It occurs primarily in the right heart, but may involve the left side to a minimal degree. The fibrous deposition does not penetrate the internal elastic membrane. Distortion of the valve cusps, chordae tendineae, and papillary muscles interferes with valvular function in the right heart and may lead to regurgitation, stenosis, or combined functional lesions. There is, however, a tendency for the fibrosing process to produce incompetence at the tricuspid valve and stenosis of the smaller pulmonary orifice, a deleterious hemodynamic combination. The vasomotor changes in carcinoid syndrome may lead to a high cardiac output, with its attendant imposition on cardiac function.

PULMONARY SYMPTOMS. Bronchoconstriction is a less common feature of the syndrome, but it may be severe. It is usually most pronounced during flushing attacks.

GENERAL. In addition to the endocrine effects, the tumors themselves may cause intestinal obstruction or bleeding. Necrosis of intestinal or hepatic tumor masses may produce abdominal pain, tenderness, fever, and leukocytosis. Hepatomegaly from the metastatic disease is usually present with the syndrome. Extensive metastatic involvement of the liver by these slowly growing tumors may occur before the liver function tests become abnormal.

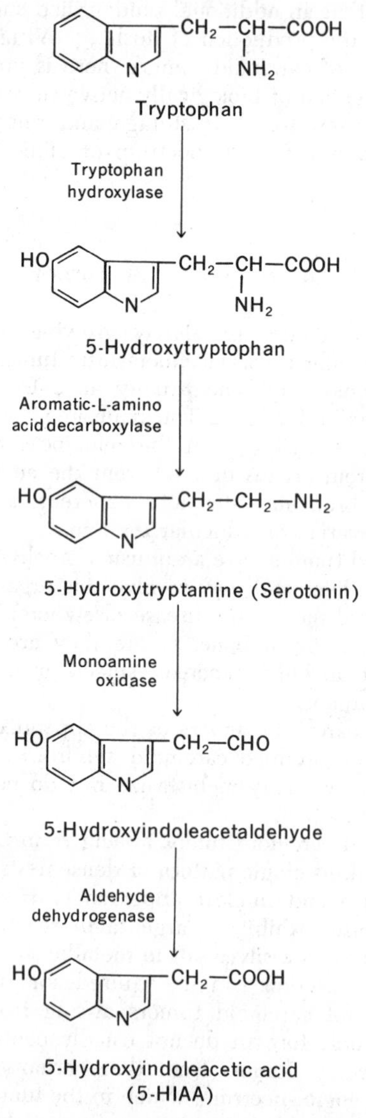

Endocrine Function of the Tumors

SEROTONIN. The most constant biochemical characteristic of carcinoid tumors is the presence of tryptophan hydroxylase, which catalyzes the formation of 5-hydroxytryptophan (5-HTP) from tryptophan (Fig. 105-1). Most tumors also contain the enzyme aromatic L-amino hydroxylase, which catalyzes the formation of 5-hydroxytryptamine (serotonin). Carcinoids from the stomach and from other organs derived from the embryonic foregut, however, are frequently deficient in this decarboxylase and release 5-HTP from the tumor.

Following its release from the tumor, serotonin is inactivated primarily by the enzyme monoamine oxidase; uptake into platelets also contributes to this inactivation. Monamine oxidase oxidizes serotonin to 5-hydroxyindoleacetaldehyde, which is rapidly converted to 5-hydroxyindoleacetic acid (5HIAA) by aldehyde dehydrogenase.

Fig. 105-1. Metabolic pathway of serotonin.

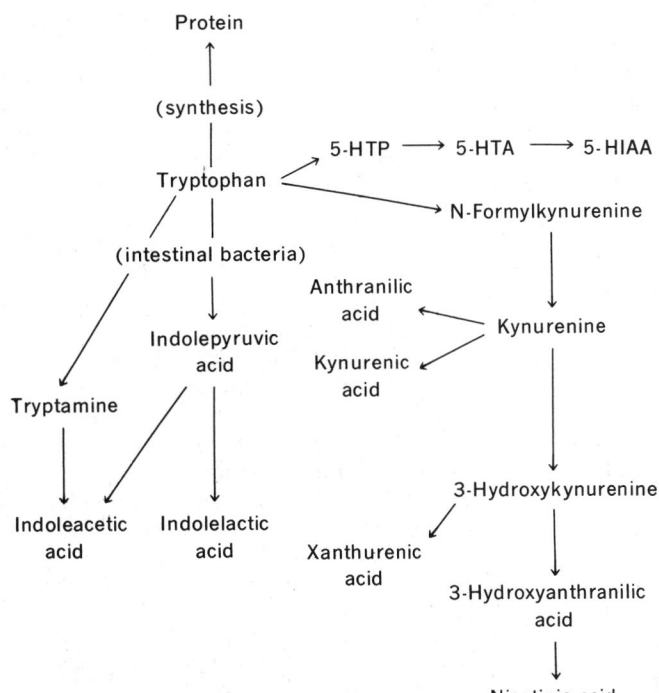

Fig. 105-2. Metabolic pathways of tryptophan.

This acid is rapidly excreted in the urine, and almost all circulating serotonin can be accounted for as urinary 5HIAA.

Carcinoid tumors vary widely in their capacity to store serotonin, with concentrations of the amine in tumors ranging from a few micrograms per gram to 3 mg per Gm. The concentration in the tumor appears unrelated to the rate of synthesis of serotonin as reflected by urinary 5HIAA. Generally, tumors from the ileum have a much higher storage capacity for serotonin than do tumors from organs of the embryonic foregut.

BRADYKININ. A potent vasodilator, bradykinin is released during flushes in some cases of carcinoid syndrome. In a few of these, excessive amounts continue to be released between flushes. Bradykinin and related kinins are formed by the action of a group of enzymes (kallikreins) which split these peptides from kininogen, a plasma globulin. It is thought that bradykinin formation in carcinoid syndrome results from release of a kallikrein from the tumor by catecholamines and possibly other stimuli. In the plasma, this kallikrein then acts on kininogen to form lysyl-bradykinin (a decapeptide), which is rapidly converted to bradykinin (a nonapeptide).

OTHER BIOLOGICALLY ACTIVE SUBSTANCES. Some carcinoid tumors, particularly those of gastric origin, produce and release excessive amounts of histamine. This can be detected by an increased excretion of this amine in the urine.

Carcinoid syndrome has been associated with hyperadrenocorticism in a number of instances. This results from ectopic production of an adrenocorticotropic hormone by the tumors which usually originate from sites other than the ileum (bronchus, pancreas, ovary, and stomach).

In a few cases, "multiple endocrine adenomas" have been seen in conjunction with carcinoids arising from organs of the embryonic foregut. The associated tumors have included parathyroid adenomas and pancreatic tumors producing Zollinger-Ellison syndrome.

Pathophysiology

Serotonin can account for those aspects of the syndrome related to intestinal hypermotility, and there is evidence that the fibrous deposits on the endocardium also result from increased levels of circulating serotonin.

A secondary effect of serotonin overproduction occurs when more than half of dietary tryptophan is shunted into the hydroxylation pathway (Fig. 105-2). This leaves less tryptophan available for the formation of nicotinic acid and protein; when urinary excretion of 5HIAA exceeds 200 to 300 mg daily, low levels of plasma tryptophan and evidence of nicotinamide deficiency are seen.

MECHANISM OF THE FLUSH. The mechanism of the flush is unclear. Release of the flush-provoking substance(s) can be triggered by the catecholamines, and this probably accounts for the association of flushing with excitement and emotional stimuli. For experimental induction of flushing, injection of isoproterenol in amounts as little as 0.5 μg may be effective. Serotonin was originally thought to be the mediator of flushes, but injection of this amine does not mimic the carcinoid flush and patients may exhibit flushes without increased levels of plasma serotonin. Bradykinin is a potent vasodilator, and its injection will simulate one type of carcinoid flush which is characterized by erythema in association with tachycardia and hypotension. Release of this peptide, however, could not be detected in a number of patients during flushing. While bradykinin, serotonin, and histamine may contribute to the varied types of flushes observed in the carcinoid syndrome, there appears to be an additional flush substance which has not yet been identified.

Diagnosis

With its full constellation of clinical features, carcinoid syndrome is easily recognized. The diagnosis also must be considered when any one of its features is present.

The diagnostic hallmark of carcinoid syndrome is *overproduction of 5-hydroxyindoles* with *increased urinary excretion of 5-hydroxyindoleacetic acid*. Normally, excretion of 5HIAA does not exceed 9 mg daily. Ingestion of foods containing serotonin may complicate the biochemical diagnosis of carcinoid syndrome; both walnuts and bananas contain enough serotonin to produce abnormally elevated urinary excretion of 5HIAA after their ingestion. Some drugs also interfere with the analysis of urinary 5HIAA; cough syrups containing guaicolate cause falsely elevated values, and phenothiazines interfere with the colorimetric test. When dietary 5-hydroxyindoles are excluded, a urinary excretion of more than 25 mg of 5HIAA daily is diagnostic of carcinoid. Elevations in the range of 9 to 25 mg can be seen with either carcinoid syndrome, nontropical sprue, or acute intestinal obstruction.

Measurement of *serotonin in blood* or platelets is of interest, but has less diagnostic value than assay of the major metabolite of serotonin in the urine.

Measurement of an increased concentration of *serotonin in tumor tissue* is a useful and sometimes necessary supplement to histologic examination. A portion of suspected tumor should always be frozen for serotonin analysis.

Variants of the Syndrome: Relations to Sites of Tumor Origin

The origin of the tumor influences the biologically active substances produced and their storage and release. Carcinoid tumors arising from organs derived from the embryonic foregut (bronchus, stomach, and pancreas) tend to differ from those arising distal to the midduodenum (midgut). The typical carcinoid syndrome usually results from tumors of midgut origin, which almost invariably secrete serotonin and rarely release 5-HTP. Tumor serotonin content is likely to be high, and the tumor usually contains dense nests of argentaffin positive cells. Metastasis to bone and skin is infrequent.

In contrast, tumors arising from the embryonic foregut contain fewer argentaffin cells, have lower serotonin content, and may secrete 5-HTP. Hyperadrenocorticism and multiple endocrine adenomas are more likely to be associated with this group, and metastasis to bone and skin is more frequent.

In addition to the general characteristics of the foregut group, certain clinical and biochemical features have been associated with gastric and bronchial carcinoids. Patients with gastric carcinoids frequently exhibit unique flushing which begins as a bright-red patchy erythema with sharply delineated serpentine borders; these patches tend to coalesce as the blush heightens. Food ingestion is especially prone to produce flushes. The tumors usually are deficient in decarboxylase enzyme and secrete 5-HTP; histamine secretion is also common as is a high incidence of peptic ulceration. Diarrhea and heart lesions are not prominent features in the patients who secrete largely 5-HTP from the tumor without much preformed serotonin.

When the carcinoid tumor arises from the bronchus, attacks of flushing tend to be prolonged and severe and may be associated with periorbital edema, excessive lacrimation and salivation, hypotension, tachycardia, anxiety, and tremulousness. Nausea, vomiting, explosive diarrhea, and bronchoconstriction may progress to a severe degree. This group is therapeutically unique in that the severe flushes often can be prevented by corticosteroids, and chlorpromazine may be helpful in relieving the symptomatology.

Treatment

Recognition of the carcinoid syndrome has led to the complete surgical cure of a few patients with tumors arising in ovarian or testicular teratomas or in the bronchus; by releasing their secretions directly into the systemic circulation, tumors from these locations can produce the syndrome before metastatic disease occurs. Because the humoral substances released by tumors draining into the portal circulation are largely metabolized by the liver, tumors arising in this location do not produce the syndrome until hepatic metastases occur. Resection of large isolated hepatic metastases has led to amelioration of symptoms in certain cases.

Pharmacologic therapy directed at the humoral mediators of the syndrome is of benefit in some cases. Methysergide, a serotonin antagonist, will improve the diarrhea, but prolonged therapy with this agent can produce retroperitoneal fibrosis. Blockade of serotonin synthesis with the tryptophan hydroxylase inhibitor *p*-chlorophenylalanine also ameliorates the diarrhea. Nicotinic acid should be given to those patients who shunt a large fraction of dietary tryptophan into the hydroxyindole pathway. The prevention of severe flushing by corticosteroids and amelioration of the syndrome by phenothiazines are limited largely to patients with tumors arising from the bronchus and other organs derived from the embryonic foregut.

Hypotensive episodes should not be treated with catecholamines; by stimulating the release of vasoactive substances from the tumor, norepinephrine and other agents with β adrenergic activity can exaggerate and prolong the circulatory disturbance. If pressor agents must be used, angiotensin or methoxamine are preferred.

Of the numerous approaches to chemotherapy of the

tumor, the most promising appears to be regional arterial perfusion with agents such as 5-fluorouracil.

REFERENCES

Oates, J. A., and T. C. Butler: Pharmacologic and Endocrine Aspects of Carcinoid Syndrome, Advances Pharmacol., 5:109, 1967.

Robertson, J. I. S., W. S. Pearl, and T. M. Andrews: The Mechanism of Facial Flushing in the Carcinoid Syndrome, Quart. J. Med., 31:103, 1962.

Sjoerdsma, A., H. Weissbach, and S. Undenfriend: A Clinical, Physiologic and Biochemical Study of Patients with Malignant Carcinoid, Am. J. Med., 20:520, 1956.

Thorson, Å., G. Biörck, G. Björkman, and J. Waldenström: Malignant Carcinoid of the Small Intestine with Metastases to the Liver, Valvular Disease of the Right Side of the Heart (Pulmonary Stenosis and Tricuspid Regurgitation without Septal Defects), Peripheral Vasomotor Symptoms, Bronchoconstriction and an Unusual Type of Cyanosis, Am. Heart J., 47:795, 1954.

106 GOUT AND OTHER DISORDERS OF URIC ACID METABOLISM

James B. Wyngaarden

Primary gout is an inborn metabolic disorder manifested by hyperuricemia, recurrent attacks of a characteristic acute arthritis, and tophaceous deposits of sodium urate. Nephrolithiasis and parenchymatous renal disease commonly develop during the course of the illness. Gout is not a single disease, but rather a syndrome resulting from different biochemical abnormalities which lead to hyperuricemia. Secondary gout is an acquired form of the disease which supervenes in the course of a number of disorders in which hyperuricemia occurs.

A classification of gout is presented in Table 106-1.

History

In the fifth century B.C., gout was described as podagra, cheiagra, or gonogra by Hippocrates, depending on whether the big toe, wrist, or knee was involved. Tophi were first described by Galen. The term *gout* is derived from the Latin *gutta*, a drop, and reflects an early belief that the disease was caused by a poison, falling drop by drop into the joint. A drug, probably identical with colchicine, was described in the Ebers Papyrus (1500 B.C.). The agent was known to Byzantine physicians in the fifth century A.D., and was brought to this country from Europe by Benjamin Franklin, who was himself a sufferer from gout. An astonishing list of men of royalty and genius have been afflicted with gout.

The modern clinical history of gout began with Thomas Sydenham, whose surpassing description of the disease (1683), based on 34 years of personal affliction, first clearly differentiated gout from other articular disorders. Uric acid was discovered in a kidney stone by Scheele in 1776. Twenty years later Wollaston and Pearson demonstrated urate in the tophi of patients with gout. Hyperuricemia was discovered by A. B. Garrod in 1848.

When the structure of uric acid was established by Emil Fischer in 1898, its relationship to the purine bases of nucleic acids was at once apparent. The pathways of enzymatic synthesis of purine compounds were elucidated by Buchanan, Greenberg, and others during the 1950s. The first specific enzymatic defect responsible for one subtype of adult primary gout was discovered by Seegmiller and associates in 1966.

Prevalence and Incidence

The prevalence of gout varies from about 0.3 percent in Europe and the United States to 8 percent in adult male Maori of New Zealand. During World Wars I and II acute gouty arthritis was uncommon in Europe. When protein again became plentiful, the incidence returned to prewar levels. Although traditionally considered a disease of middle and upper social classes, gout involves all nationalities and income groups.

Primarily gout is a disease of the adult male. In large series, only 3 to 7 percent of cases of primary gout are found in women, and these are chiefly in the postmenopausal group. Gout is very rare in prepubertal children and, when it occurs, may represent a specific form of gout associated with choreoathetosis, self-mutilation, and mental deficiency (Lesch-Nyhan syndrome), or with glycogen storage disease, type I (von Gierke's disease, Chap. 111).

Secondary gout comprises 5 to 10 percent of cases of gout, and, especially in those instances complicating myeloproliferative disorders or hypertensive cardiovascular disease may involve women in as many as 30 percent of cases.

Inheritance

The familial incidence of gout is generally reported as 6 to 18 percent in the United States, but may be much higher as reflected in figures ranging up to 75 percent in English series. The incidence of hyperuricemia among asymptomatic blood relatives of gouty subjects is about 25 percent. The genetic determinants of hyperuricemia are now thought to be multifactorial. Population studies have suggested that some are autosomal dominant and others are sex-linked dominant factors. The latter postulate is of particular interest, since it is now known that hypoxanthine-guanine phosphoribosyltransferase, an enzyme missing or defective in certain types of gout, is controlled by a gene on the X chromosome. The metabolic and genetic heterogeneity of gout underscores the need for definition of specific subtypes so that genetic patterns of transmission of each may be determined. In addition, it is known that serum urate values are positively correlated with surface area and obesity, and that environmental factors such as age, sex, diet, and drugs,

Table 106-1. CLASSIFICATION OF GOUT

Type	Metabolic Disturbance	Specific Defect	Inheritance
Primary gout:			
Adult primary gout:			
Normal excreter of uric acid (75–80% of primary gout)	Overproduction of uric acid Underexcretion of uric acid often both in same subject	Undefined	Polygenic ? Autosomal dominant forms
Overexcreter of uric acid (20–25% of primary gout)	Overproduction of uric acid	1. Hypoxanthine-guanine phosphoribosyltransferase: defective enzyme of low activity (rare)	X-linked
		2. Glutamine-PRPP amidotransferase: feedback resistance (rare)	Unknown
		3. Others undefined	Unknown
Childhood or juvenile gout:			
Associated with glycogen storage disease, type I (von Giercke's disease)	Overproduction of uric acid, plus underexcretion of uric acid; excessive deposition of glycogen and lipids; hypoglycemia	Glucose 6-phosphatase: deficiency or absence	Autosomal recessive
Associated with cerebral palsy, mental deficiency, and self mutilation. (Lesch-Nyhan syndrome)	Overproduction of uric acid	Hx-G phosphoribosyltransferase: deficiency or absence	X-linked
Secondary gout:			
Hematologic disorders:			
Myeloproliferative diseases; chronic hemolytic anemia	Excessive production of uric acid	Accelerated turnover of nucleic acids	
Chronic renal diseases			
Glomerulonephritis, pyelonephritis, polycystic kidney disease	Reduced excretion of uric acid	Reduced renal functional mass.	
Lead nephropathy	,, ,,		
Hypertensive cardiovascular disease	,, ,,	? Role of hyperlacticacidemia in suppression of tubular secretion of urate	
Hyperuricacidemogenic drugs	Reduced excretion of uric acid	? Suppression of tubular secretion of urate by drug or metabolite	
Starvation, especially in treatment of obesity	Reduced excretion of uric acid	Suppression of renal tubular secretion of urate by β-hydroxy butyric acid and other ketone bodies	

operate in conjunction with genetic factors in determining hyperuricemia.

Pathogenesis of Hyperuricemia

The concentration of uric acid in body fluids will be determined by the balance achieved between rates of production and rates of elimination of urate. Uric acid is formed by oxidation of purine bases, which are of both exogenous (dietary) and endogenous (biosynthetic) origins. The latter source is quantitatively the more important in man, except under unusual dietary circumstances. Normally, the body contains about 1200 mg uric acid and turns over about 700 mg per day. Two-thirds of this amount is excreted in the urine, whereas one-third enters the gastrointestinal tract in bile, gastric, and intestinal secretions, where it is destroyed by bacterial action. The accumulation of excessive quantities of urate in the gouty subject could theoretically result from increased dietary absorption of purines, endogenous overproduction, diminished renal or gastrointestinal excretion, or diminished endogenous destruction of urate, or a combination of these factors. Abnormalities of absorption or of intestinal uricolysis have been excluded, and endogenous uricolysis is not a significant process in human tissues because they lack uricase. In contrast, *abnormalities* of *endogenous purine production* and of *urate excretion* are important in the pathogenesis of hyperuricemia of both primary and secondary gout. The normal range of uric acid excretion in American males is about 250 to 600 mg per day on a low purine diet. About 20 or 25 percent of gouty subjects consistently excrete excessive amounts of uric acid and may be assumed to manufacture abnormally large quantities of purines. Tracer studies of the rate of turnover of the urate pool or of incorporation of labeled precursors, such as glycine, into urinary uric acid have confirmed this. Such studies have also indicated excessive purine production in one-half to two-thirds of gouty subjects who excrete normal amounts of urinary uric acid. However, a significant minority remains in whom present methods of study do not disclose excessive purine synthesis.

The structure of the purine ring and the metabolic precursors of individual atoms are shown in Fig. 106-1, and the major intermediates of nucleotide synthesis and uric acid production in Fig. 106-2. The key reaction in

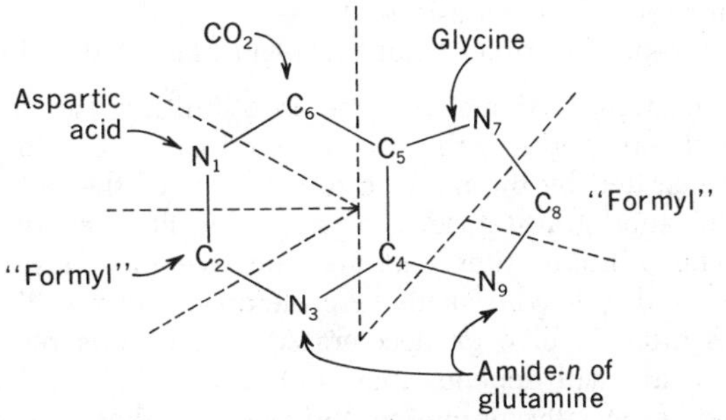

Fig. 106-1. Metabolic donors of atoms of the purine ring.

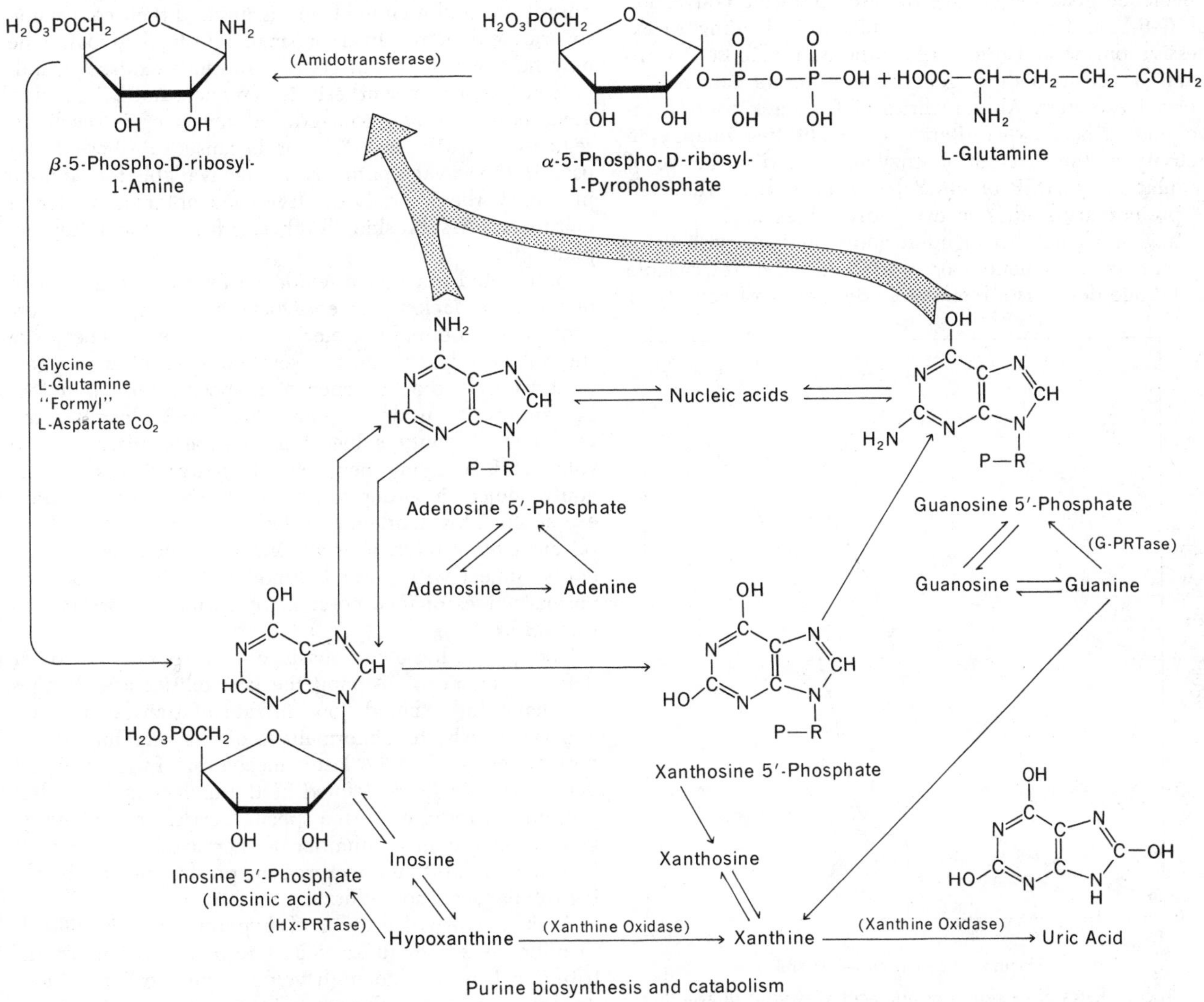

purine biosynthesis is the initial step in which L-glutamine and α-phosphoribosyl pyrophosphate interact irreversibly to form β-phosphoribosylamine, the first specific purine precursor.

Purine biosynthesis and catabolism

Fig. 106-2. Purine Biosynthesis and Catabolism. The first reaction of the pathway is under inhibitory control of adenosine and guanosine 5'-phosphates. Key enzymes are indicated in parentheses.

L-glutamine + α-PP-ribose-P + H₂O →

$$\text{L-glutamine} + \alpha\text{-PP-ribose-P} + \text{H}_2\text{O} \rightarrow$$
$$\beta\text{-phosphoribosylamine} + \text{L-glutamic acid} + \text{PP}$$

This reaction is thought to be rate-limiting for the entire pathway, and it is the site of a feedback regulatory process operated by the nucleotide products of the pathway. The amidotransferase catalyzing this first reaction has special inhibitor sites that are sensitive to levels of adenylic and guanylic acids. Accelerated purine biosynthesis must involve an accelerated rate of this reaction. The rate will depend upon (1) the availability of substrates, especially glutamine and phosphoribosylpyrophosphate, (2) the activity of the first enzyme, and integrity of its regulatory mechanisms and (3) the concentrations of regulatory nucleotides at the enzyme sites.

In gouty subjects, excessive incorporation of ^{15}N from glycine into N-3 and N-9 of urate has been observed, and has been interpreted as signifying an abnormality of glutamine metabolism in gout. In glucose-6-phosphatase deficiency glycogen storage disease, excessive conversion of G-6-P to PP-ribose-P is postulated as leading to excessive purine and uric acid synthesis. PP-ribose-P turnover is accelerated in gouty overexcreters but not in normal excreters. Abnormalities of feedback control, involving either a quantitative or qualitative change in activity of the first purine enzyme, or a disturbance of regulation of AMP or GMP levels have been detected in preliminary studies on two gouty subjects.

In a small number of adult gouty subjects with flamboyant overproduction of uric acid, the responsible metabolic defect is a remarkable deficiency of activity of the enzyme which catalyzes the reconversion of hypoxanthine and guanine to their respective ribonucleotide forms by condensation with phosphoribosylpyrophosphate.

$$\text{Hypoxanthine} + \text{PP-ribose-P} \rightarrow \text{Inosinic Acid} + \text{PP}$$
$$\text{Guanine} + \text{PP-ribose-P} \rightarrow \text{Guanylic Acid} + \text{PP}$$

Hypoxanthine-guanine phosphoribosyltransferase is the same enzyme in which activity is even more severely reduced or absent in children with the Lesch-Nyhan syndrome. In the adult gouty subject the enzyme is apparently structurally abnormal and retains only 2 to 10 percent of normal activity against hypoxanthine and guanine, but in different ratios in different patients. Other adult gouty subjects with equally accelerated rates of purine production and urate excretion (1,200 to 1,500 mg per day) have shown normal activity values of this enzyme, as assayed in erythrocytes. Deficiency of H-G-PRTase presumably allows the continuous escape of hypoxanthine and guanine from tissues and their conversion to uric acid in the liver or small intestinal mucosa, the only human tissues that contain xanthine oxidase. Simultaneously, purine synthesis is "compensatorily" accelerated, either because of reduced levels of intracellular regulators, AMP or GMP, or because PP-ribose-P not used in the salvage pathway is now available for de novo purine synthesis, or both. Evidence obtained in tissue culture studies of skin fibroblasts favors the latter explanation.

As pointed out above, evidence for overproduction of uric acid is lacking or equivocal in a substantial percentage of "normal-excreter" gouty subjects. These are the subjects whose urate excretion data often suggest most strongly the existence of a specific tubular defect in handling of urate in gout. Fig. 106-3 illustrates the tendency of gouty subjects to require a plasma urate value of 2 or 3 mg per 100 ml greater than the nongouty subject in order to achieve a given rate of urate excretion. This tendency is least evident in the flamboyant overexcreter, if at all, and most prominent in the gouty subject with normal turnover of the urate pool or normal values of incorporation of purine precursors into uric acid.

The pathophysiologic basis of this putative tubular defect is unknown. Among the possibilities are changes in renal tubular blood flow, in rate of transfer of urate into renal cells, or abnormalities of the secretory transport system itself. The latter mechanism for a transport defect has not been defined at the molecular level, but presumably requires both a specific carrier and an energy generating system. A number of chemical substances are known to inhibit urate excretion, presumably by blocking tubular secretion of urate.

A satisfactory definition of hyperuricemia is difficult to offer, as serum urate values form a continuous distribution from low to high values. Statistical definitions depend on the populations examined and methods employed. In the United States normal ranges (mean ± SD) in males are approximately 2.2 to 7.5 mg per 100 ml and in females, 2.1 to 6.6 mg per 100 ml. In epi-

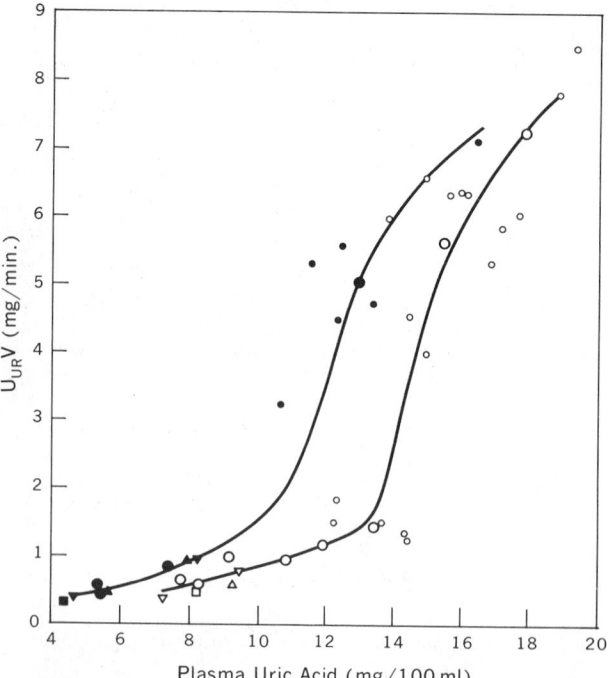

Fig. 106-3. Rates of excretion of uric acid at various plasma urate levels in control and gouty subjects. The urate levels have been raised in both groups by feeding of RNA or by infusion of lithium urate. The gouty group includes asymptomatic hyperuricemic, normal excreter, and overexcreter subjects.

demiologic surveys, values of 7.0 and 6.0 mg per 100 ml respectively are often used as discriminants. The physicochemical solubility of uric acid in body fluids is about 6.4 mg per 100 ml. Only a rare gouty subject will have serum urate values of less than 7 mg per 100 ml when reliable methods, such as the uricase differential spectrophotometric method, are employed.

Pathology

The pathognomonic lesion of gout is the *tophus*, a urate deposit surrounded by tissue exhibiting an inflammatory and foreign body reaction. Because urate crystals are water-soluble, nonaqueous fixatives are necessary to preserve urate deposits in histologic sections. Urate crystals are brilliantly anisotropic when viewed with polarized light under the microscope. In gout, urates tend to deposit in cartilage, epiphyseal bone, periarticular structures, and kidneys. The deposits produce local necrosis and (unless the tissue is avascular) an ensuing foreign body reaction with proliferation of fibrous tissue.

Tophi commonly occur in the helix or antihelix of the ear, the olecranon and patellar bursae, and tendons. Less commonly, they occur in skin of fingertips, palms, or soles, the tarsal plates of the eyelids, the nasal cartilages, in the cornea or sclerotic coats of the eye, or along nerves, causing compression syndromes. Rarely they develop in the myocardium, aortic or mitral valves, vocal cords, and arytenoid cartilages.

In the joint cartilaginous degeneration, synovial proliferation and pannus, destruction of subchondral bone, proliferation of marginal bone, and sometimes fibrous or bony ankylosis may develop. In vertebral bodies, urate deposits are found in marrow spaces adjacent to intervertebral disks, as well as in disk tissue itself. The punched-out lesions of bones commonly seen in roentgenograms of gouty patients represent marrow tophus deposits, which in most instances communicate with the urate crust on the articular surface through erosions and defects in articular cartilage (Fig. 106-4).

The only distinctive histologic feature of the *gouty kidney* is the presence of urate crystals in the medulla or pyramids and surrounding giant-cell reaction. These may be associated with pyelonephritic or vascular changes or both. The pyelonephritic changes are both acute and chronic; the vascular changes include arterial and arteriolar sclerosis.

The traditional view has been that the renal lesions stem from deposition of urates in collecting tubules with resultant obstruction, atrophy of the more proximal tubules, and secondary necrosis and fibrosis. The associated interstitial inflammatory process has been attributed to complicating pyelonephritis. More recent studies have shown that the earliest structural abnormality in the kidney is tubular damage associated with interstitial reaction. There is a distinctive glomerulosclerosis, with uniform fibrillar thickening of glomerular capillary basement membranes, different from that of nephrosclerosis or diabetic glomerulosclerosis. The Henle loops show early atrophy and dilatation, occasionally

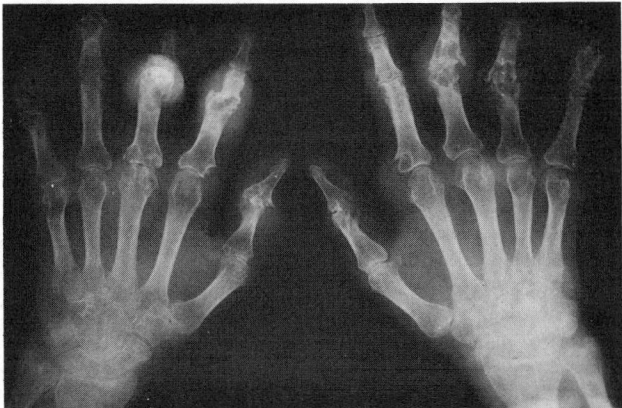

Fig. 106-4. Advanced chronic gouty arthritis of the hands, showing extensive destruction of bone by urate deposits and large asymmetrical soft-tissue tophi.

associated with brown pigment degeneration of epithelium. The interstitial reaction is maximal in the region near the changes in the Henle loops. In kidneys without tophi this reaction tends to spare the medulla and juxtamedullary cortex. The changes of chronic pyelonephritis may therefore not be of infectious origin. The vessels, both arteries and arterioles, show increased basophilia and degenerative changes which are out of proportion to the parenchymal changes.

Clinical Manifestations

The natural history of primary gout consists of three phases: asymptomatic hyperuricemia, acute gouty arthritis (which is characteristically recurrent with asymptomatic intervals), and chronic gouty arthritis.

ASYMPTOMATIC HYPERURICEMIA. This phase begins as an accentuation of the normal rise in serum uric acid value that occurs at puberty in the male and at the menopause in the female. Only a limited number of hyperuricemic subjects develops symptomatic gout, urolithiasis, or renal or vascular injury. The majority live their lifetimes with no detectable ill effects of this biochemical abnormality.

In the population study in Framingham, Mass., the cumulative incidence of gouty arthritis in men with serum uric acids of 7.0 mg per 100 ml or above was 2 percent at mean age thirty-four years and 23 percent at mean age fifty-eight years. The likelihood of developing gout increased with the degree of hyperuricemia. With levels of 10.0 mg per 100 ml or greater, the probability approached 50 percent. The peak age of onset of acute gout is about forty years, although first attacks have occurred in men eighty years or older.

ACUTE GOUTY ARTHRITIS. When gout finally becomes clinically manifest, it usually appears abruptly, as fulminating arthritis of a peripheral joint. It is difficult to improve on Sydenham's description of the acute attack:

The victim goes to bed and sleeps in good health. About two o'clock in the morning he is awakened by a severe pain in the great toe; more rarely in the heel, ankle or instep. This pain is like that of a dislocation, and yet the parts feel as if cold water were poured over them. Then follow chills and shivers, and a little fever. The pain, which was at first moderate, becomes more intense. With its intensity the chills and shivers increase. After a time this comes to its height, accommodating itself to the bones and ligaments of the tarsus and metatarsus. Now it is a violent stretching and tearing of the ligaments—now it is a gnawing pain and now a pressure and tightening. So exquisite and lively meanwhile is the feeling of the part affected, that it cannot bear the weight of the bedclothes nor the jar of a person walking in the room. The night is passed in torture, sleeplessness, turning of the part affected, and perpetual change of posture; the tossing about of the body being worse as the fit comes on. Hence the vain effort, by change of posture, both in the body and the limb affected, to obtain an abatement of the pain.

The initial attack usually subsides spontaneously in a few days to a few weeks, and recovery is generally complete. About 50 percent of initial attacks involve the great toe (podagra), and occasionally the initial attack is bilateral. Ninety percent of gouty patients experience podagra during the course of their disease. Next as sites of initial involvement are the instep, ankle, heel, knee, and wrist. Recurring bursitis of shoulder or elbow may be a manifestation of gout. Hench has emphasized that the more distal the site of involvement, the more typical is the character of the attack.

There are no characteristic changes of plasma uric acid levels that precede, accompany, or follow an acute attack of gouty arthritis. There may be an elevation of urinary uric acid excretion values during the acute attack, perhaps mediated by the uricosuric action of corticosteroids secreted during the stress of gouty inflammation. This sequence could explain the normal serum uric acid values occasionally observed during acute attacks. Garrod proposed in 1876 that the acute gouty paroxysm was triggered by precipitation of sodium urate crystals in the joint or neighboring tissues. In 1899, Freudweiler reproduced acute gouty attacks by injection of microcrystals of sodium urate, hypoxanthine, or xanthine. These observations have been confirmed by others with both purine and nonpurine microcrystals. A proposed pathogenetic mechanism involves crystallization of sodium urate from supersaturated body fluids, activation of Hageman factor by crystal surfaces, production of vasoactive kinin-like peptides in synovial fluid, induction of an inflammatory response involving leukotaxic factors,

leukocytosis, ingestion of microcrystals by leukocytes, enhanced production of lactate as a product of anaerobic glycolysis of leukocytes resulting in a drop of local pH and a tendency toward further crystal formation (Fig. 106-5).

The events leading to the initial crystallization of monosodium urate from the supersaturated fluid, after an average of 30 years of asymptomatic hyperuricemia, are poorly understood. Attacks may be precipitated by stress of many kinds, dietary, physical, and emotional. One patient may indict fatiguing travel, another unusual walking or hiking (e.g. "pheasant hunter's gout"), or celebrations such as holiday dinners or alcoholic sprees. Operative procedures are particularly prone to induce acute gout in hyperuricemic individuals, generally on the third to seventh postoperative day.

INTERVAL GOUT. The asymptomatic phase following the acute attack may last from a few weeks to many years. Generally in 6 months to 2 years the patient will suffer another episode in the same or another joint. With time, attacks tend to recur with increasing frequency. Later attacks are often polyarticular, more severe, longer, and accompanied by fever. Roentgenographic changes may develop, and the attacks may abate more gradually than before, but the joints may recover complete function.

CHRONIC GOUTY ARTHRITIS. Before effective control of hyperuricemia became possible, 50 to 60 percent of gouty patients developed visible tophi, permanent joint changes, or chronicity of symptoms. The incidence of tophi now ranges from 13 to 25 percent in various studies. Development of tophi is correlated with height of serum uric acid concentration, severity of renal involvement, and duration of the disease. The time from the initial attack to the beginning of chronic symptomatic or visible tophaceous involvement is usually many years, and ranged from 3 to 42 years in one large series, with an average of 11.6 years (Hench).

Chronic gouty arthritis is a consequence of the progressive inability, in some patients, to dispose of urate as rapidly as they produce it. The urate pool expands and crystalline deposits of urate appear in articular cartilage, synovial membranes, tendons, soft tissues, and elsewhere. In 1 or 2 percent of patients, tophi may be present at the time of the initial acute attack. At later stages, tophaceous enlargement of Achilles tendons, or saccular distensions of olecranon bursae are common and characteristic. Eventually the tophaceous deposits may produce irregular asymmetrical, moderately discrete tumescences over joints, requiring larger shoes or gloves. The classic gouty shoe is one with a window cut out to accommodate an irregularly prominant joint, usually the first metatarsophalangeal.

The process of tophaceous deposition advances slowly and insidiously, and although the tophi themselves are relatively painless, frequently there is progressive stiffness and persistent aching of affected joints. Eventually extensive destruction of joints and large subcutaneous tophi lead to progressive crippling, particularly of hands and feet, and to grotesque deformities (Fig. 106-4). The

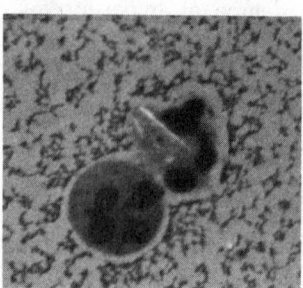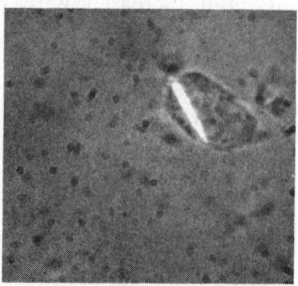

Fig. 106-5. Crystals of sodium urate monohydrate in leucocytes of synovial fluid in acute gouty arthritis, as viewed under partially polarized light. (*Courtesy, Dr. Daniel J. McCarty, Jr.*)

tense, shiny thin skin overlying the tophus may ulcerate and extrude white chalky or pasty material composed of myriads of fine, needlelike crystals.

Not uncommonly as chronic gouty changes advance, there is a tendency for acute attacks to occur less frequently; those that occur may be superimposed upon the indolent soreness of an involved joint, or may seek out new locations of previously uninvolved sites.

No joint is exempt from chronic gouty involvement, although those of the lower extremity and hand are most commonly involved. The hip and spinal joints are rarely involved in the absence of extensive tophaceous disease elsewhere.

UROLITHIASIS. The incidence of renal stone is about a thousandfold higher in gouty subjects than in the general population. Approximately 20 percent of gouty patients with normal urinary uric acid excretion values and 40 percent of those with elevated excretion values develop stones. Of those who pass stones about 20 percent have had their first episode of urolithiasis before the onset of gouty arthritis. The stones are composed of uric acid, not sodium urate, but in about 80 percent of instances they are mixed and contain in addition calcium phosphate, oxalate, or rarely, carbonate. Such stones are radiopaque, whereas pure uric acid stones are radiolucent. Some gouty subjects pass uric acid sludge, gravel, or sand, occasionally almost daily.

Several factors are at play in the pathogenesis of stones. In 20 to 25 percent of gouty patients, urinary uric acid excretion values are excessive. Also, as a group, gouty subjects tend to produce acid urines, and do not show normal postprandial alkaline tides. Renal ammonia production is subnormal in response to a given acid load. The deficit in ammonia is compensated by an increase in titratable acidity.

RENAL DISEASE IN GOUT. Many gouty subjects show evidence of renal disease. Also, 20 to 40 percent show albuminuria, which is rarely heavy in quantity and is often intermittent. Hypertension is frequent and is usually benign. Concentrating ability may be impaired. Mild degrees of nitrogen retention are common and often stable or only slowly progressive. Renal dysfunction does not shorten life expectancy in the average gouty subject, even though uremia is reported to be the eventual cause of death in 22 to 25 percent of gouty subjects. The majority of gouty patients die of cardiac or cerebral vascular disease, or malignancies, which occur in about the same incidence and at about the same time of life as in nongouty American males.

SECONDARY GOUT. Any acquired hyperuricemic state may be complicated by secondary gout. This disorder occurs in 5 to 9 percent of patients with polycythemia vera, especially those cases merging into the phase of myeloid metaplasia, occasionally in secondary polycythemia complicating congenital heart disease or chronic pulmonary disease, in chronic myelogenous leukemia, acute leukemia, multiple myeloma, or chronic hemolytic anemias. In such instances the mean age of onset is later, women are more commonly involved, and both serum and urinary uric acid values tend to be higher than in primary gout. Acute gouty arthritis may occasionally antedate evidence of the myeloproliferative disorder by many months.

In all the instances mentioned above, hyperuricemia appears to result from an increased turnover of nucleic acid. Hyperuricemia may also result from reduced renal excretion of urate, either because of chemical interference with tubular secretion of urate or because of reduced renal mass due to parenchymal disease.

Typical gouty attacks may occur in patients receiving such drugs as hydrochlorothiazide or pyrazinamide, which interfere with urate excretion. Extreme obesity may be associated with renal hyperuricemia. Total caloric restriction may result in extreme hyperuricemia, which is correlated with serum levels of β-hydroxybutyric acid and is not infrequently associated with severe attacks of acute gouty arthritis involving especially the knees and ankles. In patients with hyperlipoproteinemias there is a direct correlation between serum triglyceride and uric acid levels.

Chronic renal disease is a frequent cause of hyperuricemia, but apparently few patients with glomerulonephritis, pyelonephritis, or polycystic renal disease live long enough to develop gout. The number may increase with chronic dialysis programs, and acute gouty arthritis has complicated the course of patients so managed. Gout continues to be found in patients who survive lead exposure early in life and go on to develop the slowly progressive vascular nephritis of plumbism.

Hyperuricemia complicates benign essential and renal hypertension in 40 percent of cases, and malignant hypertension in 65 percent of cases and has been attributed provisionally to renal anoxia and local lactic acid excess. Gout occurs in 10 percent or more of patients previously subjected to sympathectomy of adrenalectomy for hypertension. In the absence of family data it may be difficult to distinguish between sporadic primary gout and gout secondary to hypertensive renal disease.

CHILDHOOD AND JUVENILE GOUT. Hyperuricemia is found in patients with glycogen storage disease due to glucose-6-phosphatase deficiency, and those children who survive the early hazards of hypoglycemia may be counted upon to develop severe tophaceous gouty arthritis. The hyperuricemia is of mixed origin: these children overproduce uric acid and also underexcrete it because of the persistent hyperlacticacidemia and triglyceridemia that characterize the disease. The condition is inherited as an autosomal recessive disorder.

Recently a new disease, characterized by cerebral palsy, choreoathetosis, self-mutilation, and mental deficiency associated with extreme hyperuricemia, uricosuria, and gout, has been described by Lesch and Nyhan. Milder variants of this syndrome have been recognized in which self-mutilation is absent, mental deficiency is mild, and the patient has been thought to have a cerebral palsy until gout supervenes. All reported patients are males, although some abnormalities of purine metabolism may be present in the mothers. The disease obeys the laws of X-linked transmission with full expression only in the hemizygous state. The purine abnormalities are attributable to the complete absence or severe deficiency of hypoxanthine-guanine phosphoribosyltransferase.

Diagnosis

Acute gouty arthritis is readily diagnosed by its typical explosive onset, the characteristic severity of involvement of the peripheral joint, the presence of hyperuricemia, and the rapid response to treatment with colchicine. Less typical presentations may be difficult to distinguish from other arthritides on clinical grounds. If present, tophi or typical roentgenologic findings of punched-out, destructive lesions will suggest the correct diagnosis. In patients lacking such lesions, the only pathognomonic finding is the presence in the leukocytes of the synovial fluid, of urate crystals which are needle-like and birefringent under polarized light (Fig. 106-5). Valuable clues in the diagnosis are a history of renal stones or of antecedent mild trauma or surgery in the patient or a history of gout, arthritis, or renal stones in the family.

Chronic gouty arthritis may be diagnosed by the presence of urate deposits in or near the affected joints or bursae or of soft-tissue deposits in the helix of the ear, the finger tips, the Achilles tendon, or other locations. The diagnosis may be confirmed by removal of the chalky contents of a tophus, microscopic identification of sodium urate crystals by optical means, or chemical identification by the murexide test or, preferably, by ultraviolet spectrophotometry and degradation by uricase.

Differential Diagnosis

Acute gout must be differentiated from acute rheumatic fever, rheumatoid arthritis, traumatic arthritis, osteoarthritis, pyogenic arthritis, sarcoid arthritis, cellulitis, bursitis, tendonitis, and thrombophlebitis. *Reiter's syndrome* in men and *palindromic arthritis* in women may present similar clinical manifestations of episodes of acute arthritis followed by periods of complete remission, but hyperuricemia will not generally be present, joint fluid will not contain urate crystals, and colchicine is ineffective. *Pseudogout*, which is chiefly a disorder of elderly persons and is manifested by acute attacks of arthritis of knees and other joints, is always accompanied by calcification of joint cartilage; and the synovial fluid contains nonurate crystals of calcium pyrophosphate or apatite. The patients are not usually hyperuricemic.

Chronic gouty arthritis must be differentiated from all other chronic arthritides which cause deformities of joints, chiefly rheumatoid arthritis, osteoarthritis, traumatic arthritis, and residua of pyogenic arthritis. The history of onset, of progression, of response to colchicine and demonstration of hyperuricemia, of asymmetrical tumescences, typical roentgenographic changes, of tophi or of crystals of urate in synovial fluid and leukocytes, should establish the diagnosis.

Treatment

The therapeutic aims in gout are (1) to terminate the acute gouty attack as promptly as possible; (2) to prevent recurrences of acute gouty arthritis; (3) to prevent or reverse complications of the disease resulting from deposition of sodium urate in joints and kidneys; and (4) to prevent formation of uric acid kidney stones. Treatment depends on the stage at which the patient is seen.

ACUTE ATTACK. Colchicine is the only treatment for acute gout of specific diagnostic value. It should be given as soon as the diagnosis is suspected. The initial dose of 0.5 to 1.2 mg colchicine is followed by 0.5 or 0.6 mg every hour for 8 hr, then every 2 hr until pain is relieved or until nausea, vomiting, cramping, or diarrhea develops. Maximum tolerated doses range from 4 to 10 mg. In most patients dramatic relief of pain and gastrointestinal side effects occur simultaneously. The diarrhea may be treated with paregoric, 4 cc, or kaopectate, 30 cc, after each loose stool. Colchicine should be discontinued until gastrointestinal symptoms subside. Since the effective dose of colchicine varies, each patient should learn his own tolerance dose and stop treatment just short of this in treatment of subsequent attacks. Colchicine usually affords relief within 24 to 48 hr; a second full therapeutic dose should not be repeated sooner than 72 hr.

Colchicine may also be given intravenously. The usual initial dose is 1 to 2 mg in 20 ml saline solution given slowly, and if a single dose is not effective, the injection may be repeated once in 4 to 5 hr (maximum intravenous dose, 3 to 4 mg). Gastrointestinal symptoms are uncommon with intravenous administration.

Phenylbutazone is also effective in acute gouty arthritis, and may be preferred when the gouty attack has proceeded for some time, or when the attack does not abate completely with colchicine. The initial dose is 400 mg orally, followed by 100 mg every 4 to 8 hr for 2 to 3 days. Oxyphenbutazone, a metabolite of phenylbutazone, is also effective in acute gout. The dose is the same as that of phenylbutazone, and the same precautions should be taken.

Patients who recognize prodromal symptoms may abort acute attacks by prompt institution of colchicine or phenylbutazone therapy and frequently require only a few tablets to achieve success.

Indomethacin is sometimes dramatically effective in acute gout. It is given orally in doses of 100 to 150 mg every 6 hours. Larger doses may cause severe headache and a transient depersonalization reaction.

If full doses of colchicine or phenylbutazone are contraindicated, or ineffective, ACTH gel may be employed. Doses of 40 to 80 USP units are given intramuscularly every 6 to 8 hr for 2 to 3 days, rarely longer, following which the doses are reduced in stepwise fashion and discontinued. To avoid rebound attacks of gout after ACTH therapy, 0.6 mg colchicine should be given two or three times daily during and after administration of ACTH for at least 7 days.

Hydrocortisone in a dose of 25 to 50 mg injected intra-articularly into the involved joint is useful in treating acute gout limited to a single joint or bursa, and relief from pain is usually prompt and complete within 24 to 36 hr. Steroid hormones are not recommended for parenteral use in acute gout, as the effects are inconsistent and rebound attacks frequent.

During the acute attack, bearing weight on the involved joints should be avoided. In severe attacks the patient will invariably immobilize himself voluntarily, but in milder attacks it is necessary for the physician to insist on this. Mobilization is permitted as soon as the joint is no longer painful.

INTERVAL PHASE. The patient with gout should avoid high purine foods so as to lessen the burden of uric acid excretion. A severe limitation of purine-containing foods is rarely indicated, unless renal function and the ability to excrete urate are reduced significantly. Many gouty patients are overweight, and gradual weight reduction is indicated. Sudden weight reduction may precipitate gouty attacks and should be avoided. In general, diets of moderate protein content, somewhat low in fat, are preferred.

A high fluid intake is advisable to maintain a urinary output of 2,000 ml per day. Urate excretion is thus promoted, and the dangers of crystal formation in the kidney or ureter are reduced. Alcoholic beverages, especially beer, ale, and wine, should be avoided if possible, as they may precipitate attacks. Distilled alcoholic beverages, in moderation, generally have little influence on the gouty process.

The daily ingestion of 0.6 to 1.8 mg colchicine is generally effective in reducing the number of acute gouty attacks in patients who are subject to frequent episodes. Maintenance colchicine therapy is particularly important during the first year or two after institution of uricosuric drugs.

CHRONIC GOUTY ARTHRITIS. Use of a drug to lower the serum level of uric acid to 6 mg per 100 ml or less is indicated in all gouty patients with visible tophi, with roentgenographic evidence of urate deposits, with serum uric acid levels above 8.5 mg per 100 ml, or with a history of four or more major attacks of acute gouty arthritis per year. The drug of choice is allopurinol, but uricosuric agents may be used. None of these agents is of any value in the immediate treatment of the acute attack. With both types the number of acute gouty attacks may be increased during the first 6 months unless maintenance colchicine therapy is given, whereas after 12 to 18 months the number may be decidedly reduced. Uricosuric drugs block tubular reabsorption of filtered urate. Those of use in gout are probenecid, sulfinpyrazone, and salicylates.

Probenecid is given in doses of 0.5 to 3 Gm daily in two or three evenly spaced doses (average dose, 1 to 1.5 Gm). This drug may produce gastrointestinal upsets, headaches, or skin rash.

Sulfinpyrazone may be given in doses of 100 to 600 mg daily in three or four divided doses (average dose, 300 mg). This drug is related to phenylbutazone and can cause untoward reactions, but is generally somewhat better tolerated than probenecid.

Salicylates block the uricosuric action of both probenecid and sulfinpyrazone and must not be used concurrently. Salicylates are uricosuric when given in high doses (4 to 6 Gm daily), but few patients can tolerate these quantities.

With all uricosuric agents the doses should be low initially, so as to avoid sudden mobilization of large quantities of urate. Fluids should be forced so as to prevent formation of concentrated urine, especially during the late hours of the night. During the first days or weeks of therapy the urine should be alkalinized; this may be difficult to achieve, as gouty patients tend to produce acid urine. In patients who are mobilizing urate, and especially those who form urate gravel, alkalinization during the night, when fluid intake is reduced, is important. A single 250 mg tablet of acetazolamide (Diamox) taken at bedtime will serve to keep the urine alkaline and dilute throughout the night.

A second approach toward controlling serum urate levels is that of regulating production of uric acid, rather than (or in addition to) augmenting its excretion. Allopurinol is a potent inhibitor of xanthine oxidase, which prevents the conversion of hypoxanthine and xanthine to uric acid and permits these uric acid precursors to be excreted instead. Its use results in reduction of levels of uric acid in serum *and in urine*. The drug is effective even in the presence of renal failure, when uricosuric agents are generally ineffective. Its action is not blocked by salicylates. The usual dose is 100 mg, given orally three or four times a day. It is usually well tolerated, but rarely may cause gastric irritation, diarrhea, or skin rash, or induce an attack of gout. Uricosuric agents may be used concurrently to hasten mobilization of urate deposits. Since allopurinol decreases uric acid excretion, it is also very useful in controlling uric acid stone formation, especially in patients who are overproducers of uric acid, but also in nongouty subjects.

In selected patients surgical removal of large extra-articular urate deposits, such as those in olecranon bursae, may be advisable. Occasionally amputation of irreparably damaged digits, especially those containing draining sinuses, is indicated. Physical therapy and appropriate self-help devices are indicated in patients who are partially disabled.

ASYMPTOMATIC HYPERURICEMIA. Asymptomatic hyperuricemia is frequently encountered in family members of patients with gout and in the general population. One must exclude hyperuricemia as a manifestation of reduced renal function or of action of certain drugs. Asymptomatic hyperuricemia generally requires no therapy, as only about one-third of patients will ever develop articular attacks, and adequate therapy can be instituted when these supervene. However, exceptions do exist, as in patients with serum levels of uric acid above 8.5 or 9 mg per 100 ml, especially if the urinary excretion levels are low and there is a family history of tophaceous involvement. In such circumstances the asymptomatic subject should be treated with allopurinol before articular or renal complications develop. It is essential that frequent close observation of the patient by the physician be maintained.

SECONDARY GOUT. Treatment of gouty arthritis occurring secondary to hematopoietic disturbances is the same as for primary gout except that one must be especially alert to potential renal and ureteral complications. The basal uric acid excretion may be high, and use of uricosuric agents may intensify the risk of urate crystalluria and of tubular or ureteral blockade. High fluid intake and alkalinization become of great importance. The drug of choice for control of hyperuricemia is allopurinol.

REFERENCES

Gonick, H. C., M. E. Rubini, I. O. Gleason, and S. C. Sommers: The Renal Lesion in Gout, Ann. Intern. Med., 62: 667, 1965.

McCarty, D. J., Jr.: Crystal-induced Inflammation; Syndromes of Gout and Pseudogout, Geriatrics, 18:467, 1963.

Rosenbloom, F. M., J. F. Henderson, I. C. Caldwell, W. N. Kelley, and J. E. Seegmiller: Biochemical Bases of Accelerated Purine Biosynthesis *de novo* in Human Fibroblasts Lacking Hypoxanthine-Guanine Phosphoribosyltransferase, J. Biol. Chem., 243:1166, 1968.

Rundles, R. W., H. R. Silberman, G. H. Hitchings, and G. B. Elion: Effects of Xanthine Oxidase Inhibitor on Clinical Manifestations and Purine Metabolism in Gout, Ann. Intern. Med., 60:717, 1964.

Seegmiller, J. E., F. M. Rosenbloom, and W. N. Kelley: An Enzyme Defect Associated with an X-linked Human Neurological Disorder and Excessive Purine Synthesis, Science, 155:1682, 1967.

Wyngaarden, J. B.: Gout, in "The Metabolic Basis of Inherited Disease," 2d ed., J. B. Stanbury, J. B. Wyngaarden, and D. S. Fredrickson (Eds.), New York, McGraw-Hill Book Company, 1966.

——, R. W. Rundles, and E. N. Metz: Allopurinol in the Treatment of Gout, Ann. Intern. Med., 62:842, 1965.

Yu, T. F., and A. B. Gutman: Uric Acid Nephrolithiasis in Gout. Predisposing Factors, Ann. Intern. Med., 67:1133, 1967.

107 HEMOCHROMATOSIS
George E. Cartwright

Definition

Idiopathic hemochromatosis (bronze diabetes, pigment cirrhosis) is characterized pathologically by excessive deposits of iron in the body and clinically by hepatomegaly with eventual liver insufficiency, pigmentation of the skin, diabetes mellitus, and frequently cardiac failure.

History

The first clinical description of the disease was given by Trousseau in 1865. In 1889 von Recklinghausen named the disease *hemochromatosis* and described the iron-containing pigment, hemosiderin. Sheldon, in a now classic monograph, reviewed the world's literature in 1935. Finch and Finch in 1955 reviewed the literature since 1935 and added 80 cases of their own. More recently, MacDonald has made important contributions by emphasizing the role of excessive dietary iron and preexisting portal cirrhosis in the pathogenesis of acquired hemochromatosis.

Incidence

Hemochromatosis is a rare disease, recognized in approximately 1 in 20,000 hospital admissions, and 1 in 7,000 hospital deaths. It is observed ten times as frequently in males as in females. Nearly 70 percent of all patients with this disease develop their first symptoms between the ages of forty and sixty years. Hemochromatosis is rarely recognized below the age of twenty years.

Pathogenesis

One of the earliest measurable alterations in iron metabolism in hemochromatosis is the elevation of the plasma iron and saturation of the plasma iron-binding protein, transferrin. As the disease progresses, the amount of storage iron increases. In advanced disease, the tissues contain over 20 Gm of iron; total body iron in normal persons is in the range of 3 to 5 Gm. The excess iron is deposited primarily in parenchymal cells in the form of ferritin and hemosiderin. Increased amounts of iron are found in almost all body tissues, especially those in which there is organ dysfunction. Iron in the liver and pancreas is increased fifty to one hundred times; in the heart, ten to fifteen times; in the spleen, kidney, and skin, about five times.

Since iron is not excreted from the body in appreciable amounts even in normal persons, the conclusion that iron absorption is increased in idiopathic hemochromatosis is inescapable. There are two quite differing explanations as to why this occurs. The classical concept is that idiopathic hemochromatosis is due to an inherited inborn error in metabolism in which the basic abnormality is the increased absorption of iron. According to this view the excessive deposition of iron is the cause of the tissue damage. The other point of view is that hemochromatosis is a variant of portal cirrhosis of the liver. A high incidence (30 to 85 percent) of alcoholism has been observed in patients with idiopathic hemochromatosis, and it has been noted that the iron content of alcoholic beverages, particularly various wines, is high.

Hemochromatosis has been observed (1) as a familial occurrence without apparent cause other than an inherited inborn error of metabolism; (2) in alcoholic subjects with a high dietary intake of iron; (3) in malnourished

Bantu subjects in South Africa secondary to long-term iron overload ("Bantu siderosis"); (4) in isolated instances of parenchymal iron overload following intake of medicinal doses of iron over many years; (5) in association with various types of refractory anemia; and (6) in a few patients given 100 or more transfusions of blood. Therefore, it would seem that hemochromatosis is a syndrome with several possible causes. The common denominator in all cases is the presence of excessive iron in parenchymal tissues.

Pathology

At autopsy the enlarged, nodular liver and pancreas present a striking ochre color. Histologically, hemosiderin is deposited in many organs, particularly the liver and pancreas. The liver shows considerable fibrosis. Testicular atrophy is frequently present, both grossly and histologically. There are hemosiderin deposits in the myocardium, and they may be associated with myocardial edema, fibrosis, and necrosis. The epidermis of the skin is thin, and melanin pigment is found in the cells of the basal layer. Hemosiderin is deposited almost entirely in the corium.

Clinical Manifestations

The symptoms and signs of hemochromatosis are related to the *skin pigmentation, diabetes, liver impairment, and cardiac disease*. Of these the cirrhosis of the liver is the most constant abnormality.

The initial symptoms most frequently encountered are related to the onset of *diabetes*. Weakness, lassitude, weight loss, change in skin color, abdominal pain, dyspnea, edema, ascites, loss of libido, and peripheral neuritis are also frequent initial symptoms. Hepatomegaly, pigmentation, spider angiomas, splenomegaly, ascites, evidences of congestive failure or cardiac arrhythmias, loss of body hair, testicular atrophy, jaundice, and hypertension are the most prominent physical signs, given in decreasing order of frequency.

The liver is the first tissue known to be damaged, and hepatomegaly is present in about 93 percent of symptomatic cases. Hepatic enlargement may exist in the absence of symptoms or in the presence of normal liver function tests. Indeed, over half the patients with symptomatic hemochromatosis have little or no laboratory evidence of functional impairment of the liver in spite of hepatomegaly and proved fibrosis. Loss of body hair, palmar erythema, testicular atrophy, gynecomastia, spider angioma, and, particularly, loss of libido are often seen and are related to the severity of the liver damage. Manifestations of portal hypertension and esophageal varices may occur but are less commonly observed than in Laennec's cirrhosis. A nontender, slightly enlarged spleen is present in approximately half the cases. Primary carcinoma of the liver develops in about 14 percent. The incidence of this last complication increases greatly with age.

Excessive *skin pigmentation* is present in about 90 percent of the patients at the time the diagnosis is established. Pigmentation may be due to deposition of melanin or iron or both. In general, melanin deposition gives rise to bronzing, iron deposition to a metallic gray hue. Pigmentation usually is diffuse and generalized, but frequently it is deeper on the face, neck, extensor aspects of the lower forearms, dorsae of the hands, lower legs, genital regions, and in scars. In only 10 to 15 percent of cases is there demonstrable pigmentation of the oral mucosa.

About 82 percent of all patients develop *diabetes mellitus* and symptoms therefrom. The diabetes may appear rapidly, and insulin requirements may increase rapidly. About 72 percent of the patients require insulin for the control of the diabetes. In some instances severe insulin resistance develops, in others there may be sensitivity to insulin. In most instances, the diabetes is controlled with little difficulty. Since the diabetes is usually present for less than a decade, the late degenerative sequelae of this complication are not prominent.

Approximately one-third of patients with idiopathic hemochromatosis die of *cardiac failure*. The heart disease is extremely common in young adults, and symptoms may develop suddenly, with rapid progression to death. The most important manifestations of heart disease are congestive failure and cardiac arrhythmias, particularly ventricular extrasystoles and paroxysmal atrial tachycardia. Other arrhythmias may occur as well.

Diagnosis

The classical *triad of skin pigmentation, diabetes mellitus, and hepatomegaly*, especially in the presence of heart disease and evidence of hypogonadism, should always suggest the diagnosis. Confirmation of the presence of liver, pancreatic, heart, and gonadal disease should then be obtained by customary tests of the functions of these organs. It then remains to demonstrate that there is excessive storage iron.

The diagnosis is enhanced considerably if the plasma iron level is found to be elevated (above 150 μg per 100 ml) and the iron-binding protein of the plasma is 75 to 100 percent saturated. However, the only definitive test is liver biopsy. Other procedures which indicate an excess of body iron stores are bone marrow aspiration for hemosiderin, examination of the urine sediment for hemosiderin, skin biopsy, and gastric mucosal biopsy.

Finch and Finch state that there are no unique features in idiopathic hemochromatosis by which it may be distinguished pathologically from the terminal stage of other iron-storage diseases, such as dietary or transfusion hemochromatosis. They define *hemosiderosis* as a focal increase in tissue iron or a general increase in iron stores without associated tissue damage, and *hemochromatosis* as a general increase in body iron stores with resultant tissue damage. From these definitions, the differentiation of hemosiderosis from hemochromatosis can be easily made by the presence or absence of organ dysfunction. Dietary and transfusion hemochromatosis can be differentiated from idiopathic hemochromatosis on the basis of a history of excessive iron intake by mouth, by injection, or intravenously in the form of blood. In evaluating dietary iron exposure, the dietary iron content, type of diet, type of cooking utensils, intake of medicinal iron, and iron content of the drinking water or other beverages must be considered.

Prognosis

The life expectancy of patients after signs of clinical hemochromatosis have become manifest averages 4.4 years, but several instances have been recorded of patients living up to 20 or 30 years after manifestation of signs. The average duration of life after diabetes has developed is 3 years. The principal causes of death are cardiac failure (30 percent), hepatic coma (15 percent), hematemesis (14 percent), hepatoma (14 percent), and pneumonia (12 percent). The most recent advance in the therapy of this disease, the introduction of methods for the removal of iron, is expected to increase life expectancy further.

Treatment

The therapy of idiopathic hemochromatosis involves removal of the excess body iron by phlebotomy and supportive treatment of damaged organs. The management of the hepatic failure, cardiac failure, and diabetes differs little from the conventional management of these conditions. Loss of libido and change in secondary sex characteristics are relieved by testosterone therapy. Iron is best removed from the body by a weekly or twice weekly phlebotomy of 500 ml. Since the average amount of iron in a patient with hemochromatosis is approximately 25 Gm, about 2 years of weekly bleeding will be required to deplete the iron stores. Chelating agents such as EDTA and desferrioxamine are of little or no practical value in the management of hemochromatosis.

REFERENCES

Bothwell, T. H., and C. A. Finch: "Iron Metabolism," Boston, Little, Brown and Company, 1962.

Charlton, R. W., and T. H. Bothwell: Hemochromatosis: Dietary and Genetic Aspects, in E. B. Brown and C. V. Moore (Eds.), "Progress in Hematology," vol. 5, p. 298, New York, Grune and Stratton, Inc., 1966.

Finch, S. C., and C. A. Finch: Idiopathic Hemochromatosis: An Iron Storage Disease, Medicine, 34:381, 1955.

MacDonald, R. A.: "Hemochromatosis and Hemosiderosis," Springfield, Ill., Charles C Thomas, Publisher, 1964.

———: Primary Hemochromatosis: Inherited or Acquired?, in E. B. Brown and C. V. Moore (Eds.), "Progress in Hematology," vol. 5, p. 324, New York, Grune and Stratton, Inc., 1966.

Sheldon, J. H.: "Hemochromatosis," Fairlawn, N. J., Oxford University Press, 1935.

108 DISORDERS OF PORPHYRIN METABOLISM

George E. Cartwright

DEFINITIONS

Porphyrins are pigments that possess a basic structure of four pyrrole rings linked by methene ($=CH—$) bridges (Fig. 108-1). The individual porphyrins differ from each other according to the nature of the eight possible side chains. Each porphyrin has a number of stereoisomers. *Porphyrinogens* are colorless compounds (reduced porphyrins) with a basic structure of four pyrrole rings linked by methane ($—CH_2—$) bridges.

Porphyrin pigments are widely distributed throughout the plant and animal worlds in chlorophyll, hemoglobin, catalase, and a number of cytochrome and peroxidase enzymes.

The term *porphyrinuria* refers to excessive excretion of porphyrins in the urine. *Coproporphyrinuria*, the excretion of increased amounts of coproporphyrin, is not uncommon and occurs in a variety of conditions. The term *porphyria* embraces a group of diseases, each with unusual and characteristic manifestations, which have in common the excessive excretion of one or more of the porphyrins, porphyrinogens, and/or porphyrin precursors (Δ-aminolevulinic acid and porphobilinogen) in the urine and/or feces.

HISTORY

Congenital porphyria was first described by Günther in 1911. Much of the knowledge of the chemistry of the porphyrins came from Hans Fischer and his school in Munich. In 1915, these workers described, named, and isolated in crystalline form the uroporphyrins and coproporphyrins from the urine of the patient in their famous case of congenital porphyria (Petry). Shemin and Granick and their groups in New York have made substantial contributions to knowledge of the biosynthesis of the porphyrins. Contributions to the understanding of the types and manifestations of porphyria have come from Waldenström in Sweden, Rimington in England, Barnes and Dean in South Africa, and Watson, Schwartz, and Schmid in the United States.

BIOSYNTHESIS

The rather complex porphyrin molecule is synthesized in the body from two simple precursors, acetate and glycine (Fig. 108-2). Acetate enters the Krebs tricarboxylic acid cycle (Chap. 75) and is converted into succinate. Succinyl CoA (active succinate) is then formed in the presence of Mg^{++} ion, adenosine triphosphate (ATP), and coenzyme A (CoA). The activated form of succinate condenses with a pyridoxal phosphate-glycine enzyme (glycine-PE) to form the 5-carbon compound, Δ-aminolevulinic acid (Δ-ALA), and carbon dioxide by the decarboxylation of glycine. This step is enzymatically controlled (ALA synthetase), and several intermediate compounds have been suggested. Two molecules of Δ-aminolevulinic acid, in the presence of glutathisone (GSH) and an enzyme, Δ-aminolevulinic acid dehydrase (Δ-ALA DH), condense to form a substituted monopyrrole, porphobilinogen, which contains acetic acid (A) and propionic acid (P) side chains. In the next step in heme synthesis, four molecules of porphobilinogen condense to form the reduced tetrapyrrolic structure, uroporphyrinogen. This step is catalyzed by at least two enzymes, porphobilinogen deaminase (PD) and uroporphyrinogen isomerase (UI). Details of the action of these enzymes and the sequence of reactions leading from porphobilinogen to uroporphyrinogen types I and III are not known. Uroporphyrin III is not in the direct pathway of heme synthesis, as was formerly assumed, but is a by-product. Uroporphyrinogen III (reduced uroporphyrin) is converted to coproporphyrinogen by the enzyme, uroporphyrinogen decarboxylase (UD). Coproporphyrinogen III is then converted to protoporphyrin III in the presence of the enzyme coproporphyrinogen oxidase. Coproporphyrin III is a by-product, whereas the available evidence suggests that protoporphyrin III is in the direct pathway of heme synthesis. Protoporphyrin III is converted to hemoglobin in the presence of iron, glutathione, globin, and the enzyme heme synthetase (HS). The intermediate steps between protoporphyrin and hemoglobin have not been identified. It is not known whether heme or a porphyrin-globin compound is an intermediate in this reaction, although the former possibility seems more likely.

METABOLISM

The most important of the naturally occurring porphyrins are uroporphyrin (isomer types I and III), coproporphyrin (types I and III), and protoporphyrin (type III).

Protoporphyrin III is present in hemoglobin and is, therefore, the most important of the porphyrins from the physiologic standpoint. It is absent from urine. The concentration of fecal protoporphyrin is related to the amount of blood in the gastrointestinal tract, the rate of liberation of protoporphyrin from hemoglobin by fecal bacteria, and the excretion of protoporphyrin by the liver.

Coproporphyrin is the predominant porphyrin in urine and feces under normal circumstances. Coproporphyrinuria occurs in a variety of clinical conditions, such as lead poisoning, poliomyelitis, liver disease, acute alcoholism, hemolytic anemia, and Hodgkin's disease. In all these disorders the increased coproporphyrinuria accompanies the underlying disease, and it is unlikely that the abnormality in porphyrin metabolism contributes significantly to the clinical picture. Coproporphyrinuria is also found in patients with certain types of porphyria. Abnormally high fecal coproporphyrin values are found in patients with hemolytic anemia, and low values occur in patients with liver disease.

Uroporphyrin is normally excreted in urine in only

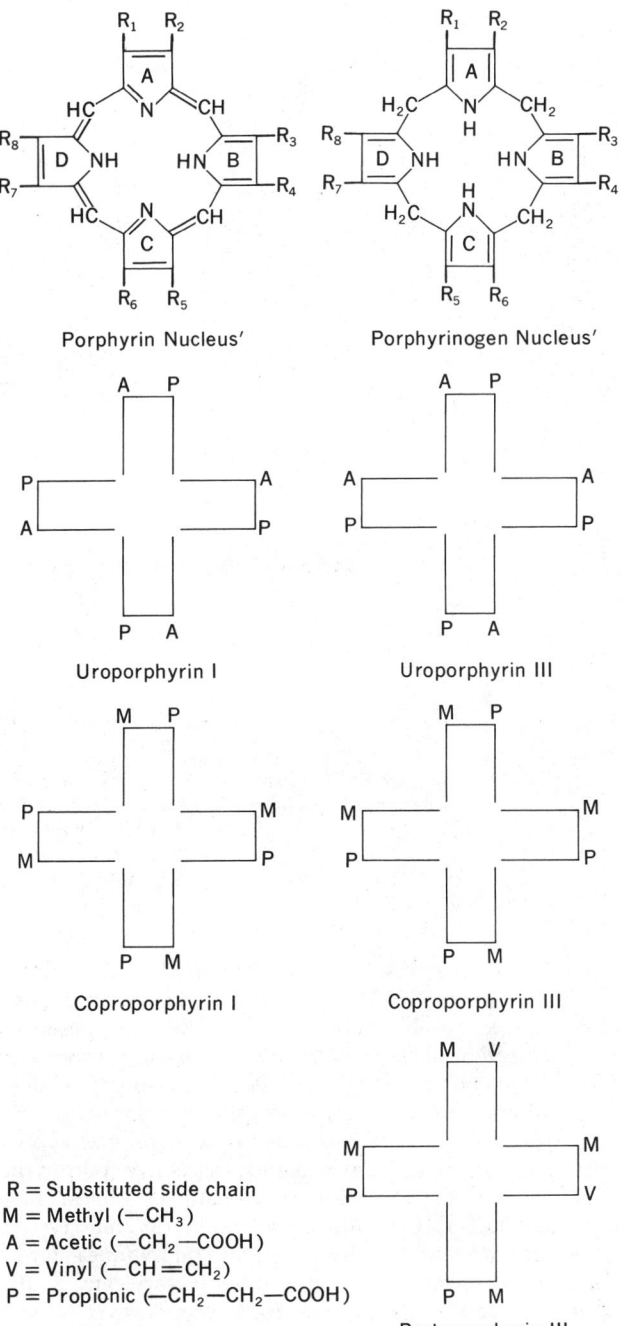

R = Substituted side chain
M = Methyl (—CH$_3$)
A = Acetic (—CH$_2$—COOH)
V = Vinyl (—CH=CH$_2$)
P = Propionic (—CH$_2$—CH$_2$—COOH)

Fig. 108-1. The structural formulas of the porphyrin and porphyrinogen nuclei and diagrammatic formulas of the important naturally occurring porphyrins.

trace amounts. The urinary excretion of this porphyrin is moderately increased in lead poisoning and is greatly increased in patients with certain types of porphyria.

PORPHYRIA

Porphyria may be divided into two general groups (Table 108-1). In erythropoietic porphyria, excessive

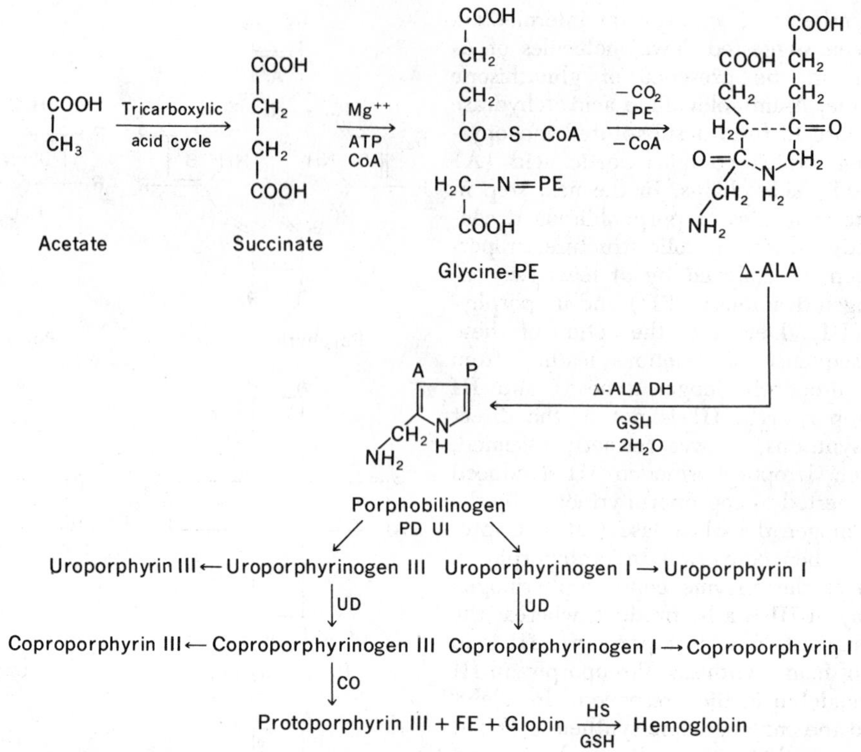

Fig. 108-2. The biosynthesis of the porphyrins from acetate and glycine and the biosynthetic pathway of hemoglobin. CoA, coenzyme A; ATP, adenosine triphosphate; PE, pyridoxal phosphate enzyme (ALA synthetase); Δ-ALA, delta-aminolevulinic acid; Δ-ALA DH, delta-aminolevulinic acid dehydrase; GSH, glutathione; PD, porphobilinogen deaminase; UI, uroporphyrinogen isomerase; UD, uroporphyrinogen decarboxylase; CO, coproporphyrinogen oxidase; HS, heme synthetase; A, acetic; P, propionic.

quantities of porphyrins accumulate in the normoblasts and erythrocytes. Under these circumstances, red fluorescence may be observed when the cells are exposed to ultraviolet light. The predominant porphyrin synthesized in erythropoietic uroporphyria (congenital porphyria) is uroporphyrin; in erythropoietic protoporphyria, protoporphyrin; and in erythropoietic coproporphyria, coproporphyrin. In porphyria hepatica, excessive porphyrin production occurs in the liver. Hepatic porphyria may be subdivided further into at least four different types: acute intermittent porphyria, porphyria cutanea tarda hereditaria (mixed porphyria, porphyria variegata, South African Caucasian porphyria, protocoproporphyria), porphyria cutanea tarda symptomatica, and hereditary coproporphyria. Not all patients with hepatic porphyria can be so classified and there is some degree of overlapping. It is quite possible that more than a single entity is included in each subtype of hepatic porphyria.

PORPHYRIA ERYTHROPOIETICA
Erythropoietic Uroporphyria

This is a very rare disorder, inherited probably as a recessive mendelian characteristic. The clinical manifestations occur very early in life, sometimes even a few days after birth, but often they are not observed until after an interval of a year of two. *The disease is characterized by the excessive deposition of porphyrin in the tissues, leading to pronounced photosensitization.* The early lesions of photodynamic origin are the blisters of hydroa estivale (hydroa vacciniforme) on skin surfaces exposed to light, especially of the face and hands. In time, scarring and mutilation occur. After years of continued photosensitivity, the mutilation becomes extensive, with loss of fingers, portions of the nose, ears, scarring of the cheeks and about the mouth, ectropion, or symblepharon. Skin not exposed to light remains unaffected. Hemolytic anemia and splenomegaly are an integral part of the disease. Erythrodontia may be observed in those cases in which sufficient porphyrin has been deposited in the teeth to make them grossly red or reddish brown. Teeth which do not show erythrodontia in ordinary light may exhibit red fluorescence in Wood's light. Red fluorescence may be seen in the phalangeal bones if a strong source of ultraviolet light is allowed to shine through the fingers. There is no marked disturbance of the nervous system, nor is there abdominal colic.

Because of the demonstration of large quantities of *uroporphyrin* and *coproporphyrin* in the normoblasts in the bone marrow, it has been suggested that in this type

Table 108-1. DISTINGUISHING FEATURES OF THE SEVERAL TYPES OF PORPHYRIA

Characteristics	Erythropoietic			Hepatic			
	Uro-porphyria	Proto-porphyria	Copro-porphyria	Acute inter-mittent	Cutanea tarda hereditaria	Cutanea tarda sympto-matica	Hereditary coproporphyria
Inheritance	Recessive	Dominant	Dominant	Dominant	Dominant	Acquired	Dominant
Sex	Both	Both	....	Both	Both	Both	Both
Age of onset, years ..	0–5	0–5	....	15–40	10–30	Any age	Any age
Phase of disease	....	....	....	*latent* *acute*	*latent* *acute*	....	*latent* *acute*
Photosensitivity and cutaneous lesions ..	++++	++	++	0 0	0 + or 0	++	0 0 or +
Abdominal, psychic, and/or neurologic symptoms	0	0	0	0 ++	0 +	0	0 +
RBC:							
Uroporphyrin	++++	++	++	N N	N N	N	N N
Coproporphyrin ...	+++	++	++++	N N	N N	N	N N
Protoporphyrin ...	++	++++	+	N N	N N	N	N N
Urine:							
Color	Red	N	N	N* Red	N* N or red	Red	N N or red
Δ-ALA.†	N	N	N	+ ++	N ++	N	+ ++
PBG.‡	N	N	N	++ ++++	N ++	N	+ ++
Uroporphyrin	++++	N	N	++ ++	N +++	++++	N ++
Coproporphyrin ...	++	N	N	++ ++	N +++	++	N or + +++
Feces:							
Coproporphyrin ...	++	N	N	N +	++++ +++	+++	++ ++++
Protoporphyrin ...	++	N to ++	N	N +	++++ +++	++	N +

0, absent; N, normal; +, increased; ++++, greatly increased.

* Freshly voided. On standing, the urine may become deep brownish-red or black.

† Δ-aminolevulinic acid.

‡ Porphobilinogen.

of porphyria the excessive quantities of uroporphyrin are formed in the marrow. It is for this reason that the disease had been called *erythropoietic uroporphyria* rather than congenital porphyria.

The color of the urine varies from pink to red. Uroporphyrin I and coproporphyrin I are the predominant porphyrins excreted. If the concentration of uroporphyrin is sufficiently great, the urine, on the addition of hydrochloric acid, exhibits an intense band at about 552 mμ and a weaker band at 596 mμ when viewed in a hand spectroscope. The excretion of porphyrin precursors, Δ-aminolevulinic acid and porphobilinogen, is not increased.

The disease is slowly progressive, and death is usually due to an intercurrent infection or severe hemolytic anemia. At autopsy there is extensive deposition of porphyrins in the skeleton and tissues. This may be so pronounced as to color the bones red. Erythroid hyperplasia of the bone marrow and splenomegaly are additional pathologic features.

TREATMENT. Exposure to sunlight should be avoided. The harmful and disfiguring effects of light may be ameliorated by the use of quinine cream. Splenectomy is indicated if there is evidence of increased erythrocyte destruc-tion. Splenectomy may be associated not only with amelioration of the hemolytic anemia but also with a reduction in photosensitivity and porphyrin excretion.

Erythropoietic Protoporphyria

Erythropoietic protoporphyria, the most common form of erythropoietic porphyria, is transmitted as an autosomal dominant characteristic. The disease usually becomes manifest in childhood and is characterized clinically by *skin photosensitivity with intense, painful itching, edema, and erythema of the exposed parts.* Chronic skin changes may develop on the dorsa of the hands, especially over the knuckles, but may also be observed on the nose, cheeks, and lips. Biochemically, the disorder is characterized by an increase in the *protoporphyrin content of the normoblasts and erythrocytes,* an increased level of plasma protoporphyrin, and an increased excretion of protoporphyrin in the feces. The urinary excretion of Δ-ALA, porphobilinogen, coproporphyrin, and uroporphyrin is not increased. However, several patterns of chemical abnormality have been demonstrated in patients with the disease and in members of their families. Elevation of free erythrocyte protoporphyrin may occur with no increase in plasma or fecal protoporphyrin. Fecal protoporphyrin may be increased with no abnormalities of plasma or erythrocyte protoporphyrin. The complete biochemical stigmata of the disease have been observed in the absence of skin photosensitivity.

Erythropoietic Coproporphyria

This disorder is less well defined than the two previous disorders, having been described in only two members of one family. Swelling of the skin and itching after exposure to sunlight were the only clinical manifestations in the propositus. The erythrocytes contained large amounts of coproporphyrin III, a moderate increase in protoporphyrin, and a relatively marked increase in uroporphyrin, in comparison with the normal. Urine and fecal porphyrin concentrations were within normal limits and the excretion of porphyrin precursors was not increased.

PORPHYRIA HEPATICA
Acute Intermittent Porphyria

This is an uncommon but not a rare disease which affects both sexes, with a slight predilection for the female. Young adults or the middle-aged are most frequently affected. Acute porphyria is extremely rare below the age of fifteen and after the age of sixty. The familial occurrence of the disease is marked. It is probably transmitted as a mendelian dominant characteristic. The disease is characterized clinically by (1) periodic attacks of intense abdominal colic, usually accompanied by nausea and vomiting; (2) obstinate constipation; (3) neurotic or even psychotic behavior; and (4) neuromuscular disturbances. The mortality rate is high.

Abdominal pain is frequently the presenting complaint. The pain is usually colicky in nature and may be extremely severe and associated with spasm without localizing signs but with fever, tachycardia, and leukocytosis. The abdominal signs may be, and frequently are, mistaken for manifestations of renal colic, acute appendicitis, cholelithiasis, or pancreatitis. It is not uncommon for patients with porphyria to have multiple surgical scars on the abdomen. The neurologic manifestations are quite varied and may include neuritic pain in the extremities, areas of hypoesthesia and paraesthesia, and foot and wrist drop. Paraplegia or a complete flaccid quadriplegia may ensue and may be followed by bulbar paralysis and death. Except for pain in the extremities, sensory changes are usually not prominent and signs of upper motor neurone changes are usually absent. The neurologic manifestations may simulate a wide variety of conditions, including poliomyelitis, encephalitis, and arsenic or lead poisoning. A true ascending paralysis of the Landry type is not observed.

The patients frequently have many vague "neurotic" complaints, even when in remission from an attack. With an attack they may become confused or even psychotic. Hypertension may accompany an attack, there may be temporary loss of vision, and convulsions have been described.

The course of the disease is extraordinarily variable. Recurrent abdominal crises may be present for years, or the patient may die in the first attack. It is not at all uncommon to find in one parent or in several siblings of a patient with porphyria that porphobilinogen, the diagnostic feature of porphyria, is present in the urine, even though they have never had active symptoms of the disease. This condition is called *latent poryphyria*. In general, the neuromuscular and psychotic symptoms are late manifestations, and with their appearance the prognosis becomes more grave. Between attacks there may be no symptoms. The mechanism by which the latent disease is converted to manifest disease, i.e., an attack of acute porphyria, is unknown, but it is known quite definitely that attacks may be provoked by the administration of certain drugs, particularly barbiturates. Menstruation, pregnancy, infection, alcohol, or lead may be the precipitating factor in a few patients.

The freshly voided urine is frequently normal in color and on standing in the sunlight turns to a Burgundy wine color or even black. This color change can be hastened by adding a small amount of acid to the urine and boiling for 30 min. The explanation for these color changes is that porphobilinogen (colorless) and not uroporphyrin (red) is excreted in the urine. Heating of porphobilinogen in an acid medium results in the nonenzymatic formation of uroporphyrin, together with a dark-brown or reddish-brown nonporphyrin pigment.

In acute intermittent porphyria during relapse the presence of porphobilinogen is a constant feature. During remission the porphobilinogen reaction is usually positive, but a negative test does not exclude the diagnosis of this type of porphyria. The qualitative determination of porphobilinogen by the Watson-Schwartz modification of the Ehrlich reaction is, therefore, a simple and valuable screening procedure. In this test 5 ml freshly voided urine is mixed with 5 ml Ehrlich's reagent (0.7 Gm paradimethylaminobenzaldehyde, 150 ml concentrated hydrochloric acid, and 100 ml water). After mixing, 10 ml aqueous saturated sodium acetate is added. The solution is then extracted successively with 10 ml chloroform and 10 ml n-butanol. A positive test for porphobilinogen gives an intense red color remaining in the aqueous layer. This test is quite specific for acute intermittent porphyria. The test is negative in erythropoietic porphyria and in porphyria cutanea tarda symptomatica. It is positive in patients with porphyria cutanea tarda hereditaria during acute attacks but is negative in the interval between such episodes.

In addition to porphobilinogen, patients with acute intermittent porphyria excrete excessive quantities of uroporphyrin (types I and III), coproporphyrin (types I and III), and other as yet unidentified porphyrins. As mentioned previously, the porphyrins are formed in the renal tubules by the nonenzymatic transformation of porphobilinogen into uroporphyrin at an acid pH. Examination of the tissues of such patients, in contrast to the findings in erythropoietic porphyria, has revealed that the porphorin content of the bone marrow is normal. The liver, on the contrary, regularly exhibits increased quantities of porphyrin, especially porphyrin precursors. For this reason, acute intermittent porphyria is classified among the hepatic porphyrias.

ALA synthetase has now been shown to be an inducible enzyme in both man and animals. Induction can be augmented by barbiturates, estrogens, certain 5β-H steroid metabolites, and a variety of chemical compounds. Induction can be inhibited by high carbohydrate intake. Thus, the major chemical manifestations of acute intermittent porphyria are best explained as resulting from overproduction of porphyrin precursors, secondary to induction of hepatic ALA synthetase. The genetic lesion in acute intermittent porphyria is most likely in the operator gene mechanism for ALA synthetase.

TREATMENT. Drugs such as barbiturates and estrogens which induce Δ-ALA synthetase must be avoided. There is a theoretical basis for recommending a high carbohydrate intake. In acute attacks, opiates such as meperidine (Demerol) or ganglioplegics such as tetraethylammonium may be used for relief of pain. Chloralhydrate or paraldehyde may be used for sedation. Neostigmine may be of value in treating severe constipation. Chlorpromazine, in doses of 50 to 100 mg, may affect rapid relief of acute symptoms, but without change in the underlying process. Hyponatremia and hypochloremia secondary to inappropriate secretion of antidiuretic hormone may occur in some patients during acute attacks and require therapy. Respiratory support may be needed in some patients. ACTH and corticosteroids and chelating agents such as BAL (2, 3-dimercaptopropanol), EDTA (disodium ethylenediaminetetraacetate), and penicillamine have not been shown definitely to be of value.

Porphyria Cutanea Tarda Hereditaria

Porphyria cutanea tarda hereditaria is characterized clinically by cutaneous lesions or acute attacks of abdominal colic and not infrequently by both. The disease is inherited as a non-sex-linked mendelian dominant. The onset of symptoms is usually between the ages of ten and thirty years. The outstanding biochemical feature of the disorder is the increased excretion of coproporphyrin and protoporphyrin in the feces *at all times* in the course of the disease.

During the latent phase of the disease the patients are entirely asymptomatic. Porphyrinuria is usually absent and the porphyrin precursors, Δ-aminolevulinic acid and porphobilinogen, are not excreted in increased amounts. The disease can be diagnosed only during the latent phase by examination of the stools for porphyrins. A simple screening test can be done by obtaining a small specimen of stool on a glove. The specimen is extracted with about 2 ml of solvent containing equal parts of glacial acetic acid, amyl alcohol, and ether. The supernatant solution is then extracted with 1.5 N HCl and viewed in a Wood's lamp. Red fluorescence in the acid layer is proportional to the porphyrin content.

In a number of patients, particularly males, the skin is unusually sensitive to light and blisters and abrades easily. Healed depigmented scars may be present over the exposed surfaces, particularly the hands. Hyperpigmentation of the skin may occur, and hirsutism has been observed in females. The photosensitivity and cutaneous deformities are not so great as in erythropoietic porphyria.

Acute attacks of jaundice and abdominal colic accompanied in some cases by psychotic manifestations and motor paralysis may intervene in the course of the disease. Indeed, any or all of the manifestations of acute intermittent porphyria may make their appearance. As in acute intermittent porphyria, death or recovery may occur. During the acute attacks the excretion of porphyrins in the feces frequently decreases and the excretion of coproporphyrin and uroporphyrin in the urine increases. Both Δ-aminolevulinic acid and porphobilinogen are usually excreted in increased amounts in the urine during acute attacks. It has been suggested that the disease remains asymptomatic as long as the liver is capable of excreting the porphyrins in the bile (latent phase); when this capacity is impaired bilirubinemia, porphyrinemia, porphyrinuria, and cutaneous lesions appear (cutaneous phase); and finally when porphyrin metabolism is greatly disturbed, Δ-aminolevulinic acid and porphobilinogen appear in the urine and all the manifestations of acute intermittent porphyria may develop (acute phase). Porphyria cutanea tarda hereditaria is not an entirely suitable name for this disorder since not all patients develop cutaneous lesions. It is for this reason that the designation *porphyria variegata* has been suggested.

Porphyria Cutanea Tarda Symptomatica

This type of porphyria is characterized clinically by cutaneous lesions, hyperpigmentation of the skin, evidences of liver disease, and hypertrichosis; and chemically by the excretion of large amounts of uroporphyrin and lesser amounts of coproporphyrin in the urine. Abdominal pain and neurologic complications are conspicuously absent. The urine does not contain increased quantities of Δ-aminolevulinic acid or porphobilinogen. The excretion of protoporphyrin in the feces is normal; the excretion of coproporphyrin in the feces is usually increased.

The skin lesions are indistinguishable from those observed in porphyria cutanea tarda hereditaria. The skin is usually sensitive both to light and to mechanical trauma. Blisters appear on the exposed skin areas, frequently ulcerate, and finally lead to scar formation. The photosensitivity is similar to that in erythropoietic porphyria but not as marked.

This disorder has been described (1) in male subjects, forty to seventy years of age, with alcoholic cirrhosis of the liver; (2) in Bantu subjects in South Africa with nutritional cirrhosis of the liver; (3) in children and adults in Turkey who have ingested the fungicide hexachlorobenzene; (4) in three elderly subjects with a tumor of the liver; and (5) in an occasional young adult without a history of alcoholism or drug exposure. Porphyria cutanea tarda symptomatica is probably acquired, but constitutional factors may be involved in some cases.

Hereditary Coproporphyria

The unique feature of this disease is an increased excretion of coproporphyrin, isomer type III. In the latent phase, the patients are asymptomatic and the only abnormality usually detectable is an increased excretion of coproporphyrin III in the urine and feces, particularly the latter. Urinary Δ-ALA and porphobilinogen may be normal or slightly increased. Acute attacks, similar to those which occur in acute intermittent porphyria, can be provoked by the ingestion of barbiturates and possibly by certain tranquilizers and anticonvulsants. During these attacks there is an excessive excretion of Δ-ALA and porphobilinogen in the urine, in addition to a massive excretion of coproporphyrin in both urine and stool. About 30 cases of this disorder have been reported. Psychiatric symptoms may be present without other clinical manifestations of porphyria. Skin photosensitivity has been described in one case. The disease is inherited as a dominant characteristic and occurs in both sexes. The neurologic and psychiatric aspects of porphyria are discussed further in Chaps. 354 and 30 respectively.

REFERENCES

Donaldson, E. M., A. D. Donaldson, and C. Rimington: Erythropoietic Protoporphyria: A Family Study, Brit. Med. J., 1:659, 1967.

Goldberg, A., and C. Rimington: "Diseases of Porphyrin Metabolism," Springfield, Ill., Charles C Thomas, Publisher, 1962.

——, C. Rimington, and A. C. Lochhead: Hereditary Coproporphyria, Lancet, 1:632, 1967.

Heilmeyer, L., and R. Clotten: Congenital Erythropoietic Coproporphyria, Ger. Med. Mon., 9:1, 1964.

Kappas, A., and S. Granick: Steroid Induction of Porphyrin Synthesis in Liver Cell Culture, J. Biol. Chem., 243:346, 1968.

Tschudy, D. P.: Biochemical Lesions in Porphyria, J.A.M.A., 191:718, 1965.

Watson, C. J., L. Taddeini, and I. Bossenmaier: Present Status of the Ehrlich Aldehyde Reaction for Urinary Porphobilinogen, J.A.M.A., 190:501, 1964.

109 DISORDERS OF MELANIN METABOLISM

Thomas B. Fitzpatrick

DEFINITION OF MELANIN

Melanin is the principal basis of the coloration of human skin, hair, and eyes. In man, it functions primarily as a screen that shields the dermis from the deleterious effects of solar radiation. Since the amount and distribution of melanin in skin and hair are changed in a number of diseases, a detailed study of the irregularities of pigmentation may provide important diagnostic clues to diseases in other organs.

The term *melanin* is derived from the Greek word *melas,* black, and is the name given to a biochrome of high molecular weight formed by enzymatic oxidation of the phenol tyrosine, by the action of tyrosinase. The biochrome is therefore often referred to as *tyrosine melanin.* Tyrosine melanin is the product of unique unicellular glands, *melanocytes,* that secrete melanin particles into epidermal cells. The exact chemical nature of melanin has not been determined, because tyrosine melanin (both natural and synthetic) is so extremely insoluble that all attempts to degrade it into identifiable fragments have failed until now. However, it is now known that all animal melanins are "indole" in type and are composed basically of indole-5,6-quinone units, in contrast with melanins of plant origin, which are "catechol" in type. Also, studies using radioactive dopa (dihydroxyphenylalanine) have revealed that melanin appears to be a copolymer of dopa-quinone, indole-5,6-quinone, and indole-5,6-quinone-2-carboxylic acid in the ratio of 3:2:1.

BIOSYNTHESIS OF MELANIN

Melanocytes are situated at the dermoepidermal interface, in the hair bulb, the uveal tract, retinal pigment epithelium, and the leptomeninges. These scattered groups of cells are known as the *melanocyte system.* They may be considered to constitute a unit, because the melanocytes in all these locations are derived from the neural crest (Fig. 109-1) and can hydroxylate tyrosine to dopa and, ultimately, to the pigment, tyrosine melanin. The melanocyte system is analogous, but not known to be related, to the chromaffin system. Like melanocytes, the cells of the chromaffin system are derived from the neural crest and possess biochemical mechanisms for the hydroxylation of tyrosine to dopa, but by the action of tyrosine hydroxylase, not tyrosinase; unlike melanocytes, they convert dopa to adrenochrome and not to tyrosine melanin. Benign and malignant neoplasms arise in all parts of the melanocyte system except the retinal pigment epithelium and the hair bulbs.

The melanocytes present at the dermoepidermal interface form a horizontal network that is closely connected to the epidermal cells by means of numerous cytoplasmic processes, or dendrites. This intimate relationship permitting cytocrine transfer of melanin particles (melanosomes —see definition below) from melanocytes to malpighian cells has been clearly demonstrated by electron microscopy in a study of the fine structure of cortical cells and hair melanocytes and by tissue culture studies of human epidermis.

It has been possible to demonstrate by electron microscopy that melanocytes contain specialized organelles with a distinctive internal structure. These organelles, known as *melanosomes,* contain tyrosinase, the melanin-synthesizing enzyme. Under normal conditions, melanin is progressively formed and deposited on the surface of melanosomes until they become amorphous particles without detectable tyrosinase activity (Fig. 109-2). Melanosomes are believed to originate in the Golgi area, appearing first as unmelanized vesicles that gradually increase in size and become dark in color and increasingly dense.

Tyrosinase is one of a large group of copper-containing aerobic oxidases that catalyze the oxidation of both monohydroxy and *o*-dihydroxy phenols to orthoquinones. In man and other mammals, this oxidase catalyzes the hydroxylation of the melanin precursor tyrosine to dopa and dopa-quinone (Fig. 109-3). Tyrosinase is required only for the first step in the biosynthesis of tyrosine melanin, i.e., the orthohydroxylation of tyrosine. It is noteworthy that zinc ions catalyze the conversion of dopa-chrome to 5,6-dihydroxyindole and that melanosomes have been shown to contain zinc in high concentration.

In the hair and skin of the various races, characteristic coloration is thought to be determined not by variations in the number of melanocytes present but by variations in the number and type of melanosomes produced by existing melanocytes. The amount of pigment present in individual melanosomes is related to their tyrosinase content; for example, melanosomes that lack tyrosinase remain unpigmented, as in some types of albinism.

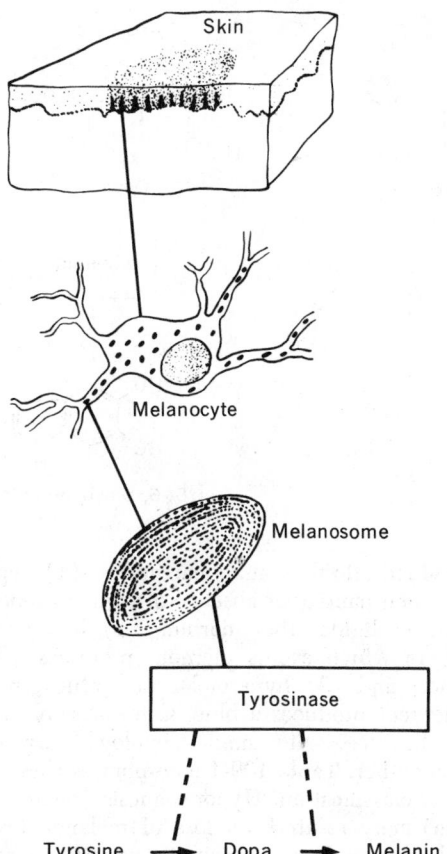

Fig. 109-2. Melanogenesis in human skin, as seen in the light microscope and the electron microscope and at the molecular level.

PATHOGENESIS OF PIGMENTARY DISORDERS

To explain the pathogenesis of a disturbance of melanin pigmentation, it is necessary to evaluate the rate at which tyrosinase is synthesized on the ribosomes, to determine the rate at which melanosomes progress through successive stages to full melanization, to understand the role played by factors that regulate the biosynthesis of melanin, and to examine the transfer of melanosomes to epidermal cells.

Availability of free tyrosine is essential for the biosynthesis of melanin. Tyrosine that is bound in a peptide linkage cannot act as a substrate if the amino group is blocked.

Aggregation and dispersion of melanosomes probably play no part in the pigmentary anomalies of man. Such movement has thus far been observed only in specialized effector cells, *melanophores*, present only in vertebrates below mammals in the phylogenetic scale.

CLINICAL DISORDERS

Disorders of melanin pigmentation that involve the melanocyte system may be classed as *hypomelanoses* and *hypermelanoses*. On a morphologic basis, these disorders

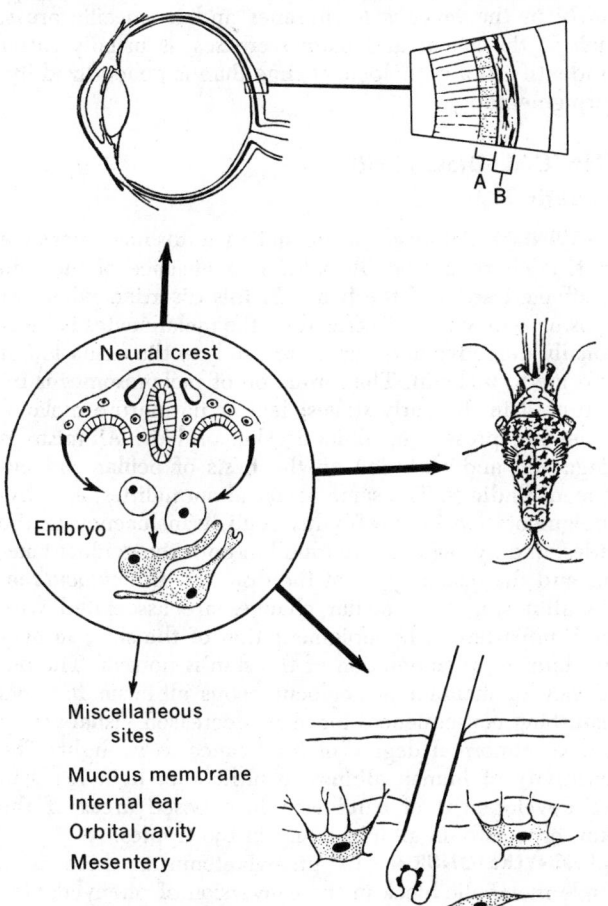

Fig. 109-1. Diagram showing the embryonic origin, dispersal, and developmental fate of melanocytes in man. (*By permission, from J. B. Stanbury et al. (Eds.), "The Metabolic Basis of Inherited Disease," 2d ed., New York, McGraw-Hill Book Company, 1966.*)

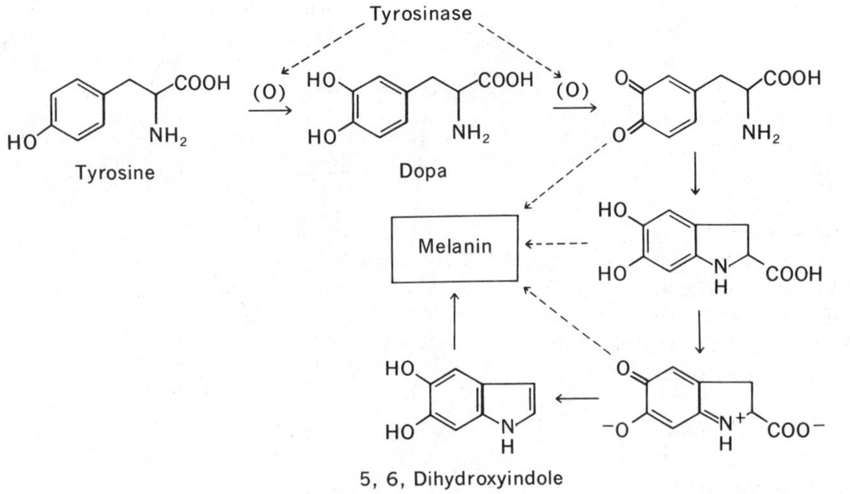

Fig. 109-3. Biosynthesis of tyrosine melanin.

can be divided into three main categories: (1) hypomelanosis, in which paucity or absence of pigment renders the skin white or lighter than normal; (2) hypermelanosis (brown), in which excess pigment produces a brown-black color; and (3) hypermelanosis (blue), in which excess pigment produces a blue, slate, or gray hue. Pigmentary disorders with similar etiology may also be grouped together. Table 109-1 incorporates these various methods of classification. Hypomelanosis (decreased pigmentation) may result from loss of melanocytes, as in thermal burns, or from absence or paucity of melanin. In the disorders listed under the heading of Brown hypermelanosis in Table 109-1, the brown pigmentation results, in most instances, from an increase in the *activity* of epidermal melanocytes and not from an increase in the number of these cells. Gray, slate, or blue hypermelanosis results from the presence of melanin within dermal phagocytes or ectopic dermal melanocytes. The blue, slate, or gray hue is related to the Tyndall light-scattering phenomenon.

Recognition of hypomelanosis and of gray, slate, or blue hypermelanosis is usually not difficult. When the degree of hypomelanosis is very slight, diagnosis may be facilitated by the use of black light.[1] Differentiation between abnormal diffuse brown hyperpigmentation and normal pigmentation frequently poses a problem because there is such a wide range of coloration in different individuals. It is usually possible, however, to determine whether the patient has observed an unusual or progressive change in coloration that has had no obvious cause. A summer tan may not have faded, or the patient's associates may have detected a gradual deepening of his skin color. The degree of brown hypermelanosis that develops appears to be related to the basic skin color of the patient. For example, a patient of Mediterranean extraction (Italian, French, Spanish) may become intensely

pigmented with the onset of primary adrenocortical insufficiency, whereas a light-skinned patient will have only a minimal degree of hypermelanosis that may or may not be detectable. Localized pigmentation that develops newly in the mucous membranes and in specific areas, such as the axillas and palmar creases, is usually easier to identify as a pathologic change than is generalized hyperpigmentation.[2]

CLINICAL DISORDERS
Genetic

ALBINISM. Albinism, a mendelian autosomal recessive trait, is characterized by paucity or absence of melanin in affected areas of the body. In this disorder, whatever tyrosinase may be synthesized by the melanocytes is functionally defective and unable to catalyze the oxidation of tyrosine to melanin. The formation of melanosomes is interrupted in the early stages; few or no mature melanosomes are present in albinotic skin or hair. Albinism is diagnosed and classified on the basis of ocular and cutaneous findings. The same ocular abnormalities, e.g., hypopigmentation of the fundus oculi, translucency of the irides, and nystagmus, are found in both the oculocutaneous and the ocular types of the disorder. In *oculocutaneous* albinism, these ocular changes are associated with total, unpatterned hypopigmentation of the skin; in *ocular* albinism, pigmentation of the skin is normal. The deficiency of melanin in oculocutaneous albinism has two disturbing consequences for man: decreased visual acuity and an abnormal degree of intolerance to sunlight. The sensitivity of human albinos to ultraviolet light leads to the development of carcinoma in exposed areas of the skin, especially in albinos living in the tropics.

PHENYLKETONURIA. In phenylketonuria, there is a single metabolic block in the conversion of phenylalanine to tyrosine. The condition is associated with subnormal

---

[1] Melanin pigment appears darker in black light than in normal light. Black light, which emits 3,660 Å, primarily emphasizes the contrast between hypopigmented and normal skin.

[2] Pigmentation of the gums, tongue, and buccal mucosa is a normal finding in Asiatics, American Indians, and Negroes and often in East Indians.

Table 109-1. DISTURBANCES OF HUMAN MELANIN PIGMENTATION[1]

Causative factors	Classification		
	Hypomelanosis (white) *in association with*	Brown hypermelanosis *in association with*	Gray, slate, or blue hypermelanosis[2] *in association with*
Genetic disorders	Piebaldism Waardenburg's syndrome Vitiligo[3] Albinism, oculocutaneous[4] Albinism, ocular Hypomelanotic macules in tuberous sclerosis[5] Phenylketonuria[6,7]	*Café au lait* macules in neurofibromatosis Melanotic macules in polyostotic fibrous dysplasia (Albright's syndrome) Lentigenes with cardiac arrhythmias Neurocutaneous melanosis Xeroderma pigmentosum Acanthosis nigricans, juvenile type Peutz-Jeghers syndrome	Oculodermal melanocytosis (nevus of Ota) Dermal melanocytosis (Mongolian spot)
Metabolic diseases		Hemochromatosis[4] Hepatolenticular disease (Wilson's disease)[4] Porphyria (congenital erythropoietica and porphyria variegata and cutanea tarda[4] Gaucher's disease[4] Niemann-Pick disease	Hemochromatosis[4]
Endocrine disorders	Hypopituitarism[4] Addison's disease Hyperthyroidism	ACTH-producing and MSH-producing pituitary and other tumors[4] ACTH therapy[4] Pregnancy[9] Addison's disease[4] Estogen therapy[10] Melasma[11]	
Nutritional disorders	Chronic protein deficiency or loss, as in kwashiorkor, nephrosis, ulcerative colitis, malabsorption syndrome; the hair is gray or reddish[6] Vitamin B_{12} deficiency[6]	Kwashiorkor Pellagra[12] Sprue[12] Vitamin B_{12} deficiency[6]	Chronic nutritional insufficiency
Chemical and pharmacologic agents	Monobenzyl ether of hydroquinone Chloroquine and hydroxychloroquine[6] Arsenical intoxication	Arsenical intoxication[4] Busulfan administration[4] Photochemical agents (topical or systemic drugs, tar) Dibromomannitol administration[4]	

Physical agents	Burns:
	    Thermal, ultraviolet, ionizing
	    Radiation[8]
	Trauma
		Ultraviolet light
		Heat
		Alpha, beta, and gamma radiation
		Trauma (e.g., chronic pruritus)	

Inflammations and infectious diseases	Pinta
	Leprosy[5]
	Fungous infections (tinea versicolor)[5]
	
	Miscellaneous dermatoses:
	    Psoriasis
	    Lupus erythematosus, discoid
		Postinflammation pigmentation (exanthems, drug eruptions)
		Miscellaneous dermatoses:
		    Lupus erythematosus, discoid
		    Lichen simplex chronicus
		    Atopic dermatitis[4]
		    Psoriasis
			Pinta in exposed areas

Neoplasms	In sites of melanoma after disappearance (therapeutic or spontaneous) of tumor	Mastocytosis (urticaria pigmentosa) Adenocarcinoma with acanthosis nigricans	Dermal-pigmentation syndrome with metastatic, melanoma and melanogenuria[4]
Miscellaneous disorders	Vogt-Koyanagi syndrome Scleroderma, circumscribed or systemic Horner's syndrome, congenital and acquired[7]	Scleroderma, systemic[4] Chronic hepatic insufficiency[4] Whipple's syndrome[4] Melasma (chloasma) Lentigo, senile ("liver spots")	

[1] This classification includes disorders of interest to physicians in general; many pigmentary disorders not listed are of special interest to dermatologists.

[2] Gray, slate, or blue color results from the presence of *dermal* melanocytes or phagocytized melanin in the dermis.

[3] Total loss of pigment in the skin and hair may occur.

[4] Pigment change is diffuse, not circumscribed, and there are no identifiable borders.

[5] Loss of pigmentation is usually partial; viewed with Wood's light, the lesions are not snow-white, as in vitiligo.

[6] Pigment is decreased in the hair.

[7] Pigment is decreased in the iris.

[8] There is a loss of melanocytes.

[9] Pigment change may be diffuse or circumscribed.

[10] Nipples are affected.

[11] Idiopathic or due to progestational agents.

[12] May be diffuse.

SOURCE: 1968 revision of table from T. B. Fitzpatrick, in T. R. Harrison et al., "*Principles of Internal Medicine*," 5th ed., Chap. 102, p. 565, New York, McGraw-Hill Book Company, 1966.

pigmentation of the hair and the iris. The hair of patients with phenylketonuria ranges in color from light blond to dark brown, and it is only by comparison with the hair of siblings that the characteristic dilution of color becomes evident. The diminution of melanin formation results from the fact that the large amounts of phenylalanine and its metabolites present in serum and extracellular fluid act as competitive inhibitors of tyrosinase activity, thus blocking melanin synthesis (Chap. 102).

PIEBALDISM. Piebaldism, an autosomal dominant trait, involves the skin and the hair only. In piebaldism, there are hypomelanotic patterned areas on the extremities and anterior surface of the thorax, and there is commonly a white forelock. The melanin content of the eyes, however, usually remains normal. Piebaldism is associated with congenital deafness in a syndrome known as Waardenburg's. Electron microscopic studies have revealed that the areas of skin lacking in pigment lack melanocytes, as in vitiligo (see below).

VITILIGO. Vitiligo may be localized or generalized. When localized, the hypomelanosis of the skin and hair may be restricted to one region, such as the genitalia or perianal area or scalp area. When generalized, the pattern of hypomelanosis is quite typical, with lesions particularly on the face, axillas, neck, and extremities, and with loss of pigment in the hair. Idiopathic vitiligo is fairly common, affecting 1 percent of the population. The lesions are completely lacking in pigment, and this snow-whiteness is distinctive and serves to differentiate vitiligo from other hypomelanoses. Vitiligo is inherited as an autosomal dominant trait with irregular penetrance. In the majority of cases, the vitiligo is idiopathic, but typical vitiligo, as just described, is known to occur with a variety of diseases, such as Addison's disease, hyperthyroidism, hypo-

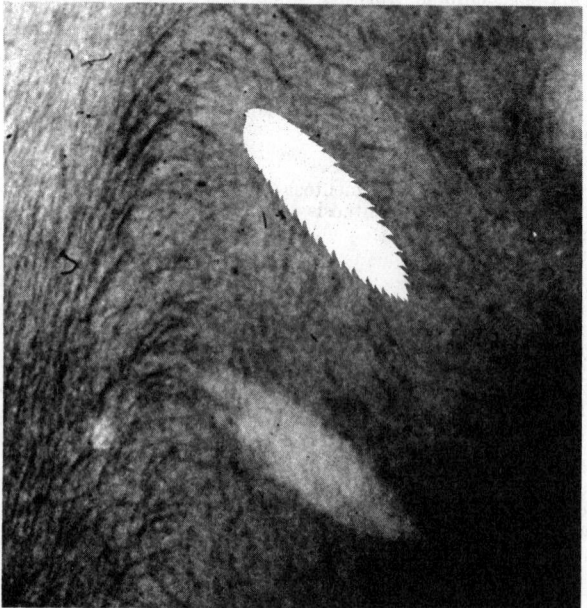

Fig. 109-4. A 4-cm lesion showing the typical configuration of a leaf from a mountain-ash tree. A projected outline of an actual leaf is shown next to the lesion.

parathyroidism, pernicious anemia, and alopecia areata. Electron microscopic studies of vitiligo of the skin reveal a severe reduction or, more commonly, a total absence of melanocytes so that the hypomelanosis is the result of a structural defect, rather than a metabolic change, in the existing melanocytes.

TUBEROUS SCLEROSIS. (See Chap. 365.) Tuberous sclerosis, a serious autosomal dominant trait usually causing mental retardation and convulsions, is associated with characteristic white macules in 67 percent of the patients. These white macules are present at birth and therefore constitute an important sign that permits the physician to establish an early diagnosis in an infant and to forewarn the parents about a possible genetic defect in any other children that they might have. These white macules are present when other diagnostic skin signs of tuberous sclerosis are not evident, because the typical facial lesions do not appear until the second to the sixth year after birth. The lesions are not snow-white, as in vitiligo, but are off-white. The white lesions are usually larger than 1 cm in diameter and are more easily detected with the aid of a black or Wood's light, especially in fair-skinned infants. Although the predominant outline of the lesion is similar to that of a mountain-ash leaflet, from which it takes its name (Fig. 109-4), other configurations occur, such as round or oval; sometimes the distribution follows a dermatomal pattern. The ash-leaf spots vary in number from 3 to 100, and may be present on any part of the skin surface, but are more common on the trunk and lower extremities. Histochemical and electron microscopic studies reveal that there is not an absence of melanocytes, as in vitiligo, but a marked reduction of melanin deposition on the melanosomes within the melanocytes present in the affected areas, with resultant hypomelanosis.

NEUROFIBROMATOSIS (VON RECKLINGHAUSEN'S DISEASE). This condition is inherited as a dominant trait. It is characterized by the presence, primarily on the trunk but also on the extremities, of numerous pale yellow-brown macules, so-called *café au lait* spots, that vary in diameter from less than 1 to more than 15 cm. Spotty generalized pigmentation may also be present, especially in the axillas. Often, but not always, a few or myriads of soft, rounded, cone-shaped or pendulous cutaneous tumors covered by normal skin are seen. Nerve-sheath tumors may occur.

The presence of six or more *café au lait* spots with a diameter greater than 1.5 cm is diagnostic of neurofibromatosis even when there is no familial history of the condition. In *polyostotic fibrous dysplasia*, there are rarely more than three or four macules, unilaterally distributed usually on the buttocks or cervical area (Chap. 384). Clinically, the single large isolated *café au lait* spot of neurofibromatosis resembles the pigmented macule of *polyostotic fibrous dysplasia* (*Albright's disease*). It is possible, however, to detect peculiar large extracellular globules of melanin in whole mounts of epidermis prepared from the *café au lait* macules of neurofibromatosis; these extracellular melanin globules are not found in the macular pigmented areas present in polyostotic fibrous dysplasia.

Metabolic

Generalized brown hypermelanosis of the skin is a characteristic manifestation of *hemochromatosis* and *cutaneous porphyria (porphyria cutanea tarda)* (Chap. 108). The hyperpigmentation observed in hemochromatosis (Chap. 107) may have a grayish-brown hue or be indistinguishable from that of Addison's disease (Chap. 92). The diagnosis of hemochromatosis is established by the presence of hemosiderin in the sweat glands of the skin. Porphyria may be recognized by the abnormally large amounts of *uroporphyrin* in the urine, stools, and plasma and by other characteristic clinical features, such as the presence of bullae, atrophic scars, and milia on the exposed surfaces of the face and hands.

Nutritional

CHRONIC PROTEIN DEFICIENCY. Chronic protein deficiency, as, for example, in kwashiorkor, chronic nephrosis, ulcerative colitis, and malabsorption syndrome, is sometimes associated with a change in hair color, first to a reddish-brown and eventually to gray. In chronic nutritional insufficiency, splotches of dirty-brown hyperpigmentation appear, especially on the trunk. In *sprue*, brown hypermelanosis may be generalized. In *pellagra*, hypermelanosis is limited to areas of skin that have been exposed to light. *Vitamin B_{12} deficiency* leads to loss of hair color and intense brown hypermelanosis around the small joints and a generalized Addisonian type of hypermelanosis.

Endocrine

Diffuse brown hypermelanosis is a striking feature of primary adrenocortical insufficiency (Chap. 92). Although this hypermelanosis is diffuse, there is marked accentuation of pigmentation in certain areas, namely, on the pressure points (vertebras, knuckles, elbows, knees), and in the body folds, the palmar creases, and the gingival mucous membrane. An identical type of diffuse hyperpigmentation has also been reported to follow adrenalectomy in patients with Cushing's disease. In these patients, there are usually signs and symptoms of pituitary tumors; all the tumors recorded have been chromophobe adenomas. A third example of the Addison type of melanosis described above has been reported in patients with tumors of organs other than the adrenal or pituitary glands. The generalized brown hypermelanosis found in all these conditions results from overproduction of two hormones: alpha-melanocyte-stimulating hormone (MSH) and ACTH. Both peptides, MSH and ACTH, share common peptide sequences. It appears that an excess of alpha-melanocyte-stimulating hormone plays the dominant role in the pigmentation that occurs in adrenocortical insufficiency. Both MSH and ACTH are increased as a result of the decreased output of hydrocortisone by the adrenals. Hypermelanosis of the Addison type can be produced in adrenalectomized human subjects by administering large amounts of homogeneous ACTH and alpha-MSH.

Chemical

Chemicals can induce both hypomelanosis and hypermelanosis. Hydroquinone and 4-isopropylcatechol prevent the formation of melanin and are of therapeutic value in treating hypermelanosis. Striking generalized Addisonian hypermelanosis of the skin follows busulfan therapy; the mechanism of action of this drug is not known. Inorganic trivalent arsenicals produce both generalized Addisonian hypermelanosis and scattered macular hypomelanosis, as well as punctate keratoses on the palms and soles.

Physical

Mechanical trauma, as well as burns caused by heat, ultraviolet light, or alpha-, beta-, and gamma-radiation, can lead to hypomelanosis or hypermelanosis. The effect of these physical agents on pigmentation is determined by the intensity and duration of exposure and is limited to the site of injury. The hypomelanosis results from destruction of melanocytes.

Chronic pruritus, such as that associated with chronic biliary-tract disease and lymphoma, may lead to generalized brown hypermelanosis.

Inflammatory and Infectious

Circumscribed hypomelanosis is a characteristic feature of tuberculoid leprosy. It occurs in areas of anesthesia, and the degree of pigment loss is only partial; the lesions are lighter in color than the areas of surrounding skin but are not snow-white as in vitiligo. Generalized spotty hyperpigmentation not uncommonly follows *exanthems* and *eruptions due to drugs;* it usually disappears spontaneously within 2 or 3 months.

Neoplastic

Hypomelanosis is seen in rare instances at the site of a primary or a metastatic *malignant melanoma* that has undergone remission spontaneously or as the result of chemotherapy. During the terminal stages of malignant melanoma, striking generalized blue hypermelanosis sometimes develops, and large amounts of a conjugated derivative of 5,6-dihydroxyindole are excreted in the urine ("melanogenuria"). This intermediate in the metabolic pathway from tyrosine to melanin can be oxidized to melanin in the absence of tyrosinase, and therefore melanin can be synthesized at almost any site in which oxidation can take place. Consequently, diffuse black pigmentation may develop in the peritoneum, liver, heart, muscle, and dermis of patients during the late stages of malignant melanoma. The brown melanin present in the dermal phagocytes appears as blue in the skin, because of the Tyndall light-scattering phenomenon.

The multiple, irregular, round or oval, yellow-brown-to-red-brown macules and papules characteristic of *urticaria pigmentosa* are related to the presence in the dermis of clusters of mast cells. Urticarial wheals develop when the individual lesions are stroked vigorously. In rare instances (*systemic mastocytosis*), mast cells infiltrate diffusely into the liver, spleen, gastrointestinal system, and bones, as well as into the skin.

Miscellaneous

Generalized brown hypermelanosis of the type seen in Addison's disease is not infrequently associated with *systemic scleroderma* and may appear very early in the course of the disorder. Generalized hyperpigmentation occasionally develops in patients with *chronic hepatic insufficiency*, especially that due to portal cirrhosis. The pathogenesis of the pigmentation in both these conditions is unknown.

Melasma (chloasma) is seen most commonly in pregnant women, but it also occurs in men and in nonpregnant women. The lesions consist of large macules with irregular borders on the exposed areas of the face and vary in color from yellow-brown to red-brown and very dark brown. Melasma is sometimes observed in women receiving oral progestational agents.

REFERENCES

Della Porta, G., and O. Mühlbock (Eds.): "Symposium on Structure and Control of the Melanocyte: Proceedings of the International Pigment Cell Conference," sponsored by the International Union against Cancer, Sofia, Bulgaria, May 1965, Berlin, Springer-Verlag, 1966.

Fitzpatrick, T. B., M. Miyamoto, and K. Ishikawa: The Evolution of Concepts of Melanin Biology, pp. 1–30 in W. Montanga and F. Hu (Eds.), "Advances in Biology of Skin: Volume VIII: The Pigmentary System," Oxford, Pergamon Press, 1967.

—— and W. C. Quevedo, Jr.: Albinism, in "The Metabolic Basis of Inherited Disease," 2d ed., J. B. Stanbury, J. B. Wyngaarden, and D. S. Fredrickson (Eds.), New York, McGraw-Hill Book Company, 1966.

——, M. Seiji, and A. D. McGugan: Melanin Pigmentation, New Engl. J. Med., 265:328, 374, 430, 1961.

Jeghers, H., and H. Mescon: Pigmentation of the Skin, in C. M. MacBryde (Ed.), "Signs and Symptoms: Applied Pathologic Physiology and Clinical Interpretation," 4th ed., Philadelphia, J. B. Lippincott Company, 1964.

Lerner, A. B.: Melanin Pigmentation, Am. J. Med., 19:902, 1955.

—— and J. S. McGuire: Melanocyte-stimulating Hormone and Adrenocorticotrophic Hormone; Their Relation to Pigmentation, New Engl. J. Med., 270:539, 1964.

Riley, V., and J. G. Fortner (Eds.): The Pigment Cell: Molecular, Biological and Clinical Aspects, Ann. N. Y. Acad. Sci., 100, pts. I and II, February, 1963.

110 HEPATOLENTICULAR DEGENERATION (Wilson's Disease)

George E. Cartwright

Definition

Hepatolenticular degeneration (progressive lenticular degeneration, Wilson's disease, pseudosclerosis of Westphal and Strümpell, tetanoid chorea of Gowers) is an uncommon, familial, progressive, fatal disease which becomes manifest usually in the first three decades of life and is characterized by the triad of basal ganglion degeneration, cirrhosis of the liver, and a ring of brown pigment at the corneal margins known as the Kayser-Fleischer ring.

History

Kinnier Wilson, in 1912, in his classic monograph "Progressive Lenticular Degeneration," first clearly defined the disease entity to which his name is now affixed. A similar condition had previously been described in 1883 by Westphal and later by Strümpell. The symptoms resembled those of multiple sclerosis, but no demyelinative plaques were observed. For that reason it was called *pseudosclerosis*. The cirrhosis of the liver was overlooked until Spielmeyer reexamined the cases many years later. His studies and the clinical observations of Hall left little doubt that hepatolenticular degeneration and pseudosclerosis were the same disease. The corneal ring was described in 1902 by Kayser in a case diagnosed as "multiple sclerosis," but to Fleischer is due the credit for appreciating its significance in relation to the disease as it is now known.

A marked increase in the copper content of both the brain and the liver was demonstrated by Haurowitz in 1930 and was later confirmed by Glazebrook and Cummings. Mandelbrote and his associates in 1948 observed by chance that the urinary output of copper was high and that this output is increased by the administration of BAL (British antilewisite). In the same year Uzman and Denny-Brown found that a persistent aminoaciduria is associated with the disease. Ceruloplasmin deficiency was recognized as a feature of the disease by Scheinberg and Gitlin in 1952. An effective treatment of the disease was introduced by Walshe in 1956.

Inheritance

The condition is inherited as an autosomal recessive trait, the affected individuals inheriting the gene from both parents who, while phenotypically normal, are heterozygous for the abnormal allele. Since the frequency of the abnormal gene is low in the general population, affected individuals may be expected to be, most often, the products of consanguineous marriages. This has proved to be the case.

Pathogenesis

Two different types of metabolic disturbance have been described, namely (1) abnormalities in the metabolism of copper and (2) impairment in renal tubular reabsorption.

A number of alterations in the metabolism of copper has been described (Table 110-1). The amount of copper in the tissues, particularly in the liver and brain, is increased about tenfold above the normal. The golden-

Table 110-1. BIOCHEMICAL ALTERATIONS IN
WILSON'S DISEASE

Determination	Normal subjects*	Wilson's disease
Total plasma copper, μg/100 ml	114 (81–147)	60 (19–103)
Direct-reacting plasma copper, μg/100 ml	7 (0–20)	26 (12–40)
Ceruloplasmin, mg/100 ml	33 (25–43)	9 (0–19)
Urine copper, μg/24 hr	15 (5–25)	522 (95–1,300)†
Liver copper, μg/Gm wet tissue	5 (3–10)	79 (53–100)†
Urine α-amino nitrogen, mg/day	164 (118–204)	337 (90–519)

* The figures in parentheses refer to ±2 standard deviations.
† Determined range.

brown pigment of the Kayser-Fleischer ring contains copper. The amount of copper excreted in the urine is increased. The specific copper protein of plasma, ceruloplasmin, is almost invariably decreased. On the other hand, the "direct-reacting" fraction of plasma copper, the copper which is probably loosely bound to albumin, is increased. Since there is a greater reduction in ceruloplasmin copper than there is increase in direct-reacting copper, the net effect on the total plasma copper is such that there is usually hypocupremia. In an occasional patient the total plasma copper concentration may be as high as 116 μg per 100 ml. Patients with this disease retain more than the normal amount of copper in the body. This is apparently because of an increased rate of absorption of copper from the gastrointestinal tract. Whether or not copper is excreted by the liver into the bile at the normal rate has not yet been determined with certainty. There may be a normal copper content in the bile, but this is not normal when the total copper content of the liver is considered.

Renal dysfunction which is present in many, but not all, patients includes abnormalities in tubular reabsorption manifested by aminoaciduria, peptiduria, proteinuria, glucosuria, uricosuria, or phosphaturia. The aminoaciduria involves most of the amino acids found in normal urine and, in addition, proline and citrulline. Taurine, aspartic acid, isoleucine, methyl histidine, and arginine are excreted in amounts close to the normal range. The urinary amino acid pattern and the severity of the aminoaciduria depend in part on the amount and type of protein ingested and vary considerably from patient to patient without relation to the type, duration, or stage of disease. The aminoaciduria is not accompanied by any significant elevation in the blood α-amino nitrogen level. The uricosuria may be associated with a diminished level of uric acid in the serum. The phosphaturia may result in hypophosphatemia and eventually in osseous changes.

The pathogenesis of the metabolic and pathologic changes is not fully understood. Because of the excessive deposition of copper in the tissues of patients with Wilson's disease, it has been suggested that the lesions in the liver and in the lenticular nuclei are the consequence of the excessive deposition of copper in these tissues and that the accumulation of copper in the kidney causes a functional impairment in the reabsorption of amino acids, peptides, and other substances. In support of this concept is the observation that excessive deposition of copper in the liver precedes the development of significant parenchymal damage. Furthermore, in most patients with the disease, the mobilization of copper from the body is associated with dramatic improvement in the clinical state of the patient.

Copper absorbed from the gastrointestinal tract enters first into the direct-reacting fraction of plasma copper. Therefore, the increase in this fraction reflects the increased turnover of copper between the gastrointestinal tract, the tissues, and the excretory routes. The copper in this fraction is easily dissociable from the albumin, and the increase in the direct-reacting fraction probably accounts for the increased excretion of copper by the kidneys.

The most widely held concept of the disease is that the inherited defect is an inability to synthesize ceruloplasmin. However, some individuals heterozygous for the gene may have as low a ceruloplasmin concentration as some patients with the disease. Furthermore, there is a poor correlation between the ceruloplasmin level and the severity or duration of the disease. An additional difficulty with this theory is that a mechanism whereby a deficiency of ceruloplasmin can lead to excessive tissue deposits of copper is not known.

Another theory which has been proposed is that the genetically determined abnormality in protein metabolism results in the formation of abnormal tissue proteins which have a high avidity for copper. The difficulty with this theory is that it does not explain the low concentrations of the plasma copper protein, ceruloplasmin.

Pathology

The characteristic pathologic findings are in the liver and the brain. The liver is usually small, firm, and coarsely nodular. It may or may not be bile-stained. Nodules of regenerating liver cells are separated by trabeculae of fibrous connective tissue. The picture is that of healed subacute yellow atrophy or the nonalcoholic variety of Laennec's cirrhosis. The most striking gross finding in the brain is cavitation of the putamen on each side and rarely of cerebral cortex and white matter. In many cases, probably more than half, the putamen and caudate nuclei are atrophic and of light grayish-brown color, and there is no evidence of cavitation. Microscopic examination almost invariably reveals a remarkable hyperplasia of protoplasmic astrocytes in the cerebral cortex, lenticular and caudate nuclei, subthalamic nuclei of Luys, substantia nigra, dentate and red nuclei. Nerve cell loss is widespread but is most pronounced in the lenticular and dentate nuclei and cerebral cortex. The protoplasmic astrocytosis does not differ from that observed in hepatic coma. Splenomegaly is a common finding.

Clinical Manifestations

The disease usually begins in adolescence, but it may appear as early as the age of four or as late as age forty. The mode of onset is somewhat variable. In a few cases the first manifestation is related to liver insufficiency, i.e., jaundice, ascites, or splenomegaly. More often the initial symptom is related to the neurologic system: tremor, dysarthria, ataxia, incoordination, or personality change. The disease may run an acute course of several months' duration associated with fever, rapid emaciation, and mental deterioration, or an extremely chronic afebrile course of 30 or 40 years' duration. The usual course in the untreated patient is 5 to 10 years.

The clinical picture of a well-developed case is quite characteristic. *Tremor* of one or both of the upper extremities is an outstanding as well as an early manifestation. The tremor consists of regular, rhythmic, alternating contractions and may occur in the earliest stages only on movement of the extremity. Later it is also present when the arm is maintained in an attitude of repose. It is accentuated by excitement or by attention being drawn to it. One of the most certain ways of demonstrating the tremor is by having the patient extend the arms in front of the body. In this position "flapping" or "wingbeating" may be noted. The tremor may also increase during fine volitional movements, taking a form that resembles intention tremor. Indeed, in some cases cerebellar ataxia and tremor are the principal neurologic manifestations. In severe cases a tremor of the mandible or even of the entire head is present. *Abnormal movements* of choreic or choreoathetoid type are present in some patients but are not frequent. *Rigidity* of the skeletal muscles, often reaching an extreme degree, is another characteristic. The rigidity may be intermittent or constant, and the resulting clinical state may vary from transient spasms in the acute cases to permanent *contractures* and *deformities* in the chronic. In the late stages of the disease the facial muscles become set in a stiff, vacuous smile, the neck and trunk become rigid, the upper extremities are held rigidly in flexion at the elbow, wrist, and metacarpal joints, and the lower extremities are held in a position of extension. *Dysarthria* or even anarthria in advanced cases is an almost constant finding. *Cachexia* and muscular wasting may be extreme. Some form of *mental disturbance* is common, and in severely affected patients changes in character and personality and terminally marked mental deterioration may be present. The sensory system is intact, and the reflexes are essentially normal. Pyramidal signs are usually absent.

The clinical course of the liver disease is extremely variable. In many patients signs of liver insufficiency are completely lacking, even though the liver function tests are abnormal and cirrhosis can be demonstrated by needle biopsy. In other patients the signs of liver insufficiency, such as splenomegaly, ascites, jaundice, hepatomegaly, hematemesis, and spider angiomas, dominate the clinical picture. When liver function is markedly impaired, anemia, leukopenia, and thrombocytopenia may be found to accompany the splenomegaly.

The most remarkable, unique, and consistent feature of the disease is the Kayser-Fleischer ring (see Chap. 401), a golden-brown or greenish-brown ring of pigment located at the periphery of the cornea in Descemet's membrane. The pigment usually goes completely around the cornea; occasionally there may be only a crescent-shaped distribution. Although the rings are frequently visible in ordinary light, in the early stages of the disease or in patients in whom the color of the iris is brown, it may be necessary to use a slit lamp to visualize the rings. Under slit-lamp examination, the ring is seen to be composed of a multitude of granular specks. The rings are pathognomonic of the disease and are present in all patients with neurologic manifestations. Failure of an experienced observer to demonstrate rings by slit-lamp examination of a patient with neurologic abnormalities virtually rules out Wilson's disease. Although the rings may be present in some patients long before the appearance of other clinical abnormalities, they are usually absent in asymptomatic subjects. They are occasionally absent in children whose only manifestations of Wilson's disease are those of hepatic involvement.

Skeletal abnormality, manifested by roentgenographic evidences of osteomalacia, cartilage injury, or bone fragmentation, is a frequent finding in the disease. Azure lunulas, bluish crescent areas at the nail bases, have been observed in several patients.

Diagnosis

The triad of Kayser-Fleischer rings, cirrhosis of the liver, and signs of basal ganglion disease is pathognomonic of this condition.

The various clinical findings combine to form several different clinical pictures, the most frequent of which is Parkinson's syndrome. Occasionally cerebellar ataxia, chorea, choreoathetosis, or dystonia predominates. If signs of liver insufficiency are not evident from physical examination, liver function studies or needle biopsy of the liver will demonstrate the presence of liver disease. Rubeanic acid stain may be used to demonstrate the excessive deposition of copper. In young patients in whom neurologic disease is not manifest and the signs of liver disease are marked, the condition has been confused with "juvenile" or "familial" cirrhosis.

The presence of hypocupremia, hypoceruloplasminemia, hypercupruria, and hyperaminoaciduria confirms the diagnosis, although it is rarely necessary to perform the difficult laboratory examinations in order to establish the diagnosis. In a rare patient with the disease, hypocupremia and hypoceruloplasminemia may not be present. Hypocupremia and hypoceruloplasminemia may be present in some normal individuals who are heterozygous for the gene. These two biochemical alterations are also present in all normal newborn infants and in at least some patients with kwashiorkor, sprue, celiac disease, and the nephrotic syndrome. Hypercupruria may be present only in the last condition mentioned. Hypercupruria may be present in patients with alcoholic cirrhosis of the liver, but the copper excreted rarely exceeds 200 μg per day; in this condition the concentration of copper and ceruloplasmin in the plasma is either normal or increased.

Prognosis

The disease is progressive and invariably fatal if untreated; death usually results from hepatic failure or intercurrent infection. There is now little doubt but that the early, continuous, and energetic therapy outlined below is associated with prolongation of life.

Treatment

The therapy of Wilson's disease is directed toward (1) the prevention of the continued accumulation of copper in the body and (2) the removal of copper already deposited.

Potassium sulfide (potash sulfurated technical, 20 mg three times daily with meals) prevents the absorption of copper by the formation of insoluble unabsorbable copper sulfide in the gut. This therapy is continued for 6 to 12 months and then discontinued. No undesirable side effects have been observed when such therapy has been given continuously for periods up to 5 years.

The administration of the copper chelating agent, penicillamine (β,β-dimethyl cysteine), results in the mobilization of copper from the tissues and an increase in its excretion in the urine. Therapy is started with 2 to 4 Gm daily in four divided doses on an empty stomach. Acute "sensitivity" reactions manifested by fever, skin rash, adenopathy, severe leukopenia, or thrombocytopenia develop in about one-third of patients. Desensitization, sometimes with corticosteroids, is required in such cases. Maintenance therapy with 1.5 Gm D-penicillamine daily should be given for the lifetime of the patient. Chronic administration of less than 2 Gm D-penicillamine is rarely associated with toxicity other than minor skin changes. Reversible optic neuritis and the nephrotic syndrome have followed the administration of the DL isomer but not the D isomer.

Therapy as outlined above results in clinical improvement beginning in several months and continuing for 6 to 12 months when stabilization occurs. If mental changes are present, they may revert toward normal, while the tremors and rigidity become less pronounced, sometimes to a remarkable degree. Liver function may improve and the Kayser-Fleischer rings diminish in intensity, but the plasma copper aberrations remain unchanged.

REFERENCES

Scheinberg, I. H., and I. Sternlieb: The Pathogenesis and Clinical Significance of the Liver Disease in Hepatolenticular Degeneration (Wilson's Disease), Med. Clin. N. Am., 44:665, 1960.

—— and I. Sternlieb: Wilson's Disease, Annual Rev. Med., 16:119, 1965.

Sternlieb, I., and I. H. Scheinberg: Penicillamine Therapy for Hepatolenticular Degeneration, J.A.M.A., 189:748, 1964.

Walshe, J. M., and J. N. Cumings: "Wilson's Disease: Some Current Concepts," Oxford, Blackwell Scientific Publications, Ltd., 1961.

Wilson, S. A. K.: Progressive Lenticular Degeneration: A Familial Nervous Disease Associated with Cirrhosis of the Liver, Brain, 34:395, 1912.

111 DISORDERS OF GLYCOGEN SYNTHESIS AND MOBILIZATION

Richard A. Field

The glycogen deposition diseases occupy a noteworthy place in the evolution of the conceptual approaches to the modern methods of study of disease. In 1952, Dr. Gerty T. Cori demonstrated by specific enzymatic studies of tissue from patients that von Gierke's disease is due to the loss of activity of a single tissue enzyme, and thus she provided a prototype for the study of genetically determined metabolic aberrations. Since the points of enzymatic abnormality of most of the syndromes to be discussed in this chapter concern the steps of synthesis and degradation between glucose 6-phosphate and glycogen, a working schema of these pathways is presented in Fig. 111-1. The Cori classification of glycogen deposition diseases is shown in Table 111-1.

Glucose 6-Phosphatase Deficiency Hepatorenal Glycogenosis

First described pathologically by von Gierke in 1929, this condition, characterized by enlargement of liver and kidneys and bouts of severe hypoglycemia, is probably the most frequent form of glycogenosis. Symptoms and recognizable clinical signs usually appear in the first year of life, and hepatomegaly may be detectable at birth. The disorder is transmitted as an autosomal mendelian recessive characteristic.

PATHOLOGIC PHYSIOLOGY. Under normal conditions hepatic glycogen serves as the main reservoir compound in the overall economy of blood glucose homeostasis. During and after ingestion of carbohydrate foods, a major portion of the glucose arriving in the liver via the portal system is phosphorylated and, by several intermediary steps, is stored as the regularly branched polysaccharide, glycogen (Chap. 75). During the postcibal period, peripheral utilization of glucose depletes circulating glucose, with the result that liver glycogen is depolymerized and free glucose is released into the hepatic vein (Chap. 75). The overall intracellular reactions in this process are called glycogenolysis, and the final enzymatic step is the hydrolytic dephosphorylation by the specific enzyme, hepatic glucose 6-phosphatase (Fig.

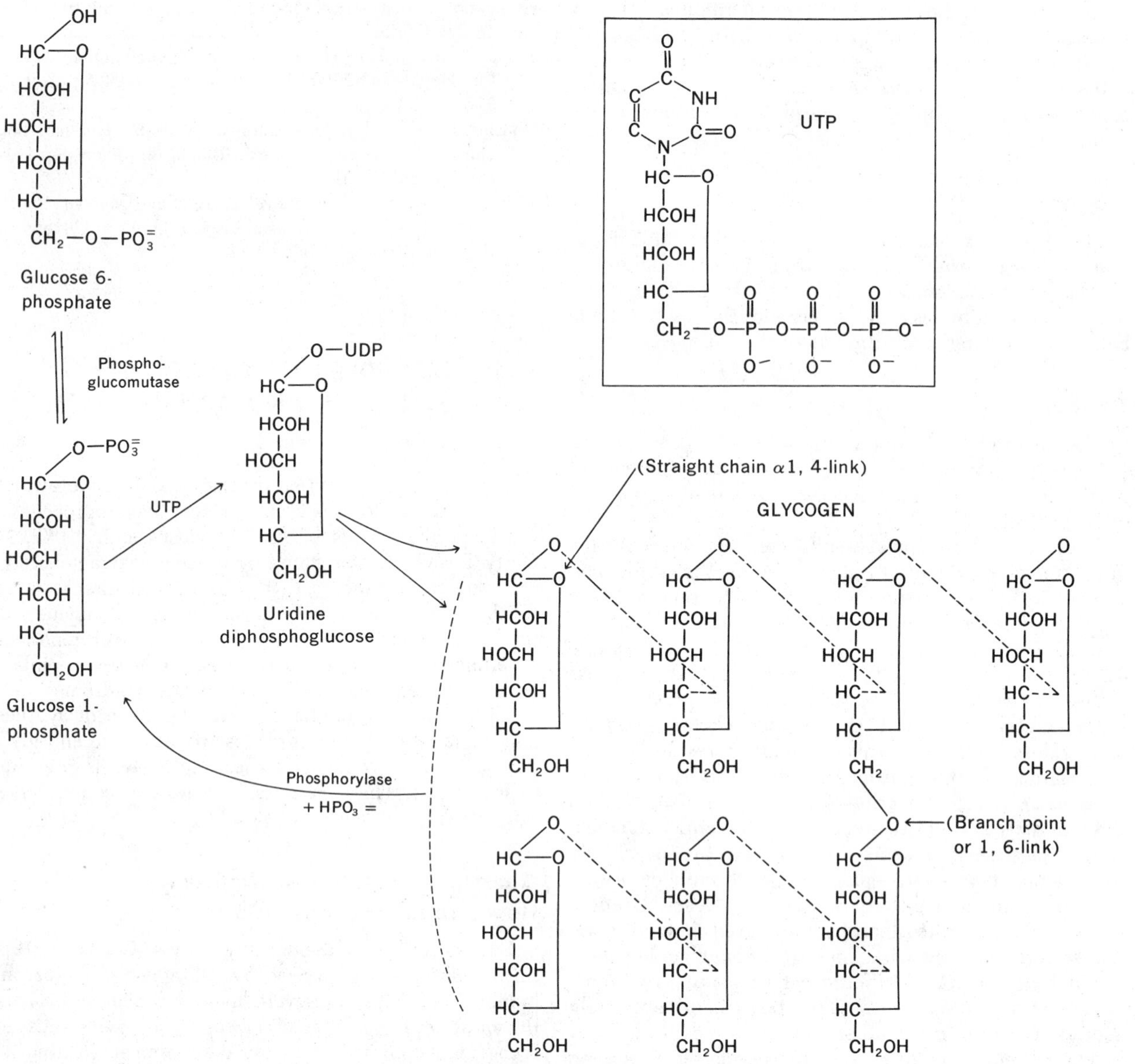

Fig. 111-1. Pathways of glycogen synthesis and breakdown.

111-1). Absence or marked reduction of this enzyme activity can be demonstrated by direct tissue assay in hepatorenal glycogenosis and accounts for most, if not all, of the metabolic disturbances noted in patients with this condition. The central feature of this limitation of hepatic glucose release is hypoglycemia, and it follows that little or no elevation of blood glucose concentration occurs following the injection of glucagon or epinephrine. Likewise, the normal expected rise in blood glucose level is not observed in patients with this hepatic enzyme deficiency following the intravenous administration of fructose or galactose. For all intents and purposes, these hexoses are metabolized solely by the liver and ultimately are converted intracellularly to glucose 6-phosphate, which, like the molecules of the same compound derived from glycogen depolymerization, cannot be dephos-

phorylated in the absence of glucose 6-phosphatase so as to appear in the bloodstream as free glucose. Apparently large quantities of glucose 6-phosphate are disposed of by increasing the amounts carried through the steps of anaerobic glycolysis resulting in an increased production and release of lactic and pyruvic acids; thus, hyperlacticacidemia is a characteristic finding in the syndrome and can be strikingly augmented by the administration of glucagon or other stimuli of hepatic glycogenolysis. Although ketonemia, lipemia, and keto-nuria are frequently observed, because of the relative un-availability of glycogen stores and the resultant hypo-glycemia which triggers mobilization of fat to meet energy requirements, marked and dangerous lacticacido-sis is also frequent and may supervene precipitously. It is believed that the chronic hyperlacticacidemia is respon-

Table 111-1. DISORDERS OF GLYCOGEN DEPOSITION AND MOBILIZATION

Cori type	Enzyme defect	Organ	Glycogen structure	Eponymic name	Suggested clinical name
1	Glucose 6-phosphatase	Liver, kidney, intestine (?)	Normal	von Gierke's disease	Glucose 6-phosphatase deficiency hepatorenal glycogenosis
2	α-Glucosidase (maltase)	Generalized	Normal	Pompe's disease	α-Glucosidase deficiency generalized glycogenosis
3	Amylo-1,6-glucosidase (debrancher)	Liver, heart, muscle, leukocytes	Abnormal; missing or very short outer chains	Forbes's disease	Debrancher deficiency limit dextrinosis
4	Amylo-(1,4:1,6) transglucosidase (brancher)	Liver, probably other organs	Abnormal; very long inner and outer unbranched chains	Andersen's disease	Brancher deficiency amylopectinosis
5	Muscle phosphorylase	Skeletal and cardiac muscle	Normal	McArdle-Schmid-Pearson disease	Myophosphorylase deficiency glycogenosis
6	Liver phosphorylase	Liver	Normal	Hers's disease	Hepatophosphorylase deficiency glycogenosis

sible for disturbance in renal clearance of water and accounts for the hyperuricemia seen in this condition. Chronic acidosis on a cellular level may play a role in the generally retarded growth, mild normochromic unresponsive anemia, hypophosphatemia, and generalized decreased bone density with mushrooming of the metaphyses and frequent fractures observed in these patients. Glycosuria and nonspecific aminoaciduria without aminoacidemia also occur and may be striking. It has been suggested that these findings correlate with the severity of glycogen infiltration and the hypothetically intracellular accumulation of phosphorylated hexoses in the renal tubular cells; but other impairments of renal function are not prominent.

PATHOLOGY. The liver is markedly enlarged, smooth, firm, and brownish in color. Microscopic study shows the liver cells to be enlarged up to three times the normal size and to be filled with glycogen and at times excessive amounts of fat. In the kidneys, which are usually at least double normal size, intracellular excess of glycogen is found in the cells of the proximal tubules. That the excess of glycogen persists in these organs long after death is not surprising when the nature of the biochemical defect is recalled.

CLINICAL PICTURE. The child is pale and undersized, with a fat face and neck and a markedly distended abdomen containing a huge, easily palpable liver without associated ascites or splenomegaly. Xanthomas with prominent lipemia may be a feature. Occasionally, epileptiform seizures and vomiting occur; however, more often the gravity and prevalence of the low blood sugar level are not appreciated until serious central nervous system deterioration has resulted.

LABORATORY EXAMINATIONS. These examinations reveal fasting hypoglycemia, hyperlipidemia, hyperlacticacidemia, anemia, and, at times, ketonemia and ketonuria. After glucose ingestion or infusion, the fall of blood levels may be delayed, yielding a pseudodiabetic curve. This may be explained as impaired capacity to increase the already superabundant stores of liver glycogen, rather than as a failure to utilize glucose at a normal rate in peripheral tissues. There is hypersensitivity to insulin, and severe prolonged hypoglycemia may follow its administration. Suspicion of this disorder is warranted when typical clinical characteristics are present and consonant results with glucagon or epinephrine challenge tests and of galactose or fructose infusion have been obtained. Final diagnosis, as with all glycogenoses, rests on biochemical assay of enzyme activity in biopsy material, in this instance, liver. In typical cases, liver glucose 6-phosphatase activity is found to be absent or reduced to less than 10 percent of normal. There is no ready explanation for the three cases reported in which glucose 6-phosphatase activity was either normal or only moderately reduced despite the careful characterization of the cases as clinically and pathophysiologically entirely consistent with the diagnosis.

DIFFERENTIAL DIAGNOSIS. The sporadic reports of cases of liver glycogenosis in which multiple enzymatic abnormalities in the glycogen pathways can be demonstrated and other cases in which members of the same kinship have distinctly different enzymatic lesions have given rise to both diagnostic and conceptual confusion. At present, it is not clear whether such cases result from secondarily induced adaptations, a close relationship of chromosomal genetic loci for determining and controlling the formation of the different enzymes, or from the influences of environmental factors. Until further investigations clarify these situations or augment the details of pathways of glycogen metabolism, the nonrestrictive labeling of cases that do not fit, either biochemically or functionally, into the classical groupings as simply "liver glycogen disease" seems wise.

TREATMENT. Although no means of increasing tissue activity levels of glucose 6-phosphatase in typical cases is available, earlier diagnosis, combined with recognition of hypoglycemia, acidosis, and intercurrent infection as the causes of morbidity and mortality, has markedly improved the life expectancy in this disease. The observation that the disturbances in metabolism and function in patients who survive beyond the fifth year tend to ameliorate provokes inquiry into the biochemical mechanisms by which such could occur and points to the necessity for assiduous care of the afflicted infant. It appears that in cases with prolonged survival the hyperuricemia and urate deposition which result, especially in the kidneys, become the major causes of difficulties. For this the daily administration of 0.5 to 2.0 Gm probenecid (Benemid) may be employed (Chap. 106).

The use of allopurinol, an inhibitor of urate formation, can also be recommended when secondary complications of hyperuricemia are manifested.

In a small number of cases, surgical transposition of the vena cava and the portal vein has been performed with clinical improvement in hypoglycemia. Diazoxide, a thiazide compound with capability of inhibiting insulin release, has been shown to improve hypoglycemia in one case.

α–Glucosidase Deficiency
Generalized Glycogenosis

This disorder, the most devastating form of glycogenosis, causes death within the first 2 years of life. It is marked by a generalized deposition of glycogen and by striking cardiomegaly. Symptoms and signs appear within 1 or 2 months after birth and quickly produce an infant with marked muscular hypotonia, enlarged tongue, cretinoid appearance, cardiomegaly, and neurologic deficits. Increased susceptibility to recurrent respiratory infections is based on poor ventilative and tussive efforts.

The structure of isolated glycogen is normal, and hyperglycemia promptly follows glucagon or epinephrine administration or the infusion of galactose or fructose. Glycogen accumulation in vacuoles located in the cytoplasm of almost all body cells occurs to a variable degree and is a process in which the leukocytes participate. The principal mechanisms of death are cardiac failure and aspiration pneumonitis. The disease is familial in occurrence, and the mode of inheritance appears to be through a single recessive autosomal gene.

Hers has demonstrated in the tissues of five affected infants the absence of a normally ubiquitous α-$(1 \rightarrow 4)$ glucosidase which has optimum activity in the acid range.

The enzyme characteristically hydrolyzes maltose and glycogen to glucose and can catalyze the transglucosylation from maltose to glycogen. Present hypotheses regarding glycogen metabolism do not provide a locus of influence at which this enzyme could effect glycogen deposition. Furthermore, spontaneous glycogenolysis occurs in excised tissues. Hers emphasizes the possible lysosomal nature of the enzyme and suggests that the polysaccharide accumulation is the result of a failure of physiologic digestion of areas of cytoplasm by the defective lysosomes. This interpretation is in agreement with the clinical observations of an absence of hypoglycemia, ketosis, and hyperlipidemia and the concept that the manifestations are the result of disruption of muscle fibers by the progressive glycogen accumulation. Although the clinical picture is highly characteristic, diagnosis depends on the demonstration of the absence of the acid α-$(1 \rightarrow 4)$ glucosidase in biopsy material.

Electron microscopic studies have demonstrated two forms of cytoplasmic glycogen aggregates, a monogranular and a multigranular. The ensacculated membrane-limited vacuoles found only in this condition probably represent lysosomes which have autophaged large amounts of monogranular glycogen and are unable to digest it because of their deficiency of acid maltase.

Treatment is unavailing, although chemotherapy of intercurrent bacterial respiratory infections appears to prolong life.

Debrancher Enzyme Deficiency (Limit Dextrinosis) and Brancher Enzyme Deficiency (Amylopectinosis)

These two conditions are the result of defects of the enzymes concerned with the formation and the disengagement of the branch points of the typically arborized glycogen molecule (3 and 4 in Table 111-1). In the first instance, there is a deficiency of the specific enzyme required for cleavage of the branch point bond, and therefore glycogenolysis is interrupted as the first branch point is reached and a glycogen of abnormal structure with excessively frequent branch points and shortened inner and outer chains results. When the branching enzyme is deficient, an unusually structured glycogen which possesses excessively lengthened inner and outer chains and a paucity of branch points is produced. Apparently, this structure formation, which resembles that of plant starch, gives the polysaccharide the physical characteristics which lead to its sequestration within the cells, where it acts as an irritative nidus, producing a characteristic increase in periportal connective tissue.

Limit dextrinosis is a relatively frequent type of glycogenosis; amylopectinosis is exceedingly rare, only two cases having been recognized. Since the clinical picture of the debrancher deficiency disturbance (limit dextrinosis) so closely resembles a mild form of the glucose 6-phosphatase deficiency, many cases of the former were mistakenly diagnosed as the latter before precise enzymatic assay techniques were available. The confusion need no longer arise even on clinical grounds or on the basis of functional tests, for in limit dextrinosis infusions of galactose lead to prompt intrahepatic conversion to glucose, with prompt hyperglycemia, there being no impediment to dephosphorylation and release. In the differential diagnosis in cases with equivocal hyperglycemic responses to glucagon or epinephrine and in which hepatomegaly, growth retardation, and a tendency to hypoglycemia and ketonuria contribute uncertainty, a liver biopsy need not be done, since it has been demonstrated that the debrancher enzyme is also absent in leukocytes, muscle, and erythrocytes. Furthermore, fasting levels of lactate and pyruvate are likely to be normal, in contrast to the situation with the type I case (glucose 6-phosphatase deficiency), where they are distinctly elevated. In the type III case, erythrocyte glycogen content is elevated, but again this is not so in the type I individual.

Prognosis for the type III defect appears to be relatively good, and at least two patients with this condition have reached the fifth decade of life. Logical treatment consists of a high protein, relatively low fat diet, with frequent feedings, prompt treatment of intercurrent infections, and prohibition of strenuous exercise, cardiodepressant drugs, and anesthetics, since the myocardium is involved.

Glycogen Deposition Syndromes Due to Deficiencies of Glycogen Phosphorylases

Glycogen phosphorylase (5, Table 111-1) catalyzes glycogen depolymerization by phosphorylytic cleavage to yield glucose 1-phosphate and thus mediates the major initiating step in making the glucose moieties available for metabolism. In the liver the bulk of the glucose derived from the action of this enzyme ultimately defends the level of blood sugar and maintains an adequate supply for the peripheral tissues, while in the muscle the phosphorylase-produced hexose phosphate provides an immediate fuel source for the energy demanded by quick, sharp increases in contractile activity. Muscle and liver phosphorylase are distinctly different proteins immunologically, structurally, and functionally, and it appears that each has its own genetic determinant. Both enzyme activities are enhanced by epinephrine, while only liver phosphorylase responds in vivo to injections of glucagon.

Myophosphorylase Deficiency Glycogenosis (McArdle)

A group of patients consisting of members of several unrelated families have been shown to be lacking in muscle phosphorylase activity. None has any growth retardation, disturbance in carbohydrate economy, or abnormality of response to glucagon or epinephrine administration. However, they have in common an incapacity to perform prolonged or strenuous muscle work and are excessively sensitive to ischemic conditions in this regard because of the occurrence of weakness, pain, and spasm of the exercised muscle. The demonstration of the isolated absence of muscle phosphorylase adequately explains the clinical phenomena when the importance of brisk glycogenolysis in supplying substrate for anaerobic glycolysis during ischemic muscle work is recalled. The impediment limiting the acceleration and augmentation of anaerobic glycolysis thus curtails increased lactate production. The failure to detect a significant rise in lactate concentration in the venous return from a muscle working under imposed ischemic conditions is a useful diagnostic test. A modest excess of glycogen in the muscles has been described, and in some cases prolonged exercise may cause breakdown of muscle cells and myoglobinuria. Although it has been shown that cardiac muscle shares the defect, no cardiac disturbance on this account has been described.

Since liver phosphorylase is normal in amount and activity, patients do quite well provided they accept limitations in excertion, protect themselves from tight garments that produce muscle ischemia, and fortify themselves with exogenous carbohydrates before attempting unusual physical tasks.

Hepatophosphorylase Deficiency Glycogenosis (Hers)

Isolated development of hepatomegaly in infancy or childhood with a tendency to fasting hypoglycemia due to excessive accumulation of hepatic glycogen of normal structure characterizes this condition. Little in the way of other metabolic or developmental disturbance accrues as a consequence of the sluggish glycogenolysis which results from the absent or markedly reduced hepatophosphorylase activity. The deficiency of the enzyme can be demonstrated biochemically in hepatic tissue or in leukocytes. A possibly contingent deficiency of glucose 6-phosphate dehydrogenase has been described in some cases. No therapy beyond avoidance of prolonged fasting and the administration of a high protein diet with frequent feedings appears to be necessary. The mechanism of failure of hyperglycemic response to glucagon or epinephrine is obvious, and the normal response to galactose infusion as well as the normal serum lactate level and lack of hyperlipemia allows easy differentiation of this disease from the more devastating glucose 6-phosphatase deficiency. Transmission appears to be by means of an autosomal recessive gene.

REFERENCES

Cori, G. T.: Glycogen Structure and Enzyme Deficiencies in Glycogen Storage Disease, Harvey Lectures, 48:145, 1952–1953.

——: "Glycogen Metabolism," Ciba Symposium, Boston, Little, Brown and Company, 1964.

Hers, H. G.: Glycogen Storage Disease, in "Advances in Metabolic Disorders," Vol. 1, Academic Press Inc., New York, 1964.

Stanbury, J. B., J. B. Wyngaarden, and D. S. Fredrickson: "The Metabolic Basis of Inherited Disease," 2d ed., New York, McGraw-Hill Book Company, 1966.

Van Creveld, S.: Glycogen Disease, Arch. Dis. Child., 34:298, 1959.

112 GALACTOSEMIA
Kurt J. Isselbacher

Galactosemia is an inborn error of metabolism associated with an impairment in the conversion of galactose to glucose and its derivatives. The disease is due to a congenital absence of a specific enzyme, galactose 1-phosphate uridyl transferase.

Clinical Features

The disease manifests itself shortly after birth when the afflicted infant is exposed to galactose (in the form of lactose) in cow's milk or breast milk. Vomiting and diarrhea occur, and as a result there is an impairment in nutrition or failure to thrive. Jaundice may then become evident, together with enlargement of the liver and spleen. The clinical picture at this point may readily be confused with that of hepatitis. If the dietary ingestion of milk or galactose continues, cataracts are likely to form, followed by the development of mental retardation. Cataracts may be evident at three or four weeks of age; several months may elapse before mental retardation is recognized. When blood galactose levels are very high, episodes of hypoglucosemia may occur and may be associated with convulsions.

If the infant is examined shortly after the ingestion of milk, galactose will be found in the blood as well as in the urine. The urine will also show an increase in amino acids (predominantly of the neutral type), and occasionally albuminuria is observed. It must be remembered that if, because of vomiting, no milk has been ingested, galactosuria will probably not be found.

All the clinical features except for mental retardation may regress completely when galactose is removed from the diet. The jaundice will readily subside, together with a diminution of the hepatosplenomegaly. Although cirrhosis of the liver may occur in the untreated galactosemic patient, only a residual fibrosis may remain in later years in patients who have been treated. Cataracts may improve greatly and, in fact, have been known to disappear completely on a galactose-free diet. Unfortunately, mental retardation is a lifelong feature, and once it has developed it is not reversible.

Pathologic Physiology

Both breast milk and cow's milk have as their sole content of carbohydrate the disaccharide lactose. This sugar is split within the intestinal epithelial cell into its component monosaccharides, namely, galactose and glu-cose. The infant with galactosemia has difficulty in converting the galactose that is liberated to glucose and its derivatives. The main enzymes and the reactions involved in galactose utilization by the mammalian organism are as follows:

1. Galactokinase:
   $$\text{Galactose} + \text{ATP} \rightarrow \text{galactose 1-phosphate} + \text{ADP}$$
2. Galactose 1-phosphate uridyl transferase:
   $$\text{Galactose 1-phosphate} + \text{UDP-glucose} \rightarrow$$
   $$\text{UDP-galactose} + \text{glucose 1-phosphate}$$
3. UDP-galactose-4-epimerase:
   $$\text{DPN}$$
   $$\text{UDP-galactose} \rightleftharpoons \text{UDP-glucose}$$
4. UDP-galactose-pyrophosphorylase:
   $$\text{UTP} + \text{galactose 1-phosphate} \rightleftharpoons \text{UDP-galactose}$$
   $$+ \text{pyrophosphate}$$
5. Direct oxidation of galactose:
   $$\text{Galactose} \rightarrow \text{galactonolactone} \rightarrow \text{galactonate} \rightarrow$$
   $$\rightarrow \beta\text{-keto-galactonic acid} \rightarrow \text{xylulose} + CO_2$$

It is seen from these reactions that the first step in galactose utilization consists in its conversion to galactose 1-phosphate by the enzyme galactokinase. The galactose 1-phosphate must then be converted to glucose 1-phosphate; this is accomplished by the second reaction, catalyzed by the enzyme galactose 1-phosphate uridyl transferase. It is this enzyme and this reaction which are deficient in galactosemia. As a consequence, galactose 1-phosphate accumulates in the tissues. The epimerase serves to interconvert UDP-galactose and UDP-glucose and is a mechanism whereby normally in a galactosemic individual, galactose-containing substances, especially those found in brain lipids, may be synthesized from glucose even in the absence of dietary galactose. The fourth enzyme occurs mostly in liver, and it will be observed that it allows for some conversion of galactose 1-phosphate to UDP-galactose by a mechanism other than the transferase reaction. A fifth enzyme system has also been shown whereby galactose is directly oxidized by galactose dehydrogenase leading eventually to the liberation of CO_2 and xylulose. It has been suggested that one or both of these latter two pathways may account for the partial oxidation of galactose in patients with galactosemia and perhaps in part for the improved galactose tolerance which occurs in some of these patients with increasing age.

The present evidence indicates that a number of the toxic symptoms found in galactosemia may be related to the accumulation of galactose 1-phosphate in the tissues. This sugar accumulates in lens, liver, and red cells and has been shown to inhibit the enzyme phosphoglucomutase. However, the mechanism whereby this accumulation and subsequent enzyme inhibition lead to changes such as hepatic fibrosis and central nervous system damage has not yet been determined. One observation suggests that cataract formation may be related to the accumulation of a nonphosphorylated derivative of galactose (galactitol) in the lens. The reduction in blood glucose levels in association with elevated galactose levels in the blood appears to be due to a decreased hepatic output of glucose. The basis for the aminoaciduria is not completely understood, but in animal studies (with intestine and kidney slices) it has been observed that sugars such as galactose tend to inhibit the transport of certain groups of amino acids.

Diagnosis

The usual clue to the diagnosis consists of the clinical picture described above, together with the finding of a reducing sugar in the urine. Such a urine will give a positive reaction to Benedict's test (copper reduction) but a negative glucose oxidase test. If the urine is chromatographed, it shows predominantly galactose rather than glucose. If these initial screening tests suggest the diagnosis of galactosemia, then more specific tests are necessary.

In the past galactose tolerance tests have been performed which typically show a delayed clearance of galactose from the bloodstream when the sugar was given by mouth or intravenously. However, because of the toxicity of this sugar in the patient with galactosemia and because of the availability of more specific tests, this procedure is no longer recommended. The specific diagnostic test for this disease consists in the demonstration of the absence of galactose 1-phosphate uridyl transferase in the patient's red blood cells. In this test, the cells are incubated together with the two substrates, galactose 1-phosphate and UDP-glucose. After a period of incubation, the amount of uridine diphosphate glucose remaining is determined. In the normal individual the UDP-glucose disappears, because of the presence of the transferase in the red cells, but in galactosemia no utilization of UDP-glucose occurs when it is incubated in the presence of galactose 1-phosphate.

It is also possible to measure the transferase deficiency indirectly by a number of other procedures. For example, one may incubate red cells with galactose and demonstrate either enzymatically or chromatographically that galactose 1-phosphate accumulates. One may also incubate red cells or whole blood with radioactive galactose. Normal cells will oxidize the galactose, and, thus, radioactive carbon dioxide (CO_2) will be produced, but in the galactosemic cells, very little of any radioactive CO_2 will be liberated because of the defect in the oxidation of galactose.

Differential Diagnosis

The most important condition from which galactosemia needs to be differentiated in the neonatal period is primary liver disease, either acute or chronic. It must be recalled that in the presence of decreased liver function, galactose removal from the bloodstream is impaired, and as a consequence, both elevated blood galactose levels and galactosuria may be found. However, in liver disease (either hepatitis or cirrhosis) normal levels of red cell transferase are found and galactose utilization and oxidation by red cells or whole blood are completely normal.

Since these patients are often seen when nausea, vomiting, and diarrhea have developed and therefore dietary intake of galactose may be minimal, it must be emphasized that neither elevated blood nor urine galactose levels will be found in the absence of recent dietary intake of this sugar. Hence, an analysis of the blood and urine at these times may be misleading.

Treatment

The treatment of this disease consists in the exclusion of galactose and galactose-containing foods from the diet. In early infancy this involves the elimination of lactose as well as galactose. The milk substitutes which have been used effectively are Dextri-Maltose and Nutramigen. Soybean preparations have been used in the past, but they possess galactose-containing polysaccharides and should be avoided. As indicated above, fairly dramatic improvement will occur when the infant is placed on a galactose-free diet, and all symptoms except for the mental retardation may improve completely. These patients must remain on very restricted galactose diets until they have reached adequate physical and neurologic development.

Genetics

Abundant evidence has been obtained to indicate that this is a disorder transmitted by an autosomal recessive gene. Specific enzyme studies have demonstrated both parents to be heterozygous with respect to galactose 1-phosphate uridyl transferase activities in their red cells. The exact incidence of this disease has not been determined, but the most recent data indicate that cases may be as frequent as 1 in 18,000 births. The occurrence of the carrier state is believed to be 1 out of 130 individuals.

REFERENCES

Hansen, R. G., R. K. Bretthauer, J. Mayes, and J. H. Nordin: Estimation of Frequency of Occurrence of Galactosemia in the Population, Proc. Soc. Exp. Biol. Med., 115:560, 1964.

Isselbacher, K. J.: Galactosemia, pp. 178–188 in J. B. Stanbury, J. B. Wyngaarden, and D. S. Fredrickson (Eds.), "The Metabolic Basis of Inherited Disease," 2d ed., New York, McGraw-Hill Book Company, 1966.

Kalckar, H. M., E. P. Anderson, and K. J. Isselbacher: Galactosemia: Congenital Defect in a Nucleotide Transferase, Biochim. Biophys. Acta, 20:262, 1956.

113 DISORDERS OF LIPID METABOLISM AND XANTHOMATOSIS

Donald S. Fredrickson

Lipidosis is a general term applied to disorders characterized by abnormal concentrations of lipids in tissues

Table 113-1. LIPIDOSES AND XANTHOMATOSES

I. Abnormal plasma lipoprotein concentrations (dyslipo-
proteinemias)
  A. Hyperlipoproteinemia
    1. Type I (hyperchylomicronemia; exogenous hyper-
glyceridemia)
      a. Familial lipoprotein lipase deficiency
      b. Acquired with dysproteinemias
    2. Type II (hyperbetalipoproteinemia; hypercholes-
terolemia)
      a. Familial (familial hypercholesterolemia)
      b. Acquired
    3. Type III (beta-lipoproteins of abnormal density)
      a. Familial ("broad beta disease;" "xanthoma
tuberosum")
      b. Acquired
    4. Type IV (hyperprebetalipoproteinemia; endog-
enous hyperglyceridemia)
      a. Familial
      b. Acquired
    5. Type V (hyperchylomicronemia and hyperprebeta-
lipoproteinemia; mixed hyperglyceridemia)
      a. Familial
      b. Acquired
    6. Other (including hyperlipidemia of obstructive
jaundice)
  B. Hypolipoproteinemia
    1. Abetalipoproteinemia (familial absence of low-
density lipoproteins)
    2. Hypobetalipoproteinemia
      a. Familial
      b. Acquired
    3. Tangier disease (familial alpha-lipoprotein defi-
ciency)
    4. Familial deficiency of lecithin: cholesterol acyl-
transferase (with alpha-lipoprotein deficiency)
II. Primary tissue lipid storage diseases
  A. Sphingolipidoses
    1. Glucosylceramidoses
      a. Gangliosidoses ("familial amaurotic idiocies")
        1) G_{M_1} gangliosidosis (generalized gangliosido-
sis)
        2) G_{M_2} gangliosidosis (Tay-Sachs disease)
        3) G_{M_3} gangliosidosis
      b. Glucosylcerebrosidoses (Gaucher's disease)
        1) Infantile (CNS involvement)
        2) Juvenile (CNS involvement)
        3) Adult (no CNS involvement)
      c. Trihexosidosis (Fabry's disease; angiokeratoma
corporis diffusum)
    2. Galactosylceramidoses
      a. Galactosylsulfatidosis (metachromatic leuko-
dystrophy; Scholz's disease; Greenfield's disease)
      b. Galactosylcerebrosidosis (Krabbe's disease)
    3. Phosphorylceramidoses (sphingomyelin lipidoses)
      a. Sphingomyelinase deficient
        1) Classical infantile form (Niemann-Pick dis-
ease)
        2) Visceral form without CNS involvement
      b. Sphingomyelinase present
        1) Late CNS involvement
        2) Nova Scotia variant

  B. Storage of less polar lipids
    1. Phytanic oxidase deficiency (storage of 3,7,11,15-
tetramethyl hexanoic acid; Refsum's disease)
    2. Cholesterol ester and triglyceride storage with
adrenal calcification (Wolman's disease)
    3. Hepatic cholesterol ester storage disease
    4. Ceroid storage
III. Granulomatous diseases with lipid storage
  A. Histiocytosis X (xanthoma disseminatum, eosinophilic
granuloma, Hand-Schüller-Christian disease, Letterer-
Siwe disease)
  B. Lipoid proteinosis (Urbach-Wiethe disease)
  C. Lipoid dermatoarthritis
  D. Disseminated lipogranulomatosis (Farber's disease)
  E. Hereditary tendinous and tuberous xanthomatosis
without hyperlipidemia
  F. Cerebrotendinous xanthomatosis
IV. Xanthomas
  A. Simple (xanthelasma, juvenile xanthoma)
  B. Associated with trauma and chronic infections
V. Adipose tissue disorders
  A. Relapsing panniculitis (Weber-Christian disease)
  B. Lipodystrophy
    1. Lipomas
    2. Adiposis dolorosa (Dercum's disease)
    3. Insulin lipodystrophy
  C. Lipoatrophy
    1. Partial (progressive lipodystrophy)
    2. Total (lipoatrophic diabetes mellitus)

or in extracellular fluid. Sometimes it is restricted to only those abnormalities of lipid metabolism that are inheritable. *Xanthomatosis* is a morphologic term referring to lipid accumulation in tissues in association with large "foam cells." The list of lipidoses and xanthomatoses in Table 113-1 encompasses most of the *primary* disturbances in lipid metabolism and includes some disorders in which secondary lipid storage is prominent and some of the disorders of adipose tissue. Omitted are several disorders in which lipids accumulate concomitant with primary abnormalities in metabolism of other substances. Noteworthy among these are mucopolysaccharidoses (gargoylism) and the glycogen storage diseases.

PLASMA LIPOPROTEIN ABNORMALITIES

The commonest of the lipidoses are those associated with primary alterations in concentrations of the plasma lipids. These can be better understood when considered in terms of lipoproteins, the form in which nearly all lipids, except for free fatty acids, are present in plasma. Both selective increases or severe deficiency and absence of some of the groups or classes of lipoproteins can occur. Abnormalities in the lipoproteins themselves may characterize a few disorders.

HYPERLIPOPROTEINEMIA

Increased concentrations of plasma lipids and lipoproteins represent metabolic problems that are difficult both to classify and to treat. Diagnosis requires two major steps: (1) Reasonable delineation of the dominant abnormality in the lipoprotein pattern. This may usually be estimated from measurement of plasma cholesterol *and* triglyceride concentrations; further qualitative information about the four major lipoprotein classes (Table 113-2) may be required and obtained by either electrophoresis or ultracentrifugation. The former is more practical, the latter more quantitative. (2) Separation of secondary (acquired) from primary (mainly, inheritable or familial) hyperlipoproteinemia. For this purpose evidence of familial involvement and a careful examination of skin and tendons for xanthomas are essential. Helpful ancillary information can also be gained by a careful history of diet, estimates of glucose tolerance, response of lipoproteins to controlled diets, and measurements of plasma postheparin lipolytic activity (PHLA).

The classification of hyperlipoproteinemia is undergoing rapid evolution. At present a useful method is

Table 113-2. CLASSIFICATION OF LIPOPROTEINS

Lipoproteins*	Synonyms	Component lipids† Cholesterol phospholipids triglyceride		
Chylomicrons	Exogenous glyceride in particles of $S\hat{f} > 400$; primary and secondary particles	+	+	++++
β-lipoprotein	Low-density lipoproteins (LDL) of $S\hat{f}$ 0–20; density 1.006–1.063	++++	+++	+
Pre-β-lipoprotein	Very low-density lipoproteins (VLDL) of $S\hat{f}$ 20–400; density < 1.006; α_2-lipoprotein; "hyperlipemic" particles of endogenous origin	++	++	+++
α_1-lipoprotein	High-density lipoproteins (HDL); density 1.063–1.21	+++	++++	+

* As defined by paper electrophoresis according to technique of Lees and Hatch (J. Lab. Clin. Med., 61:518, 1963).

† Indicating the relative degree to which the concentrations of plasma lipids will be altered by an increase in the species of lipoproteins.

based on five major types of abnormal lipoprotein patterns (Table 113-1).

These patterns usually do not represent specific diseases and require modifiers for proper diagnostic use, e.g., "type I hyperlipoproteinemia, familial"; "type II hyperlipoproteinemia, familial, heterozygote with xanthoma tendinosum"; or "type V hyperlipoproteinemia, secondary to diabetes mellitus." Each major type is associated with particular clinical manifestations and responds to different forms of therapy. The index lipoprotein patterns described below are those obtained in the postabsorptive state (12 to 14 hr after the last meal) and while the patient is eating a normal diet (approximately 20, 40, and 40 percent of calories coming from protein, fat, and carbohydrate, respectively).

Type I Hyperlipoproteinemia

DEFINITION. Normally, chylomicrons are not visible on paper electrophoresis in the postabsorptive state and less than 30 mg per 100 ml are obtained by ultracentrifugation. In the type I pattern there is marked hyperchylomicronemia and a decrease in all other lipoproteins. The plasma is milky and, after standing overnight at 4° centigrade, contains a cream layer over a clear infranatant layer. The triglyceride concentration ranges between 1,500 to 15,000 mg per 100 ml; cholesterol is abnormally high when the glycerides exceed 1,000. The ratio of cholesterol to glyceride concentrations is very low, <0.15. Within 3 to 5 days after institution of a fat-free diet, chylomicrons disappear, a modest increase in prebeta lipoproteins occurs, and beta- and alpha-lipoproteins increase but remain low; the plasma clears, glycerides are in the range of 200 to 400, and cholesterol is <150. Classical type I is seen under two conditions: one, a familial syndrome; the other, in association with dysglobulinemia.

FAMILIAL TYPE I. Hyperlipemia (lactescent plasma or serum due to hyperglyceridemia) dependent upon dietary fat intake was first reported in a child by Bürger and Grütz in 1932; and familial incidence was recorded by Holt, Aylward, and Timbres shortly thereafter. About 100 cases have since been discovered. This exogenous, or *fat-induced, hyperlipemia* is due to an inherited defect in removal of chylomicrons from plasma. The enzyme lipoprotein lipase probably plays an important role in this process in adipose tissue and perhaps at the endothelial wall in other tissues. The enzyme is "released" into plasma by heparin, and patients with this syndrome have uniquely low postheparin lipolytic activity and low levels of lipoprotein lipase in adipose tissue. The metabolic defect in the disease must still be demonstrated precisely, but all examples thus far appear to be homozygous for a relatively rare mutant gene.

Clinical picture. The disease is usually detected within the first decade, although sometimes not until early adulthood, usually when marked hyperlipemia is discovered during work-up for either sudden appearance of eruptive xanthomas, moderate hepatosplenomegaly, or bouts of severe abdominal pain. These abnormalities are only suggestive and not diagnostic for this type of hyperlipemia. The episodic abdominal pain usually follows a period of high fat intake. It is usually epigastric or midabdominal, rarely radiates to the back, and can be associated with signs of peritoneal irritation and fever, mimicking a number of "acute abdominal emergencies." Pancreatitis may develop, although, when associated with chronic pancreatitis, hyperlipemia may often be the result rather than the cause. There is no evidence that familial hyperchylomicronemia is associated with accelerated vascular disease, and the major hazard appears to be accumulation of fat in reticuloendothelial tissues and the precipitation of abdominal crises. Glucose tolerance is usually normal.

Diagnosis. The typical lipid and lipoprotein pattern and other manifestations in an otherwise healthy child or young adult provide a presumptive diagnosis if the acquired form has been specifically excluded. A fat-free diet should be administered for 1 week; the predicted changes in lipoproteins should occur rapidly. A *modest reduction* of hyperlipemia, which occurs in many patients on low-fat diets, is not diagnostic of this particular syndrome. Postheparin lipolytic activity should be demonstrated to be deficient by one of several in vitro tests. Parents will have low normal PHLA and usually normal plasma lipids. One or more siblings may have the type I pattern and low PHLA. The full-blown disease occurs in either sex.

Treatment. To avoid the crippling attacks of abdominal pain, pancreatitis, and foam cell accumulation in liver, spleen, and bone marrow seen in most cases, it is recommended that the daily intake of fat not represent more than 25 percent of calories, or 50 Gm fat per day. Both saturated and unsaturated fats are cleared poorly. Commercial preparations of medium chain glycerides, such as Protagen, offer means of occasionally satisfying craving for fat without inducing chylomicronemia, since these glycerides go directly to the liver in the portal vein.

ACQUIRED TYPE I. The typical lipoprotein pattern and other manifestations have been found in patients with systemic lupus erythematosus, myeloma, macroglobulinemia, lymphomas, or other diseases in which there are abnormal circulating globulins or other proteins. Heparin resistance, possibly due to heparin binding by the abnormal protein, is manifested by decreased prolongation of thrombin time. PHLA is abnormally low unless the usual test dose of 10 units per kg is greatly increased. The hyperlipoproteinemia fluctuates with changes in the plasma protein abnormality. Treatment is directed toward the underlying disease.

Type II Hyperlipoproteinemia

DEFINITION. This common pattern is characterized by increased concentrations of beta-lipoproteins. Both S_f 0 to 12 and 12 to 20 classes may be increased. Plasma cholesterol is elevated, and usually the plasma is quite clear. Particularly in familial cases there may be accompanying modest increases in prebeta-lipoproteins with associated elevation in plasma triglycerides, usually not above 300 mg per 100 ml. In the latter event the plasma may be slightly turbid. The C/T ratio is nearly always > 1 and can sometimes be > 10. Lipoprotein and lipid levels are relatively constant. The influence of dietary cholesterol, saturated fat (S), and polyunsaturated fat (P) upon plasma cholesterol concentrations is mainly expressed in changes in beta-lipoproteins. The definition of hypercholesterolemia or hyperbetalipoproteinemia is arbitrary due to the spread of usual lipoprotein levels in Americans. In young men, cholesterol concentrations > 260 mg per 100 ml are clearly associated with increased incidence of premature atherosclerosis.

FAMILIAL TYPE II (Familial Hypercholesterolemia). History and Clinical Picture. This syndrome was first described in the latter half of the nineteenth century in terms of its usual xanthomatous and atheromatous manifestations. Once called *xanthoma tendinosum* and sometimes termed *essential hypercholesterolemia,* it appears to represent the expression of a highly penetrant mutant at an autosomal locus primarily regulating plasma beta-lipoprotein concentrations. The heterozygote may have normal cholesterol concentrations in cord blood and during the first year. By age one the type II pattern is evident. In the first or second decade, xanthomas may begin in the Achilles or extensor tendons of the hands. Later these may involve plantar or other tendons and tibial tuberosites, and tuberous xanthomas may appear on the elbows. Ankles, knees, toes, or other joints involved with xanthomas may become tender and inflamed. The attacks usually last a few days, regress spontaneously, and can be confused with gout. Xanthelasma or arcus cornea is common. Some heterozygous patients never have xanthomas. The homozygous abnormal patient generally has higher beta-lipoprotein and cholesterol concentrations (> 500 mg per 100 ml) and will usually develop xanthomas between birth and age ten. These are generally florid and often include chamois-colored skin xanthomas on the hands, plantar, or (rarely) palmar surfaces, in the popliteal space, and on the buttocks. Homozygotes particularly are prone to premature ischemic heart disease, aortic stenosis, and atherosclerosis in peripheral and cerebral vessels. Abnormal glucose tolerance and hyperuricemia are not distinguishing features. The genetic expression varies considerably, xanthomatosis and the degree of hyperbetalipoproteinemia tending to be more similar within than between affected families.

Diagnosis. There is no absolute test for phenotype, but diagnosis can be fairly precise. All possible acquired causes must first be excluded. The heterozygote usually has a cholesterol concentration between 300 and 500 mg per 100 ml (>250 before age ten) and beta-lipoprotein cholesterols are usually >250. Diagnosis requires the type II pattern plus either (1) typical xanthomas or (2) the type II pattern in at least one parent or sibling. The homozygote usually has about double the lipoprotein abnormality of the heterozygote; at present ascertainment of this genotype requires demonstration of type II in both parents or, at least, both parental lines. The association of increased prebeta-lipoproteins and triglycerides in some patients varies in the same sibship and does not now constitute evidence of a different disease.

It may be due to concomitant presence of other genes, particularly that for diabetes.

Treatment. The first step in treatment of any primary hyperlipoproteinemia is diet. Reduction to ideal body weight does not influence familial type II patterns; it is nevertheless advisable, considering the increased hazard for vascular disease. A diet designed to increase polyunsaturated fatty acids and decrease saturated fatty acids and cholesterol to the maximum practical extent should be rigorously followed. It is most effective in children, will decrease lipoprotein levels in nearly all patients, but rarely, if ever, normalizes them. The total amount of fat or carbohydrate in the diet does not have a significant relationship to lipoprotein levels in most familial type II patients. Following achievement of maximum effect by diet, a drug may be used. The agent of choice is cholestyramine given in three divided doses to a total of 24 to 48 Gm per day (adult dose). If the chief but uncommon side effects, nausea, constipation, or steatorrhea, prove uncommon side effects, nausea, constipation, or steatorrhea, prove unmanageable, clofibrate (2.0 Gm per day) or d-thyroxin (4 to 8 mg per day) may be substituted. Failure of a drug to lower cholesterol concentrations by less than 15 percent in 4 to 6 weeks is an indication for its discontinuance. Exceptions are younger xanthomatous patients who may be mobilizing tissue lipid stores without changes in plasma lipid levels. In these cases drugs may be maintained if xanthomas appear to be softening.

ACQUIRED TYPE II. Acquired type II hyperbetalipoproteinemia may reach levels seen in hetrozygotes for the familial disorder, but usually the plasma cholesterol levels are below 300 mg per 100 ml. Xanthelasma may be seen in patients with normolipoproteinemia, but tendon and tuberous xanthomas usually occur only in familial hyperlipoproteinemia. The diagnosis of acquired type II requires the elimination of familial involvement. If both parents are clearly normal, familial type II is excluded. The acquired pattern must then be differentiated into primary or secondary forms. The type II lipoprotein pattern can be seen in hypothyroidism, the nephrotic syndrome, some dysproteinemias including macroglobulinemia, diabetes mellitus, and possibly other diseases. The commonest cause of primary nonfamilial type II is dietary excess. Many Americans normally eat twice the average intake of 600 mg of cholesterol per day, associated with high amounts of saturated fats. A prompt fall to normal cholesterol levels on a diet restricted in cholesterol and saturated fats and high in polyunsaturated fats is both a good diagnostic test and adequate therapy (Table 275-6). It has not yet been proved that hypolipidemic agents are useful or necessary in treatment of acquired type II.

Type III Hyperlipoproteinemia

DEFINITION. This pattern is characterized by a heavy broad beta-lipoprotein band on electrophoresis. The unique feature is the presence of beta-migrating lipoproteins of density < 1.006, a test which requires preparative ultracentrifugation. The profile in the analytical ultracentrifuge is characterized by a bizarre increase in lipoproteins from about S_f 12 to 70. There are usually increased prebeta-lipoproteins and often very modest hyperchylomicronemia. The cholesterol and glyceride concentrations fluctuate considerably and often are very similar, lying usually between 200 and 1,000 mg per 100 ml. Type III hyperlipoproteinemia is almost always due to a familial disorder, apparently a recessive gene, requiring the homozygous phenotype for clinical expression. It has only recently been established as a disease, the first cases being described as *xanthoma tuberosum* by Gofman and co-workers in 1954.

FAMILIAL TYPE III. Clinical Picture. The disorder is usually detected after age twenty, earlier in men than in women. In addition to the typical lipoprotein pattern, two-thirds of patients have peculiar raised yellow plaques (plane xanthomas) in the palmar creases or on the fingers. Most of these also have soft, reddish-yellow, single or confluent xanthomas on the elbows. Some have pedunculated xanthomas on the buttocks, elsewhere on the limbs, and a few have tendon xanthomas. The majority of patients have intermittent claudication and evidence of decreased blood flow in the lower extremities; some have premature ischemic heart and cerebrovascular disease. The majority of patients have glucose intolerance, many are hypersecretors of insulin. Practically all are abnormally "carbohydrate-inducible," in terms of an exaggerated rise of plasma glycerides on high carbohydrate feeding. Hyperuricemia may be present.

Etiology. The basis for the disorder is not known. Triglycerides appear to associate with beta-lipoproteins in such a way that their efflux from plasma is retarded, and abnormal very low density lipoproteins with a peculiarly high cholesterol content persist in plasma. The beta-lipoproteins appear to be identical in immunochemical behavior to those in normals or other types of hyperlipoproteinemia.

Diagnosis. The ascertainment of the anomalous lipoprotein pattern is necessary for absolute diagnosis. However, the lipid pattern combined with other clinical features, particularly palmar xanthomas and the response to therapy, allow a presumptive diagnosis, and this is enhanced if a parent, sibling, or adult offspring can be demonstrated to have the same abnormalities. Due to the recessive character or low penetrance, both parents are usually normal, as are the majority of other first-degree relatives. The frequency of type IV patterns is also abnormally high in affected families. Familial types II and III have not been observed in the same kindreds.

Treatment. The lipoprotein pattern and plasma lipids can usually be returned to normal in type III with appropriate treatment. The skin xanthomas also disappear, allowing a presumption that treatment may desirably affect the hazard for premature vascular disease. Treatment consists sequentially of (1) reduction to ideal weight; (2) institution of a rigorous diet, with special attention to keeping carbohydrate intake below 5 Gm per kg per day by increasing the intake of polyunsaturated fat if necessary; and (3) clofibrate, 2 Gm per day. The therapeutic effect of these steps is additive. Lipids should be monitored not less than every 3 to 6 months and even closer surveillance maintained for side effects of clofibrate, including muscle pain and creatine phosphokinase elevations. Nicotinic acid, 3 Gm per day, or *d*-thyroxin may be tried in place of clofibrate; the latter is the drug of choice.

ACQUIRED TYPE III. Transient lipoprotein abnormalities of the same type have been seen in diabetes mellitus during recovery from coma. The anomalous flotation of beta-lipoproteins is also seen in Tangier disease, but in this instance alpha-lipoproteins are absent, and the differential diagnosis is no problem.

Type IV Hyperlipoproteinemia (Endogenous Hyperglyceridemia)

DEFINITION. Excessive endogenous glycerides, synthesized mainly in the liver, cause an increase in prebeta-lipoproteins. All but 30 to 50 mg per 100 ml of plasma glycerides circulate in pre-beta or very low-density lipoproteins, small amounts of which are normally present. Since an excess of chylomicrons (mainly exogenous glyceride) is relatively uncommon, hyperglyceridemia usually signifies hyperprebetalipoproteinemia. Glyceride elevations between 180 and 300 mg per 100 ml occur with normal cholesterol concentrations. The plasma is not usually turbid until glycerides exceed 300, when they are also accompanied by hypercholesterolemia. Type IV hyperlipoproteinemia is not a specific disease; it is a sign of a variety of metabolic defects, some related to abnormal carbohydrate metabolism. When all well-defined diseases have been excluded, there remain many patients with unexplained type IV; frequently, screening of the families reveals more adults with the same lipoprotein abnormality.

ETIOLOGY. Many, but not all, cases of endogenous hyperglyceridemia are probably related to exaggerated *carbohydrate induction.* This is the conversion of excess starches or sugars to glyceride in amounts that maintain a higher than normal plasma glyceride level. Sometimes the rate limit may be in removal rather than overproduction. All normal subjects have transient rises in glycerides in switching from a regular diet to one in which 60 percent or more of calories comes from carbohydrate. Some patients who have type IV patterns on regular diets, particularly those who are overweight and have abnormal glucose tolerance with abnormally low or high insulin responses to glucose, over-respond to high carbohydrate feeding. If possible, such exaggerated carbohydrate induction should be sought for by dietary trials. If this cannot be excluded as an etiologic factor, patients with type IV are arbitrarily restricted to 40 percent or less of calories from carbohydrate. Other mechanisms include chonic increases in free fatty acid concentrations, sometimes related to stress or poor management of diabetes, and excess alcohol intake.

FAMILIAL TYPE IV. When all secondary causes have been eliminated, type IV should be looked for in adult relatives. Frequently one parent and half the siblings may have the same pattern, suggesting that one or more dominant genes may be involved. Children in such families below age twenty are usually normal, indicating factors associated with adulthood that determine expression. These include caloric excess and maturity onset diabetes, common in affected adults. Insulin secretion may be low, normal, or high. Primary type IV hyperlipoproteinemia has been found in a high percentage of patients with premature ischemic heart disease and is considered an important risk factor for atherosclerosis in young adults. PHLA is normal in familial Type IV.

ACQUIRED TYPE IV. This lipoprotein pattern may be seen with dysglobulinemias such as myeloma or macroglobulinemia, hypothyroidism, nephrotic syndrome, idiopathic hypercalcemia, Werner's syndrome, glycogen storage disease, and other disorders, as well as during administration of progestational hormones for contraception. The latter may enhance a familial abnormality.

TREATMENT. Management of primary type IV consists of (1) reduction to ideal weight, (2) maintenance of a diet generally high in P/S ratio and low in cholesterol with care to maintain carbohydrate between 30 and 40 percent of calories; then, if response is inadequate, (3) use of one of several drugs. Clofibrate or nicotinic acid may be effective in helping to lower glycerides, but in some patients there is little response. In patients with mild or minimal diabetes, tolbutamide (0.5 to 1.5 Gm) may help control both hyperglycemia and hyperglyceridemia. Drug or diet therapy must be followed initially by weekly glyceride measurements to establish effectiveness of regimen. Discontinue a drug if no response is obtained in 4 weeks, provided diet is followed carefully.

Type V Hyperlipoproteinemia

DEFINITION. This is mixed hyperlipemia in which chylomicrons and prebeta-lipoproteins are in excess. The plasma is turbid and, after standing overnight in the cold, contains a creamy layer over a milky infranatant layer. Triglycerides are usually between 500 to 5,000 mg per 100 ml, and cholesterol between 200 and 1,000, the C/T ratio usually lying between 0.2 and 0.4. The type V pattern occurs in many disorders and implies defective metabolism of glycerides that are either synthesized in the body or eaten. Some patients who usually have the type IV pattern will also accumulate chylomicrons when levels of endogenous hyperglyceridemia become very high. The resulting Type V pattern is thus a function of diet and the degree of saturation of glyceride-clearing mechanisms. Transient type V patterns occur in temporary deficiency of PHLA associated with insulin-deficient diabetes, acute or chronic pancreatitis, and alcoholism. The mechanisms are vague, but recognition of the pattern has clinical value, for it is commonly associated with a predictable constellation of signs and symptoms.

CLINICAL PICTURE. Usually type V hyperlipoproteinemia occurs in adults, many of whom are overweight and have glucose intolerance or a family history of diabetes. The presenting symptom is frequently bouts of abdominal pain indistinguishable from that seen in type I except that transient amylase elevations are more common. Lipemia retinalis, eruptive xanthomas, and hepatosplenomegaly may be present; and there are frequent complaints of paresthesias or painful extremities. Recurrent abdominal attacks frequently lead to laparotomy, when milky peritoneal fluid and sometimes chalky deposits on the pancreas may be found. Hyperuricemia is common especially if heavy alcoholic excess has preceded the attack.

DIAGNOSIS. Type V is both acquired and familial. After establishment of the typical pattern, insulin-deficient diabetes, acute pancreatitis, and dysglobulinemia must be excluded as well as other disorders commonly associated with hyperlipemia. Adult family members must then be examined; more than half may have type IV or type V patterns. Relationship to mutants causing type IV hyperlipoproteinemia is not clear; and type V may be the expression of one or more aberrant genes, possibly related to both diabetes and hyperlipoproteinemia. Glucose tolerance should always be examined; test of response to high carbohydrate feeding is useful; high fat test diets must be tried cautiously, for they often precipitate abdominal crises.

TREATMENT. The prognosis of type V hyperlipoproteinemia depends on the cause. The primary forms probably carry a hazard for accelerated atherogenesis, but pancreatitis and abdominal pain are the more immediate threats. The sequence of treatment is (1) reduction to ideal body weight; (2) adjustment of diet empirically by response of plasma glycerides, generally using the highest practical protein intake to avoid excesses of either carbohydrate or fat, and severe restriction of alcohol; and, if necessary, (3) trial of drugs. Clofibrate or nicotinic acid will usually effect some reduction in glycerides in type V. Tolbutamide may be helpful, especially if insulinopenia is present. Their use must be accompanied by close followup of plasma lipids. The acute abdominal crises are usually adequately managed by parenteral fluids for 24 to 48 hr. The high protein diet is then cautiously resumed.

Other Hyperlipoproteinemias

All hyperlipidemia is not encompassed in the five major lipoprotein patterns. A notable exception is hypercholesterolemia and massive hyperphospholipidemia associated with obstructive liver disease. This is usually accompanied by marked increase of alpha-lipoproteins with both unusual electrophoretic mobility and abnormally low density. This is best detected by the combination of jaundice, hypercholesterolemia, and a great increase in *unesterified* plasma cholesterol. In otherwise normal subjects, high doses of estrogens may also raise alpha lipoproteins sufficiently to cause modest hypercholesterolemia.

HYPOLIPOPROTEINEMIA
Beta (Low Density) Lipoprotein Deficiency

ABETALIPOPROTEINEMIA. Abetalipoproteinemia is a rare familial disease, uniquely characterized by complete absence of beta-lipoproteins. The plasma contains only alpha-lipoproteins; no chylomicrons or prebeta (very low density) lipoproteins are present. The syndrome follows a fairly uniform course, beginning before the age of one year, with *malnutrition* and growth retardation, lordosis, abdominal distension, and steatorrhea. *Ataxia*, nystagmus, weakness and areflexia, and other signs of progressive neurologic dysfunction, particularly involving the posterolateral columns and spinocerebellar tracts, then appear. *Pigmentary retinal degeneration* develops during adolescence. The erythrocytes have a crenated appearance (*acanthocytosis*). The esterified lipids of these cells and of the plasma are deficient in both lecithin and linoleic acid. Dietary fat is assimilated but is held up in the intestinal mucosal cells, creating a pathognomonic picture detectable by peroral biopsy. Some fat is absorbed, possibly by direct passage through the portal system into the liver.

The disease may occur in siblings and is likely due to a double dose of a mutant autosomal gene, since the consanguinity rate in affected families is high. Most relatives have normal concentrations of plasma lipoproteins. Whether the primary defect is related to formation of beta-apoprotein, beta-lipoprotein, or some other aspect of fat absorption is not known. The prognosis is guarded; patients may succumb relatively young, sometimes from cardiac arrhythmias. Familial instances of acanthocytosis and neurologic abnormalities without abetalipoproteinemia have also been reported.

Diagnosis. The diagnosis is suspected when a plasma cholesterol concentration less than 100 mg per 100 ml is associated with the above clinical picture. It must be confirmed by immunochemical evidence of the absence of plasma beta-lipoprotein.

Treatment. There is no definitive therapy. Medium-chain triglycerides may help provide some fat intake in the absence of chylomicron formation, and low vitamin A levels have been increased with supplements.

HYPOBETALIPOPROTEINEMIA. Abnormally low cholesterol and glyceride concentrations with decreased, but not absent, beta- and very low density lipoproteins are common in malnutrition or malabsorption due to a variety of causes. Remissions are promptly associated with a rise in cholesterol and beta-lipoproteins. There are also *heritable* forms of hypobetalipoproteinemia, at least one due to a dominant gene.

Alpha (High Density) Lipoprotein Deficiency and LCAT Deficiency

Familial high density lipoprotein deficiency is also called *Tangier disease*, after the island home of the first cases. The disease has been detected in other children and adults and must be suspected when hypocholesterolemia is associated with orange or yellowish-gray discoloration of the tonsils and pharyngeal or rectal mucosa or *enlargement* of *spleen, liver,* or *lymph nodes.* Reticuloendothelial tissues are infiltrated with *foam cells* containing large amounts of cholesterol esters. In adults *corneal infiltration,* hypersplenism, papular skin lesions containing foam cells, peripheral neuropathy with loss of tendon reflexes and abnormal electromyograms, and possibly premature coronary artery disease have been seen as complications.

Parents and other relatives of patients with Tangier disease have lower than normal amounts of plasma high-density (alpha$_1$) lipoprotein. The propositi are probably homozygous for a mutant gene that normally governs the synthesis of this lipoprotein.

DIAGNOSIS. Diagnosis is suspected when plasma cholesterol is between 50 and 125 mg per 100 ml with normal or slightly elevated glycerides. It is established by immunochemical evidence that the alpha-polypeptide characteristic of plasma high-density lipoprotein is present in only trace amounts and as an immunochemically different form. Carriers also have similar amounts of the abnormal alpha lipoprotein in plasma. Splenectomy may be required for hypersplenism. There is no definitive therapy.

Deficient Plasma Lecithin: Cholesterol Acyltransferase

LCAT is a familial disorder discovered in a Norwegian family. The clinical manifestations include proteinuria, anemia, and arcus cornea. Plasma alpha lipoproteins are severely deficient, although total cholesterol and glyceride concentrations may be normal or elevated. *Diagnosis* is suspected when the clinical picture is accompanied by absence of *esterified* cholesterol in plasma. Assay of the enzyme is required for confirmation.

LIPID STORAGE DISEASES

The Sphingolipidoses

There are other storage diseases characterized more by tissue rather than plasma lipid abnormalities. *In all it is exceedingly important that specimens of tissues obtained for diagnostic purposes be retained frozen without fixatives for chemical and enzymatic analyses. Histochemical diagnosis is usually not definitive.* The sphingolipidoses represent one group of these disorders and are so called because they have in common the accumulation of a different derivative (—R) of ceramide (acyl-sphingosine).

$$CH_3(CH_2)_{13}CH\!=\!CH\!-\!\overset{\overset{\displaystyle H}{\overset{\displaystyle O}{|}}}{C}\!-\!\overset{\overset{\displaystyle}{|}}{C}\!-\!C\!-\!O\!-\!R$$

$$\underbrace{CH_3\!-\!(CH_2)_n\!-\!CO\!-\!NH}$$

Ceramide

These are all inheritable disorders; each may involve the nervous system. Most occur in several clinical forms or syndromes, possibly reflecting mutations at different loci. Specific enzyme deficiencies have now been identified in some and probably represent the genetically-determined defects.

Glucosylceramidoses (Gangliosidoses, Gaucher's Disease, Fabry's Disease

GANGLIOSIDOSES. (See Chap. 364). *Gangliosidoses* (*amaurotic family idiocy*) is a generic term for several familial neurologic disorders associated with varying degrees of blindness and dementia. Three of these diseases have been identified as characterized by accumulation, and presumably defective metabolism, of a different ganglioside, the major lipid in gray matter. G_{M_1}-*gangliosidosis,* or *generalized gangliosidosis,* or *pseudo-Hurler's disease,* involves both brain and viscera. The tissues contain abnormal amounts of galactosyl-galactosaminyl-(N-acetylneuraminido) galactosyl-glucosylceramide. A galactosidase attacking the terminal glycosidic bond is deficient. G_{M_2}-*gangliosidosis* is classical *Tay-Sachs disease,* which fatally involves only the central nervous system. The excess ganglioside is N-acetyl-galactosaminyl-(N-acetylneuraminido)galactosyl-glucosyl-ceramide. A G_{M_3}-*gangliosidosis* has also recently been identified. Other forms of amaurotic idiocy, such as Batten's disease (Vogt-Spielmeyer or juvenile amaurotic idiocy), and the Bieloschowsky, Kufs, or Hallevorden types have not been chemically differentiated as lipidoses.

GLUCOSYLCEREBROSIDOSIS (see Chap. 350) (Gaucher's Disease). First described by Gaucher in 1882, these disorders represent storage of glucocerebrosides (ceramide-glucose) in reticuloendothelial cells, producing marked splenomegaly and hepatomegaly. In adults there are often bone lesions, associated skin pigmentation, and characteristic pingueculas of the scleras. In infants progressive neurologic disturbances usually occur and are associated with a rapidly fatal course. There is also a juvenile form. Deficient glucocerebrosidase has been found in spleen, liver, and white cells of patients with infantile and adult varieties.

GLUCOSYLCERAMIDETRIHEXOSIDOSIS (see Chap. 347) (Fabry's disease). In this sex-linked disorder, the manifestations are usually only seen in males and are due to deposition of glycolipids, mainly a trihexoside (ceramide-glucose-galactose-galactose), in blood vessels and nerves. Galactosyl-galactosylceramide also accumulates. The disease is also known by its unusual skin manifestations, *angiokeratoma corporis diffusum.* Deficient galactosidase which normally cleaves the terminal galactose from the trihexoside has been detected in this disease.

Galactosylceramidoses (see Chap 364)

GALACTOSYLSULFATIDOSIS. Galactosylsulfatidosis, or *metachromatic leukodystrophy* is a disorder of children in which abnormal amounts of cerebroside-sulfatide (ceramide-galactose-SO_3H) accumulate in the brain and kidney. The material is also excreted in bile, causing fibrosis of the gallbladder, and in urine, where it may be detected as an aid to diagnosis. Deficiency of an arylsulfatase appears to be the genetic abnormality.

Galactosylcerebrosides accumulate in the brain in *Krabbe's disease*, although this disorder is not yet proved to be a genetically determined lipidosis.

Phosphorylceramidoses (see Chap 350) (Niemann-Pick Disease)

Accumulation of massive amounts of sphingomyelin and cholesterol characterize lipidoses that take several forms. They may be partially distinguished by measurement of sphingomyelin-cleavage enzyme in liver, spleen, or fibroblasts in tissue culture. The enzyme is deficient in both the classical infantile form or Niemann-Pick disease and in older children with visceral but not CNS involvement. The enzyme has been normal or low normal in tissues examined from most of the older patients with late CNS involvement or those with the so-called "Nova Scotia" variant. Sphingomyelin lipidoses appear to result from several mutations.

OTHER RARE TISSUE LIPID STORAGE DISEASES
Phytanic Oxidase Deficiency

In addition to the sphingolipidoses, there are other rare disorders in which less polar lipids pile up in tissues apparently because of enzymatic defects. In *Refsum's disease* there is accumulation of phytanic acid (3,7,11,15-tetramethyl hexadecanoic acid) in the esterified lipids present in both tissues and plasma. This familial disease is characterized by ataxic neuropathy, anosmia, retinitis pigmentosa, dry skin, skeletal deformities, and ichthyosis and is commonest in children or young adults of Scandinavian ancestry. Parents may have high levels of phytanic acid in plasma without other abnormalities. The prognosis is guarded, with the symptoms sometimes progressing to complete blindness and deafness, but often waxing and waning, relapses being irregular correlated with the degree of increase in CSF protein. Phytanic acid, which may make up 10 to 30 percent of total plasma fatty acids in the patients, is normally present only in very small amounts. It is derived from dietary phytols, and present therapy consists of a low-phytol diet. The inherited defects include a block in the alpha oxidation of the phytanic acid derived from phytols. The relationship of phytanate accumulation to the nervous disorders is unknown. Diagnosis is usually made by chromatographic analysis of plasma.

Familial Xanthomatosis with Adrenal Calcification (Wolman's Disease)

This disease resembles Niemann-Pick disease in the presence of hepatosplenomegaly, foam cell deposition in tissues, and death in early childhood. The stored lipids are mainly triglycerides and cholesterol, much of it esterified. The etiology and effective treatment are unknown.

Hepatic Cholesterol Ester Storage Disease

This is a disorder seen in siblings in which the liver is selectively enlarged, butter-yellow in color, shows slight cirrhosis, and has a very high content of cholesteryl esters, predominantly cholesteryl oleate. Plasma lipids are not altered in a diagnostic fashion and the diagnosis must be made by liver biopsy. The parenchyma stains very deeply with Oil-Red-O and the Schultz technique; lipid analyses must also be made. The ultimate prognosis and treatment are not established.

Ceroid Storage Disease

Ceroid storage disease, or the accumulation of ceroid, a pigmented lipid of unknown chemical composition, may also include sufficient organ involvement to produce a clinical picture similar to severe Niemann-Pick disease. It may also be associated with cirrhosis of the liver and intestinal malabsorption. Ceroid may be identified histochemically by the combination of red periodic acid-Schiff stain, acid-fastness, and fluorescence. Deposition of this material has also been seen in aorta, liver, intestinal musculature, and other tissues in a variety of conditions, including tocopherol deficiency. The biochemical basis for ceroid formation and storage is not known.

GRANULOMATOUS DISEASES WITH LIPID STORAGE

Frequently considered among the lipid storage diseases are certain tissue proliferative disorders sometimes accompanied by lipid deposition.

Histiocytosis X

Histiocytosis X (see Chap. 350) is the generic term for a group of disorders that affect the reticuloendothelial system and which may be either different stages or forms of the same disease. *Letterer-Siwe disease* and *xanthoma disseminatum* may be the two extremes of such abnormalities, with *eosinophilic granuloma* and *Hand-Schuller-Christian disease* representing intermediate and special forms. The usual order of progression of the pathologic lesions is reticuloendothelial cell proliferation and hyperplasia, granulomatous changes featuring eosinophils and giant cells, conversion of reticulum cells and histiocytes to foam cells or xanthomas, and finally, fibrosis. These disorders do not appear to be hereditary.

Several other uncommon diseases are associated with proliferation of histiocytes and deposition of material considered to represent both lipid and carbohydrate because it stains by both the Sudan and periodic acid-Schiff techniques. The chemical composition of the lesions has not been characterized. It is likely that any faulty metabolism of lipid is secondary to some other processes, perhaps involving mucopolysaccharide metabolism.

Lipoid Proteinosis

In *lipoid-proteinosis* (cutaneous-mucosal hyalinosis; Urbach-Wiethe disease) the lesions share enough histologic features of *histiocytosis X* to suggest an etiologic relationship. The skin and mucous membranes of the pharynx and larynx are infiltrated by extracellular deposits of hyaline material. Clinical manifestations include hoarseness or aphonia, widely distributed skin papules, dental anomalies, and symmetric calcifications in the region of the sella turcica as seen by x-ray. The disease is not incompatible with long life. This disorder may be inheritable.

Lipoid Dermatoarthritis

In *lipoid dermatoarthritis* polyarthritis is associated with multiple nodular or papular skin lesions. In both skin and synovial tissues there is an infiltration of histiocytes, eosinophils, lymphocytes, red blood cells, and multinucleated giant cells. The joint changes may be extremely destructive, producing *arthritis mutilans,* or the "opera-glass hand." Serologic reactions for rheumatoid arthritis are negative. Familial occurrence has not been reported.

Disseminated Lipogranulomatosis (Farber's Disease)

This is a rare disease that appears in infancy as generalized nodular periarticular swelling and dysphonia. There is progressive systemic involvement with widespread proliferation of histiocytes and neuronal abnormalities. Storage cells appear containing both mucopolysaccharide and lipids. The basic disorder probably involves the metabolism of certain acid mucopolysaccharides similar to those in Hurler's disease (Chap. 399).

Hereditary Tendinous and Tuberous Xanthomatosis without Hyperlipidemia

This disorder has been reported in siblings who had multiple xanthomas of the Achilles tendons and subcutaneously over the knee, elbow, and shoulder, and diffuse pulmonary infiltration. Giant cells but no eosinophils are present.

Cerebrotendinous Xanthomatosis

The preceding disorder bears an uncertain resemblance to cerebrotendinous xanthomatosis, which is a familial disease in which cholesterol deposits in tendons, pulmonary parenchyma, and the cerebellum and other areas in the brain are associated with progressive spastic ataxia, large xanthomas, and sometimes, dementia and cataracts. Hyperlipidemia may or may not be present. The proper etiologic classification of these two disorders is not established.

XANTHOMAS

Many chronic infections, particularly accompanied by exudates, and other proliferative processes, such as osteitis fibrosa cystica or traumatic lesions, may be associated with collections of foam cells (*xanthomas*) and sometimes crystals of cholesterol. Most skin xanthomas are secondary to hyperlipoproteinemia, but *juvenile xanthomas* (nevoxanthoepithelioma) are benign skin lesions that can appear without abnormal plasma lipids. *Xanthelasmas* need not always be associated with hyperlipoproteinemia and sometimes occur in family members who are normolipoproteinemic.

ADIPOSE TISSUE DISORDERS

Adipose tissue can be a site of expression of many disorders including those of connective tissue, lipid, and carbohydrate metabolism. There is therefore no simple classification of the adipose tissue diseases.

Relapsing Panniculitis (Weber-Christian Disease)

This classification may represent several diseases that share similar but rather nonspecific histologic changes (see Chap. 394).

Lipodystrophy

Although the term *lipodystrophy* is sometimes used to describe *lipoathrophy,* it also has a generic meaning that allows it to encompass several disorders in which adipose tissue is abnormal but not necessarily absent. Several abnormalities may properly be considered forms of lipodystrophy.

LIPOMAS. These are benign mesenchymal tumors consisting of circumscribed masses of adipose tissue. There is usually a capsule, but the cells are histologically indistinguishable from ordinary fat. They may occur nearly anywhere in the body, singly or as multiple fatty growths (lipomatosis), most commonly in subcutaneous tissues. They also arise in retroperitoneal or peritoneal areas, in breast, mesentery, and mediastinum, and in other body cavities and organs. Lipomas have caused intestinal obstruction or dyspnea by superior mediastinal obstruction and may embarrass the function of other vital tissues. Rarely they may calcify, and it has been presumed that they may on occasion give rise to liposarcomas or other malignant tumors, but there is no general agreement on this. Multiple lipomas may be symmetrically placed and may run in families. The therapy is surgical excision; occasionally they will recur in the same site.

ADIPOSIS DOLOROSA (Dercum's Disease). *Adiposis dolorosa* refers to a poorly defined disorder in which painful subcutaneous lipomas, often widely and symmetrically situated, are sometimes associated with asthenia, decreased cutaneous sensation, motor weakness, or other evidence of peripheral neuropathy. Some patients have also had adenomas in the pituitary, thyroid, or adrenal glands. There may or may not be accompanying generalized obesity. Siblings may be similarly involved. The interstitial neuritis observed in the original adipose tissue nodules by Dercum has not been seen in many subsequent cases. There is no specific therapy.

INSULIN LIPODYSTROPHY. This term refers to changes in subcutaneous fat at the site of insulin injection (see Chap. 94) and may involve either localized hypertrophy or atrophy of adipose tissue.

Lipoatrophy

Lipoatrophy may be partial or complete.

PARTIAL LIPOATROPHY. Also called *progressive lipodystrophy*, partial lipodystrophy is characterized by the absence of subcutaneous fat over wide, symmetric areas of the body. The remaining parts of the body have normal or sometimes increased subcutaneous fat deposits. It occurs predominantly in females and often begins in childhood. The onset is usually insidious and may begin with loss of subcutaneous fat in the face and subsequently involve that of the upper extremities and upper trunk. In other instances the disorder may begin at the level of the iliac crest and extend downward. There are no subjective symptoms. The cause is unknown. There is no known therapy.

TOTAL LIPOATROPHY. In total lipoatrophy (lipoatrophic diabetes mellitus), generalized atrophy of body fat occurs gradually. In addition to subcutaneous fat deposits, nearly all other body fat, excepting that in the breasts, may disappear. This is usually but not always associated with diabetes, which may precede or follow the onset of lipoatrophy. There is also hyperlipoproteinemia with types IV or V patterns, decreased postheparin lipolytic activity, hepatomegaly, and sometimes acanthosis nigricans; serious nephropathy, including both nephritic and nephrotic manifestations, may occur whether the patient has diabetes or not. Some patients may also have hypermetabolism, others have features suggestive of "leprechaunism," and the syndrome undoubtedly results from several different causes. The diabetes is associated with high plasma insulin levels and may be very difficult to control. The course of the disease may be either indolent or rapidly progressive. No therapy is known.

REFERENCES

Abul-Haj, S. K., D. G. Martz, W. F. Douglas, and L. J. Geppert: Farber's Disease, J. Pediat., 61:221, 1962.

Bortz, A. I., and M. Vincent: Lipoid Dermato-arthritis and Arthritis Mutilans, Am. J. Med., 30:951, 1961.

Brady, R. O., Jr.: The Sphingolipidoses, New Engl. J. Med., 275:312, 1966.

Fredrickson, D. S., R. I. Levy, and R. S. Lees: Fat Transport in Lipoproteins—An Integrated Approach to Mechanisms and Disorders, New Engl. J. Med., 276:34, 94, 148, 215, 273, 1967.

Harlan, W. R., Jr., and W. J. S. Still: Hereditary Tendinous and Tuberous Xanthomatosis without Hyperlipidemia, New Engl. J. Med., 278:416, 1968.

McCusker, J. J., and R. M. Caplan: Lipoid Proteinosis (Lipoglycoproteinosis), Am. J. Pathol., 40:599, 1962.

Norum, K. R.: Biochemical Study of New Familial Syndrome Characterized by a Marked Reduction of Esterified Cholesterol in Serum, Scand. J. Clin. Lab. Invest., 19 (suppl. 100):102, 1967.

Oppenheimer, E. H., and E. C. Andrews, Jr.: Ceroid Storage Disease in Childhood, Pediatrics, 23:1091, 1959.

Schiff, L., W. K. Schubert, A. J. McAdams, E. L. Spiegel, and J. F. O'Donnell: Hepatic Cholesterol Ester Storage Disease, A Familial Disorder, Am. J. Med., 44:538, 1968.

Schimschock, J. R., E. C. Alvord, Jr., and P. D. Swanson: Cerebrotendinous Xanthomatosis, Arch. Neurol., 18:688, 1968.

Schwartz, R., I. A. Schafer, and A. E. Renold: Generalized Lipoatrophy, Hepatic Cirrhosis, Disturbed Carbohydrate Metabolism and Accelerated Growth (Lipoatrophic Diabetes), Am. J. Med., 28:973, 1960.

Senior, B., and S. S. Gellis: The Syndromes of Total Lipodystrophy and of Partial Lipodystrophy, Pediatrics, 33:593, 1964.

Stanbury, J. B., J. B. Wyngaarden, and D. S. Fredrickson (Eds.): "The Metabolic Basis of Inherited Disease," 2d ed., chaps. 22–29, New York, McGraw-Hill Book Company, 1966.

Tedeschi, C. G., and W. H. Lyon: Fat Tissue Growths, J. Mt. Sinai Hosp., 24:1272, 1957.

Wolman, M., V. V. Sterk, S. Gatt, and M. Frenkel: Primary Familial Xanthomatosis with Involvement and Calcification of the Adrenals, Pediatrics, 28:742, 1961.

114 AMYLOIDOSIS
Evan Calkins

Introduction

Although amyloidosis has been recognized as a clinical and pathologic entity for over 100 years, our knowledge about the nature, pathogenesis, distribution, and possible clinical importance of amyloid is still in a state of evolution.

The hyaline, apparently amorphous, eosinophilic material known as *amyloid* was named by Virchow because of its affinity to iodine, a property which suggested a resemblance to starch. Although amyloid was at first recognized in association with tuberculosis, and other prolonged septic processes, it soon became apparent that material indistinguishable from amyloid could be identified in the myocardium and other tissues of certain individuals who had never had chronic infections. Although this group of patients has been considered relatively infrequent, there is evidence that, at least in elderly patients, the incidence of *primary amyloidosis* may be frequent.

Sensitive histologic techniques, utilizing polarization and fluorescence microscopy, have detected what appears to be amyloid in a high percentage of people over sixty; and in a recent study amyloid was detected in the meningeal vessels and brain substance (senile plaques) in one-half of the patients over sixty and in 63 percent of the patients over seventy years of age. Cardiac amyloid deposits were present in 30 percent of patients over sixty and aortic deposits in over 39 percent of patients in the same age group. Pancreatic islet hyalin, commonly attributed to diabetes mellitus, is also common in elderly patients. Recent studies have indicated that this islet deposition is similar if not identical to amyloid.

Further studies utilizing electron microscopy and immunochemistry will be required before senile amyloid can be considered identical with the more classical form of amyloid. Electron microscopy of pancreatic hyalin and senile cardiac amyloid has, however, shown the presence of the fibrillar component which has been regarded as specific for amyloid. The clinical implications of this sort of amyloid infiltration are not yet clear. The close association of this connective tissue change with atherosclerotic plaques raised the possibility, as yet unproved, of a relationship between amyloidosis and atherosclerosis. The association with hyalin or amyloid infiltration of the pancreatic islets with diabetes mellitus has long been recognized. Preliminary studies have also indicated a relationship between amyloid infiltration of the brain and behavioral abnormalities in elderly patients without otherwise demonstrable cerebral pathology.

The concept that amyloid accumulation is an age-related process has strong support from studies in experimental animals. It has been shown that certain animal species and certain strains within a given species have a greatly enhanced predilection for developing senile amyloidosis.

These findings provide increasing support for the hypothesis that amyloidosis may represent a nonspecific phenomenon of ageing. According to this hypothesis, genetic factors and certain diseases (prolonged infections, neoplasms, etc.) enhance the development of an apparently common biologic process which results in the disease state of *secondary amyloidosis* and the various syndromes of primary amyloidosis (see below).

Physical and Chemical Characteristics

Amyloid has been shown to consist of a relatively amorphous ground substance, containing a high concentration of fibrils. The characteristics of these fibrils have been fairly well defined by electron microscopy. They are long, ranging from 300 to 100,000 Å in length, non-branching, and undulant as opposed to straight. Their diameter appears to range from 70 to 100 Å, and they may occur singularly or in bundles of varying number. They appear irregularly beaded at intervals of 35 to 100 Å. The fibrils are predominantly protein. The content of amino acids and carbohydrate components has been well defined. By all criteria amyloid fibrils are distinct from collagen, elastin, fibrin, and other known body fibers. It has been shown that the fibrils themselves do not contain gamma-globulin. On the other hand, gamma-globulin (IgG), several components of complement (C'1, C'3, and C'4), fibrinogen, and a component of normal

tissue protein appear to be adsorbed onto or closely associated with amyloid fibriles.

The nature of amyloid ground substance has not been well defined. Extracts of amyloid have shown, in addition to the fibrils, a relatively small concentration of a second, apparently unique globular component, 80 to 100 Å in diameter, resembling and referred to as "doughnuts." The relationship of this component, if any, to the amyloid fibril is not known. Preliminary analyses indicate that it has a somewhat different chemical composition from the fibril.

The precise events which lead to the accumulation of amyloid are not known. It is not known with certainty, for example, whether the formation of the amyloid fibril represents the initiating process or whether the fibril is synthesized in response to a primary change in the ground substance. It has been suggested that the amyloid fibril is synthesized by mesenchymal cells in a fashion analogous to the synthesis of collagen fibers. Immunochemical studies have failed to disclose any component of amyloid, including the fibril and doughnut, which is clearly abnormal. It seems probable that amyloidosis represents excessive accumulation of normal components.

Clinical Classification

It appears from the above discussion that amyloidosis, defined most broadly, is the tissue accumulation of detectable amounts of extracellular hyaline material which has certain rather unique tinctorial characteristics and contains characteristic fibrils which can be identified by electron microscopy. Using this definition, the incidence of amyloidosis is probably extremely high, and may be almost universal in the ageing human population.

A more practical clinical definition is that amyloidosis is the accumulation of amyloid in amounts that result in interference with normal bodily function. According to this definition the entity is probably quite rare, except in certain countries, such as Israel and Turkey, in which there appears to be a striking genetic predisposition. The remainder of this discussion will focus on amyloidosis as defined in this more restricted clinical sense.

SECONDARY AMYLOIDOSIS

Secondary amyloidosis is that which may accompany prolonged inflammatory or infectious diseases. Histologic evidence of amyloidosis is seen in approximately 25 percent of all patients with rheumatoid arthritis, dying of any cause. It becomes clinically manifest in only a small percentage of these cases however. Secondary amyloidosis is a common cause of death in paraplegics who have developed decubitus ulcers and urinary tract infections. It is seen in approximately one-third of patients with leprosy at the U.S. Public Health Service Hospital in Carville, La., and is one of the chief causes of death at that hospital. Secondary amyloidosis is manifested chiefly by nephrosis and subsequent azotemia; hepatomegaly and splenomegaly may also be seen. At autopsy the predominant sites of involvement are the kidney, spleen, liver, and adrenal glands. Microscopic traces of amyloid may be widely distributed, especially in blood vessel walls.

AMYLOIDOSIS ASSOCIATED WITH MULTIPLE MYELOMA

A second category of amyloidosis is that which accompanies multiple myeloma. Between 10 and 20 percent of patients with multiple myeloma are known to develop this complication. Clinical involvement may resemble that seen in secondary amyloidosis. More widespread manifestations, such as neuropathy of the ulnar nerve resulting in the carpal tunnel syndrome, may also be seen. The manifestations may be indistinguishable from those of primary amyloidosis (see below).

PRIMARY AMYLOIDOSIS

In the third and probably most common category of amyloidosis seen today the disease develops without any known predisposing disease. Recent studies have provided increasing evidence that this so-called "primary" form of amyloidosis is, in turn, comprised of a number of relatively discrete syndromes, each with characteristic clinical expression and pattern of occurrence.

In several of these entities the involvement resembles that seen in the secondary form. One example is the amyloidosis which often occurs in association with *familial Mediterranean fever* (FMF), primarily in members of the Sephardic and Iraqui Jewish races. The two disorders appear to be inherited as independent recessive traits; amyloidosis may be seen in members of a family who do not have FMF and vice versa (Chap. 256).

Other varieties of primary amyloidosis are manifested by more widespread evidence of the disease. One example is the primary familial amyloidosis described by Andrade. In this entity, which occurs predominantly in individuals of Portuguese ancestry, severe impairment of the sensory function of the peripheral nerves, as well as less severe impairment of motor function is encountered. This is often accompanied by involvement of the sympathetic ganglions, with postural hypotension, impotence, absence of sweating, and intestinal hypermotility and malabsorption. Adie's pupil is apt to be present. The patients usually die from severe malnutrition and inanition. Another example of primary amyloidosis occurring in families is that described by Rukavina et al. in a family of Swiss ancestry. Although some members of the family resembled the patients described by Andrade, others exhibited a variety of different clinical manifestations. Other family constellations, yielding a variety of syndromes, have also been described.

Despite the increasing awareness of the familial incidence of amyloidosis, many patients who develop the disease, without known predisposing cause, do not appear to have any genetic or familial predisposition. In some of these cases the distribution of the amyloid resembles that seen in the secondary form of the disease; others exhibit diffuse involvement, especially of the skin or the heart. In many patients the accumulation may be localized to a single area, such as the respiratory passages, without evidence of widespread involvement.

Clinical Manifestations

The clinical manifestations of amyloidosis depend on the organ or system involved. Since the symptoms may resemble those of a variety of other disorders, amyloidosis must frequently be considered in differential diagnosis.

Amyloidosis of the skin is most typically characterized by hyaline plaques, occurring chiefly in or near the folds of the skin, as in the inguinal regions. Occasionally, the disease results in widespread purpura.

Although in most cases this purpura is thought to be due to involvement of the walls of small blood vessels, other mechanisms may be involved. These may include thrombocytopenia, deficiencies of several different clotting factors, and increased plasmin activity. As a result of the defects in hemostasis, prolonged bleeding may follow such minor surgical procedures as a gingival biopsy. Other parameters of coagulation are usually within normal limits. The bleeding time may be prolonged, presumably because of increased rigidity of small blood vessels.

Ocular involvement may consist of diffuse infiltrates in the posterior chamber, discrete deposits of amyloid beneath the bulbar conjunctiva, and an Adie pupil.

Amyloid infiltration of the heart classically results in enlargement, which is due to an increased thickness of the myocardial wall, without change in intracardiac volume. The resultant syndrome, due to a stiffened myocardium, may yield results on cardiac catheterization which closely resemble those seen in constrictive pericarditis. In other cases, the clinical picture may more nearly resemble that seen in diffuse arteriosclerotic heart disease, with an enlarged and inefficient myocardium. Electrocardiogram often reveals low voltage in the QRS complex. Arteriovenous block and arrhythmias may also be seen. Amyloidosis is one of a group of conditions which may cause cardiac failure, without detectable murmurs. Unfortunately, it is very seldom correctly diagnosed ante mortem.

Amyloid involvement of the liver is characterized primarily by hepatomegaly. Clinical evidence of hepatic dysfunction and jaundice is rare. Liver function tests characteristically show minimal abnormalities, which are usually suggestive of biliary obstruction. Although liver biopsy has been recommended and often yields diagnostic information, it has been followed in a few instances by intractable bleeding and/or rupture of the liver. For this reason liver biopsy should probably be avoided when amyloidosis is suspected.

Renal amyloidosis is manifested predominantly by the nephrotic syndrome. The appearance of progressively severe proteinuria in patients with chronic inflammatory diseases such as rheumatoid arthritis should always lead to a suspicion of amyloidosis. In attempting to differentiate renal amyloidosis from chronic pyelonephritis, the size of the kidneys, as seen on x-ray, may be helpful. In pyelonephritis the kidneys are usually reduced in size; amyloid-laden kidneys are likely to be normal in size or may be enlarged. Hypertension is not commonly observed in amyloidosis. Azotemia is a very late manifestation. Kidney biopsy is a satisfactory method of confirming the diagnosis of renal amyloidosis in cases in which the clinical syndrome, plus rectal or gingival biopsy, has not already led to a definite diagnosis.

Amyloidosis may result in a variety of *neurologic lesions.* Diffuse motor and sensory neuropathy, together with interference with function of the sympathetic nervous system, is characteristic of the primary familial amyloidosis of Andrade. Sensory involvement may also be seen in amyloidosis secondary to multiple myeloma, because of diffuse involvement of the sheaths of the peripheral nerves.

Accumulations of *amyloid* in the *trachea* or bronchi may result in serious obstruction to the respiratory passages. Local excision, often with epithelial grafting, is the preferred form of treatment. Recurrences are frequent but by no means invariable.

Amyloid may infiltrate any portion of the *gastrointestinal tract,* resulting in a variety of syndromes, ranging from esophageal obstruction to malabsorption syndrome. Infiltration of the endocrine organs may also ensue. This rarely results in insufficiency of function of the involved gland, however.

Diagnosis

Confirmation of the diagnosis is best obtained by biopsy. Gingival biopsy has been helpful, permitting confirmation of the diagnosis in between one-half and two-thirds of the cases. In the experience of Sohar and his associates, the rectal biopsy has proved even more sensitive. Skin biopsy may be positive in patients with primary or secondary amyloidosis even in the absence of clinical evidence of dermatologic involvement. Renal and hepatic biopsy carry a higher risk of bleeding, and consideration should be given to this when such diagnostic studies are contemplated.

Histologic examination of biopsy specimens must be conducted with great care. Traces of amyloid should be sought in the walls of small blood vessels. In specimens of skin, deposits may also be seen in sweat glands, sebaceous glands, and surrounding the fat cells in the subcutaneous tissue (amyloid rings). Tissue should be fixed in formalin and stained with hematoxylin and eosin, crystal violet, Congo red (preferably the alkaline Congo red method of Puchtler) and thioflavine T or S. Sections should be examined under regular, ultraviolet, and polarized light. The appearance of traces of brilliant greenish-yellow fluorescence with thioflavine T or S permits identification of areas for further study, but is not, in itself, specific for amyloid. On a section stained with Congo red, the appearance of areas exhibiting a characteristic green color, together with dichroism, provides what is, in all probability, specific histologic evidence for the presence of amyloid. Definitive confirmation of this diagnosis, however, requires electron microscopy.

The Congo red test has been almost entirely abandoned as an aid in the diagnosis of amyloidosis due to occasional incidence of severe toxic reactions and greatly improved sensitivity and specificity of histologic methods.

Course and Treatment

The course of amyloidosis is usually progressively downhill, especially if the organs involved include the kidneys, heart, or gastrointestinal tract. Of the fifty odd cases studied by the author, none has exhibited a remission, except for those cases of localized amyloidosis in which surgical extirpation has been possible. The course may be prolonged, however, lasting for periods of many years. Treatment with large doses of ascorbic acid (1,000 mg per day) or of lightly seared liver (¼ lb per day) has been attempted, chiefly on empirical grounds, but there is no sound clinical evidence, to date, to support this program. If amyloidosis accompanies other inflammatory conditions, vigorous efforts to treat the underlying condition should be initiated. If these efforts are successful, remission of the amyloidosis may ensue. This outcome is rarely seen, however, chiefly because potentially treatable chronic inflammatory conditions usually receive treatment prior to the onset of amyloidosis.

REFERENCES

Bladen, H. A., M. U. Nylen, and G. G. Glenner: The Ultrastructure of Human Amyloid as Revealed by the Negative Staining Techniques, J. Ultrastruct. Res., 14: 449, 1966.

Cohen, A. S.: Amyloidosis, New Engl. J. Med., 277:522, 1967.

———: Constitution and Genesis of Amyloid, pp. 159–243 in G. W. Richter and M. A. Epstein (Eds.), "International Review of Experimental Pathology," Vol. 4, New York, Academic Press, 1965.

Heller, H., E. Sohar, J. Gafni, and J. Heller: Amyloidosis in Familial Mediterranean Fever: An Independent Genetically Determined Characteristic, Arch. Intern. Med., 107:539, 1961.

Kenney, J. D., and E. Calkins: Clinical Aspects of Amyloidosis, in A. St. J. Dixon (Ed.), "Progress in Clinical Rheumatology," London, J. and A. Churchill, Ltd., 1965.

Wright, J. R., E. Calkins, W. Breen, G. Stolte, and R. T. Schultz: Relationship of Amyloid to Aging, Medicine, 48:39, 1969.

Part Six

Disorders due to Chemical and Physical Agents

Section 1

Chemical Intoxications

115 GENERAL CONSIDERATIONS AND PRINCIPLES OF MANAGEMENT

Jan Koch-Weser

Poisoning by chemical agents is a common and serious medical problem. In the United States accidental poisonings cause at least 4,000 deaths each year. Suicides by chemical agents annually number more than 6,000. Malicious poisoning has become less common since the development of scientific toxicology, but toxic chemicals administered by homicides and abortionists are responsible for more deaths than is generally appreciated. In addition to fatal poisonings there is a much greater number of persons who are made seriously ill by chemical agents but recover after appropriate therapy. Unfortunately, some such victims are left with permanent sequelae of their intoxication. Finally, chemical agents impair the health of very many people by mechanisms not generally thought of as intoxications. Chemical carcinogenesis and mutagenesis, chronic pulmonary disease due to common inhalants, chronic alcoholic liver disease, allergic reactions, and chemical addiction and withdrawal syndromes are the most important examples.

Accidental poisonings may occur in the home or through industrial exposure. The former are far more frequent and usually acute; industrial intoxication is ordinarily the result of chronic exposure. Accidental poisoning is most commonly due to ingestion of toxic substances and involves children in the majority of cases. Each year 1 to 2 million American children accidentally swallow toxic materials, and approximately 1 ingestion in 1,000 is fatal. Aspirin is involved in 25 percent of all ingestions, other medicines in another 25 percent. Cleaning and polishing agents are ingested by 15 percent, while cosmetics, pesticides, petroleum products, and turpentine paints account for 6 percent each. Younger children tend to ingest household products, older children are more likely to choose drugs.

The frequency of accidental poisonings reflects the enormous number of toxic substances found in the American home. Many such accidents could be avoided by simple preventive measures. Physicians can play an effective role in safety education. All toxic substances must be kept out of the reach of small children. Household chemicals and medicines should be kept in the original containers, and all such containers should be labelled. Before taking or administering any medicine the label should be checked carefully.

Despite all precautions, accidental, suicidal, and criminal poisonings will remain an important problem which every physician must be prepared to treat promptly and effectively. Besides their immediate therapeutic responsibilities, physicians have legal obligations in cases of attempted suicide, homicide, or criminal abortion and of industrial exposure. The physician should also obtain psychiatric care for any patient who has attempted suicide by poison.

DIAGNOSIS OF CHEMICAL POISONING

Optimal management of the poisoned patient requires a correct diagnosis. Unfortunately, in many such patients poisoning is initially not even considered as a possible cause of the clinical picture. The patient may be unaware of exposure to poison or, as after attempted suicide or abortion, he may be unwilling to admit it. Although the toxic effects of some chemical substances are quite characteristic, most poisoning syndromes can simulate other diseases.

Poisoning is usually included in the differential diagnosis of coma, convulsions, acute psychosis, acute hepatic or renal insufficiency, and bone marrow depression. It may not be considered when the major manifestation is a mild psychiatric disturbance or neurologic disorder, abdominal pain, bleeding, fever, hypotension, pulmonary congestion, or skin eruption. Chronic, insidious intoxications are much more frequently missed than acute poisonings whose symptoms appear suddenly and may be immediately related to a specific event. Physicians should always remember the variegated manifestations of poisoning and maintain a high index of suspicion.

In every case of poisoning identification of the toxic agent should be attempted. Specific antidotal therapy is obviously impossible without such identification. In cases of homicide, suicide, or criminal abortion the identity of the poison may be of legal importance. When poisoning results from industrial exposure or therapeutic mishap, accurate knowledge of the responsible agents is essential for future prevention.

In acute accidental poisoning the offending substance may be known to the patient. In many other cases information can be obtained from relatives or acquaintances, by a search for containers at the scene of the poisoning, or by questioning the patient's physician or pharmacist. Frequently such procedures yield only the trade name of a product, which gives no clue to its component chemicals. A number of books which identify the active ingredients of household products, agricultural compounds, proprietary medicines, and poisonous plants are listed in the references to this chapter. A small handbook of this type should be carried in every physician's bag. Poison control centers and manufacturers' representatives are other useful sources of such information. When poisoning is chronic, rapid identification of the toxic agent from the history is frequently impossible. It is therefore fortunate that the lesser therapeutic urgency of such cases usually permits the required painstaking exploration of the patient's habits and environment.

Some poisons can produce clinical features characteristic enough to strongly suggest the diagnosis. Careful examination of the patient may reveal the unmistakable odor of cyanide; the cherry-colored flush of carboxyhemoglobin in skin and mucous membranes; the pupillary constriction, salivation, and gastrointestinal hyperactivity produced by cholinesterase-inhibitor insecticides; or the lead line and extensor paralyses of chronic lead poisoning. Unfortunately, these features are not always present, and in any case telltales are the exception in chemical poisonings.

Chemical analysis of body fluids provides the most definite identification of the intoxicating agent. Some common poisons, such as aspirin, bromides, and barbiturates, can be identified and even quantitated by relatively simple laboratory procedures. Others require more complex toxicologic techniques, such as gas chromatography or bioassay, which are performed only in specialized laboratories. Furthermore, the results of toxicologic determinations are rarely available in time to guide the initial treatment of acute poisoning. Nevertheless, specimens of vomitus, gastric aspirate, blood, urine and feces should always be saved for toxicologic study if diagnostic or legal questions are likely to arise. Chemical analyses of body fluids or tissues are of particular value in the diagnosis and evaluation of chronic intoxications. Finally, they are useful in following the success of some forms of therapy.

TREATMENT OF CHEMICAL POISONING

Although the physician should always try to identify the poison, such attempts must never delay vital therapeutic measures. Most poisons do not have specific antidotes. Essential supportive care must be given as indicated by the patient's clinical state and does not require knowledge of the toxic agent. Symptomatic treatment of circulatory, respiratory, neurologic, and renal function should be immediately administered as to any other seriously ill patient.

Correct treatment of the poisoned patients thus requires knowledge both of the general principles of management and of the details of therapy for specific poisons. Treatment may be divided into four approaches: (1) prevention of further absorption of the poison, (2) removal of absorbed poison from the body, (3) symptomatic or supportive therapy, and (4) administration of systemic antidotes (Table 115-1). The first three ap-

Table 115-1. TREATMENT OF ACUTE CHEMICAL POISONING

I. Prevention of further absorption of poison
   A. Poisoning by ingestion
      1. Emptying the stomach
         a. Induction of vomiting
         b. Gastric lavage
      2. Minimizing gastrointestinal absorption
         a. Neutralization and precipitation
         b. Adsorption
         c. Catharsis
   B. Poisoning by other routes
II. Removal of absorbed poisons from body
   A. Detoxification—enzyme induction?
   B. Biliary excretion—interruption of enterohepatic circulation
   C. Urinary excretion
      1. Osmotic diuresis
      2. Alteration of urinary pH
   D. Dialysis
      1. Peritoneal dialysis
      2. Hemodialysis
   E. Exchange transfusion
   F. Chelation and chemical binding
III. Supportive therapy
IV. Administration of systemic antidotes
   A. Chemical agents
   B. Pharmacologic antagonists

proaches are applicable to most types of poisoning, the fourth can be used only when the toxic agent is known and a specific antidote is available. Success often depends upon speed of treatment and, when indicated by the clinical situation, several approaches should be used simultaneously.

Prevention of Absorption of Ingested Poisons

If appreciable amounts of a poison have been ingested, one should always attempt to minimize its absorption from the gastrointestinal tract. The success of such endeavors depends upon the time elapsed since ingestion and upon the site and speed of absorption of the poison. Prompt action is essential, and it is better to proceed with makeshifts than to waste time while waiting for special equipment or drugs. Conversely, it is unwise to temporize with unpredictable remedies when reliable and effective methods for removal of poison from the gastrointestinal tract are available. When skillfully applied, these methods do not lead to such complications as pulmonary aspiration, gastrointestinal perforation, or convulsions.

EVACUATION OF THE STOMACH. Attempts to empty the stomach are always worthwhile unless specifically contraindicated. They may be highly successful if made soon after ingestion. Significant amounts of poison may be recovered from the stomach hours after ingestion because gastric emptying may be delayed by gastric atony or pylorospasm.

Emesis occurs spontaneously after the ingestion of many poisons. It may be induced in the home by mechanical stimulation of the posterior pharynx or by administration of gastric irritants such as a strong solution of salt or mustard. The emetic action of syrup of ipecac (not the fourteen times more concentrated fluid extract) in 10 to 20 ml dosage is more effective and is safe enough for home use. Regrettably its action has an average latent period of 20 min and depends in part on gastrointestinal absorption, so that it cannot be used in conjunction with other measures intended to minimize absorption of the poison. Apomorphine, 0.06 mg per kg intramuscularly, acts within 5 min but may cause prolonged vomiting. When given intravenously in doses of 0.01 mg per kg, apomorphine tends to produce almost immediate vomiting which is not followed by any other central nervous system effects. All attempts to induce emesis are more often successful if large amounts of fluid have been administered, but these may also hasten passage of the poison through the pylorus. Fluids with high fat content are preferable, since they enter the duodenum more slowly. Not uncommonly it is impossible to induce vomiting, and valuable time should not be lost with hopeful waiting. Induction of vomiting should not be attempted after ingestion of antiemetic drugs, in severely depressed or convulsing patients, or, because of the danger of gastroesophageal perforation or tracheal aspiration of vomitus, in patients who have ingested strong caustics or liquid hydrocarbons which are potent lung irritants (e.g., kerosene, furniture polish).

Unlike emesis, *gastric lavage* is predictably and immediately effective in removing poison from the stomach. Furthermore, it can be employed in unconscious patients, and removal of gastric contents reduces the risk of aspiration of vomitus in such patients. It is, however, contraindicated after the ingestion of strong corrosives because of danger of perforating injured tissues. When properly performed, gastric lavage carries little risk of aspiration of gastric contents into the lungs. The patient should be prone with head and shoulders lowered. A mouth gag is placed and a gastric tube of sufficient diameter to permit withdrawal of particulate matter (size 30) is passed into the stomach. If central nervous system function is depressed and introduction of the tube produces retching, or if pulmonary irritants have been ingested, it is wise to place a *cuffed endotracheal tube* before lavaging. Gastric contents are withdrawn with a large syringe and usually contain most of the poison that will be removed. Thereafter 200 ml (less in children) of warm water or other lavaging solution are alternately

instilled and withdrawn until the aspirate becomes clear.

INTERFERENCE WITH GASTROINTESTINAL ABSORPTION. Since neither emesis nor gastric lavage empty the stomach completely, one should also minimize absorption by administering substances which inactivate or trap ingested poisons. If mineral acids, alkalis, or other corrosives have been swallowed, water, milk, or a neutralizer (aluminum hydroxide, milk of magnesia, dilute vinegar) is given. Some toxic alkaloids can be precipitated and rendered insoluble by the administration of sulfate. Many other poisons are effectively adsorbed by powdered, activated charcoal. A good grade of activated charcoal can rapidly adsorb as much as half its weight of many common poisons. It is more effective than the so-called "universal antidote" which should be relegated to oblivion. Administration of 100 to 200 ml of a slurry of activated charcoal should be alternated with evacuation of the stomach.

Adsorption by charcoal is reversible, and the effectiveness of adsorption of many poisons varies with the pH. Acidic substances are adsorbed better in acid solutions and may therefore be released in the small intestine. It is desirable to speed the charcoal with its adsorbed poison through the intestine as quickly as possible. This will also decrease intestinal absorption of any unadsorbed poison which has passed beyond the pylorus. It is best accomplished by oral or gastric administration of an osmotic cathartic. Sodium sulfate in 10 to 30 Gm dosage is the cathartic of choice, since, unlike magnesium sulfate, it produces no symptoms after systemic absorption. Cathartics are generally contraindicated after the ingestion of strong corrosives.

Prevention of Absorption of Poison from Other Sites

Most topically applied poisons can be removed by copious flushing with water. In certain instances weak acids or bases or appropriate organic solvents are more effective, but rapid and voluminous washing with water should always proceed while they are being obtained. Chemical antidotes can be hazardous because tissue injury may result from the heat of the chemical reaction.

The systemic distribution of injected poisons can be slowed by the application of cold to the injection site or by the proximal application of a tourniquet. Cruciate incision and suction is generally ineffective except after poisonous bites.

Following inhalation of toxic gases, vapors, or dusts, the victim should be removed into clean air and adequate ventilation maintained. If the patient cannot be moved, a protective mask should be applied.

Removal of Absorbed Poison from the Body

Unlike prevention or retardation of absorption, measures to speed removal of the toxic agent from the body rarely have much influence on the peak poison concentration. However, they can significantly abbreviate the time during which the concentration of many poisons remains above any given level and thereby greatly reduce morbidity, avoid complications, and save lives. In judging the need for such measures one must consider the patient's clinical state, the properties and metabolic fate of the poison, and the amount absorbed as judged by the history and the blood level. Removal of some poisons can be accelerated by several methods; selection depends on the clinical urgency, the amount in the body, and the skills and equipment available.

DETOXIFICATION. Since many poisons are metabolically inactivated in the body, it is regrettable that no clinically effective measures to accelerate detoxification are known. Induction of hepatic enzymes would seem to hold some promise in the treatment of poisonings by certain long-acting drugs whose inactivation depends on the activity of inducible enzymes. The clinical usefulness of this approach remains to be shown. At present, therefore, one must rely on measures capable of accelerating excretion of the poison.

BILIARY EXCRETION. Certain organic acids and active drugs are secreted into the bile against large concentration gradients. Again, this process cannot presently be accelerated. However, the intestinal resorption of substances already secreted into the bile can be decreased by duodenal suction or osmotic catharsis. These procedures are useful in poisonings by substances such as glutethimide and chlortetracycline, the action of which is significantly prolonged by their enterohepatic circulation.

URINARY EXCRETION. Acceleration of renal excretion is applicable to a much larger number of poisons. Renal excretion of toxic substances depends on glomerular filtration, active tubular secretion, and passive tubular resorption. The first two processes should be protected by maintenance of adequate circulation and renal function, but for practical purposes they cannot be accelerated. On the other hand, passive tubular resorption of many poisons plays an important role in the prolongation of their action and can frequently be decreased by readily available methods.

Passive resorption of most filtered poisons occurs largely in the proximal tubules because their concentration in the filtrate increases as salt and water are reabsorbed. It can be partly prevented by inhibiting water resorption at this site. This is best accomplished by the administration of osmotic diuretics such as mannitol or urea. By infusing 10 to 20 Gm per hour of mannitol or urea after a loading dose of 25 to 50 Gm, urine volumes up to 1 liter per hour can be achieved. Great care must be used to supply water and electrolyte needs at the same time. Osmotic diuretics should not be used in the presence of congestive heart failure, shock, or renal failure. The effectiveness of osmotic diuretic therapy in increasing renal excretion has been demonstrated for salicylates, barbiturates, meprobamate, and glutethimide but is potentially applicable to all ultrafiltered poisons which are passively reabsorbed.

Alteration of the urinary pH can also inhibit passive back-diffusion of some poisons and increase their renal clearance. The renal tubular epithelium is more permeable to uncharged molecules than to ionized solutes. Weak organic acids and bases readily diffuse out of the tubular fluid in their unionized form but are trapped in it when ionized. Acidic poisons are largely ionized only at pHs above their pK_a. Alkalinization of the urine greatly increases the ionization in the tubular fluid of such organic acids as phenobarbital and salicylate. In contrast, the pK_a of pentobarbital (8.1) and secobarbital (8.0) is so high that renal clearance is not greatly increased by raising the urinary pH into the physiologic alkaline range. Alkalinization of the urine is achieved by the infusion of sodium bicarbonate, sodium lactate, or tromethamine (which also acts as an osmotic diuretic) at a rate determined by the urinary and blood pH. Excessive systemic alkalosis or electrolyte disturbances must be carefully prevented. A combination of osmotic diuresis and alkalinization of the urine can raise the renal clearance of some acidic poisons tenfold or more and has been found highly effective in poisoning by salicylate and phenobarbital. The full range of its clinical applicability is undoubtedly much wider but remains to be established. Depression of the urinary pH beyond its usual range may increase the renal clearance of some weakly basic poisons, but clinical data are lacking.

Finally, the renal excretion of certain poisons can be increased in a highly specific fashion. An example is the removal of bromide by administration of chloride and chloriuretics. Such methods will be discussed with the individual poisons.

DIALYSIS. The relative effectiveness of osmotic diuresis at favorable urinary pH and of dialysis must differ widely among drugs but has been established for very few. For barbiturates and some other poisons which are not actively secreted by the renal tubules, maximal clearance rates during extracorporeal dialysis are considerably greater than during peritoneal dialysis or forced diuresis. The latter two maneuvers appear about equally effective. Of course, a skilled team can proceed simultaneously with dialysis and solute diuresis. Dialysis has been found effective in the removal of barbiturates, borate, bromide, chlorate, dimercaprol, diphenylhydantoin, ethanol, ethinamate, glutethimide, glycols, isoniazid, methanol, salicylate, sulfonamides, and thiocyanate. Beyond these, it should theoretically accelerate the removal from the body of any dialyzable toxin which is not irreversibly bound to tissues.

Peritoneal dialysis can be easily performed in any hospital and may be continued for long periods. It is particularly valuable for the removal of poisons if renal function is impaired. Obviously, its effectiveness does not extend to large-molecule, nondialyzable poisons and is decreased by a high degree of protein binding or lipid solubility of the toxic substance. Peritoneal clearance can be increased if the dialyzed poison can be trapped chemically in the dialysis fluid so that a high gradient of the dialyzable portion is maintained from blood to peritoneal cavity between fluid changes. A percent concentration of albumin in the dialysis solution acts as an effective ligand during the dialysis of salicylate and should be similarly useful for the removal of other albumin-bound poisons. Another approach to prevent back-diffusion consists of making the pH of dialysis fluid sufficiently greater or less than 7.4 to ionize poisons which are dialyzable only in the undissociated form. Finally, the addition of various drugs to the dialysis fluid can increase peritoneal dialysis, presumably by increasing peritoneal blood flow or mesothelial permeability. The clinical value of this approach has not yet been defined.

Hemodialysis is unquestionably the most effective procedure for removing large amounts of dialyzable poisons. For barbiturates dialysance rates of 50 to 100 ml per min have been achieved, a removal rate two to five times faster than during peritoneal dialysis or osmotic diuresis. Dialysis against solutions containing albumin or lipids or perfusion of the blood through activated charcoal further speed removal of certain poisons. Extracorporeal dialysis is clearly the procedure of choice for the rapid removal of dialyzable poisons from patients who have absorbed amounts which make survival unlikely even under the best supportive care. Since the required equipment and skilled personnel are available only in a few hospitals, the possibility of transfer of such patients to one of these institutions should be considered.

EXCHANGE TRANSFUSION. Withdrawal and replacement of blood is an effective procedure for the removal of those poisons which are not highly tissue-bound or lipid-soluble and therefore remain in the blood in appreciable concentration. It has obvious advantages in poisoning by nondiffusible and particularly by highly albumin-bound toxins. While it requires little specialized equipment, its applicability to adults is limited by the requirement of large amounts of blood.

CHELATION AND CHEMICAL BINDING. The removal of some poisons is accelerated by chemical interaction with other substances followed by renal excretion. These substances are usually considered specific antidotes and will be discussed with the individual poisons.

Supportive Therapy

Most chemical poisonings are reversible and self-limited disease states. Skillful supportive therapy can keep many seriously poisoned patients alive and their detoxifying and excretory mechanisms functioning until the concentration of poison in the body has fallen to safe levels. Symptomatic measures are especially important when the poison is one of the many compounds for which no specific antidote is known. Even when an antidote is available, disturbances of vital functions must be prevented or controlled by appropriate supportive care.

The poisoned patient may suffer a variety of physiologic disturbances. Most of these are not peculiar to chemical intoxications, and their therapeutic management is described elsewhere in this text. Only those aspects of supportive therapy specially relevant to poisonings are briefly discussed here.

CENTRAL NERVOUS SYSTEM DEPRESSION. Specific therapy directed against the depressant effects of poisons on the central nervous system is usually both unnecessary and difficult. Most poisoned patients will emerge from coma as from a prolonged anesthesia. During the period of unconsciousness meticulous nursing care and close observation are essential. If depression of medullary centers results in circulatory or respiratory failure, these vital functions must be immediately and vigorously supported by chemical or mechanical means.

The use of analeptics in the treatment of poison-induced central nervous system depression is being increasingly abandoned. First, their effect is unpredictable and their use in intoxicated patients produces an abnormal pattern of nervous activity in which paroxysmal excitation and convulsions may be superimposed on depression. Secondly, the availability of artificial ventilation and of effective measures to support the circulation has lessened the need for rapid restoration of normal medullary function. It is doubtful that analeptics shorten the duration of coma sufficiently to justify their risks, and they have not been shown to improve prognosis. Certainly these agents should never be employed to restore consciousness, but under some circumstances their use to hasten the restoration of spontaneous breathing and active reflexes may be justified. Picrotoxin, pentylenetetrazol, bemegride, and ethamivan are the most useful analeptics.

CONVULSIONS. Many poisons (e.g., chlorinated hydrocarbons, insecticides, strychnine) cause convulsions by their specific excitatory effects. Poisoned patients may also convulse because of hypoxia, hypoglycemia, cerebral edema, or metabolic disturbances. In such cases these abnormalities should be corrected as far as possible. Regardless of the cause of the convulsions, anticonvulsant drugs are often required. Short-acting compounds, such as intravenously administered thiopental or amobarbital, are preferable, because in poisoned patients profound depression may accompany or quickly follow convulsions.

CEREBRAL EDEMA. Intracranial hypertension due to cerebral edema is also a characteristic effect of some poisons and a nonspecific result of other chemical intoxications. Cerebral edema is characteristically seen in poisoning by lead, carbon monoxide, and methanol. Symptomatic treatment consists of adrenocortical steroids and, when necessary, the intravenous administration of hypertonic solutions of mannitol or urea.

HYPOTENSION. The causes of hypotension and shock in the poisoned patient are legion, and often several of them coexist. Poisons can depress the medullary vasomotor centers, block autonomic ganglia or adrenergic receptors, directly depress the tone of arterial or venous smooth muscle, reduce myocardial contractility, or induce cardiac arrhythmias. Less specifically, the poisoned patient may be in shock because of tissue hypoxia, extensive tissue destruction from corrosives, loss of blood or fluids, or metabolic disturbances. When possible, these abnormalities should be promptly corrected. Vasopressor drugs are helpful and often essential in the hypotensive poisoned patient, particularly in shock resulting from central depression. As in shock of other etiologies, choice of the most appropriate agent requires an analysis of the hemodynamic disturbance which goes beyond determination of the arterial pressure.

CARDIAC ARRHYTHMIAS. Disturbances of cardiac impulse generation or conduction in the poisoned patient arise from the effects of certain poisons on the electrical properties of cardiac fibers or from myocardial hypoxia or metabolic disturbances. The latter should be corrected and antiarrhythmic agents administered as indicated by the nature of the arrhythmia.

PULMONARY EDEMA. The poisoned patient may develop pulmonary edema because of depressed myocardial contractility or because of alveolar injury from irritant gases or aspirated fluids. The latter type is less responsive to treatment and may be associated with laryngeal edema. Therapeutic measures include suctioning, high concentrations of oxygen under positive pressure, aerosols of surface-active agents, bronchodilators, and adrenocortical steroids.

HYPOXIA. Poisoning may cause tissue hypoxia by various mechanisms, and several of these may operate in one patient. Inadequate ventilation can result from central respiratory depression, from muscular paralysis, or from airway obstruction by retained secretions, laryngeal edema, or bronchospasm. Alveolar-capillary diffusion may be impaired by pulmonary edema. Anemia, methemoglobinemia, carboxyhemoglobinemia, or shock can interfere with oxygen transport. Cellular oxidation may be inhibited by cyanide, fluoroacetate, or general protoplasmic poisons. The highest priority in treatment must be given to maintenance of an adequate airway. The clinical situation and the site of obstruction may indicate frequent suctioning, insertion of an oropharyngeal airway or of an endotracheal tube, or a tracheotomy. If despite a clear airway ventilation remains inadequate as judged by clinical appearance or by measurement of minute volume or blood gases, artificial ventilation by appropriate mechanical means is imperative. Administration of high concentrations of oxygen is indicated whenever tissue hypoxia occurs. When the central nervous system is severely depressed, oxygen administration often results in apnea and must be combined with artifical ventilation. Hyperbaric oxygen may be helpful in some situations. The treatment of methemoglobinemia, carboxyhemoglobinemia, and inhibition of cellular oxidation is discussed under the specific poisons which produce these changes.

ACUTE RENAL INSUFFICIENCY. Renal failure with oliguria or anuria may occur in the poisoned patient because of shock, dehydration, or electrolyte disturbances. More specifically, it may be due to the nephrotoxic potential of poisons (e.g., mercury, phosphorus, carbon tetrachloride, bromate) many of which are concentrated and excreted by the kidney. Renal damage due to poisons is usually reversible. The management of acute renal insufficiency is outlined in Chap. 300.

ELECTROLYTE AND WATER DISTURBANCES. Imbalance of fluid and electrolytes are common features of chemical poisoning. They may result from vomiting, diarrhea, renal insufficiency, or from therapeutic maneuvers such as catharsis, osmotic diuresis, or dialysis. These disturbances are corrected or ideally prevented by appropriate therapy. Certain poisons produce more specific defects such as metabolic acidosis (e.g., methanol, phenol, salicylate) or hypocalcemia (e.g., fluoride, oxalate). These abnormalities and any specific treatment will be described under the individual poisons.

ACUTE HEPATIC INSUFFICIENCY. The primary manifestation of some poisonings (e.g., chlorinated hydrocarbons, phosphorus, cinchophen, certain mushrooms) is acute hepatic failure. Its management is described in Chap. 326.

Administration of Systemic Antidotes

Specific antidotal therapy is available for only a few poisons. Some systemic antidotes are chemicals which exert their therapeutic effect by reducing the concentration of the toxic substance. They may do this by combining with the poison (e.g., ethylene diaminetetraacetate with lead, dimercaprol with mercury) or by increasing its excretion (e.g., chloride or mercurial diuretics in bromide poisoning). Other systemic antidotes compete with the poison for its receptor site (e.g., atropine with muscarine, nallorphine with morphine, vitamin K_1 with coumarins). Specific antidotes will be discussed with the individual poisons.

REFERENCES

General

Arena, J. M.: "Poisoning," 2nd ed., Springfield, Ill., Charles C Thomas Publisher, 1969.

Coleman, A. B.: Accidental Poisoning, New Engl. J. Med., 277:1135, 1967.

Corby, D. G., R. C. Lisciandro, R. H. Lehman, and W. J. Decker: The Efficiency of Methods Used to Evacuate the Stomach after Acute Ingestions, Pediatrics, 40:871, 1967.

Dabbous, I. A., A. B. Bergman, and W. O. Robertson: The Ineffectiveness of Mechanically Induced Vomiting, J. Pediat., 66:952, 1965.

Deichmann, W. B., and H. W. Gerarde: "Symptomatology and Therapy of Toxicological Emergencies," New York, Academic Press, Inc., 1964.

De Myttenaere, M. H., J. F. Maher, and G. E. Schreiner: Hemoperfusion through a Charcoal Column for Glutethimide Poisoning, Trans. Am. Soc. Artificial Internal Organs, 13:190, 1967.

Done, A. K.: Clinical Pharmacology of Systemic Antidotes, Clin. Pharmacol. Therap., 2:750, 1961.

Dreisbach, R. H.: "Handbook of Poisoning, Diagnosis and Treatment," 6th ed., Los Altos, Calif., Lange Medical Publications, 1969.

Gosselin, R. E., and R. P. Smith: Trends in the Therapy of Acute Poisonings, Clin. Pharmacol. Therap., 7:279, 1966.

Holt, L. E., Jr., and P. H. Holz: The Black Bottle, a Consideration of the Role of Charcoal in the Treatment of Poisoning in Children, J. Pediat., 63:306, 1963.

Maher, J. F., and G. E. Schreiner: Current Status of Dialysis of Poisons and Drugs, Trans. Am. Soc. Artificial Internal Organs, 15:461, 1969.

Matthew, H., and A. A. H. Lawson: "Treatment of Common Acute Poisonings," Edinburgh, E. & S. Livingstone Ltd., 1967.

Milne, M. D.: Potentiation of Excretion of Drugs, Proc. Roy. Soc. Med., 57:809, 1964.

Myschetzky, A., and N. A. Lassen: Urea-induced Osmotic Diuresis and Alkalinization of Urine in Acute Barbiturate Intoxication, J. Amer. Med. Ass., 185:936, 1963.

Picchioni, A. L.: Activated Charcoal versus "Universal Antidote" as an Antidote for Poisons, Toxicol. Appl. Pharmacol., 8:447, 1966.

Shinaberger, J. H., L. Shear, L. E. Clayton, K. G. Barry, M. Knowlton, and L. R. Goldbaum: Dialysis for Intoxication with Lipid Soluble Drugs, Enhancement of Glutethimide Extraction with Lipid Dialysate, Trans. Am. Soc. Artifical Internal Organs, 11:173, 1965.

Shirkey, H. C.: Ipecac Syrup, Its Use as an Emetic in Poison Control, J. Pediat., 69:139, 1966.

Strickler, J. C.: Forced Diuresis in the Management of Barbiturate Intoxication, Clin. Pharmacol. Therap., 6:693, 1965.

Thienes, C. H., and T. J. Haley: "Clinical Toxicology," 4th ed., Philadelphia, Lea & Febiger, 1964.

Verhulst, H. L., and J. J. Crotty: Childhood Poisoning Accidents, J.A.M.A., 203:1049, 1968.

Toxic Product Information

Adams, W. C.: Poison Control Centers: Their Purpose and Operation, Clin. Pharmacol. Therap., 4:293, 1963.

Brown, R. L.: "Pesticides in Clinical Practice," Springfield, Ill., Charles C Thomas, Publisher, 1966.

Directory, Poison Control Centers, U.S. Public Health Service, Publ. No. 1278, 1967.

Gleason, M. N., R. E. Gosselin, H. C. Hodge, and R. P. Smith: "Clinical Toxicology of Commercial Products," 3d ed., Baltimore, The Williams & Wilkins Company, 1969.

Goodman, L. S., and A. Gilman: "The Pharmacological Basis of Therapeutics," 3d ed., New York, The Macmillan Company, 1965.

Kingsbury, J. M.: "Poisonous Plants of the United States and Canada," Englewood Cliffs, N.J., Prentice-Hall, Inc., 1964.

"The Merck Index," 8th ed., Rahway, N.J., Merck & Co., Inc., 1968.

Sax, N. I.: "Dangerous Properties of Industrial Materials," 3d ed., New York, Reinhold Book Corporation, 1968.

"Toxicants Occurring Naturally in Foods," Washington, National Academy of Sciences, Publication No. 1354, 1966.

Wilson, C. O., and T. E. Jones: "American Drug Index," Philadelphia, J. B. Lippincott Company, 1969.

116 COMMON POISONS
Jan Koch-Weser

The poisons discussed in this chapter are those which are encountered by the general population such as commonly used drugs, household products, solvents, pesticides, and poisonous plants. It has been necessary to disregard many uncommon toxic materials as well as products to which exposure occurs only in specialized industrial environments. Details concerning poisoning by such compounds may be found in some of the references following Chap. 115. Toxic effects of many drugs are considered throughout this text in conjunction with their therapeutic use. Manifestations of hypersensitivity to chemicals are described in Chap. 73. The following discussions of specific poisons stress those details of their action which are pertinent to the recognition or treatment of clinical poisoning.

ACIDS

Corrosive acids are used widely in industry and laboratories. Ingestion is almost always with suicidal intent. Death has occurred after an oral dose of 1 ml of a corrosive acid.

Toxic effects of corrosive acids are largely due to their direct chemical action. They convert tissue protein to acid proteinate which is soluble in the acid. Irritation, bleeding, sloughing, and perforation of the esophagus and stomach are common. Mouth and pharynx are brownish-black and may have a charred appearance. Yellow staining is seen after ingestion of nitric and picric acids. Severe pain in mouth, pharynx, chest, and abdomen is the rule and is soon followed by vomiting and diarrhea of coffee grounds appearance. Frequently profound shock develops. About half of those who ingest significant amounts of acid die from its immediate effects. The survivors often develop mediastinitis or peritonitis from esophageal or gastric perforation. Delayed perforation of the esophagus or stomach also occurs. Recovery from acid ingestion is often associated with esophageal stricture.

Ingested acid must be immediately diluted a hundred fold by water or milk or neutralized with weak alkali. Milk of magnesia or magnesium and aluminum antacids are excellent for the purpose. Sodium bicarbonate should be avoided because the evolved carbon dioxide may rupture an eroded viscus. The danger of perforation also contraindicates the use of emesis or gastric lavage except during the first 30 min after ingestion. Following the emergency measures, appropriate supportive therapy is administered for the relief of pain and the treatment of shock, perforation, and infection.

Certain gases found in industry may combine with water in the lungs to form corrosive acids. During rapid decomposition of plant material in silos, oxides of nitrogen are released which form nitric acid in the lungs. Inhalation of such gases causes coughing and choking sensations which are followed after a latent period of 6 to 8 hr by pulmonary edema. Treatment is supportive. Symptoms of dyspnea and hemoptysis may be prolonged and frequent relapses may occur.

ALKALIS

Strong alkalis such as ammonium hydroxide, potassium hydroxide (potash), potassium carbonate, sodium hydroxide (lye), and sodium carbonate (washing soda) are widely used in industry and in cleansers and drain cleaners. Sodium and potassium phosphates find use as water softeners. Strong alkalis form soaps with fats and proteinates with proteins, resulting in penetrating necrosis of tissues. Fatalities have occurred from the ingestion of 5 to 30 Gm of such compounds.

The toxic effects of alkalis are almost entirely due to irritation and destruction of local tissues. Ingestion is followed by severe pain in mouth, pharynx, chest, and abdomen. Vomiting of blood and sloughed mucosa and diarrhea are common. Reflex loss of vascular tone frequently leads to profound shock. Perforation of the esophagus or stomach may be immediate or delayed for several days. Mouth and pharynx show erythema and gelatinous necrotic areas. After ingestion of water softeners profound reduction in serum calcium may be seen and lead to tetany and hypotension. Ingestion of strong alkali is rapidly fatal in about 25 percent of cases. Survivors usually suffer from esophageal strictures.

Treatment consists of immediate administration of large amounts of water, milk, fruit juices, or 10 percent vinegar. The volume of liquids should exceed that of the ingested alkali a hundred fold. Vomiting should be allowed to occur and gastric lavage may be performed during the first half hour after ingestion. Because of the danger of perforation both are contraindicated thereafter. After the ingestion of water softeners (phosphates), calcium gluconate should be administered intravenously as needed. Treatment is otherwise symptomatic and directed at the relief of pain, respiratory obstruction due to edema of the hypopharynx, fluid loss, and shock.

Inhalation of ammonia, which is used as a refrigerant, results in irritation of the upper and lower respiratory tract. Laryngeal and pulmonary edema may occur and must be treated symptomatically.

ANILINE

This substance is used in printing and cloth-marking inks, crayons, paints, and paint removers. Both aniline and its derivatives, such as toluidine, nitroaniline, and nitrobenzene, are widely used in industrial synthesis. Aniline is absorbed from the gastrointestinal tract and through the lungs or skin. Ingestion of 1 Gm aniline has been fatal. Methemoglobinemia is the most important manifestation. Headache, dizziness, hypotension, convulsions, and coma may occur. If the acute period is survived, jaundice and anemia may appear. Treatment consists of correction of methemoglobinemia (see Chap. 61) and supportive measures.

ANTIHISTAMINES

The common and unprescribed use of antihistamines makes them readily available for accidental overdosage and suicidal attempts. There is wide variation from patient to patient in tolerance to these drugs and in the manifestations of poisoning. A dose of 200 mg diphenhydramine has been fatal in one adult, whereas another tolerated 2 Gm. Manifestations of poisoning are central nervous system excitement or depression. In children the usual toxic manifestations are excitement, hyperthermia, hyperreflexia, tremors, and convulsions, followed by central nervous system depression. In adults depressive manifestations with drowsiness, stupor, and coma predominate, but convulsions followed by further depression may occur.

Treatment is supportive and directed toward removal of the unabsorbed drug and maintenance of vital functions. Stimulants should be avoided. Convulsions may be controlled with short-acting barbiturates, ether, or succinylcholine. Some antihistamines have prominent atropine-like properties. Patients poisoned with these drugs may show manifestations of atropine poisoning and are treated correspondingly.

ANTIMUSCARINIC COMPOUNDS

Atropine, related belladonna alkaloids (hyoscyamine, scopolamine), and synthetic substitutes (e.g., benztropine, cyclopentolate, homatropine, methantheline, propantheline) are widely prescribed drugs and occur in many proprietary mixtures used in the treatment of gastrointestinal and upper respiratory diseases, asthma, and parkinsonism. Poisoning, especially in children, may also occur from the excessive use of ophthalmic solutions containing such compounds. Finally, children may be intoxicated by eating plants containing up to 0.5 percent of atropine or related alkaloids. Such plants are *Atropa belladonna* (deadly nightshade), *Hioscyamus niger* (henbane), and *Datura stramonium* (Jamestown or Jimson weed).

Individual sensitivity to the toxic effects of belladonna alkaloids varies widely: fatalities have occurred from as little as 10 mg atropine, but doses of 500 mg have been survived. Young children are particularly susceptible to poisoning with belladonna alkaloids. Old people appear to be more sensitive to the central nervous system effects of these drugs. Since atropine is both hydrolyzed in the liver and excreted unchanged in the urine, insufficiency of hepatic or renal function may lead to poisoning on therapeutic dosage.

The most characteristic manifestations of atropine poisoning are those of parasympathetic blockade: dryness of mucous membranes, thirst, dysphagia, hoarseness, xerophthalmia, dilated pupils, blurring of vision, rise in intraocular tension, flushing, dryness and increased temperature of the skin, fever, tachycardia, hypertension, urinary retention, and abdominal distension. This widespread parasympatholysis is almost diagnostic of belladonna poisoning, but the diagnosis can be further confirmed by the absence of any parasympathomimetic effects following the intramuscular injection of 10 mg methacholine.

Central nervous system symptoms are also very common during belladonna intoxication. Atropine and scopolamine produce similar toxic psychoses. Restlessness, excitation, confusion, and incoordination precede mania, hallucinations, and delirium. Patients intoxicated by scopolamine not infrequently show lethargy and somnolence rather than excitement. In severe intoxication with belladonna alkaloids central nervous system depression and coma are the rule. Death occurs due to circulatory collapse and respiratory failure.

In the treatment of belladonna poisoning gastric lavage with an aqueous slurry of activated charcoal should be initiated quickly. Symptomatic treatment is directed at the reduction of body temperature, the moistening of mucous membranes, and, when necessary, urethral catheterization. Excitement, convulsions, or depression may require appropriate pharmacotherapy. Parasympathomimetic agents, such as methacholine or pilocarpine, are of little value, since they cannot be given in concentrations sufficient to overcome the peripheral cholinergic blockade. Furthermore, they have no effect on the potentially lethal central nervous system toxicity of the belladonna alkaloids.

Death occurs in fewer than 1 percent of cases of atropine or scopolamine poisoning. No permanent sequelae have been observed, but manifestations may persist for several days.

BARIUM

Poisoning may be due to the ingestion of rodenticides which contain soluble barium salts or of depilatories that contain barium sulfide. Intoxication may also occur in industry or from the accidental use of a soluble barium salt as a radiopaque contrast medium. Barium is extremely toxic, producing intense stimulation of muscles of all types. Its action on the gastrointestinal musculature causes vomiting, colic, and diarrhea. Skeletal muscle tremors and spasm are commonly seen. Arteriolar spasm results in marked hypertension. Cardiac arrhythmias may proceed to ventricular fibrillation. Anxiety, weakness, and convulsions may occur. Death is usually due to cardiac arrhythmia or respiratory arrest.

Treatment consists of the oral administration of 250 ml of 10% sodium sulfate or 5% magnesium sulfate. This will precipitate and remove any unabsorbed barium in the gastrointestinal tract. A dose of 10 ml of a 10% solution of sodium sulfate should be slowly administered intravenously every 30 min until symptoms subside. Procainamide may be used to reduce the danger of fatal cardiac arrhythmias. If necessary, pain should be relieved and artificial ventilation with oxygen administered.

BENZENE, TOLUENE

These solvents are used in paint removers, dry-cleaning solutions, and rubber or plastic cements. Benzene is also present, to some extent, in most gasolines. Poisoning may result from ingestion or from the breathing of concentrated vapors. Toluene is the major ingredient in the cement used by teen-age glue sniffers.

Acute poisoning by these compounds causes central nervous system manifestations. With sufficient exposure, symptoms progress from an initial period of restlessness, excitement, euphoria, and dizziness to coma, convulsions, and respiratory failure. Ventricular arrhythmias may occur.

Chronic poisoning by benzene or toluene results from repeated exposure to their vapors in low concentration. Central nervous system symptoms include irritability, insomnia, headache, tremors, and paresthesias. Anorexia and nausea are also common. Fatty degeneration of the heart, liver, and kidneys may occur. By far the most important manifestation of chronic exposure to benzene is bone marrow depression, which may progress to aplastic anemia and complete aplasia of the bone marrow. Individual susceptibility to this effect varies greatly and may not become apparent for months after the initial exposure to the poison.

Treatment of both acute and chronic poisoning is symptomatic. After ingestion emesis must not be induced, and gastric lavage should await placement of an endotracheal tube with an inflatable cuff. Neurologic, pulmonary, or cardiovascular problems are treated as in poisoning by petroleum distillates.

BLEACHES

Clorox, Purex, Sanichlor, and other bleaching solutions contain 3 to 6 percent sodium hypochlorite. Their corrosive action in mouth, pharynx, and esophagus is similar to that of sodium hydroxide. Acid gastric juice releases hypochlorous acid from such solutions. This compound is very irritating to mucous membranes, and inhalation of its fumes causes severe pulmonary irritation and pulmonary edema. However, the systemic toxicity of hypochlorous acid is low. Perforation and stricture formation is rare after the ingestion of bleaching solutions. The fatal dose is approximately 30 ml.

Treatment consists of emesis or gastric lavage with water, milk, milk of magnesia, aluminum hydroxide, or sodium bicarbonate solution. Acid antidotes should not be used. If available, 200 ml of a 5% solution of sodium thiosulfate should be administered by mouth, since this will immediately reduce hypochlorite to nontoxic products. Supportive measures may be needed as in alkali poisoning.

BORIC ACID

This compound is a very weak germicide and has been widely employed in powders, lotions, solutions, and ointments. While not highly toxic, boric acid is not nearly as benign as widely assumed. The lethal dose is approximately 15 Gm in adults and 5 Gm in infants. Such amounts can be easily absorbed through abraded skin, from serous cavities, and after ingestion. Furthermore, accumulation of the compound occurs because of slow renal excretion.

Regardless of the route of administration, the first symptoms of poisoning are nausea, vomiting, and diarrhea. This is followed by headache, weakness, restlessness, and an erythematous rash which may progress to desquamation of skin and mucous membranes. Renal toxicity and shock are common, and more than 100 fatalities have occurred. Treatment is entirely supportive. Boric acid should always be labeled as a poison and must not be applied to extensive skin lesions.

BROMATES

These compounds are used as neutralizers in cold wave preparations. They produce widespread tissue injury, particularly in central nervous system and kidneys. The fatal oral dose of bromates is approximately 5 Gm. On contact of bromate with gastric acid, hydrogen bromate, an irritating acid, is formed. Ingestion of bromates is followed by vomiting, diarrhea, abdominal pain, drowsiness, coma, convulsions, hypotension, hematuria, oliguria, anuria, and hemolysis.

Treatment consists of emesis or gastric lavage with sodium bicarbonate solution followed by catharsis. A dose of 250 ml of a 1% sodium thiosulfate solution should be administered intravenously. Peritoneal dialysis or hemodialysis effectively removes bromate from the body. Appropriate supportive therapy should be given.

CANTHARIDIN

This active principle of Cantharis vesicatoria (Spanish fly) is not a useful therapeutic agent. Poisoning is due to the unfortunate and wishful reputation of cantharidin as an abortifacient or aphrodisiac. The compound is a very potent irritant to all tissues, and ingestion of 10 mg may be fatal. Initial symptoms after ingestion are severe burning pain in the upper gastrointestinal tract, hematemesis, and bloody diarrhea. This is rapidly followed by burning urethral pain, priapism, hematuria, oliguria, anuria, uremia, hepatic failure, myocarditis, shock, delirium, and coma. Death may occur within a few hours or up to 1 week after poisoning. Treatment is entirely symptomatic and supportive.

CARBON MONOXIDE

Carbon monoxide is a colorless, odorless, tasteless and nonirritating gas produced by the incomplete combustion of carbonaceous materials. Almost any flame or combustion device emits carbon monoxide. The gas is present in the exhaust of internal combustion engines in a concentration of 3 to 7 percent. Much higher concentrations are present in most illuminating and heating gases, but not in natural gas. Carbon monoxide is annually responsible for hundreds of accidental and suicidal deaths.

The toxic effects of carbon monoxide are the result of tissue hypoxia. Carbon monoxide combines with hemoglobin to form carboxyhemoglobin. Since carbon monoxide and oxygen react with the same group in the hemoglobin molecule, carboxyhemoglobin is incapable of carrying oxygen. The affinity of hemoglobin for carbon monoxide is two hundred times greater than for oxygen, and at equilibrium 1 part of carbon monoxide in 1,500 parts of air will result in 50 percent conversion of hemoglobin into carboxyhemoglobin. Carboxyhemoglobin also interferes with the release of oxygen from oxyhemoglobin. This further reduces the amount of oxygen available to the tissues and explains why tissue anoxia appears in the carbon monoxide poisoned individual at levels of arterial oxyhemoglobin concentration well tolerated by the anemic patient.

The extent of saturation of hemoglobin with carbon monoxide depends on the concentration of the gas in inspired air and on the time of exposure. The severity of hypoxic symptoms depends further on the state of activity of the individual, his tissue oxygen needs, and his hemoglobin concentration. As a general rule, no symptoms will develop at a concentration of 0.01 percent carbon monoxide in inspired air, since this will not raise blood saturation above 10 percent. Exposure to 0.05 percent for 1 hr during light activity will produce a blood concentration of 20 percent carboxyhemoglobin and result in a mild or throbbing headache. Greater activity or longer exposure to the same concentration causes a blood saturation of 30 to 50 percent. At this point headache, irritability, confusion, dizziness, visual disturbances, nausea, vomiting, and fainting on exertion may be observed. After exposure for 1 hr to concentrations of 0.1 percent in inspired air the blood will contain 50 to 80 percent carboxyhemoglobin, which results in coma, convulsions, respiratory failure, and death. On inhalation of high concentrations of carbon monoxide, saturation of the blood proceeds so rapidly that unconsciousness may occur suddenly and without warning symptoms. When poisoning is more gradual, the individual may notice decreased exercise tolerance and dyspnea on exertion or even at rest. Excessive sweating, fever, hepatomegaly, skin lesions, leukocytosis, bleeding diathesis, albuminuria, and glycosuria have also been described. Cerebral edema and intracranial hypertension may result from the increased permeability of hypoxic capillaries. Myocardial hypoxia is reflected by electrocardiographic abnormalities.

The most characteristic sign of carbon monoxide poisoning is the cherry color of skin and mucous membranes, which is due to the bright red carboxyhemoglobin. If the characteristic flush is not present, 5 ml of 40% sodium hydroxide may be added to 5 ml of a 5% solution of blood in water. An oxyhemoglobin solution will turn brown, but a carboxyhemoglobin solution remains red.

Treatment of carbon monoxide poisoning requires effective ventilation in the presence of high oxygen tensions and in the absence of carbon monoxide. If necessary, ventilation should be supported artificially. Pure oxygen should be administered. This will result not only in the replacement of carbon monoxide by oxygen in the hemoglobin molecule but also in the partial relief of tissue hypoxia by oxygen dissolved in the plasma. For the same reasons hyperbaric oxygen is helpful in seriously poisoned patients. Transfusion of blood or packed cells is also of value. In order to reduce tissue needs for oxygen the patient must be kept absolutely quiet. The induction of hypothermia may further reduce oxygen requirements.

During the recovery from carbon monoxide poisoning symptoms regress gradually. If severe tissue hypoxia has obtained too long, neurologic symptoms such as tremors, mental deterioration, and psychotic behavior may persist.

Histologic changes characteristic of hypoxia may be observed in cerebral cortex, medulla, myocardium, and other organs.

CASTOR BEANS

The castor bean plant (*Ricinus communis*) is grown for commercial and ornamental purposes. The beans contain ricin, an extremely toxic albumin, which causes agglutination and hemolysis of red cells and injury to all other cells. After a delay of several hours to 2 days following ingestion abdominal pain, vomiting, and profuse diarrhea appear and produce severe dehydration. Extreme weakness, drowsiness, disorientation, stupor, coma, convulsions, respiratory depression, and circulatory collapse may develop. Intravascular clotting and hemolysis have been observed. If the patient survives the acute symptoms, oliguria may progress to anuria and uremia, with death after several days. Treatment consists of fluid replacement, alkalinization of the urine with sodium bicarbonate to prevent precipitation of hemoglobin in the kidneys, and supportive measures.

CATHARTIC RESINS

Colocynth, croton oil, gamboge, and podophyllum are drastic cathartics due to their content of highly irritating plant resins. These compounds have no therapeutic use; poisoning is usually the work of ignorant pranksters. Oral administration of 1 Gm of these substances has been fatal. Symptoms are burning pain in mouth, esophagus, and stomach, hematemesis, watery or bloody diarrhea, dehydration, shock, coma, and death. Treatment consists of removal of the irritant from the gastrointestinal tract and supportive measures. Large amounts of parenteral fluids, blood replacement, and morphine and atropine to quiet the bowel may be required.

CHLORATES

Sodium and potassium chlorates are strong oxidizing agents and are found in gargles, mouthwashes, matches, and weed killers. After oral ingestion, 2 Gm has been fatal for children and 10 Gm for adults. Chlorate ion acts as a catalyst in the production of methemoglobinemia, and absorption of a small amount can result in a high methemoglobin concentration. The symptoms of chlorate ingestion are those of local mucosal irritation and of methemoglobinemia (see Chap. 61). Renal toxicity is common. Treatment is directed at the methemoglobinemia and is otherwise supportive.

CHLORINATED INSECTICIDES

These compounds are common ingredients of dusts, sprays, and solutions used as insecticides. The great majority of these compounds are chlorinated diphenyls (e.g., DDT, TDE, DFDT, DMC, Neotran) or chlorinated polycyclic compounds (e.g., Aldrin, Chlordane, Dieldrin, Endrin, Heptachlor). Lindane is a hexachlorbenzene. The toxic effects of all these agents are similar. The chlorinated insecticides are soluble in lipid and organic solvents but not in water. They are poorly absorbed unless dissolved in a vehicle such as kerosene, petroleum distillates, or other organic solvents. Under these circumstances they readily enter the body through the skin, lungs, or gastrointestinal tract. These compounds vary considerably in toxicity, and the toxicity of the dissolving vehicle must also be considered. The effects of the solvent may overshadow or modify those of the insecticide.

The initial symptoms of acute poisoning are nausea, vomiting, headache, dizziness, apprehension, excitement, and muscular tremors and weakness. These symptoms progress to generalized central nervous system hyperexcitability with delirium and clonic or tonic convulsions. This stage is in turn followed by progressive depression with paralysis, coma, and death. In chronically poisoned patients cerebellar symptoms and evidence of liver damage may develop. Hepatic toxicity is particularly prominent in poisoning by hexachlorbenzene. Treatment consists of gastric lavage and catharsis, anticonvulsive therapy with short-acting barbiturates, artificial ventilation, and other supportive measures. Sympathomimetic compounds should be avoided, since chlorinated insecticides apparently increase susceptibility to ventricular fibrillation.

CHOLINESTERASE INHIBITOR INSECTICIDES

Many substances used in agriculture for control of soft-bodied insects are potent inhibitors of cholinesterase. Most of these compounds are organic phosphates (e.g., Parathion, Malathion, Systox, TEPP, HETP, OMPA), others are carbamates (e.g., Dimetan, Matacil). The toxicity of these compounds varies widely. They are usually prepared for use by dilution with powders, organic solvents, or water. Formulations containing 1 to 95 percent of the active ingredient are available. The cholinesterase inhibitor insecticides are rapidly absorbed through the intact skin and after inhalation or ingestion.

The organic phosphate esters act by combining with and inactivating acetylcholinesterase. Since this enzyme normally breaks down the acetylcholine liberated by the central nervous system, autonomic ganglia, parasympathetic nerve endings, and motor nerve endings, its inactivation allows the accumulation of large amounts of acetylcholine at these sites. In the central nervous system initial stimulation is followed by depression of cells, resulting in convulsions followed by coma and respiratory depression. Initial stimulation and later blockade of autonomic ganglia results in multiple and variable dysfunctions of structures innervated by the autonomic nervous system. Accumulation of acetylcholine at parasympathetic nerve endings produces pupillary constriction and blurring of vision; stimulation of intestinal muscle resulting in abdominal cramps, vomiting, and diarrhea; stimulation of secretory glands causing rhinorrhea, salivation, sweating, and bronchorrhea; constriction of the bronchial musculature with symptoms of respiratory distress; depression of the cardiac sinus pacemaker activity; and impairment of atrioventricular conduction. Persistence of acetylcholine at the neuromuscular junction results in muscular tremors, cramps, and fasciculations which are followed by neuromuscular block and flaccid paralysis. Other important clinical manifestations of these poisons are cyanosis, and pulmonary edema.

Management consists of emesis or lavage, catharsis, and washing of contaminated skin with soap and water. Atropine should be given immediately to block the parasympathetic and central nervous system effects. A dose of 2 mg is injected intramuscularly and repeated every 10 min until parasympathetic manifestations are controlled and signs of atropinization appear. The same dosage must be repeated frequently to maintain xerostomia and mild tachycardia. Fatal respiratory failure or pulmonary edema may occur quickly upon cessation of atropine therapy. Atropine is virtually ineffective against the autonomic ganglionic actions of acetylcholine and against the peripheral neuromuscular paralysis. Certain oximes act as cholinesterase reactivators. Pralidoxime is useful in the treatment of organic phosphate cholinesterase inhibition but should not be used if the inhibition is due to a carbamate. A dose of 1 Gm pralidoxime in aqueous solution is administered intravenously over a 5 min period and may be repeated twice each day. Supportive therapy includes administration of oxygen with artificial ventilation if necessary, removal of pulmonary secretions by suction, and treatment of convulsions with short-acting barbiturates. Energetic therapy with artificial ventilation, atropine, and pralidoxime allows survival of doses of organic phosphate esters vastly exceeding the usual fatal dose.

CYANIDE

The cyanide ion is an exceedingly potent and rapid acting poison, but one for which specific and effective antidotal therapy is available. Cyanide poisoning may result from the inhalation of hydrocyanic acid and from the ingestion of soluble inorganic cyanide salts or cyanide-releasing substances such as cyanamide, cyanogen chloride, and nitroprusside. Parts of many plants also contain substances such as amygdalin which release cyanide on digestion. Among these are the seeds of certain stone fruits (choke cherry, pin cherry, wild black cherry, peach, apricot, bitter almond), cassava roots, the berries of the jet berry bush, the leaves and shoots of elderberry, and all parts of hydrangea. Cyanides are widely used in industry and for fumigation and may reach the home in photographic chemicals or silver polishes. As little as 300 mg potassium cyanide may cause death.

The extreme toxicity of cyanide is due to its ready reaction with the trivalent iron of cytochrome oxidase. The role of the enzyme in cellular oxygen utilization is inhibited by the formation of the cytochrome oxidase-cyanide complex. The resultant cytotoxic hypoxia leads to cellular dysfunction and death.

Inhalation of hydrogen cyanide may cause death within a minute. Oral doses act more slowly, requiring several minutes for the appearance of symptoms and up to several hours for death. The first effect is an increase in ventilation because of the blockade of oxidative metabolism in the chemoreceptor cells. As more cyanide is absorbed, there is headache, dizziness, nausea, drowsiness, hypotension, profound dyspnea, characteristic electrocardiographic changes, coma, and convulsions. Death always occurs within 4 hr.

Cyanide poisoning is a true medical emergency. Treatment is highly effective if given rapidly. The chemical antidotes should be immediately available wherever emergency medical care is dispensed. The diagnosis may be made by the characteristic "bitter almond" odor on the breath of the victim, and physicians should familiarize themselves with this smell. Since the saturation of hemoglobin is not disturbed by cyanide, cyanosis is not seen until respiratory depression supervenes. The objective of treatment is the production of methemoglobin by the administration of nitrite. The trivalent iron of methemoglobin competes with cytochrome oxidase for the cyanide ion. The cytochrome oxidase-cyanide complex dissociates and enzymatic function and cell respiration are restored. Further detoxification is then achieved by the administration of thiosulfate. Under the influence of the tissue enzyme rhodanese thiosulfate reacts with cyanide liberated by the dissociation of cyanmethemoglobin to form thiocyanate. This substance is relatively nontoxic and readily excreted in the urine.

Since speed is of the essence, nitrite should be immediately administered by inhalation of amyl nitrite perles, one every 2 min unless blood pressure is below 80 mm. This is followed as soon as possible by the intravenous injection of 10 ml of 3% sodium nitrite over a 3-min period. An intravenous infusion of norepinephrine may be necessary to maintain blood pressure during this injection period. After the administration of sodium nitrite, 50 ml of 25% sodium thiosulfate should be administered intravenously over a 10-min period. Supportive measures, especially artificial respiration with 100% oxygen, should be instituted as soon as possible, but, unless methemoglobinemia is produced promptly, other forms of treatment are of no value. Administration of sodium nitrite and sodium thiosulfate may have to be repeated. If the patient survives 4 hr, recovery is likely but residual cerebral symptoms may persist.

DETERGENTS AND SOAPS

These substances fall into the three groups of anionic, nonionic, and cationic detergents. The first group contains common soaps and household detergents. They may cause vomiting and diarrhea but have no serious effects, and no treatment is required. However, some laundry compounds contain phosphate water softeners whose ingestion may cause hypocalcemia. The ingestion of nonionic detergents is harmless and requires no treatment.

Cationic detergents, such as benzalkonium chloride (Zephiran) and many others, are commonly used for bacteriocidal purposes in hospitals and homes. These compounds are well absorbed from the gastrointestinal tract and interfere with cellular functions. The fatal oral dose is approximately 3 Gm. Ingestion produces nausea and vomiting, and shock, coma, convulsions, and death may occur in a few hours. Treatment consists of minimizing gastrointestinal absorption by emesis or gastric lavage with ordinary soap solution, which rapidly inactivates cationic detergents. If significant absorption has occurred, intensive supportive therapy may be required.

ERGOT

This fungus (*Claviceps purpurea*) grows on rye and contains a number of highly toxic alkaloids (e.g., ergotamine, ergonovine) which are used in the treatment of migraine or as uterine stimulants. Poisoning may be due to therapeutic overdosage, particularly in patients with severe infections or liver disease, but more commonly results from the use of ergot as an abortifacient. The epidemic form of chronic ergot poisoning due to the ingestion of contaminated grain is now rarely seen. Ingestion of 1 Gm ergot has been fatal, ergotamine has caused gangrene in doses of 10 mg per day. Symptoms of acute or chronic ergot poisoning are vomiting, diarrhea, burning abdominal pain, severe muscle pains, ischemic peripheral gangrene, headache, psychotic behavior, muscle tremors, convulsions, and coma. Circulatory disturbances are due both to prolonged vasoconstriction and to intimal hyperplasia and thrombosis. Treatment of ergot poisoning is symptomatic. Vigorous vasodilator and analgesic therapy should be employed.

FLUORIDES

Fluoride salts are widely used in insecticides. The gases fluorine and hydrogen fluoride are used in industry. The latter is a strong corrosive. Fluorine and fluorides are cellular poisons which block the glycolytic degradation of glucose. Fluorides also form an insoluble precipitate with calcium and cause hypocalcemia. Finally, in an acid medium fluorides form the corrosive hydrofluoric acid. Ingestion of 1 to 2 Gm sodium fluoride may be fatal.

Inhalation of fluorine or hydrogen fluoride produces coughing and choking. After an asymptomatic period of a day or two, fever, cough, cyanosis, and pulmonary edema may develop. Ingestion of fluoride salts is followed by nausea, vomiting productive of corroded tissues, diarrhea, and abdominal pain. Consequent to the decrease in serum calcium the victim develops muscular hyperirritability, fasciculations, tremors, spasms, and convulsions. Death is due to respiratory paralysis or circulatory collapse. If the patient survives the acute period, jaundice and oliguria may appear. Chronic fluoride poisoning (fluorosis) is characterized by weight loss, weakness, anemia, brittle bones, and stiff joints. Mottling of teeth is seen when exposure occurs during enamel formation.

Acute fluoride poisoning is treated by immediate administration of milk, lime water, calcium gluconate, or calcium lactate solution. Following lavage or emesis 10 Gm calcium gluconate and 30 Gm sodium sulfate should be administered to precipitate and remove fluoride from the intestine. Then 10% calcium gluconate or 1% calcium chloride should be slowly injected intravenously and repeated as needed to prevent a positive Chvostek sign. Symptomatic and supportive therapy is administered as indicated.

FORMALDEHYDE

This gas is available as a 40% solution (Formalin) which is used as a disinfectant, fumigant, or deodorant. Poisoning by Formalin may be diagnosed by the characteristic odor of formaldehyde. Formaldehyde reacts chemically with cellular constituents, depresses cellular functions, and causes cell death. The fatal dose of Formalin is about 60 ml.

Ingestion of Formalin immediately causes severe abdominal pain, nausea, vomiting, and diarrhea. This may be followed by collapse, coma, severe metabolic acidosis, and anuria. Death is usually due to circulatory failure.

Treatment consists of immediate administration of activated charcoal followed by emesis and gastric lavage with a solution containing 1% ammonium carbonate and 2% sodium bicarbonate. Parenteral administration of sodium bicarbonate is indicated to combat acidosis. The treatment is otherwise supportive.

GLYCOLS

Ethylene glycol and diethylene glycol are commonly used in antifreeze solutions. The more than 50 annual deaths from these compounds usually result from intentional drinking of antifreeze by alcoholics. The fatal dose of ethylene glycol is about 100 Gm, that of diethylene glycol somewhat lower. Both compounds are metabolized to oxalate in the body.

The initial symptoms of acute poisoning by these glycols resemble alcoholic intoxication. They may progress to vomiting, stupor, coma with absent reflexes and anisocoria, and convulsions. Tachypnea, bradycardia, and hypothermia are commonly seen. After massive ingestion death may occur from respiratory failure within a few hours or from pulmonary edema within a day or two. If the patient survives the acute stage, hepatic and renal necroses manifest themselves with jaundice, anuria, and uremia.

Treatment is largely supportive. The administration of ethyl alcohol and of intravenous calcium gluconate may be helpful by slowing the oxidation to oxalic acid and by precipitating the acid. However, the effectiveness of these procedures has not been definitely established. Dialysis is highly successful in the removal of ethylene and diethylene glycol from the body.

HALOGENATED HYDROCARBONS

Halogenated hydrocarbons (carbon tetrachloride, ethylene chlorohydrin, ethylene dichloride, methyl halides, tetrachloroethane, trichloroethylene) find wide industrial use as solvents, refrigerants, fumigants, and in chemical synthesis. They enter the home in household cleaners, floor waxes, fire extinguishers, and rubber or plastic cements. These compounds are highly fat-soluble and produce cell damage either directly or after conversion in the body to other compounds. Individual halogenated hydrocarbons differ considerably in the degree and the exact manifestations of their toxicity, but in sufficient concentration all these compounds are capable of inducing central nervous system depression and varying amounts of hepatic and renal toxicity. Myocardial depression, vascular damage, and pulmonary edema may also occur.

The most important halogenated hydrocarbon is carbon tetrachloride, widely employed as a nonflammable solvent and fire extinguisher fluid. Poisoning may occur from inhalation of the vapor, ingestion, or, rarely, percutaneous absorption. An oral dose of as little as 4 ml may be fatal. Absorption from the gastrointestinal tract is slow and unpredictable but is increased by the presence of fats and alcohol. Abdominal pain, hematemesis, and hepatic damage are more common and severe after ingestion than when the poison is inhaled. Inhalation may lead to irritation of the upper respiratory tract.

Acute systemic absorption of carbon tetrachloride results in nausea, dizziness, confusion, and headache within a few minutes. Depending upon the quantity absorbed, the symptoms may quickly progress to stupor, coma, convulsions, respiratory failure, hypotension, or ventricular fibrillation. The patient may recover from these immediate manifestations until evidence of hepatic or renal toxicity appears several hours to several days after the exposure. Liver and kidney damage may also occur in the absence of any severe early central nervous system effects. Initially tender hepatomegaly may be present, jaundice may be rapidly progressive, and death due to severe centrilobular necrosis may occur within days. The renal lesion has the characteristics of acute tubular necrosis and manifests itself by proteinuria, hematuria, oliguria, or anuria. Uremia, acidosis, hypertension, and pulmonary edema may develop as complications of renal failure. Optic neuritis, pancreatitis, and adrenal cortical necrosis are less common manifestations of carbon tetrachloride intoxication.

Chronic poisoning may occur after repeated exposures to low concentrations of carbon tetrachloride and may also lead to liver or kidney damage. More usually it manifests itself by vague symptoms of fatigue, weakness, mental confusion, abdominal pain, anorexia, nausea, blurring of vision, and paresthesias.

Treatment of acute poisoning by halogenated hydrocarbons includes vigorous effects at minimizing gastrointestinal absorption by lavage or emesis and catharsis. Treatment is otherwise symptomatic. Sympathometic drugs should be avoided because of the danger of inducing ventricular arrhythmias in the sensitized myocardium. Acute renal and hepatic failure must be carefully managed. Hemodialysis is often required and may be lifesaving until kidney function returns 3 or more weeks after poisoning.

IODINE

The traditional antiseptic Iodine Tincture is an alcoholic solution of 2% iodine and 2% sodium iodide. Strong Iodine Solution (Lugol's solution) is an aqueous solution of 5% iodine and 10% potassium iodide. Tincture of iodine is often taken for suicidal purposes. The fatal dose of iodine is approximately 2 Gm. Iodides are very much less toxic and no fatalities have been reported.

The diagnosis of iodine poisoning is suggested by the brown staining of the oral mucous membranes. The effects are largely due to the corrosive effects of the compound on the gastrointestinal tract. Burning abdominal pain, nausea, vomiting, and bloody diarrhea may occur soon after ingestion. If the stomach contained starch, the vomitus is blue or black. Tissue trauma from corrosive gastroenteritis and fluid loss by vomiting and diarrhea may result in shock. Severe edema of the glottis, fever, delirium, stupor, and anuria have also been observed.

Treatment consists of gastric lavage with a starch solution made by adding 15 Gm flour or cornstarch to 500 ml water. Thereafter, catharsis should be induced, and milk should be given orally to relieve gastric irritation. Sodium thiosulfate will reduce iodine to less toxic iodide; 100 ml of a 5% solution should be given orally and 10 ml of a 10% solution intravenously every 4 hr. With appropriate treatment most patients poisoned by iodine survive, but esophageal strictures may complicate their recovery.

IPECAC, EMETINE

Emetine is the major alkaloid of ipecac (dried roots or rhizomes of *Cephaelis ipecacuanha*) and is used for the treatment of amebiasis. Syrup of ipecac is used as an emetic or expectorant. Poisoning may be accidental or suicidal but most commonly results from overdosage during therapy, at times due to the erroneous substitution of the much more potent fluid extract of ipecac for syrup of ipecac. Emetine and other alkaloids of ipecac have serious toxic gastrointestinal, central nervous, and myocardial effects. The fatal oral dose of emetine is about 1 Gm.

Manifestations of poisoning begin with nausea, vomiting, diarrhea, and abdominal pain. Cardiac effects are heralded by electrocardiographic changes, and the depression of myocardial contractility leads to dyspnea, tachycardia, shock, and congestive heart failure. Coma and convulsions may occur, but death is usually due to heart failure. Treatment is symptomatic. Administration of digitalis may be of value.

IRON SALTS

Ferrous or ferric salts produce gastrointestinal corrosive damage. Following mucosal damage, large amounts of iron may be absorbed, particularly in children. The fatal oral dose in children is 5 to 10 Gm.

Very soon after ingestion nausea, vomiting, diarrhea, and abdominal pain appear. Systemic effects include acidosis, shock, drowsiness, coma, and respiratory failure.

These initial symptoms may partially clear but then recur with increased severity. In the later stages signs of hepatic and renal toxicity may appear.

The absorption of ingested iron should be minimized by the usual measures. Gastric lavage with a 10% sodium bicarbonate solution will precipitate the ferrous ion. Edetate calcium disodium 30 mg per kg daily in divided doses should be administered intravenously or orally. Deferoxamine methane sulfonate (Desferal) is even more effective as an iron chelating agent than edetate. Use of chelating agents is guided by determinations of serum iron and iron-binding capacity. Peritoneal dialysis and hemodialysis effectively remove iron from the body. Acidosis, shock, and renal or hepatic toxicity must be treated supportively.

ISOPROPYL ALCOHOL

This compound is used as a sterilizing agent or as rubbing alcohol. Ingestion produces gastric irritation and raises the danger of vomiting with aspiration. The systemic effects of isopropyl alcohol are similar to those of ethyl alcohol, but it is approximately twice as potent as the latter. Coma is readily produced but rarely lasts longer than 12 hr. Isopropyl alcohol is oxidized to acetone in the body, and transient acetonuria is common, but significant acidosis does not occur. Gastric lavage should always be performed to minimize the danger of aspiration following vomiting in the unconscious patient. Supportive therapy is required only after ingestion of massive amounts, and there are no sequelae other than transient gastritis.

MAGNESIUM

Magnesium sulfate is used intravenously as a hypotensive agent and orally as a cathartic. The magnesium ion is a profound depressant of the central nervous system and of neuromuscular transmission. Poisoning after oral or rectal administration is unlikely in the presence of normal renal function, because the kidney removes magnesium more rapidly than it is absorbed by the gastrointestinal tract. In the presence of impaired renal function an oral dose of 30 Gm may be fatal. Symptoms begin at a serum magnesium level of 4 mEq per liter and concentrations of over 12 mEq per liter may be fatal. Oral ingestion of concentrated solutions may cause gastrointestinal irritation. Manifestations of systemic poisoning are depression of reflexes, flaccid paralysis, hypotension, hypothermia, coma, and respiratory failure. Respiratory death usually precedes significant myocardial depression. The actions of magnesium on neurologic and neuromuscular function are antagonized by calcium. Treatment of magnesium poisoning therefore includes the intravenous administration of 10 ml of a 10% solution of calcium gluconate, which may be repeated as necessary.

METHYL ALCOHOL

This simplest of the alcohols, also called wood alcohol or methanol, is used as a solvent, antifreeze, paint remover, and as a denaturant in ethyl alcohol. Denatured ethyl alcohol preparations, such as Sterno or Solox, contain 5 to 15 percent methyl alcohol as well as other denaturants. Methyl alcohol poisoning is due almost entirely to its ingestion as a substitute for ethanol or to the drinking of denatured ethyl alcohol. The toxic dose is very variable: death has occurred after a dose of 20 ml but 250 ml have been ingested with survival. As little as 15 ml of methanol has caused permanent blindness.

Methanol is less inebriating than ethyl alcohol, and inebriation is not a prominent symptom of methyl alcohol intoxication. Methanol is oxidized in the body to formaldehyde and to formic acid. The rate of its metabolism is independent of the concentration in the body and is only 15 percent that of ethanol. The enzyme alcohol dehydrogenase appears to be responsible for the first step in oxidation. The enzyme system will preferentially utilize ethyl alcohol if this compound is also available. Thus ethyl alcohol may depress the rate of metabolism of methanol. The manifestations of methanol poisoning are largely due to the accumulation of its toxic metabolites. These products, especially formaldehyde, have toxic actions on many cells, and the retina and optic nerve are specifically damaged. The toxic metabolites of methyl alcohol are also responsible for the severe acidosis, which is the most prominent feature of methyl alcohol poisoning. This acidosis is partly due to the accumulation of formic acid, but formate also appears to exert an inhibitory effect upon enzymes involved in the oxidation of carbohydrate with consequent accumulation of acid intermediates.

Symptoms of methanol poisoning usually do not appear until 12 to 24 hr after ingestion, when sufficient toxic metabolites have accumulated. Manifestations consist of headache, dizziness, nausea, vomiting, severe abdominal and back pain probably due to pancreatitis, vasomotor disturbances, central nervous system depression, and respiratory failure. Visual disturbance is almost universal and ranges from mild blurring of vision to total blindness. Impairment of vision may be transient, but permanent blindness may follow survival of the acute intoxication. The pupils are dilated and nonreactive and there is hyperemia of the optic disc and retinal edema. Severe abdominal tenderness and spasm or nuchal rigidity may be present. Acidosis is commonly severe, but Kussmaul respiration is absent in many severely acidotic patients (plasma carbon dioxide–combining power below 20 mEq per liter).

In the treatment of methyl alcohol intoxication gastric lavage is of use only during the first hour or two. The mainstay of treatment is intravenous administration of large amounts of sodium bicarbonate. Return of acidosis is frequent after initial correction, and additional alkali must be administered as indicated by close observation of the patient and laboratory determinations. Peritoneal dialysis and hemodialysis effectively remove methanol from the body and are useful in view of its slow oxidation. The administration of 0.5 ml per kg of ethyl alcohol every 2 hr may inhibit the metabolism of methyl alcohol and is useful in conjunction with dialysis. Supportive therapy must be administered as required by the patient's clinical state.

MUSHROOMS

There are many species of poisonous mushrooms, but in the United States most poisoning is due to *Amanita muscaria* (fly agaric) or *Amanita phalloides* (destroying angel). More than 100 deaths result each year from consumption of wild poisonous mushrooms, 90 percent are due to *A. phalloides*. Fatalities have occurred after ingestion of only part of one mushroom.

Amanita muscaria contains the parasympathomimetic alkaloid muscarine, as well as variable amounts of a substance active on the central nervous system and a parasympatholytic alkaloid. Symptoms are largely those of parasympathetic stimulation: lacrimation, pupillary constriction, perspiration, salivation, nausea, vomiting, diarrhea, abdominal pain, bronchorrhea, wheezing, dyspnea, bradycardia, and hypotension. Muscular tremors, confusion, excitement, and delirium are common in severe poisoning. Very rarely symptoms of atropine poisoning have predominated. After ingestion of *A. muscaria* symptoms appear within minutes to 2 hr. The patient may die within a few hours, but with appropriate therapy complete recovery in 24 hr is the rule

Amanita phalloides, some other *Amanita* species, and *Galerina venenata* contain heat-stable polypeptide cytotoxins which are rapidly bound to tissues. Severe cell damage and fatty degeneration may occur in liver, kidneys, striated muscle, and brain. Ingestion of these dangerous mushrooms is followed by a latent period of 6 to 20 hr. Manifestations of cytotoxicity may then appear suddenly and consist of severe nausea, violent abdominal pain, bloody vomiting and diarrhea, and cardiovascular collapse. Headache, mental confusion, coma, or convulsions are common. Painful and tender hepatomegaly, jaundice, hypoglycemia, dehydration, and oliguria or anuria frequently arise on the first or second day after ingestion. The victim may die from acute yellow atrophy within 4 days. About one-half of all poisonings with *A. phalloides* have a fatal outcome in 5 to 8 days. Recovery tends to be slow.

Ingestion of other poisonous mushrooms may cause gastrointestinal symptoms, visual disturbances, ataxia, disorientation, convulsions, coma, fever, hemolysis, and methemoglobinemia.

Treatment of mushroom poisoning depends upon the species ingested. If parasympathomimetic manifestations are prominent, atropine in doses of 1 to 2 mg is given intramuscularly and repeated every 30 min until symptoms are controlled. Poisoning by cytotoxic mushrooms can only be treated symptomatically. Fluid and electrolyte balance must be carefully maintained. Hypoglycemia should be avoided, and large quantities of carbohydrate may exert some protective effect on the liver. Excitement, convulsions, pain, hypotension, and fever may need symptomatic therapy. Hemodialysis is of no value in removing the toxin but may be required to maintain renal function until recovery occurs.

NAPHTHALENE

Poisoning by this substance is almost always due to ingestion of moth repellents. An oral dose of 2 Gm has been fatal. Nausea, vomiting, and diarrhea are the initial symptoms. Larger doses may produce hepatic damage with jaundice and renal toxicity which may progress to hematuria, oliguria, or anuria. Depending upon the amount ingested, central nervous system manifestations may range from headache, mental confusion, and excitement to coma and convulsions. In individuals with glucose 6-phosphate dehydrogenase–deficient red cells the ingestion of naphthalene will produce hemolysis. Treatment consists of emesis or gastric lavage and catharsis and supportive measures.

NICOTINE

This alkaloid is an exceedingly potent and rapidly acting poison. It is a component of many insecticides. Nicotine is readily absorbed from the oral and gastrointestinal mucosa, from the respiratory tract, and through the skin. The lethal dose for an adult is approximately 50 mg, the quantity contained in two cigarettes. However, tobacco is much less toxic than would be anticipated on the basis of its nicotine content. Nicotine is poorly absorbed from ingested tobacco, and on smoking, most of the nicotine is burned. Nicotine acts on chemoreceptors, on synapses in the central nervous system and in autonomic ganglia, on the adrenal medulla, and on neuroeffector junctions. Furthermore, its initial stimulant effects are followed by a depressant phase of action. It is not surprising that the manifestations of nicotine poisoning are highly complex and somewhat unpredictable.

Small doses of nicotine produce nausea, vomiting, diarrhea, headache, dizziness, and neurologic stimulation manifested by tachycardia, hypertension, hyperpnea, tachypnea, sweating, and salivation. Larger doses also cause cortical irritability progressing to convulsions, and myocardial arrhythmias. Finally coma, respiratory depression and arrest, and cardiac arrest or fibrillation may supervene. Severe poisoning may cause death within a few minutes.

Treatment consists of gastric lavage with activated charcoal or with a 1:10,000 solution of potassium permanganate, which oxidizes nicotine. Atropine, 2 mg, and phentolamine, 5 mg, may be given intramuscularly or intravenously and repeated as often as required to control signs and symptoms of parasympathetic or sympathetic hyperactivity. These compounds are ineffective in preventing paralysis of the respiratory muscles and disturbances in cardiac rhythm. Careful attention must be given to artificial ventilation with oxygen and to therapy of active, catecholamine-induced cardiac arrhythmias. Propranolol is probably the drug of choice for the latter purpose. Nicotine is rapidly detoxified in the liver and recovery will be prompt if the patient can be tided over the initial period.

NITRITES

Poisoning by the nitrite ion may result from the ingestion of large amounts of drugs such as amyl nitrite or sodium nitrite. Nitrites are also used to preserve the color of meat, and amounts in excess of the allowable residue of 0.01 percent may appear in food. Ingested nitrates may be reduced to nitrite by intestinal bacteria, especially *E. coli.* Except after the ingestion of very large amounts adults usually absorb all nitrate before this reduction takes place. However, in children nitrite poisoning may result from the ingestion of nitrates or nitrate-containing well water. Fatalities have occurred from the oral ingestion of 2 to 4 Gm of nitrites.

Acute nitrite poisoning may lead to severe headache, flushing, dizziness, hypotension, and syncope. Usually the patient need only be positioned to facilitate venous return to the heart. Pressor agents are seldom required. The most important toxic effect of the nitrite ion is its ability to oxidize hemoglobin to methemoglobin (Chap. 61).

OXALIC ACID

This acid is found in ink eradicators and stain removers. It is corrosive and combines with calcium to form insoluble calcium oxalate. Ingestion causes irritation and corrosion of mouth, esophagus, and stomach followed by vomiting and abdominal pain. After absorption the reduction in serum calcium leads to muscular tremors, tetany, convulsions, and cardiovascular collapse. Ingestion of 5 Gm may cause death within minutes. Following recovery from the acute episode there may be renal failure due to blockage of renal tubules by calcium oxalate crystals.

Treatment consists of induction of emesis or gastric lavage with milk, limewater, chalk, or calcium salts. A dose of 10 ml of 10% calcium gluconate should be given intravenously and repeated as required to maintain normal serum calcium and prevent tetany. In supportive therapy the maintenance of a high urine output is essential.

PETROLEUM DISTILLATES

Petroleum distillates (diesel oil, gasoline, kerosene, paint thinner, solvent distillate) are liquids with a boiling point between 50 and 325°C. They contain variable amounts of branched or straight-chain aliphatic and aromatic hydrocarbons. Kerosene is widely used as a fuel and as a vehicle for cleaning agents, furniture polishes, insecticides, and paint thinners. Not surprisingly, each year petroleum distillates cause about 100 accidental deaths in the United States, 90 percent of these in young children. Furthermore, these products are annually responsible for almost 20,000 hospitalizations. Ingestion of

10 ml kerosene has been fatal, but adults have recovered from as much as 250 ml. Petroleum distillates are central nervous system depressants and damage cells by dissolving cellular lipids. Pulmonary damage manifested by pulmonary edema or pneumonitis is a common and serious complication.

Inhalation of gasoline or kerosene vapors induces a state resembling alcoholic intoxication. Headache, nausea, tinnitus, and a burning sensation in the chest may also be present. When aliphatic hydrocarbons are inhaled, these symptoms may progress to profound drowsiness or coma with absence of deep reflexes. If the distillate contains a high proportion of aromatic hydrocarbons, the coma is characterized by tremors, muscle jactitations, hyperactive reflexes, and convulsions. Death is usually due to respiratory depression, rarely to ventricular fibrillation.

The oral ingestion of petroleum distillates causes irritation of the mucous membranes of the upper intestinal tract. When large amounts have been ingested, the same manifestations as after inhalation may appear. Frequently eructation or vomiting results in aspiration of petroleum distillates into the trachea. Because of their low surface tension, minute amounts of these substances may then spread widely throughout the lungs and produce pulmonary edema and pneumonitis. Pulmonary damage may also arise due to absorption of ingested petroleum distillates from the gastrointestinal tract. However, kerosene is at least one hundred times more toxic by the intratracheal route than when ingested.

In the treatment of poisoning by petroleum distillates extreme care must be used to prevent aspiration. When large amounts have been ingested, gastric lavage should be performed but only after insertion of an endotracheal tube with an inflatable cuff. A vegetable oil and a saline cathartic may be administered to decrease the absorption of the poison. All cases of kerosene poisoning should be hospitalized for at least 24 hr for observation. If signs or symptoms of pulmonary irritation appear, adrenal steroids, oxygen under positive pressure, and antibiotics to prevent bacterial pneumonia are often of value. Symptomatic therapy for central nervous system depression or convulsions may be necessary. Sympathomimetic amines should be avoided because of the danger of inducing ventricular fibrillation in the hydrocarbon-sensitized heart.

PHENOL

Phenol and related compounds (creosote, cresols, hexachlorophene, hydroquinone, Lysol, resorcinol, tannic acid) are widely used as antiseptics, caustics, and preservatives. These substances poison all cells by denaturing and precipitating cellular proteins. The approximate fatal oral dose ranges from 2 ml for phenol and cresols to 20 ml for tannic acid.

Ingestion of phenolic compounds produces erosion of mucosa from mouth to stomach. The corroded areas may have a characteristic dead-white appearance. Hematemesis and bloody diarrhea may occur. After an initial phase of hyperpnea due to stimulation of the respiratory center, stupor, coma, convulsions, pulmonary edema, and shock are seen. The initial respiratory alkalosis is soon followed by a profound acidosis. The latter results from the renal excretion of base during the alkalotic stage, from the acidic nature of the phenolic radical, and from disturbances in carbohydrate metabolism presumably due to defects in enzymatic function. If the patient survives the acute stage, acute tubular necrosis may lead to oliguria or anuria and hepatic toxicity to jaundice.

Poisoning by phenolic compounds may often be diagnosed by their characteristic odor. Development of a violet or blue color of the urine after addition of a few drops of ferric chloride indicates the presence of a phenolic compound.

Treatment is directed at decreasing the absorption of ingested poison by administration of water, milk, or activated charcoal slurry and their removal by emesis or gastric lavage. Olive oil or castor oil dissolve phenol and retard its absorption. Supportive therapy consists of correction of the acidosis, the control of shock and convulsions, and the maintenance of a patent airway in the face of glottal edema by intubation or tracheotomy.

PHOSPHORUS

Phosphorus occurs in two forms: a red, nonpoisonous form and a yellow, fat-soluble, highly toxic form. The latter is used in rodent and insect poisons and in fireworks. Yellow phosphorus and phosphides cause fatty degeneration and necrosis of tissues, particularly of the liver. The lethal ingested dose of yellow phosphorus is approximately 50 mg.

Ingestion of yellow phosphorus is followed within 1 hr by burning pain in the upper gastrointestinal tract, vomiting, diarrhea, and a garlic odor of the breath and excreta. The patient may die in coma during the first day or two, or symptoms may subside after a few hours. Then, 1 to 2 days later, the victim may develop tender hepatomegaly, jaundice, hypocalcemia, hypotension, oliguria, and die following convulsions and coma. Death from acute yellow atrophy may occur in a few days.

Treatment consists of vigorous and repeated induction of emesis or gastric lavage. Calcium gluconate is given intravenously to maintain serum calcium. Treatment is otherwise supportive and a protective regimen for the liver should be instituted.

SALICYLATES

Each year 30 million pounds of aspirin are consumed in the United States, and salicylates can probably be found in every American household. It is therefore not surprising that salicylates (aspirin, methyl salicylate, salicylic acid, sodium salicylate) are more commonly involved in poisonings than any other agent. Aspirin is found in almost all compound analgesic tablets. Methyl salicylate (oil of wintergreen) is present in most skin liniments, and salicylic acid is used in ointments and corn plasters. The ingestion of 10 to 30 Gm aspirin or sodium salicylate may be fatal to adults, but survival has been reported after an oral dose of 130 Gm aspirin. On the other hand 3 Gm salicylate in a teaspoon of methyl salicylate has been fatal in children.

Salicylate intoxication may result from the cumulative effect of therapeutic administration of high doses. There is considerable individual variation: toxic symptoms may begin at dosages of 3 Gm per day or may not appear when 10 Gm per day are given. Toxic symptoms are also poorly correlated with the serum salicylate concentration, but few patients become intoxicated at levels less than 15 mg per 100 ml and most at levels over 35 mg per 100 ml. Therapeutic salicylate intoxication is usually mild and is called "salicylism." The earliest symptoms are vertigo, tinnitus, and impairment of hearing. Further overdosage causes nausea, vomiting, sweating, diarrhea, fever, drowsiness, headache, dimness of vision, and mental aberrations. The latter may be characterized by confusion, excitement, restlessness, and talkativeness; this "salicylate jag" resembles alcoholic intoxication without the euphoria. The central nervous system effects may progress to hallucinations, convulsions, and coma. Toxic doses of salicylates also have a direct stimulant effect on the respiratory center resulting in hyperventilation, loss of carbon dioxide, and respiratory alkalosis. Renal excretion of bicarbonate may partially compensate for this.

In acute salicylate poisoning due to accidental or suicidal ingestion of massive amounts, the same manifestations may be seen in more rapid succession. However, they are usually overshadowed by severe disturbances in the acid-base balance which follow a definite sequence. Early in the course of intoxication there may be only hyperpnea, and the seriousness of the poisoning may not be appreciated at that time. The hyperventilation causes a fall in blood P_{CO_2} and an increase in pH. Renal excretion of bicarbonate, sodium, and potassium will bring the pH back toward normal and produce a compensated respiratory alkalosis. At that point the buffering capacity of the extracellular fluid will have been significantly decreased. In young children and after large doses in adults further developments may then produce a combination of respiratory acidosis and metabolic acidosis which stem from a number of factors. High concentrations of salicylate depress the respiratory center and cause CO_2 retention. Renal function becomes impaired because of dehydration and hypotension, and inorganic, metabolic acids accumulate. Furthermore, salicylic acid derivatives may displace several mEq of blood bicarbonate. Finally, salicylates impair carbohydrate metabolism and cause accumulation of acetoacetic, lactic, and pyruvic acids. Severe acidosis and disturbances in electrolyte balance are most commonly seen in febrile young children.

Blood salicylate levels are of value in the estimation of the severity of poisoning. Serious poisoning is rare at levels less than 50 mg per 100 ml but usual at levels between 50 and 100 mg per 100 ml. Levels above 100 mg per 100 ml during the first 6 hr after poisoning signify severe intoxication and may be fatal. Excretion of salicylates is renal, and in the presence of normal renal function about 50 percent will be excreted in 24 hr. Addition of a few drops of ferric chloride solution to 5 ml of boiled acidified urine containing salicylate yields a violet color and may aid in diagnosis.

Treatment of salicylate poisoning is largely supportive. In order to decrease absorption, activated charcoal is administered and emesis is induced or lavage with sodium bicarbonate solution is performed. Disturbances of acid base or electrolyte balance and hypoglycemia are corrected by the intravenous administration of appropriate solutions. Respiratory depression may require artificial ventilation with oxygen. Convulsions may best be treated by the administration of succinylcholine and artificial ventilation with oxygen. Central nervous system–depressant agents should not be used. In order to increase renal excretion of salicylate, osmotic diuresis is induced and the urine is alkalinized. Peritoneal dialysis and hemodialysis are also highly effective in removing salicylate from seriously poisoned patients.

SMOKE

Poisoning by smoke is usually due to carbon monoxide inhalation. However, burning material may also release irritant fumes. Many irritant gases combine with water to form corrosive acids or alkalis and cause chemical burns of exposed skin and of the upper respiratory tract. Such gases (and the corrosives formed) are: ammonia (ammonium hydroxide), nitrogen oxide (nitric acid), sulfur dioxide (sulfurous acid), and sulfur trioxide (sulfuric acid). These irritating gases as well as hydrogen sulfide may also be present in smog. Another highly toxic gas which may be inhaled by firefighters or victims is phosgene. This compound is formed by the high-temperature decomposition of chlorinated hydrocarbons and is released when carbon tetrachloride from fire extinguishers comes into contact with hot surfaces.

After inhalation of irritant gases the victim may notice burning pain in throat and chest and severe coughing. These symptoms may subside completely, but from several hours to a day after exposure dyspnea and cyanosis may appear and progress rapidly to severe pulmonary edema and death from respiratory and circulatory failure. Treatment consists of administration of oxygen and adrenal steroids and appropriate therapy of pulmonary edema should that develop.

In many localities the term *smoke* is used to describe paint removers, lacquer thinners, antifreezes, and other solvent mixtures which are ingested for their supposed alcohol content. The toxicity of these compounds depends on their ingredients. Some such materials have caused profound hypoglycemia by a poorly understood mechanism. This possibility should be considered in the differential diagnosis of what appears to be alcoholic coma. Intravenous administration of glucose as a therapeutic test may be indicated.

SULFIDES

Hydrogen sulfide is a gas released by the decomposition of organic sulfur compounds and is widely used in industry. Carbon disulfide is an industrial solvent. Other sulfides have industrial uses and release hydrogen sulfide in contact with water or acids. Significant concentrations of hydrogen sulfide may be present in smoke or smog. Inhalation of hydrogen sulfide in concentrations above 50 ppm (50 times the minimum detectable by smell) causes conjunctivitis, headache, nausea, soreness of the upper respiratory passages, pulmonary edema, and drowsiness. Concentrations in excess of 300 ppm may cause coma, respiratory depression, and death. Ingestion of carbon disulfide or soluble sulfides is followed by vomiting, headache, hypotension, respiratory depression, tremors, coma, convulsions, and death. The fatal oral dose of carbon disulfide is approximately 1 Gm. Treatment of sulfide intoxication is supportive. Administration of sodium nitrite may promote the binding of sulfide in sulfmethemoglobin.

VOLATILE OILS

The volatile or essential oils (citronella oil, eucalyptus oil, menthol, pine oil, turpentine) are colorless liquids which irritate all tissues. Poisoning may result from occupational exposure (painters) and accidental or suicidal ingestion. Unfortunately, some volatile oils also have an undeserved reputation as abortifacients. Absorption occurs from skin, intestine, or lungs; the less volatile oils are more slowly absorbed. Ingestion of 15 Gm turpentine has been fatal.

Ingestion is rapidly followed by abdominal burning, nausea, vomiting, and diarrhea. Inhalation produces severe bronchial irritation and may be followed by delirium, coma, and convulsions. If the patient survives the acute stage of poisoning, evidence of renal damage may appear and progress to acute tubular necrosis with anuria.

Treatment is entirely supportive. When gastric lavage is undertaken, aspiration must be prevented with extreme care. Since the renal lesion is reversible, treatment for renal failure should be vigorous and include dialysis if necessary.

REFERENCES

Antimuscarinic Compounds

Hoefnagel, D.: Toxic Effects of Atropine and Homatropine Eyedrops in Children, New Engl. J. Med., 264:168, 1961.

Weintraub, S.: Stramonium Poisoning, Postgrad. Med., 28: 364, 1960.

Barium

Dean, G.: Seven Cases of Barium Carbonate Poisoning, Brit. Med. J., II:817, 1950.

Benzene, Toluene

Browning, E.: Toxic Solvents: A Review, Brit. J. Indust. Med., 16:23, 1959.

Brozovsky, M., and E. M. Winkler: Glue Sniffing in Children and Adolescents, N.Y. J. Med., 65:1984, 1965.

Glaser, H. H., and O. N. Massengale: "Glue-Sniffing" in Children. Deliberate Inhalation of Vaporized Plastic Cements, J.A.M.A., 181:300, 1962.

Boric Acid

Rosen, F. S., and R. J. Haggerty: Fatal Poisoning from Topical Use of Boric Acid Powder, New Engl. J. Med., 255:530, 1956.

Valdes-Dapena, M. A., and J. B. Arey: Boric Acid Poisoning, J. Pediat., 61:531, 1962.

Cantharidin

Oaks, W. W., J. F. DiTunno, T. Magnani, H. A. Levy, and L. C. Mills: Cantharidin Poisoning, A.M.A. Arch. Intern. Med., 105:574, 1960.

Carbon Monoxide

Anderson, R. F., D. C. Allenworth, and W. J. DeGroot: Myocardial Toxicity from Carbon Monoxide Poisoning, Ann. Intern. Med., 67:1172, 1967.

Cosby, R. S., and M. Bergeron: Electrocardiographic Changes in Carbon Monoxide Poisoning, Am. J. Cardiol., 11:93, 1963.

Craig, T. V., W. Hunt, and R. Atkinson: Hypothermia. Its Use in Severe Carbon Monoxide Poisoning, New Engl. J. Med., 261:854, 1959.

Lilienthal, J. L., Jr.: Cabon Monoxide, Pharmacol. Rev., 2:324, 1950.

Meigs, J. W., and J. P. W. Hughes: Acute Carbon Monoxide Poisoning. An Analysis of 105 Cases, A.M.A. Arch. Ind. Hyg., 1:90, 1950.

Smith, G., I. M. Ledingham, G. R. Sharp, J. N. Norman, and E. H. Bates: Treatment of Coal Gas Poisoning with Oxygen at 2 Atmospheres Pressure, Lancet, I:816, 1962.

Castor Bean

Brugsch, H. G.: The Castor Bean, New Engl. J. Med., 262:1039, 1960.

Caustics

Haller, J. A., and K. Bachman: The Comparative Effect of Current Therapy on Experimental Caustic Burns of the Esophagus, Pediatrics, 34:236, 1964.

Yarington, C. T., Jr.: Ingestion of Caustic; a Pediatric Problem, J. Pediat., 67:674, 1965.

Chlorinated Insecticides

Finley, A. H., and R. J. Haggerty: Toxic Hazards, Insecticides. Chlorinated Hydrocarbons, New Engl. J. Med., 258:812, 1958.

Zavon, M. R.: Chlorinated Hydrocarbon Insecticides, J.A.M.A., 190:595, 1964.

Cholinesterase Inhibitor Insecticides

Heath, D. F.: "Organophosphorus Poisons," Oxford, Pergamon Press, 1961.

Hobbiger, F.: Reactivation of Phosphorylated Acetylcholinesterase, in "Cholinesterases and Anticholinesterase Agents," Handb. Exp. Pharmak., Suppl. 15:921, 1963.

Mann, J. B.: Diagnostic Aids in Organophosphate Poisoning, Ann. Intern. Med., 67:905, 1967.

Quinby, G. E.: Further Therapeutic Experience with Pralidoximes in Organic Phosphorus Poisoning, J.A.M.A., 187:202, 1964.

Wyckoff, D. W., J. E. Davies, A. Barquet, and J. H. Davis: Diagnostic and Therapeutic Problems of Parathion Poisonings, Ann. Intern. Med., 68:875, 1968.

Cyanide

Chen, K. K., and C. L. Rose: Treatment of Acute Cyanide Poisoning, J.A.M.A., 162:1154, 1956.

Cope, C.: The Importance of Oxygen in the Treatment of Cyanide Poisoning, J.A.M.A., 175:1061, 1961.

Pijoan, M.: Cyanide Poisoning from Choke Cherry Seed, Am. J. Med. Sci., 204:550, 1942.

Detergents

Arena, J. M.: Poisonings and Other Health Hazards Associated with Use of Detergents, J.A.M.A., 190:56, 1964.

Cann, H. M., and H. L. Verhulst: Toxicity of Household Soap and Detergents and Treatment of their Ingestion, Am. J. Dis. Child., 100:287, 1960.

Fluorides

Peters, J. H.: Therapy of Acute Fluoride Poisoning, Am. J. Med. Sci., 216:278, 1948.

Glycols

Haggerty, R. J.: Toxic Hazards, Deaths from Permanent Anti-freeze Ingestion, New Engl. J. Med., 261:1296, 1959.

Peterson, D. I., J. E. Peterson, M. G. Hardinge, and W. E. C. Wacker: Experimental Treatment of Ethylene Glycol Poisoning, J. Am. Med. Ass., 186:965, 1963.

Pons, C. A., and R. P. Custer: Acute Ethylene Glycol Poisoning: A Clinicopathologic Report of Eighteen Fatal Cases, Am. J. Med. Sci., 211:544, 1946.

Halogenated Hydrocarbons

Browning, E.: Toxicology of Organic Compounds of Industrial Importance, Ann. Rev. Pharmacol., 1:397, 1961.

Myatt, A. V., and J. A. Salmons: Carbon Tetrachloride Poisoning, Arch. Ind. Hyg. Occup. Med., 6:74, 1952.

Oettingen, W. F. von: "The Halogenated Hydrocarbons of Industrial and Toxicological Importance," Amsterdam, Elsevier Publishing Company, 1964.

Ipecac, Emetine

Smith, R. P., and D. M. Smith: Acute Ipecac Poisoning, New Engl. J. Med., 265:523, 1961.

Welchman, J. M.: The Cardiac Toxicity of Emetine, J. Trop. Med. Hyg., 60:296, 1957.

Iron Salts

Covey, T. J.: Ferrous Sulfate Poisoning: Review, Case Summaries and Therapeutic Regimen, J. Pediat., 64:218, 1964.

Jacobs, J., H. Greene, and B. R. Gendel: Acute Iron Intoxication, New Engl. J. Med., 273:1124, 1965.

Leikin, S.: Deferoxamine as a Chelating Agent, J. Pediat., 72:148, 1968.

Isopropyl Alcohol

Freireich, A. W., T. J. Cinque, G. Xanthaky, and D. Landau: Hemodialysis for Isopropanol Poisoning, New Engl. J. Med., 277:699, 1967.

Methyl Alcohol

Bennett, I. L., Jr., F. H. Cary, G. L. Mitchell, Jr., and M. N. Cooper: Acute Methyl Alcohol Poisoning: A Review Based on Experiences in an Outbreak of 323 Cases, Medicine, 32:431, 1953.

Cooper, J. R., and M. M. Kini: Biochemical Aspects of Methanol Poisoning, Biochem. Pharmacol., 11:405, 1962.

Setter, J. G., R. Singh, N. C. Brackett, Jr., and R. E. Randall, Jr.: Studies on the Dialysis of Methanol, Trans. Am. Soc. Artificial Internal Organs, 13:178, 1967.

Smith, M. E.: Interrelations in Ethanol and Methanol Metabolism, J. Pharmacol., 134:233, 1961.

Mushrooms

Buck, R. W.: Mushroom Toxins—A Brief Review of the Literature, New Engl. J. Med., 265:681, 1961.

Grossman, C. M., and B. Malbin: Mushroom Poisoning: A Review of the Literature and Report of Two Cases Caused by a Previously Undescribed Species, Ann. Intern. Med., 40:249, 1954.

Naphthalene

Haggerty, R. J.: Naphthalene Poisoning, New Engl. J. Med., 255:919, 1956.

Nicotine

Oberst, B. B., and R. A. McIntyre: Acute Nicotine Poisoning, Pediatrics, 11:338, 1953.

Nitrites

Bucklin, R., and M. K. Myint: Fatal Methemoglobinemia due to Well Water Nitrates, Ann. Intern. Med., 52:703, 1960.

Petroleum Distillates

Browning, E.: "Toxicity and Metabolism of Industrial Solvents," Amsterdam, Elsevier Publishing Company, 1965.

Jacobziner, H., and H. W. Raybin: Kerosene and Other Petroleum Distillate Poisonings, N.Y. J. Med., 63:3428, 1963.

Lawton, J. J., Jr., and C. P. Malmquist: Gasoline Addiction in Children, Psychiat. Quart., 35:555, 1961.

Mayock, R. L., N. Bozorgnia, and H. F. Zinsser: Kerosene Pneumonitis Treated with Adrenal Steroids, Ann. Intern. Med., 54:559, 1961.

Subcommittee on Accidental Poisoning: Cooperative Kerosene Poisoning Study, Pediatrics, 29:648, 1962.

Phosphorus

Arena, J. M.: Phosphorus Poisoning, Clin. Ped., 2:132, 1963.

Diaz-Rivera, R. S., P. J. Collazo, E. R. Pons, and M. V. Torregrosa: Acute Phosphorus Poisoning in Man; a Study of 56 Cases, Medicine, 29:269, 1950.

Fletcher, G. F., and J. T. Galambos: Phosphorus Poisoning in Humans, Arch. Intern. Med., 112:846, 1963.

Salicylates

Done, A. K.: Salicylate Intoxication; Significance of Measurements of Salicylate in Blood in Cases of Acute Ingestions, Pediatrics, 26:800, 1960.

———: Salicylate Poisoning, J.A.M.A., 192:770, 1965.

———: Treatment of Salicylate Poisoning, Mod. Treatment, 4:648, 1967.

Dukes, D. C., J. D. Bainey, G. Cumming, and G. Widdowson: Treatment of Severe Aspirin Poisoning, Lancet, II:329, 1963.

Segar, W. E., and M. A. Holliday: Physiologic Abnormalities of Salicylate Intoxication, New Engl. J. Med., 259:1191, 1958.

Singer, R. B.: The Acid-Base Disturbance in Salicylate Intoxication, Medicine, 33:1, 1954.

Summitt, R. L., and J. N. Etteldorf: Salicylate Intoxication in Children. Experience with Peritoneal Dialysis and Alkalinization of the Urine, J. Pediat., 64:803, 1964.

117 HEAVY METALS

Ivan L. Bennett, Jr. and David C. Poskanzer

Three highly effective chemicals, BAL, Versene, and penicillamine, are now available for treatment of systemic poisoning with heavy metals by forming nontoxic, stable cyclic compounds with polyvalent metallic ions, thus permitting the offending material to be excreted safely in the urine.

The first to be developed was BAL (British antilewisite, 2,3-dimercaptopropanol, dimercaprol), which was originally intended as an antidote against the arsenical war gas, lewisite. Its tendency to combine with certain metallic ions such as arsenic, mercury, cobalt, nickel, antimony, and gold is so great that it can remove them from combination with the enzymes whose function they impair in the body. BAL is not useful in the treatment of lead poisoning. Because the effectiveness of BAL depends to some extent upon the speed with which its administration is begun, every attempt should be made to avoid delay in its use. For serious systemic intoxications, BAL should be given in doses of 4 mg per kg body weight intramuscularly as a 10% solution in oil and 20% benzyl benzoate. No single dose should exceed 300 mg. This dose should be repeated every 4 hr on the first day and every 6 hr on the second day. Thereafter, it should be given three times daily for several days; doses should then be tapered and discontinued about 10 days after acute poisoning. When the dose of poison has been relatively small, the schedule of BAL administration may be reduced by one-third. Because BAL is excreted in part by the kidneys, it can accumulate to toxic concentrations in anuric patients. Overdosage results in nervousness, hyperactivity, muscle twitching, and hyperreflexia. Large doses may produce convulsions. The presence of the material in tears sometimes causes blepharospasm. In patients with anuria or oliguria, therefore, BAL should be administered with caution and at a lower dosage than outlined above. If too much is given, sedatives should be administered.

The second antidote to metal poisons is the chelating agent Versene (ethylenediaminetetraacetate, EDTA), which forms cyclic, stable, soluble, nontoxic compounds with most metals. Because Versene reacts with calcium in the same way as with other metals, it must be given as the calcium salt (Calcium Disodium Versenate; calcium disodiumedetate) to avoid hypocalcemia. The material has been used with notable success in the treatment of lead poisoning.

It is given in a dosage of 500 mg in 250 ml of 5% glucose IV every 12 hr for 5 days. After a pause to allow for further solution of metal from body stores a second and even a third course may be given.

Penicillamine (cuprimine, beta, beta-dimethylcysteine) is an excellent chelating agent for copper, mercury, and lead, promotes their excretion in the urine, and has the additional advantage of being well absorbed from the gastrointestinal tract. It may be given orally, while BAL and Versene require systemic injection. N-acetyl-*dl*-penicillamine is even more effective than penicillamine in protecting against the effects of mercury, probably because it is more resistant to metabolic degradation and is less toxic. Penicillamine is administered orally in a dose of 1 to 4 Gm daily on an empty stomach to avoid chelation of dietary metals. It has much lower toxicity compared to BAL, the only other agent which is effective in the treatment of Wilson's disease (hepatolenticular degeneration), in which toxic amounts of copper are deposited in various tissues, but has the disadvantage of acute sensitivity reactions. It has also been shown to be useful in lead poisoning, but the excretion of urinary lead may not be as high after oral penicillamine as after intravenous Calcium Disodium Versenate.

N-acetyl-*dl*-penicillamine, though still an investigational drug, has been demonstrated to be effective in mercury poisoning and has the advantage of allowing much higher doses with fewer toxic effects. It has less effect on copper levels than penicillamine and is therefore used in the treatment of mercury poisoning when one would wish to maintain copper levels. Courses of 10 days of 1 to 2 Gm daily in divided doses have been employed in patients with good results.

ANTIMONY

Symptoms of poisoning after the ingestion of antimony may occur when an acid food is allowed to stand in cheap enamelware or "graniteware" for a sufficient time to allow solution of antimony, which is used in the manufacture of these products. The symptoms are similar to those produced by arsenic, except that antimony causes a more rapid onset of gastrointestinal symptoms. Treatment is the same as for arsenic, including BAL. Circulatory collapse occurs early and requires vigorous supportive treatment. The therapeutic injection of antimony (tartar emetic, etc.) may result in severe coughing, muscle and joint pains, or bradycardia. The last is an indication for stopping medication (See Chap. 267).

ARSENIC

Arsenic poisoning is usually the result of accidental or suicidal ingestion of insecticides or rodenticides containing Paris green (copper acetoarsenate) or calcium or lead arsenate. Pesticides containing arsenic are a frequent source of poisoning in rural areas of the United States. Medications such as Fowler's solution (potassium arsenite) and the organic arsenicals (arsphenamines and arsenoxides) were once common causes of intoxication.

The toxic dose of inorganic arsenic varies considerably and seems to depend upon individual susceptibility. Orchardists have been found to ingest as much as 6.8 mg arsenic a day without any signs of intoxication. On the other hand, as little as 30 mg arsenic trioxide has been fatal. Arsenic has a predilection for keratin, and the concentration of arsenic in the hair and nails is higher than that in other tissues. Arsenic reacts with the —SH groups in certain tissue proteins and thus interferes with a number of enzyme systems essential to cellular metabolism. Pathologic changes in fatal inorganic arsenical poisoning are fatty degeneration of the liver, hyperemia and hemorrhages of the gut, and renal tubular necrosis. The peripheral nerves often show fragmentation and resorption of myelin with disintegration of axis cylinders.

The symptoms of acute poisoning by the oral route are nausea, vomiting, diarrhea, severe burning of the mouth and throat, and agonizing abdominal pains. The vomitus often contains blood. Circulatory collapse is frequent, and death may ensue within a few hours. With chronic exposure, the first signs of poisoning are usually weakness, prostration, muscular aching, or nervous system involvement; gastrointestinal symptoms are minimal. In patients exposed to arsine gas (hydrogen arsenide), the outstanding features are hemolysis, chills, fever, and hemoglobinuria.

Patients who recover from acute poisoning and those with chronic intoxication usually develop skin and mucosal changes, peripheral neuropathy, and linear pigmentations in the fingernails (see Chap. 354). The *cutaneous manifestations* appear within 1 to 4 weeks and consist of a diffuse, dry, scaly desquamation, occasionally with hyperpigmentation, over the trunk and extremities. Hyperkeratoses of the palms and soles and edema of the face and extremities may also occur. The mucous membranes also show evidence of irritation, with conjunctivitis, photophobia, pharyngitis, or irritating cough. About 5 weeks after exposure to arsenic, a transverse white stria, 1 to 2 mm in width, appears above the lunula of each fingernail (*Mees lines*). Patients with more than one exposure to arsenic may show double lines several millimeters apart.

Symptoms of headache, drowsiness, confusion, and convulsions are seen in both acute and chronic intoxication. Evidence of peripheral neuropathy usually appears 1 to 3 weeks after exposure. There are numbness, tingling, and burning of the feet and hands followed by muscular weakness. The extremities show a decrease in touch, pain, and temperature sensations, in a symmetrical "stocking-glove" distribution, and distal weakness with inability to walk or stand, weakness of grip, and wrist drop. Tendon reflexes are absent or diminished, and atrophy of the affected muscles develops rapidly.

The laboratory findings usually consist of moderate anemia and a leukopenia of 2,000 to 5,000 white blood cells with mild eosinophilia. There is slight proteinuria, and liver function tests show mild abnormalities. The spinal fluid is normal.

None of the clinical or laboratory manifestations of arsenic poisoning is specific, and the diagnosis depends upon analysis of the hair and urine for arsenic. Normal individuals have an average concentration of 0.05 mg arsenic per 100 mg of hair, with a range of 0.025 to 0.088 mg. Concentrations of arsenic greater than 0.1 mg per 100 mg of hair are indicative of poisoning. The minimal level of arsenic in the urine indicating intoxication is difficult to establish. Normal persons have been found to excrete between 0.01 and 0.06 mg of arsenic per liter, and a few individuals as much as 0.2 mg per liter. Although there is considerable overlap, most patients with evidence of arsenic intoxication will be found to excrete more than 0.1 mg per liter; soon after acute exposure, many will show levels greater than 1 mg per liter.

The treatment for acute ingestion is gastric lavage (see Chap. 115). Replacement of lost fluids and elevation of blood pressure by vasopressor agents is often indicated. Immediate treatment with BAL should be instituted. Patients with peripheral neuropathy rarely show significant improvement with BAL and continue to have sensory disturbances and weakness for many months. Dramatic responses, however, have been observed with the use of BAL in the treatment of exfoliative dermatitis, bone marrow depression, and encephalopathy caused by the arsphenamines and the organic arsenicals. BAL is of little value in the treatment of the hemolysis caused by inhalation of arsine.

BISMUTH

Poisoning by bismuth is almost entirely a complication of antisyphilitic therapy. Toxic manifestations may appear in the mouth (gingivitis, followed by stomatitis), the kidneys (albuminuria and nephrotic syndrome), or the skin (exfoliative dermatitis), requiring immediate interruption of bismuth injections. The development of a bluish stippled line of pigmentation just at the margin of the gums is not dangerous but suggests that oral hygiene should be improved. Bismuth subnitrate occasionally gives rise to methemoglobinemia (Chap. 344).

CADMIUM

Poisoning is likely to occur after ingestion of an acid food prepared in a cadmium-lined vessel. The classic example is lemonade served from metal cans. Symptoms of nausea, vomiting, diarrhea, and prostration usually develop within 10 min after ingestion. Treatment is symptomatic, and symptoms ordinarily subside within 24 hr. The short incubation and the typical circumstances suggest the diagnosis. Inhalation of cadmium fumes in industry produces an acute, extremely severe pneumonitis (Chap. 288). The use of BAL is not recommended for cadmium intoxication, as the BAL-cadmium complex dissociates in the kidneys and cadmium is nephrotoxic.

COPPER

Acute poisoning due to ingestion of copper salts is rare. Copper sulfate (blue vitriol) is the chief offender, in which case the vomitus has a characteristic blue color. Manifestations are nausea, vomiting, bloody diarrhea, headache, severe thirst, and tachycardia. In fatal cases, death is preceded by convulsions. Treatment consists of gastric lavage with 1% solution of potassium ferrocyanide, fluid replacement, and control of pain and diarrhea with opiates.

GOLD

Because practically all cases of poisoning by gold are associated with its use in the treatment of arthritis, diagnosis is usually easy. Manifestations are skin rashes of various types, bone marrow depression, icterus, oliguria, nausea, vomiting, and gastrointestinal bleeding. Treatment consists of symptomatic relief of discomfort and the use of BAL, an effective antidote.

LEAD

Poisoning results from ingestion of lead-containing materials such as paint or water which has stood in lead pipes or from inhalation of fumes from burning storage batteries, solder, etc. Illicit whiskey contaminated by lead solder in the pipes of stills has been responsible for many cases of poisoning. Bullets or buckshot containing lead can cause poisoning years after becoming embedded in a serous cavity. Absorption is slow by any route, and prolonged exposure is required for the development of symptoms. Lead is a cumulative poison, excreted slowly. Acute poisoning is virtually nonexistent, although it was observed when lead was used for the treatment of malignant disease. Symptoms may develop suddenly after chronic exposure. Most of the absorbed lead is deposited in the bones; blood, urine, and feces contain only small amounts.

Manifestations of poisoning are colic, encephalopathy, peripheral neuritis, and anemia.

Lead colic, or painter's cramps, is characterized by agonizing, wandering, poorly localized abdominal pain, often with spasm and rigidity of the musculature of the abdominal wall. There is no fever or leukocytosis. Needless surgery has been carried out in these patients for supposed perforation of peptic ulcer or other catastrophe. Morphine has surprisingly little effect upon the pain; intravenous injection of calcium salts affords relief within a short time, although pain may recur. Attacks of colic seem to be brought on by intercurrent infection or alcoholic overindulgence.

Encephalopathy occurs chiefly in children and is manifested by convulsions, somnolence, mania, delirium, or coma. Mortality is high when convulsive seizures and coma occur. Mental enfeeblement is a common sequel.

Peripheral neuritis with paralysis, characteristically involving the muscles most used (e.g., wrist drop in painters, etc.), occurs in patients exposed to lead, often in the absence of other symptoms. It is rare in children. (See Chap. 354.)

Mild anemia, probably the result of increased brittleness of the erythrocytes as well as of a defect in cell maturation, is common. Pallor is out of proportion to anemia in patients with chronic plumbism and is attributed to spasm of small vessels in the skin. Anemia is almost never severe and is characterized by the presence of large numbers of erythrocytes with basophilic stippling. This is seen in other hematologic disorders, but a smear showing stippling should arouse suspicion of lead poisoning. In patients with poor oral hygiene a "lead line" of black lead sulfide may develop along the gingival margins. This is not seen in edentulous persons and is rare in children.

Patients with lead poisoning excrete increased amounts of coproporphyrin III in the urine (see Chap. 108). This is so consistent that examination of a urine specimen for porphyrin is the best screening test in suspected cases. A few milliliters of urine should be acidified with acetic acid and shaken with an equal volume of ether. Exposure of a specimen prepared in this manner under a Woods lamp will reveal reddish fluorescence of the ether layer if coproporphyrin is present. A positive test is strongly in favor of lead intoxication. Urinary lead determinations are of aid in confirming the diagnosis; a level of 0.2 mg per liter or more is usually regarded as significant, although interpretations vary.

Lead encephalopathy occurs chiefly in children, has a significant mortality, and causes severe permanent brain damage in 25 percent of survivors. Encephalopathy in adults is rare and usually results from consumption of lead-contaminated illicit liquor (moonshine). Once minor symptoms of poisoning are present, acute encephalopathy can develop with unpredictable rapidity. Any child with symptoms suggestive of lead poisoning should be considered a medical emergency and hospitalized immediately. The onset of encephalopathy is signaled by the development of gross ataxia, persistent vomiting, and intermittent lethargy and stupor. These symptoms are followed by convulsions, mania, and coma.

The most important single feature of treatment is removal of the patient from further exposure to lead. Once abnormal absorption is terminated, virtually all the lead in the body is shifted into bone. Chelating agents do not remove significant quantities of lead from bone. It takes approximately twice as long to excrete a given burden of lead as it does to accumulate it. As long as significant quantities of lead remain in bone any intercurrent illness which causes demineralization can cause mobilization of toxic quantities of lead into soft tissues and exacerbate plumbism.

The treatment of lead encephalopathy is begun once adequate urine flow is established. A combination of BAL and Calcium Sodium Versenate is employed, and the Versene therapy continued for 5 to 7 days. If Calcium Disodium Versenate is given alone in the presence of very high tissue concentrations of lead, some of the toxic effects may be intensified. Acute symptoms usually subside within 48 to 72 hr after Versene is begun. Within 2 weeks urinary excretion of copro-

porphyrin ceases, and there is sometimes a dramatic improvement in neuritis.

Symptoms of acute increased intracranial pressure are best treated with repeated doses of mannitol intravenously. Evidence for the use of high potency steroids to relieve cerebral edema in patients with lead encephalopathy is incomplete. Treatment of increased intracranial pressure by surgical decompression is no longer indicated.

In adults combined therapy with BAL and Calcium Disodium Versenate followed by oral penicillamine is probably indicated whenever blood levels exceed 100 mg lead per 100 Gm blood even in the absence of symptoms. Evidence of lead toxicity is usually present at this level, and the risk of symptomatic episodes is considerable. The use of oral penicillamine alone in a dose of 1 to 1.5 Gm daily for 3 to 5 days in mildly symptomatic cases has been suggested and has the advantage of easy administration and the avoidance of painful injections.

MERCURY

Poisoning occurs chiefly as a result of the acute ingestion of a soluble salt, usually mercuric chloride (bichloride of mercury). Toxic symptoms may occur with 0.1 Gm, and 0.5 Gm is almost always fatal unless immediate treatment is instituted. The mercuric ion is corrosive and produces severe local inflammation. Oral, pharyngeal, and laryngeal pain are severe; abdominal cramps with nausea and vomiting occur within 15 min. As mercury is absorbed, it is concentrated in the kidneys, where it poisons the tubular cells, producing a tendency to diuresis within the first 2 to 3 hr. The combination of vomiting, dehydration, shock, and progressive tubular damage, however, soon leads to anuria and uremia. The poison is also excreted into the colon and produces severe enteritis with bloody diarrhea and tenesmus. Death is usually from uremia. The chief objectives of treatment are to prevent the shock of dehydration and to remove mercury from the body. Early in treatment, copious quantities of fluid should be infused intravenously to prevent dehydration and to reduce the concentration of mercuric ion in the renal tubules. That the patient is anuric early is often simply the result of dehydration and shock. In such instances, forcing fluids is advisable. However, the gradual development of oliguria and anuria in a hydrated patient indicates renal damage by mercury, and at this stage a regimen for acute renal shutdown should be instituted (Chap. 300).

Chronic poisoning from metallic mercury vapor occurs in individuals exposed to large amounts of the metal in laboratories or in industry and occasionally as a result of prolonged therapeutic use, as in vaginal douches. Manifestations may be those of subacute poisoning, with salivation, stomatitis, and diarrhea or primary neurologic signs, including tremors of the extremities, tongue, and lips, ataxia and dysarthria, erethism, a state of easy embarrassment, irritability, apprehension, withdrawal, and depression.

Some poison can be removed from the body by gastric

lavage, but more important in treatment is the binding of the mercuric ion in a harmless compound by BAL. The therapeutic usefulness of BAL depends on its immediate administration. In chronic mercury poisoning, N-acetyl-*dl*-penicillamine may well be the drug of choice. It can be administered orally and appears to selectively chelate mercury with considerably less effect on copper, which is essential to many metabolic processes.

SILVER

Most poisoning by silver involves silver nitrate, a caustic salt. There are intense nausea, vomiting, and diarrhea after swallowing nitrate (lunar caustic), and death from shock may occur within a few hours. The mouth is usually deeply stained by silver nitrate. Treatment is entirely supportive, with fluid replacement and control of pain.

Chronic exposure (usually to nose drops) produces a peculiar bluish skin discoloration (argyria).

THALLIUM

Thallium is a component of certain rodenticides and depilatories, and clinical poisoning is usually a result of accidental ingestion of these materials. The fatal dose is approximately 1.0 Gm. Manifestations are vomiting, diarrhea, and leg pains, followed by weakness and paralysis of the legs. There may be visual and mental disturbances. About 3 weeks after poisoning, the patient's hair falls out, providing a strong diagnostic clue if the cause has not previously been determined. Treatment is symptomatic. The alopecia is temporary if the patient recovers.

REFERENCES

Levine, W. G.: Heavy-Metal Antagonists, pp. 929–942 in *The Pharmacological Basis of Therapeutics,* 3d ed., Louis S. Goodman and Alfred Gilman (Eds.), New York: The Macmillan Company, 1965.

Arsenic

Jenkins, R. B.: Inorganic Arsenic and the Nervous System, Brain, 89:479, 1966.
Keusler, C. J., J. C. Abels, and C. P. Rhoads: Arsine Poisoning, Mode of Action and Treatment, J. Pharmacol. Exp. Therap., 88:99, 1946.
Longcope, W. T., and J. A. Luetscher: The Use of BAL (British Antilewisite) in the Treatment of the Injurious Effects of Arsenic, Mercury, and Other Metallic Poisons, Ann. Intern. Med., 31:545, 1949.

Bismuth

Heyman, A.: Systemic Manifestations of Bismuth Toxicity; Observations on 4 Patients with Pre-existent Kidney Disease, Am. J. Syph., Gonor., Vener. Dis., 28:721, 1944.

Cadmium

Ross, P.: Cadmium Poisoning, Brit. Med. J., 1:252, 1944.

Gold

Strauss, J. F., Sr., R. M. Barrett, and E. F. Rosenberg: BAL Treatment of Toxic Reactions to Gold: A Review of the Literature and Report of Two Cases, Ann. Intern. Med., 37:323, 1952.

Lead

Aub, J. C., L. T. Fairhall, A. S. Minot, and P. Reznikoff: Lead Poisoning, Medicine, 4:1, 1925.
Chisolm, J. J., Jr.: Treatment of Lead Poisoning, Mod. Treatment, 4:710, 1967.

Mercury

Arena, J. M.: Treatment of Mercury Poisoning, Mod. Treatment, 4:734, 1967.
Doolan, P. D., W. C. Hess, and L. R. Kyle: Acute Renal Insufficiency Due to Dichloride of Mercury: Observations on Gastrointestinal Hemorrhage and BAL Therapy, New Engl. J. Med., 249:273, 1953.
Hirschman, S. Z., M. Feingold, and G. Boylen: Mercury in House Paint as a Cause of Acrodynia, New Engl. J. Med., 269:889, 1963.

Thallium

Munch, J. C.: Human Thallotoxicosis, J.A.M.A., 102:1929, 1934.

118 ALCOHOL

Maurice Victor and Raymond D. Adams

Intemperance creates many problems in modern society, the importance of which can be judged by the repeated emphasis they receive in contemporary writings, both literary and scientific, as well as from health, social, and religious agencies. These problems may be divided into three categories—psychologic, medical, and sociologic. The main psychologic problem is why a person drinks excessively, often with full knowledge that such action will result in physical injury to himself and irreparable harm to his family. The medical problem embraces all the diseases which relate to overindulgence in alcohol. The sociologic problem comprises the effects of sustained inebriety on the family and community.

The various problems raised by excessive drinking cannot be separated from one another, and the physician must therefore be conversant with all aspects of the subject. He may be asked to help the patient conquer his alcoholic tendency or to diagnose and to treat the numerous diseases to which he is subject; often he must admit or commit the patient to a general or mental hospital, according to the nature of the presenting clinical disorder; and lastly, he may be required to enlist the aid of available social agencies when their services are needed by either the patient or his family.

Alcoholism has been defined as both a chronic disease and a disorder of behavior, characterized in either context by the repeated drinking of alcoholic beverages to an extent that exceeds customary dietary use or surpasses the social drinking customs of the community and that interferes with the drinker's health, interpersonal relations, or economic functioning. Stated more succinctly, it is alcoholic addiction. The precise number of such individuals, commonly known as alcoholics, in the United States is not known. The estimate is 5 million—approximately 4 percent of the total adult population. It requires little projection of the imagination to conceive the havoc wrought by alcohol in terms of decreased productivity, accidents, crime, mental and physical disease, and disruption of family life.

PHARMACOLOGY AND METABOLISM OF ALCOHOL

Ethyl alcohol, or ethanol, is the active ingredient in beer, wine, whiskey, gin, brandy, and other less common alcoholic beverages. In addition, the stronger spirits contain enanthic ethers, which give the flavor but have no important pharmacologic properties, and impurities such as amyl alcohol (fusel oil) and acetaldehyde, which act like alcohol but are more toxic. Contrary to prevailing opinion, the content of B vitamins in American beer and other liquors is so low as to offer little or no protection against avitaminosis.

Alcohol is absorbed unaltered from the gastrointestinal tract, about 80 percent from the intestine and the remainder from the stomach. Its presence may be detected in the blood within 5 min after ingestion, and the maximum concentration is reached in ½ to 2 hr. The ingestion of milk and fatty foods impedes and water facilitates its absorption. In habituated persons the blood alcohol concentration rises somewhat faster and reaches a higher maximum than in abstainers.

Alcohol is carried chiefly in the plasma and enters the various organs of the body, as well as the spinal fluid, urine, and pulmonary alveolar air, in concentrations which bear a constant relationship to that in the blood. Elimination of alcohol is accomplished chiefly by oxidation, 5 percent or less being excreted chemically unchanged in the urine, sweat, and breath. The energy liberated by the oxidation of alcohol (7 Cal per Gm) can be utilized as completely as that of fats, sugars, and proteins, which it replaces isodynamically. It should be emphasized that alcohol cannot be stored in the body or used in the replacement of destroyed tissue. Unless, therefore, the protein intake is adequate, a state of negative nitrogen balance will develop, a common finding in chronic alcoholics.

The first step in the metabolism of alcohol is accomplished mainly in the liver, where alcohol dehydrogenase oxidizes alcohol to acetaldehyde. The latter substance may be further metabolized in the liver or carried to other tissues, where it is converted, possibly via the stage of free acetate, to acetyl coenzyme A, of which the acetate portion can be oxidized completely to carbon dioxide and water.

For all practical purposes it may be accepted that once absorption is ended and an equilibrium established with the tissues, ethyl alcohol is oxidized at a constant rate, independent of its concentration in the blood. Actually, slightly more alcohol is burned per hour when the initial concentrations are very high, but this increment is of little clinical significance. On the other hand, the rate of oxidation of acetaldehyde does depend on its concentration in the tissues. This fact is of importance in connection with the drug disulfiram (Antabuse), which increases the tissue concentration necessary to metabolize a certain amount of acetaldehyde per unit of time. The patient taking both Antabuse and alcohol will accumulate an inordinate amount of acetaldehyde, resulting in nausea, vomiting, and hypotension, sometimes pronounced and even fatal in degree. This pharmacologic principle underlies the treatment of alcoholism with Antabuse.

Very few factors capable of increasing the rate of alcohol metabolism are known. There is some evidence that repeated ingestion induces an increased rate of metabolism of alcohol, and this holds true for both normal and alcoholic subjects. The rate of alcohol metabolism may also be increased by the administration of insulin and perhaps amino acids, but neither of these has proved to make a significant difference in the treatment of intoxication. On the other hand, starvation slows the rate of alcohol metabolism in the liver, although this varies greatly in degree from one individual to another.

PHYSIOLOGIC AND PSYCHOLOGIC EFFECTS OF ALCOHOL

The immediate effects of alcohol on organs other than the central nervous system are relatively unimportant. There appears to be a direct action on the excitability and contractility of heart muscle. With intoxicating doses there is a rise in cardiac rate and output, systolic and pulse pressures, and there is cutaneous vasodilatation at the expense of splanchnic constriction. Prolonged intoxication has led on occasion to cardiac and skeletal myopathy, a degeneration of fibers due, it is said, to suppression of myophosphorylase activity. Increased sweating and vasodilatation cause a loss of body heat and a fall in temperature. In low concentrations, by whatever route it is administered, alcohol is capable of stimulating the gastric glands to produce acid, apparently by causing the tissues to form or release histamine. With the ingestion of alcohol in concentrations of over 10 to 15 percent the secretion of mucus is increased, the stomach mucosa becomes congested and hyperemic, and the secretion of acid then becomes depressed. This is a state of acute gastritis, from which recovery is relatively rapid. The increase in appetite following ingestion of alcohol is due to the stimulation of the end organs of taste and to a general sense of well-being. Similarly, the reviving effect of alcohol in fatigue states is a cerebral one, not due to a direct stimulating effect on muscle or other organs.

Alcohol has an effect on intermediary metabolism in the liver cells, particularly lipid metabolism (see Chap.

323), and also exerts a distinct effect on the renal excretion of water and electrolytes. The ingestion of 4 oz 100 proof bourbon whiskey, for example, results in a diuresis qualitatively indistinguishable from that which follows the drinking of large amounts of water. This diuresis is most likely due to the transient suppression of the release of antidiuretic hormone (ADH) from the neurohypophysis, since a relatively small amount of alcohol injected directly into a carotid artery evokes a prompt diuresis without a detectable rise in the concentration of alcohol in the systemic blood. The exact locus of action within the supraopticohypophyseal system is unknown. Alcohol does not alter the sensitivity of the kidney tubules to endogenous or exogenous ADH (Pitressin) and has no discernible effect on renal hemodynamic function in normal persons. The degree of diuresis seems to be more closely related to the duration of the rising blood alcohol level than to the rate of increase or the absolute level attained. In recumbent persons, the water diuresis following the ingestion of alcohol is associated with a diminished excretion of electrolytes (Na, K, Cl), presumably because of vasodilatation and the consequent redistribution of the circulating blood volume. There is also an increased urinary excretion of ammonium and titratable acidity following alcohol, owing to a mild degree of both metabolic and respiratory acidosis. The former is presumably due to an accumulation of acid metabolites and the latter to the direct action of alcohol on the respiratory center.

If the period of alcohol intoxication is sustained, the effects are somewhat different. Diuresis occurs only during the initial phase of alcohol administration and does not persist during prolonged drinking. However, hematocrit levels decrease and serum osmolality and sodium levels rise, even if dietary and vitamin intake is adequate. These derangements tend to resolve spontaneously after cessation of drinking and cannot be explained by the known diuretic or hormonal changes induced by ethanol ingestion.

Apart from the derangements noted above, the obvious effects of acute, nonlethal doses of alcohol are those exerted on the nervous system, constituting the characteristic symptoms and signs of alcohol intoxication. A large body of data has accumulated regarding the psychomotor effects of alcohol, the nature of tolerance, and the relation of blood alcohol levels to various manifestations of intoxication. Only the most pertinent data are presented here.

It is now generally accepted that alcohol is not a stimulant of the central nervous system, but a depressant. Some of the early effects of alcohol, manifested by garrulousness, aggressiveness, excessive activity and increased electrical excitability of the cerebral cortex, suggest a state of stimulation. There is evidence, however, that the initial action of alcohol is to depress certain subcortical structures (?high brainstem reticular formation) which ordinarily modulate or inhibit cerebral cortical activity. Similarly, the initial hyperactivity of tendon reflexes may represent a transitory escape of spinal motor neurons from higher inhibitory centers.

With increasing amounts of alcohol, however, the depressant action spreads to involve the cerebral cortical neurones directly, as well as other cerebral and spinal neurones.

All manner of motor performance, whether simply the maintenance of a standing posture, the control of speech and eye movements, or highly organized and complex motor skills are adversely affected by alcohol. The movements involved in these acts are not only slower than normal, but more inaccurate and random in character and therefore less well adapted to the accomplishment of specific ends.

Alcohol also impairs the efficiency of mental function by interfering with the learning process, which is slowed and rendered less effective. The faculty of forming associations, whether in the form of words or of figures, tends to be hampered, and the power of attention and concentration is reduced. The individual is not as versatile as usual in directing thought along new lines appropriate to the problems at hand. Finally, alcohol impairs the faculties of judgment and discrimination and all in all the ability to think and reason clearly.

A scale relating the various degrees of clinical intoxication to the blood alcohol level in nonhabituated persons has been constructed by Miles. He found that at blood alcohol levels of 30 mg per 100 ml, a mild euphoria was detectable, and at 50 mg per 100 ml, a mild incoordination. At 100 mg per 100 ml, ataxia was obvious; at 300 mg per 100 ml, the patient was stuporous; and a level of 400 mg per 100 ml was accompanied by deep anesthesia and could prove fatal. These figures are valid, provided that the alcohol content rises steadily over a 2-hr period.

It should be emphasized that such a scale has virtually no value in the chronic alcoholic patient, for it does not take into account the adjustment which the organism makes to alcohol, i.e., the phenomenon of tolerance. It is common knowledge that a habituated individual can drink more and show fewer effects than the moderate drinker or abstainer. Talland studied a series of alcoholic subjects during a period of sustained inebriation, when they were ingesting between 30 and 40 oz 86 proof alcohol per day, and found practically no decrement in the performance of tasks designed to measure attention, motor skills, and reaction time to visual or auditory stimuli; the blood alcohol levels, at the time of testing of these subjects, ranged from 60 to 200 mg per 100 ml.

This phenomenon of tolerance accounts for the surprisingly large amounts of alcohol that can be consumed by the chronic inebriate without significant signs of drunkenness. Three patients studied at the Addiction Research Center in Lexington, Ky., for example, consumed 397 to 466 ml of 94 percent alcohol per day without showing any significant amounts of alcohol in the blood or clinical evidence of intoxication. In these patients, there was a very narrow margin between the doses associated with low blood alcohol levels and sobriety and the doses (430 to 479 ml daily) associated with high blood levels and drunkenness. Observations such as these would tend to invalidate the use of a single estimation of alcohol concentration as a reliable index of drunkenness. The organism is capable of adapting itself to the presence of alcohol after a very short exposure. If the alcohol concentration in the blood is raised very slowly, no symptoms appear, even at quite high levels. It would appear that the important factor in this rapid adaptability is not so much the rate of increment or the height of the blood alcohol level, but the length of time the alcohol had been present in the body. It has also been shown that, if the dosage of alcohol which just causes blood levels to be high is held constant, the blood alcohol concentration falls and clinical evidence of intoxication disappears. The cause of this fall in alcohol concentration is not clear. This type of tolerance has been referred to as "metabolic" in contrast to "tissue tolerance," which refers to the adjustments made by the nervous system to long-continued exposure to alcohol. The latter seems to depend on an altered nervous tissue response, i.e., a biochemical adaptation of the habituated individual enabling him to function more effectively at a given alcohol concentration. The precise nature of the adaptation is still a matter of conjecture. Undoubtedly some inborn factor plays a part in determining relative susceptibility. It is also conceivable that there is a psychologic adjustment to high concentrations of alcohol in nervous tissues. The habituated individual may learn to compensate for his lack of coordination and the removal of his inhibitions in a manner that would be impossible for the abstainer.

CLINICAL MANIFESTATIONS OF ALCOHOLISM

The clinical effects of alcohol are mainly on the digestive organs and on the nervous system. Each of these will now be considered.

EFFECT OF ALCOHOL ON THE DIGESTIVE ORGANS. Symptoms of disordered gastrointestinal function are particularly common in alcoholics, and of these the most distinctive are morning nausea and vomiting. Characteristically, the patient can suppress these symptoms by taking a drink or two, after which he is able to consume large quantities of alcohol without recurrence of nausea and vomiting, until the following morning. Since sufficient alcohol actually relieves these symptoms, they are probably not due to the local effects of alcohol on the stomach. Indeed, gastroscopic studies indicate that they are not related to gastritis but instead probably have a "central" origin and represent the mildest manifestations of the withdrawal syndrome (see below).

Other complaints referable to the gastrointestinal system are abdominal distension, epigastric distress, belching, typical or atypical ulcer symptoms, and hematemesis. The most common pathologic basis for these symptoms is a superficial gastritis which is an almost invariable sequel to prolonged drinking. Most instances of gastritis are benign, and the symptoms subside in a matter of days, but more severe forms are associated with mucosal erosions or ulcerations and may be the source of serious bleeding. The incidence of peptic ulcer is exceptionally high in the alcoholic population. A less frequent but serious cause of hematemesis is the so-called "Mallory-Weiss syndrome," which is characterized by lacerations of the gastric mucosa, occurring at or just below the gastroesophageal junction. In many of these cases bleeding is preceded by an episode of forceful vomiting or protracted retching; in others, the presence of a hiatus hernia or mucosal atrophy appears to be the predisposing factor. The typical lesions have been produced experimentally, in the cadaver, by occluding the esophagus and antrum and raising the intragastric pressure to 100 to 150 mm Hg, i.e., to the range of pressure attained by normal subjects during a period of induced straining and retching.

Patients admitted to the hospital following a period of prolonged drinking and severe dietary depletion almost invariably show enlargement of the liver due to infiltration of the parenchymal cells with fat. *Fatty hepatosis,* as this is called, is essentially a reversible state, providing the patient remains abstinent and receives a nutritious diet. About 10 percent of patients with severe alcoholism develop a permanent form of liver disease, i.e., *cirrhosis,* in which a diffuse proliferation of fibrous tissue destroys the normal lobular architecture of the organ. The alcoholic variety of cirrhosis (also referred to as *Laennec's* or *portal cirrhosis*); its complications and possible relationship to fatty liver are discussed in Chap. 328.

The excessive use of alcohol is also a significant factor in the causation of *pancreatitis.* The mildest form of this disorder may be attributed to gastritis or may go unnoticed, unless detected by a transient elevation of the serum amylase. Sometimes pancreatitis presents as an acute abdominal catastrophe, i.e., with epigastric pain, vomiting, and rigidity of the upper abdominal muscles. These symptoms closely simulate those of perforated peptic ulcer, so that an operation may be performed needlessly. In these circumstances the pancreas appears tense and edematous, often with a serosanguineous exudation of fluid on its surface. The most severe form of acute pancreatitis is characterized by widespread necrosis and hemorrhage (see Chap. 334).

It is generally believed that acute pancreatitis is caused by the activation of proteolytic enzymes with consequent autodigestion of the pancreatic tissue. Two factors are probably important in the pathogenesis: (1) the powerful stimulating effect of alcohol on the gastric acidity, which stimulates the production of secretin and which in turn provokes an increase in the formation of pancreatic enzymes; (2) obstruction to the flow of pancreatic enzymes, the result of inflammatory changes in the duodenum with edema and spasm of the sphincter of Oddi.

Alcoholics are also likely to develop a *chronic relapsing form of pancreatitis.* The type associated with irregular calcification of the pancreas is practically always associated with alcoholism. The etiology of this disorder is obscure, but the occurrence of chronic pancreatic changes in human nutritional disease (Kwashiorkor), as well as in certain experimental animals (rats given a methionine-deficient diet), suggests that it may be a deficiency disease. This subject is discussed further in Chap. 333.

THE EFFECT OF ALCOHOL ON THE NERVOUS SYSTEM. A large number of neurologic disorders are associated with alcoholism. The factor common to all of them, of course, is the abuse of alcohol, but the mechanism by which alcohol produces its effects is quite different from one group of disorders to another. The classification which follows is based on these mechanisms, insofar as they are known.

I. Alcohol intoxication—drunkenness, coma, excitement ("pathologic intoxication")

II. The abstinence or withdrawal syndrome—tremulousness, hallucinosis, "rum fits," delirium tremens and auditory hallucinosis

III. Nutritional diseases of the nervous system secondary to alcoholism
   A. Wernicke-Korsakoff syndrome
   B. Polyneuropathy
   C. Retrobulbar neuropathy ("tobacco-alcohol amblyopia")
   D. Pellagra

IV. Diseases of uncertain pathogenesis, associated with alcoholism
   A. Cerebellar degeneration
   B. Marchiafava-Bignami disease
   C. Central pontine myelinolysis
   D. Cerebral atrophy
   E. "Alcoholic" cardiomyopathy and myopathy

V. Neurologic disorders consequent upon Laennec's cirrhosis and portal-systemic shunts
   A. Hepatic stupor and coma
   B. Chronic hepatocerebral degeneration

ALCOHOLIC INTOXICATION. Drunkenness is such a common phenomenon that its psychologic and physical manifestations require little elaboration. The signs consist of varying degrees of exhilaration and excitement, loss of restraint, irregularity of behavior, loquacity, slurred speech, incoordination of movement and gait, irritability, drowsiness, and, in advanced cases, stupor and coma. On rare occasions acute intoxication is characterized by an outburst of irrational, combative and destructive behavior, a state referred to as "pathologic intoxication" or "acute alcoholic paranoid state." Allegedly the latter reaction may follow the ingestion of small amounts of alcohol, and it has been variously ascribed to constitutional differences in susceptibility to alcohol, previous cerebral injury, and "an underlying epileptic predisposition." However, there are no critical data to support any of these contentions. An analogy may be drawn between this state of alcoholic excitement and a similar reaction which occasionally complicates the administration of barbiturates.

The symptoms of intoxication are caused by the depressant action of alcohol on nerve cells, acting in a manner akin to that of the general anesthetics. Unlike the general anesthetics, however, the margin between the dose of alcohol that produces surgical anesthesia and that which dangerously depresses respiration is very narrow, a fact which accounts for the occasional fatality in cases of alcoholic narcosis.

The signs of alcohol intoxication are quite distinctive and as a rule present no problem in diagnosis or management. On the other hand, coma due to alcohol may present difficulties in differential diagnosis. It should be stressed that the diagnosis of alcoholic coma is made not merely on the basis of a flushed face, stupor, and the odor of alcohol, but only after the careful exclusion of all other causes of coma (see Chap. 26). Furthermore, alcoholic coma is not always benign, as are the more common manifestations of intoxication. Serious depression of respiration, heralded by a loss of corneal and pupillary reflexes, calls for the use of respiratory stimulants and the treatment of peripheral vascular collapse, if this should manifest itself.

THE ABSTINENCE OR WITHDRAWAL SYNDROME

Of more serious consequence than the states of intoxication are the tremulous, hallucinatory, epileptic, and delirious states. Although a sustained period of chronic intoxication is the underlying factor in these illnesses, the symptoms become manifest only after a period of relative or absolute abstinence from alcohol—hence the designation *abstinence or withdrawal syndrome.* Each of the major manifestations of the withdrawal syndrome may occur distinct from the others and will be so described; more frequently, however, they occur in various combinations. The prototype of the patients afflicted with these symptoms is the spree or periodic drinker, although the steady drinker is not immune if, for some reason, alcohol is withdrawn.

TREMULOUSNESS. By far the most common manifestation of the abstinence syndrome is a state of tremulousness, commonly referred to as "the shakes" or "the jitters," combined with general irritability and gastrointestinal symptoms, particularly nausea and vomiting. The symptoms first show themselves after several days of drinking, in the morning, after the short period of abstinence that occurs during sleep. The patient needs to "quiet his nerves" by a few drinks; his symptoms are in fact relieved by alcohol, only to return on successive mornings with increasing persistence and severity. The usual spree lasts about 2 weeks, but the duration varies greatly. It is terminated not only because of recurrent tremor and vomiting, but for one or more other reasons such as lack of funds, weakness, self-disgust, or collapse. The symptoms then become greatly augmented, reaching their peak intensity 24 to 36 hr after the complete cessation of drinking.

At this stage, the patient presents a distinctive clinical picture. He is alert and startles easily. His face is deeply flushed, the conjunctivas are injected, and there is usually a tachycardia. Anorexia, nausea, and retching are always in evidence. He may complain of insomnia and craves rest and sleep. He is preoccupied with his misery, inattentive, and disinclined to answer questions; or he may respond in a rude or perfunctory manner. The patient may be mildly disoriented in time and have a poor memory for events of the last few days of his drinking spree but shows no serious confusion, being generally aware of his surroundings and the nature of his illness.

Generalized tremor is an outstanding feature of this illness. It fluctuates widely in severity, being hardly recognizable when the patient is calm, becoming gross and irregular upon attempted activity and during periods of emotional stress. The tremor may be so violent that the patient cannot stand without help, speak clearly, or feed himself. Sometimes there is little objective evidence of tremor, and the patient complains only of being "shaky inside."

Although the flushed facies, anorexia, tachycardia, and tremor subside to a large extent within a few days, the patient does not regain his full composure for a much longer time. The overalertness, tendency to startle easily, and jerkiness of movement may persist for a week or longer; the curious feeling of uneasiness may not leave the patient completely for 10 or 14 days, and only at the end of this time is he able to sleep undisturbed, without sedation. An attempt should be made to keep the patient in hospital for this length of time; to discharge him after a few days increases the likelihood that he will turn to alcohol to suppress his still-present tenseness and sleeplessness.

HALLUCINOSIS. Symptoms of disorder perception occur in about one-quarter of the tremulous patients. The patient may complain of "bad dreams"—nightmarish episodes associated with disturbed sleep, which are difficult to separate from real experience. Sounds and shadows may be misinterpreted, or familiar objects may be distorted and assume unreal forms. Although these are not hallucinations in the strict sense of the term, they represent the most common forms of disordered sense perception in the alcoholic. Hallucinations may be purely visual or auditory in type, mixed visual and auditory, and occasionally tactile or olfactory. There is little evidence to support the popular belief that certain visual hallucinations are specific to alcoholism. They are more commonly animated than inanimate and may comprise various forms of human, animal, or insect life. They may occur singly or in panoramas; they may appear shrunken or enlarged; they may be natural in appearance or take distorted and hideous forms (see Chap. 30).

ACUTE AND CHRONIC AUDITORY HALLUCINOSIS. This phenomenon merits separate consideration. For many years, an alcoholic psychosis has been recognized in which vivid auditory hallucinations are the major abnormality. Kraepelin referred to this as the *hallucinatory insanity of drunkards* or *alcoholic mania,* and Wernicke, as the *acute hallucinosis of drunkards.* The central feature of the illness, in the beginning, is the occurrence of auditory hallucinations in the face of an otherwise clear sensorium, i.e., the patients are not confused, disoriented, or obtunded and have an intact memory. The hallucinations are almost always vocal in nature, although there may be other auditory phenomena, such as the sound of running motors, buzzing, music, ringing of telephones, or dogs barking. When the voices can be identified, they are attributed to the patient's family, friends, or neighbors, rarely to God, radio, or radar. The voices may be

addressed directly to the patient, but more frequently they discuss him in the third person. In the majority of cases the voices are maligning, reproachful, or threatening in nature and are disturbing to the patient; a significant proportion, however, are not unpleasant and leave the patient undisturbed. The voices are intensely real and vivid, and they tend to be exteriorized; i.e., they come from behind the door, from the corridor, or through the floor. Another quality of these hallucinations (and of visual ones) is the appropriateness of the patient's emotional response to the hallucinatory content. He may call on the police for protection or barricade himself against invaders; even more dramatically, he may attempt suicide to avoid what the voices threaten. The hallucinations are most prominent during the night, and their duration varies greatly—they may be momentary or they may recur intermittently for days on end and, in exceptional instances, for weeks or months.

Most patients, while hallucinating, have no appreciation of the unreality of their hallucinations. As improvement occurs, the patient begins to doubt their reality, is reluctant to talk about them, and may even question whether he had been sane during the episode. Full recovery is characterized by the realization that the voices were imaginary and by the ability to recall, sometimes with remarkable clarity, the abnormal thought content of parts of the psychotic episode.

A unique feature of this psychosis is the evolution of a chronic auditory hallucinosis in a small proportion of the patients. At the outset, these patients show the characteristics of the more transient form of the illness, but after a variable period of time (as short as 1 week) the patient becomes quiet and resigned, despite the fact that the hallucinations remain threatening and derogatory. Ideas of reference and influence and other poorly systematized paranoid delusions become prominent. At this stage these patients show many of the symptoms of schizophrenia—illogical thinking, vagueness, tangential associations, and a dissociation of affect and of thought content. There is some evidence that repeated attacks of acute auditory hallucinosis render the patient more vulnerable to this chronic form of the illness. Despite the similarities to schizophrenia, there are also points of difference. In the alcoholic illness there is no family history, the age of onset is considerably beyond that of "classic" schizophrenia; the past history reveals no evidence of schizophrenia or "schizoid" personality traits, and the symptoms develop in close temporal relationship to a drinking bout.

ALCOHOLIC EPILEPSY. In this particular setting (i.e., where relative or absolute abstinence follows a period of chronic inebriation) there is a marked liability to develop convulsive seizures. Characteristically, these seizures occupy a discrete period (usually 12 to 48 hr) following the cessation of drinking, after which the patient remains free of seizures until the next cycle of drinking and abstinence. During the period of seizure activity of electroencephalogram may be abnormal, particularly in response to stroboscopic stimulation and other activating procedures, but it reverts to normal in a matter of days, even though the patient may go on to develop delirium tremens.

Seizures occurring in the abstinence period have a number of other distinctive features. There may be only a single seizure, but in the majority of cases they occur in short bursts of two to six, or even more, and an occasional patient develops status epilepticus. The seizures are grand mal in type, i.e., major generalized convulsions with loss of consciousness. If they are focal in nature, then it is likely that a focal lesion (usually traumatic) will be found in addition to the factor of alcohol. Almost one-third of the patients with generalized seizure activity go on to develop delirium tremens, in which case the seizures invariably precede the delirium. The postictal confusional state may blend imperceptibly with the onset of the delirium, or there may be a clearing of the postictal state, over several hours or even a day or two, before the delirium sets in. Seizures of this type occur in patients who have been drinking for many years, so that they have to be distinguished from other forms of epilepsy beginning in adult life.

It is suggested that the term *rum fits*, i.e., the words used by the alcoholic himself, be reserved for seizures which possess the attributes described above. This would serve to distinguish this form of seizure activity, which occurs only in the immediate abstinence period, from that which occurs in the interdrinking period, long after withdrawal has been accomplished. This is not to deny that the "idiopathic" or posttraumatic forms of epilepsy may be influenced by alcohol; indeed, it has been shown that the incidence of both these types of epilepsy is increased if the patient drinks. In patients with idiopathic or posttraumatic epilepsy, a seizure or seizures may be precipitated by only a short period of drinking (e.g., a weekend, or even one evening of heavy social drinking); interestingly, in these circumstances, the seizures occur not when the patient is intoxicated, but usually the morning after, in the "sobering-up" period.

Electroencephalographic (EEG) findings in alcoholic subjects with "rum fits" do not support the notion that the seizures merely represent latent epilepsy made manifest by alcohol, or that alcohol precipitates convulsive attacks in patients who are subject or constitutionally predisposed to seizures. Instead, the EEG reflects a sequence of changes engendered by alcohol itself—a decrease in the frequency of brain waves during the period of chronic intoxication; a rapid return of the EEG to normal immediately after cessation of drinking; the occurrence of a brief period of dysrhythmia (sharp waves and paroxysmal changes) which coincides with the flurry of convulsive activity; and again, a rapid return of the EEG to normal. Except for the transient dysrhythmia in the withdrawal period, the incidence of EEG abnormalities in patients who have had "rum fits" is not greater than in the normal population, in sharp contrast to patients who are indeed subject to seizures (see Chap. 353).

DELIRIUM TREMENS. This is the most dramatic and grave of all the alcoholic complications. It is characterized by a state of profound confusion, delusions, vivid hallucinations, tremor, agitation, and sleeplessness, as well as by increased activity of the autonomic nervous system, i.e., dilated pupils, fever, tachycardia, and profuse perspiration. The clinical features of delirium have been presented in detail in Chap. 30; only those features peculiar to the alcoholic variety (delirium tremens) are considered here. Delirium tremens develops in one of several settings. The patient, an excessive and steady drinker of many years' duration, may have been admitted to the hospital for an unrelated illness, accident, or operation, and 3 to 4 four days later becomes delirious. Or, following a prolonged spree, he may have already experienced several days of tremulousness and hallucinosis, or one or more seizures, and may even be recovering from these symptoms, when he suddenly develops delirium tremens.

In the majority of cases delirium tremens is benign and short-lived, ending as abruptly as it begins. Consumed by the relentless activity and wakefulness of several days' duration, the patient falls into a deep sleep; he awakens lucid, quiet, hungry, and exhausted, with virtually no memory for the events of the delirious period. Less commonly, the delirious state subsides gradually; more rarely still, there may be one or more relapses, several discrete episodes of delirium being separated by lucidity, the entire process lasting for as little as several days or as long as 4 or 5 weeks. The recurrent type presents the most confusing picture of all, for the delirious periods may be of varying severity and duration, and the lucid intervals of varying degrees of completeness. Where the delirium occurs as a single episode, the duration is 72 hr or less in over 80 percent of the cases.

About 15 percent of cases of delirium tremens end fatally. In many of these there is an associated infectious illness or injury, but in others there is no discernible complicating illness. Frequently, these patients die in a state of hyperthermia or peripheral circulatory collapse; in some, death comes so suddenly that the terminal events cannot be discerned.

Closely related to typical delirium tremens and about as common are the *atypical delirious-hallucinatory states*, in which one facet of the delirium tremens complex assumes prominence to the practical exclusion of the other symptoms. The patient may simply exhibit a transient state of quiet confusion, agitation, and peculiar behavior, or he may become violent and disturbed. Other patients present a vivid delusional state and abnormal behavior, consistent with their false beliefs. Such a patient may relate a loosely connected and fantastic tale of fighting pitched battles, participation in the Indian wars or bank robberies, or the like, although he may be superficially oriented and may later recall his delusions to some extent. Several of these symptoms may be combined, and these states blend imperceptibly with fully developed delirium tremens. Unlike typical delirium tremens, the atypical states always present as a single circumscribed episode without recurrences, are only rarely preceded by epilepsy, and do not end fatally. This may be another way of saying that they are a partial or less severe form of the disease.

Pathologic examination is singularly unrevealing in patients with delirium tremens. Edema and brain swelling have been absent in the authors' pathologic material except when there was shock, terminal hypoxia, or electrolyte imbalance, and there have not been any significant microscopic changes in the brain. Abnormalities of the blood nonprotein nitrogen, carbon dioxide, spinal fluid, serum sodium, chloride, sugar, potassium, and magnesium occur unpredictably. The electroencephalographic findings have been discussed in relation to alcoholic epilepsy.

The *pathogenesis* of the tremulous-hallucinatory-delirious state has been a matter of considerable controversy. The idea that it simply represents the most severe form of alcohol intoxication is not tenable. The symptoms of toxicity, consisting of slurred speech, uninhibited behavior, staggering gait, stupor, and coma are distinctive and different from the symptom complex of tremor, hallucinations, fits, and delirium. The former symptoms are associated with an elevated blood alcohol level, whereas the latter become evident only when the blood alcohol is reduced. Finally, the toxic symptoms increase in severity as more alcohol is consumed, whereas tremor and hallucinosis and even full-blown delirium tremens may be nullified by the administration of alcohol.

A specific adrenal deficiency has been postulated as the cause of delirium tremens and its variants, but it is now clear, from several critical studies, that the administration of ACTH or adrenal corticosteroids does not alter the course of the illness in any way that could not be accounted for by its natural history. Since many alcoholics eat poorly, nutritional deficiency has been invoked as a cause, but this factor is not of fundamental importance, since delirium tremens may develop in patients taking a normal diet, and it may subside uneventfully, even though the patient is denied all food and vitamins.

As has been indicated, the tremulous-hallucinatory-epileptic-delirious states depend not only on chronic intoxication but on the relative or absolute withdrawal of alcohol. The mildest degree of this syndrome, tremor and nausea, may arise after only a few days of drinking and after a relatively short period of abstinence. These symptoms may be controlled by reestablishing the blood alcohol level. The most severe form of this syndrome, delirium tremens, requires a background of months of inebriation and becomes manifest only after several days of abstinence. Any given patient may show one or all of the symptoms of abstinence, but in the latter instance they become manifest in a predictable sequence—first tremulousness and hallucinosis (and/or seizures), followed by delirium tremens.

That withdrawal of alcohol, following chronic intoxication, is an essential factor in the genesis of this syndrome has been confirmed by experimental observations in human volunteers as well as in dogs and monkeys. The exact mechanisms involved in the production of withdrawal symptoms are poorly understood. Recently it has been shown that the early phase of alcohol withdrawal (beginning 7–8 hr after cessation of drinking) is regularly attended by a drop in serum magnesium levels and a rise in arterial pH values, on the basis of respiratory alkalosis. It is possible that the compounded effect of these two factors, both of which are associated with nervous system hyperexcitability, may be responsible for seizures and perhaps other symptoms which characterize the early phase of withdrawal. Probably neither of these factors is important in the causation of delirium tremens, since the hypomagnesemia and alkalemia are transient, and frequently have been restored to normal before the onset of delirium tremens.

NUTRITIONAL DISEASES OF THE NERVOUS SYSTEM

Nutritional diseases of the nervous system comprise a relatively small but serious group of illnesses in chronic alcoholics. In contrast to the abstinence syndrome, the role of alcohol is purely secondary, serving mainly to displace food in the diet. These illnesses and the role of alcohol in their production are discussed in Chap. 363, Metabolic and Nutritional Disorders of the Brain, and Chap. 354, Diseases of Peripheral Nervous System.

ALCOHOLIC DISEASES IN WHICH THE PATHOGENESIS IS UNCERTAIN

Included in this category are several diverse disorders which are practically always encountered in alcoholic patients. The relationship of these disorders to the excessive use of alcohol is not fully understood and probably not crucial, since all of them have been described in nonalcoholic patients. There is a considerable amount of indirect evidence that these disorders are nutritional in origin, but as yet this etiology must be regarded as unproved.

ALCOHOLIC CEREBELLAR DEGENERATION. This term is applied to a nonfamilial type of cerebellar ataxia which occurs in adult life against a background of prolonged ingestion of alcohol. The symptoms may progress slowly over a long period, but more frequently they evolve in a subacute fashion (several weeks or months), after which they remain stationary for many years. The signs are those of cerebellar dysfunction, affecting stance and gait predominantly. The legs are involved more frequently and severely than the arms, and nystagmus and speech disturbances are rare. Once established, the signs change very little, although some improvement of gait (due mainly to recovery from complicating polyneuropathy) may follow cessation of drinking. The essential pathologic changes consist of degeneration of varying severity of all the neurocellular elements of the cerebellar cortex, particularly the Purkinje cells, with a striking topographic restriction to the anterior and superior aspects of the vermis, and hemispheres. The disorder of stance and gait seems to be related to the vermis lesion, and the ataxia of the limbs to the hemispheral involvement. A similar clinical syndrome has been observed in a few nutritionally depleted nonalcoholic patients.

MARCHIAFAVA-BIGNAMI DISEASE (Primary Degeneration of the Corpus Callosum). This is a rare complication of alcoholism originally described in Italian men addicted to crude red wine. The symptoms are diverse and include psychic and emotional disorders, delirium and intellectual deterioration, convulsive seizures, and varying degrees of tremor, rigidity, paralysis, apraxia, aphasia, and sucking and grasping reflexes. The duration is variable, from several weeks to months, and recovery is possible. The pathologic picture is more constant than the clinical one. It consists of symmetrically placed areas of demyelination in the corpus callosum, particularly the middle lamina, and less consistently of the anterior commissure and other parts of the white matter. Axis cylinders are better preserved than medullated fibers in these areas, and there are appropriate reactions in the macrophages and astrocytes. Various degrees of recovery may occur if alcoholic abstinence and good nutrition are established and maintained.

PONTINE MYELINOLYSIS. This term refers to a unique pathologic change affecting the center of the basis pontis, in which the medullated fibers are destroyed in a single symmetric focus of varying size. In contrast, the axis cylinders, nerve cells, and blood vessels are relatively well preserved. The disease may manifest itself by pseudobulbar palsy and quadriplegia, but usually the lesion is so small that it causes no symptoms and is found only at postmortem examination. The relationship of this condition to either alcoholism or malnutrition is obscure, but most of the cases have occurred in patients with prolonged and severe nutritional depletion.

CEREBRAL ATROPHY. The pathologic examination of relatively young alcoholic patients not infrequently discloses an unexpected degree of convolutional atrophy, most prominent in the frontal lobes, and a symmetric enlargement of the lateral and third ventricles. The ventricular enlargement may also be found on pneumoencephalography. In some patients these findings are associated with overt complications of alcoholism, such as the Wernicke-Korsakoff syndrome, but in many of them no other abnormalities can be found, and the history discloses no symptoms of neurologic disease. The nature of this disorder is quite unclear.

"ALCOHOLIC" MYOPATHY. In recent years attention has been drawn to several disorders of skeletal and cardiac muscle, apparently primary in nature, in association with chronic alcoholism. One type of myopathic syndrome, which may be generalized or focal, is characterized by the acute onset of severe pain, tenderness and edema of muscles, accompanied by myoglobinuria, renal damage and hyperpotassemia in severe cases. Another type is characterized by the subacute development of weakness and atrophy of the proximal limb and girdle muscles, without local pain or edema and without evidence of polyneuropathy, and by myopathic changes in the electromyogram and serum enzymes. Muscle power is slowly restored in these patients following abstinence from alcohol and improvement in nutrition. "Alcoholic cardiomyopathy" is the name given to a nonspecific affection of cardiac muscle, which allegedly has a higher incidence in patients with chronic alcoholism than in the nonalcoholic population. The role of alcohol or malnutrition, or some hitherto unsuspected factor in the genesis of these disorders, is not known, and the structural and biochem-

ical basis of these syndromes requires further study (see Chap. 373).

THE NEUROLOGIC DISORDERS CONSEQUENT UPON CIRRHOSIS AND PORTAL-SYSTEMIC SHUNTS

Hepatic coma refers to an episodic disorder of consciousness which frequently complicates (or terminates) advanced liver disease and/or portal systemic shunts. It is associated with typical electroencephalographic abnormalities and a peculiar intermittency of sustained muscular contraction which presents as an irregular flapping movement of the outstretched limbs (asterixis). Patients dying in hepatic coma consistently show an increase in the number and size of the protoplasmic astrocytes throughout the central nervous system, but particularly in the deep layers of the cerebral and cerebellar cortex, the basal ganglia and dentate nuclei.

Less frequently, cirrhosis is complicated by a chronic and largely irreversible form of hepatocerebral disease, the main symptoms of which are dementia, dysarthria, ataxia, and athetosis. The brain in such cases shows not only an astrocytic hyperplasia but also a degeneration of nerve cells and fibers, the distribution of the destructive lesions following closely that of the astrocytic changes. Both hepatic coma and the chronic form of hepatocerebral disease are characterized by hyperammonemia, which is probably important in their pathogenesis. Ammonium is derived from the bacterial action on intestinal proteins and normally is converted to urea in the liver. A failure to metabolize ammonium, or perhaps some other substance absorbed from the bowel, may be the result of either hepatocellular disease or of shunting of blood around the liver. Presumably, the acute and rapidly developing effect of this toxin on the brain is episodic stupor or coma, which is reflected pathologically by a diffuse astrocytic hyperplasia; a prolongation of this effect may lead to irreversible neurological symptoms and parenchymal lesions.

The treatment of recurrent hepatic stupor and coma consists essentially of the use of a low protein diet and neomycin. Intractable cases of coma and protein intolerance, as well as the chronic form hepatocerebral disease cannot, as a rule, be controlled by these medical means alone; such cases have been improved by surgical means, either by colectomy or by exclusion of the colon. However, the number of patients treated in this way is still small, and the precise indications and effectiveness of the surgical measures remain to be determined. The neurologic complications of liver disease are considered further in Chaps. 328 and 363.

MANAGEMENT OF THE ALCOHOLIC PATIENT

The management of the various gastrointestinal complications of alcoholism is considered in the section dealing with these diseases. The management of the neurologic complications, coma, delirium tremens, and status epilepticus is discussed in Chaps. 26 and 368. Here a few remarks will be made about alcohol habituation. This presents quite a different and often a more difficult problem in management than the medical or neurologic illnesses associated with alcoholism. The patient may not have any disease that requires admission to a hospital but may nevertheless be seriously disabled in his marital, social, and economic life.

The problem of excessive drinking is a formidable one, as every physician knows. However, it is not necessarily hopeless, and an attitude of complete pessimism is not justified. It is also a common misconception among physicians that specialized training in psychiatry and an inordinately large amount of time are required to deal with the addictive drinker. Actually, a successful program treatment can be initiated by any physician with an interest in this problem, using the standard techniques of history-taking, establishing rapport with the patient, and seeing the patient frequently, though not necessarily for prolonged periods. A useful point at which to undertake this task is during convalescence of the patient from a serious medical or neurological complication of alcoholism or in relation to loss of employment, arrest, or threatened divorce. Such a crisis may help convince the patient, better than any argument presented by family or physician, that his alcoholism has attained serious proportions and that his drinking does indeed constitute a serious problem.

A number of premises about alcoholism and the alcoholic are generally accepted as prerequisites for successful treatment. The most important one is total abstinence from alcohol, and for all practical purposes, this represents the only permanent solution to the problem. It is generally agreed that any attempts to curb the drinking habit will fail if the patient continues to drink. There are said to be cases in which the patient has been able to reduce his intake of alcohol and eventually to drink in moderation, but such instances must be extremely rare.

A number of other commonly held notions about the treatment of alcoholism require qualification. It is frequently stated that the patient must recognize that he is an alcoholic, i.e., that his drinking is beyond his control, and he must express willingness to be helped. Undoubtedly there is truth in both of these statements, but they should not be interpreted to mean that the patient must gain this recognition and willingness entirely on his own initiative and that he will be helped only after he does so. Actually, the physician, or for that matter, any other interested person, can do a great deal to help the patient understand the nature of his problem and thus to motivate him to accept treatment. Every device of logic and reasoning must be used to convince the patient that abstinence is preferable to chronic inebriety. The patient must be made fully aware of the medical and social consequences of continued drinking and must also be made to understand that because of some constitutional peculiarity (like the diabetic who cannot handle sugar) he is incapable of drinking in moderation. These facts should be presented in a forthright manner, in much the same

way as one would explain the essential features of any other disease. There is nothing to be gained from adopting a punitive or moralizing attitude; nor should the patient be given the idea that he is in no way blameworthy for his illness. There appears to be an advantage in making the patient feel that he is responsible for doing something about his drinking.

The prevalent belief that an alcoholic will not stop drinking under duress also requires qualification. In fact, one of the few careful studies of this matter disclosed that relatively few patients would have sought help unless pressure had been exerted by family or employer; furthermore, patients who came to the clinic under duress of this sort did just as well as those who came voluntarily.

If an earnest and sustained effort by the physician fails to convince the patient that alcohol offers a problem, it is usually impossible to modify his alcoholic tendency. The only way to make such an individual discontinue drinking is to commit him to a psychiatric hospital or special institution for the management of alcoholism in the hope that with forced abstinence and improvement in his physical state he will gain insight and later accept psychiatric or other forms of therapy.

On the other hand, if the patient comes to realize that his drinking is beyond control and that he needs to do something about it, his chances of being helped are considerable. Indeed, under these circumstances, many individuals stop drinking of their own volition. Some of these patients, despite the best of intentions, will relapse. However, this should not serve as an excuse to abandon the therapeutic program, and there are many examples of patients who have attained a state of prolonged sobriety after several false starts. A number of methods have proved valuable in the long-term management of these patients. The most important of these are the use of Antabuse, aversion treatment, psychotherapy, and the participation in social organizations for combating alcoholism.

Antabuse (tetraethylthiuram disulfide, disulfiram) interferes with the metabolism of alcohol, so that a patient who takes both alcohol and Antabuse accumulates an inordinate amount of acetaldehyde in the tissues, resulting in nausea, vomiting, and hypotension, sometimes pronounced in degree. It is no longer considered necessary to demonstrate these effects to the patient; it is sufficient to warn him of the severe reactions that may result if he drinks while he has the drug in his body. Treatment with Antabuse is instituted only after the patient has been sober for several days, preferably longer. It should never be given to patients with cardiac or liver disease. The drug is taken each morning, or at another suitable time daily, in a dosage of 0.5 Gm, preferably under supervision. This form of treatment is of particular value in the spree or periodical drinker, in whom relapse from abstinence usually represents an impulsive rather than a carefully planned or premeditated act. The patient taking Antabuse, aware of the dangers of mixing liquor and the drug, is "protected" against the impulse to drink, and this protection can be renewed every 24 hr by the simple expedient of taking a pill. The willingness with which the patient accepts this form of treatment also serves as a rough index of his motivation. Should the patient drink when he is taking Antabuse, the ensuing reaction is usually severe enough to require medical attention, and a protracted spree can thus be prevented. Antabuse may lead to a mild polyneuropathy if continued over a long period of time (months or years).

The aversion treatment consists of the simultaneous administration of a drink of alcohol and an injection of emetin. The violent nausea and vomiting which ensue are intended to create in the patient a strong revulsion for alcohol. This form of treatment as well as other types of conditioned reflex treatment have been successfully employed in special clinics, but have not gained widespread popularity.

Alcoholics Anonymous (AA), an informal fellowship of former alcoholics, has proved to be the single most effective force in the rehabilitation of alcoholic patients. The philosophy of this organization is embodied in their so-called "twelve steps," a series of propositions about alcohol and alcoholism which guide the patient to recovery. The AA philosophy stresses in particular the practice of making restitution, the necessity to help other alcoholics, trust in God, the group confessional, and the belief that the alcoholic is powerless over alcohol. AA philosophy also embodies the 24-hr plan, in which the alcoholic strives for but 24 hr of abstinence (a concept inspired by the Sermon on the Mount) as a means of facilitating the maintenance of sobriety. Although accurate statistics are lacking, it is stated that about half of the members who express more than a passing interest in the program have no relapses, and that a significant additional number relapse, but eventually recover.

The methods used by AA are not suited to every patient, and some prefer the more personalized approach offered by special clinics and centers for the treatment of alcoholism. The physician should, therefore, be fully aware of all the community resources which are available for the management of this problem, and should be prepared to take advantage of them in appropriate cases.

It is not possible, within the confines of this chapter, to discuss the numerous theories of the etiology of alcohol addiction, and the various forms of treatment based on these theories. Alcoholism has been attributed to endocrine or other biochemical abnormalities, a biologic predisposition, special types of personality structures or racial and sociocultural factors, and an infinite number of psychologic defects. The multiplicity of theories in itself suggests that no single one of them adequately explains why some people become addicted to alcohol. There is no conclusive evidence that a difference in personality or any other factor distinguishes the alcoholic from the nonalcoholic, or that any particular form of psychotherapy accomplishes more than a regimen which utilizes the principles of therapy outlined above. In a certain proportion of alcoholic patients (the exact proportion has not been determined) drinking is symptomatic of manic-depressive disease; in such patients, treatment must be directed to the latter disorder.

REFERENCES

Alcohol and Alcoholism, U.S.P.H.S. Publ. No. 1640, Washington, D.C.

Isbell, H., H. F. Fraser, A. Wikler, R. E. Belleville, and A. J. Eisenman: An Experimental Study of the Etiology of "Rum Fits" and Delirium Tremens, Quart. J. Stud. Alc., 16:1, 1955.

Victor, M.: The Pathophysiology of Alcoholic Epilepsy, in "The Addictive States," Res. Publ. Assoc. Res. Nervous Mental Disease, 46:431, 1968.

Victor, M., and R. D. Adams: The Effect of Alcohol on the Nervous System, in "Metabolic and Toxic Diseases of the Nervous System," Res. Publ. Assoc. Res. Nervous Mental Disease, 32:526, 1953.

——, and J. Hope: The Phenomenon of Auditory Hallucinations in Chronic Alcoholism, J. Nervous Mental Disease, 126 (Nos. 5 and 6):451, 1958.

——, R. D. Adams, and E. L. Mancall: A Restricted Form of Cerebellar Cortical Degeneration Occurring in Alcoholic Patients, A.M.A. Arch. Neurol., 1:579, 1959.

——, and R. D. Adams: On the Etiology of the Alcoholic Neurologic Diseases: With Special Reference to the Role of Nutrition, Am. J. Clin. Nutrition, 9:379, 1961.

119 OPIATES AND OTHER SYNTHETIC ANALGESIC DRUGS

*Maurice Victor and
Raymond D. Adams*

The drugs included in this category are morphine, opium, heroin (diacetylmorphine), Dilaudid (dihydromorphinone), codeine (methylmorphine), Pantopon, dihydrocodeinone (Hycodan), dihydroxycodeinone (Eucodal), and 14-hydroxydihydromorphinone (Numorphan). The synthetic analgesics meperidine (Demerol), the meparidine derivatives anileridine and alphaprodine (Nisentil), methadone (Dolophine or amidone), metopon (methyl-dihydromorphinone), racemorphan (Dromoran), levorphan (*l*-Dromoran), *d*-propoxyphene (Darvon), diphenoxylate (Lomotil), and phenazocine (Prinadol) should also be listed here, since they are similar to the opiates both in their pharmacologic effects and in the patterns of abuse, the differences being mainly quantitative. In fact, *d*-propoxyphene and diphenoxylate have such low addiction liabilities that they are not controlled by the Federal Narcotic Laws. A knowledge of the properties of these analgesic agents is important for the prevention of medical addiction, which is a lesser problem than social addiction, but far from negligible.

Like alcohol and the barbiturates, the opiates may suitably be considered from two points of view: (1) acute poisoning, and (2) addiction.

OPIATE POISONING

Severe poisoning with morphine or related alkaloids is not a frequent accident, but moderate degrees are relatively common, the result of ingestion with suicidal intent, errors in the calculation of dosage, or unusual sensitivity. In children as well as in adults with myxedema, Addison's disease, chronic liver disease, or pneumonia, there may be an increased susceptibility to opiates, and relatively small doses may prove toxic. Acute poisoning may occur in addicts who are unaware that tolerance for opiates declines quickly after the withdrawal of the drug and who resume the habit at a formerly well-tolerated dose.

The clinical manifestations of acute poisoning are varying degrees of unresponsiveness, shallow respirations, miosis, bradycardia, and hypothermia. Mild intoxication is manifested by anorexia, nausea, vomiting, constipation, and loss of sexual interest. In the most severe degrees of intoxication, the pupils are dilated and cyanosis and circulatory collapse occur. The immediate cause of death is usually respiratory depression, with consequent asphyxia.

Treatment consists of gastric lavage if the drug was taken orally. This procedure may be efficacious many hours after ingestion, since one of the toxic effects of opiates is severe pylorospasm, which may cause much of the drug to be retained in the stomach. Other measures are directed toward the maintenance of an adequate airway and oxygenation, as described in the section dealing with barbiturate intoxication. If the patient does not respond rapidly to these measures, N-allylnormorphine (Nalline) should be administered. This is a specific antidote to the opiates and also to the synthetic analgesics. It is given in doses of 5 to 10 mg subcutaneously or intravenously. The improvement of circulation and respiration is usually dramatic; in fact, failure of Nalline to produce a striking improvement in respiration should cast doubt on the diagnosis of opiate intoxication. Nalline does little to restore consciousness, however, and the patient may remain drowsy for many hours. This is not harmful, provided that respiration is well maintained. Since the duration of action of Nalline is shorter than that of all the analgesics except Dilaudid and meperidine, respirations may again become depressed an hour or so after the administration of the antidote. It should then be given a second time, in smaller dosage.

Once the patient regains consciousness, usually in about 8 hr, other complaints such as severe pruritus, sneezing, persistent obstipation, and urinary retention may necessitate symptomatic treatment. Nausea and severe abdominal pain, due presumably to pancreatitis resulting from spasm of the sphincter of Oddi, are other troublesome symptoms. Nalline must be used with great caution in the case of an addict who has taken an overdose of opiate because in this circumstance the withdrawal symptoms may be particularly severe.

OPIATE ADDICTION

It is estimated that there are about 60,000 persons addicted to narcotic drugs in the United States, apart from patients who are addicted because of hopeless medical illnesses. This is a relatively small number, considering the numbers who abuse barbiturates and alcohol. Nevertheless, the problem of narcotic addiction is important for several reasons. To the patient and his family it is a tragedy which often brings about complete physical, social, and economic ruin. The physician must be constantly alert to the dangers of the long-term use of narcotic drugs and the synthetic analgesics and aware of the methods of legal control and treatment of addiction. Without the restraining influence of public health measures, addiction could conceivably assume epidemic proportions.

ETIOLOGY AND PATHOGENESIS. A number of factors, socioeconomic, psychologic, and pharmacologic, all contribute to the genesis of opiate addiction. In our culture, the most susceptible subjects are young men or delinquent youths living in the economically depressed areas of certain large cities—New York, Chicago, Los Angeles, Washington, D.C., and Detroit. A disproportionately large number of addicts are American Negroes and persons of Puerto Rican or Mexican descent. Most of these individuals show psychiatric disorders, psychoneurosis and psychopathy being the most common. However, the precise "personality" factor which renders them vulnerable to addiction has not been defined. Association with addicts is the chief reason for beginning addiction. A relatively small proportion of all addicts are introduced to drugs by physicians in the course of an illness. Judging from the studies at the Addiction Research Center, Lexington, Ky., only a few of these "medical" or "accidental" addicts can be regarded as normal, well-adjusted persons. The majority have psychologic abnormalities similar to those of the "social" addicts, the only difference being the original mode of contact with the drug.

According to Wikler, the abuse of opiate drugs evolves in three successive phases: (1) episodic intoxication, or euphoria, (2) pharmacogenic dependence, or addiction, and (3) the propensity to "relapse after cure," or habituation.

Some of the symptoms of opiate intoxication have already been considered. Of equal importance are the symptoms designated as *morphine euphoria,* a term which refers to the pain- and anxiety-reducing abilities of this drug, as well as to the state of elation or sense of unusual well being which it produces and which is especially prized by psychopathic thrill seekers. Individuals who take opiates for their euphoria-producing effects quickly discover the need to increase the dose in order to obtain an effect which approaches that of the original dose. Although the intensity of the initial "euphoria" is not fully recaptured, the progressively increasing dose of drug does ablate the discomfort which arises as the effects of each injection wear off. In this way the use of opiates becomes self-perpetuating and a marked degree of tolerance is produced, so that enormous amounts of drugs, e.g., 5,000 mg morphine daily, have been administered without the development of toxic symptoms. The mechanism of tolerance is not understood. There is some experimental evidence that during addiction there is a progressive decrease in the capacity of the liver to N-demethylate morphine and other opiates.

With the continued administration of the drug, an

altered physiologic state develops, such that if administration of the drug is suddenly terminated, a drug-specific illness develops, termed the *abstinence syndrome*. This, strictly speaking, is the definition of *addiction*, alternate terms being *physical* or *pharmacologic dependence*. This definition distinguishes between "addicting" drugs (opiates, alcohol, barbiturates) and "habit-forming" drugs (bromides, amphetamine, cocaine, and marijuana), since no abstinence symptoms follow the discontinuation of the latter group, even after prolonged exposure. Stated in another way, all addicting drugs are habit-forming, but the opposite is not true.

The intensity of the abstinence syndrome depends mainly on the dose of the drug and duration of addiction, but also on individual factors. In respect to morphine it has been found that the majority of individuals receiving 240 mg daily for 30 days or more will show moderately severe abstinence symptoms following withdrawal, whereas mild grades of abstinence may be detected following as little as 80 mg daily for a similar period.

The abstinence syndrome which occurs in the morphine addict may be taken as the prototype of the opiate group. The first 8 to 16 hr of abstinence usually pass asymptomatically. At the end of this period yawning, rhinorrhea, sweating, and lacrimation become manifest. These symptoms are at first mild, but they increase in severity over a period of several hours and then remain constant for several days. The patient may be able to sleep during this early period but is restless, and thereafter insomnia remains a prominent feature. Dilatation of the pupils, recurring waves of gooseflesh, and twitchings of the muscles appear. The patient complains of severe aches in the back, abdomen, and legs and of hot and cold "flashes," so that he covers himself with blankets. By the end of about 36 hr the restlessness becomes more extreme, and nausea, vomiting, and diarrhea usually develop. The temperature, respiration, and blood pressure are slightly elevated. All these symptoms reach their peak intensity 48 to 72 hr after withdrawal, and then gradually decline. After 7 to 10 days, all objective signs of abstinence have disappeared, although the patient may complain of insomnia, nervousness, weakness, and muscle aches for several more weeks.

Wikler speaks of two types of abstinence changes—"nonpurposive" and "purposive." The former comprise the various automatic and neuromuscular signs and are relatively transient in nature. That these symptoms represent an altered physiologic state and are not psychic in origin has been clearly demonstrated experimentally; physical dependence on morphine and other opiate drugs develops even in the isolated segment of the spinal cord in chronic spinal and in chronic decorticated dogs. The flexor and crossed extensor spinal reflexes are depressed or abolished during continued administration of opiate and become remarkably hyperirritable when the drug is withdrawn. The purposive changes refer to the patient's craving for the drug and the manipulative activity directed toward obtaining it. These symptoms may persist indefinitely and are important in relation to that characteristic of addiction referred to as *habituation, emo-*

tional dependence, or *psychologic dependence*. These terms are used interchangeably and refer to the substitution of drug-seeking activities for all other aims and objects in life. Habituation is regarded by psychiatrists as the most important quality of addiction, since it is this feature which governs the initial use of the drug and relapse following apparent cure of addiction. An individual takes drugs initially not because he needs the drug to prevent withdrawal symptoms but because of its euphoria-producing effect, i.e., the relief of pain and emotional discomfort. Similarly, relapse to the use of the drug may occur long after the nonpurposive abstinence changes seem to have disappeared. The cause for relapse is imperfectly understood. It has been theorized by Wikler that fragments of the abstinence syndrome may remain as a conditioned response, and that these abstinence signs may be evoked by the appropriate environmental stimuli. Thus, when a "cured" addict finds himself in a situation where narcotic drugs are readily available, or in circumstances that were responsible for the initial use of drugs, the incompletely extinguished drug-seeking behavior reasserts itself.

The characteristics of addiction and of abstinence are qualitatively similar with all the drugs of the opiate group as well as the related synthetic analgesics. The differences are mainly quantitative and are related to the differences in potency and length of action. Heroin is two to three times more potent than morphine but otherwise the same. Dilaudid and metopon are more potent than morphine and have a shorter duration of action; hence the addict requires more doses per day, and the abstinence syndrome comes on and subsides more rapidly. The length of action of Dromoran is somewhat longer than that of morphine, but withdrawal phenomena are similar to those of morphine in temporal course and intensity. Abstinence symptoms from codeine, while very definite, are less intense than those from morphine. The addiction liabilities of Darvon are even less than those of codeine. Abstinence symptoms from methadone are less intense than those from morphine and do not become evident until 3 or 4 days after withdrawal; furthermore, this drug is qualitatively different from morphine insofar as autonomic signs are less severe in the abstinence period. For these reasons methadone is used in the treatment of morphine addiction. Demerol addiction is of particular importance because of the high incidence among doctors and nurses and because there is still a widespread belief that this drug is nonaddicting. Tolerance to the toxic effects of Demerol is not complete, so that the addict may show tremors, twitching of the muscles, confusion, hallucinations, and at times convulsions. Signs of abstinence appear 3 to 4 hr after the last dose and reach maximum intensity in 8 to 12 hr, at which time they may be worse than those of morphine abstinence.

DIAGNOSIS. This is usually made by the patient's statement that he is addicted to and needs drugs. If the patient conceals his addiction, the diagnosis may be difficult. Miosis, needle marks, emaciation, or abscess scars are suggestive but not specific signs. Demerol addicts are likely to show dilated pupils and twitching of muscles. Test procedures for opiates in the urine are difficult and usually unavailable. Formerly it was necessary to isolate questionable cases and to observe the patient over a period of at least two days for signs of abstinence. By using the specific antagonist N-allylnormorphine (Nalline) a diagnosis of addiction to opiates and related analgesic drugs can be made within an hour.

Nalline should be administered only in the presence of another physician or nurse, with the full understanding and permission of the patient. A dose of 3 mg of the antidote is given subcutaneously, and if no signs of abstinence have appeared in 20 min, an additional 5 mg is given. If no signs have appeared in another 20 min, a final dose of 8 mg is given. Provided that the patient has taken more than occasional doses of the drug within a week of the test, the administration of Nalline will precipitate symptoms of abstinence. These become evident within 5 min of the first injection, reach their peak intensity in 20 min, begin to decline in 60 min, and disappear after 3 hr. Curiously, Nalline does not precipitate abstinence symptoms in Demerol addiction, unless the patient has been taking more than 1,600 mg daily.

The diagnosis of drug addiction or the suspicion of this diagnosis should always prompt a search for infectious complications, which are due to the frequent contamination of illegally procured drugs by various organisms and to the unsterile practices of the addict in taking drugs. The usual forms of infection in the addict are abscesses at injection sites and hepatitis; occasionally tetanus and bacterial or mycotic endocarditis occur.

MANAGEMENT AND AVOIDANCE OF ADDICTION. The ambulatory treatment of addiction never succeeds and should therefore not be undertaken. Addicts who are refused opiates may ask for methadone, Demerol, or Dromoran, on the grounds that these drugs are synthetic and nonaddicting. These drugs are addicting and have been legally defined as opiates. The physician should also be aware that he is breaking both the letter and the spirit of the regulations if he prescribes narcotics for an addict, merely for the purpose of preventing abstinence changes. Occasional exceptions may be made in cases of seriously ill addicts who are awaiting hospital treatment, or in patients who are suffering from incurable painful disease.

Treatment of the hospitalized patient consists of the administration of morphine in doses just sufficient to prevent nonpurposive abstinence changes. Usually 30 mg four times daily suffices. After 3 days on this dosage, the drug is withdrawn by the so-called "rapid reduction" method, in which successively smaller doses are administered over a 5- to 10-day period. A much longer time is required in the presence of serious medical disease. Flow baths, aspirin, intravenous fluids, and the cautious use of barbiturates help to control the abstinence symptoms.

An alternate method, once the patient has been stabilized on morphine, is to substitute methadone for morphine, in the ratio of 1 to 3 mg. After a period of a week, in which the patient receives 10 mg methadone two to four times daily, the drug is rapidly withdrawn. With this method the abstinence symptoms are relatively mild but long-lasting, so that some patients prefer the first method.

Regardless of the method of drug withdrawal employed, treatment is best carried out in an institution with proper facilities for postwithdrawal rehabilitation in a drug-free environment. If such institutional facilities are not available locally (private, municipal, or state), the patient may apply to the U.S. Attorney in his community for commitment to a Federal institution (Lexington, Ky. or Fort Worth, Texas) under the Narcotic Addict Rehabilitation Act ("NARA") of 1966. Acceptance of the patient under the provisions of this act entails institutional treatment for up to 6 months after admission, followed by after-care in the patient's community for 3 years.

In recent years, attention has centered on the use of drugs in the ambulatory treatment of narcotic addiction. One of these is the narcotic antagonist, cyclazocine, which effectively blocks the pharmacologic effects of opiates and which may serve, if taken for prolonged periods, to extinguish the addict's drug-seeking behavior. In other patients, an impressive degree of social adjustment has been achieved by the oral administration of methadone (80 to 120 mg orally, once daily), which blocks the action of heroin through cross-tolerance. Both of these therapeutic methods are promising but experimental in nature, and their ultimate utility in the long-term management of the narcotic addict remains to be determined.

The physician must be constantly alert to the dangers of addiction, particularly in susceptible individuals, i.e., in those with psychoneurosis, psychopathic personality, or alcoholism. The use of opiates should be limited to cases where pain is the chief problem; they should not be used primarily as sedatives, or for the relief of asthma, or even in chronic pain until all other measures have been exhausted. It follows that it is most important to make a precise diagnosis of the cause or causes of pain, since in some cases measures other than opiates will suffice, while in others, such as hysteria and depression, narcotics are contraindicated.

If narcotics have to be used for the relief of pain, then consideration should be given to the choice of the appropriate drug and to the mode of administration. Morphine is still the drug of choice for most patients requiring relief of severe pain for short periods. Demerol may be useful in patients who cannot tolerate morphine. Patients with chronic pain should be managed with the least potent and smallest dosage of drug that will do the job; doses should be spaced as far apart as possible and discontinued as soon as the need for pain relief has passed. In general, the opiates should be administered orally whenever possible and the intravenous route should be avoided, since the latter method produces maximum euphoria and, hence, the greatest danger of addiction. The oral administration of codeine and aspirin is a useful way to begin treatment of the patient with chronic pain. If these drugs fail to control the pain, the parenteral administration of codeine should be tried. If more potent opiates are needed, methadone and levorphan should be used, because of their effectiveness by the oral route and the relatively slow development of tolerance. Should long-continued injections of morphine or meperidine become necessary, it should be kept in mind that maximum analgesic effect is obtained with 10 mg morphine rather than with 15 mg, as is often prescribed, and with 60 to 70 mg rather than with 100 mg of meperidine. In these cases, the use of the new narcotic antagonist, pentazocine (Talwin) might be considered. This drug, administered parenterally in doses of 40 to 60 mg, is said to have analgesic effects comparable to morphine and other opiates, but less of the addicting properties, features which are still under investigation. However, the respiratory depression produced by pentazocine is not counteracted by Nalline, a serious disadvantage in some patients.

REFERENCES

Dole, V. P., and M. E. Nyswander: Methadone Maintenance and Its Implication for Theories of Narcotic Addiction, Res. Publ. Assoc. Res. Nervous Mental Disease, 46:359, 1968.

Isbell, H.: Perspectives in Research on Opiate Addiction, Brit. J. Addict., 57:17, 1961.

——, and W. M. White: Clinical Characteristics of Addiction, Am. J. Med., 14:558, 1953.

Martin, W. R.: The Basis and Possible Utility of the Use of Opioid Antagonists in the Ambulatory Treatment of the Addict, Res. Publ. Assoc. Res. Nervous Mental Disease, 46:367, 1968.

Wikler, A.: Narcotics: The Effect of Pharmacologic Agents on the Nervous System, Res. Publ. Assoc. Res. Nervous Mental Disease, 37:334, 1959.

——: Drug Addictions, in F. Tice (Ed.), "Practice of Medicine," Hagerstown, Md., W. F. Prior Co., 1962.

120 BARBITURATES AND OTHER NONBARBITURATE HYPNOTIC-SEDATIVE DRUGS

Maurice Victor and
Raymond D. Adams

The high incidence of addiction, suicides, and accidental deaths attributable to the improper use of the barbiturate drugs is a matter of continuing concern to the medical profession. The production of barbiturates greatly exceeds the amount needed for therapeutic purposes. It is estimated that barbiturates account for 20 percent of acute poisonings admitted to general hospitals and that they are responsible for 6 percent of suicides and 18 percent of accidental deaths, figures exceeded by no other single poison. Despite an estimated mortality rate of only 8 percent of hospitalized cases, barbiturates reportedly cause about 1,500 deaths annually in the United States. This figure is probably a gross underestimation, since in 1964 there were over 2,200 registered deaths in Great Britain due to barbiturate poisoning.

About fifty barbiturates have been marketed for clinical use, but only the following are encountered with any frequency: barbital (Veronal), phenobarbital (Luminal), diallylbarbituric acid (Dial), amobarbital (Amytal), aprobarbital (Alurate), pentobarbital (Nembutal), secobarbital (Seconal), and thiopental (Pentothal). In the United States, pentobarbital, secobarbital, and amobarbital are the most commonly abused barbiturates. These drugs are similar pharmacologically and differ only in their speed of onset and duration of action.

In addition to the barbiturates, a number of nonbarbiturate sedative and hypnotic drugs have to be considered, since they have been shown to possess very much the same intoxicating and addicting properties as the barbiturates.

The clinical problems posed by the barbiturates differ considerably, however, depending on whether the intoxication is acute or chronic, and these two types will be treated separately.

ACUTE BARBITURATE INTOXICATION

Acute barbiturate intoxication results from the ingestion of large amounts of the drug either accidentally or with suicidal intent, the incidence of the two types being about equal. An uncommon form of accidental poisoning occurs in individuals who are intoxicated with barbiturates or with alcohol and who, being confused, ingest more of the drug. This type of poisoning has been termed *involuntary suicide* or *automatism*.

The ingestion of barbiturates with suicidal intent is most frequently the act of a depressed person. An individual with hysteria or psychopathic personality may take an overdose as a suicidal gesture and sometimes become seriously intoxicated because of a miscalculation or ignorance of the toxic dosage. At times, no psychiatric disease is present, the drug being taken impulsively or while the patient is inebriated. The combination of alcohol and barbiturate intoxication is frequent and particularly dangerous, since these drugs have an additive effect.

SITE AND MODE OF ACTION OF BARBITURATES. Barbiturates decrease the excitability of nerve cells, although the mechanism is not fully understood. Attempts have been made to localize the action of barbiturates to certain anatomic regions, or even to specific nuclei within the nervous system, but it would appear that all parts are to some extent sensitive to the drug. Nevertheless, the reticular formation of the thalami and midbrain are particularly susceptible. There is little experimental evidence to support the clinical impression that with the administration of barbiturates the cerebral cortex is affected first and that lower centers are then successively affected. Reflex and other activity of the nervous system are probably depressed at all levels simultaneously and progressively, although in the early stages of poisoning, spinal reflexes may be accentuated.

SYMPTOMS AND SIGNS. The symptoms and signs of acute barbiturate intoxication vary with the type and the amount of drug, as well as with the length of time that has elapsed since it was ingested. Pentobarbital and secobarbital produce their effects quickly, and recovery is relatively rapid. Phenobarbital induces coma more slowly, and its effects tend to be prolonged. The duration of action of these drugs can be judged from the hypnotic effect of an average oral dose. In the case of the long-acting barbiturates, such as phenobarbital, barbital, and diallylbarbituric acid, it lasts 6 hr or more; with the intermediate-acting drugs, amobarbital and aprobarbital, 3 to 6 hr; with the short-acting drugs, secobarbital and pentobarbital, less than 3 hr.

In general, much larger doses of long-acting barbiturates are required to produce a depth of unconsciousness comparable to that produced by the short-acting ones. The ingestion by adults of more than 3.0 Gm secobarbital, pentobarbital, amobarbital, or diallybarbituric acid at one time may be fatal unless intensive and skillful treatment is applied promptly; in series of cases, it has been estimated, the usual intake of drug is 6.0 to 9.0 Gm phenobarbital, 5.0 to 20.0 Gm barbital, and 15.0 Gm aprobarbital. Because of the serious complications of prolonged coma, the fatalities are greater with the long-acting than with the short-acting drugs.

Clinically, it is useful to recognize three grades of severity of acute barbiturate intoxication, particularly in regard to prognosis and treatment. Mild intoxication follows the ingestion of approximately 0.6 Gm pentobarbital or its equivalent. The patient is drowsy or asleep, a state from which he is readily roused by calling his name loudly or by shaking him. The symptoms resemble those of alcoholic inebriation, except that the face is not flushed, the conjunctivas are not suffused, and there is no odor of alcohol. The patient thinks slowly, and there may be mild disorientation, lability of mood, impairment of judgment, slurred speech, drunken gait, and nystagmus. Reflex activity and vital signs are not affected.

Moderate intoxication follows the ingestion of five to ten times the oral hypnotic dose. Here the state of consciousness is more severely depressed and is usually accompanied by depressed or absent deep reflexes and slow but not shallow respiration. Corneal reflexes are retained, with occasional exceptions. At times the patient can be roused by vigorous manual stimulation; when awakened, he is confused and dysarthric, and after a few moments he drifts back into coma. At other times the patient cannot be roused by this means. In the latter cases the depth of coma and seriousness of the respiratory depression may be roughly judged by the response of respiration to painful stimulation such as the application of firm pressure to the sternum or supraorbital ridge, or to the inhalation of 10% carbon dioxide. If these stimuli cause an increase in the depth and rate of respiration, the outlook for recovery is good, and only symptomatic treatment is indicated.

Severe intoxication occurs with the ingestion of fifteen to twenty times the oral hypnotic dose. The patient cannot be roused by any of the means indicated. Respiration is slow and shallow or irregular, and pulmonary edema and cyanosis may be present. The deep tendon reflexes are usually but not invariably absent. Most often, the patients show no response to plantar stimulation, but in those who do, the plantar responses are extensor. In the most advanced cases the corneal and gag reflexes may also be abolished. Ordinarily the pupillary light reflex is retained in severe intoxication and is lost only if the patient is asphyxiated. In the early hours of coma, there may be a phase of rigidity of the limbs, hyperactive reflexes, ankle clonus, extensor plantar signs, and decerebrate posturing; persistence of these signs indicates a severe degree of anoxia. The temperature may be subnormal, the pulse thready and rapid, and the blood pressure at shock levels.

DIAGNOSIS. The diagnosis of barbiturate intoxication is made from the history and physical findings. If a reasonable suspicion of the diagnosis exists, then a careful search for drugs or their containers may be rewarding. One should also examine the mouth and gastric contents for any characteristically colored capsules. Acute barbiturate intoxication which presents as a state of coma must be distinguished from other forms of coma by the method outlined in Chap. 26, Coma and Related Disturbances of Consciousness. Actually there are few conditions other than barbiturate intoxication which cause a flaccid coma with reactive pupils, hypothermia, and hypotension. Glutethimide poisoning may produce an identical clinical picture, excepting that the pupils are fixed (a parasympathomimetic action). In the differential diagnosis, hysteria presents the main problem.

Reliable methods are now available for the *estimation of amount of barbiturates in the blood*. The ultraviolet spectrophotometric method of Goldbaum is most widely used. The major virtue of this test is in identifying the cause of coma, when this is in question. The blood level also helps to identify the drug as long- or short-acting, thus giving information as to whether the therapeutic problem will be short or prolonged. A blood barbiturate level of 2 mg per 100 ml in a *comatose* patient is usually due to poisoning with secobarbital or pentobarbital; although the immediate mortality is high in such instances, the therapeutic problem will be short. A level of 11.5 to 12.0 mg per 100 ml is usually due to poisoning with barbital or phenobarbital, and the comatose state will be prolonged. Because of the potentiating effects of alcohol, a patient who has ingested both drugs may be comatose with relatively low blood barbiturate levels. For this reason, and also because of differences in individual tolerance, the correlation between blood barbiturate levels and depth of coma is not entirely dependable.

The *electroencephalogram* may also be useful in diagnosis, since characteristic patterns accompany barbiturate intoxication. In mild intoxication, the normal activity is replaced by fast activity, in the range of 20 to 30 per sec, most prominent in the frontal regions. In more severe intoxication, the fast waves become less regular and interspersed with 3- to 4-per-sec slow activity. In the most advanced cases, there are short periods of suppression of all activity, separated by bursts of slow (delta) waves of variable frequency.

MANAGEMENT. The management of acute barbiturate intoxication depends on its severity. In mild or moderate intoxication, recovery is the rule and no vigorous treatment is required. The mildly intoxicated patient should be watched closely for signs of deepening coma, and analeptics such as coffee or parenteral caffeine sodium benzoate may be used. If the patient is unresponsive, special attention should be given to maintaining respiration and urinary excretion and to the prevention of infection. It is most important to maintain a patent airway, at first usually by the insertion of an endotracheal tube; suctioning should be used when necessary, and the patient should be turned frequently. Tracheotomy and bronchoscopic suctioning should be resorted to if atelectasis becomes manifest, or if intubation must be maintained for longer than 48 hr. If there is any risk of respiratory depression or underventilation, it is advisable to treat the patient with a positive pressure ventilator, so as to provide adequate oxygenation and minimize the risk of atelectasis.

Cases of severe respiratory depression, with cyanosis and pupillary dilatation, represent a serious medical emergency. A clear airway should be secured immediately and artificial respiration begun, preferably utilizing an automatic intermittent positive-pressure respirator. If the patient is in shock, the foot of the bed should be elevated, and norepinephrine and whole blood or plasma administered. Catheterization is required to determine the adequacy of urinary output, to obtain samples for laboratory examination, and to prevent distension of the bladder. Since the amount of barbiturate cleared by the kidney is directly proportional to the amount of urine formed, 8 to 10 liters of 5% glucose in saline solution should be given daily. Forced diuresis is also important because toxic amounts of barbiturate have an antidiuretic effect. Coma of any significant duration requires the administration of other electrolytes as well, the amounts being governed by their serum and urinary values. The occurrence of pulmonary and urinary infections calls for the use of appropriate antibiotic treatment.

If ingestion has been recent, gastric lavage may be a therapeutic as well as a diagnostic measure. It must be performed within several hours of ingestion of the drug, since barbiturates are absorbed rapidly and completely. Laryngospasm may complicate this procedure but can be avoided by preliminary endotracheal intubation; the stomach must be entirely emptied to prevent aspiration.

Dialysis of the blood by means of the artificial kidney has proved to be an effective form of therapy. This measure should be reserved for cases of profound intoxication due to long-acting barbiturates, in which a trial of symptomatic measures has failed, and in which uremia or anuria develops.

The treatment of severe barbiturate intoxication with analeptic drugs (metrazol, picritosin, Megimide), which enjoyed a brief period of popularity, has been generally abandoned. These drugs are antagonistic to barbiturates only insofar as they are powerful cortical stimulants as well as overall nervous system excitants; they do not affect the rate of metabolism or excretion of barbiturate. Their effectiveness could never be substantiated, since there was no precise way of quantitating the depth of central nervous system depression in any particular patient, and hence no way of predicting whether or not recovery would have occurred without analeptic therapy. Because of this uncertainty, as well as the danger of convulsions with the use of these stimulants, clinicians now agree that therapy should consist of constant attention to and support of respiration, circulation, and excretion, and the prevention of infection. The mortality has been greatly reduced by the use of such methods alone. The use of nonconvulsive electrical stimulation also has no proven value in the severely intoxicated patient. Recent reports have stressed the value of alkalinization of the blood, by the use of large amounts of bicarbonate solution, as a means of mobilizing the barbiturate and increasing its rate of excretion. This method of therapy does seem to be useful, particularly where phenobarbital is the responsible agent.

Occasionally, in the case of a barbiturate addict who has taken an overdose of the drug, recovery from coma is followed by the development of an abstinence syndrome, which has to be managed by the methods outlined below.

CHRONIC BARBITURATE INTOXICATION (Barbiturate Addiction)

The problem of chronic barbiturate intoxication is quite different from that of acute intoxication, for it embraces the phenomena of tolerance and addiction as well as the effects of ultimate withdrawal of the drugs. In these respects there is a remarkable similarity to the problem of chronic alcoholism. This concept of chronic barbiturate intoxication has gained credence only in recent years, mainly through the work of Isbell and his associates at the Addiction Research Center in Lexington, Ky. The following remarks are based largely on their studies.

Chronic barbiturate intoxication, like other addictions, usually develops on a background of some psychiatric disorder, most commonly psychoneurosis with symptoms of anxiety and insomnia, or a so-called "character disorder." The patients with symptoms of anxiety and insomnia are originally given the drug by their physicians; and as the desired sleep-producing effect of the barbiturate is lost, the dose is slowly increased until the patient is taking an amount sufficient to produce symptoms when it is withdrawn. Individuals with character disorders are usually introduced to the drug by associates; since the drug is taken for its intoxicating effect, the dose tends to be increased rapidly. Addiction to alcohol or to opiates may predispose to barbiturate addiction. Alcoholics find that barbiturates effectively relieve their nervousness and tremor and then may continue to take both alcohol and barbiturates, or the barbiturate may replace the alcohol. Morphine addicts may turn to barbiturates when they are unable to obtain opiates. As with other addicting drugs, the incidence of barbiturism is particularly high in individuals with ready access to drugs, such as physicians, pharmacists, and nurses.

The symptoms and signs of chronic barbiturate intoxication may be described in relation to (1) the toxic effects of the drug, (2) the development of tolerance, and (3) the effects of sudden withdrawal of the drug after a period of prolonged intoxication.

The toxic symptoms of chronic barbiturism are much the same as those of mild acute intoxication or of alcoholic inebriation. The barbiturate addict thinks slowly, shows an increased emotional lability, and becomes untidy in his dress and personal habits. The neurologic signs are quite characteristic and include dysarthria, nystagmus, and cerebellar incoordination. Both the mental and neurologic signs fluctuate greatly in the same individual, being more severe if the drug is taken in the fasting state and tending to increase during the day as more of the drug is ingested. If the dosage is elevated rapidly, the signs of moderate or severe intoxication become manifest.

A characteristic feature of chronic barbiturate intoxication is the development of tolerance, sometimes striking in degree. The average addict will ingest about 1.5 Gm daily of a potent barbiturate and will not develop signs of severe intoxication unless this amount is exceeded. Individual variations in the degree of tolerance make it difficult to state precisely the minimal amount of drug which must be ingested before the resulting condition is designated as chronic barbiturate intoxication. Most persons can ingest 0.4 Gm daily for years without developing major withdrawal signs (seizures or delirium), although epileptic patients accustomed to this dosage may develop continuous seizures when the drug is withdrawn. With a dosage of 0.8 Gm daily, the efficiency at all tasks is greatly reduced, and after a period of 2 months on this dosage, abrupt withdrawal will result in serious symptoms in the majority of patients. Even after 2 weeks of this dosage some patients will show mild withdrawal symptoms and paroxysmal electroencephalogram changes with photic stimulation. Individuals taking 0.4 to 0.7 Gm daily fall into an intermediate category; practically all show some mental dulling, and occasionally severe withdrawal symptoms may occur.

THE ABSTINENCE OR WITHDRAWAL SYNDROME. Following the withdrawal of barbiturates from addicted individuals, characteristic symptoms occur. Immediately following withdrawal the patient seemingly improves, as he loses the symptoms of intoxication over 8 to 12 hr. After this short period a new group of symptoms appears, consisting of nervousness, tremor, and weakness. Generalized seizures, with loss of consciousness, may then occur, usually between the second and fourth days of abstinence, occasionally as long as 6 or 7 days after withdrawal. There may be a single seizure, or several, or rarely status epilepticus. A varying degree of improvement follows the convulsive phase, to be followed by a delusional-hallucinatory state or a full-blown delirium,

indistinguishable from delirium tremens. Death has been reported under these circumstances. The abstinence syndrome may occur in varying degrees of completeness; some patients have seizures and recover without developing delirium and others have a delirium without preceding seizures. The abrupt onset of seizures or an acute psychosis in adult life should always raise the suspicion of addiction to barbiturates or other sedative-hypnotic drugs.

The *electroencephalogram* shows a number of changes in chronic barbiturate intoxication and following withdrawal. During chronic intoxication, the predominant pattern is that of fast activity of moderate voltage, interspersed with short bursts of high-voltage 6- to 8-per-sec rhythms, chiefly in the frontal and parietal regions. The electroencephalogram does not correlate closely with the degree of intoxication, nor does it reflect the development of tolerance. On withdrawal of barbiturates the fast activity diminishes. Also in the first few days of abstinence, paroxysmal bursts of mixed spike and slow waves or 4-per-sec spike and dome paroxysmal discharges occur, and these may or may not be associated with seizures. These changes disappear after 4 or 5 days, the record returning to a normal pattern. The most characteristic electroencephalogram findings which follow the withdrawal of barbiturates, according to Wulff, are paroxysmal changes evoked by photic stimulation.

INTOXICATING AND ADDICTING EFFECTS OF OTHER SEDATIVE-HYPNOTIC DRUGS. In recent years a large number of nonbarbiturate sedative-hypnotic drugs have been introduced into medical practice. At least seven of them have the same intoxicating and addicting effects as barbiturates. These drugs are meprobamate (Miltown, Equanil), glutethimide (Doriden), ethinamate (Valmid), ethchlorvynol (Placidyl), methyprylon (Noludar), chlordiazepoxide (Librium), and diazepam (Valium). Like the barbiturates, each of these drugs can cause slurred speech, nystagmus, ataxic gait, drowsiness, confusion, and coma. Furthermore, if the daily dose exceeds a minimal safe range, a state of physical dependence develops, so that withdrawal of excessive dosages can result in abstinence symptoms. These include hallucinations, seizures, and delirium, and closely resemble those observed with barbiturates and alcohol. The seriousness of the abstinence syndrome in these cases is emphasized by reports of death following withdrawal of meprobamate and methyprylon. In view of these observations, physicians might well be skeptical of the new sedative drugs which are continually being introduced and which are said to possess no addicting or habit-forming properties. Treatment of the symptoms which result from withdrawal of the nonbarbiturate sedative drugs requires barbiturate substitution, followed by its gradual withdrawal at a rate not to exceed 0.1 Gm daily. It should be noted that diphenylhydantoin (Dilantin) and phenothiazine derivatives are not effective against the abstinence convulsions.

TREATMENT OF CHRONIC BARBITURATE INTOXICATION. This should always be carried out in the hospital. If the diagnosis of addiction is made before signs of abstinence have appeared, the first step in treatment should be the determination of the "stabilization dosage." This is the amount of short-acting barbiturate required to produce mild symptoms of intoxication (nystagmus, slight ataxia, and dysarthria). Usually 0.2 Gm pentobarbital given orally every 6 hr is sufficient for this purpose. The patient is examined 1 hr after each dose. If the signs of intoxication are severe, the next scheduled dose is reduced or omitted. If, instead, tremulousness and postural tachycardia appear, an additional 0.1 Gm of pentobarbital is given and the next scheduled dose is increased. This method is preferable to a blind reduction of dosage, since patients frequently underestimate the amount of drug taken. In such patients, establishment of the "stabilization dosage" may have diagnostic as well as therapeutic value. A patient who can take 0.8 Gm or more of pentobarbital daily, without developing signs of intoxication, is probably physically dependent on drugs of this type. Then a gradual withdrawal of the drug is undertaken, 0.1 Gm daily, the reduction being stopped for several days if abstinence symptoms appear. In this way a severely addicted person can be withdrawn in 14 to 21 days. Patients undergoing withdrawal treatment require careful observation for symptoms of abstinence, and special precautions have to be taken to prevent the smuggling or concealment of drugs.

If the patient comes to the physician with severe symptoms of abstinence, such as seizures, he should be given 0.3 to 0.5 Gm sodium Luminal intramuscularly and then enough to maintain mild intoxication. Most anticonvulsant medicines have been shown, both in animals and in man, to be ineffective against barbiturate withdrawal convulsions. Withdrawal should then be carried out as indicated above. If the abstinence symptoms are not severe, it is not necessary to reintoxicate the patient, but treatment can proceed along the lines laid down for the delirious and confused patient (Chap. 30).

The same principles of treatment apply to patients who are addicted to nonbarbiturate hypnotic-sedative drugs. Thus, if the drug and its dosage can be determined, it should be withdrawn at the rate of one therapeutic dose per day. Should abstinence symptoms appear, the reduction in dosage is stopped for several days. If the offending drug cannot be identified, a barbiturate such as Seconal can be administered to the point of mild intoxication and then withdrawn, in the manner indicated above.

After recovery has taken place, whether from the symptoms of chronic intoxication or of abstinence or from acute intoxication due to attempted suicide, the psychiatric problem requires evaluation and an appropriate plan of therapy. Many of the considerations in the management of alcoholism are equally applicable to the patient addicted to barbiturate or nonbarbiturate hypnotic drugs (Chap. 118, Alcohol).

BARBITURATE PROVOCATION OF OTHER DISEASES. At times the administration of one of the barbiturates may induce an attack of another disease. The most striking example of this is hereditary porphyria where a severe and sometimes fatal outbreak of abdominal pain, psy-

chosis, and polyneuropathy may follow the ingestion of a few capsules of Seconal (see Chap. 101). With severe liver disease detoxification of barbiturates may be impaired, as will be discussed in Chap. 323.

REFERENCES

Clemmesen, C., and E. Nilsson: Therapeutic Trends in the Treatment of Barbiturate Poisoning: The Scandinavian Method, Clin. Pharmacol. Therap., 2:220, 1961.

Essig, C.: Sedative Drugs that Can Cause States of Intoxication and Dependence of Barbiturate Type, J.A.M.A., 196:714–717, 1966.

Fraser, H. F., A. Wikler, C. F. Essig, and H. Isbell: Degree of Physical Dependence Induced by Decobarbital or Pentobarbital, J.A.M.A. 166:127–129, 1958.

Plum, F., and A. C. Swanson: Barbiturate Poisoning Treated by Physiological Methods, J.A.M.A., 163:827, 1957.

Wulff, M. H.: "The Barbiturate Withdrawal Syndrome," Copenhagen, Ejnar Munksgaard, 1959; Suppl. No. 14, Electroencephalography Clinical Neurophysiology, 1959.

121   DEPRESSANTS, STIMULANTS, AND PSYCHOTOGENIC DRUGS

Maurice Victor and Raymond D. Adams

DEPRESSANT DRUGS

These drugs may be divided into two main classes, according to the pattern of the sedative and hypnotic responses when the dose of drug is progressively increased. One class, which may be designated *general depressants,* is exemplified by the barbiturates; these drugs cause a more or less progressive depression of central nervous system excitability in response to increasing dosage, until death ensues. A second class of *special depressants,* generally referred to as tranquilizers, is exemplified by chlorpromazine, chlordiazepoxide, and meprobamate. These drugs also reduce hyperexcitability of the nervous system, but the sedative-hypnotic effects fail to keep pace with the increase in dosage, and excitability may remain at relatively normal levels over a wide range of dosages. Thus, the special depressants have the capacity to suppress symptoms of anxiety, irritability, and so forth, leaving the patient alert enough to work and function in an acceptable manner. An added advantage of these drugs is that large single doses, ingested with suicidal intent, may cause no serious depression of nervous system function.

General Depressants

The most important members of this group, the barbiturates, have been fully discussed in the preceding chapter. Other general depressants of clinical importance are the bromides, paraldehyde, and chloral hydrate.

Bromides are seldom prescribed by physicians at the present time, but are contained in many "nerve tonics" and proprietary headache remedies (such as Bromo-Seltzer), so that cases of bromide intoxication are encountered with some regularity. Acute poisoning with bromide is rare because large doses of the drug are irritating to the gastric mucosa and vomiting prevents the attainment of significant blood levels. Taken in smaller doses, however, bromide tends to accumulate in the body because of its slow excretion by the kidney, and toxic symptoms may appear in a matter of weeks. These symptoms are caused by the bromide ion itself and do not simply reflect a decrease in chloride, caused by displacement of the chloride by the bromide ion.

The symptoms of chronic bromide intoxication are predominantly in the mental sphere and range from dizziness, drowsiness, irritability, and emotional lability to a quiet confusional state, with impairment of thinking and memory, and in severe cases, to delirium and mania or to stupor and coma. Skin manifestations are associated in many cases, taking the form usually of an acnelike eruption and less frequently of proliferative nodular lesions, resembling those of tertiary syphilis. Headache, mild conjunctivitis, gastric distress, anorexia, and constipation may be associated as well. The blood bromide levels and the severity of toxic symptoms do not necessarily correspond. As a general rule, levels of 75 mg per 100 ml (9 mEq per liter) or more are considered abnormal and diagnostic of bromism, if the clinical picture suggests it. However, higher levels are sometimes well tolerated, and symptoms of bromism may persist even after the blood levels have been reduced to normal or near normal levels.

Treatment consists of removing the source of the bromide and administration of sodium chloride (at least 6 Gm daily, in divided doses). Ammonium chloride may be substituted if an accumulation of sodium is to be avoided and if there is no danger of an uncompensated acidosis. Confused or delirious patients require sedation, paraldehyde being the drug of choice, and the anorectic and emaciated patients need careful nursing care and special attention to diet. The administration of a mercurial or thiazide diuretic serves to promote a bromide diuresis. Hemodialysis is an effective means of removing bromide and should be utilized in the most severe cases of intoxication.

Chloral Hydrate is the oldest and at the same time one of the safest, most effective, and cheapest of the sedative-hypnotic drugs. After oral administration, chloral is reduced rapidly to trichloroethanol, which is the agent responsible for the depressant effects on the central nervous system. A significant portion of the trichloroethanol is excreted in the urine as the glucuronide, which may give a false positive test for glucose.

In large doses chloral is toxic to the heart, kidneys, and liver, but only in the presence of preexisting disease in these organs. Chloral is a strong gastric irritant, so that it should be diluted sufficiently and not taken on an empty stomach. Tolerance and addiction to chloral develop only rarely, and for these reasons it is an appropriate medication for the management of insomnia, particularly the type which is associated with the alcohol

withdrawal syndrome and depression. Poisoning with chloral is a rare occurrence and resembles acute barbiturate intoxication, except for the finding of miosis, which is said to characterize the former. Death from poisoning is due to respiratory depression and hypotension, and patients who survive these events may show signs of liver and kidney disease.

Paraldehyde is also an effective and safe hypnotic, providing that certain precautions are taken in its preparation and administration. On exposure to light paraldehyde decomposes to acetaldehyde, which is very toxic, and oxidizes to acetic acid. It must be freshly prepared, therefore, and stored in tightly stoppered, amber-colored bottles. Paraldehyde is unique in that a significant proportion is excreted unchanged through the lungs; the remainder is detoxified in the liver, so that it should be used cautiously in patients with liver disease.

Paraldehyde has a wide margin of safety when administered orally (or rectally) and even three or four times the usual dose (8 to 10 ml) causes no more than prolonged sleep or mild stupor. Intramuscular and intravenous use of the drug should be avoided because of its propensity to produce sterile abscesses and to damage the sciatic nerve and because of its unpredictable effects on respiration. The main objections to this drug are its bitter taste (this can be obviated by diluting in fruit juice) and its lingering, unpleasant odor.

Paraldehyde has its greatest value in the treatment of the alcoholic patient, following a period of prolonged intoxication. It is very effective in suppressing the tremulousness, restlessness, and insomnia that characterize the early phases (6 to 72 hr) of the withdrawal period. It remains to be proved, however, that the administration of paraldehyde (or any other depressant drug) can prevent delirium tremens or reduce the duration of or the mortality from this disorder.

The use of paraldehyde in the alcoholic patient allegedly carries the risk of replacing an addiction to alcohol with one to paraldehyde. Patients with symptoms of alcohol withdrawal do make repeated demands for the drug, which is not surprising, in view of the pharmacologic similarities between paraldehyde and alcohol and the effectiveness of both drugs in suppressing withdrawal symptoms. This does not present a problem in management, however, if the need for the drug is determined before each dose is given and the drug is withdrawn as soon as the agitation and tremor are under control. Should a relapse from abstinence then occur, some patients are said to substitute paraldehyde for alcohol, but such an occurrence must be extremely rare.

Special Depressants

Since the mid-1950s, a large new series of pharmacologic agents, generally referred to as tranquilizers, has come into prominent use, mainly for the control of nervousness, agitation, apprehension, anxiety, and depression. Their application in medical practice, which has been on an enormous scale, is fraught with difficulty. Since the symptoms for which they are prescribed are manifestations of many conditions, some of them being normal reactions to trying environmental circumstances and others being symptoms of a disease state such as anxiety neurosis or depression, the physician should be certain of the diagnosis before using them. These drugs are not curative, but only suppress or partially alleviate the symptoms, and they should not serve as a substitute for or divert the physician from the use of other measures for the relief of the abnormal mental state. They are so toxic and expensive that they should not be used indefinitely.

At the time of writing this chapter, more than 50 of these tranquilizing agents are on the market. No attempt will be made here to describe or even list all of them. Some have had only an evanescent popularity and others have yet to prove their value. Chemically these compounds form a heterogeneous group, four categories of which are of particular clinical importance: (1) the ethylamine group of drugs (including the phenothiazines), (2) the rauwolfia alkaloids, (3) the bensodiazepine compounds, and (4) the carbonic acid or urea derivatives.

The *phenothiazines* comprise some of the most widely used tranquilizers, such as chlorpromazine (Thorazine), prochlorperazine (Compazine), perphenazine (Trifalon), fluphenazine (Permatil), and thioridazine (Mellaril). In addition to sedative effects, this group of drugs has a number of other actions, so that congeners of these compounds are used as conduction anesthetics (procaine), cardiodepressants (procaine amide), antiemetics (prochlorperazine), and antihistaminics (promethazine).

The phenothiazines have had their widest application in the treatment of the psychoses. Under the influence of these drugs, many patients who would otherwise be hospitalized are able to live at home and even work productively and the hospital care of hyperactive and combative patients has been greatly facilitated.

Side effects of the phenothiazines are frequent and often serious. All of them may cause a cholestatic type of jaundice, agranulocytosis, convulsive seizures, orthostatic hypotension, skin sensitivity reactions, mental depression, and disorders of the extrapyramidal motor system. Jaundice and blood dyscrasias have occurred less often with prochlorperazine, perphenazine, and fluphenazine than with other members of the group, but the extrapyramidal side effects have been relatively more pronounced. Several types of extrapyramidal symptoms have been noted: (1) A parkinsonian syndrome—masklike facies, tremor, generalized rigidity, shuffling gait, and slowness of movement. These symptoms usually appear after several weeks of drug therapy. (2) Muscle spasms and dystonia, taking the form of involuntary protrusion of the tongue, dysphagia, torticollis and retrocollis, oculogyric crises, and tonic spasms of a limb; these complications usually occur early in the administration of the drug, sometimes after the initial dose, and often can be improved dramatically by the intravenous administration of diphenhydramine hydrochloride (Benadryl). (3) An inability to sit still and an inner restlessness or turmoil, so that the patient paces the floor constantly

(*akathisia*); involuntary movements of a choreathetotic type may be added.

These reactions must be recognized at once and the medication discontinued, but even then the extrapyramidal disorder may persist for weeks or months, *and exceptionally, even for years.* Administration of antiparkinsonian drugs (trihexyphenidyl, procyclidine, benztropine) hastens recovery. Chlorprothixene (Taractin), a thioxanthene drug with effects similar to the phenothiazines, and thioridazine (Mellaril), although not the best tranquilizing agents, are favored by some because of their lesser tendency to produce symptoms of extrapyramidal motor disorder. The latter drug, however, if given in large doses over a period of time, may cause retinal deposits with resulting visual impairment.

Reserpine is the prototype of the rauwolfia alkaloids; these drugs, so effective in controlling hypertension, are no longer to be recommended as tranquilizing agents. When given in doses adequate to attain this effect, they often provoke a parkinsonian syndrome or a serious depression of mood, which may prove more troublesome than the anxiety for which they were prescribed.

Two agents of the *benzodiazepine* group, chlordiazepoxide (Librium) and diazepam (Valium), have been used extensively to control anxiety, overactivity, destructive behaviour in children, and the symptoms of alcohol withdrawal. These drugs possess anticonvulsant properties, and the intravenous use of diazepam is a very effective means of controlling status epilepticus. In addition, diazepam has been used with moderate success in the treatment of extrapyramidal movement disorders and dystonic spasms. The benzodiazepine drugs, while comparatively safe in the recommended dosages, frequently cause unsteadiness of gait and drowsiness and at times hypotension and syncope, particularly in the elderly. In severely disturbed schizophrenic patients, rage, hostility, uncontrollable excitement, confusion, and depersonalization may develop. Nausea, diminished libido, headache, skin rashes, leukopenia, eosinophilia, agranulocytosis, and enhancement of the effects of alcohol have all been reported but are rare. Additional central nervous disorders are slurred speech, dysphagia, ataxia, confusion, and faulty memory.

The *carbonic acid or urea derivatives* are capable of modest depressant action and are appropriate for relieving mild degrees of nervousness, anxiety, and muscle tension. Maximal action occurs with reatively small doses of these drugs. Ataxia, drowsiness, autonomic and extrapyramidal effects are singularly absent with therapeutic doses. *Meprobamate* (Equanil, Miltown) is the best known but a somewhat anomalous member of this group; in its pharmacologic actions it resembles the barbiturates much more than the other special depressants. With average doses (400 mg, three or four times a day) the patient is able to function quite effectively; large doses cause drowsiness, stupor, coma, and vasomotor collapse. Hypersensitivity reactions in the form of fever, pruritis, and erythematous, maculopapular and occasionally urticarial or bullous eruptions have been reported. Cutaneous petechiae or ecchymoses may also occur without thrombocytopenia. Diplopia, syncope, menstrual irregularities, angioneurotic edema, peripheral edema, leucopenia, thrombocytopenia, and pancytopenia are other rare complications.

It is important to note that addiction to meprobamate does occur and if four or more times the daily recommended dose is administered over a period of weeks to months, withdrawal symptoms (including convulsions) may appear, resembling those which follow withdrawal of barbiturate in a chronically intoxicated patient. Several other special depressant drugs, described in the preceding chapter, have the same liability.

It hardly need be pointed out that the tranquilizing drugs have been much abused. This would be suspected just from the frequency with which they are being prescribed (it is stated that in the past decade 50 million patients have received chlorpromazine alone). Often these toxic and expensive agents are prescribed when safer and less expensive drugs, such as phenobarbital, in small sedating doses would accomplish the same purpose.

STIMULANTS

Drugs that act primarily as stimulants of the central nervous system can be divided into two general groups, based on differences in their pharmacologic actions and clinical use. (1) The first group is exemplified by analeptics such as picritoxin, which produce a prompt and short-lived effect on the nervous system and a grossly recognizable increase in motor and electrical activity, often taking the form of convulsive seizures. The effects of these drugs can be readily reproduced in animals and have been of great interest to pharmacologists and physiologists but of little clinical value. (2) The monoamine oxidase inhibitors and dibenzazepine compounds, which comprise the second group of stimulant drugs, have considerable clinical usefulness, mainly in elevating mood and ameliorating the symptoms and signs of mental depression. The effects of these drugs on the nervous system, in contrast to the more direct acting stimulants, are slow to appear, persist for long periods after their administration has been stopped, and cannot be assessed in animals.

Such a division, though clinically useful, is far from absolute. Certain of the direct acting stimulants, e.g., amphetamine, may have a beneficial effect on mental depression. Also, certain drugs that are useful in the treatment of depression (e.g., amobarbital) are not central nervous system stimulants, but depressants. In the latter case, a depressant acts as an antidepressant. These commonly used terms must not be confused—the former referring to a drug that reduces nervous system excitability and the latter to the capacity of the drug to ameliorate the symptoms of mental depression.

Direct-acting Stimulants

Amphetamine (benzedrine) and its *d*-isomer, *dextroamphetamine,* are powerful analeptics and in addition have significant hypertensive, respiratory stimulant, and appetite depressant effects. These drugs are useful in the management of narcolepsy, but they are much more widely and indiscriminately used for the control of obesity and the abolition of fatigue. Undoubtedly they are able to reverse fatigue, postpone the need for sleep, and elevate mood, but these effects are not entirely predictable and certainly not indefinite, and the user must pay for the period of wakefulness with even greater fatigue and often with depression. Because of the popularity of the amphetamines and ease with which they can be procured, instances of acute and chronic intoxication are observed frequently. The toxic signs are essentially an exaggeration of the analeptic effects—restlessness, speech and motor overactivity, tremor, and insomnia. In severe cases, a schizophrenia-like picture may occur, with hallucinations, delusions, and changes in affect and thought processes. Treatment consists of removal of the offending drug and the administration of barbiturates. Nitrites may be useful if the blood pressure is markedly elevated.

Picritoxin is a powerful nervous system excitant, the main effects of which are to produce convulsive seizures and to reverse respiratory depression induced by drugs, particularly by barbiturates. However, the modern treatment of barbiturate intoxication does not include the use of picritoxin or other analeptics, because of their epileptogenic properties and because barbiturate intoxication can be managed successfully by other means (see Chap. 120).

It has been shown by Eccles and his colleagues that picritoxin increases neuronal activity by blocking presynaptic inhibition, i.e., blocking the action of inhibitory fibres that synapse with the presynaptic terminals of excitatory fibres. *Strychnine,* on the other hand, increases neuronal excitability by interfering with postsynaptic inhibition. The therapeutic value of strychnine is negligible, but in children accidental poisoning may occur from ingestion of "A.S. & B." cathartic pills or "rat biscuits." Very rarely, strychnine is taken with suicidal intent. After a period of heightened irritability and muscle twitching, tonic seizures occur, characterized by opisthotonus, rigid extension of the legs, facial tetanus, and apnea due to spasm of the muscles of respiration. Death from anoxia may follow several seizures.

The immediate need, in the treatment of strychnine poisoning, is to control the convulsions. This calls for the intravenous administration of a short-acting barbiturate or the application of inhalation anesthesia if the appropriate drug is not immediately available; endotracheal intubation is an important safeguard. The patient must then be observed carefully, and if any signs of irritability recur, more sedative should be given. During this period, supportive care is indicated, as for any comatose patient. Morphine, which is a medullary depressant but a spinal cord stimulant, is contraindicated.

Pentylenetetrazol (metrazal, cardiazol) is a potent stimulant of all parts of the nervous system. For a number of years it served as the convulsive agent in the "shock treatment" of depression and schizophrenia but was abandoned in favor of less dangerous and more effective forms of convulsive therapy. The use of this drug to activate latent epileptogenic foci or to reproduce convulsions, with the purpose of studying the underlying cerebral mechanisms, is restricted to a few clinical centres.

The actions of *bemegride* and *nikethamide* (Coramine) are much like those of pentylenetetrazol. For many years it was common clinical practice to administer nikethamide as a final therapeutic gesture in patients dying of cardiac and respiratory failure, but there is little evidence that this drug has a significant stimulant effect on either heart or respiration. Poisoning with these drugs, which is usually due to parenteral overdosage, is best treated with barbiturates.

Caffeine and other xanthine derivatives do have therapeutic value, by virtue of their diuretic effects and their ability to stimulate the heart and nervous system. The major use of these agents is to abolish fatigue and maintain wakefulness, and the usual mode of administration is in coffee, a cup of which contains 100 to 150 mg caffeine. Overdosage leads to insomnia, mild delirium, tinnitus, tachycardia, prominent diuresis, and cardiac arrhythmias. The excitatory effects are easily controlled with barbiturates, and fatalities due to caffeine poisoning are extremely rare.

Camphor (camphorated oil) was formerly a popular stimulant, but is now rarely used therapeutically; however, occasional cases of poisoning are still seen as a result of ingestion of liniment or moth flakes. The manifestations of poisoning are headache, sensation of warmth, confusion, clonic convulsions, and terminal respiratory depression; the characteristic odor of camphor facilitates the diagnosis. Treatment consists of supportive care and the cautious use of barbiturates to combat convulsions.

Indirect-acting Stimulants

MONOAMINE OXIDASE (MAO) INHIBITORS. The observation that iproniazid, an inhibitor of monoamine oxidase (MAO), had a mood-elevating effect in tuberculous patients initiated a great deal of interest in compounds of this type, and led to their quick exploitation in the treatment of depression. Iproniazid (Marsilid) proved exceedingly toxic and was taken off the market, as have several more recently developed MAO inhibitors; but other drugs, much better tolerated, have become available. These include isocarboxazid (Marplan), nialamide (Niamid), phenelzine (Nardil), and tranylcypromine (Parnate), the latter two being the most frequently used. Tranylcypromine has proved to be the most potent of these agents, but it has also produced the most serious toxic effects.

The exact mode of action of the MAO inhibitors has not been determined. They have in common the ability to block the oxidative deamination of naturally occurring amines (norepinephrine, epinephrine, and serotonin), and it has been suggested that the accumulation of these neurohormonal substances is responsible for the antidepressant effect. However, these drugs inhibit many enzymes other than monoamine oxidases and have numerous actions unrelated to enzyme inhibition. Furthermore, many agents with antidepressant effects like those of the monoamine oxidase inhibitors do not inhibit this enzyme. At the present time, one cannot assume that the therapeutic effect of these drugs has a direct relationship to the property of MAO inhibitors.

These drugs must be dispensed with great caution and a constant awareness of their potentially serious side effects. Patients taking the drugs must be warned against the use of sympathomimetic amines and tyramine, for this may induce a severe hypertensive episode and cerebral vascular accident, headache, atrial and ventricular arrhythmia, pulmonary edema, and even death. Orthostatic hypotension of a serious degree may also develop. Sympathomimetic amines are taken in the form of nasal sprays, nose drops, and in so-called "coryza" tablets and the common tyramine-containing compounds are cheeses, yogurt, beer, and wine.

The MAO inhibitors may at times cause excitement, restlessness, agitation, insomnia, and anxiety, and occasionally, with the usual dose and more often with an overdose, mania and convulsions may occur (especially in epileptic patients). Other side effects are increased neuromuscular activity in the form of muscle twitching and involuntary movement of an extremity, urinary retention, skin rashes, tachycardia, hepatic disturbance, jaundice, visual impairment, enhancement of glaucoma, impotence, sweating, muscle spasms, and a variety of parasthesias.

Since the MAO inhibitors have such widespread possibilities of causing toxic effects and potentiating the effect of other drugs, it is wise not to give them concurrently with other medications. In particular, the phenothiazines and other powerful central nervous system stimulants should not be used with the MAO inhibitors, since occasional fatalities and severe reactions have followed their concomitant use. Exaggerated responses to the usual dose of meperidine (Demerol) and other narcotic drugs have also been observed; respiratory function may be depressed to a serious degree, and hyperpyrexia, agitation, and pronounced hypotension also may occur, sometimes with fatal issue. Unpredictable side effects may also accompany the simultaneous administration of barbiturates, alcohol, anesthetics, and insulin.

DIBENZAZEPINE DERIVATIVES. Soon after the first convincing successes in the treatment of depression with MAO inhibitors, a new class of antidepressant compounds appeared. The first of this group was imipramine (Tofranil), which was soon followed by amitriptyline (Elavil), and more recently by desipramine (Norpramine) and nortryptyline (Aventyl). The first two members of this group have proved to be the most popular.

The exact mode of action of these agents is unknown, but they produce a central stimulating effect. In the absence of other considerations, they are presently the most effective drugs for the treatment of depressive illnesses that are associated with anxiety and agitation. Persistence of their pharmacologic effects after the drug is stopped is very short in comparison with the MAO inhibitors, and their side effects are far less frequent and serious.

All of the dibenzazepine compounds are capable of

causing orthostatic hypotension, urinary bladder weakness, dizziness, and occasionally, ataxia and blood dyscrasias. They may produce central nervous system excitement, leading to insomnia, agitation, and restlessness, but usually these effects are controlled readily by the use of phenothiazines or chlordiazepoxide given concurrently or in the evenings. The dibenzazepine drugs should never be given with an MAO inhibitor, since the reactions which may occur are frequently serious; hypertensive seizures and lethal hyperpyrexia have been reported. These reactions have allegedly occurred when small doses of imipramine were given to patients who had discontinued the MAO inhibitor one week previously.

PSYCHOTOGENIC DRUGS

Included in this category are a heterogeneous group of drugs, the primary effect of which is to alter perception, mood, and thinking out of proportion to other aspects of cognitive function and consciousness. Tolerance to these drugs and addiction (i.e., the occurrence of abstinence symptoms when the drug is withdrawn) do not develop, although users may become dependent upon them for emotional support. This group of drugs comprises lysergic acid derivatives, e.g., lysergic acid diethylamide (LSD); phenylethylamine derivatives (mescaline or peyote); psilocybin; certain indolic derivatives, cannabis (marihuana), and a number of less important compounds. They are also referred to as psychotomimetic drugs, hallucinogens and psychedelics but none of these names is entirely suitable.

LSD, mescaline, and psilocybin produce much the same clinical effects if given in comparable amounts. The somatic symptoms consist of dizziness, nausea, drowsiness, paresthesias and blurring of vision. The perceptual abnormalities are the most dramatic—the user describes vivid visual hallucinations, alterations in the shape and color of objects, unusual dreams, and feelings of depersonalization. An increase in auditory acuity has been described but auditory hallucinations are rare. Cognitive functions are difficult to assess because of inattention, drowsiness, and inability to concentrate and to cooperate in mental testing. Sympathomimetic effects—pupillary dilatation, piloerection, hyperthermia, and tachycardia are prominent, and the user may also show hyperreflexia, incoordination of the limbs, and ataxia.

The effects of *marihuana*, when taken by inhaling the smoke from cigarettes, are prompt in onset and evanescent. In low doses the symptoms are like those of mild intoxication with alcohol. With increasing amounts of drug, the effects are similar to those of LSD, mescaline,

and psylocybin, and they may be quite disabling for many hours. Very large doses result in severe depression and stupor, but death is unusual.

The fact that small quantities of these drugs can produce gross mental aberrations has stimulated the search for similar endogenous substances that may be responsible for schizophrenia and other psychoses. The mechanisms involved in producing and antagonizing the "psychotomimetic" effects are also being studied intensively, in the hope of elucidating the mechanisms of the psychoses and finding improved psychotherapeutic agents. Doubtless these studies are adding greatly to our knowledge of abnormal behavior, but the fundamental problems remain to be solved.

Numerous claims have been made that LSD and related drugs are effective in the treatment of mental disease and a wide variety of social ills and that they have the capacity to increase one's intellectual performance, creativity, and self-understanding. At this time, there are no acceptable studies that validate any of these claims.

LSD is not yet an approved drug, and marihuana falls under the federal narcotic laws. Nevertheless, these drugs are very widely used. They are taken by narcotic addicts as a temporary substitute for more potent drugs, by "drug heads," i.e., individuals who use literally any agent that alters consciousness, and by many college and high school students, for reasons that are not easy to define.

The unsupervised use of these drugs is attended by a number of serious adverse reactions, taking the form of acute panic attacks, long-lasting psychotic states resembling paranoid schizophrenia, or serious physical injury, consequent upon impairment of the user's critical faculties. Recent reports have suggested that LSD may cause chromosomal damage. A discussion of the legal implications of the illicit use of these drugs and their social impact is beyond the scope of this chapter.

REFERENCES

Hollister, L. E.: "Chemical Psychoses. LSD and Related Drugs," Springfield, Ill., Charles C Thomas, Publisher, 1968.

———: Symposium on adverse drug reactions. Psychopharmacological drugs, J.A.M.A. 196:411–413, 1966.

Jarvik, M. E.: Drugs used in the treatment of psychiatric disorders, pp. 159–214 in "Pharmacological Basis of Therapeutics," 3d ed., L. S. Goodman and Alfred Gilman (Eds.), New York, The MacMillan Company, 1965.

"Psychopharmacology. A Review of Progress, 1957–1967." U.S.P.H.S. Pulb. No. 1836. Washington, D.C., 1968.

Section 2

Disorders Caused by Venoms, Bites, and Stings

122 SNAKE AND LIZARD BITES
Ivan L. Bennett, Jr.

SNAKE BITES

Fewer than one-tenth of the nearly 2,500 known species of snakes are venomous. These poisonous varieties belong to five families or subfamilies: Elapidae (cobras, kraits, coral snakes), found in all parts of the world but Europe; Viperinae (true vipers), found in all parts of the world but the Americas; Hydrophidae (sea snakes); Crotalinae (pit vipers), found in Asia and the Americas; and Colubridae, represented by a few rear-fanged species of Africa. The poisonous varieties of the United States, with the single exception of the coral snake of the Elapidae, are pit vipers and include the rattlesnakes, the water moccasin, and the copperhead. This discussion will center around these species, but the therapeutic measures outlined are applicable to snake bites in all parts of the world.

The number of individuals bitten by poisonous snakes in the United States is estimated at 2,000 to 3,000 per year; deaths are not reported separately but are undoubtedly rare, numbering fewer than 20 per year. In many European countries, deaths from snake bite have averaged only one every 3 to 5 years for the last half-century. In contrast, the estimate of annual deaths from snake bite in Brazil is 2,000 (4 per 100,000 population), and 2,000 in Burma (15.4 per 100,000).

ETIOLOGY. The coral snake is found in the Southern states from Florida to Arizona. It is marked by alternating red and black bands separated by yellow rings. Coral snakes are nocturnal and placid and rarely bite man. The fangs are short and permanently erect; the highly toxic venom is injected into multiple puncture wounds produced by a series of chewing movements.

The pit vipers are so named because of a small pit between the eye and the nostril. Large venom glands in the temporal region give the head a triangular appearance. They are generally aggressive and likely to strike if disturbed. The fangs are long and hinged, folding posteriorly when the mouth is closed. Pit vipers strike suddenly with a forward thrust of the head, and the instant that the erect fangs make contact, venom is expressed by sudden muscular contraction.

The rattlesnakes, recognized by the horny rattle on the tail which buzzes when the snake is disturbed, are widely distributed. The diamondbacks (*Crotalus adamanteus* in the Southeast and *C. atrox* in the Southwest) are the largest and most dangerous snakes in this country. Others include the prairie rattler (*C. confluentus*), the timber rattler (*C. horridus*), and the pigmy rattlers.

The water moccasin, or cottonmouth (*Agkistrodon piscivorus*), is found in swampy areas or along the banks of streams. It is a strong swimmer and can bite under water. This snake is notorious for inflicting severe facial bites when disturbed in the branches of small trees. The copperhead, or highland moccasin (*A. mokasen*), is a closely related species. Its bite is painful but rarely fatal.

PATHOGENESIS. Snake Venoms. The venoms of many species have been analyzed; invariably each proves to be a mixture of several toxic proteins and enzymes. As an example, the venom of the Indian cobra (*Naja naja*) contains these distinct and separate substances: a neurotoxin, a hemolysin, a cardiotoxin, a cholinesterase, at least three phosphatases, a nucleotidase, and a potent inhibitor of cytochrome oxidase. Several venoms, including those of the pit vipers, contain hyaluronidase and numerous proteolytic enzymes. Although opinions differ about the exact role of these components in toxicity, the action of the venom of a given species is usually predominantly *neurotoxic* or *necrotizing;* frequently associated changes are hemolysis and changes in blood coagulation. The venom of elapids, including the coral snake, is neurotoxic, and death results from respiratory paralysis, probably caused by damage to brain centers, and a curariform interference with transmission at the neuromuscular junction. The venom of crotalid snakes produces local tissue injury, hemorrhage, and hemolysis; death is preceded by circulatory collapse, the mechanism of which is poorly understood. Systemic absorption of venom occurs through lymphatics, and therapeutic measures designed to reduce lymphatic function are helpful in controlling symptoms. On rare occasions, when venom is discharged directly into a blood vessel, death occurs in less than 10 min.

Factors Affecting Severity. Several factors affect the outcome of snake bite:

1. The age, size, and health of the patient. Envenomation in children is usually serious and a fatal outcome more likely.

2. Bites on extremities or into adipose tissues are less dangerous than those on the trunk or face or penetrating a vessel. A direct stroke of the fangs is more dangerous than a scratch, a glancing blow, or one hitting a bone. The discharge orifice of the fang is well above its tip, and the point of the fang can penetrate the skin without envenomation. Even a thin layer of clothing may afford great protection.

3. The size of the snake, the extent of its anger or fear (if hurt it may inject a large dose of venom), the condition of the venom glands (recently discharged or full), and the condition of the fangs (broken, recently renewed) are all important.

4. The presence of various bacteria in the mouth of the snake or on the skin of the victim (especially clostridia) may lead to serious infection in the necrotic tissues at the local site.

5. Exercise or exertion, such as running, immediately after the bite speeds sytemic absorption of toxin.

MANIFESTATIONS. The bite of a pit viper produces severe pain at the local site within a few minutes. There is rapid swelling; ecchymoses and bullae appear over the involved areas, and as the edema spreads, serosanguineous fluid oozes from the puncture wounds. Systemic effects include circulatory collapse with hypotension, clammy skin, tachycardia, intense thirst, nausea, hematemesis, bloody diarrhea, icterus (rarely intense), hemorrhages from the nose and into the skin, and convulsions. Death may occur after 6 to 48 hr. Survival may be attended by massive local tissue loss from gangrene and secondary infection; amputation of an extremity is sometimes necessary. Fever with a temperature of 101 to 104°F, polymorphonuclear leukocytosis of 20,000 to 30,000, and albuminuria appear within a few hours in severe cases.

The bite of a coral snake causes little pain, and local swelling is slight. There are usually multiple fang marks. Numbness and weakness begin in the region of the bite within 10 to 15 min and are followed by ataxia, ptosis, pupillary dilatation and loss of reaction to light and accommodation, palatal and pharyngeal palsies, slurring of speech, salivation, and, occasionally, nausea and vomiting. The patient becomes comatose, respirations falter, there are convulsions, and death occurs within 8 to 72 hr.

Cobra bites are painful, and, in general, the clinical picture is a combination of neurotoxic and hemolytic manifestations.

TREATMENT. An attempt should be made to determine with certainty that the patient has been bitten by a poisonous snake. Absence of distinct fang punctures and failure of local pain, edema, numbness, or weakness to appear within 20 min are strong evidence against a bite's having been inflicted by a venomous species.

Treatment consists of immobilization, application of a tourniquet, incision and suction, antivenin, local hypothermia, measures to combat infection, and general support. All patients should be transported to a hospital as quickly as possible.

Local Measures. A tourniquet, preferably flat, should be placed a few centimeters above the bite (if anatomically feasible) and made tight enough to allow one finger to pass beneath it with difficulty. The purpose is to impede lymph flow, and it is not necessary to obstruct venous return; the tourniquet should be loosened and moved proximally at hourly intervals when local swelling causes it to tighten. Using whatever antisepsis is available, 1-cm linear (*not cruciate*) incisions about 0.5 cm deep should be made through each fang mark and suction applied for at least 30 min. A rubber bulb for this purpose is contained in first-aid kits, but a breast pump, funnel attached to a vacuum line, or heated jar can be used. Mouth suction is permissible if no oral lesions are present. Suction should be carried out for 15 min every hour, then every 2 hr, as long as fluid is obtainable. As the swelling progresses, successive rings of radiating, linear, shallow incisions at the advancing edge of the edema are useful; such cuts will be expanded by the progressive swelling. Once a patient has been hospitalized, a pavex boot is a convenient means of applying suction to an extremity. Extensive or deep slashes over the area are unnecessary. Incision and suction are extremely important and should be carried out diligently in every poisonous snake bite. Antivenin is not a substitute for them and should not be relied on alone.

Immobilization of the affected part during transportation is important in controlling lymph flow; splinting is useful in achieving this. The application of ice packs to the affected area reduces inflammation and swelling, slows drainage by lymphatics, relieves pain, and curtails local necrosis. Care should be taken to avoid freezing the tissues.

Antivenin. Many of the components of venom are antigenic, and effective antiserum can be prepared by inoculation of horses with graded doses. In the United States, polyvalent antivenin, effective against all American pit vipers, is available commercially. Kits contain lyophilized antivenin (reconstituted with distilled water to 10 ml per ampul), syringe, normal horse serum for prior sensitivity testing of the patient, and detailed instructions. The initial dose for a serious bite should be 5 ampuls intramuscularly or intravenously. It is not advisable to infiltrate antivenin at the local site. Further antivenin can be given as indicated by progression of swelling or systemic symptoms.

No antivenin for other snakes is manufactured in the United States, but antiserum of various types is usually kept on hand at large zoos all over the world.

Other Measures. The maintenance of respiration by manual or mechanical aids is important in patients bitten by the elapine snakes. It has been suggested that the cholinesterase of cobra and coral venom is responsible for much of the neurotoxicity and that neostigmine and atropine given as for myasthenia gravis might help. This has not been tested clinically.

Tetanus toxoid or antiserum should be given. If pyogenic infection develops, antibiotics should be used.

Alcohol has no place in the treatment of snake bite. Opiates are contraindicated. Relief of pain with salicylates or Demerol, sedation, maintenance of fluid intake, measures to combat shock, and appropriate management of coma or convulsions are all important.

Limited trials of ACTH and adrenal steroids have not shown any great usefulness of these hormones in lessening local necrosis or systemic intoxication.

PREVENTION. In snake-infested regions, long trousers, high shoes, boots or leggings, and gloves should be worn. Most important of all is to look where one steps or reaches. A sharp knife or lancet, tourniquet, suction bulb, and antiseptic suffice for an emergency kit, and in inaccessible areas, antivenin also should be carried.

GILA MONSTER BITE

The Gila monsters include the large orange and black lizard (*Heloderma suspectum*) of the arid Southwest and *H. horridum*, a closely related Mexican species. These reptiles are not aggressive, and virtually every instance of their attacking man has involved teasing or handling the animals in captivity. The venom is elaborated in eight glands in the floor of the mouth and secreted directly into the oral cavity, where it bathes the teeth, which are grooved posteriorly. The lizard clings tenaciously and is often dislodged only after considerable effort; envenomation occurs by contamination of the wound. The venom contains a potent neurotoxin which is undoubtedly responsible for its lethal effect in experimental animals. Death in man has been reported as occurring within a few hours (in one case, 30 min) after a bite. The venom also produces local tissue injury, excruciating pain, massive edema, and patchy erythema. In recovered patients, acute symptoms have lasted for 3 to 4 days and include nausea, vomiting, hematemesis, blurred vision, dyspnea, dysphonia, and profound weakness. Intense hyperesthesia of the bitten extremity may persist for several weeks. There is no antivenin available. Treatment should consist of tourniquet, incision, suction, refrigeration of the bitten area, measures to prevent or combat infection, including tetanus, and supportive measures. Because Demerol has been shown to potentiate the venom's action in animals, some other analgesic should be used to relieve pain.

REFERENCES

Buckley, E. E., and N. Porges (Eds.): "Symposium on Venoms," Am. Assoc. Advan. Sci., Publ. 44, Washington, 1956.

Ellis, E. F., and R. T. Smith: Systemic Anaphylaxis after Rattlesnake Bite, J.A.M.A., 193:401, 401, 1965.

Klauber, L. M.: "Rattlesnakes, Their Habits, Life History and Influence on Mankind," vol. 2, Berkeley, University of California Press, 1956.

Lockhart, W. E.: Treatment of Snakebite, J.A.M.A., 193: 336, 1965.

National Research Council: Ad Hoc Committee on Snakebite Report, Toxicon, 1:81, 1963.

Russell, F. E., and R. S. Scharffenberg: "Bibliography of Snake Venoms and Venomous Snakes," Oxford, Pergamon Press, 1965.

Shannon, F. A.: Case Reports of Two Gila Monster Bites, Herpetology, 9:127, 1953.

123 SPIDERS, SCORPIONS, INSECTS, AND OTHER ARTHROPODS

Ivan L. Bennett, Jr.

The bite of many spiders is locally irritating, and several species can cause severe, even fatal systemic poisoning in man. The most numerous and important of the venomous spiders are members of the genus *Latrodectus*, widely distributed throughout the world. In the United States and Canada, *Lat. mactans*, the black widow or shoe-button spider, causes a majority of clinically significant arachnidism. In Florida, *Lat. bishopi*, the red-legged widow spider, has been reported to produce human poisoning resembling mild black widow bite. From the Southern and Midwestern states, there are increasing numbers of reports of poisoning from the bite of common brown spiders, including *Loxosceles reclusa* and *Lox. unicolor*. These are characterized by pain, local necrosis, and, occasionally, a hemolytic syndrome, which can be fatal.

The symptoms and mortality from bites of large, hairy spiders, the tarantulas, such as *Lycosa raptoria* and *Phoneutria fera* in Brazil or *Glyptocranium gastereanthoides* in Peru, and of such spiders as *Loxosceles laeta* in Chile are similar, with severe ulceration, necrosis, and hemolysis. Neurotoxic manifestations of the type produced by *Latrodectus* are sometimes admixed with local necrosis and hemolysis.

It is the female *Lat. mactans*, the black widow, that bites man. She is glossy black with a body 1 cm in diameter, a leg span of 5 cm, and a characteristic red "hourglass" mark on her abdomen. She spins her web in wood-piles, sheds, basements, or outdoor privies, is very aggressive, and will bite on slight provocation. The venom produces diffuse central and peripheral nervous excitement, autonomic activity, muscle spasm, hypertension, and vasoconstriction.

In the United States, most spider bites occur between April and October, and many patients are males bitten on the genitalia or buttocks while using a privy. After a momentary sharp pain at the site, there is cramping pain that begins locally within 15 to 60 min and gradually spreads. It may involve all extremities and the trunk. The abdomen is boardlike, and the waves of pain become excruciating, causing the patient to turn, toss, and cry out. Respirations are often labored and grunting. There are also nausea, vomiting, headache, sweating, salivation, hyperactive reflexes, twitching, tremor, paresthesias of hands and feet, and, occasionally, systolic hypertension. A mild polymorphonuclear leukocytosis is usual, and many patients have slight fever. After several hours, the pains subside, although mild recurrences for 2 or 3 days are common. It may be a week before well-being is restored. Deaths have occurred, mostly in children and the aged. In an analysis of nearly 1,300 cases from the United States and Canada, the mortality rate was found to vary from 2.4 to 6.0 percent. This is higher than is usually stated.

Because the bite itself is not prominent, patients are often thought to have some abdominal catastrophe such as perforated ulcer, pancreatitis, or volvulus. Renal colic, coronary occlusion, tetanus, strychnine poisoning, tabetic crisis, lead colic, and porphyria are other conditions to be ruled out. The abdomen is not tender to palpation in arachnidism, and pains in the extremities are not typical of most of these other disorders.

TREATMENT. This consists of antiserum and measures to relieve pain. A single intramuscular injection of 1 ampul (2.5 ml) of reconstituted antiserum is all that is needed in most cases; relief is gradual. Hot baths alleviate pain temporarily, and intravenous calcium gluconate or magnesium sulfate usually produces dramatic, but transient, cessation of cramps. Opiates are sometimes necessary. Neostigmine, epinephrine, ACTH, and adrenal steroids have all been reported to give relief in isolated cases and are worth trying.

SCORPION STING

Scorpions are eight-legged arthropods. Glands in the terminal segment produce venom, which is injected into the victim by a stinger located on the tip of the tail. Scorpions often enter dwellings. During the day they retreat into crevices; emerging at night, they often get into shoes and clothing and even into bedding. They do not deliberately attack man, but accidental contact results in a sting.

Of about 650 species, roughly 40 occur in the United States, distributed over three-fourths of the nation. They are most numerous in the South from Florida to California, but the only two lethal species, *Centruroides sculpturatus* and *C. gertschi,* are limited to Arizona and portions of neighboring states.

Dangerous species found in the United States, *C. sculpturatus* and *C. gertschi,* reach a maximal length of about 7 cm. Their sting may be fatal to young children or old people, but seldom to a healthy adult. In the years 1929 to 1948, 68 deaths from scorpion sting were reported from the state of Arizona.

Most of the nonlethal species of scorpions in the United States cause only minor reactions, like a bee sting. Some in the Southwest, however, produce local edema and ecchymosis, with burning pain. In contrast, many species whose venom has potentially dangerous systemic effects, including the Arizona *Centruroides,* evoke little or no visible reaction at the site of the sting. There is an immediate burning sensation followed by local paresthesia ("pins and needles"), hyperesthesia, or numbness. These sensations spread to involve the whole extremity, and within an hour or two, malaise, restlessness, lacrimation, rhinorrhea, salivation, perspiration, nausea, and vomiting appear. Transient hypertension, glucosuria, premature ventricular contractions, and feeble pulse may be noted, or there may be bradycardia and irregular or Cheyne-Stokes breathing. Pulmonary edema develops terminally. The patient passes from an agitated state with hyperactive reflexes into coma; convulsions follow. Death usually occurs within 12 hr, but sometimes as late as 2 days after the sting.

TREATMENT. This consists of immediately placing a tight ligature on the extremity just proximal to the sting, followed by application of ice and, as soon as possible, immersion of the involved member above the ligature in ice water. The ligature must be removed in 5 to 10 min, but the limb is kept refrigerated for at least 2 hr.

After this time, if treatment has been applied promptly, it is said that no serious effects are experienced following the sting of *C. sculpturatus* or *C. gertschi.* If the sting is on the head, trunk, or genitalia, of course, the ligature cannot be used, but the area may be chilled with an ice pack.

Although tourniquet, incision, and suction as in the treatment of snake bite have been recommended, the amount of venom is minute; it produces no local necrotizing effect and is absorbed very rapidly.

Supportive therapy is directed at combating shock and dehydration. Barbiturates in large doses are useful in reducing restlessness.

PREVENTION. This depends upon alertness in avoiding contact with scorpions in infested areas. Clothing and shoes should be well shaken before being put on in the morning. Towels and bedclothes should be inspected. A house infested with scorpions can in time be rid of them by closing all obvious ways of ingress; picking up debris in the environment, such as piles of brush, logs, stones; introducing a mixture of fuel oil or kerosene, containing a small amount of creosote, between the earth and the house foundation; and spraying with a mixture of 2 percent Chlordane, 10 percent DDT, and 0.2 percent pyrethrins in an oil base.

BEES, WASPS, AND ANTS

Bee or wasp venom is hemolytic and neurotoxic and has a histamine-like action. Multiple stings in man cause pain and discomfort, but only in enormous numbers (500 to 1,000) can they cause death. Apiarists often become immune to the venom and can sustain many stings without effect.

The usual reaction to a single bee or wasp sting is sharp pain, local wheal and erythema, intense itching, and, in loose tissues such as the eyelid or genitalia, considerable edema which subsides in a few hours. Only in the rare case when a bee is inhaled or swallowed and edema of the laryngopharynx or glottis develops is there danger. A sting directly into a peripheral nerve may destroy its function for a time, much as does an injection of alcohol. Bell's palsy has followed a sting into the trunk of the facial nerve.

In hypersensitive individuals, a single sting may produce serious anaphylaxis with urticaria, nausea, abdominal cramps, asthma, massive edema of the face and glottis, dyspnea, cyanosis, hypotension, coma, and death. Sensitization is usually a result of previous stings. Beekeepers who develop allergic rhinitis followed by asthma when near bees or objects that have been in contact with bees are likely to have serious reactions to a sting.

Many ants can produce stinging bites with local redness and swelling, including the notorious "fire ant" whose bite may result in vesiculation.

The usual sting is treated by local cool applications and antipruritic lotions or oral antihistaminics. Epinephrine, 0.3 to 0.5 ml of 1:1,000 aqueous solution subcutaneously, repeated every 20 to 30 min, may be lifesaving in patients allergic to bees and/or wasps. This drug may be given as 1:100 solution in oil intramuscularly. Oxygen, antihistaminic drugs, and other supportive measures should be used. Desensitization by injections of extracts of whole bees and wasps is effective. If this is not practical, contact with these insects should be avoided and, if exposure seems likely, epinephrine or sublingual Isuprel tablets should be kept on hand.

TICK BITE AND TICK PARALYSIS

The local reaction to the bite of a tick may be nothing more than an itching papule which subsides within a few days unless there is secondary bacterial infection. However, incomplete removal of a tick, with retention of the mouthparts may result in the local formation of a nodule which continues to grow and is sometimes annoyingly pruritic. The definitive treatment is surgical excision of the nodule. Histologically, the nodule is a granuloma, but the inflammatory response is sometimes so bizarre and changes in the overlying epithelium are so striking that, in the absence of a history of tick bite, a mistaken diagnosis of malignant tumor may be made.

Removal of a tick by steady pulling is preferable to crushing. Touching with a glowing cigarette, freezing, or application of a drop of oil facilitates removal without leaving embedded remnants.

TICK PARALYSIS. Tick paralysis is a reversible disorder of the nervous system which sometimes develops in the host while a tick is engorging. It occurs in man and animals. The disease has been reported from many countries and has long been recognized in the northwestern United States and western Canada, where the wood tick, *Dermacentor andersoni* Stiles, is responsible. The dog tick, *D. variabilis* Say, has been identified in a number of cases occurring in the Eastern states. *Amblyomma americanum*, the lone star tick, and *A. maculatum*, the Gulf Coast tick, have also been incriminated.

While engorging, the tick apparently injects a neurotoxin which acts upon the spinal cord and bulbar nuclei, causing incoordination, weakness, and paralysis. It has been shown in animals that there is failure of neuromuscular transmission and striking impairment of stretch reflexes. The toxin appears to be destroyed or excreted rapidly, for when the tick is removed the nerve cells soon regain normal function.

Tick paralysis has been produced in experimental animals only with gravid female ticks, suggesting that the toxin might be elaborated by the ova. However, injection of extracts prepared from tick eggs has failed to reproduce the clinical picture in convincing fashion.

The tick must feed for several days before symptoms develop. Female ticks commonly remain attached for 7 to 9 days or longer. Paralysis is seen in experimental animals after 5 to 7 days of engorgement. Male ticks feed for a shorter period, a fact which may explain why they are less likely to cause paralysis.

Experimental confirmation of the hypothesis that the toxin is produced in tick salivary glands is also lacking. It has been found that not all gravid female ticks of incriminated species cause paralysis. In short, the nature, site of production, and mode of action of the toxin are still unknown.

Most human cases occur in children, generally in young girls. The tick is usually attached to the scalp and hidden by the hair, but may be found on any part of the body, especially the ear, axilla, groin, vulva, or popliteal region.

The patient may be irritable and have mild diarrhea for 24 hr before frank motor involvement appears. There are weakness and poor control of the legs, the tendon reflexes in the legs are diminished or absent, and the Romberg sign is positive. Temporary improvement may occur, and if the tick is removed at this stage, true paralysis may never develop. Otherwise the symptoms recur within 24 hr, with flaccid paralysis which extends in 24 to 48 hr to involve the trunk, arms, neck, tongue, and pharynx. Sensory changes are usually absent, but there may be paresthesia and hyperesthesia in the affected extremities. Nystagmus, strabismus, and facial paralysis are sometimes noted. The respirations become shallow, rapid, and irregular. The patient sinks into stupor, cyanosis appears, and death results from respiratory paralysis or from obstruction of the airway by aspirated material.

There is little or no fever unless a secondary infection is present. The leukocyte count is usually not elevated, but moderate leukocytosis may occur. The spinal fluid is almost always normal.

Tick paralysis is apt to be confused with poliomyelitis, the more so because ticks are active in warm weather when poliomyelitis is most prevalent.

Among other diseases which might be considered in differential diagnosis are polyneuritis, transverse myelitis, and infectious neuronitis (Guillain-Barré syndrome).

Definitive treatment is removal of the tick. Mouthparts retained in the skin should be promptly excised. The patient's body should be searched for other ticks. There is striking improvement within a few hours after removal of ticks.

If the tick is removed before bulbar involvement develops, the paralysis subsides, and recovery is complete in a few days, sometimes within 24 hr. The patient should be observed until the recovery trend is established, because if other ticks or retained mouthparts have been overlooked, the paralysis may progress. When bulbar or respiratory paralysis is present, death may occur if the tick is not removed in time. Other treatment is supportive.

OTHER ARTHROPODS

FLEA BITE. There are many fleas that attack man, including *Pulex irritans* and chicken fleas. In sensitive individuals, the salivary secretion of these bloodsuckers produces large, itching papules. Treatment is symptomatic only. Elimination of fleas in an environment may be very difficult, but persistent treatment of animals and of premises with appropriate insecticides is usually successful.

CENTIPEDE BITE. Local irritation is the usual reaction to centipede venom, although extensive necrosis and systemic illness have followed severe poisoning by tropical species. Treatment is purely symptomatic.

CATERPILLAR URTICARIA. Contact with hairy caterpillars of many species produces irritation of skin or mucous membranes. The type of venom involved is not known, but severe pain, erythema, urticaria, and even blister formation may come on rapidly after direct contact with caterpillars, after handling cocoons, or on being exposed to windblown fuzz. There are often a regional lymphangitis and transient eosinophilic leukocytosis. The discomfort subsides within 24 hr, but local soaks, oral antihistaminics, and when pain is severe, oral codeine are often indicated.

BEDBUG BITE. Members of the genus *Cimex* inflict bites that leave reactions varying from a simple puncture to large urticarial lesions, apparently depending on the sensitivity of the bitten individual. There is no specific treatment.

CHIGGERS OR REDBUGS. These are tiny mites which are commonly found in foliage, grass, etc., in many parts of the world. In the United States, the larval form of *Eutrobicula alfreddugesi* attacks the skin by secreting a substance which digests tissue, creating a red papule that itches intensely. The tiny reddish larva can be seen in the center of the lesion. Treatment is palliative with antipruritic applications. There is no better example of the virtues of prevention than this annoying affliction. The use of insect repellents, appropriate protective clothing, and prompt bathing after exposure reduce the risk of infestation considerably.

MYIASIS. There are, generally speaking, three ways in which human tissues may become infested by maggots. Species of flies which usually deposit eggs in carrion, feces, or garbage may lay eggs in an open wound or ulcer, usually a lesion that is necrotic and suppurating. When the larvae hatch, they feed upon the dead tissue, and despite the unesthetic aspects, the deliberate introduction of maggots has been used to supplement surgical debridement.

Occasionally, food containing fly eggs will be ingested, and when the larvae hatch, *intestinal myiasis* can result in nausea, cramps, and diarrhea. The larvae are passed in the feces.

Finally the larvae of many flies, including the sheep fly and horsefly, will attack living, viable tissue. If eggs are laid in the eyes, nose, ears, mouth, or vagina, an event that usually occurs in sleeping infants, the larvae hatch out and can produce extensive destructive lesions; indeed, fatalities have been reported.

The treatment for maggot infestation is surgical removal by irrigation and mechanical extraction. Obviously, control of fly populations by appropriate sanitary precautions is the important step in prevention. Protection of infants by screening and of wounds by bandaging is indicated in infested areas.

REFERENCES

Bee Sting

Helm, S.: Severe Anaphylactic Reaction to a Bee or Wasp Sting, Mil. Surg., 92:64, 1943.

Perlman, F.: Desensitization to Wasp Sting, J.A.M.A., 156: 1470, 1954.

Caterpillar Urticaria

McMillan, C. W., and W. R. Purcell: Health Hazard from Caterpillars, New Eng. J. Med., 271:147, 1964.

Scorpion Sting

De Magalhaes, O.: Scorpionism, J. Trop. Med. Hyg., 41:393, 1938.

Essex, H. E.: Animal Venoms and Their Physiologic Action, Physiol. Rev., 25:150, 1945.

Waterman, J. A.: Some Notes on Scorpion Poisoning in Trinidad, Trans. Roy. Soc. Trop. Med. Hyg., 31:607, 1938.

Spider Bite

Dillaha, C. J., et al.: North American Loxoscelism. Necrotic Bite of the Brown Recluse Spider, J.A.M.A., 188:33, 1964.

Nance, W. E.: Hemolytic Anemia of Necrotic Arachnidism, Am. J. Med., 31:801, 1961.

Thorpe, R. W., and W. D. Woodson: "The Black Widow: America's Most Poisonous Spider," Chapel Hill, N.C., University of North Carolina Press, 1945.

Tick Paralysis

Ransmeier, J. C.: Tick Paralysis in the Eastern United States, J. Pediat., 34:299, 1949.

Stanbury, J. B., and J. H. Huyck: Tick Paralysis: A Critical Review, Medicine, 24:219, 1945.

124 MARINE ANIMALS
Ivan L. Bennett, Jr.

The elaboration of substances that are poisonous for man is by no means an exclusive property of reptiles and arthropods. Several plant and animal products that are toxic when ingested are described in Chap. 116. Here, discussion will center around venoms of marine animals known definitely to cause illness in man after injection or inoculation under naturally occurring conditions. Information about these toxins is limited, a few isolated clinical observations being the only data available about some of them. An excellent compilation and bibliography will be found in the reviews listed at the end of the chapter.

SEA ANEMONE STING (SPONGE DIVER'S DISEASE). Contact with certain sea anemones (especially *Sargatia elegans*) in Mediterranean and African waters produces extensive dermatitis with chronic ulceration. Occasionally, especially during August and September, systemic symptoms of headache, sneezing, nausea, chills, fever, and collapse are noted. Rare fatalities have occurred. No specific therapy is known; the skin lesions have been thought to benefit from local x-ray irradiation. The disease confers no immunity.

SPONGE POISONING. Direct contact with several species of sponge results in a painful dermatitis. It is known that extracts of the sponges are lethal for mice. Dilute acetic acid ameliorates local pain strikingly, and alkali will intensify it. The lesions are self-limited.

PORTUGUESE MAN–O–WAR AND JELLYFISH STINGS. The burning discomfort induced by contact with "sea nettles" or jellyfish is familiar to most surf bathers. Contact with the tentacles of the colorful Portuguese man-o-war (*Physalia* species) or more toxic jellyfish (*Chiropsalmus* of the Indian Ocean and *Rhizostoma* of the Atlantic) is followed by severe pain, swelling, and erythema. Muscle pain, weakness, abdominal cramps, nausea, dyspnea, cyanosis, and collapse may persist for several days, and fatalities have occurred, sometimes within hours after contact.

Treatment consists of local application of ammonia, alcohol, or calamine, oral or parenteral antihistaminics, and systemic support. Cortisone has been thought to help in a few cases.

CONE SHELL POISONING. The colorful cone shells are highly prized by collectors. Many species in the Pacific are venomous, a great danger to unwary hobbyists who pick them up. The poison is delivered into a wound inflicted by pointed hollow teeth resembling darts in the long proboscis of the animal. Local manifestations include sudden intense pain, swelling, and cyanosis followed by numbness. The venom is apparently a neurotoxin and produces muscular incoordination, weakness, confusion, tachycardia, and dyspnea. Death may occur within 3 to 5 hr, but recovery within 24 hr is the rule. Recommended treatment is the use of tourniquet, incision, and suction (as for snake bite) and supportive measures which may include artificial respiration and administration oxygen.

SEA URCHIN STING. Contact with the spines of some species of sea urchin results in painful erythema and ulceration with or without neurotoxic symptoms of weakness and frank paralysis of lips, tongue, and face lasting for several hours. Treatment is purely symptomatic and supportive. The toxins isolated from sea urchins have produced paralysis in animals and are notably resistant to heat. Deaths from paralysis and drowning have been reported.

FISH STINGS. The dorsal fins or spines of bullhead sharks, dogfish (the familiar *Squalus acanthias* of biology classes), and ratfish and the dorsal and other fins of the scorpion fish, weeverfish, toadfish, and catfish are grooved, and at their bases are found venom glands. Injury by these spines results in severe pain and swelling and, in some instances, neurotoxic manifestations. Local gangrene with extensive tissue loss is a complication of catfish stings that may prolong convalescence. Little or nothing is known of the venoms involved. Suction and hot applications are advocated immediately after injury. Tetanus toxoid or antitoxin should be given also. Narcotics are often required to control the pain. Secondary pyogenic infection is a frequent complication.

Probably the most frequent type of venomous fish injury in the United States is that produced by the lashing tail of the stingray of the California coast (*Urobatis halleri*). The bony spine is encased in a sheath of epithelial cells containing venom which is expressed into the puncture wound. The wound may be several centimeters deep; portions of the bony spine may break off in it, or, more often, the integumentary sheath remains in the wound. The venom is a circulatory depressant in animals, but local injury predominates in man. There are immediately severe pain and cyanosis followed by erythema and edema. Weakness, rarely, convulsions, and death may ensue. Treatment consists of application of a tourniquet (the vast majority of these injuries occur on the legs) and copious syringing of the wound with salt water to remove fragments of sheath followed by immersion in water as hot as the patient can stand for 1 hr. The venom is heat-labile, and extensive trials have indicated the usefulness of this last procedure. Tetanus toxoid or antiserum is indicated; as with other fish stings, pyogenic infection is a frequent complication.

REFERENCES

Abbott, R. T.: "Mollusks and Medicine in World War II," Smithsonian Annual Report for 1947, p. 325, Washington, 1948.

Halstead, B. W.: Animal Phyla Known to Contain Poisonous Marine Animals, p. 9 in Symposium on Venoms, American Association for the Advancement of Science, Washington, 1956.

Keegan, H. L., and W. V. Macfarlane (Eds.): "Venomous and Poisonous Animals and Noxious Plants of the Pacific Region," Oxford, Pergamon Press, 1965.

Russell, F. E.: Marine Toxins and Venomous and Poisonous Marine Animals, Advance. Marine Biol., 3:255, 1965.

Section 3

Physical Agents

125 DISORDERS DUE TO ENVIRONMENTAL TEMPERATURES

John H. Talbott

Three clinical syndromes are associated with high environmental temperature: heat cramps, heat exhaustion, and heat pyrexia. Although each entity may be identified clinically, there is considerable overlapping of the internal changes produced by a high environmental temperature, sequelae of excessive or prolonged physiologic responses. The alterations are especially prevalent during the first days of a heat wave before effective acclimatization. Prophylaxis, by augmented sodium chloride intake prior to exposure or by restoration of the physiologic balance prior to the onset of overt morbidity, is helpful in preventing dire consequences. The child and the older person are more susceptible to heat stress. Strenuous physical activity or the presence of an acute or chronic disease may hasten the development of any one of the morbid states.

Acclimatization

The basic mechanism remains obscure, although more is known of acclimatization of man to heat than to cold. The threshold for onset of sweating is not increased. Sweating is the most effective natural means of combating heat stress with little or no change in the core temperature of the body. As long as sweating continues, provided water and salt are replaced, man can withstand remarkably high temperatures. Two, three, or more liters of sweat may be lost per day. Water and sodium chloride are the most important physiologic constituents of sweat. The concentration of sodium chloride may be low; at other times, it may approach that of interstitial body fluid. Since the sodium chloride concentration of sweat is less than that of body fluid, the excess salt must be retained in the body during the initial stages of sweating. Studies reveal the skin to be the repository. Dilatation of the peripheral blood vessels is a well-known phenomenon in high environmental temperatures. Histamine and histidine in the sweat may participate in the vasodilatation. Other alterations include a decrease in total circulating blood volume, a decrease in renal blood flow, and an increase of the antidiuretic substance in the urine (ADH). Aldosterone, the most potent mineralocorticoid, has been detected in increased quantities in the urine following exposure. Vasodilatation, with an increased circulation in the blood vessels of the skin, permits dissipation of heat. The cardiac output is increased initially. As the stress persists, there is diminished venous return with the peripheral type of forward failure. Failure of dissipation of heat with persistence of environmental temperatures greater than the temperature of the body leads to retention of heat and development of hyperpyrexia.

Heat Cramps

"Miner's cramps" and "stoker's cramps" describe the heat syndrome associated with painful spasms of the voluntary musculature following strenuous exercise. Only persons in good physical condition are victims. External temperatures need not exceed the body temperature. Direct exposure to the sun is not necessary. Muscle cramps have been observed following excessive sweating, precipitated by strenuous exercise in cold environments in untrained persons heavily clothed. Muscles of the extremities bear the brunt of physical activity and show the highest incidence of cramps. Excruciating pain accompanies the spasms and subsides with cessation of cramps. Physical examination is essentially normal between the paroxysms. Examination of the blood reveals a concentration of the formed elements and a decreased concentration of total base, especially sodium. A diminished excretion of sodium chloride in the urine is characteristic. Cessation of cramps with *replacement of sodium chloride and water* is striking and supports the hypothesis that the cause of heat cramps is associated with body depletion of these essential electrolytes.

Heat Exhaustion

Heat prostration, or heat collapse, is probably the most common heat syndrome. Weakness, vertigo, headache, nausea, anorexia, and faintness may precede collapse or participate as predisposing factors. The physically active as well as the sedentary person is susceptible. Onset may be sudden and the duration of collapse brief. During the acute stage, evidence of peripheral vascular failure and poor venous return may be detected from the ashen-gray appearance. The skin is cold and clammy. The pupils are dilated. The blood pressure may be decreased, with a significant increase in the pulse pressure. Since prostration develops before exposure is prolonged, body temperature is subnormal or normal. The duration of exposure and the extent of sweat loss determine the degree of hemoconcentration. *Treatment* embraces supporting measures and removal to a cool area. Intravenous administration of saline solution or whole blood usually is not necessary. Although the pathogenetic mechanism of prostration is not primarily a depletion of water and salt, there are theoretical and practical reasons for maintaining optimal concentration of these essential body constituents in persons exposed to high temperatures.

Heat Pyrexia

Heat hyperpyrexia, heat stroke, or sunstroke is most common in the person with a preexisting acute or chronic malady. Direct exposure to the sun is not a necessary prerequisite. A high relative humidity is an important predisposing factor. Heat pyrexia may develop during any period of hot weather, but the incidence in temperate climates increases with the prolongation of a heat wave. A diminution or cessation of sweating before onset of acute symptoms may be observed and is indicative of a breakdown of the heat regulatory mechanism. The exact cause of the cessation of sweating is not known. Persons mildly afflicted may reveal no premonitory symptoms. Others may complain of headache, vertigo, faintness, or abdominal distress. Delirium may develop in the severely afflicted patient.

Pyrexia and prostration are significant findings on physical examination. A rectal temperature greater than 106°F is a grave prognostic sign. Internal body temperatures as high as 110°F have been observed. The skin is hot and dry, and sweating is absent. The pulse rate is increased, and respirations are rapid and weak. Systolic blood pressure may be elevated. The tendon reflexes may be diminished. Clinical evidence of circulatory collapse may be observed. Examination of the blood and urine may show few alterations from the normal. A leukocytosis is characteristic. A temporary retention of nitrogenous products with albumin and casts in the urine may be noted, as well as a decrease of total body potassium. The electrocardiogram may show, in addition to tachycardia and sinus arrhythmia, flattening and subsequent inversion of the T wave and depression of the S-T segment. The roentgenogram may show a detectable decrease in the size of the cardiac silhouette. Venous pressures more than double the control level have been noted in normal persons exposed to high temperatures. The extent to which such elevations are due to increase venous return to the heart, or to early failure of this organ, or to a combination has not been clearly defined. It has been suggested that the elevation of venous pressure may be responsible for the diminished sweating, but proof for this concept is lacking.

If the patient survives 24 or 48 hr of pyrexia, and acute renal failure does not develop, recovery may be anticipated. One attack of heat pyrexia renders a person susceptible to future attacks. Extensive parenchymal damage to various organs, either from hyperpyrexia per se or from petechial hemorrhages, may complicate recovery. The brain, heart, kidneys, and liver have been the sites of petechial hemorrhages. Shibolet et al. reported increased fibrinolysis, afibrinogenemia, and especially brain damage in fatal cases of heat stroke which showed multiple hemorrhages. Low prothrombin valves have been observed by several investigators.

MANAGEMENT. Heat pyrexia requires heroic emergency measures. Time is most important. The patient should be placed in a cool place with adequate circulation of fresh air and with most of the clothing removed. Since the pathogenesis of the condition involves a failure of the heat-regulating mechanism with cessation of sweating, external means of heat dissipation must be substituted for those temporarily absent. An ice water bath is drastic treatment for an acutely ill person, but there is no effective substitute. Immersion in ice water does not induce shock or stimulate significant cutaneous vasoconstriction. An ice tub bath should be given with a minimum of delay. The patient should be watched constantly by a nurse or physician, and the rectal temperature should be taken repeatedly. The bath may be discontinued when the core temperature falls below 103°F. The treatment should be resumed if it recrudesces. Ice water sponge baths, rubbing with ice, wet sheets, and an electric fan are ineffective substitutes. Following the bath the patient should be placed in a cool, well-ventilated room. Massage of the skin aids in the acceleration of heat loss and stimulates return of the cool peripheral blood to the overheated brain and viscera. Stimulants such as epinephrine and narcotics are contraindicated. Intravenous saline solution may be recommended if the patient is not in cardiac failure and if the prepyrexic clinical state does not contraindicate it. Fresh blood, fibrinogen solutions, and possibly glucocorticoids should be prescribed (without waiting for laboratory confirmation) if afibrinogenemia is suspected. Several days of convalescence may be required after such an insult.

Although most patients die or recover completely, occasionally survivors have severe and permanent brain damage.

REFERENCES

Clinicopathologic Conference: A Sixty-Five-Year-Old Woman with Heat Stroke, Am. J. Med., 43:113, 1967.

Collins, K. J., and J. S. Weiner: Endocrinological Aspects of Exposure to High Environmental Temperatures, Physiol. Rev., 48:785, 1968.

Knochel, J. P., W. R. Beisel, E. G. Herndon, Jr., E. S. Gerad, and K. G. Barry: The Renal, Cardiovascular, Hematologic and Serum Electrolyte Abnormalities of Heat Stroke, Am. J. Med., 30.299, 1961.

Leithead, C.: Prevention of the Disorders Due to Heat, Roy. Soc. Trop. Med. Hygiene, 61:739, 1967.

Menard, D.: Evaluation of Heat Stress under Working Conditions, Industry and Tropical Health VI: Proc. of the Sixth Conference of the Industrial Council for Tropical Health, Oct. 25–27, 1966, Boston, Harvard School of Public Health, 1967.

Shibolet, S., S. Fisher, T. Gilat, H. Bank, and H. Heller: Fibrinolysis and Hemorrhages in Fatal Heatstroke, New Engl. J. Med., 266:169, 1962.

Yoshimura, H., K. Ogata, and S. Itoh (Eds.): "Essential Problems in Climatic Physiology: A Tribute to Professor Yaskuno," Kyoto, Nandodo, 1960.

126 COLD INJURY AND HYPOTHERMIA

Albert R. Behnke and
Ralph W. Brauer

COLD INJURY

In warfare, cold has been of prime concern as the most disabling environmental stress. In Korea during the winter of 1950–1951, there were approximately 8,000 injuries due to cold; about two-thirds of these were evacuated to Japan and the United States for continued treatment. Exposure to both wet and dry cold, not only of ground troops but also of aviators and shipwreck survivors, emphasizes the importance of protection, particularly of hands and feet, and of acclimatization.

In biology and medicine, dynamic progress has been made in cryobiology and in applications of hypothermia in surgery and in therapy. Hypothermia combined with hyperbaric oxygenation shows promise of eliminating complications arising from hypoxia.

The temperature ranges of concern are (1) very low temperatures, often associated with freezing of some water in tissues, (2) hypothermic temperatures which are in the range of a few degrees above freezing to a level below deep body temperature, and (3) reduced temperatures which are compensated for by physiologic adjustments. At freezing and hypothermic levels, cold injury embraces frostbite and immersion foot.

Local Cold Injury

DIRECT AND INDIRECT MECHANISMS OF INJURY. Frostbite and other lesions due to cold have been intensively studied in man and animals but the results of these investigations have not resolved controversies in regard to underlying pathology and therapeutic measures. Mechanisms of freezing injury can be separated into phenomena which affect cells and extracellular fluids (direct effects) and those which disrupt the function of organized tissues and integrity of circulation (indirect effects).

Certain *direct effects* have been delineated with unequivocal clarity. When tissue freezes, ice crystals form, and concomitantly, solutes in the residual liquid become concentrated. It is clear from a study of a histologic section of tissue fixed while frozen to preserve distortion by ice crystals that the physical dislocation during slow freezing is extreme. Ice crystals many times the size of individual cells form, but only in the extracellular spaces. There is ample evidence that large ice crystals can develop between cells in soft tissue without producing irreversible injury as long as the percentage of water frozen does not exceed a critical amount. In hamster experiments it has been demonstrated that freezing at temperatures as low as −6°C for periods up to 1 hr and the presence of large quantities of ice crystals in the skin and subcutaneous tissue are compatible with full recovery and absence of peripheral lesions. Of prime importance clinically is the observation that trauma induced by bending a frozen extremity resulted in lesions which grossly and microscopically resemble frostbite in man.

A major source of damage to living cells during freezing and thawing appears to be the deleterious effect of strong salt solutions which develop during formation and dissolution of ice; changes in the proportions of lipids and phospholipids in the cell membrane are also of great importance. The discovery of the protective value of such substances as glycerol and dimethylsulfoxide, which enter cells and prevent freezing injury during comparatively slow cooling to and rewarming from low temperatures, represents a significant advance. This method has been used extensively in banking spermatoza for subsequent artificial insemination in the bovine species. It has not been possible, however, to protect organs in this manner since the protective substance must be delivered to all cells.

Turning now to the *indirect effects* of cold on organized tissue, vascular stasis and ensuing derangements appear to be the major cause of tissue injury. There is abundant experimental evidence that the fulminating vascular reaction and stasis which supervene are associated with production of histaminelike substances which increase the permeability of the capillary bed. Within blood vessels, cellular elements aggregate. Irreversible occlusion of small blood vessels by cell masses has been demonstrated in thawed tissue following freezing injury. Structural damage of the frozen tissue simulates damage produced by burns.

CLINICAL CONSIDERATIONS. Local cold injury may be divided into freezing (frostbite) and nonfreezing (immersion foot) injuries. The two types may be observed in the same extremity or in different extremities in the same individual, e.g., trench foot, freezing of the hands and nonfreezing of the feet of shipwreck survivors. It is important to recognize differences in clinical appearance, signs and symptoms; underlying pathologic derangements; and sequelae of the two entities which may require divergent courses of therapy. The diagnosis of freezing versus nonfreezing injury can be made generally on the basis of history and clinical manifestations.

Immersion Foot

In this entity, observed in shipwreck survivors or in soldiers (trench foot) whose feet have been wet but not freezing cold for prolonged periods, there is primarily injury to nerve and muscle tissue, with no gross or irreparable pathologic changes in blood vessels and skin. The clinical picture reflects primary hypoxic trauma giving rise to three clearly recognizable conditions: (1) *ischemia*, denoted by a pale pulseless extremity; (2) *hyperemia*, characterized by a bounding pulsatile circulation in red swollen painful feet; and (3) *posthyperemic* recovery period. The initial cold-induced vasoconstriction, increased blood viscosity, and impaired oxygen transport in the ischemic state are aggravated by such factors as undernutrition, general hypothermia, dehydration, and trauma from relatively fixed, pendant extremities. The problem of rewarming is critical in these patients during the stage of ischemia, when overheating of tissue may lead to gangrene. In the state of hyperemia, the red swollen feet require judicious cooling. Severe cases may show muscular weakness, atrophy, ulceration, and gangrene of superficial areas. The sequelae of even milder injuries are sensitivity to cold and pain on weight bearing, which may be severe and last for many years.

Frostbite

In true frostbite, in contrast with immersion foot, the blood vessels may be severely or irreparably injured, the circulation of blood ceases, and the vascular beds of the frozen tissues are occluded by agglutinated cell aggregates and thrombi. The cutaneous injury consists in part of separation of the epidermal-dermal interface. There is a distinction between direct injury to cells and the subsequent fulminating vascular reaction and stasis which precede tissue necrosis. In the early postthawing stage much of the intravascular clumping is reversible. However, with the passage of time, clumped red cells within vessels in injured tissue lose their morphologic identity and take on the appearance of a homogeneous, hyalinaceous plug. It has been shown experimentally that much of the intravascular aggregation following freezing injury can be reversed, and microcirculatory perfusion improved when low molecular weight dextran is given intravenously shortly after injury.

The discouraging clinical aspects of cold injury, which present a myriad of pathologic derangements, stem from its origin. In the military, cold injury is often the badge of depression, demoralization, and defeat. It afflicts isolated scattered units with their heavy toll of wounded. Lack of food, equipment, shelter, and warmth make inevitable the disastrous injury inflicted by cold. Civilians, apart from persons who engage in expeditions which take them into snow and ice and to hypoxic altitudes, are frequently victims of circumstances associated with vagrancy and alcoholism. In both military and civilian life the physician will be confronted with tissues not frozen, but in a thawed, macerated condition. The manner of rewarming, slow or rapid, generally may be irrelevant. If thawing becomes necessary, the consensus is to use well-stirred water at about 40°C (140°F) until flushing extends to the distal parts but no longer. The rationale that led to immersion at above body temperature was based on experimental work with animals in which the conditions of the tests were not those which usually pertain to freezing in man. German experience in World War II and Swiss experience in treatment of Alpine cold exposure placed emphasis on warming the "core" of the body before treating the local area of frostbite. Heat was applied to the trunk of the body and subsequently the frozen part was placed in water at 10 to 15°C, then increased 5°C every 5 min up to 40°C but no higher.

Sympathectomy is a specific measure for the treatment of frostbite. Shumacker believes that operative sympathetic denervation is indicated as soon after injury as is possible in any good-risk patient who has sustained frostbite of such severity as to indicate likely development of gangrene and loss of tissue. For the late sequelae of frostbite, the benefits of sympathectomy are well established.

SEQUELAE OF FROSTBITE INJURY. A follow-up of 100 Korean cold-injury casualties revealed that both after 4 and after 13 years, there was excessive sweating, pain, cold feet, numbness, abnormal color, and joint symptomatology. Symptoms were more severe during the winter months or on exposure to cold. Characteristic physical findings (after 4 years) were tissue loss and scarring, abnormal nails, discoloration and depigmentation, hyperhydrosis, and on x-ray, osteoporosis and cystic defects in bone near joint surfaces. Patients who had had sympathectomy were almost free of complaints.

Prevention of Cold Injury

Assiduous effort has been made to develop protective equipment and to indoctrinate personnel by "hardening" in cold environment. Although a period of several generations is perhaps required to confer a "Patagonian" ability to exist with little protection in subzero weather, nevertheless, a degree of acclimatization is possible over a period of months to graded exposure to cold which should render individuals resistant who otherwise might become casualties.

COLD ACCLIMATIZATION. Cold acclimatization represents a state of increased resistance to cold injury and is the result of exposure to a cold but tolerable environment. Adaptative responses are *circulatory adjustments* protecting the temperatures of exposed portions of the body; *metabolic adaptation* results in greater heat production to compensate for increased heat loss; and *behavioral and neural adaptations* which minimize either the actual cold stress or the discomfort resulting from physiologically tolerable hypothermia. In contrast with heat acclimatization, it is not possible to delineate adaptive physiologic changes to cold. Nevertheless, primitive peoples live at zero temperatures wearing little or no clothing; pain perception is less in persons who work periodically with their hands in ice water such as fishermen; and military personnel shiver less during test cold exposure after training in the arctic. Comparison of temperature patterns and incidence of shivering during sleep show two distinct adaptive responses. In one, displayed by cold-acclimatized young Norwegian subjects, relatively high skin temperatures are maintained at the expense of intense shivering throughout the night, but ability develops to sleep despite bouts of shivering. The second response, displayed in extreme degree by Australian aborigines, entails marked temperature drop of the body as a whole accompanied by minimal shivering. For restoration, the natives depend upon heat absorption in the morning; hence, a tendency to welcome or worship the sun.

HYPOTHERMIA

Levels of Hypothermia and Metabolism

The moderate range of hypothermia, useful in general surgery and relatively safe, is about 28 to 34°C; deep or profound hypothermia is in the range below 28°C to about 0°C, which is compatible with survival of small mammals for limited periods of time. In man, not until cooling has reduced deep body temperature to less than 30°C is contact with the environment lost. Lowering the body temperature decreases oxygen consumption without jeopardizing vital functions. For every degree of centigrade reduction in body temperature, metabolism decreases 6.5 percent. Thus at 30°C, oxygen consumption is about 50 percent of normal, and at this temperature complete circulatory arrest can be maintained for as long as 8 to 10 min. In man, there is a high incidence of ventricular fibrillation at temperatures below 28°C. It is possible that the heart with its high extraction requirement for oxygen may be inadequately supplied by cold oxygen-bound hemoglobin. There is some evidence that hyperbaric oxygen greatly reduces the tendency of the hypothermic heart to fibrillate.

Immersion Hypothermia

Responses to cold water immersion may be classified as (1) stimulatory, deep body temperature normal to 35°C (95°F); (2) depressant, deep body temperature 35 to 30°C; and (3) critical, deep body temperature 30 to 25°C (86 to 77°F).

CARDIOVASCULAR RESPONSES. The long-distance swimmer is able to maintain a normal deep body temperature for periods of 15 to 25 hr or more under conditions in which water and skin temperatures (15°C, 59°F, or lower) are some 38°F less than deep body temperature. Such data lend support to the useful concept of a body core insulated by a body shell, which in the case of the distance swimmer consists of a substantial thickness of fat. With vasoconstriction operative in cold water, there is a virtual cutoff of peripheral circulation, which greatly reduces heat loss. There is great individual variability in heat loss when the body is immersed in cold water. The relatively obese swimmer may maintain a normal rectal temperature for 2 hr without shivering in 16°C water. A lean man under the same conditions, despite violent shivering, may experience a fall in rectal temperature of several degrees and become incapacitated from rigor. In hypersensitive persons, immersion in cold water may be followed by vascular spasm, vomiting, and syncope—a histamine-type reaction.

In tests of volunteers immersed to the neck in cold water (5 to 15°C), there was initial vasoconstriction and slight rise of rectal temperature, blood pressure, and pulse rate. The heart rate then decreases, presumably an effect of lowered temperature on the pacemaker. In contrast with bradycardia associated with inhalation of oxygen at normal and high pressures, bradycardia in the cold bath is not abolished by atropine or vagotomy. At a rectal temperature of 30°C (86°F), arrhythmias may appear, and atrial fibrillation is observed. In the dog, when deep body temperature declines to about 25°C (77°F), blood pressure may fall sharply, and at 22°C, ventricular fibrillation brings about death.

REWARMING. In contrast to the equivocal procedure of rapid rewarming of a frozen extremity in man is the mandatory (which may be lifesaving) measure of rapid rewarming in water (45°C, 113°F) of persons removed from cold water. Otherwise, a precipitous fall in deep body temperature of several degrees may follow return of blood flow through the cold peripheral tissues. It was observed, for example, that a volunteer removed from a cold bath and warmed in air on a hot Washington summer day shivered for a period of about 2 hr. An individual rewarmed in the bath, however, must be removed prior to return of deep body temperature to normal, in order to forestall circulatory collapse from vasodilatation and excessive diversion of cardiac output to peripheral tissues.

Clinical Uses of Low Temperatures

LOCALIZED APPLICATION. Extensive application of low temperatures has been made in recent years, notably in preservation of viability and banking of cells and tissues. Two basic uses of cryogenic temperatures encompass selective destruction by freezing in cryosurgery as well as preservation of biologic material. A system, for example, for cryogenic surgery has been developed which can be applied to any part of the body. Practical advantages are safety and hemostasis; the results in therapeutic management of tumors have been encouraging. If blood is cooled ultra-rapidly to the temperature of liquid nitrogen and then rapidly thawed, only a few cells are hemolyzed. This technique has been employed routinely on Naval hospital ships serving the battlefield. Mention has been made of the notable discovery that glycerol protects certain cells from freezing. This has made possible preservation of red blood cells, spermatozoa, and other viable materials in their native condition.

Hypothermia combined with hyperbaric oxygenation has been employed with notable success in harvesting, preserving, and transplanting organs, chiefly the kidney.

Local gastric hypothermia has been used effectively to control upper gastrointestinal bleeding from esophageal varices, hemorrhagic gastritis, and gastric and duodenal ulcers. This form of treatment is primarily useful in patients for whom definitive surgery must be delayed or avoided.

Medical Problems Relating to the Use of Hypothermia in Surgery

Periods of ischemia sufficient to permit surgical intervention can be tolerated by critical organs such as the brain and heart, provided that tissue temperature has been lowered to reduce metabolism before blood supply is interrupted. Hypothermia can be induced with light anesthesia and surface cooling or, more effectively, by means of pump-oxygenators to provide extracorporeal circulation. Prior to the introduction of this technique, surgical hypothermia was limited to temperatures of about 28°C; temperatures below 25°C were dangerous. At present, extracorporeal circulation has extended the application of hypothermia to temperatures of 10°C or lower. The principal medical problem arises from disturbances in acid-base balance. One aspect of this complicated problem, apart from large fluctuations in dissolved CO_2 in relation to temperature change, is an oxygen debt incurred by some tissues and an excess lactic acid production. The oxygen debt is present not only during induction of hypothermia but even more so during the period of recovery when cardiac function is less than optimal. The body's buffer mechanisms may be wholly inadequate to regulate pH. Intravenously administered buffers of the amine type (Tris or THAM) have given encouraging results. Coupling of these methods for the induction and maintenance of hypothermia with hyperbaric oxygenation may not only correct the difficulties of pH control, but enhance as well the period during which ischemia may be safely maintained.

With surface cooling the high incidence of ventricular fibrillation at temperatures below 28°C is the most serious complication of hypothermia. A contributing factor is the use of citrated blood; with heparinized blood irreversible ventricular fibrillation is not a problem. In view of the effectiveness of hyperbaric oxygenation in controlling ligature-induced ventricular fibrillation in dogs, it would appear that this modality may well diminish hypothermic cardiac irritability related to tissue hypoxia. With employment of the pump-oxygenator, however, the problem of ventricular fibrillation appears to have been circumvented.

Gastric hemorrhage occurs in animals cooled to low temperatures, and this condition may occur in man. In the rabbit, massive hemorrhage occurs from the fundus of the stomach. A similar hemorrhagic lesion is induced in rabbits at normal temperature after injection of posterior pituitary extract. It is due to intense gastric vasoconstriction and resultant reduction in volume and increase in acidity of gastric juice secreted. *It can be prevented by neutralizing gastric contents.*

Lastly, at temperatures around 10°C, with circulatory arrest, conditions favor intravascular clumping of cellular elements, which was mentioned earlier in connection with freezing injury. Cellular aggregates as part of a "sludging" phenomenon may deprive the brain of blood supply and lead to neurologic damage and possibly death.

REFERENCES

Brown, I. W., Jr., and B. G. Cox (Eds.): "Hyperbaric Medicine," Third Internat. Congress, Publ. 1404, Nat. Acad. Sci. Nat. Res. Council, Washington, 1966.

Burton, A. C., and O. G. Edholm: "Man in a Cold Environment," London, Edward Arnold & Co., 1955.

Hart, J. S. (Ed.): Proceeding of the International Symposium on Altitude and Cold, Federation Proceedings, 28:933–1321, 1969.

Taylor, A. C. (Ed.): Hypothermia, Ann. N.Y. Acad. Sci., 80:285–550, 1959.

Viereck, E. (Ed.): IV. Frostbite. Proc. Symposia Arctic Med. and Biol., Arctic Aeromedical Lab, Fort Wainwright, Alaska, 1964.

127 DISORDERS DUE TO ALTERATIONS IN BAROMETRIC PRESSURE

Albert R. Behnke

Introduction

Since 1958, man has landed on the moon, orbited the earth in excursions as long as 2 weeks, explored the ocean floor to depths of 650 ft (20.7 atm), and extended his ability to work effectively in the dry, pressurized environment to simulated depths of 1,000 ft (31.3 atm). The hyperbaric oxygen environment is being exploited in medicine through operation of numerous single- and multiple-unit pressure chambers. Pressurized tunneling is required routinely for the construction of sewage conduits, vehicular tunnels, and underground rapid transit systems. The recreational and exploratory aspects of *scuba* diving (self-contained underwater breathing apparatus) claimed the interest of several million enthusiasts. These dynamic developments make it necessary for the physician to be aware of the physiologic problems, hazards, and therapeutic measures connected with alterations in barometric pressure in the effort to control potential accidents.

Injury arises from too rapid ascent (aeroembolism, decompression sickness); indirectly from cold, hypoxia, nitrogen narcosis, hyperventilation tetany, and overexertion; and in closed breathing systems from oxygen toxicity and carbon dioxide excess. Mishaps are caused by logistic failure (the empty gas bottle); equipment deficiencies, notably lack of recompression chambers; and casual organization. Always in imminent danger of drowning, the scuba diver (breathing unnaturally through a mouthpiece and with head surrounded by water) often complicates the environmental hazard with his obsession to establish new records with diving gear which for the novice should be restricted to "free ascent" depths (without need for recompression). The practice, particularly among adolescents, of breath holding underwater is conducive to hypoxic heart failure, especially during the course of heavy exertion required in swimming. Too rapid ascent of scuba divers may overexpand the lungs and give rise to air embolism, pneumothorax, and subcutaneous emphysema. "Squeeze" effects may involve the eye, middle ear and mastoid cells, and paranasal sinuses, and occasionally produce minute gas aggregates in pulp of diseased teeth. Rapid decompression after sojourn at diving depths, and even following rapid ascent to simulated or actual high altitude, may initiate bubble evolution and decompression sickness. Diving tables evolved on an empirical basis, for the most part from fragmentary tests, afford high (96 to 99 percent) but not complete protection against decompression sickness. In carefully supervised decompressions of personnel attending a hospital hyperbaric chamber, the complication of scotoma was observed in 3 out of 1,000 otherwise uneventful decompressions. Oxygen inhalation during at least part of the decompression period provides adequate safeguard.

Experience with work in compressed air dictates the likelihood that all decompressions (not employing oxygen inhalation) conducted in accord with current diving tables are attended by some degree of nascent bubble evolution in circulating blood. Of importance to hospital personnel is the abrupt onset of post-decompression malaise, which may be related to liberation of painless "silent bubbles" but which nevertheless may induce hypoxic liberation into the circulation of such substances as proteolytic enzymes, peptides, and potassium ions. In rapidly decompressed animals, and occasionally in man at autopsy, fat emboli and even bone marrow cells are seen in the lungs and brain.

Advances in recompression therapy emphasize the value of oxygen inhalation at tolerance pressures (27 psi) without resorting to high air or helium-oxygen atmospheres except in unusual circumstances. Dramatic recoveries have occurred when prompt treatment has been accorded seemingly moribund divers. Even divers rendered paraplegic as a result of delay in treatment due to lack of on-site pressure chambers nevertheless may recover motor function following prolonged pressurization and appropriate follow-up hospital therapy. Promising advances in treatment relate to the value of fluid (dextran) administration to counteract hemoconcentration frequently observed in serious cases, notably in aviation personnel who have not been recompressed to hyperbaric atmospheres. Further, success in promoting survival of rapidly decompressed animals has followed inhalation of aerosols which incorporate heparin and antispasmolytic drugs.

It is essential that the physician have available a schedule of emergency procedures when calls are received to care for injured divers. Despite the absence of "on-the-spot" recompression chambers, it may be lifesaving to administer oxygen immediately and fluids at the first sign of hemoconcentration. Some benefit may accrue from a lowered head position to minimize brain embolization and from the recumbent position to ensure rest in the effort to minimize growth of bubbles.

Hyperbaric Chambers

Catastrophic fires have occurred in oxygen-enriched atmospheres at normal and even hypobaric pressures, but the hazard is compounded in the hyperbaric chamber. In a fire costing two lives, the pressurized chamber (3.9 atm, 95 ft) contained 36 percent helium, 36 percent nitrogen, and *28 percent oxygen*. To remove carbon dioxide, a scrubber system utilizing an electric motor was employed to circulate an oxygen-enriched atmosphere. Spontaneous combustion occurred in the scrubber filter and within 15 sec the chamber was enveloped in flame; within 1 min the pressure had increased to 7.9 atm (260 ft) due to the intense heat. *In an oxygen-enriched atmosphere in contrast with air atmospheres, there are no immediately effective measures to quench a fire.* In large chambers in which attending personnel are present, it

is mandatory that oxygen be administered to patients by means of closed systems which cannot enrich the ambient air. There is danger of implosion if sealed capsules or containers are brought into the pressurized chamber.

With reference to the physical examination, it is essential that personnel be free from pulmonary pathology (cysts, chronic bronchiolitis) conducive to aeroembolism. To ensure symptom-free decompression, oxygen inhalation is effective. The National Research Council brochure provides guidelines for safe operation of hyperbaric chambers, but indoctrination at successfully operating installations is strongly recommended.

PRIMARY PRESSURE PHENOMENA

Effect of Pressure per se and of Barotrauma

Normally some tissues of the body are subjected to compressive or distending pressure (the arteries, vertebras, and lower extremities) of the order of 100 to 200 mm Hg (1 to 2 psi). Pressure gradients may also exist in an individual who is immersed in water up to his neck. By contrast, the pressure of the atmosphere (sea level, 760 mm Hg, 14.7 psi, equivalent to 33 ft of seawater) can be increased to more than 30 atm in the hyperbaric chamber without gross signs of impairment. Some individuals, however, may experience *compression* joint pain, which subsides with slower application of pressure. Initially during rapid compression when equilibration is incomplete between inert gas in blood and tissue, there may be an "osmotic" effect affecting hydration of joint cartilage which may account for compression pain in susceptible individuals. At extreme pressures (31.3 to 37.5 atm, 1,000 to 1,200 ft) compression of protoplasm (pressure per se) may be responsible for tremors and somnolence reported in human tests, which are not attributable to narcosis. Small animals tolerate much higher pressures (100 atm) without gross impairment.

Density of inhaled gas increases linearly with pressure, but the work of breathing is roughly proportional to the square root of pressure. Compared with air, the equivalent pressure breathing helium-oxygen is reduced by a factor of 7. Respiratory impairment is not a limiting factor at deep depths. Test data show that man can spend long periods of time at the depths of the continental shelves and perform moderate work.

In air (3 atm) despite the increased density, emphysematous patients may report improvement during and following sojourn under pressure. However, respiration conducted with valvular systems may cause respiratory distress. Hence, it is mandatory *that there be physician-technician trial of all respiratory equipment prior to patient usage at all pressures.*

In contrast to innocuous application of great external forces, equally distributed over the body, is the small pressure difference (50 to 100 mm Hg) which serves to distend blood vessels and induce edema in occluded sinal (aerosinusitis) and aural (aerotitis media) spaces.

Following hyperbaric oxygen therapy, patients may experience this cupping effect during sleep, when the auditory tubes are not opened periodically by swallowing. The most frequent cause of blockage of auditory tubes (which usually is only relative in relation to rate of pressure application) is acute and chronic infection of the nasopharynx. At any one time as many as one-third of submarine personnel may show varying grades of barotrauma. A convenient classification employed in the U.S. Navy is *grade* 0 (normal), 1 (redness of Shrapnell's membrane and along the manubrium), 2 (redness of entire membrane), 3 (same as grade 2 plus fluid or fluid and bubbles in the middle ear), and 4 (blood in the middle ear, perforation of the tympanic membrane or both). These changes are clearly apparent on routine otoscopic inspection. Remarkably there is no residual impairment of auditory acuity in the speech range incurred by this type of trauma. Deafness for higher tones is frequent in divers and implicates noise as the etiologic factor. *Specific therapy is not required for barotrauma;* healing in the author's experience is spontaneous and rarely complicated by secondary infection. In grade 4 (blood in middle ear) the otologist should be consulted.

Complications Arising from Overinflation of the Lungs

If a diver holds his breath on ascent to the surface, the intrapulmonic pressure tends to increase relative to hydrostatic pressure. Excess pressures of 80 mm Hg or higher overinflate the lungs, rupture blood vessels, and force gas along dissecting planes. With the first inhalation of air by the diver on reaching the surface, gas is aspirated into pulmonary veins and disseminated to the central nervous system to bring about collapse. This type of accident has occurred 23 times in 150,000 submarine training escapes. In one instance death followed a too rapid ascent from the shallow depth of 15 ft. It is not an uncommon accident in scuba diving. Acute collapse during decompression has been reported in tunnel workers. The signs and symptoms were those of aero-embolism, not decompression sickness. In several of the patients lung cysts were identified. Treatment of aero-embolism calls for immediate recompression with oxygen inhalation. This disability can be prevented by physical examination to exclude pulmonary pathology (cysts, costophrenic adhesions, bronchiolitis) and by proper training. Routine free ascents can be made from depths of 100 ft if exhalation is continuous. The practice, however, is not encouraged.

SECONDARY PRESSURE PHENOMENA RELATED TO INCREASED PARTIAL PRESSURE OF GASES

Narcotic Action of Nitrogen

When the air pressure in a chamber is raised above 3 atm, the increased partial pressure of nitrogen is associated with changes in mood, notably euphoria, and impaired judgment and motor performance. The effects are similar to those induced by intoxicants, such as alcohol. Although all individuals are in varying degrees narcotized at diving depths, emotionally stable persons react to the stress by compensatory effort and are able to carry out an assigned task (slowly at high pressures) until consciousness is lost. The unstable person is incapable of purposeful effort and gives way to emotional aberrations characteristic of some alcoholics. Sophisticated studies have provided quantitative assessment of the impairment. If, for example, the electroencephalogram is recorded at normal pressure when a subject is attempting to solve an arithmetical problem, there is a blocking of occipital alpha rhythm which at increased pressure ("nitrogen threshold") disappears after a latent period. The period of latency is inversely proportional to the square of the pressure. Of interest is the fact that at relatively low pressures (2.5 atm, 50 ft) not associated with overt impairment, a nitrogen effect on the brain may be detected. The nitrogen narcotic phenomenon, as an innocuous stress without residual impairment, may be applied in psychic evaluation of individuals. The lack of narcotic effect of helium makes diving to depths of 1,000 ft feasible.

Oxygen Poisoning

Although inhalation of oxygen at high pressures (OHP) may give rise to limiting pulmonary and CNS alterations, it has been breathed routinely up to 3 atm during decompression of divers, in the treatment of decompression sickness, and in hyperbaric chambers in hospitals. Oxygen (OHP) therapy is possible because there is a latent period preceding overt signs and symptoms, during which cardiac function is not impaired, and initial untoward reactions are reversible when air breathing is resumed. Tolerance time for inhalation of oxygen at higher pressures is greatly extended by short intervals of air inhalation in accord with the outline in Table 127-1.

Table 127-1. GUIDE FOR ADMINISTRATION OF HYPERBARIC OXYGEN DURING DECOMPRESSION AND IN RECOMPRESSION THERAPY
Based on U.S. Navy experience

Pressure, psi	Unit exposure (U.E.) intervals, min		No. of U.E. for routine inhalation*
	Oxygen	Air	
27	20	5	1, 2, 3
27 to 13	40	...	1
13	20	5	1, 2, 3
13 to 0	40	...	1

* Depending upon duration of previous hyperbaric air exposure (decompression), or the condition of the patient during recompression.

Subjectively, inhalation of oxygen (OHP) is stimulating and may be similar to an adrenergic response. Adrenal, thyroid, and pituitary hormones, exercise, increased CO_2 tensions, elevated metabolism, and apprehension shorten the latent period of comparative well-being. On the other hand, individuals *at rest*, following overnight fast, and phlegmatic in disposition have tolerated the inhalation of oxygen (99 percent) for periods of 30 min at the usually convulsive level of 4 atm. Of clinical importance are experimental data which support a durable impression that hypoxemic patients tolerate unusually high pulmonary oxygen tensions. Venous admixture of arterial blood of dogs produced by surgical shunt, for example, prevented the pulmonary damage observed in control animals (Winter et al.). Pulmonary injury (OHP) may not be a direct (phosgene) effect but a response mediated by the same endocrine factors which augment neurotoxic reactions. Notably, cardiac function is not impaired as is respiration, despite the inhibitory action of OHP on many enzyme systems, particularly those containing essential sulfhydryl groups. Thus the heart in anesthetized dogs may beat for periods of 1 hr or longer following respiratory paralysis, and succumbs only after asphyxial concentrations of CO_2 ($+100$ to 200 mm Hg) have accumulated in the lungs.

Limitations to OHP therapy pertain to toxic pulmonary effects and striking CNS response. A serious drawback is not only lack of knowledge of the specific etiology, but also the variability of individual response and unpredictability of tissue oxygen tensions. At 3 atm (oxygen) arterial blood may contain 6 vol percent of oxygen in solution (pO_2: 2,000 mm Hg). As a result of vasoconstriction (a direct oxygen effect) or vasodilation (a CO_2 effect), there may be widely fluctuating tensions (70 to 1,400 mm Hg) of oxygen in mixed venous blood withdrawn from the right ventricle. The inference is that O_2 tensions at the cellular level also fluctuate widely.

In man, pulmonary (and tracheal) irritation is elicited at lower pressure levels (0.6 to 2 atm), while neurotoxic effects are observed at higher pressures. In carefully monitored studies, it was found that healthy men could breathe oxygen (2 atm) for about 8 hr before significant (5 to 10 percent) decreases in vital capacity occurred. After 8 to 12 hr of inhalation, the symptoms, progressive in intensity, were burning sensation on deep inspiration, carinal irritation, cough, and dyspnea. At higher pressures, the pulmonary limit for oxygen inhalation has not been determined. In earlier tests there were no pulmonary symptoms at the end of 4 hr of oxygen inhalation at 3 atm (Behnke).

Neurotoxic effects terminate the relatively benign latent period after about 2 hr of oxygen inhalation at 3 atm. Untoward responses at from 3 to 4 atm are twitching or tremors of facial muscles (notably lips and eyebrows), restlessness, anxiety, periodic waves of nausea, occasional vomiting, diminished visual acuity, narrowing of visual fields, numbness of fingers and toes, reversal of pulse rate, sharp rise in diastolic pressure, auditory hallucinations and other aura, fainting (occasionally), and violent convulsive seizures. Residual effects following seizures have not been observed in man. In small animals (which have severe limitations for comparative studies, e.g., high metabolic rates, chronic pulmonary disease), neuromuscular impairment and brain lesions have been reported following extreme exposures.

Physical examination of persons subjected to OHP should include tests of visual and pulmonary function, EEG, and for monitoring purposes, pulse rate and blood pressure.

Alteration of Carbon Dioxide Tension

Carbon dioxide not only enhances the toxicity of oxygen (a specific CO_2 effect independent of the lowering of pH), but the narcotic effect of nitrogen and other inert gases as well. An elementary assessment of this phenomenon relates CO_2 enhancement to increased cerebral blood flow. During rapid descent in deep sea diving, momentary vertigo and confusion are in part attributed to inadequate exhalation of CO_2 as a result of rapid compression. The effective CO_2 percentage should not exceed 1.5 percent, although percentages of CO_2 up to 5, are fairly well tolerated in submarines for at least 60 hr. There are no reliable data for extended periods of inhalation of high concentrations of CO_2 ($+3$ percent).

In the presence of elevated concentrations of CO_2 during inhalation of oxygen at 1 atm or higher pressures, consciousness may be lost suddenly (oxygen blackout) without onset of dyspnea. Divers working in air at high pressures have tolerated some remarkably high pCO_2 levels (e.g., 57 mm Hg) in arterial blood without distress when using breathing apparatus which prevented adequate pulmonary ventilation. A critical consideration is that warning signs of CO_2 excess at normal pressures may be absent in the pressurized environment. Hyperventilation may induce respiratory alkalosis and tetany. The danger of hypoxemia is greatly enhanced when hyperventilation in air removes the CO_2 stimulus during breath holding.

Uptake of Nitrogen at Increased Pressure

At atmospheric pressure (pN_2: 570 mm Hg) about 9 ml of nitrogen is dissolved per kg of body fluid, and about 55 ml per kg of body fat. In a lean, 70-kg man (7 kg fat) about 400 ml of nitrogen is in body fluids, 100 ml in bone and spinal cord, and 400 ml in fat. About 5.2 liters of blood per min perfuses the nonlipid cellular mass, and only about 0.7 liter of blood perfuses bone and adipose tissue. The half-time for N_2 uptake of various nonlipid tissues varies from 2 to 20 min (98.5 percent saturation in 12 to 120 min), and for organs containing large amounts of lipid (adipose tissue, long bones, spinal cord), half-time uptake may vary from 60 to 120 min (1 to 2 hr) in a lean man. In the United States, the duration of stay of personnel in diving and tunnel operations in air is such that nitrogen uptake is restricted mainly to nonlipid, rapidly saturating tissues. This is not the case in England where operational schedules are more rigorous.

Decompression Procedures

It is evident that decompression time following prolonged exposures will be greatly influenced in air dives by the amount of fat in the body. If exposures are of short duration, the amount of fat is not important as a decompression hazard. Haldane's ratio principle applies to short exposures in compressed air, and it is relatively safe to halve the absolute pressure to permit rapid ascent to the first stop. However, after prolonged (saturation) exposures in the hyperbaric environment, it is becoming increasingly evident that the ratio principle does not apply to *successive stages* of decompression and that only a small pressure head (ΔP) governs inert gas transport from tissues to lungs. In accord with the isobaric ("oxygen window") principle of decompression, ΔP is the difference between arterial and venous oxygen pressures. Hence safe decompression following helium-oxygen saturation exposures at deep depths requires from 10 to 15 min per ft of ascent. The time required for decompression is measured not in hours, but in days. Based on the hypothesis that ΔP can be appreciably elevated above isobaric tissue levels (i.e., inert gas pressure in tissue is never allowed to exceed ambient pressure during decompression), diving tables become in effect "treatment" tables applicable to a state of gas transport not in solution but, in part at least, in bubble form.

Factors Affecting Bubble Formation

After exposure to high pressure or high altitudes (in chambers, unpressurized aircraft), factors conducive to decompression sickness fall into two groups. In the first are conditions which increase gas content of tissues, namely, the amount of fat, degree and duration of exposure, intensity of work, and, in rapid ascent to high altitudes, exercise, which expands the gaseous reservoir with CO_2 accretion and facilitates cavitation. In the second group are variables affecting tissue perfusion and diffusion of gas in transport from tissue as well as surface tension and other biophysical factors affecting blood. Thus age, time of day, disruption of circadian rhythms, dehydration, fright, injury, and postalcoholic residuum seemingly affect gas transport.

Acclimatization

Divers subjected to older decompression schedules for tunnel workers developed a high incidence of bends. It appears that men who expose themselves regularly to compressed air day after day become less susceptible to attacks of decompression sickness. About 14 days are required for maximal effect. Acclimatization is gradually lost when men cease to work in compressed air. The recognition of this phenomenon by Paton and Walder is of practical importance.

DECOMPRESSION SICKNESS

Etiology

The preponderance of experimental data implicates intravascular bubbles as the initiating causal agent. In rapidly decompressed animals circulating bubbles can be observed in arteries and veins; subsequently sequestered bubbles accumulate in veins. Secondary phenomena complicate the simple etiology. Thus fat particles may enter the bloodstream from gas-distended adipose tissue, bone marrow, or even fatty liver cells when present as in alcoholics. The hypothesis has been mentioned that hypoxic cellular destruction may explain such symptoms as malaise or give rise to delayed febrile response.

Signs and Symptoms

Sequestration of nascent gas bubbles in vascular beds of tissues and organs gives rise to a remarkable array of dissimilar syndromes (Table 127-2). In British classifica-

Table 127-2. SIGNS AND SYMPTOMS OF DECOMPRESSION SICKNESS

Central nervous system	Cardiorespiratory	Extremities	Skin; systemic
Loss of consciousness	substernal distress	pain	pruritus
Scintillating scotomata	paroxysmal coughing	paresthesia	mottling
Mèniére's syndrome	tachypnea	numbness	rash
Vertigo, aphasia	asphyxia (chokes)	weakness	pallor
Staggering gait	shock	bone necrosis	
Spastic paralysis	hemoconcentration	cartilage destruction	lowered temperature
Sensory loss		edema	fever, sweating
Bladder, bowel paralysis			malaise

tion, pain in the region of joints (bends) is designated Type I (mild); respiratory, cardiovascular, and neurologic involvement is designated Type II (serious), which includes *aeroembolism* arising as explained previously from gas introduced extraneously into the circulation. Type I cases may progress to Type II. The chief problem concerns the early recognition of signs and symptoms and application of recompression therapy.

BENDS. The bends may be described as an aching, radiating type of pain, occasionally synchronous with pulse beat, of gradual onset, progressive in intensity, and felt in the joints, muscles, and bones of the extremities. Response to recompression therapy is immediate (occasionally there is exacerbation of pain if pressure is applied too rapidly), and there is no residual disability with the reservation that the relationship of bends to aseptic bone necrosis remains to be clarified.

CHOKES AND THE SHOCK SYNDROME. A type of asphyxia referred to by early workers as "chokes" may be preceded by several hours of well-being following decompression. An early symptom is a sensation of substernal soreness elicited by deep inspiration which may provoke paroxysmal coughing. Inhalation of cigarette smoke aggravates the untoward reaction. Hemoconcentration and classical signs of circulatory shock are associated with this disability, particularly if onset is gradual.

NEUROLOGIC INVOLVEMENT (CNS). Scintillating scotomata and transient episodes of vertigo and dizziness are not uncommon. The staggering gait and slurred speech simulate drunkenness, and recompression must be resorted to for differential diagnosis. Ménière's syndrome, presumably resulting from infraction of blood supply to the inner ear, was not uncommon in early tunnel workers. In recent decompressions following saturation dives, nerve deafness has been reported. Aeroembolism usually can be recognized as distinct from the neurologic sign of decompression sickness, by abrupt onset, unconsciousness with convulsion, usually focal, and independence of duration of exposure.

Paralysis of spinal cord origin, manifest as a spastic monoplegia or paraplegia, is usually confined to the lower extremities. Areas of hypersensitivity are present above the site of the cord lesion, and paresthesia of sensory paralysis occurs below. *An early premonitory sign is numbness*, which should alert the physician to anticipate a Type II condition rather than bends. There is incontinence of urine and feces following involvement of the lower part of the spinal cord. The imperative requirement to catheterize the bladder in the acute condition may be overlooked. Recovery or at least considerable improvement may occur following prolonged recompression with oxygen, even though many hours may elapse between onset of disability and recompression therapy. Prognosis for ultimate restoration of function cannot be made early since improvement may continue over a 2-year period following injury. Gas bubbles impair blood supply but do not transect the spinal cord!

BONE LESIONS. A serious complication associated with work in pressurized tunnel operations is aseptic bone necrosis, and as many as 75 percent of oldtime workmen show radiographic bone pathology. Frank lesions have not been observed in our Navy divers but have been reported occasionally in divers from other countries. Aseptic bone necrosis is related to the number of times a man has been decompressed, to the pressure level at which he has worked, and to the number of reported bends. Accepted decompression procedures in England, where hours of work are relatively long, are not adequate to prevent bone lesions. Innovations in decompression practice as incorporated into Washington State Tables (1963) greatly extend decompression time by stage rather than uniform decompression. There is good reason to believe that the extended decompression time and *shorter daily exposures* will prevent occurrence of crippling lesions.

Crippling lesions which are the result of juxtaarticular infarction and subsequent deformity and destruction of the joint surface are confined to shoulder and hip joints. By contrast, the knee joint, which is the most common site of bends, is not disabled. *A prime consideration is that the lesions are asymptomatic unless joint surfaces are involved.* The vivid x-ray-visualized lesions in the medullary shaft of long bones are innocuous. An impediment in diagnosis is a latent period of a year or longer before pathologic change becomes manifest. Our lack of definitive knowledge of aseptic bone necrosis is reflected by inability to explain why similar workmen in the same environment remain free from joint and medullary lesions. An essential part of the physical examination *prior to work in compressed air* and at yearly intervals during work in compressed air is radiologic survey of the long bones.

Recompression Treatment of Decompression Sickness and Air Embolism

The value of oxygen therapy without the need for higher air or oxygen pressures has been confirmed for Type I cases (bends), and shows promise also in management of Type II cases including aeroembolism. However, with availability of proper gas mixtures, in the author's opinion, high pressures should be utilized for treatment of serious cases. The outline of oxygen decompression and recompression procedures (Table 127-1), adapted from earlier and current U.S. Navy experience, is a guide for employment of hyperbaric oxygen inhalation. Recompression procedure in the U.S. Navy Diving Manual is to be regarded as standard practice. Occasionally long periods of time measured in days are required for compression therapy to be fully effective. Patients can be kept for weeks (if necessary) at 2.52 atm (50 ft) if there is indication that pressure decrement will cause further deterioration. Occasionally a puzzling relapse may occur during the course of treatment which is not responsive to additional pressure (occasionally to 10 atm). Errors in treatment relate to (1) inadequate time spent at peak pressure when patients are seriously ill—*the condition of the patient must regulate decompression therapy*, (2) failure to apply the compression test to doubtful cases, (3) inadequate medical monitoring during the recompression period, and (4) failure to keep the treated patient near the recompression for a 24-hr period.

ADJUVANTS TO RECOMPRESSION. Oral administration of fluid in the recompression chamber may be followed by return of blood hematocrit to normal. Intravenous fluids may be required to prevent onset of shock. The guidelines by Malette and coworkers (1962) have proved effective in restoration of normal rheology in serious cases of altitude dysbarism which are remarkable often for the many hours that patients have survived during a state of shock. For reasons unknown, heart failure does not occur even when gas embolization is extensive, and aviation patients apparently in extremis have responded quickly to recompression therapy. Follow-up investigations of Cockett have demonstrated the effectiveness of dextran in promoting recovery of rapidly decompressed dogs who otherwise would die.

An emergency tray should provide catheters, tracheal airways, instruments for myringotomy and for relief of pneumothorax, sedative drugs, and needles and syringes (see National Research Council brochure).

Special Problems

SCUBA AND SKIN DIVING. The problems are chiefly administrative, not medical, and require a "tightly-run ship." Instructors should be trained to administer resuscitation in water and to give oxygen. They should be delegated the authority to disqualify the obviously unfit. Under the initial supervision of the physician, the instructors should administer timed pulmonary function and step-up tests of not more than 5-min duration and record the results to provide evaluation of fitness on an individual basis. Divers must be good swimmers ("fit to swim, fit to dive"). Apart from the hazard of drowning, there is the matter of air purity, which is not always easy to ensure if "smog" is compressed. Maximum permissible levels of noxious substances must be reduced proportionately to pressure. Thus carbon monoxide is restricted to 20 ppm, which is one fifth of the permissible level for an 8-hr exposure in vehicular tunnels.

The skin diver must rely upon breath holding. As he descends to depths, the volume of the thorax is diminished. At 100 ft (4 atm) oxygen and nitrogen pressures have increased about threefold and elevated alveolar pO_2 (200 mm Hg) permits extended bottom time. On ascent to the surface the expansion of the thorax reduces the oxygen tension precipitously to hypoxic levels of 25 to 35 mm Hg, and the diver faces imminent collapse. *Competitive breath holding and swimming underwater are dangerous.* Man shows the bradycardic response during apneic underwater diving, which is not prevented by vigorous exercise, and serious arrhythmias have been recorded in healthy men.

MONITORING OF PRESSURIZED TUNNEL WORKERS. Medical monitoring of rugged independent workers who build tunnels is feasible if a small group of men (sometimes no more than three per shift) will report weekly to the physician for definitive but brief tests of fitness (similar to the physical evaluation for divers) and for systematic survey of compression and postcompression responses. These should include the deep inspiratory test and inhalation of cigarette smoke, examination of the skin to detect mottling, and questioning about postpressure malaise in the effort to ascertain presence of "silent" bubbles and adequacy of decompression.

DERANGEMENTS AT HIGH ALTITUDE

Physiologic Considerations

Altitudes of 3,500 to 7,000 ft are noted for salubrious climate. At higher altitudes the decreased partial pressure of oxygen gives rise to arterial hypoxemia. In response to hypoxic stimulation of aortic and carotid chemoreceptors, hyperventilation lowers alveolar CO_2 and brings about respiratory alkalosis. The newcomer to high altitude is thus affected by both hypoxia and alkalosis, which account for typical symptoms and signs of dyspnea, tachycardia, malaise, headache, and insomnia. Maximal heart rate in response to strenuous exertion decreases and pulmonary arterial pressure increases, and these changes are correlated with altitude level.

Acclimatization

The symptoms of acute mountain sickness usually disappear within 3 to 10 days, and their amelioration is hastened by graded exercise. The mountain climber may acclimatize sufficiently during a period of 1 to 3 months at intermediate altitudes so as to enable him to climb Mt. Everest (29,002 ft) with the aid of supplemental oxygen, and Nanga Parbat (26,660 ft) without added oxygen. These feats represent the exceptional acclimatization, but it is limited to about 10 days since rapid deterioration ensues after longer periods at elevations above 25,000 ft. Despite extreme difficulties, physicians and physiologists have spent more than 5 months conducting cardiopulmonary tests at altitudes of 19,000 ft and higher. In regard to permanent residence man cannot live above 18,000 ft. However, Andeans are well adapted to perform strenuous work and to engage in football games for recreation in the hypoxic atmosphere of 15,000 ft.

Characteristics of the Andean

Hurtado and Hultgren and Grover have enumerated morphologic and functional characteristics of the resident reared at high altitudes, namely, (1) decreased weight relative to stature; (2) increased vital capacity and pulmonary ventilation; (3) hypertrophy of the free wall of the right ventricle, increased thickness of the muscle mass of smaller pulmonary vessels, and sustained, hypoxic arteriolar vasoconstriction; (4) increased blood volume, hematocrit, and myoglobin; and (5) greatly increased tissue vascularization. In the above-listed adaptations, attention focuses on the unique properties of the pulmonary circulation. "The vascular wall or 'the container' of the arterial side of the pulmonary circulation is less compliant than that of sea level dwellers. . . . A rigid, fluid-filled system is more responsive to alterations in blood volume, blood flow, and vascular tone in terms of changes in intravascular pressure than is a more compliant system such as the normal pulmonary circulation of the sea level resident."

The Andean descended from generations of inhabitants living continuously at high altitude has attained nearly complete adaptation to a lowered alveolar oxygen tension of 45 mm Hg. He is able to perform strenuous physical labor as exemplified by the incredible cultivation of the slopes of the Andes. Despite the arduous life and deprivations, it is uncommon to find peripheral hypertension, coronary thrombosis, myocardial infarction, or peripheral arteriosclerosis. Blood viscosity associated with the hematocrit range of 40 to 60 percent does not significantly affect blood flow or coagulation. The erythrocytosis is stabilized and differs from the erythremia and attendant thrombocytosis of polycythemia vera. The hypoxic stimulus, specifically erythropoietin, affects strictly erythropoiesis. General myeloid hyperplasia has not been reported.

Chronic Mountain Sickness (Soroche, Monge's Disease)

The Andean, however, is affected by a clinical condition which represents a breakdown in compensation and adaptation to low oxygen tension. Loss of tolerance to the altitude environment, as pointed out by Monge in 1928, may be observed in the striking accentuation of the "normal" erythrocytosis. Hurtado has reported in detail derangements associated with this pathologic condition. In comparison with values (N) characteristic of the healthy native resident at high altitude, hemoglobin values increase to 25 Gm/100 ml (N 21 Gm), and blood hematocrit to 80 (N 60). Blood volume is increased about 50 percent chiefly as a result of erythrocytosis. Plasma volume however is decreased. There is hyperplasia and hyperactivity of bone marrow erythroid cells and increased red cell destruction, but no derangements in leukocytogenesis. The severely impaired ability to work is associated with cyanosis, hypoventilation, lowered alveolar pO_2 and pCO_2, increased cardiac output, and greater pulmonary hypertension and lower systolic blood pressure than are found in the healthy residents. Electrocardiographic findings are consistent with a diagnosis of cor pulmonale.

The features of Monge's disease have much in common with Ayerza's syndrome, or cardiaco negro (erythrocytosis, hyperplasia of bone marrow, cyanosis, dyspnea, and notably pulmonary arterial and arteriolar sclerosis). This entity appears to have a multiple etiology. Of extrinsic interest is similarity of vascular pathology (with pulmonary hypertension) in chronic oxygen poisoning affecting rats exposed to 4 atm air (0.83 atm O_2) for 3 months.

High-altitude Pulmonary Edema

Pulmonary edema occurs in persons who travel within a day or two to elevations of over 9,000 ft and also in acclimatized mountain residents who visit a low altitude for 1 to 3 weeks and then return to a higher elevation. Symptoms usually occur 6 to 36 hr after arrival and consist of dry cough, dyspnea, and a feeling of pain in the lower substernal area. X-rays of the chest in severe cases demonstrate confluent or nodular densities throughout all lung fields. Altitude pulmonary edema is distinct from acute mountain sickness in which symptoms appear promptly on reaching altitude, and do not include cough, dyspnea, or rhonchal respiration. Treatment includes rapid removal to a lower elevation if transportation is available, or hospitalization with bed rest and oxygen therapy. Prevention consists in taking adequate time for altitude ascent, and upon reaching altitude, it is important to avoid overexertion, which may precipitate pulmonary edema in well-acclimatized persons.

CONCLUDING NOTE. The studies of man and lower animals at high altitude present many challenging problems. The remarkable physical feats of the Andean, who subsists largely on a diet of vegetable protein and carbohydrate and does not get peripheral vascular disease despite the stress of heavy work, have no precedent in a European population at sea level. An intriguing problem is whether or not acclimatization (one generation) is associated with the same degree of tissue vascularization conferred by adaptation (several generations).

REFERENCES

Bennett, P. B.: "The Aetiology of Compressed Air Intoxication and Inert Gas Narcosis," New York, Pergamon Press, 1966.

Brown, I. W., Jr., and B. G. Cox (Eds.): "Hyperbaric Medicine," Third Internat. Congress, Publ. 1404, Nat. Acad. Sci. Nat. Res. Council, Washington, 1966.

Cockett, A. T. K., R. M. Nakamura, and J. J. Franks: Recent Findings in the Pathogenesis of Decompression Sickness (Dysbarism), Surgery, 58:384, 1965.

Hart, J. S. (Ed.): Proceedings of the International Symposium on Altitude and Cold, Federation Proceedings, 28:933–1321, 1969.

Hultgren, H. N., and R. F. Grover: Circulatory Adaptation to High Altitude, Annual Rev. Med., 19:119, 1968.

Lambertsen, C. J. (Ed.): "Underwater Physiology," Third Symposium, Baltimore, The Williams & Wilkins Company, 1967. See J. M. Clark and C. J. Lambertsen, p. 439; P. B. Bennett, p. 327; E. E. P. Barnard, p. 156; and M. W. Goodman, p. 165.

Lanphier, E. H., and H. W. Gillen: Management of Sports Diving Accidents, New York J. Med., 63:667, 1963.

McCallum, R. I. (Ed.): "Decompression of Compressed Air Workers in Civil Engineering," Newcastle upon Tyne, Oriel Press, Ltd., 1967.

Malette, W. G., J. B. Fitzgerald, and A. T. K. Cockett: Dysbarism, A Review of Thirty-five Cases with Suggestion for Therapy, Aerospace Med., 33:1132, 1962.

Miles, S.: "Underwater Medicine," 2d ed., Philadelphia, J. B. Lippincott Company, 1966.

Nat. Acad. of Sci. Nat. Res. Council: "Fundamentals of Hyperbaric Medicine," Washington.

U. S. Navy Diving Manual, NAVSHIPS 250–538, Navy Dept., Washington.

128 PROBLEMS OF AIR AND SPACE TRAVEL

Stuart Bondurant

Ordinary air travel imposes so little physiologic stress that most patients who can be moved at all can be moved by air if proper equipment and attendants are available.

Medical problems unique to air travel may be caused by unusual environmental conditions which may be encountered because of limitations of equipment or abnormal operating circumstances.

Many modern aircraft fly at altitudes of 20,000 to 40,000 ft, with cabins pressurized to maintain an effective cabin altitude of less than 7,500 ft (jets) or 9,000 ft (reciprocating engines). Unusual accelerations may be encountered and the normal metabolic diurnal rhythm may be disturbed by rapid movement between time zones.

Altitude

An increase in altitude is equivalent to a decrease in barometric pressure. There is a consequent reduction in the partial pressure of oxygen and an increase in the volume of any gas trapped within the body (Table 128-1).

Table 128-1. REPRESENTATIVE VALUES OF ARTERIAL OXYGEN AND THE RELATIVE VOLUME OF GAS AT VARIOUS ALTITUDES

Altitude, ft	Pressure, mm Hg	Arterial blood		Relative volume of gas
		Oxygen tension, mm Hg	Oxygen saturation, %	
0	760	94	98	1.0
5,000	632	66	92	1.2
8,000	564	60	89	1.25
10,000	523	53	86	1.5
14,000	446	44	79	1.7
18,000	379	36	71	2.0
37,500 with 100% O_2	159	74	94	4.8
44,000 with 100% O_2	116	36	72	6.5

The normal person acclimatized to sea level tolerates oxygen tension equivalent to that at altitudes of 10,000 to 12,000 ft with little change in arterial oxygen saturation. At altitudes above 12,000 ft, hypoxia becomes more marked and supplementary oxygen is usually used. By breathing 100 percent oxygen, one can maintain normal oxygen saturation at altitudes of 30,000 to 35,000 ft. An ascent of 5,000 ft or more may be followed by a period of lethargy, sleepiness, and headache. These symptoms usually subside within 24 hr.

A second consequence of decreased barometric pressure is expansion of gas trapped in body cavities. In the normal person, intestinal gas is passed as it expands and middle-ear and sinus air escapes without difficulty during ascent. Gas which cannot escape (pneumothorax, pneumoperitoneum) may cause pain, injury, or death. Patients with trapped gas in body cavities should not be exposed to a significant decrease in barometric pressure.

Acceleration

Acceleration is the instantaneous rate of change of velocity. The unit of acceleration *g* is the acceleration of a body which is falling freely *in vacuo* due to earth's gravity. It represents a change in velocity of 32.2 ft per sec each second. Most of the physiologic consequences of acceleration are due to the force (inertia) which is equal in magnitude but opposite in direction to that causing the acceleration. Thus, headward acceleration causes footward displacement of soft tissues and blood. Duration, magnitude, direction, and rate of onset of acceleration determine the physiologic effects. In general, the longer and greater the acceleration, the less well it is tolerated. Prolonged forward or backward acceleration is tolerated better (approximately 14 to 20*g*, limited by apnea) than headward acceleration (4 to 7*g*, limited by blackout and cerebral ischemia); footward acceleration (3 to 5*g*, limited by asystole and conjunctival and mucous membrane bleeding) is tolerated least well. Brief headward accelerations of 25*g* and backward accelerations of 40*g* are tolerated by normal subjects when well positioned and supported. In ordinary flight, linear accelerations greater than 1*g* are not encountered. Turbulent flight may cause brief linear accelerations of 10 to 12*g*, which are great enough to cause fractures in persons who are not restrained. Angular accelerations of turn and the linear-angular accelerations of turbulent flight are important causes of motion sickness.

Diurnal Rhythms

A dissociation between metabolic diurnal rhythms and actual local time may occur following longitudinal flight or flight over the poles in high-speed aircraft. From 3 to 5 days may be required for diurnal metabolic rhythms to come into phase with the new local time. There are no proved adverse clinical or physiologic effects of changing the diurnal rhythm. However, the management of diseases with diurnal manifestations, such as peptic ulcer, and the scheduling of all important medications should be carefully planned in preparation for a trip to another time zone.

Miscellaneous

Some fuels and lubricants and their combustion products are toxic and may, with equipment failure, become concentrated in closed cabins. Reciprocating engines produce large quantities of carbon monoxide. Jet engines use fuels which are vesicants, with fumes that may cause nausea, vomiting, and headache. Pyrolysis of lubricating oils produces fumes which cause conjunctival irritation. Ozone has not accumulated in toxic quantities.

Flight line personnel develop hearing loss after prolonged exposure to jet noise unless protected by position or by mechanical devices. Noise levels inside aircraft are very low, and those in terminals and around airfields are apparently insufficient to cause hearing loss.

Supersonic Transport

Supersonic transports cruise at speeds of Mach 2 to Mach 3 (1,300 to 1,800 mph) at altitudes of 50,000 to 70,000 ft. Flight characteristics are well known from extensive experience in military aircraft. Cabin pressure, oxygen content, and temperature will be similar to those of current jet aircraft. There are two environmental hazards which are not present in ordinary subsonic air travel: ozone and radiation.

Ozone is present in the toxic concentration of 6 to 9 ppm at the operational altitude of the supersonic transport. For this reason, the cabin atmosphere control system includes thermal or catalytic devices for the dissociation of ozone to maintain concentrations below 0.2 ppm.

Passengers and crew will be exposed to galactic cosmic radiation and to solar flare radiation. Under the most adverse ordinary circumstances galactic cosmic radiation, composed of protons, alpha particles, and a few heavy nuclei, will be less than 2 millirem per hr or approximately 6 millirem for a single intercontinental flight. The aircrew may receive 2 rem per year from this source. Solar flares produce protons and heavy nuclei. During a major solar flare, the dose rate for a passenger may reach 2 millirads per hr. For this reason, the aircraft will carry radiation monitoring equipment and will descend to lower altitudes when major solar flares occur.

The supersonic transport will cause a sonic boom, or wave of overpressure, of approximately 2.0 lb per sq ft at ground level along a corridor of 25 miles on each side of the flight path. Overpressure of this magnitude will not cause physical or physiologic damage but does cause psychological reactions.

Aircrew Selection

Physical requirements for aircrews are described in appropriate governmental and airlines literature. Absence of circulatory, pulmonary, neurologic, visual, and auditory defects is of particular importance.

Air Transportation of Patients

Since it is now possible to fly without experiencing physiologically significant departure from the usual environmental conditions, there are no absolute medical contraindications to moving patients by air. However, in many instances patients should not be moved at all, and in others, adequate aircraft with pressurized cabin and attending personnel may not be available. Commercial airlines will carry many patients subject to the discretion of the airline medical director. In addition to the condition of the patient, the comfort and convenience of other passengers must be a major factor in the decision of the commercial airlines. The following points apply to air transportation in general. Specific advice concerning commercial air transportation should be obtained from the appropriate airline medical director.

CIRCULATORY DISEASE. The lower partial pressure of oxygen which may be encountered constitutes the major deterrent to flight for patients with circulatory diseases. With oxygen breathing, normal arterial oxygen saturation can be maintained at all altitudes encountered in routine flight (Table 128-1). There is no evidence that ordinary flying is associated with an increased incidence of angina, myocardial infarction, or cerebral vascular accidents. Coronary artery disease manifested by occasional angina or old myocardial infarction, minimal cerebral or peripheral vascular disease, hypertension, and compensated congenital or rheumatic heart disease appear to entail no added risk in flying. Patients with angina related to emotional stress may benefit from preflight sedation.

Patients with severe or frequent angina, severe hypertension, recent vascular accidents, or cardiac decompensation at rest or with moderate exercise should fly only when a pressurized aircraft or supplementary oxygen is available to maintain ambient oxygen tension at levels of 150 mm Hg (sea level equivalent) or more. It is probably preferable to forego unnecessary flying for 6 weeks after a myocardial infarction or a cerebral vascular accident.

PULMONARY DISEASE. Persons with pulmonary decompensation at rest or with very mild exercise should fly only if ambient oxygen tension is maintained at levels of 150 mm Hg or more and facilities and personnel are available to treat acute decompensation. Persons with pulmonary decompensation with moderate (two flights of stairs) or severe exercise usually fly without difficulty to altitudes of 10,000 ft. Asthmatic patients who do not respond well to self-administered treatment should not fly unattended during acute episodes. The likelihood of rupture of an emphysematous bleb does not appear to be increased by ordinary flight. Because of the increase in volume of bullae as altitude increases (Table 128-1), patients with marked bullous emphysema are not advised to fly above 6,000 ft. Individuals with pneumothorax should not fly unless the cabin pressure is maintained at ground-level equivalent. Expansion of the trapped gas causes, in effect, a tension pneumothorax. Several patients with therapeutic pneumothorax have died in flight.

HEMATOLOGIC DISEASE. In the absence of cardiopulmonary disease, patients with a hemoglobin of 7 to 9 Gm per 100 ml usually tolerate flight at 4,000 to 6,000 ft without difficulty. If greater cabin altitudes are to be encountered, hemoglobin should be above 10 Gm per 100 ml.

Hypoxia causes increased sickling of erythrocytes containing hemoglobin S. There have been many well-documented reports of splenic infarction in patients with hemoglobin S during flights which usually exceeded 10,000 ft and lasted for several hours. Two patients with SC hemoglobin have had splenic infarctions during flights which did not exceed 6,000 ft. If ambient oxygen tension cannot be maintained at 150 mm Hg, flying is contraindicated for patients with SS (sickle-cell anemia) and

SC hemoglobin and for those with SA (sickle-cell trait) who have large quantities of hemoglobin S. Others with hemoglobin S should be restricted to cabin altitudes below 10,000 ft. Symptoms of splenic infarction, nausea, vomiting, left upper quadrant pain, and shock should be treated with supplemental oxygen and immediate return to ground level.

PREGNANCY. A large amount of experience has accumulated which suggests that ordinary flying has no adverse effects on the normal pregnant woman or fetus. Pregnant women should sit, when possible, facing the rear of the plane and should place the seat belt over the upper thighs and hips rather than around the abdomen. When pregnancy is complicated by preeclampsia or cardiopulmonary or hematologic disease, considerations similar to those discussed above for the nonpregnant patient apply.

EAR, NOSE, AND THROAT DISEASE. Acute infections of the upper part of the respiratory tract and chronic sinusitis may obstruct the eustachian tubes or sinus ducts with barotitis or barosinusitis resulting when external pressure is increased during descent. If flight is necessary, use of a nasal spray [½ percent phenylephrine (Neo-Synephrine)] 6, 3, and ½ hr before flight and ½ hr before descent may help to maintain patency of the ducts. A swallow or a Valsalva maneuver with the nose occluded will usually open the ducts. Children may be fed during descent to encourage swallowing. The treatment of barotrauma depends on its severity and the underlying cause. Intubation of the eustachian tubes is not advised. In most instances, conservative treatment with decongestants will suffice. Severe barotitis may be associated with hemorrhage into the middle ear, requiring myringotomy and aspiration of blood to prevent ossicular ankylosis. Plastic repair of the ducts may be required to prevent recurrence.

METABOLIC DISEASE. Control of diabetes may be complicated by rapid movement from one time zone to another and by motion sickness. Careful planning of the flight in terms of elapsed rather than local time, with consideration of the meals to be served and appropriate management of motion sickness, should enable the patient with well-controlled diabetes to fly without difficulty. Patients in diabetic acidosis may be transported after treatment is started if in-flight medical facilities are adequate.

COMMUNICABLE DISEASE. Persons known to have a communicable disease may not enter a state or nation without the consent of the local health department.

POSTOPERATIVE CONDITIONS. Because of the expansion of abdominal gas with decrease in barometric pressure, it is generally considered preferable to forego flying for 10 days after abdominal or other major surgery. However, experience with air evacuation of military casualties suggests that, with proper facilities and personnel, practically all patients whose condition is stable can be moved by air if necessary. Most persons with fractures are flown without difficulty. Fracture of the mandible, particularly when the mandible is immobilized, constitutes a special problem because of the possibility of vomiting

and aspiration. A quick-release wire support has been designed for in-flight use.

EPILEPSY. Most patients with well-controlled epilepsy fly to altitudes of 10,000 ft without difficulty. Flight to greater altitude in unpressurized aircraft may precipitate seizures.

Motion Sickness

The use of modern aircraft has considerably reduced the incidence of motion sickness. The problem remains because of occasional turbulent flights and persons who are extremely susceptible to motion sickness. Such persons should sit over the wings of the aircraft where motion is least. Cyclizine (Marezine) 50 mg, meclizine (Bonine) 25 mg, and dimenhydrinate (Dramamine) 50 mg are effective prophylactic agents.

Space Travel

The medical problems of space flight relate in part to the design of spacecraft and propulsion systems and in part to the characteristics of the space environment.

With design and engineering improvements it will be possible to build spacecraft which require only a small departure from man's ordinary environment. For example, the accelerations of launch and reentry which are of the order of 4 to 8g in present systems could be reduced to a fraction of a g by prolonging the time of acceleration. Present Soviet manned space systems operate with a cabin atmosphere which is very near to that at sea level or earth. To avoid the effects of weightlessness, an acceleration equivalent to that of the earth's gravity can be produced by rotating the spacecraft if this should prove necessary. Radiation shielding can be provided, albeit with a weight penalty. Present space systems represent a series of engineering compromises which are necessary largely because of the limitations of the propulsion systems.

During the flights of the Mercury and Gemini series, several adaptations were observed. Human performance, eating, drinking, urination and defecation, respiration, heart rate, and blood pressure showed no important changes. Weight loss occurred predominantly during the first few days of orbital flight. It was related in part, at least, to negative water balance associated with decreased fluid intake. Several astronauts have had leukocytosis of 20,000 to 30,000 upon return to earth, presumably due to stress and immobilization. There is evidence that red blood cell mass was reduced during orbital flight, possibly related in part to the high ambient oxygen tension. Astronauts manifest orthostatic hypotension after return to a gravitational field. This may be due to reduced blood volume as well as impaired cardiovascular response to gravity. Weightlessness is expected to be associated with a negative calcium balance. There is limited evidence that negative calcium balance and bone demineralization occur, but the effect has not been important in flights of less than 2 weeks' duration.

REFERENCES

Armstrong, H. B.: "Aerospace Medicine," Baltimore, The Williams & Wilkins Company, 1960.

Gauer, O. H., and G. W. Zuidema: "Gravitational Stress in Aerospace Medicine," Boston, Little, Brown and Company, 1961.

Gerathewohl, S. J.: Aeromedical Aspects of the Supersonic Transport, Aerospace Med., 38:1225, 1967.

Gullett, C. C.: Aeromedical Aspects of Turbo-jet Commercial Aircraft, Aerospace Med., 32:818, 1961.

Lafontaine, E., J. Lavernhe, J. Courillon, M. Medvedeff, and J. Ghata: Influence of Air Travel on Circadian Rhythms, Aerospace Med., 38:944, 1967.

129 RADIATION INJURY
Eugene P. Cronkite

Types of Radiation

The types of ionizing radiation most often causing injury are x-rays, gamma rays, alpha and beta rays, protons, and neutrons. X-rays and gamma rays are identical; a separate name was given because of their difference in origin. The former are produced by x-ray machines and as secondary emissions from particle accelerators or electron tubes. The latter are produced by radioactive decay. In general, gamma radiations are more energetic than x-rays; however, the energy spectrum of x-rays is continuous. Beta rays are electrons. Ordinary electrons originate from the shells surounding the atomic nucleus, and beta rays originate only from within the nucleus. Alpha rays are the stripped nuclei of the helium atom with a mass of 4 and a charge of 2+. Protons are stripped nuclei of hydrogen atoms with a mass of 1 and a charge of 1+. Protons are becoming of more interest because of their common use as primary particles in accelerators and their prevalence as an extraterrestial space radiation as described by Van Allen. Protons are of additional interest since they are usually the secondary damaging particle produced by neutron interaction with tissue or other materials. Neutrons have a mass of 1 and charge of 0. Biologic injury is produced primarily by ionization from secondary charged particles. Neutrons produce the secondary charged particles in diverse ways. Fast neutrons react principally with the hydrogen atoms, and as a result of the collision a portion of the energy is imparted to the hydrogen atom and a proton is ejected which does the damage. With thermal or slow neutrons the damage is done by actual capture of the neutrons and a secondary emission of ionizing radiation as the transmuted hydrogen, nitrogen, or other substance in tissue decays and emits radioactivity. These are the basic types of radiation with which a physician may be concerned.

Mechanism of Action

Historically the theories and concepts for mechanism of action of ionizing radiation on living things are discussed in the classic volume by Lea. The concepts of direct hits on the target molecules versus the indirect action mediated through products of reaction with the protoplasmic solvent water are analyzed lucidly. The most acceptable current view to account for a major part of the biologic effects of radiation may be divided into three interlinked steps. First, photons, or particles, penetrate the protoplasm, interacting to produce ion pairs. This reaction takes of the order of 10^{-13} sec. The second step is a primary radiochemical reaction of these ions primarily with water, producing free radicals such as H and OH. These reactions take about 10^{-9} sec. These free radicals produce a further chain of reactions with themselves and tissue water to produce further reactive forms such as H_2O_2 and HO_2. These products persist for microseconds or in part a few seconds. The last reaction is between these products and critical protoplasmic molecules. The nature of this last reaction is not known, but since the actual amount of energy imparted to the system is small, it is generally thought that the damage must involve substances of low concentration but major importance to the living system, for example, nucleic acids or enzymes. It is of interest that the amount of energy deposited to produce 100 percent mortality in animals will raise the body temperature only 0.001°C. Whatever the mechanism may be, it sets into motion a series of observable histologic or chemical lesions that unfold with time. In addition to the effects observable within days, "bad invisible information" may be stored in the proliferative or nonproliferative cells, presumably in DNA, that may not be manifested as a disease process for several years.

Dose Units

In pharmacology, standardization of drugs becomes scientific only when the structure is known and one can measure the drug in an appropriate unit such as a milligram. With ionizing radiation one is concerned not with the mass of the agent administered but with the *amount* and the distribution of energy that has been absorbed by tissue at the *point of interest* (tumor, tissue essential for life, gonads, etc.).

Two dose units are essential for the understanding of the quantitative effects of radiation. The *roentgen* (R), a measure of total dose in air, is defined as the quantity of x-ray or gamma radiation such that the associated corpuscular emission per 0.001293 Gm of air at standard conditions produces in air ions carrying one electrostatic unit of either sign. For energy to be deposited, there must be an interaction with matter. Hence, with x-rays passing through a vacuum, no radiation dose is delivered. In practice we are interested in the energy imparted to various tissues from a number of different types of radiation, and it is therefore essential to have a second unit of radiation which overcomes the limitation of the roentgen. This second unit, the *rad,* is a unit of absorbed dose equal to 100 ergs per Gm of absorbed energy which applies to any type of radiation in any tissue. For small pieces of tissue in an x-ray beam of 1 r per min, the absorbed dose is very close to 1 rad per min. However, as irradiated objects become larger and change in composition, one must consider the diminution in intensity due to the interaction of radiation with matter (buildup and then exponential attenuation) and the changing types of interaction (photoelectric effect, Compton effect, etc.). In tissue of uniform density this leads to a decreasing absorbed dose at successive levels after equilibrium is attained. However, at interfaces such as soft tissue and bone, the absorbed dose may sharply increase. Thus, in addition to the exposure dose in roentgens and the absorbed dose in rads, one must be concerned with the distribution of the absorbed dose in the areas of interest. For example, if there is sufficient protection of bone marrow by shielding of one's own tissues to permit marrow regeneration and survival from what is considered an otherwise fatal *exposure dose,* one may ascribe incorrectly some great benefit to a procedure used therapeutically. Unfortunately, failure to consider the critical influence of the distribution of absorbed dose at the site of interest on the outcome of radiation injury has resulted in ascribing therapeutic benefit to various agents of no value at all.

The *density of ionization* in tissue varies with the energy and type of radiation as well as the tissue composition. The density of ionization is referred to as *specific ionization* (ions per unit track length) or as *linear energy transfer* (LET, kiloelectron volts deposited per unit track length). Among other factors, the density of ionization influences the biologic effect for equivalent amounts of energy deposited, in general the effect being greater with more densely ionizing radiation. This leads to consideration of the relative biologic effectiveness (RBE), which is defined as the ratio of the dose in rads of standard radiation (usually x-ray or gamma radiation of 250 to 400 kv energy) to produce a given degree of biologic effect, to the dose in rads of an unknown radiation to produce the same degree of biologic effect. For example, if the LD-50 dose of x-rays is 600 rads and for neutrons 300 rads, the RBE will be 2. The RBE may vary with the biologic response or the conditions of irradiation. For example, when the same radiations are used, a different value may be obtained for mortality, cataract, or tumor development. Another useful unit is the rem, which stands for roentgen equivalent mammal. Numerically, rem = rads × RBE.

Also of importance is the *dose rate.* In general, the lower the dose rate, the less will be the acute somatic effect. In a crude sense, dose rates in excess of approximately 5 r per min give essentially the same result. However, as the dose rate falls below 5 r per min, the effect per unit of radiation becomes less. In the past, genetic effects were believed independent of dose rate. This implies that all increments of radiation received by the gonads, irrespective of when or how, would add up directly as mutations, to give a total effect ultimately to be measured as detectable effects in succeeding generations. However, it is now known that there is a dose-rate dependence in respect to the production of mutations by irradiation of spermatogonia in mice and also for leukemogenesis in mice, which is considered to be a somatic genetic effect of bone marrow irradiation.

If the dose of radiation is sufficiently high, actual death of any living cell can be observed promptly in terms of classical pathologic criteria of cell necrosis. However, after lower doses of radiation (precise values vary with the tissue), only disturbances in cell proliferation are seen. The rate at which cells divide is decreased. DNA synthesis is impaired in two manners: (1) the rate of synthesis is slower; (2) cells may continue DNA synthesis and become polyploid. It is reasonably certain that radiation has effects other than the outright killing of cells and the interference with mitosis and DNA synthesis. Among the less well understood manifestations of radiation exposure are those dealing with the effects of rather small doses of radiation on the nondividing central nervous system. This work, pioneered by the Russians, has in recent years received more attention from Western radiobiologists. However, it is still not completley understood.

The diminution in the production of new cells in these tissues that are undergoing continual renewal (mucosa, blood, gonads, etc.) results in a progressive hypoplasia to total atrophy, depending on dose. Some cells still capable of mitosis that are not killed outright may be so injured that they will go through one or two generative cycles, producing abnormal progeny, such as giant metamyelocytes and hypersegmented neutrophils, before dying. The atrophy of these steady-state cell renewal systems and direct injury of other tissues produce clearly defined clinical syndromes.

Clinical Phenomena in Relation to Dose and Time after Exposure

Human experience is based on the effects of atomic bombs; accidental exposure to fallout from a hydrogen bomb; laboratory and reactor accidents in the United States, U.S.S.R., and Yugoslavia; and on *whole-body* clinical radiotherapy. After any radiation accident close cooperation of the physician and health physicist is essential to obtain the best estimate of the radiation dose and to evaluate its probable effect in terms of the likely *distribution of the absorbed dose* in rads. However, clinical signs and symptoms remain paramount in the management of human disease and injury. Physical estimates of dose never substitute for clinical judgment and experience.

For teaching purposes three acute radiation syndromes may be classified generally as *cerebral, gastrointestinal,* and *hematopoietic.*

The *cerebral* syndrome is produced by extremely high doses of radiation, i.e., following exposure to several thousand roentgens. It is always fatal, whether the radiation is delivered to the brain alone or to the whole body. Three processes have been described: a prodromal phase of nausea and vomiting; then listlessness and drowsiness ranging from apathy to prostration (probably traceable to nonbacterial inflammatory foci in the brain); and finally, a more generalized component characterized by tremors, convulsions, ataxia, and death. This sequence was observed in an industrial accident, death occurring 36 hr after exposure.

The *gastrointestinal* syndrome occurs when the dose of radiation is lower, in the range of 600 to 1,500 r. It is characterized by intractable nausea, vomiting, and diarrhea; these lead to severe dehydration, diminished plasma volume, vascular collapse, and death. The syndrome is initiated by a pronounced "intoxication," arising presumably from diffuse necrosis of tissue throughout the body; it is extended by severe injury to the gastrointestinal tract. The latter development is caused by two factors: direct killing of a fraction of the crypt cells and inhibition of mitosis. The mature epithelial cells continue to migrate out on to the villus in an orderly fashion, eventually being lost from the tip of the villi; this produces a progressive diminution in the number of cells covering the villi. The epithelial cells progressively become cuboidal and then squamous in appearance and ultimately the intestinal villi become denuded, with massive loss of bloody plasma into the intestine. The usual 3- to 4-day death from the gastrointestinal syndrome can be prevented by massive plasma replacement during the first 4 to 6 days after irradiation. After doses greater than circa, 1,300 r, regeneration is poor and slow. After doses below roughly 1,300 r, regeneration commences around the sixth day with complete restoration of the gastrointestinal epithelium. However, the respite is only temporary, since hematopoietic failure will ensue, commencing within 2 to 3 weeks.

The *hematopoietic syndrome* which occurs following whole-body exposure in the midlethal range is accompanied by temporary anorexia, nausea, and vomiting which is maximal between 6 and 12 hr after exposure to doses of radiation between 600 and 800 r. Thereafter, the gastrointestinal symptoms rapidly subside so that within 24 to 36 hr after exposure the subject is usually asymptomatic. These symptoms have been correlated with a period of rapid necrosis of radiosensitive tissues. The prodromes must be distinguished from the gastrointestinal syndrome described earlier and from that which occurs later on. After subsidence of the prodromes, a period of relative well-being is experienced, during which atrophy of lymph nodes, spleen, and bone marrow progresses, leading to a pancytopenia. This atrophy is the result of two clearly defined processes—direct killing of radiosensitive cells and inhibition of new cell production. In the peripheral blood, lymphopenia commences immediately, becoming maximal within 24 to 36 hr. Thereafter, the lymphocytes remain at low levels for weeks and recover over several months. Within a few hours after irradiation a neutrophilic leukocytosis appears. Following this an oscillation in the neutrophil count occurs, the rate at which it falls to the minimum being a function of the dose of radiation. After sublethal and low lethal doses, the minimal values occur in 4 to 6 weeks; after high lethal doses granulocytes

diminish more rapidly and minimal values approaching zero appear within 7 to 10 days.

Thrombopenia and its relation to radiation bleeding have been studied exhaustively. After single doses of radiation a close correlation with the decrease in the platelet count and the tendency to bleed is evident. In animals and after various accidents, significant purpura was seen only when the platelet counts fell below 20,000 per cu mm. The platelets remain steady or increase for 2 to 3 days after irradiation and thereafter diminish more or less linearly with time, the ultimate minimum and the rate attained being dose-dependent. After about 200 rads, it takes about 30 days for minimum platelet levels to develop. After 600 to 800 rads, minimal levels were observed within 10 to 12 days. Earlier observations in which bleeding in radiation injury was attributed primarily to hyperheparinemia have been refuted. Today there is no evidence of hyperheparinemia; consequently the use of antiheparin agents in the therapy of bleeding induced by radiation is not indicated. Fresh viable platelet transfusions will stop bleeding, and maintenance of platelet levels by platelet transfusions will prevent development of bleeding in animals.

Decreases in the red blood cell count are prominent only after large doses of radiation that significantly interfere with new cell production and produce bleeding.

Studies of *decreased resistance to infection* have resulted in the conclusion that there are (1) a dose-dependent decrease in circulating granulocytes and lymphocytes; (2) a dose-dependent impairment of antibody production; (3) impairment of granulocyte migration and phagocytosis; (4) decreased ability of the reticuloendothelial system to kill phagocytized bacteria; (5) diminished resistance to diffusion in subcutaneous tissues; and (6) hemorrhagic areas of the skin and bowel that present foci for entrance and growth of bacteria. Obviously an increased susceptibility to infection by both commensals and pathogens must be present.

The preceding syndromes may be produced when the whole body is uniformly exposed to radiation or if there is a substantial inhomogeneous exposure of the whole body. An expression of the lethal dose range for man is desirable to assist in the management of casualties. In the case of inhomogeneous exposure, one can see how misleading any single air or exposure dose may be. There is a hierarchy of effects that vary with time, dose, and organs involved. Although 10,000 rads to the brain will be fatal, 10,000 rads to a hand may only necessitate amputation. Since the bone marrow is somewhat more sensitive than other tissues, ultimate survival is determined in large part by the dose to this tissue. For uniform whole-body exposure *without therapy* it has been estimated that the lethal dose curve will commence at about 200 rads and that survivals will be rare after doses in excess of 800 rads. Between these limits the percentage mortality dose curve is sigmoid. Even if the dose to an individual is known with precision, the prognosis must remain probable because one can never predict whether an individual belongs on the sensitive or resistant portion of the curve.

Inhomogeneous Exposure to Radiation

The preceding description of radiation injury was based primarily on human clinical experience and animal experimentation in which the distribution of dose absorbed by tissues was relatively uniform. However, in actuality, conditions of exposure may be such that there are marked inhomogeneities in absorbed dose. For example, the geometry of an exposure may result in almost no exposure to the lower part of the body and very heavy exposure to the abdomen and hands, resulting in extensive necrosis of the skin of these areas in addition to the fatal injury to deeper tissues. In one accident, the direction of the beam resulted in severe exposure to the head, but the low energy permitted marked attenuation of the beam within the head, so that the absorbed dose through the brain decreased markedly from the side closest to the beam to the side farthest from it. The superficial layers of the brain were injured badly, but death did not ensue because vital centers were not destroyed. In evaluating any radiation accident, one must reconstruct the geometry and consider the probable distribution of absorbed dose within the body. What may initially appear as a fatal accident in terms of air exposure dose may turn out to be sublethal when effects of distribution of the absorbed dose are considered.

Management of Acute Human Radiation Injury

Presumptive evidence of exposure to radiation and signs or symptoms described earlier must be recognized before there need be cause for concern. No therapy is available for the cerebral form of radiation injury after uniform brain exposure. Whereas a small percentage of persons with the gastrointestinal syndrome may be kept alive until the affected tract regenerates, they must also face the hematopoietic syndrome; hence that is the real therapeutic problem. Therapy rests on the control of the sequelae of marrow aplasia and thus is similar to management of drug-induced and idiopathic marrow aplasia, suggesting that combined use of antibacterials and transfusions would be useful. The spontaneous course of radiation injury in man has clearly shown that signs and symptoms develop at different times in different subjects after identical doses of radiation. Accordingly, the time of institution and type of therapy should be individualized. The following general therapeutic regimen is outlined.

1. *Maintain rigid asepsis* until one is confident that a sublethal exposure to radiation has been experienced. All medical staff involved in the care of irradiated individuals must have negative cultures of the nasopharynx for pathogenic organisms. Physicians and nursing staff with any evidence of respiratory or other infections are forbidden entrance to the rooms of irradiated patients. If at all possible, reverse isolation should be instituted to prevent introduction of pathogens into the environment of the patient. This requires either the use of plastic rooms in which the patient is placed or the sterilization of a room and the institution of laminar flow air barriers and appropriate ultraviolet light sources to prevent the introduction of pathogens into the patient's environment.

2. Observe *fluid and electrolyte balance* closely and restore as necessary with appropriate replacement solutions.

3. *Provide sterile, bland diet* prepared in the patient's room.

4. Administer *nonabsorbable intestinal antibiotics* such as neomycin to sterilize the gastrointestinal tract and minimize the probability of invasion by commensal organisms in the gastrointestinal tract.

5. *Treat infection* when it develops or relapses, using various antibiotics sequentially in doses two to three times the usual size. Use sulfonamides when antibiotics are exhausted. One is fighting for additional time to permit spontaneous regeneration.

6. *Use fresh whole blood* to control bleeding and/or to restore adequate red cell levels. Fresh blood is defined as that which has been taken from the donor not more than 1 hr previously and placed in plastic bags with Na_2EDTA. When the hematocrit is returned to normal range, to control bleeding use fresh platelet-rich plasma as clinically indicated, not on an inflexible schedule. Despite many claims concerning the value of lyophilized and frozen platelets, radiation bleeding has been successfully managed to date only by the use of fresh viable platelets that circulate in adequate numbers.

The preceding therapy has increased the survival rate of animals. Unless infection or serious hemorrhage develops, therapy is not needed. Prophylactic therapy other than the use of nonabsorbable intestinal antibiotics is believed to be contraindicated. Many human beings with epilation, severe pancytopenia, and purpura have recovered without therapy from doses of radiation ranging from 200 to 300 r. Recently individuals who received 400 to 500 r inhomogeneous irradiation have recovered when treated in accordance with this therapeutic regimen despite near-zero granulocyte and platelet counts.

Syngenesious and autologous bone marrow transplantation will prevent death in almost all otherwise fatally irradiated animals up to doses of about 1,200 r. In fatally irradiated animals saved by allogenic bone marrow transplantation, the transplanted marrow may eventually produce a reaction (presumably against the host) of immunologic nature, resulting in a severe late degenerative disease of the skin, kidneys, liver, and lymph nodes. A similar late fatal effect has been observed in children treated for leukemia with extensive chemotherapy and whole-body irradiation in whom allogeneic marrow transplantation was successful.

Although marrow transplantation has been widely acclaimed as the solution to fatal whole-body radiation, the results in human beings so far do not warrant optimism. This author believes it should be reserved for patients in whom there is a progressive deterioration of the hematopoietic system with granulocytes falling below 500 per cu mm in the first 2 weeks after exposure and an early rapid decline in the platelet count. The profile scoring method of Thomas and Wald may be useful on a day-to-day basis of evaluating the severity and may give some indication as to when one may be forced to resort to allogeneic marrow transplantation. In the rare case in which there is an identical twin, bone marrow transplantation should be lifesaving following fatal radiation injury up to a maximum exposure of about 1,200 r. Rigid rules cannot be formulated in advance. Decisions can be made only at the bedside.

Prevention

Nothing can substitute for prevention. Shielding, distance, and limiting of exposure time are the only effective preventive measures against exposures from radiation sources, whether in industry, medical practice, military action, or civil defense. A series of drugs, primarily sulfhydryl groups, that will protect against radiation by an effective dose reduction up to 50 percent are available. However, these must be administered within minutes preceding exposure. Accidents and warfare are not predictable. The severe toxic effects of these drugs prevent continuous prophylactic administration.

Long-term Effects

Radiation alters the "information system" of proliferating somatic and germ cells. Thus the perpetuating cells of the blood, gastrointestinal tract, skin, lens, gonads, and other areas pass on either "bad or inadequate information," presumably in altered DNA, to their progeny, resulting in late somatic disease, e.g., cancer, cataracts, degenerative disorders, or nonspecific shortening of life. Leukemia yield from radiation in human groups has been quantified. It is asserted, but not proved, that there is no threshold and that the yield of leukemia increases with dose. However, the greatest exposure of the American public comes from the medical uses of diverse types of radiation (predominantly diagnostic x-rays). If the assumption of no threshold dose for leukemia is correct, the medical uses of radiation are producing their small toll in an additional burden of leukemia and probably other disease also. Therefore, it behooves the practitioner to be exceedingly cautious and to expose patients to radiation only when it is clearly indicated and needed for diagnosis.

Radiation can produce mutation of genes, the information and transmission centers for heredity. Of this there is no doubt. Not all mutations are harmful, but the chances are overwhelming that a change will be detrimental to the species. Not all mutations produce visible immediately detectable effects. The concern is not only with an increase in the number of obvious freaks or cripples but with changes that will lead to such undesirable characteristics as lowered life expectancy, decreased fertility, a general increase in physical and mental disease, and an increase in fetal or neonatal death rates. It is the less obvious changes that are of the greatest importance. The more obvious changes usually lead to early death in the individual and reduced fertility in those that survive. Thus the harmful mutant is relatively quickly deleted from the population. The more subtle changes, however,

are propagated longer and affect a very large number of persons. The mutation may be dominant or recessive. Most dominant mutations are also lethal, and many such mutations may be missed because the fertilized egg never develops far enough to be recognized as a new individual. If the mutation is recessive, the mutant will not become evident unless both parents of the individual have the same mutant genes and transfer these to the individual concerned. It is extremely difficult to quantify these considerations. If the mutation rate were increased by a single exposure of the population to radiation, the effects would be spread through many generations. Half the total damage produced would not be observed until some 30 to 50 generations had been born. These are the practical considerations that make the problem particularly difficult to analyze. Damage that is inflicted now cannot be detected now and will only become evident many generations hence. These considerations also indicate why it is not possible to take negative evidence in populations that have been exposed to date as an indication that the degree of genetic damage is small. If, for instance, an effect was already obvious in the children born of individuals irradiated in Japan by the atom bombs, it would mean that the total genetic effect would be great indeed. These are sobering considerations for thoughtful persons. Since exposure to irradiation cannot be avoided in our modern industrial society and in the practice of medicine and because of the uncertainty about the quantitative effect in producing somatic or genetic effects, it is mandatory that exposure be minimal and rigidly controlled in order to protect the present generations from somatic effects and future generations from genetic effects.

Radium Poisoning

Today it appears strange that radium water was used as a therapeutic agent only three decades ago and resulted in poisoning. In addition, radium watch dial painters were poisoned during World War I. The radium (often mesothorium) is deposited primarily on the surface of the bones, and its distribution changes with the slow rebuilding of the osseous structure. Histologically one sees Havarsian systems plugged with highly calcified material; gross regions of resorption; and osteocyte death as evidenced by empty and highly calcified lacunae. Autoradiographs show both a "diffuse" distribution and "hot spots" of radioactivity. Pathologists consider the characteristic bony injury almost pathognomic of chronic radium poisoning. Many of the effects are due to direct radiation injury; some are secondary to vascular injury. Bone necrosis and interference with normal processes of internal reconstruction of bone result in the formation of small and large cavities, which give the characteristic radiolucency in radiographs of bone. Fibrosis of the bone is a constant feature, usually limited to the endosteal surfaces of cortical and trabecular bone. The marrow may be spottily fibrotic. The disturbed structure of bone may so weaken it as to permit pathologic fractures. The long-term irradiation is carcinogenic. Malignant bone tumors arise. The induction time is long—greater than 10 years, with an average of about 20 years. The types of tumors are not different from human bone tumors in general. In addition to bone tumors, carcinomas of the sinuses and nasopharynx have been seen in greatly increased numbers over the rare expected incidence. Leukemias have been conspicuous by their almost total absence. Aplastic anemia has also been observed as a cause of death. There is no satisfactory treatment of early or late radium poisoning. Prevention is the cure. Although these cases are mainly of historical interest, many elderly persons are still alive with significant body burdens of radium from therapy and employment in the watch dial industry. It is not possible to construct a dose-effect curve for radium poisoning. An estimate of the numerator of the incidence ratio is possible, since the diseases are brought to the attention of physicians. However, the denominator is sadly lacking since those who did not develop a disease that necessitated medical care are absent from most serious studies of the problem.

Microwaves

Microwave frequency extends from 300 to 200,000 megacycles, with wavelengths from about 1 to 50 cm.

Microwaves are the output of radars; they are used to accelerate nuclear particles in accelerators, for cooking, for industrial heating problems, and in medical diathermy for local heating of tissue. A common diathermy today utilizes a magnetron tube which operates at 2,450 megacycles and 12 cm wavelength. Numerous applicators are available for heating surfaces, within the rectum, vagina, etc. Medically the local heating of tissue at depths apparently increases blood flow and promotes more rapid healing of traumatized or inflamed areas.

Harmful effects are produced from deposition of energy too rapidly, producing excessive local heating of tissue. Deposition of energy varies with the type of tissue and the reflection from interfaces. Experimentally, bone growth has been impaired, testicles have been destroyed, and cataracts have been produced. Very high intensity radar exposure for 1 min 10 ft from the antenna resulted in sufficient injury to the bowel to produce an acute abdominal emergency, necessitating laparotomy and followed later by intestinal perforations, peritonitis, and death. Presumably the bowel was "cooked" in part. A few servicemen looked down the wave guide of a radar and later developed cataracts. Cataracts also developed in an employee who worked near an operating microwave antenna. A hazard is known to exist. Injuries can be avoided by educating those who work near and plan the propagation of microwaves so that the beam is directed away from human beings.

Ultrasound

Ultrasound consists of sound waves from a few hundred kilocycles per second to many megacycles per second. The passage of the sound wave through tissue produces successive positive and negative pressures which increase molecular motion and then generate heat via frictional forces. With large intensities (greater than 1 watt per sq cm), cavities are produced during the negative phase which become filled with gas dissolved in the medium. Cavitation produces large local temperatures, electrical discharges, and intense mechanical movement. Chemical reactions involving "free radicals" produced by the electrical discharges may occur, depending on the chemical nature of dissolved gases which may enhance or suppress the free radicals.

Ultrasound can kill cells, disrupt bacteria, etc., but local heat may inactivate enzymes and disturb subsequent chemical studies.

Ultrasound has been used in therapy, with some success, to produce local heating, as in diathermy for the treatment of arthritis, painful neuromas, and myositis. There is little danger since destruction of tissue takes about fifty times as much energy as production of pain; hence there is a built-in physiologic safeguard.

Unique ingenious multiple-port focusing devices have been built to focus ultrasonic energy in distinctly circumscribed volumes to destroy tissue. Such devices are being developed for neurosurgical work. Bone overlying the area at which the sound is focused must be removed. It is possible to destroy all neural components in a specific region without interrupting the capillary network. Ultrasonic neurosurgery is being evaluated in the treatment and relief of the hyperkinetic, hypertonic, and intractable pain disorders. It has also been used for prefrontal lobotomy instead of the usual surgical approach.

Ultrasound can also be used to localize foreign bodies and some tumors.

See Chap. 59. Sunlight and Photosensitivity Reactions.

REFERENCES

Bond, V. P., T. M. Fliedner, and J. Archambeau: "Mammalian Radiation Lethality," New York, Academic Press Inc., 1965.

Casarett, A. P.: "Radiation Biology," Englewood Cliffs, N.J., Prentice-Hall, Inc., 1968.

Cronkite, E. P., and V. P. Bond: "Radiation Injury in Man," Springfield, Ill., Charles C Thomas, Publisher, 1960.

——, W. C. Moloney, and V. P. Bond: Radiation Leukemogenesis, Am. J. Med., 28:673, 1960.

Elkind, M. M., and G. P. Whitmore: "The Radiobiology of Cultured Mammalian Cells," New York, Gordon and Breach, Science Publishers, Inc., 1967.

Hempelmann, L. H., H. Lisco, and J. G. Hoffman: The Acute Radiation Syndrome: A Study of 9 Cases and a Review, Ann. Intern. Med., 36:279, 1952.

Knauff, G. M.: Biological Effects of Microwave Radiation on Air Force Personnel, A.M.A. Arch. Indust. Health, 17:48, 1958.

Lea, D. E.: "Actions of Radiation on Living Cells," New York, The Macmillan Company, 1947.

McLaughlin, J. T.: Tissue Destruction and Death from Microwave Radiation (Radar), Calif. Med., 86:336, 1957.

Report of U.N. Scientific Committee on the Effects of Atomic Radiation, 19th Session, Suppl. 14 (A/5814), Chap. 3: Radiation Carcinogenesis in Man, 1964.

Rubin, P. R., and G. W. Casarett: "Clinical Radiation Pathology," Philadelphia, W. B. Saunders Company, 1968.

Schwan, H. P.: Biophysics of Diathermy, p. 55 in S. Licht (Ed.), "Therapeutic Heat," New Haven, Conn., S. Licht Publisher, 1958.

130 ELECTRICAL INJURIES
Ivan L. Bennett, Jr.

The first human fatality from accidental electrocution occurred in 1879 and was produced by an alternating current of 250 v. Since that time, continuing increase in household and commercial uses of electrical power has made accidents almost inevitable. Injury and death from lightning have occurred, of course, since time immemorial.

ETIOLOGY AND PATHOGENESIS. The end result of passage of an electrical current through the human body is unpredictable in the individual case. Certain generalizations are possible, however, and many of the factors that influence severity of injury by electricity are known. *Alternating currents* tend to produce tetanization of muscles and sweating (which lowers skin resistance), and *direct currents* produce electrolytic changes in the tissues. It has been estimated that alternating is about four or five times as dangerous as direct current; fatal electrocution from exposure to household circuits of 115 v at 60 cycles is relatively common.

The conductivity of tissues parallels their water content; consequently, the vascular system and musculature are good conductors, whereas bones, peripheral nerves, and skin offer high resistance. The resistance of normal skin is lowered by *moisture*, and this factor alone may convert what might ordinarily be a mild injury to fatal shock. The *grounding* of the body at the time of contact is important. It is well known that a person in water or on a wet surface is more susceptible to electrical injury. The *pathway of the current* through the body is crucial. Obviously, an accident involving passage of current between a point of contact on the leg and the ground is likely to be less injurious than one in which the poles of the circuit are the head and a foot. The *duration of contact* influences the outcome. Because, as mentioned, an electrical current can stimulate skeletal muscle to contract, a victim who has grasped an uninsulated wire may be unable to release it; this is far more likely with alternating than with direct currents and accounts in part for the greater danger of alternating circuits. Sudden convulsive contraction of muscles can result in fractures of bone; sometimes, however, it throws the individual clear of contact. This may lead to additional mechanical trauma if the victim is thrown from a high place.

In traversing the skin, energy of high-tension currents is converted to heat. When one considers that electric arcs with temperatures as high as 8000°C may be generated, it is not surprising that fourth or fifth degree burns often result. The term *electrical necrosis* is probably more

appropriate than *burn* for this injury. It has been suggested that the immediate damage is aggravated by vasospasm in adjacent tissues.

The systemic effects of electricity are incompletely understood, but, in general, low voltage produces ventricular fibrillation and death from circulatory failure, and high voltage produces respiratory arrest. High-tension currents produce cardiac standstill, but ventricular function resumes when the current stops, and death is presumably attributable to injury of medullary centers. Whether this neurologic damage results from vasospasm, increase in temperature of the brain, or direct injury to neurones is not known.

A lightning flash is a rush of electrical energy (about 1 billion v and 20,000 amp) along a path more than a mile long and 18 to 20 ft in diameter. The duration of the current is about 0.001 sec. When the bolt reaches the earth, secondary flashes occur and objects within a radius of 100 ft may be struck. Direct contact usually results in immediate death. Persons nearby may be injured by the electrical current, by burning from heated air, or by the concussive force of compressed air.

If patients die immediately, autopsy findings are limited to burns and generalized petechial hemorrhage. If patients survive for a period of days or longer, postmortem examination reveals focal necroses of nerve, spinal cord, or brain, involving both neurones and white matter, with appropriate glial and vascular reactions. Acute renal failure is an occasional complication if tissue destruction is extensive, as from high-tension accidents.

MANIFESTATIONS. Immediately after severe shock, patients are usually comatose and apneic, although the heart may continue to beat until anoxia leads to circulatory failure. Surviving this stage, patients are often disoriented and combative; convulsions are frequent. Blackened, charred areas at the points of entrance and exit of the current may appear to be relatively small and well localized. After a few days, however, huge sloughs, often involving major blood vessels, reveal the true extent of the destruction. A frequent finding in victims of lightning is a characteristic, lacy network of superficial "arborescent burns," or "lightning prints," on the skin. These fade within 24 to 48 hr. Late effects include various neurologic disabilities, visual disturbances, and, of course, the residual damage left by burns. A curious finding in many victims of lightning is temporary flaccid paralysis of the lower extremities with loss of sensation, so-called "keraunoparalysis," which passes off in 12 to 24 hr. This condition is often accompanied by blanching and coldness of the legs and is believed to be a result of severe vasoconstriction. Hemoglobinuria, oliguria, and acute renal failure may complicate massive injury to soft tissues. Injuries to the nervous system can leave symptoms resembling peripheral neuritis or multiple sclerosis. The development of cataracts has been reported as a late complication.

As many as 50 percent of persons who survive severe electrical accidents may develop a "post-electric shock syndrome," characterized by dull pain in the shoulders and chest, unrelated to exertion but aggravated by moving the arms or by deep breathing. This apparently results from traumatic myositis after severe muscular contraction during exposure to the electric current. It may produce considerable apprehension and concern about heart disease in tense or nervous individuals.

The use of electrical shock in psychiatric treatment has led to occasional accidents of two types. Sudden death, attributed to ventricular fibrillation, has been observed in elderly patients. Fracture of vertebral bodies during the convulsion has occurred; this is preventable by use of relaxant drugs.

LABORATORY FINDINGS. Leukocytosis with many large, immature granulocytes in the peripheral blood is common after severe electrical shock. Albuminuria is the rule; hemoglobinuria has been reported in many cases, probably secondary to severe burns. Although elevation of cerebrospinal fluid pressure is often mentioned in electrical shock, it is an inconstant finding; bloody spinal fluid occurs in some cases as a result of widespread vascular injury.

MANAGEMENT. Immediate *removal of the victim from contact* with the current is obviously important; this should always be preceded by cutting off the source of the current, when possible. Rescuers should be insulated by rubber gloves or a thick layer of dry cloth or newspapers. Many needless deaths have followed ill-planned attempts to rescue the body of a person already dead from electrical shock.

Artificial respiration should be instituted immediately if the victim is not breathing. The importance of this maneuver cannot be overemphasized. In one series of 700 cases of electrical injury (Maclachlan), there were 479 with respiratory arrest, of which 323 responded to artificial respiration. Most patients who respond do so within 20 min, but recovery after longer periods is frequent enough that manual or mechanical respiration should be continued for a minimum of 4 hr. It has been estimated that a delay of 6 min in the institution of resuscitative measures increases the death rate by 80 percent. External cardiac massage, coupled with defibrillation, if indicated, is extremely important in emergency management.

Other treatment is supportive. Stimulants should be used with caution during the first few hours because of the tendency of many patients toward convulsions. There is no evidence that the frequently advocated procedure of cerebrospinal fluid drainage is beneficial. Survivors of the acute episode often require extensive treatment for burns, infection, and hemorrhage as the devitalized tissues slough. If acute renal failure occurs, it should be managed as described in Chap. 300.

PREVENTION. Proper insulation of appliances, grounding of telephone lines and radio or television aerials, and the use of rubber gloves and dry shoes when working with circuits should be routine.

In a thunderstorm, the safest shelter is a closed house; an automobile, cave, or ditch is relatively secure. Hilltops, riverbanks, hedges, and wire fences should be avoided.

Ventricular fibrillation in patients undergoing electrocardiography, cardiac catheterization, angiocardiography, pacemaking, etc., has been reported often enough to indicate the need for stringent precautions as electronic equipment is used with increasing frequency in hospitals. Almost all accidents have involved a leakage of 60-cycle "house" current through the patient. Personnel should be aware of the hazards involved, the wiring of apparatus including oxygen machines and electrically operated beds should be checked carefully, and equipment should always be grounded *before* a patient is connected to an instrument.

REFERENCES

Fischer, H.: Pathologic Effects and Sequelae of Electrical Accidents, J. Occup. Med., 7:564, 1965.

Jude, J. R., W. B. Kouwenhoven, and G. G. Knickerbocker: Cardiac Arrest, J.A.M.A., 178:1063, 1961.

LaJoie, R. J.: Post-electroshock Syndrome, Indust. Med. Surg., 31:354, 1962.

Lightning Injuries, Lancet, I:351, 1946.

Maclachlan, W.: Electrical Injuries, J. Indust. Hyg., 16:52, 1934.

Ravitch, M. M., R. Lane, P. Safar, F. M. Steichen, and P. Knowles: Lightning Stroke, New Engl. J. Med., 264:36, 1961.,

131 IMMERSION INJURY AND DROWNING

Russell S. Fisher

About 7,000 deaths by drowning occur in the United States each year. This represents about one-fifteenth of the total number of fatal accidents.

Diagnosis

The term *drowning* is used to categorize a series of related phenomena resulting from submersion in a liquid medium that is per se innocuous. It, therefore, includes asphyxial changes as well as complex acute hemodynamic alterations and disturbances of the biochemical equilibrium of the blood.

Pathogenesis

Knowledge of the sequence of phenomena that occur in drowning is based upon a number of observations on humans and on experimental drowning in animals. Submersion is usually followed by an intensive and panicky struggle in an effort to reach the surface. Breath holding for varying lengths of time has been recorded to occur in the next stage, possibly lasting until the accumulating CO_2 in blood and tissues stimulates the respiratory center sufficiently to lead to an inevitable inhalation of considerable volumes of water. Swallowing of water, coughing and vomiting, loss of consciousness, and terminal gasping with flooding of the lungs and death then take place in rapid succession. When the process is interrupted before terminal gasping has set in, spontaneous recovery sometimes occurs. It has commonly been asserted that drowning essentially involves asphyxia resulting from obstruction of the airway by the drowning fluid. More recent investigations, however, show that asphyxial death in drowning is limited to between 10 and 15 percent of all cases and is due to laryngospasm and closure of the glottis. Moreover comparative enzymologic studies in rats of fresh and salt water drowning and asphyxia by exclusion of air indicate significant statistical differences between test and control groups. This seems to further stress the distinction between the mode of death in asphyxia versus that of drowning. In the majority of fatalities, death results from complex pathophysiologic events differing widely according to the chemical composition of the submersion liquid. For purposes of illustration, drowning in fresh water and sea water may be considered as separate entities.

Drowning in Fresh Water

Large amounts of water enter the lungs and due to the hypotonicity of fresh water, rapid absorption into the circulating bloodstream takes place. This results in a sudden and violent increase in blood volume with hemodilution and hypervolemia. Using deuterium oxide in the water as a tracer, Swann and Spafford have demonstrated that after 2 min submersion, a dog's blood may be diluted by as much as 51 percent of its original volume. This hemodilution is associated with massive hemolysis and an inevitable upset of the normal balance of the blood constituents. Sodium, chloride, calcium, proteins, and hemoglobin are all diluted, and the level of potassium rises. Ventricular fibrillation is often considered to be a characteristic feature of fresh water drowning. When it occurs, expulsive heartbeats are arrested at once. Ventricular fibrillation is believed to be directly related to the dilution of the blood electrolytes, in particular sodium. It cannot, however, be produced experimentally by injecting large volumes of water intravenously. The precedent condition is anoxia; the animal must be anoxic for an experimental hydremic plethora to cause fibrillation. The original hypothesis, based upon animal experiments, of "potassium intoxication" secondary to massive hemolysis as the underlying factor causing ventricular fibrillation has proved erroneous. The main intracellular cation in dog erythrocytes is not potassium as in man, but sodium, and fresh water drowning and hemolysis in the dog does not release a flood of potassium ions. The slight increase observed in plasma potassium after fresh water drowning may be accounted for by prolonged anoxia, as described by Fenn. These speculations do not answer the question of whether ventricular fibrillation occurs in fresh water drowning in man, but it would appear desirable to include defibrillation in the emergency treatment of a drowning victim.

Drowning in Sea Water

Sea water is strongly hypertonic. Its salt concentration, mainly sodium chloride, is over 3.0 percent. Submersion in sea water results in a rapid diffusion of salts into the bloodstream. The concentration of sodium, chloride, magnesium, etc., in the plasma rise conspicuously, while water moves from the circulation into the pulmonary alveoli—thus reestablishing the osmotic equilbrium. The consequences are marked hemoconcentration and fulminant pulmonary edema. Hypotension and hypovolemia accompanied by considerable bradycardia develop, and death supervenes within a few minutes. Ventricular fibrillation is not usually observed in experimental salt water drowning in spite of the adverse prevailing electrolyte environment, probably because the plasma sodium level is elevated rather than low.

Death Associated with Diving

(Refer also to Chap. 127.) In the case of divers, death is often the result of underwater asphyxia following hyperventilation; the latter leads to a sharp fall in blood carbon dioxide and to vasoconstriction, which in turn brings about a decrease of the cerebral circulation. Diminished cerebral blood flow is followed by loss of consciousness, which leads to inhalation of water. Involuntary exhalation against a closed glottis resulting in hypotension and diminished cardiac output further aggravate the condition. In diving with a scuba (self-contained underwater breathing apparatus) the cause of death is usually closely associated with the overconfidence of the diver in his breathing machine. *Nitrogen narcosis* occurs commonly, resulting from the increase of nitrogen concentration in the tissues as evident from Henry's law, according to which the solubility of a gas is directly proportional to the absolute pressure upon it. There is an increase of 1 atm of pressure for each 33 ft of water depth. Barotrauma and air embolism are second in frequency and occur during the ascent of the diver, when the air inhaled from the scuba expands proportionately as the pressure decreases (Boyle's law). An ascent, for instance, from 33 ft results in a twofold increase in volume due to the decrease in pressure from 2 to 1 atm. At this point any interference with expiration prevents release of this increased volume and results in acute pulmonary emphysema with tears in the lungs, hemoptysis, hemothorax, air embolism, and often death.

Resuscitation from Drowning

The main objective of adequate resuscitation in drowning is to institute such measures before circulatory failure sets in. Resuscitative procedures currently employed consist of clearing the airway by postural drainage, suction, etc., and giving artificial respiration, supplemented by closed-chest cardiac massage if no heart sounds are obtainable and the pulse is absent. Intermittent positive-pressure breathing with air, or preferably with oxygen, should be employed when such is available, and external electrical defibrillation should be carried out as soon as feasible after the condition arises. Plasma infusion to correct hemoconcentration is often thought to be of great value in salt water drowning, while in fresh water drowning it may be expected that an exchange transfusion, which in itself is a relatively harmless procedure, will be effective in reestablishing a normal circulating blood volume and in correcting an upset electrolyte balance. So-called "semi-" or "near drowning" in which death occurs suddenly several hours or longer after submersion has been repeatedly reported, but the mechanism of death in such cases remains obscure. Treatment should be directed to maintaining high cerebral oxygen supply and preventing pneumonia. Lower nephron nephrosis may also be anticipated in survivors of fresh water submersion due to hemoglobinemia; if oliguria or anuria develops, appropriate therapy should be initiated.

REFERENCES

Denny, M. K., and R. C. Read: Scuba-diving Deaths in Michigan, J.A.M.A., 192:220, 1965.

Kvittingen, T. D., and A. Naess: Recovery from Drowning in Fresh Water, Brit. Med. J., 1:1315, 1963.

Spitz, W. U.: Recovery from Drowning, Brit. Med. J., 1:1678, 1963.

Swann, H. G.: Mechanism of Circulatory Failure in Fresh and Sea Water Drowning, Circ. Res., 4:241, 1956.

Part Seven

Disorders Caused by Biologic Agents

Section 1

Basic Considerations

132 AN APPROACH TO INFECTIOUS DISEASES

Ivan L. Bennett, Jr., and
Robert G. Petersdorf

The vast majority of human and animal diseases of known etiology are produced by biologic agents, viruses, rickettsias, bacteria, mycoplasma, fungi, protozoa, or nematodes. No small part of the past and present importance of infectious diseases in medical practice is attributable to their enormous frequency and the public health implications of the contagiousness of many of them. However, development in sanitary engineering, vector control, techniques of immunization, and specific chemotherapy have modified the situation favorably. Although important exceptions remain, infectious diseases as a class are more easily prevented and more easily cured than any other major group of disorders. Despite the virtual elimination of certain infectious diseases and profound reduction in the morbidity and mortality of many, man is by no means free of infection. In fact, the *total human load of disease produced by microbial parasites has been only moderately, if at all, decreased.* As certain specific microbial infections have been controlled, others have emerged as troublesome therapeutic and epidemiologic problems. With the introduction of cytotoxic drugs in the treatment of malignant diseases and of immunosuppressive agents to control the rejection of transplanted organs, infections due to organisms previously considered saprophytic or commensal have increased. As Dubos has pointed out, microbial infections appear to form an inherent part of human life.

Because better environmental sanitation and other measures now prevent contact with many microbial agents and the development of acquired immunity early in childhood, certain infections have been seen more frequently in adults. For example, as contact with poliomyelitis virus in childhood declined in many countries, paralytic poliomyelitis became more common in young adults. Similarly, decreasing infection with the tubercle bacillus raises questions about the status of antituberculous immunity in adults.

As antimicrobial agents reduce the mortality associated with certain common infections, other microbes emerge as important causes of human disease. It is relatively unusual nowadays for patients to die of uncomplicated pneumococcal pneumonia—a disease readily handled with available antimicrobials. However, it is common to see serious disease produced by microorganisms which form part of man's normal microbial flora. These include infections produced by staphylococci, enteric bacilli, and fungi.

THE PARASITE AND THE HOST

The complex interaction between microorganism and man that results in infection and disease has been subjected to extensive study. Much has been learned about the initiation of the process, the ways in which microbes produce tissue injury, the influence of specific immunity and "nonspecific" resistance of the host, and mechanisms of recovery. Unfortunately, it is not yet possible to transfer in any specific way much of the information that has been acquired to the individual patient with an infection. In a textbook of medicine, therefore, it seems appropriate to emphasize those general aspects of the host-parasite relationship that form a basis for diagnostic procedures, that are of importance in deriving therapeutic principles, or that help explain the epidemiology of infection. This necessitates omitting from these pages discussion of many highly significant and interesting experimental studies, controversial issues, and theoretical or incompletely established concepts. The bibliography at the end of the chapter contains excellent reviews of these important subjects.

Infection and Clinical Disease

It is well known that microorganisms of different species or different strains of the same species vary widely in their capacity to produce disease and that human beings are not equally susceptible to the disease caused by a given bacterium or virus. Furthermore, while a specific infectious disease will not occur in the absence of the causative organism, the mere presence of the organ-

724

ism in the human body does not lead invariably to clinical illness. Indeed, the production of symptoms in man by many parasites is an exception rather than the rule, and a *subclinical infection* or the "carrier state" is the usual host-parasite relationship. *Disease* in a clinical sense is not synonymous with the presence of the organism or *infection* in a microbiologic sense. The ratio of subclinical infection to overt clinical disease varies widely for different microbial species. For example, subclinical infections with the agent causing infectious hepatitis are the rule. By contrast, active human infection with the rabies virus probably always produces progressive fatal disease and subclinical infections with rabies have not been observed.

Mechanisms of Injury

It is customary to refer to bacteria or other microorganisms that are capable of producing disease as *pathogenic*. *Virulence*, the *degree* of pathogenicity, should be distinguished from *invasiveness*, the ability to spread and disseminate in the body. For example, *Clostridium tetani* is pathogenic and, by virtue of its exotoxin, highly virulent, but it is almost completely lacking in invasiveness. These distinctions are valuable in microbiology and experimental pathology, but they often mean relatively little at a clinical level. Under certain circumstances and in certain anatomic locations, mildly "pathogenic" organisms can produce fatal disease, or highly "pathogenic" species can dwell and multiply without producing any harmful effect.

A few parasites produce *toxins* that account for the tissue damage and physiologic alterations of infection. *Hypersensitivity* to components of the parasite is demonstrable in several infections to account for the manifestations of disease. For many pathogenic agents, an explanation of their damaging effects upon the host is incomplete or wholly lacking. Generally, therefore, the aim of therapy is to stop multiplication or to kill the parasites with appropriate drugs; in diseases caused by toxin-producing organisms, the use of antiserum (as in tetanus or diphtheria) is the definitive procedure and chemotherapy is secondary.

The tendency of certain pathogenic organisms to *localize in certain cells or organs* and to produce damage is also unexplained in most instances. Clinically, however, the presence of disease in a specific anatomic site or a combination of symptoms referable to certain organs often suggests the identity of the causative organism. For example, the pneumococcus usually causes infection in the lung but almost never in the kidney, and *Hemophilus influenzae* infections are confined almost solely to the respiratory tract and meninges. Similarly, in the presence of disease known to be caused by a given agent, complicating involvement of other tissues can be anticipated or predicted. Examples include the multiple lung abscesses which are so characteristic of hematogenously disseminated staphylococcal disease and metastatic skin lesions which complicate *Pseudomonas* bacteremia.

Frequently, the proper management of infectious disease involves the use of techniques completely unrelated to microbiology or chemotherapy, in an effort to support the function of damaged organs. Survival in poliomyelitis may depend upon treatment of respiratory failure, the management of heart failure in endocarditis is sometimes a greater problem than the eradication of the causative organism, and in epidemic hemorrhagic fever, or Weil's disease, maintenance of fluid and electrolyte balance, with peritoneal dialysis or hemodialysis during the stage of acute renal failure is the important therapeutic objective.

Resistance and Susceptibility

Many so-called "host factors" are known to influence the likelihood that disease will occur if organisms enter the tissues or, if infection becomes established, to play a determining role in the outcome of infection—recovery or death. These include natural antibodies, interferon, phagocytic activity, and the level of the general inflammatory response.

In experimental animals, *sex, strain, age, route of infection,* the presence of *specific antibody, other diseases, nutritional state,* and the use of such procedures as exposure to ionizing radiation or high environmental temperature or administration of mucin, nitrogen mustard, adrenal steroids, epinephrine, xerosin, and metabolic analogues can be shown to exert a profound effect upon infection by bacteria, viruses, and other agents.

In man, these factors are no less impressive, although controlled studies are lacking for many. Alcoholism; diabetes; deficiency or absence of immunoglobulins (Chap. 69); defects in cellular immunity (Chap. 69); malnutrition; chronic administration of adrenal hormones; chronic lymphedema; ischemia; the presence of foreign bodies such as bullets, calculi, or bone fragments; obstruction of a bronchus, the urethra, or any hollow tube; agranulocytosis; various blood dyscrasias, and many other circumstances influence susceptibility to systemic or local infection. Furthermore, in those instances where the extenuating condition is remediable, the probability of recovery is enhanced.

Racial differences in susceptibility, such as the poor resistance of dark-skinned people to tuberculosis, their predilection for developing disseminated coccidioidomycosis, and the resistance of Negroes to malaria caused by *Plasmodium vivax,* are well established in several infections. Resistance to infection may be determined genetically, at least in part. The relationship of sickle-cell trait to malaria is one example. The increased frequency and severity of some infections in children, others in pregnant women, and still others in the aged are familiar clinical facts.

Prior contact with an organism or its products, whether by active infection or by artificial immunization, increases resistance to some infections, such as measles, diphtheria, and pertussis by stimulating antibody production, but seems to have little influence on resistance to others, such as gonorrhea.

Present knowledge of the factors involved in human

resistance and susceptibility is incomplete. Explanations such as changes in physical or chemical activity of phago-cytes; antibacterial substances such as lysozyme, phago-cytin, or lysozomal enzymes; qualitative or quantitative alterations in serum proteins; disordered metabolism at the cellular level; "products of tissue injury" that influ-ence vascular permeability, and the effects of tissue pres-sure remain to a considerable extent in the realm of hypo-thesis.

The profound influence of host factors upon the in-fectious process makes it clear, however, that if under-standing them ever reaches a point that permits their control in predictable fashion, a new era in the manage-ment and control of infectious disease will be at hand. There is no more important and fertile field for investi-gation in medicine.

PATHOGENESIS OF INFECTION

With relatively minor variations, the development of an infectious disease follows a consistent pattern. The parasites enter the body through the skin, nasopharynx, lung, intestine, urethra, or other portal, and a regular se-quence ensues. Once established in the host, the organ-isms can multiply and, in so doing, establish a *local* or *primary lesion*. From this site, there may be *local spread* along fascial planes or tubular structures, such as a bron-chus or ureter. The next step is *systemic spread* of the microorganisms by the circulating blood, which they reach by direct invasion of vessels (a relatively unusual occurrence) or by the common method of being borne in lymph to the thoracic duct and entering the venous system. In the bloodstream, they spread to other tissues and can produce *distant*, or *secondary*, *lesions*. In infec-tions such as tetanus and diphtheria, distant lesions are produced by toxins elaborated at the primary lesion with-out systemic spread of the parasites. The infectious proc-ess may terminate in recovery or death at any stage: the local lesion, systemic spread, or distant lesion.

The apparent inconsistency of this pattern in clinical medicine is attributable to the fact that the infection has been recognized as a *clinical entity* only at the stage when symptoms are most likely to appear. For example, pneu-mococcal pneumonia is a local lesion, and the distant le-sion, pneumococcal meningitis, is referred to clinically as a *complication*. In meningococcal infections, the local lesion, a nasopharyngitis, is rarely symptomatic and has no status as a clinical entity, but the stage of spread, meningococcemia, and the commonest distant lesion, meningitis, are clinical entities. A rarer distant lesion, ar-thritis, is called a complication. In a patient who has osteomyelitis, a clinical entity, a recent furuncle may be referred to as a *predisposing factor*. In another patient with extensive furunculosis who develops osteomyelitis, the infection in bone may be regarded by the clinician as a complication of the superficial infection. The stages mentioned are in no way limited to bacterial diseases; the primary lesion of poliomyelitis is intestinal, viremia may occur without neurologic involvement, or a distant lesion, the classic "infantile paralysis," may be established.

Because of established clinical usage and terminology based upon the symptomatic illness that leads patients to seek medical aid, the consistency of this general sequence in the pathogenesis of infection is often not recognized. However, the concept is useful to the clinician and offers some basis for systematizing what may otherwise seem to be a miscellaneous collection of unrelated clinical signs and symptoms.

CLINICAL MANIFESTATIONS OF INFECTIONS

So varied are the disorders attributable to infection or infestation of man by lower organisms that generalization about them is difficult. The clinical manifestations of in-fection can duplicate those of diseases of any other etiol-ogy. Certain clinical features are highly suggestive of infection, including abrupt onset, fever, chills, myalgia, photophobia, pharyngitis, acute lymphadenopathy or splenomegaly, gastroenteritis, and leukocytosis or leuko-penia. It is obvious that the presence of one, several, or all of these features does not constitute proof of the microbial origin of illness in a given patient. Conversely, serious, even fatal, infectious disease may exist in the absence of fever or the other signs and symptoms men-tioned.

Although there is no infallible clinical criterion of in-fection, it is still possible to recognize accurately many specific infectious diseases from information obtained by *history, physical examination, blood count,* and *urinalysis.* The importance of interrogation about past illness, pre-disposing factors such as alcoholism, familial disease, ex-posure to ill persons, contact with animals or insects, in-gestion of contaminated food, type and order of onset of symptoms, and recent or remote residence in endemic areas is discussed in subsequent chapters for specific dis-eases and etiologic agents. Cardinal physical signs are also described for each entity.

It is fitting to acknowledge ignorance of the mecha-nisms that produce most of the signs and symptoms of human infection. As discussed in Chap. 16 the pathogene-sis of fever is understood incompletely. The physiologic alterations underlying "malaise," "postinfectious asthe-nia," "toxicity," and other common complaints are com-pletely mysterious. The factors responsible for the leu-kocytoses or leukopenias that characterize certain infec-tions are only partially understood (Chap. 64). Why the rash of typhus begins on the trunk while that of another rickettsiosis, Rocky Mountain spotted fever, begins on the extremities is unanswered. It cannot be said that fail-ure to understand the production of these manifestations impairs their clinical usefulness in differential diagnosis, but it is probable that understanding would bring with it clues to more accurate diagnosis and better manage-ment.

DIAGNOSTIC PROCEDURES

When dealing with diseases produced by living agents, it is soon evident that confirmation of a presumptive diagnosis, or sometimes the first suggestion as to the etiology of illness, depends upon laboratory procedures. The availability of a multitude of laboratory tests in the modern hospital has not made it possible to substitute a "routine lab work-up" for history, physical examination, and observation of a patient's course. Indeed, the information derived from these procedures is the only reasonable basis for selecting the tests to be performed by the laboratory.

The importance of roentgenographic changes, alterations in chemical constituents of the blood, and tests of the functional capacity of organs such as the liver and kidney is as great in infectious disease as in illnesses of other etiologies and needs no discussion here.

The specific procedures for the diagnosis of infectious disease involve *direct demonstration of the causative organism* or *proof of its presence by indirect means.*

Demonstration of the Organism

In bacterial diseases, it is often possible to find the causative organism by *microscopic examination of properly stained preparations of sputum, spinal fluid, and other body fluids.* This simple procedure is often neglected as an unnecessary bother when material is being sent for bacteriologic culture, but it is a most valuable source of immediate information. In many diseases, the etiologic agent cannot be cultured (bartonellosis), and in others, isolation is time-consuming (tuberculosis, blastomycosis). The diagnosis of meningococcal infection by finding the organism in fluid from skin lesions or in the buffy coat or the finding of *H. influenzae* in stained smears of cerebrospinal fluid enables the clinician to initiate specific chemotherapy immediately with assurance that the regimen is the proper one.

Direct examination of bone marrow is a useful method for demonstrating organisms in some diseases, kala-azar, histoplasmosis, and tuberculosis being examples. In protozoan (amebiasis, malaria) and parasitic diseases (schistosomiasis, filariasis), *direct examination of blood, feces, or urine* is the only feasible method for establishing a diagnosis.

There are also infections in which the *detection of characteristic cytologic changes or the causative organism itself in smears or histologic sections of biopsy material* may be the quickest method for diagnosis. Tubercles and tubercle bacilli in lymph nodes or liver biopsy material, leprosy bacilli in skin or nasal scrapings, inclusion bodies in the skin lesions of varicella or variola and the exudate of inclusion blenorrhea, "Warthin" cells from the nasal mucosa in measles, schistosome ova in pinch biopsies of rectal mucosa, and the Councilman bodies of yellow fever in liver are examples. In addition, characteristic histologic changes make it feasible to identify the lesions of chancroid, syphilis, lymphogranuloma venereum, or viral hepatitis in biopsy specimens. Indeed, even in diseases where other reliable tests are available, diagnosis by histologic examination is sometimes the most rapid method, an example being the characteristic muscle lesion of Weil's disease (Chap. 181).

Special Microscopic Techniques

Dark-field examination of material from genital lesions for the spirochete of syphilis is a well-known but often neglected procedure. In several other spirochetal diseases, including leptospirosis, the dark-field technique can be useful, but experience in recognition of the organisms is necessary for correct interpretation of findings.

Fluorescence microscopy, in which the causative organisms can be recognized and identified rapidly by the use of fluorescent-antibody preparations (the Coons technique) is being applied increasingly in the diagnosis of streptococcal pharyngitis, gonorrhea, and pertussis. With continuing refinement and simplification, it may be expected to be extended to other infections including those viruses which carry specific antigens.

Culture and Animal Inoculation

Specimens for bacteriologic culture should be collected before the *initiation of chemotherapy.* The material to be cultured—sputum, pus, blood, or bone marrow—should be selected on the basis of the suspected infections, and the precise cultural techniques employed—media, CO_2 incubation, anaerobic incubation, etc.—must be decided upon in a similar fashion. New developments in tissue culture techniques have facilitated the isolation and identification of a wide range of viruses, and refinements in these techniques are increasing the value of tissue culture in clinical diagnosis.

In several infections, including Weil's disease, rat-bite fever, certain mycoses, tuberculosis, and the rickettsioses, the etiologic organism can be isolated by *inoculation of appropriate material into mice or guinea pigs.* This is a cumbersome procedure for routine use, but should be employed in selected instances. Many viruses can also be isolated by inoculation of appropriate animals. This is rarely feasible for ordinary clinical diagnosis and, for several agents, is hazardous.

Blood Cultures and Bacteremia

Because of the peculiar clinical importance of demonstrating bacteria in the bloodstream and because there are varying opinions about optimal timing and sites of sampling for blood cultures, it is of practical importance to understand something about the mechanisms of bacteremia.

Excepting intravascular infections (bacterial endocarditis or endarteritis, mycotic aneurysm, suppurative thrombophlebitis), bacteria enter the circulation almost invariably through the lymphatic system. Consequently, when bacteria multiply at a site of local infection in the tissues, the likelihood of bacteremia parallels the occurrence of local conditions that favor drainage of lymph from the area to the thoracic duct and eventually, the venous blood. These factors include the number and anatomic arrangement of local lymph vessels, accumulation of fluid and increase in tissue pressure, and manipulation of the part.

Once bacteria enter the blood, they are removed rapidly by the fixed phagocytes of the reticuloendothelial system in the liver and spleen and by engulfment in polymorphonuclear leukocytes in capillaries, especially those of the lung.

Clinically, bacteremia can be transient, intermittent, or continuous. Many transient bacteremias result from manipulation of infected or contaminated tissues, common examples being instrumentation of the genitourinary tract, tonsillectomy, dental procedures, and massage or surgical incision of furuncles or abscesses. In the vast majority of instances, the sudden discharge of bacteria into the blood produces no symptoms or, at most, a rigor and brief fever, and the organisms are promptly dealt with by the removal of mechanisms already mentioned. The great danger of these "man-made" bacteremias is their role in producing bacterial endocarditis in patients with endocardial damage.

Transient bacteremia accompanies the early phase of many infections. In pneumococcal pneumonia, the typical rigor at onset is a result of transient bacteremia. In most cases, with localization of the pulmonary lesion, blood cultures rapidly revert to negative. The poor prognosis of patients with pneumonia who continue to have positive blood cultures is not based on the danger from the mere presence of organisms in the blood as much as it is on bacteremia as a reflection of spreading infection in the lung itself.

A sudden single influx of microorganisms into the bloodstream may be followed by a shaking chill and fever. However, there is a "lag period" of 30 to 90 min before the febrile response (Chap. 16). During this delay, the bacteria are usually promptly removed from the circulation by phagocytosis and, consequently, a blood culture taken at the time of the rigor may be negative.

Continuous bacteremia is a feature of the first several days of typhoid fever, of brucellosis, and of intravascular infections such as endocarditis.

Blood cultures should be taken at frequent intervals in patients with febrile disease of unknown cause; in general, an attempt should be made to obtain blood *before* an expected rise in fever or chill. When a patient is suspected of bacterial endocarditis, or another of the diseases in which bacteremia is constant, two to four cultures daily for 2 to 3 days are more than sufficient to establish diagnosis, and treatment in such cases should not be withheld for a longer period.

There is no evidence that arterial blood possesses any advantage over blood from the antecubital veins for culture. Suspected bacteremia is sometimes mentioned as a contraindication to diagnostic lumbar puncture because of the possible development of meningitis, but clinical evidence does not support this idea. Culture of bone marrow is occasionally superior to peripheral blood for recovery of organisms in typhoid, brucellosis, and rare cases of subacute bacterial endocarditis. While it is common practice to make pour plates of blood and to quantify bacteremia in terms of a certain number of colonies per milliliter of blood, the results of this rather cumbersome procedure have no diagnostic or prognostic significance. Colony counts may be useful, however, to distinguish contaminating organisms. When blood cultures are taken for diagnostic purposes, some should be incubated in carbon dioxide, and a sample of blood should also be cultured in thioglycollate broth or some other anaerobic medium. Anaerobic cultures are especially important in women with puerperal or postabortal infections.

Immunologic Methods

These diagnostic methods are intended to supply evidence of past or present infection by demonstrating antibodies in serum or other body fluids, by showing changed reactivity of the host (hypersensitivity, allergy) to products of the organism, or rarely, to detect components of the causative organism in the body (Chaps. 68 to 70). Emphasis here is directed toward the interpretation of immunologic tests commonly used for clinical diagnosis.

SEROLOGIC TESTS. The finding on a single occasion that a patient's serum contains antibody that reacts with a certain antigen merely indicates that the patient has had previous contact with the antigen or a closely related substance. For this reason, with rare exceptions, the clinical interpretation of serologic tests depends on serial determinations. If the antibody titer is found to *rise or fall significantly,* it is likely that the response is a result of recent contact with the antigen. In subsequent chapters, the need for serologic testing of acute phase and convalescent serum is emphasized repeatedly. *In any patient with a puzzling illness, a sterile specimen of serum should be preserved in a frozen state so that it can, if necessary, be studied and compared with serum collected at a later date.*

Prior contact with an antigen may be the result of past artificial immunization with vaccines; interpretation of serum agglutinin titers for typhoid bacilli is often made difficult by prior immunization. The so-called "anamnestic reaction," a nonspecific stimulation of antibody formation by an acute illness (e.g., a rise in brucella agglutinins in a patient with acute tularemia), occurs only when the two organisms are antigenically related and rarely presents a serious problem.

The methods employed for detecting antibody rises in various infections have been selected empirically on the basis of the ease of performing the test and careful study to correlate the results of the test with other diagnostic criteria in patients. Therefore, the fact that antibodies against one agent are detected by a precipitin technique, another by agglutination of whole organisms or the production of capsular swelling, another by indirect fluorescent-antibody methods, and still another by complement fixation is a practical matter and bears no necessary relationship to the agent, the type of infection, or its pathogenesis. By coating some particulate material, such as erythrocytes or latex with antigen derived from a certain organism, antibody can sometimes be demonstrated by an agglutination test rather than by some more complex method.

Particular properties of the causative organism can sometimes be utilized to devise a simplified clinical test for antibody. Two striking instances of this are widely used. The ability of influenza and related viruses to clump erythrocytes makes possible the demonstration of antibody to virus by merely testing the capacity of a patient's serum to prevent the agglutination of red cells by suspensions of virus, the so-called "hemagglutination-inhibition" reaction. Similarly, because many microorganisms possess hemolytic components or toxins, the assay of a patient's serum for capacity to prevent lysis of red cells is a convenient and simple clinical test for antibody. The antistreptolysin O test in group A beta-hemolytic streptococcal infections is an example of this.

In a few infections, predominantly those caused by viruses, the only reliable serologic test is a *neutralization or protection* test, an assay of the protection afforded by the patient's serum against active infection in tissue culture or in experimental animals. This technique is time-consuming and is usually performed only in diagnostic virology laboratories.

Some mention of "nonspecific" serologic changes may serve to emphasize again that clinical laboratory tests have come into use *only because they have been found to correlate reasonably well with clinical findings.* In several diseases, it has been found, often accidentally, that serum antibody develops that will react with antigens derived from sources other than the etiologic agent (which may actually be unknown). Common examples are heterophil agglutinins in infectious mononucleosis, cold agglutinins in some forms of nonbacterial pneumonia, and the agglutination of certain strains of proteus bacilli by serum of patients with rickettsial diseases. The Wassermann test for syphilis and related flocculation tests are performed with antigens derived from sources completely unrelated to *Treponema pallidum.*

The results of serologic tests must be interpreted in the light of other information about the patient, including such factors as previous immunizations and illnesses, the possibility of exposure to chemically but etiologically unrelated antigens, and the importance of a changing titer in serial tests as opposed to a single isolated observation.

SKIN TESTS. Exposure to antigens of certain types, by various routes, and under circumstances not completely understood often results in the development of *immediate (anaphylactic, atopic) hypersensitivity* or *delayed (bacterial, tuberculin) hypersensitivity.*

Active infection with some, but not all, bacteria and viruses results in delayed hypersensitivity to the infecting agent in some, but not all, individuals. Clinically, this allergic state is detected by intradermal injection of the organisms or some component of them; in a sensitive person, induration and erythema will appear at the local site within 24 to 48 hr. If an individual is highly sensitive or if the amount of antigen injected is excessive, there may be extensive local inflammation with necrosis, vesicle formation, edema, regional lymphadenopathy, and

even malaise and fever. Antigens prepared in concentrations unlikely to provoke severe reactions are generally available for intradermal testing for tuberculosis, leprosy, mumps, lymphogranuloma venereum, cat-scratch disease, chancroid, brucellosis, tularemia, glanders, toxoplasmosis, blastomycosis, histoplasmosis, coccidioidomycosis, and many other infections. The "immune reaction" to vaccination (Chap. 223) is also an example of delayed dermal hypersensitivity.

The reliability, specificity, and usefulness of the individual tests differ and are discussed in the chapters on specific infections. However, certain general principles apply to their use and interpretation:

1. They are highly useful in epidemiologic surveys as indicators of the incidence of infection in a population.

2. In most individuals, dermal reactivity persists for many years or for life. A single positive test means only that at some past time the individual was exposed to the organism (or a closely related one). Unless supplementary information in the form of clinical findings, cultural studies, or more specific serologic data bear out the presence of active infection, a diagnosis of the disease is not justified.

3. The appearance of a positive dermal reaction in an individual known to have been nonreactive a short time before is good evidence of recent infection; this is a useful method for detecting tuberculosis.

4. A *negative intradermal test does not rule out past or present infection.* For unknown reasons, patients with measles, Hodgkin's disease, or sarcoidosis often develop a state of "anergy," or inability to react to intradermally injected antigens. In several diseases, dermal sensitivity develops after weeks or months of infection; an important example of this is acute histoplasmosis, in which patients can be ill for many weeks without showing a positive skin test. The skin test to coccidioidin is always negative in disseminated coccidioidomycosis, and in far-advanced or miliary tuberculosis in elderly patients, failure to react to intradermal tuberculin in the usual amounts employed for testing occurs in as many as 10 to 15 percent of the cases.

Intradermal injection of antigens derived from sources other than microorganisms usually produces an immediate "wheal and erythema" reaction which subsides promptly. The greatest clinical usefulness of this type of reaction is in the detection of allergy to foreign serums, pollens, and animal dander (Chap. 72). The skin tests for demonstrating infestation with helminths (trichinosis, filariasis) produce reactions of the immediate type in allergic individuals, but many of the antigens employed are so nonspecific that they are of little use in diagnosis.

THE IMPORTANCE OF SPECIFIC DIAGNOSIS IN INFECTIOUS DISEASES

Medicine and Microbiology

The diagnostic procedures employed for infectious diseases are no more absolute than those in other diseases; they cannot be blindly equated with the science of microbiology. The responsibility for interpreting the facts supplied by the bacteriologist, immunologist, and virologist in the total context of a patient's illness remains that of the physician. A positive tuberculin skin test certainly does not indicate that a patient has active tuberculosis. The finding of *Candida albicans* (monilia) in a stool culture does not necessarily mean that a patient's diarrhea is caused by intestinal moniliasis. The presence of staphylococci in nasal cultures from a patient with headaches does not establish a diagnosis of staphylococcal sinusitis. A throat culture containing beta-hemolytic streptococci does not rule out diphtheria; nor does such a culture establish that a febrile illness in a patient with mitral stenosis is a recurrence of acute rheumatic fever rather than bacterial endocarditis. A positive serologic test for syphilis, which measures Wassermann-type antibodies, may be the first sign of incipient lupus erythematosus.

The Etiologic Agent

From a practical point of view, two important steps are vital to the correct diagnosis of infection: (1) The organ(s) or organ systems involved must be found; (2) the etiologic agents causing the infections must be identified precisely. A previous section has dealt with the diagnostic approaches that are available and the following three chapters describe some important problems in infectious diseases, namely, complicated infections, which, by and large, occur in debilitated patients in the hospital, endotoxin shock, and antimicrobial therapy. The remaining chapters take up the specific bacteria, spirochetes, fungi, rickettsias, viruses, mycoplasma, and protozoa which cause infections. The common syndromes caused by these agents are described in the individual chapters. For example, bacterial pneumonia is discussed in detail in the chapter on pneumococcal infections

Table 132-1. THE SYNDROMIC APPROACH TO INFECTION

Type of infection	Etiologic agents		
	Common	Relatively common	Unusual but important
Skin and subcutaneous tissue	*Staphylococcus aureus*	Group A streptococcus, *candida* and superficial fungi	Gram-negative bacilli (burns, wounds)
Sinusitis	*S. aureus*	Group A streptococcus, *Diplococcus pneumoniae*	Mucor
Pharyngitis	Respiratory viruses, Group A streptococcus	*Hemophilus influenzae* (children), fusiform bacilli	*Corynebacterium diphtheriae*
Otitis, mastoiditis	*D. pneumoniae, H. influenzae* (children)	*S. aureus*, Group A streptococcus	*Pseudomonas, Proteus*
Pneumonitis	*D. pneumoniae, Mycoplasma pneumoniae, Mycobacterium tuberculosis*	*S. aureus, Klebsiella*, respiratory viruses	Group A streptococcus, gram-negative enteric bacilli, psittacosis, systemic mycoses, pneumocystis
Empyema and lung abscess	*S. aureus*, anaerobic streptococcus, *Bacteroides*	*Klebsiella* (abscess)	
Bacterial endocarditis	*Streptococcus viridans, S. aureus*, enterococcus	*D. pneumoniae*, anaerobic streptococcus	Gram-negative bacilli, *Candida*
Gastroenteritis	Enteroviruses, *Salmonella, Shigella*	*S. aureus, Escherichia coli* (infants), *Clostridia*	*Pseudomonas, Endamoeba histolytica*
Peritonitis, cholangitis, intraabdominal abscess	*E. coli*, enterococcus, *Bacteroides*	*Klebsiella-Aerobacter, Proteus* species, paracolon, anaerobic streptococcus	*Clostridia, S. aureus*
Urinary infection (cystitis, pyelonephritis)	*E. coli, Klebsiella-Aerobacter*, paracolon, *Proteus*, enterococcus	*Pseudomonas*	*S. aureus*
Urethritis	Gonococcus, ?*Mycoplasma*, ?*Mima-Herellea*	*Treponema pallidum*	
Pelvic inflammatory disease	Gonococcus, *E. coli*	Klebsiella-*Aerobacter, Bacteroides*, anaerobic streptococcus, enterococcus	*Clostridia, S. aureus*
Bones (osteomyelitis)	*S. aureus*	*Salmonella*	Group A streptococcus
Joints	*S. aureus*, gonococcus, *D. pneumoniae*	Group A streptococcus, *Neisseria meningitidis*	*E. coli, Proteus, Pseudomonas*
Meninges	*D. pneumoniae, H. influenzae* (children), *N. meningitidis*, ECHO and mumps viruses	*E. coli*, Klebsiella-*Aerobacter, Proteus, Pseudomonas*	Group A streptococcus, *M. tuberculosis, Cryptococcus, S. aureus, Listeria monocytogenes*

(Chap. 138), osteomyelitis is described with staphylococcal infections (Chap. 139), the manifestations of bacteriuria are described in Chap. 144 and 303, and those of meningitis in Chap. 142, 360, and 361. Nevertheless, when confronted with specific organ involvement, it is important to know the most common pathogens which cause disease in the involved organ. Table 132-1 provides a listing of these pathogens. Used in conjunction with the individual chapters dealing with specific agents and the summary of chemotherapy (Chap. 135), the table should provide a rational guide to treatment which often must be instituted before the results of antimicrobial sensitivity tests are available.

Chemotherapy

The impact of chemotherapy upon mortality and morbidity from infection and upon epidemic disease is now a matter of historical record. These therapeutic agents, however, have in no way lessened the importance of specific diagnosis; indeed their availability has increased the need for obtaining exact etiologic information. It requires but a moment's reflection to realize that the substitution of a prescription for a broad-spectrum antibiotic or a quick injection of penicillin for the systematic collection of facts and thoughtful consideration of diagnostic possibilities is a fallacious, unwise, and dangerous practice. Numerous antibiotics with overlapping spectrums are now available, dosages for different infections vary widely, the drugs themselves are potentially dangerous, and their administration entails considerable expense. They should never be prescribed as placebos, antipyretics, or substitutes for diagnosis. In the vast majority of instances in which this is done, patients recover just as they would if no "therapy" had been given and the drugs are wasted. More important, inadequate dosage or the wrong agent may suppress symptoms temporarily without curing, make isolation of the etiologic agent difficult, delay the recognition of the true nature of an illness, and postpone the institution of curative treatment. Furthermore, antibiotics may select out resistant variants or facilitate spread of infection by conferring resistance to bacteria due to R factors with subsequent hazard that these resistant organisms may spread to others. Finally, to expose a patient to the risk of drug reaction without proper indication is inexcusable, whether the drug is an antibiotic, a sedative, a laxative, or a narcotic.

Epidemiologic and Other Considerations

Just as the decision to administer antibiotics to a patient with a febrile illness of presumed infectious etiology must be made on an individual basis, the selection of cases in which extensive cultural and serologic testing is required is a matter of judgment. The majority of common "grippelike" illnesses subsides spontaneously, and symptomatic treatment is sufficient. However, because of this tendency toward spontaneous recovery and also because the results of serologic tests may not be available until a patient is convalescent, there are many who regard continued effort to determine the specific etiology of illness as an impractical, "academic" procedure. Such an attitude fails to recognize that the responsibility of the physician extends beyond the individual patient to include the community. For example, a patient recently recovered from "viral pneumonitis" may feel that his physician has cared for him competently and well. The doctor himself may feel that he has discharged his professional duties properly and that his having refrained from giving the patient antibiotics for what was clinically a virus disease and therefore unlikely to benefit from chemotherapy was a laudable act of forbearance. However, if a serologic test is reported a few days later as showing that the patient's serum has shown a rise in complement-fixing antibody against psittacosis, the situation might change. The patient himself would continue to be well, but a search for the source of the disease, such as the patient's pet parakeet, would certainly be indicated, and further illnesses in others might be prevented.

Despite the fact that pursuing diagnosis of obscure, often self-limited, illnesses may be academic, this approach has led to clarification of some important etiologic relationships. For example, the syndrome of infectious mononucleosis has been linked with development of antibody to a herpeslike virus, the EB virus, as well as cytomegalovirus (Chap. 255); some cases of erythema multiforme may be due to herpes simplex virus; several patients with encephalitis have been found to have central nervous system infections with myxoviruses. Some congenital anomalies have been related to prenatal viral infections; the relationship of subendocardial fibroelastosis to mumps is just one example (Chap. 231). The finding of bacterialike bodies in the intestinal mucosa of patients with Whipples disease and the improvement of these patients with tetracycline therapy provides another example of an entity of unknown etiology entering the realm of infectious diseases. Finally, the possibility has been raised that the Chediak-Higashi syndrome, a rare familial disorder characterized by albinism, photophobia, nystagmus, anomalous cellular granules, marked susceptibility to infection, and development of lymphoma, is caused by a virus. This association, among others, relates the field of infection to that of oncogenesis.

These discoveries clearly are the result of academic procedures which might have little immediate applicability to infection in a particular patient, yet few can question the fundamental biologic importance of these observations; moreover, it is conceivable that they will assume practical importance in the future.

REFERENCES

Bennett, I. L., Jr., and P. B. Beeson: Bacteremia: A Consideration of Some Experimental and Clinical Aspects, Yale J. Biol. Med., 26:241, 1954.

Burnet, M.: "Natural History of Infectious Disease," New York, Cambridge University Press, 1953.

Davis, B. D., R. Dulbecco, H. Eisen, H. S. Ginsberg, and W.

B. Wood, Jr.: "Microbiology" New York, Harper and Row, Publishers, Incorporated, 1968.

Dubos, R. J.: "Biochemical Determinants of Microbial Diseases," Cambridge, Mass., Harvard University Press, 1954.

——: The Evolution of Microbial Diseases, p. 20 in "Bacterial and Mycotic Diseases of Man," 4th ed., Philadelphia, J. B. Lippincott Company, 1965.

Horsfall, F. L., Jr.: Cancer and Viruses, Bull. N.Y. Acad. Med., 42:167, 1966.

—— and I. Tamm (Eds.): "Viral and Rickettsial Diseases of Man," 4th ed., Philadelphia, J. B. Lippincott Company, 1965.

MacLeod, C. M., and L. E. Cluff (Eds.): Symposium on Non-specific Resistance to Infection, Bacteriol. Rev., 24:1, 1960.

Rich, A. R.: "The Pathogenesis of Tuberculosis," 2d ed., Springfield, Ill., Charles C Thomas, Publisher, 1951.

Rogers, D. E.: The Changing Pattern of Life-threatening Microbial Disease, New Eng. J. Med., 261:677, 1959.

White, J. G.: Virus-like Particles in the Peripheral Blood Cells of Two Patients with Chediak-Higashi Syndrome, Cancer, 19:877, 1966.

Wilson, G. S., and A. A. Miles: "Topley and Wilson's Principles of Bacteriology and Immunity," 5th ed., Baltimore, The Williams and Wilkins Company, 1965.

Wood, W. B., Jr.: Studies on the Cellular Immunology of Acute Bacterial Infections, Harvey Lectures, 47:72, 1951–1952.

133 COMPLICATING INFECTIONS
Robert G. Petersdorf

A complicating infection is defined here as an infection occurring in a patient with a defect in host resistance or one which develops during hospitalization. Most of this chapter will deal with *hospital-acquired* (nosocomial) infections, because numerically they represent the most significant problem. Infections occurring in the host whose resistance has been altered by another disease or drug will be listed briefly.

EPIDEMIOLOGY. Hospital-acquired infections occur in 4 to 5 percent of all patients admitted to a general hospital. Moreover, at any one time approximately 5 percent of all patients in a general hospital will have such an infection, and among patients in the hospital with infections, fully one-third will have acquired their infection while in the hospital. The most common nosocomial infections encountered are postoperative infections, urinary tract infections, pneumonia, septic thrombophlebitis, and bacteremia.

PREDISPOSING FACTORS. Defects in Host Resistance. Certain infections occur with increased frequency with particular diseases. For example, patients with diabetes mellitus are prone to development of cutaneous infections, bacteriuria, tuberculosis, moniliasis, and, when ketoacidosis is uncontrolled, mucormycosis. Monilia infections have a predilection for patients with hypopara-

thyroidism; nocardiosis is more common in alveolar proteinosis; salmonella infections are more prevalent in patients with sickle-cell disease, schistosomiasis, malaria, and bartonellosis; pneumococcal infections occur often in very young children who have undergone splenectomy, in individuals with hypogammaglobulinemia (Chap. 69), and in association with multiple myeloma; cryptococcosis tends to infect patients with Hodgkin's disease and sarcoidosis; and a variety of bacterial infections complicates diseases associated with granulocytopenia. The reasons for the coexistence of these infections and the underlying diseases are largely unknown. In a sense, however, these associations represent peculiar experiments of nature and are overshadowed by infections resulting from the iatrogenic alterations in host resistance that follow the use of corticosteroids, antimetabolites, and radiomimetic, immunosuppressive, and antimicrobial drugs. Corticosteroids not only favor acquisition of new infections but may result in reactivation and dissemination of latent disease. Why these hormones increase susceptibility to infection is unknown; perhaps they depress the reticuloendothelial system, impair the development of immunity by decreasing antibody formation, and stabilize lysozomal membranes. Usually steroids produce infections in patients with those underlying diseases for which they were given, but because of their antiinflammatory effects, the hormones may mask the signs and symptoms of the complicating infections until they are relatively far advanced. The increased incidence of infection following cytotoxic drugs is probably a consequence of these agents' ability to produce granulocytopenia and lymphopenia and to decrease antibody production (Chap. 71).

Superinfections. Superinfections may be defined as infections which occur when antimicrobial therapy is administered for both therapeutic and prophylactic purposes. Their incidence is approximately 2 percent of all patients treated with antibiotics, and they are more common when such drugs are given in large doses, when several antimicrobials are administered concurrently, or when broad-spectrum agents are employed.

Clinical superinfections must be distinguished from the normal ecologic change in bacterial flora which accompanies all antimicrobial therapy. Most antibiotics lower the number of resident microorganisms and occasionally eradicate them entirely; the normal flora is then replaced by resistant exogenous or endogenous bacteria. In the vast majority of instances the number of bacteria replacing those eradicated by the drug is small and clinical disease does not take place. However, when the concentration of the superinfecting organisms is high, a clinical superinfection is more likely to occur.

Superinfections are particularly common with certain drugs; the tendency for *Pseudomonas* to colonize and infect patients receiving one of the cephalosporins is a notable example. Clinically significant superinfections usually appear 4 to 5 days after chemotherapy is instituted and must be watched for especially in patients being treated for pneumonia, chronic obstructive lung disease, otitis, and urinary tract infection, when a urethral catheter is in place. They often complicate the course of patients with respiratory viral diseases who are given antibiotics to prevent bacterial complications.

As a rule, they are caused by organisms that are resistant to the drug the patient is receiving, and penicillinase-producing staphylococci, gram-negative enteric bacilli, and fungi are the most common superinfecting microorganisms. The usual clinical manifestations include recrudescence of fever and other signs and symptoms at the site of the initial infection.

Other Diagnostic and Therapeutic Measures Resulting in Infections. The hospitalized patient is subjected to a variety of diagnostic and therapeutic procedures which predispose to infection. These include insertion of intravenous catheters and urethral catheterization, particularly if an indwelling catheter is left in place; uncommonly injections, thoracenteses, paracenteses, aspiration of joints, lumbar punctures, and tissue biopsies may be incriminated. At least 2 to 3 percent of operative procedures are complicated by infections; the rates vary with the type of operation. Infections are common in association with the use of equipment for inhalation therapy, and may be spread in the hospital by a variety of inanimate vehicles. The risk of complicating infections depends on the number and complexity of therapeutic or diagnostic manipulations and is enhanced by the concomitant indiscriminate use of antibiotics.

ETIOLOGY. The bacteria usually responsible for complicating infections are penicillinase-producing staphylococci (Chap. 139), *Escherichia coli* (Chap. 144), *Klebsiella-Aerobacter* (Chap. 148), *Proteus* (Chap. 145), *Pseudomonas* (Chap. 146), *Mima-Herellea* (Chap. 160), and less commonly, group D streptococci, enterococci (Chap. 141), and *Clostridia* (Chap. 172). Among the fungi, monilia (Chap. 190), mucor (Chap. 191), and aspergillus (Chap. 193) are frequent pathogens implicated in secondary infections. Cytomegalovirus (Chap. 232) and pneumocystis (Chap. 245) are common causes of complicating infections in patients with depressed host resistance.

MANIFESTATIONS. Obviously, the clinical picture of a complicating infection will vary with its site and, to a lesser extent, the microorganisms causing it. In most instances, the major sign is fever, which usually occurs after patients have been in the hospital 4 to 5 days or longer. However, in some patients the diagnosis rests only on signs of local inflammation such as phlebitis, cellulitis, or evidence of a deep-seated infection. Sometimes a complicating infection may be heralded by no more than unexplained hyperventilation, confusion, or disorientation. Specific types of infection will be considered below.

Postoperative Infections. These consist primarily of wound infections or collections of pus which form in and around the operative site. Although urinary tract infections and pneumonia are common in patients who have undergone surgery, postoperative infections are usually related to the surgical locus rather than an unrelated organ system.

Relatively few surgical procedures are responsible for the majority of wound infections, and these infections are particularly likely to occur when operations are long or require extensive resection and when contamination is unavoidable. Abdominal perineal resections, wounds involving arterial bypass grafts, insertion of cardiac prostheses, and portacaval shunts are associated with a relatively high rate of complicating infections. Most postoperative wound infections are caused by staphylococci and gram-negative enteric bacteria. Although group A streptococcal infections are averted with most chemoprophylactic regimens, wound infections which develop in patients receiving postoperative chemoprophylaxis usually are caused by organisms resistant to the drug being given. In general, chemoprophylaxis has not been successful in preventing wound infections, although the regimen which involves the administration of 10 million units of penicillin G at 2-hr intervals beginning immediately prior to and continuing throughout the operation has been shown to reduce postoperative wound sepsis.

Cutaneous, Subcutaneous, and Soft-tissue Infections. While wound sepsis comprises the major part of superficial infections, other sites are involved. These include abscesses in the skin, subcutaneous tissues and muscle, cellulitis, decubitus ulcers, vascular stasis ulcers, and lesions secondary to diminished arterial blood supply. Most often staphylococci are the causative organisms, but group A and anaerobic streptococci, gram-negative enteric bacilli, and even clostridia may be pathogenic under these circumstances. These infections may follow subcutaneous or intramuscular injections or extravasation of intravenous infusions. Although the infections usually remain localized, they may involve contiguous structures and may produce bacteremia. Gas in soft tissues should call to mind infection with *E. coli* (Chap. 144) as well as anaerobic organisms. Antimicrobial therapy should be directed at the specific organism. Staphylococcal infections should be treated with a penicillinase-resistant penicillin until the organism is shown to be sensitive to penicillin G. Surgical drainage and debridement are often essential to recovery.

Burns regularly become infected secondarily. Most of these patients are receiving systemic or local chemoprophylaxis, and usually infection develops after the gram-positive flora has been replaced by gram-negative organisms, particularly *Pseudomonas*. These organisms are usually acquired from the environment and have been shown to survive on the floors, walls, and equipment used on burn wards. The sudden development of shock in a patient with a burn is almost certain evidence that pseudomonas bacteremia is present. Treatment is discussed in Chaps. 134 and 146.

Urinary Tract Infections. Urinary tract infections usually are associated with instrumentation of the urethra, bladder, or ureters, and most often are due to insertion of an indwelling urethral catheter, which permits entry of bacteria from the external environment into the bladder. Nosocomial urinary infections do not occur without predisposing instrumentation. The organisms are usually *E. coli, Klebsiella-Aerobacter,* paracolon, *Proteus, Pseudomonas,* and enterococci and tend to be resistant to one or several antibiotics. Epidemics of *Klebsiella-Aerobacter* and *Pseudomonas* urinary infections following spread of bacteria from contaminated equipment have been reported. Most patients with hospital-acquired bacteriuria are asymptomatic, some have cystitis, and others have clear-cut evidence of pyelonephritis which may be associated with bacteremia. Treatment should be reserved for patients with symptoms and for those suspected of bacteremia. Patients with indwelling catheters who have asymptomatic bacteriuria should not receive antibiotics because it is unlikely that the organisms will be eradicated; instead, superinfections will develop.

Considerable progress has been made in preventing hospital-acquired urinary infections by maintaining a system of closed drainage. In this fashion, the urine can be kept sterile for 5 to 7 days after insertion of the catheter. Failure to maintain closed drainage will result in infection in almost all patients within 48 hr after catheter drainage is instituted.

Pneumonia. Pulmonary infections are common events in hospitalized patients with a variety of severe medical or surgical diseases. They may follow aspiration from any cause, atelectasis, heart failure, tracheostomy, and therapy with drugs that depress respiration. In a general hospital, pneumonia occurs commonly as a complication of cardiac or neurosurgery, but these infections are also seen in debilitated general medical patients, particularly when respiratory assistance devices have been employed. Mainstream reservoir nebulizers containing saline solutions are often heavily contaminated with *Pseudomonas,* flavobacteria, *Herellea,* and *Achromobacter* and are capable of producing severe pulmonary infections when nebulized directly into the tracheobronchial tree. This risk can be reduced sharply by bubbling a 0.25 percent acetic acid solution through the nebulizing equipment for 5 min prior to use. Gram-negative enteric bacteria usually are implicated in complicating pulmonary infections, particularly when patients have received antimicrobials. Although tracheostomies are often necessary to maintain adequate ventilation, they are almost invariably associated with infections. These infections can only be prevented by meticulous aseptic technique during suctioning and the use of sterile suction catheters. The major therapeutic problem in many patients with complicating infections of the lung is mechanical; positive pressure breathing, postural drainage, frequent suctioning, and sometimes bronchoscopy are at least as important in the treatment of these infections as appropriate antibiotics.

Bacterial Endocarditis. Patients undergoing open-heart surgery have a relatively high incidence of wound, urinary, and pulmonary infections, but the most dreaded complication of open-heart surgery is endocarditis on a prosthetic valve. It occurs predominantly in patients whose operation is conducted on cardiopulmonary bypass, and surgery on the aortic valve is complicated by endocarditis much more frequently than surgery on the mitral valve. *Staphylococcus aureus* and *S. albus* are the most common pathogens. Clinical signs of endocarditis are often absent, and fever during the first 4 postoperative weeks provides the best clue to infections which follow in the wake of surgery. However, in some instances the prosthetic valve becomes infected years after its insertion, emphasizing the importance of preventing bacteremia in the patients. The prophylactic regimens for preventing endocarditis are detailed in Chap. 137.

The diagnosis depends upon isolation of the organism in blood cultures. Treatment of endocarditis on intracardiac prostheses have been notoriously unsuccessful, and although the infection may be suppressed with antibiotics, reoperation, which often eventuates fatally, is usually necessary. Therefore, to prevent endocarditis, antimicrobial administration to patients undergoing open-heart surgery has become routine practice. It is clear that administration of a penicillinase-resistant penicillin will prevent postoperative pneumococcal endocarditis, but the efficacy of these drugs in preventing endocarditis with other organisms, including staphylococci, is less certain.

Bacteremia. Invasion of the bloodstream can occur in any nosocomial infection, and among the various foci, the urinary tract predominates. However, the indwelling venous catheter is fast becoming the most common source of bacteremia in hospitalized patients, particularly when it is left in place longer than 48 hr. Many of these patients develop phlebitis before bacteremia, and the catheter should be removed from all patients with inflammation at the catheter site. Staphylococci are implicated most often in catheter-associated infections, but *Mimaherellea* and other gram-negative organisms have been cultured from both the local site and the bloodstream.

Treatment of catheter-induced bacteremia requires removal of the catheter and systemic antimicrobial therapy; the treatment of staphylococcal bacteremia is discussed in Chap. 139 and that of gram-negative sepsis in Chap. 134. These infections can be prevented by (1) use of the catheter only when absolutely necessary; (2) strict aseptic technique during placement of the catheter; (3) application of bacitracin-neomycin-polymyxin ointment to the catheter site; and (4) removal of the catheter within 48 hr, or sooner if phlebitis or cellulitis is present.

Miscellaneous Complicating Infections. *Staphylococcal parotitis* is common in debilitated patients with a variety of medical diseases; it often follows in the wake of dehydration (Chap. 231). *Septic arthritis* is not uncommon in patients with antecedent rheumatoid or degenerative joint disease who are subjected to diagnostic aspiration of the joint or who are treated with intraarticular drugs, usually corticosteroids. Pneumococcus, group A streptococcus, and staphylococcus are the most common pathogens. *Iatrogenic meningitis* is a rare complication of spinal anesthesia, epidural block, injection of the stellate ganglion, diagnostic lumbar puncture, and myelography. Pneumococcus, staphylococcus, and pseudomonas have been cultured from these patients. Staphylococcal enterocolitis occurs primarily in patients who have had gastrointestinal surgery and who were given antibiotics preoperatively. It is also common in patients with liver disease who are treated with neomycin to reduce ammonia production by the bowel flora. Oral vancomycin (0.5 Gm every 6 to 12 hr for four doses) or systemic penicillinase-resistant penicillins or cephalosporins are all effective modes of treatment.

Infections Occurring During Organ Transplantation.
Aside from host versus graft reactions (Chap. 71), infections pose the most serious threat to patients undergoing organ transplantation. These patients all receive immunosuppressive drugs and large quantities of adrenal cortical hormones and have readily available portals of entry for a variety of microorganisms. Multiple infections are common. Coagulase-positive staphylococci are the most common bacteria isolated, but pseudomonas, gram-negative enteric bacilli, and streptococci other than group A are also cultured. The organisms are often present in the nasopharynx or on the skin of patients prior to transplantation, and for this reason, it is recommended by some authorities that all staphylococcal carriers be treated with a penicillinase-resistant penicillin for several days prior to the procedure and afterward until the wound has healed. Likewise, bacteriuria should be eradicated before surgery. When transplantation is performed for pyelonephritis, the ureters should be excised in their entirety along with the kidneys.

Patients who have undergone transplantation are particularly susceptible to fatal pulmonary infections which may produce few symptoms and signs. In addition to the bacteria mentioned above, cytomegalovirus (Chap. 232), monilia (Chap. 190), aspergillus (Chap. 193), and pneumocystis (Chap. 245) are found at autopsy. These infections are characterized by little in the way of an inflammatory response, and the fungi, in particular, tend to produce a necrotizing reaction. Although no definitive information is available, it is likely that pulmonary superinfections with fungi or cytomegalovirus in these patients have an almost uniformly fatal prognosis.

LABORATORY FINDINGS. Cultures of pus, appropriate body fluids, and blood form the cornerstone of treatment and always should be obtained, even in patients receiving chemotherapy. Antimicrobial sensitivity tests should be performed when indicated. Gram stains of pus or secretions are helpful when only one or two types of bacteria are present in large numbers, but may be misleading and should be interpreted with caution. Superinfections usually are accompanied by leukocytosis, but granulocytopenia may be seen because of previous drug therapy or underlying disease. Moreover, many patients have a leukocytosis to begin with, and an elevated leukocyte count is of value as a clue to a complicating infection only if it was normal previously.

THERAPEUTIC CONSIDERATIONS. Because most complicating infections are caused by bacteria, treatment depends upon identification of the organism but must not be delayed until the results of cultures and sensitivity tests are at hand. Hence, the antibiotic must be chosen on the basis of previous cultures, the gram-stained smear, and the clinical picture. For example, patients with subcutaneous and soft-tissue infections should be treated with a penicillinase-resistant penicillin and those with bacteriuria with a drug active against enteric bacteria or enterococci. Patients with pneumonia or sepsis may require treatment with several drugs pending identification of the pathogen. The appropriate regimens are found in chapters dealing with the specific organisms and in the chapter on chemotherapy (Chap. 135). A general approach to therapy of undiagnosed bacteremia is provided in Chap. 134. Removal of the mechanical factors which are often the basis for complicating infections is as important as chemotherapy. This may involve withdrawing intravenous or urethral catheters, drainage of pus, debridement of a burn eschar, removal of sutures, aspiration of bronchial secretions, a change in inhalation equipment, and even, occasionally, removal of a cardiac prosthesis.

CHEMOPROPHYLAXIS AND COMPLICATING INFECTIONS.
Most patients who develop a complicating infection are receiving antibiotics, providing *prima facie* evidence that these drugs are not successful in preventing these infections. The experience with chemoprophylaxis in many clinical situations is summarized in Chap. 135. With a few notable exceptions, antibiotics have been incapable of preventing infection in patients with depressed host resistance and have usually been the primary factors leading to infections by resistant organisms.

PROGNOSIS. Most complicating infections occur in patients being treated for another disease which is often chronic, disabling, and potentially fatal. While these secondary infections demand vigorous treatment, they may be only incidental to the patient's primary problem. For example, a patient with disseminated carcinomatosis will die even if his complicating infection is contained; and conversely, a complicating infection often will not respond to therapy unless a remission is produced in the underlying disease.

REFERENCES

Barrett, F. F., J. I. Casey, and M. Finland: Infections and Antibiotic Use among Patients at Boston City Hospital, February, 1967, New Engl. J. Med., 278:5, 1968.

Beaty, H. N., and R. G. Petersdorf: Iatrogenic Factors in Infectious Disease, Ann. Intern. Med., 65:641, 1966.

Bentley, D. W., and M. H. Lepper: Septicemia Related to Indwelling Venous Catheter, J.A.M.A., 206:1749, 1968.

Goodman, J. S., W. Schaffner, H. A. Collins, E. J. Battersby, and M. G. Koenig: Infection after Cardiovascular Surgery: Clinical Study Including Examination of Antimicrobial Prophylaxis, New Engl. J. Med., 278:117, 1968.

Kunin, C. M., and R. C. McCormack: Prevention of Catheter-induced Urinary Tract Infections by Sterile Closed Drainage, New Engl. J. Med., 274:1155, 1966.

Moser, R. H.: "Diseases of Medical Progress," Springfield, Ill., Charles C Thomas, Publisher, 1969.

Petersdorf, R. G.: "The Prophylaxis of Infection," London, Pergamon Press, 1964.

Reinarz, J. A., A. K. Pierce, B. B. Mays, and J. P. Sanford: Potential Role of Inhalation Therapy Equipment in Nosocomial Pulmonary Infection, J. Clin. Invest., 44:831, 1965.

Rifkind, D., T. L. Marchioro, W. R. Waddell, and T. E. Starzl: Infectious Diseases Associated with Renal Homotransplantation, J.A.M.A., 189:397, 1964.

Thoburn, R., F. R. Fekety, Jr., L. E. Cluff, and V. B. Melvin:

Infections Acquired by Hospitalized Patients, Arch. Intern Med., 121:1, 1968.

Weinstein, L.: Superinfection: Complication of Antimicrobial Therapy and Prophylaxis, Am. J. Surg., 107:704, 1964.

134 SEPTIC SHOCK
Robert G. Petersdorf

DEFINITION. Septic shock is characterized by inadequate tissue perfusion, usually following bacteremia with gram-negative enteric bacilli. This circulatory insufficiency is a consequence of increased peripheral vascular resistance, pooling of blood in the microcirculation, diminished cardiac output, and tissue anoxia.

ETIOLOGY. Shock is sometimes associated with gram-positive infections, in which there are usually hypotension, peripheral vasodilatation, normovolemia, and normal cardiac output—so-called "warm shock" that is readily corrected with fluids and appropriate antibiotics. For practical purposes, septic shock follows bacteremia with gram-negative enteric bacilli: *E. coli* (Chap. 144), paracolon species, *Klebsiella-Enterobacter* (Chap. 148), *Proteus* species (Chap. 145), *Pseudomonas* (Chap. 146), and *Mima-Herellea* species (Chap. 160). Furthermore, the vasoactive phenomena collectively termed septic shock are probably not due to bacteremia per se but are related to release into the circulation of endotoxin, the lipopolysaccharide moiety of the organisms' cell walls.

EPIDEMIOLOGY. Gram-negative bacteremia and endotoxin shock occur primarily in hospitalized patients who usually have an underlying disease which renders them susceptible to bloodstream invasion. Predisposing factors include diabetes mellitus; cirrhosis; leukemia, lymphoma, or disseminated carcinoma; childbirth; and a variety of surgical procedures and antecedent infections in the urinary, biliary, or gastrointestinal tracts. Most adults with gram-negative sepsis are elderly males, but neonates are also prone to develop endotoxin shock. There has been an appreciable increase in the prevalence of serious gram-negative infections among hospitalized patients since 1935. Moreover, concurrent with the introduction and widespread use of antibiotics, cytotoxic agents, adrenal steroids, intravenous catheters, humidifiers, and other hospital equipment (Chap. 133) and the increasing longevity of patients with chronic diseases, this upward trend has gained momentum and in most hospitals gram-negative are now more common than gram-positive bacteremias.

PATHOGENESIS AND PATHOLOGY. With the exception of *Pseudomonas* and *Mima-Herellea*, which are ubiquitous in the hospital environment, most of the bacteria causing gram-negative sepsis are normal commensals in the gastrointestinal tract. From there they may spread to contiguous structures, as in peritonitis following appendiceal perforation, or migrate from the perineum into the urethra or bladder. Gram-negative bacteremia follows infection in a primary focus, usually in the genitourinary tract, biliary tree, gastrointestinal tract, and adjoining structures, or lungs and, less commonly, the skin, bones, and joints. In many patients, however, particularly those with chronic disease, cirrhosis, and tumors of the reticuloendothelial system, no primary focus is apparent. When bacteremia is followed by metastatic lesions in distant sites, classical abscess formation occurs. More often, however, the autopsy findings in gram-negative sepsis are scanty or nonspecific and reflect primarily the infection at the primary locus. This lack of concrete morphologic data has led some investigators to question the role of endotoxin in gram-negative shock in man. On the other hand, damage to the endothelial lining of capillary walls has been demonstrated early in experimental endotoxin shock, and many patients who die with gram-negative shock have been treated intensively, which would tend to obfuscate the pathologic findings that are often clear-cut in experimental animals.

PATHOPHYSIOLOGY. General Considerations. Endotoxin exerts its major effects on small blood vessels with sympathetic (alpha-receptor) innervation. The toxin causes intense arteriolar and venous spasm leading to significant immobilization of blood in the pulmonary, splanchnic, and renal capillaries and to stagnant anoxia in these tissues. Local acidosis develops and promotes relaxation of the arteriolar sphincter while the venule remains constricted. Blood pools in the capillary bed, and the increased hydrostatic pressure results in leakage of plasma into the interstitial fluid. This, in turn, causes a sharp decrease in effective circulating blood volume, lowered cardiac output, and systemic arterial hypotension. These result in stimulation of the baroreceptors, further sympathetic activity, vasoconstriction, and selective reduction of blood flow to visceral organs and skin. If ineffective perfusion of vital organs is permitted to continue, metabolic acidosis and severe parenchymal damage ensue and shock is then irreversible. In man, the kidneys and lungs are the organs particularly susceptible to endotoxin; oliguria as well as tachypnea and, in some instances, pulmonary edema, develops early. On the other hand, the heart and brain are spared in the early stages of shock; myocardial failure and coma are late and often terminal manifestations of the shock syndrome.

Hemodynamic Alterations in Man. Many of the observations dealing with the pathophysiology of endotoxin shock were made in animals, and the hemodynamic data often varied according to the species studied and the dose of endotoxin administered. The establishment of centers for the study of shock has permitted detailed pathophysiologic studies in man, and several hemodynamic patterns have appeared:

1. Shock characterized by a normal cardiac output, normal blood volume, normal circulation time, normal or high central venous pressure, normal or high pH, and *reduced* peripheral resistance. These patients have warm dry skin and may have bacteremia with both gram-positive as well as gram-negative organisms; many have cirrhosis; their prognosis is generally good. Hypotension, oliguria, and lactic acidemia are present. Shock in this

group has been attributed to shunting of blood through arteriovenous communications, making it unavailable for perfusion of vital organs.

2. Shock characterized by normal blood volume, high central venous pressure, normal or high cardiac output, reduced peripheral resistance, but *marked metabolic acidosis*, oliguria, and very high blood lactate indicating ineffective tissue perfusion or impaired oxygen utilization. These patients generally have bacteremia with gram-negative organisms, and despite the presence of warm dry extremities, their prognosis is extremely poor.

3. Patients with low blood volume, low central venous pressure, high hematocrit, increased peripheral resistance, low cardiac output, hypotension, oliguria, but only a moderate elevation of blood lactate and normal or slightly high pH. These patients may be hypovolemic prior to bacteremia, and their prognosis is reasonably good provided blood volume is restored, bacteremia is treated with appropriate antibiotics, septic foci are removed or drained, and vasoactive drugs are given.

4. Shock characterized by low blood volume, low central venous pressure, low cardiac output, marked decompensated metabolic acidosis, and lactic acidemia. In these patients the extremities are cool and cyanotic, and all forms of therapy fail to reverse shock.

Although these observations suggest that there are various forms of septic shock, for the most part the data are consistent with the hypothesis that the basic abnormality in endotoxin shock is *vasoconstriction, reduction in cardiac output, hypotension,* and *oliguria*. When peripheral resistance is low and cardiac output is normal or high, other explanations are available to explain these deviations from the more typical findings. For example, arteriovenous shunts occur in cirrhosis or in the inflamed peritoneum or lung and prevent perfusion and oxygenation of vital organs. Sometimes, seemingly high cardiac output is insufficient to meet the needs of the body, and occasionally, because of cell death, oxygen utilization at the cellular level does not occur despite minor alterations in blood volume.

Coagulation Defects in Shock. In most patients with septic shock there is a deficiency in several clotting factors, probably due to consumption of these factors by disseminated intravascular coagulation. Usually, there is no clinical bleeding, although hemorrhagic phenomena due to thrombocytopenia or deficiency in clotting factors occur occasionally. A more important effect of disseminated intravascular coagulation is development of capillary thrombi, particularly in the lung. Unless there is bleeding, the coagulopathy requires no therapy and disappears spontaneously as shock is treated.

The Lung in Septic Shock. Respiratory failure is the most important cause of death in patients with shock, particularly after the hemodynamic aberrations have been corrected. The respiratory lesion has been called the "shock lung" and is characterized by pulmonary congestion, hemorrhage, atelectasis, edema, and formation of capillary thrombi. This lesion may develop and progress even as other abnormalities return to normal. Pulmonary surfactant decreases, and pO_2 progressively falls.

Renal Failure. Oliguria occurs early in shock and is probably due to inadequate perfusion of renal capillaries. If renal perfusion remains inadequate, acute tubular necrosis develops.

CLINICAL MANIFESTATIONS. Usually gram-negative bacteremia begins abruptly with chills, fever, nausea, vomiting, diarrhea, and prostration. When septic shock develops, there are, in addition, tachycardia, tachypnea; hypotension; cool, pale extremities, often with peripheral cyanosis; mental obtundation; and oliguria. When present in its full-blown form, gram-negative shock is detected readily, but occasionally the findings are quite subtle, particularly in old debilitated patients or in infants. Unexplained hypotension, increasing confusion and disorientation, and hyperventilation may be the only clues to gram-negative shock. Jaundice occurs occasionally and signifies infection in the biliary tree or intravascular hemolysis. As shock progresses, oliguria persists, and heart failure, respiratory insufficiency, and coma supervene. Death usually occurs from pulmonary edema, generalized anoxemia secondary to respiratory insufficiency, cardiac arrhythmia, disseminated intravascular coagulation with bleeding, cerebral anoxia, or a combination of these factors.

LABORATORY FINDINGS. The laboratory data in septic shock vary greatly and depend in many instances on the cause of the shock syndrome and on the stage of shock. The volume of packed red cells is often elevated and falls to below normal as the volume deficit is repaired. There usually is *leukocytosis* of between 15,000 and 30,000 with a shift to the left. However, the white blood cell count may be normal, and some patients have leukopenia. The *platelet count* is usually decreased, and a variety of *clotting factor defects* is present.

The *urinalysis* shows no specific abnormalities. Initially, the specific gravity is high; as oliguria persists, isosthenuria develops. The *blood urea nitrogen* and *creatinine* are elevated, and creatinine clearance is reduced. Electrolyte patterns vary considerably, but there is a tendency to *hyponatremia* and hypochloremia. The serum potassium may be high, low, or normal. The *bicarbonate concentration* is usually low, and *blood lactate* is elevated.

Early in endotoxin shock there is *respiratory alkalosis* manifested by a low pCO_2 and high arterial pH—probably an attempt to blow off CO_2 to compensate for developing lactic acidemia and because of progressive anoxemia. As shock progresses, *metabolic acidosis* develops. There often is striking *anoxemia*, and pO_2 values below 70 mm Hg are common. Hemodynamic measurements usually show a low *central venous pressure, low cardiac output* and cardiac index, high *peripheral resistance*, and slow circulation time. *Blood volume* is usually low, but this determination is notoriously unreliable in septic shock and should not be trusted. The *electrocardiogram* generally shows depression of the S-T segment, inversion of the T waves, and a variety of arrhythmias, and may mistakenly suggest the diagnosis of myocardial infarction.

In untreated gram-negative shock, the blood cultures should reveal the causative pathogens, but bacteremia is often intermittent and the blood cultures may be negative. Furthermore, many patients will have received antimicrobial agents when they are first seen, masking the bacteriologic diagnosis. *A negative blood culture does not exclude the diagnosis of septic shock.* Culture of the primary septic focus may aid in the diagnosis, but the bacteriology may have been altered by prior chemotherapy.

DIAGNOSIS. The diagnosis of septic shock is not difficult in the presence of chills, fever, and an overt focus of infection. However, none of the obvious clues may be present. Elderly debilitated patients, in particular, may have severe infections in the absence of fever. Unexplained confusion and disorientation and hyperventilation without abnormal chest x-rays should call the diagnosis to mind. Pulmonary embolism, myocardial infarction, cardiac tamponade, aortic dissection, and silent hemorrhage are entities often confused with septic shock.

COURSE. The rational treatment of septic shock depends upon careful monitoring of patients. Specifically, four parameters need to be followed at the bedside:

1. The *central venous pressure* (CVP) should be measured. Insertion of a catheter into the great veins or right atrium provides an accurate index of the relationship between right ventricular competence and effective blood volume and should be used as a guide to fluid replacement therapy. When the CVP exceeds 10 to 12 cm of water, there is some danger of overloading the circulation and precipitating pulmonary edema. It is important to be sure that the flow through the catheter is free and that the catheter is not in the right ventricle. *The CVP is the cornerstone of managing shock and should be measured in every patient.*

2. The *pulse pressure* serves as an estimate of stroke volume.

3. *Cutaneous vasoconstriction* provides a clue to peripheral resistance although it does not reflect accurately blood flow to kidney, brain, or gut.

4. Hourly *urine output* should be used to monitor splanchnic blood flow and visceral perfusion. Usually this requires placement of an indwelling urethral catheter.

With these four measurements the patient with shock can be followed carefully and managed intelligently. Arterial blood pressure does not provide an accurate picture of the hemodynamic situation, and perfusion of vital organs may be adequate in patients with hypotension; conversely, some patients with normal blood pressures may have marked pooling and inadequate visceral blood flow.

In units organized for treatment of shock, frequent measurements of pulmonary artery and systemic pressures, arterial and venous pH, blood gases, blood lactate, renal function tests, and electrolytes are performed.

TREATMENT. Support of Respiration. In many patients with septic shock arterial pO_2 is markedly depressed. It is essential to establish an airway at the outset and to administer oxygen nasally or by mask. Tracheal intubation or tracheostomy and use of respiratory assistance devices usually are necessary.

Volume Replacement. Using the CVP as a guide, blood volume should be replaced with blood (if anemia is present), plasma, dextran (molecular weight 70,000 or 40,000), human serum albumin, and appropriate electrolyte solutions, primarily dextrose-saline and bicarbonate (which is preferable to lactate for treating the acidosis). The quantity of fluid required is often far in excess of "normal blood volume" and may amount to 8 to 12 liters in only a few hours. Large quantities may be required even when the cardiac index is normal. *Oliguria in the presence of hypotension is not a contraindication to continued vigorous fluid therapy.* Some investigators feel that the pulmonary artery pressure is the best indicator of incipient pulmonary edema and that a sharp rise in it calls for a reduction in fluid administration.

Antibiotics. Blood cultures and cultures of relevant body fluids or exudates should be taken before instituting antimicrobial therapy. Drugs should be given intravenously and bactericidal agents used when possible. When the results of blood cultures and sensitivities are known, one of the appropriate drugs recommended in the chapters dealing with the specific infections and discussed in Chap. 135 should be given. Usually cultures and sensitivities are not at hand at the onset of shock and the etiologic diagnosis entails an educated guess based upon culture from the primary focus—urine, bile, pus, or sputum; or on the setting in which the infection occurs. For example, a young woman with dysuria, chills and flank pain, and septic shock is likely to have *E. coli* bacteremia, while gram-negative sepsis in a burn patient is probably caused by *Pseudomonas.* The drugs of choice for gram-negative bacteremia are:

E. coli:	ampicillin
Klebsiella-Enterobacter:	kanamycin or gentamicin
Proteus mirabilis:	ampicillin
Proteus rettgeri, Pr.	
morganii, or *Pr. vulgaris:*	kanamycin or gentamicin
Mima-Herellea:	kanamycin
Pseudomonas:	polymyxin B or E
	(colistin) or gentamicin

The dosages and routes of administration for these agents are detailed in Chap 135. Cephalothin can be substituted for ampicillin in patients with a history of penicillin allergy. Because of its ototoxicity, kanamycin should be given cautiously to oliguric patients; a single dose of 1.0 Gm achieves blood levels which should suffice throughout the period of oliguria. The central nervous system toxicity of the polymyxins also is accentuated in patients with poor renal function. A new drug, Gentamicin, has been effective in *Proteus* and *Pseudomonas* bacteremia.

When the cause of septic shock is unknown, therapy should be initiated with both kanamycin and a polymyxin, or gentamicin; and if the possibility of gram-positive sepsis cannot be ruled out, a penicillinase-resistant penicillin or cephalothin should be given in addition. As soon as culture results become available, the agents which are unnecessary should be deleted from the regimen.

Surgical Intervention. Many patients with septic shock have an abscess, an infarcted or necrotic bowel, an inflamed gallbladder, an infected uterus, pyonephrosis, or other local situations which lend themselves to surgical drainage or excision. As a rule, successful treatment of shock requires surgical intervention even if the patient is desperately ill. Operations should not be postponed "to get the patient in shape" because these patients' condition will continue to deteriorate unless the septic focus is removed or drained.

Vasoactive Drugs. Septic shock is accompanied by maximal stimulation of alpha-adrenergic receptors, and pressor agents which act by stimulating these receptors such as norepinephrine, levarterenol, and metaraminol are contraindicated. The two groups of drugs which have been of value in septic shock are alpha-receptor blocking agents, exemplified by phenoxybenzamine, and beta-receptor stimulants, notably isoproterenol. *Phenoxybenzamine* (dibenzyline), an adrenolytic agent, effects a central phlebotomy by reducing resistance and increasing intravascular capacity. Hence, there is a redistribution of blood. Blood leaves the lungs, relieving pulmonary edema and enhancing gas exchange. Central venous pressure and left ventricular end-diastolic pressure fall, cardiac output rises, and peripheral venous constriction regresses. The recommended dose is 0.2 to 2.0 mg per kg intravenously. Small doses can be injected instantaneously and large doses over a period of 40 to 60 min. Fluids must be given simultaneously to compensate for the increment in venous capacitance; failure to do so aggravates shock. *Chlorpromazine* in multiple small doses of 2.5 to 5 mg also relieves vasoconstriction through its direct adrenolytic effect and by ganglionic blockade.

Isoproterenol (Isuprel) counteracts arteriolar and venous constriction in the microcirculation by its direct vasodilating effect. In addition, the drug exerts a direct inotropic effect on the heart. Cardiac output is increased by stimulating the myocardium and by reducing cardiac work as peripheral resistance decreases. The dose of isoproterenol is 2 to 8 μg per min for the average adult. Ventricular arrhythmias may result from this drug and shock may be made worse if fluid administration does not keep pace with relieved vasoconstriction.

Digitalis. A rapidly acting preparation of digoxin or Cedilanid (lanatoside C) should be given when the CVP or pulmonary artery pressures remain high in the face of systemic hypotension.

Adrenal Cortical Hormones. In large doses these agents overcome peripheral resistance and mitigate the cellular injury evoked by endotoxin. Although their use has been controversial, it seems reasonable to institute therapy with these drugs when the CVP has reached 10 to 12 cm of water and hypotension persists. Hydrocortisone in dosage of 50 mg per kg should be given intravenously in the first 12 hr. This dose may be repeated during the next 24 hr, but often shock is reversed with a single course.

Other Measures. In some patients with oliguria and a high CVP, infusions of mannitol or administration of ethacrynic acid has initiated diuresis; more often than not these maneuvers have failed. Hemorrhage as a consequence of clotting-factor deficiencies has been controlled with fresh frozen plasma, but when thrombocytopenia is the cause of bleeding, whole-blood transfusions must be given. Hyperbaric oxygen has been tried in gram-negative bacteremia with indifferent results.

PROGNOSIS. The measures described above usually will resuscitate most patients, at least temporarily. The ultimate outcome is dependent upon several factors:

1. Ability to eliminate the source of infection with surgery or antibiotics. The prognosis of urinary tract infections, septic abortion, abdominal abscess, gastrointestinal or biliary fistula, and subcutaneous or anorectal abscesses is better than that of primary foci in the skin or lungs.

2. Previous contact with the organism. Patients with chronic urinary tract infections who develop bacteremia rarely have severe gram-negative shock, perhaps because they have become tolerant to the endotoxin.

3. Underlying disease. Patients with lymphoma or leukemia who develop endotoxemia while their hematologic disease is out of control rarely recover; conversely, if hematologic remission is achieved, the shock is more likely to respond to therapy.

4. Metabolic status. The development of severe metabolic acidosis and lactic acidemia—irrespective of cardiac output—is associated with a poor prognosis.

5. Development of pulmonary insufficiency even after the hemodynamic abnormalities have been corrected.

The overall mortality of septic shock has been between 50 and 90 percent.

PREVENTION. The poor results in the treatment of septic shock are not due to lack of potent antibiotics or vasoactive agents. Rather, *failure to institute therapy sufficiently early* is a major roadblock to success. Septic shock usually is recognized too late, all too often after irreversible changes have taken place. Because many patients who are likely to develop septic shock are in the hospital *before* signs and symptoms of shock appear, it is essential to watch patients who are candidates for development of shock assiduously, to treat their infections vigorously and early, and to perform appropriate surgery before catastrophic complications occur.

REFERENCES

Clauss, R. H., and J. F. R. Ray: Pharmacologic Assistance to the Failing Circulation, Surg. Gynecol. Obstet., 126:611, 1968.

Hardaway, R. M., P. M. James, R. W. Anderson, C. E. Bredenberg, and R. L. West: Intensive Study and Treatment of Shock in Man, J.A.M.A., 199:799, 1967.

Lillehei, R. C., R. H. Dietzman, S. Movsas, and J. H. Bloch: Treatment of Septic Shock, Modern Treatment, 4:321, 1967.

MacLean, L. D., W. G. Mulligan, A. P. H. McLean, and J. H. Duff: Patterns of Septic Shock in Man: A Detailed Study of 56 Patients, Ann. Surg., 166:543, 1967.

Maiztegui, J. I., J. Z. Biegeleisen, W. B. Cherry, and E. H. Kass: Bacteremia Due to Gram-negative Rods: Clinical, Bacteriologic, Serologic and Immunofluorescent Study, New Engl. J. Med., 272:222, 1965.

Petersdorf, R. G., and H. N. Beaty: The Role of Antibiotics,

Vasoactive Drugs and Steroids in Gram-negative Bacteremia, Ann. N. Y. Acad. Sci. 145:319, 1967.

Udhoji, V. S., and M. H. Weil: Hemodynamic and Metabolic Studies on Shock Associated with Bacteremia: Observations on 16 Patients, Ann. Intern. Med., 62:966, 1965.

Waisbren, B. A., and J. Arena: Shock Associated with Bacteremia Due to Gram-negative Bacilli: Autopsy Findings, Arch. Intern. Med., 116:336, 1965.

135 CHEMOTHERAPY OF INFECTION

Louis Weinstein

The use of substances elaborated by one organism to kill or inhibit the growth of another is centuries old. Over 2,500 years ago, the Chinese treated carbuncles, boils, and similar infections by applying moldy curd of soybean to such lesions. The clinical possibilities of this phenomenon were first clearly recognized in 1877 by Pasteur and Joubert, who noted that the anthrax bacillus grew well in sterile urine but failed to multiply when other bacteria were present in the urine. Similar results were observed in animals, leading them to suggest that this observation held "great promise for therapeutics."

Although numerous attempts were made over the years to develop agents that might exert a beneficial effect in bacterial, mycotic, and rickettsial infections, the era of effective chemotherapy of such disease began with the discovery and first application of the sulfonamides in 1936. The "golden age" of antimicrobial therapy was initiated by the commercial production of penicillin, an agent first discovered in 1929. Since then, the number of drugs of value in the management of a variety of infections has multiplied rapidly. The agents now available are of three types: (1) biosynthetic compounds of which penicillin G is an example; (2) semisynthetic substances such as some of the more recently developed penicillin derivatives; (3) purely synthetic agents such as the sulfonamides and some of the tuberculostatic drugs. Those derived in part or as a whole from the fermentative activity of microorganisms are classified as *antibiotics*.

THE CHEMOTHERAPEUTIC AGENTS

To be of practical value in the therapy of infection, an antimicrobial agent must exert its effect on the invading organism without seriously damaging the cells of the host. It is remarkable that so many compounds with these characteristics have been developed. As far as is known, all these drugs are effective because they act directly on the parasite and not because they enhance the natural defenses of the host. The principal result of their activity is retardation of bacterial growth. Some of them are bactericidal while others exert only a bacteriostatic effect in vitro. When these substances are administered in large doses, especially in the course of some infections, depression, delay, or abolition of the immune response to the invading microorganism may follow.

Sulfonamides

The sulfonamide compounds have been used in clinical medicine since 1937. The important members of this group are sulfadiazine, sulfisoxazole (Gantrisin), succinylsulfathiazole (Sulfasuxidine), and phthalylsulfathiazole (Sulfathalidine).

Despite the availability of newer antimicrobial agents, the sulfonamides are still very valuable in the management of some infections. Although they have been the drugs of choice for the therapy of meningococcal infections in the past, the isolation of sulfonamide-resistant strains of *Neisseria meningitidis* has decreased the universal applicability of these drugs (Chap. 142). Some but not all cases of bacillary dysentery respond to treatment with sulfonamides (Chap. 151). These compounds are very useful in uncomplicated urinary tract infections, especially those due to *Escherichia coli* and those in which instrumentation and obstruction are not problems. They also can be employed for the prophylaxis of recurrences of rheumatic fever.

The sulfonamide compounds presently employed to treat systemic infections are readily absorbed from the gastrointestinal tract and are probably best administered by this route to conscious patients. Sodium salts for either intramuscular or intravenous use are also available. Liquid preparations made palatable by the addition of flavoring materials are useful in treating young children. For most of the infectious diseases in which the sulfonamides are of value, the duration of therapy should be no less than 1 week.

When the rapidly absorbed and excreted sulfonamides (sulfadiazine or sulfisoxazole) are administered orally to adults, a "loading" dose of 4 Gm is given; this is followed by 1 Gm every 4 hr. The loading dose for parenteral injection of sodium sulfadiazine or sulfisoxazole is 5 Gm; 1 Gm may be given subcutaneously thereafter every 4 to 6 hr. As soon as patients are able to take drugs by mouth, the parenteral route need no longer be employed. Determinations of sulfonamide blood levels are of little or no value in estimating therapeutic effects; they are helpful in indicating excessive and potentially dangerous blood levels or in establishing that the drug is being taken by a patient.

Most of the sulfonamide compounds are widely distributed in the body. After absorption, the major metabolic alteration is acetylation of the primary amino group. Sulfonamides are excreted by the kidney, chiefly by glomerular filtration. Derivatives not firmly bound to plasma or tissue proteins tend to be distributed evenly in total body water and thus reach high concentrations in cells, whereas those with a tendency to be bound are concentrated in the plasma.

The bacteriostatic activity of the sulfonamides is dependent upon their antimetabolic action. Para-aminobenzoic acid (PABA), which impairs the antibacterial effect of most of these drugs, is an essential metabolite of many bacteria and is part of the molecule of folic acid. It has been suggested that sulfonamides prevent the incorporation of PABA into folic acid, but it is probable that they inhibit several steps in enzymatic activity. The principal toxic effects are hypersensitivity reactions and renal injury. These may develop any time after the first week of therapy, or even earlier in patients who have received the drugs previously. Sensitivity to one type of compound frequently confers sensitivity to others. Crystallization of the drug in the renal tubules is most likely to occur when an inadequate quantity of fluid has been ingested or when the reaction of the urine is acid, since the solubility of both acetylated and free forms is considerably greater in neutral or alkaline medium. The best method of avoiding renal injury is to maintain a copious urine output—at least 1,200 ml per day. Another method of preventing precipitation of sulfonamide crystals in the urinary tract is to administer two or three sulfonamides concomitantly because the solubility of each is independent of the presence of the others. Among other reactions observed with sulfonamides are hemolytic and aplastic anemia, thrombopenia, vascular lesions resembling those of polyarteritis nodosa, erythema multiforme including the Stevens-Johnson syndrome, Behçet's syndrome, contact dermatitis, serum sickness, hepatitis, arthritis, insomnia, confusion, vertigo, ataxia, tinnitus, peripheral neuritis, anorexia, nausea, vomiting, and hypersensitivity myocarditis (sulfamethoxypyridazine).

Sulfadiazine (2-sulfanilamidopyrimidine) is absorbed from the gastrointestinal tract slowly and incompletely, and renal excretion is relatively slow. The tissue concentration is 60 to 75 percent of that in the plasma. Sulfadiazine appears in the urine in both free and acetylated forms; neither is very soluble, and crystalluria is common. For most systemic infections in adults, sulfadiazine is administered in a dosage of 4 to 6 Gm per day after an initial dose of 4 Gm. In young children, 0.065 to 0.1 Gm/lb body weight/24 hr usually produces an adequate effect; the initial dose should be about one-half this quantity.

Sulfisoxazole (3,4-dimethyl-5-sulfanilamidoisoxazole) is more soluble than sulfadiazine. The administration of the same quantity of drug will yield a plasma concentration of sulfisoxazole three times that for sulfanilamide and about twice that for sulfadiazine and sulfamerazine. The dosage and clinical effectiveness of sulfisoxazole are of the same order as those of sulfadiazine.

Succinylsulfathiazole (2-N⁴-succinylsulfanilamidothiazole) and *phthalylsulfathiazole* [2-(N⁴-phthalylsulfanilamido)thiazole] are absorbed poorly from the intestinal tract and are used primarily to suppress bacterial growth in the intestine.

ANTIBIOTICS

The development of antibiotics for the treatment of infections represents one of the most important developments in modern medicine. The presently available agents of this class may be classified into several groups on the basis of their mechanism of action, as follows: (1) *Agents acting on bacterial cell wall synthesis*—penicillins, cephalosporin derivatives, vancomycin, and bacitracin. (2) *Agents affecting cell membranes and exerting a detergent effect*—polymyxin, colistin, novobiocin, and the polyene antifungal drugs nystatin and amphotericin. (3) *Agents producing suppression or abnormalities of protein synthesis*—chloramphenicol, tetracyclines, kanamycin, neomycin, streptomycin, and the macrolide antibiotic erythromycin. Although these mechanisms of action appear valid as of 1968, continued study may modify these concepts. Secondary changes in the anatomy or metabolism of the bacterial cell often follow the primary effect of an antimicrobial drug; the two may be easily confused. Some agents may have more than one primary site or mode of action, especially when present in high concentration. The antibiotics are classified, for clinical purposes, on the basis of the "spectrum" of organisms against which they act. For example, penicillin G is considered to have a narrow spectrum because, in conventional doses, it affects primarily gram-positive bacteria and *Neisseria*. On the other hand, antibiotics such as the tetracyclines and chloramphenicol are classified as broad-spectrum agents because they inhibit the growth of gram-positive and -negative organisms, rickettsia, Tric (TRachoma and Inclusion Conjunctivitis) agents, the psittacosis-lymphogranuloma group (*Bedsonia*), and some *Mycoplasma*.

Testing Organisms for Sensitivity to Antibiotics

The sensitivities of bacteria to chemotherapeutic agents are usually determined by bacteriologic techniques. The most accurate method for routine use involves inoculation of the organism into serial dilutions of the drug. After a suitable period of incubation, the lowest concentration of antibiotic that inhibits growth of the bacteria is expressed as the "sensitivity." A more rapid method utilizes filter paper disks impregnated with a known quantity of drug; these are applied to the surface of agar plates over which the organism is heavily streaked. The smallest quantity of antibiotic around which a given zone of inhibition of growth is present is the level of sensitivity of the bacteria. This procedure is relatively crude, but it is useful in clinical practice for the rapid determination of relative sensitivities. These tests are not necessary in all cases, but, if performed correctly, there is a good correlation between clinical response to drug and the test. Often the procedure is invaluable in indicating which therapeutic agent to employ.

Resistance of Bacteria to Antibiotics

All antibiotics are not effective against all microorganisms. The spectrum of activity of each drug is probably related to several factors among which are the availability of appropriate binding sites on the organism, the presence of essential microbial enzyme systems that can be inhibited by the drug, and the elaboration of substances, either intra- or extracellular, that inactivate the antimicrobial agent. Drug resistance is not universal, and even after 25 years, no significant degree of resistance to penicillin G has developed in group A *Streptococcus pyogenes* or *Diplococcus pneumoniae*. On the other hand, shortly after this antibiotic came into use, it became apparent that an increasing number of strains of *Staphylococcus aureus* insensitive to it were being recovered from human infections. In some instances, species of bacteria isolated prior to the availability of an antimicrobial compound have been found to be resistant, while in others the resistance seems to have become prominent only after the drug had been used for a varying period of time. Resistance of bacteria to antibiotics is, therefore, of two types—*naturally occurring* and *acquired*.

Naturally occurring drug resistance may be due to one of three mechanisms.

1. *Spontaneous mutation.* Some species of organisms, many strains of which are sensitive to a specific antimicrobial agent, may mutate spontaneously and become resistant. This is not due to exposure to the drug. When mutation occurs during therapy, it may be misinterpreted as induction of resistance because of activity of the antibiotic. This is not the case, however. The action of the antimicrobial agent is merely to *select* out the resistant mutant, as it eliminates the sensitive clones. The spontaneous mutants resist the activity of the antibiotic either by elaborating substances which degrade it or by developing alternate pathways of essential metabolic activity. An example is strains of *S. aureus* resistant to penicillin G, which produce penicillinase, a β-lactamase which inactivates the antibiotic by splitting its β-lactam ring.

2. *Failure of an antibiotic to affect essential enzyme systems.* This is the probable explanation for the selective activity of antibiotics. Some species of organisms possess enzyme systems necessary for growth and multiplication that are totally insensitive to the effects of certain drugs but not those of others. This determines the spectrum of activity of an antibiotic in many cases.

3. *Absence of appropriate binding sites* may be responsible for failure of an antimicrobial agent to inhibit microbial growth despite the fact that sensitive essential enzyme systems may be present in the organism.

Acquired drug resistance may appear in several ways.

1. Organisms cultured in vitro in media containing increasing concentrations of an antibiotic frequently become resistant to the drug either by a one-step process or gradually. The mechanisms responsible for this phenomenon are not clear, but the possibility that alternate but inactive metabolic pathways, unaffected by the antimicrobial agent, become active and take over for suppressed ones during exposure to increasing quantities of the drug, seems likely. "One-step" resistance is exemplified by streptomycin. This agent causes misreading of the genetic code leading to the production of abnormal proteins lethal to the organism. The development of resistance to the drug involves a mutation that results in a second misreading of the genetic code and the synthesis of new proteins compatible with cell life. That the mechanism involved in resistance developing as a result of spontaneous mutation is not the same as that operating when bacteria are made insensitive in vitro is illustrated

by *S. aureus*. Spontaneous mutants of this organism elaborate penicillinase, while those made penicillin-resistant in the laboratory do not produce this enzyme.

2. *Transduction* is another mechanism involved in the acquisition of acquired drug resistance. In this instance, a piece of DNA carrying a gene for resistance to a specific antibiotic is enclosed within the coat of bacteriophage and passed from the resistant organism to a sensitive one which then becomes insusceptible to the antibiotic.

3. *Episome transfer* has recently been demonstrated to be an important mechanism in the development of bacterial drug resistance. This phenomenon involves only gram-negative bacilli, primarily the *Enterobacteriaceae*. Episomes may be part of and replicate with chromosomes, or be separate from them and replicate autonomously. This genetic material is transferred from one organism to another in the process of conjugation. The resistance factor (R) consists of 2 parts, (*a*) resistance transfer factor (RTF) and (*b*) attached genes for drug resistance (R genes). In addition to transmitting other characteristics, resistance to one or more antibiotics may be transferred from the insensitive organism to the sensitive one as they come in contact with each other either in the test tube or in the intestinal tract. Insensitivity to more than one antibiotic may be induced simultaneously. Resistance to streptomycin, sulfonamides, tetracycline, and chloramphenicol may develop after a single contact. Insensitivity to ampicillin and other antimicrobial compounds may also be initiated by this mechanism. Episomal transfer occurs between organisms of the same or unrelated species. A relatively common phenomenon of considerable therapeutic importance is the development of chloramphenicol or ampicillin resistance or both in strains of *Shigella* or *Salmonella* as they become the recipients of episomes carrying such R genes from *E. coli* with which they come in contact and conjugate in the human intestinal tract.

The isolation of a sensitive organism prior to the initiation of chemotherapy, followed by the appearance during treatment of the same species now insensitive to the drug, may be interpreted erroneously as representing selection of a resistant mutant. This may be due to the implantation of a new strain of the same species, usually from the external environment, that is drug-resistant. For example, it has been demonstrated occasionally that relapse of wound infection due to penicillin G–sensitive *S. aureus* during treatment with this drug is due to invasion by a strain of different bacteriophage type of an entirely different range of sensitivity than the one recovered initially.

The general problem of bacterial drug resistance continues to be important. Solutions to it, achieved by the development of new and effective antimicrobial agents, are often only temporary. Staphylococci resistant to the penicillinase-resistant semisynthetic penicillins and the cephalosporin derivatives are presently being recovered from infections. Such strains were present prior to the development of these drugs, but the use of these agents appears to have selected out the resistant mutants. Usually *S. aureus* insensitive to methicillin is also not inhibited by oxacillin, nafcillin, and cloxacillin; a varying number are not suppressed by cephalothin or cephaloridine.

As a rule, organisms insensitive to a particular antibiotic tend to be resistant to all other chemically related antimicrobial agents. Bacteria unaffected by tetracycline are usually unresponsive to chlortetracycline, oxytetracycline, and demethylchlortetracycline. Some strains of *Pseudomonas* are an exception and are sensitive only to oxytetracycline, while being resistant to tetracycline, chlortetracycline, and other congeners. Occasionally, cross resistance may involve two agents that are chemically dissimilar; erythromycin and oleandomycin are examples. These agents have unrelated molecular structures; despite this, some erythromycin-resistant staphylococci are also insensitive to oleandomycin. In addition to inducing resistance, streptomycin may be an essential growth factor for some organisms (streptomycin dependence).

Combinations of antimicrobial agents may diminish the speed with which bacterial resistance to any of the drugs in the mixture develops. Resistance of the tubercle bacillus to a single tuberculostatic compound, such as isoniazid, is appreciably delayed when this drug is given together with another effective agent such as streptomycin or para-aminosalicylic acid (Chap. 174).

Penicillins

Penicillin is an antibacterial substance produced by various strains of *Penicillium*. Although this mold elaborates several penicillins closely related in chemical and biologic activity, the one used most extensively in clinical practice at the present time is penicillin G, or benzylpenicillin. Several modifications of the drug have been produced primarily for the purpose of prolonging the duration of antibacterial activity or increasing resistance of the drug to gastric acidity; these include the procaine ester dibenzylethylenediamine dipenicillin (Bicillin), and phenoxymethyl penicillin (penicillin V).

Penicillin G is highly effective in vitro against many but not all gram-positive and -negative cocci. Among the streptococci, groups A, C, G, H, L, and M are highly sensitive; groups B, E, F, K, and N are moderately resistant; enterococci are the least susceptible. From 85 to 90 percent of *S. aureus* isolated from infections are resistant to penicillin in ordinary dosage (600,000 to 1,200,000 units per day). Although gonococci are still relatively susceptible to penicillin, they are less sensitive than they were when this antibiotic first came into use. Pneumococci and meningococci remain highly susceptible to the drug. Most but not all strains of *C. diphtheriae*, *B. anthracis*, *Clostridia*, *Actinomyces*, *Streptobacillus* (*Haverhillia*), *Leptospira*, and *Listeria* are inhibited. One of the most exquisitely sensitive organisms is *Treponema pallidum*. Although many species of gram-negative bacilli are resistant to relatively low concentrations of penicillin G, some strains of *E. coli*, *Proteus mirabilis*, *Salmonella*, *Shigella*, *Aerobacter*, and *Alcaligenes* are suppressed in the presence of the high blood levels that follow the

administration of large doses of the antibiotic (20 to 80 million units per day).

Several semisynthetic penicillins, which are compounds made up of the basic nucleus (6-aminopenicillanic acid) to which a variety of side chains have been attached, are available. Among these are methicillin (2,6-dimethoxybenzamido penicillanate), oxacillin (5-methyl-3-phenyl-4-isoxazolylpenicillin), cloxacillin (5-methyl-3-o-chlorphenyl-4-isoxazolylpenicillin), dicloxacillin [3-(2, 6-dichlorphenyl)-5-methyl-4-isoxazolylpenicillin sodium monohydrate], nafcillin [6-(2-ethoxy-1-napthamido) penicillanic acid], and ampicillin (alpha-aminobenzylpenicillin). Some of these are resistant to penicillinase (methicillin, oxacillin, nafcillin, cloxacillin, dicloxacillin), some are acid-stable (oxacillin, nafcillin, cloxacillin, dicloxacillin, ampicillin), and one has a broad spectrum of activity but is penicillinase-sensitive (ampicillin).

Penicillin in low concentrations is bacteriostatic; large quantities are bactericidal. Organisms are killed only if they are exposed to the drug while in an active phase of multiplication. The mode of action of the antibiotic is interference with the formation of bacterial cell walls by inhibiting the incorporation of a compound containing a uridine nucleotide, an acetyl amino sugar, and a peptide of three amino acids (DL-alanine, D-glutamate, and lysine) that is an intermediate in cell wall production.

BIOSYNTHETIC PENICILLINS

Penicillin G can be administered by several routes: orally, intramuscularly, subcutaneously, or intravenously. It has also been applied topically. Application to the skin is to be avoided wherever possible, because the degree of sensitization to the drug produced by this type of therapy is very high. The procaine salt of the antibiotic is an extensively used preparation because absorption is slowed and detectable blood levels may be present for as long as 24 hr. The addition of aluminum monosterate to procaine penicillin may allow detectable blood levels to be maintained for as long as 48 to 72 hr.

Benzathine penicillin (Bicillin) may be administered either orally or parenterally. When given by mouth, however, the absorption of this agent is more erratic than that of buffered penicillin G, which yields three to six times the penicillin activity of Bicillin. Intramuscular injection of Bicillin has the advantage over penicillin G of prolonging blood levels; the administration of 1.2 to 2.4 million units may produce a detectable concentration of antibiotic in the blood for as long as 4.5 weeks. The free acid and potassium salt of phenoxymethyl penicillin (penicillin V) are more stable and less soluble at the pH of gastric juice than is penicillin G. It is rapidly dissolved in alkaline solution and is readily absorbed from the upper small intestine. Taken by mouth, penicillin V produces higher and more prolonged blood levels than the same quantity of penicillin G. It produces adequate blood levels even when taken shortly after a meal.

Much larger doses of penicillin G are needed for oral than for parenteral therapy. When penicillin is injected subcutaneously or intramuscularly, it causes little local irritation and is absorbed rapidly into the bloodstream. Normally, only minute amounts penetrate into the cerebrospinal fluid, but in the presence of meningeal inflammation, appreciable levels of the drug may be obtained.

Penicillin G is excreted by the kidneys with great rapidity, mainly by a tubular mechanism. Renal excretion is delayed by concurrent administration of substances that compete for available tubular excretory structures. Benemid [probenecid, *p*-(di-*n*-propylsulfamyl)-benzoic acid] appears to be the most effective in reducing the rapidity of excretion of penicillin; the dose is 0.5 Gm four times a day.

SEMISYNTHETIC PENICILLINS

Dimethoxyphenyl penicillin (Methicillin) is effective both in vitro and in vivo against most strains of penicillinase-producing *S. aureus*. The drug, is, however, only one-twentieth to one-fortieth as active against group A beta-hemolytic streptococci and *Neisseria* and about one-tenth as active against *D. pneumoniae* and *Streptococcus viridans* as penicillin G. It is inactive against gram-negative bacilli, even those moderately sensitive to penicillin, and only slightly inhibitory for *H. influenzae*. It is at least fifty times more active than benzylpenicillin for penicillinase-elaborating straphylococci, but probably only one-fiftieth as effective for strains that do not produce this enzyme. A few methicillin-resistant strains of *S. aureus* have recently been recovered from human infections. Dimethoxyphenyl penicillin is little, if at all, inactivated by staphylococcal penicillinase, but it is inhibited by the penicillinases of *Bacillus licheniformis* and *B. cereus* (Neutrapen).

The recommended dose for adults is 1 Gm every 3 to 4 hr, and for children, 100 mg/kg body weight/day in equally divided quantities. The agent must be given parenterally; intramuscular or intravenous injection leads to rapid excretion, adequate blood levels being demonstrable for 4 hr when the intramuscular and for 3 hr when the intravenous routes are employed.

Because methicillin is acid-labile, it should *not* be given as a slow drip dissolved in large volumes of physiologic saline or dextrose in water. The pH of both of these solutions is acid. The drug is best administered by dissolving each dose in 30 to 40 ml of either of these solutions and infusing into a vein over a period of 20 to 30 min. Methicillin is excreted very rapidly; Benemid retards the rate of loss in the urine. Large quantities must be administered before the antibiotic will diffuse into the cerebrospinal fluid.

Oxacillin is less active in vitro against pneumococci, staphylococci, and streptococci than penicillin V or penicillin G. Its minimal inhibitory concentration for these organisms is considerably lower than that of methicillin. The drug is penicillinase-resistant. Penicillinase-producing staphylococci are more susceptible, in general, to oxacillin than to methicillin. Oxacillin is acid-stable and may be administered orally or parenterally. About 80 percent of the drug is bound to serum protein. A dose of 0.5 Gm intramuscularly yields plasma concentrations

equivalent to those produced by 1 Gm administered orally. Benemid blocks the renal excretion of oxacillin. The daily dose in adults is 2.0 to 4.0 Gm.

Cloxacillin has a range of antibacterial activity similar to that of oxacillin. It is equally effective against penicillinase-producing staphylococci and strains that do not elaborate this enzyme. It possesses a greater degree of antistaphylococcal activity than methicillin. Plasma concentrations of cloxacillin after oral administration are higher than those that develop after an equal dose of oxacillin. The drug is not available in parenteral form.

Dicloxacillin, like oxacillin and dicloxacillin, is acid-stable and penicillinase-resistant. It appears to be more active against staphylococci than the other agents of the group. Methicillin-resistant *S. aureus* are generally resistant to dicloxacillin as well. This drug is ineffective against enterococci and gram-negative bacilli. It appears to be more active than cloxacillin but less inhibitory than oxacillin for pneumococci. It has the same degree of suppressive effect as the other isoxazolyl penicillins against group A streptococci. Patterns of blood levels of dicloxacillin after oral administration differ little from those that result from intramuscular injection of the drug. Serum concentrations are four times higher than those produced by oxacillin and twice as high as those following cloxacillin, when equal doses of all these agents are administered by mouth. Protein binding is approximately the same for all these drugs, 80 to 85 percent. About 65 to 75 percent of an administered dose is excreted in the urine in 24 hr. The recommended oral dose of dicloxacillin for adults with mild to moderate infections is 250 mg every 6 hr; for more serious disease, this should be increased to 500 mg every 6 hr. Children should receive 50 mg/kg/day divided into equal doses every 6 hr. Larger quantities may be required for severe infections. Children weighing more than 20 kg are treated with the adult dose.

Nafcillin, acid-stable and insensitive to penicillinase, is highly active against penicillinase-producing staphylococci. It is more effective than methicillin against such organisms but is not as potent as penicillin G for staphylococci sensitive to this agent. Its antistaphylococcal effects approximate those of oxacillin. In general, the antibacterial spectrum of nafcillin for other organisms is similar to that of penicillin G. Orally administered nafcillin yields lower plasma concentrations than an equivalent dose of cloxacillin; however, on a weight-for-weight basis, nafcillin is more active than cloxacillin against streptococci, pneumococci, and staphylococci. Only about 10 percent of an oral dose of nafcillin is excreted by the kidney, and about 90 percent of a single intravenous injection is excreted in the bile and reabsorbed from the intestine; the enterohepatic circulation of the drug probably accounts for its persistence in the body. Benemid also retards the excretion of nafcillin.

Ampicillin is termed broad spectrum in its antimicrobial activity because it inhibits a number of both gram-positive and -negative bacteria. It is destroyed by contact with penicillinase and is, therefore, ineffective against penicillin G–resistant staphylococci and all gram-negative species that elaborate this enzyme. Ampicillin is somewhat less inhibitory than penicillin G for gram-positive cocci highly sensitive to this agent. It is highly effective for *H. influenzae* and enterococci, moderately active against *E. coli*, mildly active against most strains of *Aerobacter* and *Alcaligenes fecalis,* and inactive against *Pseudomonas* and indole-producing strains of *Proteus.* Indole-negative *Proteus* are highly susceptible to the drug as are most *Salmonella* and *Shigella.* The incidence of drug-resistant strains of *Salmonella, Shigella, E. coli,* and *Aerobacter* has been increasing. Ampicillin is acid-stable; it is absorbed after oral administration to about the same extent as phenoxymethyl penicillin (penicillin V). Food appears to retard absorption of the drug. Higher and more rapidly attained blood levels follow intramuscular administration. The renal excretion of the drug is retarded by probenecid. The drug appears in active form in the bile, in concentrations very much higher (approximately 30 times) than those concurrently present in the serum. Ampicillin diffuses poorly into cerebrospinal fluid in normal individuals, but appreciable quantities can be attained in meningitis. About 20 percent of the agent is bound to plasma protein. The dose of ampicillin varies with the severity of the infection; 100 to 200 mg per kg has been employed for serious disease in children; 2 to 10 or 12 Gm per day has been administered to adults.

The penicillins are responsible for a number of untoward effects. Some result from sensitization, others are related to toxic and irritative properties, and still others are induced by the development of biologic alterations in the host other than allergy or toxicity. Among the reactions that have been observed in patients receiving the penicillins are skin eruptions including morbilliform, scarlatiniform, urticarial, and purpuric lesions; fever; angioedema; contact dermatitis; erythema multiforme, including the Stevens-Johnson syndrome; anaphylaxis, with death in some instances; glossitis; brown or black discoloration of the tongue; cheilosis; eosinophilia; Arthus' phenomenon; allergic vasculitis; pain at site of injection and sterile or infected abscesses in muscles in which the drug is injected; arachnoiditis and encephalopathy when excessive doses are injected intrathecally; thrombophlebitis following intravenous infusion; Herxheimer reactions in the early therapy of syphilis; and superinfection (discussed below). Hematuria, albuminuria, pyuria, renal cell casts, increase in serum creatinine, and oliguria have been observed rarely in patients receiving methicillin. This agent has also been responsible for a few instances of bone marrow depression.

The clinical uses and dosage schedules of the penicillins are discussed in detail in the chapters dealing with the management of specific infections.

Streptomycin

Streptomycin, an antibiotic produced by *Streptomyces griseus,* is active against the tubercle bacillus and both gram-positive and gram-negative bacteria. For antibacterial activity to be present, the exposed organisms must be metabolically active but do not have to be growing. The drug causes misreading of the genetic code, resulting in the formation of abnormal proteins which are lethal for bacteria.

Streptomycin is poorly absorbed from the gastrointestinal tract but when given parenterally is well absorbed and distributed evenly in extracellular fluids. It penetrates the blood–spinal fluid barrier poorly unless meningeal inflammation is present. Renal excretion is largely by filtration, and 80 percent of the antibiotic appears in the urine over a period of 24 hr.

The main route of administration of streptomycin is intramuscular. When a local effect in the intestinal tract is desired, the drug is given orally. The infections in which streptomycin is of value are those produced by *H. influenzae, Pasteurella tularensis,* some strains of *E. coli, A. aerogenes,* the tubercle bacillus, and some strains of enterococci (together with penicillin). The usual dose for adults is 1 to 2 Gm per day in equally spaced and divided quantities; in tuberculosis, the entire daily dose may be given as a single injection; administration of 1 Gm twice a week is common practice in this disease.

The reactions that accompany the use of streptomycin may include various types of skin eruptions, fever, eosinophilia, angioedema, exfoliative dermatitis, stomatitis, anaphylaxis, contact dermatitis, lymphadenopathy, neutropenia, agranulocytosis, aplastic anemia, thrombopenia, pain at sites of injection, nausea, vomiting, diarrhea (oral therapy), labyrinthine damage, deafness, scotomas, peripheral neuritis, paresthesias, acute encephalopathy (intrathecal injection), neuromuscular paralysis with cessation of respiration (parenteral or intraperitoneal instillation), renal irritation, and superinfection.

Specific indications for the use of streptomycin in various diseases are discussed in other chapters.

The Tetracyclines

CHLORTETRACYCLINE (AUREOMYCIN)

This antibiotic, a product of *S. aureofaciens,* has a wide range of activity, encompassing not only many gram-positive and gram-negative bacteria but also the *Rickettsia, Mycoplasma,* and *Bedsonia.* Many strains of *S. aureus* and some of the gram-negative bacteria such as *Proteus vulgaris* and *Pseudomonas* may become rapidly resistant to the drug. After a single oral dose, the antibiotic can be demonstrated in the urine for as long as 24 hr, but only a small proportion of a parenteral dose of the drug can be demonstrated in the urine. Aureomycin diffuses into the spinal fluid in smaller amounts than into the plasma. Subcutaneous and intramuscular injections are not practical because of local irritation. When the drug is given by mouth, nausea and vomiting occur occasionally. Attempts to overcome this gastric irritation by the administration of magnesium salts, aluminum hydroxide, or milk lead to a reduction of the serum concentration. Mild diarrhea, with bulky stools, may be caused by local irritation or alteration in the bacterial flora of the intestinal tract due to the antibiotic.

The oral dose of Aureomycin is 1 to 2 Gm per day,

given in divided doses at 6-hr intervals. No more than 2 Gm per day should be given intravenously because of the risk of "toxic" hepatitis.

OXYTETRACYCLINE (TERRAMYCIN)

Terramycin, an antibiotic produced by *Streptomyces rimosus,* is very closely related chemically to Aureomycin. It may be administered orally or intravenously. Intravenous injection of this antibiotic should be reserved for instances of severe illness or for cases in which it cannot be taken by mouth. Solutions of Terramycin must be properly buffered. A single oral dose may produce detectable concentration in the blood for as long as 24 hr. When 250 mg of the drug is given at 6-hr intervals, blood levels are usually in the range of 5 to 10 μg per ml.

The clinical applications of Terramycin are practically the same as those of Aureomycin, except for an occasional case of *Pseudomonas* (see above).

TETRACYCLINE (ACHROMYCIN)

Achromycin is closely related chemically to both Aureomycin and Terramycin. It contains the skeleton structure of these two antibiotics and is prepared synthetically. The biologic activity of Achromycin is equal to that of Aureomycin and Terramycin. Achromycin is useful in the same infections that are known to respond favorably to either of the other tetracyclines. The incidence of side reactions, such as nausea, vomiting, and diarrhea, is said to be lower following Achromycin than has been observed with the other related drugs.

Intravenous therapy should be employed only in patients who are unable to take medication by mouth. The average adult dose is 500 mg intravenously at 12-hr intervals. For oral treatment, 1 to 2 Gm, divided into four doses per day, is usually adequate.

DEMETHYLCHLORTETRACYCLINE (DECLOMYCIN)

Demethylchlortetracycline is a fermentation product of a mutant strain of *S. aureofaciens.* It differs from chlortetracycline in the absence of a methyl group. Declomycin is very stable and is about twice as active as Achromycin against most organisms. The rate of renal excretion is less than half that of Achromycin. Smaller doses of Declomycin are required than of Achromycin to obtain the same clinical result. The demethylated compound needs to be given less frequently; two doses per day are said to suffice.

METHACYCLINE (RONDOMYCIN)

Methacycline (6-methylene-5-hydroxy tetracycline) is a semisynthetic compound derived from oxytetracycline. Its antibacterial spectrum approximates that of the other tetracyclines except for somewhat greater potency. With some methods of assaying antimicrobial activity, no differences between this drug and tetracycline, chlortetracycline, and oxytetracycline can be detected. Equivalent doses of methacycline and demethylchlortetracycline produce approximately the same serum concentrations. The administration of 150 mg of methacycline orally every 6 hr leads to the development of lower blood levels than those that result from giving 250 mg of tetracycline at the same interval. Because of its prolonged half-life, the recommended dose of methacycline is 150 mg every 6 hr or 300 mg every 12 hr; therapeutic activity may be demonstrable in the blood for 24 to 36 hr after treatment is stopped.

DOXYCYCLINE (VIBRAMYCIN)

Doxycycline (6-deoxy-5-hydroxytetracycline) is a synthetic derivative of methacycline. Its activity against group A streptococci and staphylococci is the same as that of demethylchlortetracycline. The drug appears to be better absorbed than the other tetracyclines when administered orally. Its activity is decreased to a much lesser degree than that of demethylchlortetracycline by the ingestion of food or dairy products. Because of its prolonged half-life, the daily and total dose requirements are lower than those for other tetracyclines. The administration of 100 mg of doxycycline produces serum concentrations only slightly lower than those attainable with 300 mg of demethylchlortetracycline. The urinary excretion of doxycycline is slower than that of demethylchlortetracycline. The urinary excretion of both agents, in percentage of the dose given, is the same during a 72-hr period. About 90 percent of the drug is bound to serum protein. The recommended dose of doxycycline for adults is 200 mg the first day (100 mg every 12 hr), followed by 100 mg per day (single dose or 50 mg every 12 hr). In severe infections, the administration of 100 mg every 12 hr has been suggested. The administration of aluminum hydroxide decreases absorption of the drug, leading to decreased blood and tissue fluid levels.

REACTION TO THE TETRACYCLINES

With few exceptions, all the tetracycline compounds produce the same untoward effects. Because they resemble each other very closely chemically, hypersensitivity reactions initiated by one may appear when another tetracycline is used at a later date. Organisms resistant to one of these compounds are usually resistant to the others. Among the reactions that have been observed in patients receiving tetracyclines are various rashes; exfoliative dermatitis; angioedema; anaphylaxis; cheilosis and discoloration of the tongue; glossitis; proctitis; pruritus ani or vulvae; fever; gastrointestinal irritation with nausea, vomiting, or diarrhea; thrombophlebitis (intravenous infusions); leukocytosis; leukopenia; atypical lymphocytes in the peripheral blood; photosensitivity (primarily demethylchlortetracycline); onycholysis (demethylchlortetracycline); liver damage (cases of renal insufficiency and pregnancy); increased intracranial pressure in young infants; discoloration of the teeth when the drugs are given to babies or to women in the early months of pregnancy; superinfections; and a variant of the Fanconi syndrome (administration of outdated drug).

Chloramphenicol (Chloromycetin)

Chloramphenicol, a fermentation product of *Streptomyces venezuelae,* has been isolated in pure crystalline form and synthesized. There is no difference in the anti-bacterial activity of the synthetic and the natural products. The drug inhibits protein synthesis in sensitive organisms.

Chloramphenicol is administered orally or by intravenous injection. The maximal plasma concentration after an oral dose occurs at the end of 2 hr, but some activity remains after 16 or 24 hr. About 80 percent of an oral dose can be demonstrated in the urine; however, only about 15 percent is biologically active.

Many organisms are susceptible to chloramphenicol. Although it is active against some types of gram-positive bacteria, it is most effective against the rickettsias and gram-negative organisms. *Staphylococcus aureus,* coliform bacilli, and other enteric organisms are known to become resistant to this antibiotic.

The most serious reaction produced by chloramphenicol is depression of the bone marrow, with agranulocytosis or pancytopenia. This phenomenon is not dose-related and may be an allergic response to the drug. It is observed most frequently when therapy is given over an extended period or repeated exposure to the antibiotic takes place. It is imperative that all patients receiving chloramphenicol have a white blood count and differential determination carried out every 48 hr during the entire course of treatment and for several days after it is discontinued. Decrease of the total number of white blood cells below 4,000 per cu mm or a fall in the percentage of neutrophils below 40 makes cessation of therapy mandatory; exercise of this precaution prevents the development of serious and potentially lethal bone marrow depression. Anemia with failure of reticulocyte response is common in individuals receiving chloramphenicol. This reaction is dose-related and usually disappears within a short time after treatment is stopped; it is not an indication for withdrawing the drug unless the anemia becomes severe.

Another potentially fatal reaction to the drug is observed in neonates, especially premature infants. This is the so-called "gray syndrome," characterized by weakness, listlessness, pallor, hypotension, and death; an inadequate quantity of glucuronyl transferase, the enzyme involved in conjugation of the antibiotic with glucuronic acid, is thought to be responsible for this reaction. Treatment with quantities no larger than 25 mg/kg/day in this age group avoids this reaction. Among other untoward effects observed with chloramphenicol are skin eruptions, fever, atrophic glossitis, Herxheimer reaction, nausea, vomiting, diarrhea, optic neuritis, blurred vision, digital paresthesias, decrease in prothrombin, superinfections, inhibition of mitosis in phytohemagglutinin-stimulated lymphocytes, and chromosome breaks.

Erythromycin

Erythromycin is an antibiotic elaborated by *Streptomyces erythreus.* The usual route of administration is by mouth. Peak serum concentrations appear 1 to 2 hr after ingestion of a dose and decline rapidly over 4 to 6 hr.

Gram-positive organisms, including many strains of *S. aureus,* are highly sensitive to erythromycin and are inhibited by concentrations of less than 1 μg per ml.

In clinical practice, the use of erythromycin should be restricted to infections due to sensitive staphylococci or other penicillin-resistant gram-positive organisms that occur in patients allergic to penicillin and cephalosporin derivatives. It is of value in the treatment of pneumococcal and group A beta-hemolytic streptococcal infections. The drug is therapeutically effective in pulmonary infection due to *Mycoplasma pneumoniae.* It is also active against some species of atypical *Mycobacteria.*

Bacteria exposed to erythromycin either in vitro or vivo may become resistant to the drug.

Erythromycin administration is accompanied by a small risk of untoward effects. Among the commonest reactions are skin eruptions, fever, and eosinophilia. Epigastric burning is common when the drug is taken orally in moderate amounts. The intramuscular injection of the antibiotic is so irritating that quantities larger than 100 mg should not be given. Intravenous infusion is frequently accompanied by venous irritation or thrombophlebitis. Erythromycin estolate may produce cholestatic hepatitis in some patients; this reaction does not appear to be induced by the antibiotic itself but seems to be associated with the administration of this particular ester. Superinfections by organisms resistant to erythromycin may occur.

Novobiocin

Novobiocin is an antibiotic derived from *Streptomyces niveus* and *S. spheroides.* It has an antimicrobial spectrum very similar to that of penicillin G and erythromycin; *S. aureus* and pneumococci are the most sensitive organisms. Group A *S. pyogenes, S. viridans, H. influenzae, H. pertussis,* and *N. meningitidis* are sensitive to the drug. Although a few strains of *Proteus* are susceptible to novobiocin, the majority are resistant.

Novobiocin is well absorbed from the gastrointestinal tract; peak plasma concentrations are reached at about 2 hr after an oral dose, and blood levels are higher when the drug is given in the fasting state.

The incidence of reactions to novobiocin is relatively high; commonest are extensive skin erruptions (12 percent) and fever (1 percent). Among other untoward effects are leukopenia, eosinophilia, pancytopenia, allergic pneumonitis, myocarditis, angioedema, exudative erythema multiforme, serum sickness, nausea, vomiting, diarrhea, jaundice, alopecia, intestinal hemorrhage, and superinfections. Yellow discoloration of the skin, plasma, and scleras, due in most instances to a circulating lipochrome pigment that is a degradation product of the antibiotic, is commonly present.

The oral dose of novobiocin for adults is 0.5 Gm every 6 hr; in severe infections, this may be increased to 1 Gm every 6 hr. The quantity recommended for intravenous or intramuscular injection is 1 to 2 Gm per day; intramuscular administration is usually painful.

Lincomycin (Lincocin)

Lincomycin, a fermentation product of *Streptomyces lincolnensis,* is a monobasic substance that differs chemically from all other antibiotics available for clinical use. The majority of strains of S. *aureus* are sensitive to the drug. *Diplococcus pneumoniae,* group A. S. *pyogenes,* S. *viridans, Bacillus anthracis, C. diphtheriae,* and *Clostrisium welchii* are highly susceptible to the antibiotic. Most enterococci are resistant. Gram-negative bacteria, fungi, and viruses are not inhibited by lincomycin. Some but not all erythromycin-resistant strains of staphylococci are also insensitive to lincomycin.

Plasma concentrations are maintained at higher levels than the minimal inhibitory quantities for most gram-positive organisms for 6 to 8 hr after oral ingestion of a single dose of 0.5 Gm; detectable antibacterial activity is demonstrable for 12 to 24 hr when 1 Gm is given by mouth. Intramuscular injection produces peak plasma concentrations in about ½ hr. Intravenous infusion yields levels in the therapeutic range for about 14 hr.

Diarrhea may occur in 10 to 20 percent of patients. Nausea, vomiting, abdominal pain, urticaria, skin eruptions, generalized pruritus, rectal irritation, vaginitis, transient jaundice, and neutropenia have also been noted.

The recommended oral dose of lincomycin for adults is 500 mg every 6 to 8 hr; for children, it is 30 to 60 mg/kg/day given in three or four equal doses. The intramuscular dose for adults is 600 mg every 12 to 24 hr. Intravenous therapy requires the infusion of 600 mg (in 250 ml of 5 percent dextrose or 0.85 percent saline solution) every 8 to 12 hr.

Cephalothin (Keflin)

Cephalothin is a semisynthetic derivative of cephalosporin C, a fermentation product of *Cephalosporium.* Group A S. *pyogenes,* S. *viridans, D. pneumoniae,* penicillin G–sensitive and –resistant S. *aureus, Cl. welchii, N. gonorrheae, N. meningitidis, C. diphtheriae,* and *Actinomyces* are highly sensitive to the agent. Gram-negative organisms are, in general, less susceptible, but most strains of *Salmonella, Shigella,* all *Proteus mirabilis,* 70 percent of *E. coli,* and many strains of *H. influenzae* are inhibited by concentrations readily produced by conventional doses of the drug. *Proteus vulgaris, Pseudomonas, Herellea,* and enterococci are resistant to the antibiotic. Cephalothin is not inactivated by penicillinase. Its activity is destroyed in vitro by cephalosporinase, an enzyme elaborated by some gram-negative bacteria and by enterococci; production of cephalosporinase is not always associated with resistance to cephalothin.

Cephalothin is not absorbed when given orally. It is rapidly absorbed after intramuscular injection and reaches peak plasma levels in about ½ hr. Therapeutic levels of the drug are present in cerebrospinal fluid. Cephalothin may accumulate in the blood of patients with poor renal function.

Among the untoward effects that have been related to the administration of cephalothin are fever, eosino-philia, neutropenia, hemolytic anemia, urticaria, anaphylactic reactions, and serum sickness and pain on injection. Superinfections have occurred in some patients.

The dose of cephalothin for adults is from 6 to 12 Gm per day administered intramuscularly or intravenously in equal-sized and -spaced doses.

Cephaloridine (Loridine)

Cephaloridine [7-(2-thenyl acetamido)-3-pyridylmethyl cephalosporanic acid] is another semisynthetic derivative of cephalosporin C. Its activity against penicillin G–sensitive and –resistant strains of S. *aureus* is about the same as that of cephalothin. *Diplococcus pneumoniae,* S. *viridans,* group A streptococci and most S. *fecalis* are highly sensitive to the drug. Enterococci are not inhibited. Sensitivity to cephaloridine and cephalothin distinguishes *Klebsiella,* which is sensitive, from *Aerobacter* which is resistant. Among other gram-negative organisms susceptible to cephaloridine are indole-negative *Proteus,* most *E. coli,* and *Salmonella.* Many strains of *H. influenzae* are moderately sensitive. Indole-positive *Proteus* and *Pseudomonas* are totally resistant. The minimal inhibitory and bactericidal concentrations for both gram-positive and -negative bacteria are, with few exceptions, approximately the same. The intramuscular injection of 0.6 Gm of cephaloridine leads to peak blood levels within ½ hr; small but detectable amounts are present in most instances after 8 hr. The administration of probenecid together with the antibiotic produces higher maximal serum concentrations and longer persistence of antibacterial activity. Cephaloridine is excreted primarily by the kidneys; 70 percent appears in the urine within 24 hr after a single dose. The recommended dose is 1 Gm every 6 hr for adults. Doses above 4.0 Gm per day in adults have been associated with both tubular and glomerular damage and are contraindicated. Intramuscular injection produces much less discomfort than does cephalothin.

Polymyxin (Aerosporin)

Polymyxin is a polypeptide antibiotic obtained from *B. polymyxa.* The principal effect is upon gram-negative bacilli, for which it is one of the most potent chemotherapeutic agents; strains of *Proteus* are, however, resistant. The drug can be administered intramuscularly at intervals of 8 to 12 hr with a total daily dose no larger than 2.5 mg per kg. It is not absorbed from the bowel, but eliminates sensitive organisms from the intestinal flora when given orally. It does not pass into the cerebrospinal fluid and cannot be detected in the bile or in the urine in biologically active form. Although highly effective against many species of gram-negative bacteria, polymyxin is most useful for the management of infections due to *Ps. aeruginosa,* practically all strains of which are sensitive to the agent. The untoward effects of this agent are similar to those of colistin and are described below.

Colistin

Colistin, and antibiotic produced by *B. colistinus,* is a basic polypeptide, the salts of which are water-soluble. The antimicrobial spectra of colistin and polymyxin B are very similar; there is complete cross resistance between these compounds.

Colistin is not absorbed from the gastrointestinal tract. After parenteral injection, peak plasma concentration develops at about 1 hr; at 3 hr, the blood level is about 25 percent of peak. Patients with renal insufficiency excrete this antibiotic poorly and exhibit high and sustained antimicrobial activity in the circulation. Colistin does not appear in significant quantities in cerebrospinal fluid.

Among the untoward effects associated with the administration of colistin are skin eruptions, pruritus, transient paresthesias, dizziness, speech abnormalities, fever, apnea, leukopenia, ataxia, partial deafness, gastrointestinal disturbances, superinfection, and reduction of renal function. The renal effects are usually transient and disappear when therapy is discontinued.

The parenteral dose of sodium colistimethate for the treatment of urinary tract infections is 2 to 3 mg per kg divided into four equal injections. For disease involving other organs, doses of 5 mg per kg for adults and 7 to 10 mg/kg/day for children may be given when the kidneys are normal. Great care must be exercised in the parenteral use of colistin when renal insufficiency is present and in older adults in whom kidney function appears to be normal.

Neomycin

Neomycin, an antibiotic derived from a strain of *Streptomyces* closely related to *S. fradia,* is bactericidal for many gram-negative and gram-positive organisms. Absorption from the intestinal tract is relatively poor. The usual oral dose of neomycin is 4 to 8 Gm in divided doses per day. The antibiotic may also be administered intramuscularly; the daily dose is 1 to 2 Gm.

The usefulness of neomycin is sharply limited by high toxicity when it is given parenterally. Kidney and eighth nerve damage occur in a significant number of patients. In view of these untoward effects, neomycin should never be the first drug employed in the treatment of any infection. It should be reserved for those diseases in which no other antibiotic is effective and in which the infection threatens life. This agent is used only infrequently by the parenteral route. Two other significant reactions may be produced by neomycin. When the drug is instilled into the peritoneal cavity, especially in anesthetized patients who have been given a muscle-relaxing agent such as succinyl choline, a curarelike reaction may ensue and paralyze respiration; the same phenomenon occurs rarely when the antibiotic is administered parenterally. Neostigmine reverses the reaction rapidly. Individuals who receive neomycin orally for prolonged periods may develop steatorrhea and a sprue-like syndrome. Acute staphylococcal enterocolitis has occurred in patients receiving this agent to "prepare" the bowel for surgery. In cases of renal insufficiency, enough of the antibiotic may be absorbed from the intestine to cause accumulation of concentrations in the blood that may be harmful to the ears and kidneys.

Kanamycin (Kantrex)

Kanamycin is a fermentation product of *Streptomyces kanamyceticus.* It is distinct from but related closely to neomycin and has a lesser relationship to streptomycin. It is active against gram-negative bacteria such as *E. coli, A. aerogenes, Salmonella;* gram-positive organisms such as *S. aureus;* and the tubercle bacillus. It is ineffective against streptococci, *D. pneumoniae,* and *Clostridia.* In high concentrations the drug is bactericidal.

Kanamycin has been shown to be of use in urinary tract infections, shigellosis, bacteremia due to gram-negative bacteria, peritonitis, and systemic staphylococcal infections. Although kanamycin is called a broad-spectrum antibiotic, it is not a substitute for all other antimicrobial agents; it should be reserved for the management of infections due to organisms not susceptible to those antibiotics which are potentially less toxic. In particular, there are many better antistaphylococcal agents than kanamycin; thus, it should rarely be used in staphylococcal infections.

For the treatment of systemic infection in adults, the recommended dose of kanamycin is 0.5 Gm every 6 to 8 hr intramuscularly. When this antibiotic is given orally, the suggested dose is 4 to 12 Gm per day. Intramuscular injection of the drug yields peak blood levels at 1 to 2 hr. The total dose administered should not exceed 15 Gm.

The two most dangerous side effects of treatment with kanamycin are damage to the eighth nerve, with permanent deafness, and nephrotoxicity, which varies from abnormalities of urine sediment to severe kidney involvement with renal failure and death. The drug should be used with caution in individuals with any degree of renal insufficiency. Other untoward effects that have been observed include various rashes, pruritus, pain at sites of injection, stomatitis, diarrhea, proctitis, and paresthesias. Like neomycin, kanamycin may produce myoneural junction dysfunction with paralysis of respiration when given intraperitoneally or parenterally.

Gentamicin (Garamycin)

This aminoglycoside antibiotic is derived from a species of the genus *Micromonospora,* and is closely related to streptomycin, neomycin, and kanamycin. It has a wide antibacterial spectrum, including staphylococci and many gram-negative bacteria such as *E. coli, Klebsiella-Enterobacter, Proteus mirabilis,* and, in particular, indole-positive species of *Proteus* and *Pseudomonas.* The drug has been useful in urinary tract infections, gram-negative pneumonia and bacteremias, and some have suggested that it will become the drug of choice in gram-negative sepsis. The recommended dose is 3.0 to 5.0 mg/kg/day given intramuscularly at 6 to 8 hr intervals in patients with normal renal function. Inasmuch as the drug is excreted by the kidneys, the dose should be reduced in patients with renal failure. The major toxic effect of gentamicin is on the vestibular portion of the eighth nerve, although hearing loss occurs occasionally. Careful adjustment of the dose, particularly in patients with impaired renal function, can minimize these side effects.

Vancomycin (Vancocin)

Vancomycin, a water-soluble antibiotic elaborated by *Streptococcus orientalis,* is active mainly against group A beta-hemolytic streptococcus, *S. fecalis, D. pneumoniae, N. gonorrheae, C. diphtheriae, Cl. tetani,* and staphylococcus, including strains resistant to semisynthetic penicillins; it is ineffective against all gram-negative bacilli.

The drug is not absorbed from the gastrointestinal tract and must be administered intravenously. The administration of 500 mg intravenously every 6 hr is recommended for the treatment of staphylococcal bacteremia. This is increased to 1 Gm every 6 hr in cases of endocarditis or meningitis.

Pain at the site of intravenous injection of vancomycin is relatively frequent. Thrombophlebitis is common. Skin eruptions may result from sensitization to the drug. Most patients receiving vancomycin show hyaline and granular casts and albumin in the urine; nitrogen retention can occur. Among other reactions induced by the antibiotic are nerve deafness, chills, fever, a shocklike state, and superinfections.

Paromomycin (Humatin)

Paromomycin, an oral antibiotic produced by a strain of *Streptomyces,* is employed to reduce the number of bacteria in the intestinal tract and to treat intestinal infections due to *Salmonella, Shigella,* and *Endamoeba histolytica.* The drug is effective in vitro against gram-positive organisms including *C. diphtheriae, S. aureus,* and *S. fecalis* and gram-negative bacilli such as *E. coli, A. aerogenes,* paracolon bacillus, *Klebsiella pneumoniae, Pasteurella multocida, Brucella* and some species of *Proteus.* It is also active both in vitro and in vivo against the tubercle bacillus. *Pseudomonas aeruginosa* is not affected. The drug can also be administered orally in cases of hepatic coma, for preparation of the bowel for surgery, for the treatment of Salmonella and Shigella carrier states, and in amebic colitis. The dose is 0.5 Gm every 6 hr; a parenteral dosage form is not available. Outside of bulky soft stools, there are no major toxic reactions. Paromomycin is not absorbed from the intestinal tract except in very tiny quantities. Nevertheless, it should be given with care to patients with significant renal insufficiency in whom it may produce damage to the ears and kidneys.

Nystatin (Mycostatin)

Nystatin is elaborated by *Streptomyces noursei.* It is poorly absorbed from the gastrointestinal tract. High blood levels follow intravenous injection. This antimycotic agent is employed for local application in the form of ointments, solutions, powders, suppositories, and gels. Topical use in the treatment of *Candida* infections of the skin and vagina has been reported to be successful.

The usual oral dose of nystatin is 150 mg (500,000 units) three times a day. Although an occasional case of disseminated mycotic infection has been treated parenterally with nystatin with reported good results, the place of this agent in the therapy of deep-seated mycoses is questionable.

When nystatin is administered orally, nausea and vomiting may occur. Local application may be irritating to skin and mucous membranes.

Amphotericin B (Fungizone)

Amphotericin B is the best agent available for the treatment of deep-seated mycotic infections. It produces cure in many cases of cryptococcosis, histoplasmosis, blastomycosis, disseminated candidiasis, and coccidiomycosis; it may have a beneficial effect in some instances of aspergillosis and mucormycosis. Amphotericin B is usually administered intravenously, dissolved in 5 percent dextrose. It should not be dissolved in saline because it precipitates in this medium. Fresh solutions should be prepared for each dose. The recommended dose for intravenous administration is 0.25 mg per kg the first day, followed by an increase of 0.25 mg per kg each succeeding day. When 1 mg/kg/day is reached, this dose is continued for the rest of the treatment period. Infusion of the drug should be carried out over a period of 6 hr.

After the maximal dose has been reached, an alternative regimen is to give 1.5 mg per kg every other day. Another method is to administer 1 mg of amphotericin B dissolved in 250 ml of 5 percent dextrose solution on the first day and increase this to 5 mg (in 500 ml of 5 percent dextrose) on the second day and 10 mg (in 1,000 ml of 5 percent dextrose) on the third day; the dose is then increased by 5 to 10 mg each day until 1 mg per kg is being administered daily. At this point, the dose may be changed to 1.5 mg per kg every other day. Treatment is continued for 6 weeks to 3 to 4 months, depending on the nature and severity of the infection.

The intravenous infusion of amphotericin B is often accompanied by chills, fever, vomiting, and headache; the frequency and intensity of these manifestations may be reduced by prior administration of an antipyretic or an antihistamine. A procedure that may control these reactions in some instances is the infusion of 25 mg hydrocortisone sodium succinate directly into the tubing of the intravenous set immediately after injection of the antibiotic has been started.

Among other untoward effects that may follow the systemic administration of amphotericin are phlebitis, hepatitis, anaphylaxis, thrombopenia, flushing, hypokalemia, hypomagnesemia, electrocardiographic abnormalities, and superinfections.

Nitrofurantoin (Furadantin)

Nitrofurantoin [N-(5-nitro-2-furfurylidene)-1-aminohydantoin] is an antibacterial agent of value primarily in the treatment of some types of urinary tract infection. It is poorly soluble in water. The drug is most active against E. coli (bactericidal), of intermediate effectiveness against A. aerogenes, and without effect against Pseudomonas. The activity of the drug against Proteus is variable, although many strains are quite sensitive. Staphylococcus aureus and enterococci are inhibited by low concentrations.

Nitrofurantoin is administered orally, usually in a dose of 7 to 10 mg per kg body weight (100 to 200 mg four times a day). Useful blood levels cannot be produced. The drug is excreted in the urine. Within 4 to 6 hr after a maximal dose, the concentration in the urine is 25 to 50 mg per 100 ml; 8 hr after a dose, the levels are low. With highly alkaline urine, the effect of nitrofurantoin appears to be depressed; for this reason, the simultaneous administration of an acidifying agent has been suggested. The development of bacterial resistance to the drug has not been noted.

The infections of the urinary tract that respond most favorably to therapy with nitrofurantoin are the acute and uncomplicated ones produced by E. coli.

Nitrofurantoin is relatively nontoxic. Nausea, with or without vomiting, is the commonest untoward reaction. Various types of rashes have been described. Leukopenia occurs rarely. A syndrome resembling acute pulmonary edema has been reported.

Nalidixic Acid (Neggram)

Nalidixic acid is a naphthyridine derivative active against many gram-negative bacilli including E. coli, Aerobacter, Klebsiella, and Proteus, organisms commonly involved in infections of the urinary tract. Pseudomonas is resistant to the drug. The drug is administered orally. Blood levels are inadequate for the control of systemic infections. Sensitive bacteria may become resistant rapidly, sometimes in as short a period as 5 days after exposure. For this reason, follow-up urine cultures should be obtained within a few days after instituting therapy. Organisms developing resistance to nalidixic acid remain sensitive to other agents. Side reactions include nausea, vomiting, skin eruptions, and in a few instances, convulsive seizures. The dose recommended for adults is 4 Gm daily in divided doses for 1 to 2 weeks, followed by 2 Gm per day.

TUBERCULOSTATIC DRUGS

Although streptomycin is effective in the treatment of tuberculosis, the use of this agent alone leaves much to be desired in the way of maximal antibacterial effect as well as in preventing the emergence of drug-resistant strains of Mycobacterium tuberculosis. For these reasons, attempts have been made to develop other compounds possessing tuberculostatic activity that might be given concurrently with streptomycin. Among such agents are para-aminosalicylic acid (PAS), isonicotinic acid hydrazide (INH), cycloserine, pyrazinamide, ethambutol, and ethionamide.

Para-aminosalicylic Acids (PAS)

Para-aminosalicylic acid, a white crystalline powder, is sparingly soluble in water but easily dissolved in the form of its sodium salt. This agent has a bacteriostatic effect in vitro against many strains of M. tuberculosis, even those which have become streptomycin-resistant.

Para-aminosalicylic acid and its sodium salt, when given orally, are rapidly absorbed and quickly excreted. A single dose produces maximal serum concentration within 30 to 60 min of administration; thereafter, there is a gradual fall, with disappearance in 2 to 3 hr.

Para-aminosalicylic acid is usually given orally, but preparations for intravenous use are also available; these should be reserved for patients in whom severe gastric distress prohibits oral use or for those in coma. The daily dose of the drug is 8 to 12 Gm. Among the untoward effects of this drug are gastrointestinal irritation with anorexia, nausea, vomiting, abdominal distress, and increased frequency of bowel evacuation. Epigastric burning and pain are common. Hypersensitivity phenomena include fever, joint pain, lymphadenopathy, various skin eruptions and, eosinophilia. Other reactions that have been noted are peptic ulceration, renal irritation, meningitis, myeloradiculoneuritis, hepatic necrosis, a clinical picture resembling infectious mononucleosis (atypical lymphocytes, negative heterophile agglutination), acute hemolytic anemia, leukopenia, agranulocytosis, perifocal infiltrations in the lungs, and Loeffler's syndrome.

Isonicotinic Acid Hydrazide

Of all the tuberculostatic agents, isonicotinic acid hydrazide has the highest activity in vitro. It is not effective against organisms other than Mycobacteria. The drug is administered orally, as a rule, and is almost completely absorbed from the digestive tract. Peak serum concentrations may occur 1 to 3 hr after administration, and minimal detectable concentrations persist for 6 to 24 hr.

Cultures of tubercle bacilli readily acquire resistance to isonicotinic acid hydrazide. Resistant strains are recovered from some patients who receive this drug alone. There is no cross resistance between isonicotinic acid hydrazide and streptomycin or PAS.

Isonicotinic acid hydrazide should be given in combination with streptomycin, PAS, or another tuberculostatic agent.

There is a great deal of variation in the metabolism of isonicotinic acid hydrazide in man. Some individuals inactivate the drug slowly, others rapidly. Individuals who inactivate the drug slowly are autosomal homozygous recessives; rapid inactivators are heterozygotes or homozygous dominants. The process of inactivation is enzyme-mediated and consists in facilitation of or speeding in acetylation of the drug. The development of poly-neuritis and the reversal of infectiousness are more frequent and occur earlier in slow than rapid inactivators. There is no association between the type of isonicotinic acid hydrazide inactivator and the appearance of drug resistance in tubercle bacilli.

The incidence of reactions to isoniazid varies with the dose. When 3 mg/kg/day are given, untoward effects occur in less than 1 percent of cases; with 10 mg/kg/day, these may develop in 15 percent or more of cases. Some of the reactions are the result of sensitization to the drug. These include fever, various types of skin eruptions, eosinophilia, and hepatitis. The toxic effects are manifested primarily by nervous system abnormalities among which are peripheral neuritis, muscle twitching, convulsions, dizziness, ataxia, paresthesias, stupor, toxic encephalopathy, euphoria, transient loss of memory, separation of ideas and reality, loss of self-control, florid psychosis, and optic neuritis. Dry mouth, epigastric distress, urinary retention in men, methemoglobinemia, agranulocytosis, jaundice, pellagra, vasculitis, and pyridoxine deficiency have also been noted in persons taking this agent. The nervous system difficulties are largely prevented by the administration of 100 mg pyridoxine per day. All the reactions tend to be more frequent in slow inactivators of INH.

Cycloserine

Cycloserine is an antibiotic produced by *Streptomyces orchidaceus.* It is active against *M. tuberculosis,* including strains resistant to other tuberculostatic agents. In vivo, the drug is effective in infections due to enterococci, strains of paracolon bacilli, *E. coli, S. aureus,* and agents of the psittacosis-ornithosis-lymphogranuloma venereum group. Cycloserine is rapidly absorbed from the stomach and small intestine. Peak blood levels are reached within 3 to 4 hr after a single dose. Multiple doses lead to accumulation of the drug in the circulation after 3 days. Cycloserine is highly diffusible and is distributed throughout the body fluids and tissues. Cerebrospinal fluid levels in patients with normal or inflamed meninges are approximately the same as in the blood. About 50 percent of a parenteral dose of this antibiotic is excreted in unchanged form in the urine in the first 12 hr; a total of 65 percent is recoverable in urine over a period of 72 hr. Urine concentrations are high. Excessive blood levels develop in patients with decreased renal function.

Reactions to cycloserine tend to appear in the first 2 weeks of therapy and involve the central nervous system primarily. Among these are somnolence, headache, tremor, dysarthria, vertigo, confusional and other abnormal behavioral states, paresis, acute psychotic episodes, and seizures. The oral dose of the drug is 250 mg twice a day.

Pyrazinamide

Pyrazinamide (pyrazine-2-carboxyamide), a synthetic agent, is more active against the tubercle bacillus than para-aminosalicylic acid or cycloserine but less effective than streptomycin or isonicotinic acid hydrazide. Bacterial resistance to pyrazinamide develops in 6 to 8 weeks in patients treated with this agent alone. When given with another tuberculostatic agent, good therapeutic results are produced. The drug is well absorbed from the gastrointestinal tract. Peak plasma levels are reached about 2 hr after oral administration. Excretion is primarily by the kidneys. The dose for adults is 25 to 35 mg/kg/day given in 3 or 4 equally divided and equally spaced doses. A total quantity of 3 Gm per day must not be exceeded.

Injury to the liver is the most common and serious side effect of pyrazinamide; elevations of SGOT and SGPT are the earliest abnormalities. With a dose of 3 Gm per day, manifestations of liver disease develop in about 15 percent of patients; jaundice appears in 2 to 3 percent and death from hepatic necrosis results rarely. All individuals receiving this agent must have studies of liver function carried out before and during therapy. Among other untoward effects of the drug are arthralgia, anorexia, nausea, vomiting, dysuria, malaise, and fever.

Ethambutol

Ethambutol (ethylene diamino-di-1-butanol dihydrochloride) is active in low concentrations against most strains of *M. tuberculosis.* Bovine tubercle bacilli and group I atypical *Mycobacteria* (photochromogens, *M. batteyi*) are also highly sensitive to the drug. However, *M. avium* as well as scotochromogens and nonchromogenic *Mycobacteria* are less predictably affected. Ethambutol suppresses the growth of isoniazid-and streptomycin-resistant tubercle bacilli. Bacterial resistance develops in vivo when the compound is given alone. About 75 to 80 percent of an orally administered dose of ethambutol is absorbed from the gastrointestinal tract. Plasma levels are maximal 2 to 4 hr after the drug is taken orally. About 50 percent of the peak concentration is present in the blood at 8 hr and less than 10 percent at 24 hr after a dose. From 80 to 95 percent of an oral dose of ethambutol is excreted in the urine and feces within 1 to 4 hr after it is administered. In 24 hr, 50 percent of the ingested drug is present in the urine; 8 to 15 percent is excreted in the form of two metabolic products, an intermediary aldehyde and a terminal butyric acid derivative. The oral dose of ethambutol is 25 to 50 mg per kg once a day.

Loss of vision is the outstanding untoward effect produced by ethambutol. It occurs in about 10 percent of patients receiving 25 to 50 mg/kg/day of the drug. Evidence of visual difficulty first appears 1 to 7 months after therapy is started. The intensity of visual loss is related to the duration of treatment after decrease in visual activity becomes apparent. Recovery occurs when ethambutol is withdrawn; the time required is a function of the degree of visual impairment present when therapy is stopped.

Ethionamide

Ethionamide (2-ethylthioisonicotinamide), a derivative of isonicotinic acid, suppresses the growth of *M. tuberculosis* and is effective against strains resistant to streptomycin, para-aminosalicylic acid, isonicotinic acid hydrazide, and cycloserine. About 75 percent of photochromogenic *Mycobacteria* are suppressed by a concentration of 10 mg per ml or less; the scotochromogens are more resistant.

The oral administration of 1 Gm of ethionamide yields peak plasma levels of about 20 mg per ml in 3 hr. Slightly higher and more sustained levels follow rectal instillation of the drug, although absorption from this site may be delayed. Ethionamide is present in significant quantities in the cerebrospinal fluid.

Among the commonest reactions to ethionamide are anorexia, nausea, and vomiting. Manifestations resembling those resulting of ganglionic blockade—severe postural hypotension, mental depression, drowsiness, and asthenia—are common. Among other untoward effects are convulsions, peripheral neuropathy, allergic skin rashes, purpura, stomatitis, gynecomastia, impotence, menorrhagia, and difficulty in control of diabetes mellitus. Hepatitis may occur in diabetics but disappears when therapy is stopped.

The initial dose of ethionamide for adults is 250 mg orally twice a day. This is increased by 125 mg per day every 5 days until 1 Gm is being given daily; this dose must not be exceeded.

Ethionamide should not be used alone to treat tuberculosis. In various combinations with para-aminosalicylic acid, isoniazid, streptomycin, cycloserine, and pyrazinamide, ethionamide has produced good results.

SELECTION OF A CHEMOTHERAPEUTIC AGENT

When faced with the necessity of treating an infection, the physician finds that an ever-increasing number of antibacterial drugs is available. Bacterial cultures are desirable in most infections, but are not always practicable. In many instances, the etiology can be inferred from the mode of onset, the clinical features, and the epidemiologic background of the disease. Nevertheless, there are situations in which careful bacteriologic studies are essential to proper treatment.

Even when the etiology of an infectious process is determined, selection of an appropriate drug does not follow automatically, because there may be wide variations in susceptibility among organisms of the same or related species. The cost of the different drugs also has to be considered at times, since there are enormous differences. In addition, the nature of the illness may affect the choice of agent; for example, an orally administered drug may be unsatisfactory in a patient who is vomiting. In critically ill patients, it is sometimes safest to give a combination of drugs until cultural and sensitivity studies reveal which agent is specifically indicated.

In such cases, cultures should always be taken *before initiation of therapy.* If an individual has previously shown hypersensitivity or any other serious reaction to a drug, or if he develops a reaction during therapy, a different agent should be used, if possible. Therapy of specific infections is discussed in other parts of this book, where the agents of primary and secondary value in treatment are indicated.

COMBINATIONS OF ANTIBACTERIAL AGENTS

TREATMENT OF MIXED BACTERIAL INFECTIONS. In bronchiectasis, peritonitis, and some cases of acute or chronic otitis media and urinary tract infection, two or more organisms may sometimes be involved. In some instances, the responsible bacteria, although of different species, are sensitive to a single antimicrobial agent; in others they have distinctly different drug susceptibilities. This emphasizes the need to determine the drug sensitivity of each of the components of a mixed flora individually before therapy is initiated. The antibiotics to be given are selected on the basis of these studies and administered in *full doses.* In some cases, it may be unnecessary and even dangerous to delay initiation of treatment until definitive bacteriologic data are available. Peritonitis is an outstanding example. Because both gram-positive and gram-negative organisms may be acting synergistically to produce this disease and because delay in therapy may result in a rapidly fatal outcome, treatment should be started immediately with maximal quantities of the antibiotics known to be most effective against these bacteria.

DELAY IN RATE OF EMERGENCE OF RESISTANCE. The emergence of antibiotic resistance is delayed by combinations of antimicrobial drugs in some but not in all infections. For example, the concomitant administration of two or more drugs suppresses strikingly the development of resistance in the tubercle bacillus. Tuberculosis is best treated, therefore, with at least two, and in some instances (miliary tuberculosis and tuberculous meningitis), three, tuberculostatic agents simultaneously.

"FIXED-DOSE" COMBINATIONS. These encourage inadequate treatment, because there is an inevitable tendency to use the same total dose of the combination as of the single agent, which does not provide the expected effective quantity of either, particularly of the inferior drug. Fixed-dose combinations provide a false sense of security because they are alleged to offer wider coverage, when in fact, they provide a narrower effective spectrum by substituting less active agents and smaller amounts of individual agents than would be the case if most active antibiotics were used in the proper dosage individually. If combined therapy is necessary at all, each of the drugs should be selected on the basis of its activity and the results of sensitivity tests and should be given in full dosage.

THERAPY OF SEVERE INFECTIONS IN WHICH SPECIFIC ETIOLOGY IS UNKNOWN. The commonest use of antibiotic combinations is for the therapy of infections in which the etiology is not immediately apparent, but where the possibility that bacterial infection is present is sufficiently great to make chemotherapy necessary. Because the exact cause cannot be immediately determined, more than one agent is given in the hope that this will "cover" the situation; fixed-dose mixtures are used all too often. In a large number of cases, the infectious process is viral and an antimicrobial agent is not indicated.

When full-dose combinations are given in the absence of a specific bacteriologic diagnosis, it must be determined, on the basis of the clinical features of the disease, a detailed history, and laboratory investigations (including examination of stained preparations, if possible), not only that a patient has a bacterial infection but also what type of organism is most likely to be involved. *Under no circumstances should chemotherapy be initiated until all the necessary bacteriologic investigations have been started.* However, in many instances, treatment need not and should not be delayed until the results of these studies become available.

ALTERATION OF ANTIBACTERIAL ACTIVITY BY COMBINING ANTIBIOTICS. A number of studies indicate that the antimicrobial activity of antibiotic combinations may be unpredictable and that in vitro activity may be unrelated to therapeutic effectiveness in vivo. Enhancement, depression, or no change in activity of the combination, when compared with single drugs, have been demonstrated. However, antibiotic combinations usually have a broad-spectrum effect in vivo if the organisms being treated are sensitive to the compounds. Clinical experience has indicated those infections in which combined therapy appears to be more effective as well as those in which such treatment produces inferior results. Enterococcal infections appear to respond better when treated with a combination of penicillin and streptomycin than with either of these antibiotics alone (Chaps. 137 and 141). Combined treatment also seems to be superior to the use of single drugs in *K. pneumoniae* pneumonia (chloramphenicol and streptomycin—Chap. 148), tuberculosis (two or sometimes three effective tuberculostatic agents—Chap. 174), and brucellosis (tetracycline and streptomycin—Chap. 154). On the other hand, the use of tetracycline plus penicillin in pneumococcal meningitis produces a much lower recovery rate than does penicillin alone. This is probably also true for the treatment of this disease with a combination of chloramphenicol and penicillin. The results of therapy for streptococcal pharyngitis are better with penicillin than with erythromycin, and intermediate when these antibiotics are given together.

HOST DETERMINANTS OF RESPONSE TO ANTIMICROBIAL AGENTS

The nature of an infection determines to a great degree the kind of antimicrobial therapy to be employed. However, innate host factors, completely unrelated to the acute disorder, are often the prime determinants not only of the type of antibiotic selected but also of its dose, route of administration, risk and nature of untoward effects, and therapeutic effectiveness. Among such factors are age, genetic factors, pregnancy, metabolic abnormalities, atopic allergy, nervous system disorders, indigenous microbial flora, hepatic function, renal function, electrolyte balance, and host defense mechanisms.

AGE. Although the dose of many commonly used antibiotics may be calculated on the basis of body weight or surface area, that of others, especially those excreted in unchanged form by the kidney, exemplified by the penicillins, is determined almost entirely by the state of renal function. In addition to dose of antibiotics, age also plays an important role in conditioning the risks of some types of reactions, route of administration, and therapeutic activity.

Renal function is relatively poor in newborn children, especially premature infants, and in older persons. Although renal function increases markedly from birth, complete maturity is probably not reached until the age of one year. With advancing age, glomerular function, effective blood flow, and tubular excretion diminish. Because of these renal changes, the dose of a number of antimicrobial agents, especially those excreted in biologically active form by the kidney, needs to be relatively low in the first month of life, particularly in premature babies, considerably higher in young children, and reduced considerably in individuals over the age of fifty, even when BUN and serum creatinine are within the normal range. Among these drugs are penicillin G, methicillin, oxacillin, ampicillin, cephalothin, streptomycin, tetracycline, and kanamycin. Although the dose of colistin does not vary in children of different ages, its excretion is relatively slow in the elderly and necessitates the administration of smaller than conventional quantities despite normal BUN and creatinine.

Because the level of gastric acidity is relatively low during the first month of life and with advancing age (one-third of individuals aged sixty to sixty-nine years have achlorhydria), adequate blood levels of penicillin may follow oral administration of this antibiotic in these age groups.

The type of reaction to an antimicrobial agent is determined by age, in some instances. The livers of newborn babies produce only small quantities of glucuronyl transferase, the enzyme involved in the inactivation of chloramphenicol by conjugation with UDP glucuronic acid. Because of this, these children develop excessively high circulating levels of unconjugated biologically active drug which is toxic. This is responsible for the "gray syndrome" (abdominal distension, progressive pallor and cyanosis, vasomotor collapse, and death) which may appear when a dose in excess of 25 mg/kg/day is given. The immaturity of the acetylation process in the newborn liver also may expose babies to high blood levels of sulfonamides. Sulfisoxazole predisposes to the development of kernicterus when administered to very young infants. This drug competes effectively with bilirubin for binding sites on albumin and displaces the bile pigment. The central nervous system lesion is due to exposure to excessive concentrations of bilirubin. The teeth of young children may exhibit discoloration and enamel hypoplasia when treated with tetracycline compounds between the ages of two months and two years when the permanent dentition is undergoing calcification. Disturbances in bone growth may also be produced in youngsters receiving this group of antibiotics.

GENETIC FACTORS. The rate at which isonicotinic acid hydrazide is inactivated in the liver by conjugation with acetyl radical is genetically determined. About 50 percent of Americans are rapid inactivators; the other half are slow inactivators. This varies with race; about 95 percent of Eskimos are rapid inactivators. There is no good evidence that rapid acetylation of the drug is responsible for therapeutic failure when standard doses are employed. However, standard doses of the drug have been shown to produce toxic reactions to INH more often in persons who acetylate it slowly.

Acute hemolysis may develop in individuals given some antimicrobial compounds in the presence of glucose 6-phosphate dehydrogenase (G-6-PD) deficiency. Although common in Negro males, the defect may be expressed more actively in white people in whom the incidence is lower. The drugs which have provoked episodes of hemolytic anemia in such individuals are sulfanilamide, sulfacetamide, sulfamethoxypyridazine, sulfamethoxypyrimidine (Madribon), sulfisoxazole, chloramphenicol, salicylazosulfapyridine (Azulfidine), nitrofuration, and diaminodiphenyl sulfone (dapsone). Patients with hemoglobin Zurich and hemoglobin H may also develop hemolysis when given some of these agents.

PREGNANCY. Pregnancy imposes an increased risk of reactions to some antimicrobial agents on both the mother and the fetus. The drugs that cross the placental barrier include penicillin G, streptomycin, chloramphenicol, methicillin, oxacillin, ampicillin, cephalothin, sulfonamides, and tetracyclines. The embryo may be exposed to some degree of hearing loss when streptomycin is given to its mother. Sulfonamides and INH have produced fetal injury when administered during pregnancy. The tetracyclines pose a special danger to pregnant women. The developing teeth of the embryo may be injured if one of these compounds is given from midpregnancy on, the period when the crowns of the teeth are being formed. The pregnant patient with pyelonephritis who is treated with a tetracycline, especially if it is given intravenously in a dose of more than 2 Gm a day, may develop fatal hepatic toxicity. Pancreatitis also has been noted even when only 1 to 2 Gm per day is administered parenterally. These problems are greatest in the presence of significant renal insufficiency.

METABOLIC ABNORMALITIES. Penicillin G and sulfonamides are absorbed from intramuscular and subcutaneous sites to a lesser degree in persons with *diabetes mellitus* than in those who do not have this metabolic defect. This results in lower maximal serum concentrations than is the case in normal individuals. Poor response to treatment with vitamin B_{12} has been noted in patients with *pernicious anemia* and to iron administra-

tion in those with *iron-deficiency anemia* when they are receiving chloramphenicol simultaneously.

ATOPIC ALLERGY. Persons with a history of atopic allergy are highly susceptible to the development of hypersensitivity to antimicrobial agents whether or not they have been exposed to them previously (Chap. 73).

NERVOUS SYSTEM DISORDERS. Patients with either localized or diffuse central nervous system disease are more prone to the development of seizures than are normal individuals when treated with "massive" doses (40 to 80 million units per day) of penicillin G. These are more apt to occur when the antibiotic is administered as a continuous drip than when it is given as multiple single injections. Penetration of chloramphenicol into cerebrospinal fluid is impaired by the presence of hydrocephalus. Streptomycin, kanamycin, neomycin, polymyxin, and colistin may cause respiratory arrest in anesthetized patients, especially if they have received a muscle relaxant such as succinylcholine. This reaction also may occur in patients with myasthenia gravis and is a special problem in the presence of renal failure.

INDIGENOUS MICROBIAL FLORA. The organisms responsible for superinfections are, for the most part, members of the normal microbial flora that inhabit various areas of the body such as the intestinal and upper respiratory tracts. In some cases, the organisms are derived from the external environment and become part of the indigenous microflora. Exposure to antimicrobial agents allows the members of the bacterial population that are resistant to the drug being given to flourish and, in some instances, to produce disease. The normal microflora may condition response to treatment in special situations. Therapeutic failure or relapse of S. pyogenes pharyngitis treated with penicillin G may be due to the presence of penicillinase-producing S. aureus, E. coli, Ps. aeruginosa or Klebsiella in the throat.

HEPATIC FUNCTION. Antimicrobial agents metabolized by, inactivated by, or concentrated in the liver may behave abnormally when administered to persons with impaired hepatic function. For example, blood levels of chloramphenicol are elevated in such patients, and toxic reactions may supervene. Persons with cirrhosis or chronic or convalescent hepatitis may develop untoward effects when given 2 Gm of tetracycline orally per day. The half-life of lincomycin is almost doubled in the presence of hepatic dysfunction. Antibiotics concentrated in the liver (methicillin, ampicillin, and nafcillin) may be absent or present only in reduced quantities in the bile in the face of hepatic disease. Erythromycin and novobiocin must be used with caution when liver dysfunction is a problem.

RENAL FUNCTION. Renal function is one of the most important determinants of response to antimicrobial agents. It not only is a major consideration in the choice of a drug, but also influences selection of dose and the risk of reactions involving the kidney and other organs. The extent to which elimination of an antibiotic is affected by the presence of kidney disease depends on whether it is cleared by this organ, the rate at which this is accomplished, clearance or inactivation by other mechanisms, and the degree of renal impairment. The drugs that are removed entirely by the kidney include penicillin, streptomycin, cephalothin, kanamycin, vancomycin, and polymyxin. The renal excretion of other commonly used agents is as follows: tetracycline, 20 to 60 percent; oxytetracycline, 10 to 35 percent; chlortetracycline, 10 to 15 percent after oral and 60 percent in 12 hr after intravenous administration. The clearance of demethylchlortetracycline is about one-half that of tetracycline. Some antibiotics are excreted in only low concentrations in the urine; erythromycin, 2 to 5 percent of an oral and 12 to 15 percent of an intravenous dose; lincomycin, 4 percent when the drug is given by mouth and 15 percent when it is administered parenterally. The kidney excretes 80 percent of para-aminosalicylic acid and 50 to 70 percent of isonicotinic acid hydrazide. Retention of oxacillin, methicillin, cephalothin, and colistimethate sodium occurs in the presence of decreased renal function. Chloramphenicol and erythromycin present no important problems in patients with impaired activity of the kidneys. Lincomycin, however, may produce elevated serum concentrations when renal disease is present. It is clear that antimicrobial agents excreted to a significant degree by the kidney must be given cautiously to patients with dysfunction of this organ and, in some cases, must be avoided completely. On the other hand, those drugs which are not handled by renal mechanisms may, with few exceptions, be given in conventional doses even when the kidneys are virtually functionless. A very important aspect of penicillin G therapy that is often overlooked and that may be responsible for serious difficulty and even death is the fact that most commercially available compounds are in the form of potassium salts. Extreme care must be exercised, therefore, in the use of this drug in the presence of renal impairment, particularly if hyperkalemia is present. It is important that the status of renal function be determined not only before but also during the entire period of treatment, if serious or even lethal effects are to be avoided when potentially toxic antibiotics, especially those which may injure the kidney, are administered. Even when BUN and creatinine are normal, older individuals may accumulate antibiotics and show toxic reactions if the agents are excreted mainly by the kidney.

HOST DEFENSE MECHANISMS. Probably the most important determinant of the therapeutic effectiveness of antimicrobial agents is the functional state of the defense mechanisms of the host. Both humoral and cellular phenomena are involved. Inadequacy of type, quantity and quality of the immunoglobulins (Chap. 70), alterations in delayed hypersensitivity, and ineffective phagocytosis, acting independently or in varying combination, may result in therapeutic failure despite use of a potent antibiotic to treat an infection produced by a highly sensitive organism. This may occur in Hodgkins' disease, lymphoma, leukemia, cancer of various types, uremia, vasculitis, and granulomatous disease of childhood, which are all disorders in which immunosuppression, abnormal activity of immunoglobulins, or inadequate phagocytosis are problems. In addition, some of the drugs commonly employed to treat these disorders (cytotoxic agents,

antimetabolites, and corticosteroids) as well as to prevent rejection of transplanted organs, may add to the difficulty because they are immunosuppressive (Chap. 71).

That the normal activity of defense mechanisms is a requirement for the therapeutic effectiveness of all antimicrobial agents is frequently overlooked. The tetracyclines, sulfonamides, and chloramphenicol, which are all bacteriostatic, should, by definition, never completely eradicate sensitive organisms. However, *cure* of some infectious diseases is accomplished by these drugs, and relapse does not occur when treatment is stopped. This is strong evidence for the role of effective host defenses, which, acting on microorganisms after they have been injured by one of these compounds, are finally responsible for the eradication of infection. Clinical experience suggests that even bactericidal antibiotics probably require the adjunct activity of cellular and humoral defenses to dispose of bacteria.

THE PROPHYLAXIS OF INFECTION

The available chemotherapeutic agents offer an excellent means of prophylaxis in some but not all infectious diseases. Chemoprophylaxis has been used primarily for four purposes: (1) to protect healthy individuals, whether singly or in groups of varying size, against invasion by specific microorganisms; (2) to prevent bacterial infection in individuals acutely ill with diseases, often of viral origin, for which antimicrobial agents are not effective; (3) to reduce the risk of infection in patients with various types of chronic illness; and (4) to inhibit the spread of disease from areas of localized infection or to prevent infection, in general, in persons who have been subjected to accidental or surgical trauma. Experience has indicated the areas in which chemoprophylaxis is of value and those in which it is ineffective and may, in fact, increase the risk of infection. There still remain, however, instances in which opinion concerning the efficacy of antimicrobial agents in preventing bacterial invasion is unsettled. In general, when chemoprophylaxis is used to prevent implantation or to eradicate a single specific organism by the use of a single potent drug, it has had a high degree of success. If, on the other hand, the purpose is to prevent implantation of any or all bacteria that happen to be in the patient's internal or external environment, failure is the rule.

Table 135-1 lists the diseases or situations in which chemoprophylaxis is of proved or unsettled value and those in which experience has indicated lack of success. The antibiotics listed are not necessarily the ones recommended, but merely indicate that some success in preventing infection with them has been reported. In some instances, for example, shigellosis and meningococcal infections, many strains are resistant to sulfonamides, and prophylaxis with these agents is no longer effective. The dosage and methods of administration for each drug are discussed in the sections dealing with the specific diseases.

DANGERS OF CHEMOPROPHYLAXIS. It is important to point out that the same untoward effects that occur when

Table 135-1. VALUE OF CHEMOPROPHYLAXIS

I. Chemoprophylaxis of proved value
  A. Streptotoccal (group A) infections and rheumatic fever recurrences: sulfonamides, various forms of penicillin, erythromycin
  B. Bacillary dysentery: sulfonamides, chloramphenicol, ampicillin
  C. Diarrhea due to enteropathogenic *E. coli:* neomycin orally
  D. Gonorrhea, acute urethritis, and ophthalmia: penicillin
  E. Congenital syphilis (treatment of mother): penicillin
  F. Meningococcal infections: sulfonamides in selected cases (Chap. 142)
  G. Dental extraction in presence of heart disease: penicillin, vancomycin
  H. Mucoviscidosis: tetracycline compounds
  I. Hepatic coma: neomycin or paromomycin orally
  J. Contaminated or infected wound surgery: penicillin plus streptomycin, ampicillin, tetracyclines
  K. Labor when membranes ruptured over 24 to 48 hr: penicillin plus streptomycin, ampicillin, tetracyclines
  L. Steroid therapy in patients with high risk of tuberculosis: tuberculostatic drugs
II. Chemoprophylaxis of no value
  A. Viral infections of upper respiratory tract including common cold, influenza, and rhinovirus, ECHO, Coxsackie, and adenovirus infections
  B. Childhood viral diseases: mumps, measles, rubella, chickenpox, vaccinia
  C. Poliomyelitis
  D. Infectious mononucleosis
  E. Smallpox
  F. "Clean" surgical and obstetric procedures
  G. Pertussis
  H. Burns
  I. Shock
  J. Coma
  K. Cardiac failure
  L. Catheterization or other instrumentation of urinary tract
  M. Premature infants
  N. X-ray irradiation
  O. Administration of steroids, except in instances with high risk of tuberculosis
III. Chemoprophylaxis of unsettled value
  A. Surgical procedures on heart or urinary tract in presence of valvular heart disease
  B. Acute diffuse glomerulonephritis
  C. Syphilis—venereal contact
  D. Chronic nontuberculous pulmonary disease
  E. Tuberculin-negative contacts of active case of tuberculosis
  F. Staphylococcus carrier state
  G. Transmission of *S. aureus* in nurseries and other hospital areas
  H. Reduction of number of intestinal bacteria before bowel resection
  I. Cardiac catheterization
  J. Exchange transfusion

antibiotic agents are used for therapeutic purposes are observed when patients who have no active infection are

given these drugs. The risk of reactions as well as the cost of the drug must always be taken into consideration in planning a program of chemoprophylaxis. When there is no evidence that chemoprophylaxis will be effective, it should not be used.

SUPERINFECTIONS

These occur with all chemotherapeutic agents and are due to invasion by normal endogenous flora or by organisms acquired by contact with other patients or attendants. They may result from the accidental introduction of bacteria during injection of the drug; in all instances, the new infections are produced by strains of organisms insensitive to the antibiotic being administered at the time they first appear. Infections due to organisms of the genus *Candida (Monilia)* may also occur during chemotherapy; they may involve the mouth, pharynx, or lung, or they may spread systemically. This type of superinfection is being reported more frequently and is particularly important because systemic candidiosis is difficult to treat.

Superinfections occur in about 2 percent of patients who receive a chemotherapeutic agent. The organs involved in the secondary infection are most frequently those affected by the primary disease. The organisms responsible for superinfections are often difficult to treat with the presently available antibacterial drugs. The factors that predispose to the development of superinfection are (1) age of three years or less, (2) primary disease of the lower respiratory tract, (3) infection of the middle ear, and (4) the use of a drug or combination of antibiotic agents which tend to have a broad antibacterial effect; the wider the antimicrobial spectrum, the greater the danger of secondary bacterial invasion. Superinfections appear most frequently on the fourth or fifth day after initiation of chemotherapy and may convert a benign self-limited disease into a serious, prolonged, or even fatal one. It is essential to carry our frequent bacteriologic studies, whenever possible, to determine changes in bacterial flora that may subsequently be responsible for a secondary infection, and to treat this infection promptly when it appears (Chap. 133).

MISUSES OF CHEMOTHERAPY

There is little doubt that the antimicrobial agents are used in many situations in which they are not required and that, even when they are indicated, failure to utilize them properly may lead to poor clinical results. Listed below are the commonest misuses of the chemotherapeutic compounds.

1. Treatment of fever of obscure origin
2. Choice of ineffective antibiotic
3. Inadequate or excessive doses
4. Improper route of administration
5. Continuation of therapy with drug to which bacterial resistance develops
6. Failure to stop treatment in presence of serious toxic or allergic reaction
7. Failure to alter therapy when superinfection occurs

8. Prophylaxis of unpreventable secondary bacterial infection (see above)

9. Therapy of insusceptible infections—infections produced by true viruses

10. Use of combinations of drugs when not specifically indicated

11. Reliance on chemotherapy or prophylaxis to the exclusion of necessary surgical intervention, e.g., drainage of localized areas of infection

Probably the most frequent misuse of antimicrobial drugs is in the therapy of fever of unknown origin. The mere presence of fever, in the absence of localizing signs, does not necessarily indicate an infectious process (Chap. 16). In the absence of strong clinical evidence that a febrile episode is infectious in origin, particularly when there is no detectable focus, chemotherapy should be delayed until adequate clinical and laboratory studies have been performed.

REFERENCES

Abraham, E. P.: The Cephalosporins, Pharmacol. Rev., 14:473, 1962.

Anderson, K. N., R. P. Kennedy, J. J. Plorde, J. A. Shulman, and R. G. Petersdorf: Effectiveness of Ampicillin against Gram-negative Bacteria, J.A.M.A., 187:555, 1964.

Andriole, V. T., and H. M. Kravetz: The Use of Amphotericin B in Man, J.A.M.A., 180:269, 1962.

Chang, T. W., and L. Weinstein: A Comparison of the in Vitro and in Vivo Activity of Methacycline and Other Tetracycline Compounds, Antibiot. Chemotherap., 12:671, 1962.

Coles, H. M. T., B. McNamara, L. Mutch, R. J. Holt, and G. T. Stewart: Paromomycin in the Treatment of Shigella and Salmonella Infections in Children, Lancet, II:944, 1960.

Dowling, H. F.: "Tetracycline," New York, Medical Encyclopedia, Inc., 1955.

Feingold, D. S.: Antimicrobial Therapeutic Agents: The Nature of Their Action and Selective Toxicity, New Engl. J. Med., 269:900, 957, 1964.

Finland, M.: Chemoprophylaxis of Infectious Disease, Disease-a-Month, Chicago, Year Book Publishers, Inc., December, 1959, July, 1960, September, 1960.

——: The Symposium on Gentamicin, J. Infec. Dis., 119:537, 1969.

——and L. P. Garrod: Demethylchlortetracycline, Lancet, II:959, 1960.

—— and R. L. Nichols: Novobiocin, Practitioner, 179:84, 1957.

—— and L. Weinstein: Complications Induced by Antimicrobial Agents, New Engl. J. Med., 248:220, 1953.

Gale, E. F.: Mechanism of Antibiotic Action, Pharmacol. Rev., 15:481, 1963.

Gravenkemper, C. F., J. V. Bennett, J. L. Brodie and W. M. M. Kirby: Dicloxacillin: In Vitro and Pharmacologic Comparisons with Oxacillin and Cloxacillin, A.M.A. Arch. Intern. Med., 116:340, 1965.

Herrell, W. E.: "Erythromycin," New York, Medical Encyclopedia, Inc., 1955.

Hirsh, L. H., and L. E. Putman: "Penicillin," New York, Medical Encyclopedia, Inc., 1956.

Jawetz, E.: "Polymyxin, Neomycin, Bacitracin," New York, Medical Encyclopedia, Inc., 1956.

Kaplan, K., B. E. Reisberg, and L. Weinstein. Cephaloridine: Antimicrobial Activity and Pharmacologic Behavior, Am. J. Med. Sci., 253:667, 1967.

—— and L. Weinstein: Lincomycin, Pediat. Clin. N. Am., 15:131, 1968.

Klein, J. O., and M. Finland: The New Penicillins, New Engl. J. Med., 269:1019, 1963.

Kunin, C. M., and M. Finland: Restrictions Imposed on Antibiotic Therapy by Renal Failure, A.M.A. Arch. Intern. Med., 104:1030, 1959.

Lepper, M. H.: "Aureomycin (Chlortetracycline)," New York, Medical Encyclopedia, Inc., 1956.

Musselman, M. M.: "Terramycin (Oxytetracycline)," New York, Medical Encyclopedia, Inc., 1956.

Nord, N. M., and P. D. Hoeprich: Polymyxin B and Colistin: A Critical Comparison, New Engl. J. Med., 270:1030, 1964.

Place, V. A., and J. P. Thomas: Clinical Pharmacology of Ethambutol, Am. Rev. Resp. Dis., 87:901, 1963.

Richards, W. A., E. Riss, E. H. Kass, and M. Finland: Nitrofurantoin: Clinical and Laboratory Studies in Urinary Tract Infection, A.M.A. Arch. Intern. Med., 96:437, 1955.

Robson, J. F., and F. M. Sullivan: Antituberculous Drugs, Pharamacol. Rev., 15:169, 1963.

Utz, J. P.: Chemotherapeutic Agents for the Systemic Mycoses, New Engl. J. Med., 268:928, 1963.

Weinstein, L.: The Chemoprophylaxis of Infection, Ann. Intern. Med., 43:287, 1955.

——: A Clinical Evaluation of the Therapeutic Application of Antibiotic Combinations, Conn. State Med. J., 24:87, 1960.

——: Sulfonamides, Antibiotics and Other Antimicrobial Agents, in L. S. Goodman and A. Gilman (Eds.), "The Pharmacological Basis of Therapeutics," New York, The Macmillan Company, 1965.

—— and A. C. Dalton: Host Determinants of Response to Antimicrobial Agents, New Engl. J. Med., 279:467, 524, 580, 1968.

—— and N. J. Ehrenkranz: "Streptomycin and Dihydrostreptomycin," New York, Medical Encyclopedia, Inc., 1958.

——, M. Goldfield, and T. W. Chang: Infections Occurring during Chemotherapy: A Study of Their Frequency, Type and Predisposing Factors, New Engl. J. Med., 251:247, 1954.

——, K. Kaplan, and T. W. Chang: Treatment of Infections in Man with Cephalothin, J.A.M.A., 189:829, 1964.

——, M. A. Madoff, and C. M. Samet: The Sulfonamides, New Engl. J. Med., 263:793, 842, 900, 952, 1960.

——, C. A Samet, and R. H. Meade, III: Effect of Paromycin on the Bacterial Flora of the Human Intestine, J.A.M.A., 178:891, 1961.

Wolinsky, E.: Modern Drug Treatment of Mycobacterial Diseases, Med. Clin. N. Am., 47:1271, 1963.

Woodward, T. E., and C. L. Wisseman, Jr.: "Chloromycetin (Chloramphenicol)," New York, Medical Encyclopedia, Inc., 1958.

Section 2

Infections of Specific Tissues and Anatomic Sites

INTRODUCTION

Ivan L. Bennett, Jr.

It is traditional and convenient to classify bacterial diseases in terms of etiologic agents. This is adequate for those that follow more or less consistent patterns as do typhoid, anthrax, brucellosis, tularemia, or tetanus, but there are other important disorders that lend themselves poorly to this categorization. Because many microbial agents are able to invade and to localize in almost any tissue, they are not regularly associated with a single symptom complex. Furthermore, infection of an anatomic site such as the urinary tract or the meninges by any one of a wide variety of unrelated bacterial species produces essentially the same symptoms and clinical signs. Recognition of the basic pathologic process by the clinician is, in most instances, independent of microbiologic techniques, although specific identification of infecting bacteria is the basis for choosing the appropriate antimicrobial drugs.

In this section, many clinical entities are described. Several are more likely to be caused by certain microorganisms than others, but all can be produced by many species. Most of them can be recognized in their typical forms by history, physical examination, and clinical tests of blood and urine. Final identification of the infecting agent may depend on time-consuming bacteriologic tests, but a knowledge of the likely pathogens often enables the physician to initiate appropriate therapy before this information is available. Surgical drainage is an essential part of proper management for several of the disorders; indeed, surgery may be an emergency procedure for many of them, necessitated not by the species of the infecting organisms but by the anatomic location of the infection.

For these reasons, it seems logical to describe these diseases in terms of their manifestations in the patient. Cross references to other sections of the book have been given where specific causative organisms are mentioned or where descriptions of related entities have been included under an organ system. Pyelonephritis and cystitis are described in Chap. 303, and suppurative disorders of the central nervous system are covered in Chap. 360.

136 LOCALIZED INFECTIONS AND ABSCESSES

Ivan L. Bennett, Jr., and
Robert G. Petersdorf

Localized pyogenic infection can develop in any region or organ of the body, and may be initiated by *trauma* and secondary bacterial contamination, by some *alteration in local conditions* that renders a tissue susceptible to organisms already present as part of the "normal flora" to which it is ordinarily immune, by *contiguous spread* from a nearby lesion, or by *metastatic implantation* of microorganisms carried in blood or lymph.

The definitive treatment of many circumscribed infections, particularly if abscess formation occurs, is primarily surgical. Most often, however, infections are complications of diseases that are ordinarily cared for by the internist, and their treatment calls for careful integration of medical and surgical measures. It is important, therefore, to recognize the major types of localized suppurative disease and know something of the principles of their management.

ETIOLOGY. Under appropriate conditions of lowered tissue resistance, almost any of the common bacteria can initiate an infectious process. Cultures from open lesions such as those of the skin or from intraabdominal foci arising from perforations of the gastrointestinal tract frequently contain several bacterial species; as might be expected, the organisms found most frequently are the "normal flora" of these regions.

Infection in some areas is more likely to be caused by certain organisms (e.g., staphylococci in the skin and coliform bacteria in the urinary tract), and special features of the tissue reaction produced by some bacterial species make it possible to recognize infection by them with considerable accuracy. The *staphylococci* produce rapid necrosis and early suppuration with large amounts of creamy yellow pus (Chap. 139). Group A beta-hemolytic streptococcal infections (Chap. 140) tend to spread rapidly through tissues, causing intense edema and erythema but relatively little necrosis and thin, serum-like exudates; anaerobic streptococci (Chap. 141) and members of the *Bacteroides* group (Chap. 147) produce necrosis and profuse, brownish, foul-smelling pus. *Pseudomonas* infections (Chap. 146) are often rather indolent, and their thick, bluish green exudate is familiar to most clinicians; the *pneumococcus* (Chap. 138) stimulates the production of viscid greenish pus containing large plaques of fibrin and denatured protein.

The causative agents of many other diseases are capable of producing localized infection in tissues that are not usually involved in the specific "clinical entities" ascribed to them. Examples include the typhoid bacillus, *Corynebacterium diphtheriae* (cutaneous ulcers), the *brucellas*, and *Pasteurella tularensis*.

The identification of infecting organisms is important in the choice of local or systemic chemotherapy. However, when infection occurs in an area where there is constant exposure to the microflora, as in sputum, paranasal sinusitis, and cutaneous ulcers, it is unlikely that the site will ever become *sterile*, and serial cultures during therapy must be interpreted in the light of this knowledge.

PATHOGENESIS. Factors predisposing to the initiation and persistence of infection in a tissue include trauma, obstruction of normal drainage (sweat glands, biliary tract, bronchial tree, urinary tract), ischemia (infarction, gangrene), chemical irritants (gastric contents, bile, intramuscularly injected drugs), hematoma formation, accumulation of fluid (lymphatic obstruction, cardiac edema), foreign bodies (bullets, splinters, sutures), and others such as the occurrence of turbulence in the vascular system.

Infection in soft tissue usually begins as a *cellulitis,* a diffuse acute inflammation with hyperemia, edema, and leukocytic infiltration but little or no necrosis and suppuration. With some organisms, this is followed by necrosis, liquefaction, accumulation of leukocytes and debris, suppuration, loculation and walling off of the pus, and formation of one or more *abscesses.* Abscess formation is particularly likely to follow infection in a preexisting space or cavity, examples being the fallopian tubes, lung cysts, and renal pelvis (*pyonephrosis*).

The local spread of infection generally follows the path of least resistance along fascial planes; proper surgical treatment is based upon a knowledge of these routes, which will be described for specific infections later in this chapter. Lymphatic spread may lead to lymphangitis, lymphadenitis, or, if the regional nodes suppurate, to the formation of a *bubo.* Involvement of local venules or large veins may lead to infective thrombophlebitis with resulting bacteremia, septic embolization, and systemic dissemination of infection. Staphylococci, streptococci, and bacteroides are notorious for the frequency with which they produce vascular lesions of this type.

Depending upon the infecting organism and the anatomy of the affected region, a small abscess may subside completely, there may be gradual encapsulation of the accumulated pus and persistence of the focus in a quiescent state, or the lesion may "point" and rupture into adjacent tissues or to the outside surface of the body, as usually happens with furuncles. Spontaneous drainage ordinarily leads to subsidence and healing of a superficially situated suppurative focus. However, if the abscess is deeply situated and well encapsulated, there are often persistence of a fistulous tract and the formation of a chronic, draining sinus. *The development of persistent sinuses over an area of suppuration produced by ordinary pyogenic bacteria should always suggest involvement of underlying bone or the presence of a foreign body.* Fistulas that open onto the skin are, of course, soon colonized by microorganisms from the external environment. Ordinary bacterial cultures of drainage fluid almost invariably show a mixed flora and should never be relied upon for the etiologic diagnosis of the underlying disease. This is particularly important in disorders that characteristically lead to persistent sinus formation: tuberculosis, mycotic infection (actinomycosis,

blastomycosis), melioidosis, glanders, tularemia, and, rarely, amebic abscess of the liver or cecum.

THERAPEUTIC CONSIDERATIONS. Recognition of the striking symptomatic improvement that follows spontaneous evacuation of a suppurative focus led long ago to the adoption of *surgical incision* for the treatment of abscesses. The exact reasons for the amelioration of local and constitutional manifestations that results from drainage of pus are unknown, but, clinically, the benefits of adequate incision and drainage are unequivocal.

Incision of infected tissue before the stage of liquefaction and accumulation of pus is often deleterious and fails to relieve discomfort. Premature incision may even at times facilitate spread of infection. For this reason, it is sometimes necessary to wait until an abscess "ripens," i.e., localizes and "comes to a head." The *application of heat* to an area of inflammation will relieve pain and often speed the subsidence of cellulitis without suppuration. If necrosis of tissue is already under way, hot applications appear to facilitate localization of the process and accumulation of pus, making incision and drainage feasible at an earlier time. Another procedure that aids in reduction of swelling and relief of pain is *elevation of the affected part.*

The availability of specific chemotherapeutic drugs has modified the need for heat, elevation, and incision surprisingly little. The early administration of chemotherapeutics has reduced the incidence of suppurative complications in many disorders, but once suppuration has appeared, antimicrobial drugs become remarkably incapable of eradicating the infecting organisms, although they may mask the classical clinical features of abscess formation.

Antibiotics can be demonstrated in vitro to retain their antibacterial activity in the presence of pus and necrotic tissue, and failure of the drug to penetrate into an area of suppuration is rarely the reason for therapeutic failure. Although this possibility exists in some infections, such as osteomyelitis, it is usually overcome by increasing dosage. Because direct instillation of the antibiotic into an infected area is not, by itself, a curative procedure, other factors are probably more important than faulty diffusion of the agent into the focus. Nevertheless, in some infection such as empyema or pyarthrosis, and with some agents which provide poor tissue levels, such as the polymyxins, direct instillation of an antimicrobial into an area of suppuration is distinctly worthwhile.

The experiments of Eagle and Wood have shown clearly that an established inflammatory exudate is a relatively poor environment for bacterial multiplication. Because the bactericidal action of penicillin is exerted only against multiplying organisms, it is believed that failure of this antibiotic to eradicate bacteria in an abscess is related to their inactive metabolic state. Bacteriostatic agents such as tetracycline or chloramphenicol also are incapable of eradicating bacteria in the static phase of growth. Furthermore, by definition, these drugs are capable only of inhibiting multiplication of bacteria and usually exert no direct lethal action; the death of organisms in any infection treated with bacteriostatic agents is dependent on other mechanisms. For most pyogenic bacteria, phagocytosis is one of the most important of these mechanisms (although there must be others that have not been studied so carefully), and it is known that in the absence of phagocytes or in circumstances which inhibit their activity, bacteriostatic drugs are relatively ineffective. In fluid-filled cavities, particularly in the metabolically unfavorable milieu of an abscess, phagocytosis is greatly reduced. Consequently, despite inhibition of bacterial multiplication, organisms can remain dormant and survive for long periods of time. It is probably a combination of these two circumstances, decreased multiplication of bacteria and decreased phagocytosis, that makes infection on the heart valves, in the kidney, or in the meninges so relatively resistant to antimicrobial therapy. Large doses of bactericidal drugs for long periods are needed to achieve cure.

Antimicrobial drugs may be expected to prevent suppuration if given early or to prevent spread of an existing abscess, but cannot be substituted for surgical drainage. Indeed, their use in the face of a lesion requiring evacuation of pus is one of the most common serious errors in treating infections.

In empyema, suppurative pericarditis, or pyarthrosis, excellent therapeutic results are sometimes achieved by aspiration of pus and instillation of antibiotics into the infected area. The success of this procedure, however, is fully as dependent on the adequacy of drainage as it is upon the instillation of the antibiotic, and if there is loculation or the exudate becomes too viscid to allow removal, surgical incision becomes mandatory.

In the presence of infective thrombophlebitis, surgical interruption of the veins by ligation or, in certain instances, by total excision of an infected segment is often indicated to prevent seeding of other organs by infected emboli.

MANIFESTATIONS. Secondary infection of wounds and cutaneous ulcers is usually recognizable by inspection. Infections of the skin and subcutaneous tissues almost invariably produce the classic manifestations, *redness, tenderness, heat,* and *swelling.* Reddish streaks extending proximally and associated with tender enlargement of regional lymph nodes indicate lymphangitis. Systemic symptoms may be absent or mild, or there may be fever, malaise, prostration, and leukocytosis.

Infection and suppuration in deeper tissues or in body cavities are often manifested by local pain and tenderness, but the task of locating and determining the exact nature of the lesion may be difficult. The palpation of a tender mass is helpful, but muscle spasm and intervening structures often interfere. Abdominal or pelvic examination under anesthesia is sometimes useful in these circumstances.

Auscultation may reveal a friction rub over an abdominal viscus, the pleura, or the pericardium. The rapid development of an effusion in the pericardium, pleura, abdomen, or a joint should suggest infection. Similarly,

fluid detected by transillumination of paranasal sinuses or inspection of the tympanic membrane may be the first sign of infection.

Depending on the location of an abscess, symptoms and signs referable to encroachment upon adjacent structures may dominate the picture. Respiratory obstruction may be the first sign of mediastinal abscess; dysphagia often first calls attention to peritonsillar or retropharyngeal abscesses; and tamponade is sometimes the initial clue to pericardial infection. Localizing signs of dysfunction are especially striking and important with brain and spinal cord abscesses, although brain abscesses may be clinically silent (Chap. 360).

Local pain and tenderness or signs of dysfunction are mild or equivocal in some patients, and fever, prostration, and weight loss dominate the picture. The fever may be low-grade but is often hectic, with repeated rigors and drenching night sweats. Fatigue and anemia are frequent, and weight loss may be so rapid as to result in emaciation within a few weeks. A patient with these symptoms and signs may have chronic subphrenic, perinephric, or other abscess in the complete absence of any detectable physical sign pointing to the location of a large accumulation of pus.

Fluctuation of a mass on palpation is a reliable sign that it contains fluid, perhaps pus, but failure to detect this sign when deeper structures are examined is no guarantee that suppuration is absent and should not be taken by itself to indicate that the mass is noninfectious in origin or that drainage is not required.

LABORATORY FINDINGS. Peripheral polymorphonuclear leukocytosis is frequent with abscesses, and unexplained elevation of the white blood cell count in any patient should lead to a search for localized suppuration. Depending on the severity and duration of infection, there may be a chronic normocytic, normochromic anemia. Mild albuminuria, occasionally noted in febrile patients, has no diagnostic import.

Pus or fluid obtained by needle aspiration or incision of a suspected lesion should *always* be stained and examined directly in addition to being cultured aerobically and anaerobically. Pus is a poor metabolic substrate, and bacteria may fail to grow in cultures from an abscess of long standing. In such instances, the findings on microscopic examination may be the only guide in choosing proper chemotherapy. Failure to gram-stain exudates is the single greatest deterrent to appropriate antimicrobial therapy; it is the responsibility of the internist as well as the surgeon to see that this procedure is performed.

Blood cultures are often positive in intravascular infections such as endocarditis (Chap. 137), and in pyogenic infections in which localized abscesses are metastatic, as in staphylococcal, streptococcal, and salmonella bacteremias. Moreover, manipulation, including surgical incision, of any localized infection may be followed by transient bacteremia.

X-ray examinations are of great help in detecting localized collections of pus, primarily because they show atypical collections of gas, displacement of organs, and tissue densities in abnormal locations. Angiography of visceral organs and scintiscans using radioactive materials are also helpful in localizing abscesses.

CLINICAL FEATURES OF INFECTIONS IN VARIOUS REGIONS

The pathogenesis, diagnosis, and treatment of several important infections in specific anatomic sites and organs are discussed in detail in other parts of this book. These include lung abscess (Chap. 291), mediastinitis (Chap. 293), bacterial endocarditis (Chap. 137), pericarditis (Chap. 272), infections of the brain and spinal cord (Chap. 360), osteomyelitis (Chap. 139), pyelonephritis (Chap. 303), appendicitis and appendiceal abscess (Chap. 319), pyelophlebitis and hepatic abscess (Chap. 330), pancreatic abscess (Chap. 334), and diverticulitis (Chap. 320).

The remainder of this chapter is devoted to some features of dermal infection, chronic ulcerations, and a number of other regional infections.

Skin and Subcutaneous Tissues

Impetigo is a superficial infection caused by hemolytic staphylococci and group A hemolytic streptococci. It is primarily a disease of children, common in warm weather, characterized by multiple erythematous lesions which vesiculate and are intensely pruritic. Local spread occurs through scratching and release of infected vesicle fluid. Serious complications are metastatic abscesses and hemorrhagic nephritis. Treatment consists of local and general cleansing of the skin, application of bacitracin-neomycin ointment, covering with a loose dressing to prevent further contamination, and appropriate systemic antibiotics.

Deeper infections of the skin are almost invariably staphylococcal in origin and are described in Chap. 139. Erysipelas, a characteristic dermal lesion produced by group A streptococci, is described in Chap. 140.

Lymphadenitis with or without suppuration may complicate any pyogenic skin lesion and is often striking with superficial streptococcal infections. Specific diseases characterized by suppurative regional lymphadenitis include lymphogranuloma venereum (Chap. 229), cat-scratch disease (Chap. 230), tularemia (Chap. 155), and bubonic plague (Chap. 156).

Infections of the Hand

These are almost invariably secondary to trauma and are very common. Because of the rapidity with which infection can spread through the complex fascial spaces of the hand, wrist, and forearm, with the production of irreparable functional damage, *any deep infection in this area should receive expert surgical attention immediately.* The importance of such care has in no way been lessened by the availability of antibiotics.

The ordinary *paronychia*, or "run-around," is a superficial infection of the epithelium lateral to a nail, usually a result of tearing a "hangnail" and most frequently caused by the staphylococcus. Hot applications will lead to subsidence of paronychial cellulitis, but often a superficial blister of pus appears or the infection burrows beneath the nail to form a painful *subungual abscess.* Incision and drainage with partial or complete removal of the nail are then necessary. Recurrence is common, especially in nail biters, and this seemingly trivial infection can cause painful disability. Chronic paronychial inflammation produced by various fungi occurs in diabetics, and a similar lesion is seen in psoriasis and some types of pemphigus.

What appears to be a small furuncle of the webs of the fingers sometimes produces a *collar-button abscess,* consisting of a superficial and a deep compartment connected by a narrow tract. Evacuation of the shallow pocket without emptying the deeper abscess can lead to puzzling persistence of infection. Sometimes a foreign-body granuloma forms in the skin of the digital webs. This is most common in barbers, in whom a hair is the core of the foreign-body granuloma, the "barber's interdigital pilonidal sinus."

Infection of the distal phalanx of a finger, usually acquired by pinprick, thorn prick, etc., may lead to the formation of a *felon* or *whitlow.* This is a suppurative infection in the tightly enclosed fibrous compartments of the finger pulp (the "anterior closed space") which can compromise the distal blood supply by compression of the digital arteries, with consequent necrosis of bone and the development of osteomyelitis. The manifestations are swelling, extreme pain, and tenderness of the palmar surface of the finger tip. The treatment is immediate incision, using a lateral approach and cutting all the fibrous septums that radiate from the periosteum to the subcutaneous fascia.

Suppurative tenosynovitis, usually a complication of a puncture wound, is an even more serious infection of the hand from the point of view of functional damage; early diagnosis and treatment are mandatory to prevent permanent disability from destruction of the tendon or its sheath. The three cardinal manifestations of tenosynovitis are (1) exquisite tenderness limited to the course of the sheath; (2) the fingers held in flexion; and (3) extension of the involved finger, producing excruciating pain, most marked at the base of the digit. *Immediate incision* of the sheath is indicated, not only to prevent damage to the tendon itself but to avoid proximal extension of the process into the major fascial spaces of the hand or forearm. Vigorous antibiotic treatment should accompany surgery. The definitive treatment of any serious infection of the hand is a matter for a skilled surgeon, but the early recognition of the need for surgery often falls to other physicians.

Human bites are very important hand infections, which, if neglected almost invariably produce a highly destructive, necrotizing lesion contaminated by a mixture of aerobic and anaerobic organisms. A deliberately inflicted bite on the hand or elsewere is usually recognized as dangerously contaminated, but wounds on the knuckles produced by striking an opponent's teeth with the fists may not be recognized as potentially dangerous. In general, bite wounds should be cleaned thoroughly and not sutured. Patients should be given prophylaxis for tetanus and antibiotics, preferably a penicillinase-resistant penicillin.

Chronic Cutaneous Ulcers

A partial list of the causes of chronic ulcers of the skin includes circulatory disturbances such as varicose veins and obliterative arterial disease, extensive injury from frost bite or burns, trophic changes accompanying many neurologic disorders, bedsores, or decubiti, systemic diseases such as sicklemia and myxedema, neoplasms, and various infections. No matter what the underlying disease, secondary infection is very likely to occur and to interfere with healing, complicate grafting or other restorative procedures, or produce extension of the process.

The management of secondary bacterial infection in skin ulcers associated with obliterative arterial disease, a common problem in diabetics, is especially important, because infection is frequently the factor that precipitates spreading gangrene and makes amputation necessary.

Studies of the microflora of chronic cutaneous ulcers have almost invariably shown bacteria of many species, including staphylococci, aerobic and anaerobic streptococci, coliform bacilli, and members of the *Proteus* and *Pseudomonas* groups. Depending on the patient's environment and on systemically or locally administered antimicrobial drugs, the predominating bacterial species show great variation when lesions are cultured serially. Particularly noteworthy is the replacement of sensitive organisms by resistant strains or species during the course of chemotherapy.

Treatment of chronic dermal ulcers should be directed toward the underlying disorder but should also include *local debridement* and *chemotherapy*. Debridement by surgical excision is often needed, but the local application of proteolytic enzymes such as Varidase, a mixture of streptokinase and streptodornase, or trypsin, so-called "chemical or medical debridement," is sometimes sufficient. Intensive systemic administration of antibiotics should be carried out only in conjunction with definitive surgical procedures or when infection can be controlled in no other way, but the prevention of infection by "prophylactic" administration of antimicrobial drugs is futile because it results in the development of a flora resistant to the drugs being used. The *local application of antibiotics* is sometimes highly effective, and it is in the management of chronic mixed infections of this type that several potent but toxic antibiotics have great value. An ointment or solution containing neomycin, bacitracin, and polymyxin exerts a bactericidal effect against a wide variety of organisms and will sometimes temporarily sterilize a chronic lesion. Other useful topical medications are Furacin and 3 percent acetic acid, which is especially helpful in pseudomonas infections.

Diphtheritic ulcer of the skin is discussed in Chap. 169.

Infections of the Head and Neck

Pustules of the nose and upper lip may be particularly dangerous because they are likely to extend intracranially through the angular vein to the cavernous sinus. These lesions should be treated conservatively, manipulation or incision should be avoided if possible, and systemic antibiotics should be used if local swelling or redness appears.

Suppurative parotitis, which is usually a complication of chronic debilitating disease or blockage of Stensen's duct by a calculus, is largely avoidable by maintenance of hydration and oral hygiene. Its onset is heralded by local pain and swelling; fever and chills are frequent. Frank pus can sometimes be expressed from the duct, and the gland itself is firm and tender, often with pitting edema of the overlying skin and facial palsy. Most cases of suppurative parotitis are caused by hemolytic *Staphylococcus aureus*. Treatment consists of removal of obstructing calculi, but its mainstay is antimicrobial therapy with a penicillinase-resistant penicillin, cephalothin or vancomycin. Incision and drainage of a septate gland such as the parotid has not been particularly effective. Despite chemotherapy and drainage, the mortality rate of suppurative parotitis is 30 to 50 percent, perhaps because this infection occurs in patients with debilitating disease.

The use of penicillin and other antibiotics has reduced the incidence of many formerly common suppurative complications of streptococcal pharyngitis. However, as a result of streptococcal sore throat, bacteroides infections of the pharynx, or introduction of infection by trauma to the floor of the mouth or the pharyngeal wall, abscesses of the deep cervical structures still occur. *Suppurative cervical adenitis*, once an all-too-common sequel to streptococcal pharyngitis in children, is now rare. *Peritonsillar abscess*, or *quinsy*, is manifested by fever, sore throat, unilateral pain radiating to the ear on swallowing, and enlargement of the tonsil with redness and swelling of the adjacent soft palate. Treatment with penicillin and irrigations of warm saline solution sometimes lead to subsidence of the process, but if digital palpation reveals fluctuation, surgical drainage with or without tonsillectomy is indicated.

The course of *deep cervical infections* is fully as dependent upon the anatomic arrangement of fascial planes as is that of infections of the hand. Infection in this area is serious and is attended by fever, prostration, and leukocytosis. A tender mass may be palpated, but *surgical evacuation of such an infection should not be delayed because of failure to detect fluctuation,* which is usually absent because of the dense fascial layers.

Infection of the *sublingual space,* so-called "Ludwig's angina," is characterized by brawny induration of the submaxillary region, edema of the floor of the mouth, and elevation of the tongue. There are severe pain, dysphagia, and, within hours, dyspnea from respiratory obstruction. The usual causative organism is the streptococcus. Mortality was formerly about 50 percent. *Treatment* consists of large doses of penicillin and careful observation. If there is significant progression of obstruction during the 4 to 6 hr after treatment is instituted, wide incision is indicated and tracheostomy may need to be performed.

The retropharyngeal space lies between the muscles anterior to the cervical vertebrae and the pharyngeal mucosa. *Retropharyngeal abscess,* formerly common in children, is manifested by dysphagia, progressive stridor, pain, and fever. The bulging mass is easily seen and can completely occlude the airway within hours. Incision and drainage are mandatory; spontaneous rupture may lead to death by aspiration. Tuberculous abscess, secondary to spinal disease, occasionally appears in the retropharyngeal space; it is painless, and relief of obstruction follows surgical incision. Suppuration in the submastoid space, *Bezold's abscess,* is usually secondary to otitis and produces nuchal rigidity, which may lead to a mistaken diagnosis of otogenous meningitis. Infection can extend down the carotid sheath to the mediastinum. A suppurative thrombophlebitis of the jugular vein usually accompanies this infection, and the vessel is easily felt as a tender cord. Bacteremia and systemic spread of infection are common, and the involved venous segment may need to be excised. Spontaneous rupture of the carotid artery with rapid death from exsanguination is a rare complication.

Splenic Abscess

Splenic abscess occurs by several mechanisms: (1) dissemination via the bloodstream during bacteremia; primary foci include the endocardium, lung (lung abscess or pneumonia), pleural cavity (empyema), skin and soft tissues, ear and nasopharyngeal structures, and pelvis (pelvic inflammatory disease and septic abortion); (2) infection in a spleen damaged by bland infarcts (sickle-cell disease, leukemia) or more rarely other diseases such as malaria, typhoid, hydatid or dermoid cysts, and ameboma and trauma (following subcapsular hematoma formation); (3) extension from a perforated or diseased stomach, colon, or tail of the pancreas, as in carcinoma; and (4) rarely, without apparent cause. Onset is sudden, with chills, fever, and left upper quadrant pain. There are tenderness and muscle spasm, and the skin and subcutaneous tissues overlying the spleen may be edematous. Involvement of the upper pole commonly leads to left pleuritic pain, radiating to the shoulder, with elevation of the diaphragm or left pleural effusion. Lower pole abscess gives signs of tender splenomegaly and peritoneal inflammation. Splenic friction rub is often audible. Disorders to be considered in differential diagnosis are subphrenic abscess, infection of the left lung, bland infarction of the spleen, pancreatic pseudocyst, pyelonephritis, and abscess secondary to perforation of the transverse colon. X-ray examinations are an important adjunct in the diagnosis. Abnormal radiographic findings include (1) soft-tissue mass in left upper quadrant; (2) extraintestinal gas, which may occur even in the absence of gas-forming bacteria; (3) downward displacement of the splenic flexure of the colon; (4) inferior dis-

placement of the left kidney, best visualized on an intravenous pyelogram; (5) displacement of the stomach bubble medially; (6) elevation of the left hemidiaphragm; and (7) left pleural effusion. Spleen scan is also of great value in localizing the mass.

Treatment consists of administering antibiotics and performing splenectomy. The splenic artery and vein should be ligated prior to splenectomy. Small or multiple abscesses during bacteremia may subside with antibiotics alone, and abscess in a very ill patient may require splenotomy and drainage, with more definitive surgery at a later time. Splenic abscess is particularly common in patients with sickle-cell disease, but splenic infarction in subacute bacterial endocarditis caused by *Streptococcus viridans* almost never suppurates. Infected splenic infarcts are a rare cause of continued bacteremia in the face of massive chemotherapy, and splenectomy may then be necessary to achieve the final eradication of the organism.

Subphrenic Abscess

Peritoneal infections show a striking tendency to localize the upper part of the abdomen between the transverse colon and the diaphragm. True subphrenic abscesses are located between the liver and diaphragm on the left or right; and many so-called subphrenic infections are, in fact, subhepatic. Most of these infections are related to perforations of a disease in the gastrointestinal or biliary tracts, and over half of them follow operations on the gallbladder, duodenum, or stomach. Subphrenic abscesses following perforated appendicitis occur rarely nowadays. Closed blunt trauma following laceration of the liver is an important cause, and a few abscesses occur without predisposing neighborhood infection. These may occur on the left and may be caused by *Salmonella.* The most common organisms are *Escherichia coli,* non-group A streptococci, and staphylococci; mixed infections are common. Most abscesses occur on the right and are more common in males and elderly patients, who often have a debilitating disease such as cancer. *Any patient with persistent fever and a history of recent intraabdominal sepsis should be suspected of having a subphrenic abscess.*

The *manifestations* include fever, upper quadrant pain, and tenderness, usually along the costal margin. Shoulder pain, dyspnea, dullness, and rales at the lung base are more common than abdominal signs and symptoms, and emphasize the location of a true abscess between the liver and the diaphragm. Foul sputum connotes perforation of the abscess into the lung. The localizing signs are by no means striking in all cases, however. The widespread practice of "covering" postoperative patients with antibiotics prophylactically can attenuate subphrenic infection without eradicating it, and may result in an insidiously progressive illness with weight loss and low-grade fever beginning weeks or months after a laparotomy. Roentgenograms may show gas, sometimes with an air-fluid level beneath the diaphragm. The gas is usually from a perforated viscus or enters through an external sinus; it is only rarely the result of bacterial multiplication.

Other radiographic findings include pleural effusion, which is usually sterile, basilar infiltrates, and elevation —but not necessarily fixation— of the diaphragm. Combined lung-liver scintiscan is a considerable advance in the diagnosis of subphrenic abscess. Pneumoperitoneum may be helpful occasionally.

The outlook in subphrenic abscess is poor because so many patients have cancer as an underlying cause. Even with surgical drainage, the mortality rate approaches 40 percent; without it, nearly 80 percent of patients die. Drainage should be extraperitoneal, usually through the bed of the twelfth rib. Appropriate antibiotics should be given, both locally and systemically.

Retroperitoneal Infections

Strictly speaking, all perinephric and many subphrenic abscesses are located outside the peritoneum, but the term *retroperitoneal abscess* usually refers to infection in the lumbar and iliac regions. Suppuration in these areas is relatively rare, but the importance of recognizing its existence in patients with fever and low-back pain is great. In one series, the average duration of illness in 65 patients before diagnosis was approximately 1 month.

Infection in the retroperitoneal space may arise as a complication of staphylococcal bacteremia, but more often it reflects extension from posterior perforations of the appendix or colon, renal or spinal infections, and suppurative lymphadenitis in the iliac area, usually secondary to streptococcal infections of the lower extremities in children.

In *lumbar abscess*, there are tenderness and spasm of the back muscles on the affected side, and a mass is usually palpable in the lumbar region, or there may be a prominent, tender abdominal mass without lumbar pain or spasm. Flexion of the hip (psoas sign) occurs in a few cases but is more often present with infections lower in the retroperitoneal area. *Fever, leukocytosis,* and *lumbar spasm* should suggest the diagnosis. The absence of a palpable mass may lead to protracted observation, and it is in these instances that palpation under anesthesia is often helpful.

In *iliac abscess*, there is abdominal pain in the iliac or inguinal region and, particularly when the psoas muscle is involved, severe pain may be referred to the hip, thigh, or knee. Careful palpation of the lower part of the abdomen usually reveals a mass, and fullness and tenderness on rectal examination are common. Hip spasm (psoas sign) is often present.

Roentgenograms may delineate the inflammatory mass; pyelography shows displacement of the kidney or ureter in some cases, and scoliosis with concavity on the side of the infection and blurring of the psoas shadow are also useful findings.

Treatment consists of surgical drainage and appropriate antibiotic therapy.

Renal Abscess

Single or multiple abscesses of the renal *cortex* are almost invariably the result of metastatic implantation of staphylococci from another focus. There is no relationship to previous renal disease; the infection occurs in younger individuals, is usually unilateral, and occurs on the right side oftener than on the left. Many patients give a history of recent skin infection such as furuncle. Although acute pyelonephritis is a diffuse disease with foci of cellular infiltrates in the interstitium of the renal medulla, these inflammatory foci may coalesce to form a distinct abscess cavity. This situation probably ensues more frequently than is generally appreciated.

The onset of renal abscess is abrupt, with chill and fever, followed by costovertebral pain and tenderness. If the abscess is cortical, the urine contains *no white blood cells;* medullary abscesses are usually accompanied by pyuria. The stained urinary sediment will show myriads of gram-positive cocci in cortical abscesses, and gram-negative organisms in medullary abscesses. Transient gross or microscopic hematuria may occur at the onset. The white blood cell count is usually elevated and may exceed 30,000 cells per cu mm. Physical signs are usually localized to the region of the kidney, but abdominal spasm may lead to confusion with appendicitis, cholecystitis, or pancreatitis. Early in the disease, ureteral calculus or acute hydronephrosis may be considered as possible diagnoses. Sudden onset of *fever, leukocytosis, and renal pain in the absence of pyuria* should suggest the diagnosis of kidney abscess, especially in a patient with infection elsewhere. Obstruction of the ureter by pus or cellular debris may also yield a urine sediment sparse in white blood cells and bacteria. *Treatment* consists of appropriate antibiotics, adequate fluids, and relief of pain. An abscess may suddenly discharge into the renal pelvis, with relief of pain and the passage of cloudy urine containing enormous numbers of leukocytes and bacteria. *Complications* include formation of a thick-walled chronic renal "carbuncle," requiring surgical removal, rupture into the perirenal space, and secondary pyelonephritis, usually produced by coliform bacilli. Recovery is ordinarily prompt, and chronic sequelae are rare.

In the past, *perinephric abscess* was most often due to hematogenous dissemination during streptococcal or staphylococcal infection, but at present it more often follows calculi in the ureter and hydronephroses, noncalculous renal infection, tuberculosis, and actinomycosis. Diabetics are particularly susceptible. The causative organisms are those which are primarily responsible in acute pyelonephritis—*E. coli, Proteus* species, and *Klebsiella aerogenes.* Flank pain with radiation to the upper part of the abdomen, back, or even the shoulder, nausea, vomiting, fever, malaise, leukocytosis, tenderness with spasm of flank and upper abdominal muscles, and a palpable mass which moves with respiration are the main manifestations. Symptoms referable to the urinary tract are present when perinephric abscess is associated with pyelonephritis or stone. In a few patients, elevation of the diaphragm on the diseased side occurs and leads to confusion with subphrenic infection. The psoas muscle is involved by the inflammatory process, and patients are frequently more comfortable with the thigh held in flexion. The roentgenogram occasionally will reveal a mass; there is usually blurring of the kidney silhouette; and the psoas shadow is indistinct on the involved side. There may also be scoliosis to the side of the lesion, fixation of the kidney, anterior displacement of the organ on lateral pyelograms, and gas formation within the perinephric mass, or total nonvisualization of the kidney. Chest roentgenograms often show basal infiltrates and pleural effusions. Complications include perforation into adjacent organs, particularly the colon. *Treatment* by surgical drainage and systemic administration of antibiotics (*not* urinary antiseptics) is usually followed by dramatic subsidence of pain and fever, and unless intrinsic renal disease is present, recovery is complete. Nevertheless, the overall outcome is poor, in part because the diagnosis is often made too late or is missed altogether, and also because of the generally poor condition of many of these patients.

Rectal Abscess

Suppurations of the anorectal region have been classified anatomically in several ways, most of the classifications being based on the surgical approaches required for drainage. Infection in the apocrine glands (hidradenitis) or folliculitis in the perianal region, extension of cryptitis or obstructions in the "anal glands" which open into the crypts of Morgagni, and contamination of submucosal hematomas, sclerosed hemorrhoids, or anal fissures may lead to abscess formation. These are usually painful, easily palpable, often visible on inspection. Superficial rectal abscesses also may be confused with Bartholin's cysts, sebaceous cysts, tuberculosis, actinomycosis, urethroperineal fistulas, carcinoma of the anus, foreign body, and pilonidal sinus. Treatment is application of heat and appropriate drainage or excision. Antibiotics may be indicated in some instances.

Difficulties in diagnosis are more likely to arise with infections higher in the rectum, especially those above the pelvic diaphragm, the so-called *supralevator abscess*. Patients with this type of infection often have fever, malaise, and leukocytosis for several days or even weeks before any symptoms referable to the rectum develop. There is vague pelvic discomfort, relieved by defecation, and constipation punctuated by short episodes of diarrhea is common. In males, the inflammation often involves the base of the bladder, and urinary urgency or retention is not infrequent, falsely centering attention on the urinary tract as the source of fever and malaise. Eventually, the abscess produces severe pain, chills, and fever; palpation and instrumentation will reveal the swelling in the rectal ampulla. Such an abscess may surround the rectum and produce narrowing that is differentiated from that caused by neoplasm by the fact that the mucosa remains intact. A useful sign of deep rectal abscess is eliciting of severe pain by pressure in the region between the anus and the coccyx. The supralevator space is continuous with the ischiorectal space, with both the gluteal and obturator regions, and with the retroperitoneal space. In neglected cases, the abscess may drain through the skin of the perineum, the groin, or the buttock or may extend as high as the perirenal areas. Rectal abscesses are not uncommon in patients with diabetes, and infections in this area are also peculiarly frequent in patients with monocytic leukemia. Because the clinical picture may be that of "fever of unknown origin" for a long period, it is important that thorough digital and endoscopic examination of the rectum be carried out in febrile patients. A rectal examination should be made in all patients with diabetes, especially if ketosis is present; failure to observe this rule has more than once led to delay in detecting the infection responsible for diabetic ketosis or coma.

Rectal abscesses may be a forerunner of both ulcerative colitis and regional enteritis, and may occur months and even years before other overt manifestations of these diseases. For this reason, proctosigmoidoscopy, barium enema, and, often upper gastrointestinal roentgenograms, are indicated in nonhealing rectal lesions.

Treatment of high rectal abscesses consists of incision and drainage, hot sitz baths, analgesics, and antibiotics as indicated by culture of the exudate.

REFERENCES

General

Bunnell, S.: "Surgery of the Hand," 4th ed., T. H. Boyes (Ed.), Philadelphia, J. B. Lippincott Company, 1964.

Eagle, H.: Experimental Approach to the Problem of Treatment Failure with Penicillin: I. Group A Streptococcal Infection in Mice, Am. J. Med., 13:389, 1952.

Plorde, J. J., D. Hovland, M. Garcia, and R. G. Petersdorf: Studies on the Pathogenesis of Meningitis: V. Action of Penicillin in Experimental Pneumococcal Meningitis, J. Lab. Clin. Med., 65:71, 1965.

Smith, M. R., and W. B. Wood, Jr.: An Experimental Analysis of the Curative Action of Penicillin in Acute Bacterial Infections: III. The Effect of Suppuration upon the Antibacterial Action of the Drug, J. Exp. Med., 103:509, 1956.

Specific Infections

Barnhill, J. F.: Deep Abscess of the Neck: Surgical Treatment, Am. J. Surg., 42:207, 1938.

Burger, R. H., J. N. Ward, and J. W. Draper: Perinephric Abscess with Gas Formation, Am. Surgeon, 30:302, 1964.

Curreri, W. P., J. A. Coller, and H. MacVaugh, III: Subphrenic Abscess Secondary to Salmonellosis, Arch. Surg., 95:189, 1967.

Eisenhammer, S.: The Internal Anal Sphincter and the Anorectal Abscess, Surg. Gynecol. Obstet., 103:501, 1956.

Frankel, A., H. Ashikari, D. A. Dreiling, and A. E. Kark: Splenic Abscess, J. Mt. Sinai Hosp., 33:404, 1966.

Gaston, E. A., and L. O. Warren: Supralevator Abscess, New Engl. J. Med., 229:613, 1943.

Janke, W. H., and M. A. Block: Chronic Retroperitoneal Pelvic Abscesses, Arch. Surg., 90:389, 1965.

Magilligan, D. J., Jr.: Suprahepatic Abscess, Arch. Surg., 96:14, 1968.

Neuhof, H., and E. E. Arnheim: Acute Retroperitoneal Abscess and Phlegmon: A Study of Sixty-five Cases, Ann. Surg., 119:741, 1944.

Ozeran, R. S.: Subdiaphragmatic Abscess, Am. Surgeon, 33:64, 1967.

Petersdorf, R. G., B. A. Forsythe, and A. D. Bernanke: Staphylococcal Parotitis, New Engl. J. Med., 259:1259, 1958.

Richards, L.: Retropharyngeal Abscess, New Engl. J. Med., 215:1120, 1936.

Salvatierra, O., Jr., W. B. Bucklew, and J. W. Morrow: Perinephric Abscess, J. Urol., 98:296, 1967.

Vicher, E. E., J. W. Soska, and G. G. Jackson: Microbiologic Flora of Chronic Cutaneous Ulcers: *In Vitro* Sensitivity of Microbiologic Flora to Three Antibiotics—Penicillin, Streptomycin, and Bacitracin, A.M.A. Arch. Surg., 66:283, 1953.

137   BACTERIAL ENDOCARDITIS

Leighton E. Cluff and F. Robert Fekety

DEFINITION. Bacterial endocarditis is a microbial infection of the heart valves or of the endocardium in proximity to congenital or acquired cardiac defects. A similar clinical illness develops when there is infection of arteriovenous fistulas or aneurysms. The infection may develop abruptly or insidiously, may pursue a fulminant or prolonged course, and is fatal unless treated. The infection caused by indigenous microorganisms with low pathogenicity is ordinarily subacute, whereas infection by microorganisms with high pathogenicity is often acute. Fever, cardiac murmurs, splenomegaly, anemia, hematuria, mucocutaneous petechiae, and embolic manifestations are characteristic of the disease. *Streptococcus viridans* is the commonest cause of bacterial endocarditis when superimposed upon congenital or acquired endocardial lesions and usually is associated with a subacute course.

ETIOLOGY AND EPIDEMIOLOGY. *Acute bacterial endocarditis* is caused by relatively pathogenic microorganisms, exemplified by *Staphylococcus aureus,* pneumococcus, group A streptococcus, gonococcus, and less often *Histoplasma capsulatum, Brucella,* and *Listeria.* Endocarditis attributed to these organisms usually follows dissemination from an infected focus, which is often insignificant. Gonococcal, staphylococcal, and monilial endocarditis has been described frequently in narcotic addicts. Staphylococcal, monilial, and coliform bacilli infection of the heart resembling endocarditis has become a serious complication of surgery in which sutures or prostheses are placed in the heart or peripheral arteries. Endocarditis is sometimes observed in association with pneumococcal meningitis and bacteremia (Chap. 138). Staphylococcal endocarditis can result from bacteremia associated with septic thrombophlebitis or complicating a cutaneous, bone, or pulmonary infection. Group A streptococcal endocarditis is probably never a complication of septic sore throat, but it may follow the bacteremia of streptococcal skin or puerperal infection.

Subacute bacterial endocarditis develops usually in persons with acquired valvular or congenital cardiac lesions. It is most commonly caused by *S. viridans,* which is part of the normal upper respiratory bacterial flora. *Streptococcus faecalis* (enterococcus), indigenous to the fecal and perineal flora, is also an important cause of subacute bacterial endocarditis, particularly in elderly men, and often occurs in association with prostatism or other genitourinary conditions. *Staphylococcus aureus* may produce subacute as well as acute bacterial endocarditis. Suppuration, cellulitis, or other infected foci may precede subacute bacterial endocarditis but are recognized infrequently. *Streptococcus viridans* is commonly found in the blood immediately after dental extractions. Tonsillectomy is also occasionally associated with transient bacteremia. Chewing of food may result in bacteremia in patients with gingival disease or dental infection. Transient bacteremia of this sort is probably an important initiating factor in subacute bacterial endocarditis.

PATHOGENESIS. Subacute bacterial endocarditis occurs most frequently in persons with preexisting heart disease in the absence of congestive cardiac failure or chronic atrial fibrillation. Valvular stenosis without insufficiency is infrequently associated with bacterial endocarditis. Infection most commonly involves the left side of the heart. The mitral valve, aortic valve, pulmonary valve, and tricuspid valve may be involved, in the order of frequency as listed. Valves damaged by rheumatic fever are most commonly involved, but valves damaged by syphilis and arteriosclerosis are also susceptible to bacterial endocarditis. Enterococcal endocarditis in elderly men is associated with involvement of the aortic valve, and frequently results rapidly in marked valvular damage. Subacute bacterial endocarditis rarely involves interatrial septal defects. Infection in patients with interventricular septal defects often involves the endocardium opposite the septal defect in the direction of the shunt. Infection associated with patent ductus arteriosus develops in the pulmonary side of the ductus when the shunt is from the aorta to the pulmonary artery, but is on the aortic side of the ductus when the shunt is reversed. Valvular infection in association with rheumatic heart disease is usually on the valve edge along the line of closure.

Hemodynamic events are important in the pathogenesis of the disease. Alterations in blood flow can cause marked changes in vascular endothelium. It has been demonstrated experimentally that bacteria are deposited on the endothelium in areas of high flow with decreased lateral pressure. These factors are undoubtedly important in determining the situations and location where bacterial endocarditis develops. Infection in the heart is most often at a site of a structural change or abnormality. Thrombi developing on endocardial irregularities have been implicated as foci for bacterial implantation, and infection has been shown in thrombotic endocardial lesions. It seems unlikely, however, that endocardial thrombi are commonly involved in the pathogenesis of bacterial endocarditis, except as a feature of the infection.

Serum antibody in high titer against the infecting microorganism is often found in patients with bacterial endocarditis. Pneumococci found in the blood during pneumococcal endocarditis usually show pronounced capsular swelling attributable to serum antibody and intravenous injection of pneumococci into hyperimmunized horses can result in bacterial endocarditis. Immunity to the bacteria may facilitate localization of infection in the endocardium, but whether this mechanism plays a role in bacterial endocarditis of man is not known.

Bacterial endocarditis leads to deposition of fibrin and platelets at the site of infection, producing a *vegetation*. Highly pathogenic microorganisms often cause valvular destruction and ulceration. Less pathogenic microorganisms usually cause less valvular destruction or ulceration but can lead to development of large polypoid vegetations. The infection may extend from the valve to the mural endocardium. Involvement of chordae tendineae may lead to rupture and profound valvular insufficiency. Acute bacterial endocarditis, particularly when caused by S. aureus, often is associated with abscesses in the valve ring. Vascularization of involved valves may increase during endocarditis but rarely extends into the area of infection. Phagocytes are not prominent in the area of bacterial growth, which may explain why infection by microorganisms of low pathogenicity progresses uncontrolled without bactericidal antimicrobial therapy. The lack of vascularization of the granulation tissue in the vegetation also may account for ineffectiveness of host defenses and the requirement for intensive and prolonged treatment of the infection.

The bacteremia of bacterial endocarditis is ordinarily continuous. For this reason very few blood cultures are required to demonstrate the microorganisms. The microorganisms are primarily cleared from the blood by the reticuloendothelial cells of liver and spleen. There is no obvious reduction in the number of bacteria in the blood during circulation through the extremities. Arterial blood cultures, therefore, are no more likely to show bacteremia than are venous blood cultures.

Embolization is a characteristic feature of bacterial endocarditis. The friable fibrin vegetations may separate

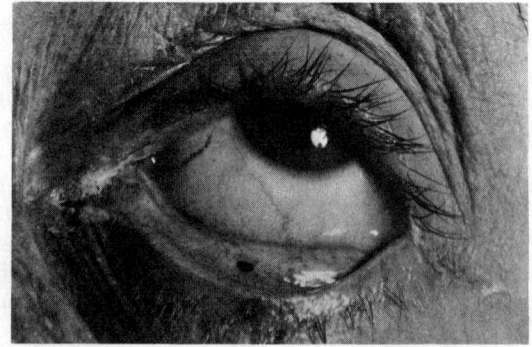

Fig. 137-1. White-centered conjunctival petechia in a patient with subacute bacterial endocarditis. (*Courtesy Dr. John Wedgwood, Cambridge, England.*)

from the site of infection and be propelled as emboli into the systemic or pulmonary circulation, depending on whether the endocarditis involves the left or right side of the heart. Emboli vary in size but may involve the brain, spleen, kidney, gastrointestinal tract, or extremities. Pulmonary infarction is common in right-sided endocarditis. Septic infarction is uncommon in subacute bacterial endocarditis caused by microorganisms of low pathogenicity, and suppurative complications are rarely seen at these sites when S. viridans is the offending agent. Osteomyelitis has been described, however, as an embolic complication of endocarditis due to S. viridans and enterococci. Septic infarction is common in acute bacterial endocarditis attributable to bacteria of high pathogenicity as are metastatic abscesses. Involvement of vasa vasorum in major arteries by emboli produces mycotic aneurysms, which may rupture. Myocardial infarction may develop after coronary embolization. In addition, focal myocarditis is common in subacute bacterial endocarditis and may be embolic.

The spleen is almost always enlarged, particularly in subacute cases. Three types of renal lesions may be produced. When large emboli find their way into the kidney, infarction may develop. Smaller emboli may produce a focal glomerulitis. In some instances there is a diffuse glomerulonephritis that is difficult to distinguish from that seen after streptococcal infection. Petechial skin lesions, characterized histologically by acute vasculitis, are probably not embolic and may be immunologic in origin. Other skin lesions associated with pain, tenderness, and cellulitis, however, may be embolic.

MANIFESTATIONS. Subacute Bacterial Endocarditis. Patients ordinarily cannot date the onset of the infection. Symptoms begin insidiously, and gradually the illness becomes apparent. In some individuals, however, the onset of infection can be related to a recent dental extraction, urethral instrumentation, tonsillectomy, acute respiratory infection, or abortion.

Weakness, fatigability, weight loss, feverishness, night sweats, anorexia, and arthralgia are the usual symptoms of subacute bacterial endocarditis. Emboli may produce paralysis, chest pain, acute vascular insufficiency with pain in the extremities, hematuria, acute abdominal pain, or sudden blindness. Painful fingers or toes and painful skin lesions may also be important symptoms. Chills are not common.

Physical examination may reveal a variety of findings, none of which alone is pathognomonic of subacute bacterial endocarditis. The association of the different manifestations, however, usually provides a characteristic picture of the disease. The patient usually appears chronically ill and pale and has an elevated temperature. The fever is most often remittent, with afternoon or evening peaks. The pulse is usually rapid, and if cardiac failure complicates the infection, it may be greater than expected with the degree of fever.

Mucocutaneous lesions are common and vary in type. Petechiae are most frequent and may be found in the mucosa of the mouth, pharynx, or conjunctivas. These small red hemorrhagic-appearing lesions do not blanch on pressure and are not tender or painful. On the mucous membranes or conjunctivas these petechiae may have a pale center (Fig. 137-1). Small, occasionally flame-shaped, hemorrhages are found in the retina, and may also have pale centers (*Roth's spots*). Petechiae may be found anywhere on the skin and are frequently difficult to distinguish from angiomas, but they gradually become brownish and disappear. Frequently, petechiae continue to appear, even during convalescence. Linear hemorrhages (splinter hemorrhages) may be found under the nails, but these are difficult to differentiate from traumatic lesions, particularly in manual laborers. These mucocutaneous lesions are not specific for bacterial endocarditis but may be found in patients with other diseases such as profound anemia, leukemia, trichinosis, and sepsis without endocarditis.

The pulp of the fingers may show tender subcutaneous papules which are purplish or erythematous (*Osler's nodes*). Larger erythematous, painful, and tender nodules may develop on the palms of the hands or soles of the feet. These are probably embolic lesions. Emboli to larger peripheral arteries may result in gangrene of fingers, toes, or larger portions of the extremities.

Clubbing of the fingers is uncommon but is observed in long-standing or prolonged bacterial endocarditis. Mild jaundice is found occasionally.

Findings in the heart are usually those of the underlying heart disease. Major changes in cardiac murmurs may be attributable to ulceration of a valve, dilatation of the heart or valve ring, rupture of chordae tendineae, or development of a very large vegetation. In rare instances, no cardiac murmurs are detected. In this situation, right-sided endocarditis or an infected pulmonary or peripheral arteriovenous fistula should be suspected.

Splenomegaly is common in subacute bacterial endocarditis. Rarely is the spleen tender, but a friction rub may be heard over it when there is infarction. Hepatomegaly is not characteristic unless heart failure develops.

Arthralgia is relatively common, and arthritis resembling acute rheumatic fever may occur.

Embolic phenomena may precipitate awareness of the infection. Sudden development of hemiplegia, flank pain with hematuria, abdominal pain with melena, pleuritic pain and hemoptysis, left upper abdominal pain with splenic friction rub, blindness, or monoplegia in a patient with fever and cardiac murmurs makes bacterial endocarditis suspect. Pulmonary emboli in right-sided endocarditis may be confused with pneumonia.

Acute Bacterial Endocarditis. Infectious endocarditis caused by highly pathogenic microorganisms usually begins abruptly. Suppurative infection commonly antedates the onset of endocarditis. For example, infection of the heart may develop as a complication of pneumococcal meningitis, septic thrombophlebitis, group A streptococcal cellulitis, or staphylococcal abscesses. The source of cardiovascular infection, therefore, is often evident.

Acute bacterial endocarditis often involves the normal heart, in contrast to the subacute infection, which almost invariably involves the abnormal heart. The acute infection is fulminant and pursues a rapid course. Fever is often greater, may be intermittent, and in certain instances (as in gonococcal endocarditis) may be characterized by a double quotidian temperature curve. Chills are common. Petechiae may be numerous, and embolic phenomena are prominent. Osler's nodes and painful erythematous nodules of palms and soles are uncommon. Hematuria is seen with embolic lesions of the kidney, but diffuse glomerulonephritis is less common than in subacute bacterial endocarditis. Destruction of the cardiac valves can be complicated by rupture of chordae tendineae or perforation of cusps, leading to rapidly progressing cardiac failure. Metastatic abscesses are frequent following septic emboli.

Because of the abrupt onset of acute bacterial endocarditis, anemia and weight loss are absent when the illness is first recognized. These changes, however, develop rapidly.

LABORATORY FINDINGS. Leukocytosis with neutrophilia is the rule but is by no means an invariable finding. Macrophages (histiocytes) may be found in the blood, particularly in the first drop of blood obtained from the earlobe. Normocytic, normochromic anemia is almost always found in subacute bacterial endocarditis, but it may not be present early in acute bacterial endocarditis. The erythrocyte sedimentation rate is increased, and the C-reactive protein test is markedly positive. Serum immunoglobulins are increased but return to normal during convalescence. The anti-gamma-globulin latex fixation test is commonly positive, and the Rose-Waaler test is negative. The thymol turbidity and cephalin flocculation tests are usually abnormal, and mild bilirubinemia is detected occasionally. Proteinuria is common, and microscopic hematuria is frequent.

Blood cultures are positive in the majority (85 percent) of cases. Three to five cultures of 10 ml blood taken at short or long intervals, depending on the patient's clinical status, are usually adequate to demonstrate the bacteremia, if it is demonstrable at all. Blood cultures may not become positive for seven or more days, however, in patients who have been receiving penicillin prophylactically for rheumatic heart disease. Similarly, the cultures may be temporarily negative or growth may be delayed in patients who have received antibiotics prior to the time when cultures are obtained. Failure to demonstrate bacteremia also may be attributable to infection by an unusual microorganism such as *H. capsulatum, Brucella,* or anaerobic streptococci which require special nutrient media or culture methods. Endocarditis of the right side of the heart seems to be as likely to produce bacteremia as endocarditis involving the left side of the heart.

DIFFERENTIAL DIAGNOSIS. When several of the manifestations of bacterial endocarditis occur together, the diagnosis is not difficult. In particular, the presence of fever, petechiae, splenomegaly, microscopic hematuria, and anemia in a patient with cardiac murmurs is most suggestive of the cardiovascular infection. When few manifestations are present, however, the diagnosis is not simple. Prolonged fever in the patient with rheumatic heart disease is particularly troublesome, but the diagnosis of bacterial endocarditis should be considered in every patient with fever and a heart murmur. The diagnosis becomes even more difficult when blood cultures show no growth.

Acute rheumatic fever with carditis is often difficult to distinguish from bacterial endocarditis, and in a few instances, active rheumatic fever has been found to coexist with the valvular infection. The diagnosis of rheumatic carditis hinges on a combination of clinical and laboratory criteria (Chap. 269).

Subacute bacterial endocarditis is a common cause of "fever of undetermined origin" (Chap. 16). It may be mistaken for a hidden neoplasm, systemic lupus erythematosus, periarteritis nodosa, poststreptococcal glomerulonephiritis, and intracardiac tumors such as myxoma of the atrium. Dissecting aneurysms with acute aortic insufficiency also may mimic bacterial endocarditis. Drug fever may be erroneously diagnosed as bacterial endocarditis.

Development of fever, anemia, and leukocytosis after cardiovascular surgery may indicate development of intracardiac infection about a suture or prosthesis. This infection is identical to that of bacterial endocarditis but usually cannot be controlled unless the foreign body is removed. In these postoperative patients, the various postthoracotomy and postcardiotomy syndromes must also be considered.

PROGNOSIS. Recovery from untreated bacterial endocarditis is rare. With appropriate antibiotic therapy, however, over 70 percent of patients survive the infection. The infection has a poor prognosis when complicated by congestive heart failure, when unassociated with demonstrable bacteremia, when produced by antibiotic-resistant microorganisms, or when therapy is delayed. Acute bacterial endocarditis is associated with the poorest prognosis.

The commonest cause of death in treated endocarditis is congestive heart failure, attributable either to valve destruction or myocardial damage. Additionally, death may be precipitated by embolization to vital organs, by renal insufficiency, or by rupture of a mycotic aneurysm. Many patients recover completely without apparent worsening of the underlying cardiovascular disease. When recurrent endocarditis develops, it usually involves the same valve and is due to failure to kill microorganisms in an environment of suboptimal host resistance.

PROPHYLAXIS. Patients with congenital, syphilitic, arteriosclerotic, and rheumatic valvular heart disease should be given antibiotics before and immediately after dental manipulation, urethral catheterization, or other forms of intubation. Procaine pencillin G, in a dosage of 600,000 units 1 hr before dental manipulation and 12 and 24 hr later, is preferred, although erythromycin, tetracycline, and other antibiotics may be used to prevent infection by S. viridans. Penicillin in the same dosage plus streptomycin (1.0 Gm), or ampicillin, might be used similarly before and after urethral or pelvic manipulation so as to prevent infection by S. faecalis. *The prophylactic doses of penicillin used to prevent group A streptococcal infection and recurrent rheumatic fever will not prevent*

bacterial endocarditis. Furthermore, these doses of penicillin (200,000 units once or twice daily) do not predispose to bacterial endocarditis caused by penicillin-resistant microorganisms.

TREATMENT. Successful therapy of bacterial endocarditis is assured when treatment is begun early in the illness, when an effective *bactericidal* antimicrobial is selected, and when treatment is continued over a long period of time.

Selection of the most effective antibiotic for treatment of bacterial endocarditis depends on the sensitivity of the infecting microorganism. When bacteremia is not demonstrated, selection of the therapeutic agent depends on understanding the probable infecting bacteria and their probable antibiotic sensitivity.

Administration of penicillin G in dosage of 12 to 20 million units per day plus streptomycin 1.0 Gm daily is the treatment of choice in most instances, and should be continued for at least 4 weeks.

Bacterial endocarditis in young persons with rheumatic or congenital heart disease is most often due to S. *viridans.* These microorganisms are usually very sensitive to penicillin G. Administration of 2.4 to 6 million units of penicillin daily to these patients is usually effective in eliminating the infection when therapy is continued for 4 weeks. The penicillin should be given parenterally, either intramuscularly or intravenously. There is a synergistic effect of streptomycin with penicillin on S. *viridans,* and it has been suggested that streptomycin in a dose of 0.5 Gm twice a day should be administered in addition to penicillin. The superiority of this regimen over penicillin alone, however, has not been demonstrated. When patients with S. *viridans* endocarditis respond promptly, some authorities recommend that parenteral therapy be discontinued after 2 weeks; an additional 2-week course of an oral acid-resistant penicillin (phenethicillin, or V-cillin) may be given with safety.

Bacterial endocarditis in older men and in women after abortion or endometritis is often due to S. *faecalis* (enterococci). These microorganisms are either resistant to penicillin alone or acquire resistance during penicillin treatment. The combination of penicillin with streptomycin is synergistic against these bacteria, however, and administration of these two antibiotics together is the treatment of choice in the infection. Penicillin G should be given parenterally in a dose of 6 to 20 million units a day, together with streptomycin in a dose of 0.5 to 1.0 Gm twice a day. Ampicillin in dosage of 6 to 12 Gm a day may be substituted for penicillin G. Treatment must be continued for a minimum of 4 weeks.

Penicillin G, 3 to 6 million units a day given parenterally, is satisfactory for treatment of pneumococcal and group A streptococcal endocarditis. Treatment should be continued for 4 weeks. Penicillinase-resistant penicillin analogs are preferred initially in treating staphylococcal endocarditis, because of the possibility that the infection is due to a penicillin-resistant organism. Methicillin should be given parenterally in a dose of 12 Gm per day, intramuscularly in divided doses or intravenously. If injected intravenously, the antibiotic should be given in divided doses in 50-ml volumes injected over 5 to 10 min. Methicillin is unstable in acid solutions and should not be given by continuous intravenous drip unless the suspending medium is brought to pH 7.0. Oxacillin, nafcillin, and cephalothin may be administered in lieu of methicillin. If the staphylococcus is found to be sensitive to penicillin G, this antibiotic should be given rather than methicillin, in a dose of 6 to 10 million units per day. Treatment should be continued for at least 4 weeks. In staphylococcal endocarditis, in particular, attention must be given to possible metastatic abscesses requiring surgical drainage.

In patients allergic to penicillin, cephalothin, erythromycin, vancomycin, and lincomycin are alternative drugs. If an allergic reaction to penicillin develops during the course of therapy, suppressant drugs such as antihistamines may be used to alleviate the manifestations of the reaction. In several instances, corticosteroids have been employed to suppress allergic drug reactions during treatment of bacterial endocarditis without deleterious consequences, as long as an effective antimicrobial drug is used to treat the infection.

At times, Probenecid in dosage of 0.5 Gm twice daily, may be given with penicillin or its analogs to slow renal excretion of the antibiotic and to increase blood levels. This regimen may be employed to provide a margin of safety but should not be substituted for adequate doses of the antibiotic.

Fever begins to disappear usually within 3 to 7 days after beginning treatment of bacterial endocarditis. Embolic complications of the disease, heart failure, and infection by insusceptible microorganisms, however, may delay defervescence. Drug fever may occasionally supervene and complicate the febrile course. Cessation of all therapy for 72 hr is not hazardous and may identify such a drug reaction readily.

Some patients with arteriovenous fistulas and infected cardiac prostheses may require surgical intervention before the infection can be controlled. In addition, early corrective surgery should be considered in patients who develop marked valvular damage (particularly aortic regurgitation) as a consequence of bacterial endocarditis. Valve replacement has been lifesaving and must be effected before intractable heart failure ensues.

When bacterial endocarditis recurs, it usually develops within 4 weeks after treatment stops. Reinstitution of antibiotic therapy will be required, but the sensitivity of the microorganism to the antibiotic must be reevaluated. Relapse may indicate inadequate or inappropriate therapy. If bacterial endocarditis develops more than 6 weeks after cessation of treatment, it usually is a new infection.

REFERENCES

Bashour, F. A., and C. P. Winchell: Right-sided Bacterial Endocarditis, Am. J. Med. Sci., 240:411, 1960.

Braniff, B. A., N. E. Shumway, and D. C. Harrison: Valve Replacement in Active Bacterial Endocarditis, New Engl. J. Med., 276:1464, 1967.

Goodman, J. S., W. Schaffner, H. A. Collins, E. J. Battersby, and M. G. Koenig: Infection after Cardiovascular Surgery: Clinical Study Including Examination of Antimicrobial Prophylaxis, New Engl. J. Med., 278:117, 1968.

Green, G. R., G. A. Peters, and J. E. Geraci: Treatment of Bacterial Endocarditis in Patients with Penicillin Hypersensitivity, Ann. Intern. Med., 67:235, 1967.

Hook, E. W., and D. Kaye: Prophylaxis of Bacterial Endocarditis, J. Chronic Dis., 15:635, 1962.

Kerr, A. J., Jr.: "Subacute Bacterial Endocarditis," Springfield, Ill., Charles C Thomas, Publisher, 1955.

Lord, J. W., A. M. Imparato, A. Hackel, and E. F. Doyle: Endocarditis Complicating Open-heart Surgery, Circulation, 23:489, 1961.

Section 3

Diseases Caused by Gram-positive Cocci

138 PNEUMOCOCCAL INFECTIONS
Robert Austrian and Ivan L. Bennett, Jr.

ETIOLOGY. The pneumococcus is a gram-positive encapsulated coccus that usually grows in pairs or short chains. In the diplococcal form, the adjacent margins are rounded and the opposite ends slightly pointed, giving the organisms a "lancet" shape. In stained preparations of exudate, gram-negative forms are sometimes present. Because pneumococci produce greenish discoloration of blood agar, they are sometimes confused with alpha-hemolytic streptococci to which they are closely related. The two organisms can be distinguished by the bile solubility and mouse virulence of the pneumococcus or by serologic typing. Another method, utilizing inhibition of pneumococci by Optochin-impregnated paper disks, is less cumbersome and very effective.

The capsular substances are complex polysaccharides and are the basis for dividing pneumococci into serotypes. Organisms exposed to type-specific antiserum show a positive capsular precipitin reaction, the *Neufeld quellung reaction;* by this means, 82 serotypes have been identified. All are pathogenic for man, but types 1, 3, 4, 7, 8, and 12 are encountered most frequently in clinical practice. Types 6, 14, and 19 often cause pneumonia in children but are less common in adults.

Specific typing of pneumococci remains of great clinical importance if pneumococcus is to be identified with regularity, but has been largely abandoned since the introduction of sulfonamides and antibiotics which are effective against pneumococci of all types. Recognition of pneumococcus has decreased significantly since the abandonment of pneumococcal typing by many clinical laboratories.

EPIDEMIOLOGY. Pneumococci are normal inhabitants of the human upper respiratory tract in 5 to 60 percent of the population, depending upon the season. Pneumococcal infection occurs predominantly during the winter and early spring; the ratio of infection in males and females is 3:2, and morbidity and mortality are higher for Negroes than whites. Person-to-person transmission by droplets is undoubtedly common, but true epidemics of pneumococcal pneumonia are rare, even in closed populations. Patients with pneumococcal infection need not be isolated because the risk of cross infection is relatively small.

PATHOGENESIS. The mechanism by which pneumococci damage tissue is obscure. It is conceivable that toxic substances may be elaborated, but no such toxin has been demonstrated. It has been suggested that rapid growth of pneumococci interferes with essential metabolic processes in the host, but this hypothesis is not supported by firm evidence. The capsular substances, though nontoxic, are known to be necessary factors in virulence, and protect the organism to a certain extent from engulfment by phagocytes.

Invasion of the tissues of the nasopharynx rarely, if ever, occurs, and "pneumococcal pharyngitis" is a doubtful entity. The organisms multiply readily in vivo, however, and may produce acute inflammation in the lungs, serous cavities, and the endocardium.

The normal human respiratory tract is provided with a variety of mechanisms which act to protect the lungs from infection. The lower respiratory tract is protected by the glottis and larynx and material passing these barriers stimulates the expulsive cough reflex. Removal of small particles impinging on the walls of the trachea and bronchi is facilitated by their mucociliary lining; and growth of bacteria reaching normal alveoli is inhibited by their relative dryness and by the phagocytic activity of alveolar macrophages. Any anatomic or physiologic derangement of these coordinated defenses tends to augment the susceptibility of the lungs to infection. Anesthesia, alcoholic intoxication, convulsions and disturbed innervation of the larynx depress cough reflex and may permit aspiration of infected material. Alterations in the tracheobronchial tree leading to anatomic changes in the epithelial lining or to localized obstruction increase the vulnerability of the lungs to infection. Pulmonary edema, local or generalized, resulting from viral infection, inhalation of irritant gases, cardiac failure, or contusion of the chest wall, provides a fluid menstruum in the alveoli for the growth of bacteria and their spread to adjacent areas of the lung. Viral infection of the respiratory epithelium with concomitant disruption of its component cells interferes significantly with the clearance of bacteria from the lungs, an observation in accord with the high incidence of pneumococcal pneumonia during epidemics of viral influenza and its frequent clinical association with sporadic viral respiratory infections.

Pneumonia begins usually in the right lower, right middle, or left lower lobe, those areas to which gravity is most likely to carry upper respiratory secretions aspirated during sleep. Bronchial embolization with infected mucinous secretions during the course of an upper respiratory infection appears to be the initiating factor in many cases of pneumococcal pneumonia. Protected initially from phagocytosis by mucinous material, the bacteria multiply and, in infected alveoli, evoke the outpouring of proteinaceous fluid which serves both as a nutrient and as a vehicle for spread to adjacent alveoli. Soon thereafter, polymorphonuclear leukocytes migrate from the pulmonary capillaries to phagocytize a part of the pneumococcal population before the appearance of detectable antibody. Delay in the polymorphonuclear leukocytic response occurs during alcoholic intoxication and certain forms of anesthesia, permitting spread of infection. Adrenocortical steroids and their congeners may also interfere with leukocyte migration. Later, as the pneumonic lesion evolves, macrophages appear in the exudate and remove the debris of fibrin and cells. It is probable that antibody to the capsular polysaccharide of the invading pneumococcus makes its appearance locally in the lung before being detectable in the circulation. Such antibody increases the efficiency of phagocytosis approximately twofold and causes agglutination of the organisms and their adherence to alveolar walls, thereby slowing their dissemination in the lung. The outcome of infection depends, therefore, on the rate at which bacteria can multiply in the edema fluid and spread and the host's ability to immobilize and destroy them by phagocytosis. Individuals with hypogammaglobulinemia and patients with multiple myeloma incapable of producing anticapsular antibody are prone to recurrent attacks of pneumococcal pneumonia. Repeated infection with the same pneumococcal type should always prompt a search for dysgammaglobulinemia.

Failure of local defense mechanisms in the lung results in lymphatic spread of pneumococci to the hilar lymph nodes. In the sinusoids of these organs, a sequence of events not unlike that in the lung ensues. If infection is not checked in this secondary line of defense, organisms find their way into the thoracic duct and then into the circulation. Although transient bacteremia may occur at the onset of many cases of pneumococcal pneumonia, it is detectable in only 25 to 30 percent of cases. Bacteremia, which reflects the body's inability to localize the pulmonary infection, is a poor prognostic sign and carries with it the danger of metastatic infection. The mortality of treated or untreated bacteremic pneumococcal pneumonia is four times that resulting from comparably managed nonbacteremic infections. Metastatic infection secondary to bacteremia may occur in the meninges, joints, or peritoneum or on the endocardium. Direct spread from the infected lung may give rise to pleural empyema or to pericarditis.

Natural recovery from pneumococcal infection coincides usually, but not invariably, with the appearance of detectable type-specific antibody in the circulation and is often accompanied by a dramatic and abrupt fall in temperature, the so-called "crisis." Antibody aids recovery by increasing the efficiency of phagocytosis and by limiting dissemination of the organisms. Bacteriostatic drugs, such as sulfonamides, facilitate control of the infection by limiting the size of the pneumococcal population, but the host's defense mechanisms are still required for the elimination of the bacteria. Bactericidal agents, such as penicillin, cause the death of pneumococci in the lung and are effective when some of the host's defense mechanisms are inoperable. With the arrest of infection, the alveolar exudate undergoes liquefaction, the inflammatory debris is removed by expectoration and via the lymphatic channels, and the lung is restored to its normal state. Necrosis of pulmonary tissue as a result of pneumococcal infection is distinctly uncommon. Primary pneumococcal lung abscess is a rare clinical entity, although the diagnosis is mistakenly made at times when pneumococcal infection complicates lung abscess of other origins.

In addition to causing pneumonia and its metastatic sequelae, pneumococcus can extend from the nasopharynx to its adjacent structures, giving rise to otitis media, mastoiditis, paranasal sinusitis, or conjunctivitis.

PNEUMOCOCCAL PNEUMONIA

Pneumococcal pneumonia is a disease remarkable for its uniformity, in contrast to other infections such as typhoid fever and tuberculosis. The diseases produced by different pneumococcal serotypes show little variation in severity or in clinical manifestations. The prognosis in type 3 pneumococcal pneumonia is usually regarded as poor, probably because type 3 infections occur frequently in the aged and in patients with other debilitating diseases such as diabetes and congestive heart failure. The type 3 pneumococcus possesses, however, an unusually large capsule, is especially difficult for neutrophils to engulf, and is most likely to produce abscesses in the lungs of man and experimental animals, suggesting that its virulence is partly intrinsic and not wholly the result of its attacking susceptible hosts. It is customary to classify pneumococcal pneumonias as *lobar*, when the process involves one or more large segments or lobes of the lung, or as *bronchopneumonia*, in which there is patchy involvement, often of both lungs. This distinction has little clinical importance; the treatment is the same for both types, and the prognosis depends upon other factors. The usual lesion in adults is lobar in distribution, but in children and the aged, bronchopneumonia is frequent.

MANIFESTATIONS. Pneumonia is often preceded for a few days by coryza or some other form of common respiratory disease. The onset is usually so abrupt that patients frequently can state the exact hour that illness began. There is a sudden *shaking chill* in more than 80 percent of the cases, a rapid rise in temperature, and a corresponding tachycardia. Most patients with pneumococcal pneumonia have a single rigor unless antipyretic drugs are administered, and repeated chills should suggest another etiologic agent.

About 75 percent of patients develop severe *pleuritic pain* and *cough*, productive of pinkish or "rusty" mucoid sputum within a few hours. The chest pain is agonizing, and respirations become rapid, shallow, and grunting as the patient tries to splint the affected side. Many patients are mildly cyanotic as a result of reduced alveolar ventilation, which accompanies altered respiration, and show dilatation of the alae nasae when first seen. Patients appear acutely ill; but nausea, headache, and malaise are not prominent, and most individuals are alert. Pleuritic pain and dyspnea are the dominant complaints.

In the untreated disease, there are sustained fever of 102.5 to 105°F, continued pleuritic pain, cough, and expectoration; and *abdominal distension* is frequent. *Herpes labialis* is a common complication. After 7 to 10 days, there are diaphoresis, abrupt defervescence, and dramatic improvement in well-being, the "crisis."

In cases which terminate fatally, there is usually extensive pulmonary involvement, and dyspnea, cyanosis, and tachycardia are prominent. Circulatory collapse or a picture resembling heart failure is common. Death in a few patients is associated with empyema or some other suppurative complication such as meningitis or endocarditis.

Physical examination reveals restricted motion of the affected hemithorax. Tactile fremitus may be decreased during the initial day of illness but is usually increased when consolidation is fully established. Deviation of the trachea away from the affected lung suggests pleural effusion or empyema. The percussion note is dull, and if the lesion is in an upper lobe, impaired motion of the diaphragm can be detected on the affected side. Very early in the course of infection, breath sounds are diminished, but as the lesion evolves, they become tubular or bronchial in quality and bronchophony and whispered pectoriloquy can be elicited. These findings are accompanied by fine crepitant rales.

EFFECT OF SPECIFIC CHEMOTHERAPY. Pneumococcal pneumonia usually improves promptly when an appropriate antimicrobial drug is given. Within 12 to 36 hr after initiation of treatment with penicillin, temperature, pulse, and respiration begin to fall and may reach normal values in that period, pleuritic pain subsides, and the spread of the inflammatory process is halted. The temperature of approximately half the patients so treated, however, requires 4 days or longer to become normal, and failure of the patient's temperature to reach normal in 24 to 48 hr should not prompt a change in antibacterial therapy in the absence of other indications.

COMPLICATIONS. The typical course of pneumococcal pneumonia can be modified by the development of one or more local or distant complications:

In the Lung. *Atelectasis.* Atelectasis of all or part of a lobe may occur during the active stage of pneumonia or after treatment has been instituted. The patient may complain of sudden recurrence of pleuritic pain and show rapid respirations. Small areas of atelectasis are often detected by x-ray in the absence of symptoms. These areas usually clear with coughing and deep breathing, but bronchoscopic aspiration is occasionally necessary. If atelectasis is allowed to persist, the affected area becomes fibrotic and functionless.

Delayed Resolution. The removal of exudate from the lung following pneumococcal infection is usually complete within 2 to 3 weeks, at which time the x-ray of the chest appears normal; but, occasionally, especially in elderly individuals and in alcoholics, consolidation persists for longer periods. Sometimes the involved area never becomes reaerated, and fibrosis results.

Abscess. Lung abscess is a rare sequel to pneumococcal infection, although pneumococcal pneumonia is a not uncommon complication of lung abscess of other origins. It is manifested by continued fever and profuse expectoration of purulent sputum. X-ray shows one or more cavities. This complication is exceedingly rare in patients who receive penicillin therapy and is most likely to follow infection with pneumococcus type 3.

In Adjacent Structures. Pleural Effusion. Pleural effusion occurs in about 5 percent of patients with pneumococcal pneumonia, even with specific therapy. The amount of fluid is usually not sufficient to cause obvious displacement of mediastinal structures. Usually the effusion is sterile and is reabsorbed spontaneously within a week or two. Sometimes, however, the effusion is large and becomes loculated. In these instances it should be aspirated by needle and occasionally tube drainage must be used.

Empyema. Prior to the introduction of effective chemotherapy, empyema occurred in 5 to 8 percent of patients with pneumococcal pneumonia; it is now observed in less than 1 percent of treated cases. It is manifested by persistent fever or pleuritic pain, together with signs of pleural effusion. In the early stages, the gross appearance of infected fluid may not differ from that of a sterile pleural effusion; later, there is a profuse outpouring of polymorphonuclear leukocytes and fibrin, resulting in an exudate of thick greenish pus containing large clots of fibrin. The quantity of exudate may become large enough to displace mediastinal structures. In neglected cases, this process leads to extensive pleural scarring, with limitation of thoracic movement. Rupture and drainage through the chest wall (*empyema necessitatis*) occurs but is rare. Metastatic *brain abscess* is an occasional complication of chronic empyema. This lesion is caused by passage of septic thrombi through the intercostal and vertebral veins.

Pericarditis. A particularly serious complication is spread of infection to the pericardial sac. This lesion is characterized by pain in the precordial region, a friction rub synchronous with the heartbeat, and distension of cervical veins, although one or all of these findings is not always present. The possibility of coexisting purulent pericarditis should be considered whenever a very ill patient with pneumonia develops empyema.

Metastatic Infections. *Arthritis* occurs more often in children than in adults. The affected joint is swollen, red, and painful, with a purulent effusion. It usually subsides promptly with systemic administration of penicillin, although intraarticular injection of penicillin may be necessary in adults.

Acute bacterial endocarditis complicates pneumococcal pneumonia in less than 0.5 percent of cases. Its manifestations and treatment are discussed below. *Meningitis,*

another complication of pneumococcal pneumonia, is also discussed subsequently.

Paralytic Ileus. Gaseous abdominal distension is commonly present and in severely ill patients may assume such serious proportions that the term *paralytic ileus* is justified. This complication further impairs respiratory movement by elevation of the diaphragm and constitutes a difficult problem in management. A rarer and more serious gastrointestinal complication is acute gastric dilatation.

Impaired Liver Function. Alterations in liver function are very common during the course of pneumococcal pneumonia, and mild jaundice is not at all rare. The pathogenesis of the jaundice is not entirely clear.

LABORATORY FINDINGS. X-ray of the chest reveals a homogeneous density in the affected area of lung. In well-established cases, the density may occupy one or more entire lobes. The white blood count usually shows a polymorphonuclear *leukocytosis* ranging from 12,000 to 25,000 cells per cu mm. A normal leukocyte count or leukopenia is sometimes observed in patients with overwhelming infection and bacteremia, in the aged, and in alcoholics. The *blood culture* is positive for pneumococci during the first 3 or 4 days of the untreated illness in 20 to 25 percent of cases. The *sputum,* when stained by Gram's method, shows polymorphonuclear leukocytes and variable numbers of gram-positive cocci, singly and in pairs. These can be typed directly, by the Neufeld quellung, or capsular precipitin reaction technique, and this procedure should be employed to facilitate diagnosis whenever possible.

DIFFERENTIAL DIAGNOSIS OF PNEUMONIA

Fever, cough, and pulmonary consolidation on physical or x-ray examination form a symptom complex that can be produced by many diseases of infectious, toxic, or other etiology.

Staphylococcal Pneumonia (Chap. 139). Staphylococcal pneumonia is likely to be encountered in children, in adults during or after an epidemic of influenza, and in debilitated elderly individuals as a nosocomial infection. The clinical picture is less uniform than that of pneumococcal pneumonia, varying from bronchitis with few systemic symptoms to a fulminating infection. Multiple chills, hectic fever, early formation of lung abscesses, empyema, and in infants, pneumatoceles or pyopneumothorax, suggest the diagnosis. The sputum is often grossly bloody or purulent and contains myriads of staphylococci readily detectable in stained smears of sputum. Culture of sputum and blood confirms the diagnosis.

Hemolytic Streptococcal Pneumonia (Chap. 140). Hemolytic streptococcal pneumonia can also occur in association with influenza or as a complication of measles. The clinical picture closely resembles that of pneumococcal pneumonia, but multiple chills, hectic fever, early prostration, and rapid pleural involvement with accumulation of fluid, or associated streptococcal pharyngitis, are distinctive signs. The diagnosis can be made by blood and sputum culture or, inferentially, by finding a rise in anti-streptolysin 0 titer in convalescent serum.

Friedländer's Bacillus (Klebsiella) Pneumonia (Chap. 148). Klebsiella is commonest in adult men, especially alcoholics, although 50 percent of these infections occur in those who do not use alcohol to excess. The patients are usually severely ill, and the sputum tends to be thick and tenacious. Physical findings in the chest are often surprisingly scanty despite massive consolidation by x-ray; nausea, diarrhea, jaundice, and delirium are more frequent than in pneumococcal infections, and large numbers of gram-negative bacilli are usually present in stained smears of sputum.

Tularemia. (Chap. 155). Tularemia is often accompanied by pulmonary lesions. There may be no respiratory symptoms and a paucity of physical signs, or pleurisy, hemoptysis, and consolidation may dominate the clinical picture. Patients are usually very ill, often delirious, with temperatures of 104 to 106°F. The disease does not respond to penicillin but does to streptomycin. Agglutinins for the organism may not appear until the third week. A history of contact with wild rabbits, ticks, or deer flies or the finding of a cutaneous ulcer and regional lymphadenitis is helpful in diagnosis.

Other Bacterial Pneumonias. Infection by other bacteria can produce pneumonia. Pulmonary involvement is frequent in patients with salmonella bacteremia, especially in *Salmonella choleraesuis* infections (Chap. 150). Pneumonia caused by other enterobacteria (*Escherichia coli, Proteus* species, *Pseudomonas*) occurs usually in the debilitated and the aged, in alcoholics, and in those with deranged defenses against infection. In most instances these patients have received antimicrobials for other infections. Necrotizing pneumonia caused by one of the several species of the anaerobic genus *Bacteroides* is seen occasionally. *Hemophilus influenzae* is a common cause of pulmonary disease in children; in adults it occasionally produces a necrotizing bronchiolitis or lobar pneumonia, and in elderly patients with chronic lung disease, it may produce bronchopneumonia (Chap. 152). The diagnosis is usually made only by culture of sputum. Pulmonary lesions with cough and hemoptysis can be prominent in Weil's disease (Chap. 181), and the plague bacillus can cause an overwhelming and rapidly fatal pneumonia, especially when plague becomes epidemic (Chap. 156).

Mycoplasma Pneumoniae Infection (Chap. 207). This infection is usually more insidious in onset than bacterial pneumonia. Chills are infrequent, fever is usually lower and falls by lysis, pleuritic pain and effusions are unusual, headache and malaise are prominent, and the cough is hacking, irritating, and productive of small amounts of mucoid sputum. Physical signs are scanty in comparison with x-ray changes. Herpes labialis is unusual.

Viral Pneumonias (Chap. 206). Viral pneumonias may result from infection with a variety of agents including myxoviruses, respiratory syncytial virus, adenoviruses, Coxsackie, ECHO, and reoviruses and those of measles and varicella. Although many of these illnesses are mild and resemble that caused by *Mycoplasma pneumoniae*, occasional infections caused by influenza virus may be difficult to distinguish from bacterial pneumonia. Secondary bacterial pneumonia is a not uncommon complication of influenza viral infection and of severe measles.

Psittacosis (Ornithosis) (Chap. 209). Psittacosis is characterized by systemic symptoms of headache, fever, lethargy, and malaise for several days before pulmonary lesions develop. The pulse is usually slow in proportion to fever, and patients are sometimes suspected of having typhoid. The leukocyte count may be normal or moderately elevated.

Q Fever (Chap. 201). Q fever is characterized by severe headache, sustained fever, and, usually, minimal symptoms of respiratory disease, although a large proportion of patients show roentgenographic evidence of patchy pulmonary involvement.

Tuberculosis. *Acute tuberculous pneumonia* (Chap. 174) may be difficult to recognize because, early in the disease, tubercle bacilli may not be demonstrable in the sputum; the first consolidation is often the result of an inflammatory response to discharge of tuberculin-containing material into the lung. Fever is usually remittent or intermittent, and the temperature may not exceed 102°F. Many patients with tuberculous pneumonia feel surprisingly well, despite consolidation of an entire lobe. *Pleurisy with effusion* is seldom abrupt in onset, its course is prolonged, and physical and x-ray findings are those of accumulating pleural fluid rather than parenchymal consolidation. Cough is usually nonproductive. The leukocyte count is frequently normal. Herpes labialis is rare in tuberculosis.

Mycotic Infections. *Blastomycosis* (Chap. 186) can produce acute lobar or bronchopneumonia, with high fever, pleuritic pain, dyspnea, and pleural fluid. The organisms usually are found easily in the sputum, and cavitation develops early in the illness. The usual course of pulmonary blastomycosis is less acute than that of bacterial pneumonia, with low-grade fever and slow evolution of the pulmonary findings. *Actinomycosis* of the lung (Chap. 184) is usually a more chronic disease than bacterial pneumonia and is more likely to be confused with tuberculosis or lung tumors. Other mycotic infections of the lung include *primary histoplasmosis* (Chap. 188), which can produce an acute illness that lasts for several weeks with fever, cough, and multiple nodular pulmonary densities; and primary coccidioidomycosis (Chap. 187), distinguishable in endemic areas by pulmonary infiltration, fever, eosinophilia, and, often erythema nodosum.

Lung Abscess (Chap. 291). Lung abscess may have an abrupt onset, with chill, fever, and pleuritic pain and can be confused with acute pneumonias. Pneumococcal pneumonia at the site of the lesion may complicate the course of any stage prior to treatment. The development of cavitation in a well-circumscribed pulmonary density and profuse, purulent, often foul-smelling sputum make the diagnosis clear. In individuals with chronic abscess, weight loss is prominent and cavitation readily apparent. There is usually intermittent or remittent fever. A history of epilepsy, alcoholic intoxication, anesthesia, dental extraction, tonsillectomy, or aspiration of a foreign body may be elicited. Abscess may be the first sign of bronchogenic carcinoma.

Atelectasis (Chap. 291). Atelectasis may occur in patients confined to bed, especially if respiratory motion is limited (as after an abdominal operation) or when the cough reflex is depressed by drugs or central nervous system disease. Infection of the collapsed pulmonary segment leads to fever, pleuritic pain, and purulent sputum. There is often a shift of the mediastinum toward the affected side. Tumor, enlarged hilar nodes, and foreign body are important causes of persistent collapse, although plugging of bronchi by inspissated mucus is by far the most frequent cause.

Neoplasms (Chap. 292).

Pulmonary Adenomatosis (Chap. 292). Pulmonary adenomatosis, a diffuse neoplastic disease, can be accompanied by fever, profuse glairy sputum, and hemoptysis, with various x-ray findings, and is sometimes mistaken at first for acute bacterial pneumonia. Much more commonly a bronchogenic carcinoma, at or near the hilum, presents as pneumonia. Failure of any "lobar pneumonia" to resolve should lead to vigorous search for malignant disease.

Pulmonary Infarction (Chap. 285). Pulmonary infarction is especially frequent in patients with congestive heart failure and after surgical procedures. Prostatic surgery and pelvic infections in women as well as delivery are particularly likely to lead to embolization from the pelvic veins. Pulmonary embolization may be asymptomatic, but in many patients, there are sudden pleuritic pain, dyspnea, anxiety, transient hypotension, and hemoptysis. Fever is common, but true chills are rare. Icterus may accompany pulmonary infarcts in individuals with congestive heart failure. Signs of consolidation and pleural fluid are common, and often evidence of phlebothrombosis can be detected in the legs. In women, *septic pulmonary infarcts* with abscess formation and cavitation should always suggest puerperal sepsis or infected abortions with pelvic thrombophlebitis. For reasons that are obscure, phlebothrombosis and pulmonary infarction are relatively frequent complications of convalescence from psittacosis.

Other Differential Diagnostic Points. The lungs of patients with *uremia* sometimes show x-ray changes consisting of infiltrations that flare toward the periphery from both hilar areas. Roentgenographically, the changes in the lungs of patients with *acute pulmonary edema* and *heart failure* are sometimes surprisingly well localized to a segment or lobe of one lung.

The inhalation of *noxious materials or irritants* (Chap. 116), including smoke, chlorine, phosgene, cadmium fumes, bagasse fibers, and other organic dusts, can lead to bronchitis, bronchiolitis, patchy or even lobar infiltration in the lung, dyspnea, and low-grade fever. The diagnosis is usually made by eliciting a history of exposure. The ingestion of gasoline or kerosene is almost invariably complicated by severe chemical bronchopneumonia. A more benign and chronic pneumonia known as *lipoid pneumonia* may follow the nocturnal ingestion of mineral oil or the use of nose drops containing oil.

Pneumonitis is detectable by physical examination or x-ray in some patients with erythema multiforme, lupus erythematosus, rheumatic fever, or intestinal helminthiasis. Infectious mononucleosis and lymphocytic choriomeningitis are sometimes accompanied by pulmonary infiltrations and, occasionally, by signs of respiratory irritation with cough and sputum. Pulmonary lesions, usually in the form of scattered nodular densities, with accompanying cough, dyspnea, and cyanosis, occur in a small proportion of patients with smallpox, chickenpox, or measles; the involvement in these diseases is believed to be caused by the virus rather than by secondary bacterial invaders. Rupture of amebic abscess into the pleural cavity can be mistaken for acute pneumonia, and in a few patients with estivo-autumnal malaria, blockage of pulmonary capillaries by parasites can lead to confusion with respiratory infections.

PNEUMOCOCCAL MENINGITIS

The pneumococcus is second only to the meningococcus as a cause of purulent meningitis in adults; in children, meningitis caused by *Hemophilus influenzae* is also more frequent than pneumococcal infection.

Pneumococcal meningitis can develop as a "primary" disease without preceding signs of infection elsewhere; as a complication of pneumococcal pneumonia; by extension from otitis, mastoiditis, or sinusitis; or following a skull fracture which creates an opening between the subarachnoid space and the nasal cavity or paranasal sinuses. Patients with pneumococcal endocarditis frequently develop meningeal infection. Patients with multiple myeloma seem to be prone to pneumococcal infection of the meninges, just as they are to pneumonia.

The *manifestations* are those of any acute pyogenic meningitis (Chap. 360) and include chills, fever, headache, nuchal rigidity, Kernig's and Brudzinski's signs, delirium, and cranial nerve palsies. Evidence of otitis, sinusitis, or pneumonia should be carefully sought by physical and roentgenographic examination in all patients.

The *spinal fluid* is under increased pressure, appears cloudy, often with a greenish tint, and shows a high protein and low glucose content. Stained smears usually reveal gram-positive diplococci and polymorphonuclear leukocytes; in some patients, the number of cells in the spinal fluid is surprisingly small, and much of the cloudiness is produced by the bacterial content. The diagnosis can be established rapidly by identification of pneumococci in the spinal fluid by Gram stain and by direct typing with the Neufeld quellung reaction.

With appropriate chemotherapy, recovery can be expected in 50 to 70 percent of cases; the prognosis is better in children than in infants or in adults. Before penicillin was available, the mortality rate exceeded 95 percent, and sulfonamides did little to reduce it. Relapse may occur but is unusual if adequate treatment is carried out. Subarachnoid block, the result of accumulation of large amounts of thick exudate in the meningeal space and at the base of the brain, is now an unusual complication.

PNEUMOCOCCAL ENDOCARDITIS

Endocarditis is usually a complication of pneumonia or meningitis. The clinical picture is that of acute bacterial endocarditis (Chap. 137), with remittent fever, splenomegaly, and metastatic infection of the lungs, meninges, joints, eye, and other tissues. Petechiae are uncommon. The infection can attack normal valves and is particularly likely to occur on the aortic valve. The valvular infection is destructive, and loud murmurs and heart failure develop rapidly. Rupture or perforation of cusps or even rupture of the aorta may occur. The blood culture is consistently positive for the pneumococcus in the absence of treatment with antimicrobial drugs; yet at the same time antibodies to the infecting organism may be demonstrable in the blood, a combination of findings seldom observed except in endocarditis or brucellosis. Although the infection is relatively easy to cure with penicillin, damage to valve leaflets, especially to the cusps of the aortic valve, may be followed by rapidly progressive heart failure. Surgical repair or replacement of damaged valvular structures should be carried out early, before heart failure becomes intractable.

PNEUMOCOCCAL PERITONITIS

Pneumococcal peritonitis is a rare disease which occurs in young girls; presumably the vagina and fallopian tubes are the portal of entry. Symptoms are fever, pain, abdominal distension, vomiting, and accumulation of peritoneal fluid. The diagnosis is made by examination of the purulent ascitic fluid; blood cultures are often positive, and a polymorphonuclear leukocytosis is the rule. In adults, the disease may occur in association with cirrhosis or with carcinoma of the liver. Peritonitis used to be a common complication of the nephrotic syndrome, particularly in children, but is rare nowadays.

TREATMENT

SPECIFIC ANTIMICROBIAL THERAPY. Penicillin G (benzathine penicillin) is the drug of choice for all pneumococcal infections. The minimum curative dose for *pneumonia* is less than 60,000 units daily, and a total dose of 600,000 units daily provides a good margin of safety for bacteremic and nonbacteremic infections in adults in the absence of an extrapulmonary focus of infection. Treatment may be administered at 12-hr intervals in doses of 300,000 units aqueous crystalline penicillin G or procaine penicillin. Therapy should be continued until the patient has been afebrile for 48 to 72 hr. The response is usually dramatic, and relapse is extremely uncommon. Pneumococcal pneumonia can be treated adequately with oral penicillin (preferably one of the drugs resistant to gastric acid, see Chap. 135) in dosage of 1.2 to 2.4 million units daily. *Peritonitis* usually responds within 36 to 48 hr to 2 to 4 million units of pencillin daily.

Pneumococcal *meningitis* should be treated with 12 to 20 million units aqueous penicillin G daily intrave-nously in adults. In many clinics, even larger amounts are used, though care must be taken to avoid neurotoxicity from excessive dosage. Intrathecal administration of penicillin is of no value. The addition of sulfadiazine to this regimen affords no advantage, and supplementary administration of chlortetracycline (and presumably, of other broad-spectrum drugs) actually exerts a deleterious effect. In the presence of sinusitis, otitis, or mastoiditis, surgical drainage should be carried out as soon as is feasible. The response of meningitis is usually less dramatic than that of pneumonia; patients often remain febrile and disoriented, and signs of meningeal irritation may persist for several days, but improvement becomes gradually evident with continued treatment.

Large doses are required in pneumococcal endocarditis also—12 to 20 million units daily by intravenous injection. Rapidly developing heart failure in these patients and the tendency to form myocardial abscess, however, often lead to a fatal outcome despite large doses of antibiotics. Surgical repair or replacement of damaged heart valves should be considered when cardiac failure develops.

Sulfonamides are effective in pneumococcal pneumonia but less so than antibiotics, and their action is not as prompt or dramatic as that of penicillin. They are useless in meningitis and endocarditis. The *tetracyclines* in doses of 1.0 to 2.0 Gm daily, *erythromycin* in doses of 1.6 Gm daily, and *Lincomycin* in doses of 1.2 Gm daily are effective treatment of pneumococcal pneumonia, but are recommended only for patients who have had untoward reactions to penicillin. Mutants of pneumococcus resistant to each of these antibiotics have been isolated from man; and, if one of these drugs is to be employed, it is essential that the organism be sensitive to the agent administered. Despite its efficacy, chloramphenicol should not be used to treat pneumococcal infections, except when unusual circumstances exist.

Pneumococcal arthritis responds to systemic penicillin, but aspiration and intraarticular instillation of the drug may be necessary.

Empyema should be detected and treated as early as possible. When an effusion is found, the fluid should be examined for organisms; and if they are present, 50,000 to 200,000 units of penicillin G should be injected intrapleurally. In addition, the same antibiotic should be administered systemically in doses of 6 to 8 million units a day. Aspiration of fluid and instillation of penicillin should be carried out at 1- to 2-day intervals until cultures are persistently negative and fever disappears. Fluoroscopic guidance may be needed for aspiration of small empyema pockets. If the exudate is especially thick or viscid, streptokinase-streptodornase (Varidase) may facilitate its withdrawal. When definite improvement is not evident in 4 to 6 days or when the empyema is of long duration, a large-lumen intercostal tube should be placed in the pleural cavity to facilitate drainage. Failure to effect prompt cure of empyema may be followed by pleural fibrosis and necessitate subsequent surgical decortication of the lung to restore pulmonary function. Aspiration of exudate and instillation of penicillin may also be used to treat *pericarditis,* but when cardiac tamponade is present, pericardiotomy may be preferable. Although medical treatment of emypema and of pericarditis is successful in some patients, there should be no hesitation in employing surgical drainage when rapid and steady improvement is not observed.

OTHER MEASURES. *Oxygen* should be used to treat intense cyanosis in pneumonia but may aggravate abdominal distension. Codeine, 30 to 60 mg every few hours, will usually control cough and mild *pleuritic pain.* A chest binder may diminish pain but may also increase the likelihood of atelectasis. When pain is severe, intercostal nerve block by injection of 2.0 ml of 1 percent procaine beneath the rib margins proximal to the site of pain is usually effective and is not technically difficult or dangerous. Other methods of relieving pleuritic pain are usually transient in their effect but are sometimes worth trying; they include ethyl chloride spray over the painful area and intravenous injection of calcium gluconate.

PROGNOSIS

With proper antimicrobial therapy, the mortality from all cases of pneumococcal pneumonia has fallen to approximately 5 percent, but that of patients with bacteremic infections is 17 percent. The recovery rate in meningitis is 50 to 70 percent; the prognosis is better in childhood. Pneumococcal endocarditis is still fatal in at least half the cases; death results from valvular damage and cardiac failure more often than from infection.

Signs of poor prognosis in pneumonia include leukopenia, bacteremia, multilobar involvement, any extrapulmonary focus of pneumococcal infection, presence of preexisting systemic disease, circulatory collapse, and occurrence of the infection in the first year of life or after the age of fifty-five. Infection with pneumococcus type 3 has a higher mortality than that caused by other pneumococcal types.

REFERENCES

Austrian, R.: Pneumococcal Endocarditis, Meningitis, and Rupture of Aortic Valve, A.M.A. Arch. Intern. Med., 99:539, 1957.

——, and J. Gold: Pneumococcal Bacteremia with Especial Reference to Bacteremic Pneumococcal Pneumonia, Ann. Intern. Med., 60:759, 1964.

Dowling, H. F., and M. H. Lepper: The Effect of Antibiotics (Penicillin, Aureomycin, and Terramycin) on the Fatality Rate and Incidence of Complications in Pneumococcic Pneumonia, Am. J. Med. Sci., 222:396, 1951.

Finland, M., and H. I. L. Lovernd: Massive Atelectatic Collapse of the Lung Complicating Pneumococcus Pneumonia, Ann. Intern. Med., 10:1828, 1937.

Heffron, R.: "Pneumonia with Special Reference to Pneumococcus Lobar Pneumonia," New York, The Commonwealth Fund, 1939.

Lepper, M. H., and H. F. Dowling: Treatment of Pneumococcic Meningitis with Penicillin Compared with Penicillin plus Aureomycin, A.M.A. Arch. Intern. Med., 88: 489, 1951.

Shulman, J. A., L. A. Phillips, and R. G. Petersdorf: Errors and Hazards in the Diagnosis and Treatment of Bacterial Pneumonias, Ann. Intern. Med., 62:41, 1965.

Wood, W. Barry, Jr.: Studies on the Mechanism of Recovery in Pneumococcal Pneumonia: I. The Action of Type Specific Antibody upon the Pulmonary Lesion of Experimental Pneumonia, J. Exp. Med., 73:201, 1941.

Zimmerman, H. J., and L. J. Thomas: The Liver in Pneumococcal Pneumonia: Observations in 94 Cases on Liver Function and Jaundice in Pneumonia, J. Lab. Clin. Med., 35:556, 1950.

Zinneman, H. H., and W. H. Hall: Recurrent Pneumonia in Multiple Myeloma, Ann. Intern. Med., 41:1152, 1954.

139 STAPHYLOCOCCAL INFECTIONS
David E. Rogers

Staphylococci cause most superficial suppurative infections in man. They also produce certain serious infections of the lungs, pleural space, endocardium, myocardium, long bones, kidneys, and surgical wounds.

While serious staphylococcal infections have always produced problems in hospitalized patients, they have much greater clinical importance since the development of antibiotics. The majority of life-threatening staphylococcal infections now arise within hospitals. Certain characteristics of staphylococci appear to have led to this situation: (1) the frequency of potentially pathogenic strains as part of man's normal flora, (2) the maintenance of staphylococci resistant to many antimicrobials in wide use in hospitals and hospital personnel, (3) the tendency of staphylococci to produce disease in debilitated patients, and (4) the rapid tissue destruction, abscess formation, and sluggish response of staphylococcal disease to antibacterial therapy.

BACTERIOLOGY. Staphylococci are members of the genus *Micrococcus.* This genus includes many morphologically similar saprophytic microorganisms which do not cause human infection. The parasitic micrococci of primary concern in medicine are grouped in the species *Micrococcus pyogenes.* Through established usage, these pathogenic micrococci are termed *staphylococci.*

Staphylococci are spherical gram-positive cells which grow abundantly in the usual meat extract or infusion media. On solid agar media, staphylococcal colonies develop characteristic pigmentation by which three species can be differentiated: *M. pyogenes* var. *aureus* (*Staphylococcus aureus*), golden yellow; *M. pyogenes* var. *albus* (*S. albus*), ivory white; and *M. citreus,* lemon yellow. Most human infections are caused by *S. aureus,* a few by *S. albus.* The name staphylococcus derives from the characteristic grapelike clusters of organisms seen in stained smears prepared from colonies on solid media (Greek *staphule* = "grape"). In stained smears obtained from pus, smaller clusters, diploids, and short chains are seen. In such preparations, staphylococci characteristically retain their uniform round shape, in contrast to the boat-like forms assumed by pneumococci. Staphylococci may be seen within the cytoplasm of polymorphonuclear cells in pus, a finding not common in other gram-positive coccal infections.

In general, pathogenic strains possess a broader complement of biochemical activity than do nonpathogenic strains. Most staphylococci isolated from human infections produce yellow pigment and hemolyze rabbit, sheep, and human red blood cells in blood agar plates. The ability to produce coagulase, a substance which clots the plasma of certain animals and man, the elaboration of *alpha toxin*, the fermentation of *mannite*, and the hydrolysis of *phenolphthalein phosphate* are characteristics of infection-producing strains. The ability of a given strain to produce coagulase is generally considered the best evidence of pathogenicity.

Different strains of pathogenic staphylococci can be recognized by the patterns of lysis produced by staphylococcal bacteriophages. Although the technique is cumbersome, phage typing of staphylococci has allowed more precise strain characterization and is commonly used in studies of intrahospital disease and epidemics of staphylococcal infection.

PATHOGENESIS. Little is known of the events which allow staphylococci to invade host tissues. While strains of staphylococci capable of producing infection are common skin and mucous membrane inhabitants, an enormous number of bacteria must be used to establish experimental infections in animals or man. Over 50 percent of serious staphylococcal infections of deep tissues arise from cutaneous foci. A lesser number of staphylococcal infections originate in the respiratory or genitourinary tract.

Staphylococcal disease appears more common in patients with *diabetes, liver disease, renal failure,* under circumstances of severe *debilitation* and/or *malnutrition,* or when skin continuity is broken. *Abrasions, wounds, burns,* and skin areas denuded by *exfoliative dermatitis* are commonly infected with staphylococci. Individuals who work with greasy skin irritants have a greater incidence of superficial staphylococcal infections. *Influenza, measles,* and *mucoviscoidosis* appear to predispose to primary staphylococcal invasion of the lung. Patients receiving *broad-spectrum antimicrobial therapy* also appear to have a higher incidence of staphylococcal disease.

Staphylococci invade the integument via hair follicles and sebaceous glands. When skin continuity has been breached, local microbial multiplication is accompanied by inflammation and tissue necrosis at the site of infection. Polymorphonuclear leukocytes rapidly enter the area and ingest large numbers of staphylococci. Thrombosis of surrounding capillaries occurs, fibrin is deposited about the periphery, and later, fibroblasts create a relatively avascular wall about the area. The fully developed staphylococcal lesion consists of a central core of dead and dying leukocytes and bacteria which gradually liquefies to form characteristic thick creamy staphylococcal pus, surrounded by a fibroblastic wall, the *pyogenic membrane.*

When host mechanisms fail to contain the cutaneous or subcutaneous infection, staphylococci may enter the bloodstream. Common sites of metastatic seeding are the diaphyseal ends of long bones in children, lungs, kidneys, endocardium, myocardium, liver, spleen, and brain.

Certain biologic properties of staphylococci appear to contribute to pathogenicity. Many pathogenic strains elaborate an *exotoxin* (alpha toxin) capable of causing dermal necrosis in animals. Fever, tachycardia, cyanosis, shock, and death ensue when exotoxin is administered to experimental animals, a picture similar to that seen occasionally in certain fulminating cases of staphylococcal bacteremia in man.

The high correlation between *coagulase* production and virulence suggests that this substance is important in the pathogenesis of staphylococcal infections. Coagulase has been said to protect staphylococci from phagocytosis by polymorphonuclear leukocytes, to promote abscess formation in man and animal species who have coagulable plasmas, or to protect staphylococci from bacteriostatic substances present in normal serum. However, none of these postulates has proven that coagulase per se is a determinant of pathogenicity, and its precise role has not been established.

Certain pathogenic staphylococci produce a *leukocidin* which destroys human and rabbit leukocytes in vitro. Some strains elaborate *hyaluronidase*. Many staphylococci produce an *enterotoxin* which produces nausea, vomiting, and diarrhea in certain experimental animals and man.

In vitro and in vivo studies have indicated that pathogenic staphylococci can survive within human leukocytes while nonpathogenic strains do not. Such intracellular survival may be a means of transporting staphylococci and spreading them to distant tissues.

IMMUNITY. Some degree of resistance to staphylococcal infections develops with age and the host's experience with staphylococci. Primary staphylococcal pneumonia is common in infants, but rare in adults. Acute staphylococcal osteomyelitis is almost exclusively a disease of children. Abscess formation appears less common and bacteremia more frequent in infants than in adults.

Coagulase-positive staphylococci have a characteristic cell wall teichoic acid which may be antiphagocytic. Certain unusual strains possess a definite capsular structure which impedes phagocytosis, and specific opsonizing antibody is required for the ingestion of these unusual strains. A number of antistaphylococcal antibodies have been shown to pass from mother to fetus, and the incidence of a variety of antibodies rapidly rises with age. Virtually 100 percent of adults possess antibodies to several staphylococcal antigens in their serum. Nevertheless, the role of humoral immunity in modifying or protecting against staphylococcal infection is uncertain. Immunization of animals with alpha toxin, toxoids, coagulase, or whole staphylococci may prolong experimental staphylococcal infection, but does not protect against eventual death. At present there has been no satisfactory demonstration that human staphylococcal disease is followed by immunity or that infection can be modified significantly by vaccination.

EPIDEMIOLOGY. Pathogenic strains of staphylococci reside in the anterior nares and upon the skin of 20 to

60 percent of humans. Hospital patients and personnel have significantly higher staphylococcal carrier rates than the general population. Over 90 percent of newborns acquire staphylococci within the anterior nares within 2 weeks. These infants are commonly colonized by the same staphylococcal phage types carried by nursery personnel.

While staphylococci remain viable for long periods in dust, blankets, or clothing, and viable staphylococci are often demonstrable in the environment by air-sampling techniques, the significance of airborne transmission remains uncertain, and the best evidence suggests that direct person-to-person contact is the most important means of transmission of staphylococci. Active staphylococcal infections are probably a more serious source of cross infection than the simple carrier state.

Certain phage types of staphylococci cause the majority of intrahospital infections. Some strains, particularly antibiotic-resistant strains in phage group III, appear to have greater "epidemic virulence" than other staphylococci. In specific hospitals, one phage type often emerges to prominence and may cause most of the serious intrahospital infections. Such "epidemic strains" have shifted from time to time and vary from hospital to hospital. The high incidence of active staphylococcal disease in carriers of certain strains (for example, the 80/81 strains) suggests that some staphylococci may possess higher virulence for humans than others.

ANTIMICROBIAL RESISTANCE. The introduction of new antibiotics active against staphylococci has generally been followed by the appearance of staphylococci specifically resistant to that agent. When penicillin was first introduced, less than 10 percent of staphylococcal strains isolated from patients or carriers were resistant to penicillin. Now 60 to 90 percent of staphylococci isolated from hospitalized patients throughout the Western world are resistant to penicillin G and the incidence of infection due to penicillinase-producing strains in nonhospitalized individuals is almost as high as in hospitalized patients. The incidence of resistance to a specific antimicrobial has correlated closely with the frequency of its administration, and the emergence of resistant strains has followed the use of streptomycin, the tetracyclines, chloramphenicol, erythromycin, oleandomycin, novobiocin, and kanamycin. Vancomycin, first employed in 1958, and the penicillinase-resistant penicillins and the cephalosporins, both introduced in the 1960s, have been exceptions to this rule. Although some strains of S. *aureus* resistant to the penicillinase-resistant penicillins have produced infections in England, France, and the United States, such strains have been unusual and, in general, all these agents have retained a high degree of activity against both penicillin-sensitive and penicillin-resistant staphylococci.

Most observations on the incidence of antimicrobial-resistant strains have been made within hospitals where antimicrobial use is heaviest. It has been shown that drug-susceptible strains carried by patients may be replaced by drug-resistant phage group III staphylococci present in the hospital environment during antimicrobial treatment. These strains are in turn acquired by hospital personnel who serve as reservoirs of potentially pathogenic, antimicrobial-resistant strains. Staphylococci isolated from population groups outside the hospital have shown a slower increase in the incidence of antimicrobial-resistant strains, but in many communities the incidence of extra-hospital infections caused by penicillin-resistant strains is now similar to that found in hospitalized patients.

SUPERFICIAL INFECTIONS

Simple infection of hair follicles manifested by a minute erythematous nodule without involvement of the surrounding skin or deeper tissues is termed *folliculitis*. Chronic recurrent folliculitis of the beard area is termed *sycosis barbae*.

A more extensive and invasive follicular or sebaceous gland infection with some involvement of subcutaneous tissues is termed a *furuncle* or *boil*. Itching and mild pain are followed by progressive local swelling and erythema. The overlying skin becomes thin, tense, shiny, and exquisitely painful on pressure or motion. Relief of pain occurs promptly after spontaneous or surgical drainage.

Furuncles occur most commonly on the face, neck, axillas, forearms, buttocks, thighs, breasts, upper back, and labia. The acne of adolescence is frequently complicated by secondary furunculosis. Staphylococcal infection may involve the sweat glands in the axillas (*hidradenitis suppurativa*). These infections may be deep-seated, slow to localize and drain, and are prone to recurrence and scarring.

Staphylococcal infections within the thick, fibrous, inelastic skin of the back of the neck and upper back lead to formation of a *carbuncle*. The relative thickness and impermeability of the overlying skin leads to lateral extension and loculation, and a large indurated, painful lesion with multiple ineffective drainage sites results. Carbuncles produce fever, leukocytosis, extreme pain, and prostration. Bacteremia is common.

OSTEOMYELITIS

Staphylococci are responsible for the majority of cases of *acute osteomyelitis*. This infection occurs almost exclusively in children under the age of twelve and has dropped sharply in incidence since the introduction of antibiotics. Men are affected more commonly than women. Approximately 50 percent of patients give a history of a furuncle or superficial staphylococcal infection preceding osteomyelitis. Bone involvement follows hematogenous dissemination of bacteria. The frequent localization in the diaphyseal end of long bones is thought to be due to the endarterial circulation of the diaphysis. Many patients give a history of preceding trauma to the involved area.

Once established, infection spreads through the newly formed juxtaepiphyseal bone to the periosteum or along the marrow cavity. If the infection reaches the subperiosteal space, the periosteum is lifted, a subperiosteal abscess forms, and rupture with infection of the subcutaneous tissues may occur. Rarely, the joint capsule is penetrated producing a pyogenic arthritis. There is death of bone producing a *sequestrum* followed by new bone formation (the *involucrum*).

Occasionally indolent staphylococcal infections of bone remain localized within dense granulation tissue about a central necrotic cavity. Such a local infection may persist for years as a so-called "Brodie's abscess."

Osteomyelitis in children usually begins abruptly with chills, high fever, nausea, vomiting, and progressive pain at the site of bony involvement. Muscle spasm about the affected bone is a common early sign of osteomyelitis, and the child may refuse to move the affected limb. Leukocytosis is the rule. Blood cultures are positive for staphylococci in 50 to 60 percent of cases early in the disease. The tissues overlying the involved bone become edematous and warm, and the skin becomes erythematous and shiny. Anemia develops during the course of untreated disease. Roentgenograms are usually normal during the first week. Bony rarefaction, local periosteal elevation, and new bone formation can frequently be seen during the second week.

DIAGNOSIS. Osteomyelitis should be suspected in any child with fever, limb pain, and leukocytosis. History of a preceding cutaneous infection, local tenderness over the end of a long bone, and the finding of S. *aureus* in blood cultures are confirmatory. In early stages, osteomyelitis must be differentiated from acute rheumatic fever, poliomyelitis, pyogenic arthritis, scurvy, and syphilitic periostitis.

PROGNOSIS. Prior to the advent of antimicrobials, the overall mortality was approximately 25 percent. Death was more common in individuals with demonstrable bacteremia. Chronic osteomyelitis with recurrent activation and metastatic foci in other bones was common. Today acute staphylococcal osteomyelitis is declining in incidence, death is rare, and chronic osteomyelitis is disappearing.

STAPHYLOCOCCAL PNEUMONIA

Staphylococci are the cause of 1 to 5 percent of bacterial pneumonias. This disease occurs sporadically except during epidemics of influenza when staphylococcal pneumonia is more common.

Primary staphylococcal pneumonia in infants and young children is a frequent cause of pyopneumothorax. This complication occurs early and should suggest S. *aureus* infection. In older children and adults, primary staphylococcal pneumonia is usually secondary to influenza or measles. More recently, staphylococcal pneumonia has been seen with increasing frequency in hospitalized patients with mucoviscidosis, leukemia, diffuse collagen disease, or other chronic debilitating disease.

In healthy adults, staphylococcal pneumonia is generally preceded by an influenza-like respiratory infection. Onset of staphylococcal involvement is abrupt with chills, high fever, progressive dyspnea, cyanosis, cough, and pleural pain. Early peripheral vascular collapse is common, and examination frequently reveals a patient who seems sicker than his physical findings would suggest.

Sputum in the early phases is not characteristic, but may be bloody or frankly purulent. Admixture with blood may produce a thick, creamy pink sputum.

Staphylococcal pneumonia arising in hospitalized patients is a common problem. This illness usually begins more insidiously. Increasing fever, tachycardia, and an elevated respiratory rate may be the only indications of infection. Typical pneumonic symptoms may be absent. This is also true when metastatic pulmonary involvement occurs during the course of staphylococcal bacteremia. Staphylococci generally produce patchy, centrally located areas of pneumonia. Pleural involvement and empyema are common.

Because of the central pulmonary involvement, chest findings are variable. Signs of frank consolidation are rare. Scattered fine to coarse rales and rhonchi may be heard over the involved areas. Empyema produces typical signs of pleural fluid. Signs of abscess may appear late in the course of the disease. Bacteremia is unusual (less than 20 percent of patients), and *its presence should suggest that the pneumonic involvement is metastatic and secondary to foci of infection elsewhere.* Chest x-rays commonly reveal a patchy pneumonic process about the hilar area and may show early evidence of pleural fluid accumulation.

The course of staphylococcal pneumonia may be stormy despite adequate antimicrobial therapy. Gradual defervescence starting 48 to 72 hr after the initiation of therapy is the rule. Pulmonary abscesses or empyema cavities may require local surgical treatment.

DIAGNOSIS. Staphylococcal pneumonia must be differentiated from other pneumonias. The preceding influenza-like illness, rapid onset of pleural pain, cyanosis, and prostration out of proportion to physical findings should suggest primary staphylococcal pneumonia. The finding of masses of polymorphonuclear leukocytes and gram-positive intraleukocytic cocci strongly suggests the diagnosis. The blood leukocyte count is generally above 15,000. The sudden or insidious development of pneumonia with higher fever, tachycardia, and leukocytosis in debilitated hospitalized patients receiving antimicrobials should be considered to be staphylococcal in origin.

PROGNOSIS. Prior to 1942, mortality ranged from 50 to 95 percent. The presence of bacteremia was almost invariably associated with a fatal outcome. The prognosis has improved with the use of antimicrobials but continues to range from 15 to 20 percent in primary staphylococcal pneumonia. Higher mortality is seen in debilitated individuals acquiring staphylococcal pneumonia in the hospital. Abscess formation and pleural involvement often prolong convalescence.

STAPHYLOCOCCAL BACTEREMIA

Staphylococcal bacteremia may arise from any local staphylococcal infection. Infections of the skin (including infections about inlying venous cutdowns or catheters), respiratory tract, long bones, or genitourinary tract precede bacteremia in descending order of frequency. Trauma to local lesions, such as pinching, or surgical drainage before adequate localization may precipitate bacteremia.

Rarely, patients with bacteremia die in 12 to 24 hr, with high fever, tachycardia, cyanosis, gastrointestinal symptoms, and vascular collapse. More commonly, the disease is slower, with hectic fever and metastatic abscess formation in the skin, bones, kidneys, brain, myocardium, spleen, or other tissues. *Meningitis* is an occasional complication.

Endocarditis occurs in 20 to 60 percent of patients with protracted bacteremia. Normal heart valves are frequently involved. Typically, staphylococcal endocarditis runs an acute course with high fever, progressive anemia, and metastatic abscesses in the skin and deeper structures. Rupture of the valve leaflets and valve ring abscesses are common. Specific diagnosis of endocardial involvement is difficult and because of its frequency, should be assumed to be present in patients with staphylococcal bacteremia with demonstrable cutaneous lesions (petechiae or cutaneous pustules) and a significant heart murmur. Both coagulase-positive and coagulase-negative staphylococci have been a major cause of endocarditis in patients undergoing cardiac surgical procedures, particularly valve replacement, and both coagulase-positive and coagulase-negative staphylococci occasionally produce a subacute endocarditis indistinguishable from that produced by *Streptococcus viridans*. Persistent *Staphylococcus albus* bacteremia has also been common after ventriculoatriostomy. These clinical settings should be remembered when blood cultures are reported as "contaminated" with *S. albus* strains.

Staphylococcal bacteremia is generally accompanied by a polymorphonuclear leukocytosis of 12 to 20,000, but a normal leukocyte count or leukopenia is occasionally seen. Anemia develops rapidly during the course of the illness.

PROGNOSIS. Staphylococcal bacteremia is an extremely serious disease. Prior to the development of antimicrobials, over 80 percent of individuals died, the majority within 10 days of the onset of illness. The development of endocarditis or meningitis during bacteremia was almost invariably fatal. The sulfonamides produced little alteration in this mortality. With the administration of effective antibiotics and appropriate surgical treatment of local sites of infection, 50 to 70 percent of patients survive. However, when staphylococcal endocarditis has occurred on a prosthetic cardiac valve, the outcome has been almost invariably fatal.

STAPHYLOCOCCAL FOOD POISONING

Certain strains of staphylococci produce an enterotoxin which is responsible for many outbreaks of acute gastroenteritis. Foods are commonly contaminated from superficial infections in food handlers or by nasal droplets containing pathogenic staphylococci. Cream-filled pastries, custards, cottage cheese, milk products, or meats subjected to improper refrigeration allowing staphylococcal multiplication are the common offenders.

Symptoms typically appear 1 to 6 hr after ingestion of enterotoxin—contaminated food. Onset is usually abrupt, with severe nausea, vomiting, cramping abdominal pain, diarrhea, and prostration. The disease is brief and requires only rest and sedation. Rare fatalities have occurred in the aged. The diagnosis is based on the short incubation period, the epidemic nature of the disease, the short duration of symptoms, and the lack of fever. The etiology can be established only if specimens of ingested food can be shown to contain large numbers of enterotoxin-producing staphylococci.

STAPHYLOCOCCAL ENTERITIS

Staphylococcal enteritis, a true infection of the gut that sometimes complicates antimicrobial therapy, is described in Chap. 133 and 320.

MISCELLANEOUS INFECTIONS

Staphylococci may cause otitis, sinusitis, or mastoid infections. Certain strains elaborate on erythrogenic toxin that results in a rash indistinguishable from streptococcal scarlet fever. Epidemics of staphylococcal pyoderma in newborn infants and maternal breast abscesses are a recurring problem in maternity units.

THE CURRENT PATTERN OF STAPHYLOCOCCAL INFECTIONS

In prolonging the life span of many patients with serious illnesses, a group of individuals with increased susceptibility to many infections has emerged. These individuals are congregated in the modern hospital. The adrenal steroids, corticotropins, nitrogen mustards, or other cytotoxic chemotherapeutic agents appear to alter host defense mechanisms. Many surgical procedures create portals of entry for microorganisms. The use of broad-spectrum antimicrobials often alters normal host flora, and hospital staff have higher carrier rates of antimicrobial-resistant microorganisms. In this setting, staphylococcal infections (along with gram-negative bacillary infections and certain fungal infections) have become an increasing problem.

Staphylococcal infections now fall into two relatively distinct groups. Individuals who develop infections *outside* the hospital commonly present with the typical acute staphylococcal syndromes already discussed. Individuals who acquire staphylococcal infections *inside* hospitals often develop atypical disease. Staphylococcal pneumonia, formerly rare, now occurs as a terminal complication of many diseases. Postoperative wound infections due to staphylococci have continued to plague major hospital centers. Staphylococcal bacteremia is a common problem, staphylococcal endocarditis is a much-feared complication of cardiac surgery when prostheses are inserted, and staphylococcal enteritis is almost exclusively a hospital disease.

There is little to suggest that staphylococcal strains resistant to antimicrobials are any more invasive than those which have always been prevalent. Nevertheless, the disease states in which staphylococcal infections commonly arise are themselves so severe that staphylococcal infections in these situations continue to have a high mortality.

TREATMENT

FEATURES OF STAPHYLOCOCCAL INFECTION WHICH INFLUENCE THERAPY. While the development of penicillinase-resistant penicillins, cephalosporins, and vancomycin has simplified treatment, certain characteristics of staphylococcal disease should be borne in mind in designing therapy.

1. The host setting in which infection occurs. Acute staphylococcal infections arising outside the hospital in otherwise healthy adults have a better prognosis than intrahospital infections arising in sick individuals with compromised host defense mechanisms.

2. The rapid necrosis of tissues produced by staphylococci. Delays in effective therapy may allow a progressing infection to advance to frank abscess formation. While many antimicrobials reach abscess cavities in adequate concentrations, the physiologic insusceptibility of microorganisms residing in areas of extensive necrosis or suppuration render antibiotic therapy quite ineffective in this situation. Surgical drainage of such lesions is often required.

3. The sluggish response to therapy. Staphylococci are killed slowly by antimicrobials and relapses are frequent. Hence antimicrobial therapy must be continued longer than in many bacterial infections.

4. The problem of antimicrobial resistance. While treatment must be initiated empirically when serious staphylococcal infection is suspected, rational therapy requires that the antibiotic susceptibility of the infecting strain be known.

5. Bactericidal versus bacteriostatic antimicrobials. It is generally believed that the so-called "bactericidal" antimicrobials (the penicillins, cephalosporins, vancomycin, bacitracin) are more effective than the "bacteriostatic" agents (erythromycin, lincomycin, novobiocin, chloramphenicol) in treating serious staphylococcal disease.

TREATMENT OF SERIOUS STAPHYLOCOCCAL INFECTIONS. The increasing incidence of penicillin-resistant strains as a cause of extrahospital infections, coupled with the effectiveness of the penicillinase-resistant penicillins, makes it reasonable to use one regimen for initial therapy for all life-threatening staphylococcal disease no matter where it arises. Two methods of initiating treatment when serious staphylococcal disease is suspected have been proposed.

1. Following appropriate cultures, treatment with large doses of both aqueous penicillin *and* methicillin (or parenteral oxacillin or nafcillin) should be instituted immediately. In adults, aqueous penicillin, 20 million units, should be given by continuous intravenous drip. The companion penicillinase-resistant penicillin can be given intravenously or intramuscularly. Methicillin is rapidly eliminated from the body, and initial doses of at least 2 Gm every 4 hr are indicated. When given intravenously,

this drug should be diluted in 50 to 100 ml of 5 percent dextrose and water and given over a 10- to 30-min period because of its tendency to deteriorate when left in intravenous infusion bottles. Parenteral oxacillin or nafcillin in doses of 1 or 2 Gm every 4 hr can be substituted for methicillin.

If in vitro sensitivity studies show the infecting strain to be sensitive to penicillin G, therapy with methicillin can be discontinued and treatment maintained with aqueous penicillin alone. If the strain is penicillin-resistant, the penicillinase-resistant penicillins alone should be continued, and, if necessary, doses as high as 30 Gm per day can be employed.

The above regimen may be advantageous because penicillin-sensitive strains of staphylococci are twenty- to fiftyfold more susceptible to penicillin G than to methicillin, and it seems reasonable to obtain this advantage from the outset in treating penicillin G–susceptible staphylococcal disease.

2. The other alternative is to use a penicillinase-resistant penicillin alone. All strains of staphylococci are susceptible to penicillinase-resistant penicillins, and because of the high incidence of penicillinase-producing staphylococci as causes of infection, some authorities initiate treatment with methicillin, oxacillin, or nafcillin alone, shifting to aqueous penicillin G if the strain is subsequently proven to be susceptible to that drug.

Despite differences in structure, the major allergenic properties of the penicillins reside in the basic 6-aminopenicillanic acid molecule. There is significant cross allergenicity between penicillins, and patients who have had well-established allergic reactions to penicillin G should not receive penicillinase-resistant penicillins. Further, there is increasing evidence that a significant number of these individuals may be allergic to the cephalosporin derivatives as well. These agents, which are good antistaphylococcal drugs, have a 7-aminocephalosporanic acid nucleus quite similar to that of penicillins.

In dealing with such allergic patients, two courses of action are open. If the use of a penicillin or cephalosporin is deemed imperative, skin testing can be performed with cephalothin and the major and minor penicillin antigens. If the skin tests are negative, therapy can be instituted. If skin tests to the agent of choice are positive, desensitization can be attempted. This procedure is not of established value, however, and the use of vancomycin, an agent which has produced therapeutic results quite comparable to the penicillins, seems preferable.

Cephalothin and cephaloridine are semisynthetic derivatives of cephalosporin C. Cephalothin is highly active against both penicillin-sensitive and penicillin-resistant strains. Cephaloridine appears more susceptible to staphylococcal penicillinase and should not be used in treatment of infections by penicillin-resistant strains unless the organism is shown to be sensitive to it. Intramuscular or intravenous doses of 1.0 to 2.0 Gm cephalothin every 4 hr are recommended; the dose of cephaloridine is limited to 1.0 Gm every 6 hr by regulation.

Vancomycin is uniformly active against coagulase-positive staphylococci regardless of their sensitivity to penicillin. It should be given intravenously in doses of 1.0 to 1.5 Gm over a 30- to 40-min period every 12 hr.

The development of these new agents has relegated several antibiotics formerly used in treatment to minor or secondary roles. These include bacitracin and kanamycin, both bactericidal drugs with good antistaphylococcal activity, and the bacteriostatic drugs erythromycin, chloramphenicol and novobiocin. Despite the fact that many strains of staphylococci remain susceptible to these agents, they appear less effective in treating serious staphylococcal disease.

CHANGES IN THERAPY. Established staphylococcal infections respond slowly even to the most effective antimicrobial regimens, making it difficult to know when therapy should be considered inadequate. Characteristically, 24 to 48 hr elapse before a decline in fever is noted, and recovery is accompanied by slow return of the temperature to normal in 7 to 10 days. If the infection shows evidence of rapid progression during the first 24 to 48 hr of treatment, or if fever remains high for over 96 hr in the absence of detectable abscess formation, dosage levels of the penicillins should be increased. Other antimicrobials may be added, but there is little evidence that this practice is helpful. Treatment should be continued for a minimum of 4 to 6 weeks. If the response appears inadequate or staphylococcal endocarditis is suspected, treatment should be prolonged to 8 weeks to 4 months.

Special Therapeutic Situations

ASYMPTOMATIC NASAL CARRIER STATE. The role of asymptomatic carriers in hospital transmission of infection remains controversial. However, it is generally agreed that hospital personnel who harbor in their anterior nares strains of coagulase-positive staphylococci which are producing intrahospital disease must be removed from nursery units, operating theaters, delivery rooms, and surgical floors. Although no method of treatment has been uniformly satisfactory, the following regimens have had limited success in treatment of nasal carriers.

1. Simple removal from the hospital environment for 3 to 4 weeks
2. Frequent baths with germicidal soaps
3. The use of topical antibiotics of low sensitizing potential in a water soluble base (i.e., bacitracin, neomycin, or a combination of these agents) four to five times daily for 2 weeks.

If the carrier state returns, a second course of treatment is indicated. In infants, colonization with disease-producing strains may be prevented by deliberate implantation of a staphylococcal strain of low virulence. This approach has been applied to adult carriers in a limited way, but evidence regarding its efficacy is not yet available.

SUPERFICIAL INFECTIONS. Superficial infections frequently do not require the use of antibiotics. There is no adequate therapy for recurrent furunculosis, but if the disease is severe, antimicrobial treatment may be attempted. Antibiotics to which the strain is susceptible should be administered systemically for a minimum of 10 to 14 days. Local moist heat, immobilization of the infected part, and incision and drainage should be utilized. The surrounding skin should be protected with a coating of zinc oxide to prevent maceration. Treatment of the nasal carrier state by the local application of topical antibiotics (see above) may be advisable. Careful daily baths with germicidal soaps, attention to personal and family hygiene, and the passage of time appear to be measures most likely to interrupt the process. Attempts to prevent recurrence by autogenous or other vaccines have not proved effective.

EMPYEMA. Empyema should be treated by aspiration. In penicillin G–sensitive infections the installation of 200,000 to 500,000 units of penicillin may be worthwhile. Local instillation of methicillin or oxacillin may be utilized in penicillin G–resistant infection. Loculation and thick exudate may prevent adequate needle drainage. While the local instillation of proteolytic enzymes may occasionally aid in liquefying the exudate, surgical drainage is generally necessary and should be performed promptly.

OSTEOMYELITIS. The initial regimen already outlined for other serious infections is recommended and treatment should be continued for 14 to 28 days. Local drainage of abscess cavities in soft tissues or bones should be considered in all patients in whom therapy is initiated after the third day, when severe pain persists, or when response to antimicrobials is inadequate. If sequestration occurs, devitalized bone should be removed. Lincomycin has been reported to be superior to other agents in the treatment of chronic osteomyelitis, but the evidence for this is not convincing.

NURSERY EPIDEMICS. The hazards of epidemic staphylococcal disease in newborn nurseries are well recognized. Pediatric texts should be consulted for full discussion of the special techniques employed in prevention and management of nursery infections. The use of deliberate colonization of newborns with a staphylococcus of low disease potential to prevent colonization with more pathogenic strains has important biologic implications.

REFERENCES

Elek, S. D.: "Staphylococcus Pyogenes," Edinburgh, E. & S. Livingstone, Ltd., 1959.

Koenig, M. G.: Staphylococcal Infections: Treatment and Control, Disease-a-Month, April, 1968.

Morse, S. L.: The Staphylococci and Other Micrococci, chap. 17 in "Bacterial and Mycotic Infections of Man," 4th ed., R. Dubos & J. Hirsch (Eds.), Philadelphia, J. B. Lippincott Company, 1965.

Nahmias, A. J., and T. C. Eickhoff: Staphylococcal Infections in Hospitals, New Engl. J. Med., 265:74–81, 120–128, 177–182, 1962.

Rogers, D. E.: Staphylococcal Infections, Disease-a-Month, pp. 1–48, April, 1958.

Shinefield, H. R., J. C. Ribble, M. Boris, and H. Eichenwald: Bacterial Interference: Its Effect on Nursery Acquired Infection with Staphylococcus Aureus, Am. J. Dis. Child., 105:646, 1963.

Whipple, H. E. (Ed.): The Staphylococci: Ecologic Perspectives, Ann. N.Y. Acad. Sci., 128:1–456, 1965.

140 HEMOLYTIC STREPTOCOCCAL INFECTIONS

Charles H. Rammelkamp, Jr.

Aerobic streptococci, as a group, are among the most important bacterial pathogens of man. They can invade any tissue or organ and, depending on the site of invasion and the parasite-host relationship, produce different clinical syndromes. Streptococcal infections may be divided into two large groups. The acute and often dramatic illnesses, such as sore throat, scarlet fever, erysipelas, puerperal fever, and lymphangitis, are included in the first group. These infections occur frequently and are characterized by certain toxic, septic, or suppurative features. The second group of diseases have been called the late, nonsuppurative complications of streptococcal infections. These illnesses, which include acute glomerulonephritis and acute rheumatic fever, commonly become manifest 2 and 3 weeks, respectively, after an acute streptococcal infection. They assume major importance because they may be followed by chronic valvular heart disease or possibly by chronic nephritis. Acute glomerulonephritis is covered in Chap. 304, and rheumatic fever in Chap. 269.

HISTORY. Although scarlet fever was recognized in 1676 by Sydenham, rheumatic fever and acute nephritis were not well described until 1805 and 1836, respectively. The role of the streptococcus as the inciting agent of scarlet fever was established in 1924. With the realization that rheumatic fever and nephritis were related to streptococcal infections, methods for the control and management of these complications developed rapidly.

BACTERIOLOGY. Streptococci are gram-positive and tend to form chains. When grown on a sheep blood agar plate, they can be divided into three groups. *Alpha* colonies show a zone of incomplete or green hemolysis; *beta* streptococci exhibit a clear zone of complete hemolysis; and *gamma* streptococci produce no hemolysis. Streaking a culture on a blood agar plate is sufficient to indicate the important pathogenic streptococci, because those exhibiting beta hemolysis are responsible for the majority of infections in man.

On the basis of a specific carbohydrate, 12 groups of streptococci have been identified and designated Lancefield groups A through N. Respiratory infections are caused by group A and only rarely by groups C and G streptococci. Group D streptococcus, previously referred to as *Streptococcus faecalis* or enterococcus, inhabits the gastrointestinal tract and is responsible for infections of the abdominal cavity and the urinary tract.

Group A comprises at least 40 specific types. Typing is determined either by an agglutinin reaction based on the T-substance or by the precipitin test, for which the M-substance is the type-specific antigen.

By grouping and typing streptococci, considerable information has been accumulated concerning streptococcal infections. The carbohydrate responsible for the group characteristics is nontoxic and unassociated with virulence or immunity. In contrast, the M-protein is probably responsible in part for the virulence of the organism as well as for type-specific immunity. Glossy forms of group A streptococci which contain no M-substance are avirulent whereas virulent organisms always contain this specific protein. The T-substance is not related to virulence.

Several substances produced during the growth serve to differentiate these organisms from other streptococci, as well as to explain, in part, their pathogenic effects. The type of hemolysis has been used for classification of these bacteria. Of the various hemolysins produced by streptococci, at least two types have been recognized and termed *streptolysin O* and *streptolysin S*. They are produced by streptococci of Lancefield groups A, C, and G, the three organisms which cause the majority of human infections. The role of these hemolysins in infections in man is not known. Approximately 85 percent of patients develop antistreptolysin O antibody during the second to third week of convalescence, and the determination of the antistreptolysin titers of acute and convalescent serums may establish the diagnosis of a streptococcal infection.

Another filtrable toxin produced by group A streptococci is the erythrogenic or *scarlatinal toxin,* which causes a scarlatiniform rash when injected into man and, if sufficient quantities are given, fever and nausea. That this toxin is responsible for the rash and toxic features of scarlet fever is well established. Trask and Blake were able to demonstrate a toxin in the circulating blood of patients with scarlet fever and showed that it was neutralized by specific antitoxin. Using the erythrogenic toxin as an antigen, a skin test for susceptibility to scarlet fever was developed by the Dicks. When one skin test dose is injected intradermally, persons susceptible to the erythrogenic toxin respond with an area of erythema which reaches its maximum within 24 hr. Persons in whom this skin reaction is positive are susceptible to scarlatiniform rashes when infected by streptococci which produce erythrogenic toxin. The occasional occurrence of second attacks of scarlet fever may be explained by the fact that there are at least two types of immunologically distinct erythrogenic toxins.

In 1933, it was observed that hemolytic streptococci rapidly liquefied human fibrin. The extracellular substance responsible for this action is termed *streptokinase*. Streptokinase does not lyse fibrin directly but activates a serum enzyme, plasminogen, which in turn lyses the clot. Streptokinase is produced by strains of Lancefield groups A, C, and G, and only occasionally in small amounts by groups B and F. The spreading nature of streptococcal infections has been thought to be due to streptokinase which breaks down the fibrin barrier.

Following infection in man by a strain of group A streptococcus which produces large amounts of streptokinase, antibody usually develops which specifically prevents the lysis of fibrin. Measurement of antistreptokinase may aid in diagnosis, but this serologic test is not as useful as the antistreptolysin test because not all group A streptococci produce sufficient streptokinase to stimulate antibody formation.

Streptodornase (deoxyribonuclease) is an enzyme produced by several groups of streptococci. Group A organisms produce three (A, B, and C) immunologically distinct deoxyribonucleases which depolymerize deoxyribonucleoprotein and deoxyribonucleic acid, the two substances which account for the high viscosity of exudates. A preparation of streptokinase-streptodornase (SK-SD) is available for injection into body cavities containing pus or blood and may result in liquefaction of fibrin and cellular debris.

Other substances produced by streptococci are leukocidin, hyaluronidase, and streptococcal proteinase. Leukocidin, which is probably identical with streptolysin O, is able to inhibit phagocytosis in vitro. The enzyme hyaluronidase, or spreading factor, facilitates the spread of bacteria by increasing tissue permeability. It is produced in large quantities by types 4 and 22 of group A streptococci.

ACUTE STREPTOCOCCAL INFECTIONS

Epidemiology

Aerobic streptococcal infections are observed in all races, in both sexes, and at all ages and occur during any season of the year throughout the world. The *incidence* and the *clinical manifestations* are altered by certain of the above factors. For example, streptococcal respiratory infections, including scarlet fever, are encountered especially during the colder months of the year. Scarlet fever is rare in the tropics. Under the age of three months, streptococcal infections are rare and, when they occur, are associated with a high mortality. Between the ages of six months and ten years, scarlet fever occurs frequently. Tonsillitis and pharyngitis are especially prevalent throughout childhood and early adult life. In women during the childbearing period, puerperal infections caused by streptococci occur occasionally. Finally, erysipelas, which may occur at any age, appears to be more prevalent in infants and the older age groups.

Soon after birth, alpha streptococci appear in the upper part of the respiratory tract and may be isolated therefrom throughout life. Streptococci of Lancefield groups C and G and, more rarely, organisms of groups other than A may be isolated from the oropharynx of 5 percent or more of the normal population. Occasionally group C and G streptococci cause tonsillitis.

The group A flora of the oropharynx is made up of many different specific types, but usually several types predominate. In general, at least 5 percent of the people of any community harbor group A streptococci. The prevalance varies and depends upon the cultural methods used as well as upon environmental, host, and bacterial factors. Persons under twenty years of age are most likely to harbor group A streptococci, especially if the tonsils are present.

Following either apparent or inapparent infection, the carrier state usually persists for several months and occasionally for longer periods. Throat cultures, which are inoculated directly on blood agar plates during the first, fourth, eighth, and eleventh weeks following infection, show 10 or more colonies of streptococci in 90, 65, 25, and 10 percent of patients, respectively. Carriers of non-group A streptococci usually show only a few colonies on culture. In addition, as the carrier state progresses, the streptococci lose their ability to produce M-protein, so that by the eleventh week, about 40 percent of strains cannot be typed. Thus, quantitative examination of cultures and typing provide important data regarding the possible duration of the carrier state, and this information is valuable in determining whether or not therapy should be instituted.

Ability to spread disease appears to be an attribute of individuals who have been infected recently. Whether such persons harbor numerous streptococci in the nose and throat or whether the organisms are especially capable of parasitizing another person cannot be determined from the available evidence. It is established that nasal carriers of group A streptococci are likely to spread disease. The spread of streptococci in any population group is related to the degree of exposure, and, during the winter months when people are confined to enclosed areas, and under crowded conditions, dissemination of bacteria is especially likely to occur.

Group A streptococci naturally deposited in dust and on blankets will not produce respiratory infections in man. The evidence implicates the direct mode of transfer as primarily responsible for dissemination of such infections.

Outbreaks of streptococcal infection occasionally occur following the contamination of food. These outbreaks are dramatic because a large number of persons are affected almost simultaneously. Formerly this type of infection was termed *septic sore throat;* except that the infection is caused by a single type of streptococcus, it varies clinically in no way from other streptococcal epidemics.

Primary infection of the upper part of the respiratory tract is undoubtedly the most common form of streptococcal infection in man. It is doubtful whether anyone in the United States escapes one or more of these infections. The disease occurs especially in individuals between the ages of one and twenty years, but it may develop at any age. It is especially prevalent in the temperate zones during the winter and early spring seasons. In most areas the disease is endemic. Epidemics are usually due to one or, at the most, several types of group A streptococci, while many different types are responsible for cases of pharyngitis and tonsillitis occurring sporadically.

Tonsillitis and pharyngitis due to the beta streptococcus are characterized by an acute sore throat which may or may not be accompanied by a cutaneous rash. If a rash is observed, a diagnosis of *scarlet fever* is made. The incidence of scarlet fever has not changed significantly in the past 30 years, but there has been a spectacular decline in mortality. Top reports a fatality rate in Detroit of 2.7 in 1920, 1.3 in 1930, and 0.3 in 1940. The reason for the apparent decreasing severity of scarlet fever is not entirely clear.

Infections of the *paranasal sinuses* and middle ear often develop following infection of the tonsils or pharynx. Not only may they occur as a complication of streptococcal sore throat, but they are also commonly seen following measles, influenza, pertusis, and other respiratory infections.

Bacterial pneumonia caused by aerobic streptococci accounts for less than 5 percent of all cases of pneumonia. The disease is almost invariably caused by group A streptococci and may arise secondarily to an infection of the upper respiratory tract. Epidemics have been observed following influenza and measles. Streptococcal empyema, a complication of pneumonia in most instances, is observed most frequently in patients under thirty years of age.

Formerly it was thought that *erysipelas* was caused by a specific strain of beta-hemolytic streptococcus, but it is now known that group A, C, or G streptococci may be isolated from the skin lesions. Group A organisms are responsible for the majority of infections, and the organisms may belong to any of the various types in this group. Erysipelas tends to occur in the older age groups, especially in those individuals with chronic disabling diseases. Immunity does not develop; in fact, individuals who have had one attack are more susceptible than the normal population. In some of the recurrences, however, the organisms cannot be isolated from the skin lesions but may be found in the oropharynx. In these instances the disease may be due to absorption of some streptococcal toxin, which, in turn, causes the local inflammatory lesion in the skin that has altered its reactivity.

Wounds may be infected by droplet contamination at the time of dressing. *Lymphangitis* may arise from a minute abrasion.

Numerous studies have indicated that either aerobic or anaerobic streptococci cause *puerperal sepsis*, but approximately 70 percent of fatal cases are due to beta-hemolytic streptococci, usually group A. Because the group A streptococcus is rarely isolated from the genital tract either before or after labor, infection probably is contracted from an outside source and occasionally from the respiratory tract of the patient herself.

Pathogenesis

Streptococci gain entrance to the body primarily through the upper respiratory tract. The organisms lodge on the mucous membranes or on other tissues and probably remain viable for relatively short periods unless they actually invade the tissues. They usually gain entrance through the lymphoid tissues of the throat, especially the tonsils. Occasionally the primary infection may be in the paranasal sinuses.

Multiple factors determine whether an infection follows exposure to the organism. The *dosage*, or number of streptococci, is apparently decisive; infection usually results when there is exposure to large numbers of group A streptococci, as occurs in food-borne outbreaks. A second factor is the *virulence* of the organism. Streptococci of groups other than A may be considered relatively avirulent when implanted in the lymphoid tissues of the throat. Whether there is variation in the virulence of group A streptococci according to the specific type is not

known, nor is there much evidence that rapid passage of a given type from man to man increases the virulence of the organisms.

Perhaps as important as the organism itself is the susceptibility of the host. It is stated that a recent or simultaneous infection with one of the common respiratory viruses renders the host more susceptible to bacterial invasion. Experience during World War I indicates that influenza does indeed increase susceptibility to bacterial infections. Whether the common cold or acute respiratory disease acts in a similar fashion is not known.

Whether the group A streptococcus gains a foothold in the tissues is also governed by the immune status of the host, and the presence of type-specific antibodies undoubtedly protects him against infection.

The organisms may invade the bloodstream if the local defense mechanism is not functioning adequately and cause either metastatic infections, such as meningitis, brain abscess, and endocarditis, or a generalized infection, which without treatment almost invariably results in death. In fulminating streptococcal infections the streptococci may be seen in blood vessels throughout the body, as well as in the endothelial cells of the endocardium and in the perivascular areas. There is little cellular reaction around the organisms, but their distribution is similar to that of lesions observed in patients dying several days after onset of the infection, in whom foci of lymphocytes, plasma cells, and histiocytes commonly are found in the heart, especially just under the surface endothelium, and endocardium. Occasionally some of the foci show polymorphonuclear leukocytes. In the kidneys, there are focal areas of round-cell infiltration in the tissue surrounding the tubules, glomeruli, and blood vessels. Similar lesions may be observed in other organs.

Most streptococcal infections are of short duration, and the acute phase ends within 5 to 7 days. The exact mechanism for recovery at this time has not been defined, but, as in other bacterial infections, it is assumed that antibodies develop which aid in the destruction of the organism.

Acute Tonsillitis, Pharyngitis, and Scarlet Fever

The terminology used to classify streptococcal infections of the upper respiratory tract was introduced before it was realized that *scarlet fever, septic sore throat, acute tonsillitis,* and *pharyngitis* with or without exudate were all caused by any of the numerous types of group A streptococci. In these diseases the organism establishes itself in the lymphoid tissue; *streptococcal lymphoiditis* might well be substituted for the above names.

SYMPTOMS. The incubation period varies from 1 to 10 days but is usually 3 to 5 days. The illness begins abruptly with symptoms of feverishness, chilliness, headache, and sore throat. Nausea and vomiting are especially common in children. A few patients complain of diarrhea. Within a period of 24 to 48 hr the disease reaches its maximum intensity. Chilliness is a constant symptom, but true rigors are rare. Approximately 75 percent or more of the patients complain of headache, malaise, and loss of appetite.

Sore throat is almost constantly present within 24 hr of onset. The soreness is aggravated by swallowing and may be referred to the neck, so that even turning of the head is accompanied by pain. Nasal obstruction and discharge are minor complaints but occur in 60 percent of patients. About half the patients develop very mild symptoms referable to the lower part of the respiratory tract, including cough and hoarseness. The cough is not productive and is rarely associated with chest pain. Loss of voice due to laryngitis does not occur. Earache is common and may last a few hours to several days. Occasionally, epistaxis is observed.

During the period of maximum temperature there may be a diffuse blush of the skin. In some cases it becomes more pronounced, and a diagnosis of *scarlet fever* is made. The rash appears 1 to 5 days after onset of illness and is first noticed over the neck and upper part of the chest. It spreads rapidly to include the skin over the abdomen and upper and lower extremities. The face appears flushed, and circumoral pallor is prominent. Itching occasionally occurs but is rarely severe.

PHYSICAL SIGNS. The degree of prostration varies, but the majority of patients appear mildly or moderately ill. The temperature is usually elevated to 102 to 104°F; occasionally it may be as high as 106°F. A few patients

have no fever. In children the pulse rate is between 140 and 160, in adults between 120 and 140 per min.

Various degrees of diffuse redness of the mucous membranes of the posterior pharynx, faucial tonsils, and soft palate are invariably present. The uvula is frequently edematous, as are the tonsils and pharynx. Lymphoid hyperplasia and edema give the posterior pharynx a cobblestone appearance. Characteristically there is discrete to confluent exudate on the tonsils, and variable numbers of pinhead-size areas of exudate appear on the pharynx. In severely ill patients these are seldom seen, because nasal secretions cover the posterior wall. The exudate is often yellow, sometimes gray or white, and is relatively easily removed by swabbing. In about 20 percent of adults, and more frequently in infants, exudative lesions on the mucous membranes do not develop. If sinusitis and rhinitis are present there is a thick mucopurulent nasal discharge which may be tinged with blood. In children the nares may be excoriated. The cervical lymph nodes are swollen and frequently tender. The lymph nodes just below the angle of the jaw are the first to enlarge; rarely they attain such size that the head is thrown back. Marked adenopathy is frequently followed by suppuration.

In those patients with *scarlet fever* the signs include both an enanthem and an exanthem. The appearance of the throat is similar to that seen in tonsillitis and pharyngitis without rash, except that diffuse redness is more intense and has been described as "boiled-lobster" red. There may be punctate redness of the soft and hard palate. The buccal mucous membranes appear red and swollen, as do the lips. About the second to fifth day, small milk-white patches may be seen on the buccal mucous membranes. They represent desquamation of the epithelium and are easily peeled off.

Early in the course of the infection the tongue is heavily coated and grayish. Soon the tip and edges become an angry red. Fungiform papillae become swollen and emerge through the gray surface of the tongue. By the fourth to fifth day there is complete lingual desquamation, which leaves multiple papillary elevations, the so-called "strawberry tongue."

The color of the exanthem varies and has been described as scarlet, bright red, rose-colored, or dull, dusky red. At a distance there appears to be a uniform blush, but upon close inspection innumerable small reddish points are seen. Because of pinpoint elevations at the site of the hair follicles, the skin may feel like sandpaper. This sign is of special importance in races where the skin is heavily pigmented. When the eruption is intense, there may be many small miliary vesicles over the chest and abdomen. The face may be free of rash, but ordinarily the temples and cheeks are deep red, leaving an area of pallor around the mouth and nose. The rash is due to hyperemia, and pressure causes it to fade. In some areas there may be punctate hemorrhages which do not fade; these are commonly seen in the creases at the elbow flexure (Pastia's sign), groin, and axillary folds.

COURSE OF ILLNESS (Fig. 140-1). The majority of upper respiratory illnesses caused by group A streptococci are

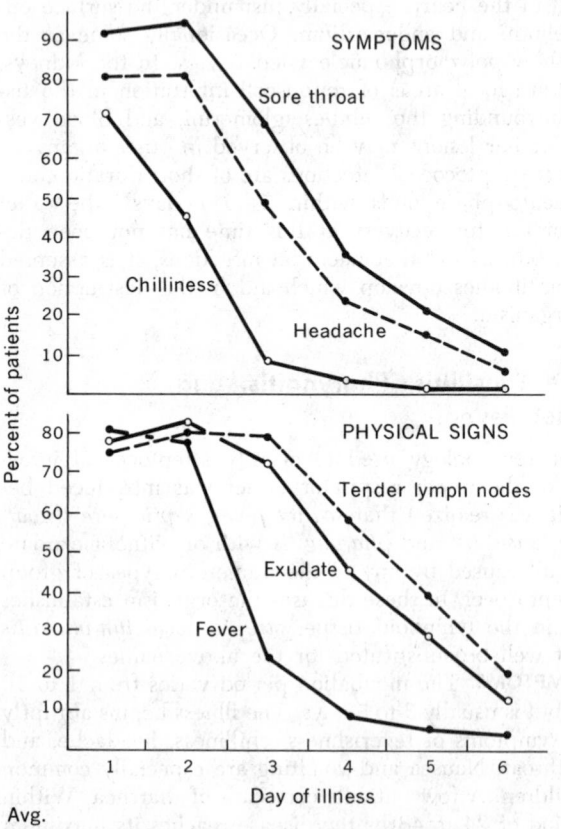

Avg.
WBC· 14,500 14,250 12,300 10,700

Fig. 140-1. The natural course of group A streptococcal tonsillitis.

self-limited. In adults the temperature usually returns to normal by the third to fourth day; in children fever may persist for 5 to 9 days. The temperature curve is not characteristic, although there is usually a slight morning remission. In patients with scarlet fever the temperature remains elevated until the rash has reached its maximum intensity. Fever may last for several weeks, but in such instances it is well to search for some suppurative complications. The constitutional symptoms, as well as the localizing symptom of sore throat, usually disappear shortly after the fever subsides.

The edema, redness, and exudate disappear rapidly, and except for a few small isolated spots of exudate and a slight degree of redness, the throat appears normal shortly after the fever subsides. The lymphoid tissues of the posterior pharynx as well as the tonsils decrease in size and by the third to sixth week appear to be normal. The lymph nodes may not return to normal size for 6 weeks.

When rash does occur, it usually makes its appearance on the second day, reaches its maximum intensity shortly thereafter, and then begins to fade. The exfoliation of the epithelium begins during the decline of the eruption and is seen first in those areas where the rash originally appeared. By the sixth to seventh day it is more or less generalized. On the hands and feet the skin sheds in flakes or, more rarely, as an entire cast of the hand or foot. The skin in these areas becomes dry, hard, and wrinkled. The most typical form of desquamation is seen beneath the free edge of the fingernails. A fissure appears under the edge of the nail and then widens, revealing the soft, pinkish underlying skin.

LABORATORY FINDINGS. In 80 percent of patients the total leukocyte count is increased. During the first 2 days of disease the average count is 14,000, and as the illness progresses, it returns to normal values. If the number of leukocytes remains elevated after 1 week, evidence of a complication may be found. During the first 2 days of illness eosinophils are rarely seen, but convalescence is characterized by an increase of these cells. Patients with scarlet fever are especially likely to have eosinophilia. Not frequently a trace of albumin may be found in the urine during the acute phase of the illness, and rarely, such specimens show a few red cells or casts. Proteinuria during the first 5 days of illness is transient and is not attended by serious sequelae.

DIAGNOSIS. Important features in the diagnosis of streptococcal pharyngitis and tonsillitis are the history of an acute onset of soreness on swallowing, associated with feverishness and other constitutional symptoms. The physical signs of diffuse redness and edema of the mucous membranes of the oropharynx, tonsils, and soft palate, the presence of discrete to confluent exudate, and the enlargement and tenderness of the lymph nodes at the angle of the jaw are especially helpful. These findings, together with a leukocyte count of at least 12,000, suggest a streptococcal infection. If the culture of the local lesion shows a predominant growth of beta streptococci, the diagnosis is established with certainty. When only a few colonies grow on the blood agar plate, it is

impossible to be sure whether the patient is a carrier or actually has an infection due to the streptococcus. In such cases it is of considerable help to obtain acute and convalescent blood specimens for determination of antistreptolysin titers.

When a rash is associated with the above clinical and laboratory findings, the diagnosis is scarlet fever. Confirmation is obtained if the skin desquamates.

DIFFERENTIAL DIAGNOSIS OF SORE THROAT. *Nonbacterial exudative tonsillitis and pharyngitis* must be differentiated from streptococcal infections of the oropharynx (Chap. 206). Adenoviruses will produce respiratory infections associated with exudate lesions, and in some outbreaks there is involvement of the conjunctiva. In general the onset of illness is not rapid, sore throat is seldom marked, and constitutional symptoms are mild. Hoarseness and cough are likely to occur several days after the onset. The exudate is rarely confluent. The lymph nodes may be slightly enlarged, but are not remarkably tender.

The leukocyte count is usually normal, although in a few cases it may be slightly elevated. Cultures of the throat fail to show beta-hemolytic streptococci. Occasionally a few streptococci are recovered, but these organisms usually belong to groups other than A and occur only in small numbers.

Infectious mononucleosis is most frequently observed in young adults and, because of the local reaction in the throat, is likely to be confused with streptococcal pharyngitis (Chap. 255). The onset may be insidious, and malaise is prominent. Sore throat with exudative lesions of the tonsils is observed in over half the cases. Fever is more prolonged than is usual in streptococcal infections. Lymph node enlargement is more generalized, but suppuration is not observed. The spleen may be palpable. In 10 to 15 percent of cases a fleeting skin rash occurs, which may be identical with that seen in scarlet fever. The blood changes are characteristic, and a positive heterophil antibody test is usually obtained.

Vincent's angina (Chap. 168) is not easily confused with streptococcal infections. The disease is characterized by insidious onset without constitutional symptoms. Fever is rare. The area surrounding the exudate shows little inflammatory reaction, generally only one tonsil is involved, and cervical adenopathy is usually unilateral.

In contrast to streptococcal pharyngitis, the onset of *diphtheria* is rarely sudden and the symptoms are not severe (Chap. 169). Sore throat is not a constant feature of the disease. The exudate is smooth and cream-colored and appears to be incorporated in the mucous membranes. The membrane is removed with difficulty, leaving a bleeding bed. Cutaneous rashes are absent. Cultures show *Corynebacterium diphtheriae*.

In patients with a rash, the disease must be differentiated from *rubella* (Chap. 221) and *rubeola* (Chap. 220). In German measles the posterior cervical lymph node enlargement is helpful, as well as the fact that the rash tends to be macular and discrete. The tongue never peels, and a leukopenia is characteristic. In measles there are prodromal respiratory symptoms, and the maculopapular rash occurs chiefly on the face and neck. The presence of Koplik's spots aids in establishing the diagnosis.

Streptococcal infections without exudate or a cutaneous rash must be differentiated from *influenza virus infection* (Chap. 208) and *common respiratory diseases* (Chap. 206). In general, this differentiation cannot be made on clinical evidence alone, and the leukocyte count, culture studies, and serologic tests must be employed.

Primary *herpes simplex pharyngitis* (Chap. 226) and *herpangina* (Chap. 210) are characterized by vesicles which rupture and produce small ulcers covered with exudate. Herpetic lesions are scattered over all mucous membranes of the mouth, and the kissing ulcer under the tip of the tongue is typical. The ulcers of herpangina, caused by Coxsackie A viruses, are observed on the anterior pillars and the soft palate. In both diseases the leukocyte count is usually normal.

Sinusitis, Otitis Media, Mastoiditis, and Peritonsillar Abscess

Infection of the paranasal sinuses probably occurs to a minor degree in all patients with streptococcal respiratory infections. Sinusitis and otitis media presenting overt clinical signs develop in approximately 3 percent of patients whose tonsils and adenoids are intact. Mastoiditis is observed in less than 1 percent of patients. Peritonsillar cellulitis is observed in 2.5 percent of patients with tonsils, but it rarely occurs in those whose tonsils have been removed or in those patients who receive proper therapy with antibiotics. The diagnosis and management of these suppurative complications are described in Chap. 282.

Pneumonia and Empyema

The natural course of pneumonia caused by Lancefield group A streptococci is extremely variable, probably because in many instances it is secondary to such infections as influenza, tonsillitis, measles, and erysipelas. It may occur as the sole manifestation of streptococcal infection or may arise as a metastatic complication of streptococcal bacteremia. Although it is not a common complication of streptococcal sore throat, about 25 percent of cases follow this infection. Characteristically, this organism produces an interstitial or confluent pneumonia. The reported mortality rate varies from 15 to 60 percent.

The onset of pneumonia may be abrupt, with such constitutional symptoms as chills, feverishness, anorexia, and vomiting. Symptoms include cough, expectoration of purulent sputum, and chest pain. The pulse and respiratory rates are increased, and cyanosis may be prominent. The temperature tends to be high (104°F), and the fever is intermittent. Examination reveals local signs of pneumonia, with scattered fine rales and occasional areas of dullness. Frank signs of lobar consolidation are rare.

The leukocyte count is almost invariably elevated to 20,000 to 30,000, and the sputum is found to contain large numbers of group A organisms. Usually the blood cultures are sterile; when bacteremia occurs, the prognosis is poor.

The untreated disease runs a variable course. In most instances recovery is delayed for several weeks, and lung abscess and bronchiectasis are not uncommon complications. In fatal cases mediastinitis and pericarditis may occur. The most frequent complication is empyema, which occurs in 20 percent of the cases.

Streptococcal *empyema* is usually secondary to pneumonia caused by the same organism, but occasionally arises following other infections of the lung, infarcts, or lung tumors. The mortality rate in untreated cases is high. Early in the disease the pleural fluid may be hemorrhagic, and it becomes thick and purulent slowly, in contrast to the exudate seen in pneumococcal empyema.

Pericarditis, Arthritis, Peritonitis, and Meningitis

Streptococcal infections of the various body cavities result from bacteremia or from extension from a local lesion. *Pericarditis,* a rare complication, is especially likely to occur during the course of pneumonia or empyema. The diagnosis is difficult, because the symptoms arising from pericarditis are overshadowed by the primary disease. The first sign may be a sudden increase in pulse rate and the development of an audible pericardial friction rub.

Suppurative arthritis is secondary to bacteremia or to extension of a local cellulitis. It is a rare complication of streptococcal sore throat. Pain is the most common symptom, and usually only one joint is involved. The pain is first noticed on motion, but within a short period redness, swelling, and tenderness develop and the pain becomes intense. Aspiration reveals a fluid containing polymorphonuclear leukocytes and streptococci. Nonsuppurative arthritis seen in patients with scarlet fever during the first week of illness indicates the onset of rheumatic fever and should not be considered a manifestation of erythrogenic toxin.

Infection of the peritoneum with the hemolytic streptococcus is rare but is especially apt to be associated with such local infections as erysipelas and scarlet fever. In these cases the organism belongs to Lancefield group A. Symptoms develop rapidly, and in addition to fever and other constitutional symptoms, prostration, abdominal pain, and vomiting are prominent. The pulse is rapid and weak. The abdomen is distended, tender, and rigid to palpation.

Streptococcal *meningitis* is usually caused by group A organisms, but occasionally members of other groups may be isolated from the spinal fluid. In most instances the meningitis arises by extension from otitis media, mastoiditis, or petrositis, which are especially likely to develop following infection of the respiratory tract and are seen most frequently in the young. Prior to the introduction of specific therapy these infections were always fatal. The symptoms are not distinguishable from those of other types of bacterial meningitis. All patients, especially infants, with infections of the middle ear should be watched for signs of meningeal irritation.

Wound and Skin Infections, Lymphangitis, Puerperal Fever, and Erysipelas

Wound and skin infections are usually the result of contamination. Children with chickenpox, impetigo, and other skin lesions may become infected with group A and C streptococci. *Impetigo* caused by group A streptococci is sometimes followed by acute nephritis.

Hemolytic streptococci are responsible for the majority of cases of *lymphangitis*, characterized by the rapid development of one or more fine red streaks extending upward from the hand or foot. Usually the process continues up to the axilla or groin, and the lymph nodes in these areas become enlarged and tender. Associated with the spread of the infection in the lymphatics, such symptoms as rigor, fever, malaise, headache, and vomiting occur. Occasionally the bloodstream is invaded. The original site of infection in these cases of lymphangitis may not be apparent. Although these infections may be serious, the course of the illness is usually short, and suppuration along the course of the lymphatics seldom occurs. Within 2 weeks after a streptococcal respiratory infection, some children develop persistent *lymphadenitis*. In children with enlarged cervical nodes 75 percent of the cases are secondary to a streptococcal infection. In these patients aspiration of the node will usually reveal the organism.

Puerperal infections caused by hemolytic streptococci are always serious. Following abortion or delivery, the streptococci invade the endometrium and lymphatics. The infection may spread to the surrounding structures, producing cellulitis, phlebitis, abscess, peritonitis, or bacteremia. The patient develops a high irregular fever associated with rigors. The pulse is rapid. The diagnosis is based on local signs of infection as well as on such laboratory findings as leukocytosis and isolation of streptococci from the bloodstream or from the cervical discharge.

Erysipelas is an acute streptococcal infection of the skin and, to a lesser extent, of the mucous membranes. The onset is usually abrupt, after an incubation period of 1 to 4 days. A history of preceding respiratory infection is sometimes obtained. The initial symptoms include chilliness, feverishness, headache, malaise, anorexia, and vomiting. At the onset the local cutaneous lesion may not be apparent. The skin may itch and feel sore around the point of entry of the organisms. Within a few hours, the cutaneous lesion becomes obvious.

The face is most commonly involved, but any area of the body may be infected. The point of entry may be just anterior to the ear, at the inner canthus of the eye, around the lips and nose, or over the cheeks. From these points the lesion spreads rapidly, reaching its maximum extent within 3 to 6 days. Erysipelas frequently involves the butterfly area of the cheeks and nose. The lesion consists of an advancing border which is raised from the surrounding normal skin and may be purple. Within this border the skin is tense and usually a dark dull red. If the infection occurs in areas where the skin is lax, such as around the eyes, edema is pronounced. The eyelids frequently become so swollen that they cannot be opened. Blebs or necrotic areas may appear as the disease progresses.

At the height of the infection the temperature is usually high (104 to 105°F), although occasionally the febrile response is slight. The bloodstream is not uncommonly invaded during this period. In most instances recovery is apparent by the sixth to seventh day. The local lesion begins to fade in the center, with some desquamation and pigmentation. No scarring results unless abscesses develop.

Before the introduction of chemotherapy, the fatality rate was about 15 percent. During the first 6 months of life approximately 65 percent of patients die, while in older children and young adults the death rate is low. In patients with fatal infections the lesion is likely to involve the trunk.

Bacteremia

Streptococci are a common cause of bacteremia, but in uncomplicated tonsillitis and pharyngitis the organisms rarely invade the bloodstream. Bacteremia occurring under the age of twenty usually is secondary to otitis media, mastoiditis, or thrombosis of the lateral or cavernous sinuses. In adults, invasion of the bloodstream is especially likely to occur in puerperal infections, whereas after the age of forty bacteremia is usually secondary to cellulitis and erysipelas. Metastatic abscesses are infrequent.

The diagnosis of bacteremia is difficult and can be made only by culturing the organisms from the blood. The sudden development of chills and high fever suggests invasion of the bloodstream. There may be arthritis, signs of pneumonia, petechiae, or skin eruptions. In fulminating cases, anemia develops rapidly and jaundice may occur. Without specific therapy the mortality rate is 70 percent.

Treatment

There are now several agents which may be employed in the therapy of aerobic streptococcal infections. The sulfonamides exert a bacteriostatic effect against all Lancefield groups except D. However, some strains of group A streptococci have acquired resistance. Most antibiotics have some antistreptococcal activity, but penicillin clearly is the best antistreptococcal drug because it kills group A organisms. If it is administered for at least 10 days, in most instances all streptococci are eliminated. Therapeutic measures which do not result in the eradication of the infecting organism do not alter the attack rate of rheumatic fever.

The administration of penicillin or other antibiotics

within 24 hr of the onset of streptococcal respiratory infections results in definite improvement of the symptoms and signs. When therapy is instituted after 48 hr, a favorable effect is difficult to demonstrate, but suppurative complications, including sinusitis, otitis media, and peritonsillar cellulitis are prevented. The time that treatment is started is not decisive in the reduction of rheumatic fever; however, early therapy may be important in the prevention of nephritis. In general, proper therapy instituted during the first 24 hr of illness will reduce the predicted rheumatic fever attack rate by 95 to 98 percent. If therapy is started 1, 2, or 3 weeks after the onset of sore throat, the reduction in attack rates is 90, 67, and 42 percent, respectively. Therefore to prevent rheumatic fever, a full course of therapy should be given to those individuals who have recovered from acute phase symptoms and received no therapy even though the onset was 3 weeks previously.

In the average case of streptococcal infection, whether scarlet fever, tonsillitis, or erysipelas, sufficient concentration of antibiotic can be maintained readily by a single injection of 600,000 to 1,200,000 units of benzathine penicillin. In patients with rheumatic heart disease who develop a streptococcal infection, it is advisable to administer 600,000 units of procaine penicillin twice daily for 2 weeks.

Oral therapy may be prescribed, but many patients discontinue the medication when the acute symptoms subside. Under these circumstances, the organism frequently invades the tissues again, and a clinical relapse occurs. More important, the attack rate of the nonsuppurative complications is not altered. All forms of oral medication must be taken in full doses for at least 10 days and preferably for 2 weeks. Oral penicillin G should be given in doses of at least 250,000 units four times daily. Penicillin V in dosage of 1 to 2 Gm daily or phenethicillin may be preferable because these agents resist degradation by gastric acid. Patients sensitive to penicillin may be given erythromycin in doses of 0.25 Gm every 6 hr. Tetracycline drugs should not be employed because of the high prevalence of resistant strains.

The *sulfonamides* should never be employed in the treatment of streptococcal infections because they fail to eliminate the infecting organism and do not alter the subsequent attack rate of rheumatic fever. Penicillin troches or sprays have little effect on the local inflammatory lesion or on the infecting organism. Penicillin appears to decrease the incidence of suppurative complications of tonsillitis and pharyngitis.

Infections of the mastoid and paranasal sinuses should be treated by the parenteral administration of 1.2 to 2.4 million units penicillin G every day. Streptococcal pneumonia should be treated with somewhat larger amounts of penicillin. Empyema, purulent pericarditis, and arthritis are treated best by local instillation of 10,000 to 50,000 units penicillin G every 48 to 72 hr until cultures are sterile. In addition, full doses of parenteral penicillin should be administered. In these infections early treatment is required if surgical drainage is to be avoided.

Prevention

There is no completely adequate method for the prevention of streptococcal infections. A number of procedures will limit the spread of the organism. The problem is exceedingly complicated because group A streptococci occur in the upper part of the respiratory tract of many individuals.

In the past it was customary to isolate all patients with scarlet fever, but this seems unwarranted, particularly because no precautions are taken for sore throat without a rash caused by the same bacterium. Any patient with a streptococcal infection of the upper respiratory tract may be a source of infection. During the acute stage of all such illnesses the patient should be advised against intimate contact with others.

Approximately 90 percent of patients with streptococcal infections continue to carry the organism in the pharynx 3 months after the acute infection. Usually the number of organisms is small. Individuals with suppurative sinusitis are likely to harbor large numbers of streptococci and are a dangerous source of infection. Proper therapy of acute infections with penicillin prevents the development of the carrier state and promptly eliminates the organism.

Individuals or groups can be protected from streptococcal infections by the prophylactic use of sulfonamides. For this purpose 1 Gm sulfadiazine or sulfisoxazole is administered daily. When given to populations already experiencing an epidemic, this prophylactic measure will control the outbreak as long as the drug is administered. When therapy is discontinued, streptococcal infections again occur because of the failure of sulfonamides to eliminate the infecting organism. For this reason, oral penicillin in doses of 250,000 units two or three times daily for 10 days or a single injection of 1,200,000 units of benzathine penicillin is a preferred form of prophylaxis in large groups. Benzathine penicillin in doses of 600,000 and 1,200,000 units will protect the individual from new infections for 3 or 4 to 6 weeks, respectively.

Tonsillectomy has been employed widely as a prophylactic measure against streptococcal infections because tonsillitis cannot occur if the organ is removed. However, no protection is afforded against streptococcal pharyngitis. Indeed, tonsillectomy makes subsequent recognition of the cause of the respiratory illness more difficult.

Many attempts have been made to control respiratory disease by altering certain environmental factors, by using ultraviolet light, aerosols, and various dust-holding procedures, and by treating bed clothing with oils. It has been demonstrated that these methods decrease the contamination of the air, but their effectiveness in preventing infection is slight.

REFERENCES

Dajani, A. S., R. E. Garcia, and E. Wolinsky: Etiology of Cervical Lymphadenitis in Children, New Engl. J. Med., 268:1329, 1963.

Denny, F. W., L. W. Wannamaker, and E. O. Hahn: Comparative Effects of Penicillin, Aureomycin and Terramycin on Streptococcal Tonsillitis and Pharyngitis, Pediatrics, 2:7, 1953.

Rammelkamp, C. H., Jr.: Epidemiology of Streptococcal Infections, Harvey Lectures, 51:113, 1957.

—— and B. L. Stolzer: The Latent Period before the Onset of Acute Rheumatic Fever, Yale J. Biol. Med., 34:386, 1961–62.

141 OTHER STREPTOCOCCAL INFECTIONS

Leighton E. Cluff

Group A streptococci account for the majority of streptococcal infections in man. Group C, D, and G streptococci, identifiable by antigenically different cell wall C polysaccharides, have also been identified as occasional causes of human infection. Other streptococci, including *Streptococcus viridans* and *anaerobic streptococci*, not characterized antigenically, also cause infection in human beings. Many of these streptococci are indigenous to the respiratory, genital, or gastrointestinal tract. They are commonly opportunistic and produce infection particularly in patients with reduced natural resistance. Contrasted with group A streptococci, these other streptococcal infections are not followed by late consequences such as rheumatic fever and glomerulonephritis.

Streptococci other than group A may or may not produce hemolysis when cultured on blood agar. Certain strains of *groups C and D* are nonhemolytic; others cause beta or complete hemolysis. Strains of *S. viridans* are usually alpha-hemolytic, producing a green zone about colonies on blood agar. Some strains of *S. viridans*, however, are nonhemolytic (gamma). *Group D streptococci* also may cause alpha hemolysis.

Streptococci of all types characteristically grow in chains, but under certain culture conditions and in clinical specimens they may be found in clusters or pairs of gram-positive cocci.

Group C strains have a low pathogenicity for man. They may be isolated from the normal respiratory tract but have been associated with acute pharyngitis, sinusitis, and rarely bacteremia. *Group G streptococci* also have been isolated from the normal nasopharynx but have produced tonsillitis, endocarditis, and urinary tract infections in man.

The prevalence of streptococci other than group A in the normal oropharynx, genital mucosa, and gastrointestinal tract complicates the problem of relating them specifically to disease. Identification of the organisms in pure culture or from pus, blood, or urine, however, is indicative of their pathogenicity.

STREPTOCOCCUS VIRIDANS. These bacteria are occasionally called alpha, or green, streptococci. Streptococci other than strains belonging to this group, however, may cause alpha, or green, hemolysis on blood agar. *Streptococcus viridans* is most commonly confused on culture with pneumococci. In some instances these bacteria are differentiated into strains referred to as *S. mitis* and *S. salivarius*. For practical purposes, however, these bacteria may be considered the same. *Streptococcus viridans* is important largely as a cause of subacute bacterial endocarditis (Chap. 137), but it has been associated with "mixed" pulmonary infections and sinusitis. It is a part of the normal bacterial population of the oropharynx. These bacteria are usually sensitive to penicillin. Some strains of oropharyngeal *S. viridans* in persons receiving penicillin prophylaxis for rheumatic fever may become resistant to penicillin, but this has not yet presented a serious problem in management of patients with bacterial endocarditis.

GROUP D STREPTOCOCCI. These bacteria possess group-specific C polysaccharide and are frequently designated as *enterococcus* or *Streptococcus faecalis*. These microorganisms are characterized by their ability to grow in 6.5 percent NaCl and to reduce methylene blue. Many strains cause alpha hemolysis and for this reason may be confused with *S. viridans*. Group D streptococci are often resistant to, or acquire resistance to, penicillin. They are of greatest importance as causes of urinary tract infection, purulent infection involving the peritoneal cavity, and bacterial endocarditis. The presence of the bacteria in the normal gastrointestinal tract and on the genitalia is significant in their relationship to both these infections. Bacterial endocarditis due to group D streptococci is commonest in elderly men with prostatism and in women with valvular heart disease following abortion. Urinary tract infection develops usually in persons with recurrent or chronic pyelonephritis or in persons with structurally abnormal urinary tracts. Septic endometritis and parametritis following abortion or prolonged and difficult labor have been associated with group D streptococcal infection, usually in combination with other microorganisms.

Administration of penicillin G or ampicillin combined with streptomycin is the preferred treatment of group D streptococcal infection. However, many strains are sensitive to the tetracyclines, erythromycin, and vancomycin (Chap. 135), and these agents have been effective in many clinical situations.

ANAEROBIC STREPTOCOCCI. Among the body's normal inhabitants are many streptococci that cannot be cultured at atmospheric concentrations of oxygen, although most of them are not obligate anaerobes and are properly termed microaerophilic. They are often found in exudates with other organisms, especially *Bacteroides*, coliform bacilli, and clostridial species.

They infect soft-tissue wounds and compound fractures, sometimes producing a crepitant myositis that resembles clostridial gas gangrene (Chap. 172). Post-abortal and puerperal sepsis with pelvic thrombophlebitis and septic pulmonary infarcts, peritonitis, empyema, abscesses of the lung, liver, and brain, perirectal abscesses, mastoiditis, dental infections, and wounds produced by human bites are the most frequent lesions from which anaerobic streptococci are isolated in pure or mixed cultures.

Certain characteristics of anaerobic streptococcal infections are distinct enough to arouse strong suspicion clinically. They cause the production of copious amounts of brown thin pus. Gas-producing infections in wounds may mimic clostridial gangrene. The pus, lochia in uterine infection, and breath of patients with lung abscess attributable to group D streptococcal infection possess a penetrating, overwhelmingly foul odor. The fetor often ascribed to colon bacillus exudates is a result of the concomitant presence of anaerobic streptococci or *Bacteroides* bacilli. Some strains (*Streptococcus foetidus*) are sometimes recognizable in stained smears by the tendency to grow in parallel chains; others (*S. parvulus*) produce black pigment on agar plates.

Patients with empyema caused by anaerobic streptococci often develop painful areas of cellulitis around the site of thoracentesis needle punctures; this is rare in other empyemas.

Two more or less distinct clinical entities have been attributed to anaerobic streptococci: *burrowing ulcer* and *progressive bacterial synergistic gangrene*. Both are unusual but sufficiently characteristic to be recognized by inspection. Burrowing ulcer occurs on the trunk or extremities and consists of a ragged ulceration from which necrotic sinuses extend subcutaneously, occasionally breaking through to the surface. The process is chronic and is accompanied by pain, fever, and emaciation; occasionally death occurs from necrosis of a major blood vessel. It does not attack muscle, and stops at the fascial layer. Anaerobic streptococci in pure culture are usually obtained from the exudate. Progressive bacterial synergistic gangrene usually complicates surgical operations on the abdomen and consists of progressive spreading ulceration, often around a stay suture. It is caused by a mixture of *Staphylococcus aureus* and anaerobic streptococci. The lesion is discolored, with a gangrenous granulating center.

Surgical drainage and debridement are important in the management of anaerobic streptococcal infections. Penicillin and its analogues in large doses are the drugs of choice; tetracyclines, erythromycin, and vancomycin may be effective in certain cases.

REFERENCES

Evan, A. C., and A. L. Chinn: The Enterococci: With Special Reference to Their Association with Human Disease, J. Bacteriol., 54:495, 1947.

Feingold, D. S., N. L. Stagg, and L. J. Kunz: Extrarespiratory Streptococcal Infections: Importance of the Various Serologic Groups, New Engl. J. Med., 275:356, 1966.

Fisher, A. M., and T. J. Abernathy: Putrid Empyema with Special Reference to Anaerobic Streptococci, Arch. Intern. Med., 54:552, 1934.

Heineman, H. S., and A. I. Braude: Anaerobic Infection of the Brain: Observations on 18 Consecutive Cases of Brain Abscess, Am. J. Med., 35:682, 1963.

Rantz, L. A., and W. M. M. Kirby: Enterococcic Infections, Arch. Intern. Med., 71:516, 1943.

Reinarz, J. A., and J. P. Sanford: Human Infections Caused by Non-group A or D Streptococci, Medicine, 44:81, 1965.

Reynolds, R. C., F. I. Catlin, and L. E. Cluff: Bacteriology and Antibiotic Treatment of Acute Maxillary Sinusitis, Bull. Johns Hopkins Hosp., 114:269, 1964.

Smith, L. D. S.: "Introduction to the Pathogenic Anaerobes," Chicago, University of Chicago Press, 1955.

Section 4

Diseases Caused by Gram-negative Cocci

142 MENINGOCOCCAL INFECTIONS

Harry N. Beaty and
Robert G. Petersdorf

DEFINITION. Meningococcal infections are defined as the varied manifestations which result from entry of meningococci into man. Characteristically, these organisms infect the nasopharynx of many individuals, but produce illness in only a few. Serious meningococcal disease occurs when there is invasion of the bloodstream and development of meningitis or fulminating bacteremia with circulatory collapse and death.

ETIOLOGY. The organism responsible for "cerebrospinal fever" was first described by Weichselbaum in 1887. It was subsequently assigned to the genus *Neisseria*, and is now designated by the binomial *Neisseria meningitidis* and the common name meningococcus. In stained smears, meningococci are gram-negative and characteristically appear as single cocci or diplococci with flattened adjacent sides. They grow well on solid or semisolid media containing blood, serum, or ascitic fluid, and thrive best at temperatures between 35 and 37°C in an atmosphere reduced in oxygen and containing 5 to 10 percent CO_2. The organism is recovered readily from biologic fluids when fresh specimens are inoculated on warm chocolate agar plates which are incubated 18 to 24 hr in a candle jar or in a more sophisticated apparatus which provides a suitable environment.

The biochemical reactions of the *Neisseria* are relatively limited, but they do contain cytochrome oxidase, which is responsible for the positive "oxidase" test, and clinically significant species usually are differentiated by their ability to produce acid in glucose, maltose, and sucrose. Although the typical meningococcus ferments glucose and maltose and the gonococcus ferments only glucose, the value of fermentation reactions for the identification of the pathogenic *Neisseria* has become limited because naturally occurring maltose-negative meningococci are being recovered with increasing frequency, probably because of the organism's progressive development of resistance to sulfonamides.

Meningococci can be divided into serologic groups on the basis of agglutination reactions with immune serum. The present classification into groups, A, B, C, and D was agreed upon in 1950, but since 1960, increasing numbers of nontypable strains have been recovered, and grouping sera X, Y, Z, and Boshard have been developed as additional serologic markers.

EPIDEMIOLOGY. The natural habitat of meningococci is the nasopharynx of man, and no other reservoir or vector has been recognized. The principal means of spread is through inhalation of droplets of infected nasopharyngeal secretions, and it is unlikely that the disease is spread by contact with contaminated fomites. Meningococci cause either epidemic or sporadic disease, and there is a cyclic variation in the prevalence of meningococcal infection, with peaks of increased frequency occurring every 8 to 12 years and lasting 4 to 6 years. The most recent upward trend of this cycle began in 1962; early in 1968, the attack rate was 2.23 per 100,000. The prevalence of meningococcal infection is also subject to seasonal influences; the lowest attack rate occurs in midsummer and the highest in late winter and early spring. This seasonal variation follows that of other bacterial and viral respiratory infections and probably reflects crowded living conditions encountered during the winter months.

Meningococcal disease occurs most frequently in children and adolescents. There is no clear-cut tendency for racial or sexual predominance, but presumably because of an increased opportunity to acquire infection, males develop meningitis and meningococcemia more frequently than females. Military recruits are particularly susceptible, and worldwide epidemics of meningococcal disease have occurred during most major wars. The military is not the major source of meningococcal infection, however, because epidemiologic studies indicate that outbreaks among military personnel usually parallel less apparent trends in the civilian population.

Since 1915, most epidemics of meningococcal disease have been caused by group A meningococci, and strains of groups B and C have been associated with sporadic, interepidemic infections. However, in the outbreaks of 1963 and 1964 a major shift in the pattern of meningococcal infection became apparent as group B meningococci were isolated from the majority of clinical infections in both civilian and military populations. In 1967, over 70 percent of meningococci isolated were group B. However, early in 1968, another shift in serogroup occurred,

and 43 percent of the meningococcal strains submitted to the National Communicable Disease Center were group C. The significance of these epidemiologic shifts is enhanced by the fact that a high proportion of the meningococci in groups B and C are resistant to 1 mg per 100 ml sulfadiazine, and prophylaxis with this drug, which was successful in aborting epidemics during World War II, has been relatively ineffective since 1960. Group A meningococci recovered in this country have retained their sensitivity to sulfonamides, but in Africa, sulfonamide-resistant strains have been isolated.

Carriers. Between epidemics, 2 to 5 percent of the individuals in urban centers harbor meningococci in the nasopharynx. When sporadic cases of meningococcal disease occur, the carrier rate in close contacts may rise to 25 percent, and in closed populations or during epidemics, it may be as high as 40 to 90 percent. Although some individuals harbor meningococci for months or years, nasopharyngeal infection is usually transient, and in 75 percent of carriers, the organism disappears within 2 weeks. The relationship between the proportion of carriers in a population and the occurrence of meningococcal disease is unclear. Case to case transmission of infection is documented rarely, and carriers, not patients, are the foci from which disease is spread. It appears that the prevalence of meningococcal disease can be attributed to the prevailing carrier rate only in a general way, and that the occurrence of clinical disease is most dependent on unknown circumstances within the host which lead to spread of infection beyond the nasopharynx. Factors which may promote dissemination include (1) failure of nasopharyngeal infection to confer immunity; (2) in vivo development of invasive mutants; (3) concomitant viral infection of the upper respiratory tract.

Immunity. The role of acquired immunity in recovery from illness or protection against infection is not known. Some degree of immunity must develop because the attack rate of meningococcal infection is much higher in young children than it is in adults. However, antibody formed during clinical infection or the asymptomatic carrier state does not provide lifelong protection against reinfection.

PATHOGENESIS. Meningococci usually enter the body through the upper respiratory tract and infect the nasopharynx. In most instances, this infection is subclinical, but occasionally, localized inflammation occurs and mild symptoms develop. Dissemination of meningococci from the nasopharynx occurs via the bloodstream and generally is followed by clinical manifestations of meningococcal disease. Purulent meningitis is the most common form of metastatic infection and is either associated with signs and symptoms of meningococcemia or constitutes the predominant clinical expression of illness. Organisms in the meninges induce an acute inflammatory reaction, and purulent exudate spreads across the surface of the brain. Rarely, a more extensive inflammatory reaction in the brain produces an acute diffuse encephalitic syndrome.

Although the mechanisms responsible for the pathologic changes associated with meningococcal infection have not been explained entirely, early investigations indicated that the tissue injury observed in laboratory animals was caused by a toxic substance liberated from dead bacteria. This substance is presumed to be an endotoxin that has not been characterized biochemically, but which produces physiologic effects similar to endotoxins of other gram-negative bacteria. It may be responsible for hypotension and vascular collapse observed in fulminant meningococcemia and may also play a role in the pathogenesis of the purpura and visceral hemorhages associated with meningococcal bacteremia. Thrombosis of dermal venules, adrenal sinusoids, and renal glomerular capillaries is commonly seen in patients who die of fulminant meningococcemia and is strikingly similar to the pathologic changes observed in experimental Shwartzman reactions (Chap. 74). It is postulated that endotoxin either induces a Shwartzman reaction directly or effects the release of clotting factors which initiate intravascular coagulation and produce these characteristic pathologic changes.

CLINICAL MANIFESTATIONS. Of patients with meningococcal disease, 90 to 95 percent have meningococcemia and/or meningitis.

Meningococcemia. Of those patients who develop overt disease, 30 to 50 percent have meningococcemia without meningitis. The onset of clinical illness may be abrupt, but patients usually have nonspecific prodromal symptoms of cough, headache, and sore throat followed by the sudden development of spiking fever, chills, arthralgia, and muscle pains which may be particularly severe in the lower extremities and back. Patients usually appear acutely ill, with an inordinate degree of prostration. In addition to high fever, tachycardia, and tachypnea, mild hypotension may be present. However, clinical shock does not occur unless fulminant meningococcemia supervenes. In the course of meningococcal bacteremia, about three-fourths of the patients develop a characteristic petechial rash. Lesions are frequently sparse, and the axillas, flanks, wrists, and ankles are the most commonly involved sites. Typically, lesions are 1 to 3 mm in diameter, deep red in color, and do not blanch with pressure. Often, petechiae are located in the center of lighter colored macules, and they may become nodular as the disease progresses. The diagnosis of meningococcemia occasionally can be established by demonstrating gram-negative diplococci in scrapings from these nodular petechiae. In severe cases, purpuric spots or large ecchymoses develop, and a widespread petechial or purpuric eruption suggests fulminating disease. However, the absence of rash does not necessarily indicate that the illness will be mild.

Fulminant meningococcemia. Also known as the Waterhouse-Friderichsen Syndrome, this is meningococcemia associated with vasomotor collapse and shock. It occurs in 10 to 20 percent of patients with generalized meningococcal infection and is associated with a high fatality rate. The onset is abrupt, and profound prostration frequently occurs within a few hours. Petechiae and purpuric lesions enlarge rapidly, and hemorrhage into the skin may be extensive. Early in the preshock stage, there is generalized vasoconstriction; patients are alert and pale, with cir-

cumoral cyanosis and cold extremities. Upon entering the shock stage, however, coma develops, the cardiac output decreases, and the blood pressure drops. Unless incipient shock is recognized and appropriate therapy instituted early, death from cardiac and/or respiratory failure almost invariably occurs. Patients who recover may have extensive sloughing of skin lesions and even loss of digits because of gangrene.

Chronic meningococcemia. This is a rare form of meningococcal infection which lasts for weeks or months and is characterized by fever, rash, and arthritis or arthralgia. Typically, the fever is intermittent, and during afebrile periods, which may last several days, patients appear remarkably well. The usual rash is a maculopapular or polymorphous eruption which waxes and wanes with the fever, but petechial or nodular lesions may be seen. Joint involvement is present in two-thirds of the patients, and splenomegaly is detected in about 20 percent. If the diagnosis is not suspected or treatment is otherwise delayed, complications such as meningitis, carditis, or nephritis may occur.

Meningitis. Meningitis is a common form of meningococcal disease which occurs primarily in adolescents and children over six months of age. Fever, vomiting, headache, and confusion or lethargy are the commonest symptoms; in about one-fourth of the patients, they begin abruptly and rapidly increase in severity. The more typical patient, however, has symptoms of an upper respiratory tract infection followed by an illness which progresses over several days. Because 20 to 40 percent of patients have meningitis without clinical evidence of meningococcemia, the diagnosis depends upon bacteriologic examination of the cerebrospinal fluid. However, when meningitis occurs in association with a petechial or purpuric rash, a presumptive diagnosis of meningococcal disease is warranted, since this pattern of illness is seen only rarely in other infections.

Rarer Manifestations. The meningococcus is a rare cause of purulent conjunctivitis or sinusitis, and it has been reported to cause lobar or bronchopneumonia in patients without evidence of meningitis or meningococcemia. Bacterial endocarditis also has been reported.

LABORATORY FINDINGS. Aside from bacteriologic data, laboratory studies are of little value in establishing the diagnosis of meningococcal infection. Polymorphonuclear leukocyte counts usually range from 12,000 to 40,000 cells per cu mm, but in meningococcemia, normal or low leukocyte counts may be encountered. Anemia is uncommon, and levels of serum electrolytes and blood urea nitrogen are normal unless shock develops. Patients with prominent hemorrhagic manifestations may have low platelet counts and decreased levels of circulating clotting factors as a result of intravascular coagulation. In meningitis, the cerebrospinal fluid pressure is increased, and the fluid usually contains from 100 to 40,000 polymorphonuclear leukocytes per cu mm. The protein content of the fluid is increased, and the concentration of glucose is almost always less than 35 mg per 100 ml and often is between 0 and 10 mg per 100 ml.

Meningococci can be recovered readily from cultures

of blood or spinal fluid, and on occasion, material aspirated from skin lesions or joints yields the organism. In addition, gram-negative diplococci may be seen in stains of nodular petechiae or the buffy coat of blood from patients with meningococcemia. In meningococcal meningitis, a smear of the spinal fluid is diagnostic in about half the patients but often shows only a few intracellular bacteria which are located with difficulty.

COMPLICATIONS. *Herpes labialis* occurs in 5 to 20 percent of patients with meningococcal disease. Other complications, which result from neurologic damage or secondary foci of infection, are uncommon following appropriate treatment and are often transient. Seizures or deafness occur in 10 to 20 percent of patients during the acute stages of meningitis, but postmeningitic epilepsy is rare and the frequency of permanent eighth-nerve damage is probably less than 5 percent. Peripheral neuropathy, cranial nerve palsies, and hemiplegia are seen occasionally, but usually clear completely within 2 to 4 months. Hydrocephalus and thrombosis of venous sinuses, once frequent sequelae of meningococcal meningitis, are encountered rarely. A number of patients complain of recurrent headache, emotional lability, insomnia, backache, memory loss, and difficulty in concentrating for months after an episode of meningitis. The organic basis for these symptoms is obscure, but they usually disappear a year or two after the infection.

Arthritis is a common metastatic complication of meningococcemia and occurs in 2 to 10 percent of patients. As a rule, multiple joints are involved, and signs and symptoms of joint involvement may not appear until after treatment of meningitis or meningococcemia has been instituted. Joint fluid usually contains many granulocytes, but meningococci are recovered infrequently. Antibiotic therapy does not appear to influence the course of the arthritis, and permanent joint changes are rare. Other purulent complications have become extremely uncommon since antibiotics have gained widespread use. Pneumonia occurs occasionally, but it is uncertain whether it is caused by the meningococcus or coexistent infection with other bacteria. Bacterial endocarditis is quite rare, but a high proportion of patients who die of meningococcal infection have myocarditis. The etiology of these myocardial changes is uncertain, but cardiac failure may be an important factor in the pathogenesis of the shock syndrome in meningococcemia.

DIAGNOSIS. The diagnosis of meningococcal disease depends upon recovering *N. meningitidis* from cultures of blood, spinal fluid, or petechial scrapings from patients with a typical clinical picture. Recovery of meningococci from the nasopharynx does not, in itself, establish the diagnosis of meningococcal disease.

Few diseases need to be seriously considered in the differential diagnosis of meningococcal infection. If meningococcal meningitis is not accompanied by manifestations of bacteremia, it is indistinguishable from meningitis caused by other common pathogens. Occasionally, the common viral exanthems, certain rickettsial infections, particularly Rocky Mountain Spotted Fever (Chap. 195), and vascular purpuras (Chap. 345) may be confused with meningococcemia, and their differentiation depends upon demonstration of the organism and knowledge of the epidemiology and clinical manifestations of each disease.

TREATMENT. Antimicrobial therapy of suspected or documented meningococcal disease should be instituted as early as possible. Penicillin G is the drug of choice, and should be administered intravenously. The dosage for the treatment of meningitis in adults is 12 to 24 million units per day, and in the pediatric age group, 16 million units/sq m/day. Meningococcemia can be treated with 5 to 10 million units a day because it is not necessary to achieve high levels of antibiotic in the spinal fluid. If treatment with these doses is continued for a minimum of 7 days, or 4 to 5 days after the patient becomes afebrile, relapse is extremely rare. Ampicillin in doses of 200 mg/kg/day is as effective as penicillin G, and it has been recommended for initial treatment of meningitis in children because it is effective against *H. influenzae*. Meningococci are susceptible to other antimicrobial agents such as chloramphenicol and tetracycline, but they should not be used unless a patient is allergic to penicillin. Under these circumstances, chloramphenicol hemisuccinate 4.0 to 6.0 Gm per day in divided doses (in adults) is an acceptable regimen. Because a significant proportion of meningococci isolated are resistant to sulfonamides, these drugs should not be used in the treatment of meningococcal infections. The combination of sulfonamides with penicillin offers no advantage and should not be used.

Patients with meningococcal infections require supportive treatment as well as antimicrobial therapy. Maintenance of fluid and electrolyte balance and prevention of respiratory complications in comatose patients are of primary concern. When shock occurs, visceral perfusion must be improved by maintenance of an adequate intravascular volume, treatment of heart failure when it is present, and support of the blood pressure. Vasopressors may produce temporary improvement, but agents which block alpha adrenergic receptors (Dibenzylene) or which stimulate beta receptors (isoproterenol) have been promising, and deserve further trial (Chap. 134). If central venous pressure is elevated, digitalis should be given, and when intravascular coagulation is recognized, treatment with heparin, whole blood, or fibrinogen is indicated. Adrenal cortical steroids are often used, but are of uncertain value, and dramatic results should not be expected.

PREVENTION. There is little likelihood that meningococcal infections can be prevented entirely. Effective chemoprophylaxis depends upon first treating an entire population at risk with a drug capable of eradicating the carrier state and then isolating the group to prevent further introduction of meningococci. This is not only impractical when applied to the general public, but the majority of carriers now harbor strains which are resistant to sulfonamides, and other drugs do not eradicate the carrier state permanently. Nevertheless, under certain circumstances, such as epidemic outbreaks in military populations, these measures may have to be instituted.

Treatment of contacts of sporadic cases with a 2-day course of a sulfonamide (on the assumption that the organism is sensitive) or a 7-day course of oral penicillin has been advocated, but the usefulness of this practice has not been documented. Attempts at development of a meningococcal vaccine are under way, but no trials have been reported in man.

PROGNOSIS. Before the introduction of antibiotics, meningococcal meningitis, and meningococcemia were almost invariably fatal. With prompt and appropriate chemotherapy, the mortality rate of meningitis without fulminant meningococcemia has dropped to less than 10 percent in the United States, and neurologic sequelae are rare. The mortality of fulminant infection remains high primarily because patients are often in irreversible shock when treatment is instituted. Chronic meningococcemia is cured readily if the disease is recognized.

REFERENCES

Banks, H. S.: Meningococcal Fever, in "Modern Practice in Infectious Fevers," vol. 1, New York, Paul B. Hoeber, Inc., 1951.

Benoit, F. L.: Chronic Meningococcemia, Am. J. Med., 35:103, 1963.

Eickhoff, T. C., and M. Finland: Changing Susceptibility of Meningococci to Antimicrobial Agents, New Engl. J. Med., 272:395, 1965.

Feldman, H. A.: Recent Developments in the Therapy and Control of Meningococcal Infections, Disease-a-Month, February, 1966.

Levin, S., and M. B. Painter: The Treatment of Acute Meningococcal Infection in Adults, Ann. Intern. Med., 64:1049, 1966.

Pinals, R. S., and M. Ropes: Arthritis in Meningococcal Infection, Arthritis Rheum., 7:241, 1964.

143 GONOCOCCAL INFECTIONS

*Harry N. Beaty and
Robert G. Petersdorf*

INTRODUCTION. Gonorrhea, an infection of columnar and transitional epithelium of the genitourinary tract, is the principal infection caused by the gonococcus. It is transmitted almost exclusively by direct sexual contact and is the commonest venereal disease of man. Most other clinical manifestations of gonococcal infection are relatively uncommon today and develop as a result of contamination with infected secretions or as a complication of venereal infection.

ETIOLOGY. *Neisseria gonorrhoeae,* or the gonococcus, is a gram-negative spherical organism which closely resembles the meningococcus in its morphology and growth requirements. In stained preparations of infected secretions, gonococci appear as reniform diplococci which often are located within granulocytes. Their recovery from infected genitourinary sites is facilitated if a selective medium containing 25 units per ml polymyxin B and 10 μg per ml ristocetin is used for initial cultures.

The biochemical reactions of these organisms are limited, but they are "oxidase positive" and usually can be distinguished from other species of *Neisseria* by their ability to ferment only glucose. Confusion arises when an occasional gonococcus which produces acid very slowly in glucose is mistaken for *N. catarrhalis,* or when a sulfonamide-resistant meningococcus is classified as a gonococcus because it fails to ferment maltose. Final identification of these strains can be accomplished with immunofluorescent techniques.

Gonococci are a heterogeneous group of organisms, and at least four morphologically distinct colonial types have been recognized. Type 1 cells are recovered only from the purulent exudate of acute gonorrhea, but on subculture, other types appear. After passage in vitro, certain of these types lose their virulence, but type 1 cells always retain their ability to infect male volunteers. Serologic heterogeneity has also been documented, but classification of gonococci on the basis of agglutination reactions is not practical.

EPIDEMIOLOGY. Man is the only host in whom infection with *N. gonorrhoeae* occurs naturally; the major reservoir is the asymptomatic female. With the exception of ophthalmia neonatorum, which results from contamination of the conjunctiva during parturition, gonococcal infection is transmitted almost exclusively by sexual contact. Gonorrhea is worldwide in distribution, and most countries reporting to the World Health Organization have documented a progressive increase in the disease rate since 1960. In the United States, it is estimated that 1.5 to 2 million new cases occur annually, but only 10 to 20 percent of these cases are reported, and approximately 70 percent are treated outside of public clinics. The disease is most common in lower socioeconomic groups, but susceptibility to infection is quite general, with no recognizable predilection for either race or sex. The highest incidence of infection is in the twenty to twenty-four-year-old age group, but the frequency of gonorrhea among teen-agers has reached alarming proportions.

Many females harbor asymptomatic infection for weeks to months, but a more prolonged true carrier state is relatively uncommon. Not all males exposed to a female with gonorrhea become infected, but those who do almost always develop acute urethritis. This is usually a self-limited infection and although asymptomatic male carriers have been recognized, they are distinctly uncommon. Individuals of either sex with asymptomatic infection can transmit the disease for months or years unless they receive effective therapy.

One of the major factors which has prevented successful control of gonorrhea is the lack of natural or acquired resistance to infection. The antibody response to acute gonorrhea is minimal and provides no significant protection against reinfection. To date, immunologic studies of this disease have had little practical value. However, attempts to develop a skin test or serologic reaction which will identify patients with active infection continue because these tests would have great epidemiologic importance.

PATHOGENESIS. Gonococci cannot penetrate stratified squamous epithelium, but they are able to infect columnar or transitional cells. Three to four days after organisms come in contact with susceptible epithelium, bacteria can be identified in subepithelial spaces. Leukocytes accumulate in these regions, and soon, granulocytes containing organisms migrate into the urethral lumen and form a purulent exudate. In males, the urethral glands are usually involved, and prostatitis or epididymitis may develop as a result of direct extension or lymphatic spread of infection. Urethritis is usually transient in females, but infection of Skene's or Bartholin's glands is common. The epithelium and glands of the endocervix also are involved frequently, and as infection spreads along the endometrium, it causes congestion, edema, and formation of a purulent exudate. The disease may continue to spread to the endosalpinx where plicae become swollen, hyperemic, and heavily infiltrated with leukocytes. Extension of the infection through the mucosa to involve the muscularis sometimes leads to abscess formation or pelvic peritonitis. Proctitis is present in about 40 percent of women with gonococcal infection of the urogenital tract, and occasionally may be recognized in males. It is likely that transient subclinical gonococcemia occurs in many patients with either acute or asymptomatic urogenital infections, but the mechanisms responsible for dissemination are unknown.

Untreated gonococcal infections tend to heal with the formation of dense scar tissue. Urethral strictures and sterility, resulting from stenosis of the epididymis or fallopian tubes, were fairly common sequelae of gonorrhea before the availability of effective antimicrobial agents.

CLINICAL MANIFESTATIONS. Genital infections and the clinical manifestations of associated bacteremia are the most likely forms of gonococcal disease to be encountered. Metastatic infections such as visceral abscesses, meningitis, endocarditis, and purulent myocarditis or pericarditis are extremely rare.

Gonorrhea in the Male ("Clap" or "Strain"). The incubation period of naturally acquired infection is 2 to 8 days, but in experimental infection of humans it has been as long as 31 days. The onset of symptoms is usually abrupt, and patients complain of urinary frequency and urgency, dysuria, and a profuse mucopurulent urethral discharge. Urinary retention, perineal pain, and hematuria may be seen occasionally. Acute prostatitis and seminal vesiculitis are uncommon, but if treatment is delayed, unilateral epididymitis complicates 5 to 10 percent of cases. In these patients, systemic manifestations such as fever and chills may occur. Untreated disease usually subsides within 6 weeks, and with rare exception, organisms cannot be recovered from the urogenital tract. Occasionally, however, gonococci persist despite apparently adequate therapy, presumably because they are sequestered in mucosal folds or the prostate. Urethral dilatation or prostatic massage may activate latent gonorrhea in these patients. A significant proportion of individuals have either pyuria or a slight urethral discharge for weeks to months after the successful treatment of gonorrhea. This postgonococcal urethritis (PGU, "gleet") may be due to latent or coexistent mycoplasma infection and can be eradicated with tetracycline. Urethral stricture is a common sequel of genital gonococcal disease if treatment is inadequate or a patient has repeated infections.

Gonorrhea in the Female. Women with acute gonorrhea are often completely asymptomatic and first come to attention as contacts of males with venereal infections. Transient urethritis may cause mild urinary symptoms, and involvement of the cervix often produces a copious, irritating vaginal discharge. If the infection spreads to the endosalpinx and produces acute salpingitis or pelvic peritonitis (pelvic inflammatory disease, PID), patients may complain of chills, fever, malaise, myalgia, anorexia, nausea, vomiting, and lower abdominal pain. Depending on the extent of the infection, the physical examination may be negative or nonspecific. However, if there is an abscess of Skene's or Bartholin's glands, or if there is pain on movement of the cervix, with or without signs of peritoneal irritation, gonococcal infection should be suspected. Proctitis, often manifested by tenesmus and bloody mucoid stools, may be caused by the gonococcus, and persistence of the organisms in this site may be responsible for treatment failures.

Prior to the availability of antimicrobials, conception after bilateral gonorrheal salpingitis was exceptional. Today, approximately 80 percent of patients have at least one patent tube after effective therapy. The duration of the infection prior to treatment is of major importance in determining the outcome.

Unlike the situation in adults, gonococcal infection of prepubescent females usually causes vulvovaginitis. The exterior cervix may be infected, but salpingitis and pelvic peritonitis are rare. The reason for this unusual expression of gonococcal disease in children is probably due to anatomic and biochemical factors, but acquisition of infection still seems to be the result of voluntary or involuntary sexual contact.

Arthritis. Arthritis occurs as a manifestation of gonococcemia in about 1 percent of patients with genital infection. In the past it occurred primarily in males and frequently destroyed the involved joints; today, it is seen predominately in females and male homosexuals, responds well to antibiotics, and leaves no residual joint damage. Symptoms usually develop after acute gonorrhea, but particularly in females, may follow exacerbation of an indolent or subclinical infection. The onset is often abrupt, and the clinical picture consists of fever, arthralgia, and painful arthritis. About 50 percent of patients develop a sparse rash which is most commonly seen over the distal portion of the extremities. The typical lesion is an erythematous papule with a hemorrhagic or vesiculopustular center. Although gonococcal arthritis has been characterized as monoarticular, it is actually polyarticular in 80 percent of cases. The knee is the most frequently involved joint, followed in order of frequency by wrists, ankles, hands, elbows, hips, and shoulders. Tenosynovitis occurs in 50 to 75 percent of cases, and should call attention to the possibility of gonococcal infection.

Patients usually have a mild leukocytosis, and fluid aspirated from involved joints may contain only a few granulocytes or may be frankly purulent. Careful bacteriologic study of joint fluid fails to reveal gonococci in the majority of cases, particularly if patients are seen relatively early in the course of their illness. Joint symptoms usually begin to improve a few days after treatment is started, and complete recovery occurs within 1 to 2 weeks. In an occasional patient, however, the response to treatment may be less dramatic and symptoms will persist for much longer.

Ophthalmitis. Gonococcal keratoconjunctivitis is rare in adults, but is one of the commonest forms of gonococcal infection in children. *Ophthalmia neonatorum,* ophthalmitis in the newborn, formerly was responsible for 12 percent of all blindness, but with the advent of effective prophylaxis, this figure has been reduced to less than 0.3 percent. Infection occurs when the conjunctiva is contaminated during birth or by the hands of infected adults with poor personal hygiene. Three to four days after the gonococcus comes in contact with the corneal epithelium, acute purulent conjunctivitis develops. It usually begins unilaterally, but soon becomes bilateral, and if untreated, most cases rapidly progress to corneal ulceration, perforation, and scarring. Gonococci are readily apparent on a gram stain of the purulent exudate, and if treatment is instituted early, results are satisfactory. The best agent for prophylaxis has not been determined, but a 1 percent silver nitrate solution may be superior to penicillin G, which, however, is also highly effective.

Perihepatitis (Fitzhugh-Curtis Syndrome). This is an unusual complication of genital infection in the female. It occurs when gonococci spread from the fallopian tube and produce a localized peritonitis. Any area of the peritoneal cavity can be involved, but the right upper quadrant is the commonest site. Patients usually present with fever and abdominal pain and have signs of peritonitis on physical examination. A friction rub is heard over the liver in some patients. Usually, liver function studies are normal, but jaundice and other mild abnormalities have been reported. Liver biopsies have been normal in most cases, but thickening of the capsule and mild subcapsular hepatitis may be seen occasionally. Perihepatitis is often confused with acute cholecystitis because of its clinical presentation and the fact that the gallbladder may not be visualized on cholecystograms until after the inflammation subsides. Specific therapy results in prompt improvement, but even without treatment, symptoms usually disappear within 2 weeks. Untreated, this form of gonococcal infection leads to the formation of "violin-string" adhesions between the liver and the anterior abdominal wall.

Gonococcemia and Endocarditis. Very rarely, gonococcemia produces a febrile illness which is so similar to meningococcemia that differentiation on clinical grounds is not possible. Otherwise, the manifestations of gonococcal bacteremia are those discussed in the section on arthritis.

Endocarditis due to the gonococcus has virtually disappeared with the availability of effective treatment of gonorrhea. Gonococci usually attack normal valves, but the course of the infection borders between acute and subacute. Left-sided endocarditis, with involvement of the aortic valve, is the commonest form of this infection, but the gonococcus is one organism which is particularly likely to infect the tricuspid or pulmonic valve. In addition to petechiae, glomerulonephritis, embolic phenomena, anemia, and splenomegaly, two clinical features of gonococcal endocarditis may suggest the diagnosis. Jaundice, presumably due to "toxic" hepatitis, is very common, and a majority of patients have two distinct spikes of fever during a 24-hr period (the double quotidian pattern).

DIAGNOSIS. A definitive diagnosis of gonococcal infection is established by demonstrating *N. gonorrhoeae* in cultures of infected secretions or biologic fluids. In males, a presumptive diagnosis of gonorrhea can be made if typical organisms are seen on gram stain of the urethral discharge. However, a negative smear does not rule out gonococcal disease, and false-positive results may be due to infection with *Mima polymorpha.* The bacillary nature of these organisms can quickly be determined, however, by culture on eosin-methylene blue or meat-broth media. The diagnosis of gonorrhea in the female often has been difficult to establish because demonstration of the gonococcus on routine smears or cultures has been inconsistent. However, use of the selective Thayer-Martin medium or the delayed fluorescent-antibody technique has simplified the task of diagnosis. Carefully obtained cultures also can be used to assess the effectiveness of therapy, but since nonviable gonococci fluoresce, the fluorescent antibody test is not a good measure of successful treatment.

The diagnosis of gonococcal arthritis often must be made on the basis of clinical data alone. Blood cultures are positive in only 10 to 20 percent of patients with presumed gonococcemia, and bacteriologic study of fluid from involved joints often fails to reveal organisms. The presence of tenosynovitis in patients with evidence of gonorrheal infection and arthritis which responds promptly to penicillin should suggest the diagnosis.

TREATMENT. Despite the fact that surveillance studies of *N. gonorrhoeae* sensitivity have revealed a steady increase in resistance in vitro to penicillin, this drug remains the preferred choice for management of gonococcal infections. However, the dose required to produce acceptable results has required repeated upward adjustments, and it is possible that sometime in the future, further increases will be impractical.

In males, gonorrhea should be treated with a single injection of 2.4 million units of procaine penicillin. Gonorrhea in females requires more drug, 4.8 million units in one dose, to achieve an 85 to 90 percent cure rate. Treatment failure may occur when organisms are sequestered in a site where antibiotics cannot reach them, when there is a concommitant infection with penicillinase-producing organisms, or when the infecting gonococcus is relatively resistant to penicillin. Only the last possibility is of major clinical significance. A variety of drugs, including kanamycin, chloramphenicol, erythromycin, ampicillin, and the cephalosporins, have been used effectively in the treatment of gonorrhea, but tetracycline seems to provide a particularly good alternative to penicillin therapy and it reduces the incidence of postgonococcal urethritis.

Gonococcal arthritis should be treated with 2 to 4 million units of penicillin per day parenterally for 10 to 14 days. Intraarticular penicillin is not recommended. Endocarditis should be treated with 4 to 10 million units of penicillin daily for 4 to 6 weeks. Pelvic inflammatory disease and perihepatitis usually respond to 1.2 million units of penicillin a day for 7 days. Ophthalmitis is best managed with topical penicillin G plus parenteral drug.

Simultaneous acquisition of gonorrhea and syphilis occurs in about 3 percent of patients. The gonococcal infection usually becomes evident first, and therapy for that alone may abort the clinical manifestations of syphilis without effectively treating the disease. Therefore, all patients with gonorrhea should have serologic tests for syphilis before treatment and at intervals for 6 months. The onset of fever and chills in a patient given penicillin for gonorrhea is highly suggestive of a syphilitic Herxheimer reaction.

PREVENTION AND CONTROL. Effective prophylaxis against infection can be achieved with a single 250-mg tablet of penicillin G taken just before or just after exposure. A condom also provides protection against gonorrhea because it prevents contact of organisms with susceptible epithelium. In women, mechanical cleansing may help prevent infection.

Control of gonorrhea as a public health problem can-not be accomplished so readily. Thayer and Garson pointed out four principles necessary for the control of contagion: quarantine, immunization, eradication of animal reservoirs or vectors, and specific therapy. When applied to gonorrhea, it is apparent that *quarantine* is out of the question. Artificial *immunization* is not available, and more important, an attack of gonorrhea confers no significant resistance to reinfection. Man is the only *reservoir*, so the end result of *specific treatment* is the return of nonimmune susceptibles to the population within a few days. These patients can be reinfected almost immediately, which makes evaluation of treatment very difficult, and the disease maintains itself in the population. There is probably no more striking illustration than gonorrhea of the failure of specific treatment alone to eradicate a communicable disease.

REFERENCES

Ashamalla, G., N. R. Walters, and M. Crahan: Recent Clinicolaboratory Observations in the Treatment of Acute Gonococcal Urethritis in Men, J.A.M.A., 195:1115, 1966.

Keiser, H., F. L. Ruben, E. Wolinsky, and I. Kushner: Clinical Forms of Gonococcal Arthritis, New Engl. J. Med., 279:234, 1968.

Lucas, J. B., E. V. Price, J. D. Thayer, and A. Schroeter: Diagnosis and Treatment of Gonorrhea in the Female, New Engl. J. Med., 276:1454, 1967.

Thayer, J. D., and W. Garson: The Gonococcus, p. 451 in "Bacterial and Mycotic Infections of Man," 4th ed., Philadelphia, J. B. Lippincott Company, 1965.

Vickers, F. N., and P. J. Maloney: Gonococcic Perihepatitis: Report of Three Cases with Comments on Diagnosis and Treatment, Arch. Intern. Med., 114:120, 1964.

Section 5

Diseases Caused by Enteric Gram-negative Bacilli

144 COLIFORM BACTERIAL INFECTIONS
(*Escherichia coli Infections*)

Marvin Turck and
Robert G. Petersdorf

ETIOLOGY. The most important "coliforms" medically, are *Escherichia coli* and organisms of the *Klebsiella-Aerobacter* group (Chap. 148). The coliforms do not constitute a distinct nosologic entity and are a group of gram-negative nonsporing rods which belong to the tribe *Enterobacteriaceae*. Coliforms generally ferment lactose, as opposed to the medically significant non-lactose-fermenting organisms, *Salmonella*, *Shigella*, and *Proteus*. The so-called "paracolon" bacilli are organisms which ferment lactose late, irregularly, or not at all, and on more careful biochemical and antigenic testing are found to belong to one or another of the genera of the tribe *Enterobacteriaceae*, which is comprised of *Salmonella*, *Arizona*, *Citrobacter*, *Shigella*, *Escherichia*, *Klebsiella*, *Aerobacter*, *Hafnia*, *Serratia*, *Proteus*, and *Providence*. All of these organisms are readily culturable on ordinary media and are aerobic and facultatively anaerobic. All species ferment glucose, reduce nitrates to nitrites, and are oxidase-negative and catalase-positive. They are differentiated among members of their own tribe by biochemical and serologic tests. It is important to make this differentiation, not only from the point of view of taxonomy, but also because of epidemiologic and therapeutic implications.

PATHOGENESIS. *Escherichia coli* is regarded generally as a normal commensal in the gastrointestinal tract, from which it may spread to infect contiguous structures if normal anatomic barriers are interrupted, as occurs in appendiceal perforation. It is believed that the urinary tract is infected from without via urethral contamination, but direct hematogenous or, rarely, lymphatic spread accounts for renal infection. Once infection has occurred in a primary focus, further spread to distant organs occurs via the bloodstream. There is experimental and clinical evidence that *E. coli* tends to settle in avascular or necrotic tissue. In more than 50 percent of *E. coli* infections the urinary tract is the portal of entry; infections of the hepatobiliary tree, peritoneal cavity, skin, and lung are not uncommon. A number of patients with *E. coli* bacteremia have no demonstrable portal of entry; they often have neoplastic and hematologic diseases, and *E. coli* is considered an "opportunistic" invader. There may be other defects in host resistance, including diabetes mellitus, cirrhosis, and sickle-cell anemia, or recent administration of irradiation, cytotoxic drugs, adrenal steroids, or antibiotics. Morphologically the lesions produced in various tissues show typical acute inflammation with pus and abscess formation. There is a common misconception that *E. coli* bacterial infections are characterized by a foul-smelling, feculent exudate. Such an odor is caused by anaerobic streptococci or *Bacteroides* species, which are often associated with coliform bacteria in mixed infections. In fact, organisms of the genus *Bacteroides* frequently far outnumber *E. coli* as the most prevalent gram-negative flora in the intestine.

EPIDEMIOLOGY. Strains of *E. coli* are characterized by their somatic (O), flagellar (H), and capsular (K or B) antigens, and there are hundreds of different serologic varieties. Any of the strains is capable of causing disease. Clinical and epidemiologic studies have demonstrated that certain specific *E. coli* serotypes are more frequently incriminated in diarrheal disease of the infant and newborn, i.e., 026:B6, 055:B5, 0111:B4, and 0127:B8. It is less clear whether certain strains are also more commonly associated with nonenteric infections.

Some epidemiologic studies performed between 1960 and 1965 suggested that *E. coli* 04, 06, and 075 were responsible for most *E. coli* infections other than infantile diarrhea. In particular, these strains appeared to colonize more avidly and more commonly infect hospital patients. With the passage of time the epidemiologic virulence of these organisms may have become attenuated, and they are no more likely to cause infections than other strains. A similar ecologic change has been observed with staphylococci of phage type 80/81.

Strains incriminated in infantile diarrhea probably are disseminated within nurseries by symptomatic or asymptomatic infant carriers, mothers, and nurses. Although fecal contamination is the usual mode of spread, airborne contamination of the environment and fomite spread may also occur.

MANIFESTATIONS. Urinary tract infections. *Escherichia coli* account for well over 75 percent of urinary tract infections, including cystitis, pyelitis, pyelonephritis, and asymptomatic bacteriuria. Strains cultured from patients with acute, uncomplicated urinary tract infections are almost invariably *E. coli*, whereas other *Enterobacteriaceae* and strains of *Pseudomonas* become prevalent among patients with chronic infection. Urinary tract infections are discussed in Chap. 303.

Peritoneal and Biliary Infections. *Escherichia coli* can usually be cultured from a perforated or inflamed appendix or abscesses secondary to perforated diverticuli, peptic ulcers, subphrenic or lesser sac abscesses, mesenteric infarction, etc. Often, other organisms, including anaerobic streptococci, clostridia, and bacteroides, are found along with *E. coli*. Acute cholecystitis with gangrene and perforation is often associated with *E. coli* infection. An air-fluid level associated with stones or a circumferential layer of gas in the wall of the gallbladder may be detectable by x-ray and is characteristic of acute emphysematous cholecystitis. From the gallbladder, infection may ascend via the biliary tree to produce cholangitis and multiple liver abscesses. More rarely *E. coli* infection in the peritoneal cavity may produce a septic thrombophlebitis of the portal vein (pylephlebitis), which in turn is followed by liver abscesses.

BACTEREMIA. Invasion of the bloodstream is the most serious manifestation of *E. coli* infection; it is characterized usually by the sudden onset of fever and chills, but sometimes only by mental confusion, dyspnea, or unexplained hypotension. It is most common in patients with urinary tract infection and biliary or intraperitoneal sepsis, and following abortions or pelvic surgery. In some patients no portal of entry is evident. Most cases occur in elderly males, presumably because of the high incidence of urethral instrumentation and catheterization in this group. Fever ranges between 100 and 106°F and is higher in younger patients. Hyperventilation may be an early sign. Hypotension may be present from the onset but usually occurs within 12 to 16 hr after bacteremia, if it is persistent; it is accompanied by oliguria and often by mental confusion, stupor, and coma. The skin is warm and dry initially, but most patients develop some evidence of peripheral vasoconstriction characterized by cold and cyanotic extremities. Fortunately hypotension is transient and self-limited in most patients with *E. coli* bacteremia and is absent altogether in some. However, about 25 percent of patients with bacteremia develop more prolonged hypotension, a syndrome known as gram-negative or endotoxin shock, which is discussed in Chap. 134.

Occasionally *E. coli* bacteremia develops in patients with cirrhosis without an overt portal of entry. This has been variably attributed to portosystemic shunts, impaired reticuloendothelial function, and diminution in humoral defense mechanisms.

Other Manifestations. *Escherichia coli* may produce abscesses anywhere in the body. Subcutaneous infections are common at the site of insulin administration in diabetics, in extremities with ischemic gangrene, or in surgical wounds. Perirectal phlegmons are not uncommon in patients with leukemia. Subcutaneous abscesses are often characterized by formation of gas in tissues, which may be detected by crepitation or by x-ray and which must be differentiated from clostridial infection. From 5 to 10 percent of patients with *E. coli* bacteremia develop metastatic infection in bone, brain, liver, and lung. *Escherichia coli* rarely causes pneumonia *de novo*, although coliform bacilli are often cultured from sputum in pulmonary superinfections.

Neonatal infection. Neonates, particularly premature infants, often develop *E. coli* bacteremia associated with meningitis and blood-borne pyelonephritis. Fecal soiling and absence of maternal IgM antibody are two of the factors which render this group particularly susceptible to coliform infections.

Gastroenteritis. Children under two years of age develop gastroenteritis, typified by nausea, vomiting, and diarrhea. Most outbreaks have occurred in nurseries and have been due to specific strains of enteropathogenic *E. coli* (EPEC). Fluorescent antibody techniques have been most useful in the rapid identification of these organisms. The rapid dehydration, with its attendant high mortality, demands prompt recognition of this condition, isolation of the infants, and treatment of both patients and contacts with the appropriate antibiotic. *Escherichia coli* per se has not been incriminated in diarrheal disease in adults, although certain strains of Arizona have presumably been responsible for benign outbreaks of gastroenteritis.

LABORATORY FINDINGS. There are no characteristic laboratory abnormalities. The white blood cell count is usually elevated, and there is a preponderance of granulocytes. At times, however, the white count is normal or low. When *E. coli* infection occurs in previously healthy individuals, anemia is absent, but more commonly there is anemia which is usually related to the patient's underlying disease. *Escherichia coli* grows readily in a variety of bacteriologic media and should be cultured from appropriate secretions and blood. In the presence of gram-negative shock, there are often profound metabolic derangements, including azotemia, metabolic acidosis, hypokalemia, and hyperkalemia, as well as a variety of coagulation defects (Chap. 134).

DIAGNOSIS. *Escherichia coli* cannot be differentiated from most other gram-negative bacteria on gram stain, and culture followed by appropriate biochemical characterization is necessary to identify the organism precisely. Flourescent antibody techniques are valuable for identifying EPEC. Serologic typing is of no value in individual patients, although it is essential for gathering epidemiologic data.

TREATMENT. As with other infections, drainage of pus and removal of foreign bodies are essential. If *E. coli* is suspected as the etiologic agent in a particular infection, choice of an appropriate antimicrobial will depend upon the site and type of infection as well as upon its severity. Often the outcome of the infection depends upon the status of the associated disease, rather than on eradication of bacteria. For example, in acute uncomplicated urinary tract infection in females, the disease is frequently self-limited even without antimicrobial therapy, and there is no evidence that antibiotics are superior to

sulfonamides. Conversely, *E. coli* bacteremia in a patient with leukemia may not respond to antimicrobials unless a hematologic remission is achieved simultaneously.

In most situations, antibiotics should be selected, when possible, on the basis of their in vitro sensitivity tests. Although no drug is uniformly active against all strains of *E. coli*, a number of agents are effective against the majority of clinical isolates. If average obtainable plasma concentrations become the criteria for in vitro susceptibility, approximately 75 percent of *E. coli* strains is likely to be sensitive to the tetracyclines, 85 percent, to chloramphenicol or ampicillin, and 90 percent, to kanamycin, polymyxin B, or colistin; 50 percent of *E. coli* isolated from hospitalized patients will be inhibited by streptomycin, and 65 percent by cephalothin. Many strains of *E. coli* are sensitive to high concentrations of penicillin G (50 to 100 μg) and this drug may be used in dosage of 10 to 40 million units intravenously daily, particularly if probenecid is given concomitantly. This regimen has been largely superseded by ampicillin, 2 to 4 Gm per day intravenously or intramuscularly; in some instances the dose can be raised to 6 to 12 Gm per day. The antibacterial spectrum of ampicillin against *E. coli* is probably identical to that achieved with very high concentrations of penicillin G, and to the spectrum covered by the tetracyclines or chloramphenicol. However, the bactericidal properties of ampicillin may be a distinct advantage over these two drugs, particularly in deep seated, gram-negative infections. Kanamycin sulfate is most useful for the initial treatment of serious *E. coli* infections. Severe urinary tract infections refractory to other antimicrobials have responded to 15 mg/kg/day, intramuscularly, in divided doses every 12 hr. In life-threatening infections, kanamycin can probably be used for 24 to 48 hr with little hazard of ototoxicity or nephrotoxicity, even in patients with concomitant renal impairment, pending results of in vitro sensitivity tests. However, some recent isolations of specific serologic strains of hospital-derived *E. coli* from newborn with diarrheal disease have been resistant to kanamycin and neomycin. Cephalothin in concentration of 25 μg per ml is effective against many *E. coli* strains. This serum concentration can be obtained only with 1.5 to 2.0 gm dosages at 3- to 4-hr intervals. Although cephalothin is highly effective against many common pathogens, peak serum concentrations after standard doses barely reach or may fall short of requirements for *E. coli*. Another cephalosporin antibiotic, cephaloridine, has become available for the treatment of *E. coli* infections. This agent yields higher and more sustained levels than does a comparable amount of cephalothin and is more active against *E. coli* in vitro. However, because of potential nephrotoxicity, the total daily dose of cephaloridine is limited to 4.0 Gm per day by law. Tetracyclines and chloramphenicol are still widely used in the treatment of *E. coli* infection, but better drugs are now available. Polymyxin B and colistin are also highly effective in vitro against the majority of *E. coli*. However, it is difficult to obtain adequate tissue and serum concentrations with these agents, and they should probably not be used for treatment of systemic *E. coli* infections. Although combinations of antimicrobials, i.e., streptomycin and tetracycline or streptomycin and chloramphenicol, have been recommended, there is little need to employ more than one agent in most situations. Nitrofurantoin (400 mg) and nalidixic acid (2 to 4 Gm) are reserved for treating patients with *E. coli* bacteriuria, and are not employed when infection is suspected outside of the urinary tract.

PREVENTION. Isolation and antimicrobial therapy of infants and contacts are essential to abort epidemic infantile diarrhea. In adults, many *E. coli* infections are hospital associated, and their incidence can be reduced by limiting use of indwelling urinary catheters, careful surgical aseptic technique, appropriate isolation of infection-prone patients, and judicious use of antibiotics, steroids, and cytotoxic agents. There is mounting evidence that the promiscuous employment of antibiotics may propagate the transfer of resistance factors among intestinal *E. coli*. These organisms may in turn transmit their resistance to other virulent *Enterobactericae*, such as, *Salmonella*.

REFERENCES

Kennedy, R. P., J. J. Plorde, and R. G. Petersdorf: Studies in the Epidemiology of *Escherichia coli* Infections: IV. Evidence for a Nosocomial Flora, J. Clin. Invest., 44: 193, 1965.

McCabe, W. R., and G. G. Jackson: Gram-negative Bacteremia, A.M.A. Arch. Intern. Med., 110:847, 856, 1962.

Marshall, T. F., and D. C. Hartzog, Jr.: Acute Emphysematous Cholecystitis, Ann. Surg., 159:1011, 1964.

Neter, E.: Enteropathogenic *Escherichia coli* Enteritis, Pediat. Clin. N. Am., 7:1015, 1960.

Studdiford, W. E., and G. W. Douglas: Placental Bacteremia: A Significant Finding in Septic Abortion Accompanied by Vascular Collapse, Am. J. Obstet. Gynecol., 71:842, 1956.

Sweet, A. Y., and E. Wolinsky: An Outbreak of Urinary and Other Infections Due to *E. coli*. Pediatrics, 33:865, 1964.

Tisdale, W. A.: Spontaneous Colon Bacillus Bacteremia in Laennec's Cirrhosis, Gastroenterology, 40:141, 1961.

145   PROTEUS INFECTIONS
Marvin Turck and
Robert G. Petersdorf

ETIOLOGY. The genus *Proteus* consists of gram-negative bacilli which do not ferment lactose and are characterized by their active motility and spreading growth on solid media. There are four pathogenic species: *P. mirabilis*, *P. vulgaris*, *P. morganii*, and *P. rettgeri*. *Proteus mirabilis* causes 75 to 90 percent of human infections and is distinguishable from the other three species by its inability to form indole. All four split urea, with production of ammonia. Some strains of *P. vulgaris* share a common antigen with certain rickettsia, accounting for the appearance of antibodies against proteus organisms (Weil-Felix reaction) in typhus, scrub typhus, and Rocky

Mountain spotted fever. The Providence group of organisms resembles those of the genus *Proteus* closely except that it fails to produce a urease.

EPIDEMIOLOGY AND PATHOGENESIS. Members of the genus *Proteus* are normally found in soil, water, and sewage and are part of the normal fecal flora. Occasionally, they have been implicated as a cause of epidemic diarrhea in infants, but the evidence for this is inconclusive. The organism is frequently cultured from superficial wounds, draining ears, and sputum, particularly in patients who have received antibiotics, and replaces the more susceptible flora eradicated by these drugs. Proteus organisms often localize in already damaged tissues, where they produce a typical exudative inflammatory reaction.

MANIFESTATIONS. Proteus organisms are rarely primary invaders but produce disease in locations previously infected by other organisms. These locations include the skin, ears and mastoid sinuses, eyes, peritoneal cavity, urinary tract, meninges, lung, and bloodstream.

Cutaneous Infections. Proteus organisms are frequently isolated from surgical wounds, particularly following antimicrobial therapy, but they do not interfere with normal wound healing provided that the tissues are viable and foreign bodies are not present. Burns, varicose ulcers, and decubiti may become contaminated with proteus organisms, often in company with other gram-negative organisms or staphylococci.

Infections of the Ears and Mastoid Sinuses. Otitis media and mastoiditis in which proteus organisms are present can result in extensive destruction of the middle ear and mastoid sinuses. Fetid otorrhea, cholesteatoma, and granulation tissue constitute a chronic focus of infection in the middle and inner ears and mastoid, and deafness ensues. Paralysis of the facial nerve is an occasional complication. The great danger of these infections lies in intracranial extension, leading to thrombosis of the lateral sinus, meningitis, brain abscess, and bacteremia.

Ocular Infections. Proteus infection may cause corneal ulcers, usually following trauma to the eye, which occasionally terminate in panophthalmitis and destruction of the eyeball.

Peritonitis. Being part of the normal intestinal flora, proteus organisms may be isolated from the peritoneal cavity following perforation of viscera or mesenteric infarction.

Urinary Tract Infections. Proteus organisms are a common cause of urinary tract infections, usually in patients with chronic bacteriuria, many of whom have had obstructive uropathy, a history of instrumentation of the bladder, and repeated courses of chemotherapy. The organism is rarely a pathogen in anatomically normal urinary tracts except occasionally in patients with diabetes mellitus. Proteus organisms are also often cultured from bacteriuric patients with renal or bladder calculi. This may be related to the ammoniagenic property of this organism, which renders the urine alkaline and provides a fertile medium for formation of ammonium-magnesium-phosphate stones.

Bacteremia. Bloodstream invasion is the most serious

manifestation of infection with this organism. In 75 percent of cases, the urinary tract serves as the portal of entry; in the remainder, the biliary tree, gastrointestinal tract, ears and sinuses, and skin are the primary foci. Proteus bacteremia is frequently preceded by cystoscopy, urethral catheterization, transurethral prostatic resection, or other operative procedures. Clinically, the signs, symptoms, and laboratory findings of proteus sepsis—high fever, chills, shock, metastatic abscesses, leukocytosis, and rarely thrombocytopenia—are indistinguishable from those of bloodstream infections with other gram-negative bacteria (Chaps. 134 and 144).

DIAGNOSIS. The diagnosis of proteus infection depends on culture of the organism from blood, urine, or exudate and its identification by appropriate biochemical tests. It is especially important to separate *P. mirabilis,* the indole-negative species, from *P. morganii, rettgeri,* and *vulgaris,* which are indole-positive, because only *P. mirabilis* is susceptible to the action of penicillin and most other antibiotics. Proteus organisms are often present in mixed infections with other pathogens. Particular care should be exercised in the isolation of other organisms growing in the same medium with members of the genus *Proteus* lest they be masked by its spreading growth. The spreading character of this organism may also make antibiotic sensitivity tests difficult to interpret.

TREATMENT. Most strains of *P. mirabilis* are sensitive to penicillin in high concentration (10 units per ml or greater), ampicillin, kanamycin, cephalothin, and chloramphenicol. Proteus bacteriuria can be readily eradicated with any of these drugs during treatment; ampicillin in dosage of 0.5 Gm every 4 to 6 hr is highly effective. In severe infection, therapy should be parenteral: 6 to 12 Gm ampicillin or 20,000,000 units of penicillin G plus kanamycin 1.5 to 2.0 Gm per day, if renal function is adequate. There is good evidence that kanamycin is synergistic with ampicillin and penicillin G in proteus infections, and that chloramphenicol may be ineffective despite the results of in vitro tests. In view of the numerous more effective agents, there is no reason to use chloramphenicol in proteus infections. In general, all strains of *P. mirabilis* are resistant to tetracycline. Most strains other than *P. mirabilis* and Providence bacilli are sensitive only to kanamycin. A newer agent, gentamycin, appears to be very effective against indole-positive proteus organisms in vitro and in vivo. In addition, although ampicillin and penicillin G alone are ineffective against indole-positive proteus, a combination of either drug and kanamycin or gentamycin displays synergism. Carbenicillin is also effective against the majority of indole-positive proteus species. As with all other gram-negative infections, appropriate attention must be given to drainage of pus, maintenance of fluid and electrolyte status, and treatment of circulatory collapse.

REFERENCES

Anderson, K. N., R. P. Kennedy, J. J. Plorde, J. A. Shulman, and R. G. Petersdorf: In Vitro and in Vivo Activity of Ampicillin in Gram-negative Infections, J.A.M.A., 187: 555, 1964.

Chin, V. S. W., and P. D. Hoeprich: Susceptibility of Proteus and Providence Bacilli to 10 Antibacterial Agents, Am. J. Med. Sci., 242:309, 1961.

Kaye, D., M. G. Koenig, and E. W. Hook: The Action of Certain Antibiotics and Antibiotic Combinations against *Proteus mirabilis* with Demonstration of in Vitro Synergism and Antagonism, Am. J. Med. Sci., 242:321, 1961.

McCabe, W. R., and G. G. Jackson: Gram-negative Bacteremia, A.M.A. Arch. Intern. Med., 110:847, 856, 1962.

Tillotson, J. R., and A. M. Lerner: Characteristics of Pneumonias Caused by Bacillus Proteus, Ann. Intern. Med., 68:287, 1968.

146 PSEUDOMONAS INFECTIONS
Marvin Turck and Robert G. Petersdorf

ETIOLOGY. *Pseudomonas aeruginosa* is a gram-negative motile rod which generally is not encapsulated and forms no spores. It grows readily in all ordinary culture media, and on agar it forms irregular, soft, irridescent colonies which usually have a fluorescent yellow-green color because of diffusion into the medium of two pigments, pyocyanin and fluorescin. *Pseudomonas* produces acid but no gas in glucose, and it is proteolytic. It is oxidase-positive and produces ammonia from arginine. A number of different strains have been identified by immunofluorescent techniques or bacteriophage typing. There is no evidence that these strains vary in their virulence for man.

EPIDEMIOLOGY. Pseudomonas organisms are present on the skin of some normal persons, particularly in the axilla and anogenital regions. They are uncommon in the stools of adults not receiving antibiotics. In the majority of instances, pseudomonas organisms are cultured as avirulent secondary contaminants in superficial wounds, or from the sputum of patients treated with antibiotics. Ordinarily this is of little consequence because the organisms merely fill the bacteriologic vacuum left by the elimination of more sensitive bacteria. Occasionally, however, superinfections with pseudomonas organisms occur in the ear, lung, skin, or urinary tract of patients whose primary pathogen has been eradicated by antibiotics. Serious infections are almost invariably associated with damage to local tissue or with diminished host resistance. Premature infants; children with congenital anomalies, patients with leukemia, usually receiving antibiotics, adrenal steroids, or antimetabolites; patients with burns; and geriatric patients with debilitating diseases are likely to develop pseudomonas infections. Most often these infections occur in the hospital environment, and the organisms have been cultured from a variety of sources in hospitals, including water from laboratory sinks and washbasins, antiseptic solutions, including benzalkonium chloride (Zephiran) and hexachlorophene soap, ophthalmic fluorescein and contact lens solution, saline, penicillin, procaine, and a variety of other medications. Other sources are incubators, humidifying equipment, air-cooling systems, forceps, and syringes. The organism is prevalent in urine receptacles and catheters, and on the hands of orderlies, nurses, and surgeons on urologic wards; in several outbreaks, pseudomonas urinary tract infections have presumably been transmitted from patient to patient by human carriers. Similar epidemics have been reported in nurseries among premature infants, and cross infection on burn wards is also common.

PATHOGENESIS. The portal of entry of pseudomonas organisms varies with the patient's age and underlying disease. In infancy and childhood, the skin, umbilical cord, and gastrointestinal tract predominate; in old age, the urinary tract is more often the primary focus. Often the infections remain localized in the skin or subcutaneous tissues. In burns the region below the eschar may become massively infiltrated with bacteria and inflammatory cells, and usually serves as the focus for bacteremia, the single most lethal complication. Hematogenous dissemination is characterized by hemorrhagic nodules in many areas, including the skin, heart, lungs, kidneys, and meninges. The histologic picture is one of necrosis and hemorrhage. Typically the walls of arterioles are heavily infiltrated with bacteria and the vessels are partially or wholly thrombosed.

MANIFESTATIONS. Pseudomonas infections occur in many locations, including the skin, subcutaneous tissue, bone and joints, eyes, ears, mastoid and paranasal sinuses, meninges, and heart valves. Bacteremia without a detectable primary focus may also occur.

Infections of the Skin and Subcutaneous Tissues. Pseudomonas organisms are frequently cultured from surgical wounds, varicose and decubitus ulcers, and burns, particularly following antibiotic therapy. Draining tuberculous or osteomyelitic sinuses may become secondarily infected. The mere presence of pseudomonas in these sites is of little significance provided that bacterial multiplication deep in subcutaneous tissues does not occur and bacteremia does not ensue. Cutaneous infections usually heal following removal or slough of devitalized tissue. Pseudomonas organisms may be responsible for green nails in persons whose hands are excessively exposed to water, soap, and detergents, who have onychomycosis, or whose hands are subject to mechanical trauma. The organism can usually be cultured from the nail plate.

Infections of the Ear, Mastoid, and Paranasal Sinuses. Otitis externa is the most common form of pseudomonas infection involving the ear. It is particularly troublesome in tropical climates and is characterized by chronic serosanguineous and purulent drainage from the external auditory canal. Otitis media or mastoiditis usually occurs as a superinfection following eradication of pneumococci, streptococci, or staphylococci by antimicrobial agents. Frequently pseudomonas organisms are present in association with other gram-negative or gram-positive organisms.

Infection of the Eye. Corneal ulceration is the most severe form of ocular pseudomonas infection. It usually follows a traumatic abrasion and may terminate in panophthalmitis and destruction of the globe. Purulent conjunctivitis occurs as a manifestation of pseudomonas infection in premature infants. Contamination of contact lenses or lens fluid may be an important means of infecting the eyes with pseudomonas organisms.

Urinary Tract Infections. Pseudomonas organisms are common pathogens in the urinary tract and are usually found in patients with obstructive uropathy who have been subjected to repeated urethral manipulations or to urologic surgery. They are rarely cultured from the urine of patients who have not seen a urologist. At times *Pseudomonas* is one of several pathogenic genuses in the urine, the others being *Escherichia coli, Aerobacter-Klebsiella, Proteus,* and enterococci. Pseudomonas bacteriuria is in no way unique and cannot be distinguished from infection with other organisms on clinical grounds.

Gastrointestinal Tract. Pseudomonas organisms have been implicated as a cause of epidemic diarrhea of infancy. In addition, a number of infants dying from neonatal sepsis have the classical necrotic, avascular ulcers of pseudomonas bacteremia in the bowel at autopsy. A "typhoidal" form of pseudomonas infection characterized by fever, myalgia, and diarrhea occurs predominantly in the Tropics. This illness, also called *13-day fever* or *Shanghai fever,* is self-limited, and the prognosis is good.

Respiratory Tract. Primary pseudomonas pneumonia is infrequent, and culture of this organism from the sputum usually is indicative of aspiration of gastric contents with secondary infection or of superinfection following eradication of a more sensitive flora with antibiotics. Pulmonary infection is often associated with microabscesses. The organism is often isolated from the sputum of patients with bronchiectasis, chronic bronchitis, or cystic fibrosis who have lingering infections punctuated by multiple courses of chemotherapy. Pseudomonas bronchitis and bronchiolitis may be the terminal event in cystic fibrosis.

Meningitis. Spontaneous pseudomonas meningitis is most unusual, but the bacilli may be introduced into the subarachnoid space by lumbar puncture, spinal anesthesia, intrathecal medication, or head trauma. Ventriculomastoid or ventriculoatrial shunts performed for hydrocephalus may become contaminated with pseudomonas organisms. Usually revision or removal of the shunt offers the best hope of cure. Meningitis may be a terminal phenomenon in pseudomonas bacteremia and in this instance represents a metastatic infection in the meninges.

Bacteremia. Bloodstream invasion tends to occur in debilitated patients, premature infants, children with congenital defects, patients with lymphomas, leukemias, or other malignant tumors, and elderly patients who have undergone surgery or instrumentation of the biliary or urinary tracts. Pseudomonas bacteremia is an important cause of death in patients with severe burns. In adults, pseudomonas bacteremia is indistinguishable from bloodstream infection with other bacterial species except for two findings (1) *ecthyma gangrenosum,* the classical skin lesion, often located in the anogenital region as a round, indurated, purple-black area about 1 cm in diameter with an ulcerated center and a surrounding zone of erythema; and (2) the passage of green urine, presumably due to the hemoglobin pigment, verdoglobin. Other features of pseudomonas sepsis include hectic fever, shaking chills, hyperventilation, confusion, delirium, and circulatory collapse. Hypothermia, leukopenia, and thrombocytopenia are more common in pseudomonas bacteremia than in other gram-negative bacteremias but are often related to an underlying blood dyscrasia. In addition to ecthyma gangrenosum, other skin lesions consist of hemorrhagic cellulitis and macular lesions on the trunk similar to "rose spots." Organisms usually can be cultured from cutaneous lesions and may provide an early clue to the diagnosis. Pseudomonas organisms may be in the bloodstream concomitantly with other organisms, notably *Enterobacteriaceae* or staphylococci. More often, however, pseudomonas bacteremia follows staphylococcal sepsis in patients with burns.

Bacterial Endocarditis. A number of cases of pseudomonas subacute bacterial endocarditis have followed open-heart surgery. Usually the organisms become implanted on a silk suture or a synthetic patch employed for closure of septal defects. Reoperation with removal of the vegetation and foreign bodies offers the best hope of cure. Pseudomonas endocarditis has been found on normal heart valves in patients with burns; it has been postulated that staphylococcal endocarditis develops first and that the vegetation is secondarily infected with pseudomonas organisms. Metastatic abscesses in bone, joints, brain, adrenal glands, and lungs are frequent consequences of pseudomonas endocarditis.

TREATMENT. Localized infections should be treated by irrigation with 1 percent acetic acid or topical therapy with colistin or polymyxin B. The administration of colistin subconjunctivally has been of value in ocular infections. Drainage of purulent material and removal of devitalized tissues are essential. The outcome of pseudomonas bacteremia is more dependent on the underlying disease than on the chemotherapy. For example, in patients with leukemia, remission must be attained before sepsis can be controlled. In burns, wound infection must be eradicated before the bloodstream can be cleared of organisms. Most strains of *Pseudomonas* are sensitive to polymyxin B and colistin, and a number of strains respond to oxytetracycline. These drugs should be used in full dosage of 30 to 50 mg every 6 hr for polymyxin B (in adults) and 75 to 100 mg every 6 hr (in adults) for colistin in life-threatening pseudomonas bacteremia. Both drugs are excellent for eradicating bacteriuria, but because blood levels exceed minimal inhibitory concentrations only two- or threefold, the results in bacteremia are inconsistent. Gentamycin, an aminoglycoside antibiotic, inhibits a number of strains of *Pseudomonas*. Carbenicillin, a new semisynthetic penicillin, is also active against many isolates and may be useful. Further experience with these drugs is necessary. Asymptomatic bacteriuria, particularly when confined to the bladder, should be treated with the least toxic and least painful agent, which, at times, may be a sulfonamide.

The prognosis has been improved in burned patients with pseudomonas sepsis as well as in a few other patients with endocarditis and with necrotizing papillitis by the use of large doses of hyperimmune γ-globulin in addition to antimicrobials.

PROPHYLAXIS. Pseudomonas cross infections in hospitals can be reduced by careful attention to aseptic techniques, particularly in nurseries for premature infants, operating rooms, and urologic wards; avoidance of cold sterilization procedures wherever possible; and scrupulous attention to clean plumbing fixtures, humidifying equipment, etc. Judicious use of antibiotics, steroids, and cytotoxic agents should also diminish the incidence of pseudomonas infections. Systemic antibiotic prophylaxis aimed at preventing colonization and infection with pseudomonas organisms has been notoriously unsuccessful and should be interdicted.

PROGNOSIS. The mortality rate in pseudomonas bacteremia is 75 percent and is highest in patients with shock or severe associated disease such as massive third degree burns, leukemia, or prematurity. When bacteremia originates in the urinary tract and is not accompanied by shock, the prognosis is considerably better. Localized pseudomonas infections do not present a threat to life unless hematogenous dissemination occurs.

REFERENCES

Curtin, J. A., R. G. Petersdrof, and I. L. Bennett, Jr.: Pseudomonas Bacteremia. Review of 91 Cases, Ann. Intern. Med., 54:1077, 1961.

Fierer, J., P. M. Taylor, and H. M. Gezon: *Pseudomonas Aeruginosa* Epidemic Traced to Delivery-Room Resuscitators, New Engl. J. Med., 276:991, 1967.

Forkner, C. E.: *Pseudomonas Aeruginosa* Infections, Modern Medical Monographs, No. 22, New York, Grune & Stratton, Inc., 1960.

———, E. Frei, III, J. H. Edgcomb, and J. P. Utz: Pseudomonas Septicemia, Am. J. Med., 25:877, 1958.

Rabin, E. R., C. D. Graber, E. H. Vogel, Jr., R. A. Finkelstein, and W. A. Turnbush: Fatal Pseudomonas Infection in Burned Patients, New Engl. J. Med., 265:1225, 1961.

Tillotson, J. R., and A. M. Lerner: Characteristics of Nonbacteremic Pseudomonas Pneumonia, Ann. Intern. Med., 68:295, 1968.

147 BACTEROIDES INFECTIONS
Edward W. Hook

ETIOLOGY. The genus *Bacteroides* includes a group of gram-negative, non-spore-forming, strictly anaerobic bacilli that are normal inhabitants of the mouth, intestinal tract, and vagina. These organisms are found in large numbers in human feces in an average concentration of about 10^9 viable units per gram, and often outnumber coliform bacilli by one-hundredfold.

Bacteroides funduliformis (*B. necrophorus*), *B. fragilis*, and *B. nigrescens* (*B. melaninogenicus*) are the species usually responsible for local or systemic infection of man.

PATHOGENESIS. Species of bacteroides are not highly invasive microorganisms, and infection is usually secondary to an underlying disease, a surgical procedure, or drug or radiation therapy which impairs the normal defenses of the host. The initial reaction to infection results in a localized suppurative lesion characterized by the formation of fetid pus. Infection usually remains localized, but bloodstream invasion may occur. In instances of bacteremia, suppurative thrombophlebitis adjacent to the site of initial infection is a frequent occurrence, and emboli harboring viable bacilli may be dislodged, resulting in septic pulmonary infarction. Organisms of the genus *Bacteroides* elaborate a heparinase, but the role of this enzyme in the formation of thrombi is unknown. Localization of blood-borne organisms at distant sites is not unusual and may result in abscess formation in brain, lung, liver, joints, kidneys, or other organs.

Although bacteroides may be isolated in pure culture from infected tissue or pus, other organisms are present in the majority of cases, usually anaerobic or aerobic streptococci, coliform species, or staphylococci. Bacteroides and anaerobic streptococci have been shown to act synergistically in the induction of abscesses in mice.

CLINICAL MANIFESTATIONS. Local Infections. Species of bacteroides are frequently isolated from local suppurative lesions of any tissue liable to contamination with the flora of the mouth, intestinal tract, or vagina. For example, members of this genus have been isolated from peritonsillar, appendiceal, ischiorectal, or pelvic abscesses, and from infected Skene's or Bartholin's glands. These organisms may be associated with sinusitis and otitis media, and can also be cultured from the surfaces of acutely inflamed appendices, from exudate in localized or generalized peritonitis, and from purulent discharge in patients with endometritis. Surgical wounds of the gastrointestinal or genitourinary tract may be complicated by bacteroides infection.

Local infection is usually manifested by pain and tenderness, and the course and outcome depend on the site of involvement and extent of infection. Necrosis of blood vessels in an abscess cavity occasionally results in severe hemorrhage.

Systemic infection. Invasion of the bloodstream by bacteroides is usually secondary to local infection of the tonsils, female genital tract, or peritoneum. The initial manifestations are determined by the portal of entry and may be those of peritonsillar abscess, endometritis, or appendicitis. When bloodstream invasion occurs, the patient becomes extremely ill. Severe chills, hectic fever ranging from 101 to 106°F, and severe diaphoresis are common. When bacteremia complicates tonsillar infection, the internal jugular vein may be the site of suppurative thrombophlebitis, and in pelvic infections the iliac and femoral veins may be involved. Palpation along the course of an involved vein, such as the internal jugular, may disclose a firm, tender cord, indicating the presence of a thrombus. Emboli may be dislodged, resulting in multiple septic pulmonary infarcts manifested by rales, dyspnea, cough, hemoptysis, pleurisy, and roentgenographic evidence of consolidation. Lung abscess and empyema often complicate pulmonary infection. Metastatic infection at other sites is not unusual, and may be manifested as brain abscess, liver abscess, or septic arthritis. A diffuse hepatitis may develop, leading to en-

largement and tenderness of the liver and jaundice. The prognosis in systemic bacteroides infection is grave, and death may occur in a few days.

The genus *Bacteroides* has also been implicated in certain other serious systemic infections. Meningitis or brain abscess occasionally results from direct extension of infection from the middle ear or sinuses. Aspiration of secretions harboring bacteroides may lead to pneumonia, lung abscess formation, or empyema. Transient bacteroides bacteremia may occur after dental extraction, and a few cases of subacute bacterial endocarditis have been described. These organisms occasionally cause infection of the urinary tract.

LABORATORY FINDINGS. Leukocytosis of 12,000 to 25,000 cells per cu mm may occur in localized bacteroides infections and is almost always present in systemic infection. Patients with liver abscesses or hepatitis have elevated serum bilirubin values and other aberrations of hepatic function. Gas formation at sites of infection occasionally results in air-fluid levels detectable by roentgenography.

Bacteroides infection should be considered whenever pus with an extremely foul odor is encountered, and anaerobic cultures should be made. A smear of the pus reveals slightly elongated gram-negative bacilli, and often another organism, usually a gram-positive coccus. Definitive diagnosis depends on isolation of the organisms from infected tissue or blood. Bacteroides grow slowly and may be difficult to detect when associated with another organism. Agglutinins against the strain responsible for an infection develop during the second or third week of infection, but because of the variable antigenic composition of these organisms, serologic methods are not of diagnostic aid.

TREATMENT. Surgical drainage of abscess cavities is of prime importance and should be carried out as soon as fluctuation and localization occur. Antimicrobial therapy is indicated when infection is not localized. Tetracycline in dosage of 2 Gm per day is the antibiotic of choice. Penicillin G in doses of 20 million units intravenously per day may be used as an alternative to tetracycline. Species of bacteroides are not highly sensitive to penicillin G, but most strains are inhibited in vitro by concentrations that are achieved in the blood of patients receiving massive penicillin therapy. Ampicillin in doses of 6 gm per day parenterally can be used instead of penicillin G. Chloramphenicol is also active against the majority of isolates from human infections, and cephalothin is inhibitory for some strains. Many strains of *Bacteroides* are highly resistant to the penicillinase-resistant penicillins and practically all isolates are resistant to streptomycin and neomycin.

Anticoagulant therapy and venous ligation should be considered in patients with thrombophlebitis and multiple septic pulmonary infarctions.

REFERENCES

Alston, J. M.: Necrobacillosis in Great Britain, Brit. Med. J., II:1524, 1955.

Bornstein, D. L., A. N. Weinberg, M. N. Swartz, and L. J. Kunz: Anaerobic Infections—Review of Current Experience, Medicine, 43:207, 1964.

Gunn, A. A.: Bacteroides Septicaemia, J. Roy. Coll. Surg. Edinburgh, 2:41, 1956.

Heineman, H. S., and A. I. Braude: Anaerobic Infection of the Brain, Am. J. Med., 35:682, 1963.

Keusch, G. T., and C. J. O'Connell: The Susceptibility of Bacteroides to the Penicillins and Cephalothin, Am. J. Med. Sci., 251:428, 1966.

McHenry, M. C., W. E. Wellman, and W. J. Martin: Bacteremia Due to Bacteroides, Arch. Intern. Med., 107:572, 1961.

Tillotson, J. R., and A. M. Lerner: Bacteroides Pneumonias, Ann. Intern. Med., 68:308, 1968.

Tynes, B. S., and W. B. Frommeyer, Jr.: Bacteroides Septicemia, Cultural, Clinical, and Therapeutic Features in a Series of Twenty-five Patients, Ann. Intern. Med., 56:12, 1962.

148   KLEBSIELLA (Aerobactor) INFECTION

*Marvin Turck and
Robert G. Petersdorf*

ETIOLOGY. Next to *Escherichia coli*, strains of *Klebsiella-Aerobacter* are the most important enteric organisms infecting man. In many laboratories *Klebsiella-Aerobacter* is not differentiated from *E. coli*. This is potentially a serious error because strains of *Klebsiella-Aerobacter* are, in general, more resistant to antibiotics and their isolation from blood, purulent exudates, and urine is of more serious prognostic significance. The Friedländer bacilli (*Klebsiella pneumoniae*) are encapsulated gram-negative bacilli, found among the normal flora of the mouth and intestinal tracts. *Klebsiella pneumoniae* has been considered to be a virulent respiratory pathogen since first described by Friedländer in 1882. *Klebsiella* is closely related to the genera *Aerobacter* (*Enterobacter**) and *Serratia* and may be differentiated only by certain amino acid decarboxylase tests. The significance of *Aerobacter* and *Serratia* in human infections has been less well clarified than infections secondary to *Klebsiella*, but all are potential pathogens, especially as opportunistic invaders in the compromised host. The strains of *Klebsiella* isolated from respiratory infections usually are nonmotile and form large mucoid colonies on solid media. *Aerobacters* on the other hand, tend to be motile. Klebsiellas are usually sensitive to the antibiotic cephalothin, to which *Aerobacters* are resistant. These characteristics, however, are not invariable enough to differentiate respiratory from intestinal isolates.

Klebsiella rhinoscleromatis, is probably the causative agent of rhinoscleroma, and *Klebsiella ozenae* has been isolated occasionally from the nose of patients with ozena (Chap. 282).

PATHOGENESIS. *Klebsiella, Aerobacter,* and *Serratia* are all capable of causing disease in diverse anatomic

---

* This name is now also acceptable.

sites. However, results of clinical and epidemiologic studies suggest that differences in pathogenicity do exist among these genera and that precise taxonomic identification is of value. Although infections of the respiratory tract with *K. pneumoniae* have been emphasized most in the past, the urinary tract presently accounts for the majority of clinical isolates. In this site clinical manifestations and pathogenesis are similar to infections produced by *E. coli*, but Klebsiellas are more frequently found in patients with complicated and obstructive urinary tract disease. Infections of the biliary tract, the peritoneal cavity, the middle ear, mastoids, paranasal sinuses, and meninges also are not uncommon. In these locations, Klebsiellas are more frequent than either *Aerobacters* or serratias and are more likely to produce an illness of greater severity. The apparent increased frequency of infection by serratias represents an increase primarily due to nosocomial spread of this organism.

MANIFESTATIONS. Symptoms and signs of common infections caused by *Klebsiella-Aerobacter*—namely those involving the urinary tract, biliary tree, peritoneal cavity —are indistinguishable from those caused by *E. coli* (Chap. 144). These infections commonly occur in diabetics and in the form of superinfections in patients who have received antimicrobials to which these organisms are resistant. Klebsiella-aerobacter infection is also an important etiologic factor in septic shock (Chap. 134).

Acute Pneumonia. *Klebsiella* is well recognized as a pulmonary pathogen, but probably accounts for less than 1 percent of all cases of bacterial pneumonia. The disease is most common in men over forty years of age and is more frequently found in alcoholics. Other factors associated with increased susceptibility include diabetes mellitus and chronic bronchopulmonary disease. Aspiration of oropharyngeal secretions containing klebsiella organisms is the likely inciting factor among alcoholic patients. The clinical manifestations are indistinguishable from those of pneumococcal pneumonia (Chap. 138), with sudden onset of chills, fever, productive cough, and severe pleuritic chest pain. Patients are frequently delirious and prostrated, but this may also occur with pneumococcal infection. A "characteristic" clinical feature, which occurs in only 25 to 50 percent of patients, is the dark brown or red currant-jelly sputum which may be so tenacious that the patient has difficulty in expelling it from his mouth and lips. The pulmonary lesion is most frequent in the right upper lobe but often rapidly progresses and if untreated, may spread from lobe to lobe. Cyanosis and dyspnea develop rapidly, and jaundice, vomiting, and diarrhea may be present. Physical findings consist primarily of signs of consolidation unless pleural effusion or necrotizing pneumonitis with rapid cavitation have intervened. The blood leukocyte count may be elevated but is often low, which probably is merely a reflection of severe infection in an alcoholic patient with poor bone marrow reserve. Lung abscess and empyema are much more frequent than in pneumococcal pneumonia and are related to the destructive capabilities of this organism. So-called "characteristic" radiographic features such as bulging fissures and loss of lung volume occur only in varying frequency, and also may be found in pneumococcal infection.

Chronic infection of the lung. Rarely, infection with *Klebsiella* may progress, often in indolent fashion, to a chronic necrotizing pneumonitis resembling tuberculosis. It may follow acute Friedländer pneumonia but is also seen in patients who give no history of acute onset. The principal symptoms are productive cough, weakness, and anemia. Hemoptysis, chronic empyema, or sterile serous effusions are also encountered. Cavitation, frequently with thin walls, occurs primarily in the upper lobes.

DIAGNOSIS. Diagnosis is established by an awareness of the clinical setting in which Klebsiella infections occur and by isolation of the organism. A presumptive diagnosis of klebsiella pneumonia should be made on the basis of gram stain of the sputum which shows a predominance of short, plump, gram-negative bacilli, frequently surrounded by a clear space because of the capsule. Often these gram-negative organisms occur together with gram-positive cocci and because the gram-positives are easier to see, the gram-negative bacteria may be ignored and the diagnosis may be missed, which in turn, may lead to potentially serious delays in instituting therapy. Additional proof of klebsiella-aerobacter infection in the lung is afforded by isolation of the organisms from blood and pleural exudate. In extrapulmonary infections, the organisms are readily seen in and cultured from pus or secretions of involved organs.

TREATMENT. Klebsiellas have variable susceptibility to antimicrobial drugs, but the majority of strains is susceptible to kanamycin, streptomycin, cephalothin, tetracycline, chloramphenicol, or polymyxin B or colistin. The organism does not respond to penicillin and its analogues. A popular regimen employs streptomycin in large doses (2 to 3 Gm daily) with chloramphenicol or a tetracycline. Kanamycin (25 mg/kg/day) is probably more active than streptomycin and has been advocated along with cephalothin (6 to 12 Gm per day). It is of clinical importance that most strains of *K. pneumoniae* are sensitive to cephalothin, but most enterobacter are highly resistant. Because of the relative poor blood and tissue levels achieved with the polymyxins, they should probably not be employed as first line agents in the treatment of klebsiella infections. Regardless of the antimicrobial regimen employed, treatment should be continued for a minimum of 10 to 14 days and prolonged if there is extensive cavitation. Pleural effusion must be drained appropriately; antibiotic therapy alone is not sufficient treatment for closed-space infections of the pleural cavity. At times, rib resection with open drainage may be necessary, and should be considered if effusions recur.

PROGNOSIS. Prior to the introduction of antimicrobials, the fatality rate reported in different clinics varied from 50 to 80 percent and death within 48 hr was not infrequent. Even with antimicrobial treatment the course of the disease is quite variable and the prognosis must be guarded. For the most part, this reflects the age group involved and the frequent association of klebsiella infection

with alcoholism, malnutrition, and severe underlying disease.

REFERENCES

Edmondson, E. G., and J. P. Sanford: The Klebsiella-Enterobacter (Aerobacter)-Serratia Group, Medicine 46:323, 1967.

Eickhoff, T. C., B. W. Steinhauer, and M. Finland: The Klebsiella-Enterobacter-Serratia Division. Biochemical and Serologic Characteristics and Susceptibility to Antibiotics, Ann. Intern. Med., 65:1163, 1966.

Manfredi, F., W. J. Daly, and R. H. Rehnke: Clinical Observations of Acute Friedländer Pneumonia, Ann. Intern Med., 58:642, 1963.

149 TYPHOID FEVER

Richard B. Hornick and
Theodore E. Woodward

DEFINITION. Typhoid fever is a systemic infection unique to man. Following ingestion of *Salmonella typhosa* no other animal develops prolonged remittent fever, characteristic rash (rose spots), splenomegaly, lymphadenopathy, or intestinal complications. Predominant symptoms include fever, headache, abdominal pain, disturbances in bowel function, anorexia, and lassitude. Diagnosis is confirmed by isolation of the causative organisms from the blood, feces, or urine and by demonstrating rising titers of agglutinins to the somatic (O) and flagellar (H) antigens of the bacillus.

HISTORY. In 1829, Louis studied 158 cases and described intestinal lesions, enlarged mesenteric lymph glands, splenomegaly, rose spots, and intestinal hemorrhage and perforation. This great clinician first employed the term *typhoide*. The British, however, continued to view the intestinal lesion as an incidental complication of typhus. In 1836 William Gerhard of Philadelphia, a former student of Louis, clearly defined differences between typhus and typhoid based on precise clinical and anatomic findings.

Budd, an English practitioner, in a series of publications from 1856 to 1870, suggested the contagiousness of typhoid and stressed the importance of spread by the bowel discharges of infected persons. His hypothesis was not verified until 1885 when Pfeiffer reported the first stool isolation. The discovery of the organism is credited to Eberth, who in 1880 reported the presence of bacteria in stained smears of mesenteric lymph nodes and spleen. Widal in 1896 described the test for agglutinins in the serum of patients.

EPIDEMIOLOGY. *Salmonella typhosa* resides solely in man and is perpetuated in nature by its transmission to healthy persons from patients or carriers. Water, milk, and food are contaminated from infected feces. It is an epidemiologic axiom that for every outbreak or sporadic case of typhoid fever there must be a carrier that is, an individual who sheds virulent organisms in spite of apparent good health. Once identified, typhoid carriers should be prevented from handling food until they have been freed of S. *typhosa.*

Flies have been incriminated in the transmission of typhoid fever because of their ability to carry the bacilli from feces to food or liquids.

The incidence of typhoid fever in the United States has declined steadily in the past century. Occupational control of carriers and improvement of water supply and sewage disposal have been the major contributors to this decline. From 1962 to 1966, the annual median number of cases reported in this country was 461. Formerly the majority of cases occurred during the summer months, but seasonal variation has disappeared as the number of carriers has lessened. The disease has not been controlled in some countries, primarily because of crowded living conditions and poor sanitation.

Typhoid fever emerges as a significant cause of disability and death among civilian and military populations during war or following severe natural catastrophes. Major epidemics have occurred in recent years in Switzerland and Great Britain, emphasizing the ability of this disease to spread unexpectedly when defects in sewage disposal or food handling occur.

PATHOGENESIS. As in other enteric infections, causative organisms gain access to the host via the oral cavity. Studies of infectivity in human subjects have failed to confirm that S. *typhosa* invade via the lymphoid tissue of the pharynx and have also ruled out the respiratory tract as a significant portal of entry. Rather, typhoid bacilli survive the acidity of the stomach, pass on into the small and large intestine, multiply, and invade the mucosal barrier. It is during the critical 24 to 72 hr after ingestion that the outcome of the infection is decided. If the organisms overcome inhibitory influences of commensal bacteria and reproduce in sufficient numbers to overwhelm the phagocytic activities of intestinal mucosa, successful entry can be made into the host. Once the intestinal barrier has been penetrated, stool cultures, which have been positive for S. *typhosa* for the few days after swallowing the organisms, usually become free of the pathogen. The bacteria probably enter the systemic circulation by way of the mesenteric-thoracic duct lymphatic drainage. From this stage in the incubation period until overt disease occurs, typhoid bacilli reside within the reticuloendothelial system, mainly the liver. Subsequent bacteremia heralds the onset of clinical signs and symptoms of typhoid fever. Shortly thereafter S. *typhosa* reappears in stool cultures, having escaped from the liver and perhaps local foci in the intestine.

Clinical manifestations and pathologic findings of typhoid fever have been attributed to the effects of circulating endotoxin. Endotoxin of S. *typhosa* is a lipopolysaccharide-protein complex with toxic activities identical to those of other endotoxins. It is derived from the cell wall and evokes numerous pharmacologic actions. Intravenous infusion of endotoxin in man produces fever, chills,

headache, nausea, backache, and abdominal pain. Volunteers could not differentiate these symptoms from those subsequently produced in the course of induced typhoid fever.

Despite this circumstantial evidence, certain well-known effects of endotoxin are inconsistent with the thesis that attributes the manifestations of typhoid fever to endotoxemia. For example, from three to five daily intravenous infusions of endotoxin result in development of tolerance to its pyrogenicity, i.e., chills and fever are no longer induced unless dosage is markedly increased. This tolerance differs from the sustained febrile course which typifies typhoid fever. Moreover, recent studies indicate that endotoxin tolerance continues to operate effectively in volunteers with induced typhoid fever. In addition, deliberate activation of tolerance either before or during induced typhoid did not mitigate the febrile or toxic course of disease. It appears, therefore, that circulating endotoxin does not play a major role in the pathogenesis of typhoid fever.

PATHOLOGY. Early in the disease, a nonspecific enteritis is present in the jejunum. Mesenteric adenopathy is striking in chimpanzees sacrificed 48 hr after ingestion of typhoid bacilli. Other components of the reticuloendothelial system (RES) are involved during the first few days of disease. Pharyngeal lymphoid tissue and peripheral nodes are enlarged; later the spleen and liver become palpable. Using ^{131}I-aggregated albumin in volunteer typhoid subjects, increased phagocytic activity of the RES, coinciding with the overt hypertrophy, was demonstrable by the third to the fifth day of disease.

The Peyer's patches are initially swollen and ultimately undergo necrosis, forming oval-shaped ulcers most numerous in the terminal 24 in. of the ileum. Ulceration may occur in the jejunum and lymphoid follicles of the cecum and colon. Necrosis of these lesions, usually during the third febrile week, leads to the common complications of hemorrhage and perforation. The intestinal ulcer eventually heals without scarring.

Histologic changes in the intestinal lesions are proliferation of large mononuclear cells and edema. Similar alterations occur in mesenteric nodes, spleen, bone marrow, and liver (typhoid nodules). Lymph nodes often exhibit necrosis and marked proliferation of the sinusoidal cells; sinusoids are filled with macrophages. Skin lesions (rose spots) consist of clumps of typhoid bacilli in the dermis, with round-cell infiltration and dilated vascular spaces.

Focal metastatic infection may be responsible for cholecystitis, osteomyelitis, chrondritis, meningitis, endocarditis, or nephritis. The gallbladder is frequently infected, although acute cholecystitis is less common. Bronchitis is not uncommon, and pneumonia due to S. *typhosa* occasionally occurs.

The intestinal lesions subside ultimately, whereas the infection in the liver and biliary tract may continue indefinitely, characterizing the carrier state. Fully developed, this chronic infection produces no symptoms, and reinfection of the host does not occur despite constant presence in the intestine of millions of typhoid bacilli.

MANIFESTATIONS. Unrecognized and inadequately treated typhoid infection may persist as a continuous or remittent fever for 3 or more weeks, with a prolonged period of convalescence.

The incubation period averages about 10 days, with a range of 3 to 25 days, which probably depends on the infecting dose. In volunteer studies, the largest number of organisms produced illness in the shortest period of time.

Onset of illness in a typical case is gradual, with symptoms appearing and increasing in severity over a 2- to 3-day period. Headache, the most common initial complaint, is generalized and constant, and worsens as the fever rises. Headache, plus the associated malaise, chilly sensations, and fever, cause the patient to take to bed. Intestinal complaints develop rapidly, beginning with continuous abdominal pain, frequently in the lower quadrants. Mild ileus occurs with associated constipation, anorexia, and nausea. Palpation elicits the feeling of gas-liquid-filled loops of intestine being compressed and displaced. Cough and bronchitic symptoms are common. Conjunctival injection occurs early in the febrile course. Sudden and unprovoked epistaxis may occur.

Fever increases in stepwise fashion for 2 to 3 days and then plateaus, with a continuous febrile pattern in the range of 103 to 105°F. It maintains this level for 2 to 3 weeks in untreated cases before abating slowly during the third and fourth weeks of disease. Many patients react to this debilitating febrile course with frank psychosis, delirium, or mania, which complicates management. Chills and sweating are not a regular accompaniment of the fever. As the temperature wanes, symptoms disappear.

The increment in pulse rate is usually inconsistent with the elevated temperature early in the course of typhoid. Etiology of this relative bradycardia has not been ascertained. Myocarditis, a not-infrequent complication, occurs later.

Some patients have diarrhea early in the disease, and in many it is a late manifestation.

Rose spots, the characteristic exanthem of enteric forms of salmonellosis, appear in only 10 percent of cases, and early therapy may reduce the incidence. Rose spots appear on the anterior thorax and abdomen early in the second week as rose-pink hyperemic papules 2 to 4 mm in diameter, that blanch on pressure. They are usually few in number, persist for only 2 to 3 days, and are detected with great difficulty in darkly pigmented patients. As they regress, the reddish color changes to a faint brown discoloration which does not blanch with pressure. Only careful scrutiny utilizing good lighting will reveal this delicate rash.

The spleen is frequently enlarged late in the first week of illness. Occasionally there is splenic tenderness, and rarely a friction rub appears, because of perisplenitis.

COMPLICATIONS. Formerly, numerous complications were associated with the prolonged convalescence of typhoid fever. Appropriate antibiotic and supportive care has eliminated the profound weakness, weight loss, and abnormalities due to nutritional deficiencies. However, patients occasionally will have thrombophlebitis, arthral-

gia, and peripheral neuritis despite adequate nursing and dietary management.

Gastrointestinal Hemorrhage. Gross hemorrhage of typhoidal ulcers occurs in approximately 10 percent of cases; occult bleeding is present in about 20 percent. Characteristically, hemorrhage occurs during the second or third week of disease, either as sudden gross hemorrhage or as continuous slow oozing. Clinical signs indicative of blood loss are apprehension, sweating, pallor, depression of cutaneous temperature, rapid weak pulse, hypotension, and narrow pulse pressure. Chloramphenicol therapy has reduced but not eliminated the incidence of this serious complication.

Intestinal Perforation. Intestinal perforation occurs in about 3 percent of untreated patients and was formerly an important cause of death. Rupture of the intestinal ulcer with peritonitis still occurs, although antibiotics have reduced the number of fatalities sharply. In most instances perforation of an ulcer in the lower ileum occurs early in the third week. Patients manifesting tympanites, diarrhea, and hemorrhage are likely to suffer this complication; it may strike unexpectedly in convalescent patients. Sudden, sharp pain in the right lower quadrant, soon associated with abdominal distension, muscle rigidity, rebound tenderness, and diminished peristalsis, is a characteristic sign. Obliteration of liver flatness on percussion, with excessive tympanites, is a valuable sign of free abdominal air. Pallor, clammy perspiration, tachycardia, and lowered pressure all herald impending shock. At this stage there is hypothermia and the blood leukocyte count ranges from 9,000 to 13,000 cells per cu mm. Perforation may be mistaken for appendicitis, acute cholecystitis, or merely an accentuation of the abdominal pain in the debilitated typhoid patient. Frequent examination and upright abdominal x-ray to demonstrate air under the diaphragm provide very helpful diagnostic clues. Rarely, typhoidal peritonitis may result from rupture of an enlarged softened mesenteric lymph gland.

Other Complications. Bacterial or lobar pneumonia developing at the height of the disease was formerly a serious complication of typhoid fever. Cultures of sputum or consolidated lungs have yielded predominantly pneumococci or occasionally typhoid bacilli. Other pyogenic complications include parotitis, sinusitis, and furunculosis. Folliculitis is a common sequel, despite early chloramphenicol therapy, but tends to be mild and disappears spontaneously within several weeks. Typhoidal meningitis is rare but serious. Chondritis and periostitis are indolent focal infections from which S. typhosa may be isolated. Monoarticular and polyarticular arthritis are rare complications. Cholecystitis may occur during the acute disease, creating a confusing diagnostic problem because of physical findings similar to those seen with intestinal perforation. Months or years later there may be chronic cholecystitis with calculi from which viable typhoid bacilli can be isolated. Acute nephritis or pyelonephritis is seen occasionally at the height of the illness or during convalescence. Deafness is common but seldom permanent. Herpes labialis is rare in typhoid patients. Severe hemolytic anemia has occurred during the acute phase of the illness, with patients showing positive Coombs tests or red cells deficient in glucose 6-phosphate dehydrogenase. Whether hemolysis is due to an enzymatic defect in the red cell, drug therapy, or typhoid per se is not clear.

Relapse. The incidence of relapse varies from 5 to 15 percent. Antibiotic therapy appears to have altered the host's recuperative powers adversely in this disease, since relapse rates are greater (20 percent) in groups of patients treated with chloramphenicol. On an average, relapse occurs approximately 15 days after cessation of chemotherapy, regardless of the duration of treatment or the stage at which the antibiotic is first given. Onset of the relapse is usually associated with recurrent bacteremia and symptoms similar to those of the primary disease. As a rule, the manifestations are milder and may abate without specific therapy. The cause of the relapse is not the emergence of chloramphenicol-resistant organisms and does not appear to be correlated with the presence or absence of somatic (O) or flagellar (H) antibodies. Cultivation of typhoid bacilli in tissue culture cells has revealed the persistence of viable, but nonmultiplying, intracellular *S. typhosa* despite presence of antibiotic. Removal of chemotherapeutic agents (3 weeks later) from the medium resulted in reactivation of the tissue culture infection. Persistence of organisms in the hepatic cells of patients treated with therapeutic doses of chloramphenicol may explain the development of relapses as well as carrier states. Reasons for the "microbial indifference" are unknown.

The Typhoid Carrier. Typhoid bacilli persist indefinitely in the bile passages and in the intestines of about 3 percent of patients who recover from the disease. Many carriers have no history of prior infection, and all are in apparent good health. A carrier is defined as one who excretes *S. typhosa* in the stools beyond 1 year following the acute infection. Most typhoid patients will have negative stool cultures after 4 months; persistence beyond this period usually indicates a carrier. The carrier state is three times as common in women as in men. The incidence increases with advancing age, suggesting that the greater frequency of biliary tract disease in older females favors development of a carrier state. Removal of a diseased gallbladder, with or without stones, eradicates the carrier state in a significant number of patients. The gallbladder is not the sole source for this persistent infection, since typhoid bacilli can be isolated from bile obtained from the T tube left in the common duct following cholecystectomy. Cultures of bile and stools usually become negative when the T tube has been removed and complete healing occurs. Typhoid carriers with cholelithiasis should be treated by cholecystectomy and antibiotics. Those without stones can often be cleared with intensive chemotherapeutic regimens. The following schedules have been successful in reported series of treated carriers: (1) Ampicillin 3 to 6 Gm per day for as long as 84 days. (2) Penicillin in a dosage of 12 million units daily, supplemented with Benemid for 14 days. (3) Combined treatment with chloramphenicol (1.0 Gm every 8 hr) and streptomycin (1.0 Gm twice daily) for 3 weeks.

Urinary tract carriers are infrequent and represent a minor health hazard in this country. Chronic bladder scarring, with pseudoabscess and stone formation secondary to *Schistosoma haematobium* infection, predisposes to development of the urinary carrier state following acute typhoid fever.

LABORATORY DIAGNOSIS. One of the distinctive hematologic features of typhoid fever is leukopenia, with cell counts ranging from 4,000 to 6,000 cells per cu mm during the first 2 weeks and 3,000 to 5,000 cells per cu mm during the third and fourth weeks. In the presence of intestinal perforation or pyogenic complications, the leukocyte count rises moderately, to 10,000 to 14,000 cells per cu mm. Normocytic anemia is present in many patients; with blood loss the anemia becomes hypochromic and microcytic. Except for transient albuminuria during the febrile stage, the urine is normal. Occult blood may be present in the feces beginning the second week.

Isolation of *S. typhosa* from the blood and feces is the most dependable diagnostic test. Blood cultures are positive in most cases during the first and early in the second febrile week. Bacteremia is also demonstrable during relapse. Typhoid bacilli are usually present in fecal cultures after the tenth day; the incidence of isolates increases up to the fourth or fifth week. Bone marrow aspirations and culture of rose spots have yielded the organism, but they offer no advantage over blood cultures. Likewise, in a small percentage of patients, *S. typhosa* can be detected in urine during the second or third week of disease.

The readily available Widal test aids in the diagnosis of typhoid fever. Specific agglutinins appear in the serum after 7 to 10 days of illness. The titer rises steadily to a peak during the third to fifth week and falls gradually over several weeks. It does not rise appreciably during relapse. The titer of the flagellar (H) antibody is usually higher than the somatic (O) agglutinin. Measurement of Vi (capsular) antibody by the agglutination of sensitized red cells has been used in conjunction with stool cultures to determine the presence of or the cessation of the carrier state. Many carriers will have elevated Vi hemagglutination titers, but this antibody should not be used as a single criterion to evaluate the activity of the typhoid carrier.

DIFFERENTIAL DIAGNOSIS. No single symptom or clinical feature is pathognomonic at the time of onset. Manifestations such as headache, fever, malaise, weakness, anorexia, cough, and abdominal pain are common to many diseases. These include the major rickettsioses, brucellosis, tularemia, leptospirosis, psittacosis, infectious hepatitis, infectious mononucleosis, primary atypical pneumonia, miliary tuberculosis, malaria, lymphoma (including Hodgkin's disease), and rheumatic fever. The rose spot is the most valuable single sign and, when coupled with fever, splenomegaly, and leukopenia, usually clinches the diagnosis. Differentiation of typhoid fever from diseases which it resembles depends on laboratory confirmation by (1) culture of the blood, feces, and urine, and (2) the demonstration of a positive Widal test. Repeatedly negative cultures of the blood and feces and negative agglutination tests should suggest other illnesses. Rarely are the bacteriologic and serologic tests entirely negative.

MANAGEMENT. The mortality and prolonged morbidity of typhoid fever have been reduced effectively by antibiotics and other supportive measures. In spite of specific therapeutic advances, intestinal hemorrhage and perforation occur in a small percentage of patients. The incidence of relapse has not been significantly reduced and, in fact, may be greater as a result of chloramphenicol therapy. Nonetheless, it is advisable to begin specific therapy as early as possible, with the aim of preventing the development of serious complications.

Specific Treatment. Although many antibiotics show excellent in vitro bacteriostatic action against S. *typhosa*, chloramphenicol gives the most consistent therapeutic results. Ampicillin therapy has been reported to be effective; but the accumulated evidence indicates that patients do not respond as uniformly or as rapidly as with chloramphenicol therapy. The delay in clinical response and the high relapse rate following chloramphenicol treatment stress the need for a more effective antisalmonella drug.

Following institution of chloramphenicol, patients are subjectively improved, with lessened headache and toxemia within 48 hr and normal temperature in less than 4 days. At this stage the patient is more vigorous, appetite has returned, and abdominal pain has abated. Bacteremia is no longer demonstrable several hours after beginning treatment, although stool cultures may be intermittently positive throughout the course.

Failure of typhoid patients to respond to chloramphenicol is unusual. Recommended administration of this drug is as follows: a loading dose comprised of 50 mg per kg of body weight, followed by the same amount divided into three doses daily given at 8-hr intervals. After the patient has become afebrile, the dose can be reduced to 2.0 Gm per day. Chloramphenicol should be continued for a total of 14 days. If nausea and vomiting obviate the oral route, the sodium succinate ester of chloramphenicol can be given intravenously or intramuscularly, on the basis of a daily dose of 25 mg per kg. Daily intravenous doses exceeding 3.0 Gm are not advised, and the oral route is preferred. In the rare situations where chloramphenicol proves to be ineffective, ampicillin can be tried, using 6 to 8 Gm per day and continuing therapy for 2 weeks.

Antitoxemic Effects of Steroids. In severely ill patients 3 to 4 days elapse after institution of chloramphenicol therapy before toxemia and pyrexia disappear. This interval can be shortened appreciably if chloramphenicol is supplemented with steroids.

Cortisone, 200 to 300 mg, or prednisone, 40 to 60 mg, is given daily. Three days of treatment with steroids are sufficient. European investigators have reported a "typhoid shock" syndrome following chloramphenicol treatment, presumably as a result of excessive endotoxin release. Under these conditions steroid treatment may exert a protective effect. Steroids should be reserved for those clinical situations associated with severe typhoidal toxemia.

Supportive Therapy. General supportive care is a vital supplement to antibiotic therapy. Bed rest extending into early convalescence is essential. Ambulation should be gradual, to avoid undue fatigue or exertion. Laxatives and promiscuous use of enemas are ill advised because of the danger of perforation or hemorrhage. Analgesics aid in ameliorating headache, although salicylates should be avoided because of the propensity of typhoid patients to show exaggerated reactions to the antipyretic action of these drugs. Tepid sponge baths are effective in lowering body temperature and should be employed when fever in excess of 104°F appears.

Good nursing care is essential and includes special attention to oral hygiene and adequate bathing. The observations of pulse rate, onset of severe abdominal pain, the presence of tarry or bloody stools, or the occurrence of vomiting are of utmost importance in the early recognition of complications.

A bland or liquid diet is prescribed until the appetite improves. Attention to fluid and electrolyte balance is essential. The judicious transfusion of whole blood given slowly and in small amounts may be lifesaving in severely ill, anemic patients.

Intestinal Hemorrhage. An awareness of this complication and its early detection are essential for proper management. The prevention of shock or its early treatment by blood transfusions is of prime importance. The extent and duration of bleeding should be assessed by frequent determinations of hematocrit and stool guiacs. Adequate reserves of blood should be readily available. Strict bed rest should be enforced, and oral alimentation should be restricted. Under these conditions the antibiotics may be given parenterally.

Intestinal Perforation. A severely damaged intestine requires time for healing. Hence the threat of intestinal perforation exists for several days after specific therapy is instituted. The debilitated toxic condition of the patient and the friability of the intestinal lesion make the typhoid patient a poor surgical risk. It is justified to place greater emphasis on medical management, i.e., to combat shock, to decompress the bowel, and to continue antibiotic treatment. Should the process fail to localize, as evidenced by abdominal examination, persistence of shock, continued leukocytosis, and other signs, surgical intervention may be indicated.

Relapses. The greatest incidence of relapse occurs about 2 weeks after the cessation of chloramphenicol therapy. Patients should be followed for 3 weeks after becoming afebrile. Specific treatment should be reinstituted and continued for a week when symptoms and fever persist beyond 24 hr.

CONTROL AND IMMUNIZATION. All typhoid patients should be reported to appropriate health authorities in order that the source of illness and infection among contacts can be investigated. Patients' stools should be cultured frequently during convalescence to determine if S. *typhosa* is being shed. Usually three consecutively negative stool cultures obtained at weekly intervals indicate that a carrier state has not developed. Convalescent carriers continue to have organisms in stool cultures for 3 months, occasionally for a year. These patients and chronic carriers should be carefully controlled to ensure that they do not engage in occupations that would allow dissemination of typhoid bacilli through accidental contamination of food or water. It is perfectly safe with modern plumbing and sewage disposal to discard stools in flush toilets. Typhoid carriers should be instructed in adequate hand-washing techniques.

The patient should be isolated during the acute phase of the disease, and hospital personnel in attendance should be gowned to protect their clothing. Bed pans, urinals, linens, and eating utensils should be sterilized in boiling water or by autoclaving.

The effectiveness of typhoid vaccines has been a debated point and recently their relative efficacy has been quantitated in volunteers. Inactivated vaccines administered to adult males induce significant but not complete resistance to an inoculum of S. *typhosa* which cause disease in 25 percent of a healthy unimmunized population. Larger numbers of organisms overcome vaccine associated immunity. The number of bacteria ingested under natural circumstances can only be estimated with retrospective analysis. It appears likely from such evidence water-borne outbreaks are caused by small numbers of bacteria, while food contaminated by a carrier may contain 10 to 1,000 times as many organisms. In these settings vaccine may cause an individual to be protected against the smaller but not the larger inoculum. The large-scale field trials conducted by the World Health Organization in Yugoslavia, Poland, and British Guiana produced results consistent with this thesis. In these countries the main method of spread of typhoid has been by impure water supply. Population groups in these studies who received typhoid vaccine were protected for as long as 7 years. However, the disease rate was many times greater in the populace that received no vaccine of any sort (including placebo), suggesting that individuals volunteering for the vaccine trials were more careful and had less exposure. Nevertheless, typhoid vaccines can reduce the incidence of disease in endemic areas but prior vaccine administration does not ensure protection.

Currently, TAB (typhoid, paratyphoid A and B) vaccine is commercially available, but it will be replaced by a monovalent preparation containing only typhoid bacilli inactivated by acetone. This preparation is rich in Vi antigen and without the paratyphoid antigens and phenol causes much less systemic and local reactivity. The schedule of vaccine administration should be 0.5 ml for adults given subcutaneously followed in 1 to 2 weeks by a second dose. TAB vaccine can be given in the same fashion. Yearly booster doses are indicated for those persons at great risk because of occupation or travel. Reactions are common with TAB vaccine and somewhat less with the newer monovalent preparation. Pain and/or swelling at site of injection, chills and fever occurring several hours after administration, myalgia, arthralgia, nausea, and occasional vomiting can be anticipated. Salicylatis may ameliorate these reactions.

PROGNOSIS. The mortality rate in typhoid fever in the United States prior to the introduction of antibiotic therapy was about 12 percent. Most deaths occurred from intestinal perforation, hemorrhage, or both. Toxemia, with resultant inanition, was responsible for some fatalities. Despite the therapeutic efficacy of chloramphenicol, 2 to 3 percent of patients now die of typhoid fever. Most deaths are in the aged, in infants, and in malnourished and anemic patients. Early diagnosis and prompt institution of treatment, reduce mortality to nil.

REFERENCES

Freitag, J. L.: Treatment of Chronic Typhoid Carriers by Cholecystectomy, Public Health Rept. U.S., 79:7, 1964.

Greisman, S. E., R. B. Hornick, and T. E. Woodward: On the Role of Endotoxin during Typhoid Fever and Tularemia in Man: III. Hyperreactivity to Endotoxin during Infection, J. Clin. Invest., 43:9, 1964.

McCrae, T.: The Symptoms of Typhoid Fever, chap. 4 in "Modern Medicine," vol. 2, "Infectious Diseases," p. 104, W. Osler and T. McCrae (Eds.), Philadelphia, Lea Bros. and Company, 1907.

Robertson, R. P., M. F. A. Wahab, and F. O. Raasch: Chloramphenicol and Ampicillin in Salmonella Enteric Fever, New Engl. J. Med., 278:171, 1968.

Stuart, B. M., and R. L. Pullen: Typhoid: Clinical Analysis of 360 Cases, Arch. Intern. Med., 78:629, 1946.

Woodward, T. E., J. E. Smadel, R. T. Parker, and C. L. Wisseman, Jr.: Treatment of Typhoid Fever with Antibiotics, Ann. N.Y. Acad. Sci., 55:1043, 1952.

150   OTHER SALMONELLA INFECTIONS
Edward W. Hook

INTRODUCTION. Since the isolation of the first member of the genus *Salmonella* from swine in 1885 by Salmon and Smith, more than 1,200 different serologic types have been identified. Although there is striking variation in the pathogenicity of the various serotypes, almost all are capable of producing human disease. The infections in man are *acute gastroenteritis, enteric* or *paratyphoid fever, bacteremia,* and *localized infections* ranging from osteomyelitis to endocarditis.

ETIOLOGY AND EPIDEMIOLOGY. The salmonellas are motile gram-negative bacilli that do not ferment lactose or sucrose but utilize glucose, maltose, and mannitol. All serotypes produce gas with the exception of S. *typhosa* and S. *gallinarum-pullorum*. These organisms are typed by immunologic methods on the basis of antigenic components in the cell body (O, or somatic antigens) and flagellar (H antigens). Specific serotyping is necessary for epidemiologic studies.

Salmonellas can be isolated from the intestinal tracts of man and many lower animals. The incidence of asymptomatic excretors of these organisms in the general population is about 0.2 percent, but the most important reservoir of infection is in domestic and wild animal species in which infection rates vary from less than 1 to more than 40 percent. An incomplete list of animals from which salmonella species have been isolated includes chickens, turkeys, ducks, pigs, cows, dogs, cats, rats, parakeets, as well as certain cold-blooded animals and insects. Animals sold as pets especially baby chicks, ducks, and turtles, may also harbor salmonella and serve as sources of infection.

Salmonella infection is almost always acquired by the oral route, usually by ingestion of contaminated food or drink. Any food product, especially those of animal origin, is a potential source of human infection. Meat or egg products obtained from animals harboring salmonellas, and food, dried or fresh milk, or water contaminated by excreta of man or animals may serve as vehicles of infection. Salmonellas may survive cooking at low temperature or food may be recontaminated after cooking by organisms from personnel or kitchen equipment.

Salmonella species may also be transmitted directly from man to man or from animals to man without the intervention of contaminated food or drink, but the latter method of spread is not common. Cross infection of this type has been shown to be responsible for a number of outbreaks of salmonellosis among patients in nurseries and hospitals. A few outbreaks apparently have been related to spread of infection by the aerial route.

Fish meal, meat meal, bone meal, and other by-products of the meat-packing industry are often contaminated with salmonella organisms. Their products are incorporated in animal and poultry feeds and apparently play an important role in the spread of infection among domestic animals.

The true incidence of salmonella infection is difficult to determine. The number of reported isolations of salmonellas from humans in the United States from 1964 to 1967 was about 20,000 isolations per year, or about 10 cases per 100,000 population. However, reported cases represent only a small proportion of the actual number of cases because bacteriologic studies are usually performed only on patients with severe or protracted diarrhea, and many outbreaks are not investigated. Although salmonella infection occurs throughout the year, the Salmonella Surveillance Unit of the National Communicable Disease Center has observed a distinct seasonal pattern with the greatest number of isolations reported from July through October for each year.

In the United States the serotypes most often responsible for human infection are S. typhimurium, S. heidelberg, S. enteritidis, S. newport, S. infantis, S. saint-paul, S. blockley, S. thompson, S. oranienburg, S. anatum, S. derby, and S. montevideo. Salmonella typhimurium is the most prevalent type throughout the world and accounts for about 30 percent of isolates from man in the United States. There is a close correlation between the species of Salmonella isolated from man and animals in any specific geographic area.

PATHOGENESIS. The course of events after salmonella organisms have gained access to the gastrointestinal tract is determined by the dose, serotype, and invasive potential of the organism, and by the resistance of the host. Multiplication of ingested organisms in the intestinal tract may be followed by symptoms of gastroenteritis. The intestinal irritation and inflammation are produced by a true infection of the mucosa; ingestion of billions of dead organisms causes no ill effects. Bloodstream invasion may occur as a complication of gastroenteritis but usually develops without preceding intestinal symptoms. Bacteremia may be transient or prolonged, and may be accompanied by recurrent chills and fever or manifestations of paratyphoid fever. Blood-borne bacteria may localize at any site and lead to suppuration in bone, joints, meninges, pleura, or other tissues.

Studies in volunteers are limited but indicate that large numbers of viable organisms must be ingested to produce clinically apparent disease. However, a transient carrier state can be produced with doses 10 or 100 times smaller than those required to evoke symptoms of infection. The minimal infectious dose varies markedly among different serotypes.

Salmonella serotypes also show marked variation in invasive potential and capacity to produce disease. For example, S. anatum characteristically produces asymptomatic intestinal infection and only rarely invades the bloodstream. In contrast, S. choleraesuis frequently produces bacteremia and metastatic infection.

The bacterial flora of the intestine is apparently important in determining the fate of ingested salmonellas. This suggestion is based on the observation that administration of certain antibiotics to mice results in a 100,000-fold increase in susceptibility to infection with S. enteritidis. The effect of antibiotic therapy may be related to a marked diminution in number of bacteroides organisms which produce butyric and acetic acids that are lethal for salmonellas. Although salmonella enteritis has been reported as a rare complication of antimicrobial therapy in man, adequate clinical documentation of the phenomenon does not exist. Alteration in intestinal flora also has been suggested as a mechanism of the increased susceptibility of patients with previous major gastric surgery, especially gastrectomy and gastroenterostomy, to intestinal infection with salmonellas. However, reduced acidity or rapid emptying time consequent to gastric surgery also may play a role by increasing the number of viable organisms reaching the small intestine.

About one-third of patients who are hospitalized because of salmonellosis have some type of major underlying disease, such as leukemia, lymphoma, lupus erythematosus, or aplastic anemia. This may be coincidence but more often reflects a decrease in resistance to bacterial infection in general. In a few diseases there is evidence to indicate an almost specific predisposition to infection by salmonellas that exceeds susceptibility to other bacterial species. Patients with sickle-cell anemia and other sickle hemoglobinopathies are unusually susceptible to bloodstream invasion by salmonellas. In these patients there is a strong tendency for localization in bone, and salmonellas, not staphylococci, are the most common cause of osteomyelitis in patients with sickle-cell diseases. Salmonella bacteremia is also an unusually frequent complication of the acute hemolytic phase of bartonellosis.

Infants are more susceptible to salmonella infection

and remain convalescent carriers for a longer period of time than adults. The mortality rate from the disease is also higher in infants than in adults.

CLINICAL MANIFESTATIONS. Gastroenteritis. Although gastroenteritis often occurs in large epidemics among individuals who have eaten the same contaminated food, family outbreaks and sporadic cases are even more common. After an incubation period of 8 to 48 hr, there is sudden onset of colicky abdominal pain and loose, watery diarrhea, occasionally with mucus or blood. Nausea and vomiting are frequent but are rarely severe or protracted. Fever of 101 to 102°F is common, and there may be an initial chill. Symptoms usually subside promptly within 2 to 5 days and recovery is uneventful. However, illness is occasionally more protracted, with persistence of diarrhea and low-grade fever for 10 to 14 days. Fatalities rarely exceed 1 percent of the affected population and are limited almost entirely to infants, the aged, and debilitated patients.

The causative organism can often be isolated from the suspected food and from feces during the acute illness. Stool cultures usually become negative for salmonellas within 1 to 4 weeks, but occasional patients continue to excrete organisms for months. The blood leukocyte count is usually normal.

Enteric or Paratyphoid Fever. Certain species can produce an illness which is clinically indistinguishable from typhoid fever, i.e., a prolonged febrile illness with rose spots, splenomegaly, leukopenia, gastrointestinal symptoms, and positive blood and stool cultures (Chap. 149). The organisms most likely to produce this picture are *S. paratyphi A, S. paratyphi B* (*S. schottmuelleri*), and *S. choleraesuis* (*S. suipestifer*). Occasionally a typical attack of food poisoning is followed in a few days by manifestations of paratyphoid fever. Generally, paratyphoid fevers tend to be milder than *S. typhosa* infections, but differentiation on clinical grounds alone is not possible in the individual case. Recovery may be followed by continued excretion of the causative organism in the stools for several months, but the chronic carrier state is less frequent than in typhoid fever.

Bacteremia. Salmonella species may produce a syndrome characterized primarily by prolonged fever and positive blood cultures. Although symptoms of gastroenteritis can precede bacteremia, they are usually lacking, and most cases arise sporadically. In many instances, the only manifestations are prolonged fever, sometimes low-grade, but often spiking and accompanied by repeated rigors, sweats, aching, anorexia, and weight loss. The characteristic features of typhoid and paratyphoid fever, such as rose spots, persistent leukopenia, and sustained fever, are absent. Stool cultures are usually negative. In contrast to the constant bacteremia of typhoid fever, discharge of organisms into the bloodstream is intermittent, and repeated blood cultures are often required to demonstrate the causative organism. At some time in the course of the illness, localizing signs of infection appear in about one-fourth of the cases. Pulmonary infection in the form of bronchopneumonia or abscess, pleurisy, empyema, pericarditis, endocarditis, pyelonephritis,

meningitis, osteomyelitis, and arthritis are relatively common. The blood leukocyte count is usually normal, but with the development of focal lesions, polymorphonuclear leukocytosis as high as 20,000 to 25,000 cells per cu mm occurs. Salmonella bacteremia can be a very puzzling disorder, especially before localization takes place, and should be considered in cases of fever of unknown origin.

Local Pyogenic Infections. Salmonella organisms can produce abscesses in almost any anatomic site, and these can occur independently of previous symptoms of gastroenteritis or other systemic illness, or as complications of bacteremias. There is nothing characteristic about the suppurative lesions, and the correct etiologic diagnosis is rarely made on the basis of clinical findings alone. There is a strong tendency for salmonellas to localize in tissues that are the site of preexisting disease. Localization has been described in aneurysms, bone adjacent to aortic aneurysms, hematomas, and many different tumors, including hypernephroma, ovarian cyst, and pheochromocytoma. Meningeal localization of infection is common in newborns and infants, and occasional small outbreaks of salmonella infection in nurseries have consisted almost entirely of meningitis.

DIAGNOSIS. Febrile gastroenteritis produced by presumed viral agents and shigellosis can be distinguished from salmonella gastroenteritis only by appropriate stool cultures, especially in sporadic cases. Staphylococcal food poisoning usually is not associated with fever, and vomiting is a more prominent feature than in most salmonella infections. Systemic manifestations are usually absent in patients with gastroenteritis caused by *Clostridium welchii*. Many toxic agents and drugs can produce diarrhea, nausea, and abdominal pain, but fever is rarely a feature of these disorders, and the diagnosis depends upon a history of exposure or ingestion.

The diagnosis of paratyphoid fever or salmonella bacteremia depends upon isolation of the causative organism. Agglutination tests with acute and convalescent sera as performed in the usual clinical laboratory are not very helpful.

TREATMENT. The treatment of salmonella gastroenteritis is supportive. Dehydration should be corrected by parenteral administration of fluids and electrolytes. Abdominal cramps and diarrhea can be alleviated by small doses of morphine or paregoric and often are much improved if the patient takes nothing by mouth for 8 to 12 hr. There is no convincing evidence that antimicrobial drugs modify the course of salmonella gastroenteritis.

Chloramphenicol in doses of 3 Gm daily in adults is the antibiotic of choice in systemic infections including salmonella bacteremia, metastatic infection, and paratyphoid fever. Response is characteristically slow, and the temperature rarely returns to normal until 3 to 4 days after beginning therapy. Therapy should be continued for at least 2 weeks, but in certain infections, such as osteomyelitis or meningitis, the duration may have to be extended.

Ampicillin is also effective in systemic infections caused by salmonella strains sensitive to the action of this antibiotic. However, a significant proportion of salmonella strains are highly resistant in vitro to ampicillin. For this reason, ampicillin should not be used in therapy of serious infections unless it is known that the causative organism is sensitive. The tetracycline derivatives have sometimes appeared to exert a beneficial effect, but streptomycin, polymyxin, neomycin, kanamycin, and the sulfonamides are generally ineffective.

Antimicrobial therapy is usually not indicated in convalescent or asymptomatic transient carriers of salmonella species. The carrier state will spontaneously cease in 1 to 3 months in the vast majority of individuals.

The chronic carrier state with localization of infection in the gallbladder and positive stool cultures for a period of time exceeding 1 year is rarely caused by salmonella serotypes other than *S. typhosa* and *S. paratyphi A* and *B*. The therapy of the chronic carrier is discussed in Chap. 149.

Surgically accessible suppurative lesions should be drained.

REFERENCES

Bennett, I. L., Jr., and E. W. Hook: Some Aspects of Salmonellosis, Ann. Rev. Med., 10:1, 1959.

Black, P. H., L. J. Kunz, and M. N. Swartz: Salmonellosis—A Review of Some Unusual Aspects, New Engl. J. Med., 262:811, 864, 921, 1960.

Gezon, H. M.: Salmonellosis, Disease-a-Month, July, 1959.

Hook, E. W.: Salmonellosis: Certain Factors Influencing the Interaction of Salmonella and the Human Host, Bull. N.Y. Acad. Med., 37:499, 1961.

Proceedings of the National Conference on Salmonellosis, March 11–13, 1964: Washington, D.C., Public Health Service Publ. No. 1262, 1965.

Prost, E., and H. Riemann: Food-borne Salmonellosis, Ann. Rev. Microbiol. 21:495, 1967.

Robertson, R. P., M. F. A. Wahab, and F. O. Raasch: Chloramphenicol and Ampicillin in Salmonella Enteric Fever, New Engl. J. Med., 278:171, 1968.

van Oye, E. (Ed.): "The World Problem of Salmonellosis," The Hague, Dr. W. Junk Publishers, 1964.

151 SHIGELLOSIS (Bacillary Dysentery)

*Harry N. Beaty and
Robert G. Petersdorf*

DEFINITION. *Shigellosis* is an acute, self-limited, infectious disease of man which is restricted to the intestinal tract and is characterized by diarrhea, fever, and abdominal pain. The disease is usually called *bacillary dysentery*, but the term *shigellosis* is preferred.

ETIOLOGY. The genus *Shigella* includes a group of more or less closely related species which are members of the family *Enterobacteriaceae*. Shigella organisms are nonmotile, nonencapsulated, slender, gram-negative rods which may appear as coccobacilli on initial isolation.

They are aerobes or facultative anaerobes and grow best at 37°C. Nutritional requirements are relatively simple, and the ability of these organisms to grow in the presence of bile salts is used in devising selective media which facilitate their isolation from the intestinal tract. Fermentation of carbohydrates differs according to the species, but all strains produce acid in glucose and either fail to ferment lactose or do so only slowly. The classification of shigellas depends upon a combination of biochemical and antigenic characteristics. The most important species from a clinical viewpoint are *Shigella dysenteriae* (*S. shigae*), *S. flexneri*, (*S. paradysenteriae*), *S. boydii* and *S. sonnei*. Antigenically, the shigellas are extremely complex. Strains of *S. sonnei* are fairly homogeneous, but the other groups contain from 6 to 11 different types which are identified with specific antigens. There is significant serologic overlap between species, and some strains share group antigens with other enteric bacilli.

The somatic antigen of the shigellas is an endotoxin which is chemically and biologically similar to the endotoxins of other gram-negative bacilli. *Shigella dysenteriae* type 1 (Shiga bacillus) also produces an exotoxin which causes neurologic abnormalities when injected into experimental animals. The role of this neurotoxin in the pathogenesis of shigellosis is unknown, and there is no evidence that other species of shigella produce a similar substance.

EPIDEMIOLOGY. The principal habitat of the shigellas is the gastrointestinal tract of higher primates. However, on rare occasions dogs and other mammals have been found to excrete organisms. Natural disease is limited almost entirely to man, and the convalescent or asymptomatic carrier is the only recognized reservoir. Infection is transmitted predominantly by contact with inanimate objects which are contaminated with fecal material containing dysentery bacilli. Waterborne outbreaks are uncommon, but food is readily contaminated by careless personnel or flies which have fed upon infected human feces.

Bacillary dysentery is worldwide in distribution, and is particularly common in countries where effective sanitation is lacking. There are between 10,000 and 15,000 cases reported in the United States each year, but this probably represents only a small fraction of the total number. The common organisms encountered in this country are *S. flexneri* and *S. sonnei*; *S. dysenteriae* type 1 is rarely the cause of infection outside Asia. Shigellosis is extremely rare during the first month of life, but is very common in children over six months of age. In adults, clinical illness occurs in about 50 percent of persons infected. Major epidemics of bacillary dysentery are rare nowadays, but in closed populations, such as mental institutions, jails, and orphanages, outbreaks develop over a period of several weeks. Poor sanitation, low standards of personal hygiene, crowded conditions, and a high proportion of children in a population favor spread of the infection. For the most part, shigella species do not persist in the stool for more than a few days, possibly because they are susceptible to the action of bacteriophage. Organisms may be excreted intermittently during convalescence, but the carrier state rarely persists longer than 3 months.

The role of immunity in the recovery from clinical infection or protection against reinfection is not known. Humoral antibodies appear in response to infection, but there is no evidence that they influence the course of the disease. Coproantibodies are also present, but their significance is unknown. Repeated attacks of bacillary dysentery are not uncommon, but persons living in endemic areas seem to develop immunity to recurrent episodes of clinical disease. Polyvalent shigella vaccines protect mice against intraperitoneal infection, but their effectiveness in man has not been established.

PATHOGENESIS AND PATHOLOGY. The pathogenesis of shigellosis is poorly understood, in part because it is difficult to produce the infection in laboratory animals. Studies in volunteers have shown that it is necessary to ingest very large numbers of bacilli to establish infection in man. Organisms presumably multiply in the lower gastrointestinal tract, where they produce an inflammatory reaction which usually involves the entire colon and may extend into the terminal ileum. The mucosa becomes uniformly inflamed and edematous and often is covered by a fibrinous exudate. Necrosis of the mucosa produces shallow ulcers which bleed readily. Microscopic examination shows that the submucosa and muscularis are infiltrated with bacteria and polymorphonuclear leukocytes. Ulcers are sharply outlined and are not undermined. The mechanisms responsible for these pathologic alterations are unclear. Shigella endotoxin is often implicated, but a variety of enteric bacteria elaborate endotoxins without producing disease.

The systemic manifestations of bacillary dysentery are primarily due to the fluid and electrolyte disturbances consequent to the diarrhea. Bacteremia in shigellosis is rare, and fever is often attributed to "toxins" which presumably are absorbed from the intestinal tract.

CLINICAL MANIFESTATIONS. Shigella infections are characterized by fever, abdominal pain, and diarrhea. However, mild diarrhea alone or asymptomatic infection occurs in a significant proportion of individuals infected. The incubation period is usually 24 to 48 hr, and the first symptom is often colicky abdominal pain, which is followed within an hour by high fever and diarrhea, often accompanied by tenesmus. Other symptoms include nausea, vomiting, headache, convulsions in children, and myalgia. The stools are liquid, greenish in color, contain shreds of mucus, and in 20 to 30 percent of cases contain various amounts of gross blood. Depending upon the severity of diarrhea and the height of fever, patients may become profoundly dehydrated, and circulatory collapse can occur. Lower abdominal tenderness and hyperactive bowel sounds are common, but there is no peritoneal irritation. Splenomegaly has been reported, but is rare. Sigmoidoscopic examination reveals diffuse mucosal inflammation, often with multiple ulcerations.

LABORATORY FINDINGS. Blood leukocyte counts usually range between 5,000 and 15,000 per cu mm, and anemia is uncommon. Microscopic examination of the stool reveals shreds of mucus, erythrocytes, and many polymorphonuclear leukocytes. Stool culture is positive, but blood cultures rarely are. Electrolyte abnormalities depend upon the degree of vomiting and diarrhea.

COURSE. Shigellosis is generally a self-limited disease, and patients usually become afebrile within 2 to 3 days. Diarrhea may continue a few days longer, but within a week most patients have recovered and no longer excrete organisms in their stool. In about 10 percent of cases a clinical or bacterologic relapse occurs unless antibiotics are given. In the United States, the overall mortality rate associated with bacillary dysentery is less than 0.1 percent. However, among young children and elderly patients, the illness is often more severe and the prognosis poorer. *Shigella dysenteriae* produces particularly severe infections, and mortality rates of 25 to 50 percent have been recorded in epidemics produced by this species.

Complications of *Shigella* infections are encountered infrequently. Chronic bacillary dysentery occurs in the tropics, particularly after *S. dysenteriae* infections, but is rare in this country. Perforation of the colon is uncommon. Hematogenous dissemination of the shigellas is also rare, but these organisms have been recovered from metastatic foci of infection such as abscesses or meningitis. In some series, bacteremia due to other gram-negative bacilli has been seen in association with shigellosis. An acute, nonsuppurative arthritis involving large, weight-bearing joints, may occur during convalescence, but in patients given chemotherapy this complication is unusual. Conjunctivitis, iritis, and peripheral neuropathy accompany bacillary dysentery on rare occasions.

DIAGNOSIS. A definitive diagnosis of shigellosis can only be established when pathogenic members of the genus *Shigella* are isolated from cultures. These organisms survive for only a short time in feces, and fresh stool specimens or rectal swabs should be cultured promptly. Recovery of the shigellas is facilitated if saline suspensions of the material to be cultured are streaked directly onto selective media such as SS agar or desoxycholate citrate agar. Selenite broth is of limited usefulness in the isolation of the shigellas. Agglutinating antibodies can be detected in the serum of a majority of patients with positive cultures, but serologic tests are of little value in establishing the diagnosis of shigellosis. Immunofluorescent techniques have been developed, however, which allow rapid detection of organisms in the stool.

Shigella infection should be considered in every febrile illness associated with diarrhea. Occasionally, children with infections such as tonsillitis or otitis have diarrhea, but the major differential diagnosis of shigellosis includes viral enteritis, amebic dysentery (Chap. 240), salmonellosis (Chap. 150), and staphylococcal food poisoning (Chap. 139). In viral infections, fever is uncommon, and the stool does not contain gross blood or pus. The onset of amebic colitis is gradual, and the diarrhea is relatively mild. Staphylococal food poisoning is associated with more nausea and vomiting, and usually is not associated with fever. Salmonella infections can be differentiated with certainty only by bacteriologic studies.

TREATMENT. The treatment of shigellosis is primarily supportive, and the major goal is correction of fluid and electrolyte abnormalities. Antibiotics are of secondary importance and are used chiefly to shorten the duration of illness and to prevent relapse. Sulfonamides formerly were effective in the treatment of bacillary dysentery, but in 1968, almost two-thirds of shigellas isolated are resistant to these drugs. More significantly, since 1955, epidemics of shigellosis in various parts of the world, including the United States, have been caused by organisms resistant to multiple antibiotics. The molecular basis for multiple drug resistance involves the episomal transfer of drug resistance determinants between enteric bacilli.

Although some strains of shigella resistant to ampicillin and tetracycline have been identified, these drugs are preferred for the treatment of bacillary dysentery, and in adults should be given in dosage of 2.0 Gm per day. Chloramphenicol is also likely to be effective, but should be given only in severe cases where other agents cannot be used. Kanamycin, neomycin, and streptomycin are often administered orally for the treatment of shigel-losis, but absorbable agents are probably more effective.

PREVENTION. The most important prophylactic measures are the maintenance of proper sanitation and adequate sewage disposal. The detection and elimination of carriers is difficult and rarely practical. Methods for increasing resistance to infection have not been developed.

REFERENCES

Farrar, W. E., and L. C. Dekle: Transferable Antibiotic Resistance Associated with an Outbreak of Shigellosis, Ann. Intern. Med., 67:1208, 1967.

Garfinkel, B. T., G. M. Martin, J. Watt, F. J. Payne, R. P. Mason, and A. V. Hardy: Antibiotics in Acute Bacillary Dysentery: Observations in 1,408 Cases with Positive Cultures, J.A.M.A., 151:1157, 1953.

Haltalin, K. C., J. D. Nelson, L. U. Hinton, R. W. Kusmiesz, and B. S. Sladoje: Comparison of Orally Absorbable and Nonabsorbable Antibiotics in Shigellosis, J. Pediat., 72:708, 1968.

Morgan, H. R.: The Enteric Bacteria, p. 634 in "Bacterial and Mycotic Infections of Man," 4th ed., Philadelphia, J. B. Lippincott Company, 1965.

Section 6

Diseases Caused by Other Gram-negative Bacilli

152 HEMOPHILUS INFECTIONS
Louis Weinstein

The genus *Hemophilus* consists of nonmotile, gram-negative rods or coccobacilli which require specific growth factors (X and V) for multiplication. The organisms of importance in human disease are *H. influenzae,* *H. pertussis, H. ducreyi,* the Koch-Weeks bacillus, and *Moraxella lacunata.* Two other species are found in the pharynges of normal individuals and, rarely, may produce pharyngitis (*H. hemolyticus*) or endocarditis (*H. parainfluenzae*). The site invaded most frequently is the respiratory tract, and the organisms responsible for the bulk of infections are *H. influenzae* and *H. pertussis.*

HEMOPHILUS INFLUENZA INFECTIONS

Hemophilus influenzae produces a wide variety of diseases in many organ systems. The organism was first isolated by Pfeiffer during a pandemic of influenza in 1890, and was thought to be the causative agent of this disease. During the 1918 influenza pandemic, extensive bacteriologic investigations revealed a high incidence of *H. influenzae* in the nasopharynges and lungs of patients in many parts of the world.

ETIOLOGY. *Hemophilus influenzae* is a gram-negative, nonsporulating, pleomorphic rod. In exudates, the organisms are usually predominantly coccobacillary and can be mistaken for pneumococci or meningococci. Some strains demonstrate bipolar staining, and bacillary forms that vary from short rods to long filamentous ones occur.

Hemophilus influenzae grows well on chocolate agar and Levinthal's medium, which has the advantage of being transparent. On Levinthal's agar, typical colonies are iridescent when viewed by obliquely transmitted light when they are about 4 to 6 hr old; this property disappears after 24 hr.

Although it had been thought that strains without capsules were nonpathogenic, these strains have been implicated in infections of the respiratory tract. On the basis of specific capsular polysaccharides, *H. influenzae* may be classified into six types. Type B produces about 95 percent of human infections.

EPIDEMIOLOGY. *Hemophilus influenzae* infects only man. It is not ordinarily invasive for any of the smaller animals, although monkeys can be infected experimentally.

The incidence of *H. influenzae* infections is greatest in the winter and early spring. Nose and throat cultures during these seasons reveal the organisms of many asymptomatic individuals. Penicillin therapy increases the incidence of positive throat cultures in a population.

Children in the first 2 months of life have a high level of passively transferred bactericidal antibody. Between the ages of two months and three years, most children show little antibody, but with aging, the levels increase.

PATHOLOGY. The characteristic tissue response to *H. influenzae* is acute suppurative inflammation. Infections of the larynx, trachea, and bronchial tree are characterized by edema of the mucosa and thick exudate, and invasion of the lungs results in a bronchopneumonia. Particularly in young children, a severe, diffuse bronchiolitis can occur. In influenzal meningitis, the vertex of the brain is covered with thick, greenish-yellow exudate.

Microscopic examination of the lesions produced by *H. influenzae* reveals an exudate consisting primarily of polymorphonuclear leukocytes and large numbers of organisms enmeshed in fibrin.

CLINICAL MANIFESTATIONS. Severe *H. influenzae* infections are usually accompanied by high fever, usually without rigors, and generalized malaise. In milder infections, fever is inconstant. The commonest diseases produced by *H. influenzae* are pharyngitis, epiglottitis, laryngotracheitis, pneumonia, bronchitis and bronchiolitis, otitis media, and meningitis. The symptoms and signs of influenzal invasion of the respiratory tract or meninges are similar to those of infection of these areas by other organisms, and differential etiologic diagnosis depends upon epidemiologic background, the age of the patient, and demonstration of the causative agent.

Pharyngitis. *Hemophilus influenzae* is a relatively common cause of pharyngitis in children, and acute influenzal pharyngitis is also observed in adults, where it often occurs as a complication of the chemotherapy of other infections. Examination of the throat usually reveals only marked redness and injection. Very rarely, patches of soft yellow exudate may be present. The pharyngitis tends to persist for many days unless properly treated. Dissociation between the appearance of the pharynx and the intensity of local discomfort is common in adults. The pharyngeal mucosa frequently appears normal or shows only slight diffuse redness at the same time that pain is so severe that swallowing of saliva is difficult and eating impossible.

Epiglottitis. Disease of the upper part of the respiratory tract produced by *H. influenzae* is sometimes limited to the epiglottis, which becomes reddened, swollen, and stiff. Discomfort in the hypopharynx and "croupy" breathing may progress to a point at which tracheotomy becomes necessary. This disease is rare in adults.

Laryngotracheobronchitis. The entire laryngotracheobronchial tree may be the site of infection, with resulting rapidly progressive obstruction of the airway. "Croupy" cough is accompanied by increasing signs of respiratory embarrassment, and tracheotomy is sometimes necessary. Influenzal laryngotracheitis is very rare in adults. The disease can lead to death within 18 to 24 hr.

Pneumonia. Primary pneumonia due to *H. influenzae*, with rare exceptions, is a disease of children. In the adult, it is usually secondary to viral influenza, measles, or bacterial pneumonitis. It may complicate rubeola or pertussis in the young. Bacteremia occurs in approximately one-third of the cases.

Bronchitis and Bronchiolitis. Severe, diffuse bronchiolitis characterized by persistent nonproductive cough, wheezing, and dyspnea occurs in children. Physical examination usually reveals lowering and fixation of the diaphragm, prolonged expirations, and typically asthmatic breathing. Roentgenographic examination of the chest reveals increased radiolucence, and flattening of the diaphragm consistent with emphysema. This is an extremely serious illness and unless promptly recognized and treated may be rapidly fatal.

The factor of infection contributes significantly to the clinical manifestations and progressive deterioration in established chronic bronchitis or "senile emphysema" in adults. Among the bacteria involved, the pneumococcus and *H. influenzae* are the commonest. *Hemophilus influenzae* has been isolated from the respiratory tracts of 80 to 90 percent of patients in some studies.

Otitis Media. *Hemophilus influenzae* is a common cause of suppurative otitis media in children; the infection is uncommon in adults. In some instances, middle ear disease due to this species is indistinguishable from that produced by *Staphylococcus aureus, Diplococcus pneumoniae* or group A *Streptococcus pyogenes*. In many cases, however, the appearance is that of serous otitis media and leads to a misdiagnosis of nonbacterial disease. Aspiration of fluid from the middle ear and culture may be necessary to establish the diagnosis of the presence of *H. influenzae* and to dictate appropriate chemotherapy.

Meningitis. The influenza bacillus is the commonest cause of meningitis between the ages of six months and two years and is frequent in later childhood. In adults, it may follow operation on or injury to the head. In rare instances, *H. influenzae* may be responsible for acute meningitis in otherwise healthy adults of any age. Next to pneumococcus, *H. influenzae* is the organism most likely to cause recurrent bacterial meningitis. Of these cases, 95 percent are produced by type B organisms, a few by type A, and a rare one by nonencapsulated strains. About two-thirds of the patients have a preceding infection of the upper respiratory tract, and about one-third have bronchopneumonia. Signs of meningeal irritation are usually prominent, except in very young babies in whom bulging of the fontanels may be the only sign. The diagnosis should be suspected because of the age of the patient and the frequent prodrome of respiratory infection.

Other Diseases. Subacute and acute bacterial endocarditis may be produced by *H. influenzae*, although more infections of the heart valves have been due to *H. parainfluenzae*. The influenza bacillus is a rare cause of suppurative pericarditis. In the winter, acute conjunctivitis may be due to *H. influenzae*. Although no clinical features distinguish it from "pink eye" produced by the Koch-Weeks bacillus, epidemics of conjunctivitis due to this organism are most common in the summer. Although *H. influenzae* and the Koch-Weeks bacillus are antigenically related, they are distinct species. *Moraxella lacunata* is also an occasional cause of acute purulent conjunctivitis. Acute pyogenic arthritis due to *H. influenzae* has been reported. Among other diseases produced by this organism are cystitis, pyelonephritis, osteomyelitis, paranasal sinusitis, appendicitis, cellulitis, and infections of the liver, genital tract, and skin.

LABORATORY FINDINGS. As a rule, infections due to *H. influenzae* are accompanied by polymorphonuclear leukocytosis ranging from 15,000 to 30,000 per cu mm. In young children with severe disease, leukopenia (2,000 to 3,000 leukocytes per cu mm) with a deficiency of polymorphonuclear leukocytes can occur. Bacteremia is rare in influenzal infections of the respiratory tract but is demonstrable in about 50 percent of cases of meningitis.

COURSE AND COMPLICATIONS. The course of *H. influenzae* infections is determined by the location of the disease. Epiglottitis, laryngotracheobronchitis, bronchiolitis, or pneumonia may be fulminating. Some of these patients die because of uncontrolled infection, but in many, the cause of death is obstruction of the airway, which cannot always be relieved by surgical methods, because impediment to flow of air is most marked in the smaller radicles of the bronchial tree. Virtually 100 percent of untreated cases of influenzal meningitis terminate fatally. Internal and external hydrocephalus, brain abscess, subdural empyema, diffuse cortical necrosis, and shock are possible complications. With specific therapy, the incidence of complications is sharply reduced. However, if subdural aspiration is carried out routinely in children with influenzal meningitis which is responding to antibiotics, sterile fluid is demonstrable in about half the cases. Neurologic disturbances from subdural effusions are uncommon. Epileptiform seizures can occur while the disease is responding favorably to chemotherapy.

TREATMENT. *H. influenzae* is susceptible in vitro to several antimicrobial agents including streptomycin, the tetracyclines, chloramphenicol, and the sulfonamides. Most strains are inhibited by 0.6 μg penicillin G or less per ml. All appear to be highly sensitive to ampicillin, a drug which has simplified greatly the management of disease produced by this organism. The dose of ampicillin in *H. influenzae* meningitis is 100 to 200 mg/kg/day, given parenterally in equal sized and spaced quantities; the larger dose is preferred. The management of otitis media or pharyngitis often requires no more than 100 to 150 mg/kg/day given by mouth. For adults respiratory infections, 2 to 4 Gm per day orally for 7 to 10 days usually suffices. Ampicillin therapy may fail in influenzal meningitis when complications, e.g., subdural empyema, supervene. Although the *H. influenzae* organism has been resistant to ampicillin only rarely, continued surveillance of this problem is indicated because of the increasing frequency with which other gram-negative bacilli resistant to this agent are being recovered. Despite the fact that practically all strains of *H. influenzae* are sensitive to very small quantities of penicillin G, the therapeutic effects of this antibiotic are poor, and it must not be used as the sole agent for the treatment of meningitis due to this organism. The results with the tetracyclines are too variable to recommend their use. An alternate regimen is chloramphenicol (50 mg per kg in equal sized and spaced doses per day) intramuscularly plus sulfisoxazole or sulfadiazine (100 mg/kg/day). Regardless of the drug employed, *H. influenzae* meningitis should be treated for 2 weeks. Chloramphenicol alone or a tetracycline is usually sufficient to treat upper respiratory tract infections, pneumonia or otitis media in penicillin-sensitive children or adults allergic to penicillin.

PERTUSSIS

Whooping cough affects about 85 percent of all unimmunized children. It is characterized by an inflammation of the entire respiratory tract which produces paroxysmal cough and the typical inspiratory stridor, or "whoop."

ETIOLOGY. The causative agent is *Hemophilus pertussis* (also called *Bordatella pertussis*), a short or ovoid gramnegative, nonmotile, nonsporulating, facultatively anaerobic bacillus. Bipolar staining is frequent, and encapsulation can be demonstrated by special stains.

The pertussis bacillus requires both the X and V factors for growth, especially for initial isolation, and multiplies best on Bordet-Gengou medium. The organism contains two antigens, the heat-stable O, common to all strains, and the heat-labile specific agglutinogens K (1,2,3,4,5). All strains contain two or more of these antigens. This is of clinical importance because, in some areas of the world, the infecting strain has been found to have different K agglutinogens than those present in the vaccine being used to prevent the disease, resulting in failure of immunization.

Other infectious agents rarely produce the syndrome of whooping cough. Among these are *Bordetella parapertussis*, *B. bronchisepticus*, and adenovirus type 12, which is responsible for a contagious disease featured by paroxysmal coughing, whooping, lymphocytosis, and eosinophilia.

EPIDEMIOLOGY. Pertussis is worldwide. Where the disease has not been present for several years, it tends to assume epidemic proportions when it reappears. In some locations, the disease is most common during the winter, and in others it is seen with greatest frequency in the late summer and fall. The index of contagion is 80 to 100 percent; about 200,000 cases occur in the United States each year.

Approximately 40 percent of cases of pertussis occur in the first 2 years of life; the same number is observed between the ages of two and five. At least 50 percent of all children have had whooping cough before they reach the age of five and 75 percent by the age of seventeen.

Pertussis is spread by droplets from the respiratory tract. Rarely, the organisms may be transmitted by fomites. Infectivity during the incubation period is questionable; the disease is most contagious during the catarrhal stage. Healthy carriers play no role in dissemination, but mild or missed cases are of great importance.

PATHOLOGY. The initial lesion in whooping cough is hyperplasia of the peribronchial and tracheobronchial lymphoid tissue. The bronchi, trachea, larynx, and nasopharynx are then involved in a necrotizing inflammatory reaction. The organisms are present in large numbers between the cilia of the trachea, and desquamation of the alveolar epithelium occurs.

CLINICAL MANIFESTATIONS. The incubation period of whooping cough averages 12 to 15 days, although it can be as long as 20 days. The first clinical manifestations are slight nasal discharge, conjunctivitis, and mild cough without fever. This catarrhal stage lasts for 7 to 14 days.

The paroxysmal phase of pertussis follows and is characterized by paroxysms of coughing ending in a loud, crowing inspiratory noise (the whoop), the expulsion of varying quantities of thick, mucoid sputum from the respiratory tract, and vomiting. Episodes of cough may be as few as 1 or 2 or as many as 40 to 50 per day. Children under the age of six months frequently do not whoop. The mere presence of a whoop is in itself not diagnostic of pertussis. Rarely, the paroxysms of coughing are replaced completely by sneezing.

Fever does not occur in the paroxysmal phase unless complications are present. Soreness over the trachea and main bronchi is common. Spasm, ulcer, or edema of the glottis sometimes occurs. In cases with severe vomiting and inability to retain food, serious inanition, wasting, and tetany may appear.

There is a bleeding tendency in pertussis. Hemoptysis, epistaxis, purpura, and subconjunctival or intestinal hemorrhages occur but are usually of little clinical significance. The mechanism of bleeding is not known.

Physical examination in pertussis is often entirely normal, but there may be injection of the blood vessels of the nose and pharynx. Although there are usually no abnormal findings in the lungs, fine, crackling, "sticky" râles are sometimes present. There are ulcers of the frenum of the tongue in about 20 percent of cases; these occur only when the lower central incisor teeth are present.

The paroxysmal stage of pertussis usually lasts from 1 to 6 weeks. When coughing persists beyond 6 weeks, it is usually due to the development of a so-called "habit whoop," not to continuation of the disease.

LABORATORY FINDINGS. The total peripheral leukocyte count may be over 100,000 cells per cu mm, and mature lymphocytes may constitute 90 percent of the cells. This helps to distinguish the blood picture from that of acute leukemia but not from acute lymphocytosis. The lymphocytosis appears to be induced by a constituent of the organism; most of the cells are released from lymphoid tissue, including the thymus. Blood cultures are sterile. Cultures of the upper part of the nasopharynx reveal *H. pertussis;* the incidence of positive isolations varies with the stage of the disease. X-ray of the lungs in the uncomplicated case usually reveals only hilar lymphadenopathy and increase in the density of the bronchovascular markings.

COMPLICATIONS. Bronchopneumonia occurs in from 1 to 10 percent of cases; the organisms most frequently involved are the beta-hemolytic streptococcus, *Diplococcus pneumoniae, Staphylococcus aureus, H. influenzae,* and *H. pertussis.* When pneumonitis appears during the course of chemotherapy, the bacteria most often responsible are *Escherichia coli, Proteus* strains, *Aerobacter aerogenes,* or *Pseudomonas aeruginosa.* Another important complication is atelectasis; small areas of collapse are an almost constant finding, but major portions or a whole lung may be involved. Pneumothorax is rare.

The severe coughing of pertussis can lead to several complications. Hemorrhage may appear in the anterior chamber of the eye or in the retina. Detachment of the retina and blindness develop in rare cases. Prolapse of the rectum and inguinal or umbilical hernias have been noted.

Nervous system manifestations are not rare in pertussis. The commonest is convulsions; they often come with the sudden fever of secondary bacterial infection. Other causes of seizures are encephalopathy (1 to 14 percent of cases), multiple petechial or gross hemorrhages of the brain, and cerebral hypoxia due to the combined effect of anoxic anoxia and venous stasis. The encephalopathy is characterized by an increase in the protein and cell content of the spinal fluid. Its etiology is unknown. Hyperreflexia, nuchal rigidity, cranial nerve palsies, areflexia, extensor plantar responses, flaccid hemiplegia, spasticity of the extremities, opisthotonos, difficulty in speaking, twitching, papilledema, nystagmus, blindness, strabismus, and dysphagia can all occur. Some of the more important residua are mental retardation, recurrent convulsions, personality disorders, amnesia, aphasia, diffuse cerebral atrophy, chorea, and athetosis.

DIAGNOSIS. The diagnosis of pertussis can frequently be made on clinical grounds alone. A known contact is helpful, but the appearance of paroxysms of typical coughing and whooping after a short period of upper respiratory symptoms is strongly suggestive. In babies under the age of six months there is usually only paroxysmal coughing, without the characteristic whoop.

An increased lymphocyte count is characteristic.

Isolation of *H. pertussis* from the respiratory tract establishes the diagnosis. Using cough plates and nasopharyngeal swabs, positive cultures can be obtained in 90 percent of patients in the catarrhal stage of the disease. The incidence of positive cultures is lower after paroxysmal coughing appears, and decreases with the duration of symptoms. Serologic studies are of little or no help in establishing the presence of pertussis.

PREVENTION. Active immunization is effective in preventing pertussis in the majority of individuals, and may be started at the age of three months; both antibody production and protection against invasion by *H. pertussis* result. If the procedure is carried out at this early age, a "booster" injection should be administered at the end of the first year of life and again just before the child starts to school. Although it is not commonly practiced, passive immunity can be conferred on the newborn child by active immunization of the mother beginning in the sixth or seventh month of pregnancy. Vaccine should not be given in the presence of the active disease; not only is it useless, but it may provoke serious neurologic reactions. There is evidence that the administration of "quadruple" vaccine—poliomyelitis virus, tetanus and diphtheria toxoid, and *H. pertussis*—leads to some degree of suppression of the response to the pertussis bacillus. For this reason, when poliomyelitis vaccine (formalinized) is used, it should be given separately from the "triple" vaccine.

In children who have been exposed to pertussis but have not been actively immunized, passive protection may be given by the injection of 20 to 30 ml human hyperimmune pertussis antiserum, or 2 ml immune γ-globulin as soon as possible after exposure and again 1 week later. This type of prophylaxis is 75 to 85 percent effective. The use of γ-globulin is preferable because hyperimmune serum has been associated with the subsequent development of infectious hepatitis.

TREATMENT. Although most of the antimicrobial drugs have been employed in the treatment of pertussis, there is no incontrovertible evidence that they are beneficial. Chlortetracycline, chloramphenicol, oxytetracycline, and erythromycin have been used, but the results obtained in controlled studies are not convincing.

There are few controlled studies of serum therapy in whooping cough, but in many clinics it is the practice to administer human hyperimmune serum (20 ml every 48 hr for three doses), or immune γ-globulin (2 ml every 48 hr for three doses) to all children with pertussis under the age of two years.

Most important in therapy is repair of the water and salt loss which follows severe and frequent vomiting. Prompt refeeding is necessary in order to maintain or gain weight.

Early detection and treatment of complications is one of the most important factors in the reduction of mortality in pertussis. The prompt recognition of secondary bacterial infections of the lungs or middle ear and therapy with a properly selected antibiotic agent lead to cure in practically all cases. When atelectasis occurs, correction by tracheal catheter suction or bronchoscopy may be lifesaving. Little can be done to influence the course or outcome of such complications as gross cerebral hemorrhage or encephalopathy.

Proper management of whooping cough has made the outlook for complete recovery excellent.

REFERENCES

Hemophilus Influenzae

Baty, J., and M. Kriedberg: Acute Laryngotracheobronchitis, Med. Clinics N. Am., 37:1279, 1952.

Collier, A. M., J. D. Connor, and W. L. Nykan: Systemic Infection with Hemophilus Influenzae in Very Young Infants, J. Pediat., 70:539, 1967.

Feingold, M., and S. S. Gellis: Cellulitis Due to Hemophilus Influenzae Type B, New Engl. J. Med., 272:788, 1965.

Goldstein, E., A. K. Daly, and C. Seamans: Haemophilus Influenzae as a Cause of Adult Penumonia, Ann. Intern. Med., 66:35, 1967.

Holdaway, M. D., and D. C. Turk: Capsulated Haemophilus Influenzae and Respiratory-tract Disease, Lancet, 1:358, 1967.

Kaplan, N. M., and A. I. Braude: Hemophilus Influenzae Infection in Adults. Observations on the Immune Disturbance, A.M.A. Arch. Intern. Med., 101:515, 1958.

Patterson, R. L., Jr., and D. B. Levine: Hemophilus Influenzae Pyarthrosis in an Adult, J. Bone Joint Surg., 47A:1250, 1965.

Turk, D. C., and J. R. May: Hemophilus Influenzae. Its Clinical Importance, London, English Universities Press, Ltd., 1967.

Walker, S. H.: The Respiratory Manifestations of Systemic Hemophilus Influenzae Infection, J. Pediat., 62:386, 1963.

Wehrle, P. F., A. W. Hathies, J. M. Leedom, and D. Ivler: Bacterial Meningitis, Ann. N.Y. Acad. Sci., 145:488, 1967.

Pertussis

Brooksaler, F., and J. D. Nelson: Pertussis. A Reappraisal and Report of 190 Confirmed Cases, Am. J. Dis. Child., 114:389, 1967.

Eldering, G., C. Hornbeck, and J. Baker: Serological Study of *Bordetella Pertussis* and Related Species, J. Bacteriol., 74:133, 1957.

Morse, S. I.: Studies of the Lymphocytosis Induced in Mice by Bordetella Pertussis, J. Exp. Med., 121:49, 1965.

Preston, N. W.: Type-Specific Immunity Against Whooping Cough, Brit. Med. J., 2:724, 1963.

Weinstein, L., R. Seltser, and C. T. Marrow: The Treatment of Pertussis with Aureomycin, Chloramphenicol and Terramycin, J. Pediat., 39:549, 1951.

White, R., L. Finberg, and A. Tramer: The Modern Morbidity of Pertussis in Infants, Pediatrics, 33:705, 1964.

Wilson, A. T., I. A. Henderson, E. J. H. Moore, and S. N. Heywood: Whooping Cough: Difficulties in Diagnosis and Ineffectiveness of Immunization, Lancet, 2:623, 1965.

153 CHANCROID
Albert Heyman

DEFINITION. Chancroid is an acute, localized, venereal disease caused by the Ducrey bacillus (*Hemophilus ducreyi*). It is characterized by ulceration at the site of inoculation and by enlargement and suppuration of the regional lymph nodes.

ETIOLOGY. The etiologic agent of chancroid, the Ducrey bacillus, is a short, plump, gram-negative organism with rounded ends. When stained by special methods, the bacillus exhibits bipolar staining. In the stained smears of genital lesions the organisms usually appear singly or in small clusters, but they may be arranged in long parallel columns between cells or shreds of mucus. Occasionally, the bacilli are situated intracellularly. The organism can be cultivated in whole defibrinated blood or nutrient broth containing blood. When grown in pure culture in a liquid medium, the Ducrey bacillus appears in long, tangled chains composed of both coccal and bacillary forms.

INCIDENCE. The number of cases of chancroid occurring every year cannot be determined satisfactorily, since accurate diagnosis of this condition is not generally attempted. A diagnosis of chancroid is frequently applied to genital lesions improving with sulfonamide therapy in which the *Treponema pallidum* cannot be demonstrated. The disease is encountered in the West Indies, North

Africa, and the Orient, particularly in the lower economic groups of the population. It is also prevalent in the Southeastern part of the United States and is more frequent in Negroes than in whites. Approximately 950 cases were reported in the United States in 1966; the true incidence is probably considerably higher.

PATHOGENESIS. Chancroid is usually contracted by sexual intercourse, and the lesions are almost always located about the genitalia. The disease can apparently be acquired from sexual partners who show no evidence of an active chancroidal infection. The organism has been cultivated from the smegma and vaginal secretions in patients without clinical manifestations of the disease. Such individuals may be carriers of the Ducrey bacillus. The organism readily produces an infection when inoculated into open or slightly abraded areas of the skin or mucous membranes. Chancroidal ulcerations frequently occur in areas of the genitalia, where minor abrasions may be present (fourchette of the vulva, edge of phimotic prepuce, and frenum). After an incubation period of 2 to 5 days, a localized ulceration appears at the site of inoculation. This may be followed later by inflammation and suppuration of the regional lymph nodes.

Chancroidal infection produces a distinct histologic appearance. The base of the ulcer is a shallow zone made up of polymorphonuclear leukocytes, fibrin, red blood cells, and necrotic tissue. Below this is a fairly wide layer, consisting chiefly of proliferating endothelial cells and newly formed blood vessels, some of which show degeneration of their walls. Finally, there is a deep zone in which a dense infiltration of plasma cells and lymphocytes occurs. This histologic pattern is sufficiently characteristic to permit differentiation from other genital lesions. Biopsy is a valuable diagnostic procedure.

CLINICAL MANIFESTATIONS. The typical chancroidal lesion is a painful, shallow, irregular ulcer with ragged undermined edges, a granular, friable base, and a dirty-yellow exudate. The lesion is characteristically nonindurated and for this reason has been called *soft chancre*. The size of the ulceration varies but seldom exceeds 2 cm in diameter. Multiple lesions resemble a folliculitis or pyogenic infection. Almost any portion of the genitalia may be involved, but extragenital lesions are rare. In about 50 percent of the patients inflammation and suppuration of the inguinal lymph nodes will occur. The term *bubo* is given to this type of lymphadenitis. The chancroidal bubo develops rapidly and becomes a very painful, inflammatory inguinal mass. When suppuration occurs, the mass may become tensely fluctuant and may rupture spontaneously, leaving a large, single, craterlike abscess. Mild constitutional symptoms may accompany the involvement of the inguinal lymph nodes, and the patient may complain of headache, malaise, fever, or anorexia.

DIAGNOSIS. Although the clinical appearance of chancroid is often sufficiently characteristic to suggest the correct diagnosis, laboratory confirmation is desirable. Stained smears or culture of the exudate taken from the undermined edge of the lesion will reveal the Ducrey bacillus in the majority of the early cases. The organism is not easily demonstrated, however, in larger lesions when secondary bacterial contamination has occurred. Biopsy is feasible in such cases and is an efficient method of diagnosis. Attempts to demonstrate the organism in the buboes by either culture or smear usually are not successful. The majority of patients with chancroidal infection will exhibit a positive skin reaction to an intradermal injection of killed Ducrey bacilli. The value of this skin test is limited by the fact that a positive reaction persists for years after exposure to the infection. One cannot be certain, therefore, whether a positive skin test in an individual patient represents the existing chancroidal infection or a previous one. Early syphilis may be present concurrently with chancroid in these patients. Serologic tests and dark-field examination of the lesions and regional lymph nodes should be done to rule out this possibility.

TREATMENT. Sulfisoxazole (Gantrisin) is the drug of choice in the treatment of chancroid; doses of 4 Gm a day for 7 to 12 days are usually curative. Local medication is not necessary, but saline soaks and cleanliness are advised. Although the buboes usually subside with sulfonamide therapy, fluctuation may persist, and the node should be aspirated in order to prevent spontaneous rupture. Streptomycin, chloramphenicol, and the tetracyclines in doses of 2 Gm a day for 7 to 10 days will each produce satisfactory healing of the lesions of chancroid. The use of these agents is rarely necessary because sulfisoxazole is equally effective. The antibiotics with treponemicidal properties should not be used in the treatment of chancroid until repeated dark-field examinations and serologic tests have ruled out the possibility of early syphilis.

REFERENCES

Heyman, A., P. B. Beeson, and W. H. Sheldon: Diagnosis of Chancroid, J.A.M.A., 129:935, 1945.

Sullivan, M.: Chancroid, Am. J. Syph., Gonor., Vener. Dis., 24:482, 1940.

154 BRUCELLOSIS (Undulant Fever)
Wesley W. Spink

DEFINITION. Brucellosis is caused by microorganisms belonging to the genus *Brucella*, and is transmitted to man from lower animals. The acute illness is frequently characterized by fever without localized findings, while the chronic form is featured by fever, weakness, and vague complaints, which may persist for months and years.

HISTORY. The first clear-cut picture of the disease was presented in 1863 by Marston, who, as a British Army surgeon in Malta, detailed his own case and those of others. The etiologic agent was discovered by Bruce in 1886. The outstanding clinical description of the disease is contained in the monograph by Hughes published in 1897. Wright and Semple in 1897 demonstrated agglutinins for brucella in human blood. In the same year, Bang reported that *Bacillus abortus* was the cause of contagious abortion in cattle in Denmark. The Mediterranean Fever Commission Reports of 1905 to 1907 detail the classic studies on epidemiology. The first recognized human case of brucellosis in the United States occurred in a nurse in Washington, D.C., and was described by Craig in 1906. In 1911 brucellosis was found to be endemic in the goats of Texas, and Gentry and Ferenbaugh traced human cases to this source. Traum first identified brucella organisms from aborting sows in 1914, and Evans in 1918 distinguished the difference between *Brucella melitensis* and *Brucella abortus*, and suggested that raw milk from infected cows could be the source of human cases. In 1924 Keefer described the first human case of brucellosis in this country due to organisms other than *B. melitensis*. A new species, *Brucella canis*, was described in 1966, causing abortions in dogs, especially the Beagle breed. In 1956, Spink described the over-all position of brucellosis in the United States.

ETIOLOGY. Human brucellosis is due to one of three species of *Brucella*: *B. melitensis* (goats), *B. suis* (hogs), and *B. abortus* (cattle). Several subtypes have been described under each of these three main categories. Brucellas are small, nonmotile, non-spore-forming rods staining gram-negative. Growth is best supported at 37°C in trypticase soy broth or tryptose phosphate broth having a pH of 6.6 to 6.8. The primary isolation of *B. abortus* requires displacement of 10 percent of the air by carbon dioxide. The differentiation of the three species is dependent upon biochemical and serologic reaction. *Brucella canis* differs from the foregoing species in that the isolates are rough colonies and lack lipopolysaccharide in the cell wall. No recognized human cases have been caused by this species.

EPIDEMIOLOGY. The natural reservoir of brucellosis is in domestic animals, particularly cattle, swine, goats, and sheep. The disease is very rarely transmitted from human to human.

Studies in the United States and elsewhere indicate that the majority of cases are acquired through contact, and fewer and fewer cases are caused by the ingestion of milk or milk products. This trend is due to the enactment of local and state ordinances requiring all milk sold for human consumption to be pasteurized. There is some evidence that brucellosis may be air-borne, with the disease resulting from the inhalation of brucella. Infections caused by *B. abortus* are spread through cow's milk or through dermal contact with brucella. Epidemics of brucellosis traced to raw cow's milk have been caused by *B. suis*. Contact with infected porcine tissue is a common cause of infections due to *B. suis*. It is readily appreciated why brucellosis is primarily a disease of rural areas and why it is considered an occupational disease involving meat-packing plant employees, farmers, veterinarians, and livestock producers.

PATHOGENESIS. Following invasion of the body by brucellas through the oropharynx or through the skin, the organisms tend to localize in tissues of the reticuloendothelial system, such as the bone marrow, lymph nodes, liver, spleen, and also the kidneys. A characteristic but nonspecific reaction of these tissues to the brucella is the appearance of epithelioid cells, giant cells of the foreign body and Langhans' types, and lymphocytes and plasma cells. Necrosis and caseation rarely occur in these granulomatous areas. When caseation is encountered, it is usually caused by *B. suis*. The granulomas are similar to those of sarcoidosis and tuberculosis. Other less frequent sites of localization of brucella organisms are the bones, especially the spine, the endocardium, and the testes. Although the central nervous system and peripheral nerves are commonly affected deleteriously by brucellas, the mechanism whereby this takes place is not known. Like other blood-borne infections, brucellas may on occasion localize in any tissue or organ in the body. Though brucellosis is a common cause of abortions in cattle, swine, and goats, authentic human abortions occur no more frequently with this disease than with other bacteremias. Orchitis in the male is rarely the cause of subsequent sterility.

MANIFESTATIONS. The incubation period varies between 5 and 21 days, though many months may elapse between the time of infection and the first appearance of symptoms. The onset in many instances may be insidious, the patients exhibiting a low-grade fever with no localized findings, and complaining of headache, weakness, insomnia, sweats, anorexia, constipation, pain over the spine, and generalized aches and pains. Less frequently, the disease may be ushered in by chills, high fever, and prostration, but, again, localized abnormal physical findings may be absent. In general, about 50 percent of the patients exhibit enlarged lymph nodes, especially of the cervical region, and splenomegaly is detected in about one-third of the cases. An enlarged and tender spleen is usually associated with the more severe cases. Pain on pressure over the vertebras occurs occasionally. Pain distributed over the course of the peripheral nerves, particularly the sciatic nerve, is encountered. Orchitis appears after several days of illness and, like the orchitis of mumps, is ushered in with a chill or chilliness, high fever, and tender and enlarged testes. Painful and swollen joints are seen occasionally, but persistent and deforming arthritis is not specific for the disease. Signs and symptoms referable to the lungs and pleurae are uncommon. A rare but serious complication is subacute bacterial endocarditis. Ocular disorders are associated with the more chronic forms of the disease.

The initial febrile stage of the illness may endure for only a few days or up to several weeks. The persistence of fever and symptoms is definitely related to physical activity. Rest in bed during the acute illness is frequently associated with prompt improvement. The natural course of the disease in the majority of patients is marked by a permanent remission of fever and symptoms within 3 to 6 months. A small number of patients with bacteriologically proved cases may have an illness that persists longer than 1 year.

The status of chronic brucellosis is extremely difficult to assess. There is no doubt that the infection may persist in a relatively small number of individuals for months and years. Such patients exhibit a state of ill health manifested by weakness, fatigue, mental depression, vague aches and pains, and no abnormal physical findings. Intermittent fever may occur. Of considerable importance in the suspected chronic case is the investigation of possible sites of chronic suppuration manifested by calcified caseating areas in the liver and spleen that can be detected by careful x-ray films of the abdomen. "Abacteric pyuria" should suggest, among other causes, renal suppuration due to brucellas.

LABORATORY FINDINGS. A precise diagnosis of brucellosis is dependent upon the results of laboratory procedures.

Blood. The total leukocyte count is usually normal or slightly reduced but is rarely over 10,000 cells per cu mm. The differential count reveals a relative lymphocytosis. The erythrocyte sedimentation rate is of no specific diagnostic aid, the rates being normal or accelerated.

The most practical method for screening suspected cases of brucellosis is the *agglutination* reaction. Agglutinins usually appear during the second or third week of illness. If proper techniques and antigen are employed, agglutinins are demonstrated in the vast majority of bacteriologically proved cases. Active brucellosis is usually associated with titers of 1:100 or above. On rare occasions, the titer may be depressed by "blocking antibodies" in chronic illness. Only very rarely are agglutinins absent in patients with bacteriologically proved disease. Agglutinins for brucellosis are not always specific, since cross reactions occur with the cholera vibrio and with *Pasteurella tularensis*. Agglutinins may persist in the blood long after the patient has recovered. One of the most critical diagnostic problems in the sporadic case of brucellosis is the interpretation of an agglutination titer of 1 to 100 or lower in the absence of both definitive bacteriologic data and localizing signs. Brucella-agglutinating immunoglobulins in serum consist of both 7S and 19S globulins, but only 7S has been associated with active disease in acute and chronic cases, providing a stimulating dose of antigen (skin test) has not been given prior to obtaining blood from the patient.

At least one *culture* of blood, and preferably more, should be carried out in every suspected case of brucellosis. *Brucella* have been isolated from aspirated sternal bone marrow, when simultaneous blood cultures remained sterile. It is too impractical for routine purposes to attempt to isolate brucellas from the urine, bile, or feces.

The *opsonocytophagic test,* which is a measure of the phagocytosis of brucellas by polymorphonuclear neutrophil leukocytes, is of no diagnostic value.

Intradermal Tests. A positive reaction to brucella antigen has no more significance than that obtained with tuberculin in suspected cases of tuberculosis. A positive reaction indicates previous invasion of the body by brucellas and does not mean that active disease is present. When agglutinins are absent and cultures remain sterile, considerable caution must be exercised before making a diagnosis of brucellosis, even though the skin test is positive.

DIFFERENTIAL DIAGNOSIS. Brucellosis must be differentiated from other acute febrile illnesses such as *influenza* and other *upper respiratory diseases* of doubtful etiology. Brucellosis is not commonly associated with coryza or pharyngitis. Other diseases from which it must be differentiated include *malaria* and *typhoid fever.* Brucellosis may be confused with *infectious mononucleosis,* but the characteristic blood picture and the elevated titer of heterophil antibodies in this disease are helpful differential aids.

Chronic brucellosis simulates *psychoneurosis, anxiety states,* and *chronic nervous exhaustion.* Indeed, a patient with brucellosis may suffer from the foregoing nervous disorders. Some confusion may arise in differentiating it from other diseases, including tuberculosis and lymphoblastoma, especially Hodgkin's disease.

TREATMENT. Patients with acute brucellosis should be reassured that a large majority of those with the disease recover spontaneously. Rest and psychotherapy are important during the febrile illness.

The course of acute brucellosis can be shortened and complications prevented by the prompt use of tetracycline, with an oral dose of 0.5 Gm four times daily for at least 3 weeks. In case of a relapse, this dose schedule can be repeated. Except in rare instances there is no advantage in more than two courses of tetracycline therapy. For the more seriously ill patients some authorities recommend the simultaneous use of streptomycin in dosages of 0.5 Gm twice daily and tetracycline. Tetracycline therapy, with and without streptomycin, is also effective in proved chronic brucellosis.

Febrile patients with either acute or chronic brucellosis can suffer from a severe toxic state with anorexia, depression, and a generalized debilitated condition. Such individuals should receive an adrenocorticoid steroid preparation in addition to antibiotic therapy. Prednisone in oral dosage of 20 mg can be given twice daily for 72 to 96 hr, or 100 mg of hydrocortisone can be administered intravenously followed by 50 mg orally twice daily.

A common therapeutic practice in the more chronic cases is to attempt desensitization to brucella organisms by treating patients with one of the several antigenic preparations, such as heat-killed brucella cells or filtrates of brucella cultures. Although hypersensitivity to brucellas is a factor in the symptomatology, and the use of ascending doses of antigenic material may be sound therapy, the results are difficult to evaluate, and treatment must often be continued for several months. Violent local and systemic reactions often occur, even following the injection of minute amounts of antigen.

For the relief of headache and the generalized aches and pains, salicylates may be prescribed; the occasional use of barbiturates is desirable for the insomnia which is so commonly a part of the disease.

PROGNOSIS. Although brucellosis may be a chronic and disabling disease, the overall mortality rate is not more than 2 percent and is negligible when appropriate antibiotic therapy is promptly employed. The physician today may learn a great deal about the prognosis of this disease by turning back and looking over the rich experience of the Mediterranean Fever Commission, which was recorded in 1905 to 1907. Without the aid of effective drug therapy, only 15 percent of patients had an illness exceeding 3 months.

Over the succeeding years, it has been observed that a relatively small, but important, number of patients will have a protracted illness. Cases of bacteriologically proved brucellosis in which the disease has continued for up to 25 years have been studied at the University of Minnesota Hospitals, but such cases are not commonly encountered. One cannot escape the conviction that so-called "chronic brucellosis" is being mislabeled too often on the basis of procedures of doubtful value, especially the intradermal test with brucella antigen.

Relapses do occur in the more chronic cases of brucellosis. These recurrences are manifested by fever and by mental and physical disability, with generalized aches and pains. But too little attention has been given to the problem of reinfections. Clinical observations in meat-packing plant employees have confirmed studies made with experimentally infected animals, in that the immunity induced by one attack of brucellosis is only relative. Second and third infections do take place. In individuals who continue to be exposed to the disease, it may be quite difficult to differentiate between relapses and reinfections. Furthermore, patients having recovered from brucellosis have an acquired brucella hypersensitivity that may render them extremely susceptible to the effects of contact with brucella antigen. This is particularly applicable to veterinarians who have accidentally injected viable brucella antigen into their skin while immunizing animals. Violent local and systemic febrile reactions follow such an incident within a few hours.

PREVENTION. As long as the reservoir of brucellosis persists in domestic animals, human brucellosis will occur. The only practical means of eliminating the disease in human beings is to eradicate the disease from cattle, hogs, sheep, and goats. Control measures in animals are being worked out in several areas in the United States. Since human brucellosis is contracted through the ingestion of contaminated milk and milk products, it is essential that only properly pasteurized milk be utilized for human consumption. Brucellosis is an occupational disease involving farmers, livestock workers, veterinarians, and those working in meat-packing plants and there is no entirely safe means for immunizing these groups against the disease.

REFERENCES

Carmichael, L. E., and R. M. Kennedy: Canine Abortion Caused by *Brucella canis*, J. Am. Vet. Med. Assn., 152: 605, 1966.

Eyre, J. W. H.: Melitensis Septicemia, Lancet, I:1677, 1747, 1826, 1908.

Hughes, M. L.: "Mediterranean, Malta or Undulant Fever," London, The Macmillan Company, Ltd., 1897.

"Reports of the Commission for the Investigation of Mediterranean Fever," pts. 1 to 7, London, Harrison & Sons, Ltd., 1905–1907.

Reddin, J. L., R. K. Anderson, R. Jenness, and W. W. Spink:

Significance of 7S and Macroglobulin Brucella Agglutinins in Human Brucellosis, New Engl. J. Med., 272:1263, 1965.

Spink, W. W.: "The Nature of Brucellosis," Minneapolis, University of Minnesota Press, 1956.

155 TULAREMIA
Leighton E. Cluff

DEFINITION. Tularemia (rabbit fever, deer-fly fever, Ohara's disease) is an infectious disease of animals transmitted to man by direct contact or by insect vectors. A cutaneous or mucous membrane lesion at the site of inoculation and regional lymph node enlargement are the characteristic manifestations of the disease in man.

HISTORY. The microorganism responsible for tularemia was identified by McCoy and Chapin in 1912 among infected ground squirrels in Tulare County, California. The first description of tularemia in man was by Wherry and Lamb in 1914.

ETIOLOGY. *Pasteurella tularensis* is a pleomorphic, nonsporulating, gram-negative bacillus. It can be cultured only on media containing glucose, cystine, and serum. Thorough cooking renders meat from infected animals safe for consumption, but tularemia can develop in persons handling carcasses that have been frozen for many days. *Pasteurella tularensis* is related antigenically to the causative organisms of brucellosis and plague and posesses an endotoxin similar to those of many other gram-negative bacteria.

EPIDEMIOLOGY AND PATHOGENESIS. Contact with infected animals is the commonest source of tularemia in man, but the disease also may be acquired from insects or by exposure to the organism in the laboratory. A variety of rodents, carnivores, ungulates, birds, and arthropods is naturally infected by *P. tularensis,* including rabbits, squirrels, woodchucks, muskrats, skunks, coyotes, foxes, opossums, mice, rats, quail, chickens, pheasants, snakes, ticks, and flies. The Rocky Mountain tick, western wood tick, eastern dog tick, and the Lone Star tick (*Dermacentor andersoni, D. variabilis, D. occidentalis,* and *Amblyomma americanum*) may act as reservoirs of infection. One species of deer fly (*Chrysops discalis*) and, in Sweden, a mosquito (*Aëdes cinereus*) can transmit tularemia to man. Ticks are an important reservoir of the disease because the microorganism is transferred transovarially from the female to her progeny. Sporadic episodes and epidemic tularemia have occurred following contact with water and fish contaminated by infected animal carcasses. However, human-to-human transmission of infection does not occur. Wild cottontail rabbits are the principal source of tularemia in the United States.

Man is highly susceptible to tularemia; the organism usually invades through the skin, mucous membrane, gastrointestinal tract, or respiratory tract. Hunters, butchers, and housewives are most often affected.

PATHOLOGY. Microscopically, the primary cutaneous lesion shows neutrophilic infiltration, granulomatous reaction, and necrosis. The regional lymph nodes develop similar changes and often suppurate. The granulomatous reaction in tularemia resembles tubercles in liver, spleen, lung, and kidney. *Pasteurella tularensis* has been recovered from lymph nodes many days after apparent subsidence of the disease.

MANIFESTATIONS. The incubation period is 3 to 7 days. Because a typical lesion of skin or mucous membranes is not invariably present, tularemia classically has been separated into several clinical types.

More than 80 percent of infections by *P. tularensis* produce a lesion of the skin or mucous membranes which begins as a reddened papule that may be pruritic and soon ulcerates. The primary lesion in this *ulceroglandular* form of the disease is rarely very painful, is usually present before onset of systemic symptoms, and may not heal until convalescence is well under way. Frequently it is overlooked, or its relationship to severe systemic symptoms is not recognized. Regional lymph node enlargement is usually more prominent than that accompanying infections of similar severity produced by other microorganisms. The involved nodes are often exquisitely tender, fluctuant, hot, and reddened. Drainage can occur spontaneously. Generalized lymphadenopathy is present in some cases, but the regional nodes are most prominently involved. There is considerable variation in the intensity of the systemic symptoms of ulceroglandular tularemia; the patient may be almost asymptomatic or severely prostrated. Clinical and roentgenographic evidence of pneumonitis may accompany this form of the disease, illustrating its disseminated character, but bacteremia is rarely demonstrable.

Localized lymph node enlargement without detectable skin lesion is referred to as *glandular* tularemia. The pathogenesis of this form of the disease is probably identical with that of ulceroglandular tularemia, and the features of the illness are also the same.

Rarely, the portal of entry of the organism is the conjunctiva, where there develops an ulcer, with edema, congestion, lacrimation, photophobia, and pain. In this *oculoglandular* type of tularemia the preauricular, submaxillary, and anterior cervical lymph nodes may enlarge. Corneal ulceration and scarring or perforation of the globe may occur.

Ingestion of contaminated meat or water may result in primary lesions in the *gastrointestinal* tract. This rare form of the disease produces diarrhea, abdominal pain, nausea, vomiting, melena, and hematemesis, but otherwise differs little from tularemia introduced through other portals. Ulcerative lesions are often found in the buccal mucosa, pharynx, or intestine, and the mesenteric or cervical lymph nodes are involved early in the disease.

Tularemia without obvious primary ulcer or localized lymphadenitis is referred to as *typhoidal*. Constitutional symptoms in typhoidal tularemia differ in no way from those in other types of the disease, although there is usually more prostration. In the absence of localized manifestations, the diagnosis of tularemia is more difficult and depends on serologic tests, isolation of the organism, or a strong epidemiologic history.

Pneumonia may accompany tularemia. Involvement of the lung is secondary to hematogenous dissemination, even when infection is acquired by inhalation of the organism (as in bacteriology laboratories). Pneumonitis in tularemia may cause cough, mucoid sputum, hemoptysis, pleuritic pain, dyspnea, and cyanosis, but extensive x-ray evidence of pneumonitis is sometimes present in the absence of any symptoms of pulmonary disease. Physical findings often correlate poorly with the roentgenologic changes, which consist of diffuse patchy or lobar infiltrations and inconstant hilar adenopathy. Pleural effusion may occur, but lung abscess is rare.

Rarely *P. tularensis* causes endocarditis, pericarditis, peritonitis, appendicitis, osteomyelitis, or meningitis.

Fever in tularemia develops abruptly, often with rigors, and in untreated patients may persist with temperatures of 104 to 106°F for as long as 4 weeks. The fever is sustained or mildly remittent, and defervescence is by lysis.

Splenomegaly is detectable in many patients. An evanescent macular or papular *rash* is sometimes present on the trunk and extremities early in the disease.

Convalescence in untreated tularemia is prolonged, and fever, lassitude, fatigability, myalgia, irritability, or anorexia may persist or recur for many months. Recovery is usually prompt if acute tularemia is treated with antibiotics. When therapy is delayed, however, patients are more likely to be left with mild debilitation that is unresponsive to further administration of antimicrobial drugs.

Recovery from tularemia is usually followed by immunity to recurrence of disease. However, immunity is not complete, and several instances of second, even third attacks of tularemia have been recorded. Almost invariably, they have consisted of the development of a local lesion and mild regional adenopathy without systemic symptoms and with little or no fever.

LABORATORY FINDINGS. Serum agglutinins for *P. tularensis* are present after the second week of illness. Cross agglutination may occur with antigens of *Brucella*, but this is not a constant finding.

Pasteurella tularensis can be recovered by appropriate cultures or animal inoculation. It is rarely found in blood but can be isolated from the mucocutaneous ulcer or regional lymph nodes with regularity. The organism has been cultured from the sputum and gastric washings even in patients without roentgenographic evidence of pneumonitis. Accidental infection of personnel in diagnostic laboratories may occur.

Skin test with a diluted suspension of killed *P. tularensis*, or purified antigen, becomes positive during the first week of disease. The cutaneous hypersensitivity response is "delayed" and resembles the tuberculin reaction.

The total blood leukocyte count is usually normal. The erythrocyte sedimentation rate is normal in ulceroglandular or mild disease but is frequently elevated in severe typhoidal tularemia.

DIFFERENTIAL DIAGNOSIS. Brucellosis, typhoid fever, disseminated tuberculosis, the early stage of several rickettsial diseases, and infectious mononucleosis may closely resemble typhoidal tularemia. History of possible contacts is important, and appropriate serologic and cultural studies are usually successful in differentiating these infections. Pneumonic tularemia must be distinguished from viral, mycotic, and other bacterial infections of the lung. The differential diagnosis of pneumonia is discussed in Chap. 138. Oculoglandular syndromes likely to be confused with tularemia are described in Chap. 230.

Ulceroglandular tularemia must be distinguished from a variety of infections in which a *local cutaneous ulcer with regional lymphadenopathy* may occur. Besides pyoderma caused by streptococci or staphylococci, these infections include lymphogranuloma venereum, cat-scratch fever, rat-bite fever, bubonic plague, anthrax, glanders, several rickettsioses of which the important one in this country is rickettsialpox, several viral infections of the skin such as orf and cowpox, and inoculation syphilis or tuberculosis. In all these, with the exception of lymphogranuloma venereum and cat-scratch fever, the regional lymph node involvement is usually proportional to the size of the cutaneous ulcer. Extragenital lymphogranuloma is rare; fever and systemic symptoms in cat-scratch fever are rarely severe for more than a few days.

TREATMENT. Streptomycin is the antibiotic of choice for tularemia. The dosage is 0.5 to 1.0 Gm every 12 hr for 10 days. *Pasteurella tularensis* cannot be recovered from lymph nodes or skin lesions after 24 to 48 hr of therapy. However, the regional lymph nodes may continue to enlarge and suppurate for several days. Pulmonary lesions usually subside rapidly, although the evolution of the cutaneous lesion is not interrupted. The tetracycline antibiotics and chloramphenicol, also are effective, although fever and other manifestations may recur 7 to 14 days after cessation of therapy. Recrudescent illness, however, responds rapidly to readministration of the antibiotic. Aspiration of pus from suppurating nodes rarely is necessary; but if fistulas persist, total surgical removal of the involved tissue can be carried out. Surgery may be followed by transient recurrence of fever despite failure to demonstrate the organism in excised tissues.

PROPHYLAXIS. A killed bacterial vaccine developed by Foshay has been shown to stimulate serum agglutinins and induces positive skin reactions to the bacterial antigens, but it produces little immunity to infection with *P. tularensis*. An attenuated live bacterial vaccine has been developed, however, and is effective in inducing protection against infection.

Antibiotic prophylaxis with streptomycin following exposure to tularemia will protect against infection. Chloramphenicol and tetracycline, however, only prolong the incubation period of the disease and do not prevent its occurrence.

Avoidance of contact with possible sources of infection is important in prevention, and the incidence of tularemia in several localities has fallen sharply with the introduction of laws prohibiting the sale of wild rabbits by butchers.

PROGNOSIS. The mortality rate in untreated tularemia is 6 to 7 percent. With antimicrobial therapy, death is rare.

REFERENCES

Foshay, L.: Treatment of Tularemia with Streptomycin, Am. J. Med., 2:467, 1947.

Francis, E.: Tularemia, in "Oxford Medicine," Fair Lawn, N.J. Oxford University Press, 1948.

McCrumb, F. R., Jr., M. I. Snyder, and T. E. Woodward: Studies on Human Infection with *Pasteurella tularensis:* Comparison of Streptomycin and Chloramphenicol in the Prophylaxis of Clinical Disease, Trans. Assoc. Am. Physicians, 70:74, 1957.

Stuart, B. M., and R. L. Pullen: Tularemic Pneumonia: Review of American Literature and Report of Fifteen Additional Cases, Am. J. Med. Sci., 210:233, 1945.

Woodward, T. E., W. T. Raby, W. Eppes, W. A. Holbrook, and J. A. Hightower: Aureomycin in Treatment of Experimental and Human Tularemia, J.A.M.A., 139:830, 1949.

156   PLAGUE
Joseph E. Johnson, III

DEFINITION. Plague is an infectious disease of animals (principally wild and domestic rodents) which is transmitted to man through the bite of infected ectoparasites (especially the rat flea). Disease in man is usually characterized by the abrupt onset of high fever, lymphadenopathy and suppuration of regional lymph nodes draining the exposure site, bacteremia, and prostration. This clinical form of the disease is known as *bubonic* plague because of the presence of enlarged suppurating lymph nodes, or *buboes*. Secondary pneumonia may occur and lead to direct respiratory transmission by infectious aerosols from man to man. This primary *pneumonic* type of human disease is highly fatal.

HISTORY. Plague was known and feared in ancient times and has been the subject of dread as well as a source of literary stimulation to authors from Dionysius in the third century to Camus in the present. It has undoubtedly been endemic in Asia and Europe for centuries. At least three major pandemics have occurred in which large segments of the population were destroyed. The first authentic pandemic was recorded in the sixth century A.D., and is estimated to have claimed 100 million victims. The second great pandemic occurred in the fourteenth century and was known as the "Black Death," presumably because of the severe cyanosis produced in some of its victims. Fifty million persons, including onequarter of the population of Europe, died. In subsequent centuries, consecutive outbreaks of plague ravaged Europe and Africa. The last major pandemic originated in China in 1894, spread eventually to all continents, and was first recognized in the United States in 1900. It is likely, however, that the disease was present in the wild rodent population (sylvatic plague) in California long before this. The disease is now well established in wild rodents in many parts of the world, including the western United States. It is present on every continent except

Australia. Human disease is endemic in parts of Asia, Africa, and South America, and sporadic human cases still occur in the United States.

ETIOLOGY. The causative agent, *Pasteurella pestis*, is a gram-negative, nonmotile, and non-spore-forming bacillus which grows both aerobically and anaerobically. It is pleomorphic in exudate or sputum, and may appear bacillary, ovid, or coccal. When stained with Giemsa or Wayson's stain, it displays a bipolar "safety pin" structure. *Pasteurella pestis* grows readily although somewhat slowly on ordinary culture media, forming small, round, transparent colonies which assume a "beaten-copper" appearance after 48 hr. At least two types of toxins have been identified, including a soluble exotoxinlike protein, and an insoluble endotoxic lipopolysaccharide. Although readily killed by sunlight, organisms have been shown to survive in sterile soil for 16 months and in nonsterile soil for as long as 7 months, and it is likely that organisms may be present in rodent burrows in the absence of fleas and rats for long periods.

Pasteurella pestis is generally susceptible to streptomycin, chloramphenicol, and the tetracycline antibiotics. A few streptomycin-resistant strains recently have been isolated in Vietnam, but no therapeutic failures have been attributable to drug-resistance. Drug resistance may pose a threat in the future, however, because transfer of drug-resistance factors (R factors) from *E. Coli* to *P. Pestis* has been demonstrated.

EPIDEMIOLOGY. Plague is firmly entrenched as an enzootic among approximately 200 species of rodents in many parts of the world. While the disease in wild rodents (sylvatic plague) is not usually a direct threat to man, it nevertheless serves as a vast reservoir for infection of domestic rats (murine or rat plague) which, along with their ectoparasites, live in close association with man. The endemic reservoir of sylvatic plague includes wild rats, ground squirrels, mice, marmots, owls, gophers, badgers, rabbits, prairie dogs, and chipmunks; in the Western Hemisphere the disease is firmly entrenched in the wild rodent population of California, Oregon, Washington, Utah, Idaho, Nevada, New Mexico, Texas, Louisiana, Florida, Michigan, Arizona, Colorado, Montana, Wyoming, Kansas, North Dakota, Hawaii, western Mexico, and western Canada. The principal murine hosts are the domestic rats, *Rattus rattus* and *R. norvegicus,* which are found throughout the world. Although ticks, lice, and bedbugs may occasionally serve as vectors, the principal ectoparasite vector is the oriental rat flea, *Xenopsylla cheopis.*

Between epidemics the infection persists as a chronic disease of wild rodents which is maintained by the insect vector. Although occasionally acquired through contact with wild rodents and their parasites, human disease is usually a result of association with domestic rats and occurs in urban areas in the wake of rat epizootics. When the concentration of people and of rats under circumstances of poor sanitation provides opportunity for the migration of fleas from rats to man, an outbreak is likely to occur. Because sylvatic plague appears virtually impossible to eradicate, it will continue to pose a constant threat of extension into urban rat populations and thence to man. Infection of the flea takes place through ingestion of blood of a bacteremic animal. After multiplication in the intestinal tract of the flea, the organisms are regurgitated when the flea attempts to ingest another blood meal. Because rat fleas will attack man if rats are not immediately available, the infection is likely to be transmitted as the rat population decreases and the fleas transfer from dead hosts to human beings. Plague can be acquired by direct contact with the tissues of an infected animal, by its bite, or by scratching of infected material into the skin.

The bubonic form of the disease rarely results in transmission from man to man because bacteremia in human disease is rarely of a level sufficient to allow infection of fleas. The principal mode of spread from man to man is by the pulmonary route, which occurs when a patient with bubonic disease develops secondary plague pneumonia and thereafter excretes large quantities of organisms in the sputum. Airborne infection by droplet nuclei is highly contagious, and primary pneumonic plague is common among those attending such a patient. Although asymptomatic oropharyngeal carriers have been identified among healthy family contacts of bubonic plague patients in Vietnam, the role of these carriers in the transmission of the disease has not been determined.

PATHOGENESIS. In the more common bubonic form of disease, *P. pestis* gains entry into the human host through the bite of an infected flea. Organisms are carried to the local lymphatics, then to the bloodstream and finally are disseminated. The prominent clinical manifestations are usually in the lymphatic system. In bubonic plague, a hemorrhagic zone of edema surrounds an inflamed and suppurating group of regional lymph nodes. The glands are hyperplastic and show multiple areas of necrosis, in which there are swarms of organisms. Metastatic lesions sometimes develop in other lymphatics or in the viscera. Particularly likely is the occurrence of secondary pneumonia, which constitutes a potential source of pneumonic spread. Hemorrhages are numerous, probably as a result of a toxin produced by *P. pestis,* and it is not unusual for individuals given chemotherapy at a late date to die of toxemia when plague bacilli can no longer be cultured from any organ. Primary pneumonic spread occurs through the inhalation of infectious aerosols emanating from another case or, rarely, from infected fomites. It is apparent that the tonsils and/or oropharyngeal mucous membranes may occasionally serve as portals of entry resulting in a cervical bubonic-septicemic form of the disease. Rarely a skin papule forms at the site of entry of the bacillus, and may develop into a pustule or a carbuncle.

Bacteremia is a constant feature of bubonic and pneumonic plague. The precise mechanisms by which the plague bacillus and its toxic factors produce severe tissue injury are not understood completely.

MANIFESTATIONS. After an incubation period of 1 to 12 days (usually 2 to 4 days), the patient develops an acute and often fulminant illness. In the more common *bubonic* variety, symptoms begin abruptly with chills, a rise in temperature to 102 to 105°F, tachycardia, headache, vomiting, uncertain gait, marked prostration, and delirium. The spleen is sometimes palpable. The fleabite at the portal of entry rarely can be seen; if present, it is marked by a papule or vesicle which ultimately becomes pustular. Pain and tenderness are present in the infected regional lymph nodes. Of the buboes, 60 to 75 percent are in the inquinal or femoral regions because the lower extremities are more commonly the site of the initial fleabite. Less often, especially in children, buboes are found in the axillary or cervical regions. Infection may extend to other superficial or deeply situated groups of glands. The bubo consists of a firm, matted group of glands measuring 2 to 5 cm in diameter and is surrounded by a boggy and frequently hemorrhagic zone of edema. It usually suppurates and drains spontaneously after 1 or 2 weeks, although in some instances there is complete resorption.

There is a marked hemorrhagic tendency, presumably because of the effect of plague toxin on blood vessels. Petechiae or ecchymoses occur often. Bleeding may occur into a viscus or a serous cavity, or from the nose and alimentary, respiratory, or urinary tracts.

The course of bubonic plague is marked by an irregular or remittent fever, which often drops at the time of appearance of the bubo, only to rise again. In favorable cases, the temperature falls gradually during the second week concomitant with improvement in the general clinical condition. A rise to hyperpyrexic levels or a precipitous fall to normal or to subnormal, frequently heralds approaching death. Most fatalities occur during the first week of illness. Although bubonic plague is usually severe, mild cases called *pestis minor* are sometimes seen during epidemics.

The "primary septicemic" form of plague is actually a variant of bubonic disease. The patient experiences a sudden and overwhelming systemic illness. There is a marked constitutional reaction, with chills, fever, rapid pulse, severe headache, nausea, vomiting, and delirium. Death ensues within a few days, before localizing lesions become clinically apparent. Nevertheless, autopsy usually reveals inflammation in some part of the lymphatic system.

Plague also may take the form of pneumonia. The initial cases appear in patients with bubonic plague, of whom as many as 5 percent develop secondary lesions in the lungs. These individuals may provide the starting point for a man-to-man epidemiologic cycle of airborne primary pneumonic plague. It is a fulminating infection accompanied by great prostration, cough, dyspnea, and in the later stages, cyanosis. The sputum is abundant, bloodstained, and teeming with *P. pestis*. Often there are no clear-cut pulmonary signs, though scattered râles or areas of dullness may be found. In the absence of specific therapy, plague pneumonia invariably ends fatally within 1 to 5 days.

Infection may localize in other regions of the body. Subcutaneous abscesses and cutaneous ulcerations sometimes occur, and occasionally the meninges are involved.

LABORATORY FINDINGS. Laboratory confirmation of plague is relatively simple, although the disease is often misdiagnosed in the United States because of its rarity. Consideration of epidemiologic and clinical features provide highly characteristic leads, and once a suspicion of plague is entertained, it can readily be verified by smear, culture, and animal inoculation of appropriate specimens. The technique of staining a suspected specimen with fluorescent specific antiserum provides an elegant method for rapid identification of *P. pestis*. If a bubo is present, a small quantity of interstitial fluid should be aspirated from its center. Large numbers of morphologically characteristic bacilli are usually seen in a stained smear. Infected sputum likewise contains many organisms. Bacteremia of varying degrees occurs at some time during the course of the disease in nearly all cases. Pus and sputum should be cultured on blood agar plates, while blood is inoculated into nutrient broth. Organisms are identified by their morphologic and colonial characteristics and by agglutination with specific antiserum. Guinea pig inoculation is the final step in identification. In this animal the gross and microscopic lesions are highly characteristic. Caution should be observed in handling infected materials or animals, because of the great danger of infection to laboratory workers.

Specific antibodies appear in the serum of patients convalescing from the disease and can usually be detected early in the second week by complement fixation, agglutination, passive hemagglutination, or immunoelectrophoretic agar-gel precipitation methods. A passive mouse-protective test serves to indicate the immune status of a convalescent or vaccinated individual.

The white blood cell count is elevated to levels often above 20,000 cells per cu mm, and there is a predominance of polymorphonuclear leukocytes. The red blood cell count usually is normal.

DIAGNOSIS. Early in the acute phase of illness, before the appearance of localizing signs, plague may be confused with severe systemic illnesses such as typhoid, typhus, or malaria. The presence of buboes may suggest other forms of infectious lymphadenitis, including tularemia, syphilis, and lymphogranuloma venereum, as well as lymphadenitis of staphylococcal or streptococcal origin. Pneumonic plague must be distinguished from tularemic, pneumococcal, and other gram-negative pneumonias as well as from anthrax, psittacosis, and mycoplasma pneumonia. The consideration of epidemiologic factors, plus bacteriologic studies, will aid in the differentiation. Serologic diagnosis is of aid only for retrospective confirmation. When plague is suspected, it is imperative to begin treatment as soon as adequate specimens have been taken for culture because early institution of therapy is essential to ensure recovery. To delay treatment may risk toxemic death in the face of a bacteriologic cure.

TREATMENT. When antibiotic treatment is instituted early in the course of the disease, the response is usually dramatic and complete. Even patients with pneumonic or septicemic disease can be cured if treatment is initiated within the first 15 to 20 hr after onset. Streptomycin is the drug of choice and is given in divided doses of 4 Gm daily for 48 hr followed by 1.5 Gm daily for a total of 7 to 10 days or until the patient has been afebrile at least 3 days. Chloramphenicol and tetracyclines are also potent antiplague agents. Chloramphenicol should be given in initial doses of 6 to 8 Gm daily intravenously, and the dose should be reduced to 3 to 4 Gm when improvement occurs. Tetracyclines are given in initial doses of 2 to 3 Gm daily intravenously, and the dose is reduced to 2 Gm daily orally when improvement occurs. Sulfadiazine has been somewhat less effective, particularly in pneumonic plague, but can be used when the other antibiotics are not available. Buboes are treated with hot, moist applications. Incision and drainage should be postponed until the lesion becomes well localized and the patient has been treated with antibiotics.

CONTROL. Prevention of plague must be directed toward elimination of endemic rodent foci, and in endemic urban areas constant vigilance is required in detecting and combating rodent epizootics. Prevention includes extermination of rats, eradication of ectoparasite vectors, and sometimes the immunization of the human population. Rats are attacked by poisoning and trapping, by elimination of harborage areas, and by separating them from their food supplies. Unfortunately, rodent control has proved to be most difficult in the endemic areas because of generally poor living standards. Vector control with DDT has been used with brilliant success in diminishing the flea population infecting both rodents and human beings, but recent studies in southeast Asia unfortunately show a significant incidence of DDT-resistant fleas, but these may yield to other insecticides such as Aldrin, Dieldrin, and Chlordane. The complete elimination of sylvatic plague appears to be impossible in the foreseeable future, and the control program must be aimed at eradicating foci of wild rodent infection around areas of human habitation. In these peripheral zones, the wild and the domestic rodents live commensally, exchange fleas, and threaten the human community.

Patients must be disinfested and carefully isolated, while other intimately exposed persons should be quarantined. Prophylaxis has been achieved effectively in the past by administering sulfadiazine in a dose of 3 Gm per day for 1 week. Recent southeast Asian studies, however, have revealed significant in vitro resistance to sulfadiazine. Alternatively, prophylaxis with streptomycin in a dose of 1 Gm per day is often effective.

Vaccines have been used for many years and apparently provide limited and transitory immunity. Three types of vaccines have been available. A formalin-killed vaccine approved for use in the United States has been advised for all persons traveling to Vietnam, Cambodia, and Laos, for those whose vocations bring them into frequent and regular contact with wild rodents in plague enzootic areas, and for all laboratory personnel working with *P. pestis* or with plague-infected rodents. Although the precise effectiveness of this vaccine has not been measured satisfactorily, it appears to reduce the incidence and severity of the disease. A second promising vaccine is a living attenuated strain of the organism which may be particularly suitable for endemic areas in Asia. Russian studies indicate that the attenuated vaccine administered by the aerosol route may be especially valuable in prevention of pneumonic plague. A third vaccine consisting of a chemical extract has been effective in experimental laboratory infections. Immunity is relative, and protection is not always conferred by the active disease, since a number of reinfections have been described. Although general vaccination may be worthwhile in an area threatened by an epidemic, the results are too slow for immediate prophylaxis. In such epidemic situations, combined use of all available control measures is indicated.

PROGNOSIS. The availability of effective antibiotic therapy has improved the prognosis in this formerly highly fatal disease. In the past the mortality rate of bubonic plague varied from 50 to 90 percent, and the pneumonic, septicemic, and meningitic forms were almost invariably fatal. In treated cases the mortality is 5 to 10 percent and even the gravest varieties of infection respond to chemotherapy if treated early enough.

REFERENCES

Cavanaugh, D. C., H. G. Dangerfield, D. H. Hunter, R. J. T. Joy, J. D. Marshall, D. V. Quy, S. Vivona, and P. E. Winter: Some Observations on the Current Plague Outbreak in the Republic of Vietnam, Am. J. Public Health, 58:742, 1968.

Gilbert, D. N., W. L. Moore, L. L. Hedberg, and J. P. Sanford: Potential Medical Problems in Personnel Returning from Vietnam, Ann. Intern. Med. 68:662, 1968.

Girard, G.: Plague, Ann. Rev. Microbiol., 69:253, 1955.

Hirst, L. F.: "The Conquest of Plague: A Study of the Evolution of Epidemiology," Fair Lawn, N.J., Oxford University Press, 1953.

Kartman, L., F. M. Prince, S. F. Quan, and H. E. Stark: New Knowledge on the Ecology of Sylvatic Plague, Ann. N.Y. Acad. Sci., 70:668, 1958.

Meyer, K. F., S. F. Quan, F. R. McCrumb, and A. Larson: Effective Treatment of Plague, Ann. N.Y. Acad. Sci., 55: 1228, 1952.

Pollitzer, R.: "Plague," World Health Organ. Monograph Series, No. 22, Geneva, 1954.

——: A Review of Recent Literature on Plague. Bull. World Health Organ, no. 23, pp. 313–400, Geneva, 1960.

157 GLANDERS
Jay P. Sanford

DEFINITION: Glanders is a serious infection of equine animals caused by *Malleomyces mallei*, which is transmitted occasionally to other domestic animals and to man.

ETIOLOGY. *Malleomyces mallei* is a small, slender, nonmotile, gram-negative bacillus. When stained with methylene blue, marked irregularities in staining are observed. Organisms grow on most common meat infusion media, but require glycerol for optimum growth.

EPIDEMIOLOGY. Glanders was at one time widespread throughout Europe, but due to the introduction of control measures, its incidence has decreased steadily in most countries. The disease still occurs in Asia, Africa, and South America, but not in the United States. Glanders has never been common in man, but the occasional infection may be very serious. There have been no naturally acquired infections in the United States since 1938, but with increasing international travel, patients with glanders may be encountered.

Glanders is primarily a disease of horses, mules, and donkeys, although goats, sheep, cats, and dogs sometimes naturally contract the disease. Rabbits, guinea pigs, and hamsters are susceptible to experimental infection. Pigs and cattle are said to be absolutely resistant. In horses, the disease may be systemic with prominent pulmonary involvement, *glanders,* or characterized by subcutaneous ulcerative lesions, and lymphatic thickening with nodules, *farcy.* The route of infection in animals remains controversial; inhalation, ingestion, or inoculation through breaks in the skin have been suggested. In man, the disease occurs primarily in individuals with close contact with horses, mules, or donkeys through inoculation or a break in the skin or by exposing the nasal mucosa to contaminated discharges. A number of instances of airborne infection have been reported in laboratory workers.

PATHOLOGY. The acute lesion is characterized by nodules consisting of polymorphonuclear leukocytes surrounded by a zone of congestion. A characteristic histologic feature is a peculiar nuclear degeneration known as chromatotexis which occurs early and is extensive. Small foci of deeply staining detritus within the abscess result from this degeneration. In older nodules, the reaction is characterized by epithelioid cells surrounding an area of central necrosis. Giant cells may be present. Occasionally calcification may occur. Virtually any organ may be involved.

CLINICAL MANIFESTATIONS. The manifestations in man are protean and are determined in part by the route of infection. Nearly 60 percent of patients have been between the ages of twenty and forty years. The disease has been rare in women, probably because of less opportunity for contact. The manifestations which frequently overlap may be categorized as (1) acute localized suppurative infection, (2) acute pulmonary infection, (3) acute septicemic infection, and (4) chronic suppurative infection.

Infection acquired by inoculation through an abrasion or scratch in the skin usually results in a nodule with an area of acute lymphangitis. The incubation period is probably 1 to 5 days. In all types of acute glanders, there is usually fever and extreme generalized malaise and prostration.

Infection of the mucous membranes may result in mucopurulent discharge involving the eye, nose, or lips followed by extensive ulcerating granulomatous lesions which may or may not be associated with systemic reactions. With systemic invasion, a generalized papular eruption which may become pustular is frequent. This septicemic form of disease is usually fatal in 7 to 10 days.

Infection by inhalation is followed by an incubation period of 10 to 14 days. The more common symptoms include fever, occasionally associated with rigors, generalized myalgia, fatigue, headache, and pleuritic chest pain. Other symptoms consist of photophobia, lacrimation, and diarrhea. Examination is usually normal except for fever and occasional lymphadenopathy, especially in the cervical chain, and splenomegaly. Laboratory findings include mild leukocytosis with 60 to 80 percent neutrophilic leukocytes, but leukopenia with relative lymphocytosis has been recorded. In the acute pulmonary form, chest radiographs characteristically reveal circumscribed densities which suggest early lung abscesses. Other findings may include lobar or bronchopneumonia. In the chronic suppurative form of disease, the most frequent finding is multiple subcutaneous and intramuscular abscesses which most often involve the arms or legs. Approximately one-half of the patients will have associated fever, lymphadenopathy, and nasal discharge or ulceration. Pain at sites other than developing foci and skin eruptions occur in one-third. Visceral involvement including pulmonary or pleural, ocular, skeletal, hepatic, splenic, and meningeal or intracranial involvement occurred in one-fourth or less of the 156 patients summarized by Robins.

DIAGNOSIS. Microscopic examination of exudates may reveal small gram-negative bacilli which stain irregularly with methylene blue; however, organisms are generally very scanty and it is often difficult to find them even in acute abscesses. Giemsa or other modifications of the Romanowski stain may be the best way to identify organisms. *Malleomyces mallei* and *Pseudomonas pseudomallei* cannot be distinguished morphologically from one another. Culturing is often avoided because of the hazard to laboratory personnel; however, if cultures are made, growth occurs on most meat infusion nutrient media. The material often is contaminated with other microorganisms and incubation with benzyl penicillin G (1,000 units per ml) prior to culturing may be helpful. Subcutaneous inoculation of material into a guinea pig or hamster affords an alternative means of isolation. Blood cultures are usually negative except in the terminal stages of disease. Serologic tests show a rapidly rising agglutination titer, which reaches levels of 1:640 within 2 weeks. Serum from normal persons has been reported to show agglutination titers in dilutions up to 1:320. The complement fixation test is less sensitive but more specific and usually becomes positive during the third week; it is considered positive in dilutions of 1:20 or greater. The mallein skin test is of help diagnostically; 0.1 ml of a 1:10,000 dilution of commercial mallein is injected intradermally. Erythema exceeding 10 mm in 48 hr is considered to represent a specific test. The test becomes positive in most patients by the third or fourth week of disease and remains positive for years.

TREATMENT. The limited number of infections in man has precluded evaluation of most of the antibiotic agents. Sulfadiazine has been found to be an effective agent in experimental animals and in man. The dosage utilized has been approximately 100 mg per kg administered in divided doses. In experimental infections, 3 weeks of therapy gave better results than 1 week. Benzyl penicillin is ineffective in vitro and in experimental infections. Streptomycin is bacteriostatic in vitro but was ineffective in experimental infections in hamsters. Broad-spectrum antibiotics such as tetracycline, chloramphenicol, and kanamycin have not been evaluated. In the acute infections, appropriate supportive measures are essential, and in the chronic suppurative infections, the usual principles of surgical drainage should be followed.

PROGNOSIS. The prognosis depends upon the type of infection. The acute septicemic form has been uniformly fatal. The localized or chronic forms have a much better prognosis.

PREVENTION. Next to acquisition from diseased horses, the commonest source of natural disease in man has been contact with human glanders. Isolation is indicated.

REFERENCES

Bernstein, J. M., and E. R. Carling: Observations on Human Glanders with a Study of Six Cases and a Discussion of the Methods of Diagnosis, Brit. Med. J., I:319, 1909.

Howe, C., and W. R. Miller: Human Glanders: Report of Six Cases, Ann. Intern. Med., 26:93, 1947.

Robins, G. D.: A Study of Chronic Glanders in Man with Report of a Case, Studies from Royal Victoria Hospital, Montreal, 2, No. 1, 1906.

158 MELIOIDOSIS
Jay P. Sanford

DEFINITION. Melioidosis is a glanderslike infection of man and animals with a protean clinical spectrum. It was described first by Whitmore and Krishnaswami in 1912. Stanton and Fletcher chose the name *melioidosis*, meaning "a resemblance to distemper of asses." Melioidosis bears a striking resemblance to glanders both clinically and pathologically, but it is epidemiologically dissimilar.

ETIOLOGY. Melioidosis is caused by a gram-negative motile bacillus, *Pseudomonas pseudomallei*, which can be differentiated from *Malleomyces mallei* by bacteriologic and serologic means. *Pseudomonas pseudomallei* (also known as Whitmore's bacillus, *Malleomyces pseudomallei*, or *Pfeifferella whitmori*) is a small gram-negative motile aerobic bacillus with occasional filamentous chains. When stained with methylene blue, Wayson's, or Wright's stain, marked irregularities with a bipolar "safety pin" pattern are observed. It grows well on standard bacteriologic media.

EPIDEMIOLOGY. The disease is endemic in southeast Asia, with the greatest concentration of cases reported from Vietnam, Cambodia, Laos, Thailand, Malaysia, and Burma. Cases in humans have also been reported from adjacent areas including India, Borneo, the Philippines, Guam, Indonesia, Ceylon, New Guinea, and North Queensland. Cases in man or animals have been reported from Madagascar, Chad, and Turkey. Human melioidosis has been described only rarely in the Western Hemisphere, and confirmed melioidosis has occurred in United States or European residents only when they have traveled in endemic areas. Even when fatal, melioidosis is quite rare; in an autopsy series from Malaya the incidence was 1.5 per 1,000 deaths. Since the original report, cases have been reported from southeast Asia, and by 1953 over 300 human cases were described, including approximately 100 cases in French troops in Indochina between 1948 to 1954. From the early 1960s through January 1968, a total of 80 cases of melioidosis including 9 fatalities have been reported in active duty Army personnel in Vietnam. Of particular interest, but not yet explained, is the observation that at least one-fifth of the cases reported in Army personnel have occurred in patients with moderately severe thermal burns; the majority of these had the acute septicemic form of the disease.

Pseudomonas pseudomallei is a natural saprophyte which can be isolated from soil, stagnant streams, ponds, rice paddies, and market produce in endemic areas. Its ubiquitous nature is illustrated by its isolation as a laboratory contaminant. *Pseudomonas pseudomallei* is capable of causing disease in epizootic form among sheep, goats, swine and horses. Occasional isolates have also been reported from cows, rodents, and cats. Although animals are susceptible to the disease, they apparently do not represent a reservoir for human disease. Attempts to culture *P. pseudomallei* from the urine and feces of a large variety of healthy animals have been unsuccessful. Arthropod-borne infection does not occur naturally, although guinea pigs have been infected experimentally by the bite of both the mosquito (*Aëdes aegypti*) and the rat flea (*Xenopsylla cheopis*). French researchers concluded that man contracts melioidosis by soil contamination of skin abrasions. Ingestion, nasal instillation, or inhalation are other possible methods of spread. In contrast to glanders, infections have been rare in laboratory workers. Man to man transmission of melioidosis has not been described.

PATHOLOGY. The gross and microscopic anatomic findings are fairly consistent for the acute and subacute forms of the disease. In acute infections, the majority of lesions occur in the lungs with occasional abscesses in other organs. In subacute infections, lung abscesses tend to be more extensive and lesions are found throughout the body, in the skin, subcutaneous tissue, meninges, brain, eye, heart, liver, kidney, spleen, bone, and lymph nodes. The acute abscesses are characterized by an outer border of hemorrhage, a medial zone heavily infiltrated with polymorphonuclear leukocytes and an inner core of necrotic debris containing large histiocytes with two or three nuclei that have been termed "giant cells." As in glanders, a striking histologic feature has been the marked karyorrhexis. In chronic infections, the lesion consists of a central area of caseation necrosis, mononuclear and plasma cells, and granulation tissue. Calcification does not occur.

CLINICAL MANIFESTATIONS. The clinical manifestations of melioidosis are variable. The illness can present as an acute, subacute, or chronic process. The incubation period has not been defined; however, based upon the development of infection following injury, it may be as short as 2 days. Following a laboratory accident, an incubation period of 3 days ensued. Clinically inapparent infections may remain latent for a number of years after an individual leaves an endemic area before disease appears. Males are more often affected than women, which is thought to represent occupational exposure. Melioidosis may be recognized as inapparent infection, asymptomatic pulmonary infiltration, acute localized suppurative infection, acute pulmonary infection, acute septicemic infection, or chronic suppurative infection.

Inapparent Infection. Using the complement fixation test, 8.3 percent of apparently healthy adult Thai males gave positive reactions, while only 1 percent of Thai women had positive reactions. None of the sera from a control group from the United States was positive. The incidence of inapparent infections in United States personnel is unknown, but in a recent study, 1.3 percent of a group of patients evacuated for other medical conditions had a significant hemagglutination titer for melioidosis. Occasionally, asymptomatic infections have been discovered by routine chest x-ray.

Acute Localized Suppurative Infection. Infection by inoculation of a break in the skin usually results in a nodule with an area of acute lymphangitis and regional lymphadenitis. There is usually fever and generalized malaise. This form of infection may rapidly progress to the acute septicemic form.

Acute Pulmonary Infection. The most common form of the disease has been pulmonary infection, which may represent a primary pneumonitis or hematogenous spread. The acute pulmonary infection can vary in severity from a mild bronchitis to overwhelming necrotizing pneumonia. The onset may be abrupt without prodromal symptoms or more gradual with headache, anorexia, and generalized myalgia. Fever occurs in almost all patients, is often in excess of 102°F, and may be associated with rigors. Dull or pleuritic chest pain is common. Cough, with or without sputum, occurs. There may be mild pharyngitis. Tachypnea may be out of proportion to the fever and findings on physical or x-ray examination. Chest findings may be minimal but usually consist of râles in the area of pneumonitis. In the absence of dissemination, the spleen and liver are not palpable. Laboratory findings include total leukocyte counts ranging from normal to 20,000 per cu mm. Mild normochromic, normocytic anemia may appear during the illness. The pneumonia usually involves the upper lobes with the radiographic appearance of consolidation. Cavitation frequently occurs. Without specific therapy, the temperature may become normal within a few days; however, the upper lobe cavitation persists, resulting in a radiographic appearance of tuberculosis. In some instances there is progressive pulmonary spread or hematogenous dissemination with the development of septicemic manifestations.

Acute Septicemic Infection. This is the form originally described by Whitmore primarily among narcotic addicts. Subsequent reports, however, have not shown a predilection for debilitated patients. The onset may be abrupt with the dominant symptoms depending upon site of major involvement. In individuals with bacteremia complicating pneumonitis, symptoms may include disorientation, extreme dyspnea, severe headache, pharyngitis, diarrhea, and development of cutaneous pustular lesions on the head, trunk, or extremities. There is high fever, extreme tachypnea, a flushed skin, and cyanosis. Muscle tenderness may be striking. On examination of the chest, signs may be absent or râles, rhonchi, and pleural rubs may be heard. The liver and spleen may be palpable. Signs of arthritis or meningitis may appear. Patients with the septicemic form usually have a rapidly progressive fatal course which in some instances may be too fulminant to affect with therapy. The leukocyte count may be normal or slightly increased. Chest radiographs most commonly show irregular nodular densities 4 to 10 mm in diameter disseminated throughout the lungs. These enlarge, coalesce, and often undergo cavitation as the disease progresses. Pleural effusion is rare. Other radiographic patterns include unilateral irregular mottled densities which became confluent.

Chronic Suppurative Infection. In some patients secondary abscesses develop which dominate the clinical picture. Organs involved include skin, brain, lung, myocardium, liver, spleen, bones, joints, lymph nodes, and even the eye. Such patients may be afebrile.

DIAGNOSIS. Melioidosis should be considered in the differential diagnosis of any febrile illness in an individual who has been in an endemic area, especially if the presenting features are those of fulminant respiratory failure, if multiple pustular or necrotic skin or subcutaneous lesions develop, or if there is a radiographic pattern of tuberculosis in a patient from whom tubercle bacilli cannot be isolated.

Microscopic examination of exudates will reveal poorly staining small gram-negative bacilli which show the characteristic staining irregularities and "safety pin" bipolar staining with methylene blue or Wright's stain. For rapid screening of suspected specimens the direct fluorescent antibody technique is the procedure of choice. *Pseudomonas pseudomallei* will grow on most laboratory media, including eosin-methylene blue agar (EMB) or MacConkey's agar, in 24 to 48 hr. The organisms can be readily differentiated from *M. mallei* and *P. aeruginosa* by standard bacteriologic procedures, which include the hanging drop test for motility. The characteristic wrinkling of the colonies may require 72 hr or longer. The hemagglutination, direct agglutination test, and complement fixation tests are an aid in diagnosis if a fourfold or greater rise in titer is demonstrated in paired sera. Single low titers are difficult to interpret because of nonspecific responses. The complement fixation test is said to be specific with titers above 1:8 during the acute illness, but may cross-react with *M. mallei*. A negative complement fixation test does not exclude disease. The hemagglutination and agglutination tests show more cross-reactions. Titers of 1:40 or more suggest infection.

TREATMENT. The treatment regimen should vary with the form of the disease. Individuals with low titer positive serologic tests, but with no clinical evidence of infection do not require therapy. The choice of antibiotics in active infection should be based upon sensitivity studies, and therapy should be given for a minimum of 30 days. *Pseudomonas pseudomallei* is usually sensitive in vitro to the tetracyclines, chloramphenicol, novobiocin, kanamycin, and sulfadiazine or sulfisoxazole, and in most instances is resistant to benzyl penicillin G, ampicillin, streptomycin, and colistin. In patients with pneumonitis or chronic suppurative lesions who are not too ill, effective therapy has included tetracycline, 2 to 3 Gm daily (40 mg per kg); chloramphenicol, 3 Gm daily (40 mg per kg); or sulfisoxazole, 4 Gm daily (70 mg per kg). If the patient is severely ill, two of these antimicrobials in combination have been recommended for 30 days followed by another 30 to 60 days of tetracycline alone. In patients with extrapulmonary suppurative lesions, prolonged therapy for 6 months to 1 year should be considered. In addition, the usual principles of surgical drainage should be followed. In desperately ill patients with severe pneumonitis or the septicemic form of melioidosis, multiple antibiotics should be administered by the parenteral route. One such regimen has included the use of chloramphenicol, 12 Gm per day; novobiocin, 6 Gm per day; and kanamycin, 4 Gm per day (Chap. 135). In view of the severe potential toxicity of this regimen, its use should be considered only in extremely ill patients, and then only on a short-term basis. Current recommendations for antibiotics in the septicemic form of melioidosis are tetracycline, 4 to 6 Gm per day (80 mg/kg); chloramphenicol, 4 to 6 Gm per day (80 mg/kg); and one of the following: sulfisoxazole (140 mg/kg); or kanamycin (30 mg/kg); or novobiocin (60 mg/kg). The dosage should be tapered rapidly as clinical improvement occurs.

PROGNOSIS. Prior to antimicrobials, the mortality of apparent infection was 95 percent. French experience in Indochina indicated that with chloramphenicol therapy the mortality was 20 percent. With better diagnosis and more prolonged appropriate therapy, the mortality in all except the septicemic form is low. Even with vigorous appropriate antibiotics and supportive therapy, the mortality rate in patients with melioidosis septicemia is greater than 50 percent. Very few patients have had long-term follow-up, and the incidence of late relapses cannot be predicted.

PREVENTION. There is no means of active immunization. In endemic areas, vigorous cleansing of abrasions and lacerations is recommended.

REFERENCES

Brundage, W. G., C. J. Thus, Jr., and D. C. Walden: Four Fatal Cases of Melioidosis in U.S. Soldiers in Vietnam, Am. J. Trop. Med. Hyg., 17:183, 1968.

Gilbert, D. N., W. L. Moore, Jr., C. L. Hedberg, and J. P. Sanford: Potential Medical Problems in Personnel Returning from Vietnam, Ann. Intern. Med., 68:662, 1968.

Nigg, C.: Serologic Studies on Subclinical Melioidosis, J. Immunol., 91:18, 1963.

Prevatt, A. L., and J. S. Hunt: Chronic Systemic Melioidosis, Am. J. Med., 23:810, 1957.

Rubin, H. L., A. D. Alexander, and R. H. Yager: Melioidosis —A Military Medical Problem?, Mil. Med., 128:538, 1963.

Spotnitz, M., J. Rudnitsky, and J. J. Rambaud: Melioidosis Pneumonitis, J.A.M.A., 202:950, 1967.

159 VIBRIO FETUS INFECTIONS

Robert G. Petersdorf and Marvin Turck

DEFINITION. *Vibrio fetus* infection is economically the most important cause of infectious abortion in cattle. In man, this organism may be associated with obscure febrile illnesses, subacute bacterial endocarditis, meningoencephalitis, and perhaps, abortion.

ETIOLOGY. *Vibrio fetus* is a motile, comma-shaped or spirillar, gram-negative rod with a single unipolar flagellum. It is best identified by its appearance in smears made from cultured material. The organism is slow-growing and microaerophilic, and grows best in liquid media incubated under increased CO_2 tension. Several serotypes have been isolated by agglutination with antiserums from human and bovine strains. Cross agglutination reactions occur with other bacterial species, particularly *Brucella abortus*.

EPIDEMIOLOGY AND PATHOGENESIS. Vibriosis is a venereal infection of cattle, sheep, and goats; when transmitted to gravid heifers or ewes, it results in abortion. The male acts as an asymptomatic carrier of the infection, and the organism has been isolated from the genitalia and semen of bulls. Although vibriosis has been thought to occur only rarely in man, reports of this disease are appearing with increasing frequency. Vibriosis in man may result from direct contact with the organism, as happens in laboratory-acquired infection, or from direct contact with infected cattle. Food and water have been implicated, without convincing evidence, as vehicles for infection. The mouth has been postulated as a portal of entry because cases of *V. fetus* endocarditis have followed dental extractions. Because *V. fetus* has been isolated from several aborted fetuses and has been the cause of neonatal meningitis, a venereal route of infection has been postulated. It is presumed that, as in cattle, the male acts as an asymptomatic carrier who transmits the infection to a pregnant partner. The relationship of *V. fetus* to prematurity, abortion, and neonatal meningitis requires further documentation. In most instances of vibriosis, the portal of entry is not known.

MANIFESTATIONS. Fever is the only characteristic sign of vibriosis in adults, and may be relapsing in character. Thrombophlebitis involving both arms and legs is not uncommon. The disease may also present as classical subacute bacterial endocarditis; septic arthritis; chronic, indolent meningoencephalitis; and fever and abortion in pregnant women. A number of patients have had co-existing disease, including cirrhosis, cardiac amyloidosis, and chronic lymphatic leukemia, or antecedent gastric surgery. Several neonates with a fulminating, lethal meningoencephalitis have been reported. It has been postulated that infection was transmitted to these infants via the placenta. A mild, self-limited diarrheal disease in which vibrios closely related but not identical to *V. fetus* have been isolated from the stool has also been reported in infants.

DIAGNOSIS. Lack of awareness of vibriosis by both the bacteriologist and the clinician has resulted in mistaken diagnosis in most instances. The organisms have been erroneously described as "fastidious strains of *Hemophilus*." Recovery of spirillar organisms in blood cultures should suggest the diagnosis because other spirochetes causing relapsing fever usually do not grow in artificial media. Failure to incubate blood cultures under increased CO_2 tension may delay growth. Identification of the organisms in smears of cultures is the only definitive method of making the diagnosis, which should then be confirmed by agglutinating the vibrios with specific antiserums. Complement-fixing antibody may be present in high titers in the active phase of the disease. Clinically, vibriosis should be suspected in obscure febrile illnesses associated with thrombophlebitis or abortion and premature delivery in pregnant women.

TREATMENT. There are few reports of antibiotic sensitivity of the organisms and various antibiotics, alone or in combination, have been used. A 10-day course of tetracycline or chloramphenicol in dosage of 2.0 Gm per day, alone or coupled with streptomycin, 1.0 Gm per day should eradicate the organisms in most instances. In cases of endocarditis antimicrobial therapy should be extended to 6 weeks. Kanamycin and erythromycin have also been effective in vitro. Penicillin, novobiocin, vancomycin, and polymyxin B are ineffective.

REFERENCES

Collins, H. S., A. Blevins, and E. Benter: Protracted Bacteremia and Meningitis Due to *Vibrio fetus*, A.M.A. Arch. Intern. Med., 113:361, 1964.

Jackson, J. F., P. Hinton, and F. Allison, Jr.: Human Vibriosis, Am. J. Med., 28:986, 1960.

Kahler, R. L., and H. Sheldon: *Vibrio fetus* Infection in Man, New Engl. J. Med., 262:1218, 1960.

Lawrence, G. D., R. D. Biggs, Jr., and T. E. Woodward: Infection Caused by Vibrio Fetus, Arch. Intern. Med., 120:459, 1967.

White, W. D.: Human Vibriosis: Indigenous Cases in England, Brit. Med. J., II:283, 1967.

160 MIMA-HERELLEA INFECTIONS

Robert G. Petersdorf and
Marvin Turck

DEFINITION. Organisms of the tribe *Mimae* are pleomorphic, gram-negative bacilli which are easily confused with members of the genus *Neisseria*. Severe infections with these organisms, including meningitis, bacterial endocarditis, pneumonia, and bacteremia, are being described with increasing frequency.

ETIOLOGY. *Mima polymorpha*, described by DeBord in 1939, is one of two well-characterized species within the tribe Mimae, the other being *Herellea vaginicola*. Organisms formerly described as *Bacterium anitratum* and B5W are synonymous with *H. vaginicola*. These organisms are pleomorphic, gram-negative, encapsulated, and nonmotile. They grow well on ordinary media, forming white, convex, smooth colonies. Diplococcal forms predominate in colonies grown on solid media; rods and filamentous forms are more common in liquid media. The species can be differentiated from the Enterobacteriaceae by their negative nitrate reaction and from members of the genus *Neisseria*, which they may resemble morphologically, by their simple growth requirements, their bacillary form in liquid media, and their usually negative oxidase reaction. *Herellea vaginicola* may be distinguished from *M. polymorpha* by its capacity to ferment 10 percent lactose.

EPIDEMIOLOGY AND PATHOGENESIS. Mimae are ubiquitous and have been cultured from a variety of human sources, including urethral, vaginal, and conjunctival secretions, sputum, pleural fluid, blood, cerebrospinal fluid, feces, cutaneous ulcers, abscesses, chancroid lesions, joint fluid, ascitic fluid, and bone marrow. In addition, these organisms have been found in river water, humidifiers, and oxygen tents. Recent observations indicate that 25 percent of normal subjects are skin carriers of *H. vaginicola*, and 10 percent of *M. polymorpha*. The striking association of mima-herellea bacteremia with cutdowns or indwelling intravenous catheters favors the skin as a major portal of entry in man. The increasing incidence of mima-herellea pneumonia, both as a primary infection and as a superinfection, also points to the respiratory tract as an important portal of entry. It is most likely that the mima organisms are normal human commensals of relatively low virulence which produce serious infections under conditions of decreased host resistance, or in the presence of local tissue trauma, and in this way resemble the *Enterobacteriaceae*. Although members of the mima tribe have been implicated as an important cause of penicillin-resistant venereal urethritis, the evidence for this relationship is not convincing. Similarly, the role of these organisms as a cause of conjunctivitis and vaginitis requires documentation.

MANIFESTATIONS. Serious infections caused by mima organisms include (1) meningitis, (2) subacute and acute bacterial endocarditis, (3) pneumonia, (4) urinary tract infections, and (5) bacteremia. Usually, the signs and symptoms associated with infections in these sites are no different from those produced by other pathogens. For example, subacute bacterial endocarditis has usually been reported in patients with congenital or rheumatic heart disease and pursues an indolent course, while urinary tract infections may be manifested by asymptomatic bacteriuria, cystitis, or pyelonephritis. Pneumonia often occurs in the form of a superinfection in patients who have received antibiotics, but occasionally herelleae may be primary pathogens in the lung. Occasionally, *M. polymorpha* may be the cause of a fulminating bacteremia, with high fever, vascular collapse, petechiae, and ecchymoses, indistinguishable from fulminant meningococcemia (Chap. 142). More often, however, bacteremia is associated with an overt portal of entry, such as infected cutdowns or indwelling intravenous catheters, surgical wounds, or burns, or it may follow urethral or other surgical instrumentation. These patients usually have severe debilitating disease or have undergone surgery. Many times they have received antibiotics, adrenal cortical hormones, irradiation, or tumor chemotherapy and have had infections with other organisms, usually gram-positive, prior to development of sepsis with mimae. The clinical picture presented by these patients is dominated by endotoxemia (Chap. 134), and the prognosis is very poor.

DIAGNOSIS. The diagnosis of herelliosis is usually missed because the clinical bacteriology laboratory is unfamiliar with these organisms and reports them incorrectly or because they are considered contaminants. The confusion attending the taxonomic classification of these organisms has not simplified matters. For practical purposes, isolation of mimae-herelleae (or their synonyms, *B. anitratum*, B5W, *Diplococcus mucosus*, or *Neisseria winogradskyi*) from blood, spinal fluid, sputum, urine, or pus should be considered significant unless there is no evidence of infection on clinical grounds. Since mimae are resistant to penicillin and members of the genus *Neisseria* are sensitive, differentiation of these organisms is of obvious importance.

TREATMENT. Antibiotic sensitivities of *Mima* and *Herellea* strains vary, but most strains are inhibited by kanamycin, colistin, or polymyxin B. Sensitivity to the tetracyclines is unpredictable and most strains are also resistant to penicillin, ampicillin, cephalothin, erythromycin, and chloramphenicol. For serious systemic infections, kanamycin should be administered in doses of 0.5 Gm intramuscularly every 8 to 12 hr (in adults). Since these organisms may produce localized abscesses, surgical drainage may be necessary.

REFERENCES

Daly, A. K., B. Postic, and E. H. Kass: Infections Due to Organisms with the Genus *Herellea*, A.M.A. Arch. Intern. Med., 110:86, 1962.

King, O. H., Jr., G. D. Copeland, and W. M. Berton: Cardiovascular Lesions of Mimae Organisms, Am. J. Med., 35:241, 1963.

Reinarz, J. A., B. B. Mays, and J. P. Sanford: In Vitro Sensitivity Determinations on *Herellea* and *Flavobacterium* Species, Antimicrob. Agents Chemo., 4:451, 1964.

Reynolds, R. C., and L. E. Cluff: Infections of Man with Mimae, Ann. Intern. Med., 58:759, 1963.

161 | PASTEURELLA MULTOCIDA INFECTION

Leighton E. Cluff

DEFINITION. *Pasteurella multocida* (*Pasteurella septica*) is a gram-negative, nonsporulating bacillus belonging to the same genus as *Pasteurella pestis*. *Pasteurella multocida*, however, differs in its cultural characteristics, antibiotic sensitivity, antigenicity, and pattern of animal parasitism. All strains are sensitive to penicillin. *Pasteurella multocida* is a respiratory or intestinal commensal in several animals, including cattle, horses, swine, sheep, fowl, dogs, cats, and rats. The bacteria produce fatal disease, so-called "hemorrhagic septicemia," in animals with lowered resistance to infection. Chronic pulmonary infection also may develop. *Pasteurella multocida* is not a common human pathogen but has been isolated from the blood of patients with bronchopulmonary disease. The source of infection in human beings is not clearly identified, but in some instances it has been related to animal contact.

MANIFESTATIONS. Localized infection with cellulitis, suppuration, and adenitis has been described after dog and cat bites. Osteomyelitis has followed such infections. Chronic pulmonary infection has been demonstrated, particularly in patients with bronchiectasis. The respiratory tract may be infected by *P. multocida* alone or in company with other pathogens. Rarely, empyema has been caused by the bacillus. The microorganism has been isolated from the nasal sinuses, but its relationship to infection of the upper part of the respiratory tract is not clear. Veterinarians and other animal handlers have been found to harbor *P. multocida* in the upper part of the respiratory tract without disease. Bacteremia with fever and chills may develop after an animal bite, occasionally without an apparent local lesion. Meningitis, brain abscess, pyogenic arthritis, endocarditis, and pyelonephritis may occasionally complicate the bacteremia.

Not all *P. multocida* infections follow documented animal bites or animal contact. The source of these infections remains unidentified.

DIAGNOSIS. There is nothing specific about the characteristics of infection by *P. multocida*, other than its relationship to animal, particularly cat, bites. Involvement of joints, brain, meninges, and pleural space is associated with abscess formation. The local skin lesion with adenitis may be confused clinically with cat-scratch fever, tularemia, or staphylococcal or streptococcal infection. Leukocytosis is the rule in *P. multocida* infection but is uncommon in tularemia and cat-scratch fever.

Gram stain of infected material shows pleomorphic gram-negative bacilli, usually extracellular. The bacteria may have bipolar staining and can be mistaken for gram-negative diplococci. *Hemophilus influenzae* and neisseria and mimae organisms are most often confused with *P. multocida* but are easily differentiated by cultural characteristics, fermentation reaction, and serology.

TREATMENT. *Pasteurella multocida* is invariably sensitive to penicillin, and administration of this antibiotic in a dosage of 600,000 to 1,200,000 units daily is the preferred regimen. The microorganism is also sensitive to many other antibiotics, however, which can be substituted effectively for penicillin. The variation in sensitivity to antibiotics other than penicillin makes it desirable to test the organism in vitro if other drugs are to be used.

REFERENCES

Bearn, A. G., K. Jacobs, and M. McCarty: *Pasteurella multocida* Septicemia in Man, Am. J. Med., 18:167, 1955.

Morris, A. J., G. B. Heckler, I. G. Schaub, and E. G. Scott: *Pasteurella multocida and* Bronchiectasis, Bull. Johns Hopkins Hosp., 91:174, 1952.

Olsen, A. M., and G. M. Medham: *Pasteurella multocida* in Suppurative Diseases of the Respiratory Tract, Am. J. Med. Sci., 224:77, 1952.

Swartz, M. N., and L. J. Kunz: *Pasteurella multocida* Infections in Man: Report of Two Cases—Meningitis and Infected Cat Bite, New Engl. J. Med., 261:888, 1959.

162 STREPTOBACILLUS MONILIFORMIS INFECTION

Edward W. Hook

Streptobacillus moniliformis causes an acute febrile disease characterized by skin rash and arthritis. Infection is usually transmitted to man through the bite of a rat, and the disease acquired in this manner is termed *rat-bite fever*. Infection is occasionally acquired by ingestion of food or drink contaminated with the streptobacillus. *Spirillum minus* is also responsible for certain cases of rat-bite fever, and the clinical manifestations of *S. moniliformis* and *S. minus* infections (Chap. 183) are sometimes indistinguishable.

ETIOLOGY. *Streptobacillus moniliformis* is a microaerophilic, pleomorphic, gram-negative bacterium that grows in artificial media as tangled chains of bacilli of variable length with beaded or fusiform swellings. Long filamentous forms in interwoven masses may be observed. Primary isolation is best achieved in a fluid medium such as tryptose phosphate broth enriched with 10 to 20 percent blood, serum, or ascitic fluid. In blood cultures, growth usually appears after 48 hr as minute "fluff balls" on the surface of sedimented red blood cells.

A pleuropneumonia-like L (L = Lister Institute) variant can be isolated from the bacterial phase of most strains of *S. moniliformis*. The L form can be maintained in pure culture and transformed back to the bacterial phase. The L variant has been isolated from the blood of man as long as 10 weeks after onset of *S. moniliformis* infection.

The organism is highly pathogenic for mice and for chick embryos, and in these hosts shows a striking affinity for joints and periarticular tissues. Abortion and arrested pregnancy have also been described in mice with streptobacillus infection.

EPIDEMIOLOGY. *Streptobacillus moniliformis* is a normal inhabitant of the nasopharynx of wild or laboratory rats; the carrier rate sometimes exceeds 50 percent. Although most sporadic cases of streptobacillus infection follow the bite of a wild rat, infection may be transmitted by the bite of a laboratory rat, mouse, squirrel, cat, or weasel. Frequently there is no history of rodent bite or direct animal contact. Infection with this organism occurs primarily in infants and children and in men and women whose occupations involve exposure to rats or rat-infested areas. The incidence of the disease is highest in urban areas with poor sanitation and large populations of rats.

Streptobacillus moniliformis infection may occur in an epidemic form related to ingestion of contaminated food or milk. The outbreak in Haverhill, Mass., in 1926 involved 86 persons and was apparently caused by streptobacillus in raw unpasteurized milk or ice cream. The names *Haverhill fever* and *erythema arthriticum epidemicum* have been applied to cases in which there is no history of rodent bite.

CLINICAL MANIFESTATIONS. The incubation period is short, usually 1 to 3 days, although extremes of a few hours to 22 days have been described. The onset of the disease is sudden, with fever, headache, myalgia, and malaise. Chills occur in about 60 percent of patients. A healing puncture wound or ulcerative lesion may be observed at the site of the rat bite, which is usually on an extremity, the face, or tongue. Regional lymphadenopathy may be present but is usually not a prominent feature. A discrete macular rash which fades on pressure develops 1 to 3 days after onset of symptoms in 75 to 80 percent of the patients. The rash is most marked on the extremities, sometimes involves the palms or soles, and may be generalized. The cutaneous lesions may occasionally become confluent, papular, pustular, or petechial. Arthritis of multiple joints appears in about 50 percent of patients during the first week of disease. Large joints are usually involved, but small joints such as those of the fingers and toes may also be affected. The joints are swollen, hot, and tender, and effusions may occur, especially in the knee joints.

Manifestations of disease usually subside after about 1 to 2 weeks, although in the absence of antimicrobial therapy convalescence may be prolonged because of arthritis and recurrent fever.

Bacterial endocarditis and abscess formation in brain, myocardium, or other tissues are rare but serious complications.

The clinical manifestations of food-borne infection are similar to those after rat bite except for the absence of a local lesion.

LABORATORY FINDINGS. The blood leukocyte count ranges from 6,000 to 30,000 cells per cu mm, but the average count is about 12,000. Differential leukocyte count may reveal an increase in the proportion of neutrophils. *Streptobacillus moniliformis* can usually be isolated from blood, joint fluid, or pus during the acute febrile phase of the disease and occasionally for 1 to 2 weeks after subsidence of fever. Agglutinins against the organism develop during the second or third week of illness and are of diagnostic importance if an increasing titer is demonstrated. A false positive serologic test for syphilis occurs in about 15 percent of the cases.

DIFFERENTIAL DIAGNOSIS. *Streptobacillus moniliformis* and *S. minus* infections both occur after rat bite and present remarkably similar manifestations. Differentiation on the basis of clinical data is difficult, sometimes impossible. However, S. *moniliformis* infection is characterized by an incubation period that is usually less than 10 days, prompt healing of the primary lesion without flare-up at the onset of systemic symptoms, a high incidence (50 percent) of arthritis, and a low incidence (15 percent) of false positive serologic tests for syphilis. In contrast, S. *minus* infection is distinguished by an incubation period of 1 to 4 weeks, recurrence of pain, induration, or ulceration at the site of the bite during the acute phase of illness, a very low incidence of arthritis, and a high incidence (50 percent) of false positive tests for syphilis. A relapsing febrile course is typical of S. *minus* infection and is observed only occasionally in streptobacillus infection.

Streptobacillus moniliformis infection must also be differentiated from other forms of acute infectious arthritis, rheumatic fever, meningococcemia, and many other processes characterized by macular eruption and fever.

TREATMENT. *Streptobacillus moniliformis* infections usually respond promptly to therapy with penicillin in moderate doses. A suitable schedule for an adult is procaine penicillin, 600,000 units intramuscularly twice daily for 7 to 10 days. The organism is also sensitive to most of the other commonly used antimicrobials, and erythromycin can be substituted if penicillin is contraindicated. Therapy of endocarditis should be with penicillin, or perhaps penicillin in combination with streptomycin, in dosages similar to that given for streptococcal endocarditis (Chap. 137).

PROGNOSIS. The mortality rate in sporadic cases prior to the advent of effective antimicrobial therapy was about 10 percent. Death was usually related to the presence of bacterial endocarditis, and occasionally to myocarditis, myocardial abscesses, or bronchopneumonia. In patients treated with penicillin or other effective antibiotics the mortality rate approaches zero.

REFERENCES

Brown, T. McP., and J. C. Nunemaker: Rat-bite Fever: A Review of the American Cases with Re-evaluation of Etiology, Bull. Johns Hopkins Hosp., 70:201, 1942.

Dolman, C. E., D. E. Kerr, H. Chang, and A. R. Shearer: Two Cases of Rat-bite Fever Due to *Streptobacillus moniliformis*, Can. J. Public Health, 42:228, 1951.

Hamburger, M., and H. C. Knowles: *Streptobacillus moniliformis* Infection Complicated by Acute Bacterial Endocarditis, A.M.A. Arch. Intern. Med., 92:216, 1953.

Levine, B., and W. H. Civin: *Streptobacillus moniliformis* Bacteremia with Minor Clinical Manifestations, A.M.A. Arch. Intern. Med., 80:53, 1947.

McCormack, R. C., D. Kaye, and E. W. Hook: Endocarditis Due to *Streptobacillus moniliformis*. A Report of Two Cases and Review of the Literature, J.A.M.A., 200:77, 1967.

Roughgarden, J. W.: Antimicrobial Therapy of Rat-bite Fever. A Review, A.M.A. Arch. Intern. Med., 116:39, 1965.

Watkins, C. F.: Rat-bite Fever, J. Pediat., 28:429, 1946.

163 BARTONELLOSIS

*Ivan L. Bennett, Jr., and
Robert G. Petersdorf*

DEFINITION. Bartonellosis (Carrion's disease) is an infection with *Bartonella bacilliformis*. Two well-defined clinical types may develop—an acute febrile anemia of rapid onset and high mortality, designated *Oroya fever;* and a benign eruptive form with chronic cutaneous lesions, called *verruga peruana*. Either of these types may be mild, and asymptomatic cases constitute the greatest epidemiologic hazard.

ETIOLOGY. *Bartonella bacilliformis* is a small, motile, pleomorphic, gram-negative bacillus which stains reddish violet with Giemsa's stain. It can be cultured on enriched media and chick embryos. The organisms are sensitive to several antibiotics in vitro.

EPIDEMIOLOGY. The disease is limited to certain valleys in the Andes Mountains comprising parts of Peru, Ecuador, and Colombia. It occurs in regions between the altitudes of 2,400 and 8,000 ft where the sandfly vector, *Phlebotomus*, propagates. The reservoir of infection in nature is not known, but certain plants and lower animals have been suspected because the disease is often contracted in regions which are practically uninhabited. Epidemics occur more frequently during the rainy season and often coincide with immigration of workers from uninfected areas. In 1966 an acute febrile anemia associated with bartonella-like erythrocytic structures was reported from northern Thailand, the first time this disease has been demonstrated outside western South America. The organisms were similar but not identical to bartonella.

MANIFESTATIONS. The incubation period is approximately 3 weeks but may be longer. The initial symptoms are fever and pains in the bones, joints, and muscles. In the early stages, the disease often resembles influenza or malaria, but blood cultures are positive even in the absence of anemia. Following this initial stage, the patient develops one of the two classic types of the infection.

Oroya Fever. This type is characterized by sudden onset of high fever, extreme pallor, weakness, and a precipitous drop in the number of red blood cells. The count may fall from normal to 1 million per cu mm within 4 or 5 days. The anemia is characterized by normochromic macrocytes in the peripheral blood, striking polychromasia and polychromatophilia, nucleated red cells, Howell-Jolly bodies, Cabot rings, and basophilic stippling. There is also leukocytosis with a shift to the left. Organisms are numerous in the blood, and stained smears may show 90 percent of the erythrocytes heavily invaded. They are also present in the circulating monocytes and fixed phagocytes of the reticuloendothelial system. Secondary infection with salmonellas is an important factor in fatal cases. Neither hemolysins nor agglutinins for bartonellas are found in the serum of patients.

Muscle and joint pain and headache are severe, and insomnia, delirium, and coma are the terminal manifestations. Death can occur within 10 days to 4 weeks. With treatment, or sometimes spontaneously, recovery results if the organisms decrease and fever abates. The red cell count stabilizes, then approaches normal values in about 6 weeks, when convalescence begins.

Verruga Peruana. This form of the disease, characterized by a profuse skin eruption, may follow the anemic form or may occur in patients without previous symptoms. The verrugas vary in color from red to purple. They may be miliary, nodular, or eroding, and they range in size from 2 to 10 mm up to 3 or 4 cm in diameter. The three types of verrugas may occur together, since eruption takes place in successive crops; verrugas of all types and in all stages of development may be found on the same patient. The chief sites involved are the limbs and face, and less frequently the genitalia, scalp, and mucosa of the mouth and pharynx. They may persist for 1 month to 2 years. The eruption is accompanied by pain, fever, and moderate anemia. Bartonellas may be demonstrated in the lesions and cultured from the blood.

TREATMENT. Chloramphenicol, orally or intravenously, is highly effective, particularly when salmonella infection is also present.

REFERENCES

Cuadra, M. C.: Salmonellosis Complication in Human Barto-nellosis, Texas Rep. Biol. Med., 14:97, 1956.

Ricketts, W. E.: Clinical Manifestations of Carrion's Disease, A.M.A. Arch. Intern. Med., 84:751, 1949.

Schultz, M. G.: Daniel Carrion's Experiment, New Engl. J. Med., 278:1323, 1968.

Ureteaga, O. B., and E. H. Payne: Treatment of the Acute Febrile Phase of Carrion's Disease with Chloramphenicol, Am. J. Trop. Med. Hyg., 4:507, 1955.

164 GRANULOMA INGUINALE
Albert Heyman

DEFINITION. Granuloma inguinale is a chronic, ulcerative granulomatous disease, usually confined to the skin and mucous membranes of the genitoinguinal area but occasionally appearing in other portions of the body.

ETIOLOGY. The etiologic agent of this disease is the Donovan body (*Donovania granulomatis*), a nonmotile, gram-negative bacillus. In stained smears of the lesions the organisms appear as encapsulated, bipolar bodies situated within large mononuclear cells. In chick embryo cultures, the morphology of the organism is variable and may consist of bipolar forms, curved rods, chains, or unencapsulated bodies. The organism is not pathogenic for laboratory animals and can be cultivated only in artificial media containing yolk material.

INCIDENCE. Granuloma inguinale was once regarded as occurring only in tropical or subtropical areas, but it has been shown to exist in almost every country and climate. The majority of the cases in the United States are found in the Southeastern section, usually among Negroes. The incidence of the disease has decreased significantly in this country during recent years. Approximately 165 cases were reported in 1966.

PATHOGENESIS. Granuloma inguinale is generally believed to be acquired by sexual intercourse. The disease is apparently not highly infectious, however, since it is frequently not transmitted to sexual partners. The factors predisposing to invasion of the organism are not definitely known, but the disease is found most frequently among sexually promiscuous individuals and in association with other venereal diseases. The incubation period varies from 3 to 40 days. Although the majority of infections appear on or near the external genitalia, lesions about the face, hands, and neck are not uncommon. Systemic complications of granuloma inguinale (such as invasion of the bones, joints, and viscera) have also been noted, suggesting that the infecting agent can spread throughout the body by way of the bloodstream.

CLINICAL MANIFESTATIONS. The lesion of granuloma inguinale usually is a painless, sharply demarcated ulcer having an exuberant, red, granulating base which bleeds easily on trauma. The disease is extremely chronic, and the ulcers slowly enlarge and coalesce. Secondary infection frequently is present and produces a foul-smelling, seropurulent discharge. Interference with lymphatic drainage may occur, leading to swelling and elephantiasis of the genitalia, similar to that caused by lymphogranuloma venereum. When healing occurs, further scarring and deformity may appear. Lesions of the cervix of the uterus are frequent and sometimes are mistaken for carcinoma. Lesions about the perianal area closely resemble condylomata lata of secondary syphilis, and dark-field examinations and serologic tests for syphilis are often necessary to differentiate the two conditions.

The disease occasionally produces widespread manifestations such as arthritis and osteomyelitis. In such instances there may be general debility, anemia, and malnutrition; occasionally, these have resulted in death.

DIAGNOSIS. The diagnosis of granuloma inguinale is based upon demonstration of the presence of Donovan bodies. Impression smears of early lesions stained by Wright's method usually will show Donovan bodies lying within the cytoplasm of large mononuclear cells. The smear is of less value in chronic cases. The diagnosis can also be made by histologic examination of fixed tissues. The microscopic appearance of granuloma inguinale is essentially that of a richly vascularized granulation tissue with marked inflammatory cell infiltration. Polymorphonuclear leukocytes are scattered throughout the tissue and form small microabscesses. Numerous large mononuclear cells are also present and show finely reticulated or vacuolated cytoplasm. Phagocytosis of polymorphonuclear leukocytes and other cellular debris by these cells is common. Intracellular or extracellular Donovan bodies are readily seen in tissue sections, particularly in acute cases. In chronic cases they may be found only after considerable search, but the histologic pattern is sufficiently characteristic to permit a tentative diagnosis, even when organisms are not found. Specific serologic tests (complement fixation) and skin tests have been developed, but their diagnostic value is yet to be determined.

TREATMENT. Healing of granuloma inguinale will usually occur promptly following treatment with streptomycin, chloramphenicol, or the tetracyclines. Streptomycin has the disadvantage of requiring parenteral administration. The other antibiotics seem to be more effective and are given orally in doses of 2 Gm a day for approximately fifteen days. These antibiotics have treponemicidal properties and should not be given until repeated darkfield examinations and serologic tests have excluded the diagnosis of early syphilis.

REFERENCES

Pariser, H., and H. Beerman: Granuloma Inguinale, Am. J. Med. Sci., 208:547, 1944.

Rajam, R. V., and P. N. Rangiah: "Donovaniosis (Granuloma Inguinale and Granuloma Venereum)," World Health Organization Monograph Series, no. 24, 1954.

Sheldon, W. H., B. R. Thebaut, A. Heyman, and M. J. Wall: Osteomyelitis Caused by Granuloma Inguinale, Am. J. Med. Sci., 210:237, 1945.

Stewart, D. B.: The Gynecological Lesions of Lymphogranuloma Venereum and Granuloma Inguinale, Med. Clinics N. Am. 48:773, 1964.

Section 7

Miscellaneous Bacterial Diseases

165 ANTHRAX

Leighton E. Cluff

DEFINITION. Anthrax (malignant pustule, charbon, splenic fever, milzbrand, woolsorters' disease) is a disease of wild and domesticated animals that is transmitted to man by contact with infected animals or their products and, rarely, by insect vectors which act as mechanical carriers of the etiologic organism. The characteristic lesion of human anthrox is a necrotic cutaneous ulcer, the *malignant pustule*.

HISTORY. The anthrax bacillus was identified by Royer and Davaine in sheep in 1849 and was, therefore, the first causative agent of an infectious disease ever demonstrated. The classic studies of Robert Koch in 1877, showing that *Bacillus anthracis* was the cause of anthrax, serve as the prototype for the establishment of causation of infectious diseases.

ETIOLOGY. *Bacillus anthracis* is a large, encapsulated, gram-positive, aerobic, spore-forming microorganism that grows well in most nutrient media. Its pathogenicity for laboratory animals differentiates it from *Bacillus subtilis*, which it closely resembles. The spores are killed by boiling for 10 min but can survive for many years in soil and animal products, an important factor in persistence and spread of the disease. The anthrax bacillus possesses a capsule of glutamyl polypeptide, which interferes with phagocytosis of the microorganism. In addition, it contains an anticomplementary substance and elaborates a "protective" antigen and a toxin which is probably of importance in determining virulence.

EPIDEMIOLOGY. Anthrax is worldwide; repeated outbreaks have occurred in Southern Europe, Africa, Australia, Asia, and on both American continents.

Cattle, horses, sheep, goats, and swine are most commonly infected. There have been outbreaks of anthrax among animals in the United States, centering mostly in South Dakota, Nebraska, Arkansas, Mississippi, Louisiana, Texas, and California. The disease tends to occur in animals in late summer and early fall.

The disease in man is acquired by butchering, skinning, or dissecting infected carcasses or by handling contaminated hides, wool, hair, or other materials. It is seen principally in agricultural and industrial employees. The majority of cases of human anthrax involves workers handling imported and unprocessed wool, hair, or hides. The disease usually follows inoculation of bacilli or spores into the skin, often through a wound or abrasion. Intestinal infection has followed ingestion of contaminated meat, and anthrax may develop after inhalation of spores.

PATHOGENESIS. The malignant pustule which follows cutaneous inoculation of anthrax organisms is characterized by vesiculation, neutrophilic infiltration, gelatinous edema, and necrosis. Suppuration is rare in the absence of secondary pyogenic infection. Spread of the bacilli to the regional lymph nodes may be followed by systemic dissemination. Examination of tissues from fatal human cases reveals masses of the bacteria in blood vessels, lymph nodes, and the parenchyma of various organs. There is scanty or absent cellular exudation at these foci, but hemorrhage and edema are widespread. So-called "anthrax pneumonia" and "anthrox meningitis" are, in all probability, an expression of this generalized hemorrhage and edema.

The blood of fatally infected experimental animals contains a lethal toxin, which can be neutralized by specific antiserum. This toxin has been isolated in vitro, but its exact role in the pathogenesis of the disease requires further study.

MANIFESTATIONS. The malignant pustule of human anthrax begins usually on an exposed body surface, as a painless, pruritic, erythematous papule, which vesiculates and ulcerates to form a black eschar. Tiny satellite vesicles are frequent. The ulcer may be surrounded by extensive edematous swelling, which is nontender, nonpitting, and so characteristic of anthrax that it is a valuable diagnostic sign. After about 5 days the ulcer begins to subside, but edema may persist for many days or weeks. Mild tenderness and enlargement of regional lymph nodes are frequently present. Constitutional symptoms are often absent despite extensive local changes, but there may be mild fever, headache, and malaise. In disseminated anthrax, high fever, prostration, and a rapidly fatal course are seen. So-called "woolsorters' disease," a highly fatal disseminated infection, is characterized by cyanosis, dyspnea, mediastinitis, and hemoptysis and is probably dependent on the pulmonary route of inoculation. Human infection may occur from ingestion of the uncooked meat of infected animals; however, enormous numbers of organisms are probably necessary to produce disease by this route.

LABORATORY FINDINGS. The fluid from the cutaneous lesion frequently contains many bacilli, demonstrable by the Gram stain and culture. Bacilli may be found on direct examination or culture of the blood of patients with bacteremia. The blood leukocyte count is normal in mild cases, but there is polymorphonuclear leukocytosis in severe disease. Similarly, the erythrocyte sedimentation rate may be increased. Patients with meningeal involvement show bloody spinal fluid in which the organisms are easily found by direct examination or culture.

DIAGNOSIS. A serologic agar-gel precipitin inhibition test has been devised which has proved useful in epidemiologic studies of anthrax, showing that subclinical infection may occur in persons exposed to the microorganism in industry and demonstrating increasing serum antibody titers following vaccination. A positive diagnosis of anthrax can be made by isolation of the organism in culture. A history of occupational exposure and characteristic eschar and edema should suggest the proper diagnosis. Pyogenic infections of the skin are usually painful; the malignant pustule is not. In addition, cutaneous anthrax is rarely purulent. The differential diagnosis of other diseases characterized by local ulceration at the portal of entry is discussed in Chap. 155.

TREATMENT AND PROPHYLAXIS. Many antibiotics are effective in the treatment of human anthrax, including penicillin, chloramphenicol, tetracycline, erythromycin, and streptomycin. A dosage of 600,000 units of penicillin should be given once or twice daily until the local edema subsides. The eschar goes through its natural evolution in spite of treatment, and lymph node enlargement may persist for several days. *Bacillus anthracis* cannot be recovered from the skin lesion after 24 to 48 hr of penicillin therapy, but it may persist for a longer period when chloramphenicol or tetracycline is used.

Infection of personnel in industrial plants where contaminated animal products are handled still occurs. An outbreak of inhalation anthrax with a high mortality rate was reported in a goat hair processing mill in the United States in the late 1950s. Sterilization of all raw wool, mohair, etc., would probably remove this hazard but has

had only limited use. A vaccine prepared from the "protective" antigen of *B. anthracis* is available and is effective in reducing the incidence of infection in an exposed population. Spore vaccines of various types are used with good effect in domestic animals in endemic areas but are not suitable for use in human beings.

Transmission of anthrax from one human being to another has never been recognized. The cutaneous disease was fatal in 20 to 30 percent of cases before antimicrobial drugs were available. The mortality now is less than 1 percent with proper treatment.

REFERENCES

Brachman, P. S., S. A. Plotkin, F. H. Bumford, and M. A. Atchison: An Epidemic of Inhalation Anthrax: II. Epidemiologic Investigation, Med. J. Hyg., 72:6, 1960.

Gold, H.: Anthrax: Report of 117 Cases, A.M.A. Arch. Intern. Med., 96:387, 1955.

Howe, C.: Anthrax, in "Oxford Medicine," New York, Oxford University Press, 1950.

Norman, P. S., J. G. Ray, P. S. Brachman, S. A. Plotkin, and J. S. Pagano: Serologic Testing for Anthrax Antibodies in Workers in a Goat Hair Processing Mill, Am. J. Hyg., 72:32, 1960.

Smith, H., and J. Keffie: Observations on Experimental Anthrax: Demonstrations of a Specific Lethal Factor Produced *in Vivo* by *Bacillus Anthracis*, Nature, 173:869, 1954.

166 LISTERIA INFECTIONS
Paul D. Hoeprich

Listeria monocytogenes is known to cause infection and/or reside in 34 kinds of mammals (including man) and 17 kinds of birds, as well as ticks and crustaceans. Genital tract involvement of the fertile female with consequent perinatal infection of offspring is the most characteristic of the many clinical syndromes collectively known as *listerosis*.

ETIOLOGY. On isolation from nature, listeria are grampositive, microaerophilic, motile bacilli. Serotypes 1 and 4b account for virtually all listerosis in man. Typing serums are not generally available; however, the definitive, epidemiologically essential aid of typing is provided by reference laboratories (Communicable Disease Center, U.S. Public Health Service, Department of Health, Education, and Welfare, Atlanta, Georgia). The usual clinical laboratory can distinguish between *Listeria* and *Corynebacterium*, *Erysipelothrix*, and *Streptococcus*—the bacteria most often confused with listeria—by testing for motility, ability to reduce 2,3,5-triphenyltetrazolium chloride, and animal pathogenicity. In the classic ocular test of Anton, keratoconjunctivitis develops 3 to 5 days after conjunctival inoculation of listeria into a rabbit or guinea pig. Generalized listerosis in the rabbit is associated with monocytosis, which is maximal 3 to 7 days after inoculation.

EPIDEMIOLOGY AND PATHOGENESIS. Worldwide in distribution, listeria have been isolated not only from a variety of animals but also from stream water, mud, sewage, silage, and dry vegetation. Such broad distribution is at variance with the infrequent occurrence of overt disease. Contact with the fluids of infected animals, ingestion of contaminated milk, and inhalation of infected dust have all been implicated as means for infecting human beings on the basis of a few proved cases of listerosis.

Whatever the route of infection, when the gravid female is infected, listeria infection of her offspring can occur either (1) prepartum, via the placenta, or (2) during parturition. In the former situation, dissemination of listeria within the fetus is assured by bacteremia originating in the infected placenta; the fetus is stillborn or is prematurely ejected, virtually always with lethal listerosis. Intrapartum listeria infections may also be associated with premature delivery, but often do not become clinically manifest for 1 or 2 weeks post partum, and then usually present as a meningitis.

Listerosis in other than pregnant women occurs most commonly in persons debilitated by other diseases. There appears to be a predisposition to listerosis in patients with neoplasia—particularly, when it involves the lymphoreticular system, alcoholism, cardiovascular disease, diabetes mellitus, tuberculosis, and any condition requiring treatment with pharmacologic doses of adrenocorticosteroids, irradiation, or cytotoxic agents. Culturally proved listerosis is preponderantly a disease of individuals under one month (about 38 percent) and over forty years (about 32 percent) of age.

MANIFESTATIONS. *Leptomeningitis* accounts for about three-fourths of the cases verified by culture and is the predominant clinical form of listerosis in the United States. Clinically, meningitis caused by *L. monocytogenes* cannot be distinguished from meningitis caused by other kinds of bacteria.

Listerosis of the newborn, the most nearly unique clinical form of listerosis, ranges from meningitis that is clinically apparent within one month post partum, to diffuse disseminated disease in aborted, premature, and stillborn infants and neonatal children who die within minutes to days after birth. In newborn infants listerosis becomes overt 1 to 4 weeks post partum. They, like children one month to six years of age, generally have listerosis localized in the central nervous system.

Infants born alive with listerosis may or may not have fever; yet these babies are critically ill with cardiorespiratory distress, vomiting, and diarrhea. Dark-red skin papules are frequent, particularly on the lower extremities. Hepatosplenomegaly may be present. This form of listerosis, also known as septic or miliary granulomatosis, granulomatosis infantiseptica, argentophile-rod infection, or pseudotuberculosis, was described as a pathologic entity by Henle in 1893.

The findings at postmortem examination are characteristic and mimic those seen in listerosis of rodents: widely disseminated abscesses varying in size from grossly visible to microscopic, involving (in decreasing frequency) liver, spleen, adrenal glands, lungs, pharynx, gastrointestinal tract, central nervous system, and skin. Typically, the lesions are abscesses, but classic granuloma formation may be seen, depending principally on the duration of infection before death. Microscopic examination of a gram-stained smear of meconium from the normal newborn infant does not disclose bacteria; fetal listerosis results in meconium laden with gram-positive bacilli. For this reason, examination of meconium by gram-stained smear and by culture should be carried out whenever there is gross soiling of the amniotic liquid with meconium, prematurity, or unexplained fever in the mother before or at the onset of labor. This recommendation is reasonable because listerosis in the pregnant woman may be asymptomatic. At most, a week to a month prepartum there may have been malaise, a shaking chill, perhaps diarrhea, pain in the back or flanks, and itching of the skin. Even when symptomatic, the disease is benign and self-limited in the mother; however, as symptoms subside, decrease or cessation of fetal movement may be noted. Infection of the fetus may occur as early as the fifth month of gestation.

The possibility has been considered that repeated abortion is caused by chronic, asymptomatic genital tract listerosis. However, there has been no support from studies of women who had repeated abortions, and *L. monocytogenes* has not been cultured from currettings, lochia, and cervical swabbings, nor have antilisteria antibodies been found in the serum. Furthermore, following delivery of infants with proved fetal listerosis, cervical cultures are, or soon become, negative for listeria; subsequently, conception, gestation, and delivery of normal offspring are usual.

Oculoglandular listerosis is the rare human analogue of the illness initiated in the rabbit by conjunctival inoculation of listeria. There is a purulent conjunctivitis, which may lead to corneal ulceration. Regional node involvement usually limits the spread from the eye. However, listeria meningitis has been reported as a complication of oculoglandular listerosis.

Other rare syndromes caused by listeria include generalized illness with bacteremia and high fever, endocarditis, polyserositis, and cutaneous infection.

LABORATORY FINDINGS. The major difficulty in the laboratory identification of listeria lies in distinguishing it from diphtheroids. Listerias grow well on the usual laboratory media. However, specimens from sites where many other kinds of bacteria are normally present are best cultured on selective enriched media. If the numbers of listerias in a specimen are likely to be few, greater success in isolation may result when the specimen is kept in glucose broth at 4°C and is subcultured weekly.

Serologic methods, using the patient's serum, are not sufficiently specific to be useful to diagnosis.

Monocytosis is not common in human listerosis. Leukocytosis with neutrophilia, as in any acute bacterial infection, is seen in listeria meningitis, oculoglandular infection, bacteremia, and endocarditis. Other laboratory findings, e.g., cerebrospinal fluid in meningitis, are in keeping with the clinical syndromes.

DIFFERENTIAL DIAGNOSIS. Abortion, premature delivery, stillbirth, and neonatal death are more often due to causes other than listerosis—Rh incompatibility, syphilis, or toxoplasmosis.

In patients with leptomeningitis, conjunctivitis, endocarditis, bacteremia, or polyserositis, reports of isolation of "diphtheroids" or "nonpathogens" must always be challenged with the possibility that these may be listerias.

TREATMENT. *Listeria monocytogenes* is susceptible by in vitro testing to sulfonamides, penicillins (of the two most active penicillins, benzylpenicillin, i.e., penicillin G, is significantly more active than ampicillin), cephalosporins, streptomycin, chloramphenicol, the tetracyclines, erythromycin, kanamycin, and novobiocin in concentrations attainable in the blood of patients. Sulfonamides, penicillin, streptomycin, the tetracyclines, and erythromycin have had most frequent clinical trial. On the basis of potency, bactericidal potential, safety, and cost, a combination of penicillin G and erythromycin appears most reasonable. Extensive clinical experience attests to the value of the tetracycline group of antibiotics. Dosage and duration of therapy should vary according to the kind of infection. In fetal listerosis, where therapy must be rapidly effective to be of value, a successful regimen is yet to be devised, although 150 to 200 mg penicillin G per kg body weight per day, by intravenous infusion, merits trial. For listeria meningitis in adults, 12 to 20 million units potassium benzylpenicillin by continuous intravenous infusion per day plus 3 to 4 Gm erythromycin estolate by mouth (or one-half as much erythromycin by intravenous injection) per day are given for 5 to 7 days beyond defervescence. Alternatively, tetracycline, 2 Gm per day by mouth (or one-third as much by intramuscular or intravenous injection), may be used in combination with erythromycin.

Listerosis in the pregnant female requires prompt effective treatment lest the fetus be infected. Tetracycline, 1 Gm per day, plus erythromycin estolate, 2 Gm per day by mouth, should be given for 2 weeks.

Oculoglandular listerosis warrants less massive therapy: 600,000 units procaine benzylpenicillin by intramuscular injection twice daily plus 2 to 3 Gm erythromycin estolate by mouth per day, for 10 days.

Endocarditis and bacteremia from an unknown site have been infrequently treated but are justification for vigorous therapy: 10 to 20 million units potassium benzylpenicillin by intravenous injection per day plus 2 to 3 Gm erythromycin estolate by mouth per day for 6 weeks.

PROGNOSIS. Prompt antibiotic therapy of the acute forms of listerosis, excepting fetal listerosis, is highly effective. On the basis of agglutinin titers, circulating antibody disappears during the months following cure of listeria infections.

REFERENCES

Gray, M. L. (Ed.): Second Symposium on Listeric Infection, Aug. 29–31, 1962, Bozeman, Mont., Montana State College, 1963.

Hoeprich, P. D.: Infection Due to *Listeria Monocytogenes*, Medicine, 37:142, 1958.

Seeliger, H. P. R.: "Listerosis," Basel, S. Karger AG, 1958.

Simpson, J. F., J. P. Leddy, and J. D. Hare: Listeriosis Complicating Lymphoma: Report of Four Cases and Interpretive Review of Pathogenic Factors, Am. J. Med., 43:39, 1967.

167 ERYSIPELOTHRIX INFECTIONS
Paul D. Hoeprich

The parasitic incursions of *Erysipelothrix insidiosa* (*E. rhusiopathiae*) are more frequently expressed in some 20 species of animals than in man. Clinically, unique cutaneous infection is the most common form of human illness; although endocarditis and arthritis have been described, they are encountered but rarely.

HISTORY. Although isolated from mice by Koch in 1880 and from pigs (swine erysipelas) by Loeffler in 1882, erysipelothrix was first related to human disease in 1884 when Rosenbach cultured the bacillus from the skin lesion of erysipeloid in a patient.

ETIOLOGY. As isolated from human disease, erysipelothrix are gram-positive, microaerophilic, nonmotile bacilli. Confusion with nontoxinogenic bacilli of the genus *Corynebacterium* or *Listeria* is not certainly resolved on morphologic grounds alone. Serologic differentiation is reliable when available. Generally, animal inoculation is required: conjunctival inoculation of erysipelothrix in the rabbit only rarely leads to a conjunctivitis; generalized infection in the rabbit may cause a mild monocytosis—a much less marked reaction than is caused by listeria; intraperitoneal injection in mice leads to death in 2 to 4 days, with purulent conjunctivitis the most notable lesion.

EPIDEMIOLOGY AND PATHOGENESIS. Widespread in nature, erysipelothrix gain a foothold through injuries to the skin. Erysipeloid is the usual result and is virtually restricted to persons who in their occupations handle animals, fish, shellfish, or materials derived from animals. The incidence of erysipeloid parallels the incidence of swine erysipelas, being highest in summer and early fall. Yet, persons who tend pigs, even pigs ill with porcine erysipelas, do not commonly develop erysipeloid. If dermal containment of erysipelothrix is not accomplished, bacteremia in persons with damaged heart valves may result in endocarditis.

MANIFESTATIONS. From 2 to 7 days after injury, which has usually healed, a maculopapular, nonvesiculated, sharply defined, raised, purplish-red zone surrounds the site of entry. An itching, burning, painful irritation may precede, and always accompanies, this typical skin lesion. There is local swelling, and when, as is usual, a finger or the hand is involved, nearby joints may become stiff and painful. Centrifugal spread from the site of inoculation is apparent in a day or so. Movement is slow, ½ in. per 24 hr maximally, and more rapid proximally than distally; involvement of the terminal phalanx of a finger is rare, while spread to other fingers and the hand below the wrist is common. With extension, the original center subsides, without desquamation or suppuration. There are usually no systemic signs or symptoms; regional lymphangitis and lymphadenitis are rarely seen. Untreated, the disease heals within 3 weeks in most patients, although relapse has been observed.

The manifestations of erysipelothrix endocarditis may be either acute or subacute, depending on the virulence of the infecting strain of bacilli and on the state of resistance of the host. Usually there are no classic erysipeloid skin lesions to suggest the disease at the time that endocarditis is clinically evident. However, a history of recent erysipeloid, when obtained, may be helpful.

Erysipelothrix arthritis is not clinically characteristic but usually can be related to erysipeloid or erysipelothrix bacteremia. Isolation of erysipelothrix from synovial fluid has not been reported.

LABORATORY FINDINGS. Isolation of erysipelothrix depends primarily on awareness of the possibility of the presence of these bacteria. The usual laboratory culture media are adequate for growth of erysipelothrix, but recognition of their significance on culture requires distinction from diphtheroids and listeria. In erysipeloid, organisms are best recovered by incubating a full-thickness biopsy of skin removed from the advancing edge of a lesion in broth containing glucose. Culture of aspirate obtained after injection of sterile, normal saline solution into the periphery of a lesion may also yield erysipelothrix.

With endocarditis and arthritis, the clinical findings are in keeping with the respective clinical syndromes and are in no way characteristic for *E. insidiosa*.

DIFFERENTIAL DIAGNOSIS. The appearance and location of erysipeloid, its slow and limited spread, the lack of constitutional reaction, the history of occupation and injury all serve to identify this disease. The afflicted skin in erysipelas is very erythematous and the face and scalp are affected; there are regional lymphangitis and lymphadenitis, leukocytosis, fever, and malaise. Eczematous lesions may itch, but they display vesicles and little abnormal color. The various erythemas have a different location and do not usually itch or burn; they are more apt to be chronic and nonmigratory.

TREATMENT. Erysipelothrix are inhibited by penicillin, the tetracyclines, chloramphenicol, erythromycin, and novobiocin. The agent of choice is penicillin G. Erysipeloid is adequately treated by injection of 1,200,000 units benzathine penicillin G. Cure of erysipelothrix endocarditis has followed benzylpenicillin therapy in dosages of 2 to 20 million units per day for 4 to 6 weeks.

PROGNOSIS. Prompt antibiotic therapy is highly effective in eradicating erysipelothrix. Second attacks of erysipeloid have been reported. As with bacterial endocarditis from any cause, the prognosis depends on the extent of valvular dysfunction.

REFERENCES

Nelson, E.: Five Hundred Cases of Erysipeloid, Rocky Mountain Med. J., 52:40, 1955.

Wilson, G. S., and A. A. Miles: "Principles of Bacteriology and Immunology," 5th ed., Baltimore, The Williams & Wilkins Company, 1964.

168 FUSOSPIROCHETAL INFECTIONS
John C. Ribble

Fusospirochetal infections are characterized by gangrenous foul-smelling ulcers containing large numbers of spirochetes and bacteria. The lesions are usually located in the mouth and pharynx but may occur in the respiratory tract, the genitalia, surgical wounds, or human bites.

ETIOLOGY. The term *fusospirochetal infection* has been used to indicate that both fusobacteria and spirochetes are found in the lesions. In addition to these organisms, common mouth bacteria such as bacteroides, anaerobic streptococci, anaerobic vibrios, and spirilla are also present. Smith demonstrated that individual strains of bacteria or spirochetes isolated from mouth ulcers did not produce disease after subcutaneous injection into guinea pigs. However, administration of mixed cultures of spirochetes and bacteria resulted in necrotic lesions resembling those found in human disease, making it probable that fusospirochetal disease results from synergistic action of several organisms.

The bacteria and spirochetes associated with fusospirochetal disease are found as normal flora in the mouths of most adults and grow best under anaerobic conditions. Fusobacteria are gram-negative, unencapsulated, nonmotile, spindle-shaped bacilli. The spirochetes associated with the disease are identifiable by a rapid, characteristic motility and can be cultured in artificial media under strict anaerobiasis.

CLINICAL MANIFESTATIONS. Acute Ulcerative Gingivitis (Trench Mouth, Vincent's Stomatitis). The onset of disease is usually sudden and is associated with tender bleeding gums, fetid breath, and a bad taste. The gingival mucosa, especially the papillae between the teeth, becomes ulcerated and may be covered with gray exudate which is removable with gentle pressure. Although involvement of the gums is usually patchy, the process can extend to most of the gingival tissue. If the ulceration is extensive, there are fever, cervical lymphadenopathy, and leukocytosis. The disease may spread to involve other tissues of the oropharynx; it may become less severe and chronic; or it may subside spontaneously. Recurrent ulceration has been described. Most patients who develop fusopirochetal infection have poor oral hygiene. Tartar deposits and eruption or extraction of teeth may damage the gums and allow for bacterial invasion. Edentulous persons almost never develop the disease. Ulcerative gingivitis is prevalent in wartime when nutritional deficiency, crowding, and emotional upsets are common, but the role of these factors in pathogenesis is not known.

Cancrum oris (Noma). Occasionally, ulcerative gingivitis spreads to involve the buccal mucosa, the cheek, and the mandible or maxilla, resulting in widespread destruction of bone and soft tissue. The first indication of cancrum oris is usually slight inflammation of the skin of the cheek. The destruction of tissue proceeds very rapidly. The teeth may fall out, and large areas of bone, even the whole mandible, may be sloughed. A strong putrid odor is present. The lesions are not usually painful, and children may push their fingers through the necrotic areas. The gangrenous lesions eventually heal, but large disfiguring defects are left. Cancrum oris is seen most commonly in severely malnourished children in underdeveloped areas of the world.

Fusospirochetal Pharyngitis (Vincent's Angina). Fusospirochetal infections of the pharynx may occur alone or in association with ulcerative gingivitis. The main complaints are an extremely sore throat, foul breath, bad taste in the mouth, sensation of choking, and fever. The pharynx in the area of the tonsillar pillars is swollen, red, and ulcerated and is covered with a grayish membrane which peels easily. Lymphadenopathy and leukocytosis are common. The disease may last for only a few days or persist for weeks if not treated. The lesion begins unilaterally but can spread to the other side of the pharynx or to the larynx. Aspiration of infected material may result in lung abscess.

Infections of Human Bites. Gangrenous lesions resulting from human bites commonly contain fusospirochetal flora, and fusobacterial septicemia following an infected human bite has been reported. Human bites are much more likely to become infected than dog bites, possibly because of the large number of bacteria and spirochetes surrounding the teeth of human beings and the relative lack of the organisms in dogs and other animals with widely spaced teeth.

Infection of Genitalia. Gangrenous balanitis and ulcers and gangrene of the vulva have been associated with the fusospirochetal flora.

DIAGNOSIS. The diagnosis can be made with certainty only by demonstrating the typical bacteria and spirochetes in sections of necrotic lesions. In clinical practice the diagnosis is made by the appearance and putrid odor of the lesions. Smears of material from mouth ulcers are not usually helpful because fusospirochetal flora are found in the mouths of healthy persons. Ulcerative gingivitis can be distinguished from herpetic gingivostomatitis by the absence of vesicles and the tendency to involve mainly the gingival papillae. In suspected cases of fusospirochetal pharyngitis, diphtheria and streptococcal pharyngitis must be excluded by appropriate cultures.

TREATMENT. Treatment of ulcerative gingivitis consists of local measures and antibacterial therapy if the disease is severe and painful. During the acute phase the patient should avoid brushing his teeth or other trauma to the gums. A 3 percent solution of hydrogen peroxide diluted with equal amounts of warm water should be used as a mouthwash several times a day. Tartar and necrotic debris should be removed from the gum margins by a dentist. In severe painful cases of gingivitis 600,000 units procaine penicillin twice a day or 1.0 Gm tetracycline a day should be used until improvement is evident. Metronidazole, a drug with some activity against spirochetes and fusobacteria, administered in dosage of 200 mg three times a day for 3 to 7 days is as effective as penicillin in promoting healing of gingival lesions and is considered by some to be the most satisfactory drug for the treatment of fusospirochetal gingivitis. Patients with fusospirochetal pharyngitis or infections of the genitalia should receive 600,000 units procaine penicillin twice a day or 1.0 Gm per day of tetracycline. The treatment of cancrum oris consists of antibiotic therapy with penicillin or tetracycline, debridement of necrotic tissue, and eventual repair of damaged structures. Human bites should be cleansed thoroughly, and obviously necrotic tissue should be removed. The wounds should not be sutured but should be left open and irrigated frequently. Antibiotic therapy should be given to all patients with human bites.

REFERENCES

Glenwright, H. D., and D. A. Sidaway: The Use of Metronidazole in the Treatment of Acute Ulcerative Gingivitis, Brit. Dental J., 121:175, 1966.

Rosebury, T.: "Microorganisms Indigenous to Man," New York, McGraw-Hill Book Company, 1962.

Smith, D. T.: "Oral Spirochetes and Related Organisms in Fusospirochetal Disease," Baltimore, The Williams & Wilkins Company, 1932.

Uohara, G. I., and M. J. Knapp: Oral Fusospirochetosis and Associated Lesions, Oral Surg. Oral Med. Oral Pathol., 24:113, 1967.

Section 8

Diseases Caused by Toxin-producing Bacteria

169 DIPHTHERIA
Louis Weinstein

DEFINITION. Diphtheria is an acute infectious disease produced by *Corynebacterium diphtheriae*, which is characterized by a local inflammatory lesion in the upper part of the respiratory tract and by remote effects resulting from toxin which affects particularly the heart and peripheral nerves.

HISTORY. The earliest precise description of diphtheria

is attributed to Bretonneau, who, in 1821, separated diphtheria from other clinical entities with which it had been grouped together as "the croup." Klebs reported the morphologic appearance of *C. diphtheriae* in 1883, and the next year Loeffler isolated the organism in pure culture. The toxin of diphtheria was defined in 1888 by Roux and Yersin. Diphtheria antitoxin was produced by von Behring in 1890 and was soon followed by application of serotherapy in the human disease. The skin test for susceptibility to diphtheria was developed by Shick in 1913. In 1923 Ramon developed the first diphtheria toxoid.

ETIOLOGY. *Corynebacterium diphtheriae* is a gram-positive, nonsporulating, nonmotile rod. Pseudobranching and "palisade" formations are often seen in stained smears. Characteristically, there is a swelling at one end of the bacillus, which gives it a club shape. Diphtheria bacilli have been classified into mitis, gravis, and intermedius groups on the basis of their colonial appearance on tellurite medium, their fermentation reactions, and their ability to produce hemolysis. Some European workers believe that there is a significant difference in the clinical manifestations and severity of the disease related to the strain; gravis and intermedius infections are thought to be accompanied by more severe toxic manifestations and a higher death rate. In the United States, the gravis strain is comparatively uncommon, and less significance is attached to the relationship of the type of organism to the clinical form of the disease.

Corynebacterium diphtheriae produces a toxin which is responsible for many of the clinical manifestations. This material is a protein; as little as 0.0001 mg is a lethal dose for guinea pigs. Strains of diphtheria bacilli which elaborate exotoxin are lysogenic; i.e., they carry bacteriophage ("prophage"). Absence of lysogeny is associated with lack of toxin formation and virulence. The lysogenic state results in a metabolic alteration manifested by toxin production. In the presence of a cofactor, nicotinamide adenine dinucleotide, diphtheria toxin inactivates soluble transferase II, which results in failure to transfer amino acids from soluble RNA to the growing polypeptide chain. Nicotinamide blocks the inhibitory effect of the toxin. The mechanism thought to be involved in the development of diphtheritic myocarditis is interference with the metabolism of carnitine, leading to a decrease in the rate of oxidation of long-chain fatty acids with accumulation of triglycerides and fatty degeneration of the myocardium.

EPIDEMIOLOGY. Diphtheria occurs primarily in the Temperate Zone and is still very common in Europe and Asia. The number of cases of diphtheria in the United States and the British Isles had been decreasing steadily. In 1959 and 1960, however, this falling trend was reversed and 1,741 cases were recorded from 45 states in the United States. The largest number was observed in the South, and more than 80 percent of the patients had never received primary immunization.

Since 1927, the highest frequency has been in children over six years of age, and adults have been involved with

increasing frequency. Another striking change has been a decrease in the incidence of laryngeal involvement.

Diphtheria is acquired by droplet transmission from active cases or carriers. Fomites play little role in spread of the infection, but *C. diphtheriae* may remain alive and virulent in the dust of a darkened room for several weeks.

PATHOGENESIS AND PATHOLOGY. The commonest portal of entry for the diphtheria bacillus is the upper part of the respiratory tract. The skin, genitalia, eye, or middle ear may also be primary sites. Growth of the organism is superficial in most cases, and there is little tendency to invade the lymphatics or bloodstream except in the terminal stages. The exotoxin elaborated in the local lesion is carried by the blood to all parts of the body. Dissemination of toxin with damage to remote areas appears to be greater when the primary lesion is in the nasopharynx, less when it is limited to the larynx, and least when it is confined to the nasal mucous membrane; the most intense intoxication is observed when lesions are present in the pharynx, larynx, trachea, and bronchial tree simultaneously.

The primary lesion of diphtheria is the membrane. It is thick, leathery, and blue-white and is composed of bacteria, necrotic epithelium, phagocytes, and fibrin. The membrane is surrounded by a narrow zone of inflammation and is firmly adherent to the underlying tissues; when it is removed forcibly, bleeding follows. Ulceration is not a regular feature; when it occurs, it is very superficial. Regional lymphadenitis is frequent, especially with gravis infections.

The systemic lesions of diphtheria are primarily in the heart, kidneys, and peripheral nerves. The brain is rarely affected. Cardiac enlargement is frequent and appears to be related to myocarditis and not to myocardial hypertrophy. The kidneys reveal cloudy swelling and interstitial changes; they may be quite enlarged. In some cases, particularly those with laryngeal involvement, there is a bronchopneumonia which may be due to *C. diphtheriae* or to secondary invading organisms. When the pneumonitis is caused by the diphtheria bacillus, membrane is present throughout the bronchial tree. The peripheral nerves may reveal fatty degeneration, breaking up of the medullary sheaths, and involvement of the axis cylinder. Both motor and sensory fibers are affected, but the main impact is on motor innervation. The anterior horn cells and the posterior columns of the spinal cord may be damaged. Other central nervous system involvement includes cerebral hemorrhage, meningitis, and encephalitis. Petechial and purpuric lesions are occasionally present in the kidneys, skin, or adrenals. Bacterial endocarditis due to the diphtheria bacillus is extremely rare.

Death results from respiratory obstruction by membrane or edema or from the action of toxin on the heart, nervous system, or other organs.

IMMUNITY. Susceptibility to diphtheria is determined by the presence or absence of circulating antibody to exotoxin. The *Schick test* yields a rough estimate of the quantity of antitoxin in the circulation. The present method of carrying out this test is as follows: 0.1 ml purified diphtheria toxin ($\frac{1}{50}$ MLD) dissolved in buffered human serum albumin is injected intradermally in the volar surface of the forearm; 0.1 ml purified diphtheria toxoid (0.01 Lf) is injected into the other arm as a control. These areas are examined at 24 and 48 hr and between the fourth and seventh days:

1. When the reaction is positive, the site of toxin injection begins to redden in 24 hr; this increases and reaches a maximum in about a week, at which time the lesion may be as large as 3 cm in diameter and moderately swollen and tender. There is usually a small (1 to 1.5 cm) dark red central zone which gradually turns brown, desquamates, and leaves a pigmented area. The area of toxoid injection shows no reaction. A positive test indicates little or no circulating antitoxin or immunity.

2. In a negative test, there is no reaction at the site of either toxoid or toxin instillation. This is consistent with a blood antitoxin level of $\frac{1}{30}$ to $\frac{1}{100}$ unit and immunity to ordinary exposure.

3. Inflammation at both sites of injection within 12 to 14 hr, which reaches a maximum in 48 to 72 hr and then fades, constitutes a pseudoreaction. This practically always indicates immunity plus hypersensitivity to the toxin or other materials in the solution.

4. The combined reaction begins like the pseudoreaction, but the inflammatory response at the toxin site persists after that in the area of toxoid injection has faded. This type of reaction indicates delayed sensitivity to toxin or other proteins and absent or low circulating antitoxin. Combined reactions probably result from previous unapparent diphtheritic infection; their frequency increases with age and is highest in unimmunized groups living in areas where diphtheria is prevalent.

Individuals with negative Schick tests occasionally contract diphtheria, and some persons with positive Schick reactions do not develop the disease after exposure. Fewer than 50 percent of adults in some parts of the United States have "protective" levels of circulating antitoxin.

Second attacks of diphtheria are very rare despite the fact that only about 90 percent of patients who have had the disease become Schick-negative. This suggests that factors other than antitoxin may play a role in protection against infection. In general, immunized patients have a milder illness than unimmunized ones when the initial clinical picture and level of circulating antitoxin are the same. Early therapy of diphtheria with antibiotics may lead to recurrence of the disease if exposure to fresh infections occurs shortly after discontinuation of treatment, suggesting that the development of antitoxic immunity is suppressed in these instances.

CLINICAL MANIFESTATIONS. The incubation period is 1 to 7 days. The local symptoms vary with the site of the primary lesion. Systemic reactions, in the uncomplicated disease, are usually of only minor to moderate severity. Although fever may be present, it is usually low (100 to 101°F), unless infection with another organism (often the beta-hemolytic streptococcus) supervenes. When toxic manifestations are absent, patients feel well except for varying degrees of discomfort at the site of the local lesion. Pallor, listlessness, tachycardia, and weakness are common in more severe cases. Peripheral vascular collapse often develops in the terminal stages of the disease.

Nasal Diphtheria. Diphtheria is occasionally restricted to the nasal mucosa. The infection is usually localized to one side, and a unilateral serosanguineous discharge is characteristic. Membrane is present on the septum or turbinates in the anterior portion of the nose and may persist for a long time. When the disease is located in the posterior nasal areas, extension to the pharynx is frequent and is followed by absorption of toxin.

Pharyngeal Diphtheria. The very early diphtheritic membrane in the pharynx consists of small areas of soft exudate which wipe off easily and leave no bleeding points. As the disease progresses, these coalesce to form an easily removable thin sheet which spreads to cover tonsils or pharynx, or both. Later, it becomes more dense; is bluish-white, gray, or black, depending on the degree of hemorrhage; and is so firmly attached that when it is taken off bleeding occurs. If infection with organisms such as the beta-hemolytic streptococcus is superimposed, the pharynx is diffusely red and edematous. In the average case of diphtheria sore throat is mild but occasionally discomfort can be severe. There is usually a moderate leukocytosis, 15,000 or fewer white blood cells per cu mm.

Marked local spread of the pharyngeal membrane may take place, and the throat, tonsils, and soft and hard palates may be completely covered. Patients with severe disease may show the picture of so-called "malignant" diphtheria. There is great swelling of the submandibular areas and the anterior neck, giving the characteristic "bull neck" appearance. The breathing is noisy, the tongue protrudes, the breath is foul, and the speech thick. The pharyngeal tissues are red and edematous, and the cervical lmyph nodes are enlarged. The skin is pale and cool. There is marked weakness. Occasionally, purpuric eruptions of the skin may appear, particularly on the neck and anterior chest wall. Drowsiness and delirium are common.

Laryngeal Diphtheria. Involvement of the larynx in the course of diphtheria usually results from extension of membrane from the pharynx. Rarely, however, the infection may begin in and be limited to the larynx or trachea. This possibility should be considered in the differential diagnosis of all cases of "croup"; it can be ruled out only by direct examination of the airway. The clinical features of this type of disease are described below.

Skin Diphtheria. Although skin diphtheria is a problem primarily in tropical areas where it is responsible for some cases of "jungle sore" and may become epidemic, it occurs occasionally in the Temperate Zone. *Corynebacterium diphtheriae* is unable to penetrate unbroken skin and invades wounds, burns, etc. Although the lesions develop most often on the lower extremities, they may appear at any site, including the perianal region. The typical lesion is a round, deep, "punched-out" ulcer 0.5 cm to several centimeters in diameter. In the early stages, the lesions are covered by a gray, yellow, or gray-brown membrane which strips off easily to reveal a clean hemorrhagic base.

This dries quickly and becomes covered by thin, leathery, dark brown or black, adherent membrane which separates spontaneously 1 to 3 weeks after infection. The margin of the fully developed ulcer is usually slightly undermined, purple, rolled, and sharply defined. Breakdown, either after minor trauma or spontaneously, is frequent, and development of anesthesia, after a few weeks, is characteristic. Healing is usually slow, and scarring is the rule. Myocarditis occurs in about 5 percent and peripheral neuritis in about 20 percent of cases of skin diphtheria; the Guillain-Barré syndrome may develop.

Diphtheria Lesions in Other Areas. Diphtheria may involve the uterine cervix, vagina, vulva, or penis (after circumcision). Diphtheritic cystitis and urethritis have been observed following prostatectomy. These lesions are often secondary to respiratory tract involvement but may be primary. Toxic manifestations are common. The tongue, buccal mucous membrane, gums, and esophagus may also be affected. Infection of the conjunctiva occurs rarely. Otitis media may occur as an isolated syndrome or secondary to diphtheria in the upper part of the respiratory tract; aural discharge from which virulent organisms can be isolated may persist for many months.

COMPLICATIONS OF DIPHTHERIA. The complications of diphtheria are of two types: those which result from spread of the membrane in the respiratory tract and those which are due to the activity of the toxin absorbed from the local lesion.

Extension and Spread of Membrane. The membrane of diphtheria may spread from the fauces over the posterior pharyngeal wall into the nasopharynx and anterior portion of the nose. This usually produces severe illness and is accompanied by a high risk of toxic manifestations. Occlusion of the airway is first manifested by tachypnea and, as obstruction increases, restlessness, use of accessory muscles of respiration, and finally cyanosis and death. This progression of events occurs most frequently in children. In some cases, the membrane extends diffusely into the bronchial tree and produces clinical manifestations of pneumonia. Bronchopulmonary diphtheria is very serious not only because of obstruction but also because of the large surface from which toxin can be absorbed; the death rate is very high. When the pulmonary lesion regresses, pieces of membrane may break off and produce sudden occlusion of the airway; a cast of the bronchial tree may be coughed up. On occasion, pharyngeal membrane has extended into the esophagus and cardia of the stomach.

Toxic Complications of Diphtheria. Studies of the mode of action of diphtheria toxin suggest that it inhibits the transfer of amino acids from soluble RNA to growing polypeptide chains, resulting in failure of the amino acids to be incorporated into the polypeptide; a cofactor, nicotinamide adenine dinucleotide, is required for toxin activity. The effects of the toxin on the myocardium are thought to result from its production of a decrease in the rate of oxidation of long-chain fatty acids by interfering with the metabolism of carnitine. Because of this block, triglycerides accumulate in the myocardium and cause fatty degeneration of muscle.

Myocarditis develops in about two-thirds of patients with diphtheria but is clinically evident in about 10 percent. In these, softening of the heart sounds, systolic murmurs, bundle branch block, incomplete or complete heart block, atrial fibrillation, ventricular premature beats or tachycardia, or both, are detectable. Ventricular fibrillation is a constant threat and is frequently the mechanism responsible for sudden death. Ninety percent of the patients with atrial fibrillation, ventricular tachycardia, or complete heart block die. Frank congestive failure due to diphtheritic myocarditis occurs infrequently. Evidence of failure of the right side of the heart usually develops first, and the most common symptom is pain in the right upper quadrant of the abdomen due to rapid engorgement of the liver. Decompensation of the left side of the heart with dyspnea and rales may appear later. Diphtheritic heart disease is not necessarily "benign," and permanent cardiac damage can occur in survivors. Fibrosis of the myocardium has been observed in patients who have expired several weeks after mild myocarditis was detected by electrocardiographic study; the degree and extent of fibrotic change are often greater than would be predicted from the type of abnormality in the tracing.

Peripheral neuritis can occur at three different times in the course of diphtheria. Paralysis of the soft palate and posterior pharyngeal wall occasionally appears very early in the disease (2 to 3 days). Neuritis develops most frequently during the second to sixth week. At this time, cranial nerve dysfunction is most common; the third, sixth, seventh, ninth, and tenth nerves are involved most often. Loss of accommodation, nasal voice, and difficulty in swallowing are the most frequent manifestations. However, any of the peripheral nerves may be affected, with resulting paralysis of the extremities, diaphragm, or intercostal muscles; death may occur from respiratory failure. The peripheral neuritides which appear in the second to the sixth week of the disease are featured almost completely by motor loss; sensory changes are uncommon and, when present, are minor in degree. Peripheral neuritis may not appear until 2 to 3 months after the onset of diphtheria. In these cases, the clinical picture and course resemble infectious polyneuritis. The outstanding findings are loss of sensation in a "glove and stocking" distribution and albuminocytologic dissociation in the cerebrospinal fluid identical with that observed in the Guillain-Barré syndrome. Motor weakness and areflexia may develop with progression of involvement. Very rarely, a fatal ascending paralysis of the Landry type may develop. Complete recovery is the rule but may take as long as a year.

Encephalitis is a rare toxic complication of diphtheria. Shock, which develops suddenly and without warning, is an occasional cause of rapid death in this disease. In some instances, it may be a consequence of myocarditis; in others, no cause can be discovered.

Other Complications. Cerebral infarction with hemiplegia occurs rarely in diphtheria; it is probably due to embolization from atrial thrombi in patients with myocarditis and cardiac dilatation. Superinfection of the lungs is a risk in all patients with diphtheria who are given antimicrobial agents. Purpuric skin eruptions may be seen in severe cases, especially those with the malignant or "bull neck" form of the disease. Thrombocytopenia is a rare finding. A mild morbilliform rash may be present during the early stage of development of the diphtheritic membrane. Beta-hemolytic streptococcal pharyngitis is uncommon because antibiotics are usually administered from the beginning of the disease to eradicate the carrier state. Serum sickness occasionally follows the use of antitoxin. Relapses of diphtheria may occur when patients given antimicrobial agents are exposed to fresh cases soon after therapy has been discontinued. Bacteremia, endocarditis, and meningitis are rare complications.

COURSE AND PROGNOSIS. The membrane may be present for only 3 to 4 days in mild faucial diphtheria, even when no antitoxin is given; it usually lasts for about a week in cases of moderate severity. It is quite common for the pharyngeal lesion to increase in extent and thickness during the first 24 hr after the administration of antitoxin. As the disease begins to recede, the exudate softens, wipes off easily leaving no bleeding areas, becomes patchy so that it resembles the picture of "follicular" tonsillitis, and finally disappears, leaving normal underlying mucous membrane.

The fatality rate in diphtheria prior to the use of specific antitoxin was about 35 percent in average cases and 90 percent in those with laryngeal involvement. Since specific serotherapy has been employed, mortality has been reduced to a range of 3.5 to 22 percent, but it is still highest when the larynx is affected. The overall death rate in the United States is about 10 percent. Although there is no difference in the distribution of gravis and mitis strains in mild forms of myocarditis, the gravis type is three times as common as mitis in cases with severe myocardial disease and a high death rate. Age influences the outcome of diphtheria, and death is most frequent in the very young and old. Immunization is a factor of great importance in determining prognosis. The fatality rate in immunized individuals is one-tenth that in the unimmunized population. Paralysis is five times and "bull neck" fifteen times less common in immunized patients. As a rule, the longer the delay in the use of serotherapy, the greater the incidence of complications and death.

A white blood cell count higher than 25,000 per cu mm is associated with a higher risk of complications and death. This is possibly related to the fact that this degree of leukocytosis is often present in patients in whom another organism, hemolytic streptococci for example, is producing disease at the same site as the diphtheria bacillus.

DIAGNOSIS. The features of the fully developed diphtheritic membrane, especially in the pharynx, are sufficiently characteristic to suggest the possibility of the disease. However, not much reliance can be placed on the appearance of the pharyngeal exudate in establishing the diagnosis. There are a number of other infections in which pseudomembranes which may be confused with those of diphtheria are present; among these are infectious mononucleosis (Chap. 255), streptococcal pharyn-

gitis (Chap. 140), viral exudative pharyngitis, fusospirochetal angina (Chap. 168), acute moniliasis (Chap. 190), and staphylococcal infections of the pharynx which may follow chemotherapy.

The only positive method of establishing the presence of diphtheria is by demonstrating the typical organisms in stained smears and cultures. With some experience, it is possible to make a positive diagnosis from methylene blue–stained preparations in 75 to 85 percent of cases. These observations require confirmation by isolation of the organisms. Diphtheria bacilli can be recovered from patients who have not been given antibiotic agents in 8 to 12 hr on Loeffler's medium incubated at 37°C; *C. diphtheriae* also multiplies, but more slowly, on ordinary blood agar. If drugs, especially penicillin or erythromycin, have been administered prior to obtaining material for culture, the organisms may not grow out for as long as 5 days or may fail to grow at all.

Staining of suspected material with fluorescein-labeled diphtheria antitoxin may allow the microbiologic diagnosis of diphtheria to be made rapidly. All strains of the diphtheria bacillus recovered from patients should be examined for toxin production. This can be accomplished in guinea pigs or by an in vitro technique.

TREATMENT. Patients with diphtheria should be isolated and kept at strict bed rest, with reduction of physical effort during the early convalescent stages. Local therapy of the diphtheritic lesion is usually not required. A soft diet is preferred. There is no indication for parenteral feeding if the patient is able to take adequate calories and fluid by mouth.

The only specific treatment for diphtheria is antitoxin. Dosage schedules are somewhat empiric, but experience has suggested the use of certain quantities in the therapy of lesions of varying severity, extent, and location. Antiserum must never be given until the presence of sensitivity to horse serum, using the eye and skin tests, has been determined. Despite a negative test for hypersensitivity, it is probably best to administer antiserum in divided doses to all adults. The following schedule is widely used: When exudate is present on only one tonsil, 5,000 units of antitoxin are given; for lesions covering both tonsils, 10,000 units are administered. When the entire pharyngeal wall and the tonsils are involved, the quantity is increased to 20,000 to 50,000 units. Laryngeal diphtheria is treated with 50,000 to 100,000 units of antitoxin. Because of the length of time required for antibody to reach maximal levels in the blood after intramuscular injection, one-half the calculated dose is given by this route. If no reaction occurs, the rest of the antitoxin is infused slowly by vein. Desensitization should be attempted if the initial skin or eye tests are positive. A rare patient may be sensitive to such a high degree that the antiserum cannot be administered without the risk of death. Nothing is gained by repeated injections of antitoxin.

Antitoxin should be given as early in the course of diphtheria as possible. It has been suggested that larger quantities of antiserum than those recommended above should be used when therapy is given late; because toxin is fixed instantaneously to tissues and then cannot be neutralized by antitoxin, the effectiveness of this practice is questionable. Antimicrobial agents do not alter the course, incidence of complications, or outcome of diphtheria.

Patients with laryngeal obstruction should be watched very carefully. In mild cases, inhalation of warm or cool steam may be beneficial. If advancing signs of airway obstruction develop, intubation or tracheostomy should be performed. These procedures must never be delayed until cyanosis appears, because, at this point, stimulation of the pharynx or trachea can result in sudden cardiac standstill and death. Sedative or hypnotic agents should not be given because they may obscure increasing respiratory difficulty. Intubation is the preferred method of relieving diphtheritic laryngeal obstruction. However, if experienced personnel are not available, tracheostomy is probably the safer measure. Because patients with tracheal tubes in place cannot call for help, special nurses must be on duty at all times to ensure prompt and proper care. Tracheostomy or intubation has to be maintained for at least 3 or 4 days.

The pulse and blood pressure should be determined frequently. Little can be done to alter the course of the myocarditis. Quinidine has been tried to prevent arrhythmias, but with little success. This drug has also been given after abnormal cardiac rhythms have appeared; the results have not been striking, and deleterious effects have been suspected in some instances. Likewise the effectiveness of procaine amide when ventricular premature beats or tachycardia supervene has not been documented. The administration of digitalis when cardiac failure occurs in diphtheria is controversial. Some observers consider this drug completely contraindicated and employ fluid and salt restriction and diuretics. Others feel, however, that careful administration of digitalis is both safe and beneficial. The treatment of shock is discussed in Chap. 134. There is no evidence that corticosteroids or corticotropin are of value in the treatment of diphtheria or of its complications.

Treatment of the Carrier. *Corynebacterium diphtheriae* usually disappears from the upper part of the respiratory tract after 2 to 4 weeks in patients who do not receive antimicrobial drugs; in a small number of individuals the organism may persist for a long time or be present permanently. The most effective treatment of the acute and chronic carrier state is penicillin or erythromycin. The administration of 300,000 to 600,000 units penicillin G in divided doses per day for 10 to 12 days eliminates the diphtheria bacilli in practically all cases. A single injection of 600,000 units of procaine penicillin per day produces about the same results. Erythromycin, 25 to 50 mg per kg body weight per day orally, is also highly effective and is the drug of choice in persons known to be allergic to penicillin. Retreatment is indicated for carriers in whom the organisms are not eradicated after the first trial. This is preferable to tonsillectomy, which may be considered as a last resort should the carrier state persist despite repeated courses of antibiotics.

PREVENTION. Diphtheria is, for the most part, a preventable disease. Immunization at the age of three months should be routine. Diphtheria toxoid is best given together with tetanus toxoid and pertussis vaccine (DPT), because antibody titers are higher with combined immunization. Booster doses should be administered at the age of one year and again just before a child goes to school. Although it has been suggested that Schick testing is not necessary in those who have been immunized, many physicians still carry this out to determine the status of antitoxic immunity. A Schick test acts as a booster. A negative reaction does not indicate absolute protection against diphtheria. The development of highly purified toxoid has made protection possible with little or no risk of untoward sequelae. The usual procedure is to inject 0.1 ml purified toxoid subcutaneously (Moloney test). If there is no reaction in 24 to 48 hr, the regular immunization procedure is carried out.

Unimmunized persons exposed to an active case of diphtheria should be given 2,000 units of antitoxin intramuscularly, after appropriate skin and eye tests. In individuals who have been immunized previously, a booster dose of toxoid is usually sufficient. Patients with diphtheria should be quarantined until three successive cultures of the nose, throat, or other infected areas, taken at 24-hr intervals, are negative. If antibiotics have been administered, cultural studies should not be initiated until at least 24 hr after cessation of therapy.

REFERENCES

Beach, M. W., W. B. Gamble, Jr., C. H. Zemp, Jr., and M. Q. Jenkins: Erythromycin in the Treatment of Diphtheria and Diphtheria Carrier State, Pediatrics, 16:335, 1955.

Boyer, N. H., and L. Weinstein: Diphtheritic Myocarditis, New Engl. J. Med., 239:913, 1948.

Doege, T. C., C. W. Heath, Jr., and I. L. Sherman: Diphtheria in the United States, 1959–1960, Pediatrics, 30:194, 1962.

Goor, R. S., and A. M. Pappenheimer, Jr.: Studies on the Mode of Action of Diphtheria Toxin, J. Exp. Med., 126:899, 913, 923, 1967.

Gore, I.: Myocardial Changes in Fatal Diphtheria: A Summary of Observations in 221 Cases, Am. J. Med. Sci., 219:257, 1948.

Hollander, M. H.: Diphtheria of the Skin, U.S. Air Force Med. J., 2:229, 1951.

Ipsen, J.: Circulating Antitoxin at the Onset of Diphtheria in 425 Patients, Medicine, 251:459, 1954.

——: Immunization of Adults against Diphtheria and Tetanus, New Engl. J. Med., 251:459, 1954.

Naiditch, M. J., and A. G. Bower: Diphtheria: A Study of 1,433 Cases Observed during a Ten-year Period at the Los Angeles County Hospital, Am. J. Med., 17:229, 1954.

Parsons, E. I.: Induction of Toxigenicity in Non-toxigenic Strains of *C. Diphtheriae* with Bacteriophages Derived from Non-toxigenic Strains, Proc. Soc. Exp. Biol. Med., 90:91, 1955.

——, M. Frobisher, M. More, and M. A. Aiden: Rapid Virulence Test in Diagnosis of Diphtheria, Proc. Soc. Exp. Biol. Med., 88:368, 1955.

Scheid, W.: Diphtherial Paralysis: An Analysis of 2,292 Cases of Diphtheria in Adults Which Included 174 Cases of Polyneuritis, J. Nervous Mental Dis., 116:1095, 1952.

Weinstein, L.: The Treatment of Acute Diphtheria and the Chronic Carrier State with Penicillin, Am. J. Med. Sci., 213:308, 1947.

Witaker, J. A., J. D. Nelson, and C. W. Fink: The Fluorescent Antitoxin Test for the Immediate Diagnosis of Diphtheria, Pediatrics, 27:214, 1961.

Wittels, B., and R. Bressler: Biochemical Lesion of Diphtheria Toxin on the Heart, J. Clin. Invest., 43:630, 1964.

170 TETANUS

Edward S. Miller

DEFINITION. Tetanus is a severe intoxication characterized by generalized hypertonicity of skeletal muscles and convulsive seizures. The disease is caused by an exotoxin produced by *Clostridium tetani*.

HISTORY. Tetanus was described by Hippocrates, and has been documented over the centuries by many authors as a scourge of parturient women, newborn babies, and wounded soldiers. For example, in the eighteenth century, 1 of every 6 infants born in the Rotunda Hospital in Dublin died of tetanus neonatorum. Modern knowledge of this disease had its inception in 1884, when Nicolaier produced tetanus in animals by injecting garden soil. Subsequently, the bacillus was isolated in pure culture and found to produce an exotoxin. In 1890, Von Behring and Kitasato succeeded in immunizing animals by injecting minute amounts of toxin, and found that these animals produced antibodies. Ramon created tetanus toxoid in 1923. These studies permitted the development of immunologic methods for the prevention of the disease.

ETIOLOGY. *Clostridium tetani* is a large, motile, spore-forming, gram-positive bacillus without a capsule. It is an obligate anaerobe. The organism produces spherical terminal spores which, when protected from direct sunlight, can survive for many years. The spores are found in soil and street dust in most of the world and are often present in the intestinal contents of man and animals. Under suitable conditions, the spores germinate to the vegetative forms, which then elaborate a powerful exotoxin. At least 10 antigenic types have been distinguished, but differentiation is of no practical importance, because the exotoxins of all have the same immunologic properties. The vegetative forms and the exotoxin are destroyed in 10 min at 65°C. Spores can be eradicated with certainty only by autoclaving at 115°C for 20 min.

EPIDEMIOLOGY. Tetanus is endemic throughout the world, but has a low incidence in the cold polar regions and occurs with increasing frequency in damp, warm climates. The prevalence is greatest in developing areas of the world and is associated with lack of education, poor hygiene, deficient public health practices, poverty, and unavailability of good medical care. It has been estimated that between 1951 and 1960, 1 million people in the world contracted tetanus, and one-half of them died. The disease has become relatively rare in the United States; approximately 400 to 500 cases per year are recorded, but it is estimated that only 20 percent of cases are reported. The majority of cases occurs in the Southeast and South Central states, and fatality rates vary from 30 to 70 percent. One-third of these deaths occur in children less than one year of age, chiefly as the result of contamination of the umbilical stump at birth.

PATHOGENESIS. Tetanus organisms gain entrance to the body through wounds. The organism is so ubiquitous in nature that almost any injured part may be contaminated. Many lesions, both large and small, including lacerations, slivers, compound fractures, gunshot wounds, varicose ulcers, tooth extractions, burns, frostbites, bedsores, penetrating lesions produced by nails, and human and animal bites, offer a suitable haven for proliferation of the organisms. Cases have resulted from the use of unsterile surgical supplies and biologic materials such as catgut. Infections of the post-partum uterus and the umbilical stump are now rare where modern obstetric techniques are used, but are common where these are not available. The disease also follows piercing of earlobes and circumcision performed under unhygienic conditions.

Clostridium tetani is a strict anaerobe and proliferates only in the presence of an oxidation-reduction potential far lower than that existing in normal living tissue. A fall in potential may occur in the presence of necrotic tissue, of soil or other foreign materials, or of tetanus toxin itself. Once the organism begins to grow, it produces toxin and thereafter can maintain the conditions necessary for continued multiplication. If conditions for growth are not optimal, tetanus spores may persist in the body for many months or years, in a dormant but viable state. If tissues are traumatized later, as in a surgical procedure, tetanus may then develop.

Tetanus bacilli grow locally in a wound, show little capacity to invade, and are in themselves harmless. They cause disease only by virtue of exotoxin elaborated during growth. Two toxins are produced, tetanolysin and tetanospasmin. Tetanolysin lyses red corpuscles in vitro and may also damage leukocytes. Its clinical significance is unknown, but it may contribute to tetanus infection by causing local tissue necrosis and by antiphagocytic action. Tetanospasmin is a protein with a molecular weight of 67,000. It is a potent neurotoxin, and it is estimated that a dose of 0.13 mg is lethal for man.

The toxin acts on the internuncial cells in the vicinity of the anterior horn cells of the spinal cord, causing a reduction of the central inhibitory balancing influences on motor neurone activity. This results in intensified reflex response to afferent stimuli, leading to exaggerated motor activity, spasticity of skeletal muscles, and paroxysmal seizures. The toxin also acts on the medullary centers. Tetanospasmin has a strong affinity for certain nerve tissues, and once combined with receptor cells, it cannot be neutralized by antitoxin. Nevertheless, the toxin is inactivated eventually by some unknown mechanism because patients who recover from tetanus show no residual neurologic defects.

The route by which toxin travels from the local lesion

to the central nervous system is a matter of controversy. There is good experimental evidence to support the theory that toxin can enter the neuromuscular end organs, pass centripetally up the axones of motor nerves to the cord, and then spread throughout the central nervous system. This pathway may account for the rare case of local tetanus. Ordinarily, most of the toxin is carried from the local lesion to the nervous system via the bloodstream, and this sequence of events probably obtains in generalized tetanus.

MANIFESTATIONS. The incubation period varies from 2 days to several months, but in two-thirds of cases it falls within the range of 6 to 15 days. Some patients have prodromal symptoms of restlessness and headache. In others, the first symptoms are caused by the developing muscular rigidity, with vague discomfort in the jaws, neck, or lumbar region. Among the first muscles to show involvement are those innervated by the fifth, seventh, ninth, tenth, eleventh, and twelfth cranial nerves. Spasm of the muscles of mastication causes trismus. This highly characteristic phenomenon gives the disease its common name of *lockjaw*. Sustained contraction of the facial muscles produces a distorted grin called *risus sardonicus*. Spasm of the pharyngeal muscles makes swallowing difficult. Stiff neck and opisthotonos are also among the early signs. Progressively, other muscle groups become involved, with tightness of the chest and rigidity of the abdominal wall, back, and limbs. The distribution of muscular rigidity may vary, as may the sequence of appearance of spasm. The *period of onset* of tetanus is considered to be the elapsed time from the first symptom until the appearance of reflex convulsive spasms. If this interval is less than 24 hr, the disease is most severe, and the fatality rate high.

The patient is conscious and mentally clear, restless, and apprehensive, and has much pain from muscular spasms. Coughing and swallowing become difficult, and breathing laborious. There is profuse perspiration. Fever is usually low-grade unless complications are present. The wound through which *C. tetani* was introduced is usually evident, although in 10 to 20 percent of patients it cannot be found. The tendon reflexes are hyperactive, often with sustained clonus, but there are no sensory changes. The symptoms and signs increase in severity for several days. Generalized tonic convulsions appear in all but the milder cases and are accompanied by spasm of the larynx and the respiratory muscles. Convulsions are precipitated by various stimuli such as a sudden noise, a hypodermic injection, or a jostling of the bed. The hypertonia sometimes disappears prior to death. If the patient survives, the intensity of muscle spasm begins to diminish slowly after 2 to 3 weeks, and complete recovery may take several months. Occasionally, in mild cases, there is only muscle rigidity without seizures. Sometimes the administration of tetanus antitoxin forestalls the development of generalized tetanus but not of local tetanus involving the muscles around the site of injury.

Complications. Complications are frequent. *Atelectasis* is common and may be followed by pneumonia, which seriously lessens the chances of recovery. *Venous thrombosis* may occur and may be followed by pulmonary embolization. Acute *gastric ulcers* with hemorrhage or perforation occur. Constipation and fecal impaction, and urinary retention, are common. Urinary tract infections often develop in patients requiring catheterization. Traumatic *glossitis* is frequent and is an important cause of airway obstruction. *Compression fractures* of vertebras sometimes result from the convulsive seizures. *Decubitus ulcers* are likely to occur in patients under heavy sedation. *Serum sickness* may appear from 3 to 12 days after administration of equine antitoxin. Footdrop and muscle contractures sometimes follow prolonged unconsciousness with the limbs in poor position.

Death can result from several causes. Tetanus toxin itself can be lethal as a result of damage to the medullary centers, especially the respiratory center. Asphyxia from respiratory muscle or laryngeal spasm or from aspiration of secretions, vomitus, or food may be the immediate cause of death. Other causes include pneumonia, pulmonary embolism, and the complications of drugs used to control muscle hyperactivity, which may lead to oversedation and respiratory paralysis. Exhaustion, inanition, and electrolyte imbalance are contributory factors.

LABORATORY FINDINGS. The diagnosis of tetanus must be based on the clinical picture, and laboratory examinations are of little assistance. It is difficult to isolate the organism from the local lesion, and it is a laborious task to identify it precisely. Furthermore, the presence of *C. tetani* in a wound does not necessarily indicate that the patient has tetanus. The intoxication itself produces no change in the leukocyte count, but leukocytosis may accompany secondary infection. The cerebrospinal fluid is often under increased pressure but is otherwise not remarkable. The urine is normal in uncomplicated tetanus.

DIFFERENTIAL DIAGNOSIS. Fully developed tetanus is unlikely to be confused with other diseases. A frequent diagnostic problem is differentiation of serum sickness from early tetanus. Many injured patients are given equine tetanus antitoxin, and some subsequently develop serum sickness with temporomandibular arthralgia and trismus. Usually arthralgia of other joints is also present, together with urticaria and generalized adenitis. Other conditions in which trismus occurs include peritonsillar abscess and local infections of the mouth and cervical region. The phenothiazine group of tranquilizers may cause extrapyramidal tract symptoms with dystonic involvement of facial and pharyngeal muscles. Normal spinal fluid in tetanus eliminates confusion with meningitis. The clinical picture of strychnine poisoning, with hyperexcitability of the muscles, opisthotonos, risus sardonicus, and tonic convulsions, may mimic tetanus closely, except that the muscles are relaxed between seizures in strychnine intoxication, while spasm tends to persist in tetanus. In rabies, inability to swallow is often an early symptom, with drooling of saliva and spasms of the muscles of deglutition, followed by fever, anxiety, excitement, delirium, hyperesthesia, and convulsions.

TREATMENT. This is a grave disease for which there is no specific treatment. Nevertheless, careful and constant attention to certain supportive measures often will change the outcome from death to recovery.

Nursing Care. There is no disease in which meticulous, gentle nursing care is of greater importance, and it is essential that a trained attendant be at the bedside at all times. The patient should be in a quiet darkened room, where external stimuli are kept to a minimum. Secretions which accumulate in the pharynx must be removed by suction and postural drainage. A padded tongue depressor should be placed between the teeth to prevent tongue biting during convulsions. Bedsores can be avoided by use of a foam rubber or an alternating pressure-pad mattress, by changing the patient's position, and by special attention to skin care. Catheterization should be avoided if possible, because it precipitates convulsive seizures and inevitably leads to infection. Enemas are given as needed. Foot drop and wrist drop can be prevented by suitable positioning.

Sedatives and Muscle Relaxants. A most important feature in therapy is the use of medications to prevent acute tetanic seizures and to induce relaxation of muscle spasm. An ideal drug should also depress consciousness without rendering the patient comatose or depressing respiration. No single drug fulfills these criteria. Sedatives act by reducing sensory stimuli to the central nervous system, and several, including barbiturates, chloral hydrate, paraldehyde, and tribromoethanol, have been useful. Some of the centrally acting muscle relaxants and spinal depressants are effective because they diminish reflex activity and motor output. These include diazepam, chlorpromazine, mephenesin, meprobamate, and methocarbamol. It is recommended that at least two agents be employed, one from each group. This will permit a smaller dosage of each and will minimize toxic effects and the likelihood of tachyphylaxis. One of the drugs should be used in a relatively fixed dose as a basal medication; the dose of the second is varied to suit the immediate clinical requirements. An excellent combination is diazepam (up to 2 mg per kg in 24 hr) and thiopental sodium, given intravenously as a slow drip in a dilution of 0.5 to 1 Gm per liter of saline. The rate of flow must be titrated carefully to produce sleep without coma, but may be speeded up to control a seizure. Narcotics are contraindicated.

Another approach to control of convulsions is to use neuromuscular blocking agents of the curare group. This technique has been popular in Europe, but has found few advocates in the United States. These medications must be given in subparalyzing doses, aimed at controlling convulsions without interfering with respiration. Alternatively, the patient can be paralyzed deliberately and maintained with constant artificial respiration. These methods are obviously complex and dangerous and should be undertaken only by an experienced and skillful therapeutic team.

Antiserum. Antiserum has no curative action in tetanus, because it does not affect the toxin which has combined with nerve tissue. Its only action is to neutralize newly formed toxin as it is produced in the lesion and before it has reached susceptible nerve cells. There is actually little statistical proof that administration of antiserum materially alters the course of clinically developed tetanus; nevertheless, it should be used. Horse serum antitoxin was introduced in World War I and was the standard preparation for many years. Technical advances ultimately permitted the development of human tetanus immune globulin (TIG), which is now generally available in the United States. TIG is so far superior to equine antiserum that horse serum should be used only if TIG is unobtainable. The additional cost of TIG is more than offset by the elimination of morbidity and expense associated with the hypersensitivity reactions which were so frequent after administration of horse serum.

1. Homologous antitoxin (TIG). Allergic reactions are practically unknown, making sensitivity testing unnecessary. This material must be given intramuscularly. Being a human gamma-globulin, its predictable half-life is 25 days or more. Little experience has accumulated on the use of TIG in treatment of human tetanus, and consequently no consensus has been established regarding dosage. From 3,000 to 6,000 units appear to be more than ample, and the drop in titer is so slow that adequate protective levels are assured throughout the recovery period.

2. Heterologous antitoxin. Careful tests for horse serum sensitivity must be performed. If these are negative, 50,000 International Units of serum are given slowly intravenously in 250 ml normal saline solution, containing 1.0 ml of 1:1,000 aqueous epinephrine. The intravenous route is preferable because maximal plasma levels of antibody are achieved immediately, while following intramuscular injection, the plasma titer rises only gradually over a 2-day period. Ten thousand units of antitoxin are infiltrated around the local lesion because a considerable reservoir of toxin is present in this region. Horse serum should never be given intraspinally. Repeated doses are not necessary except in unusual cases involving extensive, slow-healing wounds. In such instances readministration may have to be considered after several weeks, but this involves a serious hazard of an allergic reaction and in this situation every effort to obtain TIG should be made. An alternative measure is to administer a unit of plasma obtained from a donor who has previously been actively immunized and has recently received a booster dose of tetanus toxoid.

Initiation of Active Immunization. There are sound reasons to advise that active immunization with toxoid should be commenced at the onset of therapy of tetanus. Even though it will be somewhat diminished by the simultaneous administration of a large excess of antiserum, an antigenic stimulus will be instituted. Consequently, toxoid should be given every 3 days over a period of 2 weeks. These injections should be considered *in toto* as the first dose of a primary immunization series. Another dose administered 3 weeks later will then stimulate production of the patient's own antibodies to replace the waning antibody introduced passively. Administration of toxoid provides protection in situations where the organism is not eradicated and where there may be late production of toxin.

Treatment of Local Lesion. The patient should receive sedatives and antiserum before the wound is manipulated. The lesion is then treated according to the same surgical principles that would be applicable if tetanus were not present. Specifically, a limb should not be amputated simply because the patient has tetanus. Meticulous debridement is essential.

Feeding. Oral feeding is usually hazardous or impossible because of trismus and dysphagia. Intravenous feeding is necessary during the first days of illness, and particularly in heavily sedated or unconscious patients. Nasogastric tube feeding should be avoided as long as danger of aspiration persists. Electrolyte balance requires careful regulation.

Management of Respiratory Tract. It is essential that respiratory tract obstruction be prevented or corrected, because this complication leads to anoxia, atelectasis, and pneumonia. Tracheostomy has proved to be a valuable therapeutic adjunct and should be used in most moderately or severely ill patients. Following this procedure convulsive spasms often diminish and less sedation is required.

Other Therapeutic Measures. The tetanal infection itself requires the use of an antibiotic, because antitoxin does not have antimicrobial properties. Conversely, antibiotics do not possess antitoxic properties. Penicillin G in dosage of 2.4 million units a day and tetracycline in dosage of 2.0 Gm per day are both useful, and one of them should be given. Corticosteroids have not been found to improve the clinical course. Several reports have indicated that hyperbaric oxygen may be of benefit, but the data are too meager to permit evaluation.

PREVENTION. Active Immunization. Tetanus toxoid is the most effective nonliving immunizing agent known. Active immunization can be achieved safely and almost infallibly, the rare exceptions being individuals who have diseases associated with deficient antibody production. The immunity is antitoxic rather than antibacterial in nature. Two types of toxoids are in general use, an alum-precipitated, or adsorbed type and a fluid type. The alum-precipitated type is the more effective immunizing agent and should be used for all primary immunization.

Primary immunization is achieved by giving two doses, interrupted by an interval of at least 3 weeks, and preferably one of 4 to 12 weeks. Permanent immunity requires a third reinforcing dose after 6 to 12 months. In experimental animals it has been shown that some resistance to infection has developed within 10 days after the initial dose of toxoid, and circulating antibody can be found in small quantity in man within 4 weeks after the first dose. The titer rises sharply within a few days after the second dose has been given, and the individual may be considered temporarily immune after 10 days. The reinforcing third dose is followed by a very high antibody titer and is necessary to induce lasting immunity. There will be an antibody response of some degree even if the interval between the first and second doses of toxoid is as long as 12 years. Once basic immunization is accomplished, the normal person has an extraordinary capacity to respond with an effective antibody titer after a booster dose. Animal studies show a protective response within 24 hr, and a measurable rise in titer appears within 4 to 7 days, even when the recall dose is given as long as 22 years after primary immunization. Some authorities speculate that immunity persists for life; nevertheless, it seems prudent to give boosters at 10-year intervals.

Active immunization is the only really effective way of contending with the problem of tetanus, and should be a universal practice. Half the cases of tetanus in the United States involve wounds so trivial that they are disregarded by the patient or are considered by the physician to be too insignificant to warrant antitoxin prophylaxis. It is especially important to emphasize immunization in certain tetanus-prone groups. Tetanus neonatorum accounts for 10 to 30 percent of all cases in many parts of the world, and these could be prevented readily by immunizing the pregnant mothers. Many people are highly exposed to injury in their occupations and urgently require protection. The potential hypersensitivity to horse serum was formerly a major problem in all patients with an allergic diathesis and in those who had previously received equine antitoxin. This danger has diminished as human gamma-globulin has come into wider use.

A good time to initiate basic immunization is at the time of treatment of an acute injury. Tetanus toxoid is given in one limb, and if TIG is necessary, it is administered in another part of the body. In this manner, they do not significantly neutralize each other, and as passive protection slowly wanes, the patient begins to produce his own antibody.

Hypersensitivity reactions to tetanus toxoid are becoming more common, probably because of repeated injections. They are rarely seen before the age of twenty and become more frequent with advancing age. Usually they are of the delayed tuberculin type and are unpleasant but not serious. More severe local reactions of the Arthus type are seen occasionally. There have been rare reports of accelerated serum sickness or anaphylactic types of response. These reactions are associated with high antibody titers in the reacting individuals. Therefore, boosters should not be given with unnecessary frequency. Routine boosters every 10 years are sufficient, and in the event of an injury, one is needed only if more than a year has elapsed since the previous booster. If a local reaction is encountered, then future injections can be administered successfully by giving an initial dose of 0.05 ml of toxoid, followed by one or more fractional doses at intervals of several days.

Passive Immunization. Tetanus-immune human gamma-globulin is much to be preferred over horse antiserum. The prophylactic dose for an adult is 250 units given intramuscularly, and for a child it is 4 units per kg body weight. The dose may be doubled in those with highly contaminated lesions. TIG will give adequate protection for at least 1 month, and can be repeated without fear of an allergic reaction. If TIG is not available, then equine antiserum must be given subcutaneously in a dose of 1,500 to 5,000 units, depending on the severity of the wound and the degree of delay in administration. Hypersensitivity reactions are reported in 2.5 to 9 percent of patients who have not had previous serum injections and in up to 24 percent of those who have. Tests for serum sensitivity are likely to identify patients who are candidates for immediate anaphylactic reactions, but will not point out those who will develop serum sickness. Plasma antibody titers may persist for only a few days in persons who have had previous experience with horse serum. Attempts to desensitize are dangerous and probably fruitless and are not recommended.

Procedure after Injury. Of first importance is thorough and prompt cleansing and debridement. Certain types of injuries are more likely to be complicated by tetanus infections, including burns, compound fractures, deep or puncture wounds, those contaminated by soil, those over 3 hr old, wounds already otherwise infected, and those containing devitalized or avascular tissue. In addition to thorough debridement, penicillin or tetracycline should be given to prevent an incipient tetanal infection.

If the patient is known to have had basic tetanus immunization, and the last booster was given more than 1 year previously, then he should receive a toxoid booster. This will suffice except under unusual circumstances, when fortifying active immunity by giving antitoxin should be considered in addition. These circumstances are last toxoid booster more than 10 years previously; treatment delayed more than 24 hr after the injury; an extensive, mutilating, tetanus-prone injury; a patient who has a disease associated with poor production of gamma-globulin.

A decision must be made concerning the administration of TIG in the patient who has not had or has not completed a primary immunization series. Frequently, the history concerning this point is uncertain and when doubt exists it should be assumed that the patient has not been immunized. TIG is not needed if the wound is clean and minor, is treated soon after the injury, and can be debrided thoroughly. Those with more serious wounds are given TIG. Active immunization is initiated in all patients immediately, whether or not TIG is given.

PROGNOSIS. Case fatality rates average 30 to 50 percent but vary markedly. The rate is much higher in the very young, in the aged, in drug addicts, and in those who develop pneumonia or other secondary infections. It is higher if the incubation period is less than 7 days or if the period of onset is less than 24 hr. Most deaths occur within the first 10 days of illness. Survivors make a complete recovery from tetanus, although there may be residual effects from the various therapeutic measures used or from complications such as compression fractures. Those who recover are not immune to reinfection.

REFERENCES

Eckmann, L.: "Tetanus Prophylaxis and Therapy," New York, Grune & Stratton, Inc., 1963.

Edsall, G.: Current Status of Tetanus Immunization, Arch. Environ. Health, 8:731, 1964.

Laurence, D. R., and R. A. Webster: Pathologic Physiology, Pharmacology, and Therapeutics of Tetanus, Clin. Pharmacol. Therap., 4:36, 1963.

Smith, L. DeS.: *Clostridium Tetani*, pp. 88–107 in "Introduction to the Pathogenic Anaerobes," Chicago, University of Chicago Press, 1955.

Wright, G. P.: The Neurotoxins of *Clostridium Botulinium* and *Clostridium Tetani*, Pharmacol. Rev., 7:413, 1955.

171 BOTULISM

M. Glenn Koenig and David E. Rogers

DEFINITION. Botulism is a specific form of poisoning which results from absorption of toxin produced by *Clostridium botulinum*. The clinical picture is characterized by dilated fixed pupils, dry mucous membranes, progressive muscular paralysis, and high fatality rate.

HISTORY. The disease was first recognized over 200 years ago by South German physicians who adopted the term *botulismus* for the often fatal syndrome which sometimes followed the consumption of spoiled sausage (*botulus* is Latin for sausage). Studies by Van Ermengem in 1895 identified a gram-positive, spore-forming anaerobic bacillus as the etiologic agent and showed that a toxin produced by these bacilli was responsible for the disease.

Botulism was rare in the United States prior to World War I. The growth of commercial and home canning at this time led to a great increase in cases. A series of studies by Dr. K. F. Meyer and his associates in the early 1920s defined the habitat of *C. botulinum*, the foods often incriminated, and the conditions necessary for the destruction of *C. botulinum* spores. This knowledge led to the virtual elimination of botulism from the commercial canning industry. Since then clinical botulism has been infrequent in the United States and has usually followed consumption of improperly canned, home-preserved foods. In 1963 several outbreaks of type E disease followed consumption of certain commercially processed fish products. The introduction of new methods of packaging may have contributed to this problem.

ETIOLOGY. Six immunologically distinct strains of *C. botulinum*, designated as types A, B, C, D, E, and F, have been described. Each type elaborates an antigenically specific toxin which is liberated during growth and autolysis. Type A, B, and E toxins have been implicated most frequently in human disease in the United States. Only two outbreaks of type F botulism have been reported. The first occurred on the Danish island of Langeland following the ingestion of homemade liver paste. The second, which has been presumptively identified as type F, involved an outbreak in California traced to home-processed venison jerky. Types C and D produce disease almost exclusively in animals including wild water fowl, cattle, horses, and mink.

Type A and B spores are widely distributed in soil throughout the world. Type A spores are most common in the United States, especially along the Pacific Coast and the Rocky Mountain states. Type B spores have been found more frequently in the Eastern states and in Europe. Type E spores have been demonstrated in lakeshore mud, coastal sand, and sea bottom silt in northern latitudes. Fish apparently contaminate their intestinal tracts with type E spores, accounting for the high incidence of type E strains in fish-borne botulism. Type F spores have been found in marine sediments collected off the coast of California and Oregon and in salmon taken from the Columbia River.

Botulinum toxins are the most potent poisons known. Types A through E have been highly purified and identified as simple proteins. Original estimations of molecular weights have ranged from 900,000 for type A toxin to 18,600 for type E. Recent studies suggest that some botulinus toxins may depolymerize into units of lower molecular weight while maintaining or even increasing in toxicity. While antigenically distinct, all the toxins appear to produce identical symptoms in man and experimental animals, although there are marked differences in specific host susceptibility to the different toxins.

Spores of *C. botulinum* can withstand 100°C for several hours. Moist heat at 120°C for 30 min will destroy spores of all types, but the toxins are considerably more heat-labile. All varieties of toxin are destroyed by boiling for 10 min, or by temperatures of 80°C for 30 min.

PATHOGENESIS. Most human botulism follows the ingestion of food stuffs contaminated with preformed botulinus toxin. Rarely, wounds secondarily infected with *C. botulinum* have been the portal of entry. There is no convincing evidence that the botulinus bacillus produces toxin in the human gastrointestinal tract. Clinical botulism can occur only when the following conditions are met: (1) a food product is contaminated with viable *C. botulinum* bacilli or spores, (2) proper conditions for germination of the spores exist, (3) time and conditions allow production of toxin prior to eating, (4) the produce is not heated or is heated insufficiently to destroy botulinus toxin, (5) the toxin-containing food is ingested by a susceptible host (Table 171-1). While a relatively anaerobic

Table 171-1. IMPORTANT FACTORS IN THE PATHOGENESIS OF BOTULISM

Spores	Toxin production	Toxin
1. Survive at 6°C (42.8°F) for several months	1. Strict anaerobic conditions not always required	1. Destroyed at 80°C (176°F) after 30 min or 100°C for 10 min
2. Can withstand boiling for several hours	2. Can occur at 6°C (42.8°F)	2. Unstable at high pH's
3. Destroyed at 120°C (248°F) after 30 min	3. Optimal temperature 30°C (86°F)	3. Type E toxin activated by trypsin
	4. Reduced at low pH's	

environment and temperatures above 80°F are optimal for toxin production, strict anaerobic conditions are not

necessary and toxin production by some type E strains has been observed at temperatures as low as 6°C (42.8°F).

Home-canned string beans, corn, beets, spinach, asparagus, chili peppers, dill pickles, olives, tomatoes, figs, apricots, okra, mushrooms, peaches, home-processed venison jerky, gefilte fish, and albacore salad have been sources of botulism in the United States. Between 1941 and 1967, commercially processed foods have been implicated in only eight outbreaks (canned liver paste, type A; cheese, type unknown; smoked ciscoes, smoked whitefish, smoked whitefish chubs, and canned tuna fish, all type E; and possibly luncheon meat, type unknown).

Many type A and B strains of *C. botulinum* are proteolytic, and food frequently undergoes obvious putrefaction during their growth. Type E strains do not elaborate proteolytic enzymes, and foodstuffs containing type E toxin may not undergo spoilage and may look and taste perfectly normal.

Botulinus toxin is primarily absorbed in the stomach and upper small bowel. Despite its protein nature, it appears relatively resistant to inactivation by proteolytic enzymes. Indeed, the toxicity of type E toxin may be enhanced by tryptic digestion during passage through the upper gastrointestinal tract. Toxin which reaches the lower small bowel and colon may be slowly absorbed from these sites and may account for the delayed onset and the prolonged symptomatology observed in many patients.

Botulinus toxins exert a highly specific pharmacologic action, blocking transmission in cholinergic nerve fibers while sparing adrenergic fibers. Experimental studies have demonstrated that small amounts of toxin interrupt neural impulses close to the point of final branching of terminal nerve fibrils, but short of the motor end plate, and prevent release of acetylcholine. Nevertheless, muscle reactivity to acetylcholine applied directly to the motor end plate remains unimpaired. This contrasts with the action of curare, which prevents muscular response to acetylcholine. Some studies have suggested that botulinus toxins may exert some central inhibitory effects on cholinergic internuncial neurones in the spinal cord, but the clinical importance of this central action is uncertain.

CLINICAL MANIFESTATIONS. Botulism may vary from a mild illness for which patients seek no medical advice to a fulminant disease which ends in death within 24 hr. Symptoms usually begin 12 to 36 hr after ingestion of toxin, although extremes of 3 hr to 14 days are recorded. In general, the earlier the symptoms appear, the more serious the disease. Nausea and vomiting occur in approximately one-third of patients with type A or B disease and are very severe with type E intoxication. Weakness, lassitude, dizziness, and vertigo are early complaints. Severe dryness of the mouth and throat, sometimes associated with pharyngeal pain, is also noted. Neurologic symptoms may occur simultaneously or may be delayed for 12 to 72 hr. Blurred vision, diplopia, dysphonia, dysphagia, and weakness are followed by involvement of the muscles of respiration.

On examination, patients are usually alert, oriented,

and afebrile even with severe disease. Rarely, marked somnolence is noted. Difficulties in speech and deglutition may be obvious. The pupils are dilated and fixed. Extra-ocular palsies may be present but are less common than pupillary signs. The mucous membranes of the mouth and tongue are dry and crusted. Weakness of striated muscle groups, particularly the neck, proximal extremities, and muscles of respiration, appears as the disease progresses, but superficial and deep tendon reflexes remain *intact.* Abdominal distension with absent bowel sounds may be marked. Urinary retention may be present.

Respiratory paralysis may occur with startling swiftness. Failure of respiration, airway obstruction, and secondary pulmonary infection are the major causes of death. Sudden cardiac arrest has occurred in some patients with severe respiratory involvement, but whether this is secondary to anoxia or a primary action of botulinus toxin is unknown.

In patients recovering from botulism, return of function of the muscles of respiration, deglutition, and speech may be rapid, and improvement is often apparent within a week. General weakness, constipation, and ocular abnormalities may persist for weeks and sometimes several months.

LABORATORY FINDINGS. Routine laboratory studies do not aid in diagnosing clinical botulism. The cerebrospinal fluid is normal. Electrocardiographic abnormalities including minor disturbances in conduction, nonspecific T-wave and S-T segment changes, and various disorders of rhythm have been described. *The diagnosis of botulism rests on clinical grounds* and can be established only by the identification of botulinus toxin in the suspected food or in the patient. If available, portions of the suspected food should be suspended in saline and injected into mice intraperitoneally. If toxin is present, the animals will develop typical botulism and usually will die within 24 hr. Mice protected with specific antiserums survive. Fresh serum from patients suspected of having botulism should also be injected intraperitoneally in 1-ml amounts into mice with and without added type A, B, E, and F antiserums. Detection of circulating toxin in this manner has been useful in diagnosing type B and E intoxications and at least one outbreak of type A disease.

DIFFERENTIAL DIAGNOSIS. When the full clinical syndrome is evident, the symptoms and signs of botulism are sufficiently characteristic to lead to prompt diagnosis. In many instances the sequential appearance of findings can be confusing, particularly when no clear-cut history of ingestion of home-canned foods has been elicited.

The cranial nerve palsies, muscle weakness, and respiratory paralysis can lead to confusion with myasthenia gravis, Guillain-Barré syndrome, acute poliomyelitis, or stroke. A negative Tensilon test, normal cerebrospinal fluid, lack of sensory abnormalities, preservation of deep tendon reflexes, mental clarity, and absence of corticospinal tract signs in patients with botulism help to exclude these other possibilities.

Certain nonneurologic phenomena also have led to misdiagnosis. The pharyngeal pain, erythema, and dysphagia seen in some patients can suggest streptococcal or viral pharyngitis. The widely dilated pupils plus a dry mouth and mucous membranes resemble signs found in atropine, belladonna, or Jimson weed poisoning. The lack of nervous system excitement and hallucinations and the delay in onset of symptoms observed in botulism should exclude these possibilities. Nausea, vomiting, abdominal distension, constipation, and ileus may lead to consideration of intestinal obstruction. The dilated pupils and general paralytic phenomena should aid in differentiation.

Unexplained postural hypotension; dilated, unreactive pupils; extremely dry mucous membranes; and progressive muscle paresis occurring in a previously healthy afebrile patient should suggest botulism.

TREATMENT. Patients with botulism die of respiratory failure. *Early* tracheostomy and prompt use of the tank or other mechanical respirator can be life-saving. Cleansing enemas should be administered to remove any unabsorbed toxin from the colon. As soon as the clinical diagnosis of botulism has been made, appropriate skin testing for serum sensitivity should be carried out; if this is negative, 100,000 units of type A and type B antitoxin and 10,000 units of type E antitoxin should be administered intravenously. Patients sensitive to horse serum must be desensitized before antitoxin is given. Because each toxin is antigenically specific, there is no cross protection between antitoxins. Only a bivalent type A, B antitoxin is made commercially in the United States, but type E antitoxin can be obtained from the National Communicable Disease Center, Atlanta, Georgia. Because botulism antitoxin remains in the circulation for over 30 days, it is recommended that the total therapeutic dose be given immediately, rather than administering it in multiple small doses over a longer period. Antitoxin in one-third to one-half the therapeutic dose should be given prophylactically to individuals who are known to have eaten contaminated food but have not yet developed symptoms.

While older reports and certain animal experiments suggest that antitoxin does not alter the course of type A botulism once symptoms have appeared, the use of type-specific antitoxin has reduced mortality significantly in several outbreaks of type E disease. These reports suggest that antitoxin therapy should be vigorous and that the antitoxin treatment of type A and B botulism should be reassessed.

Because there is no evidence to suggest that *C. botulinum* can multiply in the gastrointestinal tract in man, antibiotics should be reserved for specific infectious complications.

PROGNOSIS. Type A strains have been the most frequent cause of botulism in the United States. Mortality rates of 60 to 70 percent have been reported in most outbreaks. Type B disease, which has been more common in Europe, has had consistently lower fatality rates of 10 to 30 percent. Type E botulism has produced outbreaks in northern latitudes among people eating raw fish (Japanese, Canadian Eskimos) with mortality rates ranging from 30 to 50 percent in large series. With more rapid diagnosis, aggressive management of respiratory paralysis, and use of polyvalent antitoxin, it seems likely these figures will be improved. Once the patient has survived the paralytic illness, the outlook for complete recovery is excellent.

REFERENCES

Dack, G. M.: "Food Poisoning," 3d ed., pp. 59–108, Chicago, University of Chicago Press, 1956.

Koenig, M. G., D. J. Drutz, A. I. Mushlin, W. Schaffner, and D. E. Rogers: Type B Botulism in Man. Am. J. Med., 42:208, 1967.

——, A. Spickard, M. A. Cardella, and D. E. Rogers: Clinical and Laboratory Observations on Type E Botulism in Man, Medicine, 43:517, 1964.

Rogers, D. E.: Botulism: Vintage 1963, Editorial, Ann. Intern. Med., 61:581, 1964.

172 OTHER CLOSTRIDIAL INFECTIONS
Edward W. Hook

INTRODUCTION AND HISTORY. Bacteria of the genus *Clostridium* are normal inhabitants of soil and the gastrointestinal tracts of man and animals. Most of the 93 species that have been described are saprophytic, but some are infectious for man and animals, usually under conditions of lowered host and tissue resistance. Infections with these organisms are often associated with profound systemic manifestations, and all pathogenic clostridia, except *Clostridium tetani* and *C. botulinum*, are capable of causing extensive tissue destruction. Diseases caused by these other clostridia are gas gangrene, cellulitis, postabortal and puerperal sepsis, and on occasion pneumonia, pleurisy, peritonitis, meningitis, endocarditis, cystitis, or bursitis. In addition, ingestion of food contaminated with certain clostridia may cause enterocolitis.

Hippocrates and Celsus were aware of the relationship between penetrating wounds and gas gangrene, but the nature of this disorder was not appreciated until the discovery of pathogenic clostridia by Pasteur, Novy, and Welch. The incidence of gas gangrene diminished markedly with the advent of antiseptic surgery in the latter half of the nineteenth century, but increased again to epidemic proportions during the trench warfare of the First World War. The rarity of serious clostridial infections in United Nations troops in Korea and in United States troops in more recent military actions attests to the advances in surgical management of war wounds. Gas gangrene and clostridial cellulitis are still encountered in neglected civilian injuries, and clostridial infections of the uterus account for a large proportion of deaths from criminal abortions.

ETIOLOGY. Wounds complicated by gas gangrene usually contain a mixture of pathogenic and saprophytic clostridia, often including *C. tetani*, as well as a variety of other bacteria. *Clostridium perfringens (welchii), C. novyi (oedematiens)*, or *C. septicum (Vibrion septique)* can be cultured from most cases of gas gangrene and clostridial cellulitis, and *C. perfringens* causes virtually all clostridial infections of the uterus. *Clostridium bi-*

fermentans, C. histolyticum, and *C. fallax* are less virulent organisms that occasionally cause gas gangrene but are more commonly associated with localized cellulitis. Proliferation of *C. botulinum* in wounds occasionally leads to clinical manifestations of botulism.

The clostridia of gas gangrene and related infections are anaerobic or microaerophilic gram-positive bacilli that produce abundant gas in artificial media and form subterminal endospores. *Clostridium perfringens* is encapsulated and nonmotile, rarely sporulates in artificial media, and produces spores that can usually be destroyed by boiling.

EPIDEMIOLOGY AND PATHOGENESIS. Clostridia do not penetrate intact skin or mucous membranes, but frequently gain access to tissues through wounds or perforated abdominal viscera. Although these organisms can be cultured from one-third to two-thirds of severe traumatic wounds, gas gangrene develops in only an occasional case. The most important prerequisite for the conversion of clostridial contamination of a wound to a progressive infection is an environment with low oxidation-reduction potential, which permits spore germination and anaerobic growth. Local oxidation-reduction potential can be reduced by failure of the blood supply to a contaminated area, by the presence of foreign bodies such as clothing, dirt, or fragments of metal or wood, or by the multiplication of other bacteria in the wound. Once multiplication and toxin production are established, rapid invasion and destruction of healthy tissue follow.

The pathogenicity of clostridia is related to the capacity of these organisms to form exotoxins which destroy tissue cells. The nature and amount of toxins vary considerably for different species and strains. For example, at least 12 different extracellular "toxins" are produced by *C. perfringens*. Alpha toxin, a lecithinase, is clearly the most important and is the principal tissue-destroying, hemolytic, and lethal toxin. Other *C. perfringens* products include collagenase, hyaluronidase, hemolytic theta toxin, leukocidin, deoxyribonuclease, and fibrinolysin.

Gas gangrene is characterized by marked systemic symptoms and a local reaction with extensive necrotizing myositis, edema, thrombosis of small vessels, interstitial gas bubbles, and minimal infiltration of leukocytes. The local reaction in infected tissue can be explained by the action of clostridial toxins, especially alpha toxin, but the factors responsible for the general reaction are unknown. Alpha toxin, or other clostridial toxins, have not been demonstrated in circulating blood during the course of severe clostridial myonecrosis.

CLINICAL MANIFESTATIONS. Clostridial Myonecrosis (Gas Gangrene, Clostridial Myositis). Gas gangrene develops in anoxic devitalized tissues in which the arterial circulation has been compromised by trauma, constricting tourniquets or casts, or obliterative arterial disease. Infection is most frequent after extensive injury to skeletal muscle, particularly of the thigh and buttock, and is more common in wounds complicated by compound fractures of lodgment of foreign bodies. Once infection is established, it spreads to involve healthy muscle undamaged by previous trauma or ischemia.

The incubation period is usually 1 to 4 days but may vary from 3 hr to 6 weeks or longer. The earliest symptom is sudden, severe pain in the injured part. The distal portion of an involved limb becomes cold and edematous within a few hours, and eventually pulseless and gangrenous. The wound drains a watery, brown, or hemorrhagic material which may have a peculiar sweet odor. The appearance of the wound is usually not that of a pyogenic inflammatory lesion. Depending on the duration of the process, the surrounding skin may be normal, white, and tense, or dusky brown and reddish. Vesicles or hemorrhagic bullae may develop, particularly in *C. septicum* infections. Gas is usually not detectable in the tissues by palpation except in advanced lesions; although it is visible easily by x-ray. Occasionally, tiny bubbles may be seen in the discharge from the wound, and rarely, crepitation can be detected at an early stage by auscultation with the stethoscope. The involved muscle appears dark red or black and may herniate through the wound.

Systemic manifestations developing shortly after onset of severe pain and swelling of an injured extremity strongly suggest gas gangrene. The patient is prostrated, pale, and motionless but is usually well oriented, alert, and extremely apprehensive. The temperature usually does not exceed 101°F and may be normal. As the illness progresses, there may be anorexia, vomiting, profuse watery or bloody diarrhea, and eventually circulatory collapse. The pulse rate usually exceeds 120 beats per minute and is elevated out of proportion to the temperature. Massive intravascular hemolysis is rare in patients with clostridial myositis. Pericardial effusion is sometimes noted. Delirium and coma may precede death, but more commonly the patient dies suddenly several days after onset of illness, often during surgery or anesthesia. Acute renal failure is occasionally a late complication.

Gas gangrene has been described after hypodermic injection, especially injection of epinephrine. Minor trauma also occasionally activates clostridial spores dormant in scar tissue and leads to development of myonecrosis years after original injury.

Gas gangrene must be differentiated from nonclostridial infections of gangrenous limbs caused by anaerobic streptococci or aerobic gas-forming coliform bacilli.

Clostridial Cellulitis. This is a relatively benign infection of skin and subcutaneous tissues that occurs in a small proportion of wounds contaminated with pathogenic clostridia. The disease is characterized by spreading necrosis of superficial tissues and a profuse, foul-smelling, brown seripurulent exudate. Gas, which crepitates on palpation, invariably forms in the subcutaneous tissues and may involve an entire limb or form a localized gas pocket. In clostridial cellulitis, the underlying skeletal muscle is not involved, pain is not severe, and the only systemic manifestations are slight fever and moderate tachycardia. It can usually be differentiated from group A streptococcal cellulitis by the presence of subcutaneous gas and the absence of erythema.

Postabortal and Puerperal Sepsis. Uterine infections with *C. perfringens* usually occur after incomplete abortions induced under unsterile conditions and occasionally after spontaneous abortions, prolonged labor at term, ruptured membranes, or operative interference with pregnancy. The organisms presumably invade the damaged endometrium through the retained products of conception. The earliest symptoms may be related to instrumentation and consist of metrorrhagia, suprapubic and back pain, chills, and fever. Fever of 100 to 103°F, often with chills, usually recurs several days after abortion, but the incubation period can be as short as 6 hr. Vaginal bleeding is almost invariably present, and there is often a brown, foul-smelling vaginal discharge containing necrotic tissue. The cervix is soft and patulous, and the uterus and adnexae are usually very tender. The lower abdominal wall is often tense, or signs of generalized peritonitis may be present, secondary to perforation of the uterus or parametrial extension of infection. Nausea, vomiting, and profuse diarrhea are often prominent.

Systemic manifestations usually appear with dramatic suddenness. Massive intravascular hemolysis, accompanied by hemoglobinemia, hemoglobinuria, and jaundice, is often the most striking feature of the disease. Icterus may appear within hours after onset of illness. As in gas gangrene, the clinical picture may be dominated by circulatory collapse with hypotension, extreme tachycardia, cyanosis, hyperpnea, and pulmonary edema. Despite severe prostration, the patient is frequently well oriented, alert, and apprehensive. The mortality rate in postabortal or puerperal sepsis caused by *C. perfringens* is 40 to 70 percent. Death may occur a few hours after onset or be delayed for several days. Acute renal failure secondary to shock, dehydration, or hemolysis occurs frequently.

Unusual local complications of the uterine infection are gas gangrene of the vagina and rectum and clostridial cellulitis of the anterior abdominal wall following cesarean section or hysterectomy. At times, the infectious process is confined to the endometrium and myometrium with intrauterine gas formation (physometra).

Diseases to be considered in the *differential diagnosis* include perforated uterus, ruptured ectopic pregnancy, ingestion of toxic abortifacients, streptococcal or staphylococcal puerperal sepsis, pelvic thrombophlebitis with septic pulmonary emboli, acute hepatic necrosis of pregnancy, and sickle-cell crisis.

Clostridium Perfringens Food Poisoning. Meat and meat products contaminated with *C. perfringens* are frequently responsible for outbreaks of acute gastroenteritis. The strains of *C. perfringens* that cause food poisoning differ from those causing gas gangrene by forming spores that resist boiling for 1 to 4 hr. These strains are widespread in nature, and have been isolated from a high proportion of raw meat samples, from animal feces, and from stools of 2 to 5 percent of normal human beings.

Typical symptoms of diarrhea with abdominal pain develop 8 to 24 hr after ingestion of meat, stew, or soup which has been stored at a warm temperature for several hours after cooking. Nausea is common but vomiting is rare. Systemic manifestations are usually absent, and recovery is uneventful after 12 to 24 hr.

Clostridium perfringens food poisoning can be reproduced experimentally in man by feeding the actively growing organisms. However, gastroenteritis does not occur after ingestion of bacteria-free filtrates of cultures of food-poisoning strains.

A severe form of clostridial infection termed "enteritis necrotans" was observed in Germany after World War II. This disease was characterized by hemorrhagic necrosis of the small intestine, bloody diarrhea, severe dehydration, shock, and death. A similar infection termed "necrotizing jejunitis" has been described in natives of New Guinea who had eaten inadequately cooked pork.

Miscellaneous Clostridial Infections. Clostridia can be isolated not infrequently from bile obtained at elective cholecystectomy in patients without symptoms of clostridial infection. Clostridial cellulitis or myonecrosis may occasionally follow surgical procedures, particularly surgery on the gastrointestinal tract or gallbladder. Pathogenic clostridia are occasionally introduced into the abdomen, thoracic cavity, or cranium through penetrating wounds. Primary pneumonia in the absence of a penetrating wound or distant focus has been described. Clostridial pleurisy may involve the underlying lung but is usually an indolent localized infection with minimal systemic manifestations. Meningitis is usually secondary to a puncture wound of the skull and is often associated with a necrotizing cerebritis. Clostridial peritonitis may follow perforation of the gallbladder, appendix, or other viscus and is usually rapidly fatal. Clostridial septicemia occurs occasionally in patients with leukemia or other neoplastic processes who are treated with antimetabolites and antiinflammatory glucocorticoids. The primary infection is in the gastrointestinal tract, which is usually the site of extensive neoplastic disease. Cystitis with pneumaturia, gaseous cholecystitis, endocarditis, and bursitis after needle aspiration are other examples of rare clostridial infections.

LABORATORY FINDINGS. The diagnosis of gas gangrene, clostridial cellulitis, postabortal sepsis, or other clostridial infections is based primarily on clinical criteria. Smears of wound exudate, uterine scrapings, or cervical discharge may show abundant large gram-positive rods, as well as other organisms. Spores are rarely observed in smears of exudates. Thioglycollate broth, deep meat broth, and blood-agar plates incubated in an anaerobic jar should be inoculated for definitive identification of specific clostridia. However, interpretation of positive wound cultures is difficult because clostridia are frequent contaminants. *Clostridium perfringens* bacteremia is common in postabortal infections but rare in gas gangrene.

Polymorphonuclear leukocytosis occurs frequently in gas gangrene and invariably in postabortal sepsis; total blood leukocyte counts range from 15,000 to 40,000 cells per mm and occasionally exceed 60,000 cells per mm. Marked thrombocytopenia develops in about 50 percent of patients with clostridial sepsis. The urine frequently contains protein and casts. Renal insufficiency may lead to severe uremia.

X-ray examination sometimes provides the first clue leading to the correct diagnosis by revealing the presence of gas in muscle, subcutaneous tissue, or uterus; however, demonstration of gas in tissues is not diagnostic

of clostridial infection. Other bacteria, especially *Aerobacter* or *Escherichia,* may be responsible for gas production, and occasionally air is sucked into a wound at the time of penetrating injury.

Profound alterations of circulating erythrocytes are common in postabortal sepsis but are much less frequent in other clostridial infection. Hemolytic anemia may develop with almost unbelievable rapidity; the red blood cell count occasionally decreases by 2 million cells per cu mm in less than 24 hr and is associated with hemoglobinemia, hemoglobinuria, and elevated levels of serum bilirubin. Spherocytosis, increased osmotic and mechanical fragility of the red blood cells, erythrophagocytosis, and methemoglobinemia have also been described.

TREATMENT. The traditional therapeutic approach to serious clostridial infection, such as diffuse, spreading myositis, is immediate surgical intervention with wide radical debridement followed by open drainage without closure. Early surgery not only aids diagnosis, but permits decompression of fascial compartments and excision of devitalized muscle and may obviate amputation. A number of authorities feel that hyperbaric oxygen therapy has modified this traditional approach to gas gangrene by assuming priority over radical surgical debridement. Hyperbaric oxygenation produces impressive, almost immediate improvement in patients with gas gangrene with rapid disappearance of systemic toxicity and prompt arrest of local spread of the gangrenous infection. Opinion differs about whether conservative debridement should be carried out before or after hyperbaric oxygen therapy. There is uniform agreement in recommending that patients with serious clostridial infections be transported immediately to a facility equipped to administer hyperbaric oxygen therapy. Oxygen toxicity consequent to hyperbaric oxygenation may lead to convulsions in some patients.

Curettage of the uterus should be performed for diagnosis and treatment of postabortal clostridial infections. Hysterectomy should be considered if metritis is present and if the condition of the patient is deteriorating. Perforation of the uterus may be present in some cases despite the lack of typical clinical findings.

Simple excision and adequate drainage usually suffice for treating clostridial cellulitis.

Penicillin is the antibiotic of choice for all clostridial infections and should be administered in doses of 20 million units a day. Tetracycline is also active against most strains of *Clostridium* and has been recommended as an adjunct to penicillin therapy.

The efficacy of polyvalent gas gangrene antitoxin is controversial. Many centers have discontinued the use of antitoxin in the management of patients with suspected gas gangrene or clostridial postabortal sepsis.

Intravenous infusions of blood, plasma-volume expanders, fluids, and electrolytes are required to combat shock, anemia, and dehydration. Renal insufficiency should be treated in the same manner as acute tubular necrosis from other causes.

The most reliable protection against gas gangrene is early and adequate wound debridement. Antitoxin is ineffective as a prophylactic agent. The use of clostridial toxoids for prophylactic immunization of individuals in hazardous occupations awaits evaluation.

REFERENCES

Boggs, D. R., E. Frei, and L. B. Thomas: Clostridial Gas Gangrene and Septicemia in Four Patients with Leukemia, New Engl. J. Med., 259:1255, 1958.

Clostridium Welchii Food-Poisoning, Editorial, Brit. Med. J., 2:1604, 1963.

Hitchcock, C. R., J. J. Haglin, and O. Arner: Treatment of Clostridial Infections with Hyperbaric Oxygen, Surgery, 63:759, 1967.

MacLennan, J. D.: The Histotoxic Clostridial Infections of Man, Bact. Rev., 26:177, 1962.

Mahn, E., and L. M. Dantuono: Postabortal Septicotoxemia Due to *Clostridium Welchii.* Seventy-five Cases from the Maternity Hospital, Santiago, Chile, 1948–1952, Am. J. Obstet. Gynecol., 70:604, 1955.

Murrell, T. G. C., L. Roth, J. Egerton, J. Samels, and P. D. Walker: Pig-Bel: Enteritis Necroticans: A Study in Diagnosis and Management, Lancet, 1:217, 1966.

Trippel, O. H., A. N. Ruggie, C. J. Staley, and J. VanElk: Hyperbaric Oxygenation in the Management of Gas Gangrene, Surg. Clin. N. A., 47:17, 1967.

173 CHOLERA
Charles C. J. Carpenter

DEFINITION. Cholera is an acute illness which results from colonization of the small bowel by *Vibrio cholerae.* The disease is characterized by its epidemic occurrence and the production of massive diarrhea with rapid depletion of extracellular fluid and electrolyte.

ETIOLOGY AND EPIDEMIOLOGY. *Vibrio cholerae* is a curved, aerobic, gram-negative bacillus with a single polar flagellum. It is rapidly motile and possesses both O and H antigens. Serologic identification is based on differences in the polysaccharide O antigens.

Cholera has been endemic in the Gangetic Delta of West Bengal and East Pakistan, and is often epidemic throughout South and Southeast Asia. The most recent pandemic spread of this disease, from 1961 to 1966, extended from the Celebes northward to Korea and eastward to Iraq and Southern Russia. The last major epidemic of cholera in the Western Hemisphere occurred during 1866–1867.

Several well-studied epidemics have clearly been waterborne, but direct contamination of food by infected feces probably contributes to spread during major outbreaks. Poor sanitation appears to be primarily responsible for the continuing presence of cholera, but as yet undefined host factors may also play an important role.

A chronic gallbladder carrier state has been observed in 4 to 5 percent of convalescent cholera patients. These chronic vibrio carriers may explain the persistence of the disease in endemic areas and also may provide a vehicle for spread outside of these areas. The basis for the annual cholera epidemics throughout the Gangetic Delta

and for the periodic outbreaks throughout the remainder of South and Southeast Asia has, however, not been clearly delineated.

PATHOGENESIS. *Vibrio cholerae* produces an exotoxin which appears to be responsible for all known pathophysiologic aberration in cholera. This exotoxin causes secretion of isotonic fluid by all segments of the small bowel, but has no major effect on electrolyte absorption from the gut. The exotoxin-induced electrolyte secretion occurs in the absence of any demonstrable histologic damage to gut epithelial cells or to the capillary endothelial cells of the lamina propria. The former erroneous belief that extensive gut mucosal sloughing was a primary lesion in cholera was based upon autopsy studies. It is now clear that the observed intestinal denudation was secondary either to postmortem autolysis or to hypovolemic shock and played no etiologic role in fluid loss from the gut. Precise studies have demonstrated that the adult cholera stool is nearly isotonic, with sodium and chloride concentrations slightly less than those of plasma, a bicarbonate concentration approximately twice that of plasma, and a potassium concentration three to five times that of plasma. Disease caused by all known strains of V. *cholerae* results in the same stool electrolyte pattern. The basic pathophysiologic defect in cholera is extracellular fluid depletion with resultant hypovolemic shock, base-deficit acidosis, and progressive potassium depletion. There is no convincing evidence that the cholera vibrio invades any tissue, nor has the exotoxin been shown, in human disease, to affect any organ other than the small intestine.

MANIFESTATIONS. The extent of incubation period has not been defined, but generally is from 6 to 48 hr. This is followed by the abrupt onset of watery, generally painless diarrhea. In the more severe cases, the initial diarrheal stool may be in excess of 1,000 ml, and several liters of isotonic fluid may be lost within hours, leading rapidly to profound shock. Vomiting generally follows, but occasionally precedes the onset of diarrhea; the vomiting is characteristically effortless and not preceded by nausea. As saline depletion progresses, severe muscle cramps, commonly involving the calves, occur.

When first seen, the typical cholera patient is cyanotic, with pinched facies, scaphoid abdomen, poor skin turgor, and thready or absent peripheral pulses. The voice is faint, high-pitched, and often inaudible, and there are tachycardia, hypotension, and varying degrees of tachypnea. In all epidemics there are mild cases in which gastrointestinal fluid loss is not severe enough to require hospitalization.

The disease runs its course in 2 to 7 days, and subsequent manifestations depend on the adequacy of electrolyte repletion therapy. With prompt fluid and electrolyte repletion, recovery is remarkably rapid, and mortality exceptionally rare. However, if therapy is inadequate, the mortality is quite high. The important causes of death are hypovolemic shock, uncompensated metabolic acidosis, and uremia, which may follow acute tubular necrosis.

LABORATORY FINDINGS. In epidemics or in endemic

areas, the clinical picture should arouse strong suspicion immediately. The most reliable technique for identification of *V. cholerae* consists of direct plating of a sample of cholera stool on bile salt, gelatin-tellurite-taurocholate (GTT), or thiosulfate-citrate-bile salt-sucrose (TCBS) agar. On bile salt or GTT agar the organisms appear as typical translucent colonies within 24 hr. On TCBS agar, *V. cholorae* appears as distinct large yellow colonies at 24 hr. Further classification requires agglutination with type-specific antiserums. In mild or convalescent cases recovery of vibrios may be important to initial enrichment for 6 hr in alkaline peptone water followed by subculture on bile salt, GTT, or TCBS agar. Rapid diagnosis is possible either by directly observing immobilization of vibrios by type-specific antiserums with dark-field or phase microscopy or by identifying the organisms by immunofluorescent methods.

THERAPY. Successful therapy requires only prompt and adequate replacement of gastrointestinal losses of saline and alkali. Isotonic saline solution and isotonic sodium lactate (or bicarbonate), administered in a 2:1 ratio, should be rapidly infused, at 50 to 100 ml per min, until a strong pulse has been restored. The same fluids should subsequently be infused in quantities equal to the gastrointestinal losses. If losses cannot be measured accurately, intravenous fluids should be given at a rate sufficient to maintain a normal radial pulse and normal skin turgor. Overhydration can be avoided by careful observation of neck venous filling and auscultation of the lungs. Close observation is mandatory during the acute phase of the illness, because the cholera patient can lose as much as 1 liter of isotonic fluid per hr during the first 24 hr of the disease. Inadequate or delayed restoration of fecal fluid losses may result in a very high incidence of acute renal failure. Serious hypokalemic symptoms are rare in adults, and potassium repletion can usually be carried out orally; the dose is approximately 15 mEq potassium for each liter of stool produced. Hypokalemia contributes significantly, however, to the morbidity and mortality in inadequately treated pediatric cholera, and potassium, 8 to 12 mEq per liter, should be included in the intravenous fluids administered to pediatric patients.

Although adequate intravenous saline and alkali repletion alone results in rapid recovery of virtually all adult cholera patients, a dramatic reduction in the duration and volume of the diarrhea, and early eradication of vibrios from the stool, may be effected by antibiotic therapy. Oral tetracycline, 500 mg every 6 hr for the first 48 hr of treatment, has been most successful. Other antibiotics, including chloramphenicol and furazolidone, are also of value, but both appear to be slightly less effective than tetracycline.

PROGNOSIS. Under ideal conditions and with prompt and adequate fluid replacement, mortality approaches zero and significant sequelae are rare. Unfortunately, death rates as high as 60 percent still occur, especially during the initial phases of certain outbreaks. This high mortality reflects lack of pyrogen-free intravenous fluids in remote areas, the difficulties of initiating treatment promptly when large numbers of cases are occurring in poverty-striken populations, and the compromises which may have to be made under emergency conditions.

PREVENTION. Immunization by standard commercial vaccine, containing 10 billion killed organisms per ml, provides significant protection for a limited (4- to 6-month) period. Immunization with toxoid provides significant protection in experimental animals, but toxoid has not yet been tested in man. Careful hygiene provides the only sure protection against cholera.

REFERENCES

Carpenter, C. C. J., P. P. Mitra, and R. B. Sack: Clinical Studies in Asiatic Cholera I–VI, Bull. Johns Hopkins Hosp., 118:165, 1966.

Gangarosa, E. F., W. R. Beisel, C. Benyajati, H. Sprinz, and P. Piyaratn: The Nature of the Gastrointestinal Lesion in Asiatic Cholera and Its Relation to Pathogenesis: A Biopsy Study, Am. J. Trop. Med., 9:125, 1960.

Greenough, W. B. III, R. S. Gordon, Jr., I. S. Rosenberg, and B. I. Davies: Tetracycline in the Treatment of Cholera, Lancet, 1:335, 1964.

Wallace, C. K., P. N. Anderson, T. C. Brown, S. R. Khanra, G. W. Lewis, N. F. Pierce, S. N. Sanyal, G. V. Segre, and R. H. Waldman: Optimal Antibiotic Therapy in Cholera, Bull. World Health Organ., 39:239, 1968.

Watten, R. H., F. M. Morgan, Y. N. Songkhla, B. Vanikiati, and R. A. Phillips: Water and Electrolyte Studies in Cholera, J. Clin. Invest., 38:1879, 1959.

Section 9

Mycobacterial Diseases

174 TUBERCULOSIS

William W. Stead

DEFINITION. Tuberculosis is a necrotizing bacterial infection with protean manifestations and wide distribution.

In man, the lungs are most commonly affected, but lesions may occur also in the kidneys, bones, lymph nodes, and meninges or be disseminated throughout the body. Two stages of the infection are recognized: (1) primary tuberculosis, in which tubercle bacilli invade a host which has no specific immunity and which undergoes at least partial spontaneous healing as specific immunity develops; (2) postprimary or adult tuberculosis (often erroneously called "reinfection tuberculosis"), which is the result of progression of the infection in spite of specific immunity. Progression may occur shortly after primary infection or after a delay of years or even decades. In the Western world, where bovine tuberculosis has been controlled, the portal of entry in man is almost exclusively the lung.

HISTORY. Some human races (Caucasian, Mongolian) have lived with tubercle bacilli throughout much of their evolution. Lesions of bone typical of tuberculosis were noted in Neolithic man and Egyptian mummies. This is indicative of a cardinal feature of the infection: a tendency toward healing in its primary stage and chronic tissue destruction in its later stage. African, American Indian, and Eskimo peoples have had contact with the disease over a much shorter period. In them, it behaves much more like an acute infection and has a higher mortality in the primary and early postprimary phases and less tendency to develop an equilibrium between the host and parasite.

Tuberculosis was named because it tends to form nodules, or "tubercles," on serous surfaces and in tissues. For many years the chronic form (then often called phthisis or consumption) was thought to be a degenerative or hereditary disease unrelated to primary tuberculosis, which was obviously an infection. Laennec was the first to consider the chronic form as merely a later development in the same infection, but even Villemin's demonstration (1865) that material from both types of disease produced tuberculosis in animals and Koch's identification of the organism (1882) failed to convince their contemporaries. The validity of Laennec's clinical observations has been born out, and the "unitary concept" of tuberculosis is now accepted.

There has been a great drop in the prevalence of tuberculosis in the economically developed countries. The death rate from tuberculosis had already begun to fall by 1900 coincident with improvement in nutrition and standard of living. For the individual with active tuberculosis, however, the most important development occurred in 1944 with the discovery of streptomycin by Waksman and his associates. Hinshaw and Feldman showed the effectiveness of streptomycin against tuberculosis in animals and man. Lehmann discovered para-aminosalicylic acid (PAS), which was shown later to have an effect upon the disease when used with other agents. Isoniazid (INH) was discovered independently in 1951 by three groups of chemists and subsequently has been the most effective tuberculostatic agent discovered. Ethambutol (EMB) appears to have great potential in the treatment of cases in whom the bacilli have developed resistance to the other drugs.

ETIOLOGY. *Mycobacterium tuberculosis* is a rod of 2.0 to 4.0 μ in length and 0.3 μ in thickness. Its distinguishing staining property, i.e., resistance to decolorization by acid alcohol when stained with basic fuchsin, is related to the waxy component of the cell wall, probably specifically to its content of mycolic acid. "Acid-fastness" is dependent upon the structural integrity of the bacillus because it is lost when the organisms are damaged by grinding but is not affected by prolonged extraction with fat solvents.

Tubercle bacilli are strict aerobes and thrive best when there is a PO_2 of 100 mm Hg or more and a PCO_2 of about 40 mm Hg, and the organs most commonly affected by tuberculosis are those with relatively high oxygen tension. Metastatic foci are most common in the apexes of the lungs, where the PO_2 is in the range of 120 to 130 mm Hg in the upright position, followed by the kidney and the growing end of bones, where the PO_2 approximates 100 mm Hg. The liver and spleen, where the PO_2 is quite low, are rarely affected except in overwhelming disseminated infection.

Three strains of tubercle bacilli infect man: human, bovine, and avian. By far the greatest number of cases in the United States are caused by the human strain. Programs for eradication of bovine tuberculosis have been carried out with such vigor over the past 60 years that the disease now appears only sporadically in this country. Avian bacilli have little invasiveness for man.

Within the last 15 years several varieties of mycobacteria which resemble *M. tuberculosis* have been associated with chronic pulmonary infection (Chap. 176). The most common are *M. battey* and *M. kansasii*. In addition, certain pigmented mycobacteria (scotochromes) produce cervical adenitis in children (scrofula) and occasionally also chronic pulmonary lesions. These mycobacteria can be recognized in the laboratory by biochemical tests (nicotinic acid negative, catalase positive) and by lack of virulence for the guinea pig. The pathology in man produced by these related mycobacteria is indistinguishable from that of tuberculosis. However, they differ from *M. tuberculosis* in two important ways: transmission appears not to be airborne and they show little response to antituberculosis drugs.

TRANSMISSION. Most cases of tuberculosis among adults develop because of late recrudescence of dormant infection and are quite independent of recent exposure. The liquid caseum from a cavity in such a case abounds with tubercle bacilli, which are excreted in aerosolized droplets during coughing, sneezing, and talking. Droplets larger than 10 μ are usually caught on the mucociliary blanket and cleared from the lung without harm, but droplets of smaller size may reach the respiratory bronchiole and deposit the bacilli beyond the protective mucous blanket. There the organisms may invade tissues and establish an infection in the susceptible host. Persons who have been infected previously are sufficiently immune that naturally acquired inocula can be handled effectively by immune macrophages which lyse the invading organisms.

Transmission is usually due to close indoor contact of a susceptible (tuberculin-negative) host with a patient who is excreting tubercle bacili in large numbers (positive sputum smear). *Persons with primary tuberculosis excrete very few organisms and need not be considered contagious.* Bacilli often can be cultured from the dust in the room of a person with cavitary tuberculosis, but house dust is a very poor vehicle because of its large and irregular particles and their electrostatic charge. There is no evidence that tuberculosis is spread by hands, eating utensils, or fomites.

Tubercle bacilli are killed readily by boiling and by pasteurization at 60°C for 20 min. In countries where bovine tuberculosis has not been eradicated, pasteurization is especially important. Milk from a tuberculous cow often contains millions of bacilli per milliliter. In all likelihood the small number of organisms sprayed on food by a tuberculous food handler is no more dangerous than those from any other person excreting tubercle bacilli into the environment.

PREVALENCE AND INCIDENCE. There has been a great fall in prevalence of tuberculosis in the United States during the last 60 years. Early in this century surveys using the tuberculin skin test and autopsies indicated that over 80 percent of the population was infected *before* the age of twenty. In an autopsy study in 1946, Medlar found evidence of tuberculosis in 80 percent of the persons over the age of fifty living in New York City. In 1968 only 5 to 10 percent of young adults reacted to tuberculin (except in some urban areas), whereas about 50 percent of the persons over the age of fifty react. The declining incidence of the infection is most apparent among children and young adults and is due to a reduction in the number of open infectious cases, which, in turn, is attributable to an improved standard of living, reduced risk of late progression of infection, and prompter recognition and treatment of contagious cases.

LATENT INFECTION. The majority of persons who harbor tubercle bacilli have latent or dormant ("healed") tuberculosis. The terms *latent* or *dormant* are preferable to "healed," because in most instances the "scars" retain the potential for reactivation. Scars within the lung may remain dormant for many years and show no changes for years on roentgenogram only to reactivate and produce active infection. Figure 174-1 illustrates the most common sites in which dormant metastatic lesions may persist after the primary infection and undergo late progression to produce chronic postprimary tuberculosis.

MORBIDITY AND MORTALITY. The incidence of clinical disease must be distinguished from prevalence as shown by the tuberculin reaction. Of the 25 million persons in the United States who react to tuberculin, only 90,000 are known to have active tuberculosis and 230,000 have recovered from clinically apparent tuberculosis and are classified as "inactive" cases. Many of the remainder harbor dormant viable bacilli in latent foci but have not developed active disease. The morbidity rate in the United States was 24 per 100,000 in 1966, a reduction from 29 in 1961 and 53 in 1953.

Figures 174-2 and 174-3 illustrate some important facts concerning the natural history of tuberculosis in man. In the analysis of mortality from tuberculosis by 10-year cohorts (Fig. 174-2), it can be seen that the only significant mortality occurs among the older persons in the community, those who were most commonly infected early in life. Furthermore, the mortality experienced by

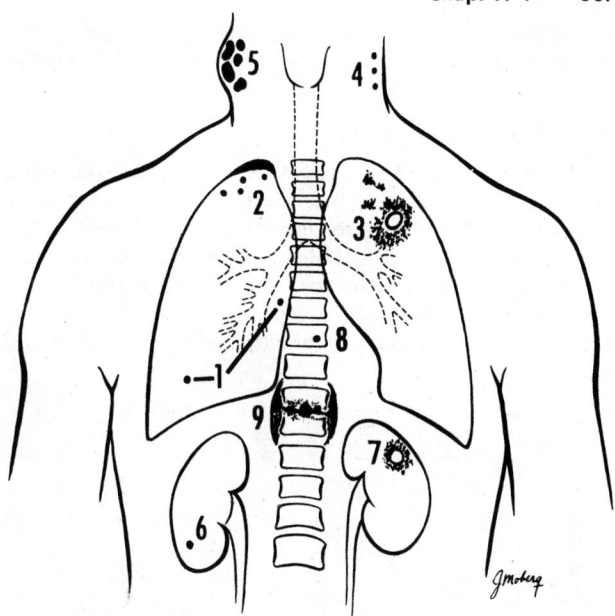

Fig. 174-1. Sites most commonly affected by tuberculosis:

1. Healed, calcified primary infection in right lung and hilar node (Ghon complex).

2. "Apical cap" and nodular scars (Simon foci) in right upper lobe due to hematogenous seeding during primary infection.

3. Recrudescence and coalescence of Simon foci, producing chronic inflammation and caseation necrosis (cavitation).

4. Dormant focus of tuberculosis in cervical lymph nodes, seeded by lymphatic drainage during primary infection.

5. Active tuberculosis in cervical lymph nodes, producing chronic inflammation and caseation necrosis.

6. Dormant focus of tuberculosis in kidney, seeded during primary infection.

7. Recrudescence of dormant renal focus producing inflammation and caseation necrosis. The male genital tract may become infected by organisms shed by a renal cavity.

8. Dormant focus of tuberculosis in vertebra.

9. Recrudescence of focus in vertebra, producing inflammation and caseation necrosis, with destruction of intervertebral disc.

(W. W. Stead: "Understanding Tuberculosis Today: A Handbook for Patients," Milwaukee, Marquette University Press, 1968.)

the cohorts to which these older persons belong was even greater in earlier years, particularly in their young adult life (Fig. 174-3).

Figure 174-2A shows the morbidity (active cases) from tuberculosis in Wisconsin in 1963, and morbidity was greatest in the older members of the population. However, when the age-specific morbidity is plotted against the age-specific prevalence (tuberculin reactors), there is a sharp peak in young adult life. The reduction in the number of tuberculin reactors among young adults accounts for the elimination of the peak of morbidity for that period in the general population. These data suggest that late reactivation of the original tuberculous infection is important in the pathogenesis of chronic tuberculosis.

Mortality has fallen steadily over the past 65 years. Tuberculosis has dropped from the leading cause of death with over 200 deaths per 100,000 in 1906 to 3.8 per 100,000 in 1966. Tuberculosis contributes to more deaths than the figures indicate because pulmonary scarring is important in the pathogenesis of cor pulmonale.

IMMUNITY

NATURAL RESISTANCE. The Caucasian and Mongolian races have a distinct natural resistance to tuberculosis consisting of the ability to develop an immune response to the infection, which enables them to recover from the primary infection. In them, primary infection usually subsides spontaneously; and reactivation generally produces a chronic disease which is characterized by cavitation and scarring.

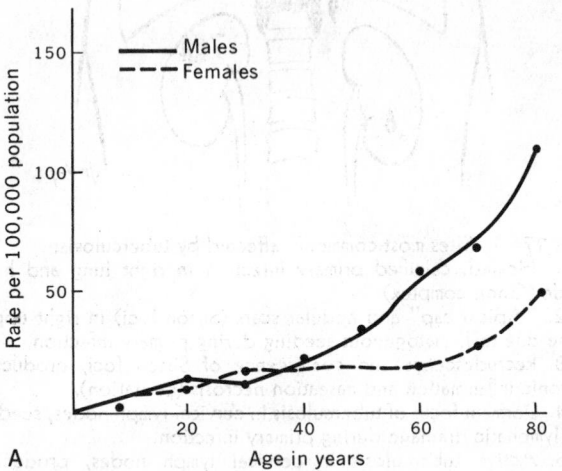

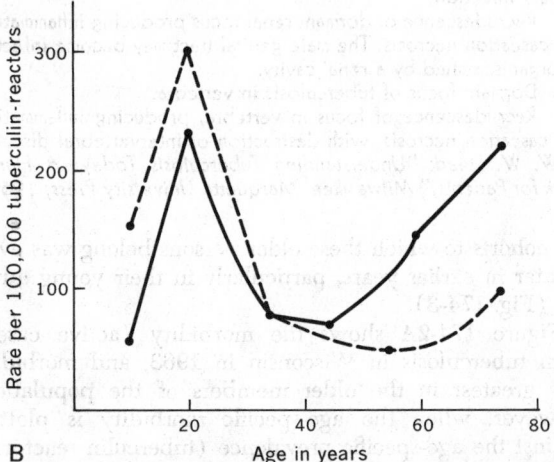

Fig. 174-2. *A.* Tuberculosis case rate per 100,000 population for each age group in Wisconsin, 1963. There is no peak in the young adult period because of the paucity of reactors to tuberculin of this age in Wisconsin today. (*Wisconsin Board of Health, Madison.*)

B. Tuberculosis case rate per 100,000 *tuberculin reactors* in each age group for Ontario, 1960. The predilection for reactors to develop active tuberculosis in young adult life and in old age can readily be seen. (*Grzybowski and Allen: Amer. Rev. Resp. Dis., 90:707, 1964; reproduced with permission of author and publisher.*)

Africans, American Indians, and Eskimos were spared tuberculous infection until extensive contact began with members of the white race in whom chronic tuberculosis was common. These people have less ability to develop an effective immune response to primary infection, and in them the infection tends to be more rapidly progressive.

SPECIFIC (ACQUIRED) IMMUNITY. Despite the immunity that infected animals have against reinfection, specific antibodies to tubercle bacilli have been difficult to demonstrate, and one of the unsolved problems in tuberculosis is why immune individuals develop progressive infection years or even decades after recovery from primary infection. Various metabolic and nutritional factors appear to impair immunity and release long-dormant bacilli.

TUBERCULIN HYPERSENSITIVITY. The most readily obtained evidence of a past or present infection with tubercle bacilli is the finding of hypersensitivity to tuberculin (protein derivative of the broth in which tubercle bacilli have been grown). Epidemiologic evidence strongly suggests that tuberculin hypersensitivity indicates that living tubercle bacilli are present. Whether the lesion in which they lie is active or inactive is often difficult to determine with certainty.

PATHOGENESIS AND PATHOLOGIC ANATOMY

PRIMARY TUBERCULOSIS. In the nonimmune subject tubercle bacilli can gain entrance to the body by several routes: lung, gastrointestinal tract, and direct cutaneous or percutaneous inoculation (as with an accident at the autopsy table). For practical purposes the only route that is of importance in the United States is the lung. The majority of primary lesions are in the lower two-thirds of the lungs, where ventilation is best and exposure to contamination of inspired air the greatest. Because they produce no toxins and no tissue reaction, tubercle bacilli initially are free to multiply without deterrence. They reach regional (hilar) nodes and even the bloodstream before their progress is inhibited by the gradual development of specific immunity over a period of several weeks. At this time the characteristic tissue reaction develops with epithelioid cell granulomata and caseation necrosis in the primary lesion, regional lymph nodes, and any site to which the bacilli have spread. The number of bacilli drops drastically with the appearance of caseation necrosis, suggesting that the process of caseation is important in the defense of the host. Thereafter the usual course of the primary infection is healing by a combination of resolution, fibrosis, and calcification.

SECONDARY STAGE. In the course of primary infection tubercle bacilli reach the general circulation in varying numbers. This event is marked only by fever and mild symptoms and is recognized as tuberculosis only when a patient is being observed closely because of a known recent exposure to tuberculosis. This stage is important in the pathogenesis of tuberculosis because it is the time when bacilli reach distant sites to establish metastatic foci of infection, which are the seeds from which post-primary chronic tuberculosis appears.

While bacilli presumably reach all organs in the secondary stage, they establish lesions with frequency in only a limited number of sites, which have one feature in common: a high tissue oxygen tension. The apex of the lung has the highest oxygen tension in the body and is the most frequent site for development of significant metastatic foci. It seems paradoxical that such a high PO_2 should exist in the poorly ventilated apexes, but this is due to a paucity of pulmonary circulation to that region when the body is in the upright position resulting in a high ventilation-perfusion ratio. Occasionally such metastatic foci progress and produce destructive tuberculosis in a short time, but more commonly the appearance of specific immunity causes the lesions to regress, scar, and become dormant. Such localized apical scars are often referred to as *Simon foci*.

Other sites at which distant metastatic lesions may develop with some frequency are the kidney, brain, and spine and long bones if infection occurs before closure of the epiphyses. Lesions in lymph nodes are probably the result of heavy seeding due to local drainage of the site of primary infection.

LATENT (DORMANT) INFECTION. Whenever a tuberculous lesion regresses and heals, the infection enters a latent phase in which infection persists without producing illness. Latent infection may remain dormant for life but may develop into active disease at any time.

TERTIARY STAGE (POSTPRIMARY TUBERCULOSIS). Chronic fibrocaseous tuberculosis may develop whenever a dormant lesion persists (Fig. 174-1). The most common site is the apical portion of the lung. At this stage bloodstream invasion is uncommon; the disease is characterized by localized areas of inflammation, necrosis abounding in bacilli, and proliferation of fibrous tissue.

OUTLOOK FOR PERSONS INFECTED WITH TUBERCULOSIS

Of new tuberculous infections, revealed by conversion of tuberculin reaction from negative to positive, 5 to 15 percent progress to serious disease within 5 years if left untreated. The risk of direct progression varies with age: it is greatest when infection begins in the first year of life or in young adults and adolescents. Among those remaining well for 5 years, a further 3 to 5 percent may be expected to develop late recrudescence at some time during life. The total morbidity in persons infected with *M. tuberculosis* is 8 to 20 percent. Both the early and the late appearance of chronic tuberculosis can be prevented if prompt treatment with INH is given when tuberculin "conversion" is discovered.

MANIFESTATIONS

I. Primary Infection

Uncomplicated primary tuberculosis often produces no significant clinical illness. It is usually diagnosed only

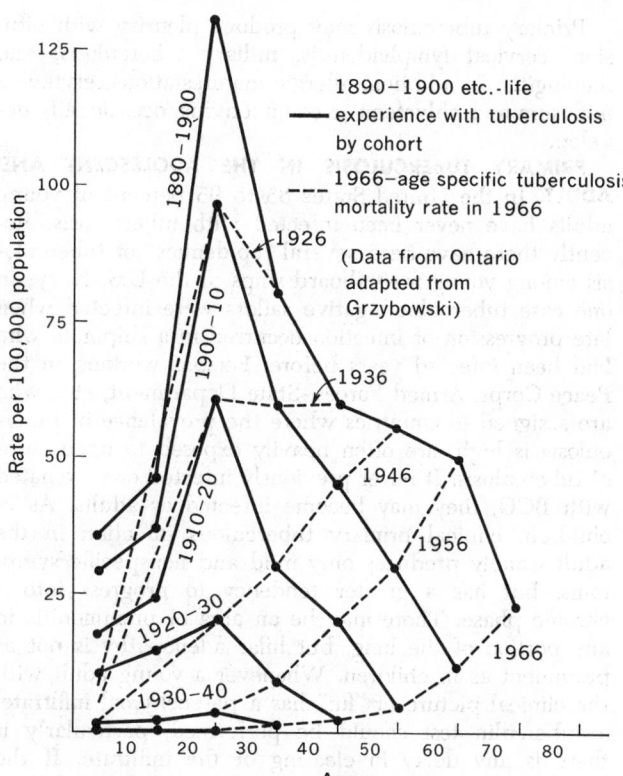

Fig. 174-3. Age-specific mortality from tuberculosis by 10-year cohorts, beginning with that of 1890–1900 (persons who were age 70–80 in 1966). Among earlier cohorts when the majority were infected in childhood, the peak death rate occurred during early adult life and declined steadily thereafter. In the later cohorts when few were infected during childhood, not many died as young adults. As shown also in Fig. 174-2A, the highest mortality rate was among the oldest persons in 1966. Tuberculosis should disappear as a health hazard in economically developed countries with the death of the oldest cohorts, who serve as the major reservoir of infection. The paucity of infection in later cohorts will furnish fewer cases of active tuberculosis. (*Adapted from S. Grzybowski, and J. Marr: Can. Med. Assoc., 89:737, 1963; published with permission.*)

when contacts of an open case are examined or when it progresses to a serious form of disease. The incubation period is 4 to 6 weeks from the time of inoculation to appearance of mild fever and malaise and tuberculin hypersensitivity. Symptoms usually subside without specific therapy because of the appearance of adequate specific immunity. Occasionally, however, the infection progresses either in the lung or by dissemination through the bloodstream. This turn of events is extremely serious unless detected and treated without delay.

Massive hematogenous dissemination is most common in very young children. For this reason any child under the age of three years who reacts to tuberculin should be given appropriate long-term antituberculosis chemotherapy. In older children primary infection only rarely progresses to a fatal form and usually passes totally unnoticed. The principal danger arises later during adolescence or early adulthood when the infection may undergo late progression.

Primary tuberculosis may produce pleurisy with effusion, cervical lymphadenitis, miliary tuberculosis, and meningitis. In addition, allergic manifestations, erythema nodosum and phlyctenular conjunctivitis, occasionally develop.

PRIMARY TUBERCULOSIS IN THE ADOLESCENT AND ADULT. In the United States 85 to 95 percent of young adults have never been infected with tuberculosis. Recently there have been several "epidemics" of tuberculosis among young men aboard ships of the U.S. Navy; in one case tuberculin-negative sailors were infected when late progression of infection occurred in a shipmate who had been infected years before. Persons working in the Peace Corps, Armed Forces, State Department, etc., who are assigned to countries where the prevalence of tuberculosis is high, are often heavily exposed to open cases of tuberculosis. If never previously infected or vaccinated with BCG, they may become infected as adults. As in children, clinical primary tuberculous infection in the adult usually produces only mild and nonspecific symptoms, but has a greater tendency to progress into a chronic phase. There may be an area of pneumonitis in any portion of the lung, but hilar adenopathy is not as prominent as in children. Whenever a young adult with the clinical picture of "flu" has a parenchymal infiltrate, a tuberculin test should be performed, particularly if there is any delay in clearing of the infiltrate. If the skin test is positive, the possibility of primary tuberculosis should be considered strongly because of the low incidence of positive reactions among young persons. The source of infection is usually an adult associate with cavitary tuberculosis.

II. Postprimary Tuberculosis

A. OF THE LUNGS. Chronic pulmonary tuberculosis may follow the primary infection directly or after a short, long, or very long period of dormancy (see Tertiary Stage in section on Pathogenesis and Pathologic Anatomy). Progressive disease has been observed to develop after 60 years of clinical dormancy. The most striking features of postprimary tuberculosis are (1) absence of recent exposure to an open case of tuberculosis (except in cases of direct progression from primary infection in adolescents and adults), (2) tendency to chronicity with liquefaction necrosis, and (3) production of fibrous tissue of repair. The last two phenomena are characteristic of the tissue responses in persons sensitized to tubercle bacilli. While the caseation necrosis of the primary stage is solid and paucibacillary, caseation produces liquefaction when it occurs in tissues previously sensitized. This liquid material contains abundant bacilli and may spread infection to other portions of the lungs and be aerosolized to contaminate the environment.

Symptoms. In most instances the onset of chronic pulmonary tuberculosis is insidious and the patient may be entirely asymptomatic. Many cases are discovered because a routine roentgenogram is taken as a part of a periodic health examination or upon admission to a hospital for some other illness.

The earliest symptoms are constitutional and probably result chiefly from the absorption of tuberculoprotein from the active lesion by the hypersensitive host. Abdominal symptoms may dominate the clinical picture. Fever is often present in the late afternoon or evening, but it is common for the patient to be unaware of it. A history of night sweats is merely a clue to the presence of an afternoon fever. It is common for the patient to be unaware of a fever as high as 102 to 103°F.

While fatigue and malaise may be noted by the patient, irritability, depression, or a need to rest at the end of the day, ascribed to excessive work, may be the only complaints.

Weight loss may precede symptoms, but is often passed off as being due to overwork or to voluntary caloric restriction. Often weight is well maintained until late in the course of the illness. When abdominal symptoms are present, anorexia may give rise to a rapid weight loss.

Headache may be noted occasionally, especially in the evening. Palpitation may occur during mild exertion. Menstruation is usually not disturbed until the disease is fairly far advanced when amenorrhea may develop.

Cough is frequent but not invariable and is often passed off as a "cigarette cough." When sputum is produced, it is usually odorless and green or yellow in color and is raised principally upon arising in the morning. Hemoptysis may accompany the cough and usually consists of streaked sputum with small amounts of blood.

In some patients the onset of pulmonary tuberculosis is relatively sudden, because of a rapid progression from a primary infection or from a massive spread from an area of liquefaction necrosis. A characteristic story is that the patient experiences a "bad cold" or "influenza" without awareness of any prior lung disease. The productive cough then persists while the constitutional symptoms partially abate, so that the patient feels that he is recovering. This situation may persist for several months before the patient notices enough constitutional symptoms to cause him to seek medical aid. When he does so, he may place more stress upon loss of weight or abdominal symptoms than upon the cough which he may attribute to smoking. Green or yellow sputum is often a clue that the cough is due to infection and not simply to smoking.

Physical and Roentgen Examinations. Early asymptomatic infiltrations due to tuberculosis are usually undetectable by physical examination, but may be extensive by x-ray. Crepitant inspiratory rales may be detected, especially when inspiration is preceded by full expiration and a small cough (posttussive rales). When larger lesions are present, especially with chronic cavitation, dullness to percussion and amphoric bronchial breath sounds may be elicited, but areas of recent excavation do not produce these signs. In tuberculous pneumonia the classical signs of pneumonia are present and even the white blood cell count may be elevated.

Long-standing tuberculosis with extensive fibrosis causes contraction and distortion of pulmonary tissue and of bronchi. In such instances, a wide variety of physical signs, such as bronchial breath sounds, coarse rales, deviation of the trachea, spasm and atrophy of various chest and neck muscles, and diminished movements of one hemithorax, may be noted. There is likely to be dullness over the apex of the involved lung.

However, because examination of the lungs in the early stages is so frequently unremarkable and the blood count and sedimentation rate are normal, *the importance of the chest roentgenogram in diagnosis of tuberculosis cannot be overemphasized.* In chronic tuberculosis the early infiltrate is usually in the apical and subapical areas. Cavitation is common but may require the use of planigraphy to demonstrate it. Because the chronic form of the disease is often a late manifestation of disseminated primary infection, nodular lesions are often present in the contralateral lung as well.

Of particular importance in the roentgen diagnosis is the comparison of the film with one or more examinations made months or years earlier, so that subtle changes can be detected in clinically dormant lesions. Because fibrous tissue does not change appreciably with time, any change in the lesions on serial films must be taken to indicate activity of the disease. Among 90 patients over the age of fifty with newly active chronic pulmonary tuberculosis, over 70 percent showed evidence of preexisting tuberculous scars. Comparison of films with previous examinations should become routine practice because it would permit detection and prophylactic treatment of slightly active lesions before liquefaction and spread of bacilli to other portions of the lungs and into the environment occur.

Other radiographic techniques which are of value in the proper evaluation of the lungs include *pulmonary oblique* views (taken at 20 to 25° rotation instead of 45 to 60°, as used for cardiac evaluation), sectional radiography (tomograms or planigrams), and the *apical lordotic* view, which shows the posterior segment of the upper lobe more clearly than the standard roentgenogram. The tomogram is of particular value in revealing the nodular and cavitary nature of indistinct pulmonary infiltrates.

Complications of Pulmonary Tuberculosis. Cavitation. When nodular lesions of tuberculosis become active and coalesce, areas of liquid necrosis develop. When necrosis includes a small bronchus, liquid material escapes into the bronchial tree and is expectorated, leaving a cavity within the lung parenchyma. At this stage, the sputum usually contains numerous tubercle bacilli.

Hemoptysis. In the majority of instances of bleeding from the lungs in tuberculosis, the blood arises from an ulceration of the bronchial mucosa and usually presents as streaks of bright red blood on the sputum. Bleeding usually subsides spontaneously if the patient lies quietly. Codeine in a dose of 15 mg or morphine, 8 mg, may be used to control cough. Many remedies have been advocated, but because bleeding usually stops spontaneously, it is difficult to demonstrate real effectiveness of any particular measure.

There is one type of hemoptysis which has a very different prognosis. When the blood is copious and dark (bluish red), its source is more likely a branch of the pulmonary artery, usually within the wall of a cavity. In the majority of instances the branches of the pulmonary artery in the vicinity of tuberculous cavities are thrombosed, but occasionally one remains open in the wall of a cavity, is eroded by the infection (Rasmussen's aneurysm), and may rupture. The majority of patients in whom this occurs exsanguinate before treatment can be administered, but if copious dark blood is expectorated and the patient survives, immediate resection of the cavitary area is indicated to prevent exsanguination.

Pleurisy with Effusion. The pleura overlying a tuberculous focus may become involved, resulting in pain on inspiration ("catch" in the side). Fibrous adhesions between the visceral and parietal pleural surfaces are usually the only residuals of such "dry pleurisy." A small caseous focus may erode through the visceral pleura and, in a hypersensitive host, produce pleurisy with effusion.

Tuberculous pleural effusion is most common in young adults between the ages of fifteen and twenty-five and occurs most commonly within the first 9 months after implantation of the primary infection. It frequently clears spontaneously, but this should not give a false sense of security because such a course is consistent with a tuberculous effusion. Pleural effusion may also develop in the course of chronic pulmonary tuberculosis (late recrudescence). The fluid is usually clear and light yellow in color. It is an exudate, which is characterized by lymphocytosis and high protein content (> 3 GM per 100 ml). The diagnosis is made best by needle biopsy of the parietal pleura. The management of unilateral tuberculous pleural effusion consists of the administration of effective antituberculous chemotherapy. When tuberculous effusion is bilateral, it is usually the result of disseminated tuberculosis and calls for prompt and vigorous chemotherapy with three effective agents.

The diagnosis of tuberculous pleural effusion is difficult because only about 20 to 25 percent of effusions yield tubercle bacilli upon culture and about an equal number of positive cultures result from gastric washings or sputum induced by inhalation of heated aerosol. Thus, in over 50 percent of the patients with tuberculous pleural effusion, bacteriologic proof of diagnosis is lacking at the time when therapy is most effective in preventing later development of overt tuberculosis. The percutaneous pleural biopsy has made a great contribution to the recognition of tuberculosis in the etiology of otherwise undiagnosed pleural effusion.

Tuberculous Pneumonia. The onset of tuberculosis occasionally is quite acute, resembling that of bacterial pneumonia. This form of tuberculosis is seen most often in Negroes, persons with diabetes, children with overwhelming primary infection, and elderly individuals in whom the lungs are flooded with bacilli discharged from an area of liquid necrosis. Chills, fever, productive cough, and pleuritic chest pain occur. Smear of the sputum usually reveals numerous tubercle bacilli.

Bronchopleural Fistula and Empyema. When a large caseous lesion erodes into the pleural space, the gross contamination often produces tuberculous empyema. The mechanism is the same as the production of exudative pleural effusion, but the extent of contamination is much greater. The caseous lesion may also erode a bronchus, giving rise to a *bronchopleural fistula* in addition to the empyema. Management is largely surgical and consists of establishing adequate drainage, in combination with the administration of three effective antituberculosis drugs.

Tuberculosis of Large Bronchi, Trachea, and Larynx. These organs are protected from implantation of *M. tuberculosis* by a covering of mucous secretion and become involved in advanced cavitary pulmonary tuberculosis with excretion of numerous tubercle bacilli. Ulceration of the bronchus may result in hemoptysis and a localized wheeze during respiration. The bronchial lumen also may be compromised without ulceration due to pressure of enlarged hilar lymph nodes associated with primary infection.

Prolonged hoarseness and pain in the throat accentuated by swallowing suggest tuberculous laryngitis. The abnormality is relatively easily detected by inspection of the vocal cords by indirect laryngoscopy. However, the lesion is fairly easily mistaken for a carcinoma of the larynx, even upon histologic examination. For this reason, a roentgenogram of the chest should be routine practice before performing a laryngectomy for carcinoma. Chemotherapy is highly effective for tuberculosis of mucous membranes.

Bronchiectasis. The smaller branches of the bronchial tree may be affected by tuberculosis either in the primary phase or in the chronic pulmonary phase. Localized dilatation of the bronchi may develop as a result of weakening of the bronchial wall and fibrous contraction of the parenchyma, just as happens with postviral suppurative pneumonia in childhood. Local obstruction by hilar nodes may also be present but is not a requisite for the development of bronchiectasis. When bronchiectasis occurs in an upper lobe, where drainage is good, it usually produces no symptoms. However, primary tuberculosis may damage bronchi in the lower portion of the lung, where poor drainage may permit pyogenic infection to occur years after the primary process has healed, resulting in a chronic cough productive of purulent sputum, often marked by periodic hemoptysis.

Gastrointestinal Tuberculosis. The gastrointestinal tract is relatively resistant to tuberculosis, but in advanced cavitary pulmonary disease associated with the excretion of numerous bacilli in the sputum, the gastrointestinal tract becomes infected usually in the ileocecal region. Symptoms consist chiefly of intermittent abdominal pain, cramping, and diarrhea. Occasionally the infection spreads through the wall of the intestine to give rise to tuberculous peritonitis, which is considered below.

Differential Diagnosis. The clinical picture presented by pulmonary tuberculosis varies widely and may simulate a great number of other diseases.

Carcinoma of the Lung. Tuberculosis is most commonly confused with carcinoma of the lung because the highest incidence of both diseases is in the upper lobe and in older men. Both cause loss of weight, chronic cough, blood-streaked sputum, and mild fever. In addition to bacteriologic studies for tubercle bacilli, sputum cytology and bronchoscopy should be employed to aid in the dif-

ferentiation. Comparison of prior roentgenograms may be of considerable help, but in some instances nothing short of a diagnostic thoracotomy will serve to make the distinction. When tuberculosis is considered among the diagnostic possibilities, antituberculosis chemotherapy should be instituted a few days before thoracotomy in order to avoid infectious complications in the event the lesion is tuberculous.

Mycotic Infections. Whenever tubercle bacilli cannot be isolated from a patient suspected of having tuberculosis, appropriate tests should be made for the various fungous infections, any of which may present a clinical picture indistinguishable from pulmonary tuberculosis. Reliable skin and serologic tests are available for coccidioidomycosis and histoplasmosis. Blastomycosis, actinomycosis, aspergillosis, nocardiosis, cryptococcosis, and sporotrichosis can be diagnosed only by demonstrating the organisms in a biopsy specimen or on culture.

Sarcoidosis. The typical patient with sarcoidosis is afebrile and has a negative tuberculin test and a roentgen picture of diffuse pulmonary infiltrations and hilar adenopathy, but the disease is very protean in its manifestations and may mimic tuberculosis. Scalene node and liver biopsies, as well as determination of serum protein and serum calcium, are of value in establishing this diagnosis. The Kveim test is of some value, but the antigen is not yet available commercially.

Aspiration Pneumonia, Lung Abscess. Pulmonary infection which is introduced by the drainage of contaminated saliva from a focus of pyorrhea during sleep occurs predominantly in the upper and midposterior segments of the lung and can mimic tuberculosis closely. The distinction can usually be made eventually, but much valuable time may be lost while the patient is erroneously treated for the wrong disease. The presence of foul sputum, hemoptysis, fever, and leukocytosis in a patient who has pyorrhea and has recently undergone surgery or who drinks to excess suggests a pyogenic lung abscess. While lung abscess is usually relatively acute, it may mimic tuberculosis in chronicity. If the differentiation cannot be made readily, it may be advisable to treat the patient with high dosages of intravenous penicillin for 1 to 2 weeks *before* initiating antituberculous chemotherapy. If the response is adequate and prompt, and there is some clearing by x-ray, a tentative diagnosis of lung abscess can be made. If not, antituberculous therapy can be instituted while the search continues for the etiologic agent.

Other Forms of Pneumonia. Several organisms (mycoplasma—(Chap. 207); adenovirus—(Chap. 206) can present clinical and roentgenologic appearances which at first are indistinguishable from pulmonary tuberculosis. Cold agglutinins and precipitin and complement fixation tests often establish the correct diagnosis. Cavitation is rare, and sputum examination does not yield tubercle bacilli. Primary tuberculosis may present with a localized infiltrate in the lung and slowly subside spontaneously coincident with tetracycline therapy, suggesting the diagnosis of mycoplasma pneumonia. However, tuberculous lesions usually fail to clear completely. A tuberculin skin test should be performed in all cases of "viral pneumonia," particularly if a pleural effusion, which is extremely rare in viral pneumonia, is present. A positive skin test in an adolescent or young adult with pneumonitis should be viewed seriously, in light of the infrequency of reactors at this age.

Pneumoconiosis. Pulmonary infiltrations associated with exposure to silicon dioxide (silicosis), beryllium, and cosmetic hair spray may present a roentgenographic appearance suggestive of tuberculosis. Silicosis can present great difficulty in diagnosis because it may produce conglomerate nodules and even cavitation that mimics tuberculosis. However, when the tuberculin skin test is positive in a patient with silicosis, smoldering tuberculosis is so likely to be present that prophylaxis with isoniazid is justified even in the absence of bacteriologic or clinical evidence of the infection.

Bronchiectasis. A productive cough due to infection in chronically dilated bronchi occurs much less frequently than formerly because of more effective antibiotic therapy for necrotizing pneumonias of childhood and the reduction in the number of children whose bronchi are damaged by primary tuberculosis. The lower and middle lobes (or lingula on the left) are most often involved, and a bronchogram effectively demonstrates the pathology. Tuberculosis should be considered as one possible cause of bronchiectasis. If the tuberculin test is positive, isoniazid should be administered prophylactically to prevent late progression of tuberculosis from coexistent Simon foci in the apexes whether or not these are visible radiographically.

Confusion Caused by Systemic Effects of Tuberculous Infection. Because of the insidious nature of tuberculosis, the clinical picture may be mistaken for that produced by several other disorders. Malaise, easy fatigability, inability to concentrate, anorexia, and weight loss may be mistaken for psychoneurosis. The tuberculin skin test and roentgenogram of the chest are usually of great aid in making this distinction. The symptoms may suggest *hyperthyroidism* or *diabetes mellitus,* but with a little care the distinction can be made. Tuberculosis should always be considered in the differential diagnosis of fever of unknown origin (Chap. 16). If the roentgenogram reveals a pulmonary infiltrate, the possibility of tuberculosis is increased, but in cases of disseminated or extrapulmonary tuberculosis, the chest roentgenogram may be normal. In these cases biopsy of an enlarged lymph node, bone marrow, or liver may be of help. Disseminated tuberculosis may present as *aplastic anemia,* particularly if associated with an obscure fever. Formerly, tuberculosis was overdiagnosed in patients presenting with general systemic symptoms. Today, however, because of a lessening awareness of tuberculosis, the principal danger is that tuberculosis will be overlooked. Furthermore, *tuberculosis may appear without reexposure in anyone who has ever been infected with it.*

B. CHRONIC TUBERCULOSIS OF OTHER ORGANS. Localized tuberculous infection may occur in a number of other organs, notably the lymph nodes, kidney, long bones, genital tract, brain, and meninges. Organisms reach these sites from the primary lesion either by lymphatic spread or by way of the bloodstream.

Tuberculosis of Lymph Nodes. The most common involvement of lymph nodes occurs in the hilus draining the lung involved with a primary infection. The enlargement is usually modest, but may be massive and give rise to obstruction and even ulceration of a major bronchus. The prognosis is good with proper chemotherapy, but the nodes may be slow in returning to normal. Surgical excision is indicated occasionally.

Cervical Adenitis. Cervical adenitis, or scrofula, has become relatively uncommon in the United States as a result of the elimination of tuberculous cattle and pasteurization of milk. Scrofula may present as a manifestation of the primary infection with human tubercle bacilli also. In Negroes, tuberculous cervical lymphadenitis occasionally appears as a late manifestation. The nodes may be quite large (several centimeters in diameter) and matted together in a mass with an area of soft fluctuation. The skin over the area is not usually red, hot, or tender. Swelling begins insidiously and usually is not accompanied by systemic symptoms. The skin may perforate with drainage of caseous material. Therapy consists of multiple-drug chemotherapy (see below). In some cases the offending organisms are unclassified mycobacteria, and for this reason cultures should be made of any pus.

Tuberculosis of the Kidney. Second to the upper lobes of the lungs, the kidney is the most common site for the late appearance of localized tuberculous infection. The mechanism of implantation is the same as that of the pulmonary apexes, namely, by hematogenous spread at the time of the primary infection. The oxygen tension in the cortical portion of the kidney approaches that in arterial blood, which enhances the growth and survival of tubercle bacilli for long periods of time. As in the lungs, foci of tuberculosis may remain dormant for many years and produce clinical disease late in life. The pathology is the same as is found in the lung: inflammation occurs, followed by caseation, liquefaction, and discharge of contaminated material into the collecting system and down the ureter to the bladder and in the male, to the genital tract.

Symptoms of renal infection are usually insidious and are often overlooked completely until the appearance of cystitis or epididymitis. Microscopic hematuria and pyuria with a "sterile" urine on culture for routine organisms should always call to mind tuberculosis and should lead to performance of a tuberculin test. If this is positive, the urine should be examined for tubercle bacilli by smear and culture of several early morning specimens. Painless gross hematuria from a chronic cavity in the kidney may occur on several occasions before the proper diagnosis is suspected and established. Intravenous pyelography may reveal a tuberculous cavity of the kidney connecting with the collecting system. Therapy consists of a multiple-drug regimen, including daily streptomycin and isoniazid. Therapy should be continued for 18 to 24 months to allow time for as complete healing as possible. The symptoms usually subside promptly with chemotherapy, and the patient may return to gainful employment when he feels clinically well. Resection of residual areas of destruction is only rarely necessary.

Genital Tuberculosis, Male. Infection of the genital tract in the male is probably always secondary to renal tuberculosis. Bacilli which are discharged from a cavitary lesion in the kidney may reach the seminal vesicles, prostate gland, and epididymis through their connections with the excretory tract. Symptoms begin insidiously, most commonly with pain in the scrotum due to inflammation of the epididymis and vas deferens or pain with ejaculation. On examination, the epididymis is found to contain one or more tender nodules. The prostate and/or seminal vesicles may be tender also. Therapy is the same as for tuberculosis of the kidney.

Genital Tuberculosis, Female. Tuberculosis of the female genital tract usually begins in the fallopian tube and is most common when the primary infection occurs during the childbearing period of life. It is uncommon in women whose primary infection occurred before puberty. Infection spreads from the tube into the uterus and may give rise to metromenorrhagia. Symptoms are usually mild and insidious and consist of abdominal pain, white vaginal discharge, and dyspareunia. Systemic symptoms and signs are uncommon, probably because the infection is indolent and localized. The most common manifestation is sterility, but ectopic pregnancy may also occur. Tuberculosis of the fallopian tube may contaminate the peritoneum and result in a tuberculous pelvic abscess or generalized peritonitis. Therapy consists of long-term multiple-drug chemotherapy.

Skeletal Tuberculosis. When primary tuberculosis occurs during childhood at the time of great metabolic activity and high oxygen tension at the epiphyseal lines, the chances for hematogenous lesions in the bones are increased. The greatest incidence of tuberculous osteomyelitis and arthritis is within 3 years after a primary infection in childhood, but late recrudescence may occur. The joints most commonly involved are the hip, knee, elbow, and wrist. Tuberculous tenosynovitis is most common about the wrist. Trauma may precipitate late activation of a dormant infection.

Tuberculous Spondylitis (Pott's disease). Implantation of bacilli in the vertebras may take place by the hematogenous route (if infection occurs before epiphyses close) or by spread of infection from a paraspinal lymph node draining tuberculous pleurisy or empyema. As with other forms of tuberculosis, lesions may not become manifest until late in life. The intervertebral disk is destroyed early, and narrowing of one such space on lateral x-ray of the spine may be the only detectable abnormality. A paravertebral abscess may be seen as a fusiform density extending the length of several vertebras. Chemotherapy with at least three drugs is usually quite effective, but the patient must be kept flat on an orthopedic bed to prevent damage to the spinal cord. Surgical drainage of the abscess and bony fusion of the involved vertebral bodies may be necessary to stabilize the spine and control the infection.

Tuberculous Peritonitis. The peritoneum may be implanted with tubercle bacilli by at least four mechanisms: (1) Spread through the wall of the infected intestine; (2) from a mesenteric lymph node; (3) from an infected fallopian tube; (4) from hematogenous seeding in the course of disseminated tuberculosis. Symptoms are insidious, but ultimately the patient has fever, night sweats, weakness, gastrointestinal symptoms, and abdominal pain. The disease occurs with increased frequency in alcoholics with cirrhosis in whom a clear tuberculous peritoneal exudate may be mistaken for ascites. Whenever ascitic fluid shows a lymphocytosis and a protein in excess of 3 Gm per 100 ml, tuberculous peritonitis should be considered. The diagnosis is most easily made by biopsy. Chemotherapy is highly effective but must be prolonged.

Tuberculous Pericarditis. Tuberculous infection may spread from the mediastinal lymph nodes or contiguous segments of lung to the pericardium in the same manner as to the pleura. The pathology is the same as with tuberculous pleurisy, with outpouring of a clear exudate from the serous surface, formation of granulomata, and subsequent fibrosis. The clinical picture is that of chronic pericardial tamponade, with hepatomegaly, edema, friction rub, cardiac enlargement during the active phase, and constriction during the phase of fibrosis. When such an illness is accompanied by afternoon fever or night sweats and a positive tuberculin reaction, tuberculosis should be strongly considered. The diagnosis is usually made by study of aspirated fluid or by open pericardial biopsy. Tuberculous effusion contains more than 3 Gm per 100 ml of protein and an increased number of white blood cells, predominantly lymphocytes. Therapy consists of a multiple-drug regimen as outlined below. Occasionally pericardiectomy is required if the process has become chronic and the pericardium fibrotic and unexpandable. However, adequate therapy early in the course of the disease usually obviates the need for pericardiectomy.

If tuberculous pericarditis has undergone spontaneous healing, the patient may present years later with the picture of chronic constrictive pericarditis (Chap. 272). Pericardiectomy is usually necessary at this stage to improve cardiac function but may be technically difficult due to extensive calcification extending into the myocardium.

Tuberculosis of the Adrenals. Occasionally hematogenous tuberculosis localizes in the adrenal glands and results in total destruction of the organs, giving rise to adrenal cortical insufficiency (Addison's disease). The condition must be differentiated from adrenal cortical atrophy, which is more common, and from other causes of adrenal destruction such as histoplasmosis. Therapy consists of the use of three antituberculosis agents plus adrenal hormone replacement therapy (Chap. 92).

Tuberculous Meningitis. Tuberculosis may involve the meninges either as a part of miliary tuberculosis or through reactivation and extension of infection from an old focus within the brain. In areas with a high incidence of tuberculosis, tuberculous meningitis is seen most commonly in young children in the first year of infection. In areas of low incidence, such as the United States today, meningitis is more common among adults as a result of late reactivation of dormant infection. Pathologically, the meninges contain small tubercles and a fibrinous exudate over the base of the brain.

Symptoms consist of headache, restlessness, and irritability usually accompanied by fever, malaise, night sweats, and loss of weight. Nausea and vomiting may be prominent. Stiffness of the neck and Brudzinski's sign are usually present. Spinal puncture usually reveals increased pressure, clear fluid containing an increased protein, reduced glucose (less than half the blood glucose), and 100 to 1,000 white blood cells, 80 to 95 percent of which are lymphocytes. Upon standing in a tube overnight a fine web of protein (pellicle) may form. A smear of this pellicle may reveal acid-fast bacilli, but culture of the fluid is often necessary to recover the organisms.

The differential diagnosis includes partially treated bacterial meningitis, fungal meningitides, and carcinomatosis of the meninges. There is considerable urgency in establishing the correct diagnosis because specific therapy is highly effective only if given early in the course of the illness. Irreversible brain damage can result from waiting 6 to 8 weeks for cultural proof of the diagnosis. When the diagnosis cannot be established readily, specific antituberculous chemotherapy should be instituted if the tuberculin is positive and the CSF findings are consistent with tuberculous meningitis. Therapy consists of at least two drugs including isoniazid, and steroids may be helpful in mitigating the inflammatory process. Intrathecal therapy is not indicated.

Low Sodium Syndrome. Older persons with tuberculous meningitis or overwhelming pulmonary tuberculosis occasionally manifest somnolence or coma associated with a very low serum sodium concentration (110 to 125 mEq per liter). This is probably due to inappropriate secretion of antidiuretic hormone, but this is not always demonstrable. It must be distinguished from adrenal insufficiency, which depresses the serum sodium concentration in concert with an elevated serum potassium. In addition to three antituberculosis agents, adequate sodium chloride should be administered, and water should be restricted.

III. Disseminated Tuberculosis

SILENT DISSEMINATION. Hematogenous dissemination of small numbers of tubercle bacilli is common during the primary infection, but usually produces little clinical illness. The principal importance of this event is the seeding of bacilli to sites far removed from the primary infection.

MASSIVE DISSEMINATION (MILIARY TUBERCULOSIS). When a liquid caseous focus empties its contents into a vein, there is a massive dissemination of tubercle bacilli throughout the body. The defense mechanisms are overwhelmed, and tubercles become established in all organs of the body. Without specific therapy death is almost certain.

Miliary tuberculosis is the most dreaded manifestation of tuberculosis. It may arise shortly after primary infection (progressive primary tuberculosis) or by reactivation of a dormant focus years or decades later. Because the resistance of the body is overwhelmed, lesions are not limited to those organs with an elevated PO_2 but are found in the liver, spleen, bone marrow, and meninges. One of the best diagnostic tests for miliary tuberculosis is biopsy of the liver, lymph node, or bone marrow in search of caseating granulomata.

Symptoms are usually nonspecific and consist of weight loss, weakness, gastrointestinal disturbances, fever, and sweats. The patient has usually had a course of penicillin or broad-spectrum antibiotics without control of the fever before the diagnosis comes to mind. Cough is not a prominent feature, but dyspnea may be. The correct diagnosis is often not suspected until the typical "miliary" pattern appears on the roentgenogram of the lungs. The white blood count may be normal or low, or may show a leukemoid pattern. One useful feature of the blood count is the finding of a decreased ratio of lymphocytes to monocytes (normal, 3:1). Proper therapy is dependent upon early and accurate diagnosis. Because histoplasmosis, coccidioidomycosis, blastomycosis, cryptococcosis, and other chronic infections may present similarly, it is imperative to obtain any material possible by biopsy or aspiration and perform appropriate stains and cultures.

SUBACUTE AND CHRONIC HEMATOGENOUS TUBERCULOSIS. Instead of a single massive invasion of the bloodstream, smaller numbers of tubercle bacilli may escape intermittently into the circulation and give rise to a variety of clinical manifestations including aplastic anemia, low-grade fever, lymphadenopathy, effusion into pleural and peritoneal cavities, and splenomegaly. There may be destructive lesions of bones, kidneys, subcutaneous tissue, or skin. This clinical picture is most common among Negroes of any age and in Caucasians of advanced years, and the process represents an overwhelming of immunity during reactivation of tuberculosis after years of dormancy.

The protean manifestations and bizarre clinical pictures caused by subacute and chronic forms of hematogenous tuberculosis provide a tremendous diagnostic challenge. To add to the confusion, the tuberculin reaction is often suppressed in persons with overwhelming infection. The solution to the clinical problem most commonly comes when the possibility of tuberculosis is considered. Confirmation must be sought from appropriate histologic and bacteriologic studies. Prognosis is uniformly bad without specific therapy, but improves with a multiple-drug regimen including INH.

DIAGNOSIS

TUBERCULIN SKIN TEST

Tuberculin (or its purified protein derivative—PPD) is derived from broth in which *M. tuberculosis* has been cultivated. It contains enough specific antigen to elicit a skin reaction in persons who are hypersensitive to tubercle bacilli whether from vaccination or from harboring the infection.

TECHNIQUE. The most reliable method of performing this test is to inject 0.1 ml of suitably diluted tuberculin intradermally, usually on the volar aspect of the forearm. An area of induration of 8-mm diameter at the site after 48 to 72 hr represents a positive result. The area is often erythematous, but only the diameter of the induration is considered significant. The usual *initial* dose is 5 tuberculin units (TU), or 0.0001 mg PPD (intermediate strength PPD), and should not exceed 10 TU in order to avoid large reactions accompanied by lymphangitis and systemic symptoms. This dose is the equivalent of a 1:1,000 dilution of "old tuberculin" (OT). If there is no reaction (or less than 8-mm induration), the test is read as negative and a stronger dose applied in the same manner, using second strength PPD or 1:100 OT, which gives a dose of 100 TU. If this test is also negative, the diagnosis of tuberculosis can be excluded with an accuracy of about 99 percent except in debilitated persons with overwhelming infection.

A positive reaction, particularly when elicited only by the stronger dose, does not necessarily indicate an infection with *M. tuberculosis,* but may be caused by an infection with one of the "unclassified" mycobacteria, i.e., *M. battey, M. kansasii,* or a scotochromogenic mycobacterium. However, a strong reaction to 5 TU of PPD usually indicates that the subject harbors an infection with *M. tuberculosis* which may be either dormant or active.

A positive tuberculin reaction can be suppressed temporarily by various factors: pneumonia, fracture of a hip, steroid therapy, or a severe toxic reaction from any disease, including overwhelming tuberculosis. Various studies have shown that as many as 15 to 30 percent of persons with bacteriologically active tuberculosis show no reaction to 5 TU of PPD. Furthermore, if there is reason to suspect an active tuberculosis or if the tuberculin is known to have been positive in the past, even a negative second strength PPD does not exclude tuberculosis. The diagnosis may be revealed by bacteriologic study.

BACTERIOLOGIC DIAGNOSIS

The only absolute proof of active tuberculosis is the cultural identification of *M. tuberculosis* from tissue or appropriate secretion: sputum, gastric washing, urine, CSF, serous effusion, or pus from an abscess or sinus. A useful preliminary examination, however, is to make a smear of the material and stain it for microscopic examination. Kenyon or Ziehl-Neelsen stain is used for standard microscopy and auromine-rhodamine stain for the more sensitive fluorescence microscopy. The smear is not a very sensitive method at best, but it has the virtue of giving immediate results and of identifying the contagious case who is excreting great numbers of organisms into the environment. For positive identification, cultures must be made on either solid egg medium (Löwenstein-Jensen) or Middlebrook 7H-10 medium using CO_2 (20 to 40 mm Hg) in the atmosphere to speed growth.

The most commonly examined material is sputum. When it can be produced spontaneously (usually in the early morning), it makes the most satisfactory material for both smear and culture. If none can be produced spontaneously, the patient may be asked to inhale a heated aerosol containing 10 percent each of glycerin and sodium chloride, which stimulates production of bronchial secretion. Sputum should never be collected over a 24-hr period because of the increased contamination associated with such prolonged collections. Guinea pig inoculation is no longer widely used for identification of *M. tuberculosis* because of the economic and technical advantages of culture methods.

When no sputum can be collected, as in young children or senile or psychotic persons, morning gastric contents may be aspirated and cultured. Diagnosis by smear of this material is less reliable than of sputum because of the occasional presence of saprophytic acid-fast bacteria in the stomach.

Multiple specimens may be needed before the organisms are recovered. This is particularly true in cases of primary tuberculosis, tuberculous pleurisy with effusion, and chronic tuberculosis of minimal extent. Also, old chronic tuberculous lesions may shed organisms only intermittently.

OTHER LABORATORY FINDINGS

HEMATOLOGY. The white blood cell count is usually not significantly elevated, except in tuberculous pneumonia, where it may suggest a pyogenic infection, and in miliary tuberculosis, where it may suggest leukemia (leukemoid reaction). Hemoglobin and hematocrit are usually normal unless a prolonged period of active disease has produced anemia of infection. The presence of 10 to 20 percent monocytes (equal to or greater than the number of lymphocytes) suggests severe and overwhelming tuberculosis. An elevated erythrocyte sedimentation rate indicates probable active infection, but a normal one is of little help in excluding activity. The ESR is usually elevated in advanced active tuberculosis, but is often normal with active lesions of lesser extent.

URINALYSIS. There are no specific changes except when a urinary lesion is present. Renal tuberculosis is not rare, and most often appears as "sterile" pyuria and hematuria. Cultures may have to be repeated several times before revealing *M. tuberculosis.*

MISCELLANEOUS. There is no satisfactory serologic test for diagnosing active tuberculosis such as exists for histoplasmosis and coccidioidomycosis. Biopsy of the liver, bone marrow, or lymph node can be of great aid in reaching a presumptive diagnosis of disseminated tuberculosis by revealing caseating granulomata. This finding may enable initiation of specific therapy in time to save a life; awaiting the results of culture may allow the situation to pass beyond the point of no return before the diagnosis is made and therapy is initiated.

TREATMENT

The availability of several effective chemotherapeutic agents during the past 20 years has completely changed the treatment of all forms of tuberculosis. While the healing of the lesions still must be accomplished by the processes of repair inherent in the host, inhibition of the organisms by properly selected drugs virtually assures a successful outcome providing that the offending organisms are susceptible to the drugs employed and the patient is not completely overwhelmed by infection.

Because healing depends upon host defenses aided by specific drug therapy, the total period of therapy must be quite long, that is, 18 to 24 months. However, only a small portion of this time need be spent in the hospital. For the remainder of the time the patient may live a rather normal life at home and may even return to work.

CHEMOTHERAPY

Ehrlich defined chemotherapy as the use of a chemical which would kill microorganisms without harm to the host. None of the agents used against tuberculosis would meet this criterion, because they merely inhibit growth or reproduction of the organisms. When streptomycin was first used in 1946–1947, it was frequently followed by relapse and the appearance of resistant bacilli because its action was bacteriostatic and served only as an aid to host defense mechanisms in overcoming the infection. From this observation stemmed the rational approach of using several drugs simultaneously in order to mitigate development of resistance and to achieve long-term inhibition of organisms while the body's rather slow defense mechanisms controlled the infection, permitting resolution of exudate and repair of tissue damage.

CHEMOTHERAPEUTIC AGENTS. The most widely used and valuable agents are streptomycin (SM), isoniazid (INH), para-aminosalicylic acid (PAS), and ethambutol (EMB), a new synthetic agent released late in 1967.

It may seem a little surprising that the tubercle bacilli from the majority of "new" cases of tuberculosis in this country still show complete susceptibility to all these agents although SM and PAS have been in general use for 22 years and INH for 18. The reason for this is that the majority of cases of active tuberculosis among adults represent reactivation of foci of infection implanted years before the advent of chemotherapy. Furthermore, most new primary infections arise from implantation of organisms from such recently reactivated cases and not from patients who have received chemotherapy. The incidence of primary antibiotic resistance can be expected to rise in the United States as the few new infections caused by resistant organisms emerge from dormancy and reactivate.

Isoniazid. INH is the keystone of antituberculosis therapy, because it is very effective, is nontoxic, and is administered orally. In adults, it is most often given in a dose of 300 mg once a day (about 5 mg per kg). In children, larger doses are advisable (10 to 20 mg/kg/day). A few years ago, a controversy raged concerning the need for larger doses in certain adults who inactivate the drug rapidly, but clinical advantage of such large doses has been demonstrated.

Streptomycin. Streptomycin was the first effective agent discovered for the treatment of tuberculosis and remains one of the most effective. It should only be used in conjunction with another agent, because organisms readily become resistant to it when it is used alone. The dosage is 1 Gm per day for most adults (0.5 Gm per day over the age of sixty) and 20 mg/kg/day in children. At the start of therapy it should always be given daily. After about 2 months, the frequency of administration may be changed to two or three injections each week in order to prolong the total period over which the drug can be administered without encountering serious vestibular toxicity. Several years ago it was the practice to administer streptomycin at these less frequent intervals from the start, but there are now adequate data to show that this practice results in a higher proportion of treatment failures and an increased number of cases with resistant organisms. Dihydrostreptomycin is no longer used because of its effects upon the auditory nerve producing deafness.

Para-aminosalicylic Acid. Para-aminosalicylic acid is of considerable value, but only as a companion agent for one or both of the drugs mentioned above. It may be given as the uncombined acid or as a sodium, potassium, or calcium salt. The dosage for adults is 12 Gm of the acid per day in divided doses (the salts must be administered in sufficient dosage to provide 12 Gm of the acid radical). All forms of PAS may be irritating to the gastrointestinal tract, and cause anorexia, nausea, cramping, and diarrhea. The sodium salt is contraindicated in patients with heart disease and hypertension in whom sodium needs to be restricted. The potassium salt is contraindicated in renal disease in which potassium may be retained. A more pure form of the acid (crystalized in the presence of ascorbic acid) is now available for which the daily dose is 6 Gm. This form produces considerably less gastric irritation, is better tolerated by patients, and is marketed as "PAS-C."

Ethambutol. Ethambutol is the most recent antituberculosis agent to receive FDA approval. Early results are very encouraging, particularly in the retreatment of tuberculosis in which the organisms are resistant to the more commonly used drugs. Optic toxicity presently limits its wide adoption for initial treatment regimens.

INDICATIONS FOR CHEMOTHERAPY

Because of the availability of several drugs, each with advantages and disadvantages, skill and experience are required to tailor therapy to each situation. The following is intended as a guide to choice of therapy.

ISONIAZID. INH may be given alone in several situations where the bacillary population is not great, no cavity is demonstrable by planigraphic radiograms, and in which the risk of producing strains of bacilli resistant to it is minimal:

1. Recent "converters" from negative to positive tuberculin skin test in whom there is no clinical or radiographic evidence of the infection

2. Young children who react to tuberculin and must be presumed to have been infected recently

3. Household contacts of an open case of tuberculosis

4. In postprimary tuberculosis of very minimal extent and questionable activity

5. As prophylaxis against the development of dormant infection into active disease when the tuberculin test is positive and the chest radiogram reveals Simon foci or other evidence of scarring from a previous infection

Chemoprophylaxis with INH is indicated when any of the following is also present because of their importance in late recrudescence of dormant infection: alcoholism, diabetes, debility due to age or any chronic disease, history of gastrectomy, silicosis, or prolonged steroid therapy for arthritis, asthma, sarcoidosis, etc.

ISONIAZID PLUS ANOTHER DRUG. When the tuberculous process is of somewhat greater extent and appears active, INH should be used in combination with at least one other effective agent in order to reduce the chance of emergence of strains resistant to INH. The most common regimen in use today is INH-PAS because of its demonstrated efficacy and the ease with which it can be given orally. Some prefer INH-SM despite the necessity of giving SM parenterally. It is likely that INH-EMB will gain in popularity because it is quite effective and not unpleasant to take. Two drugs should be continued for several months until resolution of the disease is well under way and the cultures of secretions are negative. Then INH should be continued alone for a total of 18 to 24 months, in order to permit solid healing.

ISONIAZID PLUS TWO DRUGS. Simultaneous use of three effective agents is indicated in far advanced or cavitary pulmonary tuberculosis, miliary tuberculosis, and in tuberculosis of the kidney, bone, spine, or meninges. These are all situations in which it is imperative to gain as rapid control of the infection as possible in order to prevent emergence of drug-resistant bacilli which may lead to relapse. Drugs may be used in combinations such as INH-SM-PAS, INH-SM-ENB, or INH-EMB-PAS. Because of its potency, INH should always be included in the regimen.

RETREATMENT OF "RESISTANT CASES." When the initial course of treatment has failed to eliminate organisms, several other agents are available which may be used in various combinations either alone or in combination with resectional surgery. Drugs should *never* be added one at a time to combat failure of therapy but in pairs to avoid emergence of resistant bacilli. "Secondary drugs" should be used only under experienced supervision in order to take full advantage of them along with resection or thoracoplasty, which must be timed properly to be effective. The drugs used in retreatment of "resistant cases" include ethambutol, viomycin, pyrazinamide, cycloserine, and ethionamide.

STEROID THERAPY. Therapy of arthritis, etc., with cortisone and its derivatives has been shown to increase the chance of reactivation of dormant tuberculosis. Yet, in patients who are very seriously ill with active tuberculosis, these agents may themselves be lifesaving. They should be used only when there is an immediate threat to life as shown by hypotension, debilitating fever, dyspnea, or an impending subarachnoid block in tuberculous meningitis. Prednisone should be used in dosage of 40 mg per day for 1 to 2 weeks and then 20 mg for another 8 weeks before gradual withdrawal. The effect upon temperature and general well-being may be dramatic, but there is little long-term benefit because patients who recover without steroids show no advantage. The frequency of side effects contraindicates the routine use of steroids in conjunction with chemotherapy. These agents should be reserved for patients in whom the infection poses an immediate threat to life and in whom the organism can be treated with effective agents simultaneously. There may be an exacerbation of signs and symptoms when steroid therapy is withdrawn, the "steroid rebound phenomenon."

TOXICITY. Reactions to INH are rare, but it occasionally produces peripheral neuropathy, especially in the feet, hepatitis, shoulder pain, skin rash, fever, anemia, and psychologic abnormalities. Pyridoxine in dosage of 50 to 100 mg per day may be used to counteract the neuropathy.

Streptomycin may produce vestibular damage with vertigo, which is noted first for a short time after each dose and later continuously. Impairment of hearing also occurs occasionally following prolonged usage. These symptoms require discontinuance of streptomycin. Circumoral paresthesia is common after each injection of the agent but is a side effect and not a toxic reaction. Streptomycin also has a mild toxic effect upon the renal tubules and should be used in reduced dosage in older persons and in those with borderline renal function. Blood urea nitrogen and vestibular function should be monitored in such cases.

The most serious toxic reactions occur with PAS. The gastrointestinal symptoms are more accurately termed side effects, but true toxicity is also common and may be serious. PAS becomes quite toxic if it is allowed to turn brown with age. For this reason, only fresh white (and dated) preparations should be used. Hypersensitivity reactions occur after about 15 to 30 days of administration and consist of gradually rising fever, malaise, generalized pruritic rash, and rising SGOT. Continuation of the drug in the face of such a reaction may give rise to serious hepatic toxicity or exfoliative dermatitis. The best course of action when fever develops in the course of chemotherapy is to stop all drugs until the reaction has completely subsided. Therapy then can be reinstituted one drug at a time, beginning with INH, then giving SM, and holding PAS until last. Desensitization to PAS can sometimes be accomplished, but it is usually advisable to substitute another agent such as ENB for it.

SURGICAL TREATMENT. Surgical resection of localized areas of diseased lung is of great importance in the management of selected cases of tuberculosis. The principal indications for resection are (1) persistence of cavity and excretion of bacilli, (2) persistence of bacilli in the sputum of a patient with a localized lesion, even in the absence of a demonstrable cavity, (3) drug-resistant bacilli if the infection is sufficiently localized, (4) need for a positive diagnosis where other methods have failed, and (5) bleeding or persistently positive sputum associated with tuberculous bronchiectasis.

These indications are gradually being modified. For

example, many patients with large "open negative cavities" are being discharged on medication if the sputum is repeatedly free of tubercle bacilli. The number of persons with an open negative status is increasing steadily, especially when resectional surgery carries an increased risk. Prolonged chemotherapy is particularly important in these patients to prevent reactivation.

Following a period of several months of chemotherapy, the inflammatory reaction is usually controlled and necessary resection of a localized area of disease can be accomplished with little risk. The dangers which attend resection of untreated tuberculosis, i.e., empyema, bronchopleural fistula, or spread of infection to another area of lung, are minimized by adequate preoperative chemotherapy.

Cavitary lesions which are removed following prolonged chemotherapy are usually positive for tubercle bacilli on both smear and culture. Residual closed necrotic foci, on the other hand, are often positive on smear and negative on culture and guinea pig inoculation. Failure of the organisms to grow does not indicate that they are dead but suggests that they are merely damaged by the combined effects of prolonged chemotherapy and the physicochemical properties of caseous material.

OUTMODED FORMS OF THERAPY. Therapeutic measures which are now largely of no more than historical interest are bed rest, removal to a salubrious climate, a diet rich in dairy products, collapse of the involved portions of lung by induction of pneumothorax, resection of ribs to permit collapse of underlying lung (thoracoplasty), pneumoperitoneum, surgical interruption of the phrenic nerve to allow the diaphragm on the involved side to rise, and introduction of masses of foreign materials (i.e., paraffin, lucite balls, or plastic sponge) into the extrapleural fascial plane adjacent to a cavitary lesion in the lung. A limited thoracoplasty is still used occasionally in the therapy of persistent tuberculous empyema and to lessen the risk of empyema developing in a large unfilled space after resection of a large amount of lung.

OVERALL PLAN OF MANAGEMENT AND PROGNOSIS. Because experience with the therapy of tuberculosis often is limited to tuberculosis hospitals or clinics, brief description of an overall therapeutic program seems appropriate. Usually it is desirable for patients with minimal noncavitary disease to be admitted to hospital or sanatorium for the initial laboratory and radiographic studies and initiation of therapy while they can be observed closely for signs of adverse reactions. The patient with minimal disease and negative sputum smears often can be discharged after this short initial period to continue chemotherapy at home.

In the case of moderately and far advanced cavitary tuberculosis in which bacilli are seen in the smear of the sputum, three drugs are often employed at first and the period of isolation must be longer. These patients, if cooperative, are usually ready for discharge home on therapy (usually on INH and PAS) after a few months. PAS is stopped after several more months and INH continued for about 2 years. In some instances the time required to achieve negative sputum may be prolonged, and resection of a cavity is necessary in about 5 percent of cases to stop excretion of tubercle bacilli. When all goes well, the majority of patients can return to their occupation shortly after discharge. When persistence of positive bacteriology or cavitation necessitates resectional surgery, the course is prolonged.

A favorable prognosis is dependent upon several factors: (1) Absence of other serious disease which may have been the trigger mechanism for development of dormant infection into active tuberculosis, (2) administration of adequate initial chemotherapy to control the active infection, and (3) cooperation of the patient in the prolonged chemotherapy necessary to permit healing. Alcoholism not only sets off late reactivation of dormant lesions but also serves as a serious handicap to patient cooperation in both the early intensive and the prolonged phases of therapy. The aid of social workers in the hospital and various social agencies is of great importance in the overall plan of treatment and rehabilitation.

PREVENTION AND ERADICATION OF TUBERCULOSIS

The decline in mortality from tuberculosis, which began with the improvement in living conditions which accompanied the industrial revolution, led several physicians early in this century to predict the eradication of tuberculosis by 1945. This prediction was based on the theory that the widespread infection with tuberculosis was harmless and that the danger lay in reinfections. Therefore, if reinfections could be prevented by isolation and treatment of contagious cases, the disease would rapidly disappear. It is clear, however, that active tuberculosis develops among adults largely from reactivation of old dormant foci acquired in earlier years rather than from reinfection, and eradication must await the natural disappearance of the organisms from the population through death of those who now harbor them, as well as prevention of contagious late recrudescence. This can best be accomplished by careful surveillance and prophylactic therapy with INH for those who harbor this infection. From study of Fig. 174-2, it can be seen that the disease is steadily disappearing in Western countries as the older, heavily infected segments of the population die off.

The major deterrent to the rapid disappearance of tuberculosis in the United States is the fact that such a high proportion of older persons harbor the infection in a dormant form. Such lesions may reactivate, cavitate, and disseminate as general health is impaired by old age, debility, alcoholism, steroid therapy, diabetes, gastrectomy, silicosis, or malignancy. These individuals may infect several grandchildren before active tuberculosis is detected. It is for this reason that many hospitals require routine chest roentgenograms on all hospital admissions. The most tuberculosis is no longer found among young women but in older men with chronic cough but little illness. Roentgenograms should be saved so that comparisons with subsequent films can be made in order to detect evidence of activity, before the sputum is positive for tubercle bacilli.

BIOLOGIC PROPHYLAXIS

BCG vaccine (Bacillus Calmette-Guérin), a live, attenuated strain of bovine tubercle bacilli, has been widely used in many countries to induce specific immunity against tuberculosis. In addition to reducing susceptibility to initial infection, BCG also prevents the serious effects of infections which do occur. There have been and still are conflicting opinions on the efficacy of BCG. Some authorities found no benefit from it, but most have shown the protection to be in the range of 80 percent. Its use is certainly warranted in countries where the prevalence of tuberculosis is high. In the United States today the prevalence is so low that vaccination is advisable only for tuberculin-negative persons in whom exposure is unavoidable: Peace Corps, State Department, and Armed Forces personnel assigned to countries of high prevalence and nursing and medical personnel in large city hospitals where tuberculosis continues to be common among older persons.

The question whether it is preferable to be tuberculin-negative or -positive often is raised. In the United States today, the chances for the reactor to develop a late recrudescence of dormant infection is greater than that of the nonreactor to contract an infection. On the other hand, if exposed to tuberculosis in a country of high prevalence, the nonreactor would have a greater risk of contracting a new active infection than the healthy reactor would have of developing a late recrudescence.

REFERENCES

Barry, V. C.: "Chemotherapy of Tuberculosis," Washington, Butterworth Scientific Publications, 1964.

Bentley, F. J., S. Grzybowski, and B. Benjamin: "Tuberculosis in Childhood and Adolescence," London, NAPT, 1954.

Canetti, G.: "The Tubercle Bacillus in the Pulmonary Lesion of Man," New York, Springer Publishing Co., Inc., 1955.

Dubos, R.: Acquired Immunity to Tuberculosis, Am. Rev. Resp. Dis., 90:505, 1954.

Gedde-Dahl, T.: Tuberculous Infection in the Light of Tuberculin Matriculation, Am. J. Hyg., 56:139, 1952.

Groth-Petersen, E., J. Knudsen, and E. Wilbek: Epidemiologic Basis of Tuberculosis Eradication in an Advanced Country, Bull. World Health Organ., 21:5, 1959.

Grzybowski, S., and E. A. Allen: The Challenge of Tuberculosis in Decline: A Study Based on the Epidemiology of Tuberculosis in Ontario, Canada, Am. Rev. Resp. Dis., 90:707, 1964.

——, and W. B. Marr: The Unchanging Pattern of Pulmonary Tuberculosis, J. Can. Med. Assoc., 89:737, 1963.

Pagel, W., F. A. H. Simmonds, N. MacDonald, and E. Nassau: "Pulmonary Tuberculosis," London, Oxford University Press, 1964.

Poulsen, A.: Some Clinical Features of Tuberculosis (No. 1), Acta Tuberc. Scand., 24-311, 1950; (No. 2) Acta Tuberc. Scand., 33:37, 1957.

Rasmussen, K. N.: The Apical Localization of Pulmonary Tuberculosis, Acta Tuberc. Scand., 34:245, 1957.

Smith, D. T.: Diagnostic and Prognostic Significance of the Quantitative Tuberculin Tests, Ann. Intern. Med., 67:919, 1967.

Stead, W. W.: Pathogenesis of a First Episode of Chronic Pulmonary Tuberculosis in Man: Recrudescence of Residuals of the Primary Infection or Exogenous Reinfection? Am. Rev. Resp. Dis., 95:729, 1967.

——: Pathogenesis of the Sporadic Case of Tuberculosis, New Engl. J. Med., 277:1008, 1967.

——, G. R. Kerby, D. P. Schlueter, and C. W. Jordahl: The Clinical Spectrum of Primary Tuberculosis in Adults: Confusion with Reinfection in the Pathogenesis of Chronic Tuberculosis, Ann. Intern. Med., 68:731, 1968.

175 LEPROSY (Hansen's Disease)
Charles C. Shepard

DEFINITION. Leprosy is a chronic granulomatous infection of man, which, in its various clinical forms, attacks superficial tissues, especially the skin, peripheral nerves, and nasal mucosa. The two major clinical types are *lepromatous* and *tuberculoid;* when the disease has features of both of these types it is called *borderline.* In addition an early *indeterminate* form is seen, which can later develop into one of the three types mentioned.

The earliest references to authentic leprosy are probably those in Indian and Chinese literature from about 1000 B.C. Møller-Christensen's archeo-osteological investigations indicate that leprosy was not present in the eastern Mediterranean area until 500 to 600 A.D. and that the disease then spread to western Europe in the following centuries. It remained a frequent disease in Norway less than a century ago.

At present there are probably 10 to 20 million patients with leprosy in the world. The disease is more common in tropical countries, in many of which 1 to 2 percent or more of the population is affected. It is also common in certain regions with cooler climates, such as Korea, China, and central Mexico. In the United States the chief leprosy areas are Texas, California, Hawaii, Louisiana, Florida, and New York. Part of the cases are acquired domestically, and part are acquired abroad, reflecting the increasing movement of people between the United States and the tropics.

ETIOLOGY. *Mycobacterium leprae,* or Hansen's bacillus, is the causal agent of leprosy. It is an acid-fast rod, found in enormous numbers in leprimatous lesions. Although it has not been cultivated in artificial medium, nor convincingly in tissue culture, it can be propagated in cooler tissues of small rodents, most consistently in the foot pads of mice. This development has made possible much recent experimentation, especially on drugs and vaccines. Because the organism grows slowly in mice, experiments usually require 6 to 12 months. A convenient and rapid method for estimating viability is the determination of the "solid ratio" or "morphologic index." Rationale for this measurement comes from the observation that only completely and solidly stained bacilli are infectious for mice.

Lepromin is a suspension of killed *M. leprae* prepared from the tissues of lepromatous patients. Intradermal injection elicits, somewhat irregularly, a tuberculinlike reaction at 48 hr (Fernández reaction) and, more consistently, a papular reaction at 4 weeks (Mitsuda reaction). The Mitsuda reaction is usually positive in tuberculoid patients and negative in lepromatous patients and is therefore an aid in clinical classification. However, because it is also positive in nearly all normal adults, it has no diagnostic value.

EPIDEMIOLOGY. Leprosy is frequently a family infection. Many patients give a history of prolonged exposure, and in close family contact (spouse-spouse) of untreated lepromatous patients the attack rate is 5 to 10 percent. Among young children of untreated lepromatous parents, 30 to 50 percent develop a mild, single-lesion type of leprosy which heals spontaneously. After the index case is under treatment, spread within the family apparently does not occur. Transmission from patients with tuberculoid leprosy is uncommon. The portal of entry is a matter of conjecture, but is probably either the skin or the nasal mucosa. The chief portal of exit is thought by some to be the ulcerated nasal mucosa of lepromatous patients.

The *incubation period* is frequently 3 to 5 years, but it has been reported to range from 6 months to several decades.

CLINICOPATHOLOGIC CLASSIFICATION. As is true of other chronic infections, such as syphilis and tuberculosis, the manifestations of leprosy are many and variable. The classification now in general use is based on clinical findings, histopathologic changes, and the lepromin test.

Lepromatous leprosy is one of the polar forms. The involvement is extensive, diffuse, and bilaterally symmetrical. Histologically there is a diffuse granulomatous reaction with the presence of large foam (Virchow) cells and many intracellular bacilli, frequently in spheroidal masses ("globi"). The lepromin reaction is usually negative.

Tuberculoid leprosy is the other polar type. Skin lesions are usually much fewer, and they are sharply demarcated. Neurologic involvement is relatively pronounced and may be severe. The histologic response contains epithelioid cells, and bacilli are few and sometimes difficult to demonstrate. The lepromin reaction is usually positive.

Borderline or *dimorphous* leprosy is a form in which the clinical features and histologic changes are a combination of the two polar types. The disease may change to the lepromatous or to the tuberculoid form (change from one polar type to the other is exceedingly rare, however).

In all types of leprosy peripheral nerve involvement is a constant feature. In any histologic section involvement of nerves will tend to be more severe than other tissues, and in some sections the nerves may be the only tissues involved.

PATHOGENESIS. *Mycobacterium leprae* probably enters the body through skin or upper respiratory mucosa. The early stages of infection have not been described accurately. There is evidence that the infection spreads through branches of the peripheral nerves. In lepromatous leprosy bacillemia is frequent and often so profuse that the organisms can be stained in smears of peripheral blood. Even in the most advanced lepromatous cases, destructive lesions are limited to the skin, peripheral nerves, anterior portion of the eye, upper respiratory passages above the larynx, testes, and structures of the hands and feet. The probable reason for the predilection of all these tissues is that they are all usually several degrees cooler than 37°C. Two sites of preferential involvement are the ulnar nerves near the elbow and the peroneal nerves where they pass around the head of the fibula; above and below these levels where these nerves take deeper courses, they are much less severely involved. In mice that have been experimentally infected in the foot pads, bacillary multiplication is maximal when the mice are kept at air temperatures at which the foot pad tissues are about 30°C; this is also the usual temperature of the most severely involved tissues of humans. In patients with lepromatous leprosy, collections of bacilli are also found in the liver and spleen, but these are probably scavenged from the blood.

Lepromatous leprosy is commonly held to be the result of a poor immune response and tuberculoid leprosy the result of strong immune response, but whether these different immune states precede the infection is not clear. Lepromatous patients have been shown to be deficient in the ability to develop delayed hypersensitivity, and their lymphocyte transformation in response to general stimulants is weak. Also mice that have been rendered immunologically deficient by thymectomy and irradiation respond to inoculation of *M. leprae* by developing a heavily bacilliferous infection which is histologically identical to lepromatous leprosy in man (and which spreads to the ears, nose, and uninoculated feet, i.e., the cooler tissues).

CLINICAL MANIFESTATIONS. Early Leprosy. The first signs of leprosy are usually cutaneous. One or more hypopigmented or hyperpigmented macules or plaques may be seen. There is little to distinguish them from other conditions, but they are frequently anesthetic. Often an anesthetic or paresthetic patch is the first symptom noted by the patient on careful examination, and skin involvement can also be found. When contacts are being examined, a single skin lesion is often noted, especially in children; usually a hypesthetic macule, the lesion is reported to clear in a year or two without treatment, but specific treatment is usually recommended. The earliest loss of sensation is that of temperature, followed by light touch (wisp of cotton) and then by pain (sharp or dull end of pin).

Tuberculoid Leprosy. Early tuberculoid leprosy is frequently seen as a hypopigmented macule, sharply demarcated and hypesthetic. Later the lesions are larger, and the margins are elevated and circinate or gyrate. There is peripheral spread and central healing. The lesions are usually few and not symmetrical. Nerve involvement occurs early, and the nerves leading from the lesions may be enlarged. The larger peripheral nerves may be palpably and visibly enlarged, especially the ulnar, peroneal, and greater auricular nerves. There may be severe neuritic pain. Muscle atrophy is frequent and especially involves the small muscles of the hand. Contractures of the hand are frequent, as is foot drop. Trauma, especially from burns and splinters and from excessive pressure, leads to secondary infection of the hands and to plantar ulcers. Later resorption and loss of phalanges is frequent. When the facial nerves are involved, there may be lagophthalmos, exposure keratitis, and corneal ulceration leading to blindness.

Lepromatous Leprosy. The skin lesions are macules, nodules, or papules. The macules are more often hypopigmented. The borders of the lesions are not sharp, and the raised lesions are convex (rather than concave as in tuberculoid disease). There is also diffuse infiltration between the lesions. The sites of predilection are the face (cheeks, nose, brows), ears, wrists, elbows, buttocks, and knees, and the involvement is often bilaterally symmetrical. In one form diffuse involvement with little or no nodulation progresses so subtly that the disease goes unnoticed. Loss of the eyebrows, especially the lateral portions, is common. Much later the skin of the face and forehead becomes thickened and corrugated ("leonine facies"), and the earlobes become pendulous.

Nasal symptoms (nasal "stuffiness," epistaxis, and obstructed breathing) are common and are sometimes presenting symptoms. Complete nasal obstruction, then laryngitis and hoarseness are frequent. Septal perforation and nasal collapse lead to saddle nose.

In adult males infiltration and scarring of the testes lead to sterility. Gynecomastia is common. Invasion of the anterior portion of the eye leads to keratitis and iridocyclitis. Painless inguinal and axillary lymphadenopathy occurs.

Neurologic involvement, of the same type as that seen in tuberculoid disease, tends to be less frequent in the lepromatous form. A "glove and stocking" type of hypesthesia is common in advanced lepromatous disease.

Reactional States. The general course of established leprosy is leisurely, but it is typically interrupted by episodes of rapid worsening. Several types are differentiated.

Erythema nodosum leprosum occurs only in lepromatous patients. It is particularly frequent during chemotherapy, especially toward the end of the first year of treatment. Painful, inflamed subcutaneous nodules develop, usually in crops. Each nodule subsides in a week or two, but more develop. Often there are fever, lymphadenopathy, and arthralgia. The reaction may last only a few weeks or may continue for long periods.

The bacilli of patients undergoing the reaction have greatly reduced viability as indicated by lack of infectivity for mice and by low "solid ratios."

Lepra reaction is an exacerbation of existing lepromatous lesions and fever. Probably most of the lepra reac-

tions in the older literature were in fact erythema nodosum leprosum.

The *Lucio phenomenon* is limited to patients with a diffuse nonnodular lepromatous disease; it is seen more often in Mexico, especially in Sinaloa, but has been observed in patients infected in the United States. In the reactions an arteritis leads to ulceration of the skin in a characteristic angular shape and subsequently to angular thin scars.

The reactional state in tuberculoid leprosy consists of exacerbation of skin lesions and worsening of neurologic disease, often with severe neuritic pain. Bacilli are said to become more numerous during these periods.

Complications. The crippling that follows involvement of the peripheral nerves has been mentioned. Leprosy is probably the most frequent cause of crippling of the hand in the world. Blindness also is common.

Amyloidosis is a frequent complication of lepromatous disease in the United States, but is less common elsewhere.

Patients with leprosy are said to be prone to develop other chronic infections. Tuberculosis is the chief cause of death in many leprosaria.

LABORATORY FINDINGS. There are no diagnostic blood changes. Lepromatous patients frequently have mild anemia, elevated erythrocyte sedimentation rate, and hyperglobulinemia. From 10 to 40 percent of lepromatous patients have false positive serologic tests for syphilis.

The differential diagnosis includes conditions such as lupus erythematosus, lupus vulgaris, sarcoidosis, yaws, dermal leishmaniasis, and the host of banal skin diseases. The skin lesions of leprosy, especially of tuberculoid disease, are characterized by hypesthesia, however, and peripheral nerve involvement can always be demonstrated. Peripheral neuropathy from other causes and syringomyelia are often confused with leprosy.

The combination of a chronic skin disease and peripheral nerve involvement should always lead to the consideration of leprosy.

The demonstration of acid-fast bacilli in the skin smears made by the scraped-incision method is required for diagnosis in many clinics. However, in tuberculoid disease, bacilli may be too few for demonstration. Wherever possible, a skin biopsy specimen, confined to the affected area, should be sent to a pathologist or dermatopathologist knowledgeable in leprosy.

The *lepromin* reaction has no diagnostic value.

TREATMENT. The discovery in 1943 that Promin, a sulfone, is effective against *M. leprae* ushered in a new era in the management of leprosy. Leprologists all over the world are able to use specific chemotherapy in the form of sulfones to cure or arrest the progress of the disease, to render the patients noninfectious, and to eliminate the need for segregation of leprosy patients from the general population. Just as chemotherapy alone has not eradicated tuberculosis, syphilis, or malaria, however, the sulfones have not ended leprosy as a world health problem. Even in parts of the world where chemotherapy is readily available, rehabilitation of patients with arrested leprosy for return to useful productive life has become a major concern. Physiotherapy and reconstructive surgery have assumed great importance in the management of leprosy.

Specific Chemotherapy. Promin, a conjugate of dapsone, was given intravenously, but it has been almost entirely replaced by the parent sulfone dapsone. The treatment of leprosy is largely in the hands of specialists, and hospitalization is advantageous for the first few months while the treatment is being established.

Dapsone (4,4'-diaminodiphenylsulfone, DDS, diaphenylsulfone) is effective and cheap. Oral treatment is begun with small doses and raised during the first few weeks to a maintenance dose of about 50 mg a day in adults. In a few months the bacilli lose infectivity for mice. The response of patient's bacilli to drugs can be observed by determinations of the solid ratio ("morphologic index"). When carefully done, this measurement is an accurate reflection of the viability of the bacilli. However, in lepromatous disease nonviable bacilli in large numbers (and probably a few viable bacilli) persist for many years, and treatment should be continued a year or two after the bacilli are no longer demonstrable in skin smears. Often this amounts to 6 years or more. In tuberculoid disease, especially in the milder cases, treatment is often discontinued after 2 years if the disease is clinically quiescent. Regularly scheduled follow-up is needed to detect possible relapses.

Other sulfones, such as Diasone or Sulphetrone, are used at times.

Sulfone resistance has been demonstrated by tests in mice on isolates from patients who had been treated many years with sulfone unsuccessfully. Apparently in these patients the initial response was favorable, but treatment was interrupted or irregular, and after 10 to 15 years there is no longer any response to therapy. Fortunately sulfone resistance is rare in patients treated initially with dapsone. Patients with sulfone-resistant bacilli are best treated with B663, a rimino-phenazine compound.

If given in the dosage mentioned, dapsone toxicity is rare. Dermatitis and hepatitis occur. With higher doses, anemia and methemoglobinemia are seen regularly.

The clinical response to adequate therapy is gradual, and the picture may be confused by reactional conditions (see below). However, progression of the disease stops and there is gradual improvement of skin lesions. Recovery from neurologic impairment is usually limited.

Some other drugs that have been recommended in leprosy are thiambutosine (a thiourea called SU 1906), Etisul (a mercaptan compound), isoniazid, streptomycin, and cycloserine. The precise value of these drugs is difficult to determine because of the complexities involved in clinical trials. These and other drugs are being investigated actively in experiments in mice.

Treatment of Reactional States. Moderate *erythema nodosum* (ENL) is managed by antipyretics and analgesics. If severe, it can be treated with corticosteroids and ACTH; the dosage is adjusted to alleviate severe distress but not to eliminate all signs of reaction. Sulfone therapy should be continued, if necessary in reduced dosage. In the past some leprologists have discontinued sulfone therapy at the first signs of ENL, but many now feel that such action is not warranted because it allows the emergence of viable bacilli. Corticosteroid therapy promotes the viability of *M. leprae* in mice not given antileprosy drugs.

Corticosteroids are helpful in severe reactional tuberculoid states also, but analgesics and antipyretics may be sufficient.

Several reports in the literature attest to the usefulness of thalidomide in reactional states. Because of its teratogenicity, however, the drug will not be released in the United States for many years. In countries where it is not banned, its use may be difficult to control, and for this reason its potential hazards outweigh its benefits.

Other Measures. Many of the deformities and disabilities of leprosy are preventable through proper attention from the beginning of treatment. Plantar ulcers, which are very common, may be prevented by rigid-soled footwear or walking plaster casts, and contractures of the hand may be prevented by physical therapy and application of casts. Reconstructive surgery is frequently necessary. Nerve and tendon transplants and release of contractures can give patients much more functional ability. Vocational retraining is often necessary for those with permanent disability. Plastic repair of facial deformities assist patients' acceptance in society. The psychologic trauma, which resulted from the prolonged segregation formerly practiced, is now minimized by permitting patients to continue therapy at home as soon as possible.

CONTROL. Early detection and treatment of the disease, which prevents the further development of deformities and which simplifies sulfone therapy, can be aided by education of physicians and laity in endemic areas. Because the disease is best treated by specialists, the establishment of clinics is helpful. Regular and complete skin examination of family contacts is essential. Field trials of BCG vaccination in endemic areas are showing favorable results, and BCG vaccination of family contacts even in nonendemic areas seems indicated. Chemoprophylaxis with low dosages of DDS may also be considered for family contacts. Removal of patients from the family and surroundings is probably not necessary, except perhaps in the first few months when therapy is being established, unless the patient does not follow regular treatment.

REFERENCES

Cochrane, R. G., and T. F. Davey (Eds.): "Leprosy in Theory and Practice," Baltimore, The Williams & Wilkins Company, 2d ed., 1964.

Fasal, P.: "Leprosy Occurs Everywhere," GP, 32:95, 1965.

Panel Reports from VIIIth International Congress on Leprology, Internat. J. Leprosy, 31:473, 1963.

Proceedings of Symposium on Sulfones by the U.S.-Japan Cooperative Medical Science Program, Internat. J. Leprosy, 35(4, pt. 2):563, 1967.

Wolstenholme, G. E. W., and M. O'Connor (Eds.): "Pathogenesis of Leprosy," Boston, Little, Brown and Company, 1963.

176 OTHER MYCOBACTERIAL INFECTIONS

Charles C. Shepard

Species of acid-fast bacteria morphologically similar to tubercle bacilli are widely distributed in nature as saprophytes or as pathogens of lower animals. Many examples are known of parasitism of amphibians and fishes by mycobacteria that cannot multiply at mammalian body temperatures. Among mammalian diseases that have been studied extensively are a chronic enteritis in cattle and sheep caused by *Mycobacterium paratuberculosis* (Johne's bacillus), a leprosylike disease of water buffalo and oxen called *lepra bubalorum* or *lepra bovinum,* and murine leprosy (of wild rats). The long-standing view that all other acid-fast bacilli were of importance in clinical medicine only because they might be confused with *M. tuberculosis* or *M. leprae* in smears or cultures has gradually given way to the realization that many other mycobacterial species are pathogenic for man, producing chronic *cutaneous disease, pulmonary disease,* or *lymphadenitis.*

Mycobacterium marinum (Balnei) **("SWIMMING-POOL BACILLUS").** This acid-fast organism inhabits swimming pools and gains entry to the human body through cutaneous abrasions on rough concrete. A few weeks later papules or nodules develop at the site and frequently ulcerate and enlarge to form superficial granulation tissue. The involved area usually is not extensive. Originally confused with skin tuberculosis, "swimming-pool granuloma" has now been described in many parts of the world including the United States. In Hawaii a much more chronic form lasting many years has been reported; exposure to swimming pools had usually not occurred. *Mycobacterium marinum* grows optimally at 25 to 35°C and poorly if at all at 37°C. This temperature range probably accounts for the lack of systemic spread; indeed regional lymph nodes remain uninvolved unless secondary pyogenic infection occurs.

The diagnosis is made by culturing the organism, usually from biopsy material on mycobacterial media at appropriate temperatures. Although it grows slowly on primary isolation, on transfer the organism is seen to be a rapid grower and photochromogenic (develops pigment only after exposure to light). Histologically the lesion is a nonspecific granuloma in which acid-fast bacilli can often be detected. Many, but not all, patients convert to tuberculin positivity during infection.

Treatment with antituberculous drugs, especially streptomycin, often appears to speed healing. Tests of antibiotic sensitivity are helpful in selecting drugs.

Prevention of the swimming pool outbreaks requires disinfection of the pool; reconstruction of the pool and elimination of rough surfaces may be necessary.

Mycobacterium ulcerans. This acid-fast organism produces extensive granulomatous ulceration which destroys subcutaneous tissue down to the muscle or fascia and extends peripherally under a characteristic undermined edge. Extensor surfaces of arms and legs are most often affected, but the trunk may also be involved. Histologically necrosis is prominent, and epithelialization of the ulcer floor extends under the overhanging margins. Systemic dissemination does not occur, although new lesions may develop at distant sites. In its natural course the disease may heal spontaneously in a year or two or may persist for many years with extensive ulcerations and contractures. Originally observed in southern Australia, the disease has since been described in central Africa and southeast Asia. Isolated cases and localized outbreaks, especially near rivers, have been described, but little is known of the distribution of the organism in nature.

Mycobacterium ulcerans grows optimally at 30 to 33°C and poorly if at all at 37°C. The organism grows very slowly, and colonies require 7 weeks to develop at optimal temperatures. Inoculation of mice foot pads is helpful in the isolation and identification of the organism. *Mycobacterium marinum* is easily differentiated on bacteriologic media because it is photochromogenic, grows rapidly and produces disease when inoculated into foot pads of mice much more rapidly than does *M. ulcerans.*

Treatment has been carried out with such antituberculosis drugs as streptomycin and isoniazid and the antileprosy drug dapsone. However, the rimino-phenazine compound B663 is the drug of choice. Surgical extirpation of the necrotic tissue and overlapping margins of the ulcer, followed by skin grafting, may be required.

PULMONARY DISEASE PRODUCED BY "ATYPICAL" ("Anonymous," "Unclassified") MYCOBACTERIA

DEFINITION. Mycobacterial species other than *M. tuberculosis* are known to be capable of causing chronic progressive pulmonary disease with fibrosis and cavitation closely resembling that of pulmonary tuberculosis.

ETIOLOGY. For a time the isolation from chronic pulmonary infections of mycobacteria other than *M. tuberculosis* or *M. bovis* caused widespread confusion. Fortunately recent taxonomic studies have brought order into the chaos. The nontuberculosis mycobacteria isolated from clinical sputum specimens were divided by Runyon into four groups. Of these group I (photochromogenic) is now given the species name of *M. kansasii.* Group III (nonphotochromogenic) includes several kinds of mycobacteria, but that responsible for human pulmonary disease is known as "*M. battey.*" Although closely related to *M. avium,* differences are usually distinct, and the species name *M. intracellularis* has been proposed for it. Of the nontuberculous mycobacteria isolated under circumstances that indicate their etiologic role in chronic pulmonary disease, about 90 percent are either *M. kansasii* or Battey mycobacteria. Group II (*scotochromogens,* produce pigment when grown in the dark) and group IV (rapid growers) are isolated from clinical disease less frequently. Isolation of nontuberculosis mycobacteria from clinical specimens does not have the same etiologic significance as the isolation of *M. tuberculosis,* because similar organisms can be isolated from sputum, saliva, etc., of healthy persons. Therefore it is necessary that before a nontuberculosis mycobacterium is accepted as the cause of the illness, it be isolated from several specimens and in significant numbers (more than 10 colonies per culture). However, when *M. kansasii* and Battey cultures are identified by appropriate additional tests, single isolations often have etiologic significance.

EPIDEMIOLOGY. The mode of transmission is unsettled. There is cross-sensitization between antigens of tubercle bacilli and other mycobacteria, but sensitization to the etiologic organism is usually greater. Comparative skin tests utilizing antigens from Battey bacilli and tuberculin indicate that many healthy individuals in the southeastern United States have been infected by organisms related to Battey bacilli, and in these areas chronic pulmonary disease that is not caused by *M. tuberculosis* is usually caused by Battey bacilli. In Texas and in Chicago *M. kansasii* is a more frequent causative agent than Battey bacilli. The proportion of new cases of chronic pulmonary disease caused by mycobacteria other than *M. tuberculosis* is not more than a few percent, but may be expected to increase as the number of infections due to *M. tuberculosis* decreases. In contrast to the experience with *M. tuberculosis* infections, multiple cases in the same family are very rare, and consequently enforced isolation is not indicated.

PATHOLOGY. Comparative studies of pulmonary tissue have failed to reveal consistent and reliable distinguishing features from infections due to *M. tuberculosis*. However, in *M. kansasii* infections the demarcation between diseased and normal lung is less distinct, and submucosal endobronchitis is more common. Extrapulmonary lesions are rare. Cervical adenitis due to *M. kansasii* or the scrofula type of group II is seen in children.

MANIFESTATIONS AND DIAGNOSIS. The symptoms and signs are those of pulmonary tuberculosis (Chap. 174), although there is some tendency for the disease to be more indolent. The diagnosis should be considered in single cases (without associated cases in the family). However, the diagnosis is established by isolations of the mycobacteria from the sputum. The laboratory should carry out tests for the production of nicotinic acid, at least on all isolates from new patients, because only *M. tuberculosis* consistently produces nicotinic acid. Differentiating tests can then be carried out in nicotinic acid–negative cultures.

TREATMENT. *Mycobacterium kansasii* infections usually respond to intensive antituberculous chemotherapy with isoniazid, streptomycin, and *para*-aminosalicylic acid. The cultures should be studied for drug susceptibility because many organisms are also susceptible to viomycin and ethionamide so that treatment can be adjusted in patients who respond poorly. Pulmonary resection has been found to be a valuable aid to chemotherapy, *after* the sputum cultures have become negative for *M. kansasii*.

Battey bacillus infections usually do not respond to antituberculosis chemotherapy. Fortunately, however, even though sputum cultures remain positive, pulmonary resections can be carried out with minimal risk of complication if the character and distribution of disease is suitable.

REFERENCES

Clancey, J. K., O. G. Dodge, H. F. Lunn, and M. L. Oduori: Mycobacterial Skin Ulcers in Uganda, Lancet, 2:951, 1961.

Clark, H. F., and C. C. Shepard: Effect of Environmental Temperatures on Infection with *Mycobacterium Marinum* (Balnei) of Mice and a Number of Poikilothermic Species, J. Bacteriol., 86:1057, 1963.

Kestle, D. G., V. D. Abbot, and G. P. Kubica: Differential Identification of Mycobacteria. II. Subgroups of Groups II and III (Runyon) with Different Clinical Significance, Am. Rev. Resp. Dis., 95:1041, 1967.

Lester, W.: Unclassified Mycobacterial Diseases, Ann. Rev. Med., 17:351, 1966.

Linell, F., and A. Norden: *Mycobacterium Balnei:* A New Acid-fast Bacillus Occurring in Swimming Pools and Capable of Producing Skin Lesions in Humans, Acta Tuberc. Scand., Suppl. No. 33, 1954.

Mollohan, C. S., and M. S. Romer: Public Health Significance of Swimming Pool Granuloma, Am. J. Public Health, 51:883, 1961.

Section 10

Spirochetal Diseases

177 SYPHILIS
Albert Heyman

DEFINITION. Syphilis is a chronic, infectious disease caused by *Treponema pallidum* and usually transmitted by sexual contact. It is capable of producing tissue destruction and chronic inflammation in almost any organ in the body and can produce a great diversity of clinical manifestations.

HISTORY. Considerable knowledge of the pathology and clinical aspects of syphilis was accumulated in the sixteenth to nineteenth centuries, but it was not until early in the present century that most of the fundamental information about the disease was uncovered. The etiologic agent, *T. pallidum,* was discovered by Schaudinn and Hoffmann in 1905. Soon afterward, Wassermann and his associates introduced serologic methods of diagnosis. In 1949, Nelson and Mayer introduced the *T. pallidum* immobilization test, following which other tests for demonstrating humoral antibodies were subsequently developed.

In 1910 Ehrlich announced the discovery of arsphenamine, and in 1917 Wagner von Jauregg demonstrated the value of malarial therapy for paresis. These were the two most important advances in the treatment of syphilis until 1943, when penicillin was found by Mahoney and his associates to be effective in the early stages of the disease. This drug has replaced the other forms of chemotherapy in syphilis.

ETIOLOGY. The *T. pallidum* is a slender spirochete with regular, evenly spaced spirals. It varies in length from 5 to 20 μ. When viewed under the dark-field microscope, *T. pallidum* shows characteristic motility, rotating on its long axis and moving slowly backward and forward. The spirals usually keep their uniform shape and size, although the body of the organism may bend at the middle. It does not have the quick, whipping movements of other spirochetes which are found in ulcerative lesions. The organism does not stain well with ordinary dyes and is best seen by silver impregnation methods in fixed tissues. For clinical purposes it can be demonstrated by dark-field microscopy.

Treponema pallidum is readily killed by soap, ordinary antiseptics, drying, and heat. It resists cold, however, and can be frozen and stored for long periods without loss of virulence. The organism does not remain viable, however, in whole blood or plasma which has been stored at refrigerator temperature for more than 96 hr.

Pathogenic forms of *T. pallidum* have not been cultivated and passed serially on artificial media. Strains of the organism which have been cultured are not virulent in animals and differ morphologically from pathogenic *T. pallidum.* Rabbits and monkeys can be experimentally infected with syphilis.

FREQUENCY. Although cases of primary and secondary syphilis in the United States are reportable by law, it is estimated that only a third of such patients treated by private physicians are reported to the local departments of health. For this reason exact information is not available as to the number of persons infected with syphilis in the United States (i.e., *prevalence*) or the number of new infections occurring each year (i.e., *incidence*). Both the incidence and prevalence of the disease have decreased considerably since World War II. In 1947, approximately 108,000 cases of primary and secondary syphilis were reported in this country to the Public Health Service, whereas in 1957 only 6,250 cases were reported. In the following 7 years, however, a disturbing rise in the incidence of new cases of syphilis appeared, and in 1966, more than 22,000 cases of primary and secondary syphilis were reported. The dramatic postwar decline in the incidence of syphilis was largely the result of the development of rapid-treatment methods, mass blood testing, and large-scale epidemiologic measures. Another factor responsible for the decline was the widespread use of penicillin for other diseases. As a result of this decrease in syphilis case rates, many of the states abandoned their public health control measures. The rise in the incidence of new cases leaves no doubt about the need for continuing intensive control programs. The incidence of new cases of syphilis has risen in the teen-age population, particularly in certain racial groups and in the lower socioeconomic classes.

PATHOGENESIS. Syphilis is usually transmitted by direct and intimate contact with moist infectious lesions in the skin and mucous membranes. Sexual contact is by far the commonest means of infection, but transfer of the disease by kissing or biting occasionally occurs. Indirect tranmission—i.e., by contaminated objects—is exceptional, because the organisms quickly die if allowed to dry. The disease can be spread by inoculation with infected blood, as in transfusion syphilis. Infection is transmitted to the fetus through the placenta. *Treponema pallidum* is apparently capable of penetrating the intact mucous membrane, but a small abrasion is probably required for inoculation to occur through the skin.

The natural resistance of man to virulent *T. pallidum* has been determined in volunteer subjects, in whom it was found that the ID_{50} for intracutaneous inoculation was approximately 57 organisms. Larger inocula produced larger ulcerative lesions and shorter incubation periods. Once the spirochete has penetrated the epithelium, it enters the lymphatics and can be demonstrated in the regional lymph nodes a few hours after experimental inoculation. From the lymph nodes the organism spreads rapidly throughout the body by way of the bloodstream. This spirochetemia may occur several weeks before appearance of the primary lesion at the site of inoculation. The early seeding of *T. pallidum* in various tissues is the basis for many of the later manifestations of the disease.

About 3 to 6 weeks after the organism has entered the body, a primary lesion, the *chancre,* develops at the site of inoculation. The chancre is usually a single ulceration of the skin or mucous membrane; it heals spontaneously. About 6 weeks after its appearance a generalized skin eruption, known as *secondary syphilis,* develops. In this stage, systemic manifestations are common. The signs of secondary syphilis also disappear spontaneously.

This sequence of events in early syphilis is variable. Infection without noticeable lesions probably occurs in a high percentage of cases, and many individuals with late syphilis are unable to recall either primary or secondary manifestations.

Following healing of the primary and secondary manifestations, the patient may show no outward signs of the infection (*latent syphilis*). Nevertheless, chronic, progressive, inflammatory changes may be taking place in the visceral organs or in the cardiovascular or central nervous system. Clinical evidence of cardiovascular syphilis or neurosyphilis may not develop for 10 to 20 years or more after the onset of the disease. Occasionally, the tissues of the host seem to become sensitized to the spirochetes, and large destructive lesions, called *gummas*, result. These lesions, which contain very few spirochetes, can occur in almost every organ of the body but are most frequent in the skin or bones.

Many patients with latent syphilis do not develop late manifestations and show no evidence of syphilis at autopsy. A study of patients with untreated early syphilis followed for a number of years showed that approximately one-third of them achieved spontaneous cures with the development of negative serologic tests. An equal number died of causes other than syphilis or developed latent syphilis with no clinical evidence of the disease other than a positive serologic test. The remaining third developed serious lesions of the cardiovascular or central nervous system or benign gummatous lesions of the skin or bones.

HISTOPATHOLOGY. The early lesions of syphilis are characterized by infiltration of the blood vessel walls and perivascular spaces with plasma cells, large mononuclear cells, and lymphocytes. Spirochetes can be demonstrated by silver impregnation stains. In the late lesions of syphilis there may be necrosis with granuloma or gumma formation. The necrosis is thought to be the result of an exaggerated or hypersensitivity response to a small number of organisms. Spirochetes are rarely found. These lesions heal slowly and often produce large scars.

IMMUNITY AND RESISTANCE. The development of immunity in a syphilitic patient may be considered from two standpoints: the resistance the patient develops to his own infection and the immunity he develops to reinfection.

Practically every patient with syphilis develops some resistance to his own infection. The degree of immunity determines whether the patient will achieve a spontaneous cure, the disease will remain latent, or late complications will develop. The factors responsible for the development of this type of immunity and the destruction of spirochetes are largely unknown. The serum of experimentally infected animals and patients with syphilis contains antibodies which immobilize and render noninfectious virulent strains of *T. pallidum*. These antibodies can be demonstrated in vitro by means of the *T. pallidum* immobilization (TPI) test. In human beings this immobilizing antibody appears during the early stages of syphilis and will usually persist indefinitely unless early adequate treatment for syphilis is instituted. The antibody is not present in the serum of normal persons nor in those with nonspirochetal diseases, but it occurs in the serum of patients with various treponematoses, such as bejel, yaws, and pinta. Although some workers have found a correlation in rabbits between the level of immobilizing antibody and the degree of immunity, other investigators have not confirmed their findings. The exact relationship between this antibody and the development of immunity, therefore, has not been established.

Humoral antibodies in syphilis have also been demonstrated by newer techniques such as the fluorescent antibody test and the Reiter protein complement fixation test. These procedures for detecting syphilitic antibodies are being used as diagnostic tests, particularly in cases in which there is doubt about the validity of the routine serologic methods.

Apparently the outcome of the syphilitic infection is influenced to some extent by the sex and race of the individual. Neurosyphilis, for example, occurs more frequently in men than in women, and in a higher proportion of whites than Negroes. Bone and cardiovascular syphilis are more common in Negroes.

Immunity to reinfection develops soon after the onset of the disease. In animals, immunity has been found to appear within 3 weeks after the initial infection and to increase progressively during a period of 6 months. In man, reinoculation usually results in a chancre if carried out within 15 days after the appearance of the primary lesion of the initial infection. Later than this a chancre seldom develops, but this resistance is relative. In rabbits with experimental syphilitic infection, resistance to reinfection increases with time during a 24-week period, as indicated by the need for an increasing number of virulent *T. pallidum* to produce infection.

Adequate treatment of patients with early syphilis may abort the development of immunity, and reinfections can occur. If treatment is delayed until after this period, immunity to reinfection becomes established and may remain throughout the lifetime of the individual. The question arises whether such immunity is caused by the persistence of treponemes or treponemal antigens in antibody-forming tissues. Recently, spirochetes having the characteristic motility and morphology of *T. pallidum* have been found in the anterior chamber of the eye in elderly patients with interstitial keratitis due to congenital syphilis and in other tissues in late syphilis. These organisms are also said to react to fluorescent antibody stains. Further investigations are necessary to establish whether such organisms are indeed *T. pallidum*.

If inadequate treatment is given during early syphilis and the patient's spirochetes are not completely destroyed, redissemination of the organisms may occur and produce infectious skin and mucosal lesions. This is the basis for the statement that poor treatment is worse than none at all. Once the patient has developed immunity to his own infection (usually within 4 years after the onset of the disease), inadequate treatment does not result in redissemination of organisms.

CLINICAL MANIFESTATIONS OF EARLY ACQUIRED SYPHILIS

PRIMARY STAGE. The period of incubation may vary from 10 to 90 days. The typical chancre is a solitary, indurated, nonpainful ulcer, which heals slowly with scar formation. It is often accompanied by painless enlargement of the regional lymph nodes, the *satellite bubo*. Primary syphilis is often atypical and may be manifested by small, multiple, or painful lesions which resemble many other conditions. Because of the frequent atypical appearance of the chancre, the clinical diagnosis or exclusion of primary syphilis can never be relied upon, and every genital lesion should have a dark-field examination.

Approximately 95 percent of primary lesions are found on or near the genitalia. In the male, the chancre frequently appears on the coronal sulcus or on the prepuce. Any part of the genitalia may be involved, however. Chancres of the external genitalia must be differentiated from chancroid, granuloma inguinale, lymphogranuloma venereum, carcinoma, and many other lesions which appear in this area. In the female, the primary lesion often appears on the labia and in the fourchette, but the perineum, pubis, clitoris, or urethra may be involved. Chancres of the cervix are frequent and are often mistaken for nonspecific erosions. About 5 percent of primary lesions occur on the lips, female breasts, or in the mouth.

In the diagnosis of primary syphilis, serologic tests cannot be relied upon entirely, because they are often negative in this stage of the disease. Moreover, a positive serologic reaction in a patient with a genital lesion may represent either latent infection associated with a nonsyphilitic lesion or else a biologic false positive reaction caused by another disease (i.e., lymphogranuloma venereum or chancroid). For this reason, a dark-field examination is of greatest importance in the diagnosis of this stage of the disease and should be done on the first visit of every patient suspected of having primary syphilis. If the initial dark-field examination is negative, material from the regional lymph nodes should be aspirated and examined. All local medication as well as antibiotics with treponemicidal activity should be withheld, but oral sulfonamides may be administered during this period of time. If the dark-field examinations and serologic tests for syphilis are negative, the serologic test should be repeated several times during the first 2 or 3 weeks and every few weeks thereafter for 3 months after the appearance of the lesion. If the patient develops a positive serologic reaction in a high or rising titer (with or without evidence of secondary manifestations), then antisyphilitic therapy should be begun. A single serologic test of low titer is not sufficient evidence for beginning antisyphilitic treatment if dark-field examinations are negative. Such tests should be confirmed several times for at least 2 weeks before treatment for syphilis is justified.

Penicillin or other spirocheticidal drugs should not be given as a therapeutic test to patients suspected of having primary syphilis. Healing of the genital lesion following such tests does not necessarily indicate the presence of syphilis, because nonsyphilitic lesions sometimes heal spontaneously. Biopsy of the genital lesions is often of value in the diagnosis of these patients.

SECONDARY STAGE. The secondary stage of syphilis usually develops about 6 weeks after appearance of the chancre and is manifested by a generalized skin eruption and systemic symptoms. Some patients have secondary lesions without ever being aware of a primary; others never develop secondary manifestations and enter the latent stage directly following the healing of the chancre.

The appearance of the *cutaneous lesions* of secondary syphilis varies considerably, so that they may be confused with many other skin eruptions. The lesions most often found are papules, maculopapules, or follicular papules. Occasionally, annular, pustular, or rupial lesions occur. Indeed, almost any type of skin eruption may appear except a vesicular one. The rash is usually widespread and frequently involves the palms, soles, and face, in addition to the trunk and extremities. The lesions are sometimes pruritic.

The *mucous membranes* of the mouth and genitalia are often involved in secondary syphilis. Syphilitic lesions of the mouth appear as painless, superficial erosions on the buccal surfaces, on the tongue, or inside the lip. When these lesions are covered with a thin, grayish exudate, they are known as *mucous patches*. They contain a large number of spirochetes but may be very inconspicuous, and the patient may not be aware of them. Lesions of the palate and tonsillar area can cause a persistent *sore throat*. So-called *split papules* are occasionally seen in secondary syphilis and may be mistaken for herpes, benign fissures, or the lesions of riboflavin deficiency.

Syphilitic mucosal lesions of the genitalia or perianal regions often become hypertrophic and are called *condylomata lata*. These lesions are broad, flat, wart-like excrescences which are found on the labia majora, perineum, and anal region. They are highly infectious and should be differentiated from condylomata acuminata, which are nonvenereal, pedunculated lesions (Chap. 227).

Although the clinical findings of secondary syphilis are often confined to the skin and mucous membranes, many patients will present evidence of *constitutional symptoms* and widespread spirochetal dissemination. Malaise, lassitude, headaches, fever, and myalgia are often noted. There may be a *generalized lymphadenopathy*. Localized areas of *alopecia* also occur, causing a "moth-eaten" appearance of the scalp.

Approximately 4 percent of patients with secondary syphilis have involvement of the eye, usually *iritis* or *neuroretinitis*.

Skeletal lesions occasionally occur in secondary syphilis and are manifested by localized areas of swelling and tenderness. *Arthralgia* and *hydrarthrosis* also occur, but changes in the joints cannot be detected by x-ray examination. An acute *nephrosis* with marked proteinuria, edema, and hypercholesterolemia is sometimes seen in secondary syphilis. Evidence of *central-nervous-system involvement*, such as paralysis of the cranial nerves or meningitis, may also appear in this stage of the disease.

It is apparent from the above description that secondary syphilis may be manifested by a great variety of apparently unrelated clinical symptoms. Although isolated lesions, such as iritis or periostitis, may not in themselves suggest the diagnosis, the recognition of other symptoms, such as sore throat, lymphadenopathy, or skin lesions will often make the diagnosis of secondary syphilis obvious. Whenever secondary syphilis is suspected, blood should be taken for a serologic test. This will be positive in practically 100 percent of the cases.

Conversely, if the serologic test is negative (and the possibility of technical errors has been excluded), secondary syphilis can be ruled out.

INFECTIOUSNESS AND EPIDEMIOLOGY

Syphilis is most infectious during the primary and secondary stages, when there are moist skin or mucosal lesions. The genital condylomas and the oral mucosal lesions contain large numbers of spirochetes and are more infectious than the dry skin lesions. The transmission of the disease by individuals or marital partners who deny having had open lesions is probably by way of small mucosal lesions which appear during the recurrent episodes of spirochetemia. Some secretions, such as saliva and semen, are frequently in contact with infectious mucosal lesions and may contain *T. pallidum*. The blood of patients with early syphilis has been shown to contain spirochetes and should not be used for transfusion. The serologic test is not always an indication of the infectiousness of the blood, because syphilis can be transmitted by transfusion from patients in the incubation period or in the sero-negative primary stage of the disease. The danger of transmitting syphilis either by transfusion or by direct contact is greatest in the first 4 years of the disease and is negligible after this period. In pregnancy, however, the disease can apparently be transmitted to the fetus for as long as 10 years or more after the onset of the disease, although the vast majority of congenital infections are acquired during the first 4 years of maternal infection.

It is important to determine the source of infection of patients with syphilis, particularly those with primary and secondary manifestations. It is equally important that the individuals to whom the patient may have transmitted the infection be located.

LATENT SYPHILIS

Latent syphilis is that stage of the disease in which there are no clinical signs or symptoms of the infection. Patients without signs or symptoms but with abnormal spinal fluid findings have a much more serious prognosis and are not regarded as having latent syphilis but are classified instead as having asymptomatic neurosyphilis.

Latent syphilis is by far the most frequent type of syphilis. Routine serologic testing is the only way in which the majority of patients with latent syphilis can be recognized.

Although the syphilitic infection is not clinically evident during the latent period, it may be producing serious changes in the viscera. Often the spirochete exists within the body throughout the entire lifetime of the host without producing any apparent effects upon health and longevity. Most patients with late latent syphilis develop sufficient resistance to their infection to prevent late clinical manifestations.

The diagnosis of latent syphilis is one of exclusion, and a careful history and physical examination should be made for clinical evidence of this disease. Because the diagnosis of latent syphilis is dependent upon the serologic test, false positive reactions must be ruled out. *Treponema pallidum* immobilization (TPI) tests or the newer treponemal antigen tests should be carried out routinely in patients with positive serologic tests in whom there is no history or clinical evidence of syphilis and in whom the diagnosis seems unlikely.

CLINICAL MANIFESTATIONS OF LATE ACQUIRED SYPHILIS

SKIN AND MUCOUS MEMBRANES. Late syphilis of the skin may appear as either small nodules or ulcerating gummas. The gumma begins as a painless, subcutaneous tumor which gradually softens and ruptures, exuding a viscous, gummy material. Spirochetes are seldom found in these lesions. The nodular form of late syphilis consists of slightly raised, reddish-brown lesions on the skin, which often coalesce to form arciform or serpiginous configurations.

Gummas also occur in the mucous membranes of the nose and throat, and may produce painful destructive lesions in the palate and nasal septum.

SKELETAL SYSTEM. Late osseous syphilis often presents a difficult diagnostic problem. The chief symptoms are pain, tenderness, and local warmth. The bones usually involved are the skull and tibia, although the clavicle, humerus, ribs, and nasopalatine structures are sometimes affected.

Syphilis of the skeletal system is often confused with other types of subacute or chronic osteomyelitis, primary or secondary neoplasms, or Paget's disease. The diagnosis can usually be made by close correlation of the serologic, clinical, and roentgenographic findings. In some instances, biopsy may be necessary.

The most common joint manifestation occurring in late syphilis is the *Charcot joint*, which is not caused directly by *T. pallidum* but develops as a consequence of destruction of the proprioceptive nerves in tabes dorsalis. It also occurs in other neurologic disorders, such as syringomyelia. The Charcot joint is usually confined to a single weight-bearing joint, such as the knee, ankle, or hip, and occasionally the spine. It begins as a painless swelling of the joint and is later manifested by hypermobility and loss of contour. The joint surface disintegrates, so that fragments of bone and cartilage can be felt within the joint capsule. Charcot joints often appear in arrested or "burnt-out" cases of tabes dorsalis—i.e., patients with normal blood and spinal fluid findings. Antisyphilitic drugs are of little value in treatment, and orthopedic measures are usually necessary.

LIVER. In patients with late syphilis the liver may contain multiple, minute, gummatous lesions or several very large ones. On healing, these lesions produce scarring and contraction of the surface, giving the liver the appearance of having several additional lobes—hence the name *hepar lobatum*. The most common finding on physical examination is a large, coarsely nodular, irregular liver. Ascites, jaundice, and splenomegaly are occasionally present. The serologic test for syphilis is almost always positive. Response to treatment is often dramatic, with rapid reduction in liver size and relief of symptoms.

STOMACH. Late syphilis of the stomach consists of a diffuse granulomatous infiltration of the stomach wall or a localized annular constriction about the pyloric area. Secondary ulceration and obstruction may occur, so that differentiation from carcinoma by roentgenographic examination is often impossible. Syphilis of the stomach may be suspected in young individuals on the basis of the roentgenographic appearance of the lesion and a positive serologic test, but exploratory laparotomy is usually indicated to confirm the diagnosis.

LARYNX. Syphilis of the larynx produces hoarseness without pain. Laryngoscopic examination may reveal gummatous infiltration of the vocal cords with secondary ulceration. The lesions may simulate carcinoma or tuberculosis, and biopsy is necessary for differential diagnosis. Treatment of this condition should be cautious, because intensive therapy has been known to produce edema, stridor, and suffocation. Patients with late syphilis may also develop hoarseness without pain as a result or recurrent nerve paralysis caused by aneurysm of the aorta.

KIDNEY AND GENITOURINARY TRACT. An acute nephrotic syndrome occasionally appears in early syphilis. In late syphilis, a specific type of interstitial nephritis may be present on postmortem examination without having produced a characteristic clinical picture. Gumma of the kidney is rare, but late syphilis of the bladder, testes, and penis is occasionally reported. Paroxysmal hemoglobinuria is sometimes caused by syphilis (Chap. 338).

In the female, late syphilis rarely involves the internal genital organs, but gummatous lesions sometimes appear in the breast.

Involvement of the endocrine glands, such as the adrenals, thyroid, and pituitary gland, is also infrequent.

CARDIOVASCULAR SYPHILIS. Cardiovascular syphilis is discussed fully elsewhere (Chaps. 270 and 277) and will be mentioned only briefly at this point. Cardiovascular syphilis is one of the most important of the late lesions of syphilis and probably accounts for the majority of deaths resulting from this disease. It is much more common in men than in women and seems to be more frequent in Negroes than in whites. It usually appears in the second to third decade after infection and may be associated with neurosyphilis and other late manifestations.

The fundamental lesion of cardiovascular syphilis is *aortitis. Treponema pallidum* causes destruction of the media, fragmentation of the elastic material, and eventual dilatation of the vessel. The base of the aorta is often involved, with dilatation of the valve ring and *aortic regurgitation.* If the weakening is localized, a saccular *aneurysm* may develop. The intima of the aorta becomes thickened, and occlusion of the orifices of the coronary arteries may occur. A few cases of multiple gummas of the myocardium have been reported, but the existence of a diffuse syphilitic myocarditis is a matter of controversy.

CENTRAL NERVOUS SYSTEM. Neurosyphilis, together

with cardiovascular syphilis, accounts for about 90 percent of deaths caused by syphilis. Although all the tissues of the central nervous system are invaded by the spirochetes, the clinical symptoms may be arbitrarily divided into meningeal, vascular, and parenchymatous. Meningeal and vascular symptoms usually develop early in the course of the disease, whereas parenchymatous involvement, as manifested by tabes dorsalis and paresis, usually does not appear until 10 to 20 years after primary infection. Meningeal lesions are inflammatory and often reversible. Parenchymatous lesions, however, are likely to be degenerative with irreversible damage. The type of lesion which predominates, the structures involved, and the exact location of the lesion within the central nervous system are the three important factors which influence prognosis and response to treatment.

Gummas of the brain and spinal cord are occasionally observed. They produce symptoms similar to those caused by tumors of the central nervous system, and differentiation is difficult.

Asymptomatic Neurosyphilis. Asymptomatic neurosyphilis is that stage of the disease in which an abnormal spinal fluid exists without clinical signs or symptoms to indicate that the function of the central nervous system has been affected.

The outcome of asymptomatic neurosyphilis and the extent of the spinal fluid abnormalities appear to be definitely related, because patients with marked changes are more likely to develop signs and symptoms. The activity of the neurosyphilitic process is often related to the spinal fluid cell count and protein level. The presence of a positive spinal fluid Wassermann reaction indicates that infection of the central nervous system has occurred; the cells and protein indicate the activity of the condition. This concept maintains that if the spinal fluid is inactive —i.e., if the cell count and protein are normal—the syphilitic infection in the central nervous system has been arrested and no further therapy is needed. Although this concept is not completely accepted, it seems to hold true in the majority of patients.

The serologic reaction of the blood does not always parallel the spinal fluid findings. Patients with previous treatment may have a negative blood test and a strongly positive spinal fluid. This combination seldom occurs in untreated cases.

If the spinal fluid is completely negative 5 years after the onset of the disease, it rarely if ever becomes positive again.

Meningitis. In a small number of patients, involvement of the central nervous system may be manifested by an acute meningitis. This condition usually appears within the first 2 years after the onset of syphilis. It nearly always occurs in patients who have previously had inadequate therapy and may be associated with an infectious or mucocutaneous relapse.

The symptoms usually consist of headache, cranial nerve lesions, delirium, convulsions, or signs of increased intracranial pressure. *Papilledema* is frequently found in patients with syphilitic meningitis, and these cases are often diagnosed erroneously as brain tumors.

The serologic test for syphilis and the spinal fluid Wassermann are usually strongly positive. The spinal fluid may show a marked lymphocytosis, counts as high as 2,000 cells per cu mm having been observed. This condition is often confused with other forms of lymphocytic meningitis, such as tuberculous or virus meningitis. The immediate prognosis is good, but the ultimate prognosis is much more serious. If the patient does not receive adequate treatment, late manifestations of neurosyphilis or paresis are likely to develop.

Meningovascular Syphilis. Meningovascular syphilis is usually manifested by signs of thrombosis of one or more of the branches of the cerebral or spinal arteries. Because there is almost always some evidence of leptomeningitis, the term meningovascular syphilis is used to describe these cases.

The symptoms of this condition depend upon the location and size of the vessels involved. Monoplegia or hemiplegia, hemianesthesia, aphasia, or hemianopsia may occur. Cranial nerve palsies are frequent, and convulsions are often observed. Syphilitic endarteritis may also involve the cerebellar vessels. Patients with meningovascular syphilis sometimes develop psychotic behavior, and differentiation from paresis is often difficult.

In older patients it is often impossible to differentiate clinically between syphilitic vascular disease and a cerebral thrombosis of other etiology. In these cases the blood and spinal fluid findings provide the only means of differentiation. The blood serologic test is positive in the majority of patients with vascular neurosyphilis, and the spinal fluid usually shows a moderate increase of cells and protein with a positive serologic reaction. A diagnosis of meningovascular syphilis should not be made if the spinal fluid is normal.

The vessels and meninges of the spinal cord undergo changes identical with those in the brain. With thrombosis of the anterior spinal artery, the patient may suddenly develop signs of an acute *transverse myelitis* with paraplegia, loss of sensation, and fecal or urinary incontinence. Usually, however, meningovascular lesions of the spinal cord are insidious and produce chronic progressive paralyses and sensory disturbances. A number of neurologic syndromes result from more or less localized spinal cord lesions: syphilitic involvement of the pyramidal tract produces the so-called *Erb's spastic spinal paraplegia;* anterior horn cell degeneration causes a picture similar to *progressive muscular atrophy;* while a single localized *gumma* may simulate cord tumor.

The term *meningovascular syphilis* is also employed for a large group of patients with diverse signs and symptoms, such as *epilepsy, eighth nerve deafness,* other cranial nerve lesions, or chronic headaches. Pupillary abnormalities are frequently present and may consist of a variety of changes, such as miosis, dilatation, anisocoria, fixed pupils, or typical Argyll Robertson phenomena.

Tabes Dorsalis (Locomotor Ataxia). Tabes dorsalis is a form of neurosyphilis in which there is selective degeneration in the posterior roots of the spinal nerves and the posterior columns of the spinal cord. Microscopically the dorsal roots may appear completely demyelinated, and

there is marked loss of nerve fibers. The posterior columns of the spinal cord also show a loss of myelin and degeneration of the axones. Spirochetes are rarely found in these lesions. In the majority of cases tabes appears 20 to 30 years after the initial infection. It is found more commonly in men than in women.

Patients with tabes frequently develop severe, agonizing *shooting* or *"lightning"* pains in the legs. Girdle pains also occur in tabetics, along with paresthesias, numbness, and tingling of the trunk, hands, or feet. Another type of severe pain occurs in attacks of *gastric crisis.* About 10 percent of tabetic patients develop severe episodes of abdominal pain associated with nausea and vomiting. These attacks may last for days, resulting in dehydration and exhaustion. Patients with gastric crises are sometimes diagnosed as having acute surgical conditions, and unnecessary operations have been performed on them.

Ataxia is a major symptom in tabes and may be so severe that the patient is unable to walk or stand. Some patients develop a typical tabetic gait, which consists of slapping of the feet and walking on a broad base. The ataxia is worse in the dark, and the patient may sway or fall when standing with his eyes closed (Romberg's sign). The damage to the nerve fibers in the posterior columns not only results in ataxia but also produces loss of position sense, and the patient does not know without visual assistance the exact position of his toes or feet. Vibratory sensation in the legs is diminished or absent. There may be diminution of deep pain sensation to pressure on the testes or Achilles tendon, and areas of hypesthesia may be present on the trunk or in the hands and feet. The patella and Achilles tendon reflexes are sluggish or absent. Patients with tabes often show evidence of hypotonia and hyperextensibility of the joints. Degenerative lesions, such as chronic, nonhealing lesions of the skin and *Charcot joints,* are also found.

Involvement of the autonomic nervous system may occur in patients with tabes, and *postural hypotension* is occasionally present. Severe *paroxysmal hypertension,* associated with gastric crises, has also been observed and may simulate paroxysmal hypertension caused by pheochromocytoma.

Urinary difficulties occur in approximately 50 to 60 percent of patients with tabes. These often appear early in the disease and consist of hesitancy or difficulty in starting micturition. Later the patient develops complete loss of bladder sensation. Patients with tabetic bladder often give no history of urinary symptoms, and catheterization for residual urine should be done in all who have evidence of tabes. *Impotence* and loss of sexual desire are frequently noted.

Paralysis of the oculomotor nerves is common in tabes, resulting in diplopia, ptosis of the lids, or ophthalmoplegia. Pupillary abnormalities are also extremely common and may be manifested by the classic *Argyll Robertson phenomena,* i.e., miosis, reaction to accommodation but no reaction to light, poor response to atropine, and absence of ciliospinal reflex. This condition must be differentiated from *Adie's pupil,* which is usually unilateral, is larger than the normal pupil, and reacts slowly to both light and accommodation. Patients with Adie's pupils may also have absent or diminished tendon reflexes.

Atrophy of the optic nerve occurs in about 10 to 15 percent of patients with tabes. Seventy percent of patients with untreated optic atrophy become blind in 3 years and 90 percent in 5 years. On ophthalmoscopic examination the optic disk appears white and sharply defined. The physiologic cup is prominent, and the lamina cribrosa is abnormally conspicuous. Visual field defects and diminution of vision may be present with only slight changes in the color of the disks. To detect such cases of optic atrophy early, careful perimetry and visual acuity examinations should be made in all cases of neurosyphilis. Although improvement in vision is not to be expected in patients with optic atrophy, arrest of the atrophic process can usually be obtained by penicillin therapy in patients with early involvement.

In early cases of tabes the serologic test for syphilis is often strongly positive, and the spinal fluid may show definite abnormalities, such as increased cells and protein and a positive Wassermann reaction. In patients with long-standing tabes, however, the blood and spinal fluid findings may be misleading. Approximately one-fourth of such patients have negative blood serologic tests, while as many as 20 percent have normal spinal fluids. Tabes dorsalis must be differentiated from numerous other diseases of the spinal column, such as cord tumor, combined system disease, and syringomyelia, as well as various types of peripheral neuritis (particularly diabetic neuropathy). The response of tabes to treatment is often poor, and symptoms may progress despite all forms of therapy.

Paretic Neurosyphilis (Dementia Paralytica, Paresis, General Paralysis of the Insane). General paresis is a psychosis caused by extensive spirochetal invasion of the brain. On histologic examination the most prominent feature is degeneration of the nerve cells. Perivascular infiltration and endothelial proliferation of the small vessels are seen. *Treponema pallidum* can be demonstrated in the cerebral cortex and other portions of the brain.

Paretic neurosyphilis is more common in men than in women and usually develops between the ages of thirty-five and fifty. The onset is most often insidious; prodromal symptoms consist of headache, insomnia, difficulty in concentration, and easy fatigability. As the disease progresses, a gradual change in personality takes place, with increased irritability, memory loss, poor judgment, lack of personal care, and deviations in character. These alterations may occur over a period of several months. Many of them are noted by the patient's family only in retrospect and elicited only by close questioning. The onset of paresis is sometimes sudden and may be ushered in by convulsions, syncope, or a cerebral vascular accident.

The simple, demented type of psychosis is the most common. These patients show confusion, apathy, impaired memory, and defects in judgment. Memory is particularly poor for recent events. They are often unable to concentrate on simple calculations and show

little insight or concern about their illness. The grandiose form of paresis is manifested by euphoria, overactivity, ideas of grandeur, and megalomania. Auditory and visual hallucinations are not common in these patients, but delusions of wealth and prowess are frequent. The type of psychosis that prevails in a given case depends to a great extent upon the preparetic personality of the individual. As the disease progresses, however, the symptoms of euphoria, paranoia, or mania recede, and simple deterioration and dementia become the outstanding features.

Eventually the patients become completely bedridden and are unable to move and feed themselves.

On neurologic examination these patients may present various motor disturbances, such as *tremors* of the facial muscles, tongue, and outstretched hands. The patient's handwriting is altered because of the tremors and incoordination. The speech becomes slurred, and test phrases are mispronounced. Pupillary abnormalities are common, and deep reflexes are usually exaggerated. Some patients with paresis also have signs and symptoms of tabes—i.e., *taboparesis*.

The demented form of paresis must be differentiated from senile dementia and Alzheimer's disease. The manic and paranoic types must be distinguished from manic-depressive psychoses and schizophrenia. In the early stages of paresis, differentiation from neurasthenia is sometimes difficult, and spinal fluid examination may be the only means of diagnosis.

The spinal fluid in general paresis shows marked changes, with increased cells and protein, positive serologic test, and first-zone colloidal reaction. The diagnosis of paresis should never be made in the presence of a normal spinal fluid; a positive spinal fluid is present in 100 percent of untreated cases.

The course of untreated paresis is progressive, and death usually occurs within a few years after the onset of symptoms. The prognosis improves considerably with therapy, but the chances for complete recovery are at best about 50 to 60 percent.

SYPHILIS IN PREGNANCY

Syphilis in pregnancy is a special problem, because the fetus becomes infected after the fifth month of pregnancy by passage of *T. pallidum* through the placenta. This usually occurs in women with early untreated syphilis, but is sometimes observed in late syphilis. Pregnancy complicated by syphilis may terminate in a spontaneous abortion, a stillborn infant, or a premature or full-term infected child. The maternal infection, however, becomes attenuated as the duration of the disease increases, and the chances of the fetus being infected are less with each succeeding pregnancy.

Pregnancy is believed to have a beneficial influence upon the course of the syphilitic infection, and late manifestations of the disease seem to occur less frequently in multiparous women than in others. A serologic test for syphilis should be taken routinely at the first prenatal visit of every pregnant woman. The early recognition of syphilis in pregnancy followed by adequate treatment will prevent congenital syphilis in almost every instance.

CONGENITAL SYPHILIS

Infantile congenital syphilis is often an overwhelming infection; such infants are severely ill, malnourished, and dehydrated. The most common manifestations of the disease in infants are skin lesions, fissures, condylomas, persistent rhinitis, tenderness over the long bones, and pseudoparalysis.

The diagnosis of syphilis in the infant is best established by dark-field demonstration of *T. pallidum* from the cutaneous or mucosal lesions. A positive serologic test in the first 2 months of life does not always indicate syphilis in the infant, because reacting substances may have been transferred from the maternal circulation. A very high titer of the serologic reaction or a steady rise in titer, however, is indicative of congenital syphilis. Roentgenographic examination of the long bones may show characteristic areas of bone destruction and *osteochondritis*.

Late congenital syphilis frequently manifests itself in the second decade with signs of central-nervous-system involvement, such as eighth nerve deafness, optic atrophy, and *juvenile paresis*. The prognosis of congenital neurosyphilis is serious; these patients commonly show little response to treatment. Cardiovascular syphilis is rare in the congenital infection.

Patients with late congenital syphilis often exhibit typical stigmas, such as hypoplasia, wide spacing and notching of the central incisors (*Hutchinson's teeth*), frontal bossing, a highly arched palate, and *saber shins*. The first permanent molar is also frequently affected in congenital syphilis and shows a characteristic appearance, with several small atrophic cusps on the occlusal surface. This is known as a "mulberry molar." *Interstitial keratitis*, a frequent complication, usually appears in the second decade. It is characterized by pain, lacrimation, circumcorneal injection, and corneal opacity. The response to therapy is poor, and serious impairment of vision often results. Occasionally, hydrathrosis of the knee joint (*Clutton's synovitis*) is associated with interstitial keratitis.

LABORATORY DIAGNOSIS

Dark-field demonstration of *T. pallidum* is most useful in the early stages of syphilis. It should be employed routinely on every genital lesion and on all cutaneous and mucosal lesions suspected of being syphilitic. In the hands of a competent microscopist, dark-field examination is reliable and establishes without doubt the diagnosis and stage of the infection.

SEROLOGIC TESTS. Serologic tests for syphilis (STS) are the most commonly used diagnostic procedures. In latent syphilis they are the only means by which the diagnosis can be made. The serologic tests are based upon the presence of an antibody-like substance (sometimes called *reagin*), which appears in the patient's serum soon after the onset of the disease. Syphilitic serum reacts with a lipoidal antigen made from an alcoholic extract of beef heart. Various modifications of flocculation tests for syphilis have been named after their originators (Kahn, Kline, and Hinton). The complement fixation technique or Wassermann test employs the same type of antigen, the Kolmer modification being the most commonly used in this country. The VDRL (Venereal Disease Research Laboratory) test is a rapid slide technique employing cardiolipin antigen. It has a high degree of sensitivity and specificity and has become the flocculation test of choice in most state laboratories and hospitals.

In addition to these serologic tests for syphilis using lipoidal or cardiolipin antigens, a number of other techniques have been developed which employ antigens made from whole-body virulent *T. pallidum* or from chemical fractions of this organism.

The most useful of the various tests to detect treponemal antibodies has been the *T. pallidum* immobilization test (TPI), which uses a live virulent strain of the organism as an antigen. It demonstrates a circulating treponemal antibody which persists for many years after the onset of the original infection and is little influenced by treatment unless this was carried out early in the course of the disease. Although the test is difficult to perform, it has been of value in distinguishing late syphilis from conditions causing biologic false positive reactions and in the diagnosis of patients who have clinical signs of late syphilis and in whom the tests for reagin are negative or inconclusive. Various other tests using treponemal antigens that were developed later include the *T. pallidum* agglutination (TPA), complement fixation (TPCF), and immunoadherence tests (TPIA). A standardized antigen of Reiter's strain of the cultivated spirochete is also commercially available and is being used in agglutination as well as complement fixation tests.

Perhaps the most practical of these methods has been the fluorescent treponemal antibody test (FTA). Investigations with this test have shown that syphilitic serum contains antibodies specific for *T. pallidum* as well as a low-titered nonspecific treponemal antibody which is also found in normal serums. False positive reactions to normal serums could, however, be avoided by testing the serum at a dilution of 1:200 (FTA 200 test). The FTA test has been refined further by removing the nonspecific group antibody from the serum by absorption with material derived from Reiter's strain of the cultivated spirochete. This improved technique, designated as the fluorescent treponemal antibody absorption test (FTA-ABS), has become a valuable addition to the current serologic methods for the diagnosis of syphilis. The FTA-ABS test has been shown to be more sensitive and more specific than the TPI in all phases of syphilis and promises to become the treponemal test of choice for differentiation of chronic biologic false positive reactions. It also appears to be of considerable value in the diagnosis of treated and untreated cases of late syphilis, even when the serologic tests using lipoidal or cardiolipin antigens are nonreactive. The fact that patients with such conditions maintain treponemal antibodies many years after supposedly adequate therapy has been related to the recent demonstration by fluorescent antibody stains that treponemes may be present in various body fluids and tissues such as aqueous humor and cerebrospinal fluid.

Although these and other new serologic procedures are now available, it is recommended that the standard reagin tests continue to be used for the routine serologic diagnosis of syphilis, because they are highly standardized, adequately sensitive, and inexpensive. Moreover, they are widely used and the results are readily understood and interpreted. Although treponemal tests such as the FTA-ABS may eventually supplant the standard reagin test as a primary screening device if the techniques can be simplified, in general they should be used primarily as confirmatory tests for the diagnosis of biologic false positive reactions. When the results of the various standard serologic tests are inconclusive and a biologic false positive reaction is considered, the patient's serum should be tested by one of the treponemal procedures. A close correlation has been shown between the results of the FTA-ABS and TPI tests. The FTA-ABS test is technically much simpler to perform, however.

It has been recommended that the results of serologic tests be reported as "reactive," "weakly reactive," and "nonreactive" in place of the previous terms "positive," "doubtful," or "negative." A nonreactive or negative standard reagin test does not always exclude syphilis, nor is a reactive or positive test always proof of the existence of the disease. The reagin serologic tests are nonreactive in the incubation period of syphilis, during the early weeks of the primary stage, and in many of the late manifestations such as cardiovascular disturbance and neurosyphilis (tabes dorsalis in particular). In approximately one-fourth of the patients with "adequately" treated late syphilis, the serologic tests using cardiolipin antigens may be nonreactive, whereas the TPI and FTA-ABS continue to be reactive. Reversal of the standard reagin tests from reactive to nonreactive may be indicative of the disappearance of nonspecific antibodies only, whereas the more specific treponemal antibody seems to persist despite presumably adequate therapy.

The height of the titer in serial serologic tests is of value in the diagnosis and management of the various stages of the disease. A sharply rising titer is usually found in recently acquired syphilis, while a stationary titer indicates an infection of some duration. A rapidly falling titer in the absence of therapy is evidence against the diagnosis of syphilis and may indicate a false positive reaction. The height of the titer has no bearing on the prognosis or outcome of the disease. Carefully titered tests are also important in determining the results of therapy; a continuing falling titer indicates a satisfactory response.

BIOLOGIC FALSE POSITIVE SEROLOGIC TESTS FOR SYPH-ILIS. Serologic tests for syphilis using lipoidal or cardiolipid antigens may be reactive in a great variety of non-spirochetal illnesses. These biologic false positive reactions are due presumably to the appearance in the patient's serum of substances which act like reagin and give positive flocculation and complement fixation reactions for syphilis. These reactions are usually transient, but in some instances may be positive for months or years.

Biologic false positive reactions are frequently observed in patients with vaccinia, infectious mononucleosis, malaria, leprosy, and upper respiratory diseases, as well as in spirochetal infections, such as yaws, pinta, and relapsing fever. Other infections which are occasionally associated with false positive reactions are lymphogranuloma venereum, chancroid, measles, chickenpox, atypical pneumonia, infectious hepatitis, rat-bite fever, and disseminated lupus erythematosus. In fact, any febrile disease or immunization is a potential cause of false positive tests. There is evidence that individuals with biologic false positive reactions of long duration may have autoimmune diseases or dysproteinemia. The biologic false positive STS has been shown to be associated with systemic lupus erythematosus and Hashimoto's thyroiditis. A false positive STS may serve as a forerunner to the eventual development of one of these autoimmune disorders.

The TPI test and other treponemal tests such as the FTA-ABS are often of considerable aid in the diagnosis of false positive reactions. These tests are almost always positive in late syphilis. A negative treponemal test is, therefore, of value in excluding the diagnosis of syphilis. A positive test, on the other hand, indicates the existence of a syphilitic infection even if the standard serologic tests are negative. In most cases, the false positive reaction will become negative within 6 months. If the patient continues to show a positive serologic test and if appropriate diagnostic procedures do not indicate a false positive reaction, antisyphilitic therapy should be instituted. If the patient becomes pregnant or is to be married, immediate treatment is indicated.

SERORESISTANCE. In many patients with syphilis the serologic test remains positive despite prolonged, intensive therapy. These patients are called seroresistant, or Wassermann-fast. One of the aims of therapy in early syphilis (particularly during the first 2 years of the disease) is to procure and maintain a negative serologic reaction. In late syphilis, however, seroresistance is of little clinical importance and has no relationship to the outcome of the disease.

In most patients with early syphilis the serologic test becomes negative within 6 months after therapy is begun. Occasionally the titer of the serologic reaction falls very slowly and the tests remain positive in low titer (i.e., less than 1:4 dilution) for as long as 1 to 2 years. In some patients with early syphilis there is very little serologic response to treatment, and the titer remains high for 6 to 9 months or more. This type of seroresistance is usually followed by clinical relapse, and these patients should be re-treated.

Neurosyphilis is frequently associated with seroresistance in both early and late cases, and the spinal fluid should be examined in every patient with a persistently positive serologic reaction.

The seroresistant patient is often discouraged over the failure to reverse the serologic test and becomes deeply concerned for fear that the infection is not arrested. In addition, he may be embarrassed in applying for a marriage license or employment when blood tests are a part of the premarital or preemployment examination. These patients should be reassured that the outcome of the disease is not related to the persistence of a positive serologic test. Seroresistance should not be an obstacle to marriage.

SPINAL FLUID TESTS. The spinal fluid must be examined in every patient with syphilis. This is the only method of detecting involvement of the central nervous system in the asymptomatic stage, of determining the efficacy of treatment, and of confirming the diagnosis of symptomatic neurosyphilis.

The spinal fluid cell count should be done within an hour after the fluid is withdrawn. A count of more than 8 lymphocytes per cu mm is considered abnormal. Even a small amount of blood in the spinal fluid will affect the accuracy of the various examinations. A quantitative determination of the spinal fluid protein should be done in every case.

Complement fixation tests for syphilis are generally regarded as being more sensitive than flocculation tests for examination of spinal fluid. The spinal fluid of patients with neurosyphilis has been found to contain immobilizing antibodies for *T. pallidum.*

The spinal fluid may also show biologic false positive complement fixation or flocculation reactions. This may be caused by a bloody tap or any condition which produces an increased protein in the spinal fluid. Brain tumor, bacterial or virus meningitis, encephalitis, or subarachnoid hemorrhage can produce a false positive test for syphilis in either syphilitic or nonsyphilitic patients.

The value of colloidal precipitation tests (gold and mastic reactions) has been overemphasized in the diagnosis of neurosyphilis. The zone of precipitation or the shape of the colloidal curve has little diagnostic significance

BIOPSY. Biopsy is a valuable diagnostic procedure, especially for cutaneous lesions. In late syphilis involving the lymph nodes, testes, or larynx, it is indispensable.

TREATMENT

In patients with early syphilis adequate treatment can produce an absolute, or biologic, cure, with complete healing of lesions and reversal of serologic tests and spinal fluid findings. These patients become entirely well, are not infectious, and do not develop any of the late manifestations of the disease.

Treatment of late syphilis may not achieve these goals. Despite long and vigorous therapy the serologic tests in late syphilis often remain positive. Late syphilitic lesions are often associated with permanent damage, and treatment may produce little or no return of function.

EARLY SYPHILIS. In 1943 penicillin was found to be effective in the treatment of syphilis. The use of arsenicals, bismuth, or mercurials is rarely, if ever, indicated. Other antibiotics, such as chloramphenicol and the various tetracyclines have treponemicidal activity and produce healing of both early and late syphilitic lesions. The ultimate place of these drugs in the treatment of syphilis has not been established. They are probably not as effective as penicillin. Erythromycin and the tetracyclines have also been shown to have treponemicidal action, and doses of 20 to 30 Gm are recommended over a period of 10 to 15 days in patients in whom penicillin is contraindicated.

Procaine penicillin and benzathine penicillin G have generally replaced crystalline, aqueous penicillin, except perhaps in the very serious or far-advanced stages of infection. The minimal effective total dosage of penicillin is approximately 2.4 million units. Increasing the total amount of penicillin from 2.4 to 9.6 million units does not decrease the failure rate in early syphilis.

The total dosage of depot (procaine) penicillin usually prescribed is approximately 4.8 to 6 million units given in injections of 1.2 million units at 2- or 3-day intervals for a period of 8 to 12 days. This schedule will produce satisfactory results in about 90 percent of patients. The remaining 10 percent will show clinical or laboratory changes of either relapse or reinfection. Benzathine penicillin G is also effective in early syphilis when given in a single dose of 2.4 million units (1.2 million units in each buttock) or in 2 or 3 weekly injections of 1.2 million units each. It has the advantage from the public health standpoint of completing treatment in a minimum period of time but is not recommended as a routine method. Oral penicillin is not recommended for the treatment of syphilis. The other antibiotics with treponemicidal activity should be used only in patients in whom penicillin is contraindicated.

Jarisch-Herxheimer Reaction. Within a few hours after the first injection of either an arsenical or penicillin, about 50 percent of patients with early syphilis experience fever, malaise, headache, myalgia, and a flare-up of cutaneous lesions. This is presumed to be caused by release of breakdown products of spirochetes following the injection of treponemicidal agents. In early syphilis these symptoms disappear within several hours and leave no permanent tissue damage. In late syphilis such reactions can be disastrous if the lesions are located in such areas as the ostiums of the coronary arteries, the wall of an aneurysm, or the central nervous system.

Posttreatment Observation. After completing treatment, patients should return every month during the first year for quantitative serologic tests and examination for relapsing lesions. If the patient develops a recurrence of syphilitic lesions or evidence of neurosyphilis, or if there is a birth of a syphilitic child, retreatment is necessary. If the serologic test in patients with early syphilis shows no appreciable decrease within 6 months or if the titer is elevated (arbitrarily a dilution of 1:4 or higher) 1 year after completion of therapy, further treatment is indicated. A positive reaction in any dilution 18 months or more after completion of treatment of primary or secondary syphilis should be considered as evidence of treatment failure, and another course of penicillin is indicated.

Serologic tests should be taken at 3-month intervals during the second year after treatment and at 6-month intervals during the third, fourth, and fifth years. If at the end of 5 years the patient has no clinical evidence of syphilis and has a normal blood and spinal fluid, he may be considered completely cured.

A spinal fluid examination should be performed 6 months after the completion of treatment for early syphilis. If the spinal fluid is normal at this time and if the patient continues to show no evidence of clinical or serologic relapse, the examination need not be repeated until approximately 2 years following treatment. Patients having positive spinal fluid tests for syphilis 6 months or more after treatment for early syphilis should be re-treated.

Relapse and Reinfection. Evidence of relapse in early syphilis may occur as early as 4 weeks or as late as 2 years after treatment.

The prognosis of relapsing syphilis is more serious than the initial infection, and these patients should be re-treated with twice the original dose of penicillin, given over a longer period of time. Many patients with recurrent syphilis actually have a new infection rather than a relapse of their original infection. Although various criteria have been set up to distinguish relapse from reinfection, differentiation is often impossible.

SYPHILIS IN PREGNANCY. Congenital syphilis can be prevented by proper treatment of syphilis in pregnancy. Although women with syphilis of many years' duration are not likely to bear syphilitic children, further treatment of such patients during pregnancy is recommended. Although treatment with penicillin is of considerable value when given during the last months of pregnancy, it is best given before the fetus becomes grossly infected, i.e., before the last trimester.

All patients treated for syphilis in pregnancy should be observed very closely, and quantitative serologic tests for syphilis taken at least every month. Re-treatment during pregnancy is indicated if there is a rise in serologic titer following therapy, if a definite decrease in titer fails to occur in patients with early syphilis, or if the patient develops recurrent syphilitic lesions. A positive serologic test at the time of delivery does not necessarily indicate that treatment has been inadequate. The child born of a mother treated for syphilis should have a serologic test every 2 to 4 weeks until it is at least six months of age. Once the woman has received adequate amounts of penicillin for syphilis, it is not necessary to re-treat her during succeeding pregnancies if the titer of the serologic test is negative or remains low (less than 1:4).

CONGENITAL SYPHILIS. Infants with congenital syphilis should receive careful supportive care and adequate nutrition, in addition to antisyphilitic treatment. Penicillin is very effective; a total dosage of 200,000 units per kg body weight given in equally divided amounts every 3 hr to 7 to 10 days is adequate. Although the use of procaine penicillin in a large series of these cases has not been reported, this type of penicillin should also give satisfactory results. Doses of 150,000 units of procaine penicillin in aqueous solution given every day for eight injections are recommended. Follow-up blood tests and the indications for re-treatment in early congenital syphilis are the same as in early acquired syphilis.

Treatment of interstitial keratitis is not altogether satisfactory. Penicillin therapy is recommended, but it does not always result in reduction of the inflammation or clearing of the corneal opacities. Occasionally, interstitial keratitis appears for the first time during, or immediately after, what appear to be adequate dosages of penicillin. It seems probable that this ocular manifestation represents a type of hypersensitivity phenomenon. Cortisone in aqueous suspension (5 mg per ml) or in ointment form should be applied to the involved eye every few hours day and night for several weeks. The inflammatory reaction often recurs, however, after the drug is discontinued, and repeated courses may be necessary until spontaneous regression appears. Hydrarthrosis (Clutton's synovitis) responds slowly to penicillin therapy.

LATE SYPHILIS. Latent Stage. The chief purpose in treating late latent syphilis is to prevent the development of gummatous lesions and cardiovascular syphilis. Patients with late latent syphilis have negative spinal fluids and rarely, if ever, develop neurosyphilis.

The value of penicillin has not been fully assessed in late latent syphilis. Because the prognosis of this stage of the disease is so good and the drug is known to be effective in both early and late symptomatic syphilis, it is presumed to be of value in patients with latent infection. The treatment schedules suggested for early syphilis, employing 4 to 6 million units of penicillin, are recommended. Failure of the serologic test to revert to negative after adequate treatment—i.e., *seroresistance*—is not necessarily a forerunner of late complications. Once the patient with late syphilis has had adequate treatment, additional penicillin therapy will not contribute significantly toward reversal of the blood test.

Skin, Bones, and Viscera. Gummatous lesions of the skin, mucous membranes, bones, and viscera usually respond promptly to penicillin therapy. The recommended total dosage of penicillin is greater than that employed in early syphilis and should be approximately 10 million units. This can be administered as 900,000 units of procaine penicillin given every 48 hr for 12 injections. The posttreatment observations and indications for re-treatment of these patients are the same as those recommended above. A high percentage of patients with late syphilitic lesions have abnormal spinal fluid findings, and a lumbar puncture is indicated in every patient before treatment is instituted.

Cardiovascular Syphilis. The value of antisyphilitic therapy in late cardiovascular syphilis is difficult to determine. Many syphilologists believe that treatment does not delay the ultimate development of myocardial failure or aneurysmal rupture. Treatment appears to be of some value, however, in early aortic regurgitation, uncomplicated aortitis, or small asymptomatic aneurysms. The risk of a serious Herxheimer reaction following initiation of penicillin treatment has been minimal. Preparatory bismuth therapy is probably of little value in preventing this type of reaction, and most workers begin treatment with penicillin. The total dosage is 10 to 15 million units of penicillin, given in schedules similar to those recommended for gummatous lesions. As in other types of late syphilis, the serologic test often remains positive after therapy. Proper management of congestive failure and restriction of physical activity of these patients are of paramount importance.

Neurosyphilis. The results of treatment of neurosyphilis depend largely upon the type and duration of the neuropathologic process. If the predominant lesion of the central nervous system is degenerative, as in tabes and optic atrophy, little response to any form of treatment can be expected. If the tissue reaction is chiefly inflammatory, as in syphilitic meningitis, rapid and almost complete return of function will occur.

Penicillin treatment of neurosyphilis is often followed by dramatic clinical response with prompt and favorable changes in the spinal fluid. Shortly after penicillin therapy, there is a rapid reduction in the spinal fluid cell count and protein. The spinal fluid serologic reaction, however, may not become negative for 5 years or more. Penicillin produced normal spinal fluid cell counts in 85 to 90 percent of patients treated for various types of neurosyphilis. The remaining 10 to 15 percent showed abnormal spinal fluid cell counts 6 to 12 months following treatment and were considered treatment failures.

It is generally agreed that the improvement in the clinical manifestations of neurosyphilis and in the spinal fluid abnormalities following penicillin is as good as that obtained with fever therapy. Penicillin alone is the treatment of choice in patients with asymptomatic neurosyphilis, syphilitic meningitis, meningovascular syphilis, and tabes. The optimum dosage schedule has not been definitely established, but doses of 10 to 15 million units are usually recommended either as the aqueous solution, 100,000 units every 3 hr, or as repository penicillin 900,000 units a day.

Treatment of the tabetic bladder may be very discouraging. Drugs, such as Mecholyl chloride and ergotamine, have been employed to increase bladder tone and contraction, but the results are variable. In early cases the patient can be trained to micturate at regular intervals and empty the bladder by pressure on the lower part of the abdomen. In late cases, surgical procedures (transurethral resection of the vesical neck, suprapubic cystotomy) may be necessary. Urinary tract infection should be prevented and instrumentation avoided as much as possible. Charcot joints are rarely improved by antisyphilitic therapy, and special orthopedic treatment is necessary. The management of patients with gastric crisis is sometimes very difficult. In the acute attack the patient should be heavily sedated. Morphine should be avoided. Large doses of atropine are said to be of value in relieving the symptoms of gastric crisis.

In most cases of advanced optic atrophy the use of penicillin or fever, alone or in combination, does not prevent the development of blindness. Patients with optic atrophy should be admitted to the hospital and given penicillin in aqueous solution, 200,000 units every 4 hr for 13 to 17 days, for a total dosage of 15 to 20 million units.

In paresis, penicillin alone often results in marked improvement in tremor, mental state, and speech and writing defects. It has been reported to produce entirely satisfactory results in about 20 percent and significant improvement in an additional 35 percent of a large series of patients with paresis treated in general hospitals. Early penicillin treatment of incipient paresis has resulted in clinical remission and ability to return to work in more than 80 percent of patients. Large amounts of penicillin —15 to 20 million units—are generally recommended, but doses as low as 6 million units have been found to be of value. Although the repository type of penicillin is said to be as effective as aqueous penicillin in paresis or optic atrophy, the aqueous preparation is preferred in moderately or severely affected patients. It should be given in schedules similar to those recommended for optic atrophy.

Fever therapy should not be used initially in either optic atrophy or paresis because its possible additive effects are not sufficient to justify the hazards associated with it. In selected patients in whom the neurosyphilitic process progresses despite adequate initial penicillin therapy, re-treatment with fever therapy and penicillin should be considered. Retreatment with penicillin alone, however, is indicated in progressive paresis if the initial course of treatment consisted of less than 6 million units. Penicillin alone should also be used to re-treat patients who show elevated spinal fluid cell counts a year or more after the initial therapy or in whom there was temporary clinical improvement after treatment but subsequent progression of the disease.

Careful neuropsychiatric and spinal fluid observations should be made following treatment of all patients with neurosyphilis. These should be done every 4 months during the first year, twice during the second year, and once a year thereafter, or until the spinal fluid is completely negative and permanent regression of symptoms seems apparent. In late neurosyphilis the spinal fluid serologic reaction often remains positive for many years, despite repeated courses of chemotherapy or fever; this does not in itself indicate progression or relapse of the neurosyphilitic process.

Herxheimer Reactions in Late Syphilis. Exacerbations of late syphilitic lesions are not infrequently observed following the initial administration of arsenicals or penicillin. Approximately one-half the patients treated for paresis become temporarily worse and show increased agitation and mental confusion during the first 24 hr of penicillin treatment. Other manifestations of Herxheimer's reaction, such as myelitis, convulsions, and exacerbation of lightning pains, have been reported.

There have been very few cases in which penicillin

therapy has produced an acute exacerbation of clinical manifestations of cardiovascular syphilis. Neither the use of small initial doses of penicillin nor preparatory treatment with bismuth seems indicated in an attempt to prevent Herxheimer's effects.

EFFECT OF PENICILLIN AND OTHER ANTIBIOTICS WHEN USED FOR OTHER DISEASES. The widespread use of penicillin and antibiotics with treponemicidal properties in the treatment of various other infections has created confusion in the diagnosis and management of syphilis. This is particularly true when gonorrhea is treated. Patients with gonorrhea may have acquired syphilis simultaneously. Although there is reason to believe that the use of penicillin and perhaps of the other antibiotics frequently aborts the syphilitic infection completely, they may at times only delay the appearance of the lesions or prevent their development. For these reasons it is recommended that all persons with gonorrhea treated with penicillin or the other spirocheticidal antibiotics should have serologic tests for syphilis at monthly intervals for at least 4 months. The appearance of fever several hours after the administration of penicillin for gonorrhea is suggestive of Herxheimer's reaction and of syphilis.

The management of patients with positive serologic tests who have had previous penicillin therapy for other nonrelated infections is sometimes difficult. If syphilitic infection is thought to be present, the decision as to further therapy should be based upon the amount of penicillin already administered, the type and duration of syphilitic infection, the result of the spinal fluid examination, and the titer of the serologic test.

PROPHYLAXIS

Syphilis and the other venereal diseases can be prevented in most instances by the proper prophylactic measures during and following sexual intercourse. Protection from contact with infectious genital lesions can be obtained to some degree by the use of a condom. The danger of infection can also be reduced if the genitalia are washed thoroughly with soap and water immediately after exposure. Although ointments containing various treponemicidal substances have been employed for many years as local prophylactic agents, the use of these compounds is no longer recommended. In small series of cases, penicillin has been shown to prevent infection in individuals who are known to have been sexually exposed to patients with primary or secondary syphilis. The use of penicillin in these cases is justified not only as an attempt to abort the infection in the exposed individual, but also to prevent reinfection of the original patient who often maintains sexual relations with the contact despite instructions to the contrary.

Procaine penicillin or benzathine penicillin G in doses of 2.4 million units should be given soon after exposure to persons who have had sexual contact with known or suspected cases of infectious syphilis. The administration of penicillin as a routine prophylactic measure following every extramarital sexual exposure is neither practical nor advisable. Persons receiving prophylactic treatment should be kept under observation and should have repeated serologic tests for at least 6 months.

The prophylactic treatment of nurses, physicians, or laboratory workers accidentally exposed to, or inoculated with, infectious material will depend largely upon the risk of infection in the individual case. Another indication for prophylactic treatment is in pregnant women who are sexually exposed to infectious patients. A full course of penicillin treatment in these cases is indicated in an effort to prevent fetal infection.

PSYCHOTHERAPY

There are still considerable stigma and psychologic trauma attached to the diagnosis of syphillis, and proper treatment requires more than the mere administration of chemotherapeutic agents. The sociologic and psychologic aspects of this disease are considerable. Patients often have a sense of shame and guilt, and some postpone or discontinue medical care. Others develop serious anxiety states and return repeatedly for reassurance that the disease has been arrested. Some individuals develop syphilophobia as a result of having heard or read of the serious effects of the disease. Every effort to relieve these patients of their anxiety by correcting mistaken ideas regarding the infection and by emphasizing the good prognosis should be made.

Upon learning the diagnosis, many patients either condemn their marital partners and threaten divorce or separation or else refuse to impart the information to their spouse. It is essential, however, that the marital partners of patients with infectious syphilis be examined at regular intervals for evidence of the disease.

REFERENCES

Atwood, W. G., J. L. Miller, G. W. Stout, and L. C. Norins: The TPI and FTA-ABS Tests in Treated Late Syphilis, J.A.M.A., 203:549, 1968.

Cannefax, G. R., L. C. Norins, and E. J. Gillespie: Immunology of Syphilis, Ann. Rev. Med., 18:471, 1967.

Harvey, A. M., and L. E. Shulman: Connective Tissue Disease and the Chronic Biologic False-positive Test for Syphilis (BFP Reaction), Med. Clinics N. Am., 50:1271, 1966.

Magnuson, H. J., E. W. Thomas, S. Olansky, B. I. Kaplin, L. deMello, and J. C. Cutler: Inoculation Syphilis in Human Volunteers, Medicine, 35:33, 1956.

Nicholas, L., and H. Beerman: Late Syphilis: A Review of Some of the Recent Literature, Am. J. Med. Sci., 254:549, 1967.

Tuffanelli, D. L., K. D. Wuepper, L. L. Bradford, and R. M. Wood: Fluorescent Treponemal-antibody Absorption Tests, New Engl. J. Med., 276:258, 1967.

178 YAWS
Albert Heyman

DEFINITION. Yaws is an infectious tropical disease caused by the *Treponema pertenue*. It is characterized by a primary cutaneous lesion, which is followed by a granulomatous skin eruption and, in some instances, by late destructive lesions of the skin and bones. The disease is also known as *frambesia, pain, bouba,* and *parangi.*

ETIOLOGY. The etiologic agent of yaws, the *T. pertenue,* is morphologically indistinguishable from *Treponema pallidum.* It further resembles the spirochete of syphilis, in that it produces a positive reaction with the Wassermann and flocculation tests for syphilis and is also susceptible to arsenicals, bismuth, and penicillin. Cross immunity between the two diseases has been observed in both man and experimental animals. There has been considerable controversy as to whether the two diseases were at one time identical and have been modified over the years by climate, race, and other factors.

EPIDEMIOLOGY. Yaws is confined entirely to the Tropics and is prevalent in the West Indies, South Pacific islands, equatorial Africa, and South America. The disease is usually acquired before puberty and is spread by direct contact with open lesions containing the spirochete. Transmission of the disease occurs rarely by sexual contact. Certain species of flies are also thought to be vectors of this infection. The disease is more common in natives with poor personal hygiene.

MANIFESTATIONS. Following an average incubation period of 3 to 4 weeks, a primary lesion, the *mother yaw,* appears at the site of inoculation. This is almost invariably extragenital and usually occurs on the legs. This lesion is a granuloma, which later ulcerates and heals with scar formation. About 6 to 12 weeks after the appearance of the lesion, a generalized eruption develops, consisting of large papules or granulomas on the face, neck, extremities, and buttocks. These lesions often occur about the mucocutaneous junctions, such as the mouth, nose, and rectum, and resemble condylomas of secondary syphilis. They heal slowly, but relapses may occur months or years after the onset of the initial yaw. The lesions of yaws often appear on the soles of the feet and produce painful ulcerations, so-called "crab yaws."

After several years, late destructive lesions may appear in the skin and bones. Periostitis and osteitis are found in the bones of the hands, arms, and legs, producing characteristic dactylitis and "saber shins." Destructive lesions appear about the nose and result in severe ulcerative areas (*gangosa*). Proliferative exostoses develop in the nasal portion of the maxillary bones; this is known as *goundou.* Juxtaarticular nodules are also seen in the late stage of the disease. Involvement of the aorta and the central nervous system has been reported, but these complications are rare.

DIAGNOSIS. The diagnosis of yaws can often be made on the appearance of the generalized skin eruption alone, but *T. pertenue* is easily demonstrated in the lesions. The Wassermann and flocculation tests for syphilis are usually positive. The lesions of yaws may be confused with those of leishmaniasis, leprosy, and tuberculosis. It is often impossible to differentiate between late lesions of yaws and late gummatous syphilis.

TREATMENT. Penicillin, the drug of choice in the treatment of yaws, produces prompt disappearance of the treponemes on dark-field examination and rapid healing of the lesions. The recommended dosage is a single injection of 1.2 million units of procaine penicillin in adults with early active lesions and proportionally less in children and in those with latent cases. The tetracyclines are thought to be less effective in the management of this condition. The World Health Organization has conducted large-scale campaigns to eradicate the disease in endemic areas, and some 40 million persons have been treated under its auspices. In high-prevalence areas, treatment has been given to the total population, with dramatic reduction in the incidence of new cases. As a result of these control measures and improvement in living standards of the native populations, yaws is rapidly receding in the equatorial portions of the world. The extensive and rapid travel now prevalent throughout the world and the large migration of West Indian and Middle Eastern natives to the English-speaking countries has led to the appearance of sporadic cases of infectious yaws and other types of treponematosis in several large cities in the United Kingdom.

REFERENCES

Hackett, C. J.: "An International Nomenclature of Yaws Lesions," World Health Organization Monograph Series, no. 36, 1957. (An atlas containing numerous photographs illustrating recommended terminology.)

———, and T. Guthe: Some Important Aspects of Yaws Eradication, Bull. World Health Organ., 15:869, 1956. (This reference is part of a symposium on treponematoses as a worldwide problem.)

Lanigan-O'Keefe, F. M., J. G. Holmes, and D. Hill: Infectious and Active Yaws in a Midland City, Brit. J. Dermatol., 79:325, 1967.

Turner, T. B., and D. H. Hollander: "Biology of the Treponematoses," World Health Organization Monograph Series, no. 35, 1957.

179 PINTA
Albert Heyman

DEFINITION. Pinta is an infectious disease of the skin caused by *Treponema carateum.* It is characterized by an initial papular lesion of the skin, followed by depigmented areas on the extremities and hyperkeratosis on the soles and palms. The disease is also known as *mal del pinto, azul,* and *carate.* Pinta is found almost entirely in the Western Hemisphere and is especially prevalent in Mexico and Colombia.

ETIOLOGY. *Treponema carateum,* the etiologic agent of pinta, is morphologically indistinguishable from *Treponema pallidum.* The exact relationship of this disease to other treponematoses (syphilis, yaws, and bejel) has not been definitely determined, and there are many similarities in the clinical manifestations of these infections. Pinta is usually transmitted from person to person by direct contact. It may also be spread by an insect vector.

MANIFESTATIONS. The primary lesion of pinta appears after an incubation period of 7 to 20 days as a non-ulcerative papule at the site of infection. This is followed 5 to 18 months later by a secondary eruption characterized by flat erythematous and hyperpigmented lesions, called *pintids*. Late lesions develop after several years and appear as vitiligoid, slate blue, or variously colored patches of the skin. The hands, wrists, knees, and ankles are commonly involved, and hyperkeratoses of the palms and soles are also seen. Aortitis and spinal fluid abnormalities similar to those found in neurosyphilis have been observed in some pinta patients. The Wassermann reaction of the blood and flocculation tests for syphilis are usually positive in the late stages of the disease.

TREATMENT. A single injection of 1.2 million units of procaine penicillin or benzathine penicillin G produces rapid disappearance of the *T. caratum* from the lesions of pinta and a decline in serologic titer. It is the treatment of choice in this disease and is more effective than chloramphenicol or the tetracyclines.

REFERENCES

Beerman, H.: Pinta: A Review of Recent Etiologic and Clinical Studies, Am. J. Med. Sci., 205:611, 1943.

Hume, J. C.: Worldwide Problems in the Diagnosis of Syphilis and Other Treponematoses, Med. Clinics N. Am., 48:721, 1964.

Marquez, F., C. R. Rein, and O. Arias: Mal del Pinto in Mexico, Bull. World Health Organiz., 13:299, 1955.

180 BEJEL
Albert Heyman

DEFINITION AND ETIOLOGY. Bejel is a chronic infectious disease caused by a spirochete indistinguishable from *Treponema pallidum*. It is found chiefly among the children of Arab tribes in the Eastern Mediterranean area, being particularly prevalent in some sections of Iraq, Syria, and Jordan. The illness is first manifested by ulcerations of the mucous membranes in the mouth and is thought to be spread by the use of common drinking utensils. It is rarely transmitted by sexual contact and is usually acquired by adults through close contact with an infected child as by kissing and fondling.

Treponemes are readily found on dark-field examination of the lesions of the skin and mucous membranes. The disease is thought by Hudson to be an example of nonvenereal syphilis, the causative organism and the clinical manifestations having been modified for many generations by special epidemiologic and climatic factors.

Bejel resembles in many respects the cases of endemic syphilis which appeared for many years in certain areas of South Africa and Yugoslavia.

MANIFESTATIONS. The illness begins with ulcerations in the mouth and lips, but there may also be a diffuse papular eruption with moist lesions on the mucocutaneous surfaces and skin folds. The late lesions resemble gummatous syphilis and are manifested as ulcerations in the skin and mucous membranes. Osteitis and periostitis of the long bones and skull may develop. The nasal bones, palate and pharynx, particularly, may be involved in a destructive process. The heart and nervous system are rarely, if ever, affected. The illness also differs from venereal syphilis in that it is apparently not spread to the child in utero from an infected mother. The diagnosis can be made by dark-field examination of the lesions or by the usual serologic tests for syphilis.

TREATMENT. A single injection of 1.2 million units of procaine penicillin seems to be effective. In patients with late osseous or ulcerative lesions, additional penicillin may be required.

REFERENCES

Hudson, E. H.: "Non-venereal Syphilis," Edinburgh, E. S. Livingston, Ltd., 1958.

Hume, J. C.: Worldwide Problems in the Diagnosis of Syphilis and Other Treponematoses, Med. Clinics N. Am., 48:721, 1964.

Wray, P. M.: Bejel in Sheffield, Brit. J. Venereal Dis., 42:25, 1966.

181 LEPTOSPIROSIS
Fred R. McCrumb, Jr., and T. E. Woodward

ETIOLOGY. The genus *Leptospira* comprises a large group of microorganisms possessing a high degree of antigenic specificity which forms the basis of their classification. Leptospiral serotypes pathogenic for man are indistinguishable morphologically and, in general, have similar biochemical activities and cultural requirements. The organisms show a delicate spiral configuration about an axial filament which is readily demonstrated by electron microscopy. Examination of the organisms in a fluid medium by dark-ground illumination reveals active motility with characteristic hooklike bending at one end or both ends. Within the genus there are at least 18 serogroups composed of a total of 124 serotypes. Among the 22 serotypes known to occur in the United States, 13 have been associated with human infection.

EPIDEMIOLOGY. The natural reservoir of leptospirosis is found among a broad spectrum of lower animal species; wild and commensal rodents are the major sources of infection in the classical endemic areas of the world. Leptospirosis is worldwide in distribution; however, the widest variety of serotypes is found in tropical or subtropical regions with an abundance of rainfall and a rich rodent fauna. Wherever agricultural practices have resulted in the emergence of a few rodent species, the spectrum of leptospiral serotypes becomes restricted. Natural infection of rats, mice, voles, opossums, cattle, swine, and dogs leads frequently to the development of a renal carrier state and the shedding of leptospiras in the urine of these hosts. Man may become infected whenever his activities bring him into an area frequented by animal carriers. Infected rodents rarely show any evidence of disease, and adult domestic swine may experience only an increased incidence of abortion. In contrast, well-defined clinical illness occurs in dogs and cattle, which may die from the infection.

Leptospiras are transmitted to man most frequently through water contaminated by the urine of carrier animal hosts, although direct contact with infected tissues is important among veterinarians, abbatoir workers, and farmers. The occupational hazard of leptospirosis is greatest among rice-field workers, cane cutters, miners, sewer workers, operational military personnel, farmers, veterinarians, and employees of animal processing plants. The age and sex distribution of leptospirosis is determined largely by occupational or avocational risk rather than by age or sex influences on susceptibility to infection. A notable exception to the general preponderance of leptospirosis among adult males is the high attack rate in female rice-field workers in Italy.

Recognition of leptospirosis as a human health problem in the United States is a recent medical achievement. By 1956, fewer than 500 cases of this disease in man had been reported in this country. The total number of cases reported by 1961 still numbered under 1,000; however, additional serotypes had been associated with human infections. Among the 22 serotypes associated with infections in lower animals, *L. icterohaemorrhagiae, L. canicola, L. pomona, L. grippotyphosa, L. autumnalis, L. australis, L. bataviae, L. hebdomadis, L. ballum,* and *L. pyrogenes* have been identified as causes of human infection in this country. The first three of these serotypes are most frequently associated with infection in man.

PATHOGENESIS. Leptospiras gain access to the body by way of the skin and mucous membranes. Cutaneous transmission of leptospiras must occur commonly because skin is exposed frequently to the media through which this disease is acquired, particularly in workers whose occupation results in trauma to skin of the hands and lower extremities. Accidental contamination of the buccal mucous membranes or conjunctivas has been followed by leptospiral infections in laboratory workers, and outbreaks of this disease have been related to the consumption of contaminated food or water. Transmission from man to man is rare, probably because leptospiras are unable to survive in acid urine.

Infection in man is regularly associated with entry of leptospiras into the blood and dissemination to various organs. Adequate histopathologic studies have been limited to fatal cases wherein tissue changes were extreme. Renal changes consist of cloudy swelling of tubular epithelium and focal areas of interstitial nephritis characterized by infiltration with lymphocytes and plasma cells. Dissociation of hepatic cords and cloudy swelling of parenchymal and Kupffer cells are frequent in patients dying of leptospirosis. Obstruction of bile capillaries may be observed but is not a consistent finding. Hepatic dysfunction may be much more severe than the histopathologic abnormalities would suggest. The mechanism of hemorrhagic manifestations in leptospirosis is not clearly understood. Inflammatory lesions are observed in skeletal muscle as well as in myocardium. Perivascular inflammation is present in the brain and meninges of patients with signs of central-nervous-system involvement. Leptospiras are demonstrated irregularly in renal and hepatic tissues by silver impregnation staining, but this procedure is not a suitable substitute for cultural methods.

CLINICAL MANIFESTATIONS. Leptospirosis was first recognized and described as a distinct clinical entity in 1883 by Landouzy. Three years later, Weil observed several patients with fever, jaundice, and hemorrhages associated with hepatic and renal failure. This form of leptospirosis, since known as *Weil's disease*, is characterized by unusual severity and a high mortality rate. In contrast to the leptospiras producing Weil's disease, most serotypes produce self-limiting disease of varying severity, rarely lasting more than 7 days. The vast majority of infections are benign and do not conform to Weil's description of severe leptospirosis.

Leptospiral infections in man are characterized by the abrupt onset of high fever, prostration, headache, nausea and vomiting, conjunctival injection, and myalgia after an incubation period of 3 to 19 days, usually 7 to 13 days. The febrile phase of the illness usually ends after 1 week, and in milder infections, other evidence of disease subsides with defervescence. Mild relapses lasting 2 to 3 days are not uncommon. Although the term Weil's disease is used to describe severe leptospiral illnesses caused by *L. icterohaemorrhagiae,* milder infections with this organism are not rare, and other leptospiral serotypes can produce severe and even fatal forms of the disease. The frequency with which icterus and renal failure occur varies with the geographic area, because certain serotypes commonly associated with severe infections are more prevalent in some countries than in others.

Headache is present in nearly all patients with leptospirosis, and about 50 percent of patients complain of severe retrobulbar pain. *Conjunctival injection* is noted in 85 percent of patients, and is marked in the severely ill. *Rash* appears between the fourth and eighth days of disease in about 25 percent of patients, and there is a tendency for it to become hemorrhagic in those with a serious infection. The eruption usually consists of small macules or maculopapules distributed over the trunk and extremities. *Gastrointestinal disturbances* consisting of anorexia, nausea, vomiting, and abdominal pain occur in nearly all patients with leptospirosis, and protracted vomiting and headache frequently constitute the most distressing features of the illness. *Cough* is a common complaint and is productive of blood-streaked sputum in about 25 percent of those with this symptom. Roentgen examination of the chest may reveal pneumonitis, a feature which has not received much attention.

Severe *hemorrhagic manifestations* of leptospirosis are

uncommon except in profoundly ill patients; however, some evidence of bleeding is observed in 30 to 50 percent of all patients. Hematemesis and hemoptysis are the most common hemorrhagic manifestations, followed in frequency by conjunctival hemorrhage, epistaxis, petechiae, and melena. There may be moderate lymphadenopathy, but splenomegaly is rare.

Nuchal rigidity occurs in 30 to 40 percent of patients. In some instances, the clinical picture is that of aseptic meningitis and may be indistinguishable from the same syndrome caused by mumps, lymphocytic choriomeningitis, and certain enterovirus infections. When other evidence of leptospirosis is inconspicuous or absent in patients with aseptic meningitis, some time may elapse before the true cause is suspected. Iridocyclitis manifested by photophobia and circumcorneal injection occurs in fewer than 5 percent of patients with leptospirosis.

The incidence of clinically overt jaundice varies considerably, depending on the infecting serotypes encountered. Icterus is found in 75 percent of patients infected with *L. icterohaemorrhagiae* but only in 5 to 10 percent of persons infected with serotypes such as *L. grippotyphosa*, *L. canicola*, and *L. pomona*. Jaundice usually appears toward the end of the first week of illness as the fever is subsiding. Those with marked liver involvement show evidence of progressive hepatic dysfunction, and recovery may not occur for 2 or 3 weeks. Hepatomegaly and liver tenderness are common findings in patients with jaundice.

Severe leptospiral infections are also characterized by renal failure manifested by oliguria, proteinuria, and azotemia. Fatal leptospirosis is almost always ascribable to renal failure, although hepatic insufficiency complicates the illness, and massive hemorrhage may cause death. Mortality rates range from less than 1 percent to as high as 10 percent in different regions, depending on the incidence of severe forms of the disease.

LABORATORY FINDINGS. Although normal peripheral blood leukocyte counts are the rule in uncomplicated leptospirosis, neutrophilic leukocytosis of 12,000 to 15,000 cells per cu mm may be observed in severely ill patients, and counts of 25,000 to 40,000 cells per cu mm occur in Weil's disease. Urinary abnormalities are noted in about 80 percent of patients with leptospirosis; proteinuria, cylindruria, pyuria, and hematuria are frequent and constitute important diagnostic clues. Return to normal renal function usually is rapid, and there is no evidence that permanent renal damage results from leptospiral infections.

Hyperbilirubinemia, abnormal flocculation tests, hypoalbuminemia and hyperglobulinemia, and abnormalities in alkaline phosphatase, SGOT (serum glutamic oxalic transaminase), SGPT (serum glutamic pyruvic transaminase), and LDH (lactic dehydrogenase) can be demonstrated in over 50 percent of patients without clinical evidence of liver disease. Recovery of normal liver function is rapid as the clinical manifestations of the illness subside.

Leptospirosis has been shown to be the cause of approximately 4 percent of all cases of aseptic meningitis in several well-studied series (Chap. 361). However, the frequency with which the central nervous system is involved in leptospirosis is not known. Mild pleocytosis (40 to 500 cells) with mononuclear cells characterizes leptospiral aseptic meningitis. Modest elevation of cerebrospinal fluid protein is usual, but glucose and chloride concentrations remain normal. The cerebrospinal fluid quickly reverts to normal during early convalescence.

LABORATORY DIAGNOSIS. Leptospiras can be isolated from the blood of most patients during the acute phase of the illness. Many leptospiral serotypes do not produce overt disease in guinea pigs and hamsters, and isolation of these organisms ultimately requires the use of cultural techniques. For this reason, the use of laboratory animals to diagnose leptospirosis should be limited to situations in which the only material available for isolation of the causative organism is contaminated. The simplest artificial medium for culturing of leptospiras is prepared by mixing a small amount of peptone with distilled water and adding sterile inactivated rabbit serum in a final concentration of 7 to 10 percent. This medium is dispensed in 10-ml amounts into screw-capped tubes or rubber-stoppered bottles and may be stored in a refrigerator for several months. It is imperative to use small inoculums when attempting to recover leptospiras to avoid inhibition of these organisms by excessive quantities of blood. When single drops of whole venous blood are inoculated into each of five tubes at the bedside, positive results may be expected in 75 to 90 percent of cultural attempts made during the first 3 days of illness. As the disease progresses, the intensity and regularity of leptospiremia decrease. Because of the intermittent nature of leptospiruria and the adverse effect of low pH and bacterial contamination, culture of urine is not recommended. Leptospiras also have been recovered from cerebrospinal fluid.

Incubation of cultures is carried out at 32°C, and in order to avoid the risk of contamination of the medium, dark-field examination of the cultures is performed at weekly intervals, beginning 10 days after inoculation.

Several serologic tests may be employed in the diagnosis of leptospirosis. The classical microscopic agglutination-lysis test is cumbersome because of its type specificity and the need to maintain a large number of stock cultures. In addition the use of viable antigens creates a risk of laboratory infection. For these reasons this procedure should be confined to reference centers and research laboratories where serotyping of leptospiral isolates is a major activity.

Tests employing antigen pools or broadly reactive antigens with generic specificity, permitting the recognition of antibody against most leptospiral serotypes, should be employed by diagnostic laboratories. The slide agglutination test developed by Galton employs formolized antigens in four pools representing 12 serotypes. In recent years this procedure has been widely used and is probably the best diagnostic test. Two other serologic tests with broad reactivity have been employed successfully in the diagnosis of human infection. Complement-fixing antibodies can be detected in the serum of patients convalescing from leptospirosis using sonicated antigen derived from *L. icterochaemorrhagiae*, *L. grippotyphosa*, and *L. tarassovi*. Antigen with similar group reactivity prepared from *L. biflexa* permits detection of antibody resulting from infection with a wide variety of serotypes. In this procedure, antigen adsorbed onto sheep erythrocytes will cause hemolysis of these cells in the presence of complement and leptospiral antibody. The hemolytic test has the attributes of broad reactivity and a high degree of sensitivity in the detection of antibody in man but is relatively insensitive when employed with bovine or porcine serum. Measurement of antibody using an indirect immunofluorescent technique has been reported. However, its utility as a routine diagnostic procedure is not established.

DIFFERENTIAL DIAGNOSIS. Leptospirosis should be considered a possible cause of any febrile disease characterized by headache, gastrointestinal symptoms, conjunctival injection, and myalgia. The presence of urinary abnormalities and a history of contact with water frequented by rodents or domestic animals should arouse further suspicion. The diagnosis should not be reserved for patients with jaundice, because a majority of leptospiral infections is not associated with clinically overt icterus. Leptospirosis should be considered in the differential diagnosis of all cases of aseptic meningitis. Other acute febrile illnesses with which leptospirosis may be confused include influenza, the rickettsioses, enteric fevers, brucellosis, and dengue. Late manifestations of leptospirosis may resemble infectious hepatitis, hemolytic and obstructive jaundice, and acute glomerulonephritis.

TREATMENT. Evaluation of antibiotics in human leptospirosis is complicated by the relatively short course of the acute infection and the lack of suitably controlled studies. Penicillin, streptomycin, and the tetracyclines inhibit the growth of leptospiras in vitro and will control experimental infections in hamsters and guinea pigs. Streptomycin and tetracyclines eliminate leptospiras from the kidneys of canine carriers of *L. canicola*.

Opinions differ regarding the usefulness of penicillin and tetracyclines in the treatment of human leptospirosis. It is agreed that chloramphenicol does not favorably alter the course of this disease. The use of tetracyclines, penicillin, streptomycin, and chloramphenicol in one controlled study failed to reveal a shortening of the febrile course or a reduction in the incidence of complications as a result of antibiotic therapy. Other evidence supports the concept that penicillin results in a shorter febrile course and in a lower incidence of complications. On the basis of most studies, the use of 4 to 6 million units of penicillin G daily in divided dosage during the febrile phase of the illness is probably indicated.

Most leptospiral infections are not severe and subside without complications even in untreated patients. Because acute renal failure in leptospirosis is reversible, its management should make use of all available therapeutic aids, including hemodialysis. Rarely, hemorrhage may result in enough blood loss to warrant replacement.

REFERENCES

Alston, J. M., and J. C. Broom: "Leptospirosis in Man and Animals," London, E. & S. Livingstone, Ltd., 1958.

Doherty, R. L.: A Clinical Study of Leptospirosis in North Queensland, Australasian Ann. Med., 4:53, 1955.

Edwards, G. A., and B. M. Domm: Human Leptospirosis, Medicine, 39:117, 1960.

Fairburn, A. C., and S. J. G. Semple: Chloramphenicol and Penicillin in the Treatment of Leptospirosis among British Troops in Malaya, Lancet, 1:13, 1956.

Hall, H. E., J. A. Hightower, R. Diaz-Rivera, R. J. Byrne, J. E. Smadel, and T. E. Woodward: Evaluation of Antibiotic Therapy in Human Leptospirosis, Ann. Intern. Med., 35:981, 1951.

Heath, C. W., A. D. Alexander, and M. M. Galton: Leptospirosis in the United States, Analysis of 483 Cases in Man, 1949–1961, New Engl. J. Med., 273:857, 1965.

McCrumb, F. R., Jr., J. L. Stockard, C. R. Robinson, L. H. Turner, D. G. Lewis, C. W. Maisey, M. F. Kelleher, C. A. Gleiser, and J. E. Smadel: Leptospirosis in Malaya: I. Sporadic Cases among Military and Civilian Personnel, Am. J. Trop. Med. Hyg., 6:238, 1957.

World Health Organization Tech. Rep. Ser., no. 380, 1967.

182 RELAPSING FEVER
E. H. O. Parry and Robert G. Petersdorf

DEFINITION. Relapsing fever, an acute infectious disease caused by spirochetes of the genus *Borrelia*, has two varieties which depend on the vector—the louse-borne disease and the tick-borne.

ETIOLOGY. Spirochetes of the genus *Borrelia* are 10 to 20 μ long and slender, and move in a corkscrew fashion. *Borrelia recurrentis* is the causative organism of louse-borne relapsing fever. Many strains of *Borrelia* have been found in the tick-borne disease, and they are known by their vector. Culture of the organisms is difficult.

EPIDEMIOLOGY AND PATHOGENESIS. The louse-borne disease is disappearing rapidly but is still endemic in Ethiopia, and may occur in East Asia also. Major epidemics followed World War I, when millions of cases were seen in Eastern Europe. Soldiers returning home introduced the disease to the Sudan belt of Africa; from there it moved slowly eastwards, with the mortality rate reaching 30 percent in some areas. A similar but less-virulent epidemic crossed Africa after World War II. In a small epidemic in Kenya in 1945 the mortality rate was 40 percent in untreated cases.

The tick-borne disease appears sporadically in many parts of the world, probably as a manifestation of an endemic focus in each place. It is the form which is sometimes seen in the United States.

Infection of man occurs if an infected louse is crushed against an abrasion or wound, or if a person is bitten by an infected tick. In both types, the organism enters the bloodstream and is able to spread via the hematogenous route.

MANIFESTATIONS. In general, patients with louse-borne disease are more seriously ill than those with the tick-borne disease. The incubation period varies between 4 and 12 days. Symptoms are not specific: fever, sweating, headache, and upper abdominal discomfort are the commonest. Cough, painful limbs, and bleeding—particularly epistaxis—also occur. Pregnant women often abort. The clinical picture varies from mild fever only, to one of severe toxicity characterized by confusion, jaundice, and purpura. The liver and spleen are enlarged and tender in about 20 to 80 percent of cases; jaundice, often accompanied by purpura, is seen in 10 to 70 percent. A gallop rhythm, low arterial pressure, and tachycardia are found; tachypnea, sometimes as high as 70 breaths per min, is characteristic of most cases. Tender skeletal muscles and, more rarely, neck stiffness, confusion, and even transient focal neurologic signs may be seen. The temperature may be as high as 105°F when the patient is first seen. Very rarely the picture of hypovolemic "endotoxin shock" occurs.

The term *relapsing fever* was introduced to describe the cycles of fever, i.e., periods of fever lasting for 7 to 10 days and separated by fever-free intervals of from 4 to 7 days. Relapses are rarely seen now that antibiotics are used.

PATHOLOGIC PHYSIOLOGY. In the louse-borne disease, cardiorespiratory changes, which may be very severe, occur in most cases. The electrocardiogram reveals evidence of myocardial damage in 30 percent of patients; a prolonged QTc interval, ventricular ectopic beats, and nonspecific S-T segment and T-wave changes are seen. After spirochetes disappear and the peak of the reaction is over, electrocardiographic evidence of acute right-sided heart strain may be found, and the pulmonary arterial pressure may rise transiently. The central venous pressure, which may also rise about 4 hr after spirochetes disappear, can be lowered by rapidly acting intravenous digitalis preparations. Overt pulmonary edema is rare.

At the peak of the reaction, marked overbreathing causes respiratory alkalosis. Arterial oxygen saturation decreases because of maldistribution of pulmonary blood flow. The increase in venous admixture coincides with a sudden fall in pulmonary vascular resistance. Cardiac output and systemic arterial pressure are greatly increased at this time. These changes are not related simply to the rise in body temperature, and there is no cerebrospinal fluid acidosis to explain the respiratory stimulation. Hydrocortisone suppresses the fever before the onset of rigors but does not prevent or modify the systemic reaction after tetracycline.

After the peak there is a progressive fall in arterial pressure to very low levels. The hypotensive phase lasts many hours and is the result of a decrease in cardiac output and of persistent peripheral vasodilatation. Ventilation gradually decreases and metabolic acidosis develops, while arterial glucose, lactate, and pyruvate concentrations increase. Continuous "100 percent" oxygen therapy is clinically beneficial and prevents these metabolic abnormalities.

The fully established syndrome of disseminated intravascular coagulation has been reported but is rare. However, thrombocytopenia is seen in most cases.

LABORATORY FINDINGS. The hemogram varies. Moderate anemia is common; its mechanism is uncertain. The leukocyte count is not normally raised before treatment: an "overshoot" leukocytosis, with many immature forms, occurs after the leukopenia which accompanies treatment. The sedimentation rate is elevated. The thrombocytopenia is associated with normal megakaryocytes in the bone marrow. The prothrombin time is often prolonged. Hepatic function tests reveal abnormal hepatocellular function. In severe cases, the total serum bilirubin level may reach 16 mg per 100 ml. Azotemia, apparently unrelated to extracellular fluid depletion, is common among jaundiced patients. The first investigation, and the only one essential to the diagnosis, is examination of thick and thin blood films, stained with Fields', Giemsa, and Leishman's stains. In the louse-borne disease, spirochetes are easily visible; in tick-borne disease their identification may be more difficult. Spirochetes may also be seen by phase-contrast microscopy with dark-field illumination.

DIFFERENTIAL DIAGNOSIS. Many infections in which the first symptom is fever of unknown origin, including malaria, salmonellosis (including typhoid), typhus, dengue, rat-bite fever, and Weil's disease, must be considered. Practically, the issue should not remain long in doubt if blood films are repeatedly searched for spirochetes, an essential practice in patients with fever of unknown origin in areas where the louse- and tick-borne diseases occur.

TREATMENT. The peripheral blood is quickly cleared of spirochetes by penicillin, tetracycline, and chloramphenicol. The best initial dose and the duration of treatment are not yet known.

Repeated small doses, e.g., 80,000 to 100,000 units, of penicillin clear the blood slowly and with a less-severe systemic reaction than the more usual 500,000 units, but spirochetes may persist in the brain after penicillin therapy. Tetracycline, probably the best drug, should be given in dosage of 250 mg on the first day and continued for 4 days in a daily dose of 1 Gm; however, this long a course may be unnecessary.

During epidemics, when economic factors may be important and follow-up may be impossible, a single dose of 1.2 million units of crystalline-procaine penicillin, or 1.5 Gm chloramphenicol on the first 2 days only, probably will be curative in the vast majority of patients.

The more ill patients should be hospitalized and, ideally, should receive intensive care during and after the reaction to treatment. At this time continuous oxygen therapy to prevent lactic acidosis and a digitalis preparation to support the myocardium are desirable. The patient should be nursed lying flat; hypotension can be corrected by raising the foot of the bed, but vasopressor drugs may be needed. In the face of possible myocardial damage, rapid infusion of plasma expanders may be dangerous, but it is important to maintain extracellular volume and to replace fluid lost through sweating and overventilating.

Vitamin K should be given parenterally to all patients.

Heparin is indicated if intravascular coagulation is found.

Any patient with a prolonged QTc interval on the electrocardiogram should be kept at bed rest until the QTc interval is normal.

EFFECTS OF TREATMENT. Spirochetes disappear from the peripheral blood about 1 hr after an adequate dose of penicillin or tetracycline. The arterial pressure, heart rate, respiratory rate, and temperature rise abruptly and transiently at this time, and there is a profound leukopenia. About 4 hr later, the arterial pressure has fallen substantially and the leukocyte count has returned to, or above, normal again.

This Jarisch-Herxheimer reaction is alarming; the patient shivers and groans and may vomit; transient neurologic signs may occur also. The calm which follows it may be deceptive because the marked pathophysiologic alterations, as described above, may be masked.

PROGNOSIS. When epidemics strike a nonimmune population, the high mortality rate due to the louse-borne disease shows the potential menace of this disease. Most patients, however, recover quickly and completely; relapses do not occur if antibiotic therapy is adequate. Adverse signs are deep jaundice, uncontrolled bleeding, and a grossly prolonged QTc interval.

Typhus and enteric fever may occur simultaneously with louse-borne relapsing fever, and they probably contribute to the mortality rate, particularly during epidemics.

REFERENCES

Bryceson, A. D. M., E. H. O. Parry, C. S. Leithead, P. L. Perine, D. Vukotich, and D. A. Warrell: Louse-borne Relapsing Fever in Ethiopia, Quart. J. Med. (in press).

Felsenfeld, O.: Borreliae, Human Relapsing Fever, and Parasite-Vector-Host Relationships, Bacteriol. Rev., 29: 46, 1965.

Heisch, R. B.: Studies in East African Relapsing Fever, E. African Med. J., 27:1, 1950.

183 RAT-BITE FEVER
(Spirillum minus Infection)

*Ivan L. Bennett, Jr., and
Robert G. Petersdorf*

DEFINITION. Rat-bite fever (sodoku) is an acute infectious disease caused by *Spirillum minus* and characterized by relapsing fever and a skin eruption.

ETIOLOGY. The causative organism is a spirillum 2 to 5μ in length; it has two to five broad spirals and is propelled by flagella. The organism is easily identified in dark-field preparations by its quick, darting motility. It is found occasionally in the blood of apparently healthy rats, mice, guinea pigs, and monkeys.

EPIDEMIOLOGY. In man, infection by *S. minus* is almost always acquired through the bite of a rat. It is commonest in infants and young children but may also occur in adults, particularly in laboratory workers. Rats may attack sleeping persons and will bite anyone attempting

to catch or handle them. Documented examples of infection from the bite of a mouse are known.

MANIFESTATIONS. Because of the long incubation period (1 to 6 weeks), the initial lesion may have healed before the onset of systemic symptoms. Often, however, one finds swelling and redness at the site of the eschar and swelling of regional lymph nodes. A chill may occur at the onset of a febrile period. Bouts of fever last 2 to 4 days and are separated by afebrile periods, also lasting 2 to 4 days. During febrile episodes there are malaise, headache, sweating, photophobia, nausea, and vomiting. In 75 percent of cases a *skin eruption* occurs, usually on the extremities. The rash is frequently asymmetric in its distribution and most commonly consists of reddish or purplish macules, which may become large and confluent. Arthritis is rare; if present it usually involves the large joints. The disease tends to run a prolonged course, usually 4 to 8 weeks, but cases have been reported in which clinical manifestations continued for more than a year. Subacute bacterial endocarditis due to this organism has been observed.

LABORATORY FINDINGS. The total leukocyte count may be normal, or there may be a leukocytosis up to 20,000. Biologic false positive serologic tests for syphilis occur in 50 percent of patients. The *S. minus* seldom can be found in the blood or tissues of patients by direct dark-field examination and cannot be cultured. Mice or guinea pigs should be inoculated intraperitoneally with the patient's blood. *Spirillum minus* can usually be found in the blood or peritoneal fluid of the animal by dark-field examination 5 to 15 days later. Laboratory animals may be naturally infected with *S. minus,* and precautions must be taken to ensure that the animals are free of infection before inoculation.

DIFFERENTIAL DIAGNOSIS. It is important to inquire about rat bite in all patients with a relapsing type of fever. In patients with a history of rate bite, the principal problem is in differentiating between infection with *S. minus* and that with *Streptobacillus moniliformis.* This cannot be done with certainty on clinical grounds, but a prolonged incubation period, relapsing instead of sustained fever, and few or no manifestations of arthritis suggest a diagnosis of *S. minus* infection. Laboratory tests should be made for both organisms. The significance of a previous rat bite may not be appreciated in cases with a long incubation period, and the disease may be confused with other infections characterized by relapsing fever, such as malaria, meningococcemia, and *Borrelia recurrentis* infection.

TREATMENT. Penicillin, in dosage of 300,000 to 600,000 units twice a day intramuscularly, is the drug of choice. In patients allergic to penicillin, a tetracycline in dosage of 2 Gm a day for 7 days may be used.

PROGNOSIS. Patients treated with penicillin become afebrile within 24 to 72 hr, and complete recovery is the rule.

REFERENCES

Roughgarden, J. W.: Antimicrobial Therapy of Rat-bite Fever, Arch. Intern. Med., 116:39, 1965.

Section 11

Diseases Caused by Fungi

INTRODUCTION

Abraham I. Braude

Except for their etiology, fungous infections differ little from bacterial infections. The close relationship between bacteria and fungi is apparent from transitional forms connecting the two classes, and from the similarity of the pathologic changes and clinical manifestations induced by them.

The intermediate, or transitional, forms are represented by the *Actinomycetes*. These possess the characteristic branched mycelium of fungi but divide by segmentation into gram-positive bacillary or coccoid forms. The acid-fast property of one species, *Nocardia asteroides,* indicates a relationship to the tubercle bacillus. The *Actinomycetes* also differ from fungi in their susceptibility to phages, their unorganized nuclei, and their sensitivity to antibiotics, which attack bacteria, but not to the antifungal polyene antibiotic amphotericin B. The *Actinomycetes* do not possess the sterols which complex with polyene antibiotics and injure the cell membranes of fungi. Finally, actinomyces, like bacteria but unlike fungi, contain neither chitin nor cellulose in their cell walls. Although actinomycosis and nocardiosis are placed among the fungous diseases in this book, the causative agents are unequivocally classed with the bacteria.

An important characteristic of pathogenic fungi is dimorphism, growth in two distinct forms under different environmental conditions. The fungi responsible for blastomycosis, sporotrichosis, and histoplasmosis assume unicellular "yeast" forms in infected tissues but grow as mycelia and produce asexual spores on Sabouraud's agar. The reverse is true for the fungus causing moniliasis. Another type of dimorphism is found in coccidioidomycosis. The organism responsible for this infection is multicellular in vivo and in vitro, but its form differs under the two conditions. In tissues it is a sac filled with spores, but on agar it grows as a segmented mycelium. *Cryptococcus neoformans* is the only pathogenic fungus that fails to change form when environmental conditions vary.

Mycotic diseases are not transmitted from one person to another. Many fungous infections are acquired by inhalation of spores growing freely in nature. These spores may be rectangular unicellular mycelial fragments known as *chlamydospores,* or spherical bodies borne on thin mycelial stalks and called *conidia.* Some infections, such as sporotrichosis, result from inoculation of spores directly into the skin.

A few fungous diseases are endogenous in origin.

Actinomyces israeli and *Candida albicans* are normal residents of the bowel and mouth. When resistance is lowered, endogenous infection with either agent can develop. Actinomycosis is often preceded by tooth extraction, and overgrowth of normal saprophytic bacteria by *C. albicans* in the course of antibiotic therapy can lead to moniliasis.

The mechanisms whereby fungi produce disease are obscure. *Cryptococcus neoformans* has a polysaccharide capsule similar to that of the pneumococcus which seems to protect the yeast from phagocytosis. This capsular material also produces mechanical injury in the nervous system. It is possible that the thick walls of other fungi such as *Blastomyces dermatitidis* and *Coccidioides immitis* also protect against leukocytes. Some fungi are ingested by phagocytes but seem to flourish within them. In histoplasmosis, for example, the parasites are found in enormous numbers within reticuloendothelial cells. The endothelium of small vessels can become so packed with histoplasma organisms that blood flow is compromised.

Another possible factor in the pathogenesis of these infections is hypersensitivity. In most fungous diseases the patient exhibits marked local or even systemic reactivity to intradermal injection of the causative organism. In coccidioidomycosis this type of reaction is closely associated with the development of erythema nodosum and pleural effusions. The occurrence of necrosis at the site of injection of fungous antigens suggests that hypersensitivity may be responsible for necrosis of infected tissues. In other patients, however, widespread destruction of tissue may occur despite absence of dermal sensitivity.

Despite the differences in morphology and life cycle of fungi and bacteria, both elicit similar pathologic changes and clinical manifestations. For this reason, specific diagnosis can seldom be made without demonstration of the causative organism. Fortunately, most pathogenic fungi are easily seen in infected tissues or exudates. In a few circumstances, however, it is necessary to rely upon epidemiologic and immunologic methods for diagnosis.

The following chapters deal only with those infections in which fungi penetrate beneath the skin and mucous membranes to involve the underlying tissues and viscera.

184 ACTINOMYCOSIS
Abraham I. Braude

DEFINITION. Actinomycosis is a noncontagious suppurative infection produced by an anaerobic organism normally resident in the mouth. The disease is characterized by chronic inflammatory induration and sinus formation.

ETIOLOGY. The causative agent is a branching gram-positive filamentous organism. Two separate anaerobic species of the genus *Actinomyces* have been recognized: *Actinomyces bovis* is responsible for actinomycosis in cattle, and *A. israeli*, for human actinomycosis.

Actinomyces israeli and *A. bovis* differ from other actinomyces in their intolerance of free oxygen and failure to grow on Sabouraud's medium. On blood agar, colonies require 4 to 6 days of anaerobic incubation at 37°C to reach a size of 1 to 2 mm. Although most strains require anaerobic conditions for isolation, some can be subcultured aerobically in 10 to 20 percent carbon dioxide. *Actinomyces israeli* has never been found outside man or animal, and case-to-case transmission is unknown.

PATHOGENESIS. The oxidation-reduction potential of normal tissues is probably too high for multiplication of *A. israeli*, but devitalized tissues allow it to reproduce, gain a foothold, and spread. The frequency of actinomycotic lesions of the face and neck may be explained by the greater population of *A. israeli* on surfaces of teeth, in carious teeth, and in tonsillar crypts and by the frequent trauma to which these tissues are subjected by eating, by dental procedures, or by infection with oral bacteria. Anaerobic conditions also prevail in atelectatic areas of the lung after aspiration of *A. israeli* so that pulmonary actinomycosis can develop. It is also possible that pulmonary actinomycosis may arise hematogenously from an infected focus in the mouth. The mediastinal form of thoracic actinomycosis probably spreads from the esophagus into the superior or posterior mediastinum, quickly involving the pleura to produce early pleural effusion or empyema, and then tends to attack the adjacent ribs and vertebral bodies. Eventually mediastinal actinomycosis produces abscesses which point in the paravertebral region. The exact mode of development of abdominal actinomycosis is unknown, but the frequency with which the cecal region is involved suggests that the conditions here favor devitalizing injury. Occasionally, perforation by a foreign body precedes infection.

From foci in the jaw, lung, or bowel, actinomycosis may spread by contiguity or through the bloodstream to the liver, spine, brain, kidneys, genitalia, spleen, and subcutaneous tissues. Lymphatic spread is rare.

The inflammatory reaction to *A. israeli* is characterized by three features: (1) chronic suppuration, (2) extensive necrosis, and (3) intense fibrosis. The so-called "sulfur granules" which are prominent in the inflammatory lesion of actinomycosis are composed of intertwined mycelial filaments.

CLINICAL MANIFESTATIONS. The essential feature of actinomycosis is a painful, indurated swelling. This lesion may appear over the jaw a week or more after such trauma as tooth extraction or compound fracture of the mandible. As it increases in size, points of suppuration, the openings of fistulas, appear on the bluish-red surface of the edematous skin. Cervical lymphadenopathy is rare.

The lower lobes of the lung are frequently affected; then the disease suddenly becomes evident when the pleura and chest wall are involved by direct extension from the lung. Until then the patient may notice only fever, cough, and expectoration. Physical examination at this time reveals a diffuse, tender, indurated thoracic swelling with pulmonary consolidation and empyema.

Abdominal actinomycosis is often mistaken for appendicitis, carcinoma of the cecum, tuberculosis, or amebiasis. Patients with abdominal actinomycosis are subjected to surgery for drainage of a supposed appendiceal abscess, and the true nature of the disease is recognized only when an indurated draining sinus remains and stubbornly refuses to heal. Actinomycosis may also be mistaken for tumor of the reproductive organs in women or for tuberculous psoas abscess. Peritonitis is rare.

In the rare case of hematogenous disseminated actinomycosis, lesions appear in all parts of the body. Painful indurated nodules under the skin of the legs, arms, back, and scalp are prominent and nonsuppurative effusions of the pleura or pericardium develop.

DIAGNOSIS. The disease is easily recognized by detecting *A. israeli* in pus obtained from sinuses, empyema fluid, or abscess cavities. Interpretating actinomyces in sputum is difficult because the organisms are normal inhabitants of the mouth. Sulfur granules vary in size from several microns to 3 mm in diameter. Large granules are nearly always found if a thorough search is made by diluting the pus with saline solution and filtering through gauze. They are white, yellow, or brown and stand out sharply against the background of blood-tinged pus. The conclusive finding is the demonstration of gram-positive filaments or bacilli which fail to grow aerobically. Granules of other organisms (staphylococci, nocardias, monosporia), fragments of caseous material, and clumps of pus cells or fibrin may be confused with actinomycotic granules. The technique for recovery of *A. israeli* from the infected material differs from that of other pathogenic fungi in two important respects: (1) animal inoculation is of no value, and (2) Sabouraud's medium will not support its growth. Cultural isolation of *A. israeli* is not difficult if anaerobic methods are used. A small microaerophilic gram-negative bacillus, *Actinobacillus actinomycetemcomitans*, is often associated with *A. israeli* in actinomycosis. Anaerobic streptococci, *Bacteroides*, and other anaerobes are also present frequently. Hence actinomycosis is characteristically a mixed anaerobic infection.

Biopsy may establish the diagnosis if the actinomycotic colony ("ray fungus") is observed microscopically. Demonstration of the organism may be difficult, requiring careful search of many sections.

Intradermal or serologic tests with *A. israeli* or its fractions are of no diagnostic aid. Radiologic examination may suggest actinomycosis if consolidation of the lungs and periosteal proliferation of the ribs are found because this combination rarely occurs in other conditions. The appearance of the spine in lateral views may be almost pathognomonic because the areas of absorption and newly formed bone give a picture of a coarse sieve not seen in any other vertebral disease.

TREATMENT. Penicillin and the tetracycline antibiotics are so effective that the disease is disappearing through the wide use of these drugs in conditions that would otherwise evolve into actinomycosis. When either is administered in large doses over long periods of time, remarkable improvement may be expected even when the purulent foci are inaccessible to surgical drainage. Many reports indicate that the tetracycline drugs (chlortetracycline, oxytetracycline, tetracycline) are superior to penicillin. When the tetracyclines are given in doses of 500 mg every 6 hr, there is a reduction in pain and swelling within a few days as well as gain in strength, increase in weight, and prompt defervescence. Treatment should be continued for several weeks after the patient appears cured. Because penicillin is no more effective than the tetracyclines and because it requires repeated intramuscular or intravenous injection of large doses for long periods of time, it should be reserved for patients who cannot tolerate tetracycline drugs. The optimum dose of penicillin is not known, but at least 4 million units daily should be given intramuscularly.

Surgical drainage or excision of accessible actinomycotic lesions is a valuable adjunct to chemotherapy, although surgery alone is of little value. Older treatments such as iodides, irradiation, or the sulfonamides have no place in the treatment of actinomycosis, and amphotericin B is of no value.

REFERENCES

Cope, V. Z.: "Actinomycosis," London, Oxford University Press, 1938.

Drake, C. H., M. T. Sudler, and R. I. Canuteson: A Case of Staphylococcic Actinophytosis (Botryomycosis) in Man, J.A.M.A., 123:339, 1943.

Garrod, L. P.: Actinomycosis of the Lung: Etiology, Diagnosis, and Chemotherapy, Tubercle, 33:258, 1952.

Lane, S. L., A. Kutscher, and R. Chaves: Oxytetracycline in the Treatment of Orocervical-Facial Actinomycosis: Report of Seven Cases, J.A.M.A., 151:986, 1953.

McVay, L. V., Jr., and D. H. Sprunt: A Long-term Evaluation of Aureomycin in the Treatment of Actinomycosis, Ann. Intern. Med., 38:995, 1953.

Nichols, D. R., and W. E. Herrell: Penicillin in the Treatment of Actinomycosis, J. Lab. Clin. Med., 33:521, 1948.

Rosebury, T.: The Parasitic Actinomycetes and Other Filamentous Microorganisms of the Mouth: A Review of Their Characteristics and Relationships of the Bacteriology of Actinomycosis and of Salivary Calculus in Man, Bacteriol. Rev., 8:189, 1944.

185 CRYPTOCOCCOSIS
Abraham I. Braude

DEFINITION. Cryptococcosis is a highly fatal infection caused by *Cryptococcus neoformans*, an encapsulated yeast with a special predilection for the central nervous system. Cryptococcosis may also involve the lungs, bones, and skin and occurs with increased frequency in patients with leukemia or lymphoma.

ETIOLOGY. Members of the genus *Cryptococcus*, to which *C. neoformans* belongs, form neither mycelia nor spores and reproduce entirely by budding. The cells of *C. neoformans* are spherical, measure 5 to 15 μ in diameter, retain the Gram stain, and are surrounded by a capsule which may have a diameter three times that of the cell. The capsular material contains a polysaccharide which is responsible for the slimy appearance of the yeast in culture and for the myxomatous character of cryptococcal lesions.

The organisms grow readily on various media at room temperature and at 37°C. On Sabouraud's glucose agar, visible growth appears within a few days at 37°C and gradually becomes brownish and slimy. Unlike other pathogenic yeastlike fungi, cryptococci never form mycelia. Most cells of *C. neoformans* are killed in 24 hr at temperatures of 40.6°C or higher.

PATHOGENESIS AND PATHOLOGY. Cryptococci resembling *C. neoformans* have been isolated from soil, pigeon droppings, the surface of fruit, and from the skin and intestinal tract of normal man. Hence it is possible for infections to be of either endogenous or exogenous origin. The organism reaches the nervous system in most cases. Although neurologic disturbances overshadow others, there is good evidence that infection is usually established in the lung and other viscera before dissemination to the brain and the meninges occurs. Often the pulmonary foci give rise to no clinical findings, although they can be detected if a careful search is made at postmortem examination.

The cryptococcus does not evoke the active inflammatory response observed with other fungi or bacteria. The cellular reaction is very slow to develop and is seldom intense. The cryptococcus seems to meet little resistance and frequently proliferates so freely that macroscopic masses of gelatinous yeasts fill the lesions. Older lesions occasionally show granulomatous reactions. The small number of cryptococci observed within granulomas suggests that mononuclear cells can destroy the organism. This may account in part for the fact that lymphomatous diseases involving the mononuclear cells lower resistance to cryptococcal infection. At other times, however, many cryptococci are present within mononuclear and giant cells. It is unusual to see necrosis in cryptococcosis.

Granulomas or gelatinous cryptococcal masses may appear in the nervous system, lungs, bones, or skin. In the nervous system, lesions usually develop in the meninges at the base of the brain, with resulting involvement of the brain stem, cranial nerves, and cerebellum. Large masses of yeast may accumulate in the subarachnoid space and extend diffusely along perivascular spaces into the brain substance to produce cystic nodules. Because the fungal masses shrink after fixation of the brain in formalin, cyst-like spaces remain. In the lung, scattered miliary nodules, diffuse pneumonic infiltrations, or solitary masses easily mistaken for pulmonary neoplasms may occur. Calcification or hilar lymphadenopathy is extremely rare. These characteristics of the cryptococcal pulmonary lesions are helpful in distinguishing the disease from tuberculosis, sarcoidosis, and other mycoses. In contrast to cryptococcal meningoencephalitis, serious predisposing diseases accompany pulmonary cryptococcosis in only 10 percent of patients.

CLINICAL MANIFESTATIONS. Most patients with cryptococcal infection present only after the onset of neurologic manifestations. Complaints of severe headache, diplopia, dizziness, ataxia, vomiting, tinnitus, memory disturbances, or Jacksonian convulsions are common. Fever is usually low-grade or may be absent. Many patients die within a few months, but some have lived for many years as the disease undergoes remissions and relapses.

When pulmonary infection is present in the absence of meningoencephalitis, the patient is generally free of constitutional symptoms. The disease is detected when roentgenographic examination of the chest shows a dense, usually solitary infiltration of the lower portions of the lung. Cough may be a prominent feature of diffuse cryptococcal pneumonia. Cavities are not rare.

Involvement of bones in the absence of disseminated disease is rare, and cryptococcosis of joints is almost always secondary to adjacent osseous lesions.

Disseminated infection may also produce multiple nodules or papules in the skin. These range from a few millimeters in diameter to masses resembling strawberries in size and color.

The possibility of underlying Hodgkin's disease, lymphosarcoma, leukemia, or diabetes should be considered in every patient with cryptococcosis.

DIAGNOSIS. Cryptococcal meningitis must be distinguished from other diseases which present as aseptic meningitis, including brain abscess, tuberculous meningitis, coccidioidal meningitis, and carcinomatous meningitis. In each of these, the spinal fluid is sterile by ordinary cultural methods and may contain from a few to several hundred mononuclear cells, an increased amount of protein, and a reduced concentration of glucose. Because *C. neoformans* is recovered with much greater ease than the etiologic agents of the other diseases, culture of the spinal fluid is the decisive procedure in differential diagnosis. The cryptococcus is isolated on Sabouraud's agar at room temperature and usually grows after 1 to 2 weeks. In tuberculous and coccidioidal meningitis positive cultures are much less common, and in uncomplicated brain abscess the spinal fluid is sterile. Cryptococcal cells may also be found by direct microscopic examination of sediment from centrifuged spinal fluid. Mixing a drop of sediment with India ink facilitates the recognition of the mucinous capsule. The organism can be cultured from the blood and urine in 25 to 35 percent of patients with cryptococcal meningitis. Lung biopsy is essential for diagnosis in most cases of pulmonary infection. In tissue removed by biopsy, intracellular forms with small capsules may resemble *Histoplasma capsulatum* but can be differentiated by mucicarmine, which stains the capsular mucopolysaccharide peculiar to *C. neoformans*. Biopsied material should also be inoculated onto Sabouraud's glucose agar and intraperitoneally in white mice. *Cryptococcus neoformans* is highly pathogenic for these animals and is readily demonstrated microscopically in sections or smears of their brains. In many cases, the patients' serums give positive complement fixation tests for either cryptococcal antigen or antibody. Circulating antigens appear to indicate continuing disease, while antibodies are found only after treatment, when the cryptococcus and its antigens are disappearing from the body fluids.

TREATMENT. All forms of cryptococcosis usually improve after intravenous infusions of 75 to 100 mg amphotericin B daily. These maximum daily doses are reached only after gradual increments of the initial dose of 1 mg. When maintenance levels are reached, the drug should be given every other day. Patients without meningoencephalitis can be cured with total doses of less than 1.5 Gm, but 3.0 Gm is probably required for infections of the nervous system. If relapse occurs after intravenous treatment, amphotericin B may be dissolved in the spinal fluid and 0.5 mg injected intrathecally on alternate days in conjunction with intravenous administration. Strict precautions must be taken during intrathecal injection to avoid bacterial contamination and drug overdosage. One milligram amphotericin B intrathecally may cause fever, temporary paralysis of the bladder and legs, and arachnoiditis. The chief dangers of intravenous amphotericin B are anemia, hypokalemia, and renal damage. The anemia frequently occurs after prolonged treatment and is normocytic, normochromic, and reversible. The hypokalemia develops with or without impaired renal function and requires prophylactic potassium supplements. Disturbances in renal function should be expected. Azotemia, impaired urine concentration, and microscopic hematuria with granular casts are the main findings but are reversible if caught in time. Treatment should be discontinued if the blood urea nitrogen exceeds 40 mg per 100 ml and resumed when it approaches normal levels. Serious and permanent renal damage with nephrocalcinosis has occurred in patients given a total dosage greater than 5.0 Gm.

REFERENCES

Butler, W. T., D. W. Alling, A. Spickard, and J. Utz: Diagnostic and Prognostic Value of Clinical and Laboratory Findings in Cryptococcal Meningitis, New Engl. J. Med., 270:59, 1964.

Campbell, G. D.: Primary Pulmonary Cryptococcosis, Am. Rev. Resp. Dis., 94:236, 1966.

Littman, M. L., and L. E. Zimmerman: "Cryptococcosis," New York, Grune & Stratton, Inc., 1956.

Walter, J. E., and R. D. Jones: Serodiagnosis of Clinical Cryptococcosis, Am. Rev. Resp. Dis., 97:275, 1968.

186 BLASTOMYCOSIS
Abraham I. Braude

DEFINITION. Blastomycosis is a fungous infection of the skin and viscera, caused by *Blastomyces dermatitidis* in North America and by *Paracoccidioides brasiliensis* in South America. South American blastomycosis (paracoccidioidal granuloma) produces massive lymphadenopathy and destructive lesions of the nasopharynx and bowel not found in its North American counterpart.

ETIOLOGY. In infected tissues *B. dermatitidis* has the appearance of a yeast, forming single buds from 3 to 24 μ in diameter. Two features aid in recognition: (1) its thick wall, spoken of as "double-contoured," because the inner and outer margins can be seen, and (2) the wide opening between parent cell and bud at the base of attachment.

In culture, *B. dermatitidis* is dimorphic and appears as the wrinkled, waxy yeast form on blood agar incubated at 37°C, or as a mold with branching hyphae on Sabouraud's agar at room temperature. On microscopic examination the cultured yeast may be identical with that in the infected lesions or may have abortive mycelia. The mycelia give rise to oval or pear-shaped exogenous spores.

Multiple buds on the yeastlike cell of *P. brasiliensis* distinguish it morphologically from *B. dermatitidis*. The tiny multiple buds have the appearance of a crown of small beads attached to the cell wall. The fungus reproduces by budding both in tissues and when cultured at 37°C. At room temperature it produces mycelia but not true spores.

PATHOGENESIS AND PATHOLOGY. The skin has been proposed as a portal of entry in North American blastomycosis because cutaneous lesions are prominent and because infections may follow injury to the skin. The lung is also a likely portal, but the fungus has never been cultured from the soil.

In most cases of South American blastomycosis the portal of entry is the nasopharynx. Here the fungus produces a destructive lesion with gross swelling and ulceration and eventual extension to the cervical lymph nodes. Occasionally, the primary lesion is inconspicuous and massive enlargement and suppurative necrosis of the regional lymph nodes predominate. In addition to the nasopharynx, primary lesions may occur in the lymphoid tissue of the cecal and appendiceal regions.

Characteristic pathologic features are found in the lung and skin in both North and South American forms. Pulmonary lesions vary in size from miliary granulomatous nodules to confluent areas of diffuse pneumonia involving an entire lobe. The granulomas may undergo caseation and fibrosis. Differentiation from tuberculosis is facilitated by finding the yeast in giant cells or other phagocytes.

In the skin, microabscesses lie just beneath the epidermis and are surrounded by a granulomatous reaction. The epidermis itself often becomes so hyperplastic that it resembles an epithelioma.

In both North and South American varieties, the infection may spread to the lymph nodes, brain, bones, urogenital tract, liver, spleen, and adrenals.

CLINICAL MANIFESTATIONS. In the typical case of systemic North American blastomycosis the onset is insidious. The patient may seek medical attention because of a persistent "chest cold," low-grade fever, weight loss, or progressive disability. Physical examination and roentgenogram of the chest disclose evidence of pneumonia, which may involve any segment or lobe of the lung. Cavitation is frequent, and mediastinal lymph nodes may

be prominent. Hemoptysis, purulent sputum, chest pain, and dyspnea appear as the disease progresses. Although the pulmonary infection may subside spontaneously, extrapulmonary lesions of the skin, bones, joints, and viscera eventually call attention to dissemination. These metastatic suppurative lesions are accompanied by an increase in fever, sweats, chills, and weakness. Death in the untreated infection sometimes occurs in less than 6 months, but most patients live for a year or two. The overall mortality in systemic blastomycosis is said to be 92 percent in patients who have been followed for 2 years or longer without specific therapy.

Primary infection of the skin by *B. dermatitidis* (Gilchrist's disease) first appears on unclothed areas such as the hands, face, or forearm but not the scalp, palms, or soles. The infection begins as a firm nodule surrounded by similar lesions which tend to coalesce. Suppuration in the center of the nodule is followed by partial healing and fibrosis as extension occurs peripherally. The hyperplastic epithelium gives these lesions a hard, raised, wartlike margin. When fully developed, blastomycosis of the skin presents the appearance of one or more ragged ulcers with partially healed centers and thick raised margins. The primary cutaneous infection may be confined to the skin for months or years.

The first symptoms in South American blastomycosis usually result from painful ulcers of the mouth or nose, although loss of appetite, abdominal pain, vomiting, and diarrhea may be the first complaints. In other cases, massive lymphadenopathy is the first manifestation. In the usual infection, however, there is a progressive extension of lesions from the mouth and neighboring skin. The lymph nodes undergo suppurative necrosis, and sinuses rupture through the overlying skin. The patient has severe pain, fever, inability to eat, and cachexia. Depending on the rapidity of spread to the viscera, bones, and central nervous system, the untreated disease is fatal after a few months or several years.

DIAGNOSIS. Pulmonary blastomycosis closely resembles tuberculosis, carcinoma of the lung, aspiration pneumonitis, and other fungous infections, including coccidioidomycosis, actinomycosis, nocardiosis, and histoplasmosis. Differentiation must be based on the recovery of the etiologic agent, because neither clinical nor epidemiologic features are specific. Most cases of North American blastomycosis are found in the Southeastern United States and in the Mississippi River Valley, but the disease occurs throughout the United States and Canada. Occupational history, sex, race, and age are of no diagnostic aid.

It is usually possible to find either *B. dermatitidis* or *P. brasiliensis* by microscopic examination of biopsied material, sputum, or pus. The yeastlike forms can be observed if a drop of purulent material is first mixed on a slide with a drop of 10 percent potassium hydroxide and kept at room temperature for 30 min. The multiple buds covering the entire surface of *P. brasiliensis* are connected by a narrow neck to the parent cell, while buds of *B. dermatitidis* are connected by a wide communication. *Blastomyces dermatitidis* is isolated by culturing pus on Sabouraud's agar at room temperature and on blood agar at 37°C. *Paracoccidioides brasiliensis* can also be isolated on blood agar at 37°C but grows so slowly that more than a month may elapse before colonies appear. Inoculation of mice or other animals is usually not successful in recovering either fungus.

The diagnostic value of the skin test for blastomycosis is limited. The complement fixation test in both North and South American blastomycosis is positive in high titer with serums of patients who have systemic infections. The results of intradermal and serologic tests may be of prognostic value. Patients with marked dermal hypersensitivity and low serum titers of complement-fixing antibody are said to have a better prognosis in North American blastomycosis than those with negative skin tests and high complement fixation titers.

TREATMENT. Amphotericin B is curative in both North and South American blastomycosis. North American blastomycosis also responds, but less favorably, to 2-hydroxystilbamidine, while South American blastomycosis is reitant to it. Either drug is given daily or every other day by slow intravenous drip in increasing doses. The maximum daily dose of amphotericin B is 75 to 100 mg, and that of 2-hydroxystilbamidine is 250 mg. Complete arrest of North American blastomycosis has been observed after a total of 1.0 Gm amphotericin B; 4 to 10 Gm of 2-hydroxystilbamidine may be required. Anesthesia over the distribution of the trigeminal nerve is the main untoward reaction from 2-hydroxystilbamidine; it persists after treatment. Surgical excision of pulmonary cavities or destroyed tissues is sometimes necessary in addition to chemotherapy.

In South American blastomycosis the sulfonamide drugs produce dramatic clinical remissions of most forms of the disease, but relapses invariably occur unless the patient is maintained on continuous therapy. Sulfadiazine in doses of 4 to 6 Gm daily has been successful in arresting the disease.

REFERENCES

Harrell, E. R., and A. C. Curtis: North American Blastomycosis, Am. J. Med., 27:750, 1959.

Lacaz, C. S.: South American Blastomycosis, Anales Fac. Med. Univ. São Paulo, 29:1, 1955–1956.

Martin, D. S., and D. T. Smith: Blastomycosis (American Blastomycosis, Gilchrist's Disease): Review of the Literature, Am. Rev. Tuberc., 39:257, 1939.

Smith, J. G., J. S. Harris, N. F. Conant, and D. T. Smith: An Epidemic of North American Blastomycosis, J.A.M.A., 158:641, 1955.

187 COCCIDIOIDOMYCOSIS
Abraham I. Braude

DEFINITION. Coccidioidomycosis is an infection acquired by inhalation of *Coccidioides immitis*, a fungus existing only in the mycelial phase in nature and converted to a spherule in tissues. Although most infections are mild or unapparent, *C. immitis* may produce a fatal disseminated disease with destructive lesions in the lungs, lymph nodes, spleen, liver, bones, kidneys, and brain.

ETIOLOGY. *Coccidioides immitis* grows readily at room temperature or at 35°C and produces white, cottony mycelia. As the culture ages, the segmented mycelium breaks up into thick-coated rectangular *arthrospores*, $2 \times 4 \mu$ in size. These arthrospores can survive in stored cultures and are highly infectious for laboratory personnel. The mycelium and its spores are pathogenic for various laboratory animals. The mycelial form is converted to a thick-walled spherule filled with endospores in animal tissues and under special cultural conditions.

PATHOGENESIS AND PATHOLOGY. Coccidioidomycosis is acquired by inhalation of *chlamydospores* in endemic areas in the semiarid regions of the Southwestern United States and the Chaco district of Argentina. The majority of infections occur during the dry seasons, particularly after exposure to dust storms. The fungus grows in the soil in rainy weather and becomes disseminated in dust during dry weather. *Coccidioides immitis* is isolated from soil and from desert rodents.

The inhaled spores are carried to the terminal bronchioles and alveoli, where the first reaction is an outpouring of polymorphonuclear leukocytes, fluid, and a few mononuclear cells. In most cases, the organism is probably killed, or at least arrested, at a stage when the lesion is too small to be detected by clinical means. In others, the organisms proliferate and elicit an inflammatory response which appears to depend on the rate of multiplication of the fungus. The phase of rapid multiplication is manifested by frequent discharge of endospores from the ripened spherules and elicits suppuration and an exudate rich in polymorphonuclear leukocytes. The phase of slow multiplication, with infrequent rupture of spherules, produces a granulomatous reaction in which epithelioid cells and giant cells predominate. Although polymorphonuclear leukocytes congregate about the point of rupture of a spherule and actually invade the broken capsule, attempts at phagocytosis by these cells are unsuccessful. As the released endospores develop into spherules, the neutrophilic reaction gives way to proliferating mononuclear cells which often are able to ingest the fungus.

Either phase of this inflammatory cycle may predominate, or a mixture of the two may be found. Rapidly progressive infections produce large areas of confluent suppurative pneumonia and necrosis. In contrast, granulomatous lesions contain exudates composed almost exclusively of mononuclear cells and giant cells which fill alveoli but leave their walls intact. Both reactions are accompanied by involvement of the overlying pleura and of the hilar and mediastinal lymph nodes. Ultimately the bronchopneumonia in most patients resolves or heals by fibrosis; in others, the lesions are permanently arrested but persist as cavities or solid nodules.

Recovery is accompanied by the development of hypersensitivity to the fungus. This hypersensitivity is apparently responsible for at least two special manifestations: (1) *erythema nodosum*, a sterile, focal, nodular granulomatous reaction usually limited to the skin of the lower extremities and characterized by extravasation of red cells into the lesion; (2) *pleural effusion*. It is believed that rupture of a pleural granuloma discharges antigenic material onto the sensitized pleural membranes.

In patients who do not develop dermal hypersensitivity, the infection spreads systemically to involve lymph nodes, spleen, bones, liver, kidney, meninges, skin, adrenals, and pericardium. In the meninges, the reaction may take two forms: (1) the granulomatous reaction is commoner and produces a firm plastic lesion which encloses the brainstem and other structures in a rigid mass of tissue; (2) the suppurative reaction results in outpouring of polymorphonuclear leukocytes with little granulomatous change. In either type, but especially in the granulomatous, involvement of the brainstem may lead to severe hydrocephalus.

CLINICAL MANIFESTATIONS. The infection may be either benign or disseminated. The benign infection, so-called "desert fever," is self-limited, and as many as 50 percent of benign infections are asymptomatic. The remainder are accompanied by influenza-like symptoms. After an incubation period of 1 to 3 weeks, the patient experiences fever, chills, fatigue, headache, severe arthralgia, and symptoms of respiratory infection. The most frequent complaint is poorly localized chest pain, aggravated by breathing or coughing. A nonproductive cough is common, but hemoptysis is infrequent. Physical findings are scant except in patients who develop erythema nodosum or pleural effusion. Although hydrothorax may be massive and require repeated thoracenteses, it eventually resorbs without further difficulty.

Despite the paucity of signs in the chest, prominent abnormalities are found in roentgenograms. These include focal areas of infiltration, hilar and mediastinal lymphadenopathy, nodules or cavities, and pleural effusion. The commonest are single or multiple infiltrates which may appear in any segment and can simulate tuberculosis if the upper lobe is involved. They usually resolve after several weeks.

In about 2 percent of benign infections a solid or cavitary pulmonary lesion remains. The typical cavity of coccidioidomycosis is peripheral, has a thin wall, and gives a cystlike appearance in roentgenograms. Bronchoscopic examination may disclose stenosis and ulceration of the bronchus. Residual solid lesions may be as large as 3 cm in diameter. Both solid and cavitary lesions are commoner in the upper lobes. Calcification is rare.

In a few individuals (0.05 to 0.2 percent), the primary infection progresses to the disseminated form of the disease. Dissemination usually occurs within a few months of infection. Dark-skinned persons and pregnant women are more vulnerable. Among Negroes and Filipinos, 85 to 90 percent with dissemination die, as compared to 50 percent of whites. Patients who develop progressive coccidioidomycosis do not give a history of erythema nodosum.

The course of disseminated infection is marked by fungating or ulcerating skin lesions, multiple pulmonary nodules or cavities, widespread destructive lymphadenopathy, osteomyelitis, and meningitis. Weight loss, fever, and weakness are the outstanding systemic manifestations, and the course is often rapid, with death occurring in less than a year. If vital organs are spared, however, patients with disseminated coccidioidomycosis may feel surprisingly well, continue to work, and even gain weight despite the presence of large numbers of *C. immitis* in the sputum or subcutaneous abscesses. The meningeal form is invariably fatal, but even it is compatible with survival for several years. In the presence of meningitis with progressive hydrocephalus, patients experience severe headaches, cranial nerve palsies, memory disturbances, and disorientation. The spinal fluid shows 100 to 200 cells, mostly mononuclear, elevated protein levels, and frequently a reduction in glucose concentration.

DIAGNOSIS. Except in meningitis, *C. immitis* is easily recovered from the lesions of disseminated coccidioidomycosis by direct examination and cultures of exudates or biopsied tissues. The characteristic spherule with endospores is seen best in purulent material treated with 20 percent potassium hydroxide. Occasionally, in biopsied tissue, spherules may all be immature and contain no endospores, making them indistinguishable from *B. dermatitidis*. Cultural identification becomes essential for diagnosis. On Sabouraud's agar, mycelial growth appears in 4 to 8 days, and inoculation of mice produces multiple necrotic lesions containing spherules. In meningitis, only a few spherules appear in the spinal fluid, despite the presence of large numbers in the granulomatous exudate around the brain stem. Occasionally, the culture of 20 to 30 ml of spinal fluid yields positive results, but sometimes the diagnosis can be based only on serologic tests.

Serologic tests are performed with coccidioidin, a filtrate from cultures of *C. immitis*. By the third week of primary infection, precipitins are found in the serum of 91 percent of patients with symptomatic infection but in only 7 percent of asymptomatic individuals. Complement-fixing antibodies appear later and persist longer than precipitins in nondisseminated coccidioidomycosis; they are almost always present in the disseminated disease. Intradermal tests with coccidioidin are of value in the recognition of primary benign infections because they become positive before precipitins appear, but in disseminated infection the skin test is frequently negative.

The roentgenographic appearance of pulmonary lesions is suggestive of primary coccidioidomycosis if hilar lymphadenopathy progresses while the parenchymal infiltrate is subsiding or if the adenopathy is associated with multiple areas of pneumonitis. A residual smooth, thin-walled cavity without surrounding parenchymal infiltration is also characteristic of the primary form of the disease. Other residual lesions include calcified or noncalcified nodular foci and localized bronchiectasis. In disseminated pulmonary infection the commonest picture is that of multiple infiltrates accompanied by pleural involvement and prominent hilar or mediastinal lymphadenopathy.

The only remarkable hematologic finding is eosinophilia, which may reach 35 percent of the total leukocyte count in the primary disease, especially if erythema nodosum is present.

TREATMENT. Intensive intravenous treatment with amphotericin B in daily doses of 1.0 mg per kg body weight appears to be effective in some cases of extrameningeal coccidioidomycosis. Coccidioidal meningitis is extremely resistant to amphotericin B therapy and should be treated with repeated intrathecal injections of 0.5 mg of this drug. The total dose necessary varies from less than 1.0 Gm to more than 10.0 Gm intravenously and as much as 45 mg intrathecally. Severe nausea, venous thrombosis, and reversible impairment of renal and hepatic function often interrupt the treatment schedule, but persistent administration of amphotericin B in the face of troublesome side effects has occasionally produced improvement. A fall in titer of complement-fixing antibodies and a return of coccidioidin skin sensitivity are evidence of effective treatment. Drug therapy may have to be supplemented by surgical removal of peripheral granulomas.

Primary surgical excision of residual pulmonary foci is indicated if these lesions become troublesome because of secondary infection or hemoptysis. Dissemination of the disease from these foci almost never occurs.

REFERENCES

Baker, O. B., and A. I. Braude: A Study of Stimuli Leading to the Production of Spherules of Coccidioidomycosis, J. Lab. Clin. Med., 47:169, 1956.

Emmons, C. S.: Isolation of *Coccidioides* from Soil and Rodents, Public Health Rept. U.S., 57:109, 1942.

Fiese, M. J.: "Coccidioidomycosis," Springfield, Ill., Charles C Thomas, Publisher, 1958.

Forbus, W. D., and A. M. Bestebreurtje: Coccidioidomycosis: A Study of 95 Cases of the Disseminated Type with Special Reference to the Pathogenesis of the Disease, Mil. Surg., 99:654, 1946.

Harris, R. E.: Coccidioidomycosis Complicating Pregnancy, Obstet. Gynecol., 28:401, 1966.

Peck, W. A., and S. S. Romendick: Coccidioidomycosis: A Roentgen Study, Texas State J. Med., 52:86, 1956.

Smith, C. E., M. T. Saito, and S. A. Simons: Pattern of 39,500 Serologic Tests in Coccidioidomycosis, J.A.M.A., 160:546, 1956.

Taylor, A. B., and A. K. Briney: Observations on Primary Coccidioidomycosis, Ann. Intern. Med., 30:1224, 1949.

188 HISTOPLASMOSIS
Abraham I. Braude

DEFINITION. Histoplasmosis is a protean infection caused by the dimorphic fungus *Histoplasma capsulatum*, an organism found as a tiny body within reticuloendothelial cells. The disease varies from mild or unnoticed respiratory infection to widely disseminated lethal disease characterized by fever, anemia, hepatomegaly, splenomegaly, leukopenia, pulmonary lesions, ulcerations of the gastrointestinal tract, and adrenal necrosis.

ETIOLOGY. Although *H. capsulatum* grows on Sabouraud's agar at room temperature as a spore-bearing mold, it is transformed after animal inoculation into nonencapsulated oval yeastlike cells measuring 2×4 μ. In histologic section the protoplasm is shrunken so that the unstained space beneath the cell wall has the appearance of a capsule. The name *capsulatum* is based on a misinterpretation of the nature of this unstained space. The fungus also grows in the yeastlike phase if incubated at 37°C in sealed tubes of blood agar. The most distinctive cultural feature, however, is the tuberculate *chlamydospore* found only on mycelia; it is round, 10×20 μ in diameter, and covered with warty projections. Another smaller spore, not distinguishable from that of *Blastomyces dermatitidis*, is also present on the mycelium. A newly recognized species, *Histoplasma duboisii*, resembles *B. dermatitidis* and is responsible for an infection in Africa that involves the skin and bones but not the lung.

PATHOLOGY AND PATHOGENESIS. The source of human infection is probably soil containing spores of *Histoplasma*. Several studies have emphasized the isolation of the fungus from soil in areas inhabited by chickens, birds, and bats. City dwellers are often exposed to histoplasma growing in soil under trees which shelter starlings. In most cases the portal of entry is the lung, where a primary complex may be formed by extension of infection from the pulmonary focus to the regional lymph nodes. Infection through the gastrointestinal tract probably occurs in patients whose initial lesions are in the mouth and pharynx.

The basic pathologic process is multiplication of *H. capsulatum* in cells of the reticuloendothelial system. The yeast form multiplies extensively and greatly distends the cells. As proliferating histiocytes encroach on parenchymal cells, the infected organ becomes enlarged. The liver, lymph nodes, lung, spleen, adrenal glands, bowel, and marrow may be affected in disseminated histoplasmosis.

In addition to the diffuse lesions of the reticuloendothelial system, the tissues contain nodular accumulations of epithelioid cells and giant cells of the Langhans type. The noncaseous granuloma probably represents an effective defensive action, and histoplasma organisms are difficult to demonstrate in the epithelioid cells of such a lesion.

Caseous necrosis may accompany both types of lesion. The adrenals, which are involved in nearly all disseminated infections, are often massively enlarged. Caseous necrosis is usually present in the center of the pulmonary granulomas, which resemble those of cavitary pulmonary tuberculosis. Necrotizing histoplasmosis may also take the form of renal papillitis. Extracellular forms of histoplasma are readily found in the necrotic areas of all organs by special stains (periodic acid–Schiff, Gridley). These extracellular organisms may be much larger than the intracellular ones, appear distorted, and occasionally assume the mycelial form.

CLINICAL MANIFESTATIONS. The signs and symptoms of histoplasmosis range from those of a slight self-limited infection to fatal disseminated disease. The high incidence of positive intradermal reactions to histoplasmosis in healthy persons in many parts of the world indicates that most infections by *H. capsulatum* are inapparent or very mild. This variability in severity is observed among different persons involved in the same outbreak. Severe infections are characterized by prolonged fever, dyspnea, chest pain, weight loss, prostration, widespread pulmonary infiltrates, hepatomegaly, and splenomegaly. Other infected persons may have only a benign acute pneumonitis lasting a week or less, while still others are entirely free of symptoms. Widespread ill-defined noncalcified pulmonary infiltrates of miliary size or larger are found in symptomatic infections and may also be present, although less extensively, in the asymptomatic ones. Eventually, pulmonary lesions either disappear or calcify. In the east central part of the United States there is a high incidence of pulmonary calcification in persons who have negative tuberculin and positive histoplasmin skin tests. In some epidemics of acute histoplasmosis, erythema nodosum and erythema multiforme have been prominent in middle-aged women.

Least resistance to histoplasmosis is encountered in young infants and in adults after the fifth decade. Most cases of disseminated infection have occurred at these extremes of life, but with somewhat different clinical manifestations in the two groups. In the infant there are fever, emaciation, anemia, and leukopenia, and evidence of widespread involvement of many viscera including the liver, spleen, lung, bowel, lymph nodes, adrenals, skin, kidney, brain, eye, or endocardium. Although the same degree of dissemination may occasionally occur in the adult, usually visceral involvement is less widespread. Unlike the disease in infancy, adult histoplasmosis shows a marked predilection for men. Histoplasmosis of the lips, mouth, nose, and larynx occurs almost exclusively in adults and is the initial manifestation in about one-third of the fatal cases. Among the various syndromes encountered are subacute vegetative endocarditis, massive lymphadenopathy resembling tuberculosis or lymphoma, various forms of pneumonia, cerebral histoplasmoma, and meningitis. The last is characterized by signs of basilar localization with spinal fluid findings and a clinical course identical with those of tuberculous meningitis.

In addition to the acute benign and disseminated infections, chronic localized histoplasmosis occurs in adults. Although frequently accompanied by necrosis or ulceration, this form is basically a granuloma, with a tendency to remain localized.

Two main clinical types of chronic localized histoplasmosis are encountered: (1) *Pulmonary*. This may resemble pulmonary tuberculosis in all respects. The patient may be asymptomatic or may complain of a chronic and occasionally productive cough. Roentgenograms will show lesions identical with those of reinfection tuberculosis, sometimes with cavitation, and accompanied by consistently positive cultures of sputum for *H. capsulatum*. (2) *Mucocutaneous*. Ulcers of the mouth, tongue, pharynx, gums, larynx, penis, or bladder are rare lesions found only in adults. Regional lymphadenopathy is common in these types.

In African histoplasmosis, the predominant lesions are in the skin. These may rupture through the epidermis or encroach on underlying bone. In the disseminated form, multiple lesions involve the lymph nodes, bone, skin, liver, and spleen, but, in contrast to *H. capsulatum* infections, the lungs are spared.

DIAGNOSIS. Isolation of *H. capsulatum* is not difficult in disseminated or chronic localized infections if cultures are made of bone marrow, blood, biopsied lesions, sputum, or exudate from an ulcer. After incubation of infected material on Sabouraud's agar at room temperature there appears a white cottony colony which later turns brown and produces the diagnostic tuberculate chlamydospores. Material may also be cultured at 37°C on Francis' medium or blood agar, but the growth is yeastlike, and the diagnostic spores are not found. Isolation from sputum is best accomplished in mice, because contaminants are suppressed and the mouse is extremely susceptible to infection by histoplasmas. The animal does not die, but subculture of the spleen 1 month later on Sabouraud's agar yields the organism. Histoplasmas may also be seen in bone marrow, material from open or biopsied lesions, and occasionally in blood smears of terminally ill patients. Special fungous stains (periodic acid–Schiff, Gridley) should be used. Certain intracellular forms of *Cryptococcus neoformans* may be indistinguishable from histoplasma in histologic sections, unless strains for the cryptococcal mucinous capsule are employed.

In cases from which *H. capsulatum* cannot be isolated, indirect clues to identification are (1) history of exposure to soil or dust in an endemic area, (2) positive complement fixation tests, (3) positive histoplasmin skin tests, and (4) development of miliary calcifications in the lung. Although these criteria are not dependable individually, they appear to be reliable when used together. The serologic and skin tests are frequently negative in culturally proved cases of histoplasmosis, and their specificity is not fully established. Histoplasmin skin tests may confuse the serologic picture by producing complement-fixing antibodies to mycelial antigens, but not to yeast-phase antigens.

Histoplasmosis must be differentiated from tuberculosis, sarcoid, leukemia, infectious mononucleosis, Hodgkin's disease, brucellosis, and kala-azar. Because cortisone is frequently of value in sarcoid but can cause dissemination in histoplasmosis, differential diagnosis between these two diseases is critical. Biopsied tissue in both diseases contains morphologically identical granulomas. For this reason the diagnosis of sarcoid should be withheld until tissues have been examined with special fungous stains. In kala-azar the intracellular Leishman-Donovan body bears a close resemblance to *H. capsulatum*, and cultural isolation of the fungus may be important in distinguishing between the two.

TREATMENT. Amphotericin B, in intravenous doses of 50 to 100 mg daily, is effective in all forms of histoplasmosis. Treatment given daily, or on alternate days, must be continued for periods varying from 1 to many months. Sulfadiazine has also been effective in adults in oral doses of 6 Gm daily and may be given in conjunction with intravenous amphotericin B.

REFERENCES

Binford, C. H.: Histoplasmosis: Tissue Reaction, and Morphologic Variations in the Fungus, Am. J. Clin. Pathol., 25:25, 1955.

Loosli, C., J. T. Grayston, E. R. Alexander, and F. Tanzi: Epidemiological Studies of Pulmonary Histoplasmosis in a Farm Family, Am. J. Hyg., 55:392, 1952.

Parsons, R. J., and C. J. D. Zarafonetis: Histoplasmosis in Man: Report of Seven Cases and Review of Seventy-one Cases, Arch. Intern. Med., 75:1, 1945.

Sellers, T. E., Jr., W. N. Price, Jr., and W. M. Newberry, Jr.: Epidemic of Erythema Multiforme and Erythema Nodosum Caused by Histoplasmosis, Ann. Intern. Med., 62:1244, 1965.

Shapiro, J. L., J. J. Lux, and B. E. Sprofkin: Histoplasmosis of the Central Nervous System, Am. J. Pathol., 31:319, 1955.

Sweany, Henry C.: "Histoplasmosis," Springfield, Ill., Charles C Thomas, Publisher, 1960.

189 SPOROTRICHOSIS
Abraham I. Braude

DEFINITION. Sporotrichosis is a chronic infection due to *Sporotrichum schencki*. It is characterized by the formation of suppurating nodules along the lymphatics of the skin and subcutaneous tissues. Hematogenous dissemination is rare.

ETIOLOGY. The fungus *S. schencki* is dimorphic. On Sabouraud's agar at room temperature its growth is mycelial, but in the tissue it takes the form of tiny, cigar-shaped yeast cells. The yeast phase also develops in vitro by incubation at 37°C on blood agar containing cystine.

PATHOGENESIS AND PATHOLOGY. The fungus lives as a saprophyte on vegetation and penetrates the hands when the skin is broken. Many cases have followed injury by thorns, and an outbreak of sporotrichosis occurred among South African natives exposed to *S. schencki* growing on timbers supporting a gold mine. In this country, it is primarily an occupational disease in people working with plants. Sphagnum moss is an important source of infection, and its increased use as mulch may lead to a greater occurrence of sporotrichosis.

After penetrating the skin, the fungus spreads up the extremities and evokes nodular lesions along the thickened lymphatics. Microscopically the nodules are granulomas with central necrosis. In exceedingly rare infections the organism may become disseminated throughout the subcutaneous tissues, the liver, testicles, bone, and kidney. Disseminated disease is not usually accompanied by primary infections of the extremities, and its portal of entry is believed to be the gastrointestinal tract.

CLINICAL MANIFESTATIONS. There is a marked disproportion between symptoms and findings. A chain of hard, reddened discrete lumps extends up the arm or leg to the axilla or groin, and the intervening lymphatics are red and thickened, but there is no pain, fever, or other constitutional symptom. Older nodules may rupture to produce fistulas or ulcers. In the rare patient with disseminated

sporotrichosis, constitutional symptoms may be marked and the disease is rapidly fatal. Unlike other disseminated mycoses, sporotrichosis almost never involves the lungs or central nervous system. Instead, it has a predilection for bone, joints, periosteum, and muscle.

Without treatment, sporotrichosis does not heal, and the lesions often become secondarily infected with bacteria.

DIAGNOSIS. The fungus cannot be seen upon microscopic examination of biopsied material or pus in most cases. Cultural isolation is invariably successful, however, if pus is aspirated from an unbroken nodule and inoculated onto Sabouraud's agar. The growth at first has the soft creamy character of bacterial colonies and later develops a wrinkled dark-brown appearance without the cottonlike filament of most molds. Microscopically, typical clusters of pear-shaped spores are found at the tips of conidiophores arising from the tangled mass of delicate branched mycelia. If the mold or the pus is inoculated intraperitoneally into mice or rats, numorous yeast forms will be seen in lesions of the peritoneal cavity or testicle, where they take the form of gram-positive cigar-shaped rods within polymorphonuclear leukocytes.

Recovery of the organism by these techniques permits ready differentiation of sporotrichosis from other chronic infections of the subcutaneous tissues such as syphilis, tularemia, blastomycosis, coccidioidomycosis, and tuberculosis. The hard sporotrichotic lesions are sometimes mistaken for syphilitic gummas, and their response to iodides is interpreted as therapeutic proof of the diagnosis.

TREATMENT. The common lymphangitic form of sporotrichosis is almost invariably dramatically cured by saturated potassium iodide. This should be given orally in starting doses of 10 drops t.i.d. after meals and gradually increased to the point of maximum tolerance. Treatment should be continued for a month after lesions disappear. Additional local therapy may be required for cutaneous ulcers, which should be painted with tincture of iodine. It may also be necessary to excise the epidermal lesions, because these may not subside with oral iodides. Systemic sporotrichosis is also resistant to iodides, but it responds well to intravenous treatment with amphotericin B, given in a total dose of 1.5 to 2.0 Gm over a period of 6 to 8 weeks.

REFERENCES

Kedes, L. H., J. Siemienski, and A. I. Braude: The Syndrome of the Alcoholic Rose Gardener: Sporotrichosis of the Radial Tendon Sheath, Ann. Intern. Med., 61:1139, 1964.

Wilson, D. E., J. J. Mann, J. E. Bennett, and J. P. Utz: Clinical Features of Extracutaneous Sporotrichosis, Medicine, 46:265, 1967.

190 MONILIASIS (Candidiasis)
Abraham I. Braude

DEFINITION. Moniliasis is a common mild mucocutaneous infection due to *Candida albicans*. This fungus is also an unusual cause of widespread visceral infection.

ETIOLOGY. Among the many species of *Candida*, only *C. albicans* is a common pathogen for man. On the usual nutrient laboratory media *C. albicans* grows as a budding yeast in creamy white colonies, but it produces both mycelia and yeastlike cells in infected tissues. *Candida parapsilosis* is only important as a cause of endocarditis. *Candida guilliermondii* and *Candida tropicalis* have also been isolated rarely in endocarditis.

PATHOGENESIS. *Candida albicans* resides normally on the mucous membranes and is frequently cultured from the mouth and feces of persons in good health. The rate of cultural isolation from feces in numerous surveys has ranged from 14 to 19 percent. In debilitated infants, and sometimes in adults, the fungus may produce white patches on the buccal mucosa and initiate mild inflammatory reaction in the underlying tissues. At times chronic moniliasis of the oral mucosa induces chronic hyperplastic changes that resemble leukoplakia. In pregnancy and diabetes, *C. albicans* frequently causes a mild superficial infection of the vagina. Presumably, the high glycogen content of the vaginal mucosa in pregnancy and the glycosuria of diabetes favor its growth. Candida multiplies excessively in the bowel or mouth if the normal bacterial flora is suppressed by chemotherapy. Although true infection seldom accompanies this overgrowth of candida, the large inoculum provides a threat in debilitated persons, who may develop aspiration pneumonia or even candidemia. The kidney and brain bear the brunt of hematogenous infection, but lesions also occur in the thyroid, myocardium, endocardium, pancreas, adrenals, and liver. The visceral lesions are granulomatous nodules or abscesses containing both mycelia and yeastlike cells.

A striking susceptibility to moniliasis of the skin and nails is seen in children with congenital hypoparathyroidism. Extensive cutaneous moniliasis occurs in infants with the Swiss type of agammaglobulinemia (alymphocytosis), but not in those with the Bruton form (Chap. 69).

CLINICAL MANIFESTATIONS. No systemic disturbances accompany the local signs of mucocutaneous infection. Infection of the mucous membranes, known as *thrush*, gives rise only to soft white patches on the tonsils, cheeks, gums, and tongue. These patches are easily removed and leave a reddened surface. Although usually self-limited, the disease may become chronic and spread to other mucosal surfaces or intertriginous areas in the groins, the antecubital fossae, the interdigital folds, the inframammary areas, the umbilicus, and the axillas. Eczematoid lesions and vesicles are also found in vulvovaginal moniliasis of pregnancy or diabetes.

Aspiration pneumonia is probably the chief form of visceral moniliasis. It is seen in debilitated persons, often in the course of intensive therapy with tetracycline or other antibiotics, and may be accompanied by mixed infection with bacteria. Cough, chest pain, and high fever are prominent.

Bloodstream infections are seen in the late stages of severe debilitating disease and seem to occur most commonly in children receiving intensive antibiotic therapy. Acute disseminated moniliasis may be suspected in debilitated adults who suddenly develop fever, shock, azotemia, depressed sensorium, and gastrointestinal bleeding after receiving continuous antibiotic treatment. Monilia also may cause vegetative endocarditis, a disease that has been described mainly in narcotic addicts. Meningitis is another rare form of moniliasis; it produces a clinical syndrome similar to tuberculous meningitis.

DIAGNOSIS. In thrush, the organisms are seen upon microscopic examination of the white patches as a tangled mass of mycelia and yeastlike cells. They grow readily on Sabouraud's agar. In fungemias the fungus can be isolated repeatedly from the blood. Pulmonary moniliasis may be difficult to recognize, because *C. albicans* is a normal resident of the oropharynx and may appear in the sputum in the absence of respiratory infection. For this reason, it is often impossible to be certain of the diagnosis of pulmonary moniliasis unless the organism is demonstrated in pulmonary lesions at autopsy or surgery.

TREATMENT. Oral and vaginal thrush are best treated topically. Nystatin oral suspension is used in the mouth and nystatin or candicidin tablets in the vagina. Topical therapy with nystatin ointments, amphotericin B lotion, or alcoholic solutions of gentian violet is effective in cutaneous moniliasis. Nystatin oral tablets may also be of some benefit in preventing candidal pneumonia or septicemia in debilitated persons whose mouth and intestines have become overgrown with candida during treatment with antibiotics. Intravenous amphotericin B in doses of 1.0 mg per kg body weight daily is effective in treating systemic moniliasis.

REFERENCES

Benham, R. W., and A. M. Hopkins: Yeast-like Fungi Found on the Skin and in the Intestines of Normal Subjects, Arch. Dermatol. Syphilol., 28:532, 1933.

Braude, A. I., and J. Rock: The Syndrome of Acute Disseminated Moniliasis in Adults, A.M.A. Arch. Intern. Med., 104:91, 1959.

Merchant, R. K., D. B. Luria, P. H. Geisler, J. H. Edgcomb, and J. P. Utz: Fungal Endocarditis: Review of the Literature and Report of Three Cases, Ann. Intern. Med., 48:242, 1958.

Winner, H., and R. Hurley: "Candida Albicans," Boston, Little, Brown and Company, 1964.

191 MUCORMYCOSIS
Abraham I. Braude

DEFINITION. Mucormycosis (phycomycosis) is a rare but malignant infection of cranial, pulmonary, and abdominal blood vessels due to fungi of the order Mucorales. The most frequent manifestations are ophthalmoplegia and meningoencephalitis.

ETIOLOGY. The etiologic agent has rarely, if ever, been cultured from the brain or spinal fluid even when expert mycologic techniques were used with fresh cerebral tissues known to harbor the characteristic mycelium. The mycelium is broad, branching, and aseptate, with a diameter of 6 to 15 μ. The fungus *Rhizopus oryzae*, a species of the order Mucorales, has been recovered from the paranasal sinuses of patients with fatal mucormycosis, and the mycelia in culture were identical in appearance with those in the brain. Because known members of the order Mucorales grow readily on ordinary media, the failure of cultural isolation from the brain remains a puzzle. In addition to *R. oryzae*, it has been possible to isolate *Absidia corymbifera*, *Rhizopus arrhizus*, and *Mucor pusillus* from infected foci outside the nervous system. A benign form of tropical subcutaneous phycomycosis is caused by *Basidiobolus ranarum*.

PATHOGENESIS. These fungi abound in soil, manure, and starchy foodstuffs, but become pathogenic for man only in rare cases of diabetic acidosis and even less commonly in patients debilitated by uremic acidosis, leukemia, irradiation, or radiomimetic drugs. The usual portal of entry appears to be the nasal turbinates or paranasal sinuses; from there the organism is thought to extend along the invaded vessels to the retroorbital tissues and cerebrum. Thrombosis of arteries and veins leads to multiple infarcts throughout the brain, but only a minimal inflammatory response is found. Cerebral mucormycosis may be associated with hematogenous spread to pulmonary and intestinal vessels. Pulmonary and intestinal infarction may also develop as a primary infection apparently after inhalation or ingestion of the fungus. Organisms probably penetrate the walls of bronchi or intestine and infect the adjacent hilar or mesenteric vessels. Intestinal mucormycosis takes the form of hemorrhagic segmental infarction of the ileum or colon. Invasion of coronary arteries may produce myocardial infarction.

CLINICAL MANIFESTATIONS. Cerebral mucormycosis is characterized by three features: (1) uncontrolled diabetes with acidosis, (2) ophthalmoplegia, and (3) signs of acute diffuse cerebrovascular disease. If the portal of entry is the nose, a fourth feature is a black nasal turbinate and malar anesthesia. When the patient is first seen, drowsiness and semistupor are usually attributed to the metabolic disturbance, but the cerebral manifestations persist and progress after the acidosis is corrected. Headache and fever are prominent, and paranasal sinusitis is frequently present.

In addition to complete internal and external ophthalmoplegia, there may be edema of the eyelids and retina, proptosis, and signs of retinal vascular occlusion. Nuchal rigidity and mild mononuclear pleocytosis in the spinal fluid have also been described. Pulmonary mucormycosis may start gradually or suddenly with chest pain, fever, hemoptysis, and a friction rub. A few cases have been described in which the orbit or sinuses were infected without extension to the brain. In tropical Africa, subcutaneous phycomycosis is relatively common. This benign disease is caused by fungi belonging to the genus *Basidiobolus* and produces a woody-hard, freely movable lump in the thighs, buttocks, and forearms, with no constitutional disturbances. Most patients are children. The Sassoon Hospital syndrome, a remarkable disorder attributed to the toxin of *Rhizopus nigricans*, is characterized by epidemic polyuria and polydipsia.

DIAGNOSIS. The syndrome of cerebral mucormycosis is so characteristic that it can be recognized by its clinical features alone. The fungus can be found in sections and cultures of the infarcted nasal turbinate or paranasal sinus.

PROGNOSIS. Untreated cerebral mucormycosis is almost invariably fatal. Rare cases of recovery have followed control of diabetic acidosis.

TREATMENT. A few patients with cerebral mucormycosis have recovered after treatment with amphotericin B in doses of 50 to 70 mg intravenously daily. The total doses were approximately 2.2 Gm. Treatment should also be directed toward rapid correction of the hyperglycemia and acidosis as well as local excision of infected tissue in the nose, paranasal sinuses, or orbit. Surgical removal of infected lung has been successful. Subcutaneous African phycomycosis has improved during treatment with oral potassium iodide.

REFERENCES

Baker, R. D.: Mucormycosis—a New Disease? J.A.M.A., 163:805, 1957.

Bauer, H., L. Ajello, E. Adams, and D. Hernandez: Cerebral Mucormycosis: Pathogenesis of the Disease: Description of the Fungus *Rhizopus oryzae* Isolated from a Fatal Case, Am. J. Med., 18:822, 1955.

Burkitt, D. P., A. M. M. Wilson, and D. B. Jelliffe: Subcutaneous Phycomycosis: A Review of 31 Cases Seen in Uganda, Brit. Med. J., 1:1669, 1964.

Burrow, G. N., R. B. Salmon, and J. P. Nolan: Successful Treatment of Cerebral Mucormycosis with Amphotericin B, J.A.M.A., 183:370, 1963.

192 NOCARDIOSIS
Abraham I. Braude

DEFINITION. Nocardiosis, an infection caused by an aerobic actinomycete, may produce lung abscesses and spread to the brain and elsewhere; or it may appear as a chronic deforming granulomatous infection limited to the foot (maduromycosis).

ETIOLOGY. Pulmonary and disseminated nocardiosis usually result from infection with *Nocardia asteroides*. This organism is relatively acid-fast, and its bacillary form resembles the tubercle bacillus. The following properties of *N. asteroides* permit easy differentiation from the tubercle bacillus: (1) rapid growth on Sabouraud's medium or on 10 percent blood agar with colonies appearing in 3 to 14 days at room temperature; (2) the presence in exudates of long-branched mycelial forms in addition to the bacillary forms; (3) rapid killing of guinea pigs and rabbits inoculated intraperitoneally and the recovery of *N. asteroides* from miliary nodules in the abdominal viscera; death of guinea pigs occurs in less than a week from pathogenic strains; (4) intense gram-positive staining reaction.

PATHOGENESIS. *Nocardia asteroides* can be recovered readily from soil. Nocardiosis appears, therefore, to be an exogenous infection usually having its portal of entry in the lungs. In almost every patient with nocardiosis (other than maduromycosis) the earliest and most extensive lesions are pulmonary acute suppurative foci containing acid-fast, branching nocardial filaments. A well-defined wall is absent, a fact which probably accounts for the marked tendency of nocardial abscesses to spread to the brain and to a lesser extent to the spleen, skin, peritoneum, and kidney. Occasionally noncaseating granulomas are found. Susceptibility to nocardiosis is increased in Cushing's syndrome, in pulmonary alveolar proteinosis, and in some patients with lymphomas or leukemia after antitumor chemotherapy.

CLINICAL MANIFESTATIONS. The chief symptom is cough, usually productive of a thick, sometimes bloody, sputum. Chest pain and dyspnea are common. These symptoms are usually accompanied by fever, sweats, chills, leukocytosis, weakness, anorexia, and weight loss. The illness may be prolonged and present the picture of a chronic pulmonary infection resembling tuberculosis, lung abscess, or unresolved suppurative pneumonia. In nearly one-third of the patients this syndrome is interrupted suddenly by the acute neurologic changes of metastatic brain abscess. At this time the patient may have severe headache and focal sensory or motor disturbances. The protein, cells, and pressure of the spinal fluid are increased, but the concentration of glucose is not reduced unless the meninges are also infected. Occasionally, symptoms of brain abscess are the first clinical manifestations of nocardiosis, especially in patients with Cushing's syndrome secondary to adrenal steroid therapy. Infection of the skin is frequent and produces numerous scattered abscesses or single draining sinuses of the hand, chest wall, or buttocks.

The disease is usually fatal, but the duration varies from months to years.

DIAGNOSIS. Because patients with nocardiosis are usually suspected of having tuberculosis, their sputums are likely to be examined for tubercle bacilli. The usual methods for concentrating tubercle bacilli often inactivate *N. asteroides,* however, and the fungus may not be recovered after such treatment despite the readiness with which it otherwise grows on a variety of media. *Nocardia asteroides* may also be overlooked in smears stained by the Ziehl-Neelsen method, because it is less resistant than the tubercle bacillus to the decolorizing action of acid alcohol. If nocardiosis is suspected on clinical grounds, precautions must be taken, therefore, against killing the organism by sputum concentration methods and against overdecolorizing it. The first can be avoided by concentrating with trisodium phosphate; the second by using a weak solution of acid alcohol.

Although sulfur granules are not found in pulmonary or disseminated nocardiosis, the gram-positive filamentous organisms in nocardial exudates often resemble *Actinomyces israeli.* The two pathogens can be distinguished, however, by the ease with which *N. asteroides* is cultivated on Sabouraud's medium or blood agar aerobically,

by its acid-fast staining characteristics, and by its pathogenicity for guinea pigs and rabbits. If biopsy material is available, the nongranulomatous and minimally fibrotic character of the nocardial suppurative reaction also helps to distinguish it from that seen in infections due to *A. israeli.* The absence of tubercles, of course, is valuable in differential diagnosis from tuberculosis.

TREATMENT. Sulfadiazine is sometimes successful in the treatment of nocardiosis. Penicillin and the tetracycline derivatives appear ineffective, and resistance of nocardiosis to these drugs may be used in distinguishing it from actinomycosis due to *A. israeli* and from other pulmonary infections which respond to these antibiotics. Patients with nocardiosis should receive 8 to 12 Gm sulfadiazine daily. Despite the poor clinical results with penicillin and tetracycline, in vitro tests are warranted to determine the sensitivity of each new strain of *N. asteroides* to various antibiotics. An antibiotic selected on this basis can be used to supplement the sulfonamides.

REFERENCES

Andriole, V. T., M. Ballas, and G. L. Wilson: The Association of Nocardiosis and Pulmonary Alveolar Proteinosis, Ann. Intern. Med., 60:266, 1964.

Danowski, T. S., W. M. Cooper, and A. I. Braude: Cushing's Syndrome in Conjunction with *Nocardia Asteroides* Infection, Metabolism, 11:2, 1962.

Henrici, A. T., and E. L. Gardner: The Acid-fast Actinomycetes: With a Report of a Case from Which a New Species Was Isolated, J. Infect. Dis. 28:232, 1921.

Weed, L. A., H. A. Andersen, C. A. Good, and A. H. Baggentos: Nocardiosis: Clinical, Bacteriologic and Pathologic Aspects, New Engl. J. Med., 253:1138, 1955.

193 OTHER DEEP MYCOSES
Abraham I. Braude

ASPERGILLOSIS

DEFINITION. Aspergillosis is an infection produced by *Aspergillus fumigatus* and other species of *Aspergillus,* a group of fungi of low pathogenicity for man unless resistance is overcome by an overwhelming inoculum or debilitating illness. The disease may become disseminated or remain localized to the lung, ear, orbit, or paranasal sinuses.

ETIOLOGY. Asperigilli assume the mycelial form both in culture and in infected tissues. They are hardy, widely prevalent organisms and grow rapidly on all culture media at room temperature or 35°C as colored woolly colonies peppered with dark dots. They are composed of segmented mycelia that bear masses of small round spores on a knoblike swelling at the end of specialized mycelial stalks known as conidiophores.

PATHOGENESIS AND PATHOLOGY. Primary infection of the lung sometimes develops after inhalation of massive numbers of spores from mycelia growing on grain. Pulmonary aspergillosis was an occupational disease in persons who fattened squabs by forcing masticated grain from their mouths into the esophagus of the birds. Secondary pulmonary infection may be superimposed on tuberculous cavities, bronchiectasis, and bronchogenic carcinoma or may become established after resistance is lowered by leukopenia, Hodgkin's disease, irradiation, and other debilitating processes. Excessive use of adrenal steroids or antibiotics is also thought to favor secondary invasion by aspergillus. The most distinctive pulmonary lesion is the aspergilloma, a mycelial mass in a fibrous cavity lined with bronchial epithelium. Chronic granulomatous lung lesions resembling tuberculosis have also been described. More destructive infections take the form of bronchopneumonia and lung abscesses. Thrombosis of pulmonary vessels by invading mycelia leads to local necrosis with hemorrhage and to hematogenous abscesses in the brain, lung, kidney, spleen, heart, and thyroid. Primary infections of the ear, orbit, and nasal sinuses may also be invasive and extend locally into the middle ear and brain. In all lesions, mycelia are prominently observed in tissues stained with Schiff's periodic acid or hematoxylin and eosin.

CLINICAL MANIFESTATIONS. In pulmonary aspergillomas the chief symptom is hemoptysis. Aspergillus lung abscesses and granulomas are associated with cough and fever. In fulminating disseminated infections, pulmonary manifestations are often overshadowed by coma and other signs of cerebral infection. Fever, joint pains, and skin eruptions lasting for a few weeks or months may also accompany disseminated aspergillosis. A syndrome of allergic aspergillosis occurs in asthmatics who develop hypersensitivity to aspergillus antigens. These patients are subject to recurrent episodes of localized pulmonary infiltrations with blood eosinophilia, increased wheezing, cough, fever, and pleuritic pain. Allergic aspergillosis is said to be the most frequent cause in Great Britain of transient lung infiltrates with eosinophilia. A form of allergic aspergillosis, known as hemp disease, produces asthma in people working in rope factories.

DIAGNOSIS. Cultures of aspergilli have no diagnostic value unless they are obtained directly from infected tissues. They may be present in the mouth and in sputum cultures in the absence of aspergillus infection, and they may contaminate uninfected biopsy specimens unless strict sterile precautions are observed. Cultural findings should be confirmed by demonstration of the characteristic septate mycelia in biopsy material. Diagnosis should not be based alone on the morphology of the fungus in tissue section without simultaneous culture, because its mycelia may be confused with those found in the tissues in candidiasis and mucormycosis. In chronic aspergillomas the sputum cultures may sometimes become negative after the fungus loses its ability to sporulate.

Aspergillomas of the lung can usually be recognized by the unique appearance in roentgenograms of a crescentic radiolucency surrounding a circular mass. In other forms of pulmonary aspergillosis the roentgenogram is not diagnostic and may resemble that of bronchogenic carcinoma, bacterial lung abscess, and tuberculosis. In allergic aspergillosis, the sputum may contain small plugs composed of eosinophilic and mycelial fragments, and serum precipitins against aspergillus antigens are found by double diffusion in agar gel. Such precipitins are also present constantly in pulmonary aspergillomas.

TREATMENT. Localized lesions have been successfully excised from both the lung and the brain. The value of chemotherapy has not been established in systemic infections, but intravenous amphotericin B shows enough promise to warrant its use.

GEOTRICHOSIS

DEFINITION. Geotrichosis is the name given to certain disorders of the mouth, bronchi, and intestinal tract from which *Geotrichium candidum* has been isolated. This fungus has not been established as a human pathogen, and the validity of geotrichosis as a disease entity remains questionable.

ETIOLOGY. The fungus *G. candidum* may resemble *Coccidioides immitis* in culture because its septate mycelium fragments into large square-ended arthrospores. *Geotrichium candidum* does not form sporangia in vivo, however, and its soft creamy colonies on solid medium are easily distinguished from those of *C. immitis*.

PATHOGENESIS. Geotrichium is a normal inhabitant of the pharynx and bowel and may proliferate locally to produce visible white colonies on the mucous membranes. It may also appear in devitalized tissues and secretions of the nasopharynx, bronchopulmonary tree, and colon but probably not as a primary pathogen.

CLINICAL MANIFESTATIONS. Geotrichosis is reported to cause pulmonary cavities and colitis. In bronchopulmonary geotrichosis, the patient coughs up gelatinous sputum tinged with blood, and in rare cases thin-walled cavities like those of coccidioidomycosis have been described.

DIAGNOSIS. In secretions and exudates, *G. candidum* has the appearance of oval or barrel-shaped spores measuring up to 8 to 10 mm in diameter. They are easily recovered on Sabouraud's agar at room temperature.

TREATMENT. Lesions resembling thrush respond to local application of 1:10,000 solution of gentian violet. Bronchopulmonary geotrichosis is said to respond to oral treatment with potassium iodide, and intestinal geotrichosis is treated by oral administration three times daily of capsules containing 0.32 mg gentian violet.

MYCETOMA

DEFINITION. Mycetoma is a chronic destructive infection of the skin, subcutaneous tissues, fascia, and bone. The infection produces a localized swelling containing multiple fistulas which extrude mycotic granules.

ETIOLOGY. The most frequent cause of mycetoma in the United States is a higher fungus known as *Monosporium apiospermum*, the "imperfect" form of the ascomycete *Allescheria boydii*. It grows rapidly on Sabouraud's agar as a cottony mycelium bearing asexual spores either singly or in small groups at the tips or sides of conidiophores. Other higher fungi isolated in mycetoma include members of such diverse genera as *Aspergillus, Penicillium, Madurella, Cephalosporium,* and *Phialophora.*

Members of the genus *Nocardia* are important causes of mycetoma outside the United States. *Nocardia madurae* is found in southeastern Asia and *N. brasiliensis* in South America and Mexico.

PATHOGENESIS AND PATHOLOGY. The fungi found in mycetoma are inhabitants of the soil and enter the tissues of the bare foot and leg, presumably after trauma. The chest wall is infected by sacks, contaminated with soil, and carried over the shoulder. The buttocks, abdomen, and arm are also infected.

The infection begins in the outer tissues and burrows through to destroy bone, muscle, and connective tissue indiscriminately. The areas of destruction show chronic suppuration with fibrosis and are connected by multiple fistulas which rupture to the outside. Mycotic granules are seen in the suppurative foci. The prolonged proliferation of granulation and scar tissue leads to enlargement of the affected part.

CLINICAL MANIFESTATIONS. The earliest sign is usually a small swelling on the sole or dorsum of the foot which undergoes a recurring cycle of swelling, suppuration, and healing. Later, similar lesions appear on other parts of the foot, and over a period of months destruction of deeper tissues is manifested by slight or moderate pain, generalized swelling, and redness. The course is intermittently progressive, and there may be periods of remission. Ultimately the foot becomes a swollen, deformed mass of destroyed tissue with many fistulous openings through which mycotic granules are discharged. The infection does not spread hematogenously to other parts, but in rare instances there is direct extension along lymphatics. Death may occur from secondary bacterial infection.

DIAGNOSIS. The characteristic granules are 0.5 to 2 mm in diameter and may be white, yellow, black, or red. Nocardial granules are easily distinguished from those of *Aspergillus boydii* and other higher fungi by direct microscopic examination. They are masses of radiating grampositive filaments; those of higher fungi contain large segmented hyphae and numerous chlamydospores. Either type of granule grows rapidly on Sabouraud's agar.

Roentgenograms disclose destruction of bone which is more extensive than the external appearance and pain might indicate.

TREATMENT. Nocardial mycetomas should be treated with oral sulfonamides, and those due to higher fungi with intravenous and local amphotericin B. Antibacterial chemotherapy is valuable in arresting secondary infection. There is no dependable cure, however, and many cases eventually require amputation.

CHROMOBLASTOMYCOSIS

DEFINITION. Chromoblastomycosis is an infection of the skin produced by several species of the genus *Phialophora* and characterized by slowly progressive cauliflower-like lesions of the skin of agricultural workers in tropical or subtropical regions.

ETIOLOGY. The three species *P. pedrosi, P. compactum,* and *P. verrucosa* cannot be distinguished upon microscopic examination of infected tissue, in which all appear as small clusters of spores with thick, dark-brown walls. On culture, however, the three differ in their methods of sporulation. The species most commonly found, *P. pedrosi,* exhibits three types of spore formation: (1) branching chains of spores borne at the tips of long conidiophores, (2) clusters of spores forming sleeves about the hyphae, and (3) balls of spores arising in the cuplike ends of very short flask-shaped conidiophores. *Phialophora verrucosa* forms only the third type of spore, and *P. compactum* is recognized by chains of spores arranged in compact masses. On Sabouraud's agar all three grow very slowly and will produce deeply pigmented olive or black colonies.

PATHOGENESIS AND PATHOLOGY. The fungi undoubtedly live in the soil or vegetation and enter the skin of agricultural workers. The disease occurs mostly on the lower extremity of barefoot workmen, but sometimes on the upper extremity or buttocks.

Three pathologic processes are found: (1) microabscesses in the dermis containing numerous fungi, (2) extensive fibrosis, and (3) epidermal hyperplasia and hyperkeratosis. The lesions progress along the lymphatics but only rarely beyond them, and they do not penetrate deeply to involve bone. A few cases of brain abscesses have occurred.

CLINICAL MANIFESTATIONS. The earliest lesion is a papule, which develops into a well-circumscribed bluish lesion with a warty, raised margin. Although it resembles the cutaneous form of North American blastomycosis at this early stage, it does not spread peripherally. Instead, adjacent new lesions appear over a period of years and, as the epithelial hyperplasia and hyperkeratosis increase, the entire area assumes a cauliflower-like appearance. Eventually the whole extremity is covered. Pain and constitutional symptoms are absent unless secondary bacterial infection occurs or elephantiasis develops as a result of lymphatic scarring.

DIAGNOSIS. The typical dark-brown septate bodies are seen in large numbers in biopsied tissue or pus, and brown hyphae can be found in crusts treated with 10 percent potassium hydroxide. For specific identification, however, it is necessary to culture the slowly growing fungus on Sabouraud's agar.

TREATMENT. Early in the disease, the lesions may be destroyed by electrocoagulation or removed by surgical excision. Later in the course, excision of the larger nodules leaves indolent ulcers which heal very slowly.

Saturated solution of potassium iodide, given to tolerance orally, as in sporotrichosis, is said to be effective when combined with weekly injections of calcipherol. Local injection into the lesions of 0.035 mg amphotericin B in 7 ml of 2 percent procaine solution at weekly intervals has been used because the organisms are resistant to the levels achieved after intravenous injection. This local treatment produced complete resolution of lesions in a limited trial and should be tried. In general, the treatment of chromoblastomycosis has been disappointing. The disease is never fatal, however, and the usefulness of the limb is retained despite its unsightly appearance.

RHINOSPORIDIOSIS

DEFINITION. Rhinosporidiosis produces small tumorlike masses usually confined to the nose and nasopharynx. An endosporulating fungus seen in the tissues cannot be cultured on laboratory media.

ETIOLOGY. The fungus *Rhinosporidium seeberi* is placed in the class Phycomycetes and family Coccidioidaceae because characteristic giant sporangia develop in the tissues. These thick-walled endospore-filled sporangia may reach 500 μ in diameter but otherwise resemble the smaller spherules of *Coccidiodes immitis*.

PATHOGENESIS AND PATHOLOGY. The disease is probably acquired by bathing or diving into infected water. In India, where rhinosporidiosis reaches endemic proportions, its rarity in women is attributed to social taboos that prohibit their bathing in open places. The characteristic lesion is a vascularized papillomatous proliferation of the nasal or pharyngeal mucous membrane containing sporangia in various stages of maturity. Red cells, inflammatory cells, and extruded endospores fill the interstitial tissue. As sporangia enlarge they compress the columnar epithelium of the nose or the squamous epithelium of the pharynx and allow endospores to escape and reinoculate the adjacent tissue.

CLINICAL MANIFESTATIONS. Single or multiple pedunculated fleshy red masses appear in the nares or pharynx and produce symptoms of rhinitis, epistaxis, and nasal obstruction. In exceptional cases hoarseness may develop from laryngeal infection. The conjunctivas and lacrimal sac may also be involved.

DIAGNOSIS. The characteristic sporangia are easily identified in biopsied tissue section. Because the only endemic foci are in India, most patients are Asiatic.

TREATMENT. The lesions can be completely removed surgically or by electrocautery. Electrocautery is preferred because surgery leaves open incisions in which spores can be implanted.

REFERENCES

Aspergillosis

Finegold, S. M., D. Well, and J. F. Murray: Aspergillosis: A Review and Report of Twelve Cases, Am. J. Med., 27:463, 1959.

Grcevic, N., and W. F. Mathews: Pathologic Changes in Acute Disseminated Aspergillosis, Am. J. Clin. Pathol., 35:536, 1959.

Naji, A. F.: Bronchopulmonary Aspergillosis, A.M.A. Arch. Pathol., 68:282, 1959.

Pepys, J., R. W. Reddell, K. M. Citron, Y. M. Clayton, and E. I. Short: Clinical and Immunological Significance of *Aspergillus Fumigatus* in the Sputum, Am. Rev. Resp. Dis., 80:167, 1959.

Chromoblastomycosis

Barwasser, N. C.: Chromoblastomycosis: Thirteenth Reported Case in the United States, J.A.M.A., 153:556, 1953.

Binford, C. H., G. Hess, and C. W. Emmons: Chromoblastomycosis, Arch. Dermatol. Syphilol., 49:398, 1944.

Conway, H., and W. Berkeley: Chromoblastomycosis (Mycetoma Form) Treated by Surgical Excision, A.M.A. Arch. Dermatol. Syphilol., 66:695, 1952.

Geotrichosis

Kunstadter, R. H., A. Milzer, and F. Whitcomb: Bronchopulmonary Geotrichosis in Children, Am. J. Dis. Child., 79:82, 1950.

Smith, D. T.: Geotrichosis, J. Chronic Dis., 5:532, 1957.

Mycetoma

Ajello, L.: Soil as Natural Reservoir for Human Pathogenic Fungi, Science, 123:876, 1956.

Rhinosporidiosis

Purandare, N. M., and S. M., Deoras: Rhinosporidiosis in Bombay, Indian J. Med. Sci., 7:603, 1953.

Section 12

The Rickettsioses

194 GENERAL CONSIDERATIONS AND PATHOLOGY

Theodore E. Woodward and Elizabeth B. Jackson

The rickettsial diseases of man consist of a variety of clinical entities caused by microorganisms of the family *Rickettsiaceae*. The rickettsias are obligate intracellular parasites about the size of bacteria and are usually seen microscopically as pleomorphic coccobacilli. Each of the rickettsias pathogenic for man is capable of multiplying in one or more species of arthropod as well as in animals and man. Indeed, the majority of the rickettsias are maintained in nature by a cycle which involves an insect vector and an animal reservoir, and infection

Table 194-1. RICKETTSIAL DISEASES

| Group | Disease | | Geographic distribution | Natural cycle | | Transmission to man | Serologic diagnosis | |
	Type	Agent		Arthropod	Mammal		Weil-Felix reaction	Complement fixation
Spotted fever	Rocky Mountain spotted fever	R. rickettsii	Western hemisphere	Ticks	Wild rodents; dogs	Tick bite	Positive OX-19 OX-2	Positive group- and type-specific
	Boutonneuse fever	R. conorii	Africa, Europe, Middle East, India					
	Queensland tick typhus	R. australis	Australia		Marsupials, wild rodents			
	North Asian tick-borne rickettsiosis	R. sibirica	Siberia, Mongolia		Wild rodents			
	Rickettsial-pox	R. akari	United States, Russia, Africa(?)	Blood-sucking mite	House mouse, other rodents	Mite bite	Negative	
Typhus	Endemic (murine)	R. mooseri	Worldwide	Flea	Small rodents	Infected flea feces into broken skin	Positive OX-19	Positive group- and type-specific
	Epidemic	R. prowazeki	Worldwide	Body louse	Man	Infected louse feces into broken skin	Positive OX-19	
	Brill-Zinsser disease	R. prowazeki	Worldwide	Recurrence years after original attack of epidemic typhus			Usually negative	
	Scrub	R. tsutsuga-mushi	Asia, Australia, Pacific islands	Trombiculid mites	Wild rodents	Mite bite	Positive OX-K	Positive in about 50% of patients
Q fever		R. burnetii	Worldwide	Ticks	Small mammals, cattle, sheep, goats	Inhalation of dried infected material	Negative	Positive
Trench fever		R. quintana	Europe, Africa, North America	Body louse	Man	Infected louse feces into broken skin	Negative	None available

of man is unimportant in the cycle. Epidemic typhus presents a number of points of dissimilarity to most of the other rickettsioses, because the natural cycle of infection involves only man and the louse. Moreover, the agent of epidemic typhus has not established a well-organized parasitic relationship which ensures its perpetuation either in its mammalian host and reservoir (man) or in its arthropod host (louse). Man frequently dies from epidemic typhus; only rarely do recovered patients serve as a reservoir and infect their body lice.

Furthermore, the louse is relatively poorly adapted to perpetuation of the rickettsias, which induce a fatal disease in this arthropod. In contrast, most rickettsias cause only a mild disease in their mammalian hosts and do not affect their vector adversely; indeed, a number are transmitted transovarially in arthropods from one generation to the next.

A compendium of information on the rickettsial diseases is presented in Table 194-1. Because each of the rickettsioses responds therapeutically to tetracyclines or chloramphenicol, the table mentions no therapy. Procedures for diagnostic isolation of the rickettsias are omitted because they generally are less useful than serologic methods, and the techniques which they require are highly specialized and hazardous. Information on isolation may be found in textbooks devoted to viral and rickettsial diseases.

HISTORY OF THE RICKETTSIAL DISEASES.

Of all the afflictions of mankind the rickettsial diseases, particularly epidemic typhus, rank among the foremost as a cause of human suffering and death. Classical typhus fever undoubtedly existed during ancient times, although Zinsser cites an outbreak of illness in 1083 in a monastery near Salerno, Italy, as the first probable recorded incidence of this disease. Typhus fever, through its able transmitter, the body louse, has always identified itself intimately with wars, famines, and human catastrophes of all kinds. Alone it has cast a decisive vote in the outcome of many military campaigns.

The record of deaths from epidemic typhus in this century in the Balkan countries and in Poland and Russia reaches astounding figures. Serbia in 1915 suffered an epidemic of major proportions, with 150,000 dead and a mortality rate ranging from 20 to 60 percent. Typhus ravaged Russia and eastern Poland from 1915 to 1922, infecting 30 million of the inhabitants and causing an estimated 3 million deaths.

The past two decades have seen the development of excellent methods for the prevention and treatment of the rickettsioses of man. In fact, these measures have been so successful that the rickettsioses have become of minor importance in the United States and in many other countries. Although conquered, the rickettsioses have not been eliminated, and they could again become rampant if the will to control them, the present high standards of sanitation, and the necessary industrial capacities for production of effective insecticides and therapeutic agents should be decreased through war or disaster. It is worthwhile to review the classical milestones representing the clinical and scientific contributions which have resulted in the understanding and conquest of the rickettsial infections.

Gerhard in 1836 differentiated typhoid fever from louse-borne typhus fever. In 1899, Maxcy described the clinical manifestations of Rocky Mountain spotted fever. In a series of studies from 1906 to 1909, Ricketts, for whom the rickettsial microorganisms are named, successfully transmitted this disease to guinea pigs, incriminated the wood tick as a vector, and observed rickettsias in smears prepared from tick tissues.

Nicolle in 1909 reproduced typhus fever in monkeys and demonstrated transmission by the body louse. Von Prowazek in 1914 and Da Rocha-Lima in 1916 demonstrated small microorganisms in the tissues of lice taken from typhus patients.

Brill in 1910 recognized a febrile disease in patients in New York City as an example of mild epidemic typhus unassociated with lousiness. Zinsser in 1934 postulated that this disease was a recurrent form of typhus occurring in patients during periods of stress or waning immunity. Subsequent studies have confirmed Zinsser's hypothesis. This entity is now called Brill-Zinsser disease.

Weil and Felix, working with typhus patients in Poland in 1915, recognized that agglutinins for certain proteus organisms appeared in the serum of convalescent patients. The Weil-Felix reaction, although nonspecific, affords a simple and valuable screening method for several rickettsioses.

In 1926 Maxcy, on purely epidemiologic evidence, surmised that typhus in the United States had its reservoir in rodents and was transmitted to man by ticks or fleas. Confirmation of Maxcy's hypothesis was obtained in Baltimore in 1930 by Dyer and others when they isolated rickettsias from the brains of rats and shortly thereafter incriminated the flea as a vector. This disease, caused by *Rickettsia moorseri* and now designated endemic or murine typhus, is distinct from epidemic typhus and Brill-Zinsser disease.

The development of suitable vaccines and specific diagnostic antigens was impeded until it was possible to prepare appreciable quantities of highly infectious rickettsial material in the laboratory. The most important steps were (1) the Weigl vaccine (1930), a phenolized suspension of gut tissue obtained from body lice which had been injected intrarectally with the rickettsias of epidemic typhus; (2) the killed murine typhus vaccine prepared by Casteneda (1939) from lung tissues of rats injected intranasally; and (3) the inactivated Rocky Mountain spotted fever vaccine obtained by Cox (1941) from infected yolk sacs of embryonated hen eggs. Each of the developments was applied in principle to other rickettsial agents, but the low cost and relative simplicity of the egg techniques have led to their general use for preparation of vaccines and diagnostic antigens. The specific diagnostic complement fixation tests for the rickettsial diseases now used in the United States stem directly from the pioneering work of Bengston on Q fever and of Plotz on the spotted and typhus fevers during the early 1940s.

The years of World War II saw many strides in the conquest of the rickettsioses; perhaps greatest among these were the highly successful attacks on the arthropod vectors. The lousicide DDT proved to be ideal for control when dusted on the clothes of infested persons. The epidemic at Naples during the winter of 1943 to 1944 established a milestone, because it was the first to be suppressed by the use of insecticides. On the other side of the world, scrub typhus (mite-borne typhus) was creating a major problem in military medicine in the Pacific area. Here, too, the major contributions to successful control were concerned with application of miticidal chemicals to the person and his clothes.

Hyperimmune rabbit serum (Topping, 1939) ameliorated the course of Rocky Mountain spotted fever if given during the early stages, and para-aminobenzoic acid (Yeomans, 1944) was found to be effective in typhus fever, but the advent of broad-spectrum antibiotics, first chloramphenicol, then chlortetracycline in 1948, and later oxytetracycline, provided dramatic therapeutic results in each of the rickettsoses.

Table 194-1 includes several rickettsial diseases which have not been mentioned in this historical review. Although important in themselves, none except Q fever has been the subject of work which contributed broad principles applicable to the group.

PATHOGENESIS. Rickettsial diseases of man develop following infection through the skin or the respiratory tract. Agents of the typhus and spotted fever group are introduced through the bite of the infected arthropod vector. Ticks and mites, which transmit the spotted fevers and scrub typhus, inoculate the rickettsias directly into the dermis during feeding. The louse and flea, which transmit epidemic and murine typhus, respectively, deposit infected feces on the skin; infection occurs when organisms are rubbed into the puncture wound made by the arthropod. The rickettsia of Q fever gain entry through the respiratory tract by inhalation of infected dust; moreover, the respiratory route is occasionally implicated in epidemic typhus when infection results from inhalation of dried infected louse feces.

Although organisms probably multiply at the original site of entry in all instances, local lesions appear with regularity only in certain diseases, namely, the initial cutaneous lesions of scrub typhus, rickettsialpox, and boutonneuse fever and the pneumonitis which develops in about half the persons infected with Q fever.

Volunteers infected with either scrub typhus or Q fever develop rickettsemia late in the incubation period, often some hours before the onset of fever. Similar events probably occur in all the rickettsial diseases; certainly circulating rickettsias can be detected during the early febrile period in practically all patients. Little is known about the pathogenesis of infection during the midportion of the incubation period. However, it is reasonable to assume that, during this time in patients with typhus or spotted fever, a transient low-grade rickettsemia results from release of organisms multiplying at the initial site of infection and that this seeds infection in the endothelial cells of the vascular tree. Vascular lesions developing at such sites could account for the pathologic changes, including the rash.

Rickettsia apparently invade and proliferate in the endothelial cells of small blood vessels. Endothelial cell destruction occurs from the proliferation of organisms and eventual disruption. Rickettsia may exert a cytotoxic effect on endothelial cells; in mice the rickettsial toxin causes remarkable increase in capillary permeability, independent of proliferation. Whether later manifestations in rickettsial diseases result from immunopathologic mechanisms is unknown.

The underlying cause of the toxic-febrile state which characterizes the rickettsial diseases remains unknown. Several rickettsial species contain type-specific toxins which are lethal for mice; these may play a role.

PATHOLOGY. The basic lesions in the spotted and typhus fever groups are in the small vessels. The most diverse and extensive of these are found in Rocky Mountain spotted fever. Here swelling, proliferation, and degeneration of the endothelial cells occur, frequently with thrombus formation which partially or completely obliterates the lumen. The muscle cells of the arteriole undergo swelling and fibrinoid changes. The adventitial tissues are infiltrated with mononuclear leukocytes, lymphocytes, and plasma cells. The vascular damage is scattered along the arteries, veins, and capillaries, with normal architecture prevailing throughout most of the vascular bed. The changes in murine, epidemic, and scrub typhus fevers resemble those in Rocky Mountain spotted fever, but thrombosis is uncommon and involvement of the musculature is rare.

The vascular changes, with resultant lesions in adjacent parenchymatous tissues, occur throughout the body but are most conspicuous in the heart, lung, and brain. Interstitial myocarditis occurs in each of these diseases but is usually most extensive in Rocky Mountain spotted fever and in scrub typhus. In the brain, the glial nodule is found in all members of the group; but microinfarcts in the brain tissue or in the myocardium are most often observed in spotted fever.

A rickettsial pneumonitis occurs, at least to some extent, in many patients with spotted or typhus fever and is the characteristic pathologic change in patients with Q fever. The process is patchy and consists macroscopically of areas of congestion and edema with gray granular consolidation. Microscopically, in the consolidated areas the alveoli are filled with compact fibrinocellular exudate containing lymphocytes, plasma cells, large mononuclear cells, and erythrocytes, but few if any polymorphonuclear leukocytes.

Rickettsias can occasionally be observed microscopically in sections of tissue. However failure to demonstrate rickettsias in histologic section is of no diagnostic significance.

LABORATORY DIAGNOSIS. Diagnostic procedures which depend on isolation of the etiologic agent from blood or other clinical material are expensive, time-consuming, and hazardous to laboratory personnel. Except in unusual circumstances the currently available serologic tests are adequate for laboratory confirmation of the clinical diagnosis in each of the rickettsial diseases.

As in most serologic diagnostic procedures the demonstration of a rise in titer of specific antibody during convalescence is of prime importance in establishing the laboratory confirmation. Table 194-2 summarizes the serologic results usually encountered in persons who suffer from rickettsial diseases in the United States. The Weil-Felix test employing Proteus strains OX-19 and OX-2 gives positive results in patients with spotted fever and murine typhus and negative results in those with rickettsialpox and Q fever. It is useful as a screening proce-

Table 194-2. SEROLOGIC DIAGNOSIS OF RICKETTSIAL DISEASES OF THE UNITED STATES

Group	Disease	Weil-Felix reaction				Complement fixation tests with type-specific antigen				
		Proteus	Illustrative titer		Cases with diagnostic titer	Rickettsial antigen	Illustrative titer			Cases with diagnostic titer
			10th day	20th day			10th day	20th day	30th day	
Spotted fever	Rocky Mountain spotted fever	OX-19	40	320	Most	*R. rickettsii*	20	160	80	Most
		OX-2	20	160						
	Rickettsialpox	OX-19	0	0	None	*R. akari*	0	64	128	Most
		OX-2	0	0						
Typhus.....	Murine typhus	OX-19	160	640	Most	*R. mooseri*	0	160	160	Most
		OX-2	10	40						
	Brill-Zinsser disease	OX-19	160	20	Infrequent	*R. prowazeki*	1,280	640	320	Most
		OX-2	0	0						
	Q fever	OX-19	0	0	None	*R. burnetii*	10	80	160	Most
		OX-2	0	0						

dure but cannot be relied upon to differentiate spotted fever from murine typhus. In patients with Brill-Zinsser disease the *Proteus* OX-19 reaction is usually negative or low in titer.

Complement fixation tests employing group-specific rickettsial antigens provide data which clearly differentiate the most common infections, i.e., murine typhus, Rocky Mountain spotted fever, and Q fever. Moreover, if type-specific rickettsial antigens are employed, it is generally possible to distinguish rickettsialpox from spotted fever and Brill-Zinsser disease from murine typhus.

Antibodies during response to a primary infection of epidemic typhus or Rocky Mountain spotted fever are usually 19S globulins. In patients with Brill-Zinsser disease, which is a recrudescence, antibodies occur more quickly—within several days after onset of illness—rise to a higher titer, and are 7S globulins.

Specific antibiotic therapy has little effect on the time of appearance of antibodies or on their ultimate titer, provided treatment is instituted some days after onset of the illness. However, if the illness is cut short by early and vigorous treatment, antibody production may be delayed for a week or so, and also the maximal titers attained may be below those illustrated in Table 194-2. Under these circumstances a sample of blood taken 4 to 6 weeks after onset of illness should also be tested.

An additional serologic test is based on the agglutination of sheep or human O erythrocytes after sensitization with a serologically active fraction of rickettsias designated ESS (erythrocyte-sensitizing substances). Erythrocytes exposed to the typhus ESS are specifically agglutinated by serums of patients as early as the eighth febrile day. The ESS test is simple and inexpensive.

The immunofluorescent antibody test is a very useful procedure for detecting rickettsia in the tissues of pa-tients with the typhus group of rickettsioses, the spotted fevers, and Q fever. The technique also visualizes rickettsia in ticks and the tissues of animals.

Except for normochromic anemia, which occurs in patients severely ill with rickettsial diseases, there are no other distinctive alterations in the hematologic picture. The white blood cell count in Rocky Mountain spotted fever, rickettsialpox, murine and epidemic typhus, Brill-Zinsser disease, Q fever, and others is usually within the normal range: 6,000 to 10,000 cells per cu mm. Leukopenia is occasionally observed, and in the presence of complications, such as superimposed infections and extensive vascular lesions, moderate leukocytosis occurs. The differential blood count is usually normal.

195 ROCKY MOUNTAIN SPOTTED FEVER

Theodore E. Woodward and Elizabeth B. Jackson

DEFINITION. Rocky Mountain spotted fever is an acute febrile illness caused by *Rickettsia rickettsii,* transmitted to man by ticks. The disease is characterized by sudden onset with headache and chills and by fever which persists for 2 to 3 weeks. A characteristic exanthem appears on the extremities and trunk about the fourth day of illness. Delirium, shock, and renal failure occur in the severely ill.

ETIOLOGY AND EPIDEMIOLOGY. The causative microbe *R. rickettsii* is the prototype for the rickettsial group of agents. The minute organisms are purple when stained by Giemsa's method or red by Macchiavello's technique; most are gram-negative. They are surrounded by a halo as if encapsulated. These organisms often occur in pairs and possess a cell wall similar in structure and chemical composition to that of gram-negative bacteria; there is a cell membrane, cytoplasmic granules corresponding to ribosomes, and procariotic organization of nuclear material. The cell membrane is selectively permeable; the cell wall is the focus of important antigens and an endotoxin-like substance.

The rickettsias grow in the nucleus and the cytoplasm of infected cells of ticks, mammals, and embryonated eggs; the intranuclear situation of the organisms is shared by the other members of the spotted fever group, but not by rickettsias of the typhus group. *Rickettsia rickettsii* is readily disinguishable from the agents of the typhus fevers by cross-immunity tests in guinea pigs and by complement fixation tests employing antigens prepared from infected yolk sac tissues. The differentiation of *R. rickettsii* from closely related members of the spotted fever group frequently requires elaborate procedures. Strains of the agent of Rocky Mountain spotted fever vary considerably in their virulence for man and animals.

The first reports of spotted fever in Idaho and Montana during the final decade of the last century led to the name Rocky Mountain spotted fever. However, the disease has been reported in all states except Maine and Vermont, as well as in Canada, Mexico, Colombia, and Brazil. Although related diseases are found on other continents, this particular infection is limited to the Western Hemisphere. Formerly about 500 but currently about 200 cases of spotted fever occur annually in the United States. The mortality in the days before specific therapy was about 20 percent but has decreased to about 5 percent. Although the attack rate per unit of population is highest in Wyoming, almost half the cases occur in the South Atlantic states, with the greatest number of these in Virginia, North Carolina, Georgia, and Maryland.

A number of species of ticks are found infected with *R. rickettsii* in nature, but only two are important in transmitting spotted fever to man. These are *Dermacentor andersoni,* the wood tick, which is the principal vector in the West, and *D. variabilis,* the dog tick, which assumes this role in the East. Infected female ticks transmit the agent transovarially to at least some of their offspring. Ticks which become infected, either through the egg or at one of the stages during their development cycle by feeding on an infected mammal, harbor the rickettsias throughout their lifetime, which may be several years. Thus, the tick serves as a reservoir in addition to being a vector. Small wild mammals are suspected of playing an important role in spreading the rickettsias in nature by infecting ticks which feed on them during rickettsemia.

Disease in man is generally acquired from the bite of an infected tick. Transmission is unlikely unless the tick remains attached for a number of hours. Infection may also be acquired through abrasions in the skin which become contaminated with infected tick feces or tissue juices; hence, the hazard associated with crushing ticks between the fingers when removing them from persons or animals.

There are seasonal variations in the incidence of cases of spotted fever, as well as differences in age and sex distribution of cases. In each instance these differences are related to exposure to ticks. Most cases are seen during the period of maximal tick activity, i.e., late spring and early summer. About half the cases in the Western states occur in men over forty, whereas half those in the Eastern states were in children under fifteen. This age distribution is undoubtedly influenced by propinquity to the wood and dog ticks, respectively. Mortality increases with age of the patient.

CLINICAL MANIFESTATIONS. Incubation Period and Prodromata. A history of tick bite is elicited in approximately 80 percent of patients. The incubation period varies between 3 and 12 days with a mean of 7. A short incubation period usually indicates a more serious infection.

Onset. In nonvaccinated persons, the onset is usually abrupt, with severe headache, a sudden shaking rigor, prostration, generalized myalgia, especially in the back and leg muscles, nausea with occasional vomiting, and fever which reaches 103 to 104°F within the first 2 days. Pain in the abdominal muscles may be severe, and arthralgia is not uncommon. Deep muscle palpation often elicits tenderness. Occasionally the debut of illness in children and adults is mild, accompanied by lethargy, anorexia, cephalgia, and low-grade fever. These symptoms are similar to those of many acute infectious diseases, making specific diagnosis difficult during the first few days.

Pyrexia. Fever continues for approximately 15 to 20 days in untreated cases. The febrile course in children may be shorter. Hyperthermia of 105°F or greater is of unfavorable prognostic significance, although fatalities may occur when the patient is hypothermic, with concurrent vasomotor collapse. Fever generally terminates by lysis over a period of several days, but rarely does so by crisis. Recurrent fever is uncommon except in the presence of secondary pyogenic complications.

The *headache* is generalized and excruciating, and frequently more intense over the frontal area. It persists throughout the first and second week of illness in untreated cases. Malaise continues for the first week; irritability is notable, and the patient shuns distractions such as questioning and examination.

Cutaneous Manifestations. The rash which is present in practically all cases is the most characteristic and helpful diagnostic sign. It usually appears on the fourth febrile day; the range is 2 to 6 days. The initial lesions are on the wrists, ankles, palms, soles, and forearms. The first lesions are macular, nonfixed, pink, irregularly defined, and measure 2 to 6 mm. A warm compress applied to the extremity accentuates the rash in the early stages. The exanthem is most prominent when the temperature is elevated. After 6 to 12 hr, the rash extends centripetally to the axilla, buttocks, trunk, neck, and face. (This is in contrast to the eruption of typhus fever, which begins on the trunk and spreads centrifugally, rarely involving the face, palms, or soles.) The rash becomes maculopapular after 2 to 3 days (it may be felt by light palpation) and assumes a deeper red hue. By about the fourth day it is petechial and fails to fade on pressure. Not uncommonly, the hemorrhagic lesions coalesce to form large ecchymotic blemishes; these lesions tend to form over bony prominences and may ultimately slough to form indolent, slow-healing ulcers. Patients who have had the typical rash show brownish discolorations at the site for several weeks during convalescence. In milder cases, the rash does not become purpuric and may disappear within a few days. Antibiotic therapy may abort the early exanthem; the later fixed lesion fades less rapidly with specific therapy.

The application of tourniquets for several minutes, or the occasional taking of the blood pressure, may provoke additional petechiae (Rumpel-Leede phenomenon), further evidence of capillary abnormalities.

Cardiovascular and Respiratory Features. During the early stages, the pulse is full and regular but accelerated in proportion to the height of the temperature, and the blood pressure is well sustained. During the peak of illness in seriously ill patients, the pulse is rapid and feeble, and hypotension of 90 mm Hg is common. If circulatory failure is sustained, the resultant hypoxia and shock lead to agitation and delirium and contribute to the formation of ecchymoses and gangrene of fingers, toes, genitalia, buttocks, earlobes, and nose. Cyanosis of the peripheral parts of the body is common. Venous pressure determinations show no elevation. A reduction of the total blood volume is occasionally found, as are evidences of myocardial impairment as shown by low voltage of ventricular complexes, minor S-T segment deflections, and occasionally delay in atrioventricular conduction on the electrocardiogram. These changes are transient and nonspecific. Severely ill patients have a puffy appearance of the face, hands, ankles, feet, and lower sacrum.

Respirations are either normal or slightly accelerated. Cough may be harassing and nonproductive, and localized pneumonitis may occur, but pulmonary consolidation is extremely rare. Pulmonary edema may develop after injudicious use of intravenous fluids.

Hepatic and Renal Manifestations. In the majority of patients, there is little alteration in renal or hepatic function. The liver may be enlarged, but jaundice is unusual. Oliguria commonly occurs in the seriously ill, and anuria may mark the critically ill patient. Azotemia is common and when marked, is a very unfavorable sign. Abnormalities in liver function are probably responsible for the hypoproteinemia, with reduction in the albumin fraction.

Neurologic Manifestations. The principal neurologic manifestations are headache, restlessness, and varying degrees of insomnia. Stiffness of the back is common. The cerebrospinal fluid is clear, with normal dynamics and normal chemical constituents. Coma and muscular rigidity may occur. Athetoid movements, convulsive seizures, and hemiplegia are grave manifestations. Deafness during the active stages of the disease is not uncommon. As a rule, all neurologic signs abate without residua. Findings based upon follow-up examinations and electroencephalograms may be interpreted as indicative of minor residual brain damage for a year or more following recovery of certain patients from Rocky Mountain spotted fever.

Other Physical Manifestations. Patients become dehydrated, with extreme dryness of lips, gums, tongue, and pharynx. The skin is hot and dry, the conjunctivas are frequently injected, and the eyes suffused. Photophobia is common in the early stages of illness. Petechial hemorrhages may be noted in the conjunctivas or in the retina. The spleen is enlarged in approximately one-half the cases and is firm and nontender. Abdominal distension is frequent, and occasionally some degree of intestinal ileus is observed. Constipation is usual.

COURSE OF DISEASE. In mild and moderately severe cases given no specific antibiotic therapy, the disease abates within 2 weeks, and convalescence is rapid. In fatal cases death usually occurs during the latter part of the second week as a result of toxemia, vasomotor weakness, and shock or renal failure.

In vaccinated individuals who contract the disease, the illness is mild, with a short febrile course and an atypical rash.

COMPLICATIONS AND PROGNOSIS. If the serious manifestations of spotted fever mentioned above are regarded as intrinsic parts of the disease, then complications are uncommon and consist mainly of secondary bacterial infections, namely, bronchopneumonia, otitis media, and parotitis. Thrombosis of major blood vessels may result in gangrene of a portion of an extremity. Hemiplegia and peripheral neuritis are rare sequelae.

The overall mortality rate for spotted fever was formerly about 20 percent. Death occurred in more than half of persons over forty years of age but mortality was much lower in children and young adults. Since the introduction of the broad-spectrum antibiotics and the development of more precise knowledge regarding correction of the physiologic abnormalities which develop during the disease, fewer deaths occur from this infection. Some of the fatalities can be attributed to failure to consider spotted fever in the differential diagnosis.

DIFFERENTIAL DIAGNOSIS. During the early stages of infection before the rash has appeared, differentiation from other acute infections is difficult. History of tick bite while living or traveling in a highly endemic area is helpful. The rash of meningococcemia (Chap. 142) resembles Rocky Mountain spotted fever in certain aspects, because it is macular, maculopapular, or petechial in the chronic form, and petechial, confluent, or ecchymotic in the fulminant type. The meningococcic skin lesion is tender and develops with extreme rapidity in the fulminant form, whereas the rickettsial rash occurs on about the fourth day of disease and gradually becomes petechial. The exanthem of rubeola rapidly becomes confluent, while that of rubella almost never becomes petechial.

Murine typhus is a milder disease than Rocky Mountain spotted fever; the rash is less extensive, nonpurpuric, nonconfluent; and renal and vascular complications are uncommon. Not infrequently differentiation of these two rickettsial infections must await the results of specific serologic tests. Epidemic typhus fever is capable of causing all the pronounced clinical, physiologic, and anatomic alterations seen in patients with Rocky Mountain spotted fever, i.e., hypotension, peripheral vascular collapse, cyanosis, skin necrosis and gangrene of digits, renal failure with azotemia, and neurologic manifestations. However, the rash of classical typhus is noted initially in the axillary folds and on the trunk and later extends peripherally, rarely involving the palms, soles, or face. The serologic patterns in these two diseases are distinctive when specific rickettsial antigens are employed in tests. Moreover, louse-borne typhus is not recognized in the United States except in the form of Brill-Zinsser disease (recurrent typhus fever). Rickettsialpox, although caused by a member of the spotted fever group of organisms, is usually readily differentiated from Rocky Mountain spotted fever by the initial lesion, the relative mildness of the illness, and the early vesiculation of the maculopapular rash. The Weil-Felix reaction is positive in Rocky Mountain spotted fever and in murine and epidemic typhus, but is negative in rickettsialpox. Agglutinins against *Proteus* OX-19 and OX-2 appear in the serum of patients with spotted fever, but only those against OX-19 are generally found in murine and epidemic typhus.

THERAPY. General. Certain physiochemical changes occurring in the patient seriously ill with one of the diseases of the typhus–spotted fever group should be understood before outlining a therapeutic regime. These changes are circulatory collapse, coma, oliguria and anuria, azotemia, anemia, hypoproteinemia, hypochloremia, and edema of the underlying tissues. These alterations are often absent in the mildly ill, and in them management is much less complicated. The therapeutic principles necessary for the treatment of all rickettsioses are (1) specific chemotherapy and (2) supportive care. Attention to both is mandatory for the seriously ill patient first recognized late in the disease. During the first week in the moderately ill patient, supportive therapy may be less energetic, because specific chemotherapy usually suffices. The early mild case may be successfully treated at home, while the later case should receive hospital care.

Therapeutic measures advisable for the management of Rocky Mountain spotted fever will be described in detail. Variations of this regimen which apply to the other rickettsioses are described in subsections relegated to other diseases of the typhus–spotted fever group and Q fever.

Specific Therapy. Specific therapy is most effective when initiated during the early stages of disease coincident with the appearance of the rash. When therapy is delayed until the rash has become hemorrhagic and widespread, the response is less dramatic. The antibiotics of choice are chloramphenicol and the tetracyclines, which are effective because of their rickettsiostatic properties. They are not rickettsiocidal.

The following antibiotic regimen is considered optimal: For chloramphenicol, an initial dose of 50 mg per kg body weight, and for tetracycline, 25 mg per kg body weight. Subsequent daily doses are the same as the initial loading dose, with the requirement divided equally and

given it at 6- to 8-hr intervals. Antibiotic treatment is continued until the patient is improved and has been afebrile approximately 24 hr. In patients too ill to take oral medication, an intravenous preparation of one of the antimicrobials may be employed for the loading dose.

Adrenal cortical hormones may need to be utilized for their antitoxemic effects, in patients first observed late in the course of severe illness. Large doses for brief periods (5 to 7 days) are recommended.

Table 195-1 summarizes information on the duration of disease and the mortality in the major rickettsioses prior to and since the introduction of specific antibiotic therapy.

Table 195-1. EFFECT OF SPECIFIC ANTIBIOTICS ON THE COURSE OF THE MAJOR RICKETTSIOSES

Disease	Untreated		Treated	
	Average duration of fever, days	Mortality, %	Average duration of fever after start of treatment, days	Mortality, %
Rocky Mountain spotted fever.......	16	21	3	0
Epidemic typhus.....	14	30	2	0
Murine typhus	12	2	2	0
Scrub typhus .	14	15	1	0

Duration of Therapy and Therapeutic Response. Therapy with antibiotics is continued until the toxemia has abated, the general condition has markedly improved, and the temperature has remained at normal levels for 24 hr. In uncomplicated cases of spotted fever, there is symptomatic improvement within 24 hr and temperature becomes normal in 60 to 72 hr.

SUPPORTIVE CARE. Nursing Care. Frequent turning of the patient relieves pressure from prominent bony parts and also militates against the development of aspiration pneumonia. Proper mouth care with frequent swabbing of the oral cavity may avert the development of parotitis and gingivitis. Sucking of the juice of a lemon or the oral use of glycerin or mineral oil is helpful.

Protein Balance. A generous intake of protein should be provided by frequent feedings as soon as the disease is suspected, in order to avoid subsequent protein deficiency. Usually food is well tolerated by patients with rickettsial disease, and the daily diet should provide 3 to 5 Gm protein per kg normal body weight, with adequate carbohydrate and fat to make it palatable. When the patient is uncooperative, the diet may be supplemented by hourly liquid protein feedings via stomach tube, provided that there is no abdominal distension.

At the critical stage, when hypoproteinemia is present and changes in capillary permeability lead to edema and vascular embarrassment, careful attention is given to the parenteral administration of protein supplements. When indicated by hematologic studies, whole-blood transfusions given slowly are helpful, or if the total red cell mass is adequate, one of the preformed protein supplements is beneficial. Intravenous albumin may be particularly useful, because it also aids in the reduction of tissue edema. The judicious administration of one of the plasma expanders at this stage may have a definite favorable effect upon impending circulatory collapse. If the patient is anuric and azotemia is pronounced, overloading the circulation with protein supplements and fluids should be avoided. The type and amount of parenteral therapy should be governed by clinical judgment and very careful laboratory studies. Frequent determinations of hemoglobin, hematocrit, electrolytes, and protein, sometimes at intervals of a few hours during crucial periods, are necessary in order to ascertain abnormalities and to permit institution of corrective measures.

COMPLICATIONS. *Pyogenic complications,* including otitis media and parotitis, are encountered in patients severely ill with Rocky Mountain spotted fever and other rickettsioses. These localized infections respond to therapy with appropriate antibiotics combined with ordinary supplemental surgical measures.

Pneumonitis usually develops as a result of specific rickettsial action. The sputum is scant but should be examined to determine whether superimposed infection is present. Specific therapy is guided by the results of these laboratory studies. The pneumonitis generally responds to the antibiotic therapy the patient is receiving, but if staphylococcal pneumonia is suspected, a penicillinase-resistant penicillin should be added to the broad-spectrum drug.

Circulatory failure of peripheral or central origin is combated by careful administration of electrolytic and protein supplements. Heart failure may develop rarely from the disease or as a result of overzealous intravenous alimentation and is recognized by the common signs of rapid pulse, gallop rhythm, increase in venous pressure, and muffled cardiac sounds. When the clinical signs reveal unmistakable evidence of cardiac failure, digitalis may be employed in the usual manner. Oxygen therapy by nasal tube, mask, or tent improves the cardiac and circulatory status and is helpful in hypoxic patients with involvement of the central nervous system.

PREVENTION. Prevention is attained primarily by avoidance of tick-infested areas. When this is impractical, prophylactic measures include (1) spraying the ground with dieldrin or Chlordane for area control of ticks, (2) application of repellents such as diethyltoluamide or dimethylphthalate to clothing and exposed parts of the body, or in very heavily infested areas the wearing of clothing which interferes with attachment of ticks, i.e., boots and a one-piece outer garment, preferably impregnated with repellent, and (3) daily inspection of the entire body, including the hairy parts, to detect and remove attached ticks. In removing attached ticks great care should be taken to avoid crushing the arthropod, with resultant contamination of the bite wound; touching the tick with gasoline or whisky encourages detachment but gentle traction with tweezers applied close to the mouth parts may be necessary; the skin area should be disinfected with soap and water or other antiseptics. Similarly, precautions should be employed in removing engorged ticks from dogs and other animals, because infection through minor abrasions on the hands is possible. Vaccines containing *R. rickettsii* are available commercially and should be used for those exposed to great risk, namely, persons frequenting highly endemic areas and laboratory workers exposed to the agent. Because the broad-spectrum antibiotics are such excellent therapeutic agents in spotted fever, there has been less impetus for vaccination of persons who run only a minor risk of infection.

196 OTHER TICK-BORNE RICKETTSIAL DISEASES

*Theodore E. Woodward and
Elizabeth B. Jackson*

DEFINITION. Boutonneuse fever, North Asian tick-borne rickettsiosis, and Queensland tick typhus, three diseases occurring in the Eastern Hemisphere, are caused by rickettsias closely related to one another and to the agent of Rocky Mountain spotted fever. Each is transmitted by the bite of an ixodid tick. These mild to moderately severe illnesses are characterized by an initial lesion (called *tache noire* in boutonneuse fever), a fever of several days to 2 weeks, and a generalized maculopapular erythematous rash which appear on about the fifth day and usually involves the palms and soles. Specific complement-fixing antibodies appear in the patients' serums during convalescence, but agglutinins to *Proteus* OX-19 (Weil-Felix reaction) are frequently found only in low titer.

ETIOLOGY AND EPIDEMIOLOGY. The etiologic agents of these three diseases are all members of the spotted fever group of rickettsias. Together with *Rickettsia rickettsii* and *R. akari* they possess common group antigens which are readily demonstrated by agglutination and complement fixation.

Boutonneuse fever, which may be regarded as the prototype of the three, is caused by *R. conorii.* Modern serologic methods employing specific rickettsial antigens have shown this rickettsia to be the causative agent for a single widely disseminated disease known by various local names. Information on the distribution and etiology of the various tick-borne rickettsial diseases is contained in Table 194-1.

In general, the epidemiology of these tick-borne rickettsioses resembles that of spotted fever in the Western Hemisphere. Ixodid ticks and small wild animals maintain the rickettsias in nature; man, if he intrudes accidentally into the cycle, is a dead end in the transmission chain. In certain areas, the cycle of boutonneuse fever involves domiciliary environments, with the brown dog tick *Rhipicephalus sanguineus* as the dominant vector.

CLINICAL MANIFESTATIONS. These three tick-borne rickettsioses, which occur in different parts of the Eastern Hemisphere, resemble one another closely. The clinical course is usually milder than that of spotted fever, with a shorter febrile period and fewer severe complications; fatalities are rare and generally limited to the aged and debilitated. The initial lesion, which is present in most cases at the onset of fever, heals slowly; the regional lymph nodes are enlarged. The rash usually remains papular and only in severe cases becomes hemorrhagic.

The clinical picture, including the primary lesion, the geographic location, and epidemiologic considerations are helpful in establishing the diagnosis. The typhus fevers, meningococcal infections, and measles must be considered in the differential diagnosis; the serologic reactions, i.e., Weil-Felix and complement fixation tests, are of value here.

TREATMENT AND PREVENTION. Chloramphenicol and the tetracyclines are effective therapeutic agents for boutonneuse fever. Patients generally become afebrile after 2 to 3 days of treatment, and recovery is rapid. The therapeutic procedures are comparable to those used in spotted fever (Chap. 195). Presumably these measures are also applicable to North Asian tick-borne rickettsiosis and Queensland tick typhus.

The major effective methods of control are concerned with avoidance of tick bites; these include application of newer repellents and prompt removal of attached ticks. Effective vaccines are not available commercially.

197 RICKETTSIALPOX

*Theodore E. Woodward and
Elizabeth B. Jackson*

DEFINITION. Rickettsialpox is a mild, nonfatal, self-limited, febrile illness caused by *Rickettsia akari*, which is transmitted from mouse to man by mites. It is characterized by an initial skin lesion at the site of the mite bite, a week's febrile course, and a papulovesicular rash.

ETIOLOGY AND EPIDEMIOLOGY. Rickettsialpox was first recognized in New York City in 1946, and about 180 cases were reported annually for several years thereafter. It has been diagnosed in several other areas of the United States, and outbreaks have been reported in European Russia. The vector is a small, colorless mite, *Allodermanyssus sanguineus* (Hirst), which infests small mice and rodents. House mice serve as the reservoir of infection.

Rickettsia akari is morphologically and biologically similar to other rickettsias and is antigenically related to, but distinct from, *R. rickettsii*, the cause of Rocky Mountain spotted fever. Mice, guinea pigs, and fertile hen eggs are susceptible to experimental infection. Diagnostic antigens prepared from infected yolk sacs are used in complement fixation tests.

CLINICAL MANIFESTATIONS. The initial skin lesion appears about 7 to 10 days after the mite bite as a firm red papule 1 to 1.5 cm in diameter. In a few days, the center vesiculates, and the papule is sourrounded by an area of erythema. The regional lymph glands are moderately enlarged. The primary lesion, which is never painful, becomes covered with a black scab; it heals slowly, and a small scar is visible on separation of the crust.

The febrile phase begins 3 to 7 days following the initial lesion, and exanthem may accompany the fever or begin several days later. The onset of fever is sudden, with chilly sensations or frank chills, headache, sweats, myalgia, anorexia, and photophobia. The pyrexia ranges from 103 to 104°F and continues for about a week, occasionally with morning remissions.

The exanthem is maculopapular-vesicular, generalized in distribution, and may be abundant or scant. The lesions may involve the oral cavity but not the palms or soles. In a week, the vesicles dry and form scabs which eventually scale but leave no scar.

The constitutional symptoms are generally mild, and the course of illness is uncomplicated. No fatal cases have been reported.

The disease may be confused with varicella (chickenpox—Chap. 224), which is different because it occurs usually in childhood and has no initial lesion and the papular cutaneous lesion is entirely transformed into a vesicle. Variola (smallpox—Chap. 223) is accompanied by a more severe constitutional reaction, and the vesicles become pustules. The skin lesions of the other rickettsioses differ in their lack of vesiculation. The Weil-Felix reaction is usually negative in this rickettsial disease, but the specific complement fixation test is a useful laboratory diagnostic aid even though there is considerable crossing with materials from Rocky Mountain spotted fever.

TREATMENT AND PREVENTION. Chloramphenicol and the tetracycline antibiotics are all effective for treating patients with rickettsialpox. The temperature reaches normal levels in about 2 days, and recovery is rapid.

Control measures should be directed toward elimination of house mice and the vector mites responsible for transmitting the disease.

198 MURINE (Endemic) TYPHUS FEVER

*Theodore E. Woodward and
Elizabeth B. Jackson*

DEFINITION. Murine typhus fever is an acute febrile disease caused by *Rickettsia mooseri* and transmitted to man by fleas. The clinical illness is characterized by fever of 9 to 14 days, headache, a maculopapular rash appearing on the third to fifth day, and myalgia.

ETIOLOGY AND EPIDEMIOLOGY. *Rickettsia mooseri* resembles other rickettsias in morphologic properties, staining characteristics, and intracellular parasitism. Under the electron microscope *R. mooseri* contains dense masses of nuclear material in a less dense homogeneous protoplasmic substance, the whole of which is surrounded by a limiting membrane. It differs from *R. rickettsii* in that it always multiplies within the cytoplasm of cells, in contrast to the intranuclear and cytoplasmic positions of spotted fever rickettsias.

Invasion of the body by *R. mooseri* provokes specific and nonspecific immunologic responses. Utilizing highly purified antigens, specific antibodies may be demonstrated readily by complement fixation and agglutination reactions. The positive Weil-Felix reaction which occurs in this disease is nonspecific, because it is attributable to the presence of a common carbohydrate antigen in *Proteus* OX-19 and *R. mooseri* and because the reaction is also positive in epidemic typhus and spotted fever. A number of investigators have demonstrated group-specific rickettsial antigens common to both *R. mooseri* and *R. prowazeki,* namely, a heat-stable complement-fixing substance. Furthermore, both murine and epidemic rickettsias possess toxic factors which are lethal to mice and rats and can be neutralized by convalescent serum from man or lower animals.

The common vector of *R. mooseri* for rats and man is the rat flea (*Xenopsylla cheopis*). In nature, the rat louse (*Polypax spinulosis*) may transmit the agent among rodents. Customarily, rat fleas become infected on ingestion of blood from diseased rats; the rickettsias multiply within the intestinal cells of the arthropod and are excreted in the feces. Infection in man occurs following the flea bite and contamination of the broken skin by rickettsia-laden feces. Dried flea feces may also infect via the conjunctivas or the upper part of the respiratory tract.

Rats and mice are naturally infected with murine typhus, and although the rodent disease is nonfatal, viable rickettsias persist in the brain for variable periods.

Murine typhus is one of the most benign and widespread of the rickettsioses in the United States. Prevalent in the Southeastern and Gulf Coast states, it has been identified in most of the other states and in harbor centers throughout the world wherever rats and fleas abound. Through control of rats and their fleas a sharp decline in incidence has occurred since 1951, particularly in the Southern United States; about half the cases reported annually now occur in Texas. In urban areas the disease is more prevalent during the summer and fall months and occurs predominantly among persons working in proximity to granaries or food depots. Recently there has been an extension to certain rural areas because changing agricultural practices have provided rats with ready access to adequate food supplies.

CLINICAL MANIFESTATIONS. Incubation Period and Prodromata. According to experimental observations, the incubation period ranges from 8 to 16 days, with a mean of 10. Common prodromata are headache, backache, arthralgia, and chilly sensations. Nausea, malaise, and transient temperature rises may precede the true onset of disease.

Onset and General Symptoms. A frank shaking chill and often repeated rigors are present at the onset, associated with a severe frontal headache and fever. This triad of headache, chill, and pyrexia is usually followed within a few hours by nausea and vomiting. Prostration, malaise, and weakness are sufficient to enforce cessation of activity in adults, in contrast to the course in children, whose illness is less severe. Occasionally, mild symptoms make it difficult to define the actual onset.

Pyrexia. The usual febrile course in murine typhus lasts for about 12 days in adults, and the temperature ranges from 102 to 104°F but may reach 105 to 106°F in children. The temperature may reach high levels abruptly after onset or ascend in a stepwise manner during the first few days. With the appearance of the rash, fever is usually sustained, with partial daily remissions which occasionally reach normal levels in the morning. Defervescence is generally by lysis over several days but sometimes occurs by abrupt crisis. Transient mild fever of 100°F is not uncommon during early convalescence. A few patients experience only low-grade fever throughout, but this does not necessarily connote a mild illness.

Cutaneous Manifestations. The early lesions, which are sparse and discrete, are hidden in the axillas and inner surface of the arm. Most patients then develop with surprising suddenness a generalized, dull red macular rash of the upper part of the abdomen, shoulders, chest, arms, and thighs. The individual lesions are discrete and pea-size, with an ill-defined border, and fade on pressure during the first 24 hr. They later become maculopapular, in contrast to the exanthem of epidemic typhus, which is persistently macular. The distribution over the trunk with sparse involvement of the extremities, palms, soles, and face differs from the peripheral distribution and facial involvement of Rocky Mountain spotted fever. The murine rash generally appears initially on the fifth febrile day, but rarely it is seen concurrently with the onset of fever or developing as late as the seventh day.

Eighty percent of patients develop a rash which persists for 4 to 8 days and fades before defervescence. The cutaneous manifestations vary greatly in intensity and duration and may be fleeting. They are readily overlooked in dark-skinned patients, in whom they should be searched for by light palpation and indirect lighting.

Cardiovascular and Respiratory Features. An irritating, nonproductive cough is frequent and is occasionally associated with moderate hemoptysis. Early in the second week, rales may be detected in the basilar lung areas. These changes are generally rickettsial rather than bacterial in origin and respond to the broad-spectrum antibiotics but not to penicillin or sulfonamide therapy. Pulmonary congestion occurs in extremely ill and elderly patients.

Accelerated pulse, hypotension, and general circulatory weakness occur in this disease, although less frequently than in patients with epidemic typhus or Rocky Mountain spotted fever (Chap. 195).

Neurologic Manifestations. Headache is the most common neurologic manifestation of murine typhus and may dominate the clinical picture. It is frontally localized and continues into the second week of illness. In the early stages the facial expression is strained, and the patient resents distraction. Stupor and prostration may occur in the second week, and in severe cases, there may be muttering delirium, extreme agitation, or coma. Coma in elderly patients after 2 weeks of illness presages death. Nuchal rigidity and general spasticity often suggest meningitis, although the spinal fluid is normal except for slight increases in pressure and lymphocytes (5 to 30 per cu mm). Transient partial deafness occurs occasionally in murine typhus patients, but rarely is there localized neuritis or hemiplegia. Neurologic sequelae are unusual. Children experience minimal neurologic changes.

Other Physical Manifestations. During the first 2 days of illness the patient may be nauseated and vomit, but vomiting later in the illness should arouse suspicion of an intercurrent complication. Abdominal pain, particularly in dehydrated patients, is bothersome; when associated with diarrhea it responds to intravenous alimentation. A sluggish, constipated bowel is occasionally observed. Hepatomegaly and jaundice are unusual. There is splenomegaly in approximately 25 percent of patients.

Photophobia, retroocular pain, suffusion of the eyes, and congestion of the conjunctivas are common manifestations but are less severe than in the other typhus and spotted fevers.

Renal function is usually unaltered except in elderly patients with prolonged hypotension. Under these circumstances, in seriously ill patients, azotemia may develop to the degree observed in epidemic typhus. The blood chloride level is low in severe murine typhus, as in the epidemic type; hypochloremia of 80 mEq per liter may be observed. Hypoalbuminemia is also encountered.

COURSE OF DISEASE AND COMPLICATIONS. After defervescence, murine typhus patients recover rapidly. Fatalities occur between the ninth and twelfth days in elderly or debilitated patients, usually as a result of circulatory and renal failure or intercurrent bacterial infection.

PROGNOSIS. The mortality in murine typhus was low even before the introduction of modern specific therapy. Only one death occurred in 114 cases studied by Maxcy and none in the 180 reported by Stuart and Pullen.

DIFFERENTIAL DIAGNOSIS. Because murine typhus and Rocky Mountain spotted fever occur in many of the same states, the problem of differential diagnosis often arises. Flea-borne murine typhus, which is predominantly an urban disease, is more likely to occur in late summer and autumn. In contrast, spotted fever is a rural and suburban disease in which exposure to ticks is important. Most cases occur in the spring and summer.

TREATMENT AND PREVENTION. The therapeutic procedures are comparable to those used in spotted fever. Both chloramphenicol and the tetracycline antibiotics have controlled the disease.

Prevention of murine typhus in man is attained by reducing the natural reservoir and vector by applying measures for eliminating rodents and employing DDT in rat-infested areas to control fleas.

199 EPIDEMIC (Louse-borne) TYPHUS FEVER AND BRILL–ZINSSER DISEASE (Recrudescent Typhus)

*Theodore E. Woodward and
Elizabeth B. Jackson*

EPIDEMIC (Louse-borne) TYPHUS FEVER

DEFINITION. The classical epidemic form of typhus is a severe, febrile disease caused by *Rickettsia prowazeki* and transmitted to man by the body louse. Intense headache, continuous pyrexia of about 2 weeks, a macular skin eruption appearing on about the fifth febrile day, malaise, and vascular and neurologic disturbances represent the principal clinical features. Confirmation of the diagnosis is made by demonstration of *Proteus* OX-19 agglutinins and of specific complement-fixing antibodies in convalescence. The broad-spectrum antibiotics are specific therapeutic agents.

ETIOLOGY AND EPIDEMIOLOGY. The causative microbe, *R. prowazeki*, is closely related to *R. mooseri*, which causes murine typhus; indeed, the two have a number of common antigens. *Rickettsia prowazeki* was the first of the rickettsias shown to have its own enzyme system, which permits it to respire independently of the host cell.

Man generally is infected when rickettsia-laden louse feces are rubbed into the broken skin; scratching the louse bite facilitates this process. *Pediculus humanus corporis*, which is peculiarly adapted to man, is the only important vector of epidemic typhus. It dies of its infection and fails to transmit rickettsias to its offspring. There is no known animal habitat of *R. prowazeki*; it is maintained by a cycle involving man-louse-man. New epidemics apparently originate from patients with Brill-Zinsser disease (recurrent epidemic typhus). Inhalation of dust containing dried louse feces may rarely cause infection.

Epidemic typhus, if uncontrolled, behaves as a cyclic disease in a susceptible population, extending over a 3-year period. During the first year there is a gradual seeding of cases throughout the group; during the second there is epidemic spread; and during the third the epidemic tapers off, because the majority of persons have become immune. Outbreaks of epidemic typhus last occurred in the United States in the nineteenth century, and its presence is now recognized only in the form of Brill-Zinsser disease.

CLINICAL MANIFESTATIONS. A classic clinical description of Old World typhus is provided in the 1922 monograph of Wolbach, Todd, and Palfrey. Epidemic typhus resembles murine typhus but is more severe. After an incubation period of about 7 days an abrupt onset of headache, chill, and rapidly mounting fever ushers in the illness. Cephalgia, malaise, and prostration continue unabated until the rash appears on the fifth febrile day. It is initially macular in the axillary folds but ultimately invades the trunk and extremities as a pink, irregular macular lesion which becomes fixed, petechial, and confluent in the later stages.

Neurologic features range from headache and general spasticity to extreme agitation, stupor, and coma. Circulatory disturbances consisting of tachycardia, hypotension, and cyanosis are more profound than those observed in murine typhus and are almost as severe as in Rocky Mountain spotted fever. Ultimately, in untreated cases azotemia often reaches high levels as a result of vascular and renal failure, and death occurs late in the second week of illness. Furthermore, thrombosis of major blood vessels and cutaneous gangrene develop in a manner similar to that seen in the virulent form of Rocky Mountain spotted fever.

The complications and sequelae of epidemic typhus are more severe than those in murine typhus, but not as severe as those in Rocky Mountain spotted fever. However, during certain outbreaks, epidemic typhus was fatal in 60 percent of those infected, and convalescence in survivors was prolonged. Broad-spectrum antibiotics have eradicated mortality in this dread disease, provided therapy is instituted before irreversible changes have been established in the tissues.

DIFFERENTIAL DIAGNOSIS. Differentiation of epidemic typhus from the various rickettsioses and other diseases with which it may be confused is described in Chap. 195. The disease in epidemic form never occurs in the absence of lousiness in the general population. Under the conditions in which typhus epidemics are likely to occur, other diseases which may cause confusion include malaria, relapsing fever, pneumonia, and tuberculosis. Classic typhus contracted by a previously vaccinated person is usually mild and may be clinically indistinguishable from murine typhus except by serologic methods.

TREATMENT AND PREVENTION. Both chloramphenicol and the tetracycline antibiotics have been found to be highly efficient therapeutic agents in epidemic typhus. Usually the patient becomes afebrile after 2 days of treatment. The therapeutic procedures are comparable to those used in spotted fever.

The most effective measures for controlling epidemic typhus are those which eliminate lousiness. DDT or lindane powder when dusted into clothing is suitable for this purpose. If resistant lice are found, malathion may prove effective.

A commercially available vaccine prepared from formalin-treated suspensions of infected yolk sac tissue is an effective immunizing agent.

BRILL-ZINSSER DISEASE

(Recrudescent Typhus)

DEFINITION. Brill-Zinsser disease is a recrudescent episode of epidemic typhus fever which occurs years after the initial attack. Nathan Brill in 1898 observed a sporadic disease which resembled typhus fever among non-lousy inhabitants of New York City. Zinsser, in 1934, suggested on the basis of epidemiologic and immunologic considerations that this was a recurrent form of typhus encountered in persons who had recovered from the epidemic disease while residing in countries where it was prevalent. Additional information has gradually accumulated in support of this hypothesis.

Murray and Snyder were successful in regularly isolating rickettsias indistinguishable from *R. prowazeki* from lice fed on patients during the active stages of illness.

CLINICAL MANIFESTATIONS. The clinical entity, not always mild, resembles epidemic typhus in the character of the rash, circulatory disturbances, and hepatic, renal, and nervous system changes. Recovery is the rule. The Weil-Felix reaction with the various *Proteus* antigens is usually negative, or positive in very low titer. The specific complement fixation reaction is valuable in establishing the diagnosis. In Brill-Zinsser disease the specific complement-fixing antibodies appear as early as the fourth day after the onset of illness; the peak response is attained by the eighth to tenth days. Specific antibody titers in the primary attack of epidemic typhus begin later, about the eighth to twelfth day, with maximum titers on about the sixteenth day after onset. Antibodies in Brill-Zinsser disease and the primary attack are associated with 7S and 19S globulins, respectively.

The therapeutic procedures are comparable to those used in spotted fever.

200   SCRUB TYPHUS

*Theodore E. Woodward and
Elizabeth B. Jackson*

DEFINITION. Scrub typhus is limited to eastern and southeastern Asia, India, northern Australia, and the adjacent islands. It is caused by *Rickettsia tsutsugamushi* and characterized by a primary lesion at the site of the bite of an infected mite, a fever of about 2 weeks' duration, a cutaneous rash which develops about the fifth day, and the appearance late in the second week of agglutinins against the OX-K strain of *Proteus* bacillus. The broad-spectrum antibiotics are specific therapeutic agents.

ETIOLOGY. The agent of scrub typhus resembles other rickettsias in its physical properties but differs from them in antigenic structure, vector, and reservoir. The disease is transmitted by larvae of several species of mites, especially *Trombicula akamushi* and *T. deliensis*. These tiny chiggers attach themselves to the skin and during the process of obtaining a meal of tissue juice may acquire infection from the host or transmit rickettsias to the vertebrate. The infection is maintained in nature by a cycle involving mites and small rodents and by transovarial transmission in mites; human infection represents an accident attributable to propinquity.

CLINICAL MANIFESTATIONS. About 10 to 12 days after infection, illness begins abruptly with chilliness, severe headache, fever, conjunctival injection, and moderate generalized lymphadenopathy which is most prominent in the nodes draining the area of the primary lesion. The initial lesion at the beginning of fever is evidenced by an erythematous indurated area 1 cm in diameter, surmounted by a multiloculated vesicle; within a few days the vesicle ulcerates and becomes covered with a black crust.

Fever increases progressively during the first week, generally reaching 104 to 105°F, but the pulse remains relatively slow, 70 to 100 per min. The red macular rash, which begins on the trunk about the fifth day and spreads to the extremities, sometimes becomes maculopapular but usually fades in a few days. The course of the disease and the complications resemble those of endemic and epidemic typhus; however, interstitial myocarditis is more prominent than in the other typhus fevers.

PROGNOSIS. Prior to the introduction of the broad-spectrum antibiotics the mortality varied from 1 to 60 percent, depending on the geographic area and the virulence of the local strains of *R. tsutsugamushi,* and convalescence was prolonged. With modern therapeutic methods, deaths are extremely rare and convalescence is short.

DIFFERENTIAL DIAGNOSIS. Scrub typhus is to be differentiated from the other members of the typhus and the spotted fever group of diseases as well as from measles, typhoid fever, and meningococcal infections. The geographic localization of scrub typhus, the primary lesion, and the occurrence of OX-K agglutinins are especially useful in establishing the diagnosis.

TREATMENT AND PREVENTION. Chloramphenicol and the tetracycline antibiotics are valuable specific therapeutic agents in scrub typhus. The therapeutic procedures are comparable to those used in spotted fever. In fact, scrub typhus is more amenable to drugs than are the other rickettsial infections, and patients with this disease regularly become afebrile and are decidedly improved within 24 to 36 hr after beginning treatment, irrespective of the stage of disease.

Prevention of disease in the individual is accomplished by the application of miticidal chemicals (dibutyl phthalate, benzyl benzoate, diethyltoluamide, and others) to clothing and the skin. There is no satisfactory vaccine.

201 Q FEVER

Theodore E. Woodward and Elizabeth B. Jackson

DEFINITION. Q fever is an acute infectious disease caused by *Coxiella burnetii* and characterized by a sudden onset of fever, malaise, headache, weakness, anorexia, and interstitial pneumonitis. Rickettsemia occurs during the febrile period, and specific complement-fixing antibodies are present during convalescence. In contrast to the other rickettsioses, the disease is not associated with a cutaneous exanthem or agglutinins for the *Proteus* bacteria (Weil-Felix reaction).

ETIOLOGY AND EPIDEMIOLOGY. *Coxiella burnetii* possesses the general properties of other rickettsias but is somewhat more resistant to inactivation in unfavorable environments and more pleomorphic than the others. Its infectivity after drying under natural conditions is of importance in the spread of infection to man. Its pleomorphism, which ranges from diplobacillary structures measuring 1.5 μ in length to tiny spheres about 0.2 μ in diameter, contributes to its filtrability through Berkefeld N candles. This filtrability led Cox (1939) to suggest the name *Rickettsia diaporica* for the first American isolate, but the name was subsequently abandoned when this agent was found to be identical with that causing Q fever in Australia. *Coxiella burnetii* has a wide host range in nature, but guinea pigs and embryonated eggs are the common laboratory hosts employed for its propagation.

Strains of *C. burnetii* differ in their ability to fix complement in the presence of serums from convalescent patients. This phenomenon is explained by "phase variation" of *C. burnetii*, and organisms may convert from one phase to another. Newly isolated strains from animals and ticks are characteristically in phase I. After passage in embryonated chicken eggs, phase I strains are converted to phase II strains. Any phase II strain of *C. burnetii* can be converted to phase I by passage in a susceptible animal. Knowledge of phase variation is pertinent to the interpretation of serologic reactions. Also phase I rickettsias are used for prophylactic vaccines.

Human cases of Q fever are contracted by inhalation of infected dusts, by handling infected materials, and possibly by drinking milk contaminated with *C. burnetii*. The disease in Australia is enzootic in animals, especially bandicoots, and is transmitted in nature by ticks. Rickettsia-laden tick feces may contaminate cattle hides, and inhalation of this material has caused infection in man. In the United States, a number of species of ticks are naturally infected, among them *Dermacentor andersoni* and *Amblyomma americanum,* and in North Africa transovarial transmission of the agent in indigenous ticks has been demonstrated. Sheep, goats, and cows have been found to be naturally infected in North America and in Europe, and *C. burnetii* has been recovered from the milk of such animals. Milk, as well as infected excretions from livestock, probably accounts for certain outbreaks of human disease following inhalation by cows of infected dust from barns and pens. The method of spread of Q fever was not clearly established among stockyard workers in Texas and Illinois, wool processors in Pennsylvania, employees in a rendering plant in New York, and laundry workers in Montana, who hauled dirty linen from a laboratory engaged in studies in Q fever; however, the air-borne route of dried contaminated material seems the most likely. A number of epidemics have occurred among laboratory workers engaged in studies on *C. burnetii*. The disease is not transmitted from man to man.

CLINICAL MANIFESTATIONS. After incubation of approximately 19 days (the range is 14 to 26), the disease begins with headache, chilly sensations, fever, malaise, myalgia, and anorexia. For several days, the temperature ranges from 101 to 104°F; the entire course rarely exceeds 2 weeks and usually ranges from 3 to 6 days. There may be wide fluctuations in the fever. Respiratory and gastrointestinal symptoms are not conspicuous in the early stages. Headache and fever predominate. A dry cough and chest pain occur after about 5 days, when rales are usually audible. Roentgenographic findings indistinguishable from those of primary atypical pneumonia are present usually by the third to fourth day of disease, first as patchy areas of consolidation involving a portion of one lobe, giving a homogeneous ground-glass appearance. These manifestations persist beyond the febrile period and may appear in patients who are unaware of pulmonary involvement. Complications are rare, and coincident with defervescence the appetite begins to return. Convalescence progresses slowly for several weeks, during which time the principal disability is weakness. It is not uncommon for patients to lose 15 to 20 lb during the active stages of disease. Several investigators have emphasized that the disease may be protracted in approximately 20 percent of cases, with fever persisting for longer than 4 weeks, particularly in elderly patients. Occasionally relapse occurs, especially in patients treated with antibiotics during the first several days of disease.

Hepatitis, with the development of clinically detectable icterus, occurs in approximately one-third of patients with the protracted form. This form of Q fever is characterized by fever, malaise, absence of headache or respiratory signs, and hepatomegaly with right upper quadrant pain. Liver biopsy specimens show diffuse granulomatous changes with multinucleated giant cells (see Fig. 201-1) and scattered infiltrations of polymorphonuclear leukocytes, lymphocytes, and macrophages. *Coxiella burnetii* may be demonstrated in such specimens with the fluorescent antibody technique. Therefore, Q fever must be included in the differential diagnosis of liver granulomatas such as tuberculosis, sarcoidosis, histoplasmosis, brucellosis, tularemia, syphilis, and others.

Endocarditis also has been reported, and *C. burnetii* has been identified by smear and isolation in vegetations on the heart valves obtained at operation or autopsy. The aortic valve is most commonly involved. It is important, therefore, to suspect the possibility of Q fever in cases of apparent subacute bacterial endocarditis with persistently negative blood cultures. Operative intervention with replacement of damaged valves is necessary for recovery because the available antibiotics are not rickettsicidal. A high complement-fixing antibody titer is present in both endocarditis and granulomatous hepatitis.

PROGNOSIS. Few fatalities have been recorded and, except for the patient with protracted illness and hepatic involvement or endocarditis, the course of disease is generally uncomplicated and benign.

TREATMENT AND CONTROL. The tetracycline antibiotics and chloramphenicol are effective in the treatment of patients with Q fever. Most patients, when treated early in the course of disease, respond promptly and recover without relapses. The therapeutic procedures are comparable to those used in spotted fever.

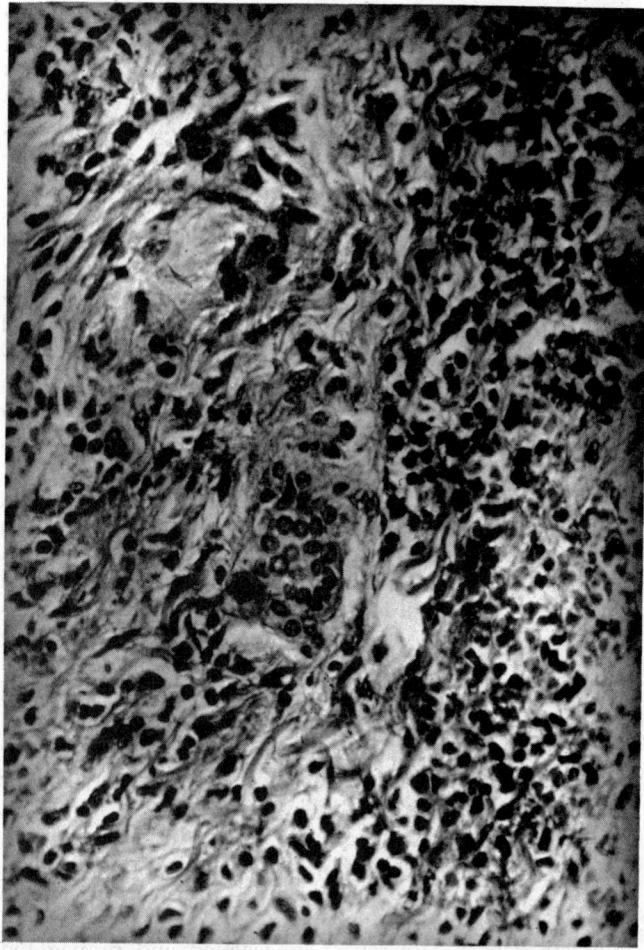

Fig. 201-1. Q fever hepatitis showing granulomatous changes in an adult male with fever, myalgia, and right upper quadrant pain. Note multinucleated giant cell. *Coxiella burnetii* was demonstrated by fluorescent antibody test, and complement fixation reaction was positive.

Chloramphenicol has been uniformly effective in treatment of patients with granulomatous hepatitis.

Control of Q fever depends primarily on immunization of susceptible persons with specific vaccines. Vaccines made from phase I rickettsias are potent and afford considerable protection to slaughterhouse and dairy workers, herders, rendering-plant workers, woolsorters, tanners, laboratory workers, and others at risk. Measures should be taken to avoid exposure to infected aerosols; milk from infected domestic livestock must be pasteurized or boiled.

202 TRENCH FEVER

Theodore E. Woodward and Elizabeth B. Jackson

DEFINITION. Trench fever is a febrile disease transmitted from man to man by the body louse, *Pediculus* *humanus corporis.* It is characterized by a sudden onset with headache and severe pain in the muscles, bones, and joints. In most cases the fever and other symptoms assume a relapsing character. Fatalities are rare. The disease is also known as Shin bone fever, Wolhynian fever, His-Werner disease, and Quintan fever.

HISTORY. Trench fever, first described as a distinct clinical entity in 1915, was widespread on the Eastern and Western fronts during World War I, constituting one of the major medical problems. Intensive investigation by British and American commissions as well as by German workers provided much basic information. In the years between the two world wars the disease ceased to be recognized, but it reappeared in epidemic form during World War II among German troops on the Eastern front.

ETIOLOGY AND EPIDEMIOLOGY. *Rickettsia quintana,* the etiologic agent, grows extracellularly in the louse gut, in contrast to other pathogenic rickettsias which can only multiply within cells. Although a subclinical infection can be produced in several species of monkeys by inoculation of *R. quintana,* until 1961 this agent had not been cultivated in the laboratory. Hence, the classic method of identification of trench fever has been by xenodiagnosis. In this test, "clean" laboratory-bred lice which ingest blood from a trench fever patient develop a characteristic histologic picture of extracellular rickettsias in the lumen of their gut.

In 1961 Vinson and Fuller reported the cultivation of a European strain of *R. quintana* on blood agar inoculated with blood from a volunteer patient with trench fever. Later, Vinson induced typical trench fever in volunteers with a Mexican strain isolated and propagated on blood agar. *Rickettsia quintana* grown in vivo in the louse gut and in vitro on blood agar are identical morphologically and tinctorially.

Man is the only known reservoir of infection. The louse does not transmit the organism transovarially but acquires its infection by ingesting the blood of a person with rickettsemia. The organisms multiply extracellularly in the louse gut, without injury to this host, and are excreted in large numbers with the feces. Man becomes infected by the inoculation of the contaminated feces into his abraded skin or conjunctivas. *Rickettsia quintana* may be recovered periodically from human blood for several years after convalescence from an acute attack. Trench fever is known to exist in Mexico, Tunisia, Eritrea, Poland, the U.S.S.R., and possibly China.

PATHOLOGY. Since there have been no recorded fatalities, histologic examination has been confined to excised macules of the skin, which have shown nonspecific perivascular infiltrates without the involvement of the vessel walls that is seen in typhus fever.

CLINICAL MANIFESTATIONS. A variety of clinical manifestations is displayed in trench fever, ranging from a mild afebrile disease to a debilitating illness with a protracted clinical course involving numerous relapses. Following an incubation period of 10 to 30 days the onset may be insidious or dramatically abrupt. The acute disease is characterized by malaise, headache, fever, and bone and body pain, especially severe in the shins. In some cases only one fever peak occurs; in others the fever continues for from 5 to 7 days; and in others there is an initial febrile episode lasting 1 to 3 days followed by relapses which characteristically occur at 4- to 5-day intervals. In some cases the fever and symptoms are continuous for 2 or 3 weeks. Enlargement of the spleen and a red macular rash occur in 70 to 80 percent of the cases. Pain and soreness in the muscles usually recur with each febrile relapse.

The disease is marked by a persistent rickettsemia, which is present during the initial attack and which continues during the relapses, throughout the asymptomatic periods between relapses, and for months or even years after cessation of physical symptoms. A relapse has been reported 10 years after the original attack.

PROGNOSIS. The disease has no known mortality, but its duration is quite variable. About 85 percent of patients are able to return to work within 2 months of onset, but about 5 percent of all cases become chronic. Recovery is even more delayed in the aged and debilitated.

DIFFERENTIAL DIAGNOSIS. During epidemics, typical cases are easily diagnosed on the basis of symptoms. The disease may be differentiated from influenza, typhoid, typhus, dengue, and relapsing fever by the specific laboratory tests available for the diagnosis of each of these diseases.

TREATMENT AND PREVENTION. *Rickettsia quintana* is highly sensitive in vitro to the broad-spectrum antibiotics, but no reliable information has been obtained about the value of these drugs in treating trench fever. The treatment is symptomatic. Aspirin is used to control pain and discomfort, but codeine may be necessary. The patient should remain in bed for a week or more after complete cessation of subjective and objective evidence of infection. He should be kept under observation for several months and returned to bed at the first sign of relapse.

The methods employed to control epidemic typhus should be equally efficacious in controlling trench fever. These are based on the elimination of lousiness and the improvement of living conditions with provision for frequent bathing and washing of clothing. DDT or lindane powder should be applied by a hand or power duster at appropriate intervals to clothes and persons of populations living under conditions favoring lousiness. If resistant lice are found, malathion or other effective lousicides may be substituted as a dusting powder.

REFERENCES

Allen, A. C., and S. Spitz: A Comparative Study of the Pathology of Scrub Typhus (Tsutsugamushi Disease) and Other Rickettsial Diseases, Am. J. Pathol., 21:603, 1945.

Andrew, R., J. M. Bonin, and S. Williams: Tick Typhus in North Queensland, Med. J. Australia, 2:253, 1946.

Audy, J. R., and J. L. Harrison: A Review of Investigations

on Mite Typhus in Burma and Malaya, 1945–1950, Trans. Roy. Soc. Trop. Med. Hyg., 44:371, 1951.

Blake, F. G., K. F. Maxcy, J. F. Sadusk, Jr., G. M. Kohls, and E. J. Bell: Studies on Tsutsugamushi Disease (Scrub Typhus, Mite-borne Typhus) in New Guinea and Adjacent Islands: Epidemiology, Clinical Observations and Etiology in the Dobadura Area, Am. J. Hyg., 41:243, 1945.

Derrick, E. H.: The Epidemiology of Q Fever: A Review, Med. J. Australia, 1:245, 1953.

Ferguson, I. C., J. E. Craik, and N. R. Grist: Clinical, Virological and Pathological Findings in a Fatal Case of Q Fever Endocarditis, Brit. J. Clin. Pathol., 15:235, 1962.

Freyche, M. J., and Z. Deutschman: Human Rickettsioses in Africa, Epidemiol. Vital Statistics Rept. (WHO), 3:160, 1950.

Gear, J.: The Rickettsial Diseases of Southern Africa: A Review of Recent Studies, South African J. Clin. Sci., 5:158, 1954.

Greenberg, M.: Rickettsialpox in New York City, Am. J. Med., 4:866, 1948.

Harrell, G. T.: Rocky Mountain Spotted Fever, Medicine, 28:333, 1949.

——: Rickettsial Involvement of the Nervous System, Med. Clin. N. Am., 37:395, 1953.

Harris, B. P.: Aureomycin in Tick Typhus, East African Med. J., 29:403, 1952.

Huebner, R. J., W. L. Jellison, and C. Pomerantz: Rickettsialpox, a Newly Recognized Rickettsial Disease: IV. Isolation of a Rickettsiá Apparently Identical with the Causative Agent of Rickettsialpox from *Allodermanyssus Sanguineus*, a Rodent Mite, Public Health Rept. U.S., 61:1677, 1946.

Lennette, E. H.: Epidemiology of Q Fever, Arch. Inst. Pasteur (Tunis), 36:521, 1959.

Ley, H. L., Jr., and J. E. Smadel: Antibiotic Therapy of Rickettsial Diseases, Antibiot. Chemotherapy, 4:792, 1954.

Lillie, R. D., T. L. Perrin, and C. Armstrong: An Institutional Outbreak of Pneumonitis: III. Histopathology in Man and Rhesus Monkeys in the Pneumonitis Due to the Virus of "Q" Fever, Public Health Rept. U.S., 56:149, 1941.

Marmion, B. P., and M. G. P. Stoker: The Epidemiology of Q Fever in Great Britain: An Analysis of the Findings and Some Conclusions, Brit. Med. J., 2:809, 1958.

Maxcy, K. F.: Typhus Fever in the United States, Public Health Rept. U.S., 44:1735, 1929.

Mohr, C. O., and W. W. Smith: Eradication of Murine Typhus Fever in a Rural Area, Bull. World Health Organ., 16:255, 1957.

Moulton, F. R. (Ed.): "The Rickettsial Diseases of Man," Washington, American Association for the Advancement of Science, 1948.

Murray, E. S., G. Baehr, G. Shwartzman, R. A. Mandelbaum, N. Rosenthal, J. C. Doane, L. B. Weiss, S. Cohen, and J. C. Snyder: Brill's Disease: I. Clinical and Laboratory Diagnosis, J.A.M.A., 142:1059, 1950.

—— and J. C. Snyder: Brill's Disease: II. Etiology, Am. J. Hyg., 53:22, 1951.

Ormsbee, R. A., E. J. Bell, D. B. Lackman, and G. Tallent: The Influence of Phase on the Protective Potency of Q Fever Vaccine, J. Immunol., 92:404, 1964.

Parker, R. R.: Rocky Mountain Spotted Fever, J.A.M.A., 110:1185, 1938.

Plotz, H., B. L. Bennett, K. Wertman, M. J. Snyder, and R. Gauld: Serological Pattern in Typhus Fever: I. Epidemic, Am. J. Hyg., 47:150, 1948.

Pratt, H. D.: The Changing Picture of Murine Typhus in the United States, Ann. N.Y. Acad. Sci., 70:516, 1958.

Price, E. G.: "Fighting Spotted Fever in the Rockies," Helena, Mont., Naegele Printing Co., 1948.

Ricketts, H. T.: "Contributions to Medical Science by Howard Taylor Ricketts 1870–1910," Chicago, University of Chicago Press, 1911.

Rose, H. M.: The Clinical Manifestations and Laboratory Diagnosis of Rickettsialpox, Ann. Intern. Med., 31:871, 1949.

Smadel, J. E.: Influence of Antibiotics on Immunologic Responses in Scrub Typhus, Am. J. Med., 17:246, 1954.

——: Status of the Rickettsioses in the United States, Ann. Intern. Med., 51:421, 1959.

—— (Ed.): "Symposium on Q Fever," Med. Sci. Publ. 6, Walter Reed Army Institute of Research, Washington, U.S. Government Printing Office, 1959.

—— and E. B. Jackson: Rickettsial Infections, pp. 743–772 in "Diagnostic Procedures for Viral and Rickettsial Diseases," 3d ed., New York, American Public Health Association, 1964.

Snyder, J. C.: Typhus Fever Rickettsiae, pp. 1059–1094 in "Viral and Rickettsial Infections of Man," 4th ed., F. L. Horsfall, Jr., and I. Tamm (Eds.), Philadelphia, J. B. Lippincott Company, 1965.

Stoker, M. G. P., and P. Fiset: Phase Variation of the Nine Mile and Other Strains of *Rickettsia Burnetii*, Can. J. Microbiol., 2:310, 1956.

—— and B. P. Marmion: The Spread of Q Fever from Animals to Man: The Natural History of a Rickettsial Infection, Bull. World Health Organ., 13:781, 1955.

Strong, R. P.: Trench Fever, pp. 984–996B in "Stitt's Diagnosis, Prevention and Treatment of Tropical Diseases," 7th ed., New York, McGraw-Hill Book Company, 1944.

Stuart, B. M., and R. L. Pullen: Endemic (Murine) Typhus Fever: Clinical Observations of One Hundred and Eighty Cases, Ann. Intern. Med., 23:520, 1945.

Vinson, J. W.: Etiology of Trench Fever in Mexico, pp. 109–114 in "Industry and Tropical Health: V," Boston, Harvard School of Public Health, 1964.

Section 13

Introduction to Viral Diseases

203 PROPERTIES AND CLASSIFICATION OF VIRUSES

Robert R. Wagner

VIRUS STRUCTURE AND FUNCTION. The viruses occupy a special taxonomic position as the simplest and most distinctive forms in the biologic universe. Separate classes of viruses infect bacteria (the bacteriophages), plants, or animals. Unlike true organisms, such as bacteria or fungi, viruses are obligate intracellular parasites which derive energy exclusively from metabolism of the cells that they infect. Two stages occur in the life cycle of all viruses: the replicative (intracellular) and the infectious (extracellular). Extracellular virus particles, *virions,* are metabolically inert, consisting of an internal core of nucleic acid surrounded by a protein coat or *capsid.* The capsid is made up of symmetrically arranged subunits known as *capsomeres.* The size, shape, number, and spacing of capsomeres can be determined by electron microscopy and x-ray diffraction. Two major groups have been recognized on the basis of capsid morphology: (1) The *helical viruses* appear as hollow rods in which the capsomeres are radially distributed around a single coil, or helix, of nucleic acid; (2) the *polygonal viruses* assume a perfect geometric shape, usually an icosahedron (a symmetric 20-sided structure), in which the capsomeres are arranged in a shell around a molecule of nucleic acid. The capsids of larger and more complex animal viruses, both helical and polygonal, may be surrounded by a lipid-containing envelope derived from the host cell. The known functions of capsids are to protect the nucleic acid from nucleases and to initiate infection by providing specific receptors for virion attachment to corresponding sites on the surface of cells. In contrast to animal and plant viruses, many bacteriophages are equipped with a tail which injects viral nucleic acid through the rigid bacterial cell wall.

The true infectious moiety of any virus is a giant molecule of deoxyribonucleic acid (DNA) or ribonucleic acid (RNA), never both. Nucleic acid alone, stripped of its protein capsid, can infect cells, although less efficiently than intact virions. Viruses vary considerably in their complexity and content of nucleic acid. The RNA of the tiny f_2 bacteriophage contains approximately 1,600 nucleotides and provides genetic information for synthesis of only three or four proteins. In contrast, the DNA of the large vaccinia virus is composed of almost 500,000 nucleotides, considerably greater than the nucleotide content of organisms of the genus *Mycoplasma.*

Viral nucleic acid has three major functions: (1) It is a template on which nucleic acid is replicated. (2) It contains the genetic information for manufacture of enzymes required for the synthesis of viral nucleic acid and protein. Protein synthesis by double-stranded DNA viruses is mediated by transcription of messenger RNA that is complementary in base sequences to viral DNA. Protein synthesis by viral RNA is preceded by formation of a complementary RNA species (minus strand) to form a double-stranded RNA "replicative form" and a "replicative intermediate" composed of double-stranded and single-stranded regions. (3) Viral nucleic acid can mutate and can also mate with nucleic acid of a homologous virus by recombination, giving rise to progeny that differ from the parents. In addition, the DNA of certain bacteriophages can become integrated with the DNA of bacterial cells, a process known as lysogeny, during the course of which new information may be imparted to the cell by genetic transduction. Malignant transformation of animal cells by DNA tumor viruses may involve a similar process.

INFECTION AT THE CELLULAR LEVEL. Viral infection is initiated after random collision between one or more virions and a susceptible cell. The concept of virus *tropism,* implying attraction of virus to a particular cell, is no longer tenable and should be discarded. The initial stage of infection is *adsorption* (physical attachment) of virion capsid to cell membrane at specific receptor sites. The nature of the chemical bonds between the capsid and cell membrane is unknown, but the receptor for myxoviruses has been identified as neuraminic acid. The absence of cellular receptors precludes infection, which explains, for example, the complete resistance of most nonprimate cells to intact polio virions. Following adsorption, *penetration* of animal viruses takes place by dissolution of the outer envelope of the virus fused at the cell surface or by phagocytosis of the entire virion. Large animal viruses can be seen by electron microscopy to be transported across the cytoplasmic membrane engulfed in a cytoplasmic vacuole. At this stage, the outer envelope is stripped off (presumably by lysosomal enzymes), freeing the viral nucleocapsid. During penetration by poxviruses, a new "uncoating enzyme" is synthesized by the viral genome, which digests the capsid and frees the viral DNA.

After penetration and decapsidation, there is always an *eclipse* period, of variable duration for each virus-cell system, during which time no infectious virus can be detected in the cell. *Biosynthesis* of viral proteins and nucleic acid begins during this stage of infection and continues in an orderly sequence. The first products synthesized under genetic control of viral DNA or RNA are nucleotide kinases, synthetases, polymerases, and other enzymes required for synthesis of viral nucleic acid. Synthesis of viral nucleic acid then begins, accompanied by, or followed by, onset of synthesis of viral structural protein. Ribosomes, amino acids, nucleotides, transfer RNA, activating enzymes, and energy all are supplied by the infected cell. Viral nucleic acid condenses with structural protein in a poorly understood and inefficient process called *maturation*. Among every population of animal viruses are many "incomplete" or noninfectious forms which result from inefficient incorporation of viral nucleic acid within the capsid. Bacteriophage can also incorporate cellular genes, which can then be transferred to other bacterial cells, a process known as *transduction*. The final step in the infectious process is *release* of virions by leakage from the living cell or by lysis of the cell. The released virus can then infect other cells, and the cycle is repeated.

Different viruses multiply and mature in different parts of the cell. Herpes simplex virus and adenoviruses, for example, form within the nucleus as a crystalline array. These crystals are the intranuclear inclusion bodies seen in stained infected cells. Intranuclear viruses are released from cells slowly and poorly. In contrast, influenza and other myxoviruses mature at the periphery of the cell just under the cytoplasmic membrane. Mature myxovirus particles protrude from the cell surface as fingerlike projections enveloped by cytoplasmic membrane, which then pinch off to become free virions almost as soon as they are formed.

Certain other cytopathologic changes appear to be common to many viral infections. Dissolution of nucleoli and clumping and margination of nuclear chromatin are frequently seen. RNA granules often appear in the cytoplasm and are extruded into the surrounding medium. Eventually, the cytoplasm may disappear, leaving a pyknotic nucleus. However, not all viral infections result in cell death. There is considerable variation in the degree to which viruses compromise the normal metabolism of infected cells. The RNA of poliovirus, for example, can code for proteins that cut off cellular RNA and protein synthesis. The tumor viruses, on the other hand, can induce malignant transformation that results in enhanced cellular proliferation and DNA synthesis. These "transformed" cells also acquire new virus-specific nuclear and cytoplasmic membrane antigens and, in some cases, can be transplanted to animals where the cells grow as malignant tumors. Measles and herpes simplex viruses alter cytoplasmic membranes,

causing them to fuse with adjacent uninfected cells, with formation of giant cells (syncytia, polykaryocytes) that are characteristic of infection with these viruses.

CHEMOTHERAPY. An important characteristic of all true viruses is their complete insusceptibility to antibiotics commonly used for treatment of bacterial infections. Contrary to popular belief, however, many antibiotics and other chemical compounds are known to inhibit viral multiplication. The main difficulty is that most of these agents also compromise the integrity of the cell to varying degrees. Nevertheless, specific inhibitors of nucleic acid or protein biosynthesis have been valuable tools in studying viral multiplication and hold out promise for eventual chemotherapy of human viral infections. Several compounds inhibit multiplication of DNA viruses without affecting most RNA viruses:

1. Mitomycin C is an antibiotic that causes depolymerization of viral and cellular DNA in a manner reminiscent of ionizing radiation.

2. Actinomycin D specifically binds to viral or cellular DNA and blocks transcription of messenger RNA. Most RNA viruses synthesize RNA by a pathway independent of DNA and, therefore, are not influenced by actinomycin D. Exceptions to this rule are the reoviruses, which contain double-stranded RNA, and influenza virus and Rous sarcoma virus, which appear to require the transcriptive function of cellular DNA for replication.

3. Halogenated pyrimidines, the best known of which is 5-iodouracildeoxyriboside (IUdR), act primarily as competitive antagonists of thymidine incorporation into DNA. IUdR may be partially effective in treatment of herpes simplex keratitis, although the results of clinical trails are equivocal and resistant mutants are common.

Competitive antagonists of viral (and cellular) protein synthesis also inhibit viral multiplication. Puromycin, a structural analogue of aminoacyl–soluble RNA, reversibly blocks incorporation of amino acids into the growing peptide chain on mammalian or bacterial ribosomes. The antiviral action of puromycin is similar, in some respects, to that of chloramphenicol on bacterial growth. Substituted amino acids, such as *p*-fluorophenylalanine, are incorporated into peptide chains, resulting in formation of "fraudulent" proteins. Isatin β-thiosemicarbazone inhibits transcription of late messenger RNA of poxviruses and is partially effective in chemoprophylaxis of smallpox.

Little success has been achieved in the search for compounds that selectively inhibit viruses without altering nucleic acid or protein metabolism of cells. Two that have been studied in the laboratory are guanidine hydrochloride and α-hydroxybenzylbenzimidazole, both of which inhibit multiplication of polioviruses, a few other enteroviruses, and some rhinoviruses. These compounds are thought to block synthesis of poliovirus RNA by interfering with the specific viral RNA polymerase. Unfortunately, resistant mutants soon outgrow the susceptible viruses.

Generic name and properties†	Prototype viruses (common name)	Major antigenic types	Best available methods of virus isolation	Principle modes of transmission	Usual clinical manifestations
Mycoplasma (PPLO)* DNA + RNA 125 × 250 mμ Protoplast-like	*M. pneumoniae* (Eaton agent) *M. hominis* *M. salivarium*	1 2 1	Enriched cell-free medium, chick embryos	Respiratory Genitourinary Oral	Pneumonia, URI, myringitis Urethritis Saprophyte
Psittacosis (*Chlamydozoaceae*) DNA + RNA 250 × 400 mμ Complex, cell wall	Psittacosis Lymphogranuloma Trachoma Inclusion conjunctivitis	1 1	Yolk sac of chick embryo, mouse Yolk sac of chick embryo	Respiratory Venereal Eye Eye, venereal	Pneumonia Bubo, proctitis Keratitis Conjunctivitis
Poxvirus DNA 200–300 mμ Complex structure Enveloped	Smallpox Vaccinia-cowpox Molluscum contagiosum Myxoma (rabbits) Orf-Milker's nodules	1 ? 1 2	Chick embryo, mouse, rabbit, cell cultures Human volunteers Rabbit (European) Cell cultures	Respiratory Skin Skin Skin Skin	Pustular exanthem Local papule, pustule Papules Hemorrhages, tumors Papules, pustules
Herpesvirus DNA 100–200 mμ Polygonal Enveloped	Herpes simplex Monkey B Chickenpox-herpes zoster Cytomegalovirus Epstein-Barr (EB) virus	1 1 1 1 ?	Cell cultures Monkey cell cultures Human cell cultures Human cell cultures Leukocyte cultures	Mucous membranes Skin (monkey bite) Respiratory latent Transplacental, respiratory(?) Not known	"Cold sores," stomatitis Encephalitis Vesicles, pneumonia Radiculitis, vesicles Hepatitis, pneumonia encephalitis Burkitt lymphoma Infectious mononucleosis
Myxovirus and *Paramyxovirus* RNA 100–200 mμ Helical Enveloped	Influenza A, B, C Parainfluenza Mumps Measles German measles (rubella) Respiratory syncytial (RS virus)	3 4 1 1 1 1	Chick embryo Human cell cultures Chick embryo, cultures Human cell cultures Monkey cell culture interference Human cell cultures	Respiratory Respiratory Respiratory Respiratory Respiratory Respiratory	Influenza, pneumonia URI, croup, pneumonia Parotitis, orchitis, meningitis Macular rash, pneumonia Macular rash, congenital malformations Bronchiolitis, croup, pneumonia
Reovirus RNA, 75 mμ, polygonal	Reoviruses	3	Various cell cultures	Respiratory, enteric	URI, fever, hepatitis, encephalitis
Rhabdovirus‡ RNA 65 × 180 mμ Helical Enveloped	Vesicular stomatitis Rabies	2 1	Cell cultures Mouse	Skin and mucosa Animal bites	Vesicles Encephalitis
Adenovirus DNA, 70 mμ cubic	Adenoviruses	44+	Human cell cultures	Respiratory, eye, enteric(?)	Pharyngitis, pneumonia, conjunctivitis
Arborvirus (Arbor, arthropod-borne viruses) RNA 50–100 mμ Polygonal Enveloped(?)	Equine encephalitis Semliki Forest Japanese B Russian tick-borne Yellow fever Dengue Morituba, Oriboca Rift Valley Colorado tick fever Sandfly fever	1 Group A 1 or more Group B Group C Many ungrouped	Cerebral injection of newborn mice, some in tissue culture	Mosquito bite Mosquito bite Tick bite, oral Mosquito bite Mosquito bite Mosquito bite Mosquito bite Tick bite Sandfly bite	Encephalitis, dengue-like fever, mild fever, hemorrhagic fever, hepatitis or asymptomatic
Papovavirus DNA 25–45 mμ Polygonal	"Warts" (human) Papilloma (rabbit) Polyoma (mouse) Simian virus 40	1 1 1 1	Human volunteers Rabbit skin Mice, hamsters Monkey cell culture	Skin Skin Unknown, enteric(?) Unknown	Warts (verrucae) Papilloma of skin Sarcomas Sarcomas (hamsters)
Picornavirus RNA, 15–30 mμ, polygonal *Enterovirus* *Rhinovirus* Others	 Poliovirus Coxsackie A Coxsackie B ECHO Common cold Encephalomyocarditis Foot-and-mouth disease	 3 24+ 6 30+ Many 1 7	 Primate cell culture Infant mouse Cell culture, mice Human cell culture Primate cell cultures Mouse, cell cultures Cell cultures	 Enteric Enteric Enteric Enteric, respiratory Respiratory Unknown Skin and mucosa	 Paralysis, encephalitis Herpangina, fever Pleurodynia, meningitis Meningitis, macular rash Afebrile URI Fever, encephalitis Vesicles, fever
Unclassified viruses	Lymphocytic chorio-meningitis Human hepatitis	1 2(?)	Adult mouse Human volunteers	Respiratory Enteric, injection	Meningitis Hepatitis

* *Mycoplasma* and psittacosis groups are bacteria rather than viruses but cause viruslike illnesses.

† Classification of true viruses is based on content of either DNA or RNA, diameter in millimicrons, polygonal or helical symmetry of capsomeres, presence or absence of outer envelope. These properties have not been thoroughly investigated for those viruses listed in "unclassified" group.

‡ Tentative terminology.

CLASSIFICATION. The primary bases for virus classification are chemical composition, morphology, size, physical properties and antigenicity. Biologic properties of viruses are neither distinctive nor stable enough to serve as criteria. All viruses can be divided into two major categories, depending on whether their genetic information is in the form of DNA or RNA. Each of these two categories can be further subdivided into those with polygonal or helical arrangement of protein capsomeres. The presence or absence of an outer envelope derived from the host cells is also useful but not always definitive. The number of capsomeres has also been proposed as a basis for classification. The size of viruses must also be considered, but this criterion is also of limited value because of wide variation among certain groups of viruses. The typing of viruses within major groups or subgroups is largely based on antigenicity.

The viruses infectious for man are classified in Table 203-1 under the generic names that are widely accepted. Eight major groups are listed, along with their distinguishing characteristics, as well as several viruses not yet classified because of insufficient information. Also included under the heading *pseudoviruses,* because of prevailing clinical custom, are the true microorganisms of the *Mycoplasma* group and the agents that cause psittacosis, lymphogranuloma venereum, and trachoma, which belong more properly with the rickettsias and bacteria.

Viruses continually undergo mutations to forms which lose the capacity to infect certain types of cells or to cause disease but which in other respects remain indistinguishable from the original strains. However, it is feasible and convenient to categorize viruses that infect man by their portal of entry and initial site of multiplication. Such a system has the advantage of characterizing viruses by their usual mode of transmission and epidemiology. Table 203-1 summarizes the salient epidemiologic, cultural, and clinical features of viruses of real or potential medical significance. These characteristics conform reasonably well to the group classifications based on physicochemical properties.

REFERENCES

Andrewes, C. H., and H. G. Peirera: "Viruses of Vertebrates," 2d ed., Baltimore, The Williams & Wilkins Company, 1967.

Davis, B. D., R. Dulbecco, H. N. Eisen, H. S. Ginsberg, and W. B. Wood, Jr.: "Microbiology," New York, Harper and Row Publishers, Incorporated, 1967.

Fenner, F.: "The Biology of Animal Viruses," vol. I., "Molecular and Cellular Biology," New York, Academic Press, Inc., 1968.

Morgan, C., and H. M. Rose: Structure and Development of Viruses as Observed in the Electron Microscope. VIII. Entry of Influenza Virus, J. Virol., 2:925, 1968.

Stent, G. S.: "Molecular Biology of Bacterial Viruses," San Francisco, W. H. Freeman and Company, 1963.

Tamm, I., and H. J. Eggers: Specific Inhibition of Replication of Animal Viruses, Science, 142:24, 1963.

Wagner, R. R.: Chemical and Biologic Approaches to the Therapy of Viral Diseases, Am. Rev. Resp. Dis., 88:404, 1963.

204 PATHOGENESIS OF VIRAL DISEASES

Robert R. Wagner

The events that occur during the course of viral infection in a single cell (Chap. 203) differ in no important respect from the sequence that leads to infection of multicellular organisms, including man. To initiate infection, a virus must make contact with a susceptible cell in the respiratory tract, intestine, skin, or eye. Newly formed virus is released and transmitted to adjacent cells at the primary focus. Certain viruses remain localized to the original site of infection and draining lymph nodes. Others invade the blood directly from infected capillary endothelium or by way of lymphatic vessels, and are disseminated to distant organs. Viremia is detectable when the rate of invasion exceeds the rate of clearance by reticuloendothelial cells. Most viruses are carried in plasma, but certain myxoviruses and arborviruses are attached to erythrocytes; the poxviruses and measles virus are transported in or on circulating monocytes, lymphocytes, and platelets. Plasma-borne viruses are rapidly cleared; viruses associated with formed elements persist in the circulation for a longer time.

Whether infection remains localized or becomes generalized and whether localized or systemic infection results in disease are largely determined by the genetic constitution of the virus and of the host. Most viral infections of man do not cause recognizable disease. *Virulence* is the disease-producing capacity of a particular virus in a particular host. It usually reflects the degree of tissue damage, which, in turn, is a function of the degree to which the virus multiplies. A strain of poliovirus, for example, is said to be virulent for man if infection of the intestine leads sequentially to viremia, dissemination to the central nervous system, multiplication of virus in anterior horn cells, cell death, and paralysis in a high proportion of cases. Immunologic responsiveness, other host factors, the infecting dose, and environmental conditions also determine the outcome of infection.

TISSUE REACTIONS TO VIRAL INFECTIONS. These vary from rapid cell destruction to indetectable changes. Cellular necrosis may be the result of virus-induced rupture of lysomes and intracellular discharge of autolytic enzymes. Inflammation is usually characterized by the presence of macrophages, but polymorphonuclear leukocytes may predominate if infection causes extensive tissue necrosis or hemorrhage. Although the extent of damage, and hence the severity of the disease, varies considerably, the types of responses to different viruses are often quite similar. For example, many viruses can infect the meninges and produce the syndrome of aseptic meningitis (Chap. 215). Conversely, a virus such as Coxsackie B can cause a variety of illnesses, including fatal myocarditis, pleurodynia, meningitis, and encephalitis.

Certain viruses stimulate cellular proliferation. Vaccinia virus sometimes induces hyperplasia, and influenza virus regularly causes squamous metaplasia of bronchial epithelium. Hundreds of viruses, among them certain strains of human adenoviruses, have now been found to be capable of causing neoplasms in animals. The Stewart-Eddy polyoma virus has been particularly well studied and has been shown to be responsible for widespread epizootics of malignant tumors in mice. Polyoma virus also infects other rodents, including newborn hamsters. Neoplastic viruses with widely varying biologic properties have been isolated from vertebrate species ranging from fish to primates. Thus far, only warts have been proved to be virus-induced tumors of man. However, a herpesvirus-like agent, the Epstein-Barr (EB) virus, present in cultured leukocytes may be the cause of Burkitt lymphoma and infectious mononucleosis. It will not be surprising if more human neoplasms are found to be caused by viruses.

Certain chronic neurologic diseases in domestic animals have been attributed to an ill-defined group of agents known as "slow viruses" (Chap. 219). A filtrable, transmissible agent with unusual physical properties has been isolated from sheep dying with scrapie, a demyelinating encephalopathy. Similar pathologic lesions are seen in sheep infected with a myxovirus-like agent known as the Visna virus. Both of these diseases bear certain resemblances to multiple sclerosis. These observations coupled with indirect evidence that measles virus can cause allergic encephalitis have stimulated a search for viruses as potential causative agents of multiple sclerosis and similar neurologic diseases of man.

IMMUNITY TO VIRAL DISEASES. Acquired resistance to viral infections takes several forms. Probably the most important is specific immunity induced by natural exposure to a virus or by vaccination. Injection of a sufficient antigenic mass of virus induces the formation of rapidly sedimenting (19S or γM) antibody within several days, followed by the appearance of smaller, more slowly sedimenting (7S or γG) antibody. Although identical in specificity, 7S antibody is more efficient than 19S antibody in neutralizing the same virus. The predominant antiviral antibody present on mucosal surfaces is γA globulin. Antibody in the circulation and extracellular fluid is a barrier to cross infection of cells. If reinfection with the same or an antigenically related virus occurs even after a long interval, a prompt anamnestic response often prevents spread of infection from the primary focus and the host's reaction to infection is mild or asymptomatic. The content of antibody (γA) in nasal secretions is thought to be one factor in immunity to rhinoviruses and other respiratory viruses. Similarly, viruses that persist in the tissues for many years after a primary infection are prevented from causing widespread disease by continual formation of antibody.

Secondary herpes simplex, for example, usually remains localized to the lips rather than becoming disseminated, as may occur in primary infection (Chap. 226).

Factors other than antibody production also influence the outcome of infection on first exposure to a virus. It is common for the acute manifestations of a viral disease to abate before neutralizing antibody can be detected in the circulation. Children with hypogammaglobulinemia have been noted to recover from measles, mumps, chickenpox, poliomyelitis, and viral respiratory infections in a normal manner. Furthermore, these children rarely show evidence of reinfection with a virus, in contrast to their tendency to undergo repeated infections by the same bacteria. However, vaccinia gangrenosa (Chap. 223) and severe viral hepatitis are unusually frequent in children with hypogammaglobulinemia.

A form of immunologic tolerance may play a significant role in resistance to congenital viral infections. Mice infected in utero, or a few hours after birth, with lymphocytic choriomeningitis virus resist reinfection with the same virus for many months. These resistant animals form little or no circulating antibody to the virus, but viral antibody and antigen-antibody complexes are found sequestered in the kidney, sometimes associated with glomerulonephritis. An analogous situation may obtain in congenital infections of man with salivary gland virus (Chap. 232). This virus often lies dormant in the tissues for many years without causing cytomegalic inclusion disease or other manifestations of infection.

Infection with one virus may also confer resistance to infection with an antigenically related or unrelated virus, a phenomenon known as *viral interference*. This observation is of practical significance in scheduling the sequence of oral vaccination with the Sabin strains of attenuated polioviruses. If all three poliovirus types are administered together, type 2 may inhibit enteric multiplication of the other two types, with consequent depression of antibody response to them. Latent enteric infection with ECHO or other enteroviruses has also been noted to prevent infection with virulent polioviruses. Experimental studies indicate that one type of viral interference is caused by a nonviral protein, called *interferon*, which is produced by infected cells. The suggestion has been made that recovery from certain viral infections may be attributable to endogenous production of interferon.

VACCINATION. Purified concentrated virus inactivated by formalin or attenuated infectious virus can be used as vaccines. Their success depends, in large measure, on the antigenic mass originally injected or on the multiplication of attenuated virus to equivalent titers. Repeated administration is often required and, even then, immunity is likely to be less pronounced and of shorter duration than that following recovery from natural infection.

The efficacy of a vaccine is judged from several standpoints. The first consideration is its safety for those receiving it and for their contacts. Secondly, a vaccine must induce a significant antibody response and, in so doing, reduce morbidity and mortality after natural exposure to the virus. Rarely is prevention of infection per se considered to be an important goal of vaccination. In fact, asymptomatic infection after vaccination can serve to enhance and prolong the immune response.

PERSISTENCE AND LATENCY. Many viruses persist in host tissues for months or years without causing overt disease. A flare-up of these latent infections may be induced by trauma, intercurrent disease, decline in antibody titers, or unknown stimuli. Experiments with tissue cultures and laboratory animals reveal that persistence of virus in tissue results from an interplay of various factors peculiar to each virus and its host. Latency is promoted by the presence of antibody or other viral inhibitors that prevent extensive cell-to-cell spread of virus. If antibody is withdrawn, viral multiplication often resumes, with concomitant cellular necrosis. Congenital viral infections tend to be latent for long periods of time, possibly through the mechanism of immunologic tolerance. One of the most important causes of virus persistence is thought to result from endogenous production of interferon by chronically infected cells. An equilibrium can be established in tissue culture when a small proportion of the cells in a population produces infectious virus and the same or different cells produce interferon.

DIAGNOSIS. Although similar in principle to diagnostic bacteriology, laboratory diagnosis of viral diseases often entails procedures that are far more time-consuming and costly. Therefore, the decision to undertake virus diagnostic studies must be based on sound clinical judgment and a carefully reasoned evaluation of the public health implications of the disease in question. Specimens sent to the virus laboratory as part of a "complete" diagnostic work-up are usually valueless. The laboratory procedures to be followed vary considerably for different viral diseases and frequently depend on the duration of illness and whether the infection has occurred sporadically or during an epidemic. The virologist relies heavily on knowledge of diseases endemic in a community, their seasonal incidence, the geographic distribution of certain viruses, and the potential animal reservoirs and insect vectors of an area. The presence of characteristic histopathologic lesions may contribute more to a retrospective diagnosis of diseases such as rabies, yellow fever, measles, cytomegalic inclusion disease, and poliomyelitis than will be gained by virus isolation and serologic studies. The diagnosis of infectious hepatitis is based entirely on clinical or pathologic findings.

The advent of tissue culture and cell culture methods has greatly facilitated isolation of certain viruses (see Table 203-1), but because of variation in cellular susceptibility to viral infection, it is often essential to choose the type of tissue culture on the basis of the virus anticipated to be present. Despite continuing advances in technique, viruses are generally difficult to isolate and even more difficult to identify. Some cause characteristic cytopathologic changes in culture, but cellular reactions to others often lack specificity. The histochemical technique of immunofluorescence is another reliable means for rapid identification of viral antigen within cells.

A serious problem in diagnostic virology is the frequency with which uninoculated tissue cultures are contaminated with latent viruses that may induce cytopathic effects indistinguishable from those caused by the virus one is attempting to isolate. For example, cultures of renal epithelium from presumably healthy monkeys often contain measles or other viruses. Another major difficulty stems from the observation that feces and nasopharyngeal secretions may contain viruses other than, or in addition to, those originally suspected of causing a patient's illness. To cite but two examples, the ECHO viruses were discovered during studies of poliomyelitis, and some of the parainfluenza viruses were originally isolated during an influenza epidemic. In several instances, identification of new viruses has led to recognition of new disease entities, the existence of which had not been suspected on clinical grounds alone.

Final identification of viruses and the diagnosis of viral diseases almost invariably depend on immunologic tests. Each diagnostic laboratory maintains a supply of viral antigens and standard reference antiserums. When a virus is isolated, it is identified in terms of its immunologic reactivity compared with known viruses. The most useful serologic procedures in virology are complement fixation and neutralization of infectivity. Virus neutralization is the most sensitive immunologic test yet devised. Precipitin reactions in fluid medium or by agar gel diffusion can be performed only with highly concentrated preparations of virus and specific antibody. For those viruses which readily agglutinate erythrocytes, such as the myxoviruses, antibody can be assayed by hemagglutination inhibition or by hemadsorption inhibition. It is important to keep in mind that different serologic tests may measure different antigenic components of the same virus. All members of the adenovirus group, for example, share a common complement-fixing antigen, but each can be typed by specific neutralizing antibody.

In the final analysis, only an antibody response in the host constitutes definitive evidence of infection with a specific virus. Therefore, it is essential to obtain serum specimens at properly spaced intervals. The result of a single serologic test is often misleading because it may be impossible to determine whether the antibody represents a response to infection in the recent or distant past.

REFERENCES

Burdette, W. J. (Ed.): "Viruses Inducing Cancer," Salt Lake City, University of Utah Press, 1966.

Fenner, F.: "The Biology of Animal Viruses," vol. II, "The Pathogenesis and Ecology of Viral Infections," New York, Academic Press, Inc., 1968.

Finter, N. B. (Ed.): "Interferons," Amsterdam, North-Holland Publishing Company, 1966.

Mims, C. A.: Aspects of the Pathogenesis of Virus Diseases, Bacteriol. Rev., 28:30, 1964.

Svehag, S. E., and B. Mandel: The Formation and Properties

of Poliovirus-neutralizing Antibody, J. Exp. Med., 119:1, 21, 225, 1964.

Section 14

Viral Diseases of the Respiratory Tract

205 GENERAL CONSIDERATIONS OF RESPIRATORY VIRAL DISEASE

Vernon Knight

The viral respiratory diseases as a group are responsible for one-half or more of all acute illnesses, and although influenza virus is the only agent among them which causes significant mortality in adults, several different viruses make a large contribution to the 20 percent of childhood mortality due to respiratory disease. Respiratory disease morbidity, due primarily to virus infections, causes 30 to 50 percent of time lost from work in adults, and from 60 to 80 percent of time lost by children from school. These diseases are worldwide, and although studies in many areas are scanty, reports from Great Britain, Western Europe, U.S.S.R., Czechoslovakia, Latin America, and the Orient indicate many common denominators in the problems of etiology, prevalence, and severity.

Viral respiratory diseases are associated with a spectrum of host responses ranging from asymptomatic carriers to severe and sometimes fatal pneumonias. There is a recurring pattern of severe illness in infants and young children and milder disease with increasing age. There are a few clinical and epidemiologic entities which can be recognized without laboratory aids, such as acute respiratory disease (ARD) in military recruits, caused by adenovirus type 4, and rhinovirus coryza in adults. The causative agent in a large proportion of cases, however, cannot be identified without virologic study. Although it is presently impractical and unnecessary to diagnose the etiology of most respiratory viral illnesses in individual patients, an understanding of this group of diseases is best when based on etiologic relationships.

EPIDEMIOLOGY IN THE UNITED STATES

There are at present at least 153 serotypes, representing 12 groups of viruses, which have been or may be associated with acute respiratory illness in man. With the capacity to isolate this large group of agents and with the recognition of the importance of the pleuropneumonia-like organism (PPLO), *Mycoplasma pneu-*

moniae (Chap. 207) in respiratory illness, it has been possible in some studies to define the cause of many respiratory illnesses. In all studies, a majority of illnesses was caused by viruses. It seems probable that the inability to identify etiologic agents is greater than can be accounted for by lack of efficient application of known diagnostic methods and that additional viral and possibly other causes of respiratory illness remain to be discovered. For example, agents with morphologic characteristics similar to the infectious bronchitis virus of chickens (IBV) have been isolated from man, and were associated with mild respiratory illness. They may represent an additional etiologic category of human respiratory disease.

NATIONAL HEALTH SURVEY. There has been considerable progress in determining the cause of respiratory disease chiefly resulting from the National Health Survey, which, since 1957, has made annual estimates from selected population samples of the incidence of acute respiratory illness in the United States. These studies were designed to show the socioeconomic impact of illness, and cases were reported only if they caused restriction of daily activity or required medical care. There were 259 million cases of acute respiratory illness in the United States between July 1, 1961, and June 30, 1962, an average of 1.4 illnesses per person per year. A similar incidence has been noted in every year of the survey. The percentage distribution of these illnesses according to clinical diagnosis (International Classification of Diseases, 1955 revision) is shown in Table 205-1.

Except for streptococcal sore throat, some cases of bacterial pneumonia, sinusitis, etc., the remaining cases were undoubtedly largely of viral origin. It seems that some illnesses were incorrectly reported as influenza, but in other respects, the diagnostic categorization correlates well with smaller studies in which the specific cause of respiratory disease has been determined.

ETIOLOGY. An example for comparison of the specific causes with the descriptive diagnoses above is a study of acute respiratory illness in university students and military personnel in Louisiana and Mississippi. Cases were admitted to the study on the basis of a request for medical care at a dispensary. Diagnostic categories consisted of mild or acute febrile upper respiratory illness, with or without pharyngitis. These would include

Table 205-1. PERCENTAGE DISTRIBUTION BY DIAGNOSIS
OF 259 MILLION ACUTE RESPIRATORY CONDITIONS:
UNITED STATES, JULY, 1961, TO JUNE 1962

Condition	Percentage of total
Common cold	43.1
Influenza	28.6
The "virus"	9.6
Sinusitis, pharyngitis, tonsillitis, laryngitis, etc.	11.3
Pneumonia Bronchitis Influenza with digestive manifestations Other	6.1
Streptococcus sore throat	1.3
Total	100.0

SOURCE: Condensed from National Health Survey.

a large majority of the illnesses described in Table 205-1. No cases of pneumonia were included. The etiologic

Table 205-2. ETIOLOGY OF ACUTE RESPIRATORY ILLNESS
IN MILITARY RECRUITS AND UNIVERSITY STUDENTS,
NEW ORLEANS, 1958–1960

Agent	Students, %	Recruits, %
Rhinovirus	45.0	38.7
Parainfluenza type 1, 2, 3	9.4	6.8
Influenza (A_2, B)	9.2	5.8
Respiratory syncytial virus	5.3	7.9
Herpes simplex	4.1	2.9
Adenovirus	1.3	11.4
	74.3	73.5
Beta-hemolytic streptococci	3.6	5.7
Mycoplasma pneumoniae	5.5	7.0
	9.1	12.7
Unknown	16.6	13.8
Total	100.0	100.0

diagnosis was made in about 85 percent of cases (Table 205-2). Rhinovirus illness was most frequent (45.0 percent of students and 38.7 percent of recruits). Adenovirus illness was uncommon in students (1.3 percent) in contrast to 11.4 percent in recruits. Respiratory syncytial, parainfluenza, and influenza viruses made up the remainder of the illnesses, except for the small percentage of beta-hemolytic streptococcal and *M. pneumoniae* infections. The small percentage of herpes simplex infections represented cases in which illness was associated with a fourfold or greater rise in titer of antibody to this agent. Whether these rises represented primary or secondary infection is uncertain. The frequency of herpes labialis complicating febrile illness, the regular isolation of herpes simplex from asymptomatic persons, and the uniform presence of serum antibody to this agent in the adult population make it difficult to interpret the role of this virus in respiratory infection in the adult. Acute respiratory illness probably occurs as a consequence of primary herpes simplex infection in children.

The distribution of the virus-caused illnesses in this study is not representative of all population groups. Nevertheless, in other studies with differences in age, sex, locale, and severity of cases, these six groups of viruses have been responsible for a great majority of the diagnosed illness. They represent at least 90 different serotypes, but a much smaller number of serotypes is responsible for most of the cases in any one area at any one time.

A classification and summary of characteristic properties of these agents appear in Table 205-3 (see also Table 203-1). It is remarkable that agents of such widely varying properties can produce respiratory illnesses in man which are so clinically similar.

FREQUENCY AND SEVERITY. The National Health Survey and the above study included only cases in which there was an appreciable severity of illness. For example in the National Health Survey in the period of July 1961 to June 1962, loss of time from work or school

Table 205-3. CLASSIFICATION AND CHARACTERISTIC PROPERTIES OF HUMAN RESPIRATORY VIRUSES

Nucleic acid core	Capsidal symmetry	Enveloped	Ether and/or chloroform sensitivity	pH 3.0 liability	Virus particle size, mμ	Virus group
DNA (deoxyviruses)	Cubic	Naked Enveloped	Resistant Sensitive	Stable Labile	60–85 180–250	*Adenoviruses* *Herpesviruses*
RNA (riboviruses)						*Picornaviruses:*
	Cubic	Naked	Resistant	Stable	28	Enteroviruses (Coxsackie virus, ECHO virus, and poliovirus)
				Labile	17–18	Rhinoviruses
						Myxoviruses:
	Helical	Enveloped	Sensitive	Labile	80–120 150–250 90–120	Influenza Parainfluenza Respiratory syncytial

SOURCE: Condensed from B. I. Wilner, "A Classification of the Major Groups of Human and Lower Animal Viruses," 2d ed., Berkeley, Calif., Cutter Laboratories, 1964.

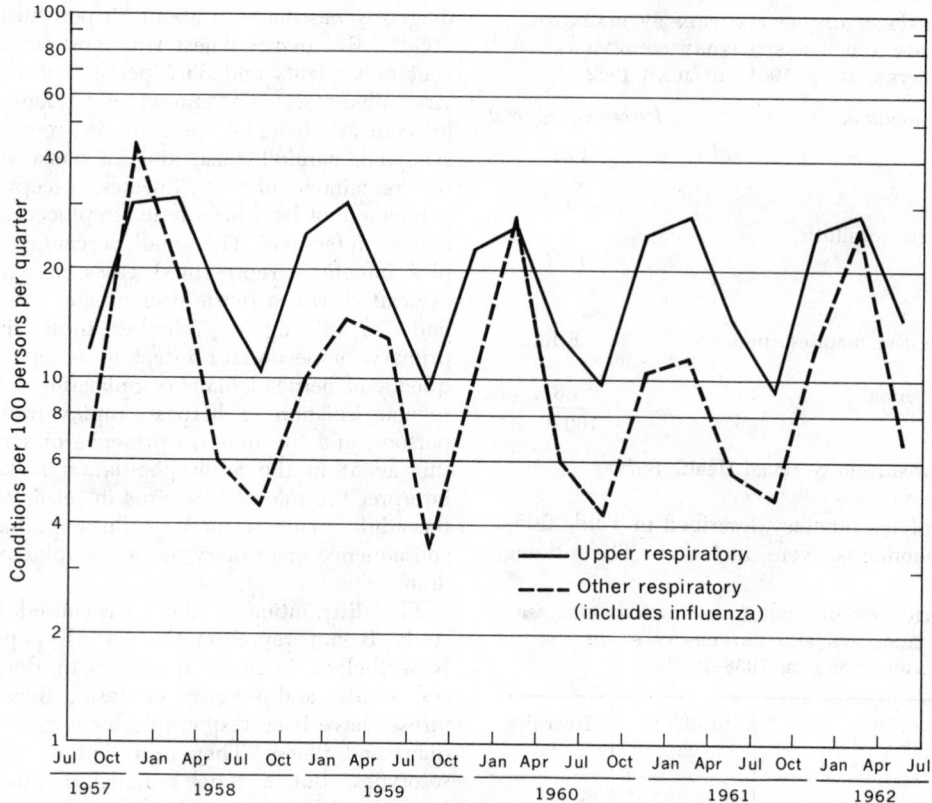

Fig. 205-1. Incidence of acute upper and other respiratory conditions per 100 persons per quarter. (*National Health Survey, U.S. Public Health Service, Publ. 1000, 1963.*)

averaged 4.2 days for the 80 percent (207 million) of cases in which some restriction of activity was reported. About 50 percent, or 130 million, of persons sought medical attention although at least 52 million reported no restriction of activity.

In other studies, milder illness has been included, with a corresponding rise in annual frequency of reported cases. The Cleveland Family Study found an annual rate of illness of 6.2 per person per year, amounting to an estimated more than 1 billion cases annually in the United States. The greatest proportion of these illnesses were so mild that they constituted no hazard to health, but they are of significance in the spread of infection. In addition, it is known that wholly asymptomatic virus infections occur.

AGE, SEX, AND SEASONAL VARIATION. All studies have been in agreement that infants and young children have the greatest number of viral respiratory infections and children under six may have twice as many illnesses per year as the average of the population. Females have more illness than males; the excess is most marked during adult years and amounts to about 25 percent. There are prominent seasonal differences in the frequency of acute respiratory illness; these are shown in Fig. 205-1 from the National Health Survey. In the January-March quarter, the rates are highest (solid line), with values approximating 30 cases per 100 persons. Illness is least frequent during the summer, about

one-third of the maximum at 10 per 100 persons. The characteristic 2- to 3-year epidemic pattern of influenza is also shown.

In the following chapter (Chap. 206) consideration is given to four of the six groups of viruses chiefly responsible for respiratory disease, i.e., rhinoviruses, adenoviruses, respiratory syncytial viruses, and parainfluenza viruses. Included also is a description of the small contribution to respiratory illness of the enteroviruses, Coxsackie virus A and B, ECHO virus, and poliovirus (these viruses are discussed in detail in Chaps. 210 to 212). Influenza is described separately in Chap. 208. Pneumonia due to *M. pneumoniae* (Eaton agent) will be considered in this section (Chap. 207) for clinical reasons, although the causative agent is a pleuropneumonia organism, not a virus. Psittacosis has been included in this section in Chap. 209 for clinical reasons, although the causative agent is not a virus.

REFERENCES

Acute Conditions, Incidence and Associated Disability, United States, July 1961–June 1962, National Health Survey, U.S. Public Health Service Publ. 1000, Series 10, No. 1, 1963.

Dingle, J. H., G. F. Badger, A. E. Feller, R. G. Hodges, W. S. Jordan, and C. H. Rammelkamp: A Study of Illness in a Group of Cleveland Families: I. Plan of Study and

Certain General Observations, Am. J. Hyg., 58:16, 174, 1953.

Loosli, C. G. (Ed.): Conference on Newer Respiratory Disease Viruses, Am. Rev. Resp. Dis., 88(Suppl):1–419, 1963.

Mogabgab, W. J.: Viruses Associated with Upper Respiratory Illnesses in Adults, Ann. Intern. Med., 59:306, 1963.

206 COMMON VIRAL RESPIRATORY ILLNESSES
(Rhinoviruses; Adenoviruses; Respiratory Syncytial Virus; Parainfluenza Virus; Coxsackie Virus, ECHO Virus, and Polioviruses)

Vernon Knight

RHINOVIRUS INFECTIONS

ETIOLOGY. Pelon and Mogabgab and associates in 1956 described a new agent isolated from recruits with respiratory illness which was subsequently designated *ECHO virus, type 28*. In 1960, Hitchcock and Tyrrell isolated new agents from cases of common cold which they named *rhinoviruses*. Subsequently a large number of agents with properties similar to ECHO virus, type 28, and rhinoviruses have been isolated. At present, 55 types are known, and others are certain to be found. Some of the properties of rhinoviruses are shown in Table 205-3. Some rhinoviruses produce cytopathic effects in monkey kidney cell culture (M strains); others are not cytopathic for monkey cells but will grow in cells of human origin (H strains).

EPIDEMIOLOGY. As much as 40 percent of acute respiratory illness in adults may be caused by rhinoviruses. On the basis of the large number of serotypes, it can be presumed that the recognized contribution of these agents to acute respiratory illness will increase. Infections occur throughout the year but are most frequent in the late winter and early spring. In a limited study of the distribution of serotypes over a continuing period of observation in children, university students, and industrial employees, multiple serotypes were found to circulate simultaneously. Individual types usually persist for only a few months, however, and do not recur during succeeding seasons. Adults commonly exhibit antibody against several serotypes, whereas young children (except for the very young with maternal antibody) are relatively free of antibody. In studies in children and adults a small percentage of non-ill controls have yielded positive cultures for rhinoviruses, but in the main, the presence of rhinoviruses in the respiratory tract is associated with illness.

Most patients develop appreciable titers of type-specific antibody, and measurable levels persist for 2 to 4 years. In screening of prisoner volunteers for participation in experiments with rhinoviruses, it was found that only one-third of men are entirely free of antibody to four rhinovirus serotypes. However, illness and virus shedding can be readily induced in volunteers unless very high titers of antibody are present. Clearly, then, a high proportion of children and adults are susceptible to infection and illness with rhinoviruses. However, with some homologous and heterologous types of rhinovirus there is almost complete resistance to reinfection for several weeks following infection which is not dependent on serum antibody.

CLINICAL MANIFESTATIONS. The incubation period for rhinovirus infections in volunteers is 1 to 2 days. The common cold syndrome induced in volunteers resembles naturally occurring cases in adults. Within 24 hr of inoculation there are scratchy throat, nasal congestion and discharge, malaise, and mild headache. There is no fever, as is usual in the disease. Nasal secretions measured in grams increase sharply between day 1 and 2 and then as promptly return to preillness values. Recovery is rapid and complete. Virus shedding begins a few hours after inoculation and continues for almost 2 weeks. Type-specific neutralizing antibody rises to 1:128 at 21 days.

Table 206-1. ILLNESS ASSOCIATION WITH RHINOVIRUS INFECTIONS

Diagnosis	Adults (61)	Children (32)	Adult volunteers with nasopharyngeal inoculation (31)
	%	%	%
Common cold	58 (92)	14 (44)	26 (84)
Croup		1 (3)	
Bronchitis	1 (2)	7 (23)	2 (6)
Bronchiolitis		3 (9)	
Bronchopneumonia		3 (9)	
No disease	2 (3)	4 (12)	3 (10)

SOURCE: Hamparian et al., Proc. Soc. Exp. Biol. Med., 117:469, 1964; and Cate et al., J. Clin. Invest., 43:56, 1964.

Table 206 summarizes clinical experience with naturally occurring rhinovirus infections in adults and children and artificial infection in volunteers. The great majority of adults have only a common cold syndrome, with a rare case of bronchitis as the only other form of illness. In contrast, more than one-half of children develop bronchitis, bronchiolitis, or bronchopneumonia. Although these findings resemble those of respiratory syncytial (RS) virus infection, rhinovirus disease is generally milder than that due to RS virus.

LABORATORY FINDINGS. In illness with rhinovirus there is usually a slight neutrophilia, which is the only significant alteration in leukocyte count which has been observed in this infection. Similar leukocyte responses are found in illness with rhinovirus, influenza virus, Coxsackie virus A, type 21, and adenovirus type 4. About one-third of volunteers develop elevations in sedimentation rates ranging from 27 to 50 mm per hr.

COMPLICATIONS. No serious complications have been reported with rhinovirus infections.

DIFFERENTIAL DIAGNOSIS. Among the respiratory viruses, rhinovirus infection most consistently results in coryzal illness. In any one case, however, the illness cannot be distinguished from coryza due to other agents. Except for rare confusion with an atypical case of streptococcal sore throat, only respiratory viral diseases need be considered in differential diagnosis.

TREATMENT AND PREVENTION. There is no specific treatment, and no vaccines are currently available for rhinovirus infections. Rest, analgesics, antihistamines, and nose drops are advised, depending on symptomatic needs.

ADENOVIRUS INFECTIONS

ETIOLOGY. The adenovirus group contains 31 human and 17 animal serotypes. Strains of types 3, 7, 11, 12, 14, 16, 18, 21, and 31 have been shown to cause sarcomas when injected into newborn hamsters.

Adenoviruses share a common antigen which is associated with a structural subunit of the protein coat of the virus called a hexon. An antigenic determinant on this protein is the basis for a diagnostic complement fixation test. Type specificity in neutralizing antibody tests depends on antigenic determinants present on hexons and on another protein subunit designated the fiber, which is part of another structure in the virus coat called a penton. Except for types 12 and 18, hemagglutination inhibition (HI) tests also permit type-specific identification. Adenovirus hemagglutinins, the bases for the HI test, are variably associated with fiber subunit, with the complete penton subunit, and with the intact virion. Human adenoviruses grow well in continuous cell lines of epithelial origin.

EPIDEMIOLOGY. Adenoviruses were first isolated in 1953 by Rowe and his associates from human adenoids after elective surgery. Association with respiratory illness in military personnel was described a short time later by Hillenman and Werner. Even though serologic surveys suggest an appreciable prevalence of infection with many serotypes, definite virus-associated illness is now limited to about 10 serotypes. These serotypes produce five major patterns of illness, all of which occur in epidemics. A summary of these is presented in Table 206-2.

Acute respiratory disease (ARD), a respiratory illness of military recruits, was described by the U.S. Army Commission on Respiratory Disease before adenoviruses

Table 206-2. ILLNESS ASSOCIATED WITH ADENOVIRUS INFECTION

Disease	Occurrence	Order of association (serotypes)		Respiratory tract involvement				Fever and constitutional reaction	Other
		Common	Less common	Common cold	Pharyngitis	Bronchitis	Pneumonia		
Acute respiratory disease (ARD)	Epidemic in winter and spring in military recruits	4, 7	3, 14, 21	Often present	*Most frequent,* usually with fever, often with laryngitis	Frequent, usually with fever and laryngitis	Infrequent complication of ARD, but adenovirus pneumonia is an important type of pneumonia in recruits	Headache, malaise, often high fever for several days	Usually no other involvement
Pharyngoconjunctival fever	Summer epidemics in civilians, often in school-age children related to swimming pools. Sporadic cases of conjunctivitis may occur without pharyngitis.	3, 7	4, 14	Often present	*Most frequent,* usually with fever and cervical lymphadenopathy, hoarseness	Uncommon	Rare	Headache, malaise, high fever for several days	Acute follicular conjunctivitis, usually unilateral, occurs with varying frequency. Preauricular lymphadenopathy common with conjunctivitis
Febrile pharyngitis	Sporadic or epidemic, resembles ARD, often in children	3, 7	1, 2, 5	Often present	*Most frequent,* usually with fever	Frequent, especially in older children	Infrequent but severe complications	High fever, malaise, headache	Nausea, vomiting, and diarrhea may occur, especially in infants
Pneumonia in children	Highly fatal illness in infants, sporadic or epidemic	3, 7		Occurs	Very frequent	Very frequent	Primary, with acidophilic necrosis of tracheal and bronchial mucosa resembling tissue culture CPE	High fever, prostration	Conjunctivitis, skin rash, diarrhea, intussusception, and CNS invasion in some cases
Keratoconjunctivitis (EKC)	Epidemic disease in shipyard workers; also spread from infected eye solutions	8	11	Unusual	Uncommon	Not reported	Not reported	Usually afebrile	Usually unilateral severe, acute conjunctivitis followed by corneal subepithelial keratosis; preauricular lymphadenopathy common

were discovered. Later testing of serum from some of these patients revealed that these infections were caused by adenoviruses. Other studies have shown regular winter and spring outbreaks of ARD in military recruits in the United States caused by adenovirus types 4 and 7, and with lesser frequency by type 3. Types 14 and 21 have caused similar outbreaks in military personnel in the Netherlands and elsewhere. In military groups, 15 to 50 percent of acute respiratory illness is caused by adenoviruses, but in civilian adults, only about 2 percent of respiratory illnesses are due to adenoviruses, and in children only about 6 percent.

Febrile pharyngitis due to adenoviruses is usually a disease of civilians, often occurring sporadically or in small outbreaks in children. Its manifestations are summarized in Table 206-2. *Pharyngoconjunctival fever* is febrile pharyngitis associated with acute follicular conjunctivitis. This disease occurs as summer epidemics, frequently among children in relation to exposure in swimming pools. Although it is not limited to swimming pool exposure, it is believed that eye irritation from water, sun, or chlorine may be a factor in its initiation. Conjunctivitis may occur without pharyngitis.

Pneumonia due to adenovirus infection is rare in civilian adults, but it now seems certain that an atypical pneumonia due to adenovirus infection occurs in military recruits, usually as an extension of ARD. In infants and children, sporadic and epidemic occurrence of highly fatal adenoviral pneumonia has been described in several parts of the world. These have been principally caused by types 3 and 7. The severity of disease in this young age group may reflect the lack of prior experience with these agents, but other factors such as size and route of inoculation, general health, or greater susceptibility due to immaturity may be important.

Epidemic keratoconjunctivitis due to type 8 and less often to type 11 or other serotypes is described in Chap. 228.

Incubation Period. The period of incubation for pharyngoconjunctival fever and ARD is 5 to 10 days. A similar incubation period has been noted for induced disease in volunteers. Incubation periods for the other naturally occurring syndromes have not been established but are probably similar.

PATHOGENESIS. Illness in volunteers is produced when the conjunctival sac is swabbed with suspensions of adenovirus. In these cases, conjunctivitis occurs and there is sometimes respiratory involvement. The initiation of illness appears to require a significant degree of conjunctival irritation. A second method of producing illness is administration of virus aerosol by inhalation. Volunteers inoculated in this way have developed ARD and primary atypical pneumonia.

These observations suggest the existence of at least two routes of inoculation for naturally occurring respiratory illness with adenoviruses: (1) ocular inoculation associated with eye irritation such as may occur in outbreaks around swimming pools, with the development of *pharyngoconjunctival fever;* (2) inoculation through inhalation of infectious aerosol generated by sneezing and coughing of ill recruits under the crowded circumstances incidental to recruit training. This exposure results in *ARD or primary atypical pneumonia.* The route of inoculation of infants is less likely to be limited to aerosolized virus, and the occurrence of pneumonia may represent primarily a lack of resistance in this young age group.

The regular production of virus infection without illness by nasopharyngeal inoculation in volunteers suggests that a similar circumstance may occur naturally as an explanation for the high frequency of antibody to many serotypes in the population. This antibody may also result from intragroup cross reactions among serotypes in the three broad immunologic groups of adenovirus.

CLINICAL MANIFESTATIONS. *Acute respiratory disease* is an acute febrile illness lasting about 1 week and characterized by fever, cough, hoarseness, and sore throat. Fever has gradual onset and reaches a maximum of 103 to 104°F on the second or third day. There are associated malaise and often headache. Pharyngitis is the most prominent localized manifestation of the disease, and reaches maximum severity after about 3 days. There may also be regional lymphadenopathy, pharyngeal injection, some edema, frequent lymphoid follicular hyperplasia, but little or no faucial exudate. Nasal obstruction and discharge occur in almost one-half of cases, but these abnormalities are not usually conspicuous. Cough is almost always present, and hoarseness is also frequent.

Many clinical and laboratory features of ARD are represented in Fig. 206-1, a case caused by inhalation of aerosol containing adenovirus type 4. This volunteer had no measurable antibody to the agent before inoculation. Five days after inoculation he developed a febrile pharyngitis which increased in severity for 2 or 3 days and then gradually improved. There were also cough, hoarseness, malaise, and headache. Shedding of virus from nose, throat, and rectum continued for at least 4 weeks, long after recovery from illness. The white cell count remained at preinoculation levels for the first few days of illness but declined to low values 1 week after onset of symptoms. This late leukopenia is in accord with observations in other volunteers and with limited observations on naturally occurring disease. There was also a significant rise in blood sedimentation rate.

Pharyngoconjunctival fever is usually a milder respiratory illness than ARD, although fever may be high for 5 or 6 days. Nontender submandibular lymphadenopathy is common even in the absence of sore throat. Lower respiratory tract involvement has not been described. Conjunctivitis is mild to moderate but may last longer than respiratory symptoms. It is an acute, nonpurulent, follicular conjunctivitis. In most cases, it is unilateral, and pre-auricular lymphadenopathy is rare. There is usually no involvement of the cornea or uveal tract.

Febrile pharyngitis without conjunctivitis resembles the foregoing illness, except for the absence of conjunctivitis.

Adenoviral pneumonia in children occurs as a primary illness and is associated with as much as 15 percent mortality. Pediatric texts should be consulted for further details.

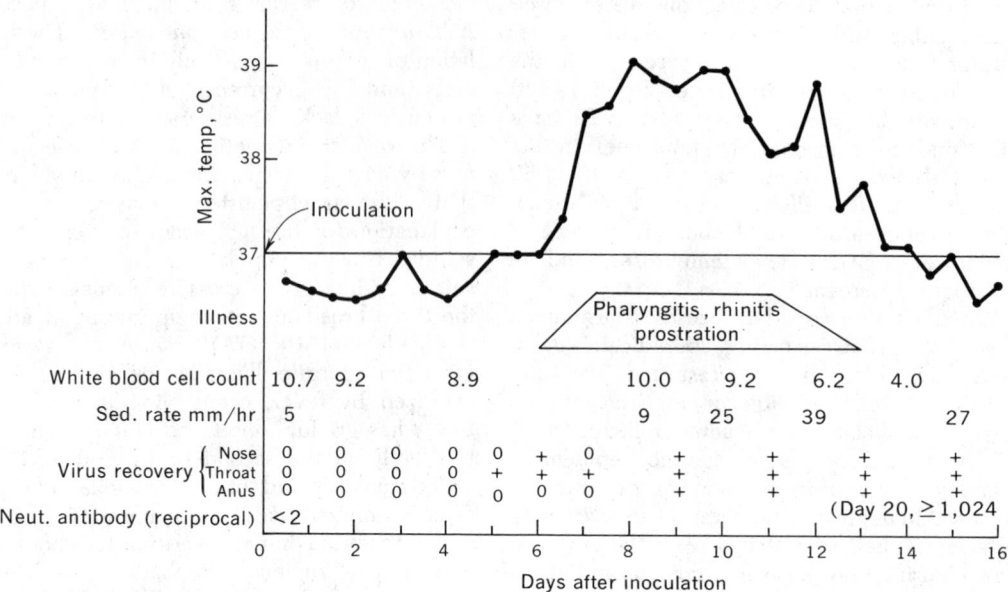

Fig. 206-1. Acute respiratory disease (ARD) produced in a volunteer by aerosol inoculation. (*Case of Dr. Robert B. Couch, National Institutes of Health.*)

DIFFERENTIAL DIAGNOSIS. The differential diagnosis of ARD should include the respiratory viral diseases described in the present chapter and influenza (Chap. 208), nonpneumonic forms of *Mycoplasma pneumoniae* infection (Chap. 207), streptococcal sore throat, and purulent sinusitis. Pharyngitis and upper respiratory illness may also accompany the onset of infectious hepatitis and infectious mononucleosis.

Differential diagnosis of *pharyngoconjunctival fever,* when conjunctivitis is prominent, includes leptospirosis, influenza, measles, herpangina, and the nonpurulent conjunctivitides, such as inclusion conjunctivitis and physical or chemical trauma to the eye.

TREATMENT. There is no specific treatment for adenovirus infection. In one study, adenovirus conjunctivitis in volunteers did not respond to 5-iodo-2′-deoxyuridine by local application. In vitro this compound prevented DNA synthesis by adenoviruses, and failure of the therapeutic trial may have resulted from inadequate contact of the drug with infected tissues. The considerable toxicity of the drug when given systemically has prevented its further study.

Treatment is limited to alleviation of general discomfort, headache, and coughing with analgesics, cough syrup containing terpin hydrate, codeine, antihistamines, or other antitussives.

PREVENTION. Communicability of adenovirus infection probably extends from a day or so before onset of illness to recovery, and conventional precautions against respiratory spread should be employed during acute illness for patients in the hospital and to the extent reasonably possible in care of patients at home.

Avoidance of swimming pools during outbreaks of pharyngoconjunctival fever is recommended. Patients with epidemic keratoconjunctivitis should be kept from work, and care should be exercised to prevent spread of discharges from infected eyes.

Early studies on volunteers revealed that type-specific antibody provided substantial protection against live virus challenge. Formalin-treated vaccines against types 3, 4, and 7 offer significant protection against infection, but their use has largely been limited to military recruits. A vaccine for type 4 adenovirus infection consisting of live virus incorporated into an enteric-coated capsule may soon become available.

RESPIRATORY SYNCYTIAL VIRUS INFECTION

ETIOLOGY. Respiratory syncytial virus (RS) is classified as a subgroup of the myxoviruses. It is of medium size (90 to 120 mμ), RNA in type, of helical symmetry, and is destroyed by ethyl ether. In tissue culture, it causes formation of giant cells, or syncytia, from which its name was derived. It grows well in several human primary and continuous cell lines and in primary rhesus monkey kidney culture. There is a soluble complement-fixing antigen which, with the neutralization test, permits virus identification and serologic studies. RS virus contrasts with other myxoviruses because it does not grow or cause detectable changes in mice, guinea pigs, rabbits, or chick embryos and does not cause hemagglutination or hemadsorption.

EPIDEMIOLOGY. Since the first recovery of RS virus from a chimpanzee with a coryzal illness by Morris and his associates in 1956, epidemiologic studies have delineated a very substantial role of this agent in acute respiratory disease in children. Illness in young children occurs most commonly in epidemics in the late winter and early spring. Attack rates are nearly 100 percent among susceptibles, who are mostly children under four years of age. In older children and adults, the disease appears in nonepidemic patterns. The limitation of epidemic disease to the younger age group is also evidence for unchanging antigenicity of the agent, in contrast to the situation with influenza virus, in which antigenic shifts are associated with recurrent epidemics in persons of all ages.

In serologic surveys of several hundred Federal prisoners for selection as volunteers, all were found to possess a measurable titer of neutralizing antibody to RS virus. Mild upper respiratory illness appears to be the only clinical manifestation of RS virus infection in adults.

It is probable that RS virus is transmitted by means of infected respiratory secretions but, as with other respiratory viral diseases, the mechanism has not been more precisely defined. The incubation period of naturally occurring disease in children is about 4 days, and in adult volunteers who developed common cold syndromes, the average incubation period was approximately 5 days. Virus was generally recovered from volunteers a day or so before the onset of illness, and throat swabs yielded a higher proportion of positive cultures than nasal swabs. Virus shedding continues for 3 to 4 days after onset of illness.

CLINICAL MANIFESTATIONS. Table 206-3 gives data on

Table 206-3. ILLNESS WITH RESPIRATORY SYNCYTIAL VIRUS IN CHILDREN AND ADULTS

Subjects	Upper respiratory illness (rhinitis, pharyngitis, cough, malaise), %	Bronchitis, %	Bronchiolitis, %	Bronchopneumonia, %
Children,* 108 cases, 8 years old and younger.........	46	16	9	21
Adults,† 20 volunteers..........	100	None	None	None

* 91% with fever, average 102°F.
† No fever.
SOURCE: McClelland et al., New Engl. J. Med., 264:1169, 1961; Reilly et al., New Engl. J. Med., 264:1176, 1961; and Kravetz et al., J.A.M.A., 176:657, 1961.

the clinical syndromes associated with RS virus infection. Somewhat less than one-half of children had symptoms defined as a common cold; the remainder had bronchiolitis or bronchopneumonia. Fever was present in 91 percent of all children, with an average elevation of 102°F. Cough was almost invariably present, and severe malaise was frequent. Pharyngitis was not usually severe. Fatalities have been reported in infants.

In contrast, naturally occurring illness or induced disease in adult volunteers is a mild syndrome characterized by rhinitis and pharyngitis. Intranasal inoculation of virus into a normal volunteer was followed in 4 days by an afebrile illness consisting of nasal obstruction, clear, profuse nasal discharge, headache, malaise, and slight cough. On the second day of illness, nasal secretion amounted to more than 30 Gm. Improvement was rapid, and recovery was nearly complete 8 days after inoculation. Virus shedding preceded symptoms by 2 days and continued during the first 4 days of illness.

LABORATORY FINDINGS. In children, leukocytosis occurs with some frequency, but no significant hematologic changes were observed in adult volunteers. Bacterial flora of the nasopharynx and other laboratory indices show no significant alterations in either age group.

COMPLICATIONS. Except for progression to overwhelming lower respiratory tract disease in a few young children, no special complications are known. There is no evidence of secondary bacterial infection or systemic invasion by the virus in children. In adults, bacterial sinusitis is occasionally encountered.

DIFFERENTIAL DIAGNOSIS. The resemblance of this disease in children to influenza has been suggested. In addition, illness with other respiratory viruses, especially adenovirus and parainfluenza, may be difficult to distinguish. Finally, *M. pneumoniae* infections or bacterial pneumonias may cause difficulty in diagnosis. In adults, the differential diagnosis should include rhinovirus and parainfluenza infection and, less often, other respiratory viral diseases and *M. pneumoniae* infection.

TREATMENT. As with the other respiratory viral diseases, treatment should include rest and palliative medications such as aspirin, nose drops, and medication for sleep when restlessness occurs. The possibility of bacterial sinusitis in adults should be kept in mind and antimicrobial treatment, drainage procedures, or other therapy instituted when necessary.

PREVENTION. No vaccine is available. The infection spreads rapidly among children in institutions and poses a threat to debilitated or very young children. Rigid isolation procedures should be enforced in such circumstances, but their effectiveness cannot be assured. Suspected cases should avoid contact with children.

PARAINFLUENZA VIRUS INFECTIONS

ETIOLOGY. The first agent of this group of myxoviruses to be isolated was the Sendai virus (parainfluenza type 1). It was obtained in mice following intranasal inoculation with material from the lung of a child with a fatal case of pneumonia. In view of later isolations of parainfluenza type 1 from mice, the human origins of this first isolate has been questioned. Subsequently, human strains were isolated in tissue culture in the period 1956 to 1960. On the basis of antigenic differences, they are divided into four types. They agglutinate avian and mammalian erythrocytes and grow slowly in tissue culture, and only type 2 produces readily visible cytopathic effects. Growth of these agents in tissue culture is detected by addition of guinea pig erythrocytes, which absorb on the surface of infected cells to form rosettes, a process known as hemadsorption. Parainfluenza viruses have antigens common to Newcastle disease and mumps viruses, but influenza virus does not share these. Parainfluenza serotypes are distinguished by complement fixation, hemagglutination-inhibition, or tissue culture neutralization tests.

Primary monkey or primary human embryonic kidney cell cultures are suitable for isolation. Other human primary and continuous lines support growth of these agents less well. They grow slowly or not at all in embryonated chicken eggs.

Animal counterparts to the first three types have been identified; type 1 (Sendai virus) has been isolated from mice and pigs, type 2 (simian viruses 5 and 41) has been isolated from monkeys, and type 3 (shipping fever virus) has been recovered from cattle.

EPIDEMIOLOGY. The first three types of parainfluenza viruses have been found in many parts of the world; type 4 has so far been isolated only in the United States. Infection with parainfluenza viruses occurs early in life. By the age of eight years, a majority of children show antibody to types 1 to 3, and, although studies are limited, it appears that most adults have antibody to all four types.

In children, illness with parainfluenza viruses occurs throughout the year, with seasonal increases in the winter and spring. Studies of institutional outbreaks suggest that type 3 virus spreads more rapidly than types 1 and 2. Heterotypic rises are frequent, with antibody to type 3 developing in half the cases with type 1 infection. In both children and adults, reinfection is frequent. In one outbreak, 96 percent of children without antibody, 67 percent with low levels, and 33 percent with high levels of antibody became infected. In adults, the disease is almost invariably a reinfection and, presumably for this reason, is much milder than in children.

The total contribution of parainfluenza infections to respiratory illness is quite variable, its frequency increasing in institutions in which general health status is lower than average and levels of sanitation and personal hygiene are less than optimum. In the United States, the percentage contribution of parainfluenza infections in several studies of children has varied from 4.3 to 17. The milder illness which occurs in adults has usually constituted less than 5 percent of respiratory illnesses.

CLINICAL MANIFESTATIONS. In all age groups, the incubation period appears to be 5 to 6 days. The disease is most serious in infants and children, the characteristic syndrome being laryngotracheobronchitis, or croup. In a study of croup in a large children's hospital, a third of the cases were due to parainfluenza infections. Much of the bronchiolitis, bronchitis, and bronchopneumonia in children was also caused by these agents. The average age of the children with croup was two years.

In older children the disease is less serious, usually without evidence of pulmonary involvment, and in adults, the virus produces a common cold syndrome with hoarseness and cough.

Fever is a constant feature of illness in children but is less frequent in adults. A description of selected febrile cases observed in a community outbreak appears in Table 206-4. Nasal discharge was a common occurrence at all ages, although this is not reflected in the small number of cases in the five- to fourteen-year age group described in the table. Cough and hoarseness were common, and stridor, indicative of croup, was present in many of the infants and children.

Table 206-4. CLINICAL FEATURES OF ILLNESS WITH PARAINFLUENZA VIRUSES

Clinical features	0–4 years, 14 cases, %	5–14 years, 7 cases, %	Adults, 11 cases, %
Fever	100	100	100
Cough	100	100	90
Hoarseness	92	86	72
Stridor	43	29	
Sore throat	36	71	72
Nasal discharge	64	28	56
Headache	7	43	72
Depression	...	...	45

SOURCE: Condensed from Banatvala et al., Brit. Med. J., 1:537, 1964.

Physical findings are not distinctive. The throat is reddened, with little or no exudate. There may be tender submandibular lymphadenopathy.

LABORATORY FINDINGS. In adult volunteers given type 2 virus, leukocyte counts were not abnormal. In children there is a considerable variation in leukocyte counts early in illness, making it difficult to distinguish this disease from pneumococcal and other bacterial infections. After a few days, however, leukocyte counts tend to become normal or low. Detailed studies of blood counts in proved cases have not been reported. No characteristic alterations have been reported in other laboratory indices such as liver or renal function tests, electrocardiograms, and urinalyses.

COURSE AND COMPLICATIONS. In children, *otitis media* has occurred as a complication more often with parainfluenza than with the other infections. It may be caused by pneumococci, streptococci, or *H. influenza.* The illness is characterized by slow resolution of pulmonary involvement and long persistence of cough and other symptoms. In very young or debilitated children, the outcome can be fatal. In adults, bacterial sinusitis may occur, and in persons with chronic bronchitis, emphysema, or bronchiectasis, the possibility of pulmonary bacterial superinfections should be considered.

TREATMENT. There is no specific treatment. Therapy is limited to symptomatic measures and efforts aimed at early detection and treatment of bacterial complications such as otitis media or pneumonia. Nursing care is important in pediatric cases, especially children with croup, and reference should be made to appropriate pediatric sources for procedures to be followed.

Table 206-5. RESPIRATORY ILLNESS ASSOCIATED WITH COXSACKIE VIRUS A AND B, ECHO VIRUS, AND POLIOVIRUS

Diagnosis	Description	Associated viruses
Herpangina..................	Febrile pharyngitis, anorexia, and discrete vesicular eruption on anterior faucial pillars. Occurs chiefly in children in summer and early fall outbreaks. Similar illnesses without eruption caused by the same viruses probably occur. An illness with nonulcerating nodules on anterior pillars caused by Coxsackie A 10 has also been described.	Coxsackie virus A 1 through 6, 8, 10, and 12
Febrile respiratory illness ("summer grippe")	Undifferentiated febrile illness marked by headache, sore throat, and anorexia occurring in summer or early fall. Includes epidemics in recruits of similar disease with Coxsackie A 21, in which illness patterns have been confirmed by experimental inoculation of volunteers.	Coxsackie virus A 21, 24, Coxsackie virus B 2, 3, 5 (?), ECHO virus 1, 3, 6, 19, 20, and polioviruses
Upper respiratory illness associated with gastroenteritis	Cases occurring largely in infants and exposed mothers.	ECHO virus 1, 11, 19, 20
Acute laryngotracheobronchitis (croup)	Winter outbreaks in nurseries and institutions. Association less definite than with other syndromes.	Coxsackie virus A 9, B 5, and ECHO virus 11
Pneumonitis and pleuritis......	Largely confined to young infants and children; of uncommon occurrence.	Coxsackie virus A 9, B 4, 5, ECHO virus 9, 19, 20

In adults, analgesics, antihistamines, and small doses of codeine for cough are generally sufficient.

PREVENTION. Vaccines against parainfluenza virus infections are not available. In hospitals, respiratory precautions should be carried out. At home, bed rest or room isolation during acute illness is advised, with special effort to avoid contact with very young children or aged persons.

COXSACKIE, ECHO, AND POLIOVIRUS INFECTIONS

Diseases produced by these agents are described in Chaps. 210 through 212 and 216. Table 206-5, however, summarizes the respiratory illnesses sometimes seen in infections by these viruses.

REFERENCES

General

Loosli, C. G. (Ed.): Conference on Newer Respiratory Disease Viruses, Am. Rev. Resp. Dis., 88(Suppl.):1–419, 1963

Adenoviruses

Bell, J. A., W. P. Rowe, J. I. Engler, R. H. Parrott, and R. J. Huebner: Pharyngoconjunctival Fever: Epidemiological Studies of a Recently Recognized Disease Entity, J.A.M.A., 157:1083, 1955.

Commission on Respiratory Diseases: Clinical Patterns of Undifferentiated and Other Acute Respiratory Diseases in Army Recruits, Medicine, 26:441, 1947.

Girardi, A. J., M. R. Hilleman, and R. E. Zwickey: Tests in Hamsters for Oncogenic Quality of Ordinary Viruses Including Adenovirus Type 7, Proc. Soc. Exp. Biol. Med., 115:1141, 1964.

Kasel, J. A., P. A. Banks, R. Wigand, V. Knight, and D. W. Alling: An Immunologic Classification of Heterotypic

Antibody Responses to Adenoviruses in Man, Proc. Soc. Exp. Biol. Med., 119:1162, 1965.

Ward, T. G., R. J. Huebner, W. P. Rowe, R. W. Ryan, and J. A. Bell: Production of Pharyngoconjunctival Fever in Human Volunteers Inoculated with APC Viruses, Science, 122:1086, 1955.

Coxsackie, Echo, and Polioviruses

Kibrick, S.: Current Status of Coxsackie and ECHO Viruses in Human Disease, pp. 27–70 in "Progress in Medical Virology, 6," J. L. Melnick (Ed.), Basel and New York, S. Karger AG, 1964.

Spickard, A., H. Evans, V. Knight, and K. Johnson: Acute Respiratory Disease in Normal Volunteers Associated with Coxsackie A-21 Viral Infection: III. Response to Nasopharyngeal and Enteric Inoculation, J. Clin. Invest., 42:840, 1963.

Parainfluenza Virus

Banatvala, J. E., T. B. Anderson, and B. B. Reiss: Parainfluenza Infections in the Community, Brit. Med. J., 1:537, 1964.

Chanock, R. M., R. H. Parrott, M. K. Cook, B. E. Andrews, J. A. Bell, T. Reichelderfer, A. Z. Kapikian, F. M. Mastra, and R. J. Huebner: Newly Recognized Myxoviruses from Children with Respiratory Disease, New Engl. J. Med., 258:207, 1958.

Johnson, K. M., R. M. Chanock, M. K. Cook, and R. J. Huebner: Studies of a New Human Hemadsorption Virus: I. Isolation, Properties, and Characterization, Am. J. Hyg., 71:81, 1960.

Respiratory Syncytial Virus

Kravetz, H. M., V. Knight, R. M. Chanock, J. A. Morris, K. M. Johnson, D. Rifkind, and J. P. Utz: Respiratory Syncytial Virus: III. Production of Illness and Clinical Observations in Adult Volunteers, J.A.M.A., 176:657, 1961.

McClelland, L., M. R. Hilleman, V. V. Hamparian, A. Keller, C. M. Reilly, D. Cornfeld, and J. Stokes, Jr.: Studies of

Acute Respiratory Illness Caused by Respiratory Syncytial Virus: 2. Epidemiology and Assessment of Importance, New Engl. J. Med., 264:1169, 1961.

Reilly, C. M., J. Stokes, Jr., L. McClelland, D. Cornfeld, V. V. Hamparian, A. Ketler, and M. Hilleman: Studies of Acute Respiratory Illness Caused by Respiratory Syncytial Virus: 3. Clinical and Laboratory Findings, New Engl. J. Med., 264:1176, 1961.

Rhinoviruses

Cate, T. R., R. B. Couch, and K. M. Johnson: Studies with Rhinoviruses in Volunteers: Production of Illness, Effect of Naturally Acquired Antibody, and Demonstration of a Protective Effect Not Associated with Serum Antibody, J. Clin. Invest., 43:56, 1964.

Hamparian, V. V., M. B. Leagus, M. R. Hilleman, and J. Stokes, Jr.: Epidemiologic Investigations of Rhinovirus Infections, Proc. Soc. Exp. Biol. Med., 117:469, 1964.

207 PNEUMONIA CAUSED BY MYCOPLASMA PNEUMONIAE

Vernon Knight

SYNONYMS. Primary atypical pneumonia, Eaton's agent pneumonia, cold agglutinin-positive pneumonia, "virus" pneumonia.

DEFINITION. Pneumonia caused by *Mycoplasma pneumoniae* is characterized by fever, pharyngitis, cough, and

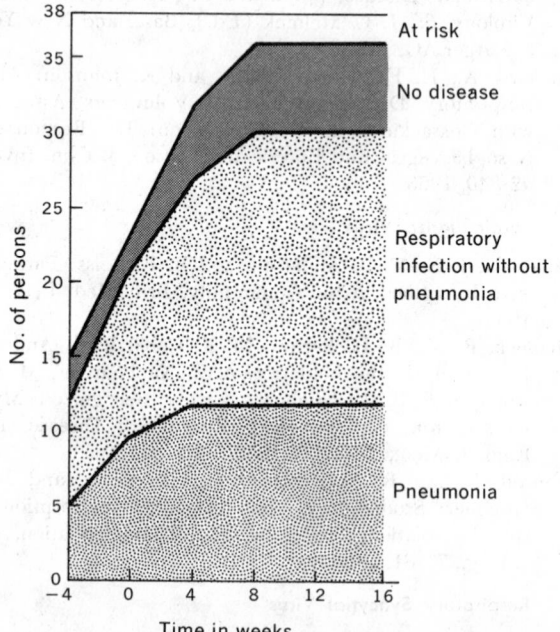

Fig. 207-1. Cumulative incidence of *M. pneumoniae* infection and clinical response in 38 exposed family members. The final case of pneumonia appeared 8 weeks after the first case. Respiratory infection without pneumonia continued to occur for 12 weeks after onset of the first case. This slow course of family spread is typical of such outbreaks. (*Balassanian and Robbins; N. Eng. J. Med., 277:719, 1967; with permission.*)

pulmonary infiltration, often multilobular, in which roentgenographic signs are more extensive than indicated by physical examination. This organism is also the cause of upper respiratory illness without pneumonia and of asymptomatic infection.

ETIOLOGY. *Mycoplasma pneumoniae*, one of several species of human and animal pleuropneumonia-like organisms (PPLO), is one of the smallest organisms (150 to 250 mμ) capable of replication in cell-free media. It lacks a cell wall, requires cholesterol for development of its limiting membrane (not a requirement for saprophyte types), and has exacting nutritional requirements. It grows on or beneath the surface of agar slants in a small, round, granular colony without the "fried egg" peripheral zone characteristic of many other PPLO. It is inhibited in vitro by tetracycline derivatives, streptomycin, kanamycin, erythromycin, oleandomycin, chloramphenicol, and gold salts. It is not inhibited by penicillin, sulfonamides, or thallium acetate. It is distinguished from other human mycoplasmas by rapid hemolysis of guinea pig erythrocytes and utilization of glucose and other sugars. It also hemolyzes human and rat erythrocytes. It may also be distinguished from other mycoplasmas by fluorescent antibody, complement fixation, growth inhibition, and indirect hemagglutination tests all of which are useful for serologic diagnosis of human infection. In addition to growth on agar, the organism grows on the surface of cells of embryonated eggs and monkey kidney cell culture with little evidence of cytopathic effect. In human cell cultures, however, there is intracellular growth with cytopathic effects.

EPIDEMIOLOGY. In the general population *M. Pneumoniae* infection is characterized by intrafamily spread. In most cases the infection is introduced into the family by a schoolchild. Once introduced, most family members become infected. The time course of the infection and associated illnesses in six involved families is described in Fig. 207-1. Spread through these families required about 8 weeks; pneumonia occurred in one-third of the infected family members. In family outbreaks, pneumonia occurs with greatest frequency among school-age children with a predominance in males. The disease is rare above age forty. *Mycoplasma pneumoniae* pneumonia occurs throughout the year, although prolonged wintertime outbreaks may occur in college groups or communities. The total incidence of *M. pneumoniae* pneumonia in a study in Seattle was 1.3/1,000/year, which constituted about 10 percent of pneumonia from all causes.

In the military, *M. pneumoniae* infections account for a small proportion of upper respiratory illness in recruits, in one study 6.3 percent. However, it accounted for almost one-half of cases of pneumonia in the same military population. The disease appears to be endemic at military bases, and onset of cases is greatest during the second to fifth months of training.

Mycoplasma pneumoniae is probably spread by means of infected respiratory secretions. The organisms can be cultured from sputum of naturally occurring cases and from volunteers inoculated artificially. Primary atypical pneumonia has been induced in volunteers both by nasopharyngeal inoculation and by inhalation of a small-particle aerosol containing the agent. Studies in volunteers reveal that naturally acquired antibody is associated with a high degree of resistance to infection.

CLINICAL MANIFESTATIONS. From studies in military recruits and normal volunteers, the incubation period appears to vary from 9 to 12 days. Illness due to *M. pneumoniae* usually begins with symptoms of upper respiratory illness, which, in a small percentage of cases, progresses to bronchitis and pneumonia. Cough is almost universal in pneumonia and is frequent in cases without pulmonary involvement. Blood-flecked sputum may occur in the more severe cases, but gross hemoptysis is rare. A variety of other respiratory and systemic complaints may occur. Fever, nasal congestion, and sore throat are common. Cervical adenopathy is not frequent. In pneumonia, harsh or diminished sounds are frequent but bronchial breathing is uncommon. Fine inspiratory rales are found in most patients but are not impressive. Pleural rubs and pleural effusion are infrequent. Studies on the distribution of pneumonia show frequent bilateral involvement in the lower lobes. Involvement of a single lower lobe is less common, and upper lobe involvement is rare. Pulmonary infiltrates may occur as an isolated area in the lung periphery but more often spread from the hilum.

The disease is variable in severity, but high fever may persist for 1 to 2 weeks in untreated cases. X-ray changes last for as long as 3 weeks in untreated cases, but for 7 to 10 days in treated cases. Even in untreated cases, complications are rare and consist of occasional purulent sinusitis, persistent cough, and, rarely, pleurisy. Prolonged weakness and malaise follow the untreated illness in adults.

Many features of naturally occurring illness are presented in a case of disease induced in a volunteer (Fig. 207-2). On day 10 after inoculation, temperature elevation was first noted; by day 12 the temperature was almost 40°C (104°F). Right lower lobar infiltration was detected on day 12. On day 13 a small area of infiltration was observed near the left cardiac border in the left lower lobe. Neither infiltrate was especially dense. Rapid recovery ensued with treatment with demethylchlortetracycline. There was no leukocytosis, but the sedimentation rate was increased on day 15 to 65 mm per hr. *Mycoplasma pneumoniae* was isolated from sputum specimens in tissue culture on four occasions. Fluorescent antibody increased from a nonmeasurable value to a serum dilution of 1:160 by day 24. Cold agglutinin titers increased from

S.m. 33YOW ♂

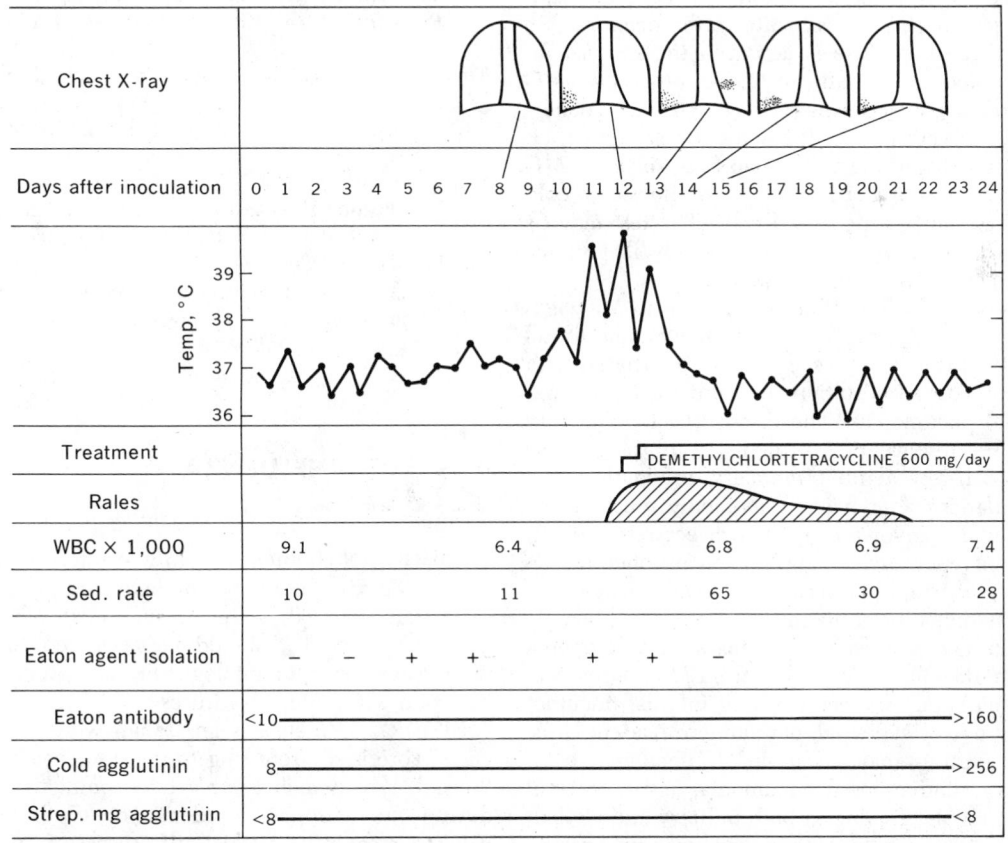

Fig. 207-2. Case of primary atypical pneumonia in a volunteer produced by inoculation with *Mycoplasma pneumoniae*. After an incubation period of about 10 days bilateral mild atypical pneumonia developed. Although the apparent response to treatment with demethylchlortetracycline in this case is not proof of drug effect, it is indicative of the favorable response seen in a large controlled study with this drug. (*Rifkind et al.: Rev. Resp. Dis., 85:479, 1962.*)

1:8 to 1:256. *Streptococcus MG* agglutinins did not appear. This patient also developed a hemorrhagic myringitis bilaterally, which healed promptly with recovery from pneumonia.

Ear involvement consisting of congestion of the tympanic membrane, bullous, and, rarely, hemorrhagic myringitis may occur in as many as 10 percent of cases, most often in children.

Studies with volunteers have revealed, in addition to pneumonia, the occurrence of febrile and afebrile upper respiratory illness characterized by nonexudative pharyngitis and tracheobronchitis, often associated with cough, headache, and nasal congestion. This disease persists for 1 to 2 weeks and is followed by uncomplicated recovery. This is a common manifestation of *M. pneumoniae* infection in the general population at all ages.

LABORATORY FINDINGS. During acute illness leukocytosis in the range of 10,000 to 15,000 per cu mm occurs in about 25 percent of cases. Increase in sedimentation rate above 40 mm per hr occurs in at least two-thirds of cases. Urinalysis, electrocardiograms, and fluid and electrolyte and liver function studies show no characteristic changes. The complement fixation, fluorescent antibody, indirect hemagglutination, and growth inhibition tests all yield highly specific diagnostic information. The simplicity of the complement fixation test recommends it for general use. Fourfold rises in titer often occur within 2 weeks, and maximum rise is achieved in 4 weeks. In atypical pneumonia, agglutinins to *Streptococcus MG* have been reported to develop in varying frequency. Higher titers are correlated with more severe illness. Of probably greater diagnostic value than *Streptococcus MG* agglutination is the appearance late in illness of cold agglutinins for human, type O red cells. The test may be positive in as high as 90 percent of severely ill patients but is less often positive in nonpneumonic cases.

DIFFERENTIAL DIAGNOSIS. Pneumonia due to *M. pneumoniae* is to be distinguished from pneumonia of all other types. It is usually less severe and is associated with less dense pulmonary infiltration than pneumococcal and other bacterial pneumonias. The discovery of pulmonary infiltrate in the absence of symptoms or physical signs may initially suggest acute pulmonary tuberculosis. In military populations adenovirus pneumonia must be excluded. Pneumonic involvement as a direct result of influenza viral infection or its complication by pneumococcal, streptococcal, staphylococcal, or *H. influenza* infection may cause difficulty in diagnosis. Q fever, psittacosis, and tularemia are less frequent causes of pneumonia which may be difficult to distinguish from *M. pneumoniae* infection. In children, especially young infants, pneumonia due to respiratory syncytial, parainfluenza, adenovirus, and influenza viruses may resemble *M. pneumoniae* infection. Cases of undiagnosed pneumonia, despite careful workup, are a regular finding in both military and civilian populations, suggesting that other causes of pneumonia remain to be discovered.

TREATMENT. Demethylchlortetracycline and other tetracycline derivatives, erythromycin, and triacetyloleandomycin are effective in treatment of pneumonia due to *M. pneumoniae*. Demethylchlortetracycline may be given to adults in daily doses of 0.9 Gm; tetracycline, 1.5 Gm; erthromycin stearate or ethyl succinate, 1.5 and 1.2 Gm per day, respectively. Response to treatment is characterized by prompt defervescence, rapid clearing of x-ray signs of pneumonia, and disappearance of malaise and weakness. Persistent cough, despite treatment, is a relatively common finding, especially in women.

Treatment temporarily reduces the frequency of positive cultures from the respiratory tract, but shedding may continue for several weeks after treatment, a finding similar to that in psittacosis pneumonia. Relapse of *M. pneumoniae* pneumonia occurs occasionally following treatment, but such cases respond to retreatment.

PREVENTION. Although antibody is apparently highly protective, effective vaccines are not yet available. For patients in the hospital respiratory precautions are advisable during the first day or so of treatment. Acutely ill patients at home should be isolated from very young children and persons in whom a complicating respiratory illness would constitute a special hazard.

REFERENCES

Foy, H. M., J. T. Grayston, G. E. Kenny, E. R. Alexander, and Ruth McMahan: Epidemiology of *Mycoplasma Pneumoniae* Infection in Families, J.A.M.A., 197:137, 1966.

Kingston, J. R., R. M. Chanock, M. A. Mufson, L. P. Hellman, W. D. James, H. H. Fox, M. A. Manko, and J. Boyers: Eaton Agent Pneumonia, J.A.M.A., 176:118, 1961.

Mogabgab, W. J.: *Mycoplasma Pneumoniae*, and Adenovirus Respiratory Illnesses in Military and University Personnel, 1959–1966, Am. Rev. Resp. Dis., 97:345, 1968.

Rifkind, D., R. Chanock, H. Kravetz, K. Johnson, and V. Knight: Ear Involvement (Myringitis) and Primary Atypical Pneumonia Following Inoculation of Volunteers with Eaton Agent, Am. Rev. Resp. Dis., 85:479, 1962.

208 INFLUENZA
Robert R. Wagner

DEFINITION. Influenza is an acute respiratory infection of specific viral etiology characterized by sudden onset of headache, myalgia, fever, and prostration. The terms *influenza* and "flu" should be restricted to those cases with clear-cut epidemiologic or laboratory evidence of infection with influenza viruses.

HISTORY. Influenza is an Italian word meaning "influence" (originally referring to the influence of the stars or the cold), which first came into common English usage during the European epidemic of 1743. In most non-English-speaking countries, the disease is referred to by the French word "grippe," or its equivalent. According to the best available records, influenza was uncommon in Europe during the nineteenth century until the pandemic of 1889. Subsequently, the frequency and severity of epidemics increased, culminating in the disastrous pandemic of 1918, which caused an estimated 20 to 40 million deaths. The isolation of the causative virus in 1933 by Smith, Andrewes, and Laidlaw led to the development of simple diagnostic tests, which have greatly advanced knowledge of the disease. The pandemic of 1957 was, perhaps, the most thoroughly studied and documented major epidemic in the annals of medicine.

ETIOLOGY. There are three distinct antigenic types of influenza virus, designated A, B, and C, in the order in which they were discovered. Infection with one type confers no immunity to infection with the other two. They are all approximately 100 mμ in diameter, visible as spheres or filaments by electron microscopy, and are biologically related by their infectivity for chick embryos, capacity to agglutinate erythrocytes, and affinity for the respiratory epithelium of various mammals. Influenza viruses are the prototypes of the myxovirus group and are related to the larger paramyxoviruses, which include mumps, Newcastle disease, measles, and the parainfluenza viruses. These viruses are composed of a helical ribonucleoprotein core wound up in a lipid-containing envelope from which protrude protein spikes that serve as attachment organs and principal antigenic sites.

EPIDEMIOLOGY. Influenza B and C usually occur sporadically or in localized outbreaks, particularly in schools and military camps. Influenza A viruses are the cause of major epidemics which tend to recur at intervals of 2 to 4 years in the winter months. The factors responsible for this periodicity are the decline in effective immunity of a population in interepidemic periods and the emergence every few years of new strains of virus. A marked change in the antigenicity of type A viruses occurred in 1946–1947, when viruses extant between 1933 and 1945 completely disappeared and were replaced by strains designated as influenza A' or A$_1$.

A further alteration in the serotype of influenza A viruses was detected in China early in 1957. These A$_2$ or "Asian" influenza viruses were widely disseminated in the Orient in the following spring, giving rise to the pandemic of 1957. On the basis of laboratory studies and international epidemic intelligence, accurate predictions were made within a month of the first outbreaks in East Asia that influenza would spread throughout the world. A second pandemic wave occurred early in 1958, and major epidemics of the same type recurred in the winter of 1959–1960. Since the pandemic of 1957, virtually everyone in urban populations has acquired antibody to A$_2$ influenza virus. A new antigenic variant of influenza virus appeared in Asia in 1968 and has tentatively been designated A$_3$.

Influenza A epidemics start abruptly, reach a peak in 2 to 3 months, and subside almost as rapidly. The attack rate is variable but was noted in 1957 to exceed 50 percent of urban populations. An additional 25 percent of individuals may show serologic evidence of infection without clinical manifestations. Experiences in 1957 proved conclusively that crowding, even in summer months or in tropical countries, is the major factor predisposing to epidemics. Schoolchildren, in particular, are the primary focus and disseminators of infection in the United States. The end of summer recess in September brings a highly susceptible population into close proximity and facilitates rapid spread. If the general immunity of a population is at low levels, community-wide epidemics may occur within a few weeks of the opening of schools. If, on the other hand, immune individuals predominate, the case rate will rise slowly and may not reach epidemic proportions, or may do so later in the winter.

PATHOGENESIS. Influenza is primarily an infection of the respiratory epithelium that is transmitted from man to man by inhalation of infective droplet nuclei. Influenza A viruses have been recovered in nature from swine and horses, but these animals probably do not transmit the infection to man. Detailed experimental studies of the pathogenesis of the disease have been made in ferrets and mice. After intranasal inoculation, the virus multiplies to maximum titers in 24 to 48 hr and rapidly involves the entire tracheobronchial tree. At first, the mucosa becomes boggy and hyperemic and loses its normal ciliary activity. This may shortly be followed by necrosis of respiratory epithelium, invasion by leukocytes, pulmonary consolidation, and abnormal regeneration of metaplastic squamous epithelium in the bronchi and bronchioles. The infection is largely confined to the respiratory tract and hilar lymph nodes of adult animals; viremia is a transient and inconstant feature. However, virus has been isolated from heart, kidney, and other extrapulmonary tissues in fatal human infections, suggesting that virus products can enter the circulation and may account for systemic manifestations of the disease.

The findings at autopsy are pulmonary hemorrhages, necrosis of bronchial epithelium, bronchiolitis, squamous metaplasia of respiratory epithelium, and marked edema of alveolar septums and spaces. Fatal human infections can be caused by the influenza virus itself or by combined viral and bacterial infections.

MANIFESTATIONS. The disease assumes its typical form during major epidemics of influenza A, but clinical differentiation between influenza A and B is not possible in localized outbreaks. Sporadic infections with either influenza A or B are likely to result in relatively minor illnesses, with predominantly respiratory symptoms, similar to those of common respiratory disease (Chap. 206). Influenza C is particularly difficult to recognize because of its mildness. Although the manifestations and severity of influenza A vary from year to year, cases in a single epidemic often follow a remarkably similar pattern. The clinical description that follows is a composite picture of epidemic influenza A of the past three decades.

The *incubation period* is usually 18 to 36 hr but may be as long as 3 days. Mild prodomal symptoms of cough, malaise, and chilliness are sometimes present, but extremely sudden onset is often such a characteristic feature that many patients can recall its exact time. The most common initial symptom is severe generalized or frontal *headache*, frequently accompanied by stabbing retroorbital pain that is accentuated by lateral or upward gaze. Diffuse *myalgia*, particularly marked in the legs and over the lumbosacral area, occurs in more than half the cases.

Pain and spasm of the abdominal muscles may simulate acute peritonitis, and incapacitating periarticular pains are sometimes confused with acute arthritis. *Feverishness* and *chilliness,* or occasionally true rigors, may be the first manifestations, but more often they are preceded by headache and myalgia. The temperature rises abruptly to a maximum of 100 to 103°F several hours after onset; rarely it may reach 106°F. Thereafter, the fever and pain usually subside over a 2- to 3-day period but may persist for as long as a week. A common variant in the temperature course is rapid defervescence after the initial peak, with a secondary rise to the original level on the following day. In general, severity of illness parallels the height and duration of the fever. The pulse rate is usually slow in relation to the fever, but marked tachycardia may occur in severely ill patients.

Prostration of some degree is almost invariable and is often the most prominent and alarming manifestation. The face is flushed, and the skin is hot and dry; however, profuse sweating and cold, mottled extremities are sometimes noted. Anorexia, nausea, and constipation are frequent secondary symptoms, but vomiting and diarrhea are rare. There is no evidence that influenza viruses infect the gastrointestinal tract, and the term *intestinal flu* is a misnomer. Meningoencephalitis, polyneuritis, cranial nerve palsies, transient nerve deafness, aphasia, hemiplegia, psychoses, and other neurologic disorders have been described in association with influenza but are very unusual. Hypotension, heart block, peripheral vasoconstriction, and fatal myocarditis have also been reported in a few cases. The exact relationship of these neurologic and cardiovascular disorders to influenza viral infection has not been determined. The incidence of abortion appears to be increased when influenza occurs during the first trimester of pregnancy.

Respiratory symptoms may be present at the onset but become most prominent when the systemic manifestations and fever begin to subside. They are frequently less pronounced than in common respiratory disease and may be entirely absent. Sneezing, watery nasal discharge, or stuffy nose occurs in most cases; hoarseness and epistaxis are less frequent. Conjunctival suffusion and burning, and itching, watery eyes are often noted. The throat may feel dry, and the pharynx often appears slightly injected. *Cough* develops during the course of the illness in more than three-fourths of the cases, and in about a third of these it is productive of small amounts of tenacious, mucoid sputum. *Chest pain,* usually substernal in location and accentuated by coughing but not by breathing, is present in almost half the patients. Pleurisy and pleural effusion are uncommon. Slight hyperpnea is often noted, but the most ominous, although infrequent, signs are dyspnea and cyanosis, which signal bronchiolar or pneumonic involvement. Physical examination of the lungs is often negative in uncomplicated influenza, but scattered rhonchi, wheezes, and showers of moist rales have been reported in 5 to 40 percent of cases in different epidemics. Influenzal bronchiolitis should be suspected if rales persist in the absence of x-ray evidence of pneumonitis and if the patient raises mucopurulent or blood-tinged sputum.

The chief *complications* of influenza are secondary bacterial infections of the paranasal sinuses, middle ear, bronchi, and lungs. The incidence of bacterial pneumonia is greatly increased during influenza epidemics; even mild or asymptomatic infections with influenza viruses predispose to pneumococcal and other types of pneumonia. The most serious complication is staphylococcal pneumonia, which tends to run a fulminant, often fatal, course.

During the 1958 epidemic a fulminating pneumonia characterized by severe dyspnea and cyanosis, scanty sputum containing gross blood, leukopenia, scanty physical findings in the lung in the face of large perihilar infiltrates, and a rapidly fatal course was described. Although staphylococci were isolated from the sputum, these patients failed to respond to appropriate antimicrobials. Furthermore, influenza virus was cultured from the lungs of some patients, suggesting that influenza virus rather than secondary bacterial infection played the major role in producing lung damage. In subsequent epidemics, this type of "influenza pneumonia" has been rare. Superinfection with *Hemophilus influenzae*, so common in the pandemic of 1918, is rarely encountered now.

Recovery from uncomplicated influenza is often complete in 2 to 3 days or, occasionally, in a week, but convalescence may be prolonged by "postinfectious asthenia" and depression, particularly in elderly persons. Minor relapses with fever can occur but are uncommon.

The *mortality* rate from all causes always increases markedly during epidemics of influenza. In the fall and winter of 1957–1958 it was estimated that 40 million persons in the United States became ill with influenza and the total numbers of influenza-associated deaths was reported to be in excess of 8,000. In addition, approximately 60,000 more deaths from various causes occurred during this period than would be expected under normal conditions. The greatest incidence of excess mortality occurred among infants under one year of age and adults over sixty years of age. Data from small series of cases clearly indicate that influenza is frequently fatal in individuals with preexisting pulmonary or cardiac disease, regardless of age. Chronic rheumatic heart disease with mitral stenosis, in particular, appears to predispose to fatal influenzal pneumonia.

LABORATORY FINDINGS. Virus is isolated most readily during the acute phase of the disease by inoculation of broth garglings into the amniotic cavity of chick embryos or into tissue cultures of monkey kidney or human cells. Serologic diagnosis can be made most reliably by hemagglutination-inhibition or complement fixation tests, using paired serum samples obtained in both the acute and convalescent phases. However, type-specific antibody against soluble complement-fixing antigens of influenza A virus often appears in the circulation of patients during the acute illness.

X-ray of the lungs in uncomplicated influenza is usually normal but occasionally reveals increased vascular markings, basilar streaking, small areas of patchy infiltration, atelectasis, nodular densities, or pleural effusion. The blood leukocyte count may be low 2 to 4 days after onset of illness, but is often normal or slightly elevated.

Leukocytosis with counts above 15,000 cells per cu mm indicates secondary bacterial infection, but leukopenia can occur in severe staphylococcal pneumonia. Slight proteinuria is common during the height of the febrile illness.

DIFFERENTIAL DIAGNOSIS. Many bacterial and viral infections simulate influenza at their onset, but few febrile diseases have such a self-limited course. The pattern of clinical manifestations becomes readily apparent during an epidemic, but many influenza outbreaks are associated with an increased incidence of other respiratory infection of viral and bacterial etiology. Noninfluenzal respiratory diseases (Chap. 206) are generally characterized by more gradual onset, milder systemic manifestations, and predominant symptoms of coryza, rhinorrhea, pharyngitis, and conjunctivitis.

TREATMENT. Antibiotics do not affect the course of uncomplicated influenza, nor is there any evidence that they prevent complications. Specific chemotherapy should be reserved for secondary bacterial infections. Clinical trials have shown some effectiveness of adamantanamine hydrochloride, a symmetrical amine which inhibits cellular penetration of influenza virus, as a chemoprophylactic agent, but the results are not impressive. Codeine affords relief from incapacitating cough and is more effective than salicylates for symptomatic treatment of headache and myalgia; salicylates often increase discomfort by causing drenching sweats and chills. Bed rest and gradual return to full activity are advisable.

PROPHYLAXIS. Formalinized egg vaccines containing a mixture of influenza A, A_1, A_2, and B viruses are the standard preparations available commercially in the United States. The British favor the use of a monovalent vaccine presently prepared from a more concentrated suspension of influenza A_2 virus. Infectious attenuated virus administered intranasally has been widely used for influenza immunization in the Soviet Union, but its safety and efficacy have not been proved. The most promising results have been obtained in the American Armed Forces by preliminary trials of adjuvant influenza vaccines emulsified with mineral oil and Arlacel A. Although they stimulate the production of serum antibodies, the prophylactic value of influenza vaccines is limited by the following factors: (1) infection can occur in spite of high levels of serum antibody; (2) antibody concentration is low at the site of infection in the respiratory tract; (3) vaccines sometimes do not contain antigens prepared from the most recent strains of virus; and (4) even under optimal conditions, their protective effect often lasts for only a few months.

The U.S. Public Health Service strongly recommends routine yearly immunization with polyvalent influenza vaccine for high-risk groups, including persons of all ages who suffer from chronic rheumatic heart disease, other cardiovascular diseases, chronic bronchopulmonary diseases, diabetes mellitus, or Addison's disease; also pregnant women and persons sixty-five years of age, or older, regardless of their previous state of health. For initial immunization it is advisable to administer the vaccine subcutaneously in two divided doses of 1 ml each, the first injection in September and the second several weeks or months later. A single subcutaneous dose of 1 ml given each autumn is satisfactory as a yearly booster. Intradermal injection of vaccine is far less satisfactory because a sufficient antigenic mass cannot be administered by this route.

Influenza vaccination is generally safe but not completely innocuous. Fatal anaphylactic reactions and purpura have been reported in individuals sensitive to egg proteins, and inactivated virus itself is pyrogenic and can sometimes produce an illness similar to active influenza. Influenza vaccine should be administered only advisedly and in much smaller doses to infants and young children, in whom severe febrile reactions may result in convulsions and death. Most influenza vaccines are contaminated with bacterial pyrogens. Large-scale purification of virus by zonal centrifugation shows considerable promise for production of vaccines from pure viral antigens.

REFERENCES

Davenport, F. M.: Factors of Importance in the Control of Influenza, Med. Clin. N. Am., 47:1185, 1963.

Loosli, C. G. (Ed.): Proceedings of the International Conference on Asian Influenza, Bethesda, Maryland, February, 1960, Am. Rev. Resp. Dis., 93:2, February, 1961.

Louria, D. B., H. L. Blumenfeld, J. T. Ellis, E. D. Kilbourne, and D. E. Rogers: Studies on Influenza in the Pandemic of 1957–1958: II. Pulmonary Complications of Influenza, J. Clin. Invest., 38:213, 1959.

Petersdorf, R. G., J. J. Fusco, D. R. Harter, and W. S. Albrink: Pulmonary Infections Complicating Asian Influenza, Arch. Intern. Med., 103:262, 1959.

Reimer, C. B., R. S. Baker, R. M. van Frank, T. E. Newlin, G. B. Cline, and N. G. Anderson: Purification of Large Quantities of Influenza Virus by Density Gradient Centrifugation, J Virol., 1:1207, 1967.

Zhdanov, V. M., V. D. Solov'ev, and F. G. Epshtein: "The Study of Influenza; A Translation from the Russian *Ucheniye o Grippe*," Public Health Service Publ. 792, Bethesda, Md., U.S. Department of Health, Education, and Welfare, 1960.

209 PSITTACOSIS
Vernon Knight

DEFINITION. Psittacosis is an infectious disease of birds caused by an organism that has a number of properties in common with gram-negative bacteria. Transmission of infection from birds to man results in a febrile illness characterized by pneumonitis and systemic manifestations. Inapparent infections or mild influenza-like illnesses may also occur. The term *ornithosis* is sometimes applied to infections contracted from birds other than parrots or parakeets, but *psittacosis* is the preferred generic term for all forms of the disease.

ETIOLOGY. The causative agent *Chlamydia psittaci* is a gram-negative obligate intracellular parasite, formerly classified as a virus. Now, along with the rickettsias, it may be considered specialized bacteria. The chlamydias, like rickettsias, synthesize RNA and DNA, reproduce by binary fission, and are susceptible to antimicrobial drugs. In contrast to rickettsias, the chlamydias are dependent on their hosts for metabolic energy. During intracellular growth, the chlamydias exhibit a large (1 μ) replicating form without a rigid cell wall, from which small (0.3 to 0.4 μ) infectious forms with a rigid cell wall are derived. The cell walls are thinner than those of bacteria, contain murein, and have a high lipid content characteristic of gram-negative bacteria. Recently, slight but definite homology of the DNA of members of the *Chlamydia* genus with the DNA of *Neisseria meningitidis* was shown. The psittacosis agent is the prototype of a biologically and antigenically homogenous class of microorganisms that includes the causative agents of lymphogranuloma venereum, trachoma, and 30 or more mammalian parasites which rarely produce human disease.

EPIDEMIOLOGY. Psittacosis is widely distributed throughout the world, and almost any avian species can harbor the agent. Psittacine birds are most commonly infected, but human cases have been traced to contact with pigeons, ducks, turkeys, chickens, and many other birds. Psittacosis may be considered an occupational disease of pet-shop owners, poultry raisers, pigeon fanciers, taxidermists, and zoo attendants. The incidence of human infection in the United States rose steadily from 1930, owing in large measure to the increasing popularity of parrots and parakeets as pets and, as subsequently recognized, transmission of infection by barnyard fowl and pigeons. The number of reported cases reached a peak in 1956 and gradually declined thereafter. By 1963 the disease had again become relatively uncommon coincident with acceptance of control measures such as incorporation of tetracyclines in poultry feed.

The agent is present in nasal secretions, excreta, tissues, and feathers of infected birds. Although the disease can be fatal, infected birds frequently show only minor evidences of illness such as ruffled feathers, lethargy, and anorexia. Asymptomatic avian carriers are common, and complete recovery may be followed by continued shedding of the organism for many months.

Psittacosis is almost always transmitted to man by the respiratory route. On rare occasions the disease may be acquired from the bite of a pet bird. Intimate and prolonged contact is not essential for transmission of the disease; a few minutes spent in an environment previously occupied by an infected bird has resulted in human infection. The severity of the disease in man bears no apparent relationship to closeness or duration of contact. Human-to-human transmission of a psittacosis-like agent has occurred particularly among hospital personnel, with severe and sometimes fatal infections. There is evidence that these "human" strains are more virulent than native avian organisms. There is no record of infection acquired by eating poultry products.

PATHOGENESIS. The psittacosis agent gains entrance to the body through the upper part of the respiratory tract and eventually localizes in the pulmonary alveoli and the reticuloendothelial cells of the spleen and liver. Invasion of the lung parenchyma probably takes place by way of the bloodstream rather than by direct extension from the upper air passages. A lymphocytic inflammatory response occurs on both the interstitial and respiratory surfaces of the alveoli as well as in the perivascular spaces. The alveoli walls and interstitial tissues of the lung are thickened, edematous, necrotic, and occasionally hemorrhagic. Histologically, the affected areas show alveolar spaces filled with fluid, erythrocytes, and lymphocytes. The picture is not pathognomonic of psittacosis unless macrophages containing characteristic cytoplasmic inclusion bodies (LCL bodies) can be identified. The respiratory epithelium of the bronchi and bronchioles usually remains intact.

MANIFESTATIONS. The clinical manifestations and course of psittacosis are extremely variable. After an *incubation period* of 7 to 14 days, or longer, the disease may start abruptly with shaking chills and high fever, but the onset is often gradual with increasing fever and malaise over a 3- to 4-day period. Headache is almost always a prominent symptom; it is usually diffuse and excruciating and often the patient's chief complaint. Generalized myalgia is also common. Spasm and stiffness of the muscles of the back and neck may lead to an erroneous diagnosis of meningitis. A faint, macular rash (Horder's spots) simulating the rose spots of typhoid fever has been described. Lethargy, mental depression, agitation, insomnia, and disorientation have been prominent features of the illness in some epidemics, but not in others; delirium and stupor occur near the end of the first week in severe cases. Occasional patients are comatose when first seen, and the diagnosis of psittacosis may be missed in this circumstance. Gastrointestinal complaints such as abdominal pain, nausea, vomiting, or diarrhea are present in some cases; constipation and abdominal distension sometimes occur as late complications. Icterus, the result of severe hepatic involvement, is a rare and ominous finding. Symptoms of infection of the upper part of the respiratory tract are not prominent, although mild sore throat, pharyngeal injection, and cervical adenopathy are often present; and on occasion may be the only manifestation of illness. Epistaxis is encountered early in the course of nearly one-fourth of the cases. Photophobia is also a common complaint.

A dry, hacking cough is characteristic of psittacosis; it is usually nonproductive, but small amounts of mucoid or bloody sputum may be raised as the disease progresses. Cough may appear early in the course of the disease or as late as 5 days after the onset of fever. Chest pain, pleurisy with effusion, or a friction rub may all occur but are not usual. Pericarditis and myocarditis have been reported. Most patients have a normal or slightly increased respiratory rate; marked dyspnea with cyanosis occurs only in severe psittacosis with extensive pulmonary involvement. In psittacosis, as in most nonbacterial pneumonias, the physical signs of pneumonitis tend to be less prominent than symptoms and x-ray findings would suggest. The initial examination may reveal fine, sibilant rales, or clinical evidence of pneumonia may be completely lacking. Rales usually become audible and more numerous as the illness progresses. Signs of frank pulmonary consolidation are usually absent.

Patients without cough or other clinical evidence of respiratory involvement present the problem of a fever of unknown origin. The pulse rate in psittacosis is slow in relation to the fever. When splenomegaly is present in a patient with acute pneumonitis, psittacosis should be considered. Inability to feel the spleen is of no diagnostic significance, however; the reported incidence of splenomegaly has ranged from 10 to 70 percent in different series of proved cases. Nontender hepatic enlargement also occurs, but jaundice is rare. Thrombophlebitis is not unusual during convalescence; indeed, pulmonary infarction is sometimes a late complication and may be fatal.

In untreated cases of psittacosis, sustained or mildly remittent fever persists for 10 days to 3 weeks, or occasionally as long as 3 months. Defervescence is by lysis, rarely by crisis, and is accompanied by abatement of respiratory manifestations. Psittacosis contracted from parrots or parakeets is more likely to be a severe, prolonged illness than infections acquired from pigeons or barnyard fowl. Relapses occur but are rare. Secondary bacterial infections are uncommon. Immunity to reinfection is probably permanent.

LABORATORY FINDINGS. The x-ray of the lungs in psittacosis mimics a great variety of pulmonary diseases. The pneumonic lesions are usually patchy in appearance but can be hazy, diffuse, homogeneous, lobar, atelectatic, wedge-shaped, nodular, or miliary. The white blood cell count is normal or moderately decreased in the acute phase of the disease but may rise in convalescence. The erythrocyte sedimentation rate is frequently not elevated. Transient proteinuria is common. The cerebrospinal fluid sometimes contains a few mononuclear cells but is otherwise normal. Cold agglutinins are rarely present in the serum of patients with psittacosis.

The diagnosis of psittacosis can be confirmed only by isolation of the causative microorganism or serologic studies. The agent is present in the blood during the acute phase of the disease and in the bronchial secretions for weeks or sometimes years after infection, but it is often difficult to isolate. Psittacosis is most readily diagnosed by the demonstration of a rising titer of complement-fixing antibody in the patient's blood. An acute

and convalescent specimen should always be tested. Even a low titer of antibody during the acute febrile phase constitutes presumptive evidence of psittacosis. The prompt initiation of treatment with tetracycline has been shown to delay antibody rise in convalescence for several weeks or months. Interpretation of a single complement fixation test may sometimes be difficult because of the antigenic cross reaction between the agents of psittacosis and lymphogranuloma venereum.

DIFFERENTIAL DIAGNOSIS. A history of exposure to birds may be the only clinical basis for differentiating psittacosis from a great variety of infectious and noninfectious febrile disorders. A partial list of pneumonic diseases that may be confused with psittacosis includes primary atypical pneumonia, Q fever, coccidioidomycosis, tuberculosis, carcinoma of the lung with bronchial obstruction, and bacterial pneumonias. In the early stages, before pneumonitis appears, psittacosis may be mistaken for influenza, typhoid fever, miliary tuberculosis, infectious mononucleosis and, less commonly, rheumatic fever or bacterial endocarditis.

TREATMENT. The tetracyclines are consistently effective in the treatment of psittacosis. Defervescence and alleviation of symptoms usually occur in 24 to 48 hr after instituting therapy with 2 Gm daily. To avoid relapse, treatment should probably be continued for at least 7 days after defervescence. The disease will usually respond to penicillin if a daily dose of at least 2 million units is used. In severe cases, oxygen and other supportive measures are indicated.

REFERENCES

Meyer, K. F.: The Ecology of Psittacosis and Ornithosis, Medicine, 21:175, 1942.

——: Psittacosis-Lymphogranuloma Venereum Agents, pp. 1006–1041 in "Viral and Rickettsial Infections of Man," 4th ed., F. L. Horsfall, Jr., and I. Tamm (Eds.), Philadelphia, J. B. Lippincott Company, 1965.

Moulder, J. W.: "The Life and Death of the Psittacosis Virus," Hosp. Practice, June, 1968.

Seibert, R. H., W. S. Jordan, Jr., and J. H. Dingle: Clinical Variations in the Diagnosis of Psittacosis, New Engl. J. Med., 254:925, 1956.

—— et al.: Epidemiological Studies of Psittacosis in Cleveland, Am. J. Hyg., 63:28, 1956.

Section 15

Enteric Viruses

INTRODUCTION

A. Martin Lerner

It has been more than two decades since Dalldorf and Sickles isolated the first Coxsackie viruses by inoculating

suspensions of feces from two children with paralytic poliomyelitis into suckling mice. Subsequently some 67 enteroviruses, including polio-, Coxsackie, and ECHO viruses, have been shown to multiply in the human gastrointestinal tract (see Table). Enteroviruses have been recovered where attempts have been made; their distribution appears global. With notable exceptions such as Coxsackie virus A, type 21, and ECHO virus, type 28 (which are predominantly respiratory pathogens and are only incidentally isolated from feces), enteroviruses, like salmonellas, periodically multiply within the human alimentary canal and sometimes concomitantly produce disease. Available information suggests there is no "normal" enteric virus flora. In addition to enteroviruses, adenoviruses (Chap. 206) and reoviruses (Chap. 214) are

CLASSIFICATION OF ENTEROVIRUSES

I. Picornaviruses of human origin
    A. Enteroviruses
        1. Polioviruses (3 types)*
        2. Coxsackie virus A (24 types)
        3. Coxsackie virus B (6 types)
        4. ECHO viruses (34 types)†
    B. Rhinoviruses (see Chap. 206)
    C. Unclassified
II. Picornaviruses of lower animals

* Typing is by neutralization of infectivity with immune serums in either suitable tissue cultures or suckling mice.

† ECHO virus, type 10, has been reclassified as belonging to another taxonomic group, now known as reoviruses.

commonly recovered from stools.

Coxsackie viruses are named for the village of Coxsackie on the banks of the Hudson River in the State of New York, where the first isolations were made. ECHO viruses are descriptively named: *E*, for their *enteric* residence; *C*, the filterable agents produced *cytopathic* effects in tissue cultures of rhesus kidney; *H*, *human*; *O*, *orphan*, indicating that their relationship to disease remained to be established. They were viruses "in search of a disease." It is increasingly evident that a wide variety of illnesses may result from enterovirus infections. As observations accumulate, the list of these illnesses is continually being refined (see table on page 963). Etiologic associations are difficult to establish because they require virologic, serologic, epidemiologic, and volunteer studies. Moreover, these are viruses often isolated from the pharynx or anus, where they multiply without causing significant injury to tissues. More meaningful are isolations from blood, vesicular fluids of patients with rashes, urine, cerebrospinal fluid, or tissues taken by biopsy or at autopsy. Coxsackie or ECHO viruses have been recovered from lung, heart, pericardial fluid, liver, spleen, testicle, kidney, muscle, and brain.

CHARACTERISTICS OF THE VIRUSES. Enteroviruses consist of a ribonucleic acid core surrounded by a capsid of protein. The outer coat determines species, tissue, and age specificities as well as antigenic quality. The RNA of the virus within infected cells transcribes and translates its own genetic information independent of the host DNA. Particle diameters are 15 to 30 mμ. Enteroviruses are quite stable in acid and in lipid solvents. They can be protected from thermal inactivation by certain cations.

When inoculated into suckling mice, group A Cox-

sackie viruses induce primarily an inflammatory myositis, whereas group B viruses cause lesions of the central nervous system and other viscera. Coxsackie virus B and ECHO viruses are cytopathogenic for cultures of monkey kidney cells, but this is not the case for Coxsackie viruses of group A. These distinctions are not invariable. Type 6 and type 9 ECHO viruses have been adapted to produce lesions in baby mice. Some strains agglutinate human erythrocytes obtained from adult or umbilical cord blood. None of the Coxsackie or ECHO viruses have been adapted to grow in embryonated eggs.

EPIDEMIOLOGY. Fecal-oral contact is the usual method of contagion and toddlers often bring enteroviruses into a household. Personal hygiene inhibits the infectious cycle. Insects may act as passive vectors. ECHO virus, type 6, can multiply in the gastrointestinal tracts of dogs. This has not been noted with other Coxsackie or ECHO viruses, and with ECHO virus 6 canine to human transmission has not been demonstrated. Respiratory transmission by droplets or their nuclei also occurs.

The incubation period is 2 to 5 days. Multiple concurrent infections within a family are not unusual. Clinical manifestations of infection vary within the family and community. For example, a two- or three-year-old child may have a mild fever with rash, while an older sibling may suffer from pleurodynia, myocarditis, or one of a number of syndromes heralding involvement of the central nervous system (see table on page 963). The mechanism of the variation in expression of enterovirus disease is not well understood, but may relate to developmental changes in the numbers or availability of specific receptors at the surfaces of susceptible cells.

Enterovirus infections are most common during summer months. Prevalence is mirrored by virus isolations from samples of sewage. Serotypes present in a community vary from year to year. The level of immunity of a populace as reflected by the prevalence of type-specific neutralizing antibodies in serums apparently determines the likelihood of infection by a particular enterovirus.

VIRUS ISOLATION. Primary multiplication occurs in epithelial and paraepithelial lymphatic cells of the pharynx. During this early period of infection the patient may be asymptomatic or have mild malaise, sore throat, or low-grade fever. Similarly virus later multiplies in the intestines. If a critical virus concentration within the pharynx results, viremia follows. During the viremic phase the patient is asymptomatic. Secondary foci of virus multiplication may occur in various tissues (skin, muscle, heart, nervous system, etc.). Major illness of moderate to serious severity sometimes results (see table on page 963). Occasionally (especially during infancy) aspirations of pharyngeal virus lead to lower respiratory infection.

Virus may be isolated from the throat during the minor illness and for as long as a week thereafter. Virus shedding persists in feces for a longer interval, but permanent fecal damage does not occur. Viremia can be documented during the incubation period until type-specific neutralizing antibodies appear.

ILLNESSES (OR SYNDROMES) ASSOCIATED WITH COXSACKIE OR ECHO VIRUS INFECTIONS

Classification	Viruses (not inclusive)		
	Coxsackie virus, group		ECHO virus, types
	A, types	B, types	
I. No Illness (probably 75% of infections).....................	1–24	1–6	1–8,* 11–34
II. Mild or moderate illness			
A. Undifferentiated mild febrile illness (nonspecific).............	1–24	1–6	1–8, 11–34
B. Upper respiratory syndromes (rhinitis pharyngitis, including herpangina and lymphonodular pharyngitis, and conjunctivitis)	1–10, 16, 21,† 22, 24	1–5	1, 3, 6, 9, 16, 19, 20, 28
C. Laryngotracheitis..	9	5	11
D. Exanthems (various)...	5, 9, 16	3, 5	2, 4, 9, 11, 16
E. Lymphadenitis, with or without splenomegaly................	5, 6, 9	5	4, 9, 16, 20
F. Pleurodynia (sometimes with pleural effusion)................	4, 6, 10	1–5	1, 6, 9
G. Orchitis..	....	1–5	9
H. Gastroenteritis...	......	3, 4	2, 3, 6–9, 11–14, 18, 19, 22–24
III. Severe or life-threatening illness			
A. Hepatitis..	4, 9	5	4, 9
B. Hemolytic-uremic syndrome...............................	4		
C. Pneumonia...	9	1, 4	3, 8, 9, 19, 20
D. Cardiac			
1. Myocarditis/pericarditis..............................	1, 4, 9, 16	1–5	3, 6–9, 22
2. Chronic myocardopathy‡			
3. Subendocardial fibroelastosis‡.......................	....	3	
4. Endocardial deformities‡			
5. Congenital malformations‡...........................	3, 4		
E. Neurologic			
1. Aseptic meningitis/encephalitis including variants (b-f).....	7, 9, 16	1–5	1–9, 11–23, 25, 30–32
2. Acute cerebellar ataxia..............................	3, 4		
3. Benign intracranial hypertension			
4. Transverse myelitis			
5. Postencephalitic Parkinsonism			

* Asymptomatic infection is less common with ECHO virus, type 9. Variation in attack rates among types (and strains of a single type) occurs.

† Coxsackie virus A, type 21, is also known as Coe virus.

‡ Suggested (and probable), but cause not established.

PROTECTIVE RESPONSES AND SEROLOGIC DIAGNOSIS. Intracellular virus multiplication stimulates the production within the infected cell of interferon, a small protein with a molecular weight of about 20,000 that inhibits virus maturation. Virulent infections lead to rapid cellular lysis and the release of lesser quantities of interferon. About 3 days after the onset of infection specific antibodies appear in saliva and serum. These immunoglobulins combine with extracellular virus to limit spread of virus; virus-antibody complexes are eliminated by phagocytosis.

Secretory immunoglobulins in saliva and succus entericus are IgA while the earliest antibodies to appear in serum are IgM (Chap. 68). Both species of macromolecules have complement- fixing and neutralizing qualities. Within 3 to 4 weeks complement-fixing antibodies reach their peak and decline. Neutralizing antibodies of higher avidity (IgG) replace the IgM molecule about 2 weeks after the onset of infection and persist, providing permanent type-specific immunity.

This information is important in practical diagnosis because IgM molecules are susceptible to reduction and resultant biologic inactivation with sulfhydryl active compounds such as 2-mercaptoethanol (2-ME). IgG immunoglobulins are resistant to 2-ME. IgG antibodies to Coxsackie and ECHO viruses traverse the placenta freely, but IgM immunoglobulins do not. IgA antibodies in colostrum and milk are not absorbed, but apparently provide some local protection in the intestines of nursing babies. Passively acquired antibodies in serum protect the newborn from viremia for 3 to 6 months, because they inhibit active synthesis of virus, but these antibodies in serum may not protect the respiratory tract where active synthesis of secretory antibody in saliva and nasal secretions is required.

A fourfold rise in neutralizing antibodies or a titer

which is diminished by 2-ME indicates recent infection. When applicable, hemagglutination inhibition tests are simple and practical. Results parallel those obtained in neutralization tests. Complement-fixing antibodies to enteroviruses are not type-specific and are less useful in diagnosis.

OTHER LABORATORY FINDINGS. Enterovirus infections are acute; persistent or chronic infections do not occur. Marked changes in concentrations of hemoglobin or plasma proteins are unusual. Occasionally hemolysis occurs (Chap. 210). White blood cell counts and the erythrocyte sedimentation rates are only mildly elevated. If there is necrosis of the liver or lung, neutrophilic leukemoid reactions may be noted. Hyperbilirubinemia, elevated transaminase and alkaline phosphatase levels, and delayed excretion of Bromsulphalein may be seen in hepatitis. Albuminuria often occurs transiently, but hematuria is rare.

TREATMENT. Antiviral chemotherapy is not available, and the 64 antigenic varieties of Coxsackie and ECHO viruses make vaccine prophylaxis impractical. Pooled human gamma globulin contains enterovirus antibodies, but during serious infections its administration has no therapeutic effect. Most human enterovirus infections are mild, and gamma globulin prophylaxis is rarely warranted. As with poliomyelitis, tonsillectomies and other inoculations probably are best delayed during an outbreak of enterovirus disease. In a murine model of Coxsackie virus A 9 myocarditis, virus was isolated in high titer from hearts of a significantly greater proportion of mice vigorously exercised daily by swimming, and rest is probably the best symptomatic therapy. It has also been shown repeatedly in the laboratory that during the acute phase of infection administration of steroids appreciably increases quantities of virus in tissues and the degree of ensuing injury. Therefore, at least during the acute phase of enterovirus infections, steroids are contraindicated.

REFERENCES

Gelfand, H. M.: Occurrence in Nature of Coxsackie and ECHO Viruses, Progr. Med. Virol., 3:193, 1961.

Horstmann, D. M.: Clinical Virology, Am. J. Med., 38:738, 1965.

Huebner, R. J.: The Virologist's Dilemma, Ann. N.Y. Acad. Sci., 67:430, 1957.

Kibrick, S.: Current Status of Coxsackie and ECHO Viruses in Human Disease, Progr. Med. Virol., 6:27, 1964.

210 COXSACKIE VIRUSES, GROUP A
A. Martin Lerner

Group A Coxsackie viruses cause herpangina, lymphonodular pharyngitis, upper and lower respiratory disease, cutaneous eruptions, hepatitis, aseptic meningitis, paralytic disease, and some sudden deaths in infancy. Pha-

ryngeal multiplication can produce diffuse moderate reddening, but purulent exudate is absent. More characteristic is herpangina (Chap. 227), a common febrile illness characterized by small papular vesicular or ulcerative lesions on the anterior pillars, solft palate, tonsils, pharyngeal mucous membrane, and posterior part of the buccal mucosa. Zahorsky in 1920 and again in 1924 described the entity, and its viral etiology was established by Huebner in 1951. Herpangina has been seen during infections with Coxsackie viruses group A, types 1 to 10, 16, and 22. Vesicular lesions of herpangina have also been described in patients with illnesses due to Coxsackie viruses group B, types 1 to 5, and ECHO viruses, types 9 and 17. Coxsackie virus A 10 may induce *acute lymphonodular pharyngitis*. Lesions here are raised, discrete, white to yellow 3 to 6-mm papules surrounded by a zone of erythema. All of the papules appear at the same time, do not ulcerate, and occur on the uvula, anterior pillars, and posterior pharynx.

Coxsackie virus A 21 (Coe virus) is predominantly a respiratory pathogen and is isolated regularly from the throat and occasionally from feces. It has been associated with several outbreaks in military recruits of a common coldlike illness.

The first enterovirus etiologically implicated in causation of pneumonias was Coxsackie virus A 9. Subsequently, a number of other enteroviruses have been implicated (see table on page 963). Fatal cases occurred in infants or young children. Hyperpnea, cyanosis hyperpyrexia, leukocytosis (or leukemoid reactions), and subsequently coma have been characteristic. Alveolar capillary block syndromes and diffuse bronchopneumonia with alternate areas of atelectasis and emphysema have been found. Histopathologic examination show mixed alveolar septal infiltration without necrosis or giant cells.

A striking cutaneous vesicular eruption, *hand, foot-and-mouth disease* (Chap. 227), has repeatedly been associated with infections due to Coxsackie virus group A, type 16, infants and children with Coxsackie virus group A, type 4, infections have been described with respiratory or gastrointestinal symptoms, acute renal disease, thrombocytopenia, and hemolytic anemia. Reticulocytosis, albuminuria, and hematuria accompany this constellation of findings, which has been described as the *hemolytic-uremic syndrome*. Aseptic meningitis with occasional paralytic disease (especially due to A 7) also occurs.

REFERENCES

Dalldorf, G., and G. M. Sickles: An Unidentified, Filterable Agent Isolated from the Feces of Children with Paralysis, Science, 108:61, 1948.

Huebner, R. J., R. M. Cole, E. A. Beeman, J. A. Bell, and J. H. Peers: Herpangina: Etiological Studies of a Specific Infectious Disease, J.A.M.A., 145:628, 1951.

Lerner, A. M., J. O. Klein, H. S. Levin, and M. Finland: Infections Due to Coxsackievirus Group A, Type 9, in Boston, 1959, with Special Reference to Exanthems and Pneumonia, New Engl. J. Med., 263:1265, 1960.

211 COXSACKIE VIRUSES, GROUP B
A. Martin Lerner

Infections with group B Coxsackie viruses cause a number of upper respiratory syndromes, exanthems, diarrheas, pleurodynia, orchitis, pneumonia, and cardiac and central nervous system disease. Pleurodynia and cardiac disease due to enteroviruses are predominantly associated with this group of enteroviruses (see table on page 963).

PLEURODYNIA (Epidemic Myalgia, Bornholm Disease, Devil's Grip). Prodromal symptoms of malaise, sore throat, and anorexia are interrupted by increasing debility, fever, and sudden onset of muscle, pleuritic, and abdominal pain. Pain is sharp, severe, and paroxysmal over the lower ribs or substernal area. It is accentuated by moving, breathing, coughing, sneezing, and hiccuping and may be referred to the shoulders, neck, or scapulas. Pain and spasm of anterior abdominal muscles occur in about half the cases, often in combination with chest pain. Muscle tenderness is usually not prominent but some patients complain of intense cutaneous hyperesthesia and paresthesia over the affected area. The illness usually lasts 3 to 7 days, but relapses may occur. Among differential diagnoses are myocardial infarction and acute surgical disease of the abdomen. Coxsackie viruses B have been isolated from striated muscle of patients with pleurodynia during epidemics. Occasionally pleuritis is accompanied by effusion, and virus has been isolated from pleural fluid. Bornholm disease may occur at any age, but is commonest in children and young adults.

Early in the course of illness, meningitis, myocarditis, or hepatitis may ensue. In patients with jaundice, liver biopsy shows subacute portal triaditis and intense cloudy swelling of central-zone hepatocytes. Orchitis is a late complication in 3 to 5 percent of cases of pleurodynia.

CARDIAC DISEASE. Acute "idiopathic" myocarditis is predominantly a disease caused by group B Coxsackie viruses. When congenital or neonatal infection occurs, the course is often rapidly fatal with concomitant myocarditis, encephalitis, hepatitis, and sometimes adrenal necrosis. Later in childhood or in adult life, the heart and pericardium usually are involved as the single site of disease. Cardiac inflammation and necrosis vary in intensity. Pericarditis may dominate the clinical picture with fever, precordial pain, friction rub, and even cardiac tamponade. There may be prominent signs of myocarditis with myocardial failure or arrhythmias. Illnesses are usually self-limited and recovery complete. Strict bed rest until all electrocardiographic changes have reverted to normal or are stationary is indicated. This may require 4 to 6 weeks. Because steroids increase virulence of Coxsackie B myocarditis in mice, they are contraindicated. Some infections heal with significant myocardial scarring. Seventeen of forty hearts from autopsies of patients dying when less than thirty years of age were positive by fluorescent antibody staining for Coxsackie virus antigen in the myocardium. Chronic focal interstitial myocarditis was present in each of the positive cases. Viral antigens were found in both the myocardium and the mitral valve in three

cases. There is epidemiologic evidence implicating Coxsackie virus B, types 3 and 4, in congenital heart disease. Most infections in pregnant mothers were subclinical and occurred in the first trimester. There are other data implicating group B Coxsackie viruses in congenital subendocardial fibroelastosis. All these findings need further study for confirmation.

REFERENCES

Bain, H. W., D. W. McLean, and S. J. Walker: Epidemic Pleurodynia (Bornholm's Disease) Due to Coxsackie B5 Virus: The Interrelationship of Pleurodynia, Benign Pericarditis and Aseptic Meningitis, Pediatrics, 27:889, 1961.

Brown, G. C., and T. N. Evans: Serologic Evidence of Coxsackievirus Etiology of Congenital Heart Disease, J.A.M.A., 199:151, 1967.

Burch, G. E., S. C. Sun, H. L. Colcolough, R. S. Sohal, and N. P. DePasquale: Coxsackie B Viral Myocarditis and Valvulitis Identified in Routine Autopsy Specimens by Immunofluorescent Technique, Am. Heart J., 74:13, 1967.

Johnson, R. T., B. Portnoy, N. G. Rogers, and E. L. Buescher: Acute Benign Pericarditis: Virologic Study of 34 Patients, Arch. Intern. Med., 108:823, 1961.

Kibrick, S.: Viral Infections of the Fetus and Newborn, Perspectives Virol. Symp. New York, 2:140, 1961.

Sutton, G. C., H. B. Harding, R. P. Trueheart, and H. P. Clark: Coxsackie B4 Myocarditis in an Adult: Successful Isolation of Virus from Ventricular Myocardium, Clin. Aviat. Aerospace Med., 38:66, 1967.

Sylvest, E.: "Epidemic Myalgia: Bornholm Disease," London, Oxford University Press, 1934.

Tilles, J. G., S. H. Elson, J. A. Shaka, W. H. Abelmann, A. M. Lerner, and M. Finland: Effects of Exercise on Coxsackie A9 Myocarditis in Adult Mice, Proc. Soc. Exp. Biol. Med., 117:777, 1964.

212 ECHO VIRUSES
A. Martin Lerner

ECHO virus infections may be asymptomatic or may cause mild, moderate, or life-threatening illness (see table on page 963). Mild to moderate are undifferentiated fevers, upper respiratory infections, various rashes (Chap. 222), pleurodynia, and diarrheas (Chap. 213). Pneumonias, myocarditis, and neurologic involvement can be serious. Illnesses due to ECHO viruses do not differ from those caused by Coxsackie viruses.

NEUROLOGIC MANIFESTATIONS. There may be a mild prodromal malaise, but major illness usually begins with increased fever, headache, and stiff neck. Papilledema, Kernig, Brudzinski, and Babinski signs may be present. Localizing sensory or motor deficits are unusual. Confusion and delirium reflect an accompanying diffuse inflammatory reaction in the substance of the brain. These acute findings may persist for 4 to 7 days. Cerebrospinal fluid pleocytosis is usually less than 500 cells per cu mm. Early there may be as many as 90 percent polymorphonuclear leukocytes, but within 48 hr the cellular response becomes completely mononuclear. Persistence of polymorphonuclear leukocytes suggests a pyogenic focus (intracerebral, subdural, or epidural) (Chap. 360). Gram stain and appropriate spinal fluid cultures must be done to exclude bacterial meningitis, tuberculosis, or mycotic meningitis. Protein concentration in the cerebrospinal fluid is moderately elevated, but glucose is normal. Early in the illness, ECHO viruses may be isolated from spinal fluid. Hospitalization for several weeks may be required, and the CSF should be checked prior to discharge. At that time, it should contain only a few lymphocytes per cubic millimeter.

Throat and rectal swabs, serum, and cerebrospinal fluid should be collected as early as possible for attempts at virus isolation. Acute and convalescent serums should be studied for type-specific neutralizing antibodies.

It is not possible clinically to distinguish aseptic meningitis due to various enteroviruses from that caused by mumps. Localizing findings, hemiplegias, prolonged fevers, oculogyric crises, coma, and bloody spinal fluid are differential features of herpes simplex encephalitis (Chaps. 218 and 361). Although ECHO virus aseptic meningitis most often is self-limited and recovery complete, about 10 percent of patients have serious involvement of the central nervous system. Minor muscle weakness with reflex changes may persist for weeks to months, but over 95 percent of patients recover completely within a year. Occasionally choreiform movements, ataxia, nystagmus, transverse myelitis, coma, bulbar involvement, and death result.

REFERENCES

Horstmann, D. M., and N. Yamada: Enterovirus Infections of the Central Nervous System, Assoc. for Res. in Nervous & Mental Dis. Res. Pub., 44:236, 1968.

Karzon, D. T., N. S. Hayner, W. Winkelstein, Jr., and A. L. Barron: Epidemic of Aseptic Meningitis Syndrome Due to ECHO Virus Type 6. II. Clinical Study of ECHO 6 Infection, Pediatrics, 29:418, 1962.

Lepow, M. L., D. H. Carver, H. T. Wright, Jr., W. A. Woods, and F. C. Robbins: A Clinical, Epidemiologic and Laboratory Investigation of Aseptic Meningitis during the Four Year Period, 1955–1958. I. Observations Concerning Etiology and Epidemiology, New Engl. J. Med., 266:1181, 1962.

Sabin, A. B., E. R. Krumbiegel, and R. Wigand: ECHO Type 9 Virus Disease: Virologically Controlled Clinical and Epidemiologic Observations during 1957 Epidemic in Milwaukee with Notes on Concurrent Similar Diseases Associated with Coxsackie and Other ECHO Viruses, J. Dis. Child., 96:197, 1958.

213   VIRAL GASTROENTERITIS
A. Martin Lerner

Sporadic endemic cases of nonbacterial diarrheas as well as acute outbreaks occur in summer or winter and have been termed "winter vomiting diseases" or "intestinal flu." There is no association of gastrointestinal symptoms with influenza virus. Diarrhea may occur as a minor manifestation of enterovirus disease during a summer outbreak, but this is not a usual occurrence. In individuals and in epidemiologically controlled series, Coxsackie viruses, types B 3 and 4, as well as ECHO viruses, types 2, 3, 6 to 9, 11 to 14, 18, 19, and 22 to 24 have been implicated etiologically. Administration of oral attenuated poliovirus vaccines also has induced gastroenteritis.

Outbreaks of vomiting and diarrhea due to ECHO viruses occurring in winter are brief but debilitating illnesses. Malaise and several watery stools may herald the onset. Fever occurs but is not always present. Within 24 hr, repeated vomiting, retching, and chilliness ensue and there may be abdominal cramps and myalgia. The disease is highly contagious, and multiple cases occur within the family at one time or following closely one upon another. Recovery from the acute episode within 48 hr is usual, but mild diarrhea may persist for several weeks. During initial chilliness and cramping, ECHO viruses have been isolated from the blood, posterior pharyngeal wall, and rectal swabs. Shedding of virus is brief, and virus isolation is often unsuccessful within 36 hr after onset.

Reoviruses and adenoviruses have been implicated in similar gastroenteritides. Nevertheless, even during epidemiologic surveillances, most episodes of nonbacterial gastroenteritis remain undiagnosed. Differential diagnosis includes staphylococcal enterotoxin diarrhea (Chap. 137), salmonellosis (Chap. 150), and shigellosis (Chap. 151). Cases of dual bacterial-viral infection have occurred, but no obvious increase in virulence has been evident.

REFERENCES

Behbehani, A. M., and H. A. Wenner: Infantile Diarrhea (A Study of the Etiologic Role of Viruses), Am. J. Dis. Child., 111:623, 1966.

Goodwin, M. H., Jr., G. J. Love, D. C. Mackel, K. R. Berquist, and R. S. Gandin: Observations on the Association of Enteric Viruses and Bacteria with Diarrhea, Am. J. Trop. Med. Hyg., 16:178, 1967.

Klein, J. O., A. M. Lerner, and M. Finland: Acute Gastroenteritis Associated with ECHO Virus, Type 11, Am. J. Med. Sci., 240:749, 1960.

Ramos-Alvarez, M., and J. Olarte: Diarrheal Diseases of Children: The Occurrence of Enteropathogenic Viruses and Bacteria, J. Dis. Child., 107:218, 1964.

214   REOVIRUSES
A. Martin Lerner

Reoviruses were discovered inadvertently in studies of the intestinal viral flora of healthy children and adults. They were initially classified as ECHO virus, type 10, but were later reclassified. They were named to emphasize their (1) *respiratory* or (2) *enteric* human origins and their (3) *orphan* status.

Reoviruses are quite different from picornaviruses. They are about 2½ times larger (70 mμ in diameter) and show icosohedral symmetry. Their RNA is unique because it is a double-stranded helix like DNA and is also resistant to ribonuclease. Reoviruses are the only animal viruses with this type of RNA. The capsid is protein and consists of 92 hollow capsomeres. Unlike that of enteroviruses, the cytopathic effects of reovirus are nonlytic. Reoviruses multiply in primate and nonprimate tissue cultures, and the particles hemagglutinate human or avian erythrocytes. On the basis of hemagglutination inhibition tests with type-specific serums, there are 3 serotypes.

Human infections with reoviruses are common, and their distribution is worldwide. Like Coxsackie and ECHO viruses, reoviruses spread by enteric and respiratory routes. By adult life, 50 to 80 percent of several widely scattered populations in this hemisphere have had reovirus infections as measured by the presence of persistent neutralizing or hemagglutinating antibodies. Infections are more frequent in winter but can occur in any season. Reoviruses have been isolated from human nasal secretions, posterior pharyngeal and rectal swabs, spinal fluid, brain, and lung. They have been recovered from tissues of Burkitt's lymphoma. In addition, reovirus isolations or serologic data indicate that natural infections occur in cattle, dogs, mice, horses, swine, and monkeys. Although animal to human contagion has not been demonstrated, its possibility is likely.

Widespread evidence of infection and few associations with disease indicate that most infections with reoviruses are probably asymptomatic. Isolations of virus and four-fold rises in HIA (hemagglutination inhibition antibodies) in individual patients with common colds, nonspecific febrile illness, exanthem, and diarrhea suggest that these viruses may be causative in these common syndromes, but adequate epidemiologic controls are not available, and these observations need to be confirmed. More provocative are data from three thoroughly studied fatal cases with encephalitis, myocarditis, hepatitis, or interstitial pneumonias. In these patients reoviruses and no other bacterial or viral pathogens were isolated.

REFERENCES

El-Rai, F. M., and A. S. Evans: Reovirus Infections in Children and Young Adults, Arch. Environ. Health, 7:700, 1963.

Gomatos, P. J. and I. Tamm: The Secondary Structure of Reovirus RNA, Proc. Nat. Acad. Sci., 49:707, 1963.

Rosen, L.: Serologic Grouping of Reoviruses by Hemagglutination-Inhibition, Am. J. Hyg., 71:242, 1961.

———, H. E. Evans, and A. Spickard: Reovirus Infections in Human Volunteers, Am. J. Hyg., 77:29, 1963.

Sabin, A. B.: Reoviruses: New Group of Respiratory and Enteric Viruses Formerly Classified as ECHO, Type 10 Is Described, Science, 130:1387, 1959.

Tillotson, J. R., and A. M. Lerner: Reovirus, Type 3 Associated with Fatal Pneumonia, New Engl. J. Med., 276:1060, 1967.

Section 16

Viral Diseases of the Central Nervous System

215 LYMPHOCYTIC CHORIOMENINGITIS

Harry N. Beaty and Robert G. Petersdorf

DEFINITION. Lymphocytic choriomeningitis (LCM) is an acute systemic viral infection which is frequently accompanied by the clinical syndrome of "aseptic meningitis" (Chap. 361) in man.

ETIOLOGY. The agent responsible for LCM has not been identified definitively. It is probably a small RNA virus which is heat labile and readily inactivated by formalin or ultraviolet light. Many different strains of the virus have been identified on the basis of tissue tropism and pathogenicity, but none is antigenically distinct. The agent can be propagated readily in chick embryo and cell cultures from chick or mouse embryo, mouse or monkey kidney, and certain established diploid cell lines.

EPIDEMIOLOGY. The virus of LCM is probably worldwide in distribution, but the disease is uncommon in man. Although natural infection occurs in a variety of animals, mice are the major reservoir for the virus and represent the only species in which latent, asymptomatic infection occurs. The latency of mouse infection depends upon immunological tolerance, and animals infected *in utero* or shortly after birth excrete the virus for life without overt disease. In man, LCM has followed direct contact with wild mice or infected rodents in experimental laboratories, and it is assumed that contact with contaminated mice or their excreta is the major mechanism for spread of this infection. Lymphocytic choriomeningitis occurs throughout the year, but is somewhat more frequently encountered in the colder months when human contact with wild rodents is greatest. Transmission of the virus by arthropod vectors has been accomplished experimentally but has not been demonstrated to occur naturally. Man-to-man transmission probably does not occur.

PATHOGENESIS. In natural infection, the portal of entry is probably through the respiratory tract. Virus multiplication occurs initially in the respiratory epithelium, and in some patients symptoms of an upper-respiratory-tract infection or influenza-like illness develop. Dissemination of virus to secondary extraneural sites of growth, possibly in reticuloendothelial cells, may be an important step in the pathogenesis of central-nervous-system disease. The virus multiplies in these sites, and when sustained viremia develops it crosses the "blood-brain barrier" and infects meningeal cells. In mice, the resulting meningitis, which is characterized by lymphocytic infiltration, is attributed to immunologic reactivity. It is postulated that this immune response is mediated by lymphocytes which were sensitized while the virus multiplied in the reticuloendothelial system and is directed against viral antigen in infected host cells. Support for this hypotesis is derived from the observation that disease can be prevented by neonatal thymectomy, irradiation, or immunodepressant drugs. There is only limited circumstantial evidence that a similar pathogenetic mechanism operates in man, but the concept that LCM is a virus-induced autoimmune disease is intriguing and deserves further study.

MANIFESTATIONS. Infection of man by the LCM virus produces a variety of clinical manifestations. Serologic surveys indicate that inapparent or unrecognized infection is common. It is also clear that symptomatic infection in man ordinarily consists of a clinically nonspecific, grippelike illness which resembles influenza. Neurologic manifestations appear only infrequently and take the form of aseptic meningitis or encephalitis.

The exact incubation period is not known, but it is probably only a few days. Initially, symptoms consist of remittent fever, anorexia, malaise, generalized aching, headache, and respiratory manifestations ranging from pharyngitis, cough, and bronchitis, to frank pneumonia. Fever and discomfort often vary in their intensity, abating somewhat and then recurring over a period of 1 to 3 weeks. Many patients then recover completely. In others, however, apparent convalescence is interrupted by a recurrence of fever and the abrupt onset of headache, photophobia, and signs of meningeal irritation. This second stage of the disease ordinarily lasts 7 to 10 days, and prompt recovery is the rule. However, relapses or recurrences of meningeal symptoms are seen occasionally. A few patients have transient erythematous or papular rashes during the meningeal phase.

Patients with aseptic meningitis almost always recover without sequelae. Fatality is also uncommon with encephalitis, but 25 to 30 percent of patients develop paralysis, and convalescence may be prolonged. Arthralgia and frank arthritis may be seen during recovery from the acute systemic illness, and in a few well-documented cases of infection with the LCM virus, orchitis has been observed.

LABORATORY FINDINGS. Leukopenia with granulocytopenia and relative lymphocytosis is commonly seen in association with the acute systemic illness. If meningitis develops, the leukocyte count is often normal, but may be elevated with a predominance of polymorphonuclear leukocytes. The cerebrospinal fluid pressure may be increased, and protein concentrations usually range from 5 to 200 mg per 100 ml. The glucose concentration in the spinal fluid is usually normal, but levels of 35 to 40 mg per 100 ml have been observed. The cell count usually ranges from 100 to 3,000 cells per cu mm with 90 percent lymphocytes.

The diagnosis of LCM often can be established with certainty by recovery of the virus from blood or spinal fluid. In most patients, however, the diagnosis is established only by serologic studies. Complement-fixing antibodies are usually detectable 1 to 2 weeks after the onset of infection, and neutralizing antibody appears after 6 to 8 weeks. Immunofluorescent studies have detected antibody to the LCM virus early in the course of the illness, and its appearance seems to parallel the development of the neurologic phase.

DIAGNOSIS. Lymphocytic choriomeningitis must be differentiated from the many other causes of the clinical syndrome of aseptic meningitis. A detailed discussion of this syndrome appears in Chapter 361.

TREATMENT. The management of infections with the LCM virus is purely supportive and symptomatic.

REFERENCES

Baum, S. G., A. M. Lewis, Jr., W. P. Rowe, and R. J. Huebner: Epidemic Nonmeningitic Lymphocytic Choriomeningitis Virus Infection, New Engl. J. Med., 274:934, 1966.

Farmer, T. W., and C. A. Janeway: Infections with the Virus of Lymphocytic Choriomeningitis, Medicine, 21:1, 1942.

Hotchin, J.: The Biology of Lymphocytic Choriomeningitis Infection: Virus-induced Immune Disease, Cold Spring Harbor Symp. Quant. Biol., 27:479, 1962.

Johnson, R. T., and C. A. Mims: Pathogenesis of Viral Infections of the Nervous System, New Engl. J. Med., 278:23, 1968.

Meyer, H. M., Jr., R. T. Johnson, I. P. Crawford, H. E. Dascomb, and N. G. Rogers: Central Nervous System Syndromes of Viral Etiology, Am. J. Med., 29:334, 1960.

216 POLIOMYELITIS
Louis Weinstein

DEFINITION. Poliomyelitis is a common acute viral infection which occurs naturally only in man and produces a wide variety of clinical manifestations. In its most severe form, it involves parts of the central nervous system. In most instances, the nervous system is not invaded; infection may take place without apparent illness, or may result in the production of nonspecific syndromes.

ETIOLOGY. The causative agent of poliomyelitis is an RNA virus of the Picorna group, 8 to 30 mu in diameter, pathogenic for man and primates. Three antigenically distinct types have been defined: type I (Brunhilde), type II (Lansing), and type III (Leon). Cross neutralization is demonstrable in highly immunized experimental animals, but infection in man with one type does not protect against invasion by another. Poliomyelitis virus grows well in tissue culture.

Under proper conditions, the virus may remain viable in water or sewage for as long as 4 months. It is not killed by ether, Merthiolate, tincture of Zephiran, ethyl alcohol, or low concentrations of mercury, oxidizing agents, 2% tincture of iodine, ultraviolet light, and 10-min exposure to a chlorine concentration of 0.05 ppm.

EPIDEMIOLOGY. Poliomyelitis is worldwide, but epidemics have been limited to a relatively small number of areas. That infection is much more prevalent than is suggested by the number of clinically recognized cases is proved by the widespread distribution of neutralizing antibody in populations all over the world. Poliomyelitis occurs with the highest frequency from July through September in the North Temperate Zone, although it may appear as early as April or as late as December. In tropical or subtropical regions, the season may be prolonged.

In areas of poor sanitation, most individuals develop neutralizing antibodies in early childhood, while in other localities, the peak of population immunity is not reached until fifteen years of age or older. Urban dwellers become immune earlier than those who live in rural areas. In lower-income groups, evidence of contact with poliomyelitis virus appears at a younger age than in individuals whose financial status is good.

Poliomyelitis was most common in the preschool child until World War II but has been increasing in older age groups. In some epidemics since the war, 25 to 30 percent of patients have been older than fifteen years of age. Paralytic disease has been described in the neonatal period and as late as the sixth decade but is very uncommon at these age extremes.

PATHOGENESIS. Man is the sole reservoir of poliomyelitis virus. Carriers, especially those with unapparent infection, are most important in transmission of the virus. A history of contact with recognized cases is uncommon. Milk was incriminated as the source of infection in one epidemic.

Virus is recoverable from pharyngeal secretions for only a few days but is demonstrable in the feces for several weeks. The intestinal tract is the main source from which virus is disseminated. The mode of infection, therefore, is fecal-oral, the same as in salmonellosis, shigellosis, and other enteric infections. Large quantities of virus are present in sewage drained from areas in which the infection is present. Flies trapped in areas close to patients with poliomyelitis may carry the virus. Attempts to reduce the spread of disease in epidemics by eradication of the fly population, however, have not been successful. Poliomyelitis is as highly communicable as measles or varicella; in individuals under fifteen years of age, infection, with or without clinical manifestations, occurs in 100 percent of household and 87 percent of daily contacts.

The following sequence of events has been postulated as the basis for infection: (1) The virus enters the body by way of the mouth, begins to multiply in the oropharynx and lower part of the intestinal tract, and can be transmitted from either area. The site of viral growth is probably extraneural. Virus is present in pharyngeal secretions and stool during the incubation period; it has been demonstrated in the feces as long as 19 days prior to onset of the disease. (2) The phase of "minor illness" (described below) develops in association with the presence of the virus in the blood, throat, and feces; the viremia persists for only a few days until antibodies make their appearance. The virus in the intestinal tract penetrates the lymphatic channels and enters the bloodstream, from which it is disseminated. (3) The final stage in the pathogenesis of poliomyelitis is invasion of the nervous system. It has been suggested that the virus enters the nervous system from the blood in the area postrema of the medulla oblongata because this is more permeable than other parts of the brain to dyes injected intravascularly; it has also been postulated, however, that viral invasion of the nervous system occurs at many points by direct passage of virus from capillaries to neurones. Once the virus has reached the nervous system, it spreads along nerve fibers.

Strains of poliomyelitis virus vary greatly in their ability to invade nervous tissue and to destroy neurones. Repeated passage in animals or tissue cultures induces changes in invasive capacity without affecting the basic antigenic character of the agent. The early presence of detectable antibody results from multiplication of virus in nonnervous tissue, and accounts for the short persistence of virus in the pharynx and blood, sites in which antibody is demonstrable. The persistence of virus in the nervous system and intestine is probably due to the difficulty which antibody has in reaching these areas.

The most important determinant of human susceptibility to poliomyelitis is serum antibody. Previous inapparent infection and illness without invasion of the nervous system are common. Many children and most adults possess neutralizing antibody for all three types of virus; this probably accounts for the relative infrequency of the disease in older age groups. Infants under six months old rarely get poliomyelitis because immunity is passively transferred from the mother. Babies born to women in the acute phase of poliomyelitis can develop the disease shortly after birth. Sex plays a role in determining susceptibility. Among children, males are affected more often than females; the opposite is true in adults. Pregnancy increases the risk of clinically apparent poliomyelitis, and multiparous females are more susceptible than primiparas. The disease is somewhat more frequent in the second than in the first or third trimesters. Menstruation or ovulation appears to heighten susceptibility. Absence of the tonsils and adenoids, regardless of the time of their removal, is associated with a marked increase in incidence of bulbar poliomyelitis. Chilling or physical exertion after invasion by the virus leads to more frequent development of paralytic poliomyelitis, especially in adults.

CLINICAL MANIFESTATIONS. The incubation period of poliomyelitis varies from 3 to 35 days; about 80 percent of cases occur 6 to 20 days after contact with the virus.

The infection may assume one of four forms: (1) inapparent infection, (2) "minor illness," (3) nonparalytic poliomyelitis, (4) paralytic poliomyelitis.

Inapparent Infection. As much as 95 percent of infection with the poliomyelitis virus occurs in this form. There are no symptoms, but the virus is present in the pharynx, intestine, and probably the blood. Type-specific neutralizing antibody usually develops.

"Minor Illness." The entire course of poliomyelitis may consist of a nonspecific illness without clinical or laboratory evidence of central-nervous-system invasion; this is "abortive" poliomyelitis. Three syndromes have been observed: (1) upper respiratory manifestations, consisting of fever of varying degree, pharyngeal discomfort, with or without coryza, and reddening and swelling of the lymphoid tissues of the throat; (2) gastrointestinal disturbances, with nausea, vomiting, diarrhea or constipation, and abdominal discomfort, accompanied by moderate fever; (3) grippelike disease with fever and generalized aching of muscles, bones, and joints, resembling influenza. Virus can be demonstrated in the pharynx, feces, and blood in the early stages of these "minor" illnesses. Type-specific neutralizing and complement-fixing antibodies develop during convalescence.

Nonparalytic Poliomyelitis. Nonparalytic poliomyelitis consists of prodromal manifestations, signs of meningeal irritation, and abnormalities of the spinal fluid. The prodrome is similar to that of the "minor" illnesses and is usually present for several days before the onset of other signs. Stiffness of the neck and back (Kernig's sign), and, with severe meningeal irritation, leg and neck (Brudzinski's sign) are present. The tripod (patient extends arms behind back with hands on bed for support when sitting up) and Hoyne's signs (head falls back when, with patient in supine position, shoulders are elevated) can be elicited in paralytic or nonparalytic poliomyelitis but are not pathognomonic.

Spinal Fluid. The spinal fluid usually contains between 25 and 500 cells, and rarely as many as 1,000 to 2,000. Very early in the disease, there is often a preponderance of neutrophils (up to 80 percent); within a few days, however, mononuclear cells predominate. The protein is normal or slightly elevated at the beginning of the illness but may increase to between 50 and 100 mg per 100 ml. The sugar content is normal. These spinal fluid findings are typical of *aseptic meningitis* (Chap. 361) and indicate an inflammatory reaction of the meninges but are not diagnostic of poliomyelitis. They are also present in healing bacterial meningitis, tuberculous meningitis, scarlet fever, pertussis encephalopathy, leptospiral meningitis, syphilis, mumps meningitis, Coxsackie virus infections, herpes simplex meningitis, infectious mononucleosis, trichinella meningitis, brain abscess, multiple sclerosis, tumors of the brain or spinal cord, allergic reactions involving the nervous system, postinfectious encephalitides, "infectious" polyneuritis, and lymphocytic choriomeningitis.

The diagnosis of nonparalytic poliomyelitis on clinical grounds alone is impossible, because the signs, symptoms, and laboratory findings are completely nonspecific. Viral and immunologic studies suggest that fewer than 40 percent of cases of "nonparalytic poliomyelitis" are actually this disease; mumps meningitis without salivary gland involvement (Chap. 231) and Coxsackie virus disease (Chaps. 210 and 211) are the two most common differential diagnoses.

The course of nonparalytic poliomyelitis is benign. Defervescence occurs in 3 to 5 days, but meningeal irritation may persist for 2 weeks. No changes in muscle and nerve function are detectable. The white blood cell count may be as high as 15,000 in the early stage of the disease but is usually normal within a week.

Paralytic Poliomyelitis. The syndrome of paralytic poliomyelitis consists of prodromal manifestations ("minor" illness), signs of meningeal irritation, abnormal spinal fluid, and signs of involvement of motor nerve cells in the spinal cord, brain, or cranial nerve nuclei, resulting in paresis or paralysis of various muscles. Lesions may also be present in parts of the nervous system other than anterior horn cells; the precentral gyrus, the reticular formation in the medulla, the roof nuclei and vermis of the cerebellum, Auerbach's and Meissner's plexuses, and sympathetic ganglions are usually involved in fatal cases. Seldom, however, are there clinical signs pointing to disease of these parts. "Skip" areas are common in spinal paralytic disease; involvement of the cervical and lumbar cord is often present with no dysfunction of the thoracic portion.

Paralytic poliomyelitis may be subdivided into the following types:

    I. Spinal
        A. Cervical
        B. Thoracic
        C. Lumbar
        D. Any combination of A, B, and C
    II. Bulbar
        A. Upper cranial nerve involvement—III, IV, V, VI, VII, VIII
        B. Lower cranial nerve involvement—IX, X, XI, XII
        C. Involvement of cardiorespiratory centers
    III. Bulbospinal
    IV. Polioencephalitis—paralytic or nonparalytic
        A. Diffuse encephalitis
        B. Focal encephalitis
        C. Cerebellar involvement (?)
        D. Bulboencephalitic disease
        E. Spinal-encephalitic disease

Prodromal manifestations are often absent in paralytic poliomyelitis. In some cases, the illness is biphasic in character. The disease starts with fever and manifestations of one of the "minor" illnesses. After several days, all symptoms disappear; in 5 or 10 days, there are recrudescence of fever, the development of signs of meningeal irritation, and the appearance of paralysis. The commonest prodromal symptoms in adults are generalized muscle and bone discomfort. In children, upper-respiratory-tract syndromes are most frequent. The spinal fluid findings in paralytic poliomyelitis are the same as those in the nonparalytic disease. Paralytic poliomyelitis may be accompanied by a completely normal spinal fluid throughout its entire course, but this occurs in no more than 0.5 percent of cases. In some patients, decrease in number of cells in the spinal fluid is accompanied by a progressive rise in protein, which may reach levels high enough to cause confusion with the cytoalbuminologic dissociation observed in "infectious" polyneuritis.

Spinal Paralytic Poliomyelitis. In the early stages of spinal paralytic poliomyelitis, cramping pain in the muscles innervated by the affected neurones and hyperesthesia of the overlying skin are present. The discomfort may be very severe; muscle "spasm," the exact mechanism of which is not clear, is usually detectable. In some instances, increase in muscle weakness is very slow; in others, it becomes widespread within 48 hr. Rarely, a rapidly ascending paralysis of the Landry type is observed. Age is one factor in determining the extent of involvement. In children less than five years old, paresis of one leg is most common. In patients between five and fifteen years of age, weakness of one arm, or paraplegia, is most frequent, while in adults (sixteen to sixty-five years old), quadriplegia is observed most often. Dysfunction of the urinary bladder is at least ten times more frequent in adults than in children. Paralysis of the muscles of respiration is most common in those older than sixteen years of age. Infants younger than one year are subject to very extensive involvement. Among adults, men develop quadriplegia, respiratory paralysis, and loss of bladder function more frequently than do women. Pregnancy does not increase the severity of the disease unless parturition takes place during the acute phase. There is a definite association of inoculation of antigenic materials ("triple vaccine," for example) with involvement of the muscles around the site of injection.

When the *cervical cord* is involved, there is paresis or paralysis of the muscles of the shoulders, arms, neck, and diaphragm. Very early in the disease, the reflexes in the arms remain intact; they diminish rapidly, however, and are usually absent by the time paralysis has become established. Coarse twitching of the affected muscles is common. With cervical cord disease, there is always danger of respiratory paralysis due to spread of the infection to the motor nuclei of the phrenic nerves and medulla.

Weakness of the muscles of the chest, upper portion of the abdomen, and spine follows involvement of the *thoracic portion* of the spinal cord. Difficulty in breathing results from dysfunction of the intercostal and other thoracic muscles. The chest wall may be in "spasm" and may appear rigid despite the presence of only a minor degree of paresis.

Disease of the *lumbar portion of the spinal cord* produces weakness of the legs and inferior portions of the abdomen and back. Again, pain, tenderness, "spasm," and twitching herald the oncoming paralysis, and the reflexes are abolished with the development of flaccid paralysis. In adults, complete paraplegia is not infrequent. Paralysis of the urinary bladder, usually temporary, occurs in about one-third of patients over sixteen years of age and is rarely observed in the absence of weakness of the legs.

The abdominal and cremasteric reflexes usually disappear before muscle weakness is marked in paralytic poliomyelitis and may be absent during the entire course of the disease. An extensor plantar response (positive Babinski's sign) is rare; its persistence is incompatible with poliomyelitis. Hyperesthesia of the skin is frequent, but sensory loss does not occur. Constipation, abdominal cramps, and metiorism are common and are due to ileus resulting from involvement of the autonomic nervous system and weakness of the abdominal muscles. When the disease is severe, sympathetic nervous system disturbances, with tachycardia, hypertension, abnormal sweating, and cyanosis and coldness of the involved extremities, are present.

Fever in spinal paralytic poliomyelitis is usually present for the first few days of the disease and disappears by lysis. In about 90 percent of cases, there is little or no extension of paralysis 48 hr after defervescence has occurred. In about 10 percent, however, considerable progression of weakness may continue for as long as a week or more.

Bulbar Poliomyelitis. The incidence of bulbar poliomyelitis differs from one epidemic to another and varies between 6 and 25 percent. In patients subjected to tonsilloadenoidectomy within 30 days of onset of the disease and in those in whom the operation was carried out years before, the bulbar form of infection is present in about 85 percent of cases. Pure bulbar involvement (without any signs of spinal cord involvement) is commonest in children; adults with bulbar disturbances usually have associated spinal paralyses. The syndromes which develop depend on the area of the brainstem involved, and result from damage to the medulla, pons, and midbrain. Signs and symptoms are produced by (1) dysfunction of the upper cranial nerve nuclei, (2) damage to the lower cranial nerve nuclei, and (3) disturbances of the respiratory and vasomotor regulating centers in the medulla. Combined bulbar and diffuse or focal encephalitis or spinal involvement may occur.

1. *Upper Cranial Nerve Nuclei—III, IV, V, VI, VII, VIII.* Isolated ocular nerve palsies, total external ophthalmoplegia, pupillary disorders, and Horner's syndrome occur. There may be unilateral or bilateral involvement of the fifth nerve, with difficulty in chewing and closing the mouth, as well as deviation of the jaws. Paralysis of the seventh cranial nerve is common and usually unilateral; the entire face or only the upper or lower parts may be affected. Disturbances of vestibular function and deafness resulting from damage to the nucleus of the eighth nerve occur infrequently.

2. *Lower Cranial Nerve Nuclei—IX, X, XI, XII.* Life may be endangered when the muscles of deglutition are paralyzed because of involvement of the nucleus ambiguus in the medulla. Hoarseness and laryngeal stridor follow weakness or paralysis of the vocal cords. Unilateral or bilateral weakness of the tongue, sternocleidomastoid, and trapezius muscles may be present. Inability to swallow results in pooling of saliva and food in the pharynx,

with obstruction to the airway. Aspiration into the larynx, reflex spasm of the glottis, and abductor paralysis of the vocal cords constitute very serious threats to life. Minor or major pareses of the soft palate and pharyngeal muscles are detectable by a nasal quality of the voice.

3. *Disease of the medullary respiratory center* produces irregularity of the rhythm, depth, and rate of breathing. Respirations are shallow, and as the disease progresses, there are progressively longer periods of apnea until breathing stops completely. The thoracic muscles and diaphragm are not weak, unless spinal involvement is present. Hiccuping is frequent in the early phase of respiratory center dysfunction. Hypoxia, without visible cyanosis, is common and contributes to the intensity of the manifestations. In the late stages, cyanosis, unresponsive to oxygen administration, is common, and temperature, pulse rate, and blood pressure are elevated. The final event is usually irreversible shock.

Involvement of the circulatory regulating center includes a cherry-red color of the lips, flushed skin, rapid, irregular pulse, small pulse pressure when the blood pressure is normal, and moderate to severe hypotension. Hyperthermia, cold, mottled, clammy skin, shallow respiration, and anxiety, restlessness, and confusion appear as the circulation becomes impaired and irreversible shock develops.

Polioencephalitis. Encephalitic symptoms occur as isolated syndromes, or together with bulbar or spinal poliomyelitis. The incidence of polioencephalitis is variable; one small epidemic in which most of the patients had this type of disease has been described. The diffuse form is characterized by confusion, agitation, anxiety with a feeling of impending doom, or somnolence. Quivering and jerking of the facial muscles and extremities, flushing of the face, tremor of the hands, and restless movements occur. Insomnia may be severe. In fatal cases, confusion is marked and progresses to lethargy and death.

In focal polioencephalitis, there may be clinical evidence of brain damage, or the lesions may be silent and demonstrable only at necropsy. Visual-verbal agnosia, myoclonic jerks, grand mal convulsions, which occasionally persist for a long time after recovery, spastic hemiparesis, ataxia of one arm or leg, and hydrocephalus have been described.

DIAGNOSIS. The diagnosis of paralytic poliomyelitis can usually be made on clinical grounds. The outstanding manifestations are a lower motor neurone lesion which develops rapidly and is characterized by flaccid weakness and hypo- or areflexia. Signs of upper motor neurone disease or decreased sensation are not compatible with poliomyelitis. Among the diseases which may cause confusion, especially in their early stages, are toxic, "infectious," or idiopathic polyneuritis, the postinfectious encephalitides, viral encephalitides, trichinosis, acute rheumatic fever, cerebrovascular accidents with paralysis, acute syphilitic meningitis (frequent cranial nerve palsies), meningomyeloencephalitis resulting from sensitization to foreign protein (horse serum, rabies vaccine,

pertussis vaccine), osteomyelitis, scurvy, acute multiple sclerosis, pseudobulbar palsy, myalgic meningoencephalitis (Iceland, Tallahassee, or Coventry disease), spinal epidural abscess or tumor, neoplasms of the brain and spinal cord, Coxsackie virus infection, the encephalitis of the preicteric phase of infectious hepatitis, infectious mononucleosis with neurologic involvement, infections due to the enteric cytopathogenic human "orphan" (ECHO) viruses, focal embolic encephalitis associated with subacute bacterial endocarditis, tuberculous meningitis with hemiplegia or cranial nerve (especially the sixth) palsies, and brain abscess. Study of these diseases over a period of a few days to a week after onset clarifies the situation in most instances. The only positive method of establishing the diagnosis of paralytic poliomyelitis is the isolation of the virus from the stool or pharyngeal secretions (spinal cord or brain at necropsy) and the demonstration of a rise in the level of neutralizing antibody to the isolated strain in acute- and convalescent-phase serums. If virus cannot be isolated, the three type strains maintained in tissue culture may be used; a significant rise in titer of neutralizing antibody against a specific serotype is diagnostic.

COMPLICATIONS. Complications occur most frequently when the respiratory muscles are involved because of involvement of spinal or bulbar motor neurones; they are, at times, the direct cause of death. Disturbances in water and electrolyte balance are common in patients receiving continuous artificial respiration. Fever and the sweating which follow enclosure in a tank respirator during the summer months, together with vomiting, diarrhea, inability to take food, and disturbances in carbon dioxide related to improperly regulated ventilation, produce a complicated series of chemical disturbances. Edema and low electrolyte levels often follow overenthusiastic hydration and have been misinterpreted as evidence of a salt-wasting syndrome. Myocarditis is not uncommon in poliomyelitis; it is probably due to direct viral invasion. ECG changes, mainly T and ST-T and P-R abnormalities, are present in from 10 to 20 percent of cases. Interstitial infiltration of the myocardium with round cells and mild muscle changes are not infrequent. Severe myocardopathy has been thought to be responsible for death in some cases. Hypertension may develop by two mechanisms: (1) transient elevation of blood pressure due to hypoxia, and (2) persistent hypertension secondary to hypothalamic involvement, which may become "malignant" and lead to severe retinopathy, convulsions, and mental deterioration.

Pulmonary edema and shock, the exact pathogenesis of which is not known, are usually the terminal events in fatal cases of poliomyelitis. Phlebothrombosis of the legs, with or without pulmonary embolism, is not uncommon, even in young adults. All methods of artificial respiration produce hemodynamic disturbances, which are countered by reflex mechanisms acting to maintain normal blood pressure and cardiac output. When patients are placed in respirators under negative tank pressure (positive intratracheal pressure) after hypotension and impending shock are already present, the peripheral vascular collapse often is made worse. Acute and marked dilatation of the stomach and large bowel, perforation of the cecum, acute ulceration of the duodenum, stomach, and esophagus, the formation of multiple erosions of the entire gastrointestinal tract with considerable bleeding and paralytic ileus have been observed. Marked depression of prothrombin, with massive spontaneous hemorrhage, occurs in individuals with severe poliomyelitis, especially if they are receiving large doses of broad-spectrum antibiotics orally. Severe bulbar (ninth and tenth cranial nerves) or bulbospinal disease with paralysis of the respiratory muscles is accompanied by the risk of major atelectasis.

Bacterial infection is one of the most dangerous complications of paralytic poliomyelitis. Pneumonia is quite common in patients with paralysis of the muscles of respiration or deglutition. The incidence of pulmonary infection is greatly increased by tracheostomy and is highest in the respirator patient subjected to this operation. The organisms involved most often are *Staphylococcus aureus* and gram-negative bacilli, many strains of which are not sensitive to the commonly used antimicrobial agents. Chemoprophylaxis is of no value in preventing secondary bronchopulmonary bacterial invasion.

The other common site of infection in poliomyelitis is the urinary tract because of the necessity for chronic catheterization in patients with paralysis of the bladder; chemoprophylaxis is usually ineffective, although closed catheter drainage may be effective in keeping the urine sterile for as long as a week. The responsible organisms are those usually found in urinary tract infections and are often insusceptible to antibiotics and sulfonamides. Renal stone formation is frequent and may be responsible for renal colic, obstruction of the pelvis, and pyonephrosis, pyelonephritis, renal decompensation, hypertension, and vascular disease. The factors which contribute to renal lithiasis are immobility with hypercalcuria, infection, stasis, dehydration, and excessive calcium intake. Attempts to control this problem consist of the liberal administration of fluids, decrease of calcium intake, acidification of the urine, administration of salicylate, and early mobilization.

A syndrome resembling rheumatoid arthritis, with redness, swelling, pain, and tenderness of the larger joints, is observed rarely in the convalescent phase of paralytic poliomyelitis. A variety of skin rashes may occur, including miliaria, seborrhea, and purpuric, morbilliform, or exfoliative eruptions due to drug sensitization. Bedsores are common in respirator patients because of the difficulty in moving them about. Markedly paralyzed individuals, especially those whose life is threatened by respiratory difficulty, frequently experience very difficult emotional problems. Disorientation, acute panic states, Korsakoff-like syndromes, and acute psychoses have been noted. Chronic anxiety and depression are almost universal in adults with severe neurologic involvement and probably reflect the sudden impact of a crippling disease, rather than brain damage due to viral invasion.

IMMUNITY. One attack of poliomyelitis usually confers lifelong immunity against reinvasion by the same sero-type. Both neutralizing and complement-fixing antibodies appear early in the disease; complement-fixing antibodies persist for several years after infection, while neutralizing antibodies persist throughout life. Theoretically, an individual could have three episodes of the disease, because immunity is strictly type-specific. Most adults and many children have poliomyelitis, without nervous system invasion, two or three times, as shown by the presence of neutralizing antibody for more than one virus type. There are, however, well-documented instances of two episodes of paralytic infection separated by a number of years in the same individual.

TREATMENT. Cases of *abortive poliomyelitis* should receive no therapy except for symptomatic relief.

The management of *nonparalytic poliomyelitis* involves primarily the relief of the headache, pain in the back, and "spasm" of the legs. Rest in bed with the mattress supported by a board may be of value in preventing paralysis and is helpful in reducing back pain. The application of wet heat, in the form of "hot packs," to the affected muscles produces considerable relief. Analgesics such as meperidine and codeine are very useful and are preferable to morphine derivatives. Antimicrobial agents are useless because they have no effect on the primary disease and do not decrease the risk of secondary infection. Neuromuscular examination should not be carried out more often than every 3 to 4 days. Bed rest is terminated as soon as severe discomfort is absent in order to reduce the risk of phlebothrombosis and pulmonary embolism. Every patient thought to have nonparalytic poliomyelitis should have careful assessment of muscle function and an orthopedic follow-up study for 2 to 3 months after recovery. The purpose of these measures is to detect and correct minor degrees of weakness which may become apparent only when muscles which appear normal at rest are taxed by the exertion of normal physical activity.

The treatment of *paralytic poliomyelitis* involves (1) the use of all measures to spare the life of the patient threatened by involvement of vital areas, (2) relief of discomfort, (3) maintenance of weak muscles in as good a condition as possible, (4) immediate recognition and treatment of medical complications, (5) prophylaxis and therapy of emotional disorders, (6) surgical treatment of correctable defects, and (7) social, economic, occupational, and physical rehabilitation.

Patients with paralysis of swallowing, loss of function of the respiratory muscles, pulmonary edema, or shock are in great danger of death. Dysfunction of the ninth and tenth cranial nerves is most important because of the danger of fatal airway obstruction. For this reason, it has been suggested that tracheostomy be performed in all such cases. However, thorough study has indicated that this operation is followed by a much higher incidence of bronchopulmonary infections due to organisms difficult to eradicate with antibiotic agents than occurs when the procedure is not carried out. In some cases, however, tracheostomy becomes necessary, despite the risk. The indications for this operation are (1) abductor paralysis of the vocal cords; (2) pneumonia with inability to clear the lungs of exudate; (3) repeated bouts of major atelectasis requiring tracheal catheterization or bronchoscopy; (4) inability to keep the airway relatively free of secretions—this is often purely a matter of availability of a sufficient complement of experienced personnel.

Decreased movement of the diaphragm or intercostal muscles dictates frequent determination of vital capacity. When this is reduced to 50 percent of normal or less, artificial respiration must be given with a tank or cuirass type of chest respirator. Details of this type of treatment are discussed in Chap. 295. An electrophrenic respirator is indicated when the respiratory center is involved because tank respiration may actually increase the difficulties imposed by respiratory center dysfunction. Indirect stimulation of one phrenic nerve through the skin is usually sufficient.

Shock is easier to prevent than to treat. Assurance of adequate oxygen saturation, prevention of dehydration, and early treatment of superimposed bacterial infection are of prophylactic value. When marked hypotension develops, vasoconstricting agents such as norepinephrine are often helpful in restoring blood pressure to normal. As a rule, however, these drugs become ineffective as their use is prolonged. Plasma infusions may be of some help. Hypotension appearing during artificial respiration may respond to alternating positive and negative tank pressures of approximately the same degree.

The relief of discomfort is one of the most important problems in paralytic poliomyelitis. Hot wet packs, diathermy, warm baths, and dry heat reduce pain due to muscle "spasm." Analgesic drugs should be used whenever necessary, but morphine derivatives should be avoided. Changing the position of paralyzed limbs and moving the patient about in bed are effective in reducing pain.

Weak muscles must be maintained in as good condition as possible until neural function returns; the time, degree, and extent of resumption of function are unpredictable, but treatment should be continued for at least 2 years and is managed best by the physiotherapist who has had experience with poliomyelitis. Daily physiotherapy is usually started 3 to 4 days after complete defervescence and after there is no further extension of weakness. Exercise against resistance is thought to be most beneficial, but in many clinics, exercise in water to remove the effects of gravity is standard practice.

The prevention and treatment of the emotional disorders which accompany severe paralytic poliomyelitis best are carried out by the attending physicians and nurses. Although the help of the psychiatrist is necessary in difficult situations, the importance of physicians, nurses, and attendants who are in constant contact with the patient and are properly oriented toward these problems cannot be overemphasized.

Maximal return of muscle function usually is established at the end of 2 years following the onset of paralytic poliomyelitis. A review of the clinical problem by an orthopedic surgeon should be carried out if residual palsies remain, and a program of surgical rehabilitation should be set in motion.

The impact of paralytic poliomyelitis on the social and economic status of adults is often very severe. Every effort must be made to enlist the cooperation of social service agencies to minimize the disruptive effects of the disease. Many patients require occupational rehabilitation because of inability to perform the work in which they were engaged prior to being crippled. For others, the use of devices, such as movable splints and hooks, is very helpful in physical rehabilitation.

PROGNOSIS. The overall mortality rate for poliomyelitis is about 5 percent. Patients with abortive or nonparalytic disease recover completely. About 2 to 5 percent of children and 15 to 30 percent of adults (increasing with age) with paralytic infection die. When bulbospinal involvement, especially with medullary or phrenic and intercostal nerve dysfunction, is present, the fatality rate varies between 25 and 75 percent and is greatly influenced by age and the presence of shock, pulmonary edema, superimposed infection, or other medical complications.

Many persons with paralytic poliomyelitis recover completely. In a considerable number, muscle function returns to some degree. Only a few remain totally paralyzed. The more life-threatening the disease in the acute stage, the more frequent is complete functional recovery, if the patient survives. For example, paralysis of the respiratory center usually disappears completely. Dysfunction of the ninth and tenth cranial nerves is followed by total recovery in most instances, although mild palatopharyngeal weakness occasionally may persist for life. Paralysis of the muscles of respiration often disappears completely. In some cases, the final vital capacity, although reduced, is adequate to maintain ventilation, even with moderate physical exertion. In very few instances is chronic respirator care necessary. Weak extremities regain about 60 percent of the total strength that they will ever recover in 3 months, and 80 percent, within 6 months. Improvement may continue for as long as 2 years. The final degree of functional return depends on the number of neurones destroyed.

PREVENTION. Because 90 to 95 percent of cases of poliomyelitis are inapparent, or "minor" infections, and are not diagnosed, the prevention of the disease by isolation is very difficult. The common practice of isolating clinically evident cases is of much greater individual than public health benefit. The usual period of isolation is about 2 weeks, although virus may be present in the feces for a much longer period. Contact with known cases should be avoided. Restriction of community activities such as swimming or gathering of people is not indicated except with large epidemics, when it is more effective in allaying panic than in reducing infection. Pregnant women should take special precaution because of the increased susceptibility to the disease during pregnancy. Tonsillectomy is contraindicated in areas where poliomyelitis is present. All individuals with "minor" illnesses during the poliomyelitis season should limit their physical activity and avoid chilling until all symptoms have disappeared.

Active immunization against paralytic poliomyelitis has been successful by means of parenteral administration of formalin-inactivated strains of the three viral serotypes grown in monkey kidney tissue culture. The vaccine is

60 to 70 percent effective against type 1 and 85 to 90 percent effective against types 2 and 3. A booster dose should be given within 2 years after initial injection series. The effectiveness of this vaccine is evidenced by the fact that, in the year (1955) in which it was introduced, there were 28,985 cases of poliomyelitis in the United States. Two years later, only 2,218 cases were reported. Formalin-inactivated vaccine does not decrease the incidence of nonparalytic poliomyelitis. It has no effect on the intestinal phase of the disease and fails, therefore, to interrupt the spread of virus from one vaccinated person to another. Another drawback is the necessity to give "booster" doses for the maintenance of a protective level of antibody. Although four doses are presently recommended, whether more injections are necessary has not been determined.

Oral administration of attenuated strains of poliovirus is highly effective in stimulating antibody production and preventing infection and is the method of choice for protecting a population. The virus preparations are easily handled and are stable. They may be stored in a conventional refrigerator up to 30 days. Once a vial has been used in part, the rest of its contents should be discarded after 7 days.

Vaccine virus multiplies in the intestinal tract and remains at this site. Viremia occurs rarely, and then only with some strains. Live vaccine virus spreads and infects contacts of vaccinated individuals. The incidence of spread is lowest in high-income groups (about 9 percent) following feeding of infants. This type of immunization in the presence of epidemic poliomyelitis may lead to replacement of the "wild" paralytogenic strain by the one in the vaccine, and may actually abort spread of the disease.

Significant levels of antibody develop in 90 to 100 percent of persons receiving live virus vacine; they develop more rapidly and persist longer than those which follow the use of formalinized vaccines. Intestinal immunity is present after feeding of the "live" preparations so that minimal or no multiplication in the bowel occurs on exposure to "wild" strains of virus.

The highest levels of poliomyelitis-neutralizing antibody appear when monovalent oral vaccines are administered. The recommended order of administration is type 1, followed within no less than 8 weeks by type 3, which, in turn, should be followed in 6 or more weeks by type 2. If the polyvalent vaccine (all three types) is given to adults, two doses are fed 8 weeks apart. If newborns are given vaccine, the viruses should be refed at a later date because about 50 percent of neonates fail to develop significant levels of immunity if treated shortly after birth. Immunization of breast-fed infants should be delayed until they are taking regular diets. It has been suggested that a community-wide program of vaccine virus feeding followed by routine immunization of infants in the first year of life may result in eradication of poliomyelitis. The efficacy of this procedure is emphasized by the fact that there were only 66 cases of poliomyelitis recorded in the United States during the first 9 months of 1966. Immunization with live vaccine is best carried out during the cooler months of the year. The widespread prevalence of other enteroviruses in the intestinal tract, especially in children, may result in a low level of immunization because these may interfere with the implantation of the vaccine strains. Although the necessity for "booster" doses of this preparation in older children and adults has not been proved, many physicians are administering the triple vaccine 1 to 2 years after primary immunization; some are giving a second "booster" 1 to 2 years after the first.

The administration of live poliomyelitis virus vaccines to millions of persons in many areas of the world has demonstrated very convincingly the very high degree of protection (over 90 percent) against paralytic poliomyelitis conferred by this preparation and a tendency for epidemic strains to be replaced by those present in the vaccine. The vaccines are remarkably safe. Although instances of the disease are thought to have been associated with feeding of each of the three strains (0.4 cases per million doses for type 3, 0.16 per million doses for type 1, and 0.02 per million doses for type 2), it has been suggested that the greatest risk of developing active disease produced by the vaccine strain is related to the administration of the type 3 preparation to individuals in the age range of twenty to thirty-nine years. However, firm proof of the association of vaccine virus and the development of poliomyelitis is lacking, and the possibility has been raised that the "compatible" cases have been caused by wild strains of poliomyelitis virus or other enteroviruses present in the intestinal tract at the time the vaccine was administered. Type 1 vaccine strain has been incriminated in a case of paralytic poliomyelitis in a young child with marked hypogammaglobulinemia. Children known to have this defect should probably not receive this agent.

REFERENCES

Grulee, C. G.: Differential Diagnosis of Poliomyelitis, J.A.M.A., 152:1587, 1953.

Henderson, D. A., J. J. Witte, L. Morris, and A. D. Langmuir: Paralytic Disease Associated with Oral Polio Vaccines, J.A.M.A., 190:41, 1964.

Hodes, J. L.: Treatment of Respiratory Difficulty in Poliomyelitis, in "Poliomyelitis, Papers and Discussions Presented at the Third International Poliomyelitis Conference," Philadelphia, J. B. Lippincott Company, 1955.

Horstmann, D. M.: The Epidemiology and Pathogenesis of Poliomyelitis, Bull. N.Y. Acad. Med., 29:909, 1953.

——, M. D. McCollum, and A. D. Mascola: The Incidence of Infection among Contacts of Poliomyelitis Cases, J. Clin. Invest., 34:1573, 1955.

Report of Special Advisory Committee on Oral Poliomyelitis Vaccines to the Surgeon General of the Public Health Service: Oral Poliomyelitis Vaccines, J.A.M.A., 190:49–51, 1964.

Sabin, A. B.: Commentary on Report on Oral Poliomyelitis Vaccines, J.A.M.A., 190:52–55, 1964.

——: Poliomyelitis. Accomplishments of Live Virus Vaccine. First International Conference on Vaccines against Viral and Rickettsial Diseases, Bull. World Health Organ., p. 171, 1967.

Symposium on Poliomyelitis, Pediat. Clin. N. Am., 1:1, 1953.

Symposium on Poliomyelitis Vaccination, J.A.M.A., 158:1239, 1955.

Weinstein, L.: Diagnosis and Treatment of Poliomyelitis, Med. Clinics N. Am., p. 1377, September, 1948.

——: The Influence of Muscular Fatigue, Tonsilladenoidectomy and Antigen Injections on the Clinical Course of Poliomyelitis, Boston Med. Quart., 3:11, 1952.

——: Influence of Age and Sex on Susceptibility and Clinical Manifestations in Poliomyelitis, New Engl. J. Med., 257: 47, 1957.

——: Cardiovascular Disturbances in Poliomyelitis, Circulation, 15:735, 1957.

217 RABIES
Robert R. Wagner

DEFINITION. Rabies (hydrophobia, lyssa) is a fatal viral infection of the nervous system transmitted in saliva of rabid animals.

HISTORY. Some of the earliest extant writings contain suggestive references to mad dogs. Aristotle (*c.* 335 B.C.) described the transmission of rabies from dogs to other animals, and Celsus (*c.* A.D. 100) recognized that hydrophobia in man was caused by the bite of a rabid dog. The prevalence of the disease in man increased markedly in the eighteenth century following a European epizootic of canine rabies. The first effective control measures were instituted in Scandinavia, resulting in elimination of the disease there by 1826. Galtier's report in 1879 of transmission of rabies to laboratory rabbits led to the classical studies by Pasteur and his associates of "fixed" virus for vaccine production. Histologic diagnosis of infection became possible after Negri in 1903 described the characteristic cellular inclusion bodies of the disease.

ETIOLOGY. Rabies is a complex, cylindrical, RNA-containing virus that has been tentatively assigned to the rhabdovirus group along with the virus of vesicular stomatitis. Rabies virus is infectious for nervous tissue of all warm-blooded animals and can also be grown in tissue culture and chick embryos. The term *street virus* is used to designate the agent of the naturally occurring disease. *Fixed viruses* are rapidly multiplying strains used in vaccine production which have lost their infectivity for salivary gland tissue after passage in laboratory animals. There is only one antigenic type of the virus.

EPIDEMIOLOGY. All mammals are potential vectors, but carnivores are responsible for most cases in man and animals. Virus is present in saliva for several days before symptoms develop and persists until the time of death. Rabies is usually contracted from bites, occasionally from scratches or abrasions contaminated with infected saliva, or rarely by penetration of mucous membranes. Although dogs were formerly the principal cause of human rabies in the United States, wild animals now constitute a more important source of infection. The usual form of the disease in dogs, called *furious rabies*, is characterized by progressive agitation, aimless wandering, difficulty in swallowing, frothing at the mouth, labored respirations,

feeble bark, ataxia, convulsions, and vicious, indiscriminate attacks on all creatures and inanimate objects. Paralysis and stupor usually develop 2 to 3 days before death and are the sole manifestations (*dumb rabies*) in about one-fifth of infected dogs.

Although quarantine, killing of stray animals, and vaccination are effective in controlling canine rabies, large reservoirs of infection exist in wild animals, such as the wolf in Eastern Europe and Western Asia, the jackal in India and North Africa, and the mongoose in South Africa. During 1964, an epizootic of rabies in foxes was prevalent in Tennessee and adjacent states, where enzootic foci still exist, and the disease is also found in skunks, raccoons, coyotes, squirrels, bobcats, mountain lions, and other animals throughout the world. Vigorous control measures have eliminated all foci of rabies in domestic and wild animals of Scandinavia and the British Isles and prevented importation of the disease into Hawaii and Australia.

The vampire bat transmits a paralytic form of the disease to cattle and horses and constitutes an important reservoir of rabies in South and Central America, Mexico, and the West Indies. Vampire bats are occasionally nocturnal predators of man, attacking silently to take their blood meal without the sleeping victim's knowledge. Human rabies acquired from bites of common bats was first recognized in the United States in 1951 to 1953, and subsequent surveys have revealed that the disease occurs in many insectivorous and herbivorous species.

Rabies is almost invariably a rapidly fatal infection in all mammals except vampire and insectivorous bats, which can continue to transmit the disease for many months. Abortive infection with subsequent immunity can be produced experimentally in mice.

PATHOGENESIS. Rabies virus spreads from the site of inoculation along sensory nerve pathways to the posterior columns of the spinal cord, if the bite is on the extremities or trunk, or by cranial nerves to the brain stem from face wounds. The salivary glands, intestine, pancreas, renal tubules, and adrenal medulla are involved by extension along the autonomic nerves. Viremia may occur. Focal inflammation, neuronophagia, demyelinization, hemorrhages, and perivascular infiltration by mononuclear cells occur throughout the nervous system, but these changes are most marked in the basal ganglia, subcortical areas, and spinal cord. Rabies can be distinguished from other viral encephalitides if the pathognomonic Negri bodies are found. These are eosinophilic inclusion bodies, 0.5 to 10 μ in diameter, demonstrable in the cytoplasm of nerve cells by special stains. In all animals, including man, they are found in greatest abundance in Ammon's horn of the hippocampus and to a lesser extent in pyramidal cells of the cerebral cortex, Purkinje cells of the cerebellum, and nuclei of the basal ganglions.

MANIFESTATIONS. The *incidence* of rabies in unvaccinated individuals bitten by rabid animals is about 15 percent, but varies from 5 to 70 percent, depending on the amount of virus in the saliva and the location and depth of the wounds. It may be difficult to obtain a history of animal exposure if the disease is acquired from minor bites or scratches. The *incubation period* is usually 30 to 70 days but can be as short as 10 days or, rarely, more than a year. Short incubation periods occur after face or arm bites, multiple wounds, or wolf bites. Prodromal symptoms of fever with temperatures of 100 to 102°F, headache, malaise, nausea, vomiting, sore throat, and persistent loose cough are often present for 1 to 4 days. The most significant early manifestations, in about 80 percent of cases, are tingling, paresthesias, and dull or stabbing pain at the site of the bite, often radiating to the hip, shoulder, or neck, and to distal parts of the involved extremity. The wound may be inflamed and excoriated by the patient's scratching. The first, or *excitement,* phase of the disease is characterized by increasing agitation, marked restlessness, excessive motor activity, aimless pacing, dysarthria, and occasionally, visual or auditory hallucinations. Episodes of unreasoning fear and rage alternate with profound depression. The patient may become destructive, wildly apprehensive, and combative if restrained but usually does not attack his attendants. Spasmodic gross muscle contractions and generalized clonic or tonic convulsions with opisthotonos develop shortly after the onset, often precipitated by loud noises, bright lights, touch, or even drafts. Respirations become shallow and irregular, the pulse becomes rapid and thready, and the temperature usually exceeds 103°F. There may be involvement of the autonomic nervous system manifested by dilated, irregular pupils, excessive lacrimation, sweating, and salivation. Many patients also exhibit vertigo, nystagmus, optic neuritis with central blindness, diplopia, strabismus, or facial palsy. Paralysis of the vocal cords results in hoarseness or aphonia. Hyperactive deep tendon reflexes, Babinski signs, and nuchal rigidity are often present.

The most characteristic feature of the disease is severe, painful *contractions of the pharyngeal muscles,* initially precipitated by attempts to swallow fluids. This usually develops 1 to 3 days after onset and progresses until the mere sight, sound, mention, or even thought of water causes reflex spasms of the muscles of deglutition and respiration, leading to bouts of apnea, cyanosis, and generalized convulsions. Most patients manifest a *fear of water* (*hydrophobia*) and to avoid swallowing allow frothy saliva to drool from the mouth. Death usually follows a generalized convulsion with prolonged apnea.

Patients who survive the excitement stage of the disease develop *generalized flaccid paralysis,* often evident at first in the bitten extremity. Muscle spasms and pharyngeal contractions cease, and agitation gives way to depression, apathy, hyporeflexia, and coma. The ability to swallow may return temporarily, and there is often transient slowing of the pulse and respirations. The bladder usually becomes atonic. Generalized paralysis, resembling the Guillain-Barré syndrome, is occasionally the only neurologic manifestation. Rabies acquired from vampire bats, which frequently bite the toes, usually takes the form of Landry's ascending paralysis without excitation or pharyngeal spasm. Death usually occurs 2 to 3 days after onset of paralytic rabies but may be delayed for several weeks.

LABORATORY FINDINGS. The blood leukocyte count may be elevated, occasionally to 30,000 cells per cu mm, with an increased number of polymorphonuclear and large mononuclear cells. Glycosuria, acetonuria, proteinuria, and oliguria are present in most cases. The cerebrospinal fluid is usually normal but may contain slightly increased amounts of protein and as many as 100 mononuclear cells per cu mm. Virus may be present in saliva or, rarely, in cerebrospinal fluid. Serum antibodies can be determined by neutralization or complement fixation tests, but serologic studies are of little value for retrospective diagnosis, because almost all surviving patients have received vaccine or immune serum. Definitive diagnosis is usually made at autopsy by demonstrating Negri bodies or by isolation of rabies virus from the brain. The histochemical technique of staining brain or parotid tissue with fluorescent antibody has proved to be an accurate and rapid method of diagnosis.

DIFFERENTIAL DIAGNOSIS. *Hysterical reactions* to dog bites and *allergic encephalomyelitis* caused by rabies vaccine are sometimes difficult at first to differentiate from rabies. Paralytic rabies may be confused with poliomyelitis or the *Gullain-Barré syndrome,* particularly when a history of animal bite cannot be obtained or the incubation period exceeds 3 months. Many of the manifestations of *tetanus,* except trismus, resemble those of rabies. *Delirium tremens* and *intoxication with belladonna alkaloids* occasionally simulate rabies.

TREATMENT. There are about 5,000 cases of rabies in animals reported annually in the United States. The incidence of recognized cases in man has declined from 56 in 1946 to a single case in 1963. However, approximately 50,000 persons each year are considered to be exposed to rabies and receive vaccine treatment. The basic principle in the treatment of individuals exposed to rabies is to furnish sufficient antibody to prevent the virus from involving the central nervous system. Semple's vaccine, prepared from fixed virus grown in rabbit brain and inactivated with phenol, was formerly used for this purpose in the United States.

A vaccine prepared in duck embryos, and free of brain tissue, is now recommended for human use in the United States. A course of 14 daily inoculations is usually given to an individual exposed to rabies. Prophylactic immunization is best accomplished in dogs and other domestic animals by injection of a single dose of live, attenuated virus of the Flury strain. Passive immunization with antirabies horse serum, used as an adjunct to vaccination, appears to afford enhanced resistance to infection, particularly in heavily exposed individuals. The local treatment of bites consists of thorough cleaning with strong soap or detergent solutions and infiltration of the area with immune serum. Cauterization or debridement of the wound is no longer recommended.

The chief hazards of Semple's vaccine are *hypersensitivity reactions* with severe local erythema, often accompanied by fever and arthralgia, in about 5 percent of cases and *peripheral neuritis* or *allergic encephalomyelitis* caused by the rabbit brain tissue in 1 of 600 to 10,000 vaccinated individuals. Encephalomyelitis usually occurs

1 to 3 weeks after the first injection of vaccine and is characterized by the sudden onset of chills, fever, headache, and vomiting, followed by disorientation, dysarthria, ataxia, paresthesias, cranial nerve palsies, visual disturbances, and, frequently, hemiparesis or paraplegia. Increased concentrations of protein in the cerebrospinal fluid and mononuclear pleocytosis are noted in the majority of cases. The mortality rate varies from 0 to 25 percent, and about one-third of patients who recover from allergic encephalomyelitis have residual neurologic disorders.

The decision to proceed with antirabies treatment must depend on the risk of exposure in individual cases. Sudden, unprovoked attacks by any animals are rare and should be considered presumptive evidence of exposure to rabies.

Vaccine should be administered promptly if a person is bitten by an animal that escapes, is clinically rabid, or shows histologic evidence of infection. However, Negri bodies are not demonstrable in 12 percent of animals with rabies proved by virus isolation. Healthy dogs or cats that inflict minor bites or scratches contaminated with saliva should be impounded and observed for 7 days. No treatment is required if the animal remains healthy. Immune serum should be administered within 24 hr to all individuals who incur severe or multiple bites, regardless of whether the animal shows signs of rabies at the time. Every bat bite should be considered to be an exposure to rabies.

Prophylactic vaccination is advisable for a small, but selected, "high-risk" segment of the population of the United States, including veterinarians, spelunkers, dog catchers, and postmen. After a primary course of duck embryo vaccine, a single booster injection induces a prompt antibody response. Semple rabbit-brain vaccine should not be used for repeated revaccination because of the increased risk of allergic encephalomyelitis in individuals sensitized to rabbit brain tissue.

No specific treatment is available if clinical manifestations develop. The patient should be kept in a quiet, darkened, draftless room and disturbed as little as possible. Large doses of barbiturates are more effective than opiates in lessening anxiety, delirium, and the frequency of pharyngeal spasms and convulsions. Parenteral administration of fluids is often required.

PROGNOSIS. Thus far, rabies has been an invariably fatal disease in man. However, every patient should receive all possible supportive treatment in the hope that the diagnosis is in error.

REFERENCES

Applebaum, E., M. Greenberg, and J. Nelson: Neurological Complications Following Antirabies Vaccination, J.A.M.A., 151:188, 1953.

Gibbs, F. A., et al.: Comparison of Rabies Vaccines Grown on Duck Embryo and on Nervous Tissue, New Engl. J. Med., 265:1002, 1961.

Hildreth, E. A.: Prevention of Rabies, or the Decline of Sirius, Ann. Intern. Med., 58:883, 1963.

Hummeler, K., H. Koprowski, and T. J. Wiktor: Structure and Development of Rabies Virus in Tissue Culture, J. Virol., 1:152, 1967.

Johnson, H. N.: Rabies Virus, pp. 814–840 in "Viral and Rickettsial Infections of Man," 4th ed., F. L. Horsfall and I. Tamm (Eds.), Philadelphia, J. B. Lippincott Company, 1965.

Koprowski, H.: Rabies. Pediat. Clin. N. Am., 2:55, 1955.

Roueché, B.: The Incurable Wound, pp. 36–67 in "The Incurable Wound and Further Narratives of Medical Detection," Boston, Little, Brown and Company, 1958.

Sulkin, S. E.: The Bat as a Reservoir of Viruses in Nature. Progr. Med. Virol., 4:157, 1962.

218 VIRAL ENCEPHALITIS
Jay P. Sanford

DEFINITION. The clinical picture of encephalitis (fever, neurologic signs indicating cerebral involvement, i.e., alterations in cerebration, seizures, cranial nerve weakness, meningeal irritation, and pleocytosis in the cerebrospinal fluid) can result from cerebral damage due to a large number of infections as well as noninfectious causes. Of the more than 3,000 patients reported with encephalitis during 1966, 34 percent were classified as postinfectious. This is a broad category which includes mumps, measles, varicella, herpes, influenza, and rubella. An enteroviral etiology (poliovirus, Coxsackie virus, and ECHO virus) was considered in approximately 4 percent, while 14 percent were due to arboviruses. In the remaining 48 percent, the etiology was not determined. Four arboviruses are presently recognized as numerically important causes of encephalitis in the United States: St. Louis encephalitis virus, Eastern equine encephalitis virus, Western equine encephalitis virus, and the California encephalitis group of viruses. With few exceptions, for the last 12 years in the United States, St. Louis encephalitis virus has been the most common cause of arboviral encephalitis in humans.

Encephalitis lethargica, or Von Economo's disease, and subacute inclusion encephalitis, diseases of presumed but not unequivocally proved viral etiology, are described in Chap. 361.

ETIOLOGY. Despite the diversity of specific viral etiologies (Table 218-1), in individual patients, the clinical manifestations of encephalitis are very similar, and preclude an etiologic diagnosis without ancillary information regarding epidemiologic and serologic features. The clinical picture for the broad entity of arbovirus encephalitis will be discussed, then the specific epidemiologic and prognostic features which characterize the major types will be presented.

CLINICAL MANIFESTATIONS. The clinical features of arbovirus encephalitis differ among age groups. In infants under one year of age, the only consistently noted symptoms are sudden onset of fever which is often accompanied by convulsions. Convulsions may be either generalized or focal. Typically the fever ranges between

Table 218-1. SUMMARY OF VIROLOGIC AND EPIDEMIOLOGIC FEATURES OF ARBOVIRUSES ASSOCIATED WITH CENTRAL NERVOUS SYSTEM INVOLVEMENT IN MAN

Virus	Serologic group	Vector	Known geographic range of infection
Eastern equine encephalitis.........	A	Mosquito	Eastern Canada, United States, Mexico, Dominican Republic, Jamaica, Panama, Trinidad, Brazil, Colombia, Argentina
Western equine encephalitis.........	A	Mosquito	Canada, United States, Mexico, Brazil, Argentina
Venezuelan equine encephalitis......	A	Mosquito	Florida, Mexico, Panama, Colombia, Venezuela, Trinidad, Brazil, Ecuador
Central European encephalitis.......	B	Tick	Central and Eastern Europe
Diphasic meningoencephalitis........	B	Tick	Central and Eastern Europe
Ilheus..............................	B	Mosquito	Northern South America, Trinidad, Central America, Florida
Japanese encephalitis..............	B	Mosquito	Japan, China, Malaya, Taiwan, Thailand, Vietnam, Burma, Guam, Philippines, Korea, Australia, New Zealand
Kyasanur Forest disease............	B	Tick	India
Louping ill........................	B	Tick	Great Britain, Eire
Medoc.............................	B		United States
Murray Valley encephalitis..........	B	Mosquito	Australia, New Guinea
Negishi............................	B	?	Japan
Powassan..........................	B	Tick	Canada
Russian spring-summer encephalitis..	B	Tick	U.S.S.R.
St. Louis encephalitis..............	B	Mosquito	United States, Caribbean Islands, Panama, Brazil, Argentina
West Nile..........................	B	Mosquito	South and West Africa, Rhone Delta, Near East, Israel, India, Malaysia, Borneo
California encephalitis.............	California complex	Mosquito	United States
Phlebotomus, Naples..............	Phlebotomus	Sandfly	Italy, Egypt, Iran, West Pakistan

SOURCE: Adapted from the World Health Organization Technical Report Series, 1961, p. 219.

102 and 104°F. Other physical findings may include tenderness of the fontanelle, rigidity of the extremities, and abnormalities in reflexes.

In children between five and fourteen years of age, subjective symptoms are more easily elicited. Headache, fever, and drowsiness of 2 to 3 days' duration before seeking medical attention are common. The symptoms may then subside or become more intense and may be associated with nausea, vomiting, muscular pain, photophobia, and less frequently, convulsions (less than 10 percent). On examination, the child is acutely ill, febrile, and lethargic. Nuchal rigidity and intention tremors are often present and on occasion, muscular weakness can be demonstrated.

In adults, the initial symptoms commonly include the fairly abrupt onset of fever, nausea with vomiting, and severe headache. The headache is most often frontal but may be occipital or diffuse in location. Mental aberrations, represented by confusion and disorientation, usually appear within the subsequent 24 hr. Other symptoms may include diffuse myalgia and photophobia. The abnormalities on physical examination predominantly relate to the neurologic examination, although conjunctival suffusion is frequently seen and skin rashes may occur. Disturbances in mentation are among the most outstanding clinical features. These range from coma through severe disorientation to subtle abnormalities detected only by cerebral function tests such as the subtraction of serial sevens. A small proportion of patients show only lethargy, lying quietly, apparently asleep unless stimulated. Tremor is common and is observed more frequently in individuals over forty years of age. The tremors vary in location and may be continuous or intention in type. Cranial nerve abnormalities resulting in oculomotor muscle paresis and nystagmus, facial weakness, and difficulty in deglutition may occur, and are usually present within the initial several days. Objective sensory changes are unusual. Hemiparesis or monoparesis may occur. Reflex abnormalities are also common; these include exaggerated palmomental reflexes, and suck and snout reflexes. Superficial abdominal and cremasteric reflexes are usually absent. Changes in the tendon reflexes are variable and inconstant. The plantar response may be extensor and fluctuates almost hourly. Dysdiadochokinesia often exists.

The duration of the fever and neurologic symptoms and signs can vary from several days to a month but usually ranges from 4 to 14 days. Clinical improvement generally follows the subsidence of the fever within several days unless irreversible anatomic changes have occurred.

LABORATORY DATA. Erythrocyte values are usually normal. Total leukocyte counts often reveal both a slight to moderate leukocytosis (occasionally greater than 20,000

per cu mm) and neutrophilia. Examination of the cerebrospinal fluid usually reveals several hundred cells per cu mm, but on occasion cloudy cerebrospinal fluid with cells in excess of 1,000 per cu mm may be seen. Within the first several days of illness, polymorphonuclear neutrophiles may predominate. The initial cerebrospinal fluid protein is often slightly elevated but may exceed 100 mg per 100 ml on occasion. The level of spinal fluid sugar is normal; a significant decrease should raise serious consideration of an alternative diagnosis. As the illness progresses, mononuclear cells in the cerebrospinal fluid tend to increase so that they predominate and the protein concentration may increase. Other laboratory studies have been performed only sporadically, but abnormalities may include hyponatremia, often due to the inappropriate secretion of antidiuretic hormone, and elevations in serum creatine phosphokinase.

DIAGNOSIS. Specific diagnosis requires the isolation of the virus or detection of antibodies with a rising titer between the acute phase of disease and convalescence. Antibodies can be detected by hemagglutination inhibition, complement fixation, or virus neutralization techniques.

TREATMENT. Treatment is entirely supportive and requires meticulous attention in the comatose patient.

EASTERN EQUINE ENCEPHALITIS

Eastern equine encephalitis, a Group A arbovirus, was first isolated in 1933 from the brain tissue of horses during an outbreak of equine illness in New Jersey. The first recognized human outbreak occurred in Massachusetts in 1938.

EPIDEMIOLOGY. The virus is distributed along the eastern coast of the Americas from northeastern United States to Argentina. Viral isolations also have been reported in the Philippines, Thailand, Czechoslovakia, Poland, and the USSR, but the question of type specificity has not been resolved. In the northeastern United States, epidemics occur in the late summer and early fall. Epizootics in horses precede the occurrence of human cases by 1 to 2 weeks. The disease affects mainly infants, children, and adults over fifty-five years of age. There is no sex preponderance. Inapparent infection occurs in all age groups, suggesting that the decreased likelihood of developing overt infection in the fifteen to fifty-four-year age group is not the result of decreased exposure. The ratio of inapparent infection to overt encephalitis approximates 25 to 1.

The natural reservoir is unknown. Isolations have been made from numerous species of wild birds and also from amphibians, reptiles, and mammals. The natural vector is the mosquito, including *Aëdes sollicitans* and *Culiseta melanura. Aëdes sollicitans,* a salt-marsh mosquito which is an avid human feeder, has been postulated as the epidemic vector, while *Culiseta melanura* is important in bird-to-bird transmission. Equine animals and man are probably "dead ends" in the transmission cycle, and infection in them is accidental.

PATHOLOGY. An outstanding feature is the predominance of neutrophilic leukocytes in the infiltrates. Foci of tissue damage represented by rarefaction necrosis are common. Neuronolysis also is very common. Large perivascular collections of neutrophiles and activated histiocytes are frequently detected in the white matter of the cortex. Other sites of predilection are the thalamus, putamen, substantia nigra, and pons.

CLINICAL MANIFESTATIONS. While human infections have been thought usually to result in serious, if not fatal, central-nervous-system involvement, the detection of inapparent infection as well as relatively mild disease establishes the occurrence of milder forms. In many patients, the cerebrospinal fluid is cloudy and contains in excess of 1,000 cells per cu mm.

DIAGNOSIS. The hemagglutination-inhibition or neutralization tests are the serologic methods of choice. The complement fixation test may be negative in patients with confirmed infections.

PROGNOSIS. The mortality in clinical infection exceeds 50 percent. In the most severe cases, death occurs between the third and fifth days. Children under ten years of age have a greater likelihood of surviving the acute illness, but also have a greater likelihood of developing severe disabling residuals: mental retardation, convulsions, emotional lability, blindness, deafness, speech disorders, and hemiplegia.

WESTERN EQUINE ENCEPHALITIS

The virus of this disease is a Group A arbovirus and was isolated in 1930 in California from horses with encephalitis. In 1938 it was recovered from a fatal human infection.

EPIDEMIOLOGY. Western equine encephalitis virus has been isolated in the United States, Canada, Brazil, British Guiana, and Argentina. Human disease has been diagnosed only in the United States, Canada, and Brazil. In the United States, the virus is found in virtually all geographic areas. The central valley of California represents an important endemic area. The disease occurs mainly in early and midsummer. Wild birds, which develop viremia of sufficiently high titer to infect mosquitoes on feeding, are the basic reservoir, although nonavian vertebrate hosts may be important. Both laboratory and field observations point to the importance of *Culex tarsalis* as the principal vector in the western United States. In areas east of the Appalachian Mountains, another vector must be operative. The virus has been repeatedly isolated from *Culiseta melanura;* however, the importance of this mosquito has been questioned, since it is not primarily a man-biting mosquito. The ratio of inapparent infection as evidenced by serologic survey studies and disease varies from 58 to 1 in children to 1,150 to 1 in adults. Approximately one-fourth of patients are less than one year of age. The highest attack rates occur in individuals fifty years or older.

PATHOLOGY. The outstanding feature is the presence of many foci of rarefaction necrosis, which are most numerous in the striatum, then the globus pallidus, cerebral cortex, thalamus, and pointine tegmentum. A number of foci contain neutrophiles and resemble "abscesses."

Perivascular collections of lymphocytes and ameboid cells are common. Occasional chronic cases have been characterized by severe cystic transformation in the basal ganglia, cerebral white matter, and cerebral cortex.

PROGNOSIS. The fatality rate approximates 2 to 3 percent in laboratory confirmed cases. The incidence and severity of sequelae are related to age. Sequelae among very young infants are frequent and severe (61 percent in a group of patients less than three months old) and consist of upper motor neurone impairment, involving the pyramidal tracts, extrapyramidal structures, and cerebellum and result in behavioral problems and convulsions. Both the incidence and severity of sequelae diminish rapidly after one year of age. Adults may complain of nervousness, irritability, easy fatigability, and tremulousness for 6 months or longer after the acute illness. Probably not more than 5 percent of adults have sequelae which are sufficiently severe to be of practical significance. Postencephalitic seizures are rare.

VENEZUELAN EQUINE ENCEPHALITIS

Venezuelan equine encephalitis virus was first reported in 1938 following studies of an epizootic disease in horses, donkeys, and mules in Venezuela known as "crazy plague."

EPIDEMIOLOGY. Disease has been confirmed in man by virus isolation in Venezuela, Colombia, and Panama. Serologic evidence of infection has also been found in persons in Trinidad, Ecuador, and Florida. The natural transmission cycle of the virus is unknown. The virus has been isolated from a variety of mosquito species, including *Aëdes taeniorhynchus* and *Aëdes escapularis*, and also from wild rodents. While several species of wild birds develop an asymptomatic viremia after experimental exposure, the role of wild birds as a reservoir is not clear. Studies on birds in Venezuela have failed to demonstrate either virus or antibodies, while in Colombia several species of wild birds have been shown to possess VEE antibodies, and the virus has been isolated from birds in Panama. During the initial 3 days of illness, viremia has been detected in approximately two-thirds of patients. The levels of viremia are sufficiently high so that man also could serve as a reservoir. VEE virus also can be isolated by pharyngeal swab in a few patients, suggesting the potential for person-to-person transmission. The available observations make it reasonable to consider that the natural vector is a mosquito, although natural infection can probably take place without an arthropod vector. Laboratory infections have occurred and are probably due to inhalation of aerosols.

PATHOLOGY. In the liver, there is focal necrosis of hepatic cells and prominence of the Kupffer's cells. The hepatic changes are similar to those in yellow fever and Bolivian hemorrhagic fever. Lymph nodes appear depleted and follicles are difficult to discern. The marked depletion of lymphoid tissues is compatible with experimental data. There may be slight turbidity of the leptomeninges with hyperemia and flattening of the cerebral convolutions. If death occurs within the first 2 days, there is swelling of vascular endothelium and transudation of fluid into Virchow-Robin spaces. Later findings include many foci of necrosis which are characterized by glitter cells and glial proliferation. The nuclei of the brainstem and surrounding tissue were most affected.

CLINICAL MANIFESTATIONS. In man, infection with Venezuelan equine encephalitis virus usually results in an acute febrile illness without neurologic complications. The illness is similar to dengue with fever of 1 to 4 days and delayed convalescence. In one case report, palatine petechiae were noted and the patient vomited "coffee grounds" material. Other hemorrhagic features were not described. In an epidemic in Venezuela in 1962, almost 16,000 cases of acute disease were evaluated; 38 percent were classified as encephalitis, but only 3 to 4 percent had severe neurologic abnormalities: convulsions, nystagmus, drowsiness, delirium, or meningitis. The mortality rate was estimated to be less than 0.5 percent, and nearly all deaths occurred in young children.

JAPANESE ENCEPHALITIS

The name Japanese B encephalitis was employed during an epidemic which occurred in 1924 to distinguish it from Von Economo's disease which was designated as type A encephalitis. The designation as Japanese B no longer seems useful, and the term Japanese encephalitis should be employed.

EPIDEMIOLOGY. Japanese encephalitis virus infection is known to occur in eastern Siberia, China, Korea, Taiwan, Japan, Malaya, Vietnam, Singapore, Guam, and India. In temperature climates, the disease shows a late summer, early fall seasonal incidence. In tropic climates there is no seasonal variation. The mosquito, *Culex tritaeniorhynchus*, is the major vector species. It is a rural mosquito which breeds in rice fields and preferentially bites large domestic animals, such as pigs, but also feeds on birds and man. Man is an accidental host in the transmission cycle. In several outbreaks, a higher incidence of cases has been reported in children than in adults.

PATHOLOGY. Japanese encephalitis is characterized by intense neuronophagia. Gliomesenchymal nodules are found in the cerebral cortex and the molecular and Purkinje cell layers of the cerebellum. In the thalamus and substantia nigra, foci of tissue breakdown are found. Perivascular infiltration adjacent to damaged nerve tissue occurs. Relatively severe involvement of the spinal cord also may occur.

CLINICAL MANIFESTATIONS. The occurrence of severe rigors at the onset has been noted in almost 90 percent of patients. Localized paresis is found more often than with other arboviral encephalitides, e.g., 31 percent, with predominantly upper extremity involvement. Weight loss has been very striking, averaging 26 lb in one report. The failure of the temperature to lyse, appearance of diaphoresis, tachypnea, and the accumulation of bronchial secretions are grave prognostic signs.

PROGNOSIS. The immediate mortality rate has varied from 7 percent to 33 percent or higher. The rate of occurrence of sequelae varies inversely with the fatality rate; in those series with high fatality rates (33 percent), sequelae occurred in 3 to 14 percent. In another series with a fatality rate of 7.4 percent, the sequelae rate was 32 percent. Sequelae consisted of neurologic or intellectual defects and psychiatric complaints.

ST. LOUIS ENCEPHALITIS

St. Louis encephalitis was first recognized as an entity during a major outbreak in St. Louis, Mo., and the surrounding area in 1933. St. Louis encephalitis is the most common type of arbovirus encephalitis in the United States.

EPIDEMIOLOGY. In the United States, epidemics of St. Louis encephalitis fall into two epidemiologic patterns. One pattern is found in the west, where mixed outbreaks of Western equine encephalitis and St. Louis encephalitis have occurred primarily in irrigated rural areas. The vector has been *Culex tarsalis*. The second pattern occurred in the original St. Louis outbreak and the numerous subsequent epidemics in the Midwest, New Jersey, and Florida. These outbreaks have been more urban in location and are characterized by a marked tendency for the development of encephalitis in older persons. In such urban-suburban epidemics, the epidemic vector has been mosquitoes of the *Culex pipiens-quinquefasciatus* complex with the exception of the Florida epidemic, in which *Culex nigripalpus* was incriminated. The presence of St. Louis virus outside of the United States has been proven by isolations in Trinidad, Panama, and Jamaica. However, except in Jamaica, no case of encephalitis due to this virus has been reported outside of the United States. The basic transmission cycle is that of wild bird-mosquito-wild bird. The mechanism by which the virus overwinters has not been defined. The disease in man usually appears in midsummer to early fall. There is no sex predominance. Man represents an accidental host and plays no role in the basic transmission cycle. Serologic studies following most urban epidemics indicate that infection rates are similar in all age groups, and the increasing age-specific attack rate for clinical encephalitis which is typical of urban St. Louis encephalitis is probably due to age differences in host susceptibility to overt disease rather than to a higher rate of infection.

PATHOLOGY. The basic lesions are small perivascular hemorrhages and cuffing by round cells. Nerve cell damage occurs in small clusters of cells in the gray matter. The lesions of St. Louis encephalitis predominate in the thalamus and substantia nigra, but the cerebral cortex may be slightly to moderately affected. There is usually little neuronophagia.

CLINICAL MANIFESTATIONS. Infection with St. Louis virus most commonly results in an inapparent infection. Of the patients with confirmed disease, approximately three-fourths have clinical encephalitis, while the remainder present with aseptic meningitis, febrile headaches, or nonspecific illness. Virtually all patients over forty years of age have encephalitic manifestations. Urinary frequency and dysuria have been symptoms in approximately 20 percent of patients despite sterile routine aerobic urine cultures. The basis for the urinary tract symptoms is not understood.

DIAGNOSIS. The occurrence of either encephalitis or aseptic meningitis as manifested by febrile illness with cerebrospinal fluid pleocytosis in the months of June through September in an adult, especially over thirty-five years of age, should raise the suspicion of St. Louis encephalitis. Because approximately 40 percent of patients with St. Louis encephalitis have antibodies detectable by hemagglutination inhibition at the onset of illness, acute serum for serologic studies should be submitted promptly to a competent laboratory.

PROGNOSIS. The case fatality ratio in the original St. Louis epidemic was 20 percent. In most subsequent outbreaks the mortality has varied from 2 to 12 percent. Subjective nervous complaints including nervousness, headaches, and easy fatigability and excitability appear to be the most common residuals. Late organic defects such as speech defects, difficulty in walking, and disturbances in vision were demonstrated in approximately 5 percent of patients 3 years following infection.

CALIFORNIA ENCEPHALITIS

A neurotropic virus which was named the California virus was isolated in 1943 and 1944 from three separate pools of mosquitoes in Kern County in the San Joaquin Valley of California. In 1945, serologic evidence of infection by this virus was demonstrated in three patients. Since 1963, a large number of isolations of what is now known to be the California group of viruses have been made. Cases of encephalitis and inapparent infection have been discovered, and the California group of viruses is now well established as a significant cause of encephalitis in the United States.

EPIDEMIOLOGY. The epidemiology has not been well elucidated. Infection has been demonstrated to occur in the Midwest, especially in Ohio, Indiana, and Wisconsin, as well as along the Eastern Seaboard. Birds do not appear to be an important host of the California viruses. Most of the potential host isolations have been from mammals. Virus has been isolated from *Aëdes triseriatus* mosquitoes. Some tick isolations also have been made. A basic transmission cycle involving small mammalian hosts and *Aëdes* species of mosquitoes has been suggested. Most of the illnesses have occurred in the late summer and early fall. One-half of the patients are children six years of age and younger. The home or recreational area of patients has been found to be in areas of high mosquito incidence.

DIAGNOSIS. Neutralizing and hemagglutination-inhibition antibodies are usually present a few days after the reported onset of disease. Complement fixing antibodies usually are detectable 10 to 12 days after the onset of illness.

PROGNOSIS. The case fatality ratio is low, and most patients recover. Follow-up studies have not been underway for sufficient time to evaluate sequelae; however, complaints of emotional lability, difficulty in learning in school, and personality problems have been frequent.

OTHER ARBOVIRUSES WITH CENTRAL-NERVOUS-SYSTEM INVOLVEMENT

There is a large group of additional arboviruses which have been associated with encephalitis or aseptic meningitis. Some of these agents are listed in the table. While the epidemiology of each of these agents differs, the general features are sufficiently similar to require laboratory support for their differentiation.

REFERENCES

Altman, R., M. Goldfield, and O. Sussman: The Impact of Vector-borne Viral Diseases in the Middle Atlantic States, Med. Clinics, No. Am., 51:661, 1967.

Briceno Rossi, A. L.: Rural Epidemic Encephalitis in Venezuela Caused by a Group A Arbovirus (VEE), Progr. Med. Virol., 9:176, 1967.

Casals, J., and D. H. Clarke: Arboviruses; Group A, p. 583 in "Viral and Rickettsial Infections of Man," 4th ed., F. L. Horsfall, Jr., and I. Tamm (Eds.), Philadelphia, J. B. Lippincott Co., 1965.

Cramblett, H. G., H. Stegmiller, and C. Spencer: California Encephalitis Virus Infections in Children. Clinical and Laboratory Studies, J.A.M.A., 198:108, 1966.

Dickerson, R. B., J. R. Newton, and J. E. Hansen: Diagnosis and Immediate Prognosis of Japanese B Encephalitis. Observations Based on More Than 200 Patients With Detailed Analysis of 65 Serologically Confirmed Cases, Am. J. Med., 12:277, 1952.

Feemster, R. F., and W. Haymaker: Eastern Equine Encephalitis, Neurology, 8:882, 1958.

Finley, K. H., W. A. Longshore, Jr., R. J. Palmer, R. E. Cook, and N. Riggs: Western Equine and St. Louis Encephalitis. Preliminary Report of a Clinical Follow-Up Study in California, Neurology, 5:223, 1955.

Johnson, K. M., A. Shelokov, P. H. Peralta, G. J. Dammin, and N. A. Young: Recovery of Venezuelan Equine Encephalomyelitis Virus in Panama, Am. J. Trop. Med. Hyg., 17:432, 1968.

Lennette, E. H., and H. Koprowski: Human Infection With Venezuelan Equine Encephalomyelitis Virus, J.A.M.A., 123:1088, 1943.

Luby, J. P., S. E. Sulkin, and J. P. Sanford: The Epidemiology of St. Louis Encephalitis (SLE): A Review, Ann. Rev. Med., 1969 (in press).

National Communicable Disease Center: Neurotropic Viral Diseases Surveillance, Encephalitis, Annual Encephalitis Summary, 1966, April 30, 1968.

Thompson, W. H., and S. L. Inhorn: Arthropod-borne California Group Viral Encephalitis in Wisconsin, Wis. Med. J., 66:250, 1967.

Weaver, O. M., S. Pieper, and R. Kurland: Japanese Encephalitis: Sequelae, Neurology, 8:887, 1958.

219 DISEASES CAUSED BY SLOW VIRUSES

Donald H. Harter

Slow virus diseases are characterized by a long asymptomatic period, often on the order of months or years, between the introduction of the infectious agent and the appearance of clinical illness.

The factors responsible for this protracted incubation period have not been defined. Viruses causing slow infections do not appear to have any unique or common features, and the slowness of the disease may be due in large measure to the manner in which the host reacts or accommodates to the virus.

Some slow viruses provoke a conventional inflammatory response during the time they are clinically silent; others are able to reside within cells for long periods without causing detectable cytopathic changes. The role of immunity in slow virus infection is largely unknown. One possibility is that the agent is kept in check by the host's immunologic defenses during the long incubation period and that disease occurs when these defenses fail.

In animals, slow viruses are known to produce a variety of pulmonary, hepatic, renal, and neurologic disorders. At present, there are only three definitely identified slow virus infections of man. These are three infrequently encountered neurologic diseases: kuru, progressive multifocal leukoencephalopathy, and subacute sclerosing panencephalitis. Of these three, only kuru has been shown to be caused by a slow virus; in the other two a "viruslike" particle or viral component have been identified, but it has not been transmitted to experimental animals.

KURU

Kuru, or "trembling with fear," is a progressive and fatal neurologic disorder which occurs exclusively among natives of the New Guinea Highland.

Difficulty in walking is usually the first sign of kuru. This usually progresses from a minor disturbance in gait rhythm to marked side to side lurching and staggering. Eventually ambulation becomes incoordinated and the patient is unable to use his limbs. As the disease progresses, cerebellar involvement (intention tremor, inability to perform rapid alternating movements, slurring of speech, hypotonia), abnormal involuntary movements resembling myoclonus, athetosis, or chorea, and convergent strabismus appear. Dementia develops in the later phases of the disease. The illness terminates fatally in 4 to 24 months, usually from decubitus ulcers or bronchopneumonia. Approximately 80 percent of adults afflicted with the disease are women.

Pathologic changes are limited to the central nervous system and include widespread neuronal loss, intense astrocytic and microglial proliferation, loss of myelinated fibers, and the presence of plaquelike bodies. Perivascular cuffing by lymphocytes and mononuclear cells has been observed occasionally.

It was the close similarity between the neuropathologic and clinical findings found in kuru and in *scrapie,* a slow infectious disease of sheep, that suggested the possibility that kuru was caused by a virus or other infectious agent. The infectious origin of kuru was confirmed subsequently by the appearance of a kurulike syndrome in chimpanzees 18 to 21 months after intracerebral inoculation of suspensions of brain from human cases. Furthermore, the kuru syndrome has been transmitted from chimpanzee to chimpanzee by intracerebral passage with shortening of the incubation period to 12 months. The chimpanzee has been the only animal found to be susceptible to experimental kuru. Although a number of known and novel viruses have been recovered from tissue explants prepared from chimpanzees with the kuru syndrome, the specific agent responsible for the disease has not yet been characterized.

Cannibalism has been considered as a possible mode to transmission of kuru. Native custom in the New Guinea dictates that marrow, viscera, and brain be cooked and eaten. The marked predilection of kuru for the adult female may be explained by the observation that cannibalism appears more prevalent among women and that males who practice cannibalism seldom eat the bodies of women. The recent influx of foreign settlers into the kuru area has led to increasing rejection of cannibalistic practices and this, in turn, may be responsible for the progressive decline in the number of cases of kuru since 1960.

PROGRESSIVE MULTIFOCAL LEUKOENCEPHALOPATHY

This rare neurologic condition first described in 1958 usually occurs in patients who have lymphomas, carcinomatosis, or sarcoidosis.

The disease affects adults of both sexes and its duration from onset of symptoms to death is 3 or 4 months. The neurologic signs and symptoms show diffuse, asymmetrical involvement of the cerebral hemispheres. Hemiplegia, hemianopsia, aphasia or dysarthria, and organic mental changes are frequent, and incomplete or complete transverse myelitis may develop. Headache and convulsive seizures are rare, but electroencephalographic abnormalities consisting of diffuse slow-wave activity are often present.

The pathologic changes consist of multiple areas of demyelination with little or no perivascular infiltration. The presence of distinctive intranuclear inclusions in oligodendrocytes first suggested that the disease was of a viral etiology. Electron microscopic observations show the intranuclear inclusion bodies to be composed of closely packed spheres which have the physical dimensions and properties of members of the polyoma, SV 40 and K virus subgroup of the papova viruses. The papova group consists of several tumor-producing virus, including the human wart virus.

The disease has not been transmitted to animals.

It has been postulated that the patient's initial underlying illness so alters immunologic responsiveness that the virus is able to enter and multiply within the central nervous system. The demyelination which occurs may be related to virus-induced damage of oligodendroglia, cells which appear to be required for the normal maintenance of myelin.

SUBACUTE SCLEROSING PANENCEPHALITIS (Inclusion Body Encephalitis)

This progressively fatal disease of children and adolescents has been suspected to be of viral origin since its initial description by Dawson in 1932. Although recent findings have given further support to a viral etiology, infective virus has not yet been recovered from the brains of patients with the disease.

Subacute sclerosing panencephalitis occurs between four and twenty years of age; 80 percent of patients are under eleven. Onset is usually insidious, and mental deterioration, often expressed by a decline in the patient's school work, is the presenting symptom. Incoordination, ataxia, and myoclonic jerks develop along with abnormalities of the pyramidal and extrapyramidal motor systems. The patient becomes bedridden within 6 to 9 months. Death occurs from superimposed pulmonary or urinary tract infections or from decubiti. Neither fever nor signs of meningeal irritation occur. The cerebrospinal fluid gamma-globulin, as determined by electrophoresis, quantitative immunochemical assay, or colloidal gold curve is elevated, but the fluid is otherwise normal. The electroencephalogram typically shows a "burst suppression" pattern characterized by synchronous and symmetrical spike and high voltage slow wave activity. Brain biopsy may be required to make a definitive antemortem diagnosis.

There is no effective treatment for the disease.

Pathologic findings include round cell infiltration about small cerebral arteries and veins, intranuclear and intracytoplasmic inclusions in neurones and glial cells, and varying degrees of demyelination.

There is considerable evidence pointing to measles virus as the etiologic agent. The electron microscope shows the intranuclear inclusions to be composed of hollow tubular filaments resembling the internal nucleic acid component of members of the subgroup II myxoviruses. Staining of brain tissue from patients with the disease with fluorescent antibody demonstrates measles virus antigen in the inclusions. Furthermore, a significant number of patients with the disease have elevated serum levels of measles antibody and increases in measles antibody titers have been observed as the disease progresses. As a group, patients with inclusion body encephalitis have higher levels of measles antibody than are found during convalescence from measles.

Attempts to transmit the disease to animals have met with variable results, and reported failures outnumber reported successes.

Subacute sclerosing panencephalitis appears many years after the patient's initial experience with rubeola and may represent an unusual response of the nervous system to viral infection. It is possible that a viral carrier state becomes established within the nervous system wherein cells may continue to elaborate intracellular viral antigen without producing detectable amounts of mature infective virus. The implications of this concept for other diseases of the central nervous system such as parkinsonism or multiple sclerosis remains in the realm of speculation.

REFERENCES

Abinanti, F. R.: The Possible Role of Microorganisms and Viruses in the Etiology of Chronic Degenerative Diseases of Man, Ann. Rev. Microbiol., 21:467, 1967.

Conference on Measles Virus and Subacute Sclerosing Panencephalitis, J. L. Sever and W. Zeman (Eds.), Neurology, vol. 18, Part 2, 1968.

Gajdusek, D. C.: Slow-virus Infections of the Nervous System, New Engl. J. Med., 276:392, 1967.

Richardson, E. P.: Progressive Multifocal Leukoencephalopathy, New Engl. J. Med., 265:815, 1961.

Section 17

Diseases with Lesions of Skin or Mucous Membranes

220   MEASLES (Rubeola)

John C. Ribble

DEFINITION. Measles (the term derives from an Anglo-Saxon word for spot) is an acute febrile eruption which for centuries has been one of the most common diseases of civilized man. With the development of effective prophylactic measures it promises to become a rarity.

HISTORY. Measles probably did not exist before the building of large cities, inasmuch as perpetuation of the disease in present day isolated communities of less than 500,000 persons does not occur. Rhazes wrote about the disease in the tenth century, but indicated that it had been described as early as the first century by a Hebrew physician. Sydenham in the seventeenth century wrote a full account of the disease as he encountered it in England and differentiated it from other exanthems. In 1905 measles was transmitted by the blood of infected persons to human volunteers and in 1911 to monkeys by both blood and nasopharyngeal secretions that had previously been passed through bacteria-retaining filters. Enders and Peebles in 1954 obtained from patients with measles an agent that produced cytopathic changes in cell cultures. This achievement has allowed the investigation of the characteristics of the measles virus and the pathogenesis of the disease and its complications and has established means for the development of diagnostic and prophylactic measures.

ETIOLOGY. The measles virion is composed of a central core of ribonucleic acid with a helically arranged protein coat encased in a lipoprotein envelope with small spike-like structures. The virion is 1,200 to 2,500 Å in diameter, and in structure and size resembles some of the myxoviruses.

The measles virus is isolated most easily from infected persons utilizing primary cultures of monkey or human kidney, although primary isolations have been accomplished using human amnion or chorion or dog kidney. After several passages, the virus can be propagated on a number of stable cell lines of human origin, human leukocytes, and primary cultures from other animals, including chick embryo cells upon which many of the vaccine strains are grown.

Measles virus infection of cells in culture results in the formation of multinucleated giant cells, many with eosinophilic intranuclear, and intracytoplasmic inclusions. The number of infectious particles of measles virus can be determined by visible plaque formation in suitably prepared cell layers or by using immunofluorescence techniques.

EPIDEMIOLOGY. Measles occurs naturally only in human beings, although infection with the virus can be demonstrated in laboratory colonies of monkeys exposed to infected individuals. Before active immunization became widespread, epidemics of measles occurred every 2 or 3 years, with the result that about 95 percent of town and city dwellers developed the disease before the age of fifteen years. The virus is transmitted by transfer of nasopharyngeal secretions, either directly or in airborne droplets to the respiratory mucous membranes or conjunctivae of susceptible individuals. Persons infected with the virus may transmit the disease during a period which extends from 4 days before, until 5 days after skin lesions have appeared. Measles is a disease of childhood in populous areas, but may occur at any age in remote isolated communities if the disease is introduced. Infants are uncommonly affected under the age of six to eight months because of the persistence for this period of time of antibody acquired by transplacental transmission from the mother.

PATHOGENESIS AND PATHOLOGY. It is probable that after infection, measles virus multiplies in the epithelium of the respiratory tract and is disseminated by way of the blood to distant sites. For a few days before, and for 1 or 2 days after the rash appears, the virus can be isolated from blood or washed white cells, conjunctiva, lymphoid tissue, and respiratory mucous membranes and secretions. The virus can be obtained from urine for as long as 4 days after the onset of the eruption.

The skin and mucous membrane lesions (Koplik's spots) consist of vesicle formation and epithelial necrosis and may be due either to direct infection of these areas or, as suggested by Enders, to the action of complexes of measles antigen and antibody. Large multinucleated cells (Warthin-Finkeldy cells) are characteristic of measles virus infection and can be found in hyperplastic lymphoid tissues, respiratory epithelium and secretions, and in urine. An unusually high number of white cells from patients with the disease contain broken chromosomes. The epithelium of the respiratory passages may become necrotic and slough, leading to secondary bacterial infection; in addition, interstitial pneumonia with giant-cell infiltration may be observed. Changes in the brain of patients with encephalitis resemble those seen in other postviral encephalitides and consist of focal hemorrhage, congestion, and demyelinization.

MANIFESTATIONS. The time from exposure to the development of the first symptoms of measles infection is usually 9 to 11 days, and from exposure to the appearance of rash is about 2 weeks. The initial manifestations of the disease are malaise, irritability, fever as high as 105°F, conjunctivitis with excessive lacrimation, edema of the eyelids and photophobia, moderately severe hacking cough, and nasal discharge. Koplik's spots, small red irregular lesions with blue-white centers, appear one or two days before the onset of the rash on the mucous membranes of the mouth and occasionally on the conjunctiva or intestinal mucosa. The findings of the prodromal illness subside or disappear within 1 or 2 days after the outbreak of skin lesions, although the cough may persist throughout the course of the disease.

The red maculopapular rash of measles breaks out first on the forehead, spreads downward over the face, neck, and trunk and appears on the feet on the third day. The density of lesions is greatest on the forehead, face, and shoulders, where coalescence of individual spots usually occurs. The lesions in each area persist for about 3 days and disappear in the same order in which they appeared, resulting in total duration of rash of about 6 days. As the maculopapules fade, a brown discoloration of the skin may be noticed, and finely granular skin may be desquamated. In adults the duration of fever may be longer, the rash more prominent, and the incidence of complications higher.

The course of measles can be altered by the administration of gamma-globulin soon after exposure. The incubation period may be prolonged for as long as 20 days. The prodromal period of the modified disease may be shorter, the fever, respiratory symptoms, and conjunctivitis milder, and the rash less marked; Koplik's spots may not be present. An atypical, severe form of measles is seen in some persons who have received inactivated measles vaccine several years before exposure. The prodromal period with prominent fever, headache, myalgias,

and abdominal symptoms lasts for 2 to 3 days and is followed by an eruption of maculopapules, vesicles, and petechiae. In contrast to natural measles, the rash begins on the feet and progresses toward the head and is especially prominent on the legs and in body creases. Peripheral edema and pneumonia have been prevalent in this form of atypical measles.

COMPLICATIONS. Measles, usually a benign self-limited disease, may be associated with a number of complicating illnesses. Viral involvement of the respiratory tract may lead to croup, bronchitis, bronchiolitis, or rarely to interstitial pneumonia, which is seen most often in children suffering from a severe systemic disease such as leukemia, and which is characterized by severe respiratory symptoms, pulmonary infiltrations, and the presence in the lungs of giant cells. It may occur in the absence of the typical measles exanthem. Conjunctivitis, which is seen regularly in the course of uncomplicated measles, may occasionally progress to permanent corneal ulceration, keratitis, and blindness. Myocarditis characterized by transient changes in the electrocardiogram occurs in about 20 percent of patients with measles, but clinical evidence of cardiac dysfunction is rare. Viral involvement of the mesenteric lymph nodes and appendix may result in abdominal pain and signs of peritoneal inflammation so severe that surgical exploration is considered. The situation is especially confusing if the evidence of appendiceal involvement become manifest during the preeruptive phase of the disease. Measles infection of pregnant women results in death of the fetus in about 20 percent of the cases; however, a teratogenic effect such as that observed in rubella has not been demonstrated.

Superimposed bacterial pneumonia caused by streptococci, pneumococci, staphylococci, or *H. influenza* is considerably more common than giant-cell pneumonia and may progress to formation of empyema or lung abscess. Bacterial otitis media is a frequent sequela of measles infection in children. In tropical areas stomatitis, probably of bacterial etiology, progressing to cancrum oris may be encountered during the course of measles.

In addition to conditions associated with consequences of viral infection and the complications resulting from superimposed bacterial infection, there are several situations which may arise after measles infection which are of uncertain pathogenesis. Clinically apparent *encephalomyelitis* occurs in every 1 of 1,000 patients with measles. It begins 4 or 5 days after the appearance of the eruption and is characterized by return of high fever, headache, drowsiness, and coma, and in some patients by focal brain or spinal cord involvement. Death occurs in about 10 percent of affected individuals, and persistent signs of central nervous system damage including mental changes, epilepsy, and paralysis are encountered. Electroencephalographic abnormalities without other signs of CNS dysfunction may be demonstrated in 50 percent of patients with otherwise uncomplicated measles. There is no evidence that encephalomyelitis is due to direct invasion of the nervous system by measles virus, and it is postulated that the disease has an allergic origin. An extremely rare condition, *subacute sclerosing panencephalitis,* is now thought to be a late complication of measles. *Thrombocytopenia* may occur 3 to 15 days after the onset of the rash and results in purpura as well as bleeding from mouth, intestine, and genitourinary tract. Measles is associated with disappearance of delayed hypersensitivity to tuberculin, exacerbation of existing tuberculosis, and an increased incidence of new tuberculous infections.

LABORATORY FINDINGS. Leukopenia is frequent in the prodromal phase of measles, and the appearance of leukocytosis suggests bacterial superinfection or another complication. During the prodrome and in the early eruptive phase, Warthin-Finkeldy cells can be identified in stained preparations of sputum, nasal secretions, or urine, and the measles virus can be isolated by inoculation of the same materials into appropriate cell cultures. Complement fixation, neutralization, and hemagglutination-inhibition tests are available for serologic confirmation of measles. Spinal fluid of patients with encephalomyelitis may contain increased protein and 500 to 1,000 lymphocytes. Bacterial infection can be identified by appropriate cultures.

DIFFERENTIAL DIAGNOSIS. Measles with its prodrome, Koplik's spots, and characteristic rash, is infrequently confused with other diseases. Rubella is a shorter, milder disease with more prominent lymphadenopathy. Infectious mononucleosis and toxoplasmosis can be identified by the presence of atypical lymphocytes and by a serologic test respectively. Drug reactions and secondary syphilis may display skin lesions similar to the measles rash. The atypical form of measles in patients previously immunized with inactivated vaccine may suggest Rocky Mountain spotted fever.

PROPHYLAXIS. Measles can be prevented by the administration of 0.25 mg per kg gamma-globulin within 5 days of exposure. Passive immunization should be considered for any susceptible person exposed to the disease, but is especially important for children under three years of age, for pregnant women, for patients with tuberculosis, and for those patients in whom immune mechanisms are impaired. A modified, less severe form of the disease which results in some degree of active immunity may be observed if 0.05 mg per kg of gamma-globulin is given within 5 days of exposure (see Manifestations). Administration of antibiotics does not decrease the frequency or severity of bacterial superinfections.

Active immunity can be induced by the use of live attenuated measles virus without spread to contacts of vaccinated individuals. The administration of Edmonston strain vaccines, prepared either in chick embryo or dog kidney cells, frequently results in a febrile illness beginning about 6 days after vaccination, a mild rash, and occasionally respiratory symptoms and Koplik's spots. To modify these manifestations of disease, gamma-globulin, 0.01 mg per kg in a separate syringe and at a different site may be given concomitantly. A further attenuated vaccine (Schwarz) is associated with fewer manifestations of disease and is administered without gamma-globulin. Vaccination with these preparations induces antibody formation in more than 95 percent of susceptible individuals. The magnitude of serologic response following use of the Edmonston strain approximates that seen after natural measles and is slightly greater than that induced by the Schwarz vaccine or Edmonston strain vaccine plus gamma-globulin. Vaccination results in protection for at least 2 or 3 years, but the total duration of immunity is not known. Live measles vaccine should not be given to pregnant women, to those sensitive to egg proteins or dog dander, to patients with tuberculosis, to patients with leukemia or lymphoma, or to those who are receiving therapy which depresses immune response.

There is no indication for the use of inactivated vaccine because of severe atypical measles which has been observed in persons immunized with it (see Manifestations).

TREATMENT. No therapy is indicated for uncomplicated measles. Gamma-globulin, although effective in prophylaxis, is of no value once symptoms are evident. Bacterial infections should be treated with appropriate antibiotics (Chaps. 135, 138, 139, 140, and 152).

REFERENCES

Enders, J. F., and T. Peebles: Propagation in Tissue Cultures of Cytopathogenic Agents from Patients with Measles, Proc. Soc. Exp. Biol. Med., 86:277, 1954.

Fulginiti, V. A., J. Eller, A. Downie, and C. Kempe: Altered Reactivity to Measles Virus, Atypical Measles in Children Previously Immunized with Inactivated Measles Virus Vaccines, J.A.M.A., 202:1075, 1967.

Katz, S. L.: Measles, Its Complications, Treatment, and Prophylaxis, Med. Clinics N. Am., 46:1163.

Krugman, S., and R. Ward: Infectious Disease of Children, 3d ed., St. Louis, The C. V. Mosby Company, 1964.

Report of the Committee on the Control of Infectious Diseases, 15th ed., American Academy of Pediatrics, 1966.

221 RUBELLA (German Measles)
John C. Ribble

DEFINITION. Rubella, a febrile disease with rash and lymphadenopathy, is usually a benign condition, but when it occurs in pregnant women it may lead to infection and serious disorders of the fetus.

ETIOLOGY. In the late 1930s and 1940s rubella was transmitted to humans and monkeys, and in 1962 a viral agent was recovered in cell cultures inoculated with nasopharyngeal secretions of infected persons. Human primary amnion cells infected with rubella virus display rounding, clumping of nuclear chromatin, and eosinophilic intranuclear inclusions. Rubella virus can be detected indirectly in monkey kidney cells by the interference or exclusion method. In this system, cells infected with rubella appear normal, but are resistant to viruses such as ECHO 11 or Coxsackie A9 that ordinarily produce cytopathic effects in monkey kidney cells. Complement-fixing antigen, and a hemagglutinin active at 4°C against red cells from young chickens have been identified.

PATHOGENESIS AND PATHOLOGY. Rubella can be induced in susceptible persons by the instillation of infected materials into the nasopharynx, and natural infection is probably induced in the same way. Virus is present in blood, throat washings, and stools for several days before the exanthem becomes apparent. It can be detected in blood for 1 or 2 days, and in throat washings and stools for as long as 2 weeks after appearance of rash. Lymph nodes show edema, hyperplasia, and loss of follicles.

Congenital rubella results from transplacental transmission of virus to the fetus from an infected mother, and may be associated with growth retardation, infiltration of liver and spleen by hematopoietic tissue, interstitial pneumonia, decreased number of megakaryocytes in the bone marrow, and various structural malformations of the cardiovascular and central nervous systems. The virus may persist in the fetus during intrauterine life and for many months after birth.

EPIDEMIOLOGY. Rubella is less contagious than measles, and large-scale epidemics are not common. In 1964, however, more than 1,800,000 cases of rubella were reported in the United States. Immunity to rubella is considered to be lifelong, but indirect epidemiologic evidence has raised the possibility that second subclinical attacks may occur.

MANIFESTATIONS. The time from exposure to the appearance of the rash of rubella is 14 to 21 days, usually about 18 days. In adults there may be a prodromal illness preceding the exanthem by 1 to 7 days and consisting of malaise, headache, fever, mild conjunctivitis, and lymphadenopathy. In children the rash may be the first manifestation of disease. It is apparent from serologic studies that rubella infection may be associated with no signs or symptoms, or may result in lymph node enlargement without skin lesions; however, rash without lymphadenopathy is uncommon. Respiratory symptoms are mild or absent. Small red lesions (Forcheimer spots) occasionally may be seen on the soft palate, but are not pathognomonic of the disease.

The rash begins on the forehead and face and spreads downward to the trunk and extremities. The small pink, maculopapular lesions, of lighter hue than those of measles, are usually discrete but may coalesce to form a diffuse erythema suggestive of scarlet fever. The rash may last from 1 to 5 days, but is most commonly present for 3 days. Enlarged, tender lymph nodes appear before the rash, are most impressive during the early eruptive phase, and may persist several days after the rash has disappeared. Splenomegaly or generalized lymphadenopathy may occur, but the postauricular and suboccipital nodes are most strikingly involved. Arthralgias and slight joint swellings may be a complication of rubella, especially in young women. The pain and swelling, usually in the small joints, are most marked during the period of rash and may persist for several days after other manifestations of rubella have disappeared. Purpura with or without thrombocytopenia may occur and be associated with hemorrhage. Encephalomyelitis following rubella resembles other postinfectious encephalitides and is much less common than encephalitis following measles.

The syndrome of *congenital rubella* has conventionally been thought to consist of heart malformations—patent ductus arteriosus, interventricular septal defect, or pulmonic stenosis; eye lesions—corneal clouding, cataracts, chorioretinitis, and microphthalmia; microcephaly, mental retardation, and deafness. In the American epidemic of 1964 thrombocytopenic purpura, hepatosplenomegaly, intrauterine growth retardation, interstitial pneumonia, and metaphyseal bone lesions were encountered frequently in association with the previously recognized manifestations, leading to the term *expanded rubella syndrome.* Any combination of lesions may be seen in an individual infant.

Congenital rubella is usually the result of maternal infection during the first trimester of pregnancy, although well documented cases have resulted from infection several days prior to conception; deafness may occur as a result of infection in the fourth month. In the 1964 epidemic, about 10 percent of women with clinically recognized rubella during the first trimester gave birth to infants with the rubella syndrome. Serologically identified, asymptomatic maternal rubella can also result in fetal disease. If exposure of a pregnant woman occurs in the first trimester, rubella antibody levels should be obtained immediately and 2 or 3 weeks later. The combination of determinations may allow the detection of seroconversion occurring in subclinical infection, aid in the diagnosis of rubella if an exanthematous disease develops, or suggest remote past infection and immunity to the disease.

DIAGNOSIS. Rubella is frequently confused with other mild diseases such as those described in Chap. 222, infectious mononucleosis (Chap. 255), or acquired toxoplasmosis (Chap. 244). A certain diagnosis of rubella can be made by virus isolation and identification, or by changes in antibody titers. Rubella antibodies may be present by the second day of rash and increase in quantity over the next 2 or 3 weeks. There are no other laboratory findings helpful in the diagnosis of rubella, although lymphocytosis with atypical lymphocytes may occur. Congenital rubella should be differentiated by appropriate serologic tests from congenital syphilis, toxoplasmosis, and cytomegalic inclusion virus disease.

PREVENTION. In adults and children rubella is usually a mild disease with infrequent complications. However, the severity of congenital infection has prompted efforts to prevent the disease. Administration of gamma-globulin to exposed persons can abort the clinical disease, but seroconversion and transmission of the disease from mother to fetus may occur despite the administration of large amounts of gamma-globulin soon after exposure.

Active immunization, as indicated by antibody response, and prevention of disease in exposed vaccinated persons has been accomplished by the administration of live attenuated rubella virus grown in monkey kidney cells. The attenuated virus is excreted in the nasopharyngeal secretion of vaccinees and the possibility of transmission to susceptible persons has led to caution in the widespread use of the vaccine. Despite the fact that rubella vaccine remains experimental, it is likely that it will be adapted to general use.

REFERENCES

Cooper, L. Z., J. Giles, and S. Krugman: Clinical Trial of Live Attenuated Rubella Virus Vaccine, Am. J. Dis. Child., 115:655, 1968.

Green, R. H., et al.: Studies of the Natural History and Prevention of Rubella, Am. J. Dis. Child., 110:348, 1965.

McCarthy, K., C. Taylor-Tobinson: Rubella, Brit. Med. Bull., 23:185, 1967.

Sever, J. L., et al.: Rubella Antibody Determinations, Pediatrics, 40:789, 1967.

——, K. Nelson, and M. Gilkeson: Rubella Epidemic, 1964. Effect on 6,000 Pregnancies, Am. J. Dis. Child., 110:395, 1965.

222 OTHER VIRAL EXANTHEMATOUS DISEASES

John C. Ribble

In addition to the diseases such as measles, rubella, and chickenpox which historically have been associated with prominent skin lesions, there are other virus infections in which skin manifestations may occur. A transient maculo-papular eruption may be seen during the course of infectious mononucleosis, cytomegalic inclusion disease, cat-scratch fever, psittacosis, and illnesses caused by arboviruses. Exanthem subitum and erythema infectiosum are mild exanthematous diseases which have been recognized by their distinctive clinical features and which are presumably of viral origin. The study of epidemics using techniques of virus isolation has identified exanthematous diseases associated occasionally with adenovirus and reovirus infection, and more frequently with illnesses caused by enteroviruses.

EXANTHEM SUBITUM (Roseola infantum)

Exanthem subitum is a benign disease of infants six to twenty-four-months of age that is characterized by a high fever and rash. The disease can be transmitted to humans and monkeys by the transfer of blood obtained from a patient during the first few days of illness. The infectious agent is probably a virus, although it has not been isolated. The first manifestation of disease, after an incubation period of 10 days, is the abrupt onset of fever which lasts for 3 to 5 days and may be as high as 105°F. There may be mild pharyngitis, slight lymph node enlargement, and convulsions may occur during the height of the fever. On the fourth or fifth day of illness, there is a sudden drop in temperature to normal or below normal. Several hours after defervescence the rash suddenly and surprisingly appears. It is characterized by faint maculopapules over the neck and trunk and may extend to the thighs and buttocks; it may last for only a few hours or may be present for a day or two. Leukopenia is frequent during the febrile period. The disease is benign and not associated with complications, although occasionally an infant may show sequelae as a result of febrile convulsions.

ERYTHEMA INFECTIOSUM (Fifth Disease)

Erythema infectiosum is a mild febrile exanthematous disease without a prodrome. The incubation period is probably 5 to 10 days, but it has not been ascertained precisely. The first manifestations are low-grade fever and a bilaterally symmetrical rash, most prominent on the face but also found on the arms, legs, and trunk but not on the palms or soles. The rash is most marked on the cheeks, giving a "slapped face" appearance. The lesions are maculopapular and tend to be confluent, forming slightly raised blotchy areas and reticular or lacy patterns. The rash usually lasts about a week, and during this time it may disappear, only to reappear in the same areas a few hours later. The waxing and waning eruption may occasionally persist for several weeks. Mild joint pain and swelling have been observed in a large proportion of adults with the disease. Erythema infectiosum affects all ages but is most common in children of school age and may occur in epidemic form. The mode of transmission of the disease is not known and an infectious agent has not been recovered.

ENTEROVIRAL EXANTHEMS

Many individual enteroviruses have been associated with rash—poliomyelitis virus only rarely, Coxsackie B5, A2, A4, and A9, and ECHO viruses 2, 3, 4, 5, 6, 11, 14, 18, 19, occasionally. Three enterovirus infections are frequently associated with rashes and have been studied extensively enough to warrant individual description.

HAND, FOOT, AND MOUTH DISEASE (COXASCKIE A16 INFECTION). (Chap. 227.)

BOSTON EXANTHEM (INFECTION WITH ECHO VIRUS 16). This is probably a common infectious disease of childhood. It was described first and most extensively during an epidemic in Boston in 1951, as a finding in many patients with ECHO virus type 16 infection. Children who were infected usually had a disease characterized by exanthem and low-grade fever, while adult family contacts developed high fever, prostration, and signs of aseptic meningitis with absent or fleeting rash. The first manifestation of the disease in children was fever of 101 to 102°F, lasting for a day or two, pharyngitis with ulcerated lesions resembling herpangina, and slight enlargement of the cervical and postauricular lymph nodes. The rash appeared during or after defervescence and consisted of small pink maculopapules on the face, upper chest, and occasionally on the whole body, including the palms and soles. The rash lasted for 1 to 5 days, and there were no important complications or sequelae. The disease resembled exanthem subitum but occurred in children of all ages and in adults.

INFECTION WITH ECHO VIRUS 9. Infection with this virus has occurred in epidemics among children and adults and has been characterized by a febrile disease with a high incidence of aspetic meningitis. The incubation period is 5 to 8 days. About 30 percent of patients have a rash which may occur with or without meningitis, is usually maculopapular, presents at the onset of the disease, appears first on the face and neck, spreads to the trunk and extremities, may involve the palms and soles, and persists for 3 to 5 days. Petechiae with or without maculopapules have been recognized, and when seen in association with meningitis, there may be confusion with meningococcal meningitis. A vesicular eruption with crusting lesions has been seen occasionally. An exanthem on the buccal mucosa and soft palate occurs in about 30 percent of patients and consists of small red areas with white centers which resemble Koplik's spots. The disease is usually benign, but rarely has been associated with permanent central-nervous-system damage.

REFERENCES

Ager, E. A., T. D. Y. Chin, and J. Poland: Epidemic Erythema Infectiosum, New Engl. J. Med., 275:1326, 1966.

Lerner, A. M., et al.: New Viral Exanthems, New Engl. J. Med., 269:678, 736, 1963.

Miller, G. D., and J. Tindall: Hand, Foot and Mouth Disease, J.A.M.A., 203:827, 1968.

Neva, F. A., R. Reemster, and I. Gorbach: Clinical Epidemiological Features of Unusual Epidemic Exanthem, J.A.M.A., 155:544, 1954.

Wenner, H. A., and T. Lou: Virus Diseases Associated with Cutaneous Eruptions, Progr. Med. Virol., 5:219, 1963.

223 SMALLPOX, VACCINIA, AND COWPOX

John C. Ribble

Poxviruses are a group of large (200 to 320 mμ), brick-shaped, DNA-containing viruses that possess a common antigen and have a predilection for skin. Many of the poxviruses, such as myxoma and fowlpox agents, cause disease mainly in lower animals. Smallpox (variola major), alastrim (variola minor), vaccinia, and cowpox agents are closely related members of the poxvirus group that cause human disease. All of these viruses grow and produce pox on the chorioallantoic membrane of chick embryos incubated at 37°C and can be cultivated in cells from various mammalian tissues with formation of intracytoplasmic inclusions, rounding, fusion, and heaping up of cells, and eventual degeneration of the infected area. The poxviruses responsible for human disease may be distinguished from each other by minor antigenic differences and by the type and severity of lesions they induce in experimental animals and man. Smallpox and alastrim viruses produce smaller pox on the chorioallantoic membrane than vaccinia. Pock production by vaccinia virus can be demonstrated at incubation temperatures of 39 to 40°C, whereas the smallpox and alastrim agents do not induce lesions at this temperature. The alastrim virus causes pock formation only below 38°C, but the variola major virus can induce lesions at temperatures above 38°C but below 39°C.

SMALLPOX (Variola)

DEFINITION. Smallpox is a severe contagious, febrile disease characterized by a vesicular and pustular eruption. Alastrim is a similar but milder illness.

PATHOGENESIS AND PATHOLOGY. The virus gains access to the body by the respiratory tract and multiples at unidentified sites, probably lymph nodes or liver. After several days, during which there are no evidences of infection, viremia ensues, with production of swelling of the endothelium of blood vessels in the corium and perivascular inflammation. Loculated vesicles are the result of cellular destruction and exudation of serum. The infected epithelial cells are swollen and contain intracytoplasmic inclusions surrounded by a halo (Guarnieri's bodies). The extent of skin involvement is greater in smallpox than in chickenpox and reaches into the corium. Pitting, most commonly seen on the face, is said to result from destruction of sebaceous glands which are abundant in this area. The liver, spleen, and lymph nodes may be enlarged and may show focal accumulations of large mononuclear cells.

EPIDEMIOLOGY. A patient with smallpox is infectious from a day before the rash appears until the lesions have healed and the scabs have fallen off. During the early phase of the illness, the virus is transmitted in nasopharyngeal secretions; when the eruption is fully formed, the lesions themselves are a major source of infectious material. Variola virus may contaminate clothing, bedding, dust, or other inanimate objects and remain infectious for months, necessitating disinfection of articles in the patient's environment. Although smallpox is usually disseminated by a patient with the disease, it is possible that the virus may be transmitted by an individual, especially a partially immune person, who has an inapparent or very mild infection. Long-term completely asymptomatic carriers have not been recognized, nor has aerial transmission over long distances been convincingly demonstrated. Smallpox is still a major world health problem and exists in endemic form in India, Indonesia, and parts of Africa; alastrim is prevalent in South America, especially in Brazil.

MANIFESTATIONS. Smallpox can be divided into a prodrome, an early eruptive phase, and a period of vesiculation and pustule formation. The prodrome is characterized by fever of 102 to 106°F, headache, myalgia especially in the back, abdominal pain, vomiting, and in some patients by a transient, blotchy, erythematous eruption. After 3 or 4 days the fever subsides, the symptoms decrease, and the patient seems to recover. It is at this time, when the patient is afebrile, that the focal eruption begins. Early manifestations are painful ulcers on the buccal mucosa, and macules which appear first on the face and forearm, and rapidly become firm, shotty papules. The papules increase in number and spread from the face and distal extremities to involve the trunk. The individual lesions may remain discrete and scattered or they may become confluent and involve most of the body. They are most concentrated on the face and distal extremities including the palms and soles and are relatively sparse in the axilla. On the third or fourth day after the appearance of the focal rash, the papules progress to vesicles containing clear fluid, which, over the next few days, becomes cloudy due to infiltration by pus cells and desquamated epithelial cells; hemorrhage into the vesicles and surrounding skin may also be seen. During the course of smallpox, the lesions at any one time, in one area, are all at the same stage of evolution. At the time the vesicles become pustular, there is recurrence of fever, which may persist until healing occurs. The pustules umbilicate and form crusts and scabs which usually fall off 3 weeks after the beginning of illness, leaving small scars or deep pits.

The above description applies to disease of moderate severity. A milder illness may occur in previously immunized persons or in some who have no history of vaccination. It is characterized by the usual incubation period and prodrome, but is followed either by focal eruption of fewer than 100 papules, or by a rash resembling chickenpox. Smallpox with prodrome, but no eruption of any kind, has been recognized (*variola sine eruptione*). The disease may also occur in a rapidly fulminating form ("sledgehammer smallpox"). After the usual incubation period, the patient develops an initial illness characterized by severe prostration, fever, bone-marrow depression, hemorrhagic skin lesions, bleeding from the mouth and intestine, shock, coma, and death. The disease progresses from inception to death within 3 or 4 days without evidence of the typical focal skin lesions.

Alastrim is similar to mild and moderate forms of variola major in that it has the same incubation period and prodromal illness, but the skin eruption is less extensive, and fatalities are extremely rare and are related to secondary infections.

COMPLICATIONS. Bacterial superinfections of the lesions, usually with *S. aureus,* may occur in the late pustular stage. Viral infections of the trachea, pharynx, and larynx, and superimposed bacterial pneumonia, may be seen in severe forms of smallpox. Mild conjunctivitis is quite common, and iritis and keratitis have been recognized. Encephalomyelitis may occur in the late stage of the disease and is similar to other postinfectious encephalitides. Osteomyelitis and joint effusions may complicate the disease.

LABORATORY FINDINGS. Leukopenia is present during the prodromal illness, and there is usually leukocytosis during the pustular stage. Rapid diagnosis of poxvirus infection can be made by finding of characteristic brick-shaped particles in preparations of vesicle fluid examined by electron microscopy. Specific precipitation in agar using antigen prepared from lesions and antivariola or antivaccinia immune serum may also allow detection of poxvirus within a few hours. These tests do not distinguish variola from vaccinia or other poxviruses but do allow rapid differentiation from herpes simplex and varicella-zoster viruses. For definitive identification the virus must be grown in cell culture or on the chorioallantoic membrane and examined for its biologic characteristics.

DIFFERENTIAL DIAGNOSIS. The major problem in differential diagnosis is in distinguishing smallpox from chickenpox. Smallpox is preceded by a longer prodrome than chickenpox and its eruption vesiculates over a period of days instead of hours. The smallpox lesions are all characteristically in the same stage of development, whereas those of chickenpox may, in one area, display all stages of evolution. Electron microscopy and agar precipitation techniques (see above) are especially useful in distinguishing between smallpox and chickenpox.

PROPHYLAXIS. Smallpox may be prevented among the patient's contacts by vaccination. Because this procedure is most successful if carried out during the early part of the incubation period, all exposed persons, regardless of previous immunization, should be vaccinated immediately upon recognition of exposure. Large controlled clinical trials have demonstrated that oral administration of 1-methylisatin-3-thiosemicarbazone (methisazone), a drug which interferes with poxvirus multiplication, can prevent smallpox and alastrim in patients exposed to these diseases. The use of the drug together with prompt vaccination results in greater chance of protection than either measure alone. A drawback to the use of methisazone is its tendency to induce vomiting. The combined use of vaccination and parenteral administration of vaccinia immune globulin early in the incubation period is effective in the prevention of smallpox in exposed individuals.

TREATMENT. There is no specific therapy for smallpox. Thiosemicarbazone, although effective in prophylaxis, has not been shown to be of value in the treatment of established cases. Fluid deficits incurred by lack of intake and by loss from affected areas should be replaced by the administration of appropriate solutions. During the vesicular and pustular phases of the disease, an attempt should be made to prevent bacterial infection by the use of sterile sheets and sterile nursing procedures. Antihistamines may be helpful in decreasing pruritus. Bathing and application of lotions or ointments should be avoided. Later in the course of the illness, when desquamation has begun, showers or baths may be helpful in removing desquamating tissue.

Administration of parenteral penicillin, beginning on the fifth day of rash, has been reported to decrease the incidence of infection of skin lesions and the formation of boils and abscesses due to penicillin-sensitive bacteria. Inasmuch as penicillin-resistant staphylococci are frequently responsible for bacterial infections, the use of penicillinase-resistant penicillin may be of value, but its efficacy as a prophylactic agent in smallpox has not been evaluated. If bacterial infection is demonstrated, an antibiotic active against the infecting organism should be given by the parenteral route. Topical antibiotics should be avoided.

VACCINIA

Vaccinia is a virus disease of the skin which is induced by inoculation for the prevention of smallpox. The exact origin of the vaccinia virus is obscure. The material used by Jenner for vaccination was derived from cowpox lesions, and the infectious agent was propagated for many years by successive passage from person to person using exudate from fresh skin lesions. The original agent possibly became contaminated with variola virus during the period when transfer was being carried out without strict controls. It has been suggested that vaccinia virus is a hybrid of cowpox and variola agents, a contention supported by the finding that laboratory-induced hybrids of variola and cowpox viruses have many of the characteristics associated with vaccinia.

VACCINATION. Live, lyophilized vaccinia virus prepared from vesicle fluid of infected calves is commercially available and maintains potency for 18 months at 46°F. It is dissolved in a diluent solution just prior to use. The usual method for vaccination is to apply a small drop of vaccine to the skin over the deltoid muscle and to press a sterile needle through the vaccine several times in such a way that only the superficial layer of skin is entered. Vaccination should always induce some form of skin reaction; complete absence of any kind of lesion indicates that the vaccine was not viable or was not administered properly. The reaction which occurs in nonimmune individuals is characterized by a red papule at the site of inoculation 3 to 5 days after vaccination. The papule becomes vesicular on about the fifth or sixth day and pustular by the ninth or eleventh day after inoculation. The vesicle and pustule may be surrounded by a large area of erythema. About 2 weeks after vaccination, the pustule dries and develops a crust which falls off by the end of the third week, leaving a scar. Fever, malaise, and irritability are common in children during the vesicular and pustular phases, and axillary lymphadenopathy may develop and persist for several months. In the partially immune person, a modified reaction develops without fever or constitutional symptoms. A papule appears on the skin within 3 days, vesiculates in 5 to 7 days, and heals without much scarring. In an immune person a small papule forms in 3 days, but it does not vesiculate or result in scarring.

COMPLICATIONS. Healing of the primary vaccinal lesion may not occur, and there may be during a period of weeks or months progressive necrosis with destruction of large areas of skin, subcutaneous tissue, and underlying structures (*vaccinia gangrenosum*). In addition to the local destruction, there may be metastatic lesions on other parts of the skin surface and in bone and viscera. Vaccinia gangrenosum occurs most frequently in persons with disorders of immunity and if untreated, is nearly always fatal. *Eczema vaccinatum* (Plate 3) is a serious complication that is seen in persons with eczema or other type of chronic dermatosis. Widespread infection in the previously affected areas, as well as in normal skin, may result from direct vaccination of an eczematous patient or from exposure to a recently vaccinated individual. *Generalized vaccinia* in patients without preexisting skin disease is characterized by a few satellite lesions surrounding the inoculation site or by widely disseminated pox resembling the primary vaccination lesion. This condition may be mild, and recovery is to be expected. Vaccinia virus may be transferred from the primary inoculation site to the eye or other sites by scratching. *Postvaccinal encephalomyelitis* appears from 2 to 25 days after vaccination. The patient becomes severely ill quite suddenly, with nuchal rigidity, drowsiness, vomiting, convulsions, coma, and signs suggesting disease of the spinal cord. The period of coma lasts for a few days, and in those who recover there are usually no permanent sequelae. Death occurs in about half of the patients with encephalo-

myelitis. *Erythema multiforme bullosum* or diffuse blotchy erythema may occur in vaccinated patients 7 to 10 days after vaccination, and are thought to be allergic reactions to the virus or other components of the vaccine.

The incidence of complications has been compiled by the National Communicable Disease Center. The frequencies of the various adverse effects per million primarily vaccinated persons are vaccinia gangrenosum, 1.1; eczema vaccinatum, 8.7; generalized vaccinia, 20.8; vaccinal lesions resulting from accidental implantation of virus, 13.6; postvaccinal encephalitis, 1.9; other complications, 6.7. The survey indicated that complications are two or three times more frequent in infants under one year of age than in any other age group, and it is recommended that first vaccination be performed sometime between the first and second birthdays. As many as two-thirds of the complications could have been prevented if vaccination had been avoided in patients with eczema, family members of patients with eczema, persons with agammaglobulinemia, blood dyscrasias, or lymphoma, or patients being treated with adrenal steroids of immunosuppressive drugs. Because of the severity and frequency of adverse effects, the rarity of smallpox in this country, and the documented efficacy of thiosemicarbazone prophylaxis, some physicians have questioned the wisdom of routine vaccination in the United States. On the other hand, the possibility of rapid spread of smallpox in a completely nonimmunized population, the difficulty in making a prompt accurate diagnosis, and the avoidability of many complications of vaccination have convinced others that routine immunization should be continued. Attenuated strains of vaccinia virus that produce fewer adverse reactions have been developed and may be generally available soon.

TREATMENT. Patients with vaccinia gangrenosum, eczema vaccinatum, generalized vaccinia, and vaccinia of the eye should be treated promptly with vaccinia immune globulin, which is available through the American Red Cross. Some experience indicates that thiosemicarbonaze, together with vaccinia immune globulin, is more effective therapy for vaccinia gangrenosum than the use of globulin alone. No specific therapy is available for patients with postvaccinal encephalitis.

COWPOX

Cowpox is primarily a disease of the teets and udders of cows. Man is almost always infected by milking, but occasional spread to contacts may occur from an infected person. The human disease is characterized by low-grade fever and by small papules on the fingers and hand which go through vesicular and pustular stages resembling the course of vaccinia infection. The lesions may be ruptured by trauma and spread to immediately adjacent areas on the hand and continue to ulcerate for several weeks. Edema, lymphangitis, and axillary lymph node enlargement are common. Very rare cases of postcowpox encephalitis and serious infections of eczematous persons have been reported. In general, the disease is benign, heals without scarring, and is usually uncomplicated.

REFERENCES

Bedson, H. S., K. Dumbell: Smallpox and Vaccinia, Brit. Med. Bull., 23:119, 1967.

Dixon, C. W.: "Smallpox," London, J. & A. Churchill, 1962.

Joklik, W. K.: The Poxviruses, Bacteriol. Rev., 30:33, 1966.

Neff, J. M., et al.: Complications of Smallpox Vaccination. National Survey in the United States, 1963. New Engl. J. Med., 276:125, 1967.

224 CHICKENPOX (Varicella)
John C. Ribble

DEFINITION. Chickenpox is a contagious disease characterized by fever and a disseminated vesicular eruption. Chickenpox and herpes zoster (Chap. 225) are different manifestations of infection with the same viral agent.

ETIOLOGY. In 1953 a virus was recovered from patients with chickenpox and herpes zoster that produced intranuclear, eosinophilic inclusions and multinucleated giant cells in lines of cells derived from various monkey and human tissues. The varicella-zoster virus in culture spreads from cell to adjacent cell by direct invasion, rather than by way of suspending medium, and can be passed to other tissue cultures only by transfer of infected cells. The structure of the varicella-zoster virion resembles that of herpes simplex; however, the difficulty in recovery of cell-free virus has hampered the investigation of its chemical composition. Complement-fixing antigens can be detected in vesicle fluid and in suitable preparations of infected cell cultures. No hemagglutinin has been identified.

PATHOGENESIS AND PATHOLOGY. Varicella is presumably transmitted by the respiratory route, although the virus has only rarely been isolated from nasopharyngeal secretions of infected persons. Virus multiplication occurs at some unidentified site and probably results in intermittent viremia, as suggested by the successive crops of widely spaced lesions. Focal viral infection of blood vessels in the corium, with intranuclear inclusions in endothelial cells, results in degeneration of epidermis and formation of vesicles containing serum, epithelial and inflammatory cells, and multinucleated giant cells. Virus can be isolated from vesicle fluid, but not from crusting lesions or scales, for 3 days after eruption. In patients with varicella pneumonia the tracheobronchial mucosa, the alveolar septa, and the interstitial areas of the lungs are edematous and contain monocytic inflammatory cells, cells with intranuclear inclusions and giant cells. The nodular areas of pneumonia may eventually become calcified. The changes in the central nervous system in patients with varicella encephalomyelitis resemble those seen in measles.

EPIDEMIOLOGY. Chickenpox is a highly contagious disease with attack rates of 70 percent or more among susceptible persons exposed to a patient with the disease. The infectious period extends from a day or two before the rash until as long as 6 days after the appearance of new skin lesions. Patients with herpes zoster may be the source of an outbreak of chickenpox among susceptible contacts. Children from five to eight years of age are most commonly affected, but younger children, including newborn infants, and adults may develop chickenpox; an estimated 2 to 20 percent of cases occur in persons over the age of fifteen years. In the United States the disease is endemic, with superimposed epidemics every 2 to 5 years, usually the winter or spring.

MANIFESTATIONS. The incubation period from the time of exposure to the appearance of rash is 10 to 21 days, most often 14 to 17 days. There may be a 1- or 2-day prodrome with fever and malaise, but these symptoms usually begin when the rash appears. The first skin manifestations are pruritic maculopapules that evolve in a few hours to thin-walled vesicles which contain clear fluid and are surrounded by a red border. During the next day the erythmea diminishes and the vesicles collapse in the center, forming annular or umbilicated lesions which dry further and form scabs that fall off after several days without scarring. New maculopapules continue to erupt during the first 3 or 4 days of illness and go through a similar evolution. The findings at one time, in one area, of skin lesions in all stages of development—maculopapules, vesicles, umbilicated lesions, and scabs—is characteristic of chickenpox. The rash is most concentrated on the trunk, but pox are frequently seen on the face and scalp, occasionally on the mucosal surfaces of the mouth or conjunctiva, and rarely on the palms or soles.

Chickenpox in adults is often more severe than the disease in children, with more profuse rash, higher fever, and greater incidence of pneumonia.

COMPLICATIONS. Hemorrhage into vesicles and surrounding skin may be seen in adults with severe chickenpox or in children receiving adrenal steroids. Infection of the varicella lesions by bacteria, most commonly S. aureus, results in delayed healing and scarring of skin, and occasionally in bacteremia.

Of adults with chickenpox, 15 percent develop *primary varicella pneumonia,* and adult patients account for 90 percent of the patients who develop this complication. Pneumonia is invariably associated with skin lesions and appears 1 to 6 days after onset of rash. The degree of pulmonary involvement is to some extent correlated with the severity of the rash; patients may be virtually asymptomatic or may develop serious, life-threatening disease. Tachypnea, dyspnea, cough, and fever of 102°F or more are present in most patients with symptomatic pneumonia; cyanosis, pleuritic chest pain, and hemoptysis each occur in 20 to 40 percent of the recorded cases. The physical examination may disclose no abnormalities, or there may be intercostal retractions, a few rhonchi, wheezes, scattered râles, and rarely, evidence of pleural effusion. In contrast to paucity of physical signs, roentgenograms demonstrate widespread nodular infiltration of both lungs, most prominent at the hila and least evident at the apices. Vital capacity is decreased, arterial oxygen saturation is diminished, and the airways may be blocked by tenacious bronchopulmonary secretions. Most patients with varicella pneumonia show symptomatic improvement at the time the rash begins to wane; however, seriously ill patients can remain febrile and dyspneic for as long as 2 weeks. Roentgenographic evidence of disease diminishes at the time of clinical improvement, but may persist for several weeks. Abnormalities of pulmonary gas diffusion have been demonstrated several months after apparent recovery.

Encephalomyelitis is a less frequent complication of chickenpox than of measles and occurs predominantly in children. It begins 3 to 14 days after the onset of rash with drowsiness and irritability progressing to vomiting, convulsions, and coma which lasts for 4 or 5 days. As the patient regains consciousness, evidence of CNS abnormalities may be apparent. Varicella encephalomyelitis is frequently associated with cerebellar dysfunction either isolated or associated with other nervous disorders such as hemiparesis, athetosis, cranial nerve abnormalities, and various spinal syndromes.

Patients who *contract varicella while receiving steroids* may have recurrent crops of new skin lesions for as long as 3 weeks. They have a higher incidence of hemorrhagic and progressive gangrenous lesions and occasionally develop a fatal disseminated disease with viral infection in all the viscera. The fatal form of the disease has been encountered most frequently in children being treated with steroids for leukemia or other disease of the hematopoietic system, but it has also been seen in those receiving therapy for rheumatic fever and allergic disorders. Other complications of chickenpox such as myocarditis, corneal lesions, iritis, nephritis, orchitis, and appendicitis have been recognized but are rare. Congenital infection with varicella can occur, and infants born of mothers with chickenpox may display the typical skin lesions. Evidence of congenital malformations as a result of infection in early pregnancy is not convincing.

LABORATORY FINDINGS. Multinucleated giant cells and epithelial cells with eosinophilic intranuclear inclusions can be identified in material scraped from the base of a vesicular lesion or in sputum from patients with varicella pneumonia. For specific diagnosis, virus can be isolated from vesicular fluid and complement-fixation tests can be performed. The white blood count in patients with uncomplicated chickenpox is normal. The spinal fluid in patients with encephalomyelitis contains increased protein and as many as 3,000 lymphocytes per cu mm.

DIFFERENTIAL DIAGNOSIS. Chickenpox can usually be diagnosed by the history of recent exposure and the character of the rash. In situations where smallpox is a possibility, differentiation from chickenpox can be attempted by noting the distribution and evolution of the rash and by examination of cells from vesicles, but definitive diagnosis can be made only by identification of the virus. Disseminated vaccinia lesions similar to chickenpox may occur in patients, especially those with disorders of immunity or eczema, who have recently been vaccinated or exposed to a vaccinated person. Herpes simplex infection in patients with chronic eczema or neurodermatitis may present as a varicelliform eruption confined to pre-viously involved areas of skin; the diagnosis can be confirmed by virus isolation. Rickettsialpox can be differentiated from chickenpox by the presence of an eschar in the area of mite bite, prominent headache, and specific complement-fixing antibodies to *R. akari*.

PROPHYLAXIS. Chickenpox can be modified but not completely prevented by the administration of 0.2 to 0.3 ml per lb gamma-globulin. If exposure occurs, passive immunization should be attempted in pregnant women without a history of chickenpox, newborn infants, and nonimmune persons on steroid therapy.

TREATMENT. The patient with uncomplicated chickenpox should receive local applications for the relief of itching. Secondary bacterial infections should be treated with appropriate antibacterial agents. Patients with varicella pneumonia require skillful nursing care, removal of bronchial secretions, administration of oxygen, and on occasion ventilatory assistance, such as positive pressure breathing. Adrenal steroids have been considered by some to be beneficial in the treatment of varicella pneumonia, but convincing evidence of their efficacy in this condition is not available. Patients suspected of having varicella-zoster infection of the eye should be promptly treated by an ophthalmologist.

REFERENCES

Brunnell, P. A.: Varicella-zoster Infections in Pregnancy, J.A.M.A., 199:315, 1967.

Gordon, J. E.: Chickenpox: An Epidemiological Review, Am. J. Med. Sci., 244:362, 1962.

Ross, A.: Modification of Chickenpox in Family Contacts by Administration of Gamma Globulin, New Engl. J. Med., 267:369, 1962.

Triebwasser, J. H., R. Harris, R. Bryant, and E. Rhoades: Varicella Pneumonia in Adults: Report of Seven Cases and a Review of Literature, Medicine, 46:409, 1967.

Weller, T. H., H. Witton, and E. Bell: Etiologic Agents of Varicella and *Herpes zoster*, J. Exp. Med., 108:843, 1958.

225   HERPES ZOSTER
Lewis L. Coriell

DEFINITION. Herpes zoster, or shingles, is an acute infectious disease of man. It is caused by a virus and is characterized by unilateral, segmental inflammation of the posterior root ganglions or extramedullary ganglions of cranial nerves and by a painful vesicular eruption of the skin along the peripheral distribution of the involved nerve.

HISTORY. The disease was called zona ("girdle") by the Greeks because of the bandlike distribution of the eruption about the trunk. Bokay (1888) suggested a possible etiologic relationship between zoster and varicella, and Lipschutz (1921) defined the specific histopathology of the skin lesions. Serial cultivation of the virus in tissue culture of human fibroblasts (1953) enabled Weller to show that the viruses of varicella and herpes zoster were identical serologically.

ETIOLOGY. The virus of herpes zoster is relatively large (204 x 240 μ). It is strictly a parasite of man. Electron micrographs of a vesicle fluid have shown it to be similar in size and shape to the virus of varicella. The virus may be plentiful in early vesicles but is typically scanty after 24 hr. Zoster is now considered to be a reactivation of a latent varicella virus in a partially immune individual, although the mechanism of reactivation is not clear.

EPIDEMIOLOGY. Infection is rare in children but increases in frequency, severity, and duration with age. It occurs in all seasons and is slightly more frequent in males than in females. In the United States the majority of patients with herpes zoster gives a history of a previous attack of varicella. Epidemics have occurred in schools and barracks but are not common. Outbreaks of herpes zoster have occurred in contacts of a patient with varicella, and vice versa. The grouping of these secondary infections suggests that zoster is infectious only during the first 2 or 3 days after appearance of the eruption. Secondary zoster following trauma such as spinal puncture, administration of arsenic or bismuth, spinal cord tumor, tabes, and lymphatic leukemia suggests that the virus may remain dormant in the tissues for long periods. The disease appears to be more common in persons who are overworked or ill.

PATHOGENESIS. Whether the virus enters the skin and travels up the sensory nerve or extends peripherally has not been established. The virus has been demonstrated only in the skin lesions, although an inflammatory reaction is a constant finding in the segmental nerve, its sensory ganglion, and the posterior horn of the spinal column (posterior poliomyelitis). The regional lymph nodes show an acute inflammatory reaction.

The skin vesicle is confined to the epidermis, while the corium is congested and infiltrated with inflammatory cells. In the margin of the vesicle are epithelial cells undergoing balloon degeneration. Some of the cells contain eosinophilic intranuclear inclusion bodies which displace the basichromatin to the periphery of the enlarged nucleus. Multinucleated giant cells may be present, each nucleus containing an inclusion body. Within 2 or 3 days, inflammatory cells fill the vesicle, and healing progresses from below, frequently with slight scarring.

MANIFESTATIONS. The incubation period varies from 7 to 21 days. The preeruptive stage consists of fever and constitutional symptoms, with pain, paresthesias, or hyperesthesia over the distribution of the involved nerve for 2 to 4 days. Following this, an erythematous dermatitis appears, which quickly becomes papular and vesiculates, with large or small grouped vesicles on an erythematous base. The vesicles, at first clear, become cloudy within 2 to 3 days, then crust and dry after 5 to 10 days. The eruption may appear first near the spinal column, with successive crops over the distal distribution of the nerve. The pain and vesicular band, following radicular lines, run transversely around the trunk or vertically over the arm and leg. The lesions are almost always unilateral. Headache and meningismus are not uncommon. Pain is frequently slight or absent in young children but may be intense and not completely controlled by analgesic drugs

in adults. It is variously described as aching, soreness, burning, gnawing, shooting, stabbing, or neuralgic.

The regional lymph nodes are enlarged and tender. Secondary bacterial infection of the ruptured vesicles is common. Over 75 percent of cases occur between the second dorsal and second lumbar vertebras; cases are rare below the elbow or knee. Involvement of the fifth cranial nerve is next in frequency, and in 50 percent the globe of the eye is affected. When the nasociliary branch of the semilunar ganglion is involved, the cornea, sclera, or ciliary body may be permanently damaged; the first branch of the fifth nerve is affected more frequently then the second or third. Disease of the geniculate ganglion may lead to zoster of the concha of the ear, the external auditory canal, or the soft palate, and to loss of taste (Hunt's syndrome); these manifestations are often accompanied by paralysis of the seventh nerve. Paralysis is not uncommon in cephalic and cervical zoster but is rare in zoster of the trunk. Second attacks of herpes zoster are exceedingly rare and should suggest the alternate diagnosis of localized herpes simplex. In some patients, a generalized vesicular eruption simulating varicella appears shortly after the appearance of the localized lesion (zoster generalisata).

The total course of the disease from onset to complete recovery is 10 days to 5 weeks. In the age group up to nineteen years, 90 percent of patients recovered within 14 days, while in the forty- to fifty-nine-year age group, only 45 percent of lesions cleared in this interval. If all the vesicles appear within 24 hr, the total illness is usually short; if crops of vesicles appear up to 7 days, the total duration was progressively longer.

A serious complication is the syndrome of postherpetic neuralgia, which is limited to aged patients with arteriosclerosis. It usually involves only the trunk or the ophthalmic division of the trigeminal nerve. Frequently there is an interval betwen the acute phase and full unfolding of severe pain, which is of such severity and intensity that the patients cannot rest or sleep, and which may persist for weeks or months.

LABORATORY FINDINGS. The fluid from unruptured vesicles is sterile bacteriologically, but a smear stained with Giemsa shows multinucleated giant cells and type A inclusion bodies. The cerebrospinal fluid is abnormal in 40 percent of cases; pressure may be increased, and a pleocytosis of up to 300 mononuclear cells has been observed.

DIFFERENTIAL DIAGNOSIS. In the preeruptive stage, the diagnosis is difficult, and the disease is usually confused with many other more common causes of pain, such as pleurisy, appendicitis, "lumbago," pleurodynia, or collapsed intervertebral disk. After the unilateral eruption appears, the clinical features are so characteristic that the diagnosis is simple. Occasionally, localized herpes simplex along the distribution of a segmental nerve may simulate zoster, including the localized pain and tenderness. The diagnosis of herpes simplex infection can be confirmed in the laboratory.

TREATMENT. Treatment is directed toward increasing the patient's comfort and preventing secondary infection.

The average case of herpes zoster is self-limited and presents no serious complications. The two unsolved problems are the syndrome of postherpetic neuralgia and ophthalmic zoster. In the acute phase, pain is usually controlled by aspirin and codeine, combined with mild sedation; local anesthetic ointments are not very effective. A petrolatum gauze pad bandage to prevent painful trauma by clothing may be helpful. The skin lesions are adequately managed with applications of calamine lotion in most cases. Adhesive tape strapping should not be applied for the preeruptive pain of herpes zoster because it will lead to extensive loss of epidermis upon removal of the tape. Antibiotics have no effect on the virus but may be indicated to control secondary infection, particularly in ophthalmic zoster or severe spinal involvement with secondary infection. In ophthalmic involvement the choice of antibiotic should be guided by bacterial cultures and sensitivity tests. Idoxuridine (IDU) is of no value. Treatment of lesions of the eye should be supervised by an ophthalmologist. Early relief of pain and inflammation follows the use of cortisone and corticotropin. Cycloplegic eyedrops are used for iridocyclitis.

Severe postherpetic pain may be resistant to all types of management. One theory advanced to explain this is the activation of self-contained pain circuits in and above the thalamus. The following procedures are based on the supposition that the defect is central: injection of dorsal root ganglion with alcohol or irradiation with x-ray, dorsal rhizotomy, cordotomy, and lobotomy. On the theory of peripheral nerve abnormality are based vitamin B therapy, procainization or excision of skin, surgical pituitrin, paravertebral block, intravenous tetraethylammonium chloride, and sympathetic ganglionectomy. Other empirical procedures which have been helpful in certain cases include autohemotherapy, sodium iodide, moccasin venom, and Protamide. The multiplicity of recommended procedures is eloquent evidence that none is entirely satisfactory.

PROGNOSIS. It is very unusual for serious complications to follow inflammation of the spinal ganglions. Partial paralysis of the third, fourth, sixth, and seventh cranial nerves, or hypesthesia, may persist for some time. Significant impairment of vision occurs in many cases of zoster ophthalmicus.

REFERENCES

Bailey, P.: Herpes Zoster, Postgrad. Med., 12:127, 1952.

Blank, H., L. L. Coriell, and T. F. McN. Scott: Human Skin Grafted upon the Chorioallantois of the Chick Embryo for Virus Cultivation, Proc. Soc. Exp. Biol. Med., 69:341, 1948.

Rake, G., H. Blank, L. L. Coriell, F. P. O. Nagler, and T. F. McN. Scott: The Relationships of Varicella and Herpes Zoster: Electron Microscope Studies, J. Bacteriol., 56:293, 1948.

Scheie, H. G., and M. C. Alper: Treatment of Herpes Zoster Ophthalmicus with Cortisone or Corticotropin, A.M.A. Arch. Ophthalmol., 53:38, 1955.

Weller, T. H.: Varicella-Herpes Zoster Virus in "Horsfall and Tamm Viral and Rickettsial Infections of Man," 4th ed., Philadelphia, J. B. Lippincott Company, 1967.

226 HERPES SIMPLEX
Lewis L. Coriell

DEFINITION. Herpes simplex is an infectious disease caused by a virus. Classically, it appears in recurrent attacks as clusters of vesicles on the face, lips, and mucocutaneous junctions. The initial infection in some individuals may be serious or even fatal. Infection of the central nervous system, the eye, the skin in eczematous patients, the viscera, or the mouth and throat in gingivostomatitis are the common forms of "primary" herpes simplex.

HISTORY. Gruter, in 1914, first transferred infection from the cornea of a patient to the cornea of a rabbit and, subsequently, back to the cornea of a blind man, reproducing a typical dendritic ulceration of the cornea. In 1938 Dodd, Buddingh, and Johnston isolated herpes simplex virus from the mouths of children suffering with febrile ulcerative stomatitis (acute herpetic gingivostomatitis).

ETIOLOGY. The virus of herpes simplex (*Herpesvirus hominis*, HVH) passes ordinary bacterial filters, measures 180 to 200 mμ in diameter, and is composed of a central core of double stranded DNA, an envelope with 162 capsomers arranged as an icosahedron, a surrounding granular zone, and an outer membrane with short projections. It is present in early vesicles. It may be propagated on the cornea or in the brain of several laboratory animals, on the chorioallantoic membrane of embryonated eggs, or in tissue culture. Two serologic types can be distinguished by microquantal neutralization tests. Type 2 isolates are usually associated with infection of the adult genital tract, and type 1 strains, with infection from all other sites.

EPIDEMIOLOGY. The serums of most adults (70 to 90 percent) contain neutralizing antibodies against herpes simplex; many of these individuals experience recurrent manifestations of disease. Fever, whether due to infectious diseases or artificially induced ("fever blister"), and the common cold ("cold sore") are probably the most frequent precipitants of recurrent herpes; emotional disturbance, physical fatigue, sunburn, menstruation, and food allergy are other incitants. The virus remains latent in the tissues between attacks but is sufficiently active to stimulate antibody production. Virus has frequently been found in the saliva when there was no clinical evidence of disease. Adults who have never been infected may contact a primary infection. Full-term newborn infants are usually immune by virtue of transplacental transfer of antibodies, which they gradually lose after the first few months of life. However, by the fifth year, the percentage of children with specific neutralizing antibodies approaches that observed in adults, indicating a high infection rate during infancy. The clinical syndromes recognized as primary infection in this age group account for only 15 percent of serologic infections. Herpes simplex has evolved an unusually successful host-parasite relationship with man. Most individuals harbor the virus from infancy to old age with little inconvenience to themselves, and even the primary contact in infancy is usually not accompanied by manifest clinical disease. The association of type 2 herpes virus with the genital tract or closely related sites suggests that it is commonly transmitted by venereal contact, whereas type 1 is spread by contact with oral secretions or from recurrent vesicles of the mucocutaneous junction about the face.

PATHOGENESIS. It is probable that during latent periods the virus lives within cells, because the extracellular fluid contains sufficient neutralizing antibody to inactivate the virus. The various precipitating factors which induce recurrent disease may have a common denominator in altered physiology of the host cell which permits the virus to multiply, but little specific information is available on this point. Skin biopsies taken during the early vesicular stage show congestion of the dermis, with swelling and ballooning degeneration of prickle cells of the epidermis. In some of these, the nuclear basichromatin is collected at the periphery and the entire central area of the enlarged nucleus is filled with a homogeneous mass which at first stains blue and later red with hematoxylin and eosin. This is the type A inclusion body, found wherever there is active herpes simplex infection. Multinucleated giant cells, with each nucleus containing an inclusion body, are frequently seen in biopsies of infected human skin.

The intraepidermal vesicle does not extend below the basement membrane and hence does not cause scarring, although depigmentation may persist for some time in dark-skinned persons. In the healing phase, the vesicle and corium are densely infiltrated with inflammatory cells.

MANIFESTATIONS. *Recurrent herpes simplex* is a circumscribed eruption, consisting of closely grouped, thin-walled vesicles on an erythematous base, which tends to recur repeatedly in the same area of the skin, particularly at mucocutaneous junctions. It begins as a mild itching or burning lesion which rapidly becomes papular and vesicular, and then passes successively through crusting, scab formation, and desiccation, the whole process taking 3 to 14 days. Typically, there is no fever, regional lymphadenopathy, or other signs of systemic illness. The disease is self-limited and is commonly identified with its anatomic location—herpes facialis, labialis, nasalis, progenitalis, or vulvovaginalis.

Herpetic keratoconjunctivitis (Chap. 228) is characterized usually by swelling and congestion of the conjunctiva, with superficial opacities in the cornea and a palpable preauricular lymph node. Bacterial cultures are sterile; hyperesthesia is a prominent sign. The presence of typical herpetic vesicles on the eyelids may aid in the diagnosis; however, the recurrent attacks are frequently confined to the cornea in the form of dendritic ulcers or, less often, as punctate, marginate, or discoform ulcers. The corneal ulcerations may persist for several weeks and respond poorly to local therapy; they are superficial, but repeated attacks pose a threat to vision.

Traumatic herpes designates those cases where the primary infection occurs at the site of a skin abrasion on the hand, elbow, finger, or other area not commonly associated with the disease. Recurrences have been observed at the same site over a period of many years.

Acute herpetic gingivostomatitis is the commonest form of primary infection and is seen most frequently in children one to four years of age, less often in adults. It is characterized by gradual or sudden onset, with fever, malaise, sore mouth and throat, and extreme irritability, sometimes alternating with lethargy. The temperature may reach 104°F, but is usually 101 to 103°F. Physical examination reveals multiple painful shallow aphthous ulcers on a red base on the buccal mucous membranes, tongue, or oropharynx. The gums are swollen, bleed easily, and are typically most inflamed at the gingival margin. The regional lymph nodes are large and tender. Fever and pain usually persist for 6 to 8 days, followed by gradual healing of the ulcers during the following week. The ulcers may be confined to, or appear first in, the pharynx (herpetic pharyngitis), and in such cases the diagnosis is commonly missed.

Eczema herpeticum (Kaposi's varicelliform eruption) is a rarer manifestation of primary infection which occurs in persons with eczema or neurodermatitis. Large areas of abnormal skin are involved, the grouped vesicles usually appearing in crops over a period of several days; hence the similarity to varicella. The temperature may reach 106°F, and marked prostration is not uncommon. The fever subsides during the second week, coincident with the crusting and healing of the skin lesions.

Meningoencephalitis was formerly thought to be a rare form of primary herpes in man, but complement fixation tests indicate that 5 to 7 percent of cases of aseptic meningitis may be due to this virus. It is accompanied by fever, headache, gastrointestinal symptoms, and signs of meningeal irritation and encephalitis. Patients with herpes encephalitis frequently manifest personality changes, bizarre behavior, hallucinations, and aphasia in the early stages of disease indicating localization in the temporal lobe.

In addition to the syndromes described above, herpes simplex has been known to occur in segmental nerve distribution simulating herpes zoster. The occurrence of repeated attacks in the same area is diagnostic.

Visceral herpes simplex, characterized by fulminating generalized infection with fever, viremia, and necrotic lesions in the liver and other viscera, and frequently terminating in death, is a clinical entity in newborn infants. Skin lesions are not always present. Most cases have been in premature infants or have occurred when the mother herself had a primary herpetic infection. In several cases the mother was known to have had repeated bouts of herpes vulvovaginitis.

LABORATORY FINDINGS. The total leukocyte count is usually normal or only slightly increased, with a normal differential. The diagnosis can be confirmed in the laboratory by (1) isolation and identification of the virus, (2) demonstration of typical eosinophilic intranuclear inclusions or fluorescence in tissue biopsy or vesicle fluid, or

(3) in primary infections, a rising titer of specific neutralizing antibodies. The acute phase serum should be collected before the fifth day of illness, because antibodies appear early. In central-nervous-system infection, the spinal fluid pressure and protein are slightly increased, and the sugar is normal. A pleocytosis up to 500 cells is observed; many polymorphonuclear leukocytes occur early, and change later to mononuclear cells; the virus may not be present in spinal fluid.

DIFFERENTIAL DIAGNOSIS. The history and clinical appearance of the recurrent skin and eye manifestations are usually sufficient to establish the diagnosis.

The laboratory tests enumerated above are confirmatory in doubtful cases and are essential for absolute diagnosis in the primary manifestations. Herpetic gingivostomatitis is often confused with Vincent's angina (Chap. 168), which responds dramatically to penicillin. Recurrent solitary aphthous ulcers in the mouth are not caused by herpes simplex.

In herpangina, caused by group A Coxsackie virus (Chap. 210), the vesicles are confined to the posterior part of the mouth, and the disease occurs in epidemics. Large bullae, recurrent attacks, and normal lymph nodes are seen in erythema multiforme (Chap. 400).

Eczema herpeticum may be easily confused with secondary bacterial infection of eczema. Extensive weeping and crusting may obscure the grouped vesicular nature of the lesion before the crusts are removed with wet dressings. Eczema vaccinatum (generalized vaccinia) (Chap. 223), usually presents with larger vesicles with a central indentation. Herpetic meningoencephalitis must be differentiated from bacterial and viral encephalitides, particularly enterovirus encephalitis, poliomyelitis, lymphocytic choriomeningitis, and postinfectious encephalitis. Early appearance of temporal lobe symptoms is suggestive.

TREATMENT. In early herpetic keratitis and dentritic ulcers, Idoxuridine (IDU) or other thymidine analogues are usually beneficial. Results are not so favorable if the stroma or iris is involved. Good results have also been reported with local application of interferon. Corticosteroids are usually contraindicated in herpes simplex eye infections, but may be helpful in stromal lesions and in herpes zoster lesions. Therapy of eye lesions should always be supervised by an ophthalmologist.

Parenteral thymidine analogues given early in encephalitis may be beneficial, but to achieve rapid confirmation of the diagnosis may require a brain biopsy and hence the frequency of temporal lobe symptoms is stressed.

Antibiotics may be helpful in controlling secondary bacterial infection. In acute gingivostomatitis, the maintenance of adequate hydration and nutrition is aided by the local application, before meals, of 1 percent Pontocaine. A detergent mouthwash helps to maintain oral hygiene and inhibits bacterial proliferation. In eczema herpeticum and visceral disease, supportive therapy, fluid replacement, blood transfusions, and appropriate antibacterial measures are indicated. Convalescent serum and γ-globulin have not been beneficial.

PROGNOSIS. Except for complications following infection of the cornea, recurrent herpes has few sequelae. The primary manifestations have a self-limited course except for meningoencephalitis and visceral disease, which are sometimes fatal, and eczema herpeticum, in which the mortality rate may be 20 percent.

REFERENCES

Dodd, K., J. Buddingh, and L. Johnston: Herpetic Stomatitis, Am. J. Dis. Child., 58:907, 1939.

Dohlman, C. H.: Annual Review—Cornea and Sclera, A.M.A. Arch. Ophthalmol., 71:249, 1964.

Dowdle, W. R., A. J. Nahmias, R. W. Harwell, and F. P. Pauls: Association of Antigenic Type of Herpesvirus Hominis with Site of Viral Recovery, J. Immunol., 99:974, 1967.

Johnson, R. T., L. C. Olson, and E. L. Buescher: Problems in Laboratory Diagnosis of Herpes Simplex Infection of the Nervous System, Arch. Neurol., 18:260, 1968.

Lynch, F. W., C. A. Evans, V. S. Bolin, and R. J. Steves: Kaposi's Varicelliform Eruption: Extensive Herpes Simplex as a Complication of Eczema, Arch. Dermatol. Syphilol., 51:129, 1945.

Marshall, W. J. S.: Herpes Simplex Encephalitis Treated with Idoxuridine and External Decompression, Lancet, II:579, 1967.

Pauls, F. P., and W. R. Dowdle: A Serologic Study of Herpesvirus Hominis Strains by Microneutralization Tests, J. Immunol. 98:941, 1967.

Scott, T. F. McN.: Infection with the Virus of Herpes Simplex, New Engl. J. Med., 250:183, 1954.

Zuelzer, W., and C. Stuhlberg: Herpes Simplex Virus as the Cause of Fulminating Visceral Disease and Hepatitis in Infancy, A.M.A. J. Dis. Child., 83:421, 1952.

227 MINOR VIRAL DISEASES OF THE SKIN AND MUCOSAL SURFACES

Alvin E. Friedman-Kien

HERPANGINA

Herpangina is a specific, benign, infectious disease of childhood, although it is not uncommon in young adults. It is caused by Group A Coxsackie viruses types 2, 3, 4, 5, 6, 8, and 10. It occurs throughout the world in epidemic form, usually in the summer and early fall. Similar disorders have been attributed to ECHO and Coxsackie B viruses (Chap. 210).

The incubation period for herpangina is about 4 to 6 days. Children between the ages of one and seven are most commonly afflicted. Immunity persists for at least 1 year; reinfection with another strain of the virus can occur.

Herpangina is characterized by sudden onset of fever, temperatures often rising to 104°F, severe sore throat, nausea, and vomiting. Anorexia, dysphagia, excessive salivation, and severe malaise are common. The throat and posterior portions of the mouth are usually quite red and injected and are covered with numerous minute vesicles (1 to 2 mm in diameter), which quickly rupture, erode and enlarge to form 3 to 4 mm punched-out, shallow ulcers with grayish centers surrounded by deep red areolas. The number and size of the lesions increase for 2 to 3 days and heal within 4 or 5 days. The anterior faucial pillars of the pharynx, the tonsils, and the soft palate are usually involved. Occasionally, similar vesicles are found in the vaginal mucosa.

The systemic and local symptoms begin to regress within 4 to 5 days, and total recovery occurs within 7 days. Headache, coryza, and other respiratory tract symptoms are absent. Myalgia and arthralgia are rare. Mild cervical lymphadenopathy is sometimes noted. Parotitis and aseptic meningitis have been reported.

Recovery from the illness is always uneventful. Treatment is confined to topical symptomatic measures; frequent mouthwashes and gargles with topical anesthetics such as Benadryl elixir or butacaine are soothing. A fluid or soft diet is advisable. Demonstration of a Coxsackie virus from one of the vesicles, or isolation from pharyngeal washing and/or stool may be helpful, especially when combined with a demonstrable rise in antibody titer in the convalescent as compared to the acute serum.

Differential diagnosis should include a primary herpes simplex infection which may produce a severe oropharyngeal eruption. However, herpes does not usually occur in epidemics and the herpetic lesions are more typically confined to the anterior portions of the mouth, such as the lips and tongue. With herpes, the gingiva are typically red and edematous. Aphthous stomatitis, bacterial pharyngitis, and the oropharyngeal lesions of viral exanthems, such as chickenpox and measles, may be confused initially with herpangina. The natural course of the disease will help clarify the diagnosis.

FOOT-AND-MOUTH DISEASE

Foot-and-mouth disease is a fairly common epidemic viral disease of farm animals in Europe, Asia, and Africa. It is rarely known to affect man. The causative agent is the smallest virus known to infect animals. A few cases have been reported in children and adults who had been exposed by contact with an infected stock of animals, by ingestion of meat or dairy products, or from exposure to the hides or excretions of sick animals. The incubation period seems to range between 2 to 18 days. Multiloculated vesicles appear on the skin and mucous membranes. Intranuclear inclusion bodies have been observed in the epidermal cells at the base of the vesicles and in the surrounding tissue.

The onset of the infection is characterized by fever, headache, malaise, and dryness and burning sensation of the oral mucosa. Within 2 to 3 days loculated vesicles develop on the lips, tongue, and buccal mucosa. The palms and soles and interdigital skin may also show such lesions. Generalized pruritus may occur. The vesicles go on to develop into irregularly shaped, painful ulcers which may become edematous and bleed easily. At times either the mouth or the hands alone may be involved. Rarely,

other areas of the skin may be affected. The course of the disease is usually mild; the temperature falls rapidly, and the lesions begin to heal after 6 or 7 days. Total healing is complete by 2 to 3 weeks, leaving no scars.

Diagnostic confirmation depends upon a rise in specific complement-fixing antibody titers. The virus can be isolated in tissue cultures, guinea pigs, and chick embryos. In the United States, strict regulations of quarantine and meat inspection have limited the occurrence to a few outbreaks near the Mexican border. Treatment is symptomatic.

HAND, FOOT, AND MOUTH DISEASE

Hand, foot, and mouth disease represents a syndrome characterized by a vesicular eruption of the skin and the mouth. It has been reported to occur in epidemics in the United States, England, and Australia. Laboratory studies suggest that the disease is associated with Coxsackie A viruses, types 16, 5, and others. The infection occurs primarily in children. The disease is mild, running its course in 4 to 8 days. A transient, low-grade fever may be present at the onset. The most troublesome symptom is stomatitis. Initially vesicles appear in random distribution on the tongue, buccal mucosa, gingiva and palate, usually sparing the pharynx. These vesicles are few in number and are somewhat larger than those seen in herpangina. The vesicles quickly develop into shallow, whitish ulcerations with red areolas.

Lesions on the skin are not always present, but are typically vesicular, approximately 4 or 5 mm in size. They are characteristically few in number, ovoid or elongated in shape, grayish in color, surrounded by a fine, red margin. These vesicles appear on the dorsum of the fingers and especially about the periungual region and the heel margin. Occasionally vesicles may be found on the palms or soles. They usually start to disappear within a few days after onset. On rare occasions a more diffuse, vesicular eruption and exanthematous rash have been reported, with particular concentration of such lesions on the buttocks.

The differential diagnosis includes herpangina, aphthous stomatitis, and other Coxsackie and ECHO virus infections. The confirmation of the exact diagnosis depends upon viral and serologic studies.

VESICULAR STOMATITIS

Vesicular stomatitis is a viral illness of horses, cattle, and pigs, but it occasionally affects man. The disease occurs in the United States and South America. The mode of natural spread among livestock is unknown, but the disease is probably transmitted by direct and indirect contact. Epidemics do not occur in freezing weather, and it is therefore assumed that the virus is arthropod-borne in nature. The virus has been isolated from flies and mosquitoes. Two antigenically distinct viruses are known to cause the disease in the United States, the Indiana type and the New Jersey type. The incubation period is 2 to 6 days. In man the disease is mild and self-limited, the symptoms are similar to those of influenza. The virus has been studied and used extensively in experimental laboratories. Consequently, several cases have been reported in laboratory personnel as well as farm workers.

The sudden onset is characterized by fever up to 104°F, lasting 24 hr, chills, and profuse sweating. Myalgias, malaise, headache, and aching of the eyes are common. The symptoms are worse on the second day. One-third of the patients develop sore throats with cervical and submandibular adenopathy. The tongue and mucous membranes may become sore as well, and conjunctivitis may occur. In a few cases, small, subcorneal, intraepithelial vesicles appear on the fingers. Symptoms last only 3 to 4 days, but relapses can occur. Inapparent infections have been demonstrated by a rise of both complement-fixing and neutralizing serum antibodies in laboratory workers. Differential diagnosis must include hand, foot, and mouth disease, herpangina, and other mucocutaneous syndromes. Viral isolation from patients is rare, but the comparison of acute and convalescent sera in a suspected case will help to confirm the diagnosis.

WARTS (Verrucae)

Warts are an infectious disease of the skin and contiguous mucous membrane. The etiologic agent is a member of the Papova group of viruses that includes the animal papilloma viruses, the polyoma, simian vacuolating viruses, such as SV_{40} and SV_5. These viruses have been shown to induce tumors in experimental animals and to cause in vitro transformation of tissue cultures.

The human wart virus, which is a DNA virus measuring about 45 mμ in diameter, has been extracted from human lesions and has been used experimentally to induce the formation of warts at inoculated sites in the skin of human volunteers. The incubation period based on the experimental inoculations varies between 1 to 20 months, averaging about 4 months. The virus has been shown electronmicroscopically to parasitize the nuclei of epidermal cells. The successful isolation of the human wart virus in tissue culture has not been accomplished conclusively.

The skin lesions induced by the wart virus are due to an abnormal proliferation of epidermal cells. The lesions, which are skin-colored, may occur as single lesions or in multiples widely disseminated over the entire body. Although the same virus is thought to cause all varieties of human warts, the character of the lesion depends upon the local response of the affected skin to the virus host. Immunity may also play a role. For convenience, lesions are classified according to location and morphology.

Common warts (verrucae vulgares) are usually seen on the hands or under and about the fingernails. These lesions are rough surfaced, horny papules which can vary in size from 1 mm to 2 cm in diameter. Confluency of clustered lesions occurs frequently. The lesions are asymptomatic.

Plantar warts occur mostly beneath pressure points on the soles of the feet and are frequently quite painful. The surface lesions are flat, firm, stippled, and horny. They may occur individually or in a mosaiclike cluster. The mass of plantar warts is beneath the skin surface. These warts are generally larger than one might expect. They have conical shape, the pointed end projected inward. This configuration is probably due to the pressure imposed by walking. Plantar warts are most common in teenagers; females seem slightly more susceptible than males.

The differential diagnosis of plantar warts includes calluses and corns. The normal epidermal ridges are continuous across the surface of calluses and corns, whereas the surface of warts disrupts the normal pattern. Local foreign body reactions and congenital keratotic lesions of the palms and soles also have to be ruled out.

Flat warts (verrucae planae) are skin-colored, smooth, flat or slightly elevated, round or polygonal papules that vary between 1 and 5 mm in diameter. They almost always occur in multiples, up to several hundred. The common sites are the face, neck, chest, dorsum of the hands, flexor surface of the forearms, and shins. The mucous membranes are rarely involved. The surface of these lesions show a stippled appearance when examined under a magnifying glass. Flat warts are most frequently confused with the lesions of lichen planus. Multiple lesions on the dorsum of the hands may be mistaken for one of the inherited disorders known as acrokeratosis verruciformis, epidermodysplasia verruciformis, or Darier's disease.

Filiform warts are most frequently seen in adult males, and usually occur in the bearded area of the face. The lips and eyelids are often involved. The lesions are horny, fingerlike projections which may grow to considerable length if left unattended. They occur in multiples, but are seen occasionally as individual lesions. Differential diagnosis includes cutaneous horns.

Digitate warts are seen on the scalp of adults as clusters of fleshy fingerlike projections. They must be differentiated from epidermal nevi.

Condylomata accuminata (moist warts), also known as venereal or fig warts, are the lesions which occur at the mucocutaneous junctions of the skin in the genital and perianal areas. Rare cases have been seen about the areola of the nipple in females, the margins of the mouth, both the inguinal and axillary folds, and in the interdigital skin between the toes.

These warts are pink-to-red in color and moist and soft. They may be pedunculated or elongated. Clusters of these warts may resemble a cauliflower in appearance. They may occur in great numbers and can become macerated and malodorous because of their location. These warts are most often seen in young adults, but children as well as adults are affected. The eruption of moist warts is frequent and more severe in pregnancy. Although the lesions have been known to be transmitted between sexual partners, it is a misconception that these lesions are usually venereal in origin.

Condylomata accuminata, unlike other warts, are most effectively treated with the repeated topical application of a 25 percent podophyllum resin in tincture of benzoin. A single, persistent, fungating lesion on the penis, resistant to this treatment, should be biopsied to rule out a malignancy, such as squamous cell carcinoma or a rare, abnormal growth, known as the Buschke-Lowenstein tumor. The more sessile condylomata lesions of secondary syphilis may be confused with viral-induced and genital warts.

Warts often tend to recur, even after apparently adequate treatment. The variety of methods used for removal are primarily destructive, such as electrodesiccation and curettage, surgical excision, x-ray, or cryosurgery by applying liquid nitrogen or dry ice. Repeated paring of warts, followed by the application of caustic agents such as mono- or trichloracetic acid, salicylic acid, phenol, or silver nitrate is very helpful. It is important to avoid radical means of therapy, because all warts will eventually disappear spontaneously, leaving no scar, suggesting the development of an immune response. However, warts may persist and spread within the same host for several years.

ORF (Ecthyma Infectiosum)

Orf is an infectious disease which primarily affects the mouth and lips of sheep. It is caused by a specific virus which has been isolated in tissue culture. The disease is transmitted between animals and also from virus-contaminated, dried crusts of lesions found in grazing pastures. The virus may remain in an infective state for several months or years. The disease has a worldwide distribution. The mouths of young lambs are most often affected; infection confers lifelong immunity. Human infection occurs in shepherds, butchers, veterinarians, and children who play with sheep.

In man, the incubation period is about 5 to 6 days. The eruption may occur as single or multiple lesions on the hands and other exposed parts of the body. Initially, a small, reddish-blue papule appears and rapidly enlarges to form a 2 to 3 cm hemorrhagic bulla. Itching is intense and the bulla ruptures to form an umbilicated, erythematous ulcer which develops a gray-white crust. Systemic manifestations are rare, except for occasional low-grade fever and mild regional lymphangitis and lymphadenopathy. A transient macular and papular red rash may occur on the trunk during the second week of the disease. Spontaneous healing occurs within 3 to 6 weeks.

The disease should be suspected when the characteristic lesions develop in individuals exposed to sheep. The diagnosis can be confirmed by virus isolation in the laboratory as well as a comparative rise of antibody titers in acute and convalescent sera.

Differential diagnosis must include milkers' nodule, anthrax, tularemia, primary inoculation tuberculosis, and cowpox.

MILKERS' NODULE (Paravaccinia, Milkers' Warts)

Milkers' nodule is a benign, poxvirus disease contracted from infected cows. The disease has a worldwide distribution. Nodules and ulcers occur on the teats of infected dairy cattle. In man, lesions appear within 5 to 7 days after milking an infected cow. They usually occur on the hands, but other exposed parts of the body, such as the face, may be inoculated. The virus has been isolated in bovine kidney tissue culture and resembles the orf virus. The early, flat, dark red papules enlarge up to 1 to 2 cm in diameter within a week and develop into solid, elastic, shiny, brownish-purple, highly vascular nodules. No pus or fluid accumulates. The nodules may be slightly tender, and mild regional lymphadenopathy may occur. Mild temperature elevations have been reported. Gradually an opaque, gray, slightly depressed eschar develops over the surface of the nodules' red granulation tissue. The lesion is surrounded by an areola of erythema. Resolution occurs within 5 to 6 weeks without scarring. One infection provides permanent immunity. The virus can be isolated in tissue culture, but this is not a practical routine procedure. There is no cross immunity between milkers' nodule, cowpox, and vaccinia.

Differential diagnosis between milkers' nodule and warts may not be possible on clinical grounds. Pyogenic granuloma and cowpox should also be considered.

MOLLUSCUM CONTAGIOSUM

Molluscum contagiosum is an infectious disease of the skin and mucous membranes caused by one of the largest known viruses. It is limited to man and most frequently occurs in childhood. Although the virus has not been grown in the laboratory, it has been classified morphologically on the basis of electronmicroscopy with the pox group of viruses. No cross-antigenicity with other pox viruses has yet been demonstrated. The mode of transmission is unknown. The disease has a worldwide distribution and has occurred in epidemics within children's institutions, between wrestlers, and members of the same family. Infections have been transmitted between genitalia during sexual intercourse and from the mouth of a suckling baby to its mother's breast. Successful experimental inoculation of lesion extracts to the skin of human volunteers has been reported. The incubation period varies between 2 weeks and 2 months. Recent fluorescent-antibody and gel-diffusion immunologic studies have shown demonstrable antibody in the serum of infected individuals.

The lesions may vary in number and size, ranging from 1 mm up to "giant" lesions of 1 to 2 cm in diameter, and average about 4 mm. They are elevated, waxy, pearly white papules which show an umbilicated central pore. By squeezing such a papule, one can express from the pore a curdlike, cheesy material, which, upon electronmicroscopic examination, proves to be loaded with virus particles. Ordinary light microscopy smears of the curd show a specific diagnostic picture of clusters of cells containing eosinophilic, giant cytoplasmic inclusion bodies. The papules may appear alone or in groups. Autoinoculation is frequent; the lesions are usually present for 6 months to a year, but may persist and spread for 3 to 4 years. The face, especially the eyelids, the trunk, and anogenital areas are most commonly involved. The conjunctiva, lips, and buccal mucosa may rarely be involved.

Molluscum lesions are frequently traumatized and become secondarily infected, but injury seems to cause individual lesions to resolve. Spontaneous regression eventually occurs without scarring.

Treatment by sharp curettage clears up the lesions with little, if any, scarring.

Diagnosis of multiple lesions is fairly simple. A single lesion may be confused with a keratoacanthoma, basal cell epithelioma, or pyogenic granuloma. The diagnosis can be made histologically.

REFERENCES

Friedman-Kien, A. E., W. P. Rowe, W. G. Banfield: Milkers'

Nodule: Isolation of a Virus from a Human Case, Science, New York, 140:1335, 1963.

Friedman-Kien, A. E., and J. Vilcek: Induction of Interference and Interferon Synthesis by Non-replicating Molluscum Contagiosum Virus, J. Immunol., 99:1092, 1967.

Huebner, R. J., R. M. Cole, E. A. Beeman, J. A. Bell, and J. H. Peers: Herpangina: Etiological Studies of a Specific Infectious Disease, J.A.M.A., 145:628, 1951.

Kibrick, S.: Current Status of Coxsackie and ECHO Viruses in Human Disease, Progr. Med. Virol., 6:27, 1964.

Nagington, J., and C. H. Whittle: Human Orf: Isolation of the Virus by Tissue Culture, Brit. Med. J., 2:1324, 1961.

Patterson, W. C., L. O. Mott, and E. W. Jenney: A Study of Vesicular Stomatitis in Man, J. Am. Vet. Med. Ass., 133:57, 1958.

Section 18

Viral Diseases of the Eye

228   VIRAL INFECTIONS OF THE EYE

J. T. Grayston

The eye and its adnexal tissues may be secondarily infected during the course of many cutaneous and systemic viral diseases. Sometimes, these infections lead only to minor disturbances, examples of which are transient loss of pupillary accommodation in dengue, and inflammatory lesions of the eyelid and conjunctiva in chickenpox and pharyngoconjunctival fever. However, serious and permanent visual disorders can result if the cornea is infected with viruses such as herpes simplex, herpes zoster, vaccinia, or smallpox. In addition, congenital rubella is an important cause of cataracts and microphthalmos, and cytomegalic inclusion disease may involve the retina and the other ocular tissues.

The diseases described in this chapter are caused by microorganisms that characteristically produce localized eye lesions without infecting other tissues. Although they are mainly of concern to ophthalmologists, they sometimes enter into the differential diagnosis of systemic disorders that involve the eye. Knowledge of the epidemiology of the diseases will aid in their recognition.

TRACHOMA AND INCLUSION CONJUNCTIVITIS (Inclusion Blennorrhea)

DEFINITION. Trachoma remains the world's most important cause of blindness and loss of sight. It has been estimated that there are 500 million cases of trachoma throughout the world. Inclusion conjunctivitis is a self-limited disease that is often not diagnosed. It occurs both in the developed western countries and in underdeveloped tropical areas.

ETIOLOGY. Although the agents that cause these diseases are obligate, intracellular microorganisms, they are not true viruses because they have cell walls with chemical and metabolic properties similar to bacteria and are affected by broad-spectrum antibiotics. They are closely related to the agents of psittacosis and lymphogranuloma venereum. The organisms causing *TR*achoma and *Inclu*sion *C*onjunctivitis (now called *TRIC* agents) are virtually indistinguishable in the laboratory. They grow only in the epithelium of the eye and the genital tract. By formation of inclusion bodies they can be identified in Giemsa-stained smears of conjunctival cells obtained from scrapings. The organisms may be isolated and grown in the yolk sacs of embryonated chicken eggs. Only primates are susceptible to eye infections with these organisms. They do not grow in mice or other laboratory animals. High-titer yolk sac material produces death in mice following intravenous injection, and can be prevented by prior immunization. This forms the basis of a mouse toxicity prevention test that permits classification of the organisms into several serologic groups.

EPIDEMIOLOGY. Trachoma is now a rare eye disease in the United States. The only important endemic focus remains in the Indians of the Southwest. Acute relapse of old trachoma may be seen occasionally following treatment with cortisone eye ointment. The disease has been most prevalent and severe in North Africa, Egypt, the Middle East, and northern India. It is prevalent in China and southeast Asia in a milder form which is characterized by prolonged low-grade activity and a relatively high incidence of late sequelae. Transmission of the disease in endemic areas is probably through close personal contact. Although hot, dry, dusty, climate and abundant flies have been implicated in the epidemiology of the disease, their role may be primarily to promote seasonal bacterial conjunctivitis and to contribute to destruction of the eye once the normal physiologic function of the lid is upset by trachoma scar formation.

CLINICAL MANIFESTATIONS. Initially, trachoma is a follicular conjunctivitis that is not different from many other follicular conjunctivitises. Epithelial keratitis is present during active disease. As the disease progresses there is pannus formation, infiltration of leukocytes, and ingrowth of new blood vessels into the cornea. These findings along with the more mature neurotic follicles permit the clinical diagnosis of trachoma. Healing of the follicles leaves characteristic scars in the conjunctiva and if severe, leads to distortion of the lid and to contractures. The lid margins may be inverted (entropion) and some eyelashes turned inward (trichiasis). Abnormal dryness (xerosis) may result from loss of secretory cells. Ingrowth of vessels may continue until the cornea is completely covered (*pannus totalis*). Loss of sight or complete blindness may be due to trauma and bacterial infections resulting from the distorted lid and dry conjunctivas or from the pannus.

DIAGNOSIS. The diagnosis is usually established on clinical grounds alone. While not difficult, demonstration of typical inclusion bodies in smears requires some experience to avoid confusion with many artifacts. In chronic inactive disease, inclusions are rare. While isolation of the organism is feasible in the acute stage, it is often unsuccessful in chronic disease. There is no useful serologic test in diagnosis. There is a tendency to overdiagnose trachoma both in endemic countries and in Westerners. Follicular conjunctivitis in Americans exposed in endemic countries is very rarely trachoma.

TREATMENT. Broad-spectrum antibiotics and sulfonamides are effective both in vitro and in vivo. Prolonged therapy usually is required to effect a cure of chronic trachoma. Reinfection, and perhaps relapse, is common in endemic areas. Tetracycline eye ointments have been used most extensively. Administration two to four times a day for 6 weeks often will result in a cure. Intermittent therapy with topical applications two times a day for 1 week each month for 6 months has been proposed as a more effective regimen. Erythromycin has also been used successfully in eye ointments. Sulfonamides have been used both orally and topically. Except for their toxicity, long-acting sulfonamides would be ideal for treatment in endemic countries. Combined oral sulfonamides and tetracycline eye ointment have been effective in curing the acute disease following experimental or laboratory infections. Because of reinfection, inadequate length of treatment, or suboptimal dosage, most treatment campaigns in countries with endemic trachoma have failed to reduce the disease significantly. Surgical repair of entropion with or without trichiasis is a useful method of decreasing the risk of visual loss.

PREVENTION. Since the organism was first isolated in 1957, there have been efforts to develop an effective vaccine. Experimental vaccines have produced short-term prevention of infection, but vaccines effective for general use are not available. General hygienic measures associated with improved living standards are effective in the elimination of trachoma.

INCLUSION CONJUNCTIVITIS

While trachoma seems to be spread from eye to eye, genital transmission of inclusion conjunctivitis has been recognized. Inclusion blennorrhea of the newborn may be differentiated from neonatal gonococcal ophthalmia by its longer incubation period (5 to 14 days versus 1 to 3 days). It invariably has an acute onset with profuse mucopurulent exudate. There may be pseudomembrane formation. In older children and adults there is prominent follicular formation in the conjunctivas. These follicles do not develop the neurotic changes seen in trachoma. The illness lasts weeks in infants or a few months in adults and does not involve pannus formation or residual conjunctival scars. Topical tetracycline therapy for 2 weeks promptly controls the disease.

A clinical form of inclusion conjunctivitis intermediate between trachoma, with punctate keratitis and micropannus, has been described in adults.

Inclusion conjunctivitis often is associated with venereal infection. Clinical conjunctivitis seems to be relatively rare, while transmission of the organism by the venereal route is not uncommon. Genital-tract disease also may be caused by TRIC agents, but they can also be isolated from normal genital tracts. The importance of TRIC agents in the etiology of nongonococcal urethritis and of cervicitis is unknown.

EPIDEMIC KERATOCONJUNCTIVITIS (EKC)

EKC is an infectious conjunctivitis with characteristic subepithelial punctate keratitis that is endemic in the Near and Far East with yearly seasonal outbreaks. The disease was unknown in the continental United States until its introduction from Hawaii during the Second World War, at which time there were large outbreaks among shipyard workers. The disease has been recognized sporadically in sailors returning from the Orient. The etiologic agent of the epidemic disease is adenovirus type 8, which may produce more serious ocular disease than the adenoviruses that cause pharyngoconjunctival fever (Chap. 206). Several other adenovirus types cause EKC but have not been associated with epidemics. In the United States, EKC occurs mainly in localized outbreaks around ophthalmologists' offices and eye clinics. This is because solutions used for sterilization of instruments do not kill the hardy adenovirus. The incubation period varies from 5 to 10 days. The disease begins unilaterally with mild or severe follicular conjunctivitis which is often associated with pseudomembrane formation and sometimes with iritis and subconjunctival hemorrhages. Transient fever, headache, and malaise are the only systemic manifestations. The preauricular lymph node on the affected side is usually enlarged. Within a few days, the cornea becomes inflamed, with resultant pain, lacrimation, photophobia, and blurred vision. The contralateral eye is involved several days after the original in about 50 percent of cases. Subepithelial punctate corneal opacities in the central area without ulceration appear 1 to 3 weeks after onset and, rarely, may persist for years. They result in surprisingly little impairment of visual acuity. Milder infections have been recognized among family contacts of affected individuals, but the incidence of secondary cases is generally low. There is no specific therapy. The disease is self-limited. Epidemics can be controlled by adequate sterilization of ocular instruments, by boiling them for 10 minutes, and strict sanitation of common use facilities in factories.

NEWCASTLE DISEASE

Human infection with this avian virus, which is related to influenza, occurs mainly in poultry workers and virologists. In man, accidental introduction of contaminated material into the eye is followed in 24 to 72 hr by conjunctivitis, edema of the lids, and profuse lacrimation. The cornea is not involved, and photophobia is unusual.

Constitutional symptoms are absent or mild. Recovery is complete in 10 to 14 days. The diagnosis may be confirmed by virus isolation in embryonated eggs.

REFERENCES

Grayston, J. T., Y. F. Yang, P. B. Johnston, and L. S. Ko: Epidemic Keratoconjunctivitis on Taiwan, Am. J. Trop. Med. Hyg., 13:492, 1964.

Hanna, L. (Chairman, program committee): "Conference on Trachoma and Allied Diseases." Am. J. Ophthalmol., 63: 1027, 1967.

Jawetz, E.: The Story of Shipyard Eye, Brit. Med. J., 1:873, 1959.

——, and P. Thygeson: Trachoma and Inclusion Conjunctivitis Agents, p. 1042 in "Viral and Rickettsial Infections of Man," Horsfall and Tamm, 4th ed., Philadelphia, J. B. Lippincott Company, 1965.

Nelson, C. B., B. S. Pomeroy, K. Schroll, W. E. Park, and R. J. Lindeman: Outbreak of Conjunctivitis Due to Newcastle Disease Virus (NDV) Occurring in Poultry Workers, Am. J. Public Health, 42:672, 1952.

Section 19

Viral Diseases Affecting Lymphoid Tissue

229 LYMPHOGRANULOMA VENEREUM

Albert Heyman

DEFINITION. Lymphogranuloma venereum is an infectious disease usually transmitted by sexual contact and characterized by a small primary lesion, regional lymphadenitis, and constitutional symptoms. The disease is known by a variety of names, such as *lymphogranuloma inguinale, lymphopathia venereum,* and *climatic bubo,* but the name generally preferred is *lymphogranuloma venereum.* This disease should not be confused with granuloma inguinale, an ulcerative infection of the skin caused by the Donovan body (Chap. 164).

ETIOLOGY. The etiologic agent of lymphogranuloma venereum is closely related to that of psittacosis (Chap. 209). When stained by special methods, the organisms can be seen with the ordinary microscope as small spherical granules or elementary bodies. The agent is also distinctive in that it is susceptible to sulfonamide therapy. It produces meningoencephalitis in mice and monkeys and can be cultured in the yolk sac of the chick embryo. Infected yolk sac tissues are used as diagnostic antigens for intradermal (Frei) tests and complement fixation reactions. There are serologic cross reactions, however, with psittacosis and certain other agents (meningopneumonitis, feline pneumonitis).

INCIDENCE. Lymphogranuloma venereum exists in almost every part of the world but is especially prevalent in tropical and subtropical countries. It is frequently seen in the southeastern portion of the United States, particularly among Negroes. There is no accurate information regarding the incidence of the disease. Only 625 new cases were reported in the United States in 1966, but it is likely that the incidence is much higher. An increased incidence has been noted recently in American soldiers returning from Southeast Asia.

PATHOGENESIS. Lymphogranuloma venereum is nearly always transmitted by sexual contact. The incubation period varies from 2 to 30 days. A small evanescent lesion may appear at the site of inoculation, but more often the first sign of the infection is inflammation and suppuration of the inguinal lymph nodes. The virus is apparently disseminated throughout the body by way of the bloodstream; it has been isolated from the primary lesion, the regional lymph nodes, the blood, and the spinal fluid. Severe systemic manifestations, such as meningoencephalitis, keratitis, cutaneous lesions, and arthritis may occur. Specific evidence of immunity to the virus, including skin sensitivity of the tuberculin type, and complement-fixing humoral antibodies, can be demonstrated in almost every patient shortly after the onset of the disease. Positive skin and complement fixation reactions persist for several years. Patients with lymphogranuloma venereum frequently have an increase in serum globulin concentrations.

Following the initial infection, the patient may remain asymptomatic for a long period of time but may eventually develop late manifestations of the disease, such as rectal strictures or elephantiasis of the genitalia.

The early histologic lesion of lymphogranuloma venereum consists of a granuloma forming about a small blood vessel and composed of large mononuclear cells. The vessel is eventually compressed and obliterated, and necrosis occurs in the center of the granuloma. The "stellate" abscesses which are formed in this manner are characteristic of the fully developed acute lesions of this disease.

CLINICAL MANIFESTATIONS. The initial lesion of lymphogranuloma venereum is seldom noted because it is transitory and inconspicuous. Those which are observed consist of single, small, shallow ulcerations on the external genitalia. Shortly after the appearance of the initial lesion there are enlargement and suppuration of the regional lymph nodes. The usual site is the inguinal or femoral region, and this lymphadenitis is called the *bubo*. The typical lymphogranuloma bubo develops slowly, is bilateral, and forms an ill-defined, lobulated mass. Suppuration usually follows, producing multilocular areas of fluctuation which may rupture spontaneously, forming one or more draining fistulas.

The majority of patients with buboes show constitutional reactions: headache, malaise, fever, and anorexia. Occasionally the virus causes inflammation of distant areas, and "aseptic meningitis," pericarditis, and conjunctivitis have been observed. Generalized skin eruptions and arthritis have also been described; these apparently have been provoked occasionally by the performance of skin tests for the disease.

Many years after the onset of the infection, the patient may develop a proctitis associated with rectal bleeding and a purulent discharge. Eventually there is scar formation, and a complete fibrous ring may develop, producing a *rectal stricture*, which may necessitate colostomy. Rectal lesions are found predominantly in women and are the result of the lymphatic drainage from the posterior part of the vulva and the vagina into the perirectal and retroperitoneal lymph nodes. In the male the lymph vessels drain from the penis to the inguinal area and thence to the deep iliac nodes.

Another late complication of lymphogranuloma venereum is elephantiasis of the external genitalia. This is known as *esthiomene* and is caused by interference with lymphatic drainage. Ulceration is frequent, and secondary infection may cause marked destruction of the genitalia.

DIAGNOSIS. Isolation of the virus is the most accurate means of diagnosis, but it is too laborious for general use. The diagnosis is usually based upon the clinical findings, together with a positive intradermal test and complement fixation reaction. Commercial antigens are available for these. A positive skin (Frei) test is of limited value, as it merely indicates that the patient has been infected with the virus at some previous time. In a recently acquired infection, the complement fixation test will usually be positive in a high titer (1:80 to 1:640). Furthermore, a change in the titer of circulating antibodies may be found in successive tests. Biopsy of the primary lesion or of a lymph node should be done whenever feasible because the histologic picture is sufficiently characteristic to permit a diagnosis and to differentiate this disease from other venereal infections.

TREATMENT. Sulfonamide therapy has been the standard treatment of the early manifestations of lymphogranuloma venereum. Sulfadiazine, in doses of 4 Gm a day for 2 to 3 weeks, usually results in disappearance of symptoms and lesions. The tetracyclines (500 mg every 6 hr) have also been found to be of value in the treatment of buboes, draining sinuses, and early proctitis, and seem to be as effective as the sulfonamides. There is evidence to suggest that sulfonamide therapy may not destroy the virus completely and that it may persist in the body after the acute infection has subsided. The late manifestations of the disease, such as rectal stricture and elephantiasis, do not usually respond to any form of medication, and treatment is chiefly surgical. Buboes which have become fluctuant should be aspirated to prevent spontaneous rupture and subsequent sinus formation.

REFERENCES

Abrams, A. J.: Lymphogranuloma Venereum, J.A.M.A., 205: 199, 1968.

Favre, M., and S. Hellerstrom: The Epidemiology, Aetiology and Prophylaxis of Lymphogranuloma Inguinale, Acta Dermato-Venereol., 34-Suppl., 30:1, 1954.

Heyman, A.: The Clinical and Laboratory Differentiation between Chancroid and Lymphogranuloma Venereum, Am. J. Syph., Gonor., Vener. Dis., 30:279, 1946.

Koteen, H.: Lymphogranuloma Venereum, Medicine, 24:1, 1945.

Sigel, M. M.: "Lymphogranuloma Venereum," Coral Gables, Fla., University of Miami Press, 1962.

230 CAT-SCRATCH DISEASE
Ivan L. Bennett, Jr. and Robert G. Petersdorf

DEFINITION. Cat-scratch disease is an infection characterized by indolent, occasionally suppurative, regional lymphadenitis, secondary to a primary cutaneous lesion at the site of inoculation, usually a minor trauma. Because more than 90 percent of the reported cases have originated from cat scratches and a history of close contact with cats is often elicited, the name *cat-scratch disease* has become popular. However, a similar disorder has been acquired from splinters, thorns, beef-bone fragments, etc., and in a fair percentage of patients no inciting trauma is recalled. Other names such as *nonbacterial regional lymphadenitis* or *benign inoculation reticulosis* have been suggested but have not been widely used.

ETIOLOGY. A specific etiologic agent has not been identified. Bacterial cultures of involved nodes are uniformly negative. The disease has been transmitted by inoculation of pus from suppurating nodes into monkeys and man, but these studies have not been confirmed, and numerous attempts to isolate a virus have failed. Intranuclear and intracytoplasmic inclusions are occasionally seen in histologic preparations of infected nodes but are absent in most specimens. Complement-fixing antibodies for lymphogranuloma venereum antigen are demonstrated in serums of about 25 percent of patients with this disease, suggesting that a virus related to the lymphogranuloma-psittacosis group may be the causative agent. Photochromogenic acid-fast bacilli have been reported to cause suppurative lymphadenitis in children, and it may be that anonymous mycobacteria are responsible for some cases of cat-scratch disease (Chap. 176).

EPIDEMIOLOGY. Careful observation of cats thought to be responsible for the disease has revealed no evidence of illness; these animals do not react to intradermal injection of antigen. These facts, together with evidence that other forms of trauma transmit the disease, indicate that the infecting agent is simply transmitted passively by the cat's claws or, perhaps, its excreta. Cats may act as long-term carriers, a hypothesis supported by the familial occurrence of several infections interspersed by months or years.

PATHOLOGY. The histopathologic appearance of lymph nodes has three characteristics: (1) Early lesions show reticulum cells hyperplasia; (2) intermediate lesions show granuloma formation; and (3) late lesions show microabscesses. These reactions are not readily distinguished from those induced by the tubercle bacillus. However, acid-fast bacilli are invariably absent.

MANIFESTATIONS. The incubation period is from a few days to several weeks. Systemic symptoms are usually mild, consisting of headache, fever, and malaise, which subside within a few days. Shaking chills and fever as high as 104°F can occur but are unusual. A transient macular or vesicular rash which subsides within 48 hr is rarely present during the early stages. Erythema nodosum and multiforme have been reported.

In a typical case the *primary* lesion consists of a raised, slightly tender papule crowned by a small vesicle or eschar; it often resembles an indolent furuncle or insect bite. Multiple primary lesions have been described. Some patients do not exhibit a lesion.

Regional adenopathy becomes evident in a few days or as long as 6 weeks after infection. The axillary and epitrochlear, femoral, or (most commonly) the cervical nodes on one side become visibly swollen and tender, often with redness of the overlying skin. The nodes occasionally suppurate, soften, and drain spontaneously; fistulas heal completely with only slight scaring. Usually the tenderness subsides gradually, and nontender, firm, enlarged nodes remain palpable for some weeks or even months. There is no generalized glandular enlargement, and the spleen is not palpable.

It seems probable that clinical forms of this infectious disease other than that described above may be delineated. A few cases of *encephalitis* associated with localized adenopathy and a positive skin test have been reported. European authors have suggested that *nonspecific*

mesenteric lymphadenitis in children is an abdominal form of cat-scratch disease, and in at least one reported case a previously negative skin test became positive after an illness diagnosed at laparotomy as mesenteric adenitis. A number of cases of so-called "Parinaud's oculoglandular syndrome," characterized by conjunctivitis and regional lymphadenopathy and previously thought to be due to infection by *Leptothrix,* have been reported to show positive skin tests for cat-scratch disease. Evidence for a primary *pulmonary* form is scant but suggestive, and at least two cases of possible bone involvement in the form of osteolytic foci have been described. Thrombocytopenic purpura has also been reported as a complication of this disease.

DIAGNOSIS. The following criteria should be fulfilled before a diagnosis of cat-scratch disease is established: (1) regional lymphadenopathy, (2) history of contact with cats, (3) positive intradermal skin test, (4) biopsy of lymph node with demonstration of histopathologic changes consistent with cat-scratch disease (this may not be necessary if the skin test is positive), and (5) failure to demonstrate other possible causative agents.

Specific diagnosis is made by means of a skin test. Antigen for this is prepared from pus aspirated from infected lymph nodes; it is inactivated by heating at 60°C for 2 hr and for 1 hr on the succeeding day. A positive reaction is of the delayed, tuberculin type, appearing in 24 to 48 hr. Patients in this country have reacted to antigens prepared from European countries, and vice versa—evidence that the disease is widespread and that strain differences in skin-test antigens are not significant. Skin reactivity to the antigen persists for at least 4 years and is probably permanent.

The skin test has several limitations: (1) Each batch of antigen must be tested against patients known to have had the disease; (2) different batches of antigen differ in potency; (3) the antigen may deteriorate with time; (4) approximately 10 percent of normal individuals have false positive reactions; (5) there is a remote chance of carrying hepatitis virus in the antigen. An alternative diagnostic test which has some promise requires incubation of the patient's blood with standard skin-test antigen. A decrease in leukocytes (cytolysis) is evidence for a positive test.

Other laboratory abnormalities include mild leukocytosis (up to 15,000), mild eosinophilia, and elevated sedimentation rate. The Frei test is negative.

Cat-scratch disease is a benign illness, and the prognosis is uniformly good. Its main clinical importance lies in its possible confusion with other more serious diseases of the lymphatics. Diseases to be considered are tularemia, lymphatic tuberculosis, sporotrichosis, lymphogranuloma venereum, and bacterial adenitis. Because of the indolent character of the adenopathy, Hodgkin's disease or other lymphomas may be suspected. Appropriate serologic and cultural tests serve to rule out other infections; biopsy may be needed to exclude tumor, but a positive skin test with cat-scratch antigen effectively rules out the necessity for such procedures.

TREATMENT. In instances of node suppuration, aspiration of accumulated pus affords relief of pain (and incidentally, serves as a source of material for the preparation of skin-test antigen). Penicillin and streptomycin are ineffective. Tetracycline drugs sometimes shorten the course of the disease, but their effect is usually not dramatic.

REFERENCES

Boyd, G. L., and G. Craig: Etiology of Cat-scratch Fever, Pediatrics, 59:313, 1961.

Brooksaler, F. S., and S. E. Sulkin: Cat-scratch Disease, Postgrad Med., 36:366, 1964.

Daniels, W. B., and F. G. MacMurray: Cat-scratch Disease, Report of 160 Cases, J.A.M.A., 154:1247, 1954.

Margileth, A. M.: Cat-scratch Disease as a Cause of Oculoglandular Syndrome of Parinaud, Pediatrics, 20:1000, 1957.

Rice, J. E., and R. M. Hyde: Rapid Diagnostic Method For Cat-scratch Disease, J. Lab. Clin. Med., 71:166, 1968.

Stevens, H.: Cat-scratch Fever Encephalitis, A.M.A. J. Dis. Child., 84:218, 1952.

Section 20
Other Systemic Viral Diseases

231 MUMPS
Robert G. Petersdorf

DEFINITION. Mumps is an acute communicable disease of viral origin characterized by painful enlargement of the salivary glands, and, sometimes, particularly in adults, involvement of the gonads, meninges, and pancreas.

ETIOLOGY. The causative agent of mumps is a virus of intermediate size which has been classified among the myxoviruses; serologic cross reactions have been demonstrated between it and some other members of this group. The virus of mumps causes agglutination of erythrocytes of certain species, produces hemolysis, and has two components capable of fixing complement, the soluble, or S, and the viral, or V, antigens. It elicits a delayed allergic reaction when used as an antigen in persons who have had mumps. The virus can be cultivated in the chick embryo and propagated in tissue cultures of HeLa cells and monkey kidney cells. In general, tissue cultures are a more sensitive means of isolating mumps virus than are chick embryos.

EPIDEMIOLOGY. Man is the only natural host for mumps. The disease is worldwide and is endemic in urban communities. Epidemics are relatively infrequent and are confined to closely associated groups who live in orphanages, army camps, or schools. The disease is most frequent in spring, and occurrence is highest in April and May. Although mumps is generally considered less "contagious" than the common exanthems, measles and chickenpox, this difference may be more apparent than real because most mumps infections tend to be inapparent clinically, at least in children, and 80 percent of an adult population had serologic evidence of previous infection with mumps.

Infections are rare before the age of two and then increase rapidly in frequency, reaching a peak at age six to ten. Clinical mumps may be more common in males than in females. Adults are usually infected through direct contact. In North American cities, most infections are contracted from schoolmates and infected family members. The virus is transmitted in infected salivary secretions, although its isolation from urine suggests that the virus may spread via this route. Mumps virus is rarely cultured from stools. The saliva is infectious for approximately 6 days prior to the onset of parotitis, and virus has been cultured for as long as 2 weeks after onset of swelling. Viruria also persists for several weeks in some patients. Despite this prolonged secretion, epidemiologic evidence suggests that the peak of infectivity occurs a day or two before onset of parotitis and subsides rapidly after appearance of glandular enlargement.

One attack of clinical or subclinical mumps confers lasting immunity, and second attacks are most unusual. Unilateral parotitis affords protection just as effectively as does bilateral disease.

PATHOGENESIS. The virus enters via the oral route; during the incubation period of 18 to 21 days, it presumably multiplies in the salivary glands, from which it is disseminated via the bloodstream to other organs, including the meninges, gonads, pancreas, breasts, thyroid, heart, liver, kidneys, and cranial nerves. An alternative, but less likely, hypothesis is that salivary adenitis is secondary to viremia and that the primary locus of multiplication is elsewhere in the respiratory tract.

MANIFESTATIONS. Salivary adenitis. The onset of parotitis is usually sudden, although it may be preceded by a prodromal period of malaise, anorexia, chilly sensations, feverishness, sore throat, and tenderness at the angle of the jaw. In many cases, however, parotid swelling is the first indication of illness. The swollen gland extends from the ear to the lower portion of the mandibular ramus and to the inferior portion of the zygomatic arch. The skin over the gland may be red, hot, and taut, and there may be reddening and pouting of the orifice of Stensen's duct. There are often considerable pain and tenderness, although at times these are absent. The edema of mumps has been described as "gelatinous," and when the involved gland is tweaked, it rolls like jelly. Swelling may involve the submaxillary and sublingual glands, and may extend over the anterior chest, as "presternal edema." Swelling of the glottis occurs rarely but may require tracheostomy. Parotitis is bilateral in two-thirds of cases and remains confined to one side in the remainder. The second gland tends to swell as the first is subsiding, usually 4 to 5 days after onset. In general, parotitis is accompanied by fever of 100 to 103°F, malaise, headache, and anorexia, but systemic symptoms may be virtually absent, particularly in children. In most patients the chief complaints refer to difficulty in eating, swallowing, and talking.

Orchitis. Mumps is complicated by orchitis in 20 percent of postpubertal males. Testicular involvement usually appears 7 to 10 days after onset of parotitis, although it may precede it or appear simultaneously. Occasionally, orchitis occurs in the absence of parotitis. Gonadal involvement is unilateral in approximately 75 percent of patients. Orchitis is heralded by recrudescence of malaise and appearance of chilly sensations, headache, nausea, and vomiting. Shaking chills and high fevers with temperatures between 103 and 106°F are frequent. The testicle becomes greatly swollen and exquisitely painful. The epididymis is often palpable as a swollen tender cord. Occasionally there may be epidydimitis without orchitis. Swelling, pain, and tenderness persist for 3 to 7 days and gradually subside; lysis of fever usually parallels abatement of swelling. Occasionally, the temperature falls by crisis. Mumps orchitis is followed by progressive atrophy of the testicle in one-half the cases. Even after bilateral orchitis, sterility is unusual, provided no significant atrophy has taken place. However, if bilateral testicular atrophy occurs after mumps, sterility or subnormal sperm counts are quite common. Pulmonary infarction has been noted to follow mumps orchitis. This may be the result of thrombosis of the veins in the prostatic and pelvic plexuses in association with the testicular inflammation. Priapism is a rare but painful complication of mumps orchitis.

Pancreatitis. Pancreatic involvement is a potentially serious manifestation of mumps, which may rarely be complicated by shock or pseudocyst formation. It should be suspected in patients with abdominal pain and tenderness, and clinical or epidemiologic evidence of mumps. It is difficult to document, since hyperamylasemia, the hallmark of pancreatitis, is also often present in parotitis. Many times the symptoms resemble those of gastroenteritis, and it is conceivable that the high incidence of gastrointestinal symptoms seen in association with the mumps epidemic in Great Britain in 1961 was due to involvement of the pancreas. Although diabetes or pancreatic insufficiency rarely follows mumps pancreatitis, several children have developed "brittle," diabetes, i.e., difficult to manage, within a few weeks after mumps.

Central Nervous System Involvement. Nearly half the patients with mumps have an increased number of cells, usually lymphocytes, in the cerebrospinal fluid, although symptoms of meningitis, stiff neck, headache, and drowsi-

ness are less common. Mumps should be recognized as capable of presenting a picture of mild paralytic poliomyelitis; definition of the cause depends on isolation of virus from the cerebrospinal fluid or serologic confirmation of mumps in the absence of changing antibody titers to poliomyelitis viruses. Rarely mumps may cause a fulminating encephalitis, transverse myelitis, or the Guillain-Barré syndrome. Although meningitis may occur in association with parotitis, it is often the sole manifestation of mumps virus infection, and some 10 to 15 percent of cases of aseptic meningitis in the United States are caused by mumps virus. Mumps meningitis is benign, and the only significant residuum, nerve deafness, is rare, and tends to be unilateral.

OTHER MANIFESTATIONS. Mumps virus tends to involve glandular tissues; inflammation of the lacrimal glands, thymus, thyroid, breasts, and ovaries occurs occasionally. *Oöphoritis* may be recognized by persistence of pain in the lower part of the abdomen and fever. It does not result in sterility. Mumps virus has been implicated in the causation of subacute *thyroiditis;* 10 of 11 patients who acquired this illness at a time when the incidence of mumps was high gave serologic evidence of infection with mumps virus, and mumps virus was isolated from the thyroid gland in two cases. A case of myxedema following mumps thyroditis has been reported. Ocular manifestations of mumps include dacryoadenitis, optic neuritis, keratitis, iritis, conjunctivitis, and episcleritis. Although these conditions interfere with vision transiently, complete resolution is the rule. Mumps *myocarditis* evidenced primarily by transient abnormalities in the electrocardiogram is relatively common, but does not produce symptomatic disease or impair cardiac function. Similarly, *hepatic* involvement may be manifested by mild abnormalities in liver function, but icterus and other clinical signs of hepatic damage are extremely rare. *Thrombocytopenic purpura* as a complication of mumps has been described, and an occasional patient has a leukemoid reaction involving predominantly lymphocytes.

A rare but interesting manifestation of mumps is *polyarthritis.* It is most common in males between the ages of twenty and thirty. Joint symptoms begin 1 to 2 weeks after subsidence of parotitis, and usually the large joints are involved. The illness lasts about 6 weeks, and complete recovery is the rule. It is not clear whether arthritis is due to viremia or whether it is a "hypersensitivity reaction."

Acute hemorrhagic glomerulonephritis in the absence of streptococcosis has been reported after mumps. The relationship of these two diseases is not clear.

LATE COMPLICATIONS. With the exception of the rare cases of encephalitis, myelitis, or polyneuritis which follow mumps, and the occasional patient who is sterile following bilateral testicular involvement or who develops nerve deafness, mumps leaves no sequelae. There is no firm evidence that stillbirths and offspring with congenital defects are more common among mothers who have mumps during pregnancy. However, the finding that infants with endocardial fibroelastosis have positive mumps skin tests (but no serologic or virologic evidence of mumps infection), raises the question of intrauterine infection, as well as the possible causal relationship of mumps virus to this lesion.

LABORATORY FINDINGS. In uncomplicated parotitis, the blood leukocyte count is normal, although there may be mild leukopenia with relative lymphocytosis. Patients with mumps orchitis, however, may have a marked leukocytosis with a shift to the left. In meningoencephalitis, the white blood cell count is usually within normal limits. The erythrocyte sedimentation rate is usually normal but may rise with testicular or pancreatic involvement. The serum amylase level is elevated both in pancreatitis and in salivary adenitis. It may also be elevated in some patients in whom the sole evidence of mumps is meningoencephalitis, and probably reflects subclinical involvement of the salivary glands. In contrast to the amylase, serum lipase level is elevated only in pancreatitis, in which hyperglycemia and glucosuria also occur. The cerebrospinal fluid contains 0 to 2,000 cells per cu mm, almost all mononuclears. The pleocytosis in mumps meningitis tends to be greater than in aseptic meningitides caused by the poliomyelitis, Coxsackie, and ECHO viruses. There is no relationship between the cell count and the severity of central nervous system involvement. Transient hematuria and mild reversible abnormalities in renal function including inability maximally to concentrate the urine, excrete PSP, and clear creatinine, occur in association with the viruria of mumps.

The definitive diagnosis of mumps depends on isolation of the virus from blood, saliva, cerebrospinal fluid, or urine. However, even with the simplification of viral isolation by means of tissue culture techniques, culture of the virus is rarely necessary. When an etiologic diagnosis is needed, as in aseptic meningitis, or atypical cases of parotitis, the complement fixation test is highly reliable, simple, and inexpensive. It becomes positive during the second week of the disease, and titers remain elevated for at least 6 weeks. Paired serums should be obtained, and a fourfold rise in titer is necessary to confirm recent infection. The hemagglutination inhibition reaction is demonstrable somewhat later and persists for several months.

The serum neutralization test is the most sensitive indicator of previous mumps infection and should replace the skin test (intradermal injection of killed mumps virus, which produces a delayed reaction of the tuberculin type). The skin test is of no value in the diagnosis of acute mumps.

DIAGNOSIS. The diagnosis of mumps during an epidemic is usually obvious. Sporadic cases, however, must be distinguished from other causes of parotid enlargement. *Bacterial parotitis* usually occurs in debilitated patients with severe underlying diseases such as uncontrolled diabetes mellitus, cerebrovascular accidents, or uremia. It may also follow surgical operations. The parotid glands are swollen and tender, and pus can be expressed from the orifices of Stensen's ducts. Marked polymorphonuclear leukocytosis is present. The disease is usually acquired in the hospital, and *Staphylococcus aureus* is the causative organism. Dehydration followed by inspissation of secretions in the salivary ducts is an important predisposing

factor. *Calculus* in a salivary duct is usually detectable by palpation or by injection of radioopaque media into Stensen's duct. *Drug reactions* may produce tender swellings of the parotid and other salivary glands. "Iodine mumps" is the commonest type. It may follow such procedures as intravenous urography; mercurialism and the antihypertensive agent, guanethidine, may also cause parotid enlargement and tenderness. Careful history usually serves to clarify the cause of these reactions. Cervical adenitis caused by streptococci, "bull-neck" diphtheria, infectious mononucleosis, cat-scratch disease, sublingual cellulitis (Ludwig's angina), and cellulitis of the external auditory canal are usually easy to distinguish from mumps by careful examination. Parotid tumors, and chronic infections like actinomycosis, tend to follow a more indolent course, with slowly progressive swelling. The common "mixed tumor" of the parotid is well circumscribed, nontender, and very firm, almost cartilaginous on palpation. Parotid swelling and fever, often accompanied by lacrimal adenitis and uveitis (Mikulicz's syndrome), may occur in tuberculosis, leukemia, Hodgkin's disease, and lupus erythematosus. The onset may be sudden, but the process is usually painless and of long duration. "Uveoparotid fever" of similar type may be the first manifestation of sarcoidosis; in this disease parotid swelling is frequently accompanied by single or multiple palsies of cranial nerves —in particular, the facial—and is referred to as Heerfordt's syndrome. Presternal edema may also be a manifestation of malignant lymphoma involving retrosternal lymph nodes. Bilateral painless parotid swelling unassociated with fever is found in patients with Laennec's cirrhosis, chronic alcoholism and malnutrition. There is a chronic inflammation of the parotid and other salivary glands which is often associated with atrophy of the lacrimal glands and occurs most commonly in women past the menopause. With cessation of lacrimal and salivary function, there may be striking dryness of the conjunctiva and cornea (keratoconjunctivitis sicca) and of the mouth (xerostomia). These patients may also have a variety of systemic manifestations, including arthritis of the rheumatoid type, splenomegaly, leukopenia, and hemolytic anemia. When dryness of the mucosal surfaces is a prominent feature, the name *Sjögren's syndrome* is often applied, although some insist that *Mikulicz's disease* (as opposed to the syndrome accompanying other diseases) is the proper term (Chap. 390). The chronicity of the process and its occurrence in elderly women make confusion with mumps unlikely. Finally, benign hypertrophy of both masseter muscles, presumably due to habitual clenching and grinding of teeth, may be confused with painless parotid swelling. The causes of aseptic meningitis are listed in Chap. 361.

Orchitis occurring in the absence of parotitis is likely to remain undiagnosed. Serologic testing may later confirm the diagnosis of mumps. Orchitis may occur in association with acute bacterial prostatitis and seminal vesiculitis. It is a rare complication of gonorrhea. Occasionally testicular inflammation accompanies pleurodynia, leptospirosis, melioidosis, relapsing fever, chickenpox, brucellosis, and lymphocytic choriomeningitis.

TREATMENT. There is no specific treatment for infections with the mumps virus. Patients with parotitis should receive mouth care, analgesics, and a bland diet. Bed rest is advisable only as long as the patient is febrile; contrary to popular belief, physical activity has no influence on the development of orchitis or other complications. Patients with epididymoorchitis may be acutely ill and in great pain. Many advocated forms of treatment, including surgical decompression of the testicle, infiltration of the spermatic chord with local anesthetics, estrogens, convalescent serum, and broad-spectrum antibiotics, have not been regularly effective. Despite failure to document their effectiveness in controlled studies, adrenal steroids have been of considerable benefit in diminishing fever, as well as testicular pain and swelling, and in restoring the sense of well-being in a number of patients. It is important to give a single large dose, corresponding to 300 mg cortisone or 60 mg prednisone, initially. During the ensuing 24 hr the same quantity should be given in divided dosage. Subsequently, administration of the hormone can be tapered over 7 to 10 days. Adrenal steroids have not exerted an adverse effect on concomitant pancreatitis or meningitis, although they have not benefited patients with meningeal involvement, and their withdrawal has usually been accompanied by a sharp recrudescence of symptoms. Adrenal steroids have not prevented the appearance of parotid involvement on the contralateral side.

Mumps arthritis is usually mild and requires no treatment. Mumps thyroiditis may subside spontaneously, but excellent relief has been obtained with adrenal hormones.

PROPHYLAXIS. A live attenuated mumps virus vaccine (Jeryl Lynn strain) prepared in chick embryo cell culture has been highly effective in producing significant rises in mumps antibody in individuals who are seronegative prior to vaccination. The vaccine also has boosted antibody levels in seropositive vaccinees, and has afforded 95 percent protection to individuals exposed to mumps. The vaccine produces an inapparent, noncommunicable infection which is not associated with fever or mumpslike symptoms. It confers excellent protection for at least 2 years, but its long-term effectiveness is not yet known. Protection has been demonstrated in both children and adults.

Live mumps vaccine should be given to children approaching adolescence, adolescents, and adults, especially men who have not had mumps. Individuals living in groups or in institutions should be vaccinated, particularly because it has been shown that isolation of mumps patients does not prevent transmission of the infection. Mumps is a mild infection in young children and vaccination of all children is not recommended. The vaccine should be given in dosage of 0.5 ml subcutaneously. A single dose suffices, and simultaneous administration of gamma-globulin does not interfere with development of mumps antibody.

Vaccination is contraindicated in babies under the age of one because of the interfering effect of maternal antibody, in individuals with a history of hypersensitivity to egg proteins, and in patients with febrile illnesses, leukemia, lymphoma, generalized malignancies or those receiving steroids, alkylating drugs, antimetabolites and irradiation.

It is not known whether the vaccine will prevent infection when administered after exposure, but no contraindication to its use in this situation exists. Specific mumps-immune globulin has been effective in aborting orchitis when given 1 to 2 days after exposure, although it may not prevent parotitis. Ordinary gamma-globulin is not effective in preventing mumps.

REFERENCES

Candel, S.: Epididymitis in Mumps, Including Orchitis: Further Clinical Studies and Comments, Ann. Intern. Med., 34:20, 1951.

Caranasos, G. J., and J. R. Felker: Mumps Arthritis, Arch. Intern. Med., 119:394, 1967.

Eylan, E., R. Zuweky, and C. Shaba: Mumps Virus and Subacute Thyroiditis: Evidence of a Causal Association, Lancet, 1062, 1957.

Hilleman, M. R., R. E. Weibel, E. B. Buynak, J. R. Stokes, and J. E. Whitman, Jr.: Live Attenuated Mumps-Virus Vaccine, New Engl. J. Med., 276:252, 1967.

Kocen, R. S., and E. Critchley: Mumps Epididymo-orchitis and Its Treatment with Cortisone, Brit. Med. J. 2:20, 1961.

Meyer, M. B.: An Epidemiologic Study of Mumps; Its Spread in Schools and Families, Am. J. Hyg., 75:259, 1962.

Petersdorf, R. G., and I. L. Bennett, Jr.: Treatment of Mumps Orchitis with Adrenal Hormones: Report of 23 Cases with a Note on the Hepatic Involvement in Mumps, A.M.A. Arch. Intern. Med., 99:222, 1957.

St. Geme, J. W., Jr., G. R. Noren, and P. R. Adams: Proposed Embryopathic Relationship Between Mumps Virus and Primary Endocardial Fibroelastosis, New Engl. J. Med., 275:339, 1966.

Weibel, R. E., J. Stokes, Jr., E. B. Buynak, J. E. Whitman, and M. R. Hilleman: Live, Attenuated Mumps Virus Vaccine, New Engl. J. Med., 276:245, 1967.

Witte, J. J., and A. W. Karchmer: Surveillance of Mumps in the United States as Background for Use of Vaccine, U.S. Public Health Reports, 83:95, 1968.

Utz, J. P., V. N. Houk, and D. W. Alling: Studies of Mumps: IV. Viruria and Abnormal Renal Function, New Engl. J. Med., 270:1283, 1964.

232 CYTOMEGALIC INCLUSION DISEASE (Salivary Gland Virus Disease)

Walter H. Sheldon

DEFINITION. Cytomegalic inclusion disease (CID) is a viral infection which may be latent or active and often reflects age-related as well as congenital or acquired changes in host resistance. This disorder at one time was regarded as an affliction of babies, but is being encountered with increasing frequency in adults, generally as a complication of severe chronic debilitating disease. Recently, a self-limited infectious mononucleosis-like syndrome attributed to CID has been described in previously healthy persons. In this form, hepatitis may dominate the clinical picture.

ETIOLOGY. Present knowledge of the infection evolved from viral isolation and serologic techniques which are more sensitive than the morphologic demonstration of the distinctive nuclear inclusions first reported in 1904. Cytomegalovirus (CMV) was isolated in tissue culture by M. G. Smith in 1956. It is included in the *Herpes virus* family, produces striking acidophilic or amphophilic intranuclear (10 to 15 mμ) and inconspicuous basophilic cytoplasmic (2 to 4 mμ) inclusions. Electron-microscopic studies reveal that the intranuclear inclusions consist of proliferating viral particles in deoxyribonucleic acid matrix, while the cytoplasmic inclusions consist of lysosomes. The inclusions occur in all types of normal and neoplastic cells including white blood cells. The agent is sensitive to temperature and other environmental changes, but sorbitol or neutral glycerin preserves specimens for storage or shipment. Several antigenically heterogenous strains have been isolated which are species-specific for man and grow in human fibroblast cultures. CMV produces neutralizing and complement-fixing antibodies. Because human strains share a common complement-fixing antigen, the complement fixation test is generally used for serologic diagnosis. Antigenically distinct, species-specific CMV occur in mice and guinea pigs. The intranuclear inclusions of CMV have been seen in tissues of many mammals.

EPIDEMIOLOGY. The infection is worldwide and more prevalent where hygiene is poor. It may be congenital or acquired, latent or clinically apparent, and occurs in localized and disseminated form. In this country autopsy data show that infection is frequent in infancy (localized 10 to 12 percent, disseminated 1 to 2 percent) and is rare though increasing in adults. Serologic data indicate that antibody, which is relatively infrequent in early childhood, is present in about 15 percent of the population at age fifteen and in about 80 percent at age thirty-five. Antibody is found in about 50 percent of women of child-bearing age, and elevated titers have been noted in pregnancy. The virus persists in the host for a long time, perhaps indefinitely, and is excreted in saliva and urine. Viral excretion in the presence of antibody often continues for months even in latent infection. Spread of the agent appears to require close and prolonged contact, which may explain the clustering of cases in families, schools, and hospitals. The importance of adult carriers is uncertain. The virus is also transmitted by transfusions. Transplacental transmission accounts for prenatal infection commonly followed by disease at birth or shortly thereafter. Newborns may also be infected by an apparently healthy contact who excretes the virus. Later in life inapparent infection appears to be common, and CID may result from either activated latent or newly acquired infection.

PATHOGENESIS AND PATHOLOGY. Localized or systemic CID is frequently associated with prolonged impaired host resistance. Latent and active infection occurs in benign and malignant disorders of the hematopoietic and lymphocytic-reticular tissues (various anemias, leukemias, lymphomas), other chronic debilitating diseases (renal failure, mucoviscidosis, malnutrition), and often after immunosuppressive measures employed for organ transplantation. It is a complication of many therapeutic measures, such as corticosteroids, antibiotics, antimetabolites, cytotoxins, and irradiation. The common denominator is a primary or acquired immunologic deficiency of immunoglobulin formation and/or cellular immunity. Serologic and some clinical data suggest that pregnancy might activate latent infection. Various forms of CID, generally with mild clinical manifestations, are being described with increasing frequency in apparently normal persons of all ages. This apparent increase in frequency may be due to improved hygiene, with less neonatal infection and an increase in the number of susceptible older persons, prolonged survival of patients with impaired host resistance, and to better diagnostic methods. The pathogenesis of the infection in infancy remains uncertain. Factors similar to those suggested in *Pneumocystis carinii* infection may be operative (Chap. 245), although prematurity and debilitation are not a frequent part of the clinical setting in which CID occurs. CID, however, may induce stillbirth or prematurity.

Enlarged cells, 25 to 40 mm in diameter, with distinctive inclusions are the morphologic hallmark of the infection. They are easily seen with hematoxylin-eosin or Papanicolaou stains and are similar in all forms and sites of infection. It has been suggested that the large inclusions begin with the formation of small, sometimes multiple, pleomorphic Feulgen-positive intranuclear inclusions. Intact infected cells are not accompanied by inflammation, which occurs only after cell death. In adults the localized form most commonly consists of interstitial mononuclear cell pneumonitis or areas of gastrointestinal ulcerations. Other less frequent sites are the nasal mucosa, salivary gland, liver, and adrenal gland. Hepatitis even in the absence of the distinctive inclusions has been attributed to CID on serologic grounds. In the disseminated form nearly every tissue and organ have been affected, including the lung, alimentary canal, adrenal, liver, spleen, lymph nodes, pancreas, kidney, thyroid, and myocardium. In infancy the localized form is largely confined to the salivary glands, hence the original designation of salivary gland virus disease. In disseminated disease the more common sites are the salivary glands, kidney, liver, lung, pancreas, gastrointestinal tract, thyroid, adrenal, and brain.

Various other, sometimes multiple infections are associated with CMV infection. Bacterial infections are most common, but *P. carinii* pneumonia is frequent, and candidiasis, aspergillosis, and nocardiosis, various forms of herpes, as well as toxoplasmosis have been seen.

CLINICAL MANIFESTATIONS. In most adults CMV infection appears to be latent and becomes clinically apparent only in persons with chronic debilitating disease in whom host responses are impaired. The clinical manifestations may be masked by the underlying disorder, are nonspecific, and vary according to the principal organ involved. The disease presents most commonly as acute pneumonia, but chronic lung disease, intestinal obstruction, malabsorption, colitis, and chronic hepatitis have been described. Rare instances of histologically proven CID manifested by either pneumonia or colitis without demonstrated underlying disease have been reported. Hepatitis and cirrhosis in infants and, on serologic grounds, chronic liver disease in normal adults have been attributed to the virus.

An *infectious mononucleosis-like syndrome* is also being ascribed to CMV infection on the basis of rising antibody titers and virus isolation. This illness was first noted after open-heart surgery where it seemed to be related primarily to transfusions with unrefrigerated blood, but has been described also in previously healthy persons. The patient is febrile and may complain of headache, back pain, or abdominal discomfort. The spleen and/or liver may be enlarged, and sometimes there is a transient maculopapular rash. Mild cervical and axillary lymph node enlargement occurs, but tonsillitis is absent. Absolute and relative lymphocytosis with atypical lymphocytes are always present. The heterophil antibody test is negative. Liver function tests are frequently abnormal. In a few instances, hepatitis with jaundice and hemolytic episodes is the presenting feature.

CMV infection is suspected as the cause of chronic cough and of an influenza-like illness in pregnancy because of the frequency with which these women subsequently deliver babies with prenatally acquired CID. If this finding is confirmed, it would be of considerable importance because surviving infants have had various grave oculocerebral abnormalities and mental retardation. Inapparent maternal infection during early gestation also has been implicated in other congenital defects. In infancy the clinical features of CID are quite constant and consist of hepatitis, hemolytic anemia, thrombocytopenia, interstitial pneumonia, and meningoencephalitis. In infants and older children with increased susceptibility to infection, a relationship between acquired hemolytic anemia and CMV infection with recurrent lymphadenitis has been described.

In adults the course of disseminated CID is generally fatal and the diagnosis is made at autopsy. The disease is often mild and self-limited when it presents as hepatitis, an infectious mononucleosis-like illness, or as a respiratory disorder. The evidence of a causal relationship of these manifestations to CMV infection is, however, not conclusive.

DIAGNOSIS. To establish the diagnosis, rising antibody titers are most useful. The virus may be isolated from tissue, blood, urine, or other body fluids, and the inclusions are sometimes demonstrated in biopsy specimens or in cell concentrates of fresh urine. While these findings are strongly suggestive of CID in the appropriate clinical setting, they do not exclude the possibility that CID may represent only coexisting latent infection. Chest roentgenograms may show interstitial pneumonitis or small nodular densities. The white blood cell count reveals no changes, with the exception of many atypical lymphocytes in the infectious mononucleosis-like syndrome. Other laboratory tests will reflect the underlying disease and the various sites of involvement but show no distinctive findings.

TREATMENT. There is no specific therapy. Beneficial effects have been attributed to the administration of interferon and particularly to the antiviral agent, floxuridine, given in combination with prednisone. The underlying disorder of which systemic CID in adults is frequently a complication should be treated vigorously.

REFERENCES

Hanshaw, J. B.: Congenital and Acquired Cytomegalovirus Infection, Pediat. Clin. N. Am., 13:181, 1966.

Klemola, E., L. Kääriäinen, R. von Essen, K. Haltia, A. Koivuniemi, and C.-H. von Bonsdorf: Further Studies on Cytomegalovirus Mononucleosis in Previously Healthy Individuals, Acta Med. Scand., 182:311, 1967.

Smith, D. R.: A Syndrome Resembling Infectious Mononucleosis after Open-heart Surgery, Brit. Med. J. 1:945, 1964.

Toghill, P. J., M. E. Bailey, R. Williams, R. Zeegen, and R. Bown: Cytomegalovirus Hepatitis in the Adult, Lancet, 1:1351, 1967.

Zuelzer, W. W., C. S. Stulberg, R. H. Page, J. Teruya, and A. J. Brough: Etiology and Pathogenesis of Acquired Hemolytic Anemia, Transfusion, 6:438, 1966.

233 YELLOW FEVER
Jay P. Sanford

DEFINITION. Yellow fever is an acute infectious disease of short duration and variable severity which is caused by a group B arbovirus, and is followed by lifelong immunity. The classical triad of symptoms, jaundice, hemorrhages, and intense albuminuria, is present only in severe infections, which are now known to comprise only a small proportion of cases.

PREVALENCE. Yellow fever remains the most dramatically serious arbovirus disease of the Tropics. For more than 200 years, after the first identifiable outbreak occurred in Yucatan in 1648, it was one of the great plagues of the world. As late as 1905, New Orleans and other southern United States ports experienced at least 5,000 cases and 1,000 deaths. Because of the existence of the sylvatic form of the disease, protective measures must be maintained against human disease, as demonstrated by recent outbreaks in Trinidad in 1954, Central America in 1948 to 1957, the Congo in 1958, and the Sudan and Ethiopia in 1959 to 1962. In 1965 an explosive epidemic erupted in Senegal.

EPIDEMIOLOGY. Human infection results from two basically different cycles of virus transmission, urban and sylvatic. The urban cycle is man-mosquito-man, *Aëdes aegypti*-transmitted yellow fever. After a 2-week extrinsic incubation period, mosquitoes can initiate infection. Sylvan yellow fever differs in various ecologic situations. In the rain forests of South and Central America, species of treetop *Haemogogus* or *Sabethes* mosquitoes maintain transmission in wild primates. Once infected, the mosquito vector remains infectious for life, and may serve as a reservoir as well as a vector. The incidence of overt disease and death in monkeys varies with the species involved. When man comes in proximity to the forest canopy mosquitoes, sporadic cases or focal outbreaks can occur. In East Africa, the mosquito-primate cycle is maintained by the forest canopy mosquito *Aëdes africanus*, which seldom feeds on man. The peridomestic mosquito *Aëdes simpsoni* feeds upon primates entering the village gardens and can then in turn transmit the virus to man. If yellow fever were reintroduced into urban areas, the urban cycle could be reinitiated with the potential for epidemic disease. Why yellow fever has never invaded Asia, despite the widespread distribution of man-biting *Aëdes aegypti* mosquitoes, has never been satisfactorily explained.

PATHOLOGY. Because of the abrupt onset and rapid course of the infection, the pathologic changes are acute. The lesions are predominantly visceral. The diagnosis of yellow fever in the experimental animal can be suspected by the presence of acidophilic degeneration in the Kupffer cells of the liver within 24 hr after inoculation. Necrobiosis and acidophilic necrosis of the parenchymal cells of the liver with the formation of *Councilman bodies* occur in a characteristically discontinuous fashion in the midzones of the liver lobules. In the kidney, the virus produces fatty changes, necrobiosis, and necrosis of the tubular epithelium. Multiple minute hemorrhages occur in the gastrointestinal tract. In the brain, the dominant lesion consists of perivascular hemorrhage, which is most frequently found in the subthalamic and periventricular region at the level of the mamillary bodies.

CLINICAL MANIFESTATIONS. The incubation period is 3 to 6 days. In accidental laboratory- or hospital-acquired infections longer incubation periods (10 to 13 days) have been reported. In *mild yellow fever* the only symptoms are the abrupt onset of fever and headache, which may last only 1 or 2 days. Additional symptoms include nausea, epistaxis, relative bradycardia (Faget's sign), and slight albuminuria. The mild illness lasts only 2 to 3 days and is like influenza. *Moderately severe* and *malignant* attacks of yellow fever are characterized by three distinct clinical periods: the period of infection, the period of remission, and the period of intoxication. Prodromal symptoms are usually absent. The onset is characteristically sudden, with headache, dizziness, and temperature elevations to 104°F without a relative bradycardia. Small children may have febrile convulsions. The headache is followed quickly by pains in the neck, back, and legs. Often there is nausea with vomiting and retching. Examination reveals a flushed face and injection of the conjunctivas. The congested eyes persist until the third day. The tongue becomes characteristic, with bright red margins and tip and a white furred center. Faget's sign appears by the second day. Epistaxis and gingival bleeding are common. On the third day of illness, the fever may fall by crisis, and the patient enters convalescence or, in the malignant form, copious hemorrhages, anuria, or delirium may occur. The stage of remission lasts from several hours to several days. In the third stage, the classic symptoms appear: the fever rises again but the pulse remains slow (Faget's sign). Jaundice becomes detectable about the third day; however, jaundice is often not a prominent symptom, even in fatal illnesses. Increased epistaxis, melena, and uterine hemorrhages are common, but gross hematuria is rare. Of the classical signs, "black vomit" is more characteristic than jaundice. It usually does not occur before the fourth day and is often associated with a fatal outcome. Albuminuria, which rarely develops before the third day, occurs in 90 percent and may be very intense (3.0 to 20.0 Gm albumin per liter). In spite of massive albuminuria, edema or ascites has not been encountered. In malignant infections, coma frequently occurs 2 or 3 days before death. Shortly before death, which usually occurs between the fourth and sixth days, the patient becomes delirious and wildly agitated. While the duration of fever in the third stage is usually 5 to 7 days, the period of intoxication is the most variable and may last up to 2 weeks. Clinical yellow fever is relatively free from complications; for some reason suppurative parotitis is the most striking. Clinical relapses do not occur.

LABORATORY FINDINGS. Early in the disease, progressive leukopenia may occur. By the fifth day, total leukocyte counts of 1,500 to 2,500 cells per cu mm are often found; the decrease is due mostly to a decrease in neutrophiles. Total leukocyte counts return to normal by the tenth day, and there may be a marked terminal leukocytosis in fatal cases. Hemoglobin values remain normal except terminally, when hemoconcentration may occur. Platelet counts are usually normal. Sophisticated coagulation studies have been performed only in rhesus monkeys experimentally infected with yellow fever. Within 72 hr after viral inoculation and prior to apparent clinical illness, a coagulation defect was observed. This was characterized by a prolonged one-stage prothrombin time and a prolonged partial thromboplastin time reflecting measured deficiencies in factors II, V, VII, VIII, IX, X, and XI. Both the euglobin lysis time and thrombin time were prolonged, suggesting a depression of plasminogen activation and accumulation of fibrinogen degradation products. At this time platelet counts and chemical measurements of fibrinogen were normal. During the subsequent 48 hr, these coagulation defects worsened as the monkeys developed clinical illness, and terminally, depression of platelet counts and fibrinogen levels occasionally were observed. The disturbances in coagulation occurred during the stage of viremia and existed before hepatic necrosis was visible in liver biopsy specimens. These data suggest that the hemorrhagic manifestations are primarily caused by a consumptive coagulopathy rather than by hepatic failure. Also, in experimental infections in primates, modest increases in total bilirubin, alkaline phosphatase, and marked increases in serum glutamic-oxalacetic transaminase occur. Electrocardiograms may show T-wave changes. Cerebrospinal fluid is normal.

DIAGNOSIS. There are three established procedures for the laboratory diagnosis of yellow fever: (1) Isolation of the virus from blood. This must be done early, preferably during the first 3 days. Caution must be exercised to avoid autoinoculation. (2) Diagnosis can also be based on the development of neutralizing antibody. (3) Diagnosis can also be reasonably based on the demonstration of the typical, although not completely specific, histopathologic lesions on liver biopsy.

TREATMENT. The management has been symptomatic and supportive. Current management should be based upon assessment and correction of the circulatory abnormalities. If evidence of disseminated intravascular coagulation is present, administration of heparin should be considered. Close attention to fluid and electrolyte balance is essential.

PROGNOSIS. The overall fatality rate in yellow fever is between 5 and 10 percent in clinical cases, and may be less because many infections are very mild or inapparent.

PREVENTION. Prophylaxis consists of vaccination and the eradication of *A. aegypti* mosquitoes. Two strains of attenuated yellow fever virus are available for the preparation of vaccines: the French neurotropic and the 17D strain. The vaccine prepared from the 17D strain consists of frozen, dried extract of infected chick embryos sealed in ampuls. For use, the virus is reconstituted by the addition of sterile physiologic saline solution. One subcutaneous injection of 0.5 ml will produce immunity in man. In rural areas, mass vaccination is the only effective protection against jungle yellow fever. The use of DDT spray on the walls of houses is effective in controlling mosquitoes, but presently no method is available for eradicating jungle yellow fever.

REFERENCES

Dennis, L. H., B. E. Reisberg, D. Crozier, and M. E. Conrad: The Original Hemorrhagic Fever: Yellow Fever, Blood, 30:858, 1967.

Kerr, J. A.: Clinical Aspects and Diagnosis of Yellow Fever, p. 389 in "Yellow Fever," G. K. Strode (Ed.), New York, McGraw-Hill Book Company, 1951.

Kirk, R.: An Epidemic of Yellow Fever in the Nuba Mountains, Anglo-Egyptian Sudan, Ann. Trop. Med. Parasitol., 35:67, 1941.

Lebrun, A. J.: Jungle Yellow Fever and Its Control in Gemena, Belgian Congo, Am. J. Trop. Med. Hyg., 12:398, 1963.

Work, T. H.: Virus Diseases in the Tropics, p. 1 in "A Manual of Tropical Medicine," 4th ed., G. W. Hunter, W. W. Frye, and J. C. Schwartzwelder (Eds.), Philadelphia, W. B. Saunders Company, 1966.

234 DENGUE FEVER
Jay P. Sanford

DEFINITION. Dengue is one of the arbovirus infections characterized by malaise, headache, generalized myalgia, lymphadenopathy, and rash. It is endemic over large areas of the tropics and subtropics. From 1963 to 1964 epidemic dengue occurred in the Caribbean, and a number of travelers returned to the United States with clinical illness. In these areas a high proportion of infections are inapparent or represent undifferentiated febrile illnesses. It is now recognized that the dengue syndrome can be caused by other arboviruses, hence the exact etiology of some of the earlier epidemics is uncertain.

ETIOLOGY. There are four distinct serogroups of dengue viruses, types 1, 2, 3, and 4, all of which are Group B arboviruses. The existence of at least two further antigenic types has been suggested. They are transmitted solely by mosquitoes of the genus *Aëdes*.

EPIDEMIOLOGY. So far as is known, dengue infections in nature involve only man and Aëdes mosquitoes. Attempts have been made to implicate lower vertebrates, especially monkeys, as reservoir sylvatic hosts, but the data are inconclusive. *Aëdes aegypti* is the most important worldwide vector species. This species, as well as the less common vector species, bite man readily or even preferentially, breed in small collections of water such as cisterns and backyard litter, and are peridomestic in nature. They fly during the day. Man appears to be uniformly susceptible, and susceptibility is not influenced by age, sex, or race. The disappearance of dengue from an area may be the result either of elimination of the vector or of exhaustion of the susceptible population. During outbreaks, attack rates may be very high: in Louisiana in 1922 the attack rate was estimated to be 1,740 per 100,000 (1.74 percent).

PATHOLOGY. The skin lesions in nonfatal uncomplicated disease produced in volunteers have been studied by biopsy. The chief abnormality occurred in small blood vessels and consisted of endothelial swelling, perivascular edema, and infiltration with mononuclear cells. Since the disease is self-limited, other studies have not been done.

CLINICAL MANIFESTATIONS. Dengue viruses frequently produce inapparent infections in man. When symptoms develop, three broad clinical patterns may be encountered: classical dengue, hemorrhagic fever (Chap. 235), and a mild atypical form. Classical dengue (break-bone fever) occurs primarily in nonimmune individuals, specifically nonindigenous adults and children. The usual incubation period is 5 to 8 days. Prodromal symptoms such as mild conjunctivitis or coryza may occur, followed in hours by the abrupt onset of a severe splitting headache, retroorbital pain, backache, especially in the lumbar area, and leg and joint pains. The headache is aggravated by movement. At least three-fourths of patients have ocular soreness with pain on moving the eyes. A few have mild photophobia. While true rigors are common during the course, they are usually not present at the onset (14 percent in one series). Additional symptoms include insomnia, anorexia with a loss of taste or bitter taste, and weakness. Mild transient rhinopharyngitis occurs in as many as one-quarter of individuals. Epistaxis has been observed. Examination reveals scleral injection (90 percent), tenderness upon pressure on the ocular globe, and nontender posterior cervical, epitrochlear, and inguinal lymphadenopathy. Over one-half of patients have an enanthem characterized initially by pinpoint-sized vesicles over the posterior half of the soft palate. The tongue is often coated. Skin rashes varying from diffuse flushing to scarlatiniform and morbilliform are frequently present over the thorax and inner aspects of the arms. These are transient and fade, only to be followed by a more apparent maculopapular rash which appears on the trunk on the third to the fifth day and spreads peripherally. The rash may be pruritic and generally terminates with desquamation. Extreme bradycardia is not observed. Within 2 to 3 days after the onset, the temperature may decrease to nearly normal and other symptoms disappear. The remission typically lasts 2 days and is followed by return of fever and the other symptoms, although they are generally less severe than during the initial phase. This "saddleback" diphasic febrile course is considered characteristic, but often is not encountered. The febrile illness usually lasts 5 to 6 days and terminates by crisis. Complaints of fatigue for several weeks after infection are common.

In addition to this "classical" syndrome, an atypically mild illness may occur. Symptoms include fever, anorexia, headache, and myalgia. On examination, evanescent rashes may be seen, but lymphadenopathy is usually absent. The course is usually less than 72 hr in duration.

At the onset both in classical and in mild dengue, the leukocyte counts may be low or normal; however, by the third to the fifth day, leukopenia, usually with counts of less than 5,000 per cu mm, and neutropenia are usually seen. Occasionally albuminuria of moderate degree occurs.

DIAGNOSIS. Virus isolation in tissue culture of serum obtained during the first days of illness is definitive. Diagnosis can be made by serologic tests employing paired sera for hemagglutination inhibition tests and complement fixation tests. Specific serologic diagnosis is complicated by cross-reactions with other group B arbovirus antibodies such as those following immunization with yellow fever vaccine.

TREATMENT. The treatment is entirely symptomatic.

PROGNOSIS. Mortality is nil.

PREVENTION. Attenuated vaccines are undergoing experimental evaluation but are not available. The hypothesis of "second infections" being responsible for the dengue hemorrhagic fever syndrome raises further questions about a program of active immunization. Control depends upon mosquito abatement.

REFERENCES

Clarke, D. H., and J. Casals: Arboviruses; Group B, p. 606 in "Viral and Rickettsial Infections of Man," 4th ed., F. L. Horsfall, Jr. and I. Tamm (Eds.), Philadelphia, J. B. Lippincott Company, 1965.

Diasio, J. S., and F. M. Richardson: Clinical Observations on Dengue Fever, Mil. Surg., 94:365, 1944.

Sabin, A. B.: Research on Dengue During World War II, Am. J. Trop. Med. Hyg., 1:30, 1952.

235 EPIDEMIC HEMORRHAGIC FEVER

Sheldon E. Greisman

DEFINITION. Epidemic hemorrhagic fever is the prototype of the viral hemorrhagic fevers, a group of illnesses characterized by an acute onset, thrombocytopenia, and widespread vascular injury with impaired vasomotor tone, enhanced capillary permeability, and a hemorrhagic diathesis. Included within this group is a variety of other distinct entities caused by viruses with no antigenic interrelationships and varying with respect to the specific clinical syndrome and pathologic findings. Certain of these entities and some important distinguishing features are outlined in Table 235-1.

HISTORY, ETIOLOGY, AND EPIDEMIOLOGY. Epidemic hemorrhagic fever was first recognized in Manchuria and Siberia by the Japanese and Russians about 3 decades ago. During the Korean War, the disease occurred among United Nations troops and was extensively investigated. It now is known to be widespread in European Russia and Scandinavia, and to extend westward as far as Hungary and Czechoslovakia.

Russian and Japanese workers have reported transmission of epidemic hemorrhagic fever to human subjects by intravenous or intramuscular injection of urine or blood taken from patients during the first 5 days of disease. Oral and intranasal routes of inoculation were ineffective. Preincubation of the acute phase with convalescent phase serum prevented transmission. The causative agent passed through filters which retained microbiologic agents larger than viruses. Neither these workers nor the Americans who investigated the Korean form were able to establish the agent in a laboratory host or in tissue culture.

Two seasonal peaks of incidence are characteristic of epidemic hemorrhagic fever, but sporadic cases occur throughout the year. Most of the 1,000 patients who were seen annually in Korea from 1951 to 1953 became ill between mid-April and early July or during October and November. The disease in Korea was limited to military personnel in rural areas north of Seoul. After the armistice, civilians of all ages contracted the disease upon returning to neglected farms in this area. In Europe, the disease affects civilians working in rural and forested areas. At least a thousand cases are reported annually in European Russia alone.

The majority of cases in Korea were isolated and widely spaced in time and place. In the small outbreaks, (1) there was no person-to-person spread of infection, (2) food and water were unimportant in epidemiology, and (3) infection followed exposure in a sharply localized area of abandoned farmland or scrub-covered terrain. It was assumed that trombiculid mites served as the vector for the agent of epidemic hemorrhagic fever and that small wild rodents provided the reservoir.

Table 235-1 indicates that epidemic hemorrhagic fever is distinct from Crimean and mid-Asian hemorrhagic fevers, which extend from the Balkans eastward across the southern U.S.S.R. These diseases do not demonstrate the renal changes typical of epidemic hemorrhagic fever, and the etiologic agents, which differ from that of epidemic hemorrhagic fever but which may be related to each other, are transmitted to man by *Hyalomma* ticks during the spring-summer season. Two other hemorrhagic fevers, also related to each other but distinct from those already mentioned, are Omsk hemorrhagic fever, which occurs in

Table 235-1. VIRAL HEMORRHAGIC FEVERS

Entity	Viral agent	Major age group infected	Vector	Renal injury	Characteristic leukocyte count	Mortality, %
Epidemic hemorrhagic fever	Not infective for animals or tissue culture	All ages	Mite (presumed)	++++	Leukocytosis	3–15
Crimean hemorrhagic fever Mid-Asian hemorrhagic fever	Not well characterized	Adults	Tick Person-to-person (minor)	±	Leukopenia	3–6 30–38
Omsk hemorrhagic fever Kyasanur Forest disease (India)	Related antigenically to Russian spring-summer encephalitis group viruses	Adults	Tick	++	Leukopenia	0.5–3 4–10
Philippine hemorrhagic fever Thailand hemorrhagic fever Malaysia hemorrhagic fever Calcutta hemorrhagic fever North and South Vietnam hemorrhagic fever Cambodian hemorrhagic fever	Dengue (usually types 1 to 4) or Chikungunya (less common)	Infants and small children	Mosquito	±	Leukopenia	1–23
Argentinian hemorrhagic fever Bolivian hemorrhagic fever	Junin Machupo (related antigenically to Junin)	Adults	Mite (presumed) Contamination of food and water by excreta of reservoir host, *Calomys callosus* (presumed) Person-to-person (minor)	++	Leukopenia	23 5–30
Yellow fever	Yellow fever virus	All ages	Mosquito	++	Leukopenia	5

western Siberia, and Kyasanur Forest disease, which is seen in central India. Both are caused by members of the Russian spring-summer group of viruses and are transmitted to man by *Dermacentor* ticks, which also serve as vectors in the natural cycle involving wild animals. Since 1950, febrile diseases with hemorrhagic manifestations have been described in the Philippines, Thailand, Malaysia, India, North and South Vietnam, and Cambodia. These are mosquito-borne infections caused by members of the dengue group of viruses. Concomitantly, viral diseases with a hemorrhagic diathesis have appeared in Argentina (initial recognized epidemic 1953) and in Bolivia (initial recognized epidemic 1959). The etiologic agents are related antigenically to each other and to the Tacaribe virus isolated from bats in Trinidad. The virus of Bolivian hemorrhagic fever has been isolated from the urine and feces of the rodent *Calomys callosus,* and although the major method of dissemination to man is uncertain, con-

tamination of food and water has been suspected. Direct person-to-person spread of infection may also occur. In contrast, mites are the presumed vector of Argentinian hemorrhagic fever. Finally, a long-recognized viral illness with a hemorrhagic diathesis, yellow fever, occurs in large areas of South America and Africa but is unrelated to any of the above illnesses.

MANIFESTATIONS. Following an incubation period of about 2 weeks (extremes of 9 to 36 days), epidemic hemorrhagic fever begins abruptly, with frontal headache, chills, high fever, anorexia, and backache. Physical findings during the first several days of fever and prostration are limited to conjunctival injection and a cutaneous flush, especially about the face and neck. About the third day, petechiae appear on the palate, conjunctivas, axillary folds, and cutaneous areas subjected to mild trauma. Increased capillary permeability becomes clinically evident about the fourth day with the rapid appearance of pathognomonic severe proteinuria and edema of the conjunctivas and periorbital tissue. Edema in the lumbar gutters and mesentery, seen at autopsy, may contribute to the back and abdominal pain.

Fever subsides about the fifth day, but the course usually progresses through additional phases: hypotensive, oliguric, diuretic, and convalescent. Manifestations of increased capillary permeability, among them a rising hematocrit, progress during the hypotensive phase but abate rapidly when the oliguric phase develops, with its associated rising blood urea nitrogen and creatinine levels. With the onset of diuresis (usually from 3 to 6 liters daily) on about the tenth day, symptoms and abnormal physiologic findings generally disappear rapidly. However, renal tubular function is restored slowly, and normal concentrating capacity usually does not return until the fourth to sixth week of convalescence. Body weight, which may decrease as much as 30 lb during acute illness, is also restored slowly. Central-nervous-system symptoms are not specific and when present, in 10 to 15 percent of confirmed cases, are usually due to hemorrhage, uremia, and/or edema. This contrasts with Argentinian and Bolivian hemorrhagic fevers, where distinctive neurologic symptoms are frequent, and 50 percent of patients with Bolivian hemorrhagic fever have intention tremors of the tongue and hands.

PATHOPHYSIOLOGY. Injury to the smaller segments of the vascular system, resulting in reduced vasomotor tone, increased permeability, and increased fragility, are the basic derangements of epidemic hemorrhagic fever. The vascular injury is characteristically more intense in certain organs than in others, and selected, rather than uniform, vascular damage accounts for the extensive retroperitoneal edema in the absence of concomitant anasarca or pulmonary edema. Several mechanisms for the vascular injury have been considered: (1) direct viral invasion of vessel walls, (2) autonomic nervous system dysfunction, (3) hypersensitivity (this mechanism is probably involved in dengue hemorrhagic fevers), (4) thrombocytopenia. Their interrelationships and relative importance are not established.

The mechanisms responsible for the thrombocytopenia during the viral hemorrhagic fevers have received particular attention. Unlike the dengue hemorrhagic fevers, depressed megakaryocytopoiesis does not contribute to the thrombocytopenia of epidemic hemorrhagic fever; indeed, megakaryocytic hyperplasia is seen. Rather, the thrombocytopenia has been linked to disseminated intravascular coagulation with associated multiple defects in the first and second stages of coagulation, hypofibrinogenemia, and accumulation of fibrinogen degradation products. This coagulopathy has been suggested as the common denominator in the hemorrhagic diathesis of the viral hemorrhagic fevers.

The decrease in cardiac output, which constitutes the basis for the hypotensive phase of epidemic hemorrhagic fever, is attributable to decreased effective circulating blood volume because of capillary leakage of plasma and dilatation of capillary and venular beds. Impaired ability to compensate by elevating peripheral resistance inten-

sifies the hypotension. In hypotensive patients with high hematocrits, tachycardia, and cold extremities, administration of concentrated human albumin is helpful. Hypotensive subjects with normal or slightly elevated hematocrits, minimal tachycardia, and warm extremities have the least increases in peripheral vascular resistance, and although treatment with vasopressor agents restores arterial blood pressure toward normal, there is no proof that these drugs reduce mortality.

During the oliguric phase, the elevated hematocrit decreases rapidly; capillary permeability is repaired, and there is resorption of the interstitial fluid lost during the hypotensive phase. Approximately 20 percent of patients develop arterial blood pressures exceeding 140/90, which results from an increased cardiac output and/or increased peripheral resistance, but the mechanisms underlying these hemodynamic alterations are uncertain. Pulmonary edema is an important cause of death at this time. Phlebotomy may be lifesaving when pulmonary edema develops in hypertensive subjects, but is of little benefit in subjects with normotension. The acute renal failure and subsequent recovery during the oliguric and diuretic phases clinically resemble those seen following exposure to a variety of other severe injurious stimuli to the kidney (Chap. 300).

LABORATORY FINDINGS AND PATHOLOGY. Clinical laboratory data in epidemic hemorrhagic fever other than those already mentioned are (1) leukopenia during the initial 2 days of illness followed by leukocytosis of 10,000 to 50,000 per cu mm, with many immature granulocytes by the end of the first week, and (2) disturbances of electrolyte balance. The characteristic lesions at autopsy are found in the kidney, right atrium, and anterior pituitary gland. Grossly, the renal cortex appears pale; the pyramids appear intensely congested. Hemorrhagic lesions can be seen in the right atrial wall. The anterior pituitary appears intensely congested. During the hypotensive phase, gelatinous edema is found in the retroperitoneal tissues and mesentery; during the late oliguric phase, these tissues are usually dry. Inflammatory lesions of small vessels and thrombosis are conspicuously lacking, but intense capillary congestion is characteristic. Indeed, most of the areas which appear grossly hemorrhagic represent sites of extreme capillary dilatation. Varying degrees of necrosis occur in the anterior pituitary.

DIFFERENTIAL DIAGNOSIS. Epidemic hemorrhagic fever may be confused with leptospirosis, the typhus fevers, hemorrhagic smallpox, meningococcemia, idiopathic thrombocytopenic purpura, leukemia, hemorrhagic dengue, or even influenza. The diagnosis must be made on epidemiologic and clinical grounds because viral isolation techniques and serologic tests available for confirmation of many of the other hemorrhagic fevers are lacking. A history of exposure in an endemic area, particularly during a seasonal epidemic, and the appearance of marked proteinuria about the fourth day of fever, associated with a rising leukocyte count and thrombocytopenia, are virtually diagnostic.

TREATMENT AND PREVENTION. The treatment of epidemic hemorrhagic fever is entirely supportive; antibiotics, cortisone, antihistamines, and convalescent serum have been tried with no success. Treatment begins with early diagnosis and prompt but gentle transfer to a hospital with adequate facilities. During the febrile phase, complete bed rest, mild sedation, fluid balance with strict avoidance of overhydration, and an adequate but light diet are important. If the evidence that disseminated intravascular coagulation constitutes a common denominator of viral hemorrhagic fevers is substantiated, anticoagulants may prove an important therapeutic adjuvant. Once diuresis is established, attention must be paid to adequate replacement of fluid and electrolytes.

Vaccines are available for dengue, yellow fever, and Omsk hemorrhagic fever and are being developed for Argentinian and Bolivian hemorrhagic fevers, but failure to isolate the virus of epidemic hemorrhagic fever precludes vaccine prophylaxis. Prevention is based on avoidance of trombiculid mites, presumed vectors of the disease. These measures are (1) use of insect repellents for impregnation of clothes (benzyl benzoate) and application to exposed skin surfaces (dimethyl phthalate), (2) clearing of all vegetation from camp sites (bulldozing) and treatment of the area with residual insecticides such as lindane, (3) rodent control in and about camps by means of rodenticides. This method resulted in dramatic reductions in Bolivian hemorrhagic fever.

PROGNOSIS. Epidemic hemorrhagic fever varies greatly in severity. It may be so mild as to make diagnosis difficult; indeed, many suspected cases are not confirmed because the patients fail to develop typical renal manifestations. About 20 percent of patients with confirmed cases become critically ill. The following factors contribute to severity and influence the prognosis unfavorably: delayed initiation of medical care, rough transportation to the medical facility, prolonged high fever, severe dehydration with ketoacidosis, early excessive fluid replacement, prolonged or recurrent hypotension, persistent hemoconcentration, anuria, and progressive severe electrolyte disturbances. The fatality rate in cases among American soldiers in Korea was between 5 and 7 percent. Of these, deaths were approximately equally distributed through the hypotensive, oliguric, and diuretic phases. Complete recovery is the rule once the convalescent phase is reached.

REFERENCES

Dennis, L. H., M. B. Garvey, N. M. Tauraso, and M. E. Conrad: Disseminated Intravascular Coagulation: A Pathogenesis for Argentinian Hemorrhagic Fever, Clin. Res., 16:330, 1968.

Entwisle, G., and E. Hale: Hemodynamic Alterations in Hemorrhagic Fever, Circulation, 15:414, 1957.

Greisman, S. E.: Capillary Observations in Patients with Hemorrhagic Fever and Other Infectious Illnesses, J. Clin. Invest., 36:1688, 1957.

Johnson, K. M., S. B. Halstead, and S. N. Cohen: Hemorrhagic Fevers of Southeast Asia and South America: A Comparative Appraisal, Progr. Med. Virol., 9:105, 1967.

Smorodintsev, A. A., L. I. Kazbintsev, and V. G. Chudakov: "Virus Hemorrhagic Fevers" (Trans. from Russian), Washington, D.C., The National Science Foundation, 1964.

Symposium on Epidemic Hemorrhagic Fever: Earle, D. P. (Ed.), Am. J. Med., 16:617, 1954.

236 COLORADO TICK FEVER
Jay P. Sanford

DEFINITION. Colorado tick fever is the only tick-transmitted virus disease of man that is recognized in the Western Hemisphere. While "mountain fever" had been described ever since the advent of immigrants to the Rocky Mountain region, Becker in 1930 differentiated it from mild Rocky Mountain spotted fever, established the clinical picture of disease, and renamed it Colorado tick fever.

ETIOLOGY. The causative agent in Colorado tick fever is an ungrouped arbovirus which has been isolated from patients with the syndrome.

PREVALENCE. The disease has been contracted only in Colorado, Idaho, Nevada, Wyoming, Montana, Utah and the eastern portions of Oregon, Washington, and California. However, the virus of Colorado tick fever has been reported to have been isolated from the dog tick, *Dermacentor variabilis,* obtained from Long Island. This observation has not been confirmed, but suggests the possibility that Colorado tick fever may occur over a wider geographic area. The actual prevalence is difficult to assess, but it is relatively common. Mild and clinically inapparent forms of the disease occur, but its frequency has never been determined. The number of cases of Colorado tick fever reported in Colorado is 20 times greater than that of Rocky Mountain spotted fever.

EPIDEMIOLOGY. Colorado tick fever is transmitted to man by the adult hard-shelled wood tick, *Dermacentor andersoni.* The virus has been found in as many as 14 percent of this species of ticks collected in endemic areas. Transovarial transmission of the virus in the tick has been established. Illness occurs primarily in the spring and summer months, with a predilection for April and May at lower altitudes and June and July at higher altitudes. Virus has been obtained from both the blood and the spinal fluid of patients during the acute illness.

CLINICAL MANIFESTATIONS. The incubation period is usually 3 to 6 days, and in most cases a history of tick bite can be obtained. Persons affected usually are those whose occupational or recreational activities bring them in contact with ticks. The disease may occur at any age. The clinical picture is characterized by the sudden onset of severe aching of the muscles of the back and legs, chilliness without true rigors, a rapid increase in temperature, which usually reaches 102 to 104°F, headache with pain on ocular movement, retroorbital pain, and photophobia. Occasionally nausea and vomiting occur. The physical findings are not specific. Tachycardia in proportion to the temperature, flushed facies, and variable conjunctival injection may be present. Occasionally the spleen is palpable. A rash is usually not present, but on occasion a petechial rash involving primarily the arms and legs or maculopapular rash over the entire body may occur. Rarely, punched-out ulcers may form at the site of tick bite. The fever with the associated symptoms lasts about 2 days, then abruptly lyses to normal or subnormal, leaving the patient very weak. After an afebrile period of about 2 days, the temperature recurs, may be higher than in the first phase, and may last as long as 3 days. Over 90 percent of patients show this saddleback pattern of temperature. Rarely there may be three febrile phases. The febrile episode may be followed by a period of weakness of several weeks' duration.

Evidence of central-nervous-system involvement has been recorded in a few patients. The findings are those of either an aseptic meningitis with stiffness of the neck or encephalitis with clouding of the sensorium, delirium and coma.

LABORATORY FINDINGS. The most important laboratory feature is moderate to marked leukopenia. On the first day of illness, the total leukocyte count may be at normal levels, but usually by the fifth or sixth day there has been a decrease to 2,000 to 3,000 per cu mm. Characteristically there is a proportionate decrease in lymphocytes and granulocytes. A moderate "left shift" in the neutrophilic series is usually apparent. Toxic changes in neutrophiles are often conspicuous and "virocyte" types of lymphocytes are frequently observed. Bone marrow examination reveals "maturation arrest" in the granulocytic series. Erythrocyte values remain normal. Thrombocytopenia has been recorded in an isolated case report. The blood picture returns to normal within a week after the fever subsides.

DIAGNOSIS. The diagnosis of Colorado tick fever is suspected on the basis of the epidemiologic history and clinical findings. The diagnosis can be established by the isolation of the virus from serum obtained during the febrile phase. Specific neutralizing or complement-fixing antibodies appear in the blood between the eighth and fourteenth days of illness. Because neutralizing antibodies persist for many years, demonstration of a rise in titer is required.

TREATMENT. Treatment is entirely symptomatic.

PROGNOSIS. The prognosis is excellent.

PREVENTION. No patients have been reported as having the disease twice. Active immunity with an attenuated virus has been produced but the immunization itself frequently produced mild disease. Prevention of Colorado tick fever is best carried out by avoiding contact with the wood tick.

REFERENCES

Becker, F. E.: Tick-borne Infections in Colorado, Colo. Med., 27:36, 1930.

Ecklund, C. M., G. M. Kohls, and J. M. Brennan: Distribution of Colorado Tick Fever and Virus-carrying Ticks, J.A.M.A., 157:335, 1955.

Florio, L., M. O. Stewart, and E. R. Mugroge: The Etiology of Colorado Tick Fever, J. Exp. Med., 83:1, 1946.

Lloyd, L. W.: Colorado Tick Fever, Med. Clinics N. Am., March, 1951.

Silver, H. K., G. Meiklejohn, and C. H. Kempe: Colorado Tick Fever, Am. J. Dis. Child., 101:30, 1961.

237 PHLEBOTOMUS FEVER
Jay P. Sanford

DEFINITION. Phlebotomus (sandfly, pappataci, or 3-day) fever is an acute, relatively mild, self-limited arbovirus infection which is characterized by malaise, headaches, and generalized myalgia.

ETIOLOGY. The disease is caused by at least two immunologically distinct ungrouped arboviruses, the Sicilian and Naples strains, but there may be additional immunologically distinct strains. The viruses have been adapted to white mice, but there is no evidence of an animal reservoir in nature.

PREVALENCE. The disease occurs throughout the Mediterranean basin, the Balkans, the Near and Middle East, the eastern part of Africa, the Soviet republics of Central Asia, West Pakistan, and possibly certain parts of southern China. In highly endemic areas, native populations acquire the disease at an early age and with repeated exposure develop and maintain high levels of immunity. The apparent absence of phlebotomus fever in indigenous adult populations residing in areas where sandflies are abundant can present a deceptive picture of the actual risk to susceptibles.

EPIDEMIOLOGY. The disease occurs during the hot, dry seasons (summer or autumn months) and is transmitted to humans by the bites of infected sandflies (*Phlebotomus papatasi*). *Phlebotomus papatasi* is a small fly which can penetrate ordinary house screens. Only the female bites and usually does so during the night. In persons who are not sensitive there is neither pain nor local irritation after the bite, hence only about 1 percent of patients will remember having been bitten. Approximately 7 days after feeding on an infected individual, the insect acquires the capacity to transmit infection. The sandflies continue to be infectious for their life span. Transovarial transmission of the virus to the next generation of insects has been demonstrated and offers the best explanation for the mechanism of over-winter survival of the virus. In man, the incubation period may be as short as 3 days. Viremia is present for at least 24 hr before and after the onset of fever, but is not detectable for more than 2 days after the onset of illness.

CLINICAL MANIFESTATIONS. The onset of symptoms is abrupt in over 90 percent of patients, with the temperature rapidly rising to its highest point, which may vary from 100 to 105°F. Headache is nearly always present, and is often accompanied by pain on moving the eyes and by retroorbital pain. Myalgia is common and may be localized to the chest, resembling pleurodynia, or to the abdomen. Other symptoms which occur (usually in less than 20 percent of patients) include vomiting, photophobia, giddiness, neck stiffness, alteration or loss of taste, and arthralgia. Physical signs include conjunctival injection in approximately one-third of patients. Small vesicles may be seen on the palate, and macular or urticarial rashes occur. The spleen is rarely palpable, and lymphadenopathy is absent. The pulse rate may be elevated in proportion to the temperature on the first day; thereafter bradycardia is often present. The fever persists 3 days in most patients, with defervescence in a staggered descent. Giddiness, weakness, and feelings of depression are frequently encountered during convalescence. Second attacks 2 to 12 weeks after the first occur in 15 percent of cases.

In common with other arbovirus infections, phlebotomus fever may be associated with aspetic meningitis. In one series, 12 percent of patients had symptoms and signs sufficient to warrant a lumbar puncture. Findings in these patients included pleocytosis, with an average cell count of 90 per cu mm and a predominance of either polymorphonuclear or mononuclear leukocytes. Spinal fluid protein concentration ranged from 20 to 130 mg per 100 ml. In another series mild papilledema was observed in a few patients with severe illness.

LABORATORY FINDINGS. The changes in leukocyte count constitute the only positive laboratory findings. Total leukocyte counts of less than 5,000 per cu mm are observed in 90 percent of patients if daily counts are done during the febrile period and convalescence. The leukopenia may not appear until the last day of fever or even after defervescence. The differential leukocyte count will reveal an absolute decrease in lymphocytes on the first day, accompanied by an increase in nonsegmented neutrophiles. During the second or third day, the number of lymphocytes begins to return to normal and may constitute 40 to 65 percent. At the same time, the number of segmented neutrophiles decreases, and immature cells increase sharply until they outnumber the segmented forms. The differential count usually returns to normal within 5 to 8 days after defervescence. Erythrocyte values remain normal, and urinalyses are usually normal.

DIAGNOSIS. In the absence of a specific serologic test, the diagnosis must be made on clinical and epidemiologic grounds.

TREATMENT. The disease is self-limited, and no specific therapy is available. Symptomatic care including bed rest, adequate fluid intake and analgesia with aspirin is recommended. Convalescence may require a week or longer.

PROGNOSIS. No fatalities are recorded among the tens of thousands of cases.

REFERENCES

Fleming, J., J. R. Bignall, and A. N. Blades: Sandfly Fever, Review of 664 Cases, Lancet, I: 443, 1947.

Sabin, A. B., C. B. Philip, and J. R. Paul: Phlebotomus (Papataci or Sandfly) Fever; Disease of Military Importance; Summary of Existing Knowledge and Preliminary Report of Original Observations, J.A.M.A., 125:603, 693, 1944.

238   WEST NILE FEVER
Jay P. Sanford

DEFINITION. West Nile virus is distributed from South Africa to southeastern India, but has been shown as a cause of significant disease only in the Near East, where it can produce a clinical picture closely resembling dengue.

ETIOLOGY. West Nile virus is a Group B arbovirus with pathogenicity for common laboratory animals. The virus multiplies and causes cytopathic effects in a variety of cells in tissue culture.

PREVALENCE. In 1940 the virus was isolated from the blood of a febrile patient. Subsequent serologic surveys demonstrated neutralizing antibodies against the virus to be widely prevalent in the native populations of Uganda, Kenya, the Congo, and the Sudan. However, the clinical manifestations were unknown until the virus was isolated from the blood of a child during an epidemic of febrile disease in Israel in 1951. Outbreaks of disease involving several hundred patients occurred in Israel in 1950 to 1952. In one outbreak, over 60 percent of the population developed overt disease.

EPIDEMIOLOGY. The disease is highly endemic in Egypt but goes largely unrecognized. Presumably the adult population is for the most part immune, and the infection in childhood is an undifferentiated mild febrile illness. The infection occurs in the summer both in Israel and in Egypt. The transmission cycle in Egypt is believed to be bird to mosquito to bird, with *Culex univittatus* as the principal vector. Although man and a variety of other vertebrates are infected by the virus, their involvement is believed to be tangential. In Israel, the most probable vectors are *Culex molestus* and *C. univittatus*.

CLINICAL MANIFESTATIONS. Most of the patients in Israel have been young adults, with neither sex predominating. The onset is usually abrupt and without prodromal symptoms. The temperature quickly rises to 101 to 104°F, with chills occurring in one-third of patients. Symptoms include drowsiness, severe frontal headache, ocular pain, and pain in the back. A small number of patients have anorexia, nausea, and dryness of the throat. Cough is uncommon (8 percent). Signs observed include flushing of the face, conjunctival injection, and coating of the tongue. The prominent finding is general enlargement of lymph nodes, which are of moderate size but are not hard and are only slightly tender. Occipital, axillary, and inguinal nodes are usually involved. The spleen and liver are slightly enlarged in a small proportion of patients. In one-half of the patients a rash may appear from the second to the fifth day of illness and persist for several hours or until defervescence. The rash occurs predominantly over the trunk and consists of pale roseolar maculopapular lesions. The illness is self-limited and lasts 3 to 5 days in 80 percent of patients.

In a few patients, transitory meningeal involvement may be encountered. Spinal fluid examinations may reveal a pleocytosis and some increase in protein concentration.

Leukopenia occurs in the majority of patients, and total leukocyte counts are lower than 4,000 per cu mm in one-third. Differential counts vary from a moderate shift to the left to a slight lymphocytosis.

Convalescence is often prolonged, lasting 1 to 2 weeks, with prominent symptoms of fatigue. Enlargement of lymph nodes subsides over several months. Only rarely have complications, sequelae, or fatalities been seen in natural infections, although in one outbreak in a group of elderly patients a high proportion of patients developed meningoencephalitis, and four fatalities ensued.

DIAGNOSIS. Accurate diagnosis rests on virus isolation, which can be accomplished because viremia persists for as long as 6 days, or the demonstration of a rising specific antibody titer.

TREATMENT. The treatment is symptomatic.

REFERENCES

Clarke, D. H., and J. Casals: Arboviruses: Group B, p. 606 in "Viral and Rickettsial Infections of Man," 4th ed., F. L. Horsfall, Jr., and I. Tamm (Eds.), Philadelphia, J. B. Lippincott Company, 1965.

Marberg, K., N. Goldblum, V. V. Sterk, W. Jasinska-Klingberg, and M. A. Klingberg: The Natural History of West Nile Fever. I. Clinical Observations During an Epidemic in Israel, Am. J. Hyg., 64:259, 1956.

Taylor, R. M., T. H. Work, H. S. Hurlbut, and F. Rizk: A Study of the Ecology of West Nile Virus in Egypt, Am. J. Trop. Med. Hyg., 5:579, 1956.

239 OTHER VIRAL FEVERS
Jay P. Sanford

Most viral infections in man are either asymptomatic or present as undifferentiated grippelike illnesses characterized by fever, malaise, headaches, and generalized myalgia. The similarities in clinical features between infections caused by viruses as dissimilar as the myxoviruses, e.g., influenza, rubella; the enteroviruses, e.g., poliovirus, Coxsackie virus, ECHO virus; some of the herpes viruses, e.g., cytomegalovirus; and the arboviruses usually preclude an etiologic diagnosis on the basis of clinical manifestations without ancillary information regarding epidemiologic features and serologic findings. The purpose of this chapter is to direct attention to the ever-expanding list of viruses, with particular attention to the arboviruses, which produce febrile disease in man. Because the number of agents is large, mention will be made of agents which have been best documented, have demonstrated unusual features, or seem to be of greatest potential significance.

ARBOVIRUSES

Arboviruses are distributed widely throughout the world and are of importance in both temperate and tropical zones. Representative viruses have been isolated in almost every geographic area outside of the polar regions. The survival of arboviruses in nature depends upon a complex cycle between the arthropod and vertebrate. The arthropod becomes generally infected, is infectious for life, and therefore serves as a reservoir as well as a vector.

Arbovirus infection of vertebrates is usually asymptomatic. The viremia which develops stimulates an immune response which sharply limits the duration of the viremia. In arbovirus infections other than urban yellow fever and dengue, infection of man represents an incidental occurrence which is tangential to the basic maintenance cycle. Hence, the isolation of virus from arthropod vectors or the detection of infection in the natural vertebrate host may provide a means for the early detection and enable the control of epizootic infection before significant spread to man occurs.

As determined by serologic evidence of host responses, at least 75 immunologically distinct arboviruses are capable of infecting man, while somewhat fewer have been incriminated as causing clinical disease. The spectrum of clinical illness produced by the arboviruses is varied both in predominant features and in severity. Five broad, often overlapping, and somewhat arbitrary clinical syndromes can be delineated (Table 239-1). Many of the more common of these infections have been considered in detail elsewhere: yellow fever (Chap. 233), dengue (Chap. 234), phlebotomus fever (Chap. 237), Colorado tick fever (Chap. 236), West Nile fever (Chap. 238), the epidemic hemorrhagic fevers (Chaps. 235), and the viral encephalitides (Chap. 218).

ARBOVIRUS INFECTIONS CHARACTERIZED PREDOMINANTLY BY MALAISE, HEADACHES, AND GENERALIZED MYALGIA

RIFT VALLEY FEVER. Rift Valley fever is an acute disease principally of sheep and cattle and first described in man during an investigation of an extensive epizotic of hepatitis in sheep in the Rift Valley in East Africa. The virus of Rift Valley fever is ungrouped and has no immunologic relationship with other arboviruses. During the extensive epizootic in sheep in 1930, workers associated with the investigations contracted a severe but limited febrile disease. A similar syndrome was common among the herders of infected flocks. More than 200 cases of human disease were originally recognized.

The infection is widespread in Africa, occurring in Kenya, Uganda, Anglo-Egyptian Sudan, French Equatorial Africa, and the Union of South Africa. Virus has been found in several species of mosquitoes: *Eretmapodites chrysogaster, Aëdes caballus, Aëdes circumluteolus,* and *Culex theileri.* Antibodies to Rift Valley fever have been found in wild field rats in Uganda. Man appears to be incidentally infected during the course of an epizootic. Although man presumably can be infected by arthropods, many human infections occur as a result of handling infected animal tissues. In addition, laboratory-acquired infections have been common, which suggests a respiratory route.

The incubation period is usually 3 to 6 days. The onset

Table 239-1. SUMMARY OF CLINICAL, VIROLOGIC, AND EPIDEMIOLOGIC FEATURES
OF ARBOVIRUSES ASSOCIATED WITH DISEASE IN MAN

Syndrome	Virus	Serologic group	Vector	Known geographic range of infection
Fever with malaise, headaches, generalized myalgia	Mayaro	A	Mosquito	Trinidad, Colombia, Brazil
	Mucambo	A	Mosquito	Brazil
	Uruma	A		Lowland Forest, Bolivia
	Kunjin	B	Mosquito	Northern Australia
	Spondweni	B	Mosquito	South Africa, Mozambique, Nigeria
	United States bat salivary gland	B	?	California, Texas, Sonora in Southwest North America
	Wesselsbron	B	Mosquito	South Africa, Bechuanaland
	Yellow fever	B	Mosquito	Africa, Central and South America
	Zika	B	Mosquito	Uganda, Nigeria
	Apeu	C	Mosquito	Brazil
	Caraparu	C	Mosquito	Brazil, Panama, Trinidad
	Itaqui	C	Mosquito	Brazil
	Madrid	C	?	Panama
	Marituba	C	Mosquito(?)	Brazil
	Murutucu	C	Mosquito(?)	Brazil
	Oriboca	C	Mosquito	Brazil
	Ossa	C	?	Panama
	Calovo	Bunyamwera	Mosquito	Czechoslovakia
	Germiston	Bunyamwera	Mosquito	South Africa, Angola
	Ilesha	Bunyamwera	Mosquito(?)	Nigeria
	Guaroa	Bunyamwera	Mosquito	Colombia, Brazil
	Tahyna	California	Mosquito	Czechoslovakia, Yugoslavia
	Catu	Guama	Mosquito	Brazil, Trinidad
	Guama	Guama	Mosquito	Brazil, Trinidad
	Oropouche	Simbu	Mosquito	Brazil, Trinidad
	Bwamba	Bwamba	Mosquito	Uganda
	Phlebotomus, Naples	Phlebotomus	Sandfly	Italy, Egypt, Iran, West Pakistan
	Phlebotomus, Sicilian	Phlebotomus	Sandfly	Italy, Egypt, Iran, Pakistan, Yugoslavia
	Chagres	Phlebotomus	?	Panama
	Candiru	Phlebotomus	?	Brazil
	Vesicular stomatitis	VSV	Sandfly, mosquito(?)	United States, Mexico, Panama, Venezuela, Colombia, Ecuador, Peru
	Colorado tick fever	Ungrouped	Hard tick	Western United States
	Nairobi sheep disease	Ungrouped	Hard tick	Kenya, Congo
	Rift Valley fever	Ungrouped	Mosquito	Africa
	Quaranfil	Ungrouped	Soft tick	Egypt, South Africa
	Piry	Ungrouped	?	Brazil
Fever with malaise, headaches, myalgia, *arthralgia*, and *rash*	Chikungunya	A	Mosquito	South, East, West, Central Africa, India, Thailand, Vietnam, Malaya
	Mayaro	A	Mosquito	Brazil, Trinidad
	O'nyong-nyong	A	Mosquito	East Africa, Senegal
	Sindbis	A	Mosquito	South and East Africa, Egypt, Israel, India, Malaya, Philippines, Australia
	Bunyamwera	Bunyamwera	Mosquito	South, East, West Africa
	Changuinola	Changuinola	Phlebotomus	Panama
Fever with malaise, headaches, myalgia, *rash*, and *lymphadenopathy*	Dengue 1	B	Mosquito	Hawaii, Oceana, New Guinea, Japan, Malaysia, Thailand, India
	Dengue 2	B	Mosquito	Circumglobal

Table 239-1. SUMMARY OF CLINICAL, VIROLOGIC, AND EPIDEMIOLOGIC FEATURES
OF ARBOVIRUSES ASSOCIATED WITH DISEASE IN MAN (Continued)

Syndrome	Virus	Serologic group	Vector	Known geographic range of infection
Fever with malaise, headaches, myalgia, *rash* and *lymphadenopathy* (continued)	Dengue 3	B	Mosquito	Caribbean, Oceana, Philippines, Thailand
	Dengue 4	B	Mosquito	Philippines, Thailand, India
	West Nile	B	Mosquito	South and West Africa, Rhone Delta, Near East, Israel, India, Malaysia, Borneo
Fever with headache, myalgia, prostration, and *hemorrhagic* signs	Chikungunya	A	Mosquito	Thailand, Malaysia, India, Vietnam
	Dengue 1	B	Mosquito	Thailand, India
	Dengue 2	B	Mosquito	Philippines, Vietnam, Thailand, Malaysia, India
	Dengue 3	B	Mosquito	Philippines, Thailand
	Dengue 4	B	Mosquito	Philippines, Thailand
	Kyasanur Forest disease	B	Tick	India
	Omsk hemorrhagic fever	B	Tick	Western Siberia, USSR
	Yellow fever	B	Mosquito	Africa, Central and South America
	Junin (Argentinian hemorrhagic fever)	Tacaribe	Rodent, mite(?)	Argentina
	Machupo (Bolivian hemorrhagic fever)	Tacaribe	Rodent, mite(?)	Eastern Bolivia
	Central Asian hemorrhagic fever	Ungrouped	Tick(?)	Central Asia, USSR
	Crimean type hemorrhagic fever	Ungrouped	Tick	Southern USSR
	Far Eastern or Korean hemorrhagic fever (hemorrhagic nephrosonephritis)	Ungrouped	Rodent, mite(?)	USSR, Manchuria, China, Korea
Fever with *central nervous system* involvement (meningitis to encephalitis)	See table in Chap. 218.			

is usually abrupt, with malaise, chilly sensation or rigors, headache, retroorbital pain, and generalized aching and backache. The temperature rises rapidly to 101 to 104°F. Later complaints include anorexia, loss of taste, epigastric pain, and photophobia. Examination is usually unremarkable except for flushing of the face and conjunctival injection. The temperature curve is often saddleback in type, with an initial elevation lasting 2 to 3 days, followed by a remission and second febrile period. Convalescence is usually rapid. Complications are rare; jaundice has not been seen in man. Macular exudates with decreased vision have been reported. One of the most characteristic findings is the initial normal total leukocyte count followed by leukopenia with a decrease in neutrophiles associated with an increase in band forms. The diagnosis is made by isolating the virus from the blood by inoculation of mice. In humans, viremia is present during the first 3 days. Neutralizing antibodies have been demonstrated as early as 4 days after onset. There is no specific treatment. The prognosis in human

infections is good. Only one fatality has been recorded, and in this instance death was not due directly to the infection.

MAYARO VIRUS. Mayaro virus was first isolated from man in Trinidad in 1954. Outbreaks involving a number of persons subsequently have occurred in Brazil and Bolivia. The virus has been isolated from a wild mosquito, *Mansonia venezuelensis*, and can be maintained serially in *Aëdes aegypti* and *Anopheles quadrimaculatus*. The mechanism of spread has not been determined, but the presence of viremia favors a biting arthropod vector. The predominance of illness and greater incidence of immunity in males suggests a forest infection. Symptoms include fever of several days' duration, which may be marked during the first 1 to 2 days. Systemic complaints include severe frontal headache, epigastric pain, backache, nausea, photophobia, and vertigo. Signs have included conjunctival injection, mild icterus in a few patients, and arthritis in at least one patient. The leukocyte count is in the range of 5,000 to 8,000 per cu mm. The illness in Bolivia was more severe, and several fatalities were reported.

BAT SALIVARY GLAND VIRUS. During the course of a survey for rabies infection in bats, an agent was obtained from the salivary glands of Mexican free-tailed bats in Texas. The virus is related to the St. Louis encephalitis complex of viruses (Group B). It is not known how the virus is maintained in nature. Five laboratory-acquired human infections have been recorded. The illnesses were characterized by fever associated with headache, myalgia, and a mild nonproductive cough. In two patients, there was evidence of central-nervous-system involvement with encephalitis and aseptic meningitis. One patient had oophoritis and two developed orchitis. By the sixth to seventh day of illness, leukopenia in the 2,000 to 3,000 per cu mm range was observed in two individuals.

ZIKA VIRUS. Zika virus was first isolated from a captive rhesus monkey in Uganda and subsequently from wild mosquitoes. Based upon serologic surveys, it is known to infect man in Uganda and Nigeria. During investigation in eastern Nigeria of an outbreak of jaundice that was suspected of being yellow fever, physicians isolated Zika virus from one patient and noted that two others had a rise in neutralizing antibodies. The symptoms in these patients included fever, arthralgia, and headache with retroorbital pain. Jaundice was present in one, and bile was demonstrated in the urine of another. Albuminuria was noted in one patient. Prothrombin times were normal. The clinical syndrome appears to simulate mild yellow fever.

BUNYAMWERA GROUP. Representative viruses of this group are found in all inhabited continents except Australia. Only four viruses of the group, Bunyamwera itself, Germiston, Ilesha, and Guaroa, have been associated with clinical disease. Based upon serologic surveys, there is evidence of a high prevalence of inapparent infection in some areas. The clinical patterns of infection due to Germiston, Ilesha, and Guaroa viruses seem similar, while infection due to Bunyamwera virus is often associated with arthralgia and may be associated with a rash. The mild clinical illness is characterized by low-grade fever, headache, and myalgia which last several days, and it may be followed by weakness during convalescence.

VESICULAR STOMATITIS VIRUS. This virus disease of animals which chiefly affects cattle, horses, and swine appears in man as an acute self-limited infection with signs and symptoms quite similar to those of influenza. Two distinct serotypes, New Jersey and Indiana, have been recognized. Most of the outbreaks, especially in North America, have been due to the New Jersey serotype. Although most commonly occurring as a laboratory infection in man, this infection is transmissible under natural conditions. In one report, three-fourths of the laboratory personnel handling experimentally infected animals or manipulating the viruses developed neutralizing antibodies. In nature, the virus has been isolated from phlebotomus sandflies collected in a tropical rain forest in Panama and from a pool of *Aëdes spp.* (prob-

ably *dorsalis*) mosquitoes during an epizootic in New Mexico. In the areas of Panama which was involved, 17 to 35 percent of the population had neutralizing antibodies against VSV. Of the laboratory workers with serologic evidence of infection, approximately one-half reported clinical symptoms. In the majority of cases the incubation period has been 2 to 6 days, although symptoms have developed within 30 hr of accidental inoculation. The onset usually is sudden, with chills, fever, profuse diaphoresis, and generalized myalgia including pain on ocular movement. One-third to one-half of patients have sore throats, and 10 percent have coryza. Physical signs include a temperature of 102 to 104°F in severe cases; fever is absent in mild cases. Conjunctivitis is noted in 20 percent, and in some patients (10 percent), small raised vesicles may be present on the buccal mucosa. Submaxillary and cervical lymphadenitis is seen in approximately one-third of patients. A diphasic course is noted in approximately 10 percent of patients. Treatment is symptomatic.

ARBOVIRUS INFECTIONS CHARACTERIZED BY FEVER, MALAISE, ARTHRALGIA, AND RASH

CHIKUNGUNYA. In 1952 an epidemic of a disease similar to dengue occurred in Tanganyika, an area in which dengue had never been observed. The disease was given the name chikungunya ("that which bends up") from the local description of the sudden onset of distinctive joint pains. A Group A arbovirus was isolated in 1956 both from serum of patients ill with the disease and from a pool of *Aëdes aegypti* mosquitoes.

Chikungunya virus is responsible for a denguelike illness in South Africa, India, and Southeast Asia, as well as a rather mild form of hemorrhagic fever in Asiatic children (Chap. 235). Outbreaks have been associated with high attack rates, with as many as 80 percent of inhabitants in some settlements becoming ill. It is not known definitely what vertebrates and arthropods are involved in the wild transmission cycle. Because the virus has been isolated from *Aëdes africanus* and antibodies against the virus can be detected in chimpanzees, these may play a role in the natural cycle in Africa.

After an incubation period estimated at no less than 8 days, the onset is typically abrupt, with a rapid rise in temperature to 102 to 105°F, often associated with a rigor and headache. Pain in large joints occurs early, incapacitating some individuals within a few minutes of onset. The pain is frequently severe enough to prevent sleep. The arthralgia is often associated with objective arthritis. Sites of involvement include knees, ankles, shoulders, wrists, or proximal interphalangeal joints. Myalgia, especially backache, and malaise occur frequently. In 60 to 80 percent of patients a maculopapular eruption, which may appear at any time during the febrile course, is noted on the trunk or on the extensor surfaces of the extremities. Mild lymphadenopathy predominantly in the axillary or inguinal areas may be evident. Pharyngitis and conjunctival suffusion may be observed in a few patients. Elevated temperatures continue for 1 to 6 days, and in some patients an afebrile interval of 1 to 3 days is followed by a secondary rise in temperature. The joint pains sometimes continue after the temperature has returned to normal. In a few individuals, joint pains have persisted for up to 4 months. Hematocrit values remain normal. Total leukocyte counts may be less than 5,000 per cu mm in some patients, while in others they remain normal. Urinalyses are normal. There is no specific antiviral treatment. Anti-inflammatory agents such as aspirin or indomethacin have been utilized. No second attacks have been recognized, and in the absence of the hemorrhagic fever syndrome, no deaths have been described.

O'NYONG-NYONG. O'nyong-nyong fever was first noted as an epidemic illness characterized by joint pains, rash, and lymphadenopathy in the northern province of Uganda in 1959. The agent is a Group A arbovirus which shows close antigenic relationships with chikungunya and Semliki Forest viruses. The original outbreak was associated with an explosive epidemic which spread to Tanzania and other areas in East Africa. By 1961, 2 million cases were recorded. In some areas, 91 percent of the population had either clinical disease or inapparent infection. Local outbreaks extended over the entire year. All age groups were affected. The most likely vector is *Anopheles funestus*. The clinical features are similar to those of chikungunya virus infection.

SINDBIS VIRUS. Sindbis virus infection in man rarely presents as a clinical disease. Of five cases from Uganda, one patient gave a history of joint pain. In the only well-studied clinical illness, a South African woman had arthritis as a prominent finding. Two days after a headache she noted swelling in her hands and feet. Soon thereafter she developed a confluent macular rash, followed by vesicle formation. The small joints of the hands and feet were swollen at the time of examination. Slight swelling of the fingers was present at 10 weeks, although she had otherwise recovered.

OTHER ARBOVIRUSES

Epidemics of polyarthritis associated with rashes have been observed in Australia since 1928. The clinical and epidemiologic features of each outbreak were quite uniform, and therefore, the name *epidemic polyarthritis* was applied. More recently, a presumed etiologic agent (designated as Ross River virus) has been isolated. The clinical features include development of a rash on the cheeks and the forehead which occasionally spreads to the trunk and lasts 2 to 10 days. Mild joint pain occurs in two-thirds of patients. Temperature elevations are rarely recorded, but a few patients give a history of feverishness.

In addition, Mayaro and Bunyamwera viruses have been associated with the syndrome of rash and arthralgia. These have been discussed under their more common manifestations, the dengue syndromes.

ENCEPHALOMYOCARDITIS VIRUSES

The encephalomyocarditis viruses, Columbia S-K, MM, Mengo, EMC, are a group of small RNA viruses which are immunologically indistinguishable from each other. Rodents, in particular certain species of wild rats, constitute the major reservoir for EMC viruses. Strains also have been isolated from primates, swine, and other rodents from many parts of the world. Strains of Mengo virus have been isolated from mosquitoes (*Taeniorhynchus fuscopennatus*) in Uganda, but the epidemiologic evidence does not suggest that EMC viruses are arboviruses. The prevalence of neutralizing antibodies in surveys of healthy individuals in the United States, Germany, Sweden, and Mexico ranges up to 7 percent.

Human infections vary from inapparent to mild febrile illness to severe encephalomyelitis. Study of an outbreak of aseptic meningitis characterized by chills, fever, headache, stiff neck, and cerebrospinal fluid pleocytosis of 50 to 500 cells per cu mm which involved a group of 44 U.S. Army personnel in the Philippine Islands revealed that during convalescence 39 percent of the individuals had high titers of specific neutralizing antibodies. In this outbreak fever lasted 2 to 3 days and all patients recovered promptly without sequelae. Sporadic EMC virus isolates have been made from adults and children with illnesses diagnosed as paralytic poliomyelitis, the Guillain-Barre syndrome, and severe meningoencephalitis. Myocarditis has not been a feature of EMC virus infection in man. Nothing is known of the pathologic findings in man. The diagnosis of human EMC virus infection depends upon isolation of the virus from blood, cerebrospinal fluid, or stool or the demonstration of a rising titer of specific antibodies during convalescence. Treatment is symptomatic and supportive.

REFERENCES

Arboviruses

Anderson, S. G., and E. L. French: An Epidemic Exanthem Associated with Polyarthritis in the Murray Valley, 1956, Med. J. Aust., 2:113, 1957.

Casals, J., and D. H. Clarke: Arboviruses; Group A, p. 583 in "Viral and Rickettsial Infections of Man," 4th ed., F. L. Horsfall, Jr., and I. Tamm (Eds.), Philadelphia, J. B. Lippincott Company, 1965.

——, and ——: Arboviruses Other Than Groups A and B, p. 659 in "Viral and Rickettsial Infections of Man," 4th ed., F. L. Horsfall, Jr., and I. Tamm (Eds.), Philadelphia, J. B. Lippincott Company, 1965.

Clarke, D. H., and J. Casals: Arboviruses; Group B, p. 606 in "Viral and Rickettsial Infections of Man," 4th ed., F. L. Horsfall, Jr., and I. Tamm (Eds.), Philadelphia, J. B. Lippincott Company, 1965.

Daubney, R., J. R. Hudson, and P. C. Garnham: Enzootic Hepatitis or Rift Valley Fever, J. Pathol. Bacteriol., 34: 545, 1931.

Deller, J. J., Jr., and P. K. Russell: Chikungunya Disease, Am. J. Trop. Med. Hyg., 17:107, 1968.

Doherty, R. L., B. M. Gorman, R. H. Whitehead, and J. G. Carley: Studies of Epidemic Polyarthritis: The Significance of Three Group A Arboviruses Isolated from Mosquitoes in Queensland, Australas. Ann. Med., 13:322, 1964.

Fields, B. N., and K. Hawkins: Human Infection with the

Virus of Vesicular Stomatitis During an Epizootic, New Engl. J. Med., 277:989, 1967.

Malherbe, H., M. Strickland-Chomley, and A. L. Jackson: Sindbis Virus Infection in Man. Report of a Case with Recovery of Virus From Skin Lesions, S. Afr. Med. J., 37:547, 1963.

Patterson, W. C., L. O. Mott, and E. W. Jenney: A Study of Vesicular Stomatitis in Man, J. Am. Vet. Med. Ass., 133:57, 1958.

Robinson, M. C.: An Epidemic of Virus Disease in Southern Province, Tanganyika Territory, in 1952–53. I. Clinical Features, Trans. Roy. Soc. Trop. Med. Hyg., 49:28, 1955.

Schrire, L.: Macular Changes in Rift Valley Fever, S. Afr. Med. J., 25:926, 1951.

Shore, H.: O'nyong-nyong Fever: An Epidemic Virus Disease in East Africa. III. Some Clinical and Epidemiological Observations in the Northern Province of Uganda, Trans. Roy. Soc. Trop. Med. Hyg., 55:361, 1961.

Smithburn, K. C., A. F. Mahaffy, A. J. Haddow, S. F. Kitchen, and J. F. Smith: Rift Valley Fever, J. Immunol., 62:213, 1949.

Sudia, W. D., Fields, B. N., and Calisher, C. H.: Isolation of Vesicular Stomatitis Virus (Indiana Strain) and Other Viruses From Mosquitoes in New Mexico, 1965, Am. J. Epidemiol., 86:598, 1967.

Sulkin, S. E., K. F. Burns, D. F. Shelton, and C. Wallis: Bat Salivary Gland Virus: Infections of Man and Monkey, Texas Rept. Biol. Med., 20:113, 1962.

WHO Technical Report 219, Report of a Study Group: "Arthropod-Borne Viruses," Geneva, 1961.

Work, T. H.: Virus Diseases in the Tropics, p. 1 in "A Manual of Tropical Medicine," 4th ed., G. W. Hunter, W. W. Frye, and J. C. Schwartzwelder (Eds.), Philadelphia, W. B. Saunders Company, 1966.

Encephalomyocarditis Viruses

Gajdusek, D. C.: Encephalomyocarditis Infection in Childhood, Pediatrics, 16:902, 1955.

Smadel, J. E., and J. Warren: The Virus of Encephalomyocarditis and Its Apparent Causation of Disease in Man, J. Clin. Invest., 26:1197, 1947.

Warren, J.: Encephalomyocarditis Viruses, p. 562 in "Viral and Rickettsial Infections of Man," 4th ed., F. L. Horsfall, Jr., and I. Tamm (Eds.), Philadelphia, J. B. Lippincott Company, 1965.

Section 21

Diseases Caused by Protozoa

240 AMEBIASIS

James J. Plorde, Harry A. Feldman, and Ivan L. Bennett, Jr.

DEFINITION. Amebiasis is an infection of the large intestine produced by *Endamoeba histolytica*. It is an asymptomatic carrier state in most individuals, but disease ranging from chronic, mild diarrhea to fulminant dysentery is frequently produced. Among extraintestinal complications, the commonest is hepatic abscess, which may rupture into peritoneum, pleura, lung, or pericardium.

ETIOLOGY. There are at least six different species of ameba that parasitize the mouth and intestine of man. Of these, *E. histolytica* is the only one that causes disease and *E. coli* is the species with which it is most likely to be confused in examination of stools.

Endamoeba histolytica exists in two forms: the motile trophozoite and the nonmotile cyst. The trophozoite is the parasitic form and dwells in the wall and lumen of the colon, divides by binary fission, grows best under anaerobic conditions, and requires the presence of either bacteria or tissue substrates to satisfy its nutritional requirements. When diarrhea occurs, the trophozoites are passed unchanged in the liquid stool, where they can be distinguished by their rapid motility, ingestion of erythrocytes, and the sparsity of vacuoles and ingested bacteria within them. In the absence of diarrhea, the trophozoites encyst before leaving the gut. The cysts are highly resistant to environmental changes and are responsible for transmission of the disease. The cysts of *E. histolytica* can be distinguished from those of *E. coli* by their thin wall and their two thick chromated bodies.

Endamoeba histolytica strains have been classified into large and small races, depending upon whether they form cysts measuring more or less than 10 μ in diameter. While it is possible that small strains (sometimes called *E. hartmanni*) are somewhat less likely to produce symptoms than are the large strains, cyst size is apparently unstable and the often-heard statement that small strains are nonpathogenic for man is not justified.

Endamoeba histolytica occurs normally in the intestines of a few dogs, monkeys, and rats; these animals, rabbits, and kittens can also be infected experimentally. Amebas can be cultivated in artificial media, a procedure that is occasionally useful in diagnosis. With rare exceptions, the presence of bacteria in the culture medium is a prerequisite to multiplication of the protozoa.

EPIDEMIOLOGY. Because trophozoites die rapidly after leaving the intestine, patients with amebic dysentery are unimportant in transmission of the disease; asymptomatic cyst passers are the source of new infections.

Amebic infection is worldwide, although both symptomatic and subclinical infection are more frequent in tropical areas. Figures obtained from local and admittedly incomplete surveys indicate that the average incidence of asymptomatic carriers is 10 percent in Europe and the United States, 16 percent in Asia, and 17 percent in Africa. Cyst passers are more frequent among children and the inmates of institutions.

Cases of amebic dysentery are usually sporadic but epidemics, usually water-borne, have occurred. Outbreaks of amebiasis are never explosive, as are those produced by pathogenic intestinal bacteria, and may not be recognized for several weeks. The cysts are often transmitted by vegetables in countries where human excreta is used as fertilizer.

Symptomatic amebiasis is unusual below the age of ten years in temperate climates, and both intestinal and hepatic lesions predominate in adult males to an extent that is not readily explainable on the basis of different rates of exposure to infection.

PATHOGENESIS AND ANATOMIC CHANGES. After ingestion, cysts pass through the stomach unchanged. In the ileum, the cyst wall disintegrates and, eventually, eight trophozoites result. These immature amebas pass to the colon, where they attack the mucosa. Mucosal lesions too tiny to be detected probably occur in all infections. The sites of involvement in order of frequency are cecum and ascending colon, rectum, sigmoid, appendix, and terminal ileum.

The factors responsible for the development of ulceration extensive enough to cause symptoms in some individuals are not understood. The size of the inoculum and the virulence of the infecting organism are both important. The virulence seems to differ among strains, and there are some studies which suggest that it is increased with rapid passage from person to person. These factors alone, however, are insufficient to explain the occurrence of disease in only a small percentage of subjects exposed naturally to the same strain or in a minority of volunteers fed cysts from a single source. Certain experimental findings suggest strongly that the bacterial flora of the intestine may be a major determinant of the extent of amebic disease. The symbiosis between bacteria and amebas in artificial media has been mentioned. When 200 strains were cultured and tested for virulence in rabbits, disease was produced by only 4 percent grown without bacteria, by 35 percent grown with a single bacterial species, and by 85 percent grown with a mixed culture of several different bacteria. Germ-free animals cannot be infected with *E. histolytica* but become susceptible if the intestine is first allowed to acquire a normal complement of bacteria.

Amebic ulceration of the intestinal wall is characteristic. A small mucosal defect overlies a larger, burrowing area of necrosis in the submucosa and muscularis, producing a bottle-shaped lesion. There is little acute inflammatory response to the damage, and, in contrast to the picture in bacillary dysentery, the mucosa between ulcers is normal, without hyperemia. In the cecum and elsewhere, chronic infection leads to the formation of large masses of granulation tissue or "amebomas." Amebas can enter the portal circulation and lodge in venules; liquefaction necrosis of liver tissue leads to the formation of an abscess cavity. Rarely, embolization results in lung, brain or splenic abscess.

Because trophozoites in histologic sections of liver or intestine are usually seen lying free in small spaces, it has been said that *E. histolytica* destroys tissue through the elaboration of a "cytolytic ferment." Not only is there no evidence whatsoever that such a substance exists, but the histologic appearance is simply a shrinkage artifact of fixation.

CHRONIC AMEBIC DYSENTERY. Most patients with this commonest type of amebic disease cannot date the onset of illness accurately. There is intermittent diarrhea consisting of one to four foul-smelling stools daily, sometimes containing mucus and blood, alternating with periods of relative normality for months or years. Vague abdominal cramping, weight loss, and mild fever are frequent. In such cases of "walking dysentery" the only findings are wasting, occasional tender hepatomegaly (not indicative of hepatic abscess), and slight pain when the cecum and ascending colon are palpated. Sigmoidoscopy sometimes reveals typical ulcerations with normal intervening mucosa, or mucosal defects may be demonstrated radiologically in the right colon. Specific diagnosis depends upon finding the organisms in the feces.

ACUTE AMEBIC DYSENTERY. This type of amebiasis is unusual but was observed in several patients during the large epidemic in a Chicago hotel in 1933 when massive contamination of the water supply occurred through defective plumbing; it is more likely to be seen sporadically in tropical areas. The onset is abrupt, with high fever (104 to 105°F), severe abdominal cramps, and profuse, bloody diarrhea with tenesmus. There is diffuse abdominal tenderness, often so severe that peritonitis is suspected. Hepatomegaly is very frequent, and sigmoidoscopy almost always demonstrates extensive rectosigmoid ulceration. Trophozoites are numerous in stools and in material obtained directly from the ulcers.

AMEBOMA (AMEBIC GRANULOMA). Chronic infection can lead to the production of large masses of granulation tissue in the colon. When the entire circumference of the intestine is involved, there may be partial obstruction and a tender, sausage-shaped mass is often palpable. This lesion is most frequent in the cecum, where a palpable mass and radiologic demonstration of a ragged encroachment upon the lumen can lead to a mistaken diagnosis of adenocarcinoma. A history of diarrhea with blood and mucus may be elicited, but this is compatible with the diagnosis of cancer. The importance of searching for amebas in the feces of any patient with these findings is very great because surgical intervention in untreated ameboma can lead to peritonitis or perforation, pericecal abscess, and sinus formation with drainage of feculent material through the abdominal wall. In addition to cancer, these lesions are likely to be confused with tuberculosis or actinomycosis.

In the tropics, amebic ulceration of the appendix is responsible for a significant proportion of cases of appendicitis. Again, operative intervention is contraindicated before specific treatment. The majority of deaths among tourists infected during the 1933 Chicago epidemic were a direct result of laparotomy carried out for symptoms of appendicitis. The operations were performed in many different towns and cities after patients had returned home and before the significance of exposure in Chicago had been widely appreciated.

HEPATIC AMEBIASIS. The parasites usually reach the liver through the portal vein; rarely, they may traverse the lymphatic vessels. It has been believed for a long time that amebas which lodged in the liver could produce a diffuse hepatitis. Careful postmortem and biopsy studies indicate that the syndrome of tender hepatomegaly, right upper quadrant pain, fever, and leukocytosis in patients with amebic colitis is not a result of the presence of amebas in hepatic tissues, is accompanied by nonspecific periportal inflammation, and is rarely, if ever, a prelude to hepatic abscess. It is evident, then, that these manifestations are best regarded as an accompaniment of colitis and do not merit a separate diagnosis of "diffuse amebic hepatitis."

Hepatic abscess may develop insidiously, with fever, sweats, weight loss, and no local signs other than painless or slightly tender hepatomegaly. In other patients, there is abrupt onset, with chills, fever to 105°F, nausea, vomiting, severe upper abdominal pain, and polymorphonuclear leukocytosis. Initially, cholecystitis, perforated ulcer, or acute pancreatitis may be suspected.

Almost invariably, amebic abscess is localized in the posterior portion of the right lobe of the liver, because this lobe receives most of the blood draining the right colon through the "streaming" effect in portal vein flow. This location is responsible for several features that aid in diagnosis. *Point tenderness* in the posterolateral portion of a lower right intercostal space is frequent even in the absence of diffuse liver pain. Most abscesses enlarge upward, producing a bulge in the diaphragmatic dome, obliteration of the costophrenic gutter, small hydrothorax, basilar atelectasis, and pain referred to the right shoulder. Radiologically, unruptured abscesses do not show a fluid level, and calcification of the liver parenchyma is very rare. Isotope liver scan is invaluable in confirming both the presence and location of a liver abscess.

Needle puncture results in the withdrawal of "pus" which consists of liquefied, necrotic liver, the classic "chocolate syrup" or "anchovy paste" exudate; the pus contains no polymorphonuclear leukocytes (barring secondary bacterial infection) and, usually, no amebas. The parasites are localized in the cyst wall and may be demonstrated at times by a Vim-Silverman needle biopsy of the cyst wall following aspiration of the abscess.

Hepatic abscess complicates asymptomatic infection of the colon more often than symptomatic intestinal disease, another factor making recognition difficult. Trophozoites or cysts are demonstrable in the feces of only about one-eighth of patients with abscess, and fewer

than one-half can recall significant diarrheal illness.

PLEUROPULMONARY AMEBIASIS. The right pleural cavity and lung are involved by direct extension from the liver in 10 to 20 percent of patients with liver abscess. Rarely, amebic lung abscess has resulted from embolization rather than direct extension.

Manifestations are those of massive pleural effusion; aspiration of chocolate fluid is diagnostic, or if the lung parenchyma is involved and perforation into a bronchus occurs, patients expectorate large amounts of the typical exudate, some patients even commenting that the sputum "tastes like liver." Cough, pleural pain, fever, and leukocytosis are the rule, and secondary bacterial infection is frequent.

OTHER EXTRAINTESTINAL LESIONS. Rupture of liver abscess into the *pericardium* has occurred; these patients are often thought initially to have tuberculous pericarditis. *Peritonitis* is a result of perforation of colonic ulcer or rupture of liver abscess. Painful ulcers of the genitalia, perianal skin, or abdominal wall (draining sinuses), vaginitis, urethritis, and prostatitis are unusual complications resulting from extension of intestinal disease. Metastatic brain abscess is rare and an etiologic diagnosis is seldom made clinically. Splenic abscess has been reported but is very unusual.

DIAGNOSIS. The diagnosis of intestinal amebiasis depends upon identification of the organism in the stool or tissues. Formed stools are examined in saline and iodine mounts for amebic cysts; concentration methods will double the yield. Liquid stools must be examined immediately (or kept at body temperature until examination) in saline solution and using a warm stage if motile trophozoites are to be detected. Fixation of specimens in polyvinyl alcohol or merthiolate-iodine-formalin will preserve amebas for later identification. Careful examination of 4 to 6 stool specimens may be required for diagnosis.

Sigmoidoscopy is of value in symptomatic cases. The mucosal lesions should be aspirated and the material examined for trophozoites. Stained sections of biopsy material obtained from such lesions also will frequently reveal trophozoites.

The diagnosis of extraintestinal amebiasis is difficult. The parasite usually cannot be recovered from stool or tissue. Serologic tests employing purified antigens are positive in nearly all patients with proved amebic liver abscess, and in the majority of those with acute amebic dysentery. However, false positive results make these tests of more value in excluding the diagnosis rather than in confirming it. Cultivation of amebas from feces or pus is possible but is not practical in most laboratories. A most important diagnostic procedure in suspected liver abscess is a therapeutic trial of antiamebic drugs. The response is often dramatic within 3 days. In the event that demonstrating parasites is difficult, a therapeutic trial should be instituted without hesitation.

TREATMENT. Treatment should be aimed at relief of symptoms, replacement of fluid, electrolyte, and blood losses, and eradication of the organism. Eradication is confirmed by healing of lesions and by disappearance of either cysts or trophozoites from the stool. Amebicidal agents may act directly on the trophozoite or indirectly by destroying the intestinal bacteria upon which it is dependent for growth. The direct-acting amebicides can be divided further into those that act systemically and those that are active only within the lumen of the bowel by direct contact with the organisms. The large number of agents available indicates the lack of a single ideal drug. While most patients are eventually cured, initial improvement in chronic cases is frequently followed by relapse. In treatment, often a combination of drugs may be necessary to achieve cure.

The available drugs fall into several different groups. *Arsenicals:* Milibis (0.5 Gm three times daily for 1 week) is the least toxic of these preparations. It is effective only against intestinal trophozoites. *Halogenated hydroxyquinolines:* Diodoquin (0.65 Gm three times daily for 21 days) is used most frequently. Like Milibis it is a contact amebicide active only within the gut. *Antibiotics:* Oxytetracycline (Terramycin) is the most effective when given in dosage of 2.0 Gm daily for 10 days. Paromomycin (Humatin) given in a single dose (4.0 Gm or 1.0 Gm three times daily for 10 days) is also used. Both are effective only in intestinal amebiasis. *Aminoquinolines:* Chloroquine diphosphate (Aralen) is a systemic amebicide which is useful in hepatic disease because of its high concentration in the liver (0.5 Gm twice daily for 2 days and 0.5 Gm once daily for 12 to 19 days). *Alkaloids:* Emetine is a relatively toxic derivative of ipecac. When given intramuscularly (65 mg daily for no more than 10 days), it is highly effective in destroying trophozoites in tissue but does not affect these organisms in the gut. Dehydroemetine is apparently less toxic. This drug must also be given intramuscularly in dosage of 80 mg daily for no more than 10 days. Oral emetine preparations are effective against intestinal organisms but are not available in the United States. *Metronidazole* (Flagyl) taken orally in dosage of 800 mg three times daily for 10 days is unique because it is active against both intestinal and extraintestinal trophozoites. A related drug, niradazole (Ambulhar) is also effective but more toxic.

In asymptomatic or mildly symptomatic patients, Milibis and Diodoquin administered sequentially give good results. Paromomycin is also effective. Stools should be examined monthly for a year to detect relapse. If relapse occurs, retreatment should consist of a combination of Diodoquin and Terramycin. Chloroquine can be added for its potentiating effect on Terramycin as well as its ability to eradicate subclinical hepatic infection.

Treatment of acute dysentery involves control of symptoms as well as eradication of the organism. A number of regimens can be used:

1. Emetine or dehydroemetine given intramuscularly will control the acute attack. Because these drugs are toxic and cannot eliminate intestinal trophozoites, therapy with these drugs should be discontinued as soon as symptoms abate and a course of intestinal amebicides should be instituted. Terramycin or a combination of Diodoquin and Milibis is satisfactory. Usually emetine or dehydroemetine need be given for only 3 to 4 days to control the attack and are also effective in treating subclinical hepatic infection.

Emetine is quite toxic and produces abdominal pain, tremor, weakness, electrocardiographic abnormalities, and orthostatic hypotension. Dehydroemetine is less toxic, but neither drug should be given for more than 10 days and the dosage should not exceed 65 mg for emetine or 80 mg for dehydroemetine or 1 mg/Kg for either drug. Neither drug should be used in patients with renal, cardiac, or muscle disease, during pregnancy, or in children, unless all other drugs fail.

2. Terramycin will bring an acute attack under control although not as rapidly as emetine. It has the additional advantage of terminating the intestinal infection. A course of choloroquine should be given with Terramycin to eradicate subclinical hepatic infection.

3. Metronidazole. This agent controls symptoms, destroys intestinal trophozoites, and eradicates hepatic infection. If more extensive experience confirms the initial results, this agent could become the drug of choice in amebic dystentery.

4. If hepatic abscess is suspected, chloroquine is the drug of choice. It is effective, nontoxic, and produces symptomatic relief in 48 to 72 hr. Even large abscesses subside, but relapse is relatively frequent. If aspiration or a dramatic response to chloroquine prove that a hepatic abscess is of amebic etiology, emetine or dehydroemetine should be given for 10 days also to prevent relapse. Drainage of an amebic abscess usually is not necessary and should be performed only if there is localized swelling over the liver, marked elevation of the diaphragm, severe localized liver tenderness, and failure to respond to systemic amebicides. Adequate drainage can usually be accomplished by needle alone and surgical drainage is rarely necessary. The greatest hazard in needling an abscess is secondary bacterial infection.

Contact amebicides must be given in combination with emetine and chloroquine, to eradicate any intestinal trophozoites that might lead to relapse.

Amebiasis in locations other than the intestine and liver should be treated like hepatic amebiasis.

PROGNOSIS. Complete cure of intestinal amebiasis occurs in 75 to 95 percent of cases with repeated courses of therapy. The relapse rate is as high as 35 percent after a single course. The fatality rate is less than 5 percent.

Hepatic and pulmonary amebiasis are still attended by appreciable mortality, but no reliable figures are available.

PREVENTION. For the individual, avoidance of contaminated food and water, scalding of vegetables, and the use of iodine-releasing tablets in drinking water (chlorine, in the form of Halazone, is ineffective) are important measures. Globaline tablets, containing tetraglycine hydroperiodide, are convenient and effective.

Improvements in general sanitation and the detection of cyst passers and their removal from food-handling duties are general measures in prophylaxis, but such segregation of carriers is rarely practiced.

INFECTIONS DUE TO *HARTMANNELLA*

The free-living amebae which commonly inhabit soil and water and are usually considered to be nonpathogenic for man are called *Hartmannella* or *Acanthamoeba.* Several species have been described under the generic name *Hartmannella,* a term which will be used pending further clarification of their taxonomy. These amebae have been grown in monkey kidney and other tissue cultures, and some animals, including primates, experience both fatal and nonfatal infections when inoculated with species of *Hartmannella.* More importantly, a number of human cases of fatal meningitis have been caused by *Hartmannella* species. Three fatal cases occurred in boys following their swimming in two small, warm, Florida lakes. Similar organisms were cultured from the lakes. Seven fatal cases of meningoencephalitis occurred in July 1951, 1952, and 1966 in the vicinity of Richmond, Virginia. Each patient had been swimming in nearby lakes. A diagnosis of purulent meningitis was usually made, and the spinal fluids had leukocyte counts ranging from 870 to 21,450, mostly granulocytes. Protein was elevated and glucose was diminished. No bacteria were demonstrated either on smear or culture. Treatment with various antibiotics and sulfonamides was to no avail. The final diagnoses were made from the microscopic examination of the brains. Within a 4-year period, 16 fatal cases of amebic meningoencephalitis were identified in northern Bohemia. The age range was from eight to twenty-five years, and no patients responded to treatment with antibiotics and sulfonamides. All patients had been swimming in an indoor pool with chlorinated water maintained at 24°C. The average incubation period was about 7 days. The clinical courses of these and other cases have lasted from 1 to 8 days. The histologic examination often suggests that infection of the brain was by way of the nose.

Several new "viruses" have been demonstrated to be *Hartmannella* species. Wang and Feldman reported the isolation of 54 strains (three species) of *Hartmannella* in tissue cultures inoculated with pharyngeal swabs that had been obtained from members of a population of "normal" families which is under continuous surveillance for respiratory infections. Most isolates were obtained from young children, often less than one year of age. Several families had multiple isolations. No evident relationship could be established between the presence of amebae and clinical disease.

The treatment of human cases of amebic meningoencephalitis with antibiotics and sulfonamides has been unsuccessful. Emetine was not very effective against the free-living amoebae in vitro, but carbarsone, a pentavalent arsenical seemed to affect them adversely. A clinical trial with this drug may be warranted should an infection of this type be recognized or suspected.

It is not possible at this time to define the spectrum of human illness which may be caused by *Hartmannella*

but it is very likely that these organisms will increase in importance.

REFERENCES

Amebiasis

Belding, D. L., and H. W. Brown: "Basic Clinical Parasitology," New York, Appleton-Century-Crofts, Inc., 1964.

Kessel, J. F., W. P. Lewis, C. M. Pasquel, and J. A. Turner: Indirect Hemagglutination and Complement Fixation Tests in Amebiasis, Am. J. Trop. Med. Hyg., 14:540, 1965.

Lamont, N. McE., and N. R. Pooler: Hepatic Amoebiasis, Quart. J. Med., 27:389, 1958.

Powell, S. J., A. J. Wilmot, and R. Elsdon-Dew: Further Trials of Metronidazole in Amebic Dysentery and Amebic Liver Abscess., Ann. Trop. Med. Parasit., 61:511, 1967.

Powell, S. J., A. J. Wilmot, I. Macleod, and R. Elsdon-Dew: A Comparative Trial of Dehydroemetine, Emetine Hydrochloride, and Chloroquin in the Treatment of Amebic Liver Abscess., Ann. Trop. Med. Parasit., 59:496, 1965.

Wilmot, A. J.: "Clinical Amoebiasis," Philadelphia, F. A. Davis Company, 1962.

Hartmannella

Butt, C. G.: Primary Amebic Meningoencephalitis, New Engl. J. Med., 274:1473, 1966.

Callicott, J. H., Jr.: Amebic Meningoencephalitis Due to Free-living Amebas of the Hartmannella (Acanthamoeba)-Naegleria Group, Am. J. Clin. Path., 49:84, 1968.

Cerva, L., and K. Novak: Amoebic Meningoencephalitis: Sixteen Fatalities, Science, 160:92, 1968.

Culbertson, C. G.: Pathogenic Acanthamoeba (Hartmannella), Am. J. Clin. Path., 35:195, 1961.

Wang, S. S., and H. A. Feldman: Isolation of Hartmannella Species from Human Throats, New Engl. J. Med., 277:174, 1967.

241 MALARIA

James J. Plorde and Ivan L. Bennett, Jr.

DEFINITION. Malaria is a protozoan disease transmitted to man by the bite of *Anopheles* mosquitoes. It remains the major infectious disease problem in the world. The increasing import of malaria into the United States by travelers and military personnel has caused a resurgence of interest in this disease. Malaria is characterized by rigors, fever, splenomegaly, anemia, and a chronic, relapsing course.

ETIOLOGY. The causative organisms are protozoa of the genus *Plasmodium.* The four species known to infect man do not produce disease in lower animals, although many species affecting animals and birds are known. *Plasmodium vivax* causes tertian malaria; *P. malariae* causes quartan malaria; *P. falciparum* causes malignant tertian (estivoautumnal) malaria; *P. ovale* causes ovale tertian malaria, a relatively rare and mild illness.

Man is the intermediate and the mosquito the definitive host. In man, after a stage of exoerythrocytic development in the liver, the parasites reproduce asexually in circulating erythrocytes. They first appear in the red cells as *ring forms;* after several divisions, daughter cells (*merozoites*) fill the corpuscle, which ruptures and releases them (sporulation) to parasitize additional erythrocytes. With repetition of this cycle, some of the red cells become filled with sexual forms (*gametocytes*); these do not induce cell lysis and are unable to undergo further development unless ingested by an appropriate mosquito during a blood meal. In the stomach of the mosquito fertilization occurs, and the resulting *ookinete* encysts on the outer surface of the stomach and releases myriads of *sporozoites*. These migrate to the salivary glands and, if inoculated into a human subject, lead to repetition of asexual multiplication. There is variation in this cycle among different species, and several intermediate stages occur.

The asexual cycle in the erythrocyte requires 36 to 48 hr for *P. falciparum*, 48 hr for *P. vivax* and *P. ovale*, and 72 hr for *P. malariae*. The periodicity of febrile paroxysms in infections by the different species coincides with the cyclic discharge of merozoites. The incubation period between bite of an infected mosquito and onset of symptoms is 10 to 14 days in vivax and falciparum malaria and 18 days to 6 weeks in quartan infections. There is good evidence for the existence of several strains of each species of human malarial *Plasmodium,* and greater virulence of some strains is suggested by the consistent severity of the clinical illnesses which they produce.

EPIDEMIOLOGY. Malaria survives only in areas where the mosquito and the infected human populations remain above a *critical density* for each. These critical densities are interdependent, but either may fluctuate in a given area. Control measures are directed toward reducing both populations to levels that are too low for the infection to survive. Important procedures include drainage or filling of breeding areas, use of residual insecticide sprays (this has largely replaced the use of oil or other antilarval measures), screening, use of skin repellents, effective treatment of cases, and large-scale suppressive drug programs in some human populations.

An active international cooperative program aimed at the eradication of malaria has resulted in a significant decline in the incidence of the disease since 1945. In over three-quarters of the original malarial areas of the world, the disease has been eradicated or active eradication programs have been instituted. The presence of mobile populations, outdoor biting mosquitoes, and high levels of disease transmission make successful eradication in the remaining areas less certain. Furthermore, the emergence of insecticide-resistant mosquitoes and drug-resistant parasites as well as a variety of administrative problems have produced serious setbacks to several previously successful eradication programs. The demonstration of naturally occurring simian malaria in man has raised the question of an animal reservoir of the disease. Although this may not prove to be a major problem, the global eradication of malaria remains today a distant goal.

PATHOGENESIS AND PATHOLOGY. The invasion, alteration, and destruction of red cells by malaria parasites, systemic and local circulatory changes, and immune phenomena are probably all important in the pathophysiology of malaria. Malaria species differ significantly in their ability to invade red cells. *Plasmodium vivax* and *P. ovale* attack only immature erythrocytes and *P. malariae,* only senescent ones. During infection with these species, therefore, no more than 1 or 2 percent of cells are involved at any one time. *Plasmodium falciparum* invades red cells regardless of age and may cause extremely high levels of parasitemia. Only the presence of certain abnormal hemoglobins, notably S, is capable of limiting parasitemia produced by the species. Whether the same protective effect is exerted in hemoglobin C, thalassemia, and G-6-PD deficiency awaits confirmation.

Once parasitized, the cells may be destroyed at the time of sporulation or phagocytosed in the liver or spleen. In the spleen the parasites are also removed from some cells, and the intact erythrocytes are returned into the circulation. However, anemia usually develops, and in the case of falciparum malaria, may be severe. This species also induces physical changes in parasitized cells resulting in intravascular agglutination and sludging.

Although paroxysms of fever coincide with sporulation and the destruction of red cells, the cause of the fever remains obscure and may be related to release of an endogenous pyrogen from injured cells.

The circulatory changes in malaria are characterized by vasoconstriction during the "cold" stage followed by vasodilation during the "hot" stage. In falciparum malaria vasodilation in the skin is accompanied by hypotension, decreased central venous pressure, increased radioiodinated serum albumin space, and increased excretion of aldosterone, suggesting a decrease in effective circulating blood volume due to enhanced vascular permeability and/or capacitance. On the other hand, there may be localized vasospasm, obstruction of capillaries with agglutinated red cells, and intravascular coagulation which may compromise perfusion to vital organs such as the kidney, brain, liver, and lung.

Normal as well as parasitized red cells are destroyed in malaria. This phenomenon occurs in all forms but is most profound during blackwater fever. Hypersplenism results in erythrophagocytosis but there is also evidence that immune mechanisms may be operative in excess red cell destruction and renal disease. Host gamma and beta-1C-globulin deposits have been noted along the glomerular capillary basement membrane of patients with the nephrosis of quartan malaria.

Negroes seem to be peculiarly resistant to *P. vivax* infection; the mechanism for this is unknown.

Immunity in malaria is mediated by species specific IgG and IgM antibodies which appear early in malaria infection in response to the erythrocytic phase of parasitemia. These antibodies have an antiplasmodial effect. The relative rarity of malaria in young infants has been attributed to transplacental passage of IgG antibodies. While immunity in malaria has been thought to be strain specific, different strains appear to share common antigens. Furthermore, there appear to be antigenic changes in the parasites during chronic simian malaria which may provide an explanation for the relapsing course of malarial infection.

MANIFESTATIONS. General. There is some variation in malaria produced by the different plasmodia, but in all, chills, fever, headache, muscle pains, splenomegaly, and anemia are common. Herpes labialis is frequent and usually appears after the infection is well established. Hepatomegaly, mild icterus, and edema are often observed, especially in estivoautumnal infections. Urticaria is common in patients with chronic malaria.

The hall mark of the disease is the malarial *paroxysm*, which recurs regularly in all but falciparum infections. The typical paroxysm begins with a rigor that lasts 20 to 60 min—the "cold stage"—followed by a "hot stage" of 3 to 8 hr with temperature of 104 to 107°F. The "wet stage" consists of defervescence with profuse diaphoresis and leaves the patient exhausted.

First attacks are often severe, but repeated episodes become milder, although debilitation may be progressive. In untreated cases, the attacks may persist for weeks. The paroxysms eventually become more irregular and less frequent and finally cease, corresponding with the disappearance of parasites from the blood and marking the end of the primary attack. Relapses occur when exo-erythrocytic parasites persisting in the liver reinvade the bloodstream.

Tertian Malaria (P. vivax or P. ovale). This infection is rarely fatal, although relapses are common, and it is the most difficult to cure. A prodrome of myalgia, headache, chilliness, and low-grade fever for 48 to 72 hr heralds the onset of the acute illness. Initially, the fever may be irregular because the maturation cycle of the parasite is not synchronized. Synchronization usually occurs toward the end of the first week, and typical paroxysms then occur on alternate days. The spleen becomes palpable at the end of the second week. Infections with *P. ovale* tend to be milder, and primary attacks shorter than those caused by *P. vivax*.

Quartan Malaria (P. malariae). Paroxysms occur every third day and tend to be regular. The disease is usually more disabling than tertian but responds well to treatment. Edema, albuminuria, and hematuria (*not* hemoglobinuria), a clinical state similar to acute hemorrhagic nephritis, occasionally appear during the course. This complication should not be confused with *blackwater fever*. Chronic *P. malariae* infection may be associated with nephrosis, which is poorly understood.

Estivoautumnal Malaria (P. falciparum). Because of an asynchronous cycle of multiplication, the onset may be insidious and fever continuous, remittent or irregular. Typical paroxysms occur in a minority of patients. Splenomegaly occurs rapidly and mental confusion, postural hypotension, edema and gastrointestinal symptoms are common. If the acute attack is treated rapidly, the disease is usually mild and recovery uneventful. If left untreated anemia becomes severe, and the decreased effective circulating blood volume results in capillary blockage that can give rise to serious complications. This feature of *P. falci-*

parum infections accounts for the protean manifestations of estivoautumnal malaria, and the high morbidity and mortality associated with it. Depending upon the organ system involved, several so-called *pernicious syndromes* are seen. *Cerebral malaria* can lead to hemiplegia, convulsions, delirium, hyperpyrexia, coma, and rapid death. When the *pulmonary* circulation is involved, there may be cough and blood-streaked sputum, leading to confusion with many other diseases of the lung. The splanchnic capillaries can be obstructed, with consequent vomiting, abdominal pain, diarrhea, or melena. Such patients are sometimes thought to have bacillary dysentery or cholera. Fever in these disorders may be low or absent. Indeed, in patients with predominantly gastrointestinal manifestations, there are usually cold clammy skin, hypotension, profound weakness, and repeated syncopal attacks, so-called *algid malaria*. Tender hepatomegaly, with or without jaundice, and acute renal failure are common. The pernicious syndromes should be anticipated if more than 5 per cent of red cells are parasitized.

Blackwater Fever. This is a disorder that occurs in association with malaria, particularly and perhaps only with *P. falciparum* infections. The usual attack begins with a rigor and fever followed by massive intravascular hemolysis, icterus, hemoglobinuria, collapse, and often acute renal failure and uremia. The pathologic findings in the kidney are necrosis of tubules and occasionally hemoglobin casts. The mortality is 20 to 30 percent, and survivors are very likely to experience hemolytic episodes with subsequent malarial infections.

Although blackwater fever is often classified as one of the "pernicious" complications of estivoautumnal malaria, its etiology is obscure. In many patients, parasitemia is absent at the time hemolysis occurs. Because blackwater fever has usually occurred in patients with chronic falciparum infections who were treated with quinine, it was suggested that the hemolysis results from an autoimmune reaction to the red cells that have been altered by the drug or parasite or both. However, blackwater fever can occur in patients not given drugs. The institution of an appropriate regimen for acute renal failure (Chap. 300) will reduce the fatality rate considerably.

Complications. In addition to the several complications already mentioned, others deserve comment. Rupture of the spleen is relatively rare, but malaria is by far the commonest cause of spontaneous rupture and predisposes to traumatic rupture of this organ.

Chronic malaria or repeated infection in an endemic area leads to anemia, debility, and cachexia. Secondary bacterial infection is often the immediate cause of death. Bacillary dysentery, cholera, and pyogenic pneumonia are common. Tuberculous foci often extend in malarial patients, and miliary tuberculosis is occasionally observed.

LABORATORY FINDINGS. The blood leukocyte count is low or normal. The erythrocyte sedimentation rate is elevated. Plasmodia are demonstrable in smears of peripheral blood from the vast majority of patients with symptomatic malaria. When the disease is suspected, appropriately stained blood films should be examined diligently. For the inexperienced examiner, a thin smear of fingertip blood on a clean glass slide should be stained with Wright, Giemsa, or Hastings stain. Parasitized erythrocytes are most frequent at the edges of a smear; extracellular parasites are not found. Thick smears should be thoroughly dried and stained with diluted Giemsa or Field stain. This method has the advantage of concentrating the parasites, but artefacts are numerous, and correct interpretation of these preparations requires much experience.

The morphology of the four species of plasmodia that infect man is specific enough to allow identification in blood smears. The parasitized red cells in *P. vivax* infections are enlarged, pale, and may contain diffuse bright red dots (Schaffner's dots), and the parasite presents in a wide variety of shapes and sizes; in *P. ovale* infections, the red cells containing parasites are oval but otherwise resemble those in *P. vivax*; in *P. malariae* the red cells are of normal size and do not contain dots. The parasites often present in "band" forms and the merozoites are arranged in a rosette around central pigment; in *P. falciparum* infections the rings are very small, may contain two rather than one chromatin dot, and often are found lying flat against the margin of the cell. Only the ring stages of the asexual forms are found in the peripheral smear, and there may be more than one ring in a single red cell. The gametocytes are distinctively large and banana-shaped.

There is no advantage over blood of material obtained by splenic or sternal puncture. The administration of epinephrine with the idea of dislodging parasites by producing contraction of the spleen has been advocated, but results are irregular. Serologic tests are used primarily for epidemiologic rather than diagnostic purposes.

DIAGNOSIS. The most important diagnostic test is the search for parasites in peripheral blood. Because the intensity of parasitemia varies greatly from hour to hour, particularly in *P. falciparum* infections, blood smears should be examined repeatedly and at frequent intervals. History of residence in an endemic area, previous attacks of malaria, typical malarial paroxysms, or some artificial exposure (blood transfusion, narcotic injections in an addict) should suggest the disease. Splenomegaly is an almost invariable finding during the second week of illness. Leukocytosis is *not* a feature of malaria.

While final cure of malaria may be difficult, particularly in *P. vivax* infections, almost all cases will respond symptomatically to quinine or one of the newer antimalarial drugs, and failure of response to a therapeutic trial argues strongly against the diagnosis.

TREATMENT. The use of appropriate chemotherapy can suppress symptoms in individuals exposed in endemic areas or cure malarial infection completely. The emergence of drug-resistent falciparum malaria in Brazil, Colombia, Venezuela, and Southeast Asia, however, necessitates the use of drug combinations in the treatment of this infection.

Treatment of Acute Attack. Treatment of an acute attack can be accomplished with chloroquine for all types of malaria except drug-resistant falciparum infection. Administration of 0.6 Gm of chloroquine base (four tablets) followed by 0.3 Gm 6 hr later and then 0.3 Gm daily for 2 days usually produces complete subsidence of symptoms and destruction of the erythrocytic forms of the parasite. If vomiting is present, chloroquine hydrochloride should be given intramuscularly in dosage of 0.2 to 0.3 Gm of base every 6 hr. Oral therapy should be resumed as soon as possible.

If the patient has contracted malaria in an area known to harbor drug-resistant *P. falciparum*, he should be treated with a combination of quinine, pyrimethamine, and one of the sulfonamides or sulfones. *Quinine sulfate,* 0.6 Gm orally three times a day, should be given for 14 days. If nausea and vomiting preclude oral therapy, quinine dihydrochloride diluted in saline or glucose can be given very slowly intravenously. The dose may be repeated every 6 hr, but oral therapy should be instituted as soon as possible. In the presence of renal failure, the dose of quinine should be limited to 0.6 Gm a day, and the drug should not be given if acute massive hemolysis occurs. An overdose of quinine produces cinchonism of which tinnitus is an early manifestation. The drug may also cause mild hemolysis, allergic purpura, and drug fever. Pyrimethamine should be given orally in dosage of 25 mg three times daily for 3 days. This is an antifolate agent and may cause megaloblastic anemia. Sulfisoxazole, 2.0 Gm initially and then 0.5 Gm every 6 hr for 5 days should be given concurrently with the other 2 drugs. Pyrimethamine with a sulfonamide may be as effective as the three-drug regimen but acts more slowly.

Patients should be followed for 1 month to detect recrudescence of the infection, and if there is evidence of recurrence, retreatment with pyrimethamine and a sulfonamide should be instituted.

Radical Cure. *Plasmodium vivax, P. ovale,* and *P. malariae* all persist in the liver in the exoerythrocytic stage and in this form are not affected by drugs used in the treatment of the acute attack. Unless destroyed, they will eventually reinvade the bloodstream. Primaquine base 15 mg by mouth daily for 14 days will effect a radical cure in most cases. If relapse occurs after primaquine therapy, a second course of the drug should be given. This agent may cause hemolysis in patients with G-6-PD deficiency, but in the dosage recommended hemolysis is rare and usually mild.

Treatment of Complications. This includes careful attention to fluid and electrolyte balance, prevention of fluid overload in patients with oliguria, and early diagnosis and treatment of renal failure. In severe hemolysis large doses of steroids may be helpful in combating hemolysis. Transfusions should be given in severe hemolysis, care being taken to match the patient's cells and plasma with that of the recipient. Dexamethasone has been helpful in management of cerebral edema.

Suppressive Therapy. Although it is not possible to prevent infection with chemotherapeutic agents, it is possible to suppress symptoms while residing in an endemic area by the administration of chloroquine base in dosage of 300 mg weekly (2 tablets Aralen). If the medication is continued for 1 month after leaving the area, sensitive strains of *P. falciparum* will be eradicated. *Plasmodium ovale, P. malariae,* and *P. vivax* will produce clinical manifestations some weeks or months after chloroquine is discontinued because of their persistence outside red cells. This can be circumvented by administration of primaquine after chloroquine is discontinued. Chloroquine is not effective in suppressing drug-resistant *P. falciparum.*

REFERENCES

Blount, R. E.: Management of Chloroquine-Resistant Falciparum Malaria, A.M.A. Arch. Intern. Med., 119:557, 1967.

Conrad, M. E.: Pathophysiology of Malaria: Hematologic Observations in Human and Animal Studies, Ann. Int. Med., 70:134, 1969.

Dukes, D. C., B. J. Sealey, and J. I. Forbes: Oliguric Renal Failure in Blackwater Fever, Am. J. Med., 45:899, 1968.

Hunter, G. W., W. W. Frye, and J. C. Swartzwelder: "A Manual of Tropical Medicine," 4th ed., Philadelphia, W. B. Saunders Company, 1966.

Maegrath, B. G.: The Physiologic Approach to the Problems of Malaria, Brit. Med. Bull., 8:28, 1951.

Malloy, J. P., M. H. Brooks, and K. G. Barry: Pathophysiology of Acute Falciparum Malaria, Am. J. Med., 43:745, 1967.

Neva, F. A.: Malaria—Recent Progress and Problems, New Engl. J. Med., 277:1241, 1967.

Russell, P. F., L. S. West, R. D. Manwell, and G. MacDonald: "Practical Malarialogy," 2d ed., Fairlawn, N.J., Oxford University Press, 1963.

242 LEISHMANIASIS

*James J. Plorde and
Ivan L. Bennett, Jr.*

DEFINITION. Leishmaniasis designates three separate disorders of man that are produced by protozoa of the genus *Leishmania.* All are transmitted by the bite of sandflies (*Phlebotomus*).

ETIOLOGY AND PATHOGENESIS. There is confusion over speciation of *Leishmania.* These organisms appear morphologically identical and must be differentiated by serologic techniques which are not entirely satisfactory. There are antigenic differences among various strains of *Leishmania* species, but the significance of these differences is not known. Four species are generally recognized: *L. donovani, L. tropica, L. mexicana,* and *L. brasiliensis.* Two others, *L. peruviana* and *L. pifanoi,* are thought to be variations of *L. brasiliensis.*

Leishmania donovani is the cause of kala-azar, the visceral form of leishmaniasis (dumdum fever, tropical splenomegaly, Burdwan fever, Sirkari disease, *Ponos, Mard el Bicha*).

Leishmania tropica causes Old World cutaneous leishmaniasis or oriental sore, also known as Delhi boil, Bagdad boil, Aleppo button, and Salek and Pendeh sore.

Leishmania mexicana produces a cutaneous leishmania-sis known as forest yaws, bay sore, and *chiclero ulcer.* *Leishmania brasiliensis* is the cause of American mucocutaneous leishmaniasis also known as *espundia. Leishmania brasiliensis* (var.) *peruviana* produces *uta,* another type of cutaneous leishmaniasis, and *Leishmaniasis tegumentaria diffusa* is caused by *L. brasiliensis* (var.) *pifanoi.*

In the sandfly, the parasites assume the flagellated leptomonas form, but in man, the organisms lose their flagella, enter mononuclear phagocytes, and multiply as small, rounded leishmanial forms 2 to 3 μ in diameter, the pathognomonic "Leishman-Donovan bodies."

In man continued intracellular multiplication of the parasite leads to rupture of the affected phagocyte and invasion of other cells, resulting in extensive histiocytic proliferation which is followed by infiltration with plasma cells and lymphocytes. The course of the disease from this point is apparently determined by the host's immunologic reaction, which is poorly understood. In cutaneous leishmaniasis the secondary cellular infiltration is associated with a reduction in the number of parasites, the development of a delayed skin (leishmanin) reaction, and spontaneous cure. In the mucocutaneous form, the spontaneous disappearance of the primary lesion may be followed by destructive metastatic mucocutaneous lesions at some later date. An interesting exception to the general pattern in cutaneous disease is *leishmaniasis tegumentaria diffusa* in which there is no infiltration of lymphocytes and plasma cells, the leishmanin reaction is negative, and the skin lesions become chronic, progressive and disseminated. In visceral leishmaniasis, the cellular changes are similar to those seen in cutaneous disease. However, the skin test remains negative, and the parasites spread to reticuloendothelial cells throughout the body. This spread is associated with development of marked hyperglobulinemia. Circulating antibodies which are rarely seen in cutaneous forms of the disease are detectable but do not seem to have a protective function. A positive skin test develops in the visceral form after successful treatment.

KALA-AZAR

DISTRIBUTION AND EPIDEMIOLOGY. Kala-azar occurs in China, Russia, India, Egypt, Sudan, East Africa, several Mediterranean countries, including Greece, Crete, and Malta, and a few areas of South and Central America. Although the manifestations of the disease throughout this area, which touches all continents but Australia, are basically similar, certain definite peculiarities in its behavior justify classification of visceral leishmaniasis into at least three main types. These differences are attributed to variations in the strains of *L. donovani* in a given area and, perhaps more important, to the length of time that the disease has been endemic in a population. It is believed that kala-azar (and also infection by *L. tropica*) is introduced into a new area from animal reservoirs and that this "primitive" or zoonotic infection is likely to result in many cases of acute, rapidly fatal illness among the population coming into contact with the parasites for the first time. After generations, kala-azar becomes endemic, the disease assumes a more chronic form, and the main or only reservoir of infection, especially in urban areas, is man.

Mediterranean, or *infantile*, *kala-azar* is primarily a disease of children under the age of two years and has its reservoir in dogs, jackals, and foxes. Adults are by no means spared, but the preceding sentence describes the predominant pattern of the disorder as it occurs in the Mediterranean area, China, Russia, and Latin America.

Indian kala-azar shows no special predilection for infants and has never been found in dogs or other animals in India, indicating that the human reservoir is responsible for perpetuation of the disease.

Sudanese, or *Egyptian*, *kala-azar* shows no predilection for children, is endemic in gerbils and other rodents in many areas, and is more resistant to therapy with antimony compounds than that found in the rest of the world.

MANIFESTATIONS. The incubation period varies from 10 days to 1 year but is usually about 3 months. No lesion appears at the site of the infecting bite in most cases, but a primary "chancre" which heals with scarring before the onset of systemic symptoms is commonly noted in the African disease. The organisms multiply extensively in the macrophages of spleen, liver, bone marrow, and lymph nodes, accounting for many of the manifestations of the disease. Organisms may be found in the blood for several months before the onset of symptoms.

Fever, which is characterized at times by two daily spikes, may be abrupt or gradual in onset. It persists for 1 to 6 weeks and then disappears only to reappear at irregular intervals during the course of the illness. Although prostration is absent even during periods of high fever, there is progressive weakness, pallor, weight loss, and tachycardia. Gastrointestinal disturbances are frequent in Indian cases. Physical findings include enormous splenomegaly, lymphadenopathy, hepatomegaly, and often, edema, which tends to conceal the extent of the wasting. The proliferation of parasite-loaded histiocytes in the bone marrow and in the enlarged spleen make anemia the rule, and thrombocytopenia with gingival and other mucosal bleeding is common. The peripheral leukocyte count is low (usually less than 4,000 per cu mm); in children, granulocytosis with cancrum oris (noma) and secondary pulmonary or intestinal infections contribute to the high mortality.

Hyperglobulinemia is universally present. Proteinuria and hematuria are frequent in the course of kala-azar, and symptoms of heart failure can occur terminally; uremia due to renal amyloidosis may complicate chronic cases.

DIAGNOSIS. The diagnosis is made by finding leishmania in stained preparations of blood (often possible in Indian but rarely so in Sudanese kala-azar), bone marrow, lymph nodes, or material obtained by hepatic or splenic puncture. The last is the best source of

organisms, but the spleen should be needled only by an expert. The organisms will grow out as flagellated forms in simple media containing blood incubated at 28°C.

A complement fixation test using an antigen from *Mycobacterium phlei* gives positive results in 95 percent of patients with kala-azar, but tuberculosis gives positive test results also. Fluorescent antibody and indirect hemagglutination tests with leishmanial antigens are more specific but are not generally available. The leishmanin skin test is negative during active kala-azar but becomes positive several months after successful treatment of the disease.

TREATMENT. Rest, good diet, transfusions, and treatment of complicating infections, of which tuberculosis, bacterial pneumonia, amebiasis, and bacillary dysentery are the more important, must supplement or precede specific therapy. Pentavalent antimony compounds are highly effective against the parasites. Neostibosan, as a 25 percent solution, can be given intravenously or intramuscularly on alternate days. A total of 3 to 4 Gm in 10 injections is needed. Urea stibamine is popular in India. Solustibosan, neostam, and Pentostam are effective antimony compounds that come as permanently stable solutions in ampuls for injection.

More than 90 percent of cases respond promptly to antimony, except in Africa, where the cure rate is as low as 70 percent. Resistant cases should be treated with 2 percent pentamidine (two courses of 5 to 10 intravenous or intramuscular injections each of 2 to 4 mg per kg on alternate days) or with the more effective hydroxystilbamidine given intravenously as 10 daily injections of a fresh solution in dosage of 0.25 Gm daily. The course may have to be repeated in African Kala-azar. Amphotericin B has been effective in some cases.

POST-KALA-AZAR DERMAL LEISHMANIASIS. Patients treated successfully with antimony compounds for kala-azar may later develop cutaneous lesions called "leishmanoids," in which *Leishmania* are demonstrable. These are rare in Mediterranean or Chinese kala-azar. They occur after a latent period of 1 to 2 years in as many as 10 percent of Indian cases, and in 30 percent of Sudanese cases, they occur almost immediately after systemic symptoms subside. The lesions range from patchy areas of depigmentation to erythematous papules and confluent nodules which may involve the ears and mucous membranes and have been mistaken for leprosy.

Antimony will cure these dermal leishmanoids, but the response is slow.

PROGNOSIS AND CONTROL. The mortality in untreated kala-azar is 95 percent in adults and 80 percent in children. This has been greatly reduced by treatment with antimony and the aromatic diamidines.

The treatment of the disease in man, the elimination of diseased dogs, and the use of DDT residual sprays against sandflies are the important preventive measures. Incidence of the disease has diminished greatly in many areas where DDT has been used to eradicate malaria—an unexpected added benefit of this program. When the vectors are exophilic, control is difficult. Attempts at vaccination with avirulent strains of *L. donovani* have been unsuccessful.

AMERICAN CUTANEOUS LEISHMANIASIS

These diseases occur in every country of Central and South America except Chile. In some areas, 10 to 20 percent of the population are infected. There are four varieties of American cutaneous leishmaniasis. All begin with a local lesion at the site of the infecting sandfly bite after an incubation period of from 10 days to 3 months.

Chiclero ulcer, which is found in Mexico, Panama, British Honduras, and Brazil is a zoonosis caused by *L. mexicana.* The disease occurs naturally in several arboreal rodents. It is occasionally transmitted to men entering forests to harvest chicle. The disease is characterized by lesions on the ear which are chronic, show little ulceration, and lead to deformities through scarring. The leishmanin skin test is positive. Spontaneous healing is the rule, and parasites are never numerous in the lesions. Mucosal ulceration does not occur. Successful treatment with both metranidazole and cycloguanil pamoate (which may also be useful as a chemoprophylactic agent) has been reported.

Uta, which occurs in cooler climates and at altitudes of more than 2,000 ft, consists of single or multiple skin ulcers in which parasites are readily demonstrable. Spontaneous healing within 3 months to a year is the rule, and mucosal spread is unusual. The etiologic agent is *L. brasiliensis* (var.) *peruviana,* and the reservoir is the domestic dog. With widespread use of insecticides in Peru, the disease has almost disappeared.

In tropical Latin America, *L. brasiliensis* causes the better-known and more serious *espundia.* The epidemiology of the lesion is poorly defined. The initial skin lesion enlarges progressively, and secondary bacterial infection is frequent. The disease may spread by direct extension or by lymphatics to the mucosal surfaces of the mouth and nose where, after the primary lesion has healed, painful, destructive, and mutilating erosions scar and distort the involved structures. Fever, anemia, and weight loss accompany these mucosal complications. Destruction of the nasal septum produces a characteristic deformity called *tapir nose* or *camel nose.* The hard palate may be destroyed, and largyngeal erosion can lead to aphonia. In Negroes, the lesion is often hypertrophic, and large polypoid masses deform the lips and cheeks, perhaps representing a type of keloid reaction. This can be mistaken for South American blastomycosis (Chap. 186). Secondary bacterial infection, inanition, and respiratory obstruction lead to death.

The diagnosis is made by finding the organisms in scrapings or by culture. The leishmanin skin test is specific and highly useful. Treatment consists of antibiotics for bacterial infections and antimonials, preferably sodium antimony tartrate, which is given intravenously as 1 or 2 percent solution, the dose being increased on al-

ternate days from 0.04 Gm initially to a maximum of 0.28 Gm, until a total of 2.2 Gm has been given. Pentavalent antimonials and Amphotericin B have also been used with some success in this disease.

The early lesions respond well, but even with repeated courses of antimony, the mucosal complications of the espundia type heal slowly; in advanced cases, the prognosis is very poor.

Leishmaniasis tegumentaria diffusa is caused by *L. brasiliensis* (var.) *pifanoi.* This remarkable disease is characterized by massive dissemination of skin lesions without visceral involvement. The clinical picture often bears a striking resemblance to lepromatous leprosy (Chap. 175). The diagnosis is not difficult because the lesion contains large numbers of organisms. In contrast to all other types of cutaneous leishmaniasis, the leishmanin skin test is negative. A similar disease caused by *L. tropica* has been described in Ethiopia. The disease is progressive and very refractory to treatment. Glucantime, amphotericin B, and pentamidine have been used to reduce remissions but cure is rare.

OLD WORLD CUTANEOUS LEISHMANIASIS: ORIENTAL SORE

This, the least serious form of human leishmaniasis, consists of localized cutaneous ulceration which heals spontaneously and is endemic in the European countries bordering the eastern Mediterranean, in North Africa, Asia Minor, Southwest Asia, and India. Two major strains of the causative organism, *L. tropica,* produce similar but distinctive clinical syndromes. Homologous immunity after recovery from infection by either strain is solid and lifelong. Infection with *L. tropica* (var.) *major* protects against *L. tropica* (var.) *minor,* but the opposite is not the case. The rural or moist type, caused by (var.) *major,* has its reservoir in gerbils and other small rodents; the ulcers usually appear on the extremities 2 to 6 weeks after the bite of the sandfly and are accompanied by regional lymphadenopathy in a majority of cases. Spontaneous healing occurs within 3 to 6 months, leaving a depigmented, pitted scar.

The incubation period in the *urban,* or *dry,* type ranges from 2 months to more than a year. The lesion is usually facial and begins as a pruritic, purplish nodule (the "Aleppo button"), which slowly enlarges and finally breaks down after 3 or 4 months. Healing of the indolent, granulomatous ulcer may require a year or more; lymphatic involvement is uncommon. Man is the only known reservoir of infection.

The typical oriental sore is a sharply punched-out, ragged ulcer about 1 in. in diameter, surrounded by an erythematous rim. Satellite lesions which fuse with the original are not rare. The center of the granulating base of the ulcer frequently contains a hard excrescence called the *Montpellier sign* or the *rake* beneath which the parasites are most likely to be found when scrapings are examined.

The wet and dry types occur together in Asia Minor;

indeed, it is not rare to find simultaneous infections in the same patient. In Africa, Southeastern Europe, and India, only the dry type is prevalent.

Diagnosis is usually made on clinical grounds and is confirmed by finding the parasites, which occur both intra- and extracellularly. Pyogenic infection makes direct visualization difficult, but *L. tropica* can be cultured in Novy-MacNeal-Nicolle medium at room temperature, and a skin test using *L. tropica* antigen becomes positive in the vast majority of patients with the disease.

Treatment should include vigorous measures for bacterial infection, such as hot soaks and appropriate systemic antibiotics. Local infiltration with a 2 percent solution of berberine sulfate weekly for 3 weeks is very effective in early lesions, but nothing seems to speed the subsidence of established ulcers except control of secondary infection. Systemic antimonials may be required where ulceration is extensive or multiple. In endemic areas the custom is to withhold treatment directed against the parasite until the initial nodule ulcerates, to assure the development of immunity against reinfection.

Prevention consists of use of insect repellents on exposed parts of the body, residual DDT sprays, and fine-mesh screening for dwellings. The lesions should be covered to prevent infection of vectors and, of course, contact with the lesion or its discharges should be avoided.

In Asia Minor, a relapsing form known as *leishmaniasis recidiva* is common. Nodules appear at the periphery of the scarred area and mimic lupus vulgaris so closely that errors in diagnosis are very frequent.

REFERENCES

Adler, S.: Immunology of Leishmaniasis, Israel J. Med. Sci., 1:9, 1965.

Convit, J., and F. Kerdel-Vegas: Disseminated Cutaneous Leishmaniasis, Arch. Dermatol., 91:439, 1965.

Faust, E. C., and P. F. Russell: "Clinical Parasitology," Philadelphia, Lea & Febiger, 1964.

Hunter, G. W., W. W. Frye, and J. C. Swartzwelder: "A Manual of Tropical Medicine," 4th ed., Philadelphia, W. B. Saunders Company, 1966.

Lainson, R., and J. Strangeways-Dixon: The Epidemiology of Dermal Leishmaniasis in British Honduras, Trans. Roy. Soc. Trop. Med. Hyg., 58:316, 1964.

243 TRYPANOSOMIASIS
James J. Plorde and
Ivan L. Bennett, Jr.

DEFINITION. Trypanosomiasis designates infection produced by protozoans of the genus *Trypanosoma*. These organisms are responsible for numerous diseases in animals and for three separate disorders in man, Gambian or mid-African sleeping sickness, Rhodesian or East African sleeping sickness, and Chagas' disease in Central and South America.

ETIOLOGY. Trypanosomes are fusiform organisms, recognized by an undulating membrane which extends along the length of the cell and terminates in an anterior flagellum. The morphologic characteristics of many species are so nearly identical that they are distinguishable only by their pathogenicity for certain animals, differences in biochemical requirements, and ability to multiply in insects.

Most species are transmitted to vertebrate hosts by insects and undergo a part of their life cycle in the vector, but direct transmission between warm-blooded hosts is the rule for others. *Tryphanosoma gambiense*, the cause of mid-African sleeping sickness, is transmitted to man by riverine tsetse flies (*Glossina*), and *T. rhodesiense* (East African) by woodland tsetse flies. *Trypanosoma cruzi*, the agent of Chagas' disease, is carried by reduviid ("assassin" or "kissing") bugs, primarily those of the genera *Triatoma, Panstrongylus,* and *Rhodnius*. Transmission of the trypanosomes of sleeping sickness occurs by what is referred to as the "anterior station;" after multiplication in the intestine of the tsetse fly, the parasites migrate to the salivary glands and are discharged when a host is bitten. The agent of Chagas' disease, however, multiplies only in the gut of the vector and is discharged in the feces, infection of man occurring through contamination of the bite wound; this is transmission by the "posterior station."

Trypanosomiasis in animals is a great economic problem in many parts of the world. Indeed, it is said that an area of approximately 4 million square miles in Africa is now essentially unpopulated because of the impossibility of keeping domestic animals in these areas where tsetse flies are infected with *T. brucei*, the cause of *nagana*, a fatal disease of cattle and horses. Among the more important trypanosomal diseases of animals are *dourine* in horses and donkeys, caused by *T. equiperdum*, which is transmitted by sexual intercourse and is worldwide; *souma*, caused by *T. vivax* in horses and cattle (Africa); *surra*, caused by *T. evansi* in horses, cattle, and dogs (Asia, Australia, Madagascar); *mal de caderas*, caused by *T. equinum* in horses and cattle (South America); and *murina de caderas*, caused by *T. hippicum* in horses and mules (Central America). The epidemiology of each of the three trypanosomiases of man is discussed separately below.

GAMBIAN SLEEPING SICKNESS. This disease occurs in tropical west and central Africa, especially along the Congo River and its tributaries. Though swine and goats are suspected of harboring *T. gambiense*, man is the only known reservoir. The vectors are the palpalis group of tsetse flies that live near water, and the highest incidence of the disease is in young men, a result of increased exposure to the flies. Less than 5 percent of flies are infected, even in the most notorious endemic foci.

The disease in man has customarily been described as proceeding through several classic "stages" interspersed with periods of remission or quiescence. Actually, there is tremendous variation in the severity, symptoms, duration, and outcome of the disease, all apparently dependent upon the resistance of the host, and the many so-called types or stages of trypanosomiasis are better understood in these terms than on the basis of duration of infection alone.

The *incubation period* is usually about 2 weeks but rarely may be as long as 3 years. The infecting bite, especially in Europeans, may show an erythematous nodule with a pale halo, the *trypanosomal chancre,* which subsides gradually. The parasites multiply locally, enter lymphatics, and appear in the blood about 3 weeks after the bite of the tsetse fly. In the usual case, the patient experiences bouts of fever for months. The temperature can exceed 106°F, and during these episodes, rashes of various types are common. These may be generalized, pruritic papular eruptions or erythema nodosum. In Caucasians, a characteristic circinate erythema resembling erythema marginatum is frequent. Transient firm areas of subcutaneous edema localized to the hands, feet, or periorbital tissue may appear. Severe headache and tachycardia accompany fever and, as the illness progresses, weight loss and progressive debilitation ensue. Tender lymphadenopathy, with gradual induration of the nodes, and splenomegaly are almost invariably present. The lymph nodes of the posterior cervical triangles are especially prominent; this is referred to as *Winterbottom's sign.* Insomnia, inability to concentrate, paresthesias, and formication are frequent, and most patients demonstrate a peculiar delayed sensation to pain combined with deep, aching hyperesthesia that can be elicited by a light blow with any hard object, known as *Kerandel's sign.* The illness can terminate spontaneously after weeks or months or can drag on intermittently for years. Death is often from intercurrent infection, of which bacillary and amebic dysentery, malaria, and bacterial (often pneumococcal) pneumonia are the most important.

Eventually, the parasites enter the central nervous system, usually about 1 year after the onset of illness, although it may occur much earlier or may be delayed for as long as 8 years. Cerebral trypanosomiasis can be explosive, causing repeated convulsions or deep coma and death within a few days. Most patients show gradual progression to the classic picture of *sleeping sickness.* Although spontaneous recovery is not rare in early trypanosomiasis, untreated *sleeping sickness* is almost invariably fatal within 4 to 8 months. The patient develops a vacant expression, the eyelids droop, the lower lip hangs loosely, and it becomes more and more difficult to gain his attention or prod him to any activity. Patients will eat when offered food, but they never ask for it or engage in spontaneous conversation, and speech gradually becomes blurred and indistinct. Tremors of the hands and tongue, choreiform movements, seizures with transient paralysis, loss of sphincter control, ophthalmoplegia, extensor plantar responses, and finally death in coma, status epilepticus, or from hyperpyrexia follow inexorably.

The overall mortality of Gambian trypanosomiasis is 25 to 50 percent; with chemotherapy, this can be reduced to 5 or 10 percent.

Anemia and *hyperglobulinemia* are invariably present, and spontaneous clumping of erythrocytes in blood speci-

mens is grossly evident in many cases. The sedimentation rate is rapid, and peripheral monocytosis is frequent.

The *cerebrospinal fluid* shows mononuclear pleocytosis and increased protein content in sleeping sickness. The colloidal gold curve is tabetic. The protein content is a better index of severity of disease and therapeutic response than is the number of cells.

Fever, lymphadenopathy, Winterbottom's and Kerandel's signs, splenomegaly, and anemia in a resident of an endemic area make the clinical diagnosis relatively easy. *Irregular fever, lymphadenopathy, and especially circinate erythema in any Caucasian who has resided in Africa within 7 years should arouse suspicion of trypanosomiasis.* Although malaria, kala-azar, Hodgkin's disease, and leprosy are sometimes confused with early trypanosomiasis, the proper diagnosis usually becomes evident within a short time.

The definitive diagnosis depends upon finding the trypanosomes in the blood, aspirate of lymph node, or cerebrospinal fluid. These should be examined first in wet mounts; actively motile organisms are seen easily under high power. For final identification thin and thick blood films should be stained with Wright's or Giemsa stain. If the blood smears are negative, citrated blood should be centrifuged at 1000 rpm for 10 min and the supernatant (including the leukocytes) recentrifuged at 2000 rpm for 15 min and the sediment examined. Cerebrospinal fluid should be centrifuged at 2,000 rpm for 15 min before examination. If these methods are negative, rats or guinea pigs may be inoculated and examined after several weeks. A severalfold increase of IgM globulins is of some confirmatory value. Complement fixation and indirect fluorescent antibody tests are used in endemic areas.

Antrypol (Bayer 205, suramin) is the most effective agent before central-nervous-system involvement has occurred. The initial dose should be limited to 1.0 ml because of possible idiosyncrasy to the drug. If red cells, casts, or protein appear in the urine, therapy should be discontinued; otherwise, 10 injections at intervals of 4 to 7 days should be given, each dose consisting of 10 ml of a fresh 10 percent solution. Pentamidine given in water either intramuscularly or intravenously on alternate days for 8 to 10 injections is effective in early disease. The dose is 2 to 4 mg per kg for each injection. When the agent is given too rapidly by the intravenous route, it may cause hypotension.

Lumbar puncture should always be performed in patients who are about to undergo therapy for trypanosomiasis. If the central nervous system is involved, agents that will penetrate the blood-brain barrier must be used; for this purpose, the most effective agent is tryparsamide given intravenously as a fresh 20 percent solution in water once weekly for 8 to 15 weeks. The initial dose should consist of 1 Gm, and subsequent doses should be 2 Gm weekly. A course of injections may be repeated after a rest of 1 month. Arsenical hepatitis or dermatitis, abdominal cramps, and most important, optic atrophy may result from tryparsamide; ocular symptoms make cessation of the drug mandatory. *Antrypol* or *pen-*

tamidine should be used in conjunction with tryparsamide. *Mel B* (*Arsobal*) an arsenical derivative of BAL, is effective both in early and late cases. It can be given intravenously in dosage of 3.6 mg per kg daily for 4 days and should be followed by 4 more daily injections after an interval of 1 week. Recovery rates as high as 50 percent have followed intensive therapy in sleeping sickness.

Prevention includes use of repellents and protective clothing (gloves, head nets) in endemic areas and chemoprophylaxis with 1.0 Gm of *Antrypol* every 2 months or pentamidine 3 mg per kg every 6 months for each member of the population. Elimination of the vector is presently a hopeless undertaking in many areas. Indeed it has been easier to move whole villages out of infested areas than to eradicate tsetse flies.

RHODESIAN SLEEPING SICKNESS. This disease is found in tropical east Africa where the etiologic agent, *T. rhodesiense,* is transmitted by woodland tsetse flies. Antelopes are known reservoirs, and other wild animals are also suspected of harboring the parasite. A recent epidemic of Rhodesian sleeping sickness in Kenya was transmitted by a peridomestic tsetse which is the normal vector of Gambian disease. More than 60 percent of human infections occur in adult males. Rhodesian trypanosomiasis is a more acute and severe disease than the Gambian form, usually terminating fatally within a year. Fever is higher, emaciation more rapid, and lymphatic involvement is less evident. Death from intercurrent infection, myocarditis, or "toxemia" usually occurs before there is appreciable central-nervous-system involvement; although lethargy and somnolence are seen, the typical sleeping sickness syndrome is rare.

Rhodesian trypanosomiasis is more resistant to treatment than the Gambian disease. *Antrypol* is effective only if given within 3 weeks of the onset of symptoms; *Mel B* can be used in cases discovered too late for treatment with Antrypol; and *tryparsamide* should be given immediately if there is any evidence of neurologic disease. No drug is really effective in advanced cases.

Prevention is complicated because of the much greater problems of eradicating woodland tsetse flies than the riverine and the need to shift populations into noninfected areas. Although chronic human cases are relatively rare, the existence of animal reservoirs makes it impossible to prevent continuing infection of the vectors. Chemoprophylaxis is the same as for the Gambian disease. Individual protection with repellents, netting, etc., is, of course, important.

The disease is almost invariably fatal if untreated. Intensive treatment results in cure of about 50 percent of early cases, but this falls to 15 percent in advanced disease.

CHAGAS' DISEASE (American Trypanosomiasis). This infection occurs from Argentina and Chile to southern Mexico, where it is a major and perhaps the primary cause of heart disease in the rural areas. The etiologic agent, *T. cruzi,* has been found in "assassin" and "kissing" bugs along our southern boundaries, but very few authenticated cases are known in which the disease was acquired in the United States. Both domestic and wild animals, especially the opossum and armadillo, may serve as reservoirs for the infection in these reduviid bugs. Infection in man usually begins with acute systemic symptoms and then becomes chronic, resembling kala-azar more than the sleeping sickness of Africa. The parasites multiply intracellularly in a leishmania form, morphologically indistinguishable from the Leishman-Donovan bodies of kala-azar, but they assume the trypanosomal form in the bloodstream.

The vector attacks man at night, usually biting the face at a mucocutaneous junction (hence the name *kissing bug*), most frequently the lip or outer canthus of the eye. An erythematous nodule, the *chagoma* appears within a few days at the initial site where the parasites have gained entrance from the infected feces of the vector. Secondary nodules are sometimes seen along draining lymphatics. *After an incubation period* of 2 weeks, there is the onset of *fever* (coincident with the appearance of parasitemia, which lasts for 30 to 60 days), and a morbilliform or urticarial *skin eruption,* which subsides after a few days. Painless *unilateral palpebral edema and conjunctivitis,* known as *Romaña's sign,* may occur during the first febrile week. The parasites spread systemically, showing a predilection for histiocytes, skeletal muscle, heart muscle, and the central nervous system, resulting in generalized lymphadenopathy and hepatosplenomegaly. Myositis may be attended by extensive gelatinous edema (pseudomyxedema) of the face and trunk, and the differentiation of Chagas' disease from cretinism and endemic goiter is sometimes surprisingly difficult. When meningoencephalitis complicates the acute illness in children, the mortality is 40 percent. An extensive acute myocarditis is sometimes accompanied by pericardial effusion and can result in heart failure. The duration of this acute stage is variable. When meningoencephalitis or severe heart disease is present, the disease may end fatally in a few days or weeks. More often it resolves slowly during a several week period. Moreover, the process usually becomes chronic and slowly progressive resulting in a number of late manifestations. Most patients presenting with these late manifestations, however, deny a history of acute illness suggesting that subclinical infections often progress to chronic disease. Chronic *neurologic* manifestations including convulsions, paresis, intention tremor, and personality disorders have been reported but have been poorly documented. Better established is the role of *T. cruzi* in the genesis of *megaesophagus* and *megacolon*. The parasite evokes inflammatory changes in and around the ganglionic nerve cells resulting in dilatation and malfunction of these organs. The most important late manifestation is *heart disease,* which may affect as many as 10 percent of the rural population in endemic areas. Symptoms and signs range from arrhythmias and heart block to chronic congestive heart failure. Sudden cardiac arrest is reportedly common. At autopsy, the hearts of patients with Chagas' disease may show a peculiar herniation of the endocardium through the apical muscle bundles. There is debate whether the heart disease is caused by an inflammatory destruction of the myocardium or by a loss of ganglion cells depriving the heart of parasympathetic innervation. Both factors may be operative.

Trypanosoma cruzi is easily grown in blood broth incubated at 28°C. The technique of *xenodiagnosis* is often used in endemic areas; a laboratory-reared vector, known to be parasite-free, is allowed to feed on suspected cases, and 2 weeks later, the insect's intestinal contents are examined for parasites. Confusion sometimes arises from the finding of trypanosomes in blood. Many children in Venezuela and other South American countries are infected with a harmless species, *T. rangeli,* which produces no symptoms but may be present in the blood for many months. Utilizing both culture and xenodiagnosis repeatedly, organisms can be recovered from most acute cases and from up to 40 percent of chronic ones. Biopsy of an involved lymph node or calf muscle may reveal the organism during the initial illness when the parasites cannot be recovered from the blood. The Machado-Guerreiro test (a complement fixation reaction) is most helpful in the diagnosis of chronic cases and in survey work. Fluorescent antibody and hemagglutination inhibition tests have been introduced which may be useful.

There is *no specific treatment* for Chagas' disease. Prevention consists of using residual insecticide sprays—of which benzene hexachloride (BHC) is the most effective—on the walls of houses, the main habitat of the vectors. Reinfestation, however, may occur within a year or two of spraying.

REFERENCES

Ashcroft, M. T.: A Critical Review of the Epidemiology of Human Trypanosomiasis in Africa, Trop. Dis. Bull., 56: 1073, 1959.

Brown, H. W., and D. L. Belding.: "Basic Clinical Parsitology," 2d ed., New York, Appleton-Century-Crofts, Inc., 1964.

Duggan, A. J.: An Appraisal of the Clinical Problems of Gambian Sleeping Sickness, J. Trop. Med. Hyg., 67:268, 1959.

Hunter, G. W., W. W. Frye, and J. C. Swartzwelder: "A Manual of Tropical Medicine," 4th ed., Philadelphia, W. B. Saunders Company, 1966.

The Etiology of Chagas' Myocarditis, Lancet, 1:1150, 1965.

244 TOXOPLASMOSIS
Harry A. Feldman

DEFINITION. Toxoplasmosis is caused by *Toxoplasma gondii,* an obligate intracellular parasite which is widely distributed among mammals and birds. It is usually, but not definitely, classified as a protozoon. In man it produces either acquired (usually asymptomatic) or congenital (generally symptomatic) infections.

HISTORY. First demonstrated in 1908 by Nicolle and Manceaux in a North African rodent, the gondii, and in the same year by Splendore in Brazil, toxoplasma were proved to cause human disease in 1939 when Wolfe, Cowen, and Paige reported that several neonatal cases of fatal encephalomyelitis had resulted from congenital infections with this parasite. A few cases of acquired infection were reported subsequently, but the parasite excited interest primarily as the cause of an uncommon congenital disease. That it did more became evident following the almost simultaneous descriptions of dye, complement fixation, and skin tests; subsequently, other serologic procedures were introduced. Their application has demonstrated that toxoplasma frequently infect man and animals and that human congenital toxoplasmosis is only one aspect of its disease spectrum.

ETIOLOGY. *Toxoplasma gondii* is considered to be a protozoon, but its taxonomic classification has not been settled. All strains are antigenically similar and of the same species. The organism measures about 3 by 6 μ and may appear crescentic, oval, or round. It divides by endodyogeny and is best stained with either Wright's or Giemsa stains. Toxoplasma are unique in that they may infect any mammalian or avian cell, except nonnucleated erythrocytes. They can be maintained in mice or tissue culture or embryonated eggs but do not multiply except in the presence of living cells. Under special conditions they can be frozen and stored, but ordinary freezing kills them. Live parasites persist in cysts which can be found in any tissue, but especially, in muscle and the central nervous system.

EPIDEMIOLOGY. Serologic surveys indicate that toxoplasma infections are worldwide in distribution. With the dye test, the most sensitive indicator of antibody, it has been demonstrated that approximately 33 percent of the inhabitants of several American cities and Haiti, 63 percent of Hondurans, and 70 percent of Tahitian natives had positive tests. In contrast, 1 percent of the inhabitants of several islands off of the northern coast of Australia, 4 percent of Navajo Indians, and 11 percent of a sample of Icelanders had positive reactions. Among American military recruits, marked differences were found in the prevalence of antibodies among those originating from different areas of the United States. East Coast recruits were 20 percent positive, but only 3 and 8 percent, respectively, from the Mountain and Pacific Coast regions reacted similarly. Overall, 14 percent of the American recruits were positive in comparison with 51 and 56 percent, respectively, of Colombian and Brazilian recruits.

Two longitudinal studies of seroconversions in American families are especially informative. In the one, conducted in Cleveland, it was found that during the 10-year observation period that only four individuals who had no hemagglutinating antibodies at the start acquired them subsequently. Among a group of Syracuse families, in a 4-year period, three had seroconversions, or 1 in 2392 person-months of observation. In neither study was it possible to identify an associated clinical illness.

In animal surveys, cats, goats, guinea pigs, sheep, swine, and to a lesser extent, rabbits and pigeons often have had positive tests. It is clear from these data that toxoplasma infections are frequent in man and animals, but that there is considerable variation in their prevalence from place to place and in different species.

The pathways whereby man and animals acquire parasites generally are unknown. Human-to-human transfer seems not to occur except from mother to fetus. It has long been known that animals can acquire infections by cannibalizing other infected animals. This information may be applicable to man, since Desmonts has shown that children without antibodies acquire them following the ingestion of undercooked mutton and beef. No clinical illnesses were noted. This does not explain the route by which herbivores acquire toxoplasma. Human infections are contracted in any season and with equal frequency by the two sexes.

Recent reports that *Toxocara cati* excretes toxoplasma-infected eggs following the ingestion of toxoplasma by nematode infested cats led to the conclusion that an additional transmission system existed. Subsequently it was shown that toxocara does not participate in this chain and that the cat excretes a new resistant, infectious cyst form of toxoplasma. Whether such cysts occur in other species and their relation to the pathogenesis of toxoplasmosis remains to be determined.

CLINICAL MANIFESTATIONS. Congenital Toxoplasmosis. Congenitally infected infants may be born prematurely or at term and stillborn or alive with active disease, which can be expressed by chorioretinitis, convulsions, fever, icterus, hepatomegaly, rash, splenomegaly, and xanthochromic spinal fluid in various combinations. The newborn infant may have none of these signs, but subsequently, hydrocephaly or microcephaly, chorioretinitis, psychomotor retardation, cerebral calcifications, and convulsions may appear, either singly or in combination. A fatality rate of 11 percent was noted in one series of 141 cases of congenital toxoplasmosis. The most common residuals in congenitally affected children are chorioretinitis, cerebral calcifications, psychomotor retardation, hydro- or microcephaly, and convulsions. Any or all of these may follow other congenital infections, especially those due to cytomegalic virus (Chap. 232). The mothers of congenitally damaged offspring ordinarily are unaware of having had any specific illnesses during the pregnancy and should be advised that future pregnancies can be undertaken with confidence because a repetion will not occur. This complication only occurs in a female who happens to be pregnant when she has an asymptomatic parasitemia with her initial toxoplasma infection.

Acquired Toxoplasmosis. Although the clinical features show great variability in proved cases of acquired toxoplasmosis, certain manifestations are suggestive of this disease. Maculopapular rashes often appear soon after the clinical onset of the illness and tend to disappear in 3 to 4 days. Lymphadenopathy is common and may be so prominent as to suggest primary lymphatic disease. Encephalitis may be present alone or in combination with other manifestations. Myalgias, arthralgias, myocarditis, and pneumonitis also have been noted. Siim described a syndrome which resembles infectious mononucleosis in that lymphadenopathy and lymphocytosis with atypical lymphocytes are present, but the heterophile reactions are negative. Parasites have been demonstrated in lymph nodes removed from such patients, some of whom were afebrile.

Toxoplasma have been isolated from several cases of posterior granulomatous uveitis, presumably the result of acquired infections. The proportion of such cases which is caused by toxoplasma has not been established. In contrast to congenital chorioretinitis, which is usually bilateral, the acquired form seems to be unilateral.

The incubation period, recovery and mortality rates, average duration of illness, and the residual defects resulting from acquired toxoplasmosis are unknown. Cerebral calcifications are not found in postnatally acquired infections.

LABORATORY DIAGNOSIS. A specific diagnosis may be made by serologic methods, by demonstrating the organism in smears, or by their cultivation in mice. Toxoplasma can be identified in cerebrospinal fluid sediments with Wright's or Giemsa stains, or occasionally, in biopsied lymph node or muscle. Laboratory-reared mice are best for isolation trials from fresh spinal fluid sediment (when acute central-nervous-systems signs are present) or suspensions of tissue.

Serum antibodies can be detected with the dye, complement fixation, hemagglutination, or immunofluorescence tests. The results are most helpful when they are negative or when a rising titer is demonstrated. Dye test antibodies appear early and persist for many years. Complement-fixing antibodies are slower to develop and disappear more rapidly. A high dye test titer (1:256 or more) and a negative complement fixation reaction in the same serum suggest either very recently acquired infection or the serologic residual of a previous one. Hemagglutinating antibodies seem to parallel dye test antibodies, but on occasion the results of the two tests are quite divergent.

Antibodies of the IgM class have been demonstrated by immunofluorescence and suggest a recent, active infection. This reaction should be especially useful in helping to differentiate between passively transferred antibodies and congenital infection in newborns.

Skin test antigens prepared from mouse peritoneal fluid or embryonated eggs have been used and yield reactions of the delayed type. Although still popular in some parts of the world, their use is not recommended.

TREATMENT. There is evidence from the treatment of experimental infections that a combination of sulfonamide and 5-p-chlorophenyl-2,4-diamino-6-ethylpyrimidine (Daraprim) is more effective than sulfonamide alone. Combinations of sulfadiazine or triple sulfonamides and Daraprim have been reported to yield excellent results in some cases of uveitis but have not affected others at all. Information on the effectiveness of this regimen in systemic toxoplasmosis is inadequate, but it does appear to control acute symptoms without eradicating encysted organisms. This drug combination is not specific for toxoplasmosis, and the patient's response does not prove the diagnosis. The sulfonamide should be administered in dosage of 2 to 4 Gm daily along with 50 mg

Daraprim daily in adults. Since Daraprim is an antifolic agent, leukocyte counts should be determined at least twice weekly. The dose of Daraprim probably should be halved after 2 weeks, and 1 month of treatment certainly constitutes an adequate trial. The leukopenia and thrombocytopenia which may result from Daraprim administration can be corrected by simultaneous administration of Leucovorin calcium and yeast cakes without interfering with the antitoxoplasmic effect of the drug.

REFERENCES

Feldman, H. A.: Medical Progress, Toxoplasmosis, New Engl. J. Med., 279:1370 and 1431, 1968.

Maumenee, A. E., and A. M. Silverstein: "Immunopathology of Uveitis," Baltimore, The Williams & Wilkins Company, 1964.

——: "Toxoplasmosis," Baltimore, The Williams & Wilkins Company, 1962.

Siim, J. Chr.: "Human Toxoplasmosis," Baltimore, The Williams & Wilkins Company, 1960.

245 PNEUMOCYSTIS CARINII PNEUMONIA (Pneumocystosis, Interstitial Plasma Cell Pneumonia)

Walter H. Sheldon

DEFINITION. *Pneumocystis carinii* (P.c.) pneumonia is an infection that becomes apparent clinically in patients with impaired host defenses. The disorder originally observed in premature or debilitated infants is being reported with increasing frequency in adults with either primary or secondary immunologic deficiency states, and instead of being a clinical curiosity, the disease is likely to become a common complication of transplantation surgery, tumor chemotherapy, and other states of increased host susceptibility. Pulmonary insufficiency is the cardinal clinical manifestation.

ETIOLOGY. *Pneumocystis carinii* first was seen by Chagas in 1909 and regarded as a form of *Trypanosoma cruzi* but was recognized as a different parasite by M. and Mme Delanoë, who in 1914 gave it the present name. The agent has not been cultured, and its taxonomic position remains uncertain; some consider it a protozoon, others regard it as a fungus. The consistent presence of P.c. in the pulmonary lesions of patients with the disease is the primary evidence for the causative role of the agent. Similar findings in laboratory animals with experimentally induced disease and serologic studies in man support the etiologic role of pneumocystis. The organism is best seen in smears as a minute oval or crescentic structure measuring 2 to 4 mμ with a single nucleuslike body or as a cyst ranging from 5 to 10 mμ and containing 2 to 8 bodies. Electron microscopic studies reveal a complex structure with organelles and suggest the capacity for protein synthesis and oxidative metabolism. Many

dyes, but *not* hematoxylin-eosin, stain the agent, which is also readily seen with phase microscopy and has been demonstrated with fluorescent antibody techniques. Silver impregnation methods are most useful for survey of preparations, and the structural detail is best observed with the Giemsa stain. The organism in patients everywhere is morphologically similar to that in animals but species-specific serologic differences may exist.

EPIDEMIOLOGY. In the absence of in vitro culture techniques and of readily applicable serologic tests, the incidence of P.c. infection is uncertain and epidemiologic data are based on indirect evidence. Morphologic observations supported by some serologic findings indicate that latent infection is not rare in man and is frequent in many animals including those commonly used in the laboratory. In man the disease is worldwide, and isolated cases occur in all age groups and in epidemics in nurseries. Retrospective study of autopsy files has uncovered typical instances of the infection antedating the description of the entity shortly after World War II. Clinical observations such as the reduction of nursery epidemics by isolation measures, the clustering of cases in families, and the apparently sequential occurrence in hospital room mates suggest that the disease is contagious and acquired by inhalation from patients with clinically apparent infection, asymptomatic carriers, and perhaps also from infected rodents. The incubation period is 1 to 2 months. Rare instances of P.c. pneumonia acquired in utero, probably by transplacental transmission, have been reported.

PATHOGENESIS. Clinical and experimental observations indicate that P.c. is of low virulence and slow to proliferate. It is possible that the presence of another living agent is needed for it to multiply. The frequent occurrence of progressive P.c. pneumonia in patients of all ages with primary or secondary immunologic deficiency states emphasizes the essential role of lowered host resistance in progressive infection. The disease has been encountered as a complication of neoplasia, particularly malignancies of the lymphocyte-reticular tissues, various anemias, cyclic neutropenia, collagen-vascular and autoimmune diseases, and renal failure. The common denominator in most patients has been their prolonged survival while treated with one or several agents such as corticosteroids, antimetabolites, cytotoxic substances, antibiotics, ionizing radiation, and colloidal gold. When some of these substances are administered to mice, rats, or rabbits, P.c. pneumonia will be produced or latent infection will be transformed into progressive disease. Suitable conditions for the proliferation of P.c. appear to occur in man and may be produced in animals not only by massive depression of the immune system but also by deficits which are thought to affect primarily only one aspect of the immune response such as antibody formation or cellular immunity. Fatal P.c. pneumonia, however, has also been reported in a few children and adults without demonstrated underlying disease. In some of these instances, exposure to massive doses of the infectious agent has been postulated.

The pathogenesis remains uncertain in the largest group of patients, in whom the disease was first described in Europe under the name of *interstitial plasma cell pneumonia*. These are premature or debilitated newborns in whom P.c. pneumonia occurs chiefly as epidemic outbreaks in nurseries with a peak incidence at the age of three to four months. Because this peak coincides with the period of physiologic hypoimmunoglobulinemia in the newborn, a relative or as yet unrecognized immunologic deficit has been suspected but remains unproven. However, in the absence of a correlation between the infection and immunoglobulin abnormalities a deficiency of cellular host defenses has been considered. Some evidence suggests that the mononuclear cell phase of inflammation in normal full-term infants is quantitatively less and morphologically different from that of healthy adults. A physiologic immaturity of the lymphocyte-mononuclear cell system which is involved in the cellular immune response, combined with age-related underdeveloped and incomplete immunoglobulin synthesis might in the presence of appropriate amounts of the infectious agent permit the development of P.c. pneumonia, particularly in the premature. Increased host susceptibility has also been attributed to chronic lung injury subsequent to presumably unrelated respiratory infections and to previous antimicrobial therapy which in animals activates latent P.c. infection.

Many other, often multiple infections occur in patients of all ages with P.c. pneumonia. Most common are acute and chronic bacterial infections, including tuberculosis and leprosy. Localized and disseminated cytomegalic inclusion disease is particularly frequent. Other concurrent infections are measles, vaccinia, candidiasis, aspergillosis, histoplasmosis, nocardiosis, cryptococcosis, and trypanosomiasis cruzi.

PATHOLOGIC FINDINGS. Gross findings in widespread disease show massively consolidated lungs without pleuritis. The process may be focal and confined to the central and dorsal lung areas. Histologically the alveoli are distended by a virtually typical, foamy material teeming with organisms. Hyaline membranes may be present. The sparse cellular response consists of mononuclear cells and occasionally giant cells. Alveolar septal infiltration by plasma cells, a prominent feature in many cases, is absent in others. Septal fibrosis is generally slight. These changes appear to be reversible. Granuloma formation, focal fibrosis, and calcification have been noted. Fragments of the alveolar contents in bronchi may account for dissemination throughout the lung. In latent infection the lesions are minute and generally few, foamy intraalveolar material is lacking, organisms are scant, and mononuclear cells are sparse. The infection is confined to the lung, but in a few instances organisms have been seen in regional lymph nodes. Systemic dissemination of the infection with focal lesions in distant sites is rare.

CLINICAL MANIFESTATIONS. Generally, the onset is insidious. The fully developed clinical picture is characterized by extreme dyspnea and tachypnea with respiratory rates up to and over 80 per min. Flaring of the nostrils,

sternal retraction, and pronounced use of the auxiliary respiratory muscles are present. The face is covered with perspiration, and the patient is anxious, cyanotic, and pale. Sometimes there is a dry cough which, together with the cyanosis, is made worse by any movement. When present, fever is slight. Pulmonary physical findings are scanty, which contrasts with the sometimes grave clinical state of the patient and the extensive lung involvement seen roentgenologically. Roentgenographic abnormalities may precede symptoms by months and usually consist of soft infiltrates, spreading from the hilum to the base and later to the entire lung but often sparing the upper lobes. Pleural effusions do not occur. Emphysema may be present. Laboratory studies reveal no consistent alterations of the white blood cell count, serum proteins, or any other parameters. Pulmonary function tests show primarily a diffusion defect. Complications include pneumothorax from a ruptured emphysematous bleb and rib fractures attributed to forced respiratory movements. Often the disease progresses relentlessly and death occurs by asphyxia or cardiac failure after 6 to 10 weeks.

DIAGNOSIS. The diagnosis depends on the morphologic demonstration of the agent. Material for histologic study may be obtained by aspiration of coughed-up hypopharyngeal and tracheal secretions, tracheal lavage, or by open or needle biopsy of the lung. Although successful in some hands, examination of secretions has, in general, yielded poor results. However, this procedure may become most useful if the recently reported staining of the organism by specific fluorescent antibody is confirmed and can be applied routinely. Because of possible subsequent pneumothorax and bleeding, needle biopsy involves considerable risk and open lung biopsy seems safer. A complement fixation test widely used in Europe is not available in this country, where it may not even be applicable because of possible serologic differences in the organism.

COURSE. In the absence of a simple diagnostic test, morbidity and mortality figures are uncertain. Beyond doubt, P.c. infection is not rare at any age, and P.c. pneumonia is likely to become more frequent. When associated with significant predisposing disorders, the prognosis is grave. An overall mortality of 40 to 50 percent has been suggested. Remissions and spontaneous cures (reported as 20 to 50 percent in some large series) occur, making claims of therapeutic success hard to evaluate.

TREATMENT. Recent clinical and experimental observations report distinctly encouraging results for treatment with pentamidine isothionate in dosage of 4 mg per kg body weight given in a single intramuscular injection for 12 to 14 days. In desperately ill patients the drug has been given intravenously. Combined treatment with pyrimethamine, 25 mg per day, and sulfadiazine, 1 to 4 Gm per day, both given orally, may also have beneficial effect. Megaloblastic anemia has been an occasional side effect but is correctable with folinic acid without apparently affecting the efficacy of the antiprotozoan drugs. Antibiotics, commercial immunoglobulin, and convalescent serum have had no success. Symptomatic treatment with oxygen and digitalis may be indicated.

REFERENCES

Ivády, G., L. Páldy, M. Koltay, G. Tóth, and Z. Kovács: Pneumocystis Carinii Pneumonia, Lancet, 1:616, 1967.

Ruskin, J., and J. S. Remington: The Compromised Host and Infection. I. Pneumocystis carinii Pneumonia, J.A.M.A., 202:1070, 1967.

Sheldon, W. H.: Pulmonary Pneumocystis Carinii Infection, J. Pediat., 61:780, 1962.

246 MINOR PROTOZOAN DISEASES

James J. Plorde and Ivan L. Bennett, Jr.

TRICHOMONIASIS

Of the many members of the genus *Trichomonas,* three are parasites of man: *T. hominis* in the intestine, *T. tenax* in the oral cavity, and *T. vaginalis,* the only one capable of producing disease, in the vagina and urethra. All three possess four anterior flagella, and their morphology is quite similar; *T. vaginalis* is the largest, however, and confusion in diagnosis is rare because of the anatomic specificity of their habitats.

Trichomonas vaginalis, despite some question about its role as a primary pathogen, is associated with persistent vaginitis in about 20 percent of parasitized women. Manifestations include itching, burning, and profuse, creamy, yellow, frothy leukorrhea. Examination shows inflammation ranging from mild hyperemia of the vaginal vault to extensive erosion, petechial hemorrhages, and perineal intertrigo.

The diagnosis is made by examining a fresh unstained drop of the discharge, which will be found to contain numerous motile trichomonads. The organisms are often present in urine. In males, a mild, usually asymptomatic urethritis is produced. The importance of the disease in males has to do with the transmission of infection by sexual contact, although the disease is also spread by toilet articles, fomites, etc.

Trichomoniasis is sometimes responsible for confusing changes in the cytologic pattern of exfoliated vaginal cells. However, ordinary Papanicolaou preparations are not well suited to establishing the diagnosis of this infection, and when it is suspected, fresh material should be looked at immediately.

Treatment consists of attention to personal hygiene and the local application of an appropriate compound. Floraquin and acetarsone have been used as insufflated powders or suppositories with success. Systemic therapy with metronidazole (Flagyl) has been quite effective. A dose of 1 Gm daily for 10 days will eliminate most infections in women. Infected sexual partners should be treated concurrently to prevent reinfection. Otherwise, infection in males seldom requires therapy. Tetracyclines are said to be effective but favor the development of vaginal moniliasis.

GIARDIASIS (Lambliasis)

Giardia lamblia is a pear-shaped, multiflagellar, protozoan parasite of the human duodenum. It possesses two large nuclei which give the organism the appearance of a face with two large eyes when viewed under the microscope. The parasite is capable of invading the intestinal mucosa. The response to infestation is highly variable and seems related at least in part to host factors. Children are three times more likely to be parasitized than adults and probably have more prominent clinical manifestations. Gastrectomy or decreased gastric acidity in adults may increase their susceptibility. Giardiasis also has been reported frequently in patients with immunoglobulin deficiencies.

Most often the infection is asymptomatic, but in some patients nausea, flatulence, epigastric pain, and distension occur. Sometimes patients have watery diarrhea and lose weight. These symptoms are more common in children and are usually self-limited. Rarely, fulminating and extensive duodenal ulceration have been described. Radiographically, asymptomatic carriers may show irritability of the duodenal bulb. Chronic giardiasis may lead to malabsorption, the pathogenesis of which is poorly understood. Mechanical blockage of microvilli by the parasites, competition between the organisms and host for nutrients, altered motility, and mucosal invasion have been suggested as possible mechanisms. Jejunal biopsy of patients infested with giardia sometimes shows flattening of the microvilli and an inflammatory infiltrate. Both malabsorption and the jejunal lesions have been reversed with specific treatment.

The diagnosis is made by finding the parasites in duodenal washings, jejunal biopsies, or diarrheal stools. Cyst forms are often passed; they contain two to four nuclei and are readily identified when stained with iodine.

Treatment consists of the administration of 0.1 Gm Atabrine hydrochloride three times daily for 3 days, a regimen which eliminates the organisms in 90 percent of the cases. Metronidazole (Flagyl) 250 mg twice daily for 5 to 7 days has also been effective. Treatment is necessary only in symptomatic cases. The frequency of infestation in children bears out transmission by the fecal-oral route, and reinfection will occur unless appropriate measures are taken.

COCCIDIOSIS

This is a relatively unusual disease characterized by fever, abdominal pain, and diarrhea, which results from ingestion of the oocysts or spores of *Isospora belli* or *I. hominis.* Volunteers develop symptoms about 1 week after ingestion, and the disease subsides spontaneously after 1 to 4 weeks. Infection is much more common in children and is worldwide in distribution, especially in tropical areas. The diagnosis is made by finding oocysts of the organisms in zinc sulfate concentrates of feces.

Isospora species occur in many lower animals, but only the dog is suspected of playing any part as a reservoir of the species that are pathogenic for man.

Diagnosis can be confused if oocysts of other members of the order Coccidia are ingested in fish or meat and appear in the feces without undergoing any change in the intestinal tract.

No treatment other than symptomatic is needed as the infection is self-limited.

BALANTIDIASIS

Balantidium coli, the largest protozoon of man, inhabits the large intestine. In addition to producing an asymptomatic carrier state, it elicits disease ranging from mild recurrent diarrhea to fulminant ulceration with perforation and death. In many respects the disease is similar to amebiasis in its range of manifestations, exclusive of spread to the liver.

The illness has been reproduced by feeding the organism to volunteers. The diagnosis is made by finding the parasites in the stool, but repeated examinations may be required because shedding of balantidium is intermittent. The disease is more likely to occur in tropical areas, but at least 60 cases have been reported in the United States. Swine are frequent carriers of *B. coli,* but there is great doubt about their role in the spread of the disease to man.

The tetracyclines in ordinary doses are highly effective in treatment, as is Diodoquin in a dosage of 0.65 Gm three times daily for 3 weeks.

REFERENCES

General

Brown, H. W., and D. L. Belding: "Basic Clinical Parasitology," New York, Appleton-Century-Crofts, Inc., 1964.

Balantidiasis

Shookhoff, H. B.: *Balantidium coli* Infection with Special Reference to Treatment, Am. J. Trop. Med., 34:442, 1951.

Swartzwelder, J. C.: Balantidiasis, Am. J. Dig. Dis., 17:173, 1950.

Coccidiosis

Matsubayashi, H., and F. Nozawa: Experimental Infection of *Isospora hominis* in Man, Am. J. Trop. Med., 28:633, 1948.

Smitskamp, H., and E. Oey-Muller: Geographical Distribution and Clinical Significance of Human Coccidiosis, Trop. Geog. Med., 18:133, 1966.

Giardiasis

Brandborg, L. L., C. B. Tankersley, S. Gottlieb, M. Baranick, and V. E. Sartor: Histological Demonstration of Mucosal Invasion by *Giardia Lamblia* in Man, Gastrointerol., 52:143, 1967.

Hoskins, L. C., S. J. Winawer, S. A. Broitman, L. S. Gottlieb, and N. Zamcheck, Clinical Giardiasis and Intestinal Malabsorption, Gastrointerol., 53:265, 1967.

Rendtorff, R. C.: Experimental Transmission of Human Intestinal Protozoan Parasites; *Giardia lamblia* Cysts Given in Capsules, Am. J. Hyg., 59:209, 1954.

Yardley, J. H., J. Takano, and T. R. Hendrix: Epithelial and Other Mucosal Lesions of the Jejunum in Giardiasis: Jejunal Biopsy Studies, Bull. Johns Hopkins Hosp., 115:389, 1964.

Trichomoniasis

Kotcher, E., C. A. Frick, and L. O. Giesel: The Effect of Metranidazole on Vaginal Microbiology and Maternal and Neonatal Hematology, Am. J. Obstet. Gynecol., 88:184, 1964.

Section 22

Diseases Caused by Worms

INTRODUCTION

Ivan L. Bennett, Jr.

Human diseases produced by worms, or, more properly, *helminths,* are truly global in their occurrence. In the Arctic and in most temperate countries, these parasites are a source of annoyance and discomfort but, generally speaking, they are not major health hazards. For climatic, socioeconomic, ethnic, and other environmental reasons, however, serious helminthic disorders are highly prevalent in many tropical areas. The devastating effects of such diseases as hookworm, echinococcosis, filariasis, and schistosomiasis in terms of disability, economic loss, and lagging of progress in developing countries are almost inestimable.

It is abundantly clear that the eventual control and eradication of helminthic diseases will require preventive measures on a massive scale, including broad public health measures, improvement of sanitation, water supply, and transportation, changes in agricultural methods, abolition of long-held customs of diet and daily living, and even a modification in religious practices. Though these aspects are mentioned in the chapters which follow, the main emphasis in this section is on the recognition and treatment of these diseases as they occur in the individual patient.

CLASSIFICATION. The worms of importance in human disease include the flukes (class Trematoda) and the tapeworms (class Cestoda) of the phylum Platyhelminthes (flatworms); class Nematoda of the phylum Nemathelminthes (roundworms); and class Hirudinea (leeches) of the phylum Annelida (segmented worms).

Medical helminthology is only a small fraction of the study of parasites, and a textbook of medicine cannot hope to include definitive information concerning morphologic variation and the details of identification of parasites, which, in the last analysis, depends upon special skill and long experience. References to more complete treatises are appended at the end of each chapter.

LIFE CYCLES AND THE HOST. Most helminths (as is true of other parasites) have developed life cycles involving one or more vertebrate or invertebrate hosts. The life cycle of some parasites is so complicated that it is difficult to see how they persist; indeed, for some species which produce disease in man (sparganosis), the complete life cycle is still unknown.

Lower animals harboring parasites which infect man are called *reservoir* hosts. The parasite reaches maturity in the *final* or *definitive* host. In the *intermediate* host (of which there may be more than one), the parasite passes through a larval stage. Man may develop disease as an *intermediate* or as a *definitive* host; sometimes he is a substitute or incidental host for parasites which ordinarily affect lower animals.

Programs of prevention and control depend on the discovery of those stages in the life cycle of a parasite which are vulnerable to attack by chemicals, environmental alterations, or elimination of a necessary host.

TRAVEL. Large migrations in the past have introduced helminthic diseases into new localities, examples being the spread of the fish tapeworm from Northern Europe to the United States, and the introduction of filariasis, hookworm (*Necator*), and dracunculosis (Guinea worm) into the New World by the importation of slaves from Africa.

Rapid transportation, greater travel by tourists, and increased military and civilian service in foreign countries now allow for exposure of many individuals all over the world to parasitic diseases which may not be manifested until their return to nonendemic areas and may, therefore, pose great problems in diagnosis. "Exotic" tropical diseases are now of more than academic interest to the practitioner. Furthermore, the firm commitment of the United States and other Western nations to render help to developing countries carries with it a need for special emphasis on the principal medical and health problems in all areas of the world.

MANIFESTATIONS OF HELMINTHIC DISEASE. The symptoms and signs elicited by helminths are largely dependent on the tissues and organs involved, the production of chemical or mechanical injury by the parasite, and the development of hypersensitivity of the host to components of the parasite. Systemic symptoms such as fever, weight loss, or anemia, gastrointestinal dysfunction,

a variety of cutaneous and systemic manifestations of allergy, and evidence of central-nervous-system disease are common to many of these disorders and will be detailed in the chapters to follow. Treatment often causes an exacerbation of allergic manifestations, and caution in initiating therapy is mandatory in many of these diseases.

DIAGNOSIS. Clinical diagnosis of parasitic disease in an endemic area is sometimes accurate, but even the most experienced physician must seek laboratory confirmation in view of the many overlapping syndromes which these diseases can create.

In nonendemic areas, a physician must be alert to the possibility of parasitic disease in individuals who may have been exposed in a foreign country. Once the possibility of helminthic disease is recognized, the physician must have knowledge of the proper specimens—feces, urine, blood, sputum, biopsy, etc.—to obtain or examination and must have available the services of a competent laboratory for diagnosis.

REFERENCES

Brown, H. W., and D. L. Belding: "Basic Clinical Parasitology," New York, Appleton-Century-Crofts, Inc., 1964.

Faust, E. C., and P. F. Russell: "Craig and Faust's Clinical Parasitology," 7th ed., Philadelphia, Lea & Febiger, 1964.

Hunter, G. W., III, W. W. Frye, and J. C. Swartzwelder: "A Manual of Tropical Medicine," 3d ed., Philadelphia, W. B. Saunders Company, 1960.

Lenczner, M., and T. Owen: "The Impact of Tropical and Parasitic Diseases in a Non-endemic Area, Can. Med. Assoc. J., 82:805, 1960.

Manson-Bahr, P.: "Manson's Tropical Diseases," 15th ed., London, Cassell and Co., Ltd., 1960.

Markell, E. K., and M. Voge: "Medical Parasitology," 2d ed., Philadelphia, W. B. Saunders Company, 1965.

Soulsby, E. J. L.: Immunity to Helminths—Recent Advances, Vet. Record, 72:322, 1960.

Stoll, N. R.: The Worms—Can We Vaccinate against Them? Am. J. Trop. Med. Hyg., 10:293, 1961.

Weller, T. H.: Tropical Medicine Today, New Engl. J. Med., 264:911, 1961.

247 TRICHINOSIS

Ivan L. Bennett, Jr., and Robert G. Petersdorf

DEFINITION. Trichinosis is caused by the intestinal nematode *Trichinella spiralis*. The disease is characterized by diarrhea during the development of the adults in the intestine and by myositis, fever, prostration, periorbital edema, and, occasionally, evidence of myocarditis or encephalitis during the stage of larval migration and invasion.

ETIOLOGY. Trichinosis in man is contracted by ingestion of meat containing the encysted larvae of *T. spiralis*. The meat is almost always pork, although a number of infections from bear meat have been observed, particularly in Northern Canada and Alaska. There are no intermediate hosts, and both the adult and larval stages develop in the same host. Infection has been produced or observed in the bear, wild boar, wolf, coyote, fox, musk-rat, horse, cow, dog, cat, rabbit, guinea pig, mouse, and marine mammals, in addition to the rat and the pig. Man is particularly susceptible; most fowl are resistant. Among pigs, infection is contracted following feeding of uncooked pork scraps, less often by eating infected rats. The incidence of infection in pigs has been reduced by laws requiring that garbage be cooked thoroughly before being fed. Rats also feed on uncooked pork scraps and, in addition, maintain a high incidence of infection by their cannibalism.

Soon after ingestion, the larvae are liberated from their cysts by gastric digestion and migrate into the intestinal mucosa, where copulation takes place. The male dies, and within a week, the viviparous female is discharging larvae ($100 \times 6 \mu$), which enter vascular channels and are distributed throughout the body. Larviposition continues for about 4 to 6 weeks. The larvae enter skeletal muscle and encyst. The muscles of the diaphragm, tongue, and eye, the deltoid, pectoral, and intercostal muscles are most often affected. Larvae carried to sites other than skeletal muscles do not encyst but disintegrate. The life cycle can be carried further only if a new host ingests the encysted larvae.

EPIDEMIOLOGY. Trichinosis is common in Europe and North America and uncommon in other parts of the world, including the Tropics. In the United States, the incidence of infection (as detected by finding calcified cysts at autopsy) has declined from 15.9 to 4.5 percent. This decline in incidence has been due to (1) a decrease of trichinosis in pigs, (2) a decrease in use of pork as compared with beef, (3) better techniques for deep-freezing pork, and (4) better education, which has led to more thorough cooking of pork products.

PATHOLOGY. The most striking lesions are in the skeletal muscles, where there is a severe myositis with basophilic granular degeneration of the invaded muscle fiber. Adjacent fibers exhibit hyaline or hydropic degeneration, and the focus becomes infiltrated with neutrophilic and eosinophilic leukocytes, some lymphocytes, and mononuclear macrophages. Hyperemia, edema, and hemorrhages are constant features.

Larvae do not encyst in cardiac muscle, but an intense myocarditis has been observed in fatal cases.

In cases of central-nervous-system involvement, there may be granulomatous nodules, and vasculitis involving small arterioles and capillaries of the brain and meninges. Encystment of larvae in the brain is unusual.

CLINICAL MANIFESTATIONS. The first symptoms usually appear within 1 to 2 days after ingestion of the uncooked or undercooked meat montaining encysted larvae. At that time diarrhea, abdominal pain, nausea, and sometimes prostration and fever develop. The next stage, that of muscular invasion, begins about the end of the first week and may last as long as 6 weeks. During this period, patients have fever, edema of the eyelids, conjunctivitis and subconjunctival hemorrhages, muscle pain and tenderness, and often severe weakness. There may be a maculopapular rash which lasts for several days and

subungual "splinter hemorrhages." Central-nervous-system involvement may be evident as polyneuritis, poliomyelitis, myasthenia, meningitis, encephalitis, focal or diffuse pareses, delirium, psychosis, and coma. Despite the severity of central-nervous-system involvement in some patients, the CSF (cerebrospinal fluid) remains normal.

Myocarditis is characterized by persistent tachycardia or development of congestive heart failure. There may be marked electrocardiographic alterations, including T-wave changes and conduction abnormalities.

LABORATORY FINDINGS. The most constant finding, and one of significance early in the course of the disease, is the eosinophilic leukocytosis (over 500 eosinophilic leukocytes per cu mm) which generally appears before the end of the second week. In cases of moderate severity, the proportion of eosinophilic leukocytes ranges between 15 and 50 percent. In severe cases, particularly terminally, the eosinophilic leukocytosis may disappear entirely.

The skin test to larval antigen becomes positive early in the third week of infection, with a wheal of 5 mm or more appearing within 30 min. The usual positive response is an immediate reaction, but early in the infection (before the seventeenth day) the response may be of the delayed type. The antigens vary in their sensitivity, and care must be taken to employ a potent preparation.

There is a variety of serologic tests for trichinosis, including the precipitin reaction, the bentonite flocculation test, the complement fixation test, and the indirect fluorescent antibody test. The last of these is probably the most accurate. These serologic tests all become positive by about the third week of the disease and may remain positive for several years. The serologic tests are most valuable if they are negative initially and then turn positive or if there is a change in titer.

Muscle biopsy remains the most useful site for demonstration of larvae or cysts. Myositis is a significant finding even in the absence of larvae or cysts.

In severe trichinosis there may be marked hypoalbuminemia, probably because of protein leakage from damaged capillaries. During the fourth, fifth, and sixth weeks of the disease, concomitant with a rise in antibody, diffuse hypergammaglobulinemia occurs. There may be moderate rises in SGOT (serum glutamic oxaloacetic transaminase), probably related to myositis, and the sedimentation rate is characteristically slow.

DIFFERENTIAL DIAGNOSIS. Trichinosis must be differentiated from diseases which are characterized by eosinophilia (such as Hodgkin's disease, eosinophilic leukemia, and periarteritis nodosa) and from entities which are characterized by myopathy, such as dermatomyositis. When the central nervous system is involved, the diagnosis may be very difficult.

TREATMENT. Thiabendazole, in dosage of 50 mg/kg/day for 5 to 7 days, has resulted in dramatic improvement in a number of patients with trichinosis. Within 48 hr of receiving this drug the patient has usually experienced subjective improvement, relief of muscle pain and tenderness, and lysis of fever. The drug has been associated with nausea, vomiting, abdominal discomfort, dermatitis, and drug fever, but despite these drawbacks it appears promising. It has not been uniformly larvicidal.

Patients with "allergic" manifestations of trichinosis, including angioedema and urticaria as well as central-nervous-system involvement, should be treated with ACTH and/or prednisone in dosage of 60 mg per day. Response to steroids usually has been prompt, particularly in central-nervous-system trichinosis. Not all focal lesions have resolved, however.

Other measures should be directed at relief of pain and maintenance of adequate caloric and fluid intake.

PROGNOSIS. The prognosis in trichinosis has improved markedly, and even when the central nervous system is involved, the mortality rate has fallen to under 10 percent. The overall mortality rate is probably less than 5 percent.

PREVENTION. The responsibility for control rests with the consumer. Adequate cooking of pork involves heating all portions of the meat to 55°C. Freezing procedures to kill the larvae require a temperature of −15°C for 20 days or −18°C for 24 hr. Proper smoking and pickling will also destroy the larvae. Important in control is the cooking of garbage fed to hogs. There is no practical method of inspection which will detect trichinous pork.

REFERENCES

Dalessio, D. J., and H. G. Wolff: *Trichinella spiralis* Infection of the Central Nervous System, Arch. Neurol., 4:407, 1961.

Gould, S. E.: "Trichinosis," Springfield, Ill., Charles C Thomas, Publisher, 1945.

Hall, W. J., III, and W. R. McCabe: Trichinosis. Report of a Small Outbreak with Observations of Thiabendazole Therapy, Arch. Intern. Med., 119:65, 1967.

Kagan, I. G.: Trichinosis: A Review of Biologic, Serologic and Immunologic Aspects, J. Infect. Dis., 107:65, 1960.

Kean, B. H., and D. W. Hoskins: Treatment of Trichinosis with Thiabendazole. A Preliminary Report, J.A.M.A., 190:116, 1964.

Most, H.: Trichinellosis in the United States, J.A.M.A., 193:871, 1965.

Rachón, K., J. Januszkiewicz, and H. Wehr: Serum Proteins in Human Trichinosis, Am. J. Med., 44:937, 1968.

Sulzer, A. J., and E. S. Chisholm: Camparison of the IFA and Other Tests for *Trichinella spiralis* Antibodies, Public Health Report U.S., 81:729, 1966.

Wilson, R.: Bear Meat Trichinosis, Ann. Intern. Med., 65:965, 1967.

248 OTHER INTESTINAL NEMATODES
James J. Plorde, Ivan L. Bennett, Jr., and Robert G. Petersdorf

HOOKWORM DISEASE

Hookworm disease is a symptomatic infection caused by *Ancylostoma duodenale* or *Necator americanus.*

Assymptomatic infection may be termed simply *hookworm infection,* and the individual with such infection is called a carrier.

ETIOLOGY. *Ancylostoma duodenale,* also known as the "Old World" hookworm, possesses four prominent hooklike teeth in its adult stage. The adults are about 1 cm long and inhabit the upper part of the small intestine of man, where they attach to the mucosa by means of the mouth parts and suck blood. Each adult extracts 0.15 ml blood daily. The adults migrate within the small intestine, and each site of attachment persists temporarily as a bleeding point. Following fertilization, the female liberates eggs which measure about 40 × 60 μ and are usually in the two- to four-celled stage when discharged in the feces.

Necator americanus, the "New World" hookworm, has a buccal capsule containing dorsal and ventral plates rather than teeth. It is slightly smaller and causes much less blood loss than *A. duodenale.*

The life cycles of both hookworms are similar. Development to the filariform or infective stage occurs outside the body. The larvae then penetrate the skin to enter vessels which carry them to the lungs. The larvae leave the alveolar capillaries, enter the alveoli, ascend the respiratory tree, enter the pharynx, and are swallowed. They reach the intestine about 1 week after penetration of the skin, and mature within 3 to 5 weeks. Adults have been known to survive in the human intestine for as long as 15 years.

EPIDEMIOLOGY. Conditions conducive to the development of the hookworm egg into infective filariform larvae are found in tropical and semitropical regions in which rainfall is plentiful. Hookworm infection occurs where there is opportunity for contact of the skin with contaminated soil. The disease may also be acquired by oral ingestion, but this is of little importance.

The white race is probably more susceptible to symptomatic infection than the Negro, but this is rarely of clinical significance. Probably because of greater exposure, males show a higher incidence of infection than females.

Repeated infections of hookworm in dogs results in immunity and elimination of the parasite. It seems probable that a similar phenomenon occurs in human infections. When the possibility of reinfection is eliminated, the majority of worms is eliminated spontaneously within 1 or 2 years.

In general, *Ancylostoma* presents a greater public health hazard than *N. americanus,* the species which is most prevalent in the Southern United States, because it is more persistent in the environment, more harmful to the host, and less amenable to treatment.

PATHOGENESIS AND CLINICAL MANIFESTATIONS. During the invasion of the exposed skin by the larvae, there are erythema and edema, with severe pruritus. These manifestations are more marked in *N. americanus* infection than in *A. duodenale* infection. The lesions are most common about the feet, particularly between the toes, and have been termed "ground itch."

During migration through the lungs, cough and, in

severe infections, fever are common. The pulmonary symptoms were particularly troublesome to soldiers engaged in close combat in the Asiatic campaign in World War II. Usually, however, pulmonary involvement does not give rise to clinical symptoms.

Various gastrointestinal symptoms, ranging from vague epigastric distress and picca to typical ulcer pain, have been reported in association with hookworm infection. Roentgenographic studies may reveal nonspecific changes such as excessive peristalsis and "puddling," particularly in the proximal jejunum. However, gross and microscopic examination of the bowel itself reveals conspicuously little damage. Previous reports of absorptive abnormalities in hookworm infection have not been supported.

The major clinical manifestations of hookworm disease clearly are those of iron-deficiency anemia consequent to chronic intestinal blood loss. Whether anemia develops and how severe it becomes depend on the balance between iron lost in the gut and iron absorbed from the diet. In many endemic areas, dietary iron is largely of vegetable origin and is absorbed poorly. General dietary deficiency also may lower resistance to parasitic infections. The severity of the disease and the prognosis depend on such factors as the age of the patient, the magnitude of the worm burden, the duration of the disease, and diet. Young children often have extreme anemia, with cardiac insufficiency and anasarca. Those who survive to puberty show retarded physical, mental, and sexual development. Milder degrees of the disease, as seen in older children and adults, are characterized by lassitude, dyspnea, palpitation, tachycardia, constipation, and pallor of the skin and mucous membranes. Poor diet influences the course of hookworm disease unfavorably.

Asymptomatic infections outnumber symptomatic infections, considering all age groups, twenty to forty times in endemic areas. The worm burden is small in asymptomatic infections, and the carrier state is probably indicative of some degree of acquired host resistance.

LABORATORY FINDINGS. In symptomatic infection, hookworm eggs are usually numerous enough to be detected by microscopic examination of a direct fecal smear. Abdominal and pulmonary symptoms appear before eggs are discharged, although a presumptive diagnosis may be made on the basis of the clinical history and the eosinophilic leukocytosis.

The feces seldom contain gross blood in hookworm disease, although tests for occult blood are usually positive. *Trichostrongylus* eggs are larger and in a later stage of maturation when observed in a fresh fecal specimen than are those of *Necator* or *Ancylostoma*.

Generally, the leukocyte count is normal or slightly elevated, and the percentage of eosinophils is increased to 15 or 30 percent. However, in some early cases, leukocytosis may be marked, with an eosinophilia as high as 70 or 80 percent. In general, the more severe the anemia, the less the eosinophilia. The anemia is characteristically hypochromic and microcytic.

DIFFERENTIAL DIAGNOSIS. Since hookworm disease occurs in areas in which beriberi and malaria are also more common, these diseases must be differentiated from hookworm disease, or their coexistence must be established.

TREATMENT. Specific therapy for the infection and that directed toward improvement of nutrition and the anemia should be considered simultaneously. In the usual case, anthelmintics may be administered immediately, followed by iron therapy and a high protein diet. A number of satisfactory antihelmintic agents are available, but the drug of choice is tetrachlorethylene (TCE). In most instances a single dose of this agent will decrease the worm load substantially. Complete cure may require several courses of treatment but is not necessary in endemic areas; the aim of therapy is reduction of the worm load to an asymptomatic level. Tetrachlorethylene is administered as a single 5-ml oral dose mixed in a glass of water. Children should receive 0.10 ml per kg (to a maximum of 5 ml) by the same route. The night before treatment, the patient is permitted a light, fat-free meal. The following morning, breakfast is omitted and the drug is administered. No food is permitted for 4 hr and no alcohol for 24 hr. Purgation following administration of the drug is no longer recommended. Treatment can be repeated in a week if complete cure is desired and has not been accomplished. The drug is inexpensive, nontoxic, and ideal for mass therapy. If ascariasis is also present, it should be treated first with piperazine citrate (see Ascariasis below).

Biphenium hydroxynaphthoate (Alcopar) is also a drug of low toxicity which is said to be more effective than TCE against *A. duodenale* but possibly less effective against *N. americanus*. In mixed infections with Ascaris it can be used alone because it is active against both types of parasite. A single dose of 5 Gm biphenium hydroxynaphthoate is dispersed in water and ingested in the morning on an empty stomach. No food is permitted for 2 hr, and no purgation is recommended. The dose for children is the same as for adults. In *N. americanus* infections, treatment should be repeated on three consecutive days. Another drug which has been introduced for treatment of hookworm infections is thiabendazole (Mintezal). This is a broad-spectrum drug which is effective against ascaris, trichuris, and strongyloides as well as hookworm. The dose is 25 mg per kg twice a day for 2 or 3 days. Twenty-five percent of patients treated with this agent develop nausea and vomiting.

The anemia requires iron replacement.

When anemia is severe and there is malnutrition with anasarca, blood transfusions and a high protein diet should be given before drug treatment is begun. Blood should be given in an amount sufficient to raise the hemoglobin level to 10 Gm per 100 ml. In advanced cases it may be necessary to delay drug treatment for 2 to 3 weeks.

PROGNOSIS. Generally, the immediate prognosis is good. When opportunity for reinfection persists and nutrition cannot be maintained, a state of chronic debility develops. Maturation of children is impaired, and intercurrent disease is a serious problem in adults.

PREVENTION. Many of the measures required are obvious but difficult to apply on a large scale. Even if facilities for proper disposal of feces are provided, it is no simple matter to educate the population in their use. Soil pollution must be eliminated, and until this is accomplished, avoidance of direct skin contact with the soil (by wearing shoes) is mandatory. Periodic mass treatment of the population has been used in some hookworm control programs.

CREEPING ERUPTION
(Cutaneous Larva Migrans)

DEFINITION. Creeping eruption is an infection of the skin in man caused by the larvae of the dog and cat hookworm, *Ancylostoma brasiliense*. The other dog hookworms, *A. caninum* and *Uncinaria stenocephala*, and the horse botfly, *Gasterophilus*, in their larval stage may produce a similar cutaneous infection.

ETIOLOGY. *Ancylostoma brasiliense* reaches adulthood regularly only in the dog and cat. The larvae emerging from eggs discharged in the feces develop to the filariform stage and then are capable of penetrating the skin. In man, the larvae usually remain in the skin and migrate, producing an irregular erythematous tunnel visible on the skin surface.

EPIDEMIOLOGY AND DISTRIBUTION. Transmission to man requires environmental temperature and humidity appropriate for development of the egg to the infective filariform larva stage. Beaches and other moist, sandy areas are hazardous, because animals choose such areas for defecation, and the *A. brasiliense* eggs develop well in such soil.

PATHOGENESIS AND CLINICAL MANIFESTATIONS. The site of penetration of the skin by the larva becomes apparent in a few hours. The migration of the larva in the skin is accompanied by severe itching. Scratching may lead to bacterial infection. In the course of 1 week, the initial red papule develops into an irregular, erythematous, linear lesion which may attain a length of 15 to 20 cm.

Wright and Gold have observed Loeffler's syndrome in 26 of 52 cases of creeping eruption. Transient, migratory pulmonary infiltrations associated with an increased number of eosinophils in the blood and sputum were interpreted as an allergic reaction to the helminthic infection.

LABORATORY FINDINGS. Eosinophils occur in the lesion, but eosinophilic leukocytosis is slight, except when Loeffler's syndrome appears. The percentage of eosinophils in the blood may then rise to 50 percent, and in the sputum to 90 percent.

TREATMENT. Thiabendazole is the drug of choice; it should be given orally in the dosage suggested for hookworm, or it may be applied topically as a 10 percent aqueous suspension. Topical administration avoids systemic toxicity. Carbon dioxide snow or ethyl chloride applied to the advancing portion of the lesion is effective and practical, when there are only a few lesions. Superficial bacterial infections are improved by the application of wet dressings and elevation of the extremity. For intense itching, oral antihistaminics may be of aid.

PROGNOSIS. Untreated infections last several months. Treatment, which is usually sought because of severe pruritus, is usually successful.

PREVENTION. Dogs and cats should be prevented from contaminating recreation areas.

STRONGYLOIDIASIS

DEFINITION. Strongyloidiasis is an intestinal infection of man and other mammals, caused by *Strongyloides stercoralis*.

ETIOLOGY. The adult female resides in the mucosa of the upper part of the small intestine and lays eggs which develop into rhabditiform larvae which are excreted in the feces. Further larval development may take one of several courses: (1) In a suitable external environment, the indirect, or sexual, cycle occurs. (2) Under less-suitable external circumstances, the rhabditiform larvae develop into the infective filariform stage (direct, or asexual, cycle). (3) Development to the infective stage is thought to take place in the large intestine, the filariform larvae then entering the body through the intestinal wall or the perianal skin. This type of "autoinfection" may explain the long persistence (20 to 30 years) of strongyloidiasis in patients who have left endemic areas and also may account for the extremely heavy worm loads in some individuals.

The migration of the filariform larvae of *S. stercoralis* after entering the skin, the oral mucosa, or the intestinal mucosa resembles that of hookworm larvae. In the intestine the females burrow into the mucosa, from which site embryonated eggs are discharged.

EPIDEMIOLOGY AND DISTRIBUTION. The usual mode of infection is the penetration of the skin by larvae. Some infections may result from ingestion of contaminated food and drink, and some are believed to be transmitted by contact. This disease is endemic in the Tropics, although sporadic cases appear in temperate countries.

PATHOGENESIS AND CLINICAL MANIFESTATIONS. The initial cutaneous penetration of the filariform larvae usually produces no symptoms. Cough, dyspnea, and gross hemoptysis occasionally may accompany migration through the lungs. Roentgenograms may show pulmonary infiltration at this time.

Epigastric pain and tenderness, nausea, flatulence, vomiting, and diarrhea alternating with constipation may be observed during the intestinal phase. Transitory skin eruptions characterized by blotchy erythema, serpiginous lesions, and urticaria may recur at irregular intervals and apparently are related to episodes of acute infection. As with hookworm infection, many asymptomatic infections occur, and most symptomatic infections occasion only vague abdominal complaints.

In massive infection, there may be serious complications. These are particularly likely to occur during treatment with corticosteroids. Presumably these drugs facilitate the transformation of rhabditiform larvae to the infective filariform stage within the lumen of the intestine, resulting in autoinfection. A severe form of ulcerative colitis, accompanied by intestinal perforation and peritonitis, has been encountered. In one fatal case, pulmonary hemorrhage and edema were observed and larvae were found in the myocardium, lungs, trachea, liver, gallbladder, and intestine.

LABORATORY FINDINGS. Although clinical findings may be suggestive, the definitive diagnosis can be made only in the laboratory. Fresh fecal specimens should be examined to avoid confusion with hookworm infection; generally, fresh specimens contain *larvae* in strongyloidiasis infections, while in hookworm infection they contain *eggs*. If pulmonary involvement is present, the sputum should be examined for larvae. Microscopic examination of the duodenal washings may also establish the diagnosis.

Eosinophilic leukocytosis is common, except in very severe cases. When eosinophilia occurs in association with peptic ulcer symptoms, strongyloidiasis should be suspected.

TREATMENT. Dithiazanine no longer can be recommended because it has caused fatal intoxication in several cases. The drug of choice is thiabendazole, which should be given orally in dosage of 25 mg per kg twice a day for 2 or 3 days. Light-headedness, nausea, and vomiting are common accompaniments of therapy with this agent. Hypersensitivity reactions may occur but usually respond to treatment with antihistamines.

PROGNOSIS. In the usual case, the prognosis is good. Since the occurrence of hyperinfection is unpredictable, every effort should be made to eradicate the infection in each case. In severe cases with hyperinfection, the prognosis is poor.

PREVENTION. In general, the measures are those for the control of hookworm infection. In addition, it is well to remember that infection may be contracted by ingestion of contaminated food (especially uncooked vegetables) or of contaminated drinking water and by contact.

ASCARIASIS

DEFINITION. Ascariasis is an infection of man caused by *Ascaris lumbricoides* and characterized by an early pulmonary phase related to larval migration and a later, prolonged intestinal phase. It is estimated that 25 percent of the world's population is infested with this nematode.

ETIOLOGY. The adult ascarids are large (20 to 40 cm in length) and cylindric, with blunt ends. The eggs are elliptic (30 to 40 μ × 50 to 60 μ) and have an irregular, dense outer shell and a regular, translucent inner shell. Under proper conditions of warmth and moisture the ovum develops to the infective larval stage in about 4 to 5 weeks. When the egg is ingested at this stage, the larva is liberated in the small intestine. It migrates through the wall and ultimately reaches the lungs. After about 10 days in the pulmonary capillaries and alveoli, the larvae pass in turn to the bronchioles, bronchi,

trachea, and epiglottis, are swallowed, and develop into male and female adults in the small intestine. The adult has a life span of 6 to 18 months.

EPIDEMIOLOGY AND DISTRIBUTION. Infection follows the ingestion of the embryonated egg contained in contaminated food, or, more commonly, the introduction of the eggs into the mouth by the hands after contact with contaminated soil. Since the eggs are resistant to desiccation and wide variations in temperature, the disease is worldwide.

PATHOGENESIS AND CLINICAL MANIFESTATIONS. Because of the extensive migration of which both the larvae and adults are capable, clinical manifestations may be unusually diverse. In heavy infections, severe bronchopneumonia, occasionally fatal in children, may occur during the migration of the larvae through the lungs. Adult worms may cause no symptoms if the infection is light and may be detected accidentally when an adult worm is vomited or passed in the stool. Heavier infections may cause abdominal pain, and occasionally a bolus of worms may result in partial or complete intestinal obstruction in the ileocecal area. Obstruction often follows febrile illnesses which stimulate the worms to increased motility. Rarely an adult ascarid will migrate into the appendix, bile ducts, or pancreatic ducts, causing obstruction of these organs.

LABORATORY FINDINGS. The diagnosis is usually made by finding the ova in the feces. The intact ova are characteristic and not easily confused with those of other helminths.

Symptomatic infection, especially during the phase of larval migration through the lungs, is usually accompanied by fever and eosinophilic leukocytosis.

TREATMENT. Only symptomatic treatment can be used during the period of pulmonary involvement by the migrating larvae. For removal of the adult worms from the intestines, piperazine citrate, as a flavored syrup administered in a single dose after breakfast on two successive days, will cure the majority of cases. The dose of piperazine is 150 mg per kg, with a maximum of 3 Gm. No particular dietary regulation is necessary. The drug must be administered with caution to patients with renal insufficiency, because impaired elimination may produce neurotoxic signs. In intestinal obstruction, nasogastric suction should be initiated. After vomiting is controlled, piperazine should be given through the nasogastric tube every 12 to 24 hr in dosage of 65 mg per kg (maximum 1.0 Gm) for six doses. Surgery usually is not required.

While piperazine citrate is the treatment of choice, thiabendazole (see Strongyloidiasis, above) or biphenium hydroxynaphthoate (see Hookworm Disease, above) may be used. When both ascariasis and trichuriasis are present, treatment with thiabendazole is effective. When both ascariasis and infection with *A. duodenale* are present, treatment with biphenium hydroxynaphthoate is recommended.

PROGNOSIS. The prognosis in intestinal infection is generally good. When acute or chronic obstruction of ducts or hollow viscera has occurred, the immediate prognosis is determined by the promptness of diagnosis and treatment.

PREVENTION. Ascariasis is primarily a household infection of rural areas. All infections should be treated, personal hygiene stressed, and adequate toilet facilities provided.

VISCERAL LARVA MIGRANS

This is a clinical syndrome usually, but not exclusively, seen in children. Hepatosplenomegaly, skin rash, and recurrent pneumonitis with wheezing respiratory distress are frequent. There is often a history of dirt eating and contact with dogs or cats. Ocular involvement, which may be mistaken for retinoblastoma, and convulsions may also be observed.

Leukocytosis with eosinophilia to high levels (over 60 percent) and hypergammaglobulinemia are common. Anti-IgG factors have been reported in the serum of children with this syndrome. The eosinophils are unusual in that they are large and have vacuolated cytoplasm containing granules which vary in size and are present in smaller than normal numbers.

This syndrome, with various degrees of clinical severity, follows the ingestion of the infective eggs of nematodes whose life cycle is not completed in man. It is caused most often by nematodes whose life cycle is completed in the dog (*Toxocara canis*) or in the cat (*Toxocara cati*). Larvae of the *Toxocara* become widely disseminated in the body and incite a granulomatous reaction. Lesions are prominent in the liver, lungs, skeletal muscle, and brain. Larvae with eosinophilic leukocytic and granulomatous reactions have been noted in liver biopsies.

The clinical diagnosis may be made on the basis of the findings described. A hemagglutination test employing ascaris and toxocara antigens has been demonstrated by Jung and Pacheco to be a valuable aid in the laboratory diagnosis of visceral larva migrans. This is another variety of helminthic infection capable of causing Loeffler's syndrome. When the respiratory difficulty is pronounced, administration of ACTH or adrenocortical steroids is helpful. A small number of cases has been treated successfully with thiabendazole in dosage of 25 mg per kg twice daily for 1 to 4 weeks.

Control measures are directed toward preventing ingestion of the toxocara eggs. Removal or repeated treatment of infected cats and dogs must be considered, as well as modifying the diet to reduce the temptation to ingest contaminated materials.

ENTEROBIASIS

DEFINITION. Enterobiasis (pinworm, seatworm, or threadworm infection; oxyuriasis) is an intestinal infection of man caused by *Enterobius vermicularis* and characterized by perianal pruritus.

ETIOLOGY. The female averages 10 mm in length, the male 3 mm. The eggs are deposited by the female on the perineal skin, the migration generally occurring at night. Each egg contains an embryo which, within a few hours, develops into the infective larva. After the egg has been ingested, the larva is released in the small intestine and, in less than 1 month from the time of ingestion, newly developed gravid females are again discharging eggs. They are planoconvex and measure approximately $20 \times 50 \mu$. The shell is clear and doubly contoured.

EPIDEMIOLOGY AND DISTRIBUTION. The eggs usually reach the host by way of contaminated hands, food, or drink, although airborne transmission is possible. They are relatively resistant to desiccation, and transmission within family and children's groups occurs readily. Enterobiasis is found in all climates and is probably the most common helminthic infection of man. Its low incidence in some tropical areas, however, defies explanation.

CLINICAL MANIFESTATIONS. The most common symptom is pruritus ani, which is most troublesome at night, being related to the migration of the gravid female worms. Scratching may lead to perineal eczema or pyogenic infection.

LABORATORY FINDINGS. Examination for ova of material obtained from the perineal skin by means of a cellophane or Scotch tape swab is the preferable method for the detection of enterobiasis. Searching for ova in the feces is rarely helpful. Scrapings from under the nails may reveal ova. The diagnosis is sometimes made by finding adult worms in feces following a laxative or an enema. Eosinophilic leukocytosis is not a typical finding.

TREATMENT. All infected individuals in a family or communal group should be treated simultaneously. Drug treatment must be combined with such measures as (1) providing a sleeping garment which prevents contamination of the fingers with ova from the perianal region, (2) instituting a morning shower, (3) lukewarm water enemas, and (4) local antipruritic ointments. It is relatively easy to reduce the worm burden and to make the infection asymptomatic, but eradication or cure is very difficult.

Pyrvinium pamoate (Povan) is the drug of choice. A single dose of 5 mg per kg is given orally, in tablet or liquid form. This compound turns the stool red and may stain bedclothes or undergarments. An acceptable alternative is piperazine citrate, which is highly effective when prescribed in a single course of 7 days. It is given in syrup each day before breakfast, with a total daily dose of 250 mg for children weighing up to 15 lb, 500 mg for those weighing between 16 and 30 lb, 1 Gm for those between 31 and 60 lb, and 2 Gm for those over 60 lb (Brown). When renal insufficiency is present, piperazine should be given in smaller dosage to avoid neurotoxicity.

PROGNOSIS. The prognosis with reference to the duration of infection is good, particularly when the other measures mentioned are carried out in addition to drug treatment.

PREVENTION. Methods of preventing autoinfection and dissemination within a group involving children are extremely difficult to enforce. Personal environmental hygiene should be stressed, and anthelmintic and symptomatic treatment of pruritus ani should be instituted. To control infection within a group, simultaneous treatment of all cases is mandatory.

TRICHURIASIS

DEFINITION. Trichuriasis (whipworm infection, trichocephaliasis) is an intestinal infection of man caused by *Trichuris trichiura* and is characterized by invasion of the colonic mucosa by the adult trichuris.

ETIOLOGY. The adult whipworms possess a threadlike anterior two-thirds and a stouter posterior third, giving them a whiplike structure. The eggs are characteristically barrel-shaped, brown, and translucent, with knoblike extremities.

EPIDEMIOLOGY. The mode of spread resembles that of ascariasis, the eggs generally being introduced into the mouth by contaminated fingers.

PATHOGENESIS AND CLINICAL MANIFESTATIONS. Symptomatic infection generally requires the presence of large numbers of adult whipworms and may be correlated in part with the degree of mucosal involvement. Heavy infections usually occur only in children and may be accompanied by nausea, abdominal pain, diarrhea, dysentery, and rectal prolapse.

LABORATORY FINDINGS. In symptomatic infection, large numbers of eggs are present in the feces and there may be eosinophilic leukocytosis and anemia.

TREATMENT. Thiabendazole, 25 mg per kg twice daily for 2 or 3 days, is effective, although less so in trichuriasis than in hookworm infection and strongyloidiasis. A 5-day course of pyrvinium pamoate or a 7-day course of piperazine citrate is also acceptable therapy (see Enterobiasis).

PROGNOSIS. Whipworm infection, unless characterized by severe diarrhea, blood loss, and systemic reaction, usually responds well to treatment. Serious infections may require supportive treatment as well as chemotherapy.

PREVENTION. Measures recommended for ascariasis apply also to trichuriasis.

TRICHOSTRONGYLIASIS

DEFINITION. Trichostrongyliasis is an intestinal infection of man and other mammalian hosts, including sheep, goats, and cattle.

ETIOLOGY. Almost a dozen species of *Trichostrongylus* are known to have infected man. Few human infections have been reported in the United States. In view of the high frequency of animal infections here, the low incidence of human infections is difficult to understand. The possibility exists that some such infections are mistaken for hookworm infection.

The ova resemble those of the hookworm but are larger and, when observed in a fresh fecal specimen, show a more advanced stage of segmentation (16- to 32-celled stage).

PATHOGENESIS. Infection is acquired by ingestion of the larvae, rather than by their penetration of the skin. The adult maintains residence in the intestine for long periods. Sandground, who infected himself, observed infection to last more than 8 years.

MANIFESTATIONS. Diarrhea is observed occasionally when infection is massive, but most infections are asymptomatic. The parasite owes its importance primarily to the resemblance of its ova to those of the hookworms. Moreover, because the trichostrongylidae do not respond to anthelmintics effective in hookworm infection, it may be assumed incorrectly that one is dealing with refractory hookworm infection.

LABORATORY DIAGNOSIS. The diagnosis depends on the finding of the ova in the feces. Since they are few, they are usually found only when a concentration method is used. In symptomatic infections, there may be leukocytosis with marked eosinophilia (e.g., 80 percent).

TREATMENT. These infections do not respond to tetrachlorethylene. Thiabendazole, 25 mg per kg twice daily for 2 or 3 days, or piperazine citrate as used against enterobiasis is effective in symptomatic infections.

PREVENTION. Contamination of the hands is to be avoided, as well as food grown in contaminated soil.

ANGIOSTRONGYLIASIS

The rat lungworm, *Angiostrongylus cantonensis,* is the etiologic agent of a fatal form of eosinophilic meningitis which has been reported from Tahiti, Hawaii, Vietnam, and Thailand. Living *angiostrongylus* has also been removed from the eye of patients without central-nervous-system involvement. Freshwater snails serve as the intermediate hosts of *A. cantonensis,* and man acquires the infection by ingestion of raw snails.

The nematode produces extensive tissue damage by moving through the brain when alive, and provokes a marked inflammatory reaction when dead. The inflammation is characterized by (1) dilatation of almost all blood vessels, particularly the veins, in the subarachnoid space; (2) marked eosinophilic infiltration of the meninges and brain substance, probably related to the presence of dead parasites, and (3) granuloma formation around dead parasites and the necrotic debris which ensheathes the worm. Charcot-Leyden crystals within macrophages are prominent.

Clinically, eosinophilic meningoencephalitis is indistinguishable from other meningitides. The cerebrospinal fluid contains several hundred cells per cubic millimeter, mostly eosinophils, and the cerebrospinal fluid protein level is elevated. There may not be an eosinophilia in the peripheral blood.

Although most of the reports of this disease deal with fatal cases, it is likely that nonfatal infections occur. There is no effective treatment. The best preventive approach is to warn the populace in endemic areas against eating raw snails.

INTESTINAL CAPILLARIASIS

Intestinal capillariasis is an infection of man caused by the roundworm *Capillaria philippinensis.* This species of capillaria was first discovered in 1963 from a fatal human infection occurring in the Philippines. The infection results in severe illness with a high mortality rate. Clinical studies have shown a severe protein-losing enteropathy and malabsorption of fats and sugars. This species of capillaria is the first of its genus found to infect the human intestine and the first to infect man in epidemic proportions. Of the more than 250 known species of capillaria which parasitize most classes of vertebrates, only three have been shown to infect man, and these have accounted for 16 sporadic cases reported in various parts of the world.

Capillaria are nematodes of the family Trichuroidea, and are closely related to comembers Trichuris and Trichinella. Adult *C. philippinensis* are small, measuring 2 to 4 mm in length. The peanut-shaped eggs have flattened bipolar plugs and an average size of $42 \times 20\ \mu$. The adults inhabit the mucosa of the small intestine, especially the jejunum. Adults, larval forms, and eggs are found in the stool.

The infection has been found only in persons residing in the Ilocano ethnic region in Northwest Luzon, Philippines. Since 1966 the disease has occurred in epidemic form and more than 1,000 cases and 100 deaths have been reported. Males are infected more frequently than females, perhaps because of occupational exposure. Prior to the discovery of an effective chemotherapeutic agent, the mortality rate in untreated cases was about 30 percent. With chemotherapy, the case fatality rate has been reduced to 6 percent.

The mode of transmission and life cycle of the parasite are not established. The presence of many adult worms, larviparous females, embryonated eggs, and all larval stages in human intestinal contents suggests that autoinfection may be part of the life cycle; this would allow for direct transmission by the fecal-oral route. In addition, indirect evidence indicates that man-to-man transmission occurs. The mechanism by which man originally became infected remains obscure. Because the Ilocano people of the region eat many animal foods raw or semicooked, numerous species of local fauna have been examined for capillaria, but without success. Experimental transmission studies in which embryonated eggs have been fed laboratory animals, including primates, have failed to result in infection.

Adult worms in large numbers invade the small-intestinal mucosa and cause a severe protein-losing enteropathy and malabsorption. Autopsy studies have failed to show extraintestinal spread of the parasite. Initial symptoms of intestinal "gurgling" (borborygmi) and recurrent vague abdominal pain are followed, usually within 2 to 3 weeks, by a voluminous watery diarrhea. Other findings, consistent with the basic pathophysiologic process, are anorexia, vomiting, weight loss, muscle wasting and weakness, hyporeflexia, and edema. Abdominal tenderness and distension may occur. The period between onset of symptoms and death is usually 2 to 3 months. Subclinical infection has not been noted.

The diagnosis is made by finding ova in the stool. *Capillaria philippinensis* ova must be differentiated from those of *Trichuris trichiura*, which are similar. Care must be taken that capillaria are not overlooked in patients with *Trichuris* infections because in the endemic area most patients with capillariasis have coexistent *Trichuris* infection.

Administration of thiabendazole, combined with fluid and electrolyte replacement, leads to dramatic improvement. Thiabendazole therapy must be given over a prolonged period to prevent relapse. A divided dose of 25 mg per kg body weight per day is given for 1 month. On this schedule ova disappear from the stool within 2 weeks. Stools should be examined biweekly for 2 months following cessation of treatment.

REFERENCES

Beaver, P. C.: Larva Migrans, Exp. Parasitol., 5:587, 1956.

Beck, J. W., D. Saavedra, G. J. Antell, and H. Tejeiro: The Treatment of Pinworm Infections in Humans (Enterobiasis) with Pyrvinium Chloride and Pyrvinium Pamoate, Am. J. Trop. Med., 8:349, 1959.

Brown, H. W., K. Chan, and K. L. Hussey: Treatment of Enterobiasis and Ascariasis with Piperazine, J.A.M.A., 161:515, 1956.

Chitwood, M. B., C. Velasquez, and N. G. Salazar: *Capillaria philippinensis* N. (Nematoda: Trichinellida) from the Intestine of Man in the Philippines, J. Parasitol., 54:368, 1968.

Davis, C. M., and R. M. Israel: Treatment of Creeping Eruption with Topical Thiabendazole, Arch. Dermatol. 97: 325, 1968.

Duguid, I. M.: Features of Ocular Infestation by Toxocara, Brit. J. Ophthalmol., 45:789, 1961.

Franz, K. H., W. J. Schneider, and M. H. Pohlman: Clinical Trials with Thiabendazole against Intestinal Nematodes Infecting Humans, Am. J. Trop. Med., 14:383, 1965.

Gelpi, A. P., and A. Mustafa: Ascaris Pneumonia, Am. J. Med., 44:377, 1968.

Getz, L.: Massive Infection with *Trichuris trichiura* in Children, Am. J. Dis. Child., 70:19, 1945.

Heiner, D. C., and S. V. Kevy: Visceral Larva Migrans: Report of the Syndrome in Three Siblings, New Engl. J. Med., 254:629, 1956.

Hsieh, H.-C., H. W. Brown, M. Fite, L.-P. Chow, C.-S. Cheng, and C.-C. Hsu: The Treatment of Hookworm, *Ascaris* and *Trichuris* Infections with Biphenium Hydroxynaphthoate, Am. J. Trop. Med. Hyg., 9:185, 1960.

Jung, R. C., and G. Pacheco: Use of a Hemagglutination Test in Visceral Larva Migrans, Am. J. Trop. Med. Hyg., 9: 185, 1960.

Karpinski, F. E., E. A. Everts-Suarez, and W. G. Sawitz: Larval Granulomatosis (Visceral Larva Migrans), A.M.A. J. Dis. Child., 92:34, 1956.

Markell, E. K.: Pseudohookworm Infection–Trichostrongyliasis. Treatment with Thiabendazole, New Engl. J. Med., 278:831, 1968.

Nelson, J. D., T. H. McConnell, and D. V. Moore: Thiabendazole Therapy of Visceral Larva Migrans: A Case Report, Am. J. Trop. Med. Hyg., 15:930, 1966.

Ochsner, A., E. G. DeBakey, and J. L. Dixon: Complications of Ascariasis Requiring Surgical Treatment, A.M.A. J. Dis. Child., 77:389, 1949.

Roche, M., and M. Layrisse: The Nature and Causes of

Hookworm Anemia, Am. J. Trop. Med. Hyg., 15:1029, 1966.

Stemmerman, G. N.: Strongyloidiasis in Migrants. Pathological and Clinical Considerations, Gastroenterology, 53:59, 1967.

Swartzwelder, J. C.: Clinical *Trichocephalus trichuris* Infection, Am. J. Trop. Med., 19:473, 1939.

Tangchai, P., S. W. Nye, and P. C. Beaver: Eosinophilic Meningoencephalitis Caused by Angiostrongyliasis in Thailand, Am. J. Trop. Med. Hyg., 16:454, 1967.

Whalen, G. E., E. B. Rosenberg, G. T. Strickland, R. A. Gutman, J. H. Cross, R. H. Watten, C. Uylangco, and J. J. Dizon: Intestinal Capillariasis, Lancet, I:13, 1969.

Wright, D. O., and E. M. Gold: Loeffler's Syndrome Associated with Creeping Eruption, Arch. Intern. Med., 78:303, 1946.

249 FILARIASIS

*James J. Plorde and
Ivan L. Bennett, Jr.*

DEFINITION. Filariasis is a group of disorders produced by infection with nematodes of the superfamily Filarioidea. These worms invade the subcutaneous tissues and lymphatics of man, producing reactions ranging from acute inflammation to chronic scarring. The clinical pictures produced by various species in this group are more or less specific. The term *filariasis* is commonly used to designate the disease produced by *Wuchereria bancrofti* or *Brugia malayi*, the organisms responsible for elephantiasis. The disorders associated with infection by *Loa loa* or *Onchocerca volvulus* are usually referred to as *loiasis* and *onchocerciasis*.

FILARIASIS (Bancroftian and Malayan)

ETIOLOGY AND EPIDEMIOLOGY. The threadlike adult worms live coiled together in the lymphatics of man. The male *W. bancrofti* measures 35 mm and the female 80 to 100 mm. The *B. malayi* adults are about one-half as long. Gravid females release microfilariae in large numbers into the lymphatics. These embryos, which are sheathed, measure approximately 200 to 300 μ. They eventually reach the peripheral blood, where further development depends on their ingestion by a proper mosquito vector. Species of *Culex*, *Aëdes*, and *Anopheles* transmit Bancroftian filariasis; *Mansonia* and *Anopheles* serve as vectors in Malayan disease. After further development in the vector, larvae migrate to the mouthparts and, if inoculated into a human host, reach maturity in about a year. In the absence of reinfection, man harbors microfilariae for 5 to 10 years, the reproductive life of the adult worms. In most *W. bancrofti* and *B. malayi* infections, the microfilariae are found in the blood in greatest numbers between 9 P.M. and 2 A.M. During the day, apparently in response to changes in oxygen tension, they accumulate in the pulmonary vessels and disappear from the peripheral blood. However, in some endemic areas this nocturnal periodicity is not seen and may actually be replaced with a diurnal periodicity in which the peak occurs in the early evenings (subperiodic form). Periodicity is of epidemiologic significance because it determines which species of mosquito serves as the vector. Furthermore, several nonperiodic forms of *B. malayi* have been found in animals, suggesting the possibility that this disease has an animal reservoir.

Wuchereria bancrofti infection is endemic between latitudes 41°N and 30°S. Distribution is irregular, and there are many peculiar "skip areas" in this geographic pattern, presumably because the endemic disease can be maintained only where human infection and mosquitoes are prevalent. *Brugia malayi* infection is much more restricted in its distribution and occurs in India, Ceylon, Burma, Thailand, Vietnam, China, South Korea, Japan, Malaysia, Indonesia, Borneo, and New Guinea. There were approximately 15,000 *W. bancrofti* infections among American military personnel in World War II.

A small endemic focus of *W. bancrofti* once existed near Charleston, S.C., but no new cases have been observed in several years.

PATHOGENESIS. Pathologic changes are caused primarily by the presence of the adult worm in the lymphatics and may be divided into inflammatory and obstructive. The inflammatory response, most marked around dead or dying worms, consists of infiltration with lymphocytes, plasma cells, and eosinophils. This is followed by a granulomatous reaction which may lead to lymphatic obstruction. There are hyperplasia of lymphatic endothelium, acute lymphangitis, and thrombosis. Repetition of this process over a period of years leads to permanent lymphatic obstruction. The tissues become edematous, thickened, and fibrotic. Dilated lymphatics may rupture into surrounding tissue. Elephantiasis is actually a relatively unusual complication of filarial infections. If repeated reinfections do not occur, the disease is self-limited.

MANIFESTATIONS. Symptoms may occur within 3 months of infection, but ordinarily the incubation period is 8 to 12 months. The clinical findings closely reflect the pathologic changes, with inflammation early in the disease followed by obstruction later. Inflammatory filariasis consists of a series of brief febrile attacks occurring over a period of weeks. Fever is usually low grade but may reach 104°F and be accompanied by chills and sweats. Other symptoms include headache, nausea and vomiting, photophobia, and muscle pain. If the involved lymphatics lie close to the surface, the local symptoms dominate the clinical picture. Lymphangitis is very common, involving the legs more frequently than the arms. It often begins as a tender spot in the region of the malleoli or femoral area and spreads centrifugally. The involved vessels are palpably tender and painful. The overlying skin is red and swollen. When abdominal lymphatics are involved, the picture may simulate that of an acute condition of the abdomen. In Bancroftian filariasis the vessels of the spermatic cord and testes may be involved, resulting in painful orchitis, epididymitis, or funiculitis. Lymphadenitis almost always accompanies and may sometimes precede lymphangitis. The inguinal, femoral, and epitrochelar nodes are involved. Abscesses which may form about involved lymphatics and lymph nodes may discharge to the surface, resulting in persistently draining sinus tracts. The acute manifestations last only a few days and then subside spontaneously, only to recur at irregular intervals over a period of weeks or months. Recovery finally ensues. With repeated infections, slowly progressive lymphatic obstruction may develop in areas where the inflammatory reactions have occurred previously. Edema, ascites, lymph scrotum-hydrocele, pleural effusion, or joint effusion may appear as a result of interference with lymphatic drainage. Lymphadenopathy persists. The lymphatic vessels become palpably enlarged as tense elastic masses beneath the skin, especially in the femoral, inguinal, and scrotal areas. They may rupture and form draining sinuses. Internal rupture of lymphatics may give rise to chylous ascites or chyluria. In a small percentage of cases elephantiasis develops. This complication is rare below the age of twenty even in natives of heavily infested areas. The chronic obstructive phase of the disease often is punctuated by acute inflammatory episodes.

DIAGNOSIS. A history of exposure, the long incubation period, the occurrence of typical inflammatory episodes, and the finding of regional lymphadenopathy, thickening of the spermatic cord, or swelling of an extremity should suggest the diagnosis. There is usually eosinophilia during acute episodes. Lymphangiography may reveal dilated afferent and small efferent lymphatics. The definitive diagnosis depends on demonstration of the parasite. Although adult worms can be demonstrated in biopsied lymph nodes, biopsy is not recommended because it may interfere further with lymphatic drainage. Microfilariae are found in the blood during intermediate stages but not early or late in the disease. As in malaria, they are demonstrated best in thick smears. Concentration methods may be used if the parasite is not found in thick smears. Microfilariae are motile and sometimes may be seen in wet mounts. Because the appearance of microfilariae in peripheral blood is periodic, it is essential to obtain blood at appropriate times. Microfilariae may also be found in lymphatic fluid, hydrocele fluid, ascites, and pleural fluid. Complement fixation and skin tests are available and, although not completely reliable, are helpful when microfilariae cannot be demonstrated.

TREATMENT. Diethylcarbamazine (Hetrazan) rapidly eliminates microfilariae from the blood. It probably also kills or injures adult worms, impairing their ability to reproduce, and clears microfilariae permanently from the bloodstream of many patients. The drug is given in dosage of 2 mg per kg three times a day for 3 or 4 weeks. Treatment with this agent is often followed by allergic reactions to the dying parasite. These reactions may be quite severe, especially in Malayan filariasis. They can be controlled with aspirin, antihistamines, or steroid hormones. In heavy infections, it may be desirable to begin treatment with antihistamines before administration of Hetrazan.

Antimony compounds have no place in the treatment of filariasis.

Reassurance of the patient is very important in this disease. Vaccines and antiserums are valueless. Pressure bandages and surgery sometimes benefit elephantiasis. The prognosis for life is excellent, particularly if infected individuals leave endemic areas or otherwise avoid reinfections. Disease control is accomplished by combining mass treatment with mosquito control measures.

ONCHOCERCIASIS ("RIVER BLINDNESS")

This infection is produced by *Onchocerca volvulus* and is transmitted by flies of the genus *Simulium*, which breed along fast-moving streams. The disease is widespread in southern Mexico and Guatemala and is common in Central Africa. It is estimated that at least 20 million individuals are infected and that about 5 percent of these are blind as a result of the disease. Onchocerciasis is characterized by subcutaneous nodules, a pruritic skin rash, and ocular lesions. Adult worms are found coiled together in the fibrous subcutaneous nodules. In South America the nodules are found most frequently over the head; in Africa they occur primarily over the trunk. The gravid female worms release unsheathed microfilariae which are actively motile and which migrate in the skin, subcutaneous tissue, and eye until they die or are ingested by a feeding simulium fly. The pathologic changes occur as a result of a hypersensitivity reaction to dead or dying microfilariae. The skin lesions may appear as an erysipelas-like reaction over the face or a pruritic papular rash over one extremity. In chronic cases, lichenification and depigmentation may be present. The most serious complication of onchocerciasis are eye lesions, which are usually found in patients who have been heavily infected for a prolonged period of time. A punctate keratitis and iridocyclitis may eventually lead to blindness.

The parasites may be eliminated by excision of nodules on the head and neck, a procedure which is useful in preventing ocular complications, or by chemotherapy. Hetrazan kills the microfilariae but has little effect on the adult worm. Rapid destruction of microfilariae may cause severe allergic reactions which may result in severe ocular damage if the eye is involved. Adrenal steroids are useful in minimizing these allergic reactions. Suramin is effective in killing the adult worms but is nephrotoxic and must be used with care. The prognosis is favorable unless ocular invasion occurs or the number of nodules exceeds 50.

LOIASIS

This form of filariasis is produced by *Loa loa* and is prevalent in West and Central Africa. The infection is transmitted by flies of the genus *Chrysops*. Localized areas of allergic inflammation in the subcutaneous tissues known as *Calabar swellings* are the hallmark of the disease, although infestation may be completely asymptomatic. The adult worms are sometimes visible beneath the conjunctiva, and *Loa loa* is often called the *eye worm*. Diagnosis can be made by finding the adult worm or by demonstrating microfilariae in contents of Calabar swellings or in blood smears. Treatment is symptomatic, and the prognosis is good. An association between loiasis and endomyocardial fibrosis has been reported.

REFERENCES

Adams, A. R. D., and B. G. Maegrath: "Clinical Tropical Medicine," 4th ed., Philadelphia, F. A. Davis Company., 1966.

Cahill, K. M., and R. L. Kaiser: Lymphangiography in Bancroftian Filariasis, Trans. Roy. Soc. Trop. Med. Hyg., 58:356, 1964.

Choyce, D. P.: Onchocerciasis: Ophthalmic Aspects, Trans. Roy. Soc. Trop. Med. Hyg., 60:720, 1966.

Hawking, F.: The 24-hour Periodicity of Microfilariae: Biological Mechanisms Responsible for Its Production and Control, Proc. Roy. Soc., London, Ser. B, 169:59, 1967.

Hunter, G. W., W. W. Frye, and J. C. Swartzwelder: "A Manual of Tropical Medicine," 4th ed., Philadelphia, W. B. Saunders Company, 1966.

McGregor, I. A., and H. M. Gilles: Further Studies on the Control of Bancroftian Filariasis in West Africa by Means of Diethylcarbamazine, Ann. Trop. Med. Parasitol., 54:415, 1960.

Manson-Bahr, P.: The Story of *Filaria bancrofti*, a Critical Review, J. Trop. Med. Hyg., 62:53, 85, 106, 138, 160, 1959.

Ive, F. A., A. J. P. Willis, A. C. Ikeme, and I. F. Brockington: Endomyocardial Fibrosis and Filariasis, Quart. J. Med., 36:495, 1967.

Woodruff, A. W., O. P. Choyce, F. Muci-Mendoza, M. Hills, and L. E. Pettit: Onchocerciasis in Guatemala, Trans. Roy. Soc. Trop. Med. Hyg., 60:707, 1966.

World Health Organization Tech. Rep., ser. 359, 1967. (WHO Expert Committee on Filariasis—Wuchereria and Brugia infections—2d report.)

250 SCHISTOSOMIASIS (Bilharziasis)

James J. Plorde and
Ivan L. Bennett, Jr.

DEFINITION. Schistosomiasis (bilharziasis) designates a group of diseases produced by three closely related species of digenetic trematodes, or blood flukes, belonging to the family Schistosomatidae—*Schistosoma mansoni*, *S. haematobium*, and *S. japonicum*. These flukes inhabit the circulatory system of man and animals living in tropical and subtropical countries. The organs and tissues most frequently affected are the colon, urinary bladder, liver, lungs, and central nervous system.

ETIOLOGY AND LIFE CYCLE. The adult worms which grow and mature within the portal venous system of the liver measure 1 to 2 cm in length. The male has a central trough, the gynecophoral canal, that enfolds the longer slender female during most of its life. After copulation the male carries the female against the flow of portal blood to the small mesenteric vessels. *Schistosoma japonicum* ascends the superior mesenteric vein and *S. mansoni*, the inferior mesenteric vein. Both eventually reach the submucosal vessels of the small intestine; *S. japonicum* ends up in the ascending colon and *S. mansoni*, in the descending colon and rectum. *Schistosoma haematobium* finds its way through the hemorrhoidal anastomoses to the systemic capillaries of the bladder and other pelvic organs. When they can travel no further, the female deposits her eggs one by one, slowly retreating down the vessel in front of them. As the egg matures, it secretes a lytic substance which destroys the surrounding tissue. If the egg lies close to the mucosal surface, it ruptures into the lumen of the gut (or bladder in the case of *S. haematobium*) and is carried to the outside in the urine or feces. On reaching fresh water, the eggs quickly hatch, liberating ciliated *miracidia*. These miracidia have a life span of 8 hr in which to search out and penetrate the specific snail host which is appropriate to its species. Within the snail the miracidia are transformed into thousands of infective larvae called *cercariae*. When cercariae are released 1 to 2 months after the original penetration of the snail, they swim around vigorously and if they contact human skin within 2 days, they penetrate it and become *schistosomulae*. Within 24 hr the schistosomulae work their way into the peripheral venules and are carried to the right side of the heart and then to the pulmonary capillaries. After some delay, they enter the systemic circulation. Those parasites that survive the passage through the mesenteric capillary bed finally reach the portal venous system, where they mature into adult flukes in 4 to 10 weeks.

EPIDEMIOLOGY AND CONTROL. Schistosomiasis is possibly the most important of the helminthic diseases because of its worldwide distribution and the extensive pathologic changes produced by the parasites. It is believed that about 150 million persons are affected by this condition. Control measures have been relatively ineffective.

The continuing presence of schistosomiasis depends on the disposal of human excrement into fresh water, the presence of suitable snail hosts, and the exposure of persons to water infested with cercarias. Promiscuous defecation, latrine drainage, and unsanitary sewage disposal are the more important sources of pollution of streams and rivers. The disease is contracted by persons washing clothes, bathing, wading, or working in contaminated water. Schistosomiasis is more frequently encountered in rural than in urban communities.

Of these three disease-producing blood flukes of man, *S. mansoni* is the most common in the Western Hemisphere. It was brought to the Caribbean area and South America by African slaves. In South America it is present in Venezuela, Dutch Guiana, and Brazil. In Africa, it occurs in the Nile Delta, Sudan, Zanzibar, Madagascar, and Central Africa.

Schistosoma japonicum affects the agricultural population in Japan, China, the Philippines, and Thailand. Men are more frequently infected than women. An important source of infection in the Orient is the use of human excreta as a fertilizer in vegetable gardens.

Schistosoma haematobium is distributed widely throughout the African continent and, to a much less extent, is found in Spain, Portugal, Cyprus, and Greece. In Africa, it is highly prevalent among the agricultural population of the Nile Valley.

The best attack on schistosomiasis is preventive. Public health measures, including proper disposal of human excrement, provision of pure water supplies, and anthelmintic therapy, should be carried out in endemic areas. The effectiveness of these measures is diminished if there are significant animal reservoirs of the disease, as in S. *japonicum* and possibly in S. *mansoni* infections. Extermination of the mollusk intermediate host by chemical agents in areas where the infestation rate is high is an extremely costly undertaking. Available molluscicides include copper sulfate, pentachlorophenate, and niclosamide (Bayluside). This drug appears to be the most effective, but the selection of an agent is determined in large part by the nature of the habitat.

SCHISTOSOMIASIS MANSONI
(Intestinal Bilharziasis, Schistosomal Dysentery)

ETIOLOGY. *Schistosoma mansoni* is distinguished from the two other major species by the structure of its eggs and the adult flukes. The eggs are bluntly oval, have a lateral spine, and measure about 140 by about 60 μ. They are passed in feces and, rarely, in the urine. The intermediate snail hosts belong to the genera *Australorbis* or *Tropicorbis* in America and *Biomphalaria* in Africa. Man is thought to be the principal host, but baboons in Kenya have been found to be infected naturally. It is not known as yet whether they constitute an important reservoir of the disease independent of man.

PATHOLOGY AND PATHOGENESIS. Schistosomiasis mansoni is divisible into three stages: (1) an early stage of migration, during which the schistosomulae are carried by the blood to the liver and mature into adult parasites within intrahepatic portal veins; (2) an intermediate stage, during which ova are accumulating in various viscera; and (3) a late stage, characterized by scarring and fibrosis.

The greatest damage to man is caused by the eggs or their secretions. Reactions may take the form of a hypersensitivity reaction, intravascular obstruction, granuloma formation and eventual fibrosis. However, the secretions, metabolic products, and toxins of the adult worms are believed by some investigators to play an important role. As long as they are living, the adult parasites apparently produce no reaction, but when they die numerous eosinophils gather about them.

Eggs that are passed into the lumen of the bowel cause little tissue damage, but if retained, they elicit an eosinophilic and mononuclear cell infiltration. This is followed by granuloma or pseudotubercle formation. Healing occurs by formation of fibrous tissue and calcification.

In the bowel, congestion of the colonic mucosa, punctate hemorrhages, and thickening of the wall due to edema and fibrosis of the submucosa are the main findings; in Egypt, pedunculated or sessile polyps were commonly found in the rectum, but this is now unusual. Ova transported from the colon by venous blood are retained in the hepatic portal spaces, where they may produce an endophlebitis. Pseudotubercles form around them, accompanied by eosinophils. The organ is enlarged during the intermediate stage but later contracts as a characteristic periportal fibrosis develops. The larger portal veins are surrounded by collars of fibrous tissue, resulting in a severe presinusoidal form of portal hypertension which frequently leads to marked splenic enlargement. With the development of portocaval anastomoses, some eggs are carried past the liver to the vessels of the lung, where they may produce an inflammatory endarteritis with deposition of hyaline, granuloma formation, and obstruction of pulmonary arterioles. There may be interstitial fibrosis and destruction of pulmonary capillaries. On roentgenogram the granulomas may resemble miliary tuberculosis. In time cor pulmonale may develop. Occasionally ova are carried to the spinal cord through anastomotic venous channels. The resulting inflammatory reaction may lead to various neurologic manifestations.

MANIFESTATIONS. The finding of schistosome ova in the stools of apparently healthy individuals is a relatively frequent occurrence in endemic areas. Because the parasites do not multiply within the human host, symptomatic disease is dependent on the continued exposure to infection.

Itching and urticaria, sometimes with fever, are common but not invariable after exposure. Anorexia, headache, generalized aches and pains, and diarrhea accompanied by abdominal discomfort soon follow and last 1 to 2 weeks. These symptoms occur after invasion of the parasite and during the periods of migration of the larvae. From 30 to 70 days following exposure, when the schistosomulae have become adult males and females and oviposition has occurred, more severe symptoms may appear. These apparently are caused by an allergic response to the growing antigenic mass of ova and adult parasites and consist of high fever, chills, cough, urticaria, abdominal pain, diarrhea, and occasionally melena. Physical examination shows lymphadenopathy, an enlarged tender liver, and fine scattered rales. Sigmoidoscopy reveals an inflamed, engorged mucosa with small areas of ulceration and hemorrhage. The peripheral blood shows an eosinophilic leukocytosis. Ova may not be present in the stool initially but usually appear within a few weeks. The clinical picture in severe infections resembles that of typhoid except for the eosinophilia. This acute illness may last as long as 3 months and subsides gradually. When the initial infection is not severe or when anthelmintic treatment is given, the patient may recover rapidly.

Deposition of eggs continues during the life of the female worm (which may be as long as 30 years) and recurrence of these acute symptoms is common.

The late clinical manifestations are related to granuloma formation, vascular obstruction, and fibrosis elicited by ova in the tissues. Abdominal pain, diarrhea with or without blood, intestinal obstruction, and rectal prolapse reflect the pathologic changes in the colon. The periportal fibrosis in the liver and resulting portal hypertension cause splenomegaly, anemia, leukopenia, and thrombocytopenia. Massive hematemesis from ruptured gastroesophageal varices is a common cause of death. The liver is enlarged, but hepatocellular function usually is well preserved, and spider nevi, gynecomastia, jaundice, and ascites are uncommon.

In some patients, particularly adolescents in whom irreversible vascular changes have occurred in the lungs, pulmonary hypertension associated with chronic cor pulmonale dominates the clinical picture. Deposition of eggs in the spinal cord may result in transverse myelitis.

DIAGNOSIS AND LABORATORY FINDINGS. Diagnosis depends on finding the ova in the stools or the rectal mucosa. By the use of methods for stool concentration, a greater number of eggs is picked up from a given specimen, and a larger number of cases may be detected.

By means of a Jackson's laryngoscopic forceps 35 cm long, a piece of mucosa 2 to 3 mm in diameter can readily be obtained through a proctoscope. When this unstained tissue is compressed between two glass slides, the ova can be recognized easily under the low-powered lens of a microscope. It is believed by many investigators that rectal biopsy is the most reliable method of diagnosis; a very small piece of tissue may contain up to several hundred ova. In many cases in which repeated stool examinations have been negative, rectal biopsy has shown living or dead ova. Occasionally, however, stools contain ova when biopsy is negative.

An intradermal test is available and may be helpful in diagnosis. It is quite sensitive except in children and becomes positive about 2 months after infection. It is not species-specific, however, and 25 percent of patients with a history of "swimmers' itch" also react to the antigen. Because it remains positive despite cure, it is valuable in epidemiologic surveys.

The complement fixation test is the most reliable serologic test available. It becomes positive early in the course of infection, often before eggs can be recovered. Like the intradermal test, it is not species-specific. A cercarial slide flocculation test may provide a simple reliable tool for serologic surveys. Positive serologic or skin tests should lead to a vigorous search for eggs by concentration methods or rectal biopsy, but positive tests are not themselves an indication for treatment.

TREATMENT. Certain trivalent antimony compounds are effective against *S. mansoni*. These are tartar emetic (antimony potassium tartrate), stibophen (Fuadin), and antimony dimercaptosuccinate (Astiban). *Tartar emetic* remains the most effective agent available but is also the most toxic. Antimony sodium tartrate is less toxic than the potassium salt and is the form generally used. It is administered intravenously as a freshly prepared 0.5 percent solution. The drug must be given slowly. Extravasation into surrounding tissue leads to painful necrosis. The initial dose is 0.04 Gm; subsequent doses are given on alternate days and gradually increased to a maximum of 0.12 Gm by the fifth dose. A total of 1.8 to 2.2 Gm should be given. The patient should be hospitalized during treatment and should remain at bed rest for a few hours after each injection. Temporary ECG changes are common during therapy; they consist primarily of repolarization abnormalities which disappear a few days after the drug is discontinued. However, arrhythmias, collapse, and sudden death have been reported. Antimonials also may cause hepatitis, acute nephritis, hemolytic anemia, and thrombocytopenic purpura. Any of these complications calls for immediate discontinuation of therapy. Nausea and joint pains can usually be controlled by decreasing the individual dose or increasing the intervals between doses. Heart, renal, or liver disease constitutes a contraindication to therapy with this group of agents.

Fuadin contains 6.3 percent trivalent antimony and is less toxic, but also less effective, than tartar emetic. If the drug can be given intramuscularly, then daily injections of 1.5, 3.5, and 5 ml are given for the first 3 days. 5.0 ml is then given every other day until a total of 100 ml of a 6.3 percent solution has been given. Pain at the site of administration is common.

Astiban appears to be as effective as tartar emetic but is much less toxic. It is given by intramuscular injection as a 10 percent solution for five doses, for a total of 35 to 50 mg per kg (maximum 2.0 Gm). Toxic side effects are mitigated if injections are given at weekly intervals.

Ambilhar (Niradazole) can be taken orally in dosage of 25 mg per kg every day for 5 to 7 days, and may be as effective as Astiban. Although ECG changes occur with this drug also, they are lesss common than with antimonial therapy. However, there has been a high incidence of neurologic abnormalities, and as many as 80 percent of patients receiving the drug show eletroencephalographic changes. Psychotic episodes or convulsions, which disappear when the drug is discontinued, have also been reported. This drug is not available in the United States.

Success of treatment is judged by the disappearance of eggs from the stool, reduction in eosinophils, and alleviation of symptoms. Patients should be examined monthly for 12 months to detect relapses. If living eggs are found, retreatment is indicated. In the late stages of the disease, therapeutic measures are palliative, since the patient is suffering from fibrosis of the liver, portal hypertension, or hypersplenism. The indications for surgical procedures are the same as for the other forms of portal hypertension.

PROGNOSIS. The prognosis is good when the symptoms are mainly secondary to colitis, but when the liver, spleen, and lungs are involved, the prognosis is poor.

SCHISTOSOMIASIS JAPONICA
(Eastern Schistosomiasis, Katayama Disease)

ETIOLOGY. The oval eggs are shorter, wider, and smaller than those of the other two species, measuring about $90 \times 70 \mu$. Mature eggs have a minute hook, or spine, laterally situated and smaller than that of *S. mansoni*. The ova are passed in the feces only. The life cycle is similar to that of *S. mansoni*, but various species of *Oncomelania* snails are utilized as intermediate hosts. *Schistosoma japonicum* lives in the inferior mesenteric venules but frequently migrates into the venules draining the large intestine and oviposits there. Water buffalo, horses, cattle, pigs, dogs, and cats as well as man may harbor the parasite, and some of these species serve as important reservoirs.

PATHOLOGY. *Schistosoma japonicum* resembles the mansoni type, but because of the much greater number of ova deposited by the female worms in the former disease, the manifestations are frequently more severe. Fibrosis of the liver develops earlier, and the duration of the disease is shorter—death often ensuing in 2 to 5 years. In advanced cases the gross postmortem findings are emaciation and pallor; a large or contracted liver with periportal fibrosis; splenomegaly, with fibrosis of pulp; ascites; fibrotic nodules over the colonic peritoneum; fibrous thickening and rigidity of the colon, with small polyps projecting from the mucosa; and thickening and fibrosis of the omentum. Microscopically, the tissue changes are similar to those of schistosomiasis mansoni. Eggs are more frequently found in ectopic locations, especially the central nervous system, than is the case with *S. mansoni*.

MANIFESTATIONS. Following penetration of cercarias through the skin, allergic manifestations such as urticaria, itching, localized dermatitis, cough, and angioneurotic edema accompanied by fever and diarrhea may appear. From 4 to 6 weeks after exposure, gastrointestinal symptoms are evident, a result of ulcerations produced in the intestinal walls by the large number of eggs. Bloody mucoid stools, or periods of bloody diarrhea accompanied by abdominal pain, may be present. If untreated, symptoms may last for several months. The liver enlarges and becomes tender, and splenomegaly develops.

As the disease progresses, signs of portal obstruction, such as engorgement of superficial abdominal veins, ascites, etc., appear. Some individuals present marked splenomegaly, a small contracted liver, profound anemia, leukopenia, and thrombocytopenia associated with severe malnutrition and hypoproteinemia. The majority of individuals suffering from schistosomiasis japonica die of cirrhosis and cachexia, massive hemorrhage from rupture of esophageal varices, or intercurrent infections.

Central-nervous-system lesions occur more frequently in the brain than in the spinal cord and appear clinically as an expanding tumor.

DIAGNOSIS AND LABORATORY FINDINGS. The characteristic ova must be found in the stools in order to establish the diagnosis. In established cases, ova are more difficult to demonstrate in the stools or in rectal biopsy; the intradermal and complement fixation tests are valuable in these instances.

TREATMENT. In general, *S. japonicum* infections are more difficult to treat, and relapses are more frequent. The drug of choice is sodium antimony tartrate; a total dose of 2.2 Gm should be given in the manner outlined for *S. mansoni*. If a lesion is present in the brain, prompt treatment may forestall the need for surgical intervention. Astiban may be used as an alternative drug. Portacaval shunt may be necessary to control bleeding from esophageal varices.

PROGNOSIS. If the condition is not treated early, prognosis is poor in the majority of cases encountered in endemic communities.

SCHISTOSOMIASIS HAEMATOBIA
(Genitourinary Schistosomiasis, Endemic Hematuria)

ETIOLOGY AND LIFE CYCLE. The eggs are compact, elongated spindles, dilated in the middle and measuring about 140 by about 50μ. At one pole they present a short terminal spine. The ova are passed in the urine, and occasionally in the feces. The life cycle is similar to that of *S. mansoni*. The adult worms live in the hemorrhoidal plexus of veins, some going to the rectum for oviposition but most of them passing on to the vesical plexus. The intermediate hosts are snails of the genera *Bulimus, Physopsis,* and *Ferrissia*.

PATHOLOGY. In the urinary bladder, large numbers of ova are deposited in the submucosa and give rise to dense infiltration with eosinophils, lymphocytes, and plasma cells. These foci, or "pseudoabscesses," apparently represent an allergic reaction to the eggs. The trigone is involved at first, but soon the entire mucosa is thickened and ulcerated. In chronic infections, the other coats become scarred and the muscularis hypertrophies. Pedunculated papillomas often develop at the trigone and about the urethral orifices. The bladder capacity becomes greatly reduced as the organ loses its contractility. Lesions occur in the distal third of the ureters in many cases, causing obstruction and hydronephrosis. Bacterial pyelonephritis may occur. In about 10 percent of cases, calculi develop in the bladder, renal pelvis, or ureters. Fistulas between the urogenital tract and intestines may develop. The prostate and seminal vesicles may be affected, and lymph blockage may produce an elephantoid condition of the genitalia. The cervix and vagina can be infected by extension from the bladder. Carcinoma of the bladder is a frequent late complication in Egypt but not in other areas. Because the ova are deposited in the vesical plexus, ectopic eggs are carried to the lungs rather than to the liver, resulting in the early appearance of pulmonary hypertension and cor pulmonale.

MANIFESTATIONS. Painful micturition, frequency, and hematuria are the leading symptoms. Secondary bacterial infection of the urinary tract is frequent, and repeated hemorrhages from the bladder produce severe anemia. Salmonellosis, including the carrier state and bacteremia, is frequently associated with *S. haematobium* infection.

DIAGNOSIS AND LABORATORY FINDINGS. As in the other types of schistosomiasis, diagnosis is made by finding the characteristic ova in the urinary sediment, in tissues obtained from vesical mucosa, or, less frequently, in the stools.

TREATMENT. Chemotherapy is effective early in the disease but is contraindicated when urinary obstruction and infection have supervened. The drugs are the same as those recommended for *S. mansoni*. Surgery may be required for abscesses, fistulas, strictures, papillomas, and various other complications involving the bladder. Chemotherapy is indicated for secondary bacterial infections of the urinary tract. The criteria of cure are the absence of ova in the urine and bladder wall and the disappearance of ulcerative granulomatous lesions, as revealed by cystoscopic examination.

PROGNOSIS. Provided treatment is started without further delay, prognosis is good in recent infection, fair when damage to the bladder and urinary infection have already occurred. Prognosis is very poor in chronic, late infections. After age forty-five, the mortality rate increases fourfold. The frequent coexistence of infection with *S. mansoni* aggravates prognosis and the clinical picture.

SCHISTOSOME DERMATITIS

DEFINITION AND GEOGRAPHIC DISTRIBUTIONS. Certain nonhuman schistosome cercarias may penetrate the skin of man and cause a dermatitis. This condition is known as *schistosome dermatitis*, or "swimmer's itch," and is common in many parts of the world. The condition apparently does not develop after a single contact with cercarias, but it ensues following multiple exposures. Definitive hosts of some of the schistosomes producing dermatitis are the muskrat and migratory birds. Again, snails are intermediate hosts.

Schistosome dermatitis has been reported from the freshwater areas of north central United States, Canada, Oregon, Central America, Western Europe (particularly Switzerland), and the Far East.

A seawater dermatitis believed to be produced by nonhuman schistosome cercarias has been reported in New York, Rhode Island, California, Hawaii, and Florida.

PATHOGENESIS AND CLINICAL MANIFESTATIONS. Because the dermatitis develops only after multiple exposures, the condition is believed to represent an allergic reaction, the nonhuman cercarias being the sensitizing agents. Exposed individuals show positive intradermal reaction when tested with cercarial antigen.

TREATMENT. Local application of antipruritic lotions

such as calamine with menthol or phenol is used to allay itching and thereby reduce the likelihood of secondary infection. Local treatment with antihistaminic drugs will relieve the pruritus.

PREVENTION. Immediate drying of the skin after swimming has been recommended as a prophylactic measure. This will not completely prevent lesions, since some penetration occurs during immersion. Dimethyl phthalate cream has been reported as an effective cercarial repellent.

In some areas, control has been effected by destruction of snails. Copper sulfate and copper carbonate have been used for this purpose. Treatment of shallow waters where snails are abundant has been moderately effective.

REFERENCES

Amaury, C.: Hemodynamic Studies of Portal Hypertension in Schistosomiasis, Am. J. Med., 44:547, 1968.

Cheever, A. W., and Z. A. Andrade: Pathologic Lesions Associated with *Schistosoma mansoni* Infection in Man, Trans. Roy. Soc. Trop. Med. Hyg., 61:626, 1967.

Chemotherapy of Bilharziasis. Report of a WHO Scientific Group, World Health Organ. Tech. Rep. Ser., no. 317, 1966.

Davis, A.: Field Trials of Ambilhar in the Treatment of Urinary Bilharziasis in School Children, Bull. World Health Organ. 35:827, 1966.

Diaz-Rivera, R., F. Ramos-Morales, E. Koppish, M. R. Garcia Palmieri, A. A. Cintron-Rivera, E. J. Marchand, O. Gonzalez, and M. W. Torregrosa: Acute Manson's Schistosomiasis, Am. J. Med., 21:918, 1956.

El-Din Hathout, S., Y. Abd El-Ghaffar, and A. Y. Awny: Salmonellosis Complicating Schistosomiasis in Egypt. A New Clinical Appreciation, Am. J. Trop. Med. Hyg., 16:462, 1967.

Epidemiology and Control of Schistosomiasis. Report of a WHO Expert Committee, World Health Organ. Tech. Rep. Ser., no. 372, 1967.

Garcia-Palmieri, M. R., and R. A. Marcial-Rojas: The Protean Manifestations of Schistosomiasis Mansoni. A Clinical Pathologic Correlation, Ann. Intern. Med., 57:763, 1962.

Kagan, I. G., and J. Pellegrino: A Critical Review of Immunologic Methods for the Diagnosis of Bilharziasis, Bull. World Health Organ., 25:611, 1961.

———, D. W. Rairigh, and R. L. Kaiser: A Clinical, Parasitologic and Immunologic Study of Schistosomiasis in 103 Puerto Rican Males Residing in the United States, Ann. Intern. Med., 56:457, 1962.

Marcial-Rojas, R. A., and R. E. Fial: Neurologic Complications of Schistosomiasis. Review of the Literature and Report of Two Cases of Transverse Myelitis Due to S. *mansoni*, Ann. Intern. Med., 59:215, 1963.

Orris, L., and F. C. Combes: Clam Digger's Dermatitis: Schistosome Dermatitis from Sea Water, A.M.A. Arch. Dermatol. Syphilol., 66:367, 1952.

Powell, S. J.: Natural History of Urinary Tract Bilharziasis in Durban, S. African Med. J., 41:991, 1967.

Zaki, M. H., S. DeRamos, H. B. Shookhoff, and M. Sterman: Further Trials with Astiban in *Schistosomiasis mansoni:*

The Effect of Increased Dosage, Am. J. Trop. Med. Hyg., 15:725, 1966.

251 OTHER TREMATODES OR FLUKES

James J. Plorde and
Ivan L. Bennett, Jr.

PARAGONIMIASIS

Paragonimiasis (endemic hemoptysis) is an infection of the lung caused by the trematode, *Paragonimus westermani*. The dog, cat, pig, rat, and wild carnivores are definitive hosts for the parasite, in addition to man. The infection is acquired by ingestion of cysts in the second intermediate host, a crab or crayfish. The metacercariae excyst in the duodenum, burrow through the intestinal wall into the peritoneal cavity, and migrate through the diaphragm and into the lung, where they become encapsulated. The pulmonary lesions are cysts with fibrous walls measuring up to 1 cm in diameter. Small fibrous nodules representing reaction around deposited eggs also occur. Eggs appear in the feces when sputum from pulmonary lesions is swallowed. In heavy infections, lesions are also found in the liver, mesentery, skeletal muscle, and brain, and cases are often classified as pulmonary, abdominal, or cerebral. In the pulmonary type, the clinical picture is one of chronic bronchitis or bronchiectasis with production of brownish sputum and hemoptysis. A poorly resolving pulmonary infiltrate, lung abscess, or pleural effusion may be present in heavy infections. Abdominal pain and dysentery characterize the abdominal type. Various types of paralysis and epilepsy are observed with cerebral involvement. Eosinophilia is a constant finding. In attempting to establish the diagnosis, eggs should be sought in the sputum and feces. Complement fixation and skin tests may be helpful.

Bithionol is the drug of choice. From 30 to 40 mg per kg in divided doses should be given every other day for a total of 10 to 15 treatment days. The symptoms disappear rapidly, and most infiltrates resolve within 3 months. Side effects are minor and consist of nausea, vomiting, and urticaria. Emetine and chloroquine are less satisfactory. Prevention of superinfection by the same parasite is important, because the disease is self-limiting.

Paragonimiasis has probably the widest geographic distribution of any of the diseases produced by the hermaphroditic trematodes. It is endemic in many parts of the Far East and has been reported from parts of Africa and northern South America.

The most practical control measure is the adequate cooking of all shellfish before it is eaten.

CLONORCHIASIS

DEFINITION. Clonorchiasis is caused by *Clonorchis sinensis* and is characterized by hepatic lesions produced by the adult worms in the biliary passages.

ETIOLOGY. *Clonorchis sinensis,* the most important liver fluke of man, measures about 15 × 5 mm. Infection is a result of ingestion of raw fish containing the larval clonorchis. Many mammals can serve as definitive hosts (dog, cat, pig, badger, guinea pig, and others). The encysted larva is released and migrates from the duodenum into the biliary tract, where it develops into the adult form. Judging from studies on individuals who have left the Far East, the major endemic area, the adult clonorchis is capable of living as long as 25 years.

CLINICAL MANIFESTATIONS. Most infections are asymptomatic. Although there are proliferations of the biliary epithelium, thickening and dilatation of the bile ducts, chronic pericholangitis, and atrophy of the parenchyma, the usual manifestations of cirrhosis are rare. Attacks of suppurative cholangitis following biliary obstruction with dead flukes have been reported. The adult worms may infest the pancreatic ducts, where they can cause squamous metaplasia and periductal fibrosis.

LABORATORY DIAGNOSIS. The diagnosis usually depends on the demonstration of the eggs in the feces or the duodenal contents. An antigen extracted from adult worms can be used in a complement fixation test for the detection of the host's antibody response. Skin tests are also useful.

TREATMENT. No consistently effective treatment is known, but some success has been noted with gentian violet and chloroquine diphosphate. Gentian violet is given orally in enteric-coated tablets in dosage of 60 mg three times a day with meals for 30 days. Chloroquine is prescribed in a dose of 0.25 Gm twice daily for 28 days. Infections which do not respond to this dosage should be treated for an additional 2- to 3-week period Good results have been claimed with hexachloroparaxylol (Hetol) but more experience with this drug is needed before it can be recommended for general use.

PREVENTION. Thorough cooking of freshwater fish will prevent infection.

OPISTHORCHIASIS

Opisthorchiasis is caused by *Opisthorchis felineus* or *O. viverini* and is characterized by hepatic lesions produced by adult worms in the larger bile ducts. The life cycle resembles that of *C. sinensis*, with lesions and clinical manifestations like those produced by *C. sinensis*. The geographic distribution differs in that it is endemic in Eastern and Central Europe and in Siberia and occurs in some parts of Asia. The diagnosis usually is based on the finding of the eggs in the feces or duodenal contents. Treatment as recommended for clonorchiasis may be used. Infection can be prevented by eating only well-cooked fish.

FASCIOLIASIS

Fascioliasis is caused by the hermaphroditic leaf-shaped fluke *Fasciola hepatica*, which inhabits the bile ducts of the definitive host. When fully matured, the adult measures about 3×1 cm and discharges large operculate eggs 140×70 mm.

Fascioliasis produces so-called "liver rot" in sheep, the principal definitive host. The disease is most common in sheep- and cattle-raising countries but has been reported from many parts of the world. In North America it occurs in the Southern and Western United States, Central America, and in the Caribbean Islands.

Infection is contracted by ingestion of the encysted form of the fluke attached to edible aquatic plants such as watercress. The larvae excyst in the duodenum, migrate through the intestinal wall, pass into the peritoneal cavity, penetrate the liver capsule, and finally reach the bile ducts, where they mature.

Early clinical manifestations are related to the migration of the larval form to and within the liver. Epigastric pain, fever, diarrhea, jaundice, urticaria, pruritus, arthralgia, and eosinophilia may be observed during this stage. Fibrosis of the liver similar to that found in clonorchiasis appears only after prolonged residence of many adult worms in the bile ducts. A pharyngeal form of the disease, called "halzoun," can result from eating infected raw liver, the young adults attaching themselves to the pharyngeal mucosa, occasionally interfering with respiration.

The diagnosis usually is based on the finding of the eggs in the feces or in the duodenal contents. It is difficult to distinguish the eggs from those of *Fasciolopsis buski*. Complement fixation, hemagglutination, and precipitin tests have been reported to be helpful. A skin test is also available.

Treatment is unsatisfactory. Emetine hydrochloride in dosage of 30 mg per day intramuscularly for 18 days may be helpful and at times curative. The drug should not be given to patients with chronic cardiac or renal disease or to children.

To prevent infection, aquatic plants such as watercress should not be eaten, vegetables grown in fields irrigated with polluted water should be boiled, and safe drinking water should be provided.

FASCIOLOPSIASIS

Fasciolopsiasis is caused by the large intestinal fluke *Fasciolopsis buski*, which inhabits the upper part of the intestine of its definitive host. The principal definitive host is the pig. In parts of China, India, and other areas in the Far East, infection of man is contracted following ingestion, or peeling with the teeth, of water chestnuts and other edible aquatic plants. The large adults attach themselves to the intestinal mucosa, and these sites may later ulcerate. Diarrhea and abdominal pain appear early. Later, if heavy infection continues, asthenia with ascites and anasarca occurs. Diagnosis is based upon the history and the finding of eggs in the feces. The eggs resemble those of *Fasciola hepatica*. The prognosis in untreated heavy infections, especially in children, is poor. Hexylresorcinol is the preferred therapeutic agent and can be expected to cure or markedly reduce the worm burden in the majority of cases. The drug should be given in a single dose with a glass of water on an empty stomach. The pills must be swallowed intact to prevent burning of the oropharynx. No food should be taken for 4 hr, and a saline purge should be administered 24 hr after treatment. The dose for adults is 1.0 Gm. The most practicable control measure is the brief immersion of all edible aquatic plants in boiling water.

REFERENCES

Chan, P. H., and T. B. Teoh: The Pathology of *Clonorchis sinensis* Infestation of the Pancreas, J. Pathol. Bacteriol., 93:185, 1967.

Edelman, M. H., and C. L. Springarn: Clonorchiasis in the United States, J.A.M.A., 140:1147, 1949.

Hunter, G. W., W. W. Frye, and J. C. Swartzwelder: "A Manual of Tropical Medicine," 4th ed., Philadelphia, W. B. Saunders Company, 1966.

Koenigstein, R. P.: Observations on the Epidemiology of Infections with *Clonorchis sinensis*, Trans. Roy. Soc. Trop. Med. Hyg., 42:503, 1949.

McFadzean, A. J. S., and R. T. T. Yeung: Hypoglycemia in Suppurative Pancholangitis Due to *Clonorchis sinensis*, Trans. Roy. Soc. Trop. Med. Hyg., 59:179, 1965.

Neghme, A., and M. Ossandon: Ectopic and Hepatic Human Fascioliasis, Am. J. Trop. Med., 23:545, 1943.

Ross, J. A., W. E. Kershae, and A. L. Kurowski: The Radiological Diagnosis of Paragonimiasis with Report of a Case, Brit. J. Radiol., 25:579, 1952.

Sadun, E. H., and A. A. Buck: Paragonimiasis in South Korea —Immunodiagnostic, Epidemiologic, Clinical, Roentgenologic and Therapeutic Studies, Am. J. Trop. Med. Hyg., 9:562, 1960.

Tillman, A. J. B., and H. S. Phillips: Pulmonary Paragonimiasis, Am. J. Med., 5:167, 1948.

Yokogawa, M., M. Iwasaki, N. Shigeyasu, H. Hirose, T. Okura, and M. Tsuji: Chemotherapy of Paragonimiasis with Bithionol, Am. J. Trop. Med. Hyg., 12:859, 1963.

252 CESTODES, OR TAPEWORMS
James J. Plorde and
Ivan L. Bennett, Jr.

TAENIASIS SAGINATA

DEFINITION. *Taenia saginata*, the beef tapeworm, is a hermaphroditic cestode which inhabits the intestinal tract of man, its only definitive host.

ETIOLOGY AND PATHOGENESIS. In its adult stage, *T. saginata* measures 5 to 10 m in length and possesses about 1,000 proglottids. The gravid proglottid measures about 5×20 mm and possesses 15 to 30 lateral uterine branches, thus distinguishing it from *Taenia solium*, which has 8 to 12. The head, or scolex, measures 1 to 2 mm in diameter and possesses prominent suckers but no hooks. The eggs are ovid, 30×40 μ, and are indistinguishable from those of *T. solium*. When the eggs are ingested by cattle, the embryo is released in the intestine, invades the intestinal wall, and is carried by vascular channels to striated muscle in the hind limbs, diaphragm, and tongue, the common sites for formation of the cysticercus stage (*Cysticercus bovis*). *Cysticercus bovis* measures about 5 × 10 mm and consists of a scolex held in a cystlike structure. After ingestion of the cyst in raw or undercooked beef by man, it requires about 2 months for the adult worm to develop in the intestine.

DISTRIBUTION. Taeniasis saginata occurs in all countries in which it is the custom to eat raw or undercooked beef. It has been estimated that there are about 20 million infected individuals in the U.S.S.R., and in the world's population almost 40 million. Beef tapeworm is not very common in the United States, but it is the most prevalent infection of this type in the Northern states.

CLINICAL MANIFESTATIONS. In probably the majority of cases the disease is asymptomatic. Epigastric discomfort, diarrhea, hunger sensations, weight loss, irritability, nausea, and rarely an increase in appetite have been reported in association with *T. saginata* infections.

Movements of the worm are sometimes apparent to the host. Rarely, segments become impacted in the vermiform appendix, with development of appendicitis.

LABORATORY FINDINGS. The diagnosis is usually made by the finding of proglottids in the feces. If it is believed that proglottids have been passed, but none is available for examination, the perianal region should be examined as for pinworm infection, using the Scotch tape swab. By this method 85 to 95 percent of infections may be detected, whereas by stool examination only 50 to 75 percent can be recognized. When the scolex is obtained, it may be examined for suckers and the absence of rostellum and hooks, to identify it as *T. saginata*. The above study is necessary, since the ova observed in the feces cannot be distinguished from those of *T. solium*. A slight eosinophilia may accompany this infection.

TREATMENT. Experience with Atabrine has shown it to be a highly efficacious agent. The evening before the Atabrine is to be administered, the patient takes 30 Gm sodium or magnesium sulfate in a glass of water. The following morning, while still fasting, he takes 1.0 Gm Atabrine as 2 tablets of 0.1 Gm each at 5-min intervals. Nausea, vomiting, and abdominal pain are quite common. Then 2 hr later a second dose of sodium or magnesium sulfate is taken. When successful, such treatment will remove the entire worm, which will be found to be stained yellow. If the scolex has not been removed, the tapeworm will regenerate after 2 or 3 months. A newer and highly effective taenicide is niclosamide (Yomesan), which digests the scolex and immature segments of the worm. This drug can be given without preparation or purge in two 1-Gm doses 1 hr apart. Few side effects have been reported.

PREVENTION. The only practical means of preventing infection is the thorough cooking of beef. Temperatures as low as 71°C for as little as 5 min will destroy *C. bovis*. Refrigeration and salting for prolonged periods also destroy the cysticercus. Adequate meat inspection and proper disposal of human excreta will also aid in control.

TAENIASIS SOLIUM

DEFINITION. *Taenia solium,* the pork tapeworm, usually manifests itself as a parasite of man by inhabiting the intestinal lumen. Man is the only definitive host and under some circumstances may act also as the intermediate host harboring the larval stage, *Cysticercus cellulosae.* The usual intermediate host is the hog.

DISTRIBUTION. Taeniasis solium is worldwide but is most common in the U.S.S.R., Asia, and Africa.

ETIOLOGY AND PATHOGENESIS. The hermaphroditic adult tapeworm measures about 3 m in length and possesses a globular scolex containing a rostellum with about two dozen hooklets. There are seldom more than 1,000 proglottids. The gravid proglottid measures about 6 × 12 mm and contains a uterus with 8 to 12 lateral branchings. The eggs resemble those of *T. saginata*. When ova are ingested by the hog, the embryo is released from the egg, penetrates the intestinal wall, and is carried by vascular channels to all parts of the body. Localization with development to the encysted larval stage, *C. cellulosae* ("bladder worm"), occurs predominantly in striated muscle of the tongue, neck, and trunk. The cysticerci are ovoid, gray-white, opalescent structures about 1 cm in diameter. Man becomes infected following ingestion of undercooked pork containing cysticerci. The scolex is freed and attaches itself to the intestinal mucosa, and development to the adult stage begins at this time.

CLINICAL MANIFESTATIONS. Clinical manifestations resemble those associated with *T. saginata*. The clinical picture is entirely different when man serves as the intermediate host. This form of the disease can occur after ingestion of the eggs or the return of gravid segments to the stomach by reverse peristalsis. The released embryos bore into the intestinal wall and are distributed by vascular channels to various parts of the body. Cysticerci develop in the subcutaneous tissues, in muscles, in viscera, and—of most significance—in the eye and brain. Only a moderate tissue reaction occurs while the scolex is viable. The dead larva, however, behaves as a foreign body and provokes a marked tissue response. Symptoms are related to active larval encystment only in heavy infections. Muscular pains, weakness, and slight fever may be observed. The involvement in the brain may be in the form of a meningoencephalitis when the cysticerci are widely distributed. However, epilepsy, brain tumor, encephalitis, and other types of neurologic disorder may be simulated. Degenerated cysticerci ultimately calcify.

Infection with the adult worm can be detected by finding eggs in perianal scrapings or in the feces. However, to differentiate *T. solium* from *T. saginata* infection, proglottids or the scolex must be examined. Cystercercosis should be suspected in an individual who has lived in a hyperendemic area and who develops neurologic findings. Biopsy of subcutaneous nodules may lead to the identification of typical encysted larvae. Roentgenograms of the soft tissues also often reveal calcified cysticerci. Group-specific serologic tests may aid in the diagnosis. The prognosis is in large part determined by the stage and location of the parasite. Surgery may be necessary in cerebral and ocular cysticercosis.

TREATMENT. For removal of the worm in the adult stage, see Taeniasis Saginata, above. It is well to administer an antiemetic before giving Atabrine, to prevent reverse peristalsis, with return of the eggs to the stomach and release of the embryos. Because Yomesan does not destroy the eggs, treatment with this drug should be followed with a purge to prevent autoinfection.

PREVENTION. The simplest and most effective preventive measure is the thorough cooking of pork. Treatment of recognized cases will reduce the hazard of larval stage development as well as the spread of the infection.

HYMENOLEPIASIS NANA

DEFINITION. Hymenolepiasis nana is an intestinal infection of man caused by *Hymenolepis nana*, the dwarf tapeworm.

ETIOLOGY. The life cycle is unique in that both the larval and adult phases occur in the same host. Man, mice, and rats readily contract infection upon ingestion of the eggs. The adult measures about 2 cm in length and may possess more than 100 proglottids.

DISTRIBUTION. Dwarf tapeworm infection has been reported in temperate and tropical regions around the globe. It is the most common tapeworm found in the United States, most of the infections occurring in the Southern states.

CLINICAL MANIFESTATIONS. This tapeworm infection is characterized by the presence of many adult worms in the host's intestine. When infection is massive, diarrhea and abdominal pain occur.

TREATMENT. Atabrine, as prescribed for taeniasis saginata, is moderately effective. Because various stages of the helminth are present simultaneously, it is necessary to repeat the course of Atabrine at least once, after an interval of 2 weeks. Yomesan, as given for taeniasis, is often effective. It should be followed by a purge to prevent autoinfection.

PREVENTION. This is a difficult problem, similar to that encountered in enterobiasis. Only a single host is involved, and the eggs are immediately infective. Personal hygiene should be stressed. The contamination of food by rats and mice should be prevented.

DIPHYLLOBOTHRIASIS LATUM

DEFINITION. *Diphyllobothrium latum*, the fish tapeworm or broad tapeworm, produces a disease in its definitive hosts, including man, characterized by the presence of the adult worm in the intestinal lumen.

ETIOLOGY. The adult worm may be as long as 5 to 10 m and possess between 3,000 and 4,000 proglottids.

PATHOGENESIS. Ingestion of infected raw fish results in infection by the so-called *pleroceroid larva* or *Sparganum*, for which the fish is the intermediate host. The larva matures in the intestine and after 3 weeks is an

adult, capable of discharging eggs. The adults of *D. latum* have been known to survive for 5 to 10 years.

DISTRIBUTION. The infection is common in the Baltic and Scandinavian countries, Switzerland, Italy, Russia, Japan, Chile, and Central Africa. It also occurs in the north central United States, south central Canada, and Florida.

CLINICAL MANIFESTATIONS. Most infections are asymptomatic or produce slight transient abdominal discomfort. Rarely, there may be severe cramping abdominal pain, vomiting, weakness, and loss of weight.

Tapeworm *anemia*, with erythrocyte counts ranging from half a million to 2 million, has many features in common with Addisonian pernicious anemia, including central-nervous-system involvement. Patients with the tapeworm produce intrinsic factor but do not respond when given extrinsic factor and normal gastric juice (intrinsic factor) as long as the infection persists. The location of the worm in the intestine is important, anemia occurring only when the tapeworm is in the proximal small intestine. Large amounts of vitamin B_{12} have been demonstrated in the tapeworm, presumably absorbed from the host's intestine. *Taenia saginata,* which does not produce pernicious tapeworm anemia, contains about 2 percent as much vitamin B_{12} as *D. latum.* The appearance of anemia is certainly related to vitamin B_{12} absorption and possibly also to decreased production of intrinsic factor or inadequate extrinsic factor. It is apparent that the tapeworm and the host compete for vitamin B_{12}.

TREATMENT. Atabrine as prescribed for taeniasis saginata will cure most infections. Yomesan is probably also effective. In the presence of severe macrocytic anemia, parenteral vitamin B_{12} should be given.

PREVENTION. The only practical control measure is the thorough cooking of all freshwater fish. To reduce contamination of waterways, dogs and cats should not be fed raw freshwater fish.

SPARGANOSIS

The *Sparganum*, or plerocercoid larva, of *Diphyllobothrium mansoni* will develop in man following ingestion (usually in drinking water) of a *Cyclops* bearing the procercoid larva. Sparganosis also follows ingestion of infected frogs or application of infected fresh frog flesh as a poultice. The frog tissues contain the Sparganum, which is capable of invading human tissues. The dog and cat are definitive hosts for *D. mansoni.* The location of the larvae determines the prognosis of the infection in man. Surgery and local injection of ethyl alcohol with epinephrine-free procaine to kill the worms is the preferred method of treatment. Novarsenobenzol given intravenously is also said to be effective.

ECHINOCOCCIASIS

DEFINITION. Echinococciasis may be caused by the larval stage of *Echinococcus granulosus* or *E. multilocularis.* These species of echinococcus are distinct morphologically and biologically. In man, *E. granulosus* produces cystic, expanding lesions, involving the liver and lungs primarily, whereas the lesions of *E. multilocularis* are destructive because of their invasive character.

ETIOLOGY. *Echinococcus granulosus* infection in man, cattle, sheep, horses, and hogs, the principal intermediate hosts, is contracted by ingestion of the eggs present in the feces of the dog, the principal definitive host. Following ingestion, the embryos escape from the eggs, penetrate the intestinal mucosa, and enter venous and lymphatic channels. Some soon arrive in the liver and may form hydatid cysts there, and those entering the lymphatics are carried ultimately to the lungs. There is no exogenous budding from the wall of the cyst, only endogenous. Transmission to the definitive host occurs following ingestion of the hydatid cysts which contain scolices. An adult worm may develop from each scolex in the intestine of the dog, wolf, coyote, and other of the *Canidae*. The adult is small, measuring about 5 mm in length, and consists of no more than five or six segments. *Echinococcus multilocularis* infection is manifested by the same type of invasive larval-produced lesion as is observed in the natural intermediate host for this stage, the microtine rodents. The adult, or tapeworm, stage is found in the dog and fox.

DISTRIBUTION. Echinococciasis caused by *E. granulosus* has its highest incidence in sheep- and cattle-raising countries, particularly in North and South Africa, Australia, Central Europe, and South America. In Iceland, a high incidence of infection in man and the dog has been markedly reduced by control measures. In the Southern, Western, and Southwestern areas of the United States, the infection is established, and a small number of cases is reported each year. *Echinococcus multilocularis* has been identified in Eurasia, Alaska, and the Kuriles and adjacent islands.

PATHOGENESIS AND CLINICAL MANIFESTATIONS. Two principal types of lesion develop in the intermediate host: the unilocular type of *E. granulosus* and the alveolar type of *E. multilocularis*. The former is more common, grows slowly, and consists of an external laminated cuticula and an inner germinal layer. Fluid fills and distends the cyst. Daughter cysts and brood capsules develop from the germinal layer, representing endogenous development. "Hydatid sand" found in the cyst consists of scolices liberated from ruptured brood capsules. Exogenous development results from evagination of the cyst wall and ultimately produces the multilocular or alveolar type of lesion. Metastatic lesions occur when growth extends into vessels.

Symptoms produced depend on the size attained by the cystic lesion and the amount of tissue destroyed. Unilocular lesions may become barren following resolution of secondary bacterial infection. Rupture into the peritoneal or pleural cavities may produce an anaphylactoid reaction, which occasionally is fatal. The unilocular type of hepatic lesion progresses slowly and is most amenable to surgical treatment. The alveolar type progresses more rapidly, with metastatic lesions developing in the bones, brain, and other sites. Pathologic fractures occur,

and cerebral involvement may be manifested by epilepsy.

DIAGNOSIS AND TREATMENT. Clinical manifestations seldom are characteristic enough to suggest the diagnosis, but roentgenographic appearance of the lesion, especially when calcification is present, is often helpful. Eosinophilia is suggestive, although seldom present. Inquiry should be made concerning residence in an endemic area, and skin tests (Casoni's or substitute antigen) and serologic tests performed, before exploration is considered. Of the various serologic tests, the indirect hemagglutination test seems the most sensitive. It is positive in three-quarters or more of patients with liver cysts and in one-third to one-half of patients with lung disease. The latex agglutination and bentonite flocculation tests are simpler but not as reliable. Nearly 90 percent of patients with echinococciasis will have either a positive skin test or a positive indirect hemagglutination reaction. Exploration may be required as both a diagnostic and a therapeutic measure. Because of serious reactions to the leakage of cyst fluid into the tissues and body cavities, aspiration should be attempted only during exploration. Aspirated cyst fluid should be examined carefully for scolices, hooklets, and laminated cyst wall. The size of the lesion will determine whether excision or marsupialization is the procedure of choice. Surgical treatment offers the only hope of cure. The contents of the cyst should be sterilized with 10 ml of 10 percent Formalin before an attempt to drain or excise the lesion is made.

PREVENTION. In prevention, (1) contact with infected dogs should be avoided, particularly fecal contamination of the hands and food; (2) infected carcasses and offal should be burned or buried, in order to prevent access of dogs to material containing scolices; and (3) dogs should be treated if found to be infected. The reduction of the incidence of echinococciasis in Iceland is an example of the efficacy of control measures.

REFERENCES

Bakir, F.: Serious Complications of Hydatid Cyst of the Lung, Am. Rev. Resp. Dis., 96:483, 1967.

Beaver, P. C., and W. A. Sodeman: Treatment of *Hymenolepiasis nana* Infection with Atabrine, J. Trop. Med. Hyg., 55:97, 1952.

Bonne, C.: Researches on Sparganosis in the Netherlands East Indies, Am. J. Trop. Med., 22:643, 1942.

Corkum, K. C.: Sparganosis in Some Vertebrates of Louisiana and Observations in a Human Infection, J. Parasitol., 52:444, 1966.

Dixon, H. B. F., and D. W. Smithers: Epilepsy in Cysticercosis, Quart. J. Med., 3:603, 1934.

Dungal, N.: Echinococcosis in Iceland, Am. J. Med. Sci., 212:12, 1946.

Halawani, A., et al.: Treatment of Tapeworms with Atabrine, J. Roy. Egypt. Med. Assoc., 31:956, 1948.

Hunter, G. W., W. W. Frye, and J. C. Swartzwelder: "A Manual of Tropical Medicine," 4th ed., Philadelphia, W. B. Saunders Company, 1966.

Hutchinson, W. F., and M. W. Bryan: Studies on the Hydatid Worm *Echinococcus granulosus*: I and II, Am. J. Trop. Med. Hyg., 9:606, 612, 1960.

Kagan, I. G., J. J. Osimani, J. C. Varela, and P. S. Allain: Evaluation of Intradermal and Serologic Tests for the Diagnosis of Hydatid Disease, Am. J. Trop. Med. Hyg., 15:172, 1966.

Mueller, J. F., E. P. Hart, and W. P. Walsh: Human Sparganosis in the United States, J. Parasitol., 49:294, 1963.

Newman, C. M., and B. S. Aron: Roentgen Diagnosis of Tapeworm Infestation, J. Mt. Sinai Hosp., 28:91, 1961.

Obrador, S.: Clinical Aspects of Cerebral Cysticercosis, Arch. Neurol. Psychiat., 59:457, 1948.

Powell, S. J., E. M. Proctor, A. J. Wilmott, and I. N. MacLeod: Cysticercosis and Epilepsy in Africans, Ann. Trop. Med. Parasitol., 60:152, 1966.

Rausch, R.: Studies on the Helminth Fauna of Alaska: XXX. The Occurrence of *Echinococcus multilocularis* Leuckart, 1863, on the Mainland of Alaska, Am. J. Trop. Med. Hyg., 5:1086, 1956.

Von Bonsdorff, B., W. Nyberg, and R. Grasbeck: Vitamin B$_{12}$ Deficiency in Carriers of the Fish Tapeworm, *Diphyllobothrium latum*, Acta Haematol., 24:15, 1960.

253   HIRUDINIASIS
Ivan L. Bennett, Jr.

DEFINITION AND ETIOLOGY. Human hirudiniasis results from the attachment of *Hirudinea* or leeches to the skin or, rarely, to internal mucosal surfaces. Leeches are found in lakes, ponds, and tropical forests and vary in size from a few millimeters to several centimeters in length. They attach themselves firmly to a host and suck blood. Because their salivary secretion contains an anticoagulant, the puncture wounds at the attachment site may continue to bleed freely after the dislodgment of the parasite.

Land leeches are found on bushes in tropical areas of Asia and South America, and man is infected by contact with the foliage. Attachment of aquatic species occurs during swimming or wading in infested waters. Rarely, young leeches may be ingested in drinking water, an event that can lead to serious illness.

MANIFESTATIONS. *External* hirudiniasis is painless and is called to the victim's attention by finding the parasites or the bleeding puncture wounds left when the engorged leeches detach. With heavy infestations, significant amounts of blood may be lost.

Internal or *atrial* hirudiniasis results from the attachment of small leeches to the mucosa of the upper part of the respiratory tract, larynx, trachea, or esophagus. Infestation of the vagina, bladder, or urethra has occurred in swimmers. As the leeches engorge and grow, they produce symptoms of obstruction, often with bleeding. Pharyngeal blockage is referred to as "halzoun." Hoarseness, cough, nasal obstruction, dysphagia, nausea, and dysuria are frequent, as are hemoptysis, hematemesis, melena, and hematuria. Anemia may be severe, and death has occurred from obstruction of the epiglottis.

TREATMENT. Leeches must be removed with care to avoid leaving mouth parts in the wound. Application of a lighted cigarette or vinegar will help with complete removal. Skin wounds should be cleaned and covered; secondary infection is the only complication.

Removal of leeches from the genitourinary tract is facilitated by irrigation. In the respiratory tract, endoscopy and removal are necessary with the use of topical anesthesia.

PREVENTION. Use of chemical repellents on skin and clothing and boiling of water are the only measures needed to avoid hirudiniasis.

REFERENCES

Chin, T. H.: Further Note on Leech Infestation of Man, J. Parasitol., 35:215, 1949.

Masterson, E. W. G.: Hirudinea as a Human Parasite in Palestine, Parasitology, 1:182, 1908.

Walton, B. C., R. Traub, and H. D. Newson: Efficacy of Clothing Impregnants M-2065 and M-2066 against Terrestrial Leeches in North Borneo, Am. J. Trop. Med., 5:190, 1956.

Section 23
Diseases of Uncertain Etiology

254   SARCOIDOSIS
Carol J. Johns

DEFINITION. A definition adopted by the 1960 International Conference of Sarcoidosis states:

Sarcoidosis is a systemic, granulomatous disease of undetermined etiology and pathogenesis. Mediastinal and peripheral lymph nodes, lungs, liver, spleen, skin, eyes, phalangeal bones, and parotid glands are most often involved but other organs or tissues may be affected. The Kveim reaction is frequently positive, and tuberculin type hypersensitivities are frequently depressed. Other important laboratory findings are hypercalcuria and increased serum globulin. The characteristic histologic appearance of epithelioid tubercles with little or no necrosis is not pathognomonic and tuberculosis, fungal infection, beryllium disease and local sarcoid tissue reactions must be excluded. The diagnosis should be regarded as established for clinical purposes in patients who have consistent clinical features together with biopsy evidence of epithelioid tubercles or a positive Kveim test.

There is no basis for altering this definition. Manifestations vary from incidental radiologic findings without associated symptoms to severe incapacity and death. The course may be one of complete spontaneous remission with no evidence of residual disease, of persistent abnormalities with little or no disability, or of progressive deterioration and death.

ETIOLOGY. The cause of sarcoidosis remains unknown. Originally, it was thought to be a special form of tuberculosis in which the atypical features were explained by some unusual reactivity of the host or some alteration in the tubercle bacillus. This hypothesis continues to have adherents, chiefly because of the occurrence of tuberculosis before, during, or following clinical sarcoidosis and the occasional identification of mycobacteria from "sarcoid" tissue. Also, mycobacteriophages in the absence of phage-neutralizing antibodies in some sarcoid patients have been observed. Lysogenic mutants then might be produced, but may be unrecognizable as the etiologic agent.

A second hypothesis is that one or several as yet unidentified specific inciting agents are responsible for the tissue reaction and clinical picture. These have included viruses, atypical mycobacteria, fungi, and pine pollen, but no definite relationship has been established. Support for the single agent hypothesis is found in the findings of comparable clinical disease and positive Kveim reactions when a single splenic suspension was used.

A third hypothesis favors a particular state of host reactivity to one or more agents. Altered host reactivity could be a result of genetic susceptibility as well as unidentified factors of hypersensitivity. This idea is in accord with the familial aggregations of sarcoidosis, observed immunologic abnormalities, and the occurrence in sarcoidosis of manifestations common to hypersensitivity diseases such as erythema nodosum, uveitis, arthritis, arteritis, and thyroiditis. Siltzbach has suggested that mycobacteria or other agents might act as an immunologic sensitizer in a manner analogous to Freund's adjuvant, with the later development of a granulomatous reaction.

EPIDEMIOLOGY. Sarcoidosis has been observed in virtually every country in which it has been sought. Prevalence rates are largely determined by rates of disease recognition; therefore, figures collected in different parts of the world cannot be compared. Negroes are ten times more commonly affected than Caucasians in the United States, and the incidence in females is usually double that in males. An increased incidence in relation to pregnancy and lactation has been noted, especially in patients with erythema nodosum. The disease is most frequent in the third and fourth decades of life, but the range begins in childhood, particularly around ado-

lescence, and extends to the sixth and seventh decade. Sarcoidosis has been observed in siblings and in parent and child but not in husband and wife. There is no evidence for patient-to-patient transmission.

PATHOLOGY. The granulomatous inflammatory changes of sarcoidosis may occur in almost any organ. The hard tubercles are generally sharply demarcated from surrounding tissues but may coalesce. Some central fibrinoid necrosis may occur, but caseation is usually absent, and inflammatory reaction is minimal. Giant cells containing laminated calcific Schaumann bodies or stellate "asteroid" bodies are frequent, but neither of these inclusions is found solely in sarcoidosis.

Similar histologic changes can be seen in tuberculosis, fungus infections, leprosy, tertiary syphilis, beryllium disease, "farmer's lung," foreign body reactions, lymphomas, and lymph nodes draining malignant tumors. The histologic picture in sarcoid is not specific for that disease alone, and the above-mentioned possibilities cannot be excluded in the absence of other data.

Adrenal steroids apparently cause a prompt reduction in the nonspecific cellular inflammatory reaction of an acute or subacute process and hasten involution and resorption of the "sarcoid" tubercles. It is not known whether these hormones prevent or lessen scarring.

Autopsy material on patients with long-standing sarcoidosis may reveal widespread tubercles in many organs, a few scattered tubercles or focal hyaline scarring, or rarely, no residual changes. Histologic changes have been described in cases where there has been no previous clinical suspicion of sarcoidosis.

MANIFESTATIONS. Clinical manifestations of sarcoidosis generally depend on the activity, degree, and site of tissue involvment. Impairment of function is caused both by active granulomatous disease and by secondary fibrosis.

Constitutional Symptoms. In some instances the presenting features are those of nonspecific constitutional manifestations, with fever, weight loss, fatigue, weakness, and malaise. *Fever* is generally slight and of incidental importance. However, the initial picture may be that of "fever of unknown origin" without localizing signs or symptoms, and daily temperature elevation to over 101°F may persist for months. This type of disease is often accompanied by active granulomatous changes and an inflammatory reaction in the liver. Fever in association with *erythema nodosum* is another form in which sarcoidosis may become evident. This syndrome includes transient tender erythematous subcutaneous nodules over the pretibial areas, arthralgias, and pulmonary hilar adenopathy on x-ray. Hepatic tubercles and a positive Kveim reaction are frequent. This syndrome has been regarded as an early manifestation of sarcoidosis and noted frequently in young women in Scandinavia and Great Britain. It is also observed in the United States, may be overlooked easily, and has a favorable prognosis.

Another common mode of presentation is that of asymptomatic *lymphadenopathy*, particularly involving the mediastinal and hilar nodes. Vague substernal chest discomfort may be the only complaint. Readily palpable peripheral nodes which are discrete, firm, and nontender often attract attention. There may be generalized lymphadenopathy or involvement may be localized to the cervical, axillary, and femoral nodes. Usually, the changes are symmetric, and the epitrochlear nodes are palpable.

Lungs. Pulmonary involvement is the most common and, perhaps, the most important manifestation of sarcoidosis. Serious parenchymal changes with or without hilar adenopathy are evident on x-ray in about 50 percent of all patients. Varying and impressive degrees of dyspnea and cough are noted. A discrepancy in which the radiologic changes exceed the symptoms and signs is a diagnostic clue in early sarcoidosis. In some patients, usually Caucasian, striking radiologic changes may be associated with no symptoms and ventilatory and diffusion measurements are normal. In others, often Negroes, pathologic and physiologic abnormalities may be present when the x-ray shows only hilar adenopathy without parenchymal lesions. There may be progression from mild exertional dyspnea to severe incapacity and cyanosis at rest. This results from extensive interstitial changes which impair oxygenation by destruction of effective diffusing surface. Compensatory hyperventilation is often noted. Symptoms are less severe or lacking altogether if the process chiefly involves the lymphatics in the interlobular septums. Large rounded intrapulmonary masses which may resemble metastatic tumor are probably a result of primary involvement of lymphoid tissue or localized infiltrates producing minimal physiologic disturbance and minimal symptoms despite their dramatic x-ray appearance. Pleural effusions are unusual and should lead to the suspicion that other disease is present.

Cough may be severe and incapacitating and may occur in paroxysms which can even lead to vomiting. Sputum is scanty; occasional blood streaking results from the strain of coughing or endobronchial granulomas. Wheezing is occasionally produced by localized bronchial lesions with stenosis. Physical findings are variable and nonspecific. Respiratory excursion may be restricted, crackling rales may be heard diffusely or at the lung bases, and P_2 may be accentuated or split if pulmonary hypertension exists.

Bronchoscopy generally reveals normal mucosa, although in a few cases it shows granulomatous inflammatory changes. Granulomas may be demonstrated occasionally in grossly normal appearing mucosa.

The course of pulmonary sarcoid may be one of complete and spontaneous resolution of symptoms and radiologic changes, or there may be residual impairment of pulmonary function.

In some patients sarcoidosis is a chronic progressive disease, and pulmonary insufficiency and cor pulmonale occur as late features. Bronchiolostenosis resulting from peribronchial fibrosis and mucosal changes may result in localized emphysema, giving rise to cystic changes, usually in the upper lung fields. With superimposed bacterial infection a bronchiectasis-like picture results. Large cavitary or bullous lesions are rare but can lead to large and repeated hemoptyses, which are occasionally fatal. Such lesions may also form the locus for an aspergilloma with which hemoptyses or disseminated aspergillus infection are hazards. Steroids and frequent use of antibiotics probably predispose to aspergillosis. Surgical management is rarely feasible because of the diffuse and restrictive nature of the disease. Spontaneous pneumothorax is an occasional complication of lung involvement.

Eyes. Acute granulomatous uveitis may be the initial manifestation of sarcoidosis. Ocular disease may progress to severe visual impairment and blindness with corneal and lenticular opacities and secondary glaucoma. A careful slit-lamp examination is worthwhile in all patients with sarcoid to detect early evidence of anterior uveitis. Lacrimal gland enlargement, conjunctival infiltrations, and keratoconjunctivitis sicca of the type seen in Sjögren's syndrome (Chap. 386) are common. Exophthalmos has been observed, as have retinal lesions with vasculitis producing papillitis and periphlebitis.

Skin. Lesions occur in about 30 percent of patients and vary from extensive erythematous, infiltrated, and raised lesions to small nondescript plaques and papules. Increased or decreased pigmentation is frequently noted. Sarcoid changes often occur at sites of old scars or recent injury. Subcutaneous nodular infiltrations occur, and in rare instances calcification of such lesions has been observed. Alopecia occurs if the scalp is affected. Erythema nodosum lesions in early sarcoidosis usually present a histologic picture of a nonspecific vasculitis.

Liver. Clinical manifestations of hepatic sarcoidosis are present in only about 20 percent of cases. Nevertheless, hepatic tubercles can be found by biopsy in about 75 percent and provide one of the most useful means of obtaining histologic confirmation of the diagnosis. Asymptomatic hepatomegaly is frequent. Severe jaundice is unusual, but mild increase in bilirubin and striking elevation of serum alkaline phosphatase level are seen frequently. Intense pruritus may be the presenting manifestation. The spectrum of hepatic sarcoid includes the incidental tubercle, tubercles with surrounding nonspecific inflammatory reaction, chronic active granulomatous hepatitis, postnecrotic cirrhosis with or without portal hypertension, and portal hypertension without significant cirrhosis. Esophageal varices have been demonstrated in patients with portal hypertension, and shunt procedures occasionally have been required. Response to steroids has been disappointing in severe hepatic sarcoid. In some patients the granulomatous disease is limited to the liver, spleen, and abdominal nodes without other clinical or radiographic evidence of sarcoidosis.

Spleen. Mild splenomegaly occurs in 20 to 30 percent of cases, but enlargement may be striking. Sarcoidosis can lead to "hypersplenism," with anemia, leukopenia, and thrombocytopenia. This condition may persist for 10 to 20 years without undue complications, although splenectomy will result in hematologic improvement. Response to steroids has been observed also.

Kidneys. Impaired renal function may occur secondary to hypercalcemia and hypercalcuria, hyperuricemia, and less commonly, because of direct granulomatous involvement. Nephrocalcinosis and renal calculi are common.

Heart. Effects are usually secondary to lung disease, with pulmonary hypertension and cor pulmonale. Primary myocardial sarcoidosis is most commonly manifested by conduction disturbances and paroxysmal arrhythmias.

Salivary Glands. Asymptomatic enlargement of the parotid, sublingual, and submaxillary glands occurs in about 6 percent of cases. Spontaneous regression commonly occurs. A syndrome of fever, uveitis, and lacrimal and salivary gland enlargement is known as uveoparotid fever, or Heerfordt's syndrome. Facial nerve palsies may be associated with parotid disease.

Muscle. Sarcoid granulomas occur in muscles far more frequently than is clinically indicated by pain and weakness. In a few cases symptoms may be severe and incapacitating. Muscle biopsy is likely to be positive in such patients and also in those with polyarthralgias.

Joints. Arthralgias may occur independently as an early prominent feature but are more common in association with erythema nodosum. Chronic migratory arthritis may respond to colchicine. Sarcoid tubercles have been observed in biopsies of synovium. Transient knee effusions are occasionally noted. Chronic periarticular swelling and tenderness may be associated with bony changes in the fingers and toes and skin lesions.

Bones. Asymptomatic, punched-out lesions in the distal phalanges of the hands and feet are visible in roentgenograms in about 10 percent of cases. Associated overlying skin changes are common. Radiolucent skull lesions have been noted in a few patients. "Routine" hand x-rays are not likely to be abnormal in the absence of overlying skin changes.

Nervous System. Neurologic manifestations are variable. Cranial and peripheral nerves may be affected by direct involvement of the nerve sheaths or roots. Facial nerve palsies, which may be bilateral and sequential, are the commonest neurologic finding and may undergo full remission. A granulomatous basilar meningitis can affect the cranial nerves and produce pleocytosis and elevation of the spinal fluid protein. Pituitary involvement produces diabetes insipidus. Involvement of the choroid plexuses may obstruct the ventricles. Cortical changes can result in convulsive seizures.

Other Tissues. Rarely involvement of the tonsils and laryngeal, buccal, and nasal mucosa (often with associated sinusitis) has been encountered. Mucosal lesions are usually associated with cutaneous sarcoid. Sarcoid lesions have been found in thyroid, parathyroid, and pancreatic tissues, and gastric granulomas have resulted in bleeding and perforation. Sarcoid involving the adrenal, cervix, uterus, epididymis, or testis is very unusual.

LABORATORY FINDINGS. Mild anemia, leukopenia, eosinophilia, and elevated sedimentation rate are common in active disease. Thrombocytopenia is unusual but may be severe.

Delayed Skin Reactions. Tuberculin anergy is noted in about two-thirds of patients. Associated generalized cutaneous anergy to other commonly occurring antigens such as *Candida albicans*, *Trichophyton*, and mumps virus has been noted. This depression of delayed skin reactivity is considered to be an important feature of

sarcoidosis, but it varies with the duration and activity of the disease.

Chemical Studies. Hypergammaglobulinemia and reduction of serum albumin are common. Hypercalcuria results from increased intestinal absorption of calcium, which is apparently related to increased sensitivity to vitamin D. Serum uric acid level may be elevated even in the absence of renal insufficiency. Elevation of serum alkaline phosphatase level is attributable to intrahepatic tubercles rather than to bone lesions and may reach levels of 60 to 80 Bodansky units, or more than 100 King-Armstrong units.

Roentgenographic Studies. Approximately 90 percent of patients will eventually show intrathoracic disease on chest x-ray. Bilateral hilar adenopathy, often with associated right paratracheal adenopathy, is a common feature. Unilateral hilar adenopathy is unusual and should initiate a search for other diseases. Patients may be grouped according to apparent severity and chronicity of the radiologic picture as follows: group I—hilar adenopathy with no parenchymal changes; group II—hilar adenopathy and diffuse parenchymal changes; group III—diffuse parenchymal changes without hilar adenopathy; group IV—chronic parenchymal changes of more than 2 years' duration with pulmonary fibrosis. The pulmonary changes are generally symmetrical, and may present a diffuse ground-glass appearance, fine reticular or miliary lesions, large nodular lesions, or multiple large confluent infiltrates resembling metastatic tumors. Fine diffuse interstitial fibrosis may be present. Pulmonary fibrosis may produce contraction and distortion, and extensive cystic and bullous lesions are common in the late stages. Bony changes in the phalanges and skull may occur.

Pulmonary Function Tests. These tests commonly demonstrate restriction, decreased compliance, and loss of effective diffusing surface. Vital capacity is reduced. Measurements of oxygen- and carbon monoxide–diffusing capacity are frequently reduced even in the absence of demonstrable radiologic changes or clinical symptoms. Measurements of vital capacity and diffusing capacity may serve as indicators of progression of disease. In diffuse disease, arterial blood studies reveal with exercise a reduced P_{O_2} because of perfusion of poorly ventilated areas of the lung. The arterial P_{CO_2} is commonly below normal because of contemporary hyperventilation. Because ventilatory obstruction occurs only occasionally, and then in severe, late stages of pulmonary fibrosis, carbon dioxide retention with elevation of arterial P_{CO_2} is a late and unusual feature. Significant impairment of pulmonary function frequently remains even after radiologic clearing. Following steroid therapy or a spontaneous remission, the vital capacity tends to return toward normal, but may remain somewhat reduced. The diffusing capacity may improve significantly but usually stabilizes well below normal despite complete remission of all symptoms. Improvement in diffusing capacity is less frequent than is that of the vital capacity. Deterioration of pulmonary function may occur gradually without significant radiologic detriment.

DIAGNOSIS. The diagnosis of sarcoidosis depends on

consistent clinical features together with histologic evidence of epithelioid tubercles from tissue biopsy or from a positive Kveim reaction. To exclude local sarcoid tissue reaction, as in nodes draining a malignant tumor, evidence of involvement of more than one site is desirable. Careful search for tubercle bacilli, fungi, and foreign bodies must be made in all histologic sections. A positive Kveim reaction is perhaps the most specific feature and helps to exclude other granulomatous processes. Tissue biopsy for histologic diagnosis is most readily and easily obtained from superficial or palpable lesions in skin, lymph nodes, conjunctiva, and nasal, buccal, and bronchial mucosa. Almost any palpable lymph node is likely to be positive. Epitrochlear and supraclavicular nodes will verify the diagnosis in a high percentage of cases. Liver biopsies reveal granulomas in 70 to 80 percent of cases even without clinical evidence of impaired hepatic function. Biopsy of the gastrocnemius muscle frequently reveals granulomatous changes in patients with arthralgias and erythema nodosum. In the absence of palpable peripheral lymph nodes or dermal lesions, biopsy of liver, deeper lymph nodes (as with mediastinoscopy), or muscle is in order. Lung biopsy is generally reserved for patients in whom other diagnostic maneuvers have not been successful or in whom the exclusion of other diseases is urgent.

Kveim Reaction. In 50 to 80 percent of patients with sarcoidosis, the intracutaneous injection of a heat-sterilized suspension of human sarcoid tissues (spleen or lymph nodes) produces a papulonodular lesion with epithelioid tubercles. The nodule must be biopsied in 4 to 6 weeks to confirm the histologic picture of sarcoid. Each batch of test material should be assayed in patients of known reactivity. When this type of standardized material is used, a positive reaction provides strong support for the diagnosis of sarcoidosis. Tests in patients with a variety of granulomatous and collagen vascular diseases have revealed only 2 to 5 percent false positives, but many false negatives are encountered in patients later shown to have sarcoidosis. The reaction is less likely to be positive in long-standing inactive disease, in the absence of lymph node involvement, and during steroid therapy. The Kveim test is particularly likely to be positive in the presence of significant lymphadenopathy of recent onset, in association with erythema nodosum, and when sarcoid skin lesions are present. The nature of the Kveim reaction is not understood.

PROGNOSIS. Sarcoidosis is frequently asymptomatic and often undergoes complete spontaneous remission with subsequent normal life expectancy. There may be impressive clearing of radiologic lesions, especially when the disease seems limited to the thorax. Following a spontaneous remission, recurrence is most unusual. Such remissions are most frequent in the syndrome of erythema nodosum and hilar adenopathy. This "benign" form is more common in Caucasians than in Negroes, where chronic progressive disease is more frequently encountered. Systemic manifestations which include skin, bone, eyes, salivary glands, and hepatosplenomegaly herald a less favorable prognosis. Sarcoidosis is directly responsible for death in only 10 percent of recognized cases. Death is usually related to pulmonary insufficiency and cor pulmonale.

The influence of steroids on the prognosis is not clear. Some patients remain in remission after steroids, but the disease commonly recurs as the dose is reduced, even when therapy has been continued for 2 or more years. It is thought that steroids prevent the progression of disease, but healing may occur with hyaline scarring. Steroids clearly cannot reverse a fibrotic process. Early steroid therapy offers more hope than that initiated after 1 to 2 years of disease.

TREATMENT. Relatively asymptomatic patients require no treatment. *Adrenal steroids* are the recommended agents to suppress the active inflammatory reaction and provide symptomatic improvement. Indications for treatment are (1) active ocular disease; (2) progressive pulmonary involvement; (3) persistent hypercalcemia or hypercalcuria; (4) central-nervous-system involvement with significant functional impairment; (5) persistent systemic evidence of illness such as fever and weight loss; and (6) involvement of a vital organ.

Steroids are most frequently required for symptomatic lung disease. Even relatively asymptomatic lung disease should be treated if there is no evidence of spontaneous regression in 6 months, or if there is progression in 3 months. Asymptomatic hilar adenopathy without evidence of parenchymal disease does not require therapy.

Prednisone is administered in initial divided daily doses of 40 mg, with 2-week periods on daily doses of 40, 30, and 25 mg, and then, maintenance doses of 20 to 10 mg. Symptomatic improvement occurs in 1 to 2 weeks, and the disease regresses over a period of several months. Therapy probably should be continued for a minimum of 6 months, with periodic attempts thereafter to reduce dosage or eliminate the drug. Objective criteria such as x-rays and measurements of pulmonary function are important. Some patients will remain in remission after 6 to 18 months of treatment. Maintenance therapy for many years has proved necessary in many patients in whom relapses recur at a dose below 15 mg. Tapering of the dose must be done slowly, with decrements of 2.5 mg no oftener than at 2- to 4-week intervals if long-term treatment has been used. Lifelong therapy may be required. Careful documentation and observation during tapering is essential in planning treatment. The efficacy of alternate day dosage is not well established, but this regimen can be used for maintenance therapy. It is probably not advisable for initial management. Endocrine side effects with weight gain of 20 to 50 lb have been observed in some women, and diabetes has appeared in some patients. Increased susceptibility to bacterial and fungus infection has been of some concern but is not a major problem. Local steroid therapy has been effective in ocular sarcoid with anterior uveitis or iritis, although there is the risk of glaucoma. Intradermal steroids have been used with some success for disfiguring cutaneous lesions.

Oxyphenbutasone also has been observed to produce radiologic remission comparable to that of steroids in a small series of relatively asymptomatic patients. There is less experience with this drug than with steroids.

Chloroquine (Aralen) in doses of 250 to 500 mg daily has been observed to induce improvement in skin lesions over periods of several weeks, but relapse is the rule when the drug is withdrawn. Remission may be maintained with as little as 125 mg daily. Hypercalcemia has also appeared to respond to chloroquine. Other beneficial effects of chloroquine in sarcoidosis have been less certain and slower, although temporary radiologic remissions of lung disease have been noted after 4 months of chloroquine sulfate in 400- to 600- mg daily doses.

Colchicine has been thought to provide symptomatic improvement in chronic arthritis associated with sarcoidosis.

Oxygen therapy is indicated and efficacious in severe lung disease if there is arterial desaturation. It can be safely administered because carbon dioxide retention is unlikely.

Antituberculous therapy is ineffective in sarcoidosis. However, prophylactic isoniazid is sometimes recommended for Negro patients with extensive pulmonary disease, in areas with high risks of exposure to tuberculosis, and for patients who are tuberculin positive.

COMPLICATIONS. The complications are related to the effects of severe and progressive disease in various organs, the side effects of therapy, and superimposed infection. An increased incidence of tuberculosis in association with sarcoidosis has been recognized. Superimposed fungus infections seem to be increasing. Aspergillosis with "fungus balls" developing in cysts has occurred. Candidiasis and cryptococcosis in association with sarcoidosis have also been noted. It is highly probable that long-term steroid and antimicrobial therapy predispose to these fungus infections.

REFERENCES

"Bibliography on Sarcoidosis, 1878–1963," National Library of Medicine, U.S. Dept. Health, Education, and Welfare, 1964.

Cummings, M. M., and J. F. Hammarsten: Sarcoidosis, Ann. Rev. Med., 13:19–40, 1962.

Longcope, W. T., and D. G. Freiman: A Study of Sarcoidosis: Based on a Combined Investigation of 160 Cases Including 30 Autopsies from The Johns Hopkins Hospital and Massachusetts General Hospital, Medicine, 31:1–132, 1952.

Mayock, R. L., P. Bertrand, C. E. Morrison, and J. H. Scott: Manifestations of Sarcoidosis: Analysis of 145 Patients, with a Review of 9 Series Selected from the Literature, Am. J. Med., 35:67–89, 1963.

Proceedings of the International Conference on Sarcoidosis, June 1–3, 1960, Am. Rev. Resp. Dis., 84(part 2):1–183, 1961.

Proceedings of the Third International Conference on Sarcoidosis, Sept. 11–14, 1963, Acta Med. Scand., 176(suppl. 425):1–310, 1964.

Reisner, D.: Observations on the Course and Prognosis of Sarcoidosis, with Special Consideration of its Intra-thoracic Manifestations, Am. Rev. Resp. Dis. 96:361–80, 1967.

La Sarcoidose, Rapports de la IVᵉ Conférence Internationale Paris, 12–15 Septembre, 1966, J. Turiaf, and J. Chabot (Eds.), Paris, Masson et Cie, 1967.

Smellie, H., and C. Hoyle: The Natural History of Pulmonary Sarcoidosis, Quart. J. Med., 29:539–558, 1960.

255 INFECTIOUS MONONUCLEOSIS
M. M. Wintrobe

DEFINITION. This disorder of unknown cause is usually benign and probably of infectious origin. It is characterized by irregular fever, sore throat, lymphadenopathy, and enlargement of the spleen, as well as by an absolute lymphocytosis made up of cells of a peculiar type. High concentrations of antibodies against sheep erythrocytes are demonstrable in the blood serum.

HISTORY. Since the designation "infectious mononucleosis" was first proposed by Sprunt and Evans in 1920, an ever-increasing number of cases has been observed and reported, especially since 1935. This is at least in part because of better recognition of the disease. Prior to 1920 a few sporadic cases had been observed. The relationship of epidemics in children and in adults described under the title of "glandular fever" to infectious mononucleosis is in doubt because in most instances appropriate serologic techniques were not used, and when they were, the results were indefinite and irregular.

ETIOLOGY AND PATHOGENESIS. This is a disease of young people, including children, which has now been observed practically throughout the world. In the United States, infectious mononucleosis has been less frequent in Negroes than in white persons. It is relatively common in interns, medical students, and nurses, but many cases among other persons undoubtedly pass unnoticed. The mild or nonspecific character of many of the symptoms may be responsible, or the fact that appropriate blood examinations have not been made. With increasing frequency, sporadic cases have been observed wherever young people live together, as in boarding schools, colleges, and military groups. Infectious mononucleosis is quite uncommon over the age of forty but has been encountered occasionally.

The cause is unknown, although it is generally believed that the disease is infectious in nature.

Patients with infectious mononucleosis have been shown to develop high antibody titers to a herpes-type virus. This agent, which has been called the EB virus, originally was found in cell lines derived from burkitt lymphomas. These observations strongly support the possibility that EB or a closely related virus is the etiologic agent of infectious mononucleosis.

PATHOLOGY. The outstanding features are the diffuse distribution of the tissue lesions and the involvement of the lymphoid tissue. In the latter the gross findings are observed. Histologically, widespread focal lesions are found, consisting of perivascular aggregates of normal and abnormal lymphocytes. Hyperplasia of nasopharyngeal lymphoid tissue is constant. Lymph node reactions range from a predominantly follicular hyperplasia to a blurred pattern due to proliferation of lymphocytic and reticuloendothelial elements in the medullary cords which may resemble the findings in malignant lymphoma.

CLINICAL PICTURE. In the absence of a demonstrable etiologic agent, some have assumed that the clinical manifestations of infectious mononucleosis are protean and have been willing to include under this diagnosis many cases of otherwise unexplained, self-limited febrile disorders with clinical and hematologic features somewhat resembling those of infectious mononucleosis, especially when occurring in young persons. This does not seem to be justified. For the present, at least, it would seem better to restrict the diagnosis to cases in which the lymphocytes constitute more than 50 percent of the leukocytes, "atypical" lymphocytes are present, and both these features have been present for a period of at least 10 days. In addition, the titer of heterophil antibodies, after guinea pig absorption, should be at least 1:56. The clinical picture of the disorder, so defined, is quite consistent.

Three clinical stages can be identified, namely, (1) a prodromal period of 3 to 6 days, characterized by nonspecific features similar to those of other infections and during which diagnosis may be difficult; (2) a mid-stage of 4 to 20 days during which the full-blown disease presents itself; and (3) the stage of convalescence.

The incubation period is uncertain and may be as long as 4 to 7 weeks. The onset is gradual, but ultimately bilateral *lymph node enlargement* develops in practically all cases. The cervical glands are always affected, the axillary and inguinal frequently but not invariably. Involvement of the posterior cervical nodes is of value in differentiation from other forms of pharyngitis. The glands are affected singly or in groups. Local heat, redness, and marked tenderness of the glands are conspicuously absent. The *spleen* is enlarged in at least 50 percent of cases.

The most common *syndrome* is the *pharyngeal* (80 percent of cases). Pharyngeal inflammation varies in intensity, but hyperplasia of pharyngeal lymphoid tissue is almost always present. The palatal arch and uvula often have a gelatinous appearance, but significant edema of the uvula is unusual. In some cases the throat presents the typical picture of follicular tonsillitis or that of Vincent's angina or of diphtheria. Stomatitis may be present.

The *fever* is of no characteristic type. It may be transient in degree, but in one-sixth to one-third of cases the temperature reaches a peak of 103 to 104°F; it is only occasionally higher. The temperature may rise in a remittent manner in the course of 4 to 8 days. A secondary rise after an initial drop to normal may accompany the onset of glandular swelling or sore throat.

A *typhoidal syndrome*, with fever, malaise, and headache predominating, is seen in 12 percent of cases. The headache may be so severe as to suggest meningitis. Gastrointestinal symptoms are rare.

In about 8 percent of cases *icterus* occurs and the picture of hepatitis is found. In the majority of cases, however, hepatitis without jaundice is present, as judged by liver function tests. The hepatic disease is usually mild.

Edema of the eyelids has been described in a third of the cases and a palatal enanthem in almost as many. The latter consists of 5 to 20 pinhead-sized red spots, usually at the junction of the soft and hard palates, which appear in crops, darken in about 48 hr, and disappear after 3 or 4 days. Cutaneous lesions are unusual except for faint erythema or, rarely, a maculopapular eruption. Petechial hemorrhages and purpura are encountered sometimes, and other hemorrhagic manifestations, such as epistaxis, may occur.

Other manifestations are rare. These include abdominal pain of a type to suggest acute appendicitis, possibly due to swelling of mesenteric nodes; cardiac and pulmonary manifestations, such as tachycardia, cyanosis, signs of pericarditis, transient T wave changes, and enlargement of mediastinal lymph nodes or pulmonary parenchymal changes; and a variety of neurologic manifestations. The last include headache, blurring of vision, even convulsions, stupor, coma, bradycardia, stiff neck, the Guillain-Barré syndrome, and encephalitis.

Convalescence is sometimes slow and may be associated with marked prostration. Recrudescences are very common. Relapse has occurred in about 6 percent of cases. Recovery is the rule, but death has been observed in a few instances from such complications as rupture of the spleen, respiratory paralysis in association with nervous system involvement, pneumonia, edema of the glottis, and hemorrhage from a deep tonsillar ulceration.

BLOOD PICTURE. The leukocyte count is usually increased but, in the first week especially, there may be leukopenia due to granulocytopenia. The leukocytosis is usually moderate (10,000 to 15,000 cells per cu mm), but it may sometimes be very marked. It is due to an increase in number of lymphocytes, and these, in the main, are of a peculiar type: their nucleus may be oval, kidney-shaped, or slightly lobulated, and the cytoplasm often is somewhat basophilic and may be vacuolated or foamy in appearance. The nuclear chromatin is usually coarse and irregular, and nucleoli are rarely seen. These cells make up 60 percent or more of all the leukocytes.

The characteristic changes in the leukocytes may appear as early as the second day of illness or as late as the twelfth day. They attain a peak by the seventh to tenth day and persist usually for 1 to 2 months.

Anemia is extremely rare, but several instances of hemolytic anemia complicating infectious mononucleosis have been reported. Thrombocytopenia is rare, but in a few cases the clinical picture resembled that of idiopathic thrombocytopenic purpura. The bone marrow reveals a slight myeloid hyperplasia and immaturity; there may be an increase in number of lymphocytes.

The serum characteristically contains agglutinins against sheep red cells in high titer (heterophil antibodies, Paul-Bunnell test). This has been observed, in different series and according to the diagnostic criteria of the authors, in 60 to 100 percent of cases. The Paul-Bunnell test is actually nonspecific. Anti-sheep agglutinins are present in titers up to 1:28 in most normal persons and occasionally even in a titer of 1:56. In various infections a titer of 1:112 and occasionally of 1:224 may be seen. Persons receiving injections of horse serum and horse immune serum may develop titers as high as any seen in infectious mononucleosis. For these reasons it is generally considered that in the presence of clinical and hematologic findings suggestive of infectious mononucleosis, only a titer of 1:224 or higher can be interpreted as confirming the diagnosis. When there is doubt, a differential test is required. This is based on the observation that heterophil antibodies in normal serum, in horse serum sensitization, and in a variety of infections can be absorbed completely by guinea pig kidney. On the other hand, anti-sheep agglutinins in infectious mononucleosis are never completely removed by treating the serum with guinea pig kidney although they are, as a rule, completely removed by beef red cells. The differential test is carried out by absorbing a portion of the patient's serum with guinea pig kidney and another portion with beef red cells. After this the absorbed specimens are tested for sheep red cell agglutination.

Horse agglutinins have been found to be as specific but more sensitive than sheep agglutinins, and horse erythrocytes are now used in preference to sheep erythrocytes in the differential test. Formalinized horse red cells serve as the immunologic indicator in the very simple and highly specific "mono" test.

In infectious mononucleosis, highest heterophil antibody titers are found usually during the second and third weeks of illness and, as a rule, positive reactions last 4 to 8 weeks. The titer bears no relation to the severity of the disease or the degree of lymphocytosis.

A 100 percent increase in IgM globulins and a 50 percent increase in IgG accompanies the increase in heterophil antibodies and a linear relation between IgM levels and heterophil antibody titers has been observed. It is postulated that the agent causing infectious mononucleosis shares antigenic determinants with the heterophil antigen on sheep cells. Additional serum protein alterations which may occur in this disease include the appearance of the cold agglutinating antibody anti-i, and transiently positive serologic tests for syphilis and for rheumatoid factors.

Renal function is rarely impaired, but albumin and red cells may be found in the *urine*. The *cerebrospinal fluid* pressure may be moderately elevated, and pleocytosis due to lymphocytes may be found.

DIAGNOSIS. Glandular enlargement, sore throat, fever, the characteristic cells in the blood, and an increased titer of heterophil antibodies are a combination of findings which makes recognition of infectious mononucleosis easy in most instances. Some investigators have been willing to define infectious mononucleosis quite broadly. However, it seems reasonable to require a minimum of 20 percent lymphocytes of the characteristic type at the time of the fever peak and a positive heterophil antibody reaction. In the absence of a positive heterophil antibody test, it is difficult to maintain the diagnosis. The paradox of a positive heterophil antibody test unaccompanied by characteristic clinical and hematologic features of infectious mononucleosis can be explained by persistence of antibodies from an earlier unrecognized attack and, in rare instances, by a resurgence of heterophil antibodies with another illness.

The above criteria should help to differentiate infectious mononucleosis from other infectious disorders. It may be added that certain symptoms are so unusual in infectious mononucleosis that their presence militates against the diagnosis; namely, nasal discharge or congestion, paroxysmal harassing cough, sputum, chest pain, joint pains, painful or extremely tender lymph nodes, watery diarrhea, and hematuria or dysuria.

Lymphocytosis, relative or absolute, may be encountered regularly or occasionally in a number of the diseases with which infectious mononucleosis may be confused on clinical grounds. Marked leukocytosis (40,000 cells per cu mm or even higher), chiefly due to the presence of small lymphocytes of normal appearance, characterizes a benign disorder, *acute infectious lymphocytosis*, which has been observed chiefly in children and is accompanied by only mild constitutional manifestations and no lymphadenopathy, splenomegaly, or positive heterophil agglutination reactions.

The clinical picture may be like that of serum sickness, a condition in which lymphocytes quite similar to those seen in infectious mononucleosis may be found and a positive heterophil antibody test may be obtained. The differential test is required to distinguish between the antibody reactions in infectious mononucleosis and the rise in titer produced by horse serum.

It is not rare for infectious mononucleosis to be confused with acute leukemia. Differentiation depends on the demonstration of very immature leukocytes ("blasts") in the blood or the bone marrow and the presence of anemia and thrombocytopenia, both of which are rare in infectious mononucleosis. The heterophil antibody test will be negative.

Following open-heart surgery a syndrome characterized by daily remittent fever, splenomegaly, less often adenopathy and a rubelliform rash, together with "infectious mononucleosis" cells in the blood has been observed in 3 to 11 percent of cases. The heterophil antibody test is negative. This picture also has been described following blood transfusion and in a few otherwise normal adults. The disorder is attributed to cytomegalic virus infection (Chap. 232).

TREATMENT. There is no specific therapy. Sodium perborate mouth washes are recommended since Vincent's infection is frequently associated with infectious mononucleosis. Many agents have been advocated, such as arsenicals, penicillin, the tetracyclines, and chloroquine, but such claims are difficult to evaluate. As a rule, without treatment, the irregular fever persists for 1 to 3 weeks, and subjective symptoms disappear in 2 to 4 weeks. *Relapses* are not uncommon and may be late, but recurrences are very rare. The positive heterophil antibody reaction may persist for as long as 5 or 6 months. In instances of more than average severity, adrenocorticosteroid therapy will give symptomatic relief and shorten the febrile period, but such treatment, if used, should be continued for only 5 to 10 days.

REFERENCES

Hoagland, R. J.: Infectious Mononucleosis, New York, Grune & Stratton, Inc., 1967.

Klemola, E., et al.: Further Studies on Cytomegalovirus Mononucleosis in Previously Healthy Individuals, Acta Med. Scand., 182:311, 1967.

Niederman, J. C., R. W. McCollum, G. Henle, and W. Henle: Infectious Mononucleosis, J.A.M.A., 203:205, 1968.

Wintrobe, M. M.: "Clinical Hematology," 6th ed., Philadelphia, Lea & Febiger, 1967.

256 FAMILIAL MEDITERRANEAN FEVER (Familial Paroxysmal Polyserositis)

Sheldon M. Wolff

DEFINITION. Familial Mediterranean fever (FMF) is an inherited disorder of unknown etiology, characterized by recurrent episodes of fever, peritonitis, and/or pleuritis. Arthritis, skin lesions, and amyloidosis are seen in some patients.

HISTORY. Although the first report of FMF was by Janeway and Mosenthal in 1908, it was not until the report of five cases by Siegal in 1945 that attention was focused on FMF as a distinct entity. Subsequently, some authors have not applied strict clinical criteria, however, and many patients with other diseases have been reported as having FMF. The detailed and extensive descriptions by Heller and Sohar have clarified many of the clinical aspects of FMF.

TERMINOLOGY. The variety of names given to FMF has led to confusion concerning its clinical features. None of the names, including *FMF*, is completely satisfactory, but FMF has received the widest acceptance. Such terms as *periodic disease, periodic peritonitis, la maladie periodique,* etc. are inaccurate because the disease often is not cyclical. *Benign paroxysmal peritonitis* is inappropriate because many of the patients have involvement of serosal surfaces other than the peritoneum, and some die of amyloidosis. *Familial paroxysmal polyserositis* is an acceptable alternative for the term *FMF*.

ETHNOLOGY AND GENETICS. FMF occurs predominantly in patients of non-Ashkenazic (Sephardic) Jewish, Armenian, and Arabic ancestry. However, the disease is not restricted to these groups, and has been seen in patients of Italian, Ashkenazic Jewish, and Irish descent as well as others.

The best studies of the genetics of FMF have been done in Israel, where relatively homogeneous population groups exist. In Israel, the disease appears to be inherited as an autosomal recessive. Nevertheless, a large number of patients give no family history of the disease. Consanguinity among the parents of FMF patients is as high as 20 percent, a figure which may be an underestimate because most patients came from very inbred ethnic groups. Approximately 60 percent of patients are male.

ETIOLOGY. Although numerous pathogenetic mechanisms have been suggested, the etiology of FMF is unknown. Fever and inflammation are such prominent signs that frequent attempts have been made to implicate infectious agents and/or their products. It has been suggested that FMF is a form of brucellosis or tuberculosis. Suffice it to say that extensive studies utilizing modern microbiologic and serologic techniques have failed to implicate these or any other specific infectious agents.

It has been reported that FMF is due to an allergy to milk or to hypersensitivity to tuberculoprotein, but such a hypersensitive state has not been substantiated. There is no firm evidence favoring an autoimmune etiology.

Reimann has suggested that FMF, like many other recurring illnesses ("periodic diseases"), may be a pathologic exaggeration of normal periodic temperature rhythmicity. However, extensive studies of temperature and other circadian rhythms in FMF patients have failed to demonstrate alterations from normal.

Because many FMF patients note that certain emotional or environmental changes may have profound effects on the frequency with which episodes of their disease occur, a psychosomatic basis has been suggested for the illness. There is no question that most patients eventually have transient or even permanent psychologic alterations, which probably reflect their reaction to a chronic recurring illness that is forever threatening their social, economic, and personal well-being, but there is no evidence for a functional etiology for FMF.

The demonstration that FMF is inherited as an autosomal recessive disorder has led to the thesis that it is another inborn error of metabolism. In view of initial optimistic reports that restriction of dietary fat ameliorates the course of FMF, it was thought that the disorder might be one of altered lipid metabolism. Despite extensive studies, no such error has been found. Reported instances of excessive urinary excretion of porphyrins in FMF are probably examples of true porphyria and not FMF.

Bondy and his colleagues reported that blood levels of unconjugated etiocholanolone were elevated during fever in 13 patients, 6 of whom had FMF. Subsequent studies, however, showed only inconstant correlation between levels of etiocholanolone and fever. The possible role of etiocholanolone and other steroids in FMF will be discussed below.

PATHOLOGY. Despite the striking clinical manifestations during an acute attack of FMF, no specific pathologic alterations have been found. Most FMF patients undergo at least one laparotomy, and only acute peritoneal inflammation in which the exudate contains a predominance of polymorphonuclear leukocytes is present. A disproportionately large number of male patients develops gallbladder disease with and without cholelithiasis, but extensive histopathologic examination has failed to reveal any specific pathologic changes. Pleural and joint inflammation are also nonspecific.

In the amyloidosis which accompanies FMF, amyloid is deposited in the intima and media of the arterioles, the subendothelial region of venules, the glomeruli, and the spleen. Aside from their vessels, the heart and liver are uninvolved.

MANIFESTATIONS. In the majority of patients, the symptoms of FMF begin between the ages of five and fifteen, although attacks sometime commence during infancy, and onset has occurred as late as age thirty-eight. The duration and frequency of attacks vary greatly in the same patient, and there is no set rhythm or periodicity to their occurrence. The usual acute episode lasts 24 to 48 hr, but some may be prolonged for 7 to 10 days. The attacks range in frequency from twice weekly to once a year, but 2 to 4 weeks is the commonest interval. Spontaneous remissions lasting up to 4 years have been seen. In the majority of cases, pregnancy is associated with an absence of acute episodes, and many patients note less frequent attacks in the summer than in the winter. There tends to be a decrease in the severity and frequency of the attacks with age or with development of amyloidosis.

Fever. Fever is a cardinal manifestation of FMF and is present during most but not all attacks. Rarely, fever may be present without serositis. The temperature rise may be preceded by a chill, and will peak in 12 to 24 hr. Defervescence is often accompanied by diaphoresis. The fever ranges from 38.5 to 40°C but is quite variable.

Abdominal Pain. Abdominal pain occurs in more than 95 percent of patients, and may vary in severity in the same patient. Minor premonitory discomfort may precede an acute episode by 24 to 48 hr. The pain usually starts in one quadrant and then spreads to involve the whole abdomen. The initial site is usually very tender. Tenderness may remain localized with referred pain in other areas, and there may be radiation to the back. There may be splinting of the chest and pain in one or both shoulders, typical of diaphragmatic irritation. Nausea and vomiting sometimes occur. The abdomen is usually distended, and may become rigid with decreased or absent bowel sounds. On x-ray, the wall of the small intestine may appear edematous, transit of barium is slowed, and fluid levels may be seen. Because the manifestations of an acute abdominal attack can simulate those of a perforated viscus so closely, patients should be advised to have an elective appendectomy between attacks so that acute appendicitis will not obfuscate the picture at a later date. An abdominal operation may precipitate an acute attack of FMF which may be confused with other postoperative complications.

Chest Pain. Most patients with abdominal attacks have referred chest pain at one time or another, and 75 percent also develop acute pleuritic pain with or without abdominal symptoms. In 30 percent, the attacks of pleuritis precede the onset of abdominal attacks by varying periods of time and a small number of patients never develops abdominal attacks. Chest pain is usually unilateral and is associated with diminished breath sounds, a friction rub, or a transient pleural effusion.

Joint Pain. In Israel, 75 percent of patients report at least one episode of acute arthritis. Arthritis can be distinct from abdominal or pleural attacks, can be acute or, rarely, chronic, and may involve one or several joints. Effusions are common and the large joints are involved most frequently. Radiologic findings are nonspecific. Despite careful search, frank arthritis rarely has been seen in the United States. Some patients have a history of rheumatic fever–like illness in childhood, but in a large series of patients, including 20 from the Middle East, acute arthritis was not observed. Mild arthralgia is common during acute attacks but is nonspecific and can be seen in many febrile illnesses, including experimentally induced hyperthermia.

Skin Manifestations. Skin involvement is reported by 25 to 35 percent of patients. These lesions consist of painful, erythematous areas of swelling from 5 to 20 cm in diameter, usually located on the lower legs, the medial malleolus, or the dorsum of the foot. They may occur without abdominal or pleural pain and subside within 24 to 48 hr.

Other Signs and Symptoms. Involvement of other serosal membranes has been reported, but pericarditis is rare, and it is probable that descriptions of recurrent meningitis have been diseases other than FMF. Hematuria, splenomegaly, and small white dots called "colloid bodies" in the ocular fundus are among the findings of questionable significance. Rarely migrainelike headaches accompany acute abdominal attacks, and some patients have become somewhat irrational or show extreme emotional lability during attacks. Whether these are primary manifestations of FMF or secondary effects of pain and fever is not known.

Complications. The most serious complication of FMF in the United States is drug addiction or habituation, and obviously efforts should be made to avoid use of narcotics. Depression and lack of motivation are common, and patients with FMF require considerable encouragement and support. A striking number of patients in one American series have developed gallbladder disease.

Another major complication of FMF is *amyloidosis*. Some investigators believe that few patients in Israel escape this complication and that it is an expression of the same gene that is responsible for the other manifestations of FMF. If the attacks occur first, as they do in over 90 percent of the patients, the patients are classified as being of phenotype I. Amyloidosis also occurs in siblings of FMF patients or precedes the abdominal attacks (phenotype II). The infiltration by amyloid involves the kidneys, and death is often attributable to renal failure.

Amyloidosis has been reported in Israel and North Africa, but despite careful search, there has been only one reported instance of amyloidosis complicating FMF in the United States, and that occurred in a young man of Dutch ancestry. These findings are even more striking because there are probably as many known FMF patients in the United States (400 to 500 patients) as in Israel (470 patients). These differences are unexplained and suggest that environmental or nutritional, as well as genetic, factors may play a role in the development of amyloidosis in FMF (Chap. 114).

LABORATORY FINDINGS. There is no specific diagnostic test. Polymorphonuclear leukocytosis ranging from 15,000 to 30,000 is almost invariable during acute attacks. The erythrocyte sedimentation rate is elevated during attacks but returns to normal between attacks. Plasma fibrinogen, serum haptoglobin, ceruloplasmin, and C-reactive protein increase during the episodes. Plasma lipids are normal, and there are no consistent abnormalities of hepatic or renal function. When amyloidosis is present, laboratory findings are typical of a nephrotic syndrome followed by renal insufficiency. Electrocardiographic and electroencephalographic changes are inconstant and non-specific.

DIAGNOSIS. When the typical acute attacks of FMF occur in an individual of appropriate ethnic background who has a family history of FMF, the diagnosis is easy. On the other hand, if the disease has not been present in the family and the patient resides in a community where FMF is rare, the diagnosis can be very difficult.

Most patients with undiagnosed FMF have had one or more abdominal operations with no relief of symptoms. When a patient is seen for the first time, a variety of other febrile illnesses must be excluded by appropriate study or observation. These include acute appendicitis, acute pancreatitis, porphyria, cholecystitis, intestinal obstruction, and other major abdominal catastrophes.

Some of the inherited forms of the hyperlipidemias (Chap. 113) may mimic the clinical picture of FMF, but measurement of serum cholesterol and triglycerides will eliminate them from consideration. The patient with FMF is not immune to the other diseases, and when an attack differs from the usual pattern or is more prolonged, consideration should be given to other diagnostic possibilities. The pleural form of the disease is sometimes difficult to differentiate from acute pulmonary infection or infarction, but the rapid disappearance of signs and symptoms resolves the problem. The joint manifestations may be more prolonged than other forms of FMF, and differentiation from septic arthritis, gout, and acute rheumatoid disease may be necessary. The erythema is sometimes difficult to differentiate from superficial thrombophlebitis or cellulitis.

Whether or not the patient is of the appropriate ethnic group, the most difficult diagnostic problem in FMF is the patient who presents with fever alone. In this situation, an extensive diagnostic work-up for fever of unknown origin may be required. Fortunately, such patients are rare and all eventually develop serosal involvement. Until specific diagnostic tests for FMF are available, patients with recurrent fever but without signs of inflammation of one of the serosal membranes should not be categorized as having FMF.

PROGNOSIS. The prognosis of the patient with FMF varies greatly according to the country in which he lives.

In the United States, the prognosis for long life is excellent. Despite the severity of the symptoms during some acute attacks, most patients are remarkably free of any debilitation during the intervals between attacks. With encouragement and an understanding of their disease, most FMF patients lead fairly normal lives. The greatest hazard to patients is prolonged periods of hospitalization due to erroneous diagnoses or failure to understand the disease. The liberal and injudicious use of narcotics for analgesia in these patients can lead to major psychologic and health problems. Establishment of a reasonable doctor-patient relationship and education of the patient will avoid this hazard. In the United States, the prognosis of patients with FMF does not seem to be different from that of patients with other chronic nonfatal illnesses. Death usually results from causes unrelated to the underlying disease.

The complication of amyloidosis in Israel, parts of North Africa, Turkey, and other parts of the Middle East, makes the prognosis quite different from that in America. Approximately 25 percent of FMF patients in Israel are known to have amyloidosis, and this complication usually leads to death. Because a majority of patients under observation in Israel are under forty years of age, it has been suggested that fatal amyloidosis may eventually occur in nearly all patients. This would explain the rarity of older patients in that area.

TREATMENT. Many forms of therapy have been tried in FMF, but no specific or uniformly effective therapeutic agent or regimen has been found. Antibiotics, hormones, antipyretic and anti-inflammatory agents, immunotherapy, psychotherapy, elimination diets, and many other agents and programs have been attempted. Chloroquine and phenylbutazone have been reported to be successful in treating FMF, but other investigators have failed to substantiate these findings. Adrenal cortical steroids have been used extensively to suppress some of the signs of inflammation, but attacks recur upon steroid withdrawal. In fact, some patients have noted increased numbers of attacks while taking corticosteroids. Symptomatic therapy and support are all that can be offered to FMF patients. Narcotics should be avoided whenever possible.

ETIOCHOLANOLONE AND THE PYROGENIC STEROIDS

In 1957, Kappas et al. reported that certain 5 β-H, C-19 steroids of endogenous human origin would induce inflammation and fever when administered to human volunteers. Etiocholanolone was the prototype of this group of hormone metabolites. Shortly thereafter, Bondy and his colleagues reported high levels of plasma unconjugated etiocholanolone in association with fever in two patients. Since that time, much has been written about the possible role of these steroids in the pathogenesis of certain recurrent fevers of unexplained etiology, including FMF. It is for this reason that special mention should be made of these compounds.

There is no question that many C-19, C-21, C-24 steroids with a 5-β-H configuration are potent inducers of fever, inflammation, granulocytosis, and other biologic effects when they are administered to man. Despite these observations, there is considerable doubt that these compounds play a role in human disease. Investigators have been hampered by the lack of a sensitive and reproducible method for detection of minute concentrations in biologic fluids. Nevertheless, the potential importance of compounds such as etiocholanolone in human febrile disease should not be disregarded until such techniques are at hand. When precise methodology is available, some of these endogenous human products may turn out to be important not only in the pathogenesis of FMF but in other conditions of unknown etiology which are characterized by fever and inflammation. In the light of available data, however, none of these steroids has been shown to cause human disease or its symptoms; to assign a pathogenetic role to them at this time leads to confusion and tends to impede the search for the etiology of these diseases.

REFERENCES

Bondy, P. K., G. L. Cohn, and P. B. Gregory: Etiocholanolone Fever, Medicine, 44:249, 1965.

Ehrenfeld, E. N., M. Eliakim, and M. Rachmilewitz: Recurrent Polyserositis (Familial Mediterranean Fever; Periodic Disease). A Report of Fifty-five Cases, Am. J. Med., 31:107, 1961.

Heller, H., E. Sohar, and L. Sherf: Familial Mediterranean Fever, Arch. Intern. Med., 102:50, 1958.

Kappas, A., and R. H. Palmer: Thermogenic Properties of Steroids, in "Methods in Hormone Research," vol. 4, R. I. Dorfman (Ed.), New York, Academic Press, Inc., 1965.

Reimann, H. A.: "Periodic Diseases," Philadelphia, F. A. Davis Company, 1963.

Siegal, S.: Familial Paroxysmal Polyserositis. Analysis of Fifty Cases, Am. J. Med., 36:893, 1964.

Sohar, E., J. Gafni, M. Pras, and H. Heller: Familial Mediterranean Fever, Am. J. Med., 43:227, 1967.

Wolff, S. M., H. R. Kimball, S. Perry, R. Root, and A. Kappas: The Biological Properties of Etiocholanolone, Ann. Intern. Med. 67:1268, 1967.

257 MIDLINE GRANULOMA
Lawrence E. Shulman

DEFINITION. This peculiar condition, also known as *lethal midline granuloma* or *granuloma gangraenescens,* is characterized by progressive destruction of the soft tissues and bony structures of the face, terminating almost invariably in death after several months or a few years of illness. It occurs mostly in young adults and the middle-aged, and is more common in men. The first case was described by McBride in 1897, and since then more than 200 cases have been reported, mostly in the otolaryngologic literature.

ETIOLOGY AND PATHOLOGY. Not only is the cause of midline granuloma unknown, but the category of disease in which it belongs is uncertain. There is disagreement as to whether it is primarily (1) vascular or allergic, (2) neoplastic, or (3) infectious. Only a few complete autopsy studies have been reported. In half of them, lesions have been found in skin, lungs, and mesenteric lymph nodes as well as the face.

Histologically, the lesions of midline granuloma vary from case to case and also from one area to another in the individual case. The most common finding in the facial lesion is chronic inflammation. In the face and elsewhere there are focal areas of necrosis and necrotic small blood vessels, often containing granular thrombi, suggesting that the process is primarily vascular. The vascular lesions, however, differ from those of polyarteritis nodosa because inflammatory cells are absent. Some areas contain large numbers of cells of varying sizes with large, pale, multilobulated nuclei, simulating Hodgkin's disease and mycosis fungoides. In other areas, hyperchromatic nuclei and numerous mitotic figures resemble those seen in undifferentiated tumors.

CLINICAL FEATURES. Midline granuloma begins with a prodromal period of months to years of nasal obstruction and discharge, at first mucoid and later purulent. During this time, the patient is usually thought to have allergic rhinitis or sinusitis. Progressive inflammation and ulceration follow. The first ulcerations are found in the nasal septum, the mucosa or skin of the alae nasi, or the center of the palate. The lesions invade underlying cartilage and bone, giving rise to septal or palatal perforations. The process spreads by local extension to involve the rest of the nose, paranasal sinuses, eyes, mouth, pharynx, and larynx. Eventually, the structures of the midface are totally destroyed by erosion. Gradually, the functions of sight, speech, and ventilation are impaired or lost. The end result is the formation of a large cavity, founded above by the frontal bone and superior aspect of the orbits and below by the mandible, which is never affected.

During periods of activity, and especially preterminally, the patient becomes febrile. Usually the fever does not respond to chemotherapy appropriate for the secondary bacterial infection which is almost always present. Moreover, even in the presence of obvious pyogenic infection, the patient often fails to develop leukocytosis and during the later stages may become chronically leukopenic. Another curious feature is the absence of cervical lymphadenopathy during periods of active inflammation and progression of the disease. A few patients show red, raised, indurated areas on the skin of the legs and abdomen, resembling those of erythema nodosum clinically and histologically. There is no anemia, and the bone marrow and serum proteins are normal. Microbiologic investigations have consistently failed to detect a specific virus, bacterium, or fungus.

The course of the disease varies greatly; some cases last for more than a decade with long periods of quiescence, and others are fulminant, ending fatally after a few months. Death usually results from meningitis, pneumonia, inanition, or massive hemorrhage. Rarely, the disease may be nonfatal.

DIAGNOSIS. During the early phases of midline granuloma it is important to rule out several specific nasal and facial conditons, many of which are treatable. These include leprosy, syphilis, yaws (gangosa), tuberculosis (lupus vulgaris), glanders, leishmaniasis, blastomycosis, and coccidioidomycosis; chromate poisoning; lupus erythematosus; and also lymphomas, mycosis fungoides, and other malignant tumors. Midline granuloma is differentiated from Wegener's granulomatosis by absence of generalized arteritis and glomerulonephritis. Early in the disease, the differential diagnosis between these two may be difficult. Noma is readily distinguished by its being largely restricted to children and involving the cheeks and mouth but not the nose.

TREATMENT. No effective therapy for midline granuloma has been found. The disease progresses despite administration of antibiotics or adrenocortical steroids. A few early reports of benefit following radiotherapy have not been substantiated by further experience. Recent encouraging reports of benefit from immunosuppressive agents, often with concomitant corticosteroids, require confirmation. Radical surgical excision is no more effective than conservative debridement. Various prostheses designed to maintain the integrity of the normal facial passages are helpful both functionally and cosmetically.

REFERENCES

Edgerton, M. T., and J. D. Desprez: Lethal Midline Granuloma of the Face, Brit. J. Plast. Surg., 9:200, 1956.

James, A. E., Jr.: Malignant Lymphoma as Cause of Midline Granuloma, A.M.A. Arch. Inter. Med., 115:200, 1965.

Pardo-Castello, V., F. L. Blanco, and R. Rivera del Sol: Granuloma Grangraenescens, Southern Med. J., 46:149, 1953.

Spear, G. S., and W. G. Walker, Jr.; Lethal Midline Granuloma (Granuloma Grangraenescens) at Autopsy, Bull. Johns Hopkins Hosp., 99:313, 1956.

Part Eight

Diseases of the Organ System

Section 1

Disorders of the Heart

258 APPROACH TO THE PATIENT WITH HEART DISEASE

Eugene Braunwald

The initial symptoms of the patient with heart disease result most commonly from myocardial ischemia, from disturbance of the contractile activity of the myocardium, or from an abnormal cardiac rhythm or rate. Coronary insufficiency is manifest most frequently as chest pain, while reduction of the pumping ability of the heart commonly leads to weakness and fatigability, or when severe, it produces cyanosis, hypotension, and syncope; elevated intravascular pressures upstream to a failing ventricle often result in abnormal fluid accumulation which in turn leads to dyspnea, orthopnea, and edema.

A cardinal principle in the evaluation of the patient with suspected heart disease is that myocardial or coronary function which may be totally inadequate during exertion may be quite adequate at rest. Thus, a history of the development of symptoms of chest pain or dyspnea during activity which disappear at rest is characteristic of heart disease, while the opposite pattern, i.e., the appearance of these symptoms at rest and their remission during exertion, is rarely observed in patients with true organic heart disease.

Cardiac arrhythmias often develop suddenly, and the resulting complaints—palpitations, dyspnea, angina, hypotension, or syncope—generally occur abruptly and may disappear as rapidly as they develop. Patients with cardiocirculatory disease may also be entirely asymptomatic, both at rest and during exertion, but may present with an abnormal physical finding, such as a heart murmur, elevated systemic arterial pressure, or an abnormality of the electrocardiogram or of the cardiac silhouette on the chest roentgenogram.

Diseases of the heart and circulation are so common and the laity is so well acquainted with the major symptoms resulting from these disorders, that patients, and occasionally physicians, erroneously attribute many complaints to organic cardiovascular disease. Furthermore, the combination of the widespread fear of heart disease in the Western World, as well as the deep-seated emotional connotations concerning this organ's function, re-

sults in the frequent development of symptoms which mimic those of organic disease in individuals with normal cardiovascular systems. The correct interpretation of symptoms and signs in patients with organic cardiovascular disturbances may be particularly difficult. Such individuals, in addition to having symptoms resulting from their disease, may also develop functional complaints referable to the cardiovascular system. The unraveling of symptoms and signs due to organic heart disease from those which are not directly related is an important and challenging task in these patients.

In every branch of medicine the establishment of the prognosis and development of a rational plan of management is based on a correct diagnostic appraisal. However, in the case of patients with disorders of the cardiocirculatory system, particular care must be taken to establish not only a correct but also a *complete* diagnosis. As outlined by the New York Heart Association, the elements of a complete cardiac diagnosis include consideration of (1) the underlying etiology; e.g., Is the disease congenital, rheumatic, hypertensive, or arteriosclerotic in origin? (2) the structural abnormalities; Which chambers are enlarged? Which valves are affected? Is there pericardial involvement? Has there been a myocardial infarct? (3) the physiologic disturbances; Is an arrhythmia present? Is there evidence of congestive heart failure or of coronary insufficiency? and (4) the extent of functional disability; i.e., How strenuous is the physical activity required to elicit symptoms? Two simple examples may serve to illustrate the importance of establishing a complete diagnosis. The identification of exertional chest pain caused by myocardial ischemia is of crucial significance. However, this diagnosis is insufficient, because treatment can be no more than symptomatic until the underlying disease process, e.g., coronary atherosclerosis, aortic stenosis, severe anemia, thyrotoxicosis, or atrial tachycardia, which is responsible for angina pectoris, is identified. Similarly, determining that heart disease is congenital in etiology provides an important starting point, but the decision as to whether or not surgical treatment is advisable generally depends upon the specific anatomic defect present and often upon the nature of the physiologic disturbance and the functional impairment.

The establishment of a correct and complete cardiac diagnosis often requires the use of five different methods of examination: (1) history, (2) physical examination (Chap. 259), (3) electrocardiogram (Chap. 260), (4) chest roentgenogram (Chap. 261), and occasionally (5) specialized examinations, such as cardiac catheterization or angiocardiography (Chap. 262). In order to be most effective it is helpful to employ each of these five techniques independently of one another as well as with the information derived from the other methods clearly in mind. Only in this way can one avoid overlooking a subtle, though extremely significant, finding. For example, an electrocardiogram should be obtained in every patient suspected of having heart disease. It may provide the critical clue in establishing the correct diagnosis, such as the finding of an atrioventricular conduction disturbance, in a patient with unexplained syncope, even when all other methods of examination do not reveal abnormal findings. On the other hand, when combined intelligently with the results of other methods of examination, the electrocardiogram may provide essential confirmatory data. Thus, the knowledge that a patient has an apical diastolic rumbling murmur may direct particular attention to the P waves, and the recognition of left atrial enlargement electrocardiographically would support the suggestion that the murmur is caused by mitral stenosis.

In obtaining the history of the patient with known or suspected cardiovascular disease, particular attention should be directed to the family history. Familial clustering is common in many forms of heart disease. Genetic transmission may occur, as in patients with familial hypertrophic subaortic stenosis (Chap. 273) or Marfan's syndrome (Chap. 395). In patients with essential hypertension or coronary atherosclerosis the genetic component may be less obvious but is also of considerable importance. The nature of the response of the myocardium to an increased hemodynamic load, such as hypertension, or a valvular lesion may also be conditioned by hereditary factors. Familial clustering of cardiovascular diseases may occur not only on a genetic basis but may be related to familial, dietary or behavior patterns.

When an attempt is made to ascertain the severity of functional impairment in a patient with heart disease, it is essential to determine the precise extent of activity and the rate at which it is performed before symptoms develop. Thus, breathlessness which occurs after running up two long flights of stairs denotes far less functional impairment than similar symptoms occurring after taking a few steps on the level. Similarly, the history must include a detailed consideration of the patient's therapeutic regimen. For example, the persistence or development of edema in a patient whose diet is rigidly restricted in sodium content and who is receiving optimum doses of digitalis and diuretics must be interpreted quite differently from the findings of edema in the absence of these measures.

In addition to a careful examination of the heart, a detailed general physical examination should be carried out in every patient with known or suspected heart disease. Cardiovascular manifestations of systemic illnesses are being recognized with increasing frequency, and often the precise cardiovascular diagnosis can be easily established if the associations are clearly kept in mind. Thus, the occurrence of coarctation of the aorta in patients with Turner's syndrome, of myocardial involvement in the presence of Friedreich's ataxia, of primary pulmonary hypertension in patients with Raynaud's syndrome, and of aortic regurgitation in patients with rheumatoid spondylitis, represent a small sample of a growing list of diseases which affect the cardiovascular and other organ systems. Conversely, identification of the cardiovascular disease should prompt a search for frequently associated noncardiac manifestations of the same underlying disease process.

The phonocardiogram and the graphic indirect recording of pulse tracings, such as the jugular venous pulse, the carotid arterial pulse and the apex cardiogram (Chap. 261), may in some instances provide information of considerable diagnostic value by amplifying the physical findings. It must be appreciated, however, that these techniques are primarily of aid in the precise timing of specific events, such as heart sounds, murmurs, and pulsations, which are easily elicited on physical examination.

The electrocardiogram (Chap. 260) is an invaluable and essential aspect of every cardiovascular examination. However, with the exception of the identification of arrhythmias, the electrocardiogram rarely establishes a specific diagnosis. In the absence of any other abnormal findings, electrocardiographic changes, particularly abnormalities in QRS voltages, S-T segments, and T waves must not be over interpreted. The range of normal electrocardiographic findings is wide, and the tracing can be affected significantly by many noncardiac factors, such as age, body habitus, and serum electrolyte concentrations.

Special examinations, such as right and left heart catheterization, selective angiography, and coronary arteriography (Chap. 262), entail cost, discomfort, and some risk to the patient and therefore should not be part of every work-up. These techniques provide precise diagnostic information under many circumstances. For example, they aid in establishing a specific anatomic diagnosis in patients with congenital heart disease, in patients with chest pain of uncertain etiology in whom coronary artery disease is suspected and in determining the functional significance of valvular abnormalities in patients with rheumatic heart disease being considered for surgical treatment.

REFERENCES

Friedberg, C. K.: "Diseases of the Heart," 3d ed., Philadelphia, W. B. Saunders Company, 1966.

Hurst, J. W., and R. B. Logue (eds.): "The Heart," 2d ed., New York, McGraw-Hill Book Company, 1970.

The Criteria Committee of the New York Heart Association, Inc. (C. E. Kossmann, Chairman): "Diseases of the Heart and Blood Vessels," Boston, Little, Brown and Company, 1964.

Levine, S. A.: "Clinical Heart Disease," 5th ed., Philadelphia, W. B. Saunders Company, 1958.

Wood, P.: "Diseases of the Heart and Circulation" 3d ed., Philadelphia, J. B. Lippincott Company, 1968.

259 PHYSICAL EXAMINATION OF THE HEART

T. R. Harrison, William H. Resnik, and Eugene Braunwald

Dyspnea and *ischemic pain*, which are the most important *subjective* manifestations of structural disease of the heart, are discussed in other chapters (Chaps. 32 and 11). The *objective* signs of cardiac disease fall into two general groups: those which are found mainly in organs other than the heart, and those which are due to cardiac disease and which are detected by examination of the heart itself. It is with the latter phenomena that this chapter is concerned.

CARDIAC ENLARGEMENT

Increase in the size of the cardiac shadow due to pericardial effusion, which may exist in the absence of any enlargement of the heart itself, is considered in Chap. 272, Pericardial Disease. Aside from these effusions, the x-ray is of particular value in regard to dilatation but may fail to detect hypertrophy which, when marked, usually produces characteristic alterations in the electrocardiogram. A very slight degree of hypertrophy may elude recognition by all methods, including autopsy, but moderate degrees are frequently best found by palpation unless there is deformity of the thoracic cage or displacement of the heart within the thorax.

The normal apex tap is mainly due to recoil of the ventricles as ejection starts. Left ventricular hypertrophy usually produces an exaggerated apical impulse which is felt over a larger area and is sustained longer than the normal, sharply localized, brief tap. Similar changes may occur following apical infarction, and the differentiation between the two causes will depend on the associated findings and the recording of the apex cardiogram, which reveals an early systolic bulge in hypertrophy and a sustained bulge in myocardial infarction. Less frequently, a striking but temporary exaggeration of the apex thrust appears during anginal attacks and vanishes as the pain subsides. The anginal and postinfarctional apical bulges are apparently caused by ballooning of the feebly contracting ischemic area as the remaining healthy muscle undergoes vigorous contraction. Right ventricular hypertrophy usually produces a diffuse precordial systolic lift which is more marked in the left parasternal and retrosternal than in the apical region.

Elevated cardiac output, whether due to exercise, excitement, thyrotoxicosis, anemia, or the idiopathic hyperkinetic heart syndrome may also cause a diffuse precordial impulse. Patients with emphysema and low diaphragms often exhibit a pronounced systolic footward-forward thrust of the inferior cardiac border. This can be readily felt in the epigastrium, but must be distinguished from the forward pulsation of the abdominal aorta and the right subcostal systolic movement of the liver which occurs in patients with tricuspid insufficiency.

When hypertrophy is marked, the palpatory findings may be confusing because extreme hypertrophy of either ventricle may cause exaggeration of both the apical and parasternal motions. However, when hypertrophy is of moderate degree, simple palpation is usually more trustworthy than instrumental methods, provided the other conditions which have been cited can be excluded.

ALTERATIONS IN HEART SOUNDS

The observer who desires to obtain maximal information from auscultation of the heart should keep two points constantly in mind: (1) In order to hear a faint sound or murmur it is necessary to listen specifically for it, i.e., to focus attention on that phase of the cycle during which the manifestation in question may be expected to occur. (2) The accurate timing (which is essential for correct interpretation) of a phenomenon necessarily involves relating it to known events. Frequently, the relationship to the first or second sound will suffice, but in many instances the clarification will come from simultaneous auscultation and inspection or palpation of the jugular venous pulse, the carotid arterial upstroke, the apical impulse, or the precordial heave.

The low-pitched sounds and murmurs are best heard with gentle pressure, using the bell-shaped stethoscopic endpiece. However, high-pitched sounds, such as diastolic blows, are better heard with the diaphragm stethoscope, or with firm pressure if the bell is used. The tense skin then acts like a diaphragm and tends to transmit high-frequency vibrations.

The interventricular septum often inhibits the transmission of the left-sided phenomena of the anterior precordium. Hence the signs arising at the mitral valve are best heard at the apex, which is normally part of the left ventricle. Likewise, the second sound at the apex, as well as in the right second intercostal space, is mainly due to aortic valve closure. The tricuspid component of the first sound is best heard in the fourth or fifth interspace just to the left of the sternum, while the pulmonic component of the second sound is usually maximal in the second or third interspace. However, the diastolic blow of aortic insufficiency and the opening snap of mitral stenosis are exceptions; both these phenomena are often best heard in the tricuspid area.

There is still some dispute concerning the relative significance of valvular, muscular, vascular, and pericardial vibrations in the production of the heart sounds. The best evidence indicates that abrupt change in tension or closure of the valve cusps are the sole, or the most important factors in the production of the audible components of the normal heart sounds. Under abnormal conditions, the great vessels or the pericardium may produce sounds, but there is controversy whether these sounds ever arise in the myocardium itself.

INTENSITY. The chief factors which influence the intensity of the first sound are (1) the position of the valves at the onset of ventricular systole, which is usually determined by the length of time elapsing between atrial and ventricular contraction; (2) the rate of rise of ventricular pressure; (3) the presence or absence of structural disease of the mitral valve; and (4) the amount of tissue, air, or fluid between the heart and the stethoscope. Increased intensity of the first sound is favored by a short interval between atrial and ventricular contraction, high cardiac output and myocardial contractility, mitral stenosis, and a thin chest wall. The reverse of these conditions tends to be associated with reduced intensity of the first sound.

Aside from such extracardiac factors as obesity, emphysema, and pleural and pericardial effusions, the intensity and to some extent the quality of the second heart sound may be influenced by alterations in the character of the vessel walls. Accentuation of the aortic component of the second sound is a normal phenomenon with age and occurs in such conditions as arteriosclerosis or syphilitic aortitis, which may cause diffuse change in the physical properties of the wall of the aorta. The other conditions which affect the intensity of the second heart sound are primarily those which alter pressures in the aorta and pulmonary artery, with an increase in pressure tending to be associated with accentuation of the corresponding sounds.

The loud first heart sound of mitral stenosis is probably related not only to the thickening of the cusps but to the delay in the onset of the mitral component because of the elevated left atrial pressure. Thus the normal splitting due to earlier mitral closure is absent, the mitral and tricuspid components are fused, and the first sound tends to be louder but briefer than normal. When the period between the start of excitation, i.e., the onset of the QRS, and mitral closure (Q-S^1 time) exceeds 0.07 sec, mitral stenosis is probable, and the degree of prolongation bears a general relationship to the height of the left atrial pressure and hence to the degree of stenosis.

QUALITY. Judgments concerning the state of the heart on the basis of the "quality" of the first sound are likely to be fallacious. The diminished intensity which is so common in older persons is usually the result either of such extracardiac factors as emphysema or obesity or a relatively long P-R interval caused by increased vagal tone. The functional integrity of the myocardium cannot be assessed accurately by the intensity or pitch of the first heart sound.

THREE-SOUND RHYTHMS. These fall into several general groups (Fig. 259-1). The additional sound may be heard in close approximation to the normal first or second sound, in midsystole, or in middiastole.

Splitting of the First Sound. This is a normal phenomenon because closure of the mitral valve precedes that of the tricuspid by 0.01 to 0.02 sec. This splitting is usually best heard at the tricuspid area where the second and fainter component is loudest. It may be heard in a

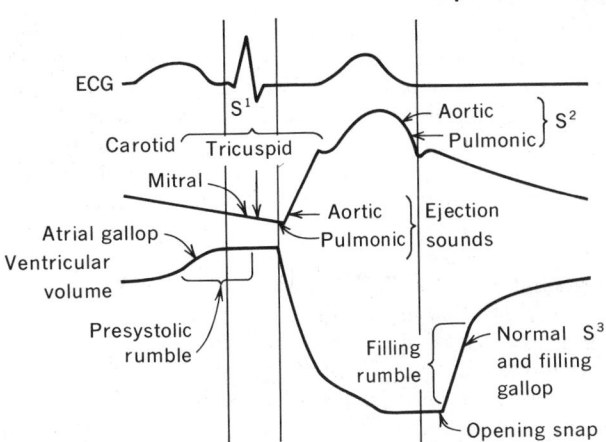

Fig. 259-1. The middiastolic sounds due to a prolonged P-R interval or to a one-sound ventricular premature beat (see text) are not shown because their times are inconstant in relation to the cardiac cycle. The midsystolic extracardiac noises are likewise not indicated.

Because of their close temporal approximation, the ejection clicks cannot be separated from splitting of the first sound by auscultation. The presystolic rumble, when very brief, may be confused with an atrial gallop, but both may usually be distinguished from the other phenomena.

During relaxation and early filling, the split second sound may be confused with the opening snap, the normal third sound, the filling (protodiastolic) gallop, or with a filling rumble of unusually brief duration. The distinction between these several phenomena, while often possible by auscultation alone, sometimes requires simultaneous phonocardiograms, electrocardiograms, pulse tracings, and records of precordial movement.

considerable proportion of healthy persons. The distinction from the less frequent ejection sound usually requires graphic methods. The latter phenomenon is apparently due either to an opening snap of a pliable but stenotic semilunar valve or to the sudden expansion of the great vessels. It may be recorded by sensitive techniques at the aortic or mitral areas in many normal persons but is rarely audible and has little practical significance.

When the P-R interval is normal, the very small vibrations of the atrioventricular cusps related to atrial activity are blended with the larger forces of the first heart sound and are usually inaudible. When, as occurs in the several types of heart block, this interval is abnormally long, the atrial (fourth heart) sounds may be heard (see below). In patients with heart failure and regular rhythm, the force of atrial contraction is nearly always increased and, even though the P-R interval is normal, an audible sound —the presystolic or atrial gallop—is commonly noted. This phenomenon, although occasionally audible in the absence of ventricular hypertrophy, usually signifies that heart failure or diminished ventricular compliance due to hypertrophy is present and is, therefore, of practical importance. Just prior to atrial contraction, the atrial pressure is equal to that in the corresponding ventricle. A slight elevation of ventricular diastolic pressure causes relatively great stretch of the thin-walled and highly distensible atrium. Thus, in accordance with Starling's law, the changes in pressure as the atrium contracts and then relaxes are greater than normal. The premature closure of the atrioventricular valves when the atrium relaxes has been postulated as being responsible for the atrial sound.

The *presystolic gallop* may usually be distinguished from a split first sound by the longer interval (ta-lubb—dup, rather than t'lubb—dup). The differentiation from an exceptionally brief presystolic rumble, a rare source of confusion, can be made by listening after exercise, which increases the duration of the murmur.

The *third sounds* occurring during midsystole are nearly always of extracardiac origin. They commonly arise from traction on pleuropericardial adhesions or motion of structures adjacent to the heart, but may be due to pneumothorax or to mediastinal emphysema. In some instances, they are associated with mitral regurgitation.

Splitting of the second heart sound. This is a normal phenomenon during inspiration, when the greater inflow into the right ventricle produces some prolongation of its ejection. The delay in pulmonic closure due to the lower pressure as compared with that in the aorta is normally very slight during expiration, and can be demonstrated only by graphic methods. Audible expiratory splitting, which is best heard in the tricuspid or pulmonary areas, is probably always abnormal when it is present in the sitting or standing position. Less frequently it is abnormal in the recumbent position. Such splitting may be due to delayed pulmonary closure because of an increased flow load involving the right ventricle only (interatrial defect or anomalous venous drainage with one or more pulmonary veins emptying into the right atrium), to an increased pressure load from pulmonic stenosis, or due to delayed activation of the right ventricle, as occurs in right bundle branch block. Unusually early aortic valve closure, such as occurs with mitral insufficiency, may also produce audible expiratory splitting.

In patients with large interatrial defects, the filling of the right atrium from the left atrium and from the venae cavae varies reciprocally during the respiratory cycle. Hence the volume and duration of right ventricular ejection are not significantly increased by inspiration. Therefore, there is no inspiratory exaggeration of the splitting of the second sound. This phenomenon, termed *fixed splitting of the second heart sound,* is of diagnostic value, i.e., a pronounced expiratory split which is not audibly greater during inspiration is suggestive evidence for the presence of an interatrial defect (Chap. 268).

When left ventricular systole is prolonged abnormally, aortic valve closure follows pulmonic valve closure, i.e., the order of semilunar valve closure is reversed. On inspiration, the normal prolongation of right ventricular systole results in fusion of the two components, i.e., a single second heart sound, with splitting during expiration. This finding is termed *paradoxical splitting of the second heart sound* and is observed in left bundle branch block, and some patients with idiopathic hypertrophic subaortic stenosis, valvular aortic stenosis, patent ductus arteriosus, and in hypertensive and ischemic heart disease with left ventricular failure.

The *opening snap* (OS) is occasionally due to tricuspid stenosis. Much more commonly, it is an important sign of mitral stenosis. Its time of onset after the second heart sound, 0.05 to 0.11 sec, is inversely related to the height of the left atrial pressure. Thus a very short S^2-OS time, like a very long Q-S^1 time, speaks for a high degree of mitral stenosis (Chap. 270).

The opening snap is of brief duration, high-pitched, and usually best heard in the fourth or fifth interspace between the left sternal margin and the apex. These features will usually distinguish it from the split second heart sound, which occurs somewhat earlier and is likely to be better heard at the pulmonic or apical regions.

The *physiologic third sound* and the protodiastolic (early diastolic or filling) gallop are apparently related to the rapid equalization of pressure between atrium and ventricle, with headward rebound of the atrioventricular cusps, and occur approximately 0.15 sec after aortic valve closure. Although they occur at the same time during the cardiac cycle, have the same low pitch, and are heard in the same (mitral or tricuspid) areas, they are not likely to be confused with each other. The physiologic third sound occurs in young persons and probably signifies rapid ventricular filling consequent upon more complete ventricular emptying. In the case of the protodiastolic gallop, the rapid filling is due not to unusually low pressure in the ventricle but to elevation of pressure in the atrium and possibly also to some dilatation of the atrioventricular orifice. Thus, we have the paradox of a similar phenomenon indicating either a vigorous or an impaired heart. The distinction is based on such associated findings as age, heart size, and the history of exercise tolerance. Furthermore, the normal third sound is usually best heard when the rate is slow, while moderate tachycardia is the rule in patients with the filling gallop. Because of this, the cadence resembling that of a cantering horse is usually present only with the gallop.

Confusion between a third heart sound and protodiastolic gallop on the one hand and a very brief filling rumble on the other can usually be settled by exercise, which tends to prolong the latter phenomenon. The filling gallop is of great practical importance. It is often the sole cardiac sign of heart failure, the other manifestations being found in the lungs or elsewhere. It may also be the earliest sign, preceding the congestive phenomena by months or even years. When, as is commonly true, it arises on the left side, it is best heard at the apex and is louder during expiration. However, right ventricular gallops occasionally occur. They are likely to be equally loud or louder during inspiration and are best heard in the lower parasternal region or, when emphysema is present, in the epigastrium.

The *protodiastolic gallop,* which occurs during early filling, may usually be separated from the split second heart sound and from the opening snap by its lower pitch and its point of maximal intensity, which is ordinarily in a more inferior interspace, as well as by its later occurrence. However, doubt may occur in a patient presenting with both mitral stenosis and insufficiency. Here, the distinction assumes great practical significance in relation to cardiac surgery. An opening snap speaks strongly for predominant stenosis, while a left ventricular filling gallop precludes marked narrowing of the valve because pronounced stenosis prevents the rapid pressure equalization which produces the gallop. Under this circumstance it may be necessary to make simultaneous recordings of heart sounds and of precordial motions in order to learn whether the sound in question precedes the onset of filling (split sound), coincides exactly with it (opening snap), or appears 0.04 to 0.06 sec later (filling gallop). Even so, caution must be exercised to avoid confusion between (1) mitral insufficiency with both a rumble due to rapid filling and a left-sided filling gallop; and (2) mitral stenosis, as the cause of the rumble, associated with a right ventricular filling gallop.

The *pansystolic murmur* of mitral insufficiency may continue during relaxation and thus mask the second sound at the apex. Under this circumstance the filling gallop may be mistaken for the second sound. Being low-pitched, the protodiastolic gallop is best heard with a bell-type stethoscope, using gentle pressure. It is ordinarily the faintest of the three sounds but may be the loudest. This confusing sign is especially common when the rate is rapid, diastole short, and the atrial and filling gallops are superimposed during rapid filling (summation gallop).

The *pericardial knock*, characteristic of chronic constrictive pericarditis (Chap. 272) also occurs at the termination of the rapid filling phase but is somewhat earlier than the protodiastolic gallop, i.e., 0.10 to 0.13 sec after aortic valve closure.

Although rubs, murmurs, or even extracardiac noises may be heard during middiastole, true heart sounds are rare at this time of the cycle. When the P-R interval is long, the faint vibrations of the valves induced by atrial activity may produce a low-pitched and faint but audible sound. It is important to separate this from the single sound caused by a very premature ventricular beat which closes the atrioventricular valves but is too feeble to open the semilunar valves and hence causes no second sound. Either phenomenon may occur in middiastole. In most instances, the premature beat has a higher pitch. However, the differentiation may be impossible by auscultation. This is almost the only situation in which the electrocardiogram will supply crucial information concerning the exact nature of heart sounds. Such a tracing should always be made because both conditions—heart block and frequent premature beats—may require treatment, and the drug which is indicated for one of them may be seriously hazardous for the other.

MURMURS

The discussion to follow is concerned primarily with the mechanisms and types of murmurs arising in the heart and their general significance, but it does not deal with the specific causative lesions, which are considered in Chaps. 268 and 270.

Most murmurs are limited to systole or diastole; a few are continuous, i.e., are heard in both phases of the car-

diac cycle. Diastolic murmurs usually mean organic disease but may be difficult to hear. Systolic murmurs are more readily heard, may or may not signify a structural disorder, and the chief question is that of interpretation. In this regard a rheumatic history, an associated thrill, or the demonstration of a calcified valve may be of crucial importance.

The precise time of onset and of cessation of murmurs depends on the instant in the cardiac cycle at which an adequate pressure difference between two chambers appears and disappears. The general principle, which is considered in some detail in subsequent pages, is illustrated in Fig. 259-2. Inspection of this diagram will reveal the reasons why murmurs are called pansystolic, ejection, late systolic, regurgitant, early filling, and presystolic.

The accentuation of a murmur during inspiration means that it almost certainly arises on the right side of the heart or the pulmonary vascular bed, with the effect of the augmented venous return predominating over the damping tendency of lung expansion. Expiratory exaggeration has less significance. It is more common with left-sided murmurs but may also occur with those arising in the right chambers if the intensifying result of reduced lung volume predominates over the hemodynamic effect of reduced venous return. Prolonged expiratory pressure against a closed glottis, i.e., the Valsalva maneuver, reduces the intensity of most murmurs by diminishing the flow rate of blood in the central circulation. The systolic murmur associated with idiopathic hypertrophic subaortic stenosis is an exception to this rule and is usually accentuated by the Valsalva maneuver (Chap. 273). Murmurs originating from the right side of the heart return immediately after release of the Valsalva, while murmurs originating from the left side return several seconds later.

There is no simple relation between the intensity of a murmur and the severity of the responsible lesion. Thus, in the advanced stages of mitral stenosis, the diastolic rumble may actually decrease because of diminished flow through the orifice. Similarly, in patent ductus arteriosus the development of secondary pulmonary hypertension, with aggravation of the patient's symptoms, may be associated with reduced intensity of the murmur as the left-to-right shunt diminishes.

The murmurs of aortic and pulmonic stenosis are low-pitched and "rough" because they are related to the low-frequency vibrations of the semilunar cusps. However, the insufficiency murmurs, being due to vibrations (eddies) of blood, are higher pitched and resemble the swishing sound of a mountain stream.

MURMURS AND TURBULENCE. When a liquid or a gas moves, not in smooth straight lines but in constantly changing directions and velocities, the flow is said to be turbulent. Cardiac murmurs result from vibrations set up in the bloodstream and the surrounding heart or great vessels as a result of turbulent blood flow, the formation of eddies, and of cavitation (bubble formation as a result of sudden decrease in pressure). Turbulence varies inversely with viscosity. Therefore, murmurs tend to occur in anemic patients, even if the volume and velocity

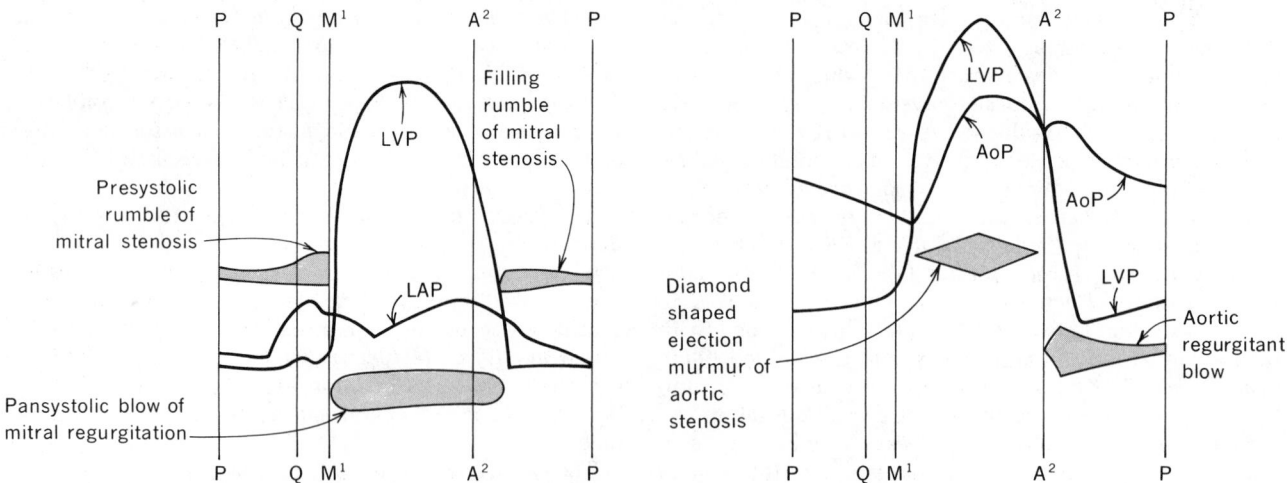

Fig. 259-2. The onset, offset, and "shape" (*crescendo, diminuendo,* or *diamond*) of murmurs in relation to the pressure differences between adjacent areas are illustrated. *P* and *Q* indicate the onset of atrial and ventricular excitation, respectively.

Note that the murmur of mitral insufficiency starts with the beginning of the first sound (*M¹*), and endures beyond the second, or until the pressure in the left ventricle (*LVP*) falls below that in the left atrium (*LAP*). In contrast, the "diamond" murmur of aortic stenosis starts later, as ejection begins. It increases and then decreases in intensity, according to the pressure gradient between the left ventricle and the aorta (*AoP*), and ceases just before the aortic second sound (*A²*) as these pressures become equalized.

The murmur of aortic insufficiency starts with the second sound because the left ventricular pressure falls below the aortic at this time. The filling rumble of mitral stenosis begins later as the ventricular pressure descends below the atrial. The presystolic accentuation of the stenotic murmurs occurs as the left atrium contracts.

of flow remain constant. Actually, they usually increase, and this also favors the production of murmurs.

These considerations explain many aspects of murmurs: their frequent occurrence during systole in vigorous young hearts (high velocity of flow); their appearance even in diastole when flow is sufficiently rapid (the "pseudostenotic atrioventricular rumbles" in patients with atrial septal defect, patent ductus, or even with uncomplicated mitral insufficiency); their presence with stenotic lesions (for a total flow the velocity is inversely proportional to the square of the orifice size). Insufficiency murmurs are related not only to the high velocity because of the large pressure difference between the respective chambers, but also to the additional turbulence caused by the convergence of two streams of blood.

The bruits heard over aneurysms are related to the increase in diameter of the vessel. The murmur caused by the increase in velocity at the site of a narrowed vessel is usually systolic only because collateral circulation above the constriction reduces the diastolic pressure gradient; when collaterals are absent, partial occlusion may cause a continuous murmur.

The energy (pressure gradient) necessary to produce a given volume flow is proportional to the velocity when the flow is laminar, but to the square of the velocity when it is turbulent. Thus a stenotic lesion exerts two harmful mechanical effects—that due to the narrowing per se and that due to the turbulence secondary to the narrowing. As the velocity of flow increases with exercise, the second effect becomes progressively more im-

portant, as shown by increasing loudness of the murmur.

SYSTOLIC MURMURS. These may be divided into three groups in relation to their timing.

Pansystolic Murmurs. This group includes those murmurs involving two chambers which have widely different systolic pressures, such as the left ventricle and either the left atrium or the right ventricle. The pressure gradient is established very early in contraction and lasts until relaxation is almost complete. Therefore, these murmurs begin during isometric contraction and at the area of maximal intensity tend to mask both heart sounds because they begin with the first and cease after the second. The pansystolic murmurs due to ventriculoatrial regurgitation may be dependent either on deformity of the cusps ("organic") or on dilatation of the rings ("relative"). The latter murmurs are associated with well-marked cardiac enlargement and become fainter with improvement of heart failure. They are rarely associated with thrills. The organic regurgitant murmurs may occur in hearts of any size, are commonly accompanied by thrills, and when accompanied by congestive failure, are likely to become louder as improvement occurs.

Pansystolic murmurs are not found in patients with interatrial defects, unless there is atrioventricular regurgitation due to associated deformities of the mitral or tricuspid valves. In the case of those interventricular shunts which are accompanied by large pressure gradients between the two ventricles, these murmurs do occur. Large openings in the interventricular septum usually lead to early pulmonary hypertension, which raises the right ventricular systolic pressure and thus tend to reduce the shunt. Furthermore, the turbulence is related to the velocity of flow which, if the pressure gradient is constant, is inversely proportional to the square of the size of the orifice. A high pressure gradient is likely to be associated with a high-pitched murmur. These considerations explain why the small and relatively innocent defects of the muscular part of the ventricular septum are likely to be associated with louder murmurs of higher pitch than the larger and more serious shunts which are situated higher and involve the membranous portion of the septum. In the latter circumstances the faint pansystolic murmur may be overshadowed by the louder ejection blow caused by the relative stenosis consequent to increased flow through the dilated pulmonary artery.

The apical pansystolic murmur of mitral regurgitation and the pansystolic murmur of ventricular septal defect are both characteristically augmented by elevating the systemic arterial pressure, as for example with phenylephrine or methoxamine, and diminished by lowering arterial pressure, as with an inhalation of amyl nitrite. The systolic murmur of tricuspid regurgitation, like that of ventricular septal defect, is heard best along the lower left sternal border, and is accentuated during inspiration, while that produced by mitral regurgitation or ventricular septal defect, is accentuated by expiration.

Ejection Murmurs. These are related to a disproportion between blood flow and the size of the orifice which it traverses. Even though the semilunar valves are normal, an excessive flow or dilated vessel beyond it may be responsible for the production of this type of murmur. Narrowing of the outflow tract or of the valves may cause such a murmur, the intensity being related to the flow. Thus, the murmur of aortic stenosis becomes faint and may disappear during heart failure and return with great intensity following digitalization (Chap. 270).

The ejection murmurs start shortly after the first sound but do not actually replace it. As the ventricular pressure rises and declines during ejection, the murmur becomes louder and then fainter. This "diamond shape" is readily seen in phonocardiograms but may not be apparent to auscultation. The second heart sound may be exaggerated or normal and is not obscured by the murmur, which ceases before semilunar valve closure occurs. However, when stenosis of one of the valves is responsible, the corresponding second sound may be faint or absent because the cusps and no longer pliable.

The age of the patient and the area of maximal intensity are of great importance in determining the significance of ejection murmurs. Thus, in a young adult with vigorous contraction and a high ejection velocity, a faint or moderate ejection blow heard only in the pulmonary area is usually without significance, while a similar murmur in the aortic area is likely to indicate stenosis of the valve or some congenital abnormality. In elderly persons, functional pulmonic blows are rare, while aortic systolic murmurs are not uncommon and may be due to dilatation or roughening of the aorta, to an important degree of aortic stenosis, or to slight narrowing of the valve. Mild narrowing, when associated with a high level of cardiac output, may produce a loud murmur even though the stenosis is of no hemodynamic importance, as shown by the lack of a significant pressure gradient between the left ventricle and the aorta. The murmur of aortic stenosis is readily audible in the second right intercostal space, but is transmitted to the apex and along the carotid vessels; it is intensified by expiration, by amyl nitrite, which increases cardiac output, and is reduced by interventions which increase arterial pressure and lower cardiac output, such as phenylephrine.

The most common ejection murmur is that heard at the pulmonary area in healthy young persons with small and vigorous hearts. It is probably due to the combination of a high velocity of flow and a thin chest wall. When it is faint (grade I or II), blowing, and unassociated with evidence of disease, the diagnosis of an innocent functional murmur will be apparent. Less frequently, the quality is rough, and the intensity may be grade III. In such patients cardiac catheterization may be necessary in order to separate such an exaggerated functional murmur from one due to a slight congenital deformity. Functional murmurs and those due to increased velocity of blood flow, e.g., as in atrial septal defect, are relatively short, while those due to organic stenosis are longer. Pulmonary ejection murmurs are increased by amyl nitrite. The systolic ejection murmur in tetralogy of Fallot, however, may be reduced by amyl nitrite.

Late Systolic Murmurs. Many patients with coronary disease present faint or moderate (rarely loud) blowing apical systolic murmurs which seem to start well after ejection and do not mask either sound. The exact mechanism responsible for them has not been clarified. These late systolic murmurs, which are almost never accompanied by thrills, are especially common in patients with myocardial infarction (old or recent) but may appear during anginal attacks and vanish as the pain subsides. There is strong evidence that they are related to papillary muscle dysfunction caused by infarction, or to ischemia of these muscles, or to their distortion induced by the ischemic ballooning of the ventricular walls, which is common in such patients.

In persons with acute myocardial infarction, it is important to distinguish these apical papillary muscle murmurs, which are relatively innocent, from the much rarer but more serious murmurs due to (1) rupture of a papillary muscle, with a rapid and usually fatal development of left-sided failure, or (2) rupture of the interventricular septum, with the sudden onset of grave left and right ventricular failure. These latter murmurs are likely to be pansystolic, louder, harsher, and associated with thrills and with greater degree of heart failure. In most instances the murmurs due to ischemia of the papillary muscles are fainter and higher pitched, are only rarely pansystolic, and usually begin after the first sound. For this reason and because they may be crescendo-decrescendo, they may be confused with the murmur of aortic stenosis.

The late systolic murmurs which occasionally occur in young subjects are usually musical or "whistling." Their mechanism is not known, but they are probably of extracardiac origin and follow a midsystolic click. In most instances, there is no evidence of cardiac disease, and the murmurs are without significance. Rarely, such a musical or squeaking late systolic murmur is seen in a young person in whom it results from mitral regurgitation, documented by cineangiography.

DIASTOLIC MURMURS. This classification also includes three main types.

Regurgitant Murmurs. The regurgitant diastolic murmurs begin with or shortly after the second heart sound, or as soon as the corresponding ventricular pressure falls sufficiently below that in the aorta or pulmonary artery. In aortic regurgitation or pulmonic regurgitation secondary to pulmonary hypertension they usually have a high-pitched swishing quality, resembling breath sounds. They are best heard during held forced expiration, with the patient leaning forward or on his hands and knees. The high-frequency vibrations are best detected by a diaphragm stethoscope, or, if a bell is used, by firm pressure. In pulmonic regurgitation without pulmonary hypertension (congenital pulmonic regurgitation), the diastolic murmur has a lower pitch and may be confused with the murmur of mitral stenosis. In contrast to the murmur of pulmonic regurgitation, the diastolic murmur of aortic regurgitation is enhanced by acute elevation of arterial pressure and may radiate to the apex.

Filling Murmurs. Diastolic murmurs during early filling are, like ejection blows, due to disproportion between orifice size and flow rate. Thus mitral and tricuspid stenosis are associated with rumbles which start soon but at an appreciable interval after the second sound. With normal or high flow, such murmurs may be loud when stenosis is slight. Conversely, a high degree of obstruction may cause a very faint or even no rumble if cardiac output is sufficiently reduced. When stenosis is marked, the diastolic murmur is inevitably prolonged. Thus the duration of the murmur is more reliable than the intensity as an index of the degree of narrowing.

Very high rates of flow may be associated with loud but brief filling rumbles, despite normal cusps, at either atrioventricular orifice. These murmurs commence at the end of the rapid filling period, i.e., immediately after the protodiastolic gallop. In the case of the tricuspid valve, the usual cause is a large interatrial defect. On the left side of the heart it is seen in patients with patent ductus and ventricular septal defect and is particularly confusing when mitral insufficiency with minimal or no stenosis is the cause. Aside from the duration of the rumble, the intensity of the first sound, the presence or absence of a well-marked opening snap, and the type of hypertrophy are important guides to the predominant lesion. A faint middiastolic murmur heard in patients with acute rheumatic fever (Carey Coombs murmur) may sometimes be heard. In these patients edema of the mitral cusps or excessive left atrioventricular blood flow as a consequence of mitral regurgitation is probably responsible (Chap. 269).

Presystolic Murmurs. The presystolic, or atrial systolic, murmur is usually due to mitral (rarely tricuspid) stenosis. It has the same quality as the filling rumble but is usually crescendo rather than decrescendo. Because of its short duration it may be confused with an atrial gallop or a split first sound. Its accentuation and prolongation by exercise, due to fusion with the filling rumble, will usually make the distinction.

When these filling rumbles, whether early or presystolic, arise at the mitral orifice, they are best heard with a bell stethoscope at the apex, while the patient lies on the left side and during expiration. Occasionally, they are audible only after exercise. The tricuspid rumbles, which are much less common, are heard in the left parasternal region and are sometimes louder during inspiration.

Despite normal mitral cusps, patients with aortic insufficiency may have a diastolic or presystolic mitral rumble (the Austin-Flint murmur). This is probably due to vibration of the aortic cusp of the mitral valve between the normal and abnormal streams of blood entering the left ventricle.

Continuous Murmurs. These signify continuous flow due to a communication between a high-pressure and a low-pressure area, without an intervening valve. The commonest cause is patent ductus arteriosus, which causes a continuous murmur as long as the pressure in the pulmonary artery is much below that in the aorta. This murmur is intensified by elevation of systemic arterial pressure, and may be reduced by inspiration. When pulmonary hypertension due to left-sided failure or to arteriolar changes in the lungs supervenes, the duration of the murmur lessens and it may eventually disappear or persist only during systole.

Less common causes of continuous murmurs include systemic, coronary, or pulmonary arteriovenous fistulas, the development of marked bronchial collateral circulation in patients with pulmonary stenosis, rupture of an aortic aneurysm into the pulmonary artery or right side of the heart, a congenital window between the roots of the aorta and pulmonary artery, or multiple stenoses of branches of the pulmonary artery with pulmonary hypertension. The murmurs produced by pulmonary arteriovenous fistulas and by multiple pulmonary artery branch stenoses are accentuated by inspiration and inhalation of amyl nitrite. Coarctation of the aorta usually causes a systolic murmur only, but when because of poor collaterals proximal to the obstruction, the pressure gradient remains large throughout diastole, the murmur may be continuous, or when the collaterals in the chest wall are prominent, flow through them causes a continuous murmur.

Rupture of a sinus of Valsalva into the right atrium or ventricle is a rare but surgically curable cause of a continuous murmur which is usually loudest in the lower sternal region.

The cervical venous hum is a faint continuous musical murmur at the base of the neck. It is accentuated by inspiration and diminishes or disappears during recumbency, the Valsalva maneuver, or digital compression of the vein. It has no significance, but may be mistaken for an organic cause of a continuous murmur.

Significance of Murmurs. Diastolic murmurs and, with the exception of the cervical venous hum, all continuous murmurs generally indicate structural disease. The systolic bruit, when very loud or associated with a thrill, has the same significance. The problem of interpretation arises with the moderately loud systolic blow, which usually is due to an organic lesion, and, especially, with the faint (grade I or II) systolic murmur. Here, the decision will depend on consideration of all of the evidence and will sometimes be in doubt, even after cardiac catheterization. In borderline instances, a faint systolic murmur, loudest at the base, should be considered innocent until proved otherwise. A similar murmur heard only at the apex is more likely to be of structural origin. Even so, if there are no other signs of organic heart disease, the only therapeutic considerations are those of prophylaxis against rheumatic fever and bacterial endocarditis.

THRILLS. In the region of the apex, thrills are of limited diagnostic import because they may be confused with vibrations set up by a vigorously beating heart. On the other hand, the presence of a thrill at the base of the heart or along the left sternal border constitutes practically conclusive evidence that the accompanying murmur is of the organic type. It is true that thrills are simply the tactile equivalent of the auditory basis of the murmur and hence have no greater significance than the murmur itself. It happens, however, that the kind of murmur which gives rise to vibrations that can be felt as a thrill is almost invariably of organic origin. Such thrills are of especial importance in the diagnosis of aortic stenosis.

The pericardial friction rub may occasionally be confused with a harsh systolic murmur or with an insignificant adventitious sound ("sternal crunch"). This uncertainty, which arises when the rub is heard only during systole, will be solved by consideration of the total clinical picture. The characteristic to-and-fro squeaking sound signifies pericarditis and is nearly always accompanied by other findings of this disorder (Chap. 272).

Discussions of electrocardiography and of other methods of examination are presented in the three following chapters.

REFERENCES

Crevasse, L., M. W. Wheat, J. R. Wilson, R. F. Leeds, and W. J. Taylor: The Mechanism of the Generation of the Third and Fourth Heart Sounds, Circulation, 25:635, 1962.

Fowler, N.: Cardiac Auscultation, chap. 3 in "Cardiac Diagnosis," New York, Harper and Row, Publishers, Incorporated, 1968.

Hurst, J. W., and R. B. Logue: (eds.): 2d ed. Part III, Section C The Physical Examination, in "The Heart," New York, McGraw-Hill Book Company, 1970, pp. 148–294.

Leatham, A.: The Place of Phonocardiography in Clinical Cardiology, Progr. Cardiovascular Diseases, 2:76, 1959.

Phillips, J. H., G. E. Burch, and N. P. DePasquale: The Syndrome of Papillary Muscle Dysfunction: Its Clinical Recognition, Ann. Intern. Med., 59:508, 1963.

Ronan, J. A., Perloff, J. K., and Harvey, W. P.: Systolic Clicks and the Late Systolic Murmur, Am. Heart J., 70:319, 1965.

Wood, P.: Physical Signs, pp. 26–84 in "Diseases of the Heart and Circulation," 3d Edition, Philadelphia, J. B. Lippincott Company, 1968.

260 PRINCIPLES OF ELECTROCARDIOGRAPHY

E. Harvey Estes, Jr.

INTRODUCTION

The aim of this chapter is to introduce the reader to some concepts underlying electrocardiographic interpretation, some techniques used in analyzing electrocardiographic waves, and some of the alterations caused in these waves by disease. The presentation is necessarily incomplete, but the bibliographic references at the end of the chapter will supply further information.

Electrocardiography began as a physiologic curiosity, but its usefulness was soon recognized, and it was quickly claimed as a tool of the cardiologist. Much useful information was gathered regarding changes in rhythm, wave form, etc., with heart disease, before there was adequate knowledge of the origin of the activity being recorded. Assumptions were made and explanations were offered for the observed changes. Much must now be discarded or drastically modified on the basis of new information and new concepts. This is a continuous process, for which no apology is necessary. One should not be upset that a concept or "method of interpretation" is no longer considered valid, but should be comforted that the empirical relationships between certain wave forms and certain disease states are rarely upset or drastically altered. Indeed, these are the factual data upon which most concepts were based. The facts do not change, but our interpretation is modified and/or the facts are refined by further observation.

At the present time, there are a number of islands of solid information which have emerged from the sea of assumptions and theories of the past. In some cases these seem isolated, since their relationship to other islands is unknown. The connections and interrelationships are slowly being explored, and it is hoped that these will eventually become a solid mass of information, so that the alterations of disease can be completely understood. Some of the areas of solid accomplishment are as follows: the electrical events in the single cell, the anatomy and blood supply of pacemaker and conducting structures, the order of spread of excitation through the heart, the distribution of electrical potential through the body, the design of lead systems, and the computer analysis of wave forms.

Each of these factual "islands" contains enough material for a volume within itself, yet some review of current knowledge in these areas is a necessary prelude to understanding the electrocardiogram.

The Electrical Events in the Single Cell

Individual cardiac cells are surrounded by a membrane composed of lipid and protein. In the resting state, a potential of about 90 mv exists across this membrane, the interior being negative with respect to the exterior of the cell. As long as a potential in excess of a critical value is maintained, this membrane remains impermeable to the passage of certain ions, such as sodium, yet permeable to others, such as potassium. When the potential falls below a critical "threshold" value, the membrane is suddenly disturbed so that it is much more permeable to sodium ion than in the resting state. This event (depolarization) initiates a cycle of events: potassium permeability is decreased, the membrane is "inactivated," and the process is reversed. The potential of about −90 mv which exists across the resting cell membrane is termed the *resting potential*. The depolarization of the membrane is accompanied by a sudden loss of resting potential and a small overshoot. This is followed by a plateau, after which the resting potential is restored. The sudden reversal in potential, the plateau, and the return to resting potential constitute the *action potential* (Fig. 260-1). Although small ionic shifts accompany these changes in the membrane, the electromotive force responsible for the resting potential and the action potential is related to the presence of differing concentrations of sodium and potassium ions in the presence of a membrane of varying permeability rather than to ionic shifts per se.

The resting potential of about −90 mv is related to the differing concentration of K^+ in the presence of a membrane permeable to this ion. The rapid reversal of polarization and the overshoot associated with membrane depolarization are probably related to the increasing permeability of the membrane to sodium, the decreasing permeability to potassium, and the dominance of the electromotive force due to the differing concentration of Na^+ across the membrane. The restoration to the resting potential is a complex process which is incompletely understood but which involves a progressive return of the membrane to the original state (permeable to K^+, impermeable to Na^+). The process involves the active extrusion of Na^+ from the interior of the cell by the "sodium pump."

Each of the various cell types which comprise the heart (sinus node, AV node, His bundle and Purkinje fiber, atrial muscle, ventricular muscle) has a characteristic value for resting potential and action potential and a characteristic shape or form. Fibers from pacemaker regions, for example, typically show a slow loss of the resting potential which begins immediately after the action potential. This "leak" causes the cell membrane to reach the threshold value (and thus initiate depolarization) spontaneously (Fig. 260-2). This feature is probably the basis of the spontaneous rhythmicity of these cell groups. In other cells, such as ventricular muscle cells, the process is apparently initiated by depolarization of adjacent fibers.

The depolarization process (the onset of the action potential and the overshoot) is associated with the QRS complex of the surface electrocardiogram, and the final phase of the action potential is related to the T wave. Drugs and electrolytes which change these phases of the transmembrane potential have a predictable effect on the corresponding portion of the surface electrocardiogram. In spite of this knowledge, there are many gaps in our understanding of the surface electrocardiogram in terms of the cell potential. The former is best considered as a resultant of the action potential of many fibers, firing in a particular sequence. At present we cannot directly relate one to the other.

The Anatomy and Blood Supply of Specialized Pacemaker and Conducting Tissues

The normal pacemaker activity of the heart is assumed by the sinoatrial node. This structure lies at the junction of the superior vena cava and the right atrium. It is best located by tracing its blood supply, which, in 80 percent of hearts, arises as the first branch of the right coronary artery. In the other 20 percent, it arises as the first branch of the left circumflex artery.

The atrioventricular node lies in the lower interatrial septum, on the right side, near the coronary sinus orifice. This structure can be clearly identified on appropriate sections. Its blood supply arises from a very constant branch from the posterior septal area, which usually arises from the right coronary artery, but in about 20 percent of hearts it arises from the continuation of the circumflex branch of the left coronary artery. The bundle of His, or common bundle, courses in the upper interventricular septum, in close proximity to the base of the aortic valve, and terminates in the right and left bundle branches. The right bundle is usually a discrete structure

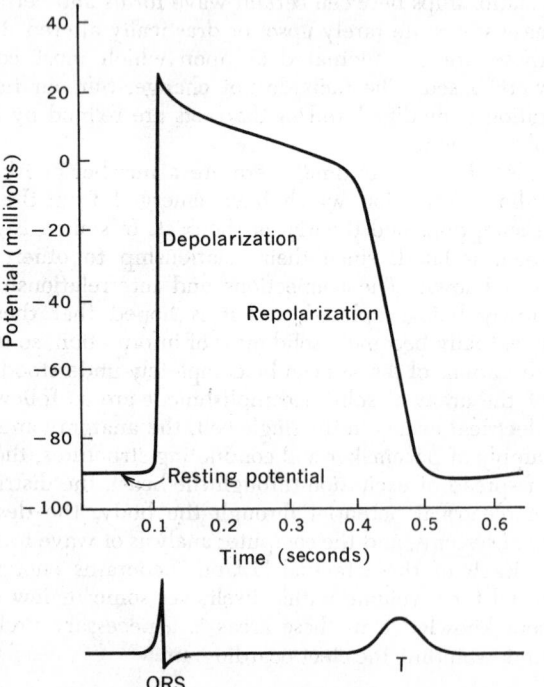

Fig. 260-1. Schematic representation of the action potential of a ventricular cell, with the surface electrocardiogram below to illustrate the time relationships between the ECG and the action potential.

which can be traced for long distances. The left bundle branch usually ends in a wide fan-shaped distribution of fibers on the left septal surface with no constant sub-branches. The bundles lie in an area of the interventricular septum in which there are considerable overlap and many anastomoses between the posterior septal branches, usually from the right coronary artery, and the anterior septal branches from the left coronary artery. The origin of the blood supply to the bundles is therefore highly variable.

The Origin and Spread of Excitation and Recovery, and Its Relation to the Electrocardiogram

Depolarization is initiated by the "leak" of resting potential in the cells of the sinoatrial node, causing these cells spontaneously to reach the threshold value. This process is propagated radially, over the right atrium, the interatrial septum, and the left atrium. The existence of conduction pathways from SA node to AV node, and from right to left atrium has been postulated.

Upon reaching the area of the coronary sinus, activation invades the area of the AV node. This structure is functionally composed of three cellular layers. On reaching the first layer, activation is slowed progressively. In the middle layer, activity reaches remarkably low propagation velocity. This is probably a result of "decremental conduction" in which the propagated action potential loses amplitude and velocity along a given path. If the process reaches the third layer with sufficient amplitude, a progressive increase in velocity of conduction occurs, carrying activation into the bundle of His and the remainder of the conduction system.

The sequence of depolarization in the ventricles is determined by the distribution of the specialized ventricular conduction system, particularly the rapidly conducting Purkinje fibers. This process has been extensively studied in the experimental animal. The earliest area of the ventricles to be depolarized is the central septal surface of the left ventricular cavity. This area of activation quickly spreads in the subendocardial layers surrounding the left ventricular cavity, and is joined by an area of activity on the right, beginning near the base of the right anterior papillary muscle and spreading around the anterior right cavity. These two areas expand rapidly, involving the septum from both sides simultaneously, and the free walls from inside to outside.

The earliest point of breakthrough to the external surface of the heart is on the right, near the base of the right anterior papillary muscle. The earlier breakthrough in this location is probably due to early activation and the thin right ventricular wall in this location. The spread of activity involves the apical area first, then spreads upward toward the AV ring. The last portions of the heart to be depolarized are the base of the interventricular septum and the basal portion of the left ventricular free wall. In the human subject, the pathway cannot be studied in the same way, but the pattern of breakthrough to the surface and the sequence of surface spread of

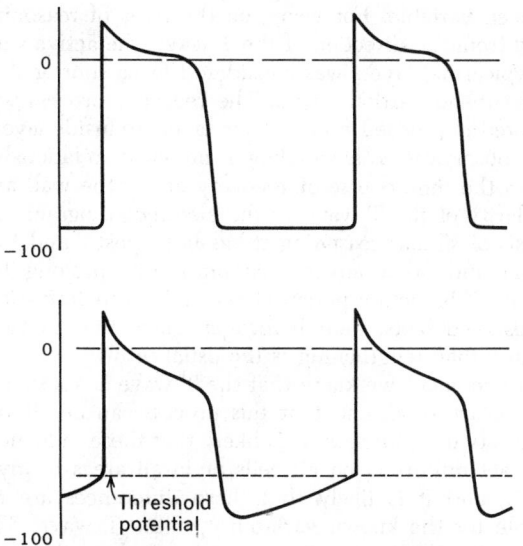

Fig. 260-2. Schematic representation of the differences in the action potential of a ventricular cell (above) and a pacemaker cell (below). Note the spontaneous "leak" of resting potential, with rapid loss of potential when the threshold value is reached.

activity are not greatly divergent from those in the dog.

The earliest forces of the QRS complex are consistently anterior in direction. This is related to the earlier activation of the left side of the interventricular septum, which does not lie in a straight anteroposterior plane, but is obliquely placed in relation to the chest, so that the left ventricle is posterior and leftward, and the right ventricle is anterior and rightward. Thus the earliest forces originating in the interventricular septum have a direction which is anterior and to the right. These forces may be slightly superior or slightly inferior in position, but their anterior position is very consistent.

Following activation of the left septum, there is activation on the right, resulting in involvement of the interventricular septum from both sides, as well as activation of the subendocardial region at the anterior apical region of the right ventricle. The resultant forces from these regions are also anterior in direction, but the center of gravity shifts toward the left as the subendocardial areas on the left are activated.

The breakthrough of activity on the anterior surface of the right ventricle, indicating completion of spread through the right ventricular wall, produces an unbalancing of forces and a marked dominance of left ventricular activity. Thus the midforces of the ventricular electrocardiogram are toward the left ventricle: in a leftward, inferior, and posterior direction.

The last area of the ventricles to be depolarized is the posterobasal area, including the high septal and high free wall areas of the left ventricle. Forces from these areas are directed posteriorly, superiorly, and usually slightly to the right. These are the forces of the terminal portion of the QRS complex.

Few studies have been made of the process of repolarization. The time course of this process in the ventricular wall has been difficult to study, and the results have been variable. For years, on the basis of reasoning derived from the direction of the T wave, the active state of subepicardial layers was considered to be shorter than that of subendocardial layers. The recovery process was considered to proceed from outside layers to inside layers. Direct observations have shown no clear relationship between the time course of recovery across the wall and the polarity of the T wave of the electrocardiogram. On the basis of similar reasoning it has been postulated that ischemia and other adverse circumstances prolong the duration of the action potential and delay repolarization. The observed facts, though meager, show that shortening rather than lengthening is the usual result.

At the moment we know that the T wave is associated with repolarization, and that this process can be altered by a variety of influences. It is likely that these influences do not act uniformly on all cells or in all areas of myocardium, and it is likely that these differences are responsible for the known variability of the T wave. The exact relationship between events in single cells, their sequence in various areas of myocardium, and the T wave as seen in the surface electrocardiogram remains obscure.

Distribution of Electrical Forces from the Heart over the Body

Early in the history of electrocardiography, attempts were made to relate the various events being recorded at the surface of the body to each other and to the events in the heart. Einthoven's concepts are the best known. He considered the body as a homogeneous conducting medium of large extent. The source of electrical activity was considered to be located in the center of the conducting medium. Electrodes on the right arm, left arm, and left leg were considered as being symmetrically placed around this source, and equidistant from it. These

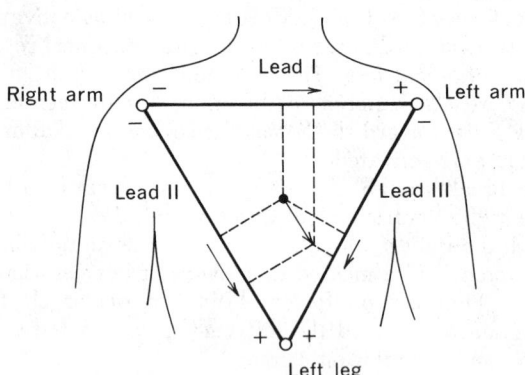

Fig. 260-3. The conventional reference frame of the Einthoven standard lead system, representing the cardiac vector as arising from a point in the center of an equilateral triangle formed by the leads between the electrodes on three extremities of the body. The components of each axis are represented for the cardiac vector. In this particular example, the three lead components will all have a positive sense because the arrows point toward the designated positive poles of the leads. These leads are one way of showing the forces in the frontal plane of the body.

electrodes were represented as forming the apices of an equilateral triangle, with the source of electromotive force (EMF) at its center, as seen in Fig. 260-3. A force represented by a vector at the center of the triangle will produce a magnitude in surface recordings between two electrodes (a "lead") proportional to the projection of this vector on the line connecting the two recording points (the lead axis).

Thus Einthoven's concepts related the magnitude and configuration of complexes recorded from extremity leads to the direction of the leads and to the direction and magnitude of EMF in the center of the thorax. These concepts were concerned with forces in the frontal plane only.

Einthoven's concepts were extended by F. N. Wilson and associates, and from this work arose the concept of the central-terminal electrode. If the assumptions underlying the Einthoven triangle are correct, a network made by connecting the electrodes on the right arm, left arm, and left leg establishes an "indifferent" electrode, whose potential is very close to zero throughout the cardiac cycle.

A series of new leads was devised, using the central terminal as the negative pole (the indifferent electrode) of each lead. The positive pole (the exploring electrode) was connected to the extremities to record "unipolar" limb leads (VR, VL, and VF), and to points on the precordium to record "unipolar" precordial leads (V_1 through V_6). In later years a modification of the Wilson central terminal has been used in recording limb leads. This modification was introduced in order to increase, or augment, the recorded amplitude of the waves. Leads recorded with this technique are called augmented unipolar leads (aVR, aVL, and aVF). The precordial electrode positions and the connections of each of the standard leads are outlined in Tables 260-1 and 260-2.

Table 260-1. PRECORDIAL ELECTRODE POSITIONS

V_1	Fourth interspace, to right of sternum
V_2	Fourth interspace, to left of sternum
V_3	Midway between V_2 and V_4 positions
V_4	Fifth interspace, in midclavicular line
V_5	Lateral to V_4, in anterior axillary line
V_6	Lateral to V_4, in midaxillary line

In introducing the precordial leads, Wilson extended the assumptions of Einthoven beyond the extremities to include leads recorded from the chest wall. It was appreciated, even by Wilson, that the assumptions of Einthoven regarding homogeneity of the body, symmetry of the leads, and the presence of a single dipolar source at the center of the conducting medium were not strictly true.

The right arm to left arm lead (lead I) is not a true horizontal lead, and the angle between the three Einthoven limb leads is not 60° as would be predicted. For example, lead I is inclined so that its axis is 10 to 15° from a true horizontal line, the left end more superior than the right end.

Table 260-2. CONNECTIONS OF THE STANDARD
ELECTROCARDIOGRAPHIC LEADS

Lead	Negative connection	Positive connection
I	Right arm	Left arm
II	Right arm	Left leg
III	Left arm	Left leg
aVR	Modified central terminal	Right arm
aVL	Modified central terminal	Left arm
aVF	Modified central terminal	Left leg
V leads (1–6)	Wilson's central terminal	Precordial positions (1–6)

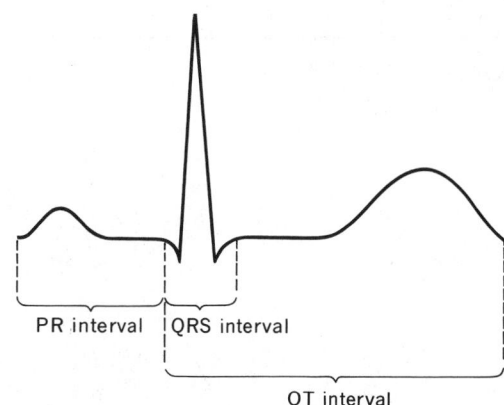

Fig. 260-5. Names and points for measurement of electrocardiographic intervals.

From a theoretical standpoint, it would be advantageous to devise three leads which would measure the projection of a given force from the heart along three mutually perpendicular axes. Not only would such a system provide a maximal amount of information utilizing a minimal number of leads, but these same leads could be used for the recording of vectorcardiograms, a technique which will be discussed more fully in another section. Over the past few years, several such systems, based largely on experiments on models of the human torso, have been devised. Although perfect systems have not been developed, reasonable approximations have been proposed. These "orthogonal" lead systems utilize resistor networks and/or multiple electrodes distributed over the body to achieve three orthogonal leads, X, Y, and Z. These developments have not yet simplified the problem, since there is some doubt that these three leads include all information contained in the conventional leads.

THE APPROACH TO INTERPRETATION OF THE ELECTROCARDIOGRAM

The usual first step in interpretation is to determine the rate and the rhythm of the heart. The rate is determined by measuring the time interval between successive P waves (for atrial rate) or between successive R or S waves (for ventricular rate), and dividing this interval, in seconds, into 60 (sec) to obtain the rate per minute (Fig. 260-4).

Since there are 300 heavy time lines per minute at the standard recording speed of 25 mm per sec, a reasonably simple approximation of the rate can be arrived at by dividing the number of large spaces between two successive cycles into 300. Two large spaces between cycles equals a rate of 150 per min; three spaces, a rate of 100 per min; four spaces, a rate of 75 per min; etc. Interpolation between these values enables one to arrive quickly at an approximation which is accurate within 5 to 10 beats per min, yet does not require more than simple calculation. The atrial and ventricular rates are usually equal, but not always, so routine measurement of both rates prevents error.

The next step in interpretation is the measurement of the various intervals. The points from which these intervals are measured are seen in Fig. 260-5. The P-R interval varies with the size of the patient and the heart rate. The upper limit of normal in the average adult is 0.20 sec. In very small patients, such as children, and in those with rapid heart rates, normal tables should be consulted. The QRS interval also varies to some extent with the age of the patient. In children the interval ranges between 0.04 and 0.08 sec. In adults, the normal interval ranges from 0.06 to 0.10 sec. The normal Q-T interval varies greatly with rate, so one must refer to normal tables to obtain the range for a given rate.

Once the intervals have been determined, the observed measurements must be compared with the normal range for these measurements. If the P-R interval is too long, one may infer that conduction through the AV node is prolonged (first degree block). A P-R interval which is too short may result from an abnormal site of initiation of the atrial impulse (such as a nodal rhythm). A prolonged QRS interval usually indicates some form of ventricular conduction disturbance, which will be discussed in a later paragraph. A shortened Q-T interval may result from digitalis administration or hypercalcemia. A long Q-T interval may result from quinidine administration or from hypocalcemia or hypokalemia.

The next step in interpretation is to consider the direction and configuration of the various waves in individual leads. As already stated, the assumptions underlying the Einthoven (Fig. 260-6) triangle are not strictly true. For this reason, calculations of direction and magnitude

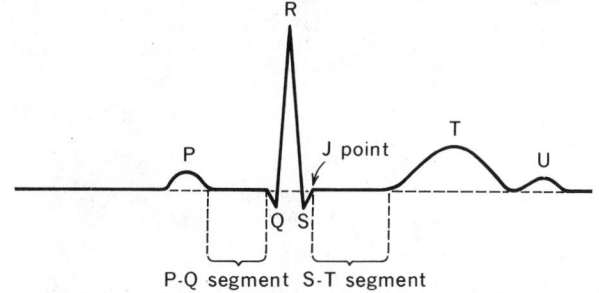

Fig. 260-4. Names of the electrocardiographic waves and segments.

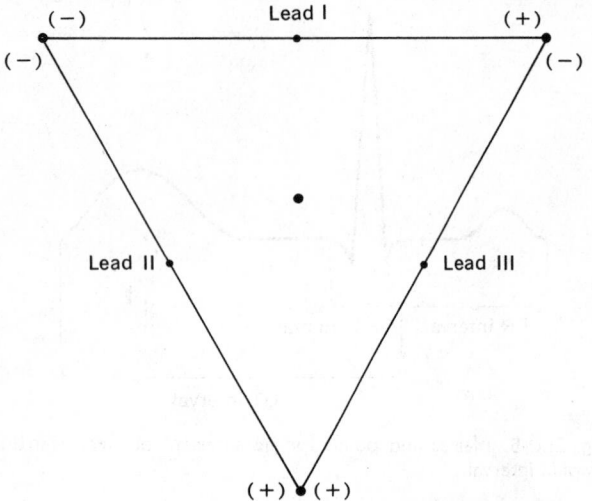

Fig. 260-6. Axes of bipolar limb leads arranged as a triangle.

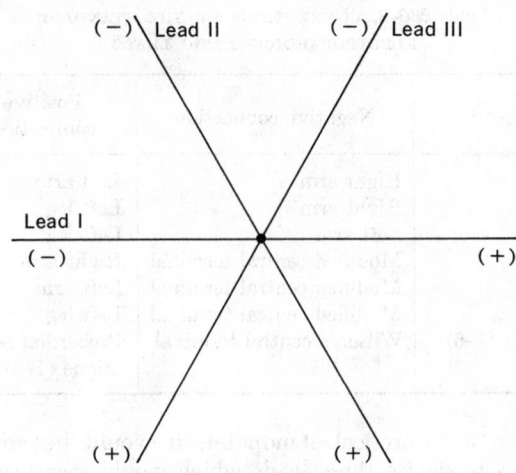

Fig. 260-7. Axes of bipolar limb leads arranged as a triaxial figure.

of forces using this reference figure, or modifications of it, are subject to error. In spite of these limitations, it is felt that consideration of the electrical events of the heart as vectorial forces in three dimensions, rather than as wave forms in individual leads, is a logical and practical approach. This "spatial vector" approach places the individual variations in waves in individual leads into a larger framework which is easier to learn and to retain, and which also incorporates the information obtained from the closely related vectorcardiographic technique.

The underlying assumptions should be reviewed. It is assumed that all activity, resulting from depolarization or repolarization, at a given instant of time, can be represented by a resultant electrical force from a single dipole, approximately in the center of the cardiac mass. This dipole is assumed to remain in one location throughout the cycle. The limb lead electrodes located on the right arm, left arm, and left leg are assumed to be symmetrically arranged around this dipolar source, and to be equidistant from it. It is also assumed that the activity recorded in the precordial leads is from the same single dipole and that the precordial leads do not "sample" the activity of the ventricular wall immediately underlying them, but record from the heart as a whole.

On the basis of the above assumptions, each electrocardiographic lead is considered as measuring the projection of the resultant electrical activity acting at any one instant along the axis of the lead. In effect, the 12 routine leads provide 12 "views" of the resultant electrical activity, and from these 12 views the size and direction of the resultant force are estimated.

Leads I, II, and III are bipolar limb leads in that they are recorded from one extremity to another. The polarity of these leads is determined by convention established by Einthoven. It has been found more convenient to arrange the axes of these leads as a triaxial figure, with the intersection at the center of the chest, rather than as a triangle. The dipole is assumed to be located at this point. These relationships and the triaxial figure are seen in Fig. 260-7.

The axis of any unipolar lead (a lead using a central terminal as the negative connection) is a line drawn from the center of electrical activity to the point at which the exploring electrode, which forms the positive connection, is placed. Leads aVR, aVL, and aVF are recorded with a modified central terminal, but their axes are drawn according to this convention. In Fig. 260-8 the axes of the bipolar and unipolar limb leads are combined in the same figure. The leads are seen to arrange themselves at 30° intervals. All these leads are in the frontal plane of the body.

The six conventional precordial leads can be considered as forming six additional axes in a horizontal or coronal plane. These leads are not actually in a single coronal plane, since the last three precordial leads are recorded several interspaces below the first two precordial leads. Errors are occasionally introduced by considering these leads as lying at a single level, but the concept is never-

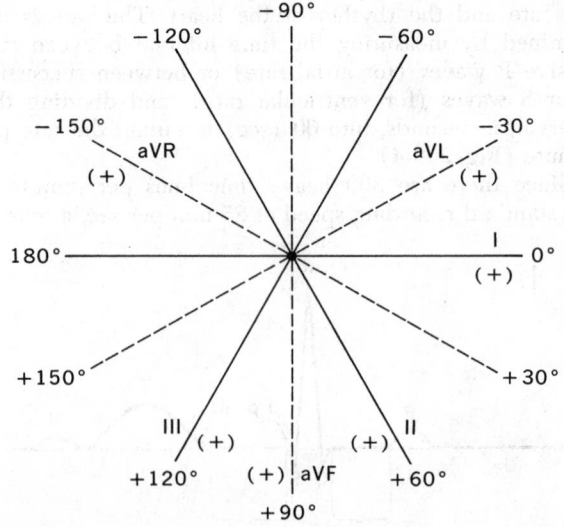

Fig. 260-8. Axes of bipolar and unipolar limb leads combined as a hexaxial figure, showing conventional directional designation in degrees.

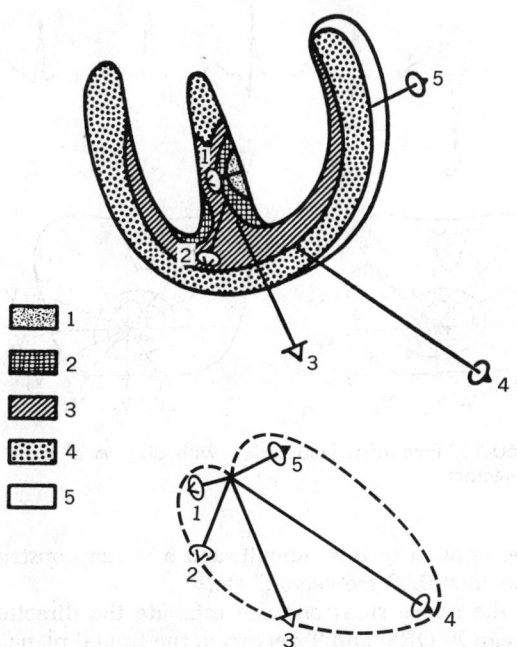

Legend:
1
2
3
4
5

Fig. 260-9. Schematic representation of the activation front at five arbitrary points during ventricular depolarization, with a vector derived from each (above). The figure below represents a combination of these same vectors at a central point. The dotted line connecting their tips represents the QRS loop of the vectorcardiogram.

theless useful. The axes of the six precordial leads are as seen in Fig. 260-12.

The resultant electrical activity at the center of the heart is often represented as a vector, a figure whose amplitude and direction represent the amplitude and direction of the resultant force. The size and direction of this vector are not constant during the cardiac cycle, but vary from instant to instant. As depolarization begins on the left septal surface, activity can be represented by a small vector directed to the right and anteriorly. In the middle of depolarization, the resultant vector would be to the left and posteriorly. Late in the depolarization process the vector would be directed posteriorly and superiorly. The process of depolarization could be broken into many time intervals, and each could be represented by a resultant vector. If this were done, and the vector tips were connected by a line, this line would form a loop-shaped figure, as seen in Fig. 260-9. This figure can be recorded by directly plotting two right-angle leads against each other using a cathode ray oscilloscope. This figure is called a vectorcardiogram.

The resultant electrical activity produced by the heart can be in any direction; thus the vector must be shown not only in a single plane but in several planes, or as a three-dimensional representation. In the presentation of the vectorcardiogram, this is accomplished by recording three views of the vector pathway—a frontal plane view, a horizontal or coronal plane view, and a sagittal plane view.

In addition to dividing the activity into a large number

of small time intervals, each represented by a resultant "instantaneous" vector, the activity during one portion of the cycle, such as the QRS or T wave, can be averaged, and the resultant can be presented as a "mean" QRS or T vector. Both techniques are used.

In estimating the magnitude and direction of the resultant vector, either as a mean vector or as an instantaneous vector at a given point in time, certain principles must be considered. A vector at the center of the electrical field will produce the largest possible deflection in that lead whose axis lies most nearly parallel to the direction of the vector. The lead whose axis is most nearly perpendicular to the vector will produce the smallest deflection. If the lead axis is exactly perpendicular, the resultant deflection in that lead will be zero (Fig. 260-10).

The magnitude and direction of the mean QRS and T vector can be determined in the frontal plane, using the limb lead recordings. One method is to measure the area under the wave in each lead, subtracting the negative areas from the positive areas and plotting the area value for each lead along the axis of this lead. A positive value is plotted along the positive end of the axis, and a negative value is plotted along the negative end of the axis. Perpendicular lines are drawn from the defined points. These lines will cross at a point, or very close to a point. This point defines the position of the head of the vector. A line drawn from the center of the figure to the point defines the vector direction and magnitude.

If a mean P, QRS, or T vector is calculated, using the above method, from leads I, II, and III, and is then recalculated using leads aVR, aVL, and aVF, the magnitude of the vector calculated using the unipolar limb leads will be found to have the same direction as that calculated from the limb leads, but to have a smaller amplitude. The amplitude units in the unipolar limb leads must be multiplied by a correction factor of 1.15 to equate the two sets of limb lead recordings in magnitude.

For most purposes, the amplitude of the electrical activity being measured can be adequately evaluated by simple measurement of amplitude of R waves or S waves in the various limb leads, and comparing these values with the normal values for these leads. For this reason, the most useful information to be gained from the mean vectors is their *direction*. This information can be quickly

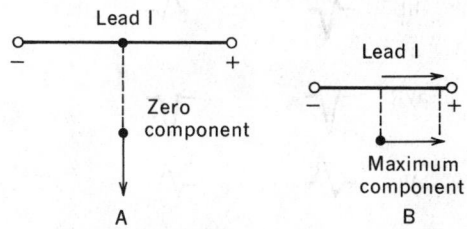

Fig. 260-10. A. When the vector force is perpendicular to the lead axis line, there will be no component on the lead line. This lead alone, therefore, will give no information about the magnitude and direction of forces perpendicular to it. B. When the vector is parallel to the lead line, the component on the lead line will be maximum.

evaluated by a procedure which does not require the determination of areas under the various waves. This technique utilizes the fact that a force, when perpendicular to a given lead, produces no deflection on that lead. Similarly, a mean vector, when perpendicular to a given lead, produces a deflection which has an equal area above and below the isoelectric line in that lead.

A quick glance at the QRS complexes in Fig. 260-11A shows that the QRS complex in lead aVF has an equal area above and below the line. This indicates that the QRS vector has a direction which is perpendicular to that lead. Another glance shows that the vector is directed toward the left instead of the right, since it is upright in lead I. These evaluations can be carried out in a very few seconds. Figure 260-11B shows another example, but there is no lead in which the areas below and above the line are equal. There are two leads, leads aVL and III, in which the complex shows almost the same area above and below the line. In this case the direction can be determined quickly by interpolation, and is found to be approximately midway between the position which would have produced an equal area in lead aVL and the position which would have produced such a complex in III.

Not only can the direction of the mean QRS be determined in this manner, but by applying the same principles to the P waves and the T waves, the direction of the mean P and T vectors can be estimated.

Once the mean vector for QRS has been determined, it is a relatively simple matter to determine the direction of smaller subdivisions of the QRS complex. This is not so precise as the estimation of mean vector direction, but can be accurate enough to be of real value. If one identifies the first portion, such as the first 0.02 sec, of the QRS complex, the same principles outlined above

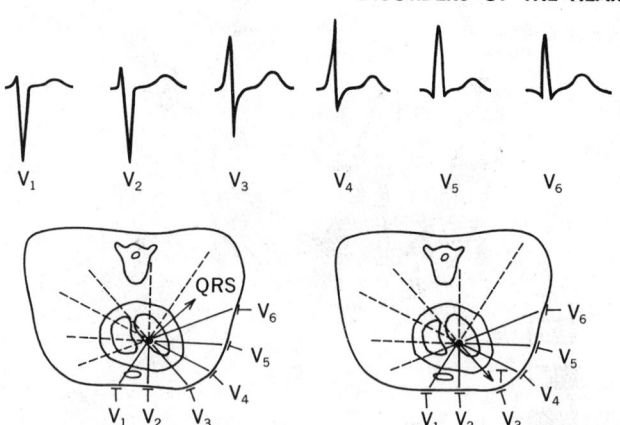

Fig. 260-12. Precordial lead series, with diagram of mean QRS and T vectors.

can be applied to this subunit, and a vector constructed for the "first 0.02-sec vector," etc.

By the above steps one can estimate the direction of the mean P, QRS, and T vectors in the frontal plane. The next step is to determine the direction of these same vectors in the horizontal plane. This is done in a manner very similar to the above, but using the precordial leads instead of the limb leads.

A quick glance at the precordial lead series in Fig. 260-12 shows that the QRS complex in V_3 has an approximately equal area above and below the isoelectric line. This indicates that the mean QRS vector has a direction perpendicular to this lead. There are two alternate possibilities, one toward the right anterior part of the chest, the other away from the right anterior part. The QRS in V_1 and V_2 is predominantly below the isoelectric line; therefore the mean QRS vector has a direction away from V_1 and V_2. With this information, the vector direction can be estimated as seen in the figure. The mean T-vector direction can be estimated in a similar fashion. Very often, the T waves in the precordial leads are all upright. In the absence of a clearly isoelectric T wave in any lead, one must infer that the T vector lies in a direction as shown in Fig. 260-12. The recording of extra leads to the right or to the left will usually locate the isoelectric T wave and enable a more precise estimate of T-vector direction.

THE VECTORCARDIOGRAM AND ITS RELATIONSHIP TO THE ELECTROCARDIOGRAM

As stated previously, the vectorcardiogram represents the pathway described by the tips of an infinite number of instantaneous vectors during one cycle. This type of recording is produced directly by plotting the amplitude obtained in one lead against that obtained in another lead with an axis at right angles to the first lead. These two leads are plotted against each other using a cathode ray oscilloscope. The resultant vectorcardiogram for one cardiac cycle consists of three loops—a P loop, a QRS loop,

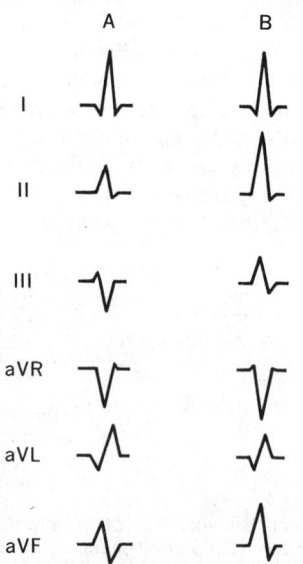

Fig. 260-11. In (A) the mean QRS vector is perpendicular to lead aVF, at 0° in the frontal plane. In (B) the mean QRS area is equally small in leads III and aVL. The means QRS vector is at +45°.

and a T loop. This type of record is a plot of amplitude in one lead against amplitude in another lead; therefore time is not a part of the record except as it is indicated by interruption of the electron beam during its sweep. This time signal is effective only when the beam is inscribing the loops. During the isoelectric periods, the electron beam remains in the center of the tube, and the interruptions cannot be appreciated.

A number of lead systems have been devised for the recording of vectorcardiograms. The ideal lead system would be one which would record along three mutually perpendicular axes, using leads of equal "lead strength" (the amplitude units along each lead are the same).

Since vectorcardiograms are recorded with leads entirely different from the routine electrocardiographic leads, it is not surprising that there are occasional discrepancies in the two systems. However, one is more impressed by the agreement between the two systems than by their discrepancies. By plotting the direction of the mean QRS vector in the frontal plane, and determining the direction of the initial and terminal vectors of the QRS, one can predict with fair accuracy the configuration and rotation of the frontal plane vectorcardiogram. The horizontal and sagittal loops are more difficult to predict, probably because of the proximity of the precordial leads. In turn, the vectorcardiogram enables one to predict with fair accuracy the configuration of the electrocardiographic leads. The appreciation of the relationship between these two systems is very useful in transferring information from one system to the other.

These two systems are complementary, and one by no means replaces the other. The vectorcardiographic method is usually very useful in those abnormalities affecting the QRS complex, but it is very poor in detecting abnormalities in the S-T-T portion of the electrocardiogram. The mean P, QRS, and T vectors usually correspond to the long axis of P, QRS, and T loops.

THE NORMAL ELECTROCARDIOGRAM

The P vector in the normal subject is directed to the left and inferiorly and is approximately parallel with the frontal plane in the anteroposterior direction. The axis lies between 0° and +75° in the frontal plane; thus the normal P wave is upright in leads I and II, and variable in lead III. The average direction is at about +60°; therefore, the P wave is usually largest in lead II. The upper limits of normal size for the P wave in this lead in normal subjects is 2.5 mm at standard sensitivity. The P wave in normal subjects is not constant in size, becoming larger with rapid rates.

The normal P vector lies near the frontal plane in its anteroposterior projection. As would be expected with this position of the vector, the P-wave direction in leads V_1 and V_2 is variable. The P loop always moves anteriorly, then posteriorly; thus the P wave in the early precordial leads always has an initial upright portion, followed by a more variable terminal portion, which may be upright, isoelectric, or inverted.

The normal mean QRS vector in the adult lies between 0° and +90° in the frontal plane. The QRS complex is usually predominantly upright in leads I and II. As with the P wave, the QRS in lead III may be predominantly upright or inverted. Lead II is usually the lead in which the upright amplitude is maximal, but this is dependent on the direction of the vector. The maximal normal QRS amplitude in the limb leads (maximal R-wave amplitude or maximal S-wave amplitude, not the sum of the two) is 20 mm at standard sensitivity.

In the newborn infant, the QRS axis in the frontal plane lies to the right, at about 135°. The axis moves to the left as the child grows older, and usually moves into the left lower quadrant at about two years of age. The QRS axis usually remains more vertical through young adulthood, after which it becomes more horizontal.

The mean QRS vector in the adult lies posterior to the frontal plane. The usual transition between predominantly negative and predominantly positive complexes is at the V_3 to V_4 position, but occasional normal individuals are seen to have transitional complexes at the V_2 position, indicating an unusually anterior position of the QRS vector.

As previously stated, the earliest forces of the QRS complex are directed anteriorly. This produces a consistent positive initial deflection of the QRS complex in V_1 and V_2. These early positive forces are usually of brief duration (0.01 to 0.02 sec) and are followed by a deep, broad S wave. In the left precordial leads the same early left-to-right forces produce a brief Q wave which precedes the large R wave. A regular progression in height of the R wave in the first three or four precordial leads is expected. The maximal amplitude in the precordial leads is 25 mm at standard sensitivity (S-wave depth in leads V_1, V_2, V_3 or R-wave height in V_4, V_5, V_6, not the sum of the two).

There is considerable variability in QRS loops recorded from normal individuals, but closer inspection reveals that normal loops may be grouped into two main groups, one with inconspicuous terminal forces (Fig. 260-13),

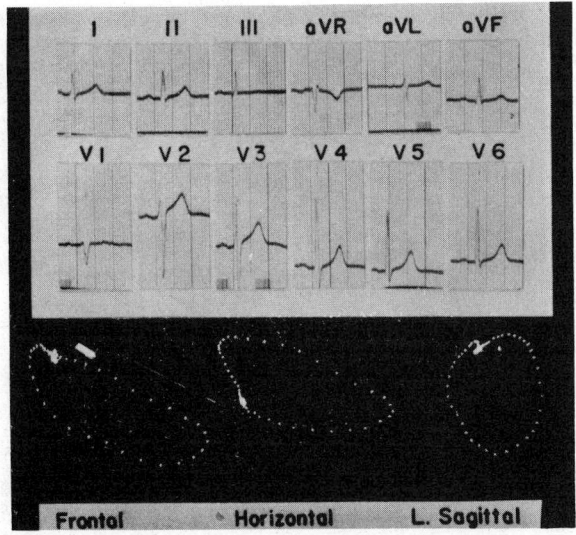

Fig. 260-13. Normal QRS loop with inconspicuous terminal forces

the other group with prominent terminal forces (Fig. 260-14). The terminal forces in the latter group are directed to the right, superiorly and posteriorly, toward the right scapular area. These terminal forces produce a large S wave in the standard limb leads and in the left precordial leads. The group with large terminal forces are termed "S_1, S_2, S_3"–type loops, indicating their usual presentation in the bipolar limb leads. This term refers to the general configuration of the loop, rather than to its specific presentation in limb leads, and an S wave in lead I or lead III may be absent. Although the S_1, S_2, S_3 type of loop is a normal finding, an exaggerated form of this same type of loop is seen in certain cases of right ventricular hypertrophy, and will be discussed further on under Right Ventricular Hypertrophy. Because of the prominent terminal forces, the S_1, S_2, S_3 type of loop is broad and the projection of the loop produces biphasic QRS complexes in many limb and precordial leads. This may lead to an erroneous location of the transitional QRS complex and a false impression of left axis deviation. When all leads appear to have biphasic QRS complexes, with large S waves in the bipolar limb leads and in V_4, V_5, and V_6, this type of loop is likely to be the cause.

In the newborn infant, the mean QRS vector is anteriorly directed, probably because of the physiologic dominance of the right ventricular mass. The QRS complex is upright in the right precordial leads. At age two to age five, the mean QRS vector moves into a posterior position, at which time the QRS configuration in lead V_1 assumes its adult configuration.

There are other, but less well-defined, changes in the electrocardiogram with age. The amplitude of all complexes tends to reach its maximum between the ages of fifteen to twenty-five years. From this time, there is a steady diminution in amplitude in most series studied. The previously stated normal amplitude limits are derived from hospitalized adult individuals. Application of these standards to healthy groups of young adults may result in a false impression of hypertrophy if this trend is not appreciated.

ABNORMALITIES IN THE P AND Ta WAVES

Right atrial enlargement is accompanied by a rightward directional shift of the P vector in the frontal plane; left atrial enlargement is accompanied by a shift to a more horizontal position. Although these trends are clearly seen in statistical comparisons of groups with and without atrial hypertrophy, there is considerable overlap with the normal range on either side. In the horizontal plane, the P vector is more anteriorly directed in right atrial enlargement, and more posteriorly directed in left atrial enlargement. The overlap with normal is not so extensive in this plane; therefore, anteroposterior leads are more useful than limb leads in detecting atrial hypertrophy.

Left atrial hypertrophy is seen with mitral stenosis and in all forms of left ventricular disease. The P wave begins to show changes long before elevation of end-diastolic pressure occurs in left ventricular disease, and at times P waves are seen to be abnormal before the QRS complex is altered. The genesis of these changes is not fully understood, but it is probably related to the fact that the atrium is contracting against a ventricle which is less compliant than the normal ventricle.

The criteria for recognition of left atrial hypertrophy have been extensively reviewed by Morris, who has established new criteria based on measurements in V_1 and V_2. The P wave can be divided into two parts, separated by a change in slope, or by a difference in direction between the initial and terminal portions. Left atrial enlargement is characterized by an increased area of negativity beneath the terminal portion of the P wave in V_1 or V_2. The area beneath the terminal portion is determined by multiplying the duration of the terminal portion (in seconds) by the height or depth of the terminal portion (in millimeters). The value for this determination in normal individuals ranges from −0.03 to +0.02 mm-sec. In those with left atrial enlargement due to mitral disease or left ventricular disease this value was −0.04 or below.

Right atrial enlargement is seen in tricuspid stenosis, in pulmonary disease, and in other conditions in which the right ventricle becomes thicker and less compliant. As mentioned above, the P vector becomes more vertical in the frontal plane and more anterior in the horizontal plane. A vertical position of the P vector, with an increased amplitude (greater than 2.5 mm at standard sensitivity) in the limb leads, and with an upright P wave in V_1 and V_2 usually suggests right atrial enlargement. Right atrial enlargement is quite reliably predicted by these criteria, but there are many cases of right atrial enlargement in which these criteria are negative.

The atrial T wave (Ta) is seldom identified in the

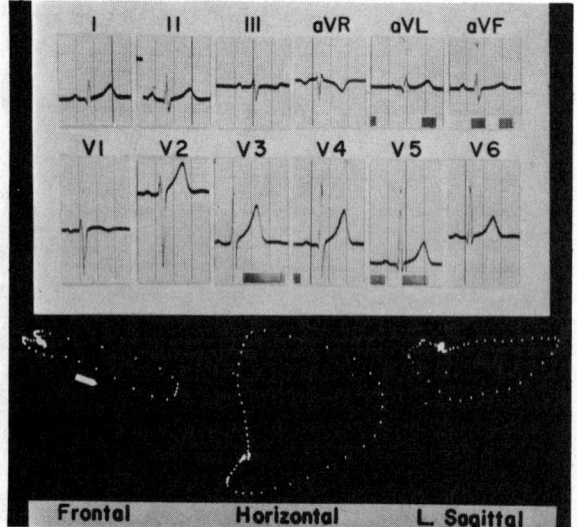

Fig. 260-14. Normal QRS loop of "S_1, S_2, S_3" type.

normal electrocardiogram. When identifiable, it is seen to be in a direction opposite to that of the P wave, and to enclose approximately the same area as the P wave. When the P wave becomes large, the Ta wave also becomes large and, under such circumstances, the Ta wave may become visible, producing deviation of the P-R and S-T segments, easily confused with the S-T segment shift of myocardial injury. The P waves become larger with a rapid rate; therefore, situations in which the P waves are large and the rate is rapid commonly produce S-T deviation due to the Ta wave. It is most frequently seen in chronic lung disease. It is identified by (1) the presence of large P waves, (2) a direction of the S-T-segment shift opposite to the P-wave direction, and (3) a curvilinear configuration of the P-R and S-T segments, as seen in Fig. 260-15, which is usually most apparent in the bipolar limb leads.

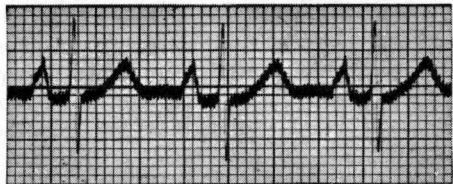

Fig. 260-15. Atrial repolarization causing a deviation of the P-R and S-T segments. Note the curvilinear configuration (lead II).

ABNORMALITIES IN THE QRS AND T WAVES

Left Ventricular Hypertrophy

The diagnosis of left ventricular hypertrophy, one of the more common electrocardiographic diagnoses, is by no means a straightforward application of clearly established criteria. The difficulty begins with the establishment of a known group of cases with pure left ventricular hypertrophy at autopsy, which can be used to test criteria. One finds that increasing hypertrophy of the left ventricle is usually joined by an increase in right ventricular wall thickness.

There is no agreement on the mechanism by which left ventricular hypertrophy produces its effect. For example, there is no correlation between amplitude of the QRS complex and heart weight until heart weight is well beyond normal. A heart of 250 Gm weight and a heart of 400 Gm weight often have the same QRS amplitude. Hugenholtz has suggested that the electrocardiographic changes which we call hypertrophy may result from the hyperplasia of cardiac fibers which has been observed to occur at heart weights beyond 450 to 500 Gm. It is also likely that some of the effects are produced by the proximity of the hypertrophied heart to the chest wall and to conduction disturbances which produce less cancellation of forces from opposite sides of the heart.

An equally difficult problem is the fact that criteria which are designed for extreme sensitivity (to detect all examples of left ventricular hypertrophy in a given population) have a low specificity and will falsely classify many normal individuals as having left ventricular hypertrophy. Thus one must consider both sensitivity and specificity of criteria and must arrive at a compromise which fits the needs most closely. For example, in a situation in which one is interested in screening a population, detecting those individuals with suggestive findings, and subjecting them to more specific follow-up examinations,

very sensitive criteria would be most useful. The false positives would be detected by further tests. On the other hand, in an electrocardiographic laboratory in which the clinical information available is minimal, and from which reports are sent to physicians with varying knowledge of the electrocardiogram, the use of very sensitive criteria would lead to much confusion and much unnecessary concern on the part of both physician and patient. In such a situation, one would choose criteria which are less sensitive and which would not result in a large number of false positive diagnoses.

A number of electrocardiographic parameters are found to correlate significantly with heart weight as determined at autopsy. Increased QRS amplitude is one of those parameters. The amplitude criteria which best separate normal and abnormal groups are as follows: R-wave height or S-wave depth of 20 mm or more in the bipolar limb leads and 25 mm or more in the precordial leads. These measurements are made in any lead, and the amplitudes above and below the line are not added. Even though these criteria correlate well with heart weight, they leave much to be desired. They are abnormal in only about one-third of patients with hypertrophy. At the same time, when applied to a series of normal young individuals, they result in a significant number of false positive diagnoses.

S-T-segment depression in the standard bipolar limb leads and in V_5 and V_6 has been found to correlate well with heart weight. This is an imperfect criterion, since digitalis administration also produces S-T-segment depression in the same leads. For this reason, this criterion can be applied only when the patient is known not to have been receiving digitalis. If S-T-segment shift of the type typical of "left ventricular strain" is seen (the J point is less depressed than the rest of the S-T segment, the S-T segment has a straight line slope downward from the J point and terminates in a T wave which is in an opposite direction from the major direction of the QRS complex), this finding has some correlation with heart weight in digitalized patients, but the correlation is much poorer than in the nondigitalized group. In addition to the confusion introduced by digitalis, the S-T segment is also involved in the electrocardiographic abnormalities seen in electrolyte disturbances and subendocardial injury. Finally, this criterion, too, is positive in only about one-third of cases of known hypertrophy.

Leftward deviation of the QRS axis is found to correlate with heart weight. An axis of −15° or more was found to separate normal and abnormal heart weights.

This criterion is imperfect too, since it is known to be influenced by diffuse left ventricular disease and coronary disease in the absence of left ventricular hypertrophy.

An increase in the "intrinsicoid deflection time" (an arbitrary measurement of the time between the onset of the QRS complex and the peak of the R wave) in V_5 and V_6 has also been found to correlate well with heart weight, but this measurement is found to correlate better with right ventricular wall thickness than with left ventricular wall thickness. Further consideration of the setting in which this criterion is positive shows that it is positive in those cases in which congestive heart failure has been present. The evidence indicates that this parameter is related primarily to the presence of a conduction disturbance, which is frequently seen in left ventricular disease with congestive heart failure and secondary right ventricular hypertrophy. Right ventricular hypertrophy in other settings does not lead to an increased intrinsicoid deflection time in V_5 and V_6.

An increased QRS duration has a modest correlation with heart weight, and a duration of 0.09 sec or greater best separates normal and abnormal groups. This criterion has a very poor sensitivity and is positive in only 10 percent of cases with known hypertrophy.

As can be seen from the above, none of the parameters mentioned is ideal. For this reason a point score system has been devised which combines the above criteria. A diagnosis of left ventricular hypertrophy is made when an arbitrary point score is reached. The parameters and their score ratings are as follows:

1. Amplitude criteria: presence of one or more of the following = 3 points.
   a. Largest R or S wave in limb leads ≥ 20 mm.
   b. Largest S wave in V_1, V_2, V_3 ≥ 25 mm.
   c. Largest R wave in V_4, V_5, V_6 ≥ 25 mm.

2. S-T-segment criteria:
   a. Any S-T-segment shift with a vectoral direction opposite to mean QRS *in the absence of digitalis* = 3 points.
   b. If digitalis *has* been administered, S-T-T segment typical of "left ventricular strain" (sloping contour, S-T and T vectors opposite to mean QRS vector) = 1 point.

3. Axis criteria: Left axis deviation ≥ −15° = 2 points.

4. Duration criteria:
   a. QRS duration ≥ 0.09 sec = 1 point.
   b. Intrinsicoid deflection in V_5 or V_6 ≥ 0.04 sec = 1 point.

Using the system, the maximum score is 10 points. A score of 4 points is interpreted as "probable left ventricular hypertrophy," and a score of 5 points is interpreted as "left ventricular hypertrophy."

The recent observations of Morris on the frequent occurrence of left atrial hypertrophy in left ventricular disease has led him to consider the abnormal terminal P wave in V_1 and V_2 (described above in the discussion of left atrial hypertrophy) as an additional criterion of left ventricular hypertrophy. Preliminary observations indicate that it is as sensitive as increased amplitude of the QRS complex, and considerably more specific. Addition of an abnormal P wave in V_1 as an additional parameter, with a score rating of 3 points, will probably increase the sensitivity of the above scoring system without adversely affecting its specificity, but this has not been adequately tested as yet.

It can be seen that any one criterion is not enough for a diagnosis of left ventricular hypertrophy using the above system. Positive amplitude criteria would not lead to a positive diagnosis unless accompanied by some other abnormality. These criteria are designed with primary emphasis on avoiding false positive diagnoses. The incidence of false positives at a level of 4 points is about 15 percent, at 5 points about 5 percent. In the clinical setting most false positive diagnoses occur in patients who have lost a great deal of body weight. Many have neoplastic diseases. False negative diagnoses are also seen in certain settings, such as pleural and pericardial fluid, and old myocardial infarction.

The most useful single criterion for the diagnosis of left ventricular hypertrophy by the vectorcardiogram is an increased amplitude of the midforces of the loop. There are differences in the configuration of the loop in various types of hypertrophy. With a volume overload there is an increase in all portions of the loop proportionately. This produces large initial and terminal forces as well as large midforces. In pressure overload, the QRS loop becomes distorted at an early stage, and assumes a figure-of-eight configuration in the horizontal plane. These features can also be recognized in the electrocardiogram. Volume overload is characterized by large Q and S waves, in addition to large R waves, in the left precordial leads. Pressure overload is likely to cause the Q and S waves to become small and to produce slurring of the QRS complex and an increased intrinsicoid deflection time in the left precordial leads. These differences are most useful in the child or in the young adult. In time, the electrocardiographic findings with both types of hypertrophy come to resemble that described under pressure overload, but this is a late development in volume overload. The S-T-T changes of left ventricular "strain" also appear at an early point in the course of pressure overload and at a later point in the course of volume overload.

Right Ventricular Hypertrophy

The criteria of Milnor are the most useful in the empirical diagnosis of right ventricular hypertrophy (they can be applied when the QRS duration is less than 0.12 sec):

1. Right axis deviation of more than + 110°
2. An R or R' wave in V_1 of 5 mm or greater with an R/S ratio in V_1 of 1.0 or greater

If the above criteria are used, one should be aware that these are relatively insensitive criteria and that many cases of known right hypertrophy will not be detected.

The vectorcardiogram has been of considerable help in the diagnosis of right ventricular hypertrophy. Again the sequence of development of abnormalities is different in volume and pressure overload of the right ventricle. Volume overload is likely to be associated with incomplete or complete right bundle branch block, with the initial and midforces in a normal direction and the terminal forces to the right and anteriorly. Pressure overload is more likely to cause the whole loop to rotate anteriorly.

Another type abnormal loop which is seen in right ventricular hypertrophy is an exaggerated form of the normal S_1, S_2, S_3 type of loop, described previously. In the adult, this type of loop is often seen in pulmonary disease, in mitral stenosis, and in the cardiopulmonary syndrome seen in extreme obesity. This loop abnormality differs from the normal S_1, S_2, S_3 loop in that it is broad, open, and clockwise in the frontal plane, and the terminal posterior forces are larger than the midforces of the loop in the horizontal plane.

Ventricular Ischemia, Injury, and Infarction

Ventricular ischemia causes the T vector to shift in a direction away from the region of ischemia. This is presumed to be related to a change in the sequence of repolarization in the layers of the ventricular wall in the ischemic area. Anterior wall ischemia causes the T vector to move to a posterior position, producing negative T waves over the anterior precordial leads. Lateral wall ischemia causes the T vector to shift to the right, producing T waves which are inverted in leads I and aVL. Posterior wall ischemia causes an anterior shift in the direction of the T vector producing very tall T waves over the right precordial leads and usually T-wave inversion in V_5 and V_6.

Myocardial injury produces a shift in the S-T segment of the electrocardiogram. In epicardial injury, the direction of the S-T-segment shift is such that the vector representing the S-T segment is directed toward the area of injury. With subendocardial injury, the direction of the S-T-segment vector is away from the left ventricular area, toward the right shoulder and anteriorly. The direction of the S-T-segment vector in subendocardial injury is such that S-T-segment depression is seen in the bipolar limb leads, maximal in lead II, and in precordial leads V_5 and V_6. In epicardial injury the direction of the S-T-segment shift in any lead depends on the location of the epicardial injury and the relation of this location to the axis of the various leads.

In anterior wall injury, the S-T-segment vector is directed anteriorly; therefore, the S-T segment is elevated in the precordial leads. In inferior (diaphragmatic surface) injury, the S-T vector is directed inferiorly, producing S-T elevation in leads II, III, and aVF.

The characteristic feature of the electrocardiogram in myocardial infarction is a distortion of the initial portion of the QRS loop in a direction away from the region of the infarct. Thus an anterior infarct causes the initial forces to move posteriorly, producing Q waves in the anterior precordial leads. An anterolateral infarct causes the initial forces to move to the right and poste-

riorly, producing Q waves in lead I, lead aVL, and in the left precordial leads. An infarct in the inferior or diaphragmatic region causes the initial forces to move superiorly, causing Q waves in leads II, III, and aVF. It should be emphasized that these distortions, which have been noted to cause Q waves in the above examples, produce an exaggeration of the R wave in leads on the opposite side of the chest. An infarct on the posterior surface of the left ventricle dramatically underlines this point. Such an infarct produces an anterior distortion of the initial loop, producing prolongation and accentuation of the R wave in the right precordial leads.

The age of a myocardial infarct is judged from the appearance of the accompanying injury and ischemia. The initial QRS deformity, which appears within minutes after the insult, persists indefinitely; therefore, it is of little value in estimating age. The S-T-segment shift of myocardial injury is a constant accompaniment of an infarct, which appears with the initial QRS deformity, and disappears over a period of 4 to 6 weeks. The T-vector shift is also a constant finding with an infarct, but its onset is often delayed for 12 to 24 hr following the insult. A QRS deformity, with striking S-T changes, but with a normal T-vector direction would be judged to be a very early infarct, probably less than 24 hr old. An infarct deformity of the QRS complex with S-T-segment shift and a T-vector direction away from the infarct (in the same direction as the abnormal initial forces) would be judged to be over 24 hr old, but less than 1½ months old.

As implied above, there are an infinite variety of locations of myocardial infarcts, and an infinite variety of electrocardiographic presentations. The recognition of initial QRS deformity is usually the key to the diagnosis. The presence of Q waves in the precordial leads is such a departure from the usual configuration that it is easily detected. The recognition of the superior and anterior distortion of the initial QRS loop in diaphragmatic and posterior infarction is much more difficult, since it requires a quantitative judgment as to whether or not the record in question differs from the "normal" tracing which may also have Q waves in leads II, III, and aVF. The abnormal initial forces usually are best detected by a duration of 0.04 sec, or more. The amplitude of these forces (as measured from the depth of the Q wave, etc.) is much less reliable. The presence of accompanying S-T and T changes adds a great deal of reliability to the diagnosis of infarction.

Ventricular Conduction Disturbances

The characteristic alteration produced by the "classic" bundle branch blocks is prolongation of the QRS interval. In left bundle branch block, the QRS interval is usually 0.12 sec, or greater, because of the greater time required for spread of depolarization into the blocked left side. The earliest forces of depolarization are altered in left bundle branch block so that depolarization begins on the right, and the earliest forces are from right to left. These early forces are seen to be anteriorly directed, though the anterior component is of brief duration (0.01 sec). This anterior component is probably contributed by the early depolarization of the anterior apical region of the right ventricle. The direction of septal activation is also altered in left bundle branch block. Instead of a double envelopment from both sides, activation proceeds from right to left. This, plus the "tilt" of the septum probably accounts for the posterior direction of the forces immediately following the brief anterior forces mentioned above. These forces also have a direction to the left. After these sharply posterior forces, the forces remain to the left, but are seen to be delayed and slurred in the electrocardiogram. These forces may represent the end of the septal phase of depolarization and the beginning of depolarization of the free wall of the left ventricle. In the loop, this phase is seen as the period of maximal slowing of the loop. The slurring may be a result of an oblique spread of the front of activation from the septum into the free wall, and an epicardial to endocardial spread.

The recognition of prolongation of the QRS interval to 0.12 sec or more, leftward spread of activation (no Q wave in leads I and V_6), and leftward and posterior orientation of mid- and late forces with slurring makes the diagnosis of left bundle branch block in most cases. It is said that the diagnosis of myocardial infarction is not possible in the presence of left bundle branch block. This is generally true, but certain findings are highly suggestive. The finding of a Q wave in leads I and V_6 in the face of left bundle branch block usually signals a clockwise rotation of the initial forces in the horizontal loop, usually related to a lateral infarct. The absence of the brief anterior forces, usually recognized as Q-S complex in V_1 and V_2, and as a totally posterior horizontal plane QRS loop in the vectorcardiogram, generally is related to an anterior infarct. The presence of atypical S-T and T-wave changes should also alert one to the possibility of infarction. The S-T and T waves with left bundle branch block should be directed away from the major terminal QRS force. An S-T segment in the same direction as the terminal QRS may be due to a current of injury.

Right bundle branch block is also associated with QRS prolongation, but there is more variability than in left block. The right bundle branch block seen with congenital heart disease in younger individuals may be 0.10 sec in duration, but the right bundle branch block seen in older individuals with coronary artery disease is usually 0.12 sec, or longer.

In right bundle branch block, the initial septal depolarization begins in the normal left midseptal region and spreads from left to right. Thus the initial forces in right bundle branch block are in a normal direction. Following these early anterior forces, depolarization spreads quickly from endocardium to epicardium on the left, producing a leftward and posterior direction of the mid-forces. The terminal forces are those directed toward the blocked right ventricle, and these forces are to the right and anterior in direction.

These anterior terminal forces are generally located at about 180° (+150° to −150°) in the frontal plane. They produce broad, slurred S waves in lead I, lead II, and the lateral precordial leads (V_5 and V_6). These forces are also anterior in direction; thus they project as prominent slurred R′ waves in V_1 and V_2.

The recognition of QRS prolongation, normal initial forces, and terminal slurred forces projecting to the right and anteriorly usually makes the diagnosis of right bundle branch block. The presence of unusually large amplitude of the R′ wave (over 15 mm) and/or the absence of an S wave in V_1 and V_2 generally signals right ventricular hypertrophy in addition. The presence of abnormal initial forces (such as broad Q waves in leads II, III, and aVF) usually signals a previous myocardial infarct. Right bundle branch block plus left axis deviation usually denotes left ventricular disease in addition to the conduction disturbance.

Peri-infarction block is a form of block produced by local delays in depolarization surrounding a myocardial infarct. The original criteria of First, Bayley, and Bedford are the most useful. They consist of an initial force deformity of an infarct, a QRS duration of 0.11 sec, or greater, and an angle of 180° between initial and terminal forces. Grant has more recently observed that left axis deviation may be seen in coronary disease. This type of conduction disturbance is also seen in other forms of diffuse myocardial disease. This nonspecificity with regard to etiology makes it seem unwise to call this electrocardiographic entity peri-infarction block. "Left axis deviation with myocardial disease" is probably the most accurate and useful term in spite of its awkward length. This type of conduction disorder may be present in the absence of QRS prolongation. In its frontal plane presentation, it may be confused with the counterclockwise QRS loop of endocardial cushion defects. In the precordial leads, the endocardial cushion defect is associated with a terminal anterior force, producing an R′ in V_1 and V_2, whereas the "left axis deviation with myocardial disease" is associated with a posterior direction of the terminal forces.

Miscellaneous

Pericarditis produces an S-T-segment vector directed toward the apex, producing S-T-segment elevation in the bipolar limb leads and in V_5 and V_6. In contrast with the changes of myocardial infarction, there is no deformity of the QRS complex. The S-T-segment elevation of pericarditis is also more transient than that of myocardial infarction. It is usually followed by T-wave alterations similar to those of myocardial ischemia.

Drugs are frequent causes of electrocardiographic changes. Digitalis causes a shortening of the Q-T interval and a shift in the S-T segment. The J point is not displaced as much as the later portion of the S-T segment; thus the S-T segment has a sloping contour. Quinidine produces a prolonged Q-T interval, a broad, prolonged T wave, and a large U wave.

Hypokalemia is associated with Q-T prolongation, a broad T wave, and a large U wave, particularly in the precordial leads. Hypocalcemia produces a prolonged Q-T interval, but the T wave is of normal duration. The prolongation is at the expense of the S-T segment. Hypercalcemia produces a short Q-T interval and S-T-segment shift which resembles digitalis effect.

REFERENCES

General

Electrical Events in the Single Cell

Hoffman, B. F., and P. F. Cranefield: "The Electrophysiology of the Heart," New York, McGraw-Hill Book Company, 1960.

Anatomy and Blood Supply of Specialized Pacemaker and Conducting Tissues

James, T. N.: "Anatomy of the Coronary Arteries," New York, Paul B. Hoeber, Inc., 1961.

Origin and Spread of Excitation

Scher, A. M., and A. C. Young: Ventricular Depolarization and the Genesis of the QRS, Ann. N. Y. Acad. Sci., 65:768, 1957.

Distribution of Electrical Forces from the Heart over the Body

Frank, E.: An Accurate, Clinically Practical System for Spatial Vectorcardiography, Circulation, 13:737, 1956.

Abnormalities in P Waves

Morris, J. J., Jr., E. H. Estes, Jr., R. E. Whalen, H. K. Thompson, Jr., and H. D. McIntosh: P-wave Analysis in Valvular Heart Disease, Circulation, 29:242, 1964.

Abnormalities in QRS and T Waves

Ainger, L., and W. R. Skinner: Normal Maturation of Spatial QRS Curve Characteristics in Early Infancy, Am. Heart J., 77:5, 1969.

Blumerschein, S. D., M. S. Spach, J. P. Boineau, R. C. Barr, T. M. Gallie, A. G. Wallace, and P. A. Ebert: Genesis of Body Surface Potentials in Varying Types of Right Ventricular Hypertrophy, Circulation, 28:917, 1968.

Cabrera, E. C., and J. R. Monroy: Systolic and Diastolic Overloading of the Heart: II. Electrocardiographic Data, Am. Heart J., 43:669, 1952.

Carter, W. A., and E. H. Estes, Jr., Electrocardiographic Manifestations of Ventricular Hypertrophy: A Computer Study of ECG-Anatomic Correlations in 319 Cases, Am. Heart J., 68:173, 1964.

Grant, R. P.: Left Axis Deviation, Circulation, 14:233, 1956.

Hugenholtz, P. G., C. E. Forkner, and H. D. Levine: A Clinical Appraisal of the Vectorcardiogram in Myocardial Infarction: II. The Frank System, Circulation, 24:828, 1961.

—— and R. Gamboa: Effect of Chronically Increased Ventricular Pressure on Electrical Forces of the Heart, Circulation, 30:511, 1964.

Sutton, R., and M. Davis: The Conduction System in Acute Myocardial Infarction Complicated by Heart Block, Circulation, 28:987, 1968.

Approach to Interpretation of the Electrocardiogram

Grant, R. P.: "Clinical Electrocardiography: The Spatial Vector Approach," New York, McGraw-Hill Book Company, 1957.

Simonson, E.: "Differentiation between Normal and Abnormal Electrocardiography," St. Louis, The C. V. Mosby Company, 1961.

Vectorcardiogram and Its Relationship to the Electrocardiogram

Massie, E., and T. J. Walsh: "Clinical Vectorcardiography," Chicago, The Year Book Medical Publishers, Inc., 1960.

261 INDIRECT METHODS OF EXAMINATION OF THE HEART

John Ross, Jr.

The indirect methods for examination of the heart include special diagnostic approaches which do not involve insertion of a cardiac catheter or injection of radiographic contrast medium into the circulation. These indirect techniques, which may be of great assistance in the evaluation of the status of the cardiac patient, include electrocardiography (Chap. 260), roentgenography, phonocardiography and external recordings of pulse wave forms, special techniques such as echocardiography, as well as certain bedside methods. The frequent and appropriate application of these indirect approaches will not only heighten the physician's clinical acumen, but often will provide important anatomic and functional information that cannot be gained on physical examination alone. Moreover, adequate interpretation of the data obtained with these methods may permit the physician to postpone, or sometimes to avoid, the necessity for the direct methods of study—cardiac catheterization and angiography (Chap. 262).

ROENTGENOGRAPHY

Roentgenographic examination of the heart and lungs is one of the most valuable indirect tools available to the physician. In some instances, standard 6-ft posteroanterior and lateral chest films may provide adequate information, but in most cardiac patients overpenetrated frontal, lateral, and oblique views obtained when the esophagus is filled with barium paste are essential for visualization of specific regions of the heart. The appreciation of selective alterations in cardiac chamber and blood vessel size is based on the varying degrees of radiopacity offered by adjacent tissues of different densities. Thus, the air-filled lungs and bronchi contrast sharply with the blood-filled cardiac chambers, pulmonary arteries, and pulmonary veins.

The posteroanterior projection is particularly useful for detecting enlargement of the aorta, right atrium, left ventricle, and left atrium (Fig. 261-1A). Enlargement of the left ventricle often causes convexity of the

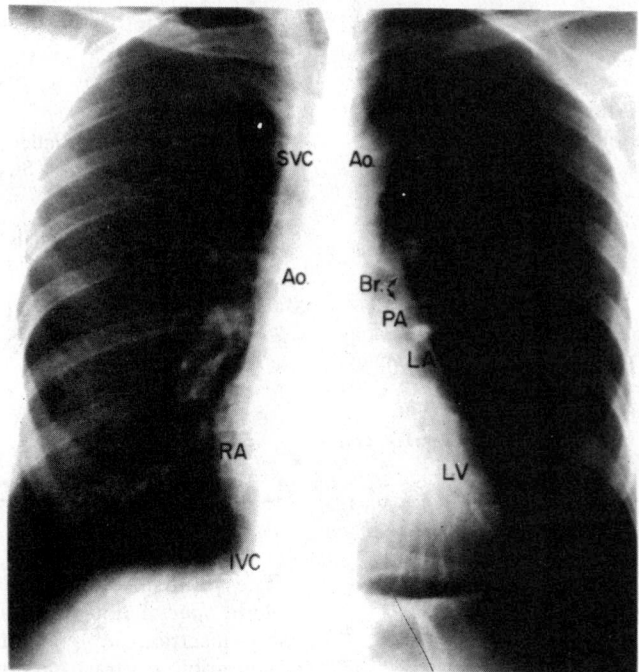

A. PA view

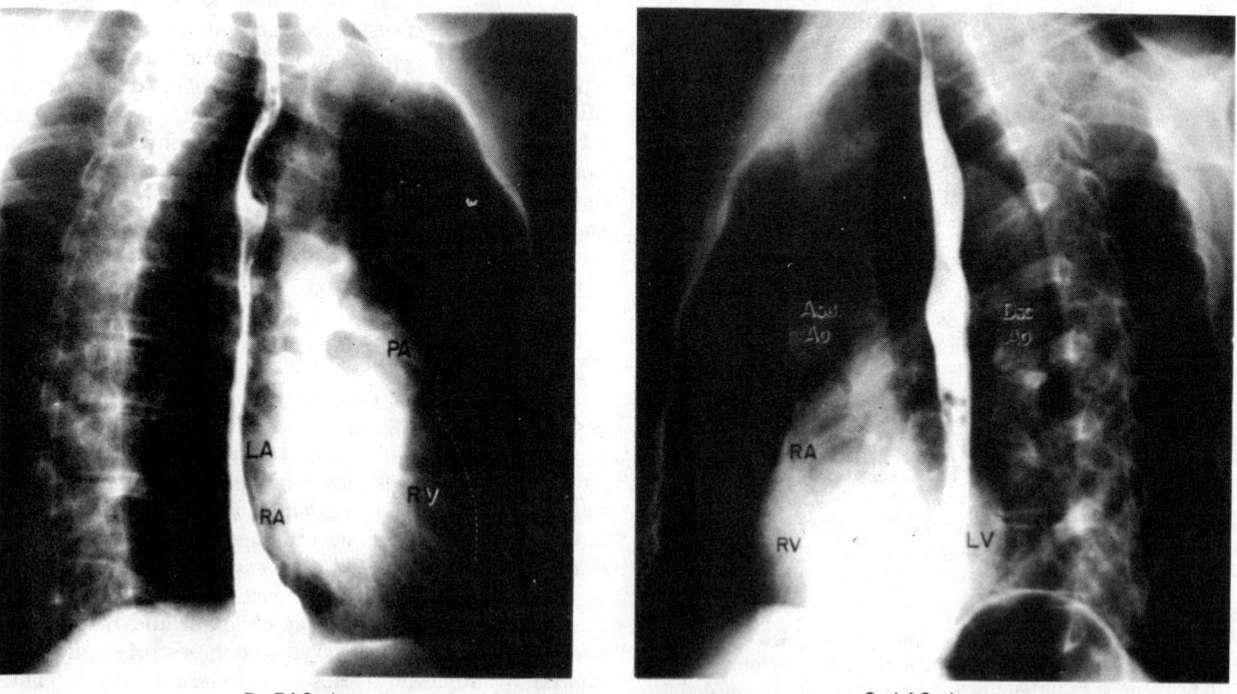

B. RAO view   C. LAO view

Fig. 261-1. Frontal projection (posteroanterior, *PA* view), right anterior oblique projection (*RAO*), and left anterior oblique projection (*LAO*) in the heart in a middle-aged woman with coronary heart disease and minimal enlargement of the left ventricle. *SVC*, superior vena cava; *AO*, aorta; *BR*, left mainstem bronchus; *RA*, right atrium; *IVC*, inferior vena cava; *PA*, pulmonary artery segment; *LA*, left atrium; *LV*, left ventricle; *RV*, right ventricle.

left cardiac border, and the cardiac apex is displaced downward, below the level of the diaphragm. The right ventricle has no representation on the cardiac silhouette in the frontal projection, but enlargement of this chamber may result in tipping upward of the cardiac apex. Left atrial enlargement produces displacement of the adjacent barium-filled esophagus and the left mainstem bronchus; abnormal elevation of this bronchus in the frontal view is present when the angle formed by the bronchus and the vertically positioned trachea exceeds 45°. In the frontal projection, an enlarged left atrium also may produce a round "double density" in the center of the cardiac silhouette.

In the right anterior oblique (RAO) projection, the patient is rotated so that the right axilla faces the x-ray film, the thorax being positioned at an angle of 45°. In this veiw, the anterior margin of the cardiac silhouette is formed by the aorta, the pulmonary artery, and the right ventricle (Fig. 261-1B), and the barium-filled esophagus courses directly adjacent to the left atrium. Therefore, this projection is of particular value for detecting compression or posterior displacement of the esophagus by an enlarged left atrium.

In the left anterior oblique (LAO) projection, the patient is rotated so that the left axilla faces the x-ray film. In this projection, the posterior aspect of the left ventricle normally clears the spine with the patient rotated to an angle of 60° or less, relative to the plane of the film. When the left ventricle is enlarged, it overlaps the spine when the patient is rotated more than 60° from the posteroanterior position, but it should be appreciated that marked right ventricular enlargement alone can cause posterior displacement of the left ventricle. This view also allows detection of an enlarged right atrium or right ventricle, which cause bulging of the anterior border of the heart. Both the ascending and descending aorta can usually be visualized, and in the presence of an aortic coarctation a characteristic "reverse 3" sign may be seen. The upper component of the 3 is formed by the anterior wall of the dilated aorta just above the coarctation, and the lower component by the poststenotic dilatation below the site of obstruction.

The dimensions of the cardiac silhouette relative to the bony thorax can be measured directly from the standard 6-ft chest roentgenogram. The measurement most commonly made is the cardiothoracic ratio, which is obtained by dividing the transverse diameter of the heart (defined as the distance from the outermost point of the right cardiac border to the midsternal line, plus the distance from the outermost point of the left cardiac border to the midsternal line) by the internal diameter of the thorax at its widest point above the diaphragm. Although the cardiothoracic ratio has limitations, being dependent on the configuration of the chest, generally it is less than 0.5 in normal subjects.

Image-intensification fluoroscopy may be employed to define further the size and the pulsations of the cardiac chambers and great vessels. It is also useful for detecting areas of calcification within the cardiac valves, coronary arteries, or pericardium. The characteristic motions of the cardiac valves observed on fluoroscopy aid considerably in identifying the site of a calcification. Often, this information is of great importance in confirming the presence of a suspected valvular lesion, or in affecting the choice of an open or closed surgical procedure upon the valve in question.

THE PULMONARY VASCULATURE. The size of the central and peripheral pulmonary blood vessels can be evaluated from the standard chest roentgenogram. The estimation of whether the pulmonary vascularity is normal, increased, or diminished may be of great diagnostic importance, particularly in patients suspected of having congenital heart disease. In addition, selective engorgement of the pulmonary veins may be observed when there is left atrial hypertension, or a disproportion between the size of the central and peripheral pulmonary arteries (enlarged main vessels that taper sharply) may suggest the presence of an elevated pulmonary vascular resistance.

An unusually prominent pulmonary vascular pattern is observed in lesions associated with a left-to-right shunt of blood. Usually, the main pulmonary artery segment is enlarged, and examination of the heart for specific chamber enlargement often aids in determining the location of the shunt. Thus, in patients with atrial septal defect there is right ventricular enlargement and the left atrium is small, because the defect allows decompression of that chamber. In contrast, in patients with ventricular septal defect, the left atrium often is enlarged and the volume overload on the left side of the heart also causes enlargement of the left ventricle. When the shunt is through a patent ductus arteriosus, the left atrium and left ventricle may be enlarged and, in addition, the aorta is prominent and exhibits increased pulsations.

A selective increase in the caliber of the pulmonary veins can be observed with lesions that produce left atrial hypertension, such as mitral stenosis or cor triatriatum. In addition, the normal pattern in the upright subject of a more prominent vascular pattern at the lung bases than at the apices may be reversed in patients with mitral stenosis, leading to more prominent vascularity in the upper lobes. Chronic pulmonary venous engorgement also may be associated with interstitial edema or fibrosis in the interlobular septa; the Kerley "B" lines, horizontal markings about 1 cm in length appearing above the diaphragm near the rib cage, represent such edema or fibrosis. Pulmonary edema (fluid within the alveoli) may be secondary to acute left atrial hypertension or left ventricular failure and is characterized by bilateral, confluent "butterfly" densities in the central lung fields.

Decreased pulmonary vascularity is observed most commonly with lesions that cause both obstruction to right ventricular outflow (pulmonic stenosis) and right-to-left shunting of blood. A reduction in pulmonary blood flow is present, and therefore the caliber of the pulmonary arteries and veins is reduced; the left atrium also may be small. Thus, in patients with tetralogy of Fallot, there is right ventricular enlargement, the main pulmonary artery segment is small, and the pulmonary vascularity is diminished. However, in patients with pure valvular pulmonic stenosis, there is poststenotic dilatation of the pulmonary artery and since the cardiac output usually is normal, the pulmonary vascularity appears normal unless the stenosis is extremely severe or unless there is an associated patent foramen ovale with right-to-left shunting of blood.

SPECIAL ROENTGENOGRAPHIC TECHNIQUES. Special roentgenographic methods sometimes are useful in resolving specific diagnostic problems. Cardiac tomography (or sectional radiography) may be helpful in identifying the site of specific vascular shadows and in localizing areas of calcification. Electrokymography is a special technique in which x-ray beams traversing the chest strike a small fluorescent screen, the light from which, in turn, strikes a photomultiplier tube. Movement of the cardiac border affects the intensity of the x-ray beams, and an analog signal can be recorded that is proportional to the cardiac excursions; the wave form so produced may reveal an abnormal pattern of cardiac motion, such as paradoxic expansion of the ventricle caused by an aneurism of its wall. Other special roentgenographic methods include angiography (Chap. 262) and the use of radioisotopes. The intravenous injection of macroaggregated ^{131}I-labeled albumin, with subsequent scanning of the lung fields for underperfused areas, is valuable in the detection of pulmonary emboli (Chap. 281). Another application of this approach is to scan the cardiac silhouette after intravenous injection of the radioisotope. The area of the cardiac silhouette occupied by the labeled intracardiac blood pool is then compared with the cardiac silhouette on the chest roentgenogram, and the presence or absence of a pericardial effusion often can be ascertained.

PHONOCARDIOGRAPHY

The phonocardiogram provides a graphic display of heart sounds and murmurs. The frequent use of this tool will enhance considerably the value of the auscultatory events available to the physician in his assessment of the nature and severity of cardiac disease. The modern phonocardiograph is capable of recording sounds in a manner that resembles their detection by the human ear. In order to simulate the relative insensitivity of the human ear to low-frequency vibrations and its great sensitivity to high-frequency signals, so-called logarithmic or high-frequency recordings are used to provide relatively greater amplification of high-frequency components. Filters also are employed to allow selective passage of low- and high-frequency sounds, perhaps the most satisfactory system consisting of a series of band-pass filters which encompass the frequency fields from 15 to 1,000 cps (cycles per second). The transducer of the phonocardiograph consists of a crystal (piezoelectric) microphone applied directly to the skin, or attached indirectly through an air-coupled diaphragm or bell. The crystals within the microphone alter their electrical properties when stressed by sound pressure waves, and the resulting electrical signal is amplified and recorded on a high-frequency oscillograph.

The phonocardiogram is useful for determining the configuration and frequency composition of individual cardiac murmurs (see Chap. 259), but perhaps its most important application is in the precise timing of cardiac sounds and murmurs. Thus, it allows clear definition of a sequence of events, such as the variation in the splitting of the second heart sound which occurs during respiration, or the differentiation of separate systolic and diastolic murmurs from a continuous murmur which continues and may be intensified throughout late systole and early diastole. The phonocardiogram also may provide some quantitative information of significance, such as the precise duration of the interval between the aortic closure sound and the opening snap in patients with mitral stenosis, an interval that correlates inversely with the atrioventricular pressure gradient (Chap. 270).

The electrocardiogram provides the basic physiologic variable which is recorded simultaneously with the phonocardiogram to provide a reference signal. The P wave of the electrocardiogram is valuable for timing atrial gallop sounds, and the QRS complex provides a reference for identifying the first heart sound. Other externally recorded variables that are extremely helpful for timing auscultatory events are the jugular phlebogram, the carotid pulse wave, and the apexcardiogram (Figs. 261-2 and 261-4).

In order to appreciate the significance of alterations in the timing of heart sounds which occur in various disease states and the relation that these sounds bear to external pulse tracings, it is essential to understand the normal temporal relations between the electrical and mechanical events of the cardiac cycle (Fig. 261-2). The normal cycle begins with the P wave of the electrocardiogram, which is followed by right atrial contraction, the initial mechanical event. Left atrial contraction occurs shortly thereafter. The QRS complex ensues, initiating the onset of isovolumetric left ventricular contraction 0.04 to 0.06 sec after the onset of the QRS complex. Right ventricular contraction then starts, and a brief period of isometric right ventricular contraction is followed by the onset of right ventricular ejection. The onset of left ventricular ejection is the next event, and since the duration of ejection is shorter on the left side than on the right, closure of the aortic valve precedes pulmonic valve closure. Isometric relaxation of the ventricles terminates earlier on the right side than on the left (at the peak of the atrial v wave). A convenient way to remember this normal sequence of mechanical events in the two ventricles (onset of isometric contraction, onset of ejection, end of ejection, end of isometric relaxation) is to recall that isometric phases of left ventricular contraction and relaxation completely encompass those of the right ventricle (Fig. 261-2).

The jugular venous pulse tracing is obtained by applying a cup transducer over the jugular bulb with slight suction; an inner chamber transmits the pressure changes induced by the venous pulsations to a crystal microphone. The nomenclature of the venous waves is the same as that employed in describing intraatrial pressure pulse contours recorded directly (Fig. 261-3; see also Chap.

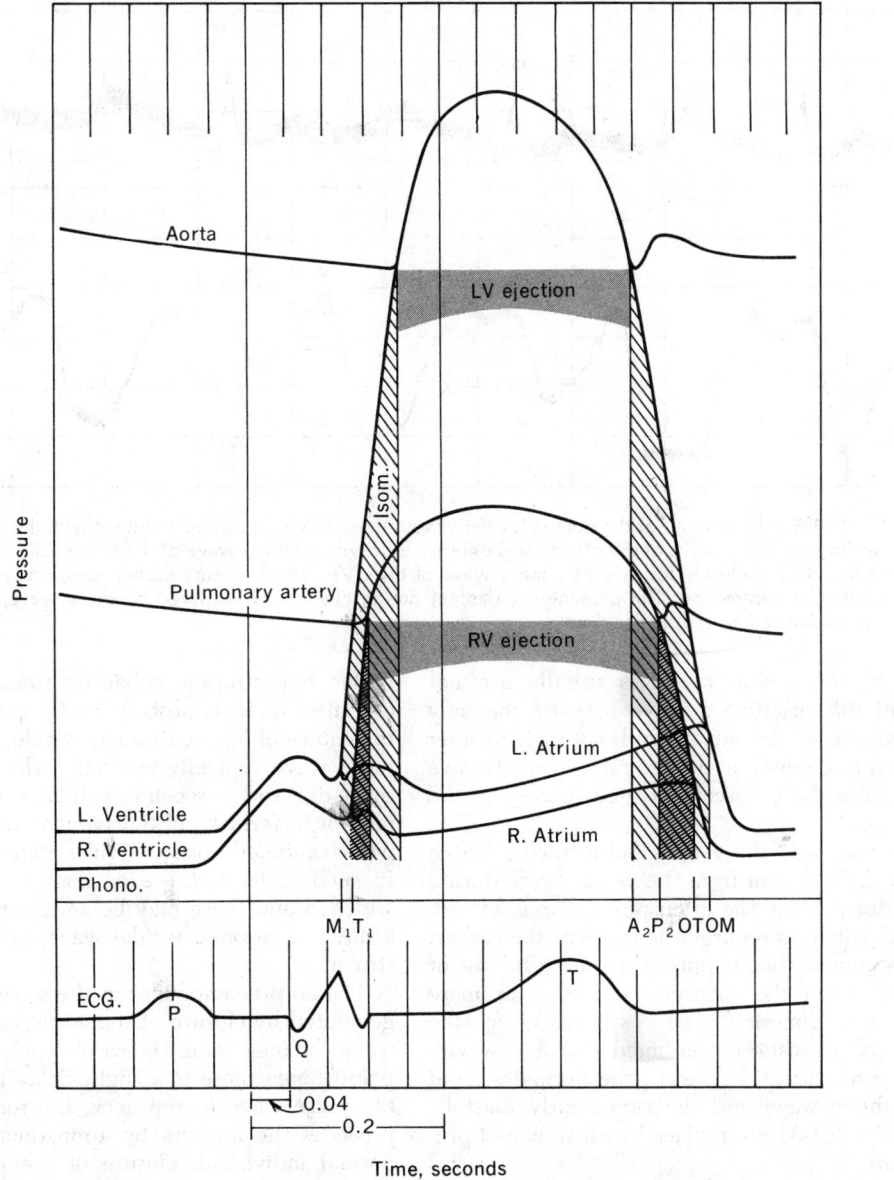

Fig. 261-2. Diagrammatic representation of pressure tracings recorded within the left and right ventricles correlated with the ECG and the phonocardiogram (*Phono*). The diagonal cross-hatched areas labeled *ISOM* represent the isometric phases of left ventricular contraction; isometric right ventricular contraction is represented by the double cross-hatching. M_1 and T_1, sounds produced by closure of the mitral and tricuspid valves, respectively; A_2 and P_2, sounds produced by the closure of the aortic and pulmonic valves; *OT* and *OM*, sounds produced by opening of the tricuspid and mitral valves, respectively.

262). Although some difficulty may be introduced by a variable delay in transmission of the venous waves to the neck (this delay generally averages 0.02 sec), the venous tracing may be extremely helpful in studying the dynamics of the right side of the heart.

The *a* wave in the jugular venous pulse, caused by right atrial contraction, normally is the dominant positive wave (Fig. 261-3). It may be enlarged when there is increased resistance to right atrial ejection, as in tricuspid stenosis, or when the right ventricular wall is thickened

and made relatively noncompliant by right ventricular hypertrophy or fibrosis. In the latter situation, an atrial gallop, or fourth heart sound, often accompanies the prominent *a* wave. In the presence of atrioventricular dissociation, atrial contraction against a closed tricuspid valve may produce giant *a* waves. The *x* descent follows the *c* wave and is associated with downward displacement of the ventricles during systole; it is responsible for the normal "systolic collapse" of the venous pulse. In patients with elevated venous pressure due to constric-

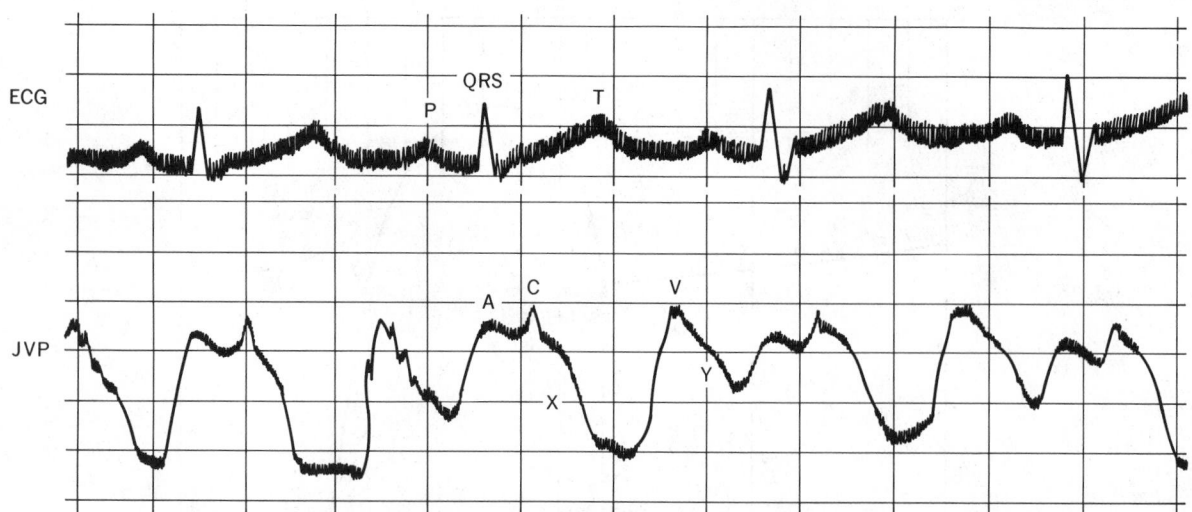

Fig. 261-3. The contour of the normal jugular venous pulse (JVP) recorded together with the electro-cardiogram. The P wave of the electrocardiogram is followed by the *a* wave of JVP. The QRS complex of the ECG is closely followed by the *c* wave of the JVP, which occurs during isovolumetric right ventricular contraction. The prominent *x* descent during ejection is followed by the *v* wave, which occurs during late ventricular systole.

tive pericarditis, the *a* and *v* waves usually are not prominent, and this negative *x* wave may be the only significant excursion of the venous pulse wave; in other patients with this disease, a prominent negative wave may occur between the *y* descent of the *v* wave and the rapid-filling wave.

The normal *v* wave in the venous pulse tracing is due to filling of the right atrium from the venae cavae during ventricular systole, when the tricuspid valve is closed. In patients with tricuspid regurgitation, one of the earliest changes in the jugular venous pulse wave may be loss of the *x* descent. When the regurgitation becomes more marked, there is an abnormally large systolic wave (the "*s*" wave), which consists of combined *c* and *v* waves. In the presence of tricuspid stenosis, the normally rapid *y* descent of the *v* wave and the rapid early diastolic filling wave (Fig. 261-3) are replaced by a slow and pro-longed *y* descent.

The indirect carotid arterial pulse wave is recorded with a transducer similar to that employed for obtaining the jugular venous tracing. This signal provides an important means of analyzing the carotid pulse contour and for timing the sounds of aortic and pulmonic valve closure (Fig. 261-4A). Normally, the ascending limb of the systolic carotid wave is steeper than the descending limb; the upstroke time from onset to peak averages 100 msec (range, 60 to 140 msec),[1] and the normal duration of ejection averages 300 msec (range, 260 to 310 msec).[1] In patients with valvular aortic stenosis, the upstroke is prolonged and interrupted by a prominent anacrotic shoulder, or notch, and with severe degrees of stenosis the ejection time is prolonged as well (Chap. 270). The carotid pulse contour in valvular aortic stenosis differs strikingly from that in patients with idio-

[1] Corrected for heart rate by dividing the measured interval by the square root of the cycle length in seconds.

pathic hypertrophic subaortic stenosis (Chap. 273). In the latter disease, obstruction to ejection develops during the course of left ventricular systole, and consequently the pulse wave typically exhibits a sharp upstroke, followed by a dip and a secondary tidal wave. Another form of bifid or bisferiens pulse wave may be observed in patients with combined aortic valvular stenosis and regurgitation. In such patients, the excursions of the carotid wave are widened and there may be an anacrotic notch, as well as a dip and secondary tidal wave, following the initial up-stroke.

The aortic component of the second heart sound (A_2), generated by closure of the aortic valve, can be identified using the incisura of the carotid pulse wave as a reference point. Since there is a slight delay in the transmission of the pulse wave to the neck, the recording of this sound precedes the incisura by approximately 0.02 sec. In the normal individual, closure of the pulmonic valve (P_2) always follows A_2 (Fig. 261-2) (Chap. 259). Although this interval is narrow during expiration (0.02 sec) and the splitting may be inaudible, it may be recorded on the phonocardiogram (Fig. 261-4A). The widening of the interval between A_2 and P_2 during inspiration, which results primarily from a transient increase in right ventric-ular stroke volume, also can be identified (Fig. 261-4A). In patients with atrial septal defect, there is wide, fixed splitting of the second heart sound during the respira-tory cycle (Chaps. 259 and 268). The pulmonic com-ponent of the second heart sound also is delayed in right bundle branch block, but P_2 moves normally rela-tive to A_2 during respiration. In patients with pulmonic stenosis, P_2 is soft and delayed by prolonged right ventric-ular ejection. When pulmonic stenosis is severe, P_2 may not be audible, but often it can be recorded as a low-frequency vibration on the phonocardiogram (Chap. 268).

Lesions that result in prolongation of left ventricular ejection may cause reversal of the normal sequence of aortic and pulmonic valve closure, termed paradoxic splitting of the second heart sound (see Chap. 259). That A_2 follows P_2 may be verified on the phonocardiogram using the carotid pulse tracing. Since the normal increase in right ventricular stroke volume occurs during inspiration, P_2 is delayed normally, and therefore the interval between A_2 and P_2 narrows or disappears.

Analysis of the carotid pulse wave also has been employed for indirectly assessing the function of the left ventricle. Thus, the ejection time, when corrected for

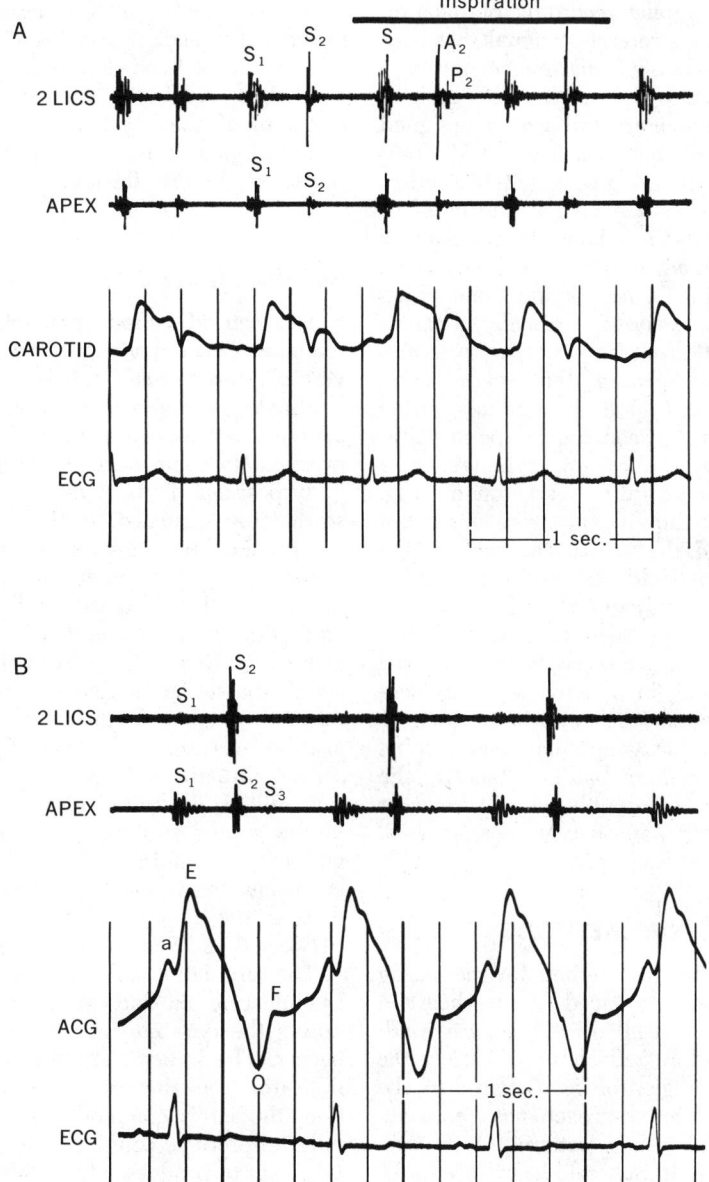

Fig. 261-4. *Panel A.* The indirect carotid pulse wave tracing exhibits two normal systolic waves, the initial percussion wave followed by a tidal wave. The incisura is then followed by the dicrotic wave. The phonocardiogram is recorded at the second left intercostal space (2LICS) and the apex, and it demonstrates the normal increase in the interval between the aortic second sound (A_2) and the pulmonic second sound (P_2) which occurs during inspiration. The diminished intensity of P_2 at the apex also may be noted.

Panel B. The apexcardiogram (ACG) in a patient having a third heart sound (S_3). The a wave of the apex cardiogram is coincident with atrial contraction, the E point shortly follows the onset of the first heart sound and coincides approximately with the onset of left ventricular ejection, and the O point corresponds to the time of opening of the mitral valve at the end if isometric ventricular relaxation. The end of the rapid-filling wave in diastole (the F point) is coincident with the third heart sound and is followed by the phase of slow ventricular filling.

heart rate, has been shown to have a significant correlation with the stroke volume measured by an independent method. In addition, the interval between the first and second heart sounds, minus the ejection time, as determined from the carotid pulse wave, provides an indirect measure of the isometric contraction period of the left ventricle.

The apexcardiogram, a graphic recording of the precordial movements, provides a reference signal that is of particular value in the analysis of diastolic events and heart sounds. The apexcardiogram is recorded using a bell-type, linear crystal microphone and a filter designed to pass only low frequencies (between 0.1 and 20 cps). The *o* point on the apexicardiogram occurs at the end of isometric left ventricular relaxation and at the onset of ventricular filling (Fig. 261-4*B*). Thus, it corresponds closely in time to the opening of the mitral valve and is useful as a reference point for identifying the opening snap in patients with mitral stenosis. Normally, a rapid-filling wave of about 0.08 sec follows the *o* point. In the presence of mitral stenosis this event is replaced by a slow-filling wave. In patients with myocardial failure, mitral regurgitation, or constrictive pericarditis, an exaggerated rapid-filling wave may terminate in a ventricular diastolic gallop or third heart sound (Fig. 261-4*B*). This sound presumably results from tensing of the chordae tendineae, and the ventricular wall, as the limit of ventricular filling, is suddenly reached.

The *a* wave of the apexcardiogram is absent in patients with atrial fibrillation and in mitral stenosis. This wave may be augmented and accompanied by an atrial gallop, or fourth heart sound, in patients with left ventricular failure and in the presence of lesions such as aortic stenosis that produce left ventricular hypertrophy. In patients with hypertrophic subaortic stenosis, the apexcardiogram often exhibits a double systolic wave, or even a triple contour if the *a* wave is prominent as well.

OTHER INDIRECT GRAPHIC METHODS

KINETOCARDIOGRAPHY. In this method for measuring the movements of the chest produced by the heart, a directly coupled rather than air-filled transducer is used; the kinetocardiogram therefore reflects more closely the absolute displacement of a region of heart than does the standard apexcardiogram. This approach has been employed in the analysis of abnormal patterns of contraction, such as those occurring in ischemic heart disease.

THE BALLISTOCARDIOGRAM. In this technique, a recording is made of small movements of the body induced by the mass movements of blood which accompany the heartbeat. Calibration of the ballistocardiographic table, together with knowledge of body mass, then allows calculation of the ballistic forces on the body. Normal and abnormal ballistocardiographic wave form patterns have been described, but considerable controversy exists as to whether these patterns primarily reflect abnormalities in ventricular ejection, or whether they are related to the physical properties of the vascular bed.

ULTRASONIC CARDIOGRAPHY. This is a means of recording the echoes produced when high-frequency (ultrasound) waves strike the boundaries between tissues of different densities (and hence different coefficients of sound absorption). An echo is produced when ultrasonic waves traverse blood-tissue, fluid-tissue or air-tissue interfaces, and several applications of ultrasonic cardiography have been reported. For example, the motion of the mitral valve leaflets has been recorded, and pericardial effusions have been detected. In the latter circumstance, two echoes can be obtained from the region of the posterior wall of the heart, one from the cardiac wall itself and the other from the pericardium, which is displaced posteriorly by the effusion.

BEDSIDE METHODS

The central venous pressure can be measured with reasonable accuracy simply by placing a centimeter ruler vertically on the sternum and directing a straight edge, held at right angles to the ruler, toward the neck. In the average patient, the center of the right atrium lies approximately 5 cm from the angle of Louis, regardless of body position. Thus, if the reclining patient is positioned so that the excursions of the top of the blood column in the jugular veins are clearly visible, the central venous pressure can be estimated by measuring the vertical distance that these excursions lie above the sternal angle and adding this value to the distance from the right atrium. In the normal patient, the height of the excursions should be no more than 3 cm above the sternal angle (3 cm + 5 cm = 8 cm blood). The venous pressure can also be measured directly in the antecubital vein by inserting into the vein an 18-gauge needle attached to a saline-filled, calibrated glass tube. The patient is placed in the supine position, with the arm slightly abducted and the antecubital surface positioned approximately 5 cm below the level of the sternum. Under these circumstances, the height of the fluid in the tube should range between 3 and 8 cm in the normal subject.

The circulation time can be estimated at the bedside by injecting an indicator substance intravenously and noting the time interval before a recognizable end point occurs. The interval represents the most rapid transit of indicator from the site of injection to the point of detection, the latter commonly being the lungs (injection of ether to produce cough or odor), the tongue (injection of Decholin to produce a bitter taste), or the earlobe (use of the earlobe oximeter to detect injected indicator dye). Occasional reactions to Decholin have occurred, and therefore this agent should be used with caution, particularly in allergic individuals. The normal arm-to-lung circulation time is 4 to 8 sec, and the normal arm-to-tongue or arm-to-ear circulation time is 10 to 16 sec. The estimation of the circulation time by these techniques can provide a relatively simple means of confirming the presence or absence of congestive heart failure. In the presence of right-sided heart failure, the arm-to-lung circulation time is prolonged, whereas with edema secondary to local venous obstruction, or ascites due to hepatic dysfunction, the arm-to-lung circulation time usually is normal. Dyspnea due to left-sided heart failure may be distinguished from that due to pulmonary disease by a prolonged arm-to-tongue circulation time, and with isolated left-sided heart failure the arm-to-lung circulation time may be normal.

REFERENCES

Roentgenography

Cooley, R. N., and R. D. Sloan: Roentgenology of the Heart and Great Vessels, in "Diagnostic Roentgenology," R. Golden (Ed.), Baltimore, The Williams & Wilkins Company, 1959.

Doyle, A. E., J. F. Goodwin, C. V. Harrison, and R. E. Steiner: Pulmonary Vascular Patterns in Pulmonary Hypertension, Brit. Heart J., 19:353, 1957.

Friedberg, C. K.: Roentgenologic Examination of the Heart, chap. 1 in "Diseases of the Heart," 3d ed., Charles K. Friedberg (Ed.), Philadelphia, W. B. Saunders Company, 1966.

Lester, R. G.: Radiological Concepts in the Evaluation of Heart Disease (I) & (II), Mod. Concepts Cardiovas. Dis., 37:113; 38:7, 1968.

Rosenthal, L.: Detection of Pericardial Effusion by Radioisotope Heart Scanning, Can. Med Assoc. J., 90:447, 1964.

Phonocardiography

Aygen, M. M., and E. Braunwald: The Splitting of the Second Heart Sound in Normal Subjects and in Patients with Congenital Heart Disease, Circulation, 25:328, 1962.

Benchimol, A., and E. G. Dimond: The Normal and Abnormal Apexcardiogram, Am. J. Cardiol., 12:368, 1963.

Hurst, W. J., (Ed.): Symposium: Physical Diagnosis, the Scientific Basis, Circulation, 30:252, 1964.

Segal, B. L. (Ed.): "The Theory and Practice of Auscultation," Philadelphia, F. A. Davis Company, 1964.

Weissler, A. M., W. S. Harris, and C. D. Schoenfeld: Systolic Time Intervals in Heart Failure in Man, Circulation, 37:149, 1968.

Special Graphic Methods

Eddleman, E. E., Jr., K. Willis, T. J. Reeves, and T. R. Hamson: The Kinetocardiogram: II, The Normal Configuration and Amplitude, Circulation, 8:370, 1953.

Hertz, C. Hellmuth: Ultrasonic Engineering in Heart Diagnosis, in Symposium on Echocardiography (Diagnostic Ultrasound), Bernard L. Segal (Ed.), Am. J. Cardiol., 19:6, 1967.

Nickerson, John L.: Circulatory System: Methods, Ballistocardiography, suppl. to vol. II, pp. 222–225, in "Medical Physics," Otto Glasser (Ed.), vol. III, pp. 131–132, Chicago, The Year Book Medical Publishers, Inc., 1960.

Bedside Methods

Ewy, G. A., and F. I. Marcus: Bedside Estimation of the Venous Pressure, Heart Bull., 17:41, 1968.

Knott, D. H., and G. Barlow: The Comparison of Fluorescein and Decholins. Circulation Times, Am. J. Med. Sci., 247:304, 1964.

262 CARDIAC CATHETERIZATION
John Ross, Jr.

In 1929, Werner Forssman described the insertion of a catheter through his own arm vein into the right atrium and proposed that the procedure might prove useful for physiologic studies. A little more than a decade later, André Cournand and his associates introduced the modern era of cardiac catheterization in man by showing that it was possible to advance the catheter with safety further into the right ventricle and pulmonary artery and to perform hemodynamic studies by measuring intracardiac pressures and cardiac output. The technique of angiography also was developed rapidly in the period between 1930 and 1940, as relatively nontoxic opaque organic iodide media were discovered, and their intravascular injection provided definition of a number of congenital and acquired cardiovascular malformations. Since then, techniques for catheterizing the left side of the heart and the coronary arteries, and for selective injection of contrast media into the cardiac chambers, have rapidly advanced knowledge of normal and abnormal cardiac structure and function. By permitting accurate anatomic and functional diagnoses of complex cardiac lesions, these procedures now have placed the selection of patients for surgical treatment on a firm, objective basis.

Important improvements in the design of radiographic equipment accompanied and facilitated these advances in cardiac catheterization methods. Improved x-ray tubes provided short exposure times and, together with apparatus for rapid sequencing of films at rates from 2 to 12 per sec, made it possible to minimize the effects of cardiac motion. However, of most significance was the introduction of image-intensification systems, in which a fluorescent screen is incorporated into a large cathode-ray tube. The light emanating from the screen falls on an adjacent photoemissive layer, which produces electrons in a quantity proportional to the intensity of the x-radiation. The electrons so released are accelerated through the vacuum tube towards the anode at the opposite end, being focused in transit by other electrodes, to strike a small fluorescent screen termed the output phosphor. This process results in an image that is several thousandfold brighter than that seen on a conventional fluoroscopic screen. Its development made possible clear visualization of catheter manipulations within the heart and allowed the expenditure of a much lower x-ray dosage than required with conventional fluoroscopy. In addition, high-speed motion pictures of the output phosphor at 15 to 80 frames per sec combined with injection of contrast medium (cineangiography) have provided understanding of the dynamic behavior of the heart and cardiac valves in a variety of acquired and congenital cardiac disorders.

INDICATIONS FOR CARDIAC CATHETERIZATION AND ANGIOGRAPHY

There are several types of problems for which hemodynamic or angiographic investigations commonly are performed, although other specific indications and contra-indications may exist in the individual patient. These broad areas may be summarized as follows:

1. In patients with acquired valvular heart disease, hemodynamic assessment and angiographic studies often are required to determine whether or not the nature and severity of a mechanical valvular defect render it amenable to surgical treatment. In particular, cardiac catheterization studies may be indicated when both the mitral and aortic valves are involved, or when associated tricuspid valve disease is suspected to be of significance.

2. In patients with congenital heart disease, hemodynamic studies and angiography usually are necessary to characterize the primary defect and to determine whether or not associated lesions are present.

3. In patients with chest pain of undetermined cause, angiographic visualization of the coronary arteries may be indicated, and in patients with known coronary heart disease such studies can determine whether or not operative treatment might be feasible.

4. In patients who have undergone cardiac operations, cardiac catheterization studies may be indicated to evaluate the success of the operation, particularly when residual symptoms are present. Such studies may reveal malfunction of a prosthetic valve or residual disease of the ventricular myocardium.

5. In patients with suspected myocardial disease, cardiac catheterization may be undertaken in an effort to exclude lesions potentially amenable to surgical treatment such as mitral regurgitation, coronary heart disease, constrictive pericarditis, and hypertrophic subaortic stenosis.

6. In patients with evidence of pulmonary hypertension, cardiac catheterization should be performed to search for such lesions as mitral stenosis, left-to-right shunts, multiple pulmonary emboli, or peripheral pulmonic stenosis.

COMPLICATIONS OF CARDIAC CATHETERIZATION

The increasingly widespread application of cardiac catheterization procedures has made it imperative to consider carefully the complications that may ensue. Although a retrospective analysis in 1953 of over 500 studies indicated that the mortality of catheterization of the right side of the heart was only 0.07 percent, the present tendency to perform more extensive and complex procedures and to study patients who are critically ill has called attention to the need for a reappraisal of this risk. Recently, a cooperative prospective study among 16 laboratories was completed on the complications of cardiac catheterization in more than 12,000 procedures. The overall incidence of major complications (including such incidents as cardiac perforation, major arrhythmia, hemorrhage, serious hypotension, infection, vascular thrombosis, as well as death) was 3.6 percent. However, when simple right-sided heart catheterization without angiography was performed, this incidence was considerably lower—1.9 percent. The overall mortality rate was 0.45 percent, but this figure, as well as the incidence of

major complications, was highly dependent on the patient's age and diagnosis. For example, in critically ill infants studied under the age of 60 days, the mortality was 6 percent, whereas it was only 0.05 percent in patients between the ages of five and fourteen years, when most of the procedures were of an elective nature. The mortality rate increased to 0.3 percent in patients aged sixty and over. These figures should be considered whenever a decision concerning the advisability of performing specialized diagnostic procedures is made, and the risks of cardiac catheterization should be weighed carefully in relation to the potential benefits to be derived from an accurate anatomic and functional diagnosis.

GENERAL METHODS OF CARDIAC CATHETERIZATION
Catheterization of the Right Side of the Heart and Angiography

Catheterization of the right side of the heart is now a well-standardized procedure. An antecubital or saphenous vein is isolated, local anesthesia is used, and a long, flexible radiopaque catheter is introduced. Alternatively, the percutaneous approach is employed, in which a needle is positioned in the vessel, a flexible wire passed through the needle, the needle removed, and a tapered-tip catheter advanced over the guide wire. Using fluoroscopic control, the cardiac catheter is guided into the right ventricle, the pulmonary artery, and the pulmonary arterial wedge position. Blood samples may then be obtained and intracardiac pressures and indicator-dilution curves determined sequentially within the chambers of the right side of the heart in the diagnosis of congenital and acquired lesions, as discussed subsequently in this chapter. The course of the cardiac catheter alone may provide a clue to the diagnosis of certain congenital malformations. The catheter may enter an anomalous pulmonary vein or left superior vena cava; it may directly traverse a patent ductus arteriosus or an atrial septal defect; and inability to cross the tricuspid valve may indicate the presence of tricuspid atresia.

Selective injection of radiopaque contrast media at various sites within the right side of the heart also may be performed during cardiac catheterization. The selective injection method accomplishes two major purposes: it allows the delivery of a high concentration of contrast medium adjacent to the area of interest, thereby providing a clear definition of structure, and it often avoids the filling of adjacent structures that may overlie the area under study. For example, with a peripheral venous injection, contrast medium retained in the right atrial appendage may obscure an area of infundibular pulmonic stenosis within the right ventricle. Venous injections are particularly useful, however, in detecting the thickened right atrial wall of constrictive pericarditis and for defining certain congenital lesions, such as Ebstein's malformation of the tricuspid valve and tricuspid atresia. Selective right ventriculography commonly is used in the delineation of congenital cardiac lesions such as pulmonic stenosis and tetralogy of Fallot. Injection into the pulmonary artery can provide adequate visualization of anomalies affecting the pulmonary venous drainage, such as cortriatriatum, and is useful in the detection of thrombi within the left atrium.

Catheterization of the Left Side of the Heart and Angiography

A variety of methods for catheterization of the left side of the heart have been devised, and each has found application under certain circumstances. Currently, the retrograde arterial approach is used most widely for catheterization of the aorta and left ventricle. The catheter usually is inserted via the femoral artery using the percutaneous method, or through a small incision directly into the exposed brachial artery. The transseptal approach often is employed to gain access to the left atrium and left ventricle, particularly when disease of the mitral valve is suspected. With this method, a catheter is inserted via the right saphenous or femoral vein, and its tip is positioned in the right atrium. A long, curved needle is introduced through the catheter and employed to puncture the intact interatrial septum in the region of the fossa ovalis. Commonly, the catheter then is advanced over the needle into the left atrium and ventricle. Other methods of catheterization of the left side of the heart are used somewhat less commonly; with the retrosternal approach, a needle is passed from the jugular fossa through the mediastinum to puncture the aorta, pulmonary artery, and left atrium, and with the anterior percutaneous approach a needle is introduced directly into the left ventricle in the region of the cardiac apex. This procedure sometimes is useful for measuring the left ventricular pressure in patients with valvular aortic stenosis.

Both the retrograde and transseptal approaches permit selective angiography to be accomplished readily. Left ventriculography now is widely employed for detecting and estimating the severity of mitral regurgitation and for the delineation of congenital and acquired lesions affecting the left ventricular outflow tract. Sites of subvalvular, valvular, or supravalvular aortic stenosis may be delineated, and the anatomy of the ventricular septum can be defined. Aortography frequently is used for assessing the severity of aortic regurgitation (Fig. 262-1), for determining the size and location of aortic aneurysms, and for the visualization of less-common malformations such as sinus of Valsalva aneurysm and coronary arteriovenous fistula. Injection into the left atrium has been used to study the movement of the mitral valve, as well as to detect thrombi within that chamber.

Several methods for angiographic visualization of the coronary arteries have been developed. Injection of acetylcholine has been employed to arrest or slow the heart temporarily during contrast injection into the aorta, a balloon has been inflated in the aorta above the site of injection, or injections have been performed through special, coiled catheters positioned within the sinuses of Valsalva. However, the most widely used method is selective coronary arteriography, in which a few milliliters of contrast medium is instilled directly into the coronary ostium while high-speed motion pictures are exposed.

THE MEASUREMENT OF INTRAVASCULAR PRESSURES

The pressures within the great vessels and chambers of the heart ordinarily are measured by means of a catheter-transducer system. The tip of the cardiac catheter is in communication with the transducer by means of the fluid column contained within the catheter lumen. A number of factors, such as movement of the catheter and the presence of air bubbles, can influence the dynamic accuracy of these catheter-transducer systems, and miniature pressure gauges attached directly to the tip of the cardiac catheter are finding increasing application. These microtransducers have frequency-response characteristics greatly superior to those of conventional catheter-transducer systems.

The Intracardiac Pressure Pulses

The upper limits of normal for intracardiac pressures and certain other hemodynamic variables are shown in Table 262-1. In understanding the contours of the intra-

Table 262-1. NORMAL HEMODYNAMIC VALUES,* mm Hg

	A wave	V wave	Mean	S/D
Right atrium............	7	5	5	
Left atrium..............	16	20	12	
Right ventricle..........	..	..	..	30/5
Left ventricle............	..	..	..	145/12
Pulmonary artery.........	..	..	20	30/16
Pulmonary artery wedge...	7	15	13	

Cardiac index = 2.5–3.6L/min/sq m BSA.

AV O_2 difference: 4.0–6.0 ml/100 ml.

Pulmonary vascular resistance: 250 dynes/sec/cm^{-5} (3 resistance units).

* The figures shown indicate the upper limits of pressure (mm Hg) and resistance in normal adult subjects. The values for the pressure waves, the mean pressures, and the systolic and diastolic pressures (S/D) are shown; in the ventricles, D = end-diastolic pressure. BSA = body surface area. The ranges for cardiac index and arterial–mixed venous O_2 differences are shown.

cardiac pressure pulses, thorough knowledge of the temporal relations between the electrical and mechanical events of the cardiac cycle is important (see Fig. 262-2, p. 1115, and 261-2). Although detailed study of the contours of the atrial pressure pulses has proved less reliable in predicting relative degrees of mitral valve stenosis and regurgitation than once was anticipated, a general understanding of the atrial pressure pulses is useful in the hemodynamic evaluation of a number of cardiac lesions.

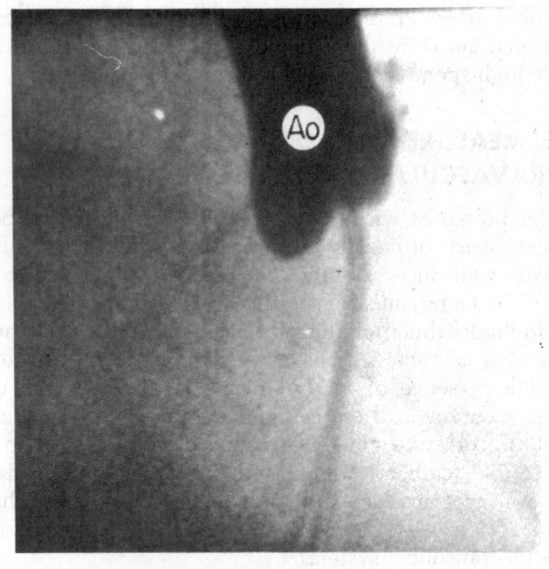

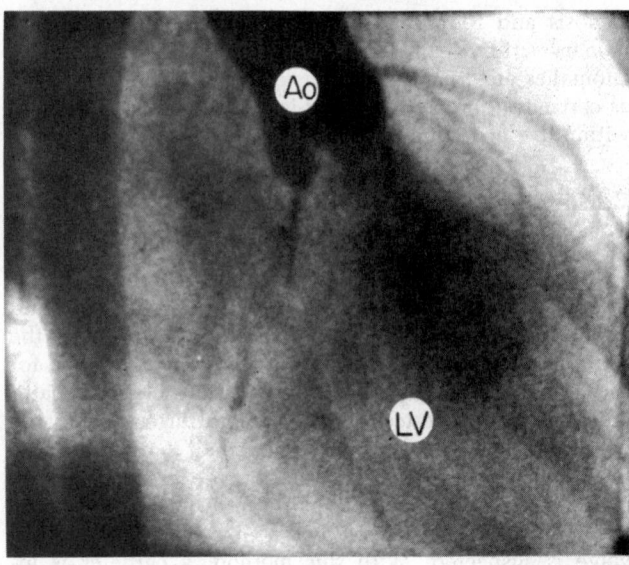

A

B

C

Fig. 262-1. Cineangiograms with injection of contrast medium into the aortic root. Studies are performed in the right anterior oblique projection in a patient with a normal aortic valve in whom the left ventricle LV is not opacified (panel A); in a patient with mild aortic regurgitation in whom the LV is slightly opacified (panel B); and in a patient with severe aortic regurgitation in whom the LV is densely opacified (panel C). Ao, aorta; LV, left ventricle.

The *A* wave in the right atrium normally is larger than the *V* wave, whereas in the left atrium the *V* wave is dominant (Table 262-1). Therefore, when the *V* wave in the right atrial pressure pulse exceeds the *A* wave, abnormal filling of the right atrium during ventricular systole, as occurs in tricuspid regurgitation or atrial septal defect, should be suspected. A characteristic right atrial pressure pulse also may be seen in the presence of tricuspid stenosis, the contour resembling that of mitral stenosis (see below), as well as in constrictive pericarditis, when an early diastolic "dip" and "plateau" elevation of pressure in mid- and late diastole occur. In many patients, the *mean* level of pressure in the left atrium is reflected with reasonable accuracy by the pulmonary artery wedge pressure (also sometimes termed the pulmonary "capillary" pressure), although the excursions of the wedge tracing often do not coincide with those measured directly within the left atrium. The characteristic contours of the left atrial pressure pulse in a normal subject and in patients with several forms of mitral valve disease are shown in Fig. 262-2. In the normal pressure pulse, or in the presence of mitral regurgitation without stenosis, there is a rapid fall in pressure during early diastole (the y descent), and a slow rise in pressure occurs during late diastole (diastasis), reflecting equilibration between the atrial and ventricular pressures during this slow phase of ventricular filling (Fig. 262-2A). In contrast, in patients with mitral stenosis the y descent is

slow and prolonged; pressure in the left atrium continues to fall throughout diastole, and evidence of diastasis on the left atrial pressure pulse is absent because of the persistent atrioventricular pressure gradient (Fig. 262-2B). When mitral stenosis is present with normal sinus rhythm (Fig. 262-2C), the A wave is abnormally prominent, and a large pressure gradient accompanies atrial contraction (often associated with a loud presystolic murmur in such patients). In patients with pure mitral regurgitation, the V wave is prominent and the descending limb of this wave (the y descent) is rapid (Fig. 262-2D).

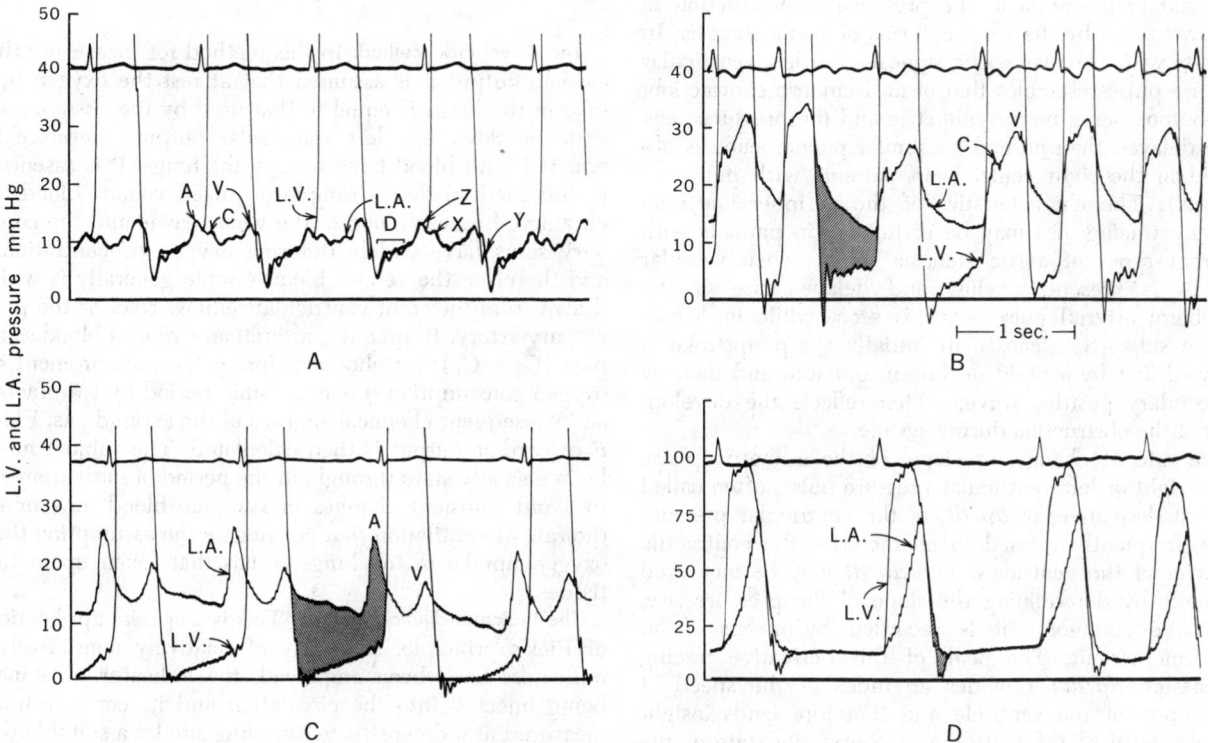

Fig. 262-2. Simultaneously recorded left ventricular (LV) and left atrial (LA) pressure tracings in a normal subject (panel A) and in patients with various forms of mitral valve disease (panels B to D). The tracings are recorded at high sensitivity (0 to 40 mm Hg), and therefore the top portion of the left ventricular pressure tracing is cut off. The electrocardiogram is recorded in the upper portion of each panel.

Panel A. In the normal heart, diastole is initiated by a rapid-filling wave, which is followed by a period of slow ventricular filling or diastasis (bracket D), in which atrial and ventricular pressure rise together slowly. This period of diastasis is followed by the atrial contraction wave (A), which precedes the onset of isometric contraction in the ventricle, the end-diastolic pressure, or the Z point in the left atrium. The C wave occurs during the phase of isometric ventricular contraction and is followed by the x descent. The V wave occurs during late systole and the downslope of the V wave, constituting the y descent, occurs immediately after opening of the mitral valve.

Panel B. Tracings obtained in a patient with mitral stenosis and atrial fibrillation. The pressure gradient from left atrium to left ventricle during diastole is indicated by the diagonally shaded area. The A wave is absent, and the CV wave is prominent.

Panel C. Tracings from a patient with mitral stenosis and normal sinus rhythm. The pressure gradient is indicated by the diagonally shaded area. A large pressure gradient occurs at the time of atrial contraction. No pressure rise during the period of diastasis is evident in the left atrial pressure tracings of panels B and C.

Panel D. Tracings from a patient with isolated, severe mitral regurgitation and atrial fibrillation. The C wave is not evident, and the giant V wave in the left atrial pressure pulse is nearly 70 mm Hg. There is a small pressure gradient during the phase of rapid ventricular filling, because of the large volume of antegrade flow across the mitral valve.

The left ventricular end-diastolic pressure immediately precedes the onset of isometric contraction in the left ventricular pressure pulse. This pressure point therefore follows the A wave and precedes the C wave, and the coincident pressure point in time in the left atrial tracing is termed the Z point (Fig. 262-2A). The left ventricular end-diastolic pressure may be elevated in several situations: (1) in the presence of heart failure, (2) when the ventricle bears a high flow load (as in aortic regurgitation), (3) when the ventricle is hypertrophied and relatively noncompliant (restrictive myocardial disease), and (4) in the presence of constrictive pericarditis.

The systolic pressure in the left ventricle is elevated over that in the aorta in the presence of obstruction to outflow caused by the various forms of aortic stenosis. In patients with valvular aortic stenosis, the left ventricular pressure pulse resembles that of an isometric contraction, the contour being more symmetric and the pressure peak more delayed than normal (a similar phenomenon is observed in the right ventricle in patients with pulmonic stenosis). The characteristics of the peripheral arterial pressure tracing also may be distinctive in patients with different types of aortic stenosis. Thus, when valvular stenosis is present, a slow and delayed rise of the peripheral arterial pulse wave is seen, while in hypertrophic subaortic stenosis an initially sharp upstroke is followed first by a rapid decline in pressure and then by a secondary positive wave, which reflects the development of the obstruction during systole.

The rate of change, or slope, of the isometric phase of the right or left ventricular pressure pulse, often called the first derivative, or dp/dt, of the ventricular pressure pulse, frequently is used to characterize the contractile behavior of the ventricles. The dp/dt may be measured manually by determining the slope of the pressure rise, but more commonly it is recorded by means of an electronic circuit. The peak of this derivative tracing (maximum dp/dt) provides an index of the speed of contraction of the ventricle and therefore lends insight into the level of the inotropic or contractile state of the heart. This measure tends to be under 1,200 mm Hg per sec in the left ventricles of patients with disease of the left ventricular myocardium, and it may be augmented strikingly by agents which improve the contractility of the heart, such as digitalis or catecholamines.

THE MEASUREMENT OF CARDIAC OUTPUT

The direct Fick and indicator-dilution methods presently are widely used in man for the determination of volume blood flow, or the cardiac output. In general, the equations used with these techniques are derived from the principle proposed by Adolf Fick which states that the rate at which a substance distributed in a fluid is delivered to an area by the moving fluid stream is equal to the product of the flow rate and the difference between the concentration of the substance at sites proximal and distal to the area. Thus,

$$q = F(C_a - C_v)$$

where q = the quantity of substance delivered per unit time

F = the flow rate

C_a and C_v = the concentrations of the substance at proximal and distal sampling sites, respectively

(The same equation is applicable to the measurement of the removal rate, or clearance, of a substance.) When flow is the quantity to be derived, the equation is rearranged to

$$F = \frac{q}{C_a - C_v}$$

The Direct Fick Method. In this method for measuring the cardiac output it is assumed that at rest the oxygen uptake in the lungs is equal to that used by the tissues, and systemic flow, i.e., left ventricular output, therefore is equated with blood flow through the lungs. It is essential to this method that a sample of mixed venous blood be obtained, because blood in the venae cavae and the coronary sinus have widely differing oxygen concentrations, and therefore the venous blood sample generally is withdrawn from the right ventricular outflow tract or the pulmonary artery. In practice, arterial and venous blood samples $(C_a - C_v)$ are obtained during the measurement of oxygen consumption q over a 3-min period by spirometry and subsequent chemical analysis of the expired gas. Flow F or cardiac output is then calculated. The subject must be in a steady state throughout the period of measurement to avoid transient changes in systemic blood flow or in the rate of ventilation that can negate the assumption that oxygen uptake in the lungs equals that taken up in the tissues.

The Indicator-dilution Method. This is a special application of Fick's principle. A variety of relatively nondiffusible indicators have been employed, the indicator substance being injected into the circulation and its concentration measured at a downstream sampling site by a suitable detector. For example, the dye indocyanine green is injected intravenously and blood is withdrawn from an artery at a constant rate through a calibrated densitometer, which provides direct measurement of the dye concentration. Generally, a single bolus of the indicator is injected rapidly and is thoroughly mixed in one of the vascular spaces such as a ventricular chamber; the concentration versus time curve then provides a measure of the rate at which indicator was washed out of the mixing site. Prior to recirculation of the indicator, the downslope of this curve is exponential, and therefore extrapolation of the curve using semilog paper permits the elimination of recirculated indicator. The mean concentration $\bar{c}$ of the dye is determined from the area of this corrected curve and its duration. The rate of blood flow F then is directly related to the quantity of indicator injected i and is inversely related to the mean concentration of the indicator $\bar{c}$ and the duration of the curve t, in seconds) by the formula $F = 60i/\bar{c}t$. A simple example will serve to illustrate this principle: if 8 mg of dye is injected and a mean concentration of 2 mg per liter is recorded, and if the indicator takes 60 sec to pass the sampling site, then the flow is 4 liters per min.

The Measurement of Pulmonary Vascular Resistance

In calculating the resistance offered by a vascular bed, blood flow is assumed to be laminar and the general resistance formula then can be employed. This formula, in simplified form which omits consideration of vessel length and blood viscosity, states that resistance is directly proportional to the pressure drop or gradient across the bed and inversely proportional to the rate of blood flow. This ratio of mean pressure gradient to volume flow is expressed in dynes/sec/cm^{-5}, the mean pressure gradient across the pulmonary bed being obtained by subtracting the mean left atrial or pulmonary artery wedge pressure from the mean pulmonary artery pressure.[1] The *resistance unit* (i.e., the pressure gradient in millimeters of mercury is divided by the cardiac output in liters per minute and expressed in arbitrary units) also is commonly employed as an index of arteriolar resistance (Table 262-1). Estimation of the pulmonary arteriolar resistance, which normally is about 15 percent of that in the systemic vascular bed, is of importance in patients with congenital heart disease and circulatory shunts, as well as in certain forms of acquired cardiac and pulmonary diseases. Its calculation provides a useful means of interpreting the level of pulmonary arterial pressure relative to pulmonary blood flow, high pressure and high flow obviously bearing a different connotation than high pressure and low flow. Pulmonary vascular resistance can be altered by varying concentrations of oxygen and by certain pharmacologic agents. For example, in patients with pulmonary hypertension secondary to congenital heart disease, the infusion of a vasodilating agent such as tolazoline into the pulmonary artery sometimes has been used to determine whether or not the pulmonary vascular resistance is fixed by irreversible changes in the pulmonary vessels, or whether the elevated resistance is potentially reversible.

Valve Orifice Size and Valvular Regurgitation

When the cardiac output is normal, the severity of a stenotic valve lesion may be estimated from the magnitude of the pressure gradient across the valve. When the cardiac output is elevated or reduced, however, reliance on the pressure gradient alone may lead to an erroneous estimate of the degree of mechanical obstruction. In addition, in patients with stenosis of the tricuspid or mitral

---

[1] Resistance =
$$\frac{PA \text{ (mm Hg)} - LA \text{ (mm Hg)} \times 1{,}332 \text{ dynes/sq cm}}{\text{cardiac output (ml/sec)}},$$
where PA and LA = mean pulmonary artery and left atrial pressures. 1 mm Hg = 1.36 cm water; 1 cm water = 980 dynes per sq cm force.

valves, it is of importance to consider the heart rate in assessing the significance of a pressure gradient. When the heart rate is rapid, systole occupies a disproportionate amount of time in each cardiac cycle, diastole filling time is limited, and a large pressure gradient across the atrioventricular valve may exist in the face of relatively mild stenosis. The application of the hydraulic formula devised by Gorlin and Gorlin to the calculation of valve orifice size has proved helpful in analyzing the degree of valve stenosis in these situations. In simplest terms, this formula states that the area of a short-bore orifice is directly proportional to the rate of blood flow across the orifice and inversely proportional to the square root of the pressure gradient. For example, if the flow rate across a narrowed valve orifice of fixed size doubles, as may occur when the cardiac output increases during exertion, the pressure gradient will quadruple. Conversely, when the flow rate is reduced, as in patients with heart failure, a small pressure gradient may exist in the presence of a severe degree of valve stenosis. This relationship differs from the general resistance equation discussed above and reflects the fact that the kinetic energy losses across a stenotic valve are high, a large pressure head being expended in developing a rapid flow velocity across the narrowed orifice.

It should be pointed out that use of the orifice formula is not valid when significant valvular regurgitation is present, and forward cardiac output alone is measured, since an unknown volume of blood is regurgitated and recrosses the valve during the cardiac cycle. Application of the formula under these circumstances leads to an underestimation of the valve orifice area, since forward flow across the valve is underestimated. The characteristics of the indicator-dilution curve are helpful in the detection of valvular regurgitation, the peak concentration being reduced and the washout slope prolonged (Fig. 262-3B). In addition, indicator may be detected by sampling from the chamber proximal to a regurgitant leak after injecting indicator into the more distal chamber (e.g., left ventricular injection with left atrial sampling for the detection of mitral regurgitation). Most commonly, the degree of valvular regurgitation is estimated by angiography (Fig. 262-1).

THE DIAGNOSIS OF CIRCULATORY SHUNTS

When a communication exists between the left and the right sides of the heart, and when pulmonary vascular resistance is lower than that in the systemic vascular bed, a left-to-right shunt of oxygenated blood will occur. Conversely, when the resistance in the pulmonary bed is higher than that in the systemic circulation, or an obstruction such as pulmonic stenosis exists distal to an intracardiac communication, a right-to-left shunt of venous blood may occur.

Many types of indicators have been employed in the diagnosis and quantification of circulatory shunts. The indicator may be oxygen in room air (Fig. 262-4), blood samples being withdrawn and analyzed manometrically

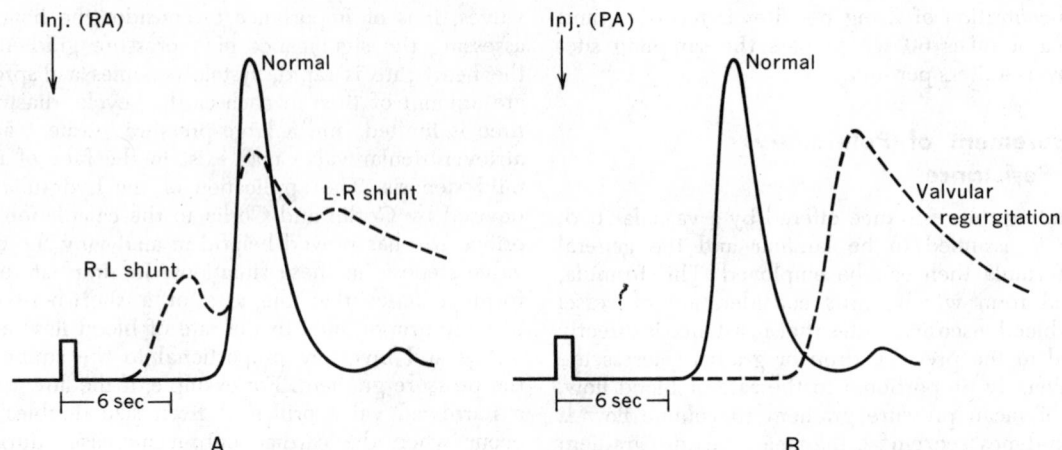

Fig. 262-3. Diagrammatic representation of indicator-dilution curves in various forms of cardiac disease. The downstream sampling method is employed. With reference to Fig. 262-4, indicator is injected with syringe No. 2 and sampled at the systemic artery (No. 1).

Panel A. The time of injection (Inj.) of an indicator, such as cardiogreen dye, is indicated by the arrow and by the square wave response on the recorded tracing. With right atrial (RA) injection and sampling at a peripheral artery, the normal appearance time is about 8 sec, and the normal contour of the indicator-dilution curve is represented by the solid line. In a patient with a right-to-left (R-L) shunt at the atrial, ventricular, or pulmonary arterial levels, early appearance time of the dye is indicated by the dashed line. In a patient with a left-to-right (L-R) shunt, the appearance time need not be altered, but there is a reduced peak concentration of dye, and a break on the downslope, indicating early recirculation of the indicator.

Panel B. The indicator-dilution curve in a normal patient with injection into the pulmonary artery (Inj. PA) shows an appearance time of about 6 sec. In a patient with severe regurgitation at the mitral or aortic valves, the appearance time is prolonged and the delayed clearance of the indicator from the left side of the heart results in a prolonged downslope of the indicator-dilution curve (dashed line).

or by an oximeter; alternatively, a fiberoptic catheter-tip oximeter system may be used. Foreign, inert gases such as hydrogen or [85]krypton may be employed; these, like oxygen, are "injected" into the pulmonary circulation by inhalation and sampled from the right side of the heart (Fig. 262-4). They may be measured by a catheter-tip sensor (hydrogen) or by withdrawal of blood samples for analysis in a Geiger counter tube ([85]krypton). In obtaining indicator-dilution curves, the substance most commonly injected is indocyanine green dye. Other injectable indicators which may be sensed by a suitable transducer include ascorbate (a reducing agent) and cooled saline solution (detected with a thermistor).

A variety of techniques have been devised for detecting, localizing, and quantifying shunts at cardiac catheterization. Basically, these methods may be divided into two categories: (1) Those methods in which an indicator is delivered distal to the site at which blood is sampled (the so-called upstream sampling method), e.g., indicator is injected into the pulmonary artery or is inhaled to enter the pulmonary veins and left side of the heart. Blood samples are then obtained upstream in the right side of the heart and analyzed for concentration of the indicator. (2) Those methods in which an indicator is delivered proximal to the sampling site (the so-called downstream sampling method), in which most frequently an indicator-dilution curve is obtained by intracardiac dye injection with sampling from a peripheral artery. This approach permits detection of right-to-left as well as left-to-right shunts.

The Upstream Sampling Method. Blood samples are withdrawn in serial fashion from the pulmonary artery, right ventricle, right atrium, and venae cavae, the indicator (or oxygen) being introduced downstream. This approach permits localization of the site of a left-to-right shunt (Fig. 262-4). With the oxygen sampling method, a step-up of 1.5 volumes percent from the venae cavae to the right atrium, or of 1.0 volume percent from the right atrium to the right ventricle, or from the right ventricle to the pulmonary artery, is considered to be evidence of a left-to-right shunt. The use of a foreign gas such as [85]krypton improves the accuracy of this approach (Fig. 262-4), since during the brief period of foreign gas inhalation the arterial level of the gas rises markedly, but because of the high solubility of the gas in the tissues, the level of radioactivity in the right side of the circulation rises slowly in the normal subject. Thus, even a small left-to-right shunt is readily detected by appropriate sampling within the right side of the heart. Upstream sampling has also been applied using two cardiac catheters, or a double-lumen catheter, one to inject indicator dye distally into a peripheral pulmonary artery, the other to draw blood continuously through a densitometer to detect early recirculation of indicator through a left-to-right shunt. The catheter-tip hydrogen electrode used during hydrogen inhalation is another variation of this approach.

For determination of the size of a left-to-right shunt, venous blood sampled proximal to the shunt, samples from the pulmonary artery, and a systemic arterial sample are obtained in close time sequence. The oxygen uptake at the lungs is measured simultaneously, or estimated, and the pulmonary and systemic blood flow rates (and hence the magnitude of the left-to-right shunt relative to systemic flow) can be calculated using Fick's equations. Generally a pulmonary to systemic flow ratio of 1.5:1 or greater is considered to indicate a left-to-right shunt of substantial magnitude.

The Downstream Sampling Method. A needle is placed into a systemic artery (usually a radial, brachial, or femoral vessel), and a time-concentration curve is recorded following upstream injection of the indicator. This technique is particularly useful for localizing the site of a right-to-left shunt. For example, when a right-to-left shunt exists at the ventricular level, an injection into the right ventricle as well as injections at all sites proximal

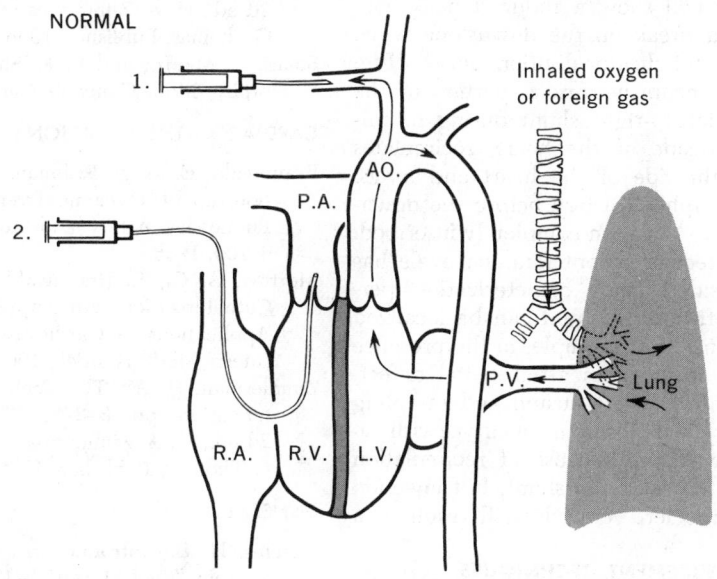

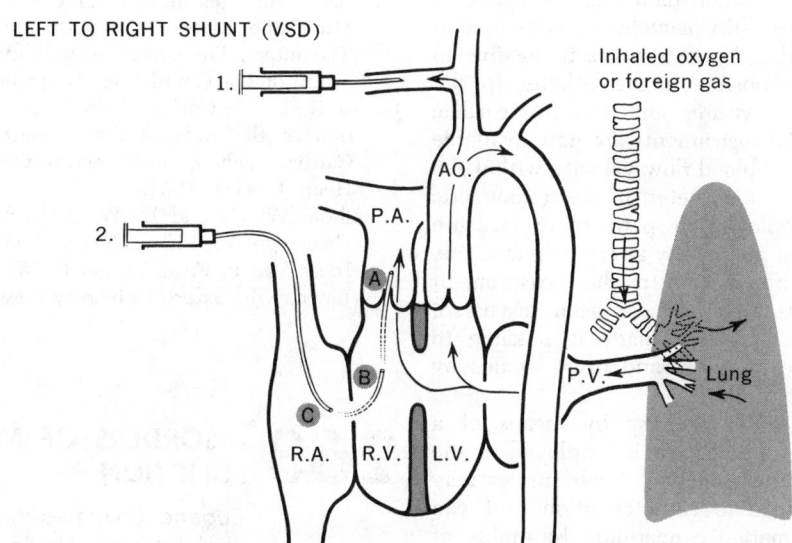

Fig. 262-4. Diagram of the upstream sampling method for detecting the presence of a left-to-right shunt.
   Upper Panel. Illustration of the normal circulation in which oxygen, or an inhaled foreign gas, traverses the pulmonary veins (P.V.), left atrium, left ventricle (L.V.), and aorta (AO). A sample obtained from a systemic artery (syringe No. 1) will contain a high concentration of oxygen or foreign gas, whereas a blood sample obtained from syringe No. 2, which is attached to a catheter the tip of which lies in the pulmonary artery (P.A.), will not contain appreciable quantities of the gas.
   Lower Panel. Illustration of the circulation in a patient with a left-to-right shunt through a ventricular septal defect (VSD). Sampling of blood in the right side of the heart with subsequent analysis of the samples for oxygen, or for foreign-gas concentration immediately after the onset of gas inhalation, will yield a high concentration of the gas in the pulmonary artery (site A), and in the right ventricle (R.V.) (site B), but normal gas concentrations at site C in the right atrium (R.A.).

to the right ventricle will result in an early appearance time of dye that has immediately traversed the defect to enter the left silde of the heart and the aorta (Fig. 262-3A). However, an injection into the pulmonary artery, distal to the right-to-left shunt, shows a normal appearance time. A left-to-right shunt also may be detected, but not localized, by injection of indicator into the right side of the heart using peripheral arterial sampling. The indicator-dilution curve will show a reduced peak concentration of dye and a break on the downslope when compared with a normal indicator-dilution curve (Fig. 262-3A). This contour occurs because a portion of the indicator traverses the left-to-right shunt during its initial passage to the left side of the heart, recirculates rapidly through the right side of the heart and lungs, and reappears at the peripheral artery before the downslope of the primary curve has been completely inscribed.

If an atrial septal defect or patent foramen ovale has been crossed, or left-sided heart catheterization performed, the site of a left-to-right shunt can be localized with downstream sampling. For example, in the presence of a left-to-right shunt through an atrial septal defect, injection of indicator into the left atrium and sampling from a peripheral artery will result in a curve with an early break on the downslope, because of recirculation of indicator which has traversed the shunt, but injection distal to the shunt in the left ventricle will result in a normal curve.

OTHER SPECIAL MEASUREMENT TECHNIQUES. A number of technical advances are gaining acceptance and improving cardiac catheterization methods. For example, use of a fiberoptic catheter-tip oximeter in combination with a video-tape recording system makes it possible to record simultaneously the position of the catheter tip, the oxygen saturation, the pressure, and the intracardiac electrocardiogram. Special instruments are now available for measurement of phasic blood flow velocity within the great vessels; for example, a catheter-tip electromagnetic flowmeter has been employed in patients to measure blood flow velocity in the pulmonary artery, venae cavae, and aorta. Catheter-tip transducers for the measurement of intracardiac pressures already have been discussed, and other special catheters have made it possible to characterize and localize murmurs and heart sounds by intracardiac phonocardiography.

EXERCISE STRESS TESTING. Exercise by means of a bicycle ergometer or treadmill often is employed in the evaluation of cardiovascular function. Such studies may be performed during cardiac catheterization and can provide important information concerning the ability of the heart to respond to this mode of stress. For example, certain patients with heart disease may have a normal cardiac output and normal intracardiac pressures at rest but exhibit a markedly impaired response of the cardiac output, or an abnormal elevation of ventricular diastolic pressure, during exercise. In addition, measurements of the cardiac output increase relative to the increase in body oxygen consumption during exercise (the so-called "exercise factor"), or relative to the level of venous blood oxygen saturation in the pulmonary artery, provide important indices of the functional reserve of the heart.

REFERENCES

ANGIOGRAPHY AND CINERADIOGRAPHY

Keith, J. D., and C. A. F. Moses: Selective Angiocardiography, pp. 225–287 in "Intravascular Catheterization," 2d ed., H. A. Zimmerman (Ed.), Springfield, Ill., Charles C Thomas, Publisher, 1966.

Sones, F. M., Jr., and E. K. Shirey: Cine Coronary Arteriography, Mod. Concepts Cardiovas. Dis., 31:735, 1962.

CARDIAC CATHETERIZATION

Braunwald, E., A. P. Fishman, and A. Cournand: Time Relationship of Dynamic Events in the Cardiac Chambers, Pulmonary Artery and Aorta in Man, Circulation Res., 4:100, 1956.

Morrow, A. G., E. Braunwald, and J. Ross, Jr.: Left Heart Catheterization: An Appraisal of Techniques and Their Applications in Cardiovascular Diagnosis, A.M.A. Arch. Intern. Med., 105:645, 1960.

Zimmerman, H. A.: The Technique of Right Cardiac Catheterization, pp. 3–37 in "Intravascular Catheterization," 2d ed., H. A. Zimmerman (Ed.), Springfield, Ill., Charles C Thomas, Publisher, 1966.

GENERAL

Abrams, H. L.: Introduction and Historical Notes, in "Angiography," vol. 1, pp. 3–12, Herbert L. Abrams (Ed.), Boston, Little, Brown and Company, 1961.

Cournand, A.: Measurement of the Cardiac Output in Man Using the Right Heart Catheterization. Description of Technique, Discussion of Validity and of Place in the Study of the Circulation, Federation Proc., 4:207, 1945.

Gorlin, R., and S. Gorlis: Hydrodynamic Formula for Calculation of the Area of the Stenotic Mitral Valve, Other Cardiac Valves, and Central Circulatory Shunts, Am. Heart J., 41:1, 1951.

Hamilton, W. F., and D. W. Richards: The Output of the Heart, pp. 71–126 in "Circulation of the Blood; Men & Ideas," A. P. Fishman and D. W. Richards (Eds.), Fair Lawn, N.J., Oxford University Press, Inc., 1964.

263 DISORDERS OF MYOCARDIAL FUNCTION

Eugene Braunwald, John Ross, Jr., and Edmund H. Sonnenblick

CELLULAR BASIS OF CARDIAC CONTRACTION

The myocardium is composed of individual striated muscle cells (fibers), 10 to 15 μ in diameter and 30 to 60 μ in length. Under the light microscope, each fiber contains multiple cross-banded strands (myofibrils), which run the length of the fiber and are composed of a serially repeating structure, the sarcomere. The remainder of the cytoplasm, lying between the myofibrils, contains other cell constituents such as the single centrally located nucleus, numerous mitochondria, and intracellular membrane systems.

The sarcomere, the fundamental structural and functional unit of contraction, is delimited by two adjacent dark lines, the Z lines (Fig. 263-1). The distance between Z lines varies with the degree of contraction or stretch of the muscle and ranges between 1.5 and 2.2 μ. Within the confines of the sarcomere, alternating light and dark bands are seen, giving the myocardial fibers their striated appearance under the light microscope. At the center of the sarcomere is a broad dark band of constant width (1.5 μ), the A band, which is flanked by two lighter bands, the I bands, which are of variable width. The sarcomere of heart muscle, like that of skeletal muscle, is made up of two sets of myofilaments. Thicker myofilaments, composed of the protein myosin, traverse and are limited to the A band. The myosin filaments are about 100 Å in diameter, with tapered ends, and they measure 1.5 to 1.6 μ in length. Thinner myofilaments, composed primarily of actin, course from the Z line through the I band into the A band. The thin filaments are approximately 50 Å in diameter and 1.0 μ in length. Thus, there is overlapping of thick and thin filaments only within the A band, while the I band contains only thin filaments (Fig. 263-1). Bridges extend between the myosin and actin filaments within the A band.

The "sliding" model for muscle rests on the fundamental observation that both the thick and thin contractile filaments are constant in overall length, both at rest and during contraction. With activation of the sarcomere, an interaction takes place between specific complementary sites on the actin and myosin filaments, and the actin filaments are propelled further into the A band. In the process, the A band remains constant in width, whereas the I bands become more narrow and the Z lines move toward one another.

Myosin is an unstable, asymmetric fibrous protein with a molecular weight of about 500,000; it is 1,500 Å in length, with a globular expansion at its end. The rodlike portion of the molecule has a diameter of 20 Å, while the globular portion, which projects laterally to the adjacent thin filament, expands to 40 to 50 Å. The globular portions are presumed to form the "bridges" which are assumed to be sites of ATPase activity, as well as part of the mechanism by which myosin filaments interact with actin to generate force and shortening. Actin has a molecular weight of 55,000. The actin myofilament is composed of a double helix of two chains of actin wound about each other. In contrast to myosin, actin has no enzymatic activity, but it does have the ability to combine reversibly with myosin in the presence of ATP and Mg^{++}. During contraction adenosinetriphosphate (ATP) is split, linkages between the actin and myosin filaments are made and detached cyclically, and directional forces are generated between these two filaments which result in shortening of the sarcomere.

The sarcoplasmic reticulum, a complex network of anastomosing, membrane-lined intracellular channels, which invests the myofibrils, has two distinct components. One portion, the longitudinal component, consists of a series of interconnecting membrane tubules closely applied to the surfaces of the individual sarcomeres and has no direct continuity with the outside of the cell. The second component, the transverse component or "T" system, is formed by tubelike invaginations of the sarcolemma, which extend into the myocardial fiber, along the Z lines, i.e., the ends of the sarcomeres.

There is evidence that once the excitatory stimulus, in the form of an electrical depolarization of the cell membrane, reaches the interior of the fiber via the transverse tubular system, it is transferred to the adjacent terminal cisternae of the longitudinal system and Ca^{++} which is contained therein is released from the sarcoplasmic reticulum. The Ca^{++} diffuses into the myofibril and activates the myofilaments to produce contraction. The sarcoplasmic reticulum then appears to reaccumulate Ca^{++}, thereby lowering its concentration in the myofibril to a level that inhibits the actin-myosin interaction which is responsible for contraction and in this manner leads to relaxation. Thus, the sarcoplasmic reticulum, with its ability to transmit an action potential, to release and then reaccumulate Ca^{++}, appears to play a fundamental role in the rhythmic contraction and relaxation of heart muscle.

The ATP formed from substrate oxidation appears to be the source of energy for all the work of the myocardial cell. Some of this energy is expended in maintenance chemical work (e.g., in modifying substrates, producing glycogen, synthesizing lipids and proteins, maintaining the integrity of the membranes), although in the normally functioning heart the major fraction of energy is expended in the mechanical work of contraction. The high-energy phosphate stores in ATP are in equilibrium with others in creatine phosphate.

In all forms of striated muscle, including cardiac muscle, the force of contraction depends on initial muscle length. The sarcomere length associated with the most forceful contraction is 2.2 μ. It is at this length that the two sets of myofilaments of the sarcomere are most ideally situated to provide the greatest area for their interaction. In support of the sliding-filament hypothesis, force development diminishes in direct proportion to the decrease in the overlap between thick and thin filaments, and the resultant decrease in the number of reactive sites. At a sarcomere length of 3.65 μ, developed tension falls to zero, and it is at this point that the thin filaments are entirely withdrawn from the A band. Similarly, when the sarcomeres are shorter than 2.0 μ, the thin filaments bypass one another, producing a double overlap of the thin filaments, a less-than-ideal arrangement for interaction between thick and thin filaments (Fig. 263-2).

The relation between the initial length of the muscle fibers and the developed force is of prime importance for the function of heart muscle. This forms the basis of the Frank-Starling relation (Starling's law of the heart),

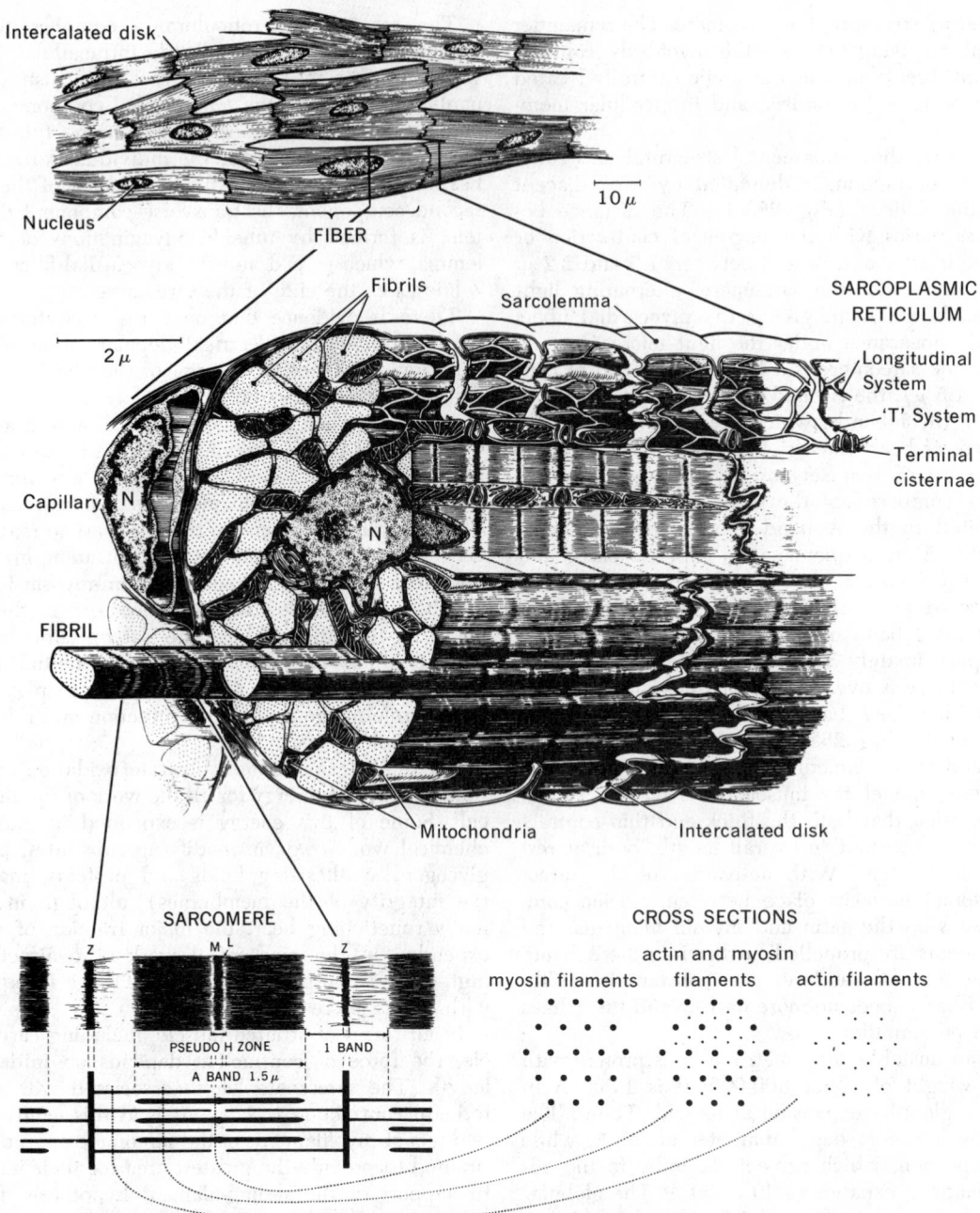

Fig. 263-1. Microscopic structure of heart muscle, showing myocardium (top) as seen under the light microscope (branching of fibers is evident, each containing a centrally located nucleus); a myocardial cell or fiber (center) reconstructed from electron micrographs (the arrangement of the multiple parallel fibrils that compose the cell and of the serially connected sarcomeres that compose the fibrils is apparent (N = nucleus) (bottom left); a diagrammatic representation of the arrangement of myofilaments that make up an individual sarcomere from a myofibril, with thick filaments (1.5 μ in length, composed of myosin) forming the A band, and thin filaments (1.0 μ in length, composed primarily of actin) extending from the Z line through the I band into the A band, and with overlapping of thick and thin filaments seen only in the A band (bottom right). Cross sections of the sarcomere indicate the specific lattice arrangements of the myofilaments. In the center of the sarcomere, left, only the thick, or myosin, filaments arranged in a hexagonal array are seen; in the distal portions of the A band, center, both thick and thin, or actin, filaments are found, with each thick filament surrounded by six thin filaments; and in the I band, right, only thin filaments are present. (From Braunwald et al., "Mechanisms of Contraction of Normal and Failing Heart," Boston, Little, Brown and Company, 1968.)

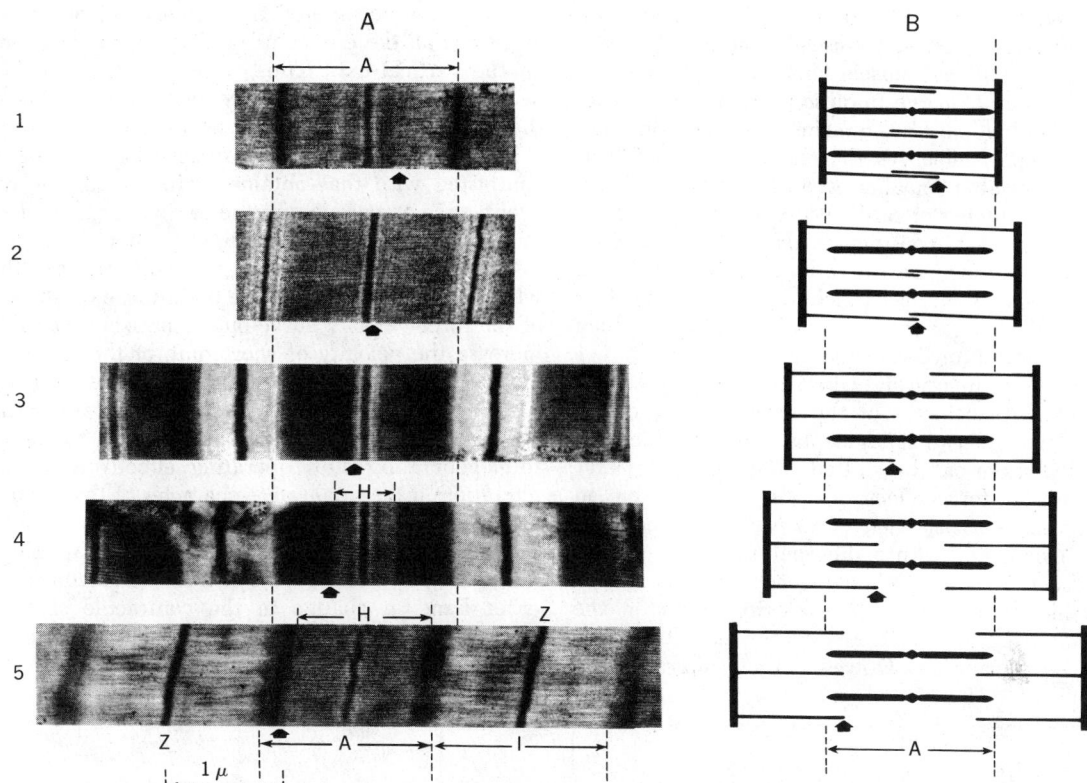

Fig. 263-2. Relation between sarcomere length and band patterns in skeletal muscle (frog sartorius). Panel A (left) shows the band patterns as seen electromicroscopically, and panel B (right) the disposition of the thick and thin filaments that create these patterns. The vertical arrows in both panels denote the ends of the thin filaments that insert at the Z line at the left. Panel A (3) represents the sarcomere at the apex of the length-tension curve, i.e., at L_{max}. In (1) and (2), sarcomere length has been progressively decreased, whereas in (4) and (5) it has been progressively elongated. Throughout, the A band remains constant in width. The placement of filaments to provide for maximum overlap is shown in B (3). (1) shows the sarcomere pattern in the contracted muscle; the I band has disappeared, and a secondary dark band has been formed at the center of the sarcomere, termed the C contraction band, which is due to the passage of thin filaments through this area as in B (1). In A (4) and (5), an expanding H zone has appeared, owing to the withdrawal of the thin filaments from the A band, as shown diagrammatically in B (4) and (5). (*From Braunwald et al., "Mechanisms of Contraction of Normal and Failing Heart," Boston, Little, Brown and Company, 1968.*)

which states that, within limits, an augmentation of initial volume of the ventricle, which is a function of the initial length of the muscle, results in an increase in the force of ventricular contraction. It has been shown for heart muscle, as well as for skeletal muscle, that sarcomere length is directly proportional to muscle length along the ascending limb of the length–active tension curve. As muscle length decreases to the point at which developed tension approaches zero and at which sarcomere length approaches 1.5 μ, the I bands at first narrow, then disappear while the A band remains constant in length. At this latter point, the Z line abuts on the edges of the A band. From these considerations it is apparent that the sarcomere length–active tension curve forms the ultrastructural basis of Starling's law of the heart. It is noteworthy that these points concerning the mechanism of contraction of the heart muscle fiber are also applicable to the skeletal muscle fiber.

MYOCARDIAL MECHANICS

Extremely helpful methods for examining the behavior of muscle were provided by the skeletal muscle physiologists early in this century. The mechanical activity of all muscle may be expressed externally in only two ways: shortening and the development of tension. A. V. Hill showed in skeletal muscle that the velocity of shortening is inversely related to the magnitude of tension development, an expression of the so-called force-velocity relation, now acknowledged to be a fundamental property of muscle. Expressed simply, the greater the load the muscle is called upon to lift, the slower the velocity of shortening and vice-versa. More recently, the concept of the force-velocity relation has been extended from skeletal to cardiac muscle. However, in this respect there is a basic difference between skeletal and cardiac muscle. Skeletal muscle has a single, essentially fixed, force-velocity curve; i.e., at any given muscle length, force and velocity are always related to each other in the same manner. The contractile activity of skeletal muscle is increased by the recruitment of additional muscle fibers, i.e., motor units, and the frequency of nerve impulses, while the contractility of each individual fiber remains constant. Although resting length also influences the characteristics of contraction, this variable remains essentially fixed in vivo. In contrast, the number of cardiac cells activated remains constant during each contraction. However, the contractile activity of the myocardium may be readily altered under physiologic conditions by changes in resting fiber length and by changes in contractility, both of which shift the myocardial force-velocity curve.

All variations in myocardial contractile activity can be expressed as displacements of the force-velocity curve. However, there are two fundamental ways in which the force-velocity curve can be shifted. Figure 263-3 (left) shows a family of force-velocity curves obtained from an isolated cardiac muscle; each curve was obtained at a different preload, i.e., with a different degree of stretch on the muscle. Note that changing the preload has altered the intercept of the force-velocity curve on the horizontal axis; i.e., it has increased the isometric force developed by the muscle. However, these alterations in

preload have not altered the intrinsic velocity of shortening, since all the curves extrapolate to the same intercept on the vertical axis. Thus, a change in initial length of heart muscle shifts the force-velocity curve by altering the total force which can be developed by the muscle.

This type of shift in the force-velocity curve may be contrasted with that obtained when a positive inotropic agent, such as norepinephrine or digitalis, is added to the muscle while the initial length is held constant (Fig. 263-3, right). These agents not only increase the force which the muscle is capable of lifting, i.e., the intercept of the force-velocity curve on the horizontal axis, but also increase the velocity of shortening of the unloaded muscle, i.e., the extrapolated intercept on the vertical axis.

It has been postulated that an increase in initial muscle length brings about an increase in the number of force-generating sites operating effectively without any alteration in the qualitative character of the cyclic process at these contractile sites. Such a change would be anticipated from a more advantageous overlap of interdigitating contractile filaments within the sarcomere. On the other hand, a change in the contractile state, characterized by an increase in the velocity of shortening of the unloaded muscle, appears to result from an increase

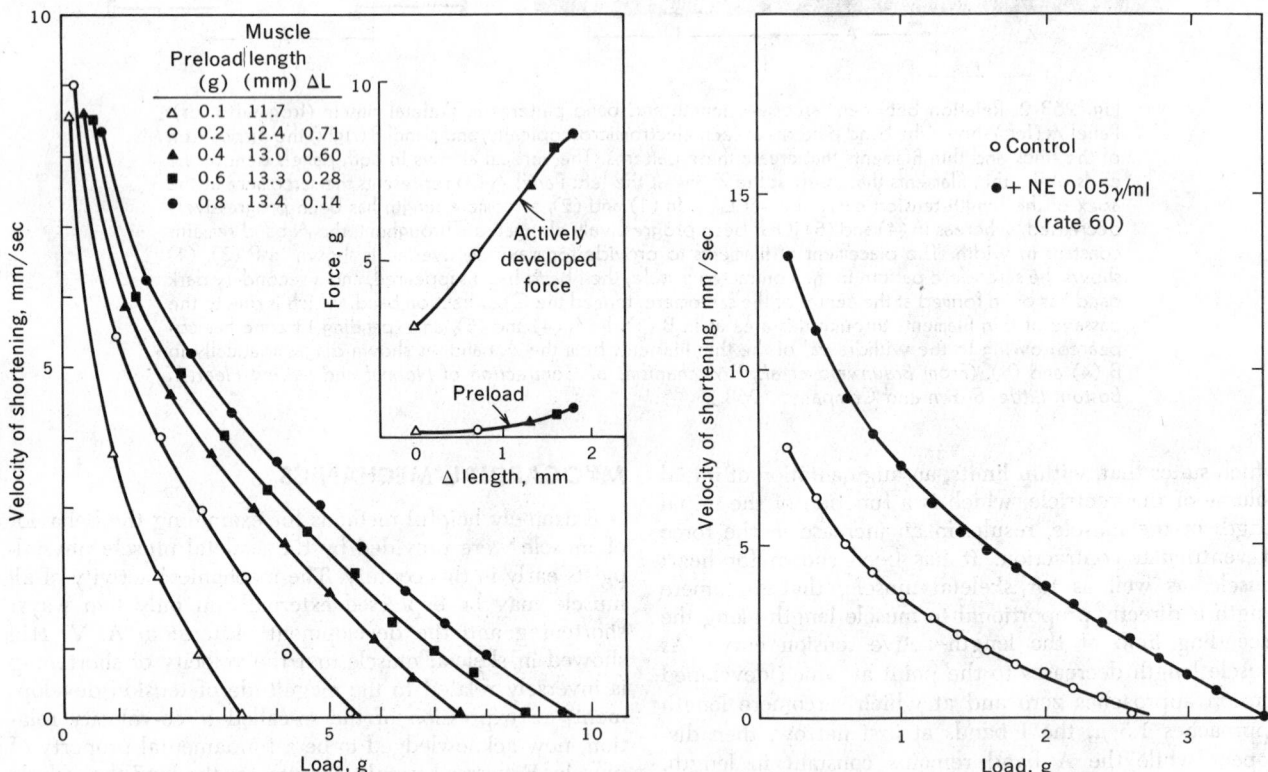

Fig. 263-3. (Left) Effects of increasing initial muscle length on the force-velocity relation of the cat papillary muscle. Initial velocity of shortening has been plotted as a function of load for five different muscle lengths. The maximum velocity of shortening (V_{max}) is essentially unchanged, whereas the maximum force of contraction (P_o) is augmented. The insert shows the places along the length-tension curves at which these force-velocity curves were determined. (Right) Effects of norepinephrine on the force-velocity relation of the cat papillary muscle. Both V_{max} and P_o have been increased. (*From Braunwald et al., "Mechanisms of Contraction of Normal and Failing Heart," Boston, Little, Brown and Company, 1968*).

in the rate of cyclic force-generating processes at the contractile sites, without a change in the number of these sites.

CONTRACTION OF THE INTACT VENTRICLE

Analysis of the heart as a pump has classically centered upon the relation between the filling pressure, or diastolic volume, of the ventricle (length of the muscle fibers) and its stroke volume (the Frank-Starling relation). It was shown clearly in the heart-lung preparation that the stroke volume is a function of diastolic fiber length, and that the failing heart delivers a smaller-than-normal stroke volume from a normal or elevated end-diastolic volume. Later, the concept of measuring stroke work (the product of stroke volume and mean aortic pressure) over a range of mean atrial or ventricular end-diastolic pressures, using one of these pressures as an index of diastolic volume, was expanded by Sarnoff and his collaborators. They concluded that this relation between the mean atrial or the ventricular end-diastolic pressure and the stroke work of the corresponding ventricle (the ventricular function curve) provided a definition of the level of the contractile state of the ventricle. Significant increases in the level of ventricular contractility were accompanied by shifts of the ventricular function curve upwards and to the left, while depression of contractility was identified by downward and rightward displacement of this relation (Fig. 263-4).

Recently considerable effort has been directed toward a study of the responses of the intact, unanesthetized animal, and it has been observed that during the adrenergic stimulation of the myocardium accompanying a stress such as exercise, no change or an actual decrease in ventricular end-diastolic size occurs while minute cardiac output, aortic flow velocity, and the rate of ventricular pressure development are augmented. Thus, reflex and humorally mediated changes in myocardial contractility, heart rate, venous return, and peripheral vascular resistance often appear to overshadow the effects of the intrinsic Frank-Starling mechanism, i.e., the relation between end-diastolic pressure or volume and stroke work.

The important influence of the neurotransmitter substance norepinephrine on the mechanical and electrical properties of the myocardium has long been recognized. Direct stimulation of the stellate ganglions and reflex stimulation of the heart consequent to hypotension in the carotid sinuses have been shown to elevate the ventricular function curve, as a consequence of the release of norepinephrine from sympathetic nerve endings in the heart. In the intact animal, these adrenergic effects are evidenced by tachycardia, a reduction in cardiac dimensions, increased velocity of ejection, and an enhanced rate of tension development. Cerebral ischemia also appears to cause a profound increase in ventricular performance.

Surgically denervated hearts *in situ*, or isolated papillary muscles taken from such hearts, do not exhibit depression of their intrinsic contractile properties despite

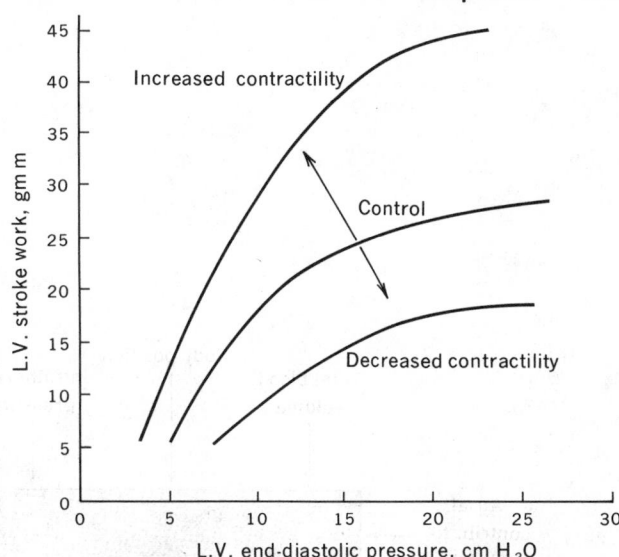

Fig. 263-4. Diagrammatic representation of ventricular function curves obtained under control conditions, during the administration of a positive inotropic agent (increased contractility), and during a negative inotropic state (decreased contractility). *LV*, left ventricular. (*From Braunwald et al., "Mechanisms of Contraction of Normal and Failing Heart," Boston, Little, Brown and Company, 1968.*)

depletion of the norepinephrine stores in the sympathetic nerve endings of the muscle. The denervated heart of the intact animal also appears capable of meeting many of the demands of muscular exercise. However, the mechanisms by which the denervated heart increases its output differ from those of the intact animal. Thus, tachycardia is less marked, and in animals subjected both to denervation and adrenalectomy, the stroke volume and cardiac output rise as a consequence of elevation of ventricular end-diastolic volume. In all these respects the activity of the heart muscle fiber differs from the activity of skeletal muscle fiber, the latter being totally dependent on its nerve supply and unable to contract effectively when denervated.

THE CONTROL OF CARDIAC PERFORMANCE AND CARDIAC OUTPUT

The extent of shortening of mammalian heart muscle and, therefore, the stroke volume of the intact ventricle are, in the final analysis, determined by three influences: (1) the length of the muscle at the onset of contraction, i.e., the preload; (2) the tension which the muscle is called upon to develop during contraction, i.e., the afterload; and (3) the contractile state of the muscle, i.e., the position of its force-velocity-length curve.

Ventricular End-diastolic Volume

At any level of its contractile state, the performance of the myocardium is influenced profoundly by ventricu-

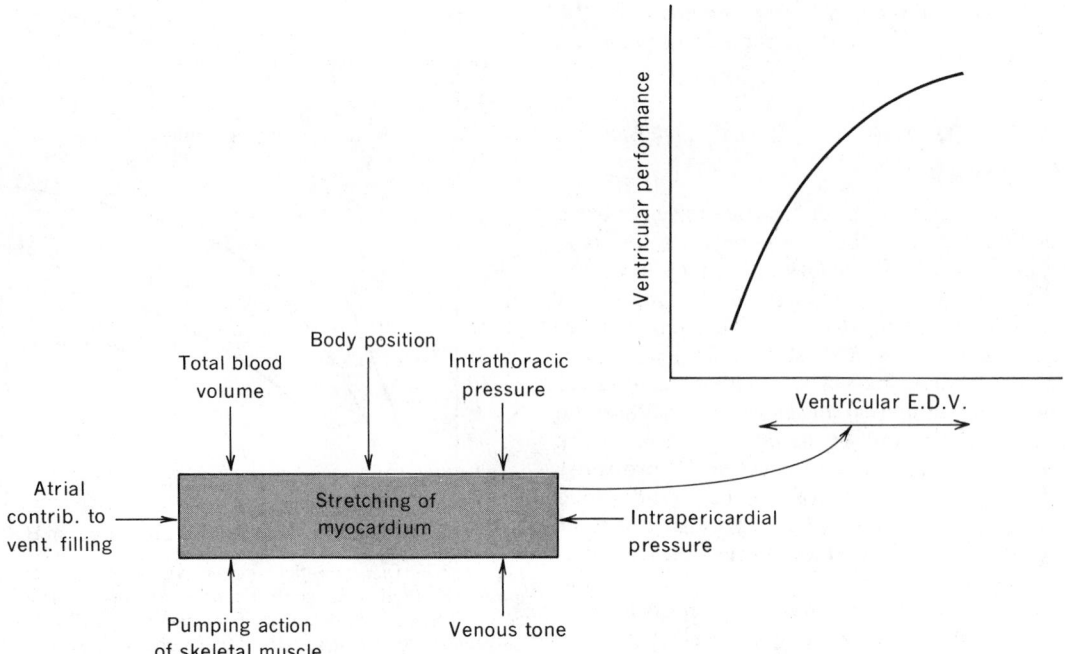

Fig. 263-5. Diagram of a Frank-Starling curve, relating ventricular end-diastolic volume (*E.D.V.*) to ventricular performance (top right) and the major influences that determine the degree of stretching of the myocardium, i.e., the magnitude of the *E.D.V.* (bottom left). (*From Braunwald et al., "Mechanisms of Contraction of Normal and Failing Heart," Boston, Little, Brown and Company, 1968.*)

lar end-diastolic fiber length and therefore by diastolic ventricular volume. The following are the major determinants of ventricular end-diastolic volume in the intact organism:

TOTAL BLOOD VOLUME. When the latter is depleted, as in acute hemorrhage, ventricular performance, as reflected in ventricular stroke work, must decline.

DISTRIBUTION OF BLOOD VOLUME. At any given total blood volume, the ventricular end-diastolic volume is influenced by the distribution of blood between the intra- and extrathoracic compartments. This distribution in turn is determined by:

Body Position. Gravitational forces tend to pool blood in the dependent portions of the body.

Intrathoracic Pressure. Normally, the mean intrathoracic pressure is negative, a factor which acts to increase thoracic blood volume and ventricular end-diastolic volume. Elevation of intrathoracic pressure, such as occurs in a tension pneumothorax, the Valsalva maneuver, or prolonged bouts of coughing, tends to impede venous return to the heart, diminish intrathoracic blood volume, and ultimately to reduce ventricular work.

Intrapericardial Pressure. When this pressure is elevated, as in pericardial effusion, there is interference with cardiac filling, and the resultant reduction in ventricular diastolic volume lowers ventricular work.

Venous Tone. The veins are not a simple system of passive conduits between the systemic capillary bed and the right atrium. Instead, the smooth muscle in venous walls responds to a variety of neural and humoral stimuli. Venoconstriction occurs during muscular exercise, deep

respiration, fright, or marked hypotension, tending to diminish extrathoracic blood volume and to augment intrathoracic blood volume.

The Pumping Action of Skeletal Muscle. During exercise the contracting skeletal muscles tend to squeeze blood out of the veins and, with the aid of the venous valves, to displace it centrally, thereby increasing intrathoracic blood volume, ventricular end-diastolic volume, and ventricular work.

ATRIAL CONTRIBUTION TO VENTRICULAR FILLING. Vigorous, appropriately timed atrial contraction augments ventricular filling and end-diastolic volume. The atrial contribution to ventricular filling is of particular importance in patients with ventricular hypertrophy, in whom the loss of atrial systole (as in atrial fibrillation) tends to reduce ventricular end-diastolic pressure and volume, ultimately lowering myocardial performance.

Myocardial Contractility

A number of factors determine the level of ventricular performance at any given ventricular end-diastolic volume (Fig. 263-6). These influences may be considered to operate by modifying the myocardial force-velocity-length relations.

SYMPATHETIC NERVE ACTIVITY. The quantity of norepinephrine released by sympathetic nerve endings in the heart is, under ordinary circumstances, dependent on the sympathetic nerve impulse traffic, and variations in the frequency of nerve impulses will modify the quantity of norepinephrine released and acting upon the beta-adrenergic receptors in the myocardium. This mechanism is probably the most important one which regulates the position of the force-velocity and ventricular function curves under physiologic conditions.

CIRCULATING CATECHOLAMINES. The adrenal medulla and other sympathetic ganglions outside the heart may, when properly stimulated by sympathetic nerve impulses, release catecholamines, which augment the contractile state of the myocardium.

THE FORCE-FREQUENCY RELATION. The position of the myocardial force-velocity curve may be profoundly influenced by the rate and rhythm of cardiac contraction; e.g., ventricular extrasystoles result in post-extrasystolic potentiation. A sustained improvement in myocardial contractility also can be induced with a bigeminal rhythm, by paired electrical stimulation, or by tachycardia.

EXOGENOUSLY ADMINISTERED INOTROPIC AGENTS. The cardiac glycosides, isoproterenol and other sympathomimetic agents, calcium, caffeine, theophylline, and their derivatives, all improve the myocardial force-velocity relation (Chap. 266) and therefore can be used therapeutically to augment ventricular performance at any given ventricular end-diastolic volume.

PHYSIOLOGIC DEPRESSANTS. Included among these are severe myocardial hypoxia, hypercapnea, and acidosis. Acting either singly or in combination, these influences exert a depressant effect on the myocardial force-velocity curve and lower the level of left ventricular work at any given ventricular end-diastolic volume.

PHARMACOLOGIC DEPRESSANTS. These include quinidine, procaine amide, and other local anesthetics (Chap. 266), barbiturates, as well as many other drugs which exert an effect analogous to that of the physiologic depressants.

LOSS OF VENTRICULAR SUBSTANCE. When a portion of ventricular myocardium becomes nonfunctional or necrotic, as occurs in myocardial infarction, total ventricular performance at any given level of end-diastolic volume is depressed, even if the remaining myocardium functions normally.

INTRINSIC MYOCARDIAL DEPRESSION. Although the fundamental mechanisms responsible for depression of myocardial contractility in heart failure still remain to be elucidated, it is now apparent that in this condition the contractile state of each unit of myocardium is depressed and that the level of ventricular performance at any ventricular end-diastolic volume is thereby lowered.

Ventricular Afterload

The volume of blood ejected by the ventricle during each contraction is ultimately a function of the extent of ventricular fiber shortening during systole. The extent of shortening at any given level of diastolic fiber length and myocardial contractile state is inversely related to the afterload imposed on the muscle. The afterload on the intact heart is dependent on the level of aortic pressure, but it may be defined as the tension or stress developed in the wall of the ventricle during ejection. Therefore, the afterload on the ventricular muscle fibers also is dependent on the size of the heart, according to the Laplace principle, which indicates that the tension of the myocardial fiber is a function of the product of intracavitary ventricular pressure and the ventricular radius. Thus, at the same level of aortic pressure, the afterload faced during systole by an enlarged left ventricle is higher than that encountered by a ventricle of normal size. The aortic pressure, in turn, is influenced largely

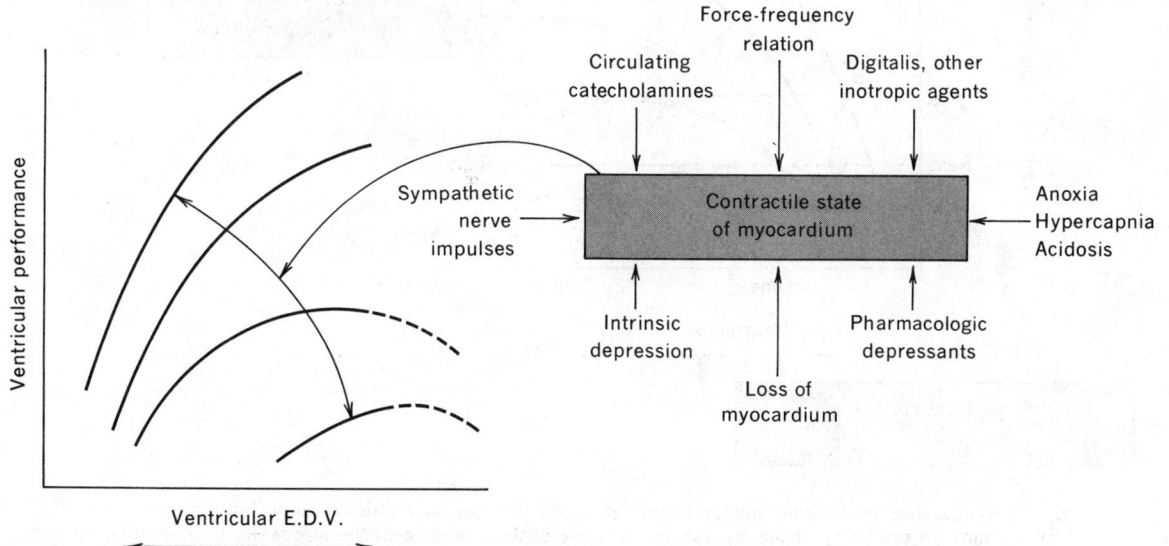

Fig. 263-6. Diagram showing the major influences that elevate or depress the contractile state of the myocardium (top right), and the manner in which alterations in the contractile state of the myocardium affect the level of ventricular performance at any given level of ventricular end-diastolic volume (bottom left). (From Braunwald et al., "Mechanisms of Contraction of Normal and Failing Heart," Boston, Little, Brown and Company, 1968.)

by the peripheral vascular resistance, the physical characteristics of the arterial tree, and the volume of blood it contains at the onset of ejection. At any given ventricular end-diastolic volume and level of the myocardial contractile state, the left ventricular stroke volume is a function of the afterload.

All the influences acting on cardiac performance enumerated above interact in a complex fashion to maintain cardiac output at a level appropriate to the requirements of the metabolizing tissues, and in a normal individual interference with one or even a few of these mechanisms may not influence the cardiac output. For example, a moderate reduction of blood volume or the loss of the atrial contribution to ventricular contraction can ordinarily be sustained without a reduction in cardiac output. Presumably other factors, such as an increase in the frequency of sympathetic nerve impulses reaching the heart, will, in the normal individual augment contractility and sustain output under these circumstances. Mechanisms are also available which prevent elevation of the cardiac output when there is no physiologic demand for augmented flow. For example, expansion of blood volume or augmentation of myocardial contractility by means of cardiac glycosides does not increase the cardiac output in normal man. Thus, in analyzing the effect of an intervention on cardiac output, it is important to recognize that the contractile state of the myocardium is not the factor that limits the volume of blood ejected by the heart in the normal individual and that an improvement of myocardial contractility by a drug which exerts a positive inotropic effect, i.e., improves contractility, such as digitalis, or by a positive inotropic influence, such as paired electrical stimulation, should not be expected to elevate the output in a normal subject. On the other hand, in the presence of congestive heart failure, the cardiac output usually is limited by the depressed contractile state of the myocardium, and a positive inotropic influence would be expected to raise cardiac output.

Exercise

The hemodynamic changes which normally occur during muscular exercise are complex (Fig. 263-7). The hyperventilation of exercise, the pumping action of the exercising muscles, and the venoconstriction which occur, all tend to augment ventricular filling. Simultaneously, the increase in the sympathetic nerve impulses to the myocardium, the increased concentration of circulating catecholamines, and the tachycardia which occur during exercise, all result in an augmentation of the contractile state of the myocardium (Fig. 263-7, curves 1 to 2), and an elevation of stroke volume, with either no change or even a decrease of end-diastolic pressure and volume (Fig. 263-7 points A to B). Vasodilatation occurs in the exercising muscles, thus reducing peripheral vascular resistance and aortic impedance. This ultimately

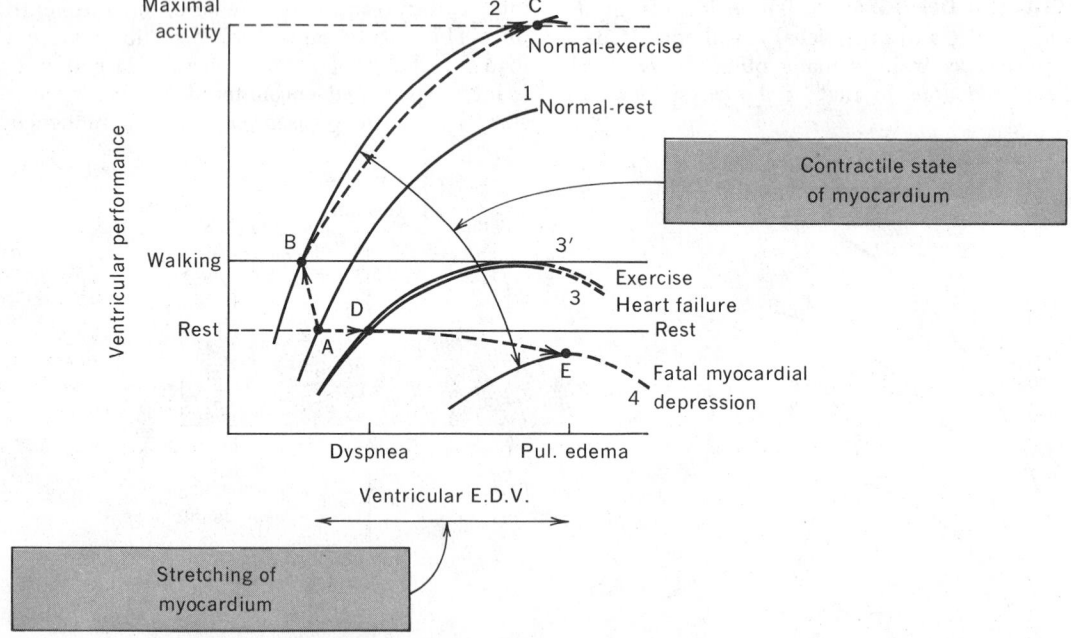

Fig. 263-7. Diagram showing the interrelations between influences on ventricular end-diastolic volume (E.D.V.) through stretching of the myocardium and the contractile state of the myocardium. Levels of ventricular E.D.V. associated with filling pressures that result in dyspnea and pulmonary edema are shown on the abscissa. Levels of ventricular performance required when the subject is at rest, while walking, and during maximal activity are designated on the ordinate. The dotted lines are the descending limbs of the ventricular-performance curves, which are rarely seen during life but which show the level of ventricular performance if end-diastolic volume could be elevated to very high levels. (From Braunwald et al., "Mechanisms of Contraction of Normal and Failing Heart," Boston, Little, Brown and Company, 1968.)

allows the achievement of a greatly elevated cardiac output during exercise, at an arterial pressure which does not differ greatly from that occurring in the resting state.

In heart failure, the fundamental abnormality resides in depressions of the myocardial force-velocity relationship and of the length–active tension curve, reflecting reductions in the contractile state of the myocardium (Fig. 263-7, curves 1 to 3). In many instances, cardiac output and external ventricular performance at rest are within normal limits but are maintained at these levels only because the end-diastolic fiber length and ventricular end-diastolic volume are above normal, i.e., through the operation of the Frank-Starling mechanism (Fig. 263-7, points A to D). The elevations of left ventricular end-diastolic volume and pressure are associated with greater-than-normal levels of the pulmonary capillary pressure, contributing to the dyspnea experienced by patients with heart failure. The normal improvement of contractility which takes place during exercise is attenuated or even prevented by the norepinephrine depletion which occurs in heart failure (Fig. 263-7, curves 3 and 3′). The factors which tend to augment ventricular filling during exercise in the normal subject push the failing myocardium even farther along its flattened length–active tension curve, and although left ventricular performance may be augmented somewhat, this occurs only as a consequence of an inordinate elevation of ventricular end-diastolic volume and pressure and therefore of the pulmonary capillary pressure. The elevation of the latter intensifies dyspnea and therefore plays an important role in limiting the intensity of exercise which the patient can perform. Left ventricular failure becomes fatal when the myocardial length–active tension curve is depressed (Fig. 263-7, curve 4) to the point at which cardiac performance fails to satisfy the requirements of the peripheral tissues even at rest, and/or the left ventricular end-diastolic and pulmonary capillary pressures are elevated to levels which result in pulmonary edema (Fig. 263-7, point E).

THE FAILING HEART

Though heart failure may be readily described as a clinical syndrome, characterized by well-known symptoms and physical signs, a precise physiologic or biochemical definition is far more difficult. However, from the clinical point of view, heart failure may be considered to be the disease state in which an abnormality of myocardial function is responsible for the inability of the heart to pump blood at a rate commensurate with the requirements of the metabolizing tissues. Though a defect in myocardial contraction always exists in heart failure, this disorder may result from a primary abnormality in the heart muscle or it may be secondary to a chronic excessive work load. It is important to distinguish heart failure from (1) states of circulatory insufficiency in which myocardial function is not primarily impaired, such as cardiac tamponade, hemorrhagic shock, or tricuspid stenosis, (2) conditions in which there is circulatory congestion because of abnormal salt and water retention but in which there is no serious disturbance of

myocardial function, and (3) conditions in which the normal heart is suddenly presented with a load which exceeds its capacity, e.g., accelerated hypertension.

The intrinsic contractile state of myocardium removed from normal, hypertrophied, and failing animal hearts has been evaluated, and both ventricular hypertrophy and heart failure were shown to reduce the maximum isometric tension and velocity of shortening to subnormal levels; the changes were more marked in the myocardium of animals in which heart failure had been present than in those with hypertrophy alone. However, ventricular hypertrophy, in the absence of heart failure, appears to be associated with a depression of the contractile state per unit of myocardium, although the absolute increase of total muscle mass maintains cardiac compensation. Papillary muscles removed from the left ventricles of patients with heart failure have also shown a depression of the maximum degree of active tension which they can develop. Electronmicroscopic analysis of failing cat papillary muscles fixed at the apices of the length–active tension curves revealed sarcomere lengths averaging 2.2 μ. Thus, the abnormalities of contractility do not appear to be produced by an alteration in the overlap of filaments within the sarcomere.

The Frank-Starling mechanism, through which an increase in the end-diastolic volume of the ventricle and in its tension are associated with an augmented force of contraction, provides the failing heart with a major compensatory mechanism. The failing ventricle may still eject a normal or nearly normal stroke volume despite considerable depression of function, when its end-diastolic volume increases. As outlined above, an increase in the initial volume of the ventricle is associated with stretching of the sarcomere, a process which augments the number of sites at which the actin and myosin filaments can interact.

Acute heart failure in the intact canine heart, studied in situ or in the heart-lung preparation, is characterized by a depression of ventricular stroke volume or stroke work at any given level of left ventricular end-diastolic volume or filling pressure. Further, as diastolic volume is augmented in the failing heart, an abnormally small increase or no change in stroke volume occurs. Thus, in order to maintain stroke volume at a normal level, the heart dilates and the Frank-Starling mechanism therefore might be considered one of the first lines of defense called upon to maintain cardiac output when myocardial contractility declines. An increase in the end-diastolic volume of the ventricle permits the ejection of a larger stroke volume, even when the extent of shortening of individual muscle fibers remains constant. The fact that in the failing heart the stroke volume is unchanged or is actually diminished when end-diastolic volume is augmented, clearly indicates that a decrease in the relative degree of muscle fiber shortening must have occurred. Thus, an important mechanical defect which can be delineated in acute heart failure is a decrease in the extent to which the cardiac muscle fibers shorten.

A number of techniques are available for defining impaired ventricular contractility in intact man. With the patient at rest, the cardiac output and stroke volume may be depressed, but not uncommonly these variables are within normal limits. A more sensitive index is the ratio of stroke volume to end-diastolic volume, which may be estimated by indicator-dilution techniques or by biplane angiography (Chap. 262), and which is frequently depressed in heart failure even when the stroke volume itself is normal. An even more sensitive method for detecting impaired ventricular performance is based on the measurement of the circulatory changes occurring during stresses such as exercise or increased afterload. Thus, left ventricular performance can be estimated accurately by studying the response of the left ventricular end-diastolic pressure, cardiac output, and total body O_2 consumption at rest and during exercise. In normal individuals, the cardiac output rises by more than 500 ml per min for each 100 ml increase in minute O_2 consumption. The left ventricular end-diastolic pressure at rest is less than 12 mm Hg and rises slightly, remains unchanged, or decreases slightly during exercise, while stroke volume usually rises. The failing left ventricle, on the other hand, is characterized by an elevation of end-diastolic pressure during exercise, which reaches a value exceeding 12 mm Hg, accompanied by either no change or a fall in stroke volume. Various degrees of impairment intermediate between the normal response and that of the failing left ventricle during the stress of exercise also have been described.

Another method, which employs standard cardiac catheterization techniques and provides a practical and useful means for evaluating the functional status of the left ventricle consists of the measurement of stroke volume, arterial pressure, and ventricular end-diastolic pressure before and after ventricular afterload is increased by means of an infusion of angiotensin. Though the normal left ventricle responds to this stress by increasing its stroke work and end-diastolic pressure, in the failing left ventricle the end-diastolic pressure rises markedly, but stroke work either remains constant or actually declines. Thus, as in the acutely failing experimental preparation, the failing human left ventricle appears to exhibit a depression of the relation between end-diastolic pressure and the stroke volume and stroke work which can be achieved. The potential value of stressing the left ventricle in some manner is emphasized by the fact that the basal values for left ventricular end-diastolic pressure, cardiac index, and ventricular stroke work may be in the same range in patients with depressed ventricular function as in normal individuals. The response to these stresses may prove useful not only in the detection of the impairment of myocardial function, but also in expressing the severity of this impairment quantitatively.

The performance of the left ventricle in man may also be characterized by examining the instantaneous myocardial force-velocity relations and the extent of shortening during individual cardiac cycles. Angiocardiographic studies have shown that depressions in the velocity and extent of myocardial fiber shortening exist in human heart failure. Further evidence for the decreases in the velocity of myocardial fiber shortening is provided by the finding of a reduced mean systolic ejection rate in patients with heart failure and a failure of the mean systolic ejection rate to rise normally during muscular exercise.

CARDIAC METABOLISM IN HEART FAILURE

The common forms of low-output heart failure, secondary to arteriosclerosis, hypertension, and certain valvular and congenital lesions, are characterized by an absolute or a relative decrease in the useful external work delivered by the heart. Considerable effort has been directed to the question of whether cardiac failure is due to a defect in the production of energy, its conservation, or its utilization. Only in isolated instances of heart failure, such as those associated with beriberi, are there clear-cut disturbances of myocardial energy production. The major pathway by which pyruvate enters the citric acid cycle and some reactions within the cycle itself are dependent on the presence of adequate concentrations of thiamine (Chap. 81). Thiamine deficiency results in diminished pyruvic acid utilization by heart slices, and in abnormally low pyruvate extraction coefficients in intact dogs and in man.

Coronary sinus catheterization, both in patients with clinical heart failure and in dogs with experimentally produced low-output heart failure, has revealed that the coronary blood flow per gram of myocardium and the myocardial extraction of various substrates and of O_2 do not differ significantly from the normal. Thus, the myocardial defect in the common forms of low-output heart failure does not appear to reside in an impairment of energy production. In the second phase of cardiac metabolism, energy conservation, the energy of substrate oxidation is converted into the terminal-bond energy of creatine phosphate (CP) and of ATP, the immediate source of chemical energy utilized by heart muscle. This process, known as oxidative phosphorylation, occurs in the mitochondria. The effectiveness of the combined energy production-conservation mechanisms may be studied by measuring the stores of ATP and CP existing in the myocardium, while energy conservation can be evaluated by determining (1) the P:O ratio, i.e., the ratio of high-energy phosphate produced to oxygen consumed in the mitochondria, and (2) the degree of coupling between electron transport and the generation of high-energy phosphate compounds. Although lively controversy exists concerning the status of this phase of metabolism in heart failure, it now appears that severe impairment of myocardial performance may occur without disturbances of mitochondrial function or reduction of high-energy phosphate stores.

In the absence of a definitive abnormality of energy liberation or conservation in the failing myocardium, attention has naturally been directed to the possibility that energy utilization is abnormal. The possibility must be considered that an abnormality of excitation-contraction coupling occurs in heart failure, although there are no experimental data available either to support or refute this hypothesis. An abnormality of energy liberation could certainly occur if the contractile proteins themselves were altered, and indeed this was once believed to be the basic biochemical abnormality occurring in congestive heart failure, a theory no longer supported. It has been shown that the ATPase activity of myofibrillar preparations is depressed in heart failure, and it is possible that this depression may be responsible for a defect in energy utilization, i.e., in the breakdown of ATP, the process which leads to the shortening and tension development by the contractile filaments.

THE ADRENERGIC NERVOUS SYSTEM IN HEART FAILURE

In view of the importance of the adrenergic nervous system in stimulating the contractility of the normal myocardium, the activity of this system has also been studied intensively in patients with congestive heart failure. An index of the activity of this system, at rest and during exercise, is provided by measurements of the concentration of norepinephrine (NE) in arterial blood. No change or very little increase in the NE concentrations occurs during exercise in normal subjects; much greater increases are seen in patients with congestive heart failure, presumably because of an increased activity of the adrenergic nervous system during exercise in these patients. Marked elevations of 24-hr urinary NE excretion occur in patients with heart failure, indicating that the activity of their adrenergic nervous systems is also augmented at rest.

The importance of the increased activity of the adrenergic nervous system in maintaining ventricular contractility when the function of the myocardium is depressed in congestive heart failure also is shown by the effects of adrenergic blockade in patients with heart failure. Antiadrenergic drugs such as propranolol or guanethidine may cause sodium and water retention, as well as intensify heart failure. The adrenergic nervous system thus plays an important compensatory role in the circulatory adjustments of patients to congestive heart failure, and caution must be exercised in the use of antiadrenergic drugs in the treatment of patients with limited cardiac reserve.

The concentration of NE in atrial and ventricular tissue removed at operation in patients with heart failure is less than one-third of that observed in the absence of failure. This is a reduction in NE content in the heart and is not the result of a simple dilution of sympathetic nerve endings in a hypertrophied muscle mass.

The biosynthesis of NE proceeds through a series of steps from tyrosine to dopa to dopamine, the immediate precursor of the neurotransmitter. It is now known that tyrosine hydroxylase, which catalyzes the first reaction (tyrosine to dopa), is the rate-limiting enzyme in the synthesis of NE. Marked reductions in the activity of this enzyme recently have been shown to accompany the NE depletion in the myocardium of dogs with experimental heart failure, and it appears likely that this reduction of enzyme concentration is responsible for the cardiac NE depletion in heart failure. It still is not clear,

however, whether or not the sustained increase in sympathetic activity which accompanies heart failure is responsible for the reduction of cardiac tyrosine hydroxylase activity.

Although the mechanism ultimately responsible for the reduction of tyrosine hydroxylase in the heart in congestive heart failure remains to be elucidated, some of the consequences of cardiac NE depletion in heart failure are evident. In view of the strongly positive inotropic effect exerted by the NE released from these nerves, the adrenergic nervous system may be considered to provide an important potential source of support to the failing myocardium. However, it has been observed that with supramaximal stimulation of the cardiac sympathetic nerves, the increments of heart rate and contractile force which occurred in animals with experimental heart failure and cardiac NE depletion are abolished or markedly reduced. Thus, it is likely that when congestive heart failure is accompanied by depletion of cardiac NE stores, the quantity of NE released by the sympathetic nerve endings in the heart is deficient relative to the impulse traffic along these nerves.

It appears that the contractile state of NE-depleted ventricular myocardium is normal and that cardiac stores of NE are therefore not fundamentally necessary for maintaining the intrinsic contractile state of the myocardium. However, if the reduction of NE stores in heart failure is associated with a diminished release of neurotransmitter, as now appears to be the case, then this depletion of NE may be responsible for loss of the much-needed adrenergic support to the congestive heart failure state.

REFERENCES

Braunwald, E., J. Ross, Jr., and E. H. Sonnenblick: "Contraction of the Normal and Failing Heart," Boston, Little, Brown and Company, 1968, 205 pp.

Braunwald, E., J. Ross, Jr., J. H. Gault, D. T. Mason, C. Mills, I. T. Gabe, and S. E. Epstein: Assessment of Cardiac Function, Annals Int. Med., 70:389, 1969.

Davies, R. E.: A Molecular Theory of Muscle Contraction: Calcium-dependent Contractions with Hydrogen Bond Formation plus ATP-dependent Extensions of Part of the Myosin-Actin Cross-bridges, Nature, 199:1068, 1963.

Gergely, J.: "Biochemistry of Muscle Contraction," Boston, Little, Brown and Company, 1964.

Hamilton, W. F., and P. Dow (Ed.), "Handbook of Physiology," Washington, American Physiological Society, 1962.

Huxley, H. E.: The Mechanism of Muscular Contraction, Science, 164:1356, 1969.

Randall, W. C. (Ed.): "Nervous Control of the Heart," Baltimore, The Williams & Wilkins Company, 1965.

Ross, J., Jr., J. W. Covell, E. H. Sonnenblick, and E. Braunwald: Contractile State of the Heart Characterized by Force-Velocity Relations in Variably Afterloaded and Isovolumic Beats, Circulation Res., 18:149, 1966.

Stenger, R. J., and D. Spiro: Structure of the Cardiac Muscle Cell, Am. J. Med., 30:653, 1961.

Tanz, R. D., F. Kavaler, and J. Roberts (Ed.): "Factors Influencing Myocardial Contractility," New York, Academic Press, Inc., 1967.

264 HEART FAILURE
Eugene Braunwald

INTRODUCTION

Heart failure may be defined as the condition in which an abnormality of myocardial function is responsible for the ventricles' inability to deliver adequate quantities of blood to the metabolizing tissues at rest or during normal activity. Although the fundamental cellular abnormality responsible for heart failure has not been elucidated (Chap. 263), the clinical manifestations resulting from this derangement are usually readily recognized, their pathogenesis is, in general, understood, and means for their alleviation in most patients are available. The underlying cause of heart failure must ultimately be traced to abnormal behavior of the myocardial cell. In many patients heart failure results from anatomic lesions of the heart valves or pericardium which interfere with cardiac filling or emptying, or from severe or prolonged disorders of cardiac rate or rhythm. In most of these instances an abnormality of myocardial function results from, or is associated with, the extramyocardial abnormality. For example, in many patients with rheumatic valvular disease and heart failure, the heart muscle has been damaged as a consequence of the rheumatic process, and/or the excessive hemodynamic burden imposed by the valvular abnormality has impaired myocardial function. In patients with chronic constrictive pericarditis, myocardial damage resulting from infiltration of the heart muscle by the pericardial inflammation and calcification is common (Chap. 272).

In some patients, however, a state which closely resembles heart failure occurs without any detectable abnormality in myocardial function. Examples of such conditions are acute pulmonary embolism, acute hypertensive crisis, severe valvular regurgitation due to bacterial endocarditis, and pericardial effusion, occurring in patients with otherwise normal hearts. In such instances, the abnormally elevated hemodynamic load exceeds the ability of even the normal myocardium to pump an adequate quantity of blood to the periphery.

The term *congestive heart failure* is frequently used in clinical medicine because so many of the clinical manifestations of heart failure result from excessive accumulation of fluid. However, effective diuretic therapy is frequently capable of eliminating or markedly reducing these congestive manifestations, while the underlying state of cardiac function may not be altered. Therefore, the simpler term *heart failure* is preferred.

CAUSES OF HEART FAILURE

It is important to identify not only the *underlying etiology* of the heart disease but the *precipitating cause*

of heart failure as well. The cardiac abnormality produced by a congenital or acquired lesion may exist for many years and produce no or only trivial disability. Frequently, however, serious manifestations of clinical heart failure appear for the first time in the course of some acute disturbance which places an additional load on the already excessively burdened myocardium, resulting in further deterioration of cardiac function. Identification of such precipitating causes is of critical importance because their prompt alleviation may be lifesaving. However, in the absence of underlying heart disease these acute disturbances in cardiovascular function do not usually, by themselves, lead to heart failure.

PRECIPITATING CAUSES OF HEART FAILURE

1. PULMONARY EMBOLISM. Patients with low cardiac output, circulatory stasis, and physical inactivity are likely to develop thrombi in the veins of the lower extremities or the pelvis. Pulmonary embolization may result in further acute elevation of pulmonary arterial pressure, which in turn may produce or intensify distension and failure of the right ventricle and may lower the cardiac output further. In the presence of pulmonary vascular congestion, such emboli may lead to infarction of the lung.

2. INFECTION. Patients with elevated pulmonary venous and capillary pressures are particularly susceptible to the development of pulmonary infections. The fever, tachycardia, hypoxemia, and the increased metabolic demands resulting from pulmonary or other systemic infections may place a further burden on the overloaded, but compensated, myocardium of a patient with chronic heart disease and may thereby precipitate heart failure.

3. ANEMIA. The rapid development of a marked reduction in the oxygen-carrying capacity of the blood may precipitate heart failure because in the presence of severe anemia the oxygen needs of the metabolizing tissues can be satisfied only by an increase in the cardiac output. While such an increase in the cardiac output might be sustained by a normal heart, a diseased, overloaded, but otherwise compensated heart may be unable to augment the volume of blood which it delivers to the periphery.

4. THYROTOXICOSIS AND PREGNANCY. Like anemia, these conditions require an increased cardiac output. The development or intensification of heart failure may actually be one of the first clinical manifestations of hyperthyroidism in a patient with underlying heart disease. Similarly, heart failure not infrequently occurs for the first time during pregnancy in women with rheumatic valvular disease, who may remain normally compensated for many years following delivery, after the excessive burden has been eliminated.

5. ARRHYTHMIAS. Persistent cardiac arrhythmias are among the most frequent precipitating causes of heart failure for a variety of reasons: *a*) tachyarrhythmias reduce the time period available for ventricular filling; *b*) the dissociation between atrial and ventricular contractions characteristic of many supraventricular and ventricular arrhythmias results in the loss of the atrial booster pump mechanism, thereby tending to raise atrial pressures; *c*) in ventricular tachycardia or any arrhythmia associated with abnormal intraventricular conduction, myocardial performance is impaired because of the loss of normal synchronicity of ventricular contraction; *d*) the marked bradycardia associated with complete atrioventricular block requires a greatly elevated stroke volume if a marked reduction in cardiac output is to be prevented

6. RHEUMATIC AND OTHER FORMS OF MYOCARDITIS. The development of acute rheumatic fever and a variety of allergic or infectious processes affecting the myocardium may further impair myocardial function in patients with preexisting heart disease.

7. BACTERIAL ENDOCARDITIS. The anemia, fever, additional valvular damage, and myocarditis which often occur as a consequence of bacterial endocarditis may, singly or in concert, precipitate heart failure.

8. PHYSICAL, DIETARY, AND EMOTIONAL EXCESSES. Sudden augmentation of sodium intake, the discontinuation of diuretics or digitalis glycosides, physical overexertion, excessive environmental heat or humidity, and emotional crises, may all precipitate cardiac decompensation.

A careful and systematic search for one or more of these precipitating causes should be made in every patient with heart failure, particularly if it is refractory to the usual methods of therapy. If properly recognized, the precipitating cause of heart failure can usually be treated more effectively than the underlying cause. Furthermore, the prognosis in patients with heart failure in whom a precipitating cause can be identified and treated is far more favorable than in patients in whom the underlying disease process has advanced to the point of producing heart failure.

FORMS OF HEART FAILURE

Heart failure may be described as *high output* or *low output, acute* or *chronic, right-sided* or *left-sided,* and *forward* or *backward.* Although these terms may be useful in a clinical setting, they are entirely descriptive and do not signify fundamentally different disease states.

HIGH–OUTPUT VERSUS LOW–OUTPUT HEART FAILURE. With the development of methods for the measurement of cardiac output, it became useful to classify patients with heart failure into those with a low cardiac output, i.e., *low-output heart failure,* and those with an elevated cardiac output, i.e., *high-output heart failure.* The cardiac output is often depressed in patients with heart failure secondary to coronary artery disease, hypertension, primary myocardial disease, valvular disease, and pericardial disease, but it tends to be elevated in patients with heart failure and hyperthyroidism, anemia, arteriovenous fistulas, beriberi, Paget's disease, and pulmonary emphysema. In clinical practice, however, it may be difficult to distinguish between low-output and high-output heart failure. The normal range of cardiac output is wide (2.6 to 3.6 liters min/m^2), and in many patients with

so-called "low-output heart failure" the cardiac output may actually be within normal limits at rest, although it may fail to rise normally during exertion. On the other hand, in patients with so-called "high-output heart failure" the output may not be excessive but rather may be close to the upper limit of normal, particularly when heart failure is severe. Regardless of the absolute level of the cardiac output, however, cardiac failure may be said to be present when the characteristic clinical manifestations described below are accompanied by a depression of the curve relating ventricular end diastolic volume to cardiac performance. (Chap. 263, Fig. 6).

An integral part of the heart failure syndrome is evidence that the heart does not deliver the quantity of oxygen required by the metabolizing tissues. In the absence of peripheral shunting of blood such inadequate delivery of oxygen to the metabolizing tissues is reflected in an abnormally widened arterial–mixed venous oxygen difference, relative to the total body oxygen consumption. However, this abnormality may not be present at rest and may become evident only during exertion. In patients with the high cardiac output states associated with conditions such as arteriovenous fistula, beriberi, thyrotoxicosis, and Paget's disease, the arterial–mixed venous oxygen difference is often abnormally low because the mixed venous oxygen saturation is raised by the admixture of blood which has been shunted past some of the metabolizing tissues, and it may be presumed that even in these patients the delivery of oxygen to the metabolizing tissues is reduced. When heart failure occurs in such patients the arterial–mixed venous oxygen difference may be normal or even subnormal, but it still exceeds the level which existed prior to the development of heart failure, and therefore the cardiac output, while normal or elevated, is lower than before heart failure occurred.

The mechanisms responsible for the development of heart failure in patients whose cardiac outputs are initially high are complex and depend on the underlying disease process. In most of these conditions the heart is called upon to pump abnormally large quantities of blood in order to deliver the normal quota of oxygen to the metabolizing tissues. This increased flow load exerts an effect on the myocardium which resembles that produced by regurgitant valvular lesions. In addition, thyrotoxicosis and beriberi may impair myocardial metabolism directly, and severe anemia and chronic pulmonary emphysema may interfere with myocardial function by producing myocardial anoxia.

ACUTE VERSUS CHRONIC HEART FAILURE. Frequently there is no fundamental distinction between these two conditions. For example, intensive efforts to prevent expansion of blood volume by means of dietary sodium restriction and the administration of diuretics will frequently delay the development of exertional dyspnea and ankle edema in patients with severe hypertension until an acute episode, such as a small myocardial infarction, an arrhythmia, or further elevation of arterial pressure, results in acute heart failure. Without intensive efforts to restrict blood volume the same patient would have been considered to have been suffering from chronic heart failure, even though his underlying myocardial disease was no further advanced.

RIGHT–SIDED VERSUS LEFT–SIDED HEART FAILURE. Many of the clinical manifestations of heart failure result from the accumulation of excess fluid behind one or both ventricles. This fluid may localize upstream to the specific cardiac chamber which is initially affected. For example, patients in whom the abnormal load is placed on the left ventricle develop dyspnea and othopnea as a result of pulmonary congestion, a condition referred to as *left heart failure*. When heart failure has existed for months or years, such localization behind the failing ventricle may no longer exist. For example, patients with long-standing aortic valve disease or systemic hypertension may have ankle edema, congestive hepatomegaly, and systemic venous distension late in their course, despite the fact that the abnormal hemodynamic burden initially was placed on the left ventricle. In contrast, when the underlying abnormality affects the right ventricle primarily, e.g., valvular pulmonic stenosis or pulmonary hypertension secondary to pulmonary thromboembolism, symptoms resulting from pulmonary congestion such as orthopnea, or paroxysmal nocturnal dyspnea are unusual, even late in the course of the disease. However, severe exertional dyspnea or even dyspnea at rest may be observed in such patients.

Thus, although specific lesions may place an abnormal load on one or the other ventricle, when this load is prolonged, failure of the heart as a whole occurs. Perhaps this is because the muscle bundles composing both ventricles are continuous and both ventricles share a common wall, the interventricular septum. Also, biochemical changes which occur in heart failure and which may contribute to the impairment of myocardial function, such as norepinephrine depletion and alterations in the activity of myofibrillar ATPase, occur in the myocardium of both ventricles, regardless of the specific chamber on which the abnormal hemodynamic burden is placed.

BACKWARD VERSUS FORWARD HEART FAILURE. For many years there has been a controversy which has revolved around the mechanism of the clinical manifestations resulting from heart failure. The concept of *backward heart failure*, originated by James Hope in 1832, contends that when heart failure occurs, one or the other ventricle fails to discharge its contents normally, the end diastolic volume of that ventricle rises, and the pressures and volumes in the atrium and venous system behind the failing ventricle become elevated. According to this concept, retention of sodium and water occurs as a consequence of the elevation of systemic venous and capillary pressures, and the resultant transudation of fluid into the interstitial space, as well as from increased renal tubular reabsorption of sodium associated with an elevation of renal venous pressure.

In contrast, the proponents of the *forward heart failure* hypothesis, expounded by MacKenzie in 1913, maintain that the clinical manifestations of heart failure result directly from an inadequate discharge of blood into the arterial system. Salt and water retention, according to this concept, is a consequence of diminished renal perfusion, which not only results in the reduction of glomerular filtration rate, but which also stimulates sodium reabsorption through activation of the renin-angiotensin-aldosterone system.

The rigid distinction between *backward heart failure* and *forward heart failure* is artificial, since both mechanisms appear to operate to varying extents in most patients with chronic heart failure. However, the rate of onset of heart failure often influences the clinical manifestations. For example, when a large portion of the left ventricle is suddenly destroyed, as in myocardial infarction, acute pulmonary edema may develop rapidly, and although stroke volume is reduced, the patient may die of acute pulmonary edema before the reduced cardiac output can be responsible for the renal retention of salt and water. However, if the same patient survives the acute insult, clinical manifestations resulting from the abnormal retention of fluid within the systemic vascular bed will develop. Similarly, the right ventricle may dilate and the systemic venous pressure may rise to high levels immediately following acute massive pulmonary embolism, but this state may have to be maintained for some days before sodium and water retention sufficient to produce edema occurs.

FLUID RETENTION IN CHRONIC HEART FAILURE

When the volume of blood pumped by the left ventricle into the systemic vascular bed is chronically reduced, and when one (or both) ventricle fails to expel the normal fraction of its end diastolic volume, a complex sequence of adjustments occurs which ultimately results in the abnormal accumulation of fluid. While, on the one hand, many of the clinical manifestations of heart failure are secondary to this excessive retention of fluid, on the other hand, this abnormal fluid accumulation constitutes an important compensatory mechanism which tends to maintain cardiac output and therefore perfusion of the vital organs. Except in the terminal stages of heart failure, the myocardium operates on an ascending, albeit depressed, function curve, and the augmented ventricular end-diastolic volume and pressure characteristic of heart failure must be regarded as aiding the maintenance of cardiac output. The expansion of the intravascular blood volume, regardless of the mechanism responsible, tends to elevate ventricular end-diastolic volume and, by the operation of the Frank-Starling principle, tends to augment ventricular performance. On the other hand, the maintenance of right ventricular end-diastolic volume and pressure at elevated levels raises systemic venous and capillary pressures, resulting ultimately in transudation of fluid from the vascular bed and edema formation (Chap. 34).

The redistribution of left ventricular output also serves as an important compensatory mechanism in the presence of severe impairment of cardiac function. This redistribution occurs when cardiac output is limited during the imposition of an additional burden, such as exercise, fever, or anemia in a patient with impaired myocardial function, but as heart failure advances, redistribution occurs even in the basal state. Blood flow is redistributed so that the delivery of oxygen to vital organs, such as the brain and myocardium, is maintained at normal or near normal levels, while blood flow to less critical areas, such as the cutaneous and muscular beds, the kidneys and splanchnic organs is reduced. Vasoconstriction mediated by the sympathetic nervous system is primarily responsible for this redistribution of peripheral blood flow. Renal vascular resistance rises, primarily as a consequence of efferent arteriolar constriction. There is a diminution of renal cortical blood flow and a drop in glomerular filtration rate, but the drop is proportionately less than that of the renal plasma flow, hence, the filtration fraction rises. The renin-angiotension system is activated, which in turn augments aldosterone secretion by the adrenal cortex. Also, in the presence of hepatic venous congestion, the metabolism of aldosterone by the liver is impaired, and therefore, in some patients with heart failure, the tubular reabsorption of sodium is increased due to augmented circulating aldosterone. While this by itself may not be sufficient to produce retention of salt and water, when accompanied by the abnormal renal hemodynamics characteristic of heart failure, the elevated aldosterone levels will result in abnormal sodium and hence fluid accumulation. The presence of augmented mineralocorticoid activity in heart failure is reflected in low concentrations of sodium in the urine, sweat, and saliva and by the finding that regardless of the total quantity of sodium presented to the proximal tubule, patients with heart failure have an enhanced tubular reabsorption of sodium.

The importance of elevated systemic venous pressure and of the aforementioned alterations of renal function vary in their relative importance in the production of edema in different patients with heart failure. In patients with tricuspid valve disease or constrictive pericarditis the elevated venous pressure appears to play the dominant role. On the other hand, severe edema may be present in patients with ischemic or hypertensive heart disease, in whom systemic venous pressure is within normal limits or is only minimally elevated. In such patients, the fluid retention is probably due primarily to a redistribution of cardiac output and a concomitant reduction in renal perfusion. Regardless of the mechanisms involved in fluid retention, patients with congestive heart failure have elevations of total blood volume, interstitial fluid volume, and body sodium. These abnormalities diminish, but may not disappear even after clinical compensation has been achieved by treatment.

CLINICAL MANIFESTATIONS OF HEART FAILURE

DYSPNEA. *Dyspnea,* or respiratory distress which occurs as the result of increased effort in breathing, is the most common symptom of heart failure (Chap. 32). It is at first observed only during activity, when it may simply represent an aggravation of the breathlessness which normally occurs under these circumstances. As heart failure advances, however, dyspnea appears with progressively less strenuous activity. Ultimately, breathlessness is present even when the patient is at rest. Thus, the chief difference between exertional dyspnea in normal individuals and in cardiac patients is the degree of activity necessary to induce the symptom. Cardiac dyspnea is observed most frequently in patients with elevations of left atrial, pulmonary venous, and pulmonary capillary pressures. In such patients there is engorgement of the pulmonary vessels and interstitial pulmonary edema, which reduces the compliance of the lungs and thereby increases the work of the respiratory muscles required to inflate the lungs. The Hering-Breuer reflex which inhibits inspiration is enhanced, resulting in the rapid, shallow breathing of cardiac dyspnea. In patients with dyspnea due to heart failure there is increased oxygen cost of breathing because of the excessive work of the respiratory muscles. This is coupled with the diminished delivery of oxygen to these muscles, which occurs as a consequence of the reduced cardiac output; hence inadequate oxygenation of the respiratory muscles may contribute to the sensation of shortness of breath.

ORTHOPNEA. *Orthopnea,* i.e., dyspnea in the recumbent position, is also characteristic of those forms of heart failure associated with elevations of pulmonary venous and capillary pressures. While orthopnea is usually a symptom of more advanced heart failure than exertional dyspnea, in patients who are physically inactive, the development of orthopnea may actually precede dyspnea. Orthopnea results from the redistribution of blood from the lower extremities and the splanchnic bed to the lungs as the result of the alteration in gravitational forces acting on vascular beds when the recumbent position is assumed. This augmentation of intrathoracic blood volume reduces the vital capacity and elevates pulmonary venous and capillary pressures.

The patient with orthopnea generally elevates his head on several pillows at night and frequently awakens short of breath if his head has slipped off the pillows. The sensation of breathlessness usually is relieved by sitting bolt upright, and many patients report that they find relief from sitting in front of an open window. As heart failure advances orthopnea may be so severe that patients cannot lie down at all and must spend the entire night in a sitting position. On the other hand, in other patients with heart failure, symptoms of pulmonary congestion may diminish as the function of the right ventricle becomes impaired.

PAROXYSMAL (NOCTURNAL) DYSPNEA. Also known as *cardiac asthma,* this term refers to an attack of severe shortness of breath which generally occurs at night and usually awakens the patient from sleep. The respirations are frequently wheezing. The attack is precipitated by stimuli which aggravate the previously existing pulmonary congestion; frequently there is augmentation of total blood volume at night due to the reabsorption of edema from dependent portions of the body which occurs with recumbency; the redistribution of blood volume which takes place results in an increase in intrathoracic blood volume and therefore produces pulmonary congestion. With the patient asleep, relatively severe pulmonary engorgement can be tolerated and he may awaken only when actual pulmonary edema and bronchospasm have developed. The patient awakens with the feeling of suffocation. While simple orthopnea may be relieved by sitting upright at the side of the bed with legs dependent, in the patient with paroxysmal nocturnal dyspnea coughing and wheezing often persist in this position. The depression of the respiratory center during sleep may reduce ventilation sufficiently to lower arterial oxygen tension, particularly in patients with interstitial lung edema and reduced pulmonary compliance. Also, ventricular function may be further impaired at night because of reduced adrenergic stimulation of myocardial function. Acute pulmonary edema is a severe form of cardiac asthma due to further elevation of pulmonary capillary pressure and associated with extreme shortness of breath, rales over both lung fields, and the transudation and expectoration of blood-tinged fluid. If not treated promptly (p. 1141) acute pulmonary edema may be fatal.

CHEYNE–STOKES RESPIRATION. Also known as periodic or cyclic respiration, Cheyne-Stokes respiration is characterized by diminished sensitivity of the respiratory center. In this form of respiration there is an apneic phase, during which the arterial P_{O_2} falls and the arterial P_{CO_2} rises. This combination of changes in the arterial blood stimulates the depressed respiratory center, resulting in hyperventilation and hypocapnia, followed in turn by apnea. Cheyne-Stokes respiration occurs most often in patients with cerebral atherosclerosis and other cerebral lesions, but the prolongation of the circulation time from the lung to the brain which occurs in heart failure, particularly in patients with hypertension and coronary artery disease and associated cerebral vascular disease, also appears to precipitate this form of breathing.

FATIGUE AND WEAKNESS. These are nonspecific but common symptoms of heart failure and are related to the reduction of cardiac output. Anorexia and nausea associated with abdominal pain and fullness are frequent complaints in patients with severe heart failure, and may be related to the enlarged, congested liver.

CEREBRAL SYMPTOMS. In severe heart failure, particularly in elderly patients with accompanying cerebral arteriosclerosis and arterial hypoxemia, there may be alterations in the mental state characterized by confusion, difficulty in concentration, and impairment of memory.

PHYSICAL FINDINGS IN HEART FAILURE

In mild heart failure the patient appears to be in no distress at rest except that he may become uncomfortable if asked to lie flat for more than a few minutes. In more severe heart failure the pulse pressure may be diminished, reflecting a reduction in stroke volume, and occasionally the diastolic arterial pressure may be elevated as a consequence of generalized vasoconstriction. There may be cyanosis of the lips and nail beds (Chap. 33) as well as peripheral pallor and diaphoresis. Sinus tachycardia is common, as well as evidence of congested neck veins, which fill from below and which become distended with sustained pressure on the liver (positive hepatojugular reflux). *Systemic venous pressure* is often abnormally

elevated in heart failure and may be recognized most readily by observing the extent of distension of the jugular veins. In the early stages of heart failure the venous pressure may be normal at rest but may become abnormally elevated during and immediately after exertion.

Early diastolic and presystolic gallop sounds (Chap. 259) are often audible, and *pulsus alternans,* i.e., a regular rhythm in which there is alternation of strong and weak cardiac contractions and therefore alternation in the strength of the peripheral pulses, may be present. Pulsus alternans may be detected by palpation or by sphygmomanometry; it frequently follows an extrasystole and is observed most commonly in patients with cardiomyopathy or with hypertensive or ischemic heart disease. It is caused by a reduction in the number of contractile units during weak contractions and/or by alternation in the ventricular end-diastolic volume.

BASAL PULMONARY RALES. Moist, inspiratory, crepitant rales and dullness to percussion over the posterior lung bases are common in patients with heart failure and elevated pulmonary venous and capillary pressures. In patients with pulmonary edema, rales may be heard widely over both lung fields, and are frequently coarse, sibilant and may be accompanied by expiratory wheezing.

CARDIAC EDEMA. Cardiac edema is usually dependent, occurring in the legs symmetrically, particularly in the pretibial region and ankles in ambulatory patients, and in the sacral region of individuals at bed rest. Pitting edema of the arms and face occur rarely and only late in the course of heart failure.

HYDROTHORAX. Pleural effusion in congestive heart failure results from the elevation of pleural capillary pressure and transudation of fluid into the pleural cavities. Since the pleural veins drain into both the systemic and pulmonary veins, hydrothorax is observed most commonly in patients with marked elevations of pressure in both venous systems, but it may also occur with marked elevation of pressure in either venous bed. Hydrothorax is noted more frequently in the right pleural cavity than the left.

ASCITES. Ascites also occurs as a consequence of transudation and results from increased pressure in the hepatic veins and the veins draining the peritoneum (Chap. 46). Ascites occurs most frequently in patients with tricuspid valve disease and with constrictive pericarditis.

CONGESTIVE HEPATOMEGALY. An enlarged, tender, pulsating liver also accompanies systemic venous hypertension and is observed not only in the same conditions in which ascites occurs, but also in milder forms of heart failure of any etiology. When systemic venous hypertension and hepatomegaly are prolonged and severe, enlargement of the spleen may also occur.

JAUNDICE. This is a late finding in congestive heart failure and is associated with elevations of both the direct and indirect reacting bilirubin; it results from impairment of hepatic function secondary to hepatic congestion and the hepatocellular hypoxia associated with central lobular atrophy.

CARDIAC CACHEXIA. With severe, chronic heart failure there may be serious weight loss and cachexia due to (1) elevation of the metabolic rate, which results in part from the extra work performed by the respiratory muscles, the increased oxygen needs of the hypertrophied heart, and the discomfort associated with severe heart failure; (2) anorexia and abdominal fullness, and (3) some impairment of intestinal absorption.

Roentgenographic Findings in Heart Failure

The chest roentgenogram is among the most important laboratory tests in the diagnosis of heart failure. In addition to the enlargement of the particular chambers characteristic of the lesion responsible for heart failure, vascular changes in the lung fields are common in patients with heart failure and elevated pulmonary vascular pressures. In *acute pulmonary edema* there usually is marked mottling which extends out from the hilar regions and may cover both lung fields. With less severe heart failure there may be increased opacity of the hilar regions and dilatation of all central vessels, particularly the veins draining the upper lung fields. Constriction of the arteries and veins to the lower lung zones may occur. The roentgenogram may also present a "ground glass" appearance with cloudy lung fields due to diffuse interstitial edema. Prolonged elevation of pulmonary venous pressure in excess of 20 mm Hg results in visible, dilated lymphatics (Kerley B Lines), i.e., thin horizontal lines most clearly evident at the bases of the lungfields. Prolonged interstitial edema may also produce nodular deposits due to pulmonary hemosiderosis. Pleural effusions may be present and associated with interlobar effusions.

In patients with heart failure associated with systemic venous hypertension, the roentgenogram may show distension of the superior vena cava, hydrothorax, and occasionally evidence of pulmonary infarction.

CLINICAL MANIFESTATIONS OF HIGH CARDIAC OUTPUT STATES ASSOCIATED WITH HEART FAILURE

THYROTOXICOSIS. In some persons, the characteristic clinical features of hyperthyroidism are so conspicuous even after the development of heart failure that the diagnosis is simple on clinical grounds (Chap. 89). In others, when eye phenomena and thyroid enlargement are not striking and other classic manifestations of thyrotoxicosis are obscured and masked by the antagonistic effects of cardiac failure, it is not surprising that the overactivity of the thyroid is hardly discernible. Nevertheless, thyrotoxicosis should be suspected as a contributing factor in patients with cardiac disease under the following circumstances: persistent tachycardia that endures after prolonged rest and during sleep; any suggestion of heart failure with a high cardiac output in the absence of other recognizable causes; lack of the usual measures in the management of failure to bring about a satisfactory response. Attacks of paroxysmal atrial fibrillation or the presence of chronic atrial fibrillation in a person without mitral stenosis, particularly when the ventricular rate is resistant to the slowing effect of full doses of digitalis, should be suspected to be due to hyperthyroidism because atrial fibrillation occurs in approximately 60 percent of patients over the age of forty-five with hyperthyroidism.

After treatment has been instituted and the euthyroid state restored, remarkable improvement in a previously intractable form of heart disease usually follows. The rhythm in about one-third of those with fibrillation reverts spontaneously to a normal sinus mechanism; angina and congestive failure disappear or become easily controllable.

Diagnosis. Estimation of the basal metabolic rate and of the serum cholesterol level is subject to so many influences unrelated to the activity of the thyroid that it is of little value. A circulation time that is within the normal range in a person suffering from congestive failure is highly suggestive of some type of high-output failure; but the most reliable methods of diagnosis are the determinations of the protein-bound iodine of the plasma and of radioiodine studies (Chap. 89). Finally, the diagnosis should be confirmed by a favorable response to therapy directed at the hyperthyroidism.

HEART FAILURE SECONDARY TO ANEMIA. The clinical picture is that of high-output failure with anemia. Cardiac enlargement, occasionally with hypertrophy; unusually pronounced systolic murmurs because of the combined effects of decreased viscosity, increased flow, and dilatation of the mitral ring; rarely an early diastolic rumbling murmur at the mitral area, due to increased flow, or an aortic diastolic blowing murmur, presumably due to dilatation of the aortic ring, may present a confusing problem of diagnosis. Furthermore, when slight fever is also present, subacute bacterial endocarditis may be mimicked. In patients with sickle-cell anemia with fever and joint pains, acute rheumatic fever may be suspected.

When there is an organic obstruction in a coronary artery, the compensatory increase in coronary flow that would otherwise take place in anemia is prevented and angina may appear; alternatively, anemia may aggravate already existing angina.

HEART FAILURE SECONDARY TO THIAMINE DEFICIENCY (BERIBERI). Thiamine deficiency (Chap. 81) leads to a deficiency of cocarboxylase and results in impaired myocardial energy production. The defect in the peripheral tissues causes a peripheral vasodilatation, increased venous return and cardiac output, and consequently, an increased load on a heart already handicapped by the metabolic defect. Cardiac failure is more likely to occur in persons who have the least involvement of the nervous system and a greater capacity for work, i.e., who have a greater opportunity to develop an increased load on the heart.

The usual clinical picture of beriberi heart disease, as seen in the Orient, is characterized by enlargement of the heart, absence of arrhythmia, systemic venous hypertension, bounding arterial pulsations, and the classical phenomena of heart failure with a high cardiac output.

This picture is rarely encountered in the occidental countries; in these areas the more common description is that of an individual who has been on a clearly deficient diet over a long period of time, who has had an excessive consumption of alcohol, who has heart disease of uncertain origin, heart failure that does not respond to the usual methods of treatment, signs of mild peripheral neuritis, or other manifestations of dietary deficiency, and whose heart failure and cardiac enlargement disappear with the administration of thiamine.

It is evident that the diagnosis depends mostly on securing a good dietary history and on observing the response to treatment. Beriberi heart disease should be suspected when heart failure with a normal or elevated cardiac output is observed in the absence of thyrotoxicosis or anemia. Furthermore, thiamine deficiency may contribute to the development of heart failure in all alcoholics.

Differential Diagnosis

The diagnosis of congestive heart failure can be established by observing some combination of the clinical manifestations of heart failure, enumerated above, together with the findings characteristic of one of the etiologic forms of heart disease. Heart failure may be difficult to distinguish from pulmonary disease. Patients with dyspnea secondary to pulmonary disease may, like patients with heart failure, be more dyspneic in the supine than in the erect position, but they do not usually have episodes of paroxysmal nocturnal dyspnea. Occasionally, a therapeutic test with dietary salt restriction, digitalis, and diuretics may be helpful in differentiating dyspnea of cardiac from that of pulmonary disease, since the latter is not alleviated by these measures. A prolonged arm-to-tongue circulation time is characteristic of low output heart failure, while in patients with pulmonary disease the circulation time is normal. The performance of pulmonary function tests, cardiac catheterization, and angiocardiography occasionally may be necessary to distinguish these two forms of dyspnea. Angle edema may be due to varicose veins, cyclical edema, or gravitational effects, but in these patients there is no generalized systemic venous hypertension, either at rest, following exertion, or with pressure over the liver. Edema secondary to renal disease can usually be recognized by appropriate renal function tests and urine analysis and is rarely associated with elevation of the venous pressure. Enlargement of the liver and ascites occur in patients with hepatic cirrhosis, but may also be distinguished from heart failure by a normal antecubital venous pressure and absence of a positive hepatojugular reflux.

Prognosis

The prognosis in heart failure depends primarily on the nature of the underlying heart disease and on the presence or absence of a precipitating factor which can be treated. When one of the latter can be identified and removed, the outlook for immediate survival is far better than if heart failure occurs without any obvious precipitating cause. The prognosis can also be estimated by observing the response to treatment. When clinical improvement occurs with only modest dietary sodium restriction and/or digitalis without the administration of diuretics, then the outlook is far better than if intensive diuretic therapy is necessary. The long-term prognosis for heart failure is most favorable when the underlying form of heart disease can be treated, as for example thyrotoxic heart disease in which thyroid suppression is effective, or constrictive pericarditis which can be corrected surgically.

TREATMENT OF HEART FAILURE

The treatment of heart failure may be divided into three components: (1) Removal of the precipitating cause of heart failure. (2) Correction of the underlying cause of heart failure. (3) Control of the congestive heart failure state. The first two are discussed elsewhere, together with each specific disease entity or complication. The third component of the treatment of heart failure can, in turn, be divided into three categories: (a) reduction of the cardiac work load; (b) enhancement of myocardial contractility; and (c) control of excessive fluid retention. The first two of these forms of therapy should be utilized simultaneously and then the third should be applied if abnormal fluid accumulation persists. The vigor with which each of these measures is pursued in any individual patient should depend upon the severity of the heart failure state. Following effective treatment, heart failure may be prevented by continuing those measures that were originally effective.

Reduction of the Cardiac Work Load

A reduction in physical activity in mild cases and rest in bed or in a chair in severe failure remain cornerstones in the treatment of heart failure. Meals should be small in quantity, and every effort should be made to diminish the patient's anxiety. Physical and emotional rest tend to lower arterial pressure, diminish the work of the respiratory muscles, slow heart rate, and reduce the load on the myocardium by diminishing the requirements for cardiac output. These influences act in concert to diminish the need for redistribution of the cardiac output, and in many patients, particularly those with mild heart failure, simple bed rest and mild sedation often result in an effective diuresis.

Rest at home or in the hospital should be maintained for one to two weeks in patients with overt congestive failure and should be continued for several days after the patient's condition has stabilized. The hazards of phlebothrombosis and pulmonary embolism which occur with bed rest may be reduced with anticoagulants, leg exercises, and elastic stockings. Heavy sedation should be avoided, but small doses of barbiturates or tranquilizers may be helpful in calming the emotionally disturbed patient with heart failure through the first few days of therapy and in allowing essential sleep. In patients with chronic, mild heart failure, bed rest on weekends will frequently allow continuation of gainful employment. Following recovery from heart failure, a careful assessment of the patient's activities must be made, and in many instances his work load and responsibilities must be reduced. Intermittent rest during the day and the avoidance of strenuous exertion are helpful.

Weight reduction by restriction of caloric intake in the obese patient with heart failure also diminishes cardiac work load and should be part of the therapeutic program in the overweight patient with heart failure.

Enhancement of Myocardial Contractility

The improvement of myocardial contractility by means of cardiac glycosides is the second of the three cornerstones in the control of the heart failure state. The pharmacology, indications, contraindications, and methods of administration of glycosides are considered in detail in Chap. 266. Digitalis is most effective in the common forms of heart failure associated with an excess hemodynamic burden, such as hypertension and valvular heart disease, as well as in ischemic heart disease. It is particularly effective in the treatment of patients with atrial fibrillation or atrial flutter and rapid ventricular rates associated with heart failure. In such patients the slowing of the ventricular rate, resulting from prolongation of the refractory period of the atrioventricular node, combined with the improved contractile state of the myocardium results in striking and rapid clinical improvement. However, even in patients without these arrhythmias digitalis produces considerable clinical improvement as a consequence of its positive inotropic action.

Cardiac glycosides are less effective in diseases primarily affecting the myocardial cell, such as the toxic and infectious myocarditis, the various forms of cardiomyopathy and fibroelastosis, and in those forms of heart failure which are precipitated by infection, fever, anemia, thyrotoxicosis, beriberi, acute rheumatic fever, complete atrioventricular block, and cor pulmonale. Digitalis is contraindicated in patients with second degree or unstable atrioventricular block and in patients with idiopathic hypertrophic subaortic stenosis (Chap. 273).

Three sympathomimetic amines which act largely on beta-adrenergic receptors—epinephrine, isoproterenol, and dopamine—have been demonstrated to improve myocardial contractility in various forms of heart failure. Dopamine, the immediate precursor of norepinephrine, appears to be most effective, since it also produces renal vasodilation by a nonadrenergic mechanism and thereby augments sodium excretion. It increases cardiac output substantially but lowers peripheral resistance slightly. It is administered by constant intravenous infusion, in doses ranging from 100 to 1,000 μg per min. It has been found useful in intractable heart failure, particularly in patients with myocardial infarction and shock or pulmonary edema.

Control of Excessive Fluid Retention

As already emphasized, many of the clinical manifestations of heart failure are secondary to hypervolemia and expansion of the interstitial fluid volume. When fluid retention due to heart failure first becomes clinically evident, considerable expansion of the extracellular space has already occurred, and heart failure is already advanced. The quantity of extracellular fluid volume is largely dependent on the extracellular sodium content, and treatment aimed at reducing extracellular fluid volume is dependent primarily on lowering total body sodium stores, while fluid restriction, per se, is of less importance. A negative sodium balance can be achieved by reducing the dietary intake and increasing the urinary excretion of this ion with the aid of diuretics. In severe heart failure mechanical removal of extracellular fluid by means of thoracentesis, paracentesis, the insertion of Southey tubes into edematous legs, thoracic duct cannulation, hemodialysis, or peritoneal dialysis may also be employed.

DIET. In patients with mild congestive heart failure, considerable improvement in symptoms may result from the simple reduction of sodium intake, particularly if this measure is accompanied by bed rest. In patients with more severe heart failure the sodium intake must be controlled more rigidly, even when other measures such as cardiac glycosides and diuretics are used, and following recovery from a bout of heart failure, at least moderate sodium restriction should be maintained. The normal diet contains approximately 6 to 10 Gm sodium chloride; this intake can be reduced by half simply by excluding salt-rich foods and salt which is added at the table. Reduction of the ordinary dietary intake to approximately one-fourth of normal may be achieved if, in addition, all salt is omitted from cooking. In patients with severe heart failure, in whom the daily sodium chloride intake is reduced to between 500 and 1,000 mg, milk, cheese, bread, cereals, canned vegetables and soups, some salted cuts of meat and fresh vegetables, including spinach, celery, and beets must be eliminated. A variety of fresh fruit, green vegetables, specially processed breads and milk, and salt substitutes are permissible, but such diets are difficult to keep palatable outside the hospital. Water intake may be ad libitum in all but the most severe forms of congestive heart failure. However, late in the course of heart failure, dilutional hyponatremia may develop in patients who are unable to excrete a water load, sometimes because of excessive secretion of antidiuretic hormone. In such cases water intake as well as sodium intake must be restricted.

Attention must also be directed to the caloric content of the diet. Substantial improvement can result from caloric restriction in obese patients with heart failure, in whom weight loss will reduce the load placed on the myocardium.

On the other hand, in individuals with severe heart failure and cardiac cachexia, an attempt must be made to maintain nutritional intake and to avoid caloric and vitamin deficiencies.

Diuretics

A variety of diuretic agents is available, and in the patient with mild heart failure almost all are effective. The choice of the particular diuretic to be employed depends to some extent on convenience. However, in the more severe forms of heart failure, the selection of diuretics is more difficult, and must take into account any existing abnormalities in the serum electrolytes. When diuretics are used in the treatment of heart failure, hypovolemia must be avoided, since excessive reduction of blood volume may reduce cardiac output, interfere with renal function, and produce profound weakness and lethargy.

THIAZIDE DIURETICS. These agents are the most widely used diuretics in clinical practice because of their effectiveness when administered orally. In patients with chronic heart failure of mild or moderate severity the continued administration of chlorothiazide or one of its many analogues abolishes or diminishes the need for rigid dietary sodium restriction. Thiazides are well absorbed following oral administration; chlorothiazide and hydrochlorothiazide reach their peak action in 4 hr, and diuresis persists for approximately 12 hr. Thiazide agents reduce the tubular reabsorption of sodium by a mechanism which appears to differ from that exerted by the mercurial diuretics. Large quantities of chloride and water follow the unreabsorbed sodium into the more distal tubule. Here, potassium-sodium exchange is enhanced, resulting in a substantial kaluresis. Unlike mercurial diuretics, thiazides fail to increase, and in some instances they reduce free water clearance, supporting the hypothesis that these drugs act on the ascending limb of the loop of Henle, at a site where the urine is normally diluted. The carbonic anhydrase-inhibiting properties of the thiazides are of limited importance and need not be invoked to account for most of the diuretic action. Chlorothiazide is administered in doses of up to 500 mg every 6 hr. Many derivatives of this compound are available but offer few, if any, significant advances over the parent compound.

Potassium depletion represents the chief adverse effect following prolonged administration of chlorothiazide, and can be prevented by the oral supplementation of potassium solutions. However, these are not palatable and may be hazardous in patients with renal failure. Therefore, to control potassium depletion produced by thiazides (as well as by ethacrynic acid and furosemide) intermittent dosage schedules, e.g., omitting the diuretic every third day, and the use of a potassium-retaining diuretic, such as spirolactone or triamterene, may be preferable. The hypokalemia produced by thiazides and other diuretics may seriously enhance the dangers of digitalis intoxication. Other side effects of thiazides include reduction of the excretion of uric acid, which may lead to hyperuricemia, and a hyperglycemic effect, which is particularly troublesome in patients with overt or latent diabetes mellitus. Skin rashes, thrombocytopenia, and granulocytopenia have also been reported.

MERCURIAL DIURETICS. Presumably these diuretics act by releasing inorganic mercury within the tubule cell, which then combines with sulfhydryl enzymes essential for sodium reabsorption. Mercurial diuretics reduce sodium reabsorption and make a greater quantity of sodium available for exchange with potassium in the distal tubule, thus tending to increase the excretion of potassium. However, since they also inhibit the secretion of potassium by the distal tubule, the kaluresis produced is not as severe as it is with the thiazide derivatives. The most commonly used mercurial diuretic, Mercuhydrin, also contains theophylline.

Mercurial diuretics are not particularly effective when given by mouth and require parenteral administration. They are usually administered intramuscularly in doses of 0.5 or 1.0 ml, but may be given intravenously in patients with severe and refractory heart failure. One commonly available mercurial diuretic, Thiomerin, may be administered subcutaneously. Mercurial diuretics result in the loss of greater quantities of chloride than of any other ion and hence may result in a metabolic alkalosis which limits the effectiveness of further administration. Effectiveness may be restored, however, in a patient who is refractory to further mercurial administration, by raising the serum chloride concentration with oral ammonium chloride, 6 to 12 Gm per mouth, in divided doses for 3 to 4 days prior to the administration of the mercurial. Mercurial diuretics may be administered daily to patients with severe heart failure until all clinical evidence of excessive fluid has disappeared, or until hypochloremia or other electrolyte imbalance results in a refractory state. Fatal reactions following intravenous injection have been reported and presumably are due to cardiac arrhythmias. Mercurial diuretics should be administered with caution to patients with renal insufficiency in whom clinical manifestations of mercurialism, i.e., stomatitis, colitis, further renal damage, and salivation have been reported. Skin rash and fever occur rarely.

ALDOSTERONE ANTAGONISTS. The 17-spironolactones resemble aldosterone structurally and act on the distal renal tubule by competitive inhibition of aldosterone. These agents produce a sodium diuresis, and in contrast to mercurial diuretics and particularly to chlorothiazide derivatives, they tend to result in potassium retention. Although hyperaldosteronism exists in some patients with congestive heart failure, the spironolactones are effective even in patients in whom the serum aldosterone concentration is within normal limits. Aldactone A may be administered in doses of 25 to 50 mg three to four times daily by mouth. The maximal effect of this regimen is not observed for approximately 4 days. Spironolactones are most effective when administered in combination with thiazide diuretics. The opposing action of these two classes of drugs on urine and serum potassium makes possible a sodium diuresis without either hyper- or hypokalemia when both agents are administered.

Aldactone should not be administered alone to patients with hyperkalemia, renal failure, or hyponatremia. Reported complications include nausea, epigastric distress, mental confusion, drowsiness, gynecomastia, and erythematous eruptions.

TRIAMTERENE. A phthalidine derivative, triamterene

exerts a renal effect similar to that of the spironolactones; i.e., it prevents sodium reabsorption and interferes with sodium-potassium exchange in the distal tubules. However, its fundamental mechanism of action differs from that of the spironolactones, since it is active in adrenalectomized animals. The effective dose is 100 mg once or twice daily. Side effects include nausea, vomiting, diarrhea, headache, granulocytopenia, eosinophilia, and skin rash. Although, like Aldactone A, the diuretic potency of triamterene is not great, it is extremely effective in preventing the hypokalemia characteristic of thiazide administration.

ETHACRYNIC ACID AND FUROSEMIDE. Ethacrynic acid is an unsaturated ketone derivative of aryloxyacetic acid, while furosemide differs from the thiazides in that the thiadiazine ring has been replaced by a furfuryl group on the amino nitrogen of the anthranilic acid.

These are extremely powerful diuretics which inhibit sodium reabsorption throughout the nephron, but especially in the ascending limb of the loop of Henle. These agents produce increases in the rate of urine formation which may be as high as one-third of the glomerular filtration rate. While other diuretics lose their effectiveness as blood volume is restored to normal levels, ethacrynic acid and furosemide remain effective despite the elimination of excessive extracellular fluid volume. The major side effects of these agents are due to this marked diuretic potency, which may result in circulatory collapse and in reductions in the renal blood flow and glomerular filtration rate. Alkalosis is produced by a large increase in the urinary excretion of chloride and hydrogen and potassium ions. Hypokalemia and hyponatremia may occur, and hyperuricemia is also observed, as with thiazide diuretics.

Both drugs are readily absorbed orally and are excreted in the bile and urine. They are usually effective by mouth, in doses of 50 mg two or four times daily, and intravenously in doses ranging from 10 to 100 mg. Weakness, nausea, and dizziness may accompany both diuretics; ethacrynic acid has been associated with skin rash and granulocytopenia.

These extremely effective diuretics are useful in all forms of heart failure, particularly in otherwise refractory heart failure and pulmonary edema. Both agents have been shown to be effective in patients with hypoalbuminemia, hyponatremia, hypochloremia, hypokalemia, and reductions in the glomerular filtration rate and to produce a diuresis in patients in whom mercurial and thiazide diuretics are ineffective.

The effectiveness of ethacrynic acid or furosemide may be potentiated by spironolactone, triamterene, a thiazide diuretic, a carbonic anhydrase inhibitor, or an osmotic diuretic, such as mannitol. In turn, when used in combination with mercurials or thiazides, ethacrynic acid or furosemide increase the effectiveness of these agents.

CHOICE OF A DIURETIC. The thiazides, administered orally, are the agents of choice in the treatment of chronic cardiac edema of mild to moderate degree in patients without hyperglycemia or hyperuricemia. Mercurial diuretics are useful when a rapid diuresis is desired, particularly in patients who do not respond adequately to orally administered thiazides, and are also valuable in patients with hyperglycemia or hyperuricemia in whom the administration of thiazide diuretics is not advisable. Spironolactones and triamterine are not potent diuretics when used alone, but they are particularly effective when administered along with other diuretics, particularly the thiazides, ethacrynic acid, and furosemide, which by themselves produce marked potassium loss. However, in patients with heart failure and severe secondary aldosteronism, spironolactone may be extremely effective. Ethacrynic acid or furosemide given alone, or with spironolactone or triamterine, are the agents of choice in patients with severe heart failure refractory to other diuretics.

Treatment of Acute Pulmonary Edema

Pulmonary edema is life-threatening and must be considered to be a medical emergency. As is the case for the more chronic forms of heart failure, in the treatment of pulmonary edema, attention must be directed to identifying and removing any precipitating causes of decompensation, such as an arrhythmia or infection. However, because of the acute nature of the problem, a number of additional measures are necessary: (1) Morphine is administered by the subcutaneous, intramuscular, or intravenous routes in doses from 10 to 20 mg, depending upon the severity of the problem. This drug reduces anxiety which tends to perpetuate pulmonary edema and thereby breaks a vicious cycle. Also, morphine exerts a positive inotropic effect and tends to reduce venous return. Naline should be available in case respiratory depression occurs. (2) High concentration of oxygen must be inhaled because the alveolar fluid interferes with oxygen diffusion, resulting in arterial hypoxemia. Therefore, 100 percent oxygen should be administered, preferably under positive pressure. The latter increases intraalveolar pressure and therefore reduces transudation of fluid from the alveolar capillaries and impedes venous return to the thorax, reducing pulmonary capillary pressure. (3) The patient should be maintained in the sitting position, also tending to reduce venous return to the heart. (4) Rotating tourniquets should be applied to the extremities and may be followed by a phlebotomy of 500 ml of blood. (5) Aminophylline (theophylline ethylene diamine) 240 to 480 mg intravenously, is effective by diminishing bronchoconstriction, increasing sodium excretion, and augmenting myocardial contractility. (6) If digitalis has not been administered previously, three-fourths of a full dose of a rapidly acting glycoside, such as ouabain, digoxin, or Lanatoside C, should be administered intravenously (Chap. 266). (7) Intravenous diuretics, such as furosemide or ethacrynic acid (25 to 50 mg.) or mercuhydrin (1 to 2 ml), will, by rapidly establishing a diuresis, reduce circulating blood volume and thereby hasten the relief of pulmonary edema.

REFERENCES

Abelmann, W. H.: Management of Congestive Heart Failure, Disease-A-Month, December, 1965.

Braunwald, E., J. Ross, Jr., and E. H. Sonnenblick: "Mechanisms of Contraction of the Normal and Failing Heart," 1st ed., Boston, Little, Brown and Company, 1968.

Fowler, N. O.: Congestive Heart Failure, chap. 11 in "Cardiac Diagnosis," New York, Harper and Row, Publishers, Incorporated, 1968.

Friedberg, C. K.: Circulatory Failure, part II, pp. 137–482 in "Diseases of the Heart," 3d ed., Philadelphia, W. B. Saunders Company, 1966.

Hurst, J. W.: Heart Failure, Chaps. 11–15 in "Diseases of the Heart and Circulation," 3d ed., Philadelphia, J. B. Lippincott Company, 1966.

Laragh, J. H.: Proper Use of Newer Diuretics, Ann. Intern. Med., 67:606, 1967.

Symposium on Congestive Heart Failure (Parts I and II), Am. J. Cardiol., 22:1, 1968.

Wood, P.: Heart Failure, Chap. 7 in "Diseases of the Heart and Circulation," 3d ed., Philadelphia, J. B. Lippincott Company, 1968.

265 CARDIAC ARRHYTHMIAS

Eugene Braunwald, E. E. Eddleman, Jr., William H. Resnik, and Tinsley R. Harrison

The term *arrhythmia*, as herein employed, is not limited to irregularities of the heartbeat but is applied also to disturbances of rate and of conduction. We shall first present certain broad considerations which apply to arrhythmias in general, and then deal with the specific disorders. Treatment by electrical methods is the topic of a separate chapter (Chap. 267); the mechanism of action of the drugs utilized in the treatment of arrhythmias is considered in Chap. 266.

GENERAL CONSIDERATIONS

ETIOLOGIC FACTORS. Certain disorders are especially likely to occur in the absence of detectable structural disease of the heart. These include sinus arrhythmia, and also sinus bradycardia or tachycardia; atrial and ventricular premature beats; milder forms of first degree block (i.e., P-R intervals of 0.21 to 0.25 sec), and paroxysmal atrial tachycardia. Although a specific agent such as tobacco or coffee can occasionally be identified in the incitement of sinus or atrial tachycardia, the cause will usually remain unknown.

Other arrhythmias are particularly likely to occur in persons with organic disease of the heart. These include fibrillation and tachycardia of the ventricles, atrial flutter and fibrillation, and second and third degrees of atrioventricular block. Although any type of structural cardiac disease may be associated with any arrhythmia, there is a strong statistical correlation between certain disturbances of rhythm and certain underlying processes. For example, atrial fibrillation is particularly frequent in patients with thyrotoxicosis, mitral valve disease, and left atrial enlargement; ventricular tachycardia is most likely to occur in persons with coronary disease, etc. Still other disturbances of the rhythm should immediately arouse the suspicion that a drug is responsible. Ventricular bigeminy—a disorder in which a ventricular premature beat follows every supraventricular beat—and atrial tachycardia with block (p. 1147) are usually due to digitalis therapy, especially when there is coexistent potassium deficiency induced by diuretics (Chap. 266).

A cardiac arrhythmia may be a manifestation of a serious circulatory or metabolic disturbance and should result in a careful, deliberate search for the underlying abnormality, which may be (1) a pathologic process in the myocardium, e.g., a myocardial infarction or myocarditis; (2) involvement of the vascular bed, e.g., leakage from an aortic aneurysm, or pulmonary embolization; (3) a sudden drop in the blood volume, as in gastrointestinal bleeding; (4) an endocrine disturbance, such as thyrotoxicosis or pheochromocytoma; (5) a disturbance in electrolyte metabolism, such as occurs with prolonged vomiting, diarrhea, or diuretic administration; (6) a systemic infection; (7) metastatic disease to the heart, such as a carcinoma of the lung, lymphoma, or melanoma; (8) the rapid development of sudden severe hypoxemia or hypercapnia. Obviously, the treatment of the arrhythmia per se, without identification and management of the underlying abnormality, is unrewarding. Also, relatively little may be gained when treatment is directed at a cardiac arrhythmia which results from a structural abnormality, e.g., a greatly enlarged left atrium in a patient with mitral valvular disease. Effective control of atrial fibrillation under these circumstances might require surgical relief of the mitral stenosis.

MECHANISM OF ARRHYTHMIAS. Many cardiac arrhythmias result from abnormalities in the automaticity of cardiac tissue. Increases in automaticity may result from (1) a more rapid rate of diastolic depolarization (Chap. 260); (2) a more negative threshold potential, i.e., a reduction in the potential which must be reached before the cell is excited; (3) a less-negative maximum diastolic potential; or (4) some combination of these effects. Reductions in automaticity are produced by the opposite changes. Certain arrhythmias, e.g., sinus tachycardia and some ectopic tachycardias, appear to result from increases in automaticity of the sinoatrial node or of pacemaker tissue elsewhere in the heart. Other arrhythmias, such as atrioventricular nodal rhythm or idioventricular rhythm, result from reduction in the automaticity of the sinoatrial node, with control of the cardiac rhythm assumed by a pacemaker which ordinarily exhibits a lower degree of automaticity.

A second important physiologic basis for cardiac arrhythmias results from a disturbance in the conduction of the action potential. Varying degrees of slowing or failure of propagation of the action potential from the atrium across the atrioventricular nodal tissue to the ventricles result in various degrees of atrioventricular block. However, slowing of conduction of the action potential may also be responsible for the development of tachyarrhythmias. Local ischemia or mechanical stresses may diminish conduction through segments of the myocardium so that when an impulse leaves the area of reduced conduction velocity it finds the adjacent myocardium no longer refractory and restimulates it. This so-called *reentry phenomenon* may be responsible for the occurrence of coupled beats, i.e., bigeminal rhythm. If, in addition, there is a unidirectional block in conduction in a diseased area, and if the proper anatomic conditions prevail, reexcitation of normal tissue may be followed by the reexcitation of the diseased area and a self-sustaining ectopic rhythm.

For a number of years the evidence supporting the circus movement as the explanation for atrial flutter and fibrillation seemed to be indisputable, but this theory was replaced by the concept that these ectopic rhythms are the result of very rapid and irregular stimuli being discharged from a single focus. Actually, this latter view was an elaboration, based on rather extensive experimental work, of a hypothesis that had preceded that of the circus movement. At the present time there is abundant evidence in favor of and in refutation of both concepts, and it is possible that each is partly true. Further evidence for any hypothesis appears necessary before the mechanism or mechanisms may be considered established.

Arrhythmias frequently occur as a consequence of *electrolyte disturbances*. In clinical situations, these are rarely isolated but usually involve a number of electrolytes, and in practice it may therefore be difficult to determine the specific ion abnormality responsible for the arrhythmia. *Hyperkalemia* leads to atrioventricular block and impairment of intraatrial and intraventricular conduction, with prolonged P waves and QRS complexes. Death occurs from ventricular fibrillation or, less commonly, from ventricular standstill. *Hypokalemia* may produce atrial and ventricular extrasystoles, coupled beats, and tachycardias, as well as mild atrioventricular and intraventricular conduction defects; severe hypokalemia may lead to multifocal premature ventricular contractions deteriorating into ventricular fibrillation. *Hypercalcemia* diminishes conduction velocity and shortens the refractory period, thereby facilitating reentry and the development of ventricular ectopic beats and ventricular fibrillation.

PATHOPHYSIOLOGY

Arrhythmias alter cardiac function by a variety of mechanisms.

EFFECTS OF CHANGES IN HEART RATE. In a resting individual with a normal heart, the cardiac output remains constant, or almost so, despite variations in heart rate from approximately 40 to 160 contractions per minute, with progressive decreases in output at lower and higher rates. In patients with significant myocardial, valvular, or coronary arterial disease, the range of heart rates at which the cardiac output is normal is much narrower. Therefore, the sudden development of a supraventricular tachycardia, with a ventricular rate of 160, or of complete atrioventricular block with a rate of 40, may not alter the resting cardiac output in the absence of serious cardiac impairment. However, such changes in rate may seriously depress cardiac output in patients with heart disease. Also, the response of cardiac output to slow heart rates is dependent on the duration of the bradycardia. Thus, in chronic long-standing heart block, cardiac output may be sustained even at rates as low as 35 beats per min. When increased demands are placed on the heart, as during exertion, infection, or anemia, the heart rate normally accelerates, and in third degree atrioventricular block with a fixed, slow ventricular rate, the cardiac output fails to rise normally.

LOSS OF AN APPROPRIATELY TIMED, VIGOROUS ATRIAL CONTRACTION. The atria are not simply structures which collect blood returning from the venous bed and conduct it to the ventricles. Rather, they should be considered as booster pumps which augment ventricular filling. In many arrhythmias the normal temporal sequence between atrial and ventricular systole is lost. These include all degrees of atrioventricular block, nodal rhythms, ventricular tachycardia, and many instances of atrial tachycardia and flutter. In atrial fibrillation, effective atrial contraction does not occur.

Simple loss of the function of the atrial booster pumps will not usually lower the resting cardiac output in individuals with otherwise normal cardiac function, since compensatory mechanisms such as augmented sympathetic stimulation of the myocardium will maintain the output. However, loss of atrial function will impair the maximal cardiac output which can be achieved during severe exertion. On the other hand, in patients with impaired myocardial function, particularly those with overt or incipient heart failure, atrial function is more critical and loss of the atrial booster pump will result in a lowering of cardiac output, an elevation of atrial pressure, or both. In patients with marked ventricular hypertrophy, such as occurs in hypertension, aortic stenosis, idiopathic hypertrophic subaortic stenosis, and related cardiomyopathies, the atrial contribution to ventricular filling is particularly important, since the thickened ventricular wall resists the inflow of blood. In patients with these lesions the sudden development of one of the aforementioned arrhythmias may seriously impair cardiac performance and depress cardiac output and arterial pressure.

EFFECTS ON MYOCARDIAL OXYGEN CONSUMPTION AND CORONARY BLOOD FLOW. The frequency of cardiac contraction is one of the major determinants of myocardial oxygen consumption (Chap. 11). Hence, when all other factors are constant, tachycardia increases and bradycardia reduces the heart's need for oxygen. Coronary blood flow occurs predominantly during diastole, and since the total number of seconds of diastole per minute is reduced during tachycardia, a rapid heart rate may precipitate myocardial ischemia in the presence of coronary arterial narrowing. In turn, the ischemia may result in angina and in impairment of myocardial function. Conversely, the development of atrioventricular block and a slow ventricular rate often diminishes the severity of angina in patients with coronary artery disease.

EFFECTS ON THE SYNCHRONICITY OF VENTRICULAR CONTRACTION. Ventricular function depends on a synchronous, nearly simultaneous ventricular contraction. Though the ventricular myocardium contracts in ventricular fibrillation, the chaotic nature of the contraction prevents the development of sufficient intraventricular pressure to propel blood forward. Lesser degrees of asynchronicity occur in arrhythmias associated with intraventricular conduction abnormalities, such as ventricular tachycardia, ventricular extrasystoles, and supraventricular tachycardias with bundle branch block. Such asynchronicity of contraction will not impair the cardiac output in an individual with an otherwise normal heart but will exert a significant depressant effect in patients with serious cardiac disease.

EFFECTS ON MYOCARDIAL FUNCTION. Although the responsible mechanism has not been identified, prolonged severe tachycardia can depress myocardial function directly, and this depression may persist even after sinus rhythm has been restored.

Methods of Examination

The most precise method of diagnosis of the various arrhythmias is by electrocardiographic examination. However, the physician who has regularly correlated his observations by simple examination with electrocardiographic tracings can usually recognize many of the arrhythmias at the bedside by physical examination.

The exact heart rate should be measured by auscultation for a full minute. Pulse rate may be misleading because of a pulse deficit. The presence or absence of irregularity should be noted. The intensity of the first heart sound and the amplitude of the peripheral pulse should be observed, and it should be especially noted whether they are constant or variable, as in arrhythmias in which the normal temporal relation between atrial and ventricular contraction is lost, e.g., in complete heart block, ventricular tachycardia, or atrial flutter. Atrial sounds independent of the first and second heart sound are frequently audible in patients with third degree atrioventricular block. If the rhythm is irregular, one should distinguish between a basic cadence that is predictable (regular irregularity, e.g., premature beats) and one that is entirely unpredictable (total irregularity, e.g., atrial fibrillation). In some instances the effect of mild exercise on the heart rate and, likewise, on the degree of irregularity should be observed; whether the deceleration immediately after exercise occurs in the normal gradual fashion (sinus tachycardia) or in one or more abrupt steps (atrial flutter), should also be noted.

Inspection of the jugular pulse will occasionally be helpful, especially when, in a patient with a very slow or rapid rate, an occasional abrupt large venous excursion—"cannon wave"—is seen. This giant "A" wave may occur when the atria and ventricles contract simultaneously. Only rarely, however, will the jugular pulse be of aid in the recognition of atrial flutter. Observation of the effect of massage of the carotid sinus on the electrocardiogram may also be valuable. Brief massage for a few

seconds may cause (1) no change in rate (ventricular tachycardia); (2) an abrupt slowing which persists after discontinuation of massage (atrial tachycardia); (3) a temporary slowing which lasts only during the massage, the rate then returning to the previous level either at once or following a brief period of irregular acceleration (atrial flutter). Carotid massage acts on the atrial mechanism (1) by gradually and temporarily slowing sinus rhythm or by abruptly interrupting a paroxysmal supraventricular tachycardia and/or (2) by increasing atrioventricular block.

Since even the most astute observer may occasionally be mistaken in his interpretation of the bedside findings, an electrocardiogram should be taken whenever there is doubt. Even so, special maneuvers, such as esophageal leads or records during carotid sinus pressure, will sometimes be necessary.

The ECG (electrocardiogram) should be studied systematically. The first and most important problem is whether the arrhythmia is ventricular or supraventricular in origin, a decision often made difficult by the presence of intraventricular conduction disturbances. The presence of P waves or flutter waves and their relation to the QRS complex in the tracing is especially important. P waves most often can be seen best in leads II, III, AVF, and/or those leads taken over the right ventricle. Occasionally, other types of tracings may be necessary. For example, paroxysmal atrial tachycardia in the presence of a bundle branch block is exceedingly difficult to distinguish from ventricular tachycardia. Similarly, flutter impulses may be superimposed on the QRS complex or upon the T wave and make the diagnosis difficult. In these instances, it may be necessary to employ esophageal electrodes or a bipolar anteroposterior lead. The right arm lead is placed over the right ventricle and the left arm lead on the back and the machine set on lead I. Another bipolar chest lead may be used by placing the left arm lead at the apex and the right arm lead over the right ventricle. These simple procedures may obviate the necessity for esophageal leads.

Therapeutic Measures

The success or failure of specific treatment by drugs or by electric shock may be conditioned by appropriate systemic management. A precipitating cause of the arrhythmia (p. 1142) should be sought and treated. Obstruction of the air passages and/or hypoxia should be corrected. The coexistence of circulatory shock, whether of cardiac or peripheral origin, may render the patient's heartbeat refractory to the usual antiarrhythmic drugs. Thus it may be necessary first to restore coronary flow by suitable infusions if the shock was initiated by loss of blood or fluid, or by means of inotropic drugs when the heart is primarily at fault, as is usually the case when a state of shock and an arrhythmia coexist. Since pressor amines tend to induce ectopic rhythms at elevated blood pressure levels, the arterial pressure as well as the ECG should be observed frequently.

Rapidly acting cardiac glycosides such as digoxin,

ouabain, or Cedilanid are useful for the treatment of any of the supraventricular tachycardias except, of course, paroxysmal atrial tachycardia with block, which is frequently caused by digitalis intoxication. The roles of antiarrhythmic drugs and of electric reversion in the treatment of arrhythmias are discussed in Chaps. 266 and 267 and in this chapter in relation to individual arrhythmias. The management of arrhythmias occurring with acute myocardial infarction is discussed in Chap. 271. In general, electrical reversion is most useful in the management of sustained tachyarrhythmias, while antiarrhythmic drugs are indicated when tachyarrhythmias recur after countershock or when there are abnormal rhythms rather than sustained abnormal rhythms.

SPECIFIC DISORDERS OF RATE AND RHYTHM

Derangements Arising in the Sinus Node

Sinus bradycardia is characterized by a slow heart rate (below 50 beats per min) with a normal spread of excitation. This condition is frequent in athletes and is usually a sign of excellent physical fitness. It may also be observed in lesions producing increased intracerebral pressure, in myxedema, and in hypothermic states.

Sinoatrial arrest is due to a sporadic failure of the sinus impulse, and, therefore, there is no ventricular excitation. The electrocardiogram shows a prolonged pause between two P-QRST complexes. It is most frequently due to digitalis or to some other cause of vagal stimulation but may result from myocardial disease. Aside from withholding digitalis and the occasional use of atropine, treatment is usually unnecessary.

Sinoatrial block is an arrhythmia in which regular sinus impulse formation occurs but in which there are no atrial or ventricular depolarizations because the impulse is blocked from reaching these structures. The P-P interval is prolonged to some multiple of the regular interval. Sinoatrial block is infrequently accompanied by atrioventricular block and may be precipitated by digitalis, quinidine, or hyperkalemia.

Sinus arrhythmia may be observed in most healthy young persons at rest; it consists of a quickening of the heart during inspiration and slowing during expiration. It tends to be intensified by deep breathing and to disappear when the breath is held or when the heart rate is increased by exercise or fever. The arrhythmia has no significance.

Sinus tachycardia (Fig. 265-1B), which is characterized by a heart rate faster than 100 beats per min, must be distinguished from the various ectopic tachycardias. The latter group will usually respond to therapy aimed directly at the heart; in sinus tachycardia, the treatment of the rapid rate depends on the management of the underlying condition. A reliable history of abrupt onset and cessation is strong evidence that the attack represents an ectopic tachycardia, rather than sinus tachycardia. However, the patient is often unable to state whether the onset of the tachycardia was absolutely sudden, and still less often is he certain that the ending was abrupt. When the rate is less than 140 beats per min, the odds favor

a sinus tachycardia, but a ventricular rate below 140 is also frequent in patients with atrial tachycardia and AV block, and is seen in some persons with atrial flutter or ventricular tachycardia. Rates of 170 or more per min are almost invariably the result of ectopic rhythms, and the difficulty in distinguishing ectopic from sinus tachycardias is chiefly in the group of patients with heart rates between 140 and 170. Sinus tachycardia also is not as constant as an ectopic tachycardia, and in the former, modest changes in rate can be brought about by exertion and rest. Anxiety, fever, blood loss, or some cause of the tachycardia is usually evident. The response to carotid sinus pressure may help in the differentiation as described above. Sinus tachycardia is slowed slightly but gradually.

Extreme sinus tachycardia is usually due to marked elevation of body temperature, to severe thyrotoxicosis, or to any condition that produces profound circulatory collapse. Frequently, patients with severe advanced obstructive pulmonary emphysema have a sustained tachycardia, usually not over 120 beats per min; however, during episodes of respiratory decompensation initiated by intercurrent pulmonary infections, heart failure, or obstruction of the airways, the tachycardia may reach 160 or more beats per min. Consequently, correcting the underlying systemic abnormality is paramount. A similar problem is often present in patients with chronic lung disease following a pneumonectomy or lobectomy. Maintaining airway patency and ventilation is of fundamental therapeutic significance. Digitalis or other cardiac therapy is of no therapeutic value in patients with sinus tachycardia unless there are manifestations of congestive failure. The problem is discovering the basic cause and correcting it.

Derangements Arising in the Atrium

Ectopic atrial beats (Fig. 265-1A) (premature atrial beats) originate from an abnormal focus in the atrium rather than from the sinus node. Ectopic atrial beats have little clinical significance, but they may precede the onset of sustained atrial arrhythmias. Also, their suppression may prevent the onset of the sustained tachyarrhythmias. Recognition of the atrial ectopic beats is important, since they may be confused at the bedside with the, at times, more serious ectopic ventricular contractions. An electrocardiogram is usually necessary to distinguish between these two disorders. Ectopic atrial beats are easily recognized on the electrocardiogram by the presence of a deformed or inverted P wave preceding a QRS complex of normal duration and configuration. They usually occur prematurely after a normal beat and are followed by an incomplete compensatory pause; however, they are not always premature, and therefore the term ectopic atrial beat is preferred. Occasionally, there may be aberrant intraventricular conduction, in that the QRS complex may be slightly altered in amplitude or configuration and may even resemble the QRS complex of bundle branch block. In these instances, the presence of the P wave preceding the beat serves as the major distinguishing feature from ectopic ventricular contractions.

Atrial rate Ventric rate Rhythm & rate disturbances

Atrial rate Ventric rate Conduction disturbances

A. Ectopic atrial contraction

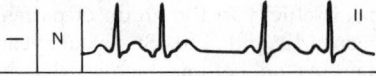

B. Sinus tachycardia

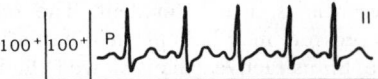

C. Paroxysmal atrial tachycardia

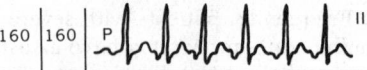

D. Paroxysmal atrial tachycardia with block (2-1)

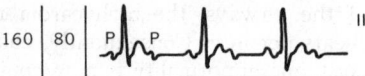

E. Atrial flutter (2:1 block)

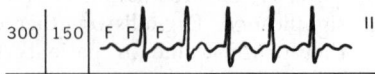

F. Atrial fibrillation

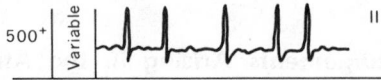

G. Ectopic ventricular contractions

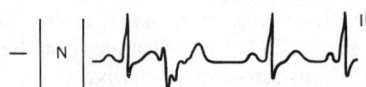

H. Ventricular tachycardia

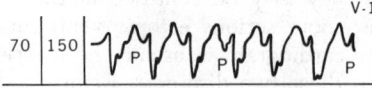

I. Ventricular fibrillation

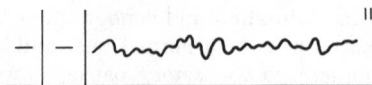

J. First degree heart block

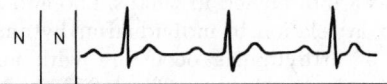

K. Second degree heart block

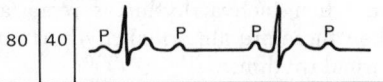

L. Third degree heart block (complete H.B.)

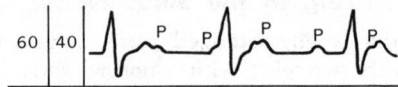

M. Wenckebach

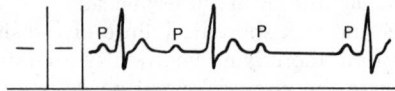

N. Wolff Parkinson White with delta waves

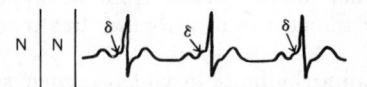

O. Wolff Parkinson White without delta waves

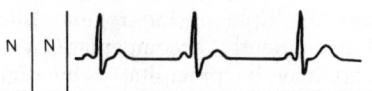

P. Right bundle branch block

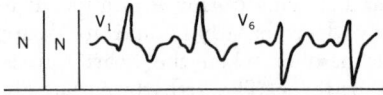

Q. Left bundle branch block

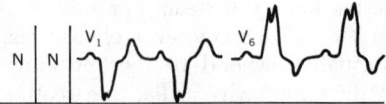

Fig. 265-1.

Paroxysmal atrial tachycardia (Fig. 265-1C) is the most common of the ectopic tachycardias aside from atrial fibrillation. It is generally attributed to rapid discharges from an abnormal atrial pacemaker. Usually it appears first in youth, and attacks may recur throughout life. The majority of patients with this disorder display no

evidence of any other cardiac abnormality, and in the absence of structural disease, atrial tachycardia should be considered a benign affection unless the rate is extremely rapid or the episodes unusually prolonged. Occasionally, the patient presents a history of precipitating events, such as emotional upset, nervousness, fatigue, indigestion, or alcohol ingestion; polyuria may occur after several hours of tachycardia. This arrhythmia may, however, produce great anxiety on the part of the patient and his family. When a patient is seen during an attack, the heart is found to be perfectly regular and the rate ranges from 140 to 250 beats per min. Procedures such as carotid sinus pressure or other types of vagal stimulation will either have no effect or will terminate the attack abruptly. Atrial tachycardia in the presence of bundle branch block may resemble ventricular tachycardia electrocardiographically, and the differentiation may be difficult. In these instances physical signs may be diagnostic. For example, a varying first heart sound and jugular cannon waves may be sufficient to make the diagnosis of ventricular rather than atrial tachycardia.

The causes of atrial tachycardia are not known, since most patients have no signs of organic disease. (However, the possibility of underlying causes, such as rheumatic heart disease and the Wolff-Parkinson-White syndrome, should be considered.) Prognosis is excellent unless the attack brings on congestive failure or myocardial ischemia. The keystone of therapy is reassurance, coupled with attempts to prevent the seizures and to terminate the disorder when it occurs. For many patients digitalis is the most effective drug for the prevention of the attacks; in others, quinidine is more useful. Certain patients notice that the attacks are regularly precipitated by certain trigger factors, such as anxiety, digestive disturbances, or hypoglycemic episodes; and avoidance of these factors will have a salutary effect. In many, the attacks occur at such long intervals that the patient himself will prefer to treat the disorder only when it transpires rather than to take a drug indefinitely to prevent the ectopic rhythm.

For the treatment of paroxysmal atrial tachycardia, the patient should assume the recumbent position and be given a sedative, such as sodium pentobarbital or secobarbital, 0.2 Gm intramuscularly. If significant hypotension is present (90 mm Hg systolic or less, slightly higher if the patient has previously been hypertensive), elevation of the blood pressure by phenylephrine or methoxamine to not more than 160 mm Hg systolic may suffice to restore a normal rhythm or to make the heart more responsive to other measures. The carotid sinuses should be massaged, each one separately, for about 15 to 20 sec, while the examiner listens to the heart and records the electrocardiogram; the massage is discontinued if the rate slows abruptly. If the ectopic rhythm persists, a rapidly acting cardiac glycoside, such as lanatoside C, 0.8 to 1.2 mg, should be given intramuscularly or very slowly intravenously, provided, of course, that the patient has not received digitalis during the preceding 2 weeks. The digitalis acts as a vagal stimulant. If after 1 hr the tachycardia continues, carotid sinus pressure should again be attempted, and if this fails, cholinesterase inhibitors, neostigmine (Prostigmine) 0.5 to 1.0 mg (intramuscularly) or Tensilon (Edrophonium sulfate) 10 mg (intravenously) may be administered, followed again by carotid sinus massage. Some physicians prefer to employ Prostigmine before using digitalis. If all these measures fail,

morphine sulfate, 10 to 15 mg subcutaneously, is given; during the ensuing sleep the attack will often cease.

Almost invariably one or more of these procedures will be effective; if not, electrical countershock may be employed. Quinidine, propranolol, or procaine amide may be given by mouth to prevent recurrences.

The treatment outlined above refers to the measures taken by the physician. Often, however, the patient has previously learned how to terminate the attack by utilizing carotid sinus pressure, or by inducing gagging and vomiting, or by the Valsalva maneuver (attempting to expire against a closed glottis). Naturally, these simple methods can also be employed by the physician before carotid sinus massage or drug therapy is instituted.

Atrial tachycardia with block (Fig. 265-1D) has certain characteristics of flutter in that the responses to vagal stimulation are similar; in other respects, it resembles atrial tachycardia in that the atrial rate is usually between 140 and 250 beats per min. It is generally considered to be a variant of flutter, and the exact mechanism is not known. Digitalis intoxication is a common cause, and on this account, this ectopic rhythm requires separate discussion because the treatment is altogether different from that of flutter or the other variety of atrial tachycardia.

Sensitivity to toxic effects of digitalis increases markedly with potassium depletion, apparently with the severity of heart failure, with hypoxia, and possibly with age. Under these circumstances, serious digitalis intoxication may ensue with doses that would ordinarily be considered therapeutic.

Paroxysmal atrial tachycardia with block should be sought in any digitalized patient who displays other symptoms of intoxication, such as nausea and vomiting, who has received vigorous diuretic treatment, who may otherwise have lost potassium as a result of vomiting or diarrhea, or whose heart rate increases after having received full doses of digitalis. The diagnosis is established by obtaining an electrocardiographic tracing displaying an atrial rate of 120 to 250 beats per min, an isoelectric line between P waves of unusual configuration, and some degree of AV block.

The earliest stage is an alteration in the form of the P wave and an increase in the atrial rate, usually with a 1:1 ventricular response. Thus the ventricular rate may increase to 120 to 140 beats per min and still resemble a normal sinus rhythm, but the impaired AV conduction remains inapparent (except when carotid sinus pressure is applied) because the P waves may be masked by the T deflections of the previous beat. At higher atrial rates, a 2:1 block usually appears. The danger of this abnormal rhythm comes from the fact that it may be a manifestation of serious digitalis intoxication, is likely to be confused with sinus tachycardia or flutter, and (because of the presence of congestive failure) may be treated with even larger doses of digitalis. The proper treatment is prompt cessation of digitalis and of potassium wasting diuretic drugs and the administration of potassium by mouth or parenterally, depending on the urgency. The serum potassium level must not be relied on as a criterion of diagnosis; most patients with this form of disturbed heart action have little or no diminution in the level of serum potassium. Dilantin (Chap. 266) may also be effective.

In about 20 percent of patients, the arrhythmia is unrelated to digitalis intoxication and potassium depletion. Procaine amide is then employed. If there is doubt about the role of potassium depletion and there is no evidence of hyperkalemia, potassium therapy may be tried. If this is ineffective, procaine amide should be given.

Atrial flutter (Fig. 265-1E) is much less common than fibrillation but is very closely allied, and the mechanism must be similar. The atria contract at a rate of 250 to 350 per min, and a 2:1, 3:1, or 4:1 AV block exists, the corresponding ventricular rates being in the neighborhood of 150, 100, or 75. When the block is constant and of high degree, the arrhythmia will usually not be suspected without an electrocardiogram; but if it is suspected, its presence can be confirmed by the fact that exercise increases the rate suddenly rather than gradually, and in the postexercise period slowing occurs suddenly, not gradually. This occurs because exercise has no influence on the rate of the fluttering atrium but the decrease in vagal tone reduces the degree of block, a 4:1 giving way to a 2:1 block, for example, and the acceleration occurs within one beat; the reverse takes place as vagal tone is restored in the postexercise period. Usually, a 2:1 block is present when the ventricular rate is between 140 and 160. This fact alone should lead to the suspicion of flutter, because other types of ectopic tachycardia are likely to be associated with faster rates. Carotid sinus pressure slows the ventricular rate in flutter by increasing vagal tone and hence the degree of AV block. The slowing is maintained only for the brief period of pressure, and both the slowing and quickening occur instantly rather than gradually, as would be the case with sinus tachycardia if there were any response at all. Occasionally, the block is so variable that the ventricular irregularity is virtually identical with that observed in atrial fibrillation. However, after exercise, the irregularity of flutter tends to disappear, whereas in fibrillation it is enhanced.

Careful auscultation will frequently reveal an appreciable difference in the intensity of the first heart sound in flutter because of slight variations in timing of the ventricular contraction in relation to the preceding atrial contraction. This variation in the intensity of the first sound is never present in sinus tachycardia or paroxysmal atrial tachycardia, but it occurs frequently in ventricular tachycardia and thus serves to limit the diagnostic possibilities. Atrial flutter is unlike paroxysmal atrial tachycardia without block, but resembles atrial fibrillation and atrial tachycardia with block because it usually occurs in patients with organic heart disease. It occurs most commonly in rheumatic mitral stenosis, but may also be seen in thyrotoxicosis, coronary disease, atrial septal defect and chronic obstructive pulmonary disease.

The usual method of treatment is to give digitalis, which slows the ventricular rate by increasing the degree of AV block, and commonly converts flutter to fibrillation. When the drug is withdrawn, atrial flutter will frequently revert spontaneously to normal rhythm; if this

does not occur, quinidine may be employed. Atrial flutter may be one of the most difficult of all arrhythmias to revert with drugs, but electrical reversion is often effective (Chap. 267). When this arrhythmia persists or recurs, increasing the AV block with digitalis (and when this is ineffective, with propranolol as well) may be necessary for long-term therapy similar to that of atrial fibrillation.

Quinidine sometimes converts atrial fibrillation to flutter, and the flutter may persist, the atrial rate decreasing from about 300 to 200 beats per min. Under these circumstances, the ventricular rate may suddenly increase paradoxically, and the previous 2:1 ratio will be replaced by a 1:1 response. Quinidine should be discontinued and digitalis administered even though fibrillation will probably be reestablished.

Atrial fibrillation (Fig. 265-1F) is an arrhythmia in which the effective contraction of the atria is abolished and the atrioventricular node and the ventricles are bombarded with a very rapid and irregular series of stimuli. Many of these impulses are blocked at the AV node, but many are passed through, so that the ventricular contractions in the untreated patient are usually rapid and completely irregular.

The untoward effects of atrial fibrillation depend on the rapidity of the ventricular rate and the extent of the pulse deficit (i.e., on the proportion of the ineffective and wasted ventricular beats), on the prior state of the affected heart, on the duration of the arrhythmia, and on the absence of effective atrial contraction. Cardiac output may be diminished and heart failure may occur. Stagnation of blood in the functionally paralyzed atria tends to predispose to the development of thrombi and hence to embolism in both pulmonary and systemic circulations. Finally, the cardiac irregularity may give rise to an unpleasant consciousness of palpitation (Chap. 35).

When the rate is rapid, 120 beats or more per min, the diagnosis is readily made by clinical examination, because atrial fibrillation is the only common condition in which one observes the combination of a well-marked tachycardia with a gross irregularity. When the rate is normal or only slightly increased, as in digitalized patients, the diagnosis is less apparent on clinical examination alone. The distinction from numerous extrasystoles can be made by noting that it is only in atrial fibrillation that abnormally long pauses occur in groups of two or more. Moreover, exercise may abolish the extrasystolic arrhythmia, whereas it exaggerates the irregularity of atrial fibrillation. More difficult, and frequently impossible, is the differentiation by physical examination of fibrillation from atrial flutter with varying block, and from a shifting pacemaker associated with multifocal atrial ectopic beats. Paroxysmal atrial tachycardia with block is also sometimes confused with atrial fibrillation.

Atrial fibrillation may be paroxysmal or persistent. Occasionally, the paroxysmal form occurs in healthy persons in whom no evidence of structural cardiac disease can be found. It is also encountered in individuals who, otherwise normal, develop acute infections such as pneumonia, or in patients with rheumatic heart disease or acute myocardial infarction. Rarely, paroxysmal atrial fibrillation may be the consequence of anesthesia, surgical manipulation within the chest, potassium deficiency, digitalis intoxication, or other forms of poisoning. Most frequently, however, paroxysmal atrial fibrillation is seen in thyrotoxicosis, mitral stenosis, or in elderly persons, many, but not all, of whom have ischemic heart disease. The paroxysmal attacks frequently occur before the arrhythmia is permanently established. The bouts may last for a few seconds to a few days, and, as is true in all types of paroxysmal rapid heart action, the onset and offset are sudden. Unless the patient happens to be observed during an attack, the physician must rely on the patient's observation that the onset was abrupt and that the heart action was highly irregular during the episode.

Permanent atrial fibrillation is confined almost exclusively to patients with myocardial disease, mitral stenosis, constrictive pericarditis, ischemic heart disease, and thyrotoxicosis. In patients with thyrotoxicosis the clinical signs may be absent and the arrhythmia may be the only feature suggesting the possibility of thyroid disease. Rarely, chronic atrial fibrillation may be the sole cause of congestive failure that persists despite full digitalization, and in such instances reversion to normal rhythm is a curative procedure. When the ventricular rate fails to slow in the usual fashion after full doses of digitalis, thyrotoxicosis, a recent silent coronary occlusion, multiple pulmonary infarcts, or acute rheumatic carditis should be suspected. The onset of the ectopic rhythm in a person who has received therapeutic doses of digitalis and of diuretic drugs, such as mercurials or chlorothiazide, may be a manifestation of potassium deficiency and an indication for potassium therapy. Rarely, persistent atrial fibrillation occurs in individuals without other evidence of heart disease.

In a patient with atrial fibrillation, several choices of therapy are available: (1) attempting to control the ventricular rate with digitalis, and letting the rhythm remain irregular; (2) abolishing the arrhythmia by quinidine or other antiarrhythmic drugs (Chap. 266); and (3) reverting the arrhythmia by electrical means (Chap. 267). In patients with mitral stenosis, or with marked cardiac enlargement with failure, it is rarely possible to restore normal sinus rhythm for more than a transient period, and in these patients, quinidine may be especially hazardous. In other patients with chronic atrial fibrillation, a normal rhythm can be restored with large, nearly toxic doses of quinidine, but usually normal sinus rhythm can be maintained only by permanent maintenance doses of quinidine, and even then, for only a variable period, before the arrhythmia returns. Electrical reversion is usually the treatment of choice (Chap. 267). However, the problem of maintaining sinus rhythm still remains. In some patients, chronic atrial fibrillation must be controlled with digitalis. Hence, reversion to sinus rhythm with electrical countershock or quinidine is likely to be of value in patients with fibrillation of recent development who are known to have had no evidence of congestive failure prior to the onset of the arrhythmia. Reversion to sinus rhythm should also be considered when the ventricular rate is not well controlled by digitalis; and it may be attempted in intractable failure provided the risk inherent in quinidine therapy under these circumstances is recognized. In patients who cannot be maintained in sinus rhythm and in whom the ventricular rate cannot be slowed sufficiently with digitalis, small doses (5 to 10 mg four times daily) of propranolol will control the ventricular rate. In all cases of atrial fibrillation, therapeutic doses of digitalis should be administered before quinidine is given, but reversion should not be attempted if the patient is near digitalis intoxication. When atrial fibrillation follows acute myocardial infarction, the first and most important objective is to slow the ventricular rate with digitalis. For the treatment of paroxysmal atrial fibrillation, a rapidly acting digitalis glycoside is preferable; for the control of established fibrillation, one of the sloweracting digitalis preparations should be used.

Although there are many instances of transient atrial fibrillation in which the administration of digitalis is followed by the disappearance of the arrhythmia, when atrial fibrillation is of long duration, digitalis rarely abolishes the ectopic rhythm. Under these latter circumstances, the ventricular rate slows and becomes less obviously irregular unless a complete AV block and a regular idioventricular rhythm develop; but electrocardiographic tracings reveal that the atria continue to fibrillate.

Thromboembolism is one of the dreaded complications in patients with atrial fibrillation, particularly when fibrillation is chronic and when mitral stenosis is present. Thromboembolism is responsible for about 20 percent of the deaths in patients with mitral stenosis. To prevent such catastrophes, long-term anticoagulant therapy has been advocated and is especially important in patients who have already experienced one or more episodes of embolism.

Derangements Arising in the AV Node

Ectopic nodal beats occur as several types. The configuration of the electrocardiogram depends on whether the nodal beat originates in the high, mid-, or lower portion of the node. In higher nodal beats, the P-R interval is short, and P waves of unusual configuration precede the ventricular complex. The QRS complex is usually normal in configuration unless there is aberrant ventricular conduction. When the impulse arises in the midportion of the node, the retrograde atrial conduction travels into the atrium presumably at the same time that the impulse goes down the conduction system, and consequently there is no visible atrial wave; again the QRS complex is normal in configuration and duration, resembling a normal supraventricular beat but without a visible P wave. Low nodal beats have rapid conduction to the ventricles, and consequently, the P wave may follow the normal QRS complex.

Nodal tachycardia usually is associated with a ventricular rate between 120 and 140. This disorder, though much rarer than paroxysmal atrial tachycardia with block, is likewise usually due to digitalis toxicity. Reversion may occur after stopping the digitalis or giving intravenous potassium. However, occasionally in critical situations, more vigorous therapy is required; in these instances procaine amide, lidocaine, Dilantin, or propranolol may be effective. When nodal tachycardia is due to digitalis toxicity it may be particularly grave, because it may lead to ventricular tachycardia and ventricular fibrillation.

Nodal bradycardia is rare but occasionally occurs in patients with diffuse myocardial disease. The ventricular rate is about 50 beats per min. No treatment is necessary as the circulation is usually adequate.

Derangements Arising in the Ventricle

Ectopic ventricular beats (Fig. 265-1G) are relatively more frequent in patients with structural cardiac disease than in healthy persons, but they are so common in the healthy person that their presence has no diagnostic significance unless they appear only, or increase in numbers, after exercise. In the absence of organic heart disease, premature beats may be due to excessive use of tobacco, coffee, tea, and occasionally alcohol or to reflexes from the gastrointestinal tract; often they are caused by emotional stress, but in many patients the cause cannot be ascertained.

Ventricular ectopic beats are often easily recognized, as the contraction occurs before the next beat would ordinarily occur and is commonly followed by a compensatory pause. The patient may or may not be conscious of the premature beat. When extrasystoles are frequent, they may be confused with atrial fibrillation on clinical examination, an error that can sometimes be avoided by noting that the rhythm becomes regular when the heart rate is accelerated by exercise. There is still uncertainty whether ectopic ventricular beats are produced by an abnormal pacemaker or by reentry (see p. 1142). In some patients ectopic ventricular beats and even ventricular tachycardia occur during episodes of severe bradycardia.

Bigeminal rhythm, a state in which every alternate beat is premature, is usually the result of digitalis overdosage and disappears within a few days after the drug has been withheld. It should not be confused with pulsus alternans or with paradoxic pulse; in these two, the rhythm remains regular. Bigeminy not due to digitalis is usually, though not always, associated with structural heart disease.

The treatment of ectopic ventricular beats depends on the circumstances. When these beats occur occasionally, and evidence of cardiac disease is lacking, no treatment is necessary. If there is reason to believe that tobacco or coffee is a precipitating factor, its use should be discontinued or curtailed. In excitable patients, extrasystoles may disappear following the administration of a mild sedative, barbiturates, reserpine, or other tranquilizers. In fully digitalized patients, ectopic ventricular beats, if caused by the digitalis, will disappear if the drug is withdrawn; or, if the irregularity occurs after the ingestion of a high carbohydrate meal, it will be abolished by the administration of potassium. The occurrence of extrasystoles in undigitalized patients does not constitute

a contraindication to the use of digitalis if the patient has congestive heart failure. Often with the restoration of myocardial function, the irregularity will disappear. Lidocaine, quinidine, procaine amide, and diphenylhydantoin are all effective in the treatment, and the relative efficacy of each drug varies in different patients. In patients in whom the development of ventricular ectopic beats or ventricular tachycardia is precipitated by bradycardia, increasing the atrial rate with atropine may be helpful.

Although ectopic ventricular beats may ordinarily be considered a benign form of irregularity, the occurrence of numerous such beats may diminish the efficiency of the heart with an impaired cardiac reserve. Moreover, the appearance of ventricular extrasystoles following an acute myocardial infarction should not be viewed with complacency, since they may herald the onset of ventricular tachycardia; or an isolated ventricular beat, occurring in the "vulnerable" period (the time during ventricular repolarization when the ventricles are especially likely to develop ventricular fibrillation) at the end of the previous systole, may initiate ventricular fibrillation and sudden death. It is for this reason that premature ventricular contractions occurring in patients with acute myocardial infarction should be treated vigorously, with intravenous lidocaine, Dilantin, or procaine amide (Chap. 271).

Ventricular tachycardia (Fig. 265-1H) is much less frequent and far more serious than paroxysmal atrial tachycardia. The commonest cause is ischemic heart disease, and this arrhythmia frequently occurs within a few days following the development of an acute myocardial infarction (Chap. 271). Less commonly, it is induced by digitalis or quinidine intoxication, and very rarely the arrhythmia appears spontaneously in healthy persons without any evidence of cardiac disease. The diagnosis should be suspected when the following clinical features are observed: (1) The patient has evidence of coronary disease or has been receiving digitalis or quinidine in large doses. (2) As a rule, there is no history of numerous previous attacks. (3) During the attack, the ventricular rate is usually between 150 and 210 beats per min, and although the rhythm is essentially regular, there are often slight variations in it. (4) Carotid sinus stimulation has no effect on the rate. (5) A jugular cannon wave is often a help in the diagnosis. (6) The first heart sound varies in intensity, because the relationship between the atrial and ventricular contractions is inconstant.

Although these clues are useful, the clinical impression should be confirmed by an electrocardiogram, but the interpretation even of the ECG may be rendered difficult because atrial tachycardia may be associated with intraventricular conduction defects (aberrant QRS complexes) which cause the tracing to resemble that of ventricular tachycardia. In other words, the electrocardiographic diagnosis cannot be made with certainty solely on the basis of the abnormal complexes. In these instances, bedside observation of a varying first heart sound and jugular cannon waves with a regular tachycardia may be diagnostic. In addition, it is necessary that the P waves be shown to occur at a rate slower than and independent of the ventricular rate, or that there be demonstrated, in the intervals between attacks, ventricular premature beats identical in form with the complexes seen during the paroxysm.

Since it is but one step removed from the almost invariably fatal ventricular fibrillation, ventricular tachycardia is the most serious of the ectopic tachycardias. If the attack occurs during a bout of acute myocardial infarction, immediate electric countershock is utilized (Chap. 267), but there is a strong probability that another episode will occur soon after the first. Hence, a maintenance dose of an antiarrhythmic drug (e.g., intravenous lidocaine, diphenylhydantoin, or procaine amide), parenteral or oral, should be continued until the healing of the infarct is complete.

When heart failure occurs in an undigitalized patient with ventricular tachycardia, digitalis should be administered, since the drug is not especially hazardous in such patients.

The cardiac rhythm of patients with ventricular tachycardia who are receiving large doses of quinidine or of procaine amide may fail to revert to the normal mechanism but the ventricular rate may still show marked slowing, to 120 beats per min or less. Under these circumstances the administration of large doses of atropine (up to 2 mg intravenously) may increase the atrial rate to a level above that of the ectopic rhythm, which may permit the sinoatrial node to resume its normal role as pacemaker and restore the normal sinus mechanism. Extracardiac toxicity of procaine amide and quinidine is not necessarily additive, and therefore it may be desirable to use the drugs simultaneously in patients who are especially liable to such side effects as diarrhea and tinnitus (quinidine) or hypotension and nausea (procaine amide).

Ventricular fibrillation (Fig. 265-1I) may occur in very brief bursts, lasting for a few seconds, and then subside spontaneously, following which the rhythm previously present is resumed. These episodes are responsible for some of the Stokes-Adams attacks that characterize high-grade AV block. Usually, however, ventricular fibrillation is synonymous with practically instantaneous death, since effective ventricular contraction and circulation cease. Aside from AV block, ischemic heart disease is the most common cause of the arrhythmia, particularly during attacks of acute myocardial infarction. There was no treatment for this calamitous disorder until introduction of externally applied countershock. Needless to say, this form of therapy must be applied promptly, because cessation of the circulation beyond 2 to 4 min leads to irreversible damage in the brain and heart. This means that in a candidate for the arrhythmia, whether he has suffered an acute myocardial infarction or has sustained a series of Stokes-Adams attacks, the heartbeat must be monitored constantly and there must be constant readiness to apply countershock. This incessant watch may be required for weeks, until the patient has been free of attacks for at least a few weeks. In the absence of the special equipment for delivering the countershock, vigorous pounding of the precordium, coupled with artificial res-

piration, preferably mouth-to-mouth, may be attempted. If the heartbeat does not return immediately, the procedure of closed chest massage should be employed. This involves manual rhythmic compression of the sternum once per second, plus mouth-to-mouth respiration. Thus it may be possible to sustain life during the crucial time required to secure and apply the apparatus needed for countershock.

Atrioventricular dissociation, as its name implies, is an arrhythmia in which the atria and ventricles are controlled by two independent pacemakers. Fundamentally, atrioventricular dissociation may occur in two forms—(1) with atrioventricular block and (2) without it. In the first type, the ventricles are excited by a pacemaker in the atrioventricular node, the bundle of His, or the Purkinje system, because impulses arising in the sinoatrial node or atria are blocked in the atrioventricular conduction system. In the second group of arrhythmias, without block, the automaticity of the AV node or ventricle exceeds that of the supraventricular pacemaker, and the impulses from the atrium, while normally conducted to the ventricles, find these tissues refractory. Occasionally, the regular ventricular rhythm may be interrupted by a normally conducted impulse which arrives fortuitously at an instant when the ventricle is not refractory. The precise term for this rhythm is "atrioventricular dissociation without antegrade block with interference." In atrioventricular dissociation without block there must be some degree of retrograde block or else the atria would be depolarized by the more rapidly firing nodal or ventricular pacemaker. Nodal and ventricular tachycardia may be considered a form of atrioventricular dissociation without antegrade block.

Abnormalities of Conduction

The sinoatrial block, which represents a disorder of excitation rather than of conduction, has been considered above (p. 1145). The unqualified term *heart block* as herein employed refers to a condition in which the wave of excitation from the atria is delayed or blocked at the junctional tissues (AV node and common bundle). The P-R interval represents the time required for the impulse to traverse the atrium and the AV node and bundles, and 0.20 to 0.21 sec is generally accepted as the upper limit of normal in adults; it is shorter in children. When the P-R interval exceeds this period of time and all the atrial beats are followed by ventricular beats, first degree block exists. A more advanced disturbance in the conduction system, second degree block, is present when from time to time the atrial impulses are incapable of penetrating the conduction systems and of exciting the ventricles. Third degree, or complete, heart block describes the condition in which the conduction system is so altered that no atrial impulses reach the ventricles, and the atria and ventricles maintain separate and independent rhythms (atrioventricular dissociation with block).

First degree block (Fig. 265-1J) may be caused by impairment of the conduction system as a result of digitalis or any of the inflammatory, toxic, degenerative, or vascular processes that may affect the heart. Prolongation of the P-R interval, such as may occur in rheumatic fever, may be suspected when the intensity of the first heart sound suddenly declines without any other change in the clinical picture and without evidence of fluid in the pericardium, or when a presystolic murmur becomes middiastolic in the absence of atrial fibrillation. It may also be due to increased vagal tone in a healthy, normal person. An Olympic champion whose P-R interval is regularly 0.26 to 0.28 sec has been described.

In the absence of any other criteria to indict the heart, this one electrocardiographic deviation from an arbitrary norm should not be construed as evidence of organic heart disease, and it requires no treatment.

Second degree, or partial, block (Fig 265-1K) may be divided into two groups. In the Mobitz type I, the P-R interval increases progressively until finally an atrial beat is completely blocked, the corresponding ventricular beat dropping out (Wenckebach's pause) (Fig. 265-1M). The P-R interval after the pause shortens to within the normal range, but each successive one lengthens, and the cycle is repeated. The dropped beat may occur after six to eight conducted beats, or it may take place after every second atrial impulse, thus giving rise to a 2:1 AV block and becoming indistinguishable at first glance from the more serious 2:1 block, to be described below. However, the differentiation can be readily made by inhibition of vagal tone, as by intravenous injection of atropine (1 to 2 mg) or exercise. In type I, the block diminishes or disappears with such a procedure, whereas it increases with Mobitz type II block and may change into a complete, though temporary, AV block. Type I, second degree block, is usually due to increased vagal tone, occurring spontaneously or after carotid sinus pressure or following digitalis therapy. It is almost always a transitory phenomenon and requires no treatment.

In the Mobitz type II form of partial heart block, a far more serious disorder, the P-R interval is either normal or increased but is always fixed and unvarying. There may be periodic dropped beats, or 2:1, 3:1, or 4:1 block. This form of heart block may be caused acutely by a myocardial infarction or by diphtheric or other forms of myocarditis. It is usually transient. Idiopathic sclerosis producing damage of the atrioventricular node is perhaps the most common cause of heart block. It may also result from coronary sclerosis in the absence of an acute episode of infarction, calcification of the mitral annulus, extension of the lesion of aortic stenosis into the septum, any of the diffuse disorders of the myocardium, or congenital heart disease, usually an interventricular septal defect. This type of second degree block is sometimes characterized by a unique phenomenon, a slowing of the ventricular rate during exercise as 2:1 block suddenly appears when the atrial rate increases.

Syncopal attacks are common in type II block, and they have the characteristics of all such syncopal attacks that are due to a sudden cessation of the circulation. The attacks occur suddenly and without warning and in both the upright and recumbent postures, in contrast to the premonitory light-headedness, faintness, and "blacking out" that always precede the simple emotional vasovagal syncope, which invariably develops in the upright position and is relieved by the recumbent posture. If patients with type II 2:1 block, for example, are carefully observed during or shortly after the lapse of consciousness, ventricular standstill or fibrillation will be recorded during the syncopal period, often followed by complete block in the early recovery state, a 2:1 block being restored after a few hours or days. When a person with a slow heart rate or with an electrocardiographic tracing of partial block develops a syncopal attack with the characteristics described above, the diagnosis should be simple. However, in a number of patients, syncopal attacks may appear at relatively long intervals over a number of years, during which time the electrocardiogram may be perfectly normal and the P-R interval well within the normal range. Nevertheless, intravenous atropine in such persons will usually unmask a concealed block. The important lesson to be drawn is that when a middle-aged or elderly person gives a history of syncopal attacks that develop without warning, one should suspect a Stokes-Adams attack even if the electrocardiogram at the time of the examination is normal in all respects. Eventually, most of the persons with type II block, whether of the overt or concealed form, will develop complete block if, prior to this development, they have not succumbed in a Stokes-Adams attack or to some other disease. One condition, less serious, that may cause identical syncopal attacks is a hypersensitive carotid sinus that is responsible for fainting attacks of the cardio-inhibitory type.

Complete or third degree block (Fig. 265-1L) is caused by any of the disorders responsible for type II partial block, as well as accidental surgical trauma to the AV node or common bundle. Occasionally, one encounters an otherwise normal person with congenital block, and rarely a patient with persistent complete block will be found at autopsy to display no demonstrable microscopic lesion in the conduction system. A transitory form, lasting a few seconds, may follow carotid sinus pressure, and it may also be a consequence of digitalis intoxication, disappearing a week or two after the drug is withdrawn. The ventricular rate is 45 beats per min or less, although following an acute posterior infarction or digitalis intoxication, and in congenital heart block, the rate may be as rapid as 60 beats per min. The rhythm is regular, and the rate increases only slightly or not at all after exercise. Congenital heart block is an important cause of complete AV block prior to the age of forty-five. It may be associated with other congenital lesions, primarily ventricular septal defect, but also occurs without other anomalies. The QRS complex is usually normal in duration in congenital heart block and abnormally prolonged in acquired heart block, suggesting that the lesion tends to occur above and below the bifurcation of the bundle of His respectively. The intensity of the first heart sound varies from beat to beat, being sometimes almost inaudible and at other times so loud as to merit the term *bruit de canon*. Faint atrial contractions can also be heard, and a short, faint, mitral diastolic blow may be heard and recorded. This, the Rytand murmur, is possibly due to diastolic mitral regurgitation caused by atrial relaxation with a momentary reduction of atrial pressure below the ventricular level.

The prognosis of first and second degree, type I, block is favorable. The outlook for high grades of block (type II, partial or complete AV block) is always uncertain, since the patient is constantly subject to the risk of Stokes-Adams attacks, any of which may be fatal. When such attacks occur frequently in patients with complete block and are uncontrolled, death usually occurs within a year. During this period the patient who is having numerous and prolonged attacks seems to alternate between the realm of the living and the kingdom of the dead. In acute myocardial infarction, the presence of high-grade block doubles the risk during the first 2 to 3 weeks. AV block occurring in the course of acute myocardial infarction is often transient, and if the patient survives with the aid of a pacemaker catheter, sinus rhythm is usually restored after several days. In addition to entailing the hazards of Stokes-Adams attacks, complete heart block may lead to impairment of cardiac reserve or frank heart failure.

Treatment of Heart Block. The important problem is the management of the Stokes-Adams attacks. The most generally effective drug is isoproterenol; however epinephrine may be occasionally necessary. In acute myocardial infarction drugs may also be employed, but all drugs used, including isoproterenol (the one most favored), increase myocardial metabolism and, hence, tend to cause hypoxia and occasionally prolonged anginal attacks. Should these signs occur, the drugs should be discontinued promptly. Corticotropin and corticosteroids sometimes are efficacious when the sympathomimetic drugs are not helpful or cannot be continued; the mechanism of their beneficial effect is not certain. Because potassium depletion accelerates conduction, chlorothiazide, 500 to 700 mg, combined with sodium bicarbonate, 10 Gm, given throughout the day, has been found to exert a favorable effect in partial heart block. In life-threatening situations, when syncopal attacks are frequent and uncontrolled, external pacemakers may be used under constant observation for ventricular standstill, and external countershock may be applied for ventricular fibrillation; these measures may tide the patient over a very stormy period. During the minutes required to initiate these procedures, life may be sustained by closed chest cardiac massage. Intracardiac pacing by means of a catheter electrode is now the most effective way of maintaining a heart beat during these critical times. For congestive failure in conjunction with the complete block, digitalis is sometimes beneficial but should be used in conjunction with an artificial electric pacemaker. When the block is partial, digitalis therapy may either improve or worsen the degree of block. Hence the drug should be withheld unless congestive failure fails to respond to other measures. Under no circumstances should quinidine, procaine amide, or beta-adrenergic blockers be used in the presence of high-grade block unless the ventricular rhythm is controlled by an artificial electrical pacemaker. In fact, those agents are useful in patients with complete heart block who manifest frequent ventricular premature contractions during ventricular pacing.

When, despite drug therapy, syncopal attacks continue, a permanent internal pacemaker should be inserted. The surgical hazard is small, and the results have been unusually successful:

Bundle branch block disorders (Fig. 265-1*P* and *Q*), which are not arrhythmias in the strictest sense, may be conveniently mentioned at this point. When the duration of the QRS complex is 0:13 sec or more, and when the main deflection is positive in leads I and V_6 and negative in leads III and V_1, left bundle branch block is said to be present. Similar prolongation but with opposite directional deflections in the leads mentioned is characteristic of right bundle branch block (Chap. 260). Lesser degrees of QRS lengthening are often designated as incomplete left or right bundle branch block. In some instances the ventricular complex may be markedly prolonged without the above-mentioned characteristic reciprocal changes in the opposite leads. Such cases are usually considered intraventricular block.

These several disorders are all related to delayed spread of ventricular excitation. The commonest causes are ischemic heart disease, inflammatory or infiltrative disease of the myocardium, and marked univentricular hypertrophy, producing delay in the onset of excitation and/or an abnormal conduction pathway.

None of the rather numerous physical signs which have been attributed to bundle branch block is wholly reliable. The electrocardiogram remains the only consistently accurate method of diagnosis.

These disturbances of conduction are usually encountered in persons with advanced myocardial disease or severe pressure loads, but they may be seen in association with volume loads, incomplete right bundle branch block in atrial septal defect being a classic example. It is probable that the abnormal sequence of contraction consequent to the disordered excitation impairs further the effectiveness of ventricular systole. In a patient with heart failure, marked prolongation of the QRS complex adds to the gravity of the prognosis. However, when right bundle branch block is encountered in an asymptomatic person under the age of forty who lacks all other objective evidence of cardiac disease, the outlook is excellent. Since right bundle branch block is probably often of congenital origin and associated with little or no structural heart disease, it has the best prognosis of the conduction defects. In asymptomatic patients of any age with left bundle branch block, and in those with right bundle branch block who are older than forty, the prognosis is less certain, because there is always the possibility that the conduction disorder may be the sole manifestation of ischemic heart disease. It is also probable that the mechanical effects of an abnormal sequence of contraction are more serious in the case of the left ventricle. Even so, any activity which causes symptoms should be permitted. The treatment of bundle branch block is that of the associated disorder.

Wolff-Parkinson-White syndrome (anomalous atrioventricular excitation) (Fig. 265-1N) is a congenital disorder characterized by the presence of normal P waves, a P-R interval of 0.1 sec or less, an increased QRS interval, a slur on the initial phase of the QRS complex (delta wave), and a pronounced tendency for the occurrence of the ectopic atrial rhythms—either paroxysmal tachycardia or atrial flutter or fibrillation. It is thought by some pathologists that the entire picture is based on the presence of an accessory conducting path (the bundle of Kent) connecting the atria with the ventricles, over which impulses bring about premature activation of a portion of the ventricular musculature. There is other evidence that the disorder is caused by accelerated conduction through some of the fibers in the AV node or bundle.

The electrocardiogram shifts between the abnormal (W-P-W type) and the "normal," intraventricular conduction, although this latter may now reveal abnormalities that have been masked by the W-P-W form. The latter may be one of two types. In group A the delta wave is directed anteriorly and there are tall R waves in right precordial leads; in some instances deep Q waves are present in lead aVF. In group B the delta wave is directed to the left and posteriorly, resulting in a Q-S wave over the right precordium and tall R waves in left precordial leads. Therefore, in both types, the tracing may be mistaken for that of myocardial infarction, especially when it is obtained from a patient in the midst of an attack of paroxysmal tachycardia, which occurs in about 75 percent of the patients with this anomaly. The shift to the anomalous conduction can sometimes be induced by vagal stimulation, as by carotid sinus pressure or by digitalis given intravenously. The normal type of conduction may be brought on by vagal inhibition, as by atropine or exercise, and also by quinidine and procaine amide. During paroxysms of tachycardia, the widened, aberrant ventricular complexes usually assume a normal configuration.

The condition should be suspected in any person subject to paroxysms of tachycardia, particularly when they have occurred from youth. The diagnosis is established by careful scrutiny of the electrocardiographic tracings for the criteria enumerated above. Digitalis appears to be less effective than usual in the treatment of the paroxysms of rapid heart action, and propranolol is much more effective. Frequent attacks of paroxysmal tachycardia may be disabling, and a few instances of sudden death during an attack have been reported. Hence, when a patient has a history of frequent bouts of paroxysmal tachycardia, maintenance doses of propranolol should be given.

Figure 265-1A–Q is a drawing of the various common arrhythmias and conduction abnormalities discussed in this chapter.

REFERENCES

Cardiac Arrhythmias and Their Management., Prog. Cardiovasc. Dis., 8:319–569, 1966; 9:1–165, 1966.

Chung, Koo-Young, T. J. Walsh, and E. Massie: Wolff-Parkinson-White Syndrome, Am. Heart J., 69:116, 1965.

Friedberg, C. D.: The Cardiac Arrhythmias, part III, pp. 483–642 in "Diseases of the Heart," 3d ed., Philadelphia, W. B. Saunders Company, 1966.

Gilchrist, A. F: Clinical Aspects of High grade Heart Block, Scot. Med. J., 3:53, 1958.

Lown, B., N. F. Wyatt, and H. D. Levine: Paroxysmal Atrial Tachycardia with Block, Circulation, 21:129, 1960.

—— and S. A. Levine: The Carotid Sinus, Clinical Value of Its Stimulation, Circulation, 23:766, 1961.

Papp, C.: New Look at Arrhythmias, Brit. Heart J. 31:267, 1969.

Watanabe, Y., and L. S. Dreifus: Newer Concepts in the Genesis of Cardiac Arrhythmias, Am. Heart J., 76:114, 1968.

Wolff, L.: Diagnostic Clues in the Wolff-Parkinson-White Syndrome, New Eng. J. Med., 261:637, 1959.

Wood, P.: Disorders of Cardiac Rhythm, chap. VI, pp. 226–290 in "Diseases of the Heart and Circulation," 3d ed., Philadelphia, J. B. Lippincott Company, 1968.

266 PRINCIPLES OF PHARMACOLOGIC TREATMENT OF CARDIOVASCULAR DISORDERS

Peter E. Pool and
Eugene Braunwald

The effect on cardiovascular function of drugs which are employed in the treatment of heart disease is understood sufficiently to allow their rational clinical use, even though knowledge of their action at the molecular level is still quite limited. The direct cardiac action of these drugs may be divided into four major areas: (1) An effect on *contractility* (inotropic effect); changes in myocardial contractility may be thought of as alterations in the force-velocity relation at any given initial muscle length (Chap. 263). (2) An effect on *heart rate* (chronotropic effect); this is expressed as an alteration in the rhythmicity, i.e., the rate of discharge of the sinoatrial node. (3) An effect on *conductivity* (dromotropic effect); this is the action of a drug which affects the velocity with which the depolarization wave travels through the myocardium, the atrioventricular node, and the specialized Purkinje fibers. (4) An effect on *excitability* (bathmotropic effect); this action refers to the alterations in the threshold with which the various cardiac tissues respond to stimulation. In addition to these direct effects, in the intact patient drugs may also alter any or all of these four properties indirectly by activation or withdrawal of autonomic influences acting on the heart.

CARDIAC STIMULANTS

Digitalis Glycosides

The digitalis glycosides have been employed for many centuries for their noncardiac actions, including their emetic effects, and as rat poisons. Although Withering first used digitalis in edematous states in 1785, he did not associate this action of digitalis with direct cardiac effects. Ferriar in 1799 was the first to postulate that digitalis affected the heart directly. Only in the present century, however, has digitalis been used for its specific action on the heart, when it began to be employed in the management of atrial fibrillation, and its usefulness in congestive heart failure, regardless of whether atrial fibrillation or sinus rhythm is present, was firmly established relatively recently.

The basic molecular structure of the digitalis glycosides is a cyclopentanoperhydrophenanthrene (steroid) nucleus to which an unsaturated lactone ring is attached at C_{17} (Fig. 266-1A). These two elements are called the *aglycone* or *genin*, and it is this portion of the molecule which is responsible for the cardiotonic activity. The addition of a sugar to this basic structure enhances both the potency of the glycoside and the duration of its action, probably as a result of increasing solubility which allows increased cell penetration. The sugar residue may prevent alterations in the steric structure of the molecule which would result in a loss of cardiotonic activity.

Though digitalis is adequately absorbed from the intestinal tract even in the presence of vascular congestion secondary to heart failure, some glycosides, including ouabain, are poorly absorbed and therefore are effective only when administered parenterally. The cardiac glycosides should not ordinarily be given subcutaneously or intramuscularly, because of irregular and uncertain absorption. When they are administered orally, absorption is close to complete within 2 hr. The fraction of orally administered glycoside which is absorbed varies; it has been calculated by comparing the effects of oral and intravenous doses of the same drug. In this manner it has been determined that approximately 20 percent of digitalis powder, 50 percent of digoxin, and almost 100 percent of digitoxin are fully absorbed. Varying degrees of protein binding occur in the bloodstream, and though these differences may account in part for the varying duration of the effect of different glycosides, they are not related to the speed of action of these drugs. The glycosides are also directly bound by various tissues, including the heart, but cardiac muscle binds no more glycoside than does kidney or skeletal muscle and actually substantially less than does the liver.

Digitoxin, with a half-life of approximately 9 days, is metabolized chiefly in the liver; digoxin (half-life of 2 days) is largely excreted in the urine in unchanged form. Both the glycosides and their degradation products are chiefly eliminated through the kidneys, and in man biliary excretion is negligible. However, both advanced hepatic and renal disease may delay the metabolism or elimination of tritiated digoxin and therefore may prolong the effects of these drugs, allowing them to accumulate to toxic levels.

The cardiac effects of digitalis glycosides are listed in Table 266-1. These effects result from positive inotropic and bathmotropic actions and from negative chronotropic and dromotropic actions. In addition, the cardiac glycosides potentiate the vagal effect on the heart. The most important effect of digitalis on cardiac muscle is to elevate its force-velocity relation. This positive inotropic effect is present in normal and nonfailing hypertrophied hearts as well as in failing hearts. In the absence of heart failure, however, when cardiac output is not limited by the contractility of the heart, the drug does not elevate the cardiac output. The finding that digitalis increases the contractility of the nonfailing heart has led logically to its increasing use prophylactically in patients with heart disease, prior to operation or other stressful situations such as serious infections, or in the presence of a chronically increased load, such as hypertension.

Digitalis exerts a negative chronotropic effect, which is in part due to a direct action on the sinus pacemaker and is in part a vagal effect. The slowing of ventricular rate in atrial fibrillation and flutter is due to prolongation of the refractory period of the atrioventricular conduction system. In heart failure, slowing of the sinus rate following the administration of digitalis results from withdrawal of sympathetic activity secondary to general improvement in circulatory status due to the positive inotropic effect of the glycoside. In the nonfailing heart the slowing effect is negligible, and digitalis should not be used for the treatment of sinus tachycardia unless heart failure is present. The apparent suppression of pacemaker activity which may take place following high doses of digitalis is probably due not to arrest of the pacemaker but rather to a sinoatrial block related to a depression of conduction.

In general, digitalis exerts a negative dromotropic effect on the heart, slowing conduction through Purkinje

Table 266-1. CLASSIFICATION OF DRUG EFFECTS ON THE HEART

Effect	Digitalis glycosides	β-Adrenergic catecholamines	Quinidine and Procaine amide	Nitrites	Propranolol
Inotropic.............	+	+	−	−	−
Chronotropic........	−	+	+(−)	0	−
Dromotropic........	−	+	−	0	−
Bathmotropic........	+	+	−	0	−
Vagal..............	+	0	−	0	0

+ = positive effect; − = negative effect; 0 = no direct effect. All effects listed represent the overall effect of the drug. Where this differs from the direct effect, the latter is shown in parentheses. Reflex vagal actions are not indicated.

fibers and through the atrioventricular nodal system. However, conduction velocity is slightly increased in the atrium and ventricle by low doses before being depressed by higher doses. Digitalis may increase automaticity sufficiently to initiate pacemaker activity in Purkinje cells and in this manner may lead to the development of ventricular premature contractions, bigeminal rhythm, atrial or ventricular tachycardia, or ventricular fibrillation.

The exact mechanism of action of the digitalis glycosides at the cellular level remains to be elucidated. Although it has been suggested in the past that digitalis glycosides may enhance energy metabolism or may directly affect the contractile proteins and thus increase the strength of contraction of the heart, the weight of evidence is against these hypotheses. The intracellular process most likely involved in producing the positive inotropic effect of digitalis glycosides is that of excitation-contraction coupling. It appears that following activation, digitalis increases the intracytoplasmic concentration of calcium, thus augmenting the contractile state.

In addition, the digitalis glycosides also have an action on the peripheral vasculature, causing venous and arterial constriction in normal individuals and reflex dilatation in patients with congestive heart failure. A direct renal action of digitalis glycosides to inhibit tubular sodium reabsorption has also been demonstrated, but this effect is probably not significant in enhancing diuresis.

The most outstanding indication for the administration of digitalis is congestive heart failure (Chap. 264). By improving the contractile function of the heart, digitalis aids in restoring normal circulatory function. Another important indication is atrial fibrillation or flutter with a rapid ventricular response (Chap. 265). Digitalis is also indicated both in the prevention and the treatment of recurrent episodes of paroxysmal atrial tachycardia.

Although digitalis is one of the cornerstones of treatment for heart failure, it is a two-edged sword, because intoxication due to digitalis excess is a common, serious, and potentially fatal complication of its use. There is no nontoxic cardiac glycoside, and in most patients with heart failure the lethal dose of most glycosides is probably five to ten times the minimal effective dose and only about twice the dose which leads to minor toxic manifestations. In addition, old age, acute myocardial infarction, cor pulmonale with hypoxemia, renal insufficiency, cerebrovascular disease, calcium administration, and hypothyroidism all may increase the sensitivity of the patient to the digitalis glycosides. The most common precipitating cause of digitalis intoxication, however, is depletion of potassium stores which occurs as a result of diuretic therapy.

Anorexia, nausea, and vomiting, which are among the earliest signs of acute digitalis intoxication, are caused by direct stimulation of centers in the medulla and are not of gastric origin. The most frequent disturbance of cardiac rhythm caused by digitalis is premature ventricular contractions, which may take the form of bigeminy due to increased irritability of the ventricle. Atrioventricular block of varying degrees of severity may occur.

Paroxysmal atrial tachycardia with atrioventricular block is quite distinctive of digitalis intoxication. Finally, sinus arrhythmia, sinoatrial block, sinus arrest with wandering pacemaker, and electrical alternans may also occur. Chronic digitalis intoxication, on the other hand, may be insidious in onset and may be characterized by exacerbations in heart failure, weight loss, and cachexia.

When arrhythmias result from digitalis intoxication, withdrawal of the drug and treatment with potassium, lidocaine, or diphenylhydantoin are indicated. Potassium administration is especially indicated if hypokalemia is present but may also be helpful when serum potassium levels are normal. Intravenous lidocaine or diphenylhydantoin (see below) are the drugs of choice for controlling serious digitalis-induced tachy arrhythmias.

Electrical conversion may not only be ineffective in treating these arrhythmias but may induce more serious arrhythmias and is, therefore, contraindicated (Chap. 267).

Catecholamines and Sympathomimetic Drugs

Catecholamines are normally found in the hearts of most animal species including man. Approximately 80 percent of the endogenous stores of catecholamines in the heart are synthesized within the nervous structures of the heart in the sympathetic postganglionic nerve endings; the remainder are taken up from the circulation. The principal catecholamine in the heart is norepinephrine, which is protected from enzymatic degradation because it is stored in granules found in the postganglionic nerve endings. The heart is capable of functioning normally in the absence of endogenous catecholamines, and in the presence of congestive heart failure, these stores are depleted (Chap. 264). However, sympathetic nerve stimulation is an important supporting mechanism for the heart in the presence of stress.

Catecholamines and other sympathomimetic drugs act upon the circulation by stimulating adrenergic receptors in the effector organs. Activation of α-adrenergic receptors results in vasoconstriction, leading to a pressor response. Stimulation of β-adrenergic receptors results in vascular dilatation and stimulation of cardiac contractility, rate, conduction velocity, and excitability (Table 266-1).

The catecholamines are based on the β-phenylethylamine molecule, an aromatic nucleus consisting of a benzene ring and an aliphatic portion, ethylamine (Fig. 266-1B). Greatest sympathomimetic activity occurs when two carbon atoms separate the aromatic ring from the amino group. Beta-receptor–stimulating activity is augmented by an increase in the size of the alkyl substituent, while alpha activity is enhanced by less substitution on the amino group. Maximal alpha and beta activity depends on the presence of OH groups in the 3 and 4 positions of the aromatic nucleus.

In general, these compounds have a brief duration of action. When administered orally they are rapidly inactivated in the gut wall and liver and are therefore ineffective. Epinephrine is rapidly absorbed after intramuscular injection. However, norepinephrine should be administered only intravenously because it tends to produce necrosis of tissue. Isoproterenol may be administered parenterally, as an aerosol, or sublingually.

Catecholamines may be inactivated by ortho-methylation by the enzyme catechol ortho-methyl transferase (COMT), or they may be deaminated by monoamine oxidase (MAO). The combined action of MAO and COMT on epinephrine or norepinephrine leads to the production of vanillylmandelic acid (VMA), elevated urinary levels of which are useful in the diagnosis of pheochromocytoma (Chap. 93).

The specific effects of catecholamine administration depend on whether the drug is of the α- or β-adrenergic type, and whether its action is direct or due to release of stored catecholamines. Certain sympathomimetic drugs, similar in structure to the catecholamines but lacking the catechol nucleus, act by a combination of a direct action on the sympathetic receptor as well as by causing the release of stored catecholamines. Examples of this type are *metaraminol* (Aramine) and *mephentermine* (Wyamine), which have both direct and catecholamine-releasing action. Tyramine acts solely by releasing stored catecholamines. In addition, sympathomimetic agents may be used for the reflex effects which they frequently induce. *Methoxamine* (Vasoxyl) and *phenylephrine* (Neo-Synephrine), for instance, are pure α-adrenergic stimulators, and are effective in the treatment of paroxysmal supraventricular tachycardias because they elevate arterial pressure directly, an effect which reflexly reduces cardiac sympathetic activity and increases parasympathetic activity. *Norepinephrine* (Levophed), on the other hand, exerts a predominant α-adrenergic action on the peripheral vascular bed but also stimulates cardiac beta receptors. Its effects include an increase in systolic and diastolic blood pressure, as well as an increase in total peripheral resistance with a compensatory reflex slowing of the heart. Stroke volume is increased and cardiac output unchanged or slightly decreased. Coronary blood flow is increased, but blood flow through kidney, brain, liver and, skeletal muscle is usually reduced.

Isoproterenol (Isuprel) has pure β-adrenergic activity. Its administration therefore leads to a decrease in peripheral vascular resistance with an increase in heart rate and contractility and, thus, an increase in cardiac output. Tachycardia and ectopic rhythms may also occur.

The exact mode of action of sympathomimetic drugs at the cellular level remains obscure. It has been suggested that the biochemical mechanism of beta-receptor stimulation may be the formation of 3'-5'- cyclic AMP (adenosine monophosphate) from ATP (adenosine triphosphate). However, the mechanism by which this leads to an increase in contractile force of the heart is not clear.

Sympathomimetic amines are useful in the management of a variety of cardiovascular disorders. Isoproterenol is indicated in the treatment of a number of arrhythmias characterized by reduced rhythmicity and conductivity. It may be administered as a continuous intravenous infusion (2 to 12 mg per 500 ml) or sublingually in patients with sinus arrest, sinoatrial block, sinus brachycardia, various forms of atrioventricular conduction defects, and Stokes-Adams attacks (Chap. 265). This amine is also indicated in a variety of low cardiac output states, including those associated with myocardial infarction and shock, following cardiac operations, and those associated with septic and hemorrhagic shock unless the peripheral vascular bed is dilated (Chap. 36). *Methoxamine* and *phenylephrine*, which act almost exclusively by stimulating alpha receptors, are indicated in hypotensive states secondary to loss of vasoconstrictor tone, in which it is desired to augment peripheral resistance without stimulating cardiac contractility. These agents are not indicated in shock due to myocardial infarction and other conditions in which depression of cardiac contractility plays an important role in the genesis of the hypotension. Agents which stimulate both alpha and beta receptors, such as norepinephrine and metaraminol, may be used to elevate arterial pressure when hypotension is secondary to depression in myocardial contractility and an inadequate vasoconstrictor response. However, in most hypotensive states peripheral vascular resistance is increased and the alpha-receptor stimulation provided by norepinephrine may actually be deleterious.

Toxic reactions to the catecholamines include headache, anxiety, severe hypertension, and the production of cardiac arrhythmias. When norepinephrine extravasates from its site of intravenous administration, tissue necrosis and sloughing may occur. Infiltration of the area with an α-adrenergic blocking agent such as *phentolamine* (Regitine) may prevent necrosis by blocking vasoconstriction. Following prolonged administration of sympathomimetics for the support of arterial pressure, the dose may have to be tapered slowly to prevent vascular collapse. The replacement of endogenous catecholamine stores with nonreleasable congeners such as *metaraminol* (Aramine) may explain in part the problems of weaning patients from the effects of these drugs.

ANTIARRHYTHMIC AGENTS

Quinidine

Quinidine is one of some twenty alkaloids derived from the bark of the cinchona tree, found in certain regions of South America and the Far East. It was noted many years ago that in patients with atrial fibrillation who were treated for malaria with the cinchona alkaloids the heartbeat would occasionally revert to sinus rhythm. Wenckebach originally used quinine in the treatment of cardiac arrhythmias, but it was Frey in 1918 who discovered that quinidine, the optical isomer of quinine, is the most cardioactive of the alkaloids. It is composed of a quinoline group attached through a secondary alcohol linkage to a quinuclidine ring (Fig. 266-1C). A methoxy side chain is attached to the quinoline ring and a vinyl to the quinuclidine group.

Quinidine may be administered orally, intramuscularly, or intravenously. Following oral administration, maximum effects occur in 1 to 3 hr. If the drug is given at intervals of 2 to 4 hr, effects will be cumulative. Effects are

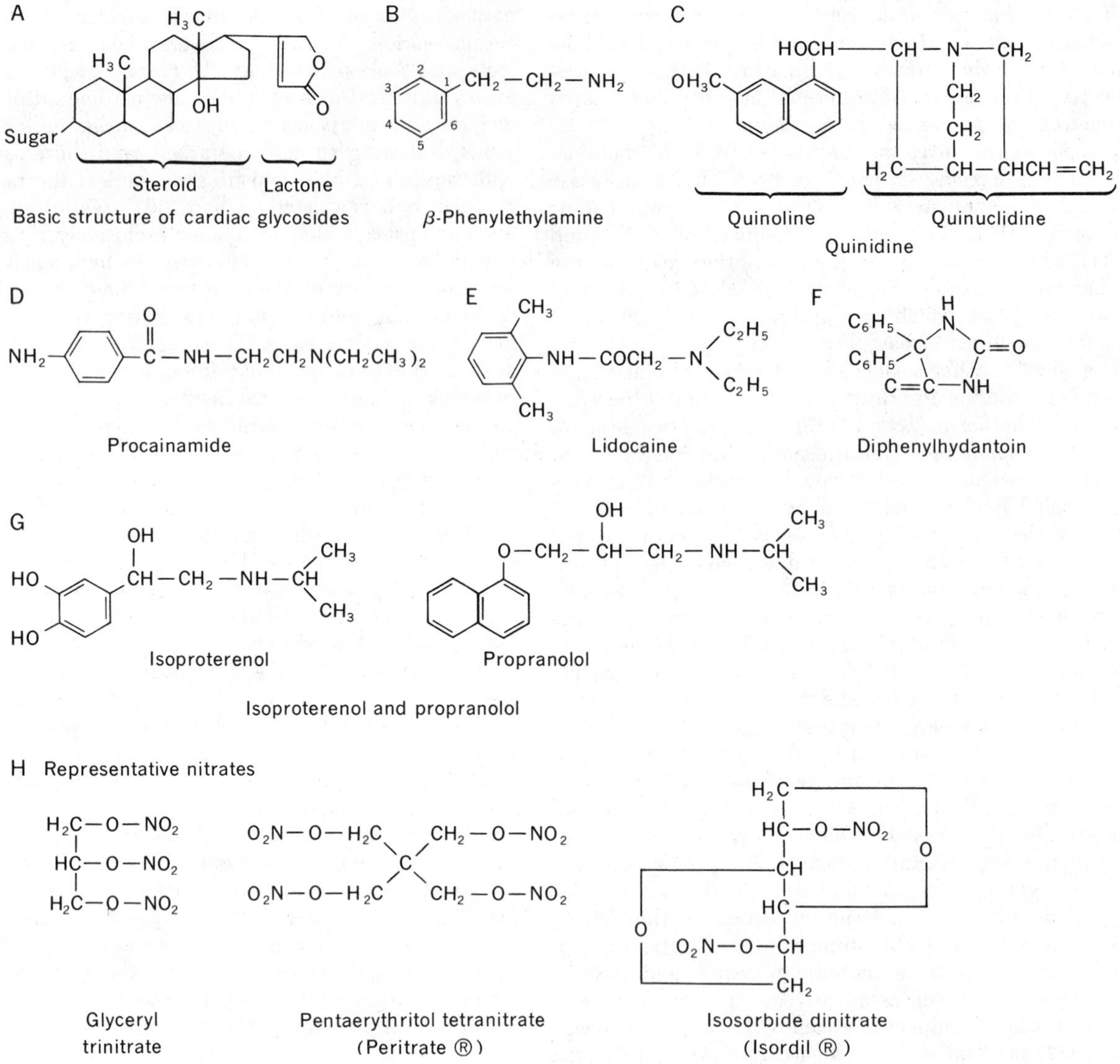

A

H₃C

Sugar — Steroid — Lactone

Basic structure of cardiac glycosides

B

$CH_2-CH_2-NH_2$

β-Phenylethylamine

C

Quinoline   Quinuclidine

Quinidine

D

NH_2 — C — NH — $CH_2CH_2N(CH_2CH_3)_2$

Procainamide

E

$NH-COCH_2-N$ $\begin{matrix}C_2H_5\\C_2H_5\end{matrix}$

Lidocaine

F

Diphenylhydantoin

G

HO ... $CH-CH_2-NH-CH$ $\begin{matrix}CH_3\\CH_3\end{matrix}$

Isoproterenol

$O-CH_2-CH-CH_2-NH-CH$ $\begin{matrix}CH_3\\CH_3\end{matrix}$

Propranolol

Isoproterenol and propranolol

H   Representative nitrates

$H_2C-O-NO_2$
$HC-O-NO_2$
$H_2C-O-NO_2$

Glyceryl
trinitrate

O_2N-O-H_2C — C — CH_2-O-NO_2
O_2N-O-H_2C — CH_2-O-NO_2

Pentaerythritol tetranitrate
(Peritrate ®)

Isosorbide dinitrate
(Isordil ®)

Fig. 266-1. Chemical structure of various cardioactive drugs.

negligible 8 hr following administration, and patients on chronic maintenance may experience no effects from the drug unless it is given more frequently or unless sustained-release preparations are employed. Peak effects occur 30 to 90 min following intramuscular administration. Intravenous administration, however, does not produce instantaneous effects, and therefore, when given by this route, the drug should be administered slowly.

In the bloodstream approximately 60 percent of quinidine is bound by plasma albumin. Blood concentrations may be measured easily; concentrations of the order of 3 mg per liter are necessary for therapeutic effects; approximately 10 mg per liter usually produces toxicity. Although metabolic degradation of quinidine, mostly to hydroxy derivatives, occurs in most tissues, particularly in the liver, hepatic injury does not appear to influence the rate at which quinidine leaves the plasma. Because most of the administered quinidine is metabolically altered prior to excretion, the optimal time interval between doses is determined by tissue metabolism rather than by the rate of renal excretion of end products.

The direct effects of quinidine on the myocardium may be thought of as negative (Table 266-1). Quinidine is a direct myocardial depressant and exerts negative inotropic effects. In addition, large doses, especially when given parenterally, produce peripheral vasodilatation, which together with a decreased cardiac output may lead to a fall in arterial pressure. The drug also has negative chronotropic effects, depressing both the sinoatrial node and ectopic pacemaker activity. However, this negative chronotropic effect of quinidine is often counteracted by its vagal blocking action, which may lead to no change or an actual increase in heart rate. Quinidine exerts a directly negative dromotropic effect, slowing conductivity in the atrioventricular nodal systems. Again, however, its potent vagal blocking action overcomes this effect, so that conduction through this system may actually be facilitated. Quinidine also has direct negative bathmotropic effects, increasing the threshold to electrical stimulation and thereby making atrial, ventricular, and Purkinje tissue less irritable.

There are various interpretations of the means by which quinidine is effective in converting atrial fibrillation to normal sinus rhythm. If atrial fibrillation is considered to result from the rapid formation of wavelets in the atrium (Chap. 265), then quinidine, by diminishing the rate of impulse formation of ectopic pacemakers, would slow this rate below the frequency at which atrial fibrillation occurs. If, on the other hand, atrial fibrillation is thought to result from a circus movement of impulses around the atrium, the prolongation of the atrial refractory period by quinidine would interrupt the circus movement, even though the velocity of impulse transmission is also decreased by quinidine.

The effects of quinidine on the heart are reflected in the electrocardiogram. Diminished intraventricular conduction velocity is reflected in an increase in the duration of the QRS complex and in delayed repolarization by prolongation of the Q-T interval. The anticholinergic action of quinidine may produce sinus tachycardia. Should paroxysmal supraventricular tachycardias occur while quinidine is being administered, sympathomimetic drugs may not terminate these tachycardias because of the vagal blocking action of quinidine. This same vagal antagonism also may increase conductivity in the atrioventricular node, which may be a hazard if quinidine is used for the treatment of atrial flutter or fibrillation before the node is sufficiently depressed by digitalis glycosides.

Though quinidine was used for years to convert atrial fibrillation to normal sinus rhythm and is still administered for this purpose, electrical countershock is now employed more frequently because of its safety and effectiveness (Chap. 267). Quinidine may also be used in atrial flutter after a trial of digitalis therapy has failed to convert this rhythm to normal sinus rhythm. In the treatment of atrial flutter, however, quinidine frequently leads to a progressive reduction in the degree of block from 4:1 or 2:1 to 1:1, and when this occurs the rapid ventricular response may be hazardous. Quinidine is frequently used to prevent ventricular tachycardia and fibrillation in patients who have had episodes of these serious arrhythmias. However, if atrioventricular block is associated with ventricular tachycardia, quinidine is contraindicated, because suppression of the ventricular focus in the presence of complete heart block may lead to ventricular standstill. Quinidine is also used in the treatment of ectopic premature atrial and ventricular contractions, but it is not indicated unless the frequency of these contractions seriously disturbs the patient or unless the onset of a more serious arrhythmia is feared, as in acute myocardial infarction (Chap. 271).

Toxic reactions to quinidine include cinchonism, consisting of ringing in the ears, headache, nausea, and distorted vision. Diarrhea, nausea, and vomiting are common side effects but may be controlled with the phenothiazines. Frequently, in order to convert atrial fibrillation to normal sinus rhythm, it may be necessary to accept moderate levels of toxicity, including some nausea, vomiting, tinnitus, and minor widening of the QRS complex. Idiosyncratic reactions, thrombocytopenic purpura, and severe hypotension may occur. The myocardial depressant action of quinidine limits its usefulness in the presence of congestive heart failure and hypotensive states. Its use is contraindicated in patients with a history of thrombocytopenic purpura or in individuals with digitalis intoxication who have an atrioventricular conduction disorder. Widening of the QRS complex by 50 percent or greater of control values and reduction of arterial pressure by more than 20 mm Hg are serious warning signs and necessitate discontinuation of the drug.

Procaineamide

In 1936 it was discovered that procaine, applied directly to the heart, elevates the threshold of ventricular muscle to electrical stimulation. Its prominent central-nervous-system–stimulating effects and rapid enzymatic hydrolysis make it undesirable clinically. Procaineamide, which differs from procaine in that an amide structure (—CONH—) is present instead of an ester linkage (—COO—) (Fig. 266-1D), has negligible central-nervous-system effects and is protected from enzymatic hydrolysis by plasma esterases.

Procaineamide may be administered by the oral, intramuscular, or intravenous routes. It is rapidly and almost completely absorbed from the gastrointestinal tract and has a peak effect in approximately 1 hr. It is concentrated in most tissues to levels greater than in the plasma. The major metabolites of procaineamide are diethylaminoethanol and para-aminobenzoic acid, which are excreted along with unchanged procaineamide in the urine. As a result, the drug may accumulate to toxic levels in patients with renal insufficiency.

The effects of procaineamide on the heart are similar to those of quinidine (Table 266-1). The excitability of cardiac tissue is depressed. Conduction in the atrium and ventricle is slowed. The refractory period of the atrium is prolonged, and contractility of the heart is depressed. The effects on the electrocardiogram are to widen the QRS complex and prolong the P-R and Q-T intervals. Clinically, procaineamide is generally used in the treatment or prevention of ventricular tachyarrhythmias in which it appears to be slightly more effective than quinidine. Procaineamide may cause hypotension, especially when given by the intravenous route, and α-adrenergic stimulators should be available to counteract this effect.

During the chronic administration of procaineamide frequent blood counts should be obtained, because this drug has caused fatal agranulocytosis. It is also frequently a cause of drug fever. Cross sensitivity to procaine and other related drugs should also be anticipated. Procaineamide is contraindicated in the presence of atrioventricular block and when there is a history of hypersensitivity to local anesthetics.

Lidocaine

Although lidocaine is similar to procaine in its antiarrhythmic action, it is not similar in the aromatic portion of its structure to procaine and the other local anesthetics (Fig. 266-1E). In addition, lidocaine lacks an ester linkage and may be given to individuals sensitive to procaine. Lidocaine is ineffective orally; when administered intravenously, it acts almost instantaneously, but its action is quite transient. Because of these properties, it is particularly useful when it may be expected that the inciting cause of the arrhythmia will disappear. Lidocaine, therefore, is widely used during cardiac catheterization and during cardiac operations when the stimuli which produce arrhythmias are short-lived. However, arrhythmias abolished by single injections of lidocaine may reappear in 10 to 20 min. A continuous intravenous infusion (2 to 5 mg per min) may be helpful in suppressing ventricular irritability (Chap. 265). Lidocaine depresses myocardial contractility only slightly and may be useful in patients with impaired cardiac function. It is contraindicated in patients with atrioventricular block.

Diphenylhydantoin

Diphenylhydantoin (Dilantin) was introduced in 1938 as an antiepileptic drug (Fig. 266-1F). During the following 20 years a number of studies in animals reported its effectiveness in experimentally produced cardiac arrhythmias, but only in the last several years has its use been extended to arrhythmias and especially to those induced by digitalis.

Soon after intravenous administration, the drug is concentrated in liver, kidney, and salivary glands and to a lesser extent in brain, fat, and muscle. Plasma concentrations decrease rapidly. The liver is the chief site of detoxification, and there is a substantial enterohepatic circulation of metabolites of the drug; urinary excretion of metabolites is also significant. Diphenylhydantoin may be administered orally, intramuscularly, or intravenously. Intravenous doses have consisted of 250 mg diluted in 5 ml solvent, and antiarrhythmic effects are usually observed between 30 sec and 4 min after administration. The duration of response to intravenous medication is not well documented, but in some patients only transient effects have occurred. While the mechanism of action of diphenylhydantoin in cardiac arrhythmias has not been established, there is evidence that the sodium content in heart muscle is reduced and that of potassium increased, an effect opposite to that of digitalis. Also, conduction velocity is reduced.

Diphenylhydantoin has been most effective in cardiac arrhythmias resulting from digitalis excess, particularly paroxysmal supraventricular and ventricular arrhythmias. It is particularly useful in these arrhythmias because, in contrast to other antiarrhythmic agents, diphenylhydantoin does not interfere with atrioventricular conduc-tion. Other antiarrhythmic agents may be capable of reducing the ventricular irritability produced by digitalis but they also exaggerate the atrioventricular block produced by the glycosides. Less success has been reported with diphenylhydantoin in the treatment of atrial fibrillation and atrial flutter. In those patients who have had a successful response to diphenylhydantoin, chronic oral administration has been used. This drug may therefore become the agent of choice in the management of digitalis excess.

Toxic reactions include transient hypotension and bradycardia; with long-term administration, ataxia, slurring of speech, mild gastric upsets, and skin rashes occur in 2 to 5 percent of patients. During chronic administration, hyperplasia of the gums develops in about 20 percent of patients.

BETA-ADRENERGIC RECEPTOR BLOCKING AGENTS

Propranolol (Inderal) is similar in configuration to the pure β-adrenergic stimulant, isoproterenol, except for the addition of a benzene ring (Fig. 266-1G). Beta-adrenergic blockade with propranolol is basically of the competitive type and is always reversible. Propranolol may be administered both orally and parenterally. It is capable of blocking the effects of catecholamines and sympathetic nerve stimulation on heart rate, cardiac output, and contractility (Table 266-1I). It reduces resting heart rate, cardiac index, and arterial blood pressure in normal subjects, but the impairment of cardiac performance during muscular exercise is even more pronounced because of the augmented sympathetic activity which occurs during exercise. In addition, propranolol reduces oxygen uptake by the myocardium and in large doses may cause sodium retention. The cellular action leading to these effects is not known with certainty but is thought to involve blockade of catecholamine-induced synthesis of 3'-5'-cyclic AMP (adenosine monophosphate).

Propranolol, alone or in combination with long-acting nitrates, may be effective in patients with angina pectoris in whom nitrates alone have failed to give relief (Chap. 271). The beneficial effects of propranolol in angina pectoris probably are achieved by preventing the increased myocardial oxygen requirements induced by sympathetic nervous discharge during exercise. Because propranolol depresses myocardial contractility, it may intensify heart failure and should be used only with extreme caution in patients with seriously diminished cardiac reserve.

A second major use of propranolol is in the treatment of cardiac arrhythmias, particularly ectopic tachycardias. Propranolol is effective in the treatment of tachyarrhythmias resulting from digitalis intoxication, where electric countershock is contraindicated (Chap. 267). It is particularly useful in reducing excessive ventricular rate in patients with atrial fibrillation. Its beneficial effects in this regard result from prolongation of the refractory period of the atrioventricular nodal conduction system by blocking adrenergic influences on this system. In this regard the effects of propranolol are additive to those of digitalis. Although only the *l*-isomer of propranolol has β-adrenergic blocking activity, *d*-propranolol is also effective against digitalis-induced arrhythmias. Therefore, the antiarrhythmic effects of propranolol may derive both from β-adrenergic blocking action and from direct antiarrhythmic activity, i.e., a "quinidine-like" effect.

Propranolol has also been effective in relieving many of the symptoms of idiopathic hypertrophic subaortic stenosis (Chap. 273). Its effects are related to a depression of the contractile state of the heart, leading to lessening of the severity of obstruction. Finally, propranolol has received a trial in the treatment of hypertension, but its efficacy in this condition is limited.

Toxic effects of propranolol, which occur in less than 2 percent of patients, include nausea, fatigue, visual disturbances, diarrhea, cutaneous eruptions, and insomnia. The serious side effects of propranolol include the production of shock and intensification of heart failure. Propranolol is specifically contraindicated in patients with second or third degree atrioventricular block, in whom it may produce serious bradycardia or even asystole. The drug is also contraindicated in patients with asthma or pulmonary insufficiency associated with bronchospasm, because beta blockade may induce bronchial constriction.

VASODILATORS

Glyceryl trinitrate (nitroglycerin) and *amyl nitrite* have been used for more than a century for their vasodilating properties. In recent years, however, numerous other nitrate compounds have been introduced which have a longer duration of action than nitroglycerin (Fig. 266-1*H*). The nitrite ion is an active vasodilator in both inorganic and organic forms. However, the nitrate ion is active only in organic form. The organic nitrates are absorbed most effectively from the sublingual or buccal mucosa. Many of the longer-acting organic nitrates, however, are also absorbed from the gastrointestinal tract and may be administered orally. However, for optimal absorption, these drugs should be ingested before meals. Once absorbed they disappear rapidly from the bloodstream. Portions of absorbed nitrite ion may be converted to ammonia, and portions are excreted in the urine, but their metabolic fate is largely unknown.

The vasodilators have only one specific therapeutic effect—to relax smooth muscle. The mechanism of this action is not known, and it cannot be blocked by any known inhibitors. For example, nitrite ion can relax smooth muscle even in the presence of the α-adrenergic–stimulating effects of norepinephrine. Administration of organic nitrates leads to generalized arterial and venous dilatation, resulting in a fall in mean systemic arterial pressure and in peripheral pooling of blood. Pulse pressure, stroke volume, and central venous pressure decline, particularly when the patient is in the erect position. The hypotension evokes a compensatory tachycardia. Dilatation of blood vessels in the skin causes marked flushing of the head, neck, and chest, and severe pounding headache may occur because of dilatation of the meningeal vessels.

Though nitroglycerin increases coronary blood flow

Table 266-2. APPROXIMATE DOSAGE SCHEDULES FOR CARDIOACTIVE DRUGS*

Drug	Initial or loading dose			Maintenance therapy
	PO	IM	IV	
Ouabain	....	....	0.5–1.0 mg	
Digoxin	1.0–3.0 mg	....	0.8–1.6 mg	0.25–0.75 mg PO daily
Digitalis leaf	1.0–2.0 Gm	....	....	0.05–0.2 Gm PO daily
Quinidine	0.2 Gm PO, q.i.d.— increase dose by 0.2 Gm until arrhythmia converted or dose of 1.0 Gm q.i.d.	....	....	0.2 Gm PO, q.i.d.
Procaine amide	0.5–1.0 Gm PO, q.2 hr	....	0.2–0.5 Gm	0.5–1.0 Gm PO, q.i.d.
Lidocaine	....	....	50 mg	
Diphenylhydantoin	....	....	250 mg	100 mg PO daily
Glyceryl trinitrate	0.3–0.6 mg sublingually	....	....	As needed
Pentaerythritol tetranitrate	....	....	....	10–20 mg PO, q.i.d.
Propranolol	10–100 mg PO, q.i.d. or greater for angina	....	0.5 mg for arrhythmias	Same as initial dose for angina

* Dosage schedules represent broad ranges and must be modified for individual patients. Initial digitalis doses are total loading doses and should be given in fractional amounts.

in normal individuals, there is considerable evidence that it does not always evoke this effect in the presence of diffuse, severe coronary artery disease. Therefore it is difficult to relate the beneficial effects of this drug in angina pectoris to a direct increase in total coronary blood flow. Coronary ischemia, however, may relate not only to the amount of blood which reaches the coronary capillaries, but also to the myocardial demands for oxygen. Since nitrates regularly reduce arterial blood pressure, the work performance and the oxygen requirements of the heart are diminished. The venous dilatation produced by these drugs leads to a reduction in heart size which also tends to reduce myocardial oxygen consumption. Coronary blood flow, however, is not diminished, and therefore the major effect of these drugs may be to improve the relationship between myocardial oxygen delivery and myocardial oxygen requirements. Also, there is some evidence that nitroglycerin dilates collateral vessels, increasing perfusion of ischemic areas.

The nitrates are primarily used for the treatment of angina pectoris; the chest pain is relieved within 1 to 3 min by sublingual nitroglycerin. Because the effects of this drug may persist for 30 min, it may also be used prophylactically to prevent angina pectoris when the patient predicts that it will occur. However, long-term prophylaxis with the long-acting nitrates has been relatively unsuccessful, perhaps because of the development of tolerance. When given in adequate doses, nitrates regularly produce cutaneous flushing and headache; if the patient fails to be relieved of angina but also fails to show any side effects, it is possible that the dose of the drug is not adequate.

Toxic effects of the nitrates include headache and hypotension as well as occasional drug rashes. In addition, the nitrate ion readily oxidizes hemoglobin to methemoglobin, which may cause severe hypoxia if large enough doses are ingested.

REFERENCES

Braunwald, E., and P. E. Pool: Mechanism of Action of Digitalis Glycosides, Mod. Concepts Cardiovas. Dis., 37:129, 1968.

Epstein, S. E., and E. Braunwald: Beta-adrenergic Receptor Blocking Drugs. Mechanisms of Action and Clinical Applications, New Engl. J. Med., 275:1106, 1175, 1966.

Friedberg, C. K.: "Diseases of the Heart," 3d ed., Philadelphia, W. B. Saunders Company, 1966.

Goodman, L. S., and A. Gilman (Eds.): "The Pharmacological Basis of Therapeutics," 3d ed., New York, The Macmillan Company, 1965.

Lyon, A. F., and A. C. DeGraff: "Digitalis Therapy: A Reappraisal of Digitalis and Cardiac Glycosides," St. Louis, The C. V. Mosby Company, 1967.

Mason, D. T., and E. Braunwald: Mechanisms of Action in Therapeutic Uses of Cardiac Drugs, in "Modern Trends in Pharmacology and Therapeutics," W. F. M. Fulton (Ed.), London, Butterworth & Co. (Publishers), Ltd., 1967.

Pitt, B. and R. S. Ross: Beta Adrenergic Blockade in Cardio-

vascular Therapy, Mod. Concepts Cardiovas. Dis., 38:47, 1969.

Thorp, R. H., and L. B. Cobbin (Eds.): "Cardiac Stimulant Substances," New York, Academic Press, Inc., 1967.

267   ELECTRICAL REVERSION OF CARDIAC ARRHYTHMIAS

Bernard Lown

Ectopic arrhythmias of the heart have generally been controlled by means of drugs. Major reliance has been on quinidine, procaine amide, and the digitalis glycosides. The use of antiarrhythmic drugs presents a number of problems. To reach an effective dose requires a time-consuming biologic titration involving frequent monitoring of the patient. There is a high incidence of mild as well as serious toxic reactions. Furthermore, a number of rhythm disorders are refractory to drugs. A method is needed that is simple in application, restores sinus rhythm consistently, and is free from untoward side effects. These requirements are satisfied by the use of a specific type of electrical discharge across the intact chest.

THEORETIC BASIS FOR USE OF ELECTRICAL DISCHARGE

The use of electrical energy for terminating ectopic arrhythmias is based on three propositions:

1. Chronic ventricular and atrial arrhythmias are initiated by a multiplicity of interacting factors, some of which are transient. Once initiated, the abnormal mechanisms are self-sustaining, perhaps because of a continuing passage of recirculating wave fronts of excitation over fixed or variable pathways (circus movement).

2. When an ectopic disorder is momentarily extinguished, the sinus node, which has the highest rhythmicity in the heart, resumes as dominant pacemaker.

3. The heart can be depolarized across the intact chest by electrical discharge. When effective, such depolarization abolishes the ectopic mechanism and permits restoration of sinus rhythm.

If electrical discharge were safe it would constitute an ideal form of antiarrhythmic therapy. Ventricular fibrillation has been terminated across the intact chest by 60-cycle alternating current (a-c) shocks. When this type of electrical discharge is administered to normal animals, it may induce cardiac arrest or ventricular fibrillation. The danger of provoking such serious disruptions in cardiac mechanism has deterred adoption of alternating current for the treatment of arrhythmias other than ventricular fibrillation.

CARDIOVERSION

Capacitor discharge, or direct current (d-c) shock, can also be employed to defibrillate the heart. A capacitor can be made to yield a great variety of wave forms, depending on the parameters of the discharge circuit. By incorporating an inductance in the circuit, the peak voltage released by a capacitor is reduced and the duration of discharge is lengthened. A single monophasic pulse resulting from the use of an appropriate capacitor and inductor is more effective in depolarizing the heart, induces fewer arrhythmias and less tissue damage than alternating current and, furthermore, does not provoke cardiac standstill. The one hazard remaining is the sporadic occurrence of ventricular fibrillation.

When the d-c pulse is delivered systematically through the cardiac cycle, ventricular fibrillation occurs only when the discharge is triggered during the final one-third of systole. This vulnerable period appears to be an essential physiologic property of the mammalian heart. It generally has a duration of 30 msec and just precedes the apex of the T wave of the surface electrocardiogram. When a d-c discharge is triggered outside this vulnerable period, ventricular fibrillation does not occur.

Thus by employing a capacitor discharge with a specific underdamped pulse and synchronizing the release of this pulse within a safe part of the cardiac cycle, the twin dangers of electricity, namely, ventricular standstill and fibrillation, can be avoided. The use of synchronized capacitor shock has been designated *cardioversion* and is employed for terminating a diversity of ectopic arrhythmias.

TECHNIQUE OF CARDIOVERSION

The technique employed is essentially the same irrespective of the type of arrhythmia. Cardioversion can be carried out as an outpatient procedure, although brief hospitalization is preferred. No special area is required. When treating atrial fibrillation or atrial flutter, quinidine in a dose of 0.3 Gm every 6 hr is initiated 24 to 48 hr prior to the procedure. The objective is fourfold:

(1) To build up an adequate level of drug in the body so that the arrhythmia will not occur soon after reversion

(2) To determine whether quinidine is tolerated

(3) To obtain a small dividend of reversion which occurs in about 10 percent of patients with chronic atrial fibrillation who are given this dose of quinidine

(4) To decrease the occurrence of postcardioversion arrhythmias

Premedication is limited to a sedative drug given about an hour before the procedure. Amnesia is induced by means of small intravenous doses of diazepam.

The electrical discharge is applied by means of two insulated electrode paddles. These are covered with thick layers of conductive paste. One electrode is placed below the angle of the left scapula, the other is applied over the right parasternal area of the third intercostal space. The instrument is automatically synchronized to deliver the discharge during inscription of the QRS complex. The initial energy setting is 5 to 10 watt-sec, depending upon the severity of heart disease and uncertainty as to the presence of overdigitalization. If reversion is not accomplished with these low-energy discharges, successive shocks are delivered without delay at increasing energies, proceeding to 25, 50, 100, 200, 300, up to 400 watt-sec. The patient's response consists of a single twitch of thoracic muscle, a slight jerk of the arms, and at times an audible sigh. Normal rhythm is restored instantly, at times a brief episode of nodal rhythm precedes establishment of sinus node dominance.

CLINICAL RESULTS

Many thousands of patients have been treated with this method. The good results that have almost always occurred have confirmed theoretic expectations. Cardioversion has been found effective in many ectopic rhythm disorders, whether of ventricular, nodal, or atrial origin.

VENTRICULAR TACHYCARDIA. In the majority of instances, ventricular tachycardia arises in patients with serious organic heart disease; usually, it occurs in the wake of a myocardial infarction. The rapid heart action and aberrant activation of the myocardium seriously compromise cardiac function. This arrhythmia frequently constitutes a dire emergency. Antiarrhythmic drugs may reduce ventricular contractility and peripheral resistance, and thus further impair cardiac function. Cardioversion is devoid of these adverse actions. Restoration of sinus rhythm is immediate (Fig. 267-1). This method is nearly 100 percent effective and constitutes a treatment of choice for ventricular tachycardia when the disorder does not respond to a 50 mg bolus of lidocaine. In the case of the oft recurring episodes of ventricular tachycardia which accompany acute myocardial infarction, the use of continuous intravenous infusion of lidocaine is the treatment of choice.

ATRIAL FIBRILLATION. This arrhythmia is the most com-

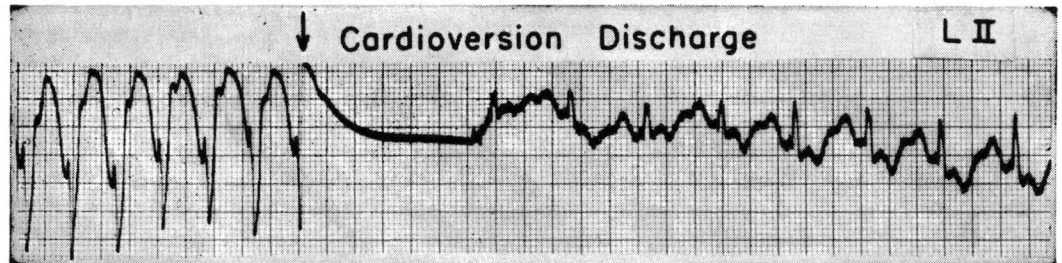

Fig. 267-1. Ventricular tachycardia in a forty-two-year-old man with acute myocardial infarction. A single cardioversion discharge restores sinus rhythm.

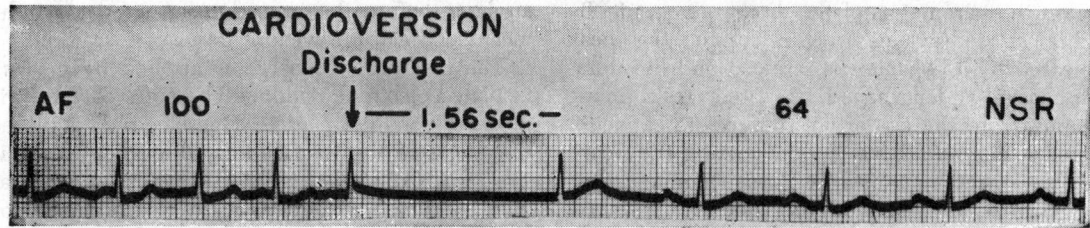

Fig. 267-2. Restoration of sinus rhythm in a patient with long-standing atrial fibrillation. The isoelectric interval of 1.56 sec represents an artifact due to the massive electrical field across the chest. Note the marked slowing in ventricular rate.

mon chronic disorder of the heartbeat. Until recently treatment has been based on the use of quinidine. Even when it is given to the point of toxicity, the heartbeat of only 50 percent of patients can be restored to sinus rhythm. With cardioversion, atrial fibrillation can be terminated in more than 90 percent of patients. Failures are encountered mainly in patients with mitral valvular disease, with giant left atria, and with continuous arrhythmia for 5 years or longer. A typical example of cardioversion is illustrated in Fig. 267-2. At times, transitional mechanisms are encountered, consisting of nodal rhythm and ectopic atrial beats which generally last for 30 to 60 sec, until the SA node "warms up." Slowing the ventricular rate is one immediate effect of restoration of sinus rhythm. The P-R interval is full, and not infrequently first degree AV block is present. In patients with congestive heart failure, restoration of sinus rhythm results in an increase in the cardiac output. The patient generally feels improved and comments on the newly sensed "calm" in the chest. Compared to the use of quinidine, cardioversion is a more efficient and safer method. Nevertheless, quinidine continues as an invaluable antiarrhythmic drug for maintenance therapy. Without its use a majority of patients would experience recurrence of atrial fibrillation.

ATRIAL FLUTTER AND OTHER ARRHYTHMIAS. Cardioversion has proved nearly 100 percent effective in chronic atrial flutter. Usually, a single low-energy discharge proves adequate. This method is also applicable to other atrial and AV nodal ectopic arrhythmias which have not responded to drug therapy.

COMPLICATIONS. Immediate complications have been limited to the development of ventricular ectopic beats, ventricular tachycardia, and, rarely, even ventricular fibrillation. Such disorders can nearly always be avoided if the lowest effective amount of energy for reversion is employed, electrolyte deficits are corrected prior to the cardioversion, and treatment of overdigitalized patients is avoided. Futhermore, the electrical discharge should not be released in the presence of artifacts in the electrocardiogram. Such artifacts may trigger the discharge to occur during the vulnerable period, thereby precipitating ventricular fibrillation. It is probable that most, if not all, of the very rare fatalities which have been reported have been due either to neglect of these precautions or to the excessive and, at times, improper use of such drugs as digitalis and quinidine.

In many patients electrical reversion is only temporarily successful and the arrhythmia soon recurs. It is, therefore, often necessary to continue the use of the drugs mentioned in the previous chapter. Moderate to large doses of quinidine, procaine amide, or both, may be needed. Agents such as reserpine or guanethidine, that deplete or antagonize catechols, may be beneficial. In refractory patients antithyroid substances such as propylthiouracil or radioiodine may be necessary as a supplement to the several antiarrhythmic drugs.

SUMMARY. Cardioversion is a simple and direct method for terminating various ectopic cardiac arrhythmias by depolarizing the heart transthoracically by means of a synchronized d-c discharge. It is based on physiologic principles and is the most effective and safest means yet devised for restoring a sinus mechanism.

REFERENCES

Lown, Bernard: "Cardioversion" of Arrhythmias (1), Mod. Concepts Cardiovascular Disease, 33:863, 1964; (2) *ibid.*, 33:869, 1964.
——:Electrical Reversion of Cardiac Arrhythmias, Brit. Heart J. 29:469, 1967.

268 CONGENITAL HEART DISEASE
William F. Friedman and Eugene Braunwald

GENERAL CONSIDERATIONS

Incidence

Approximately 1 percent of term or near-term infants are born with a structural malformation of the heart or great vessels, and over half of them die before one year of age. Moreover, various noncardiac anomalies occur more frequently in patients with congenital heart disease than in the normal population. Congenital heart disease as a whole is equally distributed between males and females, although specific defects may show a definite sex preponderance; patent ductus arteriosus and atrial septal defect are more common in females, whereas valvular aortic stenosis, coarctation of the aorta, tetralogy of Fallot, and transposition of the great arteries are more

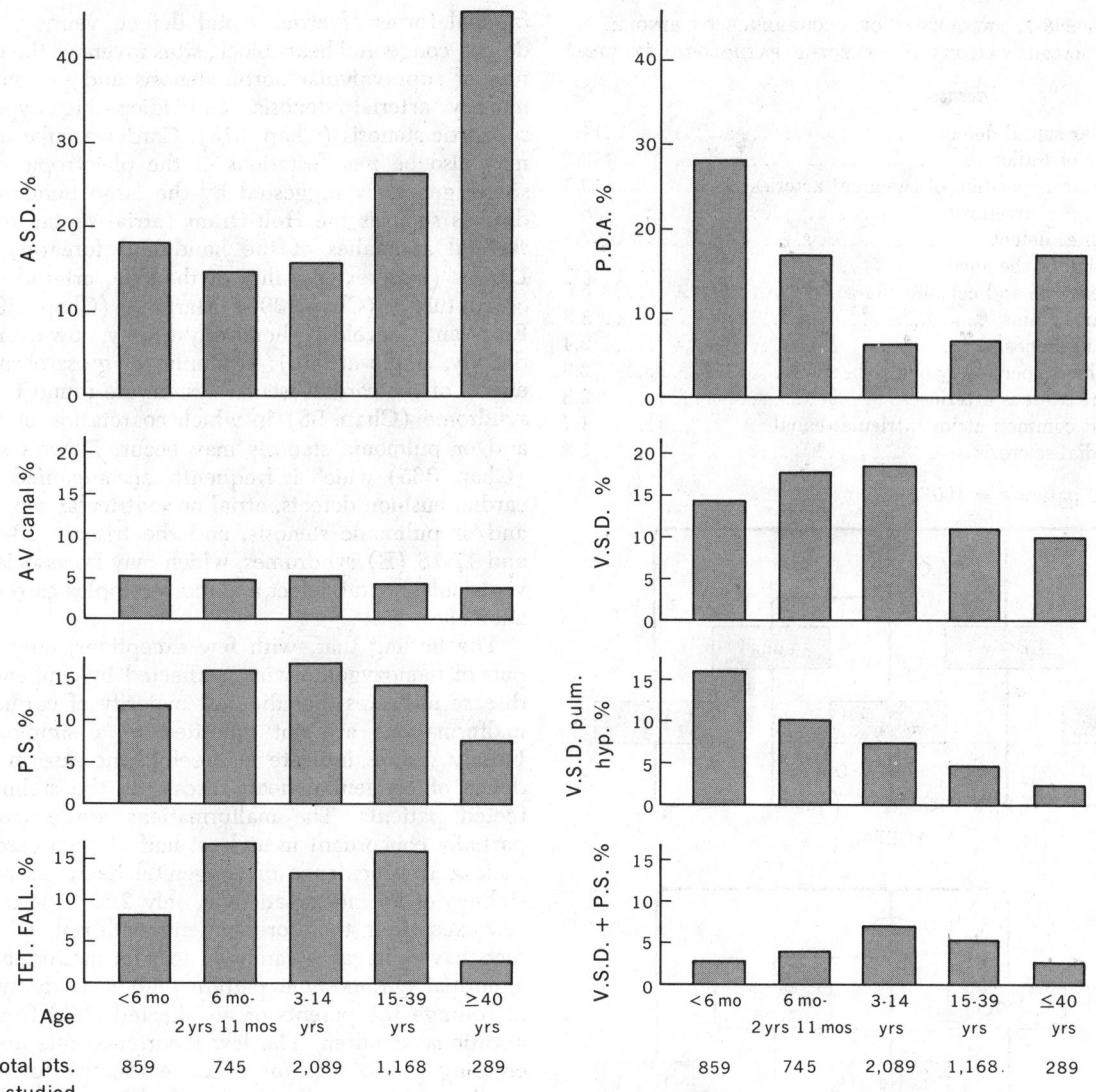

Fig. 268-1. Percentage of patients with specific congenital cardiovascular malformations studied at cardiac catheterization. *A.S.D.*, atrial septal defect; *A-V Canal*, atrioventricular canal; *P.S.*, pulmonic stenosis; *Tet. Fall.*, tetralogy of Fallot; *P.D.A.*, patent ductus arteriosus; *V.S.D.*, ventricular septal defect; *Pulm. Hyp.*, pulmonary hypertension. (*From Braunwald and Gorlin, Circulation, Suppl. III, vol. 37–38, 1968.*)

common in males. Table 268-1 and Fig. 268-1 demonstrate the frequency of occurrence of specific cardiovascular malformations in clinical and pathologic studies.

Etiology

Congenital cardiovascular malformations are generally the result of aberrant embryonic development of a normal structure or a failure of such a structure to progress beyond an early stage of embryonic development. Malformations appear to result from a complex interaction between multifactorial genetic and environmental systems that does not allow a single specification of etiology; only rarely may a causal factor be implicated in their genesis. Maternal rubella and the ingestion of thalidomide

early during gestation are two environmental insults that are known to interfere with normal cardiogenesis in man. The rubella syndrome consists of cataracts, deafness, microcephaly, and, either singly or in combination, patent ductus arteriosus, pulmonary valvular and/or arterial stenosis, and ventricular septal defect (see Chap. 221). Thalidomide is associated with major limb deformities and occasionally with atrial or ventricular septal defect, pulmonic stenosis, or persistent truncus arteriosus. Hypoxia, deficiency or excess of several vitamins, and ionizing irradiation are teratogens that are capable of causing cardiac defects in experimental animals, but their precise relation to human malformations requires further definition.

A primary genetic origin may be responsible for the

Table 268-1. FREQUENCY OF OCCURRENCE OF SINGLE CARDIAC MALFORMATIONS IN SELECTED PATHOLOGIC STUDIES*

Disease	%
Ventricular septal defect	14.1
Tetralogy of Fallot	9.8
Complete transposition of the great arteries	9.4
Patent ductus arteriosus	8.3
Atrial septal defect	7.1
Coarctation of the aorta	6.2
Single ventricle and cor biloculare	5.0
"Valvular atresias"	3.3
Pulmonary stenosis	2.4
"Idiopathic hypertrophy of the heart"	2.3
Persistent truncus arteriosus	2.3
Persistent common atrioventricular canal	1.7
Endocardial sclerosis	0.8

* 2,040 patients = 100%.

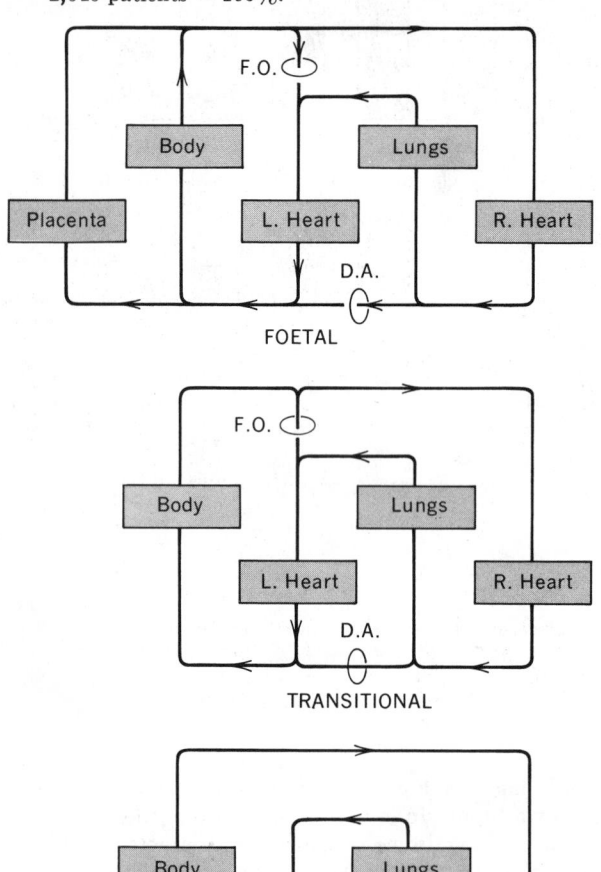

Fig. 268-2. Diagrams of the fetal, transitional (neonatal), and adult types of circulation. F.O. = foramen ovale; D.A. = ductus arteriosus. (*From G. S. Dawes, "Foetal and Neonatal Physiology," Chicago, Ill., The YearBook Medical Publishers, Inc., 1968.*)

familial forms of atrial septal defect, ventricular septal defect, congenital heart block, situs inversus, the combination of supravalvular aortic stenosis and peripheral pulmonary arterial stenosis, and idiopathic hypertrophic subaortic stenosis (Chap. 273). Cardiovascular anomalies may also be manifestations of the pleiotropic effects of single genes, as suggested by the large number of syndromes such as the Holt-Oram (atrial septal defect and skeletal anomalies of the hand and forearm), Ehlers-Danlos (hyperextensibility of the skin, arterial dilatation or rupture), (Chap. 396) Marfan's (Chap. 395), and Ellis-van Creveld (chondrodystrophy, dwarfism, polydactyly, single atrium). Examples of gross chromosomal effects of the cardiovascular system are found in Turner's syndrome (Chap. 98) in which coarctation of the aorta and/or pulmonic stenosis may occur, Down's syndrome (Chap. 365) which is frequently accompanied by endocardial cushion defects, atrial or ventricular septal defect, and/or pulmonic stenosis, and the trisomy 13-15 (D1) and 17-18 (E) syndromes, which may be associated with ventricular septal defect and more complex cardiovascular anomalies.

The finding that, with few exceptions, only one of a pair of monozygotic twins is affected by congenital heart disease indicates that the vast majority of cardiovascular malformations are not inherited in a simple manner. Family studies indicate a threefold increase in the incidence of congenital heart disease in the siblings of affected patients. The malformations are concordant or partially concordant in at least half of such cases. Nonetheless, the incidence of congenital heart disease in the siblings of an index patient is only 2 to 3 percent. With few exceptions, therefore, patients with isolated heart defects have a negative family history for malformations and a normal chromosome pattern, and it is rarely wise to discourage the parents of an affected child from having additional children. The low recurrence rate and the increasing possibilities for effective therapy for nearly all cardiac lesions usually justify a positive approach to family counseling.

The Fetal and Transitional Circulations

An understanding of the fetal and neonatal circulations is important to systematic comprehension of congenital heart disease (Fig. 268-2). The fetal circulation is a single circulation in which the pulmonary vasculature exists in parallel and not in series with the systemic circulation. Prenatal survival is not endangered by extremely severe cardiac anomalies as long as one side of the heart can drive blood from the great veins to the aorta. Blood can bypass the nonfunctioning lungs both proximal and distal to the heart. Inferior vena caval blood is deflected across the foramen ovale into the left atrium. Most of the blood that reaches the right ventricle bypasses the high-resistance, unexpanded lungs and passes through the patent ductus arteriosus into the descending aorta. In fetal life, pulmonary vessels are surrounded by a fluid medium, have relatively thick walls and small lumens, and resemble comparable vessels in the systemic circulation.

Normally, the fundamental change which occurs at birth is the division of this single circulation into two separate, interdependent circulations. Inflation of the lungs with the first breath produces a marked reduction in pulmonary vascular resistance. Fetal pulmonary vessels, heretofore supported by fluid media, are suddenly suspended in air, reducing extravascular pressure. New vessels are opened, and already patent vessels enlarge. Pulmonary arterial pressure falls, and pulmonary blood flow increases greatly. The systemic vascular resistance rises when clamping the umbilical cord removes the low-resistance placental circulation. Increased pulmonary blood flow increases the return of blood to the left atrium and raises left atrial pressure, which in turn closes the foramen ovale. The shift in oxygen dependence from the placenta to the lungs produces a sudden increase in arterial blood oxygen tension, which is one of the factors that initiates constriction of the ductus arteriosus, and total anatomic closure follows within a few days.

Pulmonary Hypertension

Pulmonary hypertension frequently complicates congenital heart disease, and the status of the pulmonary vascular bed may determine the clinical picture, its rate of progression, and whether or not corrective surgical treatment is feasible. The basis for elevation of pulmonary blood pressure frequently depends on morphologic alterations in the pulmonary vascular bed. Following the fall in pulmonary arterial pressure, resistance, and vasomotor tone shortly after birth, a gradual reduction of the ratio of pulmonary vessel wall thickness to lumen size occurs for some months postnatally. The muscular media of the pulmonary arterioles becomes thin, and their lumens widen. Hence, the pulmonary circulation of the normal adult has evolved from a high-pressure, high-resistance, highly reactive vascular bed with relatively small cross-sectional area, to a low-pressure, low-resistance, less-reactive bed with a large cross-sectional area.

As in the other vascular beds, the pressure in the pulmonary artery is determined by the relationship between the volume of blood flow, per unit of time, and the resistance to that flow. Equalization of pressures in the systemic and pulmonary circulations may be expected if a large communication exists between the two ventricles or the two great arteries in the absence of semilunar valve obstruction. For example, if a ventricular septal defect is as large as the aortic orifice, the left and right ventricles behave as a common ejectile chamber and equal systolic pressures exist in the aorta and pulmonary artery; the diastolic pressures in each circulation depend on vascular resistance and may differ. Pulmonary vascular resistance is calculated as the transpulmonary pressure difference per unit of pulmonary blood flow. When blood flow increases, existing patent vessels are distended and additional vessels are opened, so that calculated vascular resistance diminishes. Therefore, in a normal pulmonary

vascular bed, pressure will rise substantially only if flow is very greatly increased. In patients with normal pulmonary blood flow at rest, whenever the mean pressure in the pulmonary vascular bed exceeds one-fourth of that in the systemic bed, pulmonary vascular resistance is elevated. In some patients with congenital heart disease and pulmonary hypertension, the pulmonary blood flow exceeds normal; in others it is either normal or reduced. In the vast majority of patients with congenital heart disease and elevated pulmonary vascular resistance, the pulmonary arterioles are the principal locus of this abnormal resistance.

In contrast to the normal postnatal involution of the pulmonary vascular bed, the fetal pattern may persist in the presence of an intra- or extracardiac communication. However, the pattern of involution may be normal even if the size of the communication is large if the magnitude of the left-to-right shunt is small in the neonatal period, as in patients with atrial septal defect, or if the intra- or extracardiac communication, regardless of location, is small or moderate in size. In patients having high pulmonary arterial pressure from birth, anatomic changes in the pulmonary vessels, in the form of medial thickening and intimal proliferation, usually progress so that in the older child or adult the vascular resistance may ultimately be fixed by obliterative changes in the pulmonary vascular bed. However, if pulmonary arterial hypertension is not present in infancy or childhood, it is not likely to develop until the third or fourth decade, or even later. In infants and young children, elevations of pulmonary vascular resistance may be partially reversible because, prior to the development of fixed structural changes later in life, there may be significant vasoconstrictor tone in the muscular pulmonary arteries.

Because pulmonary vascular obstructive disease may be the factor limiting a decision concerning the operability of a specific cardiac malformation, it is essential to quantify and compare the ratios of pulmonary to systemic flows and resistances in patients with severe pulmonary hypertension. Furthermore, the lability of the pulmonary vascular resistance should be evaluated; a reduction with acetylcholine and tolazoline, or oxygen inhalation suggests that resistance may fall after successful operation. Some defects between the left and right sides of the heart should be closed in order to eliminate a sizable left-to-right shunt, which, in turn, may result in a significant drop in pulmonary arterial pressure because of reduction of pulmonary blood flow. Conversely, little or no benefit and high mortality rates may be expected from the closure of defects that are associated with bidirectional or predominant right-to-left shunts in patients with high resistance and obstructive pulmonary hypertension. The designation "Eisenmenger's reaction" is applied to this condition in patients who may have a large communication between the two circulations at the aortopulmonary, ventricular, or atrial levels.

The actual mechanism for the persistence, delayed reduction, or late onset of elevated pulmonary vascular resistance is not known. The separate roles of increased pulmonary blood flow, increased pulmonary arterial pressure, increased pulmonary venous pressure, and altered pulmonary vasomotor tone have not been defined precisely.

The clinical manifestations of the hyperkinetic form of pulmonary hypertension, i.e., that associated with a large left-to-right shunt, reflect the specific malformation responsible. When a significant right-to-left shunt exists in patients with pulmonary hypertension, the patient is cyanotic, and polycythemia and clubbing of the digits may be noted (Chap. 33). A dominant *a* wave in the jugular venous pulse may be seen, reflecting vigorous right atrial contraction; in some instances there are large *v* waves, which suggest tricuspid regurgitation. A prominent right ventricular parasternal lift and palpable systolic expansion of the pulmonary artery are present. On auscultation, one often hears a soft pulmonary systolic ejection murmur following a loud ejection click, marked accentuation of the pulmonic component of the second heart sound, and, often, a fourth heart sound produced by right atrial contraction. The decrescendo diastolic murmur of pulmonary valvular regurgitation and/or the holosystolic decrescendo murmur of tricuspid regurgitation may be heard. The electrocardiogram shows a QRS orientation rightward and anteriorly, an increase in the QRS voltages and R/S ratio, and a qR pattern in the right precordial leads. With severe right ventricular hypertension, the T waves may be inverted in the right precordial leads, AVF and III, and tall peaked P waves indicating right atrial hypertrophy may be observed. Roentgenologic examination reveals moderate enlargement of the right ventricle, a conspicuously enlarged pulmonary artery, prominent hilar pulmonary vascular markings, and attenuated peripheral vessels. The site of the underlying defect can be localized by means of cardiac catheterization and angiocardiography (Chap. 262). Pressures in the right side of the heart are essentially identical to systemic pressures in cyanotic patients if the shunt is at the ventricular or aortopulmonary levels, but they are usually lower than systemic pressure in patients with an interatrial shunt. No specific treatment is currently available for the obstructive pulmonary vascular disease. In a small fraction of patients with pulmonary hypertension, detailed clinical, hemodynamic, and histologic examinations do not uncover a specific cause, and such patients are considered to have *primary pulmonary hypertension* (Chap. 286).

Circulatory Shunts

Although equal quantities of blood flow through the pulmonary and systemic circulations in normal man, the systemic circulation is a relatively high-resistance system requiring a systolic pressure in the left ventricle in excess of 100 mm Hg to maintain normal blood flow. Right ventricular pressure, however, is approximately one-sixth that in the left ventricle, indicating that the resistance to flow through the normal pulmonary vascular bed is much lower than that in the systemic bed. Also, the pressure in the left atrium exceeds that in the right. Therefore, it may

be expected that, ordinarily, if an abnormal communication is present blood will flow from the left to the right side of the heart. The size of the opening and the pressures on either side of it may vary, so that shunt flow may also vary in magnitude and even direction during a single cardiac cycle. In addition, the location of the opening between the two circulations may predispose to a streamlining of shunted blood in directions not readily explained by resistance differences. A right-to-left shunt usually requires the presence of either an obstructive lesion at some point in the right-sided circulation, i.e., tricuspid stenosis or atresia, pulmonary valvular or infundibular stenosis, elevated pulmonary vascular resistance, or an obligatory mixing of systemic venous and arterial blood, i.e., total anomalous pulmonary venous drainage, a single atrium or ventricle, or a persistent truncus arteriosus. The location, direction, and magnitude of the right-to-left shunt may be determined at hemodynamic study by measuring the admixture of venous and arterial blood at various sites in the central circulation, by indicator-dilution or foreign gas techniques, and by angiocardiography, as outlined in Chap. 261.

Clinical Manifestations of Right-to-left Shunts

CYANOSIS AND POLYCYTHEMIA These signs are discussed in Chap. 33.

CLUBBING. A prominent accompaniment of arterial hypoxemia is a widening and thickening of the terminal phalanges of the fingers and toes accompanied by convex nails. Physiologic and histologic studies of clubbing indicate that these digits have an increased number of capillaries with increased blood flow through extensive arteriovenous aneurysms, and an increase of connective tissue.

SQUATTING. Patients with cyanotic heart disease, especially tetralogy of Fallot, typically assume a squatting posture after exertion to obtain relief from breathlessness. Squatting appears to hasten an increase in the arterial oxygen saturation by increasing systemic vascular resistance and thereby diminishing the right-to-left shunt and by pooling markedly unsaturated blood in the legs. In addition, the maneuver may increase systemic venous return and therefore pulmonary blood flow.

ANOXIC SPELLS. A sudden marked increase in cyanosis due to an abrupt reduction in pulmonary blood flow occurs in certain types of cyanotic heart disease, particularly tetralogy of Fallot. These alarming episodes are seen in younger children; they may lead to convulsions and may even be fatal. The spells may be precipitated by fluctuations in arterial P_{CO_2} and pH, a sudden fall in systemic vascular resistance, or increased contraction of the hypertrophied muscle in the right ventricular outflow tract. Treatment consists of oxygen administration, placing the child in the knee-chest position, and intravenous administration of sodium bicarbonate to correct the accompanying acidosis. Additional medications that may prove of value include morphine, α-adrenergic receptor stimulants such as phenylephrine or methoxamine, or angiotensin to raise peripheral resistance and to diminish right-to-left shunting, and β-adrenergic blocking agents which may relieve infundibular spasm by reducing cardiac sympathetic tone.

PARADOXIC EMBOLUS AND BRAIN ABSCESS. In patients with cyanotic heart disease, venous blood bypasses the normal filtering action of the lungs. Therefore, emboli arising in systemic veins may pass, paradoxically, directly to the systemic circulation. In addition, arterial bacteremia occurs in the absence of bacterial endocarditis. Patients with severe cyanosis or polycythemia have often had previous occlusive microcirculatory damage to the central nervous system. These predisposing factors are primarily responsible for the high incidence (2 to 4 percent of brain abscess in patients with cyanotic forms of congenital heart disease.

IMPAIRED GROWTH. Physical underdevelopment and a delayed onset of adolescence are common features of many types of cyanotic and, to a lesser extent, acyanotic forms of congenital heart disease. Mental development is rarely affected. Various explanations for the mechanisms of growth interference have implicated malnutrition, tissue anoxia, diminished peripheral blood flow, hypermetabolic state, chronic cardiac decompensation, genetic and endocrine factors, and frequency of upper and lower respiratory infections. In many instances, the underdevelopment is influenced little by operative correction of the underlying cardiac anomaly.

Specific Cardiac Defects

Various classifications of congenital cardiovascular lesions have been proposed, depending on hemodynamic, anatomic, and radiographic factors. Although there is overlapping between groups, the following arrangement of the more common anomalies has been employed.

1. Communications between the systemic and pulmonary circulation without cyanosis (left-to-right shunts)

2. Obstructing valvular and vascular lesions with or without associated right-to-left shunts

3. Abnormalities in the origins of the great arteries and veins; the transpositions

COMMUNICATIONS BETWEEN SYSTEMIC AND PULMONARY CIRCULATION WITHOUT CYANOSIS (LEFT-TO-RIGHT SHUNTS)
Atrial Septal Defect

Atrial septal defect, the most common congenital cardiac anomaly in adults, is particularly common in females. Anatomically, defects of the sinus venosus type occur high in the atrial septum and near the entry of the superior vena cava. Sinus venosus defects are associated frequently with anomalous connection of pulmonary veins from the right lung to the junctional area of the superior vena cava and right atrium. Most often, an atrial defect involves the fossa ovalis, is midseptal in location, and is of the ostium secundum type. The ostium secundum

defect should not be confused with a patent foramen ovale. Anatomic obliteration of the foramen ovale ordinarily follows its functional closure soon after birth. An opening may persist if the flap valve covering the foramen is too short or if left atrial dilatation is accompanied by stretching and enlargement of the foramen ovale. Ostium primum anomalies are a form of endocardial cushion defect that lie immediately adjacent to the atrioventricular valves, either of which may be deformed and incompetent, or which may form together a common atrioventricular canal; this defect may also involve the superior portion of the interventricular septum. Ostium primum defects occur commonly in patients with Down's syndrome (mongolism). Lutembacher's syndrome is the designation applied to the rare combination of atrial septal defect and mitral stenosis; this component of the malformation almost invariably is the result of acquired rheumatic valvulitis.

The magnitude of the left-to-right shunt through an atrial septal defect depends on the size of the defect, the relative compliance of the ventricles, and the relative resistances in the pulmonary and systemic circulations. In patients with a patent foramen ovale or a small atrial septal defect, the left atrial pressure may exceed the right by several millimeters of mercury, whereas the mean pressures are similar in both atria when the defect is large. The left-to-right shunt causes diastolic overloading of the right ventricle and increased pulmonary blood flow. The pulmonary vascular resistance is usually normal in the child and young adult with atrial septal defect, and the volume load is usually well tolerated even though pulmonary blood flow may be three to six times greater than systemic. There is a preferential shunting of the blood returning to the left atrium through the right pulmonary veins, because of their proximity to the defect. Streaming of unsaturated inferior vena caval blood from right to left is not uncommon in patients with ostium secundum defect or a prominent crista dividens of the inferior vena cava, even in the absence of pulmonary hypertension. Patients with atrial septal defect are usually asymptomatic in early life, although cardiorespiratory symptoms occur in many of the older patients. Beyond the fourth decade, a significant number of patients develop atrial arrhythmias, pulmonary arterial hypertension, bidirectional and then right-to-left shunting of blood, and cardiac failure. Patients exposed to the chronic environmental hypoxia of high altitude tend to develop pulmonary hypertension at younger ages. Features that suggest that the defect is of the ostium primum variety include the onset of disability, pulmonary hypertension, and heart failure in infancy or childhood.

Physical examination usually reveals a prominent right ventricular cardiac impulse and palpable pulmonary artery pulsation. The first heart sound is normal or split with accentuation of the tricuspid valve closure sound. A pulmonary ejection sound is rare. Increased flow across the pulmonic valve is responsible for a midsystolic pulmonary ejection murmur. The second sound is widely split and is fixed in relation to respiration, because of reciprocal changes in the magnitude of the left-to-right shunt and of the systemic venous inflow into the right ventricle during respiration, so that filling of the right ventricle remains constant throughout the respiratory cycle. A middiastolic rumbling murmur at the fourth intercostal space and along the left sternal border reflects increased flow across the tricuspid valve. In patients with ostium primum defects, an apical thrill and holosystolic murmur indicate the presence of associated mitral or tricuspid incompetence or a ventricular septal defect.

The physical findings are altered when an increase in the pulmonary vascular resistance results in diminution of the left-to-right shunt. Both the pulmonary and tricuspid murmurs decrease in intensity, the pulmonic component of the second heart sound and the systolic ejection sound are further accentuated, the two components of the second heart sound may fuse, and a diastolic murmur of pulmonic incompetence appears. Cyanosis and clubbing accompany the development of a right-to-left shunt.

The electrocardiogram in patients with an ostium secundum defect usually shows right axis deviation and a right ventricular conduction defect. A coronary sinus pacemaker is occasionally noted in patients with defects of the sinus venosus type. In patients with an ostium primum defect, the right ventricular conduction defect is characteristically accompanied by left axis deviation and by superior orientation and counterclockwise rotation of the QRS loop in the frontal plane. Varying degrees of right ventricular and right atrial hypertrophy may be seen with each type of defect, depending on the height of the pulmonary artery pressure; prolongation of the P-R interval is most common with defects of the ostium primum variety. Chest roentgenograms reveal enlargement of the right atrium and ventricle, dilatation of the pulmonary artery and its branches, and increased pulmonary vascular markings. Left atrial enlargement is extremely uncommon.

The diagnosis may be confirmed readily at cardiac catheterization by passage of the catheter across the atrial defect. The site at which the catheter crosses, if high in the cardiac silhouette, may suggest a sinus venosus defect, or, if low, a primum defect. Serial determinations of the oxygen saturation, or indicator-dilution or foreign-gas techniques, may be used to identify the magnitude of the shunt. In young patients, pressures in the right side of the heart are often normal despite a large shunt; pulmonary arterial hypertension occurs with greater frequency in the older patients. If a primum defect is present, a left ventricular angiogram will frequently demonstrate a "gooseneck" deformity of the left ventricular outflow tract caused by an abnormal anterior mitral valve leaflet; it may also show mitral regurgitation. When a high oxygen saturation is found in the superior vena cava, or when the catheter enters pulmonary veins directly from the right atrium, a sinus venosus defect is likely, and indicator-dilution dye curves and selective angiography will aid in identifying the number and location of the anomalous veins. Partial anomalous pulmonary venous connection, although generally associated with a sinus venosus defect, may occasionally accompany primum and secundum defects.

Patients with atrial septal defect rarely die before the fifth decade of life. During the fifth and sixth decades, the incidence of progressive symptoms, often leading to severe disability, increases substantially. Medical management should include prompt treatment of respiratory tract infections, antiarrhythmic medications for atrial fibrillation or supraventricular tachycardia, and the usual measures for heart failure (Chap. 264) if these complications occur. Although the risk of subacute bacterial endocarditis is low, antibiotics should be administered prophylactically prior to dental procedures (see Chap. 137).

Operative repair, ideally between five and ten years of age, should be advised for all patients with uncomplicated atrial septal defects in whom there is evidence of significant left-to-right shunting, i.e., with pulmonary-to-systemic flow ratios exceeding approximately 1.5/1.0. Excellent results may be anticipated, at low risk, even in patients beyond forty years of age. The defect is closed by suture or with a patch of prosthetic material with the patient on cardiopulmonary bypass. Special attention must be given to the atrioventricular valves in patients with primum defects, since suture repair of a cleft in either or both of them, and even replacement with a prosthetic valve, may be necessary to prevent significant regurgitation and failure in the postoperative period. The operative risk and the incidence of such complications as complete heart block and the persistence of significant mitral regurgitation are significantly higher in patients with endocardial cushion defects. Operation should not be carried out in patients with small defects and trivial left-to-right shunts, or in those with severe pulmonary vascular disease without a net left-to-right shunt.

Ventricular Septal Defect

Isolated defects of the ventricular septum are among the commonest cardiac malformations, and they are encountered as one component of a combination of anomalies more often than any other. Most frequently, the opening is single and situated in the membranous portion of the septum. The functional disturbance caused by a ventricular septal defect is dependent primarily on its size and the status of the pulmonary vascular bed, rather than on the location of the defect. A substantial left-to-right ventricular pressure gradient occurs in the presence of a small defect (maladie de Roger), and a small shunt, limited by the size of the defect, occurs throughout systole. The larger the defect, the more likely it is that both ventricles will function as a single pumping chamber with two outlets, equalizing the pressures in the systemic and pulmonary circulations. In such patients, the magnitude of the left-to-right shunt varies inversely with the pulmonary vascular resistance. In patients with large defects and large left-to-right shunts, the left ventricle is overloaded and may fail. Survival through infancy in many of these patients is predicated on persistence of the fetal pulmonary vascular pattern, the development of an elevated pulmonary vascular resistance, or the secondary development of infundibular hypertrophy and obstruction to right ventricular outflow. Irreversible obliterative changes in the pulmonary vessels with dominant right-to-left shunts and cyanosis become manifest after the second decade in many patients with large defects. Spontaneous closure of even large ventricular defects occurs in a significant number of patients, especially before the age of two years. In others, the relative size of the interventricular communication may diminish as normal growth of the heart occurs with advancing age.

The clinical picture varies greatly, depending on the patient's age, the size of the defect, and the level of the pulmonary vascular resistance. Patients with a small defect are asymptomatic; moderate left-to-right shunts are associated with effort intolerance and fatigue. Large defects are commonly accompanied by frequent pulmonary infections, growth retardation, and cardiac failure in infancy, but survival past this period is often associated with an amelioration of symptoms until adulthood. In patients with severe pulmonary vascular obstruction, symptoms develop most often in adult life and consist of exertional dyspnea, chest pain, syncope, and hemoptysis. The right-to-left shunt leads to cyanosis, clubbing, and polycythemia.

Patients with moderate-sized defects exhibit cardiomegaly with a forceful left ventricular impulse and a prominent systolic thrill along the lower left sternal border. The second heart sound is normally split, with moderate accentuation of the pulmonic component, and a third heart sound and diastolic rumbling murmur reflecting rapid ventricular filling are often audible at the cardiac apex. The characteristic holosystolic murmur results from flow across the defect; it is best heard along the third and fourth interspaces to the left of the sternum, and is widely transmitted over the precordium. A basal midsystolic ejection murmur may also be heard, because of increased flow across the pulmonic valve. In patients with pulmonary vascular obstruction and small left-to-right shunts, both the systolic thrill and murmur decrease in intensity and duration and may disappear entirely, to be replaced by a marked right ventricular precordial lift, pulmonary ejection sound and soft systolic ejection murmur, a closely split second heart sound with accentuation of the pulmonic component, and the diastolic murmur of pulmonic incompetence.

The electrocardiographic pattern, the relative size and contour of the two ventricles roentgenographically, and the appearance of the lung fields serve as indicators of the underlying pathophysiology. The electrocardiogram is generally normal in patients with small defects. Left or combined ventricular hypertrophy is seen with large left-to-right shunts; right ventricular hypertrophy occurs with pulmonary vascular obstruction. The roentgenograms may be normal in patients with small defects, whereas large defects are characterized by an enlarged left atrium, biventricular hypertrophy, a prominent pulmonary artery segment, and increased pulmonary vascular markings. Relative diminution and attenuation of the peripheral pulmonary vasculature occur in patients with obstructive pulmonary vascular disease.

In approximately 90 percent of patients with this mal-

formation, the defect occurs in the membranous septum. Defects in the muscular interventricular septum are more difficult to detect; frequently they are multiple, small fenestrations which produce a large left-to-right shunt. Their recognition is a necessary preliminary to successful operation, because incomplete repair may result in postoperative cardiac failure and death. A shunt from the left ventricle to the right atrium may occur with a defect in the most superior portion of the ventricular septum, since the tricuspid valve is lower than the mitral valve. The clinical, electrocardiographic, and radiologic findings in these patients do not differ appreciably from those with a simple ventricular septal defect, but the diagnosis can be established by left ventriculography. Prolapse of an aortic valve leaflet through a ventricular defect high in the septum beneath the right and noncoronary cusps, or the combination of ventricular septal defect and underdevelopment of an aortic valve commissure, may produce aortic regurgitation that is frequently progressive and is the most significant hemodynamic lesion. In these patients complete operative repair may necessitate insertion of a prosthetic aortic valve. The pathophysiology of single or common ventricle resembles that of a large ventricular septal defect, although the two lesions are dissimilar embryologically. There may be little or no cyanosis if selective streaming and increased pulmonary blood flow occur in patients with a single ventricle. Severe pulmonary hypertension is invariably present unless pulmonic stenosis coexists. It is imperative to differentiate single ventricle from a large ventricular septal defect by angiography because no corrective operation is available for single ventricle.

The prevention or treatment of bacterial endocarditis is part of the medical management of ventricular septal defects of any size, but the risk of this complication is highest in patients with small or moderate-sized defects. Vigorous therapy of respiratory infections is required. In the small infant with a large left-to-right shunt, congestive failure may be severe and intractable despite intensive medical management; this problem is managed best by surgical constriction of the pulmonary artery, followed when the patient is older, by a corrective operation. Closure of the defect of the ventricular septum is indicated in older children and adults when there is a moderate or large left-to-right shunt, regardless of the level of pulmonary artery pressure. Operation is contraindicated when the pulmonary vascular resistance is elevated to a level which eliminates the net left-to-right shunt. The recognition of associated cardiac anomalies is imperative if surgical treatment is contemplated. The most common of these are patent ductus arteriosus, ostium secundum atrial defects, pulmonic stenosis, coarctation of the aorta, and corrected transposition of the great arteries.

Patent Ductus Arteriosus

The ductus arteriosus is a vessel leading from the bifurcation of the pulmonary artery to the aorta just distal to the left subclavian artery. Normal closure of the ductus immediately after birth may be due to the sudden increase in arterial oxygen tension that accompanies ventilation and/or the release of vasoactive substances. Intimal proliferation and fibrosis proceed more gradually, so that total anatomic obliteration may not occur for several months after birth. Persistent patency of the ductus after birth is a relatively common anomaly, occurring more frequently in females, in the offspring of pregnancies complicated by first-trimester rubella, and in children born at high altitudes. Although this anomaly occurs most frequently in the isolated form, it may coexist with other malformations, particularly coarctation of the aorta, ventricular septal defect, pulmonic stenosis, and aortic stenosis.

The flow across the ductus is determined by the pressure relationships between the aorta and the pulmonary artery and by the cross-sectional area and length of the ductus itself. Most commonly, pulmonary pressures are normal, and a gradient and shunt from aorta to pulmonary artery persists throughout the cardiac cycle. Physical examination reveals a characteristic thrill and a continuous "machinery" murmur, with a late systolic accentuation at the upper left sternal border. The left atrium and ventricle enlarge to accommodate the increased pulmonary venous return, and flow murmurs across the mitral and aortic valves may be detected. With large or moderate left-to-right shunts, the runoff of blood through the ductus causes a widened systemic pulse pressure and bounding peripheral pulses. The hemodynamic abnormality is reflected by left ventricular and, occasionally, left atrial hypertrophy on the electrocardiogram, and by left atrial and ventricular enlargement, a prominent ascending aorta and pulmonary artery, and pulmonary vascular engorgement on the chest roentgenogram.

The clinical recognition of patent ductus arteriosus may be difficult in infancy, in pulmonary hypertension, or in heart failure. In these circumstances, the pressure gradient between the aorta and pulmonary artery is reduced or absent, as is the typical continuous murmur, and there may only be a systolic ejection murmur at the base, a diastolic blowing murmur of pulmonary regurgitation (Graham Steell), or no murmur audible at all. When severe pulmonary vascular disease results in reversal of flow through the ductus, unoxygenated blood is shunted to the descending aorta, and the toes, rather than the fingers, become cyanotic and clubbed, a finding termed *differential cyanosis.*

Although a large ductus often results in cardiac failure and pulmonary edema in infancy, this anomaly is usually compatible with survival until adult life. The leading causes of death in adults with patent ductus are cardiac failure and bacterial endocarditis. In older patients, severe pulmonary vascular obstruction may cause aneurysmal dilatation, calcification, and rupture of the ductus.

In the absence of severe pulmonary vascular disease with predominant right-to-left shunting of blood, the simple presence of a patent ductus is generally considered a sufficient indication for operation, at least in patients over three years of age. Ligation or division of the ductus is associated with a low risk (under 2 percent) when it is performed electively in an otherwise healthy individual. The operative risk is reduced if cardiac failure can be treated successfully before operation. Operation should be deferred for several months in patients treated successfully for bacterial endarteritis because the ductus may remain somewhat edematous and friable. Rarely, when the infection does not subside with intensive antibiotic treatment, surgical ligation may be necessary to eradicate the ductal endarteritis. In the occasional older patient with a calcified ductus and thin-walled, dilated pulmonary artery, surgical treatment may require patch obliteration of the aortic opening of the ductus with the patient on cardiopulmonary bypass.

AORTOPULMONARY SEPTAL DEFECT. Aortopulmonary window, partial truncus arteriosis, and aortic septal defect are other designations applied to this relatively uncommon anomaly, which consists of a communication between the aorta and the pulmonary artery just above the semilunar valves. Such defects are usually large and are accompanied by varying degrees of obstructive pulmonary vascular disease and severe pulmonary arterial hypertension. The anomaly may coexist with patent ductus arteriosus and be difficult to distinguish from it. However, the murmur of aortopulmonary septal defect is rarely continuous, and a basal systolic murmur is most common. Cardiomegaly is present, and pulmonary hypertension is reflected in a loud and palpable sound of pulmonary valve closure. The diagnosis of aortopulmonary septal defect should be suspected whenever a large shunt into the pulmonary artery is demonstrated at catheterization. Distinction from patent ductus and persistent truncus arteriosus is facilitated by selective angiocardiography, with the injection of contrast material into the left ventricle and/or the root of the aorta. Operative correction is usually indicated in children and adults with large left-to-right shunts; total cardiopulmonary bypass is required, and the defect is closed, generally with a prosthetic patch.

AORTIC SINUS ANEURYSM AND FISTULA. Congenital aneurysm of an aortic sinus of Valsalva, particularly the right coronary sinus, is an uncommon anomaly with a predilection for males; it consists of a separation, or lack of fusion, between the media of the aorta and the annulus fibrosus of the aortic valve. Progressive aneurysmal dilatation of the weakened area develops but may not be recognized until the third or fourth decade of life, when rupture into a cardiac chamber occurs. The receiving chamber of the aorticocardiac fistula is usually the right ventricle, but occasionally, when the noncoronary cusp is involved, the fistula drains into the right atrium. Associated anomalies are common and include bicuspid aortic valve, ventricular septal defect, and coarctation of the aorta.

The unruptured aneurysm generally does not produce a hemodynamic abnormality, although pressure on the intracardiac conduction system by an unruptured aneurysm occasionally causes atrioventricular block. Rupture is often of abrupt onset, causes chest pain, and creates continuous arteriovenous shunting and volume overloading of both right and left heart chambers, with resultant heart failure. An additional complication is bacterial endocarditis, which may originate either on the edges of the aneurysm or on those areas in the right side of the heart which are traumatized by the jetlike stream of blood flowing through the fistula. This anomaly should be suspected in a patient with a history of the recent onset of chest pain, symptoms of diminished cardiac reserve, bounding pulses, and a loud, superficial, continuous murmur accentuated in diastole when the fistula opens into the right ventricle, as well as a thrill along the right or left lower parasternal area. The electrocardiogram shows biventricular hypertrophy, and the chest roentgenogram demonstrates generalized cardiomegaly. The diagnosis may be established definitively by retrograde thoracic aortography. At operation the aneurysm is closed and amputated and the aortic wall is reunited with the heart, either by direct suture or with a prosthesis.

CORONARY ARTERIOVENOUS FISTULA. Coronary arteriovenous fistula is an unusual anomaly that may be seen in various anatomic patterns but most often consists of a communication between the right coronary artery and the right atrium or ventricle. Most often the shunt through the fistula is of small magnitude and myocardial blood flow is not compromised. Potential complications include bacterial endocarditis, thrombus formation with occlusion or distal embolization, rupture of an aneurysmal fistula, and, rarely, pulmonary hypertension and congestive failure when the left-to-right shunt is large. The finding of a loud, superficial, continuous murmur at the lower or midsternal border usually prompts a further evaluation of asymptomatic patients. Retrograde thoracic aortography or coronary arteriography permit identification of the size and anatomic features of the fistulous tract, which may be closed by suture obliteration.

ANOMALOUS PULMONARY ORIGIN OF CORONARY ARTERY. In this rare malformation, the left coronary artery originates from the pulmonary artery. Myocardial infarction and fibrosis commonly develop during the first 6 months of life, leading to death within the first year. Rarely, the patient lives into childhood or adolescence without surgical correction. As the elevated pulmonary vascular resistance declines immediately after birth, perfusion of the left coronary artery from the pulmonary artery ceases and the direction of flow in the anomalous vessel reverses. Thus, blood flows from the aorta to the right coronary artery, then through collateral channels to the left coronary artery, and finally to the pulmonary artery. In effect, the left coronary artery behaves as a fistulous communication between the aorta and the pulmonary artery. Total myocardial perfusion through the right coronary artery increases if adequate collateral channels develop between the two coronary circulations, but this collateral circulation may become so extensive that the patient may develop clinical manifestations of a large arteriovenous shunt, as well as a continuous or diastolic murmur.

The diagnosis of anomalous origin of the coronary artery is supported by the electrocardiographic demonstration of deep Q waves in association with S-T segment alterations and T-wave inversions in leads I, aVL, V_5, and V_6. Chest roentgenograms show moderate to severe enlargement of the left atrium and ventricle. Indicator-dilution curves and aortic root or coronary angiography demonstrate the retrograde drainage of the coronary vessel into the pulmonary artery.

Ideal operative management of these patients consists of anastomosis of the left coronary artery to a systemic artery or to the aorta via a graft. However, the disorder may also be managed by simple ligation of the left coronary artery at its origin, preventing retrograde flow and allowing perfusion of the left ventricle by blood supplied through anastomoses from the right coronary artery. The outcome of operation and ultimate prognosis are influenced significantly by the degree of myocardial damage suffered preoperatively.

PERSISTENT TRUNCUS ARTERIOSUS. Persistent truncus arteriosus is a rare but serious anomaly that often coexists with malformations of other organ systems. A single vessel forms the outlet of both ventricles and gives rise to the systemic, pulmonary, and coronary arteries. It is always accompanied by a ventricular septal defect and frequently by a right-sided aortic arch. The designation "pseudo-truncus arteriosus" refers to the condition in which a single vessel arises from the heart but is accompanied by a remnant of atretic pulmonary artery, a malformation which does not differ from tetralogy of Fallot with pulmonary atresia (p. 1175). Truncus malformations may be classified embryologically and anatomically according to the mode of origin of the pulmonary vessels from the common trunk, or from a functional point of view, by the magnitude of flow to the lungs. Pulmonary flow is governed by the size of the pulmonary arteries and the pulmonary vascular resistance. Most often, mild cyanosis coexists with the cardiac findings of a large left-to-right shunt. The most frequent physical findings include cardiomegaly, a systolic ejection sound, a loud, single second heart sound, a harsh systolic murmur accompanied by a thrill, and a low-pitched middiastolic rumbling murmur. Left ventricular hypertrophy, alone or in combination with right ventricular hypertrophy, is present electrocardiographically. Gross cardiomegaly with left or combined ventricular enlargement, left atrial enlargement, and a small or absent main pulmonary artery segment with pulmonary vascular engorgement are the usual radiographic findings. The diagnosis should be suspected at catheterization if the catheter fails to enter the central pulmonary arteries from the right ventricle; selective angiocardiography and retrograde aortography are often necessary to establish a precise anatomic diagnosis.

The early fatal course and, in patients surviving infancy, the development of pulmonary vascular obstructive disease are responsible for the poor prognosis associated with persistent truncus arteriosus. Corrective operation is difficult and has met with limited success. Palliative banding of one or both of the pulmonary arteries may be indicated when pulmonary flow is markedly excessive. In patients with inadequate pulmonary blood flow it is usually not possible to enhance pulmonary blood flow with a shunting operation.

VALVULAR AND VASCULAR LESIONS WITH RIGHT-TO-LEFT OR NO SHUNT
Pulmonary Stenosis with Intact Ventricular Septum

Pulmonary stenosis is relatively common, both as an isolated anomaly and in association with other intracardiac defects. Obstruction to right ventricular outflow may be localized to the supravalvular, valvular, or subvalvular levels, or to a combination of these sites. Multiple sites of narrowing of the peripheral pulmonary arteries are often a feature of rubella embryopathy and may be associated with both the familial and sporadic forms of supravalvular aortic stenosis. Valvular pulmonic stenosis, four times as common as the other forms of right ventricular obstruction, may also be familial.

The severity of the obstructing lesion, rather than the site of narrowing, is the most important determinant of the clinical course. In the presence of a normal cardiac output, a peak systolic transvalvular pressure gradient between 50 and 100 mm Hg is considered to be moderate stenosis; levels below and above that range are classified as mild and severe, respectively. Patients with mild pulmonic stenosis are generally asymptomatic and demonstrate little or no progression in the severity of obstruction as they grow older. In patients with more significant stenosis, the severity of the obstruction may increase with time. Progression may be relative and may reflect disproportional physical growth of the patient, infundibular narrowing due to progressive hypertrophy of the right ventricular outflow tract, or fibrosis of the valve cusps. Atresia of the pulmonary valve is commonly associated with a hypoplastic right ventricle and interatrial communication. Symptoms vary according to the degree of obstruction. Infants with pulmonary atresia often die from hypoxia. Fatigue, dyspnea, and syncope may limit the activity of older patients, in whom moderate or severe obstruction prevents an augmentation of pulmonary blood flow with exercise.

The degree of obstruction, or the effective outflow orifice area, influences both the mean transvalvular pressure gradient and the flow rate across the site of stenosis. In patients with severe obstruction, the systolic pressure in the right ventricle may exceed that in the left ventricle, since the ventricular septum is intact.

Right ventricular ejection is prolonged in patients with moderate or severe stenosis, and the sound of pulmonary valve closure is delayed and soft. Right ventricular hypertrophy reduces the compliance of that chamber, and a forceful right atrial contraction is necessary to augment right ventricular filling. A fourth heart sound, prominent *a* waves in the jugular venous pulse, and, occasionally, presystolic pulsations of the liver reflect the vigorous

atrial contraction. The clinical diagnosis is further supported by the presence of a right parasternal lift and a harsh systolic ejection murmur and thrill at the upper left sternal border, often preceded by a systolic ejection sound if the obstruction is valvular. The systolic murmur becomes louder, and its crescendo occurs later in systole as progressively more severe degrees of valvular obstruction result in increasing prolongation of right ventricular systole. The holosystolic decrescendo murmur of tricuspid regurgitation may accompany severe pulmonic stenosis, especially in the presence of congestive heart failure. Cyanosis usually reflects venoatrial shunting through a patent foramen ovale. In patients with supravalvular or peripheral pulmonary arterial stenosis, the murmur is systolic or continuous and is best heard over the area of narrowing, with radiation to the peripheral lung fields.

The electrocardiogram may be helpful in assessing the degree of obstruction to right ventricular output. In mild cases, the electrocardiogram is often normal, whereas moderate and severe stenoses are associated with right axis deviation and right ventricular hypertrophy. A right ventricular strain pattern, consisting of inverted T waves across the precordium, is associated with severe stenosis. Severe stenosis may be accompanied by high-amplitude P waves in leads II and V_1, indicating right atrial enlargement. The chest roentgenogram in patients with mild or moderate pulmonic stenosis often shows a heart of normal size and normal vascularity of the lungs. In the presence of valvular stenosis, poststenotic dilatation of the main pulmonary artery may be evident. In patients with severe obstruction and resultant right ventricular failure, right atrial and right ventricular enlargement are generally evident. The pulmonary vascularity may be reduced in patients with severe stenosis, right ventricular failure, and/or a venoarterial shunt at the atrial level.

When pulmonic stenosis is suspected clinically, cardiac catheterization and angiocardiography with right ventricular injection are indicated to localize the site of obstruction and evaluate its severity, and to document the coexistence of additional cardiac malformations. The treatment of moderate and severe degrees of pulmonary valvular and subvalvular stenosis is surgical. Direct surgical relief of the obstruction may usually be accomplished at a low risk. Although operation may reduce or obliterate the pressure gradient, the pulmonic valve is not rendered normal, and prophylaxis against bacterial endocarditis should be continued. Multiple stenoses of the peripheral pulmonary arteries are usually inoperable, but narrowing of a single branch or at the bifurcation of the main pulmonary trunk may be corrected.

Tetralogy of Fallot

The four components of this malformation are (1) ventricular septal defect; (2) obstruction to right ventricular outflow; (3) overriding of the aorta; and (4) right ventricular hypertrophy. Systolic pressures are equal in the right ventricle and aorta as a consequence of the first two components. The overall incidence of tetralogy approaches 10 percent of all forms of congenital heart disease, and it is the most common anomaly responsible for cyanosis after the age of one year. The ventricular defect is usually large, approximating the aortic orifice in size, and located high in the septum, just below the aortic valve. The aortic root may be displaced anteriorly and straddle or override the septal defect, but, as in the normal heart, it lies to the right of the origin of the pulmonary artery. The site of obstruction to right ventricular outflow is variable; infundibular stenosis occurs as the only major lesion in about one-half the patients and coexists with valvular obstruction in another 25 percent. Supravalvular and peripheral pulmonary arterial narrowing may be observed, and unilateral absence of a pulmonary artery is noted occasionally. When the main pulmonary artery, pulmonic valve, or right ventricular infundibulum is atretic, the condition may be called *pseudo-truncus arteriosus* (p. 1173). In such cases, the lungs are perfused through enlarged bronchial arteries and/or through the pulmonary arteries via a patent ductus arteriosus. A right-sided aortic knob, arch, and descending aorta occur in approximately 25 percent of patients with tetralogy of Fallot.

The relationship between the resistance to blood flow from the ventricle into the aorta and into the pulmonary vessels plays the major role in determining the hemodynamic and clinical picture. Therefore, it is the severity of obstruction to right ventricular outflow which is of fundamental significance. When right ventricular outflow obstruction is severe, the pulmonary blood flow is markedly reduced and a large volume of unsaturated systemic venous blood is shunted from right to left across the ventricular septal defect, severe cyanosis and polycythemia occur, and symptoms of systemic anoxia are prominent. The term *pink,* or *acyanotic, tetralogy of Fallot* is used often to describe an interventricular communication and a milder degree of obstruction to right ventricular outflow with no appreciable venoarterial shunting. In some patients the obstruction to right ventricular outflow is so mild that pulmonary exceeds systemic blood flow and the symptoms resemble those produced by a simple ventricular septal defect. Occasionally in such patients, progressive pulmonary infundibular obstruction leads ultimately to the typical cyanotic picture of tetralogy of Fallot.

Most children with tetralogy of Fallot are cyanotic from birth or develop cyanosis before one year of age. Dyspnea with exertion, retarded growth and development, clubbing, and polycythemia are common. When resting after exertion, patients with tetralogy characteristically assume a squatting posture. Spells of severe anoxia and cyanosis (see p. 1168) related to sudden increase in venoarterial shunting and a reduction in pulmonary blood flow constitute a major threat to survival.

Physical examination reveals variable degrees of underdevelopment and cyanosis. Clubbing of the terminal digits may be prominent after the first year of life. A right ventricular impulse and systolic thrill may be palpable along the left sternal border; there is no generalized cardiomegaly. The second heart sound is single, and the pulmonic component is rarely audible. A systolic ejection murmur is produced by flow across the narrowed right ventricular outflow tract or pulmonic valve. The intensity and duration of the murmur vary inversely with the severity of obstruction, the opposite of the relation existing in patients with an intact ventricular septum and pulmonary stenosis. Polycythemia, decreased systemic vascular resistance, and increased obstruction to right ventricular outflow may all be responsible for a decrease in the intensity of the murmur. A continuous murmur over the paravertebral area may indicate collateral circulation to the lungs through bronchial arteries.

The electrocardiogram ordinarily shows right ventricular and, less often, right atrial hypertrophy. Radiologic examination characteristically reveals a normal-sized, boot-shaped heart (*coeur en sabot*) with prominence of the right ventricle and a concavity in the region of the pulmonary conus. The pulmonary vascular markings are typically diminished, and the aortic arch and knob may be on the right side. Selective angiocardiography with right ventricular injection is necessary to evaluate the architecture of the right ventricular outflow tract, pulmonary valve and annulus, and caliber of the main branches of the pulmonary artery.

Among the factors that may complicate the management of patients with tetralogy are iron deficiency anemia, subacute bacterial endocarditis, paradoxic embolism, polycythemia, coagulation defects, and cerebral infarction or abscess. The paroxysmal cyanotic spells may respond quickly to oxygen, placing the child in the knee-chest position, and morphine. If the spell persists, metabolic acidosis will develop from prolonged anaerobic metabolism, and infusion of sodium bicarbonate may be necessary to interrupt the attack. Vasopressors, β-adrenergic blockade, or general anesthesia may occasionally be necessary.

Total correction is ultimately advisable for almost all patients with tetralogy of Fallot. However, if cyanosis or symptoms are marked in an infant or young child, the risk of primary repair is high, and a palliative operation designed to increase pulmonary blood flow is recommended. These procedures include aortopulmonary or subclavian-pulmonary arterial anastomosis or transventricular infundibulectomy or valvulotomy. Total correction can then be carried out at a lower risk later in childhood or during adolescence.

EBSTEIN'S ANOMALY. In this rare anomaly the annular attachment of the septal and posterior leaflets of the tricuspid valve is usually lower than normal; the leaflets originate from the right ventricular wall rather than from the atrioventricular ring. Hence, the portion of the right ventricle that lies between the atrioventricular ring and the origin of the valve is continuous with the right atrial chamber. The tricuspid valve is usually incompetent, and the foramen ovale is patent. In addition, the right ventricle exhibits varying degrees of hypoplasia. The clinical manifestations of Ebstein's anomaly are variable, depending on the severity of the anatomic changes. Ultimately, however, it is characterized by the development of either progressive cyanosis resulting from the right-to-left shunt across the interatrial communication, or symptoms resulting from right ventricular dysfunction. Paroxysmal arrhythmias are common.

On physical examination, a prominent systolic pulsation of the liver and large *v* wave in the jugular venous pulse are found to accompany the systolic thrill and murmur of tricuspid regurgitation. Wide splitting of the first and second heart sounds and prominent third and fourth heart sounds may produce a characteristically rhythmic auscultatory cadence. The electrocardiogram shows giant P waves, a prolonged P-R interval, and complete or incomplete right bundle branch block. Occasionally, there is a short P-R interval with the Wolff-Parkinson-White conduction anomaly. Roentgenographic and fluoroscopic studies usually demonstrate an enlarged right atrium, a small right ventricle, and pulmonary artery with reduced pulsations; the pulmonary vascularity may be reduced if a large right-to-left shunt is present. At cardiac catheterization the intracavitary electrocardiogram recorded just proximal to the tricuspid valve shows a right ventricular type of complex, while the pressure recorded is that of the right atrium.

In some patients improvement has resulted from anastomosis of the superior vena cava to the right pulmonary artery to divert systemic venous return from the right atrium and to increase pulmonary blood flow. Others have been benefited by prosthetic replacement of the tricuspid valve.

TRICUSPID ATRESIA. The features of this complex malformation include atresia of the tricuspid valve, an interatrial communication, and, frequently, hypoplasia of the right ventricle and pulmonary artery, as well as transposition of the great arteries. Extrauterine survival is dependent on a right-to-left shunt at the atrial level. Blood reaches the lungs through a patent ductus arteriosus, bronchial collateral vessels, or the right ventricle and pulmonary artery via a ventricular septal defect. The clinical picture is usually dominated by symptoms resulting from greatly diminished pulmonary blood flow, with anoxic spells and severe cyanosis.

The electrocardiogram may be of particular help in establishing the diagnosis. Left axis deviation, right atrial enlargement, and left ventricular hypertrophy in a cyanotic child strongly suggest tricuspid atresia. The prognosis for these children is extremely poor; many die in the first weeks or months of life. Palliative operations, consisting of increasing pulmonary blood flow and/or relieving significant interatrial obstruction, carry a significant risk. Total operative correction of the anomaly is not yet feasible.

Coarctation of the Aorta

Narrowing or constriction of the lumen of the aorta may occur anywhere along its length but is most commonly localized just distal to the origin of the left subclavian artery near the insertion of the ligamentum arteriosum. Coarctation is encountered in approximately 7 percent of patients with congenital heart disease and is twice as common in males as in females, although the lesion occurs frequently in patients with gonadal dys-

genesis (Turner's syndrome, Chap. 98). The clinical manifestation depend on the site and extent of obstruction and the presence of associated cardiac anomalies, which occur in about one-third of patients. These include bicuspid aortic valve, patent ductus arteriosus, ventricular septal defect, and congenital aortic stenosis. When the coarctation is located proximal to the ductus arteriosus, right ventricular hypertrophy develops in utero and pulmonary hypertension and congestive heart failure are common in early life. Differential cyanosis may result from preferential shunting of unsaturated pulmonary arterial blood through a patent ductus arteriosus to the lower part of the body.

More commonly, the coarctation is postductal and the ductus arteriosus is closed. The majority of children and young adults with isolated postductal coarctation are asymptomatic. Complaints of headache, cold extremities, and claudication with exercise may be noted, although attention is usually directed to the cardiovascular system when a heart murmur or hypertension in the upper extremities is detected on routine physical examination. Both mechanical and humoral factors, particularly of renal origin and involving the renin-angiotensin-aldosterone mechanism (Chap. 37), play a significant role in the production of hypertension in these patients.

Absence, marked diminution, or delayed pulsations in the femoral arteries and a low or unobtainable arterial pressure in the lower extremities with hypertension in the arms is the basic clue to diagnosis. In adults, enlarged and pulsatile collateral vessels may be palpated in the intercostal spaces anteriorly, in the axillae, or posteriorly in the interscapular area. A midsystolic murmur over the anterior part of the chest, back, and spinous processes is most frequent, becoming continuous if the lumen is narrowed sufficiently to result in a high-velocity jet across the lesion throughout the cardiac cycle. Additional systolic and continuous murmurs over the lateral thoracic wall may reflect increased flow through dilated and tortuous collateral vessels. The electrocardiogram reveals left ventricular hypertrophy of varying degree, depending on the height of the arterial pressure proximal to the obstruction and the patient's age; predominant right or combined ventricular hypertrophy may be seen in infants and children, and usually implies a complicated lesion. Roentgenograms may show a dilated left subclavian artery high on the left mediastinal border and a dilated ascending aorta. Indentation of the aorta at the site of coarctation and pre- and poststenotic dilatation (the "3" sign) along the left paramediastinal shadow are almost pathognomonic. Notching of the ribs is an important radiographic sign; it is due to erosion by dilated collateral vessels, increases with age, and usually becomes apparent between the sixth and twelfth years of life. Confirmation of the diagnosis by cardiac catheterization and aortography is generally unnecessary but may be indicated to localize accurately the site of obstruction, determine the length of the coarctation, and identify associated malformations.

The treatment of uncomplicated coarctation of the aorta is surgical; resection and end-to-end anastomosis can be accomplished with excellent results in most patients, although it is occasionally necessary to use a graft in the repair if the narrowed segment is long. Paradoxic hypertension of short duration is often noted in the immediate postoperative period, and occasionally a necrotizing panarteritis of the small vessels of the gastrointestinal tract of uncertain cause complicates the course of recovery. Without operative treatment, heart failure may occur during infancy in patients with severe obstruction. In those who survive the first 2 years of life complications are uncommon before the second or third decade, and operation on asymptomatic patients is advised ideally between the ages of six and twelve years. The chief hazards to patients with coarctation result from severe hypertension and include the development of cerebral aneurysms and hemorrhage, rupture of the aorta, left ventricular failure, and bacterial endocarditis.

Congenital Aortic Stenosis

Malformations that cause obstruction to the ejection of blood from the left ventricle include congenital valvular aortic stenosis, the discrete form of congenital subaortic stenosis, congenital narrowing of the supravalvular ascending aorta, and idiopathic hypertrophic subaortic stenosis (Chap. 273).

VALVULAR AORTIC STENOSIS. Valvular aortic stenosis occurs in approximately 4 percent of patients with congenital cardiovascular defects. The congenital bicuspid aortic valve, which is not necessarily stenotic, may actually be the most common congenital malformation of the heart, although it may go undetected in early life. Because bicuspid valves may become stenotic with time, the lesion may become of clinical significance only in adult life, when it may be difficult to distinguish it anatomically from acquired rheumatic aortic stenosis. Congenital valvular aortic stenosis occurs three to four times more often in males than in females. Associated cardiovascular anomalies occur in almost one-fifth of the patients; patent ductus arteriosus and coarctation of the aorta occur most frequently with valvular aortic stenosis, and all three lesions may coexist.

The basic malformation consists of thickening and increased rigidity of the valve tissue and varying degrees of commissural fusion. The dynamics of blood flow associated with a congenitally deformed aortic valve commonly leads to thickening of the cusps and, in later life, to calcification. When the obstruction is hemodynamically significant, concentric hypertrophy of the left ventricular wall and dilatation of the ascending aorta occur.

The hemodynamic abnormalities produced by obstruction to left ventricular outflow have been discussed in Chap. 264. A peak systolic pressure gradient exceeding 75 mm Hg, in association with a normal cardiac output, or an effective aortic orifice less than 0.5 sq cm per sq m body surface area, is considered to represent critical obstruction to left ventricular outflow. The resting cardiac output and stroke volume are generally within normal limits. During exercise, however, the majority of patients with critical stenosis show little elevation of the cardiac output, because an increase in blood flow across the stenotic valve can occur only if the transvalvular pressure gradient increases disproportionately.

Most children with congenital aortic stenosis are asymptomatic and grow and develop normally. Initial attention is usually called to these children when a murmur is detected on a routine examination. At least moderately severe obstruction should be suspected if there is a definite history of fatigability and exertional dyspnea. In patients with severe obstruction, the inability of the left ventricle to increase its output and the cerebral flow during exercise may result in exertional syncope, while the disparity between the oxygen supply to the left ventricle and myocardial oxygen requirements may be responsible for anginal pain. The truly symptomatic child with valvular aortic stenosis generally has critical stenosis, although a lack of symptoms does not preclude the presence of moderately severe obstruction. Sudden death, a potential threat to these patients, occurs in from 1 to 7.5 percent. Its precise cause is poorly understood, but ventricular arrhythmias, perhaps initiated by acute myocardial ischemia, may be the inciting event.

When the degree of aortic stenosis is significant, a left ventricular lift is usually palpable and a precordial systolic thrill is felt over the base of the heart with transmission to the jugular notch and along the carotid arteries. The increased force of left atrial contraction in the presence of left ventricular hypertrophy results in a palpable presystolic expansion. A systolic aortic ejection sound, signifying opening of the aortic valves, may be heard at the cardiac apex when the valve is mobile; it is heard more often in patients with mild to moderate stenosis than in those with severe stenosis. Delayed closure of the stenotic aortic valve leads to a single or a closely split second heart sound, and paradoxic splitting may be present. A fourth heart sound is generally associated with severe obstruction. The systolic murmur which is characteristic of valvular aortic stenosis starts after the completion of left ventricular isometric contraction or with the ejection sound, and is rhomboid-shaped, loud, harsh, and best heard at the base of the heart. The murmur, like the thrill, radiates to the jugular notch and carotid vessels, as well as to the apex. In some patients, an early diastolic blowing murmur of aortic regurgitation is present, but unless the valve leaflets have been eroded by bacterial endocarditis, the regurgitation is usually not hemodynamically significant.

The electrocardiographic findings produced by left ventricular hypertrophy tend to vary with the severity of obstruction, although a normal or near-normal electrocardiogram does not exclude severe aortic stenosis. The left ventricular "strain pattern," which consists of left ventricular hypertrophy combined with S-T segment depressions and T-wave inversion in the left precordial leads, generally, but not always, indicates that severe aortic stenosis is present.

Roentgenographically, the overall heart size is most often normal or slightly enlarged. Left atrial enlargement and concentric left ventricular hypertrophy accompany moderate or severe obstruction. Poststenotic dilatation of the ascending aorta is a common finding. Cardiac catheterization is indicated when the clinical diagnosis of aortic stenosis has been established and in patients in whom the history, clinical examination, roentgenogram, *or* electrocardiogram suggests the possibility of severe obstruction. The procedure may be expected to establish precisely the site and severity of obstruction, and to identify associated malformations.

The medical management of congenital valvular aortic stenosis includes prophylaxis against bacterial endocarditis, the administration of digitalis, and sodium restriction in patients with symptoms of diminished cardiac reserve. If severe aortic stenosis is present, strict avoidance of strenuous physical activity is advised even when the patient is asymptomatic, and participation in competitive sports should probably also be restricted in patients with milder degrees of obstruction. The decision concerning the advisability of operation depends on the presence of severe obstruction rather than on the symptoms described by the patient. Operation is carried out under direct vision with the aid of total cardiopulmonary bypass, and the fused commissures are opened judiciously in order to avoid the creation of significant aortic regurgitation while relieving the obstruction. Following commissurotomy the valves remain somewhat deformed, and it is possible that further degenerative changes, including calcification, will lead to significant stenosis later.

SUBAORTIC STENOSIS. The most common form of subaortic stenosis is the idiopathic hypertrophic variety, which occurs in a congenital form in about one-third of the patients and is discussed in Chap. 273. Both clinically and physiologically, however, it is the discrete form of subaortic stenosis which resembles valvular aortic stenosis. Discrete subaortic stenosis is less common than isolated valvular obstruction, but it also occurs more frequently in males than in females. The lesion consists of a membranous diaphragm or fibrous ring encircling the left ventricular outflow tract just beneath the base of the aortic valve. There are no clinical criteria which can be relied upon to distinguish the two forms of obstruction, although a systolic ejection sound is rarely heard in patients with the discrete form of subvalvular aortic stenosis and the diastolic murmur of aortic regurgitation is more common with this lesion than it is in patients with valvular aortic stenosis. Also, valvular calcification is not observed roentgenographically in patients with subaortic

Table 268-2. UNUSUAL CAUSES OF SUBAORTIC STENOSIS

1. Accessory tissue of the mitral valve
2. Restriction of movement of the anterior mitral valve leaflet
   a. Anomalous basal attachment of anterior leaflet
   b. Accessory chordae tendineae
   c. Abnormal fusion of valvular tissue to the septal wall of the outflow tract
   d. Convergence of all of mitral chordae into one or two fused papillary muscles ("parachute" deformity)
3. Deficiency of the ventricular septum (endocardial cushion defects)
4. Anomalous subaortic muscle bundle (corrected transposition)
5. Type II glycogen storage disease

stenosis. Definitive differentiation between valvular and subvalvular obstruction is best accomplished at cardiac catheterization by recording pressure tracings as a cardiac catheter is withdrawn across the outflow tract and valve, or by localizing the site of obstruction with selective left ventricular angiocardiography.

There are no differences in the indications for or risks of operation in patients with discrete subaortic stenosis and valvular aortic stenosis. Surgical correction consists of excising the membrane or fibrous ridge; it may be expected to improve the hemodynamic state substantially and frequently may be totally curative. In a small fraction of patients, secondary muscular hypertrophy of the outflow tract and a subaortic pressure gradient may persist following the operative relief of valvular or discrete subvalvular aortic stenosis. Ultimately, however, as the secondary hypertrophy regresses, this form of outflow obstruction generally resolves.

Occasionally, valvular and subvalvular aortic stenosis coexist in the same patient, producing a tunnel-like narrowing of the left ventricular outflow tract. Associated findings are often a small ascending aorta, hypoplasia of the aortic valve ring, and thickened valve leaflets. The subvalvular fibrous process usually extends onto the aortic valve cusps and almost always makes contact with the ventricular aspect of the anterior mitral leaflet at its base. The presence of "tunnel stenosis" may be suspected angiographically from the appearance of the outflow tract and the aortic root. Operative treatment is complicated by the frequent necessity for prosthetic replacement of the aortic valve, as well as for enlarging the aortic annulus, proximal aorta, and left ventricular outflow tract.

Several anatomic lesions other than a membrane, ridge, or muscular band that may produce subaortic stenosis are listed in Table 268-2.

SUPRAVALVULAR AORTIC STENOSIS. Supravalvular aortic stenosis is a localized or diffuse narrowing of the ascending aorta, originating just above the level of the coronary arteries at the superior margin of the sinuses of Valsalva. In contrast to other forms of aortic stenosis, in the supravalvular variety the coronary arteries are subjected to the elevated pressures that exist within the left ventricle, and are often dilated and tortuous. Adherence of the free edges of the aortic cusps to the site of supravalvular stenosis may interfere with coronary arterial inflow.

The designation *supravalvular aortic stenosis syndrome* has been applied to the distinctive clinical picture produced by coexistence of the cardiovascular lesion and a metabolic disorder, idiopathic infantile hypercalcemia, that is probably related to deranged vitamin D metabolism. Other manifestations of this syndrome include mental retardation, a peculiar "elfin facies," craniosynostosis, strabismus, narrowing of peripheral systemic and pulmonary arteries, inguinal hernias, cryptorchidism in males, premature development of secondary sexual characteristics in females, and abnormalities of dental development. Supravalvular aortic stenosis and peripheral pulmonary arterial stenosis are also seen in familial and sporadic forms unassociated with the other features of the syndrome. Genetic studies suggest that when the anomaly is familial it is transmitted as an autosomal dominant trait with variable expression.

The findings resemble those in valvular aortic stenosis, except that the sound of aortic valve closure is accentuated, ejection sounds are infrequent, and transmission of the thrill and murmur into the jugular notch and along the carotid vessels is more prominent. Also, the systolic pressure in the right arm tends to be higher than in the left.

The electrocardiogram generally reveals left ventricular hypertrophy, but biventricular, or even right ventricular hypertrophy may be observed if significant narrowing of peripheral pulmonary arteries coexists. Poststenotic dilatation of the ascending aorta is rarely seen roentgenographically. The diagnosis is confirmed by the demonstration at retrograde aortic catheterization of a pressure gradient just above the aortic valve and a constriction at this level by aortography.

Early recognition of the distinctive *supravalvular aortic stenosis syndrome* may prove to be a prerequisite to successful medical management, because it is conceivable that prompt diagnosis and treatment of idiopathic hypercalcemia in infancy might retard the progression of the cardiovascular lesions. The lumen of the aorta may be widened effectively by the insertion of an oval or diamond-shaped fabric prosthesis, and operative treatment is indicated when the obstruction is discrete and severe without generalized hypoplasia of the ascending aorta and arch.

HYPOPLASTIC LEFT HEART SYNDROME. This designation is used to describe patients with an obstructive lesion on the left side of the heart, associated with hypoplasia of the left ventricle and hypertrophy of the right ventricle. This syndrome, which is a significant cause of neonatal mortality, may be caused by atresia and/or hypoplasia of the aortic and mitral valves and of the aortic arch. The diagnosis should be considered in infants, particularly males, with the sudden onset of cardiac failure, hypotension, and a nonspecific murmur. The electrocardiogram frequently reveals right axis deviation, right atrial and ventricular enlargement, and ST- and T-wave abnormalities in left precordial leads. Chest roentgenograms show moderate to marked cardiac enlargement, with or without increased pulmonary vascular markings. Definitive diagnostic studies may be indicated as early as the first 24 hours of life. Most often, the anatomic lesions are inoperable, but if palliation by means of mitral or aortic valvulotomy or by enlarging an interatrial communication appears feasible, the anticipation of imminent death justifies the risk of prompt operative intervention.

COR TRIATRIATUM. In this malformation, an abnormal fibromuscular diaphragm most often divides the left atrium into a posterosuperior chamber which drains the pulmonary veins, and an anteroinferior chamber which communicates with the mitral valve and atrial appendage. The diaphragm contains an opening or, occasionally, several openings, the size of which determines the degree of obstruction to pulmonary venous return. Hemodynamically, the lesion mimics mitral stenosis, and clinically it resembles congenital mitral stenosis. There is severe pulmonary arterial hypertension, as a consequence of elevations both of the pulmonary venous pressure and of pulmonary vascular resistance. At cardiac catheterization, the lesion may be suspected if a pulmonary arterial wedge pressure is higher than a simultaneous left atrial pressure obtained by transseptal catheterization. The diagnosis is established by visualizing the obstructing lesion angiographically. Although this malformation is rare, it is important to recognize it because it may be easily correctable at operation.

TRANSPOSITION COMPLEXES

The term *transposition* identifies a complicated group of malformations that have in common abnormal relationships between the cardiac chambers and the great arteries.

Complete Transposition of the Great Arteries

In this condition, the aorta arises from the right ventricle to the right of and anterior to the pulmonary artery, which emerges from the left ventricle. This results in two separate and parallel circulations, and some communication between the two circulations must exist after birth in order to sustain life. Almost all patients have an interatrial communication, two-thirds have a patent ductus arteriosus, and about one-half have an associated ventricular septal defect. Transposition occurs more frequently in males than in females, in a ratio of approximately 2.5:1. It is the leading cause of death due to congenital heart disease in the first 2 months of life and accounts for approximately 10 percent of all patients with cyanotic heart disease. Half the patients with this malformation die by the age of six months. A few survive into childhood, and rarely a patient survives into young adult life. Those who live beyond infancy have, as a general rule, either an isolated large atrial septal defect or a ventricular septal defect and pulmonic stenosis.

The clinical course is determined by the degree of tissue hypoxia, the ability of each ventricle to sustain an increased work load in the presence of reduced coronary arterial oxygenation, the nature of the associated cardiovascular anomalies, and the anatomic and functional status of the pulmonary vascular bed. A bidirectional shunt is always present, because continuous unidirectional shunting would result in a progressive depletion of the circulating volume in either the pulmonary or the systemic vascular beds. The magnitude of both the arteriovenous and venoarterial shunts is modified by the number of intercirculatory communications that exist, the presence of associated obstructive intra- and extracardiac anomalies, and the relations between the pulmonary and systemic vascular resistances.

The usual clinical manifestations are dyspnea and cyanosis from birth, retardation of growth, and congestive heart failure. In some patients, there may be differential reversed cyanosis, in which the head, upper part of the trunk, and extremities are more cyanotic than the lower part of the body, indicating the presence of a patent ductus arteriosus with reversed (pulmonary to systemic) blood flow. Reversed flow may be associated with interruption of the aortic arch, preductal coarctation, or pulmonary vascular obstruction. Paroxysmal dyspneic attacks may occur, but not as frequently as in patients with the tetralogy of Fallot. Murmurs are often of no diagnostic significance and are absent or insignificant in approximately 30 percent of these infants.

The usual electrocardiographic findings include right axis deviation, right atrial enlargement, and right ventricular hypertrophy, reflecting the fact that the right ventricle is the systemic pumping chamber. Left ventricular hypertrophy is also present in those patients with large ventricular septal defects or significant obstruction to pulmonary blood flow. The roentgenographic findings are often diagnostic and consist of (1) progressive cardiac enlargement in early infancy; (2) characteristic oval or egg-shaped cardiac configuration in the anteroposterior view and a narrow base of the heart, created by superimposition of the aortic and pulmonary artery segments; and (3) increased pulmonary vascular markings. Cardiac catheterization always shows a lower oxygen saturation in the aorta than in the pulmonary artery. Angiocardiography is diagnostic and demonstrates that the anteriorly placed aorta arises from the right ventricle and the pulmonary artery posteriorly from the left ventricle.

Medical treatment is often of limited help but should be vigorous because all patients should be considered candidates for palliative surgical therapy now that total correction of the malformation has become a reality. Conservative measures include oxygen, digitalis, diuretics, iron if an associated iron-deficiency anemia is present, and intravenous sodium bicarbonate for severe anoxemic metabolic acidosis. The creation or enlargement of an interatrial communication is the simplest procedure for providing increased intracardiac mixing of systemic and pulmonary venous blood; it may be performed surgically or by rupturing the valve of the foramen ovale with a balloon catheter during transseptal catheterization of the left side of the heart. Pulmonary artery banding should be considered as an adjunct in infants with increased pulmonary blood flow and high pulmonary arterial pressure. Systemic-pulmonary artery or superior vena caval–pulmonary artery anastomosis may be indicated in the patient with associated severe pulmonic stenosis and diminished pulmonary blood flow. Complete intracardiac repair may be accomplished by rearranging the venous return so that the systemic venous blood is directed to the mitral valve and thence to the left ventricle and pulmonary artery, while the pulmonary venous blood is diverted through the tricuspid valve and right ventricle to the aorta. Although the risk of this corrective operation is relatively high, it is indicated in patients one year of age or older without associated severe pulmonary vascular disease.

PARTIAL TRANSPOSITION. This designation is applied to both the Taussig-Bing malformation, in which the aorta is transposed and arises entirely from the right ventricle while the pulmonary trunk communicates with both ventricles and overlies a large anterosuperior ventricular septal defect, and to the closely related anomaly referred to as "double-outlet right ventricle," or "origin of both great vessels from the right ventricle." This anomaly consists of transposition of the aorta but not of the pulmonary trunk, and a ventricular septal defect in the basal portion of the interventricular septum, caudal to the crista supraventricularis, so that the pulmonary trunk does not sit astride the defect. In both lesions, the aortic and pulmonary orifices are situated at about the same vertical level in both the frontal and horizontal planes. Both physiologically and clinically the Taussig-Bing malformation resembles complete transposition with ventricular septal defect and pulmonary vascular obstruction. In double-outlet right ventricle, the ventricular septal defect is the only route of ejection from the left ventricle. Because of the streamlining of blood flow from the left ventricle across the outflow tract of the right ventricle to the aorta, these patients may resemble clinically those with isolated, large ventricular septal defects without cyanosis. However, when there is accompanying pulmonary stenosis, the clinical findings are similar to those of cyanotic tetralogy of Fallot. Diagnosis of these lesions is dependent on careful angiocardiographic analysis, and increased preoperative recognition of the partial transposition anomalies may be expected to result in improved operative results.

CORRECTED TRANSPOSITION. The two fundamental anatomic derangements comprising this malformation are transposition, or anteroposterior reversal of the ascending aorta and pulmonary trunk, and inversion, or right-left reversal of the ventricles. This arrangement of the great vessels and ventricles (in contrast to the uncorrected transposition) permits functional correction, so that systemic venous blood passes into the pulmonary trunk while arterialized pulmonary venous blood flows into the aorta. In the heart with corrected transposition, the venae cavae and coronary sinus drain into a right atrium which is normal in position and structure. Venous blood flows from the right atrium, designated as the "venous atrium," across an atrioventricular valve, which has the structure of a normal mitral valve, into the right-sided "venous ventricle." This chamber, however, has the morphologic characteristics of a normal left ventricle, i.e., its interior lining is finely trabeculated, it has no crista supraventricularis, and the bicuspid atrioventricular valve is in continuity with a posteriorly placed semilunar valve. The venous ventricle ejects blood into the pulmonary trunk, which arises posterior to the ascending aorta. Oxygenated blood returns from the lungs to the left atrium, which is normal in position and structure, from which it flows into the left-sided "arterial ventricle" across an atrioventricular valve, which has the structure of a normal tricuspid valve. The interior lining of the arterial ventricle has the morphologic characteristics of a normal right ventricle, i.e., it has coarse trabeculations and a crista supraventricularis; the tricuspid atrioventricular valve is not in continuity with the anteriorly placed semilunar valve. The arterial ventricle ejects blood into the aorta, which arises anterior to the pulmonary trunk.

In complete, "uncorrected," transposition of the great vessels the maintenance of life is dependent on the presence of associated defects. In contrast, patients in whom corrected transposition exists as an isolated anomaly present no functional alterations and have no symptoms. When a patient with corrected transposition has symptoms and signs of congenital heart disease, it may, therefore, be assumed that one or more associated malformations is present. Ventricular septal defect, Ebstein-type anomalies of the left-sided, tricuspid atrioventricular valve, obstruction to outflow from the venous ventricle, and congenital heart block are those malformations most often associated with corrected transposition. Malposition of the cardiac apex (mirror-image dextrocardia, dextroversion in situs solitus, levoversion in situs inversus) may further complicate the altered anatomy.

In addition to the manifestations of the associated lesions, patients with corrected transposition frequently have an accentuated, single second heart sound in the second left intercostal space, representing closure of the aortic valve, which lies lateral and anterior to the pulmonic valve. Because of the inversion of the conduction system of the heart, the electrocardiogram may provide important clues to the diagnosis. An abnormal direction of initial ventricular depolarization is manifested by a reversal of the precordial Q-wave pattern (Q waves are present in the right precordial leads and absent on the left). Commonly, arrhythmias, conduction disturbances, and unusual T-wave patterns are also observed. Roentgenographic examination characteristically reveals absence of the normal pulmonary artery segment and a smooth convexity of the left supracardiac border produced by the displaced ascending aorta.

The diagnosis of corrected transposition can usually be established by selective angiocardiography, which allows visualization of the transposed great arteries and morphologic differentiation of the two ventricles. The competence of the left atrioventricular valve also may be determined by injection of contrast material into the arterial ventricle.

A high operative mortality rate has attended repair of the lesions associated with corrected transposition and is related to the elevated pulmonary vascular resistance which exists in patients with associated ventricular septal defect, and to a high incidence of surgically induced heart block. In addition, the inversion of the coronary arterial system greatly limits and may preclude an incision into the venous ventricle, thereby interfering with exposure of intracardiac defects in the usual manner. The presence of significant regurgitation from the arterial ventricle to the arterial atrium further raises the risk of operation.

TRANSPOSITION OF THE PULMONARY VEINS. When all the pulmonary veins connect either to the right atrium directly, or to the systemic veins or their tributaries, the condition is called total anomalous pulmonary venous connection (TAPVC). Because all venous blood returns to the right atrium, an interatrial communication is an integral part of this malformation. There are additional major cardiac malformations in about one-third of these patients; in two-thirds it exists as an isolated anomaly. TAPVC accounts for about 2 percent of the deaths from congenital heart disease in the first year of life. The anomalous connection is usually supradiaphragmatic and to the left brachiocephalic vein, right atrium, coronary sinus, or superior vena cava. In about 10 percent, particularly in males, the distal site of connection is situated below the diaphragm, a condition which is often unrecognized but which is hazardous because it is associated with markedly elevated resistance to pulmonary venous return.

Most infants with the more usual, unobstructed form of supradiaphragmatic TAPVC fail to thrive, are subject to repeated respiratory infections, and have congestive heart failure by the age of six months. The physiologic consequences and, accordingly, the clinical picture depend on the size of the interatrial communication and on the magnitude of the pulmonary vascular resistance. When the interatrial communication is small, systemic blood flow is markedly limited, right atrial and systemic venous pressures are elevated, and hepatic enlargement and peripheral edema are present. On the other hand, the magnitude of the pulmonary blood flow and, therefore, the ratio of the oxygenated to the unoxygenated blood which returns to the right atrium are a function of the pulmonary vascular resistance. Accordingly, the arterial oxygen saturation, which ranges from markedly reduced to normal values, is inversely related to the pulmonary vascular resistance. Therefore, cyanosis is not usually prominent in the absence of congestive failure unless the patient survives long enough to acquire secondary pulmonary vascular changes and a reduction in pulmonary blood flow.

A characteristic physical finding is the presence of multiple heart sounds, consisting of a first sound followed by an ejection click, a fixed, widely split second heart sound with an accentuated pulmonic component, and a third, and often a fourth, heart sound. The electrocardiogram shows right axis deviation, as well as right atrial and ventricular hypertrophy. Roentgenograms of the chest reveal increased pulmonary blood flow; the right atrium and ventricle are dilated and hypertrophied, and the pulmonary artery segment is enlarged. In addition, the specific site of anomalous connection may result in a characteristic appearance of the cardiac silhouette. Thus, in patients with TAPVC to the left brachiocephalic vein, the superior vena cava on the right, left brachiocephalic vein superiorly, and left vertical vein on the left produce a cardiac shadow that resembles a "snowman" or figure-of-eight. The upper right cardiac border may be prominent when the anomalous connection is to the right superior vena cava. Indicator-dilution studies at cardiac catheterization are especially helpful in determining the drainage pathways of the pulmonary veins. Indicator injected into the right ventricle or pulmonary artery takes longer to reach the peripheral arterial sampling site than indicator injected into the venae cavae or right atrium. The contour of the dilution curves obtained from a peripheral artery after injection into both the right atrium and a pulmonary vein are identical and show a large right-to-left shunt while the left atrial curve is normal.

Unless serious pulmonary vascular disease is present, results of operation for TAPVC in patients more than one year of age are good. The procedure consists of creating an anastomosis between the common pulmonary venous channel and left atrium and closing the atrial defect.

PARTIAL TRANSPOSITION OF THE PULMONARY VEINS. In this condition, one of the pulmonary veins (or more than one) is connected to the right atrium or to one or more of its tributaries. An atrial septal defect, particularly one of the sinus venosus type, often accompanies partial transposition of the pulmonary veins, and the usual connection involves the veins of the right upper and middle lobe and the superior vena cava. In the absence of associated anomalies, the physiologic disturbance is determined by the number of anomalous veins and their site of connection, the presence and size of an atrial septal defect, the state of the pulmonary vascular bed, and associated anomalies. In the usual patient with isolated partial transposition of the pulmonary veins, the hemodynamic state and physical findings are similar to those in atrial septal defect. Occasionally, drainage is into the inferior vena cava. This condition may be associated with pulmonary parenchymal abnormalities, hypoplasia of the right pulmonary artery and lung, and dextroposition of the heart. This complex has been designated the "scimitar syndrome," because of the characteristic roentgenographic findings of a crescent-like shadow in the right lower lung field which is produced by the anomalous venous channel.

Malposition of the Heart

Positional anomalies of the heart refer to conditions in which the cardiac apex is located in the right side of the chest (dextrocardia) or at the midline (mesocardia), or in which there is a normal location of the heart in the left side of the chest but abnormal position of the viscera (isolated levocardia). Knowledge of the position of the abdominal organs is important in diagnosing these malpositions. For example, a mirror-image dextrocardia is usually observed in a patient with complete situs inversus; this condition occurs more frequently in an otherwise normal individual than in one with a malformed heart. In contrast, when dextrocardia occurs without situs inversus, associated malformations are the rule. When the heart occupies its normal position, but situs inversus of the viscera is present, the heart is almost always seriously malformed. Moreover, when the visceral situs is indeterminate, there is a striking association of asplenia or polysplenia with complex, multiple cardiac anomalies which usually include a combination of systemic and pulmonary venous abnormalities, defects in the atrial and ventricular septums, and endocardial cushion defects. In addition, pulmonary arterial obstruction and maldevelopment of the great arteries may occur with both asplenia and polysplenia but are more common in the former. It is important to recognize these complex syndromes in order to distinguish them from forms of cyanotic heart disease that are amenable to corrective surgical therapy. The diagnosis is suggested by a symmetric liver shadow roentgenographically, and by the presence of Howell-Jolly and Heinz bodies as demonstrated hematologically, and confirmed by a negative or abnormal radioactive splenic scan.

Once the type of visceral situs is defined, it is necessary to describe the basic anatomic structure of the heart and its vascular connections. The atria exhibit a strong tendency to conform to the general orientation of the viscera, so that the right, or venous, atrium lies on the same side of the body as the trilobed lung, liver, and inferior vena cava, while the morphologic left, or arterial, atrium tends to lie on the same side as the stomach, spleen, and bilobed lung. The visceral situs can usually be determined by the location of the stomach bubble and liver on a routine roentgenogram, and the inferior vena cava can be located by the position of a cardiac catheter or by means of venous angiocardiography. The location of the ventricles and the relationship between the great arteries may also be demonstrated angiocardiographically. The cardiac chambers should be diagnosed positionally (left- and right-sided), functionally (arterial and venous), and morphologically (in terms of their intrinsic anatomic characteristics). The anatomic right ventricle is equipped with a tricuspid valve, is highly trabeculated, and contains the crista supraventricularis; its infundibulum always lies anteriorly to and superiorly beyond the outlet of the left ventricle. The morphologic right ventricle generally connects with whichever of the two great arteries is the more anterior. The left ventricle is guarded by a bicuspid mitral valve with an anterior leaflet which is in continuity with elements of the semilunar valve at its outlet, is smooth-walled, and contains an outlet that lies posterior to the right ventricular infundibulum. Transposition of the great arteris is an important problem in cardiac malposition, and in considering the positions of the great arteries to each other, it is important to emphasize that the anterior of the two arteries connects with the morphologic right ventricle.

Once the positional, functional, and morphologic relationships are understood, and the presence of associated anomalies has been established, the principles of medical and surgical treatment apply to these cardiac malpositions as they do to normally located hearts.

REFERENCES

General

Fontana, R. S., and J. E. Edwards: "Congenital Cardiac Disease: A Review of 357 Cases Studied Pathologically," Philadelphia, W. B. Saunders Company, 1962.

Gasul, B. M., R. A. Arcilla, and M. Lev: "Heart Disease in Children," Philadelphia, J. B. Lippincott Company, 1966.

Keith, J. D., R. D. Rowe, and P. Vlad: "Heart Disease in Infancy and Childhood," 2d ed., New York, The Macmillan Company, 1967.

Moss, A. J., and F. H. Adams: "Heart Disease in Infants, Children, and Adolescents," Baltimore, The Williams & Wilkins Company, 1968.

Watson, H.: "Paediatric Cardiology," London, Lloyd-Luke Ltd., 1968.

Atrial Septal Defect

Braunwald, N. S., and A. G. Morrow: Incomplete Persistent A-V Canal, J. Thoracic Cardiovasc. Surg., 51:71, 1966.

Gault, J. H., A. G. Morrow, W. A. Gay, Jr., and J. Ross, Jr.: Atrial Septal Defect in Patients over the Age of 40: Clinical and Hemodynamic Studies and Effects of Operation, Circulation, 37:261, 1968.

Levin, A. R., M. S. Spach, J. P. Boineau, R. V. Canent, Jr., M. P. Capp, and P. H. Jewett: Atrial Pressure-Flow-Dynamics in Atrial Septal Defects (Secundum Type), Circulation, 37:476, 1968.

Rahimtoola, S. H., J. W. Kirklin, and H. B. Burchell: Atrial Septal Defect, Circulation, 37–38 (Suppl. 5):2–11, 1968.

Ventricular Septal Defect

Bloomfield, D. K.: The Natural History of Ventricular Septal Defect in Patients Surviving Infancy, Circulation, 29:914, 1964.

Braunwald, N. S., E. Braunwald, and A. G. Morrow: The Effects of Surgical Abolition of Left-to-right Shunts on the Pulmonary Vascular Dynamics of Patients with Pulmonary Hypertension, Circulation, 26:1270, 1962.

Hoffman, J. I. E., and A. M. Rudolph: The Natural History of Ventricular Septal Defects in Infancy, Am. J. Cardiol., 16:634, 1965.

Levin, A. R., M. D. Spach, R. V. Canent, Jr., J. P. Boineau, M. P. Capp, V. Jain, and R. C. Barr: Intracardiac Pressure-Flow Dynamics in Isolated Ventricular Septal Defects, Circulation, 35:430, 1967.

Wood, P.: The Eisenmenger Syndrome, Brit. Med. J., 2:701 and 755, 1958.

Patent Ductus Arteriosus

Rudolph, A. M., F. E. Mayer, A. S. Nadas, and R. E. Gross: Patent Ductus Arteriosus: A Clinical and Hemodynamic Study of 23 Patients in the First Year of Life, Pediatrics, 22:892, 1958.

Aortopulmonary Septal Defect

Morrow, A. G., L. J. Greenfield, and E. Braunwald: Congenital Aortopulmonary Septal Defect: Clinical and Hemodynamic Findings, Surgical Technic, and Results of Operative Correction, Circulation, 25:463, 1962.

Aortic Sinus Aneurysm and Fistula

Onat, A., O. Ersanli, A. Kanuni, and T. B. Aykan: Congenital Aortic Sinus Aneurysms, Am. Heart J., 72:158, 1966.

Coronary Arteriovenous Fistula

Gasul, B. M., R. A. Arcilla, E. H. Fell, J. Lynfield, J. P. Bicoff, and L. L. Luan: Congenital Coronary Arteriovenous Fistula, Pediatrics, suppl. 25:531, 1960.

Upshaw, C. B., Jr.: Congenital Coronary Arteriovenous Fistula. Report of a Case with an Analysis of Seventy-three Reported Cases, Am. Heart J., 63:399, 1962.

Anomalous Pulmonary Origin of Coronary Artery

Wesselhoeft, H., J. S. Fawcett, and A. L. Johnson: Anomalous Origin of the Left Coronary Artery from the Pulmonary Trunk, Circulation, 38:403, 1969.

Talner, N. S., K. H. Halloran, M. Mahdavy, R. H. Garnder, and F. Hipona: Anomalous Origin of the Left Coronary Artery from the Pulmonary Artery, A Clinical Spectrum, Am. J. Cardiol., 15:689, 1965.

Truncus Arteriosus

Tandon, R., A. J. Hauck, and A. S. Nadas: Persistent Truncus Arteriosus: A Clinical Hemodynamic and Autopsy Study of Nineteen Cases, Circulation, 28:1050, 1963.

Van Praagh, R., and S. Van Praagh: The Anatomy of Common Aortico-pulmonary Trunk (Truncus Arteriosus Communis) and Its Embryologic Implications, Am. J. Cardiol. 16:406, 1965.

Pulmonary Stenosis

Levine, O. R., and S. Blumenthal: Pulmonic Stenosis, Circulation, 32:33, suppl. III, 1965.

Moller, J. H., and P. Adams, Jr.: The Natural History of Pulmonary Valvular Stenosis, Am. J. Cardiol., 16:654, 1965.

Silverman, B. K., A. S. Nadas, M. H. Wittenborg, W. T. Goodale, and R. E. Gross: Pulmonary Stenosis with Intact Ventricular Septum: Correlation of Clinical and Physiologic Data, with Review of Operative Results, Am. J. Med., 20:53, 1956.

Tetralogy of Fallot

Lev, M. G., and A. O. Eckner: The Pathologic Anatomy of Tetralogy of Fallot and Its Variations, Dis. Chest, 45:251, 1964.

McCord, M. D., J. Van Elk, and S. G. Blount, Jr.: Tetralogy of Fallot, Circulation, 16:736, 1957.

Malm, J. R., F. O. Bowman, Jr., A. G. Jameson, E. Ellis, S. P. Griffiths, and S. Blumenthal: An Evaluation of Total Correction of Tetralogy of Fallot, Circulation, 27:805, 1963.

Ebstein's Anomaly

Schiebler, G. L., P. Adams, R. C. Anderson, K. Amplatz, and R. G. Lester: Clinical Study of Twenty-three Cases of Ebstein's Anomaly of the Tricuspid Valve, Circulation, 19:165, 1959.

Vacca, J. B., D. W. Bussmann, and J. G. Mudd: Ebstein's Anomaly. Complete Review of 108 Cases, Am. J. Cardiol., 2:210, 1958.

Tricuspid Atresia

Riker, W. L., W. J. Potts, L. Grana, R. A. Miller, and M. Lev: Tricuspid Stenosis or Atresia Complexes, J. Thoracic Cardiovasc. Surg., 45:423, 1963.

Coarctation of the Aorta

Campbell, M., and J. H. Baylis: The Course and Prognosis of Coarctation of the Aorta, Brit. Heart J., 18:475, 1956.

Congenital Valvular Aortic Stenosis

Braunwald, E., A. Goldblatt, M. M. Aygen, S. D. Rockoff, and A. G. Morrow: Congenital Aortic Stenosis. I. Clinical and Hemodynamic Findings in 100 Patients, Circulation, 27:426, 1963.

Friedman, W. F., and E. Braunwald: Congenital Aortic Stenosis, in "Heart Disease in Infants, Children and Adolescents," H. J. Moss, and F. H. Adams (Eds.), The Williams & Wilkins Company, Baltimore, 1968.

Hoffman, J. I. E.: The Natural History of Congenital Isolated Pulmonic and Aortic Stenosis, Ann. Rev. Med., 20:15, 1969.

Discrete Subaortic Stenosis

Edwards, J. E.: Pathology of Left Ventricular Outflow Tract Obstruction, Circulation, 31:586, 1965.

Supravalvular Aortic Stenosis

Beuren, A. J., C. Schulze, P. Eberle, D. Harmjanz, and J. Apetz: Syndrome of Supravalvular Aortic Stenosis, Peripheral Pulmonary Stenosis, Mental Retardation and Similar Facial Appearance, Am. J. Cardiol., 13:471, 1964.

Friedman, W. F.: Vitamin D as a Cause of the Supravalvular Aortic Stenosis Syndrome, Am. Heart J., 73:718, 1967.

———, and W. C. Roberts: Vitamin D and the Supravalvular Aortic Stenosis Syndrome: The Transplacental Effects of Vitamin D on the Aorta of the Rabbit, Circulation, 34:77, 1966.

Hypoplastic Left Heart Syndrome

Sinha, S. N., S. L. Rusnak, H. M. Sommers, R. B. Cole, A. J. Muster, and M. H. Paul: Hypoplastic Left Ventricle Syndrome: Analysis of Thirty Autopsy Cases in Infants with Surgical Considerations, Am. J. Cardiol., 21:166, 1968.

Cor Triatriatum

Lucas, R. V., Jr., R. C. Anderson, K. Amplatz, P. Adams, Jr., and J. E. Edwards: Congenital Causes of Pulmonary Venous Obstruction, Pediat. Clinics N. Am., 10:781, 1963.

Complete Transposition of the Great Arteries

Lev, M., H. J. A. Rimoldi, R. Paiva, and R. A. Arcilla: The Quantitative Anatomy of Simple Complete Transposition, Am. J. Cardiol., 23:409, 1969.

Noonan, J. A., A. S. Nadas, A. M. Rudolph, and G. B. C. Harris: Transposition of the Great Arteries, New Engl. J. Med., 263:592, 637, 684, 739, 1960.

Plauth, W. H., Jr., A. S. Nadas, W. F. Bernhard, and R. F. Gross: Transposition of the Great Arteries: Clinical and Physiological Observations on 74 Patients Treated by Palliative Surgery, Circulation, 37:316, 1968.

Partial Transposition

Beuren, A. B.: A Differential Diagnosis of the Taussig-Bing Heart from Complete Transposition of the Great Vessels with a Posteriorly Overriding Pulmonary Artery, Circulation, 21:1071, 1960.

Neufeld, H. N., J. W. DuShane, and J. E. Edwards: Origin of Both Great Vessels from the Right Ventricle. II. With Pulmonary Stenosis, Circulation, 23:603, 1961.

———, ———, E. H. Wood, J. W. Kirklin, and J. E. Edwards: Origin of Both Great Vessels from the Right Ventricle. I. Without Pulmonic Stenosis, Circulation, 23:399, 1961.

Corrected Transposition

Berry, W. B., W. C. Roberts, A. G. Morrow, and E. Braunwald: Corrected Transposition of the Aorta and Pulmonary Trunk, Am. J. Med., 36:35, 1964.

Schiebler, G. L., et al.: Congenital Corrected Transposition of the Great Vessels: A Study of 33 Cases, Pediatrics, 27(suppl.): 849–888, 1961.

Van Praagh, R., and S. Van Praagh: Anatomically Corrected Transposition of the Great Arteries, Brit. Heart J., 29:112, 1967.

Transposition of the Pulmonary Veins

Bonham Carter, R. E., M. Capriles, and Y. Noe: Total Anomalous Pulmonary Venous Drainage, Brit. Heart J., 31:45, 1969.

Malposition of the Heart

Stanger, P., R. C. Benassi, M. E. Korns, K. L. Jue, and J. E. Edwards: Diagrammatic Portrayal of Variations in Cardiac Structure, Circulation, 37(suppl. 4):1–16, 1968.

Van Praagh, R., S. Van Praagh, P. Vlad, and J. D. Keith: Anatomic Types of Congenital Dextrocardia, Am. J. Cardiol., 13:510, 1964.

269 RHEUMATIC FEVER
Alvan R. Feinstein

Acute rheumatic fever is an arbitrarily designated portion of the spectrum of inflammatory complications that may follow group A streptococcal infections. As specified in the revised Jones' diagnostic criteria (Table 269-1), rheumatic fever is manifested by the appearance, either alone or in various combinations, of arthritis, carditis, chorea, or erythema marginatum. A diagnosis of rheumatic fever is usually justified if two of these manifestations are present.

ETIOLOGY. The relationship between rheumatic fever and group A streptococcal infection was obscure for many years because the antecedent infection is often clinically asymptomatic or atypical, and because the streptococcus is not always demonstrable in the throat when the rheumatic patient comes to medical attention. With the modern availability of tests for streptococcal antibodies, the organism can now be identified by its "fingerprints" in the serum after it has left the scene of its original "crime" in the throat.

Figure 269-1A shows the complex natural spectrum of patients who may have sore throats (a clinical symptom), streptococcal throats (a positive result obtained when material taken from the throat is tested by culture or by fluorescent staining), and streptococcal infections (a positive result in a test of serologic antibodies). This Venn diagram emphasizes that not all sore throats are due to the streptococcus, that not all streptococcal throats

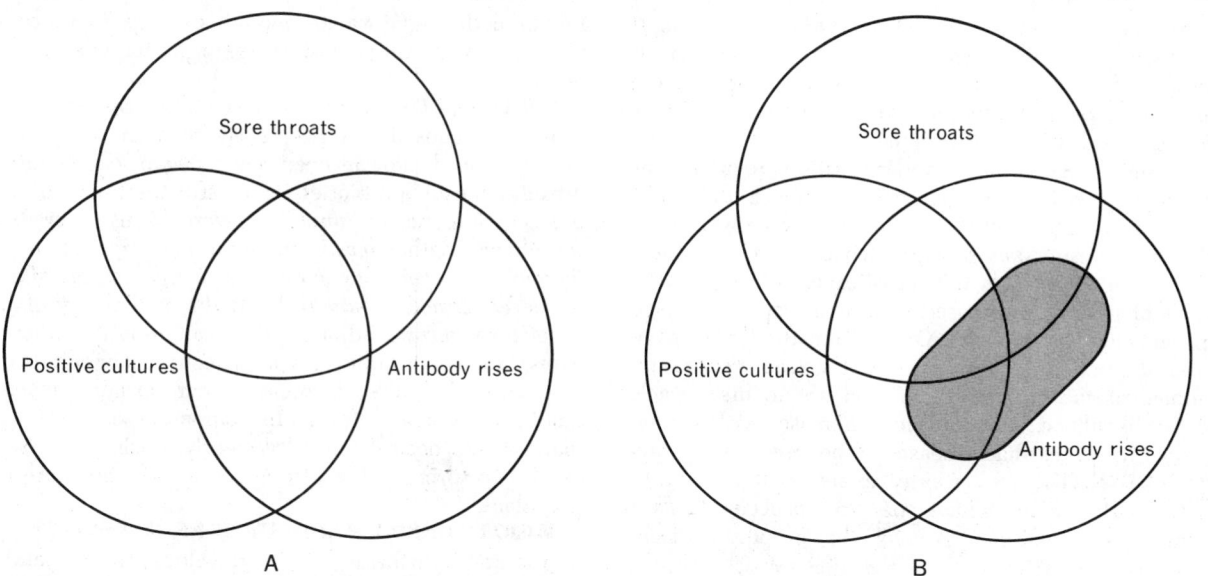

Fig. 269-1.*A*. Spectrum of sore throats, streptococcal throats, and streptococcal infections. *B*. Sources of rheumatic fever (shaded area) in the spectrum shown in *A*.

are sore, and that streptococcal infections may occur in the absence of sore throats.

Figure 269-1*B* shows the emergence of rheumatic fever from only a restricted portion of this spectrum: patients whose streptococcal infection produced an antibody rise, with or without sore throats, and with or without a positive culture. For this rise to be regularly demonstrated, testing for antibodies may have to be exhaustive, involving the use of multiple antibodies, examination of sequential specimens, demonstration of suitable increments, and concomitant comparisons. Because the antistreptolysin O titer will rise in only about 80 percent of group A infections, more than one type of antibody must be examined; among the most useful of the additional antigens are streptococcal antihyaluronidase and antideoxyribonuclease B. Evidence of a recent infection must be demonstrated by a *change* in the titer of sequential specimens rather than by any single value; the time interval between specimens need not be shorter than 2 weeks, and a significant change can usually be shown even when the specimens are separated by 2 months. Since a difference of one tube dilution may be due to nonspecific variations, a true "change" in titer should not be diagnosed unless the increment spans at least two tubes in the dilutional system used for the test; a knowledge of the laboratory's dilutional system is necessary for meaningful interpretation of the results.

Streptococcal infections that are detected and treated appropriately (Chap. 140) can be prevented from causing rheumatic fever, but when the infection is not treated, the rheumatic attack rate varies according to the clinical type of infection. With symptomatic exudative streptococcal pharyngitis, the rate is about 3 percent; in patients in whom the infection is less severe, the rate may be 0.4 percent or even lower.

In epidemics of exudative streptococcal pharyngitis,

rheumatic fever occurs about 2 weeks after the pharyngeal symptoms, but in other clinical circumstances, this latent interval is generally more variable. For chorea, and less often for erythema marginatum, the poststreptococcal latent interval is longer than for other clinical manifestations of rheumatic fever; it may be as long as 6 months. The chorea or the skin rash may appear after other rheumatic manifestations have subsided, and may suggest a spurious posttherapeutic "rebound" or a new rheumatic attack. When chorea is the only clinical manifestation, the long latent interval may preclude successful identification of an antecedent streptococcal infection, because the elevated antibody titers already have returned to normal values. The long-standing belief that "pure chorea" was an isolated disease, unrelated to rheumatic fever, has been refuted by recent examinations of sequential serums obtained in repeated periodic examinations of rheumatic patients. When some of these patients developed a recurrence of "pure chorea," the antibody rise of an earlier asymptomatic streptococcal infection could be demonstrated.

Features that influence susceptibility to a first episode of rheumatic fever are not well defined. Familial cluster-

Table 269-1. JONES' CRITERIA (REVISED) FOR GUIDANCE IN THE DIAGNOSIS OF RHEUMATIC FEVER

Major manifestations	*Minor manifestations*
Carditis	History of previous rheumatic fever
Polyarthritis	or evidence of preexisting rheumatic
Chorea	heart disease
Erythema marginatum	Arthralgia
	Fever
	Abnormal erythrocyte sedimentation
	rate or C-reactive protein test
	Electrocardiographic changes

ing has been observed, but clear evidence for genetic transmission has not been found. Acute attacks of the disease seldom occur in patients below the age of four years, are most common in the age group of five to seventeen, and decline in frequency thereafter.

Although poverty and undernutrition regularly are indicted as predisposing factors, their role is difficult to separate from that of the concomitant overcrowding that facilitates transmission of streptococci in this socioeconomic group, and from the statistical bias created when epidemiologic data are based mainly on populations seen in public clinics and wards. Once rheumatic fever has occurred, the patient is more susceptible to recurrences than members of the general population are to first attacks, and the likelihood of recurrences increases with increasing severity of cardiac disease in the preceding attack.

PATHOGENESIS. No certainty exists about the pathogenetic pathway by which the streptococcus leads to rheumatic inflammation. Among the proposed mechanisms are a direct invasion of the affected tissues either by the unaltered streptococcus or by "L forms" lacking in cell wall; a direct toxic action by substances produced by the streptococcus, such as streptolysin S; a specific allergic reaction to the organism or its products; or the development of an autoimmune reaction. The theory that supports the last of these mechanisms is currently the most fashionable, although none has been proved unequivocally.

The rheumatic inflammation has relatively few histologic characteristics that are sufficiently distinct to be pathognomonic. For this reason, biopsy of inflamed joints or of subcutaneous nodules is seldom diagnostically rewarding and is generally performed mainly to rule out other diseases. Because of the low fatality rate, the morbid anatomy of chorea is not well defined.

Although the most distinctive histopathologic characteristics of rheumatic fever are found in the heart, not all hearts are involved, and not all of those that are involved show typical lesions. The pericardial inflammation of rheumatic fever does not have a unique histologic appearance, but Aschoff bodies in the myocardium are pathognomonic of the disease. How often these occur is uncertain, because of the diverse histologic criteria used by different pathologists. Although once believed to represent *acute* rheumatic inflammation, the Aschoff body has been found in many patients with no other clinical or laboratory evidence of inflammation; conversely, Aschoff bodies have been absent from the myocardium when acute rheumatic inflammation was unequivocally present on clinical grounds. The most frequent cardiac lesions of rheumatic fever are evident as gross, rather than microscopic, lesions in the valves. Dilatation of valve rings, destruction of valve substance, or contraction of chordae tendineae produces regurgitation; and fusion of cusps or commissures leads to stenosis. The mitral valve is affected most frequently; the aortic next, more commonly in boys than in girls; the tricuspid valve is seldom involved; and the pulmonic, rarely if ever. Although progressive scarring with age can further

impair a damaged valve, enough damage may occur to produce significant stenosis or regurgitation even in childhood.

EPIDEMIOLOGY. In the United States, rheumatic fever is now diagnosed less frequently than in the past, but because the decline in occurrence began long before the introduction of antibiotics, successful treatment of streptococcal infections cannot be given exclusive credit for the change. Other reasons include more rigorous modern diagnostic criteria to eliminate many minor ailments formerly termed *rheumatic,* and the availability of more precise diagnostic adjuncts that can identify other diseases, such as lupus erythematosus, congenital heart disease, and sickle-cell anemia, that formerly masqueraded as rheumatic fever. In temperate climates, rheumatic fever occurs most frequently during late winter and early spring, when streptococcal infections are more prevalent.

MAJOR CLINICAL MANIFESTATIONS. Arthritis. The pain of rheumatic arthritis usually develops rapidly, and the affected joint may become exquisitely tender before redness, heat, or swelling has appeared. The knees and ankles are affected most frequently, and the next most common are the elbows, wrists, or hips. The shoulders and small joints of the hands or feet are involved uncommonly, and the temporomandibular or vertebral joints, rarely; a disease other than rheumatic fever should be considered when these are the *only* affected joints. Characteristically, the joint pain is migratory and fleeting. No permanent joint deformities occur.

Certain patients develop poststreptococcal arthralgia rather than arthritis. They complain of pain in the joints but have no overt evidence of arthritis, i.e., redness, swelling, or deformity of the joints. Among patients who appear clinically to have *arthralgia,* a more correct diagnosis is often *tendonalgia* or *myalgia.* In such patients, a careful examination will reveal that the pain originates in a neighboring muscle or tendon, not in the joint. With the joint held immobile, isometric tension of the associated muscle or tendon will reproduce or increase the pain, although passive movement of the joint is painless. The common "growing pains" of children and adolescents are an example of this type of musculotendonalgia, and should not be attributed to rheumatic fever.

Chorea. Chorea is more common in girls than in boys. Choreic movements are purposeless, nonrepetitive, spasmodic motions that may involve any voluntary muscle, including those of the face and tongue. Although not present during sleep, the movements persist while the patient is awake, and are partially controllable by concentrated voluntary effort, which may, however, also sometimes exacerbate them. With more severe attacks, the extremities and the trunk may be in constant motion, and the patient may need protection from injury. Choreic motions must be distinguished from habit tics or spasms, which are repetitive, and from hyperkinetic movements, which are purposeful and voluntarily controllable. The poststreptococcal episodic type of chorea, often called *Sydenham's chorea,* is also called *chorea minor,* to distinguish it from the hereditary *chorea major* (or *Huntington's chorea*, Chaps. 22 and 364), which usually begins in adult life and is relentlessly progressive.

Carditis. Since no specific objective tests are available, the clinical diagnosis of acute carditis may be difficult. Prolongation of the P-R interval on the electrocardiogram cannot be regarded as definitive evidence of carditis, because this finding is nonspecific and present in about one-third of patients with rheumatic fever. It has shown no definite relation to other evidence of cardiac damage or to the long-term cardiac prognosis. The diagnosis of carditis thus becomes dependent on the clinical recognition of four events that may occur alone or in various combinations: abnormal murmur(s), pericardial rub, cardiac enlargement, and congestive heart failure.

The clinical manifestations of congestive heart failure in rheumatic children and adolescents are often similar to those noted in adults (Chap. 264), but certain differences may exist, probably because congestive failure develops more rapidly and is detected more promptly in children than in adults. During acute decompensation due to rheumatic fever, young patients often have dyspnea without rales; an ache in the right upper quadrant or epigastrium due to tenderness of the distended hepatic capsule; and a hacking nonproductive cough, due to pulmonary congestion, that may at first be attributed to a respiratory infection. After antirheumatic treatment has been instituted, congestive heart failure may be diagnosed incorrectly if the tachypnea of salicylate toxicity is mistaken for dyspnea, or if the slight hepatomegaly that may develop with steroid therapy is mistaken for hepatic congestion.

The first heart sound in rheumatic fever is often faint or "muffled," not because of carditis but because prolonged atrioventricular conduction allows the valve leaflets to drift closer together before they close. If heart failure is present, or if a pericardial effusion has occurred, both the first and second sounds may be faint. A third heart sound is a common normal finding in children, and it is frequently audible in patients with acute rheumatic fever. If the sound is long or somewhat roughened, it may be mistaken for a pericardial rub or a middiastolic murmur; if the cardiac rate is rapid, the quick repetition of three sounds will produce a gallop cadence. The short middiastolic noise that is often heard with mitral regurgitation during acute carditis is called a *Carey Coombs murmur;* a phonocardiogram may be required to differentiate it from a third heart sound.

A systolic murmur of mitral regurgitation is the most common auscultatory finding in rheumatic carditis. It is generally at least grade III/VI in intensity, loudest at the apex and transmitted to the anterior axillary line, blowing, high-pitched, and relatively unaltered by respiration and by changes in position. The murmur commonly begins with and masks the first heart sound. Mitral regurgitation is often falsely diagnosed in patients with acute rheumatic fever and a functional systolic murmur, so common in children and young adults, particularly in the presence of fever or tachycardia. This physiologic

systolic murmur arises from the pulmonary artery and is generally loudest along the left sternal border; it is an ejection murmur (Chap. 259), rather than pansystolic, as is the murmur of mitral regurgitation, and its intensity is reduced during inspiration. A blowing, high-pitched early diastolic murmur due to aortic regurgitation is most easily audible at the left sternal border, in the third or fourth interspaces, with the patient leaning forward, in expiration, and may also be audible in patients with acute carditis.

The harsh crescendo-decrescendo systolic murmur of aortic stenosis seldom, if ever, occurs alone during rheumatic carditis in young patients. When the aortic valve is involved, the diastolic murmur is almost invariably present, and the associated systolic murmur results either from mild stenosis of the valve or from ejection through the dilated orifice. Aortic stenosis is commonly overdiagnosed when physiologic pulmonary murmurs are audible to the right of the sternum.

The classical acoustic pattern of mitral stenosis—a presystolic rumble merging with an accentuated first sound, as well as the early diastolic sound often regarded as an "opening snap" (Chap. 259)—is uncommon during acute carditis. More commonly, the presystolic rumble and accentuated first sound are detected without an "opening snap," or the mitral deformity is manifested by systolic and long diastolic murmurs.

With marked mitral regurgitation, a systolic thrill may be palpable at the apex; as the right ventricle enlarges or is pushed forward by an enlarged left atrium, a left parasternal lift or heave can be felt; with marked aortic valve damage, a systolic thrill may be palpable over the carotid arteries but is seldom felt—in young patients—at the base of the heart; an apical diastolic thrill is uncommon.

A pericardial rub is sometimes the major or sole clinical manifestation of carditis, but more frequently it occurs in patients with cardiac decompensation.

No radiographic findings are characteristic of acute rheumatic carditis, and the cardiac size may remain normal despite unequivocal acoustic evidence of mitral or aortic regurgitation. Certain cardiac chambers may enlarge in accordance with valvular hemodynamic abnormalities; and generalized enlargement of the cardiac silhouette may occur with rheumatic myocarditis, congestive failure, or pericardial effusion.

Erythema Marginatum. This nonpruritic, flat or slightly raised rash occurs in only about 5 percent of patients with rheumatic fever, and it almost always coexists with arthritis, chorea, or carditis. Serpiginous or circular shapes are formed, usually on the trunk and thighs; the rash is often evanescent.

Subcutaneous Nodules. These are firm, painless, colorless, seldom larger than 1 to 2 cm; they most commonly develop near tendons or bony prominences of joints, particularly the elbows, are found in about 5 percent of patients with rheumatic fever, and are especially likely to coexist with severe carditis.

Other Clinical Features. The fever of rheumatic fever

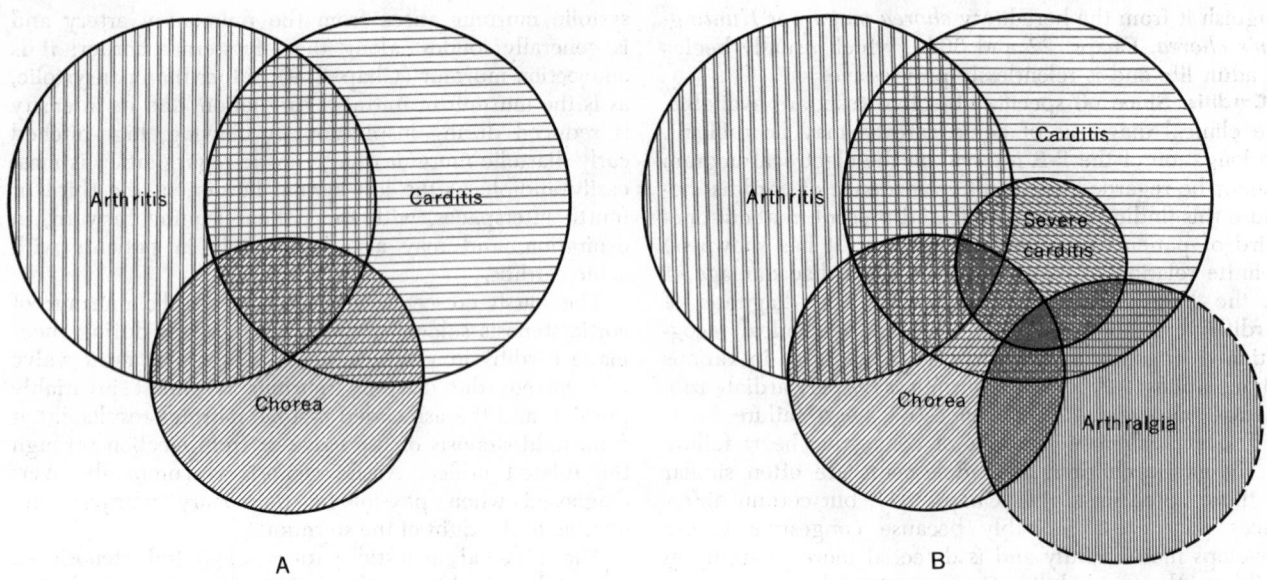

Fig. 269-2.A. Major constituent sets in rheumatic fever. B. The clinical spectrum of acute rheumatic fever.

has no distinguishing pattern. Epistaxis occurs in about 5 to 10 percent of cases, generally along with carditis. Abdominal pain appears in about 10 percent of patients; it may be due to hepatic congestion during cardiac decompensation or mesenteric lymphadenitis. Pleurisy and pneumonia, previously common manifestations, are now seldom observed. Although pulmonary infarctions and infections regularly occur in association with heart failure, "rheumatic pneumonia" as a clinical or histopathologic entity cannot be defined. Pleurisy, although sometimes found in rheumatoid arthritis and lupus erythematosus, does not occur in rheumatic fever unless heart failure, pneumonia, or pulmonary infarction is present.

PATTERNS OF CLINICAL PRESENTATION. Because erythema marginatum and subcutaneous nodules seldom occur alone, the basic clinical spectrum of rheumatic fever may be portrayed (Fig. 269-2A) as the overlap of "sets" of patients with arthritis, chorea, or carditis. In Fig. 269-2B, the complete clinical spectrum is constructed by further distinguishing a subset of severe carditis, and by adding a set of patients with poststreptococcal arthralgia. The spectrum shows the wide range of clinical manifestations—some of which are neither "rheumatic" nor "febrile"—that may be diagnosed as rheumatic fever. Arthralgia alone is shown in Fig. 269-2B with a dotted outline, because it does not fulfill Jones' diagnostic criteria. This spectrum of diverse clinical constituents shows that rheumatic fever need not have a single pattern of appearance. The presenting features may be as diverse as arthritis alone, "pure" chorea, or congestive heart failure without arthritis or chorea.

In the most common clinical situation, a child or adolescent develops nonspecific symptoms and then develops fever and painful enlargement of a large joint. Joints in other or symmetric contralateral locations then may become affected. Although the term "migratory polyarthritis" is used regularly to describe the articular events

of rheumatic fever, the arthritis is often neither "migratory" nor "poly": several joints may begin to hurt simultaneously; and only one joint may remain involved, particularly when bed rest or anti-inflammatory treatment is initiated promptly.

In about 10 percent of cases, the patient seeks medical attention because of fever or arthralgia, and a diagnosis of rheumatic fever may be established only if carditis is found or if chorea develops later. Unless one of these two major manifestations appears, the condition is defined as a poststreptococcal inflammatory state that does not fulfill the Jones diagnostic criteria for rheumatic fever. Somewhat fewer than 10 percent of patients have chorea. Its onset may be so insidious that the patient may have been regarded as behaving peculiarly for weeks before the movements become overt or severe enough to come to medical attention.

Although pericarditis may produce pain, other features of carditis per se are asymptomatic unless congestive failure occurs. Thus, in a first rheumatic episode, carditis often is detected not because of its own manifestations, but because the patient seeks medical attention for arthritis, chorea, or fever. In a patient with only mild carditis without heart failure who does not manifest arthritis, fever, or chorea, rheumatic fever may therefore escape detection during the acute rheumatic episode. In such patients (upper right, Fig. 269-2B), the valvular disease develops insidiously, primarily because medical attention is not sought by the patient. When the residual evidence of carditis is found in a subsequent examination, the patient is considered to have "rheumatic heart disease without a history of rheumatic fever." Such patients may first reach medical attention in adolescence or adult life as the result of a recurrence of rheumatic fever, manifested by arthritis.

Definite evidence of carditis occurs in about half the patients having their first attack of rheumatic fever. The percentage of cardiac abnormalities is higher in patients with recurrent rheumatic fever, because patients with previous carditis are particularly likely to develop recurrences.

LABORATORY DATA. The erythrocyte sedimentation rate and the level of serum C-reactive protein are always elevated during active rheumatic inflammation, and repeated tests of these acute-phase reactants are useful indexes of the inflammatory activity as the disease progresses. "Pure" chorea, however, may not begin until after the acute-phase reactants have reached normal values. A slight leukocytosis is usually present during the acute inflammatory phase; and in children receiving steroid treatment, the white blood cell count may reach values of 25,000 per cu mm. Because the development of heart failure alone will not return an elevated sedimentation rate to normal, decompensation is probably not due to active carditis when a normal sedimentation rate is found in patients with rheumatic heart disease and heart failure.

Mild degrees of anemia may occur, particularly after a long period of cardiac decompensation. Slight microscopic hematuria, of 2 to 6 red blood cells per high power field, is sometimes noted during repeated examination of the urine in rheumatic fever, particularly when the patient is febrile, but gross hematuria and overt glomerulonephritis seldom occur, despite their frequent provocation by group A streptococcal infection. Rarely, rheumatic fever may be followed several years later by an episode of glomerulonephritis, but the acute simultaneous occurrence of significant renal and articular inflammation suggests an alternative diagnosis, such as lupus erythematosus.

DIFFERENTIAL DIAGNOSIS. *Bacterial endocarditis* sometimes makes its appearance with articular symptoms, and the combination of fever, heart murmurs, and arthralgia may suggest rheumatic fever until positive blood cultures are obtained. A suppurative bacterial arthritis can usually be ruled out by the history of trauma or infection elsewhere and by the findings when the joint fluid is examined. The arthritis associated with gout, gonococcal infection, and sickle-cell anemia generally can be excluded by appropriate laboratory tests. Acute leukemia, which may begin with fever and articular symptoms, is identified after the white blood cells are examined. Rheumatic arthritis may be difficult to differentiate from rheumatoid arthritis or lupus erythematosus, because the diagnostic laboratory test results in the latter two diseases often are negative early in the clinical course. A "butterfly" facial rash, pleuritic involvement, and significant renal abnormalities are common in lupus erythematosus (Chap. 392) and unusual in rheumatic fever, as are the persistence of arthritis and permanent articular deformities, the hallmarks of rheumatoid disease. Furthermore, elevations in streptococcal antibody levels are characteristic of the initial episode or with a recrudescence of the arthritis due to rheumatic fever, but do not occur with systemic lupus erythematosus or rheumatoid arthritis.

Rheumatic carditis must be distinguished from congenital or less-common forms of heart disease, such as tumors or subendocardial fibroelastosis. Cyanosis suggests a congenital origin for the heart disease; otherwise, careful auscultation will often demonstrate that the murmurs are not of rheumatic origin. In doubtful circumstances, cardiac catheterization and angiocardiography are necessary to define the lesion.

A common problem is to identify a recurrence of rheumatic fever in a patient who already has rheumatic heart disease, particularly when such a patient does not develop arthritis or chorea, but rather when carditis is the only major manifestation of the recurrence. The appearance of a new murmur and a significant enlargement in cardiac size are among the features of carditis in a previously damaged heart. Congestive heart failure may sometimes be the only evidence of recurrent carditis, but it may also be precipitated by valvular dysfunction and may not be associated with "rheumatic activity." Elevations of the erythrocyte sedimentation rate, C-reactive proteins, and other acute-phase reactants may be of diagnostic value but are not specific.

CLINICAL COURSE AND PROGNOSIS. Aside from carditis, each of the major manifestations of rheumatic fever subsides after a finite interval, leaving no residual effects. Erythema marginatum lasts no more than several days; subcutaneous nodules last about 1 to 2 weeks; and arthritis lasts 2 to 3 weeks, and rarely longer than a month. Chorea has a variable course, sometimes lasting only 2 weeks, and sometimes persisting for 6 months or more.

When carditis develops, overt evidence of it is usually present by the time the patient reaches medical attention. Thereafter, the cardiac damage may increase or decrease, but manifestations of carditis will seldom appear *de novo* in a patient with acute rheumatic fever who was carefully examined after the onset of an attack and was initially found free of carditis.

The sedimentation rate returns to normal in about 2 months in the absence of carditis, and in about 3 months in patients with carditis. Occasionally, the sedimentation rate may remain slightly elevated, in the range of 25 to 35 mm per hr, for months or even years after all other clinical evidence of acute inflammation has subsided. In these patients, a normal C-reactive protein test should be taken as evidence that the inflammation has subsided.

The long-term outcome of rheumatic fever depends on the state of the patient during the acute attack. Patients who do not develop carditis almost always remain free of rheumatic heart disease thereafter. Among those with questionably abnormal murmurs, the murmur will become distinctly abnormal in about 10 percent and will disappear in the remainder. In patients with definitely abnormal murmurs but without significant cardiomegaly or congestive heart failure, residual heart disease will be found in about 50 percent. Patients with severe carditis have the worst prognosis: some die during the acute attack; about 20 percent of those who survive will die during the following decade; and residual rheumatic heart disease remains in most of the others.

Susceptibility to recurrences of rheumatic fever increases with increasing severity of cardiac damage but diminishes as the patient grows older and the preceding rheumatic episode becomes more remote. Though most recurrences take place within a few years after the previous attack, they may occur at any age. As already stated, patients who have had carditis are more susceptible to rheumatic recurrences than those who were free of carditis, and the recurrences often increase the existing cardiac damage.

After cardiac damage is established, the subsequent course of the rheumatic heart disease depends on the hemodynamic effects of the valvular deformity and on the severity of myocardial damage (Chap. 270).

TREATMENT AND SUBSEQUENT MANAGEMENT. Even though a group A streptococcus cannot always be demonstrated in the throat, once the diagnosis of rheumatic fever is established an effort to eradicate this organism is justified. A single injection of benzathine penicillin, 900,000 or 1,200,000 units, usually suffices for this purpose, although different schedules of penicillin, as well as other antibiotics, may be used in patients with penicillin hypersensitivity. In any case, the effectiveness of treatment should be followed up by a throat culture, and a second course of treatment is indicated if the streptococcus has not been eradicated.

Although long regarded as an integral part of antirheumatic treatment, bed rest has no proven value and may be psychologically deleterious if maintained too long. A patient with painful arthritis, uncontrolled chorea, or severe congestive heart failure usually will choose to limit his activity. In patients whose symptoms are not sufficiently disabling to limit physical activity, bed rest is unnecessary.

For patients without carditis, treatment with adrenocortical steroids is unnecessary. Acute arthritis can be relieved with codeine or with salicylate, the latter being preferable if fever is also present. When salicylate is used in the therapy of rheumatic fever, the dosage should be increased until the drug produces either a clinical effect, manifested by elimination of fever or joint pains, or systemic toxicity, characterized by tinnitus, headache, or tachypnea. A useful starting daily dose is 15 to 20 mg per kg in children and 6 Gm in adults, given in four or five portions. Of the various salicylate preparations, ordinary aspirin is both cheapest and most effective. Absorption of enteric-coated preparations is too erratic; buffered preparations seldom contain enough buffer to exert a physiologic effect. Gastric intolerance can usually be avoided by meals or antacids 15 to 30 min following the aspirin.

Chorea should be managed as if it were a self-limited, completely reversible form of cerebral palsy. The most critical aspect of treatment is not the administration of drugs, but the avoidance of intellectual and psychologic trauma. The patient, and all those who deal with him, should be reassured that the peculiar movements are due to a specific neurologic disorder, of finite duration, that does not lead to any impairment of the intellect. Barbiturates or tranquilizers can sometimes be helpful in reducing the intensity of the choreic movements.

Many physicians prefer steroids to salicylates for the treatment of carditis, despite the lack of a demonstrated advantage of adrenal hormones in controlled clinical trials. Although more potent anti-inflammatory agents, steroids are more likely to be followed by a posttherapeutic rebound and have the additional disadvantage of more frequent side effects, particularly acne, hirsutism, and cutaneous striae in young people during prolonged therapy. For this reason, salicylates are the drugs of choice in patients with carditis. However, if these drugs fail to reduce fever and ameliorate heart failure, therapy with steroids should be initiated promptly. Prednisone is administered in dosage of 60 to 120 mg, or higher when necessary, in four divided doses daily. After the inflammation has been brought under control by either salicylate or steroid, treatment should be continued until the sedimentation rate reaches normal values, and should be maintained for several weeks thereafter. Salicylate may then be discontinued abruptly; administration of steroid should be tapered off over a 2-week period. To prevent poststeroid rebounds, an "overlap" course of salicylate therapy should be added when the steroid tapering begins, and this program should be continued for 2 weeks after steroid therapy has been discontinued. Rebounds are usually of short duration and, when mild, are best managed without resuming anti-inflammatory treatment, because a second rebound may occur when it is discontinued.

About 5 percent of rheumatic attacks persist for 8 months or longer, either in the form of spontaneous acute recrudescences or as posttherapeutic rebounds. These "chronic" attacks, which are most likely to occur in patients with cardiac damage and with previous rheumatic episodes, occasionally may be terminated with immunosuppressive agents such as nitrogen mustard or 6-mercaptopurine.

After streptococci are eradicated at the start of treatment, a prophylactic regimen should be initiated to prevent recurrent streptococcal infections that in turn may produce rheumatic recurrences. The most effective regimen is a monthly injection of 1.2 million units of benzathine penicillin. Oral prophylactic therapy avoids the pain and inconvenience of the injections, and a single daily dose of 1.0 Gm sulfadiazine or sulfisoxazole is as effective as 250,000 units of oral penicillin twice daily, but is not as good as injected benzathine penicillin. There is no agreement about how long antirheumatic prophylaxis should be maintained. A reasonable policy for all patients is to continue prophylaxis for at least 5 years after the last acute attack and until the patient reaches the age of twenty-five years. Thereafter, prophylaxis may be discontinued in patients who have not had carditis, but should be maintained indefinitely in patients who have had cardiac involvement.

REFERENCES

Ad Hoc Committee to Revise the Jones Criteria (Modified) of the Council on Rheumatic Fever and Congenital Heart Disease of the American Heart Association: **Jones Cri-**

teria (Revised) for Guidance in the Diagnosis of Rheu-matic Fever, Circulation, 32:664, 1965.

Feinstein, A. R., and M. Spagnuolo: The Clinical Patterns of Acute Rheumatic Fever: A Reappraisal, Medicine, 41: 279, 1962.

——, E. K. Stern, and M. Spagnuolo: The Prognosis of Acute Rheumatic Fever, Am. Heart J., 68:817, 1964.

Joint Report of a U.K.-U.S. Co-operative Study: The Natural History of Rheumatic Fever and Rheumatic Heart Dis-ease. Ten-year Report of a Cooperative Clinical Trial of ACTH, Cortisone, and Aspirin, Circulation, 32:457, 1965.

Massell, B. F., D. C. Fyler, and S. B. Roy: The Clinical Pic-ture of Rheumatic Fever. Diagnosis, Immediate Prog-nosis, Course and Therapeutic Implications, Am. J. Cardiol., 1:436, 1958.

Rammelkamp, C. R., Jr., and B. L. Stolzer: The Latent Period before the Onset of Acute Rheumatic Fever, Yale J. Biol. & Med., 34:386, 1961–1962.

Taranta, A., and G. H. Stollerman: The Relationship of Sydenham's Chorea to Infection with Group A Strepto-cocci, Am. J. Med., 20:170, 1956.

Wood, H. F., A. R. Feinstein, A. Taranta, J. A. Epstein, and R. Simpson: Rheumatic Fever in Children and Adoles-cents: A Long-term Epidemiologic Study of Subsequent Prophylaxis, Streptococcal Infections and Clinical Se-quelae. III. Comparative Effectiveness of Three Prophy-laxis Regimens in Preventing Streptococcal Infections and Rheumatic Recurrences, Ann. Intern. Med., 60 (suppl. 5):31, 1964.

270 VALVULAR HEART DISEASE[1]
Eugene Braunwald

AORTIC STENOSIS

Aortic stenosis occurs in about one-fourth of all pa-tients with chronic valvular heart disease; approximately 80 percent of adult patients with symptomatic valvular aortic stenosis are male.

Pathologic Physiology

The primary hemodynamic abnormality in aortic steno-sis is obstruction to left ventricular outflow which leads to a pressure gradient between the left ventricle and aorta during the systolic ejection period. When severe obstruction is suddenly produced experimentally, the left ventricle responds to this excess afterload by dilatation and reduction of stroke volume. However, in clinical aortic stenosis, the obstruction may be present at birth or it increases gradually over the course of many years and left ventricular output is maintained by the presence of left ventricular hypertrophy. A large pressure gradient

[1] In addition to the discussion of the specific valvular ab-normalities in this chapter, the role of phonocardiography and other indirect graphic techniques in the evaluation of patients with these lesions is considered in Chap. 261, and the role of cardiac catheterization and angiocardiography in Chap. 262.

across the aortic valve may exist for many years without a reduction of cardiac output, left ventricular dilatation, or the development of any symptoms. As aortic stenosis progresses in severity, the left ventricular systolic pres-sure continues to rise but rarely exceeds 300 mm Hg.

As with any stenotic lesion in the cardiovascular sys-tem, in order to estimate the severity of obstruction, it is necessary to measure both the transvalvular pressure gra-dient and the blood flow, preferably simultaneously. A peak systolic pressure gradient exceeding 50 mm Hg in the face of a normal cardiac output or an effective aortic orifice less than 0.7 sq cm per sq m body surface area, i.e., less than approximately one-third of the normal orifice, is generally considered to represent critical ob-struction to left ventricular outflow. The left ventricular pressure pulse exhibits a rounded summit as the contrac-tion of this chamber becomes progressively more iso-metric, and pulsus alternans in the left ventricle is a common finding in patients with severe stenosis. The elevated left ventricular end-diastolic pressure observed in many patients with severe aortic stenosis does not necessarily signify the presence of left ventricular failure or dilatation, but may instead reflect diminished com-pliance of the hypertrophied left ventricular wall.

A large *a* wave in the left atrial pressure pulse is usu-ally present in patients with severe aortic stenosis, because of unusually forceful atrial contraction and diminished ventricular compliance. Atrial contraction tends to raise left ventricular end-diastolic pressure without producing a concomitant elevation of mean left atrial pressure. This "booster pump" function of the left atrium prevents the pulmonary venous and capillary pressures from rising to levels which would produce pulmonary congestion, while at the same time maintaining left ventricular end-diastolic pressure at the elevated level necessary for effective left ventricular contraction. Loss of an appropriately timed, vigorous atrial contraction, as occurs in atrial fibrillation or atrioventricular dissociation, occasionally results in a rapid aggravation of symptoms or cardiovascular collapse, even when the ventricular response is not particularly rapid.

The cardiac output and stroke volume at rest are within normal limits in the majority of patients with se-vere aortic stenosis. These variables may fail to rise normally during exercise. Late in the disease the cardiac output and stroke volume decline and the mean left atrial, pulmonary artery wedge, pulmonary arterial, and right ventricular pressures usually become elevated while the left ventricular–aortic pressure gradient falls. At this stage, a prominent *a* wave in the right atrial pressure pulse is also commonly found and hemodynamic evidence of mitral regurgitation, with a tall left atrial *v* wave and sharp *y* descent, may occur in association with marked left ventricular dilatation.

The hypertrophied left ventricular muscle mass and increased myocardial wall tension elevate myocardial oxygen requirements in the presence of aortic stenosis. In addition, there may be interference with coronary blood flow, because the pressure compressing the coro-nary arteries exceeds the coronary perfusion pressure.

A significant fraction of patients with rheumatic aortic stenosis has associated mitral valve disease. Aortic stenosis intensifies the severity of mitral regurgitation by increasing the pressure driving blood from the left ventricle to the left atrium. The dilatation of the left ventricle which occurs late in the course of the disease in some patients with aortic stenosis further intensifies the magnitude of the mitral regurgitant flow.

Etiology

Aortic stenosis may be congenital in origin, secondary to rheumatic inflammation of the aortic valve, or due to calcification of the aortic cusps of unknown cause. The congenitally affected valve may already be stenotic at birth and may gradually become calcified during the first three decades of life, becoming progressively more stenotic. The valve may also be congenitally bicuspid without serious narrowing of the aortic orifice during childhood; its abnormal architecture apparently makes the leaflets susceptible to normal hemodynamic stresses, which ultimately lead to valvular calcification, increased rigidity, and narrowing of the aortic orifice.

Rheumatic endocarditis of the aortic leaflets produces commissural fusion, resulting, at first, in a bicuspid valve. This, in turn, also makes the leaflets more susceptible to local trauma, and ultimately leads to calcification and further narrowing. By the time the obstruction to left ventricular outflow causes serious disability and the valve is examined, either at operation or at autopsy, it is usually a rigid calcified mass, and even careful examination makes it impossible to determine whether the underlying process was rheumatic or congenital. A rheumatic etiology is favored by a history of active rheumatic fever, by clinical, hemodynamic, or pathologic evidence of involvement of the mitral and tricuspid valves, and by associated severe aortic regurgitation. Idiopathic calcific aortic stenosis occurs most often in the elderly and is rarely associated with fusion of the valve cusps; although this disease may produce many of the characteristic physical signs of aortic stenosis, the valvular obstruction is usually relatively mild and of little if any hemodynamic significance.

In some patients with calcific aortic stenosis a spur of calcium extends inferiorly from the left ventricular aspect of the aortic valve to the anterior leaflet of the mitral valve. It may also invade the ventricular septum and rarely may be responsible for complete heart block.

Other Forms of Obstruction to Left Ventricular Outflow

Although valvular aortic stenosis is certainly the most common form of obstruction to left ventricular outflow, three other lesions may be responsible for this physiologic abnormality.

Idiopathic Hypertrophic Subaortic Stenosis. This is the most important of these conditions. It is characterized by marked hypertrophy of the left ventricle, involving in particular the interventricular septum of the left ventricular outflow tract, as described in Chap. 273.

Discrete Congenital Subvalvular Aortic Stenosis. Less common than hypertrophic subaortic stenosis, this condition is produced by either a membranous diaphragm or a fibrous ridge just below the aortic valve (Chap. 268).

Supravaluvlar Aortic Stenosis. This uncommon congenital anomaly is produced by narrowing of the ascending aorta or by a fibrous diaphragm with a small opening just above the aortic valve (Chap. 268).

Symptoms

Aortic stenosis rarely becomes of hemodynamic or clinical importance until the valve orifice has narrowed to approximately one third of normal. Thus, in contrast to mitral stenosis, which results in symptoms as soon as the obstruction becomes severe because the chamber just proximal to the narrowed valve provides little compensation, severe aortic stenosis may exist for many years without producing any clinical disability.

Most patients with pure or predominant aortic stenosis do not become symptomatic until the fourth or fifth decade. Exertional dyspnea, angina pectoris, and syncope are the three cardinal symptoms. Dyspnea results primarily from elevation of the left ventricular end-diastolic pressure, which in turn increases the mean left atrial and pulmonary capillary pressures. Angina pectoris usually develops somewhat later and resembles the pain of myocardial ischemia which occurs in patients with coronary artery disease. However, when severe angina pectoris is present in patients with aortic stenosis, it does not necessarily signify coexisting coronary artery disease, but more commonly reflects an imbalance between the augmented myocardial oxygen requirements and oxygen availability. Exertional syncope may result from a decline in arterial pressure caused by vasodilatation in the exercising muscles in the face of a fixed cardiac output, or from a sudden fall in cardiac output produced by an arrhythmia. If prolonged, the syncopal episode may be accompanied by convulsions and loss of sphincteric control.

Since the cardiac output is well maintained at rest until the late stage of the disease, marked fatigability, debilitation, peripheral cyanosis, and other clinical manifestations of a low cardiac output are usually not prominent until this stage is reached. Orthopnea, paroxysmal nocturnal dyspnea, and pulmonary edema, i.e., symptoms of left ventricular failure, also occur in the advanced stages of the disease. Severe pulmonary hypertension leading to right ventricular failure and systemic venous hypertension, hepatomegaly, atrial fibrillation, and tricuspid regurgitation are usually preterminal findings.

When aortic stenosis and mitral stenosis coexist, the mitral obstruction masks many of the clinical findings of aortic stenosis. The reduction of cardiac output induced by mitral stenosis lowers the pressure gradient across the aortic valve, diminishes the frequency of anginal episodes, and retards the development of aortic calcification and severe left ventricular hypertrophy. On the other hand, symptoms considered more characteristic of mitral stenosis, such as pulmonary congestion and hemoptysis, occur more frequently in patients with combined stenotic lesions than in those with isolated aortic stenosis. Careful physical, electrocardiographic, and radiologic examinations in patients with aortic and mitral stenosis generally reveal more evidence of left ventricular enlargement than in patients with pure mitral stenosis, and catheterization of the left side of the heart is helpful in defining the relative importance of each valvular abnormality.

Physical Findings

The systemic arterial pressure is usually within normal limits. In the late stages, however, when stroke volume declines, the systolic pressure may fall and the pulse pressure narrows. Severe systemic hypertension is extremely unusual in patients with marked aortic stenosis, and a basal systolic arterial pressure exceeding 200 mm Hg practically excludes severe narrowing of this valve. On palpation, the peripheral arterial pulse characteristically is found to rise slowly, with a delayed peak. Indirect recordings of the carotid pulse exhibit a gradually ascending limb, often with a prominent anacrotic notch or shoulder on the upstroke, as well as a delayed peak, with coarse systolic vibrations. A palpable double systolic wave, the so-called bisferiens pulse, excludes pure or predominant aortic stenosis, and signifies dominant or pure aortic regurgitation or idiopathic hypertrophic subaortic stenosis (Chap. 273). In the late stages of the disease, when the pulse pressure is reduced, the pulse amplitude is so small that the anacrotic nature of the pulse and the delay in its upstroke may become more difficult to appreciate. The jugular venous pulse may be normal, although in many patients the a wave is accentuated. This results from the diminished distensibility of the right ventricular cavity caused by the bulging, hypertrophied, interventricular septum and/or the presence of pulmonary hypertension. A prominent jugular venous v wave, signifying tricuspid regurgitation, is extremely rare in aortic stenosis and is observed only in the latest stages of the disease.

On palpation, the apex beat is usually found to be active and displaced inferiorly and laterally, reflecting the presence of left ventricular hypertrophy. A double apical impulse may be appreciated, particularly with the patient in the left lateral recumbent position; the first outward expansion occurs during atrial systole and reflects the important contribution made by atrial contraction to ventricular filling, while the second commences during early ventricular systole and is well sustained during ejection. The right ventricle is usually palpable only when pulmonary hypertension develops in the late stages of the disease. A systolic thrill is generally present at the base of the heart, in the jugular notch, and along the carotid arteries, but occasionally it is palpable only during expiration and with the patient leaning forward. In patients without marked pulmonary emphysema, a thick chest wall, thoracic deformity, or heart failure, absence of a systolic thrill signifies that the aortic stenosis is relatively mild.

The rhythm is generally regular, and the presence of atrial fibrillation should call to mind the possibility of associated mitral valve disease. An early systolic ejection sound, actually the opening snap of the aortic valve, is frequently audible in children and adolescents with noncalcific valvular aortic stenosis. However, this sound usually disappears when the valve becomes calcified and rigid. The sound of aortic valve closure can also be identified most frequently in patients with aortic stenosis with pliable valves, and calcification tends to diminish the intensity of this sound. As aortic stenosis increases in severity, left ventricular systole may become prolonged so that the aortic valve closure sound no longer precedes the pulmonic valve closure sound, and the two components may become synchronous, or aortic valve closure may even follow pulmonic valve closure. This is called paradoxic splitting of the second heart sound (Chap. 259) and may be recognized by finding on auscultation or phonocardiography that the two components do not widen but actually narrow during inspiration. Paradoxic splitting of the second heart sound in patients with aortic stenosis in the absence of a left intraventricular conduction defect usually signifies severe obstruction to left ventricular outflow. An atrial (presystolic) gallop, audible at the apex in many patients with severe aortic stenosis, reflects considerable left ventricular hypertrophy and an elevated left ventricular end-diastolic pressure; a ventricular (protodiastolic) gallop in adults generally occurs when the left ventricle dilates and fails.

The systolic murmur in aortic stenosis is of the ejection type, i.e., it commences not simultaneously with the first heart sound but shortly after it, increases in intensity to reach a peak toward the middle of the ejection period, and diminishes progressively thereafter to end just before aortic valve closure. The murmur is usually low-pitched, rough, and rasping in character and is loudest at the base of the heart, usually in the second intercostal space just to the right of the sternum. It is transmitted upwards to the jugular notch and along the carotid arteries. In patients with trivial degrees of obstruction or in those with severe stenosis in the late stage of the disease in whom the stroke volume is reduced, the murmur may be relatively soft and brief, and confined to midsystole. However, in almost all patients with significant obstruction, the murmur is quite loud, at least grade III/VI, and its intensity and duration are not particularly helpful in distinguishing patients with moderate stenosis from those with severe stenosis. Occasionally the murmur is transmitted downward and to the apex and may be confused with the systolic murmur of mitral regurgitation. However, this murmur is usually holosystolic, while that of aortic stenosis is diamond-shaped and of the ejection type (Chap. 259).

ELECTROCARDIOGRAM. The electrocardiogram reveals evidence of left ventricular hypertrophy in the majority of patients with severe aortic stenosis. In advanced cases, S-T segment depression and T-wave inversion in standard leads I, aVL, and in the left precordial leads are evident. However, there is no close correlation between the electrocardiogram and the hemodynamic severity of obstruction, and the absence of electrocardiographic signs of left ventricular hypertrophy does not always exclude severe obstruction. Left bundle branch block or the presence of intraventricular conduction defects with QRS prolongation suggests diffuse fibrotic involvement of the myocardium. Atrial fibrillation or electrocardiographic indication of left atrial enlargement is rarely seen in patients with pure aortic stenosis; when present they should suggest the possibility of associated mitral valve disease.

ROENTGENOGRAPHIC FEATURES. The chest rotengenogram may show no or little overall cardiac enlargement for many years, since the development of concentric left ventricular hypertrophy is the initial response to obstruction to left ventricular outflow. Considerable hypertrophy without dilatation may produce some rounding of the cardiac apex in the frontal projection and slight backward displacement in the lateral view; significant aortic stenosis is usually associated with poststenotic dilatation of the ascending aorta. Aortic calcification is usually readily apparent on fluoroscopic examination with an image intensifier; indeed, the absence of such calcification in an adult suggests that severe aortic stenosis is not present. In later stages of the disease as the left ventricle dilates, there is progressively more evidence of left ventricular enlargement, and there may also be roentgenologic signs of pulmonary congestion, as well as enlargement of the left atrium, pulmonary artery, right ventricle, and right atrium.

CATHETERIZATION AND ANGIOCARDIOGRAPHY. Catheterization of the left side of the heart should be carried out in the majority of patients suspected of having severe aortic stenosis, particularly before a final decision concerning operative treatment is made. These investigations are especially indicated in (1) young, asymptomatic patients with noncalcific aortic stenosis, in order to define the severity of their obstruction to left ventricular outflow, since operation may be indicated if severe aortic stenosis is present; (2) patients in whom it is suspected that the obstruction to left ventricular outflow may not be at the aortic valve, but rather that it is in the sub- or supravalvular regions; (3) patients with clinical signs of aortic stenosis and symptoms of myocardial ischemia, in whom associated coronary artery disease is suspected. An effort should be made to determine whether aortic stenosis or coronary atherosclerosis is responsible for the symptoms in this group of patients, and coronary arteriography may have to be carried out in addition to catheterization of the left side of the heart; and (4) patients with multivalvular disease, in whom the role played by each valvular deformity must be defined before operative treatment is planned.

Angiocardiographic studies with left ventricular injection of contrast material are helpful in defining the size of the left ventricular cavity, the thickness of the wall, the site of obstruction, the degree of deformity and mobility of the aortic valve cusps, the diameter of the ascending aorta, and the presence and degree of accompanying mitral regurgitation. In patients with severe narrowing, a jet of contrast substance passing through the aortic orifice is readily visualized. When contrast substance is injected into the ascending aorta, the aortic valve cusps can also be outlined and associated aortic regurgitation can be detected and its severity assessed.

NATURAL HISTORY. The advanced age at death of patients with severe acquired stenosis has been a remarkably consistent feature of this disease, and has averaged sixty-three years in males. In several studies, based on analysis of data obtained at postmortem examination, the average duration of various symptoms was as follows: angina pectoris, 3 years; syncope, 3 years; dyspnea, 2 years; and congestive heart failure, 1.5 to 2 years. Moreover, in more than 80 percent of these patients who died with aortic stenosis, symptoms had existed for less than 4 years. Congestive heart failure was considered to be the cause of death in one-half to two-thirds of patients.

Among patients dying with acquired valvular aortic stenosis, sudden death occurred in 15 to 20 percent, and at an average age of sixty years. Sudden death was more common in patients with symptoms, and 65 to 80 percent of patients coming to autopsy after sudden death had a history of angina pectoris, heart failure, or syncope. Thus, only 3 to 5 percent of the deaths in acquired aortic stenosis appear to occur suddenly in patients without symptoms. The incidence of significant coronary arterial disease in adults with aortic stenosis and angina pectoris is relatively high, and in addition, about one out of every six patients dying suddenly has evidence of old or recent myocardial infarction at postmortem examination.

Treatment

Because strenuous physical activity further elevates the left ventricular systolic pressure in patients with *severe* aortic stenosis, it should be avoided even in the asymptomatic stage. Digitalis glycosides, sodium restriction, and diuretics are indicated in the treatment of congestive heart failure, nitroglycerin is helpful in relieving angina pectoris. The most critical decision in the management of aortic stenosis concerns the advisability of surgical treatment. The indications and results of operation, as well as the techniques, differ considerably, depending on the patient's age and the nature of the valvular deformity.

In children and adolescents with noncalcific aortic stenosis, considerable hemodynamic improvement can be anticipated from simple commissural incision under direct vision. When carried out by an experienced surgeon, this procedure may be expected to enlarge the size of the valvular orifice significantly, without increasing the magnitude of aortic regurgitation, with a mortality rate of less than 5 percent. This operation is recommended not only for symptomatic patients but also for asymptomatic children and adolescents with hemodynamic evidence of severe obstruction to left ventricular outflow, with a peak systolic pressure gradient exceeding 50 mm Hg when the cardiac output is normal, or a calculated effective orifice less than 0.7 cm per sq m of body surface area. Though this procedure can be expected to result in complete or almost complete relief of obstruction in the majority of patients, the valve cannot be rendered entirely normal anatomically, and it is entirely possible that it will become deformed, calcified, and stenotic again in later years, entailing the possibility of reoperation, and perhaps valve replacement at some later date.

In the majority of adults with calcific aortic stenosis, satisfactory valve function cannot be restored, even by deliberate sculpturing procedures carried out under direct vision, and replacement of the aortic valve is necessary. In most instances, it seems prudent to postpone operation in patients with severe calcific aortic stenosis who are asymptomatic since they may continue to do well for many years. However, it is likely that as the results of surgical replacement of the aortic valve improve, many of these patients will become candidates for operation before their disease reaches the symptomatic stage. Replacement of the aortic valve should be undertaken in patients with symptoms believed to result primarily from aortic stenosis, and in those who have hemodynamic evidence of severe obstruction.

It is clear that when symptoms of angina pectoris, syncope, or left ventricular decompensation develop in adults with valvular aortic stenosis, the immediate outlook is poor but can be improved significantly by replacement of the aortic valve with a ball valve prosthesis or homograft. Therefore, the risk entailed by operation in this group of patients is considerably lower than the risk involved by nonoperative treatment; moreover, the symptomatic improvement in many survivors of operation has been remarkable. However, the influence of aortic valve replacement on long-term survival and disability has not been established.

, Operation should, if possible, be carried out before the development of frank left ventricular failure; the operative risk in such patients is extremely high, and evidence of myocardial disease may persist even when the operation is technically successful. Nonetheless, in view of the very poor prognosis of such patients when they are treated medically, there is usually little choice but to advise surgical treatment. In patients in whom severe aortic stenosis and coronary artery disease coexist, relief of stenosis may result in striking clinical improvement, presumably because of the diminution of the pressure load on the left ventricle and the resultant decrease in myocardial oxygen requirements. However, aortic valve replacement can relieve only one aspect of the patient's problem and the presence of associated coronary artery disease increases the risk of operation and diminishes the likelihood of complete symptomatic recovery. Since many patients with calcific aortic stenosis are elderly, particular attention must be directed to the levels of hepatic, renal, and pulmonary function before valve replacement is recommended. At the present time aortic valve replacement in symptomatic patients with severe obstruction is associated with a higher immediate mortality rate than is aortic commissurotomy in childhood (10 to 20 percent in most centers), and the long-term results and complications associated with the use of available prostheses have still not been defined completely. Accordingly, a more conservative approach to operative treatment is warranted in adults with calcific aortic stenosis than in children with noncalcific stenosis.

AORTIC REGURGITATION
Pathologic Physiology

The total stroke volume expelled by the left ventricle, i.e., the sum of the effective forward stroke volume, and the volume of blood which regurgitates back into the left ventricle are both increased in aortic regurgitation. In contrast to mitral regurgitation, in which a fraction of the left ventricular stroke volume is delivered into the low-pressure left atrium (page 1203), in aortic regurgitation the entire left ventricular stroke volume must be ejected into a high-pressure zone, the aorta. Although the low aortic diastolic pressure facilitates ventricular emptying during early systole, an increase of the left ventricular end-diastolic volume constitutes the major hemodynamic compensation to aortic regurgitation, and the total stroke volume is augmented, primarily through the operation of the Frank-Starling mechanism (Chap. 263). Measurements of aortic regurgitant flow by means of angiocardiographic techniques, as well as with electromagnetic flowmeter probes placed on the aorta during operation, have revealed that in patients with free aortic regurgitation the volume of regurgitant flow may be of the same order of magnitude as the effective forward stroke volume. The dilatation of the left ventricle allows this chamber to expel a larger stroke volume without requiring any increase in the relative shortening of each myofibril. On the other hand, through the operation of Laplace's law, which indicates that myocardial wall tension is the product of intracavitary pressure and left ventricular radius, left ventricular dilatation increases the left ventricular systolic tension required to develop any given level of systolic pressure. As left ventricular function deteriorates, the end-diastolic volume increases without further elevation of the aortic regurgitant volume. Considerable thickening of the left ventricular wall also occurs with chronic aortic regurgitation, and at autopsy the hearts of these patients may be among the largest encountered, occasionally exceeding 1,000 Gm in weight.

The reduction of the aortic diastolic pressure in aortic regurgitation shortens the left ventricular isometric contraction period, which is helpful in allowing a longer left ventricular ejection period. The reverse pressure gradient from aorta to left ventricle, which is responsible for the aortic regurgitant flow, falls progressively during diastole, accounting for the decrescendo nature of the diastolic murmur. Equilibration between aortic and left ventricular pressures may occur toward the end of diastole, particularly when the heart rate is slow, and the left ventricular end-diastolic pressure may be elevated, occasionally to extremely high levels (>40 mm Hg). Rarely, the left ventricular pressure exceeds the left atrial pressure towards the end of diastole, and this reversed pressure gradient closes the mitral valve prematurely.

In patients with free aortic regurgitation the effective forward cardiac output usually is normal or slightly reduced at rest, but often it fails to rise normally during exertion. In advanced stages there may be considerable elevation of the left atrial, pulmonary artery wedge, pulmonary arterial, and right ventricular pressures, and lowering of the cardiac output at rest. The recordings of aortic and left ventricular pressures provide only a rough estimate of the severity of aortic regurgitation. Indicator-dilution techniques with left ventricular injection and arterial sampling are helpful in the assessment of aortic regurgitation, since they show a markedly prolonged descending limb. A qualitative index of the severity of aortic regurgitation may also be obtained by determining the intensity of left ventricular opacification and the size of the left ventricle during thoracic cineaortography. In addition, this technique allows the detection of associated mitral regurgitation. However, biplane angiographic techniques are required for accurate estimates of aortic regurgitant flow.

Myocardial ischemia occurs in patients with aortic regurgitation because both left ventricular dilatation and the increased left ventricular systolic pressure tend to elevate the systolic tension developed by the myocardium, and thereby to increase myocardial oxygen requirements. However, the major portion of coronary blood flow occurs during diastole, when arterial pressure is lower than normal.

Etiology

Approximately three-fourths of all patients with pure or predominant regurgitation are males; however, females predominate among patients with aortic regurgitation who have associated mitral valve disease. In approximately 80 percent of patients with aortic regurgitation the disease is rheumatic in origin, resulting in thickening, deformation, and shortening of the individual aortic valve cusps, changes which prevent their proper closure during diastole. Less commonly, bacterial endocarditis may attack a valve previously affected by rheumatic disease, a congenitally deformed valve, or rarely a normal aortic valve, and may result in the perforation or erosion of one or more of the leaflets. Patients with discrete membranous subaortic stenosis may develop thickening of the aortic valve leaflets, which in turn leads to mild or moderate degrees of aortic regurgitation and makes these valves particularly susceptible to bacterial endocarditis. Aortic regurgitation may also occur in patients with congenital bicuspid aortic valves. Prolapse of an aortic cusp, resulting in progressive aortic regurgitation, occurs in approximately 15 percent of patients with ventricular septal defect. Traumatic rupture of the aortic valve is an uncommon cause of aortic regurgitation, but it represents the most frequent serious lesion observed in patients surviving nonpenetrating cardiac injuries. Congenital fenestrations of the aortic valve occasionally produce mild or moderate degrees of aortic regurgitation. In patients with aortic regurgitation due to primary valvular disease, dilatation of the aortic annulus may occur secondarily and intensify the regurgitation.

Aortic regurgitation may be due entirely to marked aortic dilatation, without primary involvement of the valve leaflets; widening of the aortic annulus and separation of the aortic leaflets are responsible for the aortic regurgitation. Syphilis and ankylosing rheumatoid spon-

dylitis may be associated with cellular infiltration and scarring of the media of the thoracic aorta, leading to aortic dilatation, aneurysm formation, and severe regurgitation. In syphilis of the aorta (Chap. 277), the involvement of the intima may narrow the coronary ostiums, which narrowing in turn may be responsible for coronary insufficiency. Cystic medionecrosis of the ascending aorta, which may be associated with other manifestations of Marfan's syndrome (Chap. 277), idiopathic dilatation of the aorta, and severe hypertension may also widen the aortic annulus and lead to progressive aortic regurgitation. Occasionally, retrograde dissection of the aorta involving the aortic annulus produces aortic regurgitation.

The coexistence of hemodynamically significant aortic stenosis with aortic regurgitation usually excludes all the rarer forms of aortic regurgitation because it occurs almost entirely in patients whose aortic regurgitation is on a rheumatic or congenital basis.

Symptoms

The history is often helpful in determining the cause of aortic regurgitation. A family history may frequently be elicited from patients with Marfan's syndrome, and a history of a heart murmur heard early in life may be obtained from patients with congenital aortic regurgitation. Patients with aortic regurgitation of obscure cause should also be questioned in detail about prior chest trauma; a history compatible with subacute bacterial endocarditis may sometimes be elicited from patients with rheumatic or congenital involvement of the aortic valve, and the infection often precipitates or seriously aggravates preexisting symptoms.

The interval between the first episode of acute rheumatic fever and the development of hemodynamically significant aortic regurgitation averages approximately 7 years, and this period is followed by an asymptomatic interval of approximately 10 years, during which the severity of the aortic regurgitation usually increases. Thus, severe aortic regurgitation may exist for many years without producing symptoms.

The first complaint is often an uncomfortable awareness of the heart beat, especially on lying down. Sinus tachycardia occurring during exertion or with emotion, or premature ventricular contractions may produce particularly uncomfortable palpitations, as well as head pounding. These complaints may persist for many years before the development of exertional dyspnea, usually the first symptom of diminished cardiac reserve. This is followed by angina pectoris, orthopnea, paroxysmal nocturnal dyspnea, and excessive diaphoresis.

Angina occurs as frequently in younger as in older patients with severe aortic regurgitation, and it is not necessary to invoke the presence of coronary artery disease to explain this symptom. The clinical features of angina pectoris in patients with aortic regurgitation may differ from those commonly observed in patients with coronary artery disease or predominant aortic stenosis. Thus, anginal pain may develop at rest as well as during exertion in patients with aortic regurgitation. Nocturnal angina is a particularly troublesome symptom in many patients and is frequently accompanied by marked diaphoresis. The anginal episodes may be prolonged and often do not respond satisfactorily to sublingual nitroglycerin. Late in the course of the disease, evidence of systemic fluid accumulation, including congestive hepatomegaly, ankle edema, and ascites, may develop. Patients with severe aortic regurgitation do not tolerate high fevers, infections, or cardiac arrhythmias, and may die in pulmonary edema as a result of one of these complications.

Physical Findings

The general examination should be directed towards the detection of causes predisposing to aortic regurgitation, such as Marfan's syndrome, rheumatoid spondylitis, syphilis, essential hypertension, and ventricular septal defect. Even prior to the examination of the heart of the patient with free aortic regurgitation, the jarring of the entire body and the bobbing motion of the head with each systole can be appreciated and the abrupt distension and collapse of the larger arteries are easily visible. On palpation, one finds a rapidly rising "water hammer" pulse, which collapses suddenly as arterial pressure falls rapidly during late systole and diastole (Corrigan's pulse). Capillary pulsations (Quincke's pulse), an alternate paling and flushing of the skin at the root of the nail while pressure is applied to the tip of the nail, may also be observed. A booming, "pistol-shot" sound can be heard over the femoral arteries, and a to-and-fro murmur (Duroziez's sign) is audible if the femoral artery is lightly compressed with a stethoscope.

The arterial pulse pressure is widened, with an elevation of the systolic pressure, sometimes to as high as 300 mm Hg, and a depression of the diastolic arterial pressure. The measurement of arterial diastolic pressure with a sphygmomanometer may be complicated by the fact that systolic sounds are frequently heard with the cuff completely deflated. However, the level of cuff pressure at the time of muffling of the Korotkoff sounds generally corresponds fairly closely to the true arterial diastolic pressure. The severity of aortic regurgitation does not always correlate directly with the arterial pulse pressure, and in many instances severe regurgitation exists in patients with arterial pressures in the range of 140/60 mm Hg. As the disease progresses, and the left ventricular end-diastolic pressure becomes markedly elevated, the arterial diastolic pressure may actually rise.

The apex beat is displaced laterally and inferiorly. The left ventricle is hyperdynamic in patients with free regurgitation, and the systolic expansion and subsequent retraction of the apex are prominent and contrast sharply with the sustained systolic thrust characteristic of severe aortic stenosis. A diastolic thrill is often palpable along the left sternal border, and a prominent systolic thrill may be palpable in the jugular notch and transmitted upwards along the carotid arteries. This thrill and the accompanying systolic murmur are due to the markedly increased blood flow across the aortic orifice, and do not necessarily signify the coexistence of aortic stenosis. Palpation, or indirect recording of the carotid arterial pulse, reveals it to be bisferiens, i.e., with two systolic waves separated by a trough, in many patients with pure aortic regurgitation, or with combined stenosis and regurgitation.

In patients with severe aortic regurgitation the aortic valve closure sound is usually diminished or absent, and the indirectly recorded carotid arterial pulse does not usually show a clear-cut incisura. A third heart sound is common, and occasionally a fourth heart sound may also be heard. A loud systolic ejection sound is frequently audible; it presumably results from the sudden dilatation of the aorta by a greatly increased stroke volume.

The murmur of aortic regurgitation is a high-pitched, blowing, decrescendo diastolic murmur which is usually heard best in the third intercostal space to the left of the sternum. In patients with mild regurgitation this murmur is brief and usually lasts less than one-third of diastole. However, as the severity of regurgitation increases, the murmur generally becomes louder and longer, and in patients with free aortic regurgitation it is usually holodiastolic. When the murmur is soft, it can be heard best with the diaphragm of the stethoscope and with the patient sitting up, leaning forward, and with the breath held in forced expiration. As it increases in intensity it tends to radiate widely, particularly down the lower sternal edge. In patients in whom the regurgitation is caused by primary valvular disease, the diastolic murmur is usually louder along the left than along the right sternal border. However, when the decrescendo diastolic murmur is heard best along the right sternal border, it suggests that the aortic regurgitation is caused by dilatation or an aneurysm of the aortic root.

It may be difficult to distinguish the murmur of aortic from that of pulmonic regurgitation in patients with multivalvular rheumatic heart disease. However, on a purely statistic basis, a diastolic blowing murmur along the left sternal border is much more commonly caused by aortic than by pulmonic regurgitation. Unless it is trivial in magnitude, the aortic regurgitation can also be recognized by peripheral signs such as a widened pulse pressure or a collapsing pulse. On the other hand, the Graham Steell murmur of pulmonary regurgitation is usually accompanied by clinical evidence of severe pulmonary hypertension, including a loud and palpable pulmonary component of the second heart sound. In addition, the phonocardiogram reveals that the murmur of aortic regurgitation begins with the aortic second sound and therefore commences somewhat before the murmur of pulmonary regurgitation.

A systolic ejection murmur is generally heard best at the base of the heart and is transmitted to the jugular notch and along the carotid vessels. This murmur may be as loud as grade V/VI without reflecting any organic obstruction; it is often higher pitched and less rasping in quality than the ejection systolic murmur heard in patients with predominant aortic stenosis.

The third murmur which is frequently heard in patients with aortic regurgitation is the Austin Flint murmur, a soft, low-pitched, rumbling bruit. It is probably produced by the displacement by the aortic regurgitation stream of the anterior leaflet of the mitral valve. However, this displacement of the mitral valve does not appear to be associated with hemodynamically significant obstruction to left ventricular filling. In patients with rheumatic aortic regurgitation it may be difficult to distinguish the Austin Flint murmur from the rumbling diastolic murmur of mitral stenosis. Both are loudest at the apex, but the murmur of mitral stenosis is usually accompanied by a loud first heart sound and immediately follows the opening snap of the mitral valve, while the Austin Flint murmur is usually associated with a soft first heart sound and follows the third heart sound. The Austin Flint murmur is often shorter in duration than the murmur of mitral stenosis, and in patients with sinus rhythm the latter more frequently is characterized by presystolic accentuation. A blowing holosystolic murmur at the apex, which is transmitted to the axilla, may also be heard in patients with marked left ventricular dilatation and functional mitral regurgitation.

ELECTROCARDIOGRAM. In patients with mild aortic regurgitation there may be no electrocardiographic abnormalities, but as the severity of aortic regurgitation increases, so do the electrocardiographic signs of left ventricular hypertrophy (Chap. 260). In addition to the abnormally tall R waves over the left precordium and deep S waves over the right precordium, patients with severe aortic regurgitation frequently exhibit S-T segment depressions and T-wave inversions in leads 1, aVL, V_5, and V_6. Electrocardiographic signs of previous myocardial infarction generally indicate associated coronary artery disease. Left axis deviation and/or QRS prolongation denote diffuse myocardial disease, generally associated with patchy fibrosis; these signs are usually associated with a poor prognosis.

ROENTGENOGRAM. Moderate or severe degrees of regurgitation are always associated with varying degrees of left ventricular enlargement. The apex is displaced downwards and to the left on the frontal projection, and frequently the cardiac shadow appears to extend below the left diaphragm. Left ventricular enlargement also occurs in the left anterior oblique and lateral projections, in which the left ventricle is displaced posteriorly and encroaches on the spine. In patients in whom primary valvular disease is responsible for the aortic regurgitation, the ascending aorta and aortic knob may be moderately dilated and may extend further to the right than the right atrial shadow in the frontal view. On fluoroscopic examination the aorta and left ventricle pulsate vigorously in opposite directions during systole. When aortic regurgitation is caused by primary disease of the aortic wall, aneurysmal dilatation of the aorta may be seen roentgenographically, and the aorta may fill the retrosternal space in the lateral view.

Treatment

The left ventricular failure of aortic regurgitation at first usually responds to treatment with digitalis glyco-sides, salt restriction, and diuretics. Digitalis may also be indicated in patients with severe regurgitation and dilated left ventricles without symptoms of frank left ventricular failure, since it may retard its development (Chap. 266). Cardiac arrhythmias and infections are poorly tolerated in patients with free aortic regurgitation, and must be treated promptly and vigorously. Although nitroglycerin and long-acting nitrites are not as helpful in relieving anginal pain as in patients with coronary artery disease or aortic stenosis, they are worth a trial. Patients with syphilitic aortitis should receive a full course of penicillin therapy (Chap. 177).

As in patients with aortic stenosis, the most critical decision in patients with aortic regurgitation concerns the advisability and proper timing of surgical treatment. Total replacement of the aortic valve with a suitable prosthesis is generally necessary in patients with rheumatic aortic regurgitation and in many patients with other forms of regurgitation. Rarely, when a leaflet has been perforated during an episode of bacterial endocarditis, or torn from its attachments to the aortic annulus, surgical repair may be possible. When aortic regurgitation is due to aneurysmal dilatation of the annulus and ascending aorta, rather than to primary valvular involvement, it may be possible to reduce the regurgitation by narrowing the annulus or by excising a portion of the aorta without operating on the aortic valve itself. More frequently, however, regurgitation can be eliminated only by replacing the aortic valve, excising the aneurysm responsible for the regurgitation, and replacing the latter with a graft. This formidable procedure probably entails a higher risk than aortic valve replacement alone, since the diseased, dilated aortic wall, particularly in the presence of cystic medionecrosis, will not hold sutures well.

As in patients with aortic stenosis, the risks of aortic valve replacement are largely dependent on the stage of the disease. Surgical treatment should be considered in patients who have free aortic regurgitation and who are symptomatic when engaged in ordinary activity in spite of maximal medical therapy. It is likely, however, that further reductions of the operative mortality rate and increased confidence in the long-term effects of valvular prostheses will make it possible in the future to recommend operative treatment to minimally symptomatic or even asymptomatic patients with severe regurgitation and cardiomegaly.

MITRAL STENOSIS
Pathologic Physiology

In normal adults the mitral valve orifice is approximately 4 sq cm. In the presence of significant obstruction, i.e., when the orifice is less than one-half of normal, blood can flow from the left atrium to the left ventricle only if propelled by an abnormally elevated left atrioventricular pressure gradient; such a gradient is the hemodynamic hallmark of mitral stenosis. When the mitral valve opening is reduced to 1 sq cm, a left atrial pressure of approximately 25 mm Hg is required to maintain a normal cardiac output. The elevated left atrial pressure in turn raises pulmonary venous and capillary pressures, resulting in exertional dyspnea. The first bouts of dyspnea are usually precipitated by situations associated with an increased rate of blood flow across the mitral orifice, which results in further elevation of the left atrial pressure. In order to assess the severity of obstruction, it is essential to measure the transvalvular pressure gradient and flow rate. The latter is dependent not only on the cardiac output but on the heart rate as well. An increase in heart rate shortens diastole proportionately more than systole, and diminishes the time available for flow across the mitral valve. Therefore, at any given level of cardiac output tachycardia augments the transvalvular gradient and elevates left atrial pressure.

The left ventricular diastolic pressure is normal in pure mitral stenosis; coexisting mitral regurgitation, aortic valve disease, rheumatic myocarditis, systemic hypertension, or coronary artery disease may be responsible for elevations. In pure mitral stenosis and sinus rhythm the mean left atrial and pulmonary artery wedge pressures are usually elevated and the pressure pulse shows a prominent atrial contraction (a) wave, and a gradual pressure decline after mitral valve opening (y descent). In patients with mild to moderate mitral stenosis without elevation of the pulmonary vascular resistance, the pulmonary arterial pressure may be normal at rest and may rise only with exercise. However, when mitral stenosis is severe and whenever the pulmonary vascular resistance is significantly increased, the pulmonary arterial pressure is elevated when the patient is at rest and in extreme cases exceeds even the systemic arterial pressure. The right ventricular end-diastolic and mean right atrial pressures are frequently elevated in patients whose pulmonary arterial systolic pressure exceeds 50 mm Hg.

Cardiac output varies considerably in patients with mitral stenosis. Thus, the hemodynamic response to a given degree of mitral obstruction may be characterized by a normal cardiac output and a high left atrioventricular pressure gradient or, in patients at the opposite end of the hemodynamic spectrum, by a greatly reduced cardiac output and low transvalvular pressure gradient. In some patients with moderately severe mitral stenosis, the cardiac output is normal at rest and rises normally during exertion; under these circumstances, the high atrioventricular pressure gradient elevates the left atrial and pulmonary capillary pressures, which is responsible for symptoms of pulmonary congestion. In other patients with obstruction of equal severity the cardiac output is normal at rest but rises subnormally during exertion. In patients with severe stenosis, particularly those in whom the pulmonary vascular resistance is strikingly elevated, the cardiac output is subnormal at rest and may fail to rise or even decline during activity.

The clinical and hemodynamic picture of mitral stenosis is dictated largely by the level of the pulmonary artery pressure. Pulmonary hypertension results from (1) the passive backward transmission of the elevated left atrial pressure, (2) arteriolar constriction, which presumably is triggered by left atrial and pulmonary venous hypertension, and (3) organic obliterative changes in the pulmonary vascular bed. The elevation of pulmonary vascular resistance may be considered to be a complication of mitral stenosis; in time it often results in tricuspid and pulmonary incompetence as well as right-sided heart failure. However, the changes in the pulmonary vascular bed may also be considered to exert a protective effect; the elevated precapillary resistance reduces the likelihood of pulmonary congestive symptoms by tending to prevent blood from surging into the pulmonary capillary bed and damming up behind the stenotic mitral valve.

Etiology

Mitral stenosis is generally rheumatic in origin. A history of one or more attacks of acute rheumatic fever can be elicited from approximately two-thirds of adult patients with predominant or pure mitral stenosis. The scarring of the valve leaflets leads to their retraction as active rheumatic endocarditis heals. The mitral commissures fuse, the chordae tendineae fuse and shorten, the valvular tissue becomes rigid, and these changes in turn lead to narrowing of the mitral orifice. Pure or predominant mitral stenosis is the most common chronic valvular abnormality following rheumatic fever, occurring in approximately 40 percent of all patients with rheumatic heart disease. Two-thirds of all patients with mitral stenosis are females. Rarely, mitral stenosis is congenital in origin.

Symptoms

When valvular obstruction is trivial, all the physical signs of mitral stenosis may be present in the absence of any symptoms. However, even in those patients whose mitral orifices are large enough to accommodate a normal blood flow with only mild elevations of left atrial pressure, extreme exertion, excitement, fever, paroxysmal tachycardia, sexual intercourse, pregnancy, and thyrotoxicosis may precipitate elevations of pulmonary capillary pressure and lead to dyspnea. As stenosis progresses the stresses that precipitate dyspnea become less severe and the patient becomes limited in his daily activities. Redistribution of blood from the dependent portions of the body to the lungs, which occurs when the recumbent position is assumed, leads to orthopnea and paroxysmal nocturnal dyspnea. Pulmonary edema develops when there is a sudden increase in flow rate across a markedly narrowed mitral orifice. When moderately severe mitral stenosis has existed for several years, atrial arrhythmias —premature contractions, paroxysmal tachycardia, flutter, and fibrillation—tend to occur with increasing frequency. The rapid ventricular rate associated with untreated atrial fibrillation is frequently responsible for acute exacerbations of dyspnea. The development of permanent atrial fibrillation often marks a turning point in the patient's course and is generally associated with acceleration of the rate at which symptoms progress.

Hemoptysis, a complication which is almost never fatal, results from rupture of pulmonary-bronchial venous connections and occurs most frequently in patients who have elevated left atrial pressures without markedly elevated pulmonary vascular resistances. True hemoptysis must be distinguished from the bloody sputum that occurs with pulmonary edema and pulmonary infarction, two conditions that occur with increased frequency in the presence of mitral stenosis.

When the pulmonary vascular resistance rises or when tricuspid stenosis or regurgitation develops, symptoms secondary to pulmonary congestion often diminish, and the episodes of acute pulmonary edema and hemoptysis become reduced in frequency and severity. Elevation of pulmonary vascular resistance further increases right ventricular systolic pressure, ultimately leading to right ventricular failure, fatigue, weakness, abdominal discomfort due to hepatic congestion, and ankle edema.

Recurrent pulmonary infarctions are an important cause of morbidity and mortality late in the course of mitral stenosis, occurring most frequently in patients with right ventricular failure and markedly elevated pulmonary vascular resistance. Pulmonary infections, i.e., bronchitis, bronchopneumonia, and lobar pneumonia, commonly complicate untreated mitral stenosis.

In addition to the afore-mentioned changes in the pulmonary vascular bed, extensive fibrosis of the alveolar walls and thickening of pulmonary capillary walls occur commonly in mitral stenosis. The vital capacity, total lung capacity, maximal breathing capacity, and oxygen uptake per unit of ventilation tend to be reduced, and the latter fails to rise normally during exertion in patients with severe stenosis. In advanced cases there is uneven distribution of ventilation and later of blood flow, resulting in physiologic right-to-left shunting and enlargement of the physiologic dead space. In other patients, the diffusing capacity during exertion may be lowered as a result of structural changes in the diffusing surface and reduction of the pulmonary capillary blood volume. The reduction of pulmonary compliance that occurs generally correlates directly with the severity of the dyspnea and inversely with the left atrial pressure. In some patients airway resistance is abnormally increased.

All these changes are due, in part, to increased transudation of fluid from the pulmonary capillaries into the alveolar spaces as a consequence of the elevated pulmonary capillary pressure. A combination of the above-mentioned alterations in pulmonary function, particularly the diminution of pulmonary compliance, contributes to the increase of respiratory work and plays an important role in the genesis of dyspnea in mitral stenosis. However, the thickening of the alveolar and capillary walls tends to impede the transudation of fluid into the alveoli and the development of pulmonary edema at times when the pulmonary capillary pressure exceeds the plasma oncotic pressure.

Thrombi may form in the left atria, particularly in the enlarged atrial appendages of patients with mitral stenosis. When these thrombi are discharged, they embolize to the systemic vessels, most commonly the brain, kidneys, spleen, and extremities. This complication occurs much more frequently in patients with atrial fibrillation, in older patients, and in those with a reduced cardiac output. However, it is not particularly more common in patients with extremely severe mitral valve obstruction than in those with only moderate degrees of obstruction of this valve, and systemic embolization may even be the presenting complaint in otherwise asymptomatic patients with mild mitral stenosis. At operation, thrombi are not found more frequently in the left atria of patients with a past history of embolization than in those without this complication, indicating that it is usually the freshly formed clots that break off. Patients who have had one or more systemic emboli are more likely to have further embolic episodes than are patients with stenosis of comparable severity without previous embolization. Rarely, a large pedunculated thrombus or a free-floating clot may suddenly obstruct the stenotic mitral orifice. Such "ball valve" thrombi produce syncope, angina, and changing auscultatory signs with alterations in position.

Physical Findings

Peripheral and facial cyanosis occur commonly in patients with extremely severe mitral stenosis. In advanced cases there is a malar flush and the facies appear pinched and blue. Inspection of the jugular venous pulse reveals prominent *a* waves due to vigorous right atrial systole in patients with sinus rhythm who have severe associated pulmonary hypertension or tricuspid stenosis. When atrial fibrillation is present the jugular pulse reveals only a single expansion during systole (*c-v* wave). The systemic arterial pressure is usually normal or slightly low. Examination of the heart generally reveals a right ventricular tap along the left sternal border, signifying an enlarged right ventricle, and pulmonary hypertension. In patients with associated pulmonary hypertension, the impact of pulmonary valve closure can usually be felt in the second and third left intercostal spaces just to the left of the sternum; the left ventricle is not palpable in severe, pure mitral stenosis. A diastolic thrill may frequently be felt at the cardiac apex, particularly if the patient is turned into the left lateral recumbent position. The apex cardiogram (Chap. 261), i.e., a recording of the movement of the cardiac apex, reveals a slow rate of left ventricular filling during early diastole; when a rapid left ventricular filling phase is present, either mitral stenosis is very mild or there is associated mitral or aortic regurgitation.

On auscultation, the first heart sound is generally accentuated and snapping, and since the mitral valve cannot close until the left ventricular pressure reaches the level of the elevated left atrial pressure, it is often slightly delayed, particularly in patients with severe stenosis. In patients with pulmonary hypertension the pulmonary component of the second heart sound is often accentuated, and the two components of the second heart sound may be closely split. A pulmonary systolic ejection click is heard commonly in patients with severe pulmonary hypertension and extensive dilatation of the pulmonary artery. The opening snap of the mitral valve is most readily audible in expiration at, or just medial to, the cardiac apex but may also be easily heard along the left sternal edge or at the base of the heart. This sound generally follows the sound of aortic valve closure by 0.06 to 0.12 sec, and occurs after the pulmonic valve closure sound. Since the opening snap of the mitral valve occurs at the instant at which the left ventricular pressure falls below the left atrial pressure, the time interval between aortic closure and the opening snap will tend to be short, i.e., 0.06 to 0.08 sec, in patients with moderate or severe obstruction.

The opening snap usually ushers in a low-pitched, rumbling, diastolic murmur, heard best at the apex with the patient in the left lateral recumbent position, and often accentuated by exercise carried out just before auscultation. In general, the duration of this murmur correlates with the severity of the stenosis. In patients with sinus rhythm the murmur may reappear or become reaccentuated during atrial systole, as atrial contraction reelevates the rate of blood flow across the narrowed orifice. Soft (grade I or II/VI) systolic murmurs are commonly heard at the apex or along the left sternal border in patients with mitral stenosis and do not necessarily signify the presence of mitral regurgitation. Hepatomegaly, ankle edema, ascites, and the physical finding of pleural effusion, particularly in the right pleural cavity, may occur in patients with mitral stenosis and right ventricular failure.

ASSOCIATED LESIONS. When severe pulmonary hypertension is present, a loud pansystolic murmur produced by functional tricuspid regurgitation may be audible along the left sternal border. This murmur is often accentuated by inspiration, diminishes during forced expiration or during performance of the Valsalva maneuver, may disappear as compensation is restored, and should not be confused with the apical pansystolic murmur of mitral regurgitation. This distinction is of considerable clinical importance, since surgical management may be quite different if mitral regurgitation is present.

Once the diagnosis of mitral stenosis is established, the recognition of associated mitral regurgitation is of considerable clinical importance. A presystolic murmur and an accentuated first heart sound may be taken as evidence against the presence of serious associated mitral regurgitation; when the first sound and/or the opening snap are soft or absent in a patient with mitral valve disease, it is likely that significant mitral regurgitation and/or serious calcification of the deformed mitral valve leaflets are present. A third heart sound at the apex often signifies that the degree of associated mitral regurgitation is more than trivial. This sound is generally duller and lower pitched and follows the opening snap. Occasionally, in patients with pure mitral stenosis, physical signs may falsely suggest the presence of mitral regurgitation. Thus, in the presence of severe pulmonary hypertension and right ventricular failure, a third heart sound may originate from the right ventricle and be audible along the left sternal border. In such patients the enlarged right ventricle may rotate the heart in a clockwise

direction and form the cardiac apex, giving the examiner the erroneous impression of left ventricular enlargement. Under these circumstances the rumbling diastolic murmur and the other auscultatory features of mitral stenosis becomes less prominent or may even disappear. When severe congestive heart failure exists in a patient with calcific mitral stenosis, none of the auscultatory findings typical of severe mitral stenosis may be detectable, but they may become apparent as compensation is restored. Associated tricuspid stenosis also tends to obscure many of the physical signs of mitral stenosis.

The Graham Steell murmur of pulmonary regurgitation, a high-pitched, diastolic, decrescendo blowing murmur along the left sternal border, results from dilatation of the pulmonary valve ring and occurs in patients with mitral valve disease and serious pulmonary hypertension. This murmur may be indistinguishable from the more common murmur produced by mild aortic regurgitation except that it is rarely audible at the second right intercostal space, and may disappear following successful surgical treatment of the mitral stenosis.

ELECTROCARDIOGRAM. The QRS complex may be normal, even in patients with critical mitral stenosis. However, with severe pulmonary hypertension, right axis deviation and right ventricular hypertrophy (Chap. 260) in patients with mitral stenosis generally indicate that an additional lesion that places a burden on the left ventricle, such as mitral regurgitation, aortic valve disease, or hypertension, is present. In mitral stenosis and sinus rhythm the P wave usually suggests left atrial enlargement (Chap. 260). It may become tall and more peaked in lead II and upright in V_1 when severe pulmonary hypertension or tricuspid stenosis complicates mitral stenosis and right atrial enlargement occurs. When atrial fibrillation is present in patients with mitral valve disease, the base line shows coarser undulations than when this arrhythmia occurs as a consequence of coronary artery disease.

ROENTGENOGRAPHIC FEATURES. The earliest changes are straightening of the left border of the cardiac silhouette, prominence of the main pulmonary arteries, dilatation of the upper lobe pulmonary veins, and backward displacement of the esophagus by an enlarged left atrium. In patients with mild or moderate stenosis, the overall cardiac size is not grossly enlarged. In severe mitral stenosis, however, all chambers and vessels upstream to the narrowed valve are prominent, including the pulmonary arteries and veins, right ventricle, right atrium, and superior vena cava. Kerley B lines are fine, dense, opaque, horizontal lines which are most prominent in the lower and mid-lung fields and which result from distension of interlobular septums and lymphatics with edema. These lines usually signify a resting mean left atrial pressure of at least 20 mm Hg. As the pulmonary arterial pressure rises, the smaller pulmonary arteries become attenuated, at first in the lower and then in the mid-lung fields. Deposits of hemosiderin occur in the lungs of patients who have had multiple hemoptyses; the hemosiderin-containing macrophages fill the air spaces, and if they become large enough and confluent result in a fine, diffuse nodulation most prominent in the lower lung fields. Ossified nodules are also more common in this region and are produced by true lamellar bone, which tends to develop in areas of interstitial pulmonary edema.

Differential Diagnosis

A number of cardiac and noncardiac conditions may be confused with mitral stenosis. Significant mitral regurgitation may be associated with a prominent diastolic murmur at the apex, but this murmur commences slightly later than in patients with stenosis, and there is often clear-cut evidence of left ventricular enlargement on physical examination, roentgenography, and electrocardiography. In addition, a pansystolic murmur of at least grade III/VI intensity as well as a third heart sound, should arouse the suspicion of significant associated regurgitation. Similarly, the apical middiastolic murmur associated with aortic regurgitation (Austin Flint murmur) may be mistaken for mitral stenosis. However, in a patient with aortic regurgitation the absence of an opening snap or of presystolic accentuation if sinus rhythm is present points to the absence of mitral stenosis. Tricuspid stenosis, a valvular lesion that rarely occurs in the absence of mitral valve disease, may mask many of the clinical features of mitral stenosis.

Exertional dyspnea and recurrent pulmonary infections may be falsely ascribed to pulmonary emphysema in patients with both *chronic lung disease* and mitral stenosis. Careful auscultation, however, will generally reveal the characteristic opening snap and rumbling diastolic murmur. Similarly, the hemoptysis that occurs in many otherwise asymptomatic patients with mitral stenosis may be improperly attributed to bronchiectasis or tuberculosis. Actually, the latter condition is uncommon in patients with significant mitral obstruction.

Primary pulmonary hypertension (Chap. 286) results in a number of the clinical and laboratory features of mitral stenosis. It is seen most frequently in young women. However, the opening snap and diastolic rumbling murmur are absent, there is no left atrial enlargement on the electrocardiogram or roentgenogram, and the pulmonary artery wedge and left atrial pressures are normal in primary pulmonary hypertension.

Atrial septal defect (Chap. 268) may also be mistaken for mitral stenosis; in both conditions there is often clinical, electrocardiographic, and roentgenographic evidence of right ventricular enlargement and accentuation of the pulmonary vascularity. The widely split second heart sound of atrial septal defect may be confused with the mitral opening snap, and the diastolic flow murmur across the tricuspid valve considered to be the mitral diastolic murmur. However, the absence of left atrial enlargement on the roentgenogram or electrocardiogram, the absence of Kerley B lines, and demonstration of fixed splitting of the second heart sound all favor atrial septal defect over mitral stenosis.

Cor triatriatum is an unusual congenital malformation that consists of a fibrous ring within the left atrium (Chap. 268). It results in elevation of the pulmonary venous, capillary, and arterial pressures. This lesion can be recognized most readily by means of left atrial angiography.

A *left atrial myxoma* (Chap. 274) may obstruct left atrial emptying, resulting in dyspnea, a diastolic murmur, and hemodynamic changes that resemble those of mitral stenosis. However, patients with left atrial myxoma often demonstrate findings suggestive of a systemic disease, with weight loss, fever, anemia, systemic emboli, elevated erythrocyte sedimentation rate, and increases in the serum gamma-globulin concentration. Usually an opening snap is not audible, there is no clinical evidence of associated aortic valve disease, and the auscultatory findings frequently change with body position. The diagnosis can be established by demonstrating a lobulated filling defect in the left atrium by angiocardiography.

SPECIALIZED TECHNIQUES. Catheterization of the left side of the heart is extremely helpful in deciding whether or not valvulotomy is necessary in patients in whom it is difficult to estimate the severity of obstruction by clinical means alone. Similarly, when this procedure is combined with left ventricular angiocardiography, it is particularly valuable in the detection and estimation of associated mitral regurgitation and in the detection and estimation of coexisting lesions such as aortic stenosis and regurgitation. Left atrial thrombi and tumors may be detected or excluded by angiocardiography, particularly when the contrast medium is injected directly into the left atrium. Catheterization of the left side of the heart is also helpful in the detection of conditions that impair left ventricular function and would thereby contraindicate or reduce the effectiveness of mitral valvulotomy. Detailed physiologic investigations are indicated for most patients who have undergone previous mitral valve operations and who have redeveloped serious symptoms; in such patients clinical assessment is particularly difficult, and the hemodynamic studies allow determination of the hemodynamic severity of the lesion, intelligent planning of the operative procedure when it is indicated, and aid in estimating the risk.

Treatment

In the asymptomatic adolescent with mitral valve disease, penicillin prophylaxis of β-hemolytic streptococcal infections (Chap. 269) and vocational counseling are particularly important; physically strenuous occupations should be avoided so that premature retirement will not be necessary should symptoms develop later. In symptomatic patients considerable improvement can be expected with restriction of sodium intake and maintenance doses of oral diuretics. Digitalis glycosides do not usually benefit patients with pure stenosis and sinus rhythm, but they are necessary for slowing the ventricular rate of patients with atrial fibrillation and for reducing the manifestations of right-sided heart failure in the advanced stages of the disease. Particular attention must be directed to detecting and treating anemia and infections. Hemoptysis is treated by measures designed to diminish pulmonary venous pressure, including bed rest, the sitting position, salt restriction, and diuresis. Anticoagulants are indicated in patients who have had systemic and/or pulmonary embolization.

If atrial fibrillation is of relatively recent origin in a patient whose mitral stenosis is not severe enough to warrent surgical treatment, reversion to sinus rhythm, either by means of electrical countershock (Chap. 267) or quinidine (Chap. 266) is indicated. Conversion to sinus rhythm is rarely helpful in patients with severe mitral stenosis, particularly those in whom the left atrium is especially enlarged or in whom atrial fibrillation has been present for more than one year, since it is frequently impossible to maintain sinus rhythm, and reversion to atrial fibrillation is common.

SURGICAL TREATMENT. Surgery is indicated in the symptomatic patient with pure mitral stenosis whose effective orifice is less than approximately 1.5 sq cm. Unless recurrent systemic embolization has occurred, valvulotomy is not indicated in patients who are entirely asymptomatic, regardless of hemodynamic findings. In uncomplicated cases, the surgical mortality rate should be less than 3 percent, and a comparison of the natural history of patients with serious symptoms treated by valvulotomy with those who did not receive the benefits of surgical therapy has shown considerable improvement following operation. However, there is no evidence that surgical treatment improves the prognosis of patients with slight or no functional impairment. When there is little symptomatic improvement following valvulotomy, it is likely that the procedure was ineffective or that it induced mitral regurgitation. The recurrence of symptoms several years after an excellent clinical and hemodynamic result is usually due to mitral restenosis, but myocardial failure or mitral regurgitation is occasionally responsible.

A closed operation is usually preferable for patients with pure mitral stenosis who have not been operated upon previously, who have no detectable valvular or perivalvular calcification on fluoroscopic examination and in whom there is no suspicion of left atrial thrombosis. Many surgeons have found that transventricular instrumental dilatation of the mitral valve results in more effective relief of stenosis than transatrial finger fracture, and the importance of loosening any existing subvalvular fusion of papillary muscles and chordae tendineae is now generally appreciated. In a number of patients with uncomplicated mitral stenosis, closed valvulotomy may be ineffective or may result in severe regurgitation. For these reasons, the ready availability of an extracorporeal system is helpful. Surgery for patients with extremely severe obstruction, significant associated mitral regurgitation, valvular calcification, left atrial thrombi, or a mitral valve distorted by previous operative manipulation is usually managed most effectively under direct vision, with open heart techniques utilized. Total prosthetic replacement of the valve may have to be carried out in those patients who were severely symptomatic preoperatively and in whom the surgeon does not find it possible to improve valve function significantly. Since the operative mortality rate of prosthetic replacement of the mitral valve is still approximately 10 to 15 percent in most centers, and since there is some uncertainty concerning the fate of prosthetic valves, patients in whom preoperative evaluation suggests the possibility that prosthetic replacement may be required should be operated on only if they are significantly limited and symptomatic on ordinary activity despite optimal medical therapy.

MITRAL REGURGITATION
Pathologic Physiology

The regurgitant mitral orifice may be considered to be in parallel with the aortic orifice, and therefore the resistance to left ventricular emptying is reduced in patients with mitral regurgitation. As a consequence, the left ventricle decompresses itself rapidly into the left atrium early during ejection, and with the marked reduction in left ventricular size there is a rapid decline in left ventricular tension. As a consequence a greater proportion of the contractile activity of the left ventricle is expended in shortening and thus the cardiac output may be maintained at normal levels for many years even in patients with significant regurgitation. Thus, the initial compensation to mitral regurgitation consists of more complete systolic emptying of the left ventricle. However, a progressive increase in left ventricular end-diastolic volume occurs as the severity of the regurgitation increases and the function of the left ventricle deteriorates. The atrial contraction wave in the left atrial pressure pulse (a wave) is not as prominent as it is in mitral stenosis, but the v wave is often much taller, since it is inscribed during ventricular systole, when the left atrium fills from the left ventricle. During early diastole, as the distended left atrium suddenly empties, there is a particularly rapid y descent. The left ventricular end-diastolic pressure is either near the upper limits of normal or somewhat elevated. The effective cardiac output usually declines in seriously symptomatic patients. Although a left atrioventricular pressure gradient persisting throughout diastole signifies the presence of significant associated mitral stenosis, a brief, early diastolic gradient may occur in patients with pure regurgitation as a result of the torrential flow of blood across a normal-sized mitral orifice.

The diagnosis of mitral regurgitation can be established by means of indicator-dilution curves; the prompt appearance of indicator in left atrial blood following its injection into the left ventricle signifies the presence of mitral regurgitation. When the indicator is sampled from a peripheral artery, the curve characteristically ascends rapidly but exhibits a gradual descending limb as indicator is washed back and forth between the left ventricle and left atrium. The regurgitant volume can be measured by determining the difference between the total left ventricular stroke volume estimated angiocardiographically, while simultaneously measuring the effective forward stroke volume by Fick's method. The results of such studies suggest that the regurgitant volume may be of the same magnitude as the effective forward stroke volume or may even exceed it in patients with severe regurgitation. Qualitative, but clinically useful, estimates of the severity of regurgitation may be made by cineangiographic observation of the degree of left atrial opacification following the injection of contrast material into the left ventricle.

Patients with severe mitral regurgitation may be divided into several subgroups, depending on the compliance, i.e., the pressure-volume relationship, of the left atrium and pulmonary venous bed, which appears to be capable of modifying profoundly the clinical and hemodynamic picture. Among patients with severe mitral regurgitation, three major conditions have been identified: (1) *Normal or reduced compliance.* In this group there is little enlargement of the left atrium, but marked elevation of the mean left atrial pressure, particularly of the *v* wave. In many patients in this group severe mitral regurgitation develops acutely, as in those in whom it follows rupture of chordae tendineae, infarction of a papillary muscle, or tear of a mitral leaflet. Marked elevation of pulmonary vascular resistance frequently occurs, presumably as a consequence of the left atrial hypertension, and therefore right-sided heart failure is a common clinical manifestation; sinus rhythm is usually present. (2) *Moderate increase in compliance.* By far the most common group consists of patients whose clinical and hemodynamic features are midway between those in the other two groups; i.e., they exhibit variable degrees of enlargement of the left atrium, associated with significant elevation of the left atrial pressure. (3) *Marked increase in compliance.* At the other end of the spectrum from group 1 are those patients with severe chronic mitral regurgitation, massive enlargement of the left atrium, and normal left atrial pressure. The pulmonary artery pressure and pulmonary vascular resistance are normal or only slightly elevated at rest. Clinically, these patients are usually disabled with fatigue and exhaustion, because of a low cardiac output, while symptoms resulting from pulmonary congestion are less prominent. In this group the mitral regurgitation is long-standing and atrial fibrillation is almost invariably present. The association of a normal left atrial pressure with a markedly enlarged, thin-walled left atrium indicates that this chamber must be far more compliant than normal. Thus, long-standing mitral regurgitation may, in some instances, alter the physical properties of the left atrial wall and thereby displace the atrial pressure-volume curve, allowing a normal pressure to exist in a greatly enlarged left atrium.

Etiology

In the large majority of patients, mitral regurgitation is caused by chronic rheumatic heart disease, but in contrast to mitral stenosis, pure or predominantly rheumatic mitral regurgitation occurs more frequently in males. The rheumatic process produces rigidity, deformity, and retraction of the valve cusps, as well as fusion, shortening, and contraction of the chordae tendineae. Mitral regurgitation may also occur as a congenital anomaly, most commonly as a consequence of a defect of the endocardial cushions; it may follow rupture or ischemic dysfunction of the papillary muscles after myocardial infarction or fibrosis, as well as rupture of chordae tendineae or valvular perforation consequent to bacterial endocarditis. Functional mitral regurgitation may occur with marked left ventricular dilatation of any cause, and idiopathic hypertrophic subaortic stenosis may distort the mitral valve so as to render it regurgitant. Massive calcification of the mitral annulus of unknown cause which occurs most commonly in elderly women can also be responsible for significant mitral regurgitation.

Regardless of etiology, significant mitral regurgitation tends to be a gradually progressive disease, since enlargement of the left atrium places tension on the posterior mitral leaflet, pulling it away from the mitral orifice, thereby aggravating the valvular dysfunction. Similarly, the dilatation of the left ventricle increases the regurgitation, which in turn further enlarges the left atrium and ventricle, resulting in a vicious cycle.

Symptoms

Only a small fraction of patients with rheumatic mitral regurgitation ever experience any reduction of cardiac reserve, but in patients who do become symptomatic, fatigue, exertional dyspnea, orthopnea, and nocturnal dyspnea are prominent complaints. Symptoms resulting from pulmonary congestion tend to be less episodic in nature than in mitral stenosis, since fluctuations of the mean pulmonary capillary pressure are less marked. Indeed, acute paroxysmal pulmonary edema is quite rare in patients with mitral regurgitation. Similarly, hemoptysis and systemic embolism occur far less frequently in mitral regurgitation than in stenosis. On the other hand, fatigability, weakness, exhaustion, weight loss, and even cachexia are more prominent and occur most frequently in patients with marked reduction of cardiac output. Right-sided heart failure, characterized by painful hepatic congestion, ankle edema, distended neck veins, ascites, and evidence of tricuspid regurgitation, is observed commonly in patients with mitral regurgitation who have associated pulmonary vascular disease.

Physical Findings

Although the arterial pressure is usually normal, the arterial pulse is often characterized by a sharp upstroke. The jugular venous pulse shows abnormally prominent *a* waves in patients with sinus rhythm and marked pulmonary hypertension. A systolic thrill is usually palpable at the cardiac apex, the left ventricle is hyperdynamic, and the apex beat is often displaced laterally. When the left atrium is markedly enlarged, it may extend anteriorly, and its expansion may be palpable along the sternal border late during ventricular systole. The combination of the retraction of the left ventricle and expansion of the left atrium during systole may produce a characteristic rocking motion of the chest with each cardiac cycle. A right ventricular tap and the shock of pulmonary valve closure may be palpable in patients with marked pulmonary hypertension.

The first heart sound at the apex is generally absent, soft, or buried in the systolic heart murmur, and an accentuated mitral closure sound is useful in excluding severe regurgitation. A pulmonary ejection sound is audible in patients with associated pulmonary hypertension. The splitting of the second heart sound is usually normal, although in patients with severe regurgitation, aortic valve closure may occur early, resulting in wide splitting of the second heart sound. An opening snap indicates associated mitral stenosis but does not exclude predominant regurgitation. A low-pitched, third heart sound, occurring 0.12 to 0.17 sec after the aortic valve closure sound, at the completion of the rapid-filling phase of the left ventricle, and later than the opening snap of the mitral valve, is believed to be caused by the sudden tensing of the papillary muscles, chordae tendineae, and valve leaflets, and is an important auscultatory feature of severe mitral regurgitation. The absence of a third heart sound indicates that if mitral regurgitation exists, it is not severe. The third heart sound may usher in a short, rumbling, diastolic murmur. A presystolic murmur is not ordinarily heard in patients with pure regurgitation and sinus rhythm but is present when there is significant mitral stenosis.

A systolic murmur, grade III/VI in intensity or louder, is the most characteristic auscultatory finding in patients with severe mitral regurgitation. It is usually holosystolic (Chap. 259), but in patients with papillary muscle dysfunction or mild regurgitation of nonrheumatic etiology, it may be confined to late systole and may be ushered in by a midsystolic click. Although the systolic murmur usually radiates into the axilla, in a minority of patients, particularly those with ruptured chordae tendineae or primary involvement of the posterior mitral leaflet, the regurgitant jet strikes the left atrial wall adjacent to the aortic root, and the systolic murmur is referred to the base of the heart and therefore may be confused with the murmur of aortic stenosis. However, the systolic murmur of aortic stenosis usually ends just before aortic valve closure, while that of mitral regurgitation ends with, or immediately after, the aortic closure sound. In patients with ruptured chordae tendineae the systolic murmur may have a cooing or "sea gull" quality.

ELECTROCARDIOGRAM. The electrocardiographic signs of ventricular hypertrophy are variable; in many patients, there is no clear-cut electrocardiographic evidence of enlargement of either ventricle. In severe regurgitation the signs of left ventricular hypertrophy (Chap. 260) are often present, although in many patients associated right ventricular hypertrophy is apparent. Electrocardiographic signs of pure right ventricular hypertrophy occur in patients with severe pulmonary hypertension, and, though unusual in patients with pure mitral regurgitation, they do not exclude this diagnosis. There is electrocardiographic evidence of left atrial enlargement in patients with sinus rhythm, but right atrial hypertrophy may be present when pulmonary hypertension is extreme. Prolonged, severe mitral regurgitation with marked left atrial enlargement is generally associated with atrial fibrillation.

ROENTGENOGRAPHIC FEATURES. The left ventricle and left atrium are the dominant chambers; the latter may be enlarged to aneurysmal proportions and form the right border of the cardiac silhouette. Though both mitral stenosis and regurgitation tend to increase left atrial size, extreme left atrial enlargement usually signifies that regurgitation is the predominant lesion and has existed for many years. On fluoroscopic examination the left ventricle is hyperdynamic and the left atrium exhibits vigorous systolic expansions. Marked calcification of the mitral leaflets occurs commonly in patients with combined severe regurgitation and stenosis but is uncommon in patients with pure regurgitation.

Treatment

The nonsurgical management of mitral regurgitation is directed towards restricting those physical activities which regularly produce extreme fatigue and dyspnea, reducing sodium intake, and enhancing sodium excretion with the appropriate use of diuretics (Chap. 264). Digitalis glycosides (Chap. 266) play a more important role in the treatment of mitral regurgitation than in treatment of mitral stenosis, since these drugs augment the output of the overburdened left ventricle even in the presence of sinus rhythm. The same considerations as in patients with mitral stenosis apply to the reversion of atrial fibrillation to sinus rhythm. In the late stages of the disease, anticoagulants and leg binders are used to diminish the likelihood of venous thrombi and pulmonary emboli.

Although nonrheumatic mitral regurgitation can sometimes be treated by direct surgical repair of the defective valve or by constriction of the widened annulus, effective surgical treatment of rheumatic mitral regurgitation generally requires total valvular replacement with a suitable prosthesis. The mortality rate of this procedure usually ranges from 10 to 15 percent, depending on the level of compensation and the patient's general condition. Though most patients who survive operation appear to be greatly improved, some degree of myocardial dysfunction may persist. The development of thrombi around the prosthesis, which may block the valvular orifice or result in systemic embolization, may be a serious hazard, both in the early and the late postoperative periods. The likelihood of this complication may be reduced by some of the newer valves.

When surgical treatment is contemplated, detailed hemodynamic investigations and selective left ventricular angiocardiography are indicated. These studies are helpful in confirming the presence of severe regurgitation, and they aid in the identification of patients with primary myocardial disease and relatively mild, functional mitral regurgitation, who usually do not benefit from operation. Hemodynamic studies are also helpful in detecting and assessing the severity of associated valve lesions, which may have to be dealt with at the time of operation or which might limit the patient's ultimate improvement if they are left untreated.

In the selection of patients for surgical treatment, the chronic, often slowly progressive nature of the disease must be balanced against the immediate risks and long-term uncertainties attendant upon valve replacement. Patients with hemodynamically significant mitral regurgitation who are asymptomatic or who are limited only during severe exertion are not considered to be ideal candidates for surgical treatment, since they may live for many years with relatively little deterioration. However, surgical treatment should be considered seriously in patients who are so disabled that they are no longer able to work or carry out normal household activities despite optimal medical management. The risks of valve replacement rise sharply when the patient has developed congestive heart failure which is refractory to medical therapy, or associated severe tricuspid regurgitation. However, conservative management has little to offer these patients, so that operative treatment may be indicated even at these advanced stages of the disease, and occasionally the clinical and hemodynamic improvement following surgical treatment is dramatic. It is likely that both the immediate and long-term results of surgical treatment will improve considerably and will lead to recommendations of operative treatment for selected patients with mitral regurgitation even before they become severely disabled.

TRICUSPID STENOSIS

Tricuspid stenosis, a relatively uncommon valvular lesion, is generally rheumatic in origin. It does not usually occur as an isolated lesion or in patients with pure mitral regurgitation, but most commonly is observed in association with mitral stenosis, and sometimes with combined mitral and aortic stenosis. Hemodynamically significant tricuspid stenosis occurs in 5 to 10 percent of patients with severe mitral valve disease; carcinoid heart disease, fibroelastosis, and endomyocardial fibrosis are rare causes of tricuspid stenosis.

Pathologic Physiology

A diastolic pressure gradient between the right atrium and right ventricle is the hemodynamic hallmark of tricuspid stenosis. This gradient can be recorded most accurately and conveniently with a double-lumen cardiac catheter, by placing the tip into the right ventricle and the opening of the proximal lumen into the right atrium. The pressure gradient is augmented when the transvalvular blood flow increases during inspiration, and it is reduced when flow declines during expiration. A mean diastolic pressure gradient exceeding 5 mm Hg is usually sufficient to elevate the mean right atrial pressure to levels which result in systemic venous congestion and, unless sodium intake has been restricted or diuretics have been given, is associated with ascites and edema. In patients with sinus rhythm, the right atrial *a* wave may be extremely tall and may even approach the level of the right ventricular systolic pressure. The resting cardiac output is usually depressed and fails to rise during exercise. The low cardiac output is responsible for

the normal or only slightly elevated left atrial, pulmonary arterial, and right ventricular systolic pressures despite the presence of even moderately severe mitral stenosis.

Symptoms

Since in patients with rheumatic heart disease mitral stenosis generally precedes the development of tricuspid stenosis, many patients initially have symptoms of pulmonary congestion. Amelioration of the symptoms of pulmonary congestion in a patient with mitral stenosis should raise the possibility that tricuspid stenosis may be developing. Characteristically, patients with hemodynamically significant tricuspid stenosis complain of relatively little dyspnea for the degree of hepatomegaly, ascites, and edema which they present. In some patients tricuspid stenosis may be suspected for the first time when symptoms of right ventricular failure persist after an adequate mitral valvulotomy.

Physical Findings

Severe tricuspid stenosis is associated with marked hepatic congestion, often resulting in cirrhosis, jaundice, serious malnutrition, severe edema, and ascites. The jugular veins are distended, and there may be giant *a* waves in patients with sinus rhythm. The *v* waves are less conspicuous, and since the presence of tricuspid obstruction impedes right atrial emptying during diastole, there is a slow, gentle, almost imperceptible *y* descent. In patients with sinus rhythm there may be prominent presystolic pulsations of the enlarged liver.

The right ventricle and the shock of pulmonary valve closure are usually not easily palpable. Indeed, a giant *a* wave in the jugular venous pulse without palpatory evidence of pulmonary hypertension or right ventricular enlargement suggests the possibility of tricuspid stenosis. The pulmonic closure sound is not accentuated on auscultation, and occasionally an opening snap of the tricuspid valve may be heard or recorded phonocardiographically approximately 0.06 sec after pulmonary valve closure. The diastolic rumbling murmur of tricuspid stenosis has many of the qualities of the mitral diastolic murmur, and since tricuspid stenosis almost always occurs in the presence of mitral stenosis, the less-common valvular lesion may be missed on superficial auscultation. However, the tricuspid murmur is generally most readily audible along the left sternal margin and over the xiphoid process. It is augmented during inspiration, when negative intrathoracic pressure increases the velocity of blood flow across the tricuspid orifice, and it is reduced during expiration and particularly during the Valsalva maneuver, when tricuspid blood flow is reduced. The diastolic murmur is reduced in amplitude laterally, only to intensify or reappear as the mitral murmur at the apex. In patients with sinus rhythm the presystolic component is often louder at the tricuspid than at the mitral area; the tricuspid presystolic murmur commences before the mitral, and it often is of the crescendo-decrescendo type.

ELECTROCARDIOGRAM AND ROENTGENOGRAM. The most striking features are tall, peaked P waves in lead II, as well as prominent, upright P waves in lead V_1. The absence of electrocardiographic evidence of right ventricular hypertrophy in a patient with right-sided heart failure who is believed to have mitral stenosis should suggest the possibility of associated tricuspid valve disease. The chest roentgenograms in patients with combined tricuspid and mitral stenosis show particular prominence of the right atrium and superior vena cava without much enlargement of the pulmonary artery and with less evidence of pulmonary vascular congestion than occurs in patients with pure mitral valve disease.

Treatment

Patients with tricuspid stenosis generally exhibit marked systemic venous congestion; intensive salt restriction, digitalization, and diuretic therapy are required during the preoperative period. Such a prolonged preparatory period may diminish hepatic congestion and thereby improve hepatic function sufficiently so that the risks of operation are diminished. Surgical treatment of the tricuspid valve is not ordinarily indicated at the time of mitral valve surgery in patients with mild tricuspid stenosis. On the other hand, definitive surgical relief of the tricuspid stenosis should be carried out, preferably at the time of mitral valvulotomy, in patients with moderate or severe tricuspid stenosis who have mean diastolic pressure gradients exceeding 5 mm Hg and tricuspid orifices less than 1.5 to 2.0 sq cm. Tricuspid stenosis is almost always accompanied by significant tricuspid regurgitation; simple finger-fracture valvulotomy often does not result in significant hemodynamic improvement, but may merely substitute severe regurgitation for stenosis. However, open operations utilizing cardiopulmonary bypass may permit substantial improvement of tricuspid valve function. If this cannot be accomplished, the tricuspid valve may have to be replaced with a prosthesis.

TRICUSPID REGURGITATION

Tricuspid regurgitation is usually functional and secondary to marked dilatation of the right ventricle and the tricuspid valve ring. Functional tricuspid regurgitation may complicate right ventricular failure of any cause, and is commonly seen in the late stages of heart failure due to rheumatic or congenital heart disease with severe pulmonary hypertension, as well as coronary artery disease or hypertension. Rheumatic fever may also produce organic tricuspid regurgitation, which is associated with tricuspid stenosis in some instances. Less commonly, regurgitation results from congenitally defective tricuspid valves, it occurs with defects of the atrioventricular canal, as well as with Ebstein's malformation of the tricuspid valve. Carcinoid heart disease, endomyocardial fibrosis, bacterial endocarditis, and trauma may also produce tricuspid regurgitation.

The clinical features of tricuspid regurgitation result primarily from systemic venous congestion and reduction of the cardiac output. Functional tricuspid regurgitation usually intensifies the preexisting clinical manifestations of right-sided heart failure. The neck veins are generally distended, with prominent v waves, and marked hepatomegaly, ascites, pleural effusions, edema, systolic pulsations of the liver, and positive hepatojugular reflux are common. There are a prominent right ventricular pulsation along the left parasternal region and a blowing holosystolic murmur along the left sternal margin which is generally intensified during inspiration and reduced during expiration or the Valsalva maneuver. Atrial fibrillation is usually present.

There are no electrocardiographic features characteristic of tricuspid regurgitation; roentgenographic examination reveals enlargement of both the right ventricle and right atrium, and the latter chamber expands during systole. The cardiac output is usually markedly reduced, and the right atrial pressure pulse may exhibit no x descent during early systole, but a prominent c-v wave, with a rapid y descent. The mean right atrial and the right ventricular end-diastolic pressures are often elevated.

Treatment of the underlying cause of heart failure usually reduces the severity of functional tricuspid regurgitation. In patients with mitral valve disease and tricuspid regurgitation due to pulmonary hypertension and massive right ventricular enlargement, effective surgical correction of the mitral valvular abnormality results in lowering of the pulmonary vascular pressures and gradual reduction or disappearance of the tricuspid regurgitations without direct treatment of the tricuspid valve. However, in patients with severe regurgitation secondary to rheumatic involvement of the tricuspid valve, particularly those without severe pulmonary hypertension, surgical treatment of the tricuspid regurgitation—either valve replacement or narrowing of the annulus—should be carried out.

REFERENCES

Braunwald, E.: Mitral Regurgitation; Physiological, Clinical and Surgical Considerations, New Eng. J. Med., 281:425, 1969.

Ellis, L. B.: Recurrent Mitral Stenosis, Mod. Concepts Cardiovasc. Dis., 33:851, 1964.

Morrow, A. G., W. C. Roberts, J. Ross, Jr., R. D. Fisher, D. M. Behrendt, D. T. Mason, and E. Braunwald: Obstruction to Left Ventricular Outflow: Current Concepts of Management and Operative Treatment, Ann. Intern. Med., 69:1255, 1968.

Perloff, J. K., and W. P. Harvey: Clinical Recognition of Tricuspid Stenosis, Circulation, 22:346, 1960.

Segal, J., W. P. Harvey, and C. Hufnagel: A Clinical Study of One Hundred Patients with Severe Aortic Insufficiency, Am. J. Med., 21:200, 1956.

Symposium on Mitral Insufficiency, Progr. Cardiovasc. Dis., 5:119–334, 1962.

Werko, L.: The Dynamics and Consequences of Stenosis or Insufficiency of the Cardiac Valves, in "Handbook of

Physiology," W. F. Hamilton, and P. Dow (Eds.), vol. I, "Circulation," p. 645, Washington, American Physiological Society, 1962.

Wood, P.: An Appreciation of Mitral Stenosis: Parts I and II, Brit. Med. J., 1:1051 and 1113, 1954.

——: Aortic Stenosis, Am. J. Cardiol., 1:553, 1958.

271 ISCHEMIC HEART DISEASE
Richard S. Ross

INTRODUCTION. Ischemic heart disease develops as a consequence of inadequate perfusion of a portion of the myocardium. The designation *ischemic heart disease* is preferred to other widely used terms, such as arteriosclerotic heart disease, coronary heart disease, and coronary artery disease, since it identifies the myocardium as the site of the physiologic deficit. Ischemic heart disease may occur in the absence of symptoms or may present as angina pectoris, myocardial infarction, congestive failure, or sudden death. By far, the most common cause of ischemic heart disease is atherosclerosis of the coronary arteries, but myocardium can be rendered ischemic by other coronary obstructive lesions, such as arteritis or embolism. Myocardial ischemia also may occur as a consequence of altered hemodynamics in the presence of aortic valve disease or in association with hypotension from any cause. Congenital abnormalities of the coronary circulation occasionally can result in myocardial ischemia and may be important in childhood.

Coronary atherosclerosis begins in early life, and advanced lesions have been identified in a significant number of young adult American males killed in battle. The average age of the population of 300 autopsied soldiers was 22.1 years, and 77.3 percent of the hearts showed "some gross evidence" of coronary atherosclerosis. In 3.0 percent of the cases, plaques caused complete occlusion of one or more of the vessels. The rate of progression of the atherosclerotic process is greater in males than in females; diabetes, hypertension, and certain hyperlipoproteinemias (Chaps. 113, 275) accelerate the process and result in the onset of ischemic heart disease at an early age.

Severe coronary atherosclerosis always produces ischemic heart disease, but lesser degrees of arterial involvement may exist without resulting in disease of the myocardium. The location of the atherosclerotic lesion is important in determining whether or not it will result in significant and, hence, clinically evident ischemia. The most important factor in determining whether or not ischemic heart disease develops as a consequence of coronary atherosclerosis is the presence or absence of collateral circulation. Collateral channels connecting one coronary artery with another appear in less than 10 percent of hearts in the absence of occlusive coronary artery disease, but these connections may be demonstrated in almost all hearts with evidence of coronary disease. It seems reasonable to conclude that the potential for the development of collaterals is present in many and possibly all hearts, but that they do not develop sufficiently to be visualized until the stimulus of ischemia is superimposed.

The patient may pass from the phase of asymptomatic coronary artery disease to symptomatic ischemic heart disease in several ways, as illustrated in Fig. 271-1. Angina pectoris and myocardial infarction are at the extremes of the clinical spectrum and represent the most usual clinical pictures. Another common presentation is with sudden death, presumably as a result of an arrhythmia in a patient with no history of either angina or an infarction. An alternate presentation has been referred to as the intermediate syndrome, because it shares features with both myocardial infarction and angina pectoris. Once in the symptomatic phase, the patient may die or recover and return to the asymptomatic stage.

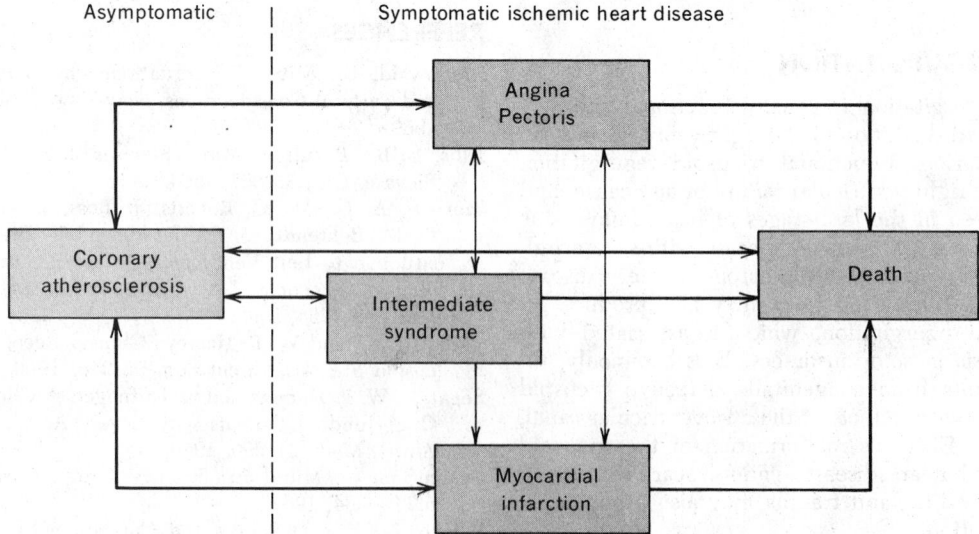

Fig. 271-1. Schematic diagram of natural history of ischemic heart disease.

Movement from one to another of the symptomatic phases, either directly or after passing through an asymptomatic interval, is also possible. The average expected duration of life following entry into the symptomatic phase of ischemic heart disease is the same whether the initial event be the development of angina pectoris or a myocardial infarction from which the patient recovers.

A *coronary artery occlusion* is the most common and easily explained event which precipitates the onset of the symptomatic phase. However, if collaterals are present or become functional rapidly, the patient may remain in the asymptomatic phase. Occlusion of the right coronary artery occurs more commonly without infarction than does occlusion of the left coronary artery.

The pathogenesis of the coronary occlusion remains a matter for debate. Clear pathologic evidence of hemorrhage into the plaque, with consequent elevation of the plaque to fill the lumen of the vessel, is seen sometimes, but this is less common than the occurrence of a thrombus superimposed on an atherosclerotic plaque of long standing.

PHYSIOLOGIC AND BIOCHEMICAL CONSEQUENCES OF ISCHEMIA

The heart depends on an adequate supply of oxygen and metabolic substrate for the generation of the energy for contraction. If blood supply is reduced by a partial obstruction in a major coronary artery, the heart extracts more oxygen from the arterial blood, and the oxygen saturation of coronary venous drainage becomes very low. This compensatory mechanism is of limited value, because under resting conditions, the heart already extracts approximately 75 percent of the oxygen contained in arterial blood, and therefore little additional oxygen is available for extraction under emergency conditions.

The major substrates utilized by the heart are glucose, fatty acids, and lactate. Under normal circumstances, glucose is converted to pyruvate, which enters the Krebs cycle, resulting in the generation of ATP (adenosinetriphosphate) in the presence of oxygen. The energy stored in the form of ATP and other phosphate-containing compounds is utilized in contraction. Lactate is also converted to pyruvate and is oxidized in the Krebs cycle. However, in the absence of oxygen, oxidative phosphorylation of pyruvate through the Krebs cycle is slowed and compensatory metabolic changes take place. The lactate-to-pyruvate reaction slows and may be reversed, so that lactate is produced by the heart. The anaerobic metabolism of glucose through pyruvate to lactate yields energy stores in the form of ATP, but the energy yield from a molecule of glucose is far less than in the case of aerobic metabolism (Chap. 75).

The physiologic counterparts of this biochemical abnormality are a reduction in the contractility of the involved portion of the heart. The ischemic process also alters the electrophysiology of the heart; the most characteristic early changes in the electrocardiogram involve the repolarization process, typified by inversion of T waves and later by displacement of the S-T segment (Chap. 260). S-T segment shifts are seen clinically in association with angina pectoris and also in the early stages of myocardial infarction. A second and important consequence of myocardial ischemia is ventricular irritability, which may result in ventricular premature systoles, ventricular tachycardia, and ventricular fibrillation. Most patients who die suddenly from ischemic heart disease do so from a ventricular arrhythmia, arising from an irritable focus produced by the ischemia.

Structural changes in the mitochondria can be seen by electron microscopy after as little as 15 min of ischemia, and these mitochondrial changes are correlated with the physiologic and biochemical changes. When ischemia is prolonged, the myocardial cells are damaged and the cell membranes become permeable to enzymes which leak into the blood, where their presence may be utilized to confirm the diagnosis of myocardial infarction. Potassium also leaks out of ischemic cells. The failure of the infarcted portion of the myocardium to contract results in a decrease in cardiac output, which may eventuate in either left ventricular failure or shock. Not only does the infarcted area fail to contribute to the contraction of the ventricle, but it may actually decrease the effectiveness of the contraction of the normal muscle by bulging outward while the remaining myocardium is contracting.

ANGINA PECTORIS

Angina pectoris is a clinical syndrome characterized by chest pain which most often is a presenting manifestation of ischemic heart disease but which may occur in other situations characterized by myocardial ischemia, such as aortic valve disease and anemia. Not all patients with ischemic heart disease develop angina pectoris, but when typical angina pectoris does develop the diagnosis of ischemic heart disease can be established with certainty.

DIAGNOSIS. Approximately three-fourths of patients with angina are males; the typical patient is in his late fifties or early sixties and seeks medical advice because of chest discomfort. The patient commonly declines to apply the word pain to his chest symptom, and has difficulty describing the sensation, but will usually select words such as heaviness, pressure, tightness, choking, or squeezing. The typical discomfort is substernal. The most important feature of angina pectoris is its relation to exertion; the discomfort comes on during activity and is relieved by rest. The discomfort may be precipitated by emotion as well as by exertion. Anger, fright, or merely enthusiastic enjoyment of a sporting event may bring on the syndrome. The threshold for the development of angina varies with the time of day more than from day to day. The typical patient may have to stop at exactly the same spot on his way to work each morning, yet by midday he may be able to cover many times that distance without discomfort. Symptoms which develop soon after arising are common, and the patient may not be able to shave without stopping; yet he may perform moderately heavy manual labor later in the day, after he has "gotten warmed up." Precipitation of angina by coitus is common, and inquiry about this may yield information of value in separating angina pectoris from other syndromes which cause similar chest discomfort but do not interrupt or prevent sexual activity.

If the chest discomfort comes on at rest but not with exertion and good exercise tolerance is maintained, the diagnosis of angina pectoris is unlikely but not excluded. In such a case, it is important to determine by direct observation that the patient actually can exercise without distress, because the patient who has true angina at rest may be unaware that he has reduced his activity to subnormal levels and he may therefore not appreciate that symptoms would be precipitated by usual activities.

ANGINA DECUBITUS. One form of angina does come on at rest; the term *angina decubitus* has been applied to this variant because it develops while the patient is in the recumbent position. The classical history is that of angina pectoris on effort which has increased in severity during the few weeks prior to the onset of the nocturnal pain. The patient reports that he is awakened at night by a sensation which is similar if not identical to that which he experiences on exertion. The syndrome of angina decubitus is similar to that of paroxysmal nocturnal dyspnea, and dyspnea actually often accompanies the chest discomfort. It is postulated but not proved that the pathophysiology is also similar and that angina decubitus is a form of left ventricular failure precipitated by the expansion of the intrathoracic blood volume which occurs with recumbency. Elevation of systemic arterial blood pressure has been demonstrated to precede attacks of pain and may be another precipitating factor. Dreaming has also been implicated in the pathogenesis of this relatively unusual variant of angina.

ATYPICAL ANGINA PECTORIS. Variation in the location and character of the discomfort may occur, so that angina pectoris·should not be ruled out just because the location of the pain is atypical, especially if there is a strong relation to exertion. Myocardial ischemia may be characterized by pain in the neck, jaw, throat, or shoulder, with no symptoms in the chest. Radiation to the arms is common in typical angina, and sometimes the only discomfort may be in the arms, where it is often described as a numbness. Sharp pains, especially those of short duration are rarely due to myocardial ischemia, but the words knifelike or cutting are occasionally utilized to describe ischemia.

PHYSICAL EXAMINATION. Physical findings are usually normal in the patient with angina pectoris between episodes, but during an attack of pain certain signs may be present and may be helpful in establishing a diagnosis. The most important of these is the fourth heart sound, which is the auscultatory manifestation of the increased amplitude of the presystolic expansion of the left ventricle. Sometimes this presystolic activity can be felt or even seen. Another manifestation of ischemia is dysfunction of the papillary muscles, which may be manifested as a systolic murmur of mitral regurgitation. For this reason, it is important to inspect, palpate, and auscultate

at the apex of the heart if the patient should happen to develop pain during the examination.

Physical examination is also valuable in detecting evidence of a systemic disease or a metabolic state which predisposes to coronary atherosclerosis. For example, systemic hypertension is a finding of great significance because it accelerates the atherosclerotic process. Xanthelasma and xanthoma may indicate an abnormality of lipid metabolism with which an increased incidence of coronary atherosclerosis may be associated (Chap. 113).

LABORATORY EXAMINATION. The electrocardiogram, especially, may be very helpful in establishing the diagnosis of ischemic heart disease if characteristic changes are present. The absence of abnormalities is, however, far less specific and does not exclude the diagnosis, because the 12-lead electrocardiogram is normal in approximately 50 percent of patients with typical angina pectoris and demonstrable coronary atherosclerosis. The most definite and diagnostic electrocardiographic changes are those of an old myocardial infarction. The characteristic Q-wave changes of a myocardial infarction, especially if they are of the anterior type with changes in leads I, II, or the precordial leads, are almost specific for myocardial infarction. The diagnosis can be made with greater certainty when a previously normal electrocardiogram is present and the appearance of the changes of myocardial infarction can be documented.

T-wave changes are more difficult to interpret as evidence of ischemic heart disease. Inverted T waves may appear as the only manifestation of ischemic heart disease, but they may also occur in other conditions which may be associated with chest pain, such as pericarditis, myocarditis, and abnormalities of vasoregulation.

Great diagnostic significance can be placed upon S-T and T-wave changes which occur during attacks of pain and which disappear thereafter. The most characteristic change is displacement of the S-T segment, with or without T-wave inversion, which is similar in every way to that which is induced during the course of an exercise test. Long-term monitoring with magnetic tape may be useful in documenting the association of ECG changes and chest pain. The S-T segments are usually depressed but rarely may be strikingly elevated, as in the early stages of myocardial infarction.

Stress Testing. This is a keystone in the evaluation of patients with chest pain which may be due to ischemic heart disease. It has a firm basis because it is designed to reveal the basic physiologic defect, i.e., the inability of myocardial blood flow to increase in proportion to the metabolic demands. The coronary circulation may be adequate to supply blood in sufficient quantity to meet resting demands and, hence, prevent ischemia, but the discrepancy between supply and demand is apparent when demand is increased by exercise or when supply is decreased by hypoxia.

Methods for the execution and interpretation of the electrocardiographic stress test vary with respect to exercise load, lead systems, and methods of recording and evaluating the records. The two-step system of exercise developed by Master has the advantage of being well standardized but suffers from the fact that the standard load may not constitute a uniform stress when patients in different states of physical condition are tested. To overcome this objection, the so-called graded exercise test has been developed. The patient is exercised at increasing loads on a treadmill or bicycle ergometer until he develops electrocardiographic signs of ischemia, pain, and fatigue or until his heart rate reaches 80 to 90 percent of the predicted maximum for his age. The graded exercise tests may be criticized on the ground that the work load is not standard, but the limit based on heart rate provides a means of equating the load to the patient's capabilities. The percentage of positive tests in a population of patients with angina is greater with the graded exercise test than with the standard double two-step test. A physician must be in attendance throughout every graded exercise test to observe the patient, to evaluate the in-exercise ECG, and to decide whether the testing should continue.

Approximately 10 percent of patients with positive tests results will have changes only during exercise, and hence, the sensitivity of the test is also improved by monitoring during exercise. Exercise testing is safer with in-exercise monitoring, because S-T segment changes or arrhythmias may develop before pain or other symptoms occur, and the stress can be discontinued before severe ischemia develops. Multiple leads should be recorded, and precordial leads should be included, because one-third of patients with a positive test result will have changes only in one lead; this one lead is most likely to be V_6.

A characteristic positive exercise response is seen in lead V_4 of the postexercise record in Fig. 271-2. The S-T segment is depressed 1.0 mm below the baseline, and this depression lasts for more than 0.08 sec. The depression is of the "square wave" or "plateau" type and is flat or slopes downwards, unlike the S-T segment depression in lead V_4 during exercise, which slopes upwards, is referred to as a junctional change, and does not constitute a positive test result. T-wave abnormalities, arrhythmias, and conduction disturbances may develop with exercise but do not constitute evidence of myocardial ischemia. If 1.0 mm or more of S-T segment depression is required before the test is considered to be positive, the percentage of false positive results will be small (less than 5 percent and only about 15 percent of patients with angina

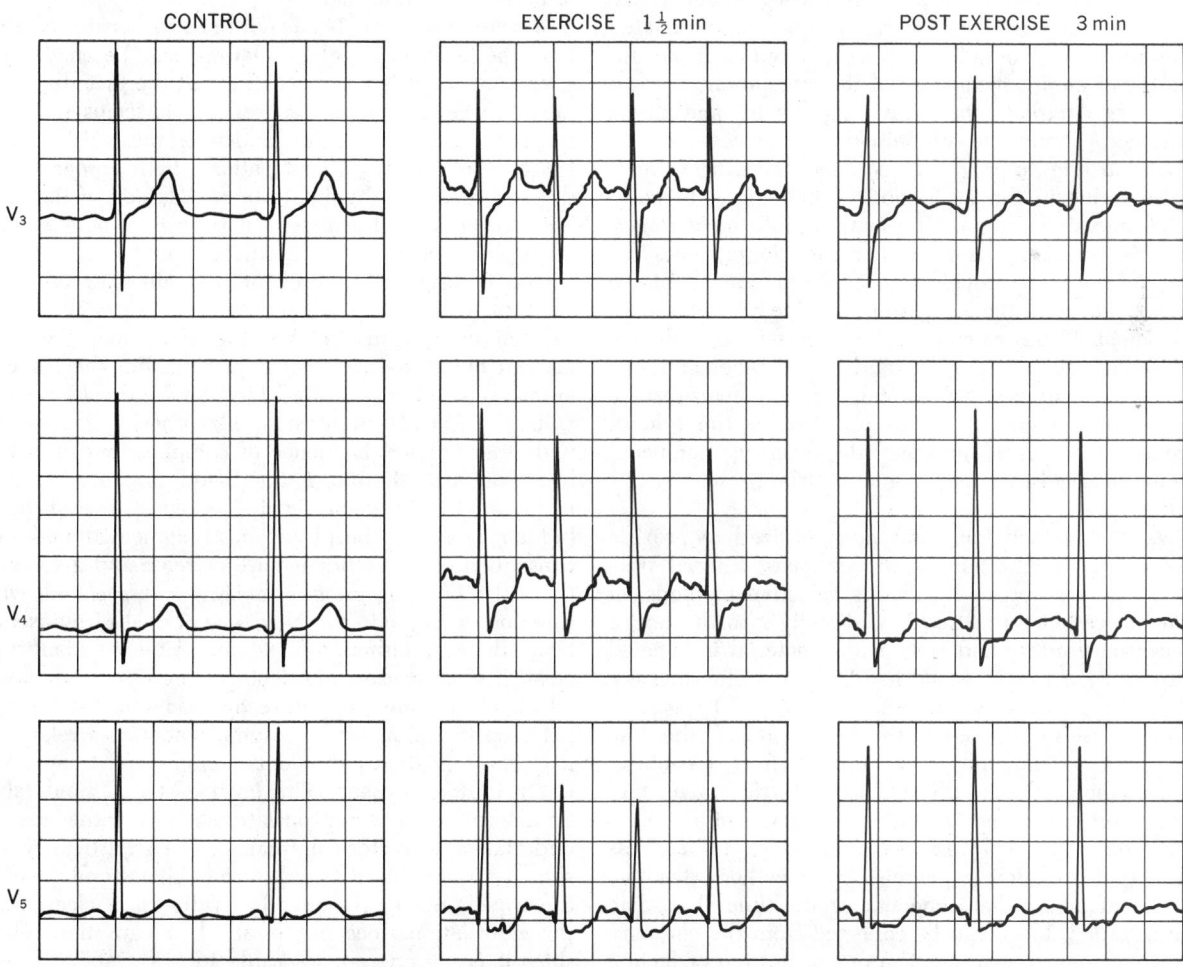

Fig. 271-2. Positive electrocardiographic exercise test. "Square wave" S-T segment displacement in lead V_4 in postexercise record. Changes in V_4 during exercise are junctional.

pectoris due to severe coronary atherosclerosis will have negative tests. If the threshold of positivity is set at 0.5 mm, there will be more false positive tests and fewer false negative ones.

Exercise electrocardiography is still the best generally available test for the detection of myocardial ischemia. The negative tests in patients with severe coronary disease and angina can be explained by the experimental observations which show that electrocardiographic changes may not be the earliest manifestation of ischemia. In other patients with severe disease, pain or fatigue causes termination of exercise before ECG changes appear. If collaterals are adequate, severe coronary atherosclerosis, as indicated by arteriography, may coexist with a negative exercise test result.

A particular form of false positive exercise test may be seen in patients who have a disorder of vasomotor control which has been termed vasoregulatory asthenia. These patients frequently develop S-T segment and T-wave changes resembling those of myocardial ischemia when they assume the erect posture prior to the onset of exercise. During the first minute of exercise, typical positive electrocardiographic changes develop, but as exercise continues they are rapidly replaced by junctional S-T segment depressions. The changes can be eliminated by β-adrenergic blockade, and are attributed to an abnormality of autonomic control of the circulation.

Coronary Arteriography. Providing precise and direct information about the atherosclerotic process in the coronary arteries during life, coronary arteriography is of great value in the evaluation of patients with chest pain of uncertain origin. The anatomy of the coronary arteries is revealed by the coronary arteriogram, but the technique does not provide direct information about the functional status of the myocardium. If the atherosclerotic involvement of the coronary arteries is severe, ischemic heart disease will be present, and at the other extreme, if the coronary arteries are normal, ischemic heart disease will not be present. Problems arise when the atherosclerotic disease is of intermediate severity; significant ischemic heart disease may or may not be present in this situation.

A variety of techniques has been utilized to provide radiographic visualization of the coronary arterial tree. Best results are obtained with the selective methods, in which the catheter is introduced directly into the orifice of a coronary artery and radiopaque material is injected (Chap. 262). In experienced hands these techniques are safe, with a mortality rate of less than 0.1 percent. Additional useful information can be obtained at the time of coronary arteriography. For example, it is possible to advance the catheter through the aortic valve and measure left ventricular pressure. Elevation of left ventricular end-diastolic pressure in response to a stress such as that provided by exercise provides hemodynamic evidence of myocardial ischemia. At the time of cardiac catheterization, blood can be collected from the coronary sinus for chemical analysis. The demonstration of lactate production represents additional evidence of an ischemic myocardium.

MANAGEMENT OF ANGINA PECTORIS. The term *management* is more appropriate than *treatment* with reference to angina pectoris because far more is required than the prescription of a drug or the recommendation of surgery. The patient must be studied with particular reference to the interaction between his disease and life pattern. The physical and emotional stresses which precipitate pain must be identified, and the pleasurable activities prohibited by angina must also be recognized. The first step in management is reassurance. The patient must be made to realize that long useful life is possible even though he has angina pectoris. It is usually not advisable to quote statistics, but the recital of case histories of persons in public life may be of great value. A realistic explanation of the pathophysiology of the disease is worthwhile for the intelligent patient and can be used as the basis for the life plan which is to be described.

The management plan has two parts: (1) general measures directed toward the prevention or progression of ischemic heart disease, and (2) measures to prevent or minimize the attacks of ischemia. The general measures also apply to patients in whom the initial presentation of ischemic heart disease is a myocardial infarction or the intermediate syndrome.

General Measures. It has not been demonstrated clearly that the lesions of atherosclerosis can be made to regress, but there is no question about the fact that certain factors accelerate their progression. It seems reasonable, therefore, to make the reduction of these risk factors a keystone of therapy in all patients with coronary artery disease. Ideal weight should be maintained; if the patient is obese he should reduce, but if he is of normal weight when he comes under medical management, his diet should be adjusted to prevent the gain in weight which so often accompanies advancing years, especially if physical activity is restricted because of angina. The caloric content of the diet is most important, but the content of animal and other saturated fats should also be restricted (Chap. 275). Hypertension, like obesity, is associated with an increased incidence of complications of ischemic heart disease; therefore, the blood pressure should be maintained at normal levels. Smoking should be forbidden, unless in the physician's judgment the emotional consequences of abstinence are extreme and greater than the risks of continuing. Smoking is associated with a threefold increase in the incidence of death from ischemic heart disease; although it is impossible to identify this clearly as a cause-and-effect relationship, the vascular effects of nicotine are well recognized and, hence, it does not seen unreasonable to assume that such a relationship may exist. Diabetes should be sought and treated effectively if it is present. The level of blood lipids should be determined and appropriate dietary or other measures undertaken to restore normalcy. The statistical relationship between an elevated serum cholesterol level and the appearance of ischemic heart disease is clear; though this correlation does not establish a causative relationship, it is considered advisable to bring about a reduction in serum cholesterol whenever possible. This can sometimes be effected by the diet, but if this is ineffective, one of the chemical agents which lowers cholesterol should be employed. The serum lipoprotein pattern should be analyzed; if a hyperlipoproteinemia exists, appropriate treatment, as outlined in Chap. 113, should be carried out. The patient should be encouraged to engage in regular exercise. The maintenance of good physical condition enables him to perform physical work more efficiently at a lower pulse rate and, therefore, reduces the frequency of anginal episodes. It has also been suggested that exercise accelerates the development of collateral circulation in the heart. The patient in good physical condition also has a better chance of surviving a myocardial infarction.

Specific Measures. The basic principle of specific management is to eliminate the discrepancy between the demand of the heart muscle for oxygen and the ability of the coronary circulation to meet this demand. The intelligent patient can be made to understand this fundamental concept and utilize it in the rational programming of activity. He must learn to pace himself so that the rate of performing physical activity is kept below the threshold of discomfort. He must appreciate the variation in tolerance with the time of day and see that the activity requirements are reduced in the morning and immediately after meals. It may be necessary to advise a change in job or residence to avoid physical stress, but with the exception of the manual laborer it is usually possible for the patient to continue to function merely by allowing more time for the completion of each task. Emotional tension is often neglected in the planning of a program for the patient with angina. In some patients, anger and frustration may be the most important precipitating factors in daily life.

The mechanism of action of *nitroglycerin,* the most valuable drug in the treatment of angina pectoris, is complex and is discussed in Chap. 266. The drug is administered sublingually in tablets of 0.4 or 0.6 mg. Patients with angina should be instructed to take the medication to relieve an attack and also in anticipation of stress which is likely to induce angina. When the patient develops pain on exertion, he should cease activity and place a tablet under his tongue. The discomfort generally disappears more rapidly with nitroglycerin than would be expected if the drug were not administered. Patients should be encouraged to anticipate stress which will produce pain and take nitroglycerin prophylactically. A flight of stairs, a walk up a hill, or sexual intercourse may produce pain consistently, but the pain can be prevented by the anticipatory use of nitroglycerin.

The dose of nitroglycerin should be large enough to relieve pain but not large enough to produce a feeling of pulsating fullness in the head or a frank headache, the most common side effect of nitroglycerin, which fortunately only rarely becomes disturbing at doses below those required to relieve angina. If nitroglycerin produces neither relief of pain nor a headache, the preparation is probably inactive.

If the patient does not experience relief after the first dose of nitroglycerin, he may take a second but should be instructed not to continue to take the medication if the first few doses prove unsuccessful. If pain continues despite nitroglycerin, the patient should consult his physician, who can evaluate him for possible myocardial infarction or intermediate syndrome. In the early stages of infarction, the administration of multiple doses of nitroglycerin may be deleterious, because the drug lowers arterial pressure, resulting in a reduction in coronary blood flow, which in turn may lead to an extension of the area of ischemia or infarction.

Unfortunately, none of the long-acting coronary vasodilators is as effective as nitroglycerin in the relief of angina pectoris. However, several of these preparations are useful in prolonging the time interval between attacks and, hence, in reducing the amount of nitroglycerin which has to be taken as therapy for acute attacks. A chewable preparation of erythrityl tetranitrate (Cardilate) combines the advantages of sublingual and oral administration. There is marked variation among patients in the necessary dose of the long-acting vasodilators, just as there is variation in the dose of nitroglycerin required for relief of an acute attack. The dosage of the long-acting vasodilators should be increased gradually until either a therapeutic or a toxic effect is encountered. Nitroglycerin ointment applied to the chest can be utilized as a slow-release preparation which is especially useful in the treatment of angina decubitus. An application of ointment at bedtime may give the patient a night's sleep which had not been possible before.

Cardiac Glycosides and Diuretics. During an attack of angina pectoris, left ventricular function usually becomes impaired and the left ventricular end-diastolic pressure rises, leading in turn to an elevation in pulmonary vascular pressures. Therefore, agents useful in the treatment of congestive heart failure (Chaps. 264 and 266) also may be valuable in the management of angina pectoris. The daily nitroglycerin requirement of a patient with stable angina pectoris, particularly one with cardiac enlargement, will frequently be significantly decreased by treatment with digitalis. The addition of an oral diuretic, such as one of the thiazides, will also prove useful in many patients. These measures are especially valuable in the prevention of attacks of nocturnal angina and of angina at rest, i.e., angina decubitus. When angina pectoris is refractory to the general measures outlined above, digitalis should be tried even though overt congestive failure may be absent.

Beta-Adrenergic Blockade. The most recent addition to the pharmacologic treatment of angina pectoris consists of the β-adrenergic blocking agents, such as propranolol. The effects of β-adrenergic blockade are described best as being the opposite of those of isoproterenol, an agent which stimulates the cardiac beta receptors (Chap. 266). Isoproterenol produces an increase in heart rate, myocardial contractility, cardiac output, and myocardial oxygen consumption, associated with a decrease in total peripheral resistance, while the β-adrenergic blocking agents prevent these changes. The effects of these drugs are most apparent during exercise; there is only a small decrease in cardiac output and heart rate at rest, but beta blockade reduces these variables significantly during exercise. Propranolol is useful in angina pectoris because it reduces the work load associated with exercise, rather than because of any direct effect on the coronary arteries. The combination of a beta blocking agent and a long-acting nitrate has been reported to be very effective. The β-adrenergic blocking agents may have their greatest usefulness in the management of patients in whom emotional and neural influences play a large role in precipitating attacks of pain.

Anticoagulants. There is little evidence that the chronic administration of anticoagulants to patients with angina pectoris is helpful. Anticoagulants are indicated in the management of the intermediate syndrome or preinfarction angina pectoris, as discussed below.

Surgery. A variety of surgical procedures has been advocated for the treatment of angina pectoris. The most direct approach to the problem is coronary endarterectomy, which is most effective in patients whose symptoms can be attributed to a single obstructing lesion in a major coronary artery. Such "ideal" surgical lesions are produced occasionally by syphilis but rarely by atherosclerosis. Coronary atherosclerosis, the most common cause of ischemic heart disease, is diffuse, and multiple lesions are usually present. Nevertheless, good results have followed endarterectomy in isolated cases of coronary atherosclerosis which have been selected carefully on the basis of coronary arteriography.

The revascularization operation, developed originally by Vineberg, is the most popular and most widely performed procedure for ischemic heart disease; it consists of the implantation of a systemic artery into an ischemic area in the myocardium. There are many variations on the basic technique, and the one used depends on which systemic vessel is selected for implantation. A single internal mammary artery may be used, or three vessels may be implanted by utilization of both internal mammary arteries and the gastroepiploic artery. Vineberg also utilizes an omental graft over the surface of the heart to provide an anastomotic distribution network.

Definitive appraisal of the clinical value of this operative procedure is not possible yet, but certain facts are established: (1) A systemic artery implanted into the ventricular myocardium will remain patent in 80 to 90 percent of patients. (2) Vascular channels develop between the implanted systemic artery and the coronary circulation. These channels can be demonstrated by the passage of radiopaque dye injected into the systemic artery. (3) Radioisotope clearance measurements indicate that the implanted vessel contributes to the functional nutritional flow to the myocardium and is not just a shunt between the systemic and coronary circulations. (4) Lactate production by the ischemic myocardium has been eliminated by operation in some patients. (5) The operative mortality rate is low, less than 5 percent. (6) Approximately 80 percent of patients experience a decrease in symptoms following the operative procedure.

On the other hand, the following important questions remain to be answered: (1) Does revascularization prolong the life of patients with ischemic heart disease?

(2) Does it decrease the likelihood of myocardial infarction? (3) Does it increase the exercise tolerance in patients? (4) How long does the period of symptomatic improvement last? (5) What is the extent of the placebo effect?

The relatively high probability of symptomatic improvement and low operative mortality rate justify the use of the revascularization procedure in the management of certain patients with ischemic heart disease. The indications for revascularization surgery will continue to change as experience increases, but certain general principles for selecting patients can be stated. Operation should be considered in all patients who have severe angina pectoris, despite vigorous medical management, which is not improving over a 6- to 12-month period. Operation is contraindicated in the first 6 months after the onset of symptoms, because spontaneous nonoperative revascularization may result in remission.

The arteriographic criteria for surgery have changed with the development of more extensive operations. When only one internal thoracic artery was implanted, operation was advised only when there was significant occlusive disease of the anterior descending coronary artery, with relatively uninvolved circumflex and right coronary arteries. The potential for three vessel implants makes it possible to adopt less-strict criteria because the operation can be tailored to each particular patient. Patients selected for operation should have at least 80 percent obstruction in one of the three major vessels. Ideally, collaterals should be seen entering the ischemic area from neighboring vessels to enable the implanted vessel to make connection with a collateral vascular network already present. Demonstration of myocardial lactate production with stress is another important criterion upon which selection for operation can be based. From the surgical viewpoint, the implants should be made into areas of ischemia, but not into an avascular scar. A preoperative ventricular angiogram may be useful in assuring that the ventricular wall is sufficiently thick to accept the implant.

Other Measures. Mechanical stimulation of the carotid sinuses and, more recently, electrical stimulation of the sinus nerves is effective in the treatment of angina pectoris. This treatment is founded on the physiologic principle that carotid sinus nerve stimulation reduces the heart rate, the arterial pressure, and ventricular contractility, all of which contribute to a decrease in the energy requirements of the heart.

MYOCARDIAL INFARCTION

Austin Flint, Osler, and others were familiar with the pathology of coronary atherosclerosis and coronary occlusion, but the pathologic and clinical features were associated for the first time in 1912 by Herrick.

CLINICAL PRESENTATION. Pain is the most frequent presenting complaint of the patient with myocardial infarction and is usually severe enough to be described as the worst pain the patient has ever experienced. It is a deep visceral pain, and adjectives commonly applied to it are "heavy," "squeezing," and "crushing." It is similar in character to the pain of angina pectoris but is more severe, lasts longer, and is usually relatively constant. The typical pain involves the central portion of the chest and epigastrium and radiates to the arms in about 25 percent of cases. Less-common sites of radiation are the abdomen, back, jaw, and neck. The location of the pain beneath the xiphoid is responsible for the mistaken diagnosis of acute indigestion. The pain is often accompanied by a feeling of weakness, nausea, vomiting, and giddiness. Usually it is not precipitated by exertion or relieved by rest.

Although pain is the most common presenting complaint, it is by no means always present, a minimum of 15 to 20 percent of myocardial infarcts may be painless. The frequency of painless infarcts is probably much higher than this estimate because the patient without pain does not come to the hospital. The incidence of painless infarcts increases with age, and in the elderly, the presenting complaint of a myocardial infarct may be the sudden onset of breathlessness, which may progress to pulmonary edema. Other less-common presentations in the absence of pain include sudden loss of consciousness, a confusional state, the appearance of an arrhythmia, or merely an unexplained drop in arterial blood pressure.

PHYSICAL FINDINGS. In most instances, the dominant feature of the patient's presentation is his reaction to the chest pain. He is typically anxious and may be restless, attempting to relieve the pain by moving about in bed, squirming, stretching, belching, or even inducing vomiting. Pallor is common and is often associated with perspiration and coolness of the extremities. The pulse is rapid except in a few patients who exhibit profound bradycardia with heart rates of 40 or 50 beats per min.

The precordium is usually quiet, and the apical impulse may be difficult or impossible to palpate. An abnormal systolic pulsation in the area between the apex and the left sternal border may be noted in a few patients. On auscultation, the heart sounds are usually of diminished intensity, but may be normal. The most common extra sound is the S_4, or atrial gallop sound, which may be detected in the majority of patients with myocardial infarction. An S_3, or ventricular gallop sound, is far less common. Occasionally, the second heart sound is paradoxically split. An apical systolic murmur of mitral regurgitation secondary to papillary muscle dysfunction is present in more than half of these patients at some time during their course.

LABORATORY DIAGNOSIS. The laboratory tests of value in confirming myocardial infarction may be divided into three groups: (1) nonspecific indexes of tissue necrosis and inflammation, (2) the electrocardiogram, and (3) the serum enzyme changes.

The nonspecific reaction to myocardial injury is associated with leukocytosis, which often reaches levels of 12,000 to 15,000. The leukocytosis appears within a few hours after the onset of the pain and persists for 3 to 7 days. The magnitude of the leukocytosis yields some information about the size of the infarct, the higher white blood cell counts being associated with the larger infarcts.

The second nonspecific change is elevation of the erythrocyte sedimentation rate, which rises more slowly than the white blood cell count, peaks during the first week, and remains elevated for several weeks.

Electrocardiographic Manifestations. The electrophysiologic process within the heart is sensitive to alterations in the perfusion of the myocardium and, hence, the electrocardiogram is of great value in the study of ischemic heart disease (Chap. 260).

Subendocardial Infarction. It is now clear that if the infarct does not involve the entire thickness of the myocardium, the characteristic ECG changes described in Chap. 263 will not occur. If only the subendocardial tissue is involved, there will be no Q waves and the characteristic changes will be S-T segment depresion, in association with tall, peaked T waves. The amplitude of the R waves in the precordial leads may also be decreased. These changes are nonspecific, and the diagnosis of infarction has to be supported by other clinical and laboratory information. Enzyme studies are especially helpful in this situation.

Serum Enzyme Studies. The discovery of increased concentration of serum glutamic oxalacetic transaminase (SGOT) in patients with myocardial infarction ushered in an era of improved accuracy in the diagnosis of the condition. It was learned that certain enzymes present in heart muscle in large quantities are released into the blood when the myocardium is infarcted. The same enzymes are present in tissues other than the heart, and they differ with respect to the rate of liberation following injury. The time course of the serum concentration of the most commonly used enzymes is shown in Fig. 271-3. Levels of two of the enzymes, SGOT and creatinine phosphokinase (CPK), rise and fall rapidly, while that of lactic dehydrogenase (LDH) rises later and stays up longer. SGOT is the most widely used enzyme in the first or rapid group, but it has several disadvantages. In the first place, the levels may have fallen to normal in 3 days and if the first blood sample is not taken until the third day following the infarct, diagnostic changes may not be present. The enzyme is also present in skeletal muscle, liver, and red blood cells and may be liberated from these extra-cardiac stores. CPK has an advantage over SGOT in that it is not present in significant concentrations in red blood cells, the kidney, liver, or lungs, but only in heart, skeletal muscle, and brain. Therefore, it is more specific and sensitive than SGOT, but its rise is also short-lived and may be missed.

In myocardial infarction, the LDH rises during the first day, with a peak at 3 to 4 days, and returns to the normal range in 14 days. There are a number of different LDH enzymes, referred to as isoenzymes, which may be separated by starch gel electrophoresis. Tissues differ with respect to the specific isoenzymes which predominate; the rapidly migrating isoenzyme predominates in heart, kidney, and erythrocyte, while the slowly migrating components predominate in liver and skeletal muscle. The rapidly migrating LDH isoenzyme is, therefore, more specific for myocardial infarction than is the total LDH concentration. The LDH isoenzymes can also be separated

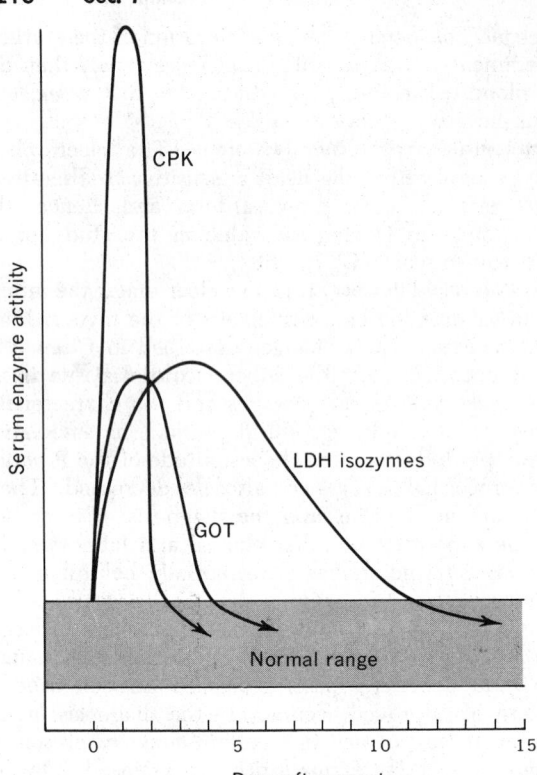

Fig. 271-3. The time course of serum enzyme concentration changes following a typical myocardial infarction. *CPK*, creatinine phosphokinase; *LDH*, lactic dehydrogenase; *GOT*, glutamic-oxaloacetic transaminase.

on the basis of differential heat stability as the rapid or "heart" fraction, which is relatively heat-stable, as compared to the slow or "liver" fraction.

It is the time course of the change which is important in establishing the diagnosis, and it is appropriate to select an "early riser" like SGOT or CPK and another enzyme with a slower time course such as LDH. The specificity of the LDH for the heart can be improved if the rapid or heart isoenzyme is identified by one of several means. The best estimates of the accuracy of enzyme diagnosis are based on the experiences with SGOT. A characteristic rise occurs in more than 95 percent of patients with clinically proved myocardial infarction, and the SGOT generally does not rise in the conditions most often considered as differential diagnostic possibilities in the case of suspected myocardial infarction. Specifically, SGOT does not rise in coronary insufficiency or the intermediate syndrome, rheumatic carditis, or pericarditis. The rise in SGOT which follows pulmonary infarction occurs later and is of a lesser magnitude than that which follows myocardial infarction. The list of conditions other than myocardial infarction which may result in elevated SGOT includes (1) right ventricular failure with hepatic damage due to acute congestion, (2) the administration of salicylates, opiates, or coumarin-type anticoagulants, (3) primary muscle disease, including muscular dystrophy and surgical trauma, (4) cardiac operations, (5) acute pancreatitis, (6) extensive central-nervous-system dam-

age, (7) toxemia of pregnancy, (8) hemolytic crisis, (9) crush injuries or burns, and (10) infarction of kidney, spleen, or intestine.

CLINICAL COURSE. In about two-thirds of patients who reach the hospital the clinical course is relatively benign and the convalescence uncomplicated following myocardial infarction. The pain generally subsides within 24 hr. As it is not possible to predict which patients will follow this benign course, the major goal of management is the early recognition and prompt treatment of arrhythmias, heart failure, and shock.

Arrhythmias. At least 95 percent of patients with myocardial infarction experience some disturbance of rate, rhythm, or conduction; this high frequency has been recognized only since the advent of monitoring in coronary care units. For example, in one series of 100 patients, 56 developed one or more serious arrhythmias, such as frequent ventricular ectopic beats, atrial tachycardia, flutter and fibrillation, nodal rhythm, ventricular tachycardia and fibrillation, and advanced heart block. The mortality rate of this 56 percent of patients with serious arrhythmias was significantly higher than in those who did not develop one of these arrhythmias.

If the patients with ventricular ectopic beats are separated into groups on the basis of frequency, it is clear that the more frequent the ectopic beats, the more serious the prognosis. This difference in prognosis reflects the increased probability of ventricular fibrillation in the patients with frequent ectopic beats. A particularly significant type of ventricular ectopic beat has been designated as exhibiting the "R on T" phenomenon, in which the ectopic beat is superimposed on the T wave of a previous sinus beat. This pattern of ventricular premature beat is especially likely to be followed by ventricular fibrillation.

Ventricular tachycardia and *ventricular fibrillation* are the most serious arrhythmias associated with myocardial infarction. Ventricular tachycardia is most likely to occur on the first day. The duration of the attack is variable; many patients have frequent short bursts of ventricular tachycardia (10 to 25 beats). The high mortality in the group with ventricular tachycardia may be attributed to the frequent association of hemodynamic alterations with ventricular tachycardia, which may initiate a deleterious cycle of hypotension, reduced coronary blood flow, increased myocardial ischemia, more irritability, ventricular fibrillation, and death.

Ventricular fibrillation accounted for approximately one-third of the deaths from myocardial infarction prior to the aggressive treatment of arrhythmias. This arrhythmia is especially likely to develop during the first 2 days but may occur at any time. Normal sinus rhythm is usually present immediately prior to the onset of ventricular fibrillation, but the majority of patients have ventricular ectopic beats or ventricular tachycardia some time before the development of ventricular fibrillation. Ventricular fibrillation is usually fatal, but there are cases reported of transient episodes of ventricular fibrillation which disappear without treatment.

A variety of supraventricular arrhythmias may be encountered, but none of them appears to be associated with a major alteration in prognosis unless it is secondary to seriously impaired myocardial function. Digitalis intoxication should always be suspected when the ectopic rhythm is atrial or nodal in character. The conduction disturbances constitute another important group of arrhythmias associated with myocardial infarction. Complete heart block occurs in less than 10 percent of patients and is more common during the first few days than later in the course. It is also more common in association with posterior than with anterior infarctions. Complete heart block is commonly transient, lasting for a period of a few minutes to several hours.

Killip has emphasized the important interrelations between arrhythmias and hemodynamic states. For example, he notes that potentially life-threatening arrhythmias occur with a frequency of 45 percent in patients *without* shock but the incidence reaches 94 percent in a group *with* shock. Both atrioventricular conduction disturbances and ventricular fibrillation are much more common when shock is present. Shock may be responsible for the development of arrhythmias, which may then result in further deterioration of cardiac performance. In other patients, the opposite sequence of events occurs, i.e., the arrhythmia is responsible for impairment of left ventricular function, with depression of cardiac output and arterial pressure.

Hemodynamics. Arterial pressure is reduced in at least 80 percent of patients after myocardial infarction; the reduction may persist for several days, and in a few patients may not return to previous levels. Shillingford and colleagues have shown that hypotension may exist in two physiologic patterns, depending on the status of the peripheral resistance. Hypotension may be clearly attributable to reduced cardiac output and reduced stroke volume with a normal or increased total peripheral resistance, as in the case illustrated in Fig. 271-4A. When first seen, patients with this hemodynamic pattern usually have cool extremities, a small pulse volume, and clouded sensorium. Other patients with myocardial infarction and hypotension have been found to have reduced peripheral vascular resistance with a normal cardiac output and stroke volume, as in the example in Fig. 27-4B. Patients in this second group with reduced peripheral resistance are found to be clear mentally and to have warm extremities and a full pulse. The clinical distinction between these two groups is often but not always possible.

It is clear that the blood pressure alone is not a good index of the patient's clinical status, that the physiologic alterations associated with hypotension in myocardial infarction are not always identical, and that a rise in blood pressure in response to therapy with pressor drugs does not always reflect clinical improvement. Hypotension may persist for many weeks after a myocardial infarction in patients with previously normal blood pressures, as well as in those with prior hypertension. This change is most often attributed to a reduction in cardiac output, which slowly returns to normal, but reflexes originating in the heart also may be important by producing peripheral vasodilatation.

Profound changes in the lungs and pulmonary circulation may occur following myocardial infarction. The pulmonary artery pressure is elevated in 80 percent of patients with myocardial infarction. Right ventricular end-diastolic pressure is also elevated commonly, and these alterations in hemodynamics of the right side of the heart usually persist for about 1 week following infarction. The pulmonary hypertension is, in all probability, secondary to left-sided heart failure and reflects an elevation of left ventricular end-diastolic pressure. The mortality rate is related to the level of pulmonary artery pressure. Although a reduction of P_aO_2 is common, it is unlikely that this hypoxia is responsible for the pulmonary hypertension. The disordered pulmonary circulation is also evident on radiologic examination of the chest. Pulmonary congestion of some degree is visible on the chest radiograph in almost all patients, even though it may not be detectable on physical examination.

The arterial oxygen tension is reduced during the first week following myocardial infarction in most patients in whom it is measured, and persists at subnormal levels for as long as 2 to 4 weeks. In some patients, this reduction in P_aO_2 lasts longer than does the elevation in pulmonary artery pressure, and is presumably due to the shunting of blood in the lung, i.e., the perfusion of under- or poorly ventilated alveoli.

The role of the autonomic nervous system in myocardial infarction has been under active investigation, and the urinary excretion of catecholamines has been found to be a function of the magnitude of the alteration in the circulatory status.

MANAGEMENT. The first objective of management of the patient with myocardial infarction is to prevent death due to arrhythmia or asystole. These complications can be managed successfully if trained personnel and appropriate equipment are available when the complication develops. The importance of rapid action to put the patient in contact with appropriate personnel and equipment can be easily appreciated by consideration of the time of death in myocardial infarction. Sixty-three percent of male subjects under fifty years of age who died of myocardial infarction, did so within 1 hour of the onset of symptoms; 85 percent died during the first 24 hr; and only 23 percent lived long enough to be examined by a physician. Experience in coronary care units indicates that the mortality rate is highest during the first few hours; therefore, there is a great urgency in bringing the patient into an environment where complications can be treated. The patient can be placed in such a protective environment by admitting him to a coronary care unit in a hospital or by bringing trained personnel and apparatus to the patient. It is possible that this scheme may prove to be the most effective way of reducing early mortality. When the mobile intensive care system comes to the patient, he is placed under observation with ECG monitoring at an earlier stage in the disease, and treatment for arrhythmias, pain, and heart failure can be instituted before the trip to the hospital commences. Furthermore, the trip to the hospital need not be hurried because the patient is already in an intensive care unit where closed-chest mas-

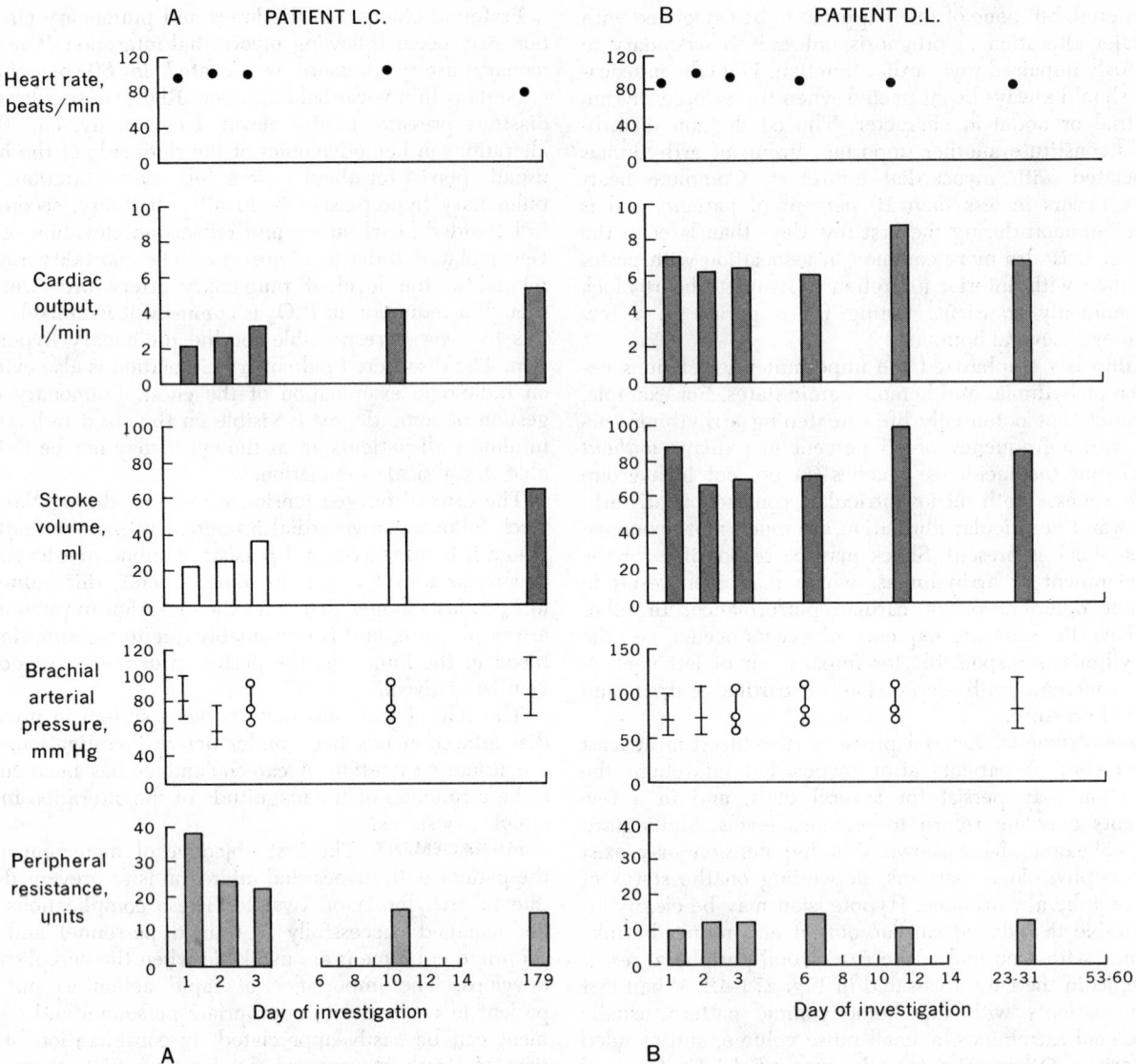

Fig. 271-4. Hemodynamic changes following myocardial infarction. A. Patient with low cardiac output and high peripheral resistance. B. Patient with normal cardiac output and low peripheral resistance. (Reproduced by permission from J. Shillingford.)

sage, defibrillation, and antiarrhythmic drugs can be used as necessary.

Coronary Care Units. The development of coronary care units has resulted in improved care of patients with myocardial infarction, a reduction in mortality rates, and also in a major increase in the body of information about myocardial infarction. The coronary care unit is a specially designed nursing unit, the most important feature of which is a staff of highly trained personnel with authority to take immediate action in emergency situations. The unit should be equipped with systems which permit the continual monitoring of the electrocardiogram of each patient for the first 5 days. Defibrillators, pacemakers, and respirators must also be available, but equipment alone will not make an effective coronary care unit. Of

prime importance is the organization of highly trained personnel with nurses who can recognize arrhythmias, adjust the dosage of antiarrhythmic drugs, and apply electroshock when necessary. A physician should be available at all times but many lives have been saved because the nurse treated ventricular tachycardia with electrical shock before the physician arrived.

The policies and procedures for admission to a coronary care unit should assure that patients are being admitted early in their illness when they may expect to derive maximal benefit from the care provided. Mortality rates for myocardial infarction in coronary care units vary from 12 to 20 percent, and this variation is probably best explained by the delay between the onset of symptoms and the admission to the unit. The earlier patients are brought under observation, the higher will be the incidence of arrhythmias discovered and the higher will be the mortality rate, as a larger fraction of patients subject to the high early mortality characteristic of this disease will be included.

Treatment. **Analgesia.** Myocardial infarction usually announces itself with severe pain, and therefore, one of the important initial therapeutic objectives is the relief of pain. Morphine, the drug traditionally used for the relief of pain, is still the most effective and remains the drug of choice. It may lower arterial pressure; this must be recognized but does not necessarily contraindicate its use. The skin may become cool and moist, and the patient may complain of nausea, but these events usually pass and are replaced by a feeling of well-being associated with the relief of pain. It is likely that the hemodynamic effects of morphine are related to the pooling of blood in the venous circulation, and the improvement which follows elevation of the legs is consistent with this explanation. It is important to recognize this syndrome as one attributable to morphine, because the hypotension and signs of peripheral constriction may be interpreted as manifestations of the shock syndrome and taken as grounds for the initiation of vasoconstrictor or other therapy which would be inappropriate. Meperidine (Demerol) has similar hemodynamic effects. There is great variability in the analgesic and hemodynamic response of patients to morphine. Because of its potential for producing hypotension, it is advisable to select the minimal effective dose for the relief of pain.

Oxygen. The use of oxygen is supported by the observation that the arterial PO_2 is reduced in many patients with myocardial infarction, and inhalation of oxygen increases the PO_2 of the blood and, hence, increases the concentration gradient responsible for the diffusion of oxygen into the ischemic myocardium from adjacent, better-perfused areas. Certain side effects of oxygen administration may be undesirable under some circumstances. Oxygen elevates peripheral resistance and lowers cardiac output, stroke volume, and heart rate slightly. Although it is possible that these effects may be deleterious, the weight of evidence indicates that oxygen should be administered, by tent, face mask, or nasal cannula for the first 4 or 5 days to the majority of patients.

Rest. It has been demonstrated that 6 to 8 weeks are required for the healing which takes place by the replacement of the infarcted myocardium by scar tissue, and the objective of rest is to provide the most favorable possible circumstances for this healing. The development of collateral circulation in and around the area of the infarction is another important and time-consuming part of the healing process. The work of the heart should be maintained at the lowest possible level while this recovery is taking place. It is no longer considered necessary to keep patients at absolute bed rest for 6 weeks, and some authorities advocate allowing the patient to sit in an armchair within 24 hr of admission. A schedule should be developed for each patient to provide as much rest as possible with minimal frustration and anxiety. Muscle tone and general body condition are better maintained

if the patient is mobilized early in his convalescence, and the incidence of thromboembolic complications is thereby reduced.

A schedule for the usual, uncomplicated convalescence is as follows:

Days 1 to 5. The patient should be under constant observation by trained personnel utilizing continual electrocardiographic monitoring. This is usually accomplished most effectively in a coronary care unit. A catheter should be introduced through a needle into an arm or neck vein, advanced into the intrathoracic veins, and kept open by the slow infusion of glucose solution. Antiarrhythmic drugs can be administered via this route, and it can also be used as a means for measuring central venous pressure at frequent intervals if necessary. The catheter can be withdrawn by the third day. The patient should be at complete bed rest, using the bedpan and being fed and bathed by a nurse. Oxygen will be administered continuously during this period. The bed should be equipped with a foot board and the patient should push his feet against the foot board firmly 10 times each hour to prevent venous stasis and thromboembolism, and to maintain the muscle tone in the legs. To help prevent atelectasis, the patient should be instructed to take 10 deep breaths during each hour.

Days 5 to 10. Complete bed rest continues, but some restrictions can be removed and the patient permitted to feed and bathe himself, especially if he feels frustrated by having these tasks performed by the nurse. If management of the bowels becomes a problem during this period, the patient may be permitted to use a bedside commode.

Days 10 to 14. The patient may be allowed to sit on the edge of the bed for increasingly longer periods, starting with 30 min, three times a day and increasing to 1 hr, three times a day, usually during meals.

Days 14 to 21. The patient may sit in a chair for 30 to 60 min, three times a day. It is advisable to check the patient's blood pressure in response to the assumption of the erect posture because he may experience postural hypotension. The tendency to hypotension may persist for 6 to 8 weeks, and it may or may not be symptomatic.

Days 21 to 28. The usual patient is discharged from the hospital during the fourth week. At home he should be confined to one floor but gradually spend more time out of bed.

Days 28 to 42. The patient is up as he desires during the day except for 1 hr in bed in midmorning and midafternoon. He should also spend at least 10 hr in bed at night.

Weeks 6 to 8. Activity is increased as tolerated during this period, and the patient is allowed to climb stairs once a day. He may begin to conduct business for a few hours each day at home.

From 8 weeks onward, the physician must regulate the patient's activity on the basis of his exercise tolerance. It is during this period of increasing activity that the patient may become aware of profound fatigue. Postural hypotension may still be a problem. Most patients will be able to return to work between 12 and 16 weeks.

Diet. During the first 5 days, a liquid diet divided into six small feedings is preferred. Four glasses of sodium-free milk are often sufficient for the first 2 days. Cardiac output increases following ingestion of food and, therefore, the quantity and frequency of feedings should be kept small. During the second week, solid food may be added. At this time, the importance of restriction of calories and saturated fat may be explained to the patient, and he can be started on an appropriate diet. His willingness to accept dietary restriction will never be greater than it is during this early period of convalesence.

Bowels. The enforced bed rest of the first 5 days added to the effect of the narcotics utilized for the relief of pain often leads to constipation; most patients require a laxative, which should be administered prophylactically. Colace in a dose of 300 mg twice daily is usually effective. Alternate regimens are either mineral oil, 30 ml, or Senokot tablets. It must be remembered that straining at stool is highly undesirable because it serves as a vagal stimulant which may produce bradycardia and provoke arrhythmias. The Valsalva maneuver associated with defecation may also lead to the release of pulmonary emboli. The patient should be reassured that it will not be deleterious to go without a bowel movement for several days, but if he is distressed and uncomfortable, he may be permitted to use a bedside commode or to receive a rectal suppository on the fourth or fifth day.

Sedation. Most patients require sedation during the period in the hospital in order to withstand better the period of enforced inactivity. Phenobarbital is utilized most frequently and is usually found to be effective in a dosage of 16 to 32 mg four times a day, but other sedatives and tranquilizers may be substituted. The only problem encountered with phenobarbital is related to its use in patients receiving anticoagulants. The destruction of warfarin-type (dicumarol and coumadin) anticoagulant drugs is increased by phenobarbital, and therefore a larger dose of the anticoagulant drugs is required if phenobarbital is given simultaneously. In patients in whom the anticoagulant dosage is regulated while they are receiving phenobarbital which is subsequently discontinued, the dosage of anticoagulant drug may be too large. It is advisable, therefore, to discontinue the phenobarbital as the patient's activity is increased and to readjust the anticoagulant dosage before discharging the patient from the hospital. A hypnotic should be given at night to ensure adequate sleep. This is especially important during the first few days in the coronary care unit, where the atmosphere of 24-hr vigilance may interfere with the patient's sleep.

It is inadvisable to use morphine or meperidine as sedatives because of their cardiovascular effects. Furthermore, morphine may depress respiration and intensify arterial desaturation. Morphine and meperidine should be reserved for use in the relief of pain.

Anticoagulant and Thrombolytic Therapy. Anticoagulant therapy has been utilized for the treatment of myocardial infarction for more than a quarter century, but unfortunately its efficacy in reducing mortality still remains in doubt because the results of well-designed clinical trials are conflicting. The lack of any statistically clear-cut, valid demonstration of a lower mortality rate suggests that the benefit, if any, of anticoagulant therapy is small. However, there is agreement that anticoagulant therapy decreases the incidence of thromboembolic complications. There is no evidence that anticoagulation is beneficial in any other way in the treatment of infarction. The incidence of myocardial rupture and of mural thrombus formation is not altered either favorably or unfavorably by anticoagulation.

Anticoagulant therapy is not without hazard and should be avoided in patients with a history of bleeding diathesis, bleeding ulcer, severe hypertension (diastolic pressure > 110 mm Hg), or cerebral hemorrhage. The patient must be willing and able to cooperate and, therefore, inadequate intelligence and an uncooperative attitude also constitute contraindications to anticoagulant therapy.

Despite some uncertainties, anticoagulant therapy is utilized in most patients with myocardial infarction. Thromboembolic complications do not appear in the first few days and, therefore, could be prevented by the use of the slower-acting anticoagulants (coumadin, etc.) alone, but many physicians prefer to administer heparin intravenously during the first 3 days. This practice cannot be supported by statistics but is defended on the theoretic grounds that heparin may reverse or at least prevent the extension of the thrombotic process in the coronary arteries.

The potential use of thrombolytic agents in the therapy of acute myocardial infarction is under active investigation. The plasminogen activator, urokinase, present in human urine has been obtained in purified form, utilized in experimental studies, and also tried in patients with thromboembolic vascular disease. Preliminary results are encouraging and it is hoped that urokinase may be useful in the treatment of myocardial infarction.

The administration of "polarizing solutions" containing potassium, glucose, and insulin has been advocated as a means whereby intracellular potassium is repleted in the cells at the margin of the infarct. However, there is no conclusive evidence that either polarizing solutions or oral potassium is of benefit in the treatment of myocardial infarction.

COMPLICATIONS. Arrhythmias—Prevention and Treatment. The improved management of arrhythmias constitutes a most significant advance in the treatment of myocardial infarction. The prevention of the serious and life-threatening arrhythmias depends on the early recognition and aggressive management of their precursors.

Ventricular Premature Systoles. These are the most frequent harbingers of more serious ventricular arrhythmias. Infrequent, sporadic ventricular premature systoles occur in almost all patients and do not require therapy, but prompt treatment is indicated if the premature systoles occur frequently or in certain patterns. In general, more than five isolated ectopic beats per minute is considered an indication for therapy. Similar indications are the occurrence of consecutive or multifocal ventricular extrasystoles. Ectopic beats occurring early in diastole and, hence, superimposed on the previous T wave are also likely to precede ventricular tachycardia and should be treated promptly. Intravenous lidocaine has become the treatment of choice for the precursors of ventricular arrhythmias, because it acts rapidly and its effects disappear soon after its administration is discontinued. Lidocaine is given initially as a single injection of 25 to 50 mg, which usually eliminates the ectopic beats; this initial dose is followed by an intravenous infusion of 1 to 2 mg per min. If the patient is able to take oral medication, he can be maintained on procaine amide (500 mg q. 4 h.) or quinidine (300 mg q. 4 h.).

Ventricular Tachycardia and Ventricular Fibrillation. Sustained ventricular tachycardia is treated first with lidocaine, and if it cannot be terminated by a 50- to 100-mg dose, electroconversion should be employed. Electroshock is used immediately in patients with ventricular fibrillation. If fibrillation has persisted for more than a few seconds, the first shock may be unsuccessful, and in this situation it is advisable to administer closed chest massage and mouth-to-mouth respiration before attempting electroconversion again. The improvement of oxygenation and perfusion increases the likelihood of successful defibrillation.

In considering the efficacy of therapy for ventricular fibrillation, it is useful to divide patients into groups based on the circumstances of origin of the arrhythmia. Primary ventricular fibrillation is defined as that which occurs in a patient without heart failure and/or hypotension. The long-term survival in this group is good; 87 percent of these patients in one series left the hospital alive. This is in sharp contrast to the prognosis in the patients who develop ventricular fibrillation as a complication of preexisting heart failure or hypotension. A far smaller percentage, 29 percent, of patients in this group was discharged from the hospital alive.

Bradycardia. Another important precursor of ventricular tachycardia is bradycardia. Lown found the incidence of ventricular tachycardia in patients with sustained bradycardia to be twice that observed in patients with normal heart rates. Atropine is useful in speeding the heart rate and should be given in adequate doses of 0.5 to 1.2 mg. Isoproterenol, administered in an intravenous infusion, in a concentration of 2 to 12 mg per 500 ml, is also useful in counteracting bradycardia.

Supraventricular Arrhythmias. Although of less potential significance than the ventricular arrhythmias, supraventricular arrhythmias are common and should be treated promptly. The common arrhythmias in this group are nodal rhythm, atrial tachycardia, atrial flutter, and atrial fibrillation. The administration of a short-acting glycoside such as digoxin or ouabain is the treatment of choice. If the abnormal rhythm persists for more than 2 hr with a ventricular rate in excess of 120 beats per min, treatment with electroshock should be utilized. If there is evidence of heart failure or shock, electroshock should be utilized sooner.

Heart Block. This condition can be treated more effectively with a catheter pacemaker which can also be used on a standby or prophylactic basis in patients likely to develop serious conduction disturbances. Transvenous catheter pacing is indicated in patients with complete heart block with an intrinsic rate of 40 beats per min or less. Certain patients with second degree block who have been observed to develop transient episodes of complete block with a slow rate will also benefit from catheter pacing on a regular or standby basis. The introduction of a catheter into the irritable ventricle of a patient in the acute phases of myocardial infarction is not without hazard and, therefore, should be reserved for those with a clear indication.

Asystole. The arrhythmia with the poorest results following treatment is asystole. It usually occurs in patients who have heart failure and/or hypotension. Asystole is treated with closed chest cardiac massage, artificial ventilation, electrical stimulation, and the intravenous administration of bicarbonate, but the salvage rate is not high.

The Shock Syndrome. With the development of effective methods for treating arrhythmias, shock or "power failure" has become the most important fatal complication of myocardial infarction. Shock occurs in about 20 percent of patients with myocardial infarction and accounts for at least 50 percent of the deaths now that the mortality rate due to arrhythmias has been reduced. The mortality rate in myocardial infarction with shock ranges from 85 to 95 percent, but the lack of uniform definition of the syndrome has made it difficult to compare the results obtained by different investigators.

Hypotension alone is not a basis for the diagnosis of the shock syndrome, because many patients who make an uneventful recovery will have hypotension (systolic pressures of 80 mm Hg) for several days. The shock syndrome is considered to be present when hypotension is accompanied by other clinical signs of circulatory inadequacy. The following criteria for the shock syndrome define a population of patients with a mortality rate of greater than 95 percent: (1) systolic arterial blood pressure of less than 80 mm Hg, (2) clinical signs of peripheral circulatory insufficiency; cold, moist skin and cyanosis, (3) dulled sensorium, (4) oliguria with urine flow of less than 30 ml per hr, and (5) failure of improvement following relief of pain and administration of oxygen.

Pathophysiology. The insult to the heart is the cause of the shock syndrome in myocardial infarction, although all organ systems are involved ultimately. The function of the heart is impaired by the initial insult; this results in a decrease in arterial pressure and, hence, in coronary blood flow because of its dependence on aortic perfusion pressure (Fig. 271-5). The reduction in coronary perfusion pressure and myocardial blood flow further impairs myocardial function and may increase the size of the myocardial infarction. Arrhythmias and metabolic acidosis also participate in this deterioration, because they are the result of inadequate perfusion and both tend to perpetuate the precipitating conditions. It is this negative feedback relationship (impaired cardiac function → arterial hypotension → reduced coronary blood flow → impaired cardiac function) which accounts for the high mortality rate associated with the shock syndrome.

Arterial blood pressure is a function of two factors—

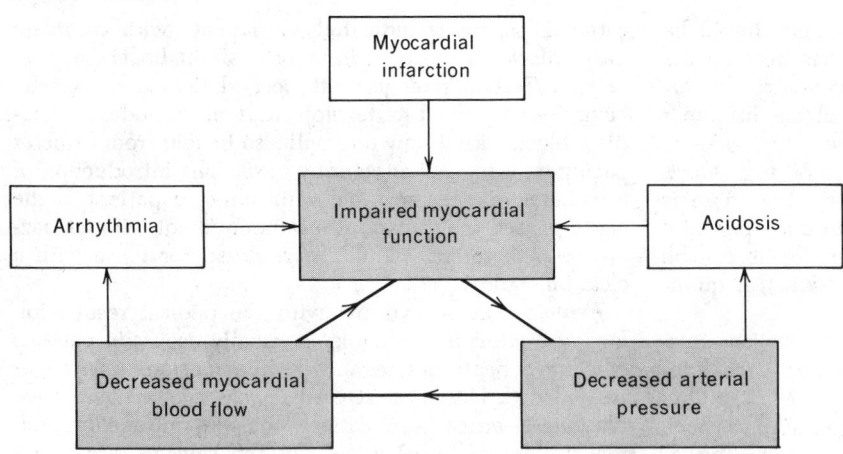

Fig. 271-5. Diagram illustrating the physiologic interrelationships in the shock syndrome following myocardial infarction.

the cardiac output (C.O.) and the peripheral resistance (TPR)—as expressed in the following simple equation:

$$BP = C.O. \times TPR$$

A decrease in either C.O. or TPR will result in a fall in arterial blood pressure and cardiac output is lower in a population of patients with shock than in those who do not have the shock syndrome, but this is by no means the whole explanation. Many patients with myocardial infarction without shock have cardiac outputs in the same range as those measured in patients with shock, and therefore it is not possible to characterize these patients on the basis of changes of cardiac output alone.

Total peripheral resistance, the other factor important in determining blood pressure, may be either normal or increased in myocardial infarction. Here again, a similar range of values for total peripheral resistance may be seen in patients in the absence of shock. Normally, a fall in cardiac output is accompanied by a compensatory rise in total peripheral resistance, but in patients with shock due to myocardial infarction the appropriate response in peripheral resistance fails to occur. It appears that the total peripheral resistance is inadequate to support blood pressure at the existing level of cardiac output.

Derangement of the autonomic control of the circulation appears to be responsible for this combination of circumstances, but the precise mechanism is still under investigation. Experimental work suggests that reflexes originating in the ischemic or infarcted myocardium may interfere with the appropriate vasomotor response. The efferent pathway responsible for the inappropriate vasomotor response to decreased cardiac output appears to be in the sympathetic fibers. An inappropriately slow heart rate in some patients with myocardial infarction and shock is consistent with the concept of impaired neural control of the circulation. In most other situations characterized by hypotension and the shock syndrome, there is tachycardia, but in myocardial infarction, hypotension is often associated with inappropriate bradycardia.

It is necessary to return to the heart itself as the site of the fundamental physiologic alteration in the shock syndrome. It is axiomatic that if the diagnosis of myocardial infarction is correct, there will be a reduction in myocardial contractile function. Moreover, it is fallacious to accept normal systemic venous pressure as evidence that there is no impairment of left ventricular function. Hence, left ventricular function may be impaired in the absence of the usual clinical manifestations of left-sided heart failure, such as pulmonary edema. This relationship is illustrated by a simple schematic diagram depicting the relationship between left ventricular work and filling pressure (Fig. 271-6). The upper curve represents the familiar Frank-Starling relationship in the normal heart; the lower curve shows the relations which might be expected in the patient with shock secondary to myocardial infarction. It is obvious that at all levels of end-diastolic pressure the left ventricular work of the patient with myocardial infarction is depressed. At point B, the end-diastolic pressure is elevated, but at point C, it may be normal, while the myocardial work is well below that expected of the normal heart at this diastolic pressure, as indicated by point A.

Treatment is directed at the interruption of the negative feedback loop (Fig. 271-5), whereby impaired myocardial function leads to a reduction in arterial pressure, decreased coronary blood flow, and a further depression of left ventricular function. This objective is approached by attempting to improve cardiac function and to raise the arterial blood pressure.

Vasopressors. A small increase in arterial pressure may result in a sizable increase in coronary blood flow. Arterial pressure can be increased by the use of vasopressor agents, which may be divided into three groups on the basis of the mechanism and site of action. The first group, which includes norepinephrine (Levophed) and metaraminol (Aramine), acts both on the alpha receptors in the arterial wall and also on the beta receptors in the myocardium. The second group, consisting of methoxamine (Vasoxyl) and phenylephrine (Neo-Synephrine), stimulates only the alpha receptors and does not stimulate myocardial contractility directly. Angiotensin is the only representative of the third group, which acts directly on the smooth muscle of the arterial wall to produce vasoconstriction.

Numerous studies indicate that the agents in group 1 are preferable to those in groups 2 or 3. Although vasoconstriction and elevation of arterial pressure may be associated with the administration of the drugs in groups 2 and 3, cardiac output often falls and clinical improvement does not follow. The practical experience with the treatment of shock in myocardial infarction is consistent with the theory of its pathogenesis which emphasizes the dual nature of the pathophysiology, because drugs which act on both the heart and the peripheral circulation are the most effective.

Norepinephrine should be administered intravenously through an indwelling catheter to avoid risk of extravasation, which results in necrosis of subcutaneous tissue. It is desirable to determine the smallest possible effective dose of norepinephrine by starting with one ampul of 4 mg dissolved in a liter of glucose solution. The infusion rate is set to maintain a systolic pressure around 90 mm Hg, which provides adequate perfusion of the coronary bed. To increase the pressure above this level imposes an unnecessary load on the heart. Should 4 μg per min (1 ml per min) prove inadequate to maintain systolic pressure near 90 mm Hg, the concentration of the infused solution should be increased, but if pressure cannot be maintained with a dosage of 48 μg per min, it is unlikely that a further increase in dosage will be beneficial. Renal blood flow is decreased early in the development of circulatory failure, and therefore urine flow constitutes a sensitive indicator of the rate of perfusion, which can be considered adequate if a urine flow of 0.5 ml per min is maintained.

Prolonged therapy with vasopressor agents has been shown to be deleterious and to lower the circulating plasma volume. Therefore, every effort should be made to use the smallest effective dose for the shortest possible time. Weaning the patient from pressors is often difficult and requires close observation and the exercise of great clinical judgment. The rate of administration must be reduced cautiously. The pressure may fall to 70 mm Hg systolic, but if there are no other clinical signs of circulatory insufficiency, i.e., cyanosis, clouded sensorium, or cold moist extremities, it is wise not to reinstitute therapy. Instead the patient should be observed closely, because the pressure may rise with the passage of time. If, on the other hand, the pressure falls further or clinical signs of circulatory inadequacy appear, therapy must be reinstituted.

Special problems may be encountered with vasopressor therapy in the previously hypertensive patient who has been treated with hypotensive agents such as rauwolfia alkaloids and guanethidine which deplete the stores of catecholamines at the effector sites. The action of the direct-acting vasopressors such as norepinephrine is not compromised, but when an attempt is made to wean the patient from these agents, he may not be able to mobilize endogenous catechols in a normal fashion in response to a falling arterial pressure.

An effective pressor response to norepinephrine may be expected in 77 percent of patients with the shock syndrome, according to a compilation of 258 patients in 17 reported series. In this same group, it was noted that clinical improvement was noted in only 51 percent, documenting the clinical observation that elevation of blood pressure is not always associated with improvement in clinical status.

Isoproterenol is a sympathomimetic amine with a profound inotropic effect (Chap. 266). It increases the vigor of cardiac contraction, but, unlike the action of levarterenol and metaraminol, its effect on the peripheral vascular bed is one of vasodilatation. It also increases heart rate and cardiac automaticity, and these effects may be deleterious. Isoproterenol may be used cautiously for its myocardial effects in selected patients, if its potential undesirable effects are clearly kept in mind.

Cardiac Glycosides. Consideration of the central role of impaired myocardial function in the shock syndrome leads to the conclusion that cardiac glycosides should be administered to all patients with this condition. Obviously, the cardiac glycosides cannot improve the function of necrotic myocardium, but a positive inotropic influence on the noninfarcted myocardium is desirable. It has been demonstrated that the incidence of arrhythmia and cardiac rupture is no higher in patients with myocardial infarction treated with digitalis than in a control group.

General Measures. All patients with the shock syndrome should receive 100 percent oxygen continuously. The addition of dissolved oxygen to the plasma helps to combat the hypoxemia which is universally present. The pressor effect of oxygen may also be desirable. The relief of pain is important, as some vasodepressor reflex activity may be a response to severe pain, but narcotics should be used cautiously in view of their propensity to lower arterial pressure.

Fluid volume replacement has a limited, but definite, place in the therapy of the shock syndrome due to myocardial infarction. It may be indicated in patients who have been receiving pressor drugs for a prolonged period, because pressor therapy results in a decrease in plasma

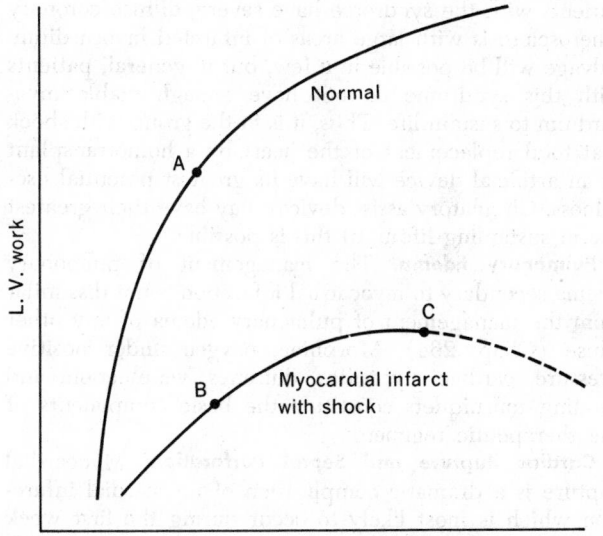

Fig. 271-6. Schematic representation of the Frank-Starling relationship as applied to patients with the shock syndrome in myocardial infarction. (*Reproduced by permission from E. Braunwald.*)

volume secondary to the movement of fluid into extravascular space. If central venous pressure is low and there is no evidence of pulmonary congestion, the blood pressure may be easier to maintain after plasma volume has been expanded by the administration of plasma or salt-poor albumin. Venous pressure should be monitored and the lungs examined frequently during the administration of plasma. Also, fluid replacement is necessary in patients who have lost extracellular fluid volume consequent to vomiting or sweating. Finally, the combination of plasma volume expansion and isoproterenol infusion, even in the absence of hypovolemia, may prove to be effective therapy.

Newer Forms of Therapy. The basic defect in the shock syndrome is impaired myocardial function; therefore, many mechanical assist devices have been developed to supplement the pumping action of the heart. With counterpulsation, a pump is connected to the arterial circulation and programmed to withdraw blood during systole and return it in middiastole, in order to raise mean arterial pressure and facilitate coronary blood flow, while reducing the pressure against which the left ventricle must work. Other systems employ balloons introduced into the aorta and inflated at the appropriate time to retard diastolic runoff and enhance coronary flow. Complete bypass of the left side of the heart by means of an external pump is also available for clinical trial.

A second technique involves use of hyperbaric oxygen therapy. High-pressure chambers have been utilized to deliver 100 percent oxygen at 2 to 3 atm (atmospheres) of pressure, and thus increase the total amount of oxygen carried in each volume of blood. Studies with experimental animals are encouraging, but clinical trials have been disappointing.

There is reason to believe that therapy of the shock syndrome secondary to myocardial infarction will continue to be disappointing because a large fraction of patients with the syndrome have severe, diffuse coronary atherosclerosis with large areas of infarcted myocardium. Salvage will be possible in a few, but in general, patients with this syndrome do not have enough viable myocardium to sustain life. Thus, it is in the group with shock that total replacement of the heart by a homotransplant or an artificial device will have its greatest potential usefulness. Circulatory assist devices may have their greatest use in sustaining life until this is possible.

Pulmonary Edema. The management of pulmonary edema secondary to myocardial infarction is not dissimilar from the management of pulmonary edema of any other cause (Chap. 264). Morphine, oxygen under positive pressure, cardiac glycosides, diuretics, venesection, and rotating tourniquets constitute the basic components of the therapeutic regimen.

Cardiac Rupture and Septal Perforation. Myocardial rupture is a dramatic complication of myocardial infarction which is most likely to occur during the first week after the onset of symptoms. Its frequency increases with the age of the patient, and it apparently is more common in women than in men. The clinical presentation may often be that of a sudden disappearance of the pulse,

blood pressure, and consciousness while the electrocardiogram continues to show sinus rhythm. The electrical activity of the heart continues, and the myocardium continues to contract, but forward flow is not maintained and blood is pumped into the pericardium instead of into the aorta. Cardiac tamponade ensues, and closed chest massage is ineffective in producing forward flow. It is conceivable that prompt recognition and surgical intervention might be effective.

The pathogenesis of perforation of the ventricular system is similar to that of external rupture of the myocardium, but the rate of progression is slower, and, hence, the therapeutic potential is greater. The clinical presentation is one of congestive failure in association with the appearance of a pansystolic murmur typical of a ventricular septal defect. This condition must be differentiated from rupture of a papillary muscle, which may present similarly. The diagnosis can be established by the demonstration of a left-to-right shunt by limited cardiac catheterization; this can be performed at the bedside using a platinum electrode and having the patient inhale hydrogen. Rupture of the ventricular septum is amenable to surgical treatment, which may be lifesaving.

Mitral Regurgitation. Apical systolic murmurs of mitral regurgitation appear in more than half the patients during the first 5 days after the onset of a myocardial infarction, but only in a minority of patients is the mitral regurgitation severe and of hemodynamic importance.

In one-third of patients the murmur is present during the acute phase and disappears with recovery. A characteristic and useful clinical sign of the appearance of mitral regurgitation is the development of P-wave changes in the electrocardiogram suggestive of left atrial overload. The most common cause of mitral regurgitation following myocardial infarction is the infarction of one or both of the papillary muscles in the left ventricle. The posterior papillary muscle is more commonly involved than the anterior, and, hence, the syndrome more commonly accompanies posterior infarction.

Other pathogenic mechanisms may contribute to or be solely responsible for the development of mitral regurgitation after myocardial infarction. Mitral valve competence depends on the normal structure and function of the left ventricle; therefore, mitral regurgitaion may be the result of ventricular dilatation due to impaired contractility or to aneurysm formation. Surgical replacement of the mitral valve may be followed by dramatic results in patients in whom heart failure results primarily from mitral regurgitation due to papillary muscle rupture or dysfunction and in whom myocardial function is maintained relatively well.

Ventricular Asynergy—Ventricular Aneurysm. Cineradiographic techniques have been responsible for the extension of knowledge of the disorders of ventricular function in ischemic heart disease. Gorlin has introduced a new term, *ventricular asynergy*, to describe disorders of ventricular function which occur in 20 to 25 percent of patients with ischemic heart disease and which may be divided into four subgroups: (1) dyskinesis: local expansile paradoxic wall motion; (2) akinesis: local absence of wall motion; (3) asyneresis: geometric distortion of inequality of wall motion; (4) asynchrony: temporal distortion of wall motion. Ventricular function is impaired by all these disorders because the normally functioning myocardial fibers must increase their degree of shortening if stroke volume and cardiac output are to be maintained.

The presence of asynergy was suspected from clinical findings alone in 19 of Gorlin's 24 patients with ischemic heart disease, while cineventriculography was required for diagnosis in the remainder. Apical aneurysms are the most common and the most easily detected by clinical examination. The physical finding of greatest value is a double, diffuse or displaced apical impulse. The standard roentgenogram frequently reveals an abnormal bulge distorting the contour of the heart, but overall enlargement is not common. The electrocardiographic finding of S-T segment elevation at rest was present in precordial leads in 60 percent of patients with either apical or anterior aneurysms.

All Gorlin's patients with ventricular asynergy had severe coronary artery disease, as shown by arteriography, and all probably had experienced myocardial infarction even though there was no history of prior infarction in some. Congestive heart failure was present in one-half of these patients.

Clinical evidence of *thromboembolism* complicates myocardial infarction in approximately 10 percent of cases, but thrombotic lesions are found in 45 percent of patients in necropsy series, suggesting that thromboembolism is often unrecognized clinically. Thromboembolism is considered to be at least an important contributing cause of death in 25 percent of patients. The left ventricle is the most common locus for mural thrombus, and the rarity of mural thrombi in the right ventricle is consistent with the belief that most pulmonary emboli arise in the leg veins. Thromboembolism most commonly occurs in association with large infarcts and in the presence of congestive failure. The high incidence of thromboembolism constitutes one of the best arguments for the use of anticoagulant therapy in myocardial infarction.

INTERMEDIATE SYNDROME— CORONARY INSUFFICIENCY

The manifestations of ischemic heart disease may be thought of as representing a spectrum ranging from angina pectoris at one end to acute myocardial infarction at the other (Fig. 271-1). In the case of angina pectoris, the myocardial blood supply is temporarily inadequate, but there is no death of tissue, as evidenced by the ECG changes of infarction or elevation of the serum enzyme levels. Myocardial infarction is characterized by death of myocardial tissue associated with the typical changes in the ECG and serum enzymes.

Some patients develop manifestations which logically place them at an intermediate position between these two extremes; hence, the designation "intermediate syndrome," which seems preferable to the alternatives of "preinfarction angina" or "acute coronary insufficiency."

The syndrome is characterized by chest pain which is of longer duration than that of angina pectoris and is not relieved by rest or by nitroglycerin. Sometimes there is a history of change in the stable pattern of angina pectoris during the weeks before the bout of severe, prolonged pain with the patient reporting that the pains have become more severe and more frequent and are precipitated by less exertion. The ECG may reveal S-T segment depression identical to that characteristic of a positive exercise test result. Slight elevations or at least abnormal variations in serum enzyme levels are common. It is clear that there is some degree of tissue necrosis in a large percentage of patients with the intermediate syndrome.

It is likely that a new occlusion or possible spasm of coronary artery is responsible for the intermediate syndrome. The collateral circulation is barely adequate to maintain viability during the critical period. If the collateral circulation is able to increase to meet the new demands, infarction will not occur, but if it fails, tissue will die and myocardial infarction will result. Sometimes the issue may hang in the balance for several days. The objective of management of the intermediate syndrome is to prevent myocardial infarction. Rest is probably the keystone of management, and activity should be reduced for from 1 to 3 weeks, depending on the response of symptoms. Anticoagulant therapy is indicated, and intravenous heparin may be given for several days. Nitroglycerin or long-acting coronary vasodilators may be used to relieve pain. The vasodilators such as erythrityl tetranitrate (Cardilate) and isosorbide dinitrite (Isordil) that are absorbed through the mucous membranes are preferable. Treatment must be geared to the specific problem posed by the patient and ranges from that of angina pectoris to that of myocardial infarction with prolonged rest and anticoagulants.

REFERENCES

General Reviews

Blumgart, H. L. (Ed.): "Symposium on Coronary Heart Disease," 2d ed., rev., New York, The American Heart Association, 1968.

Friedberg, C. K. (Ed.): Acute Myocardial Infarction and Coronary Care Units, Progr. Cardiovasc. Dis., 20:450, 1968.

Lown, B., and J. P. Shillingford (Eds.): Symposium on Coronary Care Units, Am. J. Cardiol., 20:449, 1967.

Sievers, J.: Myocardial Infarction—Clinical Features and Outcome in Three Thousand Thirty-six cases, Acta Med. Scandinav., suppl. 406, 1963.

Additional References

Brener, B. J., and R. Warren: Internal-mammary Implantation Operations for Relief of Myocardial Ischemia, New Engl., J. Med., 273:479, 1965.

Gorlin, R., M. D. Klein, and J. M. Sullivan: Prospective Correlative Study of Ventricular Aneurysm. Mechanistic Concept and Clinical Recognition, Am. J. Med., 42:512, 1967.

Heikkila, J.: Mitral Incompetence as a Complication of Acute Myocardial Infarction, Acta Med. Scandinav., suppl. 475, 1967.

Jordan, R. A., R. D. Miller, J. E. Edwards, and R. L. Parker: Thrombo-embolism in Acute and in Healed Myocardial Infarction, Circulation, 6:1, 1952.

Julian, D. G., Valentine, P. A., and G. G. Miller: Disturbances of Rate, Rhythm and Conduction in Acute Myocardial Infarction—A Prospective Study of 100 Consecutive Unselected Patients with the Aid of Electrocardiographic Monitoring, Am. J. Med., 37:915, 1964.

Lown, B., M. D. Klein, and P. I. Hershberg: Coronary and Precoronary Care, Am. J. Med., 46:705, 1969.

Mason, R. E., I. Likar, R. O. Biern, and R. S. Ross: Multiple-lead Exercise Electrocardiography: Experience in 107 Normal Subjects and 67 Patients with Angina Pectoris, and Comparison with Coronary Cinearteriography in 84 Patients, Circulation, 36:517, 1967.

Scheuer, J.: Hemodynamic and Metabolic Correlates of Coronary Insufficiency, Cardiol. Digest, 3:24, 1968.

Seaman, A. J., H. E. Griswold, R. B. Reaume, and L. Ritzmann: Long-term Anticoagulant Prophylaxsis after Myocardial Infarction, J.A.M.A., 281:115, 1969.

272   PERICARDIAL DISEASE

William H. Resnik, Tinsley R. Harrison, and Eugene Braunwald

Pericarditis may be classified according to two different methods, both of practical importance.

CLASSIFICATION

I. Morphologic and clinical classification
  A. Acute pericarditis
    1. Fibrinous
    2. Effusive
  B. Chronic pericardial effusion
  C. Chronic constrictive pericarditis
  D. Chronic adhesive pericarditis
II. Etiologic classification
  A. Infectious pericarditis
    1. Acute benign
    2. Tuberculous
    3. Pyogenic
    4. Mycotic (fungous infection)
    5. Other infections (syphilitic, parasitic)
  B. Noninfectious pericarditis
    1. Ischemic (acute myocardial infarction)
    2. Uremic
    3. Neoplastic
    4. Myxedematous
    5. Traumatic
    6. Anticoagulant therapy
  C. Pericarditis of uncertain etiology (hypersensitivity?)
    1. Rheumatic
    2. Collagen vascular disease
      a. Disseminated lupus erythematosus
      b. Periarteritis nodosa
      c. Rheumatoid arthritis
    3. Post-cardiac-injury syndrome
      a. Post-myocardial-infarction syndrome
      b. Postpericardiotomy (postcommissurotomy) syndrome
      c. Posttraumatic syndrome

ACUTE PERICARDITIS

Pain is an important symptom in various forms of acute pericarditis; it is usually present in the acute infectious types and also in those forms enumerated under "uncertain etiology." Pain is often absent in a slowly developing tuberculous or neoplastic pericarditis, and it is usually absent in the pericarditis of myocardial infarction. Pain rarely constitutes an important complaint in uremic pericarditis, probably because of the stuporous or comatose state of the patient. The character of the pain has been described in a previous chapter (Chap. 11). Any one or combination of the three components of pericardial pain may occur, but *usually* the predominant one is the pleuritic type of pain. Occasionally the steady, constrictive pain, radiating into either arm or both arms and similar to the pain of myocardial ischemia, may overshadow the pleuritic pain, or it may occur alone at the onset of the illness, with the result that confusion with myocardial infarction is not infrequent. This problem becomes even more perplexing when, with acute pericarditis the serum transaminase level rises to about 80 units, occasionally to 125 to 135. Occasionally, shock may appear, but its mechanism is uncertain. Possibly in some instances it may be caused by the same obscure reflexes that play a part in the shock of myocardial infarction; in other cases, it may be brought about by tamponade caused by the rapid development of pericardial fluid, too small in amount to be detected by x-ray. The location of pericardial pain has also been described (Chap. 11). Suffice it to say that a pain felt either in the precordium or in one or both of the shoulders or trapezius ridges and aggravated by inspiration should alert one to the possibility of an acute pericarditis.

The *pericardial friction rub* is the most important physical sign, sometimes elicited only when firm pressure with the stethoscope is applied to the chest wall. The pericardial rub is likely to be inconstant and transitory, and a loud to-and-fro leathery sound may disappear within a few hours, possibly to reappear the following day.

The *electrocardiogram* in acute pericarditis usually displays elevation of the S-T segments in several leads without reciprocal depressions in others and without significant changes in the QRS complexes. Several days later the S-T segments return to normal and the T waves become inverted; in some instances this change is permanent. Atrial arrhythmias are not uncommon.

PERICARDIAL EFFUSION. Usually associated with an enlargement of the cardiac silhouette, pericardial effusion is especially important when it develops within a relatively few days. There is no definitive contour to the cardiac shadow in effusion, and differentiation from enlargement of the heart may be difficult. A very important bedside clue to the presence of effusion is the increase in the area of cardiac flatness (not dullness) on percussion, extending to the lower half of the sternum (where, normally, the percussion note is resonant), and sometimes to the third left interspace, and to the right of the sternum from the third to the sixth interspace. The heart sounds tend to become faint; the friction rub may disappear or remain clearly audible; the apex impulse may vanish but sometimes is felt well within the left border of dullness. On fluoroscopic examination, the ventricular pulsations are usually diminished or absent. When the effusion is large, one often encounters an area of dullness and tubular breath sounds at the angle of the left scapula, probably caused by compression of the lung (Ewart's sign). The importance of this finding comes from the fact that often these signs are misinterpreted as being due to a pneumonic consolidation.

Six laboratory techniques are available for establishing the diagnosis of pericardial effusion: (1) *Cardiac catheterization:* a catheter is introduced into the right atrium and rotated so that its tip makes contact with the lateral right atrial wall. In the presence of an effusion, the tip of the catheter is seen to be separated from the radiolucent lungs by an opaque band. (2) *Angiocardiography:* contrast medium is injected rapidly into the right atrial chamber, and the lateral wall of the atrium is outlined. (3) *Carbon dioxide angiography:* the intravenous injection of carbon dioxide, with the patient in the left lateral position, also provides the contrast between the interior of the right atrium and surrounding structures that makes possible an estimation of the width of the pericardium or of the contents of the pericardial sac. (4) *Ultrasonic cardiography:* recordings of reflected ultrasound disclose two echoes from the posterior wall of the heart, one from the left ventricular wall and the other from the pericardium; the distance between these two echoes is increased in the presence of effusion. (5) *Radioisotope scanning:* following the intravenous injection of a gamma-emitting isotope which remains within the vascular bed, a pool of blood much smaller than the roentgenographic size of the cardiac silhouette may be demonstrated. (6) *Pericardiocentesis:* when examination of tissue or fluid is deemed essential, exploration of the pericardium may be required. This should be accomplished with a needle attached to an electrocardiographic lead. When an effusion develops, the fluid nearly always has the physical characteristics of an exudate. Bloody fluid is commonly due to tuberculosis or tumor, but it may also be found in the effusion of rheumatic fever or in the post-cardiac-injury syndrome (see below). Occasionally, bloody fluid may be found in the effusion of uremic pericarditis and in the hemopericardium following infarction, especially when anticoagulants have been given.

Tamponade

When fluid in the pericardium accumulates in an amount sufficient to cause serious obstruction to the inflow of blood to the ventricles, *tamponade* is said to be present. The amount of fluid necessary to produce this critical state may be as small as 250 to 300 ml, when the fluid develops rapidly; or it may be over 1,000 ml in slowly developing effusions when the pericardium has had the opportunity to stretch and adapt to the increasing volume of fluid. Tamponade is usually due to tuberculosis, pyogenic infection, or tumor, but it may occur in the pericarditis of acute rheumatic fever, acute benign pericarditis, the post-cardiac-injury syndrome, hemopericardium following trauma or that associated with anticoagulant therapy, and rarely in disseminated lupus erythematosus. The clinical manifestations are due to the sudden fall in cardiac output and to systemic venous congestion. Orthopnea, with few or no rales, is prominent; the mechanism of this symptom is not fully understood. The heart rate increases, the blood pressure and pulse pressure decline. Distension of the neck veins and rapid enlargement of the liver occur. The fullness of the neck veins is increased during inspiration (Kussmaul's sign) or when pressure is applied with the palm of the hand over the liver (hepatojugular reflux). This phenomenon is due to the inability of the chambers of the right side of the heart to accommodate the increased inflow of blood from the abdomen and the consequent reflux of blood into the veins already under increased tension. A proto-diastolic gallop sound is usually heard.

PARADOXIC PULSE. An important clue to the presence of pericardial tamponade and of constrictive pericarditis is the *paradoxic pulse*. This phenomenon consists of *a greater than normal inspiratory decrease in arterial pressure. It is often accompanied by an absence of the normal inspiratory fall in venous pressure.* Indeed, there may be an actual inspiratory rise in venous pressure, which is often visible in constrictive pericarditis, but only occasionally in tamponade.

Normally, the inspiratory decline in intrathoracic pressure enhances right ventricular filling by virtue of the increased gradient of pressure between the extrathoracic veins and the right chambers of the heart. Right ventricular output increases, but because of the delay in the transmission of this augmented output within the pulmonary vascular bed and left atrium, left ventricular output does not rise until the following expiration; indeed, left ventricular output normally declines during inspiration, following upon the decrease in right ventricular output during expiration. Thus, normally there is a slight inspiratory diminution in systemic arterial pressure.

A number of mechanisms has been suggested to explain the occurrence of a paradoxic pulse in cardiac tamponade and constrictive pericarditis. (1) The inspiratory increase in venous returns distends the right atrium and right ventricle; since these chambers share a tight incompressible covering with the left side of the heart, the volume of the latter declines reciprocally and left ventricular stroke volume falls more than normal. (2) The fall in intrathoracic pressure that accompanies inspiration is transmitted to the intrathoracic but extrapericardial pulmonary veins, but is not transmitted to the intrapericardial left atrium. Hence, the normal pressure gradient between pulmonary veins and left atrium is reduced during inspiration. This causes a greater than normal drop in left ventricular inflow and output and a corresponding decline in systemic arterial pressure (a difference of more than 10 mm Hg between inspiration and expiration).

(3) The inspiratory descent of the diaphragm stretches the already taut pericardium, causing an increase in pressure within the heart, and so obstructing still further diastolic inflow to the ventricles. On the left side, this leads to a greater than normal reduction in ventricular output and a corresponding fall in systemic arterial pressure. The elevated pressure in the chambers of the right side of the heart accounts for the equally important failure of the systemic venous pressure to decline in the normal manner.

It is important to bear in mind that the paradoxic pulse is not pathognomonic of pericardial disease because it may be observed in other forms of constrictive heart disease and, indeed, in some cases of severe heart failure without structural disease of the endocardium or pericardium, and in hemorrhagic shock (Chap. 36) and obstructive airway disease.

TREATMENT. All patients with an acute pericarditis should be observed frequently and carefully for the possibility of a developing effusion or, if effusion is already present, for signs of tamponade. Arterial and venous pressures and heart rate should be monitored and serial chest films obtained. If manifestations of tamponade appear, pericardiocentesis should be instituted at once, since relief of the intrapericardial pressure may be lifesaving.

POST-CARDIAC-INJURY SYNDROME

During the past few years, it has been recognized that a number of disorders, identical in their clinical manifestations, may appear under a variety of circumstances. They have one common feature; previous injury to the heart. The syndrome has been observed when the injury has been induced in the course of a heart operation, (postpericardiotomy syndrome or, as it was originally designated, postcommissurotomy syndrome). It may also follow myocardial infarction (Dressler's syndrome), or it may develop after trauma of the heart (stab wound, nonpenetrating blow to the chest).

The symptoms usually occur after an interval of 2 weeks or more following the cardiac injury, and sometimes may appear only after a lapse of months. Recurrences are common and may occur up to 2 years or more after the injury. Fever up to 102 to 104°F, pericarditis, pleuritis, and pneumonitis are the outstanding features, the bout of illness usually subsiding in 1 or 2 weeks. The pericarditis, which appears to be the most constant lesion, may be of the fibrinous variety, or it may assume the character of a pericardial effusion, which is often serosanguineous and sometimes causes tamponade.

The mechanism whereby the clinical manifestations are induced is not certain, but there is a strong likelihood that they are the result of an antigen-antibody reaction, in which the antigen originates from injured myocardial tissue, and the term *post-cardiac-injury syndrome* is suggested as an appropriate designation for this group of disorders. It is meant to imply only that these disorders of variable etiology have a common clinical picture and may have a common pathogenetic mechanism.

The clinical picture mimics in practically every detail the disease known as "acute benign infectious pericarditis" (see below). Moreover, it is possible that the recurrences that occur so frequently in this condition are not always caused by an exacerbation of the original viral infection. It is possible that the original viral injury may have initiated the sequence of events that culminates in the post-cardiac-injury syndrome. This concept is speculative, and further investigation is required.

"Cardiac injury" may be used in both a broad and a restricted sense. Here, the term *post-cardiac-injury* is applied to various types of heart injury: necrosis due to ischemia, the trauma of surgery, and possibly the damage resulting from a viral infection of the pericardium, such as occurs in acute benign pericarditis. It also embraces the injury caused by contusions and penetrating wounds of the heart. For this last group and the identical syndrome that may follow, we have used the term *post-traumatic syndrome* in the restricted sense and imply that it is simply one form of the post-cardiac-injury syndrome.

TREATMENT. Often no treatment is necessary aside from analgesics for pain. The management of pericardial effusion and tamponade has already been discussed. When the illness is severe and is followed by a series of disabling recurrences, steroid therapy is usually effective.

The proper approach to the clinical problems of pericardial disease is to consider that the disease consists of three syndromes: *acute fibrinous pericarditis, pericardial effusion, and constrictive heart disease.* The physician should first determine whether any of these syndromes is present; if one of these forms of pericardial disease is found, his task is then to determine the cause. To simplify the discussion and to avoid needless repetition, we have chosen to select one important example of each of the syndromes as the prototype and then to discuss the problem of etiologic diagnosis.

ACUTE BENIGN PERICARDITIS

This disorder is an important clinical entity because of its frequency and because it may be confused with other more serious affections. In some cases, a Coxsackie B, type 8 ECHO, and mumps virus have been isolated; in other instances, acute pericarditis has occurred in association with illnesses of known viral origin and, presumably, was caused by the same agent. It occurs at all ages but most frequently in young adults, and is frequently associated with pleural effusions and sometimes with pneumonitis. Often there is a history of an antecedent respiratory infection within the preceding 2 to 3 weeks. Fever and precordial pain appear at about the same time and constitute an important feature in the differentiation from myocardial infarction. The constitutional symptoms are usually mild to moderate, but occasionally the initial symptoms are stormy, the temperature rising to 104 to 105°F. The disease ordinarily runs its course in a few days to 2 weeks, but occasionally after the patient has presumably recovered, he may have one or several recurrences, weeks or even months later. Tamponade is unusual, and constrictive pericarditis rarely develops. As is true in other forms of acute pericarditis, the pain is usually exaggerated by breathing, change of position, or swallowing. A pericardial friction rub is often audible. The ST-T-wave alterations in the electrocardiogram are usually transitory, but they may persist for several years or indefinitely, constituting a subsequent source of confusion in persons without a clear history of pericarditis. Constrictive pericarditis rarely complicates acute benign pericarditis. There is no specific therapy, but corticosteroids effectively suppress the clinical manifestations of the acute illness. When repeated recurrences of acute pericarditis develop, pericardiectomy has been found to be effective in terminating the illness.

Differential Diagnosis of Acute Fibrinous Pericarditis

Since there is no specific test for acute, benign, infectious pericarditis, the diagnosis is primarily one of exclusion. Consequently, before concluding that one is dealing with this disorder, one must consider all other disorders that may be associated with an acute fibrinous pericarditis.

ACUTE MYOCARDIAL INFARCTION. When an ischemic pericarditis gives rise to pleuritic pain, confusion with an infectious form of pericarditis is common and the disease must be differentiated by the time of occurrence of fever and pain, electrocardiographic abnormalities (such as the appearance of Q waves), the extent of the elevations of serum transaminase and other myocardial enzymes, and the total clinical picture. More common is the error of assuming that acute, benign, infectious pericarditis represents an acute myocardial infarction.

POST–CARDIAC–INJURY SYNDROME. The two disorders in this category that are likely to be confused with acute, benign, infectious pericarditis are the *post-myocardial-infarction syndrome* and the pericarditis that may follow a nonpenetrating bruise to the chest. When the pericarditis occurs within a few weeks or months after the infarction or the blow to the chest, it is justifiable to conclude that the two are probably related. However, it is known that many individuals suffer a completely symptomless infarct; when an acute pericarditis occurs in such a person and when there is no reason to suspect a previous infarction, differentiation between the post-myocardial-infarction syndrome and acute, benign, infectious pericarditis is impossible on clinical grounds, although the electrocardiogram will usually show evidence of myocardial necrosis with abnormal Q waves. Subsequently, the development of angina pectoris or acute infarction may then, in retrospect, clarify the nature of the previous illness. The conclusion to be drawn is that in any person over the age of forty to forty-five, an apparently classical picture of acute, benign, infectious pericarditis may actually be the first overt manifestation of serious coronary disease. Similarly, a nonpenetrating chest wall blow may be forgotten when the acute pericarditis develops several weeks later, and the relationship between the two may not be recognized.

PERICARDITIS DUE TO COLLAGEN DISEASE. Most important in the differential diagnosis is the pericarditis due to disseminated lupus erythematosus, which occurs in more than one-third of the cases. Sometimes it appears as an asymptomatic effusion, but more often pain is present, and very rarely tamponade may develop. Very rarely, when it occurs in the absence of other evidences of the underlying disorder, differentiation from acute, benign, infectious pericarditis or a mild form of *tuberculous pericarditis* may be made only on discovery of LE (lupus erythematosus) cells, a rise in antinuclear factors, or by the specific methods of diagnosis of tuberculosis. It is well to bear in mind that the failure to find LE cells does not exclude their possible appearance later. Acute pericarditis is also an occasional complication of periarteritis nodosa, and of rheumatoid arthritis, but again other evidence of these diseases is usually present.

The pericarditis of *acute rheumatic fever* is always associated with evidences of severe pancarditis. *Pyogenic pericarditis,* usually secondary to pneumonia, is now far less common than before the advent of effective antibiotics. *Uremic pericarditis* is a common finding in patients with uremia. It may be fibrinous or associated with a serous or bloody effusion. A friction rub is common; pain and tamponade are unusual. Pericarditis due to *neoplastic diseases* results from the extension of primary or metastatic tumors of the thorax (usually carcinoma of the lung) to the pericardium, or from invasion by a lymphomatous or leukemic process. Pain, atrial arrhythmias, and tamponade are complications which occur occasionally. Unusual etiologies of pericarditis include syphilis, fungous infection (actinomycosis, histoplasmosis, coccidioidomycosis), parasitic infestation (amebiasis, toxoplasmosis), infectious mononucleosis, and familial Mediterranean fever.

CHRONIC TUBERCULOUS PERICARDIAL EFFUSION. Tuberculous pericarditis has been described in Chap. 174. The acute form has already been mentioned, and it needs to be stated here only that there may be no history of pain, and there may be no other evidence of tuberculosis. The symptoms are those of an infection in an individual with massive effusion. It is important to bear this condition in mind when a middle-aged or elderly person with fever has an apparent enlargement of the heart of undetermined origin, with or without congestive failure. Weight loss, fever, and fatigability are sometimes observed. Inasmuch as effective specific methods of therapy have now reduced the mortality rate radically from the previous figures of 50 to 80 percent, overlooking a tuberculous pericardial effusion is a serious error. Consequently, no method of examination should be omitted to establish or rule out this diagnosis. Included are chest films for pulmonary tuberculosis and a search for tuberculosis in other structures; tuberculin tests, repeated after several weeks; cultures and smears of gastric washings and of pericardial fluid. Finally, if the diagnosis is still obscure, a pericardial biopsy should be performed. If definitive evidence is then still lacking and there is good reason to be suspicious of tuberculosis, a trial of isoniazid and para-aminosalicylic acid is justified. Pericardiectomy following a 2-week course of antituberculous therapy has been successfully employed when exploration revealed a thickened pericardium. Pericardiocentesis and antituberculous therapy are indicated in patients with tuberculous pericardial effusions.

Cultures and smears of the pericardial fluid are so frequently negative in subsequently proved cases of tuberculous pericarditis, and a positive tuberculin test is so often found in persons who have no active tuberculosis, that one is sometimes faced with the dilemma of trying to decide how much emphasis to attach to each of these conflicting findings.

Differential Diagnosis of Chronic Pericardial Effusion

Myxedema may be responsible for a pericardial effusion that is sometimes massive. The other manifestations of myxedema should clarify the diagnosis, but unfortunately, even when they are present, the diagnosis is frequently overlooked. It is important, therefore, to carry out appropriate tests for thyroid function in every person with an enlarged cardiac outline of undetermined origin (Chap. 89).

Neoplasms, disseminated lupus erythematosus, rarely *polyarteritis nodosa, rheumatoid arthritis, mycotic infections, radiation therapy,* certain forms of *endomyocardial fibrosis* found in Africa, and very rarely, *severe anemia* and *scleroderma* may be the cause of a chronic pericardial effusion.

Finally, there are individuals who, without fever or other constitutional symptoms, are known to have had an "enlarged heart" for years, sometimes with, more often without, congestive failure, and who have subsequently been found to have a chronic pericardial effusion. The most exhaustive studies have failed to reveal the cause of these effusions, but all have been completely relieved by the establishment of a pleuropericardial window. Such disorders have been designated *chronic idiopathic pericardial effusion,* with full recognition that "idiopathic" merely signifies ignorance of the cause of these disorders. For example, one form of idiopathic pericardial effusion has been found to be caused sometimes by an *injury to the heart* following a nonpenetrating blow to the chest with the relationship between the injury and the subsequent effusion obscured by the lapse of weeks before the effusion develops. This type of pericardial effusion is simply another form of the post-cardiac-injury syndrome.

CHRONIC CONSTRICTIVE PERICARDITIS

This disorder results when the healing of an acute fibrinous or serofibrinous pericarditis is followed by obliteration of the cavity of the sac, with the formation of granulation tissue which gradually contracts and forms a firm scar, encasing the heart and interfering with filling. In some reports, a high percentage of all cases has been of tuberculous origin. In other series, tuberculosis has been an infrequent cause. The condition has also been known to follow pyogenic infection, trauma, radiation, histoplasmosis, neoplastic disease, and acute (so-called

benign) pericarditis, and it is occasionally associated with atrial septal defect. In many reports, the cause of the pericardial disease has been undetermined. Rarely, routine fluoroscopic or radiographic examination may reveal calcification of the pericardium in an individual who is free of all symptoms referable to the heart.

The basic abnormality in chronic constrictive pericarditis in symptomatic patients is the inability of the ventricles to fill adequately during diastole because of the limitations imposed by the rigid, thickened pericardium. Stroke volume is diminished and the end-diastolic pressures in both ventricles as well as the mean pressures in the atria, pulmonic veins, and systemic veins are elevated to about the same levels. The central venous, right and left atrial pressure pulses display an M-shaped contour, with sharp *a* and *v* waves and *x* and *y* descents; the *y* descent is the most prominent deflection and is interrupted by a rapid rise in pressure during early diastole, when ventricular filling is impeded by the constricting pericardium. During diastole, both ventricular pressure pulses exhibit characteristic "square root" signs (Chap. 262). These hemodynamic changes, although characteristic, are not pathognomonic of constrictive pericarditis, but are also observed in other lesions which produce restriction of ventricular filling, discussed on page 1234. Contrary to a widely held impression, dyspnea, though absent or minimal at rest, is present on exertion, and orthopnea is commonly present in chronic constrictive pericarditis, although it is not severe. Attacks of acute left ventricular failure (acute pulmonary edema) practically never occur. The cervical veins are distended, and in about one-half the cases, a paradoxic pulse associated with increased inspiratory venous distension (Kussmaul's sign) may be observed. Congestive hepatomegaly is pronounced, and ascites is common and is more prominent than dependent edema. In about half of the patients, the heart is normal in size; if it is enlarged, the enlargement is rarely extreme. The heart sounds are distant, and an early third heart sound, i.e., a pericardial knock, occurring 0.10 to 0.13 sec after aortic valve closure, is usually conspicuous. The apex beat is poorly defined, and cardiac pulsations under fluoroscopic examination are diminished. Because of the high sustained venous pressure, congestive splenomegaly may be sufficiently pronounced to make the spleen palpable. In the absence of evidence of bacterial endocarditis or tricuspid valve disease, splenomegaly in a patient with congestive heart failure should arouse suspicion of constrictive pericarditis. Protein-losing gastroenteropathy sometimes complicates chronic constrictive pericarditis. The electrocardiogram frequently displays low voltage and flattening or inversion of the T waves in all three limb leads. Electrocardiographic evidence of ventricular hypertrophy and prominent cardiac murmurs are unusual, but atrial fibrillation is often present.

Systemic and/or pulmonary venous congestion is initially the result of impaired filling of the ventricles caused by the restrictive action of the inelastic pericardium. However, the fibrotic process may extend into the myocardium, and venous congestion may then be due to the combined effects of the myocardial and pericardial lesions. The interference with filling reduces the work of the heart, and perhaps this leads to myocardial atrophy. The latter probably accounts for the delayed beneficial effects of operative treatment.

Inasmuch as the usual physical signs of cardiac disease (murmurs, cardiac enlargement) may be inconspicuous or entirely lacking, hepatic enlargement and intractable ascites may lead to a mistaken diagnosis of cirrhosis of the liver. This error should be avoided if the neck veins are inspected carefully in all patients with ascites and hepatomegaly. *Given a clinical picture resembling that of cirrhosis, but with the added feature of distended neck veins, careful search for calcification of the pericardium by chest films, with the patient in the oblique position, should be carried out and may disclose a curable or remediable form of heart disease.* Since calcification occurs in only about 50 percent of these patients, exploration of the pericardium is justifiable if the clinical picture is suggestive enough.

The clinical picture described above represents the full-blown and classical disorder. It is important to bear in mind that sometimes a calcified pericardium, clearly visible on the roentgenogram, may cause no symptoms whatsoever; or a patient may display symptoms of congestive failure without the classical features of constrictive pericarditis, and autopsy may nevertheless reveal this lesion.

TREATMENT. In the treatment of constrictive pericarditis, diuretic drugs and sodium restriction are useful during preoperative preparation for decortication. Digitalis, which is rarely of value in the preoperative state, may be beneficial in the prevention of heart failure when resection of the thickened pericardium permits an increased inflow into the ventricles and hence an enhanced burden on an atrophic myocardium. The benefits derived from cardiac decortication are often striking, and frequently the improvement, though slight at first, is progressive over a period of many months. Presumably, this continued improvement is due to the gradual disappearance of myocardial atrophy. The patient may be restored from a state of invalidism to one approaching normal activity.

Many instances of contrictive pericarditis are of tuberculous origin. Antituberculous therapy during the phase of effusion may prevent the development of constriction, and such therapy should be carried out before and after operation, if a tuberculous origin is suspected in a patient with chronic constrictive pericarditis (Chap. 174).

No treatment is required for those persons who are found to have a calcified pericardium but in whom there is no evidence of increased venous pressure.

Differential Diagnosis of Constrictive (Restrictive) Heart Disease

Constrictive heart disease consists of a group of disorders in which the basic hemodynamic disturbance is similar to that in chronic constrictive pericarditis, i.e., an impediment to ventricular diastolic filling due to impairment of cardiac compliance. These disorders have also been termed *restrictive heart disease.*

There are two general problems in the diagnosis of constrictive heart disease: (1) the differentiation of the constrictive from the nonconstrictive disorders that lead to congestive failure; (2) the separation of constrictive pericarditis from other forms of constrictive heart disease. The nonconstrictive type of heart disease may simulate the constrictive forms: e.g., *cor pulmonale* may be associated with severe systemic venous congestion and with little or no pulmonary congestion; the heart may not appear to be enlarged; a striking inspiratory fall in arterial pressure may be present. However, in contrast to constrictive pericarditis, there is also an inspiratory fall in venous pressure. *Tricuspid stenosis* may also simulate the picture of chronic constrictive pericarditis; congestive hepatomegaly and ascites may be equally prominent, and the manifestations of left-sided heart failure may be inconspicuous. However, the characteristic murmur, the absence of a paradoxic pulse, as well as the absence in the jugular pulse of the steep, deep *y* descent followed by a rapid ascent (manifested by the diastolic shock on palpation and its audible equivalent, the pericardial knock or third heart sound), should make the differentiation possible.

On the other hand, the same physiologic abnormalities and the same clinical picture may be induced by other forms of constrictive heart disease, such as *fibroelastosis, endocardial fibrosis,* the various forms of *endomyocarditis,* extensive involvement of the myocardium by *amyloid disease, scleroderma, fibrosis secondary to myocarditis,* and, perhaps most important, *idiopathic myocardial hypertrophy,* in which the enormous thickening of the ventricular wall is responsible for the diminished compliance. These disorders are all capable of inducing the same hemodynamic defect, leading to a disorder that is practically indistinguishable from that caused by constrictive pericarditis. It has also been shown that diffuse and severe scarring of the endocardium and myocardium caused by *coronary sclerosis,* which, in some instances, has not been associated with the pain of myocardial ischemia may mimic constrictive pericarditis.

The features favoring the diagnosis of one of the above forms of cardiomyopathy are a well-defined apex beat, conspicuous enlargement of the heart, and pronounced orthopnea with attacks of acute left ventricular failure, left ventricular preponderance in the electrocardiogram, bundle branch block, or significant Q waves.

The lesson to be learned is that when a patient has progressive, disabling, and unresponsive congestive failure, and if he displays any of the phenomena of constrictive heart disease, the most careful and detailed clinical and laboratory studies must be carried out in order to detect or exclude constrictive pericarditis; in many instances cardiac catheterization, selective angiocardiography, and coronary arteriography may be required. However, when these examinations do not yield a definitive diagnosis, the only decisive method of determining whether or not constrictive pericarditis is responsible for the clinical manifestations of heart failure is by exploration of the pericardium.

OTHER DISORDERS OF THE PERICARDIUM. *Tumors* involving the pericardium are almost always secondary to malignant neoplasms of the mediastinum. The most common primary sources are carcinoma of the bronchus or breast, lymphoma, and occasionally other malignancies of the mediastinum, such as a thymoma. Rarely, a tumor, such as a mesothelioma, may originate in the pericardium. The usual clinical picture is that of an insidiously developing pericardial effusion, often bloody, and the chief problem is differentiation from a tuberculous effusion.

A *pericardial cyst* appears as a rounded or lobulated deformity of the cardiac silhouette; its most common location is at the right cardiophrenic angle. Its only clinical significance lies in the possibility of confusion with a tumor or ventricular aneurysm.

REFERENCES

Beck, W., V. Schrire, and L. Vogelpoel: Splitting of the Second Heart Sound in Constrictive Pericarditis, with Observations on the Mechanism of Pulsus Paradoxus, Am. Heart J., 64:765, 1962.

Bedford, D. E.: Chronic Effusive Pericarditis, Brit. Heart J., 26:499, 1964.

Burwell, C. S., and E. D. Robin: Diagnosis of Diffuse Myocardial Fibrosis, Circulation, 20:606, 1959.

Dock, W.: Inspiratory Traction on the Pericardium: The Cause of Pulsus Paradoxus in Pericardial Disease, A.M.A. Arch. Intern. Med., 108:837, 1961.

Fowler, N.: Pericardial Diseases, chap. 35, pp. 593–614 in "Cardiac Diagnosis," Harper & Row, Publishers, Incorporated, New York, 1968.

Hurst, J. W., and R. B. Logue (eds.): "The Heart," New York, McGraw-Hill Book Company, 1970.

Schepers, G. W. G.: Tuberculous Pericarditis, Am. J. Cardiol., 9:248, 1962.

Spodick, D. H.: "Chronic and Constrictive Pericarditis," New York, Grune & Stratton, Inc., 1964.

Wood, P.: Chronic Constrictive Pericarditis, Am. J. Cardiol., 7:48, 1961. (In this issue of vol. 7 of the American Journal of Cardiology there is a symposium on pericarditis, containing not only the above paper but numerous others reviewing many aspects of pericarditis.)

——: Pericarditis, chap. 13, pp. 762–788 in "Disease of the Heart and Circulation," 3d ed., Philadelphia, J. B. Lippincott Company, 1968.

273 CARDIOMYOPATHY AND MYOCARDITIS

Gerald Glick and Eugene Braunwald

CARDIOMYOPATHY

Until recent years, virtually all adult patients suffering from symptomatic heart disease were classified as having ischemic, hypertensive, valvular, or congenital heart disease. When unequivocal evidence for one of these diagnoses was not present, the patient, especially if in an older age group, was frequently diagnosed as suffering from coronary artery disease, even though a history of a myocardial infarction or angina pectoris could not be elicited. With the development of newer diagnostic techniques, particularly coronary arteriography, it has become clear that ischemic heart disease is not a diagnosis of exclusion, but must meet rigorous and specific criteria (Chap. 271). With this realization, various cardiomyopathies, previously considered uncommon, have emerged as important causes of morbidity and mortality. This chapter is concerned with these important forms of heart disease.

The term *cardiomyopathy* is used here to indicate a disease entity in which the presenting signs and symptoms result entirely or predominantly from dysfunction of the myocardium. However, myocardial lesions produced by ischemic heart disease, hypertensive cardiovascular disease, cor pulmonale, valvular heart disease, congenital heart disease, and specific inflammatory lesions are excluded. The cardiomyopathies may be classified on a pathologic basis as resulting either from primary involvement of the myocardium or from secondary involvement as part of a generalized disease (Table 273-1).

Table 273-1. PATHOLOGIC CLASSIFICATION OF CARDIOMYOPATHIES

I. Primary myocardial involvement
   A. Idiopathic
   B. Familial
   C. Alcoholic
   D. Postpartum
   E. Endocardial fibroelastosis
   F. Endomyocardial fibrosis
II. Secondary myocardial involvement
   A. Amyloidosis
   B. Hemochromatosis
   C. Sarcoidosis
   D. Scleroderma
   E. Polyarteritis
   F. Lupus erythematosus
   G. Leukemia
   H. Neuromuscular disease
      1. Friedreich's ataxia
      2. Progressive muscular dystrophy
      3. Myotonia atrophica
   I. Glycogen storage disease (Pompe's disease)
   J. Hurler's syndrome

However, from a clinical point of view it is more desirable, as suggested by Goodwin, to classify the cardiomyopathies on the basis of differences in their patho-

Table 273-2. CLINICAL CLASSIFICATION OF CARDIOMYOPATHIES

I. Characterized by: Congestive heart failure, arrhythmias, emboli, and murmurs of mitral and tricuspid regurgitation
II. Characterized by: Restriction to ventricular filling
III. Characterized by: Obstruction to ventricular outflow

logic physiology and consequent differences in clinical presentation (Table 273-2).

Cardiomyopathies Characterized by Congestive Heart Failure, Arrhythmias, Emboli, and Murmurs of Mitral and Tricuspid Regurgitation

IDIOPATHIC CARDIOMYOPATHY. Many terms for this form of cardiomyopathy have been employed, and the resulting confusion has impeded understanding of this important class of disease. These terms include myocardiopathy, primary myocardial disease, idiopathic myocardial hypertrophy, and myocardosis. The term *cardiomyopathy* seems most appropriate, since it simply means "heart muscle disease."

The specific cause of this form of cardiomyopathy remains unknown. Pathologically, the hearts are dilated but they may also be hypertrophied, and mural thrombi frequently are seen in the left ventricle, left atrium, and right atrium. On histologic examination the major changes are fibrosis and myocardial degeneration and hypertrophy. Idiopathic cardiomyopathy most frequently occurs in middle-aged men, who, when first seen, have the signs and symptoms of congestive heart failure. The failure is both left- and right-sided and is manifested by dyspnea on exertion, fatigue, orthopnea, paroxysmal nocturnal dyspnea, peripheral edema, and palpitations. In addition, pulmonary emboli emanating from mural thrombi in the right atrium and the venous system and systemic emboli coming from the chambers of the left side of the heart may produce serious complications.

Physical Findings. Examination reveals that the pulse pressure is small; when failure is present, the diastolic pressure may be significantly elevated. The jugular venous pressure is raised. Protodiastolic and presystolic gallop sounds (Chap. 259) are present, and because of cardiac dilatation, the tricuspid and mitral rings are stretched, with consequent production of valvular regurgitation. Therefore, a pansystolic murmur in the tricuspid area which increases on inspiration and which is associated with a systolic wave in the jugular venous pulse is noted, as is a pansystolic murmur in the mitral area that is not affected by respiration. As the congestive failure improves with treatment, the raised venous pressure and diastolic arterial pressure return toward normal, the heart decreases in size, and the pansystolic murmurs and gallop sounds become softer or may disappear.

Roentgenologic examination reveals the heart to be grossly and diffusely enlarged, pericardial and pleural effusions may be present, and the lung fields may show evidence of venous hypertension and interstitial congestion. The most common abnormalities present in the *electrocardiogram* are premature ventricular contractions, nonspecific ST-T wave changes, sinus tachycardia, and atrial fibrillation. Left axis deviation is common, and complete left bundle branch block or, rarely, right bundle branch block may be present. Frequently, low voltage is noted, but left ventricular hypertrophy is seen in about 25 percent of cases. All degrees of atrioventricular block may also be observed.

Cardiac catheterization reveals a cardiac output that is moderately or severely reduced at rest and that does not increase normally with exertion. The end-diastolic pressures in both ventricles are elevated, and consequently the mean atrial pressures are also elevated to abnormally high levels.

Treatment. It is difficult to treat these patients because in its advanced stages the disease is frequently refractory to the standard therapeutic measures for congestive failure. Burch and associates believe that prolonged, strict bed rest for up to one year or more is important for the optimal management of these patients. However, frequently this form of therapy is not feasible and one must rely on the standard management for congestive heart failure (Chap. 264). Anticoagulants may be necessary, especially in patients with a history of embolization, atrial fibrillation, or a low cardiac output. The usefulness of steroids has not been established.

Until recently, this form of cardiomyopathy, characterized by congestive heart failure, usually has been recognized only in its far-advanced stages; as a result, treatment has been difficult and the prognosis poor. As the diagnosis of this disease is established earlier, its pernicious course may be interrupted by proper therapy, and the prognosis may be improved.

ALCOHOLIC CARDIOMYOPATHY. Increasing evidence has been brought forth to indicate that alcohol exerts a direct injurious effect on the myocardium and that the clinical entity of alcoholic cardiomyopathy is a real one. Regan has demonstrated in dogs that ethanol depresses ventricular performance, changes myocardial substrate utilization from carbohydrate to triglyceride, and causes myocardial cell injury. Counterparts to this animal model are seen in patients who repeatedly go into congestive heart failure after ingestion of large quantities of alcohol. Because successive insults to the myocardium may lead to increasing irreparable damage, these patients must be instructed to stop all alcoholic intake. Clinically, they resemble patients with idiopathic cardiomyopathy, described above. When the myocardial damage has become widespread and severe, prognosis is poor. Therefore, ingestion of alcohol must be interdicted as early in the course of the disease as possible. Although thiamine deficiency may be present in many of these patients, alcoholic cardiomyopathy is associated with a low cardiac output and systemic vasoconstriction, whereas beriberi heart disease (Chap. 264) is characterized by an elevated cardiac output and diminished peripheral vascular resistance.

POSTPARTUM CARDIOMYOPATHY. When cardiac enlargement and congestive heart failure of unexplained etiology develop for the first time in a patient during the first 4 months following delivery, the diagnosis of postpartum cardiomyopathy should be considered. This temporal relation to delivery may not represent a direct consequence of pregnancy itself, but may be conditioned by such factors as poor nutrition, familial or hereditary factors, unsuspected myocarditis, or some as yet unknown cause. Nevertheless, a clinical picture quite characteristic for this entity has emerged. The patient is usually a young multiparous Negro who has been undernourished, may have a history of hypertension, and may have suffered a pulmonary embolus. The symptoms and signs are similar to those seen in the older, male patients suffering from idiopathic cardiomyopathy, described above. The course of the disease frequently leads to death as a result of heart failure, despite intensive treatment. Therapy is the same as for patients with the idiopathic form of cardiomyopathy, although patients with the postpartum form apparently have an increased sensitivity to digitalis. Patients who recover should be encouraged to improve their nutritional state and to avoid further pregnancies.

ENDOCARDIAL FIBROELASTOSIS. This disease, also of unknown etiology, is most commonly seen in infants and is a relatively common cause of congestive heart failure in this age group. It has also been reported to occur in adults, but far less frequently. It is characterized by a thickened endocardium that shows proliferation of elastic tissue. The process generally affects the left ventricle most extensively but may also involve the mitral and aortic valves. Mitral regurgitation is often present, and it may be difficult to determine whether the clinical picture results primarily from the endocardial or the valvular lesion. Involvement of the chambers of the right side of the heart is less common. When first seen, the patient generally has congestive heart failure and shows stigmata of both the congestive and restrictive forms of cardiomyopathy. Mural thrombi are common and may lead to systemic embolization. The electrocardiogram usually shows evidence of left ventricular hypertrophy, and various forms of conduction disturbances and arrhythmias may occur. The chest roentgenogram reveals cardiac enlargement, involving primarily the left ventricle and atrium. As in the other forms of cardiomyopathy characterized by heart failure, therapy is directed at heart failure, with emphasis on adequate digitalization, but it is generally unsatisfactory.

ENDOMYOCARDIAL FIBROSIS. This is a progressive form of heart disease, seen in the tropics and especially in Africa, that is characterized by fibrosis in the inflow tract and the apex of one or both of the ventricles. Though it may occur at any age, endomyocardial fibrosis is most common in children and young adults. Although a hypersensitivity mechanism has been suggested, the cause is unknown.

Fibrosis of the endocardium begins at the apex of either ventricle and extends toward the inflow tract to involve the tricuspid and mitral valves and also toward the outflow portions of each ventricle. In addition, the disease process extends into the myocardium to produce muscle destruction, fibrosis, and occasionally calcification. As a result of the involvement of the atrioventricular valves, tricuspid and mitral regurgitation are common. When the chambers of the right side of the heart are principally involved, the patient has an enlarged tender liver and marked ascites, but relatively little dependent edema. The jugular venous pressure is elevated, with a prominent systolic wave, due to tricuspid regurgitation, a rapid *y* descent, and a right ventricular protodiastolic gallop; a pansystolic murmur along the left

sternal border can be detected. When the left ventricle is chiefly involved, the symptoms are breathlessness, orthopnea, and cough. The physical signs are those of mitral regurgitation, left ventricular failure, and resultant pulmonary hypertension; there are right and left ventricular heaves, accentuation of the sound of pulmonic valve closure, a third heart sound and a pansystolic murmur at the apex, and crepitant rales at the posterior lung bases.

The electrocardiogram generally shows low voltage, although right ventricular hypertrophy may be seen in those patients with left ventricular involvement and severe pulmonary hypertension. Roentgenologically the heart is generally enlarged, although in some instances it may appear to be of normal size. The large atria are mainly responsible for the enlarged silhouette. Intramyocardial calcium may be visualized. In patients with predominant involvement of the right side of the heart, the vascularity of the lung fields is diminished, whereas in patients with predominant left-sided lesions, the lung fields are congested and the pulmonary arteries enlarged.

The most prominent findings at cardiac catheterization are a decreased cardiac output, elevated central venous pressure, and a dip and plateau configuration of the ventricular pressure tracing during diastole. This configuration of the pressure pulse is typically seen when restriction to ventricular filling is present. Such restriction may be the result of an endocardial or myocardial fibrotic process, as seen in endomyocardial fibrosis or endocardial fibroelastosis, or it may result from constriction produced by the pericardium, as in constrictive pericarditis. Thus, endomyocardial fibrosis falls into the category of a cardiomyopathy that has features both of restrictive and of congestive disease.

NEUROMUSCULAR DISEASE. The heart is usually involved in *Friedreich's ataxia* and in the various *muscular dystrophies* by a pathologic process that causes cardiac dilatation and replacement of myocardial fibers with connective tissue, together with extensive interstitial fibrosis. The clinical picture is that of a congestive type of cardiomyopathy associated with arrhythmias.

Cardiomyopathies Characterized by Restriction to Ventricular Filling

As indicated in the discussions of endocardial fibroelastosis and of endomyocardial fibrosis, the division of cardiomyopathies into the congestive type and the restrictive type is somewhat artificial, because a given disease entity may present certain features of each, either simultaneously or sequentially; i.e., as the heart in the congestive form becomes progressively more fibrosed and therefore less distensible, it acquires some of the characteristics of the restrictive form of cardiomyopathy. In addition, an infiltrative disease such as amyloidosis may present initially as either a congestive or a restrictive cardiomyopathy. However, certain of the cardiomyopathies are dominated by the features of restriction to ventricular filling, and the pathologic physiology and clinical presentation are similar, even though the etiologies may be diverse. Thus, patients with restrictive cardiomyopathy resulting from primary amyloidosis, hemochromatosis, sarcoidosis, endocardial fibroelastosis, and Loeffler's fibroplastic endocarditis have similar cardiac findings. As a result of persistently elevated venous pressure, they commonly have dependent edema, ascites, and an enlarged, tender liver. The jugular venous pressure is elevated and does not fall normally or may rise with inspiration (Kussmaul's sign). The heart is usually enlarged, the heart sounds are distant, and third and fourth sounds are common. Murmurs are not distinctive. The electrocardiogram shows low-voltage, nonspecific ST-T wave changes, and various arrhythmias. The major radiologic feature is a moderately enlarged heart and absence of calcium in the area of the pericardium.

Cardiac catheterization shows a decreased cardiac output, elevation of right and left ventricular end-diastolic pressure, and a dip and plateau configuration of the diastolic portion of the ventricular pressure pulse. This form of cardiomyopathy may be completely indistinguishable from constrictive pericarditis (Chap. 272), both at the bedside and even with the benefit of cardiac catheterization. Certain clues to the differentiation, however, may be observed. In the restrictive cardiomyopathies, the left ventricular end-diastolic pressure is often significantly higher than the right ventricular end-diastolic pressure, whereas in constrictive pericarditis both these pressures are usually identical, or almost so. In constrictive pericarditis, pericardial calcification may be evident on the roentgenogram. However, thoracotomy and surgical exploration may be necessary to make a definitive differentiation between a restrictive cardiomyopathy and chronic constrictive pericarditis. This distinction is of importance, because the latter condition is potentially curable by operation.

DIFFERENTIAL DIAGNOSIS. *Amyloidosis* may be diagnosed by biopsy of the tongue, gums, liver, or rectal mucosa. *Hemochromatosis* should be suspected if cardiomyopathy occurs in the setting of diabetes mellitus, hepatic cirrhosis, and increased skin pigmentation. *Sarcoid* involvement of the heart is generally associated with other manifestations of generalized disease, such as uveitis, hilar lymphadenopathy, pulmonary infiltrates, and cor pulmonale (Chap. 254). In *scleroderma*, although the heart may be involved, the major symptoms result from esophageal, pulmonary, and skin involvement. *Loeffler's disease*, or *fibroplastic endocarditis*, is associated with a marked eosinophilia and must be distinguished from cardiac involvement in *polyarteritis*, *trichinosis*, and *eosinophilic leukemia*.

Cardiomyopathies Characterized by Obstruction to Ventricular Outflow

Idiopathic hypertrophic subaortic stenosis (IHSS) is another cardiomyopathy that has emerged as a distinct entity since 1957. This disease has also been referred to as hypertrophic obstructive cardiomyopathy, muscular subaortic stenosis, and asymmetric ventricular hypertrophy. The various appellations all emphasize the characteristic abnormality of this disease, namely, marked hypertrophy of the left ventricle, most striking in the interventricular septum. Obstruction to outflow occurs when the hypertrophied septum abuts against the anterior mitral leaflet during systole. In contrast to the obstruction to flow seen in patients with valvular aortic stenosis, in whom the size of the narrowed orifice is fixed, in IHSS the obstruction to outflow is dynamic and may change between examinations or even from beat to beat. The severity of obstruction is a function of the width of the outflow tract during systole, which in turn appears to be related to three major factors: (1) the left ventricular end-diastolic volume, (2) the myocardial contractile state, and (3) the pressure that distends the left ventricular outflow tract during systole. Interventions such as muscular exercise, isoproterenol infusion, and digitalis glycosides, which both increase the force of myocardial contraction and decrease the size of the ventricle, intensify the obstruction. Similarly, when the ventricular volume is decreased by the Valsalva maneuver, hemorrhage, nitroglycerin, or tachycardia, the obstruction is once again increased. Conversely, elevation of arterial pressure by phenylephrine, increasing venous return by raising the legs, expansion of the blood volume, and general anesthesia, all tend to increase the ventricular volume and, consequently, ameliorate the obstruction. Sometimes the hypertrophied septum bulges into the outflow tract of the right ventricle, thereby impeding the ejection of blood from this chamber as well. IHSS occurs in familial form in one-third of the cases, while in the remainder it occurs sporadically. In some patients the condition may be congenital, but, more commonly, the manifestations are acquired.

Physical Findings. The most common symptoms are dyspnea, angina, dizziness, syncope, and left ventricular failure. Physical examination usually reveals a prominent *a* wave in the jugular venous pulse, a double or triple apical impulse, a sharply rising peripheral pulse that is best appreciated in the carotid arteries, and a fourth heart sound. The second heart sound may be paradoxically split, and a third heart sound may be audible. A systolic ejection murmur is heard along the left sternal border or at the apex, rather than at the aortic area or along the carotid arteries, as in patients with valvular aortic stenosis. Some degree of mitral regurgitation is present in almost one-half of the patients, probably as a result of the displacement of the mitral valve by the grossly hypertrophied left ventricular myocardium, and indeed, IHSS must be distinguished both from isolated mitral regurgitation and from ventricular septal defect, conditions which it resembles superficially.

The electrocardiogram commonly shows left ventricular hypertrophy, and widespread abnormally deep, broad Q waves which suggest an old myocardial infarction but which probably result from gross septal hypertrophy. Although chest roentgenograms reveal left ventricular hypertrophy, in contrast to valvular aortic stenosis, calcification of the aortic valve is not observed and poststenotic dilatation of the aorta is only rarely present. The indirectly recorded carotid arterial pressure pulse rises unusually rapidly and often displays a double peak during systole. Generally a pressure gradient is present between the body of the left ventricle and the area directly below the aortic valve. When a gradient is not present, it frequently can be induced by provocative maneuvers such as infusion of isoproterenol or the Valsalva maneuver. In some patients symptoms may be severe but obstruction to ventricular outflow may be minimal. In these patients the left ventricular end-diastolic pressure is generally elevated, and their symptoms probably result from impedance to ventricular filling, which is a consequence of decreased ventricular compliance.

The natural history of IHSS is variable; in some patients the condition improves, in some it deteriorates, and in some it remains stable. Sudden death occurs in a small fraction of patients but does not seem related to the severity or type of previous symptoms or to the extent of obstruction. Cardiac glycosides or nitroglycerin are ordinarily not helpful. Beta-adrenergic receptor blocking agents reduce the frequency and severity of angina, but if symptoms remain intractable, surgical excision or incision of the hypertrophied portion of the outflow tract may be indicated.

Type II glycogen storage or Pompe's disease with cardiac involvement may also show features of obstruction to ventricular ejection. In addition, signs and symptoms of congestion and restriction may also be present.

MYOCARDITIS

Generally, myocarditis is the result of an infectious process, but it may also be produced by hypersensitivity states such as acute rheumatic fever (Chap. 269), by radiation therapy, chemical poisons, or physical agents. The myocarditides may be divided into the acute and chronic forms. In the United States, clinically significant acute myocarditis is caused most commonly by viruses. Thus far, the Coxsackie B viral strains and the influenza virus have been the best-documented etiologic agents, but as viral studies become more widespread, other viruses probably will be implicated. Generally, when the heart is involved in these diseases, only transient ST-T wave abnormalities are noted and the myocardial involvement does not influence the course of the disease. However, sometimes myocarditis, which may develop either during or several weeks after the respiratory illness, may lead to acute heart failure or to a variety of cardiac arrhythmias. Myocarditis is frequently associated with acute pericarditis, especially when it is caused by Coxsackie B viruses (Chap. 211).

On *physical examination*, the first heart sound is faint, a ventricular gallop (third heart) sound may be heard, and a soft apical systolic murmur is often present. A pericardial friction rub is usually heard in patients with associated pericarditis.

Viral myocarditis is most often self-limited and without sequelae, but measures to combat the congestive failure, such as digitalis, diuretics, and salt restriction, may be necessary. These patients are sometimes exceedingly sensitive to digitalis; therefore, this drug should be given cautiously and a short-acting preparation should be used. The arrhythmias are occasionally extremely difficult to manage and may be refractory to the usual treatment with drugs such as quinidine, procaine amide, diphenylhydantoin, or propranolol. When propranolol is used, care must be taken that congestive heart failure is not precipitated (Chap. 266). Deaths attributed to arrhythmias have been reported. Prolonged bed rest may prove to be a valuable form of therapy.

It is still uncertain whether or not acute viral myocarditis progresses to a chronic form. In addition, the possibility must be considered that many of the instances of idiopathic cardiomyopathy (p. 1233) arise from mild or subclinical episodes of myocarditis.

Myocarditis has been reported in association with many other viral diseases, including mumps, infectious mononucleosis, primary atypical pneumonia, measles, poliomyelitis, chickenpox, and rabies. Myocarditis is frequently observed in *acute rheumatic fever,* as discussed in Chap. 269.

Isolated Myocarditis. Also called *Fiedler's* myocarditis, this is a rare condition in which only the myocardium is involved, and the cardiac involvement cannot be related to a previous or concurrent disease. The etiology of this disease is unknown, but a viral causation has been postulated. When first seen by the physician, the patient generally has fulminating congestive heart failure; adrenal corticosteroids are occasionally effective, but in general, therapy is unsatisfactory and the patient dies after a brief illness.

Diphtheritic Myocarditis. When diphtheria was common, acute diphtheritic myocarditis was frequently encountered. Caused by an exotoxin produced by *Corynebacterium diphtheriae* (Chap. 169), this is a severe affliction. Patients may die in acute congestive heart failure or as a result of complete heart block, which is a common complication. Widespread immunization against diphtheria has virtually eliminated this disease.

Toxoplasmosis. (See also Chap. 244.) Toxoplasmosis is a relatively common cause of acute myocarditis in the newborn. The parasite *Toxoplasma gondii* can pass in utero from the mother to the fetus, so that toxoplasmosis may occur in the fetus or in the newborn; rarely it affects adults. This condition should be considered in the differential diagnosis of obscure myocarditis. A complement fixation test and the antibody dye test are valuable diagnostic aids. Therapy consists of administration of pyrimethamine and a sulfonamide.

Chagas' Disease. (See also Chap. 243.) Chagas' disease, which is caused by *Trypanosoma cruzi,* is a form of myocarditis that occurs in well-defined acute and chronic forms. It is one of the most common forms of heart disease encountered in Central and South America. The acute form is generally seen in infants and children and is characterized by a local inflammatory reaction at the site of inoculation (the chagoma), fever, generalized edema, tachycardia, lymphadenopathy, and hepatosplenomegaly. The heart is enlarged, the sounds are distant, and a protodiastolic gallop sound may be present. Lymphocytosis is common. The electrocardiogram may show first degree atrioventricular block and abnormal T waves. Immunologic tests may be negative in the early stages of the disease, and the diagnosis is established by finding the parasite in thick blood films. The acute myocarditis is usually self-limited, but some patients develop the chronic form. The latter, which may occur in patients without a history of an acute episode, is observed most commonly between the ages of fifteen and fifty years. The main pathologic features of the chronic form are dilatation of the cardiac chambers, fibrosis and thinning of the ventricular wall, aneurysm formation in the areas of thinning, especially at the apex, and mural thrombi. In the asymptomatic stage, the major manifestations are premature beats and cardiac enlargement. The electrocardiogram may show evidence of intraventricular block, mainly right bundle branch block, abnormal T waves, and frequent premature ventricular contractions. As the patient becomes symptomatic, signs and symptoms of congestive heart failure develop. Thromboembolic complications are prominent. Premature contractions become more frequent and are increased by exertion, and serious arrhythmias, such as ventricular tachycardia, may occur. The cause of death is either intractable congestive failure or an arrhythmia. In the chronic form of Chagas' disease, the complement fixation test is usually positive. Therapy is directed toward the treatment of the congestive heart failure and arrhythmias.

Radiation. Patients who receive large doses of radiation therapy to the area of the heart (generally in excess of 4,000 rads), most frequently for carcinoma of the lung or breast, may develop serious cardiac complications, including acute pericarditis, chronic constrictive pericarditis, and chronic myocarditis.

REFERENCES

Cardiomyopathy

Bajusz, E. (Ed.): Experimental "metabolic" Cardiopathies and their relationship to human heart diseases. Ann. N.Y. Acad. Sci. 156, Art. 1:1–625, 1969.

Braunwald, E., C. T. Lambrew, S. D. Rockoff, J. Ross, Jr., and A. G. Morrow: Idiopathic Hypertrophic Subaortic Stenosis. I. A Description of the Disease Based Upon an Analysis of 64 Patients, Circulation, 30 (suppl. 4):3–119, 1964.

Brigden, W., and J. Robinson: Alcoholic Heart Disease, Brit. Med. J., 2:1283, 1964.

Burch, G. E., J. J. Walsh, V. J. Ferrans, and R. Hibbs: Prolonged Bed Rest in the Treatment of the Dilated Heart, Circulation, 32:852, 1965.

Eliot, R. S., H. J. McGee, and S. G. Blount, Jr.: Cardiac Amyloidosis, Circulation, 23:613, 1961.

Frank, S., and E. Braunwald: Idiopathic Hypertrophic Subaortic Stenosis: Clinical Analysis of 126 Patients with Emphasis on the Natural History, Circulation, 37:759, 1968.

Goodwin, J. F., H. Gordon, A. Hollman, and M. B. Bishop: Clinical Aspects of Cardiomyopathy, Brit. Med. J., 1:69, 1961.

Hoffman, F. G., D. Rosenbaum, and P. D. Genovese: Fibro-plastic Endocarditis with Eosinophilia (Löffler's Endocarditis Parietalis Fibroplastica): Case Report and Review of Literature, Ann. Intern. Med., 42:668, 1955.

Lewis, H. P.: Cardiac Involvement in Hemochromatosis, Am. J. Med. Sci., 227:544, 1954.

Moller, J. H., R. V. Lucas, Jr., P. Adam, Jr., R. C. Anderson, J. Jorgens, and J. E. Edwards: Endocardial Fibroelastosis. A Clinical and Anatomic Study of 47 Patients with Emphasis on Its Relationship to Mitral Insufficiency, Circulation, 30:759, 1964.

Parry, E. H. O., and D. G. Abrahams: The Natural History of Endomyocardial Fibrosis, Quart. J. Med., 34:383, 1965.

Perloff, J. K., A. C. deLeon, Jr., D. O'Doherty: The Cardiomyopathy of Progressive Muscular Dystrophy, Circulation, 33:625, 1966.

Porter, G. H.: Sarcoid Heart Disease, New Engl. J. Med., 263:1350, 1960.

Regan, T. J., Levinson, G. E., Oldewurtel, H. A., Frank, M. J., Weisse, A. B., and Moschos, C. B.: Ventricular function in non-cardiacs with alcoholic fatty liver. J. Clin. Invest. 48:397, 1969.

Walsh, J. J., G. E. Burch, W. C. Black, V. J. Ferrans, and R. G. Hibb: Idiopathic Myocardiopathy of the Puerperium (Postpartal Heart Disease), Circulation, 32:19, 1965.

Myocarditis

Bell, R. W., and W. M. Murphy: Myocarditis in Young Military Personnel, Am. Heart J., 74:309, 1967.

Cohn, K. E., J. R. Stewart, L. F. Fajardo, and E. W. Hancock: Heart Disease Following Radiation, Medicine, 46:281, 1967.

Puigbo, J. J., J. R. Nava Rhode, H. Garcia Barrios, J. A. Suarez, and C. Fil Yepez: Clinical and Epidemiological Study of Chronic Heart Involvement in Chagas' Disease, Bull. World Health Organ., 34:655, 1966.

Sainani, G. S., E. Krompotic, and S. J. Slodki: Adult Heart Disease Due to Coxsackie Virus B Infection, Medicine, 47:133, 1968.

Woodward, T. E., F. R. McCrumb, Jr., T. N. Carey, and Y. Togo: Viral and Rickettsial Causes of Cardiac Disease, Including the Coxsackie Virus Etiology of Pericarditis and Myocarditis, Ann. Intern. Med., 53:1130, 1960.

274 CARDIAC TUMORS AND OTHER UNUSUAL FORMS OF HEART DISEASE

Gerald Glick and Eugene Braunwald

TUMORS OF THE HEART

MYXOMA. Though rare causes of heart disease, cardiac myxomas are the commonest type of primary tumor of the heart seen in adults. Despite their rarity, myxomas are of clinical importance because they represent a potentially curable form of heart disease; therefore they always present a formidable diagnostic challenge to the clinician. Myxomas, which are histopathologically benign, occur most frequently in the atria, the left atrium being involved three times as often as the right. They are generally pedunculated, with the stem attached to the interatrial septum in the region of the foramen ovale. They may be either firm and smooth or gelatinous and polypoid. When located in the ventricles, myxomas are generally sessile. The clinical manifestations produced by cardiac myxomas may be divided into three separate groups: (1) symptoms resulting from impediment to blood flow through the heart as a result of mechanical obstruction produced by the tumor itself; (2) symptoms resulting from emboli released from the tumor into the pulmonary or systemic arterial beds; and (3) generalized constitutional abnormalities.

When the myxoma is located in the left atrium, it characteristically mimics mitral stenosis, because the pedunculated mass may fall into the mitral orifice, thereby obstructing blood flow into the left ventricle. As a result, the left atrial pressure is elevated and the increased pressure is transmitted through the pulmonary vascular bed, with consequent pulmonary congestion and pulmonary arterial hypertension. All the symptoms and some of the signs of mitral stenosis therefore may be produced (Chap. 270). In addition, episodes of syncope or sudden relief of exacerbation of symptoms with changes in posture may occur as the myxoma shifts its position in relation to the valve orifice. The pertinent physical findings include splitting of the first heart sound, accentuation of the pulmonic component of the second heart sound, an early diastolic sound attributed to the hitting of the myxoma against the ventricular wall, and both apical pansystolic and middiastolic murmurs. The auscultatory findings may change with alterations in the position of the patient. Systemic emboli, resulting from the breaking off of pieces of tumor tissue or from the formation of thrombi on the tumor, may involve any organ. In fact, when many organs are involved, attention may be diverted away from the heart. Intracardiac myxomas also produce constitutional symptoms such as weight loss, fever, weakness, anemia, hyperglobulinemia, and an elevated erythrocyte sedimentation rate. These findings may also direct attention away from the heart. Coupled with the finding of changing heart murmurs, they may suggest the diagnosis of subacute bacterial endocarditis.

When the myxoma is located in the right atrium, it produces the signs and symptoms of tricuspid stenosis. Embolization from these tumors produces pulmonary hypertension as a result of widespread obstruction of the pulmonary vascular bed. Constitutional symptoms are similar to those occurring with left atrial myxomas. Ventricular myxomas are much less common and may produce aortic or pulmonic stenosis by involving these valves, as well as emboli.

The diagnosis of intracardiac myxoma is made by selective angiocardiography. Surgical removal results in a complete cure, including relief of the constitutional symptoms.

RHABDOMYOMA. This is the most common form of primary cardiac tumor in young children. It is considered to be a hamartoma, i.e., it arises from normal embryonal elements found in the heart, and is therefore benign. It is frequently associated with tuberous sclerosis, a disease in which hamartomas of many organs occur. The left ventricle is the chamber most frequently involved, and multiple nodules are present in the interventricular septum and free wall.

SARCOMAS. These comprise the malignant primary cardiac tumors. They occur most commonly in the right atrium; as a result they may occlude inflow into the atrium from either the inferior or the superior vena cava, and produce an inferior or superior vena caval syndrome. Obstruction to right ventricular outflow may also be produced. Metastases to the vertebral column and to parenchymal organs are common. The tumors are named for the dominant cellular element involved, the most common being *fibrosarcomas, rhabdomyosarcomas,* and *angiosarcomas.*

SECONDARY TUMOR INVOLVEMENT. Metastases to the heart occur most frequently from bronchial carcinomas. Other tumors that commonly metastasize to the heart are carcinoma of the breast, malignant reticulosis, renal carcinoma, and malignant melanoma. Leukemic infiltrates have been found in one-third of patients who have died of acute leukemia. The most common abnormalities produced by secondary involvement of the heart by tumor are the production of arrhythmias and bloody pericardial effusions. Atrial fibrillation is the commonest arrhythmia seen in these circumstances.

UNUSUAL FORMS OF HEART DISEASE

MALIGNANT CARCINOID. In the usual form of carcinoid syndrome with gastrointestinal tumors and hepatic metastases (Chap. 105), the lesions in the heart are mainly on the right side and consist of tricuspid regurgitation and pulmonic stenosis. The clinical manifestations consist of dilated neck veins with prominent *v* waves, hepatomegaly, ascites, and edema. Predominantly left-sided lesions of mitral stenosis have been reported in patients with bronchial carcinoid tumors and in patients with right-to-left shunts through a patent foramen ovale. It is probable that an as yet unidentified substance released by the tumor is responsible for the development of the valvular lesions, and that this substance is removed or detoxified in the pulmonary circulation.

OBESITY. In extremely obese patients, the heart may be markedly enlarged, the left ventricle showing the greatest hypertrophy. This form of heart disease must be distinguished from the Pickwickian syndrome (Chap. 284). The clinical course of obesity heart disease is marked by congestive heart failure, with both pulmonary and systemic venous congestion. Since obesity without cardiac involvement may be responsible for dyspnea and ankle edema, evidence of superimposed congestive failure may be difficult to recognize; measurement of venous pressure and circulation time may be helpful. Also, a therapeutic trial of digitalis, diuretics, salt restriction, and weight loss may be indicated.

MYXEDEMA. (See also Chap. 89.) The heart is often seemingly enlarged, and electrocardiographic abnormalities such as low voltage, prolonged P-R interval, and T-wave alterations are common. Occasionally, arrhythmias such as paroxysmal atrial tachycardia and atrial fibrillation and high-grade atrioventricular block have been reported. Disappearance of the electrocardiographic abnormalities and arrhythmias is usual after the administration of thyroid extract, and the marked decrease of the cardiac silhouette makes it likely that the apparent enlargement of the heart is caused by a pericardial effusion. A large amount of fluid may accumulate in the pericardial space, but this rarely, if ever, causes serious tamponade. Myxedema per se, rarely, if ever, causes actual myocardial failure; when heart failure is present in patients with myxedema, it is likely that some other form of heart disease, such as ischemic heart disease, is associated with the myxedema. Because of the possibility of precipitating anginal attacks or cerebral dysfunction when arteries that have been narrowed by atherosclerotic lesions cannot provide blood flow adequate to meet the increased oxygen demands of the heart and brain, thyroid replacement therapy should be carried out with great caution, and the initial dose should be quite small.

RHEUMATOID ARTHRITIS. In rheumatoid arthritis a granulomatous lesion somewhat similar to that found in the subcutaneous nodule may affect all tissues of the heart. Clinical disorders resulting from rheumatoid heart disease have been observed rarely, except for occasional instances of acute fibrinous pericarditis, of pericardial effusion or of constrictive pericarditis. Aortic regurgitation occurs in up to 5 percent of cases of ankylosing spondylitis.

TRAUMATIC HEART DISEASE. Cardiac damage may be due to both penetrating and nonpenetrating injuries. The most frequent cause of a nonpenetrating injury is impact of the chest against the steering wheel of an automobile. Serious injury of the heart may ensue even when no external sign of thoracic trauma is evident. Although the common type of injury is myocardial contusion, any structure of the heart may be affected by the trauma. If the valve cusps become ruptured, a loud heart murmur may appear, followed by the development of rapidly progressive heart failure. Hemopericardium with fatal tamponade may follow tear of the myocardium, of a pericardial vessel, or of a coronary artery. Myocardial contusion may cause arrhythmias, bundle branch block, or electrocardiographic abnormalities resembling those of

infarction. Thus, it is important to bear trauma in mind as a cause of otherwise unexplained electrocardiographic changes. The most serious consequence of nonpenetrating injury is rupture either of the atria or of the ventricles, which is generally fatal; rarely, a patient with a ruptured ventricular or atrial septum may survive. Pericardial effusion may also occur weeks or even months after the accident, as a late manifestation of a nonpenetrating injury of the chest wall. In these cases, the pericardial effusion is a manifestation of the post-cardiac-injury syndrome, which resembles the postpericardiotomy syndrome (Chap. 272).

Conservative medical treatment for acute myocardial failure resulting from rupture of a valve is rarely effective; operative correction is usually necessary. If the electrocardiographic abnormalities are those of myocardial infarction, it may be impossible to distinguish between myocardial contusion and infarction secondary to coronary artery injury; in either case, treatment is the same, namely, that indicated for myocardial infarction due to ischemic heart disease (Chap. 271). Tamponade has been managed successfully by repeated pericardiocentesis. Other authorities recommend open drainage when tamponade recurs rapidly or when bleeding takes place into the thoracic or abdominal cavities. When pericardial hemorrhage leads to constrictive pericarditis, decortication may be necessary.

REFERENCES

Tumors of the Heart

Bigelow, J. C., R. H. Herr, and A. Starr: Atrial Myxoma, Surgery, 65:247, 1969.

Obesity

Alexander, J. K., and J. R. Pettigrove: Obesity and Congestive Heart Failure, Geriatrics, 22:101, 1967.

Traumatic Heart Disease

DeMuth, W. E., Jr., and H. F. Zinsser, Jr.: Myocardial Contusion, Arch. Intern. Med., 115:434, 1965.

Goodwin, J. F. (Ed.): Symposium on Cardiac Tumors, Am. J. Cardiol., 21:307–387, 1968.

Parmley, L. F., W. C. Manion, and T. W. Mattingly: Nonpenetrating Traumatic Injury of the Heart, Circulation, 18:371, 1958.

Section 2

Disorders of the Vascular System

275 ATHEROSCLEROSIS AND OTHER FORMS OF ARTERIOSCLEROSIS

Donald S. Fredrickson

The major cause of death in the United States and most industrialized societies is vascular insufficiency on the high pressure (arterial) side of the cardiovascular system. The largest share of such arterial failure is attributed to *arteriosclerosis,* a generic term for degeneration resulting in thickening and induration of the arterial wall. One type of arteriosclerosis is *atherosclerosis,* the disorder that underlies most *arteriosclerotic heart disease* or *coronary artery disease* (in this chapter referred to as *ischemic heart disease*) and also plays a major role in cerebrovascular disease. Atherosclerosis dwarfs all other single causes of mortality in the United States (Table 275-1). The major arterial diseases other than

Table 275-1. DEATHS FROM CARDIOVASCULAR DISEASES IN THE UNITED STATES IN 1965

Causes of Death	No. of deaths, in thousands		
	All ages	Under 65 yr	
		Males	Females
All deaths.................	1,828		
All cardiovascular disease.....	1,000	179	82
Arteriosclerotic and degenerative heart disease*	612	127	39
Cerebrovascular disease......	202	20	17
Hypertensive disease..........	67	9	8
Diseases of arteries and veins..	66	7	5
Rheumatic heart disease......	16	5	6
Congenital heart disease......	10	5	4
Other heart disease..........	29	6	4

* Rubrics 420–422 in the seventh edition of the International Classification of Disease, now referred to as "Ischemic Heart Disease" (410–414 in the eighth edition) (Table 2).

SOURCE: National Center for Health Statistics, *Vital Statistics of the United States.*

arteriosclerosis include *congenital structural defects, inflammatory* or granulomatous diseases, e.g., syphilitic aortitis, and *hypersensitivity* or autoimmune diseases. The last tend to affect the smaller vessels; they include *thromboangiitis obliterans* and possibly the specific capillary lesions of *diabetic angiopathy.*

THE ANATOMY OF ARTERIOSCLEROSIS

There is no universally accepted classification of the degenerative diseases of the arterial tree. Arteriosclerosis and its subclasses result from the interplay of multiple factors upon tissues that are limited in their range of expression and whose outwardly simple structure and metabolism are inadequately understood in their finer details.

GENERAL STRUCTURE OF ARTERIES. Endothelial Layer. All blood vessels, with the possible exception of sinusoids, are lined with a continuous single-cell layer of *endothelium.* The cells all have a well-defined plasma membrane which abuts closely to the neighboring cells. Some spacing, up to 180Å, is visible in the electron microscope, but no definite pores exist between the cells. Though there is free exchange of gas across the endothelial cells, many plasma solutes, possibly molecules up to at least 40,000 mol wt, may normally pass through the endothelial junctions. Presumably some macromolecules, including lipoproteins, are moved across the cells by the process of pinocytosis. The endothelial cells, at least in smaller vessels, have a clearly defined basement membrane, below which fine elastic fibrils extend to contact the smooth-muscle cells of the media. These fibrils usually appear as a continuous refractile strand, the *internal elastic membrane.* It is particularly prominent in the muscular arteries of medium caliber, and it disappears in capillaries. The fibrils of *collagen* and *elastin* are elaborated and maintained from the surrounding amorphous ground substance, which consists mainly of acid mucopolysaccharides produced by fibroblasts or mast cells scattered throughout the arterial wall. The amount of collagen and ground substance generally increases with age.

Medial Layer. In contrast to the longitudinal orientation of the intimal layer, the media consists of smooth-muscle cells and elastic fibers arranged in concentric spirals. In *conducting* or *elastic* vessels like the aorta, brachiocephalic, subclavian, or the beginning of the common carotid and the pulmonary arteries, elastic lamellas are very prominent. Such arteries expand and increase their elastic tension with the pulse of systole. In diastole, the elastic fibers contract. This propels the blood distally and progressively dampens the pulsatile character of flow toward more terminal vessels. In *distributing* or *muscular* arteries there is a preponderance of smooth-muscle cells and often an *external elastic membrane* between the media and adventitia. The muscular arteries regulate peripheral flow by contraction (vasoconstriction) and relaxation (vasodilatation).

There is predictable local variation in the preponderance of muscle or elastic tissue in the media and between the relative thickness of media and intima. These relationships also change with age and in response to stresses or special demands. The evolution of the coronary arteries is an example. These are arteries of the muscular type, representing a sudden transition from the more elastic aorta. At birth the media is thicker than the intima. During life both layers continue to increase, particularly by accumulating elastic elements and collagen. The intima thickens more rapidly, however, and exceeds the width of the media by the thirtieth year. Sometimes, apparently as a compensatory mechanism, smooth muscle may even ultimately appear in the intima. The evolution of the coronary vessels is about the same in men and women; possibly the intimal changes are not unrelated to the predilection of these vessels for atheroma formation.

Adventitial Layer. The external coat of the arteries consists mainly of longitudinally directed bundles of collagen fibers. In addition, there are fibroblasts, some elastic fibers, nerve bundles, and small blood vessels (*vasa vasorum*).

Metabolism and Nutrition. Studies of arterial tissue or cultured endothelial fibroblasts have established their capacity for both aerobic and anaerobic metabolism (glycolysis), the presence of a number of enzymes, including lipoprotein lipase and fibrinolytic activity, and the ability of the cells to synthesize cholesterol and phospholipids, to take up various fats and lipoproteins, and to incorporate components into ground substance. They have not adequately clarified the metabolism of a structure that must accommodate to the stresses and strains of continuous flow at high pressures of a viscous and complex fluid along its surface and also meet a steady demand for energy production, both to maintain smooth-muscle tension and to replenish and repair a great many tissue elements. One of the simplest aspects of the arterial wall is presently of the most help in understanding the importance of the anatomic changes associated with arteriosclerosis. This is the presence of a nutritional "watershed" in the wall of most arteries. The flux of oxygen and substrates and the reverse flow of catabolic products are directed both from the luminal and adventitial sides. There is a division point, about midway in the media, beyond which the vasa vasorum in the adventitia do not supply. Hence the integrity of transfer across the endothelial wall is essential, and the various responses of the intima to assure the nutrition of the inner half of the arterial wall become paramount in the development of arteriosclerosis.

Intimal Response to Injury. If the intima is denuded, the endothelial cells rapidly proliferate and form a new lining on vessels or contiguous foreign substances, such as prostheses. Damage to the endothelium also promotes thrombus formation, possibly initiated by adherence of platelets. The cells undertake the rapid organization of such thrombi, including the rapid formation of new capillaries within them. At the very least, however, the ultimate reaction to thrombus formation or adherence of platelets or fibrin to the endothelial surface will be thickening of the intima. Interruption of endothelial integrity leads to other reactions, as deduced from experimental studies with arterial tissue or other models such as the cornea. Among the earliest reactions of isolated endothelial cells to injury is the accelerated formation of intracellular vesicles that may be serving to transport fat or lipoproteins across the wall. The introduction of excess lipids into the intima leads to formation of scavenger foam cells from endothelial cells or other primitive cell types. This is accompanied by increase in collagen, elastic fibrils, and ground substance. Capillaries may proceed inward from the lumen, again compensating for altered diffusion of oxygen and other nutrients. These in turn may allow intramural hemorrhage, which promotes further reaction. The end stages include calcification, sclerosis, and a distorted arterial wall, ultimately obliterating the lumen. Such intimal thickening and these subsequent alterations may also be initiated by events deeper in the wall. These include the smooth-muscle hyperplasia or hyalinoid degeneration in the media associated with hypertension, involutional or focal changes, and molecular abnormalities such as the abortive collagen formation in Marfan's syndrome.

FORMS OF ARTERIOSCLEROSIS

Atherosclerosis involves primarily the intimal layer, most commonly in the aorta, coronary, and cerebral arteries. It may accompany or accelerate the other major forms of arteriosclerosis, which consist of (1) *involutional* or *senile* changes, (2) *focal calcification*, and (3) *arteriolosclerosis*. They involve primarily the medial layer and usually affect segments of the arterial tree other than those in which atherosclerosis is most prominent.

INVOLUTIONAL CHANGES. Arteries normally undergo changes with age that are not necessarily classified as arteriosclerosis unless they occur prematurely. The walls of most arteries *thicken* up to about the age of twenty-five. Thereafter there is a gradual loss of distensibility. This implies a relative increase in the number and "slack" of collagen fibers, with resulting increase in the elastic constant of the wall. The loss of distensibility and the associated multiplication of elastic fibers (*elastosis*) are the major changes of senescence. Other involutional changes begin in midlife, especially in the abdominal aorta and its iliac, splenic, renal, hepatic, and superior mesenteric branches. Loss of elasticity is accompanied by medial atrophy, increase in collagen, and sclerosis with calcification. The vessels become dilated and elongated, and an aneurysm may form, especially if medial degeneration is accelerated by an encroaching intimal plaque. Such "wear-and-tear" lesions are frequently proportional to the vessel diameter and correlated with branching, curvature, and anatomic points of attachment. The amount of external support also determines the ability of vessels, weakened by loss of elasticity, to withstand hydrostatic pressure. The unsupported cerebral arteries are particularly vulnerable in this regard and are more subject to rupture than any other vessels. Though senescence is accompanied by the intimal thickening, medial calcification, and elastosis that are features of localized atheromatosis, all in all, there is a lack of direct correlation between many changes of senescence and arteriosclerosis.

FOCAL CALCIFICATION. Not to be confused with atherosclerosis is focal calcification of the media of smaller arteries. This includes *Mönckeberg's arteriosclerosis*, common in the lower extremities, and *Fahr's sclerosis*, calcification of the extramural branches of the cerebral arteries.

ARTERIOLOSCLEROSIS. This disorder represents alterations in small arteries that are particularly common in hypertension. Lesser degrees of sustained hypertension characteristically cause *hyaline proliferation* in renal arterioles; more severe or malignant hypertension produces a pathognomonic *fibrous hyperplasia* of the media and intima.

ATHEROSCLEROSIS

Although a scourge of modern civilizations, atherosclerosis is an ancient disease which has been detected in Egyptian mummies and described in Greek writings. The term *atheroma* (from the Greek *athere*, gruel) was revived by Albrecht von Haller of Bern (1755) to focus attention on the softening process which often accompanies the sclerosis and the aneurysms that had been emphasized earlier by Vesalius and other anatomists of the sixteenth and seventeenth centuries. For a time in the nineteenth century, it was believed that events at the endothelial blood interface might cause atheromas (Rokitansky); but by the time the term *atherosclerosis* was coined (Marchand, 1904), the dominant concept was that the lesions were intimal softenings secondary to an increase in subintimal connective tissue that in turn was due to irritative or mechanical forces. The present-day preoccupation with the etiologic importance of lipid infiltration began about 1910 with the demonstration of an increased amount of cholesterol in atheromas (Windhaus, Aschoff) and the experimental production of atherosclerosis by feeding cholesterol (Ignatowski, Anitschkow, and others). The most significant advances in understanding the disease have recently been derived from epidemiologic data. No single cause of human atherosclerosis has been rigorously demonstrated.

MORBID ANATOMY. Atherosclerosis is basically a nodular type of arteriosclerosis, grossly visible as yellow fatty plaques irregularly distributed over the intimal surface. Microscopically, the nodules appear mainly to be increased fibrous tissue in the intima or at other times to be highly cellular or granulomatous deposits containing fat. Sometimes a fresh thrombus is adherent to the surface of the plaque, or there may be evidence of an old thrombus, already organized by capillaries arising from a thickened intimal layer beneath. Capillaries may also come from deeper regions of the media, and a vascular network seeming to arise from both the lumen and the vasa vasorum may penetrate the atheroma. There is often evidence that this dual blood supply from such anastomoses is inadequate, for necrosis, presumed to be ischemic, is very common in the region between intima and media in atheromas. In addition there are often fragmentation and reduplication of elastic fibers, calcification, and eventually sclerosis of the plaque. The first lesions may consist of the *fatty streak* or *milk streak* grossly visible as a nonelevated yellow or whitish patch on the intimal surface. These lesions may appear in the aorta, the coronaries, and other arteries as early as infancy or childhood, but in locations that are sometimes dissimilar to the sites favored by atheromas. Though the fatty streak may be a precursor of the plaque, it is not always so and often completely resolves.

LOCALIZATION. The aorta and the left coronary artery are the "index vessels" for most surveys of atherosclerosis.

The *aorta* is most heavily involved in the arch, about the orifices of its branches, particularly the coronaries and intercostals, in its abdominal portion, and frequently at its terminal bifurcation into the iliacs. There is more atherosclerosis in the lower limbs than the upper ones. In the legs, the incidence decreases peripherally, as the musculoelastic vessels give way to large muscular arteries and these become smaller vessels, such as the plantar or digital arteries. Intimal thickening, plaques, and thrombosis are particularly common in the *femoral* artery, in Hunter's canal, and in the *popliteal* artery just above the knee joint. The *anterior* and *posterior tibials* are often occluded together, but in different sites—the posterior where it rounds the internal mallelous, the anterior where it is superficial and becoming the dorsalis pedis artery. The peroneal artery, which is well embedded in muscle, often escapes while other major vessels are occluded, and it may be the main blood supply to the extremity (*pero-*

neal leg). Atherosclerosis in abdominal branches, except for the renal arteries, causes much less difficulty than in coronary or cerebral vessels.

Involvement of the *coronary arteries* is sometimes out of proportion to atherosclerosis elsewhere. Atheromas are most prominent in the main stems, the highest incidence being a short distance beyond the ostiums. The epicardial portions of the vessels are much more involved than the transmuscular segments. The left coronary is usually more affected than the right. In the *cerebral vessels* the distribution of atherosclerosis is patchy, as it is elsewhere in the body. It first appears in the base of the brain in the carotid, basilar, and vertebral arteries. The proximal portion of the internal carotids in the neck is a site of special predilection. There is a concentration of lesions near bifurcations. Atherosclerosis in the *retinal vessels* may often be secondary to other arteriopathies, such as those due to hypertension or diabetes. Whether atheromas cause the common intrinsic lesions of retinal vessels that lead to decreased choroidal circulation and macular degeneration with aging has not been clarified. Atherosclerosis in the *pulmonary artery* bears no relation to the severity of the disease in the aorta or other systemic arteries. There is some involvement in about half of adults over fifty who have no reason to have pulmonary hypertension. Pulmonary hypertension per se, however, is associated with medial hypertrophy, intimal thickening, and great acceleration of atheroma formation.

THE RECOGNITION OF ATHEROSCLEROSIS. Except for angiographic visualization of the vessel lumen or perhaps the ophthalmodynametric detection of differences in retinal artery pressure due to carotid insufficiency, there is no satisfactory antemortem means of demonstrating silent atherosclerosis. Calcification in the location of coronary vessels can be demonstrated radiographically and usually indicates atherosclerosis, but complete luminal obstruction may occur in the absence of any calcification. Calcification, or beading, of peripheral arteries and funduscopic changes are not correlated directly with atherosclerosis, and no direct blood chemical indexes of the disease exist. Detection usually waits upon one of the clinical complications attending rupture or a critical decrease of blood flow in an involved vessel. Ischemic electrocardiographic changes, principally S-T segment depressions, during strenuous exercise, suggest myocardial ischemia, which most commonly results from coronary atherosclerosis.

INCIDENCE. Knowledge of the prevalence and incidence of arteriosclerosis and most of the inferences concerning its causes are derived from tabulations of the appearance of its complications. Table 275-1 shows that the majority of deaths in the United States is attributed to ischemic heart disease and cerebrovascular disease. Together they accounted for 44 percent of all deaths in 1965 and for 28 percent of the deaths under age sixty-five. The estimated cost of these 200,000 deaths occurring before age sixty-five in that year, in calculated future lifetime earnings alone, was between 10 and 15 billion dollars.

Ischemic heart disease (IHD), synonymous with coronary artery disease or arteriosclerotic heart disease, is the most useful indicator of atherosclerosis available today. Over 90 percent of patients with *coronary occlusion,* as defined by electrocardiographic and enzyme changes, incident to *myocardial infarction* have coronary atherosclerosis. At autopsy, ostial occlusion due to other types of vascular disease, emboli, aneurysms, or other structural abnormalities is rare; and one or more atheromatous plaques reducing the lumen of one or more vessels are nearly always present. The International Atherosclerosis Project has compared the incidence of deaths from IHD and the intimal surface of the left coronary artery involved by raised atheromatous lesions in autopsy samples from many United States and Latin American populations. The correlation was impressive. Nontraumatic *sudden death,* often certified as due to IHD, makes up a sizable portion (about 40 percent) of all deaths due to myocardial infarction, and presents a special problem in the epidemiology of atherosclerosis. At autopsy, evidence of fresh myocardial infarction is usually absent; and a fresh *coronary thrombosis* may not be present. Support is often not obtainable for the presumption that *cardiac arrest* was due to sudden closure of a partially compromised vessel, whether from a small thrombus or embolus that has subsequently lysed or from *spasm.* In one series over 60 percent of "cardiac sudden deaths" occurred in patients previously diagnosed as having IHD. Ten percent were diabetics and one-quarter were hypertensive. The sum of autopsy and epidemiologic studies to date indicates that at least half, probably more, of all "sudden deaths" involves atherosclerosis as an important contributing cause. Ischemic changes as seen on the electrocardiogram, without apparent infarction, and *angina pectoris* are good but less-infallible signs of atherosclerosis and are generally treated separately as "end points" in epidemiologic studies. Cerebrovascular disease includes both *cerebral hemorrhage* and *cerebral thrombosis,* the latter usually representing infarction due to atherosclerosis and softening without evidence of embolus. Cerebral hemorrhage is often due to congenital aneurysms or other vascular defects peculiar to hypertension and diabetes; on the other hand, cerebral thrombosis correlates well with atherosclerosis. It may be observed in Table 275-1 that the sex differential between cerebrovascular (and hypertensive) disease and IHD is considerable under the age of sixty-five years. Furthermore, in a country such as Japan, the death rates from cerebral hemorrhage and thrombosis are diverging rapidly. Although "strokes" are often a complication of atherosclerosis and the general incidence in the United States is correlated with certain risk factors such as hypercholesterolemia, in a manner similar to such correlation in IHD, cerebrovascular disease is an impure criterion of the prevalence of atherosclerosis in a population or in a single patient. The same is true for dissecting aneurysms, thrombosis of other major vessels, or renal ischemia. For all these reasons, the present discussion of atherosclerosis revolves about IHD. It also concentrates particularly on that which is "premature," arbitrarily defined as IHD appearing before age sixty-five.

ISCHEMIC HEART DISEASE

INCIDENCE. According to the National Health Survey, about 5 million Americans have IHD (See Chap. 271), which is second to hypertension as the most prevalent cardiovascular disease. Premature deaths from IHD occur preponderantly in men. Between the ages of thirty-five and fifty-five the death rate is nearly six times higher in white men than in white women in the United States; this difference narrows after the menopause (Table 275-2). The only exceptions are women with severe hypertension, diabetes, or premature (usually iatrogenic) menopause, who share the risk of the male. A distressing higher mortality rate in nonwhite women (Table 275-2) is

Table 275-2. DEATH RATES IN THE UNITED STATES FROM ISCHEMIC HEART DISEASE (DEATHS PER 100,000)

Sex	Age	White	Nonwhite
Male.........	25–34	10	21
	35–44	87	108
	45–54	346	322
	55–64	906	760
	65–74	1,973	1,674
Female........	25–34	2	9
	35–44	14	48
	45–54	67	162
	55–64	260	489
	65–74	911	1,048

SOURCE: *Vital Statistics of the United States,* 1965.

probably due mainly to a greater incidence of hypertension in Negroes. There is less difference between men and women in the prevalence of angina pectoris than of myocardial infarction; after age sixty-five more women than men have angina without a history of infarction. IHD accounts for practically all the excess mortality in American males below age sixty-five (Table 275-1), emphasizing again that cerebrovascular and hypertensive complications do not reflect the effects of accelerated atherosclerosis in the same manner as does IHD. The death rate from IHD has been rising in the United States since 1930. In the decade 1953–1963 it was the only major form of cardiovascular disease in which there was not a significant decline in death rate, even in persons below age sixty-five. The percentage increase in death rate in recent years has been very little. This reflects a steady decline in death from hypertension and may also indicate that the United States population is coming into equilibrium with the major factors that produce much of its premature disability and death.

INTERNATIONAL COMPARISONS. In most of those countries from which adequate statistics are available, IHD is the major single cause of premature cardiovascular deaths. A notable exception is Japan, which has the highest death rate from cerebrovascular disease and one of the lowest from IHD, the age-adjusted rate for all men thirty-five to sixty-four being only 16 percent of that in the United States. Greece and Yugoslavia have even lower IHD death rates in young men than Japan. Among industrialized societies, the United States, Finland, and Scotland have the highest death rates from IHD, followed by the rest of the United Kingdom, the Netherlands, and Scandinavia. Sweden, for example, has an age-adjusted premature death rate in males from IHD that is one-half of that in the United States. This difference results in an excess of deaths before age sixty-five of about 60,000 males in the United States. The rates in Scandinavia and Europe are converging and climbing much faster than in the United States. In the United Kingdom the death rate began to rise before or during World War II. The low rates in Norway and the Netherlands during World War II have risen rapidly (90 percent in Norway between 1953 and 1963). The trend for women in all countries has been similar to that for men.

RISK FACTORS IN IHD. Many of the theories about the origin of accelerated atherosclerosis and its prevention are derived from relating the prevalence or incidence of IHD in a population (or in more than one) with certain biologic, demographic, and social variables. From these have emerged a few variables, quantitatively assessable and mathematically correlated with increased IHD, and considered definite *risk factors*. The major ones are *hyperlipemia, cigarette smoking, hypertension,* and *obesity* (in the order of their correlation with IHD in multivariate analyses of the Framingham data in men of ages thirty to sixty-two), and *diabetes*. They are listed in Table 275-3,

Table 275-3. TEN INDEXES TO INCREASED SUSCEPTIBILITY
TO PREMATURE ATHEROSCLEROSIS (IHD)

1. Age
2. Hyperlipidemia
   a. Cholesterol or LDL (low-density lipoprotein) increase
   b. Triglyceride or VLDL (very low-density lipoprotein) increase
3. Cigarette smoking
4. Hypertension
5. Obesity
6. Diabetes
7. Physical inactivity
8. Hyperuricemia
9. Positive family history (premature IHD, diabetes, xanthoma, and hyperlipidemia)
10. Electrocardiographic abnormalities

along with five other indexes to increased susceptibility to premature IHD, a clinician's checklist for the minimum screening necessary for detection of those persons at above-average hazard for the complications of atherosclerosis. Of these other determinants, *age* and *electrocardiographic abnormalities*, particularly those of left ventricular hypertrophy, intraventricular block, and atrial fibrillation, have a strong and calculable association with increased morbidity from IHD. *Uric acid* levels greater than 6.9 mg per 100 ml carry a significantly increased risk in one or two studies. *Physical activity* and *personality type* may be assigned important but less-quantitative significance. A positive family history is a secondary

route to detection of other risk factors. There are many other possible risk factors, but as yet their implication remains on an intuitive rather than a factual basis.

Risk factors shift in their relative importance with age and tend to be additive. For example, in a cohort understudy in Framingham, Mass., the combination of hypercholesterolemia, hypertension, and cigarette smoking increased the incidence of IHD eight times over that held by men with none of these factors. The risk was five times greater than that associated with any one factor and two and one-half times that associated with any two factors.

HYPERLIPIDEMIA

The lipids in plasma of major general clinical importance are *cholesterol, triglycerides,* and *free fatty acids* (FFA). All circulate bound to protein, the FFA with albumin, the cholesterol and triglycerides along with *phospholipids* in *lipoproteins*. The FFA are most important in meeting caloric demands and have the most labile concentrations. They have not yet been directly tied to premature atherosclerosis. The normal concentration (0.3 to 0.7 μ Eq per liter) of FFA is increased when tissue insulin activity is low or glucose utilization is deficient and by the excessive sympathetic or catecholamine discharge that may arise from such diverse causes as emotional stress, nicotine, and caffeine. The FFA released from adipose tissue in excess of those utilized by muscle, liver, or other tissues mainly reappear in plasma as *endogenous glyceride*. FFA play a key role in supplying oxidizable substrate to the heart, are a delicate indicator of the state of carbohydrate metabolism, and have an indirect effect on the concentration of plasma lipoproteins. FFA may cause intravascular thrombosis, but this has been demonstrated only in concentrations exceeding those reached in health or disease.

The lipoproteins are separable by various methods into four major classes: *high-density* (HDL or alpha-lipoproteins), *low-density* (LDL, beta- or S_f 0 to 20 lipoproteins), *very low-density* (VLDL, pre-beta- or S_f 20 to 400 lipoproteins), and *chylomicrons*. HDL has some not clearly defined function in maintaining tissue levels of cholesterol and the level of cholesterol esters in plasma. HDL concentrations are higher in women than in men, and administration of estrogens raises HDL, while administration of androgens lowers HDL. Neither this knowledge nor estrogen administration to men with IHD has led to an understanding of the role of HDL or of sex hormones in atherosclerosis. Less than one-third of the plasma cholesterol is in HDL. Most of the cholesterol is carried in LDL, and this lipoprotein class correlates best with total plasma cholesterol. LDL has an important function in facilitating glyceride transport. Both HDL and LDL combine with *endogenous* glycerides to make up the very low-density lipoproteins. Chylomicrons are the large particles in which dietary or *exogenous* fat is carried from the intestinal lacteals to the bloodstream via the thoracic duct.

TYPES OF HYPERLIPOPROTEINEMIA. Rises in cholesterol generally reflect either increased LDL or VLDL or both.

Increases in plasma glycerides imply increased VLDL or chylomicrons. Both scatter light and impart the lactescence or turbidity commonly known as *hyperlipemia*. Modest *exogenous* (dietary or fat-induced) hyperlipemia due to chylomicron accumulation is normal up to 6 hr after fat ingestion. After an overnight fast the presence of chylomicrons is abnormal. Genetically determined hyperchylomicronemia (type I hyperlipoproteinemia) is not associated with accelerated IHD. Discrete elevations in LDL (type II hyperlipoproteinemia) may be due to excessive intake of saturated fats and cholesterol, hypothyroidism, liver disease, genetic abnormalities (Chap. xx), dysglobinemias, diabetes, and other causes. *Endogenous hyperlipemia* is the elevation of VLDL, and *mixed hyperlipemia* involves a combination of increased VLDL and chylomicrons. These types of hyperlipoproteinemia may be familial (types III, IV, and V, Chap. xx) or may be secondary to other diseases, most commonly those with abnormalities in glucose tolerance and insulin secretion.

Correlation with IHD. Hyperlipidemia is associated unequivocally with increased incidence of premature IHD. Hypercholesterolemia has been measured more extensively than any other lipid or lipoprotein. It correlates highly with the risk of myocardial infarction in both men and women, more highly with men. For both sexes combined over a 14-year study in Framingham, the relative incidence of infarction between ages thirty and forty-nine at starting cholesterol levels > 260 mg per 100 ml was fourfold that at cholesterols < 220; for men, the difference was sixfold. A cholesterol level between 220 and 260 was associated with twice the incidence. These data are supported by comparisons of prevalence of IHD and cholesterol in other populations, notably in Israel. LDL has the same relationship to IHD as does cholesterol. Measurements of triglycerides or VLDL also show a correlation between modest elevations and increased prevalence or incidence of IHD. One Swedish study has suggested that in young men glyceride elevations are a better index to risk than cholesterol. Moreover, risk of IHD is increased in a significant number of subjects who have elevated glyceride levels (or VLDL) and *normal* cholesterol levels. This has been shown also in a study of lipoprotein patterns in patients with abnormal coronary angiograms. The *atherogenic index* (Gofman) thus takes into account both LDL and VLDL. [Where A.I. (the atherogenic index), $= [S_f° \ 0\text{--}12 + 1.75 \ (S_f° \ 12\text{--}400)]/10$, a value over 75 to 100 is considered to represent a definitely higher risk for IHD.]

All studies indicate that hyperlipidemia is a more meaningful risk factor below age fifty and that it operates independently of obesity, hypertension, and diabetes. Considering the increased risks demonstrated for subjects with cholesterol > 220 mg per 100 ml, it is of interest to compare this figure with the mean and distribution of cholesterol levels in Americans (Table 275-4). It is apparent that much of the population falls in a range where increased risk may be determined by modest differences in cholesterol concentration.

DETECTION OF HYPERLIPIDEMIA. Screening for hyperlipidemia as a risk factor in atherosclerosis requires at least one prebreakfast sample of blood, while the subject is eating a regular diet, in which plasma (or serum) concentrations of cholesterol *and* triglycerides are determined. If both are clearly within "normal" limits (Table 275-4),

Table 275-4. PLASMA LIPID CONCENTRATIONS IN AMERICANS, MG/100 ML*

Age, yr	Cholesterol	Triglycerides
1–19	175 (120–230)	70 (10–140)
20–29	180 (120–240)	70 (10–140)
30–39	205 (140–270)	75 (10–150)
40–49	225 (150–310)	85 (10–160)
50–59	245 (160–330)	95 (10–190)

* The approximate mean and upper and lower 5 percent limits for Americans; the data are calculated from small samples and ignore significant differences between the sexes in different age groups.

further analyses are not necessary. If one or both is elevated, plasma lipoprotein patterns will be helpful in distinguishing elevations in LDL, VLDL, and chylomicrons, and perhaps the diagnosis of specific genetic defects. A precise quantification of atherogenic index is less helpful than understanding of the various metabolic abnormalities and possibly the dietary origin of the hyperlipoproteinemia.

Diet and Hyperlipidemia

Several decades of research and debate have resolved into good agreement concerning at least three dietary determinants of the plasma cholesterol concentration in "normal" subjects. These are the intake of saturated and polyunsaturated fats and of cholesterol. One formulation of their relationship is that of Keys, Anderson, and Grande:

$$\Delta C = a(2S - P) + bZ$$

where $\Delta C =$ the change in plasma cholesterol, in mg per 100 ml, due to isocaloric changes in the percentage of total calories provided by saturated (S) and polyunsaturated (P) fatty acids

$Z =$ the square root of the dietary cholesterol in mg per 1000 cal of diet

a and $b =$ constants of about equal weight

Such a formulation has been developed from metabolic experiments and confirmed in field studies, including the recent National Diet Heart Study involving 1,200 men. The clinical usefulness of such an equation is qualitative. It emphasizes that the *quantity* of S and P eaten is more relevant than the simple P/S ratio of dietary fat, that both reduction of S and increased feeding of P help to lower cholesterol, and that the influence of these modifications is greater than the actual amount of cholesterol ingested. The influential saturated fatty acids are those

Table 275-5. FAT AND CHOLESTEROL CONTENT OF THE TYPICAL AMERICAN DIET

Food	Amount, Gm/person/day	Fat consumption				Cholesterol	
		Gm fat/day	% total/day	P/S		Approx. cholesterol content of foods, mg/100 Gm	Consumption, mg/day
Meats:							
Beef, veal, lamb..........	98	19	....	<0.1		75	73
Pork, lard, lunch meat.....	90	31	....	<0.2		70	63
Liver, other organ meats...	5	≤1		<0.2		300	15
Total..................	193	50	34				151
Poultry:							
Chicken, turkey..........	39	2	1	<0.7		60	23
Fish and shellfish:							
Fish..................	18	1		<2.5		70	12
Shellfish (shrimp, crab, oyster, etc.)...........	2	≤1				160	3
Total..................	20	1	<1	<2.5			15
Dairy products:							
Milk, fresh; whole and chocolate..............	331	12		<0.1		10	33
Milk, processed; whole.....	62	2		<0.1		10	6
Cream (all kinds).........	6	1		<0.1		65	4
Frozen milk desserts.......	56	7		<0.1		45	25
Cheese (cheddar type).....	13	4		<0.1		100	13
Cheese (cottage).........	9	<1		<0.1		15	1
Butter................	8	7		<0.1		250	21
Milk, skim, buttermilk.....	36			<0.1		5	2
Total..................	521	33	23				105
Eggs: fresh and equivalent ...	48	6	4	<0.3		550	264
Margarine and shortening:							
Margarine..............	16	13		<0.4		Neg	
Shortening..............	7	7		<0.4		Neg	
Total..................	23	20	14				
Salad oil and dressing							
Oils, oil-type dressing......	9	8		>3.0		0	0
Mayonnaise type.........	9	6		>3.0		54	5
Total..................	18	14	10				5
Bakery products and cereals:							
Flour, cereals, and pastas ..	83	1		<4.0		0	0
Bread, rolls..............	93	3		<0.7		Neg	
Crackers	10	1		<0.7		Neg	
Bakery products (cake, pie, muffins)..............	48	8		Varies		Varies	22
Prepared flour mixes	9	1		Varies		Varies	5
Total..................	243	14	10				27
Other fat							
Chocolate; chocolate candy.	6	2		<0.1		Neg	
Other candy	4	<1		<0.2		Varies	
Potato chips.............	4	2		2.0		Neg	
Nuts, peanut butter.......	8	1		<1.5		0	
Other vegetables and fruit..	326	≤1		—		0	0
Total..................	348	5	3				
Totals.................		145	99%	0.3 (average)			590

SOURCE: Prepared by Miss J. L. Tillotson from the following sources: (A) *Food consumption*: "Food Consumption of Households in the United States, U.S. Department of Agriculture Household Food Consumption Survey 1965–1966, Report No. 1. Quantities reported in terms of "quantity per household per week" were used to derive average consumption (in grams) per individual per week. (B) *Food composition*: (1) Values for average fat and fatty acid composition of food were taken from: (a) "Composition of Foods," Agriculture Handbook No. 8 by Bernice K. Watt and Annabel L. Merrill, December, 1963. (b) "Fatty Acids in Food Fats," U.S. Department of Agriculture Home Economics Research Report 7, by V. R. Goddard and L. Goodall, 1959. (2) Values for cholesterol content of foods were derived from Watt and Merrill, *op. cit.*

of 12 carbons or greater, the most important in the United States diet being palmitic acid (16:0). Stearic acid (18:0) and short-chain acids, including butyric, appear to have no significant effect on cholesterol levels. The same is true for the monounsaturates (m), which in the diet consist mainly of oleic (18:1) acid, especially high in olive oil, and erucic (22:1) acid; hence the absence of an "M" term in diets dealing with hyperlipemia and a preoccupation with the P/S content of specific foods. The polyunsaturates in the diet are mainly linoleic (18:2) and linolenic (18:3) acids, an exception being fish oils, which have a higher content of longer-chain, highly unsaturated acids.

The present content of the "typical" American diet shown in Table 275-5 is broken down relative to fat and cholesterol. Immediately apparent is the dominant contribution of animal fats, which have a low P/S ratio and provide a singular source of cholesterol. It should be noted that the predominantly unsaturated vegetable fats and oils (exceptions being coconut oil and cocoa butter) in particular foods are often hydrogenated to improve their shelf life and harden their consistency. Sometimes plasticizers are used to keep relatively unsaturated margarines and shortenings solid at room temperature. There are several basic changes in diet that can be made when it is desired to conform with present-day knowledge of the determinants of plasma cholesterol concentrations. One practical approach is to base diets almost entirely on the percentage of calories provided by saturated fat (Brown et al.). Another is to pay more rigorous attention to dietary cholesterol, maintaining it as low as 100 mg per day, the stringent limit of practical dietary control. A set of menus representing one of the currently most recommended diet plans is shown in Table 275-6. Compared with the typical American food intake (Table 275-5), this diet provides a little more than half as much saturated fat, four times as much polyunsaturated fat, and about 40 percent of the usual cholesterol intake. The P/S ratio of the total fat is about 1.5, compared with the typical ratio of 0.3. Egg yolks should be limited to three a week. Beef, lamb, or pork is used only three times a week. Butter, cream, and whole dairy products are excluded. This diet also requires that four or more tablespoons of vegetable oil (other than olive oil) per day be used in salads or for baking and frying. Margarines with high P/S content may be used to provide one-fourth of this requirement. Such margarines are identifiable in the store as those which have "liquid oil" listed as the first ingredient on the label. It is emphasized that the mechanism by which such a diet tends to lower the plasma cholesterol level has not been established, although no harmful effects have been observed, provided the rest of the diet meets known nutritional requirements. These dietary modifications are applicable to most patients with hyperlipidemia, but may not have any visible effect on some types of hyperlipidemia in which glyceride elevations are extreme.

DIET AND HYPERGLYCERIDEMIA. The effect of dietary carbohydrate or protein on the plasma cholesterol level has not been established. The plasma glyceride and VLDL concentrations, however, at least in the postprandial state, are higher on very high carbohydrate diets than on high fat diets. Patients on the rice diet, for example, often have triglycerides above the normal mean, a phenomenon which led to the eventual elucidation of the phenomenon of *carbohydrate induction* of hyperlipemia. Normal subjects who are fed 75 percent of their calories as carbohydrate (7 Gm/kg/day) will usually have twice the glyceride levels they maintain on regular diets. Simple sugars and starches have about the same effect, although fructose sometimes has a brief, more dramatic effect. Obese patients, particularly those with abnormal glucose tolerance and either high or low insulin responses to glucose, or patients with familial type III or IV hyperlipoproteinemia may have exaggerated responses to high carbohydrate feeding. In particular they may fail to adapt to such diets as well as normal subjects whose glycerides usually return to lower levels despite continued high carbohydrate intake. Not all endogenous hyperglyceridemia is due to "carbohydrate induction." As a general rule, however, such patients should be brought to ideal body weight and given diets that do not contain more than 40 percent of calories in carbohydrate. The effect of dietary carbohydrate on lipid levels in the general population is not established. It has not been demonstrated that as much as 55 percent carbohydrate in the diet (as obtained with the usual limits of fat restriction) increases glyceride or cholesterol concentrations. The correlation between consumption of refined sugars and prevalence of IHD in a number of populations is as good as the correlation of IHD with saturated fat intake. The correlation between sugar and saturated fat consumption is even higher. The relationship of dietary carbohydrate to atherogenesis is complex and unresolved.

ALCOHOL. In man and animals, sustained administration of ethanol may elevate the levels of VLDL and triglycerides. "Binge drinkers" may develop sudden hyperlipemia, often with hyperuricemia and sometimes abdominal pain with or without elevated serum amylase level. The mechanism responsible for hyperglyceridemia is not known. Only the intemperate use of alcohol, especially when it contributes to caloric excess, may be considered a possible minor risk factor in atherosclerosis.

DIET AND ATHEROSCLEROSIS. A relationship of diet to plasma cholesterol level and of cholesterol to prevalence or incidence of IHD has been established. The sum of all geographic studies to date strongly indicates an association between IHD and a high intake of saturated fat and of sucrose. Still there is a paucity of published data providing a systematic correlation of the general diet of many different populations and the prevalence of atherosclerosis or IHD. The link between diet and atherosclerosis has yet to be forged from rigorous, statistically significant evidence. It must be procured using two major study designs. One is *secondary prevention,* the alteration of diet (or some other intervention) in patients who have definite atherosclerosis or, more practically, IHD, and observation of the effect on subsequent morbidity and mortality rates. A model study of this type involving drugs is the National Heart Institute's Coronary Drug

Table 275-6. SUGGESTED 2400-CAL MEAL PLAN*

Food	Typical portion size of one serving or one "exchange"	Breakfast portion	Lunch portion	Dinner portion	Snacks portion	Remarks
Milk, nonfat.............	1 cup-(8 oz)	1	....	1	....	Skim milk; buttermilk from skim milk
Vegetables:						
Low carbohydrate......	....	....	As desired	As desired	As desired	Raw vegetable salads; leafy vegetables, tomatoes, etc.
Medium carbohydrate..	½ cup	....	....	1	....	Carrots, beets, peas, etc.
Fruit..................	½ cup; 1 small apple	1	1	1	2	Fresh, frozen, canned; if sweetened, subtract 2 sugar exchanges per portion
Bread, cereals, starches....	1 slice bread, or ½ cup cereal, or potato	2	2	2	2	
Lean meat, fish, poultry...	1 oz, cooked weight	..	3	4	....	11 meals/week—poultry (no skin), veal, fish, uncreamed cottage cheese; 3 meals/week—lean beef, lamb, or pork well trimmed of fat
Eggs.................	....	..	....	....	....	3–4 per week—as substitute for meat (1 egg = 1 oz meat)
Fat..................	1 tsp.	..	6	9	....	Vegetable oil (except olive) and salad dressing from these oils
Special margarine........	1 tsp.	1	....	1	1	Margarine with 30–40% polyunsaturates; first-named ingredient on label should be "liquid oil"
Sugar, sweets............	1 tsp.	5	3	2	2	

SAMPLE MENU (2400-CAL MEAL PLAN; 35–40% OF CALORIES FROM FAT; HIGH IN POLYUNSATURATES, LOW IN CHOLESTEROL)

Breakfast	Lunch	Dinner	Snack

½ grapefruit
2 tsp. sugar
½ cup cooked cereal
2 tsp. sugar
1 slice toast
1 tsp. special margarine
1 tsp. jelly
1 cup skim milk
	Sandwich:
	  3 oz chicken
	  1 tbsp. mayonnaise
	  2 slices bread
	Salad:
	  Lettuce, celery, green pepper,
	  1 tbsp. oil, vinegar to taste
	1 small apple baked with 1 tbsp. sugar
		4 oz breaded haddock, fried in
		  1 tbsp. oil (bread crumbs
		  from 1 slice bread)
		½ cup potatoes, fried in 1 tsp. oil
		½ cup tomato & lettuce salad,
		  2 tsp. oil, vinegar to taste
		½ cup peas with 1 tsp. special
		  margarine
		1 tbsp. mayonnaise with relish as
		  tartar sauce
		1 small pear with 2 tsp. sugar (or
		  two sweetened canned pear
		  halves)
		1 cup skim milk
			2 slices cinnamon toast with
			  1 tsp. special margarine
			2 tsp. sugar
			½ cup orange juice
			½ small banana

* 35–40% of Calories from fat; high in polyunsaturates, low in cholesterol. Total fat, 115.5 Gm; saturated fat, 30.2 Gm (11% of Calories); linoleate, 44.8 Gm (17% of Calories); cholesterol <350 mg.

Source: Adapted from suggested meal plan included in the Regulation of Dietary Fat, a review prepared by the Council on Foods and Nutrition of the American Medical Association (J.A.M.A., 181:411, 1962).

Project, in which 8,500 men will be studied. The other type is a *primary prevention* study, in which diet is altered in subjects without overt IHD to observe the effect on the incidence rate. Depending on its design, a study of this type may require from 10,000 to more than 50,000 subjects to yield a significant answer in 5 to 7 years. No primary study has yet been started in a large open population, but many secondary studies are in progress. One noteworthy, well-controlled experiment, which restricted itself to the variable of diet, has recently been completed by Leren in Norway. A diet with a *P/S* ratio of about 2 was fed to 200 men. There was a comparable group of controls. The diet lowered plasma cholesterol levels about 18 percent. The treated group had a significantly lower rate of recurring myocardial infarction and angina, but not of sudden death. The average cholesterol level in Norway is about the same as in America, and the general diet is fairly saturated and high in cholesterol. The number of subjects was small, and it is possible that the management of the controls and treated groups may have been different in some more subtle variables other than diet. Overall, this excellent study requires corroboration; a major uncertainty that it and similar studies cannot resolve is how well results of such *secondary* prevention can be interpreted as applying to atherogenesis in apparently healthy subjects. All diet studies tend to be confounded by risk factors other than hyperlipidemia which are now known to be of importance and which emerge when field trials are designed properly to permit *multivariate* analyses. It is now certain that diet alone is not the only determinant of the rate of atherogenesis.

Other Risk Factors

HIGH BLOOD PRESSURE. In the Framingham study, the incidence of IHD in men age forty-five to sixty-two with blood pressures exceeding 160/95 was more than five times that in normotensive men (blood pressure 140/90 or less). Elevations in both diastolic and systolic pressures correlate positively with IHD, the diastolic pressure perhaps being more important in younger people. After the age of forty-five, hypertension has greater weight than hypercholesterolemia as a risk factor. One recent report comparing incidence of IHD in British and Americans suggests that the difference could be attributed mainly to slightly higher blood pressures in Americans. These in turn were believed to be related to a higher average body weight in Americans. In the Framingham data an increase of 20 percent above the norm for the population or significant weight gain after age twenty-five is associated with a higher incidence of angina and sudden death but not of myocardial infarction in men. In women, obesity was an added risk for IHD only if concomitant hypercholesterolemia and hypertension were present. In general, the effect of *obesity* or increased *ponderal index* is independent of hyperlipemia but is very modest when corrected for associated increase in blood pressure.

CIGARETTE SMOKING. Ample statistical evidence supports a mean increase of about 70 percent in the death rate from IHD in men who smoke one pack of cigarettes per day compared with nonsmokers. The excess morbidity ratio in some instances may be as high as 200 percent. In general, the increase in death rate is proportional to the amount smoked and decreases with age. Excess morbidity from myocardial infarction is also present in women smokers, but the relationship is somewhat less firm than in men. In men, but not in women, smoking is also associated with increased angina pectoris. Smoking involves an excess risk in younger men that is not removed by adjustment for hyperlipemia, hypertension, and other variables. The explanation for the association of smoking and increased IHD is not known. Pipe and cigar smokers do not have a greater risk of IHD than nonsmokers, presumably because less smoke is inhaled. Smokers dying of causes other than IHD have been found at autopsy to have more coronary atherosclerosis than nonsmokers. The major influence of smoking is upon the incidence of sudden death, however; and the data now appear convincing that stopping smoking rather rapidly decreases this particular risk.

ABNORMAL GLUCOSE TOLERANCE. There is at least a twofold increase in incidence of myocardial infarction in diabetics compared with nondiabetics. There is an increased tendency of cerebral thrombosis and infarction but not of cerebral hemorrhage in diabetes. Gangrene of the lower extremities has been variously estimated to be from 8 to 150 times as frequent in diabetics as in nondiabetics. Proof is lacking that increased myocardial infarction or gangrene in diabetes can be attributed entirely to accelerated atherogenesis. An approximately twofold increase in the frequency of hypertension in diabetics may be an important contributory factor. The capillary basement membrane thickening, proliferative lesions, and microaneurysms considered to be pathognomonic of diabetes have not been adequately studied in the hearts of diabetics. They have been demonstrated in peripheral arteries; these lesions may cause small infarcts in vessel walls, interfere with development of collateral circulation, and promote atherogenesis. Studies in the United States indicate that diabetics do not have consistent significant elevations in either cholesterol (or LDL) or triglycerides (or VLDL) compared with nondiabetics. Therefore, the usual forms of hyperlipidemia are not the basis for the increased risk of IHD in diabetics. Exaggerated swings in free fatty acid concentrations might have some subtle relationship, but none has been proved. Data suggesting hyperinsulinism as an atherogenic factor do not adequately support this proposition. Plasma glyceride and cholesterol levels in diabetics have been shown to decrease when a 20 percent fat, low cholesterol diet is fed. Retinal exudates may disappear on such diets. However, it has not been proved that diabetics will respond in the same way as nondiabetics to all variations of diets now employed to treat hyperlipidemia.

PHYSICAL ACTIVITY. Data seeking to relate prevalence of IHD to daily (occupational) physical activity are confounded by too many variables for clear interpretation. Among prospective studies, the Framingham data do indicate that the less sedentary an individual is, the less susceptible he is to sudden death. The continuing Health Insurance Plan experiment also indicates a favorable relation of physical activity to incidence of disease. Moderate exercise, unassociated with weight change, has not been proved to have a beneficial effect on blood lipid levels. Advocates of physical activity in primary or secondary prevention of IHD have suggested that exercise improves sympathetic tone or development of collateral circulation. Implication of these possible mechanisms, operating independently of effects on caloric expenditure or body weight, remains largely on an intuitive basis.

PSYCHOLOGIC FACTORS. A Western Collaborative Group Study has classified men into two personality types with different incidence of IHD. "Type A" is compulsive, striving, and deadline-conscious compared with the more sluggish or passive type B. In a prospective study type A men, age thirty to thirty-nine, have had nearly three times the incidence of new IHD as type B men. This difference is not clearly related to cigarette smoking or other well-established risk factors. There is a general clinical impression that psychic or other emotional stress and anxiety are associated with sudden death and even with development of IHD. In individual cases this sometimes seems incontrovertible. Except for the above-mentioned study, however, many social and demographic analyses have so far failed to reach any agreement about the relationship of occupation and similar situational factors and the incidence of IHD (Marks).

GENETIC FACTORS. The inclusion of family history among risk factors (Table 275-3) implies the value of detecting familial expression of other risk factors such as hyperlipemia, diabetes, and hypertension. Surprisingly little is known about the role of other mutations in accelerating atherosclerosis. Pertinent population studies are not yet complete. The mortality rate from IHD in mainland Japanese is much lower than in Japanese who have migrated to the United States, and the incidence among Japanese in Hawaii falls in between. Keys, in a small sample, has suggested that the difference in plasma cholesterol levels between mainland and Hawaiian Japanese could explain the difference in the prevalence of IHD. Other known risk factors, some presumably related to environmental factors, have not been excluded in the available data concerning twins or other population samples. The increased atherogenesis associated with familial hyperlipoproteinemia, especially types II and III (Chap. 113), remains the most dramatic demonstration of genetic determination of atherosclerosis. The gene frequency of these diseases is not known, and it is probably not high enough to account for major differences between populations. Diabetes, occurring in about 1 in 80 Americans, is likely to prove to be the statistically most important known genetic variable in atherogenesis.

Theories of Causation

There are many theories concerning atherogenesis. The above discussion has touched upon the manner in which variations in flow or hydraulic stresses, involutional changes, hypertension (*wear-and-tear* or *hydrodynamic*

theories), or diabetes may initiate or promote the disease. Other demonstrated risk factors, particularly hyperlipidemia, deserve consideration in the context of the two most popular concepts of how intimal events may initiate atheroma formation, the so-called *lipid-infiltration* and *thrombogenic* theories of causation.

Lipid is very early demonstrable in fatty streaks in the intima or sometimes in the media. These streaks are said to be as common in the South African Bantu as in the New Orleans white child in the United States, even though later in life these groups will differ greatly in prevalence of atherosclerosis. Below age ten, the cholesterol content of the aorta in both males and females is low (about 10 mg per Gm) and practically all is unesterified. Later, the lipid increases, and much of the cholesterol is esterified. Males, age ten to thirty-nine, have a greater amount of cholesterol in the arterial wall than females. Lipid is visible between the media and intima, or by electronmicroscopy as droplets in the endothelial cells. The distribution is spotty and related to intimal thickening and other signs of early atheroma formation; the greatest concentration is in well-developed lesions. There is thus a definite correlation between age, the total and esterified aortic cholesterol, and the amount of grossly visible atherosclerosis. Species vary greatly in the amount of spontaneous atherosclerosis and in susceptibility to its experimental induction. The direct studies in rabbits, monkeys, and some other species support the inferences drawn from man that increasing the plasma cholesterol does increase the number of atheromas. Although arterial wall and atheromas can synthesize cholesterol and other lipids, the cumulative data also suggest that the lipid in atheromas comes mainly from the lumen. Its accumulation may reflect increased inward flux, a deficient removal mechanism, or both. The infiltration of lipid doubtless is related to the plasma concentrations of particular lipoproteins, but is not solely determined by them. A normal-appearing aorta shows a poor correlation between its lipid content and age of the subject, i.e., duration of exposure of the aorta to lipoproteins. Japanese and Americans, who have very different plasma cholesterol concentrations, have similar amounts of cholesterol in the *normal* aortic wall. Differences in overall aortic cholesterol is related to great differences in the degree of atheromatosis. Enhanced movement of lipid into the wall and creation of an imbalance in its removal are likely to rest on some initiating events within or on the surface of the intima. Such injury could, of course, be partially dependent on plasma lipid concentrations.

Duguid has called attention to *fibrin deposition* on the otherwise healthy-appearing portions of arterial wall. It occurs in children, but the frequency increases with age. The fibrin becomes covered with endothelium and undergoes hyalinization, and sometimes there is organization and fatty change. This could lead to irregularity and thickening of the arterial wall, with loss of normal flexibility, and to atheroma formation, but no such sequence has been convincingly demonstrated. Test systems have shown that if the endothelium is damaged, platelets will aggregate, develop an interconnecting fibrin net, and adhere to the surface. The interplay of known factors related to *platelet aggregation,* such as ADP, fibrinogen, surface charge, fibrinolytic activity, or platelet abnormalities, has yet to be sorted out in possible relationship to the earliest stages of atherosclerosis. Many reports of platelet stickiness, decreased fibrinolysis, or other abnormal coagulation indexes in association with IHD, hyperlipidemia, or high saturated fat diets, suffer from uncertain tests or other deficiencies. There is a high probability that molecular events on the endothelial surface will someday explain a part of the problem of atherogenesis. Today's knowledge does not offer a rationale for preventive measures relating to platelets or the coagulation system.

Treatment

One may view the "treatment" of atherosclerosis as falling into four categories: (1) management of overt complications, (2) attempts to delay recurrence or retard the atherosclerotic process in patients with complications (secondary prevention), (3) corrective steps in subjects with above-average risk of developing an initial complication, (4) the extension of primary preventive measures to the general population. In the present state of knowledge, good medical practice requires diligent detection of susceptible persons and reasonable application of means to reduce known risk factors. Until this is systematically undertaken, and until interventions are proved to be effective and completely safe, they cannot be extended wholesale to all people of all ages.

The identification of risk factors (Table 275-3) for atherosclerosis should be a part of every thorough medical examination. Screening should begin at age twenty-five to thirty-five or earlier if family history dictates. Some types of hyperlipidemia and diabetes are more likely to develop after age thirty, when normal growth has ceased, physical activity lessened, and caloric excess has become a pattern.

The reduction of risk factors is a problem requiring individual attention, the stringency of recommendations depending on the degree of risk and the age of the patient. A vigorous regimen advisable at age thirty has less rationale at sixty-five. Diet changes can be more radical for a cholesterol level of 450 than for one of 250. A program of physical activity must be steady, reasonable, and not productive of hernia and sprains. The treatment of hyperlipidemia requires exclusion of diseases to which it is secondary, and is made more rational by identification of the type of hyperlipidemia, as outlined in Chap. 113. In Americans under fifty, a cholesterol concentration of >250 mg per 100 ml or of triglycerides > 170 is a mandate for preventive action. For the majority of subjects the first step is adoption of some degree of dietary modifications, as indicated in Table 275-6. Reduction to normal weight is applicable to patients with all types of hyperlipidemia. Only after diet management has been instituted and hyperlipidemia persists, should hypolipemic drugs be tried, as outlined in Chap. 113. Plasma cholesterol and glycerides must be monitored to justify continuation of any treatment. Interventions to reduce other risk factors are discussed elsewhere. Premature atherosclerosis is largely a preventable disease, seemingly born of poor adaptation to the modern environment. The ultimate control will require the general adoption of measures that are not yet completely defined. While specifics are awaited, the physician's advice, like the patient's life, had best be temperate.

REFERENCES

Adams, C. W. M.: "Vascular Histochemistry," Chicago, The Year Book Medical Publishers, Inc., 1967.

Blumenthal, H. T. (Ed.): "Cowdry's Arteriosclerosis," 2d ed., Springfield, Ill., Charles C Thomas, Publisher, 1967.

Brown, H. B., M. Farrand, and I. H. Page: Design of Practical Fat-controlled Diets, J.A.M.A., 196:205, 1966.

Epstein, F. H.: The Epidemiology of Coronary Heart Disease. A Review, J. Chronic Dis., 18:735, 1965.

Fredrickson, D. S. R. I. Levy, and R. S. Lees: Fat Transport in Lipoproteins—An Integrated Approach to Mechanisms and Disorders, New Engl. Med., 276:34, 94, 148, 215, 273, 1967.

Hodges, R. E., W. A. Krehl, D. B. Stone, and A. Lopez: Dietary Carbohydrates and Low Cholesterol Diets: Effects on Serum Lipids of Man, Am. J. Clin. Nutr., 20:198, 1967.

Kannel, W. B., W. P. Castelli, and P. M. McNamara: The Coronary Profile: 12-year Follow-up in the Framingham Study, J. Occupational Med., 9:611, 1967.

Keys, A., J. T. Anderson, and F. Grande: Serum Cholesterol Response to Changes in the Diet, Metabolism, 14:747, 1965.

Kimura, S. J., and W. M. Caygill (Eds.): "Vascular Complications of Diabetes Mellitus," Saint Louis, The C. V. Mosby Company, 1967.

Kuller, L., A. Lilienfeld, and R. Fisher: An Epidemiological Study of Sudden and Unexpected Deaths in Adults, Medicine, 46:341, 1967.

Leren, P.: The Effect of Plasma Cholesterol Lowering Diet in Male Survivors of Myocardial Infarction, Acta Med. Scand., suppl. 466, 1966.

McGandy, R. B., D. M. Hegsted, and F. J. Stare: Dietary Fats, Carbohydrates and Atherosclerotic Vascular Disease, New Engl. J. Med., 277:417, 469, 1967.

Marks, R. U.: A Review of Empirical Findings. Social Stress and Cardiovascular Disease, Milbank Mem. Fund Quart., 45:51, 1967.

Mustard, J. F., and H. C. Roswell: Platelets and Atherosclerosis, Acta Cardiol., suppl. 11:401, 1965.

Pickering, G.: Arteriosclerosis and Atherosclerosis. The Need for Clear Thinking, Am. J. Med., 34:7, 1963.

Rosenman, R. H., M. Friedman, C. D. Jenkins, R. Straus, M. Wurm, and R. Kositchek, Am. J. Cardiol., 19:771, 1967.

Shapiro, S., E. Weinblatt, C. W. Frank, and R. V. Sager: The H.I.P. Study of Incidence and Prognosis of Coronary Heart Disease. Preliminary Findings on Incidence of Myocardial Infarction and Angina, J. Chronic Dis., 18:527, 1965.

Symposium on Atherosclerosis, Am. J. Med., 46:655, 1969.

The Framingham Study, An Epidemiological Investigation of Cardiovascular Disease, Section 10, U.S. Government Printing Office, September, 1968.

Truett, J., J. Cornfield, and W. Kannel: A Multivariate Analysis of the Risk of Coronary Heart Disease in Framingham, J. Chronic Dis., 20:511, 1967.

276 HYPERTENSIVE VASCULAR DISEASE

John P. Merrill

CLASSIFICATION OF HYPERTENSION

A system of classification of hypertension is presented in Table 37-1. Marked elevation of systolic pressure with little or no elevation of diastolic pressure has a different etiologic connotation and, even more important, an entirely different prognostic significance than does elevation of the diastolic phase. As has been pointed out previously, predominance of systolic elevation depends more on the factor of cardiac output. Predominance of diastolic elevation is a manifestation of increased residual resistance in the peripheral vascular bed after systole and, as such, more closely represents the clinically significant abnormality in the hypertensive syndrome. The term *essential hypertension* has been employed to indicate those cases of hypertension for which a specific endocrine or renal basis cannot be found, and in which the neural element may be only a mediator of other influences. Since even this latter relationship is not entirely clear, it is more properly listed for the moment in the category of unknown etiology. The term *essential hypertension* defines simply by failing to define; hence it is of limited use except as an expression of our inability to understand adequately the forces at work. Nevertheless, the bulk of patients with significant and persistent elevation of diastolic pressure form a fairly uniform group for which no well-defined etiologic process has been delineated. From the standpoint of wide acceptance, the term probably should be retained. Unquestionably, cases of essential hypertension in the progressive form may develop a renal component which perpetuates this syndrome as a result of development of vascular lesions in the kidney. The development of vascular lesions here and elsewhere has served for some authors to differentiate *hypertensive disease* from *hypertension,* which latter term connotes only elevation of blood pressure without associated vascular lesions. The prognostic significance of this division is obvious, but the dividing line is often difficult to draw. Hypertension, regardless of its etiology, may be further subdivided into two types, *benign* and *malignant.* These terms should be employed only as relating to the rapidity and severity of the vascular disease accompanying increased blood pressure levels. The malignant type may be superimposed upon the benign type; occasionally, however, it may be so rapid in onset and so severe in its course as to appear a separate entity. In addition, the severity and rapid progress of vascular disease associated with hypertension primarily renal in origin may justify the term *malignant hypertension.*

Many factors involved in the hypertensive syndrome have now been delineated. It may be permissible to attempt to integrate them in a theoretic case of human "essential" hypertension in a fashion which lays much stress on the primary role of nervous vasoconstrictor influences. In this idealized view an individual, by reason of inherited traits, including race and sex, may be particularly susceptible to vasomotor reactions resulting from a stressful environment. Specific reasons for this susceptibility might include emotional instability, a labile vasomotor apparatus, possibly including the vasomotor center in the medulla, and a peripheral vasculature which hyperreacts to nervous constrictor stimuli. Such an individual would manifest early in life greater rises in blood pressure in response to environmental stimuli than his fellow born without these genetic traits. Such abnormal responses might be elicited by the cold pressor test and Valsalva maneuver. During early adult life these rises would be more frequent, reach higher levels, and tend less and less to return to so-called "normal" values. The continued stress of pressure on a genetically sensitive vasculature might then result in small blood vessel changes which would be manifest in the optic fundi and kidneys. With the involvement of the kidneys and possibly the adrenals, a second, humoral mechanism might originate which could then overlay and finally completely dominate the original neurogenic origin. At this point, although the labile vasomotor response might still be elicited, its importance from an etiologic and therapeutic standpoint would be secondary. Such a formulation is admittedly speculative. It does, however, fit many of the observed facts. There is increasing evidence both in the experimental animal and the human that hypertension of renal origin may follow a course very similar to that described for essential hypertension. Even in well-established cases of renal hypertension, vasomotor lability and hyperreactivity may be present. Although many doubt that increased pressure per se may cause vascular disease, in the author's view, the statistical correlation in mortality tables is too impressive to neglect. By analogy, too, the pulmonary vascular disease that may result from prolonged increased pulmonary arterial pressure with mitral stenosis suggests very strongly that this relationship may obtain.

A second and possibly more important classification has been constructed in Table 276-1. Such a table emphasizes the fact that the physician confronted with the problem of hypertension must think first of those situations in which the hypertension may be associated with a specific defect which may be amenable to specific therapy. A causal relationship of this type may be difficult to establish and may be defined only by the resultant success or failure of therapy. Nevertheless, the opportunity to "cure" hypertension must be sought diligently in each hypertensive patient.

Unilateral renal disease as a cause of hypertension has received increasing attention with the advent of newer diagnostic methods and forms of surgical therapy. Stenosis of one or both renal arteries due to atheromatous plaques, fibromuscular hyperplasia, and even neurofibro-

Table 276-1. CURABLE HYPERTENSION

Systolic hypertension only	Combined systolic and diastolic hypertension
Thyrotoxicosis	Brain tumor
Arteriovenous fistula	Unilateral renal disease
Anemia	Adrenal cortical hyperfunction
	Aldosteronism
	Cushing's syndrome
	Pheochromocytoma
	Pituitary tumors
	Coarctation of the aorta
	Increased intravascular volume
	Eclampsia
	Polycythemia

matosis may be "cured" by appropriate vascular surgery. Since this is a "curable" kind of hypertension, it should be carefully eliminated as a major factor in any patient with significant elevation of blood pressure. The diagnostic principles of importance are based on the following pathophysiologic observations. A decrease in blood flow to the normally functioning renal tissue may result in hypertension even in the presence of normal renal function as measured by the usual clinical tests. It has been shown that the resultant decrease in perfusion, pulsation, pressure, or all three, will result in the following: (1) The elaboration from the kidney of renin, an enzyme acting upon an α_2-globulin in the plasma to produce, after an intervening step, angiotensin-2, a potent hypertensinogenic agent. The source of renin has been thought to be the granules of the juxtaglomerular cells of the kidney, and the sequence of events described above results in an increase in juxtaglomerular granularity. Angiotensin, in turn, may stimulate the secretion of aldosterone by the adrenal cortex, with sequelae which have been described elsewhere (Chap. 92). (2) The urine volume is decreased with or without a significant decrease in filtration rate. The urinary sodium/potassium and sodium/creatinine ratios are decreased, but there is an increase in the total solute content of the urine (increased osmolality).

The application of these principles to the diagnosis of hypertension due to unilateral disease should be made by an orderly sequence of diagnostic procedures, beginning with the simplest and least traumatic tests. These should include a careful history and physical examination. Occlusion of a renal artery or one of its branches should be suspected when malignant hypertension appears suddenly in patients with no previous history, and in an age group in which "hypertension" is unlikely to make its initial appearance, i.e., below twenty-one or above forty-five. A strong family background of hypertension in a patient with long-standing disease may make the coexistence of a renal lesion and hypertension coincidental rather than causal. Evaluation should include search for history of trauma in the renal area, and cardiovascular evaluation for the possibility of renal arterial compromise or occlusion by emboli or atherosclerotic plaques. Examination of the urine may reveal evidence of renal disease, as may elevation of the serum creatinine or blood urea nitrogen

level. Secondary aldosteronism due to secretion of renin-angiotensin may result in a decreased serum potassium level and elevated serum bicarbonate concentration.

In approximately two-thirds of the patients with renal artery stenosis, abdominal bruits may be heard over the upper part of the abdomen or in the costovertebral angles. It should be remembered, however, that abdominal bruits are not infrequent in normotensive individuals. Discrepancy in renal size or in the secretion of contrast medium visualized by intravenous pyelography may be an important clue. Because the secretion of renin depends on the functional renal tissue, however, the pyelogram may be completely normal. In fact, the contrast medium may appear more concentrated on the side with the vascular lesion. Rapid-sequence films made 1, 2, 3, and 5 min after injection of the dye may reveal a delay in appearance on the affected side which is not apparent in the 15-min film.

The measurement of the uptake or excretion of radioactive iodopyracet (Diodrast) or iodohippurate sodium (Hippuran) may be made by counters placed over the renal area following the intravenous injection of the isotope; a picture of disturbed function may be elicited by plotting these functions of the two kidneys simultaneously. This has proved an innocuous and a frequently helpful screening test. When the radiohippuran renogram is completely normal, surgically curable hypertension is rarely present. On the other hand, some 10 to 15 percent of these studies may be positive for reasons other than renovascular disease.

Simultaneous comparison of the function of two kidneys by samples obtained from each ureter may yield important information, particularly when there is no discrepancy in overall function, as measured by the intravenous pyelogram. Characteristics of the urine composition on the affected side have been mentioned above. Although this "split function test" has been valuable in some hands, the discomfort, risk of infection, and misleading results due to leakage around catheter assign it secondary importance.

Translumbar aortography or preferably renal arteriograms made by the injection of contrast material directly into the renal arteries through a catheter passed up the femoral artery may directly visualize the affected vessel. It must be remembered, however, that a number of patients has been shown to have renal arterial stenosis and no hypertension.

Renal venous blood may be obtained by catheterizing a renal vein. A demonstration in these samples of substances with pressor activity for the rat or of angiotensin itself is a somewhat laborious assay but constitutes direct evidence of the participation of the kidney in the pressor mechanism. If the sample from one renal vein shows a renin concentration three times that of the other, this is strong presumptive evidence of the renal origin of hypertension. Of the tests outlined above, this correlates best with the surgical cure of renal hypertension. The measurement of renal blood flow by the xenon washout technique combined with samples of both renal arterial and venous blood enables calculation of the actual rate

Table 276-2. ROUTINE WORKUP

Uric acid	PSP	24-hr urine collection for VMA[1]
BUN	Creatinine clearance	24-hr urine collection for 17-keto and 17-hydroxysteroids[2]
Na	ECG	Intravenous pyelogram (rapid sequence)
K	7-ft heart film	
Cl	Urinalysis	
CO₂	Urine culture	

If routine workup suggests: *Additional tests required:*

1. Renovascular disease
    a. Radiohippuran renogram
    b. Selective renal arteriography
    c. Renal vein renin
    d. "Split function" study

2. Pheochromocytoma[3]
    a. Assay of urinary catecholamines
    b. Regitine test[4]
    c. Histamine or tyramine test[5]

3. Primary aldosteronism
    a. High salt diet
    b. Plasma renin concentration
    c. Aldosterone secretory rate

[1] See Chapter 93.
[2] See Chapter 92.
[3] If VMA excretion increased.
[4] If BP greater than 170/100.
[5] If BP less than 170/100.

The routine determinations are those which should be done in any patient with substantial hypertension. These tests can be done in most hospitals with the help of commercial biochemistry laboratories. Completely negative test results in conjunction with negative clinical evidence for those syndromes listed in Table 276-1, should be adequate to eliminate the various causes of "curable hypertension." If, however, the tests or clinical examination suggest presence of those syndromes listed on the left, the more complicated tests suggested on the right should be done in sequence to explore the possibility further.

of renin production. Concentration per se may not accurately reflect rate of production. This latter technique, although complicated, is also more accurate and correlates best with good surgical results in preliminary trials.

Suggestive but not conclusive are the following: (1) a decreased pressor response to the infusion of angiotensin suggesting that such patients have developed tachyphylaxis to continue endogenous angiotensin elaboration. (2) The demonstration at operation of a pressure gradient of 30 mm Hg or more across the arterial constriction. (3) Biopsy evidence of increased granularity of juxtaglomerular cells in the affected kidney.

If these criteria are rigidly applied to the selection of patients for surgery, approximately two-thirds of the patients may expect significant improvement. Of 253 such individuals culled from the literature, 191 were reported improved, 1 year after surgery; 62 were unimproved and these included 18 deaths. Several additional points may be made to supplement these data. Involvement of the contralateral side by vascular disease may mitigate against surgical cure, even with relief of the obstructive lesion. However, persistent hypertension due to diffuse

vascular changes on the contralateral side may be much more easily controlled by medical therapy. Mild nitrogen retention does not necessarily contraindicate surgery, since removal of the damaged kidney may allow compensatory hypertrophy in the contralateral kidney, which is further abetted by relief of the hypertension. It is the duty of the internist to keep in mind that mild to moderate hypertensive disease, even when conclusively due to unilateral renal disease, may respond to medical therapy. This fact must be weighed carefully against the morbidity and mortality of renal vascular surgery.

The diagnosis and treatment of *thyrotoxicosis* have been discussed in Chap. 89. The presence of an *arteriovenous fistula* may be manifested by systolic hypertension and a wide pulse pressure, and may be diagnosed by the presence of a murmur or thrill over the site of the abnormal communication. This may be over the peripheral vessels where they are involved, or a typical "machinery murmur" may be heard over the left precordium in the case of patent ductus arteriosus. Both these conditions may be amenable to surgical correction.

Adrenal cortical hyperfunction may be manifest by hypertension as well as the other signs of Cushing's syndrome (Chap. 92). Osteoporosis, hirsutism, "buffalo hump," striae, and disorders of glucose metabolism are typical. Hypersecretion of aldosterone and its relation to hypertension are discussed elsewhere in this chapter and in Chap. 92. Patients with hypertension with hypopotassemic alkalosis should be evaluated carefully for this syndrome. Two factors may confuse the diagnosis. The common administration to hypertensive patients of thiazide diuretics may cause potassium depletion. (Hyperuricemia may occur with the administration of the thiazide diuretics and not with aldosterone, and may serve as a point in differential diagnosis.) The administration of diets low in sodium may prevent hypopotassemia in hypertensive patients and alkalosis in patients with full-blown hyperaldosteronism. It, therefore, becomes important to evaluate patients suspected of this syndrome while they are ingesting an adequate sodium intake.

Pheochromocytoma, though rare, produces a completely curable form of hypertension when surgery is performed before the vascular disease has become irreversible. In spite of such diagnostic techniques as perirenal air injection and retroperitoneal insufflations with oxygen, the newer pharmacologic agents for provocative and blocking tests, the assay of urinary pressor amines and their metabolites (VMA), the diagnosis remains extremely difficult and may be established only by exploration. Pheochromocytoma, in addition to the typical intermittent attacks, may produce a steady hypertension. The problem is discussed further in Chap. 93.

The diagnosis of *coarctation of the aorta,* if considered, will usually be made by comparison of blood pressure in the arm and leg, and appropriate x-rays of the chest may show the typical notching of the ribs.

Polycythemia, as a cause of increased intravascular volume, may be diagnosed upon estimation of the hematocrit and erythrocyte count. Phlebotomy, the administration of phenylhydrazine hydrochloride, radioactive phosphorus, and x-ray have been used successfully in treatment.

Pituitary tumors, accompanied by hypertension, may be associated with the picture of hyperadrenalism or with that of acromegaly, in which case the characteristic facies, increase in head, hand, and foot size, as well as x-rays of the extremities and sella turcica, may confirm the diagnosis.

The toxemias of pregnancy are discussed in Chap. 306. Whether or not toxemia of pregnancy occurring in a previously normal woman can give rise to subsequent hypertension is still debatable.

SYSTEMIC HYPERTENSION

SIGNS AND SYMPTOMS. The signs and symptoms of hypertension can rarely be attributed to the elevated blood pressure itself. A large number of patients with elevated blood pressure may have no symptoms or signs whatever. In the more advanced stages of hypertensive disease, signs and symptoms depend on the organ involved by the vascular disease accompanying the hypertensive process. These include, of course, cerebral arterial and arteriolar disease, coronary artery disease, congestive heart failure, and renal failure, which will be discussed in separate chapters. A not infrequent early symptom is the presence of headache. This may take any form but classically is a dull, pounding occipital headache, which is present upon awakening in the morning and tends to wear off during the day. Many patients with hypertension complain of nonspecific difficulties such as weakness, nervousness, flatulence, palpitation, and dizziness. Since hypertensive patients are prone to emotional and psychic difficulties, it is frequently difficult to evaluate these symptoms. There is indeed some reason to believe that patients with labile hypertension and no evidence of vascular involvement may have a multitude of such nonspecific symptoms, while patients with sustained elevation of diastolic pressure and evidence of hypertensive vascular disease may complain only of weakness and perhaps mild headache. As hypertensive vascular disease progresses in hypertensive patients, a number of more specific signs and symptoms may result.

Epistaxis may occur, as well as microscopic and even gross intermittent hematuria accompanied by moderate proteinuria. The latter findings may signify vascular involvement of the kidney, but should alert the physician to the possibility of preexisting renal disease. An important physical finding, which may give some clue to prognosis and progress of the vascular disease, is the change in the vessels of the optic fundi. The damage caused by hypertensive disease is better recognized by a careful study of the retina than by any other means. These changes deserve careful attention and should be accurately described in the patient's record. The physician should note exactly what he sees in the retina and not use one of the grades or classifications currently employed. The grading method is useful for statistical studies by one person or group, but a subsequent ex-

aminer cannot be sure that he and the previous examiner understood exactly the same changes implied by a numerical grade. If possible, the lesions when seen should be described as to character and location and, even better, drawn. Early changes in the retinal vessels include diminution in the caliber of the smaller vessels most distal from the disk. A convenient standard of reference is to relate the arteriolar diameter to that of the vein. Generalized constriction or "spasm" of the arterioles may be seen in severe toxemia of pregnancy. A more specific lesion, however, is segmental constriction of the arterioles. This is a permanent lesion and characteristic of significant diastolic hypertension. Tortuosity of the larger vessels close to the disk appears in hypertensive disease, but may also be seen in arteriosclerosis without hypertension, and is of little significance to the hypertensive process itself. Arteriovenous nicking is characteristic of chronic moderate hypertension but may also be seen in those patients with severe elevation of diastolic blood pressure. True arteriovenous nicking requires the presence of an open space between artery and vein on both sides of the artery (Fig. 276-1). Frequently, a darker red area in that portion of the vein just peripheral to the crossing may be seen, representing stasis of venous flow at that point. To be significant, arteriovenous nicking must occur at least one disk diameter from the edge of the optic disk. Since both segmental constriction and arteriovenous nicking are permanent changes, they represent evidence of a preexisting hypertensive state. As such, they may have important diagnostic importance in a patient who at the time of examination has a drop in blood pressure secondary to myocardial infarction or hemorrhage.

An increased light reflex signifies thickening of the vessel wall. With advancing changes, small flame-shaped hemorrhages and glistening white exudates may make their appearance. A serious prognostic sign, indicative of

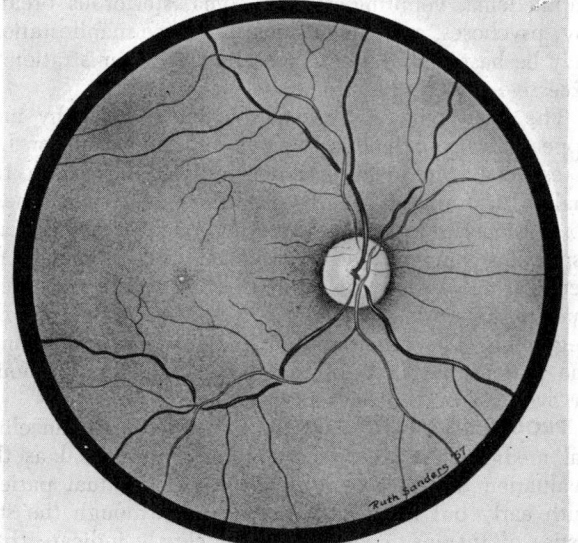

Fig. 276-1. Retinal changes of hypertension—arteriovenous compression and segmental constriction of the arterioles. (S. A. Shelburne: Ann. Intern. Med., 1957.)

advanced disease, is papilledema, manifested by blurring of the disk margins. This should be particularly evaluated at the temporal margin, since some degree of blurring of the nasal margin may be physiologic. Separation of the retina has been observed in the acute hypertensive episodes of eclampsia. Although somewhat unusual, there may be marked differences in the degree of involvement of the retinas. The visual symptoms usually depend on the degree of involvement and the location of the lesions.

Patients with hypertensive disease occasionally suffer from acute episodes characterized by marked rise in blood pressure above the previous level, and by disorders of the nervous system which last for minutes, hours, or days, and then disappear without clinical evidence of lasting damage. Such episodes, described as *hypertensive encephalopathy,* are not limited to any single etiologic type of hypertensive disease but are particularly common in association with renal disease, especially where a common factor, such as acute glomerulonephritis or disseminated lupus erythematosus, has produced both vascular lesions and hypertension. Spasm of cerebral vessels is generally thought to be the cause of these attacks, although adequate demonstration of this has yet to be made. Small thrombi and edema play a role in some cases. This syndrome may frequently simulate the hypertensive crises of pheochromocytoma or mimic brain tumor. The clinical syndrome appears in two forms, depending on whether the disturbances in the nervous system are chiefly of generalized or of focal nature.

The general form usually appears in individuals without previous long-standing hypertension. It may occur in women with eclampsia and in children and young adults with acute glomerulonephritis. Rapidly progressing malignant hypertension is frequently accompanied by hypertensive encephalopathy. Aside from a rapidly rising blood pressure, the attacks are characterized by headache, visual disturbances which may progress to blindness, papilledema, vomiting, stupor, coma, stertorous breathing, psychoses, and convulsions. All these manifestations may be hastened and enhanced by the administration of excessive amounts of fluid.

The focal type of hypertensive encephalopathy may appear in any individual with chronic hypertension but is especially frequent in older individuals and in the malignant form of the disease. Loss of consciousness, convulsions, and paralysis involving one-half the body are especially common, and the clinical picture, though reversible, may exactly resemble cerebral vascular accident due to hemorrhage, thrombosis, or embolism, at the beginning. The differentiation may be impossible until the patient has been observed for a number of hours or even for several days.

PROGNOSIS IN HYPERTENSION. Few problems in clinical medicine are as difficult or as controversial as the evaluation of the prognosis for any individual patient with early but marked hypertension. Although the statistics of the insurance companies clearly indicate that, in general, the mortality experience is increasingly unfavorable with progressive elevation of the blood pressure, individual variation in tolerance to hypertension and hypertensive disease is marked. A few of the factors affecting prognosis have already been mentioned. In Table 276-3 are listed factors which are known to affect

Table 276-3. FACTORS INDICATING AN ADVERSE PROGNOSIS IN HYPERTENSION

Negro origin
Youth and male sex
Persistent diastolic pressure > 110 mm Hg
Marked cardiac enlargement
ECG changes of ischemia or left ventricular strain
Renal functional impairment
Retinal hemorrhages and exudates
Angina pectoris
Myocardial infarction
Cerebrovascular accident
Congestive heart failure
Marked retinal arteriolar sclerosis
Nitrogen retention*
Papilledema

* Nitrogen retention, when due to vascular disease of the kidney, indicates a very grave prognosis. Its occurrence in primary renal disease with only mild hypertension may be less important.

adversely the prognosis in patients with hypertension. These are listed in order of increasing gravity. Systems of classification of hypertension, characterizing the disease in varying grades of severity and with varying prognoses, have been devised on the basis of (1) retinal changes and (2) a combination of the factors listed in Table 276-3, plus phenolsulfonphthalein excretion and response to sedation. It may be concluded that young male patients of racial origins known to be susceptible to hypertensive disease, with high, relatively fixed diastolic pressures, are apt to do badly. On the other hand, women apparently tolerate elevated blood pressure and even hypertensive vascular diseases better than do men. Every physician interested in hypertensive disease has followed women and an occasional man through many years of relatively good health with persistent diastolic pressures of 120 mm Hg or more. The degree of retinopathy may give some clue as to the prognosis, although this, in general, is a better guide to the progress than to the ultimate prognosis, since even severe retinopathy may be reversed occasionally by appropriate therapy, and rarely improves spontaneously. Papilledema and renal insufficiency are extremely grave prognostic signs in every instance. The occurrence in the hypertensive patient of myocardial infarction, congestive heart failure, or cerebral vascular accident signifies a poor prognosis, although, again, every hypertensive clinic has its share of patients constituting exceptions to this general rule. Emotional instability, while making the treatment somewhat more difficult, does not otherwise affect prognosis itself. Poor response to adequate treatment of any sort, including failure to correct obesity, frequently indicates impaired prognosis.

DIAGNOSIS. The diagnosis of hypertension may be

made with a blood pressure cuff, and the diagnosis of hypertensive vascular disease by the usual methods for evaluating the cardiovascular system, kidneys, and optic fundi. The differential diagnosis should, from the very first, include disease states giving rise to hypertension for which more specific therapy exists. A list of these, which should be considered during the first evaluation of any hypertensive problem, is given in Table 276-1.

In previous editions of the chapter, opposing viewpoints on the medical therapy of hypertension were presented. Certain arguments, e.g., that the exact level of blood pressure correlates poorly with the progress of the vascular disease, or that spontaneous remissions of hypertensive vascular disease occur, or that the lowering of blood pressure may fail to halt the progress of atherosclerotic vascular disease, were encountered. At the present time, this is a dead issue. The evidence is overwhelming that in the hands of experienced physicians the prognosis in severe hypertension is unequivocally improved by medical therapy. Since various effective hypotensive agents exist, it is now justifiable to utilize mild forms of therapy (including reassurance) for mild forms of hypertension, or drastic and hazardous therapeutic methods in the severe forms of the disease. It can no longer be said, in this light, that the danger and side effects of our nonspecific hypotensive drugs are worse than the natural courses of the disease.

Whatever the form of therapy selected, it must not be forgotten that the physician who treats hypertension is treating the patient as a whole rather than the separate manifestations of a disease.

SELECTION OF PATIENTS FOR THERAPY. In the decision to institute treatment, the factors delineated in the paragraph on prognosis must bear considerable weight. Factors of increasing gravity, shown in Table 276-3, are increasingly important indications for specific therapy. Severe nitrogen retention, however, may contraindicate and obviate any specific form of depressor therapy. Sudden, marked, and persistent elevation of diastolic pressure may precede signs and symptoms and, as such, indicates need for therapy. Marked elevation of systolic pressure, with little or no rise in diastolic, does not constitute an indication for depressor therapy. This is particularly true in the elderly or arteriosclerotic patient, even though the diastolic pressure may also be moderately elevated. A trial of mild forms of therapy, including psychotherapy, reducing diets, sedation, or mild depressor agents, which fails to improve signs or symptoms, may justify more intensive forms of therapy. The physician must, however, carefully weigh the value of making his patient "blood pressure conscious" by a specific regimen and regular follow-up, against real need for any particular form of therapy. Above all, in treatment or prognostication, he must avoid engendering in the patient a fear of the disease which may be unwarranted in our present state of knowledge. Promising therapies are available, however, and it should be remembered that the forms of treatment are not mutually exclusive. Particularly, it should be remembered that the confidence, patience, and enthusiasm of the physician are important ingredients in

any form of therapy. The hypertensive process being what it is, this factor undoubtedly accounts in large part for the varying degrees of success achieved by different investigators with the same therapeutic program.

SYMPTOMATIC THERAPY. Improvement in symptoms, as well as blood pressure levels, frequently results from adequate psychotherapy (see below). For the relief of hypertensive headache, elevation of the head of the bed during the night is usually beneficial. Thiocyanate salts have been used with some success, although the necessity for carefully checking blood levels of this drug to prevent toxicity has greatly decreased its usefulness. Not infrequently a cup of black coffee or the administration of 200 to 400 mg caffeine as the citrate or sodium benzoate salt, given on arising, may help the hypertensive headache. Periodic venesection has met with occasional success in alleviating headache and dizzy spells. Small amounts of sedation in properly selected patients may be of some value. They should be carefully evaluated after preliminary therapeutic trial for the undesirable side effects. With renal failure, the short-acting barbiturates Seconal and Amytal are preferable to phenobarbital, since they do not require the renal route for their excretion. Because sedation may play a more fundamental role in hypertension than that of symptomatic therapy, its use becomes a highly individualized problem. The administration of 30 mg phenobarbital three to four times a day to one patient may well dull the knife-edge of anxiety and result in improvement. In other individuals, the mental confusion that may result, as well as the necessity for taking medication continually, may do more harm than good. The conscientious executive, faced with a problem which he is capable of solving with a clear head, does not benefit his hypertensive disease by grappling with his problem under the influence of sedatives which cloud his thinking. Such situations must be carefully assessed on their individual merits. The tranquilizing agents (e.g., meprobamate (Miltown, Equanil), diazepam (Valium) may be useful in allaying anxiety and tension without impairing critical faculties.

PSYCHOTHERAPY. A majority of patients with essential hypertension have disorders of personality which may be aggravated by environmental or emotional stress resulting in conflicts and anxiety which may be correlated with fluctuations in blood pressure. Although there is little agreement on the specific personality patterns involved, such emotional contributions may be recognized frequently; they are particularly evidenced in the tense, anxious individual with marked fluctuations in blood pressure. In such cases, psychotherapy alone has produced results equal to the best of other forms of therapy. It is, moreover, an indispensable adjunct to them. Intensive psychotherapy may not be necessary and, indeed, should not be undertaken unless it can be followed to completion, since the early part of the exhaustive psychiatric approach may often be followed by exacerbation of hypertension. One should not underestimate the value of the psychotherapy resulting from a good physician-patient relationship. It is probable that just this resulted in the improvement in hypertension attributed to nostrums such as watermelon seed and garlic. It follows from this example, however, that an emotionally labile patient, with numerous emotional problems and psychosomatic complaints, cannot always be told—because of the absence of vascular or renal disease—simply to forget his problems. In the vast majority of instances, a discussion of the problem with reassurances fortified by mild medication and follow-up visits at infrequent but regular intervals will do more good.

DIETARY MANAGEMENT. Obesity is frequently a sign as well as a complication of the hypertensive personality. Since it has an undoubted adverse effect upon prognosis and progress of the disease, it should be specifically treated by an adequate weight-reducing regimen, such as has been outlined in Chap. 48. The patient should fully understand the necessity for this regimen without being frightened by it.

In the past, diets low in sodium and protein have in some hands unquestionably resulted in striking amelioration of hypertensive vascular disease. The low sodium content of the diet appears to have been the effective factor. The multitude of effective oral natriuretic agents available today, however, makes unnecessary diets rigidly restricted in sodium, such as the rice diet. Moderate sodium restriction and judicious use of oral diuretic agents are equally effective in the control of hypertension in individuals with normal renal function. Both rigid sodium restriction and the use of diuretics, however, may further impair kidney function in the patient with renal failure. A diet effectively low in sodium, either because of its composition or because of the use of diuretics, may potentiate the effect of other forms of treatment of hypertension, both surgical and pharmacologic.

DRUG THERAPY. The rationale for the use of drugs which lower blood pressure is based on the belief that prolonged, marked elevation of systemic arterial pressure is in itself harmful and may contribute to and hasten the vascular lesions. Although this view is regarded with skepticism by some, there can be no question but that there are well-documented cases in which the use of depressor drugs has aborted or reversed progressive changes of malignant hypertension. Furthermore, there is evidence that patients with severe hypertension whose blood pressure has been effectively lowered by drug therapy over a period of 3 to 4 years may then be maintained on gradually decreasing doses and eventually no drug at all. Since peripheral resistance is the most important of the factors which determine the level of the blood pressure, hypotensive agents, to be effective therapeutically, should act by decreasing resistance rather than by decreasing cardiac output or flow. The introduction of hypotensive agents with varying sites of action has provided the physician with a new approach to medical therapy of hypertension. These drugs, although effective, require of the physician a thorough knowledge of the disease as well as of the agent employed. It should be remembered that hospitalization alone may lower the blood pressure and increase the responsivity

to antihypertensive agents. Therefore, although drug therapy may begin in the hospital, it must be regulated on an out-patient basis when the patient has resumed activity. Finally, since most of the agents used may have alarming if not serious side effects, it may be wise to allow the patient to experience these effects (including hypotension) in the hospital under the observation of the physician so that the patient may become aware of these manifestations and how to prevent or correct them on the outside. The use of sodium thiocyanate and nitroprusside, whose actions are similar, has been found by some to be effective in the treatment of hypertensive headache and in lowering of arterial pressure. Because of the necessity for controlling blood levels, however, their use is not widespread.

In Table 276-4 is listed a number of agents of value in the treatment of hypertension, along with their sites of action and side effects. Of these, the ganglionic blocking agents are of extreme and unquestioned potency. Their side effects, however, as well as the need for frequent control by careful blood pressure readings, relegate their use to the severer forms of hypertensive vascular disease. The uncertain absorption from the gastrointestinal tract of some of the previously used blocking agents constitutes an additional difficulty. This particular difficulty is overcome by the use of mecamylamine (Inversine), which is completely absorbed. A significant advance in therapy is represented by the introduction of guanethidine, which prevents the peripheral release of catecholamines from the postganglionic sympathetic nerve fibers. In effect, the sympathetic transmission is blocked, leaving unopposed parasympathetic action, thus eliminating those side effects of the ganglionic blockers which are specifically related to parasympathetic blockade. Guanethidine appears to be preferable to other agents acting at the same site because of its more gradual and prolonged effect.

Sympathetic blockade usually results in a decrease in peripheral resistance, with decreases in cerebral and renal blood flow. Frequently, the cardiac output may fall. For this reason, these agents may be hazardous in cerebral, renal, and coronary vascular disease. Since the blood pressure fall produced by these agents is most marked in the upright position, it may be of value to test their effects upon the electroencephalogram and the electrocardiogram, when the desired fall in blood pressure is achieved by gradual assumption of the upright posture on a tilt table. Decreased sensitivity or tolerance to all these agents has been reported. Because of its effect in increasing renal blood flow, Hydralazine may be an important adjunct to the use of the blocking agent. The increase in renal blood flow which occurs with Hydralazine, however, is not entirely consistent and results in part from increased cardiac output, in which the renal share of the cardiac output may be actually increased. The production of a syndrome resembling rheumatoid arthritis and disseminated lupus erythematosus with the prolonged use of Hydralazine is now well documented. Although, usually, this syndrome is reversible with cessation of therapy, in a few instances

Table 276-4. DRUGS USED IN TREATMENT OF HYPERTENSION

Drug	Site of action	Pharmacodynamics	Dosage*	Special indications	Contraindications	Side effects
Hydralazine	Central vasodilator and adrenergic blockade	Vasodilation Increased cardiac output Increased renal blood flow (±) Tachycardia	Oral: 10–200 mg q.i.d. Tolerance + +	As an adjunct to other agents	Lupus erythematosis Coronary artery disease Peptic ulcer (?)	Arthritis, lupus Headache, edema, nausea, tachycardia Unopposed cholinergic hyperacidity
Ganglionic blocking agents	Blocks autonomic transmission at ganglion	Sympathetic and parasympathetic inhibition (orthostatic hypotension with tachycardia, decreased intestinal motility, etc.)	. . . .	Severe hypertension	Coronary artery disease Arteriosclerosis Diabetes Glaucoma Prostatism	Constipation, visual symptoms Urinary retention Impotence
Mecamylamine	. . . .	Complete absorption	SC: 2–10 mg q. 8–10 hr	. . . .	. . . .	Tremor, hallucinations
Reserpine	Central sedative effect Depletes stored catecholamines Direct vasodilation (parenteral)	Central sedation Mild hypotension Increased intestinal motility Miosis Full action requires 3–6 days	Oral: 0.1–0.5 mg t.i.d. Parenteral: 2.5 mg q 2–4 hr Tolerance ±	As adjunct to other drugs Alone, in labile neurotic hypertensives	Pheochromocytoma	Sedation Diarrhea Bradycardia Nightmares Nasal congestion Weight gain, increase appetite Depression
Phenoxybenzamine	Adrenergic blockade (alpha receptors) Blocks circulating catecholamines (epinephrine, norepinephrine)	Prevents action of adrenergic mediators (epinephrine, norepinephrine) Miosis Orthostatic hypotension	Oral: 10–20 mg q.i.d. Tolerance + +	As adjunct in hypertension with renal failure	Coronary artery disease Arteriosclerosis	Miosis Dry mouth Nasal congestion Impotence Tachycardia
Guanethidine	Blocks accumulation of amines in axon storage granule	Sympathetic inhibition (orthostatic hypotension) Parasympathetics intact Prolonged effect	Oral: 10–400 mg per day IV: 0.5 mg/kg	Moderate to severe hypertension	Coronary artery disease Glaucoma Arteriosclerosis Pheochromocytoma	Facial pain, parotitis, impairment of ejaculation, abdominal pain, visual blurring, diarrhea, neurologic disturbance, hallucinations, flapping tremor
Monamine oxidase inhibitors (iproniazid, carboxazid, pargyline)	Blocks destruction of monamines	Sympathetic inhibition (orthostatic hypotension) Mood elevation	Oral: iproniazid, 50–150 mg/day	Coronary artery disease in elderly depressed patients	Coronary artery disease Arteriosclerosis Pheochromocytoma	Flushing, dizziness, confusion Hepatotoxicity Acute hypertension (precipitation by tyramine-containing foods, e.g., aged cheese)
α-Methyl DOPA	Inhibits decarboxylation of aromatic amino acids	Catecholamine depletion "False" neurotransmitter	Oral: 0.25–2.0 Gm t.i.d.	Renal disease	Pheochromocytoma	Sedation, fatigue, fluid retention, impotence Fever, Coomb's positive hemolytic anemia
Meprobamate	Central sedative effect	Decreases centrally modulated pressor responses	Oral: 400 mg b.i.d.–t.i.d.	Mild hypertension Moderate hypertension (with thiazides)	?	Sedation
Spironolactone	Renal tubule	Block action aldosterone	Oral: 25–100 mg t.i.d.–q.i.d.	Alone, mild hypertension potentiates other depressor agents Primary and secondary aldosteronism	Renal failure	G.I. irritation Hyperkalemia
Thiazide diuretics	Distal renal tubule	Na diuresis vasodilation	Depends on compound	Alone, mild hypertension Potentiates other depressor agents	Diabetes mellitus Hyperuricemia	K depletion Hyperglycemia, Hyperuricemia
Diazoxide	Arteriole	Arteriolar dilation	IV: 5 mgm/kg Tolerance + +	Hypertensive crisis	Diabetes mellitus Hyperuricemia	Hyperglycemia Sodium retention

* Tolerance + + indicates a strong likelihood that the dose will eventually need to be increased in order to maintain a given effect.

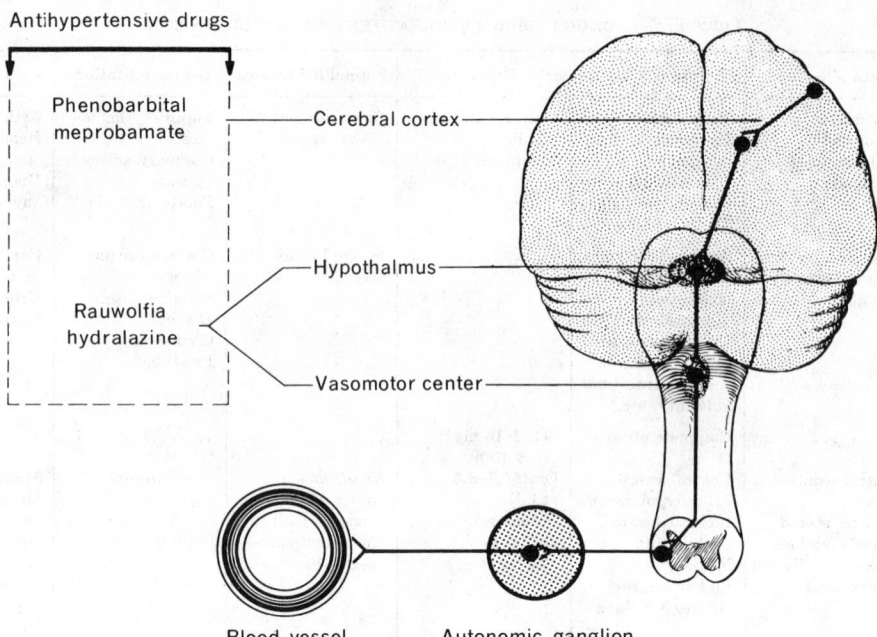

Fig. 276-2. Central action of antihypertensive drugs.

persistence of the disease has occurred following cessation of the drug.

The thiazide diuretics are among the most commonly used agents for the treatment of hypertension. In part, their action depends upon their natriuretic effect, but lowering of blood pressure can be shown to persist without significant depletion of intravascular or extracellular volume and there is probably a direct action upon the vasculature. Chlorothiazide (Diuril) is the prototype. The various substituted thiazides, hydrochlorothiazide (Hydrodiuril, Esidrex, Oretic, trichlormethiazide (Naqua, Metahydrin), and polythiazide (Renese) differ in dosage but are essentially similar in their mode of action. The one exception is chlorthalidone (Hygroton), whose action is more prolonged, requiring only a single daily dose varying from 100 to 600 mg. Nonthiazide diuretics, such as Triamterene and ethacrynic acid, are extremely potent oral diuretics. The former does not cause uric acid retention but does depress filtration rate. These agents have a mild antihypertensive effect when given alone, but their major value is through the potentiation of the action of other hypertensive agents.

The so-called "loop diuretics" ethacrynic acid (Edecrin) and furosemide (Lasix) act to inhibit sodium absorption on the ascending loop of Henle. They are of much greater natriuretic potency than the thiazides but have comparable antihypertensive properties. Unlike the thiazides, however, they are potent enough so that they may produce natriuresis in the presence of renal failure.

Spironolactone (Aldactone) blocks the peripheral action of aldosterone. It is a mild antihypertensive agent in itself and is used to prevent the rebound in sodium retention following diuretic administration as well as to prevent potassium losses during their use. The mechanism

of action of these diuretic agents is discussed in Chap. 264.

Dramatic and unquestioned therapeutic results have been obtained with the use of these substances. Most of them are toxic and dangerous in excessive dosage, however, and the margin between the toxic and the therapeutic dose is relatively narrow; hence, all such therapy should be begun in the hospital. The hypotensive agents selected should be administered initially in less than effective dosage and increased slowly, until either the desired therapeutic effect or toxicity supervenes. As with insulin therapy it may be wise, under controlled conditions in the hospital, to familiarize the patient with mild toxic effects so that they can be recognized. Alternate dosage with the initial agent and one of the others, or preferably the potentiation of the depressor effect of the initial agent by the addition of small doses of another drug, may increase the depressor effect while decreasing the side effects inherent in both. Such a combination, too, may minimize the effect of tolerance to either agent. Experience suggests that the concurrent use of two or three of these agents with different sites of action may be the method of choice. When the patient's dosage has been established in the hospital, he may be seen at less frequent intervals on the outside, and the therapeutic effects may be increased without increasing toxic effects by the addition of a third agent or by the substitution of a new agent for one of the two when tolerance becomes apparent. Potentiation of depressor effect can be achieved also by decreasing the sodium content in the diet. Cessation of therapy should never be abrupt, since dangerous hypertensive rebounds may result. The necessity for carefully controlling the use of these agents carries with it the disadvantage of making the patient drug conscious and blood pressure conscious. Once he has become familiar with the drugs, however, and confident of their therapeutic benefits he may learn to regulate them by taking his own blood pressure in the same manner that an intelligent diabetic regulates his insulin by testing his urine.

The chlorothiazide analogue diazoxide (Mutabase) is of particular interest. This agent has the advantage of causing an increase in cardiac output and cerebral blood flow and a decrease in systemic arteriolar tone. Its chronic administration is contraindicated because of its diabetogenic action. However, in many instances it has the interesting ability of causing increasing responsiveness to other agents to whose chronic administration the hypertensive patient has become refractory. A single injection of 5 mg per kg diazoxide may decrease blood pressure effectively for 5 to 6 hr. A program of 1 to 2 injections per day for a period of a week or 10 days in the hospital may permit effective and safe decrease in blood pressure for a period of months or even years with other depressor agents to which the patient had become refractory. It is possible that the action of diazoxide in this regard is to reset the baroreceptors so that pharmacologically induced drops in blood pressure no longer result in a reflex response which maintains the blood pressure at hypertensive levels.

The presence of advanced renal failure requires special caution in the use of antihypertensive agents. Dibenzyline (10 to 20 mg t.i.d.) appears to be an effective antihypertensive agent in about 20 percent of patients with renal failure, possibly through its action on unexcreted pressor amines. In mild renal failure large doses of reserpine (2 to 5 mg per day) or the combined use of ganglionic blockers and Hydralazine may be of value. However, such doses of reserpine are rarely well tolerated. Guanethidine must be administered with caution to patients with renal failure both because of the severe orthostatic hypotension that may result and because of drug accumulation. In such patients the hypotensive effect may continue for 7 to 10 days after discontinuing the drug. Alphamethyldopa (Aldomet), although ineffective in one-third of the patients with renal failure, appears to be of special benefit in others. It is more effective in lowering the blood pressure in the supine position than other agents and appears to have less adverse effect on renal function. In properly selected cases an initial increase in nitrogen retention may be followed later by improvement in renal function although at considerably decreased blood pressure levels. This may result in part from decreasing the pressure load on the left ventricle and improving cardiac output. Since some patients with renal failure may be sodium wasters, sodium depletion with its enhancement of vasodepressor action of drugs must be carefully considered. The sites of action of the various depressor agents are shown schematically in Figs. 276-2 and 276-3.

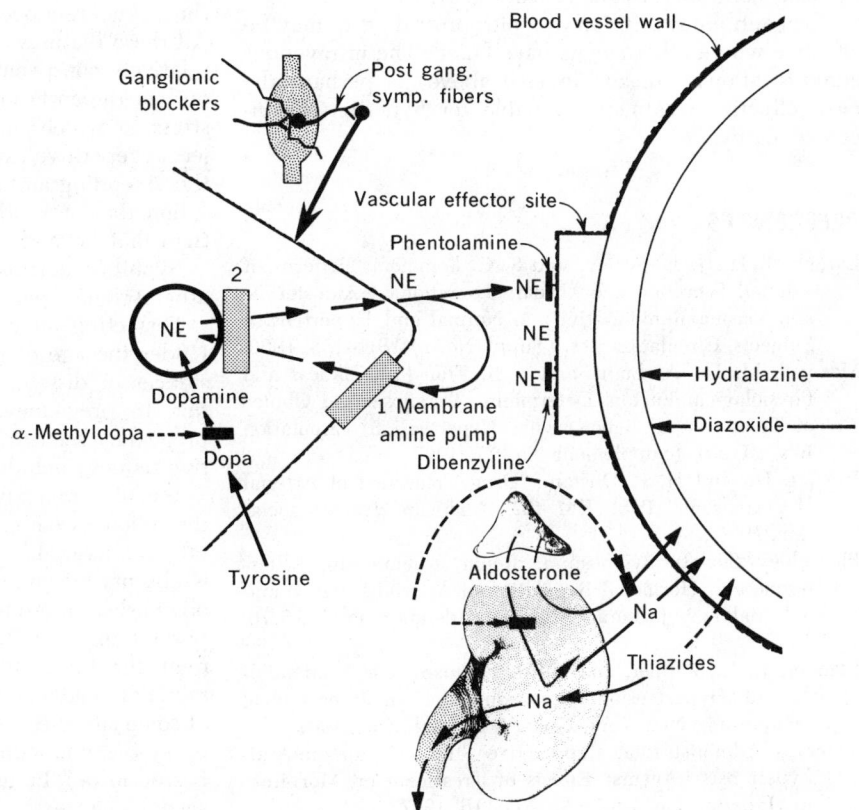

Fig. 276-3. Peripheral action of antihypertensive drugs. Guanethindine inhibits the axonal membrane amine pump. (1) Active transport of cytoplasmic amine into axonal granules is blocked by both reserpine and Guanethidine (2), thus depleting the storage granule of norepinephrine effectors. Phentolamine and dibenzyline are alpha adrenergic blocking drugs which block the effect of norepinephrine (NE) on the vascular receptor.

TREATMENT OF HYPERTENSIVE ENCEPHALOPATHY. The incidence and clinical picture of hypertensive encephalopathy have been described earlier in this chapter. Although in certain cases hypervolemia may contribute greatly to the abnormality, the common denominator is hypertension due largely to generalized vasospasm. It is rational, therefore, to attempt to lower the diastolic blood pressure by pharmacologic means. This may be done effectively in children, and in a small percentage of young adults, by the intramuscular injection of a 50% solution of magnesium sulfate, in doses of 0.2 ml per kg body weight. This may have to be repeated several times at 4-hr intervals, to keep pressure at satisfactory levels, following which the oral administration of 13 to 30 ml of 50% magnesium sulfate two to three times a day may satisfactorily control the blood pressure. If intravenous injection is necessary a 3% solution of hydrated magnesium sulfate may be given slowly; 150 mg of the salt per kilogram of body weight is given over a period of 1 hr. The effects of overdosage (somnolence, respiratory difficulty) may be counteracted by the administration of a 10% solution of calcium gluconate by vein. Oxygen therapy, sedatives, and, occasionally, venesection and spinal tap may be useful. Dramatic results have been observed with the use of intravenous or intramuscular protoveratrine or with large doses (2 to 5 mg parenteral reserpine), and with the continuous drip of an aqueous solution of trimethaphan (Arfonad), a rapidly acting, short-lived ganglionic blocking agent whose effect by this route can be easily controlled by the rate of the drip.

The continuous infusion of a nitroprusside drip may be effective where other agents have failed. The intravenous administration of diazoxide (see above) is perhaps the most effective treatment available for hypertensive encephalopathy.

REFERENCES

Laragh, J. H., J. E. Sealey, and S. C. Sommers: Patterns of Adrenal Secretion and Urinary Excretion of Aldosterone and Plasma Renin Activity in Normal and Hypertensive Subjects, Circulation Res. (Suppl. No. 1) 18:1–158, 1966.

Maxwell, M. H., A. Lupu, and S. S. Franklin: Clinical and Physiological Factors Determining Diagnosis and Choice of Treatment of Renovascular Hypertension, Circulation Res. 21:201 (Supplement No. 2), 1967.

Page, I. H., and H. P. Dustan: "Drug Treatment of Arterial Hypertension," Publ. EM 422, American Heart Association, 1966.

Physiology Society Symposium: Renin, Angiotensin, Aldosterone and Hormonal Regulation of Arterial Pressure and Salt Balance, J. Laragh (Ed.), Federation Proc. 26:70, 1967.

Stamler, J., R. Stamler, and T. M. Pullman: The Epidemiology of Hypertension—Proceedings of an International Symposium, New York, Grune & Stratton, Inc., 1967.

Veterans Administration Cooperative Study Group on Antihypertensive Agents: Effects of Treatment on Morbidity in Hypertension, J.A.M.A., 202:116, 1967.

277 DISEASES OF THE AORTA
Victor A. McKusick

DISSECTING ANEURYSM OF THE AORTA

CYSTIC MEDIAL NECROSIS. This is the most frequent morphologic substrate of dissecting aneurysm. It is not the only structural change which can lead to dissection, and conversely it can produce clinical manifestations in the absence of dissection. Cystic medial necrosis appears to be a nonspecific change in the aorta in response to hemodynamic stresses. The frequency with which it is found at autopsy increases with the age of the group studied. (The age distribution of cases of dissecting aneurysm is similar.) Its anatomic distribution is also characteristic, being most marked in the ascending aorta and decreasing progressively as one passes farther from the aortic valve, especially beyond the vessels which branch at the aortic arch. Hypertension accelerates the development of cystic medial necrosis. Furthermore, cystic medial necrosis and dissecting aneurysm are occasional complications of coarctation of the aorta. The hemodynamic changes produced by aortic stenosis and regurgitation accelerate the development of cystic medial necrosis in the ascending aorta. In the genetically defective aorta—that of Marfan's syndrome (Chap. 395) is the only clear example one can cite—the ordinary hemodynamic stresses lead to early development of cystic medial necrosis, especially in the ascending aorta, with progressive dilatation and/or dissecting aneurysm. (In all dissecting aneurysm, the intimal rent occurs most often in the ascending aorta.) All these features suggest that cystic medial necrosis is a relatively nonspecific morphologic expression of "wearing-out" of the aorta in response to hemodynamic stress. The stress to which the ascending aorta is particularly subject is repetitive expansile pulsation. With each heartbeat the ascending aorta is subjected to greater expansile pulsation than any other part of the aorta, especially more than that beyond the aortic arch.

Syphilitic aortitis does not lead to dissection, nor does atherosclerosis per se.

Dissecting aneurysm occurs more commonly in men. Under the age of forty years, approximately half the instances of dissecting aneurysm in women occur in relation to pregnancy. Hormonal changes associated with pregnancy seem to be responsible for effects on connective tissues, including those of the aorta.

Usually from an intimal rent in the ascending aorta, dissection extends proximally to the aortic ring and distally for a variable distance. (Occasionally an intimal rent is absent. Bleeding into the media from vasa vasorum is obviously important in such cases and probably is important in the initiation of most cases; hence the synonyms for dissecting aneurysm: medial hematoma and dissecting hematoma of the aorta.) "Reentry" may take place at some site such as just beyond the left subclavian orifice or in the abdominal aorta, with creation of a "double-barrel aorta." Prognosis is better in such cases. The dissection may extend for a considerable distance into one or several of the branches of the aorta, from the coronary arteries to the iliac arteries. The proximal dissection may distort the aortic ring and result in aortic regurgitation. (Cystic medial necrosis antedating the dissection may have resulted in dilatation of the sinuses of Valsalva and aortic regurgitation.) Rupture of the aorta into the pericardial or pleural cavity occurs in a majority of cases, although other sites of rupture such as the transverse portion of the duodenum are occasionally observed. Rupture into the pericardial sac is not surprising since the pericardial deflections extend high on the ascending aorta in many persons.

The clinical manifestations of dissecting aneurysm may be classified as follows: (1) pain, (2) aortic regurgitation, (3) interference with the blood supply through branches of the aorta, (4) x-ray evidence of progressive widening of the aorta, (5) rupture of the aorta.

In addition, tissue destruction may be of sufficient proportions to produce mild fever, leukocytosis, and elevation of sedimentation rate.

The pain of dissecting aneurysm is sometimes described as tearing in quality. It is questionable that its quality is truly different from that of myocardial infarction. Characteristically it attains peak intensity very shortly after onset. It may involve the anterior chest, back, lumbar area, or abdomen, sometimes in a progression. Dissecting aneurysm may occur, however, with little or nothing the patient describes as pain. The blood pressure may drop precipitously during the dissection, but maintenance of hypertension or increased blood pressure in response to the pain is often the finding.

The most frequently observed evidence of disturbance at the orifices of the branches is discrepancy in the pulses and blood pressure readings in the arms. Asymmetric diminution in these signs may occur. The same observations may be made in the carotid and femoral vessels. Myocardial infarction or changes of myocardial ischemia, neurologic signs from interference with cerebral and/or spinal blood flow, intestinal symptoms, and hematuria may occur.

Rupture of the aorta is, of course, usually fatal. However, in rare instances leakage into the pericardial cavity may be interrupted and the patient may survive for months or even years. The chest pain, together with a pericardial friction rub, may indicate the presence of leaking dissecting aneurysm hours before the leak proceeds to the point of producing cardiac tamponade.

In the differential diagnosis of dissecting aneurysm, myocardial infarction and pulmonary embolus present the greatest problems. Pain reaching a rapid peak of intensity, especially if followed within minutes or hours by signs of arterial occlusion, favors the diagnosis of dissecting aneurysm. Unconsciousness may result from involvement of the cephalic trunks in the dissection and is unusual in myocardial infarction in the absence of severe hypotension or arrhythmia. The maintenance of arterial hypertension favors the diagnosis of dissecting aneurysm, although profound hypotension may occur in both dissection and myocardial infarction.

Only a few patients survive more than a few days after an acute dissection. Most of the survivors succumb to rupture of the aorta or other complications within a year. Pharmacologic hypotension in those cases with maintained hypertension during the acute dissection has a rational place in treatment of the early stages. In normotensive patients, reserpine or propranolol in subhypotensive doses, by changing the shape of the ventricular ejection curve and reducing the abruptness of ejection, may be beneficial. (Reserpine has been effective in reducing the incidence of aortic rupture in strains of turkeys predisposed to this accident.) Significant aortic regurgitation, evidence of encroachment on the ostiums of branch arteries, especially the renals, inability to maintain a normal blood pressure, evidence of progressive dissection or of adventitial rupture are all indications that surgical intervention should be considered.

Cystic medial necrosis sometimes results in aneurysm, usually of the ascending aorta, without dissection. The clinical behavior resembles that of syphilitic aneurysm in many respects. In other cases, aortic regurgitation is the main and presenting problem. Surgical treatment has been successful in some of these instances.

SYPHILITIC AORTITIS

Syphilitic involvement is limited largely to the thoracic aorta, particularly the ascending aorta. Syphilitic cardiovascular disease rarely occurs in persons who have had syphilis for less than 10 years or in those who received even a moderate amount of antisyphilitic treatment in the early stage of the infection. On the other hand, so great is the predilection of *Treponema pallidum* for the aorta that a majority of patients with untreated cases have involvement of that vessel. Fortunately, the frequency of syphilitic cardiovascular disease has decreased markedly in the last decade.

The predominant localization of syphilitic change to the ascending aorta may be the result of the combination of the particular hemodynamic stress (see Cystic Medial Necrosis, above) with the medial damage by the treponemal infection. Other explanations are probably less satisfactory.

Aortic regurgitation, fusiform aneurysm, or saccular aneurysm may result. Syphilitic aortitis uncomplicated by any one of these three may betray its presence by a change in the quality of the aortic second sound usually referred to as "tambouric" (scarcely a pathognomonic sign, however) and by the presence of intimal, shell-like calcification in the first part of the ascending aorta. In some cases this calcification even extends proximally to outline the sinuses of Valsalva. Atherosclerosis alone usually does not produce calcification in the first part of the ascending aorta. The primary lesion of syphilitic aortitis is medial, but intimal atherosclerosis is accelerated by the damage to the media. Occlusive change in the ostiums of branch arteries, such as the coronaries with production of angina pectoris or the aortic arch vessels with production of the aortic arch syndrome, occurs through a similar mechanism.

Syphilitic aneurysms occur with diminishing frequency from the ascending aorta distally toward the abdominal aorta. They may be single or multiple, diffuse or sharply localized, fusiform or saccular, smooth-walled or thrombus-filled. Symptoms are likely to be due to compression (e.g., of the trachea, pulmonary artery, or superior vena cava) or erosion (e.g., of the sternum or vertebral column). Rupture into the superior vena cava or pulmonary artery may occur and the patient may survive for some time, with dramatic physical findings. Sudden death may result from external rupture or rupture into the tracheobronchial tree, pericardium, esophagus, etc. Happily, with improved public health control of syphilis and with better treatment, syphilitic aneurysm may soon become a matter of no particular concern to the clinician.

There has never been convincing evidence that specific treatment given after the development of clinical signs of cardiovascular syphilis prolongs life. There is evidence that aortic regurgitation is more frequent in syphilitic aortitis than previously thought; however, the prognosis in these patients is better than previously realized.

Herxheimer reactions following closely after the administration of penicillin have been observed in early syphilis, in which fever may occur, and in central nervous system syphilis, in which fever and aggravation of mental disturbances may be seen. Although the occurrence (after penicillin treatment) of Herxheimer reactions involving the coronary ostiums remains to be established, it is probably wise in a patient with cardiovascular syphilis and angina pectoris or electrocardiographic signs of myocardial ischemia to improve the myocardial status as much as possible before antisyphilitic therapy and to institute such therapy only under conditions of optimal rest and observation.

Surgical therapy for syphilitic aneurysms has made outstanding advances. With cardiopulmonary bypass aneurysms of the ascending aorta can be resected. Operation is indicated for all except small aneurysms, for which observation is warranted.

ARTERIOSCLEROTIC ANEURYSMS

Arteriosclerotic aneurysms occur most frequently, although not exclusively, in the abdominal aorta, especially in that portion between the ostiums of the renal arteries and the bifurcation. The patients are usually men in the sixth or seventh decade of life or older. Both dilatation and buckling of the aorta are usually involved, and the buckling is usually predominantly to the left.

Manifestations include primarily pain in the back or anterior part of the abdomen and a pulsatile abdominal mass which usually presents in the epigastrium. (As projected on the anterior abdominal wall, the bifurcation lies at approximately the level of the umbilicus.) The patient may discover that the knee-elbow position relieves the pain. The diagnosis may be obvious from ordinary roentgenograms of the abdomen if an eggshell-like or other calcification outlines the aneurysm. Aortograms can make the definitive anatomic diagnosis.

Rupture of arteriosclerotic aneurysms is frequently the mechanism of death. Rupture is likely to begin in the ulceration of an atheromatous plaque. There is usually no more than short medial dissection. Rupture may result in the rapid development of a mass in the left flank. The hematoma may dissect retroperitoneally into the groin and produce manifestations simulating incarcerated inguinal hernia. Rupture into the duodenum, another indication of the high location of these aneurysms, may occur.

Arteriosclerotic aneurysm of the abdominal aorta has been treated surgically with good results. Resection of the affected portion and replacement with a synthetic prosthesis have been performed successfully in literally thousands of patients. If the general condition of the patient permits, all except small aneurysms should be resected. In the minority of cases in which the renal arteries and higher branches of the aorta are involved in the wall of the aneurysm, modifications of the basic procedure are necessary.

AORTIC ARCH SYNDROMES (Pulseless Disease, Young Female Arteritis, Takayasu Syndrome, Reverse Coarctation)

Slowly progressive change may lead to partial or total obliteration of the major branches of the aortic arch. Intimal atherosclerosis alone can produce at least a partial aortic arch syndrome, and it often collaborates with other factors such as syphilis and trauma in producing obliteration. Severe trauma to the upper part of the chest, especially if the neck is extended, may rupture elements of the media in the region of the ostiums of the arch branches and thus lay the groundwork for progressive intimal atherosclerosis at these sites. An inadequately understood progressive disorder occurs especially in young females, for which reason the designation *young female arteritis* has been used. Histopathologically these cases have been characterized by collections of chronic inflammatory cells, including giant cells. In this disorder the obliteration of major branches is especially likely to be complete, and the designation *pulseless disease* is particularly appropriate. Because of the absence of pulses in the upper part of the body with normal femoral pulses and hypertension in the legs, the term *reverse coarctation* has also been applied to this group of conditions.

In addition to the loss of palpable pulses, clinical manifestations include easy fatigability of the arms, atrophy of the muscles and other soft tissues of the face, necrosis of the cartilaginous nasal septum, and cataract. Systolic murmurs may be heard just above and below the clavicles if the occlusion is partial. If the pressure proximal to the obstruction is at all times in the cardiac cycle higher than that distal to the obstruction, a continuous murmur simulating that of patent ductus arteriosus may be heard in the same area. Syncopal attacks, especially with quiet standing after exercise, also occur.

Surgical replacement of the aortic arch has been performed in a few cases and will undoubtedly become increasingly feasible in the future.

THROMBOTIC OBLITERATION OF THE BIFURCATION OF THE AORTA
(Leriche Syndrome)

The bifurcation of the aorta is, like the bifurcation of the common carotid artery and the coronary arteries, an Achilles heel of the arterial tree as far as the development of atherosclerosis is concerned. Slowly progressive thrombosis at the bifurcation can result in complete obliteration of the aorta. The patients are usually men and may be as young as in the fourth decade. Some of the patients have hypercholesterolemia. The same clinical picture may result from saddle embolism of the bifurcation, as in mitral valve disease or myocardial infarction, if the patient survives the acute episode and is not operated on early.

The clinical manifestations of Leriche's syndrome are (1) intermittent claudication, with pain in the low part of the back or *gluteal area* which may be mistaken for "sciatica"; (2) loss of the ability to maintain a stable erection, because of the poor blood supply to the penis; (3) globose, i.e., symmetric, atrophy of the legs, which may be difficult to appreciate because of its symmetry; and (4) absence of both femoral pulses. Most of the patients have manifestations of atherosclerosis elsewhere —cerebral, coronary, aortic arch ostiums—and hypertension is frequent. Differentiation from coarctation of the aorta is afforded by feeling an aortic pulse in the epigastrium and by the absence of certain other signs of coarctation such as notching of the ribs and dilated collateral vessels over the thorax. Lateral roentgenograms of the lumbar spine may reveal basket-like or other calcification in the region of the bifurcation. Aortograms can make the diagnosis definite.

Surgical replacement of the aortic bifurcation with a synthetic prosthesis has been performed in a large number of patients, with great success.

TRAUMA OF THE AORTA

Penetrating wounds of the chest may be rapidly fatal because of puncture of the aorta. Nonpenetrating trauma to the chest, most commonly the steering wheel injuries in automobile accidents, may lead to rupture of the aorta. In over one-third of cases such rupture is just beyond the mouth of the left subclavian artery. If the victim survives the acute tear, a false aneurysm may result at this site. Such aneurysms are susceptible to surgical resection. As mentioned elsewhere (p. 1264), progressive obliteration of ostiums at the aortic arch with production of the aortic arch syndrome may be a late complication of trauma of a particular type.

AORTIC SINUS ANEURYSM

Aneurysms may occur in the sinuses of Valsalva from syphilis, idiopathic cystic medial necrosis, or a presumably congenital (ill-understood) basis. Rupture into the right atrium or right ventricle may occur. Successful surgical closure has been effected in such cases. Aneurysm of the aortic sinuses, usually with symmetric involvement of all three sinuses, occurs as a characteristic feature of Marfan's syndrome. Such aneurysms rarely if ever rupture into the right side of the heart.

UNUSUAL FORMS OF AORTITIS

Unusual forms of aortitis include mycotic aneurysm, such as that produced by aortic tuberculosis, temporal arteritis with aortic involvement, and granulomatous aortitis of the proximal few centimeters in ankylosing spondylitis.

Coarctation and other congenital anomalies of the aorta are discussed elsewhere (p. 1176).

REFERENCES

Boyer, S. H., IV, and V. A. McKusick: Diseases of the Aorta, Ann. Rev. Med., 9:85, 1958.

Leriche, R., and A. Morel: The Syndrome of Thrombotic Obliteration of the Aortic Bifurcation, Ann. Surg., 127:193, 1948.

Palmer, R. F., and M. W. Wheat, Jr.: Treatment of Dissecting Aneurysms of the Aorta, Ann. Thoracic Surg., 4:38, 1967.

Ross, R. S., and V. A. McCusick: Aortic Arch Syndromes, A.M.A. Arch. Intern. Med., 92:701, 1953.

278 VASCULAR DISEASE OF THE EXTREMITIES

Eugene A. Stead, Jr.

SYMPTOMS AND SIGNS

One should suspect peripheral vascular disease in a patient with the following symptoms and signs:

1. Pain in an extremity which is induced by exercise and relieved by rest: pain which is influenced by posture, is localized to one digit, is unilateral, or is paroxysmal

2. Impaired pulsations of peripheral arteries

3. Abnormal color of the skin, particularly when affected by raising or lowering the part

4. Gangrene, ulceration, impaired nail and hair growth, scleroderma, excessive calluses, or paronychial infections

5. Abnormal pulsations, enlarged veins, or edema

6. Unusual warmth or coldness

7. Swelling, atrophy, or difference in length of extremities

8. Auscultatory evidence of arteriovenous fistula

9. Localized systolic or continuous murmur over a large peripheral artery

10. Cyanosis or unusual pallor of digits when immersed in cold water. History of "dead-white" fingers or toes

11. Peripheral neuritis

If the above signs and symptoms are absent, peripheral vascular disease need not be considered.

The arteries, capillaries, veins, and lymph vessels may be involved separately or in varying combinations. The disturbances may be due to organic disease of the vessels or to abnormal constriction or dilatation caused by dysfunction of the autonomic nervous system.

SPECIAL DIAGNOSTIC TESTS

The history and physical examination will establish the presence or absence of arterial insufficiency. When the circulation is normal, no instruments are necessary to demonstrate the fact. The skin shows no trophic changes and does not blanch abnormally on elevation. The arterial pulses are palpable. If the main artery is occluded by pressure for several minutes, release of pressure will cause bright-red reactive hyperemia. Heating of the body causes the extremities to warm, and immersion of the part in hot water brings out the capillary pulse. Histamine pricked into the skin produces a typical wheal and erythema. When there is obvious arterial insufficiency, these findings are changed as outlined further on, under Special Points in History and Physical Examination. When other signs of arterial insufficiency are present, it is not safe to attempt to demonstrate the capillary pulse by placing the involved extremity in hot water.

Special tests have been of value in understanding the normal physiology of the peripheral circulation. They have been of use in quantifying the degree of damage caused by pathologic processes and have aided our understanding of the development of collateral circulation. They have been useful in determining, in at least a semiquantitative way, the effects of therapy in occlusive vascular disease.

The following tests are useful at times:

1. *Measurement of skin temperatures.* If the findings are those of arterial circulatory insufficiency, it must be determined whether the insufficiency results from (1) occlusive disease entirely, (2) overactivity of the sympathetic nervous system, (3) abnormal reaction of the blood vessels to cold, (4) the effect of cold agglutinins or cryoglobulins on the physical state of the blood, or (5) a combination of mechanisms.

The constrictor effect of the autonomic nervous system may be removed by paravertebral block of the appropriate sympathetic ganglion with procaine or by release of vasoconstrictor tone by body heating. In either method the patient, with body exposed, is placed in a cool room (temperature of 18 to 20°C). The body temperature may be raised by enclosing the trunk in a heating cabinet or by immersing two uninvolved limbs in water baths at 43°C for 40 min. When vasodilatation is produced in the upper extremities by body warming or by blocking of the sympathetic ganglion, the temperature of the digits rises rapidly to between 30.5 and 33°C. If the temperature rises to between 27 and 29°C, there is moderate organic vascular disease. If no rise occurs or if the temperature falls, advanced local arterial disease is present. Body warming is the simplest and most effective method of relieving vasoconstrictor tone in the upper extremities. It fails occasionally in the lower extremities. Therefore, if full vasodilatation does not occur, paravertebral block in the lower extremities is indicated.

2. *Arteriography and venography.* The arterial tree is visualized by x-ray after the intraarterial injection of 50 percent Hypaque or other contrast media. When the femoral pulses are absent, injection is made into the aorta. The exact point of arterial obstruction and the pattern of the collateral circulation can be determined. This procedure is helpful in showing segmental occlusion in the iliac and femoral vessels. These lesions can now be approached surgically. Visualization of the veins by the injection of radiopaque material is occasionally useful.

3. *Circulation time to the extremities.* Several methods are available. The fluorescein test is the most objective. For this, 3 ml of a 20 percent aqueous solution of fluorescein is injected quickly into the antecubital vein, and the time of appearance of a greenish-yellow glow in various parts of the body is observed, with illumination from ultraviolet light. When arterial insufficiency is present, the appearance time of the fluorescein is prolonged. In severe ischemia no fluorescein may appear.

4. *Oscillometer.* This is a volume recorder which magnifies the changes in volume which normally occur with each cardiac cycle. The ordinary blood pressure recording apparatus may be used as a crude oscillometer. Refinements of the oscillometer have not increased its clinical usefulness.

5. *Histamine wheal test.* If the arterial circulation is inadequate, histamine pricked into the skin gives a subnormal or absent reaction.

6. *Measurement of blood flow by plethysmographic techniques* has advanced our knowledge of the circulation, but the method is not suitable for routine clinical use.

7. *Cannulation of lymph vessels* in the web of fingers and toes with injection of radiopaque substances affords good visualization of the anatomic problems in patients with edema from diseases involving the lymphatic system. Lymphatic obstruction, lymphatic varicosities, or reduction in the number of lymph channels may be the major factor in the edema.

DISTURBANCES IN ARTERIAL FUNCTION

SPECIAL POINTS IN HISTORY AND PHYSICAL EXAMINATION. Arterial insufficiency causes disturbances in nutrition to the part. The following points in the history and examination are to be noted:

Sensitivity to Cold with Blanching or Cyanosis of Digits. On examination, the part with arterial insufficiency may be colder than the corresponding part of the opposite extremity. Most normal persons have cool or cold feet in the absence of any disease of the blood vessels or nerves.

The feet warm normally when the body is heated sufficiently to cause a rise in rectal temperature.

Muscle and Nerve Ischemia. Pain which develops in the muscles during exercise and which disappears at rest is called intermittent claudication. If exercise is continued after the pain appears, the muscles may become tender. Intermittent claudication occurs most frequently in the muscles of the calves and feet. When the lower aorta is occluded, pain may involve the muscles of the buttocks and back. The patient may describe claudication as a cramping pain, but examination by the doctor reveals pain but no spasm of the muscle. Pain produced by spasm of muscles must not be confused with claudication caused by arterial disease. In more severe ischemia of the leg, pain may occur at rest and be relieved by dependency. The pain of ischemic neuritis is severe and diffuse, with severe exacerbations. Sharp shooting pains may dart through the entire extremity. The acute paroxysms are apt to occur at night. Occlusive disease of the lower aorta may cause impotence.

State of Peripheral Vessels. Presence or absence of carotid, subclavian, brachial, femoral, popliteal, dorsalis pedis, and posterior tibial pulses is noted. Gangrene of the digits may occur without disturbances in these pulses. In the absence of a palpable pulse, the skin may show no evidence of malnutrition. This indicates that the main vessels below the point of obstruction are open.

Murmurs over Peripheral Vessels. Pistol shot sounds are heard over the major vessels when the diastolic pressure is low and the stroke output is high. Localized systolic murmurs are heard over areas of narrowing, produced either by disease of the blood vessel or by external pressure. When the vessel is narrowed, the local points of stenosis produce a murmur similar to that heard in aortic stenosis. If the diastolic pressure below the point of narrowing is low, either because of poor collateral circulation or because of wide vasodilatation produced by exercise, a continuous murmur may be heard. With this exception and that of venous hums, continuous murmurs are commonly the result of an arteriovenous communication.

Blanching on Elevation; Redness and Cyanosis on Dependency. On elevation to a 90° angle, the part becomes pale and at times white. The extent of the pallor indicates the extent of the arterial insufficiency. If only the toes are involved, or a part of a toe, the pallor is limited to the ischemic area. The color returns slowly on lowering the part to heart level. The pallor occurs on elevation because the blood in the capillaries and venules drains out of the part by gravity, and because the effective arterial pressure is lowered by having to overcome the hydrostatic force of a column of blood extending from the heart level to the elevated part. Some pallor on elevation will occur in a normal foot, but the pallor of arterial insufficiency is much more marked.

When the part hangs down, the blood flow is increased temporarily over the horizontal position because the hydrostatic pressure is added to the pressure created by the heart. The increase in arterial pressure is effective until the veins fill. Then it is opposed by an equal column of blood on the venous side, and the pressure differential between artery and vein returns approximately to the differential present in the horizontal position. The minute vessels of the part, being in a state of chronic injury because of an inadequate circulation, are dilated. When these vessels first fill, they are red. Varying degrees of cyanosis gradually develop because of the slow blood flow.

Atrophic Changes in Skin and Edema. The skin becomes thin and atrophic. Slight edema with loss of normal wrinkles is common. If the patient keeps the foot dependent day and night to relieve pain, pitting edema may develop from the combination of a high capillary pressure from dependency and the damaged state of the capillaries caused by ischemia. Hair will disappear from ischemic areas.

Gangrene. Devitalized tissue offers a good place for infection to spread. When peripheral neuritis is present, infection may be more prominent than ischemia. Osteomyelitis may occur.

Arteriovenous Fistula (Direct Communication between Artery and Vein). Any object which penetrates the skin and injures both artery and vein may cause a traumatic arteriovenous fistula. Venipuncture and catheterization procedures occasionally cause arteriovenous fistula, but bullets and knives are the common offenders. The surgeon's curet also produces aortic–posterior vena cava fistulas during the removal of ruptured intervertebral disks. Traumatic compression of the chest may cause an aortic–left atrial fistula. The congenital arteriovenous communications may involve one or several areas of the body. In any one area, the communications are usually multiple and any one connection is small in comparison with the usual traumatic fistula. Congenital arteriovenous fistula may be present in the lung or other parts of the body as a part of the syndrome of familial telangiectasis. Both congenital and acquired fistulas may cause overgrowth of an extremity if the epiphyses are open.

Arteriovenous fistula, if large, may cause varicosities, edema, and a local mass which may press on adjacent nerves. Traumatic fistulas are always accompanied by a continuous murmur and usually by a thrill. If the fistula is large, the cardiac output is increased, the diastolic pressure is decreased, and the blood volume is increased. Obliteration of the fistula raises the arterial blood pressure, slows the pulse, and reduces the cardiac output. Large fistulas may cause cardiac enlargement and heart failure.

Neurologic Findings. Peripheral neuritis is a common complication of diabetes. Periarteritis nodosa and arteriosclerosis may cause neuritis because of the interference with the blood supply to the nerves. In periarteritis, motor weakness, as well as sensory loss and pain, is common.

Occupation. There may be a history of unusual exposure to cold and dampness. Use of the pneumatic hammer has been said to cause Raynaud's phenomenon.

ORGANIC OBSTRUCTION

BALANCE BETWEEN OBSTRUCTION AND COLLATERALS.
Obstruction of a large artery is a strong stimulus for new-vessel formation and collateral circulation. The symptoms produced represent the result of the balance between these two processes. Complete obstruction of the aorta below the renal vessels which occurs slowly may produce no symptoms or the picture of impotence and thigh claudication. The extremities may appear normally nourished. When skin involvement becomes marked, little blood vessels are usually thrombosed. This may be primary small-vessel endarteritis, as in diabetes, or it may be thrombosis or embolization in small vessels secondary to proximal occlusion. Gangrene with normal pedal pulses indicates small-vessel disease. Intermittent claudication may occur with absent popliteal and femoral pulses and normal skin; more rarely, with palpable pulses in the femoral, posterior tibial, and dorsalis pedis vessels. When these pulses are present at rest, they will disappear or markedly decrease with exercise.

PERIPHERAL ARTERIOSCLEROSIS. The etiology and pathology of peripheral arteriosclerosis have been discussed in Chap. 275. The history and physical findings are those of arterial insufficiency. The diagnosis is based on the following factors:

1. Age of patient. It is more frequent after fifty years of age but is not rare after thirty.
2. Sex. Males are more commonly affected than females.
3. Diabetes. The incidence of arteriosclerosis is increased in patients with diabetes.
4. Evidence of arteriosclerosis is usually present bilaterally, although the symptoms may be unilateral.
5. There are usually no symptoms of arterial disease in the upper extremities, but complete or partial obstruction of the subclavian vessels is not rare.
6. Coronary disease is common.
7. Extracerebral carotid disease is frequent.
8. Unilateral and bilateral renal arterial disease, with hypertension, may be present.
9. Aneurysm of abdominal aorta may be felt or visualized by x-ray.
10. The arteries, as seen by x-ray, are frequently calcified. Calcification may occur in the media and not cause any obstruction. The combination of the symptoms of vascular insufficiency in a part and calcification in vessels supplying the part increases the likelihood that arteriosclerosis is an important factor.
11. In patients with diabetes, the small vessels may be occluded, although the larger vessels are only moderately diseased. Local gangrene of the skin of the toes may occur, even though the rest of the foot is warm.
12. In patients with diabetes, neuropathy is common.

THROMBOANGIITIS OBLITERANS. This condition was described by Buerger in 1908 as an obliterative vascular disease affecting chiefly the peripheral arteries and veins of Jewish males in early adult life. The disease involved primarily the blood vessels of the extremities, beginning in medium- and small-sized arteries. Veins were involved less commonly. The lesion was a nonsuppurative panarteritis or panphlebitis and was segmental, leaving normal vessels between diseased segments. The lesions came in crops, producing complete and usually permanent obstruction, followed by the development of extensive collateral circulation. The history and physical findings were those of arterial insufficiency or superficial phlebitis. The diagnosis was based on these considerations:

1. Age. Onset was usually between twenty and forty-five years.
2. Sex. Males predominated in a ratio of 75:1.
3. Race. Half the patients were Jewish.
4. Migratory phlebitis preceding or accompanying arterial disease.
5. Severe pain at rest from ulceration or from ischemic neuritis.
6. Absence of calcification as seen by x-ray.
7. Small vessels of the hands might be involved. Thrombosis of mesenteric, coronary, cerebral, or renal arteries was not common.

Atherosclerosis in young men is now a well-known entity. It is a segmental disease. Thrombosis in the arteries is frequently associated with thrombosis in the veins. The arteries and veins respond to thrombosis with an inflammatory reaction, followed by various degrees of recanalization. There is little doubt that most of the patients diagnosed in the past as having thromboangiitis obliterans had atherosclerosis. Nevertheless, there is a small group of patients with recurrent inflammatory lesions involving in the beginning the small vessels of the feet and hands with local gangrene, and eventually going on to thrombosis of medium-sized arteries. In some of these patients, abstinence from tobacco results in a complete remission. These patients may well be considered to have Buerger's disease.

LESS-COMMON CAUSES OF OBSTRUCTION IN MEDIUM-SIZED ARTERIES. Narrowing or obstruction of the radial, ulnar, and posterior tibial arteries is common in patients with pseudo-xanthoma elasticum. Thromboses secondary to inflammatory changes caused by periarteritis and lupus erythematosus are not uncommon.

Thrombosis. Thrombosis of the larger arteries of the lower extremities is common in the natural course of arteriosclerosis. Whether or not dramatic symptoms of acute arterial insufficiency appear will depend on the degree of collateral circulation which has developed. Gradual narrowing of a major vessel may progress unnoticed to complete occlusion, because the symptoms of arterial insufficiency may not develop until the collateral channels begin to thrombose.

Embolus. Emboli are usually fragments from more centrally placed thrombi. The occurrence of sudden arterial insufficiency without physical findings of marked peripheral vascular disease generally indicates an embolus. The common sources are:

1. Mural thrombus from the left atrium of a patient with chronic atrial fibrillation

2. Mural thrombus from the left atrium of a patient with mitral stenosis and, commonly but not necessarily, with atrial fibrillation

3. Mural thrombus from myocardial infarction of the left ventricle or, more rarely, from acute or subacute myocarditis

4. Thrombi on valves from subacute or acute bacterial endocarditis

5. Cholesterol emboli from ulcerated atheromatous plaques

Less-common sources are:

1. Thrombi in the aorta or its large branches

2. Venous thrombosis in patients with a right-left shunt from congenital heart disease

3. Venous thrombosis, causing pulmonary embolization, right-sided heart failure, and the passage of a clot through the patent foramen ovale

4. Myxoma of the left atrium

Emboli are likely to lodge at the bifurcation of large vessels. A saddle embolus riding on the bifurcation of the aorta may cause circulatory insufficiency in both lower extremities. The signs of circulatory insufficiency are usually considerably distal to the embolus because of the presence of collateral circulation. An embolus in the common femoral artery usually shows temperature and color changes at the level of the knee, but an embolus to the popliteal artery will show similar changes if adequate collateral circulation is not present. Loss of motion and of sensation may occur rapidly. Ischemic pain in muscles supplied by vessels distal to the embolus will occur if the muscles are used. If the muscles are not used, the sensory nerves may become paralyzed before pain develops. At first there is no pain at the site of the embolus, but tenderness may develop after a few hours as the embolus sets up a local inflammatory reaction in the vessel.

Exposure to Cold; Trench Foot. Extremities with normal blood vessels are injured by prolonged exposure to cold. Dependency and wetness combined with cold cause tissue damage, even though actual freezing of the tissues does not occur. On warming, the injury results in extreme vasodilatation, with swelling of the part because the capillaries have been damaged. Later, true capillary flow in the skin may cease because of capillary stasis and thrombosis, although flow continues through small arteriovenous communications. This gives the clinical picture of superficial gangrene in a warm part. Whether complete recovery or gangrene occurs depends on the extent of the injury. Persistent tenderness because of fibrosis and ischemic neuritis may develop.

Obstruction of Main Arterial Trunks from Other Causes. Broad insertion of the scalenus anticus muscle with or without cervical rib is a rare cause of Raynaud's phenomenon or organic arterial occlusion. The vascular disturbances may be reflex from compression of a portion of the brachial plexus. At times, trauma from compression of the artery causes thrombus formation, with or without embolic phenomena distal to the area of injury.

Persons who sleep with their arms hyperabducted above the head or whose occupation causes them to work with their arms hyperabducted may develop numbness and tingling from occlusion of the subclavian axillary vessels. Usually, discomfort causes the arms to be moved to a different position, but gangrene of the fingers has been reported in some cases.

Syphilitic aneurysm or dissecting aneurysm may cause obstruction to the main artery supplying the limb.

Obstruction of Aorta below the Renal Vessels and Obstruction of the Vessels Arising from the Arch of the Aorta. These disorders are considered in chapter 277.

Obstructive Disease of the Small Vessels. Inflammatory involvement of the small divisions of the vascular tree may cause local areas of gangrene. The arteritis may be secondary to severe infection with bacteremia, or it may be part of a more generalized process such as systemic lupus erythematosus or periarteritis. At times there is no evidence of any other involvement beyond the local lesions. In time, thrombosis may occur in larger vessels. Occasionally, cigarette smoking is the cause and complete abstinence the cure.

SPASM OF ARTERIES AND ARTERIOLES

RAYNAUD'S DISEASE AND RAYNAUD'S PHENOMENON. Raynaud's disease is an idiopathic bilateral paroxysmal contraction of the arteries and arterioles of the digits, usually without local gangrene. The primary fault seems to be a local sensitivity of the digital vessels to cold. The attacks are precipitated by cold or emotion and are relieved by warming. Raynaud's phenomenon consists of paroxysmal attacks of ischemia of the digits occurring in the course of other diseases, such as scleroderma, thromboangiitis obliterans, cervical rib, arteriosclerosis, crutch paralysis, and pneumatic hammer disease.

Diagnosis of Raynaud's disease from the history and examination is made from the following points:

1. Sex. Females are affected much more often than males.

2. Age. It is less common before puberty and after forty, although it may occur at any age.

3. Bilateral and symmetric involvement of the digits. It is more common in the hands than in the feet.

4. "Dead" fingers or toes (extreme pallor followed by cyanosis) can be reproduced by immersion of the hands in cold water, by cooling the body rapidly by a cool shower, or by emotional arousal. The digital arteries and arterioles contract. The fingers become blue if the minute vessels remain dilated, pale if they contract. On rewarming, reactive hyperemia occurs.

5. If the disease is of many years' duration, small superficial areas of gangrene may occasionally be present.

Diagnosis of Raynaud's phenomenon is made if the above findings are noted in conjunction with organic arterial disease, scleroderma, cervical rib, or history of the use of a pneumatic hammer. In the beginning, it is frequently impossible to differentiate between benign

Raynaud's disease and progressive scleroderma with Raynaud's phenomenon.

SCLERODERMA. This is a diffuse disease of the collagenous system with skin and visceral manifestations. The cause is unknown. Raynaud's phenomenon is frequently seen before the characteristic skin changes occur. In many instances the skin changes are localized to the distal portions of the extremities (acroscleroderma). The skin becomes boardlike and is bound down to the underlying tissues. Decreased sweating, increased pigmentation, and calcification of the skin occur. Gangrene of the digits, with marked shortening of the phalanges, is not uncommon (sclerodactylia). Involvement of the esophagus, heart, lungs, and kidneys may occur early or late in the disease (Chap. 393).

ERGOTISM. Spasm of the arterioles, with thrombosis and gangrene, is produced by ergot poisoning. In the past, it was seen in epidemic form as the result of the contamination of rye with ergot fungus (*Claviceps purpurea*). It is occasionally seem after the repeated use of ergot to induce abortion or after the use of ergotamine tartrate for pruritus.

MERTHYLSERGIDE. This drug, a serotonin antagonist, is used in the treatment of migraine. A few patients develop marked arterial spasm with cold, cyanotic, and pulseless limbs. One or more extremities may be involved. The pulses return over a period of days when the drug is discontinued.

VASCULAR SPASM AND DILATATION. Any painful area in the extremities may cause symptoms and signs of ischemia from stimulation of the autonomic nervous system. The ischemia of embolus or thrombus is intensified by reflex activity. Ischemia from organic disease of the vessels, from arteriosclerosis, or from thromboangiitis obliterans may be intensified by active vasoconstriction mediated through the autonomic nerves.

ERYTHROMELALGIAS. Occasional patients complain of redness or burning of the skin of the feet, which is exaggerated by heat and dependency and benefited by cooling and elevation. The cause of this disturbance is not known. It may occur in other parts of the body. Local erythromelalgias may be part of the syndrome of causalgia and may persist long after other local effects of the injury have disappeared.

ACROCYANOSIS. The color of the skin is largely determined by the amount of blood in the small vessels. In some subjects arteriolar constriction, as shown by cool extremities, is not accompanied by constriction of the venules. In the presence of slow flow, the blood in these veins contains a large quantity of reduced hemoglobin, and local cyanosis may be present. These changes are accentuated by dependency and disappear when the part is warm and nondependent. No treatment is needed.

DISTURBANCES IN SMALL VESSELS FROM CHANGES IN BLOOD. Changes in the physical state of the blood may cause small-vessel obstruction. Patients with sickle-cell anemia are liable to multiple thromboses. The leg ulcers seen in this disease are probably an example of small-vessel thrombosis on the basis of mechanical obstruction caused by the sickled cells. When the titer of cold agglutinins is high, exposure to cold may cause Raynaud's phenomenon. The development of globulins which precipitate in the cold (cryoglobulins) in patients with leukemia or myeloma may also cause Raynaud's phenomenon.

PROGNOSIS IN DISEASES OF THE ARTERIES

The prognosis depends on the age of the patient, the rate of progression of the primary disease, the degree of development of the collateral circulation, and the amount of involvement of the cerebral, coronary and visceral vessels. The clinical course is very variable. Fingers are occasionally lost; the hand is almost never lost. It is more common for one or both of the lower limbs to be lost. The mortality rate and development of gangrene in embolus and thrombosis are approximately the same.

In *Raynaud's disease,* as defined in this discussion, the prognosis is good by definition. Complications are rare, and the digits are not lost. In *Raynaud's phenomenon* accompanying other disease, the prognosis is that of the primary disease. Thus, in scleroderma associated with Raynaud's phenomenon, the outlook depends on the extent and rate of progression of the scleroderma. This is true whether the sclerodermatous changes are generalized or are still localized to the extremities.

TREATMENT OF ARTERIAL INSUFFICIENCY

CHRONIC ARTERIAL INSUFFICIENCY. Since the specific cause of arteriosclerosis is not known, treatment directed toward prevention or removal of the primary factors is not possible. In segmental obstruction of the femoral and iliac arteries, intimal stripping, grafting, and bypass procedures offer new hope for improving the circulation.

General Care. The *reduction of blood cholesterol* level by dietary management and by drugs has been considered in Chap. 275. Because of the *frequency of diabetes* in persons with vascular disease, fasting and postprandial blood sugar levels should be measured routinely in all such patients. *Complete abstinence from tobacco* should be advised, but abstinence will cause dramatic results only in those few patients with inflammatory disease specifically caused by cigarette smoking.

Care of Local Areas. The care of the local area with circulatory impairment from arteriosclerosis, thromboangiitis, or damage from exposure to cold is similar. The greatest danger is gangrene of the toes. This is usually precipitated by *trauma, infection,* or *burns,* all of which can be prevented by good foot care. Care of the feet means careful washing in tepid water at night; keeping the skin pliable with lanolin; use of a bland dusting powder to absorb perspiration; use of warm, finely woven woolen socks in winter; and careful cutting of the nails, with the ends cut straight across to avoid ingrowing nails. Epidermophytosis must be treated when present, but strong ointments or solutions are to be avoided. Soaking twice daily in 1:8,000 potassium permanganate solution is satisfactory. Dry heat is contraindicated. One should remember that sensation may be impaired because of peripheral nerve involvement. Heat above the temperature of the blood raises the temperature of a part with impaired blood supply much more rapidly than that of a normal part. In this situation, the blood acts as a cooling system to lower the temperature of the tissues; if this cooling system does not function efficiently, burns occur. Heating the part by reflex vasodilatation is safe; local heat may raise the metabolism, without a corresponding increase in blood supply, and precipitate gangrene. The shoes should fit perfectly and should be broken in gradually. If any break in the skin or blister occurs from any cause, the patient should go to bed and call his physician. Reflex vasoconstriction is to be minimized. In the winter, there is need not only for adequate protection for the part itself but for attention to preserving the warmth of the body as well. No local protection will keep the extremities warm if the trunk is cool and the body is attempting to preserve heat.

Reflex vasoconstriction may accompany organic occlusive vascular disease. If body warming or paravertebral block demonstrates release of reflex tone, improvement of the circulation to the extremity by sympathectomy is indicated. Some observers have reported improvement after sympathectomy, even though paravertebral block caused no rise in temperature. Sympathectomy may be followed by gangrene in advanced disease because it may divert the greatly limited supply of blood from the severely ischemic tissues to the more normal tissues of the part.

Sympathectomy does not increase the flow of blood through muscles and has no direct effect on intermittent claudication. If sympathectomy is performed in patients with intermittent claudication, it should be more extensive than is necessary to release the vasoconstrictor tone of the vessels of the skin of the leg and foot. A higher sympathectomy may be effective in increasing the circulation in collateral vessels.

Buerger's exercises are useful. The foot is emptied by raising it just far enough above heart level to produce collapse of the veins and slight pallor. It is then returned to the dependent position. The ideal conditions are (1) maximal lowering of the foot below heart level and leaving it there until the veins are full, and (2) the least elevation for the shortest period of time which will suffice to empty the foot. They have the disadvantage of being too tiresome to continue for a long period of time. They help because when the foot is dependent the effective arterial pressure is increased until the pressure from gravity is counteracted by an equal column of blood in the veins. When the valves of the legs are competent, walking slowly is an effective form of Buerger's exercises. In many patients it appears that frequent short walks constitute the most effective of all methods of treatment. The contraction of the muscles forces blood up the deep veins, the venous pressure falls sharply as the muscles relax, and the high arterial pressure produced by gravity is effective until the veins fill. The oscillating bed can be used to perform Buerger's exercises passively and is sometimes effective in relieving pain.

Pyogenic infections of the feet and toes are common in patients with impaired blood supply. This is particularly true if peripheral neuritis is present. If an apparently gangrenous part is warm, infection is playing an important role, and intensive penicillin therapy may greatly change the picture. Each time he is confronted with an acute episode of arterial insufficiency, the physician must ask himself: is infection or ischemia the primary cause?

ACUTE ARTERIAL INSUFFICIENCY. In acute arterial insufficiency resulting from thrombosis, emergency surgery is not done unless the loss of a limb is imminent. In addition to removal of the thrombus, methods must be devised to remove or bypass the diseased area which caused the thrombus. It is desirable to determine the exact anatomy of the arterial tree and the extent of the collateral circulation before carrying out reconstruction of the artery or a bypass of the obstruction. Sensation is the best guide to viability. If feeling is present in the great toe, the limb is usually viable unless further thrombosis occurs. The absence of sensation and the development of hardening of muscles indicate that the part will not survive unless the circulation is improved quickly.

In the first few hours massive iliofemoral venous thrombosis may be mistaken for acute arterial occlusion. There may be marked pallor and absence of pulse. Sensation may be diminished but not lost. The oscillometric pulsations are diminished but not absent. After 4 hr the arterial spasm relaxes and cyanosis and edema develop.

In acute arterial insufficiency from an embolus to the brachial or femoral systems, embolectomy is performed if the limb is viable. With the use of balloon catheters, antegrade and retrograde extensions of the original clot can be extracted. Emboli to the iliac, renal, or mesenteric arteries or to the bifurcation of the aorta may be removed if the general condition of the patient permits the procedure.

Medical therapy for acute arterial insufficiency consists of the intravenous injection of aqueous heparin (5,000 USP units undiluted). This is repeated at intervals of 3 to 4 hr, keeping the coagulation time twice that found before treatment. The heparin may also be administered by continuous intravenous infusion. If the arterial insufficiency is the result of an embolus, anticoagulant therapy is usually continued for approximately 3 weeks, until there has been time for the site of origin of the embolus to be covered by endothelium.

The affected part is maintained in a slightly dependent position by elevating the head of the bed on 8- to 10-in. blocks. The skin is protected from the bedclothes by a nonheated cradle. Local heat is detrimental, since it would increase the metabolic requirement in an area of limited arterial inflow.

Two other procedures may be considered: (1) the

enhancement of fibrinolysis by the intravenous administration of purified streptokinase or human urokinase; (2) procaine block of the sympathetic nerves supplying the part. The use of fibrinolytic agents is still in the experimental stage. The sympathetic block should be carried out before heparinization, as hemorrhage may complicate the procedure after prolongation of the clotting time. Since heparinization is the most important process to accomplish quickly, paravertebral or other types of block are not usually performed.

RAYNAUD'S DISEASE. The body should be dressed warmly so that the vessels in the hands and feet will dilate to help dispose of body heat. The hands and feet should be protected with warm socks and gloves. Hand and foot warmers of the type used by hunters are useful. Minor episodes of "dead fingers" should not occasion alarm. If these measures are not adequate, the drug therapy discussed in the next paragraph may be useful.

RAYNAUD'S PHENOMENON. Adequate heat to the body and protection of the extremities from cold and trauma are important. The response of the underlying disease to therapy is more important than the treatment of the vasospasm. When associated with scleroderma, the prognosis is guarded. Tolazoline (Priscoline) 25 mg or phenoxybenzamine (Dibenzyline) 10 mg given orally three times a day may be helpful in controlling the vasospasm. The injection of 0.5 mg of reserpine into the brachial or radial arteries produces a surprisingly long-lasting effect and will frequently cause ulcers of the fingers to heal. Sympathectomy may be tried, but the effect is usually temporary.

AMPUTATION. The indications for amputation are (1) gangrene, (2) uncontrollable infection, (3) intractable pain, and (4) such complete loss of function from deformity or contracture that the limb is a burden. Amputation is a last resort, and conservative therapy has saved many limbs. The site of amputation must be at a level where tissue nutrition is good. In the last analysis, the amount of bleeding at operation and the appearance of the tissues after incision determine whether the stump will be viable. Usually, clinical observation determines the level of the trial incision, but special tests such as the appearance time of intravenous fluorescein and the effect of intradermal histamine may be helpful.

ARTERIOVENOUS FISTULA. Large traumatic fistulas are not helped by ligating the artery proximal to the fistula. If collateral vessels around the fistula have not developed, ligation may cause gangrene. If collateral vessels have developed, the fistula is fed both by the main line and by the collateral vessels. Ligation of the main vessel proximal to the fistula may cause retrograde flow of the blood from the collaterals through the fistula, with a decrease in capillary flow in the areas normally supplied by the ligated artery. Direct repair of the artery and vein or removal of the fistula after the development of the collateral vessels is effective.

The treatment of congenital arteriovenous fistulas is less satisfactory. Ligation of the main vessel and multiple ligation of communications may reduce the flow to a level where limb hypertrophy and edema are minimized.

DISTURBANCE IN VENOUS FUNCTION

VARICOSE VEINS. Dilatation and tortuosity of the superficial veins of the lower extremities result from constitutionally defective valves affected by postural strain or from enlargement of the superficial circulation to compensate for obstruction of the deep circulation. The obstruction of the deep circulation usually results from deep thrombophlebitis. Increased blood flow from an acquired or congenital arteriovenous fistula is a rare cause of varicosities. The varicosities caused by defective valves are easily treated surgically. Those resulting from deep vein obstruction are compensatory, and the extremities are not helped by ligation and vein stripping.

In a normal person who stands motionless for a short time, the hydrostatic pressure in the leg veins is equal to the height of a column of blood extending from the fourth rib to the level of the vein. In a man 6 ft in height, the pressure at the ankle is about 105 mm Hg. Blood from the heart is returned by the force of the heartbeat, and all the valves are open. These pressure relations are the same, therefore, in valved and nonvalved veins. On contracting the muscles of the leg and thigh, blood is forced up the extremity by the high intramuscular tension. With normal valves, it cannot be forced downward or outward into the superficial circulation through the communicating veins. The blood in the superficial veins of the leg is not forced upward by the contraction because the skin tension does not exceed the hydrostatic pressure. When the extremity is relaxed, blood does not flow downward into the muscles because the valves control it. Blood enters the veins in the muscles from the arteries and from the superficial veins by way of communicating veins. Backflow from the vena cava is prevented by valves, and the runoff through the communicating veins lowers the pressure in the superficial veins effectively. The fall in hydrostatic pressure in the venous system lowers capillary pressure effectively and prevents edema. When the valves of the veins are destroyed, the venous and capillary pressures are not lowered by exercise. Chronic edema, petechial hemorrhage, poor drainage, and infection frequently result.

Varicose veins fall into the following groups: (1) Simple dilatation of the veins with competent valves. The lowering of capillary pressure by exercise is maintained, and edema does not result. Superficial venous thrombosis in the dilated, tortuous vessels may be troublesome. (2) Varicose veins with incompetent valves in the superficial veins, but competent perforating and deep valves. On walking, the venous pressure is not lowered unless the superficial veins are prevented from filling from above by local pressure. When the superficial veins are correctly obstructed by a tourniquet, exercise effectively lowers the venous pressure. (3) Varicose veins secondary to occlusion of the deep femoral veins. The varicosities have resulted from thrombophlebitis of the deep veins, and the valves of the deep veins are destroyed. Exercise has no effect in lowering the venous pressure when walking. Brawny edema may mask the superficial varicosities, and their extent is rarely realized until the venous tree is visualized by the use of Hypaque. Intractable chronic ulcers are common.

Treatment. The treatment of the first two groups by the combination of high ligation and injection of sclerosing solutions, or removal by vein stripping, is satisfactory. The treatment of the last group is unsatisfactory, and prevention by more intensive treatment of the deep-vein thrombophlebitis is the most satisfactory answer. Once the condition is present, it is beneficial to prevent edema formation by application of external force to counteract the effect of gravity. Bed rest with elevation of the parts allows healing. The application of pressure bandages or of a jelly boot prevents the breakdown of the healed lesion when the patient is up. One should remember the magnitude of the hydrostatic force that one must counteract when the patient stands. Ace bandages are rarely adequate; a pure rubber roller bandage 3 in. wide and 15 ft long is much more effective.

THROMBOPHLEBITIS. Thrombus formation in veins is common. Dilated, tortuous superficial varicose veins frequently become tender and hard, with redness of the overlying skin. The inflammatory reaction usually subsides uneventfully, and embolic complications are unusual. Recurrent superficial or deep venous thrombosis is a common occurrence in the natural history of obliterative arterial disease. Local trauma from the administration of various solutions and medications is a not uncommon cause of superficial thrombophlebitis. Again, embolic phenomena are rare.

Thrombus formation in veins occurs at times in all acute and chronic infections, after operations, and after childbirth. It is common in patients with chronic debilitation, heart failure, or carcinomatosis, and occasionally occurs in apparently normal persons. Venous thrombosis is apt to occur contiguous to areas of local infection or trauma. It is seen in the pelvis in puerperal infection and in the prostatic veins after prostatectomy. In the majority of instances, the thrombus begins in the deep veins of the calf and extends proximally. The process may cause very little reaction in the vein wall (phlebothrombosis), and if this is the case, the thrombus is particularly likely to break loose and lodge in the pulmonary tree. On the other hand, the reaction may involve the veins of the entire extremity, with the inflammatory reactions extending into surrounding lymph channels (thrombophlebitis). With an extensive reaction, the clot adheres tightly to the vein wall, and then embolic phenomena are less common.

The precise cause of thrombophlebitis is unknown. Slowing of the bloodstream seems to be an important factor in thrombus formation. Acceleration of the clotting time probably plays a part. The role of changes in the vein walls has not been determined. In spite of the severe systemic reaction and the evidence of the reaction of inflammation in the extremity in the more fulminating cases, no infectious agent has been found.

Local symptoms may be absent. A rise in pulse rate or an unexplained slight fever in a patient in bed may be the only sign of phlebothrombosis, and the condition may not be recognized until an embolus has lodged in the pulmonary artery. Several days later, tenderness in one or both of the calves may occur. Tenderness in the calf and pain in the calf on dorsiflexion of the foot may be the only sign. If the foot is dependent, slight edema and cyanosis may be observed. Other findings may include a measurable, although not always visible, increase in the circumference of the calf as compared to that of the opposite leg, slight prominence of the veins, increased local warmth or diminished pulsation on the affected side, and local pain on compression with a blood pressure cuff at a pressure of 80 to 120 mm Hg.

In acute thrombophlebitis the leg may be painful, swollen and cyanotic. In this condition, the arteries are not involved directly; in the first few hours intense reflex vasoconstriction may occur, however, and at times the arterial pulse may not be palpable and pallor rather than the expected cyanosis and edema may be present. Fever and leukocytosis are common.

Treatment. The treatment is divided into three parts:

1. Prevention of clot formation in the leg veins by early ambulation or by bandaging of lower extremities when the patient is confined to bed, and by the use of heparin and bishydroxycoumarin (Dicumarol).

2. Prevention of pulmonary emboli after leg veins are involved. Anticoagulant therapy is usually successful. Pulmonary emboli continue in an occasional patient, and ligation of both common femoral veins or the vena cava becomes necessary. (Embolism and infarction of the lungs are discussed in Chap. 285.)

3. Prevention of destruction of veins which leads to persistent edema and chronic ulcers. In very acute thrombophlebitis surgical removal of clots from the femoral and iliac veins may be indicated. Anticoagulant therapy will reduce the number of vessels permanently thrombosed. Elevation and proper bandaging will minimize the edema. Particular attention to bandaging should be given when the patient is allowed to be up. If the edema becomes chronic, paravertebral blocks may be performed with procaine to determine if sympathectomy would be useful.

DISORDERS OF PERIPHERAL LYMPHATIC VESSELS

Water and electrolytes which leave the capillaries can reenter the capillaries without difficulty. Protein and various forms of particulate matter pass into the lymphatic capillaries. If the lymphatic drainage to a part is blocked, the extracellular fluid will gradually assume a high protein content. The capillary filtrate may contain very small amounts of protein, but as the water can be reabsorbed by the blood capillaries and the protein cannot, an effective concentrating mechanism is present. When the lymph vessels are normal, lymph flow depends on muscular contraction, respiratory movements, transmitted movements from arterial pulsations, and, to a certain extent, on gravity. Complete immobilization of the lower extremity in a patient sitting in a chair leads to physiologic lymphatic obstruction.

ACUTE LYMPHANGITIS. When bacterial infection in an extremity is not localized, the inflammatory products pass proximally along the lymphatic channels. The material carried in the lymph channels causes dilatation of the small blood vessels about the lymph vessels, and their courses are outlined by one or more red streaks. Before chemotherapy was available, lymphangitis always carried a serious prognosis because it is a sign of uncontrolled, spreading infection. The hemolytic streptococcus is the usual cause. Immobilization of the part greatly reduces the rate of spread of the infection by reducing the rate of lymph flow. With chemotherapy, fear of lymphangitis has largely disappeared.

CHRONIC LYMPHATIC OBSTRUCTION. Widespread obstruction of the lymph vessels may result from congenital or familial disorders of the lymph vessels. The lymphedema of the familial type is called Milroy's disease. Acquired chronic lymphedema results from obstruction of the lymph channels by neoplasm, scar, operative removal of lymph nodes, and fibrosis caused by x-ray therapy. It may follow low-grade lymphangitis from filariasis, from lymphogranuloma venereum, and from repeated streptococcal infections. It may be a complicating factor in certain instances of severe edema following thrombophlebitis.

In its early stages, lymphedema cannot be distinguished physically from any other form of soft pitting edema. On laboratory examination, the high protein concentration separates it from cardiac and nephritic edema but not from the fluid of myxedema. Lymphedema causes fibrosis in the tissues, and in time the tissue becomes hard and brawny. The skin may be thick and folded with indolent ulcerations.

Treatment of Chronic Lymphedema. Early and persistent therapy is important. If marked edema is prevented by postural drainage, by effective bandaging, and by limiting upright activity to periods short of edema formation, much of the fibrosis and recurrent infection will be prevented. In the absence of infection the limb may be placed in an appliance each night which allows the application of positive pressure throughout the night. This program calls for persistence on the part of both physician and patient. Acute attacks of lymphangitis can be controlled by appropriate chemotherapy.

LEG ULCERS IN PATIENTS WITHOUT PERIPHERAL VASCULAR DISEASE

In a normal person, an injury to the skin of the foot or ankle is much more serious than one to the hand or wrist. In the ambulatory patient, lesions on the lower leg and foot may heal slowly. If healing does not occur promptly, the patient should be put to bed and the part elevated. If the lesion is allowed to become chronic, low-grade phlebitis, lymphangitis, and arteritis develop. Even if the main vessels to the part are unaffected, these local changes cause poor tissue drainage and there is a tendency to recurrent infection and ulceration. A nonhealing, nontraumatic ulcer of the lower part of leg is an emergency and requires bed rest until healing occurs.

REFERENCES

Barker, W. F.: "Peripheral Vascular Disease," Philadelphia, W. B. Saunders Company, 1966.

Dible, J. H.: "The Pathology of Limb Ischemia," St. Louis, W. H. Green Co., Inc., 1967.

Jurgens, J. L., N. W. Barker, and E. A. Hines, Jr.: Arteriosclerosis Obliterans: Review of 520 Cases with Special Reference to Pathogenic and Prognostic Factors, Circulation, 21:188, 1960.

Lowenberg, R. I.: Early Diagnosis of Phlebothrombosis with Aid of a New Clinical Test, J.A.M.A., 155:1566, 1954.

McKusick, V. A., W. S. Harris, O. E. Ottesen, R. M. Goodman, W. M. Shelley, and R. D. Bloodwell: Buerger's Disease: A Distinct Clinical and Pathological Entity, J.A.M.A., 181:5, 1962.

Wessler, Stanford: Intermittent Claudication, Circulation, 11:806, 1955.

Winsor, T., and C. Hyman: "A Primer of Peripheral Vascular Diseases," Philadelphia, Lea & Febiger, 1965.

Section 3

Disorders of the Respiratory System

279 APPROACH TO THE PATIENT WITH DISEASE OF THE RESPIRATORY SYSTEM

Eugene Braunwald

As in other branches of medicine, a careful and detailed *history* and *physical examination* are the corner-stones in the establishment of a diagnosis in patients with diseases of the respiratory system. In addition, the *roentgenographic examination* occupies a particularly important role in the evaluation of patients with lung disease.

In eliciting the *history* of patients with pulmonary disease, it must be appreciated that an increasing fraction of the population is exposed to materials which are potentially toxic to the lung, and the history must therefore contain a description of exposure to industrial hazards such as silica, asbestos, beryllium, bagasse, iron oxide, tin oxide, cotton lint, titanium oxide, silver, and nitrogen dioxide. A history of the patient's previous residence is also of considerable importance in the diagnosis of histoplasmosis, coccidioidomycosis, or tropical eosinophilia. The family history should consider pulmonary diseases which may be familial, such as cystic disease of the lung, cystic fibrosis, and asthma, as well as infections due to the tubercle bacilli where exposure to involved family members is important.

Dyspnea is a cardinal manifestation of diseases involving the respiratory and cardiovascular systems (Chap. 32). A detailed physical examination of both organ systems is therefore mandatory in every patient with this symptom. Dyspnea secondary to cardiac disease is often recognized by the presence of other evidence of heart failure, of cardiac enlargement, and of cardiac murmurs. However, when there are no obvious findings to incriminate either organ system as a cause of exertional dyspnea, the origin is much more likely to be the heart rather than the lungs, since shortness of breath due to pulmonary disease is usually accompanied by obvious abnormal findings on physical examination. However, it may be more difficult to differentiate paroxysmal nocturnal dyspnea due to pulmonary edema of cardiac origin from the nocturnal attacks of bronchial asthma.

Patients with diseases involving the respiratory system may also present with *chest pain* (Chap. 11), which is frequently caused by inflammation of the pleura, occurring in pneumonia, pulmonary thromboembolism, tuberculosis, and malignancy. Pleuritic pain is usually localized to one side of the chest and is related to movements of the thorax and to respiration. Lesions confined to the pulmonary parenchyma do not produce pain. Chest pain may also be due to intercostal neuritis, as occurs in herpes zoster (Chap. 225) or compression of the intercostal nerves as they leave the spinal cord. Such pain is often superficial in character and may be related to coughing and straining. Thoracic pain may also be due to myositis, costochondral disturbances, myocardial ischemia, pericarditis, and aortic aneurysm (Chap. 11).

Cough and expectoration are also cardinal features of pulmonary disease (Chap. 38). Few patients can describe the severity of cough or quantity of expectoration reliably, and it is therefore extremely desirable for the physician to inspect a 24-hr collection of sputum. Cough is frequently caused by inflammation of the bronchi, which may be chronic, as in patients with a cigarette cough, or acute, as occurs in a variety of viral and bacterial infections. Bronchiectasis produces purulent sputum which may have an offensive odor or be streaked with blood. Paroxysmal cough may also be the presenting feature of patients with bronchial asthma (Chap. 72) in whom physical examination reveals wheezing respirations and musical squeaking sounds. Pulmonary tuberculosis (Chap. 174) remains a common cause of cough and expectoration, as does carcinoma of the lung (Chap. 292).

Hemoptysis is often a frightening symptom (Chap. 38). Faint streaking of the sputum with blood may be observed in acute infections of the respiratory tract. However, many patients with bloody sputum have serious disease, such as pulmonary thromboembolism, tuberculosis, mitral stenosis, carcinoma of the lung, or bronchiectasis (Chap. 291). In all instances of hemoptysis it is necessary to exclude sources of blood in the nasopharynx and bleeding of esophageal origin.

Unfortunately, in recent years, *physical examination of the chest* has been deemphasized, largely because of the recognition of the enormous value of radiographic techniques. However, abnormalities such as small or moderate amounts of fluid in the alveoli or in the mediastinal structures, bronchospasm, and pleural effusions can often be detected more accurately by physical examination than by chest roentgenography. On the other hand, gross abnormalities of thoracic structure; pulmonary, mediastinal, and pleural masses; parenchymal consolidation, cysts, cavities, and abnormalities of the pulmonary vascular bed are detected more reliably by roentgenographic than by physical examination. In the *general examination* of the patient with disease of the respiratory system it must be appreciated that pulmonary neoplasms and suppurative lesions are frequently associated with clubbing of the fingers and osteoarthropathy, i.e., new bone formation along the phalanges and long bones as well as in the peripheral joints. A careful search for infection in the teeth, gums, tonsils, or sinuses is recommended in patients known or suspected of having bronchiectasis or lung abscess. Neurological findings including headache, drowsiness, papilledema, and other evidence of increased intracranial pressure occur in patients with pulmonary disease who have hypoxia and hypercapnia. Vascular collapse is a late complication of carbon dioxide intoxication and is characterized by hypotension, flushed skin, sweating, and tachycardia.

An abnormal *chest roentgenogram* may be the presenting feature in an otherwise symptomless patient. In such circumstances the physician must make every effort to obtain earlier films in order to determine whether the lesion is new or old. Laminography, angiocardiography, and pulmonary photoscanning are additional procedures which may be helpful in establishing a diagnosis in a patient with an abnormality on the plain chest radiogram. *Skin tests* for tuberculosis, histoplasmosis, coccidioidomycosis, etc., as well as appropriate *serum complement fixation tests* are frequently helpful. Cytologic examination of the sputum and bronchial washings, bronchoscopy, bronchoscopic biopsy, scalene node biopsy, pleural or lung biopsy, may also be instrumental in establishing the diagnosis of an infiltrate in an otherwise asymptomatic patient (Chap. 281). Particularly important points which must be investigated in the history of the asymptomatic patient with a lesion discovered on a routine chest roentgenogram include exposure to individuals with tuberculosis, previous tuberculin and fungus skin tests, residence or visits to areas of the country where fungal disease is endemic, a history of smoking and of exposure to dusts, and symptoms of systemic disease such as fever, sweat, fatigue, and weight loss.

280 DISTURBANCES OF RESPIRATORY FUNCTION

John B. West

The prime function of the lung is to exchange gas between the inspired air and the venous blood. A convenient starting point, therefore, for a discussion of disturbances of respiratory function is the alveolar membrane across which gas exchange occurs (Fig. 280-1). This blood-gas barrier is less than 1 μ thick and has a surface area of some 100 sq m. It is therefore ideally suited to its gas exchange function.

Air is pumped to one side of this membrane and blood to the other. The air flows through conducting tubes, the bronchi; these are not lined with blood capillaries, with the result that no gas exchange can occur within them. These conducting airways, therefore, comprise a *dead space.* Beyond these airways is the *alveolar gas,* which makes up most of the volume of the lung. This gas is in a constant state of agitation because of molecular diffusion, and thus all the alveolar gas has access to the capillary blood via the alveolar membrane.

On the other side of the membrane, blood is pumped from the right side of the heart to the pulmonary capillaries. These delicate vessels have diameters of only about 10 μ, so that the blood is spread out in a thin film, one or two red blood cells thick, around the air sacs.

It is worth emphasizing two features of the basic lung unit shown in Fig. 280-1: (1) its symmetry, i.e., air and blood are equally important in the central process of gas exchange (this simple fact is sometimes forgotten in clinical medicine, where the patient's difficulties in moving air in and out of the lung often dominate the picture); (2) the simplicity of the lung unit compared with, say, the nephron. The structure of the lung is simple because its main role is simple, i.e., bringing together air and blood so that gas exchange can occur by passive diffusion. By contrast, the kidney carries out many functions involv-

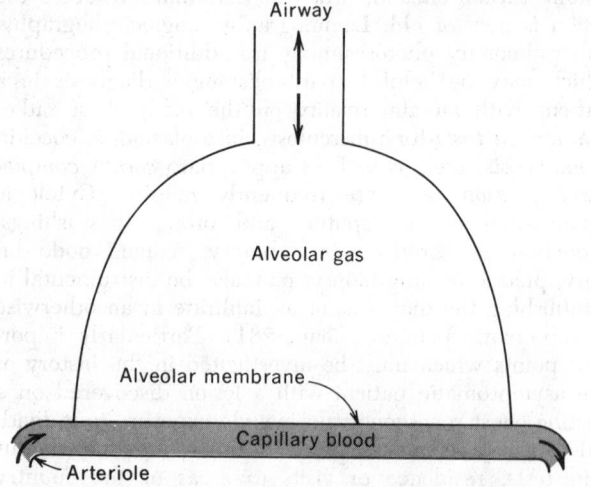

Fig. 280-1. The functional lung unit. The alveolar membrane across which gas exchange takes place has alveolar gas on one side and pulmonary capillary blood on the other.

ing active transport, and its structure is correspondingly complicated.

VENTILATION

This is the process of moving inspired air into the alveolar gas compartment (Fig. 280-1), where the gas exchange with the blood occurs. It is worth attaching some typical values for ventilation to the lung shown in Fig. 280-1. A normal breath is about 500 ml, so that with a breathing frequency of 15 per min, some 7 to 8 liters of air enter the lung each minute. However, because the volume of the conducting airways (dead space) is about 150 ml, only 350 of the 500 ml of air inhaled with each breath reaches the alveolar gas compartment. The rest remains behind in the airways and is subsequently exhaled. Thus, the volume of fresh gas entering the alveoli each minute is about 350 ml × 15, or some 5 liters. This is known as the *alveolar ventilation* and is of key importance to gas exchange. Of the 5 liters of air entering the alveoli, some 300 ml of oxygen moves across into the blood each minute to be replaced by about 250 ml of carbon dioxide. Thus less than 5 percent of the gas volume inhaled is exchanged with the gas in the blood.

The above figures apply to resting conditions. On exercise, the oxygen uptake may rise as high as 4 to 6 liters per min and the minute volume of air inspired may increase twentyfold. This is accomplished by an increase in both tidal volume and the frequency of breathing.

It should be noted that inspired air passes only a limited distance down the airways by ordinary bulk flow. Before it gets to the alveoli, its forward velocity is reduced to something like a millimeter per second, because of the enormous combined cross-sectional area of the small bronchi. In addition, the volume of gas in the small bronchi is so large that the alveoli and their ducts have completed their expansion before the fresh inspired air reaches them. The last millimeter or so of its travel is therefore accomplished by molecular diffusion within the small airways. This process is very rapid for gas molecules but exceedingly slow for dust particles if they are over ½ μ in size. For this reason most inhaled dusts and aerosols never reach the alveoli, and many are deposited in the region of the terminal bronchioles.

MEASUREMENT OF VENTILATION. The minute volume of air passing the lips is easily measured by connecting the patient to a large bag or spirometer via a mouthpiece and one-way valve. The resting and exercise ventilations are increased when disease impairs the efficiency of pulmonary gas exchange, but the measurement of ventilation by itself is rarely useful because it is partly under voluntary control and is often changed by the stress of the measurement.

The maximum ventilation, or maximum breathing capacity, can be measured by asking the patient to breathe as fast and deep as he can for 15 sec. This measurement gives information about the mechanical properties of the lungs, but it has largely been replaced by a less demanding measurement, the forced expiratory volume (see below).

HYPOVENTILATION. When inspired air reaches the alveoli, oxygen is removed from it and carbon dioxide is added. The concentrations, or partial pressures, of these two gases in the alveoli depend on a balance between two processes. On the one hand, the removal of oxygen from (or addition of carbon dioxide to) the alveolar gas is determined by the metabolic demands of the body. On the other hand, the addition of oxygen to (or removal of carbon dioxide from) the alveolar gas depends on the amount of alveolar ventilation. Thus, if the alveolar ventilation is low in relation to oxygen uptake and carbon dioxide output, the partial pressure of oxygen in alveolar gas and arterial blood falls, and the level of carbon dioxide rises. This is hypoventilation.

Hypoventilation is commonly caused by disease outside the respiratory system and may exist in the presence of normal lungs. Causes include depression of the respiratory center by drugs or anesthesia, damage to the medulla by disease, diseases affecting the nerve supply to the muscles of the thorax or the muscles themselves, injury to the chest wall, and obstruction to the airways. Because the lungs themselves are often normal, the prognosis may be excellent if the precipitating cause is removed. Note that hypoventilation always causes both hypoxemia and hypercapnia, although the first can be abolished by adding oxygen to the inspired air. The carbon dioxide retention can only be relieved by increasing the ventilation, e.g., by using a ventilator.

HYPERVENTILATION. If the alveolar ventilation is abnormally high for the carbon dioxide production of the body, the arterial carbon dioxide tension falls. This may occur in metabolic acidosis, e.g., uremia, in which the respiratory center responds to the low blood pH. Hysterical hyperventilation is also not uncommon.

DIFFUSION ACROSS THE ALVEOLAR MEMBRANE

Oxygen and carbon dioxide move across the blood-gas barrier by a process of simple physical diffusion from a region of high partial pressure to one of low, just as water runs downhill. Consider a red blood cell as it enters a pulmonary capillary. The oxygen tension in mixed venous blood (in the pulmonary artery) is typically about 40 mm Hg, and as the cell enters the capillary, it sees an oxygen tension in alveolar gas of some 100 mm Hg, less than a micron away. Oxygen therefore moves rapidly across the barrier into the cell to combine with hemoglobin, and the oxygen tension rises. As a consequence, the oxygen pressure difference between the cell and the alveolar gas falls, and the rate of inflow of oxygen is reduced. However, under normal conditions, the diffusion properties of the alveolar membrane are so good and the rate of combination of oxygen with hemoglobin so rapid that before the cell has spent more than about a third of its time in the capillary, its oxygen tension has virtually reached that of the alveolar gas. This transfer of oxygen is helped by the shape of the oxygen dissociation curve, which ensures that the driving pressure difference is maintained until almost all the oxygen is moved across. Thus,

under ordinary circumstances, there is no measurable difference between the oxygen tension of alveolar gas and that of the blood at the end of the pulmonary capillary. Indeed, the normal lung has plenty of reserve diffusion in hand.

Two factors which stress the diffusion ability of the lung are exercise and the inhalation of a low oxygen mixture. During strenuous exercise, the time spent by the red blood cells in the capillaries is greatly reduced, perhaps to a third of that at rest, so that the time available for the diffusion process is curtailed. Even so, the oxygen tension in the capillary blood almost reaches that of the alveolar gas, except possibly during the most exhausting work. Additional stress occurs if the lung inspires a low oxygen mixture, thus reducing the alveolar oxygen tension. Because the pressure difference between the oxygen in the gas and that in the red blood cells as they enter the capillary is lowered, the rate of movement of oxygen across the membrane is slowed. There is evidence that heavy work when the inspired oxygen tension is very low (e.g., at high altitude) causes lowering of the arterial oxygen tension because of inadequate diffusion into the pulmonary capillary. Note that carbon dioxide transfer is never limited by diffusion across the alveolar membrane, because of the much higher diffusion rate of this gas.

MEASUREMENT OF DIFFUSING CAPACITY. This can be done using carbon monoxide. The subject inspires a low concentration (approximately 0.1 percent) and the rate of uptake of the gas by the blood is calculated from the difference between the inspired and expired concentrations. The measurement can be made during the course of a single 10-sec breath-holding period, or over a minute or so of steady breathing. In both cases, the diffusing capacity is expressed as the milliliters per minute of carbon monoxide taken up by the lung per millimeter of mercury of partial pressure of carbon monoxide in the alveolar gas. Normal values are in the region of 20 ml/min/mm Hg at rest, rising to 60 or more on exercise.

The reason why the uptake of carbon monoxide measures the diffusing capacity is the remarkable avidity of the blood for this gas. This means that appreciable amounts of carbon monoxide can be combined with hemoglobin in the blood at an exceedingly low partial pressure. As a result, the rise in tension of carbon monoxide in the red blood cells as they pass along the pulmonary capillaries is negligible and the amount of the gas which is transferred into the blood is determined only by the diffusion properties of the alveolar membrane and the rate of combination of carbon monoxide with hemoglobin. The latter depends on the oxygen tension in the alveoli; by measuring the carbon monoxide uptake at various inspired oxygen tensions, it is possible to determine separately the diffusing capacity of the alveolar membrane itself and the volume of blood in pulmonary capillaries.

The measurement of carbon monoxide uptake is a relatively simple procedure, and there is no problem in following changes of diffusing capacity in the normal lung under a variety of conditions. Unfortunately, however, it is very difficult to say how far the carbon monoxide uptake reflects the diffusing capacity of the lung in the presence of appreciable lung disease. The reason for this is that gross inequality of ventilation and blood flow in the lung reduce the carbon monoxide uptake, even in the absence of impaired diffusion. For this reason, the test when used in the clinic is best said to measure the *transfer factor* of the lung for carbon monoxide and should be looked upon as a general index of the efficiency of gas exchange in the lung, rather than as a specific test of diffusion.

A method of measuring diffusing capacity using oxygen has also been described, but its validity is uncertain and the test is now rarely done.

IMPAIRMENT OF DIFFUSION. There are generalized lung diseases, such as diffuse interstitial fibrosis (Chap. 284), sarcoidosis (Chap. 254), asbestosis (Chap. 290), and alveolar carcinomatosis (Chap. 292), in which microscopically the alveolar wall is thickened, and it is tempting to attribute any hypoxemia to defective diffusion. The term "alveolar-capillary block" was coined for this situation, and it is certainly an easy one to remember. Recently, however, the importance of impaired diffusion as a cause of the hypoxemia in these diseases has been questioned. The chief reason for this is that it is impossible to imagine normal ventilation and blood flow in an alveolus which has a thickened wall, and indeed several studies have shown marked inequality of ventilation and blood flow in the lung in these conditions. Since it is now recognized that uneven ventilation-perfusion ratios constitute a potent cause of hypoxemia (see below), the role of impaired diffusion is not clear. Furthermore, because the uptake of carbon monoxide in these diseases is undoubtedly reduced by the presence of uneven ventilation and blood flow, it is difficult to see how the question can be resolved. It is safer, therefore, to attribute the bulk of the hypoxemia in these generalized lung diseases to ventilation-perfusion inequality and leave the question of the importance of diffusion impairment open.

BLOOD FLOW

Mixed venous blood is pumped to the pulmonary capillaries directly from the right side of the heart so that the total *pulmonary blood flow* is equal to the cardiac output, say 5 or 6 liters per min in a normal adult. We saw earlier that the volume of fresh inspired air entering the alveoli each minute, the *alveolar ventilation*, is some 5 liters. Thus, the overall ratio of ventilation to blood flow, or *ventilation-perfusion ratio*, is about 1.

Even though the volumes of fresh gas and blood reaching the alveoli each minute are about the same, the volumes involved in exchanging gas at any instant are very different. Thus, while the alveolar gas volume is 2 to 3 liters at the end of a normal expiration, the capillary blood volume is only some 70 ml. This is why the lung microscopist sees chiefly air.

The pressures in the pulmonary circulation have long been considered the domain of the cardiologist, but they have an important bearing on gas exchange in the lung. The normal pulmonary arterial pressure is only just sufficient to raise blood to the top of the upright lung; if the pressure is reduced, as in hemorrhagic shock, the upper part of the lung is unperfused and gas exchange is impaired. Alterations in the pulmonary venous pressure, too, affect the distribution of blood flow in the lung.

VENTILATION-PERFUSION RELATIONSHIPS

Up to this point, we have been assuming that all lung units behave identically. Thus, Fig. 280-1 has been taken to refer to an alveolus, a group of alveoli with their duct, a lobe, or even the whole lung. In fact, however, the lung is not homogeneous, and the differences in behavior between the millions of units are responsible for the great bulk of the hypoxemia and hypercarbia seen in clinical practice. We shall see that even in the normal lung, there are marked regional differences in blood flow and ventilation which affect gas exchange, while in diseased states, the inhomogeneity becomes so severe that respiratory failure may ultimately develop.

NORMAL DISTRIBUTION OF BLOOD FLOW. Recently, radioactive gas methods have been introduced to measure the regional distribution of blood flow and ventilation in the lung. In one technique, the inert gas ^{133}xenon is used. To measure blood flow, the xenon is dissolved in saline solution and injected into a peripheral vein. On reaching the lung, it is evolved into alveolar gas because of its poor solubility; there it remains during breath holding and can be detected by external counters. To measure ventilation, the patient inhales a single breath of the radioactive gas and again its regional distribution is measured. In both instances, a further measurement after a period of rebreathing of xenon allows a correction for lung volume to be made.

In the normal upright lung, blood flow per unit volume decreases rapidly from bottom to top, reaching very low values at the apex (Fig. 280-2). This pattern is affected by change of posture and exercise. When the subject lies supine, the apical and basal blood flows become the same, but the posterior (dependent) part of the lung has a higher blood flow than the anterior region. In the lateral position, the dependent regions are best perfused. On exercise in the upright position, both apical and basal blood flows increase, so that the proportion of the total flow going to the apex rises.

The cause of this uneven distribution of blood flow lies in the hydrostatic pressure differences within the lung. The pulmonary circulation is unique in that air and blood are separated by a very delicate membrane over a vertical distance of some 30 cm, and consequently, the hydrostatic effect of this large column of blood determines the caliber of the small vessels. It has been shown that the distribution of blood flow depends on the relative magnitudes of the pulmonary arterial, venous, and alveolar pressures. In particular, if pulmonary arterial pressure falls (as in hemorrhage, shock, and anesthesia)

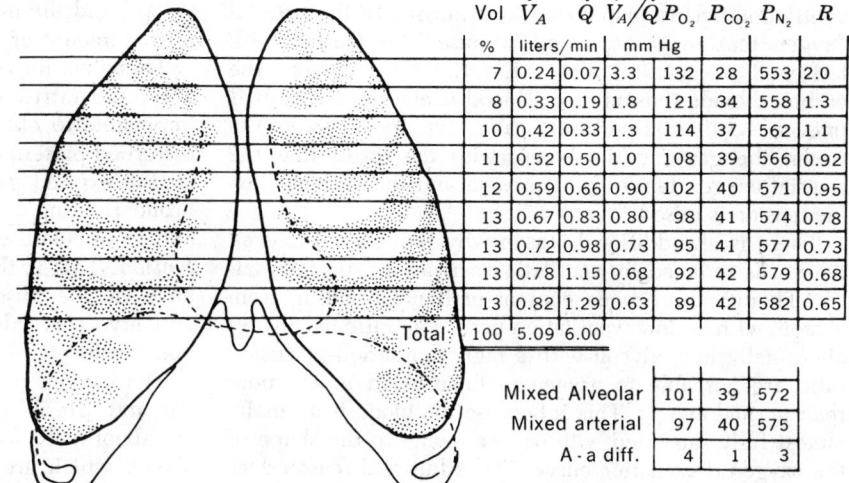

Vol	$\dot{V}_A$	$\dot{Q}$	$\dot{V}_A/\dot{Q}$	P_{O_2}	P_{CO_2}	P_{N_2}	R
%	liters/min			mm Hg			
7	0.24	0.07	3.3	132	28	553	2.0
8	0.33	0.19	1.8	121	34	558	1.3
10	0.42	0.33	1.3	114	37	562	1.1
11	0.52	0.50	1.0	108	39	566	0.92
12	0.59	0.66	0.90	102	40	571	0.95
13	0.67	0.83	0.80	98	41	574	0.78
13	0.72	0.98	0.73	95	41	577	0.73
13	0.78	1.15	0.68	92	42	579	0.68
13	0.82	1.29	0.63	89	42	582	0.65
Total 100	5.09	6.00					

	P_{O_2}	P_{CO_2}	P_{N_2}
Mixed Alveolar	101	39	572
Mixed arterial	97	40	575
A - a diff.	4	1	3

Fig. 280-2. Regional differences within the normal upright lung. Note the large inequality of blood flow $\dot{Q}$ and the smaller inequality of ventilation $\dot{V}_A$. The resulting ventilation-perfusion ratio ($\dot{V}_A/\dot{Q}$) inequality causes regional differences in gas exchange. Overall gas exchange is impaired, as shown by the tension differences between mixed alveolar gas and arterial blood.

or alveolar pressure is raised (as in positive-pressure ventilation), the distribution of blood flow becomes more uneven. The normal pattern is also commonly affected by both heart and lung disease.

NORMAL DISTRIBUTION OF VENTILATION. Ventilation also increases down the upright lung, though the changes are less marked than for blood flow (Fig. 280-2). This distribution of ventilation which is seen under normal resting conditions is altered at low lung volumes. It has been shown that when a normal subject exhales as far as he can (to residual volume) and then gradually inhales in small steps, initially very little air goes into the lower zones, but the upper zones are well ventilated. However, before he reaches his normal resting lung volume (functional residual capacity), this distribution is reversed and the lower zones are better ventilated than the upper. This pattern is then maintained right up to maximal volumes. The poor ventilation of the dependent regions of the lung at low lung volumes is seen in the erect, supine, and lateral positions, and it has important implications in clinical situations where the lung volume is low, e.g., in obesity or following abdominal surgery. Since the dependent regions are the best perfused, the impairment of gas exchange may then be severe.

The cause of the uneven distribution of ventilation has to do with the way the lung is supported inside the chest. It is known that the expanding pressure on the lung is less in the dependent zones, presumably because these regions help to support the lung above them. Thus, the intrapleural pressure is less negative at the bottom of the lung than at the top. The reason for the greater ventilation of the dependent regions at normal volumes is twofold: (1) these alveoli have a smaller resting volume, and (2) their increase in volume is relatively large because they are so distensible. By contrast, these dependent regions are poorly ventilated at low lung volumes, because the expanding forces on them are then too weak to inflate them. Indeed, under these conditions, the airways to these alveoli may close and become unventilated.

VENTILATION-PERFUSION RATIO. We have seen that

while blood flow increases greatly down the upright lung, the change in ventilation is less. As a result, the ventilation-perfusion ratio varies from a high value at the top of the lung to a low value at the bottom. The ventilation-perfusion ratio is of key importance because it determines the gas exchange which occurs in any part of the lung.

Consider a lung unit as shown in Fig. 280-1. Intuitively, it can be seen that the partial pressure of oxygen in the alveolar gas (and therefore in the end-capillary blood) will be set by a balance between the rate of its removal by the blood flow on the one hand, and the rate of its replenishment by the ventilation on the other. Thus, if the ventilation is gradually reduced but the blood flow is maintained, the oxygen partial pressure will gradually fall. The limit is reached when the unit is not ventilated and the oxygen tension becomes that of venous blood. This is a ventilation-perfusion ratio of zero. By contrast, if perfusion is gradually reduced, the oxygen tension will rise. The limit now occurs when the unit is unperfused and the oxygen tension in the alveolus is the same as inspired air. This is a ventilation-perfusion ratio of infinity.

Thus, the crucial factor determining the oxygen partial pressure is the ventilation-perfusion ratio; this is true also for the partial pressure of carbon dioxide, and indeed of any other gas that might be present. Figure 280-2 shows some of the regional differences in gas exchange which are calculated to occur in the normal upright lung as a consequence of the uneven ventilation-perfusion ratios.

OVERALL GAS EXCHANGE. Though these regional differences in gas exchange are of interest, more important is the effect of uneven ventilation-perfusion ratios on overall gas exchange, i.e., the ability of the lung to take up oxygen and put out carbon dioxide. The reason why gas transfer is impaired by uneven ventilation and blood flow is made clearer by referring to Fig. 280-2. It can be seen that the base of the lung is much more important than the apex in determining the arterial blood composition, because it contributes most of the blood. However, the base has a low oxygen tension (because of its low ventilation-perfusion ratio). Thus, inevitably the arterial oxygen tension is depressed because it is loaded with less well oxygenated blood. For the same reason, the carbon dioxide tension in the blood is elevated. It is as if uneven ventilation-perfusion ratios set up a barrier between the gas and the blood, with the result that the arterial oxygen tension is depressed and the carbon dioxide tension is raised.

There is an additional reason why the arterial oxygen tension is reduced by ventilation-perfusion ratio inequality. Though the oxygen content of blood draining from alveoli with a low ventilation-perfusion ratio is always abnormally low, alveoli with a high ventilation-perfusion ratio are not able to oxygenate their blood much more than normal alveoli. This is because the blood is normally almost fully saturated with oxygen owing to the shape of the oxygen dissociation curve. This additional reason does not apply to carbon dioxide.

In the normal lung (Fig. 280-2), the effects of uneven ventilation-perfusion ratios on overall gas exchange are trivial; the arterial oxygen tension is reduced by a few millimeters of mercury and the carbon dioxide tension is raised by less than 1 mm Hg. Both these liabilities can be met if the total ventilation of the lung and thus its overall ventilation-perfusion ratio are increased. Indeed, the level of overall ventilation is normally set by the respiratory center via the arterial carbon dioxide tension. Thus, if uneven ventilation-perfusion ratios elevate the arterial carbon dioxide tension, this is brought back by the increased respiratory drive and the consequently higher overall ventilation.

In the diseased lung, the effects of ventilation-perfusion ratio inequality on gas transfer may be very severe because the degree of uneven ventilation and blood flow is far greater than in the normal lung. The arterial oxygen tension may be depressed by 50 or more millimeters of mercury, and in practice no amount of increased ventilation can return it to its normal level. The carbon dioxide tension, however, is often brought down by an increase in total ventilation; sometimes however this is not possible and hypercapnia develops. Ventilation-perfusion ratio inequality is much the commonest cause of hypoxemia in generalized lung disease.

MEASUREMENT OF VENTILATION-PERFUSION INEQUALITY. Unfortunately, it is difficult to derive much information about the pattern of uneven ventilation and blood flow in the diseased lung. Because much of the inequality is at the microscopic level, radioactive gas detectors which "see" relatively large regions of lung give little indication of the extent of the unevenness. The best method as yet is by the analysis of expired gas and arterial blood.

We saw in Fig. 280-2 that the arterial oxygen tension is depressed in the presence of ventilation-perfusion ratio inequality because it is loaded with less-well-oxygenated blood from the well-perfused lung base. By contrast, the expired alveolar gas receives a disproportionately high contribution from the apex, where the oxygen tension is high. An alveolar-arterial oxygen difference therefore de-

velops, and the magnitude of this difference is a measure of the amount of ventilation-perfusion ratio inequality.

Though arterial blood can be collected by puncture, a representative sample of mixed alveolar gas is often impossible to obtain in the diseased lung because of its disturbed pattern of emptying. An alternative is to collect all the expired gas (including the dead space from the bronchi) using a valve box and a large bag or spirometer and to calculate what is called the *ideal alveolar oxygen tension*. This is the value which the alveolar gas would have in the absence of ventilation-perfusion ratio inequality. This calculation is made using the arterial carbon dioxide tension and the alveolar gas equation.

The oxygen tension difference between ideal alveolar gas and arterial blood chiefly reflects those alveoli with an abnormally *low* ventilation-perfusion ratio, i.e., the alveoli which are overperfused in relation to their ventilation. These alveoli cause the hypoxemia, and their presence has the same effect as the admixture of some venous blood with arterial blood. Indeed, it is possible to express their contribution as if a certain proportion of the venous blood bypassed the lung altogether and was then added to the arterial blood. This is called *venous admixture* or wasted blood flow and is calculated from the oxygen tension difference between ideal alveolar gas and arterial blood. Normally, calculated venous admixture is only about 2 percent of the pulmonary blood flow, but it may rise to 30 percent or higher in the presence of severe ventilation-perfusion ratio inequality.

The alveoli with an abnormally *high* ventilation-perfusion ratio, i.e., those which are overventilated in relation to their perfusion, mainly affect carbon dioxide elimination. They behave as if a certain proportion of the inspired gas bypassed the alveoli altogether, i.e., as if the dead space were increased in size, thus resulting in wasted ventilation. Their contribution can be calculated from the carbon dioxide tension of arterial blood and mixed expired gas using Bohr's equation. This gives a value for the *physiologic dead space*, which includes not only the volume of the bronchi but also the so-called alveolar dead space attributable to the overventilated alveoli. Normally the physiologic dead space is less than 30 percent of the tidal volume at rest, but it may rise to 50 percent or more in the presence of severe disease.

MEASUREMENT OF VENTILATION INEQUALITY. Because the measurement of ventilation-perfusion ratio inequality is a relatively difficult procedure, the simpler measurement of uneven ventilation is often made. Although theoretically it would be possible for a patient to have ventilatory inequality but no mismatch of ventilation and blood flow, this is not seen in practice.

Two methods of measuring uneven ventilation are in use. In the single breath test, the patient takes a single inspiration of pure oxygen and then exhales fully. A rapid nitrogen meter analysis of the expired nitrogen concentration at the lips and analysis of the expired volume are recorded simultaneously. After 750 ml has been expired (sufficient to clear the dead space), the rise in nitrogen concentration over the next 500 ml is measured.

This is less than 1.5 percent in normal subjects. However, in patients with uneven ventilation, the nitrogen concentration rises more rapidly because the degree of dilution of the nitrogen by the inhaled oxygen varies throughout the lung, and also because the poorly ventilated regions (which received little oxygen and therefore have most nitrogen) always empty last. This is a simple, quick, and useful test.

Uneven ventilation can also be detected by the multibreath washout method. Pure oxygen is breathed via a one-way valve, and again expired nitrogen concentration at the lips is measured. When the nitrogen concentration is plotted against the number of breaths on semilogarithmic paper, an almost straight line is found in normal subjects. This is because the successive dilution of the nitrogen in the lung by each breath of pure oxygen causes an exponential decay in nitrogen concentration. However in the presence of uneven ventilation, the line becomes successively flatter because different regions of the lung lose their nitrogen at different rates until finally only the nitrogen in the worst-ventilated spaces is being washed out. An additional check can be made after 7 min of washout. A forced expiration will show a nitrogen concentration of less than 2.5 percent in normal subjects but a higher value in patients with uneven ventilation because of delayed washout of the poorly ventilated spaces.

VENTILATION-PERFUSION RATIO INEQUALITY IN DISEASE. Virtually all generalized diseases of the lung, such as emphysema, chronic bronchitis, diffuse interstitial fibrosis, and the pneumoconioses, result in mismatch of ventilation and blood flow. Very little is known about the pattern of unevenness in these conditions, though it is not difficult to imagine that an area of fibrosis or a bulla, for example, must interfere with both ventilation and blood flow.

There is evidence that in general, areas of the lung which are poorly ventilated are also poorly perfused. One reason for this is that local pathologic change tends to disturb both processes by its mechanical effects. However, there are other physiologic mechanisms which reduce the mismatch of uneven ventilation and perfusion. One is the reduction in blood flow to a poorly ventilated, hypoxic region of lung, which has now been demonstrated on many occasions. The precise mechanism is unknown, but it appears to be a local response to alveolar hypoxia, since it occurs in the isolated denervated lung. Another mechanism is the reduction of ventilation which has been shown to follow obstruction to a branch of the pulmonary artery. This is apparently due to an increase in resistance of the small airways caused by a fall in carbon dioxide tension in the region.

How far these two mechanisms operate in practice is unknown, but it has been shown that the administration of various bronchodilator and vasodilator drugs to patients with generalized lung disease can exaggerate their hypoxemia. For example, isoproterenol (by aerosol) and epinephrine and aminophylline (by injection) have been shown to reduce the arterial oxygen tension of some patients with chronic obstructive lung disease. It is likely that one of the actions of these drugs is to interfere with these active mechanisms which reduce ventilation-perfusion ratio inequality.

MECHANICS OF BREATHING

This section deals with the forces involved in supporting and moving the lung and chest wall so that ventilation can be accomplished. The bellows function of the lung is one of the easiest to measure and also one of the most informative measurements in practice. Serious malfunction of the lung is almost always accompanied by a reduced ventilatory capacity.

LUNG AND CHEST WALL. The lung is elastic and collapses if it is not held expanded. The pressure *inside* the lung (alveolar pressure) is the same as atmospheric pressure at the end of inspiration or expiration if the glottis is open. The pressure *outside* the lung (intrapleural pressure) is less than atmospheric pressure, or "negative." This pressure keeps the lung inflated and is developed by the chest wall, which is also elastic and tends to bow outwards. If air is introduced into this space and a pneumothorax is produced, the lung collapses inwards and the chest wall moves outwards.

During quiet breathing, inspiration is produced by the action of the diaphragm and intercostal muscles, and expiration results from the passive elastic recoil of the lungs. During deep breathing, the accessory muscles such as the sternomastoids and scaleni are called upon, and patients with diseased lungs may use these even at rest. Under these conditions, expiration is often assisted by the abdominal muscles.

COMPLIANCE. This is the term used to describe the elastic properties of the lung and chest wall. The normal lungs expand by about 200 ml when the expanding pressure (intrapleural pressure) changes by 1 cm of water. Thus the compliance (or distensibility) of the lungs is said to be 200 ml per cm of water. In fact, this figure only applies at normal resting lung volumes; at high lung volumes, the lungs are less easy to expand and their compliance falls. The compliance of the normal chest wall is about the same as that of the lungs, and the compliance of both lung and chest wall together is therefore about half this value, i.e., 100 ml per cm of water.

The compliance of lung depends very much on how much tissue is present. A single lobe, for example, will clearly not change its volume by as much as a whole lung for the same change in expanding pressure. Compliance is therefore sometimes corrected for lung volume and called *specific compliance*.

The normal elastic behavior of the lungs is only partly caused by the elastic tissue within it. An important component is the surface tension of the fluid lining the alveoli. The lungs may be regarded as composed of 300 million tiny bubbles which tend to collapse for the same reason that a soap bubble on the end of a bubble pipe does. During the last few years it has been found that the cells lining the alveoli produce a phospholipid which lowers the surface tension of the lining fluid to extremely low values. The substance is known as "surfactant." This lowering of the surface tension has great physiologic importance, because it helps to maintain the stability of the alveoli and discourage atelectasis. About half the normal compliance of the lung is due to these surface forces.

The normal elastic behavior of the lung is disturbed by many diseases. Diffuse pulmonary fibrosis, pleural thickening, healed tuberculosis with scarring, and atelectasis all reduce the compliance of the lung. Heart disease, such as mitral stenosis and left ventricular failure, also commonly lowers compliance, although it is often difficult to be certain whether the volume of ventilating lung is reduced by edema in the airways, for example, or whether the elastic behavior of lung tissue itself is altered. An absence of surfactant is thought to be responsible for the alveolar collapse and the stiff lungs seen in hyaline membrane disease of the newborn. In emphysema and old age, the lungs become more compliant and have an abnormally large volume at normal expanding pressures.

AIRWAYS RESISTANCE. So far we have been looking at the static forces involved in maintaining the expansion of the lung. However, during ventilation, additional forces are required to move air along the airways, because of the resistance offered to flow. This is expressed as the pressure difference between the alveoli and the mouth per unit of airflow rate. The normal value is in the vicinity of 1 to 2 cm water/liter/min of flow at normal flow rates. The resistance rises at higher flow rates.

The airways resistance is higher during expiration than inspiration, and it is greater at small lung volumes because the airways are then not held open so much. A single deep inspiration often reduces the resistance, but the inhalation of cigarette smoke or other irritants increases it. During a forced expiration, airways resistance rises greatly, because of collapse of parts of the bronchial tree, and the expiratory resistance increases with respiratory effort. The reason for this is that the expiratory pressure is applied not only to the alveoli in an effort to empty them, but also to the outside walls of the airways which lie within the chest. As a result, the expiratory flow rate is independent of respiratory effort over a large range. In normal subjects, this is only true for forced expirations but it often occurs much more readily in patients with emphysema, because the diseased airways collapse easily.

Diseases which increase airways resistance include bronchial asthma, chronic bronchitis, and pulmonary emphysema. The resistance may rise to many times its normal value and even during clinical remissions of the disease can be shown to be abnormally high. Lung volume increases in these conditions, and this has two helpful consequences: the airways are pulled open more, thus limiting the increase in resistance, and the higher passive recoil pressure of the lung assists expiration.

WORK OF BREATHING. In order to move the lungs and chest wall and force air along the airways, work is required and the respiratory muscles must consume oxygen. In normal subjects, the work of breathing is very small except during the large ventilation of heavy exercise. In

patients with obstructive lung disease, however, the frictional resistance to airflow is high even at rest and the work of breathing is much increased, perhaps to five or ten times its normal value. Under these conditions, the oxygen cost of breathing may become an appreciable fraction of the total oxygen consumption. Occasionally patients with very severe obstructive disease have such a high metabolic cost of ventilation that when they attempt to lower their arterial carbon dioxide tension by voluntary hyperventilation, the tension actually rises. This is because the increased carbon dioxide output due to the greater work of breathing more than offsets the enhanced carbon dioxide output caused by the hyperventilation.

Patients with a reduced compliance of the lungs or chest wall have a higher work of breathing, because the stiffer structures are more difficult to move. These patients tend to use rapid shallow breaths, which reduces their oxygen cost of ventilation. However, if breathing becomes too shallow, the volume of air merely moved in and out of the bronchial dead space becomes disproportionately high, and gas exchange is consequently impaired. A compromise is therefore reached.

MEASUREMENTS OF MECHANICS. One of the most useful tests in the armamentarium of the pulmonary function laboratory is the analysis of a single forced expiration. The patient makes a full inspiration and then exhales as hard and as fast as he can into a lightweight spirometer. Typical records are shown in Fig. 280-3. It can be seen that for a normal subject the total volume exhaled, the *vital capacity* or VC, is large, and also that about 80 percent of this volume is exhaled in 1 sec. This is called the *forced expiratory volume* or FEV_1. In *obstructive lung disease*, e.g., emphysema, the vital capacity is reduced because the airways close and limit expiration before the patient has breathed out fully. In addition, the FEV_1 is grossly reduced, as is the FEV/VC percentage. This is because of the high airways resistance, which slows down the rate of expiration. In *restrictive lung disease*, e.g., ankylosing spondylitis, the VC is low because of the limited expansion of the lung or chest wall. However, the FEV_1 is often not reduced proportionately, because airway resistance is normal. Thus the FEV/VC percentage is normal or high.

The FEV_1 is closely related to the maximum breathing capacity, and since it is a much simpler test to perform, it has largely replaced it. Impaired lung function is almost always associated with a reduced FEV_1, and the test is therefore a valuable screening procedure. It is also useful in assessing the efficacy of bronchodilator therapy and in following the progress of patients in the clinic.

Other lung volumes can also be measured at the same time. The *inspiratory capacity* is the maximum volume which can be inspired from the resting volume of the lungs, which is called the *functional residual capacity*. The maximum volume which can be expired from the resting level is the *expiratory reserve volume*. This leaves the *residual volume* still in the lungs, and this can be measured only indirectly. One technique is to connect the patient to a spirometer circuit containing helium and

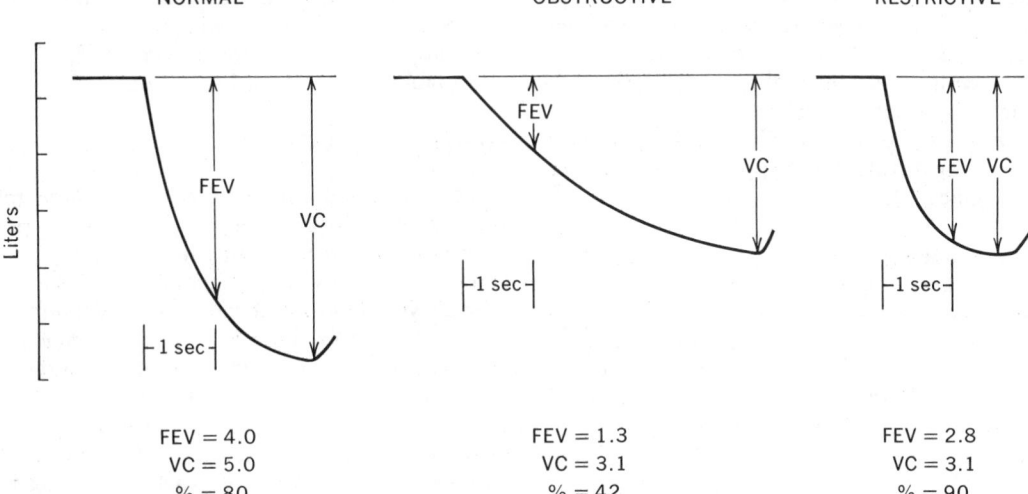

NORMAL   OBSTRUCTIVE   RESTRICTIVE

FEV = 4.0	FEV = 1.3	FEV = 2.8
VC = 5.0	VC = 3.1	VC = 3.1
% = 80	% = 42	% = 90

Fig. 280-3. Measurement of the forced expiratory volume FEV_1 and vital capacity VC. The patient makes a full inspiration and then exhales as hard and as fast as he can. As he exhales, the pen moves down. The FEV_1 is the volume exhaled in 1 record; the VC is the total volume exhaled. Note the differences between the normal, obstructive, and restrictive patterns.

measure the degree of dilution of this gas which occurs after several minutes of rebreathing. Another is to use a body plethysmograph (see below).

The measurement of compliance and airways resistance is more difficult. In order to determine lung compliance, i.e., volume change per unit of pressure change, the pressure expanding the lungs must be known. In practice this can be found by passing a small rubber balloon connected to a manometer down into the esophagus. Esophageal pressure is then taken as a measure of intrapleural pressure. To measure airways resistance, i.e., the pressure drop along the airways per unit of airflow, alveolar pressure must be known. This can be found by seating the patient in a large airtight box, or plethysmograph. First, he is asked to try to breathe against a complete obstruction, and from the change in box pressure, lung volume can be calculated. Next, he is asked to pant in and out, and again box pressure is recorded. Alveolar pressure can then be derived and airway resistance calculated. This equipment is available only in specialized centers.

ACID-BASE DISTURBANCES. If pulmonary gas exchange is impaired, carbon dioxide tension in the arterial blood may rise, thus tending to depress the pH and causing *respiratory acidosis*. The compensatory mechanisms which are then brought into play are discussed in Chap. 297.

MEASUREMENT OF BLOOD GASES. Blood gas measurements play a vital role in the management of patients with respiratory failure. Arterial blood can be obtained by direct puncture, and the oxygen and carbon dioxide tensions and the pH measured by electrodes. Oxygen saturation can be derived from the oxygen content of the blood using van Slyke's method before and after complete oxygenation, or the saturation can be calculated from an oxygen dissociation curve.

In some situations, it is valuable to know whether the arterial carbon dioxide tension is raised but it is incon-

venient to perform an arterial puncture. For example, a patient with chronic lung disease may attend the clinic because of a recent infective episode, and it may be important to rule out incipient respiratory failure. In these circumstances, a rebreathing technique for measuring the carbon dioxide tension of mixed venous blood is useful. It depends on the fact that when a subject rebreathes into a small bag, the carbon dioxide tension in the lung-bag system rapidly approaches that of the mixed venous blood, but then rises only slowly. The patient is allowed to rebreathe for 1.5 min from a rubber bag containing 100 percent oxygen, its volume being about twice the tidal volume. Then after a 3-min rest, the patient rebreathes from the same bag for a further 30 sec and the carbon dioxide tension in the bag is found, using a carbon dioxide meter. This value is almost always within 2 mm Hg of the mixed venous value, which itself is about 7 mm Hg above the arterial carbon dioxide tension. Thus the test is a useful screening procedure, and it is also valuable for following the progress of a patient with chronic carbon dioxide retention.

HYPOXEMIA

The four main causes of a low arterial oxygen tension are ventilation-perfusion ratio inequality, right-to-left shunt, hypoventilation, and impaired diffusion. In addition, living at high altitude or deliberately inspiring a low oxygen mixture causes hypoxemia. Ventilation-perfusion ratio inequality is the commonest cause and is responsible for almost all the hypoxemia seen in chronic lung disease. Specific tests of ventilation-perfusion inequality are not available; it is generally deduced by exclusion. The demonstration of ventilatory inequality (see above) is a useful pointer. Mild degrees of ventilation-perfusion ratio inequality may be present without hypoxemia, and considerable inequality may exist without hypercapnia if overall ventilation is increased. However, carbon dioxide retention almost always develops eventually. The hypoxemia is abolished by the administration of 100 percent oxygen, though with severe inequality, the arterial oxygen tension may take many minutes to rise to normal values, because of very poorly ventilated areas. Exercise may or may not aggravate the hypoxemia and hypercapnia (see Table 280-1).

Table 280-1. FEATURES HELPFUL IN DISTINGUISHING THE VARIOUS CAUSES OF HYPOXEMIA AND HYPERCAPNIA

	Hypoxemia	Hypercapnia	Hypoxemia on exercise	Hypercapnia on exercise	Hypoxemia on 100% O_2
Ventilation-perfusion ratio inequality..	Yes	Yes or no	Yes	Yes or no	No
Shunt......	Yes	No	Yes	Possible	Yes
Hypoventilation....	Yes	Yes	Often severe	Often severe	No
Impaired diffusion..	Yes	No	Often severe	No	No

Shunted blood, i.e., blood which has not circulated through ventilated areas of the lung, causes hypoxemia. Patients with right-to-left shunts through congenital heart defects belong to this group. Patients with ventilation-perfusion ratio inequality often have some parts of the lung completely unventilated, and the contribution of these regions is indistinguishable from that of a shunt. The hypoxemia due to shunt is not abolished (though it is reduced) by administering 100 percent oxygen, and this test will distinguish it from the other causes of hypoxemia. The level of the arterial oxygen tension under these conditions allows the percentage of shunted blood to be measured. The arterial tension rises to some extent because of the addition of dissolved oxygen to the pulmonary blood, and a measurement of arterial saturation may not permit detection of the hypoxemia. It is therefore important to measure oxygen tension. The hypoxemia of shunt may be exaggerated by exercise. Hypercapnia does not occur unless the shunt is very gross, because the respiratory center increases the ventilation, thus holding the arterial carbon dioxide tension down.

Hypoventilation always causes both hypoxemia and hypercapnia. Because of the shape of the oxygen dissociation curve, considerable carbon dioxide retention may be present without recognizable cyanosis. If the patient is inhaling an enriched oxygen mixture, e.g., in the anesthetic recovery room, hypoxemia is not present but the hypercapnia may be severe.

Impaired diffusion causes hypoxemia but never hypercapnia. The hypoxemia is accentuated by exercise but abolished if an enriched oxygen mixture is administered. As we have seen, diffusion impairment may occur in normal subjects during work at very high altitude, but its importance as a cause of hypoxemia in disease is disputed.

HYPERCAPNIA

The two chief causes of carbon dioxide retention are ventilation-perfusion ratio inequality and hypoventilation. Ventilation-perfusion ratio inequality is the commonest cause, although many patients have some degree of uneven ventilation and blood flow without hypercapnia. A combination of the two causes is common.

Why does a patient with chronic lung disease develop hypercapnia? Progressive lung disease (perhaps aggravated by an acute infection) causes increasing mismatch of blood flow and ventilation and greater impairment of carbon dioxide transfer. For a time, the respiratory center is able to hold the arterial carbon dioxide tension down by increasing the ventilation, but the work of breathing is usually high because of airways obstruction, so that eventually a compromise is reached and the arterial and alveolar tensions are allowed to rise. This has the advantage that more carbon dioxide tension is put out for the same ventilation, so that it may be looked upon as a compensatory mechanism, albeit a hazardous one. As the ventilation-perfusion ratio inequality becomes worse, the tendency is for the arterial carbon dioxide tension to rise further.

A particularly dangerous situation may arise if the patient is given oxygen to breathe. The chief stimulus to ventilation in these patients is often hypoxia, and when this is suddenly relieved, the ventilation may drop precipitously and the arterial carbon dioxide tension climb rapidly. The carbon dioxide retention and acidosis may then cause unconsciousness, muscular twitching, and a raised intracranial pressure. This is known as *carbon dioxide narcosis*. Drugs which depress the respiratory center may produce a similar effect. Thus while oxygen administration is generally indicated in these patients because of their severe hypoxemia, it should be given with caution.

Another hazardous situation often arises when these patients are taken off oxygen because they are retaining too much carbon dioxide. Since the body stores of carbon dioxide are so large, many minutes elapse before the alveolar carbon dioxide tension returns to reasonable levels. During this recovery period, this high alveolar carbon dioxide dilutes the alveolar oxygen and may cause profound hypoxemia.

REFERENCES

Bates, D. V., and R. V. Christie: "Respiratory Function in Disease," Philadelphia, W. B. Saunders Company, 1964.

Campbell, E. J. M., and J. B. L. Howell: The Measurement of Arterial and Mixed Venous CO_2 Tension by Rebreathing Techniques, in "pH and Blood Gas Measurement: Methods and Interpretation," R. Woolmer (Ed.), London, J. & A. Churchill, Ltd., 1959.

Comroe, J. H., R. E. Forster, A. B. Dubois, W. A. Briscoe, and E. Carlson: "The Lung: Clinical Physiology and Pulmonary Function Tests," Chicago, The Year Book Medical Publishers, Inc., 1962.

Mead, J.: Mechanical Properties of Lungs, Physiol. Rev., 41:281, 1961.

Roughton, F. J. W.: in "Handbook of Respiratory Physiology," W. M. Boothby (Ed.), Texas, USAF School of Aviation Medicine, 1954.

West, J. B.: "Ventilation/Blood Flow and Gas Exchange," Oxford, Blackwell Scientific Publications, Ltd., 1965.

281 DIAGNOSTIC PROCEDURES

Kenneth M. Moser

In seeking a definitive diagnosis in the patient with respiratory disease, a wide choice of diagnostic procedures is available. These procedures vary considerably, not only in diagnostic reliability and specificity, but also in terms of the discomfort and hazard to the patient. Hence, an orderly sequence of test selection is mandatory. This sequence should begin with procedures involving little risk and moving on to those which entail higher morbidity and mortality only if necessary.

RADIOGRAPHIC PROCEDURES

The *chest roentgenogram* serves two major roles in the search for a diagnosis in the patient with respiratory disease: *detector* and *guide*. Often, in its role as a detector, the routine chest roentgenogram initiates the diagnostic search by disclosing an abnormality in an asymptomatic individual. More commonly, it detects pulmonary involvement in someone already ill. Rarely, detection may coincide with diagnosis; for example, in spontaneous pneumothorax or when a radiopaque foreign body has been aspirated.

Far more frequently, however, the roentgenogram, having detected potential disease, provides a guide to the selection of subsequent diagnostic procedures. Many radiographic findings are quite characteristic of certain diseases. A number of radiographic patterns are sufficiently repetitive to warrant descriptive names, such as bilateral hilar adenopathy, solitary pulmonary nodule, diffuse interstitial infiltrate, alveolar filling pattern, multinodular lesion, honeycomb lung. Thus, a particular radiographic finding, combined with other pertinent data, often permits establishment of a reasonable list of possible diagnoses. For example, the roentgenographic detection of bilateral hilar adenopathy in an asymptomatic, twenty-six-year-old Negro male immediately places sarcoidosis at the top of the list. A chest roentgenogram disclosing upper lobe cavities in a febrile male whose brother recently was admitted to a tuberculosis sanitarium would make tuberculosis the most likely entity. Or a "diffuse interstitial" infiltrate—for which more than 100 etiologies exist—may yield a prompt diagnosis of varicella pneumonia when combined with the classical skin lesions.

In some instances, special radiographic technics may provide valuable diagnostic insights.

Fluoroscopy. This procedure allows visualization of the thoracic contents in a dynamic rather than static manner and also permits a wide range of special views. It also indicates whether a lesion is pulsatile, what its precise location in the thorax is, whether the hemidiaphragms move normally; i.e., whether they are fixed or move paradoxically, and how various zones of the lung behave during inspiration and expiration.

Tomography (Laminography, Planography). This is a radiographic technique by which a sequence of roentgenograms, each representing a "slice of the lung" at a different depth, is obtained. Ordinarily, "cuts" at 0.5-to-1.0-cm distances through the area of interest are made. Tomograms can identify a number of features which were not appreciated on the "routine" roentgenogram, including the presence of calcium or cavity in a lesion; the presence of hilar adenopathy; abnormalities in configuration of the trachea and major bronchi; and the contours of masses in the mediastinal area.

Skin Tests. Having arrived at a tentative list of diagnostic possibilities based on the history, physical examination, and the radiographic appearance, the physician should move to other procedures. One of the simplest and most commonly overlooked is the application of *skin tests* with specific antigens. Antigens are now available to assist in the diagnosis of tuberculosis, histoplasmosis, coccidiodomycosis, blastomycosis, trichinosis, and toxoplasmosis. A negative battery of skin tests may provide a diagnostic clue by suggesting a disorder associated with skin anergy, such as sarcoidosis.

Serologic Tests. These tests also may be useful in the diagnosis of histoplasmosis, blastomycosis, coccidioidomycosis, toxoplasmosis, mycoplasma pneumonia, and a variety of other infectious diseases involving the lungs. Often, more extensive diagnostic procedures can be avoided if appropriate serologic tests are obtained.

Sputum Examination. Another rapid, innocuous diagnostic procedure is *sputum examination*. It is important that the specimen contain sputum and not saliva. The gross nature of the sputum—color, odor, and the presence of blood—may provide valuable clues. Carefully stained smears of the sputum should be examined next, for these will disclose the causative organism in many bacterial pneumonias, in tuberculosis, and in some fungous infections. Often valuable time is lost because the sputum smear is not examined, and results of culture are awaited instead.

Sputum Culture. Culture of the sputum is not a substitute for careful microscopic examination of stained sputum specimens. Proper results from sputum culture require attention to detail. Specimens for culture should be collected and delivered to the laboratory promptly. If unusual organisms are anticipated, the laboratory should be alerted so that implantation on all appropriate media will be assured.

Exfoliative Cytology of the Sputum. This procedure is helpful in the diagnosis of carcinoma of the lung. Again, proper handling of such specimens is essential. Sputum samples often can be obtained in patients who are not coughing by inhalation of heated mixtures of mildly irritative solutions.

Examination of Pleural Fluid. Like sputum, *pleural fluid* can supply definitive information and should be examined for specific gravity, white blood cell count and differential, hematocrit and/or red blood cell count, protein and glucose concentrations, amylase, appropriate cultures, and exfoliative cytology. The gross appearance of the fluid, the quantity obtained, and the precise location of the thoracentesis should be recorded.

Pulmonary Function Tests. These tests may serve as diagnostic guides. Certain "patterns" of derangement in spirometric tests, arterial blood gases, diffusing capacity and other functional parameters are particularly suggestive of certain pulmonary diseases (Chap. 280).

Pulmonary Radiophotoscanning. This technique can provide a visual image of, and quantitative data regarding the distribution of both blood flow and ventilation in the lungs. Photoscans are obtained by a variety of "scanning" devices which record the pattern of pulmonary radioactivity after intravenous injection or inhalation of gamma-emitting radionuclides. Injection (perfusion) photoscans have proven especially valuable in detecting zones of absent or decreased blood flow compatible with embolism (Chap. 285). Inhalation scans can disclose areas of decreased ventilation.

All of the above procedures involve minimal risks and discomfort to the patient. These approaches should be exhausted before the techniques discussed below are considered unless the condition of the patient demands immediate diagnosis.

Bronchoscopy. Bronchoscopy is employed to visualize directly the trachea and its major subdivisions. A lighted mirror-lens system is introduced into the anesthetized tracheobronchial tree. In addition to observing abnormalities such as tumors or granulomatous lesions, suspicious or obvious lesions can be biopsied and bronchial washings for culture and cytologic examination can be obtained. Bronchoscopy permits visualization only of the lobar bronchi and the orifices of certain segmental bronchi. Beyond this limited range, only *bronchography* can supply visual information regarding bronchial anatomy.

Bronchography. In this method, a viscous radiopaque material is instilled into the tracheobronchial tree via a catheter. By positioning the patient properly, the material will coat all portions of the tracheobronchial tree for a sufficient period to permit their outline to be recorded on chest roentgenograms. Bronchography is required for the diagnosis of bronchiectasis, for the identification of obstruction in distal bronchi, and for the detection of other types of congenital and acquired forms of bronchial distortion or malformation.

Pulmonary Angiography. Just as bronchography outlines the tracheobronchial anatomy, *pulmonary angiography* permits visualization of the pulmonary vasculature. Radiopaque materials are injected rapidly by vein or via a catheter into the systemic veins, right chambers, or the pulmonary artery. The distribution of this material in the pulmonary vasculature is recorded on film (angiography), by a high-speed camera (cineangiography), or on videotape (Chap. 262). Angiography is frequently used to detect pulmonary emboli and a variety of congenital and acquired lesions of the pulmonary vessels.

Often, despite the application of the procedures discussed above, a definitive diagnosis is still lacking, and biopsy of tissue is indicated. If a pleural effusion exists, *pleural biopsy* is often worthwhile. This can be carried out with either a "closed" or "open" technique. In the former, a needle specially constructed for biopsy is inserted at the time of thoracentesis. All available needles have a cutting edge and some mechanism for retaining the biopsy specimen. The needle is introduced into the effusion and seated on the parietal pleura, from which a biopsy is then obtained with the cutting edge. The procedure is sufficiently safe and productive to warrant its performance in every thoracentesis done in an effusion of obscure cause. Pleural fluid should be obtained prior to biopsy because bleeding after parietal pleural biopsy may obscure the true character of the fluid. Usually, three biopsies are taken from differing sites at the same session. Care should be exercised to place the needle in a position least likely to impinge upon the intercostal vessels.

The absence of pleural fluid increases the hazard of "closed" biopsy, because the needle cannot be placed into the pleural space with assurance. Bleeding, pneumothorax, and bronchopleural fistula induced by cutting through visceral pleura are more likely, and a satisfactory biopsy specimen is less likely to be obtained. Therefore, in the absence of effusion—or when "closed" biopsy has not provided a diagnosis—"open" biopsy is indicated. This involves a limited thoracotomy, requiring anesthesia. A small intercostal incision is made, and the parietal pleura is biopsied under direct visualization. The incision is then closed, often without an intercostal tube. "Open" biopsy has several advantages because a larger specimen is obtained and the pleura and underlying lung can be seen and palpated. When pleural involvement is "spotty," open biopsy increases the possibility of establishing a diagnosis.

Another favored site for biopsy is the *scalene fat pad*. Because the lymph nodes invariably present in this fat pad receive lymphatic drainage from the lungs, they often disclose intrathoracic diseases such as carcinoma, granulomatous infections, and sarcoidosis. Scalene biopsy can be performed under local anesthesia. In some clinics, scalene node biopsy has been combined with, or replaced by, *mediastinoscopy.*

Mediastinoscopy. This involves insertion of a lighted mirror-lens system, much like a bronchoscope, through an incision at the base of the neck. The instrument is advanced under visual control into the mediastinum where inspection and biopsy can be carried out.

Lung Biopsy. Finally, if the diagnosis still remains unclear, biopsy of the lung may be required. Again, "closed" and "open" approaches are available. Closed, needle biopsies of the lung are a subject of some debate because pneumothorax and bleeding are encountered in a substantial number of patients. In addition, the pulmonary architecture leads to difficulty in cutting and retaining the specimen. Finally, because of its small size, the amount of tissue obtained may be inadequate for diagnosis. Advocates of closed lung biopsy emphasize that, in experienced hands, pneumothorax and bleeding are rare, mild, and easily controlled; and that a substantial number of diagnoses can be established without resort to open biopsy.

Those who prefer open (surgical) biopsy feel that the risk and morbidity of a limited thoracotomy are not substantially greater than those encountered in closed biopsy and are counterbalanced by the fact that an adequate, representative lung biopsy will provide a reliable answer to the diagnostic problem. The decision in favor of closed lung biopsy usually depends upon local expertise. However, there is general agreement on three points: (1) closed biopsy is particularly hazardous in patients with pulmonary hypertension; (2) prior to needle biopsy, provision should be made for prompt treatment of pneumothorax and bleeding; and (3) large solid lesions abutting, or attached to, the thoracic wall are the most favorable for closed biopsy. Needle biopsy of such lesions is safer and more likely to provide a diagnosis than is needle biopsy of lesions located deeply in the pulmonary parenchyma.

All specimens obtained by biopsy should be both cultured and processed for pathologic examination.

In summary, there are many diagnostic procedures which can be applied to patients with pulmonary disease. All options should be considered, and the hazards of each procedure must be weighed against its diagnostic efficacy. Finally, careful observation over a period of time may be the wisest course to follow in some patients.

REFERENCES

Baum, G. L.: "Textbook of Pulmonary Diseases," Boston, Little, Brown and Company, 1964.

Felson, B: "Fundamentals of Chest Roentgenology," Philadelphia, W. B. Saunders Company, 1960.

Lillington, G. A., and R. W. Jamplis: "A Diagnostic Approach to Chest Diseases," Baltimore, The Williams & Wilkins Company, 1965.

Perry, K. M. A., and T. Holmes Sellors: "Chest Diseases," London, Butterworth and Company (Publishers), Ltd., 1963.

Rubin, E. H., and M. Rubin: "Thoracic Diseases," Philadelphia, W. B. Saunders Company, 1962.

Spencer, H.: "Pathology of the Lung," New York, The Macmillan Company, 1962.

282 DISEASES OF THE UPPER RESPIRATORY TRACT

Ivan L. Bennett, Jr.
Robert G. Petersdorf

This chapter summarizes some of the diseases that are manifested in whole or in part by structural alterations or dysfunction of the nose, nasopharynx, paranasal sinuses, and larynx. In the course of their normal function of warming, humidifying, and preliminary cleansing (by impingement of inhaled particles upon the mucosa) of inspired air, these passages are exposed to a multitude of irritants and infectious agents. Their lining membranes contain many mucous glands and deposits of lymphoid tissue; the vascular bed of the nasal mucosa is capable of such rapid and extensive alterations in response to local or systemic stimuli that it is often classified as an erectile tissue. Engorgement, hypersecretion of mucus, and hyperplasia of the adenoids and other lymphatic foci in response to irritation or infection can produce acute or chronic obstruction of the passages draining the sinuses, conjunctivas, and middle ears. This leads to initiation or aggravation of bacterial infection in these areas.

The annoying and distracting discomfort occasioned by interference with inspiration and speech, coupled with the frequency of viral and allergic disorders of this region, makes upper respiratory disease a most important transient disability.

DISEASES OF THE NOSE AND NASOPHARYNX

Hay fever, vasomotor rhinitis, and complicating nasal *polyposis* are discussed in Chap. 72. Acute coryza and other forms of viral rhinitis are discussed in Chap. 206. The upper respiratory prodrome of *measles* is discussed in Chap. 220.

Among bacterial infections, the persistent rhinitis ("snuffles") of *congenital syphilis,* nasal diphtheria, and *furunculosis* of the nares (which occasionally may be complicated by *cavernous sinus thrombosis*) are the more important.

Clear, watery discharge characterizes *cerebrospinal rhinorrhea,* which may be diagnosed by instilling a dye such as methylene blue into the cerebrospinal fluid and watching it appear in the nasal secretions. Chronic mucoid, occasionally bloodstained discharge is frequent in children with enlarged *adenoids.* Unilateral purulent or sanguineous discharge suggests foreign body, diphtheria, or tumor.

Perforation of the Nasal Septum. This condition results most commonly from habitual nose picking, but syphilis and occupational exposure to chromate are other causes to be considered. Many diseases are characterized by extensive destructive and deforming lesions of the nose and adjacent structures. These include leprosy (Chap. 175), the *gangosa* and *goundou* lesions of yaws (Chap. 178), the *espundia* type of American leishmaniasis (Chap. 242), *South American blastomycosis* (Chap. 186), *midline granuloma* (Chap. 257), Wegener's granulomatosis (Chap. 394), and mucormycosis (Chap. 191), another cause of gangrene and perforation of the nasal septum.

Rhinoscleroma. In rhinoscleroma chronic obstruction of the nasal passages is produced by recurrent, indurated, nonulcerating, inflammatory nodules. Rarely, sinuses or the upper trachea are involved also. The disorder occurs primarily in the Mediterranean countries, South Asia, Indonesia, and Latin America; most cases seen in the United States are in immigrants. Rhinoscleroma is probably an infection, caused by von Frisch's bacillus, *Klebsiella rhinoscleromatis*, which is always present in the lesions, but the diagnosis is usually established by the pathognomonic histologic finding of masses of atypical plasma cells interspersed with large, foamy Mikulicz cells. Treatment is surgical excision of the recurrent nodules. Untreated, the disease can lead to enormous nasal enlargement with flared nares, the *Hebra nose*.

Rhinosporidiosis. Caused by a yeastlike organism, *Rhinosporidium seeberi*, this disease is common in India and Ceylon; sporadic cases occur in many other areas. Soft, pinkish, sessile or pedunculated polyps appear on the nasal mucosa; sometimes the conjunctivas and, rarely, other mucosal surfaces are involved. Treatment is simple excision (see Chap. 193).

Rhinophyma. Also called *Pfundnase*, this progressive, deforming, nodular enlargement of the alae nasi is due to hypertrophy of sebaceous follicles in patients with chronic, severe acne rosacea. There is no specific treatment; plastic repair may be necessary.

Ozena. This is a severe chronic rhinitis of unknown cause characterized by thick, greenish discharge, mucosal crusts, turbinate atrophy, and an offensive odor. Patients eventually become anosmic. Even when the nasal passages are widened and resistance to airflow is decreased, obstruction is a constant complaint. Cultures grow gram-negative bacilli (*Klebsiella, Pseudomonas,* etc.). Treatment, aimed at reducing the odor, includes use of local or systemic antibiotics and large doses of vasodilators (Priscoline, nicotinic acid). Local cleansing by means of repeated saline irrigation is extremely important to get rid of the foul-smelling crusts. Some patients get relief from sniffing powdered sugar. Surgically narrowing the nasal airway may afford relief in many cases.

Mycosis Leptothrica. So called because infection by Leptothrix was thought to be its cause, this is a focal hyperkeratosis of the tonsils, pharynx, and larynx that occurs in young adults. The many small, white, raised patches over the mucosa are striking and are often mistaken for exudate; removal causes no bleeding. Patients are sometimes asymptomatic but may complain of a "scratchy" throat. There is no treatment; the lesions regress after months or years.

Pharyngeal bursitis. Also called Tornwaldt's disease, this is a bacterial inflammation of a small recess in the posterior nasopharyngeal wall which sometimes persists into adulthood. Obstruction of the neck of the pouch leads to infection and abscess formation. Treatment consists of antibiotics followed by surgical excision of the bursa, rather than simple drainage.

Recurrent, profuse *epistaxes* occur with hypertensive vascular disease, familial telangiectasia, coagulation defects, and tumors.

Basal cell carcinoma of the nares and septal hemangioma. These malignant tumors are relatively common. Carci-

nomas of the nasal mucosa are unusual; they occur in elderly individuals and invade or metastasize late.

Carcinoma of the nasopharynx (so-called lymphoepithelioma) occurs in young and middle-adged adults and is especially common among Chinese. These tumors metastasize early. Large, cancerous cervical lymph nodes often result from a primary lesion so small that it is found with great difficulty. These tumors tend to occur near the orifice of a eustachian tube, and the combination of *cervical adenopathy and ipsilateral ear pain or deafness* is a signal for careful examination of the nasopharynx. These tumors are radiosensitive, and survival for several years with repeated courses of therapy is usual; complete cures are rare.

Lymphoma. Lymphoma and reticulum cell sarcoma are often first detected as nasopharyngeal masses. Isolated plasmacytomas of the nasopharynx are found predominantly in elderly males, some of whom develop multiple myeloma. Two tumors of children deserve mention. A highly malignant and rapidly fatal lesion which tends to arise in the nasopharynx or soft palate is the *sarcoma botryoides* or *embryonal rhabdomyosarcoma*. *Juvenile angiofibroma* is a benign growth that occurs almost exclusively in young boys, arising from the base of the sphenoid and filling the nasopharynx. Sometimes the tumor will regress during puberty, but excision is usually necessary. These tumors bleed spontaneously, and profuse hemorrhage is very likely to complicate surgical manipulation.

DISEASES OF THE PARANASAL SINUSES

The mucosa of the ethmoid and maxillary sinuses may become involved by the polyposis that occurs in patients with allergic rhinitis (Chap. 72). Although primary tumors of the sinus mucosa are rare, encroachment by neoplasms arising in contiguous structures is common and easily visualized by x-ray. *Osteoma of the frontal sinus* is the most frequent lesion of this type; neoplasms of the maxilla and mixed tumors of the salivary gland type arising in the palate invade the antrum.

SINUSITIS. In the vast majority of cases, acute sinusitis is a bacterial infection brought on by impairment of drainage by the boggy, engorged nasal mucosa of allergic or viral rhinitis. Occasionally, pressure changes of air travel may result in an "aerosinusitis" similar to "aerotitis media"; deviations of the nasal septum are contributory.

The manifestations are local pain and tenderness, sometimes with edema of the overlying facial skin, headache, and fever. The headache is worse in the morning, when exudate has accumulated overnight, and tends to improve with upright posture and drainage during the day. If fluid has filled the frontal or maxillary sinuses, they cannot be transilluminated. Treatment consists of administration of analgesics and appropriate antibiotics, and, most important, the establishment of adequate drainage. In the acute stage, drainage is achieved most effectively by reduction of nasal swelling by astringents such as Neo-Synephrine, ephedrine, or antihistaminics in patients with allergy. Aspiration or irrigation of the infected cavity by an otorhinolaryngologist should be avoided during the acute stage but frequently is indicated after acute symptoms subside, particularly in maxillary sinusitis. Often, however, acute sinusitis clears up promptly when acute coryza or allergic rhinitis has subsided.

About 10 percent of antral infections are secondary to dental sepsis or result from fractures of the bony floor during dental extractions.

Complications of acute sinusitis are statistically rare but may be serious. Frank suppuration and abscess may lead to osteomyelitis and spread of infection to the orbit (retrobulbar abscess, cavernous sinus thrombosis), the meninges (see pneumococcal meningitis, Chaps. 138 and 360), and brain (via the diploic veins). Surgical drainage of frontal and ethmoid abscesses is sometimes an emergency procedure. About 10 percent of brain abscesses originate from frontal sinusitis, and infection of the frontal or sphenoid sinus precedes almost every case of subdural empyema. A serious complication of frontal suppuration is osteomyelitis of the skull, recognized by doughy edema of the forehead ("Pott's puffy tumor") and rapid destruction of bone.

With repeated episodes of acute infection, there may be thickening of the sinus mucosa, continual partial obstruction, and chronic inflammation that flares up with even slight obstruction such as may follow smoking, ingestion of spicy foods, the use of alcohol, or chilly, damp weather. Each acute episode becomes more difficult to control, and the patient may be continuously miserable. Rigid control of exposure to allergens and extremes of temperature, correction of structural defects such as deviated septum, and intensive treatment of acute exacerbations will sometimes bring relief, but radical surgery to ensure free drainage is eventually necessary in many instances. Chronic sinusitis is especially common in patients with bronchiectasis (Chap. 291), but a causal relationship between lung and sinus disease has not been shown.

Cerebral *mucormycosis* in patients with diabetic acidosis (Chap. 191) usually originates as a sinusitis and invades the orbit and cranium secondarily.

When a diagnosis of "sinusitis" has been made radiologically, the distinction between acute, chronic, or inactive disease may be impossible and the diagnosis must depend on the patient's symptoms as well as on accurate bacteriologic identification of the causative organism. Nasal swab cultures are *never sterile*, and the choice of an antibiotic should be based on the predominating pathogenic organism in cultures of exudate from the sinus; usually these are group A streptococci, pneumococci, and staphylococci and may be treated with a penicillin, erythromycin, or lincomycin. Gram-negative pathogens are common in patients who have received antibiotics, and it is fruitless to change antimicrobial drugs in these patients.

DISEASES OF THE LARYNX

The two most important manifestations of laryngeal diseases are *hoarseness* and *respiratory* obstruction. Aphasia and *aphonia* do not signify a lesion of the larynx. *Hoarseness* that persists for more than 3 weeks in an adult calls for intensive investigation; tumor, chronic infection (tuberculosis, mycosis), and vocal cord paralysis are the important possibilities. Respiratory obstruction by edema, exudate, foreign body, or bilateral cord paralysis is an acute emergency.

Among infectious agents, the diphtheria bacillus, *Hemophilus influenzae,* the viral agents of croup and laryngotracheitis, *Treponema pallidum,* the tubercle bacillus, and fungi, especially monilia, are the ones most likely to attack the larynx. Laryngitis and hoarseness are not complications of streptococcal pharyngitis; their appearance in a patient with sore throat indicates a viral etiology or complicating diphtheria.

Laryngeal papillomatosis is believed by many to be a viral disease. They are multiple pedunculated growths on the cords, which are easily excised but recur. They are seen most commonly, but not invariably, in children and are rare after puberty.

Laryngeal acanthosis or *hyperkeratosis* (pachydermia laryngis) causing hoarseness may be a result of misuse of the voice, smoking, and probably of alcoholism; it is not a precancerous lesion. Leukoplakia of the larynx has the same significance in terms of later development of cancer that it has elsewhere and calls for local excision. It is important not to confuse acanthosis and leukoplakia.

The so-called *singers' nodule* is a lesion of the vocal cord that appears in individuals who have strained or misused their voices. If discovered early, the lesions may regress as proper voice modulation is practiced. Once the nodule becomes firm, treatment is excision; the lesion does not recur.

Carcinoma of the larynx is ten to twelve times more common in men than in women; it appears at an average age of sixty. Tumors arising on the vocal cords are classified as "intrinsic" and constitute 70 percent of the lesions; those extending beyond the cords are "extrinsic." Hoarseness is an early symptom of intrinsic cancer; it is often delayed in the extrinsic type. Treatment varies, but radiation alone is recommended only for small lesions of the middle third of the cord. Laryngectomy is the treatment of choice for many cancers; preoperative radiation and extensive removal of lymph nodes are used in many clinics. Partial supraglottic laryngectomy is preferable in some patients with cancer of the epiglottis and/or false cords because it permits patients to retain normal speech without jeopardizing their chances for cure.

Among the many causes of partial or complete paralysis of the vocal cords are pressure by aortic aneurysm, mediastinal tumors, metastatic esophageal cancer, postdiphtheritic neuritis, poliomyelitis, and operative trauma (especially thyroidectomy). If a nerve is cut at operation, there will be sudden stridor; if stretching and edema are affecting the nerve, the onset of stridor and hoarseness will be gradual. Bilateral injury may cause sudden obstruction, necessitating tracheostomy.

283 CHRONIC OBSTRUCTIVE PULMONARY DISEASE. BRONCHITIS AND EMPHYSEMA

John H. Knowles

The problem of chronic nonspecific pulmonary disease, consisting mainly of chronic bronchitis and obstructive emphysema, has become the most important one in the field of pulmonary disease from all standpoints, including prevalence, morbidity, mortality, and economic loss. Knowledge of these conditions has been incomplete and uncertain for a number of reasons. A persistent cough has been accepted as a normal phenomenon in the cigarette smoker, and rarely is the physician consulted for this complaint alone. Because of the length of time required for all the dire consequences of chronic bronchitis to unfold and because it frequently accompanies a more dramatic illness, such as bronchogenic carcinoma, pneumonia, or peptic ulcer, it has been relegated to a position of secondary importance by lay persons as well as the medical profession. Clinically, the differentiation of asthma, chronic bronchitis, and the various types of emphysema (e.g., senile, "compensatory," obstructive) has been difficult because of confusion concerning the etiologic significance of the barrel chest, "smoker's cough," and wheezing respiration (the patient compounds this felony by announcing that he has "asthma"), the inadequacies of radiologic diagnosis in these conditions, and generally, the unqualified use of the word "emphysema" to denote anything from the kyphotic chest deformity of old age to the hyperinflated chest of the child with acute bronchial asthma.

DEFINITIONS AND CLASSIFICATION

Chronic diffuse nonspecific lung disease refers to a condition of chronic cough with sputum production with or without paroxysmal or persistent uncomfortable shortness of breath, which cannot be attributed to localized lung disease, generalized pulmonary infection, granulomatous, fibrotic, or collagen disease of the lung, pneumoconiosis, primary cardiovascular disease, disorders of the chest wall, or psychoneurosis. It may coexist with any of these conditions and not infrequently does. In such instances two diagnoses should be made. There are two main categories of chronic diffuse nonspecific lung disease: chronic bronchitis and generalized obstructive lung disease.

Chronic bronchitis has been arbitrarily separated from recurrent acute bronchitis in epidemiologic studies as "cough with production of sputum occurring on most days for at least 3 months in the year during at least 2 years." The sputum may be mucoid or purulent. Chronic bron-

chitis predisposes to recurrent respiratory infection, particularly during the winter months, and eventually may lead to dyspnea by virtue of a gradual loss of ventilatory capacity due to the development of emphysema. The smoker's cough, when it conforms to the above description, is an example of chronic bronchitis.

Generalized obstructive lung disease is a condition characterized by increased airway resistance due to diffuse narrowing of the bronchial tree. This is the result of hypersecretion, smooth-muscle spasm, a check-valve mechanism, bronchiolar fibrosis, or all four of these factors. *It is diagnosed simply and with certainty by finding a reduction in the timed vital capacity* (1-sec forced expiratory volume—FEV_1 in British terminology) or maximal midexpiratory flow rate. The severity of dyspnea depends on the degree of obstruction.

Generalized obstructive lung disease is subdivided into reversible and irreversible forms.

Reversible obstructive lung disease is chiefly caused by bronchial asthma, which is characterized by intermittent, reversible increases in airway resistance due to excessive mucous secretion and smooth-muscle spasm and is associated with paroxysmal shortness of breath and wheezing respiration. Obstruction to airflow may vary and improve spontaneously or with the use of bronchodilator drugs, including corticosteroids. Bronchial asthma is discussed in Chap. 72 and the differential diagnosis of asthma and emphysema in Chap. 284.

Airway obstruction caused by excessive secretions as a result of infection is the other important cause of reversible airway obstruction. Varying degrees of reversible obstructive lung disease may coexist with irreversible obstructive lung disease, chronic bronchitis, or both, and the amount may be accurately quantified by simple pulmonary function tests.

Irreversible obstructive lung disease refers to irreversible generalized narrowing of the bronchial tree and increased airway resistance which have persisted for more than 1 year, unaffected by treatment including bronchodilator drugs as well as corticosteroids. The majority of such patients will be found to have emphysema at postmortem examination. A few reveal only varying combinations of chronic bronchial asthma, chronic bronchitis, or tubular bronchiectasis. The British make a diagnosis of "irreversible obstructive lung disease," appending "with emphysema" if the clinical picture warrants the anatomic statement.

The above definition and classification of chronic nonspecific lung disease was developed by British authorities to supplant the irrational use of the terms chronic bronchitis, asthma, and emphysema. It is presented here because it stresses (1) the use of functional rather than anatomic diagnosis clinically and (2) the difficulties in the accurate diagnosis of emphysema and the various combinations of bronchitis and reversible and irreversible obstructive lung disease which may occur during life. In the discussion that follows, chronic bronchitis and obstructive emphysema will be considered as such, as is the practice in the United States.

CHRONIC BRONCHITIS

OCCURRENCE. Chronic bronchitis marks its onset usually between the ages of thirty and sixty years. There is a preponderance in men of approximately 4:1. In England there exists an inverse relationship between the social scale and the incidence of the disease—the laboring classes being the most commonly afflicted, the professional classes least so. The death rate also rises steeply from rural to urban and highly industrialized areas, suggesting that atmospheric pollution plays an important role. Variations in smoking habits may prove to be the important variable, however. It is possible that the disease is more common and more severe in England than in the United States because of the damp, cold climate and degree of atmospheric pollution in England, both of which aggravate the symptoms. However, the only epidemiologic study carried out in the United States (Pemberton) indicated that the prevalence of uncomplicated bronchitis was similar in the two countries. The presently available figures indicate greater disability and far higher mortality from the disease in England than in North America. In England it is the commonest cause of death and morbidity among all respiratory diseases, including pneumonia, tuberculosis, asthma, and lung cancer.

ETIOLOGY. The disease may be insidious in onset, or it may follow a bout of acute pneumonia or bronchitis or well-established bronchial asthma. A possible etiologic relationship has been suggested for bronchiectasis and pulmonary tuberculosis, because of their frequent association with chronic bronchitis. In the United States the disease is associated with a history of heavy cigarette smoking in more than 75 percent of patients. Present evidence favors the theory that exposure to irritants (cigarette smoke, air pollutants, such as sulfur dioxide) in the susceptible individual leads to chronic hypersecretion of mucus in the bronchial tree.

PATHOLOGY. The most important lesion in chronic bronchitis is hyperplasia and hyperactivity of the mucus-secreting glands in the trachea and bronchi and of the goblet cells of the bronchial epithelium. The bronchial wall may show varying degrees of chronic inflammation with focal scars. The ratio between the size of mucous glands and submucosal tissues (the Reid index—normally less than 0.33 and usually greater than 0.60 in chronic bronchitis) is a good pathologic criterion of bronchitis. Many older patients with a long history of chronic bronchitis will show, in addition, the changes of emphysema at postmortem examination, even though this may not have been clinically manifest as breathlessness (associated with the symptoms of chronic bronchitis) during life.

CLINICAL MANIFESTATIONS. The patient consults the physician because of (1) cough and expectoration, (2) an acute respiratory infection, (3) breathlessness, which usually signifies the association or onset of complicating bronchospasm (asthma) or obstructive emphysema, or (4) fear of cancer. The chronic productive cough is usually attributed to cigarette smoking or is dated from childhood or an attack of influenza. The sputum is ropy, white, and elastic and varies in amount from a few milliliters to several ounces daily. During superimposed infections ("chest colds"), cough and sputum increase and the secretions become yellow or yellow-green and occasionally blood-streaked. The symptoms are worse in the winter, in the morning on awakening, and at the end of the day; with changes in barometric pressure and humidity; on exposure to dusts, air pollution, and cigarette smoking; in crowds and after excessive talking and alcohol ingestion. Severe paroxysms of coughing may occur nocturnally or on awakening in the morning. Postnasal drip and symptoms suggestive of chronic sinusitis are frequent. Acute chest pain may be due to rib fracture incurred during severe coughing, to pleurisy associated with a complicating pneumonia, or to muscular strain around the lower costal margins. Syncope may occur during a sudden fit of coughing (tussive syncope, Chap. 20). Vigor is usually well maintained, and there is no loss of appetite or weight. Dyspnea is not a feature of uncomplicated chronic bronchitis, although recent knowledge indicates that chronic bronchitis may lead to extremely severe obstructive disease in the absence of destructive lung changes or emphysema.

Physical examination is remarkable for the lack of positive findings. The nose may contain crusted purulent material, and the nasal and pharyngeal mucosa may be fiery red, raw, and dry appearing, and the uvula, slightly edematous. The patient clears his throat frequently, and deep breathing may result in a violent fit of coughing. The lungs may be clear, or there may be scattered basilar rales and transient rhonchi, frequently clearing up with cough. The heart is normal. There is no clubbing of the fingers.

Blood counts and radiologic examination of the chest and paranasal sinuses are usually completely normal. Culture of sputum may yield pathogenic organisms, most commonly the pneumococcus or *Hemophilus influenzae*. *Staphylococcus aureus* and gram-negative organisms are found occasionally, and the hemolytic streptococcus is remarkable for its rarity. Pulmonary function may be completely normal, or there may be slight reduction in timed vital capacity (60 to 75 percent in the first second as compared with greater than 80 percent normally) or maximal midexpiratory flow rate (e.g., 1.5 to 2.0 liters per sec as compared with greater than 3 liters per sec normally) and maximal breathing capacity (55 to 70 liters per min in contrast to 100 liters per min or more, normally).

Bronchoscopy and bronchography may be necessary to rule out other causes of chronic cough such as tumor, bronchiectasis, and foreign body. At bronchoscopy, the tracheobronchial mucosa is usually seen to be hyperemic and redundant. Bronchography may show diverticula on the inferior surface of the main stem and primary segmental bronchi which represent the filling of the dilated ducts of mucous glands. Beading of the bronchial lumen may be observed because of excessive mucus, or there may be an accordion-like appearance because of shortening of the bronchus with heaping up of redundant mucosa. Failure of peripheral filling and dilated bronchioles presenting as peripheral "pools" of dye may be seen in long-standing cases and probably indicate coexistent emphysema. Occasionally an area of tubular bronchiectasis is found. The differentiating features of bronchitis and bronchiectasis are discussed in Chap. 291. The diseases may coexist, and some observers believe that local bronchiectasis may lead to diffuse chronic bronchitis elsewhere in the lung. There is, however, no evidence that bronchitis has been cured by resection of localized bronchiectasis.

The *course of chronic bronchitis* is not completely known as there have been no studies of its natural history spanning more than several years. It seems clear, however, that subjects with chronic bronchitis often continue to have their symptoms for many years without further complication and die of some totally unrelated disease. Others suffer repeated respiratory tract infections and develop paroxysmal, reversible obstructive pulmonary disease (bronchial asthma). In this group as well as in a number of patients who remain noninfected and produce minimal sputum ("dry" bronchitis), there arise a certain number who ultimately develop obstructive emphysema.

EMPHYSEMA

The term *emphysema* is derived from the Greek and means a "blowing into" or "inflation." *Subcutaneous emphysema* occurs with soft-tissue infection with gas-forming organisms such as colon and Welch bacilli. It is also seen in the area of the incision following thoracotomy or with dissection of air from mediastinal emphysema, or after chest trauma. *Interstitial emphysema* refers to the escape of air from alveoli into the interstices of the lung where it dissects along vascular sheaths into the mediastinum to give rise to *mediastinal emphysema* (p. 1348), which, in turn, can also result from perforation of the thoracic esophagus. *Senile emphysema* refers not to a primary disease of the lungs but to a degenerative disease of the thoracic spine occurring in elderly individuals (see below).

Pulmonary emphysema is characterized pathologically by increase in the size of the air passages distal to terminal bronchioles due to *dilatation* and *destruction* of their walls. Further subdivision includes the factor of distribution, e.g., *selective*, as occurs in the focal emphysema due to dust, versus *unselective*, as with the dilatation of air spaces seen in pulmonary tissue adjacent to a resected area ("compensatory emphysema"). The classification adheres to the recommendations of the Ciba Guest Symposium and is slightly modified.

Emphysema Due to Dilatation Alone

UNSELECTIVE DISTRIBUTION—PANACINAR DILATATION EMPHYSEMA. There are two main conditions in this category: (1) compensatory or overdistension emphysema and (2) emphysema secondary to partial bronchial ob-

struction as with foreign body or bronchogenic carcinoma. The term *panacinar* means that all the air spaces distal to the terminal bronchiole are affected.

Panacinar dilatation emphysema results from expansion of lung (by virtue of negative intrapleural pressure) to fill the empty space created by removal or shrinkage of lung tissue. It has been called "overdistension" or "compensatory emphysema" in the past. It is not possible to relate pulmonary disability or insufficiency to this phenomenon, nor is there any evidence, either pathologically or by pulmonary function test, that it leads to destructive or obstructive changes in the area involved. Following pneumonectomy, for example, the remaining lung overdistends without the occurrence of dyspnea or disability.

Panacinar dilatation emphysema occurs distal to partial bronchial obstruction. Partial bronchial obstruction becomes complete with the normal narrowing of the bronchus in expiration, and air is trapped. Pulmonary function shows chiefly obstruction to airflow, which is variable in amount depending on how early in expiration the obstruction becomes complete. The main significance of this type of panacinar dilatation emphysema is that its discovery as an area of increased radiolucency in the lung fields by x-ray may be the first sign of bronchogenic carcinoma.

SELECTIVE DISTRIBUTION—FOCAL EMPHYSEMA. This is a disease of coal workers. Inhaled dust is deposited around the respiratory bronchiole, eliciting fibrosis and atrophy of smooth muscle. Coal-worker's pneumoconiosis is the only known form of dilatation emphysema localized to the respiratory bronchiole; hence the term *focal emphysema*. There may be no symptoms and minimal or no change in pulmonary function. In advanced cases, however, the clinical picture of obstructive emphysema may appear. The roentgenogram shows diffuse bilateral nodulations. The disease is described in greater detail on page 1324.

THE AGING LUNG. This third category of dilatation emphysema is added here with the presumption that aging results in loss of elasticity of pulmonary tissue, leading to dilatation of air spaces. A change in the size of air spaces with advancing age has not been demonstrated pathologically as yet; however, changes in pulmonary function as a result of aging are well established. These changes suggest a state of hyperinflation of the lung and airway obstruction. There are an increase in residual lung volume, decrease in maximal breathing capacity and mild increase in airway resistance, decrease in arterial P_{O_2}, and mild maldistribution of inspired air. More air is contained in the aged than the youthful lung at the same intrapleural pressure, indicating loss of elasticity of the lung and presumably, therefore, dilatation of air spaces. No definite symptoms or disability can be attributed to these changes alone in the otherwise healthy elderly individual.

The term "senile emphysema" has not been used above because it should be reserved to refer to changes in the thoracic cage with age, not to pulmonary changes. Loss of water and disorganization of the cartilaginous intervertebral disks result in a kyphotic distortion of the thoracic spine, in turn resulting in rotation of the ribs so that the anterior part of the chest is thrown out and up and assumes the barrel shape. Pulmonary function is unimpaired save for the minor changes expected as a consequence of normal aging (above), and dyspnea and disability should not be attributed to this skeletal deformity alone. The aged individual, although showing the functional changes described above, may or may not have an accompanying dorsal kyphosis.

Emphysema Due to Destruction of the Walls of Air Spaces

UNSELECTIVE DISTRIBUTION—PANACINAR DESTRUCTIVE EMPHYSEMA. The word *panacinar* refers to uniform dilatation of all air passages distal to the terminal bronchiole. The lesions may be localized or widespread and vary in different parts of the lung.

SELECTIVE DISTRIBUTION—CENTRILOBULAR DESTRUCTIVE EMPHYSEMA. This type of emphysema selectively affects the respiratory bronchiole, resulting in dilatation of air spaces in the proximal portion of the acinus, i.e., there exists a state of bronchiolectasis. Lesions may be local or widespread.

IRREGULAR DISTRIBUTION—IRREGULAR EMPHYSEMA. Irregular emphysema refers to the dilatation and destruction of air spaces seen adjacent to scars or in diffuse fibrotic disease such as the Hamman-Rich syndrome. As such it may occur anywhere in the acinus; hence the term "irregular." The word "focal" should not be used as it refers specifically to dilatation of respiratory bronchioles associated with coal-worker's pneumoconiosis.

Panacinar and centrilobular destructive emphysema may be seen singly or together in the same lung, and it is these pathologic forms which are demonstrated in subjects with obstructive pulmonary emphysema (see below). They cannot as yet be differentiated clinically. Blebs and bullae can be seen in any type of destructive emphysema, and therefore the term "bullous emphysema" should not be used to imply a special form of the disease.

Obstructive Pulmonary Emphysema

Obstructive pulmonary emphysema is a disease that affects predominantly men between the ages of forty-five and sixty-five years. It is usually preceded by chronic bronchitis and is characterized by dyspnea on exertion, hyperinflation of the chest, irreversible obstruction to airflow, and destruction and dilatation of the walls of air spaces.

ETIOLOGY. Because of the association of chronic bronchitis as a concomitant event or as one preceding the onset of exertional dyspnea in over 70 percent of patients, most observers have favored this disease as the inciting factor. The cause of chronic bronchitis is unknown, but because of the high association of cigarette smoking with bronchitis and emphysema, an etiologic role has been assigned to cigarettes. This may be so, just as the cold damp weather and a dusty working or polluted urban environment may also lead to hypersecretion of mucus in the bronchial tree and ultimately to obstructive emphysema, although there is increasing evidence to support air pollution as a cause of emphysema. In short, the etiologic factors of chronic bronchitis apply equally well to patients with obstructive emphysema. Dyspnea in the patient with chronic bronchitis usually signifies either reversible bronchial narrowing due to secretions or bronchospasm or irreversible obstruction to airflow due to the development of destructive emphysema. It may well be that the development of obstructive emphysema results from gradual extension of chronic bronchitis into the bronchioles, perhaps accelerated by repeated bouts of secondary bacterial infection. In some patients this sequence of events is obvious, but in others it must be assumed that the process is subclinical and smolders over a period of many years. Obstructive emphysema is due partly to the destructive effects of chronic bronchiolitis per se and partly to the distending effect of air trapped distal to the obstructing lesions. The theory that a primary degeneration of pulmonary elastic tissue initiates the disease has been abandoned.

The etiologic role of bronchial asthma remains obscure, but the few careful studies reported indicate that it rarely, if ever, progresses to obstructive emphysema. Part of the confusion on this point has arisen from the difficulties of differentiating obstructive emphysema with attacks of bronchospasm from bronchial asthma (see below).

Several investigators have pictured emphysema as an abnormal acceleration of the aging process because of the functional changes resembling a mild state of emphysema seen regularly in most elderly individuals (above).

Regardless of one's opinion concerning the role of smoking in chronic bronchitis, there remain approximately 10 percent of patients who deny chronic productive cough ("dry emphysema") and perhaps 20 percent who have never smoked. In some a family history of chronic bronchitis is obtained; in others, there have been repeated bouts of pneumonia. In some individuals, pre-existing localized bronchiectasis or long-standing pulmonary tuberculosis seems to have been complicated by slow superimposition of diffuse, chronic bronchitis and obstructive emphysema. A deficiency of the enzyme alpha$_1$-antitrypsin has been described in instances of familial emphysema, characterized by early onset of the disease between thirty and forty years of age.

Because of the many and diverse associated conditions and possible etiologic factors, it is important at the present time to consider obstructive emphysema to be a syndrome as well as a disease. In addition to the above conditions, a number of known disease processes can produce or be associated with a picture which is clinically and physiologically indistinguishable from the "idiopathic" disease. These include silicosis, coal-worker's pneumoconiosis, sarcoidosis, bronchogenically disseminated tuberculosis, and some cases of kyphoscoliosis. In these instances localization of the disease process at the level of the respiratory bronchiole or associated chronic bronchitis gives rise to chronic irreversible obstruction of airflow and the picture of obstructive emphysema. All these conditions must be considered in diagnosis when the patient with apparent chronic bronchitis and obstructive emphysema is seen.

PATHOLOGY. Classically the lungs are large and do not collapse when the thorax is opened. Blebs (subpleural air collections) and bullae (parenchymal emphysematous spaces with a diameter greater than 1 cm) may be noted, as well as generalized dilatation of air spaces. Nodular areas of scarring and fibrosis may be visible subpleurally. If the lung is fixed under a constant head of distending pressure, centrilobular or panacinar types of emphysema may be distinguished in nearly equal frequency. Microscopically there are seen chronic bronchiolitis and peribronchiolitis, ulceration of the epithelium, intraluminal granulation tissue, and fibrosis. Smooth muscle may be hypertrophied. The lumen of the bronchiole supplying areas of emphysema is often narrowed but may be normal or even dilated. The distal alveoli are obliterated and larger air spaces are formed, presumably by confluence of alveoli, and increased by air trapping due either to check-valve mechanism or collateral ventilation. Loss or degeneration of alveolar elastic tissue is seen. The number of visible capillaries is reduced because of destruction of alveolar walls. Foci of intrabronchiole mucus ("mucous plugging") and pus are seen, as are occasional areas of pneumonia. Besides reduction in capillary bed, there may be marked enlargement of the bronchial venous system. The evidence is not convincing that the bronchial arterial system is diseased.

CLINICAL MANIFESTATIONS. The typical patient gives a history of chronic bronchitis. Frequent respiratory infections have occurred, usually during the winter months, characterized by febrile episodes with increase in purulent sputum. Finally, at some point after years of bronchitic symptoms, breathlessness on exertion makes its appearance. Early in the course, dyspnea may occur only during the winter months with exacerbations of infection and is due to partially reversible ventilatory defects, i.e., bronchospasm and excessive secretions. Later, dyspnea on exertion becomes firmly established, persists the year around, and signifies the development of irreversible obstructive ventilatory defect. Of all the clinical clues, persistent breathlessness is the most reliable sign on which to establish a presumptive diagnosis of obstructive emphysema. The *clinical* diagnosis cannot be made in its absence, even though many patients with chronic bronchitis and no dyspnea may be found at postmortem examination to have mild emphysema.

The *onset* may be acute, and breathlessness is dated from an episode of pneumonia or severe, acute bronchitis. In some subjects, this is the easily remembered episode in what really is a long history of slowly progressive bronchitis. In other patients, breathlessness and cough have been accepted as concomitants of "getting old" or of smoking. The disease may come to the physician's attention in a number of ways: (1) by the development of acute respiratory failure with acute bronchitis or pneumonia, or during the postoperative period following intubation, atropine, and morphine—when the retrospective history of chronic cough and dyspnea is finally

obtained and its significance fully appreciated; (2) by the development of bronchogenic carcinoma; (3) by the development of inguinal hernia because of chronic cough; and (4) because of the occurrence of the symptoms or complications of peptic ulcer (see below). The disease may be so insidious in development that the diagnosis is not established until postmortem examination.

Other complaints are frequent. Because of limitation of activity the patient may gain weight initially, but later anorexia leads to loss of weight. Vigor is lost, and sleep is difficult. As the disease becomes more severe, changes in the arterial blood gases occur and cor pulmonale develops.

Physical signs may scarcely be more notable in the early phase of the disease than those seen in the patient with uncomplicated chronic bronchitis. In the moderately ill patient who exhibits no alteration in the blood gases at rest, the following signs are likely to be noted. The patient appears dyspneic with exertion. The fingers may be tobacco stained but are usually not clubbed. The eyes are prominent. The neck veins distend on expiration. The chest is fixed in the hyperinflated, inspiratory position, and the flesh about the neck and supraclavicular spaces is sunken. The accessory muscles of respiration, particularly the sternomastoids, are large and active during inspiration, and the trachea descends markedly on maximal inspiration. Lower rib margins may flare outward, and the subcostal angle is wide. There is frequently a dorsal kyphosis. Prominent cutaneous venules are seen anteriorly and laterally around the lower costal margins. During inspiration, the chest moves *en bloc* instead of "unfolding" from below upward during expansion. Expiration is prolonged. Cardiac and hepatic dullness are impaired or even absent, and heart sounds are distant. The pulmonary second sound is prominent and may be split, particularly on expiration. The percussion note of the chest is hyperresonant, and the diaphragms are low with minimal or absent excursion. The breath sounds are distant or even absent and when heard have a more bronchovesicular than vesicular quality. Occasional early inspiratory ("opening") rales are heard at the bases. Expiratory wheezing during spontaneous respiration is heard only if excessive secretion or bronchospasm is present. The impulse of the heart is prominent in the epigastrium, and the sounds are best heard here. The liver is displaced downward, and the edge is easily palpable. The abdominal muscles are lax. A decline in arterial pressure during inspiration may be observed, but the veins continue to display inspiratory collapse. Thus the complete picture of the paradoxic pulse (see Chap. 272) is lacking.

Roentgenography is of little help in diagnosis until the disease is advanced, at which time the following picture is seen. The thoracic cage is large with low diaphragms, an apparent horizontal position of the ribs, and wide intercostal spaces. Prominent soft-tissue shadows may indicate hypertrophy of the pectoralis muscles. The heart lies vertically and appears small. The mediastinal shadow is elongated. The hilar vascular shadows may be prominent, but the peripheral vessels are small and appear reduced in number. Thin-walled areas of translucency in which no vascular shadows can be seen represent blebs and bullae and are seen commonly at the apices and bases of the lungs. Nodular or linear areas of scarring and fibrosis may be seen, but generally the lung fields are notable for their radiolucency. In the lateral projection, an increase in size of the thoracic cage and a dorsal kyphosis are present. The retrosternal and retrocardiac air spaces are increased. Fluoroscopy is vital to the diagnosis, and the best radiologic sign is reduction in the excursion of the diaphragm. Air trapping is demonstrated on rapid expiration by areas of local radiolucency. Tomography may occasionally be helpful in delineating vascular changes such as prominent hilar vessels, small and fewer peripheral vessels, or absence of vessels in bullous lesions. It should be emphasized that even in advanced cases the chest roentgenogram may be entirely normal and, conversely, that typical roentgenographic changes may be seen in patients who do not have chronic obstructive lung disease.

Blood counts and urinalysis are normal. The electrocardiogram is normal in uncomplicated cases; it may reveal a loss of the usual tendency to left axis deviation seen in older individuals. The sputum has been described. Sputum cell counts usually reveal lymphocytes or polymorphonuclear leukocytes, but occasionally eosinophils are numerous see below). The results and use of pulmonary function tests are described below.

PATHOPHYSIOLOGY. Obstruction to airflow as a result of granulating and fibrosing bronchiolitis and expiratory closure of loosely supported respiratory bronchioles, coupled with degeneration of elastic tissue, results in hyperinflation of the lung. This is demonstrated by finding an increase in functional residual capacity, residual volume, and residual volume to total lung capacity ratio. The work of breathing is increased because of airway resistance. Timed vital capacity, maximal midexpiratory flow rate, and maximal breathing capacity are reduced in proportion to the degree of obstruction and therefore correlate well with the severity of dyspnea. If a partially reversible ventilatory defect exists because of acute infection or bronchospasm, these tests will indicate improvement with effective therapy. Obstructing lesions vary throughout the lung, and therefore abnormalities of distribution are seen, including maldistribution of inspired air, venous admixture, and dead-space effects (Chap. 280). Areas perfused with blood but poorly ventilated cause increased venous admixture of arterial blood ("physiologic shunting"); other areas, including bullous lesions, are ventilated but not perfused, leading to dead space effect. Cardiac work is wasted in the first situation and ventilatory work is wasted in the second instance. Both pumps have to increase their work to compensate. Increased ventilation of well-perfused areas can compensate for the shunted carbon dioxide and maintain a normal CO_2 tension of arterial blood. It cannot add appreciable amounts of oxygen to the blood, however, to compensate for hypoxemia (Chap. 33). This is because of the difference in the shapes of the CO_2 and O_2 dissociation curves and explains the sequence of changes in arterial blood gases, beginning first with mild arterial oxygen unsaturation and normal CO_2 contents and tension. As the disease becomes more severe, hypoxemia increases, and finally alveolar hypoventilation results in CO_2 retention, with respiratory acidosis. Earlier in the disease, the increased requirements of gas exchange necessitated by exercise may result in unsaturation of blood, normally saturated at rest.

As the disease progresses and continued destruction of pulmonary capillary bed occurs, the pulmonary diffusing capacity falls and the pulmonary vascular resistance rises. Hypoxemia stimulates erythropoiesis and causes secondary polycythemia. It also leads to pulmonary vasoconstriction and an increase in arterial resistance. The work of the right side of the heart is increased, and cor pulmonale ultimately ensues, signifying the final and most advanced stage of the illness (Chap. 287).

COURSE OF THE DISEASE. The course of the disease is extremely variable, and prognostication is difficult. At any time, superimposed pulmonary infection causes an increase in the severity of the disease due to further reduction in functioning lung tissue because of consolidation, secretions, or bronchospasm. The course may be rapidly malignant, with death in respiratory failure in a matter of several years, or the duration from onset of dyspnea may be as much as 20 or 30 years with death due to intercurrent disease. The occurrence of hypoxemia and hypercapnia or the development of cor pulmonale are bad prognostic signs, and death usually occurs within several years of their onset. Mild hypoxemia by itself does not carry such a dire prognosis.

Respiratory failure is said to have occurred when the lung can no longer provide for normal gas exchange and CO_2 retention and arterial oxygen unsaturation are the result. As hypoxemia supervenes, further weight loss may occur, and when CO_2 retention follows, headache, difficulty in concentrating, drowsiness, and confusion are common findings. In the presence of cor pulmonale with right-sided heart failure, papilledema may be seen. There may also be a curious inability to sustain a posture (asterixis, "flapping tremor"), identical with that observed in hepatic insufficiency or uremia. This is particularly common in acute respiratory failure. Respiratory failure may occur insidiously without obvious precipitating event but commonly occurs because of acute respiratory infection, administration of sedative, narcotic, or anesthetic agents, or heart failure. Administration of oxygen is absolutely necessary but may be hazardous.

The association of peptic ulcer and emphysema appears to be more than fortuitous. About 20 percent of patients with emphysema have a peptic ulcer, usually duodenal in location, and the incidence of emphysema is two or three times as common in patients with peptic ulcer as in the normal population. Whether common psychic factors, cigarette smoking, or hypoxia are important etiologic factors is unknown, but it is important to keep the relationship in mind.

DIAGNOSIS. Obstructive pulmonary emphysema is misdiagnosed frequently. Physical signs, except in advanced cases, are notoriously misleading and unreliable. The diagnosis should not be made without demonstrating obstruction to airflow. Persistent dyspnea on exertion and depression of breath sounds are the cardinal features. Restriction of diaphragmatic motion correlates best with the severity of the process. The finding of radiolucency and a large chest does not in itself establish the diagnosis.

Once the diagnosis has been established, the degree of reversibility or irreversibility must be determined by measuring the timed vital capacity before and after the use of a suitable bronchodilator such as aerosolized isoproterenol hydrochloride. In occasional patients with chronic intrinsic bronchial asthma, intensive treatment with corticosteroids may be necessary to achieve maximal reversal of the obstructive ventilatory defect.

If the patient has bronchial asthma, certain features may suggest this diagnosis, namely, family history of allergic disease, lack of smoking because of aggravation of asthmatic symptoms, positive skin tests, peripheral blood eosinophilia, and, most important, intermittency of symptoms and spontaneous reversibility to normal or near normal of abnormal pulmonary function or reversal with the use of bronchodilators, including corticosteroids. The pulmonary diffusing capacity is normal in uncomplicated asthma and reduced in obstructive emphysema; thus differentiation is possible.

The treatment of chronic nonspecific pulmonary disease (bronchitis and emphysema) and of respiratory failure is discussed in Chap. 295.

REFERENCES

Bates, D. V.: "Chronic Bronchitis and Emphysema," New Engl. J. Med., 278:546, 600, 1968.

Grover, R. F. (Ed.): "Research in Emphysema and Chronic Bronchitis: Normal and Abnormal Pulmonary Circulation," New York, S. Karger, 1962.

Knowles, J. H.: "Respiratory Physiology and Its Clinical Application," pp. 135, 142 Cambridge, Mass., Harvard University Press, 1959.

Orie, N. G. M., and H. J. Sluiter (Eds.): "Bronchitis—An International Symposium," Springfield, Ill., Charles C Thomas, Publisher, 1962.

"Pulmonary Structure and Function," Ciba Foundation Symposium, 1962, London, J. & A. Churchill, Ltd., 1962.

Reid, L.: "The Pathology of Emphysema," Chicago, The Year Book Medical Publishers, Inc., 1967.

Symposium on Emphysema and the Chronic Bronchitis Syndrome, Am. Rev. Res. Dis., 80 pt. 2:1, 1959.

Talamo, R. C., J. B. Blennerhassett, and K. F. Austen: "Familial Emphysema and Alpha₁—Antitrypsin Deficiency," New Engl. J. Med., 275:1301, 1966.

Terminology, Definitions and Classifications of Chronic Pulmonary Emphysema and Related Conditions, Thorax, 14:286, 1959.

U.S. Surgeon General's Advisory Committee: "Smoking and Health," Public Health Service Publication 1103, Washington, 1964.

284 RESTRICTIVE AND DIFFUSIONAL DISORDERS OF THE LUNG

Eugene D. Robin

RESTRICTIVE DISORDERS

Restrictive pulmonary diseases are characterized by decreased expansibility of the lung. Although restrictive factors are important in a large number of different respiratory diseases, this section will concern itself with those disorders in which a restrictive ventilatory defect is the primary abnormality.

There are two general types of restrictive disease. In one group the fundamental abnormality is neurologic, neuromuscular, or muscular and the structure of the respiratory apparatus itself is mechanically normal. In the other group restriction occurs because of some structural defect involving the respiratory apparatus, which results in a specific mechanical abnormality and in a reduction in total pulmonary compliance (lung plus thorax).[1]

Total pulmonary compliance (Chap. 280) is a measure of the elastic properties of the lungs and thorax, and may be defined quantitatively as the volume change in the lung for a unit change in pressure. Its units are liters per centimeter of H_2O. Total pulmonary compliance is equal to the total volume change divided by transthoracic pressure. Lung compliance is equal to the volume change in the lung divided by transpulmonary pressure. Thoracic compliance may then be calculated from the above two values. Decreasing values of compliance indicate increasing stiffness of the lungs and/or thorax (Chap. 280). As a result, the work required to overcome the elastic forces of the respiratory apparatus during breathing increases. Thus the characteristic symptom is dyspnea (Chap. 32).

There are four mechanisms by which compliance may be reduced:

Replacement, Infiltration, or Compression of Pulmonary Tissue by Substances Other than Lung Tissue. Since such substances, in general, have different volume-pressure relations (compliance) than lung tissue, significant amounts of these substances would be expected to modify the compliance of the respiratory apparatus. For example, replacement of a portion of pulmonary tissue by fibrous tissue would be expected to reduce pulmonary compliance because fibrous tissue has a lower compliance than lung tissue.

[1] The term *compliance* implicitly assumes that the volume-pressure curve being considered is a straight line over the entire range of lung volumes and is independent of the phase of inspiration or expiration. These assumptions are manifestly incorrect, but the term is convenient and is used here as a semiquantitative measurement of the static volume-pressure relationships of the respiratory apparatus.

Change in the Amount, Type, or Organization of Pulmonary Elastic Tissue. Since, to some extent, the elastic properties of the lung depend on the elastic fibers present in it, modification of these fibers by disease would be expected to modify compliance. For example, some of the changes in compliance in obstructive emphysema may be related to anatomic changes in pulmonary elastic tissue.

Changes in the Magnitude of Surface Tension Forces in the Alveoli. The alveolar surfaces of the lung are gas-liquid interfaces. At such interfaces, surface tension forces are generated. The predicted magnitude of these forces is considerable and, if unmodified, would be expected to produce alveolar collapse. There is evidence that the magnitude of these forces is maintained at a relatively low value by the presence, in the alveolar lining, of a surface-active material which has the property of reducing surface tension forces to low values during deflation. This material appears to be lipoprotein in nature. It serves to minimize the elastic work required to distend the lungs, and keeps the alveoli patent. A decrease in the amount of activity of surface-active material would result in decreased pulmonary compliance. For example, the respiratory distress syndrome of the newborn is believed to represent a disorder in which a decrease in surface-active material produces restrictive pulmonary disease.

A Decrease in Lung Volume. Since measured compliance is the ratio between volume and pressure, if the volume is reduced by 50 percent and the distending pressure remains the same, then compliance will be reduced by 50 percent. For example, following pneumonectomy, lung compliance may be reduced in the absence of structural change in remaining lung tissue.

The physiologic and clinical consequences of restrictive disease are as follows: There is a reduction in all lung volumes, including vital capacity, which affords a simple clinical measurement in these disorders. Evidence of airflow obstruction and abnormalities of intrapulmonary gas mixing are minimal.

A major consequence of restrictive lung disease may be the development of alveolar hypoventilation, the manifestations of which frequently dominate the clinical picture. Alveolar hypoventilation has already been discussed (Chap. 283). It exists when alveolar ventilation is insufficient to maintain normal alveolar gas tensions. It is, therefore, characterized by a low mean alveolar O_2 tension and a high alveolar CO_2 tension, resulting in corresponding abnormalities of pulmonary capillary blood, arterial blood, and ultimately, of tissue gas tensions. Since the adequacy of gas exchange is judged by measurements of arterial blood gases, the cornerstone of alveolar hypoventilation is an elevated arterial CO_2 tension (P_{aCO_2}).

The physiologic and clinical consequences of alveolar hypoventilation are related to the associated hypoxia and hypercapnia. With hypoxemia of sufficient magnitude, cyanosis is apparent. Hypoxic stimulation of the bone marrow produces polycythemia (Chap. 33). The presence of hypoxia and hypercapnia may produce an increase of cerebrospinal fluid pressure, with or without papilledema, by mechanisms which remain to be defined. Chronic hypercapnia leads to bicarbonate retention by the kidney, resulting in an increased concentration of this anion and a decreased concentration of Cl^- in intracellular fluid. Chronic hypercapnia likewise leads to a depression of respiratory center sensitivity to the normal stimuli of CO_2 and pH, thus accentuating the degree of alveolar hypoventilation. Periodic breathing of the Cheyne-Stokes variety is common and likewise reflects respiratory center depression. The combination of hypoxia and hypercapnia may lead to mental symptoms. Prominent among these is somnolence, which may constitute the patient's chief complaint. There is no clear-cut relationship between the degree of hypercapnia and the degree of somnolence. There may be marked hypercapnia without somnolence or somnolence with only minor degrees of hypercapnia. With acute rises in concentration of CO_2, delirium and even coma may occur. The electroencephalogram may show abnormalities consisting of slow-frequency, low-voltage waves. The combination of papilledema, central-nervous-system signs, and an abnormal electroencephalogram may lead to an erroneous diagnosis of brain tumor.

The combination of hypoxia and hypercapnia produces pulmonary hypertension and right-sided heart failure by mechanisms discussed later (p. 1317). This form of cor pulmonale is characterized by its reversibility when blood gases are restored to normal.

The symptoms of alveolar hypoventilation are so varied that the diagnosis can be securely established only by demonstrating a significant increase of arterial or alveolar CO_2 tension (P_{CO_2}).

In addition to alveolar hypoventilation and its consequences, dyspnea, resulting from the augmented work of breathing required to overcome the abnormally high elastic forces in the respiratory apparatus, is common in patients with restrictive disease. These patients tend to show tachypnea (rapid, shallow breathing). The relationship between rate and depth of breathing appears to be adjusted in a manner so that there is maximal ventilation for minimal work cost of breathing. Since shallow breathing decreases the elastic work cost of breathing, it is not surprising that tachypnea characterizes the breathing pattern of these patients. Specific features of the individual varieties of restrictive disease depend on the nature and extent of disease and are discussed below.

Restrictive Disease Associated with Neurologic, Neuromuscular, or Muscular Disorders

Restrictive disease may be produced by direct involvement of the medullary respiratory center by a number of different processes. The existence of hypoxemia, hypercapnia, and polycythemia in patients without clinical or physiologic evidence of primary respiratory or cardiac disease has been attributed to idiopathic disease of the medullary respiratory center. This syndrome has been called "Ondine's curse." [1] Patients with this condition are capable of restoring blood gases entirely to normal values by voluntary hyperventilation. Meticulous investigation of pulmonary and cardiac function fails to reveal any abnormalities of pulmonary mechanics, gas exchange, or perfusion. Cardiac abnormalities, when present, are related to cor pulmonale produced by the blood gas abnormalities. Inhalation of high concentrations of CO_2 (5 to 8 percent) in air by these patients fails to elicit the degree of hyperventilation seen in normal subjects or may even lead to depression of ventilation. For this reason, it has been suggested that the underlying mechanism is an injury involving the medullary respiratory center (such as tumor, inflammatory disease, or vascular accident) which results in relative insensitivity to its normal stimuli, P_{CO_2} and pH. Alveolar hypoventilation develops, with resultant hypoxemia and hypercapnia. The chemical control of breathing depends to a great extent on impulses arising from the peripheral chemoreceptors located in apposition to the great vessels (carotid body, vertebral body, aortic body), which are primarily sensitive to a fall in the oxygen tension of arterial blood (hypoxemia). The volume of involuntary ventilation achieved by the patient represents a new steady state, which depends on the degree of respiratory center depression and on the degree of respiratory stimulation arising from the peripheral chemoreceptors. This steady state operates in such a manner that the patient has persistent hypoxemia and hypercapnia.

Central-Nervous-System Abnormalities. A number of inflammatory and other diseases involving the brain often may result in alveolar hypoventilation. For example, acute bulbar poliomyelitis causes respiratory abnormalities in the absence of respiratory muscle paresis or paralysis produced by lower motor neurone lesions. Breathing becomes irregular in rate, shallow, and exceedingly slow. It is striking that such patients can breathe normally when given frequent and firm verbal orders to do so. The retention of volitional control with the loss of reflex rhythmic control is presumably caused by impaired sensitivity of the respiratory center to the $CO_2 -$ pH stimulus. Not infrequently, swallowing and coughing are likewise impaired, again suggesting brainstem localization of disease. Generally, this variety of respiratory disturbance is acute and transient, although the patient may then develop frank respiratory paralysis because of lower motor neurone disease.

Drug-induced Alveolar Hypoventilation. A number of drugs are capable of producing respiratory center depression, thereby resulting in alveolar hypoventilation. Drug-induced respiratory depression is most frequently seen during administration of anesthesia. The reduction of ventilation is noted by the anesthesiologist and is treated by assisted ventilation. However, if specific measurements of alveolar or arterial P_{CO_2} are not performed,

[1] Ondine was a water nymph in Greek mythology. Her affection having been rejected by a mortal man, she placed a spell upon him so that, according to one view, all automatic activity was suspended. When he fell asleep, his respirations ceased and he died, presumably of pulmonary insufficiency.

significant hypoventilation, during or after the operative procedure, may be overlooked. All drugs of the morphine group and the barbiturate group may produce respiratory center depression and hypoventilation. With ordinary doses in patients without preexistent respiratory center depression, the respiratory effects of these drugs are ordinarily not of great clinical significance. However, overdosage (e.g., in attempted suicide) or the administration of even modest doses to patients with established respiratory depression may result in life-threatening alveolar hypoventilation.

Hypercapneic Hypoventilation. An important variety of respiratory center depression is seen commonly in patients with prolonged hypercapnia, which occurs most frequently in obstructive emphysema. Such patients show a subnormal ventilatory response to the inhalation of CO_2-enriched air. At least two basic factors are involved. The first is related to the disordered ventilatory mechanics of diffuse obstructive disease. This factor can be demonstrated by having normal subjects inhale CO_2-enriched mixtures while airway resistance is artificially increased. Under these circumstances, there is a diminished ventilatory response to CO_2 inhalation. The second factor is related to the decreased sensitivity of the medullary respiratory center to the CO_2-pH stimulus following prolonged hypercapnia. This factor can be demonstrated by chronically exposing normal subjects to increased concentrations of CO_2 in the inspired air. After a period of several weeks under these conditions, there is a decrease in the ventilatory response to CO_2, even in the absence of obstruction.

The relative importance of mechanical and chemical factors in the genesis of CO_2 insensitivity in obstructive emphysema is not clear. However, it seems certain that chemical factors play an important role in some patients. This is best seen in the syndrome called "carbon dioxide narcosis," which occurs in patients with chronic hypercapnia with hypoxia. When the degree of hypoxia is decreased by the administration of high concentrations of oxygen, and without any change in respiratory mechanics, there follows the development of confusion, coma, and profound hypoventilation, occasionally to the point of apnea. The chemical control of breathing depends no longer on the CO_2-pH stimulus, but on the stimulus of hypoxemia acting through the peripheral chemoreceptors. When hypoxemia is relieved, the stimulus for ventilation decreases and hypoventilation is accentuated.

The term "carbon dioxide narcosis," frequently used to describe the above sequence of events, is misleading. No direct relationship exists between the absolute level of arterial P_{CO_2} and either the cerebral symptoms or the hypoventilation. Severe hypoventilation may occur following oxygen administration to patients free of pulmonary disease with only modest initial elevations of P_{CO_2} induced by narcotics. Also, some patients with marked elevations of P_{CO_2} may show little or no central-nervous-system malfunction. The exact role of CO_2 in the pathogenesis of the syndrome remains to be elucidated.

Abnormalities of neural or neuromuscular transmission

to the respiratory muscles may result in paresis or paralysis leading to alveolar hypoventilation. *Amyotrophic lateral sclerosis* is an example of an upper motor neurone lesion which may produce respiratory insufficiency. Direct involvement of the anterior horn cells by *poliomyelitis* virus represents a lower motor neurone lesion which produces respiratory insufficiency. *Infectious neuronitis* (Guillain-Barré syndrome) produces flaccid paralysis by means of an inflammatory function involving ganglion cells and peripheral nerves. *Myasthenia gravis* produces respiratory failure by abnormalities involving the myoneural junction.

Direct involvement of respiratory muscles by diseases diffusely affecting skeletal muscle, such as *progressive muscular dystrophy* and the *myotonic dystrophies,* may lead to restrictive disease. These diseases are commonly associated with reduction of vital capacity, total lung capacity, and maximal breathing capacity without obstructive disease.

The severity of respiratory involvement in any of the above diseases depends on the amount of anatomic involvement. Vital capacity is reduced in proportion to the degree of paresis of the respiratory muscles. There are generally an increased residual volume and a decreased airflow velocity. In moderately severe involvement, there may be alveolar hypoventilation with hypoxemia, hypercapnia, and respiratory acidosis. In very severe involvement, there may be total apnea, requiring assisted ventilation for survival.

Because of ineffective coughing and the limitation of respiratory excursions, recurrent bronchial infection is frequent in this group of patients. Although none of these diseases is associated with parenchymal lung damage per se, recurrent infections may result in permanent structural damage. In some patients, the neuromuscular or muscular disease may result in kyphoscoliosis, giving rise to additional pulmonocardiac abnormalities, as discussed below.

Recognition of pulmonary insufficiency may be difficult in the milder forms of these diseases. An awareness of the frequency of respiratory insufficiency is an important factor in formulating therapy. Quantitative serial measurements of vital capacity and blood gases are important guides to the intensity of disease and the degree of therapy required. When relatively specific measures are available for a given disease (e.g., anticholinesterases for myasthenia gravis), they should be energetically employed. Assisted ventilation, control of secretions, and prompt therapy of infections are frequently critical aspects of the care of these patients.

Restrictive Diseases Associated with Decreased Total Compliance

THORACIC CAGE LIMITATION. Limitation of motion of the thoracic cage may be associated with the development of severe alveolar hypoventilation. The mechanisms underlying this development may be illustrated by considering pulmonary-cardiac failure associated with kyphoscoliosis and with obesity.

PULMONARY—CARDIAC FAILURE ASSOCIATED WITH KYPHOSCOLIOSIS. Kyphosis refers to any posterior angulation of the spine. Clinically significant kyphosis is generally associated with a marked gibbus and loss of stature. Scoliosis consists of a lateral displacement of the spine with at least one other compensatory curve in an opposite direction. Of these two processes, scoliosis appears to be the more important in the genesis of pulmonary and/or cardiac insufficiency. Approximately 80 percent of cases of kyphoscoliosis are of unknown cause. The sequelae of poliomyelitis or of Pott's disease account for most of the remaining 20 percent. Although kyphoscoliosis is relatively common, existing in approximately 1 percent of the population of the United States, a deformity severe enough to produce pulmonary or cardiac insufficiency is found in only a relatively small fraction of these patients.

Kyphoscoliosis is associated with marked structural abnormality of the thoracic cage, leading to abnormal positioning and functioning of the respiratory muscles. The lungs are compressed by the thoracic deformity, leading to a small lung volume. Breathing entails a high work and energy cost, primarily because of the abnormal elastic resistance of the chest and, to a lesser degree, because of increased elastic resistance of the lung. In some unknown manner, the increased elastic work leads to the development of rapid shallow breathing, which in turn leads to alveolar hypoventilation by preferential ventilation of the anatomic dead space at the expense of alveolar ventilation. As a result, hypoxemia, hypercapnia, and respiratory acidosis develop. Prolonged hypercapnia leads to a depression of respiratory center sensitivity, accentuating the degree of hypoventilation.

The thoracic deformity leads to compression of pulmonary vessels, which, therefore, present an increased resistance to pulmonary blood flow. With prolonged pulmonary hypertension, there is damage to the intima of pulmonary vessels with the development of pulmonary arteriosclerosis, which further increases pulmonary vascular resistance and aggravates pulmonary hypertension. The combination of hypoxia, hypercapnia, vascular compression, and the intimal changes produces high degrees of pulmonary hypertension, leading ultimately to right ventricular failure.

It should be emphasized that the physiologic processes leading to alveolar hypoventilation in kyphoscoliosis are quite distinct from those seen in obstructive emphysema. In kyphoscoliosis, lung volumes are small; there are, at most, moderate disturbances in the distribution of inspired air, and airway resistance is only moderately elevated. In chronic obstructive emphysema (Chap. 283), the residual volume is abnormally large, there are marked disturbances in the distribution of inspired air, and the major defect is an abnormally high resistance in the airways.

Recurrent pulmonary infections are not uncommon in kyphoscoliosis, because of abnormal cough dynamics and inadequate bronchial drainage. Such infections may lead to parenchymal pulmonary structural abnormalities and occasionally to obstructive emphysema. In such patients diffuse obstructive disease represents a complication superimposed on the fundamental physiologic abnormalities related to the thoracic deformity.

The therapy of pulmonary and cardiac failure in kyphoscoliosis should be directed toward correcting the physiologic abnormalities, since the underlying anatomic abnormality is unfortunately almost never correctable. The periodic use of mechanically assisted ventilation decreases the work cost of breathing and increases alveolar ventilation. Control of bronchial secretions and prompt therapy of pulmonary infections decrease parenchymal pulmonary destruction. Avoidance of drugs which depress ventilation prevents additional hypoxia and respiratory acidosis. Oxygen administration relieves hypoxia and tends to decrease the right ventricular work. Cardiac glycosides, diuretics, and a low sodium diet are useful in the management of congestive heart failure.

PULMONARY–CARDIAC FAILURE ASSOCIATED WITH OBESITY (PICKWICKIAN SYNDROME). The association of obesity, somnolence, polycythemia, and excessive appetite has long been recognized. A classic description of the association of these signs and symptoms was written by Charles Dickens. In "The Pickwick Papers," he described "a fat and red-faced boy in a state of somnolency." The boy (Joe) was subsequently addressed as "Young Dropsy," "Young Opium Eater," and "Young Boa Constrictor," no doubt in reference to his obesity, his somnolence, and his excessive appetite, respectively. Because of the resemblance of Joe, the fat boy, to patients with obesity associated with pulmonary-cardiac failure, this combination has been referred to as the "Pickwickian syndrome."

In its fully developed form, the Pickwickian syndrome consists of marked obesity, somnolence, cyanosis, periodic respiration, secondary polycythemia, and right ventricular failure. Blood gas measurements reveal hypoxemia and hypercapnia, documenting the existence of alveolar hypoventilation. Measurements of lung volumes reveal a decrease of total lung capacity, a decrease of vital capacity, and a striking reduction of the expiratory reserve volume. Measurements of thoracic compliance in obesity show a reduction below normal values. The total energy cost of breathing in obese subjects is high. However, the work cost of moving the lung is not increased. This suggests either that the excess energy is used to impart motion to extrapulmonary structures or that excess energy is required by the respiratory muscles to perform a given amount of mechanical work. Obesity, like kyphoscoliosis, is associated with an increased work cost of moving the thorax and likewise with a tendency for the development of rapid, shallow breathing. A common pathogenetic mechanism responsible for the development of alveolar hypoventilation seems probable for both diseases. In the case of kyphoscoliosis, the increased work load is imposed by the thoracic deformity. In the case of the Pickwickian syndrome, the increased work load is imposed by the excessive deposition of fat. In Pickwickians, as in kyphoscoliosis, the increased work load leads to tachypnea with inadequate tidal volumes, which in turn leads to alveolar hypoventilation.

In the uncomplicated Pickwickian syndrome, there is no evidence of increased airway resistance. There is generally a decreased ventilatory response to CO_2 inhalation. This finding is consistent with a decrease in respiratory center sensitivity and tends to accentuate alveolar hypoventilation.

Intrapulmonary gas mixing may be entirely normal. Occasionally there is maldistribution of inspired air, presumably caused by the exaggeration of hypoventilation which occurs in the less-distensible perihilar areas, producing ventilation-perfusion abnormalities and accentuating arterial oxygen unsaturation.

In occasional patients, the Pickwickian syndrome is associated with diffuse obstructive lung disease or myxedema. Pulmonary vascular occlusion, resulting from either embolism or thrombosis, is common. Its pathogenesis is undoubtedly related to the relative immobility of these patients, the high viscosity of their blood, and the presence of congestive failure.

Obese patients without frank alveolar hypoventilation may also show congestive heart failure. This failure is associated with a high rather than low cardiac output and with insufficiency of both ventricles, predominantly the left.

Several clinical features of this syndrome require additional emphasis. Alveolar hypoventilation is relatively uncommon in even massively obese patients. Normal pulmonary function has been found in patients whose weight exceeded 400 lb. The exact factors which determine the development of pulmonary failure in some obese patients are not entirely understood. Among the factors favoring the development of alveolar hypoventilation are the pattern of distribution of the fat and its rate of accumulation. Pulmonary-cardiac failure occurs most commonly when the excess fat is packed tightly under the diaphragm, restricting its range of motion. Not infrequently there is a history of rapid weight gain in the immediate period preceding the development of frank pulmonary insufficiency. In some patients the rapid accumulation of intraabdominal fluid, rather than fat, may precipitate the full-blown syndrome.

The degree of somnolence is usually more severe in this syndrome than in other diseases associated with alveolar hypoventilation. At times the somnolence is truly extraordinary and the patient may find it impossible to distinguish between the waking and sleeping states. Somnolence occasionally antedates the appearance of respiratory insufficiency and may be present with only minor elevations of arterial P_{CO_2}, suggesting the importance of independent central-nervous-system disease in the pathogenesis of the syndrome. Normal sleep is known to be associated with a rise in P_{CO_2} and a decrease in respiratory center sensitivity. For this reason somnolence, per se, may increase the blood gas abnormalities.

The most remarkable aspect of both the clinical and physiologic abnormalities is that they may be completely reversed by simple loss of weight. With weight reduction, somnolence and the ventilatory abnormalities may disappear, blood gases may become normal, and pulmonary hypertension and cor pulmonale may disappear. Because of such dramatic changes, the Pickwickian syndrome represents an important example of curable lung and heart disease. However, in some patients, complicating obstructive pulmonary disease, independent heart disease, or pulmonary vascular occlusion limits reversibility.

The most important aspect of therapy is weight reduction. It is generally not necessary for the patient to lose weight to the predicted or "ideal" level. Often the loss of only 25 to 30 lb is sufficient to restore normal pulmonary function. However, excessive appetite is frequently a fundamental part of the illness (or of the patient's personality) and recurrent gain of weight is not uncommon.

Restrictive Disorders Associated with Decreased Alveolar Lining Surface Activity

RESPIRATORY DISTRESS SYNDROME OF THE NEWBORN. Newborn infants, especially if premature, may develop pulmonary insufficiency, with a relatively consistent clinical picture. This picture consists of progressive dyspnea, rapid, shallow respiration, sternal retractions during inspiration, and grunting expirations. Chest roentgenogram shows a relatively characteristic diffuse reticulogranular infiltrate and an air bronchogram (outline of small and medium bronchi by air, which is visible on routine chest roentgenogram). Physiologic measurements show hypoxemia, hypercapnia, increased blood lactic acid concentrations, and severe acidosis produced both by CO_2 accumulation and by the accumulation of organic acids resulting from hypoxia. A relatively large number of affected infants die. Postmortem examination invariably shows extensive and dramatic atelectasis. Foam is absent in the airways, and following installation of saline solution no typical pulmonary foam appears. In approximately 50 percent of postmortem examinations, hyaline membranes lining the alveoli may be present.

The pressure-volume characteristics of the lungs in these children are grossly abnormal. Not only are the lungs poorly distensible unless extraordinarily high pressures are applied (80 cm H_2O), but on deflation they trap little or no air.

Several lines of evidence suggest that the mechanical abnormalities in this disorder are related to a lack of the normal surface-active alveolar lining layer necessary to prevent atelectasis.

1. Embryologic findings suggest that alveolar surface-active material appears relatively late during fetal life. Thus the premature infant might be especially likely to demonstrate deficiencies of this material.

2. Pathologic findings show severe atelectasis and lack of pulmonary foam, indicating a lack of surface-active material.

3. Physiologic findings demonstrate the dramatic degrees of decreased compliance.

4. Biophysical findings demonstrate that extracts from the lung of these infants are deficient in surface-active substances.

In addition to the intrinsic interest and importance of the respiratory distress syndrome of the newborn, it ap-

pears to be the first clear example of surface tension abnormalities in the pathogenesis of pulmonary disease. It is anticipated that this mechanism may be important in other forms of pulmonary diseases such as pulmonary edema, various pulmonary infections, pulmonary alveolar proteinosis, and resorption atelectasis.

MISCELLANEOUS RESTRICTIVE DISORDERS. The parenchymal pulmonary diseases are described further on under Diffuse Interstitial and Alveolar Pulmonary Disorders, or are listed in Table 284-1.

A number of restrictive diseases are rarely associated with alveolar hypoventilation. These include pulmonary collapse (atelectasis) and pleural fibrosis. Pectus excavatum (funnel chest) is a congenital malformation consisting of a depression of the lower portion of the sternum and the adjacent costal cartilages. The depressed sternum may compress and restrict the lower portions of the lung or may produce restriction by distortion of the diaphragm. Restriction due to pleural fibrosis is limited to the areas of lung involved in fibrosis. Bilateral constrictive calcific fibrosis may result in virtually complete loss of thoracic motion and even in limitation of diaphragmatic motion. Rheumatoid spondylitis has been shown to result in loss of chest expansion because of immobility of the costovertebral and costosternal joints. Reduction of vital capacity and of total lung capacity with a normal residual volume results from this immobility. An interesting aspect of the impaired thoracic mobility is that painful or difficult sneezing is a common complaint. However, there is a striking absence of pulmonary signs and of pulmonary infections.

DIFFUSE INTERSTITIAL AND ALVEOLAR PULMONARY DISORDERS

There is a large number of disorders which affect the pulmonary interstitium and/or alveoli. Formerly these diseases were collectively described as disorders producing so-called "alveolar-capillary block," since it was believed that many of them produced specific impairment of pulmonary diffusion. In recent years, it has been suggested that the process of diffusion is seldom, if ever, the limiting factor involved in producing hypoxemia in patients with lung disease. It has also been suggested that hypoxemia in such patients is produced by ventilation/perfusion abnormalities. It now appears that the term "alveolar-capillary block" has outlived its usefulness. However, methods used in the past to measure "diffusion abnormalities," such as the carbon monoxide diffusing capacity, may be useful in identifying and quantifying abnormalities of gas exchange in these disorders.

This description will, therefore, focus on the nature of the pulmonary interstitium and alveoli rather than on the problem of pulmonary gas diffusion.

Anatomy and Fine Structure of the Gas Exchange Areas in the Lung

The terminal exchange areas of the lung involve four important units: (1) alveoli, (2) pulmonary exchange vessels, (3) the pulmonary interstitium, and (4) small pulmonary lymphatics.

Alveoli. The cell population of the alveoli normally consists of three cell types: (1) Membranous pneumocytes, the long, attenuated cytoplasmic extensions of which make up the major portion of the alveolar wall; their major function is to provide a structural basis for gas exchange. These cells possess distinct basement membranes, which apparently play an important role in the normal metabolism of the membranous pneumocyte, in regenerative processes, and in many pulmonary diseases. (2) The granular pneumocytes, located in irregular fashion beneath the alveolar epithelium in the interstitium. They appear to be capable of rapid multiplication and of differentiating into either fibroblasts or macrophages. (3) Alveolar macrophages, which are nonfixed cells that are actively phagocytic and play a major role in local pulmonary defense mechanisms.

Pulmonary Exchange Vessels. This includes all vessels undergoing significant exchange with the interstitial space of the lung, including not only pulmonary capillaries but almost certainly some small pulmonary arterioles and venules as well. The functional cell of the pulmonary capillary is the pulmonary endothelial cell, with its thin basement membrane. In some areas this basement membrane is fused with the basement membrane of the membranous pneumocyte. In other areas the basement membranes are not fused, increasing the volume of the interstitial space.

The Interstitial Space. The interstitial space plays a critical role in exchanges between alveoli and blood vessels. It contains predominantly connective tissue. In some areas it exists as a potential space (say, between fused basement membranes). In other areas this space is expanded and contains the small pulmonary lymphatics and pulmonary arterial and pulmonary venous branches.

Small Pulmonary Lymphatics. These vessels are generally found proximal to alveolar ducts and play an important role in regulating water and electrolyte balance at an alveolar-capillary level, as well as providing an important route for disposal of various potentially harmful substances.

Metabolic Background. Fundamental understanding of this group of disorders on a mechanistic basis will ultimately require an understanding of the metabolic processes of the individual types of pulmonary cells in health and disease. It may be visualized that each cell type has more or less specific metabolic pathways and metabolic requirements. Disorders of cellular metabolism produced by infectious agents, toxic substances, immunologic factors, and modification of the ambient microenvironment of these cells produce the structural and functional changes which make up diffuse interstitial and alveolar diseases. Some progress has been made in this area. The modification by O_2 depletion of the biochemical pathways involved in phagocytosis by alveolar macrophages, and the pulmonary basement membrane immunologic abnormalities in Goodpasture's syndrome (see p. 1308) are two examples of the usefulness of this approach. Until more specific information is available concerning the na-

ture of pulmonary cellular metabolism and its alteration by disease, knowledge of these diseases will remain superficial and descriptive.

PATHOLOGIC CHANGES. Chronic interstitial disease may occur as a result of five basic mechanisms.

1. Alveolar cell injury leading to an intraalveolar fibrinous exudate. Failure of resolution of this exudate may lead to organization of the fibrin, with incorporation into alveolar walls by overgrowth of regenerating alveolar epithelium.

2. Infiltration of alveolar walls and interstitium by a variety of cell types, depending on the nature of the exciting process.

3. Direct damage to the alveolar epithelium with the accretion of alveolar macrophages. Some macrophages may remain adherent to the damaged wall, becoming incorporated into the wall by alveolar epithelial regeneration and overgrowth and finally leading to the deposition of fibrous connective tissue.

4. Damage to the alveolar capillary endothelium from a variety of causes leading to interstitial, alveolar wall, and intraalveolar edema. This in turn may lead to increasing deposition of interstitial fibrous connective tissue and to loss of alveolar wall substance.

5. Chronic lymphedema with secondary deposition of fibrous connective tissue.

Following fibrosis, a series of secondary changes often occurs, including bronchiolectasis, honeycombing, smooth-muscle hypertrophy in the distal parts of the lung, bronchopulmonary arterial anastomoses, alveolar epithelial metaplasia, and occasionally neoplasia in the damaged segments.

PHYSIOLOGIC FEATURES. The physiologic abnormalities seen in this group of patients vary widely. To some extent the degree of physiologic abnormalities depends on the nature and extent of the abnormal pathologic processes. A number of these patients may have no demonstrable physiologic abnormalities. A restrictive physiologic defect with its concomitant decrease in vital capacity and other lung volumes and tachypnea is common. Obstructive features may be absent, and indeed maximal breathing capacities may be supranormal, possibly related to respiratory muscle hypertrophy. The patient may manifest alveolar hyperventilation either at rest or during exercise. Hypoxemia is the most important blood gas abnormality, and it commonly occurs in conjunction with arterial P_{CO_2} that is abnormally low. Measurements of "diffusion" capacity or transfer factors are frequently subnormal, and this type of measurement represents a fairly sensitive index of loss of alveolar surface or pulmonary capillary bed without necessarily reflecting the ability of the lung with respect to O_2 diffusion.

None of the physiologic abnormalities is specific, but measurements of physiologic status are useful in quantifying the degree of abnormality, in following the progress of a given disorder, in guiding therapy, and in assessing the results of therapy.

RADIOLOGIC FEATURES. Most of these disorders produce radiologic abnormalities at some point in their natural life history. These changes are seldom specific, and

Table 284-1. THE ETIOLOGIC BASIS OF DIFFUSE
PULMONARY INFILTRATION

I. Infections
 A. Bacterial, including miliary tuberculosis, staphylococcal, streptococcal, salmonellosis, shigellosis, infectious bronchiolitides, brucellosis, tularemia, glanders, plague (*Pasteurella pestis*), and *Klebsiella pneumoniae*
 B. Mycotic, including histoplasmosis, blastomycosis, coccidioidomycosis, cryptococcosis, aspergillosis, moniliasis, sporotrichosis, actinomycosis, streptotrichosis, nummulariasis, nocardiosis, geotrichosis
 C. Viral, rickettsial, and pleuropneumonia organisms, including chickenpox, measles, psittacosis (ornithosis), influenza, lymphopathia venereum, Rocky Mountain spotted fever, Q fever, primary atypical pneumonia (*Mycoplasma pneumoniae*)
 D. Parasitic, including schistosomiasis, toxoplasmosis, pneumocystis carinii, trichinosis, ascariasis, paragonimiasis, filariasis, human hookworm, dog hookworm, strongyloides, echinococcosis, amebiasis, visceral larva migrans
 E. Possibly infectious but cause unknown, including acute miliary pneumonia, diffuse miliary granulomatous pneumonia, acute diffuse interstitial fibrosis (Hamman-Rich), infectious mononucleosis, inclusion body pneumonia, erythema nodosum, Stevens-Johnson syndrome, pulmonary-alveolar proteinosis, desquamative interstitial pneumonia (DIP)
II. Pneumoconiosis, including berylliosis, asbestosis, silicosis, Shaver's disease, bagassosis, byssinosis, siderosis, welder's lung, baritosis, suberosis, Caplan's syndrome, inflammation from inhalation of tin, barium, talc, vanadium, silver, aluminum, Fuller's earth, and graphite
III. Systemic diseases of unknown cause, including collagen diseases: scleroderma, lupus erythematosus, polyarteritis, Wegener's granulomatosis, rheumatoid arthritis, rheumatic fever pneumonia, Weber-Christian disease; sarcoidosis; amyloidosis; reticuloendotheliosis, including eosinophilic granuloma, Hand-Schüller-Christian disease, Letterer-Siwe disease; hexamethonium fibrosis; Dilantin fibrosis; busulfan fibrosis; idiopathic pulmonary hemosiderosis; Goodpasture's syndrome
IV. Allergic, including eosinophilic pneumonia, Loeffler's syndrome, tropical eosinophilia; serum sickness; angioneurotic edema; reactions to drugs, including para-aminosalicylic acid, penicillin, nitrofurantoin, sulfonamides, chlorpropamide, mephenesin carbamate, 3-pentadecylcatechol
V. Congenital or familial (possibly hereditary), including congenital cystic disease of the lung, pneumatocoele, tuberous sclerosis, mucoviscidosis (cystic fibrosis of pancreas), pulmonary alveolar microlithiasis, hereditary idiopathic pulmonary fibrosis
VI. Inhalational, including farmer's lung, pigeon-breeder's lung, mushroom-compost lung, silo-filler's lung, smallpox-handler's lung, lipoidol pneumonia, lipid pneumonia, maple bark disease, elm disease, ehesauresis, sequoiosis, inhalation of acetylene, carbon tetrachloride, nitric acid, vomitus, tricalcium phosphate crysalosis, Hytrast, kerosene, sulfur dioxide, phosgene
VII. Metabolic, including uremic pneumonia, hyperparathyroidism
VIII. Neoplastic, including alveolar cell carcinoma, hema-

Table 284-1 THE ETIOLOGIC BASIS OF DIFFUSE
PULMONARY INFILTRATION (*Continued*)

togenous metastatic malignancy, lymphangitic carcinomatosis, leukemia, lymphoma, polycythemia vera, sarcomatosis, multiple myeloma, Waldenström's macroglobulinemia
IX. Physical agents, including postradiation fibrosis, uranium exposure, thermal
X. Circulatory, including pulmonary edema; multiple pulmonary emboli; mitral stenosis and left ventricular failure; bronchial artery occlusion; fat embolism; sickle-cell anemia with multiple pulmonary infarcts; diffuse pulmonary ossification secondary to mitral stenosis; postperfusion pulmonary syndrome; pulmonary fibrosis secondary to pulmonary venous occlusion.

often there is poor correlation between the degree of roentgenographic involvement and the physiologic and clinical status of the patient. However, it is frequently possible to decide on radiologic grounds whether the primary process is intraalveolar, interstitial, or both. Intraalveolar processes usually show small circular densities on the roentgenogram and are frequently accompanied by an air bronchogram (outlining of small and medium-sized bronchi on routine chest roentgenogram). Patients with pure interstitial disease frequently show blurring of hilar marking, linear densities, small-lymphatic-vessel engorgement, and a tendency toward honeycombed appearance in heavily involved areas.

CLINICAL MANAGEMENT. The differential diagnosis involved in this group of diseases is vast. Frequently, a diagnosis can be made only by means of lung biopsy, but occasionally, even lung biopsy does not permit accurate diagnosis. Table 284-1 is a partial list of the entities which may produce diffuse pulmonary infiltrations. The remainder of this chapter will be devoted to a description of some of the more important entities.

The Interstitial Pneumonias

Diffuse alveolar damage with basement membrane sparing produced by a variety of different etiologic factors results in a similar pathologic sequence (see above) and a similar clinical sequence. These disorders generally begin with necrosis of the alveolar epithelial lining, which leads to intraalveolar exudate and hyaline membranes. The disease may be acute or chronic, and the pulmonary involvement may be focal or diffuse. In some patients, these lesions may resolve completely. In other patients, they go on to organization, with interstitial proliferation. Because of the similarity of the pathogenetic sequence, the term *usual interstitial pneumonia* has been applied to this group of diseases. Within this group several pathologic variants have been described. Occasionally the interstitial cellular infiltrate consists of mature lymphocytes; the term *lymphoid interstitial pneumonia* has been used to describe this pathologic change. Patients have been described with lymphocytic interstitial infiltrates and with numerous bizarre giant cells in the alveoli; the term, *giant-cell interstitial pneumonia* has been used for this condition. In other patients diffuse interstitial infiltration with plasma cells may be present and the term *plasma cell interstitial pneumonia* may be appropriate. In some patients, the lesions noted show a relatively minor interstitial component with little evidence of cellular necrosis, and the alveoli become filled with intact granular pneumocytes. The term *desquamative interstitial pneumonia* has been given to describe this picture. It is important to point out that the primary basis for the above classification is the pathologic appearance of the pulmonary lesions. Within this broad group of diseases it is possible to describe a number of more or less clinically distinct entities, which include (1) Hamman-Rich syndrome, (2) drug pneumopathies, (3) familial idiopathic pulmonary fibrosis, (4) desquamative interstitial pneumonia, (5) pulmonary venous occlusion, (6) lymphangitic carcinomatosis, (7) pulmonary scleroderma, (8) pulmonary reticuloendothelioses.

HAMMAN–RICH SYNROME. In 1935 and, again, in 1944, Hamman and Rich reported four patients with an unusual form of pneumonia characterized by progressive interstitial fibrosis of both lungs. The disease was accompanied by progressive hypoxia and the ultimate development of right ventricular failure. In each patient the disease ended fatally within a year of onset. Since this original description, a relatively large number of patients has been described who more or less fit into this diagnostic category.

Clinical features include dyspnea, cough, and cyanosis, terminating in many patients with intractable pulmonary insufficiency and cor pulmonale.

The cause of this disorder is unknown, and indeed, it seems likely that a number of different processes may have as their end result the development of Hamman-Rich changes. Etiologic theories include viral infection with an unknown agent, infection caused by the pleuropneumonia group, the failure of resolution of acute interstitial pneumonia, a hypersensitivity reaction, and a form of collagen disease. The last two possibilities are suggested by hypergammaglobulinemia, splenomegaly, and eosinophilia, which have been reported in some patients with Hamman-Rich syndrome.

The radiographic signs vary, and severe physiologic involvement has been reported in patients with only moderate roentgenographic abnormalities. The chest films in some patients resemble those in congestive heart failure with marked cardiomegaly, and the lung lesions resemble those of pulmonary edema; or the chest roentgenogram may resemble that in diffuse bronchopneumonia; or the films may reveal diffuse interstitial fibrosis. Adrenal steroids apparently have induced remissions in some patients. Such remissions tend to be rather limited in time. Hormone withdrawal may produce a severe and unrelenting relapse.

At present the diagnosis of Hamman-Rich syndrome should be reserved for patients having acute disease with a histologic picture consistent with usual interstitial pneumonia and a rapidly fatal course. Patients with a similar histologic picture of unknown etiology but with a less-acute course also may be conveniently diagnosed as having usual interstitial pneumonia.

DRUG PNEUMOPATHIES. A number of pharmacologic agents are capable of producing generalized interstitial pulmonary fibrosis, even though they are not administered via inhalation. This association has been reported with the therapeutic use of hexamethonium, mecamylamine, busulfan, Dilantin, hydrochlorothiazide, methysergide, sulfonamides, antituberculosis drugs, and nitrofurantoin. The reaction may occur as an acute pneumonia with fever, cough, and pulmonary infiltrates or it may result in chronic interstitial pneumonia with fibrosis.

The administration of hexamethonium in the treatment of hypertension has been associated with the development of interstitial fibrosis and a rapid clinical course, with death from pulmonary insufficiency. Both the clinical course and the histologic changes are similar to those seen in usual interstitial pneumonia.

Busulfan (Myleran). This drug is widely used in the therapy of chronic granulocytic leukemia (Chap. 348). A number of patients receiving this therapy have developed diffuse interstitial pulmonary fibrosis. There may be dyspnea, cough, fever, and bilateral crepitant rales. Chest roentgenogram shows bilateral nodular infiltrations. Some of these patients show diffuse hyperpigmentation of the skin and other features suggesting adrenal insufficiency. The diagnosis of busulfan lung is complicated by the common occurrence of miliary tuberculosis in leukemia and by the occasional occurrence of leukemic infiltration of the lungs in such patients. However, in busulfan pneumopathy the infiltrations regress following the cessation of drug therapy.

Dilantin. Commonly used in the therapy of epilepsy, Dilantin has caused a variety of toxic manifestations. Recent studies suggest that chronic pulmonary fibrosis may represent one such manifestation. The fibrosis seen on the roentgenogram may vary from minimal increases in bronchovascular markings to severe, extensive diffuse involvement. Once established, the lesions do not appear reversible. It is of interest that there seems to be an inverse relationship between gingival hypertrophy and pulmonary involvement in chronic Dilantin therapy.

Most of these reactions appear to represent hypersensitivity reactions, and the development of eosinophilia in the acute stage is not unusual. Withdrawal from the offending drug and the use of adrenal steroids are the indicated forms of therapy, although the development of interstitial fibrosis may make the disease irreversible. In general, as more drugs are used in medicine, it may be anticipated that more pulmonary syndromes related to their use will become apparent.

FAMILIAL IDIOPATHIC PULMONARY FIBROSIS. The occurrence of diffuse interstitial pulmonary fibrosis on a familial basis has been described in several studies. The radiologic picture noted is that of a diffuse nodular infiltrate. Pulmonary function studies showed findings consistent with abnormal gas exchange. Some of these patients showed persistent eosinophilia. In one affected member, the disorder was associated with an unusual single gamma-globulin peak. Genetic studies in two such kindreds suggested the possibility that the disorder is heritable, being transmitted as an autosomal dominant trait.

DESQUAMATIVE INTERSTITIAL PNEUMONIA. This is a disorder of unknown etiology with some distinctive clinical features and characteristic pathologic findings. Typical symptoms include dyspnea, weight loss, and cough. There is a substantial incidence of pleural complications, including effusions and recurrent pneumothorax. Clubbing and cyanosis are occasionally present. The chest roentgenogram in most patients shows predominantly basal involvement. This consists of a slight triangular haziness radiating from the hilus along the heart borders to both bases and sparing the costophrenic angles. There is also an increase in the number and thickness of basal vascular markings. Once established, the roentgenographic abnormalities tend to stabilize. Physiologically, there are usually mild restrictive disease and hypoxemia related to an increase in venous admixture. Pathologically there are an extensive accumulation of masses of granular pneumocytes within alveoli, and minute lymphoid follicles in the periphery of the lung without evidence of alveolar necrosis, fibrin exudation, or hyaline membranes. There may be moderate thickening of isolated alveolar walls. Diagnosis is best established by lung biopsy. It is of great importance that these patients frequently show an immediate and dramatic response to adrenal steroid therapy.

PULMONARY VENOUS OCCLUSION. Complete, partial, or intermittent obstruction of the pulmonary veins may lead to the development of pulmonary fibrosis. This fibrosis appears to be independent of the cause of the venous obstruction. Unilateral venous obstruction leads to unilateral fibrosis. The clinical picture consists of cough, dyspnea, and hemoptysis as modified by the manifestations of the underlying disease producing vascular obstruction. The histologic picture closely resembles that seen in usual interstitial pneumonia. The prognosis depends chiefly on the nature of the underlying disease.

PULMONARY RETICULOENDOTHELIOSES (EOSINOPHILIC GRANULOMA, HAND–SCHULLER–CHRISTIAN DISEASE, LETTERER–SIWE DISEASE). Pulmonary involvement in these diseases produces a diffuse fibrosis associated with formation of multiple small cysts (honeycomb lungs). The clinical course varies. The occurrence of spontaneous pneumothorax is frequent. Diabetes insipidus and bone lesions are commonly associated findings. In severe forms, abnormal gas exchange is a major physiologic abnormality. Diagnosis in general depends on the presence of other stigmas of the disease, as well as pulmonary involvement. Radiation has been advocated, either with or without steroid therapy.

PULMONARY SCLERODERMA. The general manifestations of scleroderma are described elsewhere (Chap. 393). Pulmonary involvement is common. The manifestations vary, depending on the site and extent of the disease. With extensive involvement of the skin of the thorax, there may be an inability to expand the chest adequately,

leading to restrictive disease. Diffuse peribronchial fibrosis may lead to an obstructive pulmonary defect and to marked distortions of pulmonary parenchyma, with the development of honeycombing of the lung. Pleural fibrosis may produce pulmonary restriction. Diffuse interstitial fibrosis may produce the typical pathologic, physiologic, and clinical picture described above. With esophageal involvement, there may be "spillover" of esophageal contents, leading to recurrent bronchopneumonia. There may be direct involvement of the pulmonary vasculature by fibrosis, leading ultimately to the development of cor pulmonale. It has also been suggested that the proclivity of systemic vessels to show abnormal vasospasm may be shared by pulmonary vessels, so that the tendency to pulmonary hypertension and eventually to cor pulmonale is increased. Rarely, pulmonary manifestations may antedate the appearance of skin or esophageal lesions (scleroderma sine scleroderma). Under this circumstance, the diagnosis is difficult, since the histologic appearance of the pulmonary lesions is not specific. The coexistence of scleroderma and bronchiolar (alveolar cell) carcinoma occurs with sufficient frequency to suggest more than a coincidental relationship between these two relatively uncommon diseases.

LYMPHANGITIC CARCINOMATOSIS. Lymphangitic carcinomatosis (Chap. 292) is a process in which there are widespread neoplastic metastases throughout the lymphatics of both lungs. It differs from the more common varieties of pulmonary metastases in that it causes severe symptoms and is the direct cause of death in most patients.

The primary tumor may arise from any site, but bronchogenic carcinoma and carcinoma of the stomach are the most common primary tumors. The primary tumor may be small and clinically inapparent during life. The outstanding symptom is severe and rapidly progressive dyspnea. The characteristic radiologic appearance is that of stringlike shadows distinct from vascular markings, stretching from the hili to the periphery of all lung zones. Rarely the chest roentgenogram may be normal despite severe dyspnea. The possibility of lymphangitic carcinomatosis should be considered in older patients with marked dyspnea for which no other cause can be determined. It is included in this section because the two primary physiologic abnormalities, a reduced compliance and hypoxemia, are related to infiltrative changes in the pulmonary interstitium, producing pulmonary stiffness and possibly pulmonary edema because of compromised lymphatic drainage with abnormal alveolar-pulmonary capillary water exchange.

Disorders Associated with a Variety of Pulmonary Lesions Which Are Often Interstitial or Alveolar in Location

PULMONARY SARCOIDOSIS. The etiologic background and general features of sarcoidosis are discussed elsewhere (Chap. 254). This section will deal specifically with the pulmonary forms of the disease.

The lung is the organ most often involved in sarcoidosis. The pattern of pulmonary involvement varies. Granulomatous and/or fibrotic infiltration may be found involving hilar and mediastinal lymph nodes, peribronchial parenchyma, interstitial parenchyma, the pleura (very rarely), and pulmonary vasculature. Each of these areas may be involved alone or in combination with other areas.

Because of this diversity of anatomic involvement, the physiologic and clinical pictures tend to be rather diverse. Although a subdivision into distinct groups is somewhat arbitrary, patients with pulmonary sarcoidosis generally may be separated into three groups: (1) those without physiologic abnormalities; (2) those with increased airway resistance; (3) those with restrictive disease with or without impairment of gas exchange.

Patients with sarcoidosis may show no abnormalities of pulmonary function on careful testing. This may occur not only with isolated hilar or mediastinal lymphadenopathy, but also with fairly extensive intraalveolar infiltration, replacing both alveoli and pulmonary blood vessels, with sparing of the airways and interstitial area of the lung. Aside from abnormality of the chest roentgenogram, such patients commonly show no clinical evidence of lung disease. Indeed, the finding of marked pulmonary infiltration in the absence of clinical symptoms should arouse the suspicion of sarcoid. Isolated adenopathy is the most favorable form of this disease from the prognostic standpoint. A large percentage of such patients will show no progression of lesions and may have complete resolution of roentgenographic densities.

Involvement of the tracheobronchial tree produces an increase in airway resistance, leading to obstructive disease and ultimately to obstructive emphysema. The major physiologic abnormalities of obstructive disease have already been discussed (Chap. 283). In general, the most favorable response to steroid therapy in pulmonary sarcoidosis is seen in this group of patients.

Diffuse interstitial involvement by granulomatous or fibrotic tissue leads to restrictive disease with or without abnormalities of gas exchange. This form of pulmonary sarcoid produces the physiologic and clinical abnormalities already described.

There may be poor correlation among physiologic abnormalities as demonstrated by functional measurements, the clinical status of the patient, and the chest roentgenogram. In general, physiologic abnormalities tend to antedate frank clinical symptoms. Scalene lymph node or lung biopsy may be required for diagnosis.

The natural course of pulmonary sarcoidosis is characterized by variability. Remissions and exacerbations, as judged by radiologic appearance, sign and symptoms, and physiologic measurements, are not uncommon. Steroid therapy is frequently effective in inducing a clinical and physiologic remission.

MILIARY GRANULOMATOSES OF INFECTIOUS ORIGIN.
The development of abnormalities of pulmonary gas exchange has been documented in patients with diffuse miliary tuberculosis and presumably may also occur in histoplasmosis. Such patients show dyspnea, tachypnea, and cyanosis during the acute phase of their illness. Function measurements are consistent with the thesis that the major physiologic abnormality is impaired pulmonary gas exchange. Once an etiologic diagnosis is established, prompt specific chemotherapy, when available, together with adrenal steroid therapy, is appropriate. Chronic pulmonary fibrosis and insufficiency may develop in the late stages of these disorders.

CHRONIC BERYLLIUM DISEASE OF THE LUNG.
The inhalation of certain salts of beryllium (Chap. 288) leads to the development of pulmonary lesions. In the acute form of the disease one sees the development of a chemical pneumonia, characterized by cough, with occasional blood streaking of the sputum, substernal burning pain, dyspnea, cyanosis, anorexia with weight loss, progressive fatigue, and diffuse radiologic densities. In patients who recover, the lung fields generally clear up after several months.

Beryllium exposure is also capable of producing a chronic form of lung disease. This disorder develops insidiously months to years after the initial exposure. The clinical picture may be that associated with interstitial disease. The chemical demonstration of beryllium in lung or urine may help to reinforce the diagnosis. Therapy includes the use of adrenal steroids, oxygen, and measures designed to relieve cor pulmonale.

ASBESTOSIS.
The inhalation of asbestos dust (hydrated calcium-magnesium silicate) may lead to the development of a diffuse interstitial pulmonary fibrosis known as asbestosis (Chap. 288). A striking feature of the reaction to asbestos is the development of marked pleural fibrosis. Significant physiologic derangements indicating abnormalities of gas exchange have been noted even in the absence of roentgenographic changes.

SILICOSIS.
Silicosis, the disease resulting from the inhalation of silicon dioxide dust, is described elsewhere (Chap. 288). Usually it gives rise to an obstructive ventilatory defect, the end stage of which is chronic obstructive emphysema. Occasionally, patients with silicosis present physiologic abnormalities consistent with interstitial disease without significant obstruction.

SILO–FILLER'S DISEASE.
Silo-filler's disease results from the inhalation of the oxides of nitrogen (primarily nitrogen dioxide) (Chap. 288). Evolution of the various oxides of nitrogen starts within a few hours after silo filling, reaches a maximum between 1 and 2 days later, and continues at a decreasing rate for a week or longer. The disease is limited to individuals who enter silos within a day or two after filling.

Histologic examination during the acute phase reveals diffuse pulmonary edema. As the disease progresses, pathologic examination shows the lung to be filled with innumerable grossly visible, uniformly distributed lesions. Each nodule consists of a small bronchus or bronchiole filled with fibrotic exudate. This exudate becomes organized, obliterating the bronchiolar lumen. The pathologic picture is typical of what has been called "bronchiolitis obliterans fibrosa." This entity is composed of a group of diseases whose end stage is the fibrotic obliteration of significant portions of the bronchiolar tree, resulting from inhalation of toxic gases, from infection of the bronchial tree, and in some patients from unknown causes. The basic physiologic defect in fibrosing bronchiolitis is that many areas of the lung have a marked reduction in ventilation although perfusion is relatively well maintained. Under these circumstances total effective ventilation is inadequate, and hypoxia and hypercapnia result. The marked decrease in airway diameter produces greatly augmented airway resistance.

Acute Interstitial Reactions

A number of inhaled agents may produce an acute reaction involving the pulmonary interstitium and alveoli. Two typical examples are farmer's lung and maple bark disease, although similar clinical syndromes are described in pigeon breeders, mushroom-compost workers, handlers of sugar cane (bagasse), and in the cotton processing industries.

FARMER'S LUNG. Farmer's lung is related to the inhalation of spoiled ("moldy") hay (Chap. 289). Clinically, the disease is characterized by the sudden onset of dyspnea some hours after exposure to moldy hay or other vegetable materials, including stored silage. The histologic picture consists of numerous granulomas, involving the pulmonary interstitium with histiocytes, foreign-body giant cells, thickening of alveolar septums, and occasional fibrotic strands. There may be an obliterative bronchitis and pleuritis as well. Physiologic abnormalities during the acute phase include the presence of restrictive disease, with a reduction in lung compliance and in vital capacity. There may be ventilation-perfusion abnormalities and mild pulmonary hypertension.

MAPLE BARK DISEASE. Exposure to maple wood dust in the lumbering and paper mill industries may give rise to acute interstitial pneumonia with fever, chills, dyspnea, and a diffuse pulmonary infiltrate (Chap. 289). Histologic examination of the lung reveals cellular infiltration of alveolar walls with thickening. Similar syndromes have been reported following suitable exposure to sawdust from redwood trees and from elms. These syndromes appear to be related to exposure and subsequent sensitization to fungi of the genus *Graphium*.

Disorders Associated with Intraalveolar Accumulations

There are several disorders in which the major abnormality is the deposition of an abnormal material within alveoli with little or no interstitial or alveolar wall reaction. Pulmonary alveolar proteinosis and alveolar microlithiasis are typical examples of these diseases:

PULMONARY ALVEOLAR PROTEINOSIS. This term has been applied to a syndrome of unknown causation with a fairly specific pathologic pattern. The typical lesion consists of the deposition of eosinophilic material within the alveoli without serious alteration of the lung tissue structure. There is usually proliferation of the alveolar septal cells. The disease was recognized before 1953. The chief clinical symptom is progressive dyspnea associated with the signs and sequelae of hypoxia, including cyanosis, clubbing, and polycythemia. Few or no abnormal physical signs are found on physical examination of the chest. Laboratory findings, aside from those related to the pulmonary abnormality, are not remarkable. X-ray examination usually reveals a diffuse, hazy, ground-glass appearance of the lung. There is generally no hilar hymphadenopathy. In several asymptomatic patients, the disease was discovered on routine chest roentgenogram.

Physiologically these patients may show a restrictive ventilatory defect and hypoxemia which is related to the nonventilation of affected alveoli. Although the chemical nature of the intraalveolar fluid is not known, chemical studies suggest that it is rich in lipid content and that the amount of protein may be relatively insignificant. Thus, the term "proteinosis" is a misnomer.

The drug phenosulfonphthalein (PSP) appears to bind tightly to the intraalveolar material. It has been suggested that the intravenous injection of 1 mg PSP might be useful as a diagnostic test, since this substance will continue to be excreted in the sputum for long periods in patients with "proteinosis." It has also been suggested that the presence of periodic acid–Schiff positive material in the sputum may likewise be diagnostically useful. The level of serum lactic acid dehydrogenase has been reported elevated in patients with active disease. Specific diagnosis, however, requires lung biopsy.

Death usually occurs as a result of pulmonary insufficiency, but spontaneous remission with complete recovery is not rare. The etiologic basis of this disorder is unknown. In some patients coexistent fungal infection, such as nocardiosis and cryptococcosis, of the lung has been reported. The basis of this relationship is not clear.

A number of different therapeutic approaches have been advocated. The use of adrenal steroids is contraindicated because of the possibility of fungal infection. Recently the use of bronchopulmonary lavage in a previously degassed lung has been reported to produce alveolar clearing.

PULMONARY ALVEOLAR MICROLITHIASIS. This disease of unknown cause is characterized by familial occurrence and the deposition of laminated calcium stones within alveoli.

The intraalveolar concretions are similar in appearance to the corpora amylacea found in the prostate. The alveoli containing concretions are themselves normal, although there may be some small degree of interstitial cellular infiltration or fibrosis. The number of alveoli containing stones may vary from 25 to 80 percent of the total number. It seems probable that both the number of calculi and the amount of interstitial reaction increase with the age of the patient or the known duration of the disease. At postmortem examination, there may be startling increases of lung weight (to over 4,000 Gm) because of the accumulated mass of small stones.

The most specific diagnostic technique available is radiologic examination of the chest by means of overpenetrated (Bucky) films. On such films the x-ray appearance is pathognomonic, since it shows the fine sandlike particles spread uniformly through both lungs. There is little variation in particle size, and the calcific nature of the particles is unmistakable. The total density of the millions of stones may be sufficient to obscure cardiac and diaphragmatic outlines. Chemical analysis of the alveolar microliths reveals that they consist of calcium and phosphorus, with smaller amounts of magnesium and aluminum and traces of silicon and iron. The nature of the process leading to the precipitation of calcium inside apparently normal alveoli is unknown.

Although the etiologic basis of the disease is unclear, approximately 50 percent of cases have been associated with a familial incidence, suggesting a hereditary defect.

The disease is usually asymptomatic for years and is most commonly discovered on routine chest roentgenogram examination. With progressive alveolar involvement, there is the ultimate development of pulmonary insufficiency, characterized by dyspnea, cyanosis, cor pulmonale, and a fatal outcome. There is no known specific therapy for the disorder.

Disorders Associated with Intraalveolar Bleeding

Intraalveolar bleeding may occur in a number of different disease states, including uremic pneumonia, rheumatic pneumonia, hypersensitivity reactions involving the lung, and two more or less specific disease entities, Goodpasture's syndrome and idiopathic pulmonary hemosiderosis. The latter two diseases represent important examples of this general group of diseases and will be described more extensively.

GOODPASTURE'S SYNDROME. This syndrome, or basement membrane disease of lung and kidney, consists of lung hemorrhages, usually manifested by hemoptysis, and renal failure produced by nephritis. The disease generally occurs in the age group twenty-five to thirty-five years, and 75 percent of reported cases have been in males. The hemoptysis consists of bright red blood, and its origin from pulmonary capillaries seems indubitable. Clinically the renal failure is not unlike that found in other varieties of glomerulonephritis except that it often runs an accelerated course, with death occurring in several weeks. The abnormal pulmonary manifestations, including roentgenographic appearance and the presence of hemosiderin-laden macrophages in sputum or gastric washings, are simply explained on the basis of bleeding at an alveolar-pulmonary capillary level. Routine and electron microscopy reveal important changes in the basement membranes of both glomeruli and alveolar-pulmonary capillary units. Recent studies utilizing immunofluoresence demonstrate the deposition of immunoglobulins in the basement membranes of glomeruli and alveoli. This deposition occurs in a linear fashion, and indeed this peculiar type of deposition is perhaps the most specific hallmark of the disease. It has also been shown that similar linear deposition of immunoglobulins may be produced in the basement membranes of sheep glomeruli following the injection of antilung serum. It seems reasonable that the basement membranes of both organs share common antigens, thus accounting for the involvement of both organs. The localization of immunoglobulins in the basement membranes suggests but does not establish an immunologic basis for this disease, since this may merely represent a secondary phenomenon. However, it does establish that a major aspect of the disease is basement membrane involvement.

It is of interest that some patients with idiopathic pulmonary hemosiderosis have a picture which blends with that of Goodpasture's syndrome. These cases might represent a form of Goodpasture's syndrome with predominately pulmonary involvement. In similar fashion, some patients with rapidly progressive glomerulonephritis have been described with a linear deposition of immunoglobulins in glomerular basement membranes. Conceivably such patients represent the isolated renal form of Goodpasture's syndrome.

Although the mortality rate in Goodpasture's syndrome is high, significant numbers of long-term survivors have been reported. Some survivors are patients with relatively mild renal involvement and with remission of lung hemorrhages. Many of them have been on adrenal steroid therapy. The other significant group of survivors is composed of patients in whom pulmonary hemorrhage has been mild and in whom renal insufficiency has been controlled by chronic dialysis or renal transplantation, either with or without bilateral nephrectomy.

IDIOPATHIC PULMONARY HEMOSIDEROSIS. This is a relatively uncommon pulmonary disease that results from recurrent hemorrhages into the lung. The majority of patients are less than sixteen years of age, although the disease has also been described in adults. The sex distribution is approximately equal in children; in adults the male sex predominates 2:1.

The clinical picture is relatively characteristic. These patients have recurrent febrile episodes of cough, dyspnea, severe hemoptysis, hypochromic anemia, and diffuse pulmonary mottling. Hepatosplenomegaly and digital clubbing are common. Pulmonary hypertension may develop. The chest roentgenogram usually shows diffuse shadows which suggest edema or hemorrhage. These shadows may clear up or change rapidly, leaving multiple nodular areas behind. Following repeated episodes, there may be progressive increase in nodularity. The disease may also be associated with the development of diffuse myocardial fibrosis without iron deposition. Heart failure from this cause is one of the mechanisms of death. Eosinophilia has been reported in approximately 10 to 20 percent of patients. Cold agglutinins are not infrequently present. Hemosiderin-laden macrophages are commonly found in sputum or gastric washings.

The anemia found in these patients is related to the pulmonary hemorrhages. Although a shortened life span of red blood cells in these patients has been reported, it has been established that this anemia is caused by loss of red blood cells inside the pulmonary parenchyma. The mechanism of the pulmonary hemorrhages is not known. The pulmonary histologic changes are said to be relatively specific and include degeneration, shedding, and hyperplasia of alveolar epithelial cells and marked localized alveolar capillary dilatation. Changes secondary to intrapulmonary hemorrhage include diffuse interstitial fibrosis, hemosiderosis, degeneration of elastic fibers, and nonspecific pulmonary vascular abnormalities. Some of these patients may have mild variants of Goodpasture's syndrome.

Various etiologic suggestions have been advanced, including the possibility that the disorder represents an immunoallergic disease. This hypothesis suggests that an unknown sensitizing agent produces autoantibody formation and that the hemorrhages result from an immunoallergic reaction, with the lung as the shock organ. In line with this possibility are the reports of rather remarkable improvements produced by adrenal steroid therapy. Unless the disease is ameliorated by steroids, its outcome is frequently fatal, although the course of the disease is relatively slow.

The Diffuse Pulmonary Infiltrate

The preceding paragraphs have dealt with a group of diseases in which the pathologic picture and clinical manifestations are more or less specifically defined. Not infrequently, the physician is faced with the problem of the patient whose chest roentgenogram show diffuse pulmonary infiltrations of varying sizes, shapes, and degrees of opacity. Such patients represent a heterogeneous group clinically, physiologically, and etiologically. The patient may be entirely asymptomatic and have as his only abnormality the presence of abnormal roentgenographic densities; or he may have high-grade pulmonary insufficiency.

As shown in Table 284-1, the differential diagnosis of the diffuse pulmonary infiltrates is vast; resolution of the problem often requires a knowledge not only of lung disease but of general medicine as well.

REFERENCES

Diffusional Disorders

Duncan, A. D., K. N. Drummond, A. F. Michael, and R. L. Vernier: Pulmonary Hemorrhage and Glomerulonephritis, Ann. Intern. Med., 62:920, 1965.

Gaensler, E. A., A. M. Goff, and C. M. Prowse: Desquamative Interstitial Pneumonia, New Engl. J. Med., 274:113, 1966.

Liebow, A. A.: "The Lung—New Concepts and Entities in Pulmonary Disease," chap. 24, Monograph 18, pp. 332–365, International Academy of Pathology, 1962.

Rosen, S. H., B. Castleman, and A. A. Liebow: Pulmonary Alveolar Proteinosis, New Engl. J. Med., 258:1123, 1958.

Rosenow, E. C., R. A. DeRemee, and D. E. Dines: Chronic Nitrofurantoin Pulmonary Reaction. Report of 5 Cases, New Engl. J. Med., 279:1258, 1968.

Scadding, J. G.: Prognosis of Intrathoracic Sarcoidosis in England. A Review of 136 Cases after Five Years' Observation, Brit. Med. J., 2:1165, 1961.

Soergel, K. H., and S. C. Sommers: Idiopathic Pulmonary Hemosiderosis and Related Syndromes, Am. J. Med., 32:499, 1962.

Wilson, R. J., G. P. Rodnan, and E. D. Robin: An Early Pulmonary Physiologic Abnormality in Progressive Systemic Sclerosis, Am. J. Med., 36:361, 1964.

Restrictive Disorders

Avery, M. E.: Alveolar Lining Layer; A Review, and Role in Mechanics and Atelectasis, Pediatrics, 30:324, 1962.

Bergofsky, E. H., M. Turino, and A. P. Fishman: Cardiorespiratory Failure in Kyphoscoliosis, Medicine, 38:263, 1959.

Burwell, D. S., E. D. Robin, R. D. Whaley, and A. G. Bickelmann: Extreme Obesity Associated with Alveolar Hypoventilation: A Pickwickian Syndrome, Am. J. Med., 21: 811, 1956.

Comroe, J. H., R. E. Forster, A. B. Dubois, W. A. Briscoe, and E. Carlsen: "The Lung," 2d ed., Chicago, The Year Book Medical Publishers, Inc., 1962.

Fishman, A. P., G. M. Turino, and E. H. Bergofsky: The Syndrome of Alveolar Hypoventilation, Am. J. Med., 23:333, 1957.

Ratto, O., W. A. Briscoe, J. W. Morton, and J. H. Comroe, Jr.: Anoxemia Secondary to Polycythemia and Polycythemia Secondary to Anoxemia, Am. J. Med., 19:958, 1955.

Sarnoff, S. J., J. L. Whittenberger, and J. E. Affeldt: Hypoventilation Syndrome in Bulbar Poliomyelitis, J.A.M.A., 147:30, 1951.

Turner, W. A., and McD. Critchley: Respiratory Disorders in Epidemic Encephalitis, Brain, 48:72, 1925.

285 PULMONARY THROMBOEMBOLISM

Kenneth M. Moser

Pulmonary thromboembolism (PTE) is a leading cause of morbidity and mortality, and can appear in many clinical contexts. A survey in 1962 indicated that PTE was responsible for at least 6,000 deaths in that year. Autopsy statistics further emphasize the magnitude of the problem. Routine autopsies disclose evidence of recent or remote pulmonary embolism in 25 to 30 percent of all patients. When special techniques are applied at autopsy, the frequency of discovery exceeds 60 percent. The high incidence of PTE at autopsy contrasts sharply with the incidence of antemortem diagnosis. Available information suggests that an antemortem diagnosis is made in only 10 to 30 percent of all cases. One cause of this discrepancy is incomplete understanding of the pathogenesis of thrombosis.

The three factors involved in thrombogenesis are stasis, abnormalities in the vessel wall, and alterations in the blood coagulation system. Coagulation alterations have been studied extensively, but as yet, there is no reliable test for a state of "hypercoagulability" in a given patient. Conditions which are associated with a high risk of venous thromboembolism include the postoperative period; pregnancy, particularly the postpartum period; congestive heart failure; chronic pulmonary disease; fractures or other injuries of the lower extremities; chronic deep venous insufficiency of the legs; prolonged bed rest; and carcinoma.

Although there is increasing awareness of the pathogenetic and clinical substrates which lead to PTE, detection of embolism in the majority of patients remains poor. One reason is inadequate understanding of the natural history of pulmonary embolism.

Natural History of Embolism

THE ACUTE EVENTS. The immediate result of thromboembolism is complete or partial obstruction of the pulmonary arterial blood flow to the distal lung. This obstruction leads to a series of pathophysiologic events which can be categorized as the "respiratory" and "hemodynamic" consequences of PTE.

Respiratory Consequences. Embolic obstruction produces a zone of the lung which is ventilated but not perfused—an intrapulmonary "dead space" (Chap. 280). Because it cannot participate in the process of gas exchange, ventilation of this nonperfused area is "wasted," in the functional sense. Another consequence of embolic obstruction is a constriction of the airspaces and airways in the affected lung zone. This "pneumoconstriction" appears to be due to the bronchoalveolar hypocapnia that results from cessation of pulmonary capillary blood flow because experimentally it can be abolished by inhalation of carbon dioxide–enriched air. This constrictive response may be viewed as beneficial since it decreases the amount of "wasted" ventilation.

Another disturbance caused by embolic obstruction—loss of alveolar surfactant—does not occur immediately. This surface-active lipoprotein is required to maintain alveolar stability. In its absence, alveolar collapse occurs. Cessation of pulmonary capillary blood flow leads to reduction in surfactant within 2 or 3 hr, which becomes severe at 12 to 15 hr. Frank atelectasis—the morphologic expression of alveolar instability—can be detected at 24 to 48 hr after interruption of blood flow.

Hemodynamic Consequences. The primary hemodynamic consequence of thromboembolic obstruction is a reduction in the available cross-sectional area of the pulmonary arterial bed. This loss of vascular capacity increases the resistance to pulmonary blood flow which, if marked, leads to pulmonary hypertension and acute failure of the right ventricle. Tachycardia, and often a decline in cardiac output, also occur.

The factors which determine the severity of these hemodynamic changes have been a subject of continued debate. There is agreement that the *extent of embolic obstruction* is a key factor. However, the reserve capacity of the pulmonary arteriocapillary bed is so extensive that more than 50 percent of the vascular area must be obstructed before significant elevation in pulmonary arterial pressure results. Because pulmonary hypertension occurs in some patients with occlusion of lesser extent, investigators have searched for reflex or humoral vasoconstrictor mechanisms associated with embolism. Despite long and careful search for such mechanisms, their extent and fre-

quency in human PTE remains unknown. Hence, some workers maintain that the degree of embolic obstruction itself is the only determinant of hemodynamic impairment. They suggest that instances of apparent disparity between the extent of embolism and clinical response reflect only clinical underestimation of the magnitude of the embolism. Other investigators, however, have presented compelling evidence to support the occurrence of vasoconstriction with embolism. Some have demonstrated that constriction is associated with obstruction of the smaller, but not the larger, pulmonary arterial vessels. Another thesis holds that serotonin, a known pulmonary vasoconstrictive-bronchoconstrictive substance, is released from platelets coating fresh emboli as they lodge in the pulmonary tree. This thesis introduces the attractive concept that an embolus should be regarded as a packet with pharmacologic, as well as obstructive, potential. Studies which have identified fibrinopeptide B, one of the breakdown products of fibrinogen, as a powerful pulmonary vasoconstrictor, support this concept. A consensus view, then, suggests that, while the extent of embolism is a key factor, humoral and/or reflex influences probably are operative in certain patients and compromise the pulmonary circulation to a greater extent than might be expected on an anatomic basis alone.

The cardiopulmonary status of the patient prior to embolism is also critical in determining the clinical severity of embolism. A small embolus may have limited impact upon an otherwise healthy individual but may have serious consequences in someone with advanced cardiac or pulmonary disease.

Both experimental and clinical studies have established that infarction—death of lung tissue—rarely accompanies embolic occlusion. It is likely that less than 10 percent of emboli in man lead to infarction. That infarction rarely follows embolism should occasion little surprise. The lung has three avenues for obtaining its oxygen requirements: the pulmonary arterial circulation; the bronchial arterial circulation; and the airways. Thus, infarction occurs infrequently, and its appearance usually requires simultaneous compromise of bronchial arterial flow and/or airways to the involved area.

BEYOND THE ACUTE STATE. The vast majority of pulmonary emboli resolve, and resolve rather quickly. Resolution of fresh emboli begins within the first few days and is well advanced in 10 to 14 days. Two powerful mechanisms promote restoration of vascular patency: the fibrinolytic system and the process of organization. The fibrinolytic system seems specifically designed to dissolve fibrin thrombi wherever they occur in the body and is responsible for the rapid phase of thromboembolic resolution. Organization is a slower process, requiring some days. As it proceeds, the thrombus is gradually transformed into a small scar attached to the vascular wall.

The availability of these two efficient mechanisms raises the question as to why all emboli do not resolve. There may be some impairment of the intrinsic fibrinolytic system. The emboli may have been well organized prior to their lodgment in the lung so that they are neither subject to fibrinolytic attack nor further organization. Alternatively, some emboli may be recurrent so that their failure to resolve is more apparent than real.

Another important element of the natural history of thromboembolism is the development of bronchial arterial collateral circulation. If pulmonary arterial obstruction persists, bronchial arterial flow increases substantially over a period of several weeks, restoring flow to the capillary bed. With the return of flow, surfactant production is restored so that alveolar stability is regained, atelectasis resolves, and alveolar hypocapnia and its resultant pneumoconstriction also subside.

Finally, it should be recognized that many emboli are not totally occlusive. Some distal pulmonary arterial flow often persists and modifies the cardiopulmonary events described above.

DIAGNOSTIC FEATURES

Sudden onset of unexplained dyspnea should suggest the diagnosis of embolism. This symptom, related to the sudden addition of alveolar "dead space," is usually the only one which occurs. *Pleuritic chest pain and hemoptysis are present only when infarction has occurred* and, because bland embolism rarely leads to infarction, are usually absent. With extensive embolism, severe substernal oppressive discomfort may be present. Patients also may present with syncope, suggesting a neurologic disorder. The most reliable symptom, however, is breathlessness. Severe, persistent dyspnea is an ominous sign, for it usually indicates extensive embolic occlusion.

PHYSICAL EXAMINATION. The *physical examination,* like the history, may be deceptively normal. Examination of the lungs may disclose a few atelectatic rales, and localized wheezes may be heard. A pleural friction rub or evidence of pleural effusion will not be present unless infarction has occurred.

On cardiac examination, the single consistent finding is tachycardia. Only in the rare cases of massive embolism will such signs as a right ventricular gallop, a palpable "lift" over the right ventricle, a loud pulmonary closure sound, or prominent *a* waves in the jugular venous pulse be found. A scratchy systolic ejection-type murmur may be heard in the pulmonic area. Also, a systolic or continuous murmur accentuated by inspiration may be audible over the lung fields. These murmurs appear to be generated by turbulence of flow in vessels partially obstructed by emboli since they disappear after resection or resolution of emboli. They should be carefully sought in any patient suspected of PTE. Wide, often fixed, splitting of the second heart sound may be present. This indicates extensive embolic obstruction and implies both severe pulmonary hypertension and right ventricular failure. As embolic resolution occurs, this finding disappears. Absence of an accentuated pulmonic closure sound is not a reliable guide to the severity of PTE, since, when embolism is sufficiently massive to reduce cardiac output, pulmonary closure may be normal or diminished.

The detection of *deep venous thrombosis* qualifies as an excellent clue to the diagnosis of embolism, but its absence should by no means rule out the diagnosis. Even when sought with diligence, thrombophlebitis is found in less than half of patients with PTE. Not only may emboli arise from sites other than the veins of the extremities, but even when deep venous thrombosis is present, it may not be detectable. Often, the entire venous thrombus may have detached as an embolus. *Fever* in patients with pulmonary embolism is uncommon without complicating infection or infarction. With infarction, fever of 100 to 101°F (oral) is the rule; but temperature elevations to 103°F or above may occur, making difficult the differentiation between pulmonary infarction and infection.

On clinical grounds alone, then, a firm diagnosis of embolism is rarely possible, and the clinical suspicion of embolism requires confirmation by laboratory studies.

LABORATORY STUDIES. Routine laboratory studies contribute little toward the diagnosis. Leukocytosis and elevation of the sedimentation rate are rarely present in the absence of infarction. A diagnostic "triad" of elevation of serum lactic dehydrogenase (LDH) and bilirubin with a normal serum glutamic oxalacetic transaminase (SGOT) has been proposed but is of limited value.

Aside from tachycardia, the *electrocardiogram* is normal in most patients. With extensive embolization, there may be evidence of acute pulmonary hypertension: rightward shift of the QRS axis; a tall, peaked P wave; and ST-T changes indicative of right ventricular "strain" and "ischemia." These changes are often transient, lasting minutes to hours, but when persistent, suggest severe pulmonary vascular obstruction.

The *chest roentgenogram* may show a parenchymal infiltrate and evidence of a pleural effusion if *infarction* has occurred. Characteristically, the infiltrates caused by infarction abut against the pleura. However, their shape varies, and they do not usually appear until 12 to 36 hr after the infarction has occurred. The effusion, which often precedes the infiltrate, is characteristically small. Thoracentesis usually yields hemorrhagic fluid, with the characteristics of an exudate.

The radiographic findings with embolism alone are more subtle. *Differences in diameter between vessels which should be of equivalent size* should raise the suspicion of embolism. For example, embolic obstruction of the right main pulmonary artery can lead to dilation of the left main pulmonary artery because that vessel must accept the entire pulmonary flow. There may be *abrupt "cut-off"* of a vessel; i.e., as the vessel is traced distally, it suddenly disappears. Clot has the same radiodensity as blood, accounting for the proximal shadow; the absence of flow beyond the clot explains the sudden radiographic "disappearance" of the vessel.

Organization of a clot within a pulmonary artery may lead to retraction of the vessel's walls and a so-called *"rat-tail configuration,"* in which the vessel is relatively normal proximally and suddenly tapers to a sharp point. Finally, there may be *abnormal radiolucency* in some lung zones due to absent or decreased flow. Such abnormally lucent areas, indicative of proximal arterial obstruction, are best appreciated by examining comparable areas in the two lung fields.

Even in embolization without infarction, the roentgenogram may show small infiltrates, which appear in about 24 hr and reflect atelectasis secondary to surfactant depletion. Unlike those of infarction, they are not associated with effusion, may fail to touch a pleural surface, and disappear without the linear scarring characteristic of infarction. All of these roentgenographic findings are most common in the lower lung fields because embolism favors the lower lobes. Because emboli are often multiple, findings may be present in more than one area. Although these radiologic features should be sought in all patients, they are not definitive and, unfortunately, are often not present. Thus, a *normal chest roentgenogram does not exclude the diagnosis of PTE.*

Fluoroscopy. This procedure may be a useful adjunct to chest roentgenography. While clot and blood have the same radiodensity, a vessel containing clot will exhibit reduced or absent pulsations. Fluoroscopic discovery of a nonpulsatile vessel is a good clue to PTE.

Analysis of Arterial Blood Gases. This may be of diagnostic value, since massive embolism is commonly associated with arterial hypoxemia, hypocapnia, and respiratory alkalosis. In addition, the difference between alveolar P_{CO_2} and arterial P_{CO_2} ("A-a" P_{CO_2} gradient) is widened due to the increase in alveolar dead space (Chap. 280).

The laboratory tests discussed thus far are often negative in PTE and are relatively nonspecific. Therefore, it is usually necessary to proceed to two more definitive techniques: the pulmonary perfusion radiophotoscan and the pulmonary angiogram.

Pulmonary Perfusion Radiophotoscans. These scans are obtained by intravenous injection of gamma-emitting radionuclides. The most commonly used material is macroaggregated albumin (MAA), labeled with [131]Iodine or [99m]Technetium. It is obtained by treating human serum albumin to make aggregates with diameters from 20 to 40 μ. These radioactive particles are trapped in the pulmonary capillary bed because the pulmonary capillaries approximate 10 μ in diameter. Alternatively, [133]Xenon gas, dissolved in saline, may be used, but the patient must hold his breath. It has been established that the distribution of MAA particles entrapped in capillaries, or of [133]Xenon evolved from them, accurately depicts the distribution of pulmonary blood flow.

After injection, a gamma-detecting device records the pattern of radioactivity within the lungs. This radioactive image can be recorded in a variety of ways: on radiographic film, on special photographic film, as a television image, or on videotape. Normal scans exhibit homogeneous distribution of radioactivity, smooth margins, and a configuration which corresponds to the normal anatomy of the lungs. Any deviation from these characteristics requires explanation because it represents abnormalities in blood flow distribution.

The lung photoscan has been most valuable in the diagnosis of embolism. Zones of absent or sharply decreased radioactivity in the patient whose other findings are compatible with PTE provides substantial diagnostic support. Scanning is simple, safe, and rapid. It can be repeated to define the resolution, or recurrence, of obstructive vascular phenomena. Like any laboratory test, however, the photoscan must be applied and interpreted with care. It is important, for example, to obtain multiple scan views because lesions not apparent in one view may be easily detected in another. Furthermore, the lung photoscan demonstrates only abnormalities of the *distribution of blood flow.* It does not provide anatomic information. Many disorders other than PTE are associated with abnormalities in the distribution of pulmonary blood flow. Any disease process, such as pneumonia, atelectasis, or pneumothorax, which reduces the ventilation of a lung zone will decrease its perfusion. Parenchymal diseases, such as emphysema, sarcoidosis, bronchogenic carcinoma, and tuberculosis, can all produce scan defects. Furthermore, emboli may exist without producing obvious scan defects, either because they only partially obstruct the vascular lumen or because the obstructed zones are too small to be detected by current techniques. Despite these limitations, the perfusion photoscan has been invaluable in the diagnosis of embolism when interpreted properly.

Pulmonary Angiography. This is another means for providing anatomic information about the pulmonary vasculature. Injection of radiopaque material, preferably through a cardiac catheter advanced into the pulmonary artery, provides a visual image of the pulmonary vessels which may be recorded on serial roentgenograms, by cinephotography, or on video tape. Cardiac catheterization and angiography require specialized personnel, a reasonable period for preparation and performance, and do entail more risk than the procedures discussed above. However, the procedure has the advantage of providing valuable hemodynamic data which may be necessary for therapeutic decisions. Interpretive limitations of angiography are of three types: (1) *Injection artifacts* may occur which suggest absence of flow to a vessel. Injection should be repeated whenever the question of such artifacts exists. (2) The inability to evaluate the patency of small vessels is another limitation. Emboli in vessels below the resolving capability of the method cannot be detected with certainty. (3) Interpretive errors may also be a consequence of *not looking for the proper type of defect.* Classically, the angiogram shows an *abrupt "cutoff"* of a vessel at the point of embolic impaction. However, complete embolic obstruction is uncommon. Therefore, *filling defects* are the most frequent finding; i.e., the embolus creates a "negative" shadow as the radiopaque material flows around it. Also, a *decrease in filling* of a lung zone suggests embolic obstruction.

How far one should proceed down the diagnostic pathway outlined above depends on many factors, the major ones being the severity of the patient's symptoms, and therefore, the urgency of the need for prompt and precise diagnosis. There should be no complacency in dealing with this potentially lethal disease. Photoscanning should be employed in any suspected case. Furthermore, there should be no hesitancy in proceeding to catheterization and angiography when a correct therapeutic decision is at stake.

TREATMENT

Once a diagnosis of PTE has been established, management is determined by two considerations: (1) the degree to which the circulation has been compromised; and (2) the natural history of the disease. In time, most emboli will resolve. Therefore, the goals of therapy should be to sustain life until resolution can occur, and to prevent embolic recurrence. In most instances, *medical therapy* with anticoagulant drugs is adequate. Heparin is the drug of choice for several reasons: immediate onset of action; potent inhibition of the coagulation system; enhancement of fibrinolytic dissolution of fresh thrombi; inhibition of platelet breakdown (and therefore serotonin release); and prompt reversibility of anticoagulant action.

There are some differences of opinion regarding the specific techniques by which the drug should be given. A consensus would suggest that therapy should be initiated with an intravenous injection of 15,000 units, followed by intravenous administration of 5,000 to 7,500 units every 4 hr. If intravenous therapy cannot be maintained reliably, heparin should be given subcutaneously in doses of 7,500 units every 6 hr or 10,000 units every 8 hr. Intramuscular injection should be avoided because hematomas result. The need for, and utility of, clotting times to guide therapy is debated. If done improperly, this test is worthless, and may be misleading. If used appropriately, the usual objective is to keep the clotting time, measured *just prior to the next dose* of drug, 2 to 3 times the baseline clotting time (or 20 to 30 min, assuming a normal clotting time of 8 to 10 min). Heparin therapy should be maintained until the patient's cardiopulmonary status has stabilized and any evidence of venous thrombosis has resolved. Because thrombi become firmly attached to vessel wall and are well along the road toward organization within 5 to 7 days, patients should be maintained at bed rest for at least that period. If possible, ambulation is begun on heparin therapy, with elastic supports applied to the legs. If symptoms do not recur, the heparin may be tapered over the next 36 to 48 hr and then discontinued.

Prothrombinopenic drugs are not suitable for initial therapy in embolism. Their only role is in maintaining anticoagulant protection for prolonged periods. This is advisable if conditions exist which suggest that venous thrombosis and embolism are likely to recur, such as congestive heart failure, chronic venous insufficiency of the lower extremities, or the need for prolonged bed rest. In the absence of such indications, heparin alone suffices.

Thrombolytic (fibrinolytic) agents such as plasmin and urokinase have the potential of actually dissolving fresh thromboemboli. Despite extensive study, their efficacy and safety for routine clinical use remains to be established. Thrombolytic drugs should have their greatest utility in patients with massive embolism in whom surgical intervention would otherwise be contemplated.

Surgical therapy should be reserved for those patients in whom heparin therapy is deemed inadequate or impractical. Anticoagulant therapy may be contradicted by the presence of a bleeding diathesis, or the patient may be in such critical condition that it is felt unwise to await a response to medical therapy. In such instances *venous ligation* and *pulmonary embolectomy* must be considered.

The objective of venous ligation is to prevent immediate recurrence of embolism. Ligation of the superficial femoral vein offers no protection against embolization from the deep femoral venous system, and ligation of the common femoral vein is unacceptable because of severe obstruction to venous drainage. Furthermore, these procedures must be bilateral to grant protection from a suspected embolic focus in the legs. For these reasons, interruption of the inferior vena cava has replaced more distal ligation procedures. A number of surgical procedures have been applied to the inferior vena cava: simple ligation; plication, in which fine channels are preserved; and the application of totally or partially occlusive "clips." Each procedure has advantages and disadvantages. For example, total interruption leads to variable degrees of edema of the legs, while successful plication does not prevent small emboli from reaching the lungs. Unfortunately, inferior vena caval interruption does not preclude embolic recurrence. There are several reasons for this: sizable collateral channels develop weeks to months after interruption of the cava, through which embolization may recur; thromboembolism may originate at the site of caval manipulation; caval blockade does not prevent embolization from foci within the right cardiac chambers. Therefore, because most pulmonary emboli do resolve, caval surgery should be regarded as a *lifesaving procedure* to be restricted to patients who could not tolerate an *immediate* embolic recurrence. To elect this procedure, definite evidence of cardiopulmonary compromise by embolism is required, and there should be reasonable assurance that the embolic source is in the caval drainage area.

Caval interruption is not a formidable surgical procedure, but may be associated with substantial morbidity. It should be used therefore only when required, and with recognition that it does not necessarily provide long-term protection. There is one instance, however, in which prompt caval ligation is the therapy of choice: septic thrombophlebitis of pelvic origin with multiple septic pulmonary emboli. These patients may die unless caval (and left ovarian vein) ligation is carried out promptly.

The decision to carry out emergency *pulmonary embolectomy* has many features in common with the decision to interrupt the inferior vena cava. In addition, however, since embolectomy is a major, complex operation which has been associated with a 50 percent mortality, the decision to carry out this procedure is a difficult one. However, there is agreement that two criteria should be met before embolectomy is performed: (1) there must be evidence of severe hemodynamic compromise due to embolism which is not responsive to supportive measures; and (2) the personnel and equipment required for embolectomy must be available.

These criteria require angiographic confirmation of the

extent and location of the embolus except under the most unusual circumstances when a scan might suffice. Hemodynamic measurements are extremely helpful. Facilities for cardiopulmonary bypass should be available. Unless these requirements are met, the opportunity for error is great and the chances of successful embolectomy, limited —indeed, possibly less than with medical therapy.

SPECIAL CONSIDERATIONS. Total resolution of emboli does not always occur. If residual vascular obstruction is substantial, the patient may present, months or years after the actual embolic events, with dyspnea and pulmonary hypertension of uncertain etiology. Multiple undetected recurrent small emboli may produce the same picture. These patients may masquerade with the diagnosis of "chronic lung disease" or "primary" pulmonary hypertension (Chap. 286).

Such patients should be studied by appropriate techniques, since larger emboli are potentially resectable, even after having been present for months to years. These patients represent potentially curable forms of otherwise fatal pulmonary hypertensive disease.

Embolism should also be suspected in other clinical contexts: as a precipitating cause for cardiac arrhythmia; as a reason for sudden or progressive worsening of congestive heart failure (Chap. 264); as an explanation for sudden deterioration in the patient with chronic obstructive pulmonary disease; and as a possible alternative to the diagnosis of "psychic" hyperventilation.

PROPHYLAXIS. The ultimate goal in thromboembolism is its prevention, and certain measures can be invoked to limit the occurrence of venous thrombosis and pulmonary embolism. Elastic stockings or bandages should be used in any patient requiring a prolonged period of bed rest, particularly when venous stasis is present. Early ambulation should be encouraged in the postpartum and postoperative periods. Prophylactic use of anticoagulant drugs is indicated in patients over the age of forty years with fractures of the pelvis or lower extremities in whom a period of 10 days of immobilization is anticipated, and in patients with severe congestive heart failure. Truly effective prophylaxis, however, must await a better understanding of the pathogenesis of thrombosis, and tests which can identify individuals with thrombotic tendencies.

REFERENCES

Gray, F. D.: "Pulmonary Embolism," Philadelphia, Lea & Febiger, 1966.

Moser, K. M., V. N. Houk, R. C. Jones, and C. C. Hufnagel: Chronic Massive Thrombotic Obstruction of Pulmonary Arteries. Analysis of Four Operated Cases, Circulation, 32:377, 1965.

Moser, K. M., G. P. Harsanyi, G. Rius-Garriga, M. Guisan, G. A. Landis, and A. Miale, Jr.: Assessment of Pulmonary Photoscanning and Angiography in Experimental Pulmonary Embolism. Circulation 39:663, 1969.

Nasbeth, D. C., and J. M. Moran: Reassessment of the Role of Inferior Vena Cava Ligation in Venous Thormboembolism, New Engl. J. Med., 273:1250, 1965.

Sasahara, A. A., and M. Stein: "Pulmonary Embolic Disease," New York, Grune & Stratton, Inc., 1965.

Swenson, E. W., T. N. Finley, and S. V. Guzman: Unilateral Hypoventilation in Man during Temporary Occlusion of One Pulmonary Artery, J. Clin. Invest., 40:828, 1961.

Thomas, D. P: Treatment of Pulmonary Embolic Disease, Critical Review of Some Aspects of Current Therapy, New Engl. J. Med., 273:885, 1965.

Torrance, D. J: "The Chest Film in Massive Pulmonary Embolism," Springfield, Ill., Charles C Thomas Publisher, 1963.

286 PRIMARY PULMONARY HYPERTENSION

John Ross, Jr.

Primary (or idiopathic) pulmonary hypertension is an uncommon disease, the diagnosis of which can be established only after a thorough search for the usual causes of pulmonary hypertension. The patient with primary pulmonary hypertension typically is a young female between the ages of twenty and forty, although older and younger patients of either sex have been described. The clinical and laboratory features of severe pulmonary hypertension are present, but there is no evidence of parenchymal pulmonary disease or organic cardiac disease, nor is there cause to suspect the occurrence of pulmonary emboli. In the past, anatomic verification often has been necessary to distinguish clearly the primary form of pulmonary hypertension from that due to multiple pulmonary emboli, although angiography and radioisotope scanning methods have facilitated this differentiation considerably.

PATHOLOGY. The findings on pathologic examination of patients with primary pulmonary hypertension usually are confined to the right side of the heart and lungs. The right atrium often is enlarged and the right ventricle is hypertrophied. Frequently, the large pulmonary arteries exhibit atherosclerotic plaques. The disease process involves the small pulmonary arteries (between 40 and 300μ in diameter) which exhibit muscular hypertrophy and intimal hyperplasia, sometimes with fibrosis. Abnormal vascular structures or plexiform lesions also have been described and are attributed by some investigators to recanalization of thrombi, by others to abnormal vascular anastomoses. On occasion, a necrotizing arteritis may be encountered. Fowler and his associates have contrasted these pathologic findings with those in thromboembolic pulmonary hypertension, in which similar disease of the small pulmonary vessels may be observed, but in addition thrombotic material is present in the larger pulmonary vessels (300μ to 1.5 mm in diameter). Rarely, disease of the systemic arterial vascular bed resembling that found in the pulmonary blood vessels has been described. In this connection, James has attributed the syncope and sudden death which may occur in this disease to involvement of the coronary arterial branch supplying the sinoatrial node.

ETIOLOGY. The cause of primary pulmonary hypertension is unknown, but a number of possible etiologic factors have been suggested. A few patients with primary pulmonary hypertension have been reported in whom minimal changes were found in the pulmonary vessels on pathologic examination, and this observation has raised the possibility that a neurohumoral vasoconstrictor mechanism is involved. Support for this view has been provided by the observation that the pulmonary vascular resistance can be acutely reduced in some patients with this disease by the intrapulmonary injection of vasodilators, or by breathing oxygen. A febrile illness may precede the onset of the disease by a variable period and has been implicated in the etiology. The occurrence of the disease in young females has prompted the suggestion that unrecognized thromboemboli or amniotic fluid embodi during pregnancy may play a role. In other patients, it seems quite possible that the disease may represent an end stage of earlier, unrecognized emboli originating from the legs or pelvic veins.

Raynaud's disease has preceded the onset of primary pulmonary hypertensive disease by a number of years in an appreciable number of patients. This association and the occurrence of Raynaud's disease in scleroderma, disseminated lupus erythematosus, rheumatoid arthritis, and dermatomyositis has led to the speculation that primary pulmonary hypertension may represent a form of collagen vascular disease. It also has been suggested that the disease may be congenital and present from birth; however, the closely packed, parallel elastic fibers in the main pulmonary arteries in patients having Eisenmenger's syndrome from birth, described by Heath and Edwards, usually have not been observed in patients with primary pulmonary hypertension. Finally, primary pulmonary hypertension has been reported in a number of families; sometimes more than two members and up to three generations have been affected.

PATHOPHYSIOLOGY. Some studies have suggested that the response of the pulmonary vascular bed is labile early in the course of this disease, as evidenced by a response to vasodilating agents and oxygen. It also has been proposed that the disease tends to progress. Thus, serial cardiac catheterizations in several patients by Sleeper and his coworkers have shown a tendency for the pulmonary vascular resistance to increase and to become fixed. With the development of severe pulmonary vascular disease, abnormal elevation of the pulmonary arterial pressure occurs, often to a striking degree, and the pulmonary arterial pressure may be equal to that in the systemic arterial bed. The pulmonary arterial wedge pressure is normal in patients with primary pulmonary hypertension, the cardiac output is normal or reduced, and no intracardiac shunts are detected. In many patients the mean right atrial pressure is elevated, and the *a* wave in the right atrium may be markedly elevated, an indication of the forceful atrial contraction necessary to fill the hypertrophied right ventricle. With the long-standing overload on the right heart, right ventricular

failure finally develops. In some patients, peripheral cyanosis occurs secondary to reduced cardiac output, and occasionally central cyanosis becomes evident at the end stage of the disease due to right to left shunting through a patent foramen ovale. Mild systemic arterial desaturation is quite common, even in the absence of heart failure, and may be due to shunting within the lungs. Pulmonary function in patients with primary pulmonary hypertension generally is normal, although hyperventilation often is present, resulting in hypocapnia and a decreased serum bicarbonate concentration.

CLINICAL PICTURE

The patient, usually a young female, gives a history of relatively recent onset of symptoms. Ordinarily, the natural course of the disease encompasses less than 5 years. Not uncommonly, patients with primary pulmonary hypertension are classified as neurotic early in the course of their disease because of the hyperventilation, chest discomfort, and the relative paucity of objective findings. Precordial pain on exertion occurs in from 25 to 50 percent of patients, and occasionally severe chest pain has been associated with a dissection of the main pulmonary artery. Other common symptoms are weakness, fatigue, exertional dyspnea, and effort syncope. Hoarseness may be noted due to compression of the left recurrent laryngeal nerve by the enlarged pulmonary artery. Unexplained, sudden death occurs relatively often. Sudden death also has occurred during cardiac catheterization or surgical procedures and after the administration of barbiturates or anesthetic agents. The terminal course usually is characterized by right heart failure.

On physical examination, the jugular venous pulse usually shows a prominent *a* wave, there is a right ventricular heave, and an impulse may be felt over the region of the main pulmonary artery. An ejection click may be audible at the pulmonic area, the second heart sound is narrowly split, and the pulmonic closure sound is markedly accentuated. Often, an atrial gallop sound is heard at the lower left sternal border, and in some patients there is an ejection murmur at the pulmonic area, or the early diastolic murmur of pulmonic regurgitation. The chest roentgenogram may show cardiac enlargement with right ventricular and right atrial prominence, and there is marked dilatation of the pulmonary artery segment. Peripherally, the pulmonary arteries taper sharply, and the lung fields appear oligemic. The electrocardiogram almost always shows some evidence of right ventricular enlargement, with right axis deviation, right ventricular hypertrophy in the precordial leads, and sometimes inverted T waves over the right precordium. Right atrial enlargement also may be evident on the electrocardiagram.

DIFFERENTIAL DIAGNOSIS. It is imperative that the diagnosis of primary pulmonary hypertension not be made until potentially treatable causes of elevated pulmonary arterial pressure have been excluded. The presence of cor pulmonale can be established readily by finding abnormalities in pulmonary function. Cardiac catheterization studies are necessary to search for a primary cardiac defect, and angiography or radioactive lung-scanning studies also may be indicated to detect pulmonary emboli (Chap. 285). Patients having chronic emboli to the lungs are difficult to distinguish from those with primary pulmonary hypertension, but the distinction is important because anticoagulants, inferior vena caval or common femoral vein ligation, and pulmonary embolectomy sometimes have been effective in patients with embolic disease. Often a site of origin for emboli cannot be identified in the leg veins, and other possible sources should be considered, such as right atrial thrombus, or ovarian and pelvic vein thromboses.

Several congenital cardiac conditions must be considered and excluded by appropriate cardiac catheterization studies. Valvular pulmonic stenosis usually can be distinguished from pulmonary hypertension by identification of the delayed, soft pulmonic closure sound, but peripheral stenoses of the pulmonary arteries can be associated with an increased second heart sound. A left-to-right shunt at the pulmonary arterial, ventricular or atrial levels should be sought. The wide, fixed splitting of the second heart sound should be helpful in identifying patients with atrial septal defect. Eisenmenger's syndrome in a patient with ventricular septal defect or patent ductus arteriosus (Chap. 268) may be confused with primary pulmonary hypertension, but usually in Eisenmenger's syndrome cyanosis, polycythemia, and clubbing are present, and at cardiac catheterization a large right-to-left shunt at the ventricular or pulmonary arterial level can be demonstrated.

The murmurs of tricuspid or pulmonic regurgitation, and the atrial gallop sounds heard in patients with primary pulmonary hypertension may be mistaken for the murmurs of rheumatic mitral and aortic valve disease, or vice versa. Before making the diagnosis of primary pulmonary hypertension, the presence of left atrial hypertension due to undetected mitral stenosis, or to a more unusual lesion such as left atrial myxoma, should be specifically sought and excluded. This can be done by obtaining a pulmonary arterial wedge pressure tracing or by left heart catheterization, with angiography if necessary.

THERAPY. Presently, there is no definitive treatment available for patients with primary pulmonary hypertension, and therapy during their progressive downhill course therefore must be palliative. The use of anticoagulants is of doubtful value, provided chronic pulmonary embolic phenomena can be excluded. Right heart failure should be treated with a cardiotonic and diuretic regimen (Chap. 264). Since there is no hypercapnia in these patients, the hypoxia which may accompany heart failure can be treated safely with oxygen therapy.

Pharmacologic approaches to therapy have proved disappointing, and while transient reductions in pulmonary vascular resistance can be observed with intrapulmonary arterial injection of acetylcholine or talazoline, the chronic oral use of these agents has not been effective. The possibility of performing lung transplantation has, of course, been under consideration for many years, and much experimental work in animals is directed toward this goal.

REFERENCES

Fowler, N. O., B. Black-Schaffer, R. C. Scott, and M. Gueron: Idiopathic and Thromboembolic Pulmonary Hypertension, Am. J. Med., 40:331, 1966.

Heath, D., and J. E. Edwards: Configuration of Elastic Tissue of Pulmonary Trunk in Idiopathic Pulmonary Hypertension, Circulation, 21:59, 1960.

Liebow, A. A.: Cardiovascular Disease: Pulmonary Hypertension, Ann. Rev. Med., 2:95, 1960.

Melmon, K. L., and E. Braunwald: Familial Pulmonary Hypertension, New Engl. J. Med., 269:770–775, 1963.

Winters, W. L., Jr., R. R. Joseph, and N. Learner: Pulmonary Hypertension and Raynaud's Phenomenon, Arch. Intern. Med., 114:821, 1964.

Wood, P.: Pulmonary Hypertension, Mod. Conc. Cardiovasc. Dis., 28:512, 1959.

287 COR PULMONALE
Alfred P. Fishman

DEFINITION. The term *cor pulmonale* is used to indicate enlargement of the right ventricle secondary to a disorder of the pulmonary parenchyma or vasculature or a disturbance in the act of breathing. If the initiating disorder for cor pulmonale is in the lungs, the disease will be diffuse, bilateral, and extensive, in most cases affecting the airways as well as the parenchyma. Alternatively, if the pathogenetic mechanism is a disturbance in the act of breathing, the derangement may be either in the control of breathing or in the mechanical performance of the chest cage.

This definition has several practical implications. By involving the lungs and ventilatory apparatus as the major elements in the pathogenesis of cor pulmonale, it underscores the fact that prognosis and treatment of cor pulmonale depend more on the adequate treatment of the respiratory disorder than on cardiotonic or diuretic therapy. As a corollary, it excludes disorders of the left side of the heart, e.g., mitral stenosis, left-sided heart failure, and congenital heart disease, in which the pulmonary disorder and right ventricular enlargement are secondary to a disorder on the left side of the heart and in which the heart, rather than the lungs or ventilatory apparatus, is the main target of treatment. Finally, by stressing *enlargement* rather than *failure* of the right ventricle as a criterion for cor pulmonale, the definition indicates that right ventricular failure is a complication, rather than an essential feature, of cor pulmonale.

TYPES OF COR PULMONALE. By tradition, the designation "acute" is generally reserved for the dilatation of the right side of the heart which follows acute embolization of the lungs. This is a complicated process, involving nervous as well as mechanical factors (Chap. 285). The designation "chronic" is less specific. Usually it indicates an enlargement of the right ventricle in the course of a continuing pulmonary or ventilatory disorder. Just how long the heart remains enlarged depends on the natural history of the respiratory disorder and its response to treatment. Acordingly, "chronic" refers more to the "pulmonale" than to the "cor."

INCIDENCE. Because of the prevalence of diffuse pulmonary disease, cor pulmonale is a common type of heart disease. Men are more often affected than women. In parts of the world where air pollution is marked and bronchitis is severe, e.g., England or India, cor pulmonale may comprise up to one-quarter of all kinds of heart failure. It is a common complication in adult patients with cystic fibrosis and often is the cause of death. Cor pulmonale is rarely a complication of the allergic asthma of childhood, even though it often complicates asthmatic bronchitis in adults. Most chronic pulmonary disorders are too limited in extent to strain the right side of the heart. Indeed, even the great majority of those patients with the disseminated lesions of silicosis, emphysema, or diffuse fibrosis, who suffer from severe breathlessness for many years, fail to develop any clinical evidence of cardiac involvement attributable to their pulmonary disorders.

PATHOGENESIS OF COR PULMONALE

Prerequisite for cor pulmonale is an increase in the work of the right side of the heart. Regularly, the increased work load is in the form of pulmonary hypertension; occasionally, a high cardiac output also contributes. Since the increased cardiac output is of only secondary importance, the pathogenesis of cor pulmonale should be sought in mechanisms which elicit pulmonary hypertension. For convenience, these mechanisms may be divided into two groups: (1) anatomic restriction of the pulmonary vascular bed and (2) alveolar hypoventilation. Often these mechanisms coexist. Indeed, in patients with extensive anatomic curtailment of the pulmonary vascular bed, sufficient pulmonary hypertension to strain the right side of the heart rarely occurs without some degree of alveolar hypoventilation.

ANATOMIC RESTRICTION. In the normal individual, the pulmonary circulation is a highly distensible, capacious, low-pressure system. A cardiac output of 5 to 6 liters per min at rest is acommodated with pulmonary arterial pressures of 20 to 28 mm Hg in systole and 8 to 12 mm Hg in diastole; increases up to three times this blood flow, such as occur during moderate exercise, are associated with only slight increments in pulmonary arterial pressures. However, if there is sufficient restriction in pulmonary vascular extent and distensibility, even modest increments in blood flow may elicit considerable pulmonary hypertension. Such restriction may occur from extensive pulmonary resection, from a widespread destruction of small pulmonary blood vessels, from arteriosclerotic narrowing, thickening, and occlusion of pulmonary arteries and small vessels, and from multiple pulmonary emboli or thrombosis. In addition to these mechanisms, which affect the pulmonary vascular bed directly, the pulmonary

vascular bed may become more rigid and increase its resistance to blood flow as a consequence of adjacent parenchymal disease or edema, or from the extrapulmonary distortion and compression which accompany severe skeletal deformity.

The normal pulmonary vascular bed can maintain normal or virtually normal pressure-flow relations with as little as one-third of normal functioning lung. Even patients who have had a pneumonectomy can accommodate a two- or threefold increment in pulmonary blood flow with only a minimal increase in pulmonary artery pressures, as long as the remaining lung is free of fibrosis, emphysema, or pulmonary vascular change. Similarly, a considerable reduction in the pulmonary capillary bed, as occurs in emphysema, is generally insufficient to elicit pulmonary hypertension unless alveolar hypoventilation coexists.

ALVEOLAR HYPOVENTILATION. Pathologists are often disappointed by the disparity between the degrees of pulmonary hypertension and anatomic changes in the lungs and pulmonary vessels. This discrepancy is particularly marked in patients with severe bronchitis in whom the anatomic changes in the lungs and airways consistently appear to be inadequate to explain the functional abnormalities. But much of the discrepancy disappears when account is taken of alveolar hypoventilation and the corresponding changes in the blood gases.

Although both the alveolar P_{O_2} and P_{CO_2} are abnormal in alveolar hypoventilation, the arterial P_{CO_2} is the more useful clinical index of the adequacy of the alveolar ventilation. Thus, in practice, an arterial P_{CO_2} (approximately the same as the alveolar P_{CO_2}) in excess of 45 mm Hg is accepted as evidence of alveolar hypoventilation. A decrease in P_{O_2} regularly accompanies the increase in P_{CO_2}. If hypercapnia has persisted for more than hours, the serum bicarbonate level will also increase—in part because of CO_2 retention by the kidney —tending to return arterial pH toward normal values.

Recognizing that alveolar hypoventilation is the main cause of cor pulmonale is critical for two reasons: (1) elimination of the initiating mechanism (e.g., bronchitis) usually reverses the alveolar hypoventilation, and (2) unless alveolar ventilation is improved, other therapeutic measures are apt to be ineffective. On etiologic grounds, clinical instances of alveolar hypoventilation may be sorted into two groups (Table 287-1).

1. General Alveolar Hypoventilation. Either because of an inadequate ventilatory drive from the respiratory center or an unresponsive chest bellows, the lungs are not ventilated adequately. The entire lung shares in the underventilation, even though there may be regional differences in degree arising from regional differences in the mechanical properties of the normal lungs. Theoretically, as P_{CO_2} increases, P_{O_2} should decrease proportionately, milligram of mercury for milligram of mercury. Actually, the decrease in P_{O_2} is usually somewhat greater than would be predicted, because of collapse and, occasionally, infection of the most underventilated parts of the lungs.

2. Net Alveolar Hypoventilation. The fundamental defect is an imbalance between alveolar ventilation and

Table 287-1. TYPES OF CHRONIC ALVEOLAR HYPOVENTILATION

I. General alveolar hypoventilation
   A. Inadequate ventilatory drive from respiratory center
      1. Functional depression of respiratory center
         a. Sleep
         b. Carbon dioxide retention
         c. Metabolic alkalosis
            (1) Vomiting
            (2) Some diuretics
         d. Mountain sickness (seroche)
      2. Anatomic (irreversible) demage to respiratory center
   B. Poorly responsive breathing apparatus
      1. Irreversible derangement
         a. Dwarfed and deformed chest cage
         b. Neuromuscular disorders of respiratory muscles
            (1) Poliomyelitis
            (2) Muscular dystrophy
            (3) Guillain-Barré
      2. Reversible derangement
         a. Extreme obesity
         b. Myxedema
         c. Fibrothorax
II. Net alveolar hypoventilation
   A. Obstructive diseases of the airways
      1. Bronchitis
      2. Cystic fibrosis of the pancreas
      3. Asthma
   B. Distortion of pulmonary parenchyma
      1. Massive pulmonary fibrosis
      2. Healed, conglomerate tuberculosis

blood flow so that alveolar-capillary gas exchange is ineffective even though total ventilation is either normal or excessive. Because of the bronchopulmonary disease, alveolar ventilation varies enormously with respect to perfusion in different parts of the lungs: some parts are hyperventilated, but most of the lung is hypoventilated; the net result, as in general alveolar hypoventilation, is hypercapnia and hypoxia.

The clinical consequences of alveolar hypoventilation arise from the arterial hypoxemia, hypercapnia, and acidosis. The abnormal blood gases exert their adverse physiologic effects in different ways: hypoxia acts mainly on the circulation, taxing the right side of the heart chiefly by way of pulmonary vasoconstriction and, to a lesser degree, by hypervolemia, polycythemia, and occasionally by an increased cardiac output. That hypoxemia rather than hypercapnia is responsible for the load on the circulation is supported by the occurrence of pulmonary hypertension and enlargement of the right ventricle in native residents at high altitude (Morococha, Peru—14,900 ft) where hypoxemia is unassociated with hypercapnia. On the other hand, hypercapnia affects mainly the central nervous system, producing cerebral vasodilatation (and increased cerebrospinal fluid pressure) and a neurologic disorder ranging from weakness, irritability, lassitude, and a cloudy sensorium to somnolence, confusion, and coma. When severe hypoxemia and hypercapnia coexist, it may be impossible to distinguish between their neurologic effects because severe hypoxia causes anatomic damage to nervous tissues. The acidosis

which complicates the abnormal blood gases enhances the pulmonary vasoconstricting effects of hypoxia. However, it merits no special treatment, since it stimulates the ventilation.

Carbon dioxide retention, with elevated CO_2 tensions in the blood and tissues, has two untoward effects: (1) a blunting of the responsiveness of the respiratory center to the CO_2 stimulus, and (2) a retention of bicarbonate by the kidney. In turn, both these effects promote further CO_2 retention. Moreover, not only the hypercapnia from a primary disorder of the lungs or ventilation, but also the hypercapnia of metabolic alkalosis may contribute to this functional depression. Somnolence and coma are most apt to occur if hypercapnia is sudden in onset and severe in degree. Because of the respiratory depression, patients with chronic hypercapnia are particularly vulnerable to the effects of sedatives or oxygen breathing, both of which may induce calamitous increments in the degree of hypercapnia: sedatives by depressing further the respiratory centers in the brain; oxygen by abolishing the hypoxic peripheral drive to ventilation. It is usually in the severely hypoxic, hypercapnic patient that right-sided heart failure occurs.

THE HEART IN COR PULMONALE

In patients who develop cor pulmonale, pulmonary hypertension first appears either when blood flow is increased or during a bout of acute hypoxia, e.g., during exercise or pulmonary infection. In time, pulmonary hypertension may even be present at rest. At first, the pulmonary hypertension during exercise or hypoxia is associated with normal filling pressure in the right ventricle. But as pulmonary hypertension is prolonged or becomes more severe, abnormally high filling pressures (end-diastolic) develop in the right ventricle, a reflection of ventricular hypertrophy and inadequate ventricular emptying. Finally, if right-sided heart failure does occur, pulmonary arterial pressures are found to be quite high, reaching levels of 80/50 mm Hg; end-diastolic pressures in the right ventricle are high at rest (greater than 10 mm Hg), and systemic veins are congested.

In older patients who have suffered myocardial infarcts or have other reasons for left ventricular disease, the left atrial pressure may be high. But in the great majority of patients with cor pulmonale, left-sided heart pressures are entirely normal. Some confusion exists concerning involvement of the left side of the heart in cor pulmonale, largely because of the use of unreliable indices of left atrial pressure and failure to take into serious account the likelihood of independent disease of the left ventricle, particularly in older patients.

CLINICAL MANIFESTATIONS OF COR PULMONALE

Because there are no certain clinical indices of pulmonary hypertension in patients with chronic pulmonary or ventilatory disorders, cor pulmonale is often recognized for the first time only when right ventricular dilatation has progressed to the point of failure. The onset of right-sided heart failure may be insidious, with gradually increasing edema of the ankles and legs, over days or weeks. Or right-sided heart failure may appear suddenly, especially during an acute respiratory infection which further compromises gas exchange.

Suspicion of cor pulmonale depends on the recognition of an appropriate pulmonary or ventilatory disorder. These disorders are considered below. The problem is particularly troublesome and critical in the elderly patient who has had a productive cough for years and is just as apt to be suffering from combined right and left ventricular disease consequent to arteriosclerosis as from cor pulmonale. The likelihood of pulmonary arterial hypertension and normal pulmonary venous pressures is strengthened by finding clinical evidence of hypoxemia and hypercapnia, and corresponding abnormalities in the blood gases. The enlargement of the right side of the heart may be too subtle for clinical detection. Indeed, without right-sided heart catheterization, the diagnosis of cor pulmonale is more often established by roentgenogram and electrocardiogram than at the bedside.

A right ventricular protodiastolic gallop rhythm is common in cor pulmonale. Hydrothorax is uncommon, even after the advent of frank congestive failure. Permanent arrhythmias, such as atrial flutter or fibrillation, are uncommon. Transitory arrhythmias may occur when severe hypoxia or respiratory alkalosis has been induced by treatment.

The diagnostic value of the electrocardiogram varies according to the underlying pulmonary or ventilatory disorder. Thus, where cor pulmonale follows multiple pulmonary emboli, the electrocardiographic pattern may resemble that of acute cor pulmonale. On the other hand, it is least helpful in obstructive pulmonary disease, where it is complicated by changes in the position of the heart and overdistended lungs. Thus, conventional criteria allow a clear-cut diagnosis of right ventricular enlargement to be made in only one-quarter of patients with obstructive lung disease whose hearts show right ventricular hypertrophy at autopsy.

CLINICAL FORMS OF COR PULMONALE AND THEIR TREATMENT

In order to illustrate physiologic principles, the various clinical forms of cor pulmonale will be divided according to pathogenetic mechanisms.

DISEASES ASSOCIATED WITH RESTRICTION OF THE PULMONARY VASCULAR BED. Anatomic changes in the pulmonary arterial tree, if sufficiently extensive, may become associated with a sustained and progressive pulmonary hypertension. Once pulmonary hypertension from any cause is established, it tends to aggravate itself because of secondary pulmonary atherosclerotic changes. Only in the terminal stages of these diseases does appreciable hypoxia introduce a reversible element for treatment. The prototypes of pulmonary diseases that restrict the pulmonary vascular bed are occlusive disorders of the small pulmonary arteries and diffuse granulomatous

and/or fibrotic disorders; extensive bullous emphysema may have the same effect, but the patients usually die of ventilatory insufficiency rather than cor pulmonale. The dwarfed, distorted lung of the kyphoscoliotic patient may also severely compromise the pulmonary vascular bed, but alveolar hypoventilation is the predominant mechanism for cor pulmonale in such patients.

Occlusive Disease of the Small Pulmonary Arteries. In these disorders, there is widespread, usually gradual occlusion (taking place over years) of the small pulmonary vessels. The most common mechanism is multiple pulmonary emboli; less common are the multiple thromboses which complicate sickle-cell anemia and "primary pulmonary hypertension," which may be no more than a healed stage of multiple pulmonary emboli. Anatomically, there is obliteration of much of the distal pulmonary arterial tree by clotted materials and by organization.

Clinically, the outstanding features in these patients are tachypnea (even while asleep), breathlessness on mild exertion, and striking evidence of right ventricular enlargement both on the roentgenogram and the electrocardiogram. Because the lungs and chest are normal, the electrocardiogram is a valuable index of right ventricular hypertrophy. Because of the fixed changes in the vascular walls, once heart failure develops, it is rarely reversible. Cyanosis, which is rarely striking before the onset of heart failure, usually becomes intense with the advent of heart failure. The clinical impression may be confirmed by pulmonary angiography and scanning.

Of all the patients with cor pulmonale, these have the highest pulmonary arterial pressures. Levels of pulmonary arterial pressure approximating systemic arterial pressures are not uncommon. The cardiac output is low. Mild arterial hypoxemia is the rule and seems to arise from shunting within the lungs. Whether the "shunt" represents flow through recanalized vessels no longer in contact with alveoli, or too-rapid flow of the entire cardiac output through the remaining portions of the pulmonary vascular tree, or the opening of latent anatomic pulmonary arteriovenous channels is conjectural. Chronic hyperventilation, manifested by a low arterial P_{CO_2} and serum bicarbonate level, is characteristic.

Treatment is palliative because of the irreversible changes in the pulmonary blood vessels. Anticoagulation is commonly employed, presumably directed at the source of the emboli, but its value remains uncertain. Inferior vena caval ligation and embolectomy are of little value once pulmonary hypertension exists. Oxygen may be administered with impunity for relief of hypoxemia since there is no hypercapnia. Heart failure is treated with the usual cardiotonic program.

DIFFUSE GRANULOMATOUS AND/OR FIBROTIC DISORDERS. This group includes (1) the various granulomatoses of the lung, such as sarcoidosis, berylliosis, and the "nonspecific" granulomatoses; (2) scleroderma of the lung; (3) the various interstitial or alveolar-septal fibroses such as "nonspecific" infections, or pulmonary asbestosis, or the special progressive form known as the Hamman-Rich syndrome; and (4) rarely, pulmonary adenomatosis, or "alveolar cell" carcinoma. Heart failure is usually a terminal event. Unless appreciable arterial hypoxemia develops, it is more usual for such restricted vascular beds to give rise to a modest pulmonary hypertension, particularly during exercise, than to lead to cor pulmonale.

Clinically, the persistent respiratory difficulty begins with an acute respiratory illness. The roentgenogram characteristically shows fine nodular or fibrotic lesions widely distributed throughout both lung fields. Physiologically, the characteristics are a marked increase in respiratory frequency, arterial hypoxemia on exercise (later, also at rest), CO_2 levels slightly low or normal, oxygen consumption which may be normal or increased, depending on the nature of the pulmonary process, and a cardiac output which varies with the level of the oxygen consumption in the early stages but decreases, often to very low levels, when right-sided heart failure supervenes. In some patients, pulmonary hypertension and cor pulmonale may occur without appreciable hypoxemia, suggesting that the anatomic lesions are mainly responsible for the pulmonary hypertension. In most patients, however, the contribution of hypoxemia to pulmonary hypertension increases with time as ventilation-perfusion abnormalities, due to distortion of the pulmonary parenchyma, are superimposed on the original limitation in diffusion.

The success of treatment of heart failure in these disorders depends on the initiating mechanism. Rarely is the underlying lesion in the lungs reversible. In some patients with granulomatous lesions of the lungs, steroids have brought temporary or even permanent improvement. On the other hand, a pulmonary infection or bronchitis may topple a stable patient into heart failure because of the added cardiac burden from hypoxemia. Oxygen therapy rarely poses a hazard in these patients, since carbon dioxide retention is unusual except preterminally, when ventilation-perfusion abnormalities become marked.

DISEASES ASSOCIATED WITH GENERAL ALVEOLAR HYPOVENTILATION (TABLE 287-1). The overriding importance of abnormal blood gases in the pathogenesis of cor pulmonale is illustrated by those types of alveolar hypoventilation in which the lungs are entirely normal ("general alveolar hypoventilation") but are insufficiently driven as the result of some abnormality either in the regulation of ventilation or in the neuromuscular apparatus.

Inadequate Ventilatory Drive. An inadequate ventilatory drive may be either functional or organic in its genesis. Among the functional causes, carbon dioxide retention is paramount. This type of depression complicates carbon dioxide retention from a variety of causes: chronic lung disease, prolonged residence in carbon dioxide–rich environments, and the metabolic alkalosis that follows prolonged vomiting or certain diuretics. The effects of sedatives and of carbon dioxide retention on the ventilatory drive are additive. Also of clinical importance is the fact that in patients with depressed responsiveness to the CO_2 stimulus, the importance of the hypoxic drive to ventilation increases. For these reasons, sedation and uncontrolled oxygen therapy in patients with carbon dioxide retention and hypoxemia may be disastrous.

Anatomic damage to the respiratory centers is a rare cause of general alveolar hypoventilation. The types of injury to the respiratory centers may be of several different kinds, ranging from diffuse and nonspecific inflammatory lesions, such as those which have been found at autopsy in patients with a "dead" respiratory center from unknown cause ("idiopathic"), to the localized lesions which have been described in bulbar poliomyelitis or which may follow cerebral vascular thrombosis. Recent evidence also suggests that x-irradiation of the pituitary gland may cause sufficient damage elsewhere in the brain to cause alveolar hypoventilation. In recent years, the "idiopathic" group has attracted particular attention. An outstanding feature of this group is the prompt restoration of the arterial blood gases to normal by voluntary or mechanical hyperventilation.

Poorly Responsive Ventilatory Apparatus. This group includes both reversible and irreversible derangements of the chest bellows.

Among the *irreversible* types, structural disorders of the chest are the most important. Severe kyphoscoliosis, sufficient to cause dwarfing, is the main example. Because of the severely deformed, stiff chest and the small lungs, the mechanics of breathing are abnormal; the abnormal elastic resistance of the chest wall somehow sets a ventilatory pattern of rapid shallow breathing, one in which alveolar ventilation is sacrificed for dead-space ventilation.

Neuromuscular Disorders. Various kinds of neuromuscular disorders may also lead to chronic alveolar hypoventilation. These disorders, in which the muscles of respiration are either damaged or inadequately stimulated, include muscular dystrophy as well as subclinical damage to respiratory muscles and nerves after apparent clinical recovery from poliomyelitis and Guillain-Barré disease. Poliomyelitis has a more complicated basis for alveolar hypoventilation than muscular dystrophy, because not only the muscles but also the respiratory centers and nerves may suffer some permanent damage.

Extreme Obesity. A complicated but dramatic illustration of a reversible derangement in the ventilatory apparatus is provided by extreme obesity. In a few extremely fat individuals, severe alveolar hypoventilation occurs producing the "Pickwickian syndrome" of somnolence and lethargy due to carbon dioxide retention, and heart failure due largely to hypoxia. Loss of weight restores alveolar ventilation to normal and reverses the syndrome. As in the other structural deformities of the chest, an abnormal breathing mechanism seems to be involved. But why some obese individuals develop alveolar hypoventilation whereas others of comparable dimensions do not is unclear. The possibility has been raised that the occurrence of alveolar hypoventilation in so few of the extremely obese patients is attributable to their congenitally poor ventilatory response to chemical stimuli, i.e., either hypoxia or hypercapnia; this low-normal response would be of no clinical significance to normal subjects but would become important in subjects whose obesity led to inordinate work of breathing.

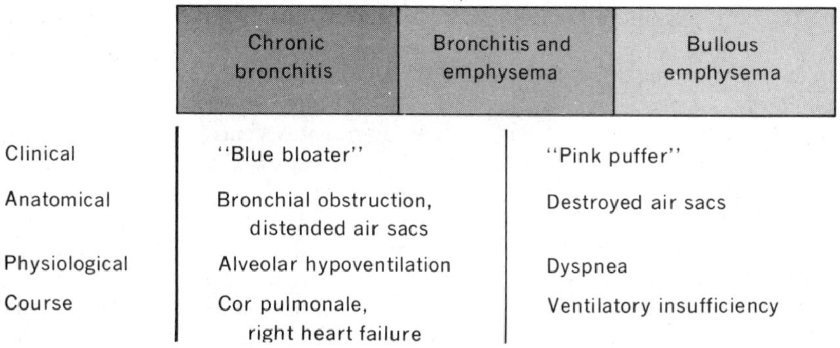

		Chronic bronchitis	Bronchitis and emphysema	Bullous emphysema
	Clinical	"Blue bloater"		"Pink puffer"
	Anatomical	Bronchial obstruction, distended air sacs		Destroyed air sacs
	Physiological	Alveolar hypoventilation		Dyspnea
	Course	Cor pulmonale, right heart failure		Ventilatory insufficiency

Fig. 287-1. Spectrum of chronic bronchitis and emphysema. Only the left side of the spectrum is associated with alveolar hypoventilation and cor pulmonale.

The left side of the heart as well as the right side is involved in the heart failure of obesity, presumably because obesity, per se, is regularly associated with a high cardiac output and a large blood volume. Accordingly, the cor pulmonale of obesity is unusual because the left as well as the right ventricle carries an excessive hemodynamic load, in large part a reflection of the adaptation of the circulation to the high metabolic needs of the large body mass. In addition, the left ventricle may be taxed further by systemic hypertension, which occurs more often in exceedingly obese persons than in the population at large.

DISEASES ASSOCIATED WITH NET ALVEOLAR HYPOVEN-TILATION (TABLE 287-1). The common denominator in this group of disorders is the imbalance between alveolar ventilation and perfusion, resulting in hypercapnia and hypoxemia. In contrast to *general* alveolar hypoventilation, in which the blood gases are abnormal despite normal lungs, abnormalities in the lungs are the cause of the abnormal blood gases in net alveolar hypoventilation. Two major categories illustrate this group: obstructive diseases of the airways and severe distortion of the pulmonary parenchyma.

Obstructive Diseases of the Airways. Such diseases comprise one end of a spectrum of diseases of the lungs ranging from pure bronchitis to pure emphysema (Fig. 287-1). At one end of the spectrum is the patient with bronchitis in whom obstructive disease of the airways has so deranged the balance between alveolar ventilation and perfusion as to cause cyanosis, somnolence, and heart failure. At the other end is bullous emphysema, in which parts of the lungs have been destroyed, decreasing alveolar ventilation and circulation in proportional amounts, so that the patient is left breathless but well oxygenated. In between are most patients, with a combination of chronic bronchitis and emphysema. Only those with net alveolar hypoventilation, the "blue bloaters," develop cor pulmonale. The others who maintain normal or near-normal blood gases by augmented breathing, the "pink puffers," usually spend their lives free of cor pulmonale except preterminally or during an intercurrent upper respiratory infection. Successful treatment of the "blue bloater" with cor pulmonale depends on appreciating the predominant role of bronchitis over anatomic changes in the lungs in providing the abnormal blood gases. Consequently, cor pulmonale can be reversed if

the bronchial obstruction is relieved. Such relief is easier in the patient with chronic bronchitis than with cystic fibrosis of the pancreas, in which most of the airways remain plugged with abnormal, thick, tenacious sputum despite the most heroic therapeutic efforts.

Severe Distortion of Pulmonary Parenchyma. Cor pulmonale is uncommon in uncomplicated silicosis or tuberculosis. On the other hand, it is not uncommon when silicosis, anthrosilicosis, or long-standing fibrotic tuberculosis is complicated by extensive, conglomerate, massive fibrosis, distorted adjacent parenchyma, shrunken lobes, and bronchitis. The likelihood of cor pulmonale is increased further by chronic pleurisy, fibrothorax, or excisional surgery. In such cases, a combination of anatomic restriction of the vascular bed and disturbances in gas exchange is involved in the pathogenesis of the pulmonary hypertension. Indeed, the disturbances in gas exchange, often brought to clinical levels by bronchitis, are the most reversible element of this disorder.

THERAPEUTIC PRINCIPLES IN THE MANAGEMENT OF COR PULMONALE SECONDARY TO ALVEOLAR HYPOVEN-TILATION. Although it is convenient to separate "net" from "general" alveolar hypoventilation on pathogenetic grounds, the principles of management are basically the same for both and are described in Chap. 295. The present section will deal only with the circulatory abnormalities.

Since the pulmonary hypertension is rarely anatomically fixed but arises mainly from hypoxia and acidosis, relief of the hypoventilation is usually remarkably successful in restoring the circulation to normal. Measures to improve alveolar ventilation vary considerably. In mild cases, simple measures often suffice; in more severe degrees of hypoxemia and hypercapnia, with heart failure, depressed respiratory center, and personality changes, mechanical aids to respiration are usually needed.

Treatment of right-sided heart failure, per se, is less important than restoring the blood gases to tolerable levels. The usual therapeutic measures for heart failure (Chap. 64) apply: low salt regimen, digitalis, diuretics. However, measures to decrease the circulating blood volume (and hematocrit) are of greater importance. Several phlebotomies of 300 to 400 ml may be needed, within a period of 2 to 3 weeks, to bring hematocrit and blood volume back to normal; repeated phlebotomies at monthly or bimonthly intervals may have to be instituted to prevent return of the hypervolemia. Diuretics have to be given with more care than usual for two reasons: (1) metabolic alkalosis, which may complicate the use of potent diuretics such as ethacrynic acid, aggravates ventilatory insufficiency by depressing the effectiveness of the CO_2 stimulus on the respiratory centers, and (2) any relief of carbon dioxide retention by promoting the renal excretion of bicarbonate is difficult to accomplish in the face of the moderate to severe depletion of potassium and chloride which often follows the use of diuretics and chlorothiazide. A new diuretic, furosemide, is particularly promising not only because of its effects on the kidney, but also because it seems to improve alveolar ventilation.

The effects of vigorous therapy, directed mainly to the pulmonary disorder, are often dramatic in relieving the blood gas abnormalities and heart failure: within 2 weeks to a month, arterial oxygen saturation at rest will be restored to over 90 percent; CO_2 levels will approach normal; blood volume, hematocrit, cardiac output, and even pulmonary arterial pressures may return to completely normal values.

REFERENCES

Alexander, J. K., K. H. Amad, and V. W. Cole: Observations on Some Clinical Features of Extreme Obesity with Particular Reference to Cardiorespiratory Effects, Am. J. Med., 32:512, 1962.

Bergofsky, E. H., G. M. Turino, and A. P. Fishman: Cardiorespiratory Failure in Kyphoscoliosis, Medicine, 38:263, 1959.

Fishman, A. P.: Dynamics of the Pulmonary Circulation, in "Handbook of Physiology," W. F. Hamilton and P. Dow (Eds.), vol. 2, "Circulation," sec. 2, Washington, American Physiological Society, 1963.

——, R. M. Goldring, and G. M. Turino: General Alveolar Hypoventilation. A Syndrome of Respiratory and Cardiac Failure in Patients with Normal Lungs, Quart. J. Med., 35:261, 1966.

Fishman, A. P., and H. Hecht: "The Pulmonary Circulation and Interstitial Space," Chicago, University of Chicago Press, 1969.

Fowler, N. O.: Editorial: The Normal Pulmonary Arterial Pressure-flow Relationships During Exercise, Am. J. Med., 47:1, 1969.

Goldring, R. M., A. P. Fishman, G. M. Turino, H. I. Cohen, C. R. Denning, and D. H. Andersen: Pulmonary Hypertension and Cor Pulmonale in Cystic Fibrosis of the Pancreas, J. Pediat., 65:501, 1964.

Harvey, R. M., and M. I. Ferrer: A Clinical Consideration of Cor Pulmonale, in "Symposium in Congestive Heart Failure," Monograph 1, H. L. Blumgart (Ed.), New York, American Heart Association, 1966.

Heath, D., D. Brewer, and P. Hicken: "Cor Pulmonale in Emphysema," Springfield, Charles C Thomas, 1968.

Peñaloza, D., F. Sime, N. Banchero, and R. Gamboa: Pulmonary Hypertension in Healthy Men Born and Living at Altitude, Med. Thorac., 19:449, 1962.

Richards, D. W.: Pulmonary Emphysema: Etiologic Factors and Clinical Forms, Ann. Intern. Med., 53:1105, 1960.

288 PULMONARY REACTIONS DUE TO THE INHALATION OF NOXIOUS AGENTS

Lloyd P. Tepper and
Edward P. Radford

GENERAL RESPONSES OF THE RESPIRATORY TRACT TO INHALED AGENTS

Injurious agents in the environment most commonly gain access to the body through the respiratory tract. Absorption of some substances is followed by systemic intoxication; the effect of other materials is restricted to the lungs. Although generalized air pollution may be an important source of chronic exposure to inhaled noxious agents, most serious acute exposures occur in special occupations where the concentration of the agent may be much higher than that associated with air pollution (Chap. 290). Accurate exposure and occupational histories with competent measurement of exposure conditions are fundamental to proper diagnosis, care, and prevention.

It is worthwhile to summarize briefly the effects that inhaled agents may have on the respiratory tract. *Gases* are absorbed in various regions of the airways or lungs, depending on the solubility of the gas in water. Highly soluble gases, such as many of the irritant gases, may be nearly completely absorbed in the oropharynx or in the trachea and larynx. Their effects, therefore, will be direct laryngospasm or reflex bronchospasm, which are characterized by changes in airflow resistance. Less-soluble gases penetrate to the alveoli, where they may produce acute pulmonary edema, or, in the case of substances such as nitrogen dioxide or ozone, more chronic changes, depending on their specific effects on the pulmonary tissue.

The size of *particles* determines the site of deposition in the respiratory tract. Particles with a mean diameter of more than about 3 μ are removed in the upper part of the respiratory tract by impaction; particles less than 1 μ in diameter are deposited primarily in the parenchyma by diffusion. Intermediate-sized particles are absorbed in the oropharynx, bronchi, and lungs by impaction and gravitational settling. Occasionally very large fibers, many microns long, are able to penetrate to the peripheral regions of the lungs. When gases and particles are inhaled together, the gases may be absorbed on the particles and reach deeper regions of the lungs than would otherwise be the case.

Dusts are cleared quite rapidly from lung tissues, usually by way of the bronchial tree and the so-called "mucus escalator," moved by ciliary action. Most dusts are presumably phagocytized and carried to the bronchi. The proportion of dusts cleared via the lymphatics varies with the kind of response elicited in the alveoli by the dust; the more fibrogenic the dust, the higher the proportion which penetrates to the lymphatics. Physiologic changes in response to dusts may include a variety of altered pulmonary functions. Bronchospasm and changes in airflow resistance are observed often, and ventilation may be distributed in a nonuniform manner. At the same time, there may be increased bronchial mucus and infection. With parenchymal disease (such as progressive fibrosis, granuloma formation, or dissolution of alveolar tissues), changes in lung compliance, altered ventilation/perfusion ratios, and lowered diffusion capacity may be present (Chap. 280). Symptoms may include dyspnea at rest or with exertion, wheezing, tightness of the chest, productive cough, cyanosis at rest or with exercise, and decreased exercise tolerance.

REACTION TO TOXIC IRRITANT GASES

AMMONIA AND ACID MISTS. Ammonia, hydrogen chloride, and other highly soluble gases or mists produce such vigorous conjunctival and upper-airway reactions that persons exposed make every possible attempt to flee a contaminated atmosphere. These voluntary efforts, breath holding, laryngeal and bronchial spasm, and the partial removal of the soluble gas by contact with moist upper-airway surfaces tend to protect the lung.

Deep lung irritation in such cases generally occurs in unconscious persons or when the route of escape is blocked. Visible and intense conjunctival, nasal, and pharyngeal reaction is invariably present, and the skin may be reddened, especially if it is wet. There are prompt, violent, and exhausting coughing, choking, a burning sensation in the pharynx, and substernal pain. Laryngeal spasm and edema of the glottis and lungs are seen. Oxygen is helpful; rinsing of the eyes and skin with water will remove residual irritant. Recovery is prompt and complete over the course of several days, although permanent damage to the eyes may occur (e.g., cataracts, iris adhesions).

CHLORINE. Chlorine produces a reaction of the respiratory tract similar to that produced by acid fumes; however the response of the lung tends to be somewhat more severe, inasmuch as chlorine is less potent as an acute irritant and therefore is more likely to be inhaled. Pulmonary edema and a necrotizing bronchitis are likely to occur. In some cases the acute episode may be followed by permanent pulmonary changes, mainly decreased diffusing capacity and compliance.

PHOSGENE. Although the injurious effects of phosgene are primarily due to deep lung irritation, this response may not be apparent for several hours. Prolonged exposure at low concentrations is consequently possible. Only when high concentrations are present is phosgene sufficiently irritating to the upper airway to cause termination of the exposure. Phosgene exposures may occur in organic synthetic processes and in unsuspected situations in which relatively nontoxic chlorinated hydrocarbon vapors are decomposed by heat to yield this toxic gas. The use of chlorinated solvents near open flames (e.g., welding) or hot metal surfaces commonly generates the gas.

At high phosgene concentrations there may be cough, chest discomfort, and nasopharyngeal irritation, and injury to the lung may occur relatively promptly. The more common situation reflects less-intense exposures and

a delay or latent period of as long as 16 hr. For that reason exposed individuals should be kept under observation for 24 hr; failure to do so has permitted pulmonary edema to develop under circumstances poorly adapted to the provision of adequate medical care. Oxygen is indicated in the treatment of patients with acute phosgene poisoning. Individuals with more than minimal symptoms should receive corticosteroids to reduce the acute inflammatory response and the tendency to chronic fibrotic changes. Because tissue necrosis is almost always complicated by bronchopneumonia, antibiotic therapy is indicated, and a penicillinase-resistant penicillin is the drug of choice (Chap. 135). Following the acute episode, survivors may develop chronic fibrotic and stenosing lesions of the bronchi and bronchioles.

NITROGEN DIOXIDE PNEUMONIA; SILO-FILLER'S DISEASE

Nitrogen dioxide is a red-brown gas associated with the action of nitric acid on metals (e.g., pickling, etching) and organic materials, the detonation of explosives, the oxidation of rocket fuels, the combustion of nitrate film, welding, and the fermentation of silage. Silo-filler's disease is the reaction among workers who are exposed to the gas in the course of entering poorly ventilated silos containing fresh ensilage (see also Chap. 284).

The clinical pattern of nitrogen dioxide poisoning shows wide variability because of varying intensities and durations of exposure. In persons with a relatively heavy industrial exposure, pulmonary edema may appear after a latent period up to 24 hr. These cases are frequently fatal, but full recovery may occur in survivors. In other cases recovery is only partial, and permanent pulmonary changes resulting from bronchial and bronchiolar narrowing occur.

In many cases with a silo gas etiology, a period of persistent cough, dyspnea, choking, and weakness commences at the time of exposure and extends throughout the period of illness. Typically a 2- to 3-week period of incomplete amelioration of symptoms is followed by a second phase in the illness, with progressive severe dyspnea and cough, cyanosis, chills, and fever. The symptoms do not respond to the usual bronchodilator drugs, but improvement after the administration of corticosteroids may be dramatic.

FIBROGENIC DUSTS; THE PNEUMOCONIOSES

The generic term *pneumoconiosis* encompasses diseases of the lung due to the inhalation of dust. In a strict sense diseases due to certain metals (e.g., cadmium, beryllium) are not pneumoconioses because the causal agents need not be dusts, and the syndromes may have prominent systemic manifestations. The designation "benign pneumoconiosis" has been applied to conditions in which an abnormal pulmonary deposition of radiopaque dust is detectable by x-ray but in which there are no associated symptoms. These include iron oxide (siderosis, as in welders) and tin oxide or barite (as seen in miners). These pulmonary phenomena are important because they must be differentiated from diseases due to fibrogenic dusts. In some exposures, dusts of silica and iron or other materials may be jointly responsible for the pulmonary changes.

Silicosis

Silicosis is caused by the inhalation of *free crystalline silica*, SiO_2 (not silicates), and is most commonly found among miners, stone workers, sand blasters, and foundry-men (often as siderosilicosis). In most cases as much as 20 years of exposure occurs prior to detectable radiographic changes. The initial pulmonary response to silica is typically a whorled nodular fibrosis, primarily in the peribronchial and perivascular portions of the lung. At this stage there is little if any pulmonary impairment, and there are no associated symptoms or signs. With termination of exposure the silicotic process may progress slightly for a year or two, but it then remains roentgenographically stationary, and the patient remains asymptomatic (Chap. 284).

Symptoms occur when silicosis advances and becomes complicated by infection and emphysema. Bronchial infection is prominent. Mechanical compression of respiratory bronchioles by enlarging nodules and distortion of bronchi increase airway resistance. Emphysematous changes are seen, especially at the apices, bases, and periphery of the lungs. Poor mixing and distribution of air and impaired pulmonary perfusion lead to hypoxia, although cyanosis and clubbing are usually absent. In the patient in whom the silicosis has become complicated by infection and emphysema, these changes are marked by intolerance to exertion, exhausting episodes of coughing, paroxysmal nocturnal dyspnea due to pooling of secretions in the tracheobronchial tree, and tenacious mucopurulent sputum. Examination reveals wheezes, rhonchi, and rales. Massive conglomerate shadows, usually in the upper lung fields, indicate complicating infection, often tuberculous, or proliferating fibrosis. "Eggshell" calcifications may be seen in the hilar lymph nodes and occasionally in the bronchopulmonary nodes. Silicosis complicated by infection and emphysema progresses in spite of termination of exposure and becomes incapacitating when pulmonary hypertension and cor pulmonale develop.

Treatment of the worker with silicosis depends on the character of the disease and the nature of the exposure. In the case of the patient who develops disease after only a few years of exposure, or who has progressive tuberculosis or conglomerate shadows, termination of exposure to dust is mandatory. On the other hand, simple silicosis after 20 or more years of exposure is not incompatible with continued work if control of exposure and medical surveillance are effective. In complicated silicosis, reversible bronchospasm, infection, and accumulations of secretions respond to bronchodilators, antibiotics, and postural drainage. Antituberculous drugs may be required (Chap. 174). Smoking should be discouraged inasmuch as it is irritating and stimulates the production of bronchial secretions.

Coal Workers' Pneumoconiosis

Pulmonary disease in workers exposed to coal dust is not entirely the result of silica present in mining situations. Though it is true that siliceous rock occurs in relation to coal seams and that sand is used to improve traction on mine haulageways, these exposures are of little significance in many instances of pneumoconiosis in coal miners.

The differences between silicosis and coal workers' pneumoconiosis relate primarily to etiology, pathogenesis, and pathology. In coal workers' disease the lungs contain large amounts of coal dust which is deposited around respiratory bronchioles. Associated fibrosis is minimal, and the dust is held in a fine mesh of reticulin fibrils. This stellate lesion contrasts sharply with the round whorled nodule of silicosis and its more extensive fibrosis. In both diseases a nodular pattern is seen on chest roentgenograms. The deposition of coal dust is associated with bronchiolar dilatation or focal emphysema.

As with silicosis, simple coal workers' pneumoconiosis is compatible with good health, and symptoms are generally due to concurrent bronchitis. The disease may be complicated by infections, but the incidence of tuberculosis does not appear to be increased, as it is among patients with silicosis. The nodular masses increase in size and coalesce in a condition often referred to as progressive massive fibrosis. Cavitation occasionally occurs within the masses as a result of ischemic or infectious necrosis.

With the onset of bronchitis, infection, and emphysema, symptoms of cough, sputum, breathlessness, and dull diffuse chest pain appear. Sputum may be stained black with coal particles. Cardiac complications of increasing pulmonary hypertension are associated with advanced disease. At that stage coal workers' pneumoconiosis can not be differentiated from silicosis. Coal workers' pneumoconiosis may progress in the absence of continued exposure to dust. There is no specific therapy. In coal workers with rheumatoid arthritis, multiple well-defined round opacities, 0.5 to 5 cm in diameter, as described by Caplan, may appear throughout both lungs.

Asbestosis

Asbestos is a generic term which refers to at least six fibrous silicate mineral species. Most asbestos minerals are used in the manufacture of wallboard, insulation, vinyl-asbestos floor tiles, brake and clutch facings, and asbestos-cement products such as siding and roofing. With prolonged inhalation of asbestos fibers, a diffuse nonnodular pulmonary fibrosis arises which affects alveolar walls, interlobular septums, and pleural surfaces. The physiologic changes are primarily those associated with impaired gas exchange and stiffening of the lung parenchyma. Disturbances in ventilation are not apparent, and the maximum breathing capacity is maintained (Chap. 284).

In contrast to silicosis, asbestosis may become symptomatic prior to the development of radiographically detectable changes. Breathlessness on exertion is the cardinal symptom, and a cough may be present. Examination typically reveals crackling basal rales and often clubbing of the fingers; cyanosis appears later. The roentgenographic pattern is variable, but a shaggy heart shadow, obliteration of the costophrenic angles, thickened interlobar septums, and a "ground-glass" appearance in the lower lobes are common. Pleural calcification may be observed; when it is present bilaterally it is almost pathognomonic of asbestosis.

Asbestosis does not predispose to tuberculosis as does silicosis. Cor pulmonale, however, is a common complication and cause of death. The relationship between asbestosis and bronchogenic carcinoma is well established, and this, too, is a common cause of death. In those workers with exposure to crocidolite or Cape blue asbestos, the incidence of pleural and peritoneal mesothelioma is striking. Sudden rapid clinical deterioration is seen in patients with this complication. There is no specific therapy for asbestosis.

SILICATOSES. Certain silicates other than asbestos produce a pulmonary fibrosis designated as silicatosis. These conditions are often marked by dyspnea, cough, infection, and the clinical phenomena associated with other pneumoconioses. Disease has been attributed to kaolin (china clay), mica, and more commonly to talc.

PULMONARY REACTIONS TO TOXIC METALS

CADMIUM. Acute cadmium pneumonitis invariably has been associated with exposure to freshly generated cadmium fumes arising from various welding, heat treating, metallizing, or metallurgic operations. During the exposure symptoms may be mild: irritation of the throat or an unpleasant metallic taste. After 2 to 6 hr the onset of cough, malaise, headache, chills, nausea, and vomiting suggests the presence of an acute viral upper respiratory infection. These premonitory symptoms are typical of metal fume fever and may in fact have the same etiologic basis.

Whereas metal fume fever resolves spontaneously within about 6 to 18 hr, cadmium poisoning progresses in 24 to 48 hr to a prolonged pulmonary reaction marked by chest pain, dyspnea, and cough. Fluid deposition within the pulmonary interstitium leads to impaired gas diffusion, and severe cyanosis is common. Because of the fibrinous character of the fluid and its location in the interstitium, findings on physical examination of the chest are often unimpressive, but the roentgenographic examination frequently shows multiple patchy bronchopulmonary infiltrates.

Although the case fatality rate in acute cadmium pneumonitis approximates 15 to 20 percent, a prolonged latent period prior to the onset of symptoms offers a better prognosis. Bacterial infection is a serious complication. In nonfatal cases recovery occurs during the second week of illness, and the chest roentgenogram returns to normal in a month.

Urinary excretion of cadmium is unrelated to the severity of the acute disease and is poorly correlated with the intensity of exposure. In cases of chronic exposure, renal disease and the excretion of an abnormal, low molecular weight protein may be observed. Chronic low-level cadmium exposure has also been associated with an increased prevalence of pulmonary emphysema. Treatment of cadmium pneumonitis consists of administration of oxygen, and when pulmonary involvement is severe corticosteroids are recommended.

Beryllium Disease

Airborne beryllium compounds may cause either an acute chemical pneumonitis or a chronic granulomatous interstitial pneumonitis. With the exception of the silicate beryllium, beryl, all respirable beryllium compounds, including the metallic dust, should be considered capable of inducing an injurious pulmonary response (Chap. 284).

Disease in the United States has occurred most commonly among employees at beryllium extraction works, among workers manufacturing fluorescent lamps (until 1949), and among those in various metallurgic, nuclear, and metal fabricating operations. Because clinical manifestations of chronic beryllium disease may be delayed for more than 20 years following cessation of exposure, careful inquiry is necessary to reveal relevant occupational factors.

The acute reaction to beryllium is a chemical pneumonitis most commonly related to exposure to acid salts (fluoride, sulfate), although other compounds have been incriminated as well. The reaction may be insidious in onset and marked by gradually progressive dyspnea, dry cough, and occasional constricting pain in the chest intensified by exertion. Paroxysms of violent coughing may be exhausting. Cyanosis and diffuse pulmonary rales are commonly noted. Chest roentgenograms may show diffuse bilateral haziness, irregular areas of infiltration, or nodularity throughout both lung fields. The spectrum of the acute response is broad and includes syndromes difficult to distinguish from common bronchitis, as well as a fulminating pneumonitis with edema which follows massive exposure by some 72 hr and may be fatal. In many cases there is associated inflammation of the eyes and upper airway, including the nose and pharynx. Most cases of acute beryllium disease are relatively benign, and total recovery occurs within 1 to 6 months. In moderate to severe cases treatment with corticosteroids is indicated.

Chronic beryllium disease ("berylliosis") is a systemic intoxication with a chronic pulmonary reaction characterized pathologically by interstitial granulomas, giant cells, and a thickening of alveolar walls. The attack pattern is spotty among exposed individuals, and a latent period prior to the onset of clinical disease is typical. The most common manifestation is progressive dyspnea, which reflects impaired diffusing capacity of the lung. A nonproductive cough, chest pain, and fatigue or weakness are common, and pneumothorax has occurred in 15 percent of known cases. The physical examination may be entirely negative, although clubbing of the fingers and cyanosis are noted in established cases. Pulmonary phenomena may be accompanied by granulomatous skin lesions, nephrolithiasis (10 percent), cachexia, and ultimately by cor pulmonale.

Laboratory studies characteristically show an increased serum gamma-globulin level, and there may be disturbed hepatic function and hypercalcuria. The chest roentgenographic changes are nonspecific, although a nodular pattern is common, and there is poor correlation between x-ray findings and the clinical status. Studies of pulmonary function show abnormal ventilation-perfusion relationships, and reduced diffusion capacity.

Chronic beryllium disease must be differentiated clinically from sarcoidosis; however, in the former disease lymphadenopathy, eye lesions, isolated hilar adenopathy, neurologic involvement, bone lesions, and leukopenia are lacking. Pathologic examination of lung tissue may be helpful in establishing the diagnosis, but the findings are not specific. A positive assay for beryllium in tissue is indicative of exposure but not necessarily of disease.

Therapy is based on the use of corticosteroids and prompt treatment of infection in persons with limited respiratory reserve. Oxygen, digitalis, and associated supportive measures may be indicated. The prognosis is much less favorable than in sarcoidosis.

REACTIONS TO OTHER METALS. Linear pulmonary markings and micronodular densities on roentgenograms have been observed among men shaping machine tools, rock drills, and dies in the "hard metal" cutting tool industry. "Hard metal" is composed of various metal carbides sintered with elemental cobalt, which is believed to be the biologically active component.

Pulmonary fibrosis also has been reported in men manufacturing "pyro," a very fine aluminum flake used in flares and fireworks. Breathlessness is the predominant symptom.

METAL FUME FEVER. Metal fume fever, brass-founder's ague, zinc fever, zinc chills, and galvo are all terms referring to a self-limited acute respiratory reaction to freshly generated metallic fume (suspended particles less than 0.1 μ in diameter). The response is not specific to any particular metal but has been associated with zinc, antimony, cadmium, cobalt, copper, manganese, and other metals. Dusts of these metals or intravenous injections are incapable of causing the response; fine fumes or sublimates are required. The reaction has most commonly occurred in workers engaged in smelting, galvanizing, brass founding, or welding.

In mild cases metal fume fever is easily confused with common viral respiratory illnesses. A patient often knows from previous experience what his trouble is and will use a diagnostic term specific to his trade. He may recall a dry irritative pharyngeal sensation during exposure and a sweet or metallic taste. Subsequently, he develops substernal tightness and a nonproductive cough. Several hours later he may experience chills, nausea and vomiting, severe sweating, generalized aches, and a fever to 103°F. Because of the delay in onset, symptoms may not appear until the evening of the work day. Rales may be heard on examination of the chest. The chest roentgenogram is usually normal but may show increased bronchovascular markings. The white blood cell count may rise to 16,000. Recovery in less than 18 hr is the rule, and there are no sequelae. With repeated exposure a temporary resistance or "immunity" is developed.

REACTIONS TO ORGANIC COMPOUNDS

The inhalation of organic compounds may irritate the lungs directly, as described below, or may result in a hypersensitivity reaction, i.e., an allergic interstitial pneumonitis, as described in Chap. 289.

Byssinosis

Byssinosis is an occupational respiratory disease among textile workers exposed to dusts of cotton, flax, hemp, and jute. The precise mode of action of these dusts is not fully established, but the leading hypothesis suggests that a biologically active, possibly histamine-releasing agent exists in the inhaled material. It appears less likely that byssinosis results from a hypersensitivity reaction to antigenic materials in or on the vegetable dusts.

Clinical manifestations generally appear after years of exposure in dusty areas of textile mills such as the carding areas and blow rooms. Initially the worker describes dyspnea, chest tightness, and cough on Monday mornings or on other days following an absence from work. Total remission of these symptoms on continuing exposure the next day is the rule in early cases, and permanent cessation of exposure to textile dusts generally results in permanent relief from symptoms. With continued exposure, however, the Monday symptoms become more severe and extend into other days of the week. Productive cough becomes prominent, and a permanent reduction in work capacity may occur even if exposure is terminated. In such cases severe chronic bronchitis and emphysema are prominent parts of the clinical picture. Asthmatic reactions and right-sided heart strain may occur.

The diagnosis of byssinosis is based on a history of exposure to cotton, flax, hemp, or jute dust over a period of years and on the characteristic occurrence of dyspnea and chest tightness after having been away from work. In contrast to patients with simple chronic bronchitis, the byssinotic worker does not experience symptoms on exposure to all dusty atmospheres. Pulmonary function tests show significant decreases in pulmonary ventilatory capacity and increases in airway resistance. Such studies may be especially revealing when they are conducted before and after a period of textile dust exposure. The roentgenographic pattern is not specific, but in early stages there may be pulmonary infiltrates which clear up rapidly but recur with further exposure.

Polymer Fume Fever

A self-limited acute systemic reaction with prominent pulmonary symptoms has been associated with exposure to certain plastic polymers or their thermal degradation products. The syndrome is indistinguishable from metal fume fever and has most commonly occurred in workers handling fluorohydrocarbons of the Teflon type. A frequent element of the exposure history is contamination of tobacco products by airborne or surface dusts, chips, or turnings of the plastic. The primary contaminants need not be of respirable size; however, the heat of the burning tobacco is sufficient to induce physical or pyrolytic changes which impart biologic properties to otherwise essentially inert materials. Other plastic materials may give rise to similar toxic fumes or gases when heat levels create fine sublimates or degradation products. Polymer fume fever is not directly related to experimental pulmonary edema or interstitial pneumonia from irritant gases which can be generated by thermally cracking fluorohydrocarbons at high temperatures. Health hazards have not been encountered in the use of Teflon-coated kitchen utensils.

Individuals who smoke or store tobacco products in areas in which Teflon is machined or in which Teflon parting compounds are used may experience tightness of the chest, dyspnea, body aches, cough, headache, chills, and fever to 104°F several hours after smoking contaminated tobacco. Roentgenograms have occasionally suggested pulmonary edema. Oxygen gives limited relief from the acute symptoms, which resolve spontaneously without known sequelae.

Pulmonary Reactions to Synthetic Resin Systems

Polyurethan and epoxy plastics are the products of polymerizing chemical reactions between resins and hardeners which are mixed at the time of final application. Toluene di-isocyanate (TDI), used in polyurethan systems, is a potent irritating and sensitizing agent that stimulates pulmonary reactions in sensitized individuals. In epoxy systems amine hardeners may also produce similar reactions, although they are much less common.

In toxic TDI exposure, the initial symptoms are those of mucosal irritation: itching of the eyes, rhinitis, and pharyngeal dryness and discomfort. With prolonged exposure and after an "incubation period" of several days to a week, a dry cough and chest pain occur. Occasionally the cough is sufficiently severe to interfere with sleep, and blood-streaked sputum may be noted. Physical examination reveals rapid pulse and respirations, a low-grade fever, rhonchi, and rales. The chest roentgenogram is usually normal, and recovery is rapid.

Most workers exposed in this fashion become sensitized, and subsequent exposures to extremely low concentrations of TDI can induce characteristic attacks of bronchospasm which are sufficiently severe to prevent return to work. Being in the room with TDI commonly results in asthmatic symptoms in sensitive individuals.

Response to Tobacco Smoke

The most important inhaled noxious agent in terms of the number of persons potentially affected is tobacco smoke, a mixture of a number of gases, such as oxides of nitrogen, carbon monoxide, and various cyanides, and an aerosol consisting of suspended droplets less than 1μ in size. The aerosol consists of condensed products of tobacco combustion, some adsorbed gases, and other volatile materials such as nicotine. Cigarette smoke is considered to be more damaging than pipe and cigar smoke, presumably because cigarette smoke usually is inhaled deeply. A smoker who inhales deeply may retain nearly 100 percent of cigarette smoke; the reason for this high degree of retention is thought to be rapid agglomeration and settling of the particles in the humid environment of the respiratory tract.

Acute effects of cigarette smoking on the lungs include a slight increase in airway resistance (depending on the degree of habituation of the smoker), perhaps some increase in bronchial mucus production, and a slowing of bronchial clearance rates for particles. Delayed effects include chronic bronchitis, emphysema, and bronchogenic carcinoma. It is probable that cigarette smoking accounts for a large fraction of all chronic lung disease in developed countries.

REFERENCES

Biological Effects of Asbestos (Conference Proceedings), Ann. N.Y. Acad. Sci., 132:1, 1965.

Bouhuys, A., L. J. Heaphy, R. S. F. Schilling, and J. W. Welborn: Byssinosis in the United States, New Engl. J. Med., 277:170, 1967.

Lowry, T., and L. M. Schuman: "Silo-filler's Disease"—A syndrome Caused by Nitrogen Dioxide, J.A.M.A., 162:153, 1956.

Tepper, L. B., H. L. Hardy, and R. I. Chamberlin: "Toxicity of Beryllium Compounds," Amsterdam, Elsevier Publishing Company, 1961.

289 ALLERGIC INTERSTITIAL PNEUMONITIS

Philip S. Norman

A series of syndromes caused by inhalation of organic dusts produce a hypersensitivity reaction in the lung manifested by fever, cough, granulomatous interstitial pneumonitis, and decreased pulmonary diffusing capacity. They are to be distinguished from asthmatic reactions to inhaled pollens, dander, and mold spores (Chap. 72), from pneumoconioses resulting from inorganic dusts, and from disorders due to directly noxious agents (Chap. 288). In allergic interstitial pneumonitis the hypersensitivity reaction results in a granulomatous reaction in alveolar septums, with collections of lymphocytes, plasma cells, poorly defined epithelioid cells, and occasionally numerous giant cells of Langhans. Ordinarily eosinophils are not part of the cellular infiltrate. In most instances, the antigens appear to be products of bacterial and fungal growth in stored vegetable materials. An exception is pigeon breeder's lung, in which animal emanations appear to initiate the reaction. Precipitating antibodies to the inciting antigen occur in most patients and appear to mediate the reaction, although some individuals who are exposed without developing disease have similar antibodies and a few individuals have disease without detectable antibodies.

In these conditions the period of exposure required to establish the specific sensitivity is uncertain, but once sensitization is established, inhalation exposure to the antigen commonly leads to a moderately acute illness in a matter of hours. The reason that only a minority of individuals develop these sensitivities when a majority of those similarly exposed have no untoward consequences is not understood.

FARMER'S LUNG

Agricultural workers may develop chills, fever, cough, and dyspnea rapidly, a few hours after exposure to moldy organic dusts (hay, grain, corn, tobacco, etc.). In nearly half the patients with farmer's lung, however, dyspnea, cough, and weight loss develop insidiously over several weeks or months. Whether the initial onset is acute or insidious, subsequent attacks may vary; acute attacks may develop in patients whose previous attacks were characterized by a gradual onset, while in patients with an acute initial episode, slow inexorable deterioration may occur as long as exposure to the antigen continues. Dyspnea often is accompanied by tightness or pain in the chest. There are occasionally small hemoptyses, but cough is usually nonproductive. There are usually loud crackling rales at the lung bases, and early in the disease, the chest roentgenogram shows diffuse interstitial or nodular infiltrates. Although the disease improves in a few days or weeks when exposure stops, recurrence upon reexposure is usual. Furthermore, prolonged or recurrent exposure may result in pulmonary fibrosis with distortion of the bronchioles and emphysema, which may not be entirely reversible.

Moldy hay is rich in the thermophilic actinomycetes, *Micropolyspora faeni* (formerly, *Thermopolyspora polyspora*) and *Micromonospora vulgaris,* as well as a number of fungal species (*Aspergillus, Cladosporium, Mucor, Penicillin,* and *Humicola*). Growth of these actinomycetes is favored by spontaneous heating during mold growth. The serum of patients with farmer's lung contains precipitating antibodies against extracts of moldy hay dust but none to clean hay dust. Furthermore, when inhaled by aerosol, extracts of moldy hay of cultures of the actinomycetes will produce typical attacks in patients with farmer's lung while extracts of clean hay will not. Precipitins against thermophilic actinomycetes and molds repeatedly have been demonstrated in the serum of patients with farmer's lung.

The *physiologic derangement* is a direct result of the interstitial infiltrate. Compliance is reduced and pulmonary gas diffusion is defective, but airway resistance is normal or nearly so.

Diagnosis depends on a history of exposure to moldy agricultural products, a finely granular reticular pattern on chest roentgenogram, pulmonary function tests showing reduced compliance and diffusion of gases, and improvement when exposure is discontinued. Eosinophilia is not part of the syndrome. A lung biopsy is not ordinarily necessary but may be required in cases which do not resolve quickly. The demonstration of precipitating antibodies to moldy hay extracts or to thermophilic actinomycetes may also be helpful. Although skin tests to mold or hay extracts are often positive, they are not useful in diagnosis because they are frequently positive not only in exposed individuals who do not have symptoms but also in some normal individuals, possibly because of endotoxin in the extract. Coworkers of patients with farmer's lung who are exposed to similar substances do not develop the illness, indicating that this is truly a disease of hypersensitivity.

If exposure is continued, the physiologic derangements, particularly the diffusion defect, may lead to right-sided heart failure, with a fatal outcome in some instances. When exposure is stopped, symptoms, pulmonary infiltrates, and physiologic derangements all tend to abate. Eventually, complete recovery occurs, although some patients, particularly those with prolonged exposure, have residual interstitial pulmonary fibrosis.

MAPLE BARK DISEASE

Sawmill or logging workers may develop typical attacks of interstitial pneumonitis after shaving or peeling bark from maple logs that have been stored for some time after cutting. Examination of the logs reveals heavy growth of the sporulating mold *Cryptostroma corticale,* just beneath the outer bark. Lung biopsies may show a number of inhaled spores; these spores have not germinated or grown mycelium, but by their presence, they initiate a strong hypersensitivity reaction. Skin tests with extract of *C. corticale* give both immediate (wheal and erythema) as well as delayed reactions. Serum precipitins to *C. corticale* also appear. Improved ventilation in sawmills and methods for storing logs to prevent continued dampness will usually eradicate the problem in a logging operation. Similar syndromes occur after exposure to redwood or elm sawdust and may be due to sensitivity to fungi of the genus *Graphium.* As in other conditions in this group, cessation of exposure usually results in complete recovery.

MUSHROOM-WORKER'S LUNG

Mushrooms are cultivated commercially on beds of aged horse manure. The manure, admixed with straw, is aged under conditions of warm temperature and high humidity which encourage the growth of the same thermophilic actinomycetes implicated in farmer's lung. When the aged manure is spread in beds to be sown with the spawn of the mushrooms or when the spent manure is removed after harvest of the mushrooms, workers may develop attacks of allergic interstitial pneumonitis. These individuals have serum precipitins against *T. polyspora* and *M. vulgaris*. A change of job usually results in complete relief.

BAGASSOSIS

Bagasse is the dried fiber of sugar cane after the sugar-bearing juice is pressed out. It is used as a source of cellulose for a variety of manufactured goods. Bagassosis results from the inhalation of the dust of bagasse when the bales are eventually opened or the fibers shredded. Fresh bagasse is not a problem, and the condition is not observed in sugar cane workers or at sugar mills. The baled bagasse is often stored, usually outdoors, without protection against moisture before being used, and there is often evident mold growth. Attacks of chills, fever, and dyspnea accompanied by granulomatous pneumonia have been described in bagasse workers in many parts of the world.

Precipitins to moldy bagasse can be demonstrated in the serum of 80 to 100 percent of patients with bagassosis but are also found frequently in bagasse workers without pulmonary disease and occasionally in individuals with no known contact with bagasse. Cultures of moldy bagasse show a variety of thermophilic actinomycetes, with *Micromonospora vulgaris* being the most frequent. Precipitins to this organism are found in a majority of bagassosis patients, but there are rarely precipitins to the other microorganisms in bagasse. Precipitins to *M. vulgaris* are rare in bagasse workers without the disease and appear to be in low titer. Immediate hypersensitivity to moldy bagasse with wheal and erythema skin reactions is clearly not diagnostic because it is as common in workers without disease as in those with disease.

The clinical picture and the physical and laboratory findings are quite similar to those of farmer's lung, and prolonged exposure may lead to pulmonary fibrosis and chronic restrictive disease. The presence of the typical clinical syndrome and of serum precipitins to *M. vulgaris* is strong presumptive evidence for bagassosis. Ordinarily the disease improves when jobs are changed. If the bagasse is moistened before handling, the exposure can be considerably reduced, and when exposure to moldy bagasse is curtailed, precipitins to *M. vulgaris* tend to disappear over several years.

PIGEON BREEDER'S DISEASE

Acute attacks of chills, fever, cough, and breathlessness recently have been observed in individuals who breed and race pigeons or keep parakeets. The attacks occur a few hours after handling the birds and are accompanied by rales at the lung bases and by a fine diffuse interstitial pneumonia which appears with each episode. As with farmer's lung, some patients have insidious onset of exertional dyspnea without dramatic episodes of chills and fever. Weight loss may be striking. Exposure to aerosols of pigeon droppings reproduces the

acute attacks and is accompanied by a drop in pulmonary diffusing capacity within 24 hr. The patient's serum contains precipitins against pigeon serum or pigeon egg white, and immunoglobulin levels are almost always elevated. Challenge with 3 ml of aerosolized pigeon serum also reproduces the disease so that it appears that molds or actinomycetes play a role. The relationship of serum precipitins to the disease is not clear because some pigeon breeders have serum precipitins to pigeon antigens but do not develop the illness after handling the birds. Symptoms disappear and precipitin levels decline when exposure is stopped. Similar conditions occur after inhalation of pituitary snuff and grain weevil dust, but in these cases the antigens are proteins not derived from microorganisms.

TREATMENT

In this group of diseases, cessation of exposure is usually the only treatment required. Acute episodes may dictate bed rest and supportive measures such as oxygen and antipyretics for fever. It is possible to hasten resolution of the process with corticosteroids, but this is not always necessary. When cor pulmonale and right-sided heart failure occur, they should be treated as described in Chap. 287.

REFERENCES

Emanuel, D. A., B. R. Lawton, F. J. Wenzel: Maple Bark Disease, Pneumonitis Due to *Coniosporium corticale,* New Engl. J. Med., 266:333, 1962.

Pepys, J.: Farmer's Lung, Brit. Med. J., 2:359, 1965.

Rankin, J., W. H. Jaeschke, Q. C. Callies, and H. A. Dickie: Farmer's Lung, Physiopathologic Features of the Acute Interstitial Granulomatous Pneumonitis of Agricultural Workers, Ann. Intern. Med., 57:606, 1962.

Reed, C. E., A. Sosman, and R. A. Barbee: Pigeon Breeder's Lung, a Newly Observed Interstitial Pulmonary Disease, J.A.M.A., 193:261, 1965.

Salvaggio, J. E., H. A. Buechner, J. H. Seaburg, and P. Arquembourg: Bagassosis: I. Precipitins against Extracts of Crude Bagasse in the Serum of Patients, Ann. Intern. Med., 64:748, 1966.

Weill, H., H. A. Buechner, E. Gonzalez, S. J. Herbert, E. Aucoin, and M. M. Ziskind: Bagassosis: A Study of Pulmonary Function, Ann. Intern. Med., 64:737, 1966.

290 MEDICAL ASPECTS OF AIR POLLUTION

John R. Goldsmith and
Edward P. Radford

In this chapter the term *air pollution* refers to the accumulation of airborne materials arising from human activities; the natural pollutants, such as pollens, are not included. With increased population density in urban centers, man-made sources of atmosphere contamination are increasing rapidly. As early as the Middle Ages, the use of coal as a fuel led to an appreciable amount of smoke in the large northern cities where it was extensively burned. Modern problems of air pollution, however, are characterized by the complexity of multiple air pollutants, the enormous number of sources from which they emanate, and the large population exposed. The most important medical problems arising from air pollution may prove to be related to a small segment of the population who, because of age or preexisting cardiopulmonary disease, is particularly susceptible to inhalation of pollutants.

Concern for the deleterious effects of air pollution became widespread following an episode in London in 1952. At that time the city experienced an unusually protracted meteorologic inversion that resulted in a buildup in the concentration of particles and gases in the atmosphere. Epidemiologic evaluation indicated approximately four thousand excess deaths. These deaths were believed to occur predominantly in patients with underlying cardiopulmonary disease and were ascribed principally to the effects of sulfur dioxide (SO_2) and smoke accumulation in the atmosphere. In addition to these effects on the lungs, attention also has been directed to community-wide or local air pollutants which are known to produce eye irritation or unpleasant odors. Although not often thought of as having major medical effects, these nuisances often can disturb sleep or evoke adverse psychologic responses.

TYPES OF COMMUNITY AIR POLLUTION

SULFUR OXIDE AND PARTICULATE TYPE. The oldest and most troublesome of the major forms of air pollution is associated with fossil fuels that are contaminated with sulfur compounds which are used for heating and generation of power. The combustion of soft coal and fuel oil in fireplaces, furnaces, and power plants produces sulfur oxides and particulates, resulting in community-wide air pollution. The severity of pollution is best estimated by the concentration of sulfur oxides in the air, although the substances which are harmful are not pure SO_2, but some combination of sulfur oxides with particulate matter.

The efficiency of a fire is inversely related to the proportion of carbon in the fuel which is emitted as soot or black smoke. The modern power plant can be designed to burn fuel oil and coal very efficiently, and the principal pollutants emitted from these relatively efficient power-generating systems are SO_2 itself, with some fine particulate matter, and oxides of nitrogen. The nitrogen oxides result from nitrogen of the air being oxidized or "fixed" by atmospheric oxygen at high combustion temperatures.

PHOTOCHEMICAL AIR POLLUTANTS. A new class of pollutant has been recognized, and because it was described first in the Los Angeles area, is known as "Los Angeles smog." This type of pollution arises from hydrocarbon vapors and nitrogen oxides in motor vehicle exhaust. When exposed to sunlight, these fumes undergo a complex series of reactions leading to four major phenomena which characterize photochemical air pollution: (1) the production of ozone; (2) a characteristic form of vegetation damage; (3) widespread eye irritation and somewhat less widespread respiratory irritation; and (4) interference with visibility. Since their discovery in the Los Angeles atmosphere, the same processes have subsequently been identified in most major cities in the United States and in several countries overseas. Photochemical damage to vegetation has been found in over half the states. A new class of compounds first identified in photochemically polluted mixtures, the *peroxyacetyl nitrates,* has been incriminated as the cause of one of the two major forms of vegetation damage. The other form is caused by ozone. Peroxyacetyl nitrate is also a potent eye irritant, but measured levels of this substance have not accounted for the magnitude of eye irritation observed in natural pollutant mixtures. Another compound emitted by motor vehicles, *formaldehyde,* is also produced by photochemical reactions and is a major contributor to the characteristic eye irritation.

CARBON MONOXIDE. This gas is another important air pollutant arising from vehicular exhaust. In many downtown areas of large cities the CO concentration has been increasing progressively, and concentrations of thirty parts per million are not unusual during periods of peak traffic. These concentrations are still low in terms of percent of hemoglobin bound by CO (about 5 percent with exposures averaging 6 to 8 hr), but chronic exposure of individuals whose oxygen transport may be impaired for other reasons may be important, particularly in supplying oxygen to brain or myocardium. While the concentration of *carbon dioxide* also has been increasing slowly, its concentration is not medically significant.

OTHER SPECIFIC COMMUNITY AIR POLLUTANTS. These pollutants include *lead,* thought to be in air primarily as a result of use of tetraethyl lead in automobile fuels, and also other metals like *beryllium* or *cadmium,* which become part of air pollution as a result of industrial operations. Another pollutant is asbestos, which may become airborne in the community as a result of wearing brake linings. Certain smelters produce trace metal contamination, particularly with *arsenic* and *lead.* For example, outbreaks of arsenical dermatitis have been reported in the vicinity of smelters in Nevada which have excessive emissions of arsenic. In the Soviet Union alterations in porphyrin metabolism have been reported in children in the vicinity of plants emitting lead.

CLASSIFICATION OF POLLUTANT EFFECTS

(See Table 290-1.) Many of the important pollutants are irritating to the respiratory tract and produce increased secretions and laryngeal or bronchial spasm because they are soluble in the secretions of the lining material of the nose and airway. Eye irritants are usually soluble in conjunctival secretions.

Some irritating pollutants including ozone and NO_2 exert their major effects within a day or two after exposure has been terminated. The effect of these substances is not immediately unpleasant. Because of this

Table 290-1. HEALTH EFFECTS OF COMMUNITY AIR POLLUTANTS

Pollutant	Concentration	Duration	Effect	Conditions
Sulfur oxides and particulates Sulfur dioxide	1.6 ppm 0.2 ppm	1 hr Daily average exceeded more than 3% of days	Increased airway resistance Cough and respiratory symptoms	Healthy experimental subjects Population surveyed in vicinity of a smelter
Sulfur oxide and particulates	>0.05 ppm SO_2 particulate measurements not standardized in U.S. units	Long-term average	Increased cough and sputum, impaired expiratory flow in children	Population surveys in United States, Japan, and United Kingdom
	>0.2 ppm SO_2 with >200 $\mu g/m^3$ of black suspended matter (smoke)	Daily average	Exacerbation of chronic bronchitis	Panel studies in London
	>0.25 ppm SO_2 with >750 $\mu g/m^3$ of black suspended matter (smoke)	Daily average	Increased mortality	General mortality studies in London
Oxidants Ozone	0.5 ppm	4 hr daily 3 days a week for 6 weeks	Diminished forced expiratory volume in 1 sec	Healthy experimental subjects (recovery in weeks)
	0.6 ppm	2 hr	Increased airway resistance and impaired diffusion capacity	Healthy experimental subjects (recovery in 2 to 24 hr)
Unspecified as found in Los Angeles area	0.1 ppm	1 hr	Increased airway resistance in emphysematous patients	Moderately advanced respiratory disease—about half react
			Impaired performance in school track team	Level producing effect based on regression over range of 0.05 to 0.35 ppm
			Increased likelihood of asthma	In a small fraction (about 5%) of asthmatic patients in a panel study
			Eye irritation	In a high proportion of exposed population
Carbon monoxide	30 ppm	8 hr	Significant impairment in oxygen transport at sea level (effects greater at higher altitude)	Produces 5% COHb in active subjects, nonsmokers. Higher values likely in cigarette smokers
			Impairs visual discrimination with minimal illumination	Additive to effects of age and altitude
	50 ppm	45 min	Impairs judgment of time intervals	Normal subjects

delayed effect, the magnitude and seriousness of the exposure are not appreciated. These reactions probably occur because of cellular responses in the target organ, which is usually the lung, and may be mediated immunologically. For example, toluene diisocyanate, a substance used in the plastics industry, is highly antigenic.

Strenuous efforts have been made to examine persons exposed to high levels of air pollution in the community in order to describe a characteristic syndrome, but these efforts have been unsuccessful. Except for the specific toxicants, such as CO or beryllium, there is no specific disease associated with community air pollution exposure.

This does not mean that there are not many effects on health, such as the production of symptoms, e.g., tearing, cough, and dyspnea, or the aggravation of preexisting pulmonary disease.

ACUTE INCREASES IN MORTALITY DUE TO POLLUTION. Under unusual meteorologic conditions, the normal exhalations of an urban area, instead of being diluted and altered to the point where they are innocuous, can accumulate, with serious results. This has been documented in London; Osaka, Japan; Donora, Pennsylvania; in the Meuse Valley (Belgium); and in New York City. No doubt similar effects will be found in other urban areas and cities. Persons with chronic obstructive pulmonary disease are usually the most severely affected, and it is among this group that the largest excess in relative mortality occurs. While these episodes are important, present control measures should be capable of preventing them. It is the more insidious effects of continuous exposure of large segments of the population to lower levels and a greater diversity of air pollutants that is of greatest concern.

ASSOCIATION OF AIR POLLUTION WITH CAUSATION OF CHRONIC DISEASE

Air pollution has been examined as a possible causal factor in a series of chronic respiratory diseases. Despite suggestive evidence, it is no longer thought likely that air pollution is a cause of *lung cancer;* cigarette smoking is a much more important etiologic factor. In contrast, cigarette smoking and community air pollution are causally important in *chronic bronchitis,* and it has been suggested that they exert a synergistic effect on bronchitic symptoms and on the associated impairment of pulmonary function. *Asthma* is often precipitated or aggravated by air pollutants (See Chap. 72).

It has been suggested that *carbon monoxide* exposures could be of sufficient magnitude to affect the survival of persons who have suffered a myocardial infarction because of the adverse effect of the gas on oxygen transport. At concentrations of about 5 percent carboxyhemoglobin, impairment of central nervous system function is detectable, and above this concentration impaired visual discrimination by the dark-adapted eye can be expected.

Asbestos. This mineral fiber is an important occupational pollutant. Excessive exposure to it is associated with pleural calcification, a higher incidence of bronchogenic carcinoma, and pleural mesothelioma. In one South African series, more than half the persons who developed mesothelioma had not worked in the asbestos industry, but only lived in the vicinity of the mines and mills. In Finland 10 percent of the adult population of one mining town had bilateral calcification of the parietal pleura which was attributed to nonoccupational exposure of anthophyllite asbestos. The diagnosis of asbestosis has been based partly upon the findings of characteristic asbetos bodies in the lungs at autopsy or in the sputum. The presence of these bodies in 25 to 33 percent of autopsies in presumably unexposed persons has raised the question as to whether bronchogenic carcinoma might be related to casual exposure to the substance, presumably from abraded brake linings.

Although the concentration of *lead* in the environment, particularly from automobile exhausts, has been rising, and the equilibrium concentration in tissues of individuals living in areas of heavy automobile traffic also may be increasing, there is no evidence that this produces significant health hazards.

REDUCTION OF AIR POLLUTION

Air pollution can be reduced by setting emission standards on refineries and power plants and by limiting the sulfur content of fuels. The elimination of open-burning dumps and control of commercial and domestic incinerators are also helpful measures. Perhaps of greatest potential importance is the control of motor vehicle emissions by establishing mandatory crankcase and exhaust controls.

REFERENCES

"Air Conservation," Report of the Air Conservation Commission of the American Association for the Advancement of Science, Publ. 80, 1965.

Boffey, P. M.: Smog: Los Angeles Running Hard, Standing Still, Science, 161:990, 1968.

"The Eighth Annual Air Pollution Medical Research Conference, Los Angeles, March, 1966." Arch. Environ. Health, Vol. 14, No. 1, Jan. 1967.

Ferris, B. G, and J. L. Whittenberger: Environmental Hazards: Effects of Community Air Pollution on Prevalence of Respiratory Disease, New Engl. J. Med., 275: 1413, 1966.

Goldsmith, J. R.: Air Pollution, chap. 14 in "Effects of Air Pollution on Human Health," vol. 1, Arthur Stern (Ed.), New York, Academic Press Inc., 1967.

291 BRONCHIECTASIS, BRONCHIAL OBSTRUCTION, AND LUNG ABSCESS

John H. Knowles

BRONCHIECTASIS

The term *bronchiectasis* refers to a state of dilatation of the bronchial tree. The disease was first described by Laennec in 1819. Extensive clinical study and description were made possible with the introduction of bronchography in 1922 by Sicard and Forestier. The incidence, prognosis, and severity of the disease have been radically altered with the advent of chemotherapy.

Bronchiectasis is a disease of *patchy* distribution in the lung. The affected segmental or subsegmental bronchus may undergo a tubular (cylindrical) or saccular dilatation. *Generalized* tubular dilatation of smaller (more peripheral) bronchi may be seen in chronic bronchitis and obstructive emphysema, but this is not of the same significance as the *localized,* more striking dilatation of larger (more proximal) bronchi seen in bronchiectasis. The differentiation of bronchitis and bronchiectasis is discussed below.

PATHOGENESIS. Prolonged bronchial obstruction and infection must be present to cause irreversible dilatation of the bronchial tubes. If uncontrolled, the infection extends into the bronchial wall, with disruption of smooth muscle and elastic tissue, and invades the adjacent peribronchial tissue. Ciliated columnar epithelium is replaced by nonciliated cuboidal epithelium, and in some instances the entire bronchial wall may be replaced by fibrous tissue, with resultant formation of saccules. With damage or loss of ciliated epithelium and loss of bronchial tone and peristaltic action there is further stasis of infected secretions. Traction by peribronchial and parenchymal scars distorts the diseased bronchus. In the region of third order bronchi, large (up to 1 mm in size) anastomotic communications between bronchial artery and pulmonary artery may be seen.

The posterior basal segments of the lower lobes are the most commonly involved. More than half of patients with left lower lobe disease also have involvement of the lingular segment of the left upper lobe. Upper lobe bronchiectasis is usually seen in the posterior or apical segment and is likely to be secondary to (old) tuberculous endobronchitis or to healed lung abscess.

ETIOLOGY. Prior to the introduction of antibiotics and extensive immunization programs, the commonest precursors of bronchiectasis were pertussis, measles, and influenza, and more than 50 percent of patients dated the onset of their symptoms from the first decade. By giving rise to peripheral bronchial obstruction and stasis, these infections set the stage for superimposition of suppurative infection and bronchiectasis. At present *bronchopneumonia* is the most likely precursor of bronchiectasis. When drainage is hindered by inspissation of secretions or treatment is inadequate, there is delay in resolution and bronchial infection persists. Similarly, aspiration of a foreign body, particularly in children, and bronchogenic carcinoma and bronchial adenoma, by partially obstructing the bronchial lumen, lead to chronic infection and the development of bronchiectasis distally.

Kartagener's syndrome consists of a triad of dextrocardia, sinusitis, and bronchiectasis. The incidence of bronchiectasis in patients with congenital dextrocardia is 15 to 20 percent. The disease may never supervene in subjects with dextrocardia or it may develop late in life, depending probably on the element of infection. The reasons for the association are obscure.

Cystic fibrosis of the pancreas is a congenital disease characterized by exocrine pancreatic insufficiency and chronic obstructive pulmonary disease. Ninety percent of deaths in cystic fibrosis are directly attributable to the pulmonary complication of obstructive emphysema, atelectasis, and bronchiectasis. Thick, tenacious secretions obstruct the bronchial lumen, resulting in atelectasis distally. If infection is superimposed (commonly with the staphylococcus or *Pseudomonas aeruginosa*), the ground is set for the development of bronchiectasis.

Bronchiectasis is a frequent complication of congenital *agammaglobulinemia* and results presumably from recurrent pulmonary infection. Only rare instances of bronchiectasis have been reported in adults in association with acquired agammaglobulinemia.

The right middle lobe bronchus is particularly vulnerable to compression by lymph nodes situated at its origin from the right bronchus. With enlargement of the peribronchial lymph nodes because of tuberculosis or nonspecific infection, the right middle lobe bronchus is compressed and stasis and infection occur distally. This has been called the *middle lobe syndrome.*

Primary tuberculosis can lead to bronchiectasis via enlarged, obstructing lymph nodes at the root of a lobar bronchus. Secondary or reinfection tuberculosis may lead to a state of bronchiectasis by (1) distortion of subsegmental bronchi adjacent to a healing cavitary or granulomatous lesion, or (2) destruction secondary to endobronchial tuberculosis.

Bronchiectasis, usually of the tubular type, may occasionally be seen in long-standing cases of bronchial asthma, chronic bronchitis, and obstructive emphysema. Presumably this has resulted from bronchial obstruction and infection due to viscid secretions and is patchy in distribution. Generalized dilatation of smaller bronchi may be seen in chronic bronchitis and emphysema (see below).

Bronchiectatic changes can frequently be demonstrated in the area of a healed lung abscess. Reepithelization of lung abscess cavities and extension of suppurative disease to surrounding segmental bronchi result in their permanent dilatation.

Anomalous pulmonary arteries arising from the aorta may be associated with sequestration of a lobe and resulting bronchiectasis commonly in the region of the posterior segment of the left lower lobe and close to the diaphragm.

Because of the frequent association of sinusitis with bronchiectasis, an etiologic role was assigned with the notion that chronic aspiration of infected sinus contents led to bronchiectasis. Similar reasoning has been applied to poor oral hygiene because of the rarity of healthy teeth and gingiva in patients with bronchiectasis. Perhaps this mechanism applies in a few individuals, but the association of upper and lower respiratory tract disease has not offered a convincing clue to the etiology of disease in either area.

CLINICAL MANIFESTATIONS. *Symptoms of bronchiectasis depend on superimposed infection, not on the bronchial dilatation per se.* Thus bronchiectasis may be continuously or intermittently symptomatic. Some individuals known to have bronchial dilatation in a lower lobe for many years have symptoms only after an infection in the upper part of the respiratory tract. Upper lobe lesions may remain permanently asymptomatic because stasis and infection of secretions do not occur.

The *cardinal manifestations* are *cough, mucopurulent sputum, hemoptysis,* and *recurrent pneumonitis.* The cough is particularly severe and productive when the subject lies down, thereby emptying the contents of the dependent lower lobes into the larger bronchi. The morning production of sputum is large, and the patient may have syncopal episodes (cough syncope) or may vomit (emetic cough) as he struggles to rid his bronchi of the overnight accumulation.

The sputum is mucopurulent and varies from 1 to 8 oz a day. It initially settles into three and finally into two layers as the frothy top layer subsides. The final two layers consist of an upper watery saline component and a lower heavier part consisting mainly of pus cells, and includes various organisms, Dietrich's plugs, and elastic tissue. The sputum (and breath) is occasionally foul smelling but usually has a sickish sweet odor and a pea-soup appearance.

Hemoptysis varies from blood streaking of the sputum to massive and rarely exsanguinating amounts. In the former instance the blood has arisen from granulation tissue in the chronically infected bronchial wall and in the latter instance from erosion of a bronchial artery or a bronchial-pulmonary arteriolar anastomosis. Commonly in upper lobe bronchiectasis and occasionally with lower lobe disease, the initial symptom may be that of hemoptysis, so-called "dry bronchiectasis." Here cough and sputum production have been minimal (or minimized by the patient) and a subclinical, smoldering infection in a bronchiectatic segment has finally eroded a vessel. Hemoptysis is said to be more common with saccular than with tubular disease.

Recurrent pneumonitis commonly punctuates the course of bronchiectasis. A high index of suspicion should be aroused when recurrent pneumonia involves the same lobe repeatedly. In this case the reservoir of infection is the underlying infected bronchiectasis, and extension from here into the surrounding parenchyma has developed. Occasionally intrapulmonary aspiration of infected secretions from a diseased area into a healthy lobe has occurred.

More than 60 percent of patients will have associated symptoms of sinusitis with postnasal drip and sinus headaches.

Dyspnea may be a prominent complaint in some patients, particularly older adults with extensive bilateral disease or an additional element of diffuse chronic bronchitis and obstructive emphysema.

On physical examination, the patient appears chronically ill. His wet cough frequently interrupts the examination. Sinus tenderness may be elicited. Clubbing of the fingers and toes is observed in 50 percent of the patients. The chest may have the emphysematous configuration if accompanying diffuse chronic bronchitis is present. The most important finding is the auscultation of persistent, wet, coarse inspiratory rales at either or both of the posterior lung bases, more frequently the left, and over the right middle lobe or lingular segment of the left upper lobe. The breath sounds may be coarse and bronchial. The findings of diffuse chronic bronchitis may also exist (see Chap. 283). Examination of the heart may rarely reveal the findings of pulmonary hypertension. One should also be alert to the possibility of dextrocardia. There may be *no* abnormal physical findings in the chest in some patients.

LABORATORY FINDINGS. There is mild normocytic normochromic anemia if infection has been prolonged and severe. Older patients with severe respiratory impairment may develop secondary polycythemia. Leukocytosis may be seen if acute bacterial infection with pneumonitis is superimposed on the chronic infection. Urinalysis may reveal persistent albuminuria if the rare complication of secondary amyloidosis has occurred. The characteristics of the sputum have been alluded to above. Only occasionally do cultures reveal a predominant pathogen, particularly during an acute pneumonitis. Study of plasma

protein electrophoretic pattern and of sweat electrolyte excretion may be useful in excluding agammaglobulinemia and cystic fibrosis, respectively (Chap. 69 and 334).

Pulmonary function is not measurably altered until the disease involves more than three segments or is bilateral. Decrease in vital capacity correlates with the extent of the disease. Some patients will show the pattern of obstructive emphysema, and their dyspnea correlates well with the reduction in ventilatory reserve. Abnormalities of distribution as regards venous admixture effect (resulting in arterial oxygen unsaturation) may be minimized by the effect of the bronchial artery–pulmonary artery precapillary anastomoses in shunting returning venous blood away from diseased, poorly ventilated areas to normally ventilated areas where gas exchange is normally maintained. Pulmonary hypertension and cor pulmonale result when extensive bilateral disease destroys excessive parenchymal vascular bed.

Although the conventional roentgenogram of the chest may be normal in some cases, it is usually abnormal. Linear shadows extending from the hilum into the periphery of the lung field probably represent peribronchial thickening. Triangular shadows of lobar collapse may be seen at either lung base, particularly in children. So-called ring shadows—air-filled areas with thin or thick walls—may represent bronchiectatic sacs or local overdistension emphysema adjacent to atelectatic areas. With lobar collapse and in the rare instance of massive whole lung involvement, mediastinal contents will be shifted toward the diseased area and the homolateral hemidiaphragm will be elevated.

Bronchoscopy is ordinarily done prior to bronchography. It is an important diagnostic adjunct and helps in localization of the disease. It is also used to rule out bronchostenosis by external compression or by intrinsic tumor, foreign body, or endobronchial tuberculosis.

Bronchography is necessary to define the extent of the disease. The bronchial tree is outlined by the use of an oily iodine preparation called Dionosil. This is completely absorbed in several days, in contrast to older oily preparations (Lipiodol) which might remain at the lung bases permanently. The bronchogram generally reveals a tubular or saccular dilatation of several or more of the proximal (second or third order) bronchi in the lung. The affected lobe is atelectatic, and the dilated bronchi are squeezed together.

A problem frequently arises in the differential diagnosis of bronchiectasis and chronic bronchitis, which may have the same symptoms and very similar bronchographic patterns and which frequently coexist. Clinically sinus disease, copious amounts of sputum, hemoptysis, clubbing, wet rales which persist in a localized area of the lung over long periods of time, all seen in a youth or young adult patient, are highly suggestive of bronchiectasis. The middle-aged or elderly man with the chronic, poorly productive "cigarette" cough, signs of hyperinflated chest with quiet breath sounds, and *generalized* squeaks but no local wet bubbling rales more likely has chronic bronchitis and emphysema. There are several important radiographic points which may help in diagnosis:

in bronchitis the volume of the lung (or lobe) is increased, whereas in bronchiectasis it is decreased even though there may be emphysematous changes peripherally. In bronchitis the bronchi fill out more peripherally, whereas in bronchiectasis only the larger and more proximal bronchi fill. Bronchial diverticula, representing filling of the dilated ducts of mucous glands, are diffuse and sparse in chronic bronchitis. In bronchiectasis they are numerous and localized to the bronchus of the involved lobe. If both situations exist, then both diseases may be present.

The *diagnosis* of bronchiectasis should be suspected in any patient complaining of chronic and usually productive cough or hemoptysis or recurrent episodes of pneumonia. The suspicion is strengthened if clubbing is found along with persistent, wet inspiratory rales at the lung bases posteriorly or over the lingular segment or right middle lobe. If radiographic abnormalities are also seen on the plain film, the diagnosis is almost certain. It is strengthened by the bronchoscopic findings and confirmed by bronchography.

The *course* of the disease is extremely variable. Known bronchial dilatation may exist without symptoms for years, only to become suddenly and persistently symptomatic. As a general rule, saccular bronchiectasis is a more serious disease than the tubular form, and bilateral involvement carries a worse prognosis than unilateral disease. It is of utmost importance to note that bronchiectasis is an acquired disease that is not, except in rare instances, progressive. It does not commonly spread and is ordinarily maximal when first seen. The typical patient *prior to the antibiotic era* was between fifteen and thirty years of age. His symptoms extended over 10 to 20 years, and their onset was usually dated from an episode of pneumonia or pertussis during the first decade of life. He was incapacitated by his foul sputum, general debility, and malnutrition. The individual whose illness began before ten years of age rarely lived beyond the age of forty, and the mortality rate of hospital patients followed for any length of time was 30 to 50 percent. The usual causes of death were pneumonia, overwhelming sepsis, brain abscess, hemorrhage, and cor pulmonale. In addition to the complications, an occasional instance of secondary amyloidosis was recorded. More recent studies have shown that those complications now are exceedingly rare and that the prognosis has improved considerably, partly because of antibiotics and partly because more recent studies have considered ambulatory groups of clinic patients. Bilateral disease, persistent large amounts of fetid sputum, frequent bouts of fever, and clubbing of the fingers are poor prognostic signs. The presence of chronic bronchitis and obstructive emphysema also worsens the prognosis. The mortality rate is now approximately 10 percent over a 10-year period. The cause of death may be pulmonary insufficiency and cor pulmonale, but intercurrent and unrelated disease are also frequent causes. Surviving subjects rarely show progression of disease and fairly frequently show improvement.

TREATMENT. The treatment of bronchiectasis combines the judicious use of antibiotics, postural drainage (see Chap. 295, Therapy), and in certain patients resection of diseased areas. Antibiotic therapy is guided during periods of acute infection by the results of sputum (or blood) cultures. In patients who suffer repeated episodes of acute infection, small doses of antibiotics may be given prophylactically during the winter months. Periodic culture of the sputum should be obtained during such therapy to detect the emergence of other, sometimes resistant, organisms.

Because the disease is usually not a progressive or spreading process, every patient at least initially deserves a course of conservative medical therapy under close observation before a decision for or against surgery is made. The most dramatic surgical cures are effected by the excision of localized, unilateral disease which has remained symptomatic despite medical therapy. Massive and recurrent hemoptysis may also necessitate surgical removal. The poorest results are obtained with the excision of local disease in the face of bilateral, extensive disease and coexistent diffuse chronic bronchitis or bronchial asthma. Bronchitis or bronchial asthma is not cured by excision of bronchiectatic segments. Surgical therapy in general is not indicated where there is too little or too much disease. A period of conservative medical therapy is nearly always indicated, perhaps even for as long as a year, not only to judge its success or failure, but to avoid the mistake of resecting reversible or pseudobronchiectasis, recalling that following the expansion of a collapsed lobe or the resolution of atypical pneumonia the bronchial tree may take months and even a year to revert to normal with disappearance of bronchial dilatation.

BRONCHIAL OBSTRUCTION AND PULMONARY ATELECTASIS

Atelectasis refers to a state of incomplete expansion and airlessness of the lung, due to failure to expand at birth (atelectasis of the newborn) or to collapse of pulmonary alveoli. This results from external compression (pleural effusion or pneumothorax) or bronchial obstruction. Collapse from external compression is ordinarily readily reversible with removal of fluid, air, or fibrous tissue (decortication) from the intrapleural space provided the underlying lung is normal. Atelectasis distal to bronchial obstruction is important for several reasons: (1) its discovery aids considerably in diagnosis as, for example, the lobar atelectasis seen in infancy associated with cystic fibrosis of the pancreas, and in childhood associated with compression of lobar bronchi by caseous nodes, or in adult life associated with bronchogenic carcinoma; (2) it is one of the prevalent causes of postoperative morbidity, and (3) it predisposes to lung abscess and bronchiectasis.

Bronchial obstruction with atelectasis may be caused by endobronchial disease such as tumor, stenosing inflammatory disease such as tuberculosis, foreign body, broncholiths, or inspissated mucous plugs; or it may be caused by extrabronchial compression by enlarged lymph nodes (middle-lobe syndrome), neoplasm, or aneurysm.

Inspissation of mucus to form an obstructing plug is particularly common in patients with bronchial asthma, cystic fibrosis of the pancreas, or chronic bronchitis, in conditions associated with decreased movement of the chest wall, e.g., poliomyelitis, and in the early post-operative period.

Aspiration of foreign body, gastric contents, or of infected material from the upper part of the respiratory tract occurs commonly and may result in pneumonia or abscess formation (see pp. 1337 and 1349) because of bronchial obstruction with distal infection. The defenses against aspiration of cough, laryngeal closure, and ciliary motion are impaired by sleep, alcohol, anesthesia, immersion and exposure, epilepsy, or coma from any cause. Aging per se results in a lessening of the airway's protective reflexes. Blood, mucus, dental deposits, or food may be aspirated, and the infected plug occludes the segmental bronchus. The right lung is more commonly involved because the right main bronchus is the straightest route for aspiration. The parts of the lung affected most often are the posterior segments of the upper lobes and superior segments of the lower lobes, as these are the most dependent areas when the patient is in the supine or lateral decubitus positions, respectively. Foreign body, lung abscess, and aspiration pneumonia are discussed further below.

Obstruction of a main stem bronchus which develops gradually may give rise to mild, vague discomfort in the chest and little or no dyspnea. Acute obstruction of the same bronchus in the postoperative period (acute massive collapse of the lung) may be accompanied by anxiety, agitation, dyspnea, tachypnea, cyanosis, fever, and tachycardia.

Postoperative atelectasis occurs in about 5 percent of patients, most commonly following upper abdominal procedures. It is more likely to be found in men, in smokers, in patients with chronic bronchitis, in the aged, obese, and debilitated, and in patients incapable of early ambulation. Minimal degrees of atelectasis are heralded by mild fever (temperatures to 101°F), tachycardia, and tachypnea within 48 hr after operation. Vague chest discomfort and mild respiratory distress and a cough, first nonproductive but later yielding tenacious mucus or mucopurulent sputum, are usual. If the collapse increases, expansion of the chest may be diminished on the affected side, and hyporesonance, inspiratory rales, and depressed breath sounds may be heard. The chest roentgenogram reveals linear shadows, usually in the lower lung fields, segmental or lobar atelectasis, or merely increased density of pulmonary parenchyma. If lobar or whole lung collapse has occurred acutely, it is heralded by severe agitation and anxiety, dyspnea, and tachypnea. Hypoxia leads to cyanosis and acute systemic hypertension, and there may be substernal oppression if the mediastinum shifts toward the affected side. The percussion note may not be dull if the lung has not had time to lose enough air, but the hemithorax moves poorly and the trachea and heart are shifted *toward* the collapsed side. The roentgenogram shows the mediastinal shift, narrowing of the intercostal spaces, a high diaphragm, and a dense lobe or lung on the affected side. If the inspissated secretions are not removed, pneumonia may develop.

Treatment of atelectasis depends on the cause of the obstruction, and for this reason diagnostic bronchoscopy is always indicated in obscure cases. This procedure is also therapeutic in instances where removal of a foreign body or inspissated secretions is feasible, and it should be done with all haste. Therapeutic bronchoscopy may be necessary in postoperative cases if suctioning, percussion therapy, and coughing do not relieve the situation. The best treatment is preventive, however, and careful pre- and postoperative care will be amply rewarded.

Foreign Bodies in the Air Passages

The importance of aspiration of a foreign body in the genesis of pulmonary disease is frequently overlooked. The physician fails to elicit the history, the patient may have forgotten the event because of a symptomless interval following aspiration, and the various clinical syndromes produced are more readily explained by invoking the commoner disease processes which are mimicked, such as asthma, lung abscess, or bronchiectasis.

In order of frequency, the foreign bodies found are nuts, hardware, pins and needles, dental material, safety pins, and bone. A variety of predisposing factors are known, such as weakening of the defenses against aspiration, bad personal hygiene (loose teeth), or hasty eating. Inhalation of vegetable material such as a peanut causes a severe local and systemic reaction because its shape allows complete occlusion of a bronchus and it also incites a chemical bronchitis. Irregular metallic objects usually produce only incomplete blockage.

A foreign body may shift its location in the lung or be passed to the opposite lung. Those which lodge in the trachea give rise to a palpable thud, an audible slap, and loud wheeze when expiration or cough forces the object against the inferior surface of the vocal cords. Death from asphyxia may occur. When a bronchus is occluded so that there is a "check-valve" effect with expiratory trapping of air, there will be distal emphysema, but complete obstruction leads to atelectasis and, finally, to drowned lung.

The initial episode may be violently symptomatic, with severe cough, wheezing, dyspnea, and cyanosis. Bronchoscopy is an immediate necessity and is successful in removing the foreign body in most cases. If the level of obstruction is in a lobar or segmental bronchus, the initial fit of coughing may be followed by a symptomless interval of days or weeks, after which chronic suppurative disease (lung abscess, bronchiectasis) develops. The patient may finally show the clinical picture of "asthma" and localized hyperinflation of the lung, lung abscess, or bronchiectasis. Bronchoscopy may not reveal the foreign body, as overgrowth of granulation tissue may have obscured it. X-ray may show the radiopaque object, which may also be confused with calcified hilar lymph nodes. Even though symptoms have been present for several years, removal of the foreign body may lead to complete restoration of apparently damaged lung. Therefore after removal, observation under medical therapy is advisable before deciding about the need for lobectomy.

LUNG ABSCESS

ETIOLOGY AND PATHOGENESIS. The commonest etiologic factor in the development of primary lung abscess is aspiration of infected material from the upper part of the respiratory tract, such as dental deposits (see above under Bronchial Obstruction). The virulence of the organisms and their ability to cause necrosis of tissue, the development of vascular occlusion due to septic endarteritis, and the pressure of increasing exudation combine to cause liquefaction of tissue within a few days. If the bronchus is eroded, partial drainage will lead to the formation of an air-fluid level. New abscesses or suppurative pneumonia may occur by direct extension or aspiration of pus into another segment. If healing is delayed, the cavity is lined by a downgrowth of cuboidal or squamous epithelium from connecting bronchi. Formerly, the differentiation of putrid (anaerobic) and nonputrid (aerobic) abscesses was stressed, but this is no longer regarded as important in therapy.

The following conditions predispose to abscess formation in the lung and should be considered in any patient with localized pulmonary suppuration.

Bronchial Obstruction. Most lung abscesses are initiated by bronchial occlusion, either by virtue of aspiration of infected material from the upper airway or the occurrence of an obstructing lesion, such as a tumor or postinflammatory bronchostenosis. Foreign body and bronchostenosis are relatively unusual. *Bronchogenic carcinoma* may be even commoner than aspiration as a condition leading to lung abscess in men beyond the age of forty-five. The abscess may be produced either by obstruction of the bronchus with distal stasis and infection of secretions or, more commonly, by necrosis and excavation within the tumor mass. Radiologically, the wall of the cavity is thick and irregular, the most important clue to the correct diagnosis.

Bacterial Pneumonia. Pneumonias due to the Friedländer bacillus, *Actinomyces bovis,* pneumococcus type III, *Staphylococcus aureus,* and *Streptococcus hemolyticus* are occasionally complicated by true abscess formation because of the ability of these organisms to cause necrosis.

Vascular Embolism. Pulmonary infarction is a rare cause of abscess formation; fewer than 5 percent of bland pulmonary infarcts are secondarily infected. Vascular embolization of infected material from osteomyelitis, suppurative pelvic disease (postabortal), or phlebitis (e.g., in a drug addict) may result in multiple small pulmonary abscesses.

Other Causes. Trauma to the chest may result in abscess formation by penetration of the chest wall by an infected foreign body, by infection superimposed on a traumatic pulmonary hematoma (a very rare event), or because of retained secretions due to reduced cough following rib fracture.

Stasis of secretions or aspiration of infected secretions into a congenital or acquired cyst may result in localized suppuration and accumulation of pus. The finding of a very thin wall with minimal surrounding inflammation may be a radiologic clue. The thin wall is also characteristic of coccidioidomycosis.

Amebic or pyogenic abscesses in the liver or beneath the right side of the diaphragm may extend into the right lower lobe of the lung and result in abscess formation. One should never forget the possibility of tuberculosis as the underlying cause of any lung abscess.

CLINICAL DESCRIPTION. The patient may present himself to the physician with acute or chronic symptoms. Following the initiating event, such as tooth extraction or an alcoholic debauch, there is a several-day period of fever and malaise (representing segmental atelectasis and pneumonitis) followed by chest pain, usually pleuritic (extension of suppurative pneumonitis to pleural surface), and a dry cough. Anywhere from 4 to 10 days after the onset, the cough and fever become more severe (gangrene of lung). Scanty amounts of purulent bloodstreaked sputum (erosion of bronchus) precede acute rupture of the abscess into the bronchial tree. When this occurs, the sputum becomes copious, and up to a liter of purulent and sometimes bloody sputum may be produced for the next several days. As free drainage continues, illness begins to abate, although the temperature may not become normal for several more days. When severe respiratory distress and prostration occur suddenly after the onset of pleural pain, rupture of the abscess into the pleural space with the formation of a pyopneumothorax has probably occurred. In acute lung abscess, if drainage of the area and antibiotic treatment are adequate, the patient will be free of cough and sputum production and constitutional debility after 10 days to 3 weeks of treatment, although complete clearing on the roentgenogram and closure of the cavity may take anywhere from 10 days to 4 months. If drainage is inadequate, the organism is resistant, or treatment is delayed, a necrotic slough forms in the cavity. Chronic cough and purulent sputum persist, with intermittent fever and cachexia.

In the acute disease physical examination reveals a febrile, anxious patient with rapid pulse and respiratory rate. The oral hygiene is usually bad, and the gag reflex may be absent or diminished. Dullness and bronchial breath sounds and rarely a pleural friction rub may be heard over the disease segment. Exquisite tenderness to palpation of the chest wall over the diseased area may be found because of pleural involvement. After bronchial communication has been established, amphoric breath sounds may be heard. Clubbing of fingers and toes is present within weeks of the onset in 10 to 20 percent of cases and regresses with resolution of the disease. Rarely, painful hypertrophic osteoarthropathy may occur, although this usually signifies underlying bronchogenic carcinoma.

Laboratory findings show a polymorphonuclear leukocytosis in the acute phase. With chronic lung abscess a normocytic normochromic anemia may develop.

The sputum is purulent and frequently bloody. Elastic fibers are present, indicating tissue destruction. Culture is essential and may reveal a single organism or varying combinations of beta- and alpha-hemolytic streptococci, staphylococci, occasionally pneumococci, *Hemophilus influenzae,* and *Escherichia coli.* Sensitivity to antibiotics must be determined. Anaerobic cultures will reveal the anaerobic streptococcus, fusiform bacilli, and spirochetal organisms. Sputum should also be examined for tubercle bacilli and malignant cells. Blood cultures obtained during the acute disease may yield the predominant pathogen.

Early in the disease the roentgenogram reveals segmental or lobar consolidation which assumes a spherical shape as the area distends with pus. Localization in the posterior segment of the right upper lobe or superior segment of the lower lobes should suggest the possibility of lung abscess. With rupture into the bronchial tree, an air-fluid level appears. The wall of the abscess cavity should be inspected carefully. If it is very thin, with minimal surrounding pneumonitis, the process may represent infection of a preexisting congenital cyst or bulla. If it is irregular and thick, cavity formation in a bronchogenic carcinoma may be at fault. Abscess due to Friedländer's bacilli may be multiloculated with many fluid levels, and staphylococcic abscess is frequently multiple, small, and thin-walled in a peripheral, subpleural location.

Bronchoscopic examination is necessary, particularly in the patient past forty or in any patient with atypical features or delayed resolution, to rule out neoplasm as the underlying cause. In the child, foreign body must be considered.

Complications of lung abscess are very rare at present, with the exception of pyopneumothorax, and include exsanguinating hemorrhage, metastatic brain abscess, and secondary amyloidosis.

Differential diagnosis of the primary lung abscess includes tuberculosis, empyema with bronchopleural fistula, infected lung cyst, and peripheral carcinoma. Abscess formation must not be confused with the rarefied areas seen in a pneumonic consolidation undergoing normal resolution. Also transient ball-valve occlusion of the bronchus in an area of pneumonia may lead to acute tension cysts, distinguished from lung abscess by their rapid onset and disappearance.

TREATMENT. The principles of treatment of lung abscess are similar to those involved in any suppuration—the establishment of adequate drainage and the eradication of infection (see also Chronic Empyema). Antibiotics and postural drainage are the mainstays of treatment. The longer the duration of symptoms prior to therapy, the less likely is medical cure, although every patient deserves a trial of medical therapy initially. Treatment is begun with 2 to 10 million units of penicillin daily. The urgency of the situation and the results of culture dictate the need for an additional antibiotic to cover gram-negative organisms (see Chap. 135). Postural drainage is instituted, and its practice is guided by the segmental localization of the abscess. A record of sputum volume is kept to follow the course of healing. Bronchoscopy may rarely be of therapeutic benefit. Tracheostomy and suctioning of secretions may be necessary in the weak or paralyzed patient. Clinical improvement occurs within days, and radiologic clearing usually becomes complete within 3 to 6 weeks. Segmental resection and lobectomy are reserved for those individuals who remain symptomatic and without continuous radiologic clearing during 3 to 6 weeks of continuous medical therapy.

In elderly patients, alcoholics, and those with low pulmonary functional reserve, Monaldi's procedure of local rib resection and drainage still has a place because it has a low mortality rate and only slightly greater morbidity rate than segmental resection and lobectomy.

REFERENCES

Bronchial Obstruction and Pulmonary Atelectasis

Churchill, E. D.: The Architectural Basis of Pulmonary Ventilation, Ann. Surg., 137:1, 1953.

Dripps, R. D., and M. V. Deming: Postoperative Atelectasis and Pneumonia, Ann. Surg., 124:94, 1946.

Knowles, J. H.: Pulmonary Function Tests and Thoracic Surgery, pp. 228–243, in "Surgery: A Concise Guide to Clinical Practice," G. L. Nardi and G. D. Zuidema (Eds.), Boston, Little, Brown and Company, 1961.

Spain, D. M.: Acute Nonaeration of Lung: Edema versus Atelectasis, Dis. Chest, 25:550, 1954.

Bronchiectasis

Mallory, T. B.: The Pathogenesis of Bronchiectasis, New Engl. J. Med., 237:795, 1947.

Perry, K. M. A., and D. S. King: Bronchiectasis: Study of Prognosis Based on a Follow-up of 400 Patients, Am. Rev. Tuberc., 41:531, 1940.

Wynn-Williaus, N.: Bronchiectasis: A Study Centered on Bedford and Its Environs, Brit. Med. J., 1:1194, 1953.

——: Observations on the Treatment of Bronchiectasis and Its Relation to Prognosis, Tubercle, 38:133, 1957.

Foreign Bodies in the Air Passages

Jackson, C., and C. L. Jackson: Foreign Bodies in the Air and Food Passages, sec. III, pp. 13, 106 in "Bronchoesophagology," Philadelphia, W. B. Saunders Company, 1950.

Linton, J. S. A.: Long-standing Intrabronchial Foreign Bodies, Thorax, 12:164, 1957.

Lung Abscess

Amberson, J. B.: A Clinical Consideration of Abscesses and Cavities of the Lung, Bull. Johns Hopkins Hosp., 94:227, 1954.

Brock, R. C.: "Lung Abscess," Oxford, Blackwell Scientific Publications, 1952.

Schweppe, H. I., J. H. Knowles, and L. Kane: Lung Abscess: An Analysis of the Massachusetts General Hospital Cases from 1943 through 1956, New Engl. J. Med., 265:1039, 1961.

292 NEOPLASMS OF THE LUNG
Gennaro M. Tisi and
David C. Sabiston

At the turn of the century Adler, in his classical monograph, was able to collect only 374 cases of cancer of the lung from the world's literature. During the past 50 years, there has been a slow but steady increase in the incidence of cancer of the lung. Currently, lung cancer is the most common form of malignancy in the male, reaching a peak between the fifth and seventh decades and accounting for 1 in 4 male cancer deaths. The sex incidence is at least 5 to 1, male to female.

EPIDEMIOLOGY

It has been approximately 30 years since Müller first drew attention to the relationship between lung cancer and heavy cigarette smoking. Extensive statistical analysis has confirmed this relationship. It has been demonstrated that the more cigarettes a person smokes, the greater is his risk of developing cancer of the lung. Hammond and Horn report the death rate in cancer of the lung per hundred thousand is 3.4 in the male nonsmoker; 59.3 for ten to twenty cigarettes daily; and 217.3 for forty or more cigarettes daily. If a person stops smoking, he is less likely to develop lung cancer than his counterpart who continues to smoke. Although smoking has attracted the principal interest in the epidemiology of lung cancer, other factors also have been implicated. Considerable attention has been directed to the potential role of air pollution, exposure to ionizing radiation, and numerous occupational hazards, including exposure to chromates, metallic iron and iron oxides, arsenic, nickel, beryllium, and asbestos. In many tissues, chronic inflammatory changes are known to precede cancer. In the lung, fibrosis may follow focal destructive and proliferative lesions. Numerous studies report an increased incidence of peripheral adenocarcinomas in such areas of chronic scarring (so-called "scar carcinoma").

PATHOLOGY

Primary cancer of the lung can be classified, in terms of its anatomic location, into *central* or *peripheral* categories. Central lesions involve the tracheobronchial tree from the primary to the distal bronchi, while peripheral lesions involve the distal bronchi and bronchioles. The relative frequency of cancer of the lung, when divided into these broad anatomic categories, is approximately equal. This simple classification helps in understanding many of the vagaries of the clinical presentation, the pattern of growth, the avenues of metastasis, and the preferential diagnostic approach.

There is not universal agreement on the histologic classification of primary pulmonary carcinoma. The classification offered here has been selected because it stresses the correlation between a histologic pattern and particular mode of clinical-pathologic behavior. Four basic histologic patterns of primary lung cancer and their approximate relative incidences are recognized: (1) *Squamous cell* carcinoma (epidermoid carcinoma)—60 percent; (2) *adenocarcinoma*—15 percent; (3) *undifferentiated* or anaplastic carcinoma including the round-cell, large-cell, and oat cell types—20 percent; and (4) *bronchiolo-alveolar* cell carcinoma (alveolar cell carcinoma)—2 percent. In some instances it is difficult to discern a uni- from histologic pattern and this leads to the diagnosis of mixed patterns.

With reference to this histologic classification, the following observations should be considered: (1) Squamous cell or epidermoid carcinoma is virtually always associated with cigarette smoking, usually occurs in central locations, produces earlier symptoms due to the potential for bronchial obstruction, spreads generally by continuity, and may undergo cavitation; (2) adenocarcinoma has been associated with focal lung scars and chronic interstitial fibrosis, occurs primarily in peripheral locations, may spread by all routes but particularly by the bloodstream, and often remains clinically silent until distant hematogenous metastases occur; (3) undifferentiated carcinoma is found in a relatively younger age group than the other types, occurs predominantly in the male (as does squamous cell carcinoma), occurs with equal frequency in central and peripheral areas, and metastasizes early; and (4) bronchiolo-alveolar cell carcinoma classically presents with a diffuse or multinodular type of lesion, significant bronchorrhea, progressive dyspnea, and increasing hypoxemia usually associated with hyperventilation. This combination of hypoxemia and hypocapnia is classical of diffuse interstitial processes. Considerable controversy centers on whether alveolar cell carcinoma has a multicentric or unicentric origin. The principal evidence favors a unicentric origin, providing philosophically a brighter approach to therapy.

Primary carcinoma of the lung may spread by any of four routes: (1) direct local extension; (2) hematogenous dissemination; (3) lymphatic spread; and uncommonly (4) transbronchial spread. The preferential sites of extrapulmonary metastasis include the prescalene lymph nodes, liver, brain, adrenal glands, and bones.

CLINICAL PRESENTATION

Primary Tumors

The clinical presentation of carcinoma of the lung depends upon many variables including cell type; site of origin; the concept of biologic predetermination of cancer behavior; and immunologic mechanisms, at present poorly understood. The resulting symptom complexes should be viewed as constituting two modes of presentation: early and late.

The *early* mode of presentation has special clinical significance because a reasonable expectation of cure can be anticipated. In this stage of the disease, a patient may present with symptoms attributable to an intrabronchial lesion, such as a mild cough or a change in the pattern of a chronic cigarette cough. He may instead have symptoms secondary to local bronchial obstruction and/or surrounding inflammation including fever, chills, sputum production, a localized wheeze, or hemoptysis. The latter is alarming but a presenting symptom in only 7 to 10 percent of patients. In many instances a patient may be entirely asymptomatic, the sole reason for referral to medical attention being an abnormal chest roentgenogram. Unfortunately, in the early cases, the physical examination may be entirely negative. A localized wheeze over a segmental bronchus brought out by a forced expiratory or panting maneuver may be an early sign. As the lesion progresses, the classical physical signs due to obstruction may develop, including those of atelectasis, pneumonitis, abscess formation, and loss of lung volume.

The *late* mode of presentation indicates that a lesion has extended beyond the stage of resectional or curative surgery. In this stage of his disease, depending upon the degree or direction of spread, a patient may present with one or a combination of the following: (1) nonspecific systemic symptoms; (2) signs and symptoms due to intrathoracic spread; (3) signs and symptoms due to extrathoracic extension; and (4) classical systemic syndromes.

A patient with advanced disease may present with *nonspecific systemic* symptoms such as weight loss, anorexia, nausea and vomiting, and weakness. The longer the duration of such symptoms, the more likely the lesion is nonresectable.

When the patient is first seen, evidence for *intrathoracic spread* already may be present. Evidence for such spread includes hoarseness, due to involvement of the recurrent laryngeal nerve; pleuritis with or without effusion, due to pleural extension; a unilaterally paralyzed diaphragm with paradoxical motion, due to involvement of the phrenic nerve; dysphagia due to esophageal involvement; Horner's syndrome, due to involvement of the cervical thoracic sympathetic nerves; and superior vena caval obstruction due to entrapment of the superior vena cava.

Symptoms of *extrathoracic spread* or distant metastasis may also be present. The symptoms in any given patient depend upon the sites of metastasis. Commonly involved are one or more of the following: prescalene lymph nodes, brain, liver, adrenal glands, and bone.

The fourth symptom complex includes numerous *systemic syndromes*. These syndromes are of diagnostic value in that, in some instances, they may antedate the roentgenographic appearance of a pulmonary lesion. The list of syndromes associated with cancer of the lung (particularly the oat cell variety) continues to grow. This intriguing array of classical systemic syndromes can be divided into six categories: (1) *metabolic* including hypercalcemia, the syndrome of inappropriate ADH secretion, Cushing's syndrome, gynecomastia, and carcinoid syndrome (the latter is usually associated with bronchial adenoma); (2) *neuromuscular* including peripheral neuropathy, corticocerebellar degeneration, and nonspecific myopathy; (3) *connective tissue* abnormalities including hypertrophic pulmonary osteoarthropathy, clubbing, and nonspecific arthralgias; (4) *dermatologic* abnormalities including acanthosis nigricans and dermatomyositis; (5) *vascular* abnormalities including thrombocytopenic purpura, leukemoid reaction, myelophthisic anemia, and nonbacterial thrombotic endocarditis.

Two modes of presentation deserve separate mention: the patient with a solitary pulmonary nodule (coin lesion) and the patient with a bronchial adenoma.

A *solitary pulmonary nodule* is one with minimal satellite lesions in the pulmonary parenchyma and normally aerated lung around it. Its shape may be round or oval; lobulations, if present, must be minimal. Its margins are circumscribed and its contour smooth, and there must be minimal, if any, associated pneumonitis, atelectasis, or regional adenopathy. Most patients with such a lesion have no symptoms on initial questioning, but upon closer interrogation, a number may admit to a slight cough. Several roentgenographic features should be stressed. The presence of indentation or umbilication of the nodule's border has been referred to as a potential sign of malignancy ("notch sign"). Review of old roentgenograms is of particular importance in the evaluation of a patient with a solitary pulmonary nodule since a demonstrable increase in size suggests that the lesion is neoplastic. The pattern of calcification within a lesion is of paramount importance. The presence of a calcific fleck or of peripheral calcification does not exclude the presence of a malignant lesion. However, centrally located or "core" calcification, lamination, and dense generalized calcification are often associated with benign lesions. In reviewing series of resected solitary pulmonary nodules, one must bear in mind that preoperative evaluation excludes the obviously benign lesions, and therefore these surgical series are weighted to favor a higher incidence of malignant lesions. In 1956, Davis collected 1,203 cases of resected solitary pulmonary nodules from the literature. Of resected lesions, 36.7 percent were malignant with bronchogenic carcinoma comprising the major subgroup. The remaining 63.3 percent were benign, with granulomas accounting for approximately two-thirds of the benign group. In the individual patient surgical excision remains the only absolute assurance of benignity.

Bronchial adenomas (carcinoid bronchial adenoma) comprise 3 to 10 percent of all surgically excised pulmonary neoplasms. They are primarily central in location with approximately 90 percent visible at bronchoscopy. The characteristics of central location, slow growth, and marked vascularity account for the common types of clinical presentation: (1) recurrent hemoptysis; (2) localized wheezing; (3) infection distal to bronchial obstruction; and (4) history often antedating diagnosis by 5 or more years. Distant blood-borne metastases are rare. Bronchial adenoma, like oat cell carcinoma, has been associated with multiple endocrinopathies.

Metastatic Tumors

The pulmonary capillaries with a mean cross-sectional diameter of 12 micra are ideally suited to the entrapment of tumor emboli. This feature and the rich lymphatic supply of the lung account, in large part, for the high incidence of metastatic (secondary) carcinoma to the lung. The great majority of pulmonary metastatic lesions are adenocarcinomas from the gastrointestinal tract, genitourinary tract, and glandular tissues. Metastases to the lung are usually spherical in shape, variable in size, multiple, and bilateral. These roentgenographic features combined with symptoms suggesting an extrapulmonary source help in the differential diagnosis of primary from metastatic carcinoma.

Early diagnosis and improved therapy have produced an increase in the number of long-term survivors of nonpulmonary, primary malignancies. If such a patient presents with a new pulmonary lesion in the course of his long-term follow-up, what are the etiologic possibilities? The problem of distinguishing among late metastasis to the lung, a new primary in the lung, or a benign pulmonary lesion has been reviewed by Adkins. The majority of such patients will present with ancillary evidence of metastatic spread from the original primary tumor. The pattern of spread will depend upon the sites of predilection of the original primary. However, if the patient is asymptomatic, and if diagnostic evaluation fails to provide evidence for other distant metastases, a substantial percentage of such lesions will prove to be either a new primary or a benign lesion.

DIAGNOSTIC EVALUATION

There are three principal aims in the diagnostic evaluation of a patient with carcinoma of the lung: (1) Identification of the lesion as a carcinoma; (2) determination whether the pulmonary lesion has extended (a) beyond the pulmonary parenchyma and (b) beyond the thoracic cavity; and (3) preoperative cardiopulmonary evaluation to determine whether the patient with an operable lesion will be able to tolerate the degree of resection anticipated.

In most instances, the initial diagnostic approach is *roentgenographic*. Many times the x-ray may provide the only abnormality in an asymptomatic patient. In all cases, inquiries about past roentgenograms should be made, and every attempt should be made to obtain these films promptly. The initial x-ray lesion may be of any size, shape, or location. Early roentgenographic signs include the solitary pulmonary nodule, areas of localized overinflation due to intrabronchial obstruction, atelectasis with unilateral loss of volume, and the appearance of localized inflammatory changes. All patients over the age of forty with pneumonia should be followed with serial chest films to the point of complete resolution. Such an approach may lead to the diagnosis of a slowly resolving pneumonia and be the first indication of carcinoma of the lung. Roentgenographic signs of intrathoracic spread include pleural thickening and/or effusion (providing an inflammatory basis is excluded), elevation of a diaphragm, rib erosion, hilar metastasis, and lymphatic obstruction with Kerley B lines. Multiple roentgenographic

views, including lateral and oblique projections, and tomography may be invaluable in defining the features described above, particularly the presence of calcification within solitary pulmonary nodules. Fluoroscopy may help in determining the mobility of a diaphragm and in differentiation of neoplastic processes from vascular lesions, granulomatous diseases, inflammatory lesions, thromboemboli, and artifacts. Common artifacts include chest wall lesions such as warts and hemangiomas, nipple shadows, and technical artifacts due to film processing.

The triad of bronchoscopy, scalene lymph node biopsy, and cytologic smear will provide information on both the tissue diagnosis and the extension of lung cancer. *Bronchoscopy* and bronchoscopic biopsy are of principal value in central epidermoid carcinomas. Lower-lobe tumors, which less commonly metastasize to the anterior scalene nodes, are usually accessible to bronchoscopy and bronchoscopic biopsy. It has been reported that a positive diagnosis of epidermoid carcinoma can be established in 26 to 60 percent of patients by means of bronchoscopy and bronchoscopic biopsy. Bronchoscopy is obviously of less value in peripheral adenocarcinomas. However, it is significant that *scalene node biopsy* is most successful in the diagnosis of those lung cancers which are inaccessible to bronchoscopy. The yield in scalene node biopsy is greater when the lesion involves the upper rather than the lower lobes, and greater when the lesion is a peripheral adeno- or undifferentiated carcinoma than when it is a central squamous cell carcinoma. The side of a scalene node biopsy should preferentially include the side of parenchymal involvement and all palpable nodes. Reports of *cytologic smears* illustrate considerable lack of uniformity and success in the detection of lung cancer. The primary variables here are the training of the cytologist and the method of sputum collection. The range of positive cytologic smears has been reported anywhere from 44 to 95 percent. Most observers have noted a decreased yield in the cytodiagnosis of peripherally situated lung carcinomas.

If a pleural effusion is observed as an isolated presentation or related to a parenchymal lesion, *thoracentesis* and *needle biopsy* of the *pleura* should be performed. The fluid should be sent for cytologic analysis. The character of the pleural fluid in malignancy is usually exudative (specific gravity greater than 1.015 and protein greater than 3.5 Gm per 100 ml) with an increased red blood cell count (greater than 10,000 red blood cells per cu cm).

When the initial clinical presentation, physical examination, or initial laboratory examination suggests one of the classical patterns of metastatic spread to liver, brain, or bone, further evaluation should include, in the instance of suspected brain metastasis, skull films, echoencephalogram, brain scan, and lumbar puncture; in the instance of suspected liver metastasis, liver function tests and liver scan and biopsy; and in the instance of bone metastases, a skeletal x-ray survey, radioisotopic bone scan, and biopsy where possible.

The efficacy of closed-chest *needle biopsy* of the lung in establishing a diagnosis of pulmonary carcinoma has been stressed by many centers. The primary use of this procedure is reserved for those patients who have probable inoperable or nonresectable lesions and in whom a tissue diagnosis should be obtained prior to institution of second-line therapy such as radiation and/or chemotherapy.

In patients with carcinoma of the lung, *pulmonary scintiphotoscans* with radioisotope-labeled macroaggregated albumin may provide nonspecific information on the status of arteriocapillary pulmonary perfusion. At the current stage of development of this technique, the scintiphotoscan cannot differentiate altered perfusion due to vascular occlusion from altered perfusion due to regional hypoventilation. It is hoped that pulmonary scintiphotoscans and pulmonary angiograms in selected patients may provide potentially valuable and reliable information on resectability and operability.

Several centers have reported their experience with *interosseous azygography*. This procedure allows roentgenographic evaluation of the mediastinal venous pattern. A definite deformity or a complete blockade may provide evidence of the mediastinal extension of an intrathoracic lesion and thus offer evidence of nonresectability. *Mediastinoscopy* with acquisition of biopsy material may provide similar evidence of extension and for nonresectability.

Although a patient may have a pulmonary lesion, which by all criteria is operable, with potential for a curative resection, a decisive problem remains. Will the patient's cardiopulmonary reserve allow him to tolerate the degree of pulmonary resection anticipated? If there are no clinical signs of cardiopulmonary disability, simple determination of static lung volumes, dynamic flow rates, and resting arterial blood gas tensions and pH is sufficient, but if these studies are abnormal, further evaluation is indicated. The patient with obvious pulmonary disability presents a more complex physiologic problem. In this group of patients the determination of the type and degree of disability is essential. The more extensive the patient's clinical disability, the more extensive and sophisticated should be his preoperative evaluation.

Indications of nonoperability include laboratory evidence of (1) a *severe* restrictive and/or obstructive defect (determined by static lung volumes, dynamic flow rates, and measurement of pulmonary compliance and total pulmonary resistance by body plethysmography, Chap. 280); (2) a *markedly reduced* functional pulmonary arteriocapillary bed (determined by a decreased diffusion capacity for carbon monoxide, an increase in calculated wasted ventilation, i.e, ventilation of nonperfused areas, and resting hypoxemia with a widening of the alveolar-arterial oxygen gradient under conditions of exercise); (3) *grossly abnormal* ventilation/perfusion relationships (determined by pulmonary scintiphotoscans with radioisotope-labeled macroaggregated albumin, Xenon (^{133}Xe) ventilation/perfusion scans, and pulmonary angiography); (4) *marked alveolar hypoventilation* (determined by a level of alveolar ventilation inadequate to maintain a normal arterial carbon dioxide tension);

(5) *serious* pulmonary hypertension and cor pulmonale (determined by right heart catheterization with measurement of cardiac output, pulmonary artery pressure, and total pulmonary vascular resistance).

TREATMENT

If a patient has had adequate diagnostic evaluation, the therapeutic approach will follow naturally. The currently preferred therapeutic approach is surgical resection of the primary pulmonary carcinoma. In most instances, in an attempt to conserve pulmonary function, lobectomy rather than pneumonectomy is the operation of choice, provided the lesion can be excised completely by lobectomy.

An operative candidate is an individual who has no demonstrable evidence of intra- or extrathoracic spread of his malignancy and whose cardiopulmonary status does not preclude resectional surgery. Accepted contraindications to thoracotomy and pulmonary resection for primary carcinoma include (1) evidence of metastatic lymph node involvement; (2) superior vena caval obstruction; (3) recurrent laryngeal or phrenic nerve paralysis; (4) pleural thickening and/or effusion, with histologic evidence of carcinomatous involvement of the pleura, and/or the presence of malignant cells in the pleural fluid; (5) distant metastasis to liver, brain, adrenal glands, or bones; (6) multicentric or multilobar distribution of the lesion; and finally (7) a *serious* cardiopulmonary functional defect.

The *classical systemic syndromes,* with which a patient may present, by themselves do not constitute contraindications to resection. To the contrary, since they may contribute significantly to the patient's discomfort and demise, resection of the pulmonary parenchymal lesion may offer significant palliation. As a rule, many of these syndromes abate with resection and recur with metastasis.

The management of a patient with inoperable pulmonary carcinoma includes *supervoltage radiotherapy* and *chemotherapy.* Radiotherapy alone is seldom curative, while chemotherapy alone is generally ineffective. However, both modalities have a definite role in the palliative treatment of some patients with distressing manifestations of pain, superior vena caval obstruction, bleeding, and bronchial obstruction. The physiologic evaluation of the candidate for radiotherapy is as critical as that of the operative candidate, for the patient with severe cardiopulmonary disability may be converted to a cardiopulmonary cripple by extensive radiation therapy as well as by resection.

There is renewed enthusiasm in the use of preoperative supervoltage radiation in an attempt to obtain sterilization of local lymph nodes and reduction in size of the primary parenchymal lesion. Both of these goals, especially with regard to superior sulcus tumors, may increase the percentage of resectable lesions and improve the survival statistics.

PROGNOSIS

The prognosis of primary carcinoma is a direct function of the cell type and the extent of the malignant process at the time of diagnosis. The statistics of survival for the patient with inoperable carcinoma are universally poor; the average survival time from diagnosis to demise has been variously reported as between 5 and 14 months. Of all patients with carcinoma of the lung, one-third are inoperable at the time of diagnosis. Of the remaining patients only 30 to 50 percent of those subjected to exploratory thoracotomy prove to be resectable. The 5-year survival of this selected resectable group is approximately 20 percent. This results in an overall 5-year survival of all patients with primary pulmonary carcinoma of approximately 5 percent. It is apparent that the major therapeutic gains and improved prognoses, at this time, hinge upon the early diagnosis of the early lesion. Jackman and associates support this tenet by reporting a resectability rate of 98 percent and a 5-year survival of 45 percent for bronchogenic carcinoma presenting as a solitary nodule (less than 4 cm in diameter).

REFERENCES

Adkins, P. C., C. W. Wesselhoeft, Jr., W. Newman, and B. Blades: Thoracotomy on the Patient with Previous Malignancy: Metastasis or New Primary, J. Thor. Cardiov. Surg., 56:351, 1968.

Beck, R. E., S. Kay and J. W. Brooks: Oat Cell Carcinoma of the Lung, Surg. Gynecol. Obstet., 122:826, 1966.

Davis, E. W., J. W. Peabody, Jr., and S. Katz: The Solitary Pulmonary Nodule, J. Thor. Surg., 32:728, 1956.

Greenberg, E., M. B. Divertie, and L. B. Woolner: A Review of Unusual Systemic Manifestations Associated with Carcinomas, Am. J. Med., 36:106, 1964.

Jackman, R. J., A. C. Good, O. T. Clagett, and L. B. Woolner: Survival Rates in Peripheral Bronchogenic Carcinomas up to Four Centimeters in Diameter Presenting as Solitary Pulmonary Nodules, J. Thor. Cardiov. Surg., 57:1, 1969.

Liebow, A. A.: Bronchiolo-alveolar carcinoma, Adv. Intern. Med., 10:329, 1960.

Smoking and Health, Report of the Advisory Committee to the Surgeon General of the Public Health Service, Pub. Health Serv. Publ. No. 1103, 1964.

293 DISEASES OF THE PLEURA, MEDIASTINUM, AND DIAPHRAGM

David C. Sabiston, Jr.

THE PLEURA

The pleura and pleural cavities are the site of a variety of medical and surgical disorders. An understanding of their development is important in consideration of the diseases related to these structures. During embryogenesis the two pleural cavities become separated from the central pericardial cavity by the pleuroperi-cardial membranes. Although initially they are continuous with the peritoneal cavity, further development of the pleuroperitoneal membrane ultimately separates these serous cavities. However, defects may remain and may be the site of a hernia connecting the pleural and peritoneal cavities. The parietal pleura covers the inner surface of the chest wall, the diaphragm, and the mediastinum, and is reflected at the pulmonary hilum to cover the entire lung. The pleura is composed of a very thin layer of connective tissue with a mesothelial surface. Both smooth-muscle and elastic fibers are present, and numerous lymphatics and small vessels form a diffuse network in the pleural wall. In addition, the pleura is supplied with many nerve fibers, a factor of considerable importance in the presence of inflammation or stretching of the pleura, either of which is apt to produce a highly *painful* response.

Several important physiologic principles affect the pleura. Normally, the intrapleural pressure is negative and varies between −4 to 8 cm of water at the end of inspiration and −2 to 4 cm at the end of expiration. In patients with severe pulmonary emphysema, the intrapleural pressure is apt to be less negative than normal; in pneumothorax the pressure is usually elevated, frequently to a high level. Air or gas in the pleural cavity produces a partial collapse of the underlying lung. The disappearance of the gas in the pleural cavity is related to the concentration of the specific gas in the blood, as well as to other factors. For example, oxygen is more rapidly absorbed than nitrogen, and with the passage of time, air in the pleural cavity has a higher concentration of nitrogen. Since carbon dioxide is present in the blood, equilibrium is established between this gas and the blood, yielding a higher concentration of carbon dioxide than is present in normal air.

In the normal pleural cavity the surfaces of the pleural membranes are moist, although no appreciable amount of fluid is present. In various disease processes, fluid may accumulate in the pleural cavities; such fluid has been arbitrarily divided into two groups: (1) transudates and (2) exudates. The transudates have a specific gravity less than 1.015 with a protein content under 2 or 3 Gm per 100 ml. Transudates are usually clear, although they may have a tinge of color and at times may contain blood. Few cells are present. Examples of transudates are the fluid accumulations in congestive heart failure, cirrhosis of the liver, and nephritis. Exudates are generally thicker and may be either clear or cloudy. They may contain a considerable number of cellular elements as well as bacteria. Such fluid is found in inflammation and infection of the pleura.

Hydrothorax

The accumulation of significant amounts of fluid in the pleural cavity may be the result of a variety of causative factors. The diagnosis may be established by abnormal physical findings which include prominence of the interspaces on the affected side, increased dullness on percussion, impaired transmission of breath sounds, and deviation of the trachea to the opposite side. The chest roentgenogram confirms the diagnosis with evidence of marked radiopacity of the involved pleural cavity. Perhaps the most common cause of noninflammatory fluid collection in the pleural cavity is congestive heart failure. Other causes include nephrosis with hypoproteinemia, trauma, and cirrhosis of the liver. Primary or metastatic neoplastic involvement of the pleura may produce a transudate or an exudate. Some females with an ovarian fibroma may also have an associated pleural effusion (Meigs' syndrome), a poorly understod transudate which disappears following removal of the ovarian neoplasm. The "phantom tumor" is an interesting form of pleural effusion which can present a diagnostic problem. This lesion is usually found on a chest roentgenogram and is actually an interlobar effusion occurring with congestive heart failure or following pleural inflammation.

CHYLOTHORAX. The accumulation of fluid in the pleural cavities may be caused by chylothorax. As the thoracic duct passes through the posterior mediastinum, it may be ruptured as a result of trauma, invaded by tumor, or injured in a thoracic surgical procedure. Chyle has a milky appearance, a specific gravity between 1.020 and 1.030, a protein content of 3 to 4 Gm per 100 ml, and fat content from 1 to 4 Gm per 100 ml. In most instances, chylothorax can be managed by aspiration or continuous catheter drainage. In refractory cases, thoracotomy with direct closure of the lymph fistula is indicated.

Another cause of pleural effusion is that which has been termed "sympathetic effusion." An inflammatory process beneath the diaphragm, such as a subphrenic abscess or acute pancreatitis, can stimulate the accumulation of fluid in the pleural cavities as a response to injury. In the early stages such fluid is usually a transudate and sterile, although later it may become thicker and infected.

Pleuritis

Inflammation of the pleura is apt to produce severe pain, which is often sharp and stabbing in quality, aggravated by deep inspiration, and augmented by coughing and sneezing. The cause of acute pleurisy may be pneumonia, viral infections, tuberculosis, and pulmonary abscess. The inflammation usually resolves with the subsidence of the primary disease. *Fibrinous pleurisy* may be a sequel and may be associated with a friction rub. The treatment of pleuritis and fibrinous pleurisy is generally directed toward the primary disease. The use of analgesics, strapping, and intercostal block may at times be symptomatically helpful. Failure of the process to resolve completely may produce chronic *adhesive pleuritis*. In this condition, marked pleural thickening may be sufficient to interfere with pulmonary function. It may be the final result of an empyema, tuberculous effusion, or unresolved hemothorax. If pleuritis is chronic, and especially when it is productive of symptoms, surgical removal of the thickened pleura (decortication) may be indicated.

Empyema

Empyema is defined as the presence of purulent fluid in the pleural cavity. It is the result of extension of infection from a contiguous structure, and may be a complication of pneumonia, pulmonary abscess, subdiaphragmatic abscess, perforation of a carcinoma into the pleural cavity, or penetration from an acute mediastinitis. In most instances, acute empyema is a serious infection and produces prominent clinical manifestations. Malaise, fever, and tachycardia are generally present and are accompanied by appropriate physical signs of fluid accumulation within the chest. The chest roentgenogram also usually shows evidence of fluid, although the definitive diagnosis rests upon thoracentesis with aspiration of purulent material and subsequent culture for the specific organism. Some of the more frequently encountered organisms responsible for empyema include *Staphylococcus aureus,* anaerobic streptococcus, *Escherichia coli. Pseudomonas aeruginosa, Klebsiella pneumoniae.*

The therapy of empyema is directed both at the control of the specific organism by appropriate use of antimicrobial drugs and at drainage of the pleural cavity. Needle aspiration of the pleural cavity is rarely effective in the management of empyema, and surgical drainage is most often required in adults. Moreover, surgical drainage is apt to be followed by rapid amelioration of symptoms and marked improvement in the clinical course of the patient. In selected patients *closed* drainage employing a trocar for introduction of a tube is satisfactory, but in the majority of patients open drainage with resection of a small portion of rib is the treatment of choice. The empyema cavity gradually becomes obliterated with expansion of the underlying lung. Occasionally, decortication for removal of a fibrous peel surrounding the lung may be necessary in order to produce expansion and obliteration and healing of the empyema cavity. In rare instances, when treatment is delayed, the empyema presents beneath the skin and drains spontaneously ("empyema necessitatis"). Treatment of empyema is more difficult in the presence of a bronchopleural fistula and requires suction under negative pressure in order to expand the lung. If the fistula is the result of a benign inflammatory process, it is likely to close spontaneously. However, should the fistula be due to neoplastic disease, spontaneous closure is very unlikely.

Chronic Empyema. If the acute process is not treated adequately, chronic empyema may result. Continuous drainage of purulent material from the chest may lead to chronic debilitation, including anemia, malnutrition, and, occasionally, secondary amyloidosis. Treatment should be directed toward the surgical closure of the empyema cavity by decortication.

Spontaneous Pneumothorax

The term *spontaneous pneumothorax* is applied to a condition frequently encountered in otherwise healthy patients who suddenly exhibit symptoms of pneumo-

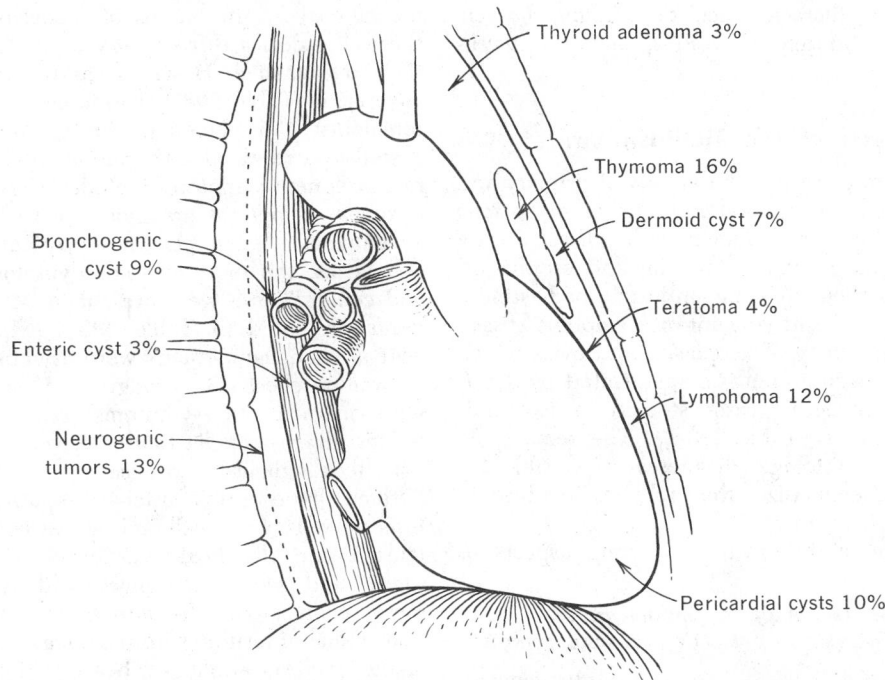

Fig. 293-1. Diagrammatic illustration of usual anatomic sites of primary cysts and neoplasms of the mediastinum. The figures given refer to those shown in the series presented in Table 293-1.

thorax. Formerly, it was thought that the onset of this condition was truly *spontaneous,* but subsequent evidence has shown that it is nearly always produced by rupture of an emphysematous bleb on the pleural surface. The severity of the clinical manifestations varies in proportion to the magnitude of the pneumothorax. At times the amount of air may be minimal, producing only slight pleural pain. In some patients the amount of air in the pleural cavity is great, collapsing the lung, with resultant shift in the mediastinum, heart, and trachea to the opposite side, and producing severe dyspnea and cyanosis. Spontaneous pneumothorax is characterized by a sudden onset of unilateral chest pain associated with dyspnea. The pain is often sharp and agonizing and produces considerable apprehension in the patient, especially during the first attack. The chest roentgenogram establishes the extent of the pulmonary collapse, and together with the gravity of the symptoms, dictates the choice of therapy. Though the majority of spontaneous pneumothoraxes result from rupture of emphysematous blebs, the condition is known to follow specific pulmonary diseases such as sarcoidosis, silicosis, infection, and neoplasms in rare instances. If the amount of air is minimal, with only slight collapse of the lung, observation alone may suffice. More commonly, it is necessary to perform a thoracentesis, removing the air, and preferably to insert an indwelling chest catheter for continuous drainage of the pleural cavity.

One of the characteristics of spontaneous pneumothorax is its *tendency to recur.* Following the first attack, a second one occurs in half the patients; there is an even higher likelihood of a third attack after a second one.

Though the first and second attacks are most often treated by removal of the air alone, either by thoracentesis or the use of an intercostal catheter, the third and subsequent attacks are generally best treated by open thoracotomy. The surgical procedure is designed to produce an adherence of the parietal pleura to the visceral pleura so that a pneumothorax cannot recur. This can be accomplished by pleurectomy or by the application of irritants to the pleural surfaces (poudrage). When pleural blebs are present, these can also be resected at the time of operation.

THE MEDIASTINUM

The mediastinum is an anatomic division of the thorax which may be the site of numerous disorders, including neoplasms, cysts, inflammation, emphysema, and aneurysms (Fig. 293-1). Anatomically, the mediastinum extends from the superior aperture of the thorax to the diaphragm; it is bounded laterally by the mediastinal pleura and posteriorly by the vertebral column. For descriptive purposes, the mediastinum is customarily divided into three major compartments: the superior, anterior (or middle), and posterior divisions. The clinical manifestations of the various disorders of the mediastinum are due in part to pressure or invasion of the multiple structures present within the mediastinum. In the *superior* division are the thymus gland, trachea, esophagus, thoracic duct, aortic arch, innominate vein, and the phrenic, vagal, and recurrent nerves. The *anterior* mediastinum contains the heart, pericardium, lymph nodes, and substernal fibroareolar tissue. In the *posterior* division are the esophagus, thoracic duct, descending thoracic aorta, intercostal and azygos vessels, and the vagus nerves.

Tumors and Cysts of the Mediastinum

The mediastinum is the site of a variety of primary and metastatic neoplasms. In addition, a number of specific cysts originate in the mediastinum, including those arising from the pericardium, thymus, bronchi, and esophagus. Lymphomas are particularly common in the mediastinum because of the significant amount of lymphoid tissue present. The large variety of neoplasms and cysts which may occur in the mediastinum is demonstrated by a collection of 330 consecutive cases studied in two university medical centers (Table 293-1). The remarkable number of specific histologic diagnoses responsible for mediastinal lesions emphasizes the problems involved in diagnosis and management.

DIAGNOSIS. One of the more interesting aspects of

Table 293-1. INCIDENCE OF VARIOUS TYPES
OF PRIMARY NEOPLASMS AND CYSTS OF THE MEDIASTINUM*

Cysts		107 (32%)
Bronchogenic	27 (25%)	
Pericardial	33 (31%)	
Dermoid	24 (23%)	
Enterogenous	10 (9%)	
Nonspecific†	13 (12%)	
Thymoma		52 (16%)
Benign	39 (75%)	
Malignant	13 (25%)	
Neurogenic		43 (13%)
Neurinoma	9 (21%)	
Ganglioneuroma	12 (28%)	
Neurofibroma	13 (30%)	
Neurogenic sarcoma	3 (7%)	
Ganglioneurosarcoma	1 (2%)	
Neuroblastoma	3 (7%)	
Paraganglioma	2 (5%)	
Carcinoma‡		34 (10%)
Teratoma		12 (4%)
Hodgkin's disease		17 (5%)
Lymphosarcoma		15 (5%)
Sarcoma		9 (2%)
Thyroid neoplasms		10 (3%)
Lipoma		6 (2%)
Parathyroid adenoma		4 (1%)
Miscellaneous neoplasms (fibroma, leiomyoma, leiomyosarcoma, mesothelioma, hemangioma, lymphoblastoma, nonspecific lymphomas, liposarcoma, fibrosarcoma, myxoma, lymphangioma, seminoma, mesothelioma)		21 (7%)
Total		330

* Summary of 330 patients observed at the Johns Hopkins Hospital and the Duke University Medical Center.

† These cysts represent benign lesions in which the lining consisted of fibrous tissue without further evidence of a specific histologic type.

‡ Patients in whom carcinoma was found in the mediastinum without evidence of a pulmonary or other primary lesion.

the clinical manifestations of mediastinal lesions is that these disorders are frequently asymptomatic, even when they are massive. However, in two-thirds of the cases covered in Table 293-1 symptoms were present. In the remainder (35 percent), the diagnosis was first suggested as a result of a routine chest roentgenogram. The most frequent symptoms included chest pain, cough, and dyspnea. Symptoms are most apt to be associated with a malignant lesion. In most patients with malignant neoplasms, the most common symptoms are chest pain and cough. These were present in 94 percent of the patients presented in Table 293-1, whereas only 6 percent of malignant lesions were asymptomatic and found on routine chest roentgenogram. A variety of syndromes with characteristic symptoms may be associated with lesions in the mediastinum. Several examples include von Recklinghausen's disease in association with neurofibroma, hypertrophic osteoarthropathy with neurogenic tumors, red blood cell aplasia with thymomas, hypertension and diarrheal syndromes with pheochromocytomas and ganglioneuromas, and hypoglycemia with mesotheliomas and teratomas. Pressure symptoms are also common, resulting from encroachment on or invasion of the trachea, esophagus, heart, various nerves, or great veins.

The diagnostic evaluation begins with a careful history to determine the site and extent of the lesion, with especial emphasis on manifestations which suggest a specific lesion. Roentgenographic studies are essential, and the chest roentgenograms in the anteroposterior, oblique, and lateral positions usually outline the size and extent of the lesion. The use of fluoroscopy (to establish the presence of intrinsic pulsations), esophagram, and tomography are helpful. Angiocardiography plays an important role in the differentiation of vascular lesions involving the great veins, pulmonary vessels, and aorta. Radioisotope scanning is helpful in the diagnosis of thyroid and perhaps parathyroid lesions within the mediastinum. Mediastinoscopy and bronchoscopy may also be useful, especially in establishing the histologic diagnosis. The differentiation between vascular lesions and primary mediastinal tumors and cysts is of considerable importance. In a recent study a distinct group of patients (8 percent) was initially thought to have primary cardiovascular abnormalities. The original diagnosis was made on the basis of chest roentgenograms and the associated clinical findings. Angiocardiography showed the mediastinal mass to be nonvascular in each case. Similarly, it is important to employ angiocardiography in the diagnosis of those lesions which indeed are vascular in order to be prepared properly at the time of surgical exploration. For example, extracorporeal circulation may be necessary in the treatment of aneurysms and other vascular abnormalities.

The anatomic site of the lesion is often of diagnostic significance. Characteristically, the superior mediastinum is the location in which substernal goiters and thymic tumors occur. The anterior (and middle) mediastinum is the most common site of teratomas, dermoid cysts, and lymphomas. Pericardial and bronchogenic cysts are also

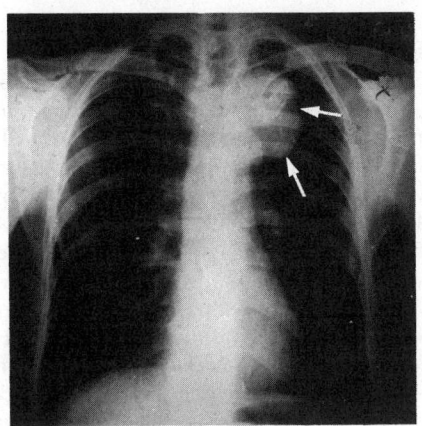 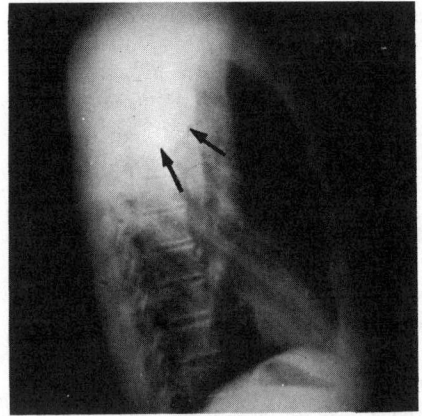

Fig. 293-2. *A.* Chest roentgenogram showing neurofibroma in left upper mediastinum. *B.* Lateral chest roentgenogram illustrating posterior position.

found in this location. The posterior mediastinum is the well-recognized site of nearly all neurogenic tumors (Fig. 293-2). It is thus possible to evaluate statistically mediastinal lesions in a meaningful manner according to their location.

Neurogenic tumors are among the most common histologic types found in the mediastinum. They occur in all age groups, but the malignant variants are most often present in childhood. Nearly all neurogenic tumors arise in the posterior mediastinum near the paravertebral gutter. These lesions arise from the intercostal nerves, the sympathetic chain, and embryonal neurogenic rests. Though many are asymptomatic, pain and/or cough are present in approximately two-thirds of neurogenic tumors. Hormonal activity may be present in ganglioneuromas and neuroblastomas, and diarrhea, hypertension, flushing, and sweating may occur in these patients. The urine may show excretion of vanillylmandelic acid (VMA). *Neurofibromas* may occur either singly or in association with von Recklinghausen's disease. Neurilemmomas arise from the sheath of Schwann. *Ganglioneuromas* originate from the sympathetic chain and have a stronger potential to become malignant, especially in children. Neuroblastomas may also occur in the mediastinum, usually in children, and are especially responsive to x-ray therapy. Pheochromocytomas may arise from sympathetic tissue along the vertebral column and are capable of secreting epinephrine and norepinephrine with corresponding symptoms. Other chromaffin tumors are also present and may be hormonally inactive.

Teratodermoid tumors characteristically occur in the anterior mediastinum. In its simplest form, the lesion is an isolated cyst with ectodermal components alone. However, the majority of these lesions, even in the cystic form, contain cells from each of the three primary germ layers and are therefore more properly called ·teratodermoids. The lesions often contain teeth, which may be seen in the chest roentgenogram. Most of the lesions become apparent in adult life and may become quite large. Unless removed, they have a tendency to become malignant. Approximately 10 percent undergo malignant change, usually in the epithelial component. *Chorio-*

epithelioma, a type of embryonal carcinoma, may rarely occur solely in the mediastinum. It is found almost exclusively in the male.

Thymomas are common mediastinal lesions, especially in association with myasthenia gravis (Chap. 377). The incidence of the latter disorder in patients with thymomas has been reported to range from 10 to 50 percent, whereas the presence of thymomas in patients with myasthenia gravis is lower (8 to 10 percent). The beneficial effects of thymectomy in patients with myasthenia gravis have been greatest in the young female without a thymoma, especially if the disease is of short duration. Similarly, patients with myasthenia gravis and a thymoma have a poorer prognosis. Thymomas are often malignant (25 percent in Table 293-1), but they rarely metastasize. Their malignant potential is demonstrated by direct invasion of the lung, pericardium, blood vessels, and lymphatics. Thus, a diagnosis of a malignant thymoma is made primarily on the basis of its gross and microscopic invasiveness, rather than on the basis of the histologic cell type. Fortunately, the malignant lesions are usually sensitive to x-ray therapy.

Lymphomas are especially common in the mediastinum, and involvement of lymph nodes with leukemia, lymphosarcoma, Hodgkin's disease, and the various types of reticulum sarcoma are well recognized. Though most of these tumors are widespread, solitary lesions also occur. The chest roentgenogram usually demonstrates multiple lesions, and the supraclavicular nodes are frequently involved as well. If the lesions are localized, surgical extirpation may be performed. Additional treatment with irradiation and chemotherapy is also indicated.

Mediastinal *thyroid* lesions usually occur in the superior mediastinum and receive their blood supply from the thyroid vessels. Totally intrathoracic thyroid (or ectopic) mediastinal lesions are rare.

Parathyroid adenoma in the mediastinum, usually within the thymus gland, has been recognized for many years. As many as 10 percent of parathyroid adenomas have been reported to occur in the mediastinum, and nearly all are associated with clinical evidence of hyperparathyroidism.

Primary *cysts* are among the most common mediastinal lesions. The vast majority of these cysts occur in the *anterior* mediastinum. In the collected series shown in Table 293-1, these lesions comprise 32 percent of the total. In this group, most of the lesions (62 percent) were asymptomatic, and the diagnosis was made on routine chest roentgenogram. Pericardial cysts are attached to the pericardium and most often occur at the inferior cardiophrenic angles. Since they contain clear fluid, they have also been termed "spring water cysts." These lesions rarely communicate directly with the pericardium. *Bronchogenic* cysts are also common and occur in close approximation to the main bronchi, usually near the carina. The cyst wall is characteristically comprised of ciliated respiratory epithelium with cartilage, smooth muscle, and mucous glands. Rarely, communication with the bronchus or trachea is present. These lesions are benign but may produce troublesome pressure symptoms, especially if the contents become infected. *Enteric* cysts occur along the esophagus and usually contain a mucosal lining more akin to gastric or intestinal epithelium. Although they rarely communicate with the esophagus, infection and abscess formation may occur. The presence of hydrochloric acid in some of these cysts may lead to ulceration, perforation, and bleeding. Mediastinal cysts are encountered which have only a fibrous wall and no specific histologic lining. These lesions have been termed *nonspecific* cysts, for lack of a more appropriate designtion. Their exact nature is poorly understood; they may actually represent lesions in which the original lining has disappeared. *Dermoid* cysts were described above.

Other types of neoplasms and cysts are rare. Among them are fibromas, leiomyomas, mesotheliomas, hemangiomas, liposarcomas, and lymphangiomas (Table 293-1). Also of importance are metastatic lesions in mediastinal lymph nodes. These occur especially as a result of primary tumors of the lungs and bronchi. Sometimes the enlarged hilar lymph nodes may be more prominent than the primary lesions. Carcinoma of the breast, lymphomas, and tumors of the intestinal tract may also metastasize to the mediastinum. Moreover, the mediastinal metastases may occur before the primary lesion appears. Therefore, in every patient with a mediastinal lesion attention should be directed toward the elimination of a distant primary site as the responsible factor.

The Superior Vena Caval Syndrome

Superior mediastinal lesions characterized by a dense infiltration and obstruction of the superior vena cava produce a characteristic clinical syndrome. These manifestations usually include marked cyanosis, swelling of the head, neck, and upper extremities, and the development of numerous superficial venous collateral vessels. Primary mediastinal tumors, particularly lymphomas, aneurysms, and carcinoma of the lung are the most common causes of this condition. Occasionally, mediastinal *fibrosis* may be responsible for this syndrome. This condition may occur at any age but is most common in middle or late life. Initial symptoms in mediastinal fibrosis include facial edema with spread to the arms, conjunctival suffusion, headache, tinnitus, and dyspnea. Nonpitting edema involving the upper thorax and arms becomes progressively more severe. A helpful roentgenographic finding associated with mediastinal fibrosis is the absence of positive changes on the chest roentgenogram. Pathologically, dense fibrosis is present in the mediastinum, involving the superior vena cava and occasionally the pulmonary veins. If the latter are involved, pulmonary hypertension may ensue. In some patients, histoplasmosis has been shown to be the cause and has been demonstrated in microscopic sections. Fortunately, in many instances spontaneous amelioration occurs because an adequate venous collateral circulation develops.

Mediastinitis

Although uncommon, acute infection in the mediastinum is usually serious. Acute suppurative mediastinitis accompanies esophageal perforation, which may be due to external trauma, esophageal erosion, or perforation, or may develop as a result of endoscopy. Symptoms usually appear promptly and consist of substernal pain, subcutaneous emphysema, fever, tachycardia, and leukocytosis. If untreated, overwhelming sepsis follows, producing prostration and collapse. Though acute mediastinitis may respond to antimicrobial therapy alone, prompt surgical drainage is also indicated in most patients.

Mediastinal Emphysema

Air within the planes of the mediastinum may produce few clinical manifestations, but in the presence of an increased pressure it can produce severe pain which may spread to the surrounding tissues. Mediastinal emphysema may result from traumatic perforation of the trachea or esophagus, from rupture of pulmonary alveoli in interstitial emphysema of the lung, from spread along the fascial planes of the neck or pharynx, or from dissection from the retroperitoneal space. Traumatic rupture of the bronchial tree in association with pneumothorax following puncture wounds or associated with endotracheal anesthesia may be the antecedent cause.

The escape of air from ruptured alveoli producing *spontaneous mediastinal emphysema* was first described by Hamman. Air dissects along the vascular structures of the lung to the hilum and thence into the various planes of the mediastinum. From the mediastinum it may spread to the subcutaneous tissues of the neck or through the diaphragm to retroperitoneal structures. If a large amount of air is involved, and especially if it is under pressure, it may produce collapse of the veins in the mediastinum, with impaired venous return to the heart.

Though small amounts of air in the mediastinum are generally without clinical consequence, severe substernal pain may result, and a characteristic crunching noise synchronous with the heartbeat is often heard over the precordium. Dyspnea, cyanosis, and distension of the cervical veins may follow. The chest roentgenogram demonstrates air shadows in the mediastinum, usually along specific planes. Moreover, air shadows are seen in the soft tissues of the neck and over the chest wall. In most instances, sedation and oxygen suffice as treatment. Rarely, surgical relief of the increased mediastinal pressure is indicated.

DISORDERS OF THE DIAPHRAGM

The most common abnormality of the diaphragm is *displacement*. The diaphragm may be displaced upward or downward by a variety of abdominal and thoracic disorders. Normally, the right side of the diaphragm is approximately 4 cm higher than the left, because of the right lobe of the liver. Upward displacement of the diaphragm may be associated with intraabdominal masses, ascites, marked obesity, or pregnancy. Disorders within the thorax can also produce displacement. The diaphragm may be depressed because of pleural effusion or pneumothorax. Phrenic nerve paralysis will produce upward displacement and paradoxic motion of the diaphragm with respiration. Phrenic paralysis is most commonly caused by direct invasion of metastatic tumor, but it may be the result of infection and trauma.

Diaphragmatic hernia may occur in several specific sites. The most common location is the esophageal hiatus through which the stomach can pass into the posterior mediastinum. The diagnosis and management of hiatus hernia are discussed in Chap. 313. In addition, congenital defects occur on either side of the sternum (foramen of Morgagni) and posterolaterally (foramen of Bochdalek). In addition, blunt trauma to the abdomen or chest may rupture the diaphragm, usually in its central portion. Direct trauma, such as incised wounds and missile wounds, may produce an opening which is followed by herniation of abdominal contents into the thorax. Traumatic diaphragmatic hernias may produce symptoms of intestinal obstruction and should be corrected surgically as soon as the diagnosis is established.

Eventration of the diaphragm is a condition in which the diaphragm is quite thin and membranous. The muscular portion of the diaphragm is usually confined to the posterior third, with a thin membrane constituting the remainder of the diaphragm. This causes marked upward displacement of the diaphragm and results in the presence of abdominal contents in the thoracic cage. Though often asymptomatic, eventration may produce pulmonary insufficiency. The chest roentgenogram, particularly following ingestion of barium, is diagnostic, and in most instances no therapy is required. However, in patients in whom symptoms are present, surgical correction is indicated.

Neoplasms in the diaphragm occur but are uncommon. Direct spread or lymphatic involvement may occur from primary neoplasms within the abdomen, e.g., in the stomach or colon. Also, direct involvement may occur from primary carcinoma of the lung. Primary tumors of the diaphragm are rare and include lipomas, fibromas, mesotheliomas, and neurogenic tumors. Approximately half are benign and the remainder malignant. Surgical removal is indicated.

REFERENCES

Barrett, N. R.: Idiopathic Mediastinal Fibrosis, Brit. J. Surg., 46:207, 1959.

Bilgutay, A. M., N. K. Jensen, W. R. Schmidt, J. J. Garamella, M. F. Lynch, and W. D. Kelly: Mediastinoscopy, J. Thoracic Cardiovasc. Surg., 57:841, 1969.

Cardon, L.: Significance of Small Pleural Effusions in Cardiopulmonary Disease, and Some Other Observations on Pleural Fluid in General, Ann. Intern. Med., 53:765, 1960.

Chin, E. F., and R. B. Lynn: Surgery of Eventration of the Diaphragm, J. Thoracic Surg., 32:6, 1957.

Gobbel, W. G., Jr., W. G. Rhea, Jr., I. A. Nelson, and R. A. Daniel, Jr.: Spontaneous Pneumothorax, J. Thoracic & Cardiovasc. Surg., 46:331, 1963.

Hamman, L.: Spontaneous Mediastinal Emphysema, Bull. Johns Hopkins Hosp., 64:1, 1939.

Oldham, H. N., and D. C. Sabiston, Jr.: Primary Tumors and Cysts of the Mediastinum: Lesions Presenting as Cardiovascular Abnormalities, Arch. Surg., 96:71, 1968.

————, and ————: Primary Tumors and Cysts of the Mediastinum, Monographs in Surg. Sci., 4:243, 1968.

Schechter, M. M.: The Superior Vena Cava Syndrome, Am. J. Med. Sci., 227:461, 1954.

294   OTHER DISORDERS OF THE LUNG

John H. Knowles

MISCELLANEOUS TYPES OF PNEUMONIA
Aspiration Pneumonia

Aspiration pneumonia usually refers to the acute parenchymal inflammation associated with aspiration of infected material from the upper respiratory passages and to the condition associated with aspiration of water, food, or vomit. The same etiologic and pathogenic considerations described for lung abscess apply here, and indeed aspiration pneumonia will result in an abscess if necrosis is extensive. Aspiration of food and drink is particularly common in debilitated, elderly individuals. Patients with obstructing esophageal disease often develop chronic, bilateral lower lobe pneumonitis because of repeated aspiration.

Aspiration of gastric contents may occur in infancy and old age, in alcoholics and epileptics, and in patients with head injuries, after the administration of drugs such as morphine, and during anesthesia. Maternal death during or following delivery may be due to aspiration of gastric contents. Rapid onset of acute toxemia occurs with high fever, tachycardia, cyanosis, tachypnea, and extreme dyspnea. Rarely, a latent period of as much as 6 hr may occur before onset of symptoms. Rhonchi and bubbling rales may be heard over the lower lobes. The roentgenogram shows bilateral lower lobe infiltrates with indistinct borders. There is necrotizing bronchopneumonia with hemorrhage, edema, and often multiple abscesses. Treatment consists of immediate suctioning of the tracheobronchial tree and bronchoscopy as soon as possible. Penicillin and streptomycin should be given. Oxygen and assisted ventilation may be needed if the disease is severe and there is evidence of respiratory insufficiency. Corticosteroids are advocated to quell the chemical inflammation.

Lipid Pneumonia

Lipid pneumonia is due to the repeated aspiration of animal oil (halibut and cod liver oil, milk, and egg yolk), vegetable oil (castor, olive, and wheat germ oil), or mineral oil. In the adult subject, the condition is almost invariably due to the chronic administration of mineral oil as a laxative or to drugs administered in an oily vehicle, such as nose drops. The condition is seen most frequently in elderly, bedridden, and chronically ill individuals, in short, those apt to have difficulty swallowing and to suffer from constipation necessitating the use of laxatives. Mineral oil apparently incites no cough reflex and moves unimpeded into the tracheobronchial tree. As it is chemically inert, it acts as a foreign body and incites a chronic inflammatory and granulomatous reaction. The disease is usually seen as a bilateral, lower lobe process but may rarely be confined to one lobe and simulate neoplasm (paraffinoma).

Clinically, nonspecific symptoms of mild cough and signs of scattered rales at the lung bases may be elicited. Most frequently the condition is asymptomatic and is discovered unexpectedly on routine x-ray examination.

The roentgenogram reveals increased lung markings, most notable at the lung bases early in the disease, and scattered nodular and irregular infiltrates, which become confluent in more advanced cases. Sometimes a local circumscribed density simulates bronchogenic carcinoma. The right lower lobe is the most frequent site of such a paraffinoma; hilar lymph nodes are not enlarged.

Examination of fresh sputum reveals characteristic macrophages filled with vacuoles which stain positively for fat with Sudan III or IV. Their appearance may be intermittent, however, and several sputum examinations should be made.

The vital capacity is reduced in patients with extensive involvement, indicating a restrictive ventilatory defect due to replacement of air spaces with fat-laden inflammatory tissue.

The only treatment is cessation of the use of oil. When the disease is localized, pulmonary neoplasm must be excluded and exploratory thoracotomy may be necessary; when the disease is diffuse, tuberculosis and the diseases associated with interstitial fibrosis should be ruled out.

One should not confuse cholesterol (or lipid) pneumonitis of endogenous origin with *lipid* pneumonia of exogenous origin.

Loeffler's Pneumonia and Pulmonary Eosinophilia

In 1932, Loeffler described a syndrome of transient pulmonary infiltration associated with peripheral blood eosinophilia and minimal or no symptoms. Mild cough, lassitude, and low-grade fever were associated with migrating, fleeting nodular pulmonary densities and mild leukocytosis with eosinophils to 20 percent of the total differential count. The disease was benign and self-limited, rarely lasted more than 3 weeks, and left no residual lesion. Although Loeffler initially thought this might be a manifestation of tubeculosis, subsequent studies by himself and others revealed infestation by ascaris in some patients.

Since that time the association of pulmonary infiltration and peripheral eosinophilia has been described in a wide variety of conditions, and the term *PIE syndrome* (pulmonary infiltration with eosinophilia) has been used. Thus collagen disease, such as polyarteritis nodosa, malignant neoplastic disease, bronchial asthma, tropical eosinophilia, the Hamman-Rich syndrome, sarcoidosis, allergic reactions to drugs such as penicillin, the sulfonamides, PAS, organic arsenicals, barbiturates, and thiouracil, certain infectious diseases such as tuberculosis, coccidioidomycosis, brucellosis, or exposure to the privet plant, mite infection, and parasitic infestation have all been described as causes. The following parasites have been associated with the syndrome: *Ascaris lumbricoides, Necator americanus, Trichinella spiralis, Fasciola hepatica, Strongyloides stercoralis,* and *Ancylostoma brasiliense.* In the case of some of these parasites, such as ascaris, larval migration through the lung doubtless gives rise to the syndrome and explains its transient, benign, and self-limited course.

The diagnosis of Loeffler's syndrome should be limited to cases conforming to his original description. In cases associated with persistence of symptoms and recurrence of roentgenographic abnormalities with marked systemic reaction, a hypersensitivity angiitis such as polyarteritis nodosa must be considered.

Tropical eosoinophilia should be considered under similar circumstances, particularly in India and Ceylon or in natives from these countries. The condition consists of cough, paroxysmal dyspnea with bronchospastic, asthmatic attacks, splenomegaly in 50 percent of cases, a positive Wassermann or Kahn reaction (which reverts after specific therapy), a high titer of cold agglutinins, and a roentgenogram showing bilateral mottled shadows. The sputum may contain many eosinophils. The white blood cell count ranges from 12,000 to 80,000, with 20 to 80 percent eosinophils. A curious subacute degenerative syndrome affecting the cerebellum has been associated with the condition, being especially well documented in the French medical literature. Over 35 percent of the cases respond to arsenical therapy, and this has been considered a diagnostic feature. It differs from Loeffler's syndrome in the presence of marked systemic reaction, persistence and chronicity of symptoms and x-ray findings, the striking response to arsenical therapy, and the occurrence of relapse in occasional cases.

Present theories of the causation of Loeffler's syndrome favor a local hypersensitivity state in the lung. Bronchial asthma, hypersensitivity angiitis, or polyarteritis nodosa may represent other more dire manifestations of similar immunologic processes.

The response of some patients with pulmonary infiltration and eosinophilia to steroid therapy may be dramatic.

BRONCHOLITHIASIS

Broncholithiasis refers to calcified concretions occurring in the tracheobronchial tree. They may arise in three ways: (1) by calcification of tracheobronchial cartilage and subsequent sequestration, (2) by secondary calcification of an exogenous foreign body, or (3) most commonly by migration and erosion of calcified material from hilar and paratracheal nodes into the tracheobronchial tree. The calcified node is the "tombstone" of the original disease, usually tuberculosis or histoplasmosis.

The condition occurs in both sexes equally and is most common between the ages of forty and sixty years. It is especially common in children as a complication of tuberculosis. Cough and hemoptysis are the commonest manifestations and are due to bronchial ulceration or to intrabronchial location of the stone, with resultant obstruction and bronchiectasis. Recurrent chills and fever and purulent sputum may be noted, and 50 percent of patients give a history of coughing up one or more stones. Some complain of wheezing or "asthma," which is due to partial bronchial obstruction by the concretion. The right bronchial tree is involved twice as often as the left. Rarely, active tuberculosis is found distal to such an obstruction, and careful examination for tubercle bacilli is essential.

The x-ray reveals calcification of hilar or paratracheal nodes, atelectasis or pneumonitis with dense calcification at the apex of the affected lobe, or bronchiectasis on plain film or bronchography. Tomography may be necessary to delineate the relationship of calcification and bronchus.

The broncholith can be removed occasionally through the bronchoscope, but thoracotomy and broncholithotomy are usually necessary. Lobectomy is reserved for those patients who have persistent or recurrent symptoms or localized bronchiectasis.

CYSTIC DISEASE OF THE LUNG

Cysts of the lung may be either congenital or acquired, solitary or multiple. The congenital origin of cystic disease has been presumed because of its occurrence in infancy and childhood and its association with congenital heart disease, polycystic disease of the liver or kidneys, dextrocardia, and aberrant pulmonary vessels (pulmonary sequestration). Congenital cysts are of bronchial origin.

Presumably, maldevelopment and failure of maturation of the terminal bronchial passages result in blind rests lined with bronchial epithelium, which usually communicate with the bronchial tree.

Acquired cysts develop from the rupture and coalescence of alveoli and are thus "alveolar in origin." When the air collection lies between visceral pleura and lung substance it is termed a *bleb*. They occur commonly at the apices and ordinarily have little functional significance. The term *bulla* refers to an air space more than 1 cm in diameter, situated in the substance of the lung, and frequently seen in association with obstructive pulmonary emphysema. Acquired cysts may be seen as a sequel to lung abscess (due to epithelialization of the cavity), pneumonia, tuberculosis, fungous disease such as coccidioidomycosis, or echinococcus disease.

Lung cysts are ordinarily asymptomatic. The patient may suffer one or more of the complications, which are (1) infection, (2) hemorrhage, (3) rupture of blebs or subpleural cysts with pneumothorax formation or rupture of bullae with interstitial and mediastinal emphysema, and (4) respiratory insufficiency. Repeated infection is what usually necessitates surgical removal of the diseased area. Communication with the bronchial tree determines the clinical behavior and functional deficit. The cyst may be air-filled and may remain stable in size over long periods if it communicates freely. If the opening is small and is intermittently occluded, the cyst may enlarge progressively, as air trapping occurs on expiration, and may intermittently become infected and fluid-filled. Progressive air trapping is most apt to occur with exercise and may give rise to substernal pain. This may be confused with the symptoms of angina pectoris.

In infancy large unilateral cysts called *pneumatoceles* may develop rapidly in association with pneumonia and occupy the entire hemithorax. In adults, a progressively enlarging bullous lesion may replace an entire lung; this is referred to as the "vanishing lung syndrome." Multiple cysts are usually bilateral and may simulate bronchiectasis in their clinical course.

The development of respiratory insufficiency depends on the communication of the cyst, its size and the degree of parenchymal replacement or compression, and the presence of obstructive emphysema. If the cyst is large and communicates freely with the bronchial tree, the effect is an increase in dead space ventilation, as the wall of the cyst is poorly vascular and gas exchange does not occur. If the cyst communicates poorly or intermittently with the respiratory tree, air trapping and, as the cyst grows larger, compression of the surrounding parenchyma occur. Obstruction to airflow and reduction in lung volume may be seen, and dyspnea is thus due to both obstructive and restrictive ventilatory defects. Arterial oxygen unsaturation occurs if ventilation to surrounding parenchyma is reduced more than perfusion, leading to a venous admixture effect.

The presence of associated obstructive emphysema must be detected prior to surgical removal of pulmonary cysts. Fluoroscopic demonstration of contralateral air trapping and restriction of diaphragmatic motion, great reduction in maximal breathing capacity, and large increase in residual lung volume may be helpful differential points. The finding of respiratory acidosis with an elevated CO_2 tension in the arterial blood nearly always indicates underlying, severe obstructive emphysema and virtually precludes surgical therapy. This is not true of oxyhemoglobin unsaturation as an isolated abnormality of the blood gases, as this may be relieved by surgical excision of a large cyst.

Findings on physical examination may be unremarkable. Tracheal deviation may be seen with large unilateral, poorly communicating cysts, as well as mediastinal shifting toward the lesion on inspiration and away on expiration. Rales may be heard if there is infection or bronchiectasis adjacent to the cyst. Large unilateral air cysts simulate pneumothorax, with hyperresonance, decreased or absent breath sounds, and tracheal deviation.

Radiologically the cysts are usually thin-walled and multiple but may be solitary and easily confused with lung abscess, bronchiectasis, chronic nonspecific pneumonitis, staphylococcic pneumonia, and tuberculosis. Pneumothorax and encapsulated empyema with bronchopleural fistula must also be differentiated. Generally the same principles of medical treatment apply here as in lung abscess (see Chap. 291).

REFERENCES

Broncholithiasis

Moersch, H. J., and H. W. Schmidt: Broncholithiasis, Ann. Otol., Rhinol. & Laryngol., 68:548, 1959.

Cystic Disease of the Lung

Baldwin, E. deF., K. A. Harden, D. C. Green, A. Cournand, and D. W. Richards, Jr.: Pulmonary Insufficiency. IV. A Study of 16 Cases of Large Pulmonary Air Cysts or Bullae, Medicine, 29:169, 1950.
Sellors, T. H.: Congenital Cystic Disease of the Lung, Tubercle, 20:49, 114, 1938.
Siebens, A. A., A. R. Grant, D. C. Kent, R. Klopstock, and J. J. Cincotti: Pulmonary Cystic Disease: Physiologic Studies and Results of Resection, J. Thoracic Surg., 33:185, 1957.

Miscellaneous Types of Pneumonia

Berg, J. R., and T. H. Burford: Pulmonary Paraffinoma (Lipoid Pneumonia), A Critical Study, J. Thoracic Surg., 20:418, 1950.
Gardner, A. M. N.: Aspiration of Food and Vomit, Quart. J. Med. (n.s.), 27:227, 1958.
Loeffler, W.: Die fluchtigen lungen Infiltrate mit Eosinophile, Schweiz. Med. Wochschr., 66:1069, 1936.
Reader, W. H., and B. E. Goodrich: Pulmonary Infiltration with Eosinophilia (PIE Syndrome), Ann. Intern. Med., 36:1217, 1952.
Viswanathan, R.: Pulmonary Eosinophilosis, Quart. J. Med. (n.s.), 17:257, 1949.
Volk, B. W., L. Nathanon, S. Sosner, W. B. Slade, and M. Jacobi: Incidence of Lipoid Pneumonia in a Survey of 389 Chronically Ill Patients, Am. J. Med., 10:316, 1951.

295 TREATMENT OF ACUTE AND CHRONIC RESPIRATORY IMPAIRMENT

Eugene D. Robin and John H. Knowles

The numerous physiologic defects present in chronic pulmonary disease have already been discussed (Chap. 280). Regardless of cause, these defects are found to a greater or lesser degree in most forms of chronic pulmonary disease. Effective therapy must obviously be based on an understanding of the physiologic aberration present and should be guided by the fact that defects due to infection, excessive secretions, bronchospasm, and alteration of the blood gases are potentially reversible. The physiologic abnormalities and their therapy are considered below. Generally, the discussion applies to chronic bronchitis and obstructive emphysema, the commonest forms of chronic pulmonary disease.

AIRWAY OBSTRUCTION

Airway obstruction in chronic pulmonary disease results from the presence of thick, viscid respiratory tract secretions; from bronchial edema, from bronchospasm, from bronchial or peribronchial fibrosis; and from parenchymal destruction, with the development of bronchiolar check valves.

SECRETIONS. The patient with chronic pulmonary disease commonly suffers from hypersecretion of mucus in the tracheobronchial tree, which leads to chronic cough, dyspnea by virtue of airway obstruction, and recurrent infection. He may be unable to dispose of such secretions because of ineffective mechanics of coughing and inadequate ciliary activity. The first principle of treatment is the avoidance of irritants, the chief offender being tobacco smoke. Cessation of smoking is essential. Careful inquiry into the presence of noxious environmental gases and dusts, both at work and in the vicinity of the patient's home, must be undertaken. A change of job or home might be indicated. Similarly, a change of climate, from one with wide swings of temperature and humidity to one which is warm and dry the year around, may be beneficial if the patient can undertake the financial and emotional burden of moving. A trial period in the chosen area should precede the patient's final decision.

Periodic increase in cough and in the volume of secretions is commonly due to superimposed bacterial infection, particularly during the winter months (see also below). Both cough and sputum production may be markedly diminished by full courses of the appropriate antibiotic dictated by the result of sputum culture.

During periods of acute infection, secretions may become particularly thick, tenacious, and viscid (in addition to their volume increase) and therefore difficult to remove. The sputum of the ambulatory patient without obvious infection may have similar characteristics, although in lesser degree. Measures to liquefy the sputum should be employed in either instance. The inhalation of warm, moist air (steam) is probably the single most effective measure in decreasing sputum viscosity.

Recently, ultrasonic nembulizers have been introduced for moist steam administration. This apparatus furnishes steam for inhalation. The mist provided has a high absolute humidity and is composed of individual droplets with small diameters, permitting deposition deep within the lung. It appears that this technique is particularly suitable for sputum liquefication and may be used both during acute infection and on a chronic basis when sputum retention is an important problem.

Agents designed to liquefy the sputum are commonly used. They include iodides, administered orally or parenterally; detergents, given by inhalation (e.g., Alevaire, which consists of glycerin, sodium bicarbonate, and Triton A-20), to lower sputum viscosity; and enzymes, by inhalation, such as aerosolized trypsin or pancreatic dornase. Definite evidence is lacking that any of these measures is effective except for the local hydration produced by inhaled solutions.

The compound acetyl cystein (Mucomist) has been introduced as an inhalable agent which theoretically decreases sputum viscosity by rupturing S—H bonds in the sputum. There is some evidence that this substance may be relatively effective in sputum liquefaction. However, it possesses several disadvantages. Relatively large volumes must be administered to produce adequate liquefaction; expensive equipment is necessary for aerosolizing the material so that it may be inhaled; and it may produce nausea and increased coughing.

Special measures designed to assist in removing secretions may be necessary. In the patient who is not acutely ill, a consistent program of postural drainage may be helpful, particularly if the volume of secretions is continuously large. The patient should be carefully instructed in the proper technique of performing postural drainage. The patient should assume the head-down, prone, right and left lateral decubitus, and sitting positions, so that all lobes are drained. Coughing in explosive style during drainage should be avoided, to prevent further lung damage. During acute respiratory infections, postural drainage may not suffice; mechanical removal of secretions is then necessary. This may take the form of tracheal suction by means of a soft catheter passed through the naso- or oropharynx. If this is not successful in the emergency situation, therapeutic bronchoscopy may be required. Finally, if none of the above measures is effective, or if they are of only transient benefit in the severely ill patient, a more long-term provision for effective tracheobronchial suction may be provided either by an indwelling endotracheal tube or by tracheostomy. The use of the former should be restricted to less than 96 hr, because of the danger of pressure ulceration or necrosis of the trachea.

Tracheal intubation by either technique also provides an effective connection with most types of ventilators which may be required for controlled ventilation in these patients.

Exact indications for either form of tracheal intubation are difficult to outline.

Certainly, inability to control secretions by more conservative methods is one indication. Continued deterioration despite intensive therapy is another indication. Such deterioration may be defined either by clinical criteria or by a rising arterial P_{CO_2}. The patient with severe pulmonary insufficiency who is about to undergo thoracic surgery may be considered a candidate for prophylactic tracheostomy. In general, if any doubt exists as to the necessity for this procedure, it should be resolved by having the procedure performed. Preferably, if indicated, the tracheostomy should be instituted early rather than late, should be done in a slow, unhurried manner, and should be performed in the operating room rather than at the bedside.

After tracheal intubation, a number of precautions are necessary to prevent complications. To avoid infection, tracheal suction should be performed with sterile precautions and disposable catheters. To prevent trauma to the tracheal mucosa, the catheter should be moistened before use. A T tube arrangement should be placed in the suction line so that negative pressure is applied only when the catheter has been positioned inside the lumen of the trachea. The catheter should not be vigorously thrust up and down within the tracheal lumen. The patient's head should be turned to the right and left during suction, so that the left and right main-stem bronchi can be reached. If available, a curved catheter for entering the left main-stem bronchus is desirable. To prevent hypoxia, hypercapnia, and fatigue, suctioning periods should be limited to 15 to 30 sec at a time. The use of very high expiratory flow rates to dislodge retained secretions (exsufflation with negative pressure) has been of value in some patients with postoperative atelectasis, but only rarely in those with chronic pulmonary disease.

DECREASED CROSS-SECTIONAL AREA OF THE BRONCHIAL TREE. The degree of reversible luminal narrowing of the bronchial tree due to bronchospasm and bronchial edema varies widely from patient to patient. It is not sufficiently appreciated that many patients with chronic obstructive ventilatory disease have a component of bronchospasm as a factor in airflow obstruction. This may be impossible to detect clinically. For this reason, the routine employment of bronchodilators is useful in the therapy of chronic pulmonary disease. Their use need not be entirely empiric. The 1-sec timed vital capacity or peak expiratory flow rate should be determined before and after the inhalation of aerosolized bronchodilator, and any increase should be noted. The drugs may be administered orally (ephedrine, 15 to 25 mg three or four times a day); by aerosol inhalation [1:200 isoproterenol hydrochloride (Isuprel) or 2.25 percent racemic epinephrine hydrochloride (Vaponephrin)]; rectally (the use of rectal aminophylline which, preferentially, is administered in water solution as an enema, resulting in relatively high blood levels); or parenterally (intravenous aminophylline). (Parenteral epinephrine is not generally suitable for use in the elderly patient.) The aim of therapy is to relieve bronchospasm for as much of the 24-hr period as possible. For this reason, bronchodilators should be administered on a consistent schedule, and around the clock, if necessary; the dosage should be increased during periods of increased bronchospasm.

Corticosteroids may be useful in the control of bronchospasm and bronchial edema in some patients. In the life-threatening situation, they may be used empirically if the condition does not respond to the usual measures outlined above and a reversible bronchospastic element is suspected. Similarly, in the occasional patient with chronic pulmonary disease whose clinical state suggests the possibility of bronchial asthma or at least a large reversible obstructive element which is not improved by the usual therapy, a diagnostic and therapeutic trial with corticosteroids may be indicated. Careful evaluation by serial test (e.g., timed vital capacity) is necessary to determine the ultimate need for such therapy. The hazards of peptic ulceration and reactivation of pulmonary tuberculosis must be recognized in such patients.

Since it has been demonstrated that cigarette smoke and other respiratory tract irritants produce an increase of resistance to airflow, cigarette smoking should be interdicted and the patient removed, to whatever degree possible, from exposure to irritant fumes.

More difficult to treat than the functional decreases in bronchial cross-sectional area are those based on anatomic damage to the bronchial tree or its loss. One major factor in this form of respiratory tract obstruction is that the application of high positive pressure across the thorax tends to collapse bronchioles and, hence, increases the degree of obstruction. The patient can be taught breathing exercises to prolong expiration by using lower intrapleural pressures. Pursed-lip breathing—pursing the lips and making an "F" sound on expiration—is taught. Expiration is made an active, prolonged effort; active use of abdominal muscles is stressed. The pressure gradient across the thoracic cage is lessened, and the amount of air trapping and of airway resistance due to early closure of bronchioles is decreased. Decrease in general physical conditioning, with loss of respiratory muscle "tone," has been suggested as an important factor in patients with chronic obstructive pulmonary disease. For meeting this problem, graded physical exercise while the patient breathes O_2-enriched mixtures may be tried. The inhalation of gas mixtures that are less dense than air (80 percent helium, 20 percent oxygen) may decrease the resistance to turbulent flow, although resistance to laminar flow may be increased because the mixture is more viscid than air.

There is no general agreement on the value of intermittent positive-pressure breathing (IPPB) as a routine measure in the day-to-day treatment of patients with chronic obstructive disease. Some workers believe that such therapy has great value in increasing alveolar ventilation, and others feel that it may represent a potentially useful technique for administering bronchodilator aerosols.

PULMONARY HOMOTRANSPLANTATION. Because of the essentially irreversible nature of some of the structural changes in chronic pulmonary disease the use of pulmonary homotransplantation has been suggested as a therapeutic measure.

The technical surgical problems have, by and large, been overcome. However, the immunologic problems have not been solved. There is also evidence in the experimental animal of progressive loss of function in the transplanted lung with time, independent of transplant rejection. Therefore, this therapeutic approach is not feasible *at this time*.

HYPOXIA

Hypoxia in patients with chronic pulmonary disease may result from generalized alveolar hypoventilation, from regional hypoventilation, or from right-to-left shunting (Chaps. 33 and 280). Aside from measures designed to produce an overall increase in total ventilation and to improve regional hypoventilation by decreasing airflow resistance, the most effective measure in the therapy of hypoxia is the inhalation of oxygen-enriched mixtures. The inhalation of high concentrations of oxygen will produce an increase in the alveolar tension of oxygen in all ventilated alveoli (i.e., those that are not totally occluded). The increase in alveolar oxygen tension will be reflected in an increase of oxygen tension in the pulmonary-capillary blood supplying these alveoli and will ultimately be reflected in an increased tissue oxygen supply (provided cardiac output remains adequate). Oxygen administration also permits an adequate supply of oxygen at a minimal work cost of breathing to the patient. This factor tends to decrease the overall oxygen consumption of the patient, and may partially explain the decrease in dyspnea that occurs during oxygen inhalation.

The administration of O_2 involves several potential hazards. In some patients with extremely severe pulmonary disease with acute or chronic hypercapnia and hypoxemia, there may be a loss of the normal respiratory center responsiveness to CO_2-pH stimulation, presumably because of narcotic levels of P_{CO_2} in the blood. In such patients the ventilatory drive appears to depend chiefly on impulses arising from the chemoreceptors of the aortic and carotid bodies, which respond chiefly to hypoxemia. Removal of the hypoxemic drive by means of oxygen inhalation may result in increasingly severe hypoventilation, with a precipitous rise in arterial blood P_{CO_2} and a drop in pH. Drowsiness and disorientation occur, and in severe cases convulsions, coma, and even apnea ensue. In such patients, oxygen administration must be carefully controlled.

There is also evidence that abnormally high alveolar oxygen tensions maintained over a period of time can produce local pulmonary damage. This damage has been demonstrated histologically by changes in the microscopic appearance of alveolar epithelial cells and subcellular tissue components. Physiologically such lungs may show progressive stiffness. Clinically pulmonary oxygen toxicity may be manifested by tachypnea, the requirement of progressively increasing inflation pressures, and by an inability to maintain adequate arterial P_{O_2} despite increasing concentrations of O_2 in the inspired air.

Thus the objective of O_2 therapy should be the maintenance of the lowest alveolar O_2 tension which results in an arterial P_{O_2} between 70 to 100 mmHg. Arterial tensions below this level may impair tissue O_2 supply, and values substantially above this level require alveolar P_{O_2} which are potentially injurious to the lung. In order to achieve such control, frequent monitoring of arterial P_{O_2} is usually required.

It should be emphasized that the relief of profound hypoxia is essential for survival and recovery of the patient. The problem therefore is not whether acutely hypoxemic patients should be treated with oxygen but how to treat them and maintain ventilation while doing so.

There are several ways in which this may be accomplished. The use of relatively low concentrations (24 to 28 percent) of O_2 in air using masks employing Venturi's principle is one such technique. The use of intermittent rather than continuous O_2 or the use of low flow rates of 100 percent O_2 may be tried. If these measures are unsuccessful, mechanical ventilators are necessary in patients developing life-threatening mechanical hypoventilation during oxygen administration. A large number of such mechanical respirators is now available.

The above considerations apply to the acutely hypoxemic patient. In recent years, the possibility of prolonged O_2 therapy in chronically hypoxemic patients has been explored. Such therapy may be given continuously or intermittently (e.g., during sleep). Some patients have shown gratifying responses to this form of chronic O_2 therapy.

ACID-BASE DISTURBANCES

The fundamental acid-base disturbance in chronic pulmonary disease is respiratory acidosis. This results from a decreased pulmonary excretion of CO_2 secondary to inadequate alveolar ventilation. Such inadequacy may result from an overall decrease in ventilation or from severe regional hypoventilation of sufficient magnitude so that CO_2 being produced metabolically cannot be disposed of in adequate amounts. Carbon dioxide retention may be treated by two general techniques: (1) reduction of the amount of CO_2 being produced metabolically, and (2) increased CO_2 excretion by the lungs.

The following techniques are available for reducing CO_2 production:

Reduction in the Work Cost of Breathing. In normal subjects the work cost of breathing amounts to less than 2 percent of total metabolism. In patients with chronic pulmonary disease, this value may increase to as much as 40 percent. Indeed, it has been suggested that the work of breathing may be so high in some patients with chronic pulmonary disease that further increase in ventilation actually causes a rise, not a fall, in arterial P_{CO_2}. The measures outlined above result in more efficient ventilation and, hence, in a decreased work cost of breathing.

Reduction in Physical Activity. Obviously a reduction in overall activity will result in a decrease of metabolism. Such reduction in activity during periods of acute illness is usually provided by hospitalization. In nonacute periods, the avoidance of severe overexertion and periodic rest intervals may help to accomplish the same purpose.

Reduction of Total Metabolism by Means of Induced Hypothyroidism. Radioactive iodine administration has been employed in an effort to induce some degree of hypothyroidism in patients with chronic pulmonary disease and in this manner to limit their metabolic requirements. This approach is as yet experimental and has not enjoyed widespread use. The unpleasant symptoms and appearance of hypothyroidism may be intolerable to the patient and his family.

The following techniques are available for increasing CO_2 output by the lung:

1. Improving the ventilatory status of the lungs by removal of secretions, treatment of infection, and the liberal use of bronchodilators, as outlined above.

2. Attempted stimulation of the respiratory center by drugs in order to induce hyperventilation. Such drugs as Coramine and Ethamivan are capable of increasing alveolar ventilation. In general, these drugs have limited usefulness because, regardless of central drive, the degree of hyperventilation is limited by the underlying abnormalities of the peripheral ventilatory mechanism, i.e., the disease of the lungs and thoracic cage.

In this regard it is useful to point out that one of the most important aids in restoring respiratory center sensitivity is to improve the blood gas composition by increasing ventilation. Either increasing oxygenation or reducing CO_2 retention (or both) of the arterial blood may result in resumption of rhythmic and efficient respiratory movement in the patient nearly apneic with uncoordinated respiratory muscle activity. It is mandatory to withhold any drugs, such as morphine, Demorol, and the barbiturates, that are capable of accentuating respiratory center depression.

3. In the acutely ill patient, assisted ventilation by means of one or another type of mechanical ventilator offers the best method of increasing alveolar ventilation and decreasing P_{CO_2}, thus increasing the excretion of CO_2. A number of different respirators is available. The one most commonly used at present employs intermittent positive pressure. With this apparatus the lungs are periodically inflated by means of positive pressure and expiration takes place passively. Such apparatus also provides facilities for the humidification of inspired air and for the administration of bronchodilators in the form of aerosol deep into the tracheobronchial tree. This type of apparatus is generally designed so that it may be activated by the patient's own respiratory efforts or may function automatically in the patient whose spontaneous respiratory drive is not sufficient to maintain ventilation.

A second acid-base abnormality may be the development of metabolic acidosis as the result of excess accumulation of organic acids, chiefly lactic acid. During severe hypoxia, particularly if the onset is acute, a relatively large portion of total-body energy requirements is met by anaerobic glycolysis. As a result large amounts of lactic acid are produced. This substance is a proton donor and thus consumes blood and tissue buffers such as HCO_3, resulting in metabolic acidosis. Since respiratory acidosis results in increased HCO_3^- concentrations and metabolic acidosis in decreased HCO_3^- concentrations, the development of metabolic acidosis may be difficult to detect by routine measurements of plasma total CO_2 content or CO_2-combining power. Although a number of techniques has been advocated for judging the degree of metabolic acidosis complicating respiratory acidosis, none of them is adequate except for direct measurement of blood lactate concentrations. If significant lactic acidosis is found, it may be treated by therapy of the underlying factors producing hypoxia and occasionally by the administration of base.

A third acid-base abnormality may be the development of alkalosis in patients with primary respiratory disease and CO_2 retention. Alkalosis may develop during therapy as a result of three mechanisms.

1. Artificial hyperventilation in patients with marked hypercapnia and moderate increases in HCO_3^- concentration. Hyperventilation rapidly reduces P_{CO_2} while HCO_3 falls slowly, thus resulting in alkalosis.

2. Cl^- deficiency resulting from increased renal excretion of this ion. In the face of Cl^- deficiency, there is decreased renal HCO_3^- excretion as plasma P_{CO_2} falls during therapy, resulting in alkalosis.

3. Alkalizing therapy such as intensive diuresis and corticosteroids which produce augmented renal H^+ excretion, either directly or secondarily as a result of K^+ depletion.

Severe alkalosis in the patient with hypercapnia may be associated with shock or the development of severe neurologic symptoms, including focal neurologic signs, fits, coma, and death. Its prevention requires frequent measurements of acid-base parameters and electrolytes during therapy of hypercapnia. P_{CO_2} should be lowered gradually rather than abruptly. Meticulous restriction of the electrolyte composition of plasma is necessary.

COR PULMONALE

The treatment of this complication is considered in some detail in Chap. 287. The problem is basically that of the vigorous management both of congestive heart failure (Chap. 264) and of pulmonary failure, as discussed above.

PULMONARY INFECTIONS

Because of the difficulties of proper drainage of secretions, recurrent infection in patients with chronic pulmonary disease is serious. Either frankly pathogenic organisms or bacteria of relatively low virulence, such as *Hemophilus influenzae*, may be responsible. Anaerobic bacteria, including bacteriodes and veillonellae, may be of importance in the pathogenesis of infection in this group of patients. The use of transtracheal aspiration for obtaining material for culture adds to the accuracy of bacteriologic diagnosis. Severe pulmonary infection may occur in this group of patients without the usual systemic indications such as fever or leukocytosis. For this reason early and vigorous chemotherapy is important. Such

chemotherapy should be guided by careful bacteriologic examination. The use of prophylactic chemotherapy is widely practiced. It should also be reiterated that postural drainage, bronchodilators, and steam inhalations are important adjuvants to the therapy of recurrent pulmonary infection.

SURGICAL THERAPY

The operative treatment of chronic pulmonary disease involves the excision of blebs and bullae which have compressed normal lung. Resection of such lesions allows adjacent normal lung tissue to reexpand and, depending on the size and location, will allow greater excursion of the diaphragm and relieve distortion of the mediastinal contents. The poorest results are achieved when a severe degree of underlying obstructive emphysema accounts for the dyspnea and disability experienced by the patient. Indications and contraindications for the removal of cysts have been discussed in Chap. 294.

A direct approach to obstructive pulmonary emphysema, per se, has centered on surgery of the autonomic nervous system and on efforts to increase the blood supply of the lung. Dorsal sympathectomy, vagal denervation, dissection of perivascular and peribronchial tissues, and parietal pleurectomy with talc poudrage have all been tried, alone or in combination. The evidence is slim that any of these maneuvers gives lasting benefit to patients with chronic pulmonary disease, and the hazards involved do not usually justify the attempts.

The use of pneumoperitoneum and of abdominal binders, in the hope of increasing the excursion of the diaphragm by upward displacement, has largely been abandoned.

THE ACUTE RESPIRATORY EMERGENCY

A number of different diseases may produce such interference with the process of ventilation that the patient's life is threatened by the resultant hypoventilation or apnea. Under these circumstances, artificial maintenance of ventilation is mandatory. The initial step is to ensure a patent airway. The patient's neck should be hyperextended, and, if they are available, either an oropharyngeal airway or, preferably, a cuffed endotracheal tube inserted. While equipment is mobilized, adequate ventilation may be maintained by means of mouth-to-mouth breathing. As soon as possible, suction should be performed to clear out respiratory secretions. Artificial ventilation over a prolonged period can be successfully carried out by a number of techniques. One commonly employed method uses an intermittent positive-pressure apparatus. This apparatus is powered by compressed air or oxygen. The lungs are inflated by positive pressure and deflate passively. Preferably, the instrument should have an automatic cycling device so that if the patient's respiratory efforts are too feeble to trigger the mechanism, ventilation will continue. Also desirable in such instruments are independent controls for the regulation of airflow and pressure, so that these parameters may be tailored to the patient's requirements. All such apparatus provides means of humidifying the inspired gas before it reaches the patient. Another commonly used variety of respirator is the piston type (Moersch), in which fixed volumes of moistened and heated air or oxygen are driven into the lung by means of a piston powered by a motor.

Ventilation may also be accomplished by means of a tank (Drinker) respirator. The patient's body (except for head and neck) is enclosed in a chamber, in which subatmospheric and supraatmospheric pressures are generated to produce volume flow of air into and out of the patient's respiratory tract.

As indicated above, when cough or swallowing is impaired, tracheostomy should be performed for the control of secretions.

Meticulous attention to hydration, electrolytes, care of bowel and bladder, infections, and orthopedic and psychologic problems is required. The patient's survival frequently depends on the degree of excellence of the nursing care provided.

REFERENCES

Comroe, J. H., Jr., and R. D. Cripps: "The Physiological Basis for Oxygen Therapy" (American Lecture Series, no. 42), Springfield, Ill., Charles C Thomas, Publishers, 1950.

Muskin, W. W., L. Rendell-Baker, and P. W. Thompson: "Automatic Ventilation of the Lungs," Springfield, Ill., Charles C Thomas, Publishers, 1959.

Pridie, R. B., N. Dotte, D. G. Massey, G. W. Poole, J. Schneeweiss, and P. Stradling: A Trial of Continuous Winter Chemotherapy in Chronic Bronchitis, Lancet, 2:723, 1960.

Robin, E. D.: Abnormalities of Acid-Base Regulation in Chronic Pulmonary Disease, with Special Reference to Hypercapnia and Extracellular Alkalosis, New Engl. J. Med., 268:917, 1963.

Rotheram, E. D., Jr., P. Safar, and E. D. Robin: CNS Disorder during Mechanical Ventilation in Chronic Pulmonary Disease, J.A.M.A., 189:993, 1964.

Sykes, M. K., M. W. McNicol, and E. J. M. Campbell: "Respiratory Failure" Blackwell Scientific Publications, Oxford, 1969, p. 333.

Section 4

Disorders of the Kidneys and Urinary Tract

296 DISORDERS OF FLUIDS AND ELECTROLYTES

Louis G. Welt

PHYSIOLOGIC CONSIDERATIONS
Volumes of Body Fluid

The total volume of body fluid is equivalent to 50 to 70 percent of the body weight. Since adipose tissue is relatively free of water, the figure is closer to 50 percent in the obese and approximates 70 percent in lean individuals. This fluid is compartmented into two major phases, the *intracellular* and the *extracellular*, and several subdivisions thereof. Approximately two-thirds of the total water is within the cells. The extracellular fluid (one-third of the total, approximately equivalent to 16 to 20 percent of the body weight) is further partitioned between the plasma and interstitial fluid. The smallest component represents about 2.5 percent of the total volume of water and is referred to as *transcellular*. It includes the fluid within the gastrointestinal tract, the tracheobronchial tree, the excretory system of the kidneys and glands, the cerebrospinal fluid, and the aqueous humor of the eye.

The volume of several of these major compartments can be estimated. The technique entails administration of some material whose distribution is considered to be uniform throughout the compartment in question. If a known amount of the test material is administered, and if the amount lost from the body during the time necessary for complete mixing can be determined and the concentration per liter at the time of equilibration can be estimated, the volume of distribution of the test substance can be calculated. The volume of total body water can be estimated by using water labeled with deuterium or tritium. A variety of substances, such as inulin, sucrose, and sulfate, have been used to define the volume of the extracellular fluid. The volume of the intracellular fluid cannot be estimated directly but may be inferred from the difference between the total volume of body water and the volume of the extracellular fluid. Plasma volume (approximately 4 percent of the body weight) has been calculated from the volume of distribution of protein-bound dyes, such as T-1824, and of albumin tagged with [131]I. However, since the proteins, particularly albumin, are not wholly confined to the vascular compartment and gain access to the interstitial spaces and the lymph, the volume of distribution of tagged albumin is likely to be in excess of the plasma volume itself. The volume of the red blood cell mass is considered to be more reliable and may be estimated utilizing erythrocytes tagged with an isotope of iron, phosphorus, or chromium. From the red blood cell mass and the hematocrit one can readily calculate the plasma volume.

Each of these measurements has been of value in investigating both normal and pathologic exchanges of water and electrolytes. There is no doubt that such measurements would provide considerable aid in managing patients whose illness is complicated by a disorder of hydration and of electrolyte imbalance.

Composition of Body Fluids

There are major differences in the composition of the intra- and extracellular fluids, and minor differences among the several components of the latter. The composition of the extracellular fluid is better understood and more precisely defined, both because it is a simpler fluid and because it is available for analysis in the form of serum and transudates into the serous cavities. The only cells that can be obtained in relatively pure form in any bulk are the erythrocytes. Generalizations from the characteristics of this unique and highly specialized cell to all cells would, of course, be most hazardous.

The *interstitial fluid* of the extracellular compartment is an ultrafiltrate of serum and differs from the latter in that it contains very low concentrations of large-molecular species such as proteins and lipids. The usually accepted normal range of values for the concentrations of electrolytes in serum is as follows:

Cations, mEq/L

Sodium................. 132–142
Potassium.............. 3.5–5.0
Calcium................ 4.5–5.5
Magnesium............. 1.5–2.0

Anions, mEq/L

Chloride................. 98–106
Total CO₂................. 26–30 (mM/L)
Phosphate and sulfate..... 2–5
Organic anions........... 3–6
Proteins.................. 15–25

The average total cation concentration approximates 150 mEq per liter, and this is considered to be identical with the total anion concentration. Although these concentrations are conventionally expressed in relation to a unit volume of serum, it is understood that these ions are for all intents and purposes distributed in the aqueous phase of the serum. The average water content of serum is about 93 percent, and hence to express these concentrations in terms of serum water, they should each be divided by 0.93. The concentrations in the water of serum can then be translated to the concentrations in the interstitial fluid by applying a correction factor to account for the asymmetric distribution of ions across the capillary membrane. This latter is related to the presence in the serum of nondiffusible ions, the proteins. The Donnan ratio that describes the relative concentrations between serum and an ultrafiltrate thereof is approximately 1.05 for the univalent cations and 0.95 for the univalent anions. For example, the calculations of the concentra-

tions of sodium or chloride in the interstitial fluid are performed as follows:

$$Na_{IF} = \frac{Na_S}{SW} \times 1.05$$

and

$$Cl_{IF} = \frac{Cl_S}{SW} \times 0.95$$

where IF = interstitial fluid, SW = fraction of serum that is water.

The compositions of joint fluid, aqueous humor of the eye, and cerebrospinal fluid are all similar to an ultrafiltrate of serum, but there are enough differences in the aqueous humor and spinal fluid to suggest that these are not pure dialysates but are, in part at least, formed by active transport processes.

The composition of the intracellular fluids cannot be examined directly, and hence the characteristics of cell fluid are inferred from analyses of whole tissue and the use of certain "reasonable" calculations. The total tissue water can be readily estimated from the difference in weight between the fresh wet tissue and the weight after it has been dried. The volume of this water that is to be ascribed to the extracellular phase is calculated from knowledge of the concentration of some substance in the tissue and serum, with the assumption that that particular substance is confined to an extracellular position. In the past, most of these calculations were made on the assumption that chloride was confined to the extracellular phase. This is obviously not true, and for more precise data one must employ other agents such as inulin. The values for the volume of the extracellular fluid and the concentrations of sodium and potassium in this fluid (as derived from their values in serum) are used to calculate the quantity of these two ions in the noncellular phase. The difference between the total tissue sodium and potassium and the quantity in the extracellular phase represents the amount in cells. The difference between the total water and the extracellular volume is the intracellular water. The concentration of sodium and potassium in the intracellular fluid can then be calculated. These details have been recited to emphasize the indirectness with which cell composition is defined.

The average data, derived largely from muscle analyses, obtained in this inferential manner are as follows:

Cations, mEq/L

Sodium.................... 10
Potassium................. 150
Magnesium................. 40

Anions, mEq/L

Bicarbonate................ 10 (mM/L)
Phosphate and sulfate....... 150
Proteins................... 40

Granting the calculations are valid, much is still unknown about the physicochemical state of these materials. For example, the characteristics of the phosphate, sulfate, and proteins in terms of valence are unknown. It is not certain that all the potassium and magnesium is in a free and ionized state. Furthermore, it is probably unrealistic to speak of intracellular fluid as an entity, since diverse tissue cells have major differences in composition. Lastly, the intracellular fluid of a single cell type is probably not an entity, since it, in turn, is compartmented into extra- and intramitochondrial fluid, nuclear fluid, etc.

Another important technique to evaluate the composition of body tissues employs radioactive isotopes. These are used to calculate a value that is referred to as the *total exchangeable quantity* of a given ion. This method involves administration of a known quantity of the particular radioactive material. After a sufficient period of time, allowing the isotope to equilibrate with as much of the stable element as it will readily exchange with (approximately 24 hr), one then determines the specific activity in serum; with this datum plus knowledge of the quantity that has been lost by decay as well as that which has been excreted in the urine, one can calculate the total quantity of the ion that is readily exchangeable. This figure is usually expressed as a unit of body mass. The data collected by Moore and his colleagues provide the following average figures:

	mEq/kg body weight	
	Male	*Female*
Sodium...........	39.5	38.3
Potassium.........	48	39.4
Chloride..........	29.3	28.6

It must be cautioned that these figures do not represent the *total* quantity of these ions in the body, since the total is not readily exchangeable. For example, approximately 75 percent of the total body sodium and 85 percent of the total body potassium are exchangeable.

The most complicated characteristics of cell composition and the marked differences between it and the environment of the cells serve to emphasize the highly specialized functions of cells, the complex mechanisms that must be available to maintain these compositional differences, and the possibilities for alterations in metabolic pathways that may result from even subtle alterations in composition.

In contrast to the marked differences in the composition of these two major phases, it is believed that the total solute concentration in these fluids is identical. This, in turn, is due to the presumed free permeability of most of the cell membranes to water. This concept has been challenged in recent years. Although a categorical statement is not appropriate, the preponderance of evidence continues to support the concept that the cellular fluids are, in fact, isotonic with respect to their environmental fluid. This may not apply for those cells which secrete a hypotonic fluid, such as the sweat and salivary glands, and for the renal tubular cells that tolerate fluids of markedly different osmolalities on each surface.

Internal Exchanges of Water

When two aqueous solutions are separated by a membrane that is freely permeable to water, molecules of water will move from one compartment to the other. There will be an equilibrium with respect to water when the same number of water molecules pass in each direction per unit of time. At such a time there is no *net* alteration in volume in either of the compartments separated by the membrane. The tendency for the molecules of water to pass from one compartment to the other is spoken of as an "escaping tendency" and is referred to as the *chemical potential* of the water. Whenever the chemical potentials of the water of two contiguous solutions differ, there will be a net movement of water from the phase with the higher chemical potential to that with the lower, until equilibrium is reached. The chemical potential of water is reduced when solutes are added, and the reduction is proportional to the concentration of solutes. In contrast, the chemical potential of water molecules is enhanced by increases in hydrostatic pressure and temperature.

Thus, the addition of a solute that can traverse a membrane with freedom will result in its uniform distribution throughout the volumes of fluid separated by that membrane. The addition of this solute will diminish the chemical potential of the water molecules, but since the water in both compartments is influenced to the same degree, there is no *net* change in the volume of water on either side of the membrane. The only effect is that fewer molecules of water, but an equal number of them, move in each direction per unit of time. In contrast, if the added solute were unable to permeate the membrane in question, it would be confined to the side to which it was added and would diminish the chemical potential of the molecules of water on that side alone. Under this circumstance molecules of water would continue to *enter* this phase at the rate which obtained prior to the addition of the solute, but water molecules would *escape from* this compartment at a slower rate and there would be a net change in volume, such that water would accumulate in the compartment to which the solute had been added. The redistribution of water would continue until a new state of equilibrium was established.

This problem may be looked at a little more carefully in terms of the pore theory of membranes. In the context of the discussion just presented, imagine a membrane separating two aqueous solutions and visualize a pore that permeates the membrane. Assume that the solutions in the two phases are pure water and that exchange (with no *net* movement) occurs owing to the random movement of molecules of water. Now if one adds to Side I a solute that cannot permeate the membrane, it is clear that more molecules of water will move from the pore at its interface with Solution I than will move from Solution I into the pore. This loss of water molecules at the interface must promote a pressure drop across the pore and be responsible for the net movement of water into Solution I. This is emphasized by pointing out that there is only pure water within the pore and, hence, no tendency for the molecules of water to move more in one direction than another. The situation that conditions the movement must, in fact, be the pressure gradient across the pore. Ordinarily these problems are discussed in terms of osmotic pressure. In this context, the addition of a solute that can permeate membranes freely, such as urea, contributes to the total osmotic pressure, but it is not effective in promoting a redistribution of water. Glucose, which is not free to enter cells by passive diffusion, not only contributes to the total osmotic pressure of a solution to which it is added, but it contributes what is referred to as an *effective osmotic pressure* (as opposed to *total* osmotic pressure) and does condition a redistribution of water.

With respect to biologic fluids and membranes, it may be said that an increase in the concentration of those solutes that permeate membranes freely augments the total osmotic pressure (decreases the chemical potential of the water molecules) in all compartments of the body fluids. However, an increase in the concentration of a solute that cannot penetrate a membrane freely will increase the *effective* osmotic pressure as well as the total (diminish the chemical potential of the molecules of water) in the fluid in which the concentration has been altered. If this fluid is separated by a membrane freely permeable to water, there will be a net alteration in volume in favor of the compartment to which the solute has been added. Despite long usage and familiarity, the terms *total* and *effective osmotic pressure* will be replaced in the rest of this discussion with the terms *total* and *effective osmolality*. This should serve to recall that it is the activity of the molecules of water that is under discussion, and not the technique (utilizing hydrostatic pressure) used to estimate these activities. However, since hydrostatic pressure increases the chemical potential of molecules of water, a change in hydrostatic pressure may counterbalance the influence of solutes so that a *difference* in total solute concentration across a membrane may be unassociated with net transfers of water.

Sodium salts represent almost all the solutes that usually contribute to the effective osmolality of the extracellular fluid. Hence, in most instances an increase or a decrease in the concentration of sodium in the serum may be equated with an increase or decrease in the effective osmolality of the extracellular fluid and, in turn, will promote movement of water from or into the cellular compartment.

There are two circumstances when depressed concentration of sodium in serum may not necessarily represent diminished effective osmolality of the serum water. It will be recalled that it would be more precise to speak of the concentration of an ion such as sodium in terms of its concentration in the water of serum. Since the determination is actually performed on a diluted aliquot of serum, and since the percentage of serum that is water is so commonly between 90 and 93 percent, the convention is to refer the concentration to a unit (usually a liter) of serum. In circumstances characterized by hyperlipemia, the lipids may occupy a significant volume of the serum, and the percentage of serum that is water

may be drastically reduced, to as low as 70 to 80 percent. An average concentration of sodium of 138 mEq per liter in a serum of which the water content was 93 percent would represent a concentration of 148.3 mEq per *liter* of serum *water* (138/0.93). If this same concentration obtained in the water of a *lipemic serum* where the water content was only 75 percent, the concentration per liter of *serum* would be 111.2 mEq (148.3 × 0.75). Thus, a striking hyponatremia in this instance would not mean a diminished effective osmolality of the water of the serum. This may also obtain with unusual hyperproteinemias.

Although glucose contributes to the effective osmolality of the extracellular fluid, the magnitude is usually small. At a concentration of 100 mg per 100 ml (1,000 mg per liter) this would amount to 5.5 mOsm per liter. However, if hyperglycemia supervenes, the corresponding increase in the effective osmolality will promote a movement of water from the cells. This will dilute the concentration of sodium and may depress the level to the point of frank hyponatremia. In this instance the interpretation that the hyponatremia signifies a decrease in effective osmolality would be in error. For these reasons the concentration of sodium in a patient with diabetes mellitus should be interpreted with knowledge of the simultaneous concentration of glucose in the serum.

SIGNIFICANCE OF HYPONATREMIA

Hyponatremia is observed frequently in hospital practice. Not all instances of hyponatremia have the same pathogenesis; many are poorly understood, and a decision about management may be difficult. This discussion excludes those instances in which hyponatremia is not equivalent to a decrease in the effective osmolality of the body fluid, such as those cited in relation to hyperlipemia and hyperglycemia.

The commonest situations in which hyponatremia is observed are those cases of dehydration or edema in which salt has been lost in excess of water or water has been retained in excess of salt. A modest deficit of sodium is frequently accompanied by an equivalent loss of water. The sequence of events may be something as follows: (1) the loss of sodium induces a mild reduction of the concentration of this cation in the extracellular fluids; (2) this, in turn, suppresses the secretion of the antidiuretic hormone (ADH) (and furthermore the loss of salt impairs the ability to elaborate an appropriately concentrated urine); (3) the excretion of water is increased until the concentration of sodium has been restored. This is frequently referred to as a "sacrifice of volume in the interests of tonicity of the body fluids." However, as the volume deficit assumes more significant proportions, equivalent losses of water no longer follow further deficits of sodium salts and hyponatremia is established. It may be that the deficit in volume, or some expression thereof, is a stimulus for the secretion of ADH despite hyponatremia, and the volume deficit may influence renal function, in some fashion independent of ADH, to conserve water. It is clear from this sequence that one very important implication of a state of dehydration accompanied by hyponatremia is that the intensity of the dehydration is probably severe. In addition, the decrease in effective osmolality of the extracellular water will have promoted movement of water into the cellular compartment. Thus, the deficit in volume of the extracellular phase is greater than the total external loss. Lastly, the dilution of the intracellular fluid may be expected to have untoward consequences with respect to cell functions. These latter are most clearly expressed on a clinical level by a clouded sensorium, which may progress to frank coma and may be accompanied by seizures. In addition, there are data that hyponatremia (with or without cellular dilution) promotes an increased rate of production of urea nitrogen and induces a rise in the serum level of potassium.

Hyponatremia may occur in the absence of dehydration. In fact, there are some indications that it may develop in patients with no apparent alteration in the volume or disposition of body water; and it may certainly occur in patients with edema. There is some value in a tentative effort to characterize the several pathogeneses of hyponatremia other than that already discussed with regard to dehydration.

Essential Hyponatremia

There is a group of patients who have hyponatremia but no other obvious disturbances in body fluid physiology. These patients have advanced and debilitating diseases and are frequently in preterminal status. They excrete in the urine the approximate quantity of salt ingested. They are able to conserve sodium when this ion is removed from their regimen, and they are able to excrete an appropriately dilute urine when a water load is administered. No aspect of their symptom complex is apparently favorably modified by attempts to restore the concentration of sodium in serum to the normal range. If this is attempted, the patient becomes thirsty, ingests water, and then excretes salt and water until the volume and tonicity of the body fluids have been restored to the level from which they began.

It is clear that the basic defect of this syndrome is mysterious, but it may be suggested that a generalized cellular disorder promotes a new "setting" of the osmolality of the body fluids. Some have referred to this as the "sick cell syndrome." It is not difficult to discriminate between this syndrome and the condition in patients with hyponatremia and dehydration or in those whose condition is deteriorating as a consequence of adrenal cortical insufficiency. The physical examination and collateral laboratory data such as a normal level of serum urea nitrogen and potassium are important clues. The disorder from which it must be differentiated is inappropriate secretion of antidiuretic hormone.

Inappropriate Secretion of ADH

More and more examples of this condition have been noted. Many of these patients have intrathoracic lesions, both benign and malignant. Some of the latter have been found to secrete a material that cannot be differentiated from lysine vasopressin. Other intrathoracic lesions may interfere with neural pathways that normally translate the message of increased volume to promote suppression of secretion of the antidiuretic hormone by the neurohypophyseal system. Many other instances are associated with intracranial lesions, including trauma, infection, and tumor. These lesions may promote the secretion of antidiuretic hormone by partial destruction of the posterior lobe of the pituitary gland, with escape of hormone; or by virtue of an irritative focus that promotes the secretion of the hormone (Chap. 88). In addition, the syndrome is noted in an odd variety of circumstances which defies a unifying concept.

The problem is that the patient is secreting antidiuretic hormone (or an antidiuretic substance of other origin) under inappropriate circumstances. This implies that ADH is secreted in abundance in the absence of an osmometric or volumetric stimulus. The consequence is that the continued ingestion of water is not followed by its excretion and the patient develops a positive balance of water and dilutional hyponatremia. This hypotonic expansion of the body fluids usually promotes an increased glomerular filtration rate and an augmented excretion of salt. At this point, the urine osmolality may not be as high as it was initially, owing to the solute diuresis and perhaps in part to some suppressive influence on the secretion of ADH by the severe hypoosmolality of the body fluids. In any event, the urine osmolality is still inappropriately high for the degree of dilution consequent to the positive balance of water.

Since there is frequently an increased rate of glomerular filtration, it is not uncommon to find that these patients show serum urea nitrogen at the lowest levels of normal. Although these patients have an expanded volume of total body water, it is distributed throughout both the cellular and the extracellular compartments, and one usually finds only the most subtle signs of edema.

The treatment of these patients is clearly aimed at dissipating the positive balance of water. This is usually accomplished by drastic restriction in the volume of water ingested until a normal concentration of sodium in serum has been achieved. Then one must find, in an empirical fashion, what food and fluid regimen will be comfortable for the patient and yet not permit a positive balance of water to be achieved once again.

There are occasional circumstances when the level of hyponatremia is so extreme as to produce clouding of consciousness, coma, or seizures. These instances demand more rapid correction, and there are two courses available. One may administer solutions of mannitol, hypertonic glucose, or urea to induce a solute diuresis that will dissipate part of the positive balance of water via the urine and restore the concentration of sodium in serum to a more nearly normal level quickly. Alternatively, one may administer a volume of hypertonic saline solution sufficient to increase the concentration of sodium to a level where the hazards attendant on hyponatremia no longer obtain. This should be employed as the last resort, since, in fact, the patient already has an expanded body fluid volume.

It is almost certain that what was formerly referred to as "cerebral salt wasting" was, in fact, misinterpreted and represented instances of inappropriate secretion of ADH.

Hyponatremia with Edema

There are many instances of patients who have hyponatremia associated with lesser or massive degrees of edema. These conditions are usually classified in two general categories: *chronic dilutional* and *acute dilutional hyponatremia*.

CHRONIC DILUTIONAL HYPONATREMIA. (1) It seems reasonable that some of these patients may well have what is called *essential hyponatremia*. In that circumstance there would obviously be no value to restoring the concentration of sodium in serum to "normal." In fact, the patient would then have the discomfort of thirst added to his other problems. (2) Some of these patients may well have *inappropriate secretion of ADH*. The best management is to dissipate the relative positive balance of water by restricting intake. As in the instances of this syndrome without edema, there may be occasions when more aggressive measures are required, such as administration of a solution to provoke a solute diuresis. There may be *rare* occasions when the administration of small volumes of hypertonic saline solution is justified if the hyponatremia per se is truly hazardous. However, since these patients are already markedly expanded with fluids and may already have congestive heart failure, it is obvious that the treatment itself is dangerous and should be employed only under the most dire circumstances. (3) Lastly, it is quite probable that in many states of edema the rate of glomerular filtration is markedly reduced. Under these circumstances the quantity of water that escapes reabsorption in the more proximal portions of the nephron may be so small that very little gains access to the more distal segments where it might escape into the bladder. Why patients in such circumstances do not lose their thirst and thereby automatically prohibit a positive balance of water is certainly not clear. Nevertheless, drinking and eating patterns in man are such that a positive balance of water can be readily achieved under these circumstances. Once again, the treatment is dissipation of the positive balance of water.

ACUTE DILUTIONAL HYPONATREMIA. (1) One example of this disorder is simply the consequence of administering water or urging a patient with edema to ingest quantities of water in excess of his ability to excrete the load. This is possible in any circumstance including health but is much more easily achieved in patients with edema who have altered renal hemodynamic and other parameters. In any event, the first point to emphasize is that this is preventable. Secondly, should it occur, the treatment again demands restriction of water to rid the body of this relative excess. Lastly, under duress the use of hypertonic solutions may be employed to encourage a solute diuresis. (2) A second example is observed in patients who develop considerable thirst after a successful therapeutic measure aimed at ridding the edematous patient of a volume of fluid. This may be noted after a brisk diuretic response and more commonly after a large abdominal paracentesis. The reasons for the intense thirst are not clear but may relate to a sudden loss of volume in some crucial segment of the vascular system. These complications are preventable. Patients should be warned that they may develop thirst, and their ingestion of water should be limited by themselves and carefully monitored and restricted when indicated by those responsible for their care.

The point of emphasis in managing patients with hyponatremia and edema is that if the concentration of sodium in serum is to be restored, it should be accomplished by dissipating the relative positive balance of water by restricting intake or by hastening excretion through the use of an osmotic load. Some patients, reflecting a state referred to as essential hyponatremia, may, in fact, be more comfortable with hyponatremia than with "normal" concentrations of sodium in serum. The indications for administration of hypertonic saline solutions are *exceedingly rare,* and the measure is only to control what are considered hazardous symptoms from the hyponatremia per se. Even under these circumstances saline solution should be administered in a small quantity sufficient only to restore the sodium concentration to levels that no longer represent a hazardous state.

Another way that hyponatremia might develop is by movement of sodium from the extracellular compartment to cells or to bone. There is some evidence that such an intercompartmental shift of sodium may occur in adrenal cortical insufficiency. Sodium may accumulate in cells deficient in potassium, and some investigators have considered that certain instances of hyponatremia are related to this transfer from the extracellular compartment.

An assessment of the pathogenesis of hyponatremia can usually be made on the basis of the above discussion, and hence the therapeutic implications can usually be arrived at according to the above criteria.

SIGNIFICANCE OF HYPONATREMIA

In contrast to hyponatremia, an increase in the concentration of sodium in the serum reflects loss of water in excess of salt or administration (or ingestion) of salt in excess of water. The hypernatremia, which is the chemical expression of a water deficit, in turn, incites the following responses, which result in the acquisition of more water, the most efficient conservation of same, and the most desirable distribution of the available water:

1. Thirst
2. Secretion of ADH, which promotes excretion of a concentrated urine
3. Movement of water from the cells to the extracellular space, thus mitigating the deficit of volume in this latter compartment
4. Diminution in the loss of insensible perspiration
5. Decrease in the rate of secretion of sweat

At least one report leaves little doubt that there may

well be circumstances in which there is hypernatremia with no other disorder in body fluid physiology and the patient appears to operate with a new "setting" of body fluid osmolality. This may be the counterpart of essential hyponatremia and perhaps should be referred to as *essential hypernatremia.*

COMMENTS ON CORRECTION OF HYPO– AND HYPERNATREMIA

One other implication of the free permeability of cell membranes to water and a uniform osmolality throughout the body fluids concerns the manner in which the concentration of sodium in the serum is restored to normal from both hypo- and hypernatremic levels.

If hyponatremia complicates an illness and it is considered advisable to correct this abnormality by administering a hypertonic solution of sodium salts, the amount of sodium required is equivalent to the deficit in concentration per liter multiplied by the estimated number of liters of *total body water.* If there is to be osmotic equality throughout the body fluids, it is implicit that the concentration of sodium in the extracellular phase cannot be increased without an equivalent increase in solute concentration in the cellular fluid. The administered sodium will increase the osmotic activity of intracellular fluid, not by entering the cells, but by promoting movement of water from the cells to the extracellular compartment as the osmolality of the latter is increased. If it is desired to restore the concentration of sodium reasonably promptly, or if it is to be accomplished with a small volume of fluid, the sodium salts must be administered in hypertonic solution. The amount of sodium that must be administered to restore the concentration to normal is equal to the nomal concentration of Na_s (138 mEq per liter) minus the current concentration of Na_s multiplied by the total volume of body water. For example, in a 70-kg adult with an assumed body water content of 60 percent (42 liters) and a concentration of sodium in the serum of 128 mEq per liter,

$$(138 - 128) \times 42 = 420 \text{ mM deficit of sodium chloride}$$

Since there are 17.1 mM per Gm NaCl, 420/17.1 or 24.56 Gm NaCl would be necessary to restore the sodium to 138 mEq per liter. This could be supplied in 500 ml 5 percent NaCl solution.

The same principles apply to estimating the volume of water that may be necessary to reduce the concentration of sodium in the serum from hypernatremic to normal levels. Since the intensity of the hypernatremia (due to the loss of water in excess of or without salt) is proportionate to the deficit of total body water, the following relationship obtains:

$$\frac{\text{Normal concentration } Na_s}{\text{Elevated concentration } Na_s}$$

$$= \frac{\text{current vol total body } H_2O}{\text{assumed normal vol total body } H_2O}$$

The value for the current volume of total body water can be calculated, and the difference between it and the assumed normal volume for total body water represents the deficit of water. For example, in the same adult mentioned above but with a concentration of sodium in the serum of 160 mEq per liter:

$$\text{Current vol total body } H_2O = \frac{138}{160} \times 42 = 36.2 \text{ liters}$$

The deficit would be $42 - 36.2 = 5.8$ liters of water.

Although these calculations are of value, it should be cautioned that there may be some danger in the too-rapid correction of the elevated or depressed concentration of sodium in extracellular fluid. This, in turn, may be related to adaptive alterations that have obtained. The important feature to be kept in mind in the management of a patient with dehydration and an abnormal concentration of serum sodium is that, in the net, the hyponatremic subject should receive salt in excess of water, and the hypernatremic patient should receive water in excess of salt.

EXCHANGES BETWEEN PLASMA AND INTERSTITIAL FLUID

The net exchange of fluid between the plasma and interstitial space is conditioned by a series of forces. Some of these forces favor transudation from the vascular system, such as the hydrostatic pressure within the vessels and the colloid osmotic pressure of the tissue fluids. The tissue tension and the colloid osmotic pressure of the plasma favor the reabsorption of fluid from the interstitium (see Chap. 34). It should be emphasized that, unlike the cell membranes, the capillary endothelial membrane is freely permeable not only to water but to all the solutes of the plasma except the large molecular species such as the proteins and the lipids. Thus, the concentration of sodium and its salts does not influence the distribution of water between these two major components of the extracellular compartment. Although the proteins do not contribute a large osmolality, they alone contribute to the effective osmolality since they are unable to permeate the endothelial membrane except in very small quantity. Thus, hypoalbuminemia may promote expansion of the interstitial fluid, with diminution in plasma volume and hemoconcentration, with normal values for the concentration of sodium.

A change in the forces governing the net exchange between the plasma and the interstitial fluid need not necessarily condition a redistribution of volume between these two compartments. A net increase in transudation could be largely compensated by the return of this increment of fluid to the vascular system by way of the lymphatic vessels. Lymphatic flow is frequently increased when the interstitial fluid volume is expanded, and this influence must be carefully considered when analyzing the forces that govern the disposition of fluid within the extracellular compartment.

INTERNAL EXCHANGES
OF ELECTROLYTES

Although it is apparent that ions such as sodium, potassium, and magnesium move in and out of cells, it is equally apparent that their net movements are not a consequence of free passive diffusion. The measurements of the electric potential differences across the membranes as well as the determination of the concentration gradients make it clear that these ions are not in a state of equilibrium but exist in what is referred to as a *steady state away from equilibrium*. This demands a series of operations dependent on sources of energy and referred to in general terms as *active transport*. The special permeability or "leakiness" characteristics of the plasma membranes of cells with regard to the several ionic species as well as the specific active transport mechanisms and the factors that regulate their rates are ultimately the determinants of the steady state composition of the several cell types. Any change in the permeability characteristics or rates of transport could readily influence the cell composition. It is presumed that metabolic reactions are necessary to maintain cell membrane structure, which, in turn, establishes the permeabilities to passive diffusion as well as the mechanisms involved in the active phases of transport. There are data which establish adenosinetriphosphate (ATP) as the ultimate source of energy for active transport, and, lastly, there is an enzyme within the membrane structure itself, ATPase, which may play an important role in making the energy available for the work of transport.

In some instances there appear to be elements of active transport in which the movement of two ionic species in opposite directions may be linked. Although hypothetical, an illustration of the manner in which muscle cells become laden with sodium in the face of potassium deficits can be offered. For example, assume that the level of potassium outside the cell is one of the factors which regulates the rate at which sodium is actively extruded from within the cell. Assume, further, that the rate of extrusion of sodium from the cells controls the inward movement of potassium from the extracellular fluid to the intracellular space. When potassium is lost from the extracellular fluid owing to augmented urinary excretion, or losses from the gastrointestinal tract, etc., the level in the extracellular fluid tends to diminish. This creates initially a larger gradient for potassium from inside to outside the cell, and perhaps more potassium leaks out by passive diffusion. However, this is still inadequate to raise the extracellular fluid concentration of potassium to normal levels. At the same time sodium is constantly diffusing into the cells only to be actively extruded. However, if the diminished level of potassium in the extracellular fluid imposes a rate-limiting influence on the extrusion of sodium from the cells, the latter should accumulate within the cells. The advantage of this is that with the higher intracellular concentration of sodium more of this ion can now be extruded (despite the lower external concentration of potassium), and restoration toward normal of the rate of sodium extru-

sion at the expense of the higher intracellular concentration of this ion promotes the ability to implement the movement of potassium back into the cell. All these alterations induce a net change characterized by a loss of cell potassium, an increase of cell sodium, and the achievement of new steady state away from equilibrium. This may very well be fanciful in detail, but it provides an overall context in which one may view some of the problems.

The most prominent hypothesis relating to a mechanism of active transport is referred to as the *carrier hypothesis*. In an oversimplified fashion this may be described as suggesting that a compound resides at one side of the cell membrane and has a particular affinity for the sodium ion. Because of this characteristic it becomes linked with this ion; it is now a new species of compound with a higher concentration at one side of the membrane than the other. As a result, it diffuses passively to the other side of the membrane, where a reaction splits the sodium ion from the carrier. This reaction again modifies the compound, and it can be postulated that it now has an affinity for potassium. The latter ion articulates with the carrier and, again, owing to the establishment of a diffusion gradient in this fashion, it moves backe to the original side of the membrane, where the potassium ion is split off and the carrier is returned to its original state with a great affinity for sodium, and the process is repeated over and over again.

This discussion of active transport has been too simple and succinct to provide more than a vague conceptual framework. The interested reader is referred to Ussing and other sources for detailed discussions of this fascinating and fundamental property. It should be emphasized that the active transport of ions is responsible at the least for the maintenance of cell volume and tissue excitability as well as what must be a vast array of phenomena that are dependent on the details of intra- and extracellular fluid composition.

Bone as a reservoir of ions other than calcium has attracted increased attention. Approximately one-third of the total body sodium is in bone, and only 15 percent of this can be ascribed to the extracellular phase. About one-half of the total body content of magnesium is in bone. Potassium is present in much smaller amounts. Deficits of sodium, potassium, and magnesium are shared by bone, and this tissue participates in exchanges that articulate with alterations in acid-base relationships. (See also Chap. 297, Acidosis and Alkalosis.)

EXTERNAL EXCHANGES OF
ELECTROLYTES AND WATER
Thirst

In considering the net exchange of water between the individual and his environment, it seems reasonable to begin with thirst. This is the sensory impression that motivates the ingestion of water. Several stimuli may give rise to the sensation of thirst, and the most important of these is an increase in the effective osmolality of the body fluids. This appears to hold true whether the hypertonicity is promoted by loss of water in excess of salt or by administration of salt in excess of water. These two circumstances differ in that in the first instance the volume of the extracellular fluid is decreased, and in the second this volume is expanded. However, in each circumstance the volume of the cells is diminished by virtue of a shift of water to the extracellular phase. A secondary stimulus is related somehow to a deficit of volume (or some expression of such a deficit) in some key portion of the extracellular space. Other factors that condition and modify the sensation of thirst include exposure of the oropharyngeal and esophageal tissues to water, the fullness of the stomach, and emotional as well as social factors. The central nervous system is responsible for the appreciation of and the response to thirst in both a specific and a nonspecific manner. There is now abundant evidence that lesions in key portions of the central nervous system—predominantly in the hypothalamus—may induce hypodipsia or polydipsia. The latter need not be accompanied by diabetes insipidus. The polydipsic center can be stimulated by exposing it to tiny volumes of hypertonic, but not isotonic, saline solutions. It can also be aroused by electrical stimulation.

In a less-specific sense the nervous system conditions the reception and response to stimuli provoking thirst in relation to the level of the state of consciousness. The frequency with which patients with a clouded sensorium or coma are allowed to develop significant deficits of water is sufficient justification for emphasizing the obvious fact that such patients can neither appreciate nor respond to their own thirst mechanism.

Potassium depletion may be accompanied by thirst and polydipsia. This may reflect, in part, the inability of the kidneys to conserve water appropriately in this condition. However, it is also possible that there may be a primary influence on some aspect of the stimulus-response pathways concerned with thirst.

Insensible Perspiration

Water is continuously lost from the body in the expired air and from the skin. The sum of these losses is spoken of as "insensible loss" of water and is equivalent to about 600 to 1,000 ml per day in the average adult. This loss is augmented with increase in metabolic activity (fever, exercise, hyperthyroidism) and respiratory exchange. The catabolism of tissues produces 200 to 300 ml water per day; hence, the *net* loss of insensible water may be considered as 400 to 700 ml per day. Since this loss is water without solutes, it should be replaced as water without salt (e.g., 5 percent glucose in water when fluid balance is being maintained by parenteral techniques).

Sweat

The production of sweat is primarily responsive to heat. The latter presumably excites afferent impulses to centers that regulate motor activities promoting the loss of heat. The important centers in the central nervous system are in the anterolateral portions of the hypothalamus. Sweat is not a simple fluid, and the details of its secretion are not well understood. It is always a hypotonic solution except in adrenal cortical insufficiency and in patients with fibrocystic disease (mucoviscidosis) of the pancreas. Among other influences, the rate of sweating is diminished by an increase in the effective osmolality of the body fluids. An average composition for sweat, in millimoles per liter, is as follows: sodium 48.0, potassium 5.9, chloride 40.0, ammonia 3.5, and urea 8.6. The characteristics of this fluid dictate the replacement of losses incurred as sweat by a solution that is one-third to one-half isotonic saline. This is readily satisfied for intravenous administration with 1 part isotonic saline to 1 or 2 parts of 5 percent glucose in water.

Gastrointestinal Tract

The exchange of water and solutes between the body fluids and the lumen of the gastrointestinal tract is large. It is contributed to by saliva and the secretions of the stomach, liver, pancreas, and intestinal mucosa. The volume of these secretions may exceed 8 liters per day under ordinary circumstances, but the net loss from the body is negligible. However, when there are losses through vomitus, diarrhea, or drainage from enterostomies, colostomies, or fistulas, the deficits of water and electrolytes may be prodigious. Loss of fluid through these routes probably represents the commonest pathogenesis of significant dehydration in clinical practice.

Aside from saliva, which is a hypotonic solution, the secretions mentioned are close to isotonicity with the extracellular fluids. However, they differ from the latter in composition. For example, the gastric secretion, if it contains free HCl, has a much lower pH, less sodium and bicarbonate, and more chloride than the extracellular fluids. In contrast, the pancreatic secretion has a higher pH and more bicarbonate. Most gastrointestinal secretions have more potassium than the extracellular fluid. Thus, although losses of gastrointestinal secretions per se represent isotonic deficits, the derangements that accompany the dehydration will be conditioned by the particular portion of the gastrointestinal tract from which the lost fluid derived. In many instances, however, these losses can be successfully replaced by equal volumes of isotonic saline solution. The potassium lost with these secretions and the consequences thereof must also be adequately managed.

Renal Exchanges of Electrolytes and Water

The kidneys represent the major organs of conservation as well as of excretion in the net balance of water and electrolytes. The kidneys can excrete large volumes of excess water and large quantities of unwanted ions and other solutes. In addition, they respond to the need to conserve water by excreting small volumes of highly concentrated urine. Their response to a sodium deficit is to excrete a urine virtually free of salt. The conservation of magnesium is also good, and subjects subsisting on a diet deficient in magnesium may excrete as little as 1 mEq of this ion per day. Although the excretion of potassium is very much diminished when there is a deficit of this cation, the efficiency with which the kidneys conserve potassium is not quite so great as it is with sodium, chloride, or magnesium.

The excretion of sodium is markedly reduced when there is primarily a deficit of water, despite the fact that this is accompanied by hypernatremia. This has the advantage of eliminating a major solute from the urine and, by reducing urine flow, furthers the conservation of water.

The kidneys display other exquisitely sensitive responses to most of the alterations in the composition, volume, tonicity, and pH of the body fluids. Details of these responses and the mechanisms involved therein are discussed in Chap. 50.

CLINICAL CONSIDERATIONS

An understanding of the pathogenesis and management of disorders of fluid and electrolyte balance depends on an appreciation of the approximate net exchanges of water and the several ions that have occurred during the course of a patient's illness. In essence, many of the problems concerning clinical disorders of hydration are resolved by the simple expediency of setting up a balance sheet in which the total estimated losses are accumulated, the total intake is summated, and the net differences are calculated. Although not quantitatively precise, this practice usually defines the qualitative nature of the alterations and provides an approximation of the quantitative characteristics. Many of these data can be obtained from the carefully taken history or the well-documented hospital chart. In addition, the physical examination, the chemical analyses of serum and urine, and other laboratory data provide additional insights. The management of the problem then becomes largely one of providing those materials which will restore the normal state of hydration. It is not an oversimplification to state that the majority of these problems are easily resolved with simple arithmetic.

In many instances a disordered state of hydration could have been avoided by provision of adequate replacement of certain predictable and mandatory losses. It is desirable, therefore, to define the characteristics of the basal requirements for water and electrolytes, and to describe how they are modified by a variety of conditioning circumstances.

Basal Requirements

For the purposes of this discussion it will be assumed that the patient must receive the necessary water, electrolytes, and other materials by parenteral routes, that he has accumulated no antecedent deficits, that he is not sustaining any unusual losses, and that he has normal renal function. One other qualification is that the problem is one of short duration and that the need for calories and protein is not a major consideration. The task then is to prescribe a regimen which will maintain a normal state of hydration, avoid depletion of the major essential minerals, and minimize the most immediate threats of starvation.

The volume of water recommended per day is the sum of (1) the probable net insensible loss, 400 ml; (2) a reasonable volume for urine, 1,000 ml; and (3) perhaps a small additional volume, 400 ml, which is provided to anticipate other losses such as sweat but which, if not lost by extrarenal routes, can be readily excreted in the urine. These total 1,800 ml.

If a patient has been previously ingesting an average diet, he has probably been receiving about 8 to 10 Gm (135 to 170 mM) NaCl per day. If the intake of salt is suddenly eliminated, the patient will probably be able to excrete a urine essentially free of sodium in about 5 days. During this interval of 5 days a negative balance of sodium is allowed to develop. This is likely to be accompanied by an equivalent loss of water in the interests of maintaining a normal concentration of sodium in the extracellular fluid. This deficit in volume is probably not harmful in itself, but it prejudices the patient's ability to withstand subsequent losses. Therefore, unless there is some specific contraindication, it is recommended that the patient receive 4 to 5 Gm (70 to 85 mM) NaCl each day.

As noted earlier, the conservation of potassium is not quite so efficient as that of salt, and unless the urinary excretion of this cation is replaced, a deficit of potassium will be ultimately achieved. From 40 to 60 mM potassium per day should be adequate to avoid a negative balance of this cation.

Although the mechanisms of conservation for magnesium are quite good, one of the settings in which depletion of this cation is observed is prolonged parenteral fluid management. The administration of as little as 2.0 to 4.0 mM magnesium per day ought to suffice under most circumstances.

It has been stated that approximately 100 Gm carbohydrate is necessary for the operation of the Krebs cycle. Unless this is made available from preformed endogenous or exogenous carbohydrate, the catabolism of protein and fat will be accelerated and 4-carbon ketones will be formed faster than they can be utilized. The acid products of protein catabolism and the excess ketones must be excreted to avoid a metabolic acidosis; they are excreted in part as sodium salts, which adds another drain to the body's store of sodium. Each of these complications can be avoided by the provision of an adequate quantity, 150 to 200 Gm, of glucose per day.

The total basal requirements are the following:

Water............	1,800 ml
NaCl............	70–85 mM (4–5 Gm)
KCl............	40–60 mM (3–4.5 Gm)
MgSO₄...........	2.0–4.0 mM (1–2 ml 50% $MgSO_4 \cdot 7H_2O$)
Glucose.........	150–200 Gm

An appropriate fluid prescription to meet these requirements is the following:

1,300 ml 10% glucose in water
500 ml 5% glucose in isotonic saline solution
4 Gm KCl (added to the total water to be administered)
2 ml 50% MgSO$_4$·7H$_2$O (added to the total water to be administered)

It should be reemphasized that this prescription is appropriate for the patient with qualifications set forth in the initial paragraph of this discussion on Basal Requirements.

Additional Requirements

There are many circumstances which would require revision of the above prescription. Fever, restlessness, and increased respiratory activity will augment the loss of water as insensible perspiration. A hot environment and fever will promote sweating. Water loss in urine will be accelerated during an osmotic diuresis due to glycosuria or unusual amounts of urea. The latter situation is observed when unnecessarily large amounts of protein are administered to patients who are experiencing a reaction to injury and hence are limited in the ability to store nitrogen. Additional amounts of salt may be lost with glycosuria. Impaired renal function will demand an increased volume of urine, and the conservation of sodium may be less efficient than in patients with normal kidneys.

Fluids Available for Parenteral Administration

There are available a number of specially prepared solutions, such as "gastric replacement fluid" and "intestinal replacement fluid," aimed at meeting the requirements of particular types of loss. Their use should be discouraged. The basic tenet of the individualization of therapy applies here, as it does elsewhere in clinical practice. The proper management of disorders in fluid and electrolyte balance demands an analysis of the specific characteristics of the distortion in the particular patient at hand. The routine use of a special solution tends to diminish the diligence with which this analysis is made through the false sense of security provided by the claims of the value of the particular solution. This is not to imply that solutions other than glucose in water and isotonic saline are not frequently needed. However, when the need arises, the appropriate fluid should be designed for the particular patient and his problem. A great variety of special problems can be met by preparation of a special solution from the following list of raw materials:

5%, 10%, 50% glucose in water
0.9% NaCl (154 mM/liter)
5.0% NaCl (855 mM/liter)
7.5% NaHCO$_3$ (900 mM/liter)
14.9% KCl[1] (2,000 mM/liter or 2 mM/ml)
50%[1] MgSO$_4$·7H$_2$O (2mM/ml)

[1] These solutions are highly concentrated and should never be administered unless they are diluted.

Lastly, it should be emphasized that the most appropriate replacement fluid for lost blood is whole blood; and where the particular need is to expand plasma volume, the use of whole blood, single units of plasma, or, preferably, 25 percent salt-poor albumin or some other plasma expander, is recommended.

Techniques of Administration of Fluids

Fluids may be given by vein, by hypodermoclysis, or by gavage into the stomach. The latter method has many advantages, especially when the problem is likely to last for some time and when considerations of calories, proteins, and other essential foodstuffs merit attention. The intravenous route is convenient, and the use of plastic tubing threaded into larger veins has eliminated some of the technical problems.[2] The rate of administration of fluid deserves some attention, and in patients with cardiovascular disease the patient should be observed carefully and frequently to ensure the earliest recognition of an untoward response. The potential hazard of cardiovascular complication may serve to modify the fluid prescription and the speed with which the fluids are administered. However, it should certainly not interfere with the proper management of dehydration.

The subcutaneous route may have some advantages in patients with heart disease. The access of fluid from the subcutaneous tissue to the bloodstream is obviously slower than when fluid is introduced directly into the vein, but, in addition, its absorption may be even further delayed if there is a rise in venous pressure. In this fashion there is an added factor of safety. If fluids are administered by hypodermoclysis, two precautions must be borne in mind:

1. The fluid should be isotonic with the plasma. If it is hypertonic, there will be a tendency initially for water to leave the plasma and enter the clysis pool. This will cause an initial decrease in plasma volume, which is undesirable, especially if the patient is already dehydrated. Moreover, a hypertonic solution may be irritating to the subcutaneous tissue and result in a bad slough of tissue.

2. A solution of 5 percent glucose in water should not be administered by clysis if the patient is dehydrated. When glucose is administered in this fashion, concentration gradients are established for the diffusion of glucose from clysis pool to plasma and for diffusion of sodium from plasma to clysis pool. Sodium diffuses more rapidly than glucose, the fluid in the pool, therefore, becomes hypertonic, and this, in turn, promotes movement of water from the plasma. This reduction in plasma volume superimposed on the antecedent deficit may be sufficient to induce a state of peripheral vascular collapse.

DEHYDRATION

The term *dehydration* continues to mislead, since it implies to many physicians the loss of water alone. Clin-

[2] The site of the plastic intravenous catheter should be changed every 48 hr if at all possible. Significant incidence of infection and phlebitis usually appears after 2 days.

ical dehydration is rarely a pure deficit of water. Dehydration is usually associated with losses of both salt and water (in proportionate or disproportionate quantities), with deficits of other ions such as potassium, and with the frequent complication of a disturbance in acid-base equilibrium. All these factors must be considered in planning appropriate management. For purposes of orientation and discussion, clinical dehydration may be classified into three major groups as follows:

1. Loss of water in excess of sodium
2. Loss of sodium in excess of water
3. Isotonic losses of sodium and water

Loss of Water in Excess of Sodium

The failure to drink is the commonest cause of a water deficit. This is observed most frequently in severely debilitated patients with clouding of consciousness or coma. Not only are these patients too weak and ill to respond to thirst, but they are even unable to communicate the fact that they are thirsty to their families or to their physicians. The size of the water deficit, though it may increase each day, may be small and hence easily overlooked. However, this deficit can achieve significant proportions and contribute greatly to the severity of the patient's illness.

Solute diureses due to glycosuria are usually characterized by a loss of water in excess of salt. This is the situation, for example, in almost all patients with significant degrees of diabetic acidosis.

Another type of solute diuresis may be responsible for a deficit of water. Many physicians have become impressed with the therapeutic value of feeding large quantities of protein. There are many situations in which this is desirable. However, in the early stages of reaction to injury, the ability to store nitrogen may be very seriously impaired, and large amounts of protein (usually administered by gavage) will find their way to urea, demanding excretion in the urine. If the patient is able, he may complain of thirst if the urine flow is large enough to induce a deficit of water. The unconscious patient cannot provide this help. Delay in recognition is due, in great measure, to misinterpretation of the significance of a large flow of urine, especially when the latter is not concentrated. This is equated with an appropriate state of hydration, whereas, in fact, the large volume of unconcentrated urine may be causing the deficit of water (see Chap. 88).

Diabetes insipidus may be responsible for large deficits of water. Unfortunately, acute diabetes insipidus is commonly associated with trauma or infection in the central nervous system, and hence a clouded or comatose state is not unusual. Major deficits of water may occur in a matter of hours. A large volume of very dilute urine should alert the clinician to this possibility. The defect in the tubular reabsorption of water is easily corrected by the administration of pitressin (see Chap. 88).

The loss of sweat contributes to a deficit of water in excess of salt loss. To the extent that water alone is ingested and retained to replace the volume of lost sweat, a dehydration characterized by a loss of water in excess of salt loss is readily converted to one characterized by a loss of salt in excess of water loss. This serves to emphasize the point that the characteristics of the net deficit are conditioned not only by the quantity and quality of the fluid lost but also by the characteristics of the replacement fluid.

The hallmark of dehydration characterized by a loss of water in excess of salt loss is an increase in the effective osmolality of the extracellular fluids. In most instances this is reflected in an increase in the concentration of sodium in the serum, and the intensity of the hypernatremia may be used as a gauge to calculate the relative deficit of water (see above).

Deficit of Salt in Excess of Water Deficit

Adrenal cortical insufficiency is probably the classic example of this type of dehydration (see Chap. 92). Although the loss of sodium may be the primary event in the pathogenesis of the dehydration in this disorder, it does not necessarily follow that the concentration of sodium will be depressed in the early phase (see Significance of Hyponatremia, earlier in this chapter). However, as the contraction of volume becomes more significant, further deficits of sodium salts are not accompanied by equivalent deficits of water and hyponatremia supervenes. The dehydration is severe, the cells are overhydrated, and the contracted volume of the plasma may compromise the renal blood flow and glomerular filtration rate, leading to azotemia and some degree of acidosis. The excretion of potassium is diminished. This is owing to the failure to reabsorb sodium at a site in the renal tubule where potassium secretion is coupled with sodium reabsorption. Hyperkalemia out of proportion to the azotemia and hyponatremia is characteristic of this disorder. Peripheral vascular collapse is common, as are hypoglycemia, restlessness, and an altered sensorium.

Patients with chronic renal insufficiency may exhibit an inability to conserve salt properly. This may be of striking proportions and has been known to mimic and be misdiagnosed as adrenal cortical insufficiency. More commonly, the defect is much less intense and may be unmasked only when such patients are advised to restrict the use of dietary salt. The loss of salt each day may not be great, but in the course of time a significant deficit may develop, accompanied by hyponatremia. The dehydration is associated with alterations in renal hemodynamics, and further reduction of an already deficient renal function is a common and dangerous complication. The hazard of a salt-poor regimen in patients with chronic renal disease should be recognized, and it is the responsibility of the physician to make certain that the patient can tolerate the treatment. Careful evaluation of daily weights, observations with respect to changes in concentration of blood urea nitrogen and the concentration of sodium in serum, and an estimation of the total 24-hr excretion of salt in the urine are helpful in evaluating the response.

Isotonic Deficits of Salt and Water

In general, these deficits are primarily incurred by losses of fluid from the gastrointestinal tract. The ultimate character of the net deficit will be determined in part by the quality and quantity of fluids that the patient may receive. If the patient refrains from taking fluid and none has been administered by a parenteral route, the continued loss of insensible perspiration, sweat, and urine will determine a net deficit characterized by the loss of water in excess of salt loss. If the patient drinks water and vomits, the net deficit will be a loss of salt in excess of water loss.

Analysis of the Characteristics of Dehydration

The discussion presented above concerns the pathogenesis of dehydration in rather isolated terms, and in the hope of achieving clarity the price of oversimplification has been paid. Most patients have experienced a variety of physiologic insults of different magnitudes and for shorter or longer periods of time. The essence of the analysis of the characteristics of the dehydration is an assessment of all the data, in both quantitative and qualitative terms. These data are derived from the history, the physical examination, and the laboratory.

HISTORY. A careful review of the sequence of events during the course of the illness provides most important information concerning the quality and magnitude of the deficits of electrolytes and water. These data should actually be tabulated, and it is most desirable to develop the habit of preparing a balance sheet to use in the analysis. A sheet with the simple headings indicated below will usually suffice:

Intake:	Output:
Date/time	Diarrhea
Weight	Vomitus
Character of fluid	Urine
Volume	Insensible loss
	Sweat
	Blood

The systematic analysis of these data should provide a fair estimate of deficits in terms of volume, salt, potassium balance, and acid-base equilibrium. In an illness of short duration, information relating to the patient's usual and current weight may be helpful in estimating the volume of fluid that has been lost. The presence or absence of fever and sweating is relevant, as are data concerning the possibility of renal insufficiency or diabetes mellitus. Information concerning the usual level of blood pressure is helpful, since a "normal" blood pressure may be hypotensive for a patient whose blood pressure is usually in the hypertensive range. The symptom of thirst is most significant and can be most helpful in calling the physician's attention to a disorder of hydration which might otherwise be neglected. Thirst is most often due to a primary deficit of water, although it may also reflect a contracted volume, even when salt has been lost in excess of water.

A disorder of hydration may develop during the course of hospitalization. The data referred to above should certainly be available in a precise fashion in the hospital chart. The administration of parenteral fluids should be recorded with as much attention to detail as in the record of drug therapy.

PHYSICAL EXAMINATION. The physical signs may provide important information for the analysis of the deficits of electrolytes and water. The appearance of the skin, its elasticity, texture, temperature, and color, the appearance of the mucous membranes, the tension of the eyeballs, the blood pressure, and the pulse rate all contribute to an estimation of the magnitude of the deficit. The state of consciousness may be related to the magnitude of the deficit. Muscle weakness and diminished-to-absent deep tendon reflexes may suggest potassium depletion.

The character of respiratory activity may suggest a disequilibrium in acid-base relationships. The respirations in metabolic acidosis, with dehydration as an almost invariable concomitant feature, are deep and eventually accelerated, and one can usually detect an effort toward the end of expiration. A systemic alkalosis is suggested by a positive Chvostek reflex; this may also be present if the patient has hypocalcemia despite a concurrent acidosis. Clinically detectable changes in respiration in alkalosis can rarely if ever be appreciated. The odor of acetone on the breath implies a ketonemia.

LABORATORY DATA. The value of the *packed cell volume* (hematocrit), the concentration of *hemoglobin*, and the concentration of *total proteins* in the serum can help in evaluating the degree of contraction (or expansion) of the plasma volume. Since this inference is dependent on *changes* in the concentrations, these data are of help primarily in evaluating those disorders that develop while the patient is under observation and in following the progress of a patient whose dehydration is undergoing correction.

It is worthwhile to reemphasize that the concentration of sodium per se cannot possibly be equated with the presence or absence of a state of dehydration. The *concentration* of sodium is merely a statement of the amount of sodium in a liter (or any other unit of volume) of extracellular fluid. The patient with a normal concentration of sodium in the serum may have no disorder of hydration, he may have gained many liters of fluid, or he may have lost a large volume of fluid.

The excretion of urea is related to the amount filtered less the amount reabsorbed through the renal tubules. This latter process is considered to be primarily passive. There are data suggesting that some component of urea reabsorption may be active. However, to the extent that it is passive it is favored by high concentration gradients between renal tubular and interstitial fluid. Therefore, it is clear that a diminished rate of filtration at the glomerulus, or a highly concentrated urine, or both will favor a diminished rate of excretion and an increase in urea concentration in the body fluids. To the extent that dehydration is responsible for these alterations in renal function, the concentration of urea in blood may serve as a gross index of the severity of the dehydration.

The urinalysis contributes considerable information. In the first place it provides information concerning the probability of renal disease. A urine of high specific gravity, in the absence of glucose or protein, suggests good renal function and an antidiuretic response. This, in turn, carries certain implications with respect to alterations in the internal environment. The excretion of salt despite hyponatremia may indicate one of the salt-wasting disorders or the syndrome of inappropriate secretion of antidiuretic hormone.

The concentrations of potassium and total CO_2 content of the serum may be altered, and these deviations are frequently accompanied by disturbances in acid-base equilibrium. These matters are discussed in more detail in Chap. 297. Hypo- or hypermagnesemia may be present. The former is not uncommon in the same situations that are characterized by deficits of potassium such as diabetic acidosis, gastrointestinal disturbances including the malabsorption syndrome, and the postoperative period.

DEFICIT OF POTASSIUM
(See Chap. 297, p. 1382)

DEFICIT OF MAGNESIUM
(See also Chap. 77)

There are approximately 2,000 mEq magnesium in the average 70-kg adult, and of this approximately one-half resides in bone. The concentration in serum is between 1.5 and 2.0 mEq per liter and is remarkably constant; approximately one-third of this is bound to protein. The residual magnesium is in the skeletal muscles and parenchymatous tissues.

Much more is known about experimental magnesium deficiency, and most of these data have been obtained in rodents. Nevertheless, a brief review of this information may provide the clues necessary to make new observations at the bedside.

Growing animals made deficient in magnesium with a diet free of this mineral develop hyperemia of the skin, appear ill, lose their appetite, and finally, startle easily and may have generalized seizures. The common chemical findings in serum include hypomagnesemia, hypercalcemia, hypophosphatemia, mild azotemia, and, significantly, normal levels of potassium and total CO_2 content. The muscle analyses reveal depressed levels of magnesium and a mild but consistent and significant deficit of potassium, even though the animals received more than what is usually considered adequate quantities of potassium in the dietary regimen. This alteration, in addition to evidence that there is a higher concentration of sodium in the erythrocytes of magnesium-deficient animals, suggests that this deficient state promotes one or more defects in the mechanisms of transport across cell membranes which are crucial to the steady state composition of cell fluid.

The hypercalcemia and hypophosphatemia are accompanied by hyperphosphaturia. The first two observations are not present when control and magnesium-deficient animals which have been parathyroidectomized are compared, but the magnesium-deficient animals still excrete more phosphorus. Thus, some but not all of these alterations reminiscent of hyperparathyroidism are dependent on increased parathyroid activity.

The pathology of this deficient state includes alterations in skeletal and cardiac muscle with myocytolysis and necrosis; and in the kidneys there is a striking nephrocalcinosis. This is unique in that it is confined to the broad ascending limb of the loop of Henle and consists primarily in the formation of microliths within the lumen, with only secondary damage to the cells as the lamellated stone expands in size.

It is, of course, not surprising that deficits of this cation should be accompanied by architectural and functional changes. This ion is known to be an important activator of many enzyme systems. In particular, attention is drawn to alkali-metal-sensitive ATPase, which demands magnesium and which may be important in the mechanisms of active transport.

The clinical circumstances in which magnesium deficiency is likely to be observed include the malabsorption syndromes, chronic alcoholism, prolonged and severe losses of body fluids, diabetic acidosis, cirrhosis of the liver, and primary aldosteronism. It is also noted following removal of a parathyroid adenoma, and this is more likely when there is evidence of bone demineralization. Lastly, patients who must be treated for long periods of time by the parenteral route may develop some deficit of magnesium when this ion is not added to the maintenance fluids.

The symptoms consist primarily of neuromuscular disorders and others related to the central nervous system. In the former area the prominent features include weakness, muscle fasciculation, tremors and occasionally a positive Chvostek's sign, and tetany. With reference to the central nervous system there may be personality changes, agitation, delirium, frank psychoses, and coma. Choreiform and athetoid movements have been noted.

It should be cautioned that the presence of hypomagnesemia does not *necessarily* imply a significant deficit of this cation. If normal subjects are provided with a diet which contains less than 1 mEq magnesium per day, the urinary excretion will diminish to this level in 4 to 5 days. The negative balance by way of the urine will be no more than 10 to 20 mEq. Despite this, the serum level of magnesium will be depressed by more than three standard deviations from the mean. Hence, a patient who has been on an alcoholic binge for 4 to 5 days with the ingestion of little or no food may have hypomagnesemia but a trivial magnesium deficit.

It is important to emphasize that it is difficult to evaluate the specific characteristics of the response to magnesium therapy. This is because magnesium in pharmacologic doses may readily improve some of the signs and symptoms noted above when their origins are not necessarily ascribable to magnesium deficit. Nevertheless, in the presence of these symptoms with evidence of magnesium deficiency, these patients should be treated with appropriate amounts of magnesium, since such treatment can be performed safely.

Since one cannot define antecedently the quantitative nature of the deficit, the repletion program must be empirical. The use of the intramuscular route for the injection of magnesium sulfate is appropriate, and if modest doses, such as 10 mEq magnesium (2.5 ml 50 percent $MgSO_4 \cdot 7H_2O$), are given at intervals and the serum levels checked, it is unlikely that one will promote hazardous hypermagnesemia. In general, levels as high as 3 to 4 mEq per liter in the serum are unassociated with untoward effects.

PRINCIPLES OF MANAGEMENT OF DEHYDRATION

The initial goals of the management of a state of dehydration are simple and include the restoration of the body fluids to normal volume, effective osmolality, composition, and acid-base relations. The quality and quantity of fluids required to satisfy these goals depend on the analysis of the characteristics of the dehydration. On the basis of this analysis it should be possible to outline a course of action. Since the analysis cannot be expected to be precise, it is wise to include in the outline a plan to interrupt therapy at an appropriate point to allow a reevaluation of the status of the patient. This reevaluation should employ all the available clinical and laboratory data relevant to the problem. The initial plan of management may then be modified in accord with this second analysis. Like the management of many other clinical problems, management of dehydration requires a combination of information, logic, and empiricism. In many instances the restoration of normal volume and tonicity of the body fluids, and the repair of a deficit of potassium, if present, will be accompanied by the coincidental correction of a complicating disturbance in acid-base balance. The administration of insulin and, at an appropriate time, of glucose and potassium is obviously necessary in a patient with diabetic acidosis. Since the alleviation of the acid-base disturbance is dependent on normal renal and respiratory function, these problems are more complex in patients with renal and pulmonary disease. The basic principles of the management of adrenal cortical insufficiency do not differ from those presented above; however, cortisone or hydrocortisone and 9-α-fluorohydrocortisone are added to the regimen. The management of the water deficit in diabetes insipidus differs from that of other deficits of water only insofar as the patient with diabetes insipidus should be given a preparation of the posterior pituitary gland to replace the deficiency of the ADH.

When these first goals have been realized, plans must be made to maintain the normal state of hydration. The fluid prescription must be developed in relation to the usual basal requirements and their possible alterations in this particular patient and to the need to replace losses other than those included in the former category.

REFERENCES

Elkinton, J. R., and T. S. Danowski: "The Body Fluids, Basic Physiology and Practical Therapeutics," Baltimore, The Williams & Wilkins Company, 1955.

Moore, F. D., H. Olesen, J. D. McMurrey, H. V. Parker, M. R. Ball, and C. M. Boyden: "The Body Cell Mass," Philadelphia, W. B. Saunders Company, 1963.

Ussing, H. H., P. Kruhøffer, J. H. Thaysen, and N. A. Thorn: The Alkali Metal Ions in Biology, in "Handbuch der Experimentellen Pharmakologie," O. Eichler and A. Farah (Eds.), Berlin, Springer-Verlag, 1960.

Welt, Louis G.: Water Balance in Health and Disease, p. 449, in "Diseases of Metabolism," 5th ed., G. G. Duncan (Ed.), Philadelphia, W. B. Saunders Company, 1964.

297 ACIDOSIS AND ALKALOSIS
Louis G. Welt

PHYSIOLOGIC CONSIDERATIONS

An understanding of the physiologic regulation and the clinical disorders of acid-base balance is often needlessly difficult because of the multiple uses and misuses of the terms *acid* and *base*. In the past these terms have been applied to anions and cations. This is not now acceptable, although the respectability of long usage has tended to perpetuate the error. Moreover, this is not a semantic quibble, since the use of these inadequate and misleading definitions creates a major handicap in the efforts to appreciate the very nature of the problem. In this discussion the term *acid* refers to any substance that can donate a hydrogen ion (H^+), and *base* means any substance that can accept a hydrogen ion. This statement may be rewritten as follows:

$$\text{Acid} \rightleftharpoons \text{base} + H^+$$

Some substances may serve as an acid *or* a base. For example, $H_2PO_4^-$ can dissociate to H^+ and HPO_4^{--}, or it can accept a hydrogen ion to form H_3PO_4. In the first instance it serves as an acid, and in the second as a base. These definitions serve to focus attention on the hydrogen ion as the significant item in acid-base balance. The manner in which the concentration of hydrogen ions may be expressed and the inferences drawn from this expression therefore become highly relevant.

The dissociation of an acid, HA, may be expressed in the following manner:

$$HA \rightleftharpoons H^+ + A^- \tag{1}$$

The rate at which this reaction proceeds to the right is proportional to the molar concentration of the acid and may be said to be equivalent to $k_1[HA]$. Likewise, the rate at which the reaction proceeds to the left is proportional to the product of the molar concentrations of H^+ and A^- and may be described as equivalent to $k_2[H^+][A^-]$. At equilibrium the two rates are equal, and therefore

$$k_1[HA] = k_2[H^+][A^-] \tag{2}$$

This equation can be rearranged to

$$\frac{k_1}{k_2} = \frac{[H^+][A^-]}{[HA]} \qquad (3)$$

The ratio of the two constants can be included in one new constant, K, and the statement can be rearranged to function as an expression of the concentration of hydrogen ions:

$$[H^+] = K \frac{[HA]}{[A^-]} \qquad (4)$$

Sorenson introduced the alternative method of expressing the concentration of hydrogen ions as the negative logarithm. The latter is denoted as pH, and the following statement emerges:

$$pH = pK + \log \frac{[A^-]}{[HA]} \qquad (5)$$

This may be stated in the more general form:

$$pH = pK + \log \frac{[base]}{[acid]} \qquad (6)$$

which is referred to as the *Henderson-Hasselbalch equation*. The logarithm of 1.0 is zero, and therefore when the concentrations of the base (the hydrogen ion acceptor) and the acid (the hydrogen ion donor) are equal to each other, the pH is equal to pK.

Buffers

A buffered solution is able to minimize the deviation of pH owing to the addition to that solution of a strong acid or a strong base. A buffer pair is composed of a weakly dissociated acid or base and a highly dissociated salt. Such a pair might be designated as HA and NaA. The addition of a strong acid, such as HCl, to this solution would promote the following reaction:

$$HA + NaA + HCl \rightarrow 2HA + NaCl$$

In this fashion a weak acid is substituted for the strong acid. The concentration of hydrogen ions will be increased to the extent that the increment of weak acid dissociates. This increase is clearly considerably less than that which would have occurred had the HCl been added to pure water.

The pH of a buffered solution will be defined by the ratio of the molar concentrations of the members of the buffer pair:

$$pH = pK + \log \frac{[NaA]}{[HA]}$$

Several characteristics of buffer activity are implicit in this equation. The deviation in pH consequent to the addition of an acid stronger than HA will be equated with a decrease in the concentration of A^- (represented by the numerator of the ratio) and an increase in the concentration of HA. This implies that, for a given increment of acid, the least change in pH will occur when the buffer ratio has a value of 1. Another implication is that at *any* specific ratio of the concentrations of the pair,

the addition of a given quantity of acid will alter the ratio less if the concentrations of the members of the pair are high rather than low. Finally, it is apparent that the capacity to buffer is lost when there is no hydrogen ion acceptor (base) left.

A solution may contain several buffers. The ratio of the concentrations of the components of each buffer pair is determined by the pH and, in turn, determines the pH. The ratios of each pair will be different at a specific pH in accordance with the individual dissociation constant for the system. Therefore, in a solution with several buffers a change in one component of any pair will dictate a change in the ratio for every other pair.

As mentioned in the preceding chapter, the body fluid most accessible for analysis is the plasma, and the pH of the extracellular fluid can be defined by the relationship between $NaHCO_3$ and H_2CO_3, or, more precisely, the tension of CO_2 (P_{CO_2}).[1] This is expressed by the equation

$$pH = 6.1 + \log \frac{NaHCO_3}{\underset{\Updownarrow}{H_2CO_3 + \text{dissolved } CO_2}}$$
$$CO_2 + H_2O$$

The ratio of the concentrations of sodium bicarbonate and the carbonic acid plus dissolved CO_2 is 20:1 at the pH of serum 7.40. This is far removed from the more efficient ratio of 1:1, and in a closed system this would be a poor buffer pair at that pH. However, the buffer is unique in that its acid component is a gas whose excretion can be rapidly accelerated or diminished by variations in respiratory exchange, and it is ubiquitous in that it is constantly being formed as a metabolic end product.

Although much of the buffer activity within the body is reflected and mirrored in the bicarbonate–carbonic acid system, this is by no means the only important buffer system in the body's fluids. The proteins of the plasma, the hemoglobin of the red blood cells, and the bicarbonate, phosphate, and proteins of the intracellular fluids all play a significant role in buffer activity. The sum total of the anions of the buffer salts capable of accepting hydrogen ions (i.e., the sum total of *base*) represents the first line of defense in absorbing the insult of the accession of an acid load in the body. The total of all body buffers (including those contributed by cations from cells and bones) cannot be estimated readily; some indication of their magnitude and a reflection of changes therein may be obtained from a consideration, as developed by Singer and Hastings, of the buffers present in whole blood alone.

The buffers in whole blood include the bicarbonate, proteins, and phosphate of the plasma and the hemoglobin, bicarbonate, and phosphate salts in the red blood cells. In addition, since the anionic properties of hemoglobin vary between the reduced and oxygenated state, the degree of saturation of hemoglobin with oxygen must be stipulated. The sum of these buffers has been referred to as *buffer base*. Initially this term was used to mean the

[1] The term P_{CO_2} refers to the partial pressure of carbon dioxide and is usually close to 40 mm Hg.

cation equivalents of the buffer anion. It is now more proper to use the term interchangeably with *buffer anion* itself. The range of normal values for the sum of the buffer base is 46 to 52 mM per liter. The values for buffer base and P_{CO_2} can be read from a nomogram prepared by Singer and Hastings if the pH of the blood, the hematocrit, the oxygen saturation of the hemoglobin, and the total CO_2 content of whole blood or plasma are known. Since the anionic properties of the proteins vary directly with pH, the primary retention or loss of carbon dioxide and bicarbonate, as in respiratory disturbances, is accompanied by reciprocal changes in the buffer base value for the proteins. Hence, the characteristic of respiratory acidosis and alkalosis will be the lack of deviation from normal in the value for buffer base. In contrast, the value for buffer base will be diminished in metabolic acidosis and increased in metabolic alkalosis.

Astrup and Siggaard-Andersen have emphasized the concept of *standard bicarbonate,* from which one can calculate a base excess or a base deficit. In a sense this represents a somewhat more refined and sophisticated method of determining what was alluded to above as the buffer base of Singer and Hastings. The essence of the concept is to remove from consideration the contribution made by the respiratory regulatory defenses. In this technique the pH of the blood is determined as drawn. Following this the pH is again measured at two different levels of P_{CO_2}, and the hemoglobin is rendered fully oxygenated. From a nomogram one can then determine the standard bicarbonate. The normal values range between 21 and 25 mEq per liter. If the determined value is greater, there is a base excess, and if lower, a base deficit. Thus, if the pH of the blood as originally drawn is depressed or elevated and there is neither a base excess nor deficit, the disturbance is respiratory in origin. Those who champion this system consider an additional advantage to be the quantitative nature of the determination and stress its usefulness in management of the clinical problem. In contrast, others have indicated that this technique offers little that is not readily available through less elaborate methods; and they point out in addition that the specific datum of base excess or deficit can be misleading.

ACIDOSIS AND ALKALOSIS

It should be clear from the above that the status of the acid-base relationship cannot be evaluated solely from knowledge of the total CO_2 content of the serum. This latter represents the sum of the members of the buffer pair and includes bicarbonate as well as carbonic acid and CO_2 gas. The total provides no information with respect to the relative proportions of the components of the buffer pair. In fact, a high or low concentration of total CO_2 is compatible with either acidosis or alkalosis. The pH of arterial blood (or blood obtained from a limb vein after warming the part at 45°C for about 10 min) is ultimately necessary to define the acid-base relationship. The pH, however, may be found to be disturbed more or less than the deviation in total CO_2

content of the serum. This depends, in part, on the sequence of events, the speed with which the distortion has supervened, and the success or failure of the compensatory mechanisms. Furthermore, in more complicated circumstances, the estimation of both P_{CO_2} and whole-blood buffer base may be necessary to unravel the nature of the disturbance in acid-base relationships.

CALCULATION OF P_{CO_2} AND PARTITION OF TOTAL CO_2 CONTENT

The quantity of carbon dioxide dissolved in a liquid is proportional to the P_{CO_2} and may be expressed in millimoles per liter as equal to alpha P_{CO_2}. The term *alpha* is equal to 0.0301 (mM/liter/mm Hg) for plasma at a temperature of 38°C. At different body temperatures an appropriate correction must be made. In turn, dissolved CO_2 is in equilibrium with H_2CO_3, and therefore the sum of dissolved CO_2 and carbonic acid may be said to be proportional to P_{CO_2}. Since the quantity of dissolved CO_2 is so much greater than the concentration of carbonic acid, this value will be used as the denominator in the Henderson-Hasselbalch equation.

In the sample calculation to follow, it will be assumed that the pH is 7.40, the total CO_2 content is 26 mM per liter, and the pK for the bicarbonate–CO_2 system is 6.10. The Henderson-Hasselbalch equation may be written as follows:

$$pH = 6.10 + \log \frac{(HCO_3^-)}{(\alpha P_{CO_2})}$$

Since the concentration of bicarbonate in plasma is equal to the difference between the total CO_2 content and P_{CO_2}, the equation may be rewritten:

$$pH = 6.10 + \log \frac{(total\ CO_2) - (\alpha P_{CO_2})}{(\alpha P_{CO_2})}$$

$$7.40 = 6.10 + \log \frac{(26) - (0.0301\ P_{CO_2})}{(0.0301\ P_{CO_2})}$$

$$7.40 - 6.10 = 1.3 = \log \frac{(26) - (0.0301\ P_{CO_2})}{(0.0301\ P_{CO_2})}$$

$$Antilog\ 1.3 = \frac{(26) - (0.0301\ P_{CO_2})}{(0.0301\ P_{CO_2})}$$

$$Antilog\ 1.3 = 19.95$$

therefore,

$$19.95\ (0.0301\ P_{CO_2}) = (26) - (0.0301\ P_{CO_2})$$
$$19.95\ (0.0301\ P_{CO_2}) + (0.0301\ P_{CO_2}) = 26$$
$$0.6306\ P_{CO_2} = 26$$

$$P_{CO_2} = \frac{26}{0.6306}$$

$$P_{CO_2} = 41.2\ mm\ Hg$$

The sum of the concentrations of dissolved CO_2 and H_2CO_3 is equal to

$$0.0301\ P_{CO_2} = 0.0301 \times 41.2 = 1.24\ mM/L$$

Since the concentration of bicarbonate ion is the difference between total CO_2 content and the value for dissolved CO_2 and H_2CO_3,

$$(HCO_3^-) = 26 - 1.24 = 24.76 \text{ mM/L}$$

REGULATION OF ACID-BASE EQUILIBRIUM

In general, the problem of regulating acid-base balance in health is to protect the pH from alterations induced by the continuous formation of acid end products of metabolism. In health the pH of the extracellular fluids is maintained at a level between 7.35 and 7.45. This is accomplished by buffer activity (discussed earlier), by exchange of ions between the two major fluid compartments, and by adaptations of respiratory and renal function.

Regulation by Ion Exchange

The exchange of *anions* across membranes appears to be most free in the red blood cells and, probably, the renal tubular cells. Chloride and bicarbonate ions can diffuse across the erythrocyte membrane, and their distribution between the red blood cell and plasma water is responsive to changes in their concentrations and pH. For example, an increase in the P_{CO_2} of the plasma due to the addition of carbon dioxide is followed by diffusion of the gas into the red blood cell, where part of it is hydrated to H_2CO_3. The dissociation of this acid increases the concentration of bicarbonate ions, and these diffuse from the cell. This, in turn, is accompanied by a movement of chloride into the red blood cells. The net effect of this redistribution of anions in terms of the acid-base relationships of the extracellular fluid is to increase the concentration of bicarbonate in this compartment. This increase in the concentration of HCO_3^- tends to offset the effect of the initial increase in P_{CO_2} on the buffer ratio of the Henderson-Hasselbalch equation.

The exchange of *cations* such as sodium, potassium, and perhaps calcium as well from muscle cells and bone for hydrogen ions in the extracellular fluid (and vice versa) plays a significant role in modifying the alterations in pH of the extracellular fluids. It has been estimated, for example, that approximately 50 percent of an acid load administered to dogs was neutralized by such an exchange of sodium and potassium for hydrogen ions. In another study it was suggested that 25 percent of the "neutralization" of an infusion of $NaHCO_3$ had been achieved by the exchange of extracellular sodium for intracellular hydrogen ions. Similar exchanges are reported in studies of both respiratory acidosis and respiratory alkalosis.

Respiratory Regulation

The lungs play a major role in the excretion of acid as carbon dioxide. Moreover, the centers that regulate the rate and depth of ventilation are exquisitely sensitive to subtle changes in the composition of the blood and extra-vascular fluids. The central chemoreceptors located in the medullary respiratory centers are responsive to the P_{CO_2} and pH of their environment in such a way that an increase in P_{CO_2} or hydrogen ion concentration promotes an increase in pulmonary ventilation. In contrast, a decrease in CO_2 tension or increase in pH tends to inhibit ventilation. In either case it is clear that the alteration in respiratory activity tends to correct the primary deviation in P_{CO_2} or pH. The P_{CO_2} appears to be the more potent stimulus of the two. In addition, there are peripheral chemoreceptors located in the carotid and aortic bodies. These are relatively insensitive to pH and P_{CO_2} but are responsive to the arterial oxygen tension (P_{O_2}).

An interesting aspect of the chemoregulation of pulmonary ventilation concerns the phenomenon of a change in the "sensitivity" of the central respiratory centers to a specific P_{CO_2}. It appears as though a period of hypercapnia diminishes "sensitivity," and hypocapnia enhances the intensity of the response to a given tension of CO_2. The precise nature of this altered response is not clear. An appreciation of this adaptation is helpful in understanding certain complications of acid-base disorders, which will be discussed in more detail later (see Chap. 33 for a more complete discussion of respiratory regulation).

Renal Regulation

The kidneys contribute to the regulation of acid-base balance by varying the net rate of excretion of hydrogen ions and by processes of selective reabsorption and rejection of cations and anions. These two processes are interdependent to the extent that the reabsorption of sodium is closely related to the secretion of hydrogen ions and potassium. The total rate of *secretion* of hydrogen ions by the tubular cells may be calculated from the sum of the titratable acid, ammonium ion, and a fraction equivalent to the difference between the filtered and excreted bicarbonate.

The rate of *excretion* of acid is calculated from the sum of the titratable acid plus ammonium ion *minus* the bicarbonate.

The titratable acid is equivalent to the quantity of NaOH that must be added to the urine to change its pH to that of the plasma. It represents the hydrogen ions present in free acid compounds and incorporated in the buffer components of the urine. Caution must be exercised to avoid the error of necessarily equating a low urinary pH with a high rate of excretion of acid. A small quantity of dissociated acid in a poorly buffered urine will lower the pH considerably. This same quantity of titratable acid in a buffered solution might be accommodated with very little depression of pH.

Pitts and his collaborators demonstrated that the urinary excretion of acid may be in excess of what can be accounted for by filtration and preferential reabsorption. They developed the hypothesis that hydrogen ions are secreted into the tubular fluid in exchange for sodium. The source of the hydrogen ions for this secretory process is not known for certain, although it is usually represented as having been derived from carbonic acid. The latter, in turn, is believed to be formed from the hydration of carbon dioxide:

$$\left. \begin{array}{c} H_2O + CO_2 \\ \Updownarrow \\ H_2CO_3 \\ \Updownarrow \\ H^+ + HCO_3^- \end{array} \right\} \text{This reaction accelerated by the enzyme carbonic anhydrase}$$

The rate of tubular *secretion* of hydrogen ions is probably conditioned by many factors, some of which include the pH of the renal tubular cell fluid, the P_{CO_2} (rather than the pH) of the extracellular fluid, the availability of buffers in the tubular fluid, the intensity of the stimuli primarily responsible for the reabsorption of sodium, and the status of the stores of potassium in the tubular cells. A decreased pH in the cell fluid, hypercapnia, and a diminished content of potassium in the renal tubular cells tend to favor the secretion of hydrogen ions. These ions cannot be secreted against a concentration gradient in excess of approximately 800:1. A diminished tubular content of buffer will therefore impose a restriction on the rate of secretion of hydrogen ions by failing to resist the decrease in pH consequent to this secretion.

In essence one may view the major role of the kidney in combating acidosis as reabsorbing all the filtered bicarbonate and, in addition, regenerating the bicarbonate that is continuously dissipated by the buffer action of strong acids with the bicarbonate–carbonic acid system. These operations may be portrayed in the following fashion:

1. The reabsorption of filtered bicarbonate

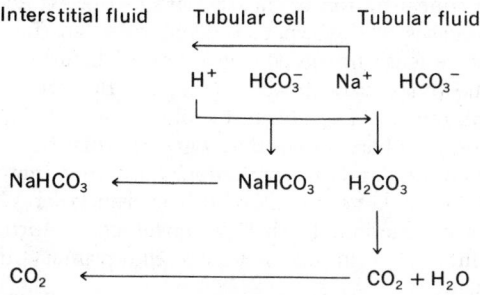

It will be noted that the reabsorption of the filtered bicarbonate is somewhat indirect. The sodium which is reabsorbed by exchange with hydrogen ion is then transported from the cell to the interstitial fluid of the kidney along with the bicarbonate remnant of the carbonic acid that donated the hydrogen ion. The carbonic acid left behind in the tubular fluid is then dehydrated to CO_2 and H_2O, and the carbon dioxide diffuses back to the body fluids.

2. The reabsorption of bicarbonate that is *not* filtered
In this fashion sodium of a salt other than bicarbonate is reabsorbed in exchange for a hydrogen ion that becomes incorporated in a buffer. In a somewhat similar fashion the following reaction may obtain when the anion accompanying sodium is relatively unable to permeate the tubular cell membrane:

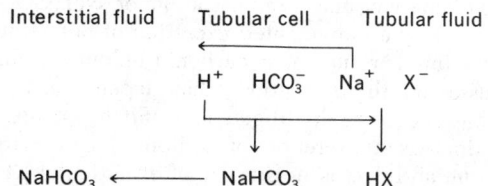

In addition to excretion as titratable acid, as illustrated above, hydrogen ions are excreted as ammonium, NH_4^+, as well. The sequence of events leading to enhanced excretion of ammonium depends in part on the reaction just described. The active transport of sodium produces a potential difference across the tubular membranes such that the lumen is negative. This creates a driving force which can be accommodated either by reabsorption of an anion with a negative charge along the established electrochemical gradient or by secretion of a positively charged cation. If the anion cannot permeate, the second alternative must obtain. Hydrogen ions can be secreted until the luminal fluid pH falls to a level against which no more hydrogen ions can be transported. Ammonia is considered to be in diffusion equilibrium between tubular cells and lumen and can move freely in either direction, but NH_4^+ cannot. Thus, if hydrogen ions are secreted and all filtered buffers are exhausted, the NH_3 in the luminal fluid can buffer the hydrogen ion. The NH_4^+ which is formed cannot diffuse back and hence is excreted into the urine. This sets the direction of the reaction pathway for ammonia, the hydrogen ion gradient is reduced, and now more hydrogen ions can be secreted. This may be illustrated in the following fashion:

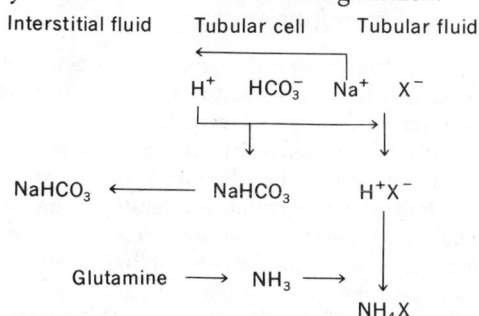

The rate of excretion of ammonia does not change as acutely as is the case with titratable acid, but in appropriate circumstances it may make a greater contribution in quantitative terms. Ammonia is formed in the tubular cells, and the largest fraction is derived from glutamine. The deamidation of glutamine is accelerated by the enzyme glutaminase, which is present in the kidneys.

Thus, in these several ways the renal tubules regenerate the bicarbonate that is dissipated (and excreted as CO_2) by the buffer activity consequent to the accession of an acid load in the body fluids.

The reabsorption of sodium may be associated with an

exchange for potassium in lieu of hydrogen ion. These alternatives are frequently pictured as competing one with the other. These interrelationships may explain, in part, the aciduria which may accompany potassium depletion despite an extracellular alkalosis; and this may also explain why the administration of $NaHCO_3$ is accompanied by an augmented excretion of potassium.

The administration of a carbonic anhydrase inhibitor suppresses all these reactions that depend on a readily available source of hydrogen ions. Such an agent promotes increased excretion of sodium, bicarbonate, and potassium and decreases the rate of excretion of titratable acid and ammonia. Some of these alterations are observed in patients with renal disease characterized by tubular dysfunction. The defect in some instances is due to inability to transport hydrogen ions against a concentration gradient.

The role of the kidneys in acid-base regulation will be discussed further later in this chapter. The nature of the specific responses in each type of acid-base disturbance will serve to illustrate the particular contributions of the kidneys.

A comment is in order concerning the significance of *compensation*. The responses just described are initiated by a distortion of one or more of the physicochemical characteristics of the body fluids. If the response were such as to efface the distortion, the stimulus for the response would be removed and the distortion would reappear. Thus, it is unlikely that compensation can ever be perfect since it would automatically be self-destructive so long as the initial basis for the disturbance persisted. Hence, if a patient with an obvious acid-base disturbance has a normal value for pH, or P_{CO_2}, or total CO_2 content, the implication is that this is almost certainly an instance of a *mixed* acid-base disturbance.

CLINICAL CONSIDERATIONS

There are four major disturbances in acid-base equilibrium, and it is convenient to discuss them individually and as separate entities. Nevertheless it should be remembered that mixed disturbances occur fairly frequently. In this discussion the aim is to analyze each disorder in terms of the primary alteration, the impact of this insult and the compensatory respiratory and renal responses on the Henderson-Hasselbalch equation, the nature of the compositional changes, and the approach to the management of the disorder. The Henderson-Hasselbalch equation is re-presented here with respect to the bicarbonate–carbonic acid buffer system. Reference to this equation, which defines the pH, is most helpful in visualizing the sequence and consequence of primary and secondary events in the pathogenesis of acidosis and alkalosis:

$$pH = 6.1 + \log \frac{NaHCO_3}{H_2CO_3 + \text{dissolved } CO_2}$$
$$\updownarrow$$
$$CO_2 + H_2O$$

The ratio of the concentrations of the buffer pair is 20:1.

Respiratory Acidosis

Respiratory acidosis is due to inadequate elimination of CO_2 by the lungs because of hypoventilation or because of uneven ventilation in relation to blood flow. It is unlikely to be associated solely with impaired diffusion across the alveolar capillary membranes, since the diffusion of CO_2 is so rapid. Respiratory acidosis is found commonly in patients with conditions such as emphysema, pulmonary fibrosis, and cardiopulmonary disease.

The retention of CO_2 will increase the P_{CO_2} and the concentration of carbonic acid. The increase in the value for the denominator of the buffer ratio will change this to something less than 20:1 and will define a decrease in the pH. The CO_2 can penetrate cell membranes freely, and in this fashion a considerable quantity of acid can be buffered in the intracellular fluids. In addition, there is evidence that hydrogen ions from the extracellular fluids exchange for potassium and sodium from cells and bone.

The increase in P_{CO_2} and the decrease in pH both serve to stimulate ventilation, and further accumulation of CO_2 may be prevented or at least retarded thereby. The renal response is characterized by increased excretion of titratable acid, ammonium, and chloride and diminished excretion of bicarbonate. The above-mentioned response clearly implies a net increase in the total rate of *secretion* of hydrogen ions by the renal tubule, which is not necessarily the case in metabolic acidosis (see below). In this manner the kidneys help eliminate acid, but, in addition, they alter electrolyte composition so that the concentration of bicarbonate in the extracellular fluid increases at the expense of chloride. To the extent that this increase in the concentration of bicarbonate restores the buffer ratio toward 20:1, the deviation of the pH is minimized. The ability to tolerate a high P_{CO_2} has an additional advantage in that a greater quantity of CO_2 is excreted per unit of ventilation. This increment may be sufficiently large to allow the excretion of CO_2 to equal its production. In this circumstance no further increase in P_{CO_2} will occur unless the primary disease worsens.

It was stated earlier that the increase in CO_2 tension stimulated respiratory activity, but as the hypercapnia is maintained the respiratory centers appear to develop decreased sensitivity to this stimulus. A diminution in the respiratory response to the next increment of P_{CO_2} will promote a more intense hypercapnia. This new level of P_{CO_2} serves to maintain some increase in ventilation until a new level of desensitization develops, and the vicious cycle is repeated. Ultimately the hypercapnia becomes extreme, and the increased P_{CO_2} no longer serves as an appropriate stimulus to increase ventilation. At this time the most important stimulus for respiratory activity is the accompanying hypoxia. It has been said that if patients with respiratory acidosis were left to their own devices, they would probably succumb to hypoxia rather than to hypercapnia or acidosis. The slower diffusion of oxygen would be expected to promote incapacitating hypoxia before the development of CO_2 narcosis or a pH incompatible with life. However, if such patients are treated by exposure to a breathing mixture with a high content of oxygen in an effort to relieve the hypoxemia, they may quickly become confused, lapse into coma, and die. The improvement in the hypoxia may remove the last effective stimulus for respiratory activity. As a result of the diminished ventilation, there is a further decline in the excretion of CO_2, leading to the grave consequences of extreme hypercapnia. This should not be interpreted to suggest that such patients should never be treated with oxygen; it emphasizes the need for close observation when oxygen therapy is used to detect the earliest evidences of this complication. If morphine is given these patients, it should be administered with caution, since this drug may affect the respiratory center in such a manner as to induce hypoventilation. This, in turn, will promote a sharp increase in the P_{CO_2}, the intensity of the acidosis, and the degree of hypoxia.

The management of these patients includes all those measures which may be expected to improve the basic disease condition responsible for pulmonary insufficiency, as discussed in Chap. 295. However, these measures may fail, and the extreme hypoxia and hypercapnia may require immediate attention. In this situation artificial respiration (by mechanical respirator) may offer a valuable therapeutic approach. The increase in ventilatory exchange induced by the respirator improves the hypoxia and promotes an increased excretion of CO_2. In the course of a few days this may be successful in reducing the P_{CO_2} to more nearly normal levels. This, in turn, may restore the sensitivity of the respiratory center to lower levels of CO_2, and a rising P_{CO_2} may again serve as a proper stimulus to respiratory activity.

The use of the carbonic anhydrase inhibitor Diamox has been recommended in the management of this problem. Although it has not been uniformly successful, some patients appear to have improved as a result of its use. The data suggest that its mode of action is most likely a consequence of an influence of the carbonic anhydrase inhibitor on the respiratory center itself, which may serve to improve ventilation. Another agent that may be useful is salicylate, which may be ingested as aspirin or administered intravenously as the sodium salt. This drug definitely increases the sensitivity of the respiratory center to carbon dioxide and may be helpful in patients with chronic hypercapnia. Progesterone has been reported to influence the sensitivity of the respiratory center to carbon dioxide. Vanillic acid diethylamide improves ventilation, primarily by increasing the depth rather than the rate of respiration. It may be useful in the management of acute as well as chronic respiratory insufficiency. One other agent has been suggested to combat respiratory acidosis, namely, THAM (tris hydroxy methyl amino methane). This agent combines with CO_2 and in this fashion aids in restoring the pH toward normal. However, this by itself might have undesirable consequences by reducing ventilation and oxygenation. Hence, its use without mechanical assistance may be harmful, and if the latter is provided, the use of THAM would appear unnecessary.

The compositional changes in the serum have been mentioned; a fairly typical pattern of concentrations of electrolytes in a patient with respiratory acidosis is

Na	137 mEq/L
K	4.5 mEq/L
Total CO_2	40 mM/L
Cl	90 mEq/L
pH	7.31
P_{CO_2}	79 mm Hg

The pattern, neglecting pH and P_{CO_2}, would also be compatible with metabolic alkalosis. The gross characteristics of the underlying clinical problem will usually dictate the appropriate selection between these two alternatives. The normal concentration of potassium suggests that this is not metabolic alkalosis. The arterial pH clearly resolves the problem in the above instance.

Metabolic Acidosis

Metabolic acidosis is due to either an accumulation of acids or a primary loss of bicarbonate. An accumulation of acids is observed classically in diabetic acidosis and in renal insufficiency, and a primary loss of bicarbonate may be observed in renal disease as well. In diabetes the offenders are the 4-carbon ketones, and if these may be represented by the expression HK, the consequences of their accession to the extracellular fluid may be visualized as follows:

$$HK + NaHCO_3 \rightleftharpoons NaK + H_2CO_3$$

If this buffering of the ketone acid is related to the effect on the Henderson-Hasselbalch equation, it is readily observed that the reduction in bicarbonate and increase in carbonic acid will decrease the ratio to something less than 20:1 and will define a decrease in the pH. The latter as well as the presumed initial increase in P_{CO_2} both serve as stimuli to increase pulmonary ventilation, the excretion of CO_2 will be accelerated, P_{CO_2} will fall, the buffer ratio will be restored toward 20:1, and the deviation in pH is minimized. The violent respiratory response to acidosis characterized by an increase first in depth and later in frequency of respirations is referred to as *Kussmaul breathing*. If one observes the characteristics of this respiratory activity closely, it is usually noted that the effort appears to be on the expiratory phase in contrast to the inspiratory effort noted in patients with oxygen lack.

Since the P_{CO_2} is depressed along with the decrease in pH, the inference is either that the latter is now solely responsible for the increased respiratory activity or that the hypocapnia has induced a state of increased sensitivity of the respiratory centers to low tensions of CO_2. The latter appears quite likely, and it has been pointed out that during the recovery phase of several types of metabolic acidosis, the pH reaches normal values while the P_{CO_2} is still depressed. This would be an unlikely event unless the respiratory center was responsive to these lower levels of P_{CO_2}.

The renal response to this metabolic acidosis includes virtual total reabsorption of filtered bicarbonate and an increase in the net *urinary excretion* of acid as titratable acid and ammonia. The increase in net excretion of acid does not necessarily imply an increase in the net *secretion* of hydrogen ions. This will be apparent if it is recalled that the secretion of hydrogen ions to effect total reabsorption of a small filtered load of bicarbonate may be considerably less than that needed for incomplete reabsorption of bicarbonate when there is a much higher filtered load, as is the case normally or in respiratory acidosis. The net rates of excretion of acid may be similar in respiratory and metabolic acidosis, although presumably more hydrogen ion is secreted in the former to effect the larger bicarbonate reabsorption. Thus, although higher levels of P_{CO_2} favor the secretion of hydrogen ions, the renal response, in terms of the *net excretion* of acid, is not jeopardized by the hypocapnia of metabolic acidosis.

A fairly typical pattern of the concentrations of electrolytes in the serum in diabetic acidosis is

Na	125 mEq/L
K	3.5 mEq/L
Total CO_2	5 mM/L
Cl	90 mEq/L
Glucose	800 mg/100 ml
pH	7.01
P_{CO_2}	19 mm Hg

It will be noted that the sum of the concentrations of CO_2 and chloride is 95 mEq per liter. The difference between this sum and the concentration of sodium is 30 mEq per liter, which is significantly higher than the usual difference of 5 to 10 mEq per liter and implies an unusual concentration of some anion other than bicarbonate and chloride. In diabetic acidosis this is likely to be almost all represented by ketones. (Although the concentration of sodium is depressed, the effective osmolality of the extracellular fluids will be found to be increased if one calculates the osmolar contribution of the elevated concentration of glucose.)[2]

The management of the acid-base disturbance in diabetic patients is not usually a primary concern. The administration of adequate amounts of insulin can be expected to promote the utilization of glucose and to decrease the production of ketones. Under these circumstances the ketonemia is soon dissipated by utilization and excretion, and as the ketonemia subsides, the concentration of bicarbonate increases and the pH is soon restored to more nearly normal levels.

Metabolic acidosis due to the loss of bicarbonate in the urine is not uncommon in chronic renal insufficiency. It is due, presumably, to inadequate reabsorption of bicarbonate by the renal tubular cells. This may, in turn,

[2] The osmolar contribution of glucose is calculated as follows: mg/100 ml glucose $\times$ 10 = mg/L; mg/L divided by 180 (molecular weight of glucose) = the number of milliosmols of glucose. Thus: $800 \times 10 = 8,000$; 8,000 divided by $180 = 44.4$ mOsm/L.

be due to one of several steps that must precede the actual secretion of hydrogen ions in the process of exchange with sodium. Since this is primarily a reflection of tubular dysfunction, it has been stated that it is seen more commonly in chronic pyelonephritis than in glomerulonephritis or other forms of chronic Bright's disease; it may occur, however, in all types of chronic renal failure. In one rather rare form of renal disease there is relatively little functional evidence of glomerular disease. In some of these disorders, the tubular defect may be congenital in origin. In this last instance the defect appears to be concerned not with the formation of hydrogen ions but with the inability to secrete these ions against the concentration gradient. The net effect of the defect is reduced concentration of bicarbonate in the extracellular fluids, accompanied by reciprocally increased concentration of chloride. The diminution in concentration of bicarbonate defines a decrease in the pH of the extracellular fluid. This latter serves as a stimulus to respiratory activity, increased excretion of CO_2 promotes a decrease in P_{CO_2}, and pH approaches a normal value as the ratio of the buffer pair approaches a value of 20:1. Since the ability to secrete hydrogen ions is not totally defunct, the excretion of bicarbonate diminishes only to the point where the filtered load of bicarbonate reaches a value no longer in excess of the residual capacity to secrete hydrogen ions. This disorder may also be associated with increased excretion of calcium and potassium. The latter is not unexpected by virtue of the competitive relationship between hydrogen ions and potassium for exchange with sodium. The reason for the augmented excretion of calcium is less clear. It may be due, in part, to the effect of systemic acidosis in mobilizing calcium from bone. It may also represent some specific renal response of an adaptive nature.

A characteristic set of concentrations of electrolytes in the serum is

Na	134 mEq/L
K	3.5 mEq/L
Total CO_2	12 mM/L
Cl	115 mEq/L
PO_4	2 mEq/L
pH	7.25
P_{CO_2}	26 mm Hg

It should be noted that the sum of the concentrations of CO_2 and chloride, 127 mEq per liter, differs only by 7 mEq per liter from the concentration of sodium and that the phosphate concentration is normal. This makes it clear that the depression of CO_2 cannot be ascribed to the accumulation of anions other than chloride. This same pattern might be observed in a patient who had received large doses of NH_4Cl or Diamox or who had respiratory alkalosis. The determination of the pH readily resolves the directional deviation in this instance. In clinical situations the history alone should reveal whether this pattern resulted from a renal lesion or from the administration of ammonium chloride or a drug.

In instances of renal insufficiency accompanied by a

significant decrease in filtration rate and renal mass, there is an inability to regenerate bicarbonate. This may be due in part to the filtration of lesser quantities of sodium salts, diminished buffer capacity in the tubules, and failure to excrete ammonia properly owing to the loss of the tissue responsible for this function. The diminished filtration rate is presumably responsible for the retention of phosphate, sulfate, and other anions of fixed acids as well. This constellation of defects is characterized by a diminution in the total CO_2 content as well as an increase in what is commonly referred to as the *undetermined anions.* Hence, the sum of the concentrations of total CO_2 and chloride subtracted from the concentration of sodium in the serum will usually equal a value in excess of 5 to 10 mEq per liter. This type of acidosis is the one most commonly encountered in chronic renal failure. A characteristic set of concentrations is

Na	130 mEq/L
K	5 mEq/L
Total CO_2	12 mM/L
Cl	93 mEq/L
PO_4	7 mEq/L
pH	7.25
P_{CO_2}	26 mm Hg

Note that the total CO_2 plus chloride subtracted from the sodium equals 25 mEq per liter. The hyperphosphatemia accounts for part of this excess, and sulfates would, if measured, probably be equally increased. Note also the slight hyperkalemia.

Metabolic acidosis due to renal insufficiency can be corrected by administering sodium bicarbonate. In this fashion the concentration of bicarbonate can be increased and the buffer ratio restored to a normal value. Correction can be made effectively in many instances simply by prescribing the ingestion of sodium bicarbonate either in addition to or in lieu of table salt. The reduction in the intake of NaCl is particularly desirable where there is some reason to avoid an excessive intake of sodium or where the substitution of sodium bicarbonate for sodium chloride is indicated because acidosis is due to a primary loss of bicarbonate and the concentration of chloride is already high. The amount of sodium bicarbonate necessary as a daily supplement must be gauged in an empirical manner by correlating the dosage with the response. The use of 2 to 4 Gm $NaHCO_3$ per day is safe to start with. Two complications may mar the success of this treatment. Since the kidneys of these patients have lost the capacity to discriminate properly, it is possible to overcorrect the acidosis. The possibility of overcorrection may be increased by the maintenance of a low P_{CO_2} due to increased sensitivity of the respiratory center to CO_2 as a stimulus. The second complication deals with the possible development of tetany. Many of these patients have hyperphosphatemia and hypocalcemia. The acidosis may protect against tetany from hypocalcemia, and this protection may be lost as the pH is corrected with $NaHCO_3$. The ingestion of several grams of calcium gluconate or lactate may prevent this complication. The obvious advantages of the correction of the metabolic acidosis include elimination of the hyperpnea which may be a troublesome symptom, in most cases some relief from subjective discomfort, and maintenance of an internal environment better able to buffer sudden increments of acid. The increase in excretion of calcium and potassium that may accompany the acidosis may be diminished as well. However, it is unnecessary to raise the level of bicarbonate in excess of 20 mM per liter.

So far this discussion has concerned management in a noncritical chronic phase of the disease. When patients with renal insufficiency experience an episode of dehydration with further decompensation in renal function, they may develop acute and more intense disturbances in acid-base balance. However, it is frequently in these very circumstances that the physician may be most effective in correcting a disabling acidosis. The efficient correction of acidosis depends on increasing the concentration of bicarbonate in the extracellular fluid. This can be accomplished most dramatically when hyponatremia accompanies the disorder, since the concentration of sodium can be raised together with the bicarbonate by administering a hypertonic solution of $NaHCO_3$. The quantity of sodium to administer is calculated as discussed in Chap. 296. This should represent too much bicarbonate, but, in fact, it rarely does. The second most dramatic correction may be accomplished when the patient with acidosis has a normal concentration of sodium but is dehydrated. The administration of an isotonic solution of a sodium salt will expand the volume of the extracellular fluid and repair the dehydration. If the salt is the bicarbonate, the concentration of this anion will be increased.

The possibility of provoking hypocalcemic tetany must always be considered when sodium bicarbonate is administered in these circumstances. It is recommended that prior to the infusion of $NaHCO_3$ the patient should receive at least 10 ml 10 percent solution of calcium gluconate intravenously. In addition, the presence of Chvostek's reflex should be checked during the administration of the bicarbonate and more calcium administered if the reflex is elicited. The solution of calcium should not be mixed with bicarbonate, since calcium carbonate will precipitate.

Respiratory Alkalosis

Respiratory alkalosis is due to hyperventilation and results from the excretion of carbon dioxide in excess of its production. This reduces the tension of CO_2, increases the value for the ratio of the buffer pair, and defines an increase in pH. This disorder may be observed in the early phases of pulmonary and cardiopulmonary disease when hyperventilation is induced by hypoxia. It is more commonly observed as a manifestation of anxiety and tension, and it may be due to a lesion in the area of the central nervous system responsible for respiratory regulation. This last is the least common variety, but it is the circumstance in which one may see the most significant deviations from normal.

The anxious and tense patient, usually a woman, who hyperventilates in response to emotional stimuli may develop acute, although transient, alkalosis accompanied by a variety of symptoms, which include giddiness and light-headedness, circumoral and peripheral paresthesias, muscle tremors, and frank carpopedal spasm. Since these episodes are short-lived, there is insufficient time for a significant renal response in the nature of a compensatory effort. For the same reasons the only compositional changes are the increase in pH and decrease in P_{CO_2}.

In those instances of relatively sustained hyperventilation, as with an irritative lesion in the reticular formation of the medulla, compensatory responses and compositional changes may be prominent. The renal responses are characterized by increased excretion of bicarbonate, decreased excretion of chloride, and augmented excretion of potassium and sodium. The diminution in renal tubular reabsorption of bicarbonate is due, presumably, to decreased secretion of hydrogen ions for the exchange with sodium. This may be due to hypocapnia. The lessened secretion of hydrogen ions may be responsible for an increase in the secretion and excretion of potassium. The most significant consequence of these renal responses is decreased concentration of bicarbonate in the extracellular fluids. This alteration tends to reduce the value for the ratio of the buffer pair toward 20:1 and hence minimizes the deviation in pH. The other alterations in composition include an increase in the concentration of chloride in the serum, along with a tendency to a lowered concentration of sodium and potassium.

These alterations in the electrolyte pattern may mimic those of metabolic acidosis. It is important to recognize respiratory alkalosis as distinct from metabolic acidosis, since the administration of bicarbonate, which may be desirable for acidosis, may be detrimental to the patient who is already alkalotic.

The management of patients with hyperventilation as a manifestation of anxiety and tension is primarily directed toward helping the patient to understand the pathogenesis of the disorder. It is frequently helpful to have the patient induce an episode by voluntary hyperventilation and then to demonstrate how this may be modified by rebreathing into a paper bag or by holding the nose and covering the mouth. This demonstration is usually quite convincing and helps to furnish the motivation for the patient to train herself to discontinue this habit. In those instances where hyperventilation has provoked carpopedal spasm, the immediate need is to use some technique to increase the P_{CO_2} of the body fluids. This is most easily accomplished by having the patient rebreathe into a paper bag.

Metabolic Alkalosis

Metabolic alkalosis is characterized by increased concentration of bicarbonate unattended by an equivalent increase in the P_{CO_2}, so that the ratio of the concentrations of the buffer pair is in excess of 20:1 and the pH is elevated. This condition may arise as a consequence of

(1) the administration of sodium bicarbonate (or sodium salts of organic acids such as citrate or lactate); (2) the loss of chloride as HCl, as in vomiting or gastric suction; (3) the loss of chloride with sodium in a ratio in excess of that which characterizes their relative concentrations in the extracellular fluid; (4) excessive excretion of acid in the urine; (5) the movement of hydrogen ions from the extracellular fluid to the cells in consequence of a deficit of potassium. The interrelationships among these possible primary events are intimate, and each of them provokes responses of an interdependent character, so it is rare to find metabolic alkalosis that is not multicausal. The interplay of primary events and subsequent responses can be illustrated by examining the sequence that may follow each of the major initiating events.

Throughout the discussion it will be well to visualize the effects of compensatory mechanisms that tend to mitigate the deviation in pH as these may be surmised from the Henderson-Hasselbalch equation. These include an increase in the CO_2 tension, which may be induced by hypoventilation, and a reduction in the concentration of bicarbonate in the extracellular fluid. Hypoventilation would, presumably, be favored by the increase in pH. However, this path of compensation is not usually of great quantitative significance. There are limiting influences on hypoventilation, which include the development of hypoxia and hypercapnia. These are both stimuli to increased respiratory activity. Reduction in the high concentration of bicarbonate may be achieved to some extent by the accelerated excretion of $NaHCO_3$ in the urine. To the extent that an increase in P_{CO_2} tends to enhance the reabsorption of bicarbonate, it may be said that a more successful hypoventilatory response would impose serious limitations on the efficiency of the renal response. Other limitations imposed on the compensating mechanisms will be illustrated in the discussions to follow. Furthermore, there may be specific deleterious effects on renal function and anatomic integrity as a consequence of certain features of metabolic alkalosis. One of these effects is potassium depletion.

ALKALOSIS INDUCED WITH SODIUM BICARBONATE. The administration of $NaHCO_3$ will induce metabolic alkalosis, which depends, in part, on the magnitude and rapidity with which a particular load of this salt is administered. However, the ability to accelerate the excretion of $NaHCO_3$ in the urine is so great that it is difficult to maintain any serious degree of alkalosis in this fashion in the absence of other conditioning influences. The ingestion or administration of $NaHCO_3$ is accompanied by an augmented excretion of potassium. If the ingestion or administration of potassium is inadequate to match the accelerated urinary loss, a deficit of potassium develops. The depletion of potassium has several consequences that tend to intensify rather than mitigate alkalosis:

1. A potassium deficit tends to diminish the secretion of potassium and enhance the exchange of hydrogen ions for sodium in the renal tubular reabsorptive mechanism. The augmented secretion of hydrogen ions promotes in-

creased reabsorption of sodium as bicarbonate, which imposes a limit on the efficiency with which bicarbonate may be excreted.

2. A large experimental literature dealing with the production of potassium depletion utilizing diets essentially free of this cation and administering $NaHCO_3$ describes an increase in the quantity of sodium in tissue cells. However, in most instances the quantitative relationship is such as to suggest that some other cation has gained access to the cell along with sodium. In some instances, at least, this appears to be hydrogen ion. To the extent that this transfer of hydrogen ions from the extracellular fluids to cells operates, the intensity of the extracellular alkalosis will be augmented.

As long as potassium depletion is avoided, large amounts of administered bicarbonate may fail to induce significant alkalosis.

METABOLIC ALKALOSIS DUE TO LOSS OF GASTRIC SECRETION BY VOMITING OR SUCTION. The primary cause of alkalosis in this instance is the loss of HCl with the consequent increase in the bicarbonate concentration and decrease in the chloride concentration in the extracellular fluids. The renal response to this alkalosis is similar to that just described and is characterized by accelerated excretion of sodium and potassium bicarbonate in the urine. The loss of potassium in the urine added to the loss of this ion in the gastric fluid represents an early potassium deficit. The nature of the primary event precludes retention of ingested food or fluid, and if potassium is not administered parenterally and the gastric losses continue, the intensity of the potassium depletion increases. Furthermore, the loss of sodium in the gastric fluid and in the urine, if unreplaced, induces a deficit of this ion as well. The deficits of potassium and sodium both impose limitations on the mechanisms that tend to compensate for alkalosis. Those related to potassium depletion have just been described. The limits imposed by sodium depletion may operate as follows: As the deficit of sodium develops, there is a loss of fluid. If no water is ingested or administered, the net deficit tends toward a loss of water in excess of sodium loss. If water is ingested and promptly vomited, or if water without salt (e.g., glucose in water) is administered by vein, the net deficit will be of sodium in excess of water. In either event, there will be a contraction of the extracellular volume. This, in turn, will promote a decreased rate of sodium excretion. To the extent that renal tubular reabsorption of sodium is increased (owing to the sodium depletion and the consequent hypovolemia) and the concentration of chloride in plasma is diminished, a set of circumstances is created that dictates an increase in acid secretion and excretion. As alluded to earlier, the reabsorption of sodium from the tubular urine will be associated with the reabsorption of the accompanying anion or the secretion of a positively charged ion such as potassium or hydrogen. One of the determinants of these options relates to the ease with which the anion can permeate the renal tubular cells. This varies, and chloride may be the most permeant, bicarbonate the least, with the others

in intermediate positions. Hence, if there is hypochloremia, virtually all the chloride may be reabsorbed along with sodium before the luminal fluid reaches more distal sites. Under these circumstances, the nonchloride salts of sodium predominate, and since their permeability is limited, the option for reabsorption of the anion may be likewise limited. The alternative of the secretion of a positively charged ion is then likely to play a more important role. If there is accompanying potassium depletion, hydrogen ion will be secreted in response to the reabsorption of sodium; and the reabsorbed sodium will then relate to bicarbonate in the cell and enter the interstitial fluid as sodium bicarbonate. These conditioning factors are, presumably, the genesis of the *paradoxic aciduria* that may be noted in clinical disorders associated with metabolic alkalosis. The paradoxic aciduria in the context of an alkalosis is presumptive evidence of sodium depletion and, probably, of potassium depletion as well. In most instances the urine will become alkaline if the sodium deficit is repaired with saline, since in the absence of volume depletion the demands for sodium reabsorption are diminished and sodium bicarbonate can then escape into the urine.

These considerations have very important therapeutic implications and serve to emphasize the need for an overall evaluation of the problem in management. For example, administration of ammonium chloride to such a patient could correct the state of alkalosis but add the complications of metabolic acidosis; it would probably enhance the loss of potassium and sodium and serve very poorly to improve the patient's status. In contrast, the clearly indicated therapeutic measures include the following:

1. Dehydration should be corrected by administration of salt and water. The proportion in which they should be administered depends on the net character of the deficits. If there is hypernatremia, the patient needs more water than salt; if he is hyponatremic, the need is for more salt than water. If one is in doubt, isotonic saline solution will usually be adequate. The amount to administer must be judged by an evaluation of the quantity of the deficit, made on the basis of history, physical examination, laboratory data, and the observed response to therapy (see Chap. 296).

2. The deficit of potassium must be corrected. The manner in which this may safely be accomplished will be discussed below under Deficit of Potassium.

3. Sufficient carbohydrate should be administered to minimize protein catabolism and ketonemia.

Once the antecedent deficits are restored, care must be taken to ensure appropriate replacement of current losses so that a new state of depletion will not obtain.

ALTERED URINARY COMPOSITION DUE TO DIURETIC AND STEROID THERAPY. The administration of many diuretic agents promotes potassium loss and alkalosis. The precise manner in which this occurs is not clear. However, it is most probably a consequence of the delivery of greater quantities of sodium to sites where its reabsorption articulates with secretion of hydrogen ions or potassium. In the first instance this would tend to induce alkalosis with its attendant consequences; and in the second instance it induces a loss of potassium, which, in turn, tends to provoke a state of alkalosis.

The naturally existing adrenal cortical hormones tend to enhance the excretion of potassium. This appears to be a secondary rather than a primary event, since it does not occur when the dietary regimen is free of sodium. The suggestion is that the steroids enhance reabsorption of sodium and to the extent that this promotes the secretion of potassium, more of this latter ion is excreted in the urine. The synthetic steroids, employed for reasons other than replacement therapy, have a considerably diminished activity in this regard.

DEFICIT OF POTASSIUM. (See also Chap. 85.) The manner in which a deficit of potassium interrelates with a state of metabolic alkalosis has already been described. There are many causes of a deficit of this ion, including prolonged periods of parenteral alimentation without addition of potassium, excessive losses in gastrointestinal fluid, diarrhea due to disease or induced with cathartics, excessive losses in the urine as with the use of organic mercurial diuretics, chlorothiazide, and steroid hormones, potassium-losing renal disease, Cushing's syndrome, and primary aldosteronism.

Potassium is the major intracellular cation, and depletion is accompanied by disorders of structure and function in various tissues. These tissues include skeletal muscle, smooth muscle of the gastrointestinal tract, myocardium, cartilage, kidneys, and gastric mucosa. Weakness of the muscles and hyporeflexia are common, alterations in the electrocardiogram are well established, and abnormalities in the motor and secretory activity of the gastrointestinal tract are well documented. Inability to concentrate the urine appropriately, decreased rate of filtration at the glomerulus, and defective transport of para-aminohippurate have all been reported.

Although a potassium deficit may have serious consequences, judgment must be exercised in the technique of repletion to avoid the complications of therapy. The most significant hazard is the possibility of administering a potassium salt in too great a quantity or too rapidly so that cardiotoxic levels are reached in the serum.

In the course of the development of a potassium deficit, the patient may become sufficiently dehydrated or acidotic that the depletion is not mirrored in hypokalemia. This is seen quite often, for example, in diabetic acidosis. It would appear to be safer under these circumstances to refrain from administering potassium until partial correction of the dehydration and utilization of the carbohydrate have induced a decrease in the concentration of potassium in the serum and there is clear evidence of satisfactory flows of urine. Potassium salts may be administered more safely by mouth than parenterally. There is sufficient delay in absorption from the gastrointestinal tract to provide some assurance that a sudden increase in the concentration of potassium in the serum will not obtain.

These precautionary comments should not be interpreted to mean that potassium salts cannot be safely administered intravenously. There are many circumstances where for obvious reasons the salt cannot be administered orally and potassium repletion is clearly indicated. However, some control should be exercised with respect to the rate of administration. It is reasonably safe to administer potassium at a rate of about 20 mEq per hr, but it would be desirable to limit the first replacement to 50 to 100 mEq. After this first phase of replacement has been completed, the level of potassium in the serum should be determined. A change in the pattern of the electrocardiogram may also be used as a guide. The change in concentration will provide some indication as to the safe dosage for the next phase of therapy. Unfortunately, there is no way to estimate the magnitude of the deficit with any precision from knowledge of the concentration of potassium in the serum. There is, of course, a gross correlation, but this is an inadequate premise on which to base a safe prediction.

Since the rate of infusion may vary with change of position of the needle, it is always possible that the plan of administration may fail. An additional safeguard is provided by limiting the concentration of potassium in the infusate to approximately 50 mEq per liter. Under this circumstance an accidental increase in the rate of administration of the infusion will have less effect on the rate of administration of potassium.

The particular salt of potassium that is used may be very important. If there is no source of chloride in the diet (as might well be the case with hypertensive or edematous patients who have become potassium-depleted), the potassium should be given as potassium chloride. Other salts of potassium such as acetate, bicarbonate, or citrate may make it difficult to retain potassium under these circumstances. The reasons for this relate to some of the earlier discussion of renal regulation of acid-base equilibrium. Chloride is quite able to permeate the renal tubular epithelium, so when sodium is reabsorbed and an electric gradient established, the reabsorption of sodium will usually be accompanied by chloride if it is present. However, when there is a deficit and no dietary source of chloride, more sodium may be reabsorbed at sites where chloride is no longer present. Since the other anions are less able to permeate, there will be a tendency for the reabsorption of sodium to articulate with the secretion of hydrogen ions or potassium. If it is the former, alkalosis will be established that promotes potassium excretion; if it is potassium, it is obvious that its excretion will be enhanced. In either event the retention of potassium is not as efficient. This has several important consequences. First, the ill effects of potassium depletion are not reversed appropriately. Secondly, if the patient has hypertension and is potassium-depleted and it appears difficult to effect repletion, the clinical state may be misinterpreted as primary aldosteronism.

Once again it must be emphasized that, although this discussion has presented the disturbances of acid-base equilibrium as four distinct and separate entities, mixed clinical pictures are common. However, these should not be too difficult to analyze if the principles described are recalled. In addition, it must be remembered that a disturbance in acid-base equilibrium may be only one aspect (and not necessarily the most important) of the patient's total disease picture. In fact, in some instances attention to the primary disorder may improve the disturbance in acid-base equilibrium so that no therapy for the disequilibrium per se is necessary. Moreover, there are circumstances in which a correction of abnormal chemical values may be undesirable in that it may destroy an adequate compensation.

REFERENCES

Davenport, H. W.: "The ABC of Acid-Base Chemistry," 4th ed., Chicago, The University of Chicago Press, 1958.

Pitts, R. F.: "Physiology of the Kidney and Body Fluids," Chicago, Year Book Medical Publishers, Inc., 1963.

Siggaard-Andersen, O.: "The Acid-Base Status of the Blood," 2d ed., Copenhagen, Munksgaard, 1964.

Singer, R. B., and A. B. Hastings: An Improved Clinical Method for the Estimation of Disturbances of the Acid-Base Balance of Human Blood, Medicine, 27:223, 1948.

298 APPROACH TO THE PATIENT WITH RENAL DISEASE

Franklin H. Epstein

The patient with renal disease may exhibit any one of a wide variety of problems. He may complain of symptoms easily recognized as originating in the urinary tract, such as dysuria, frequency, and polyuria (Chaps. 49 and 50), or of those generally (and sometimes wrongly) attributed to the kidneys, such as back pain. He or his doctor may have noticed blood in the urine. Proteinuria may have appeared on a routine examination. Often, however, the presenting complaints and signs are less overt and specific, more general, and hence more confusing. The kidneys must be suspected in cases of unexplained fever, lassitude, anorexia, nausea, weakness, and anemia. Hypertension, heart failure, or edema may dominate the clinical picture. Neurologic disturbances such as headache, tremor, coma, or convulsions often monopolize attention when the patient is first seen. Stunted growth may be the chief concern of the child or adolescent with chronic renal disease. Abnormalities in bone metabolism caused by renal insufficiency may masquerade as arthritis, gout, or rickets (see Chap. 83).

The physician should be continually alert to the possibility that certain curable but rare disorders may produce clinical pictures almost identical with those caused by more common but less treatable diseases. Thus he should consider the possibility that hypertension may be due to unilateral renal disease (Chap. 276) and the fact that drug sensitivity and syphilis are rare but curable causes of the nephotic syndrome. In a patient with renal insufficiency, the diagnosis of chronic uremia should not be adopted until all reversible disorders which depress renal function have been considered and excluded. The most

important of these are acute glomerulonephritis, acute tubular necrosis, obstructive nephropathy, circulatory insufficiency (including shock or congestive heart failure), and depletion of water and salt. Proper management of renal insufficiency requires above all an expert appreciation of the physiology of body fluids. Treatment should be individualized and animated by a concern with the specific problems of a particular patient rather than with general formulas which fit only an average.

APPROACH TO THE DIAGNOSIS OF ASYMPTOMATIC PROTEINURIA

A few points in the study of the patient with asymptomatic proteinuria deserve special emphasis. Postural proteinuria should be ruled out, as well as the proteinuria which is normally associated with exercise or which follows certain febrile diseases. A careful history should inquire into the possibility of recent respiratory or skin infections, recurrent pyelitis, edema or hypertension during pregnancy, arthritis, rash, and drug sensitivity. A history of enuresis past the age of six may suggest congenital structural or neurologic anomalies of the urinary tract or chronic childhood pyelitis. The results of prior examinations for employment, insurance, or military service should be ascertained. The family history may be positive for renal and vascular diseases; inquiry should also be made about gout and diabetes. Blood pressure should be checked in the erect as well as the supine position, and retinal as well as peripheral vessels should be examined. Amyloidosis may be suggested by an enlarged liver or spleen; palpable masses in both upper quadrants should also raise the question of polycystic kidneys. Physical examination should not overlook the possibility of a cystocele or enlarged prostate.

A fresh urine sample should be examined *by the physician* as outlined on p. 1385. Clinical tests of renal function should include a measure of blood urea or serum creatinine. Occasionally, a disproportionate elevation of blood uric acid level will suggest underlying gouty nephropathy. Examination of the blood for LE cells or of the serum for antinuclear antibodies may detect early lupus erythematosus. Electrophoresis of the serum may reveal globulins characteristic of multiple myeloma.

The size and shape of the kidneys as well as the structure of calyces and ureters may be ascertained from an intravenous pyelogram. At the conclusion of this examination, a postvoiding film of the bladder gives information about residual urine without the necessity for catheterization. The size of the kidneys can be estimated in relation to the vertebral shadows on the plain film of the abdomen; normal kidneys are approximately as long as three to three and one-half lumbar vertebral bodies. When one kidney is shrunken and the other has failed to hypertrophy, disease is usually bilateral.

Percutaneous needle biopsy of the kidney has provided much useful information for the student of renal disease, but even in the most skillful hands, it is not without hazard. It may contribute to the management of the individual patient (e.g., the unexpected finding of amyloidosis or periarteritis; the detection of advanced changes of pyelonephritis in an apparently uninvolved kidney), but its greatest value has been to illuminate the natural history of diffuse diseases of the kidney. The accuracy of needle biopsy as a diagnostic technique is limited in focal disorders of the kidneys by the smallness of the specimen and in diffuse glomerular disease by the fact that the sample obtained may contain no or few glomeruli. In most patients with proteinuria, proper use of the more conventional diagnostic methods will permit an accurate working diagnosis. Biopsy sections must be interpreted with proper regard to the rest of the clinical and laboratory findings.

Finally, the diagnostic maneuver of following the course of the patient's condition, in addition to being innocuous, has a great deal to recommend it. Acute or self-limited processes, even when the histologic picture is clear, can sometimes be diagnosed only in retrospect.

APPROACH TO THE TREATMENT OF RENAL INSUFFICIENCY

The physician's approach to the patient with chronic renal failure is shaped by the relationship between renal function and the signs and symptoms of renal insufficiency. Figure 298-1 illustrates the hyperbolic relation between the plasma level of urea or creatinine and the rate of glomerular filtration. When clearance is low, small fluctuations in glomerular filtration produce large changes in concentration of plasma urea or creatinine. The relationship between functioning renal tissue and the clinical signs of renal failure may be visualized in the same fashion, as in Fig. 298-2. This curve, illustrating the nature of the physiologic reserve of the kidneys, also clarifies certain aspects of the course of many chronic progressive renal diseases characterized by a long "latent" period and rapid terminal progression. One can visualize a slowly progressive process, relentlessly destroying renal substance, which is relatively asymptomatic for many years. When the limits of renal reserve are reached, symptoms appear in swift succession and the condition of the patient deteriorates rapidly, though there may be little

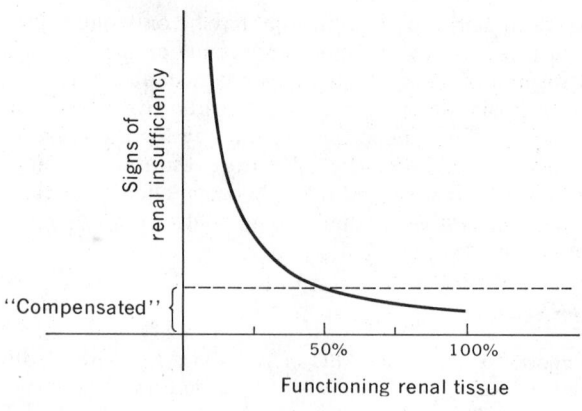

Fig. 298-2.

actual acceleration of the rate of parenchymal destruction of the kidneys.

The curve of Fig. 298-2 provides a rationale for the treatment of patients with renal disease. The less kidney tissue there is remaining, the more difference an increment in function makes to the patient. The fragility of patients with little remaining renal function is apparent. Prolonged dehydration, the depressant effects of anesthesia, or the circulatory shock of septicemia may be easily withstood by a person with normal or slightly impaired renal reserve but may be disastrous to a patient balanced on the knife-edge of renal decompensation. In treating a patient with advanced renal disease, the extent of damage *that is reversible* is obviously tremendously important. The goal of the physician is the discovery and treatment of reversible disorders, no matter how insignificant they may appear. For a patient on the steeply ascending portion of the curve, a small improvement in function may mean the difference between life and death. Treatable causes of renal failure include obstruction of the urethra or ureters, congestive heart failure, infection, dehydration, salt depletion, potassium deficiency (Chap. 296), and hypercalcemia. In addition, chronic renal disease is sometimes complicated by self-limited disorders of the kidney which will eventually resolve if the patient does not die in the meantime. These include acute glomerulonephritis, acute exacerbations of chronic glomerulonephritis, and acute tubular necrosis.

REFERENCES

Black, D. A. K.: "Renal Disease," 2d ed., Philadelphia, F. A. Davis Company, 1967.
Strauss, M. B., and L. G. Welt: "Diseases of the Kidney," 2d ed., Boston, Little, Brown and Company, 1969.

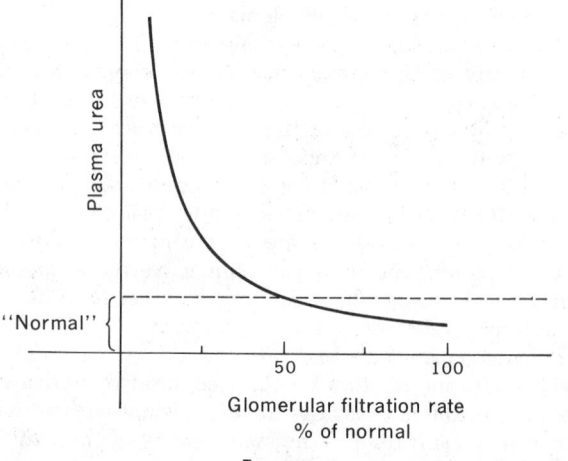

Fig. 298-1.

299 RENAL FUNCTION TESTS
Franklin H. Epstein

URINARY SEDIMENT

Perhaps the most important diagnostic maneuver in patients with renal disease is the *examination of a fresh urine sample by the physician.* Specimens suitable for quantitative culture as well as microscopic examination of the sediment can be obtained by cleansing the external genitalia, blocking vaginal contamination with a gauze tampon, and collecting the second half of the voiding in a sterile container. One then centrifuges 15 ml urine for 5 min at 3,000 rpm, discards the supernatant, and resuspends the sediment in the few remaining drops of urine. For most clinical purposes, qualitative or semiquantitative enumeration of the type and number of formed elements seen in the unstained sediment is sufficient. If possible, a concentrated urine specimen should be examined, since formed elements may be difficult to find if the urine is dilute.

Normal urine collected carefully in this way contains no more than one or two red blood cells and one or two white blood cells and epithelial cells per high-power field. An occasional hyaline cast per low-power field may be seen. The desquamation of renal tubular epithelial cells and their excretion into the urine is increased in renal disease of many types, particularly in glomerulanephritis. These cells should be distinguished from the squamous epithelium lining the bladder which may fill the urinary sediment in cystitis. Tubular cells choked with fat, called "oval fat bodies," as well as fatty casts, are characteristically found in the urine of patients with heavy proteinuria.

The composition of casts is particularly significant, since the entrapment of red blood cells or leukocytes in casts establishes their origin in the renal parenchyma. Casts are formed by the agglutination of protein, cells, or cellular debris in the lumen of renal tubules.

Hyaline casts result from the precipitation of pure protein in the renal tubules. They are clear, colorless cylinders barely seen against the usual background. When the urine contains a pigment such as bile pigment or hemoglobin, the protein making up hyaline casts will be stained this color. They are seen in concentrated acid urines in which much protein is excreted. *Broad casts,* sometimes referred to as *renal failure casts,* are characteristically found in advanced renal disease where there is hypertrophy of some remaining renal tubules and stasis of urine in lower reaches of the collecting duct system. *Leukocyte casts* and clumps of leukocytes suggest pyelonephritis or sterile interstitial inflammation of the kidneys. White blood cell casts are also found in the exudative stage of acute glomerulonephritis. *Epithelial cells entrapped in casts,* together with red blood cells, and casts containing lipid droplets, should suggest glomerulonephritis without distinguishing among its various causes. *Granular casts* are said to represent a further stage in the degeneration of cellular casts. *Red blood cell casts* often are orange or rusty brown in color, even when the cell outlines have deteriorated, but when only a few erythrocytes are present they may appear colorless. Their presence in association with hematuria almost invariably signifies a destructive lesion of the glomerulus, as an active glomerulonephritis, lupus, arteritis, or malignant hypertension. It should be emphasized that the absence of formed elements does not rule out either chronic glomerulonephritis or pyelonephritis.

When urinary infection is suspected, a Gram stain of the urinary sediment may permit prompt diagnosis and early initiation of therapy.

PROTEINURIA

Although some protein is probably filtered by normal glomeruli, and there is a small amount of protein in normal urine, protein excretion in excess of 150 mg per day or 20 mg per 100 ml urine is abnormal. Proteinuria may be induced in normal subjects by injections of epinephrine, by exercise, or by renal ischemia resulting from dehydration, hemorrhage, or salt depletion. Continuous proteinuria almost always implies disease of the kidneys.

The bulk of urinary protein in most renal diseases is albumin, which passes into the urine through damaged glomeruli. In myeloma, macroglobulinemia, and primary amyloidosis, the excretion of globulin may exceed that of albumin. This is also the case in some patients with the adult Fanconi's syndrome.

Heavy proteinuria, in excess of 4 Gm daily, signifies a gross increase in glomerular permeability, usually the result of a generalized glomerular disease. Venous congestion of the kidneys and malignant hypertension may also cause proteinuria of this degree. When such large amounts of protein are excreted into the urine, the degree of proteinuria is influenced by both the glomerular filtration rate and the level of serum albumin, so that, for example, when a dose of prednisone is given which increases filtration rate, protein excretion rises. Renal diseases that may be present without proteinuria include polycystic disease, pyelonephritis, disease of the large or small blood vessels, hypercalcemic or hypokalemic nephropathy, obstruction, stone, congenital malformations, and tumor. Proteinuria is usually absent or scant in renal insufficiency due to dehydration or "prerenal azotemia."

Orthostatic and Functional Proteinuria

In perhaps three-quarters of adolescents and young adults, proteinuria may be induced by prolonged standing in the erect position. This effect is more pronounced when a lordotic posture is assumed. In some patients lordosis has been demonstrated to result in compression of the inferior vena cava by the liver, and it has been postulated that the resulting increase in pressure in the renal veins is responsible for proteinuria. It appears more likely that changes in the renal circulation secondary to peripheral sequestration of blood are involved, since proteinuria can be produced in susceptible individuals by applying tourniquets in the supine position, prevented by having the subject stand upright in water, and aggravated by the peripheral vasodilatation induced by heat. In patients with orthostatic proteinuria, urine passed early in the morning, before arising, is free of protein, although of high specific gravity. Care must be taken to have the patient empty his bladder at midnight, without getting up, so that urine formed in the erect position during the previous evening is discarded. Urine produced after the patient has been up may contain as much as 1 to 3 Gm protein per liter, although usually less than 1 Gm protein is excreted per day. The excretion of casts and other formed elements may also increase with the appearance of protein. Often a history of easy flushing, fainting, or other evidence of autonomic instability is obtained.

In most young individuals with intermittent orthostatic proteinuria, the condition is entirely benign and unassociated with other evidence of renal disease. The fact that proteinuria is intermittent does not, however, rule out organic disease. A certain percentage of apparently healthy patients with intermittent orthostatic proteinuria are found on renal biopsy to have some form of nephritis, and they eventually develop signs of chronic renal disease.

CLINICAL MEASUREMENTS OF GLOMERULAR FILTRATION RATE

In a healthy adult, blood flow to both kidneys accounts for approximately one-quarter of the cardiac output, or about 1,250 ml per min. Renal plasma flow is about 600 ml per min, and glomerular filtration rate is 100 to 150 ml per min. The rate of glomerular filtration can be estimated by measuring the plasma clearance of a substance such as inulin or mannitol, which appears in the glomerular filtrate in the same concentration as in plasma but which is neither reabsorbed nor secreted by renal tubules.

The clearance of a substance is given by the equation,

$$\text{Clearance} = \frac{\text{excretion rate}}{\text{plasma concentration}}$$

$$= \frac{\text{mg/ml urine} \times \text{ml urine/min}}{\text{mg/ml plasma}}$$

The relationship of the plasma level of urea or creatinine to its clearance is expressed in Fig. 298-1. The clearances of urea and creatinine or their plasma levels, although determined in part by tubular processes, are related closely enough to glomerular filtration rate to make them convenient clinical indices of glomerular function. Urea is filtered at the glomerulus and variably reabsorbed, presumably as a passive consequence of the concentration gradient established by water reabsorption, so that its clearance is 40 to 70 percent of the true glomerular filtration rate. The back diffusion of urea is diminished when urine flow is increased; hence urea clearance approaches a maximum when daily urine volume exceeds 3 liters, but it decreases out of proportion to glomerular filtration when urinary output is low. Furthermore, for the same rate of urine flow and of inulin clearance, urea clearance is higher during solute diuresis than during water diuresis.

Since the blood urea varies during the course of a day and urea excretion is dependent on the rate of urine flow, tests of *urea clearance* are usually carried out over relatively short time periods. It is apparent from Fig. 298-1 that blood urea nitrogen (BUN) rises only slowly when urea clearance is first compromised but more rapidly later when renal insufficiency is advanced. In addition to changes in renal function, blood urea nitrogen is also influenced by the quantity of urea available for excretion. The BUN will tend to rise, therefore, when a diet high in protein is fed, when additional protein is digested and absorbed because of gastrointestinal bleeding, or when protein breakdown is accelerated in injuries or infections or because adrenal steroids have been administered. Contrariwise, the fall in BUN concentration which occurs when patients with renal disease are placed on a low-protein diet is usually not associated with improvement in glomerular filtration rate or urea clearance.

Because of the hyperbolic nature of the curve in Fig. 298-1, the wide range of "normal," and the influence of diet, BUN may remain below 20 mg per 100 ml even in patients whose urea clearance and glomerular filtration rate have been reduced to only 50 percent of their normal value. Conversely, if the blood urea nitrogen level is persistently elevated in what seems at first glance to be only unilateral renal disease, impaired function of the opposite kidney must be suspected.

Although when creatinine is infused in man, some tubular secretion takes place so that its clearance exceeds that of inulin, the clearance of endogenous creatinine in general approximates inulin clearance. Creatinine excretion is independent of urine flow, and its level in plasma is relatively stable. Creatinine clearance may therefore be determined over 24 hr by collecting all the urine formed during this time and drawing one sample of blood within this period. Normal values for men are 140 to 200 liters per day (97 to 140 ml per min); for women, 120 to 180 liters per day (85 to 125 ml per min). The quantity of creatinine formed and excreted per day is related to muscle mass and does not change appreciably with changes in diet or protein breakdown. Serum creatinine is therefore more reliable than blood urea as an index to serial changes in glomerular filtration when renal function is comprised. At low serum levels the usual analytic methods for creatinine in serum are less accurate, and a variable portion of the result can be ascribed to noncreatinine chromogens of plasma, unless special precautions are taken by the laboratory.

The creatinine clearance provides a convenient index against which to evaluate the excretion of other substances (e.g., phosphorus) whose excretion is influenced by changes in glomerular filtration. For any substance, that fraction of the amount filtered at the glomerulus which is excreted in the urine (E/F) is given by dividing its urine/plasma concentration ratio by that of creatinine.

$$\frac{\text{Clearance substance}}{\text{Clearance creatinine}} = \frac{U \text{ substance } V}{P \text{ substance}}$$

$$\div \frac{U \text{ creatinine } V}{P \text{ creatinine}} = \frac{(U/P) \text{ substance}}{(U/P) \text{ creatinine}}$$

where U = urine concentration
P = plasma concentration
V = urinary volume (ml/min)

MEASUREMENT OF TUBULAR FUNCTION

Phenolsulfonphthalein Excretion

Phenolsulfonphthalein (PSP), like Diodrast, para-aminohippurate, and penicillin, is secreted into the urine by the proximal tubules. Only 4 percent of the PSP reaching the bladder is filtered through the glomeruli. With the usual 6-mg intravenous dose, the plasma level of PSP is no more than one-fifth of that normally needed to saturate tubular capacity to secrete the dye. Its excretory rate is therefore usually limited by renal plasma flow, and with severely impaired kidneys by proximal tubular function. Errors in interpretation of the test may arise from incomplete emptying of the bladder; hence the patient should be loaded with water before the test is begun. Inadequate urine volumes (< 150 ml) in the 15-min sample may be avoided by injecting the dye only after the patient feels the urge to void. Normal values are given in Table 299-1. The 15-min period is the most sig-

Table 299-1. EXCRETION OF PSP BY NORMAL SUBJECTS

Time, min	Excretion of PSP, percentage	
	Minimum	Average
15	28	35
30	13	17
60	9	12
120	3	6
Total for 2 hr	53	70

nificant, since even a damaged kidney may be able to remove normal amounts of PSP from the blood in the number of circulations through the kidney afforded by the 2-hr interval. Excretion which is greater during any subsequent period than during the first 15 min should suggest hydronephrosis or incomplete bladder emptying. Urinary retention may also be suspected when substantial amounts of dye are excreted after 2 hr. In the presence of liver disease, the total excretion of PSP may be increased.

In most chronic diseases of the kidney, the excretion of PSP and the urea or creatinine clearance are reduced together as the disease progresses. In acute glomerulonephritis, however, PSP is often normal or near normal when glomerular filtration is greatly reduced and the BUN and serum creatinine levels are elevated.

Urinary Concentration

When dehydrated, normal adults can concentrate the urine to 750 to 1,400 mOsm per liter (specific gravity 1.020 to 1.032). Withdrawal of fluids for 12 to 18 hr overnight is often not a satisfactory stimulus to the kidneys to reabsorb water maximally in patients with edema who are diuresing, or in those whose diurnal pattern of

urine flow is reversed. In such cases and in other states (e.g., renal insufficiency) where dehydration may be dangerous, concentrating ability may be tested by measuring urinary specific gravity or osmolarity after an injection of 5 units of vasopressin in oil. Slightly lower values are achieved when the kidneys are induced to concentrate by an injection of vasopressin rather than by prolonged dehydration. For practical purposes, if the specific gravity of a casual urine sample or one obtained after a short period of dehydration or an injection of vasopressin reaches 1.022 or more, concentrating ability may be considered intact. The measure of specific gravity may be misleading when heavy solutes, such as glucose, protein, or contrast dyes, are excreted abundantly in the urine. Freezing-point measurements of urinary osmolarity avoid this difficulty.

The production of a concentrated urine depends on the development of a high concentration of sodium in the interstitial fluids of the renal medulla as a consequence of the active transport of sodium out of the thin medullary loops and of the countercurrent pattern of flow through loops of Henle and medullary capillaries. Disease processes which disturb the function or structure of the medulla should therefore be expected to produce early, marked, and disproportionate impairment of concentrating ability. This impairment has been noted in patients with acute tubular necrosis, pyelonephritis, papillary necrosis, obstructive uropathy, potassium depletion, hypercalcemic nephropathy, medullary cysts, and sickle-cell disease. Maximum urinary concentration is reduced by starvation and by a low protein diet, as well as by excessive water drinking and overhydration. Urinary concentration is also lowered when urinary solute is increased, e.g., by infusions of mannitol or saline solution. Because of this, the decrease in maximum urinary specific gravity which characterizes most patients with renal insufficiency has been ascribed to a solute diuresis provoked by the concentration of urea in the glomerular filtrate and the resulting increase in solute load per individual intact nephron. This is probably not a sufficient explanation for impaired concentrating ability in most cases of chronic renal disease, in which medullary tubules are damaged or destroyed.

Urinary Dilution

Normal persons can excrete 70 percent of a load of water equal to 2 percent of the body weight within 5 hr of drinking it, and can reduce urinary solute concentration to 50 mOsm per liter. Water diuresis and urinary dilution are impaired in states characterized by inappropriate liberation of antidiuretic hormone (such as severe infections, cerebral injuries, and lung carcinoma), circulatory disturbances (heart failure, hepatic cirrhosis), and adrenal insufficiency, as well as in renal insufficiency of whatever cause. Tests of urinary dilution are therefore not specific nor especially sensitive in the detection and the follow-up of patients with renal disease.

Urinary Acidification

A normal man who eats 70 Gm protein daily produces 40 to 60 mEq of H^+ each day, chiefly as sulfuric and phosphoric acids. About half this is excreted in the urine as NH_4^+ and half as titratable acid. Normal kidneys readily increase NH_4^+ excretion by five or ten times and reduce urinary pH to a minimum of 4.5 units in response to greater loads of acid. This ability is impaired in most patients with chronic renal disease and azotemia, and is specifically diminished without proportionate impairment of glomerular filtration rate in renal tubular acidosis, certain cases of acquired nephrocalcinosis, and some cases of Fanconi's syndrome.

Other Tests of Tubular Function

All the *glucose* normally present in glomerular filtrate is completely reabsorbed by the proximal tubules. *Renal glycosuria* (the appearance of glucose in the urine when the blood glucose level is below 180 mg per 100 ml) frequently signifies proximal tubular damage, as in Fanconi's syndrome, heavy metal poisoning, or certain cases of the nephrotic syndrome with glomerulonephritis. Renal glycosuria may also result, without tubular dysfunction, when the load of glucose presented to the tubules is greatly increased because of an increase in the glomerular filtration rate (GFR), as in pregnancy.

Since phosphates and amino acids are also actively reabsorbed in the proximal tubules, *phosphaturia* and *aminoaciduria* may also accompany injury to proximal tubules if filtration does not cease in the involved nephrons.

Early in chronic disease of the kidneys, each of the clinical tests of function may be impaired while the others are normal. Serial measurements of any or all functions may therefore be helpful in evaluating progress. When azotemia supervenes, PSP and concentration tests usually change in rough proportion to filtration rate. In severe renal insufficiency, urinary specific gravity becomes fixed near 1.010 and no longer reflects changes in GFR, and PSP excretion is too low to be accurately measured. Serial measurements of filtration rate, by creatinine clearance or serum creatinine level, therefore remain the most suitable way of following the course of chronic azotemic renal disease.

REFERENCES

Lippman, R. W.: "Urine and the Urinary Sediment: A Practical Manual and Atlas," Springfield, Ill., Charles C Thomas, Publisher, 1957.

Pitts, R. F.: "Physiology of the Kidney and Body Fluids," 2d ed., Chicago, Year Book Medical Publishers, Inc., 1968.

300 ACUTE RENAL FAILURE
Franklin H. Epstein

The term *acute renal failure* has been used loosely to include all forms of acute urinary suppression, generally secondary to acute parenchymal damage. *Acute tubular necrosis* (or lower nephron nephrosis) indicates the clinical and pathologic syndrome which results when renal excretory function is temporarily lost because of renal tubular degeneration caused by renal ischemia or toxic agents.

PATHOLOGY

Microdissection studies of kidneys with acute tubular necrosis reveal two types of lesions. When renal toxins (bichloride of mercury, carbon tetrachloride, diethylene glycol) have been administered, there is diffuse necrosis of the proximal tubular cells, while the basement membrane of the proximal tubules, from which a new lining may regenerate, is spared. The lesion caused by ischemia, on the other hand, occurs at random among nephrons and in any part of a nephron. It consists of complete destruction of limited stretches of tubular lining scattered along the course of an otherwise well-preserved nephron. The basement membrane is frequently disrupted. During recovery from both types of lesions mitotic cells may be seen. Except when extremely severe and prolonged ischemia has produced renal cortical necrosis, the glomeruli are intact. Casts packed with degenerating epithelial cells and hemoglobin are seen in the straight tubules of the medulla. The most important inference to be drawn from the nature of the pathologic process is that should the patient survive his other injuries, the renal lesions will be repaired.

ETIOLOGY AND PATHOGENESIS

Acute tubular necrosis typically occurs in a setting of sudden injury or illness usually associated with shock or with intense renal vasoconstriction. Even those cases which follow the administration of known tubular poisons are generally aggravated by vascular collapse and renal ischemia. Nevertheless, perhaps because of difficulty in recognizing and quantifying the ischemic state, the cause may go undiagnosed in as many as 25 percent of patients. Common causes include hemolysis and hypotension following extensive burns, rapid hemorrhage or hypotension on the operating table, bacteremic shock, crushing injuries in which the toxic effects on the kidney of myoglobin are added to those of vasoconstriction and shock, and intravascular hemolysis from transfusion of mismatched blood or rapid infusions of distilled water (e.g., during transurethral prostatectomy). Following operations on the heart, aorta, or great vessels, during which renal circulation is interrupted, some degree of acute tubular necrosis is almost invariable. Pregnancy appears in some way to predispose to ischemic renal insults; in a large proportion of most published series, acute renal failure followed placenta previa, septic abortion, post-partum hemorrhage, or eclampsia. Other conditions which have triggered tubular necrosis include sudden defervescence following salicylate administration and status epilepticus. Acute renal failure is the most important cause of death in epidemic hemorrhagic fever.

Tubular necrosis resulting from many poisons is enhanced by prior dehydration and tends to be prevented by infusions of saline solution or mannitol if these are given before the noxious agent is presented to the kidneys. Paradoxically, healthy renal tubules are more susceptible to certain types of injury than are poorly functioning ones. A dose of uranium nitrate that induces acute tubular necrosis in a healthy dog may not interrupt the urine flow when given again to the same animal during the diuretic phase of early recovery from renal insufficiency. The role of free pigments derived from blood and muscle in the pathogenesis of tubular necrosis is not clear. Infusions of purified hemoglobin decrease renal blood flow and may be toxic to tubular cells. In addition, intravascular hemolysis may liberate other vasoconstrictor substances which promote renal ischemia.

PATHOPHYSIOLOGY OF ANURIA

The formation of casts which occlude the renal tubular lumens may play some part in the pathogenesis of oliguria. In most patients, however, casts appear to be a result of diminished urinary flow, rather than its cause. An exception is the renal failure which follows dehydration in *multiple myeloma* and which is characterized by extensive gel formation by abnormal proteins in renal tubules.

Following the acute renal ischemia which usually initiates tubular necrosis, renal blood flow is decreased to approximately one-third to one-half normal during the first days of oliguria. There is some evidence that the reduction in glomerular filtration is a vasoconstrictive response mediated through the macula densa and the juxtaglomerular apparatus. Increased interstitial pressure secondary to edema probably reduces renal blood flow and filtration rate and collapses tubules. The presence of interstitial edema may be inferred from the increase in the weight of the kidneys during acute tubular necrosis. Experimental measurements of wedged renal vein pressure and of pressures at the end of a fine needle inserted directly into the kidneys have not shown elevation. The pressures may nevertheless be sufficient to collapse renal tubules which are distended with less than normal pressure derived from glomerular filtration and urine flow. In any case, much of the fluid which is filtered at the glomerulus must leak back into the substance of the kidney through the widely scattered disruptions in the denuded tubular basement membranes. As tubular repair proceeds and these leaks are mended, urinary flow improves.

CLINICAL FEATURES

In the majority of cases, acute tubular necrosis is characterized by a period of oliguria and increasing clinical and chemical evidence of renal failure, lasting from a few days to as long as 3 weeks, and averaging about 10 to 14 days. This is succeeded by a period of relatively rapid return of urine flow and improvement in renal function, while water and metabolites accumulated during the oliguric phase are excreted.

During the first few days of *oliguria,* the clinical picture is dominated by the underlying illness. The urine is scanty and usually bloody. Although the specific gravity may be high owing to the presence of red blood cells and protein, its freezing point is close to that of plasma, and the sodium concentration is usually over 50 mEq per liter. Traces of glucose may appear in the urine. Complete anuria for more than 24 hr is infrequently encountered, though it is common to see less than 30 to 40 ml urine for several days. If the condition is not recognized early, edema and/or hyponatremia may develop as a result of the unrestricted intake of fluids. If this pitfall is avoided and shock is successfully treated, the only symptoms during the first week may be lethargy and nausea. The latter is related partially to the development of metabolic acidosis. Fever is uncommon after the first day or two. Leukocytosis, on the other hand, is the rule with or without infection. It should be emphasized that severe systemic symptoms during the first several days are usually a result *not* of renal failure but of associated conditions.

Serum amylase and lipase concentrations may be elevated as a result of renal failure per se, without implying active pancreatitis. The blood urea nitrogen level rises at a rate influenced by the degree of tissue necrosis and endogenous protein catabolism. In a chronically ill patient who has had a mismatched transfusion, a daily rise of 20 mg per 100 ml might be expected; increments of 50 mg per 100 ml per day in blood urea nitrogen are not uncommon in previously healthy persons who have undergone severe crushing injuries or overwhelming infections. Disproportionate elevations in serum phosphate or serum creatine levels have been proposed as diagnostic aids in the detection of devitalized tissue.

During the second week of oliguria, nausea, weakness, and somnolence become more prominent as azotemia mounts, acidosis increases, and the serum potassium level becomes elevated. Thirst is commonly present and may be severe, although the serum sodium level is frequently depressed, extracellular fluid volume is expanded, and there are no clear signs of shock or heart failure.

Cardiovascular complications arise in most patients during the oliguric phase of acute renal failure. Although overhydration is the most important cause of pulmonary edema, signs of pulmonary congestion and cardiac failure may appear even in patients who have not gained weight, probably because water has been added to the extracellular fluid from the dissolution of tissue. Pulmonary edema may develop in the absence of hypertension and without peripheral edema. Diastolic hypertension becomes evident in about 25 percent of patients during the second week of oliguria. The fundi, however, remain normal. In exceptional instances in which the tension is very high, arteriolar necrosis develops. Arrhythmias are frequent and are not necessarily associated with potassium intoxication or removal. Pericarditis may develop but does not have the grave prognosis attached to its appearance in chronic renal disease. It may be extremely painful and simulate intraabdominal disease. Occasional patients die of acute cardiorespiratory failure characterized by apprehension, tachypnea, inconstant respiratory wheezing, progressive cyanosis, and hypotension. At postmortem examination no evidence is found of pulmonary emboli, and the lungs show mild to moderate terminal congestion.

Potassium intoxication may arise because of the liberation of large amounts of potassium from injured or infected muscle, intravascular hemolysis, or hematomas. It rarely occurs in the course of renal failure following a postoperative hemorrhage or transfusion reaction in which the rate of tissue catabolism is not increased and in which proper attention has been paid to hydration and caloric needs from the inception of the disease. The rate of rise of the serum potassium level reflects the catabolic response of the patient to injury. In addition, anoxia, acidosis, and dehydration are important determinants of the rate of loss of potassium from cells. The dangers are cardiac arrhythmias and standstill. Serious electrocardiographic abnormalities rarely occur when the serum potassium level is below 7 mEq per liter but are almost always present above 9 mEq per liter. As serum potassium concentration rises, the T waves become high and peaked. The P wave disappears, the QRS complex becomes broad and slurred, bradycardia and arrhythmias ensue, and the ventricular complexes finally resemble those of ventricular tachycardia. These changes may be modified by digitalis and by correction of acidosis and hyponatremia. Susceptibility of the heart to vagal standstill is enhanced, and sudden death may occur, even in the absence of characteristic electrocardiographic changes of potassium intoxication. The electrocardiogram, though a necessary adjunct, is not a satisfactory replacement for the flame photometer in evaluating such situations.

Infection is the most frequent complication of acute tubular necrosis and the most common cause of death. Sepsis may often be overlooked because of confusion with uremic symptoms. Pulmonary and bloodstream infections with "hospital" organisms, particularly the staphylococcus, are frequent in exhausted, semicomatose patients. Common predisposing factors are loss of ability to cough or change position, drying of the pharyngeal mucosa from constant mouth breathing, and the aspiration of inspissated mucous plugs or vomitus. Healing of surgical wounds seems to be impaired, and infection or dehiscence of incisions is common. Infection of the urinary tract, sometimes silent but often with fever, flank pain, and gram-negative septicemia, frequently results from the use of inlying catheters or repeated instrumentation of the bladder.

Neurologic manifestations are common, the two most important being coma and convulsions. Hyponatremia may be responsible for somnolence or seizures early in the course of acute renal failure and may be corrected by hypertonic saline solution, with proper regard for the complications of overhydration and heart failure. Hypo-
...a may also predispose to convulsions, as may too-...s administration of alkali without accompanying ...i in the treatment of acidosis. Seizures may be ...n nature or generalized; some presumably have a

vascular basis. They sometimes appear to be triggered by vomiting, heart failure, or the rapid changes in body volume and composition which may accompany the onset of profuse diuresis.

Anemia usually appears in the second week, even without bleeding, presumably as a result of a mild increase in erythrocyte destruction and a deficiency in erythroid hyperplasia. Defects in hemostasis are commonly encountered and include thrombocytopenia, abnormal prothrombin consumption time, and other less well-defined coagulation deficiencies.

In some patients tubular necrosis is not associated with oliguria, or the period of diminished urine flow is so short as to pass unrecognized. The urine volume in such cases is, however, not flexible or responsive to body needs and may be fixed at perhaps 800 to 1,200 ml per day. The diagnosis is appreciated only when the blood urea nitrogen level is seen to rise at the rate of 15 to 20 mg per 100 ml per day and when the patient becomes edematous owing to retention of fluids in excess of the excretory capacity of the kidneys. The urine unlike that in most other edema-forming states, contains sodium in a concentration higher than 20 to 30 mEq per liter, and the concentration of total solutes does not differ significantly from that of plasma.

After the first few days of oliguria the urine loses its grossly bloody character and becomes clear, increasing slightly in amount every day. The onset of tubular recovery is usually heralded by an increase in daily urinary output to 400 ml. At this point the urine usually contains very little protein, although the sediment may still contain red blood cells and many large dark hematin casts. Further increases in flow are sometimes dramatic, the urine volume increasing by 50 to 100 percent each day until polyuria exceeds 3,000 ml daily. In other patients daily urine volume only gradually approaches a liter over the course of a week or two. If brisk diuresis is never achieved, the blood urea concentration falls only slowly or not at all, and the urine contains more than 3 to 4 Gm protein per liter, cortical necrosis must be suspected. The blood urea *usually continues to rise* for several days after urinary output exceeds 1 liter per day, until the excretion of urea exceeds its production. In addition, during the early diuretic phase of recovery, hyperkalemia, congestive heart failure, and convulsions may complicate the clinical picture. Pyelonephritis frequently makes its appearance at this time, and death from infection, when it occurs, is commonly during diuresis. The onset of the diuretic phase, therefore, should not cause the physician to relax his vigilance.

Diuresis is usually associated with a striking weight loss, representing loss of fluid accumulated during the period of oliguria. The urinary concentration of sodium usually varies from 50 to 75 mEq per liter. Some of the excreted sodium is derived from edema fluid, but if the remainder is not replaced hyponatremia and dehydration may ensue. Elevated levels of serum sodium and chloride are observed during the diuretic phase when water replacement is inadequate and the patient is allowed to dehydrate himself through the obligatory excretion of a large volume of urine containing sodium at a lower concentration than plasma. Occasionally, urinary losses of potassium so greatly exceed intake that the serum potassium level falls below normal. Once established, diuresis proceeds smoothly unless interrupted by urinary obstruction or shock, and azotemia regresses over the course of 1 to 3 weeks. *If diuresis is interrupted by a second period of oliguria and rising blood urea concentration, obstruction to bladder or ureters must be seriously considered.*

After the patient has been discharged from the hospital, anemia sometimes persists for weeks or months, gradually disappearing without benefit of hematinics. Muscle weakness and joint stiffness slowly improve. Chronic pyelonephritis may be a major problem. Although azotemia generally disappears and renal function may be restored, renal blood flow and glomerular filtration rate usually do not return completely to normal. Hypertension is not a sequel in those who recover from acute tubular necrosis, though it may complicate the unusual case of cortical necrosis in a patient who survives anuria.

DIFFERENTIAL DIAGNOSIS

The physician is frequently faced with an oliguric patient who has just passed through an episode which might have produced tubular necrosis, but in whom this diagnosis is not yet established. Vigorous treatment of shock, congestive heart failure, dehydration, or hyponatremia frequently resolves the question by promoting diuresis. Urinary osmolarity is not appreciably higher than that of plasma after the first few hours of acute tubular necrosis, whereas it may be elevated in simple dehydration and other prerenal causes of oliguria. The sodium concentration of the urine in acute tubular necrosis is usually over 30 mEq per liter; in oliguria secondary to acute glomerulonephritis or renal arterial occlusion it is usually much less than this. Low urinary sodium concentrations may, however, be observed in tubular necrosis associated with terminal hepatic and cardiac failure. Failure of the blood urea level to rise in a stepwise fashion makes the diagnosis of tubular necrosis unlikely, even though oliguria is present. If doubt persists, a liter of glucose in water or 10 percent mannitol may be infused rapidly to determine the effect on urine flow.

Lower urinary tract *obstruction* must always be kept in mind. A plain roentgenogram of the abdomen should be obtained in all patients with acute renal failure to delineate the size of the kidneys and detect radiopaque stones. If the possibility of ureteral obstruction exists, gentle investigation of the patency of one ureter is indicated.

Complete anuria for more than 48 hr should suggest obstruction, bilateral renal arterial emboli or thrombosis, cortical necrosis, or acute glomerulonephritis. Atheromatous emboli to the small renal arteries sometimes produce irreversible anuria following attempts at aortic resection. Carcinomatous obstruction to the ureters and idiopathic retroperitoneal periureteral fibrosis are frequently associated with intermittent oliguria, alternating with periods of polyuria and diuresis. Occasionally, acute papillary necrosis is attended by oliguria. Uric acid crystals may obstruct both ureters temporarily in patients with leukemia or lymphoma who have received nitrogen mustards or x-ray irradiation. Similar obstruction may be caused by certain sulfonamides given to dehydrated individuals. The prolonged anuria which occasionally follows bilateral retrograde pyelography is probably a result of obstruction to the lower ureteral orifices by inflammatory edema.

Oliguria attending the terminal stage of chronic kidney disease can usually be distinguished by the history, presence of hypertension, abnormal fundi, and smallness of the kidneys. During the terminal stages of hepatic failure, especially in cases complicated by dehydration, hemorrhage, or low blood pressure, a syndrome of oliguria and progressive azotemia appears which is associated with the lesions of tubular necrosis at postmortem examination but differs in some respects from the course of acute tubular necrosis outlined above. The oliguria is not severe, urine flow usually exceeding 150 ml per day. Urinary osmolarity may in some instances be distinctly elevated above that of plasma, and urinary sodium concentration is low. Vigorous transfusion and the use of vasopressor agents improve urinary flow only inconstantly and transiently. Although progression of the syndrome may in rare instances be halted, a typical diuretic phase does not ensue.

TREATMENT

Perhaps more than in any other renal disease, the course of acute renal failure is determined by the therapy the patient receives. Treatment during the initial stages of the disease must be directed toward reversing circulatory failure, which may have initiated the ischemic episode. Although overhydration predisposes to later pulmonary edema if renal failure is established, too timid replacement of blood or saline solution in shocked or dehydrated patients may perpetuate oliguria and permit tubular necrosis to develop. If vasoconstrictor agents are substituted for blood in hypovolemic shock, further renal damage with ischemic coagulative necrosis of cortical tubules may result.

Once circulatory efficiency has been restored, only current losses should be replaced. The patient should receive enough water and salt to provide for obvious extrarenal (e.g., gastrointestinal) and urinary losses and, in addition, enough water to compensate for insensible perspiration and water in expired air. Under average conditions of environmental and body temperatures, normal hydration in an adult patient can be maintained by the daily administration of about 600 ml water in addition to other measured losses (since some water is provided from oxidized foodstuffs and tissue breakdown). Accurate daily weights provide a reliable index of fluid balance; ideally the patient should lose ¼ to ½ lb daily as a result of consuming his own fat calories.

At least 100 to 150 Gm carbohydrate should be given

daily, to minimize protein breakdown and prevent keto-sis. Its effect in this direction is enhanced if it is adminis-tered throughout the day rather than over a short period of time. There is no evidence that high-calorie mixtures containing more carbohydrate and much fat are appre-ciably more efficacious in reducing protein catabolism *when the intake of protein is interdicted,* as it must be in acute renal failure. When nausea is not present, 50 Gm lactose, 25 Gm sucrose, and 25 Gm glucose may be dissolved in the daily water requirement, flavored with a little lemon and served cold, to be sipped throughout the day. Ordinary food, especially juices, should not be given, since potassium intake is undesirable. *Oral feedings should not be attempted in the presence of nausea or vomiting.* Sodium lactate, accompanied by calcium, may be given in amounts of 40 to 80 mEq per day to avoid further acidosis, when the plasma CO_2 has fallen to 16 mEq per liter. Larger amounts may be indicated, espe-cially when overhydration is not apparent and congestive heart failure is not present.

Potassium intoxication is prevented in many cases by proper attention to requirements for water and glucose, as well as by the prophylactic oral administration of a teaspoon of potassium-exchange sulfonic resin, sodium polystyrene sulfonate (Kayexalate, Winthrop), three times daily. Larger amounts of the latter may be used if necessary. One tablespoon four times daily by mouth or enema usually serves to reduce an elevated serum potas-sium level by 1 or 2 mEq every 24 to 48 hr. If hyper-kalemia is associated with acidosis, it is frequently brought under control by infusions of sodium bicarbonate or sodium lactate. Infusions of hypertonic glucose solu-tions, with or without insulin, have a similar but more transient effect. The deleterious action of potassium on the heart may be counteracted to some extent by infu-sions of calcium or by the administration of digitalis. If hyperkalemia cannot be controlled by these measures, artificial dialysis is indicated.

Heart failure should be treated with digitalis in the usual doses (Chap. 264). Artificial dialysis, with the removal of several kilograms of edema fluid by ultra-filtration, may be dramatically effective in relieving pul-monary edema. Testosterone propionate or norethandro-lone, 25 to 50 mg daily, may be given during the first 2 weeks in an attempt to reduce nitrogen breakdown. Its action is frequently overwhelmed by the intense catabolic reaction to acute injury.

Scrupulous care should be taken to avoid *infection.* After the diagnosis is established, an accurate estimate of the daily output may be obtained by catheterizing the patient, using sterile precautions, only once in 24 or 48 hr, thus dispensing with an inlying bladder catheter. As the urinary volume reaches a significant level, most pa-tients will be able to void spontaneously. It is desirable for hospital personnel handling the patient to wear mask and gloves. In alert patients, deep breathing and forced coughing should be stressed to avoid atelectasis. Trache-otomy should be considered early if there is difficulty in handling bronchial secretions. Careful mouth care, with prevention of crusting and ulceration, is important in

avoiding parotitis and aspiration of infected material. Prophylactic administration of antibiotics should be avoided.

The prime indication for *artificial dialysis* in acute renal failure is uncontrollable hyperkalemia. (It should be remembered that suddenly lowering the serum potas-sium level by dialysis may induce dangerous arrhythmias in digitalized patients.) Acidosis cannot be successfully treated by measures short of dialysis without giving sodium; mounting acidosis in the presence of congestive heart failure is therefore another clear indication for dialysis. Dialysis is especially helpful in temporarily in-ducing a return of appetite and clearheadedness in azo-temic patients. Repeated dialyses may make management during oliguria simpler by permitting patients to continue to eat and drink and by preventing clinical deterioration due to uremia. Peritoneal dialysis has the advantage that if necessary large amounts of fluid can be easily removed from the body by the use of concentrated glucose in the irrigating solution. Artificial dialysis may also be used to remove exogenous toxins such as barbiturates, bromide, and salicylates. Indeed, a portion of the clinical improve-ment following dialysis in some patients with uremia may be related to removal of sedatives. Although the majority of patients in civilian practice can recover with-out dialysis if proper care is instituted from the onset of anuria, extensive wounds, severe infection, or pro-longed oliguria are likely to necessitate its use.

During the *early diuretic phase,* every effort should be made to avoid salt depletion and dehydration and to sus-tain diuresis by replacing the previous day's urinary losses. Daily weights and determinations of serum and urinary electrolytes serve as guides; a useful approxima-tion for replacement is to give one-quarter of the urine volume as 0.9 percent saline solution, one-quarter as ⅙ M sodium lactate, and one-half as 5 percent glucose in water, in addition to replacing other losses. Equiva-lent quantities of sodium and water may be provided by mouth if oral feedings are tolerated. As azotemia re-cedes, tubular ability to reabsorb salt and water im-proves, and the daily provision of large volumes of fluids becomes unnecessary. In a patient who is alert, spon-taneous intake of food and water may usually be trusted to prevent depletion after the blood urea nitrogen level has fallen below 80 mg per 100 ml. At this time protein may be allowed in the diet and will generally be well utilized in repleting tissue stores.

PREVENTION

The development of toxic or ischemic tubular necrosis in experimental and clinical situations is conditioned by the state of hydration and the concentration of the urine. Renal vasoconstriction is potentiated in dehydrated ani-mals. Hemorrhagic or tourniquet shock is enhanced by dehydration and modified by prior infusions of saline so-lution. It would seem wise to give enough saline and glucose solution before and during surgical operations to compensate for antecedent losses as well as those an-ticipated during the operative procedure. Since dehydration contributes to the production of shock, it is likely that these simple measures will reduce the necessity for transfusions and therefore the likelihood of transfusion reactions.

PROGNOSIS

Even though in most cases the damage to tubular epithelium is theoretically reparable, acute tubular necrosis is a dangerous disease with a serious prognosis. The mortality in many large series of cases is about 50 percent, in spite of the most careful attention to details of fluid and electrolyte balance and with the aid of the artificial kidney. The result depends to a large extent on the background of associated illness leading up to the acute episode and the outcome of infections acquired during its course.

When renal ischemia is extremely intense or prolonged, *acute cortical necrosis,* with destruction of glomeruli, may occur. Such lesions are not reversible, and most patients die without emerging from anuria. Most instances of acute cortical necrosis have followed complications of pregnancy, particularly premature separation of the placenta, eclampsia, and septic abortion, although the disease is also encountered following severe shock in nonpregnant patients with preexisting vascular disease. Anuria for several days is common, followed by prolonged oliguria. The protein content of the urine is elevated. In the few patients who survive, renal calcification and contraction of the kidneys may be observed and death may occur within 12 to 18 months from malignant hypertension.

REFERENCES

Bluemle, L. W., Jr., G. D. Webster, Jr., and J. R. Elkinton: Acute Tubular Necrosis: Analysis of One Hundred Cases with Respect to Mortality, Complications and Treatment with and without Dialysis, A.M.A. Arch. Intern. Med., 104:180, 1959.

Kirkland, K., K. D. G. Edwards, and H. M. Whyte. Oliguric Renal Failure: A Report of 400 Cases Including Classification, Survival and Response to Dialysis, Australian Ann. Med., 14:275, 1965.

301 CHRONIC RENAL FAILURE

Franklin H. Epstein and
John P. Merrill

CLINICAL FEATURES OF RENAL INSUFFICIENCY

The onset of chronic renal failure is usually insidious. Polyuria and nocturia may be the only signs at first. Later the patient complains of feeling weak and unwell, of easy fatigue, insomnia, and slight breathlessness. Appetite is lost, and there is a bad taste in the mouth. Intractable nausea, especially in the morning, frequently brings the patient to the physician. He looks pale and may be referred to the hematologist because of anemia. When acidosis and azotemia become more severe, the patient takes to his bed, becomes increasingly lethargic, and may be troubled by hiccups and uncontrollable twitching of the limbs. Heart failure, progressive anemia, and bleeding into the skin, mucous membranes, and gastrointestinal tract herald the final illness. The skin becomes dry, with a sallow tint, the breath uriniferous. Exophthalmos may be present. Vision is impaired as hemorrhages and exudates appear in the fundi. The urinary output becomes progressively restricted. Fibrinous pericarditis or pleurisy, usually but not always painless, may appear within a few weeks of death. Disorientation and coma mercifully precede the end.

Cardiovascular Manifestations

Although chronic renal insufficiency per se does not produce congestive heart failure, hypertension and hypertensive heart disease are so often associated with renal disease that heart failure is one of the most common complications of uremia. In addition to hypertension, anemia may aggravate heart failure. Finally, when renal failure is so severe that oliguria is present, continued intake of salt and water will expand the circulation and produce circulatory congestion with pulmonary edema that is not relieved by digitalis.

When *edema* is present in patients with renal disease, heart failure or hypoproteinemia is usually the cause. The edema of acute glomerulonephritis and toxemia of pregnancy are exceptions to this rule. Edema without heart failure or hypoproteinemia may also be seen during oliguria in acute tubular necrosis or terminal renal insufficiency, when the intake of fluid has been excessive.

The contribution of heart failure to renal insufficiency can sometimes be assessed only by a therapeutic trial of digitalis. Both digoxin and digitoxin are eliminated in the urine, the former to a greater extent than the latter. In severe renal failure one-half of the usual loading dose and one-half of the usual maintenance dose of digoxin are appropriate, while three-fourths of the usual dose of digitoxin can be given (Chap. 264). Diuretics are generally ineffective when glomerular filtration rate is greatly restricted, i.e., when the blood urea nitrogen level is over 100 mg per 100 ml, though large intravenous doses of furosemide or ethacrynic acid may cause transient increases in urine flow in patients with this degree of renal impairment.

In many patients with renal insufficiency, pulmonary edema tends to be central, producing a "butterfly pattern" on the chest roentgenogram; this condition is sometimes miscalled "uremic pneumonia." Because congestion without alveolar edema is common, rales may be absent. Increasing agitation and restlessness, coupled with accentuation of the second pulmonic heart sound, are often the first warning to the physician of an impending explosion of paroxysmal dyspnea which may be warded off with digitalis.

Pericarditis, usually painless, may sometimes produce

excruciating pain, and occasionally bloody effusion with tamponade. A coarse rub and characteristic electrocardiographic signs are commonly found. It is unusual for uremic pericarditis to be present when the blood urea nitrogen level is below 80 mg per 100 ml; signs of pericarditis in patients with lesser degrees of renal impairment should make one think of other diseases of the heart or pericardium. Although it is not clear what causes uremic pericarditis or uremic pleuritis, signs of pericardial inflammation or pleurisy disappear regularly soon after hemodialysis, though they may return later when the blood urea and serum creatinine levels rise. Occasionally tamponade develops and pericardiocentesis must be performed. Vigorous treatment of *hypertension* may be hazardous when the blood urea nitrogen level is 80 mg per 100 ml or more. Under these circumstances a small reduction in perfusion pressure and blood flow through the kidneys often precipitates renal decompensation. Hypotensive agents may be used cautiously when headache, retinopathy, or hypertensive heart failure produce symptoms (see Chap. 276). With lesser degrees of renal insufficiency, it is frequently possible to lower severely elevated blood pressure with drugs (e.g., alpha-methyl-dopa, 750 mg to 3 Gm daily) without depressing renal function. Sodium depletion with diet or diuretics, on the other hand, usually impairs the function of the kidneys. Hypertensive headaches may be treated with analgesics; when they occur on awakening, elevating the head of the bed often provides some measure of relief. In this phase of management, as in many others, *primum non nocere* should be the rule; the patient with chronic renal insufficiency and hypertension who is asymptomatic should, in general, be given no treatment.

Gastrointestinal Manifestations

The mouth ulcers and parotitis which often complicate advanced uremia are related to bacterial breakdown to ammonia of the urea present in high concentration in saliva, to mouth breathing in acidosis, and to dehydration. Careful attention to cleansing of the mouth and removal of tartar from teeth helps to prevent these complications.

Anorexia, hiccups, nausea, and vomiting are common symptoms of uremia. The vomitus usually contains no free acid and therefore seldom results in alkalosis. Bleeding from small ulcers may occur from anywhere in the gastrointestinal tract. Bloody diarrhea is a distressing complication. Abdominal pain occurs with severe vomiting and diarrhea but may also be due to pericarditis or pancreatitis. The last diagnosis is sometimes difficult to establish because serum amylase levels are often high in advanced renal insufficiency, even without pancreatitis.

The treatment of nausea should include close attention to proper hydration, correction of acidosis, and treatment of sodium depletion. Anorexia is one of the first signs of a low serum sodium concentration, and nausea often improves dramatically when hyponatremia is corrected. Sometimes, however, nausea and vomiting persist despite full correction of serum electrolyte levels. In such

cases, small doses of phenothiazine or of Benadryl several times daily coupled with small frequent feedings may prove helpful. The pattern of meals should be adjusted flexibly to take advantage of the sometimes unpredictable periods of hunger and well-being. When vomiting is persistent, all feedings should be stopped and fluids given intravenously for a few days. Nausea and vomiting usually subside after dialysis.

Neuromuscular Disturbances

Mental clouding, inability to concentrate, drowsiness, and lethargy are the rule in advanced uremia. The EEG is frequently abnormal. Psychotic disturbances may be troublesome. The patient may alternate between periods of torpor and uncontrollable restlessness. Hyponatremia, acidosis, and dehydration may cause coma, which often disappears when these are corrected. Accumulation of sedative drugs normally excreted by the kidney may cause hypotension and unconsciousness which should not be mistaken for the terminal coma of uremia. Chloral hydrate (1 to 2 Gm nightly) and Benadryl (100 mg) are useful sedatives.

Frank tetany, often brought out by alkali therapy in the presence of hypocalcemia, can be relieved by intravenous calcium salts (1 Gm Ca++ intravenously as the gluconate or chloride). Hypocalcemia or alkalosis may trigger convulsions, however, without the warning signs of tetany. The gross tremors, twitchings, and jactitations of uremia are usually not caused by hypocalcemia and are not improved by the administration of calcium. Occasionally they disappear or improve when hyponatremia is corrected. They are usually relieved by dialysis, suggesting that they have a chemical, rather than a vascular, origin. A flapping tremor may mimic that seen in liver disease. Rigidity, tremor, and even convulsive episodes sometimes follow overdoses of the phenothiazine drugs in azotemic patients. Grand mal seizures are more common when hypertension is present and are usually thought to have a vascular basis. They are best controlled by sodium phenobarbital given intravenously or intramuscularly.

Peripheral neuritis, producing pain and paralysis of the extremities, may appear in patients who have lived many months with severe renal insufficiency. Its cause is unknown. It can be prevented by intensive hemodialysis and cured by successful kidney transplantation.

Hematologic Disturbances

Normocytic, normochromic anemia is the rule, and though it is usually proportionate to the degree of azotemia, there are many exceptions. Its mechanism is discussed in Chap. 61. For the treatment of the anemia of advanced renal disease, reliance must be placed on transfusions. Although the degree of tolerance to anemia varies greatly, weakness, shortness of breath, and poor appetite are likely to be improved by transfusions when the hemoglobin is below 7 Gm per 100 ml. Strenuous efforts to maintain normal or near-normal hemoglobin levels by transfusion are, however, unwise and unnecessary. Unless serum proteins are depleted, or hemostatic defects are present, in which case whole blood should be given, transfusions should ideally be of packed red blood cells derived from fresh blood. Transfusion should be given cautiously in the presence of congestive heart failure, but treatment of severe anemia should not be neglected because the heart is failing; in such circumstances, transfusions should be of packed red blood cells given slowly in small amounts, with the patient in a sitting position. If blood is given at intervals to ambulatory patients with advanced renal disease before the red blood cell count has fallen to a critical level, general well-being and strength may be greatly improved and the remaining days made happier and more useful.

The *bleeding tendency* of uremic patients often makes venipuncture and the therapeutic use of tubes in the nose, esophagus, and bladder distressingly complicated. Ecchymoses, nosebleeds, and oozing from mucous membranes are prominent. Bleeding and clotting times are usually normal, though capillary fragility may be increased. The platelet count is often low. Abnormal prothrombin consumption and thromboplastin generation are sometimes present, suggesting a qualitative defect in platelets. The cause of these disturbances is not known, and the only treatment is symptomatic, consisting of transfusions of fresh whole blood or platelet-rich plasma.

Skin

Accumulation of carotene-like pigments in renal insufficiency combine with anemia to give the skin a sallow, yellow cast. The high concentration of urea in sweat gives rise to *uremic frost* when the sweat dries. *Itching* is an inconstant symptom, not closely correlated with the level of blood urea and contributed to by dryness and superficial irritation of the skin. It may sometimes be controlled by daily baths, bland lubricating ointments, and the use of Benadryl. Topical adrenal cortical steroids sometimes give relief. Meticulous daily cleansing with antibacterial soaps helps to reduce the tendency to superficial skin infections.

Infection

Although mildly azotemic patients do not seem to be unusually susceptible to infection, with advanced renal insufficiency septic complications are common. Poor nutrition, pulmonary congestion and edema, inanition and coma, vascular insufficiency, and the use of indwelling catheters, tubes, and cannulas undoubtedly predispose to sepsis. The necrotizing cystitis and subsequent bacteremia triggered by an indwelling bladder catheter are often fatal.

Streptomycin, colimycin, and kanamycin, normally excreted by the kidneys, may rapidly accumulate to toxic levels when given in usual doses to patients with impaired renal function. Tetracyclines and penicillins are also excreted slowly in patients with damaged kidneys.

Chloromycetin is inactivated normally, but its metabolic products are only slowly eliminated.

SOME DISORDERS OF BODY CHEMISTRY IN CHRONIC UREMIA AND THEIR MANAGEMENT

Water

Because they are unable to excrete a concentrated urine, patients with renal insufficiency must ingest and excrete more water than normal in order to handle the usual load of urinary solutes. Nocturia, polyuria, and polydipsia are therefore among the first signs of advancing impairment of renal function. Reversal of the normal diurnal pattern contributes to nocturia. Most patients with renal disease are able to excrete a urine at least as concentrated in solutes as is the glomerular filtrate. Persistently hypotonic urines unresponsive to vasopressin (nephrogenic diabetes insipidus) may be encountered, however, in obstructive uropathy, chronic pyelonephritis, amyloidosis, nephrocalcinosis, and familial nephrogenic diabetes insipidus.

Because polyuria is obligatory, dehydration may be readily produced by relatively brief abstention from fluids. Thirsting and purgation in preparation for x-ray studies may prove fatal in the delicately balanced patient with renal decompensation. In such patients it is usually unnecessary and unwise to withhold fluids before blood is drawn for chemical determinations in the morning. Even minor surgical procedures should be undertaken against a background of adequate hydration, by the intravenous route if necesary, both before and after operation. Overnight polyuria in many patients results in early morning thirst and a feeling of hunger on awakening which quickly turns to nausea and vomiting, thereby perpetuating the vicious circle of dehydration. This can sometimes be prevented by a drink of water taken after urinating at night or a small preliminary feeding immediately on awakening.

Although restriction of fluid intake is seldom indicated, there is no reason to push fluids to the point of discomfort. The efficiency of the kidney in excreting urea and other solutes appears to reach a maximum at a urine volume of about 3,000 ml; even the diseased kidney is not much more effective at higher volumes. Moreover, the ability to excrete large loads of water rapidly is impaired in most patients with azotemia. Excessive administration of water, especially when salt is limited, is therefore likely to result in hyponatremia, with its attendant symptoms of nausea, muscle cramps, and mental disturbances.

Sodium

A normal man reduces his urinary output of sodium to negligible levels within 2 or 3 days after taking a salt-free diet. Patients with renal insufficiency are unable to restrict renal losses of sodium this efficiently, and continue to leak variable amounts of sodium into the urine when salt is restricted. At first, losses of water may occur in parallel with sodium so that the serum sodium concentration is normal even though extracellular fluid is contracted. Later hyponatremia develops, as water is no longer lost proportionately. The degree of hyponatremia, then, is not a reliable guide to the magnitude of sodium deficit, but must be supplemented by a clinical estimate of extracellular fluid depletion. One mechanism contributing to the salt-wasting tendency in renal disease is the increased solute load excreted by each intact nephron, since osmotic diuresis in normal kidneys results in obligatory salt losses. Specific damage to salt-resorbing portions of the renal tubule is also responsible in many cases. Salt wasting is more common in patients with chronic pyelonephritis, interestitial nephritis, and obstructive disease than in chronic glomerulonephritis, but it may occur in renal insufficiency from any cause, especially when polyuria is prominent. In such cases the triad of asthenia, dehydration, and hyponatremia may suggest the diagnosis of Addison's disease. From 5 to 8 Gm sodium chloride daily is often required to prevent sodium depletion, and as much as 15 Gm salt may be necessary.

Salt losing may disappear or become less marked in the terminal stages of renal failure as glomerular filtration becomes progressively compromised and oliguria supervenes. The diagnosis of salt wasting can be established by measuring the urinary sodium. In the presence of obvious volume depletion or of hyponatremia, an output of more than 5 to 10 mEq sodium per day or per liter of urine is suggestive. With marked constriction of blood volume, or in heart failure, a fall in glomerular filtration rate may enable a sodium-free urine to be excreted, even when underlying renal disease is severe, by restoring glomerulotubular balance.

In addition to urinary losses, vomiting and diarrhea commonly produce sodium depletion in uremic patients. Anorexia may defeat attempts to replace deficits by oral feeding, and since hyponatremia commonly causes nausea, a vicious circle ensues. Depletion of extracellular volume, with or without hyponatremia, compromises renal function by reducing renal blood flow and glomerular filtration, even when the degree of volume depletion is not readily detected by physical examination. Although a fall in blood pressure, a dry mouth, and some loss of skin turgor are often present, listlessness, fatigue, nausea, and mental clouding may dominate the picture. As sodium depletion progresses, muscle cramps and generalized muscle twitches or convulsions may appear, and the patient becomes confused, somnolent, and comatose. It is important not to mistake these signs of sodium deficit for an inevitable progression of uremia.

In azotemic patients without edema, congestive heart failure, or oliguria, restriction of salt is unwise and unnecessary. The intake of sodium should be encouraged, preferably in the form of salty foods and drinks, rather than by use of pills of sodium chloride, which irritate the stomach. If acidosis is present, part of the sodium requirement may be taken as sodium bicarbonate or citrate. The slight expansion of extracellular fluid induced by a diet high in sodium is often reflected in improved renal blood flow and glomerular filtration. Excretion of urea, sulfates, and phosphates is augmented, and the secretion of acid and potassium is promoted. Because salt stimulates thirst, the intake of water is encouraged in a natural fashion and urinary flow is improved. The appearance of congestive failure sharply limits the extent to which an increased intake of salt can be used as a lever to improve renal function in chronic renal disease. Because of the beneficial effects of salt on renal function, an attempt should be made to control early congestive heart failure in patients with chronic renal disease with digitalis, rather than by rigid limitation of dietary sodium. Unnecessary restriction of salt and consequent salt depletion may, in fact, result in considerable further impairment of renal function in patients with renal insufficiency.

Potassium

Although the kidneys are the main route for excretion of the 50 to 80 mEq potassium in a normal diet, hyperkalemia does not commonly complicate chronic renal insufficiency so long as urinary output is well maintained. The enormous capacity of the distal tubules to secrete potassium into the urine is usually adequate to maintain the level of potassium in the serum close to normal even though glomerular filtration is greatly restricted. Tubular secretion of potassium is enhanced by a high sodium diet and depressed when sodium excretion is reduced. Serum potassium level may therefore rise in patients with chronic azotemia when they are placed on salt-free diets, especially when juices and fruits, high in potassium content, are simultaneously given in large amounts to "force fluids." If the supply of potassium from diet or breakdown of tissue is not excessive and urinary output is adequate, the cause of an elevated serum potassium level is usually found to be acidosis. Hydrogen ions are buffered by intracellular proteins, which release potassium to the extracellular fluid. Restoration of serum bicarbonate to normal usually reduces the serum potassium concentration. Persistent hyperkalemia in the absence of excessive potassium intake, salt restriction, oliguria, or acidosis should raise the suspicion of adrenal insufficiency.

When urinary output falls below 500 to 1,000 ml daily in patients with renal decompensation, serum potassium may rise to dangerous levels. Clinical manifestations and management of hyperkalemia are discussed in Chap. 300.

Inability to conserve potassium is not a feature of most primary diseases of the kidney, though hypokalemia with potassium wasting may complicate renal tubular acidosis, nephrocalcinosis, and Fanconi's syndrome, and may sometimes occur during the diuretic phase of recovery from tubular necrosis. Renal potassium losing with urinary potassium in excess of 15 to 20 mEq per day or per liter in the presence of hypokalemia is characteristic of primary aldosteronism but may also be seen in malignant hypertension, presumably because of the high level of circulating aldosterone in this condition. When patients with azotemia are depleted of potassium by vomiting or diarrhea, additional renal damage may result; repair of the deficit, with care taken not to cause hyperkalemia, is therefore indicated.

Acidosis

Failure to excrete normal amounts of H^+ as urinary NH_4^+, and inability to reabsorb all the filtered bicarbonate at normal levels of serum bicarbonate are chiefly responsible for the acidosis of chronic renal insufficiency. The excess of acid produced over that excreted is neutralized by body buffers, including bone. Acidosis therefore contributes to osteoporosis and negative calcium balance in renal disease. Systemic acidosis is often responsible for nausea, fatigue, malaise, and breathlessness on exertion, long before Kussmaul's respiration is clinically apparent. Acidosis may be avoided by prescribing an amount of alkali equal to the daily production of acid, or 40 to 60 mEq per day. This is contained in 1 to 2 tsp baking soda, or 2 to 4 tbsp 10 percent sodium citrate in syrup of wild cherry. Taken in divided doses after meals, this usually suffices to maintain serum bicarbonate at 18 to 22 mEq per liter, thereby avoiding the unpleasant side effects of acidosis. Excessive administration of alkali must be avoided, especially in the presence of hypocalcemia, when correction of acidosis without the simultaneous administration of calcium may precipitate tetany and convulsions. Large amounts of sodium bicarbonate or lactate are also contraindicated in congestive heart failure.

Calcium, Phosphorus, and Bone

As the glomerular filtration rate progressively diminishes in the course of chronic renal disease, the fraction of filtered phosphate reabsorbed by the renal tubules decreases so as to keep phosphate clearance constant and maintain a normal level of inorganic phosphorus in plasma. When creatinine clearance has decreased to about 25 ml per min, however, phosphate excretion can no longer be maintained by this method of compensation, and the serum phosphate level begins to rise. The increase in serum phosphate occurs earlier and is more striking in children than in adults.

Serum calcium level is characteristically depressed in renal decompensation. A portion of the decrement is a result of decrease in the protein-bound fraction, since serum albumin is often low, but the ultrafiltrable portion of serum calcium is also regularly reduced. Calcium and phosphate ions normally are present in extracellular fluids at concentrations close to the limit of solubility of calcium phosphate salts. When the concentration of phosphate is increased, therefore, calcium phosphate tends to be deposited in soft tissues and in bone. If the serum calcium level is low, however, it may not return to normal even when phosphorus levels are reduced by oral aluminum hydroxide gel, which retards the intestinal absorption of phosphate. Other factors must therefore be responsible for hypocalcemia in renal insufficiency. One of these is impaired absorption of calcium from the gastrointestinal tract. Increased fecal excretion of calcium

and decreased urinary calcium can in fact be detected quite early in azotemic renal disease. Calcium absorption improves in uremic patients only after very large doses of vitamin D (from 50,000 to 200,000 daily), which commonly produce hypercalcemia in normal patients. Resistance to the action of vitamin D, both in the gut and on bone, has therefore been postulated. The level of ionized calcium in plasma in uremia is further decreased by the tendency of calcium to form undissociated but soluble complexes with sulfate, citrate, and phosphate ions.

Although hypocalcemia in renal failure is frequent, tetany is rare. The reasons for this are not completely clear. Acidosis may protect against tetany by increasing the dissociation of calcium from protein complexes as well as by a direct action on neuromuscular irritability. The high levels of serum magnesium in uremia also counteract the tendency to tetany.

The tendency to hypocalcemia is resisted to a variable degree by an increase in parathyroid secretion accompanied by secondary parathyroid hyperplasia. Serum calcium may thus be maintained in the normal range, though often at the expense of osteitis fibrosa and metastatic calcification. In contrast to primary hyperparathyroidism, hypercalcemia does not occur in secondary hyperplasia of the parathyroids.

When renal insufficiency and secondary parathyroid hyperplasia have been present for a long time, however, the parathyroid activity sometimes becomes autonomous, or autonomous adenomas may develop. When this happens, the serum calcium level may rise above normal and osteitis fibrosa may be noted. Parathyroid autonomy ("tertiary hyperparathyroidism") may be unmasked by procedures, such as dialysis or transplantation, which lower the serum phosphorus level. In some cases parathyroidectomy is necessary to relieve hypercalcemia, itching, and bone pain.

The development of clinical bone disease appears to be determined by the rate of skeletal growth and the chronicity of the renal failure. Renal osteodystrophy is consequently more common in children and in patients with congenital anomalies of the kidney and with slowly progressive renal disease such as chronic pyelonephritis with normal blood pressure. Radiographic changes in bone are of three general types: (1) widening of osteoid seams at the growing ends of bones, as in rickets (hence the term "renal rickets"), (2) erosive and cystic changes of osteitis fibrosa, as in hyperparathyroidism, in which the earliest signs are of subperiosteal resorption in the phalanges and long bones, and (3) hyperostosis or osteosclerosis. The serum alkaline phosphatase level is usually high but may be normal. Retardation of growth is usual. Bones and joints are often tender. Painful, swollen joints, often with deposits of calcium in the bursae, may mimic classical gout. Proximal muscular weakness, producing a waddling gait, may be mistaken for myopathy or neuritis but improves dramatically with administration of vitamin D.

Azotemic osteodystrophy may be treated with vitamin D, 50,000 to 200,000 units daily. Elevation of the serum calcium level above 10 mg per 100 ml, the development of lassitude, anorexia, and nausea, or a rising blood urea level not attributable to other causes, warn of vitamin D intoxication and should signal the complete withdrawal of medication, since the action of vitamin D persists for about 2 weeks. Calcium lactate or citrate, in amounts of 10 to 20 Gm daily, may be given to supplement dietary calcium. Aluminum hydroxide gel, 30 to 60 ml with each meal, may be given when hyperphosphatemia is present, to reduce phosphate absorption. These medications sometimes interfere with the patient's already poor appetite. In view of the hazards of treatment, it seems wise to limit therapeutic aims to the relief of symptoms rather than attempt the cure of radiologic abnormalities.

Other Chemical Abnormalities

The serum magnesium level is usually elevated when the glomerular filtration rate falls below 30 ml per min, unless counteracted by starvation or diarrhea or accelerated by urinary excretion due to diuretics. Unless magnesium salts are administered either orally as laxatives or antacids or parenterally to control convulsions, the level of magnesium does not generally rise high enough to cause symptoms.

The blood uric acid level may be increased early in renal insufficiency but does not usually rise above 10 mg per 100 ml even in severe renal failure. Secondary gout is rare, and repeated episodes of gout in a patient with uremia suggest a gouty family background or primary uric acid nephropathy.

Indoles, phenols, guanidine, certain amino acids, and various organic acids appear in increased concentration in the blood in renal decompensation, but their contribution to the clinical syndrome of uremia is not established.

TREATMENT

Protein and Diet

When oliguria is present at any stage of renal disease, it is clear that the dietary intake of protein should be restricted, if not eliminated. Similarly, there is general agreement that protein intake should be increased in the nephrotic syndrome. Controversy still surrounds the proper prescription of protein in the diet of the large number of patients with chronic renal disease and azotemia who have an undiminished or increased urinary output. Restriction of dietary protein will reduce the blood urea nitrogen and the rate of accumulation of metabolic acids, without, however, improving renal function. Derivatives of testosterone may induce a positive balance of nitrogen and a slight fall in level of blood urea for a few weeks in some patients with renal insufficiency, but their action is self-limited and they are not generally useful in the chronic treatment of renal disease.

Protein restriction is most efficacious in reducing blood urea when the protein eaten is of high biologic value (eggs and milk) and the intake of carbohydrate and calories is sufficient to prevent ketosis and loss of weight. If these conditions are met, and protein is restricted to 18 to 20 Gm daily, the blood urea may be expected to fall to 50 to 60 percent of the level present at a daily intake of 40 to 60 Gm protein. Nausea, vomiting, and lethargy often respond temporarily to this form of dietary treatment. It is most useful in the symptomatic treatment of patients with a creatinine clearance between 10 and 3 to 4 ml per min, but it need not be resorted to if symptoms are not present or can be controlled in other ways.

The treatment of advanced renal insufficiency has been transformed by the development of techniques for *dialysis* and *kidney transplantation*. The latter is discussed in detail in Chap. 71.

Role of Dialysis in the Treatment of Renal Failure

It is now clear that intermittent dialysis of blood may rehabilitate a majority of uremic patients, although not all of them. With adequate sodium restriction or depletion hypertension and hypertensive disease may be markedly improved. In most instances peritoneal dialysis and hemodialysis with the artificial kidney are the two techniques commonly used.

PERITONEAL DIALYSIS. Physiologic fluid (dialysate) is introduced into the peritoneal cavity via an indwelling plastic catheter placed by paracentesis. The dialysate is left in place for 20 min to 1 hr, during which time solute (urea, phosphate, uric acid, etc.) diffuses from the blood across the peritoneal membrane into the dialysate. The dialysate is then removed. This process is repeated for the desired number of times, usually 30 to 40. Disposable equipment and solutions are now available commercially. There are two indications for peritoneal dialysis in the treatment of chronic renal failure: (1) As an adjunct to the conservative regimens described above. Patients critically ill with uremia but whose disease has a reversible element may be dramatically improved by 2 or 3 days of peritoneal dialysis, which enable them to take adequate amounts of fluid and electrolyte and a low protein diet. (2) As a "holding action." Peritoneal dialysis in conjunction with a diet with 20 Gm protein and adequate caloric content may be used until the patient can enter a program of chronic dialysis with the artificial kidney (hemodialysis) or receive a renal allograft. A few patients have been maintained for 1 to 2 years on a program of peritoneal dialysis performed three times a week. The long-term peritoneal dialyses are performed in the home by the family members, although a physician must insert an indwelling catheter on each occasion. With few exceptions, the use of permanently indwelling plastic prostheses providing access to the peritoneal cavity has not been successful for more than a few months at a time. The complications of peritoneal dialysis are infection, protein loss from the peritoneal cavity, pain, and occasional bleeding. In general it has not been as satisfactory a technique as long-term intermittent dialysis with the artificial kidney for the treatment of chronic renal failure.

HEMODIALYSIS. Hemodialysis with the artificial kidney is now a well-established method for treatment of chronic renal failure. The development of permanent inlying plastic arteriovenous "shunts" has made the technique a painless and relatively simple one. Cannulae placed surgically in an artery and a vein of the leg or the arm are connected by a bypass. The bypass may be removed at will so that the cannula in the artery can be connected to the inflow end of an artificial kidney and that in the vein to the outflow end to receive the blood returning from the artificial kidney after it has been dialyzed. A surgically established subcutaneous arteriovenous fistula has been used as another method of establishing portals for the connection to the artificial kidney. This requires percutaneous puncture of the proximal portion of the venous limb of the fistula for the outflow of the blood from the patient and the distal portion for the inflow. This technique has the advantage of eliminating the externalized "shunt" with the hazard of infection in the exit sites, but it has the disadvantage of requiring a percutaneous puncture on each occasion.

Two types of apparatus are in general use for hemodialysis, one in which the cellophane tubing is spirally wound between a polypropylene screen (twin-coil artificial kidney), and the other in which sheets of cellophane are compressed between plastic plates (Kiil type). The twin coil is immersed in a tank through which dialysate is pumped, whereas in the Kiil type, dialysate fluid flows in a countercurrent fashion between the cellophane and the plastic plates. Smaller, equally effective types of artificial kidney (the capillary kidney) which do not require priming with blood prior to the onset of dialysis are now under active clinical trial. A number of "centers" for the treatment of patients with chronic renal failure by hemodialysis have been established in university and Veterans' Administration hospitals throughout this country and in Europe. The centers vary in size from 4 to 30 beds. Usually patients report for treatment two or three times a week and are treated for 4 to 6 hr if the twin coil is used and for 10 to 12 hr if a Kiil type of artificial kidney is employed. Recently a number of "satellite units" to the centers have been established in nursing homes or in community hospitals.

Since the object of chronic hemodialysis is the rehabilitation of patients with debilitating chronic disease, the successful institution of self-dialysis at home has been a major advance in this field. Patients with arm shunts may be treated by spouses or nurses who have been trained in the technique of hemodialysis. Ideally, the shunts are placed in the leg so that with arms free of shunts the patients are able to use the hands to treat themselves. One of the advantages of home dialysis lies in the fact that a patient may arrange his schedule to suit himself; e.g., dialysis may be done in the evening after work.

The major criterion for the initiation of chronic hemodialysis is the inability of the patient to maintain useful comfortable existence without it. The major criterion for selection of patients is that the disability be due to primary renal failure without any underlying disease. A rare exception is the removal of localized cancer in a single kidney. Physiologic rather than chronologic age is the limiting factor for selection of patients. In general children do not adjust well to the strict routine of dialysis, although there are many exceptions. The patient and/or his assistant must be intelligent, adequately motivated, willing, and able to learn. Psychiatric problems may arise during long-term dialysis, particularly in the home. It is important, however, to remember that psychiatric findings in the patient while he is terminally ill with uremia may be quite different from those in the same individual after he has been adequately dialyzed for a period of weeks. Another problem of chronic hemodialysis is the cost, at present estimated at $14,000 (range $8,400 to $19,000) per patient per year in the centers. The cost of home dialysis is considerably less, averaging approximately $5,000 per year exclusive of the initial investment in equipment.

Management of the Patient on Chronic Dialysis

Where adequate facilities exist, the patient should be begun on hemodialysis early rather than late to prevent some of the irreversible complications of renal failure. In general with adequate dialysis dietary protein need not be restricted. In most patients, however, some degree of sodium and water restriction is necessary. Although it is possible to remove sodium and water by ultrafiltration during hemodialysis, large swings in the state of hydration make the patient uncomfortable. Moreover, edema and congestive heart failure may ensue if proper sodium and fluid restriction is not practiced. Peripheral neuropathy may be prevented and to some extent reversed by adequate dialysis, but once firmly established it is not often markedly improved. Anemia is not corrected and may require transfusion of packed red blood cells during the first year. There is increasing evidence, however, that if the patient is not transfused erythropoiesis may be improved over a period of months or years, and that he may be able to maintain an adequate hematocrit without transfusion. An occasional patient with pruritus may not respond to dialysis. Pericarditis with or without hemorrhagic effusion may occur even in patients on adequate dialysis. Although this complication may be treated with conservative measures, pericardiotomy is required in occasional cases. Osteoporosis and metastatic calcification are complications that are becoming less frequent as more careful attention is being paid to calcium intake and to the levels of calcium in the dialyzing fluid. Infection and clotting of the shunts are infrequent if care is given to the prosthesis.

In most centers approximately 15 percent of the patients per year are lost from the program, exclusive of those who receive kidney allografts. With adequate dialysis in the centers, "satellite units," or at home, restoration to full activity may be expected in approximately 75 percent of the patients treated for more than 1 year.

REFERENCES

Hampers, C. L., and E. Schupak: "Long-term Hemodialysis," New York, Grune & Stratton, Inc., 1967.

Welt, L. G.: Symposium on Uremia, Am. J. Med., 44:653–802, 1968.

302   OBSTRUCTIVE UROPATHY

Bernard Lytton and
Franklin H. Epstein

OBSTRUCTION OF THE BLADDER OUTLET

The importance of obstruction as a cause of renal failure is indicated by the fact that fully two-thirds of deaths from uremia may be attributed wholly or in part to obstructive disease. Obstruction of urinary flow occurs most frequently at or below the bladder outlet. The principal causes are meatal stenosis, congenital or acquired urethral strictures, urethral valves, bladder neck contracture, prostatic and urethral carcinoma, and, most commonly, benign overgrowth of the prostate.

Prostatic obstruction may cause frequency, slowing of the stream, hesitancy, urgency, terminal dribbling, pain, and hematuria. Sometimes, however, progressive obstruction occurs with few or no urinary symptoms and the patient presents signs of uremia or a palpable mass in the lower part of the abdomen because of a distended bladder which may be mistaken for some other abdominal tumor. It is estimated that some 30 to 50 percent of men will develop symptoms of prostatism after the age of fifty, but only 1 in 10 will require surgical relief of obstruction before reaching the age of eighty.

Obstruction of the bladder neck is a late symptom in carcinoma of the prostate, since this usually arises in the posterior part of the gland. The disease often goes unrecognized until distant metastases or ureteral obstruction appear.

An obstructive lesion of the bladder outlet may be closely mimicked by neurogenic vesical dysfunction, as in tabes, multiple sclerosis, or diabetic neuropathy. The effect of minor degrees of obstruction of the vesical neck is commonly magnified by disease of the nervous pathways supplying the bladder.

Although bladder neck obstruction is usually signaled by dysuria, frequency, and overflow incontinence, it is important to remember that nausea and vomiting may be the only outward signs of a distended bladder in a bedridden patient.

Chronic obstruction of the neck of the bladder in children is frequently associated with vesicoureteral reflux. If reflux of urine from bladder to ureters persists, it leads in some patients to progressive dilatation of the upper part of the urinary tract and to renal damage having the radiologic and pathologic characteristics of chronic pyelonephritis. This may occur without any histalogic or bacteriologic evidence of infection. In adults with obstruction of the bladder outlet, on the other hand, reflux occurs less commonly and is detectable in only about 10 percent of cases. Ureteral reflux can also be caused by anatomic abnormalities of the ureterovesical junction or by infection of the bladder, even when obstruction is not present, and in the latter case perhaps contributes to the development of parenchymal renal damage.

OBSTRUCTION OF THE URETERS

Obstruction of the ureters may be caused by calculi, congenital anomalies, cancer, or retroperitoneal fibrosis. Obstruction of a single ureter may pass unrecognized unless colic or bleeding occurs, as with a *calculus* (see Nephrolithiasis, in Chap. 307). Anomalies of the ureteropelvic junction and pressure on the upper part of the ureter by aberrant vessels or congenital bands produce hydronephrosis through the mechanism of partial obstruction. Sometimes this is intermittent, especially when the kidney is excessively mobile. Intermittent obstruction of the pelvicalyceal system can also be produced by calculi. Pain in the flank is the usual complaint, but the discomfort may be more vague, referred to the upper part of the abdomen, and confused with gastrointestinal disease. The pains of intermittent hydronephrosis may be precipitated by exercise or drinking large amounts of fluid, and relieved by recumbency. Pyelographic roentgenograms taken in the erect position and during forced diuresis are helpful in diagnosis.

Retrocaval ureter, a developmental anomaly, presents a typical I-shaped deformity of an upper ureter on pyelographic examination and is often associated with obstruction. Hypertrophy and dilatation of the ovarian vein, usually the right, may cause partial obstruction of the ureter at the pelvic brim. Temporary ureteral dilatation is sometimes associated with pregnancy and may persist for many months post partum.

After pelvic surgery, vascular or mechanical injury to a ureter may cause stenosis. Obstruction developing several months after treatment of a pelvic tumor may be the first indication of a recurrence of the growth.

Bilateral ureteral obstruction is most commonly due to malignant disease, either from local extension of tumors of the pelvic organs or from metastases in the retroperitoneal lymphatics. Occlusion of both ureters may also be caused by calculi. Congenital anomalies of the ureteropelvic and ureterovesical junctions in infants cause partial obstruction and dilatation of the upper part of the urinary tract, sometimes resulting in failure to thrive and in chronic uremia.

Retroperitoneal fibrosis is a chronic inflammation of unknown cause which involves the cellular tissue surrounding the great vessels in the lower lumbar area. It has been related in some instances to the taking of methysergide derivatives (Sansert) for the relief of migraine. The resulting fibrous constriction may obstruct the vena cava and occasionally the aorta. Rarely the process spreads to the upper part of the abdomen and mediastinum, leading to obstruction of the duodenum, bile ducts, and superior vena cava. It frequently involves the midportion of the ureters, which become drawn medially. Ureteral compression leads to hydronephrosis and finally to azotemia. Patients, usually males of middle age, complain of abdominal and low-back pain, anorexia, weakness, weight loss, and fever. Urinary symptoms include frequency, hematuria, and, depending on the degree of obstruction, either polyuria or anuria. Ureterolysis with lateral transposition or intraperitoneal placement of the ureters is the most effective treatment for the urinary obstruction. Occasional spontaneous remissions have been recorded. The condition must be distinguished from lymphomas and metastatic malignant diseases which involve the retroperitoneal tissues.

PATHOLOGIC PHYSIOLOGY

Complete obstruction of a ureter causes eventual atrophy of its kidney while the opposite kidney undergoes a conpensatory increase in growth and function. Failure of these compensatory changes to occur indicates severe disease in the contralateral kidney, although some degree of functional improvement may occur in the presence of a moderate degree of parenchymal damage.

Increases in ureteral pressure produce a fall in glomerular filtration rate and renal blood flow and impairment of renal concentrating capacity. Partial obstruction of the urethra or of both ureters may therefore result in progressive azotemia associated with an apparently adequate or even excessive urinary output. Polyuria is the result of loss of renal concentrating power from tubular damage by the obstruction. When the urinary passage is greatly narrowed, small changes in the size of the lumen produce large alterations in flow and in pressure proximal to the obstruction. *Unexplained wide fluctuations in blood urea or urinary output in patients with azotemia should always raise the question of partial urinary obstruction.*

When obstruction is relieved, a profuse obligatory diuresis may follow. The urine is dilute and alkaline, and contains much sodium. This is caused in part by an osmotic diuresis, resulting from excretion of the large amounts of urea which have accumulated during obstruction. In addition, the capacity of the renal tubules to reabsorb water and salt and to excrete acid is impaired. Adequate amounts of both water and salt must be provided to avoid dehydration during the early postobstructive period. *Rapid dehydration is probably responsible for some cases of shock following sudden decompression of an obstructed bladder.*

The special susceptibility of the obstructed kidney to infection is discussed in the chapter on pyelonephritis (Chap. 303).

CLINICAL FEATURES

The distended bladder is often felt as a cystic swelling in the lower part of the abdomen arising out of the pelvis. It may be displaced to one side either from an asymmetric enlargement or by a large diverticulum. The bladder may be difficult to detect in obese individuals or when the abdominal muscles are poorly relaxed, and the passage of a urethral catheter to establish the diagnosis may be a lifesaving procedure. Even though on rectal palpation the prostate appears normal or only slightly enlarged, it may still be causing obstruction. Conversely, a considerable degree of prostatic hypertrophy may be present

without any obstruction. The important factor is the degree of distortion of the bladder neck and intraurethral anatomy. The diagnosis of partial obstruction of the urinary tract may be suggested by the pattern of excretion of phenolsulfonphthalein dye (see Chap. 299, Renal Function Tests).

Urinary obstruction may mimic or complicate uremia due to chronic parenchymal renal disease. In the bedridden and obtunded patient, unrecognized functional difficulty in bladder emptying, often precipitated by sedatives, but treatable with urecholine or Prostigmine, may cause rapid and otherwise inexplicable deterioration. If an obstruction is suspected, delineation of the upper part of the urinary tract may be necessary to establish the diagnosis. In some cases this can be done by injecting large doses of contrast material for excretory urography; in other instances retrograde pyelography is ultimately required. *In the absence of residual urine in the bladder after spontaneous voiding, or of evidence of hydronephrosis, obstruction is unlikely to contribute to azotemia.*

Obstruction of the bladder or ureters does not usually cause hypertension unless it is complicated by renal scarring and atrophy. Simple relief of obstruction, therefore, cannot be expected to cure chronic high blood pressure when this is present in cases of hydronephrosis, although improvement has been reported in some instances.

Patients with obstructive uropathy usually improve remarkably with drainage. The greater part of the recovery of renal function occurs within 2 to 3 weeks, but improvement may continue slowly for several months after this. During the period of drainage, recurrent infections of the kidneys and the bloodstream remain as hazards. After occlusion of one ureter lasting four or more months, recovery of function is unlikely, especially if the opposite kidney has undergone compensatory growth. It may however retain its potential for recovery for a long time and this would become apparent only after loss of or injury to the normal kidney.

REFERENCES

Bricker, N. S.: Obstructive Nephropathy, in "Renal Disease," 2d ed., p. 402, D. A. K. Black (Ed.), Oxford, Blackwell Scientific Publications, Ltd., 1967.

303 PYELONEPHRITIS AND OTHER INFECTIONS OF THE URINARY TRACT, INCLUDING PROSTATITIS

Lawrence R. Freedman and Franklin H. Epstein

Bacterial infections of the urinary tract constitute one of the major medical problems encompassing all fields of practice. They are extremely common, notoriously resistant to treatment, and likely to recur. They are dangerous because of their ability to produce serious renal disease (pyelonephritis) and to serve as a source of spread of infection to the bloodstream.

It is important to define "urinary tract infection" and "pyelonephritis," since these terms do not mean the same thing to all physicians. Urinary tract infection is taken to mean the detection of significant numbers of bacteria in the urine. Pyelonephritis is considered to be disease resulting from the immediate or late effects of bacterial infection of the kidney. A person with pyelonephritis might or might not have a urinary tract infection at a given point in time. Similarly, a patient with a urinary tract infection might or might not have pyelonephritis, and might or might not develop it in the future.

The majority of persons with a urinary infection are unaware of its presence. Careful questioning and follow-up, however, reveal that symptoms have often occurred but are either intermittent or not recognized by the patient as arising from the urinary tract. These patients are sometimes referred to as having asymptomatic bacteriuria (or bacilluria). In many instances infections take the form of acute infectious disease, and rarely they are first recognized because of growth retardation in children, anemia, hypertension, or uremia—consequences of severe renal damage.

INFECTIONS OF THE URINARY TRACT

Etiology

Many different microorganisms can infect the tissues and fluids of the urinary organs, but by far the commonest are the coli-aerogenes group of gram-negative bacilli. Other microorganisms which may be found include enterococcus, proteus, pseudomonas, chromobacteria, staphylococcus, and certain yeasts. Infection by other than the coli-aerogenes organisms is generally related to previous instrumentation of the urinary tract, with or without the use of chemotherapeutic agents. Proteus and pseudomonas urinary infections, for example, are virtually never seen except in patients who have had catheters or other instruments passed through the urethra. Staphylococci play a minor role in the total problem of urinary tract infection. Their detection has been overemphasized in the past because of the use of qualitative cultural techniques which did not permit their identification as contaminants. Viruses have been shown to be able to produce pyelonephritis in animals and are effective in increasing the susceptibility of the kidney to infection with coliform bacteria. In man, viruses are commonly recovered from the urine in subjects without evidence of urinary tract disease, but recently they have been implicated as a cause of hemorrhagic cystitis.

Pathogenesis

SOURCES OF INFECTION. The common urinary pathogens are usual inhabitants of the large intestine. In the majority of instances these bacteria gain access to the bladder cavity via the urethra. Under normal circumstances bladder urine is sterile and large numbers of bacteria placed in the bladder cavity are cleared rapidly in man and animals. However, the balance between bacterial multiplication rates and host defense mechanisms is a delicate one. In animals as many as 10,000,000 *Escherichia coli* may be cleared rapidly from the bladder cavity, whereas slight physiologic alterations may permit the survival of as few as 10 microorganism which multiply rapidly and persist for prolonged periods.

The entire urinary tract must be looked upon as a single anatomic unit with a minute column of urine constantly maintaining a channel of communication between bladder and kidney. The ascent of bacteria within this channel from the bladder is the usual pathway for the majority of renal parenchymal infections. Most patients with bacteria in the bladder urine do not, however, have evidence of renal parenchymal infection, and the factors which determine whether the kidney will become infected are as a rule not clinically apparent.

Hematogenous pyelonephritis occurs most often in the late stages of terminal illness when there is general lowering of resistance to infection from either the primary illness or the use of potent agents which interfere with host antibacterial defenses. Staphylococcal pyelonephritis, however, may be seen following dissemination of bacteria from distant septic foci such as a carbuncle or osteomyelitis.

ASSOCIATED CONDITIONS. Age and Sex. Urinary infections are found in about 1 to 4 percent of females from childhood to the childbearing age. The prevalence of infection then rises, with the greatest increment occurring at about age sixty, beyond which age infections are detected in 5 to 10 percent of women. In men, on the other hand, urinary infections are rare below age fifty and even in older age groups are considerably less common than in women. There is evidence that race and socioeconomic status also influence the rates of infection.

Pregnancy. Depending on the socioeconomic status of the persons studied, urinary infections are detected in perhaps 4 to 8 percent of pregnant women. Another increment of infections occurs if bladder catheterization is performed at the time of or following delivery. The majority of infections during pregnancy are established before the time when dilatation of the ureters occurs. The infections that occur during pregnancy occur at a rate approximately consistent with that expected in the nonpregnant population.

It has been suspected that urinary infections and pyelonephritis are more common in toxemia of pregnancy. However, data utilizing modern bacteriologic techniques, although sparse, do not clearly support such a relation. There are, in addition, conflicting data concerning possible increased rates of prematurity and of newborn mortality in women with urinary infections.

Diabetes Mellitus. Despite reports that pyelonephritis at autopsy is very common in diabetics, clinical surveys of hospital and nonhospital populations have failed to document any convincing difference in the prevalence of urinary tract infections in diabetic and nondiabetic persons of the same age. This suggests either that diabetics with urinary infections are more likely to develop pyelonephritis or that in the presence of severe vascular and glomerular lesions in diabetic kidneys, morphologic changes result which are similar to those of bacterial infection. The problem requires further study. Irritation of the vulva in women with heavy uncontrolled glucosuria probably increases the rate of false positive voided urine cultures and may predispose to bladder infection. When diabetic neuropathy has interfered with normal bladder function, persistent infections of the urine are frequent.

Urinary infection may produce difficulties in the regulation of carbohydrate metabolism and may precipitate diabetic acidosis. The risk of additional renal disease caused by infection in persons already subject to severe vascular and glomerular disease is, of course, to be avoided whenever possible. Diabetics are also likely to develop *necrotizing papillitis,* a fulminating form of renal disease usually associated with infection.

Obstructive Uropathy. Any impediment to the free flow of urine—tumor, stricture, or stone—results in hydronephrosis and a greatly increased frequency of urinary tract infection. Infection superimposed on urinary tract obstruction may lead to the rapid destruction of renal tissue. It is of utmost importance, therefore, when infection is present, to repair obstructive lesions.

Instrumentation. Infection of the lower urinary passages is sometimes initiated by bacteria carried on catheters or other instruments being passed through the urethra into the bladder. Although the risk is small in normal people, it undoubtedly rises considerably in patients in hospital. Indwelling catheterization for 24 to 48 hr is usually accompanied by the initiation of a urinary infection, unless careful attention is directed to the proper use of closed drainage systems or the use of antibacterial lavage of the bladder and drainage system. These special techniques considerably lessen the risk of short-term catheterization (up to 1 week) but even with these precautions, infection rates steadily increase thereafter.

Renal Disease and Hypertension. Experimental and clinical evidence indicates that various renal diseases increase the susceptibility of the kidney to infection. In addition, persons with abnormal urinalyses or hypertension are likely to have had some diagnostic procedures involving urinary tract instrumentation, thereby providing access of bacteria to the urinary tract. A careful medical history is essential but often not sufficient to distinguish cause from effect.

In surveys of nonhospital populations it has been found that mean blood pressure levels are likely to be higher in women with urinary infections than in those without infections. The significance of this relation remains to be determined, and the data are not sufficient to ascertain whether rising blood pressure or urinary infection is primary. Too few infections have been found in men in these surveys to study the problem in that sex.

Neurogenic Bladder Dysfunction. Interference with the nerve supply to the bladder, as in spinal cord injury, tabes dorsalis, multiple sclerosis, etc., is likely to be associated with urinary tract infection. The infection may be initiated by the use of catheters for bladder drainage and favored by the prolonged standing of urine in the bladder. Additional factors which often operate in these patients are bone demineralization due to immobilization, causing hypercalciuria, calculus formation, and obstructive uropathy.

Experimental Evidence. Urinary tract infections can be produced in experimental animals by several methods, including inoculation of bacteria into the pelvis or substance of the kidney, or into the bladder urine. Certain organisms such as pseudomonas, enterococci, staphylococci, and monilias are capable of causing infection in the normal kidney when they are injected by the intravenous route. Coliform organisms will not do this as a rule, unless the kidney has previously been injured by mechanical bruising or acute obstruction of the ureter. It has also been shown that the renal damage resulting from a virus or staphylococcal infection can render the kidney susceptible to infection by colon bacilli injected intravenously.

The frequent association of urinary tract infection with an obstructive lesion has led to the widespread view that stasis of urinary flow is a prime factor in the development of infection. In support of this is the fact that urine is a good medium for growth of bacteria; hence, prolonged opportunity for multiplication during slow passage along the tract would provide a heavier inoculum to which the kidneys and other tissues of the tract are exposed. There may be an additional factor to explain the association between obstruction and urinary infection: the effect of increased hydrostatic pressure. To assess the relative importance of stasis and increased pressure is difficult, since slowing of flow of the fluid is an inevitable accompaniment of obstruction and dilatation of the passages above the level of obstruction. It may be said with assurance that even when a profuse diuresis is obtained in a patient with a partially obstructed urinary tract, this seldom achieves cure of an infection, whereas relief of the obstruction, with or without diuresis, may be followed by subsidence of infection. Even if the urinary infection is not cured, relief of obstruction materially reduces the risk of renal damage.

In urinary tract infection, two different areas are interacting: the tissues and the urine itself. On the basis of animal experiments and clinical observations it seems clear that infection beginning in one can spread to the other. The pathogenesis of chronic nonobstructive pyelonephritis is not well understood. Chronic pyelonephritis may be an indolent process consisting of many isolated microabscesses, some of them within single tubules. Here bacterial growth may be slow, phagocytosis inefficient, and antibacterial drugs incapable of acting optimally. Yet such areas may, from time to time, discharge their contents into the urinary passages, affording opportunity for rapid bacterial multiplication and spread to other parts of the system. In the urine phagocytosis is probably less effective than it is in tissues, and elimination of bacteria may call for more than simple bacteriostasis. This line of reasoning leads to the conclusion that optimal results in drug treatment require the use of an agent or a combination of agents capable of killing the infecting bacteria both in the tissues and in the urine.

In recent years clinical and experimental evidence has accumulated showing that the papilla and medulla of the kidney are particularly susceptible to bacterial infection. This is where bacterial multiplication begins in animals with pyelonephritis, and in this normally hypertonic environment host defense mechanisms such as leukocyte migration, phagocytosis, and complement activity are likely to be impaired. In addition, forms of bacteria with defective cell walls such as spheroplasts or protoplasts (a consequence of the action of antibiotics or complement and antibody) can survive and even initiate infection in the hypertonic environment of the renal medulla, whereas they would be expected to burst in tissues isotonic to plasma. Thus, in patients without urinary obstruction, decreasing the osmolarity of the papilla by drinking large quantities of water would be expected to increase the resistance of the kidney to infection. The question is unresolved as to whether water diuresis is helpful or not in the treatment of urinary infections in man.

Manifestations

CYSTITIS. This is the name used by many physicians to refer to urinary tract infection with pathognomonic local symptoms: frequency and urgency of micturition, and burning pain felt in the urethra during and immediately following the act. Prominent systemic manifestations of infection, such as fever above 101°F, muscular pain, nausea, vomiting, and prostration, should cause the physician to suspect concomitant infection in the kidney, prostate, or some other part of the body. Even in the absence of systemic manifestations of infection, it is usually not possible to be certain that infection is limited to the bladder area in patients with cystitis.

ACUTE PYELONEPHRITIS. The symptoms of acute pyelonephritis generally develop rapidly over a period of a few hours or a day or two. The characteristics are aching pain in the lumbar region, and fever which may be high (103 to 105°F), often with shaking chills. There may be nausea, vomiting, and diarrhea or, occasionally, constipation. Symptoms of cystitis are generally associated, and either one may precede the other.

On *physical examination*, in addition to fever and some generalized tenderness of the muscles, the key finding is tenderness on deep pressure in one or both of the costovertebral areas or on bimanual palpation of the kidney region. Occasionally, this sign is absent in acute pyelonephritis.

Except in individuals with papillary necrosis or urinary obstruction, *the manifestations of acute pyelonephritis usually subside within days, even without specific antibacterial therapy.* The patient becomes symptom-free, although laboratory tests may show that bacteriuria with or without pyuria is still present. When pyelonephritis is severe, fever subsides only slowly and may not disappear for several days even after appropriate antibiotic treatment has been started.

Undoubtedly some individuals recover completely and permanently after an attack of acute pyelonephritis, but in a considerable proportion of cases there are repeated attacks, at irregular intervals, sometimes over a period of many years; between these attacks the patient may be symptom-free. Bacilluria and pyuria are often demonstrable during these symptom-free intervals. The important point to be stressed is that infection in any part of the urinary tract is capable of subclinical continuation, which may persist for months or years. A patient with such a condition may exhibit no symptoms and may live an apparently normal life for long periods, even though urine cultures give continuing evidence of active infection.

Laboratory Findings

In *acute pyelonephritis* there is a polymorphonuclear leukocytosis, whereas in patients with localized or few symptoms the white blood cell picture is normal. The urine sediment in *acute pyelonephritis* or *cystitis* usually reveals numerous leukocytes occurring singly, in clumps, and in casts, and occasionally some red blood cells. Sometimes there is gross hematuria. The persistence of hematuria after localized or generalized symptoms of infection have subsided is unusual and should alert one to the possibility of tumor or tuberculosis within the genitourinary tract. In chronic infections of low-grade activity, diagnosis may be very difficult on the basis of urine sediment. There may be a few pus cells, or they may be found only intermittently during repeated urinalyses.

Enumeration of the numbers of bacteria in the urine is the most important diagnostic procedure. In symptomatic infections of the urinary tract, bacteria are virtually always easily demonstrable in large numbers in the urine. The absence of easily demonstrable bacteria in uncentrifuged bladder urine indicates that urinary infection is not likely to explain the patient's symptoms. Quantitative estimation of the number of bacteria in the urine, as a rule, makes it possible to distinguish contaminants (from the anterior urethra or elsewhere) from bacteria multiplying in the bladder urine and is, therefore, essential for the interpretation of urine cultures.

A rough quantitative estimate of the situation can be made by means of Gram's stain or microscopic examination of uncentrifuged freshly voided urine. If bacteria can be found by this method, it may be assumed that the number present is approximately 100,000 per ml. Since bacteria multiply in urine, when bacterial infection is present they usually achieve concentrations in excess of 100,000 viable units per milliliter. In culturing voided urine specimens contamination is common. It is essential, therefore, to examine two or three urine specimens bacteriologically before starting treatment in patients with few or no symptoms. In patients who are sufficiently ill to require prompt antibiotic therapy, a single quantitative estimate of the number of bacteria in the urine combined with symptoms typical of infection is sufficient to make the diagnosis of urinary infection. *If fewer than 10,000 viable bacterial units per milliliter are cultured from a voided urine specimen, they are likely to be of no significance.* Between 100,000 and 10,000 one cannot draw a positive conclusion. Since the large numbers of bacteria in the bladder urine are due in part to bacterial multiplication during residence in the bladder cavity, samples of urine from the ureters or renal pelves might contain considerably fewer bacteria and yet indicate infection. When the urine contains antibacterial substances or if the pH is low (about 5.0), inhibition of bacterial multiplication will also result in lower numbers of bacteria in the presence of the infection. For this reason, antiseptic solutions should not be used in washing the periurethral area prior to collection of the specimen urine. Intravenous pyelograms may be of value in the diagnosis of pyelonephritis, evidenced by an asymmetry between the kidneys as judged by their size and the density of the renal shadows. This, of course, is a reflection of the patchy distribution of the pyelonephritic lesion. It is said also that careful radiographic studies will show hypotony of the calyxes, pelvis, and ureters in a high proportion of these cases. Particular attention should be paid to papillary deformities and corresponding cortical scars. *Biopsy of the kidney* by needle for the purpose of demonstrating pyelonephritis is of limited value because the distribution of the lesions is spotty and because it is difficult to evaluate focal inflammatory lesions in a tiny sample of renal tissue.

Treatment

The soundest approach to treatment is based on a conception of the urinary tract as a complex system in which infection introduced into, or persisting in, any one part may spread to all the others. For example, certain drugs which have been recommended for treatment of urinary tract infection appear to be capable of acting only in urine. These, which include nalidixic acid, mandelic acid, urotropin, and nitrofurantoin, often suppress but may not eradicate infection. The antibiotics are generally also effective in tissues, although some are more likely to exert a bactericidal action than others. Sulfonamides are principally bacteriostatic. Another essential principle in management is to consider what factors in the patient may be contributing to the infection, such as obstruction, faulty bladder innervation, etc.; these were mentioned in Chap. 302. Relief of obstruction may be an essential factor in eradicating the infection. If the lesions are not progressive, it is important to weigh the risk of introducing infection during the repair procedure, against the likelihood of successfully relieving the obstruction. It is often the proper judgment to leave a nonprogressive obstructive lesion alone.

In antibacterial therapy, best results are obtained when the treatment is individualized. Advertisements and medical articles which describe the effectiveness of any one agent in the treatment of urinary infections are misleading. There is a wide choice of agents which may be used, and the best results are obtained by employing the appropriate therapy suited to the individual patient.

In view of the varying conditions under which bacteria grow in urine and in urinary tract tissues, it seems probable that the ideal chemotherapeutic attack is one which is capable of bactericidal, not simply bacteriostatic, action. The synthetic penicillins meet this requirement. Determination of possible synergistic or antagonistic effects of combinations of agents on the bacteria to be attacked is sometimes necessary. Streptomycin is a valuable agent, its main defect being the rapidity with which bacteria develop resistance to it; this defect can be lessened, however, by giving streptomycin in combination with another antibiotic such as tetracycline. Enterococcus infections may yield to a combination of penicillin and streptomycin. For proteus infections, the antibiotics most likely to be beneficial are Kanamycin, penicillin in massive doses, or neomycin. For pseudomonas infection, polymyxin or colistin may be required. Since the use, contraindications, dosages, etc., of these agents are covered in detail in another chapter, they will not be repeated here. Many antibiotics are potentially nephrotoxic. It often requires considerable clinical judgment to decide between the risk of renal damage due to treatment and that due to infection (Chap. 135).

In view of the nature of urinary tract infection, it seems possible that prolonged treatment, for about 2 weeks to several months, might be ideal. This, however, is impractical in many situations, and its efficacy has not yet been demonstrated. Nevertheless, every effort should be made to administer the appropriate drug or drugs for 7 to 10 days, no matter how prompt the symptomatic response may be. It is essential to obtain follow-up urine cultures after discontinuing treatment, to avoid overlooking smoldering asymptomatic infection with its potentialities for eventual development of serious disease. It is wise to avoid catheter specimens for urine examinations, since catheterization may actually cause reinfection of the urinary tract. With proper care it is possible to obtain suitable "clean-voided" specimens of urine from females as well as males. Since bacteria multiply rapidly in urine, a specimen should be cultured or refrigerated immediately. Specimens kept at about 4°C for as long as 1 to 4 weeks are still suitable for bacteriologic culture.

It has now been established that many patients with recurrent urinary infections can be treated effectively with very low dosages of a variety of antibacterial agents given over a long period of time. As little as 50 to 100 mg nitrofurantoin or 0.5 to 1.0 Gm nalidixic acid or 0.5 to 1.0 Gm of a soluble short-acting sulfonamide given at bedtime, with perhaps another dose upon arising, may keep the urine sterile in patients who up to the time of treatment had been subject to recurrent symptomatic infections at monthly intervals. Even patients with nonprogressive urinary obstruction, neurogenic bladder, or staghorn calculi may respond dramatically to such treatment. In most instances discontinuing antibiotics is associated with prompt reappearance of bacteriuria or recurrence of infection.

The action of antibiotics used in this way can best be understood by reference to the delicate balance between host defense mechanisms and invading microorganisms which has been demonstrated in the bladder cavity in animals. It is possible to look upon these antibacterial agents as interfering with bacterial multiplication sufficiently to permit host defenses to be effective.

Prognosis

It is usually possible to obtain a dramatic cessation of symptoms in the treatment of acute urinary infection not complicated by other diseases. The dangerous feature is persistence of relatively asymptomatic infection, which will gradually destroy the kidney. It is not possible to state which patients with urinary infections will eventually suffer renal damage and which patients may have persistent infection without significant damage to the kidney. Nevertheless, the fact that a significant proportion of patients coming to autopsy show evidence of pyelonephritis and some degree of renal damage indicates the importance of this problem. In patients with some of the complicating diseases mentioned above, particularly neurogenic bladder, irremediable obstruction, or multiple stones, eradication of urinary tract infection is exceedingly difficult, if not impossible. Even here, however, the extent of the process can be minimized by comprehensive care, including surgical measures, prevention of stone formation, and appropriate chemotherapy guided by reliable laboratory procedures.

CHRONIC PYELONEPHRITIS

In contrast to urinary tract infections, for which simple diagnostic criteria are available, the diagnosis of chronic pyelonephritis is reached only after careful consideration of nonspecific clinical and pathologic data. Because of the nonspecific nature of the diagnostic criteria, there is a great deal of debate about how frequently chronic pyelonephritis is responsible for significant renal disease. For example, autopsy surveys have found chronic pyelonephritis in from 1.6 to 35 percent of cases. Most observers report prevalence of about 3.0 percent. Aside from difficulties in making the diagnosis, other factors influence these data: nature of the hospital, age of the patients, percentage of autopsies obtained on different hospital services, etc.

Etiology

There is general agreement, however, about some facts. *Urinary obstruction* is a common accompaniment of chronic pyelonephritis, but in a large proportion of cases obstruction cannot be demonstrated anatomically. Most patients with renal lesions which fulfill criteria for chronic pyelonephritis at autopsy have sterile kidney cultures and were not known to have had clinical episodes of bacterial urinary infection. These observations have stimulated investigations into factors other than obstruction which make the kidney susceptible to infection and into other injuries which may result in morphologic changes in the kidney resembling those produced by bacterial infection.

Pathology

The kidneys are frequently asymmetric in size. The parenchyma is scarred, and the surface is coarsely and irregularly pitted. In many areas glomeruli and tubules are completely replaced by connective tissue, which may contain lymphocytes and plasma cells. Foci of active interstitial inflammation may be seen throughout the medulla and cortex, and leukocyte casts are found in some tubules. Other tubules are dilated and contain large amounts of homogeneous eosinophilic material (colloid casts). Most glomeruli appear relatively normal in comparison with the nearby atrophic tubular and inflammatory interstitial changes. The capsule of many glomeruli is disproportionately thickened and fibrotic in contrast to the relative integrity of the Malpighian tufts. Some glomerular loops may be thickened or hyalinized, probably as a result of vascular changes proximally, and cortically there are clusters of fibrotic glomeruli, especially within the wedges of atrophic areas. Often, distinctive inflammatory changes in the pelvic mucosa are lacking. A proliferative endarteritis is usually present, most marked in the areas of chronic inflammation. More generalized and severe vascular changes develop with the onset of hypertension.

It should be emphasized that even at the autopsy table, the diagnosis of chronic pyelonephritis is often not clearcut. None of the foregoing changes is pathognomonic of chronic infection of the kidneys, though when taken together they are useful in suggesting the diagnosis. Similar morphologic features may be encountered as a result of many diseases, including the nephropathy of chronic potassium depletion, nephrocalcinosis, chronic poisoning with analgesic mixtures, primary vascular disease of the kidneys, obstruction, diabetes mellitus, and tubular necrosis. The point to be emphasized is that the kidney responds similarly to a variety of insults. When the damage is principally interstitial, the reaction will take the form of what is called acute or chronic interstitial nephritis. Chronic pyelonephritis is chronic interstitial nephritis resulting from bacterial infection. Since urinary infections are common and frequently initiated by instrumentation of the urinary tract in attempting to diagnose renal disease, the determination of the contribution of infection in any particular patient with renal disease may not be possible.

Clinical Features

"Starting with a pyelitis in childhood, an infection of the urinary tract during pregnancy, or, in rare instances, an acute pyelonephritis, there may be from time to time attacks of *unexplained fever,* with or without slight or fairly severe pain in the lumbar regions. These attacks are often accompanied by the passage of cloudy urine. Occasionally there is a history of albuminuria of many years' duration. Often there is a story of malnutrition or sometimes of retarded growth in children, leading occasionally to rickety deformities. In some instances the progress of the disease is, for years, symptomless. The majority of patients fall into the last-named category. Early symptoms are particularly infrequent in the group with bilaterally atrophic, nonobstructed kidneys. A history of acute pyelitis in childhood may be especially difficult to obtain because the symptoms are mainly gastrointestinal, the physical signs are scanty, and pyuria is difficult to demonstrate; a history of persistent enuresis is sometimes the only helpful clue.

Patients often, therefore, come to the attention of the physician only when renal failure or hypertension has made its appearance, or because of the accidental discovery of proteinuria. *Fatigue* and *lassitude* associated with anemia may be the presenting complaints. If renal failure is severe, nausea and vomiting or breathlessness may be present. Edema is rare, and when it occurs it is a result of heart failure. Splenomegaly occurs in some patients with chronic pyelonephritis; when it is associated with anemia, a primary hematologic disease may be simulated.

Many patients with chronic pyelonephritis develop *hypertension* at some time in the course of their illness. It has been suggested that this is related to the contraction of scar tissue and to endarteritis obliterans with focal renal ischemia, rather than to diffuse renal damage. The blood pressure may become elevated long before there is measurable impairment of renal function, and only a persistently positive urine culture or characteristic changes in the intravenous pyelogram may distinguish the clinical picture from that of "essential" or "malignant" hypertension. The incidence of hypertension is greater in the interstitial, nonobstructive form of pyelonephritis than in the obstructive variety; in the former group rapidly progressive vascular disease occurs terminally in 15 to 20 percent of cases.

In general, glomerular filtration and renal blood flow decline together and proportionally as the disease progresses. As might be expected, there is usually more disparity between the function of the right and left kidneys than is generally the case in diffuse diseases of the kidney such as glomerulonephritis or nephrosclerosis. Maximum concentrating ability tends to become impaired earlier in the course of the disease than in patients with chronic glomerulonephritis. Occasional patients with advanced azotemia may excrete a urine hypotonic to plasma, even when they are dehydrated. Many patients are unable to conserve sodium on a low salt diet, even when only mild azotemia is present. *Polyuria* and *nocturia* are prominent in such cases. *Hyperchloremic acidosis* as a result of impaired renal excretion of acid and reabsorption of bicarbonate is more often a feature of chronic pyelonephritis than of glomerulonephritis. Proteinuria is usually less than 2 Gm (rarely as much as 4 to 6 Gm) daily, except when congestive heart failure supervenes.

Careful examination of the urinary sediment is often the key to diagnosis. Leukocytes may be numerous or infrequent, but the appearance of white blood cell casts should alert the physician to the possibility of chronic pyelonephritis. Bacteria may be present on the fresh stained smear but, together with pus cells, often appear intermittently or not at all in the chronic atrophic stage of the disease. It should be noted that the urine sediment may be normal and, especially with a dilute urine of fixed specific gravity, that no albuminuria, or only a trace, may be detected. On intravenous or retrograde pyelography, distortion, flattening, and reduction in size of the renal pelves can be seen. The renal substance may be narrowed unevenly and the underlying pyramid distorted or destroyed to produce "blunting" of the calyxes. The absence of roentgenographic changes does not, however, rule out chronic pyelonephritis.

When pyelonephritis is not accompanied by hypertension, the course may be prolonged and compatible with comfortable and useful life even after considerable encroachment upon renal function. In perhaps no other disease of the kidneys can fluctuations in renal function be so marked or so frequent. During acute infections or episodes of dehydration, renal decompensation may progress to the stage of advanced uremia; yet the patient may be able to recover and carry on with adequate though impaired renal function for years. Nonspecific complaints of fatigue, anorexia, and weakness often remit remarkably when the urine is sterilized by an appropriate course of antibiotics and if acidosis, dehydration, and salt depletion are adequately treated.

The problem of *recurrent infections*, sometimes with resistant bacteria, is important and unsolved. An effort should be made to treat urinary tract obstruction and to improve bladder emptying, when residual urine is present. Reducing the bacterial population of bladder urine by the prolonged administration of urinary antiseptics may offer some hope for halting the indolent progression of the disease.

It should be emphasized that even when one kidney appears small and the other normal in size, pyelonephritis is in most instances bilateral. Nephrectomy which is undertaken in the hope of eradicating the disease is generally doomed to failure. Excision of a hydronephrotic, pus-filled renal shell will, however, sometimes permit a successful therapeutic attack on infection in the opposite kidney with a carefully chosen antibiotic given in adequate dosage for a long period of time.

It is important to recognize that this general view of the frequency of asymptomatic destruction of the kidney in pyelonephritis may be incorrect since patients may not have had pyelonephritis but rather some other form of chronic interstitial nephritis. Proper understanding of the problem requires continued careful study with clear recognition of the possible error of traditional concepts.

PAPILLARY NECROSIS

When severe infection of the renal pyramids is present in association with vascular diseases of the kidney or urinary tract obstruction, renal papillary necrosis is likely to result. Patients with diabetes, sickle-cell hemoglobin, chronic alcoholism, and vascular disease seem peculiarly susceptible to this complication. *Hematuria, pain in the flank* or abdomen, *chills,* and *fever* are the most common presenting symptoms. Acute renal failure with oliguria or anuria sometimes occurs. Rarely, sloughing of a pyramid may take place without symptoms in a patient with chronic urinary infection, and the diagnosis is made when the necrotic tissue is passed in the urine or identified as a "ring shadow" on pyelography. If renal function deteriorates suddenly in a diabetic patient or one with chronic obstruction, this diagnosis should be entertained, even in the absence of fever or pain.

The chronic overuse of drug mixtures containing *phenacetin* and perhaps other analgesics predisposes to necrotizing papillitis which may be unassociated with renal infection or obstruction and present the picture of slowly progressive renal insufficiency. This problem is much more common than generally recognized, and diagnosis requires careful attention to historical information obtained from the patient.

PROSTATITIS

This term is loosely used to designate various inflammatory conditions affecting the prostate. These include acute and chronic infections with specific bacteria and, more commonly, instances where signs and symptoms of prostatic inflammation are present but no specific organisms can be detected. Patients in this category usually have low-back pain and perineal or testicular discomfort. They may have microscopic pyuria or hematuria without any other evidence of genitourinary disease. Such patients are generally treated symptomatically by prostatic massage and warm sitz baths, but many receive antibiotics, with variable results. In some cases infection may be secondary to the T strain of mycoplasma which has been incriminated in the pathogenesis of specific urethritis.

Acute Bacterial Prostatitis

This disease generally affects young male adults when it occurs spontaneously, but it may be associated with an indwelling urethral catheter. It is characterized by fever, chills, dysuria, and a tense or boggy, extremely tender prostate. Palpation of the prostate is the key to diagnosis. The infection is generally due to one of the common urinary tract pathogens or *Staphylococcus aureus,* and the response to antibiotics is usually prompt. The long-term prognosis is good, although in some instances, acute infection may result in abscess formation and a residual chronic bacterial prostatitis. Since the advent of antibiotics, the frequency of acute bacterial prostatitis has diminished markedly, and it is now an uncommon cause of acute urinary tract infection.

Chronic Bacterial Prostatitis

This entity is less well defined. Symptoms are usually absent, the prostate feels normal on palpation, and although many white blood cells may be seen in the urinary sediment, conventional bacteriologic studies are negative. Stamey and his colleagues have added considerably to the understanding of this problem. They have shown that chronic bacterial prostatitis is characterized by the presence of small numbers of bacteria which may be cultured from the expressed prostatic secretion. The presence of these bacteria can be determined only by careful quantitative bacteriologic techniques when the bladder urine is sterile. The usual symptoms of frequency and dysuria occur when infection spreads to the bladder urine, but infection confined to the prostate is asymptomatic. Antibiotics are of limited value in eradicating the foci of chronic infection in the prostate, even though they may relieve the symptoms of the acute exacerbations promptly. The relative ineffectiveness of antimicrobials is due in part to the poor penetration of most antibiotics into the prostate because the low pH which prevails in this organ precludes solubility of most drugs. The macrolide group of drugs (erythromycin, oleandomycin) do enter the prostatic secretions, but these agents are generally ineffective against gram-negative organisms. These patients should be managed with prolonged courses of antimicrobials with a view toward suppressing symptoms and keeping the bladder urine sterile.

Urinary infections are much less common in men than in women, perhaps because of the antibacterial properties of prostatic fluid. The pattern of recurrent bladder infection in the male with chronic bacterial prostatitis is clinically not very different from that seen in the recurrent cystourethritis of the female. It has been suggested that this pattern of infection in women is due to chronic bacterial infection of the paraurethral glands and ducts, which are in fact vestigial remnants of the prostate.

REFERENCES

Beeson, P. B.: Urinary Tract Infection and Pyelonephritis, in "Renal Disease," 2d ed., D. A. K. Black (Ed.), Oxford, Blackwell Scientific Publications, Ltd., 1967.

Freedman, L. R.: Urinary Tract Infection, Pyelonephritis and Other Forms of Chronic Interstitial Nephritis, in "Diseases of the Kidney," 2d ed., M. B. Strauss and L. G. Welt (Eds.), Boston, Little, Brown and Company, 1969.

Kass, E. H.: "Progress in Pyelonephritis," Philadelphia, F. A. Davis Company, 1965.

Meares, E. M., and T. A. Stamey: Bacteriologic Localization Patterns in Bacterial Prostatitis and Urethritis, Invest. Urol., 5:492, 1968.

Norden, C. W., and E. H. Kass: Bacteriuria of Pregnancy. A Critical Appraisal, Ann. Rev. Med., 19:431, 1968.

304 GLOMERULONEPHRITIS, ACUTE AND CHRONIC. LUPUS, SCLERODERMA, AND PERIARTERITIS

Franklin H. Epstein

ACUTE GLOMERULONEPHRITIS

Acute glomerulonephritis is an acute diffuse inflammation of the glomeruli of the kidneys. It represents about

0.5 percent of all admissions to general hospitals in the United States and is found at autopsy in 0.1 to 0.2 percent of deaths. The disease is twice as frequent in males as in females. Although it is more common in children than in adults, it is found in adults of every age.

Etiology

Acute glomerulonephritis is a pattern of reaction of the kidneys, rather than a single disease with a specific cause. Preceding infection with the group A, beta-hemolytic streptococcus is the most common cause. The infection usually arises in the upper part of the respiratory tract, and its severity is not necessarily related to the incidence or severity of the ensuing nephritis. Streptococcal infection of the skin or of wounds may also be followed by glomerulonephritis. There is considerable evidence that only certain strains of group A streptococci are nephritogenic; these include types 12, 4, 25, and Red Lake.

Acute nephritis has been reported by Bates, Jennings, and Earle as a complication of an epidemic of acute pharyngitis, presumably of viral origin, in which streptococcal infection was excluded by bacteriologic and immunologic evidence. Bacterial endocarditis is frequently complicated by acute glomerulonephritis, and glomerulonephritis has occasionally been reported to follow other acute infections.

Acute nephritis superficially resembling the poststreptococcal variety may occur in the course of lupus erythematosus, periarteritis, or erythema nodosum. It is commonly seen as a complication of the allergic purpuras, associated with joint or abdominal pain. Finally, it may be a manifestation of hypersensitivity to drugs or other foreign agents.

Pathogenesis

Glomerulonephritis is an immunologic disorder that may be produced by two quite different and distinct pathogenetic mechanisms. The first is based upon production by the patient of antibodies capable of reacting with his own glomerular basement membrane, which form a smooth deposit along the glomerular membrane, identifiable by immunofluorescent stains. The second depends upon the patient's production of antibodies capable of reacting with nonglomerular exogenous or endogenous antigens in his circulation, with the resultant formation of circulating antigen-antibody complexes that are subsequently trapped in the glomerular filter. Either process serves to concentrate an antigen-antibody reaction in the glomeruli, where it causes inflammation via mediators such as complement and polymorphonuclear leukocytes.

The first mechanism is probably operative in certain cases of Goodpasture's syndrome, as well as in experimental nephrotoxic serum nephritis. It is not the cause of poststreptococcal nephritis, but it may serve to perpetuate and extend glomerular damage in this disease when the nephritis becomes chronic. The second mecha-

nism is the likely cause of the poststreptococcal disease, as well as of the nephritis of serum sickness and lupus. Macromolecular conglomerates of antigen, antibody, and complement appear on electron microscopy as lumpy deposits within the glomerular filter. In poststreptococcal nephritis, the presumed antigen is streptococcal M protein; in lupus erythematosus it is DNA; in serum sickness and drug reactions it is, in each case, a specific exogenous antigen, usually unrelated to the kidney.

The latent period between streptococcal infection and the first symptoms of nephritis (which may last 1 to 4 weeks but averages 10 to 14 days) thus represents the time necessary for the development of circulating antibodies to the streptococcal antigens. The *fall in serum complement* characteristic of an attack of acute nephritis is a result of combination with antigen-antibody complexes in the kidney.

Pathology

The kidneys are normal in size or swollen. The surfaces are smooth and spotted with fine punctate hemorrhages; the pyramids are markedly congested. All or almost all glomeruli are generally involved; yet the degree of inflammation may vary from one to another and be focal in distribution inside the glomerular tuft. In poststreptococcal nephritis, the glomeruli are usually swollen and hypercellular, with thickened glomerular loops, infiltrating polymorphonuclear leukocytes, and proliferation of endothelial and epithelial cells. Occasionally, however, especially when function is completely recovered but while the urine sediment is still abnormal, renal biopsy will reveal glomeruli which appear normal except for occasional focal thickening of basement membranes. Red blood cells and red blood cell casts are present in the tubular lumens. Tubular cells may appear flattened or vacuolated, but pathologic changes in tubules are minimal compared with those in the glomeruli. Afferent arterioles sometimes show focal medial necrosis with perivascular cellular infiltrates, and there may be similar lesions of the interlobular vessels.

As the disease process subsides, there may be complete resolution of the inflammatory process, with restoration of normal architecture. More frequently, hyalinized glomeruli, glomerular adhesions, and vascular changes persist, with wedge-shaped areas of atrophy and fibrosis separated by areas of relatively well-preserved tissue in which the remaining tubules are dilated. Even after the urine has completely cleared, focal hypercellularity and thickening of the stalks of glomerular lobules may persist. Widespread proliferation of the capsular epithelium, producing glomerular "crescents," is a characteristic finding when the condition deteriorates rapidly, with the patient dying with hypertension and oliguria within 1 to 12 months of the onset of the disease.

Clinical Features and Pathologic Physiology

The typical patient develops a pharyngitis with fever and malaise. Microscopic hematuria may be found during the first few days of the respiratory illness when fever is present, but it then disappears. One or two weeks after the onset of the infection, when the initial symptoms have completely subsided, weakness and anorexia return. The patient awakens with puffiness of the eyes and notices shortness of breath or swelling of the ankles during the day. The urine is scanty and looks like Coca-Cola or diluted coffee. Abdominal pain, nausea, and vomiting may be prominent. High blood pressure, usually asymptomatic, may be heralded by headache or an unexpected convulsion. The clinical picture is often dominated by one or more manifestations which overshadow the rest and which initially mislead the physician who anticipates a "classical" pattern.

Fatigue and *anorexia* are almost universal; it is unusual for a patient with acute glomerulonephritis to feel as well as before the illness or to have a good appetite.

Pain in the loins or abdomen may be colicky or steady and, in exceptional instances, may be so severe as to simulate a surgical condition. Fever generally does not exceed 101°F and usually subsides within a few days. Persistent fever may be caused by residual streptococcal or other infection, by a reaction to antibiotics, or by extrarenal vasculitis.

Although facial *edema* is extremely common, edema of the legs without any swelling of the face is frequent, especially in older persons. Edema may be generally distributed and hence unapparent; and the only clue to its presence may be a 5- or 8-lb weight loss after the patient is put to bed and given a low salt diet. Localization of edema about the eyes is best explained by the low tissue turgor in this region. The absence of orthopnea, at least during the early stages of the disease, further favors accumulation of fluid in the upper half of the body during the hours of sleep.

Whether salt and water retention in acute nephritis is primarily due to renal disease per se or is secondary to other circulatory disturbances which provoke even normal kidneys to retain sodium is not entirely clear. Considerable evidence suggests that disproportionate reduction in glomerular filtration rate is responsible for the initial oliguria and subsequent retention of sodium which result in excessive accumulation of extracellular fluid. Edema formation is generally associated with some decrease in the inulin clearance and with diuresis which produces a fall in blood urea nitrogen level. Nevertheless, diuresis may be initiated in acute nephritis without any measurable improvement in a depressed filtration rate; the relationship between impaired inulin clearance and sodium retention is therefore not simple or clear-cut. Generalized capillary damage is probably *not* a cause of edema in nephritis, since the edema fluid does not contain increased amounts of protein. Although hypoalbuminemia resulting from extensive losses of plasma protein into the urine may contribute to edema in some cases, this factor cannot be the most important one in the many instances where plasma volume, by direct measurement, is increased or normal. Urinary excretion of aldosterone is low in acute glomerulonephritis in the presence of edema, even when the patient is on a salt-free diet. As might be expected in such a situation, spironolactone does not provoke diuresis. Renal retention of sodium under these circumstances is probably a result of altered renal hemodynamics, rather than of excessive secretion of salt-retaining hormone by the adrenal cortex.

Together with edema, signs and symptoms of *congestive heart failure* are often prominent, whether or not arterial hypertension is present. The sudden onset of heart failure in a previously well person may be the manifestation which brings the patient with acute nephritis to the doctor. Fatal pulmonary edema may be precipitated by convulsions. The heart is usually somewhat enlarged, and the venous pressure may be elevated. Nonspecific alterations in the electrocardiogram are common. Unlike the pattern of "low-output" cardiac failure, the circulation time is typically normal or short, and cardiac output is normal even when edema is present or increasing. Under such circumstances cardiac output does not rise further when digitalis is administered. It seems probable that, in most cases, circulatory congestion is a result of fluid retention rather than its cause. It should be emphasized, however, that heart failure responsive to digitalis (and associated with a prolonged circulation time) may at times complicate acute nephritis. When orthopnea is present, especially if accompanied by rales or gallop rhythm, digitalis should be prescribed. In other instances of edema and elevated venous pressure, a careful therapeutic trial of digitalis should be undertaken, with the knowledge that in many instances it will be found ineffective.

Hypertension is observed in approximately 50 percent of adults with nephritis admitted to a general hospital. The incidence is lower in mild cases detected in the course of a streptococcal epidemic. The onset is usually coincident with the first abnormal urinary findings, although in certain cases it may even precede and in others follow them.

The reason for the high blood pressure is not established. Though it is tempting to invoke a pressor substance liberated by the kidney, the level of renin in peripheral blood is normal in many patients with acute hypertension due to nephritis.

The *optic fundi* are generally normal but may show arteriolar narrowing and, in exceptional circumstances, papilledema, hemorrhages, and fluffy exudates.

When the blood pressure rises rapidly, headache, somnolence, and *convulsions* may develop, simulating in an occasional case the clinical picture of brain tumor. The differential diagnosis in such instances is not made easier by the fact that proteinuria and microscopic hematuria are often detected immediately following generalized seizures of any origin. Vomiting, dehydration, and heart failure appear to predispose to convulsions. They are not dependent on nitrogen retention but are probably the result of cerebral ischemia or tiny hemorrhages secondary to changes in the cerebral vasculature.

Mild *anemia* occurs frequently in acute glomerulonephritis, especially with edema. Total red blood cell mass has been found to be normal in many such patients, in whom the low hematocrit reflects dilution. In addition, depression of the bone marrow and increased destruction of red blood cells contribute to anemia in certain azotemic patients. Serum albumin level may be low as a result of urinary losses and of the excessive catabolism of protein observed in many acute diseases or injuries. Serum cholesterol level is sometimes elevated even when serum albumin is not greatly decreased. The presence of anemia and hypercholesterolemia, then, does not necessarily mean that nephritis is chronic or progressive.

Changes in renal function which occur in acute nephritis are characteristic. Glomerular filtration rate is usually depressed, and to a greater degree than renal blood flow. The latter may, indeed, be elevated, though in severe cases it falls as well. Filtration fraction is therefore reduced. Blood urea nitrogen is elevated in perhaps half the patients with glomerulonephritis. In cases of mild or moderate severity, phenolsulfonphthalein excretion is either normal or only slightly decreased, even when the blood urea nitrogen level is elevated. With more severe initial involvement, or with progression of the disease, excretion of phenolsulfonphthalein falls. Acid urine of high specific gravity may be excreted early in the course of the illness, despite pronounced azotemia. *The combination of azotemia with well-maintained phenolsulfonphthalein excretion and high urinary specific gravity is seen in few diseases of the kidney other than acute glomerulonephritis.*

The *urine* may be grossly bloody or coffee-colored; on the other hand hematuria may be apparent only on careful inspection of the spun sediment. The identification of red blood cells embedded in casts establishes the glomerular origin of the bleeding. Granular and epithelial cell casts, especially the latter, are characteristically present. Lipid droplets and fatty casts are usually not seen at the very onset of the disease, but may appear within the first few weeks, regardless of the presence or absence of hyperlipemia in the serum. Leukocytes and white blood cell casts reflect the essentially inflammatory character of the glomerular lesion. Proteinuria may reach impressive levels, over 6 to 8 Gm daily, but is more often below 2 Gm per day. Especially during recovery, protein may disappear from the urine while red blood cells and red blood cell casts continue to be excreted.

The disease is sometimes ushered in by a period of *oliguria* which sometimes progresses to complete anuria. Usually this lasts only a few days, but an occasional case has been reported of acute glomerulonephritis with anuria lasting more than 20 days, followed by complete recovery. The oliguria which occurs at the onset of acute nephritis has a much better prognosis than that which may supervene when the disease has been active for several weeks. In contrast to the condition in patients with acute tubular necrosis and oliguria, urinary sodium concentration is very low (less than 15 mEq per liter) and urinary osmolarity is usually above that of plasma.

Extrarenal vasculitis may be an important concomitant of nephritis. Its myocardial and cerebral manifestations have already been mentioned. Purpuric rashes, subungual hemorrhages, and even acute arthritis may rarely be seen in the course of severe poststreptococcal nephritis. At postmortem examination, necrotizing and organizing lesions of periarteritis may be found in the kidneys and elsewhere.

Pulmonary infiltration and *hemoptysis* occur most frequently in acute nephritis as a result of circulatory congestion and do not necessarily imply a bad prognosis. In certain cases, however, when the nephritis is of the rapidly progressive, crescentic variety, necrotizing alveolitis produces massive pulmonary hemorrhage, indistinguishable from *idiopathic pulmonary hemosiderosis.* The term *Goodpasture's syndrome* has been applied to this condition In other cases, periarteritis is present in the lung vessels, often with granuloma formation (*Wegener's granulomatosis*). In most patients with nephritis, hemoptysis is associated with foamy sputum and is the result of left ventricular failure with pulmonary hypertension and edema.

Finally, it should be emphasized that patients may develop acute nephritis with no symptoms and no abnormal physical or laboratory findings other than mild proteinuria and an abnormal urinary sediment. Several cases have even been documented in which the renal biopsy showed typical changes of acute glomerulonephritis although the urine was normal.

Differential Diagnosis

Periorbital edema, occurring as an initial symptom of urticaria, trichinosis, infectious mononucleosis, or insect bites about the face may suggest acute nephritis until the urine is examined. The finding of red blood cell casts and the coincidence of an elevated blood urea nitrogen level with normal phenolsulfonphthalein excretion serve to exclude many other diseases of the urinary tract, in which glomeruli are not primarily affected. The nephritis associated with lupus, polyarteritis nodosa, and subacute bacterial endocarditis will often be recognized as a complication of the primary disease, but sometimes may be its only manifestation. The characteristic elevation and subsequent fall of antistreptolysin titer is excellent evidence of preceding streptococcal infection, but it may not be present, especially when the infection has been treated with penicillin. Gross hematuria with lower urinary symptoms is much more likely to be due to hemorrhagic cystitis or prostatitis. In middle-aged or elderly men, azotemia and hematuria may be mistakenly ascribed to the prostate until the daily excretion of protein is found to be greater than 2 Gm, suggesting the correct diagnosis of glomerulonephritis. The presence of small kidneys or of severe anemia (less than 8 Gm hemoglobin) suggests chronic renal disease, as do the stigmas of prolonged hypertension in heart or fundi. In the elderly, acute nephritis is often misdiagnosed as heart failure, until disproportionate oliguria and the abnormal urinary sediment call attention to the kidneys.

Idiopathic malignant hypertension accompanied by hematuria and azotemia, may present diagnostic difficulties, though such patients often have a previous history of high blood pressure and the degree of hypertension is greater than in the usual case of nephritis. Spontaneous improvement in blood pressure and renal function is unlikely in malignant hypertension and favors a diagnosis of glomerulonephritis. *The appearance of acute nephritis immediately following a respiratory infection, without a latent period, suggests an acute exacerbation of chronic nephritis.* Persistent fever, cardiac murmurs, or a palpable spleen should spur a search for subacute bacterial endocarditis.

Course and Prognosis

The course and outlook of acute glomerulonephritis vary widely. In children or young adults who develop nephritis following streptococcal infection, the entire disease may be over within 2 to 4 weeks. Most children recover completely, although a small number (less than 10 percent) go rapidly downhill and die within the first few months. On the other hand, in the adult population of a general hospital the likelihood of chronicity is much greater. It has been estimated that 50 percent of adult patients hospitalized with acute glomerulonephritis either succumb to the acute episode or develop chronic disease. The latter may be quiescent for long periods and manifested only by proteinuria and an abnormal urinary sediment. The ultimate outcome bears a rough relation to the initial severity of the illness, though there are many exceptions to this rule. The most frequent duration of the disease in hospitalized adults is probably about 2 to 3 months. Blood pressure usually returns to normal before the urine clears. Heavy proteinuria lasting longer than 3 to 4 months suggests a poor prognosis, though nephritis may heal completely even after proteinuria has been present for as long as 2 years. Microscopic hematuria commonly persists for some months after proteinuria has disappeared or diminished to a faint trace. Postural dizziness, easy flushing, and other signs of autonomic instability, as well as postural proteinuria, are not infrequent during convalescence. After the urine has become completely normal on several examinations, a second attack of nephritis is extremely unlikely, probably because of the persistence of type-specific antibodies to the hemolytic streptococcus.

Acute nephritis associated with anaphylactoid purpura (Henoch-Schönlein disease) has a much worse initial prognosis and higher incidence of chronicity than the poststreptococcal variety.

Treatment

Penicillin should be given to eradicate residual streptococcal infection even when this is not proved but only suspected. It has been suggested that early treatment of streptococcal infections with penicillin may prevent nephritis, but in the only study performed to test this hypothesis the number of patients observed was too small to permit statistically valid conclusions to be drawn.

During the acute stages *bed rest* is indicated, at least until the systemic manifestations of the disease have disappeared. There is no critical evidence to establish that further rest in bed appreciably modifies the course, although most studies concerned with this problem have been carried out in children with mild nephritis in whom complete recovery is the rule. If proteinuria or microscopic hematuria is the only remaining sign after 6 weeks to 2 months of rest in bed, the patient may be allowed up.

In the presence of edema or signs of *heart failure* salt should be restricted. Treatment for congestive heart failure is discussed above. During the initial stages of the disease, when urinary output is restricted, it may be wise to limit the intake of protein as outlined in Chap. 300, Acute Renal Failure. There is no reason, however, to restrict protein during convalescence.

Hypertensive crises may be treated with 0.5 to 2.5 mg reserpine intramuscularly two to four times a day, by alpha-methyl-dopa, or by an infusion of magnesium sulfate (Chap. 276).

Adrenal steroids have no clear-cut beneficial effect in acute nephritis. When massive doses of steroids or azothioprine have been used in occasional instances of rapidly progressive glomerulonephritis with oliguria, they have failed to modify the course.

CHRONIC GLOMERULONEPHRITIS

Chronic glomerulonephritis is not a single entity but a collection of different diseases which predominantly affect the glomerular tufts, causing inflammatory changes and subsequent scarring. It may be expected that as knowledge of the nature of renal disease expands, additional nosologic entities will emerge from the group termed "chronic glomerulonephritis" as distinctly as Kimmelstiel-Wilson disease and lupus nephritis have in the past.

Incidence

Chronic glomerulonephritis affects all ages but is more frequent before forty. It is more common in men than in women. Occasionally a strong familial predisposition is apparent. Only a minority of patients have a clear-cut history of acute onset following infection or have evidence of antibodies against nephritogenic strains of streptococci. Some cases of chronic nephritis probably originate in an unapparent infection with streptococcus, following which edema or bloody urine was not noticed, but it seems likely that most instances represent some disease other than poststreptococcal glomerulonephritis.

Classical Course

The course and duration of chronic glomerulonephritis are highly varied and often unpredictable. Although in many patients the condition fits a "classical" pattern, in others it is comprised of several patterns. Many patients progress into the terminal stage without ever having experienced edema. An occasional patient develops clear-cut acute glomerulonephritis following respiratory infection, succeeded by a "nephrotic stage," which yields over a period of years to slowly progressive renal insufficiency and mounting hypertension, but it is not usual to observe this full sequence of events in one individual. Some characteristic patterns are considered below.

RAPIDLY PROGRESSIVE COURSE. The entire course lasts only a few months, usually less than a year. Sometimes the onset is explosive, originating in acute nephritis following an infection. In other instances evidence for an infectious origin is absent and the beginning of the disease can be dated only by the last normal examination. In any case, *fatigue, anemia,* and *breathlessness* quickly appear, hypertension is prominent even though the heart may initially not be enlarged, and the urine contains large quantities of protein and red blood cells and may be grossly bloody. Oliguria and rapidly advancing uremia, complicated by pulmonary edema, characterize the terminal weeks. The kidneys are usually normal in size, and the glomeruli are swollen, with intense proliferation of the capsular epithelium, resulting in widespread crescent formation.

SLOWLY PROGRESSIVE COURSE. *Abnormal urinary findings* may be detected in a completely asymptomatic patient in the course of a routine physical examination. *Renal biopsy* shows a patchy glomerulitis, with focal thickening of glomerular loops, occasional capsular adhesions, and some completely hyalinized glomeruli. Other glomeruli may appear completely normal. Alterations in arterioles of the kidney can sometimes be detected even though blood pressure is normal.

Hypertension is often absent. The fundi are normal. The usual tests of renal function may be completely within normal limits, and serial studies over many years show no or very slow progression of functional impairment. The character of the *urinary sediment* is a poor guide to prognosis; moderate proteinuria, red blood cells, and red blood cell casts may be present intermittently or continuously for years, with a normal or only slightly elevated serum creatinine level. The pathologic process is continuously active at a low level, though counterbalanced by forces of repair and renal hypertrophy. Some patients live normal lives for decades without any change, and some are cured; others eventually develop severely impaired renal function and hypertension.

Recurrent frank hematuria, occurring after exercise or within a few days of a nonspecific respiratory infection, characterizes one group of young patients, usually male, in whom renal biopsy shows only *focal glomerulitis.* Proteinuria is slight or absent. The course appears to be benign, and most cases never develop renal insufficiency, though red blood cells are seen from time to time in the urinary sediment.

NEPHROTIC SYNDROME. Glomerulonephritis in some patients begins insidiously with nightly *swelling* of the ankles and early-morning puffiness of the eyes. *Proteinuria* is in excess of 5 Gm daily, and the serum albumin level is low. Hypertension may or may not be present initially but eventually makes its appearance. *Renal biopsy* reveals diffuse thickening of all glomerular loops, with little or no cellular proliferation, capsular adhesions, or crescent formation, though all these changes may be present in occasional instances. In other cases interlobu-

lar thickening in the glomerular tufts is focal rather than diffuse (chronic interlobular glomerulonephritis), resulting in a pathologic picture that superficially resembles the nodular form of Kimmelstiel-Wilson disease. The rate of progression of the lesion is extremely variable, though within 6 years perhaps half of all patients will have developed the uremic syndrome. Occasional patients appear to recover completely. In many cases, edema remits as the glomerular filtering area is progressively restricted and the excretion of protein falls; in others, hypoalbuminemia and edema persist to the end.

HYPERTENSION. Many patients with chronic glomerulonephritis seek medical attention because of complaints associated with hypertension. Sometimes high blood pressure will be found to have developed without significant impairment of renal function. Such cases may be indistinguishable in their clinical manifestations and course from benign essential hypertension, except that proteinuria, dating in occasional instances from a clear-cut attack of acute nephritis, has antedated the hypertension. In some instances "malignant hypertension," with papilledema and extremely high diastolic blood pressure, may develop and dominate the picture. In patients in whom azotemia has not become pronounced, judicious use of hypotensive agents may produce a remission in the pattern of malignant hypertension without seriously damaging renal function.

By the time azotemia has appeared, hypertension is present in most patients with glomerulonephritis, and as the disease approaches its terminus, blood pressure is elevated in all. When progression is very slow, both azotemia and mild hypertension may be borne without symptoms for years.

EXACERBATIONS OF CHRONIC NEPHRITIS. Respiratory infections, especially with the streptococcus, sometimes cause an increase in proteinuria, hematuria, and hypertension as well as a decrease in renal function in patients with chronic nephritis. These exacerbations may be distinguished from attacks of acute nephritis, which they resemble, by the short latent period between the onset of the infection and the exacerbation. There is little evidence that the tendency to progression seen in most patients with chronic glomerulonephritis is related to infection. In some patients, reversible exacerbations of vascular disease characterized by rising blood pressure, hematuria, and retinitis occur without evidence of preceding infection and subside spontaneously.

Prognosis

It is almost impossible, except in the most advanced cases, to offer an accurate prognosis from a single set of clinical observations and tests of renal function. Serial observations of the level of blood urea nitrogen or serum creatinine, phenolsulfonphthalein excretion, the degree of proteinuria and anemia, and the blood pressure level afford an estimate of the velocity and character of the process. Anemia eventually develops in most patients by the time renal insufficiency makes its appearance. In patients in whom renal failure has developed only slowly, fatigue associated with anemia may be the presenting symptom. Severe anemia, recurrent after transfusions, implies a poor prognosis. *Probably because of the intensity of the associated vascular disease, the prognosis is much worse in glomerulonephritis with renal insufficiency than in pyelonephritis with azotemia of comparable severity.*

Regardless of the character of the glomerular involvement in the early stages of the disease, it is usually difficult to discern its nature at postmortem examination, since the kidneys are shrunken and fibrotic. Many glomeruli are completely hyalinized; in others there is only partial eccentric fibrosis, with varying degrees of adhesion of capillary loops to one another and to Bowman's capsule. The few glomeruli which are not injured are enlarged, as if stimulated to compensatory hypertrophy.

Differential Diagnosis

In patients with renal insufficiency, the possibility of other diseases of the kidney must be kept in mind. A history of acute nephritis with edema is helpful if present, but a detailed account of the illness should be obtained because what the patient refers to as nephritis may have been a urinary infection. Multiple myeloma and amyloid disease mimic chronic nephritis in the middle-aged and elderly. Hypercalcemia may produce polyuria, azotemia, and anemia, all of which are potentially reversible.

Heavy proteinuria (over 2 to 3 Gm daily) is present in most patients with chronic glomerulonephritis (and the various other disorders which cause the nephrotic syndrome) but in few other renal diseases unless heart failure or malignant hypertension is present. Epithelial cell casts, red blood cell casts, and lipid droplets in the urinary sediment are useful in distinguishing the disease from pyelonephritis or primary nephrosclerosis. The kidneys are of equal size, usually without evidence of distortion of the calyxes on pyelography, and if small, are contracted symmetrically. The possibilities of lupus erythematosus, periarteritis, and bacterial endocarditis should be kept in mind. Elderly patients with endocarditis, without fever or audible murmurs, may come to the physician with what appears to be nephritis and may die of progressive renal insufficiency without a correct diagnosis having been made.

Treatment

Restriction of activity is indicated in patients with heart failure, acute exacerbations of nephritis with hematuria, or intercurrent infections. Patients who feel well enough should be permitted to be up and about and should be encouraged to lead normal lives. Diet should not be restricted except for the clear indications mentioned in Chap. 301. Strenuous exertion leading to fatigue is probably best avoided. Pregnancy may in some cases be safely undertaken by patients in whom hypertension has not appeared and whose blood urea nitrogen level is

normal. In others the risk of preeclampsia or exacerbation of nephritis is greatly increased. Since the day of Richard Bright, moving to a warm climate has been recommended to patients with nephritis by physicians living in cold climates; there is no evidence that it influences the natural history of the disease. Prophylactic administration of penicillin has not been shown to alter the course of the disease. Treatment of the nephrotic syndrome is dealt with in Chap. 305, and management of renal insufficiency, in Chap. 301.

NEPHRITIS IN LUPUS ERYTHEMATOSUS
Incidence

In about two-thirds of all patients with lupus erythematosus there is clinical evidence of renal involvement. Nephritis is found at postmortem examination in 75 percent of these patients, the majority of whom die of renal failure. Lupus is a common cause of the nephrotic syndrome in women, the diagnosis having been made in one-third of all adult and adolescent women with the nephrotic syndrome examined at the Presbyterian Hospital of New York over the course of 20 years.

Pathology

The earliest lesion is a focal membranous glomerulonephritis involving the periphery of the glomerular tuft, usually in conjunction with small areas of endothelial proliferation. As the disease advances, the glomerular process becomes more generalized, with diffuse thickening of the basement membrane, resulting in "wire loop" formation and intense focal cellular proliferation, with capsular adhesions and epithelial crescent formation, progressing to hyalinization. Lesions are frequently seen in various stages of development. It should be emphasized that they overlap morphologically with those observed in chronic glomerulonephritis. Some of the morphologic differences may be expressions of the relatively rapid rate of progression of the disease. Thus, contracted kidneys with many fibrotic and hyalinized glomeruli are uncommon, while focal zones of necrosis in the glomeruli, with nuclear fragmentation, are frequent. Hematoxylin bodies, consisting of depolymerized ribonucleic acid, are occasionally observed in the glomeruli; they have not been reported in chronic glomerulonephritis.

Clinical Features

Lupus nephritis may present as acute glomerulonephritis, "latent" nephritis with asymptomatic albuminuria, nephrosis, or chronic glomerulonephritis with renal insufficiency. Its course may be fulminating, with death in uremia after only a few weeks of onset, or the patient may live for years, with proteinuria and microscopic hematuria regarded as merely subsidiary to the other vicissitudes of the disease. In its early phases, signs of renal disease may be remittent, but when massive proteinuria or azotemia has appeared, the course is generally rapidly downhill within 1 to 3 years. Hypertension is rare unless azotemia is present or the patient is being treated with steroids. The urinary sediment is characteristic of chronic active glomerulonephritis, with leukocytes, red blood cell casts, doubly refractile lipid granules, and broad granular casts. Other systemic signs of lupus, such as rash and arthritis, as well as a positive reaction to the LE test, may disappear while the nephritis is active; this is especially likely with the development of the nephrotic syndrome or signs of uremia.

Treatment

Treatment with relatively small doses of adrenal steroids (e.g., 1 to 20 mg prednisone daily), which may be enough to suppress fever and arthritis, rarely improves advanced lupus nephritis and does not prevent its development, though mild proteinuria and hematuria may show improvement. Larger doses of steroids (e.g., 60 to 80 mg prednisone daily) plus azothioprine, approximately 3 mg/kg/day, or cyclophosphamide in the same dose often produce remission of proteinuria and improvement in renal function. Many cases, however, continue to progress regardless of treatment. This is especially true after azotemia and hypertension have appeared.

SCLERODERMA

About one-third of patients with scleroderma die of renal failure, and in two-thirds renal changes are present at death. The characteristic lesions consist of extensive intimal thickening of the interlobular arteries, fibrinoid necrosis of the cortical arterioles, thickening of glomerular loops, and spotty ischemic cortical necrosis. These changes may be indistinguishable from those seen in malignant hypertension. Proteinuria does not generally exceed 2 Gm per day. The blood pressure is usually elevated, especially terminally. In exceptional instances, however, it may be normal, even in patients with widespread arterial and arteriolar lesions at postmortem examination. Minimal proteinuria may be the only sign for long periods. Once renal involvement is moderately advanced, the course is rapid, leading to death from renal insufficiency within a few weeks or months after azotemia has appeared. Terminal oliguria or anuria is common. The rapid progression of renal insufficiency frequently appears to be precipitated by the use of hypotensive agents. Adrenal steroids do not prevent or ameliorate the renal disease; it has been suggested that they accelerate it, but the evidence for this is not convincing.

PERIARTERITIS NODOSA— HYPERSENSITIVITY ANGIITIS

The kidney is said to be involved in approximately 80 percent of all patients with periarteritis nodosa. Precise nosology in this area is complicated by the fact that arteritic lesions nearly always occur in the course of malignant hypertension and occasionally appear in the course of glomerulonephritis.

Pathology

Renal lesions in periarteritis are of two types. The *first* is characterized by segmental fibrinoid necrosis of part or all of an arterial wall, with an inflammatory perivascular infiltrate. Usually, arteries of medium size are involved (arcuate arteries or larger), but arterioles and even capillaries may be attacked. Signs of organization are evident, with fibrous replacement of the damaged media and the formation of aneurysms at weakened spots in the larger muscular arteries. Multiple infarctions and gross cortical scars are apparent in the renal parenchyma. There may be scattered focal glomerulitis of varying age and activity. The *second* type of involvement is characterized by an active, rapidly progressive glomerulonephritis, with widespread fibrinoid necrosis of glomeruli and epithelial crescent formation. Combinations of these types of lesions may occur.

Clinical Features

With lesions of the larger renal arteries, hypertension is usual and may dominate the clinical picture. Albuminuria is always present, and the urinary sediment frequently contains red blood cell casts and fat bodies. Episodes in which the urine is grossly bloody are common. Uremia may be noted terminally, but azotemia frequently is absent or mild and only slowly progressive. Remissions and relapses often mark the clinical course. Persistent hypertension may be a serious sequel when the disease is no longer active.

When the clinical and pathologic features of acute glomerular nephritis are present (as in the variety of hypersensitivity angiitis commonly caused by reaction to drugs), hypertension is more often absent, even in the presence of marked azotemia. Although death from renal insufficiency usually takes place within 6 months to a year of onset, in milder cases permanent spontaneous remissions have been observed.

Periarteritis should be suspected in patients with renal failure or hypertension, especially when features suggesting glomerulonephritis are present, when other organ systems are involved, or in the presence of obscure fever or unexplained leukocytosis or eosinophilia.

Large doses of adrenal steroids (60 to 80 mg prednisone daily) produce improvement in renal function in some patients. In a few of these, the manifestations of renal involvement completely disappear and the remission persists after steroids are withdrawn. In others, maintenance on steroids and azothioprine is necessary to sustain the remission, and in many patients the renal lesion appears to progress in spite of treatment.

REFERENCES

Comerford, F. R., and A. S. Cohen: The Nephropathy of Systemic Lupus Erythematosus, Medicine, 46:425, 1967.

Ferris, T. F., P. Gorden, M. Kashgarian, and F. H. Epstein: Recurrent Hematuria and Focal Nephritis, New Engl. J. Med., 276:770, 1967.

Levine, R. J., and B. R. Boshell: Renal Involvement in Progressive Systemic Sclerosis (Scleroderma), Ann. Intern. Med., 52:517, 1960.

McCluskey, R. T., and D. S. Baldwin: Natural History of Acute Glomerulonephritis, Am. J. Med., 35:213, 1963.

Michael, A. F., R. L. Vernier, K. N. Drummond, J. I. Levitt, R. C. Herdman, A. J. Fish, and R. A. Good: Immunosuppressive Therapy of Chronic Renal Disease, New Engl. J. Med., 276:817, 1967.

Rusby, N. L., and C. Wilson: Lung Purpura with Nephritis, Quart. J. Med., 29:501, 1960.

Unanue, E. R., and F. J. Dixon: Experimental Glomerulonephritis: Immunologic Events and Pathogenetic Mechanisms, vol. 6, p. 1, "Advances in Immunology," New York, Academic Press, Inc., 1967.

Wilson, C.: The Natural History of Nephritis, in "Renal Disease," 2d ed., D. A. K. Black (Ed.), Oxford, Blackwell Scientific Publications, Ltd., 1967.

305 NEPHROSIS AND THE NEPHROTIC SYNDROME

Franklin H. Epstein

The nephrotic syndrome is a clinical constellation characterized by (1) massive proteinuria, (2) hypoalbuminemia, and (3) edema. Hyperlipemia is frequently but not invariably present. The term "nephrosis" is sometimes used by pathologists to indicate degenerative changes in renal tubular epithelium, but this definition should not be confused with the clinical syndrome under discussion.

Etiology

The *nephrotic syndrome* is the result of diffuse injury to the glomerulus. In most cases the origin of the disorder is uncertain. Many patients have a history of allergic disease and some show striking eosinophilia. The injury may occur in the course of poststreptococcal glomerulonephritis or in association with amyloid infiltration of the glomeruli, diabetic intercapillary glomerulosclerosis, or lupus erythematosus. It is occasionally observed in allergic reactions to plant pollens, poison ivy, poison oak, or insect stings, or as a manifestation of sensitivity to trimethadione or paramethadione. It may occur as a complication of secondary syphilis or malaria and has sometimes appeared in the course of treatment with mercurial diuretics and salts of gold and bismuth. Massive proteinuria may result from the marked elevation in glomerular capillary pressure which follows thrombosis of the renal veins or constrictive pericarditis. Uncomplicated pyelonephritis or nephrosclerosis does not cause the nephrotic syndrome.

Pathology

In patients with amyloid disease, lupus, or Kimmelstiel-Wilson disease, the characteristic glomerular changes of these disorders are present. In others, the kidneys reveal a spectrum of morphologic changes. Some glomeruli appear quite normal by light microscopy, but under the electron microscope the foot processes of glomerular endothelial cells are seen to be broadened and smudged. (There is evidence that this particular change is a result of proteinuria, rather than its cause.) When the lesion is more advanced, definite spotty or diffuse thickening of the basement membrane is apparent by the usual histologic techniques, often with little or no cellular infiltration or endothelial proliferation; hence the term *membranous glomerulonephritis*. In other patients there is an increase in glomerular cellularity, and occasional capsular adhesions may be observed. In still other cases, the process of basement membrane thickening has gone on to fusion and simplification of the glomerular loops and to partial or complete hyalinization of some glomeruli. In all instances, the proximal tubular cells are swollen with intracytoplasmic droplets and vacuoles, some of which are doubly refractile. It is not clear whether these represent protein and lipid reabsorbed in huge quantities from the glomerular filtrate or that deposited from the blood in injured cells.

Clinical Features

The disease is more common in children than in adults and is more frequent in males, but may affect any age and either sex. Occasionally a respiratory infection has occurred just before the onset, but it is uncommon to find evidence of preceding streptococcal infection. The patient usually comes to the physician because of the insidious onset of *edema*. This is often particularly noticeable in the face because of the absence of orthopnea. The edema is characteristically soft and pits easily. Ascites and pleural effusions are frequently present, but pulmonary edema does not occur without heart failure. Though edema may be the only manifestation, other symptoms are often present, vaguely suggesting the extensive depletion of body proteins that hypoalbuminemia betokens. Loss of appetite is frequent, although not so common as in poststreptococcal glomerulonephritis. A previously active child may feel tired and run-down. Amenorrhea or some irregularity in menses is the rule in women. The course is sometimes punctuated by unexplained episodes of abdominal pain, vomiting, and diarrhea.

The *blood pressure* is often normal, and in the absence of hypertension the heart is not enlarged. The fundi are normal except when diabetic glomerulosclerosis is the cause of the disorder. The skin looks puffy and pale; there may be a mild normocytic anemia, but the hematocrit is usually higher than the pasty appearance of the patient suggest. Mild generalized osteoporosis is frequently observed, especially in children.

The daily urine usually contains more than 4 to 5 Gm protein, *chiefly albumin*, but significant quantities of α_1-, β-, and γ-*globulins* are found as well. Some nephrotic patients excrete as much as 20 to 30 Gm protein each day. The serum proteins are grossly reduced in number, especially the albumin and, less predictably, the γ-globulin fraction. Serum γ-globulins are said to be normal in the nephrosis caused by lupus erythematosis or amyloid disease; they may also be found within normal limits, in the author's experience, in the nephrosis associated with membranous glomerulonephritis. α_2-Globulin levels are generally elevated, but this occurs in many chronic diseases. Serum albumin concentration is usually below 2.0 to 2.5 Gm per 100 ml when edema is present, and with massive edema it is frequently below 1.0 Gm per 100 ml. The overall increase in the lipid-carrying globulins conceals a reduction in the concentration of the smaller metal-carrying proteins, transferrin (iron) and ceruloplasmin (copper). *Serum complement* is decreased in membranous glomerulonephritis, although not in diabetic glomerulosclerosis. Serum calcium level is low, entirely as a result of a decrease in the fraction bound to albumin. The *plasma fibrinogen* level is elevated, and the sedimentation rate is greatly accelerated. The cholesterol, phospholipid, and triglyceride levels in the serum are usually elevated, and the serum is often lactescent. The low-density β-lipoproteins, to which these molecules are attached, increase in concentration. When caloric intake has been low and nutrition poor, however, serum cholesterol and triglycerides may be normal. This is frequently the case in instances of the nephrotic syndrome caused by lupus erythematosus and Kimmelstiel-Wilson disease.

The *basal metabolic rate* is usually low, perhaps as a result of malnutrition and, in some cases, of failing to correct for edema fluid in estimating weight. The impression of hypothyroidism may be strengthened by a puffy face and pasty appearance, by an elevated serum cholesterol level, and by the decrease in serum precipitable iodine, which, however, is a consequence of the low concentration of thyroxin-binding proteins in the serum, rather than of impaired thyroid function. Treatment with thyroid produces no improvement.

The *urinary sediment* is filled with granular and epithelial cell casts, and casts in which highly refractile lipid droplets are embedded. Fat bodies may be seen in the urine even when the serum cholesterol level is normal. Red blood cells are often absent, but many patients show some degree of continuous or intermittent microscopic hematuria.

Glomerular filtration rate is frequently normal or above normal early in the course of the nephrotic syndrome, and blood urea level is not elevated. Azotemia gradually develops, together with a fall in filtration rate and filtration fraction, in patients with progressive nephritis. In others renal function may remain normal, despite edema, for years, or may be depressed transiently, particularly during or immediately following infections. Tubular functions such as concentrating ability and phenolsulfonphthalein excretion are generally normal. Occasionally aminoaciduria or renal glycosuria is observed, presumably as a result of interference with proximal tubular reabsorption.

The term "pure" or "lipoid" nephrosis has been used to designate the nephrotic syndrome without hematuria, hypertension, or azotemia and without discernible cause.

Although prognosis is clearly better the longer patients escape hypertension or renal insufficiency, such patients should not be classified separately from others with membranous glomerulonephritis and the nephrotic syndrome, since glomerular lesions are observed in all by electron microscopy and some develop hematuria, high blood pressure, and azotemia later in the course of their disease.

Pathologic Physiology

The *glomerular basement membrane* is abnormally permeable to proteins. Those of low molecular weight and small size, like albumin, are lost into the urine in greatest quantity. Although it is conceivable that failure of the renal tubular epithelium to reabsorb protein might contribute to proteinuria, the massive amounts of protein excreted by some nephrotic patients and the striking increase in protein excretion observed following infusions of concentrated serum albumin suggest that increased glomerular permeability is the major determinant of the nephrotic syndrome. Indeed, there is good reason to believe that tubular reabsorption of protein is increased. There is no evidence (except in nephrosis associated with multiple myeloma) that abnormal proteins appear in plasma or urine. Hypoalbuminemia is chiefly a result of the extensive urinary losses of this protein; its synthesis is normal or even increased. In addition, in some patients the rate of catabolism of albumin is accelerated in a manner similar to that observed in a variety of acute injuries or infections. Associated with the reduction in amount of serum albumin there is usually marked wasting of tissues, which may be clinically evident only after the edema disappears. Balance studies carried out in nephrotic patients during refeeding with high protein, high calorie diets suggest that for every gram of protein added to the plasma, 20 to 100 Gm tissue protein must be incorporated in tissue.

The *decrease in plasma albumin* and consequent fall in the oncotic pressure of plasma results in an increased transudation of fluid from the bloodstream to extravascular spaces. Plasma volume falls. The reaction of the kidneys to these events is to diminish the excretion of sodium and of water, as in many other situations where the integrity of the effective circulating blood volume is threatened. Secretion of aldosterone by the adrenal cortex is augmented.

The primary role of sodium in the production of nephrotic edema is demonstrated by the fact that, when administered without salt, water may be excreted normally. When the intake of sodium is continued, it is retained by the kidneys and sequestered with water in an expanded interstitial fluid. Despite edema, plasma volume remains normal or low. If albumin is added to the bloodstream in increased amounts, or its rate of loss is diminished, the sequence of events will be reversed and diuresis will ensue.

When the quantity of circulating albumin is increased in a nephrotic patient, plasma volume is expanded by dilution with extravascular edema fluid, thereby minimizing the expected rise in albumin *concentration*. For this and other reasons, diuresis and edema formation need not be correlated with the exact concentration of albumin in the serum.

Serum cholesterol, phospholipids, and triglycerides usually are all increased in nephrotic patients. The rise in triglycerides may be so marked that the serum is milky. At least one reason for the elevation in serum cholesterol level is its increased solubility in fatty serum, though increases in amount of serum cholesterol may also be observed in the absence of lactescent serum and even when serum triglycerides are normal. Decreases of cholesterol and lipid phosphorus frequently coincide with periods of especially severe anorexia or vomiting; increases, with periods in which appetite is good. Nevertheless, the most intense lipemia may be observed in wasted patients with extreme hypoproteinemia and the most massive edema. Though hyperlipemia usually disappears when elimination of edema marks regression of or recovery from the disease, it may persist in rapidly progressive cases despite advanced azotemia and hypertension.

The cause of *hyperlipemia* is not clear. It is not secondary to increased synthesis of fat or to difficulty in disposing of fat in the diet. Infusions of albumin produce an immediate fall in serum lipid level, often, but not always, to normal. In general, elevation of serum lipid level tends to be inversely proportional to the level of serum albumin. Infusions of dextran which restore the colloid osmotic pressure of serum also result in a fall in serum lipid level in patients with nephrosis. Overproduction of β-lipoproteins may be responsible for hyperlipemia. Since albumin binds and transports unesterified fatty acids, a deficiency of binding sites for free fatty acids, with consequent "trapping" of neutral fat in the plasma, has also been suggested.

Natural History and Prognosis

The following discussion will be concerned with nephrosis of uncertain cause characterized by glomeruli which appear "normal" on light microscopy or have the morphologic changes of membranous glomerulonephritis.

A distinction should be made between the course and prognosis of the disease in children and in adults, the prognosis being appreciably better in children. Before the introduction of steroid treatment, the disease was eventually cured or arrested in about 50 percent of children, although 40 percent died within 5 years of onset. By contrast, in only one-quarter of adults with the nephrotic syndrome was a cure or spontaneous arrest of the disease observed which lasted longer than 2 years. Spontaneous diuresis is occasionally observed to follow measles, but in other instances bacterial or viral infections appear to induce a relapse. Before antibiotics were available, deaths from infections, frequently with the pneumococcus, were common. Erysipelas, pneumonia, septicemia, and peritonitis can now be avoided or successfully treated, and as a result, early mortality has been sharply reduced. The disease is frequently remittent, with intervals in which proteinuria is decreased or

absent, and cases are occasionally seen in both children and adults in whom episodes of proteinuria and edema are separated by intervals of many years. Repeated remissions and exacerbations are uncommon, on the other hand, in the course of the nephrotic syndrome which follows in the wake of acute hemorrhagic glomerulonephritis. Persistent hypertension and azotemia are associated with a poor prognosis. Mild elevation of blood urea level, intermittent hypertension, and microscopic hematuria have been observed in patients who improve spontaneously, as well as in those who develop progressive impairment of renal function. About one-quarter to one-third of children and one-half to two-thirds of adults with nephrosis develop progressive renal insufficiency and increasing hypertension and die of heart failure or uremia, generally within 2 to 5 years. In others, proteinuria is diminished but seldom disappears, renal function remains stationary at a level near normal, and the patient is asymptomatic, with or without hypertension. In patients whose dietary intake of protein is high, considerable proteinuria may be compatible with only moderate reductions of serum albumin, without edema. Edema may be precipitated by intercurrent infections which decrease appetite and promote the breakdown of protein, and may disappear when these disturbances are removed, without alterations in the urinary excretion of albumin. With the development of advancing glomerular hyalinization, proteinuria frequently diminishes in amount, serum albumin level rises, and edema disappears as azotemia progresses.

Treatment

Although a few days in bed help to mobilize edema, there is no indication for prolonged bed rest. Hospitalization is indicated at the onset of the disease to confirm the diagnosis and to obtain base-line studies but need not be prolonged.

The diet should be low in sodium and high in protein. Except in the presence of hyponatremia, water should not be restricted. Very low sodium diets (200 mg) are unpalatable, although the development of "sodium-free" milk and milk powders has made a satisfactory high protein, low salt diet more feasible. Sodium restriction should, however, be considered an emergency measure to control edema; it is not indicated during convalescence from the nephrotic syndrome or when edema is minimal. A high consumption of protein, together with adequate calories, leads to steady replenishment of wasted tissues. Since the goal is to restore body proteins, not simply to prevent further wastage, additional intake of protein above the normal requirement of 1 Gm/kg/day, plus urinary losses, is of importance. If the additional protein is to be utilized, sufficient calories must be given. The proportion of fat and carbohydrates is determined, as a practical matter, by the composition of the supplements of milk or milk powder. There seems to be no great advantage to restriction of fat. With such liberal intake of protein and calories, there is usually some subjective increase in feeling of well-being, as well as, over many months, a slow rise in plasma albumin concentration. The increase in blood urea level which invariably occurs on a high protein diet reflects the additional amount of urea presented to the kidney for excretion, rather than deterioration of renal function. Proteinuria may also increase when serum albumin level rises.

Adrenal steroids or ACTH produce improvement in about two-thirds of children but in only one-quarter to one-third of adults with the nephrotic syndrome. A reasonable plan is to give 60 to 80 mg prednisone or 40 to 80 units zinc corticotropin suspension daily until a remission occurs or treatment has been continued for 4 weeks. Daily doses of prednisone lower than 40 mg are often insufficient to control proteinuria, while amounts higher than 80 to 100 mg are unnecessary. Remission generally requires the development of Cushing's syndrome. If no improvement is observed after a month of treatment with high doses of adrenal hormones, further prolonged treatment is not likely to produce a cure, although the patient may improve spontaneously. Diuresis sometimes occurs when steroids are discontinued, without diminution in proteinuria, but this is a nonspecific and transient response probably ascribable to temporary suppression of endogenous adrenal secretion. The earliest sign of a therapeutic effect on the disease process is a diminution in the number of grams of protein excreted daily. This may be observed as early as 2 days after the beginning of treatment, but usually after 10 days to 2 weeks. Once begun, the decrease in proteinuria proceeds rapidly, succeeded by a rise in serum albumin level and loss of edema. Proteinuria may disappear completely or diminish to a constant low level. During the initial stages of therapy, blood urea concentration may rise because of the increased catabolism of protein induced by steroids. Glomerular filtration rate, however, usually is unchanged or increased by steroid treatment, so that the serum creatinine level does not rise and may even decrease. After no further improvement can be detected, the dose of steroids is gradually reduced over a period of about 4 to 6 weeks. If the drug is interrupted at this time, some patients will continue in remission indefinitely, but many relapse at varying intervals up to years following cessation of treatment. In an attempt to prevent such recurrences, it is common practice to keep patients for 6 to 12 months on some maintenance schedule of steroid, administered either daily, every other day, or 3 to 4 days per week, in a dose intermediate between that originally required to induce remission and that at which proteinuria occurs. Serial biopsy studies suggest that, when successful, such treatment decreases cellular proliferation in glomeruli and arrests the usual progression from thickening of capillary basement membrane to obliteration of the glomerular capillary.

Complications of steroid treatment include hypertension, muscular weakness and cramps, peptic ulcer, potassium depletion, diabetes, and osteoporosis (Chap. 92).

Striae which break down and become infected may be troublesome in edematous nephrotic patients. The leukocytosis which regularly accompanies administration of large doses of steroids may confuse proper evaluation of infection. Hyponatremia associated with rising serum potassium level and high blood pressure is observed in occasional unresponsive patients who have received large doses of hormone for long periods of time. The advantages of a proper dietary regimen must not be neglected in the course of treatment with steroids.

Patients with amyloid disease or the Kimmelstiel-Wilson syndrome do not respond to treatment with steroids, nor do those with the nephrotic syndrome occurring in the course of acute poststreptococcal glomerulonephritis. Treatment of nephrosis complicating lupus erythematosus is discussed in Chap. 304.

Renal biopsy is helpful in ruling out amyloid disease and diabetic nephropathy. In general, those patients with little glomerular thickening, or only slight hypercellularity of the tufts, have the best chance of improving with steroid therapy. However, it is clear that the presence of some hyalinized glomeruli, cellular proliferation, or membranous thickening of capillary loops does not rule out the possibility of a remission with steroids. A favorable response may be observed in the presence of mild hypertension, microscopic hematuria, and even moderate azotemia.

Diuretics may be used to control edema in conjunction with sodium restriction, whether or not adrenal steroids are prescribed. The action of diuretics is enhanced by infusions of albumin, plasma, or dextran. These agents raise the oncotic pressure of plasma and expand plasma volume temporarily but are rapidly lost into the urine through the leaky glomerular filter. Diuresis is not an end in itself; a little edema is often to be preferred to the complications of too-vigorous diuretic therapy.

Alklyating agents and purine antimetabolites reduce proteinuria in some patients with the nephrotic syndrome. Success is more easily achieved in patients who also respond to steroids, but improvement has also been reported in a few cases resistant to steroid therapy. When proteinuria can be controlled only by large doses of prednisone that produce distressing and dangerous signs of Cushing's syndrome, cyclophosphamide or azothioprine may be useful additions to the regimen, reducing the amount of glucocorticoid necessary to maintain a remission.

REFERENCES

Adams, D. A., M. H. Maxwell, and D. Bernstein: Corticosteroid Therapy of Glomerulonephritis and the Nephrotic Syndrome: A Review, J. Chron. Dis., 15:29, 1962.

Derow, H. A.: The Nephrotic Syndrome, New Engl. J. Med., 258:77, 1958.

Drummond, K. N., A. F. Michael, R. A. Good, and R. L. Vernier: The Nephrotic Syndrome of Childhood: Immunologic, Clinical, and Pathologic Observations, J. Clin. Invest., 45:620, 1966.

Roscoe, M. H.: The Natural History of the Nephrotic Syndrome, Acta Med. Scand., 172:79, 1962.

306 VASCULAR DISEASE OF THE KIDNEY. TOXEMIA OF PREGNANCY

Franklin H. Epstein

NEPHROSCLEROSIS (See Also Chap. 276, Hypertensive Vascular Disease)

Definition and Pathology

Although early in the course of "essential" hypertension there may be no morphologic changes in the kidney at all, structural alterations in the small arteries and the arterioles are almost always present in the kidneys of patients who die in the course of hypertensive disease. In about 10 percent of such patients the changes are severe enough to produce marked renal insufficiency. Large and medium-sized arteries show intimal thickening. This change is more ubiquitous and more severe in the small arteries and arterioles. In addition, an eosinophilic hyaline thickening frequently involves the entire wall of arterioles and prearterioles. These changes lead to mild generalized atrophy of the cortex with focal scars. Hyalinized glomeruli are a conspicuous microscopic feature.

In patients who die with rapidly progressive, "malignant" hypertension, especially after renal insufficiency has appeared, there is often intense intimal hyperplasia of the medium-sized and small arteries, so that the lumen is substanially reduced. Necrosis of the preglomerular arterioles is present, which frequently extends into the glomerular tufts. There are hemorrhages into Bowman's space and occasional crescent formation.

It is not generally realized that similar but less intense changes may be found at postmortem examination in patients without systemic hypertension. Arteriolosclerosis is observed in the renal biopsies of a few patients with normal blood pressure and mild asymptomatic proteinuria. Definite arteriolosclerosis was described by Bell in 10.6 percent of normotensive patients fifty to sixty years of age and increased in intensity and frequency in older age groups. It seems clear that renal arteriolosclerosis may occur in the absence of systemic hypertension, though it rarely produces symptoms or signs. Such vascular changes may account for the moderate decrease in renal reserve often observed in elderly patients.

Clinical Features

Hypertension antedates proteinuria by many years in most patients with "essential" hypertension. When proteinuria does appear it is usually minimal. The urinary sediment is usually not remarkable, although microscopic hematuria and occasionally gross urinary bleeding may occur in the accelerated phase, when the excretion of protein may also increase to more than 4 Gm daily, reflecting widespread necrosis of glomerular capillaries. The anemia associated with advanced renal insufficiency occurs in some patients with nephrosclerosis as in other renal diseases, although the appearance of hypertensive neuroretinopathy with azotemia *in the absence of anemia*

should suggest primary vascular disease. The patient with hypertension and uremia whose optic fundi are normal usually has glomerulonephritis or pyelonephritis. At the inception of the hypertensive process, renal blood flow is usually depressed more than glomerular filtration rate. The opposite is true in glomerulonephritis, but the difference has no important clinical significance.

The course of nephrosclerosis is extremely variable and cannot be reliably predicted from the height of the blood pressure. Proteinuria and even mild azotemia may be borne without symptoms for many years. The abrupt change in course which marks the onset of the malignant phase is characterized by an increase in proteinuria and hematuria. Extremely high blood pressure, retinal hemorrhages and papilledema, heart failure, and hypertensive encephalopathy complicate the rapidly progressive uremia, which is fatal. It is of interest that most patients in whom this syndrome occurs have been known to have hypertension for less than 8 years.

The term "malignant hypertension" has been used variously to indicate (1) hypertension with papilledema, (2) hypertension with rapidly progressive renal insufficiency, or (3) hypertension with necrotizing arteriolitis. These arbitrary definitions should not be confused or allowed to obscure the facts in individual cases. Papilledema, hematuria, weight loss, advancing uremia, and necrotizing arteriolitis usually coexist in hypertensive patients, but it is not unusual for any of these features to be absent in the presence of the others. Thus, 23 percent of 68 cases studied by Goldring and Chasis with excessively high diastolic pressure and rapidly advancing uremia did not have papilledema. In some, the fundi showed only arteriolar narrowing without hemorrhage. Contrariwise, papilledema may be present in occasional patients at intervals for many months or even years without advanced renal involvement or necrotizing arteriolitis. In some patients the uremic syndrome appears over the course of a year or two, but hematuria and proteinuria remain minimal, and neuroretinopathy may never be present. Such patients are likely to have massive cellular intimal hyperplasia of the interlobular arteries with little necrotizing glomerulitis.

In addition to "primary" nephrosclerosis, the clinical syndrome of malignant hypertension may occur in the course of chronic pyelonephritis, glomerulonephritis, periarteritis nodosa, scleroderma, pheochromocytoma, and unilateral renal arterial occlusion.

RENAL ARTERIAL OCCLUSION

Arterial infarction of the kidney is usually attended by sudden sharp unremitting pain in the upper part of the abdomen or flank. The most common cause is embolic occlusion. Fever and moderate leukocytosis are common, especially when a major branch of the renal artery has been occluded. Gross hematuria is not unusual, and microscopic hematuria is present in more than half the cases. The blood urea nitrogen usually is not abnormal unless there is contralateral disease. Shortly after a renal infarct, the kidney may not function on intravenous pyelography, although it appears normal in size and retrograde pyelograms are normal. During the ensuing days or weeks, function is slowly regained.

When occlusion of the renal artery is *incomplete* as a result of atherosclerotic narrowing, or if a branch of the main renal artery is occluded and viability of kidney tissue is preserved by collateral circulation, hypertension may ensue which is often of the rapidly progressive type, though reversible by nephrectomy. In such patients intravenous pyelograms may be normal but most often the affected kidney is contracted. In a significant minority of cases, albuminuria is absent and the urinary sediment may be completely normal. The diagnosis may be made by studies of the volume and composition of urine obtained on bilateral ureteral catheterization, by aortography, and by measurement of renal venous renin (see Chap. 276).

RENAL VEIN THROMBOSIS

Etiology

One or both of the kidneys may be involved by renal vein thrombosis. Occlusion of both renal veins usually implies thrombosis of the inferior vena cava as well. A common cause is invasion of the veins by *hypernephroma* or compression by *malignant metastases* to retroperitoneal lymph nodes at the level of the celiac axis. *Thrombophlebitis* of the legs with extension upward, *periarteritis*, *congestive heart failure*, or severe *dehydration*, especially in children, may be etiologic factors. The venous occlusion may follow an *abdominal injury* or *operation*. In adults, renal vein thrombosis may occur as a secondary and often terminal complication of renal disease which has previously caused perinephric inflammation or reduction of renal blood flow. It is particularly likely to occur in *papillary necrosis* and in renal *amyloidosis*.

Clinical Features

Sudden complete thrombosis of a renal vein causes severe lumbar pain, enlargement of the affected kidney, hematuria, and proteinuria. If the condition is bilateral, oliguria and death from uremia usually ensue. If the occlusion is more gradual, renal function may be partially preserved by the development of collateral venous channels. In a few such cases, massive proteinuria results in a full-blown *nephrotic syndrome;* in other instances, proteinuria is not prominent and is overshadowed by hematuria. The blood pressure is usually normal, and when hypertension occurs it is not severe. The presence of collateral abdominal veins with upward blood flow, unexplained edema of the legs and lower part of the trunk, or recurrent pulmonary emboli may suggest the diagnosis, which can be established by venography of the inferior vena cava.

PREECLAMPSIA AND ECLAMPSIA— TOXEMIAS OF PREGNANCY

The term *toxemia of pregnancy* includes those disorders encountered during gestation or shortly after delivery which are characterized by the appearance of hypertension, edema, and proteinuria (preeclampsia) and, in severe cases, convulsions and coma (eclampsia). There is no reason to believe that patients with convulsions suffer from a disease essentially different from that of patients with preeclampsia. Such a clinical classification usually includes many patients with diverse diseases of the kidneys and blood vessels which begin or are exacerbated during pregnancy and to which pregnancy lends a distinctive coloration. The following discussion, however, will be concerned with a specific disease affecting the kidneys and the vascular system, usually commencing in the last trimester of pregnancy, which in most cases is dramatically improved when the pregnancy is terminated.

Pathology

The most common histologic finding in the kidneys in toxemia of pregnancy is marked swelling of the endothelial and epithelial cells of the glomeruli. In severe or prolonged cases, thickening of afferent arterioles may be apparent. Generalized and focal thickening of the glomerular basement membrane and fibrinoid necrosis of glomerular tufts have been described at postmortem examination, but these changes are rarer in renal biopsies obtained from patients who recover. Tubular necrosis is present in almost all patients who die of acute toxemia of pregnancy. Necrosis of liver cells and hemorrhages in the periportal areas are present in some but not all fatal cases; it has been suggested that these as well as the necrotic lesions of the kidneys are secondary to vascular spasm and shock.

A characteristic lesion in toxemia of pregnancy is the deposition of fibrin in glomeruli. Fibrin deposits can be demonstrated by immunofluorescent techniques even when they are not apparent with the usual stains. Unlike acute glomerulonephritis, antigen-antibody complexes and complement do not seem to be involved in the pathogenesis of the disease, and the serum complement is normal. In its severe forms, when *cortical necrosis* appears, the condition bears a tantalizing resemblance to the generalized Shwartzman phenomenon, because of widespread fibrin deposits in small blood vessels.

Clinical Features

Toxemia occurs more often in women pregnant for the first time and in those in the age group over thirty-five. It is more common with twins than in single pregnancies. Interestingly, its incidence is especially high in mothers bearing hydatidiform moles, in which albuminuria and hypertension characteristically appear early rather than late in pregnancy, suggesting that the disorder is associated with the placenta, rather than the fetus. As with most vascular disorders, its manifestations are more frequent and pronounced in the obese, though paradoxically its incidence is higher in economically underprivileged segments of the population. Toxemia of pregnancy is especially frequent in patients with prior renal and vascular disease. From 35 to 50 percent of pregnant women with preexisting hypertension can expect to have their pregnancy complicated by a toxemic episode. The incidence increases in general with the height of the diastolic blood pressure and is especially high if in previous pregnancies preeclampsia was superimposed upon chronic hypertensive vascular disease. Preceding toxemia of pregnancy appears to predispose to recurrence in 30 to 60 percent of patients even if blood pressure and urine have been normal between pregnancies. Evidence of pyelonephritis is encountered clinically in about one-fifth of patients with preeclampsia. Patients with diabetes are not especially susceptible to the disorder unless vascular or renal disease is present.

The *onset* may be either insidious or shockingly abrupt. Although toxemia commonly appears after the twenty-fourth week of gestation and frequently only a day or two before delivery, it may begin earlier, particularly in patients with underlying renal disease. *Hypertension* is usually an early sign. Because of the normal decline in blood pressure during the latter two-thirds of pregnancy, the physician should not disregard the significance of a *rising blood pressure*, even though it may not exceed 140/90. With hypertension, *headaches* and visual disturbances are frequent but not universal complaints. The *fundi* often show narrowing and spasm of the retinal arterioles. The retina may appear glistening or wet, but this sign is not specific. Exudates and hemorrhage are late occurrences in severe cases.

The appearance of *proteinuria* is usually coincident with hypertension, although it may follow (less often, precede) the rise in blood pressure by a week or so. The amounts may vary from a trace of protein to 8 or 10 Gm in 24 hr. Granular and hyaline casts are found in the urinary sediment. Unlike the condition found in acute glomerulonephritis, red blood cells and cellular casts are usually not present in large numbers. Renal concentrating ability is generally unimpaired, and phenolsulfonphthalein excretion is normal except in severe cases and in patients with previously decreased renal function. The blood urea nitrogen level does not often rise above 20 mg per 100 ml. Nevertheless, glomerular filtration rate is probably diminished by the disease in most cases. Even slight nitrogen retention must be interpreted with due regard to the physiologic increase in glomerular filtration rate and fall in blood urea which characterize the normal pregnancy. Blood *uric acid* level is commonly though not invariably elevated, reflecting a decrease in renal clearance of urate. In fulminant cases, oliguria may be prominent and may presage the acute renal failure of tubular necrosis.

The *edema* which characterizes preeclampsia resembles that of acute glomerulonephritis in its distribution and probably in its pathogenesis. Edema may be absent when the toxemia has been explosive in its onset, as with convulsions. In other cases excessive weight gain with puffiness of the face, fingers, and ankles is the earliest symptom, antedating hypertension or proteinuria. Edema is usually contributed to by hypoalbuminemia; yet the serum albumin, though diminished, is not often below 2 Gm per 100 ml, and the edema of toxemia is not so dramatically relieved by injecting serum albumin as is the edema of nephrosis.

Signs of *cardiac failure* are present in a significant proportion of cases. With the appearance of edema, orthopnea and exertional dyspnea are often exaggerated. These symptoms frequently subside with bed rest, digitalis, and diuresis. As in glomerulonephritis, the circulation time may be normal while the venous pressure is elevated.

Certain patients with severe toxemia, with or without eclamptic convulsions, may develop multiple clotting deficiencies or intravascular hemolysis, often following delivery, in a syndrome of *consumptive coagulopathy*.

Convulsions are often preceded by the development of hyperactive tendon reflexes and occasionally by epigastric pain. Though they are often associated with marked hypertension, their appearance is not necessarily correlated with the height of the blood pressure. They may occur within the first day or two following delivery; as well as before or during labor. Petechial hemorrhages are observed in the brain in most patients who die of eclampsia.

Termination of the pregnancy is usually followed by prompt improvement of the mother. Proteinuria and hypertension usually disappear by the end of 1 or 2 weeks, though occasionally they persist longer. Nevertheless, in perhaps 35 percent of patients with preeclampsia, hypertensive vascular disease indistinguishable from essential hypertension develops later. The incidence of irreversible renal changes and of late hypertension increases significantly with the duration of the toxemia.

Treatment

The most effective treatment is prompt emptying of the uterus. *Ganglionic blocking agents should not be used* to treat the hypertension, since they cross the placental barrier and may injure the fetus. Abrupt and severe hypotension induced by drugs may result in fetal distress and cause acute renal failure in the mother. In mild cases, hypertension may be treated by vasodilating agents such as reserpine, hydralizine, alpha-methyl-dopa, or magnesium sulfate, and edema can be eliminated with diuretics, bed rest, and a low salt diet. Simple sedatives, such as phenobarbital, help prevent convulsions, and parenteral barbiturates are useful in controlling seizures. When proteinuria and hypertension persist, however, it is doubtful that such symptomatic treatment prevents further vascular injury to the placenta and the kidneys. In such instances attempts to prolong the pregnancy for several weeks are associated with a high fetal mortality and the risk for the mother of permanent vascular disease.

REFERENCES

Harrison, C. U., M. D. Milne, and R. E. Steiner: Clinical Aspects of Renal Vein Thrombosis, Quart. J. Med., 25:285, 1956.

Kincaid-Smith, P., J. McMichael, and E. A. Murphy: The Clinical Course and Pathology of Hypertension with Papilledema (Malignant Hypertension), Quart. J. Med., 27:117, 1958.

Pollack, V. E., and J. B. Nettles: The Kidney in Toxemia of Pregnancy. A Clinical and Pathological Study Based on Renal Biopsies, Medicine, 19:469, 1960.

Vasalli, P., R. H. Morris, and R. T. McCluskey: The Pathogenic Role of Fibrin Deposition in the Glomerular Lesions of Toxemia of Pregnancy, J. Exp. Med., 118:467, 1963.

307 NEPHROLITHIASIS

Franklin H. Epstein

Renal stones vary in size from tiny particles to large staghorn calculi which fill the entire renal pelvis. They may be asymptomatic or continue to be formed and passed for years with no deleterious effect on renal function and no discomfort except occasional renal colic. Even a large staghorn calculus may produce no symptoms save perhaps for occasional nagging abdominal or flank pain. Often, however, renal calculi are associated with infection and progressive encroachment on renal function. Stones passed from above are rarely retained in the bladder unless there are obstruction and residual urine.

Clinical Manifestations

The typical attack of renal colic is exquisitely painful, causing the patient to double up in agony. The crampy pain begins in the side or back, radiating to the lower part of the abdomen, genitals, and inner thigh. The attack usually persists for several hours, although it may be over in a matter of minutes. Dysuria is frequently present, and even after the attack has subsided, tenderness along the course of the ureter often persists. Fever and leukocytosis signal associated infection. Hematuria and proteinuria are almost always present. Sometimes the pain is not referred in the usual manner and may simulate gallbladder disease, appendicitis, peptic ulcer, or disease of the spine. Renal colic may also be produced by blood clots or pus obstructing the ureter.

Pathogenesis

Every effort should be made to obtain stones for analysis since this often provides the key to an underlying disorder. It should be appreciated that a stone consisting predominantly of calcium oxalate can have a small central nucleus of uric acid or cystine, and that magnesium ammonium phosphate may be deposited in layers around a central calcium phosphate core.

HYPERCALCURIA. In approximately one-half of all patients with renal calculi, some predisposing cause can be found. These causes include disorders that *increase the excretion of calcium* in the urine as in hyperparathyroidism, excessive ingestion of milk, alkali, and vitamin D,

bone disease producing hypercalcuria, sarcoid, and renal tubular acidosis. *Idiopathic hypercalcuria* is found in a large proportion of patients with recurrent calcium stones. In such cases urinary calcium excretion exceeds 250 to 300 mg daily in patients who seem otherwise healthy. These patients may be examples of one "tail" of the distribution of calcium excretion in the general population.

CYSTINURIA (Chap. 104). This congenital disorder is characterized by decreased tubular reabsorption of cystine, arginine, ornithine, and lysine. Owing to its relative insolubility, cystine tends to precipitate in the urinary tract to form stones, which are radiopaque on account of their high content of sulfur. The condition may be diagnosed from the hexagonal appearance of cystine crystals in the urine and their characteristic reaction with nitroprusside. Cystine stones may be dissolved or prevented from forming if the reaction of the urine is kept alkaline and the urine volume high.

GLYCINURIA. Hereditary glycinuria is a rare familial disorder associated with nephrolithiasis and excessive urinary excretion of glycine unaccompanied by other amino acids.

URIC ACID STONES. Uric acid stones are radiolucent, form most readily in acid urine, and may be prevented if the urine is kept persistently alkaline (Chap 106). They frequently complicate gout and may appear in a variety of hematologic diseases, notably polycythemia. More than half of all patients with urate calculi have neither hyperuricemia nor increased urinary excretion of uric acid. In this group of patients an unexplained tendency to excrete urine of pH below 5.5 may predispose to uric acid stones.

HYPEROXALURIA. Although most patients with calcium oxalate stones do not excrete excessive amounts of oxalate, the rare condition of primary hyperoxaluria is characterized by progressive calcium oxalate urolithiasis and nephrocalcinosis beginning in early childhood (Chap. 103).

RENAL INFECTION. Finally, primary renal infection, especially with urea-splitting organisms and in the presence of hydronephrosis, may promote the formation of renal calculi.

In most patients with recurrent kidney stones, calculus formation is not correlated with abnormal urinary excretion of calcium or phosphorus. A family history of stone is often obtained. The mucoprotein found in stone matrices may be excreted in excessive quantity by patients who form stones.

Treatment

Treatment must be individualized and governed by the patient's symptoms and the signs of associated renal disease. A small asymptomatic calculus entrapped in a renal calyx and unassociated with infection may be best left alone. Many stones pass spontaneously, but in the majority of instances special urologic and surgical procedures are eventually required. Daily urine volume should be kept over 2,500 ml. Special emphasis should be placed on drinking before retiring and once more during the night. Infection should be vigorously treated. Unless inordinate milk drinking is the cause of hypercalcuria, calcium excretion is rarely changed much by reducing the dairy content of the diet. A much easier way to decrease the tendency to crystallization is to increase water intake. Urinary calcium can be reduced by feeding phosphate. In addition, certain complex phosphates interfere with crystal formation and are excreted into the urine when phosphate is supplied in the diet. Perhaps for this reason, a mixture of sodium and potassium neutral phosphates, made isotonic to reduce the cathartic effect, and given in three divided doses totaling 1.5 Gm *phosphorus* per day, is efficacious in preventing the growth of new calculi in patients with recurrent calcium stones.

REFERENCES

Maurice, P. F., and P. H. Henneman: Medical Aspects of Renal Stones, Medicine, 40:315, 1961.

Smith, L. H., Jr.: Symposium on Stones, Am. J. Med., 45:649–783, 1968.

308 CYSTIC DISEASES OF THE KIDNEYS

Franklin H. Epstein

POLYCYSTIC KIDNEYS

In this disorder normal renal tissue is gradually replaced and encroached upon by multiple cysts of the renal parenchyma of varying size. The disease is congenital and in one-half to two-thirds of adult cases appears to be familial. The condition is bilateral, though one kidney may be involved to a greater extent than the other.

Pathology

The kidneys are enlarged to several times normal size and are filled with grapelike clusters of cysts containing clear or hemorrhagic fluid. Between the cysts islands of normal or partially fibrotic renal parenchyma persist. In infants the cysts are said to be closed and do not communicate with the renal pelvis; in adults there is evidence that the cysts are functional. In patients with polycystic kidneys, cysts of the liver may be present and, more rarely, cysts of the pancreas and spleen. These are usually asymptomatic. There is a high associated incidence of intracranial aneurysms, and death from cerebral hemorrhage occurs in about 10 percent of cases.

Clinical Features

The infantile familial form of polycystic kidney disease with enlarged kidneys and a very high perinatal mortality rate is often associated with other malformations and appears to be inherited as an autosomal recessive trait. In contrast, the adult familial disease is an autosomal dominant trait, with virtually complete penetrance if the bearers of the gene survive to the ninth decade. The two diseases appear to be distinct, since families have not been reported in which both the infantile and the adult forms have appeared. Multiple cysts observed in adult kidneys in the absence of symptoms and of a family history may represent the asymptomatic stage of the familial disease, or an unrelated and nonprogressive disorder. The condition in the adult is commonly discovered in the fourth, fifth, or sixth decade, frequently in the course of a routine physical examination or as part of an investigation of asymptomatic hematuria, proteinuria, or hypertension. Both kidneys are usually palpable; in one-fifth of the cases, only one can be felt, and occasionally no mass can be palpated. In all instances, however, intravenous or retrograde pyelography demonstrates enlarged kidneys with elongation of the pelvis, flattening of the calyxes, and indentations due to the cysts. Lumbar and abdominal ache is a frequent complaint; owing to the weight of the kidney which produces tension on the pedicle, to intracystic hemorrhages, or to pressure on other organs. The pain is often increased by exertion and relieved by lying down. Pain may also be colicky and associated with hematuria and the passage of clots or with concomitant renal calculi. Hypertension appears in the third or fourth decade, when symptoms referable to high blood pressure may predominate. After the age of forty or forty-five, the more common presenting complaints are those associated with renal insufficiency. When a patient comes to the physician with uremia and a palpable "liver" and "spleen," the diagnosis of polycystic kidneys must be considered. Polyuria is common and oliguria is rare, even terminally. The average age at death is between fifty and sixty years; several patients have lived past seventy. Although the rate of progression may be extremely slow, patients generally do not live longer than 5 years after the blood urea nitrogen level rises above 50 mg per 100 ml. Superimposed pyelonephritis occurs frequently and may induce renal decompensations, which can be reversed by appropriate treatment.

Treatment

It is important to remember that polycystic kidney disease is compatible with a normal life span. Puncture or marsupialization of the cysts has not been demonstrated to prolong life and may introduce a disastrous infection. Because of the high incidence of bilateral disease, excision of one polycystic kidney is practically never indicated unless it is irretrievably infected or causing alarming hemorrhage, and then only after the other kidney has been shown to have fair function and to be only moderately involved in the cystic process. Hematuria usually responds to bed rest but should be disregarded if it is microscopic and asymptomatic. Pregnancy may be undertaken before hypertension and azotemia have appeared.

MEDULLARY CYSTIC DISEASE

This is a rare disorder in which the kidneys are not large and may be contracted. Cysts varying in size from a few microns to a centimeter in diameter occupy what once was the corticomedullary junction and are lined with a single layer of epithelium. Completely normal as well as hyalinized glomeruli are found in the thinned cortex, together with chronic interstitial inflammation and fibrosis. Few abnormalities are seen in the urine, other than an inability to concentrate it. The blood pressure is usually normal until late in the course of the disease. Anemia, polyuria, and salt wasting are prominent. Bone disease is common. Death of renal insufficiency before the age of thirty is the rule, but patients have been reported in their fifth decade. There appears to be a familial incidence in some cases, especially those described in Europe as "familial juvenile nephronophthisis," but in others there is absolutely no evidence for familial inheritance.

MEDULLARY SPONGE KIDNEY

Medullary sponge kidney, an entirely separate condition, has been recognized primarily as a radiologic abnormality; it is usually asymptomatic and nonprogressive, with a good prognosis. The cysts, which often appear as tiny clusters of radiopaque material adjacent to the calyces on intravenous and, less commonly, on retrograde pyelography, often contain small calculi. Occasionally these calculi erode to produce bleeding, colic, obstruction, or infection. No familial incidence has been noted. The chief importance of the accidentally discovered sponge kidney is that it may be mistaken for renal tuberculosis or diffuse nephrocalcinosis.

OTHER CYSTS OF THE KIDNEY

Solitary cysts usually occur at the lower pole, projecting from the surface of the kidney. They contain a serous fluid which is not urine. They may be associated with a dull, dragging pain in the side but are most often asymptomatic unless complicated by hemorrhage or infection. Occasionally one kidney is completely replaced by *multiple congenital cysts*, while the other is uninvolved. *Multiple small retention cysts*, secondary to obstruction of tubules, are common in nephrosclerosis and pyelonephritis.

REFERENCES

Dalgaard, O. Z.: Bilateral Polycystic Disease of the Kidney, Acta Med. Scand., Suppl., 328:1, 1957.

Lagergren, C., and N. Lindvall: Medullary Sponge Kidney and Polycystic Disease of the Kidney: Distinct Entities, Am. J. Roentgenology, Radium Therapy Nucl. Med., 88:153, 1962.

Mongeau, J. G., and H. G. Worthen: Nephronophthisis and Medullary Cystic Disease. Am. J. Med., 43:345, 1967.

Osathanondh, V., and E. L. Potter: Pathogenesis of Polycystic Kidneys: Survey of Results of Microdissection, Arch. Path., 77:510, 1964.

Strauss, M. B.: Clinical and Pathological Aspects of Cystic Disease of the Renal Medulla. An Analysis of Eighteen Cases, Ann. Int. Med., 57:373, 1962.

309 OTHER CONGENITAL AND HEREDITARY DISORDERS OF THE KIDNEY AND URINARY TRACT

Franklin H. Epstein

HEREDITARY NEPHRITIS

The most widely recognized form of familial nephritis is associated with nerve deafness and sometimes with cataracts or other defects of the lens. Although it is transmitted as an autosomal dominant trait, males are affected more severely than females and usually die before the age of forty of renal failure; hence the disease is more often transmitted by the mother. Gross microscopic hematuria are common, often worse after nonspecific infections. In childhood, while renal function is normal, renal biopsy may show nothing but blood in the tubules. At autopsy, on the other hand, the picture may resemble either chronic glomerulonephritis or advanced interstitial nephritis ("pyelonephritis"). Foam cells containing anisotropic lipid are frequently found in the interstitial tissue. Families are also found with a high incidence among the members of glomerulonephritis, toxemia of pregnancy, and asymptomatic albuminuria, but without deafness or lenticular abnormalities. It is not clear whether or not these cases all represent variants of the same inherited affection of the kidneys.

ANGIOKERATOMA CORPORIS DIFFUSUM

This is a familial disorder characterized by deposition of an abnormal glycolipid in vascular smooth muscle, myocardium, cells of sympathetic ganglions and the central nervous system, and epithelial cells of the renal glomeruli. The disease is recognized by characteristic punctate skin lesions (most profuse around the genitals and buttocks), acroparesthesias, dependent edema, defective sweating, and unexplained attacks of fever and pain. Proteinuria develops in the majority of cases in the second decade. Lipid globules and foam cells may be seen in the urine. Uremia and hypertension usually supervene in the fourth or fifth decade.

NAIL-PATELLA SYNDROME
(Osteoonychodysplasia)

Transmitted as an autosomal dominant trait, this condition involves arthrodysplasia of the elbows (webbed elbows), rudimentary patellas, split deformed nails, and iliac horns. The kidneys are the site of a mild chronic glomerulonephritis that is usually asymptomatic but may progress slowly to renal insufficiency.

NEPHROGENIC DIABETES INSIPIDUS

This hereditary defect in tubular function occurs more often in males than in females. Like pituitary diabetes insipidus, it is characterized by the excretion of large volumes of dilute urine, with osmolality well below that of plasma, but is distinguished by the failure of the kidneys to respond to vasopressin. Polyuria and polydipsia are apparent early in life ("water babies"). There are no associated genetic abnormalities of tubular function, but atonic bladder and hydronephrosis often result from the high rates of urine flow with prolonged voluntary retention of urine. Treatment consists of adequate water intake combined with chlorothiazide or chlorproamide (Chap. 88), which probably acts by producing mild salt depletion, resulting in increased reabsorption of fluid in the proximal segment of the renal tubule.

OTHER MALFORMATIONS

Congenital malformations of the kidney are sometimes associated with malformations of the external ear. Complete *absence of one kidney* occurs about once in 500 births. *Unilateral hypoplasia* is a rarer congenital anomaly. *Horseshoe kidney* results from fusion of the renal blastemas, generally at their lower poles, at the eighth to tenth fetal week. The common location is close to the region of the aortic bifurcation. The anomaly is found once in every 500 to 1,000 autopsies and in most instances is asymptomatic and compatible with long life. It may, however, be complicated by renal calculi, recurrent pyelonephritis, hematuria, and abdominal pain. A few patients have nausea and vomiting associated with abdominal pain which is accentuated by hyperextension and relieved by leaning forward (Rovsing's syndrome). In some, a mass may be palpated in the lower part of the abdomen. In *crossed ectopia* the renal blastema becomes deviated to the opposite side, where it usually lies caudal to the normal kidney, with which it may fuse. Its ureter usually crosses the midline to terminate in the normal position. Such kidneys, as well as *unilateral fused kidneys,* are predisposed to hydronephrosis and pyelonephritis but not to other renal lesions. Pain is the most common symptom; many patients are entirely asymptomatic.

Anomalies of the ureter include bifurcation, complete reduplication, and abnormal implantation in the bladder, as well as stricture at the ureteropelvic or ureterovesical junction. Anomalies of the vesical neck may underlie enuresis in children, which is sometimes treated as a behavior problem, while the kidneys are irretrievably damaged.

REFERENCE

Perkoff, G. T.: The Hereditary Renal Diseases, New Engl. J. Med., 277:79, 1967.

310 TUMORS OF THE URINARY TRACT

Bernard Lytton and Franklin H. Epstein

TUMORS OF THE KIDNEY

Benign Tumors

Benign renal tumors rarely present a clinical problem, as they are usually small and asymptomatic. The majority are adenomas, but a variety of fibrolipomyomas also occurs. When they enlarge they may be difficult to differentiate clinically from malignant growth of the kidney or suprarenal gland. They have a potential for malignant change.

Malignant Tumors

Malignant tumors of the kidney occur chiefly in childhood and after the age of forty. The incidence in adults is considerably higher in men. The common malignant tumor of children is *nephroblastoma* (Wilms' tumor), which probably arises from embryonic nephrogenic tissue and may contain both epithelial and connective tissue elements. It constitutes 20 to 25 percent of all malignant neoplasms of childhood and is observed before the age of seven in 90 percent of cases. The tumor usually appears as a palpable abdominal mass and may grow to enormous size. It is associated in a high proportion of cases with hypertension, which is relieved by nephrectomy. It has to be differentiated from multicystic kidney, neuroblastoma, hydronephrosis, and renal cyst. The tumor is present bilaterally in 1 to 2 percent of cases. Treatment consists of a combination of surgery, chemotherapy, and irradiation, which has resulted in a dramatic improvement in the prognosis. Dactinomycin (Actinomycin D) administered during the first week after operation and subsequently at intervals during the next year, together with postoperative radiation of the tumor bed, has achieved a 5-year survival of 60 to 70 percent. The most favorable prognosis is in those children in whom the diagnosis is made before the age of two years. Preoperative irradiation may be employed to render a large tumor operable.

In adults, *carcinoma of the kidney* (hypernephroma, Grawitz' tumor) is the commonest neoplasm of the kidney. One or more of the classic triad of hematuria, flank pain, and abdominal mass is present in about half the cases, but not infrequently the first symptoms arise from metastases to lung, bone, liver, or brain. Obscure fever together with a moderate leukocytosis, without infection, is a common presenting symptom. Occasionally gastrointestinal symptoms are prominent. *Serum alkaline phosphatase* level is sometimes elevated even in the absence of bony metastases. Calcification within the tumor mass is occasionally seen on the plain film of the abdomen. The diagnosis of a renal mass has been greatly improved with the advent of the *renal angiogram.* The characteristic tumor stain due to pooling of the dye in the vascular sinusoids distinguishes it from a simple cyst. In a small percentage of cases, however, the appearance of the angiogram is indeterminate and precludes the differentiation between a benign and malignant lesion; surgical exploration then becomes necessary to establish the diagnosis.

Lactic dehydrogenase activity in the urine has been shown to be elevated in the presence of carcinoma of the urinary tract. It cannot as yet be regarded as a satisfactory screening test, as there appears to be a significant number of false negative results, and a high proportion of patients with pyuria have an elevated level.

In rare instances *polycythemia* may be observed, unaccompanied by leukocytosis, thrombocytosis, or splenomegaly. It is thought to be due to an erythropoietic factor produced by the tumor. A similar factor has also been detected in the fluid of some renal cysts. In such cases the polycythemia may be cured by removal of the tumor. *Polyneuritis* and *myopathy* found in association with other forms of malignant disease are occasionally seen in carcinoma of the kidney and bladder. Abnormalities may be detected in the liver function tests, in the absence of metastases, and these resolve after extirpation of the tumor. An *elevated serum calcium level* and a *low phosphorus level,* suggesting hyperparathyroidism, may be caused in occasional cases by a parathormone-like substance elaborated by the tumor. *Hypertension,* if present, is usually coincidental and is not improved by nephrectomy. Extension of the tumor into the renal veins with subsequent venous thrombosis is not infrequent. A few cases have been reported in which there has been radiologic evidence of spontaneous regression of lung metastases following nephrectomy; progression of the lesions is unfortunately more common. Long-term survival after the excision of solitary pulmonary and cerebral metastases has also been recorded. About one-quarter of the patients with renal carcinoma survive more than 10 years after nephrectomy. The value of postoperative irradiation is controversial, as the tumors are relatively radioresistant. Some of the more anaplastic tumors are sensitive, and a course of postoperative irradiation appears to be worthwhile in these cases.

Papillary transitional cell *neoplasms of the renal pelvis* are often associated with similar tumors of the ureter and bladder. Hematuria is the outstanding symptom. An association with calculi and infection is frequent in the less-common squamous cell carcinoma, which has a poor prognosis. Nephroureterectomy is the treatment of election. Carcinoma of the renal pelvis may appear deceptively benign, and failure to find infiltration at operation does not ensure prolonged survival. The prognosis is worse than with parenchymal carcinoma.

TUMORS OF THE BLADDER
Carcinoma of the Bladder

This type of tumor is seen in two main forms, papillary and solid. Where possible, surgical extirpation by partial or total cystectomy is the treatment of choice, often in combination with radiation therapy. Supervoltage irradiation offers results approaching those of surgery, but there is considerable morbidity from radiation cystitis and proctitis. The *papillary tumors* are often relatively benign and may be single or multiple. Those which show no evidence of invasion of the bladder wall are usually well controlled by fulguration, but as the entire bladder mucosa appears susceptible to the neoplastic change, the appearance of further tumors is likely, and careful follow-up by cystoscopy is essential. The local instillation of Thiotepa has been found effective in the treatment of multiple lesions. A small group of these tumors become invasive after a variable period of time and behave like the *solid lesions,* whose prognosis depends on the depth of penetration and the degree of anaplasia. A tumor which has penetrated to the perivesical tissues and is poorly differentiated is associated with a very small chance of cure with any form of treatment. The most frequent symptom is *painless hematuria. Dysuria* and *frequency* are also common even in the absence of infection. Ureteral obstruction seen on the pyelogram indicates invasion of the bladder wall. A cystogram may be helpful in the localization of the lesion. Individuals exposed to intermediate products in the manufacture of aniline dyes (1- and 2-naphthylamines, benzidine, and 4-aminodiphenyl) have been noted to have a high incidence of bladder tumor. These tumors usually develop after a long latent period of between 3 and 40 years. A higher incidence of bladder cancer has been noted in heavy cigarette smokers; in such patients there is an increase in urinary carcinogens which disappear with the cessation of smoking.

TUMORS OF THE PROSTATE

Benign overgrowth of the prostate is a result of an irregular, multifocal hyperplasia of the fibromuscular stroma, with a varying amount of secondary invasion by glandular elements, affecting principally the lateral and middle lobes. The degree of enlargement may be from one to one-half to ten times normal. The enlarging hyperplastic nodules compress the normal prostatic tissue into a thin shell, the surgical capsule, from which they may readily be enucleated, as in subtotal prostatectomy. The enlargement produces varying degrees of urethral obstruction as a result of compression, elongation, or ball valve action of the middle lobe. The cause remains obscure, but the condition is associated with senescence and is thought to be due to hormonal imbalance, the exact nature of which is undetermined. About 50 percent of men over fifty develop clinical symptoms of prostatic hypertrophy, but only 10 percent require surgical relief of obstruction. It has been thought by some investigators that benign hypertrophy is a precancerous lesion, but there is little direct evidence to support this view.

Adenocarcinoma of the prostate is one of the most common tumors in men and accounts for 10 percent of deaths from malignant disease in males in the United States. The incidence rises rapidly with advancing age and has been found microscopically at autopsy in 15 to 20 percent of men in the fifth decade, increasing to as high as 60 percent in the eighth decade. Fewer than one-sixth of these cases, however, become clinically apparent prior to death, the remainder being latent carcinoma. *Three-fourths of the tumors arise in the posterior lobe, and urinary symptoms therefore tend to occur late in the disease.* Frequent routine rectal examinations are the best means of demonstrating the early and operable tumors. A *solitary indurated nodule confined to one part of the prostate should be investigated* by open perineal biopsy in patients who are suitable for radical surgery, as this is the only reliable procedure for a definitive diagnosis. About one-half of these nodules subsequently prove to be malignant. The more advanced carcinoma is indicated by a hard irregular nodularity, generalized induration, loss of the normal contour of the prostate, and infiltration extending upwards and laterally over the vesicles with fixation of the gland. One-fifth of the patients come to the physician with symptoms due to distant metastases. Needle biopsies and cytologic studies of prostatic fluid are unreliable for the diagnosis of early cancer but are useful methods of obtaining a histologic diagnosis in the more advanced cases. *The "prostatic" fraction of the serum acid phosphatase,* though a more sensitive estimation than that of the total enzyme, is rarely elevated with tumors confined to the prostate but is elevated in a high proportion of cases when local or distant dissemination has occurred. Elevation of the prostatic acid phosphatase level may occur for 24 hr after palpation of the normal prostate, and is found in a small number of cases without evidence of carcinoma. The serum alkaline phosphatase level is frequently elevated in prostatic carcinoma, but this occurs in a wide variety of conditions so that it is of little aid in diagnosis. Biopsy of the marrow from the sternum or ilium in patients with unexplained anemia will sometimes reveal metastatic prostatic cancer in the absence of radiologic changes in the bones or elevation of the acid phosphatase level. Radioactive strontium scanning of the skeleton has proved to be helpful in the detection of bone metastases in the absence of radiologic changes.

Radical prostatectomy remains the treatment of choice for tumors confined to the gland but is applicable to only 5 percent of cases. About 40 percent of these patients live for 10 years postoperatively without evidence of recurrence. *Fibrinolysins* should be looked for in patients in whom surgery is contemplated, as they have been found occasionally in association with prostatic carcinoma and have resulted in severe and uncontrollable hemorrhage postoperatively. The use of aminocaproic acid, which inhibits plasminogen activators and plasmin, has been helpful in these cases. Orchiectomy and estrogen therapy together appear to be the most effective palliative treatment in patients with symptomatic cancer of the prostate, and are also used as an adjunct to surgery. Diethylstilbestrol 5 to 10 mg, or the equivalent dose of other estrogenic products, is administered daily. There is evidence that the mortality from cardiovascular disease may be significantly increased in patients receiving hormonal therapy for carcinoma of the prostate. *Caution should therefore be exercised in the administration of estrogens to patients with asymptomatic prostatic cancer.* Obstruction may be relieved by transurethral resection. A 2-year remission may be expected in 70 to 80 percent of patients. If dissemination is not present at the outset of treatment, 44 percent survive for 5 years, but in the presence of metastases only 20 percent survive. However, only 5 to 10 percent of all patients may be expected to live 5 years without treatment. When relapse occurs following estrogen therapy, further remissions may sometimes be obtained by adrenal suppression with corticosteroids, adrenalectomy, and hypophysectomy; such

remissions are thought to be due to suppression of extragonadal sources of androgen.

Supervoltage irradiation and direct injection of radioactive gold have been used in the treatment of tumors confined to the pelvis, with variable results. Local irradiation of skeletal metastases may effectively relieve bone pain when hormone therapy fails.

TUMORS OF THE PENIS AND SCROTUM

Penile warts or papillomas occur usually in the coronal sulcus and are often associated with poor hygiene. Occasionally they may involve the external meatus. Treatment is by fulguration or application of 25 percent podophyllum in mineral oil. The surrounding normal skin must be protected with petrolatum when the latter irritant is used. *Carcinoma of the penis* is rare and affects elderly uncircumcised men. The disease may reach a fairly advanced stage before diagnosis if phimosis is present. Small superficial tumors may be adequately treated by irradiation, but amputation is usually required. *Carcinoma of the scrotum* is primarily an occupational disease occurring as a result of contact with petroleum and its products which may soil the workman's clothes. The classic example is mule spinners' cancer. Arsenical medicines may give rise to epitheliomatous changes in the scrotal skin and elsewhere.

REFERENCES

Mostofi, F. M., and R. V. Thompson: Benign Hyperplasia of the Prostate Gland, chap. 25 in "Urology," M. F. Campbell (Ed.), Philadelphia, W. B. Saunders Company, 1963.

Nesbit, R. M., and W. C. Baum: Endocrine Control of Prostatic Carcinoma: Clinical and Statistical Survey of 1,818 Cases, J.A.M.A., 143:1317, 1950.

Riches, E.: On Carcinoma of the Kidney, Ann. Roy. Coll. Surg. Engl., 32:201, 1963.

311 OTHER DISEASES AFFECTING THE KIDNEYS

Franklin H. Epstein

DIABETIC NEPHROPATHY— INTERCAPILLARY GLOMERULOSCLEROSIS— KIMMELSTIEL-WILSON DISEASE

Pathology

In about 25 percent of patients with diabetes mellitus a distinctive nodular glomerular lesion is evident at autopsy, which was first described by Kimmelstiel and Wilson as *intercapillary glomerulosclerosis.* The typical, ball-like, hyaline, acidophilic masses are situated at the periphery of the glomerular tuft, often with an apparently intact capillary running over the surface. The mass often contains cell nuclei, but they are usually distributed around its periphery. The wall of the afferent arteriole is usually hyalinized, and hyaline change in the efferent arteriole is frequently present as well. (The latter change is said to be so characteristic of diabetes as to be almost specific.) The nodules may be sparse or frequent; they rarely involve every glomerulus but completely obliterate some. In addition, a more diffuse hyaline thickening of the glomerular basement membrane is apparent in many cases of diabetes, even when the nodules are absent, although this change is more difficult to distinguish from similar "axial thickenings" in such diseases as benign nephrosclerosis and membranous glomerulonephritis. Examination of renal biopsies from patients with diabetes by the electron microscope usually demonstrates some thickening of the glomerular basement membrane, even though the diabetes is of short duration, proteinuria and hypertension are absent, and conventional histologic sections appear normal. In patients with long-standing diabetes, three renal diseases are likely to be present: intercapillary glomerulosclerosis, arteriolar nephrosclerosis, and pyelonephritis.

Clinical Features and Changes in Function

The usual textbook description is of a patient with 10 years or more of diabetes who develops proteinuria and hypertension. Though the patient is asymptomatic at first, massive urinary losses of protein produce hypoproteinemia, and edema and anasarca follow. The blood urea slowly rises, and vision is impaired by retinopathy. Within 5 years after proteinuria is first noted, death occurs from uremia complicated by infections, anemia, and heart failure (Chap. 94).

Departures from the classic picture are legion. Although both *hypertension* and *proteinuria* are present in 80 percent of diabetic patients with eosinophilic glomerular nodules, one-fifth have normal blood pressure, and occasional patients have no detectable proteinuria. Both hypertension and proteinuria can, of course, be caused in diabetic patients primarily by pyelonephritis or nephrosclerosis rather than Kimmelstiel-Wilson disease, and if this is true, the prognosis is probably better. In some cases, slight proteinuria, with fluctuating retinopathy, may persist for years with little or no impairment of renal function. In other instances, the interval from onset of proteinuria to death is as short as 2 years, and the intensity and rapidity of the deterioration in renal function reminds one of a subacute glomerulonephritis, though at postmortem there is only widespread nodular intercapillary glomerulosclerosis.

The appearance of *heavy proteinuria* (over 4 to 5 Gm daily) usually signifies extensive involvement of the glomeruli by the diffuse or the nodular type of diabetic lesion. Heavy losses of albumin into the urine produce hypoalbuminemia, which in turn predisposes to edema and pleural effusions. Poor appetite and inadequate intake of protein and calories often contribute to the low concentration of albumin in serum. Unlike childhood nephrosis, in the nephrosis of diabetes the serum cholesterol is often normal. When much protein is excreted, the urine also contains many granular and fatty casts and epithelial cells choked with doubly refractile lipid, called *fat bodies*. Hematuria is unusual except with malignant hypertension.

As renal reserve declines, glomerular and tubular functions deteriorate in parallel, so that *blood urea nitrogen rises* while creatinine clearance, phenolsulfonphthalein excretion, and concentrating capacity fall. The kidneys are scarred and contracted somewhat in size, but very small kidneys are not characteristic of Kimmelstiel-Wilson disease, in contrast to chronic end-stage pyelonephritis. It is not uncommon to see kidney outlines normal or only slightly reduced and a creatinine clearance one-tenth normal.

With advanced renal insufficiency, *glycosuria may not be an accurate guide to levels of blood sugar*. There is no consistent change in insulin requirements with progression of renal disease, though many patients require less insulin as their appetite wanes and they lose weight.

Retinopathy precedes proteinuria in practically all cases of diabetic glomerulosclerosis. Thus, although diabetic retinopathy may be present without clinical manifestations of glomerulosclerosis, one almost never sees marked proteinuria or azotemia in Kimmelstiel-Wilson disease without retinopathy. *When the retinas are absolutely normal in a diabetic with nephrosis, the cause of the difficulty is not likely to be the diabetes.*

Because of the generalized vascular disease that is always present, *myocardial infarcts, congestive cardiac failure,* and *cerebral vascular accidents* punctuate the course of diabetic nephropathy. They are responsible for more deaths in such patients than is uremia. When edema is present, heart failure is usually a contributing cause. A sudden deterioration in renal function may be the only reflection of a critical weakening of myocardial function or a silent myocardial infarct.

Sclerosis of the intrarenal arteries, infection, and in some cases, ureteral dilatation and reflux secondary to neurogenic bladder may combine to produce papillary necrosis. This is usually asymptomatic, though it may be attended by pain, colic, hematuria, and the passage of bits of tissue in the urine. Occasionally, *papillary necrosis is the cause of rapid progression of renal insufficiency or acute oliguric renal failure.*

Factors predisposing to *urinary infection* in diabetes include incomplete emptying of the bladder because of *diabetic neuritis,* and repeated instrumentation of the bladder during hospitalization. *Uncontrolled glycosuria* with associated vaginal itching and irritation probably contributes to the incidence of urinary infections in women. It is not clear whether the metabolic defect in diabetes confers any additional susceptibility to infections of the kidney; the high incidence of positive urine cultures in elderly hospitalized diabetic patients is not greatly different from that in control patients of the same age.

Retention of urine in the bladder because of difficulty in emptying commonly causes nausea and accentuates azotemia in bedridden diabetics. In patients with neurogenic bladders, proper emptying, using suprapubic pressure and full doses of urecholine, may permit infection to be controlled. In a few patients, residual urine may be eliminated by resection of the bladder neck.

Prevention and Treatment

The development of intercapillary glomerulosclerosis does not seem to be avoided by rigid control of the blood sugar, and there are several well-documented cases in which the fasting blood sugar was normal. It seems likely, on the other hand, that prevention of urinary infection (e.g., by avoiding unnecessary catheterization of the bladder) and proper treatment and follow-up of those infections which do occur may be important in preventing ultimate renal scarring from pyelonephritis in at least some diabetic patients.

Adrenal steroids do not alter the proteinuria of diabetic glomerulosclerosis. Hypoalbuminemia may, however, sometimes be improved by a more generous intake of protein and calories. Edema can usually be eliminated by salt restriction and diuretics if renal insufficiency is not severe and heart failure is not present. Because heart failure occurs at some time in almost every patient with Kimmelstiel-Wilson disease, digitalis should be given a therapeutic trial in every patient with edema or uremia in whom the heart is enlarged. Heart failure should be controlled by digitalis if possible rather than by restricting the intake of fluid and salt or by sole dependence on diuretics. When the latter become necessary, they should not be pushed to the point of dehydration. Modest edema is often to be preferred to progressive azotemia with its attendant weakness and nausea. Dehydration procedures in the hospital such as fluid restriction and castor oil before intravenous pyelography should be carefully avoided in azotemic patients.

Alpha-methyl-dopa and reserpine are useful in moderating the blood pressure in situations where hypertension is clearly responsible for symptoms (e.g., intractable vascular headaches) or menaces vision (severe diastolic hypertension with hemorrhagic retinitis). The tendency to postural hypotension induced by drugs used to lower high blood pressure is greatly accentuated by diabetic neuropathy. When the blood urea is elevated, asymptomatic hypertension should be ignored. Efforts to lower the blood pressure by drugs or diet are almost always rewarded by an increase in the signs and clinical symptoms of uremia.

Normocytic, normochromic anemia usually appears in diabetic nephropathy when the blood urea is elevated, and contributes to fatigue and weakness. It is due to renal insufficiency and responds only to transfusions. When anemia is severe and recurrent, an attempt should be made to give blood before the critical level is reached at which the patient complains of symptoms.

Frequent feedings with adequate quantities of carbohydrate and insulin to prevent ketosis and to avoid excessive breakdown of protein are especially important in treating patients with diabetic nephropathy, since sudden increases in the load of urea and acid presented to the kidneys, which are excreted with ease in patients with normal renal function, are retained in renal insufficiency and augment azotemia and acidosis.

Peritoneal dialysis is often useful in tiding a uremic diabetic patient over a reversible episode which temporarily decreases renal function, such as, for example, systemic or renal infection, decreased cardiac output secondary to myocardial infarction; or salt depletion from vomiting or diarrhea.

AMYLOID KIDNEY (Chap. 114)

Renal amyloidosis is most commonly encountered as a complication of chronic suppurative diseases, such as osteomyelitis, tuberculosis, tertiary syphilis, and leprosy, as well as Hodgkin's disease, ulcerative colitis, regional enteritis, and rheumatoid arthritis. As the incidence of chronic infection has declined owing to the introduction of antibiotics, the amyloid kidney of "primary amyloidosis" and amyloidosis secondary to multiple myeloma (Chap. 114) and rheumatoid arthritis have become relatively more prominent. Amyloid involvement of the kidneys, as well as of other organs, commonly occurs in the course of familial Mediterranean fever, in which renal insufficiency secondary to amyloidosis is usually the cause of death. The clinical and pathologic features of the renal disease produced by "primary" and "secondary" amyloidosis are similar.

Amyloid deposition in the kidney may be most prominent in the walls of blood vessels (especially the small arteries), or in the glomeruli, or surrounding the collecting tubules and small blood vessels of the medulla. In all these locations its distribution tends to be patchy rather than diffuse and uniform.

The clinical picture is influenced by the location and degree of involvement. When amyloid deposits are limited to blood vessels and to occasional focal deposits in glomeruli, mild proteinuria, sometimes with hematuria, is the only sign. On the other hand, when glomeruli are massively infiltrated, heavy proteinuria is the rule, associated with the nephrotic syndrome. In such cases, glomerular filtration may be surprisingly well maintained despite extensive deposits of amyloid in the Malpighian tufts. The rare instance of amyloidosis confined chiefly to the medulla is marked by polyuria resistant to vasopressin. Hypertension is unusual unless the disorder has progressed to the stage of azotemia and contracted kidneys. Heart failure, purpura, generalized muscular weakness, difficulty in swallowing, and postural hypotension are frequent accompaniments of primary amyloidosis. Biopsy of the kidney, liver, or rectal mucosa is useful in establishing the diagnosis. The course of the disease is generally prolonged, but in some cases secondary to advanced tuberculosis, only 6 months may elapse from the first appearance of albuminuria to the development of advanced uremia. Death occurs from the primary disease, amyloid involvement of the myocardium, intercurrent infection, or renal insufficiency. *Renal vein thrombosis* causing anuria is a special complication of amyloidosis. The disease does not respond to steroid treatment. In those instances in which a chronic suppurative disease can be eradicated, a complete remission has occasionally been observed.

THE KIDNEY IN MULTIPLE MYELOMA (Chap. 349)

Impairment of renal function occurs in over 50 percent of patients with multiple myeloma. Proteinuria is even more common. Renal damage can be related in many cases to the excretion of abnormal proteins of low molecular weight and the injurous effect of these substances on the renal tubules and ultimately on the entire nephron. Impairment of renal function is not necessarily correlated, however, with the *degree* of albuminuria or Bence Jones proteinuria. Hypercalcemia may produce transient or irreversible renal damage. In some cases the kidney is infiltrated by amyloid. Rarely, deposits of myeloma cells diffusely infiltrate the kidneys.

The major early change produced by the Bence Jones proteins is in the tubules. Proximal tubular cells are swollen and have droplets or rodlike inclusions. Large obstructing casts form along the entire length of the renal tubule, most prominently in the straight tubules of the medulla. These are often laminated and surrounded by multinucleated giant cells possibly derived from degenerating tubular epithelium. In addition, there is usually distinct thickening of the glomerular basement membrane, without cellular proliferation or crescent formation. Vascular sclerosis is not common; when it occurs it is probably coincidental.

Alterations in renal function is most frequently characterized by nitrogen retention and loss of concentrating power, without hypertension, retinitis, or edema. Proteinuria is usually present, consisting of albumin as well as certain globulins and Bence Jones proteins which may be excreted only intermittently. Anemia may seem out of proportion to the degree of azotemia. The disease may superficially resemble the chronic forms of glomerulonephritis or pyelonephritis. The nephrotic syndrome probably does not occur in multiple myeloma unless the disease is complicated by amyloidosis. In unusual instances before azotemia has become prominent, disturbances in renal tubular function dominate the picture, with renal glycosuria, aminoaciduria, low levels of serum uric acid, and renal potassium wasting. Loss of concentrating power is common and nephrogenic diabetes insipidus has been reported. Renal loss of phosphate with consequent hypophosphatemia and elevation of the serum alkaline phosphatase level may, in rare cases, cause confusion with hyperparathyroidism. Because of the exceptional tendency to formation of obstructive casts, procedures which cause dehydration must be carefully avoided in the patient with multiple myeloma. Acute anuria has been observed in several instances following intravenous pyelography, probably as a result of the dehydration which is often induced in preparing for this procedure. Acute renal failure with anuria or oliguria which follows an episode of dehydration in an elderly person should suggest the possibility of myeloma kidney.

SICKLE-CELL NEPHROPATHY (Chap. 339)

Patients with sickle-cell anemia often develop progressive changes in renal function as a result of multiple small ischemic and hemorrhagic infarcts in the kidney. In children the principal anatomic finding is congestion of blood vessels, with sickled erythrocytes most prominent in the medulla. The glomeruli appear engorged and stuffed with red cells. In adults interstitial fibrosis and areas of cortical necrosis and hyalinization may be seen, resembling those of chronic glomerulonephritis or chronic pyelonephritis. Papillary necrosis may occur in patients with the homozygous disease or the trait. There is early impairment of renal concentrating ability, even when blood urea nitrogen, glomerular filtration rate, and renal plasma flow are normal. This selective disturbance in renal function may be present in patients with sickle-cell trait as well as in the full-blown disease. It is said to be temporarily reversed in children by transfusion of normal blood, but this is not the case in adults. Gross and microscopic hematuria occur frequently; bleeding may come from lesions in the papillae and pelvic mucosa as well as miliary infarctions in the cortex. Renal insufficiency may eventually develop in adults with sickle-cell anemia as a result of renal scarring. Despite the high incidence of at least minimal renal changes, the sickle-cell trait does not appear to predispose to toxemia of pregnancy.

CHYLURIA

The chief cause of chyluria is filariasis (Chap. 249) with obstruction between the abdominal lymphatics and the thoracic duct, producing lymph varices in the kidney which rupture into the renal tubules. The urine is milky and on standing settles into a top layer of fatty material, a middle pinkish layer, often containing a clot, and a bottom layer containing blood and debris. Hematuria is common, and pyelonephritis is almost universal. Microfilarias are usually found in the urine for about 6 weeks after an acute infection but not thereafter unless the patient is in an endemic area. The lymph and blood may coalesce into ureteral casts, causing flank pain and renal colic. Chyluria may disappear with recumbency and be aggravated by exertion. The condition is entirely suppressed in some cases by wearing a tight abdominal corset.

RADIATION NEPHRITIS (Chap. 129)

Following the administration of large doses of x-ray (2,300 r during 5 weeks) to the kidneys in the course of therapy for abdominal carcinoma or lymph node metastases from testicular tumors, a characteristic syndrome develops. The clinical disease may mimic either benign or malignant hypertension or chronic glomerulonephritis. The latent period between irradiation and the appearance of symptoms is usually at least 6 months but may be much longer. Hypertension invariably appears and may lead to congestive heart failure, retinopathy, and encephalopathy. Refractory anemia is often prominent. Uremia is usually progressive, but in some cases renal insufficiency may be reversible, improvement commencing about 6 months after the onset of symptoms. Proteinuria is present but slight; hematuria is characteristically absent. Oliguria is never observed except with heart failure. Histologic features include widespread fibrosis between atropic tubules, damage to almost all the glomeruli, and fibrinoid necrotic lesions of arterioles.

HYPERCALCEMIC NEPHROPATHY (Chap. 90)

Acute elevations of serum calcium level may be associated with marked polyuria, succeeded by dehydration, oliguria, and rapidly advancing azotemia. Prolonged hypercalcemia and/or hypercalcuria, as in hyperparathyroidism, vitamin D intoxication, Boeck's sarcoid, multiple myeloma, or carcinomatosis, may result in diffuse nephrocalcinosis and present as renal insufficiency, insidious in onset and only slowly progressive. In such cases, severe disturbances in renal function need not be associated with stones or with radiologic evidence of calcification in the kidneys. Patients who have drunk several quarts of milk daily and ingested large amounts of absorbable alkali for prolonged periods of time to assuage symptoms of peptic ulcer sometimes develop azotemia, hypercalcemia without elevation of the serum alkaline phosphatase level, and calcinosis manifested by band keratopathy (milk-alkali syndrome).

Impairment of urinary concentrating capacity is an early sign of chronic calcium nephropathy, and polyuria and polydipsia are frequent, although not invariable. In more severe cases, filtration rate and renal blood flow are depressed, with retention of nitrogen. The urinary sediment may contain red blood cells, as well as leukocytes and white blood cell casts; in many patients, however, it is remarkably free of formed elements. Unless congestive heart failure is present, proteinuria is slight. Hypertension is common when nephrocalcinosis is established and does not disappear when the serum calcium level has returned to normal, even though renal function improves. Renal insufficiency may sometimes be completely or partially reversed when hypercalcemia is eliminated. In other cases, uremia and hypertensive vascular disease progress to a fatal termination despite the disappearance of hypercalcemia. The degree of reversibility of renal impairment is related to the extent of scar formation and permanent medullary obstruction by calcium precipitates, as well as to the presence of vascular disease and infection.

THE KIDNEY OF GOUT (Chap. 106)

From 30 to 50 percent of gouty patients die of renal disease. The kidneys of most patients with gout contain characteristic fan-shaped clefts containing deposits of urate in the interstices of the medulla. Pyelonephritis is a frequent finding, and arteriolar sclerosis is almost always present.

Urate calculi occur in approximately 15 percent of patients with gout and are particularly common during uricosuric therapy if a high fluid intake is not maintained. Both uric acid stones and interstitial deposits of urate crystals in the kidney may occur in patients with hyperuricemia who have never had gouty arthritis.

The most common indications of early renal damage are mild proteinuria, decreased excretion of phenolsulfonphthalein, and a reduction in concentrating ability. Slowly progressive azotemia with minimal albuminuria and little or no abnormality in the urinary sediment characterizes the course of this disease in some patients. Though hypertension may be absent, the blood pressure is commonly elevated; in fact, it has been suggested that hypertension and vascular sclerosis, especially nephrosclerosis, occur as part of a constitutional diathesis of which gout or hyperuricemia is a component part. Hyperuricemia and evidence on renal biopsy of arteriolar sclerosis may occasionally be the only positive findings in patients with asymptomatic proteinuria.

In rare instances of gouty kidney, renal function has been reported to improve slowly and urate stones to dissolve following the long-term maintenance of a high fluid intake and use of alkali in association with uricosuric agents. Allopurinol, which blocks the formation of uric acid, is a rational treatment to use in the hope of preventing progression in gouty nephropathy (Chap. 106).

REFERENCES

Berkman, J., and H. Rifkin: Newer Aspects of Diabetic Microangiopathy, Ann. Rev. Med., 17:83, 1966.

Brandt, K., E. S. Cathcart, and A. S. Cohen: A Clinical Analysis of the Course and Prognosis of Forty-two Patients with Amyloidosis, Am. J. Med., 44:955, 1968.

Epstein, F. H.: Calcium and the Kidney, Am. J. Med., 45: 700, 1968.

Gellman, D. D., C. L. Pirani, J. F. Soothill, R. C. Muehrcke, and R. M. Kark: Diabetic Nephropathy: A Clinical and Pathological Study Based on Renal Biopsies, Medicine, 38:321, 1959.

Lindemann, R. D., R. L. Scheer, and L. G. Raisz: Renal Amyloidosis, Ann. Intern. Med., 54:883, 1961.

Luxton, R. W.: Radiation Nephritis, Quart. J. Med., 22:215, 1953.

Perillie, P. E., and F. H. Epstein: Sickling Phenomenon Produced by Hypertonic Solutions. A Possible Explanation for the Hyposthenuria of Sicklemia, J. Clin. Invest., 42: 570, 1963.

Sanchez, L. M., and C. A. Domzy: Renal Patterns in Myeloma, Ann. Intern. Med., 52:44, 1960.

Schlitt, L. E., and H. G. Keitel: Renal Manifestations of Sickle-Cell Disease: A Review, Am. J. Med. Sci., 239: 773, 1960.

Talbott, J. H., and K. L. Terplan: The Kidney in Gout, Medicine, 19:405, 1960.

Section 5

Disorders of the Alimentary Tract

312 APPROACH TO THE PATIENT WITH GASTROINTESTINAL DISEASE

Kurt J. Isselbacher

GENERAL CONSIDERATIONS

Gastrointestinal symptoms occur not only with primary gastrointestinal tract pathology but also frequently as manifestations of other systemic diseases. Thus anorexia, nausea, and vomiting may be seen in congestive failure and uremia, and diarrhea or constipation may be seen as a consequence of metabolic derangements such as electrolyte changes or alterations in thyroid function. With today's technical advances one finds too often that the physician is willing to diagnose (or misdiagnose) gastrointestinal disease simply by relying on routine x-ray studies of the upper and lower gastrointestinal tract. Such an overwhelming dependence on technical procedures often leads to great pitfalls. In order to define the most probable and profitable area of study the proper approach includes careful attention to the history and physical examination before ordering the appropriate diagnostic tests.

IMPORTANCE OF THE HISTORY

To evaluate gastrointestinal symptoms, a careful history is crucial. Pain or indigestion is the most common intestinal complaint. Correlation between pain and gastrointestinal function must of necessity be chronologic. There should be a meticulous inquiry as to the frequency and specificity of the complaint. The questioning should include the location of the pain and whether it is circumscribed or diffuse. It is important to determine what factors aggravate or relieve the discomfort. *Does eating produce the symptom?* If so, determine whether the discomfort occurs *while eating* (as in esophageal disorders and abdominal angina), shortly *after the meal* (as often occurs in biliary tract disease), or *30 to 90 min later* (as typically seen with peptic ulcer). *Does eating relieve the symptom,* and if so, for how long? Temporary relief of epigastric pain is characteristic of gastritis and peptic ulceration. Many patients have tried or taken antacids by the time they come to the physician, and a history indicating relief of epigastric pain by antacids is suggestive of peptic disease of the upper intestine. *What is the relation of pain to bowel movements?* The patient with ulcerative colitis often obtains temporary relief from his lower abdominal cramps by defecation.

Attention should be paid to *anorexia* and *weight loss;* their combined occurrence should make one suspicious of an underlying malignancy. If weight loss is accompanied by an increased appetite, one must consider the diagnosis of malabsorption or maldigestion as well as a hypermetabolic state, such as thyrotoxicosis. If *diarrhea* is present, one should determine the average number of the stools and their consistency. To some patients, diarrhea means an increased number of stools, even though they are relatively normal in consistency; to others, diarrhea means watery stools. In a patient with diarrhea one should ask about stool *odor* (malodorous stools being typical of pancreatic insufficiency and sprue), change in stool *color* (light-colored stools are seen with steatorrhea or cholestasis), and whether blood or mucus has been noted. (Blood is characteristic of ulcerative colitis but is hardly ever noted in mucous colitis.)

Finally, careful attention must be given to a "drug history." We are living in a "medicated society." Unless asked, the patient may forget to mention that he takes aspirin almost daily for headache, and this may indeed account for the occult blood in his stool. Many patients take daily laxatives, which may explain chronic diarrhea and colonic changes on x-ray. It was through a careful analysis of drug therapy that the syndrome of intestinal ulceration due to the ingestion of enteric coated KCl was recognized.

PHYSICAL EXAMINATION AND ENDOSCOPY

A vague history of abdominal distress may be brought into focus by a thorough physical examination. Upper abdominal distress together with tenderness in the right upper quadrant suggests that cholecystitis or hepatitis may be present. The history of intermittent abdominal pain together with a palpable mass or tender loop of bowel in the right lower quadrant should make one suspicious of regional enteritis. All too often, however, in gastrointestinal diseases the routine physical examination is negative and other techniques for examining the bowel are needed. Among the techniques which should almost be routine as an extension of the physical examination is sigmoidoscopy. Not only will this serve to exclude rectosigmoid tumors, but it permits inspection of the mucosa for edema, erythema, friability, or ulceration. In a patient with diarrhea due to nonspecific causes, the mucosa may be normal; with dysentery due to agents such as shigella, the mucosa may become friable, edematous, and hyperemic; if the latter findings are combined with extensive ulcerations, ulcerative or amebic colitis may be present.

With the advent of fiberoptic instruments, it has become much easier and less hazardous to perform esophagoscopy and gastroscopy. Gastroscopy is often invaluable in helping to determine whether a gastric ulcer is benign or malignant. Endoscopy is also becoming an increasingly routine technique in the approach to the patient with upper gastrointestinal bleeding.

RADIOLOGIC EXAMINATION

Perhaps in no other organ system is the use of x-ray examination as important to diagnosis as in disorders of the intestinal tract. In fact, with few exceptions investigation of the patient with gastrointestinal symptoms is not complete without appropriate x-ray examination. However, all too often x-rays are ordered by the physician without attention to a number of important factors.

INITIAL CONSIDERATIONS BY THE INTERNIST. To obtain the best and most effective use of gastrointestinal x-rays, the physician must decide (1) which organ system is most likely to be involved, (2) in what sequence to perform the x-rays, and (3) whether there are any contraindications to the proposed radiologic study.

If the physician orders an upper gastrointestinal series and the results are negative, he may decide to order a barium enema only to find that it cannot be performed because of the presence of barium from the prior study. Therefore, if a thorough study of the intestinal tract is contemplated, the sequence should be (1) oral cholecystogram, (2) barium enema, and (3) upper gastrointestinal series. Preparation or prior cleansing of the intestinal tract is important for a proper barium enema examination, but the physician must keep in mind that with obstructing lesions of the colon or small bowel or in the presence of ulcerative colitis, the use of strong cathartics may be hazardous and even life-threatening. Hence *no x-ray preparation should be considered routine.* In fact the barium examination itself may aggravate an acute ulcerative colitis or precipitate colonic perforation or the onset of toxic megacolon. Similarly, if partial obstruction of the bowel is detected by plain film of the abdomen, the physician must be wary of introducing barium from above for fear of producing further or complete intestinal obstruction.

CONSULTATION WITH THE RADIOLOGIST. One cannot overemphasize the importance of providing the radiologist with as much information as possible about the nature of the disease process under investigation. While this can be done in writing (on the x-ray requisition), it is often preferable to do this verbally. In fact in difficult cases it is advantageous for the physician to join the radiologist during the study. In addition, the radiologist may suggest, for example, that instead of barium an iodinated radiopaque dye may be preferable; that the study should be supplemented with angiography or a scinti-scan of the organ; or that the examination be repeated with more adequate preparation of the patient.

INTERPRETATION. All too often the busy physician allows a negative x-ray report to be the decisive factor in his diagnosis. If the patient has had weight loss and a change in bowel habits and the physician suspects a colonic neoplasm, inspection of the films (by himself or preferably with the radiologist) may in fact reveal that the patient had too much retained fecal material in his colon or that the area of concern was never well visualized. Similarly, if the patient has typical ulcer symptoms or a classic history of biliary colic, the physician should not discard his diagnosis only because of a negative x-ray report.

On the other hand, the physician must be able to determine whether the abnormal finding is causally related to the symptoms. This is especially true in older patients where the presence of a hiatus hernia, gallstones, or diverticulosis is not unusual and hence may be coincidental. Thus it is clear that in order to reach the correct gastroenterologic diagnosis, the physician must insist that (1) the clinical picture and the results of the technical diagnostic procedures (especially x-ray and endoscopy) are in accord and that (2) all information, whatever the source and nature, creates a reasonable whole.

DIAGNOSTIC APPROACHES

PROBLEMS OF SWALLOWING

The approach should be as follows:

1. Careful visual and *neurologic examination* of the pharynx, with tests for myasthenia gravis if indicated.

2. *Routine esophageal* x-rays in the upright and lateral or Trendelenburg position. The horizontal views are essential for demonstration of the swallowing mechanism, unaided by gravity, and of the esophagogastric junction. For details of the pharyngoesophageal area cineradiography is necessary because of the rapidity with which the contrast media passes through. Hiatus hernia is extremely common (in 15 to 35 percent of persons over fifty) and often asymptomatic unless reflux of gastric contents can be demonstrated to occur repeatedly.

3. *Esophagoscopy* is desirable to describe lesions suspected by x-ray, or unsuspected, to obtain biopsies from masses or abnormal mucosa, and to obtain washings for exfoliative cytologic study. The diagnosis of peptic esophagitis is best made endoscopically. Esophageal varices can be identified by this approach when they are too small to be seen radiologically, although the latter technique will pick up 70 percent of large varices.

4. *Manometric studies* of the pharyngoesophageal area, particularly in conjunction with cineradiography, at present offer the best differential between disorders primary in the central nervous system, primary pharyngeal muscular disease, and cricopharyngeal dystonia. Furthermore, such studies applied to the body of the esophagus clearly identify aperistalsis, diffuse spasm of the esophageal body, and the inferior esophageal sphincteric apparatus, both in the unstimulated state and in response to parenteral injections of cholinergic drugs, which in the denervated (aganglionic) esophagus of achalasia produce a tetanic contraction of the lower esophagus.

PEPTIC OR DIGESTIVE DISORDERS

The approach to this type of disorder involves:

1. *Insertion of a nasogastric tube.* This is necessary to establish whether significant gastric retention (more than 75 ml) exists, and whether there is acid, bile, blood, or other material in these contents. If pyloric obstruction or gastric atony is present, the tube is used to maintain suction while the patient's electrolyte and fluid balance is restored to normal; the stomach is kept as clean as possible so that reliable radiologic investigation may be carried out.

2. *Radiologic examination* of stomach, duodenum, and the upper part of the jejunum is the most important single procedure in this area. The single examination of the stomach carries an overall accuracy of about 80 percent if the lumen is carefully cleaned out beforehand; duodenal lesions are more precisely identified (90 percent). Puzzling lesions of the entire area are often clarified by *cineradiographic* techniques.

3. When lesions are noted radiographically in the stomach, *gastroscopy* may be very helpful in identifying the diffuseness of the mucosal response in gastritis or together with biopsy differentiate between peptic and neoplastic ulcerating lesions. It can make the diagnosis of superficial erosive gastritis as a cause of bleeding when the x-ray examination is negative. The endoscopist has difficulty in visualizing that portion of the stomach high under the diaphragm, as well as the gastric antrum along the lesser curvature. Gastroscopy is particularly helpful in inspecting the postoperative stomach, especially when stomal ulceration is suspected.

4. *Exfoliative cytologic study* of gastric contents, in the hands of those who are expert, is capable of diagnostic accuracy of 85 to 95 percent in identifying mucosal abnormalities such as malignancies and the gastric changes of pernicious anemia. The method is of value in follow-up studies of patients with high probability of developing gastric neoplasms. *Peroral biopsy* of the stomach carries a slight risk but may confirm cytologic or endoscopic findings.

5. *Gastric acid secretory studies* are of importance in establishing a diagnosis of active duodenal ulcer or of the Zollinger-Ellison syndrome, in confirming a diagnosis of pernicious anemia, in suggesting the best surgical operation for duodenal ulcer in a particular patient, and in testing the completeness of surgical vagotomy.

The only reliable technique for measuring rates of gastric acid production employs an indwelling tube and requires careful attention to detail of tube placement, handling of samples, and analysis. Presently this method is used in one of two ways: (1) "Basal secretion" is that obtained in the morning after an overnight fast in an unstimulated stomach; it measures vagal plus hormonal factors acting on the gastric mucosa. After discarding the first aspirate, four samples are taken over a period of an hour, while the patient expectorates any saliva. The absence of hydrochloric acid in any of the four samples is considered incompatible with the presence of an active duodenal ulcer. (2) "Maximum acid output" is assessed by collecting samples every 15 min for an hour in a patient who has previously received a parenteral antihistaminic drug, then an amount of parenteral histamine equal to 0.04 mg histamine acid phosphate per kg body weight, or of the safer analogue, betazole, 2.0 mg per kg body weight. This concept is based on data showing that all parietal cells are maximally stimulated by this dosage. Thus maximum output is equivalent to the total "parietal cell mass." Achlorhydria is defined as the failure of the stomach so stimulated to produce a juice with a pH less than 6.0. The normal basal fasting secretion is 30 to 70 ml per hr with acid production being 1 to 2.5 mEq per hr. Maximal acid output is 20 to 25 mEq per hr. In the Zollinger-Ellison syndrome basal acid secretion is usually greater than 10 mEq per hr.

DISORDERS OF THE MESENTERIC SMALL INTESTINE

Such problems usually present as obstructive syndromes; the plain film of the abdomen is the most important diagnostic adjunct to careful physical examination. Patterns of dilatation of individual loops of bowel may be characteristic, as in volvulus or acute pancreatitis; erect and decubitus views will often show fluid levels in the affected segments. Air under the diaphragm is diagnostic of a perforated viscus; air in the portal vein usually results from bowel necrosis secondary to mesenteric vascular occlusion. The diagnostic accuracy of the plain film in all types of intestinal obstruction is about 75 percent. Celiac artery angiography is a new method of special value in the diagnosis of mesenteric vascular disease.

INFLAMMATORY AND NEOPLASTIC DISEASES OF SMALL AND LARGE BOWEL

Patients with these conditions are usually identified by history, physical examination, and careful examination of the stools for exudate and blood. Sigmoidoscopy is valuable in identifying mucosal and neoplastic lesions of the lower 25 cm of colon; anal lesions commonly accompany inflammatory disease of the ileum and colon. The radiologic examination of the small intestine is highly reliable in identifying the prestenotic and stenotic lesions of Crohn's disease and in suggesting various malabsorptive syndromes. In the colon a single examination in a well-prepared patient has a diagnostic accuracy of 80 to 85 percent; the addition of air-contrast technique in a second examination brings the accuracy up over 90 percent, but none of these figures is meaningful if the patient is poorly prepared for the examination. In the demonstration of small polyps the degree of accuracy is understandably not so high, but for polyps larger than 1 cm it is satisfactory. The cecal area is the hardest to examine adequately because of its anatomy; flat plaquelike lesions on the posterior wall are particularly hard to demonstrate. The rectal area is usually better visualized proctoscopically than radiologically.

Peroral biopsy of the small intestine and forceps biopsy of the rectosigmoid are of considerable importance in revealing mucosal disease. Rectal biopsy is an excellent means of demonstrating amyloidosis, schistosomiasis, and amebiasis. Submucosal disease is not seen in these superficial biopsies. Hirschsprung's disease is histologically diagnosed by a deep surgical biopsy of the lower part of the rectum.

MALABSORPTION SYNDROMES

Malabsorption may be suspected on the basis of history and physical examination and is confirmed by examination of the stools. Radiologic examination is of general help in ruling out local lesions and suggesting motor and secretory dysfunction, but it is rarely diagnostic unless calcifications in the pancreas or short circuits between intestine and stomach are demonstrated.

The tests useful in the diagnosis of malabsorption are discussed in Chap. 316. Analyses of 3-day stool collections for volume, fat, and nitrogen content on a standard diet establish the diagnosis of malabsorption. The d-xylose absorption test is about 90 percent accurate in separating mucosal disease from pancreatic insufficiency. Peroral biopsy of the small intestine is of value in the diagnosis of celiac disease, and may show the less common infiltrations of the mucosa by amyloid or bacterial mucoproteins (Whipple's disease). Leakage of protein into the intestinal lumen may cause hypoproteinemia and can be demonstrated by the recovery in stools of intravenously administered markers such as ^{131}I polyvinylpyrrolidone or albumin labeled with iodine or chromium isotopes.

BILIARY TRACT

Radiologic examination is most helpful in the nonjaundiced patient, since the obstructed or diseased liver cannot adequately excrete the contrast media into the biliary tree. Oral cholecystography is a highly reliable technique, with an accuracy approaching 95 percent. In the cholecystectomized patient, intravenous cholangiography has given excellent visualization, particularly if accompanied by tomography. When air is seen in the biliary tree, it often results from gallstone ileus.

Barium studies of the duodenum for the changes produced by pancreatic masses, pancreatitis, and retroperitoneal nodes have been markedly improved in recent years, especially by the use of hypotonic duodenography, but the accuracy of such examinations is still not over 80 percent. Exfoliative cytologic studies of the second and third duodenum are reliable in expert hands, particularly when they are used after "flushing" the pancreatic ducts with secretin. The accuracy of this technique for cancer of the pancreas in the best hands approaches 80 percent; negative results thus may not have important significance. The same kind of intubation technique can be used to demonstrate cholesterol crystals and microspheroliths in aspirated bile for the positive diagnosis of gallstones, and with the addition of an indwelling gastric tube for suction, to carry out tests of pancreatic secretion as stimulated by secretin and cholinergics (see Chaps 333, 334).

REFERENCES

Cooley, Robert N.: The Diagnostic Accuracy of Radiologic Studies of Biliary Tract, Small Intestine, and Colon. Am. J. Med. Sci., 246:610, 1963.

Raskin, H. F., J. Wenger, M. Sklar, S. Pleticka, and W. Yorema: Diagnosis of Cancer of the Pancreas, Biliary Tract and Duodenum by Combined Cytologic and Secretory Methods, Gastroenterology, 34:996–1016, 1958.

Sparberg, M., and J. B. Kirsner: Gastric Secretory Activity with Reference to HCl, Arch. Intern. Med., 114:508, 1964.

Truelove, S. C., and R. C. Reynell: "Diseases of the Digestive System," Philadelphia, F. A. Davis Company, 1963.

313 DISEASES OF THE ESOPHAGUS
Thomas R. Hendrix

Although the exact correlation of anatomic, radiologic, and functional features of the esophagus and the cardio-esophageal junction in particular continue to be debated, it is useful to consider disorders of the esophagus in functional terms. In normal swallowing the activities of the striated muscle of the pharynx and upper esophagus and smooth muscle of the lower esophagus are so closely integrated that they function as a single tissue. The esophagus proper is separated from adjacent segments of the alimentary tract by two sphincters. (A sphincter is a segment that has a resting tone greater than the adjacent segments and that relaxes in response to the appropriate stimulus—swallowing in the case of the esophagus.) The upper esophageal sphincter (cricopharyngeus) separates the pharynx from the esophagus and prevents air from filling the esophagus during inspiration. The lower esophageal sphincter is the barrier to reflux of gastric juice into the esophagus. It relaxes during swallowing, regurgitation, belching, and vomiting.

Other structures illustrated diagrammatically in Fig. 313-1 have been assigned varying roles in preventing reflux. These include the infradiaphragmatic segment of the lower esophageal sphincter, the possible flap valve mechanism provided by the angle of His, and the diaphragm itself. The first phase of swallowing, the movement of the bolus from the mouth to the pharynx, is voluntary, but subsequent events are involuntary. As the upper sphincter relaxes, the bolus is propelled into the esophagus. The lower esophageal sphincter relaxes prior to the arrival of the bolus in the lower esophagus. Finally, the esophagus is swept clean by a peristaltic wave proceeding from pharynx to lower esophageal sphincter.

SYMPTOMATOLOGY. Dysphagia (See Chap. 40). Difficulty in swallowing can be produced by the derangement or incoordination of any part of the swallowing act as well as by the narrowing of the lumen by tumor or an inflammatory stricture. Dysphagia of oropharyngeal origin is characterized by failure to move a bolus out of the mouth, regurgitation into the nose, or aspiration into the trachea. Esophageal dysphagia is characterized by the complaint that food is sticking somewhere behind the sternum. Dysphagia occurs only with swallowing and must be differentiated from globus hystericus, a persistent sensation of a lump or tightness in the throat.

Dysphagia is usually localized to the level of the lower sternum corresponding to the most frequent site of esophageal disease. In other instances dysphagia is localized higher in the chest or at the base of the neck, either because the responsible lesion is situated higher in the esophagus or because in some patients sensations from the distal esophagus are referred to the level of the sternal notch.

Dysphagia may be painless, but more often it is distressing and sometimes causes pain of alarming proportions. It commonly appears gradually in intermittent attacks, although on occasion the onset is abrupt and reaches maximum intensity rapidly. Certain foods, notably beef and soft breads, are often the first offenders, probably because these elastic solids are wedged by peristalsis into the segment narrowed by esophageal disease. The impacted bolus may be forced through the narrowed area by drinking liquids, or forceful retching may be required to dislodge the food, and on occasion it must be removed through the esophagoscope.

Pain. Heartburn, or pyrosis, is the most common type of esophageal pain. Heartburn, a burning, tight, or searing sensation, appears intermittently beneath the lower sternum and spreads upward in a wavelike fashion to the throat or even into the angles of the jaw. It is often associated with increased salivation. Heartburn is most likely to occur 10 to 60 min after eating, especially after overindulging, and is accentuated by bending over or lying down. Heartburn is the consequence of reflux of gastric juice into the esophagus, and it is believed that refluxed gastric contents initiate an abnormal esophageal motor response that is appreciated by the patient as pain.

Esophageal pain frequently accompanies dysphagia and may be severe if the bolus is unable to pass the constricted segment. In addition, esophageal pain may occur in the absence of dysphagia or obvious heartburn. At times its onset is so abrupt and severe that myocardial infarction is the initial diagnosis. Esophageal pain may mimic ischemic heart pain even to the radiation of pain down the ulnar aspect of the arms. Referral of esophageal pain to the epigastrium is common, and referral to the back is encountered on occasion.

Belching. A belch is caused by the forceful regurgitation of air from the stomach or esophagus. Although belching is an esophageal phenomenon, it is, except in diaphragmatic hernia, not a common manifestation of esophageal disease. More often it is a functional disorder or is indicative of peptic, cardiac, or biliary tract disease.

Regurgitation. Regurgitation, as opposed to vomiting, means the effortless appearance of esophageal or gastric contents in the mouth. A functional disorder of esophageal motility, a retrograde flow of material forced by normal peristalsis against an obstructed segment, or a gravitational effect, as in the case of the dilated esophagus of cardiospasm, may be responsible for regurgitation.

DIAPHRAGMATIC HERNIA

Diaphragmatic hernia is usually defined as a herniation of a portion of the stomach into the chest through the

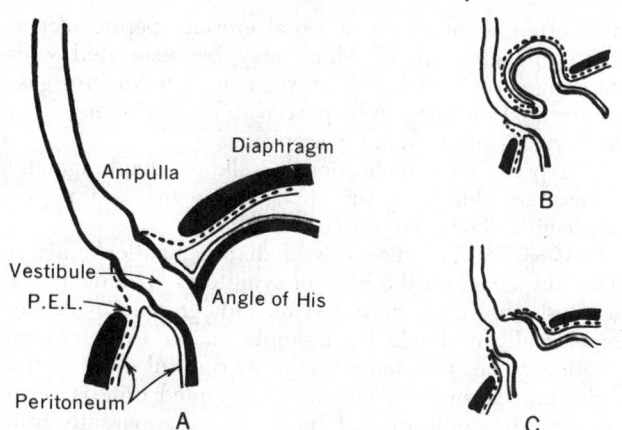

Fig. 313-1. Diagrammatic representation of the structure and relations of the lower esophagus. A. Normal esophagus. B. Parahiatal hernia. C. Sliding hernia. In this type of hernia the distinction between the vestibule and the herniated cardia is lost, and the angle of His has become obtuse. P.E.L. = phrenoesophageal ligament. The location of the gastroesophageal junction is a matter of opinion. It may be defined as located at the level where the tube of the esophagus widens into the sac of the stomach, but sometimes the transition from one shape to the other is gradual rather than abrupt. Alternatively, the junction is placed at the serrated line where squamous esophageal and glandular gastric mucosas meet, but this epithelial boundary may be located somewhat above the level of the angle of His and thus does not necessarily coincide with a division of stomach and esophagus based on gross shape and muscular function.

esophageal hiatus of the diaphragm. Clinically it is useful to classify hernias as rolling, or paraesophageal, and sliding, or direct. In the first, the gastric cardia rolls through the hiatus beside a gastroesophageal junction that is normally situated with respect to the diaphragmatic hiatus (Fig. 313-1B). In the second, the sliding, or direct, hernia, both the stomach and the gastroesophageal junction slip up into the chest, thereby placing the gastroesophageal junction above the diaphragmatic hiatus (Fig. 313-1C). This position of the junction may make the esophagus appear shortened, but actual shortening occurs rarely. Many hernias are mixed and present features of both types.

Sliding hernia is three to ten times as common as the rolling and mixed hernias combined. Paraesophageal hernias are primarily a disorder of women, being ten times as frequent in women as in men.

SYMPTOMS. The major symptoms that can be attributed to diaphragmatic hernia are those initiated by reflux of gastric juice into the esophagus. Heartburn, regurgitation, and epigastric pain associated with reflux precipitated by eating and aggravated by lying down or bending over are characteristic. Belching, vomiting, dysphagia, and anemia (because of bleeding) may also be associated with a diaphragmatic hernia.

Symptoms due to the herniated pouch of the stomach are almost exclusively limited to the rolling, or mixed, type of hernia. On rare occasion a patient with a paraesophageal hernia presents with acute prostration due to strangulation of the hernia. Although chronic and acute bleeding commonly are attributed to hernias, bleeding most often originates in mucosal erosion, peptic ulcers, and esophagitis, all of which may be associated with diaphragmatic hernia. It is uncommon, however, for gastrointestinal bleeding to be *proved* to be originating from the hernia itself or from the esophagus.

The principal complications of sliding diaphragmatic hernias are due to gastroesophageal reflux and peptic esophagitis. These are discussed below.

DIAGNOSIS. The diagnosis of diaphragmatic hernia is often suspected on the basis of symptoms. The definitive diagnosis, however, must rest on radiographic evidence. Superficially it should be a simple matter to determine whether or not the stomach is in its rightful place in the abdomen, because the commonly accepted criteria seem precise. The application of these criteria apparently presents great difficulty, and the incidence of diaphragmatic hernia has been reported to be as low as 1 percent and as high as 70 percent in routine barium meal studies performed for the investigation of dyspepsia. There is also no agreement as to the frequency with which diaphragmatic hernias produce symptoms, and it has been claimed that the incidence of symptoms varies from 30 to 97 percent. Symptoms ascribed to diaphragmatic hernia are diverse and may resemble those of coronary insufficiency, biliary colic, pancreatitis, gastric and duodenal ulcers, esophageal disorders, and functional digestive disorders. Association, however, does not establish a cause-and-effect relation. The important clinical question is not whether the patient has a hernia but whether significant reflux is present.

TREATMENT. The aim of treatment is to decrease gastroesophageal reflux. This will be discussed under Chronic Peptic Esophagitis. Operative repair of paraesophageal hernias is indicated if they have been identified as causing esophageal obstruction, respiratory symptoms, perforation, strangulation, repeated or chronic bleeding, or severe distress not affected by intensive use of medical measures.

ESOPHAGITIS

ACUTE ESOPHAGITIS. Mild acute esophagitis, with substernal pain aggravated by swallowing, may complicate infections of the upper part of the respiratory tract. Severe esophageal inflammation with variable necrosis may occur in moribund states, in diseases of the central nervous system, after extensive burns or trauma, after operations, especially if vomiting is pronounced or gastric intubation prolonged, with herpetic oral lesions that extend into the esophagus, and with monilial esophagitis that may appear in those weakened by chronic disease, especially if antibiotics or adrenocortical hormones have been used. In many of these conditions debility, ischemia, the trauma of vomiting, or exposure of the esophageal mucosa to acid gastric contents must be important pathogenic factors.

The ingestion of alkaline corrosive agents produces a form of acute esophagitis which, if not immediately fatal, may terminate in extensive esophageal stenosis. Immediate treatment consists of parenteral analgesics for pain and avoidance of oral intake for 3 to 7 days. The use of adrenocorticosteroids to contain the tissue reaction responsible for the stricture, intubation to maintain an esophageal lumen, and antibiotics to prevent mediastinitis are controversial.

CHRONIC PEPTIC ESOPHAGITIS. Esophagitis means inflammation of the esophagus; the term, however, is used commonly to indicate severe or persistent symptoms of reflux. Although esophagitis frequently accompanies severe reflux, at least one-fourth of patients with symptoms severe enough to be diagnosed as peptic esophagitis have normal esophageal biopsies. On the other hand, inflammation of the esophagus can occur without symptoms. Symptoms of reflux are frequently encountered in patients with high gastric acidity. One-third of patients with peptic esophagitis have or have had a duodenal ulcer. Because sliding diaphragmatic hernia is associated frequently with an incompetent lower esophageal sphincter, it predisposes to reflux and esophagitis. Ten to forty percent of patients with peptic esophagitis do not, however, have diaphragmatic hernias. Occasionally chronic esophagitis appears in elderly patients following an episode of severe vomiting or after intubation that has been used postoperatively or to treat gastrointestinal distention. In these cases, debility and local trauma presumably enhance esophageal susceptibility to refluxed gastric contents.

SYMPTOMS. These patients may or may not have a history of duodenal ulcer but almost invariably have suffered chronic heartburn. At first heartburn is troublesome only after overeating, soon after retiring to bed, or when bending over. In some patients heartburn worsens, cold and hot foods and slightly acid foods are increasingly painful to swallow, and eventually dysphagia appears. Dysphagia is most frequently due to acid-induced esophageal spasm. In some patients, not necessarily those with the most impressive reflux symptom, an inflammatory stricture develops causing progressive dysphagia. With advancing disease, malnutrition is inevitable, and occasionally slow blood loss occurs.

DIAGNOSIS. The diagnosis of esophagitis can be suspected on clinical, radiographic, and esophagoscopic findings but is established by demonstrating inflammatory changes in an esophageal biopsy. Of more importance is the demonstration that the patient's symptoms are due to reflux and are induced by acid. The acid perfusion test of Bernstein et al. provides the simplest and most direct demonstration that the patient's symptoms can be attributed to reflux. This test is positive if 0.1 N hydrochloric acid but not saline solution duplicates the patient's pain when dripped into the esophagus at a rate of 100 drops per min. Reflux and esophagitis are not necessarily primary processes but may be the manifestation of a variety of diseases such as peptic ulcer, cancer, and scleroderma.

TREATMENT. Medical management aims to protect the esophagus by decreasing reflux of gastric juice and by decreasing the irritant effect of the refluxed juice. The first aim may be achieved by decreasing the volume of gastric contents available for reflux, by positioning the patient so that gravity acts to impede reflux, and by improving the function of the lower esophageal sphincter. In practical terms, the patient is advised to take small meals and not to eat in the 2 to 3 hr before retiring. Patients should avoid those foods which they may have found to be associated with dyspepsia and heartburn. Four to six-inch blocks elevating the head of the bed lessen nocturnal gastroesophageal regurgitation.

Although anticholinergic drugs decrease the volume of gastric secretion, they are not indicated in the treatment of peptic esophagitis, because in effective doses they decrease tone in the lower esophageal sphincter, decrease the volume of alkaline saliva, and decrease frequency of secondary peristalsis, which functions to return refluxed gastric juice to the stomach. To aid in decreasing the irritant effect of refluxed gastric juice, 1 tsp. of a liquid, viscous antacid preparation, such as aluminum hydroxide gel, should be taken at hourly intervals while the patient is awake. The medication should be taken "straight" and should not be followed by other material.

Finally, in stocky or obese patients, weight loss is beneficial.

DIFFUSE ESOPHAGEAL SPASM

Diffuse esophageal spasm is a very common disorder of esophageal motor function. Although encountered at all ages, it is most frequent in individuals over fifty-five and increases in frequency with age. Diffuse spasm in severe form produces retrosternal pain or dysphagia or both. In patients with this disorder peristalsis is initiated normally by swallowing, but as the wave approaches the distal third of the esophagus, the progressive contraction is supplanted by "spastic" or simultaneous contractions. Unlike cardiospasm, lower esophageal sphincter function is usually normal in diffuse esophageal spasm. The nature of the underlying neuromuscular dysfunction is not known. This type of esophageal motor disorder may be induced by reflux of gastric juice and is responsible for much of the dysphagia associated with diaphragmatic hernia and peptic esophagitis.

SYMPTOMS. Dysphagia or substernal distress occur episodically. Symptoms frequently, although not necessarily, are triggered by ingestion of elastic boluses, such as meat, cold or carbonated beverages, and eating when tense or upset. On occasion a bolus becomes so firmly lodged in the "spastic" segment that relief is achieved only by retching and regurgitating the offending bolus. Often following such an episode the patient can return to the table and finish his meal without incident. Weight loss and aspiration pneumonia are not features of diffuse spasm. Substernal pain of esophageal origin may be acute and severe, and may be confused with angina pectoris, especially if symptoms are not associated with eating.

DIAGNOSIS. The diagnosis is suggested by the history of intermittent dysphagia and chest pain. X-ray findings (with barium swallow) confirm the existence of disordered esophageal motility. The mildest abnormality is tertiary or segmental contractions without a peristaltic wave in the distal esophagus. The contour of the lower esophagus may take a variety of bizarre shapes described

as curling, pseudodiverticulosis, corkscrew, or rosary bead esophagus. Symptoms, however, do not clearly correlate with the extent of the abnormality seen on barium swallow. Indeed, only a minority of patients with this disturbed motor pattern have significant symptoms. The motility abnormalities of diffuse esophageal spasm may be recorded by esophageal manometry.

TREATMENT. The first step in the treatment of diffuse spasm is to reassure the patient as to the benign nature of the disorder. The second step is to minimize the contribution of gastroesophageal reflux by giving antacids and small meals and elevating the head of the bed as described under Esophagitis.

An occasional patient obtains gratifying control of symptoms with the use of sublingual nitroglycerine at mealtime. Anticholinergic drugs, however, have not provided symptomatic relief. In patients with severe, poorly controlled symptoms forceful distension of the lower esophagus and sphincter by a pneumostatic dilator may be employed. As a last resort, a longitudinal myotomy of the entire distal esophagus has been successful in providing relief. This is, however, an extensive operation for a benign disorder.

CARDIOSPASM (ACHALASIA)

The terms *cardiospasm* and *achalasia* are used interchangeably; although well established by custom, neither describes the nature of the disorder accurately. Actually, cardiospasm is a motor disorder involving the entire distal two-thirds of the esophagus. In the esophagus above the lower esophageal sphincter there is either no motor response or nonprogressive, uncoordinated contractions following a swallow. For this reason the name *aperistalsis* is used in Brazil. The massive esophageal dilatation seen in some cases has, in turn, given rise to the name *megaesophagus*. Finally, the term achalasia (literally, "not relaxation") is used to indicate that the lower esophageal sphincter does not relax and thus creates an obstructing segment at the distal end of the esophagus. Actually, the tone within the lower esophageal sphincter is greater than normal, and it does relax in response to swallowing, but relaxation is incomplete and too brief to permit passage of much of the swallowed bolus.

The motor disorders of cardiospasm appear to reflect an impaired cholinergic innervation of the esophagus. Histologically the cells of the myenteric plexus, i.e., the parasympathetic ganglions, are damaged or absent. Pharmacologic studies have shown that administration of a cholinergic agent produces a tetanic, specific, and often violent contraction of the affected esophagus. This response, when interpreted in the light of Cannon's finding that denervated structures respond maximally to neurohumoral stimulation, provides additional evidence that in cardiospasm the cholinergic innervation of the esophagus is deficient. The ultimate cause, however, is unknown. In Brazil, the remarkable prevalence of cardiospasm in areas where Chagas' disease is endemic has fostered the strong conviction that the intrinsic esophageal denervation is a late result of esophageal infestation by the responsible agent, *Trypansosoma cruzi*, but this etiologic agent is not involved in the cardiospasm found in the United States.

SYMPTOMS. Cardiospasm affects patients of all ages and of both sexes. Its course is usually chronic, with dysphagia gradually worsening over months to years, leading to progressive weight loss. In some patients, the process is painless; in others spasms of substernal pain may follow eating. Occasionally the initial episode of dysphagia appears with dramatic suddenness, either after bolting food or after an emotional upset. In either case, however, the condition has probably been present in latent form before the acute episode. As the disease progresses, extreme and tortuous dilatation of the esophagus may develop. When the patient lies down, the copious amount of food residue, saliva, and other secretions contained in the spacious esophageal sac runs freely back into the pharynx and mouth. If the regurgitated material is aspirated, recurrent aspiration pneumonia is a potential complication. Although stagnation of food in the esophagus may be striking, esophagitis rarely if ever occurs in untreated cardiospasm. Malignant degeneration is an occasional late complication.

DIAGNOSIS. Diagnosis is usually made without difficulty on the basis of the history and the characteristic radiologic findings of abnormal esophageal motor function with smooth, beaklike narrowing of the distal esophageal segment. An occasional case presents as diffuse esophageal spasm and over many years evolves into a completely typical example of cardiospasm. In some cases, cancer originating in the gastric cardia and infiltrating the esophagus may present a somewhat similar x-ray appearance, and a variety of motor disorders of the lower esophagus have been confused with cardiospasm. These problems in differential diagnosis should be less frequent if it is remembered that the radiologic abnormalities of cardiospasm consist of deranged peristalsis as well as narrowing in the area of the sphincter.

TREATMENT. Symptomatic medical treatment consisting of sedatives, semisoft foods, nitrites, and anticholinergic drugs is not effective. The best available therapy is forceful dilation of the narrowed sphincter with the specific purpose of tearing some of the muscle fibers in this area. Passing graduated mercury-tipped bougies does not accomplish this and therefore relieves dysphagia only briefly. It is necessary to use bags that can be inflated under pressure or a mechanical (Starck) dilator. In experienced hands, these instruments, when positioned under fluoroscopic control, rarely cause esophageal rupture, and dysphagia is relieved successfully for years, or even permanently, in over 75 percent of cases. Forceful dilation does not restore normal esophageal motility, but it impairs the contractile power of the sphincter and thus permits the esophagus to empty under the influence of hydrostatic and transmitted oropharyngeal pressures. Improved esophageal emptying, in turn, prevents further distension of the lumen and aspiration of esophageal contents.

When the esophagus is extremely dilated and sufficiently tortuous to warrant the adjective *sigmoid*, mechani-

cal dilation of the narrowed area is often not feasible, and surgical intervention becomes necessary. Unfortunately any procedure that creates a new opening between the dilated esophagus and the stomach permits, when the patient lies down, reflux of gastric contents into an already damaged esophagus which cannot muster the peristaltic force necessary to return the gastric contents to the stomach. As a consequence severe esophagitis, which is often more distressing than the cardiospasm, occurs and also may be a major source of blood loss. If technically feasible, the surgical procedure favored at present is the Heller myotomy, which is based on the same principle as forceful dilation: the contractile power of the sphincter is reduced by placing a longitudinal cut through the muscle, but not the mucosa, of the narrowed segment. Myotomy is, however, not invariably successful in alleviating dysphagia or preventing reflux esophagitis. In advanced cases, with unsuccessful previous operative procedures, jejunal interposition may have to be used to replace the hopelessly malfunctioning gastroesophageal segment.

CANCER

SYMPTOMS. The importance of dysphagia as a symptom and the urgent necessity of determining its cause are no better exemplified than by the patient with esophageal cancer. Difficulty in swallowing is often the patient's first, and at times his only, complaint as the tumor encroaches upon the lumen. Although initially intermittent, the dysphagia is inexorably progressive over the course of months. In fungating tumors, the most common gross variety of esophageal cancer, pain under the sternum, in the back, or in the neck, is common and sometimes precedes dysphagia. In some cases an early symptom not to be ignored is substernal burning on swallowing hot liquids. Slow oozing of blood is a frequent complication, but brisk bleeding a rare. In about 25 percent of cases, however, particularly with infiltrative or polypoid cancers, symptoms other than dysphagia appear only terminally. When esophageal stenosis is severe, regurgitation of esophageal contents, which are sometimes blood-flecked, is common.

Approximately 20 percent of esophageal cancers are in the upper third, 30 percent in the middle, and 50 percent in the lower third of the organ. The lesions in the upper-two-thirds are derived squamous esophageal mucosa. In the distal esophagus over half the cases prove to be adenocarcinomas, indicating that many cancers in this area are gastric in origin. Origin in the stomach is, in fact, often evident at operation in cases which radiologically appear to be purely esophageal.

COURSE. Physical examination is usually negative, and even those patients with advanced disease may present no more than the signs of malnutrition. Although metastases to lymph nodes occur in three-fourths of the cases, only 5 percent have palpable nodes in the supraclavicular or other accessible areas. Because the liver and lung each are involved eventually in 20 to 25 percent of the cases, hepatomegaly or pulmonary lesions may be evident. Other organs subject to metastatic foci are bone, kidneys, and adrenal glands. Sometimes direct invasion of adjoining structures leads to dramatic complications: (1) mediastinitis with subcutaneous emphysema in the neck, (2) tracheoesophageal or bronchoesophageal fistula, with an apoplectic cough induced by swallowing liquids, or (3) aortic perforation with precipitous exsanguination.

DIAGNOSIS. Esophageal cancer occurs in the usual cancer age groups, and predominantly in males in a ratio of 4:1. It is about one-tenth as common as cancer of the stomach in either sex. X-ray often reveals the irregular and sometimes surprisingly long luminal defect caused by esophageal cancer, but supplemental diagnostic information must usually be sought by esophagoscopy and biopsy. The initial examination with either procedure is not, however, invariably adequate in differentiating cancer from inflammatory stricture. In these cases, cytologic examination of material obtained by esophageal lavage is indicated. This procedure, depending upon the interest and experience of the cytologic laboratory, yields 75 to 95 percent positive results in patients with esophageal cancer.

TREATMENT. Lesions that appear to be resectable are usually treated surgically. Calculated on the basis of all esophageal cancer patients who enter a hospital, the 5-year cure rate is still a disappointing 0 to 7 percent. In some hands, however, 5-year cure rates in patients who at operation have no gross evidence of extension are over 30 percent for cancers in the lower third of the esophagus. Successful resection of higher cancers is more difficult, and such lesions are often treated with radiotherapy. In the case of inoperable tumors of the fungating variety, a remarkable degree of palliation may sometimes be achieved by deep radiotherapy.

OTHER ESOPHAGEAL DISORDERS

DIVERTICULA. Diverticula are found in the esophagus in about 5 percent of older patients who are given a swallow of barium. Most of these pouches occur in the midesophagus and distal esophagus, but they are usually small (1 to 4 cm in diameter) and do not cause symptoms. Extremely rarely an esophageal diverticulum is subject to ulceration or becomes large enough to cause dysphagia. A diverticulum of great clinical importance, however, is Zenker's diverticulum, a pouch which actually arises in the posterior aspect of the hypopharynx but which extends downward between the spine and the esophagus. Patients with this condition—elderly men for the most part—suffer dysphagia because swallowed material tends to fill the diverticular sac, which then compresses the esophagus. Regurgitation of stagnant food and nocturnal fits of coughing may complicate the picture. The diagnosis can usually be made by x-ray provided the pharynx is adequately studied as the patient swallows barium. Surgical treatment is necessary to relieve the symptoms of Zenker's diverticulum but may be complicated by mediastinal infection, disorders of pharyngeal function during swallowing, or recurrence of the diverticulum.

LOWER ESOPHAGEAL RING. This is the name given to a thin, symmetric, diaphragmlike structure located 1 to 4 cm above the diaphragmatic hiatus. Ten to twenty percent of adults have asymptomatic rings, but if the residual lumen is less than 12 mm in diameter, the ring may cause a highly characteristic syndrome consisting of intermittent attacks of dysphagia, recurring over years, unassociated with any other esophageal abnormality and precipitated only when the patient swallows meat or other elastic chunks without proper chewing. Treatment usually consist of avoiding hasty swallowing. Dilation is inconstantly successful. In a few, unusually severe cases, surgical treatment with cutting or fracture of the diaphragm is indicated.

SCLERODERMA (Progressive Systemic Sclerosis). Scleroderma is associated with loss of esophageal peristalsis and sphincter tone in 80 percent of the cases. Although gastroesophageal reflux and esophagitis are common, heartburn is not a prominent feature, and dysphagia, which is much less striking than that encountered with achalasia, does not become prominent until esophagitis has led to stricture of the esophagus. Chronic blood loss may be an important complication. Esophageal aperistalsis is not limited to scleroderma but may be seen occasionally in other disorders, particularly those associated with Raynaud's phenomenon.

DERMATOMYOSITIS. Oropharyngeal dysphagia (see Chap. 40) complicates the course of patients with dermatomyosis because of involvement of the striated muscle of the pharynx. Difficulty propelling the bolus from the mouth into the esophagus, regurgitation into the nose, and aspiration are the consequences of pharyngeal muscle weakness. Aperistalsis of the esophagus is seen occasionally in patients with polymyositis. It is sometimes difficult to categorize these patients, because they may have features of both scleroderma and dematomyositis.

PEPTIC ULCER. A solitary peptic ulcer is occasionally found in the distal esophagus. This lesion differs from peptic esophagitis in that the ulcer is more sharply localized, penetrates more deeply, and is more apt to perforate or to cause massive bleeding. On the other hand, the ulcer is more susceptible to standard medical management with antacids (Chap. 314), produces less extensive stricture on healing, and causes less chronic dysphagia than peptic esophagitis. The solitary peptic ulcer in the distal esophagus thus resembles a benign gastric ulcer in many respects. Indeed many ulcers at the lower end of the gullet actually involve either a herniated portion of stomach or a section of the esophagus that is lined with gastric mucosa.

PERFORATION AND RUPTURE. Perforation of the esophagus may complicate esophagitis, peptic ulcer, or neoplasm. Rupture may be induced by external trauma or, more commonly, during instrumentation of the esophagus. Sometimes it develops spontaneously in a previously healthy organ. The consequences are a syndrome comprising (1) severe pain, usually substernal but occasionally epigastric or precordial, intensified by swallowing, (2) free air in the mediastinum, producing a mediastinal crunch and subcutaneous emphysema palpable within 1 to 12 hr, (3) digestion of mediastinal pleura by pressure and gastric juice with resultant hydropneumothorax or hemopneumothorax and respiratory embarrassment, (4) shock, and (5) secondary infection.

Spontaneous rupture is a specific entity that develops suddenly during vomiting or coughing, or occasionally merely after injudicious gluttony. The tear, 1 to 8 cm in length, almost invariably is in the posterolateral portion of the esophagus immediately proximal to the diaphragmatic hiatus. The diagnosis should be suspected in elderly men (80 percent of cases) who suddenly have pain while vomiting or coughing; it is established by x-ray (air in the mediastinum or neck, demonstration of laceration by having the patient swallow radiopaque material, pleuropulmonary abnormalities), detection of methylene blue in the pleural fluid after a swallow of the dye, and exclusion of myocardial infarction, pancreatitis, and ruptured abdominal viscus. Air under the diaphragm is never found in spontaneous esophageal rupture.

Perforation of the esophagus is fatal if not treated vigorously. In early cases, constant esophageal suction and parenteral administration of antibiotics, which are active against both enteric gram-negative organisms and enterococci, should be given. Surgical drainage and repair of the laceration are indicated as soon as possible.

A disorder closely allied to spontaneous esophageal rupture is vertical laceration of the gastroesophageal junction producing severe and occasionally exsanguinating hemorrhage. This so-called "Mallory-Weiss syndrome" usually develops when vomiting follows an alcoholic bout.

PATTERSON-KELLY (PLUMMER-VINSON) SYNDROME. This syndrome, also known as *sideropenic dysphagia*, is a cause of dysphagia in women with hypochromic anemia. A crescentic fold indenting the anterior aspect of the cricopharyngeal area and mucosal atrophy and inflammation of the hypopharynx are features of this disorder. A good diet and iron are usually therapeutically effective, but sometimes supplemental instrumental dilation is required. This lesion predisposes to pharyngeal carcinoma.

FOREIGN BODIES. Foreign bodies may cause dysphagia, pain, or perforation of the esophagus. Rigid bodies usually are arrested above the aortic arch, and elastic material usually is held up in the distal esophagus. Not infrequently a structural abnormality or disease or the esophagus is responsible for stopping the foreign body.

VARICES. Esophageal varices are discussed in Chaps. quently a structural abnormality or disease of the esophageal symptoms. Radiologically, however, they may be confused with cancer or esophagitis.

BENIGN INTRAMURAL TUMORS OF THE ESOPHAGUS. Tumors such as cyst (usually of respiratory tract origin), leiomyoma, fibroma, and neurofibroma may cause intermittent dysphagia and sharply defined radiologic defects with smooth margins. Some benign tumors, especially adenomas, may produce intraluminal polyps.

The esophagus may be affected by leukoplakia, acanthosis nigricans, sarcoma, Hodgkin's disease, and leukemia.

EXTRINSIC DISEASE. Diseases of the aorta, heart, respiratory tract, or mediastinal lymph nodes often displace the esophagus and may appear to narrow the lumen. Aneurysms of the aortic arch and an aberrant right subclavian artery may compress the esophageal lumen; however, dysphagia is rarely produced by extrinsic esophageal masses. Invasion of the esophagus by bronchogenic carcinoma occurs rarely.

REFERENCES

Adams, C. W. M., R. H. F. Brain, F. G. Ellis, R. Kauntze, and J. R. Trounce: Achalasia of the Cardia, Guy's Hosp. Rep., 110:191, 1961.

Allison, P. R.: Reflux Esophagitis, Sliding Hiatal Hernia, and the Anatomy of Repair, Surg. Gynecol. Obstet., 92:419, 1951.

Atkinson, M.: Mechanisms Protecting against Gastro-oesophageal Reflux: A Review, Gut, 3:1, 1962.

Bernstein, L. M., R. C. Fruin, and R. Pacini: Differentiation of Esophageal Pain from Angina Pectoris: Role of the Esophageal Acid Perfusion Test, Medicine, 41:143, 1962.

Cauthorne, R. T., J. J. Vanhoutte, M. W. Donner, and T. R. Hendrix: A Study of Patients with Lower Esophageal Ring by Simultaneous Cine-radiography and Manometry, Gastroenterology, 49:632, 1965.

Edmunds, W.: Hiatus Hernia: A Clinical Study of 200 Cases, Quart. J. Med., 26:455, 1957.

Ingelfinger, F. J.: The Physiologic Background of Heartburn, Esophagitis and Cardiospasm, Arch. Intern. Med., 105:770, 1960.

Rex, J. C., H. A. Andersen, L. G. Barlholomew, and J. C. Cain: Esophageal Hiatal Hernia: A 10-year Study of Medically Treated Cases, J.A.M.A., 178:271, 1961.

Terracol, J., and R. H. Sweet: "Diseases of the Esophagus," Philadelphia, W. B. Saunders Company, 1958.

314 PEGTIC ULCER
314 PEPTIC ULCER
William Silen

A rational understanding of the pathophysiology of gastric secretion and peptic ulcer requires a sound knowledge of the normal mechanisms which control the function of the stomach.

PHYSIOLOGY OF THE STOMACH

Gastric Secretion

MECHANISMS. It is generally accepted that gastric juice is the result of two types of secretion, a parietal component actively produced by the oxyntic cells consisting of a slightly hyperosmotic secretion of hydrochloric acid and potassium chloride, and a nonparietal component, possibly of extracellular origin and virtually identical in composition to interstitial fluid. The rate of gastric secretion is virtually linearly related to mucosal blood flow, but it is not yet clear whether agents such as histamine and gastrin exert their effect on gastric secretion primarily by producing alterations in the circulation or by acting directly on the parietal cell. The role of endogenous histamine as a final common pathway by which other stimuli act remains controversial.

THE CONTROL OF GASTRIC ACID SECRETION. The *cephalic phase* of gastric secretion consists of (1) a direct vagal stimulation of the parietal cell mediated over long vagal tracts causing elaboration of acid gastric juice rich in pepsin and (2) an indirect component also carried over long tracts of the vagus which results in the release of antral gastrin. The *gastric phase* of gastric secretion also consists of two components: (1) a direct component in which activation of local cholinergic reflexes by *fundic* distension is by itself a rather weak stimulus, although potentiation of other stimuli such as gastrin or histamine is marked, and (2) an indirect component which consists of secretion of antral gastrin in response to local antral stimuli such as distension or the presence of an alkaline solution in the lumen. The indirect component of the gastric phase is mediated by local antral cholinergic reflexes. Since all four components are thus cholinergically influenced, neurohumoral relationships are the key to the control of gastric secretion. A variety of stimuli may thus ultimately produce the same two cholinergic end effects, namely, the direct stimulation of parietal cells or the release of antral gastrin (Fig. 314-1).

Gregory has succeeded in establishing the structure of gastrin and in purifying and synthesizing it (Fig. 314-2). Gastrin is a polypeptide composed of 17 amino acids. The active moiety of the molecule is contained in the terminal tetrapeptide, and all the actions of the entire molecule can be produced by a peptide consisting of the terminal four amino acids arranged in the proper sequence. The terminal tetrapeptide is the same in the gastrin of all species identified to date. On a molar weight basis gastrin is about 500 times as potent as histamine in its capacity to stimulate gastric secretion. The actions of pure gastrin are (1) stimulation of gastric acid and pepsin secretion, (2) stimulation of gastric and intestinal motility, (3) increased volume and enzyme output by the pancreas, (4) increased flow of hepatic bile, (5) increased output of intrinsic factor. Since pancreozymin and cholecystokinin are similar to each other structurally and possess the same terminal tetrapeptide as gastrin, some of the extragastric effects of gastrin are more easily understood. The length and composition of the remainder of the molecule may thus modify the intensity of the various effects of the hormones. Several investigators have been successful in producing antibodies to gastrin or one of its analogues after coupling them with other protein moieties.

The *intestinal phase* of gastric secretion consists of a small stimulatory effect when various foodstuffs, especially peptones, are introduced into the small intestine; it is likely that this effect is mediated by a humoral substance. Of greater importance is the role of the small intestine as an inhibitor of gastric secretion. Resection of long segments of small intestine is often followed by the development of gastric hypersecretion, probably because

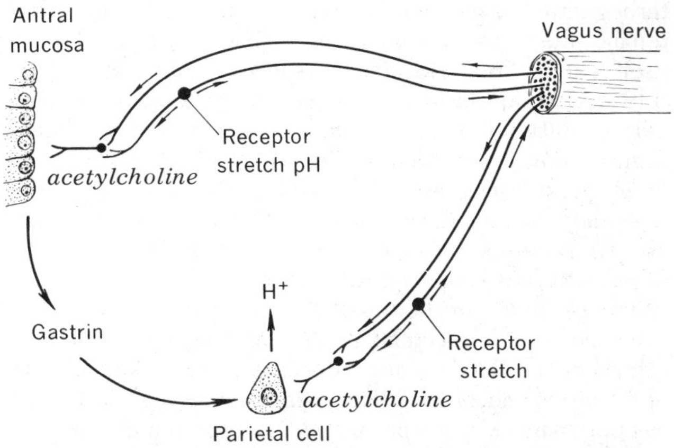

Fig. 314-1. Diagrammatic representation of neurohumoral control of gastric secretion. The two cholinergic end effects, cholinergic stimulation of parietal cells and release of gastrin, are identical for the cephalic and gastric phases. (*Modified after M. I. Grossman: Physiologist, 6:349, 1963.*)

of loss of the inhibitory influences of the small intestine. Perfusion of all portions of the small intestine with stable fat emulsions causes inhibition of gastrin-stimulated gastric secretion. It is possible but not yet proved that this inhibition is caused by the release of enterogastrone, a hormone whose structure has not been defined. Bathing the duodenum in an acid medium (pH of 2.5) similarly inhibits gastric secretion. It is tempting to postulate that such inhibition is produced by secretin and pancreozymin released from the duodenum, especially because the administration of exogenous secretin or pancreozymin also inhibits gastric secretion.

Resistance of the Mucosa to Injury

The gastric mucosa is remarkably resistant to injury. Two factors normally protect the stomach from autodigestion: (1) gastric mucus and (2) the epithelial barrier.

The application of an irritant to the gastric mucosa is followed by the outpouring of large quantities of mucus, the protective capacity of which is largely attributable to its physical characteristics. These properties are more beneficial in protecting the mucosa from thermal or mechanical trauma than from chemical injury, because acid and other chemical substances readily penetrate the mucus barrier. Only about 1 percent of fasting acid secretion can actually be neutralized by the gastric mucus. An additional protective effect of mucus is its ability to adsorb pepsin. Cortisone and acetylsalicylic acid produce qualitative changes in the gastric mucus that may facilitate its degradation by pepsin, and in addition they decrease the total output of mucus.

Mucus-producing cells are generously distributed

Fig. 314-2. Amino acid sequence of human gastrin I. The amino acids in positions 14 through 17 comprise the active tetrapeptide. Gastrin II possesses a tyrosyl o-sulfate in position 12. The leucine at position 5 is replaced by methionine in hog gastrin and by valine in sheep gastrin.

1   2   3   4   5   6   7   8   9   10 11 12 13 14 15 16   17

Glu-Gly-Pro-Try-Leu-Glu-Glu-Glu-Glu-Glu-Ala-Tyr-Gly-Try-Met-Asp-Phe-Ala-NH$_2$

throughout the gastric mucosa. This epithelial lining has remarkable properties of repair and is able to reproduce itself within 36 to 48 hours. Aspirin, alcohol, and other substances injurious to the gastric mucosa alter the permeability of the epithelial barrier, allowing back-diffusion of hydrochloric acid with resultant injury to underlying tissues, especially blood vessels. It is possible that the gastric mucosal barrier to ionic diffusion may also be disrupted in a variety of disease states, especially in gastritis and benign gastric ulcer.

The resistance of the small intestine to trauma or peptic ulceration deserves comment. The thick layer of Brunner's glands in the duodenum produces a highly alkaline (pH of 8) viscid mucoid secretion which has a high buffering capacity and which appears to have an important protective action. Possible loss of, or a defect in, these secretions requires greater attention, since the intraduodenal pH differs little between normal individuals and those with duodenal ulcers. Except for the duodenal Brunner glands, there is little if any inherent difference in susceptibility to acid peptic digestion as one proceeds distad in the small intestine.

Gastric Motility and Gastric Emptying

The musculature of the upper half of the stomach produces weak peristaltic waves which scarcely disturb its contents. The function of this portion of the stomach is mainly an adaptive one enabling great changes in volume with insignificant alterations in pressure. Thus, after a distal gastrectomy, gastric emptying must occur mainly by gravity. Studies of electrical activity indicate the presence of a "pacemaker" in the cardia from which an impulse is propagated to the remainder of the stomach.

The "gastric pump" resides in the antrum and pylorus, which should be regarded as a unit, because the pylorus is not truly a sphincter but is rather an integral part of the pumping mechanism, contracting at the culmination of a peristaltic wave and relaxing the remainder of the time. In fact, the pylorus does not act in opposition to the antrum, and because it is usually relaxed, the term "sphincter" is misleading. During its contraction at the end of a peristaltic wave, the pylorus serves to prevent reflux into the stomach when the pressure in the duodenum is raised and also turns back larger solid particles which need further gastric trituration. The action of the pyloroantrum may thus be likened to the squeezing of the gastric contents toward a pointed funnel which narrows as the squeezing proceeds.

The regulation of gastric emptying is complex. The extrinsic nerve supply to the stomach seems important, since vagotomy produces marked gastric retention, resulting not as has been commonly suggested from pylorospasm but rather from a delay in the onset of antral peristalsis. The duodenum contains osmoreceptors which when exposed to hypertonic solutions inhibit gastric emptying. The instillation of fat or acid chyme into the small intestine similarly causes gastric motor inhibition, perhaps by a humoral mechanism.

DUODENAL ULCER

INCIDENCE AND PATHOLOGY. Duodenal ulcer comprises about 80 percent of all peptic ulcers. At one time during their lives, approximately 10 percent of the population probably suffer from duodenal ulcer many of which may be asymptomatic. Mainly because of hemorrhage or perforation, as many as 10,000 lives are lost yearly in the United States as a result of this disease. Duodenal ulcer is most common in men between the ages of twenty and fifty years. The preponderance of males varies from 3:1 to 10:1, but no significant differences in occurrence between the sexes is evident before puberty or after the menopause. While gastric ulcer is relatively more common in females, the absolute incidence of duodenal ulcer in females is greater than the occurrence of gastric ulcer.

Duodenal ulcers are usually found within 3 cm of the pylorus and occur with about equal frequency on the anterior and posterior walls. The depth of the ulcer varies from a shallow erosion confined to the mucosa to a full-thickness destruction of the wall of the duodenum. Juxtaposition to adjacent organs and rapidity of destruction of the wall are the two factors which determine whether a lesion *perforates* into the free peritoneal cavity or *penetrates* into an adjacent organ. *Perforation* indicates a free communication between the gut and the peritoneal cavity and usually occurs during a period of extremely active ulceration. *Penetration* signifies that a free perforation has not occurred but that an adjacent organ, usually the pancreas, has become adherent to a slowly progressive but chronic ulcer which ultimately erodes that structure. In the process, a posterior penetrating ulcer may erode the gastroduodenal artery or one of its branches and cause sudden massive hemorrhage.

Grossly, duodenal ulcers are generally round with a slightly irregular outline. The base is white, gray, or yellow, and the surrounding mucosa is soft, pliable, and of normal color although occasionally somewhat edematous and hyperemic. Microscopically the base of the ulcer consists of mucus and necrotic debris surmounting a bed of granulation tissue and scar containing variable amounts of inflammatory reaction. Ulcers arising from exposure to gastric juice have a similar appearance whether they occur in the duodenum, stomach, jejunum, or the base of a Meckel diverticulum which contains gastric mucosa. Hence the term *acid-peptic ulceration,* or *acid-peptic disease,* can be applied correctly to all these ulcerations.

Occasionally, anterior and posterior duodenal ulcers coexist. The simultaneous occurrence of gastric and duodenal ulcers is common and may be noted in as many as one-third of patients with duodenal ulcers. It is unusual for a gastric ulcer to precede a duodenal ulcer, and it is safest from a therapeutic standpoint to assume that a patient with both has primarily a duodenal ulcer diathesis. It has been suggested that a chronic duodenal ulcer which causes delay in gastric emptying and consequent gastric stasis stimulates the production of gastrin and thus the development of a gastric ulcer.

PATHOPHYSIOLOGY. In the development of duodenal ulcer in a given patient, it is likely that a multiplicity of causative and contributing factors are involved.

Hypersecretion of Gastric Juice. Duodenal ulcer *never* occurs in the absence of acid. No single test of gastric secretion shows abnormal hypersecretion in much more than half of duodenal ulcer patients with the unexplained exception of the caffeine-stimulated test. An explanation for the absence of excessive acid secretion in some patients with duodenal ulcer is lacking. Dragstedt has proposed that duodenal ulcer arises from hypersecretion caused by excessive vagal stimulation. This thesis is based upon the fact that the nocturnal or basal hypersecretion in most patients with duodenal ulcer is abolished by complete division of the vagus nerves. Absolute proof for this theory is not available. The amount of gastrin or gastrin-like substance in the antra of patients with duodenal ulcer appears to be greater than that found in those with benign gastric ulcer or in normal persons. Whether this results from excessive vagotonia or is by itself a primary etiologic factor is unknown.

There is a linear correlation between the parietal cell mass, or the total number of parietal cells secreting acid, and the secretion achieved by maximal gastric stimulation with histamine. The factors which control the population of parietal cells are not well understood.

Tissue Resistance and Disturbances in Motility. It has been suggested that the resistance of the duodenal mucosa is diminished in patients with duodenal ulcers, but substantiation is lacking. There is no clear evidence that disturbances in gastric motility have a *pathogenetic* role in the development of duodenal ulcer.

Genetic Factor. A family history of duodenal or gastric ulcer may be striking in some patients, and endocrine factors should be sought in such families. However, familial tendency to ulcer is often absent, and the importance of genetic factors in the development of most duodenal ulcers is not clear. The blood group substances are mucopolysaccharides with antigenic properties present in the red blood cell which in certain individuals are secreted into the gastrointestinal tract (secretors) and which may protect against the development of ulceration. Duodenal and stomal ulcers are more common in patients with the O blood grouping and in nonsecretors.

Neuropsychiatric Factors. Emotional factors may alter gastric function profoundly. However, studies of patients with gastric fistulas have shown that different types of stimuli affect the stomach in varying ways which differ from one individual to another. Patients with duodenal ulcers themselves can often clearly point to an emotional upset which may have triggered the onset or exacerbation of their ulcer. Experimentally, ulcers can be produced in monkeys under the stress of being placed in an executive capacity, or it can be produced in rats by physical restraint. Although it is true that many patients with duodenal ulcer are hard-driving ambitious executives, many exceptions are found. Clearly, psychiatric factors may play a role in the pathogenesis of duodenal ulceration but are in all likelihood not the sole causative factor.

Endocrine Factors. Because peptic ulceration is far more common in males, it has been suggested that estrogenic hormones may protect against the development of ulcer. Gastric secretion is not altered by pregnancy, however, and a lesser gastric secretion in normal females than in males may indicate only a genetically determined smaller parietal cell mass rather than a primary effect of estrogens upon gastric secretion.

The role of adrenal steroids has received much attention. In the absence of the adrenal glands, in patients with Addison's disease, or in hypopituitarism, gastric hyposecretion occurs and ulcer is virtually nonexistent. Responsiveness of the parietal cells has been restored after total adrenalectomy by treatment with glucocorticoids but not mineralocorticoids. It is likely therefore that adrenal steroids play a permissive role in the regulation of gastric secretion. The acute administration of glucocorticoids or ACTH exerts no effect on gastric secretion in normal man or animals. Chronic glucocorticoid administration to dogs with intact adrenals increases acid and pepsin secretions, but evidence for this is inconclusive in man. No abnormalities in adrenal function have been detected in patients with duodenal ulcer. In patients who receive large doses of steroids for prolonged periods of time ulcerlike symptoms often develop, and peptic ulcers develop in some. Whether the true incidence of duodenal or gastric ulcers among patients receiving long-term steroid therapy is greater than the incidence occurring in the disease for which the treatment is being administered is debatable. In the presence of sepsis or burns, which of themselves are probably ulcerogenic, steroids may be dangerous. It is likely that steroids not only affect gastric secretion but also may cause serious injury to the mucosal epithelial barrier.

A high incidence of peptic ulceration has been reported in patients with hyperparathyroidism, and many studies have attempted to elucidate the reasons for this relationship. In certain cases of hyperparathyroidism, gastric acid hypersecretion has reverted to normal after surgical cure of the hyperparathyroidism, but this has by no means been uniform. The parathyroid probably acts in a "permissive" way, as do the adrenal and the thyroid, since calcium must be present in adequate amounts for the normal gastric secretory process to occur.

Other Predisposing Diseases. An increased incidence of peptic ulceration is found in cirrhosis of the liver, chronic pancreatitis or cystic fibrosis, chronic pulmonary emphysema, and rheumatoid arthritis. While gastric hypersecretion is present in some of the patients with these diseases or in animals with their experimental counterparts, it is often possibly because of a preexistent abnormality of the stomach. In cirrhosis, failure of the liver to inactivate a gastric secretagogue (histamine?) normally present in portal blood, either because of functional deterioration or because of portacaval shunting, is the probable mechanism of hypersecretion. In chronic pancreatitis or cystic fibrosis, the loss of the buffering capacity of pancreatic juice in the duodenum and of the inhibitory effect of normally digested fat upon gastric secretion may contribute to the development of ulcer. Patients with chronic pulmonary disease are subjected to stress, hypoxia, and hypercapnia, all of which may play a role in enhancing the development of peptic ulcer. The cause of the increased incidence of ulcers in rheumatoid arthritis is unknown.

CLINICAL FEATURES. Duodenal ulcer is a chronic disease characterized by exacerbations and remissions. Although many individuals have only one encounter with active duodenal ulceration, the diathesis seems to recur or persist in most. Characteristically symptoms last for a few days, weeks, or months and disappear for varying periods of time, only to reappear with or without therapy or frequently without identifiable precipitating cause. Although it has been disputed, classically exacerbations appear to occur more frequently in spring and fall. Eighty to ninety percent of patients with duodenal ulcer have a relatively benign course interrupted occasionally by the inconvenience of necessity for therapy. In the remaining 10 to 20 percent intractability or other complications develop, and these patients become candidates for operation. Many patients have ulcers sufficiently asymptomatic to evade detection, and in about 20 to 30 percent of cases of perforation or hemorrhage no antecedent symptoms can be elicited.

The symptomatology of duodenal ulcer has a remarkably uniform pattern. The development of pain followed by the relief of discomfort after ingestion of food or alkali is such a characteristic sequence that the absence of this rhythmicity or periodicity should raise serious question as to the correctness of the diagnosis. The pain is a steady, gnawing, burning, aching, or hungerlike discomfort high

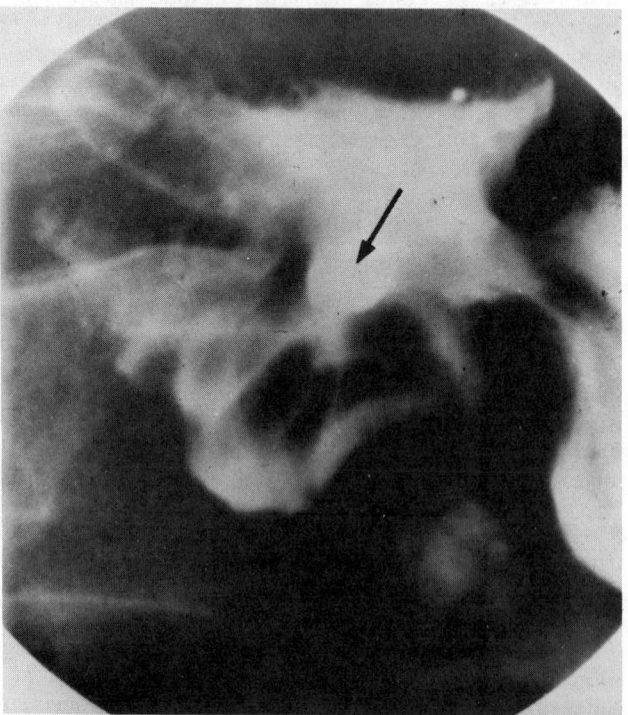

Fig. 314-3. Duodenal bulb showing persistent fleck of barium, representing a true crater with radiating folds of mucosa.

in the midepigastrium or slightly to either side of the midline, especially on the right. It is located over a limited area and does not radiate unless penetration of the pancreas has occurred, in which case spread of pain to the back is common. The pain usually begins about 2 or 2½ hr after meals and usually is relieved immediately by the ingestion of alkali or food. The pain may awaken the patient between midnight and 3 A.M., but for reasons that are unclear, it is almost never present upon awakening before breakfast. The mechanism of the pain is disputed, but most observers believe that the acid bathing the ulcer causes the discomfort, especially because buffering of acid within the stomach invariably produces relief. Some patients have no pain even prior to a major and serious complication.

A variety of other gastrointestinal symptoms may be present, many of which are often found in the general population. Heartburn, a sensation of retrosternal burning, is very common and may be especially severe in patients who have associated sliding hiatus hernia (see Chaps. 40 and 313). Alterations in bowel habits, including both constipation and diarrhea, often related to medications, are not infrequently observed. *Water brash*, the welling up, or regurgitation, of sour burning fluid in the mouth, is common, especially if a hiatal hernia is present. The appetite is usually good, and gain in weight is common, because these patients eat so frequently to relieve discomfort. Weight loss is uncommon unless chronic duodenal obstruction has been present. Physical examination of patients with active duodenal ulcers may be negative or show only mild tenderness in the epigastrium or to the right of the midline.

Atypical symptomatology occurs in certain types of duodenal ulcer. In childhood the pain is frequently bizarre in type and location and may even be accentuated by the ingestion of food. Bleeding or perforation is often the initial manifestation in children. Ulcers in the second portion of the duodenum or in the pyloric canal may have unusual pain patterns, and the pain-food-relief sequence is less common. Interference with the normal antropyloric pump by ulcers of the pyloric canal often causes nausea, vomiting, anorexia, weight loss, and cramping pain shortly after ingestion, and this constellation of symptoms has been called *syndrome pylorique*. Ulcers in this region respond poorly to medical therapy.

DIAGNOSIS. The most important criterion in the diagnosis of duodenal ulcer is the elicitation of the typical sequence of pain-food-relief. A variety of nonspecific symptoms such as heartburn, belching, intolerance to certain foods, and vague diffuse abdominal discomfort are frequent symptoms in the general population. Although they are often equated with duodenal ulcer, more frequently other diseases or no specific underlying diseases are found. The typical periodicity of relief of discomfort by the ingestion of food or alkali is usually helpful in excluding these other diseases. The presence of pain at night and its absence in the early morning are also important diagnostic features. The response of the discomfort to medical treatment is important but must be interpreted carefully, because some patients with nonspecific symptoms or other diseases also may improve. If the history is atypical and the radiologic findings do not substantiate the presence of a duodenal ulcer, further diagnostic steps including barium examination of the colon and small intestine and cholecystography should be taken lest serious lesions in other portions of the gastrointestinal tract be missed.

X-ray examination with barium is the most definitive diagnostic step. The demonstration of a crater persistent on several films is the only means by which the presence of an active duodenal ulcer can be clearly established (Fig. 314-3). Giant craters in the duodenal bulb may be missed because of their enormous size. The presence of a persistent deformity of the duodenal bulb does not necessarily indicate that *active* duodenal ulceration is present but signifies only that at one time ulceration was present which in the process of healing produced the deformity (Fig. 314-4). Not infrequently active ulcers are present in these deformed bulbs, but they may be difficult to demonstrate. Only a history compatible with active disease together with the presence of a deformed bulb can define active duodenal ulceration when a crater is not demonstrable.

Gastric analysis is generally unnecessary in patients with typical duodenal ulcer. In certain instances of fulminating or atypical disease or when the possibility of marginal ulceration exists and cannot be confirmed radiologically, examination of gastric secretion may be useful. Near-maximal output of acid in the basal state combined with a minimal increment to maximal histamine stimulation strongly suggests that the parietal cell mass is already maximally stimulated under basal conditions and that the Zollinger-Ellison (Z-E) syndrome may be present. A 12-hr nocturnal test of gastric secretion is uncomfortable and unnecessary, and careful determination of the 1-hr basal acid output coupled with the maximal histamine stimulation provides as much information. True achlorhydria excludes a benign peptic ulcer.

TREATMENT. Medical Treatment. Virtually every conceivable dietary regimen and drug has been advocated at one time or another. Yet, in controlled studies of various types of therapy, the rate of healing of ulcers has been significantly altered by few things. Certain recommendations can be made, however, which will provide greater comfort and relief of symptoms. Rather than uniformly imposing an extremely restrictive dietary and pharmacologic regimen, each patient can be treated in a manner most suitable for him without significantly altering the incidence of recurrence or complications.

Antacids. Antacids are the mainstay of therapy. The rationale of antacid therapy is to elevate the pH of the gastric contents to at least 5, where the proteolytic capacity of pepsin is virtually abolished and the damaging effect due to acidity is minimal. Some antacids also inactivate pepsin by an adsorbant effect. When given to the *fasting* patient with duodenal ulcer most antacids have an effect lasting for only 20 to 30 min. This evanescent effect is related not to the inadequacy of the buffering capacity of the antacid but rather to rapid gastric emptying. The effect of antacid therapy can be prolonged

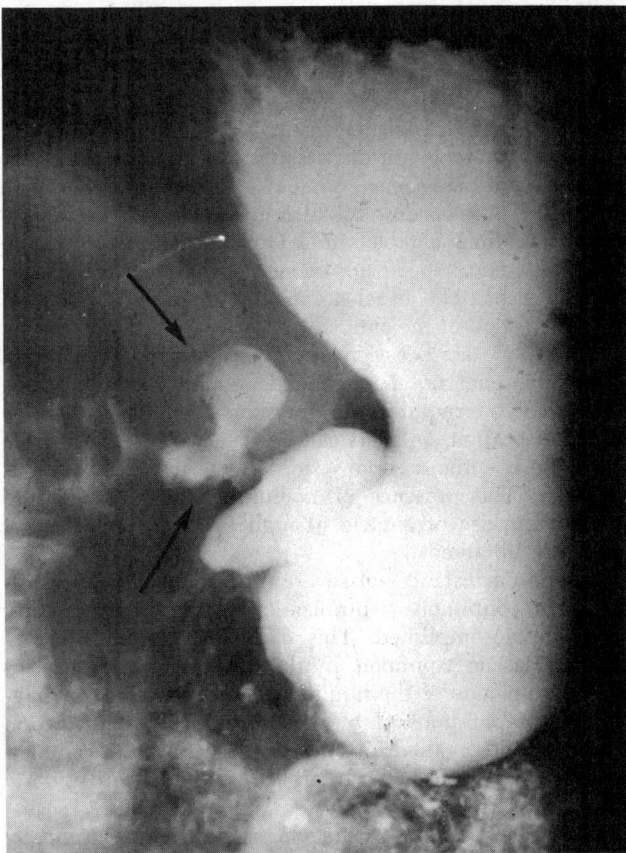

Fig. 314-4. Markedly deformed duodenal bulb with "cloverleaf" deformity.

markedly if the agent is taken 1 hr after eating, the gastric acidity decreasing to 30 to 40 percent of its control values as long as 4 hr after the meal.

The choice of antacid is important, but the ideal antacid probably does not yet exist. Absorbable antacids such as sodium bicarbonate should not be used, because they induce systemic alkalosis. Especially if combined with the prolonged ingestion of milk, absorbable antacids and occasionally even nonabsorbable agents may produce the milk-alkali syndrome, consisting of hypercalcemia, alkalosis, azotemia, and nephrocalcinosis. Nonabsorbable antacids either singly or in combination are the most frequently employed agents. Calcium carbonate is probably the most effective antacid, because its neutralizing action is prolonged and it reduces peptic activity. It should not be used for patients with a history of renal calculi, or for those with dehydration and electrolyte imbalance because of its tendency to cause hypercalcemia and hypercalcuria. Magnesium oxide is eight to ten times more potent than magnesium trisilicate or magnesium carbonate, and the aluminum hydroxide gels have little neutralizing capacity. Calcium carbonate and aluminum hydroxide have the disadvantage of producing severe constipation and fecal impaction, especially in the aged. These side effects may be countered by the replacement of one or two of the daily doses with 4 Gm magnesium oxide. The high sodium content of many alumina preparations may be disadvantageous in patients who require a low sodium intake. The binding of phosphate in the intestine by alumina preparations is usually not a severe problem, because the diet ingested by these patients is generally high in phosphorus.

Liquid antacids are dispersed more readily within the stomach and are hence somewhat more effective than tablets. The usual dose of calcium carbonate, magnesium oxide, or alumina tablets is 4 Gm, and the dose of alumina gels is 15 to 30 ml, enough to neutralize 50 mEq acid in 1 hr. The usual ambulatory regimen consists of administration of the antacid 1 hr after meals, at bedtime, and on any other occasion when discomfort arises. Should adequate relief not be obtained, a more stringent regimen may be required. In intensive therapy for active acute ulceration, antacids can be given every hour in the usual dose without serious side effects if constipation is avoided. The presence of nocturnal discomfort should dictate the use of antacid at night until complete relief of pain is obtained.

In certain instances of severe ulceration with unrelenting pain continuous neutralization of the gastric acidity must be accomplished. This can be achieved by continuous gastric aspiration, by the constant intragastric installation of one of the liquid alumina hydroxide or magnesium preparations, or by the continuous administration of a milk and cream drip. These instances are not common but are more often encountered in patients with pyloric channel ulcers.

Anticholinergic Drugs. Anticholinergic drugs theoretically not only inhibit the direct effect of the vagus nerve upon the parietal cells but also decrease the vagal release of gastrin and excessive gastric motility. These agents reduce the *output* of gastric acid but do not decrease the concentration of acid or the output of pepsin. Consequently anticholinergic drugs do *not* reduce the peptic digestive capacity of gastric juice but facilitate the neutralization of gastric juice by food and antacids. Prolonged use of anticholinergic agents probably diminishes the incidence of exacerbations of duodenal ulcer disease. However, the doses necessary to produce the desired gastric action have many undesirable side effects. They cannot be used in individuals with glaucoma or prostatic hypertrophy and should not be employed in uncomplicated pyloric channel ulcers or when pyloric obstruction is imminent or is present.

These drugs are generally given to tolerance by increasing the dose until side effects such as blurred vision and dryness of the mouth appear, and are then reduced until these symptoms become tolerable. They should be given about 30 min before meals, because their maximal activity is during the second hour after administration whereas the secretory response to food is maximal between 15 and 75 min after eating. Perhaps the most acceptable use of anticholinergic agents is at bedtime, because the side effects are less troublesome during sleeping hours. Propantheline, glycopyrrolate, and oxyphencyclimine are superior to atropine and along with isopropamide and poldine methylsulfate are the only anticholinergic drugs sufficiently potent to warrant clinical use. Until longer-acting anticholinergic drugs which produce less undesirable side effects can be developed, these agents should be used only in the most intractable and difficult cases or in those in which basal secretion exceeds 6 mEq hydrochloric acid per hr. There is no evidence that anticholinergic drugs accelerate the healing of duodenal ulcers.

Dietary Management. Controlled observations indicate that there is no clear-cut therapeutic effect of diet therapy. From a practical standpoint, frequent small bland feedings are likely to be tolerated more readily than a routine diet, because nonspecific food intolerances are common and large meals may cause discomfort to some patients, especially in the acute phases of duodenal ulcer. This is begun with six small feedings consisting of skim milk or protein snacks which have a high buffering capacity and avoidance of highly seasoned foods, roughage, and greasy or fried foods. As soon as pain is diminished or has completely disappeared, the diet is gradually liberalized.

Sole reliance upon dietary therapy for buffering the excess acid is not physiologically sound, since considerable stimulation of acid secretion occurs after the initial buffering effect of the meal has worn off. Antacid therapy 1 hr after eating should also be employed. The traditional administration of large quantities of cream and milk has recently been implicated in causing a higher incidence of atherosclerosis in ulcer patients. The high fat content of such a diet may also be contraindicated for other reasons, such as the presence of biliary tract disease.

Rest, Sedatives, and Tranquilizers. Rest and adequate sleep are strongly advised, and patients are urged to curtail their business and social responsibilities. Controlled investigations have revealed that rest in the form of hospitalization has proved beneficial in patients with gastric ulcer, but data are not available for an assessment of its effect in duodenal ulcer patients. Should symptoms from a duodenal ulcer persist despite active therapy on an outpatient basis for 5 or 6 days, the more rigid therapy and enforced rest produced by hospitalization will very frequently become effective. While sedatives and tranquilizers have not been shown to affect the course of duodenal ulcer materially, they may be helpful in the anxious and tense patient. There is no need to administer these agents routinely.

Psychotherapy. Psychotherapy has no proven beneficial effect on the healing or recurrence of duodenal ulcer. In fact, intensive psychotherapy during phases of acute activity of a duodenal ulcer is probably contraindicated, because it may result in exacerbations. However, a warm and sympathetic attitude on the part of the physician, reassurance, and support are important aspects of the care of the ulcer patient. If specific indications for psychotherapy exist, it is better carried out during quiescent phases of ulcer activity.

Interdictions. Ingestion of alcohol is strictly contraindicated. Alcohol not only produces direct stimulation of the parietal cell but may also cause the release of gastrin. In addition, it probably injures the gastric mucosal epithelial barrier. Coffee, tea, and cola drinks stimulate gastric secretion because of their caffeine content and are also interdicted. Cigarette smoking has been documented to be a definite cause of delayed healing of gastric ulcers, although the reasons for this are unclear. Cessation of smoking is similarly recommended for duodenal ulcer, but a firm rationale is lacking. In most patients the habit of cigarette smoking is so firmly ingrained, however, that absolute abstinence may be extremely disturbing. Consequently, the ideal therapeutic regimen must be tempered by the judgment of the physician. The detrimental effects of tobacco should be explained to the patient and every device used to support him in attempting to decrease if not stop his consumption of tobacco.

All drugs which may contribute to peptic ulceration such as the xanthine alkaloids, all anti-inflammatory drugs, reserpine, adrenal steroids, and salicylates should be discontinued if not absolutely necessary.

Irradiation of the Stomach. Irradiation of the stomach has a definite albeit small role in the treatment of duodenal ulcer. The administration of approximately 1,500 r in 10 divided doses with conventional therapy or 2,000 r with cobalt teletherapy generally produces marked depression of gastric secretion. True achlorhydria is rare after irradiation, and the usually resultant hypochlorhydria is frequently transient. Within 6 to 12 months, the acid secretion returns to normal in at least half of the patients. For reasons which are incompletely understood, however, rates of recurrence remain reasonably low. This mode of therapy is useful in a limited number of patients who have not responded adequately to medical therapy but who are extremely poor risks for surgical procedures.

Other Forms of Therapy. Claims of therapeutic success have been made for an enormous variety of additional therapeutic modalities, but none has survived the test of time. The remarkable tendency for spontaneous remission makes the evaluation of any form of therapy difficult at best, and only carefully controlled clinical trials can confirm the efficacy of any therapeutic regimen. A perfect example is the wave of enthusiasm which followed the introduction of gastric freezing. Only after an "excessive" period did it become clear that improvement was transient and complications frequent. Gastric freezing can be regarded as a transient curiosity with no place in our therapeutic armamentarium.

Therapy between Recurrences. Since a duodenal ulcer may take from several weeks to months to heal depending upon its size and depth, active therapy should be continued for 2 to 3 months in all patients with an acute exacerbation. Spontaneous recurrence is frequent despite continued therapy, and because most patients who are feeling well do not tolerate severe restrictions, the physician must outline an acceptable interim regimen.

That recurrent symptoms are likely should be explained to the patient, since 50 to 95 percent of duodenal ulcers will recur within 5 years. Therapy may not prevent such recurrences; hence dietary and antacid management should be liberalized after the initial 2 to 3 months of active therapy. Indeed, medications may be discarded in many patients with the admonition that gastric stimulants be avoided and that moderation be used in smoking and other aggravating factors. At the first inkling of recurrent symptoms, active therapy should be reinstituted immediately and should be continued for 2 to 3 weeks, or longer if relief is not immediate. Even in the absence of symptoms prophylactic therapy for a short period should be advised if the patient is about to enter a period of emotional stress or a potentially ulcergenic situation. An occasional party might also be covered with prophylactic therapy.

The long-term use of anticholinergic drugs has been shown in a few controlled studies to reduce the recurrence rate below 10 percent. Because of the side effects of these drugs and their poor acceptance, the routine use of anticholinergic drugs is not warranted. They should be considered, however, in severe cases.

Surgical Treatment. Indications. The indication for operation in patients with duodenal ulcer are the complications of the disease: (1) perforation, (2) organic obstruction, (3) intractable bleeding, and (4) refractoriness to medical therapy. Surgical therapy is indicated in the minority of patients. The indications are usually clear, with the possible exception of those patients with intractability to medical management. The decision to advise operation in a patient with duodenal ulcer must balance the risks of the disease with those of operation. The repeated discomfort, cost of frequent hospitalization, time lost from work, possible mortality, the threat of complications are the factors which influence the decision in favor of continued medical treatment. These must be compared with operative and anesthetic risks, the incidence of recurrent ulcers, and some of the symptoms which occur following operations for duodenal ulcer. The risks on the surgical side must be evaluated in light of the experience of the surgeons with whom the internist works closely and not solely from results reported in the literature. In many instances the results are either markedly better or worse than those which are published, a consideration generally given insufficient attention.

Acceptable Surgical Procedures. The goals of surgical therapy are identical with those of nonoperative therapy, namely, profound and lasting decrease of the secretion of hydrochloric acid and pepsin. There is probably no single operation which is suitable for all patients with duodenal ulcer, and contemplated procedures should be tailored to fit the individual patient.

Vagotomy and drainage operation are designed to ablate any direct effects of vagal stimulation upon the parietal cell as well as the vagal release of gastrin. Stimulation of the antrum by chemical means or by distension remains operative in the presence of a vagotomy. From a physiologic standpoint, pyloroplasty has theoretical advantages over gastroenterostomy for drainage purposes, because pyloroplasty maintains duodenal continuity, is less frequently associated with the dumping syndrome, and should preserve any acid inhibitory influence of the duodenum. Interestingly, however, the recurrence rate of ulceration following either of these procedures is about the same and varies between 5 and 8 percent in most series. The operative mortality rate for elective vagotomy and drainage throughout the country is approximately 1 percent, the lowest figure for any operative procedure.

Subtotal distal gastric resection is the time-honored procedure for duodenal ulcer, preferably with reconstruction by gastroduodenostomy because of nutritional advantages derived for the establishment of normal gastrointestinal continuity and because of the preservation of inhibitory influences of the duodenum. The operation removes approximately 75 percent of the stomach including the antrum and a generous portion of the parietal cell mass. In all probability, if mobilization of the stomach is extensive, nondeliberate vagal denervation may also be produced. The operative mortality rate for elective operation by well-trained surgeons is approximately 3 percent, and the recurrence rate of ulceration is also approximately 3 percent. Subtotal gastrectomy has a higher incidence of nutritional inadequacies and dumping than does vagotomy with an emptying operation.

Vagotomy and antrectomy have become an extremely popular procedure. The overall mortality rate is about 3 percent, although in selected series it has been as low as 1½ to 2 percent. Removal of the antrum and denervation of the remaining parietal cell mass carries with it the lowest rate of recurrence, less than 1 percent. The nutritional consequences occupy a position midway between those for vagotomy and drainage operation and subtotal distal gastrectomy.

Segmental gastric resection leaves the antrum in place but removes a large portion of the parietal cell mass. The recurrence rate of ulceration, the mortality rate, and the nutritional consequences are similar to those of distal gastrectomy.

GASTRIC ULCER

It is useful clinically to separate the approach to gastric and duodenal ulcers, because the implications of the two are very different, even though the ulcers are similar pathologically.

INCIDENCE AND LOCATION. Clinically gastric ulcers are less common than duodenal ulcers in the ratio of about 1:4, but autopsy studies show a roughly equal incidence of duodenal and gastric ulcer. This indicates that many gastric ulcers may be asymptomatic and also that terminal acute gastric ulcers are probably included in the autopsy studies. Males usually predominate by a ratio of 3.5:1, somewhat less than the predominance noted in duodenal ulcers. Although gastric ulcers may appear at any age, they tend to occur between forty-five and fifty-five years, whereas the maximal incidence for duodenal ulcer is about 10 years earlier.

Gastric ulcers occur most often in the antrum or at the junction of the antral and fundic tissue. They are usually single and often located on the lesser curvature or in the prepyloric area. About 20 percent of gastric ulcers occur in patients who have had past or present duodenal ulceration, but it is very unusual for duodenal ulcer to follow the onset of pure gastric ulceration.

PATHOPHYSIOLOGY. With the exception of those patients having concomitant duodenal and gastric ulceration, the average basal gastric secretion and maximally stimulated gastric secretion and, hence, parietal cell mass are either decreased or normal. True achlorhydria following maximal stimulation is so exceptional that its demonstration should virtually exclude the presence of a benign gastric ulcer.

Several theories have been proposed to explain the development of benign peptic ulceration in the stomach. Dragstedt suggested that gastric ulcers are due to hypersecretion of gastric juice of hormonal origin dependent upon prolonged or excessive liberation of the antral hormone gastrin. Although this theory may explain the ulceration which occurs secondary to gastric stasis produced by vagotomy without a drainage operation, it is by no means a satisfactory explanation for the vast majority of spontaneously occurring gastric ulcers. No proof has been provided that gastric hypomotility or stasis is more prevalent in patients with gastric ulcer than in the normal population.

Other hypotheses which have been proposed include a decreased resistance of the stomach to ulceration by injury of the epithelium or by a decrease in gastric mucus. Although qualitative and quantitative changes in gastric mucus have been described following the administration of salicylates or steroids, evidence for the exhaustion of the mucus-secreting cell or the excessive destruction of mucus in patients with gastric ulcer is not at hand. It has been suggested that regurgitation of bile into the proximal parts of the stomach is more common in patients with gastric ulcer and that such regurgitation injures the mucosa so that acid-peptic ulceration may occur. This is consonant with the findings of Davenport that injury to the gastric mucosa by various substances enhances the back-diffusion of hydrogen ion, causing destruction of blood vessels and possible ulceration. Patients with gastric ulcer may therefore actually have hypersecretion of acid which cannot be detected because of the back-diffusion of hydrogen ion, accounting for the usual clinical finding of normal or low acid secretion.

CLINICAL FEATURES. Asymptomatic gastric ulcers are common, so that some are found by chance and others are heralded only by severe complications such as perforation or bleeding. Symptomatic ulcers produce a picture not nearly as invariable as that associated with duodenal ulcer. Atypical symptoms such as vague bloating or nausea after eating are common. Although the rhythmicity of the pain-food-relief sequence may occur, it is not as frequent or as clear-cut as it is in duodenal ulcer. In fact, food often aggravates the pain. The discomfort may be burning or cramping in nature and is usually less localized and more diffuse than that found in patients with duodenal ulcers. Pain occurring at night is uncommon. Nausea, anorexia, and vomiting are not infrequent and may occur in the absence of obstruction. Weight loss is frequent. The symptoms of gastric ulcer tend to be chronic, often respond poorly to medical management, and frequently recur.

DIAGNOSIS. The history is not as informative or as diagnostic as it is in duodenal ulcer. Only a high index of suspicion will result in the proper diagnosis in patients who so frequently have vague symptomatology. The diagnosis is almost completely dependent upon radiologic and gastroscopic examinations, because the determination of gastric acid secretion is of little value. Roentgenologic examination with barium will detect a gastric ulcer in the majority of cases and is approximately 80 to 85 percent accurate in differentiating a benign from a malignant gastric ulcer. The radiologic features which allow this distinction include the smooth oval nature of the defect extending beyond the projected wall of the stomach, the absence of a mass lesion, ready passage of peristalsis through the area, and the presence of normal or slightly edematous mucosal folds to the very edge of the lesion (Fig. 314-5). Gastroscopic examination is almost as accurate as roentgenologic demonstration of the ulcer in differentiating benign from malignant lesions if the lesion can be visualized. However, many areas of the fundus of the stomach cannot be seen with the gastroscope. Gastroscopic biopsy may be useful; however, if benign tissue is obtained, it must be emphasized that the specimen represents but a very small superficial segment of the lesion in question. The major concern in the diagnosis lies in the ability to distinguish between benign and malignant ulcers.

DIFFERENTIATION OF BENIGN AND MALIGNANT GASTRIC ULCER. Although the vast majority of gastric ulcers are benign, about 7 percent of ulcerating gastric lesions which were originally indeterminate, i.e., in which a clearcut diagnosis was not evident, will prove to be carcinoma of the stomach. The diagnostic accuracy of approximately 90 percent can be improved by the rigid application of criteria to be mentioned. In case of doubt, the ulcer should be considered malignant until proved otherwise. The 5-year survival rate in patients with initially indeterminate gastric ulcers which proved to be carcinomas at operation is approximately 50 percent, roughly five times the overall survival rate in gastric cancer. It is not uncommon to see patients with operable and potentially curable lesions who have been treated nonoperatively for as long as 2 or 3 years and who later appear with either inoperable, unresectable lesions or with distant metastases. Furthermore, an error in making a diagnosis of gastric cancer when such does not exist may also be forgiven in view of the high recurrence rate of medically treated gastric ulcer. Within a 5-year period, 75 to 80 percent of patients with benign gastric ulcer will have recurrent morbidity, and 3 to 4 percent will die from complications of the ulcer, a figure quite comparable to the mortality of gastric resection for benign ulcer. Since the surgical therapy of gastric ulcer is usually successful, it cannot be emphasized too strongly that procrastination is to be clearly avoided. These statements should not be misconstrued to indicate that the majority of gastric ulcer patients should be subjected to operation. On the contrary a sober and rational approach may be achieved by utilizing the following criteria:

1. *Roentgenologic examination of the stomach.* This is probably the most important diagnostic aid. In the hands of an expert roentgenologist, the correct diagnosis can be made in 80 and 85 percent of the cases.

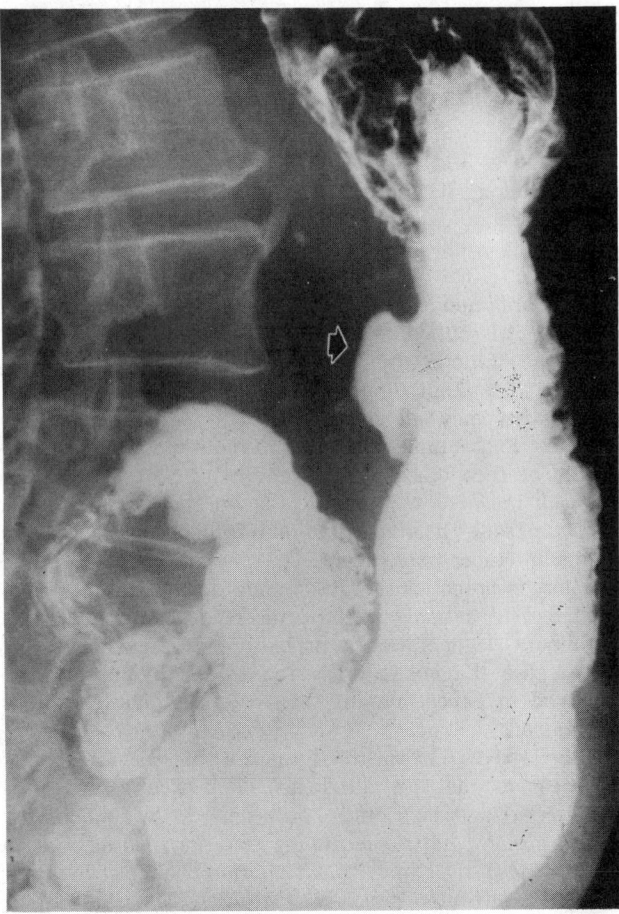

Fig. 314-5. Typical benign lesser curvature gastric ulcer. Note ulceration beyond projected margins of the stomach and collar of edema.

2. *Gastroscopy.* This may be of value in the differentiation if the lesion exists in an area which can be seen with the gastroscope. Gross appearance and gastroscopic biopsy may provide helpful clues.

3. *Cytologic examination of the gastric juice.* When properly performed, this yields a diagnostic accuracy as high as 80 to 90 percent. The errors usually encountered are in the direction of false negatives. False positive results are uncommon.

4. *Examination of the gastric acid.* This too may be of some value. If true histamine-fast achlorhydria is present, the diagnosis of carcinoma cannot be excluded no matter what other criteria are present. On the other hand, should acid be present, gastric carcinoma cannot be ruled out, because gastric secretion persists in many patients with carcinoma.

5. *Response to medical therapy.* Should one of the four criteria outlined above provide evidence of the presence of malignancy or should there be suspicious findings in two of these, operation is clearly indicated. However, if all these studies suggest that the lesion is benign, then a trial of medical therapy should be instituted, a test at least equal in importance to the other criteria. Strict rules for this test must be applied lest serious errors be made.

The patient should be placed on an intensive medical regimen similar to the one described for duodenal ulcer. Roentgenologic examination should be repeated between 2 and 3 weeks after medical therapy has begun. By this time the benign ulcer should be approximately half its original size, and a small ulcer may show virtually complete healing. If less or no improvement has occurred, operation should in general be undertaken. If healing is progressing well, the medical regimen is continued for another 2 to 3 weeks, and a second gastrointestinal series is then obtained, at which time healing should be complete. If it is not, then operation must be recommended.

If one adheres rigidly to these criteria, diagnostic errors will be kept to an absolute minimum. Undue procrastination may allow patients with carcinoma of the stomach to go untreated for inordinate periods, and it should be recognized that patients with carcinoma of the stomach improve symptomatically on a medical regimen and that some healing or diminution in the size of the malignant ulcer may occur.

There is no conclusive pathologic demonstration of the transition of a benign gastric ulcer to a malignant one. Malignant degeneration is probably a rare event. Nevertheless the diagnostic criteria outlined above must be followed to be certain that an early malignant lesion is not missed.

TREATMENT. The medical therapy of gastric ulcer is identical to that for duodenal ulcer except that anticholinergic agents should not be used. Anticholinergic drugs prolong gastric emptying and may contribute to ulcerogenesis by stimulating elaboration of gastrin. Randomized controlled prospective studies have shown that hospitalization of the patient with gastric ulcer has a beneficial effect. Consequently, hospitalization for a 2- to 3-week period will not only provide the opportunity for adequate work-up of the patient but will also permit supervision of the medical therapy. The follow-up roentgenologic examination can be obtained at the end of the second or third week of therapy, and the patient may be discharged if 50 percent healing has occurred. The rationale for antacid therapy in benign gastric ulcer lies in the protection of the diseased gastric mucosa from destruction by normal or even subnormal quantities of acid and pepsin. Carbenoxolone sodium, a hydrolytic product of glycyrrhizic acid derived from licorice, has been shown in randomized studies to have a salutary effect in patients with gastric ulcer, but it has sodium-retaining properties and may produce fluid retention. This drug has not been widely used in this country, although it has received extensive trial elsewhere. Its mechanism of action is unknown.

Surgical therapy is indicated for perforation, bleeding, obstruction, and intractability, the same indications used in the operative treatment of duodenal ulcer. Failure to heal completely in a period of 6 weeks is an important addition to this list. The surgical therapy of gastric ulcer generally consists of subtotal, distal gastrectomy which encompasses mainly the gastric antrum. Wide resection of the parietal cell–bearing areas is unnecessary, because gastric hypersecretion is uncommon and a less radical resection almost invariably is associated with an extremely satisfactory result. The recurrence rate of benign gastric ulcer after antrectomy is less than 1 percent. Reconstruction should be by gastroduodenostomy for reasons mentioned in the discussion of Surgical Treatment under Duodenal Ulcer. Lesser procedures such as pyloroplasty and vagotomy have been advocated for benign gastric ulcer, but the ultimate role of this operation in the treatment of benign gastric ulcer remains to be defined. However, recurrences have not been uncommon after pyloroplasty and vagotomy.

STRESS-INDUCED ULCERS AND DRUG-INDUCED ULCERATIONS

Stress-induced ulcers and ulcerations caused by various drugs are similar in many respects. These ulcers are usually acute, tend to be superficial, and frequently occur without symptoms. When symptomatic, bleeding or perforation are the most common manifestations. Stress ulcers are far more common in the stomach than in the duodenum. They are encountered commonly in diseases of the central nervous system, especially after trauma, operation, or vascular accidents and under these circumstances are known as *Cushing's ulcers*. They can also appear in patients with burns (Curling's ulcer), severe sepsis, or injury. The mechanism whereby stress ulceration develops is not readily apparent. However, hypersecretion of acid gastric juice is not the sole causative factor, and vascular alterations produced by changes in splanchnic blood flow or by stimulation or irritation of the hypothalamic areas may be important. Stimulation of the anterior hypothalamic nuclei is known to increase gastric secretion and blood flow, whereas the opposite effect is seen after stimulation of the posterior hypothalamus.

Drug-induced ulcerations or erosions may be caused by a variety of therapeutic agents. In many instances the exact mechanism by which these agents produce ulceration is unknown. Perhaps the most common substance known to cause ulceration or erosion is acetylsalicylic acid. Salicylates damage the mucosal epithelial barrier, allowing the back-diffusion of hydrogen ion with subsequent injury to the underlying tissue. It may be that other anti-inflammatory agents such as phenylbutazone, cincophen, acetophenetidin, and colchicine produce similar types of injury. Reserpine in large oral doses or given parenterally augments gastric secretion by accentuating the vagal release of gastrin. The role of adrenal steroids in the production of peptic ulceration has already been discussed. Although any of these agents may induce ulceration, they may, in addition, reactivate a preexisting duodenal or gastric ulcer.

Because stress and drug-induced ulcerations are often asymptomatic prior to a major complication, attempts to prevent them with antacids should be made in high-risk situations, such as burns in children, or where large doses of steroids are used postoperatively. Drugs known to induce ulceration should be avoided in situations which may enhance ulcerogenesis.

STOMAL OR GASTROJEJUNAL ULCERATION

The incidence of stomal or gastrojejunal ulceration is reasonably low in acceptable operations for duodenal ulceration, but these types of ulceration develop in approximately 20 to 30 percent of patients with simple gastrojejunostomy without vagotomy.

The causation of stomal ulcers usually is related to a defect in the original therapy, although an underlying Z-E syndrome may be present (see below). Stomal ulceration following simple gastroenterostomy is due to the direct effect of the vagus nerve upon the parietal cell and the persistent vagal release of gastrin. The regurgitation of alkaline juices into the antrum of the stomach also enhances the chemical release of gastrin. If marginal or stomal ulceration occurs following distal gastrectomy, the possibility that not all of the distal antrum was resected should be considered. This occurs if a difficult duodenum was encountered in the first operative procedure, so that closure of the duodenal stump occurred proximal to the pylorus. The constant bathing of the excluded antrum in alkaline juice produces profound hypersecretion, which may reach proportions resembling those of the Z-E syndrome.

The symptoms are often extremely vague. A poorly localized burning sensation associated with a mild degree of cramping abdominal pain is common. This discomfort is often but not always relieved by antacid therapy. Massive hemorrhage alone is commonly the sole presenting manifestation. Free perforation into the peritoneal cavity or penetration into adjacent organs producing a gastrojejunocolic fistula are also complications of stomal ulceration. The diagnosis may be extremely difficult, because approximately two-thirds to three-fourths of stomal ulcers are not visible roentgenologically because of their superficial nature. Under these circumstances gastroscopy may be of value, because the stoma usually can be visualized. An occasional marginal ulcer may occur as a result of a granuloma around a nonabsorbable suture in the gastrojejunal or gastroduodenal suture line.

Medical therapy of marginal ulceration is generally unsatisfactory, and this diagnosis is usually an indication for reoperation. All attempts should be made prior to reoperation to ascertain the possible physiologic causes for the recurrent ulcer, so that inappropriate therapy can be avoided. When the Z-E syndrome can be ruled out, vagotomy is the most successful treatment if it has not previously been carried out or if it has been shown to be incomplete in the presence of an adequate distal gastric resection. In cases of retained antrum, removal of the stump of distal gastric antrum may be all that is necessary. Occasionally resection and vagotomy are required if a gastroenterostomy alone has been previously carried out or if the resection is inadequate.

ZOLLINGER-ELLISON (Z-E) SYNDROME

The Z-E syndrome is the clinical entity of fulminant peptic ulceration associated with a non-beta cell islet tumor of the pancreas. Although most of these tumors occur in pancreas, approximately 10 percent are aberrant and are located in the region of the duodenum or within the duodenal wall itself. Microscopically, the tumors resemble either islet cells or often have a striking resemblance to carcinoid tumors. In 50 percent of the cases, metastases have already occurred at the time of operation and are located in the regional lymph nodes which drain the pancreas as well as in the liver. However, these patients rarely die from malignant spread but rather succumb to the *malignant potentialities of the ulceration* caused by the release of gastrin from the tumor or its metastases. In 20 percent of cases more than one tumor is present. In approximately 10 to 20 percent of the reported cases of the Z-E syndrome multiple endocrine adenomas have occurred, particularly in the parathyroid, pituitary, adrenal, and thyroid glands. In these instances of polyendocrine adenomatosis, familial incidence is very common. Gastrin has been isolated from these tumors, and immunoassays of plasma gastrin levels promise to provide a firm basis for accurate diagnosis.

The symptoms of the Z-E syndrome in many cases are similar to those of the common variety of duodenal ulceration. On the other hand, the tendency toward fulminant ulceration with severe complications is very great. Rapidly recurrent ulceration after previously adequate surgical therapy should raise the possibility of the Z-E syndrome, particularly if ulceration occurs in the jejunum. Profound gastric hypersecretion is present, and basal rates of secretion between 10 and 30 mEq per hr are almost invariable. Since the stomach is almost maximally stimulated at all times, further stimulation by histamine produces only a small or no increment in secretion over the basal state. A ratio of basal to maximally stimulated secretion of 0.6 or greater is considered highly suspicious.

Diarrhea and malabsorption may be the only presenting manifestation of the Z-E syndrome or may occur in conjunction with symptoms of peptic ulceration. The highly acid environment of the lower regions of the small intestine in patients with Z-E syndrome causes inactivation of pancreatic lipase and tends to precipitate bile salts; as a consequence malabsorption occurs. The enormous volume of highly acid gastric juice also contributes to the diarrhea in these patients. The diarrhea of the Z-E syndrome must be clearly distinguished from that produced by another non-beta, non-insulin-producing islet cell tumor of the pancreas. These tumors have not been associated with ulcerogenesis and do not cause gastric hypersecretion. The cause of the diarrhea in these instances is not known, although it has been suggested that these tumors elaborate a substance which alters the intestinal transport of water and electrolytes.

The ulceration present in patients with Z-E syndrome is notably resistant to both medical and ordinarily satisfactory surgical therapy. It is attractive to postulate that removal of the tumor without operation upon the stomach will cure the patient. In fact, although this sequence has been noted in a few cases, the extremely high incidence of multiple lesions, particularly of a metastatic nature, usually causes this form of therapy to fail. Despite reluctance to undertake radical therapy in these patients, they do not often die of malignant disease, and the weight of evidence is overwhelming that nothing short of total gastrectomy will suffice. Leaving only a tiny remnant of the stomach is fraught with hazard and will only result in recurrent ulceration and possibly death. The mortality rate in cases without total gastrectomy is as high as 90 percent, whereas when total gastrectomy is carried out, the mortality is about 10 to 15 percent.

COMPLICATIONS OF ULCERS

The complications of benign peptic ulceration include perforation, obstruction, and hemorrhage.

Hemorrhage

Hemorrhage is the most common complication. Any discussion of hemorrhage from peptic ulceration must necessarily include other major causes of gastrointestinal hemorhage, since the latter account for almost half the instances of massive gastrointestinal hemorrhage.

DIAGNOSTIC APPROACH (See Also Chap. 44). A vigorous diagnostic approach must be taken in all instances. For example, it is dangerous to assume that a patient with cirrhosis of the liver is bleeding from esophageal varices, since peptic ulcer is more common among patients with cirrhosis than in the general population. Similarly, a malignant lesion of the colon may be overlooked in a patient with a chronic duodenal ulcer if the assumption is made that the long-standing ulcer is the cause of the bleeding.

An initial assessment of the level of the bleeding is of the utmost importance. Hematemesis almost invariably means that the location of the bleeding point is proximal to the ligament of Treitz, although in rare instances the lesion is in the upper jejunum. Intubation of the stomach should be carried out in every patient with gastrointestinal bleeding in the absence of hematemesis, because blood in the aspirate has the same significance as does hematemesis. The intubation should be carried out *while the patient is bleeding* to increase the opportunity of localizing the site of hemorrhage. The character of the stool is helpful in deciding the location of the bleeding. A massive hemorrhage from esophageal varices may be associated with the passage of bright-red blood by rectum if bleeding has been sufficiently rapid and the transit time short. Conversely, if hypomotility is present, a lesion in the cecum may produce a rather dark, tarry stool. If gastrointestinal transit time is slow or normal, bright-red or dark-red liquid stools usually point to lesions of the terminal ileum or colon. Tarry stools in the presence of a normal transit time usually indicate bleeding from the upper tract. Tarry black stools are not to be confused with the dark, blackish-green stools of patients receiving iron or bismuth therapy.

In general, these simple measures are adequate to define the level of bleeding. *Under very special circumstances,* other methods may be employed. *Intubation of the small intestine* with a long intestinal tube can be carried out. During the passage of the tube gentle aspiration

should be done every 20 to 30 min. If bloody aspirate is obtained, a small amount of barium is given under fluoroscopic control, and careful study of the area in question is carried out. It may be necessary to withdraw the tube 6 to 8 in. prior to the x-ray examination, so that the tube does not migrate distal to the lesion. This method is generally applicable only to patients with slow and intermittent bleeding when there is adequate time for the necessary manipulations. If the site of bleeding is identified and the roentgenologic examination is normal, the tube should remain in place, so that the surgeon may more readily identify a possibly otherwise undetectable lesion at operation.

A less accurate counterpart of this test is the so-called "string test." The results of this test are often equivocal, and there are many false positive results. The patient swallows a string or umbilical tape containing lead markers. After the string has progressed well into the small intestine, an x-ray is taken to outline the location of the markers. The tape is then withdrawn and examined for gross blood stains and guaiac-positive areas. The intravenous injection of 20 ml 5% fluorescein after the tape is in place followed by examination 4 min later for fluorescence in ultraviolet light has produced slight improvement in the results of the string test, but fluorescein is rapidly excreted in the bile and may produce false positive tests. The time and discomfort of the test with a small yield of valuable results makes the string test and its modifications rarely worthwhile. Other tests including selective visceral angiography show promise for elucidation of hitherto undiscoverable sites of bleeding.

Specific diagnostic tests may reveal the exact nature of the lesion once the level of bleeding has been determined. The most important of these is the roentgenologic examination which can be done in a leisurely fashion if the patient is not bleeding rapidly. If upper gastrointestinal tract bleeding is massive, the stomach should be emptied of clots with a large Ewald tube using iced saline solution for irrigation. When the bleeding is under reasonable control, an emergency gastrointestinal series can be carried out and is rewarding in a surprisingly large number of patients. Since bleeding usually stops after irrigation of the stomach, useful information can be obtained if gastroscopy and esophagoscopy are carried out immediately before the x-rays are taken.

Complete evaluation of the patient is extremely important, since a variety of systemic diseases may be associated with hemorrhage. A bleeding diathesis must always be ruled out. Investigation of hepatic function should be included, because cirrhosis of the liver is so often associated with bleeding esophageal varices, gastritis, or peptic ulceration.

CLINICAL FEATURES. Syncope or other symptoms of acute blood loss are frequent and usually signify a blood loss of at least 1,000 to 1,500 ml. Melena alone in the absence of any other symptoms is surprisingly common. Bleeding from duodenal or gastric ulcers occurs without prior symptoms in 20 percent of patients. In individuals who have had prior symptoms of ulcer, these complaints often disappear at the onset of bleeding, because blood in the stomach and duodenum buffers the highly acid gastric juice. Hyperperistalsis and frequent bowel movements are common, because blood within the gastrointestinal tract is irritating.

TREATMENT. The treatment of gastrointestinal hemorrhage from peptic ulcer will depend upon the magnitude of the hemorrhage. In the majority of patients the therapy is nonoperative, and if the general condition permits, all patients should undergo the diagnostic tests outlined above. Surgical consultation should always be obtained from the outset. The decision to operate or not to operate should be made jointly by internists and surgeons. Occasionally, operation may be necessary as a diagnostic as well as therapeutic maneuver.

Sedation is important, because apprehension is common and may contribute to hypersecretion of acid. Replacement with blood should be early and adequate, and frequent monitoring of the physical findings and vital signs are mandatory. Careful records of the frequency, character and output of stools must be made. Continuous gastric aspiration for the first 6 to 12 hours may be helpful, not only in determining whether bleeding is continuing, but also in removing acid from the ulcerated area. This may be supplanted by a drip of milk or alkali or by the stringent antacid regimen described above. Cooling of the stomach to 10 to 14°C by insertion of a balloon perfused with alcohol and saline solution may be of value in treatment of acute massive gastrointestinal hemorrhage, but in general gastric cooling has little advantage unless operation is precluded. Thorough ice water lavage may be useful.

There is fairly universal agreement on the indication for operation in most cases of hemorrhage. Operation should be considered *urgent* when exsanguinating hemorrhage is present, and such a patient may need to be taken to the operating room under less than optimal circumstances. In patients with esophageal varices, a Sengstaken-Blakemore tube may be used when hepatic function is so poor as to preclude operative therapy. A second group of patients requiring *emergency operation* are those who have continued to bleed after initial replacement of blood loss. In general, if a patient requires as much as 500 ml blood every 8 hours after replacement of the initial blood loss, operation should be undertaken. Those patients who *rebleed* in the hospital after the initial episode constitute a third group in which there is unanimity in favor of emergency operation. Such patients are frequently individuals who have a large crater in either the stomach or duodenum. Even if bleeding stops, a previous history of multiple hemorrhages or other indications for operation should suggest that an opportune time for operation has arrived.

Factors which adversely affect the outcome of a gastrointestinal hemorrhage include age over sixty, previous massive hemorrhage, long-standing ulcer, or previous perforation. Bleeding from a gastric ulcer is much less likely to cease than is bleeding from a duodenal ulcer. Any of these factors might dictate operative therapy when other indications are equivocal.

Patients who bleed intermittently from an undeter-mined site following extensive evaluation should be operated on only when bleeding, because the chance of finding a lesion at operation in such an individual when he is not bleeding is very small.

Perforation

Perforated ulcers are usually located on the anterior wall of the duodenum but may occur either on the anterior or posterior wall of the stomach.

CLINICAL FEATURES. The onset of pain is usually sudden and severe. The pain begins in the epigastrium or right upper quadrant, is of a constant steady nature, and may radiate to the supraclavicular area if soiling of the subdiaphragmatic surfaces has occurred. The pain is accentuated by movement, coughing, or straining. Hence, the patient usually lies quietly in bed, often with flexed thighs. Vomiting of gastric content may occur once or twice, but persistent profuse vomiting is rare. On occasion, patients give a history suggesting preexisting symptoms of ulcer, but at least 10 to 20 percent of patients with perforation do not have a previous history of peptic disease. Examination shows a quiet abdomen usually with marked direct and rebound tenderness, and severe rigidity, although these findings are greatly attenuated in the elderly. Liver dullness may be absent, and there may be tenderness on rectal examination if the irritating gastric juice has migrated to the cul-de-sac. Shock is rare until late in the course of the disease and is caused by the extravasation of large quantities of fluid into the peritoneal cavity, the extent of which may be assessed by the rise in hematocrit if no significant bleeding has occurred.

DIAGNOSIS. The diagnosis rests mainly upon the clinical findings. The shift of pain from the epigastrium to the right lower quadrant may be confused with acute appendicitis, but the findings of peritoneal irritation are usually more striking in patients with perforated ulcer, and a carefully taken history is usually adequate to distinguish between these diseases. Confusion is particularly likely to occur in patients who are examined 6 to 10 hr after perforation and in whom sealing of the perforation has occured by adherence of the liver or other adjacent structures to the lesion. Rapidly progressive clinical improvement serves to differentiate this special group from patients with acute appendicitis.

Roentgenologic examination of the abdomen in the flat and upright position is often extremely helpful to detect free air under the diaphragm, though approximately 15 percent of patients with perforated ulcers do *not* show this sign. The absence of free air must not be misconstrued to indicate that perforated ulcer is not present. The white blood cell count is usually increased with a concomitant increase in the number of immature cells. An *elevated serum amylase level* is not infrequent and should not be a contraindication to operation if the clinical diagnosis suggests perforated ulcer. Intravenous cholangiography may be useful to exclude acute cholecystitis.

TREATMENT. Operation is the mainstay in the treatment of perforated ulcer. Nonoperative therapy should probably be confined to those patients in whom sealing of the perforation has already taken place and in whom marked and progressive clinical improvement has occurred when they are first seen. Nonoperative treatment consists mainly of careful continuous gastric suction to ensure complete emptying of the stomach. In addition, antibiotics and adequate fluid therapy are given. The major objections to nonoperative therapy are that intraabdominal and subphrenic abscesses are more common than after surgical treatment.

Preparation of the patient for operation should include intubation of the stomach and replacement of fluid losses. The magnitude of the "third space" losses in these patients is often underestimated, but even 3 or 4 hr after a perforation, as much as 3,000 ml fluid may be required if contamination of the peritoneal cavity has been massive. For the majority of patients simple closure of the ulcer is the safest therapy associated with the lowest mortality rate. If the patient is seen within 6 to 8 hr of the perforation and should other indications for surgical therapy of the peptic ulcer disease already exist, definitive surgical therapy of the ulcer may be undertaken, especially if peritoneal soiling is minimal. The results of definitive treatment have been gratifying in these carefully selected cases. Biopsies should always be taken of perforated gastric ulcers, but if carcinoma is likely, gastric resection is indicated.

Gastric Outlet Obstruction

Obstruction to the outlet of the stomach is most commonly associated with duodenal ulceration, but in a significant minority of cases, a distally located antral ulcer may produce the same clinical picture. Carcinoma of the stomach, congenital anomalies, and a variety of other lesions may also cause gastric outlet obstruction.

PATHOPHYSIOLOGY. Obstruction is usually the result of one of two processes, edema associated with active ulceration or fibrous stenosis. The severity of the symptoms are related to the degree and rapidity of onset of the obstruction and depend upon the competence of the antral musculature, the so-called "antral pump." An effectively compensated antral pump may overcome a high-grade stenosis for prolonged periods and may be associated with mild or no symptoms. On the other hand, less severe degrees of obstruction may produce severe symptoms if the antral pump decompensates, a more common finding when the obstruction is sudden rather than slowly progressive.

CLINICAL FEATURES. Anorexia, nausea, and fullness after eating are the most frequent symptoms. Surprisingly, vomiting may not occur until late when decompensation of the antral pump has occurred. A vague aching pain after eating associated with hyperperistalsis may also be present and is usually relieved by vomiting. Spontaneous vomiting without pain may occur only once a day, and generally the vomitus consists of the food in-gested during the previous 24-hr period. Vomiting rarely occurs more than two or three times daily despite severe obstruction. Weight loss and constipation are frequent. As the obstruction progresses, severe extracellular fluid deficits and hypokalemic and/or hypochloremic alkalosis often supervene. Roentgenologic examination of the abdomen usually shows an enormously dilated stomach, often occupying as much as two-thirds of the abdomen. Definitive examination of the upper gastrointestinal tract with barium before adequate decompression and cleansing of the stomach is unrewarding, because accurate assessment of the cause of the obstruction is difficult or impossible. Such studies are best delayed for a few days, since they often exhaust an already seriously ill patient.

DIFFERENTIAL DIAGNOSIS. In addition to gastric and duodenal ulcer, tumors of the stomach and foreshortening secondary to antral gastritis may produce gastric outlet obstruction. Occasionally, corrosive gastritis from the ingestion of alkali, postoperative stenosis of gastroduodenal anastomoses or pyloroplasties, congenital anomalies, and inflammatory disease of adjacent organs also produce outlet obstruction.

Neuromuscular defects must also be considered. Diabetic autonomic neuropathy, vagotomy without a drainage operation, anticholinergic drugs, severe postoperative ileus, potassium deficiency, hypothyroidism, and acute and chronic disease of the central nervous system may all be associated with gastric dilatation because of failure of the antral pump. Sometimes a single lesion cannot be identified, and the dilatation is attributed to severe debility, aging, and protein deficiency.

TREATMENT. The response to therapy is of great value in determining whether organic irreversible stricture or edema is the predominant cause of the obstruction. Correction of fluid and electrolyte deficits can usually be accomplished within the first 24 hr, particularly if azotemia is not present. *Continuous* gastric aspiration for 72 hr is the most important part of the therapeutic regimen and will almost always allow differentiation between organic stricture and edema. Although intermittent aspiration of the stomach is advocated by some, this method does not allow sufficient decompression of the stomach and frequently causes prolongation of nonoperative therapy because of the misleading information derived from it. Resolution of the obstruction after 72 hr of continuous aspiration is generally excellent when edema is the predominating feature, whereas large gastric residuals of over 500 ml persist in organic strictures.

Repeated attempts to produce resolution of the obstruction beyond 72 to 92 hr cause undue delay and further deterioration of the patient. If the obstruction is so marked that 5 to 6 days of aspiration is required, operation is undoubtedly indicated anyway. Following the original period of gastric suction, a stringent antacid regimen and clear-liquid diet are begun. Anticholinergic drugs are contraindicated, because gastric emptying is delayed. The gastric residual volume is determined 24 hr after the institution of such a regimen and occasionally 48 hr later. Should gastric obstruction be evident by the indication of large residual volumes, then operation is immediately indicated.

SYNDROMES AFTER GASTRECTOMY OR VAGOTOMY

The immediate postoperative complications are those which may follow any abdominal operation in addition to a small group of special complications peculiar to gastric operations. A full discussion of these is not within the purview of this chapter, and it is the late complications to which we shall direct our attention.

Anatomic and Functional Derangements

FAILURE OF GASTRIC EMPTYING. After vagotomy there is failure of the normal antral pump mechanism. Since the advent of the combination of an emptying procedure (pyloroplasty or gastroenterostomy) with vagotomy, this complication is not common. In rare instances of long-standing preoperative obstruction where decompensation of the antral pump has occurred, pyloroplasty in the presence of an elongated J-shaped stomach may fail to provide adequate gastric emptying after vagotomy. Gastroenterostomy or resection may be necessary to overcome this problem. Obstruction of a gastroduodenal or gastrojejunal anastomosis may be a delayed occurrence and usually results from faulty surgical technique, although rarely the late development of recurrent ulcer or carcinoma of the stomach may be causative factors. Obstruction of the efferent loop of a gastrojejunostomy more commonly results from adhesions or kinking, however, and may require operative intervention.

OBSTRUCTION OF THE AFFERENT LOOP. This complication occurs only in the presence of a gastrojejunostomy and is slightly more frequent when the afferent loop is anastomosed to the greater curvature of the stomach. The usual symptoms are a marked feeling of fullness, bloating, and nausea after meals. These symptoms are dramatically relieved 20 to 60 min after the ingestion of the food by the vomiting of clear bilious material not containing the ingested food. Food is absent because the efferent loop is patent, while the bilious vomiting is caused by the sudden release of the secretions from the biliary and pancreatic systems. Usually the symptoms are chronic, although occasionally acute severe complete obstruction may develop. The latter condition resembles acute pancreatitis clinically, and elevation of the serum amylase level is common. The diagnosis is usually difficult, since lack of filling of the afferent loop on radiologic examination is not infrequently observed in the absence of afferent loop obstruction. Treatment consists of surgical revision of the anastomosis. Afferent loop obstruction may be associated with the blind loop syndrome (see Chap. 316) due to bacterial overgrowth in the obstructed afferent loop.

JEJUNOGASTRIC INTUSSUSCEPTION AND RETROANASTOMATIC HERNIATION. Retrograde intussusception of the jejunum into the gastric pouch may cause acute obstruction of either the afferent or the efferent loop of the gastrojejunal anastomosis and may occur early or many years after operation. Herniation of the afferent loop or the efferent loop behind the gastrojejunal stoma or herniation of the jejunum through the mesocolon if a posterior gastrojejunal anastomosis has been carried out may also be the cause of acute obstructive symptoms. These complications are associated with repeated vomiting and require immediate surgical intervention.

GASTRITIS. In addition to the usual factors which may cause irritation of the gastric mucosa the loss of the pylorus allows almost continuous regurgitation of alkaline juices into the stomach. Consequently, microscopic gastritis is present in an extremely high percentage of patients following gastric operations. The relationship of such histologic gastritis to clinical symptoms is conjectural. It is probable that few symptoms arise from these changes, although, rarely, severe gastritis in the region of the gastrojejunal stoma may contribute to the development of obstruction in an already slightly stenotic anastomosis.

Metabolic and Other Derangements

EARLY AND LATE POSTPRANDIAL POSTGASTRECTOMY SYNDROMES. The early syndrome, often referred to in the literature as the *dumping syndrome,* is characterized by the development of weakness, nausea, a feeling of warmth, palpitation, pallor, borborygmi, diarrhea, and distension, 20 to 30 min after a meal. There is often a strong urge to assume the recumbent position, and recumbency usually relieves the symptoms. The syndrome is most violently and frequently produced by a high carbohydrate intake. The late syndrome, not truly dumping, consists of profound weakness, tremulousness, palpitation, and sweating without hyperperistalsis and diarrhea, usually occurring approximately 2 to 3 hr after the meal.

The causes of the symptoms of the early and late syndromes are different. Loss of the pylorus, by whatever surgical operation, allows the introduction of hyperosmolar substances into the small intestine with a resultant outpouring of fluid from the plasma to produce an isosmotic intestinal content. However, the lack of correlation of decreases in plasma volume with the severity of the symptomatology has led to a search for other causes of the early postprandial dumping syndrome. The release of serotonin from the small intestine, and rapid and prolonged alimentary hyperglycemia have also been implicated, but their role is uncertain. Recently, elevations of circulating kinin levels have been found to correlate with the vasomotor symptoms in these patients, but further studies are required to assess the importance of these findings. The late postprandial symptoms clearly result from a functional hypoglycemia which may be caused by excessive production of insulin or an insulin hypersensitivity. The diagnosis of the early postprandial syndrome is relatively easy if a careful history is taken. The late hypoglycemic syndrome can be diagnosed by the finding of hypoglycemia late in the course of a 6-hr oral glucose tolerance test.

Attempts at prevention of the early postprandial dumping syndrome by surgical narrowing of the original gastroenteric stoma have not been uniformly successful and may be associated with early or late stomal obstruction. Treatment consists of frequent small meals low in sugar and starch in order to decrease the osmolarity of the meal. Fluids are permitted between meals only, because the concomitant administration of food and fluids permits the production of a hypertonic solution. Anticholinergic drugs may retard the hyperperistalsis and are often helpful. Serotonin antagonists have been disappointing and probably are of little value. Excellent results have been obtained by the administration of tolbutamide in those patients with prolonged alimentary hyperglycemia. The usual dose is 0.5 to 1 Gm tolbutamide 10 to 30 min before meals. The late prandial hypoglycemic symptoms are best treated with a high protein–low carbohydrate diet.

Although any patient may develop the dumping syndrome after loss of normal pyloric function, significant symptoms occur in only about 5 to 10 percent of patients. In only 1 percent is the symptomatology sufficiently severe that operative reconstruction is contemplated. In selected instances the introduction of an antiperistaltic loop of intestine has been very helpful.

ANEMIA. Anemia is probably the most common complication of partial gastrectomy. If patients are carefully studied after gastrectomy, 20 to 50 percent will show some anemia. Anemia is more common after gastrojejunostomy than after gastroduodenostomy and is more prevalent after resection than after simple vagotomy with emptying operation. It often represents a combination of iron deficiency and vitamin B_{12} deficiency. The iron deficiency results not only from decreased oral intake but also from impaired iron absorption caused by hypochlorhydria, rapid gastric emptying, and bypass of the duodenum especially after gastrojejunostomy. Chronic blood loss from stomal gastritis may contribute to the iron deficiency. The treatment of iron deficiency anemia is discussed in Chap. 336. Vitamin B_{12} deficiency may result not only from extensive removal of the source of intrinsic factor but also from the ensuing gastritis in the gastric remnant. The afferent loop syndrome described above may be contributory. Vagotomy also reduces the amount of intrinsic factor in gastric juice. Folic acid deficiency after gastrectomy is rare. Every patient who undergoes gastrectomy should be carefully surveyed for anemia at least once yearly for the remainder of his life and appropriate therapeutic measures undertaken if anemia appears.

MALABSORPTION AND WEIGHT LOSS. Weight loss following gastric operations is common if the patient is overweight at the time of operation. On the other hand, when patients have lost a great deal of weight prior to operation, they will often gain after the procedure but do not usually reach their previous level. Weight loss is caused by poor eating habits, fear of eating because of the dumping syndrome or mechanical abnormalities, and malabsorption. The cause of the malabsorption is not completely understood, but causative factors include poor mixing of bile and pancreatic secretions with food, rapid intestinal transit, and the effects of bacterial overgrowth in the afferent loop if afferent loop obstruction is present. Osteomalacia may occur as a result of poor absorption of vitamin D and calcium. Careful demonstration of the etiologic factors is important, and treatment includes an adequate diet occasionally supplemented by pancreatic extracts and bile salts. Courses of broad-spectrum antibiotics may be dramatic in reversing the malabsorption if afferent loop obstruction accompanied by overgrowth of bacteria is an important factor. Surgical revision may be considered should these nonoperative methods fail.

POSTVAGOTOMY EFFECTS. An increasing number of instances of development of gallstones after total abdominal vagotomy are being recognized. This is probably caused by poor emptying of the gallbladder, not only from loss of its nerve supply, but also from inadequate stimulation of bile flow by secretin and cholecystokinin and lack of contraction of the gallbladder by cholecystokinin, especially if the duodenum has been bypassed. Consequently, this complication may also occur after high subtotal gastric resection with gastrojejunostomy.

Postvagotomy diarrhea has been reported in as many as 50 to 60 percent of individuals undergoing vagal resection. However, as a troublesome symptom it occurs in only 4 or 5 percent of patients. It consists of intermittent pale, greasy stools, associated with sudden explosive loose bowel movements seemingly occurring without any predisposing factor. This occurs once every week or two, lasts 1 or 2 days, and then subsides as rapidly as it commenced. The cause of the diarrhea is unknown, and even selective denervation of the stomach alone has not been uniformly successful in preventing this complication.

REFERENCES

Davenport, H. W.: Salicylate Damage to the Gastric Mucosal Barrier, New Engl. J. Med., 276:1307, 1967.

Du Plessis, D. J.: Pathogenesis of Gastric Ulceration, Lancet, 1:973, 1965.

Fordtran, J. S., and J. A. H. Collyns: Antacid Pharmacology in Duodenal Ulcer: Effect of Antacids on Poscibal Gastric Acidity and Peptic Activity, New Engl. J. Med., 274:921, 1966.

Gregory, R. A., and H. J. Tracy: Constitution and Properties of Two Gastrins Extracted from Hog Antral Mucosa, Gut, 5:103, 1962.

Grossman, M. I.: Integration of Neural and Hormonal Control of Gastric Secretion, Physiologist, 6:349, 1963.

Kirsner, J. B.: Peptic Ulcer: A Review of the Recent Literature on Various Clinical Aspects, Gastroenterology, 54: 611 and 945, 1968.

Larson, N. E., J. C. Cain, and L. G. Bartholomew: Prognosis of the Medically Treated Small Gastric Ulcer. II. Ten-year to Nineteen-year Follow-up Study of 391 Patients, New Engl. J. Med., 264:330, 1961.

Stammers, F. A. R., and J. A. Williams: "Partial Gastrectomy: Complications and Metabolic Consequences," London, Butterworth & Co (Publishers), Ltd., 1963.

Wormsley, K. G., and M. I. Grossman: Maximal Histalog Test in Control Subjects and Patients with Peptic Ulcer, Gut, 6:427, 1965.

315 CANCER AND OTHER DISEASES OF THE STOMACH

Edwin Englert, Jr.

GASTRIC CARCINOMA

Carcinoma of the stomach is asymptomatic during early growth. Later, local and systemic symptoms may appear through necrosis, bleeding, ulceration, obstruction, disturbed gastrointestinal motor function, invasion of adjacent structures, metastasis to distant organs, and the effects of advanced malignancy. Resultant clinical patterns range widely from a brief acute febrile illness to one mistaken for a mild protracted psychoneurosis, and diagnosis may be easy or extremely difficult. Clinical descriptions of gastric carcinoma relate almost exclusively to late manifestations and are not of much help to the physician who wishes to make the diagnosis early enough to effect a cure by complete excision. Such bleak features of the disease are tempered on occasion by a slow-growing tumor with low invasiveness and a reasonable chance for cure.

INCIDENCE. There has been a definite but unexplained decline in the incidence of gastric carcinoma in the past several decades. It is no longer the leading cancer of males but remains common. The reported death rate in 1964 in the United States was 9.7 per 100,000 population. Men are affected two times more often than women. The disease afflicts all races, but as in other gastroduodenal diseases, there appear to be unexplained geographic and cultural differences in incidence. It attacks at all ages although rarely before the third decade, and the risk rises progressively thereafter. The antrum is the leading site of gastric carcinoma, followed by the lesser curvature, cardia, and body of the stomach.

PREDISPOSING FACTORS. *Genetic* predisposition is evident from the striking familial incidence of carcinoma of the stomach as well as the increased inheritance of blood group A among its victims. *Alteration of the gastric mucosa* also may be determined genetically but requires special mention, because it defines patients at high risk. The cancer rate increases progressively in patients with hypochlorhydria, achlorhydria, gastric atrophy, gastric polyps, and pernicious anemia, and reaches an incidence of 6 to 12 percent in the last group. In fact, some investigators believe that every cancer begins on a patch of gastric atrophy even when the rest of the stomach is normal. It should be noted in passing that the conditions listed correlate with each other as well as with carcinoma.

Polyps are not found frequently in cancer-bearing stomachs, but in the past pathologic interpretation of the adenoma itself sometimes suggested carcinomatous degeneration, particularly when it was over 2 cm in diameter. The criteria and incidence of carcinomatous change have been challenged, however, and the precancerous role of small polyps is in doubt.

The adult form of *acanthosis nigricans,* a pigmented papillomatous skin disease of intertriginous areas, face, and flexor surfaces, confers a huge risk of subsequent visceral carcinoma, usually of the stomach. The mechanism is unknown, but again the disease is transmitted genetically.

CLINICAL FEATURES. As already mentioned, the early carcinoma is frustratingly silent, and the late manifestations are extremely variable. The course may be fulminating or insidious, short or prolonged. Anorexia is a remarkably constant feature, and in late cases there are usually abdominal discomfort, weight loss, anemia, weakness, and rapid filling on eating. Discomfort varies from mild intermittent epigastric pain to constant severe pain boring into the back. It is often poorly localized and may be a sensation of fullness, aching, or bloating initiated or aggravated by meals. In ulcerated carcinoma, the pain may mimic ulcer pain.

Gastric carcinoma *invades* locally and *metastasizes* by way of the lymphatics, by way of the bloodstream, and by free passage across the peritoneum. Commonly it extends into the lower esophagus, proximal duodenum, omentum, colon, peritoneum, or pancreas. Because pancreatic invasion can be extensive, it may be difficult to tell whether the pancreas or the stomach was the site of the primary tumor. Pulmonary metastases may be lymphangitic and diffuse or hematogenous and nodular. Local and distant spread also produces symptoms in liver, pleura, bone, nervous system, and skin. There may be diarrhea, thrombophlebitis, nausea, vomiting, backache, cough, hiccup, pleurisy, fever, and melena. Perforation and massive bleeding are unusual.

PHYSICAL EXAMINATION. Physical findings are entirely normal during the early course, but in late cases there is evidence of local and metastatic tumor. Commonly there are signs of anemia and weight loss, mass or tenderness in the epigastrium, low-grade fever, and a nodular enlarged liver. There are numerous eponymic metastases of gastric carcinoma, such as Virchow's left supraclavicular lymph node, the Irish left pectoral node, Blumer's shelf on rectal examination, and the Krukenberg tumor in the ovary, but these occur in 10 percent of cases, or fewer. There may be bone tenderness, ascites, pleural effusions, peripheral or central neurologic signs, jaundice, pericardial rub, or an umbilical mass. The wasted cachectic look of terminal malignancy is surprisingly uncommon.

ROENTGENOGRAPHIC AND GASTROSCOPIC EXAMINATION. These types of examination rarely are performed in early unsuspected carcinoma, and hence their diagnostic accuracy at that stage is unknown. In advanced cases, they reveal features of one of several types of growth which cancer of the stomach pursues: (1) polypoid mass, (2) tumor with punched-out ulceration, (3) ulcerative mass blending into adjacent stomach wall, (4) diffusely infiltrating intramural tumor, or (5) superficial spreading mucosal plaque. Diagnostic features of the mass and ulceration were described in Chap. 314, but it may be reemphasized here that x-ray examination detects abnormality in the great majority of late cases and that differentiation of benign from malignant ulcers is clearcut and easy in over 80 percent of cases. In the small remaining group, the radiologist is less certain, and while he may still prove correct in most of these, his accuracy is lessened. It is for this reason that gastric ulcers which

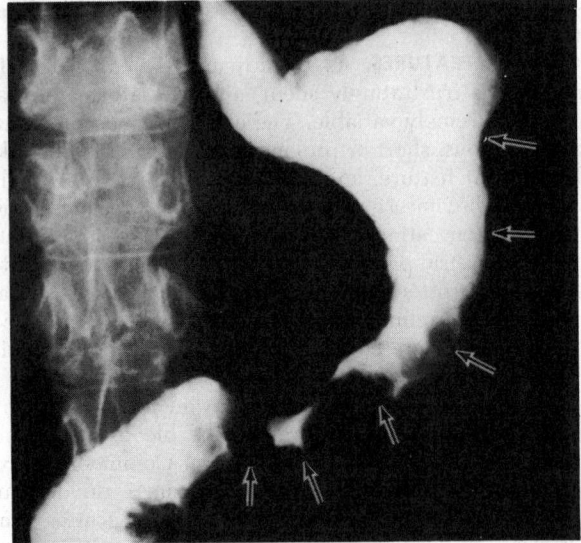

Fig. 315-1. Diffusely infiltrating gastric carcinoma (linitis plastica). The stomach is rigidly contracted to a narrow channel throughout most of its length. Note fine irregularities in the wall, absence of peristaltic contractions, and nodular tumorous masses in the distal third.

are not obviously malignant and destined for early surgical therapy should be evaluated thoroughly by the combined use of x-ray, gastroscopy, cytologic examination of the gastric juice, examination of gastric acidity, and trial of medical management outlined in Chap. 314.

Diffuse infiltrating carcinomas may not produce roentgenographic evidence of a mass. Instead, they cause concentric narrowing of the lumen or areas of flattening, rigidity, and absent peristalsis (Fig. 315-1). This variety is responsible for the "leather bottle stomach" deformity and the term *linitis plastica*, referring to dense fibrous tissue interspersed with isolated carcinoma cells. Superficial spreading carcinoma is the type most likely to be missed, since there may be only small patches of mucosal flattening, beading, or stiffness. Gastroscopy is a valuable adjunct in such varieties.

In addition to the standard barium meal, roentgenographic techniques, such as selective celiac angiography and abdominal lymphangiography, demonstrate the extent of the tumor and thus its operability, but they do not increase the yield of initial primary diagnoses.

LABORATORY FINDINGS. In late or symptomatic cancers laboratory findings include *anemia,* usually of chronic blood loss type, and *occult blood* in the stools in most patients. True *achlorhydria* to maximum betazole or histamine testing is found in half the patients and *hypochlorhydria* in another quarter of them. This leaves sizable numbers with normal secretion. Therefore, the presence of acid is of no value in differential diagnosis. Moreover, true hypersecretion, although rare, does not rule out carcinoma. *Hypoalbuminemia* due to leakage of serum albumin into the stomach is found occasionally. As in other malignant conditions, there may be elevated levels of serum haptoglobin and abnormal spikes in the serum protein electrophoretogram, usually due to an IgG globulin. *Cytology* is a valuable diagnostic aid, providing, under optimum circumstances, over 85 percent accuracy in the diagnosis of adenocarcinoma of the stomach and less than 1 percent false positive reports in normal or benign disease stomachs.

The *tetracycline fluorescence test* takes advantage of the fact that malignant cells bind tetracycline longer than do normal cells. Tetracycline is administered for 2 days; then 36 hr after the last dose the gastric washings are neutralized and centrifuged, and the sediment is spread on filter paper, allowed to dry in the dark, and examined immediately under ultraviolet light. Any yellow fluorescence is positive, and the test is reported to be 96 percent accurate with but 4 percent false positive results.

Antigens, specific for gastric carcinoma in that antibodies raised against them do not react with normal gastric tissue, have been found in some human gastric adenocarcinomas. This discovery holds promise for future therapeutic as well as diagnostic approaches to cancer of the stomach, but practical applications, such as these would be, have not yet been developed.

DIAGNOSIS. Diagnosis of advanced carcinoma may be easy. Clinical and roentgenographic findings are clear-cut in such patients. In other cases, the condition defies analysis completely or mimics many other diseases. It is wise to *insist* upon histologic diagnosis before condemning a patient to the category of inoperable terminal malignancy. This may be obtained by cytology; lymph node biopsy; blind needle biopsy of the liver (Chap. 324); needle biopsy of metastatic nodules in liver, pleura, or bone marrow; or limited surgical exploration.

Early cases are regrettably silent, but sudden changes in upper gastrointestinal function, particularly the appearance of anorexia in men over forty years of age, should always be suspected. Clinical judgment must be exercised in deciding how far to follow suspicion, but the minimum is an x-ray study of the stomach and repeated tests of the stool for occult bleeding. If any doubt exists, cytology, gastroscopy, secretory studies, repeated x-ray, and gastroscopy of any suspicious area and exploration are the next steps to be taken in sequence.

CANCER SCREENING PROGRAMS. Roentgenographic surveys of the normal population have been made to detect silent carcinomas of the stomach, but the yield of curable lesions did not justify their routine use. On the other hand, the high risk of patients with pernicious anemia, gastric polyps, and gastric atrophy suggests the desirability of semiannual examinations with alternating gastric cytology and roentgenography. In past surveys of these groups, unsuspected tumors were detected five times more often and had spread beyond the possibility of surgical cure less often than in surveys of the normal population. Periodic testing of the stool for occult bleeding also is indicated in these patients.

TREATMENT. *Surgical treatment* to attempt *complete excision* of the tumor is indicated in every patient in whom careful clinical investigation fails to reveal evidence of spread beyond the stomach. Moreover, *palliative operation* is necessary to relieve obstruction in some patients and rarely for emergencies of perforation or massive bleeding.

The natural history of the disease too often places the surgeon at the disadvantage of being able to do too little too late. Surgical statistics, on the other hand, are confusing and can raise false hopes for the patient. This results from (1) the lack of adequate controlled populations for surgical series, (2) the inevitable selection of patients that characterizes surgical series, (3) controversial pathologic criteria for the diagnosis of adenomas and low-grade malignancy, and (4) the traditional way in which surgical series are reported, whereby the patients are reanalyzed statistically several times with varying numbers of dead patients excluded for different reasons at each analysis. Consequently, it is difficult if not impossible to be certain of the real effectiveness of surgical treatment or even to compare one surgical series with another. It is believed that the overall *5-year survival rate* in patients undergoing operation for carcinoma of the stomach is 5 to 15 percent. A few reports, perhaps for reasons cited above, suggest that this should be raised to 20 percent. In unoperated patients, it is 0 to 2 percent. The *surgical mortality* of operations hopefully designed as curative is 5 to 12 percent, a figure considerably higher than that for noncancer gastric surgery (Chap. 314).

On the bright side of the statistics, high survival rates may be expected in tumors of low invasiveness and growth potential, such as small ulcerating and superficial spreading carcinomas. Although poorly understood and therapeutically unexplored, the same appears to be true for occasional patients with augmented host resistance to the tumor. Sporadic reports of prolonged survival without surgical treatment and of true recurrence (rather than an independent primary cancer) 10 or more years postoperatively also reflect these factors. This teaches us not to use the length of clinical history to diagnose widespread and incurable tumor, since a long course may mean slow growth, high resistance, and a favorable prognosis. Other factors which determine the outcome of surgical therapy are location and extent of tumor, condition of the patient, and the presence of metastases at exploration. When no metastases are found in regional lymph nodes, optimism is warranted, since 5-year survival may occur in as many as half of this highly selected and fortunate but small group of patients.

Formerly, attempts at curative operation required total gastrectomy, but comparable results have attended the use of subtotal resection for all but high gastric cancers near the cardia. The procedure is more extensive than in ulcer operations, since local and lymphatic pathways of extension are included in the resection. The incidence and types of postgastrectomy syndromes depend on the extent of resection (see Chap. 314).

Cancer chemotherapy has been tried in inoperable carcinoma of the stomach, but clear-cut long-standing palliation has been infrequent. Moreover, these agents actually may shorten the patient's course through toxic effects on other tissues, such as the bone marrow. Thus, it cannot be considered a routine therapeutic technique. The development of new agents and methods holds promise that this approach could be of value in the future.

OTHER MALIGNANT TUMORS OF THE STOMACH

Carcinoma of the stomach comprises at least 90 percent of gastric malignant tumors, and lymphoma accounts for most of the remainder. A rare group of sarcomas, the most common of which is leiomyosarcoma, includes fibrosarcoma, neurogenic sarcoma, neurofibrosarcoma, and myxosarcoma. They usually are misdiagnosed as carcinoma or found by chance, the true diagnosis coming as a surprise in either event.

LYMPHOMA OF THE STOMACH. Lymphoma of the stomach generally is a lymphosarcoma or reticulum cell sarcoma. It appears in about one-fifth of patients with systemic lymphomatous involvement and also occurs as a "primary" lymphoma without obvious disease elsewhere. There are no distinctive gastric symptoms, and indeed there often are no gastric symptoms in patients with widespread disease. Epigastric pain or mass and weight loss are frequent in the "primary" variety. Characteristically, the patient's general condition is good when first seen. Lymphoma of the stomach bleeds massively or perforates more often than carcinoma but usually presents a similar roentgenographic appearance. However, large stiff folds or a submucosal mass may be the sole finding on roentgenographic examination. So-called "primary" gastric lymphoma is often removed surgically and the patient subsequently irradiated. Initial results of such therapy or of radiation alone are good, with 5-year survival in half the patients.

LEIOMYOSARCOMAS. These tumors often ulcerate and bleed, but there are no distinctive clinical features. Long histories, however, are not at all uncommon. On x-ray examination, they appear as circumscribed globular filling defects or submucosal tumors, frequently with central ulceration, or as exogastric masses. Treatment is surgical, and because of low growth characteristics 5-year survivals may be expected in half.

BENIGN TUMORS OF THE STOMACH

The benign gastric tumors are adenomas, leiomyomas, fibromas, lipomas, and neurofibromas, and, excepting the adenomas, each is rare in clinical practice. Usually they do not produce symptoms, but those derived from mesenchyme and ectoderm may ulcerate and bleed. Although features of benignancy are generally evident on x-ray, these tumors often are removed, because carcinoma cannot be excluded with certainty.

ADENOMATOUS POLYPS. These tumors occur in the distal two-thirds of the stomach and often are multiple. They appear in about 2 percent of achlorhydric patients and in 5 percent of patients with pernicious anemia. Conversely, 85 percent of patients with polyps will be found to be achlorhydric. Roentgenographically they produce smooth, oval filling defects within the gastric lumen, and gastroscopy reveals a berrylike mass with an intact mucosa.

In the past, polyps have been removed routinely, either to be certain that they were not cancerous or to prevent carcinomatous degeneration. Since the likelihood of the latter is in dispute, this practice may be modified for small lesions which are clearly benign, particularly in aged, debilitated patients of high surgical risk. Polyps over 2 cm in diameter and those whose benignity is suspect, however, should be removed.

LEIOMYOMAS. Leiomyomas occur in the antrum and body of the stomach and bleed commonly. Roentgenographically they appear as smooth, globular filling defects, frequently surmounted by an ulcer niche, or they may grow "dumbbell" fashion exogastrically and produce little or no x-ray evidence of an intragastric mass. Although rare clinically, careful pathologic search reveals small ones in 16 to 50 percent of autopsies. There is no evidence that they undergo malignant change.

PSEUDOTUMORS. *Benign lymphoid hyperplasia,* or pseudolymphoma, may occur in the stomach as well as other organs and cause a long history of vague dyspepsia. It may ulcerate and bleed and produce a variety of appearances on roentgenographic examination simulating carcinoma or peptic ulcer. This often leads to surgical intervention, where simple excision is curative. The cause is uncertain although believd to be inflammatory. The same is said of *eosinophilic granuloma,* or inflammatory fibroid polyp, but this disease may be related to diffuse eosinophilic gastroenteritis, an alleged hypersensitivity state. Granulomas occur throughout the gastrointestinal tract but usually in the gastric antrum, where they produce episodic cramps and vomiting or ulceration and bleeding. Roentgenographic appearances mimic adenoma, carcinoma, or antral narrowing, and there may be peripheral eosinophilia. Some cases respond to corticosteroid therapy.

FUNCTIONAL DYSPEPSIA

The genesis of functional symptoms is poorly understood, but by definition they reflect *disturbances of gastrointestinal function.* These undoubtedly are affected by psychogenic factors as well as physiologic, hormonal, and pharmacologic factors, extreme aging, debility, acute illness, electrolyte factors, and nervous system influences. Functional symptoms are the *leading* reasons for which patients seek medical advice. The two most frequent functional syndromes in the gastrointestinal tract are flatulent dyspepsia and the irritable colon. The former commonly enters the differential diagnosis of gastroduodenal diseases and in fact often occurs simultaneously with one or more organic lesions of the upper gastrointestinal tract.

CLINICAL FEATURES. *Symptoms* include dry mouth, lump in the throat, difficulty in initiating swallowing, anorexia, belching, flatus, abdominal distension or rumbling, nausea, vomiting, sourness, water brash, and epigastric or midabdominal discomfort. The latter assumes a wide range of forms from vague fullness through cramps

and burning to persistent mild or moderate poorly described pain. It is usually quite diffuse and frequently aggravated or initiated by eating or by the ingestion of certain foods. However, the patient with functional dyspepsia characteristically is difficult to pin down concerning specific details of his discomfort, its timing, and its relationship to bodily functions or associated symptoms. Extremely common is flatulent indigestion after fatty foods, the so-called "fatty food intolerance" attributed erroneously by many to organic biliary tract disease. Often food idiosyncrasies are learned experiences; controlled testing rarely confirms the patient's prejudices. *Aerophagia* is so common as to be virtually universal, but many patients refuse to believe this, despite concern over gas, rumbling, and embarrassing gaseous passage from both ends of the digestive system.

The *course* of functional symptoms is chronic, with tendencies to wax and wane. Despite great concern over symptoms, the patient usually sleeps well, appears healthy, and shows no evidence of weight loss, even when he says his fear of eating or vomiting prevents adequate nutrition. Often there are *neurasthenic* symptoms in addition to gastrointestinal complaints, and many patients have *headaches,* chronic *fatigue,* and acute or chronic *anxiety* or *depression.*

Although combinations of symptoms and the patient's emphasis on certain complaints vary, the symptom patterns and associations outlined generally permit clear-cut *diagnosis.* It is therefore a *serious error* to diagnose functional disease only when organic lesions cannot be demonstrated by objective testing. Such an approach automatically misdiagnoses the many cases in which there are concomitant functional and organic disease and the many organic lesions in which initial objective testing is negative. It is also important not to jump to the conclusion, once the diagnosis of functional disease is clear, that the condition is psychogenic. It very often is, but the physician must remember to rule out the other causes of functional symptoms, such as hypothyroidism, hypocalcemia, drug side effects, and the host of others applicable to the etiologic categories noted earlier, which may be subclinical or mild and difficult to diagnose.

TREATMENT. This is not usually curative but often is effective for prolonged periods. It consists of thorough *examination* to exclude and treat accompanying and underlying organic disease, sympathetic but firm *explanation* of symptoms, strong *reassurance,* and *symptomatic* measures. Since many of the symptoms do have a physiologic basis, temporary relief often follows judicious use of agents known to influence demonstrated physiologic abnormalities, e.g., anticholinergic agents for cramps and hypermotility (Chap. 314), wetting agents to facilitate passage of aerophagic bubbles (simethicone, 50 mg q.i.d.), or alumina compounds for pain and sourness (Chap. 314), which are characteristically relieved only after eructation. With all these agents, relief is gradual rather than dramatic. Other measures to try are discussed under Nonspecific Common Gastritis, below.

Such symptomatic therapy always wears out, but reexamination often reveals changing physiologic events which justify changing the symptomatic agent. It is wise also to proscribe foods believed by the patient to cause him distress. *Sedatives and tranquilizers* usually are recommended, but there is little documentation to indicate that they alter the course of the disease. In contrast, they are very useful for any concomitant acute anxiety or insomnia. In some patients, there is a marked psychopathologic condition with gross psychiatric symptomatology over and above the functional gastrointestinal complaints. Such patients require psychiatric referral and treatment, but this is unnecessary in the majority.

One of the physician's prime responsibilities to these patients is to remain alert for the development of new symptoms, which frequently are difficult to pick out of the wondrous array of functional complaints but which may herald the onset of additional serious organic disease.

NONSPECIFIC COMMON GASTRITIS

For a large part of the present century, the existence of this disease was doubted in many segments of the medical world because of discrepancies between clinical, gastroscopic, and roentgenologic observations and postmortem or surgical tissue specimens. The advent of the peroral suction biopsy tube provided serial, well-preserved biopsies of living tissue and a firm basis for analyzing the disease. The result has been an explosive increment in investigational literature, new concepts, and increased recognition of the disease.

Gastritis is a *very common* disease, the reported incidence of the chronic variety starting at 28 percent in childhood and rising to 52 percent of the population past age sixty! It is usually *asymptomatic*, however, and its clinical significance therefore lies almost, if not entirely, in its complications: bleeding, possibly neoplasia, digestion and nutrition (loss of acid, pepsin, and intrinsic factor). The cause seems evident in some patients but is uncertain in many and is as yet unproved in most. The disease is confined to the gastric mucosa and hence cannot be detected by standard roentgenographic examinations. It may, however, affect gastroduodenal motor function with secondary nonspecific alterations of gastric rugal patterns, which are evident roentgenographically. Gastroscopy and biopsy are the only reliable diagnostic tools.

ACUTE GASTRITIS. Acute alcoholism, food poisoning, certain drug and food sensitivites, acute illnesses, uremia, and heavy metal poisoning may be accompanied by acute gastritis. *Symptoms* include anorexia, constant mild nausea, vomiting, diffuse epigastric discomfort, fever, and, in severe cases, the systemic fluid and electrolyte consequences of persistent vomiting. Brisk hemorrhage is common and in alcoholic patients often occurs suddenly without prior gastric symptoms. Physical examination reveals tenderness in the epigastrium and left upper part of the abdomen, which often corresponds to the subcostal projection of the gastric silhouette. *Pathologically* there are hyperemia, edema, erosions, hemorrhages, inflammatory cell infiltration of the lamina propria, and surface denudation and exudate. The process lasts for hours to a few days and heals rapidly, with complete

restoration of anatomic features. Therefore, the diagnosis usually is missed if gastroscopy or biopsy is delayed until symptoms abate. *Treatment* of acute gastritis is supportive, since the process heals spontaneously. Bleeding, when present, generally is self-limited. Some massive bleeders require emergency operation, which is followed by recurrence in one-third or more patients unless vagotomy is added to the surgical procedure. The reason for the vagal effect is unknown.

CHRONIC GASTRITIS. The pathology of chronic gastritis has been described in three categories: chronic superficial gastritis, chronic atrophic gastritis, and gastric atrophy. These may represent stages of progression, and it is clinically useful to consider them all as one entity. *Histologically*, there are necrobiosis in the generative layer of the mucosa (the neck cells between the gastric pits and gastric tubules), chronic inflammatory cell infiltration, erosion of surface epithelium, loss of parietal and chief cells, epithelial cell abnormalities, and metaplasia ("intestinalization"). As atrophy progresses, mucosal lymphoid follicles and patchy areas of irregular hyperplasia develop. *Gastroscopically* the mucosa appears normal or is reddened, granular, mamillated, and thinned with patches of erosions and surface exudate. As atrophy advances, the mucosa becomes dull gray-blue and transparent and permits visualization of submucosal veins. Hyperplastic zones appear as excrescences or polyps. Follow-up of atrophic gastritis for a decade or more reveals no change in two-thirds of patients and regression or progression in one-sixth each.

Chronic gastritis most often is asymptomatic, but there may be either episodic or persistent vague and annoying complaints. These include one or more of the following: constant mild nausea with resultant anorexia; nausea on seeing or smelling food; sense of distension or pain on eating, which is related to the size of the meal; easy satiety; bad taste in the mouth, particularly before breakfast; vomiting after eating; and diffuse dull epigastric discomfort or burning. At times pain may be severe and radiate into the back, but despite hypochlorhydria it is often relieved by alkali. These symptoms are difficult to differentiate from those of functional dyspepsia and indeed may all be caused by secondary alterations of gastric motor function. *Physical examination* is negative, or there may be mild epigastric tenderness. Hemorrhage is uncommon, but occult bleeding may occur and lead to hypochromic microcytic anemia.

The *cause* of chronic gastritis is unknown, but it occurs in association with carcinoma of the stomach, pernicious anemia, gastric polyps, all types of thyroid disease, sprue, chronic wasting diseases, pituitary or adrenal insufficiency, diabetes mellitus, Sjögren's syndrome, chronic iron deficiency, x-ray and surgical treatment of the stomach, chronic use of acetyl salicylic acid, and normal aging. Antibodies to the microsomal fraction of gastric parietal cells are found in 60 percent of patients with atrophic gastritis, 75 to 95 percent with pernicious anemia, 30 percent with thyroid disease, and 2 to 16 percent of the general population. Antibodies to gastric intrinsic factor are rare in gastric atrophy but very common (60 to 70 percent) in pernicious anemia. These observations along with meager experimental results in animals and the clinical association of atrophic gastritis with so-called "auto-immune" diseases, like thyroiditis, led to the suggestion of an immunologic cause for atrophic gastritis. Alternatively, the antibody responses have been considered nonspecific reactions to mucosal damage of a variety of causes.

LABORATORY FEATURES. The laboratory features of gastritis include those of *anemia* from brisk or chronic blood loss, *occult blood* in the stool, and *impaired gastric secretion,* which is transient in acute gastritis but persistent and related to the stage of histologic change in chronic gastritis. *Hypochlorhydria* is the rule in early cases; true *achlorhydria* upon maximum betazole or histamine testing is found in complete gastric atrophy. *Hypoalbuminemia* may follow leakage of proteins from the bloodstream into the stomach.

TREATMENT. Treatment is traditional, since the relationship of symptoms to the pathologic features is unproved and controlled therapeutic trials are sparse. Restoration of normal histologic characteristics (without effect on parietal cell antibody) has been reported in atrophic gastritis treated with dexamethasone, 10 to 30 mg per day for 5 months. Pain, when present, frequently responds, for unclear reasons, to antacid gels and powders. In contrast, sipping of dilute (0.1 *N*) hydrochloric acid with meals (1 to 2 tsp. in a glass of fruit juice) often aggravates it severely! Other measures are those outlined under Functional Dyspepsia as well as the avoidance of foods and spices which the patient blames for symptomatic aggravation; frequent small feedings in place of large meals; correction of anemia, chronic sinusitis, and pyorrhea if present; and the use of mucosal "coating" agents such as bismuth subnitrate and bismuth subcarbonate powder and alumina gels. The dose of powder is 1 tsp. with sufficient water to make a thick paste, and of gel, ½ oz. For demulcent usage these agents are prescribed every 2 to 4 hr and after every drink, snack, or meal which could remove them from the mucosa.

A "double-blind" study of a mixture of a topical anesthetic agent with an alumina preparation (oxethazine, 10 mg in 5 ml alumina, in a dose of 1 to 2 tsp.) gave good symptomatic results; the potential toxicity of the anesthetic limits the use of such mixtures to four daily doses. Finally, in view of the necrobiotic, atrophic, and inflammatory nature of the disease, use of cigarettes and gastric irritants is often prohibited, reduced, or restricted to use with simultaneous doses of alumina gels (see Chap. 314).

BENIGN GIANT HYPERTROPHIC GASTRITIS

This rare condition, also known as *Menetrier's disease,* is probably not a form of common gastritis but is discussed here because of its name. It must not be confused with a cobblestone appearance of the mucosa occasionally found in normal or diseased stomachs and known by the obsolete gastroscopic term "hypertrophic gastritis," or with large gastric rugae, which occur normally and can be effaced

by air insufflation during gastroscopy and by the examiner's finger during fluoroscopy.

Etiology, symptomatology, and pathophysiology are unsettled. Mucosal hypertrophy, lymphocytic infiltration, metaplasia, thickening of the muscularis mucosa, and edema produce huge convoluted and interconnecting gastric rugae, pseudopolyps, and cystic dilatations diffusely through the stomach or in localized areas, especially on the greater curvature. Alleged instances have been related to the multiple endocrine adenoma syndrome (Chap. 314), and there may be ulcerlike symptoms and severe accompanying ulcer disease. In contrast, excessive mucus secretion and achlorhydria frequently have been reported! Bleeding occurs in 40 percent. Some patients present with *idiopathic hypoproteinemia* with edema and ascites secondary to massive leakage of serum proteins into the stomach (see Chap. 316) but have unimpressive gastric symptoms. Others have had vomiting and cancerlike symptoms or diarrhea and weight loss. Roentgenographically, the gastric hypertrophy may be confused with gastric neoplasms, particularly lymphoma. Diagnosis is made gastroscopically and confirmed by biopsy, but many patients come to gastric resection because of the roentgenographic simulation of tumor or bleeding. In unoperated cases, symptoms are said to respond to ulcer-type treatment (Chap. 314). One reported case underwent spontaneous metamorphosis to atrophic gastritis.

SPECIFIC GASTRITIS

Specific gastritis is rare, resulting from known physical, microbiologic, and infiltrative processes.

CORROSIVE GASTRITIS. This type of gastritis follows ingestion of strong acids and, less often, strong alkalies. It usually affects the cardia or pylorus but occasionally involves other parts of the stomach, and in one-fifth the esophagus also is involved (Chap. 313). It may lead to perforation within hours to several days or may heal, with scarring and eventual obstruction. Such complications depend upon the concentration of acid, duration of exposure, volume and type of diluting and neutralizing gastric contents, rapidity of vomiting, and delay before therapy. Treatment is expectant, with the stomach kept empty during the acute episode. Operation is necessary if either of the complications arises.

PHLEGMONOUS AND EMPHYSEMATOUS GASTRITIS. These acute pyogenic bacterial infections of the stomach wall are very rare in the United States. Bacteria gain entry through infarction, surgical manipulation, or ulcerative disease, or through the bloodstream. These diseases constitute a serious threat to life and must be treated with gastric rest, vigorous specific antibiotic therapy based on the results of blood and gastric cultures, and good surgical principles of drainage and resection of focal abscess formation. *Nonbacterial interstitial gastric emphysema,* following rupture of a pulmonary emphysematous bleb, pyloric obstruction with vomiting, and instrumentation, or pneumatosis cystoides intestinalis (Chap. 321), causes similar roentgenographic findings but does not interfere with clinical diagnosis of bacterial emphysematous gastritis, because it is a benign, self-limited condition.

GASTRIC SYPHILIS, TUBERCULOSIS, AND MYCOSES. These conditions may produce ulcerative, diffusely infiltrative, or local granulomatous lesions in the stomach and may mimic neoplasm on x-ray examination. They are extremely rare in the United States, and there is nothing distinctive about the symptoms they produce. Usually, evidence of the disease elsewhere points to the diagnosis, or they are discovered at operation or autopsy. Syphilis and tuberculosis will respond to specific therapy, but most patients with these conditions come to resection because of the suspicion of neoplasm.

GRANULOMAS AND INFILTRATIONS. Under this heading are included sarcoidosis, eosinophilic granuloma (see under Benign Tumors, earlier in this chapter), berylliosis, Crohn's disease, primary amyloidosis, and xanthomatosis. They rarely produce symptoms and rarely are diagnosed in life. When large, these lesions may ulcerate, interfere with gastric motor function, or be detected on x-ray examination, in which event the uncertainty in distinguishing them from cancer often leads to surgical resection, much as it does in the case of the other benign "masslike" lesions described above.

ANTRAL GASTRITIS

Antral gastritis, or periantritis, is a confusing condition in its etiology and diagnosis. It produces deformities of the antrum, often a lengthy segment of persistent concentric narrowing, which lead to a roentgenographic diagnosis of carcinoma (Fig. 315-2). In contrast, gastroscopy shows no abnormality or only partial restriction of antral motility and some dulling, pitting, and reddening of the mucosa. Morphologically, fibrosis or chronic inflammation of the antral wall is common, but mucosal gastritis is variable. The patient may be asymptomatic or may have complaints of atypical ulcer pain.

The process follows repeated antral ulceration in some cases, but it is not clear if this accounts for all instances. Obstruction is uncommon, and therefore each case requires careful investigation to avoid unnecessary surgical treatment. Most helpful are the absence of complete consistency in the deformity on sequential spot films during the roentgenographic examination and the gastroscopic evidence of normal expansibility and nontumorous mucosa. Nevertheless, in cases wherein the gastroscopist sees greater motility than the roentgenologist but still feels there is some limitation, he cannot rule out an intramural neoplasm, and exploration is necessary.

MISCELLANEOUS CONDITIONS OF THE STOMACH

HYPERTROPHIC PYLORIC STENOSIS. A condition identical or closely related to congenital hypertrophic pyloric stenosis of infancy has been reported in adults. However, restraint must be exercised to avoid over-interpretation of every little muscular lump found at laparotomy, deformity on roentgenography, or long-standing muscle disuse and

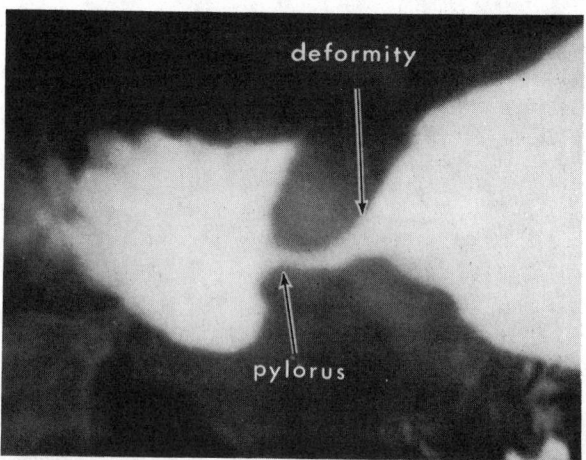

Fig. 315-2. Antral gastritis. Smooth, asymmetrical, conical, narrowed deformity of the distal antrum. Modest variation in size and shape on other films argued against a diagnosis of infiltrating carcinoma. Gastroscopy demonstrated normal expansibility and hemorrhagic erosive gastritis. The roentgenographic appearance returned to normal over a 2-year period following treatment.

foreshortening on pathologic examination as diagnostic proof of this rare disease. Strict roentgenographic and pathologic criteria are required for this diagnosis, lest common lesions, e.g. antral gastritis and neuromuscular causes of gastric retention, be missed and consequently the patient be mistreated.

Symptoms date from birth or appear at any age. Pathologically, there is pyloric muscle hypertrophy and scarring, and the clinical features are those of slowly progressive obstruction and gastric retention (Chap. 314). The characteristic olive-sized mass of neonatal patients is rare in adults. Roentgenography demonstrates persistent elongation and narrowing of the pyloric segment and establishes the diagnosis. The Fredet-Ramstedt operation of pyloromyotomy is said to be less effective than in infants, and limited gastric resection or pyloroplasty is the procedure of choice.

GASTRIC RETENTION (ATONIA AND DILATATION). This may be acute and catastrophic, chronic and mild, static or progressive. Failure of gastric motor function is neuromuscular or secondary to relative obstruction or organic stenosis (Chap. 314) at the gastric outlet. There are a host of *neuromuscular* causes, many of which are uncommon, produce only mild retention, and are rarely considered in the physician's preoccupation over organic and psychiatric alternatives. They include anticholinergic drugs, vagotomy, diabetic autonomic neuropathy (Fig. 315-3), migraine, acute and chronic diseases of the central nervous system, spinal injury, the postoperative state, fluid and electrolyte disturbances, hypocalcemia, hypothyroidism, and poorly understood effects of acute illness, abdominal trauma, protein deficiency, debilitating diseases, extreme aging, body casts, overloading of the starved stomach, and psychiatric disease. When no cause is evident, retention is said to be *idiopathic*, but similar mechanisms must be operative.

Symptoms vary with the degree and rate of develop-

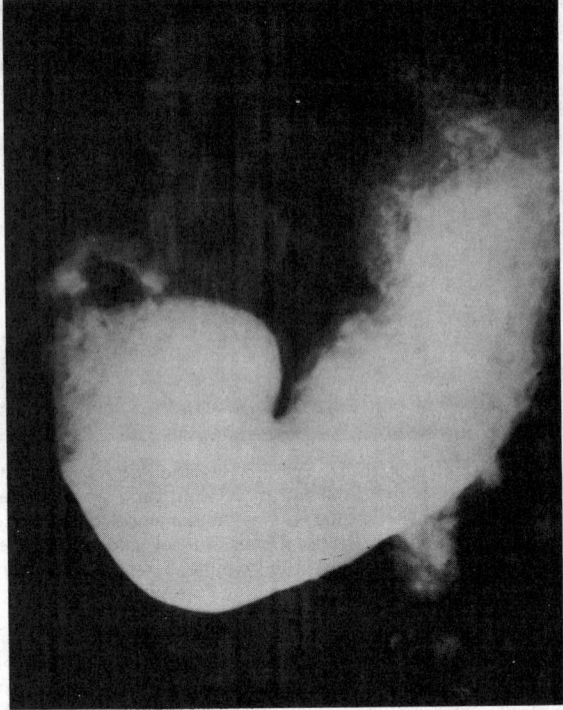

Fig. 315-3. Gastric retention due to gastric hypotonia in a patient with diabetic autonomic neuropathy. The stomach is dilated moderately, peristaltic contractions are weak, and little barium has entered the duodenum. The mottled appearance is caused by dilution and flocculation of barium by retained gastric secretions.

ment of motor failure. The clinical features and early treatment are similar to those of pyloric stenosis outlined in Chap. 314, except that operation rarely is necessary to provide adequate drainage of the stomach whose motor function is totally refractory. This occurs when the underlying disease cannot be corrected. Ambulatory measures to try include a clear-fluid diet, which is gradually augmented every few days as tolerated to full fluids, soft foods, and finally solids and motor stimulants such as methacholine in gradually increasing doses to tolerance, starting at 10 mg before meals.

PROLAPSE OF GASTRIC MUCOSA. In 1 or 2 of every 10 barium studies of the stomach, some prolapse is present. It causes the duodenal bulb and pyloric canal to appear mushroomlike on roentgenograms but virtually never causes symptoms. Prolapse must not be seized upon to account for cases of unexplained symptoms unless there is objective supporting evidence, such as massive prolapse in the presence of clinical signs of obstruction, or mucosal congestion, inflammation, and bleeding on gastroscopy.

GASTRIC TORSION AND VOLVULUS. Torsion, rotation of the stomach on its long axis (organoaxial) with the greater curvature rising anteriorly and superiorly to lie cephalad to the lesser curvature, is revealed in 0.5 percent or more of gastric x-ray examinations. Usually, it is asymptomatic. Rarely it causes twists at the cardia and pylorus or one twist in the midfundic region, which may be incomplete and recurrent or complete and disastrous. When complete

and disastrous, a twist in the midfundic region constitutes true volvulus, which produces acute obstruction and signs of an acute abdomen and is a surgical emergency. Mesenterioaxial volvulus, or a combination of the two, may also occur. The cause is uncertain, but associated hernias, lax ligaments, and anomalous spaces and mobility of stomach or duodenum frequently are blamed.

The recurrent variety frequently defies diagnostic analysis, since symptoms may be vague, variable, or intermittent. Retching which cannot yield vomitus and relationships to eating, size of meal, and posture are significant clues. Inability to pass a gastric tube beyond the cardia is the crucial physical finding. Other features are those of gastric retention (Chap. 314). Patients learn to empty the sac with the aid of position and movement or the use of a nasogastric tube. Operative correction is controversial and usually unnecessary.

CARDIOESOPHAGEAL LACERATION. Exsanguination from laceration at the junction of esophagus and stomach is known as the Mallory-Weiss syndrome, and perforation with mediastinitis or peritonitis as the Boerhaave syndrome. It is not appreciated in many quarters that nonfatal lacerations occur and indeed are relatively common causes of gastrointestinal bleeding, accounting for 5 to 15 percent of massive gastrointestinal hemorrhage in modern series. A clear historical clue is the time lag between severe retching without bleeding (presumably the cause of the laceration) and subsequent hematemesis. Rarer causes reported have been coughing, childbirth, straining at stool, chest trauma, convulsions, and accidental insufflation with compressed air. Most patients have been alcoholic, and many have had hiatus hernia. Diagnosis can be made only by esophagogastroscopy or laparotomy. Treatment of bleeding by gastroesophageal cooling is highly effective. Reported use of gastric tamponade with the Sengstaken-Blakemore tube is sparse and usually ineffective. Surgical plication is indicated in instances of perforation or uncontrolled bleeding, which are encountered in less than one-third of cases.

GASTRIC RUPTURE. Spontaneous rupture is a rare event. Since smooth muscle accommodates dramatically to pressure or volume changes, there must occur at the moment of rupture a combination of factors, including sudden or massive pressure-volume alteration, obstruction to outflow, and/or failure of muscle adaptation. In fact, prior gastric dilatation has been present in many reported cases. Because the organ is full under these conditions, rupture is catastrophic and requires emergency medical and surgical measures.

Endoscopy rarely causes gastric perforation. Since the stomach is empty at the time, minimal leakage and spontaneous closure are usual. Symptoms may be absent or mild, and treatment is constant gastric aspiration and bactericidal combinations of antibiotics. Sometimes no wound is demonstrable, even at laparotomy. This explains the belief that insufflation of air during endoscopy may force air into the mucosa through minor defects, further dissection of which results in pneumoperitoneum without anatomic perforation.

GASTRIC DIVERTICULA. These are uncommon, almost

always congenital, and posteriorly situated near the cardia. Fifteen percent appear in the pyloric region and few elsewhere. Very rarely, acquired traction or pulsion diverticula may be found anywhere in the stomach. Virtually all diverticula are asymptomatic and require no treatment, but small ones may be mistaken for ulcers on x-ray examination. Some produce mild complaints, like those in paraesophageal hiatus hernia, and may be relieved by postural maneuvers. Only when symptomatic cause and effect is objectively demonstrable can a rational case be made for surgical removal. Complications of hemorrhage and perforation are reported but are rare.

HOURGLASS DEFORMITY. Midgastric narrowing may appear to be rigid on roentgenographic examination, the general outline of the stomach vaguely resembling the shape of an hourglass. The most common cause is disordered gastric motor function adjacent to a gastric ulcer with a segment of tonic contraction forming an incisura on the contralateral curvature, which seems to point at the ulcer. Occasionally, this persists after the ulcer heals. Rarely, disease in the stomach wall, e.g., infiltrating carcinoma or gastric syphilis, produces a similar configuration.

FOREIGN BODIES AND BEZOARS. A wide variety of foreign objects may be found in the human stomach, but except in certain groups with specific predilections—psychotics, pregnant women with pica, and malingering prison inmates—all are rare. Some occur occupationally without the patient's knowledge, e.g., the sailmaker or upholsterer who swallows a needle or tack. Others follow gastric hypotonia or gastric operation after which ingested food, medicinal pills, or diagnostic agents such as barium sulfate are not passed. Gastroconiosis, foreign body granulomas in the mucosa, follows long-continued ingestion of particulate matter, e.g., chalk, kaolin, or silica. Dirt and asphalt may be eaten, and alcoholics who take to drinking alcoholic solutions of resins may retain resinous masses. Anyone may accidentally swallow a fragment of bone in a bolus of meat, and children ingest a variety of small objects such as coins and marbles.

An interesting group of foreign bodies are the *bezoars,* balls of hair from the patient's head (trichobezoar), ingested plant fibers (phytobezoar), or mixtures of hair and fiber, which assume the shape of the patient's stomach. In the United States, human hair ingestion and persimmon eating (diospyrobezoar) are the leading causes of bezoar formation.

Most foreign bodies are asymptomatic or pass through the intestinal tract without incident, but numerous complications may occur. Sharp objects may perforate, produce localized abscesses, or migrate through the peritoneum, abdominal viscera, or parietal structures. Bezoars and blunt objects may lie freely in the lumen for long periods or become embedded and cause erosions, ulcerations, and bleeding. Some cause intestinal obstruction and perforation after leaving the stomach.

Diagnosis begins with a history of ingestion or the detection of a mass on roentgenographic examination. Gastroscopy establishes the nature of the mass. Once a body has reached the stomach, it probably will pass through the gastrointestinal tract; treatment is expectant. If the mass fails to leave the stomach, progression ceases after the pylorus is negotiated, or complications of bleeding, obstruction, or penetration occur, surgical intervention is indicated. With plastic masses, cessation of oral intake of the material and restoration of gastric motility often lead to breakup and passage (Chap. 314). Repeated lavage may also be tried, in instances of diospyrobezoar utilizing papain and sodium bicarbonate if not contraindicated by associated devitalized eroded gastric tissue which also could be "digested." The physician requires great forbearance in dealing with the families of these patients, who out of awe over the drama of a foreign object loose in the mysterious "innards" of a human body are apt to be panicky and unreasonable, demanding that "something be done at once! "

REFERENCES

Avery Jones, F., and J. W. P. Gummer: "Clinical Gastroenterology," 2d ed., Oxford, Blackwell Scientific Publications, Ltd., 1968.

Hitchcock, C. R., L. D. MacLean, and W. A. Sullivan: Secretory and Clinical Aspects of Achlorhydria and Gastric Atrophy as Precursors of Gastric Cancer, J. Nat. Cancer Inst., 18:795, 1957.

Koch, J. P., and R. M. Donaldson, Jr.: A Survey of Food Intolerances in Hospitalized Patients, New Engl. J. Med., 271:657, 1964.

Monaco, A. P., S. I. Roth, B. Castleman, and C. E. Welch: Adenomatous Polyps of Stomach: Clinical and Pathologic Study of 153 Cases, Cancer, 15:456, 1962.

Roitt, I. M., D. Doniach, and C. Shapland: Autoimmunity in Pernicious Anemia and Atrophic Gastritis, Ann. N.Y. Acad. Sci., 124:644, 1965.

Taebel, D. W., J. C. Prolla, and J. B. Kirsner: Exfoliative Cytology in the Diagnosis of Stomach Cancer, Ann. Intern. Med., 63:1018, 1965.

Wells, R. F.: A Common Cause of Upper Gastrointestinal Bleeding: The Mallory-Weiss Syndrome, S. Med. J., 60:1197, 1967.

Wilken, B. J., and J. W. W. Thomson: Chemotherapy in Cancer of the Stomach, Brit. J. Surg., 53:904, 1966.

Wood, I. J., and L. I. Taft: "Diffuse Lesions of the Stomach," London, Edward Arnold (Publishers) Ltd., 1958.

316 DISORDERS OF ABSORPTION
Norton J. Greenberger and Kurt J. Isselbacher

MECHANISMS OF ABSORPTION

Diseases of the small intestine are frequently accompanied by alterations in intestinal function, and clinically this impaired function is seen as the malabsorption syndrome. In order to obtain a better appreciation of the derangements which occur in the many disorders of intestinal function the processes of normal absorption will first be reviewed.

It is important to distinguish between digestion and absorption, since an increased loss of nutrients in the stool may be a reflection of a derangement of either process. Digestion involves the breakdown or hydrolysis of nutrients to smaller molecules in order to prepare the ingested substances for absorption or transport across the intestinal cell. It will be recalled that most of the digestive process is initiated in the stomach by acid and pepsin and is continued in the upper small intestine primarily by the action of pancreatic enzymes such as lipase, amylase, and trypsin. As a result of these digestive actions carbohydrates are broken down to monosaccharides and disaccharides, proteins to peptides and amino acids, and fats to monoglycerides and fatty acids. In the adult it is in this form that nutrients are, to a large extent, transported across the epithelial surface of the intestinal cell.

Anatomic and Physiologic Factors

The intestine has an enormous surface area. This can be attributed in large part to its length, which in the adult is more than 12 ft, and to the foldings of the surface plicae. At the light microscopic level, the villi of the small intestine provide additional surface area, which is further augmented by the presence of microvilli (approximately 2×10^8 per sq cm) on the outer, or brush border, region of epithelial cells. Thus the total absorptive area of the small intestine is enormous.

Motility (contractility) of the bowel is an important process which permits nutrients to remain in intimate contact with the intestinal cells and possibly influences the continued movement of the nutrients *into* and along the absorbing channels, such as the lymphatics. Two types of motility aid in this process: the gross motility of the intestine itself and the motility of individual villi. Entrance of the nutrients into the general circulation is achieved via the capillaries into the portal system or via the lacteals into the intestinal lymphatics.

Types of Absorption

Four mechanisms have been considered to be important in the transport of substances across the intestinal cell membrane, namely, active transport, passive diffusion, facilitated diffusion, and pinocytosis (Table 316-1).

Active transport involves the transport of a substance across the cell against an electric or chemical gradient; this process requires energy, is carrier-mediated, and is subject to competitive inhibition. *Passive diffusion* is the opposite of this process; energy is not required, transport is with (rather than against) the electric or chemical gradient, the process is not carrier-mediated, and it does not show properties of competitive inhibition. Thus active transport may be viewed as "uphill" transport, whereas passive diffusion is equivalent to "downhill" transport. *Facilitated diffusion* is similar to passive diffusion except that such a process shows evidence of being carrier-mediated and frequently subject to competitive inhibition.

Pinocytosis, which literally means "cells drinking," is a process akin to phagocytosis. By this mechanism nutrients (soluble or particulate) upon entering the cell are surrounded by the components of the outer plasma cell membrane. In the intestinal tract pinocytosis has been definitely demonstrated only in the neonatal period, and the quantitative significance of this process in the adult organism seems to be limited.

It should also be emphasized that not every substance presented to the intestinal surface is subject to transport, or absorption, because the normal epithelial cell is able to exclude many substances. Generally water-soluble compounds with a high molecular weight (above 300) or with pK less than 4 or greater than 9, especially polyvalent ions, tend not to be absorbed. When the mucosa is damaged, as for example by mesenteric vascular disease, the ability to exclude substances may be lost, and compounds of high molecular weight may be absorbed.

Sites of Absorption

While many substances are absorbed throughout the length of the small intestine, certain nutrients tend to be absorbed in one region more than the others. The proximal intestine is a major area for the absorption of iron, calcium, water-soluble vitamins, and fat (monoglycerides and fatty acids). Sugars are absorbed in the proximal small intestine and also in the midintestine. While the major absorption of amino acids appears to occur in the middle of the small intestine or jejunum, some absorption also occurs in the upper and lower areas. The distal small intestine appears to be the *major* absorptive area for bile salts and vitamin B_{12}. As is emphasized below, this factor is of clinical significance in circumstances where there has been removal or disease of the ileum.

The colon is important for the absorption of water and electrolytes, a process which occurs predominantly in the cecum. Although the rectum is not a usual site for absorption of ingested foodstuffs, drugs introduced by rectum may be absorbed there. Thus drugs introduced by this route, such as salicylates or steroids, may be absorbed systemically.

Absorption of Specific Nutrients

CARBOHYDRATE ABSORPTION. Much of the carbohydrate we ingest is in the form of starch, a complex polysaccharide consisting of many hexose units (attached

Table 316-1. MECHANISMS OF TRANSPORT ACROSS THE INTESTINAL CELL

Types of transport	Properties			
	Energy-dependent	Carrier-mediated	Competitive inhibition	Electric or chemical gradient
Active.......	+	+	+	+
Diffusion:				
Passive.....	0	0	0	0
Facilitated..	0	+	+/0	0
Pinocytosis...	0	0	0	0

either in a 1, 4 or 1, 6 linkage). By the action of salivary and pancreatic amylase, starch is hydrolyzed to oligosaccharides, then to disaccharides (mostly maltose), and a small amount to monosaccharides. While monosaccharides such as glucose are readily absorbed, disaccharides are not. Disaccharides are split enzymatically into their component sugars by enzymes located on or within the microvilli of the intestinal epithelial cells. By the action of these *disaccharidases*, lactose is split into glucose and galactose, sucrose into glucose and fructose, and maltose into two molecules of glucose. The resultant monosaccharides are then transported through the cell into the portal circulation.

Sugars such as glucose and galactose are absorbed by an active transport mechanism. Most actively transported sugars possess a hydroxyl group at the C-2 position. Fructose, a hexose lacking a hydroxyl group at the C-2 position, is absorbed by passive diffusion, and after its entry there is also some conversion of fructose to glucose and lactic acid within the mucosal cell. The transport of xylose, a pentose frequently used in absorption studies, is complex. At low concentrations xylose transport is active; at higher concentrations some is by facilitated diffusion.

The exact mechanism for the active transport of sugars such as glucose and galactose has not been elucidated. However, *sodium* ions appear necessary for the *entry* of the sugar into the cell, and *energy* is required for the *accumulation* of the sugars within the cell. Glucose and galactose presumably are transported by a carrier-mediated mechanism, but the nature of this carrier remains to be determined.

PROTEIN AND AMINO ACID ABSORPTION. Dietary proteins are initially subject to degradation in the stomach by pepsin. However, complete hydrolysis is largely achieved by the action of the pancreatic enzymes trypsin, chymotrypsin, and carboxypeptidase. By these enzymatic processes polypeptides, dipeptides, and amino acids are formed. Just as there are disaccharidases in mucosal cells to digest disaccharides, there are also dipeptidases to split dipeptides. Dipeptidases are located in the cytoplasm as well as on the microvilli. In general proteins are not absorbed as such, except in the neonatal state. In the adult, absorption is primarily in the form of amino acids or dipeptides, although some larger peptides (usually no greater than eight amino acid residues) may be absorbed to a limited extent.

Most naturally occurring amino acids are L-amino acids, and these are subject to a number of different transport processes. *Neutral* amino acids seem to share a common "pump," or pathway; thus amino acids such as tryptophan and alanine show competitive inhibition. Among the *basic* amino acids which appear to have a distinct transport mechanism are arginine, ornithine, and lysine, and also cystine. There is also a separate transport system for the *imino acids* proline and hydroxyproline. Therefore, in genetic disorders, such as cystinuria, one will find impaired absorption not only of cystine but also of arginine, ornithine, and lysine. Similarly in Hartnup's disease, a defect in the transport of all neutral amino acids is found.

The actual mechanism of the absorption of amino acids by the intestine has not been elucidated. As in the case of carbohydrates, sodium ions appear to be required for entry, and energy for concentration within the cell. Since pyridoxine deficiency interferes with the transport of amino acids, pyridoxine may be involved in amino acid transport, but it exact role is not understood.

FAT ABSORPTION. Most of the ingested dietary fats are in the form of long-chain triglycerides. These triglycerides contain both saturated fatty acid acids (such as palmitic, stearic) and unsaturated fatty acids (such as oleic and linoleic). The particle size of the fat is decreased largely by the churning action of the stomach. The entry of fat into the duodenum plus the presence of acid causes release of secretin and pancreazymin-cholecystokinin, which in turn leads to a stimulation of the flow of bile and pancreatic juice.

Role of Pancreatic Lipase. For the hydrolysis of triglycerides by pancreatic lipase, the fats must be emulsified. The detergent properties of the bile salts permit the enzyme to gain access to the water-insoluble lipids. The enzymatic action of lipase results in the stepwise hydrolysis to diglycerides, monoglycerides, and fatty acids with the concomitant liberation of glycerol. Normally only 25 to 30 percent of the triglyceride is completely hydrolyzed to fatty acids. Monoglycerides constitute the major end product of hydrolysis (i.e., 70 to 75 percent of the ingested fat). Usually less than 5 percent of the fat remains in the form of diglycerides or triglycerides (Fig. 316-1).

Role of Bile Salts. Bile salts play an important role in the digestion and absorption of fat. They are synthesized in the liver (approximately 800 mg daily) from cholesterol and excreted in the bile in the form of their glycine or taurine conjugates. In man the principal bile acids excreted are the conjugates of cholic and chenodeoxycholic acid. Bile salts are good detergents, because they have both polar (hydrophilic) and nonpolar (hydrophobic) groups. During digestion the concentration of conjugated bile salts in the lumen is in the range of 5 to 15 micromoles per ml, and at these concentrations the bile salts aggregate to form *micelles*. Fatty acids and monoglycerides enter these micelles, forming mixed micelles. An emulsion of triglyceride is turbid; mixed micelles containing bile salts, fatty acids, and monoglycerides are clear solutions. The formation of mixed micelles and hence the solubilization of fatty acids and monoglycerides is much more effectively achieved with *conjugated* rather than unconjugated bile salts at the pH of the intestinal lumen.

There are additional properties of bile salts which are important in fat absorption and digestion. Bile salts shift the pH optimum of pancreatic lipase from 8 or 8.5 to 6.5. This is important because the pH in the upper small intestine is normally 6 to 6.5. Bile salts, especially conjugated bile salts, appear to enhance cellular uptake and esterification of fatty acids. Most of the conjugated bile salts are absorbed in the ileum and after entering the portal vein are subject to an enterohepatic circulation. By this process about 90 percent of the conjugated bile salts reaching the ileum are reabsorbed. As a consequence

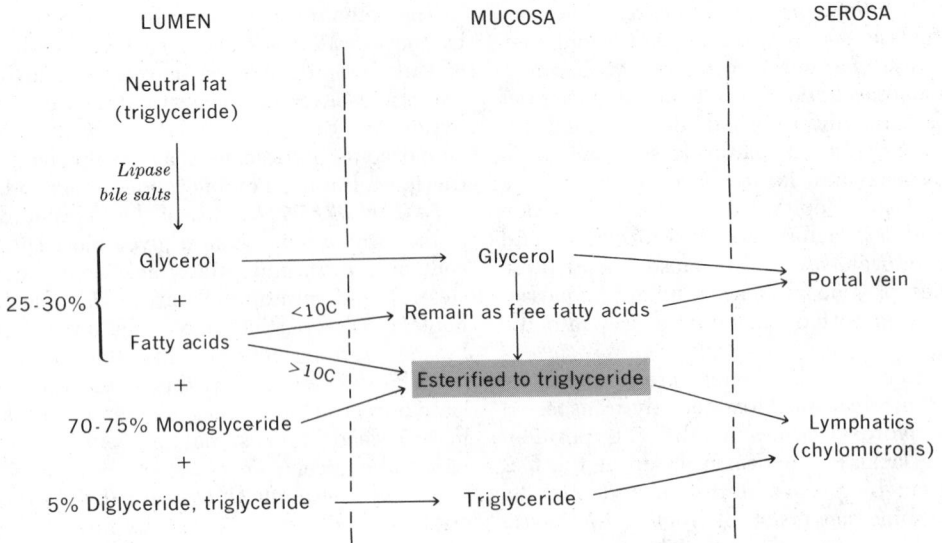

Fig. 316-1. Scheme of the intestinal digestion, absorption, and transport of ingested triglyceride. C refers to number of carbon atoms in fatty acids.

only about 800 mg bile salts is excreted in the feces per day, while, as part of the enterohepatic circulation, as much as 20 to 30 Gm bile salts recirculates daily between the liver and intestine. If the ileum is diseased or removed, absorption of bile salts is impaired, and a significant fecal loss of bile salts will occur. As a consequence of this bile salt depletion, their concentration in the intestinal lumen will also decrease, and this will further impair fat absorption. A similar result will occur if bile salt reabsorption is prevented by chelating agents, such as cholestyramine (see below).

Intramucosal Aspects of Fat Absorption. After the hydrolysis of fatty acids to monoglycerides and their interaction with bile salts to form mixed micelles, the lipids are presented to the epithelial cell surface. The mixed micelles appearently do not enter the cell, but instead the component fatty acids and monoglycerides are released from the micellar phase and then enter the cell by diffusion. The subsequent fate of the intracellular lipid is then strongly influenced by the fatty acid chain length. Fatty acids and monoglycerides derived from long-chain triglycerides (i.e., containing C-16 to C-18 fatty acids) are promptly *reesterified to triglycerides* by enzymes of the endoplasmic reticulum. These triglycerides then interact with specific proteins (lipoproteins) plus cholesterol and phospholipid leading to the formation of chylomicrons. These initially accumulate in the Golgi region of the cell and then are secreted into the lacteals and the intestinal lymph. There are thus four major steps in absorption of long-chain fatty acids and monoglycerides: (1) mucosal uptake, (2) reesterification to triglycerides, (3) chylomicron formation, and (4) secretion into lymph.

By contrast, fatty acids derived from medium-chain triglycerides (i.e., containing C-8 and C-10 fatty acids) are *not reesterified* to any significant extent within the cell and are not incorporated into chylomicrons. Instead, they rapidly enter the portal venous system, where they are transported as fatty acids bound to albumin. The major aspects of fat absorption are summarized in Fig. 316-1.

ABSORPTION OF CHOLESTEROL AND FAT-SOLUBLE VITAMINS (A,D,E,K). In addition to contributing significantly to the total body synthesis of cholesterol, the intestine also plays an active role in the absorption of cholesterol and its esters. Within the lumen, cholesterol esters from the bile and diet are hydrolyzed by an esterase secreted by the pancreas. There is also a separate cholesterol esterase in the intestinal microvilli, which completes this hydrolysis. As a result only free cholesterol appears to enter the intestinal cell. However, just as in the case of long-chain fatty acids, much of the cholesterol is reesterified and is then secreted primarily into lymph.

The absorption mechanisms of the fat-soluble vitamins A,D,E, and K are not well understood. In the case of vitamin A (or retinol), it has been clearly shown that the intestine converts beta-carotene into vitamin A. The vitamin A thus formed or absorbed from the lumen is esterified in the mucosa primarily with palmitic acid, transported in the chylomicrons of the lymph, and stored as retinyl palmitate in the liver. The other lipid-soluble vitamins also appear in lymph chylomicrons, but esterification with fatty acids does not appear to be necessary for their transport.

WATER AND SODIUM ABSORPTION. In spite of extensive investigations the main mechanisms of water and electrolyte transport are not well understood. To explain water movement across the lipid membrane of the mucosa, it is believed that this surface has aqueous-filled channels or pores. These allow diffusion of water as well as bulk flow; the latter refers to water movement in response to osmotic pressure differences. The largest fraction of net water movement appears to be the result of bulk flow.

Sodium ions seem to be absorbed largely by active transport and to be linked in some manner to the brush border ATPase; sodium movement in some manner is also linked to the transport or metabolism of glucose, since sodium transport usually ceases in the absence of glucose. Some sodium transport accompanies the movement of water (i.e., solvent drag).

CALCIUM ABSORPTION. Calcium is actively transported by the small intestine, and this process is intimately linked to the action of vitamin D. Thus vitamin D promotes the absorption of calcium, and in patients with vitamin D deficiency, calcium absorption is impaired. It has been shown that vitamin D initiates the synthesis of a protein in the intestinal mucosa which binds calcium. This calcium-binding protein appears to be intimately related to the active transport of calcium by the intestine.

IRON ABSORPTION. A regulatory mechanism for the absorption of inorganic iron appears to exist within the small-intestinal mucosal cells. Iron is actively transported by the small intestine, and the duodenum is the principal site of iron absorption. The absorption of elemental iron in man and animals involves at least two distinct steps: (1) mucosal uptake of iron from the lumen and (2) mucosal transfer of iron to the plasma. Much of the iron entering the mucosal cell is not transferred to the plasma but remains trapped within the cell and is excreted into the lumen when the cell is shed. Iron lost by this mechanism seems to vary inversely with body iron stores. However, this mucosal regulatory mechanism can be overcome when pharmacologic doses of iron are ingested. Hemoglobin iron is also absorbed by human subjects depending upon body requirements for iron; the heme is split from globin in the lumen and absorbed as an intact metalloporphyrin. The absorption of inorganic iron is increased by ascorbic acid. Similarly, the presence of anemia, liver injury, pregnancy, idiopathic hemochromatosis, a portacaval shunt, and pancreatic insufficiency may result in increased iron absorption. Conversely, the prior ingestion of large doses of iron and the presence in the lumen of phosphates, carbonates, and phytates may lead to decreased absorption of inorganic iron. Impaired absorption of iron is frequent in disorders (such as nontropical sprue) which involve the duodenal mucosa.

WATER-SOLUBLE VITAMINS. The absorption of *vitamin B_{12}* is discussed in Chap. 337. In the case of *folic acid absorption,* it must be emphasized that folates exist in food conjugated with glutamyl peptides. These *polyglutamates* must be deconjugated by a brush border deconjugase to monoglutamates for absorption to occur. Certain drugs such as diphenylhydantoin inhibit this conjugase, decrease the absorption of dietary polyglutamates, and hence can cause folate deficiency. Thiamine and riboflavin appear to be absorbed by passive diffusion.

Tests Useful in the Diagnosis of Malabsorption

Most of the tests useful in the diagnosis of malabsorption indicate the presence of abnormal absorptive or digestive function, and only a few tests may suggest a specific diagnosis. Accordingly, it is frequently necessary to employ a combination of tests to establish a diagnosis.

To illustrate the use of various tests, the characteristic findings in nontropical sprue, an example of a primary malabsorptive disorder, and pancreatic insufficiency, an example of impaired digestion, are compared in Table 316-2.

STOOL FAT. The qualitative examination of the stool for undigested muscle fibers, neutral fat, and split fat is a simple and reliable screening test for steatorrhea. The finding of an increased number of muscle fibers indicates impaired intraluminal digestion. Properly performed, the qualitative microscopic examination of a stool specimen with the Sudan III stain is of value and correlates well with the quantitative determination of fecal fat by the Van de Kamer method. The latter remains the most reliable measurement of steatorrhea. A normal fecal fat excretion is less than 6 Gm for 24 hr, or less than 5 percent of ingested fat.

XYLOSE ABSORPTION. In the most commonly employed form of the xylose absorption test, the patient ingests 25 Gm D-xylose. A 5-hr urine xylose excretion of 4.5 Gm or greater is considered normal. There is some decreased renal excretion with age, and over age sixty-five 3.5 Gm is the normal value. Falsely low values may be obtained in patients with renal insufficiency and if the urine collection is incomplete. To obviate these difficulties it is advisable to determine the blood xylose level 2 hr after ingestion of xylose. A xylose blood level of 30 mg per 100 ml or greater indicates normal absorption of D-xylose. An abnormal D-xylose absorption test is found most frequently in disorders affecting the mucosa of the proximal small intestine, such as nontropical and tropical sprue.

GASTROINTESTINAL X-RAY STUDIES. All patients with malabsorption should have radiographic examinations of the small intestine and in many cases of the esophagus, stomach, and colon. Occasionally, the latter two examinations may provide important clues to the presence of such disorders as gastroileostomy, scleroderma, Zollinger-Ellison syndrome, ulcerative colitis, and intestinal fistulas. The typical small-bowel radiographic abnormalities in patients with a malabsorption syndrome are a breaking up of the barium column with segmentation, clumping, and coarsening of the mucosal folds. Segmentation or clumping of the barium in a small-bowel loop is often termed a *moulage sign.* This results in part from an increased amount of intraluminal fluid which mixes with the barium sulfate. Less frequently there is dilatation of the proximal small bowel and loss of a normal mucosal pattern. Collectively, these changes have been referred to as a *malabsorption pattern.* The above findings are nonspecific and may be found in several of the disorders listed in Table 316-3. Some representative examples of abnormal small-bowel radiographs are shown in Fig. 316-2

SMALL-INTESTINAL BIOPSY. The most commonly used instruments for obtaining peroral biopsy specimens from the small intestine include the Rubin and Shiner tubes, and the Crosby, Carey, and Ross-Moore capsules. These instruments have been quite helpful in establishing a few specific diagnoses. Characteristic abnormalities have been described in the following disorders: nontropical sprue, abetalipoproteinemia, Whipples disease, intestinal lym-

Table 316-2. TESTS USEFUL IN THE DIAGNOSIS OF MALABSORPTIVE DISORDERS

Test	Normal values	Typical findings in		Comment
		Malabsorption (nontropical sprue)	Maldigestion (pancreatic insufficiency)	
Quantitative determination of stool fat	< 6 Gm/24 hrs; > 95% coefficient of fat absorption	> 6 Gm/24 hrs	> 6 Gm/24 hrs	Best test for establishing presence of steatorrhea.
D-Xylose absorption (25-Gm oral dose)	5-hr urinary excretion > 4.5 Gm; peak blood level > 30 mg/100 ml	↓	Normal	A good screening test for carbohydrate absorption.
Small-intestinal x-rays		Malabsorption pattern	Normal or minimal malabsorption pattern; occasionally pancreatic calcification	Moulage sign and other abnormalities may be present in several disorders (see text).
Small-intestinal mucosal biopsy		Abnormal	Normal	A specific diagnosis can be established in a small number of disorders (see text).
Schilling test for vitamin B_{12} absorption	> 8% urinary excretion in 48 hr	Frequently ↓	Usually normal	Useful in determining whether vitamin B_{12} malabsorption is due to gastric or small-intestinal disorders.
Secretin test	Volume: > 1.8 ml/kg/hr— bicarbonate concentration: > 80 mEq/L	Normal	Abnormal	See discussion of pancreatic insufficiency in Chap. 333.
Serum calcium	9–11 mg/100 ml	Frequently ↓	Usually normal	
Serum albumin	3.5–5.5 Gm/100 ml	Frequently ↓	Usually normal	Decreased levels of both serum albumin and globulins should raise the question of protein-losing enteropathy.
Serum cholesterol	150–250 mg/100 ml	↓	Frequently ↓	Usually decreased in disorders associated with significant steatorrhea.
Serum iron	80–150 μg/100 ml	Frequently ↓	Normal	Low values may reflect decreased body iron stores.
Serum carotenes	> 100 IU/100 ml	↓	Usually ↓	Fairly satisfactory screening tests for malabsorption.
Serum vitamin A	> 100 IU/100 ml	↓		
Prothrombin time	70–100%; 12–15 sec	Frequently ↓	Frequently ↓	
Urine 5-hydroxyindoleacetic acid (5-HIAA)	2–9 mg/24 hr	↑	Normal	Slightly increased level (12–16 mg/24 hr) characteristically found in nontropical sprue.
Urine indican	100 mg/24 hr	↑	Normal or ↑	Increased values found in several malabsorptive disorders as well as in bacterial overgrowth syndromes.

phangiectasia, scleroderma, and amyloidosis. Some examples of abnormal small-bowel biopsy specimens are shown in Fig. 316-3.

SCHILLING TEST FOR VITAMIN B_{12} ABSORPTION. The Schilling test is valuable in the differential diagnosis of malabsorption and is frequently carried out in three stages: (1) without intrinsic factor, (2) with intrinsic factor, and (3) after a course of treatment with antibiotics. Since vitamin B_{12} is absorbed primarily in the distal ileum, an abnormal Schilling test may indicate a pathologic condition of the distal small bowel. In disorders affecting the terminal ileum such as regional enteritis and lymphomas, the first-stage Schilling test is frequently abnormal. The ileal receptor site appears to be damaged in these disorders, and the impaired absorption of B_{12} is not corrected by the addition of intrinsic factor or the use of antibiotics. The Schilling test may also be useful in establishing a diagnosis of abnormal bacterial overgrowth of the small bowel which may be present in disorders such as blind loop syndrome, sclero-

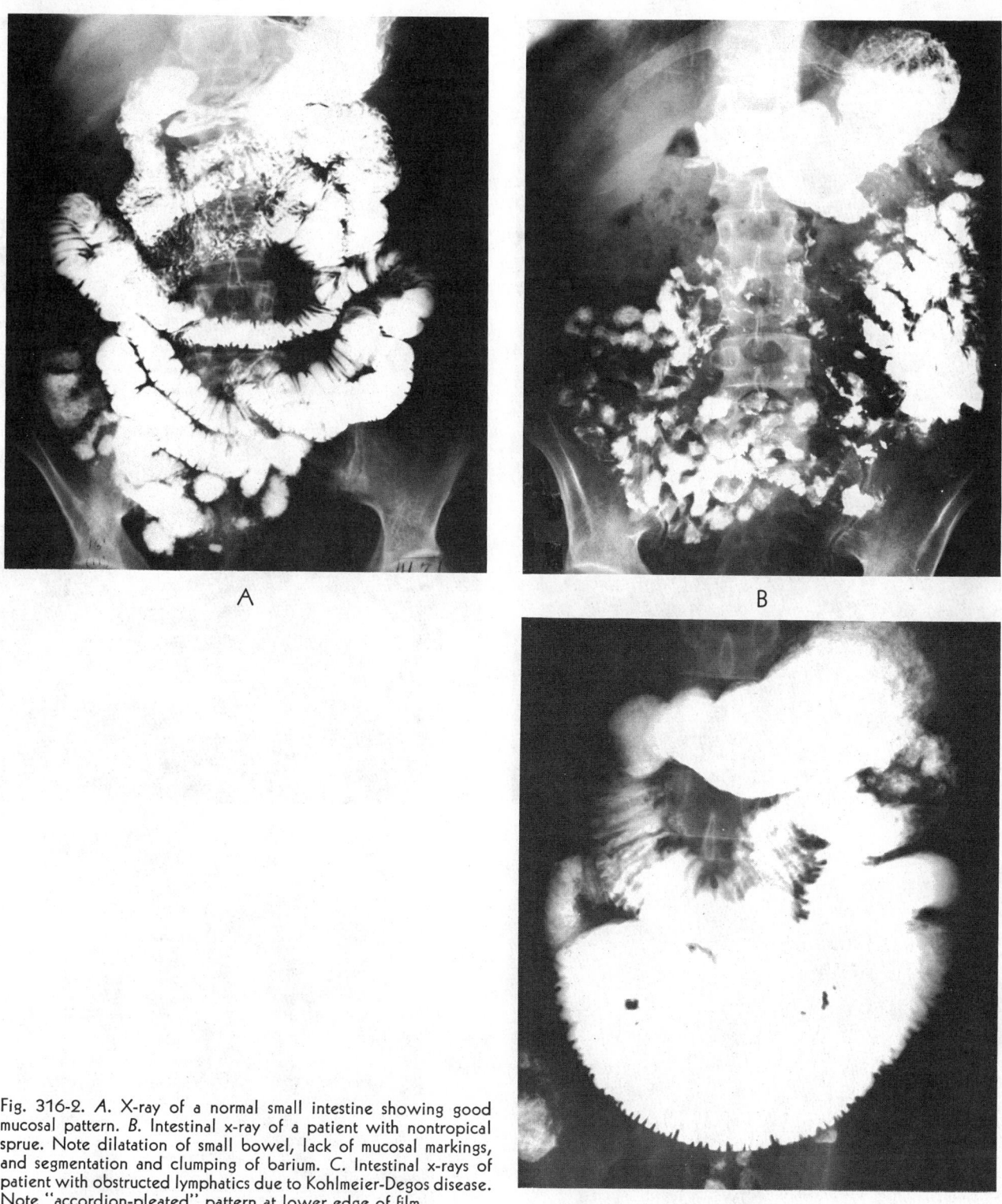

Fig. 316-2. *A.* X-ray of a normal small intestine showing good mucosal pattern. *B.* Intestinal x-ray of a patient with nontropical sprue. Note dilatation of small bowel, lack of mucosal markings, and segmentation and clumping of barium. *C.* Intestinal x-rays of patient with obstructed lymphatics due to Kohlmeier-Degos disease. Note "accordion-pleated" pattern at lower edge of film.

derma, and multiple small-bowel diverticula (Table 316-3). In the blind loop syndrome, for example, the bacteria can actually take up vitamin B$_{12}$ with resultant impaired absorption of B$_{12}$. Under these conditions the

first-stage Schilling test is frequently abnormal. After appropriate antibiotic treatment the Schilling test usually returns to normal.

SECRETIN TEST. The secretin test and the secretin-

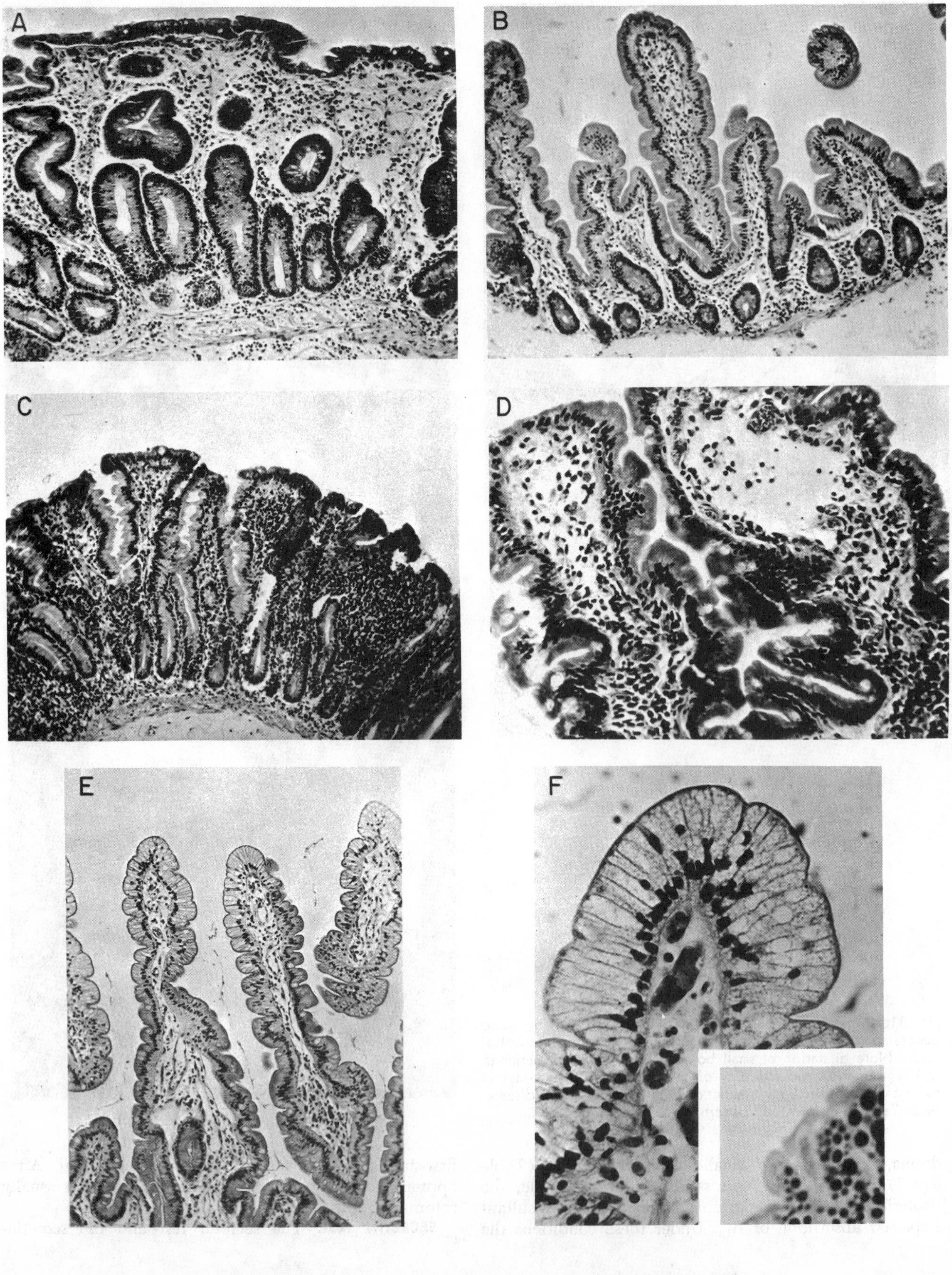

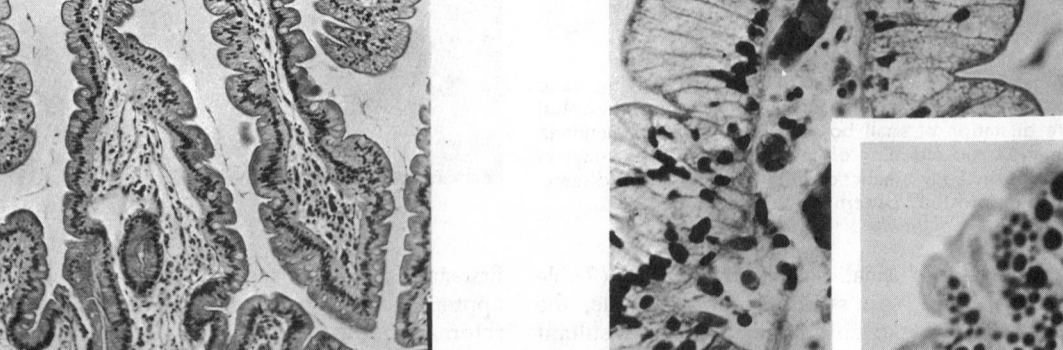

Table 316-3. PATHOPHYSIOLOGIC BASIS FOR SYMPTOMS AND
SIGNS IN MALABSORPTIVE DISORDERS

Symptom or sign	Pathophysiology
Generalized malnutrition and weight loss.......	Malabsorption of fat, carbohydrate, and protein → loss of calories
Diarrhea..............	Impaired absorption of sodium and water; effect of unabsorbed fatty acids and bile acids
Nocturia..............	Delayed absorption of water
Anemia..............	Impaired absorption of iron, vitamin B_{12}, and folic acid
Glossitis, cheilosis......	Deficiency of iron, vitamin B_{12}, folate, and other vitamins
Peripheral neuritis......	Deficiency of vitamin B_{12}
Edema...............	Impaired absorption of amino acids → protein depletion → hypoproteinemia
Amenorrhea..........	Protein depletion and "caloric starvation" → secondary hypopituitarism
Bone pain............	Protein depletion → impaired bone formation → osteoporosis
	Calcium malabsorption → demineralization of bone → osteomalacia
Tetany, paresthesias....	Calcium malabsorption → hypocalcemia; magnesium malabsorption → hypomagnesemia
Hemorrhagic phenomena	Vitamin K malabsorption → hypoprothrombinemia
Weakness.............	Anemia; electrolyte depletion (hypokalemia)

pancreozymin test, which may be useful in establishing a diagnosis of pancreatic insufficiency, are discussed in detail in Chap. 334.

SERUM CALCIUM, ALBUMIN, CHOLESTEROL, MAGNESIUM, AND IRON. Abnormal serum calcium, albumin, cholesterol, magnesium, and iron values may be found in several malabsorptive disorders. The primary value of such tests is to suggest that abnormal intestinal absorptive function may be present. These tests are usually of limited value in the *differential diagnosis* of malabsorption but if abnormal may be helpful in supporting this diagnosis.

SERUM CAROTENES, VITAMIN A, AND PROTHROMBIN TIME. Absorption of the fat-soluble vitamins A, D, K, and E is frequently impaired in patients with steatorrhea.

Measurements of serum carotene and vitamin A levels are useful as screening tests for malabsorption. However, other tests not only are more sensitive but often give more specific information than the serum carotene and vitamin A levels. The blood prothrombin time is an important test, since patients with malabsorption may present with abnormal bleeding due to vitamin K deficiency. If the decreased prothrombin activity is due to malabsorption, it should be readily correctable with parenteral vitamin K.

5-HYDROXYINDOLEACETIC ACID (5-HIAA) AND URINE INDICAN. Patients with malabsorption frequently have abnormalities in tryptophan metabolism which are reflected by an increased urinary excretion of tryptophan metabolites. Such patients frequently have a deficiency of vitamin B_6 (pyridoxine) which results in decreased conversion of tryptophan to xanthurenic acid, kynurenic acid, and nicotinamide. Consequently, increased amounts of tryptophan are converted to other metabolites such as 5-hydroxyindoleacetic acid (5-HIAA) and indole-3-acetic acid.

In untreated nontropical sprue or sprue in relapse there is characteristically a modest increase in the urinary excretion of 5-HIAA, usually in the range of 10-20 mg per 24 hr. This reverts to normal after institution of a gluten-free diet. Indican (indoxylsulfate) is another metabolite of tryptophan. Bacteria within the gut lumen cleave the side chain of tryptophan to form indole, which is absorbed, hydroxylated, and esterified with sulfate in the liver. Urine indican excretion greater than 100 mg per 24 hr is abnormal. The urine indican excretion is useful as a screening test for bacterial overgrowth in the gastrointestinal tract. Abnormal values are frequently found in the blind loop syndrome and scleroderma. An increased urine indican excretion is not specific for such disorders, and elevated values have also been found in patients with nontropical sprue, tropical sprue, and regional enteritis.

Pathophysiologic Basic for Symptoms and Signs in Malabsorptive Disorders

The common symptoms and signs found in malabsorptive disorders are listed in Table 316-3. The most frequent symptoms are those of malnutrition, weight loss, and diarrhea. However, in each of the clinical settings listed in Table 316-3, it is important to consider the cause of the malabsorption.

Fig. 316-3. (On facing page.) Typical peroral intestinal biopsies. *A.* Jejunal mucosa of patient with nontropical sprue. Note virtual absence of villi, elongated crypts (some are cut in cross section), mononuclear infiltrate, cuboidal instead of columnar epithelium on top of villi (×300). *B.* Biopsy from the same patient as in (A), after 9 months on a gluten-free diet. Note the reappearance of villi with normal-appearing columnar cells, and reduction in infiltrate and crypt height (×300). *C.* Biopsy from patient with agammaglobulinemia. The features bear a striking resemblance to those of nontropical sprue. There is a marked mononuclear infiltration, some of it in aggregates (×200). *D.* Close-up of villi of patient with protein-losing enteropathy. Tips of villi are broadened and dilated. Lymphatic spaces are present (*arrows*) (×450). *E.* Intestinal biopsy from patient with abetalipoproteinemia. The villus tips have a "lacy" appearance (*arrows*) due to retained fat (×300). [This is more apparent at the higher magnification shown in *F.*] *F.* High-power micrograph of villus from patient with abetalipoproteinemia. The vacuoles are filled with lipid (×750). Insert shows dark-staining (osmium) lipid droplets in mucosal cells (osmium counterstained with Giemsa; ×800).

Classification of Malabsorption Syndromes

A classification of the malabsorption syndromes is given in Table 316-4. The classification is based both on func-

Table 316-4. CLASSIFICATION OF THE
MALABSORPTION SYNDROMES

A. Inadequate digestion
   1. Diseases of the liver
   2. Diseases of the biliary tract
   3. Postgastrectomy steatorrhea
   4. Pancreatic insufficiency
B. Inadequate absorptive surface
   1. Intestinal resection or bypass
   2. Gastroileostomy
C. Abnormal bacterial proliferation in the small bowel
   1. Afferent loop stasis
   2. Strictures
   3. Fistulas
   4. Blind loops
   5. Multiple diverticula of the small bowel
   6. Hypomotility states (scleroderma, diabetes)
D. Lymphatic obstruction
   1. Intestinal lymphangiectasia
   2. Whipple's disease
   3. Lymphoma
   4. Kohlmeier-Degos disease (primary progressive arterial occlusive disease)
E. Cardiovascular disorders
   1. Constrictive pericarditis
   2. Congestive heart failure
   3. Mesenteric vascular insufficiency
F. Primary mucosal absorptive defects
   1. Inflammatory or infiltrative disorders
     a. Regional enteritis
     b. Amyloidosis
     c. Scleroderma
     d. Lymphoma
     e. Radiation enteritis
     f. Tropical sprue
     g. Infectious enteritis (e.g., salmonellosis)
   2. Biochemical or genetic abnormalities
     a. Nontropical sprue
     b. Disaccharidase deficiency
     c. Hypogammaglobulinemia
     d. Abetalipoproteinemia
     e. Hartnup disease
     f. Cystinuria
     g. Monosaccharide malabsorption
G. Endocrine and metabolic disorders
   1. Diabetes mellitus
   2. Hypoparathyroidism
   3. Adrenal insufficiency
   4. Hyperthyroidism
   5. Ulcerogenic tumor of the pancreas (Zollinger-Ellison syndrome)
   6. Mastocytosis
   7. Carcinoid syndrome

tional and anatomic abnormalities. In this chapter, not all the disorders listed in Table 316-4 are discussed in detail. Rather, only the more common disorders are discussed,

and, where appropriate, the pathophysiologic changes are described.

DISORDERS ASSOCIATED WITH MALABSORPTION

INADEQUATE DIGESTION

LIVER AND BILIARY TRACT DISEASE. It is not generally appreciated that patients with acute or chronic liver disease may develop malabsorption due to impaired intraluminal digestion. Steatorrhea has been described in acute viral hepatitis, chronic extrahepatic biliary tract obstruction, primary biliary cirrhosis, and postnecrotic and nutritional cirrhosis. Absorption of D-xylose and vitamin B_{12} are usually normal, and small intestinal mucosal biopsy specimens are generally unremarkable. The steatorrhea associated with liver and biliary tract disease is thought to be due to impaired hepatic synthesis or excretion of conjugated bile salts. In addition to steatorrhea, patients with liver disease may have impaired absorption of vitamin D and calcium resulting in severe metabolic bone disease. This is particularly common in patients with primary biliary cirrhosis. Skeletal roentgenograms may show increased porosity of bone, cortical thinning, vertebral compression, and spontaneous pathologic fractures. Patients with alcohol-induced liver disease may also have exocrine pancreatic insufficiency. Accordingly, pancreatic function should be evaluated in patients with liver disease and malabsorption.

POSTGASTRECTOMY MALABSORPTION. The presence of a malabsorption syndrome has been documented frequently in patients after subtotal gastrectomy. Steatorrhea is more common with a Billroth II than a Billroth I type of anastomosis. Usually the fat loss is minimal, ranging from 7 to 10 Gm per 24 hr. Patients with gross steatorrhea usually have impaired intraluminal fat digestion due to several factors: First, with a Billroth II anastomosis the duodenum is bypassed, and there is a decreased entry of stomach contents into the proximal duodenum (i.e., afferent loop). This leads to a decreased stimulus for the release of *secretin* and *pancreozymin* from the pancreas and in essence is a form of functional pancreatic insufficiency. Second, there may be *inadequate mixing* of the pancreatic enzymes and bile salts secreted into the proximal duodenum with the gastric contents entering the jejunum. Third, there may be *stasis* of intestinal contents in the afferent loop resulting in abnormal bacterial proliferation in the proximal small bowel. This in turn may lead to abnormalities in bile salt metabolism (see Pathophysiology, below). Fourth, the presence of maldigestion may lead to *protein depletion,* which in turn may produce further impairment in pancreatic function. Fifth, the *loss of the reservoir function of the stomach* may result in decreased intestinal transit time. In some patients treatment with pancreatic enzymes may lead to significant improvement. Specimens of duodenal or jejunal fluid should be obtained for culture of both aerobic and anaerobic organisms and appropriate antibiotic therapy instituted if there is evidence of abnormal bacterial overgrowth (colony count of greater than 10^5 per ml jejunal fluid). Because the duodenum is the principal site of absorption of iron and calcium, in patients with a Billroth II anastomosis impaired absorption of calcium and iron may also develop.

INADEQUATE ABSORPTIVE SURFACE

See Regional Enteritis, p. 1479.

MALABSORPTION DUE TO BACTERIAL OVERGROWTH OF THE SMALL BOWEL

The proximal small intestine is often bacteriologically sterile. When bacteria are isolated from the upper small bowel, they are frequently contaminants transported from the mouth and upper respiratory tract, and the colony count rarely exceeds 10^4 per ml jejunal fluid. The major mechanism limiting the growth of bacteria in the small intestine is normal peristalsis. Any disorder leading to impaired intestinal motility may result in abnormal stasis of intestinal contents with ineffective mechanical cleansing of bacteria. This in turn may lead to abnormal bacterial proliferation and malabsorption. Several malabsorptive disorders have been associated with bacterial overgrowth of the small bowel, and these are listed in Table 316-4.

PATHOPHYSIOLOGY. Bacterial overgrowth may result in changes in bile salt metabolism, and these are believed directly and indirectly to account for the steatorrhea. First, bacteria (especially anaerobic gram-positive bacteria) may lead to the intraluminal deconjugation of bile salts with a consequent production of free bile acids. In contrast to conjugated bile salts, unconjugated bile salts may be absorbed in the proximal small bowel by nonionic diffusion resulting in decreased intraluminal concentrations of bile salts in the jejunum. Second, the decreased bile salt concentrations, the increase of unconjugated bile salts, and the decrease of the conjugated salts all serve to contribute to impaired intraluminal micelle formation and hence fat malabsorption. Third, experimental studies have shown that mucosal uptake of fatty acids and possibly also esterification of fatty acids to triglycerides appear to be impaired. There is little evidence that decreased lipolysis of triglycerides by pancreatic lipase or increased fecal excretion of endogenous lipid are important factors in the pathogenesis of steatorrhea in the blind loop syndrome. The impaired absorption of vitamin B_{12} is not related to the disturbed bile salt metabolism but appears to be due to uptake of vitamin B_{12} by microorganisms.

Many of the above abnormalities in bile salt metabolism may be reversed by appropriate antibiotic therapy. When such treatment is instituted, unconjugated bile salts in the jejunal fluid decrease, an increase in the micellar lipid phase will occur, and steatorrhea diminishes or disappears. In addition, significant improvement in the absorption of vitamin B_{12} will occur with broad-spectrum antibiotics such as tetracycline.

CLINICAL MANIFESTATIONS. The diagnosis of a malabsorption syndrome due to abnormal bacterial overgrowth of the small intestine is usually established on

the basis of the following findings: (1) steatorrhea of a moderate degree, usually in the range of 15 to 30 Gm fecal fat per 24 hr, (2) macrocytic anemia with a megaloblastic bone marrow, (3) impaired absorption of vitamin B_{12} which is not corrected by intrinsic factor, (4) large numbers of microorganisms (greater than 10^5 per ml) in cultures of duodenal or jejunal fluid, (5) correction of steatorrhea and impaired vitamin B_{12} absorption by antibiotic therapy, together with a decrease in the number of microorganisms in the small intestinal fluid, and (6) increased urinary indican excretion which reverts to normal with antibiotic therapy. Absorption of D-xylose, peroral small-intestinal biopsy specimens, and other tests of absorptive function (Table 316-2) may be normal in these patients.

SCLERODERMA. Although there are numerous reports of small-intestinal involvement in scleroderma, frank malabsorption has been reported infrequently. It has been suggested that malabsorption may be due to several factors: (1) lymphatic obstruction; (2) reduced arterial blood supply to the gut; (3) impaired intestinal motility leading to relative stasis of intestinal contents and hence bacterial overgrowth; and (4) involvement of the intestinal wall by the disease. At present there is little data to support the first two postulated mechanisms. In some cases abnormal bacterial proliferation in the upper small bowel has been documented, and in these patients antibiotic therapy has resulted in decrease in steatorrhea, gain in weight, and increased absorption of vitamin B_{12}. In the intestinal wall there may also be extensive deposition of collagen, especially in the muscular mucosa, submucosa, and muscularis externa, with significant muscle atrophy. Electron microscopic studies have revealed a paucity of nexuses (cell junctions) between adjacent muscle cells in the small intestine of these patients. Since nexuses are important in the propagation of electric impulses, the loss of contact between muscle cells may result in impairment of muscular contraction. This may be an important factor in the dilatation, atony, and stasis of intestinal contents in scleroderma.

DISORDERS ASSOCIATED WITH LYMPHATIC OBSTRUCTION

WHIPPLE'S DISEASE. This is a rare disorder characterized clinically by arthralgia, abdominal pain, diarrhea, progressive weight loss, and impaired intestinal absorption. The disease is unusual in women and occurs predominantly in men of middle age. Wasting, low-grade fever, increased skin pigmentation, and peripheral lymphadenopathy are frequently present. In addition, there may be enlargement of mesenteric, periaortic, and celiac lymph nodes. Laboratory examination usually reveals the presence of steatorrhea, impaired xylose absorption, abnormal small-bowel x-rays, hypoalbuminemia, and anemia. Hypoalbuminemia is due to excessive loss of serum albumin into the gastrointestinal tract as well as impaired synthesis of albumin. Serum calcium, cholesterol, and iron levels are usually low and often inversely correlated with the degree of malabsorption.

The diagnosis is established by demonstrating the presence in the mucosa of macrophages containing large cytoplasmic granules which give a brilliant magenta stain with periodic acid–Schiff reagent (PAS). Such macrophages may also be seen in other tissues such as lymph nodes, spleen, or liver. The PAS-positive reaction is due to the presence of glycoproteins. The finding of PAS-positive macrophages in the lamina propria is not specific for Whipple's disease, but virtual replacement of most cellular elements in the lamina propria by these macrophages has been seen only in this disorder. In addition to the PAS-positive macrophages, jejunal biopsies frequently show dilated lymphatics and some degree of blunting of the intestinal mucosal villi.

Electron microscopic studies have revealed the presence of rod-shaped structures (or bacilliform bodies) 0.3 by 1.5 to 2.5 μ within and adjacent to the macrophages in the lamina propria as well as within epithelial cells, and polymorphonuclear leukocytes. The ultrastructural features of these bacilliform bodies suggest that they are microorganisms. It is of particular interest that after treatment with antibiotics the bacilliform bodies decrease or disappear together with a decrease in the number of PAS-positive macrophages. In addition, the reappearance of the bacteria often heralds the onset of a clinical relapse after antibiotics have been withdrawn. Despite the fact that the presence of bacilliform bodies is usually associated with active disease, the exact role of the bacilli in the pathogenesis of Whipple's disease is unclear. The microorganism has not been identified with certainty, and the disease has not been reproduced in animals.

Whipple's disease at one time was thought to be invariably fatal. However, it is now clear that therapy with antibiotics, with or without corticosteroids, will usually induce a clinical remission. In a few cases there has been complete reversal of the histologic abnormalities in the jejunal mucosa, and some of these cases have been followed for 10 years. It is recommended that patients with Whipple's disease be treated with antibiotics such as tetracycline for at least 1 year and then followed closely with serial small-bowel biopsies. The most important parameter for following the disease and predicting its course is the presence or absence of bacilli in sections of small-bowel biopsies.

INTESTINAL LYMPHOMA. Steatorrhea is an uncommon manifestation of intestinal lymphoma. The disease occurs predominantly in men, and the mean age of onset of symptoms is about fifty years. The diagnosis should be suspected in patients with malabsorption with the following findings: (1) a malabsorption syndrome in which clinical and biopsy features resemble those of nontropical sprue but in which there is an incomplete response to a gluten-free diet, (2) the presence of abdominal pain and fever, and (3) signs and symptoms of intestinal obstruction. It should be emphasized that the usual stigmas of generalized lymphoma are frequently absent. Hepatomegaly, splenomegaly, palpable abdominal masses, and peripheral adenopathy are usually not found. Lymphangiography may reveal abnormal intraabdominal nodes. The diagnosis can be established by laparotomy and often may be made by thorough examination of multiple mucosal biopsy specimens obtained perorally. There may be a total absence of villi or lesser degrees of blunting and shortening of the villi. In contrast to nontropical sprue, the lamina propria is usually massively infiltrated with lymphoid cells. Malignancy may be diagnosed by demonstrating lymphoid cells with the cytologic features of malignancy, the presence of reticulum cells outside of germinal centers, and infiltration and destruction of crypts by pleomorphic lymphoid cells.

The mechanism of malabsorption in intestinal lymphoma may be related to several factors: (1) diffuse involvement of the small intestinal mucosa; (2) involvement of the bowel wall with lymphatic obstruction; and (3) localized stenosis with stasis of intestinal contents and bacterial overgrowth. It is thus evident that it is at times difficult by clinical and morphologic features definitively to distinguish nontropical sprue from intestinal lymphoma. Indeed, there is evidence to suggest that lymphoma may develop as a late complication of nontropical sprue.

The course of intestinal lymphoma has ranged from 4 months to 4 years from the onset of symptoms. Perforation, bleeding, and intestinal obstruction are common terminal complications. There is insufficient data to determine whether radiation therapy, chemotherapy, or localized surgical resection modify the natural course of the disease.

KOHLMEIER-DEGOS DISEASE. This is a rare progressive arterial occlusive disorder involving fibrosis of small and medium-sized arteries leading ultimately to ischemia and tissue infarction. The vascular changes in Kohlmeier-Degos disease are found primarily in the skin and intestine, but multiple organ systems may be involved. The disorder usually affects males fifteen to thirty-five years of age and characteristically begins with a pathognomonic skin eruption over the trunk and extremities. The skin lesions are characterized by a distinctive central porcelain-white area about 2 to 10 mm in diameter surrounded by a narrow erythematous halo. After a variable period of time during which the patient appears well, abdominal pain, weakness, fatigue, and weight loss develop. Intestinal perforation ultimately occurs in most cases leading to peritonitis and death. Malabsorption, chylous ascites, and cerebral and renal infarcts have been described. No effective therapy has been discovered to date.

CARDIOVASCULAR DISORDERS

Steatorrhea has been described in patients with chronic congestive heart failure, superior mesenteric artery insufficiency, and constrictive pericarditis. Abnormal dilated mucosal lymphatics and excessive enteric loss of protein have been demonstrated in patients with constrictive pericarditis. The mechanism of steatorrhea in patients with chronic heart failure remains uncertain. It might be due to congestion and edema of the mucosa, mucosal hypoxia, or abnormalities in pancreatic function. Although pronounced steatorrhea is uncommon in congestive heart failure, these patients are frequently anorectic, and a low fat intake could mask a latent steatorrhea.

Defects in Mucosal Function

INFLAMMATORY OR INFILTRATIVE DISORDERS

REGIONAL ENTERITIS. The clinical features of regional enteritis are described in Chap. 317. Malabsorption in regional enteritis may result from several factors: (1) inadequate absorbing surface due to intestinal resection; (2) changes in mucosal cell structure and function; (3) inflammatory cell infiltration of the lamina propria; (4) strictures and fistulas with secondary stasis of intestinal contents and bacterial overgrowth; and (5) impaired absorption of bile salts due either to ileal resection or to the presence of active inflammatory disease in the ileum. After intestinal resection, the functional capacity of the remaining small bowel will depend on the site and extent of resection as well as the presence of residual inflammatory disease. Massive intestinal resection usually results in impaired absorption of all food constituents. Such patients should be treated with a low fat diet, and substitution of medium-chain for long-chain triglycerides may be beneficial. When the malabsorption is due to strictures and blind loops as a result of previous surgical therapy, antibiotic therapy may be helpful, but surgical removal of these areas is usually necessary for long-term improvement. With diffuse inflammatory disease a florid malabsorption syndrome may occur with steatorrhea, hypocalcemia, impaired vitamin B_{12} absorption, and hypoalbuminemia due to increased enteric protein loss. Treatment with salicylazosulfapyridine and corticosteroid drugs may be beneficial.

After *ileal resection,* patients frequently have bothersome diarrhea. This appears to be due to *interruption of the enterohepatic circulation* whereby increased amounts of bile salts reach the colon, where they interfere with water and electrolyte absorption and thus have a cathartic effect. The *bile salt–induced diarrhea* after ileal resection may respond to treatment with cholestyramine, an exchange resin which binds bile salts and causes them to lose their biochemical effect on the bowel.

AMYLOIDOSIS. This disorder is discussed in detail in Chap. 114. The intestinal tract is involved infrequently in amyloidosis. Diarrhea and steatorrhea are thought to be due to (1) infiltration of the intestinal wall with amyloid and (2) involvement of the autonomic nervous system. Metachromatic and congophilic amyloid has been demonstrated in small and medium-sized blood vessels in the intestine, in nerve bundles in Meissner's submucosal and Auerbach's myenteric plexus, and in the thoracolumbar and celiac sympathetic ganglions. With involvement of the autonomic nervous system, patients may show uncontrollable diarrhea, orthostatic hypotension, trophic ulcers, anhydrosis of the distal extremities, and impotence. The clinical features closely resemble those found in "diabetic diarrhea." The diagnosis can be established by demonstrating amyloid deposits in rectal and small-intestinal biopsy specimens. In addition to malabsorption, rare manifestations include intestinal perforation, colonic infarction, and excessive enteric loss of protein. There is no effective treatment for the disease.

RADIATION INJURY TO THE SMALL BOWEL. Extensive morphologic damage of the small-intestinal mucosa often follows after normal or excessive abdominal irradiation. These changes include a decrease in crypt mitoses, marked shortening of the villi, megalocytosis of epithelial cells, and inflammatory cell infiltration of the lamina propria. This may be associated with transient diarrhea and impaired intestinal absorption. However, restoration of normal intestinal architecture is usually complete within 2 weeks after cessation of therapy. Persistent diarrhea and malabsorption may develop shortly after x-ray therapy, or there may be a latent period of several years before the onset of diarrhea. Steatorrhea, ranging from 10 to 70 Gm per day, has been frequently observed, but impaired absorption of calcium, iron, D-xylose, or vitamin B_{12} is less common. In some patients intestinal strictures may develop following irradiation, and thus stasis of intestinal contents and abnormal bacterial proliferation may occur. In others, intestinal lymphangiectasia, presumably due to lymphatic obstruction, has been documented. Diarrhea and malabsorption may be refractory to all methods of management. Treatment with antibiotics, pancreatic enzymes, gluten-free diet, adrenal corticosteroids, anticholinergic drugs, and opiates has met with but limited success.

TROPICAL SPRUE. This is a disorder of unknown cause characterized by malabsorption, abnormal small-intestinal histologic characteristics, and the ultimate development of multiple nutritional deficiencies. The disease occurs in tropical or subtropical zones such as the Caribbean area, Indian subcontinent, and Southeast Asia. However, patients who have previously lived in the tropics may not develop overt symptoms of the disease until after return to a temperate climate. While bacteriologic and viral studies of the intestinal tract in these patients have been inconclusive, improvement often occurs after institution of antibiotic therapy, suggesting that microorganisms may play an etiologic role in this disorder. Patients frequently complain of anorexia, fatigue, diarrhea with malodorous stools, weight loss, and glossitis. There is often a megaloblastic anemia in association with lowered serum folate and vitamin B_{12} levels. Impaired absorption of D-xylose, folate, iron, and vitamin B_{12} can also be demonstrated. The intestinal mucosa shows varying degrees of villous atrophy with blunted and flattened villi, together with intense lymphocytic infiltration of the lamina propria. The changes are similar to, but generally less severe than, those observed in nontropical sprue. In addition, there may be megalocytosis, decreased mitoses in the crypt cells, and decreased overall mucosal thickness. Treatment with oral broad-spectrum antibiotics, folic acid, and vitamin B_{12} either singly or in combination results in hematologic remission as well as cessation of gastrointestinal symptoms. This is associated with improvement in small-intestinal absorptive function and reversal of histologic abnormalities. It appears that oral antibiotic therapy induces a hematologic remission by improving jejunal absorptive capacity so that sufficient quantities of dietary folic acid can be absorbed. It is not surprising, therefore, that many patients not maintained on antibiotic therapy will relapse within a 6- to 12-month period.

BIOCHEMICAL OR GENETIC ABNORMALITIES

NONTROPICAL SPRUE. Definition. Nontropical sprue is a disorder characterized by malabsorption, abnormal small-bowel structure, and intolerance to gluten, a protein found in wheat and wheat products. It has been appropriately referred to as *gluten-induced enteropathy*. Celiac disease in children and nontropical sprue of the adult are probably one and the same disorder with the same pathogenesis.

There are insufficient data to provide an accurate estimation of the incidence of nontropical sprue in any population. This is largely because the severity of the disease varies greatly and individuals may have typical mucosal change and yet have no overt symptoms. The incidence in siblings appears to be many times higher than that in the general population, and it has been suggested that sprue may be inherited through a dominant gene of incomplete penetrance. Seventy percent of the cases in most reported series are in women.

PATHOPHYSIOLOGY. Gluten and the related substance gliadin are high molecular weight proteins found especially in wheat. These proteins are unique in that glutamine accounts for about 40 percent of the component amino acids. These proteins as well as the larger peptide hydrolysis products (containing glutamine) are toxic when administered to patients with sprue in remission. The exact mechanism for this effect is not clear, but two theories have been proposed: One possible mechanism is that patients with sprue lack a specific mucosal peptidase, such that gluten or its larger glutamine-containing peptides are not effectively hydrolyzed to smaller peptides (i.e., dipeptides) or amino acids. As a consequence "toxic" peptides might accumulate in the mucosa. It has been demonstrated that patients with sprue in remission will develop steatorrhea and typical mucosal changes when they are given gluten. Similar results will occur with the administration of peptide hydrolyzates containing at least eight amino acids with a terminal glutamine residue. It has been shown that when gluten is instilled into the *ileum* of sprue patients, histologic changes begin to occur within hours, but not in the upper jejunum, suggesting that the effect is immediate and local rather than systemic. While the mucosa of patients with sprue shows many enzyme alterations, no specific and selective peptidase deficiency has been demonstrated.

It has also been suggested that gluten or gluten metabolites may initiate a hypersensitivity reaction in the intestinal mucosa. The presence of a mononuclear inflammatory cell infiltrate in the lamina propria of the mucosa, the beneficial response to corticosteroid drugs, and the finding of abnormal antibodies to gliadin in the serum of sprue patients have all been cited as evidence in support of this hypothesis. There are no firm data indicating that an abnormal (immune) mechanism is important in initiating or perpetuating this disease process.

Jejunal biopsy specimens from patients with nontropical sprue usually show a characteristic lesion referred to as *subtotal villous atrophy*. There is blunting and flattening of the mucosal surface, with villi either absent or broad and short. The crypts are elongated, and there is generally a dense infiltration of inflammatory cells in the lamina propria. The surface epithelium is altered with a sparse brush border, cuboidal rather than the normal columnar cells, and infiltration of inflammatory cells in the epithelial layer. These changes are usually most severe in the proximal small bowel, presumably because this area of the bowel is exposed to the highest gluten concentration. The typical morphologic changes are illustrated in Fig. 316-3. It should be emphasized that these changes are characteristic of nontropical sprue but are not specific. Similar changes have been described in other conditions including lymphoma, tropical sprue, and hypogammaglobulinemia associated with malabsorption. Many biochemical abnormalities have been demonstrated in mucosal biopsy specimens from nontropical sprue patients. Impaired esterification of fatty acids to triglycerides, decreased uptake of amino acids, and decreased activity of intestinal disaccharidases (especially lactase) have been well documented. The latter observation may account for the high incidence of milk intolerance in untreated sprue patients or those in relapse.

Clinical Features. Most patients with nontropical sprue will have a typical malabsorption syndrome characterized by weight loss, abdominal distension and bloating, diarrhea, steatorrhea, and abnormal tests of absorptive function. The characteristic alterations in tests of intestinal absorption are outlined in Table 316-2. It should be emphasized, however, that some sprue patients may present with isolated abnomalities which initially do not suggest the diagnosis of nontropical sprue. Thus, a patient may be admitted for investigation of iron deficiency anemia without apparent blood loss or of abnormal bleeding due to hypoprothrombinemia but not have diarrhea or overt steatorrhea. Likewise, sprue patients may present with puzzling metabolic bone disease without diarrhea or steatorrhea. Such patients usually complain of bone pain and tenderness and frequently are found to have extensive demineralization of bone, compression deformities, kyphoscoliosis, and Milkman's fractures. Emotional disturbances are common in these patients, and many individuals with a diagnosis of weight loss initially considered related to severe anxiety and depression are subsequently found to have nontropical sprue. In each of the above clinical settings, the diagnosis of sprue should be considered in the differential diagnosis.

Since there is no specific diagnostic test, three criteria should be met in order to establish a definite diagnosis of nontropical sprue: (1) evidence of malabsorption, (2) an abnormal small-bowel (jejunal) biopsy showing blunting and flattening of the villi along with changes in the surface epithelium (i.e., subtotal villous atrophy), (3) clinical, biochemical, and histologic improvement after institution of a gluten-free diet. In equivocal cases, the patient can be challenged with 30 to 50 Gm gluten orally, and if this promptly results in increased diarrhea and steatorrhea, the diagnosis of gluten-induced enteropathy is established. It should be emphasized that tests of intestinal absorption may reveal abnormalities which range from very minimal alterations to severe changes. Abnormalities in absorption tests have been shown to correlate reasonably well with the length of small-bowel involvement and to a lesser extent with the severity of the proximal lesion.

Treatment. Despite the uncertainties concerned with the diagnosis of nontropical sprue, approximately 80 percent of the patients improve after institution of a gluten-free diet. Symptomatic improvement usually occurs within a few weeks, but improvement in tests of absorptive function and small-bowel histologic characteristics may not occur for months. It has been repeatedly demonstrated that strict adherence to a gluten-free diet more consistently results in improvement than suboptimal gluten restriction. Nevertheless, even with strict diet adherence some cases show little improvement in intestinal histologic features.

If a patient with nontropical sprue does not respond to a gluten-free diet, other possibilities or complicative factors must be considered: (1) the diagnosis is incorrect, (2) the patient is not adhering strictly to the diet, (3) there may be another concurrent disease, such as pancreatic insufficiency, (4) the patient may have ulceration of the jejunum or ileum, (5) lactase deficiency may be present with resultant milk intolerance, and (6) the patient may have developed intestinal lymphoma, a disease which appears to occur more frequently in sprue than the general population. Finally, it should be emphasized that a small number of patients show a markedly delayed response to a gluten-free diet with significant improvement occurring only after 24 to 36 months of therapy.

DISACCHARIDASE DEFICIENCY SYNDROMES. As indicated above, the hydrolysis of disaccharides occurs on or within the brush border (microvilli) of intestinal epithelial cells by specific disaccharidases located there. As would be anticipated both prmiary (genetic or familial) and secondary (acquired) deficiencies of these disaccharidases have been observed.

Lactase Deficiency in the Adult. Instances of isolated deficiency of mucosal lactase occur which are associated with symptoms of lactose intolerance. Since lactose is the principal carbohydrate of milk, such individuals show milk intolerance with symptoms of abdominal cramps, bloating, or distension, and diarrhea. Similar symptoms will occur following the ingestion of lactose. The symptoms are due to the fact that lactose, when not hydrolyzed, is not absorbed and its osmotic effect in the lumen leads to shifts of fluid into the intestinal tract. The pH of the stool will also decrease because of the production of lactic acid and short-chain fatty acids from the fermentation of lactose by colonic bacteria. Although primary intestinal lactase deficiency seems to be hereditary, lactose or milk intolerance may not become clinically evident until puberty or late adolescence. There are significant racial differences in the incidence of this entity. It would appear that about 5 percent of the adult white population show intestinal lactase deficiency, but in American Negroes, Bantus, and Orientals, the incidence has been reported as high as 60 to 90 percent.

The diagnosis may be suspected by obtaining a history of gastrointestinal symptoms following milk ingestion. That these symptoms are not due to allergic reactions to the proteins in milk (i.e., milk allergy or hypersensitivity) can be demonstrated by performing a lactose tolerance test. This test consists of administering an oral dose of lactose (usually from 0.75 to 1.5 Gm per kg body weight) and obtaining serial blood samples for measurements of blood glucose. In a positive test, intestinal symptoms occur, and the blood glucose increases less than 25 mg per 100 ml above the fasting level. Because false positive tests occur in about 20 percent of normal subjects, a positive test should be confirmed by direct enzymatic measurements of lactase on peroral mucosal biopsy specimens. In primary lactase deficiency the intestinal mucosa is normal histologically.

Acquired lactase deficiency is often seen in association with a variety of gastrointestinal diseases, in many of which there is histologic evidence of mucosal damage. The disorders in which lactose intolerance and lactase deficiency may occur include nontropical and tropical sprue, regional enteritis, bacterial infections of the intestinal tract, giardiasis, abetalipoproteinemia, cystic fibrosis, and ulcerative colitis.

Deficiency of Other Disaccharidases. Damage to the intestinal mucosa may produce decreased levels of other disaccharidases such as invertase (sucrase), but usually these are not as depressed as lactase, and symptoms of specific intolerance, such as sucrose intolerance, are uncommon. There are instances of primary and apparently hereditary invertase intolerance, but these always occur in association with isomaltase deficiency. There have been no reports of maltose intolerance, perhaps reflecting the fact that there are at least four mucosal enzymes capable of hydrolyzing maltose.

HYPOGAMMAGLOBULINEMIA. There are several reports documenting the association of malabsorption in hypogammaglobulinemia or agammaglobulinemia. The hypogammaglobulinemia may be of the congenital or acquired type with the onset either in childhood or adulthood. When malabsorption has been noted, it has included impaired absorption of fat, D-xylose, and vitamin B_{12}. Peroral intestinal biopsy may reveal changes comparable to those seen in nontropical sprue, but often one finds a more striking mononuclear infiltrate giving nodular appearance to the mucosa both microscopically and macroscopically. Diarrhea and steatorrhea may precede or follow the development of hypogammaglobulinemia, and these may worsen during infections and subside after the infection is controlled with antibiotics. Arthritis, resembling rheumatoid arthritis, and thymoma have also been described in patients with this syndrome. In some patients improvement in diarrhea and malabsorption may occur spontaneously, whereas in others improvement may follow treatment with a gluten-free diet, corticosteroids, antibiotics, and injections of γ-globulin. These forms of therapy have not been uniformly successful. Although transient improvement is common, complete cessation of symptoms is distinctly unusual.

The relationship between hypogammaglobulinemia and malabsorption remains obscure. There is no evidence to date indicating that excessive enteric loss of γ-globulin or alteration of the intestinal microflora occurs, but abnormalities in IgA metabolism may be important in this syndrome. This immunoglobulin is the predominant one in the intestinal mucosa and is found in many exocrine secretions including tears, saliva, gastric juice, and intestinal juice. A few patients have been described with malabsorption and selective deficiency of IgA.

ABETALIPOPROTEINEMIA. See Chap. 113.

HARTNUP DISEASE. See Chap. 103.

CYSTINURIA. See Chap. 103.

ENDOCRINE AND METABOLIC DISORDERS

DIABETES MELLITUS. The occurrence of diarrhea and steatorrhea in patients with diabetes mellitus has been well documented. When steatorrhea accompanies diabetes, it may be due to the presence of (1) exocrine pancreatic insufficiency, (2) coexistent nontropical sprue, and (3) severe and uncontrolled diabetes per se (e.g., so-called "diabetic diarrhea"). Patients falling into the first two categories will usually respond in a satisfactory manner to treatment with pancreatic extracts or a gluten-free diet, respectively. The pathogenesis of diarrhea and steatorrhea in patients in the third category remains poorly understood, and the response to various forms of therapy has been quite variable. It has been demonstrated that patients with "diabetic diarrhea" and steatorrhea may have involvement of the autonomic nervous system with degenerative changes in the sympathetic and parasympathetic nerves and ganglions. In some patients bacterial overgrowth in the stomach and proximal small bowel may occur and contribute to the diarrhea and steatorrhea.

The clinical features in patients with diarrhea and steatorrhea due to diabetes per se seem to be fairly uniform. Diabetes usually develops at a young age and is often severe and difficult to control. There is a distinct predominance of males. Several signs of autonomic neuropathy are usually present including postural hypotension, anhydrosis, impotence, and bladder irregularities. Peripheral vascular disease and peripheral neuropathy are also common. Gastrointestinal x-rays may show delayed gastric emptying and disordered transit through the small bowel. Peroral small-bowel biopsy specimens are normal. Tests of intestinal absorptive function are normal except for steatorrhea and azotorrhea. There has been no consistent response to therapy with pancreatic extracts, gluten-free diet, corticosteroids, and cholinergic drugs such as Urecholine. When bacterial overgrowth is present, broad spectrum antibiotics may be helpful. In a few patients improvement in steatorrhea and diarrhea occurs after satisfactory control of diabetes.

HYPOPARATHYROIDISM. Steatorrhea has been documented in several patients with idiopathic hypoparathyroidism. In addition to hypocalcemia, impaired absorption of D-xylose and vitamin B_{12}, decreased serum iron values, and abnormal small-intestinal roentgenograms have been demonstrated in some cases. In such patients the serum phosphorus level is elevated (due to the hypoparathyroidism) rather than low (as in primary malabsorption). The cause of malabsorption in this disorder is unclear. It is possible that hypocalcemia causes impaired neuromuscular function, which in turn may lead to hypomotility, stasis of intestinal contents, and abnormal bacterial proliferation in the small bowel. The latter abnormality could account for the development of steatorrhea and malabsorption of vitamin B_{12}.

ADRENAL INSUFFICIENCY. Although there are few studies on fat excretion in adrenal insufficiency in man, malabsorption, especially of fat, would appear to occur more frequently than has been generally appreciated. Patients with adrenal insufficiency have been found to have steatorrhea which was corrected by therapy with adrenal corticosteroids. Jejunal biopsies in a small number of these patients were normal. It is possible that the diarrhea and weight loss seen in adrenal insufficiency may be due in part to malabsorption.

ULCEROGENIC TUMOR OF THE PANCREAS (ZOLLINGER-ELLISON SYNDROME). See Chap. 314.

MASTOCYTOSIS. See Chap. 400.

CARCINOID SYNDROME (See Chap. 105). Although diarrhea is common in the carcinoid syndrome, malabsorption with significant steatorrhea is unusual. In many of the cases of carcinoid syndrome with steatorrhea there has been a prior intestinal resection (usually ileal), and in these cases the resection is the important factor in the causation of steatorrhea. However, direct involvement of the bowel wall and mesentery by the carcinoid tumor have been well documented. That abnormalities in serotonin metabolism may also be important is suggested from the decrease in the steatorrhea observed in some of these patients when treated with the antiserotonin drug methysergide. Although side effects may occur, for control of diarrhea and steatorrhea, patients may be given a trial of 8 to 12 mg methysergide per day.

PROTEIN-LOSING ENTEROPATHY

The gastrointestinal tract has been shown to play a significant role in the metabolism and physiologic degradation of plasma proteins. The exact magnitude of the normal gastrointestinal protein loss in man has remained unclear, but studies with [131]I- or ^{125}I-labeled albumin and ^{51}Cr-labeled albumin have suggested that between 10 and 20 percent of the normal turnover of albumin may be accounted for by enteric protein loss. However, under certain pathologic conditions, excessive gastrointestinal protein loss may develop. An extensive number of disorders have been found to be associated with intestinal protein loss. Some of these are listed in Table 316-5.

PATHOPHYSIOLOGY. Several mechanisms have been proposed for the passage of plasma proteins across the gastrointestinal mucosa both normally and in certain disease states: First, plasma proteins may pass into the gastrointestinal tract through an inflamed or ulcerated mucosa and account for the protein loss occasionally seen in regional enteritis and ulcerative colitis. Second, plasma protein loss may occur as a result of disordered mucosal cell structure. For example, patients with nontropical sprue have abnormal villous structure and surface epithelium, and these changes could facilitate the diffusion of plasma protein between the cells. Third, in the presence of increased lymphatic pressure, there may be increased passage of plasma proteins into the lumen via the

Table 316-5. DISORDERS ASSOCIATED WITH
PROTEIN-LOSING ENTEROPATHY*

A. Stomach
   1. Gastric carcinoma
   2. Giant hypertrophy of the gastric mucosa
   3. Atrophic gastritis
   4. Postgastrectomy syndrome

B. Small intestine
   1. Nontropic sprue
   2. Tropical sprue
   3. Regional enteritis
   4. Whipple's disease
   5. Lymphoma
   6. Intestinal lymphangiectasia
   7. Intestinal tuberculosis
   8. Acute infectious enteritis
   9. Scleroderma
  10. Jejunal diverticulosis
  11. Allergic gastroenteropathy

C. Colon
   1. Colonic neoplasm
   2. Ulcerative colitis
   3. Granulomatous colitis
   4. Megacolon

D. Cardiac
   1. Congestive heart failure
   2. Constrictive pericarditis
   3. Interatrial septal defect
   4. Primary cardiomyopathy

E. Miscellaneous
   1. Esophageal carcinoma
   2. Gastrocolic fistula
   3. Agammaglobulinemia
   4. Nephrosis

* Modified from Waldman, T.A.: Gastroenterology, 50:422, 1966.

intercellular spaces of the mucosal epithelium. This might be expected to occur in disorders in which there is granulomatous or neoplastic involvement of lymphatics. Fourth, dilated lymph vessels in the mucosa may rupture through the surface epithelium, discharging their contents into the intestinal lumen. This is thought to be important in the pathogenesis of steatorrhea and hypoproteinemia in patients with idiopathic intestinal lymphangiectasia (see Intestinal Lymphangiectasia, below).

Several techniques have been developed for the detection and quantitation of gastrointestinal protein loss. Most of these involve the use of intravenously administered radioactive-labeled macromolecules such as ^{131}I- and ^{125}I-labeled serum albumin, iodinated polyvinylpyrrolidone (PVP), ^{51}Cr-labeled albumin, and ^{67}Cu-labeled ceruloplasmin. ^{51}Chromium-labeled albumin and ^{51}CrCl$_3$ (both of which rapidly become attached to circulating transferrin) are the compounds used most frequently. After the intravenous administration of 25 to 30 microcuries of the labeled compound to normal subjects, between 0.1 and 0.7 percent of the administered radioactivity is recov-

ered in the stool over a 4-day period. Patients with excessive enteric protein loss may excrete from 2 to 40 percent of the injected radioactive label. False positive results may be obtained if the stool specimen is contaminated with urine.

Using intravenously administered radioiodinated albumin, the decline in radioactivity in the serum and whole body can be followed and the rate of albumin synthesis and degradation determined. Such studies carried out in patients with protein-losing enteropathies have demonstrated a reduced circulating (intravascular) and total body pool of albumin, a normal or increased rate of albumin synthesis, a markedly shortened albumin survival, and increased fecal protein loss. Whereas normal subjects catabolize 5 to 10 percent of their intravascular albumin pool each day (the fractional catabolic rate), patients with excessive enteric protein loss may have fractional catabolic rates of 50 to 60 percent.

Studies utilizing radioiodinated immunoglobulins have demonstrated a decreased intravascular globulin pool and increased fractional catabolic rate. However, the synthesis of IgG is usually normal, suggesting that a decreased level of IgG and increased enteric protein loss is not a potent stimulus for IgG synthesis. The increase in fractional catabolic rate is comparable for albumin, IgG, and IgM immunoglobulins, further suggesting that there is bulk loss of plasma proteins into the intestinal tract and not a selective loss of certain proteins. The finding of decreased globulins often is an ancilliary aid in excluding renal, cardiac, and hepatic causes of hypoalbuminemia.

Several studies have demonstrated that abnormalities in albumin and globulin metabolism in patients with a protein-losing enteropathy may be reversed or diminished within a few months after the institution of appropriate therapy. It is obviously important that a specific etiologic diagnosis should be established in all patients with treatable disorders, who may be expected to have a remission induced by the appropriate therapy for the underlying disease. The intestinal protein loss in patients with nontropical sprue, Whipple's disease, constrictive pericarditis, regional enteritis, ulcerative colitis, and Menetrier's disease has been ameliorated by therapy appropriate for the underlying disorder.

INTESTINAL LYMPHANGIECTASIA. Pathophysiology. Intestinal lymphangiectasia is a disorder characterized by increased enteric loss of protein, hypoproteinemia, edema, lymphocytopenia, malabsorption, and abnormal dilated lymphatic channels in the small intestine. The high incidence of chylous effusions and abnormal peripheral, retroperitoneal, and thoracic lymphatics indicates that intestinal lymphangiectasia is part of a generalized congenital disorder of the lymphatic system. It has been suggested that the hypoplastic visceral lymphatic channels result in obstruction to lymph flow with the subsequent development of increased intestinal lymphatic pressure. This in turn may lead to dilated lymphatic vessels throughout the small-bowel wall and mesentery. Hypoproteinemia and steatorrhea are thought to be due to rupture of the dilated lymphatic vessels with discharge of lymph into the bowel lumen. In adults approximately 1,500 ml lymph, containing 70 Gm fat and 50 Gm albumin, passes through the thoracic duct each day. The leakage of a small amount of this lymph might be expected to result in considerable loss of protein and fat into the intestinal lumen. In addition, absorption of dietary long-chain triglycerides stimulates lymph flow, and this may increase further the retrograde leakage of intestinal lymph into the lumen. Three lines of evidence support the concept of intestinal leakage of lymph in intestinal lymphangiectasia: (1) chylous fluid has been recovered from the duodenum in these patients, (2) retrograde passage of contrast material from retroperitoneal lymphatics into the duodenum and jejunum has been documented, and (3) significant steatorrhea may persist in patients after institution of a completely fat-free diet, suggesting an increased enteric loss of endogenous fat present in lymph.

Clinical Features. The disease affects primarily children and young adults. All patients have edema, which may be asymmetrical because of hypoplastic peripheral lymphatics. Chylous effusions and diarrhea are common symptoms. The primary laboratory finding is hypoproteinemia with decreased serum levels of albumin, immunoglobulins IgG, IgA, and IgM, transferrin, and ceruloplasmin. Despite moderate to severe hypogammaglobulinemia there does not appear to be an increased incidence of pyogenic bacterial infections. In addition, circulating antibody response to challenge with *Brucella* and typhoid antigens is normal. Steatorrhea is usually mild, although in some instances fat loss may be as much as 40 Gm per day. Some patients have hypocalcemia and impaired absorption of vitamin B_{12}. Lymphocytopenia (due to the loss of lymphocytes in lymph) is common with lymphocyte counts ranging from 400 to 1,000 per ml (normal: 1,500 to 4,000 per ml). This is associated with abnormal delayed hypersensitivity as evidenced by prolonged homograft survival and impaired cutaneous responsiveness to antigens such as mumps and monilia.

Small-bowel roentgenograms are frequently abnormal, showing changes of mucosal edema and a malabsorption pattern. Lymphangiograms may demonstrate hypoplastic peripheral and visceral lymphatics with the absence of groups of retroperitoneal lymph nodes. Specimens of jejunal mucosa characteristically reveal dilated and telangiectatic lymphatic vessels in the lamina propria and submucosa. The villi may be club-shaped because of distortion from grossly dilated lymphatics (Fig. 316-3). Such changes in the intestinal mucosa may be reversed after appropriate therapy. The diagnosis of intestinal lymphangiectasia is, therefore, established by (1) small-intestinal biopsy and (2) demonstration of increased enteric protein loss using radioactive macromolecules.

Treatment. A low fat diet, by decreasing lymph flow, usually results in significant improvement with decreased fecal fat excretion, decreased enteric protein loss, increased serum calcium and albumin levels, and an increased half-life of injected ^{131}I-labeled albumin. Similar results may be obtained by the substitution of medium-chain triglycerides (MCT) for dietary long-chain triglyc-erides, since MCT are transported as medium-chain fatty acids by the portal vein rather than via the lymph.

REFERENCES

Benson, G. D., O. D. Kowlessar, and M. H. Sleisenger: Adult Celiac Disease with Emphasis upon Response to the Gluten-Free Diet, Medicine, 43:1, 1964.

Chears, W. C., Jr., M. D. Hargrove, Jr., J. V. Verner, A. G. Smith, and J. M. Ruffin: Whipple's Disease: A Review of Twelve Patients from One Service, Am. J. Med., 30: 226, 1961.

Conn, H. O., and R. Quintiliani: Severe Diarrhea Controlled by Gamma Globulin in a Patient with Agammaglobulinemia, Amyloidosis, and Thymoma, Ann. Intern. Med., 65: 528, 1966.

Donaldson, R. M., Jr.: Intestinal Bacteria and Malabsorption, Ann. Intern. Med., 64:948, 1966.

Donaldson, R. M., Jr.: Intestinal Bacteria and Malabsorption, Ann. Intern. Med., 64:948, 1966.

Hofmann, A. F.: The syndrome of ileal disease and the broken enterohepatic circulation: cholerheic enteropathy, Gastroenterology, 52:752, 1967.

Jeffries, G. H., E. Weser, and M. H. Sleisenger: Malabsorption, Gastroenterology, 56:777, 1969.

Kahn, I. J., G. J. Jeffries, and M. H. Sleisenger: Malabsorption in Intestinal Scleroderma, New Engl. J. Med., 274: 1339, 1966.

Kilpatrick, C. H., D. Waxman, O. Smith, and R. N. Schimke: Hypogammaglobulinemia with nodular lymphoid hyperplasia of the small bowel, Arch. Intern. Med., 121:273, 1968.

Klipstein, F. A.: Tropical Sprue in New York City, Gastroenterology, 47:457, 1964.

Krone, C. L., E. Theodor, M. H. Sleisenger, and G. H. Jeffries: Studies on the Pathogenesis of Malabsorption: Lipid Hydrolysis and Micelle Formation in the Intestinal Lumen, Medicine, 47:89, 1968.

Littman, A., and J. B. Hammond: Diarrhea in adults caused by deficiency in intestinal disaccharidases, Gastroenterology, 48:237, 1965.

Mistilis, S. P., A. P. Skyring, and D. D. Stephen: Intestinal Lymphangiectasia: Mechanism of Enteric Loss of Plasmaprotein and Fat, Lancet, 1:77, 1965.

Rosenberg, I. H., W. G. Hardison, and D. M. Bull: Abnormal Bile Salt Patterns and Intestinal Bacterial Overgrowth Associated with Malabsorption, New Engl. J. Med., 276: 1391, 1967.

Rubin, C. E., L. L. Brandborg, A. L. Flick, P. Phelps, C. Parmentier, and S. Van Niel: Studies of Celiac Sprue. III. The Effect of Repeated Wheat Instillation into the Proximal Ileum of Patients on a Gluten-free Diet, Gastroenterology, 43:621, 1962.

Trier, J. S., P. C. Phelps, S. Eidenman, and C. E. Rubin: Whipples Disease: Light and Electron Microscopic Correlation of Jejunal Mucosal Histology with Antibiotic Treatment and Clinical Status, Gastroenterology, 48:684, 1965.

Waldmann, T. A.: Protein-losing Enteropathy, Gastroenterology, 50:422, 1966.

Wruble, L. D., and M. H. Kalser: Diabetic Steatorrhea: A Distinct Entity, Am. J. Med., 37:118, 1964.

317 DISEASES OF THE SMALL INTESTINE

Albert I. Mendeloff

DIVERTICULOSIS

It is usually impossible on clinical grounds to decide whether diverticula of the intestinal tract are congenital or acquired. The rarer congenital diverticula contain the entire thickness of the intestinal wall, whereas acquired diverticula consist of mucosa and serosa alone. Probably the defect in the muscular wall through which the mucosa herniates is always potentially present, usually at the points where the nutrient arteries perforate the serosal and muscular layers. As with other forms of herniations, these potential tunnels are widened as life proceeds, so that all forms of diverticulosis are more common among persons in the later decades of life. Some individuals display great numbers of diverticula of the gastrointestinal tract, from esophagus to anus, but more often diverticula of the stomach and small intestine are solitary; they are more common in the duodenum (in possibly 5 percent of all persons having barium studies of this area), next most frequent in the jejunum, and rare in the ileum, except for Meckel's diverticulum.

Diverticula of the duodenum are most commonly found on the medial surface of the second portion of the duodenum, in close proximity to the entrance of the pancreatic and common ducts. They are usually wide-necked, about 1 cm in diameter, and appear to fill with and expel intestinal contents with ease.

The location of duodenal diverticula constitutes the main reason for suspecting their pathogenicity. Although statistically few patients harboring these common outpouchings suffer any misfortune from their presence, there are documented cases in which obstruction to the neck of the diverticulum has led to acute diverticulitis, hemorrhage, and necrosis of the wall; pressure exerted by obstructed diverticula on pancreatic ducts has definitely resulted in acute pancreatitis, pressure on the common duct in obstructive jaundice. When diverticula occur along the third portion of the duodenum they have occasionally been the site of acute inflammation and free perforation, with consequent peritonitis.

Diverticula of the jejunum, while less common, seem to be more subject to the development of acute inflammation and necrosis of the wall, with severe upper abdominal pain and occasionally massive intestinal hemorrhage ensuing. The acute process may go on to suppurate; a definite mass and localized peritonitis are the accompanying physical findings. Another way in which multiple diverticula of the jejunum may result in disease is the effective replacement of normal absorbing jejunal surface by multiple bacteria-filled sacs, resulting in a characteristic malabsorption syndrome due to loss of surface and competitive loss of nutrients to the saprophytic bacteria in the diverticula (Fig. 317-1) (see Chap. 316).

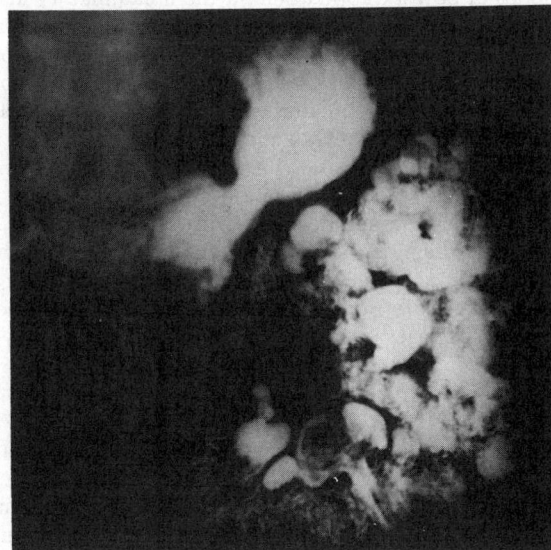

Fig. 317-1. Multiple diverticula of jejunum in 55 year-old man with macrocytic anemia.

Meckel's diverticulum, resulting from persistence of the omphalomesenteric duct, is reasonably common, occurring in about 3 percent of all laparotomized children in whom a definite search is made and in about 2 percent of autopsied adults. Even though only a small percentage of these diverticula cause trouble, the possibility must be thought of in every case of gastrointestinal hemorrhage and obstruction. The diverticula are usually found on the antimesenteric border within the last 90 cm of the ileum, and most frequently within 50 cm of the ileocecal valve. They may be wide-mouthed or narrow, short or long, sometimes a nubbin hard to find on the smooth surface of the ileum, occasionally a long 10- to 20-cm funnel attached like a stout pipe to the umbilicus. Diverticula lying within the mesentery are rare and do not arise from the omphalomesenteric duct. The diverticulum may be lined with normal ileal mucosa, or it may contain varying amounts of ectopic gastric, pancreatic, duodenal, or colonic epithelium. Symptoms are more common in males by at least 3:1. Coincident malformations are infrequently met. There is no hereditary pattern. In children and adolescents, bleeding from this epithelium is the striking clinical feature, with or without the presence of a palpable mass. The source of bleeding is almost invariably an ulceration, and this is generally of peptic origin. The gastric mucosa in Meckel's diverticulum has been shown to secrete acid peptic juice, which acts on bordering ileal epithelium to produce the ulcer. Pathologically the ulcer is always near the junction of gastric and ileal mucosa, on the ileal side; it thus resembles the usual anastomotic ulcer occurring after gastrojejunostomy. In the young adult the clinical picture begins to change, inflammatory processes becoming more prominent, and varying degrees of intestinal obstruction, either of the ileum proximal to the diverticulum or of neighboring loops of bowel trapped behind the inflammatory mass, constitute the most serious presenting symptoms. Free perforation of Meckel's diverticulum is relatively uncommon, but sealed-off localized perforations are very common once the initial inflammatory process has distorted the bowel enough to set up the pathologic requisites for cyclic bouts of inflammation. A number of these patients have repeated bouts of low-grade abdominal cramps referred to the infraumbilical area, usually aggravated by eating. The diagnosis is rarely made by x-ray studies of the small or large intestine, but these are necessary in order to eliminate other possible lesions. The treatment is entirely surgical.

BRUNNER'S GLAND HYPERTROPHY

Occasionally one notes on radiologic examination a cobblestone appearance of the duodenal bulb caused by hypertrophy of Brunner's glands, submucosal structures secreting an alkaline mucoid material of unknown function, highly viscid, and apparently affording a mechanical protective action to the duodenum as it receives acid chyme. Most patients showing this hypertrophy have no evidence of disordered duodenal function, but occasionally they have peptic symptoms.

MOTOR DISTURBANCES

OBSTRUCTIVE SYNDROMES. The natural tendency of smooth muscle when operating against a pressure gradient is to stretch and contract forcibly. This increased distension is pain-producing (see Chap. 12, Abdominal Pain). Thus all syndromes in which normal small bowel is trying to force luminal contents past nonrelaxing segments of more distal bowel, whether occasioned by a tumor, a stricture, an occluding gallstone, or a constricting band, are primarily characterized by painful cramps at the onset, progressing to loss of pain sensation as the bowel loses its viability. Associated with the progress of events are many others which may assume prominent roles in coloring the symptoms evoked. Intermittent jejunal or ileal obstruction, with poor maintenance of oil-water interfaces, will lead to malabsorption (see Chaps. 12, Abdominal Pain, and 318, Acute Intestinal Obstruction).

Motor abnormalities of the duodenum associated with many psychic disturbances (e.g., anorexia nervosa) or with generalized disorders like lupus erythematosus may result in severe bouts of nausea and vomiting. The radiologist may get the impression of an organic obstruction of the third portion of the duodenum at the point at which the superior mesenteric vessels cross anterior to the gut. Such impressions have given rise to many diagnoses of "mesenteric root compression syndrome" which fail to be borne out on surgical exploration to remove the source of the obstruction. It is important to understand that an atonic or sluggish duodenum proximal to this "compressed" area will of itself produce the apparent obstructive picture, just as gastric atony may make a normal pyloric area appear to be "obstructing." Only if the peristaltic activity of the first and second portions of the duodenum is normal or hyperactive can one suspect an organic obstruction of the third portion of the duodenum. If this is identified, exploration is indicated and a bypassing operation justified.

STASIS. Complete stasis of the duodenum occurs rarely, usually in association with mesenteric vascular catastrophes. On x-ray examination, dilatation of the duodenum with a peculiar churning of the barium meal is characteristically noted in the patient with anorexia nervosa and, occasionally, in those suffering from severe ulcerative colitis. Elsewhere in the small intestine, stasis is the result of loss of vascular integrity, and exhaustion following mechanical or paralytic ileus (Chap. 318).

SPASM. Spasm of the duodenum occurs in peptic disorders, acute pancreatitis, or in various conditions associated with severe nausea. Experimental nausea, as, for example, that produced by vestibular stimulation, gives characteristically a tetanic spasm of the duodenum.

PAIN. Migratory or steady pain around the umbilicus may result from *insufficiency of the mesenteric vessels,* usually as a result of degenerative aortic disease encroaching on the lumina of the vessels.

REGIONAL ENTERITIS (Crohn's Disease)

The most disabling and discouraging affliction of the small intestine known to the internist is regional enteritis, an unpredictable granulomatous response of the submucosa to an unknown agent or agents, in which damage is done by encroachment upon the lumen, scaring of the muscle, ulceration of the mucosa, and necrotic breakdown with fistula formation between loops of bowel, bowel and skin, and bowel and perirectal spaces. Any, all, or none of these sequelae may follow the initial bout of the disease, and single attacks are well documented. Much more common, however, is recurrence and slow spread of the lesion to involve contiguous areas of the intestine, including occasionally the duodenum. Involvement of the antrum of the stomach by a similar process has been described.

Since the original description by Crohn, Ginzburg, and Oppenheimer in 1932, in which this disorder was localized to the terminal ileum, a number of different clinical syndromes have been distinguished from the classic forms, but our knowledge is far from satisfactory as to causes, course, and proper management.

EPIDEMIOLOGY. The disorder is worldwide in distribution and occurs among all races. In the United States its exact incidence is unknown, but it appears to be about one-fifth as common as chronic ulcerative colitis. It has been reported as having its onset in every decade of life, the peak incidence being between the ages of fifteen and thirty-five. Both sexes are affected, with equal frequency; Negroes are less commonly affected than whites.

The affected subjects are more often of Jewish origin than one would expect by chance; in some series Jews appear to be about three times as commonly involved as their distribution in the population at large would

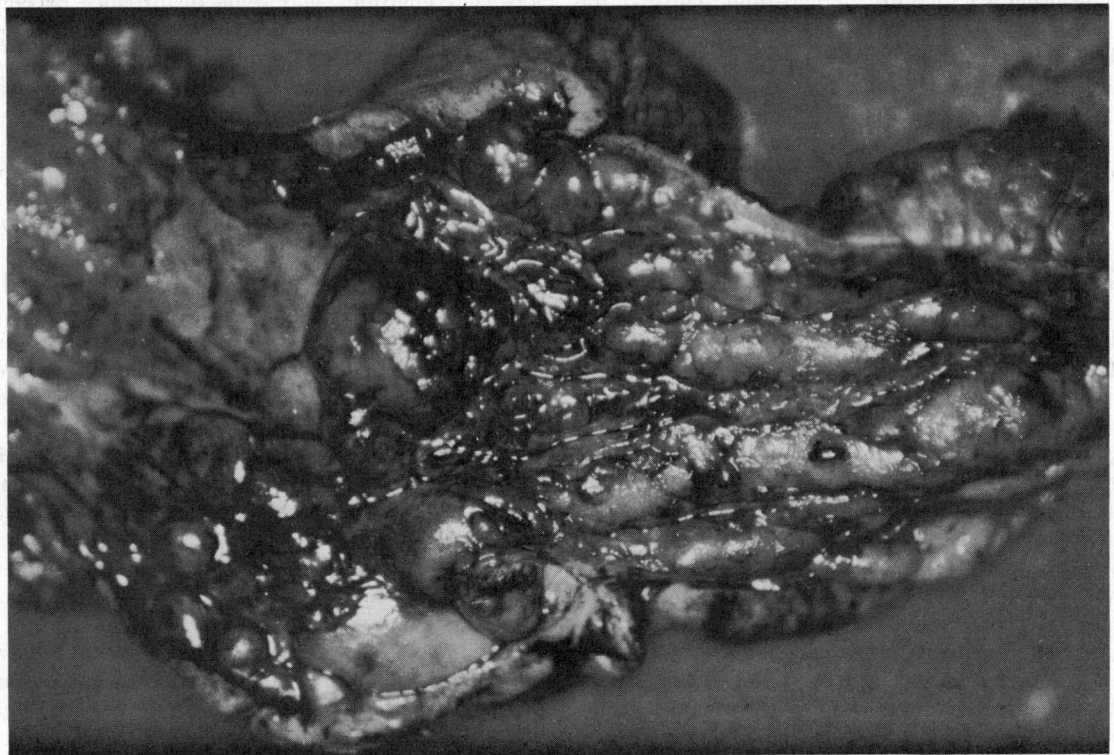

Fig. 317-2. Regional enteritis: resected specimen of ileocecal area demonstrating the hypertrophy of ileai submucosa (*right*), with nodular encroachment on the lumen and minute areas of mucosal hemorrhage.

suggest. The patients show urban backgrounds more commonly than rural and reach higher levels of schooling than usual and slightly higher economic status than ordinarily encountered. Despite some evidence to the contrary, severely disturbed personalities are not routinely met with in these patients, particularly early in the course of the disease or antedating the onset of the disease. Many such patients show remarkable fortitude in meeting the innumerable difficulties wrought by progressive destruction of the intestine; a number have distinguished themselves in the arts, sciences, professions, and business despite prolonged and progressive disease.

Familial occurrence of the disease has been recognized from the onset. In various series the percentage of cases occurring in siblings ranges from 2 to 10; father-daughter, mother-son, and father-son patterns are recorded in all large series of cases. The onset of disease in the child does not exhibit anticipation, and other associated stigmas are so rare as to make it unlikely that genetic factors are of more than predisposing importance.

ETIOLOGY AND PATHOGENESIS. No specific cause of this disease has been identified. Investigations have been carried out on the possible etiologic relationship of bacterial and viral organisms identified no more frequently in the gastrointestinal tract of these patients than in normal subjects, but all such studies have been fruitless. Certain disorders of the mesenteric arteries seen in the aging population have occasionally given rise to a sub-mucosal inflammatory and cicatricial reaction producing a picture similar to that of regional enteritis, but in the majority of cases of regional enteritis no such arterial lesions can be found. The enlarged and succulent lymph nodes of the mesentery seem to result from the submucosal inflammation rather than cause it; remarkable alterations in the autonomic ganglions of the bowel wall, frequently seen in excised specimens, are rarely present early in the course of the disease. Histochemical studies are remarkably normal, particularly with respect to the columnar epithelium of the bowel luminal surface. Noncaseating tubercles are found in about half the cases in the bowel submucosa and in the serosa; these show giant cells but no evidence of fungi or inclusion bodies. The fistulous tracts usually show only granulation tissue and a purulent response.

The earliest lesions, as seen in the terminal ileum, are rarely minute and more usually involve appreciable (6 to 20 cm) lengths of gut in a swollen beefy glistening mass, occasionally rather purplish, but more often intensely red. The serosa is often injected and the mesenteric fat edematous. Large lymph nodes in the mesentery nearby are commonly noted. The luminal surface of the bowel is thrown up into injected folds stretched over the heaped-up submucosal hypertrophy (Fig. 317-2). Ulceration of this mucosa, although common, is usually superficial in the early stages of the disease, when microscopically the nonulcerated areas of mucosa appear healthy.

There is usually a definite demarcation between the diseased and healthy bowel; the appendix may be involved by a similar process or may merely show lymphoid hyperplasia and venous congestion as a result of the adjacent inflammatory reaction. The initial process may disappear rather quickly, may remain indolent only to flare up months or years later, or may slowly progress to involve ileal segments more cephalad. "Skips" are well-documented in which an initial ileal lesion subsides and a midjejunal lesion of similar character develops later, the intervening area remaining uninvolved. Adjacent or contiguous small or large intestine may be involved, if not invaded, by this inflammatory process; cicatrization, local perforations, abscesses, and fistulas commonly characterize the development of such a process. The fistulas may go from intestine to colon, from intestine to skin, or from one loop of intestine to another. Loops low in the pelvis or involving sigmoid colon may fistulize into the adnexae or vagina and produce perirectal or ischiorectal abscesses, perirectal nodular masses seen on proctoscopy, or a patchy proctitis.

A number of changes—endothelial cell proliferation in lymphatics, giant-cell aggregations in the edematous submucosa, ischemic contraction of smaller arterioles, and increased numbers of ganglion cells and neurofibrillar accumulations—occur characteristically in surgical and autopsy material and in such profusion as to render the pathologic diagnosis of the disease easy to make. However, the primacy of any one of these changes, or even the proper sequence of lesions, is not clear.

The endothelial reaction in lymphatics and the presence of granulomas have suggested to many that the disease must be a reaction to some irritant absorbed in the lymphatics; the absence of foreign bodies in the giant cells would lead one not to suspect particulate foreign matter as the offending agent; attempts have been made to produce the disease experimentally by abnormal fatty substances, but so far these studies have been fruitless. There is little evidence that the succulent lymph nodes seen in the mesentery of cases of early acute ileitis are more than a phase of acute secondary lymphadenitis, rather than a reflection of an etiologic primary lymphangitis. Sarcoidosis, tuberculosis, and reaction to abdominal trauma seem unrelated to the characteristic forms of this disease, even though some of the granulomas may be indistinguishable from the characteristic lesions of these processes.

SYMPTOMS. These depend on the location of the inflammatory lesion, its extent, its acuteness, the amount of obstruction it produces, the peritoneal reaction, if any, and its relationship to contiguous structures. A certain number of such patients may present only with the systemic features of a febrile illness without localizing symptoms or signs. Even in these cases, a careful history will often document abdominal discomfort, loose stools, rectal urgency, and mild anorexia made worse by the feeling that abdominal discomfort increases after eating. Spondylitis occurs in a small percentage.

Acute ileitis presents as the sudden development of right lower quadrant pain and tenderness, with fever,

localized guarding, and some disturbance of bowel motility—either diarrhea or constipation. It thus presents the clinical picture of appendicitis, and the differential diagnosis can be made only at laparotomy, when the characteristic beefy red terminal ileum, boggy mesenteric fat, and succulent lymph nodes of the mesentery tell the surgeon that appendicitis alone could not produce the picture. The appendix also may be involved in the primary lesion, or it may be obstructed secondarily by the acute submucosal edema of the adjacent ileitis.

In one large series, diarrhea, colicky pain, and weight loss were encountered as presenting symptoms in over two-thirds of 600 patients. Fever occurred in one-third, and a history of bright red rectal bleeding or melena in less than one-sixth. Symptoms related to rectal and anal complications predominated in about 10 percent.

Approximately half the patients have initial involvement of the terminal ileum, another 15 percent have both ileum and cecum affected at the onset, and less than 4 percent present initial symptoms due exclusivly to jejunal or duodenal involvement. Various other combinations of jejunal, ileal, and colonic lesions may be seen at the time the patient first consults the physician.

Variants of this picture include (1) a full-blown *malabsorption syndrome* (Chap. 316) with any one or many malnutritive derangements capturing the spotlight, (2) *acute perforation and generalized peritonitis* (less than 1 percent), or (3) *massive melena*, seen in less than 2 percent of cases. The advanced case, with cutaneous fistulas, easily appreciable masses throughout the abdomen, increased pigmentation, and severe proctitis, presents little difficulty in diagnosis. Amyloidosis due to regional enteritis is becoming a more frequent complication and may be responsible for the patient's death in renal failure.

As experience with the disease as a whole has expanded, a certain number of patients have been encountered who present a diffuse involvement of jejunum and ileum when first seen. These patients have been described by Crohn as having a subtype of regional enteritis in which the lesions are more superficial but much more extensive, less prone to suppurative complications and fistula formations, but likely to lead to malabsorptive symptoms, fever, splenomegaly, and clubbing of the fingers, the reasons for which are not understood.

On physical examination these patients with enteritis characteristically display various evidences of undernutrition and malnutrition if the symptoms are of long standing. Clubbing of the fingers is frequent in this group. Special attention to the abdominal examination is necessary, since a definite mass or doughy aggregations of bowel loops can be felt in one-third of the patients. Fistulous tracts between the involved bowel and the abdominal skin are classic complications of the disease and are easily appreciated. More readily overlooked are the perirectal and ischiorectal fistulas found in nearly 10 percent of chronic cases; rectal digital examination will disclose an anorectal stricture in half of these cases and in 3 to 4 percent of those without fistulas. Proctoscopic examination is abnormal in 10 to 15 percent; the abnormalities may include nodular submucosal masses, acute proctitis, ulceration, or stricture in the rectosigmoid junction. Rectovaginal fistulas are noted in a small percentage of cases.

DIAGNOSIS. Regional enteritis should be suspected on clinical grounds in most instances when a patient presents with a history of intermittent chronic diarrhea, fever, weight loss, crampy pain, or distension and on physical examination shows abdominal masses, perianal suppuration, and anal strictures. It should be part of the differential diagnosis of all types of malabsorption (Chap. 316), fever of unexplained origin, intermittent small bowel obstruction, and secondary amyloidosis.

Laboratory features of regional enteritis parallel the severity of the (1) inflammatory reaction: leukocytosis, elevated sedimentation rate; (2) blood loss by ulceration: iron deficiency anemia; (3) undernutrition and malabsorption: hypoalbuminemia, hypocalcemia, hypokalemia, elevated serum alkaline phosphatase level, hypoprothrombinemia, and macrocytic anemia; (4) possibly more specific changes related to disturbed protein metabolism: increased seromucoids in the serum and hypergammaglobulinemia. The inflammatory lesion may cause a continual leak of albumin from the blood, leading to hypoalbuminemia. None of these laboratory tests is diagnostic.

The most helpful adjunct to the clinician suspicious of regional enteritis is the radiologist, who generally establishes the diagnosis short of histologic confirmation. Marshak and Wolf have tried to separate the nonstenotic phase of regional enteritis from the stenotic phase on radiologic grounds, despite the fact that occasionally both phases may be encountered in the same patient. In the nonstenotic phase the principal changes are loss of detail in the mucosa, stiffening of the submucosa to form a tubular pattern on the radiograph, and separation of the tubular loops by inflammation in the mesentery. The stenotic phase is characterized by narrowing of the lumen, with dilatation of normal bowel proximally. In the dilated area poor oil-water interfaces and retained mucus secretions produce abnormal puddling of the barium. Fistulous tracts are often seen, particularly in the ileocecal area, and are virtually diagnostic, the only other disease likely to produce a similar picture being actinomycosis. When the duodenum or upper jejunum is involved by regional enteritis, the stenotic phase predominates from the onset, whereas ileal involvement characteristically is nonstenotic and ulcerative early in its course (Fig. 317-3). The unoperated case usually demonstrates little radiologic change after the first studies are completed, except for fistula formation.

Definitive diagnosis on histologic grounds is established under the microscope, although most surgeons can make an accurate diagnosis by inspection at the operating table of the beefy reddish-to-bluish serosa, edematous mesentery, and large lymph nodes. Differential diagnosis in the operating room includes tuberculosis, various lymphomas, sarcoidosis, and fungous diseases. Biopsies of the bowel and lymph nodes provide adequate bases for histologic diagnosis.

COURSE AND PROGNOSIS. Acute regional ileitis appar-

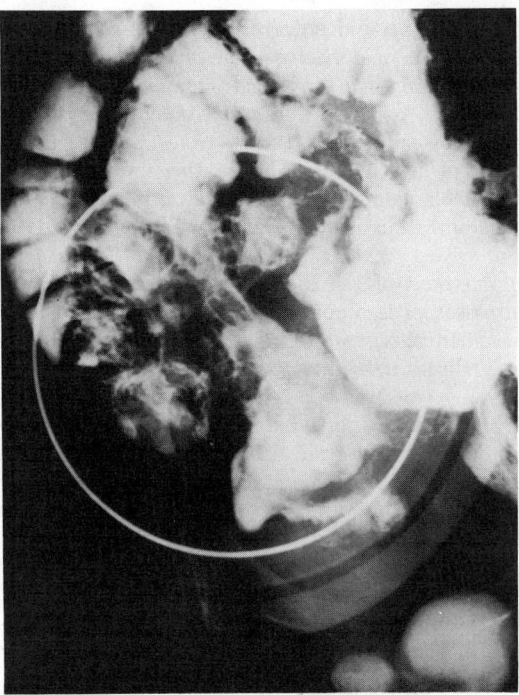

Fig. 317-3. Regional enteritis. Several involved loops of ileum communicate via multiple fistulous tracts. Small bowel proximal to involved areas is dilated (*upper*).

ently is self-limited in over two-thirds of the cases; the remaining one-third go on to develop chronic enteritis. Since many patients first operated upon for seemingly acute symptoms present to the surgeon the picture of *chronic* disease with acute exacerbation, reported differences in the course of patients so operated upon must reflect differences in the criteria for making the diagnosis of "acute" disease.

Accurate prognostication in this disease is at present impossible, largely because there exists no large body of cases treated entirely supportively in the atmosphere of a sanatorium. Almost every large series of cases consists of a heterogeneous population of enteritis of different longevity, severity, and past nutritional and pharmaceutical experience, 90 percent of whom require surgery for some complication of the original disease. Our prognostications, then, must be made on the basis of surgically treated patients subjected to a wide variety of therapeutic procedures at widely varying periods of disease, with interim periods of varying supportive therapy. The extent of the intestinal lesions in an unoperated case tends to remain at the level present when the patient was first seen, except for the development of fistulas. If operation is carried out to remove the entire diseased bowel, as was the custom soon after the disease was first identified, approximately half the cases have a recurrence of the disease within a few years of the operation. Whether this is due to failure at operation to recognize "skip" areas of enteritis proximal to the resected area or whether new foci of enteritis develop in hitherto normal bowel is not clear. In any case, the physician should expect a patient with regional enteritis to have exacerbations and remissions over a period of many years; these exacerbations usually involve the same areas of bowel established as diseased in the first attack, but ulceration, fistulas, and stenosis may supervene at any time. Extension of these suppurative and necrotic lesions to neighboring loops of small bowel, colon, bladder, and perirectal tissues may be constantly suspected and looked for by the physician.

Involvement of the colon by a granulomatous inflammatory process is reported by some workers in half their cases of enteritis, and there is no question that primary Crohn's disease of the colon is a definite entity (see Chap. 320).

Involvement of more distant organs and organ systems unrelated to the intestine has been reported with increasing frequency as these patients have been studied more closely over a long time span. Liver abnormalities and nodular pancreatitis have been reported, but their relation to the primary disease is dubious in view of the transfusions, injections, and drugs these patients receive and of the many nutritional deficiencies they incur. More significant is the incidence of arthritic symptoms which also are noted in a proportion of cases of ulcerative colitis. The arthritis involves larger joints and is often of the spondylitis type, unaccompanied by the laboratory data suggestive of rheumatoid disease.

TREATMENT. In a chronic disease of unknown cause and unpredictable course, medical management of the most comprehensive type is mandatory. Regardless of the validity of the theory that psychiatric disorder underlies or determines the onset and progression of this disease, it is clear that careful attention to personality factors must proceed *pari passu* with meticulous attempts to meet the nutritional requirements of these patients. These must be combined to assure physical and mental rest as part of the program for combating the discouraging periods during which all efforts of physician and patient seem unable to slow the progress of the process. Psychiatric assistance will be needed in evaluating a number of these cases and should form the principal management in a small percentage. Supportive care consists first of all in explaining to the patient the problem which faces him, the relatively limited areas in which pharmacologic and surgical maneuvers can aid him, and yet at the same time repeatedly pointing out that adequate hyperalimentation, rest, and the more specific measures can enable him to "ride out" the disease; it is generally true that the activity of the disease does slow down after a number of years, at which time the patient will have residua demonstrable on x-ray and physical examination but will be able to lead a reasonably normal life. For women it should be made clear that pregnancy is not something to avoid; many women with severe ileitis but with a genuine wish to have children have produced normal offspring without undue hazard to themselves. Even menstrual function seems preserved better in women with ileitis than in those with ulcerative colitis.

Specific Measures. Chemotherapeutic and antibiotic drugs are of assistance in managing the purulent complications of enteritis but have little or no effect on the primary disease process. Nonabsorbable sulfonamides have been the most beneficial of these agents.

Treatment with corticosteroids may be dramatic in the acute phase of this disease and is of value often in converting a subacute obstructing lesion into a nonstenotic one. Radiologic improvement may not parallel the clinical response. The use of corticosteroids with salicylazosulfapyridine as in ulcerative colitis should be continued in this disease if the initial response is favorable; not only can surgical intervention be postponed by the use of this form of therapy, but there is suggestive evidence that long-term administration of anti-inflammatory agents can hold this disease in check for months and perhaps years. It is certainly worth trying.

Surgical therapy, originally used solely for the complications of a then little-understood process, has gone through a number of stages only to return full circle to its original status. In the 15 years from 1932 to 1947, surgical therapy was thought to effect a cure of the disease; radical resection of the involved ileocecal area in the original group of patients with disease localized there was advocated as curative. As the years went by, however, not only did a high percentage of these patients return with a recurrent disease, but more diffuse lesions were encountered than at the first operation, making eradication surgically impossible. A more conservative surgical approach was then devised, essentially consisting of enterocolostomy without resection. Although the operative mortality and immediate postoperative morbidity from this procedure has been satisfactorily low, it is difficult to state that the recurrence rate among these patients is much lower (about 33 percent) than among those treated with radical excision (about 40 percent). Whether these recurrences result from spread outward of foci of disease not seen at the time of operation or from some ill-understood activation of the disease process by newly contiguous bowel is not clear. Unfortunately, once a recurrence has occurred following operation, every subsequent surgical maneuver tends to result in recurrence.

Since surgical measures are not curative, they have now returned to their original place in the therapy of enteritis, as a means of eliminating complications of the disease which are producing serious symptoms on their own. Among these are intermittent intestinal obstruction, blind loops leading to macrocytic anemia, ulcerating lesions in fixed stenotic bowel, and fistulas between the bowel and adjacent hollow viscera.

The sequelae of resections of the small intestine have been of considerable interest in throwing light on the mechanisms of nutrient absorption. The physician taking care of a patient with unoperated enteritis must have a good understanding of the nutritional derangements produced by the disease; when that patient has lost, in addition, a sizable segment of his small intestine by resection, the physician must be very much more alert in detecting and correcting the multitude of nutritional defects which inevitably result (see Chap. 316).

UNUSUAL DISORDERS OF THE SMALL INTESTINE

Pneumatosis Cystoides Intestinalis

This is a rare disease involving small or large intestine, predominantly the former, in a process characterized by numerous gas-filled cysts forming subserosally and occasionally in the muscularis. Some of these cysts originate because of migration of air, largely nitrogen, from other lesions of the gut, principally obstructive in type, e.g., pyloric stenosis, regional enteritis, or tumors, or from traumatic perforations, including sigmoidoscopy or biopsy. The cyst walls may contain giant-cell systems. Most, however, have been called primary; gas analyses of their endothelial-lined cysts were highly variable, and a number of theories to account for them had been invoked before Keyting called attention to the possibility that they might be produced from primary pulmonary alveolar rupture, the resulting free air tracking backward into the mediastinum and thence downward along the retroperitoneal spaces and out along the mesenteric vascular network until it reaches the intestinal wall.

Symptoms are primarily abdominal pain, bloody diarrhea, or the sudden onset of pneumoperitoneum from rupture of a cyst. Diagnosis is usually made radiologically, the cysts deforming the bowel lumen in a characteristic way.

Treatment is to attack the underlying disease when possible. Conservative management of these patients is usually successful insofar as the cystic disease is concerned, but the underlying process may require surgical intervention.

Mesenteric Arterial Insufficiency

The splanchnic area is supplied with arterial blood by the celiac axis, superior mesenteric, and inferior mesenteric arteries. In recent years, as the population of older persons has increased, a growing number of patients presenting ischemic symptoms referred to the periumbilical and general abdominal area has been observed. Gradual luminal encroachment by atherosclerotic or other degenerative changes in the aorta or in any two of these three arteries can produce these painful syndromes, initially brought on 1 or 2 hr after eating, but with further progression resulting in pain that is not only steady but often agonizing. The relationship of pain to food discourages the sufferer from eating; weight loss is therefore prominent. In addition, chronic arterial insufficiency may produce mucosal and mural deterioration, leading to malabsorption, which aggravates the weight loss. When the symptoms are intermittent, the term *abdominal angina* is often used, but this rarely remains static for long, going on either to the development of adequate collateral circulation or to the production of mesenteric infarction. The diagnosis may be confirmed by mesenteric angiography, which is not without serious risk in these patients, of course, but the disease is life-threatening. The only definitive treatment is surgical removal of the obstruction or the construction of bypass arterial grafts to the ischemic bowel.

Stenosing Ulcers of the Small Intestine

Although the existence of rare solitary and unexplained ulcers of the small intestine has been recognized for many years, a recent sharp increase in their incidence has led to studies which appear to implicate a vascular factor producing ischemic necrosis of the mucosa in one or more areas of the small bowel. Most of these newly recognized ulcers occur in patients receiving enteric-coated tablets of materials recognized to be highly caustic to mucosa; the most commonly identified material has been potassium chloride, given routinely to patients receiving chronic diuretic therapy. The symptoms are those of abdominal pain and obstruction, rarely with peritonitis and perforation. The treatment is discontinuance of the medication and surgical excision of the damaged segment if symptoms warrant. Sometimes severe atherosclerotic disease of the mesenteric vessels is the underlying cause.

Protein-losing Enteropathy. See Chap. 316.

TUMORS OF THE SMALL INTESTINE

Generally, this is an infrequently occurring group of lesions, but because of the variety of symptoms they produce, they may be very difficult to diagnose. It is perhaps best to describe them according to their pathology, since any or all of them may produce identical symptoms.

Benign Tumors

Leiomyomas of clinical significance are rare in the small intestine, but they may produce intussusception with obstruction, ulceration and hemorrhage, with fatal outcome, or varying degrees of intestinal obstruction alone. The mucosa becomes stretched tightly over these solid tumors and frequently ulcerates to produce gastrointestinal hemorrhage of mild to fatal severity. Malignant change may occur at any time.

Hemangiomas of the small intestine, although rare, are very difficult to identify by clinical methods or radiologic examination. When they bleed suddenly into the bowel wall, they often collapse, so that they do not present to radiologic study any space-occupying defect in the barium-filled bowel. Here mesenteric angiography may be very successful in demonstrating the tumor and its leakage of contrast material into the lumen. The occurrence of these various syndromes as hereditary disorders is well documented, and a hint as to the existence of an intestinal hemangioma may well be gleaned from identification of hemangiomas of the skin or mucous membrane.

Lipomas are more common than leiomyomas or hemangiomas in the small intestine and, like them, may be involved in developmental anomalies of supporting tissues in the bowel and elsewhere. Although a number of these could be considered to be hamartomas, they do exhibit the neoplastic ability to grow and expand. Characteristically, they are found in middle adult life, although they may have been growing slowly for many years before making clinical mischief. Sex incidence is probably equal. It is probable that they arise from adipose tissue anywhere in the body. Since the mesentery of the small intestine contains a large amount of such tissue, a variety of lipomas involving the wall of the bowel to produce obstruction have been documented.

Polypoid tumors of the small intestine usually turn out to be hamartomas. These have been thoroughly studied as part of the Peutz-Jeghers syndrome (see Chap. 109). Such tumors are rarely malignant but may cause intussusception and hemorrhage.

Malignant Tumors

Malignant tumors of the small intestine are not common in the United States, accounting for less than 1 percent of all digestive tract cancers. In Africa, on the other hand, primary tumors of the small intestine have been described among some races as more common than carcinoma of the stomach.

Adenocarcinoma of the duodenum is more frequent as an independent lesion than is carcinoma of the jejunum or ileum. However, in recent years diffuse carcinomas of the small bowel have been described in patients with long-standing regional enteritis. The most frequently involved area of duodenum is the second, near the papilla of Vater. The tumor usually causes ulceration with hemorrhage or high obstruction and may be easily confused radiologically with chronic peptic ulcer in the same area. Carcinoma of the jejunoileum may present as diffuse foci of intestinal obstruction due to early metastases to the peritoneum, as ascites, or as a malabsorption syndrome.

Argentaffine tumors are found in 0.5 percent of all surgically removed appendixes, as a yellowish indurated area. They are the most common epithelial tumors of the small intestine and may appear anywhere from the duodenum to the colon. They arise from argentaffin cells in the crypts of Lieberkühn and grow as clumps or strands of small closely packed polyhedral cells. The degree to which these tumors are regarded as malignant varies among pathologists, but there is increasing recognition of their invasive tendencies. They are often multiple, but when solitary some 60 percent arise in the ileum, enlarging to form plaques projecting into the muscularis and serosa. Adenofibrosis of the surrounding tissues accompanies this spread so that ulceration from the luminal spread and compromise of the lumen by pressure of the inflammatory reaction may produce the symptoms. They are tumors of middle age, more common in males. Remote spread is infrequent and late. For some reason, lesions of the duodenum tend less to invade surrounding tissues. When metastases invade the liver, the characteristic *carcinoid syndrome* results (see Chap. 105).

Lymphosarcoma, which may develop in any region where lymphoid tissue is present, is an important invader of the small intestine. Reticulum cell sarcoma usually develops in retroperitoneal lymph nodes, secondarily involving the bowel; localized lymphosarcoma usually involves the ileum as a solid bulky tumor which may cause ileal obstruction. It may remain stationary for a long time and can produce an x-ray picture simulating that of localized ileitis. When it spreads, it does so slowly, to regional lymph nodes. Hodgkin's granuloma and sarcoma may invade any organ in the body, but they rarely cause localized lesions in the small intestine. Enlarged retroperitoneal nodes may distort the x-ray picture of the upper small intestine, but localized infiltrations are uncommon.

Both *liposarcomas and leiomyosarcomas* are infrequently encountered in the small intestine. The symptoms may be the same as those of the benign tumors or of any malignant lesion.

Diagnosis

Tumors of the small intestine should be thought of in the differential diagnosis of obstructive syndromes of any type, of gastrointestinal bleeding, and of malabsorptive states. They are less likely to cause fever than is regional enteritis or tuberculosis, but in all other respects benign inflammatory disease, benign tumors, and malignant tumors of this organ can produce identical clinical syndromes. The reason for this is not hard to find, since most symptoms are due to (1) ulceration of mucosa with bleeding, (2) obstruction of the lumen behind which mucosal bowel wall contracts forcibly, giving rise to crampy pain, (3) necrosis and inflammation of the wall, giving rise to persistent pain and tender masses, (4) interference with intraluminal, mucosal, and lymphatic aspects of digestion and absorption of nutrients, producing abnormal stools, weight loss, anorexia, vomiting, and occasionally intestinal obstruction.

Radiologic techniques designed to differentiate localized from generalized lesions, pressure of enlarged nodes or inflammatory abscesses on the intestines, "deficiency patterns" and flocculation of barium in the bowel lumen, distortion of outlines of the bowel by stiffened mesentery —all these may be of the greatest diagnostic assistance or may indicate in only a general way the nature of the underlying disease.

Localization of a specific bleeding point may be achieved either by use of a long plastic tube through which intraluminal contents are aspirated and tested for blood or, especially if bleeding is brisk, by mesenteric angiography of the celiac axis or superior mesenteric artery.

Careful microscopic and chemical testing of the stools may confirm the presence or absence of an inflammatory exudate, cancer cells, and malabsorbed or maldigested foodstuffs, as well as blood, abnormal concretions, or parasites.

If a diagnosis of tumor is made presumptively or if symptoms persist and no diagnosis can be arrived at, laparotomy is indicated. Therapy for most of the tumors described is entirely surgical. In the case of lymphomas and lymphosarcomas, local removal and general irradiation or chemotherapy are employed.

REFERENCES

Bockus, H. L. (Ed.): Regional enteritis, Chap. 50, in "Gastroenterology," 2d ed., vol. 2, Philadelphia, W. B. Saunders Company, 1964.

Boley, S. J., L. Schultz, H. Krieger, S. Schwartz, A. Elguezabal, and A. C. Allen: Experimental Evaluation of Thiazides and Potassium as a Cause of Small-bowel Ulcer, J.A.M.A., 192:93, 1965.

Chanoine, F.: Contribution à l'étude des tumeurs malignes-primitives du jéjuno-ileon, Acta Gastroenterol. Belg., 18: 163, 1955.

Crohn, B. B., and H. Yarnis: "Regional Ileitis," 2d ed., New York, Grune & Stratton, Inc., 1958.

Fry, W. J., and R. O. Kraft: Visceral Angina, Surg. Gynecol. Obstet., 117:417, 1963.

Gump, F. E., M. Lepore, and H. G. Baker: A Revised Concept of Acute Regional Enteritis, Ann. Surg. 166:942, 1967.

Keyting, W. S., R. R. McCarver, J. L. Kovarik, and A. L. Waywitt: Pneumatosis Intestinalis: A New Concept, Radiology, 76:733, 1961.

Soderlund, S.: Meckel's Diverticulum, Acta Chir. Scand. Suppl. 248, 1959.

Stahlgren, L. H., and L. K. Ferguson: The Results of Surgical Treatment of Chronic Regional Enteritis, J.A.M.A., 175:986, 1961.

318   ACUTE INTESTINAL OBSTRUCTION

Albert I. Mendeloff and
Arnold M. Seligman

DEFINITION. Acute intestinal obstruction may be defined as a failure of progression of intestinal contents, whether due to mechanical causes or to inadequacy of intestinal muscular activity.

ETIOLOGY. The most useful classification is based on the immediate need for surgical or medical therapy. The *mechanical* type of intestinal obstruction usually requires surgical intervention for its correction. This type is due either to intraluminal obstruction by foreign bodies, gallstones, meconium, bezoars, enteroliths, and worms or to mural obstruction due to encroachment by compression of the intestinal wall, such as in adhesions, stenosis, hernia, volvulus, intussusception, tumors, and atresia. *Nonmechanical obstruction* is referred to as *ileus*. Ileus is either adynamic (paralytic) or dynamic (spastic).

Adynamic ileus occurs (1) reflexly after certain surgical manipulations, diagnostic studies such as retrograde pyelography, or trauma; (2) secondary to peritoneal insult by chemical agents (hydrochloric acid or blood), pancreatic enzymes, or bacterial agents; (3) as the result of metabolic changes secondary to generalized dislocation of electrolyte equilibrium, especially abnormally low serum potassium levels, interference with the enzymes and coenzymes involved in acetylcholine synthesis (pantothenic acid), or drug effects (especially ganglionic blocking agents); (4) following mechanical *hypoactivity* in which the musculature of the intestinal wall loses its functional integrity on the basis of localized hypoxia secondary to compromised blood supply. This can happen suddenly as a result of arterial spasm secondary to venous or arterial thrombosis or embolism of intestinal vasculature, or more slowly when obstructing factors progress to a degree that embarrasses the arterial or venous blood flow through localized portions of the bowel.

Spastic ileus is an uncommon form of mechanical *hyperactivity* of the normal bowel behind a spastic segment or segments of the gut. It is seen in toxic conditions such as uremia, heavy metal poisoning, porphyria, infections, and extensive ulcerations.

Untreated ileus with progressive distension enhances mechanical obstruction as well as circulatory embarrassment in the wall of the involved segment. In this way partial mechanical occlusion may progress to complete obstruction and eventually strangulation.

SYMPTOMS. Acute mechanical intestinal obstruction is characterized by colicky pain, nausea, vomiting, distension, and constipation or obstipation. Obstruction high in the intestinal tract produces earlier and more severe vomiting, whereas obstruction low in the intestinal tract produces earlier obstipation, more distension, and later vomiting. When obstruction is accompanied by strangulation, the pain is more severe and constant, and evidence of sepsis soon develops. Diagnosis of the strangulation is relatively easy when a large segment of bowel is involved, but the diagnosis of devitalized bowel, although equally important, is difficult when only a few centimeters of bowel is involved. When the obstruction is primarily due to adynamic ileus, pain is absent, obstipation is present, and discomfort results when distension is severe enough to cause a tight abdomen, at which time tachypnea, tachycardia, and oliguria are the result of pooling of fluids in the intestinal lumen and interference with diaphragmatic respiration.

Pain in acute mechanical obstruction of the small bowel is referred to the midabdomen and occurs in severe paroxysms that reach a crescendo and cease abruptly. In acute mechanical obstruction of the large bowel, colicky pain is less severe and is referred to the lower part of the abdomen. When the ileocecal valve is competent, distension is confined to the colon, and vomiting occurs late if at all. As distension progresses, the intensity of the pain decreases, and the paroxysms becomes less frequent. When strangulation supervenes, the discomfort becomes constant, and pain becomes more localized to the quadrant of the abdomen in which the strangulated loop of bowel resides.

Vomiting occurs earlier and is more severe, the higher the obstruction in the intestinal tract. High obstructions results in earlier dehydration and alkalosis due to loss of hydrochloric acid, whereas lower obstructions result in slower dehydration and loss of alkaline fluid, and they produce acidosis. Vomitus at first contains bile and mucus but later becomes brown and fecal in odor because of putrefaction of protein in the small bowel. When the ileocecal valve is competent, little or no vomiting occurs in colonic obstruction.

Obstipation results in all cases of complete obstruction after the intestinal tract distal to the obstruction is emptied. In high obstruction, the lower bowel may function quite well for a time, e.g., expelling an enema readily, whereas in low intestinal obstruction and colonic obstruction obstipation occurs early. Blood in the scanty stool suggests strangulation in low lesions. Diarrhea is not encountered, except in those rare situations where mechanical obstruction is precipitated by gastroenteritis in already mechanically embarrassed loops of intestine. When the onset of constipation is gradual but steadily increasing in severity, chronic intestinal obstruction due to encroachment on the lumen of bowel by the growth of neoplasm should be suspected. The progression of symptoms may be marked by bouts of obstipation, distension, and cramps, only to be relieved by purgation with the passage of a fecal impaction. Eventually these measures fail to give relief, and complete obstruction supervenes, with the added hazard of perforation into the peritoneal cavity of bowel proximal to the obstruction.

PHYSICAL FINDINGS. The physical findings vary from very few at the onset, to severe dehydration and alkalosis or acidosis from continued vomiting, to localized or generalized distension with abdominal tenderness after several hours of obstruction. Severe sepsis and shock revealed by pallor, sweating, cold and clammy extremities, rapid pulse, hypotension, and stupor supervene

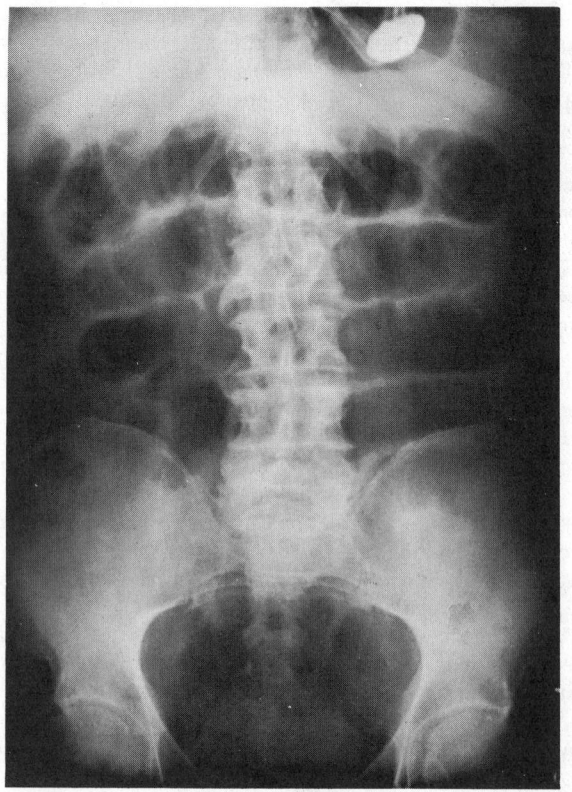

Fig. 318-1. Paralytic ileus due to thrombosis of superior mesenteric artery.

when strangulation and perforation occur. Disorientation may be one of the earliest evidences of peritonitis, especially in older persons, occurring before shock becomes manifest. Clinical evidences of shock indicate extensive fluid and blood loss into bowel lumen, bowel wall, and peritoneal cavity as well as loss of fluid by vomiting. The shock state is also produced by endotoxemia from colonic organisms in the peritoneal cavity. Shock is seen early when the intestine is infarcted, whether because of vascular occlusion or strangulation of bowel wall. Involuntary spasm of the abdominal muscles is noted only when strangulation with local peritonitis occurs and is not a prominent feature of acute obstruction. During paroxysmal painful contractions of small intestine, proximal to the point of obstruction, there is noted voluntary rigidity of the abdominal wall, but this subsides when the contraction subsides. These paroxysms of bowel contraction are accompanied by auscultatory sounds that are exaggerated, gurgle more than normal because of the abnormal amounts of fluid in the bowel, and become more high-pitched as gaseous distension increases. Sometimes one can locate the noisy proximal bowel in one quadrant of the abdomen by auscultation with a stethoscope. The sounds become more tinkling in character as the ileus progresses and distension increases. The abdomen is silent when ileus becomes adynamic, which occurs when peritonitis is superimposed or when large segments of bowel are infarcted.

Distension in high obstruction may be limited to the upper part of the abdomen and in low colonic obstruction may outline the colon. Most of the gas in the distension that accompanies acute intestinal obstruction is from swallowed air. In those who tend to swallow air readily and unconsciously, gaseous distension may develop very rapidly indeed and to a degree not only to aggravate mechanical obstruction but to endanger life by respiratory embarrassment, cardiac arrhythmias, and the precipitation of vascular insufficiency of the gut with perforation. When perforation results, it usually occurs on the antimesenteric surface.

Detection of a large heart with irregular rhythm or the definitive finding of mitral stenosis may suggest that an embolus to the superior mesenteric artery has occurred. Embolism to that artery is also suggested by a history of recent myocardial infarction, subacute bacterial endocarditis, or other embolic phenomena. In an older patient, palpation of an abdominal aortic aneurysm, evidence of defective arterial circulation to the legs, or history of diffuse abdominal pain exacerbated by eating all suggest diffuse aortic arteriosclerosis with encroachment on the lumina of vessels supplying the intestine. Rarely, periarteritis nodosa will cause thrombosis of the superior mesenteric artery or one of its branches. When portal hypertension is present, thrombosis of the portal venous bed may occur, with resultant mesenteric venous thrombosis. Polycythemia vera, postsplenectomy states, and disorders of the coagulating mechanism such as thrombotic thrombocytopenic purpura are rare but documented causes of venous mesenteric thrombosis.

ROENTGENOGRAPHIC FINDINGS. An x-ray is a very

valuable adjunct to the physical examination in demonstrating whether gas is present in loops of small bowel with or without fluid levels, whether gas is in the upper part of the small bowel or the entire small bowel, or in single loops of intestine, or primarily in the colon. A clue to the point of obstruction may be obtained often by a flat film together with a film of the patient sitting up or lying on his side. Classic radiologic evidence of obstruction of the small intestine is seen in Fig. 318-1, the stepladder distribution of distended small bowel loops being readily identified. Distension of the large bowel is usually recognized on the flat films from the distribution of the air-filled colon, the haustral markings extending not entirely down the lumen. Volvulus of the sigmoid colon presents a very characteristic radiologic picture, and various forms of internal or sliding hernias give characteristic radiologic patterns. The diagnosis may be much more difficult when low-grade or early obstruction is present or when large fecal masses obscure the picture. In low acute obstructions it is not wise to give barium by mouth, although in chronic situations contrast media can sometimes be injected through a tube in the intestinal tract to visualize the point of obstruction. If evidence points to colonic obstruction, a carefully administered barium enema will often demonstrate the point of obstruction and reveal its cause.

LABORATORY FINDINGS. Laboratory findings are usually related to the amount of necrosis, the presence of peritonitis, and other chronic diseases which may underlie the catastrophe. Leukocytosis is usually of moderate degree, the hematocrit may be high, and electrolytes are disturbed to various degrees. Lactic dehydrogenase levels in the serum are often very high in intestinal infarction. The stool may be grossly bloody if a large area of small bowel has been strangulated.

TREATMENT. Therapy consists of (1) correcting fluid and electrolyte imbalance, (2) alleviating vomiting and distension by intubation and decompression, (3) control of peritonitis, if present, and blood transfusion for shock, if present, and (4) removal of the obstruction and restoration of bowel continuity and function.

Since the efflux of fluid into the dilated gut and peritoneal cavity results in dehydration and often hemoconcentration and since chloride is lost in high obstructions and both sodium chloride and potassium chloride are lost in lower obstructions, the administration of saline solution and potassium chloride is indicated. Extra water should also be given in the form of 5 percent glucose. Because these patients have not taken anything by mouth and will not do so for several days, caloric requirements (2000 per day) must be met by continuous infusion of glucose, and parenteral vitamin preparations should be given. Adequate hydration can be gaged by measuring urinary excretion, which should be kept near a liter per day. The hematocrit is also useful in determining the results of combating hemoconcentration. Determination of sodium, chloride, potassium, and bicarbonate ionic levels in the serum twice a day in very sick patients serves as a useful guide to electrolyte therapy and control of acidosis or alkalosis. No attempt to maintain nitrogen

equilibrium other than by blood and plasma infusion is indicated in short periods of disability.

Decompression is best achieved by intubation with one of the long, weighted intestinal tubes attached to gentle continuous suction. Single-lumen tubes drain more effectively than double-lumen tubes. This method of decompression, supplemented with pantothenic acid parenterally, is useful in adynamic ileus. However, there is great danger in relying solely on this means of relieving mechanical obstruction whenever there is any question of strangulation of bowel or when large-bowel obstruction occurs in the presence of a competent ileocecal valve. Early operative intervention is required in all such cases.

In the majority of cases, surgical intervention is necessary to remove the obstructing agent and restore normal bowel continuity and function. In some cases due to adhesions and hernia, relief by decompression suffices, and in some cases of intussusception or volvulus a barium enema under fluoroscopy restores normal continuity. Many cases of adynamic ileus are cured by tube decompression alone. However, if the patient does not improve rapidly on such conservative measures, operation within 24 hr is indicated to establish an accurate evaluation of the cause of obstruction and to effect a cure. When *severe* distension is not relieved *promptly* by intubation, surgical intervention is required for immediate decompression by means of enterostomy or colostomy. However, treatment of shock, metabolic acidosis, and dehydration should be instituted before surgical therapy is undertaken in order to lessen the operative risk.

PROGNOSIS. The prognosis is always guarded, depending upon the level of obstruction, being poorer in high obstruction than in low intestinal obstruction, and upon the viability of the bowel wall, the length of time the bowel has been obstructed and strangulated, and the amount of bowel involved in the strangulation. Patients with complicating peritonitis from perforation have a poorer prognosis, and this is especially true in very young infants or in elderly patients with complicating cardiovascular or renal disease.

REFERENCES

DeMuth, W. E., W. T. Fitts, Jr., and L. T. Patterson: Mesenteric Vascular Occlusion, Surg. Gynecol. Obstet., 108: 209, 1959.

Moore, F. D.: "Metabolic Care of the Surgical Patient." Philadelphia, W. B. Saunders Company, 1959.

Tumen, H. J.: "Intestinal Obstruction," chap. 53, in "Gastroenterology," 2d ed., vol. II, H. L. Bockus (Ed.), Philadelphia, W. B. Saunders Company, 1964.

319 ACUTE APPENDICITIS

*Albert I. Mendeloff and
Arnold M. Seligman*

Inflammation of the vermiform appendix constitutes one of the most common and most important acute disease processes. Although descriptions of isolated cases of the disease had been written in the seventeenth and eighteenth centuries, and appendiceal abscesses had been described at autopsy, it was Reginald Fitz in 1886 who first collected a series of cases in which clinicopathologic correlations were established.

EPIDEMIOLOGY. The disease occurs in all age groups but appears to be productive of higher mortality rates in the group aged five to fourteen and after age fifty-five. It is estimated that in 1946, in England and Wales, one case occurred every year for every 700 of the population. The incidence of the disease is somewhat higher in males, and the death rates for the period prior to 1946 were 40 percent higher in males. A consistent feature of the disease has been its greater incidence and mortality in the upper socioeconomic stratum and its tendency to decline in frequency during periods of food shortages. In Western Europe and in the United States, the death rates for the disease have shown a steady decline, ranging from 8.1 per 100,000 of the population in 1941 to less than 1.0 per 100,000 in 1960. There is also definite evidence that the incidence of the disease has recently decreased; despite great increases in the number of admissions of surgical patients to American hospitals since World War II, the absolute number of acutely inflamed appendixes removed has steadily declined by 30 to 60 percent, and approximately at the same rates in urban and rural institutions. It is difficult to explain this decrease by single causation. Possible factors are the greater use of effective antibiotics and chemotherapeutic agents to treat upper respiratory infections, some of which undoubtedly have been associated with appendicitis, and a lessened infestation with helminths. Changes in diet have also occurred, changes which many feel have increased the incidence of degenerative disease but may have sharply reduced the incidence and the mortality from appendicitis. Surgeons are also probably more careful about removing nearly normal appendixes now than heretofore. None of these explanations is adequate to clarify in its totality what appears to be a progressive and definite decrease in the incidence of one of our most important acute inflammatory diseases.

PATHOGENESIS. Appendicitis is an inflammation of the vermiform appendix involving all layers of the organ, beginning either as a focal ulceration or as a diffuse phlegmon. Evidence of a focal point of obstruction due to fecalith or stricture is sometimes found. The appendiceal artery is an end artery, and its tributaries are susceptible to occlusion from the increased pressure within the lumen of the obstructed appendix or direct pressure of a fecalith. Infections lead to vascular thrombosis, local necrosis, and infarction resulting in perforation. Streptococcal involvement, which rises in frequency when acute respiratory infections are prevalent, adds to the necrotic process and to the virulence of the disease. The process either subsides early or progresses to gangrene or perforation with abscess or peritonitis. Chronic inflammation occurs only with the granulomatous infections such as tuberculosis, amebas, or actinomycosis. Recurring appendicitis due to spontaneous subsidence of acute attacks should not be considered chronic appendicitis. Recognition of the disease as an entity was first made by Fitz, and treatment by appendectomy was introduced thereafter by Morton, Ochsner, Murphy, McBurney, and Deaver. Since then to the present time, acute appendicitis is the most common major surgical disease.

CLINICAL PICTURE. The history of onset should be carefully obtained, for the history may be the *only* clue to a correct diagnosis of retrocecal appendicitis, when abdominal signs are absent. The first symptom in an otherwise well individual is acute periumbilical or epigastric pain. In young children the abdominal pain cannot be localized and is usually generalized. Pain varies from mild or vague to quite severe and is followed by anorexia, nausea, or vomiting. The sequence of these symptoms is very important. When the illness is initiated by nausea and vomiting, which is then followed by abdominal pain, one should suspect an infection capable of producing extensive toxic absorption such as is noted in cases of gastroenteritis, tonsillitis, scarlet fever, and pneumonia, rather than the early stage of appendiceal inflammation. Pain is the first symptom of appendicitis and is due to distension of the appendiceal serosa by edema. Stretching of the serosa stimulates sympathetic nerve endings in the wall of the appendix, producing pain first and, because of continued stimuli, anorexia, nausea, and vomiting afterward. For this reason it is important to determine whether abdominal pain preceded the nausea and vomiting. The only other mechanism for producing pain is by the acute contractions of the appendiceal musculature which occurs in appendiceal colic, when the lumen is obstructed by stricture, fecalith, worms, or foreign bodies. Since the sensory innervation of the appendix corresponds to the tenth spinal segment, the pain is referred to the periumbilical region like sensory impulses originating anywhere in the entire small bowel.

At the time of the initial symptoms, inflammation is confined to the appendix. Fever and abdominal signs are not prominent at the onset. High fever, like vomiting, as an initial symptom is suggestive of some other diagnosis. Within a few hours, when the inflammatory process has begun to involve peritoneal surfaces of neighboring loops of bowel, omentum, and the anterior parietal peritoneum, pain shifts to the right lower quadrant of the abdomen, and tenderness, spasm, and rebound tenderness become increasingly prominent. In a sixth of the patients, diarrhea may appear owing to irritation of bowel, but constipation is more common. Contralateral rebound tenderness, like pain in the right lower quadrant on sneezing, is a particularly reliable sign of peritoneal inflammation. Although direct pressure of the examining hand produces pain, it may do so in the distended gut of gastroenteritis as well. However, release of tension by the examining hand, as in demonstrating rebound tenderness, can produce pain only when peritoneal surfaces are inflamed. Sudden cessation of abdominal pain some hours after onset signifies perforation of a distended appendix, infarction of the appendix, or the accumulation of enough peritoneal fluid to lubricate the moving inflamed surfaces.

In the absence of anterior abdominal signs and a history of onset consistent with appendicitis, one must suspect that the appendix is in the retrocecal position. Evidence for inflammation in this area may be obtained by stretching the iliopsoas muscle either by passive hyperextension of the legs on the torso or by actively flexing the iliopsoas by straight-leg raising. When the appendix lies over the brim of the pelvis, evidence of inflammation is more striking on rectal examination than on abdominal examination. After 24 hr, progressive appendicitis results in localized peritonitis and abscess formation, when the signs remain confined to the right lower quadrant with the appearance of a tender mass. Diffuse peritonitis develops as a result of perforation before adequate adhesions by omentum and neighboring loops of bowel have been able to form. This is more common in children than in adults. Tenderness and spasm are generalized, ileus becomes evident, and progressively severe toxicity develops, with high fever, severe leukocytosis, vomiting, dehydration, rapid pulse, and shock. When a history of illness for 2 to 3 days is obtained, one should expect to find evidence of appendiceal abscess with mass or more generalized peritonitis with ileus, rather than signs of appendicitis alone.

Atypical clinical pictures of appendicitis are distressingly common and difficult to identify. If one remembers that appendicitis is the most common acute intraabdominal focal inflammation, the onset of unexplained weakness, anorexia, and tachycardia in the elderly may lead the physician to suspect the appendix; similarly, in patients obtunded by cerebral disease or whose pain pathways are disturbed by neurologic degeneration or whose appreciation of pain is blunted by sedatives or ganglionic blocking agents, the objective signs of early peritonitis may be the only clue that an acute appendicitis has occurred. Retrocecal appendicitis can easily be confused with disease of the right kidney or ureter or with colonic disease, as noted below.

DIFFERENTIAL DIAGNOSIS. *Gastroenteritis* may produce vomiting, abdominal pain, and fever that are difficult to distinguish from those of acute appendicitis. However, vomiting is often the first and predominating symptom in the former and is later followed by diarrhea. Sometimes diarrhea ushers in the illness. Although tenderness is sometimes present, especially after considerable retching has occurred, spasm and rebound tenderness are absent. Systemic muscle aching and prostration are common, and bowel sounds are loud and "whooshing." The illness may occur in epidemics or affect several members of a family, making diagnosis somewhat easier.

Referred pain from diaphragmatic irritation in *pneumonia* may simulate appendicitis, especially in children. This is especially the case when the signs of appendicitis are found to be higher in the abdomen than usual and are attributed to malrotation of the colon. However, fever and vomiting are more prominent at the onset of abdominal symptoms and respiration is more rapid in pneumonia. Abdominal spasm and rebound tenderness should be absent in pneumonia, unless pneumococcal peritonitis has occurred.

Abdominal pain from mesenteric *lymphadenitis* is very difficult to distinguish from acute appendicitis and is frequently a cause of illness in children. Less spasm and rebound tenderness, lower leukocytosis, and more gradual onset of symptoms help distinguish it from appendicitis.

Since free blood in the peritoneal cavity produces the symptoms and signs of peritoneal irritation, a *ruptured graafian follicle* or a *ruptured tubal pregnancy* will simulate the acute abdominal condition of appendicitis. The signs are less localized, however. Other acute processes accompanied by a mass are *torsion of an ovarian cyst* and *acute salpingitis*. These conditions are usually readily distinguished on vaginal examination by noting tenderness mainly on movement of the cervix. The local signs are usually more pronounced than the general illness of the patient would warrant.

Other acute processes such as *acute cholecystitis, diverticulitis* of the *colon,* and *perforation* of *carcinoma* of the *colon* are often difficult to distinguish, especially in older patients. The history is the most helpful means of making a correct diagnosis. Urologic conditions such as *stone* and *pyelonephritis* of the right kidney may give symptoms referred to the right lower quadrant. The urine is usually abnormal, and pain begins in the costovertebral angle and radiates to the groin or pubic area. however, a retrocecal appendicitis may also cause the appearance of blood cells in the urine.

In all these conditions, with the exception of pneumonia, it is usually safer to operate in the suspected case of acute appendicitis than to wait until the signs and symptoms of peritonitis make diagnosis relatively easy. The more patients who are operated upon after peritonitis has occurred, the higher the mortality will be.

TREATMENT. If appendicitis is considered a possible diagnosis, cathartics are absolutely contraindicated.

Once the diagnosis of acute appendicitis is made, the patient is prepared for operation by initiating parenteral administration of fluid and electrolytes, and the appendix is removed as soon as possible, at any hour of the day or night. Uncomplicated appendicitis results in prompt recovery; with early ambulation, the patient may be able to eat within 2 days and be discharged within a few days thereafter. The complications of appendicitis such as local abscess, peritonitis with ileus, and intestinal obstruction require surgical intervention such as drainage or lysis of adhesions, prolonged hospitalization, energetic treatment with gastrointestinal intubation, antibiotics, and careful control of fluid, glucose, and electrolyte balance by parenteral means.

REFERENCES

Bowers, W. F.: Appendicitis, with Especial Reference to Its Pathogenesis, Bacteriology, and Healing, Arch. Surg., 39: 362, 1939.

Castleton, K. B., C. D. Puestow, and D. Sauer: Is Appendicitis Decreasing in Frequency? Arch. Surg., 78:794, 1959.

Fitz, R.: Perforating Inflammation of the Vermiform Appendix, Am. J. Med. Sci., 92:321, 1886.

Moloney, G. E., W. T. Russell, and D. C. Wilson: Appendicitis: A Report on Its Social Pathology and Recent Surgical Experience, Brit. J. Surg., 38:52, 1950.

320 DISEASES OF THE COLON AND RECTUM

Albert I. Mendeloff

SYMPTOMS OF COLONIC AND RECTAL DISEASE. Man can exist without a colon or rectum, although with some difficulty. This basic fact has allowed important observations to be made regarding the functions carried on by the large bowel and the adjustments which result when it is no longer present. The increasing freedom with which resections of the organ, bypassing operations, and colostomies have been carried out has led to significant advances in our understanding of normal activities of the colon, although our comprehension of many of its diseased states is still rudimentary.

Pain Reference. Anatomists, experimentally minded surgeons, and gastroenterologists have established that pain of colonic origin, unlike small-intestinal pain, is lateralized by the brain to the right or left sides of the abdomen. Pain fibers from the cecum and ascending colon accompany sympathetic fibers to the lower ganglions of the celiac plexus; fibers from the transverse colon, sigmoid, and rectum accompany fibers passing into the inferior mesenteric ganglions. Interconnections of these fibers with somatic nerves permit a considerable amount of localization of pain by the brain, roughly corresponding to the festoon distribution of the colon in the peritoneal cavity. Pain from the rectum is projected low on to the sacral nerve distribution; the lower it arises, the more accurate is the localization. Anal pain has the exquisite tactile discriminative accuracy expected of skin near a mucocutaneous junction.

Pain stimuli from the noninflamed large bowel, as from other areas of the normal intestinal tract, consist almost exclusively of distension of the bowel musculature. In the uninflamed gut most forms of trauma result in no appreciable pain, stretching of the muscularis layer of the bowel wall being alone adequate to excite this sensation. When the wall is stiffened by an inflammatory response, however, the threshold for pain stimuli is lowered, and many previously subliminal impulses are perceived as pain. In the presence of peritoneal inflammation, pain previously lateralized on the abdominal wall in a general way becomes much more sharply localized and may be accompanied by spasm of the abdominal muscles and rebound tenderness upon pressure.

Thus it is evident that pain from the uninflamed colon really results from distension of normal bowel proximal to an unrelaxing segment. If the unrelaxing segment is inflamed or infiltrated, pain arises from this area as well as from the contraction of the normal bowel proximal to it; if the inflammation or infiltration penetrates through the serosa of the gut to involve the parietal peritoneum, the more localized and sharper pain of spastic striated muscle and overlying skin becomes prominent.

Motor Disorders. The colon is a rather sluggish organ, contracting desultorily at rates not exceeding 1 per min, compared to regular contraction frequencies in the small intestine ranging from 10 to 12 per min in the duodenum to 3 to 4 per min in the ileum. The transition between the innervation of the ascending colon and that of the transverse colon occurs just distal to the hepatic flexure, where radiologists often note irregular propulsion of barium (Cannon's point). The colon husbands its motor activity for the processing of ileal contents, waiting until a certain volume has accumulated in the cecum. Gas delivered into the cecum from the small intestine, which is intolerant of air and passes it rapidly downward, diffuses into the colon and distributes itself along the length of that organ. About 100 ml gas is contained in the large intestine, obeying the law of gravity, rising to the most superior portion of the colon—the flexures—when the subject is erect, the transverse colon when he is supine, the rectum when he is in the knee-chest position. Since most colonic motility is uncoordinated segmental churning of the fecal contents for the purpose of their partial desiccation, symptomatic disturbances of motor activity tend to be related rather to the infrequent mass propulsive waves which deliver the fecal bolus to an adjacent and more distal colonic region. The same types of disturbance which cause motor difficulties in the small intestine are also seen in the colon —intraluminal obstruction, destruction or paralysis of muscle, compromise of vascular integrity, pressure from neighboring masses, or infectious processes. The colon differs from the small intestine, however, in its more successful accomodation to these processes, distending to much greater degrees without serious symptoms than the small bowel can. In particular, obstructive lesions of the left colon characteristically produce gradual enlargement of the right colon of astonishing magnitude, occasionally to the point of cecal perforation.

Defecation Patterns. These have been described in Chap. 43. It is still not common knowledge among physicians how varied are the defecatory habits of their fellow citizens, how fanciful their interpretation of deviations from those habits. It is well to ask the patient to describe in some detail what he regards as his normal defecatory pattern, with particular attention to time of day or night, relation to meals, sensation during actual expulsion of stool, and aftersensations. Cardinal symptoms of serious disease are the inability to exert adequate expulsive pressure, a sense of incomplete evacuation, an intolerable urgency, and the presence of blood or of mucopus in the stools.

Bleeding. Bleeding from the colon may be occult, massive, or of any grade between. Most often it is occult, an important early sign of malignancy, often of the right colon. Melena and tarry stools rarely result from colonic bleeding. Bright-red blood, either by itself or coating the stools, may originate from any portion of the lower ileum as well as from the colon. Bleeding results from localized lesions such as polyps, Meckel's diverticulum, hemangiomas, other tumors, from generalized blood dyscrasias, from uremic states, from inflammatory lesions—ulcerative colitis, regional enteritis, bacillary dysentery, diverticulitis—from diverticulosis on occasion, or from vascular anomalies such as hereditary telangiectasia. Hemorrhoids are so common that their presence can never allow the physician to abandon the search for other bleeding lesions.

DIAGNOSTIC PROCEDURES. Examination of the Abdomen. Careful examination will often disclose masses or palpable colonic contents strongly suggesting more distal narrowing. Colonic outlines distended by gas have similar significance in leading one to the diagnosis of a more distal obstructing lesion. Spasm and guarding in the left lower quadrant are characteristic of an acute diverticulitis; a distended loop of sigmoid percussed in the midline at the level of the umbilicus may represent a sigmoid volvulus. Generalized hypogastric tenderness is associated with acute inflammations of the colon, the dysenteries and ulcerative colitis, both of which may also be accompanied by abdominal distension out of proportion to the habitus of the patient.

Digital Examination. This is a cheap and highly efficient procedure provided that the finger's education is maintained by steady use. Proper routinization of this examination should permit recognition of perianal, sphincteric, and ampullary lesions, gross deformities of prostate and cervix, and perception of even small neoplastic masses in the rectum. Two-thirds of all rectal carcinomas lie within reach of the inquiring index finger; when one considers that these cancers not only account for 12 percent of all gastrointestinal cancers but have a favorable prognosis if removed early, the importance of digital rectal examination is easily appreciated. Examination of the material coating the gloved finger on its withdrawal from the rectum is often of diagnostic importance, and all physicians should form the habit of routine testing of the finger specimen for occult blood.

Proctosigmoidoscopy. The proctosigmoidoscope is an inexpensive instrument of extraordinary importance in the detection of colonic disease. Contrary to the general impression, it is not difficult to master, and it can be introduced into the rectum as the examining finger is removed without discomfort to the patient. As experience accrues in its use, this examination becomes very informative. The physician should learn to evaluate friability of the mucosa, one of the earliest signs of proctitis and colitis, abnormal vascular patterns, edema, ulcerations, and polyps. Ninety percent of tumors of the rectum and rectosigmoid can be directly visualized with this instrument; seventy percent of all tumors of the large intestine lie within the terminal 25 cm of the colon which it can bring into view. This area is particularly difficult to visualize radiographically, so that the proctosigmoidoscope is the most important diagnostic instrument in this region. In addition, radiography in the pelvis carries a radiation hazard to the gonads which can frequently be minimized or avoided by making the diagnosis endoscopically.

In addition to the visual inspection of the area, bacteriologic, parasitologic, and cytologic studies can be made on washings obtained through the instrument, and biopsy of a suspicious lesion is easy to perform. Routine proctosigmoidoscopy of all patients past the age of forty produces a substantial yield of "precancerous" lesions, since most such surveys have identified adenomatous polyps in 5 to 8 percent of these individuals.

Stool Examination. Stools constitute important objective evidence of disease processes; some of the difficulties in obtaining them and describing them are discussed in Chap. 43. One must distinguish blood streaking on otherwise normal stools from dark stools containing blood, tarry stools from the gray-black formed stools passed by patients ingesting iron, and, most importantly, the inflammatory mucopurulent exudate passed by patients with inflammatory rectal and sigmoid disease from true diarrheal stools. Microscopic examination of the freshly passed stool or rectal swab is useful not only for parasitologic study but for demonstration of the characteristic exudate of ulcerative colitis and bacillary dysentery and the presence of malignant cells (Papanicolaou technique). Tests for occult blood employ gum guaiac, benzidine base or benzidine dihydrochloride, or orthotoluidine. Of these, the modified Gregersen test using benzidine dihydrochloride, barium peroxide, and 50 percent acetic acid is the most satisfactory screening test, being roughly five times as sensitive as the guaiac test and yet not producing a significant number of false positive reactions.

To summarize, the digital examination should be a routine feature of the general physical examination of all adults. Finger specimens obtained during the examination should be inspected and tested for blood. Whenever abdominal complaints, stool abnormalities, unexplained weight loss, changes in defecation patterns, or a strong family history of colonic disease are features of the history, proctosigmoidoscopy should be carried out. Any patient with anorectal disease should have routine proctosigmoidoscopy prior to surgical treatment for the same.

When these procedures have been carried out, it is usually necessary to visualize the colon proximal to the rectosigmoid by radiologic techniques. The routine barium enema is a very accurate diagnostic tool for the identification of structural abnormalities of the colon; for detection of mucosal abnormalities such as small polyps or early ulcerative colitis, it is often necessary to follow it with an air-contrast enema. The combined use of the digital examination, proctosigmoidoscope, and radiologic investigation of the colon will identify 95 percent of inflammatory, neoplastic, congenital, and vascular diseases of this organ. Negative results of these procedures constitute strong evidence that disorders of a functional type are producing symptoms. Routine employment of these measures in the periodic health examination of all persons over forty years of age will disclose frequent evidence of serious disease in an early and treatable stage.

DEVELOPMENTAL DISORDERS

Malrotations of the colon produce no disease states, but the abnormal location of the organ and its attachments (e.g., appendix) produces serious confusion in the pain reference pattern when any of the usual colonic diseases are present. Barium enema studies are usually necessary to identify the abnormally placed organ and make possible a more rational interpretation of the symptoms and physical findings.

Megacolon

Aganglionic megacolon, or Hirschsprung's disease, is a congenital disorder manifesting symptoms in early infancy, occurring more often in boys, often in familial clusters. There is abdominal distension occasionally reaching massive proportions; the sigmoid colon is the earliest segment to be distended, and visible peristalsis is common. The stools consist of characteristically very small pellets or ribbons of pasty consistency. On rectal examination the ampulla is empty of feces, and the anal sphincter feels normal. X-ray examination, when properly carried out, shows a narrowed lumen in the rectosigmoid area, with a distended sigmoid colon above the constricted area. Swenson and others have now established that the narrowed area results from a lack of functioning ganglion cells in Auerbach's plexus; this area is thus unable to relax in advance of the normal peristaltic activity of the colon proximal to it (Fig. 320-1). Diagnosis is made by deep surgical biopsy under anesthesia or by special rectal balloon motility patterns in the unanesthetized patient.

The condition may also be acquired; in Brazil a large number of acquired megacolon cases have been reported in the aged; pathologic specimens show all degrees of degeneration of the ganglion cells of Auerbach's plexus, and in some cases a relationship to infection with *Trypanosoma cruzi* (Chagas' disease) has been demonstrated. In a small number of patients generalized aganglionosis of the esophagus, ureters, and colon has been described, and thiamine deficiency has been incriminated as the etiologic agent.

Treatment of this condition is largely surgical, although a number of borderline cases may be carried along on measures designed to empty the colon. Definitive diagnosis is made by a rectal biopsy deep enough to include the muscularis layer of the rectum; failure to find adequate numbers of ganglion cells indicates that the most effective treatment is resection of the aganglionic segment and a "pull-through" anastomosis to the intact and sphincter.

Chronic idiopathic megacolon has its onset later in childhood, usually at the time toilet training begins; it is characterized more by constipation than by distension, and the rectal ampulla is invariably found distended with feces. X-ray examination shows the entire colon to be distended from the anal sphincter cephalad; no narrowed segment is seen, and rectal biopsy discloses the normal complement of ganglion cells in Auerbach's plexus. The treatment is based on education in normal bowel habits, but a long course of enemas may have to be carried out concomitantly. It should be pointed out that water intoxication may occur in small children whose enormously dilated colons are vigorously irrigated with tap water; saline enemas are probably safe.

Diverticulosis

Saccular outpouchings of the colon are more common than those of the small intestine, occurring probably in 10 percent of all persons over fifty years of age. The outpouchings are nearly always made up of mucosa and serosa following the course of a nutrient artery perforating the muscularis layer of the organ. There is a definite increase in the frequency of the findings as one follows patients into the later decades of life; indeed, there is an increase in frequency of diverticula in the same individual as he ages. It is probable that straining at stool has some role in increasing the rate at which diverticula develop, since the potential tunnel along the nutrient arteries is present in everyone. Diverticula are most frequently found in the sigmoid colon, least commonly in the ascending colon. Recently hypertrophic changes in sigmoid muscle have been shown to permit diverticula on the antimesenteric border to form and enlarge, a mechanism totally distinct from the usual one described above.

These diverticula are occasionally associated with diverticula elsewhere in the stomach or small intestine (see Chap. 317); in themselves they can hardly be called pathologic, but the peculiarities of their structure and location provide the basis for two serious complications:

1. Acute inflammation of the diverticular sac, known as diverticulitis (see under Inflammatory Disorders, below).

2. Hemorrhage into the colon. This may occur in the absence of an acute diverticulitis, although the association

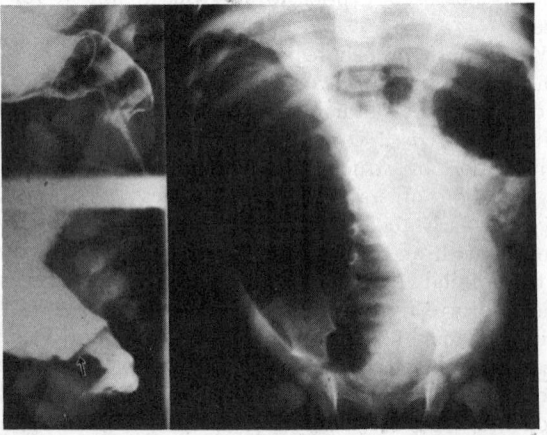

Fig. 320-1. Aganglionic megacolon. The contracted rectal segment is seen on the left, the dilated colon on the right.

is much more common. The anatomic basis for the bleeding in uninflamed diverticulosis consists of the glomus-like capillary and arteriolar vascular network left unprotected in the lumen of the colon when the diverticular sac pushes out along the nutrient artery of the mucosa and serosa. In older patients these vessels, presumably damaged by contact with hard fecal aggregates, may be ruptured and bleed furiously. Such catastrophes, seen with increasing frequency as the population ages, often require emergency operation for their amelioration.

Polyposis

Polypoid lesions of colon and rectum may be *hamartomatous* (as in the retention polyp seen commonly in children or in the Peutz-Jeghers polyp), *inflammatory* (as in ulcerative colitis and Crohn's disease), or *neoplastic*. The neoplastic lesions may be epithelial or nonepithelial. The word *polyp* is a clinical term referring to a structure which can be seen by proctoscopy or x-ray examination and which cannot be given a histologic dimension until it is removed and sectioned or unless cells exfoliating from its surface can be recovered and stained.

In adults, single polyps of the adenomatous type are identified in 2 to 8 percent of the population. Small mucosal tags are very common and have no particular significance. True adenomatous polyps are more common in men than in women and are found more commonly with increasing age. The lobulated surface of adenomatous polyps is in contrast to the smooth vascular surface of childhood retention polyps or to the frondlike, soft appearance of papillary or villous adenomas. All such adenomatous polyps are rare in patients under thirty; when one is discovered, more should be sought, since familial polyposis does occur in this age group and almost always bespeaks prospective malignancy. In children polyps are frequently large, vascular, and on long pedicles, and may produce intussusception or massive hemorrhage. In adults the polyps are more frequently sessile, arise from the glandular epithelium of the crypts, and bleed less frequently. Less often, polyps arising from the surface epithelium may form villous masses which secrete watery discharges rich in potassium. Such villous adenomas, although infrequent, can lead to watery diarrhea of remarkable magnitude, but the primary danger they pose is their high capacity for malignant transformation. (Probably 50 percent of these polypoid tumors will become cancers if not totally removed; fulguration is usually followed by prompt recurrence.)

The relationship of adenomatous polyps, whether sessile or pedunculated, to the development of cancer of the colon is at present a subject of hot debate among pathologists. There is dispute as to whether the distribution of such polyps in the colon is parallel to or totally unlike that of the distribution of rectal and colonic cancers, the evidence favoring the latter idea. Colonic specimens resected for cancer frequently show adenomatous polyps in close proximity to the malignant tissue; polyps removed from noncancerous patients have been observed

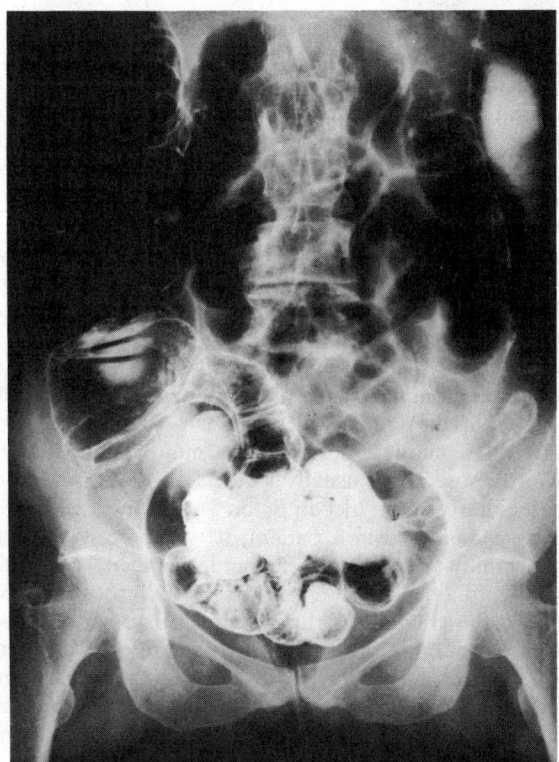

Fig. 320-2. Two adenomatous polyps in the sigmoid.

to show all grades of differentiation known to occur in the progression from benignancy to frank malignancy.

Clinically, polyps are usually silent. When they do give rise to symptoms, these are intermittent episodes either of bleeding, manifest or occult, or of intermittent obstruction. The latter occurs when a large sessile polypoid mass weakens the wall to which it is attached or a pedunculated polyp flips caudad, causing the wall from which it arises to buckle. In either case a partial intussusception may result, with the production of crampy pain, occasionally an abdominal mass, and often a bloody exudate.

Treatment of polyps in adults is influenced by this debate as to their possible malignant transformation. Unfortunately, there is no certain way of determining whether a given polyp is benign or malignant when *first* identified until it has been studied microscopically. Exfoliative cytologic examination of colonic contents obtained by repeated enemas may assist, but the procedure is tedious and at present not well standardized. Polyps less than 1 cm in diameter, or those on long pedicles, are rarely malignant; they may be followed radiologically at yearly intervals if their removal requires a laparotomy otherwise contraindicated (Fig. 320-2). Larger lesions, all villous adenomas, and polyps in areas hard to define radiologically will require laparotomy and resection of the involved bowel. Inspection by sigmoidoscopy at the operating table of the area above and below the resected bowel will often reveal hitherto unrecognized lesions, although it should be said that often small polyps readily demonstrated by barium enema prove hard to find in the operating room.

Sufficient information is now at hand to disclose the remarkably high incidence of recurrence of adenomatous polyps after fulguration and excision. In approximately 40 to 50 percent of patients who have had polyps removed from the colon and rectum new polyps will develop in the decade following the polypectomies. Although most of the new polyps will be of the same type as the original polyps, about 15 to 20 percent of the new polyps will be malignant when the original polyps were benign.

Multiple congenital polyposis of the colon, inherited as a simple dominant gene and thus characterizing many members of the families affected, is a disorder in which many adenomatous polyps are found from ileocecal valve to anus. These usually give rise to some symptoms, usually diarrhea or bleeding, but once such a disorder has been identified in a patient, it is imperative that the entire family be examined sigmoidoscopically and radiologically to detect the characteristic polyps. The probability of malignancy supervening in these polypoid colons is so high that present reasoning requires each sufferer from this disorder to have a total colectomy; since sigmoidoscopic follow-up can be effectively and easily carried out, some surgeons elect to perform ileoproctostomy, leaving the rectum intact.

FUNCTIONAL DISTURBANCES

Irritable Colon Syndrome

This name is applied to a triad of symptoms—abdominal distress following the colonic distribution of pain, variations in defecatory habits from constipation to diarrhea, and the passage of stools which are of small caliber at the time when abdominal distress is at its worst. The stools may be hard and pelletlike or soft and pasty, but they are characteristically of smaller size than when the patient is not complaining of distress. The physiologic basis for most of these symptoms has been dealt with in Chap. 43. Over the years many different terms have been applied to this syndrome: some, such as "unstable colon" or "colonic neurosis," stress the anxiety which characterizes these patients; others, like "spastic colitis," lay emphasis on the pain and distress experienced; still others, such as "mucous colitis," describe the increased mucus content of the stools and the pain which is usually relieved by defecation. In its milder forms the syndrome is extremely common, being more frequently seen in women aged fifteen to forty-five but commonly observed in both sexes under conditions of emotional tension. Constipation, with pain in the left lower quadrant relieved by defecation, is the most common symptom when the disorder is mild. Extremely severe pain, diarrheal stools accompanied by much mucus, and various degrees of generalized disability are much less common and carry a rather serious prognosis, patients with such complaints being severely psychoneurotic. Vasomotor instability and disabling headaches are frequently noted to occur in many patients even when the colonic symptoms are minimal. Aerophagia is a frequent accompaniment of the attacks, the swallowed air producing further difficulties when irregularly handled by the "irritable" colon. Bloating, borborygmi, explosive flatulence, and low backache are often described during the days or weeks when the symptoms are at their worst.

On *physical examination* these patients are anxious, often sweaty, but otherwise normal. During intense pain the abdomen may be distended, but no visible peristalsis is noted, the abdominal musculature is relaxed, and in the left lower quadrant a tender sigmoid full of feces may be palpated. Characteristically, the rectal ampulla is empty of feces. Proctoscopic examination usually is entirely normal or may show prominent vascular patterns in an otherwise unremarkable mucosa. Large amounts of clear mucus are frequently encountered during the examination, and there is often difficulty in negotiating the rectosigmoid curve at 13 to 15 cm from the anus because of violent spasm of the rectosigmoid.

The *diagnosis* of the irritable colon syndrome is suggested by the length of the history without obvious signs of physical deterioration, the intermittent character of the disability, and the relationship of distress to periods of environmental or emotional stress. Nevertheless, each patient presenting such symptoms deserves not only a careful history but also a complete physical examination including proctosigmoidoscopy, stool examinations for blood, parasites, and pathogenic bacteria; a barium enema is also indicated. The radiographic study serves to rule out other lesions, since there are no findings diagnostic for this syndrome, although spasticity of the sigmoid, accentuated haustra, and tubular descending colon may be observed if the patient is having symptoms at the time of the examination.

The *differential diagnosis* includes all disorders of the colon, female genital tract diseases, regional enteritis, malignant tumors of stomach or pancreas, and those common disorders which are often associated with the irritable colon—gastric and duodenal ulcer and cholelithiasis.

Treatment of the irritable colon syndrome is that of any chronic anxiety neurosis, with more specific symptomatic medication. The relationship between patient and physician can be established on the firm grounds of reassurance that the syndrome does not lead to the development either of ulcerative colitis or colonic malignancy, although it should be stated that it confers no protection against these eventualities. From this point the patient should receive a sympathetic ear from the physician as he talks over the circumstances surrounding the onset of his symptoms and those characterizing his present difficulties. Attempts should be made to discover in what way situational and emotional stresses differ when symptoms are present and when they are absent. The emphasis is placed on the patient and his relationship to others in his environment rather than on the symptoms and long discussions of what is "normal" bowel physiology. Repeated x-ray examinations are avoided insofar as possible, but general physical examinations, hemograms, and stool examinations are carried out at regular intervals.

During the acute attacks it is generally best to limit the diet to frequent bland feedings, with emphasis upon relatively even temperatures of liquids. Many patients find sweet whole milk troublesome at these times; skimmed milk, buttermilk, and cheeses are better tolerated. The cabbage and turnip families should be avoided, as well as coffee, alcoholic drinks, and tobacco. Hydrophilic colloid laxatives are often very helpful; other laxatives and cathartics are best avoided. Fecal impaction is a very infrequent complication of this syndrome unless the patient has taken to his bed unexpectedly for some disorder which prevents his customary posture at stool.

Although anticholinergic drugs are less effective in controlling colonic motility than they are in decreasing tone and amplitude of contractions of the stomach and small intestine, when given in doses sufficient to produce dry mouth and blurring of accomodation they often prove helpful in relieving colonic pain. Sedatives of barbiturate or other types are usually indicated during the acute attacks. An occasional patient is remarkably helped by cyproheptadine, and some patients believe diphenoxylate, which acts primarily on the small bowel, is more easily tolerated than a comparably effective anticholinergic. Although opiates are very effective in controlling the diarrheal phase of this disease, they also produce an increase in rectosigmoidal tone.

Constipation and Urgency of Rectal Origin

In Chap. 43 the mechanism of defecation is discussed. Disorders involving the sensory or motor components of this mechanism may arise from destruction of the nerves subserving these functions, from invasion or inflammation of the rectosigmoid itself, or from central nervous system dysfunction based on conditioning abnormalities or structural disorganization. If the afferent stimulus from the rectal wall cannot reach the brain or if, upon reaching it, no efferent action occurs, defecation is not initiated. If defecation is initiated but muscular power is lessened or lost, the act is not carried to completion. If all anatomic pathways are intact but habitual neglect of the afferent impulses is established, defecation is not initiated. The result of all these disorders, regardless of cause, is failure of the rectum to empty its contents. Accordingly, physical examination of such patients reveals the rectal ampulla to be full of stool, often to the astonishment of the patient.

Aside from degenerative disease of the central nervous system, severe psychoses, the use of ganglionic blocking drugs, and morphine addiction, the most common cause of this type of rectal or "simple" constipation is voluntary suppression of the defecation reflex. Such inhibitory activity is essential in the daily routines of civilized society; disordered bowel habits are therefore very common in civilized life. Toilet training in infancy leads to a powerful development of these inhibitory actions; repeated experiences in suppressing defecation because of social impropriety, unaccustomed surroundings, uncomfortable commodes, or intercurrent factors lead to a habit pattern in which suppression of defecation becomes simpler than its achievement. When constant distension of the rectum with feces becomes habitual, anorectal disorders, in particular hemorrhoidal itching and bleeding and anal fissures, make defecation painful, thus reinforcing the inhibitory impulses. The next step for the patient is the use of laxatives, which soon becomes as much a constant feature of the regimen as is the voluntary suppression of defecation.

TREATMENT. The principal bulwark of therapy for rectal constipation is education. The chain of events leading up to the ineffective rectum is evaluated by careful physical examination of the status of the abdominal musculature, neurologic defects, drug effects, postural abnormalities, and accompanying local lesions of the anus and rectum. Such lesions as can be treated are taken care of, but the therapy may take a long time and usually must be carried out concomitantly with efforts to modify anal sphincteric spasm when it is present. Attention to regular habits of diet and time of defecation is most important; although defecation for most persons is best accomplished following meals, particularly breakfast, in these patients it is more important to select for evacuation whatever time is as free as possible from the pressure of daily events. Habit patterns of many years' standing may have to be altered, one may need to force the patient to get up earlier in the morning, to take some form of physical exercise—for older patients walking briskly outdoors is often helpful—to abandon the usual laxatives and cathartics, to pay more attention to defecatory urges (without becoming excessively bowel-conscious), and to space out the workday in such a way as to honor these urges when they arise.

The elderly patient may be feebly motivated to make such sweeping changes; under such circumstances one must proceed cautiously, making sure impactions are broken up by the physician's finger, that oil retention enemas at night are utilized, that sigmoidoscopy above the impaction reveals no tumor or diverticulitic encroachment on the lumen. The use of hydrophilic colloid laxatives or enemas of tap water may be required for the remainder of the patient's life, if motivation for more drastic alteration of living, eating, and defecatory habits cannot be stimulated or if poor muscle tone, difficulties in ambulation and in achieving a comfortable posture at stool, or cerebral arteriosclerosis are major factors.

As described in Chap. 43, the presence of unaccustomed fecal masses in the rectosigmoid may produce rectal urgency in the patient who has always had normal defecatory responses to such masses. Sudden onset of rectal urgency in a previously healthy person demands immediate investigation. Usually it is seen in young adults required by emergency surgical indications to lie very still in bed (classically, in ophthalmologic, orthopedic, or neurosurgical disorders); intolerable urgency accompanied by the passage of watery exudate of small quantity suggests that an impaction has occurred. Severe urgency accompanied by the frequent passage of an exudate rich in blood, pus, or mucus usually signifies the presence of an acute proctitis (see below).

INFLAMMATORY DISORDERS

Acute Diverticulitis

Acute diverticulitis is an acute inflammation of colonic diverticula, the origin of which has been described above. (Inflammation of Meckel's diverticulum has been discussed in Chap. 317.) The causes of the acute inflammation of single or multiple diverticula usually are mechanical, related to the plugging of the neck of the outpouching by undigested food residues. Under such conditions the blood supply to the thin wall of the diverticular sac, made up of mucosa and serosa only, is easily compromised, and colonic bacteria can invade these tissues and produce a purulent reaction. Mild attacks of this type are probably quite frequent in the elderly population; dislodgment of the obstructing plug by the increased pressure in the sac is followed by evacuation of its contents into the bowel lumen, thus resolving the process uneventfully. When this does not occur, however, the purulent sac enlarges and causes an inflammatory reaction in neighboring structures, including the colonic wall. As this latter becomes edematous, other diverticular necks are blocked, and a number of adjacent diverticula become the site of abscess formation. If no other egress is afforded and the process enlarges, the sacs may rupture into other hollow viscera to which the inflammatory reaction has attached them; fistula formation follows, most frequently into the bladder in men, into the bladder and pelvic organs in women. Not only is diverticulitis of the colon more common in men, but it is at least three times as often encountered in the descending colon as in the right colon. This is probably explainable because of the higher intraluminal pressures developed in the sigmoid and rectosigmoid, the less fluid character of the fecal contents in this area, and the anatomic fixation of the organ at the apex of an intraperitoneal pressure cone during defecation.

The *clinical features* of acute diverticulitis are lower abdominal pain, made worse by defecation, and the signs of peritoneal irritation—muscle spasm, guarding, fever, and leukocytosis. The disease has long been called "left-sided appendicitis," with good reason; diverticulitis of the transverse colon or ascending colon, although less common, presents similar findings; such a process in the cecal area may be impossible to distinguish from true appendicitis. The attendant spasm of the colonic wall in patients with diverticulitis usually produces constipation; the stools may be fluid or pasty. Rectal bleeding occurs in one-fourth the cases of sigmoid diverticulitis and is usually gross. Occasionally it is massive and life-threatening. As the process develops, the inflammatory reaction produces a tender mass appreciated on abdominal examination; behind the obstructing mass partial large-bowel obstruction may develop, and in low-grade or recurrent diverticulitis the entire picture cannot be distinguished from that due to a rectosigmoid carcinoma.

The *differential diagnosis* is principally that of neoplasm in the area of known or detected diverticulosis. Proctoscopy may show an acutely inflamed mucosa pushed into the lumen by an extrinsic mass; it is usually impossible to force the instrument through the spastically contracted lumen. Cytologic studies of rectal exudate may show carcinoma cells. Radiologic findings on barium enema may be diagnostic (see Fig. 320-3), but often the distortion of the area by the inflammation prevents a clear distinction between cancer and diverticulitis. The same difficulty confronts the surgeon at operation; he sometimes cannot make this distinction even when looking directly at the specimen. Occasionally a patient presents generalized peritonitis, acute paralytic ileus, and shock. Differential diagnosis here is that of any ruptured viscus or of any intraabdominal catastrophe producing such manifestations—acute pancreatitis, mesenteric infarction, mechanical forms of intestinal obstruction, or acute pyelophlebitis.

Treatment in the usual case comprises bed rest, heat to the tender abdominal area, and the administration of antibiotics, usually penicillin plus tetracycline or chloramphenicol. Warm cottonseed oil enemas and a very soft diet complete the management of the mild acute attack. Once the attack is over, the patient is cautioned to avoid eating nuts, seeds, and fibrous foods, and any constipation is treated as described previously.

The principal danger of such repeated attacks is the development of fistulous tracts between the diverticula and neighboring structures, in particular the bladder and vagina. These are extremely difficult to manage surgically. A preliminary colostomy has to be created before any attack on the primary disease can be undertaken; the ensuing postoperative period may be prolonged, numerous surgical attempts may have to be made, and the general health of the patient may deteriorate, thus preventing adequate healing.

Because of the dangers of such complications, as well as the possibility of peritonitis and acute perforation, current opinion is in favor of primary resection of the diverticulitic segment of colon if it is subject to recurrence of the disease despite adequate medical management.

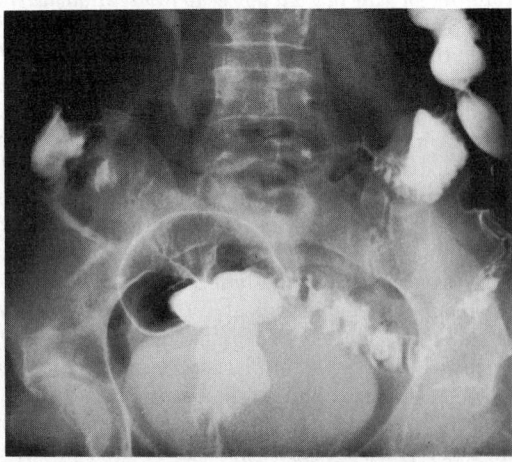

Fig. 320-3. Diverticulitis of the sigmoid colon.

Chronic Nonspecific Ulcerative Colitis

This disorder or group of disorders is characterized pathologically by an inflammatory reaction involving the mucosa and submucosa of the colon and/or rectum, not ascribable to invasion of these tissues by specific bacteria, parasites, or viruses. The clinical expression of the inflammatory response is the passage of an inflammatory exudate—blood, pus, fibrin, and mixtures thereof—into the lumen, where it may coat an otherwise normal stool, be admixed with unformed stools, or be excreted as a pure exudate. The absence of parasites (*Endamoeba histolytica* in particular), bacteria (of the genus *Shigella* or *Salmonella* in particular), mycobacteria (*Mycobacterium tuberculosis* in particular), and the virus of lymphogranuloma venereum in stools, exudates, or biopsies of the colonic mucosa suggests the diagnosis, although certain characteristic findings allow the experienced physician to classify the disorder in the idiopathic group *despite* the presence of these organisms.

The disease is worldwide in distribution, although there are marked differences in the reported frequency from country to country. The reported mortality from the disease is remarkably similar in the United States, Canada, and Denmark, about 0.5 per 100,000 population. It is much higher in England and Wales, and distinctly lower in Norway. All ages are affected, from infancy to the ninth decade, and both sexes are affected approximately equally; about half the cases are recognized in the patient under forty. In the United States the disease is more common in the city than in the country, in the North than in the South, in the wards of private voluntary hospitals than in those of city and county hospitals, among those of better-than-average incomes and educational backgrounds. As with regional enteritis, the frequency with which the disease is seen in the United States in those of Jewish extraction is three times the expected; the disease is about one-third as frequent among Negroes as among whites. A family history of ulcerative colitis can be elicited in 5 to 10 percent of all cases. The number of reported cases is highest where the reported frequency of shigellosis and salmonellosis is least. There is little doubt that it is becoming increasingly frequent, so that it now constitutes one of the commonest forms of serious bowel disease encountered in United States medical practice.

ETIOLOGY AND PATHOGENESIS. There is no known single cause of ulcerative proctitis or colitis. Not only are no specific viruses or bacteria associated with its onset, but no other disorders—irritable colon syndrome, longstanding constipation, attacks of gastroenteritis—seem to predispose the patient to the later development of ulcerative colitis. Although a few patients give a story of precipitation of symptoms by ingestion of whole milk or other foods, food allergy is generally not regarded as of etiologic significance, nor do various nutritional disturbances play a causative role.

The primary pathologic lesion in this disease is not understood. Far-advanced lesions removed by colonic resection or at autopsy show varying degrees of abscesses in the crypts of Lieberkühn and some degree of vascular injury, expressed as thrombosis, hyaline change, or perivascular inflammation. Some pathologists believe there is evidence of defective epithelial regeneration. Specimens removed from less ill patients by rectal or colonic biopsy show principally an intense inflammatory reaction, acute, chronic, or mixed; in early acute cases the lamina propria is often full of eosinophils, and the goblet cells appear abnormal. In recurrent cases of longer duration, such biopsies often reveal plasma cell infiltration, small granulomas, dilatation of lymphatics, and vascular thrombosis.

In all stages of the disease, however, small abscesses in the lamina propria are seen breaking through epithelium. The nature of the exudate seen in the colonic lumen reflects accurately the primacy of this ulcerative process, which spews forth blood, pus, fibrin, and mucus. As the disease waxes, wanes, and becomes chronic, plasma cell invasion, histiocytes, and crypt abscesses are seen. The mucosa and submucosa take on the general characteristics of granulation tissue—telangiectasis, fibrosis, conversion of colmnar to cuboidal epithelium, and disappearance of the crypts. As this process becomes generalized, the total colonic bulk shrinks and is replaced by fibrous tissue, and the mucosa exhibits the characteristic pseudopolypoid appearance of normal or abnormal mucosa projecting from the diseased bowel.

Attempts to produce experimental ulcerative colitis have employed chronic overstimulation of the parasympathetic nervous system, postganglionic splanchnicectomy, inoculations with many different bacteria, and a variety of hyperimmunizing systems. All these have been followed irregularly by a hemorrhagic colitis which resembles to some degree the human lesion.

The systemic effects of the disease in patients carefully followed for a number of years, plus the tissue responses involving eosinophils and plasma cells, have led many investigators to postulate an autoimmune origin for this disease. However, early enthusiasm for this concept of pathogenesis has not been justified by subsequent work, nearly all of which would indicate that the immunologic abnormalities demonstrated are clearly secondary to colonic injury rather than primary. Electron microscopic studies have identified the epithelial cell as the primarily damaged tissue. Hay fever, asthma, and drug sensitivity seem no more common among these patients than among controls.

CLASSIFICATION. *Clinical classifications* of ulcerative colitis have been based on the presenting features—these depend on the area of the colon or rectum involved—and the acuteness of the inflammatory process. Thus a sudden *acute ulcerative proctitis* involving the lower rectum might be manifest solely by a bloody exudate on otherwise normal stools, unaccompanied by fever, anorexia, or any signs of systemic toxicity. Proctoscopy reveals an intensely red and edematous mucous membrane, the normal vascular pattern completely disappearing from view until the proctoscope reaches 10 to 12 cm from the anal margin, at which point all inflammatory changes subside. The intense friability of the involved mucosa, bleeding at the slightest touch of a cotton swab, cannot be identified above this point; biopsies from the involved and uninvolved areas are strikingly different. If the proctitis is most active in the upper rectum, intolerable rectal urgency may be the presenting sign. Under such circumstances the rectal mucosa may not appear so abnormal near the anus but reaches its most friable and edematous appearance at 5 cm or so from the skin, abruptly receding at 15 cm, so that the visible rectosigmoid appears normal.

Patients with this type of ulcerative proctitis have been considered to differ from those patients whose colons are the site of disease, although the appearance of the lesions in the rectum via proctoscopy and on microscopic inspection via biopsy cannot be distinguished. It is generally agreed that the course of the disease is definitely milder, systemic symptoms being absent, and response to local therapeutic measures more gratifying, but recent follow-up studies suggest that these patients have the same familial aggregates of colitis, similar age and sex distribution, and similar types and degrees of personality maladjustments. It is the feeling of most authorities in the field that in at least 10 percent of these patients extension of the inflammatory process into the rectosigmoid will develop.

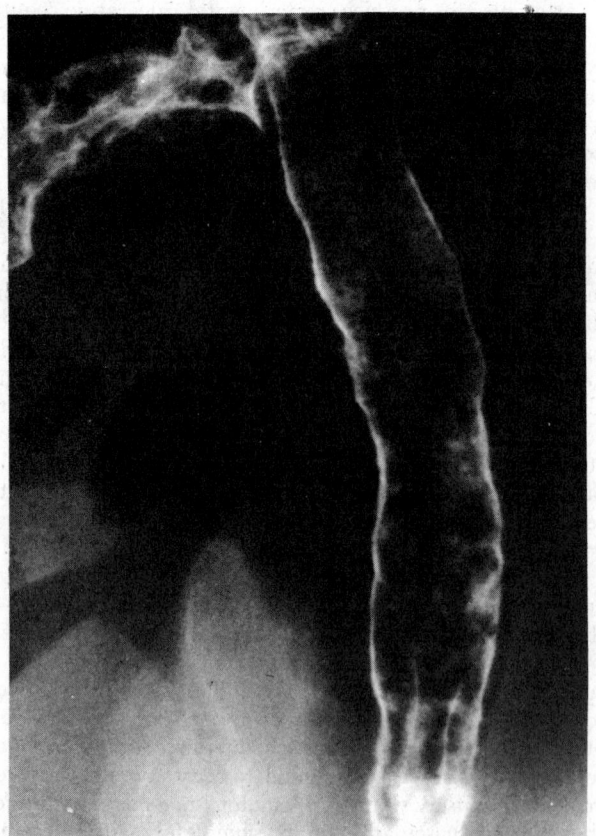

Fig. 320-4. Acute ulcerative colitis of the transverse and descending colon.

Acute ulcerative colitis is the term given to an acutely developing pancolitis, characterized by toxicity, fever, abdominal pain, distension, and tenesmus. The sigmoidoscopic picture shows uniform involvement for the length of the instrument (25 cm); the mucosa bleeds easily and is covered by a purulent exudate full of neutrophils and eosinophils. When the rectum and rectosigmoid are both involved maximally, as is most frequently the case, diarrhea and tenesmus are usually present, and the sigmoidoscopic appearance is similar throughout. The muscular contractions of the sigmoid make sigmoidoscopy above 13 cm difficult to perform; ulcerations are usually quite evident under the exudate one swabs away, and friability is extreme.

As a general rule, the larger the area of involvement, the greater the systemic toxicity, the more diffuse the cramps, and the more abnormal the stools. Exceptions are not rare, however; *an ulcerative pancolitis* from the ileocecal valve to the anus, demonstrable by barium enema in terms of innumerable ulcerations, spasm, and contraction, may rarely be accompanied by little clinical evidence of active inflammation; conversely, some patients are prostrated despite the involvement of only a few inches of colon.

The clinical course is sometimes used as the basis for classification of this disease, but this is, naturally, not known when the patient is first seen. The only rationale for this is to characterize those few unfortunate patients who suffer from *fulminant ulcerative colitis;* in these the disease is maximal at its onset and literally overwhelms the patient with the dissolution of his colon, massive colonic hemorrhage, or generalized sepsis. Such patients, accounting for perhaps 1 percent of all cases of the disease, either die within 1 to 8 weeks of the onset or survive emergency colectomy and ileostomy.

Chronic Intermittent Colitis. The course of the disease is unpredictable, but the majority of patients have a chronic intermittent colitis once the initial episode has been weathered. As described above, of this group the majority has disease localized in the descending colon and rectum; no evidences of toxicity may ever be noted, and blood on the stool, rectal urgency, and the characteristic proctoscopic findings may constitute all the evidence of disease. For *most* patients the initial bout is accompanied by fever, malaise, anorexia, and weight loss; the stools contain blood before they become unformed. Cramping abdominal pain aggravated by eating, severe urgency, and tenesmus are more prominent than nausea and vomiting. If properly managed medically, such patients undergo a slow subsidence of symptoms over a period of weeks or months; usually a definite remission of months or years ensues before another exacerbation comes on to plague them. The recurrences may be as severe as the original bout or more severe and may follow an upper respiratory infection or an emotional upset. The succession of remissions and exacerbations over the years often results in a prematurely aged appearance of the patient, in the production of damage to other organ systems, in conditioned malnutrition, and in severe depression. Specific complications are considered below.

Crohn's Disease of the Colon. Although ulcerative colitis may involve selectively the ascending colon as one form of segmental colitis, the majority of inflammatory lesions of the right colon now being seen in the Western world have the histopathologic characteristics noted by Crohn and his colleagues in the ileum. In order to avoid confusion in terminology, it would be advisable to call such lesions "Crohn's disease" of the colon, of colon and ileum, or of colon and small intestine. The clinical features of this disorder are not totally agreed upon, but the clinical course is less often marked by severe bleeding than is ulcerative colitis, malignant change seems less frequently to occur, and the frequency of anal lesions is higher, often in the absence of rectal mucosal change. Fistulous tracts from the colon suggest this entity rather than ulcerative colitis, but both diseases may give rise to rectovaginal fistulas. Proctoscopically there are none of the usual findings of ulcerative colitis, and the biopsy may show the characteristic sarcoid reaction if taken from the edge of a lesion. Radiologically there are many points of difference, although these points are at present still being contested. Both tuberculosis and diverticulitis may be difficult to separate from Crohn's disease, but tuberculous lesions are now rare, and diverticulitis involves predominantly the sigmoid colon. Treatment is as in Chron's disease of the intestine (see Table 320-1).

PSYCHOLOGIC FEATURES. The psychologic features of patients with ulcerative colitis, although largely ignored in the medical literature prior to 1932, have enlisted intense interest in recent years. Some workers believe that a larger proportion of patients with ulcerative colitis resemble each other psychologically, and even physically, than is the case with many other chronic disorders. The patients who fall into this category are juvenile in appearance, hostile and depressed, guarded in their relationships with physicians, and very easily wounded by verbal and attitudinal disparagement. They seem to maintain their interpersonal contacts only by devious and tenuous means, erecting a system of interdependent relationships which seem preposterous to the physician and disheartening to the psychiatrist. On the other hand, more than half the patients with this disorder cannot be distinguished from the general population; these subjects have a resilient personal and work history, often have been successful at school, trade, or profession, have maintained strong interpersonal attractions and defenses, and to the careful historian present many facets of character which provide clear guides to proper supportive psychotherapy. The disease itself, however, with its chronicity, relapses, and remissions and cost in time and money, usually is associated in all patients with some degree of depression and anxiety, and these reactions influence both the course of the disease and its therapy.

LABORATORY STUDIES. These comprise radiologic, chemical, and bacteriologic techniques. Sigmoidoscopy usually makes the diagnosis, but the barium enema is employed to determine the extent of the lesions above the reach of that instrument, to identify segmental disease when the sigmoidoscopy is negative, and to follow the course of the disease and detect the presence of complications. No formal preparations are needed before sigmoidoscoping a patient with ulcerative colitis; for the barium enema any preparation more violent than a low-pressure warm saline enema is best avoided. It is important to obtain good delineation of mucosal relief by the barium enema; air-contrast studies are helpful if the patient is not too spastic to prevent a successful visualization of pseudopolyps and other abnormalities often overlooked in the routine examination.

The radiologic findings in the disease may bear little relationship to the clinical severity or course of the

Table 320-1. INFLAMMATORY DISEASES OF THE COLON

Characteristics	Ulcerative colitis	Crohn's disease
Clinical features:		
Rectal urgency	Very common	Rare
Rectal bleeding	Usual	Infrequent
Anal disease	Not prominent	Often severe
Fistulas	Rare	Common
Radiologic features:		
Type of involvement	Continuous	Discontinuous
Right colon affected	Only if pancolitis present	Common
Opposing borders of inflamed colonic segment	Symmetrically involved	Asymmetrically involved
Terminal ileum, if involved	Widened, patulous	Narrowed, stiff
Sigmoidoscopic features:		
Extent of rectal and rectosigmoidal involvement	Diffuse	Patchy
Friability	Always present	Uncommon
Histopathologic features:		
Involved colonic layers	Mucosa and submucosa, with thinning and fibrosis	All layers, with hyperplastic response
Granulomas	Rare	Common (25–75%)
Fissuring and fistulas	Rare	Common
Mesenteric fat and lymph nodes	Not remarkable	Markedly edematous and hyperplastic

disease. Characteristically, in early ulcerative colitis irritability of the rectosigmoid is combined with demonstrations of hairline projections of barium from the wall of this spastic area; more irregular serrations and even flask-shaped ulcerations may be seen as the disease progresses (Fig. 320-4). The entire colon is abnormal on barium examination in a large number of patients, even though their symptoms may be minimal or confined to the rectosigmoid. In patients with fulminant colitis or in aged persons who display rather marked lack of resistance to the process, the entire colon may be dilated—so-called "toxic megacolon." In long-standing disease the entire organ may appear contracted and irregular, with a totally disorganized mucosal pattern. Pseudopolyps, which may occasionally be visualized sigmoidoscopically, more often are in the descending and transverse colon and seen only in the barium enema (Fig. 320-5). The terminal ileum may be involved in an ulcerative process which renders it dilated and patulous in contrast to the constricted lumen noted in regional enteritis. Localized masses may be fecaliths, localized constrictions, or carcinoma of the colon, a recognized complication of this disorder. When the right side of the colon and the terminal ileum bear the brunt of the disease process, a small-intestinal barium series is mandatory to investigate the jejunoileal area.

Chronic intermittent forms of colitis are identified primarily by history and radiologic abnormalities, as described above. On sigmoidoscopy these patients usually show at all times the scars of their disease, presenting an abnormal mucous membrane which bleeds very

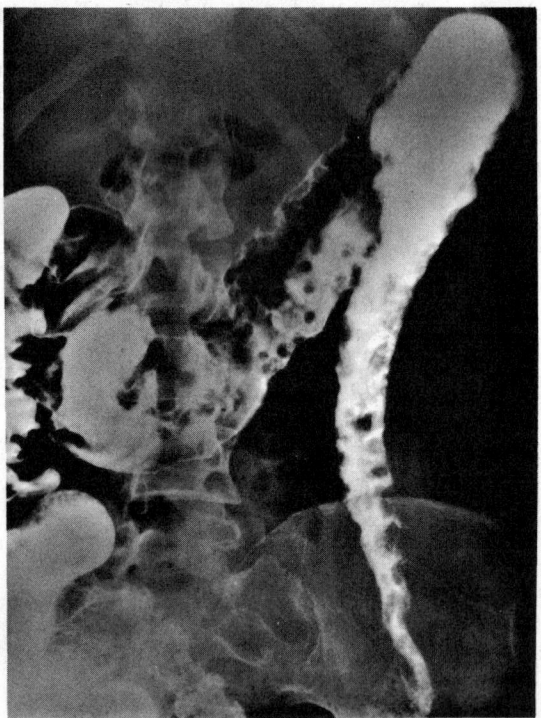

Fig. 320-5. Pseudopolyposis of the entire colon secondary to chronic ulcerative colitis of 12 years' duration.

easily, has lost its normal vascular patterns, and may vary in consistency from an edematous beefy involvement of superficial submucosa and mucosa to a leathery violaceous colonic wall, studded with scar tissue and pseudopolyps. Characteristically, a fibrinopurulent exudate is present, and broad, flat ulcerations may be seen. Biopsies in this stage usually reveal areas of granulation tissue, containing very few crypts; the lamina propria is thickened and infiltrated with plasma cells and lymphocytes. Small blood vessels are prominent.

Strictures of the rectum are frequent in the long-standing case, being encountered about midrectum.

DIFFERENTIAL DIAGNOSIS. This includes the following entities: Specific colonic infections are identified by culture and examination of the stools or rectal exudate and by sigmoidoscopic appearance. *Amebic disease* characteristically presents as deep ulcerations in an otherwise nearly normal mucosa, which is not friable or granular. Swabs or biopsies from the edges of these ulcers give a good yield of the trophozoites of *Endamoeba histolytica;* the exudate contains few nutrophils but much frank blood. *Bacillary dysentery* can present as an acute ulcerative colitis; the exudate is very rich in neutrophils, but friability is not striking in the rectum. Cultural identification of the organisms makes the diagnosis. *Tuberculosis* involves the cecum and ileum; if ulcerative it is usually associated with active pulmonary tuberculosis; if hyperplastic it produces obstructive symptoms rather than bloody diarrhea, and the sigmoidoscopy is negative. *Lymphogranuloma venereum* may rarely produce a mild acute colitis, but under such circumstances the venereal characteristics of the disease are prominent. The proctitis associated with the long-standing case is secondary to chronic lymphadenitis; it is thus more common in women and associated with rectal stricture, usually just inside the anus; the blood shows hyperglobulinemia, and the skin gives a positive reaction to the Frei antigen.

Nonspecific involvement of the colon may be produced by Crohn's disease, in which case the colon is infiltrated by a hyperplastic submucosal granulomatous process, friability of rectal mucous membrane is absent, and small-intestinal disease is usually identified by radiologic examination (see Table 320-1). The *uremic patient* may have a bloody rectal or colonic discharge, because of the vascular fragility produced by that condition; there is little difficulty in identifying the accompanying stigmas of uremia. *Diverticulitis* of the sigmoid may cause spasm, fever, and rectal bleeding, but the sigmoidoscopic appearance is entirely unlike that of ulcerative colitis, and the exudate usually is much less purulent. A segmental colitis localized to the rectosigmoid may, however, be impossible to differentiate from this disorder. Cancer of the colon may give many of the symptoms of colitis but usually is easy to distinguish from it. However, cancer of the colon supervening on a chronic colitis may be impossible to identify except by surgical biopsy, and rarely a mild ulcerative colitis seems to occur proximal and secondary to a slowly obstructing carcinoma of the left colon.

COMPLICATIONS, SEQUELAE, AND ASSOCIATED DISORDERS. These may be *local:* perianal abscesses, rectovaginal fistulas, strictures, sealed-off perforations, pseudopolyposis, localized peritonitis, and carcinomatous changes; if one excludes those patients presenting ulcerative proctitis alone, the incidence of carcinoma of the colon in patients with chronic ulcerative colitis is 3 to 5 percent, or an incidence forty to fifty times that of the general population. Or they may be *systemic:* patients with colitis may have the entire disease confined to the colon or may exhibit a wide range of symptoms and signs, suggesting that many distant organ systems reflect to some degree the underlying inflammation. Such occurrences are considered evidence of an underlying systemic hyperimmune response of patients with this disorder. The most important of these is arthritis, particularly of the large joints in both sexes and of the spine in men. The symptoms primarily are those of periarthritis; rheumatoid factor is absent from the serum, and the severity of the process usually parallels that of the colitis. The skin shows a number of abnormalities, usually forms of erythema nodosum, erythema multiforme, and rarely, the very dangerous pyoderma gangrenosum. The eyes may be the seat of chorioretinitis or iridocyclitis; thrombophlebitis may be present in a migratory form, and endocrine abnormalities, particularly amenorrhea, are common. Liver disease, either postnecrotic cirrhosis or chronic pericholangitis, seems to be more common in these patients than one would expect, and varying degrees of pancreatic fibrosis have been described. Most of the patients with these complications have had a severe illness, characterized by long periods of malnutrition, have received multiple transfusions and intensive chemotherapy, and have suffered severe electrolyte disturbances. Amyloid disease may also complicate the course of long-standing and severe colitis but more commonly is seen in Crohn's disease.

TREATMENT. The treatment of patients with this disease comprises both medical and surgical management. Since there is no truly specific form of therapy medical regimens of treatment aim to correct nutritional and electrolyte loss, control diarrhea, discourage bacterial invasion, and minister to the psychologic needs of the patient. When fever, anorexia, severe diarrhea, and increasing blood loss are present, hospitalization is necessary, and a very careful watch over daily changes in status must be maintained. The disease is very treacherous in that perforations and massive hemorrhage may occur without warning.

Most ill patients are best treated by parenteral alimentation on admission to a hospital. Complete parenteral supplementation can be achieved for 3 or 4 days, at which time a low-residue but highly nutritious regimen is instituted.

Oftentimes it is wise to allow the patient to eat foods he particularly craves. There is no evidence that any articles of food influence the disease, but it is felt that some foods, especially whole milk, increase diarrhea and abdominal gaseousness. Lactose intolerance is apparently common in these patients. Small, frequent feedings are usually better tolerated than larger meals, but this is not always the case. It is best not to give very cold liquids, which stimulate small-bowel propulsive activity. Vitamin preparations should be added to both the parenteral and oral intakes; preparations containing fat-soluble vitamins dispersed in watery vehicles are preferred to capsules or tablets. Blood transfusions should be given for anemia and hypoproteinemia. Anabolic steroid preparations are often useful (testosterone propionate in men, 25 mg two to three times weekly; norethandrolone, 30 mg daily).

These patients put out only small quantities of fecal material by rectum; most of the discharges are exudate and blood. In very toxic subjects it is not wise to attempt to control this "diarrhea" by large doses of opiates, since there is a danger of producing acute or toxic dilatation of the colon when neural elements are so greatly defunctionalized. The same objection may be raised to the very large doses of anticholinergic medications needed to produce an effect on this badly damaged colon. In the less toxic case, particularly when ambulatory, the judicious use of tincture of opium to control urgency until other measures reduce the inflammatory response can be very helpful.

Chemotherapeutic and antibiotic drugs are very useful in managing certain stages and complications of ulcerative colitis. In milder forms of colitis, in which high fever and toxicity are not prominent, salicylazosulfapyridine (Azulfidine) (1.0 Gm three to four times a day) has been proved able to control friability and bleeding and to lessen markedly the rectosigmoid irritability responsible for urgency and tenesmus. It can be given continuously or in courses lasting 3 to 6 weeks followed by intervals of several months, then reinstituted as a prophylactic. In the acutely ill patient in the hospital, penicillin and chloramphenicol are usually administered concomitantly in an attempt to halt or prevent acute peritonitis. Other sulfonamide drugs and broad-spectrum antibiotics, although not without usefulness, have been less specific than those described.

Adrenal steroid hormones and ACTH have become very important in the medical management of ulcerative colitis. For acute proctitis and proctosigmoiditis, where urgency is very severe despite the absence of generalized illness, rectal instillations of soluble corticosteroids have been remarkably effective. They are usually given as retention enemas of small volume (100 ml aqueous or oily suspension containing 20 mg prednisolone) morning and at night until symptoms have been brought under control; then only the nightly instillation is continued, the frequency of administration gradually diminishing. In the acutely ill patient with life-threatening colitis, parenteral administration of ACTH (40 to 80 mg daily) for a 10-day period usually effects an improvement in appetite, a decrease in toxicity, and a gradual improvement in sigmoidoscopic appearance of the involved bowel Cortisone, hydrocortisone, or prednisolone in adequate doses may produce similar effects in the acutely ill patient, but seem rather less reliable than ACTH. On the other hand, in the less severely toxic patient or in the toxic patient as he recovers, oral steroids are easy to administer and are quite effective. Many patients have now been maintained for years on oral doses of these hormones, either alone or combined with Azulfidine, with a low incidence of complications of therapy. The use of intermittent corticosteroids every 48 hr has in some instances proved effective in controlling the inflammation and in preventing many undesirable side effects of these agents.

Psychiatric approaches to the patient with ulcerative colitis are not generally agreed upon. It is the opinion of most psychiatrists that the acutely ill patient is approachable only by the most superficial forms of supportive psychotherapy. In the more usual types of the disease the physician managing the case can supply the needed support by searching the patient's history and behavior for indications of inner resources and motivations which can be converted to therapeutic use. Attempts to manipulate the immediate home and work environment of the patient are necessary but may require professional assistance beyond the scope of the physician's training and resources. Pregnancy frequently mobilizes severe stress and can aggravate or ameliorate the disease. When ulcerative colitis begins during pregnancy, it is usually very severe.

Professional psychiatric assistance should not be neglected when indicated. An attitude of optimism, warm concern, and patience, tempered with frequent medical examinations of the patient, his rectum, and his stools seems the best armamentarium of the physician caring for patients suffering from this disorder.

Surgical measures are absolutely indicated for several local complications and for certain catastrophic events which may complicate the course of the disease. In the presence of a diseased colon it is almost impossible to heal perianal and perirectal abscesses, fistulas, and rectal strictures. Furthermore, it is not possible to make use of a rectum deformed by these processes after localized lesions of the colon have been resected, so that ileostomy and total colectomy are the treatment of choice. Similarly, massive hemorrhage from the diseased bowel and acute toxic dilatation of the colon are best handled as emergencies by ileostomy and colectomy.

The principal areas of disagreement as to the proper time for or advisability of surgical therapy concern patients with chronic recurrent disease of more than 2 years' duration and those who are disabled by chronic anemia, arthritis, or pseudopolyposis. Increasingly, and in particular as surgical techniques for ileostomy and colectomy have improved, more of these patients are being subjected to this treatment earlier in the course of their disease. Attempts to preserve the rectal area by ileorectal anastomosis and the French techniques for electrocoagulative prefrontal lobotomy are as yet improved methods to modify the surgical approach. Any patient with ulcerative colitis of 10 years' activity must be considered to have a 3 to 5 percent risk of malignancy of the colon; the presence of pseudopolyposis or the slightly less common adenomatous polyposis complicating the disease is probably an indication for colectomy. The

ileostomized patient has now a much better outlook for a normal life than ever before; the formation of ileostomist clubs has stimulated interest in the intelligent design and management of ileostomy appliances; reanastomosis of the ileum to partially resected colons has proved so often disastrous that it is better to offer the patient no unrealizable picture of the ileostomy as a temporary measure, but rather to concentrate his attention on the fuller life he will be able to lead with his diseased bowel totally removed.

SUMMARY. Ulcerative colitis is, then, a chronic inflammatory disease of the colon, encountered in all age groups, affecting any portion or all of the large bowel. About 75 to 80 percent of all patients with the disease will be able to cope medically with its ravages, despite the remissions and exacerbations which characterize its course. There is some evidence that the disease is more severe when its onset is in young children or in those over sixty. The case fatality rate is hard to determine, since so many patients with ulcerative proctitis alone never come into hospitals, but for those ill enough to warrant hospitalization, approximately 10 percent now die of the disease or its complications, including carcinoma of the colon. Surgical intervention at present is necessary for approximately 20 percent of patients in whom the disease involves more than the rectum. Unless some newer medical or psychiatric therapy is devised, it is probable that this figure will increase.

ISCHEMIC COLONIC DISEASE (Segmental Infarction, Ischemic Colitis)

As the population ages, atheromatous involvement of visceral arteries increases in frequency and degree. The left side of the colon, and particularly the splenic flexure, depends on a long and rather nonbranching vasculature from the middle and left colic arteries, which atheromatous disease can easily compromise. Whenever an older patient or one with heart disease suddenly experiences acute abdominal pain, usually on the left side, with fever and the passage of bright-red blood or clots per rectum, a *segmental infarction* of the colon should be suspected. Barium enema usually shows a narrowed splenic flexure or thumbprint defects in the descending colon over a short segment; the patient is carefully watched for signs of gangrene or peritonitis; if these do not ensue, barium enema studies several weeks later show a gradual return of the narrowed bowel toward normal or toward a smooth, often asymmetrical constriction involving several inches of bowel.

The differential diagnosis on clinical grounds is most commonly acute diverticulitis; the x-ray differential also includes Crohn's disease of the colon, but the lack of previous history makes this not difficult to exclude. Diverticulitis occurs, unfortunately, often in the same age group, and it is probable that many such attacks of ischemic colitis have been labeled as acute diverticulitis in the past.

Treatment is usually that of close observation, with

laparotomy dictated by signs of gangrene or peritonitis. Most patients recover spontaneously.

TUMORS OF THE COLON AND RECTUM

Neoplasms of the large intestine and rectum account, in the United States, for 15 percent of all deaths due to malignant disease. These lesions represent 45 percent of all deaths due to neoplasms of the digestive tract, being nearly twice as frequent as the number of deaths due to cancer of the stomach. They occur equally among males and females and in all age groups but of course are most frequently encountered in persons forty-five to seventy-five years of age.

ETIOLOGY. Although the true causes of colonic malignancy are not established, there appears to be an intimate relation between the adenomatous polyp and the development of carcinoma. All stages of carcinomatous change have been recognized in polyps, and there appears to be a definite risk of malignant polypoid growth and of malignancy in the colons of patients who have polyps, whether or not the tumor originates in or near the polyps. Congenital multiple polyposis of the colon has an astonishingly high malignant potential; chronic inflammatory disease of the colon, as seen in ulcerative colitis, also seems to potentiate or stimulate the development of carcinoma in the diseased bowel. Other lesions of the large intestine seem to bear no relationship to cancer, although in no case is it possible to demonstrate that they offer protection against its development. As with malignant disease generally, familial aggregates of the disease are well documented, and multiple malignant lesions have been shown to occur in certain members of such families.

PATHOLOGY. The vast majority of tumors originating in the colon and rectum are of epithelial origin. Those which are not are usually benign; they include lipomas, endometriosis, benign lymphomas, leiomyomas, enterocytomas, and hemangiomas. Nonepithelial malignant lesions are infrequent but should be mentioned because of the necessity for recognizing them in a treatable stage of their development. *Carcinoids* of the rectosigmoid and rectum ordinarily form yellowish elevations between the muscularis mucosae and mucosa; they are usually discovered by chance sigmoidoscopy, although a few have been indicted as causing bleeding. If the muscularis is invaded, the tumor is malignant and will require wide excision. It is estimated that 10 percent of rectal carcinoids will metastasize. Those beginning in the ileocecal valve or in the cecum, although not ulcerating deeply, metastasize early to regional nodes and the liver; radiologically they may present as a rounded filling defect. *Leiomyosarcomas* are almost never found elsewhere in the colon than in the sigmoid or rectum, where they may grow to large size and produce mucosal ulceration with bleeding. *Lymphosarcomas* of the colon and rectum may present exactly as do carcinomas, but there is less fixation of the wall as the tumor grows, so that intussusception is occasionally the presenting syndrome. Colon

carcinomas affect women more often than men, whereas rectal carcinomas are seen more commonly in men. They have been recorded at all ages, but with their peak incidence in the fifth, sixth, and seventh decades. The cecum and ascending colon are involved in 15 percent of all carcinomas of the large bowel and rectum, the transverse colon in 10 percent, and the sigmoid colon, rectosigmoid, and rectum in 75 percent. Thus, nearly two-thirds of all cancers of the large intestine are within reach of the sigmoidoscope. In most series of cases, multiple primary colonic cancers are found in about 3 percent of patients operated on or autopsied. Lesions of the colon which seem statistically to favor the development of carcinoma are multiple polyposis, adenomatous polyposis, and chronic ulcerative colitis of over 10 years' duration. In addition to the statistical "precancerousness" of these lesions, indubitable malignant transformation of villous adenomas, single adenomatous polyps, multiple adenomatous polyps, and multicentric foci in ulcerative colitis have been observed.

In the colon above the rectum, adenocarcinoma is the common cell type. Classifications of the tumors according to their microscopic appearance—papillary, medullary, scirrhous, or colloid—are not of great assistance to the physician. Obviously, scirrhous carcinomas tend to constrict the lumen of the bowel, thereby producing obstructive syndromes, especially in the sigmoid area. Colloid tumors, most common in the right colon, can grow to enormous bulky mucinous masses, often forming mucous fistulas to the overlying skin. The common medullary tumor grows as a solid mass, the bulk of which may produce intermittent obstructive symptoms. Papillary tumors of the distal colon usually bleed early. All these tumors invade the regional lymph nodes and spread through the lymphatics and portal veins to the liver; direct spread into the paravertebral venous plexus is occasionally seen.

Symptoms of colonic carcinoma are usually vague and nonspecific at the outset. Rarely an acute perforation with peritonitis or a massive hemorrhage will call attention to the disease while it is still in an early stage, but much more often many months elapse before the symptoms finally bring the patient to the physician.

1. Changes in bowel habits are most frequent when carcinoma affects the left colon; these changes are often minimal but progressive alterations in frequency or in time of evacuation, in the size of the stool, and most significantly, in a sensation that evacuation has been incomplete.

2. Bleeding is complained of by the patient with a left-sided lesion in about 70 percent of cases; when the lesion is in the ascending colon or cecum, fewer than 25 percent of patients notice any blood in or with the stools, no doubt fewer because the blood is thoroughly admixed with the fecal slurry in the right colon. It is urgently important that the physician *not* attribute to hemorrhoids or anal fissures bleeding that is dark, associated with clots, well-mixed with mucus, or adherent to the stool.

3. Pain in the lower part of the abdomen is common

in lesions of the cecum or ascending colon; the pain is characteristically severe on climbing stairs or on bending forward; pain in left colonic lesions is often felt in the right side as a vague distension, or as a dragging sensation low in the pelvis toward the left inguinal ligament. Low-back pain is frequently present later in the course of the disease.

4. Pallor and anemia are classic presenting syndromes of right-sided colonic cancer; cardiac insufficiency and angina may be striking manifestations of the anemia, which reaches a remarkably severe degree in the absence of symptoms calling attention to the diseased bowel.

5. Anorexia, weight loss, and malaise may occur at any time or be absent.

PHYSICAL EXAMINATION. As with most malignant tumors early signs are not found. Aside from the characteristic pallor of anemia and the wasting suggestive of chronic disease, the signs are principally those due to masses, partial obstruction of the bowel, fistulas, and invasion of abdominal wall, bladder, uterus, and liver. Fecal masses are often felt behind partially obstructing neoplasms or inflammatory aggregates which have surrounded a perforation due to tumor. Rectal examination with the patient in the lithotomy or right decubitus position will often detect an intussuscepting lesion of the rectosigmoid. Marked distension in the right lower quadrant may represent an accommodation of bowel contents to incomplete obstruction by carcinoma of the left colon; caution should be exercised in palpating the cecal area under such circumstances, as perforation, always imminent, may be precipitated by digital manipulation from either the abdominal or the intrarectal areas.

LABORATORY FINDINGS. There are no diagnostic laboratory procedures. Detection of occult blood or gross blood in the stools is the most important laboratory technique for early identification of the possibility that malignancy of the colon exists. Other findings occur as

the tumor spreads locally to provoke an inflammatory response (increased sedimentation rate, leukocytosis), invasion of the liver (increased serum alkaline phosphatase, Bromsulphalein retention), hemolytic anemia, or direct bone marrow invasion. The anemia is usually hypochromic and is present in over half the patients with right-sided lesions, even when occasional stool specimens do not contain occult blood. Patients with left-sided lesions may also be anemic, but to a much less severe degree and not so frequently, since their blood loss is more easily appreciated in the appearance of the stools and they see physicians earlier.

DIAGNOSIS. Carcinoma of the colon is one of the most common malignant tumors and therefore must be thought of whenever a patient complains of changes in bowel habits, regardless of the kind of change. The finding of gross or occult blood in the stools or of a mass or distended colon on routine physical examination or of definite abnormalities on rectal examination or of evidences of weight loss and chronic illness should make one consider the diagnosis very seriously. Vague dyspeptic symptoms, especially when hypochromic anemia is present, also should lead the physician to investigate the right colon in particular.

The combination of digital and proctosigmoidoscopic examination should bring two-thirds of all cancers of the colon and rectum into direct view. The lesion may present itself directly as a polypoid or solid mass, frequently ulcerated, or as a large ulcer with a rolled margin or as a deformity of the colonic wall producing obstruction to the passage of the instrument. Instillation of Ringer's solution through the sigmoidoscope and centrifugation of the returning fluid will yield exfoliative cytologic smears of diagnostic value in many cases. Biopsy of suspicious lesions should be carried out whenever possible.

Radiologic diagnosis of lesions above the peritoneal reflection is highly accurate, but not infallible. In the presence of rectal bleeding it is important to follow a barium enema which has been reported as normal with an air-contrast study; such air-contrast enemas may reveal small lesions (greater than 5 mm in diameter) as well as nondistensible portions of the bowel wall. A cecal area which does not respond satisfactorily to preparative enemas and laxatives and shows poor radiologic detail should be particularly suspected of harboring a tumor.

The radiologist looks for structural and physiologic abnormalities reflecting the various ways these tumors may present, as described above under Pathology. (1) Tumors may project into the bowel, giving rise to a filling defect in the barium column (Fig. 320-6). (2) They may partially or completely encircle the bowel, producing a narrowing of the barium column proximal to which the bowel is often dilated (Fig. 320-7). (3) They may, by contiguous infiltration, distort the position of the colon, so that it is not free to follow gravity during the radiologist's maneuvering of the patient. (4) After the patient has expelled the barium, films of the mucosal relief may show defects due to tumor which has not penetrated the muscular coat. (5) Some tumors give rise to no defects

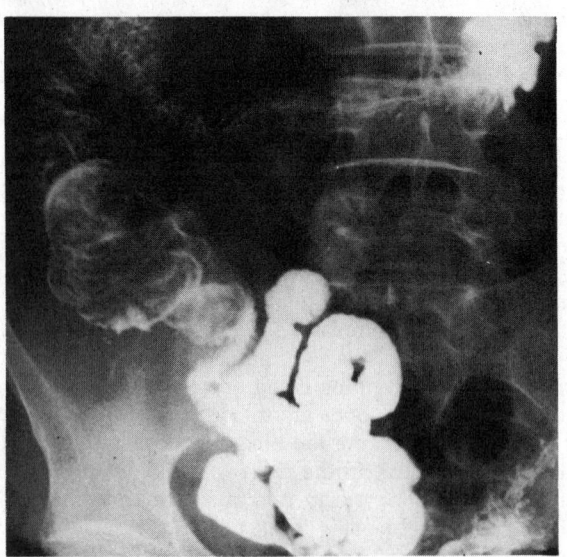

Fig. 320-6. Filling defect in the cecum produced by a carcinoma.

as such but interfere with neuromuscular integration, so that irritability, fluid retention, and spasticity may be noted.

Differential diagnosis of carcinoma of the ascending colon includes (1) benign lesions: gastric and duodenal ulcer, cholecystitis and cholelithiasis, liver disease; (2) inflammatory processes: appendiceal abscess, amebiasis, regional enteritis, segmental colitis, tuberculosis; (3) other tumors, such as carcinoids, lymphomas, lipomas, gastric cancer, renal cancer; (4) blood dyscrasias and uremia. In the descending colon carcinomas must be distinguished from diverticulitis, endometriosis, ulcerative colitis, lymphogranuloma venereum, and benign tumors.

Carcinoma of the rectum and anus presents more specific early symptoms than do the lesions discussed above. Bleeding, intolerable rectal urgency, pain, and soiling are the most frequent symptoms. The principal difficulty occurs when preexisting abnormalities have been present for so long a time that the patient and his physician do not detect subtle changes in them. Most frequently such problems arise when the patient has had an irritable colon syndrome, ulcerative colitis, simple constipation, or a variety of anorectal disorders, often complicated by surgical procedures.

These carcinomas are more frequent in men than in women (5:4) and comprise both adenocarcinoma in the rectum and squamous carcinoma in the anal skin, as well as mixed tumors in the anal canal. Malignant melanoma and basal cell carcinoma may arise in the anal skin, lymphoma, carcinoids, tumors arising from neighboring structures—prostate, cervix, ovary—as well as the seeding of upper abdominal carcinoma into the pelvic peritoneum may present as though they were primary lesions of the rectum.

Diagnosis is made by inspection, digital examination, anoscopy, proctoscopy, biopsy, and exfoliative cytology. Radiologic accuracy in the rectum is only fair and should not be necessary for identification of these low lesions.

COMPLICATIONS. Since it is the character of tumors to invade, many tumors of the colon, like tumors elsewhere, may first be diagnosed because of a complication of the original lesion; i.e., the tumor may perforate the bowel wall, giving rise to acute peritonitis, may perforate slowly and wall itself off, giving rise to local inflammatory mass and localized peritonitis, or may invade blood vessels to produce a brisk episode of rectal bleeding. More often, the tumor partially obstructs the bowel lumen for a long period of time, during which the colon proximal to the tumor dilates slowly without dramatic change in symptoms until a fecal impaction occurs, converting the proximal bowel into a large distended sac which may very well produce symptoms in the right lower quadrant, as noted previously. This occurs most often when the tumor is in the sigmoid, where the stool is driest. Tumors also weaken the colonic wall in such a way that an intussusception may occur, the tumor leading the intussusception. Similarly, fixation of the bowel wall by a tumor may produce a volvulus, which is most frequently seen in the sigmoid colon. Very large

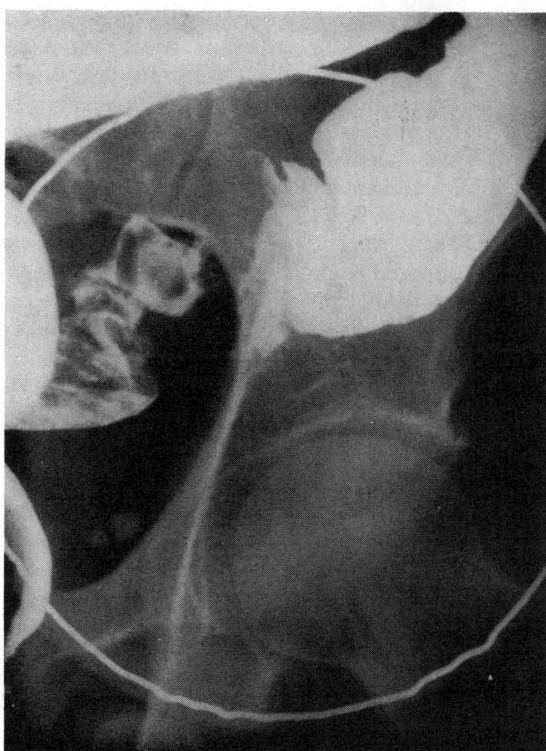

Fig. 320-7. Obstructing carcinoma of the sigmoid.

and slowly growing tumors may produce symptoms by pressure on neighboring organs; in particular, the uterus and the ureters may be involved, and, conversely, tumors of the uterus may compress the colon. Inguinal hernias may become apparent as the first sign of such increased pressure. Fistulas between the colon and pelvic organs suggest a thorough search for an underlying neoplastic infiltration. Abscesses inside the peritoneal cavity and cellulitis of the abdominal wall secondary to tumor infiltration are not infrequent.

TREATMENT. Although the only readily available therapeutic techniques are surgical, there are indications that radiotherapy combined with surgical therapy and some new chemotherapeutic means may significantly improve the outlook for patients with colonic and rectal cancer. Surgeons generally prefer abdominoperitoneal resection and colostomy for tumors located below the peritoneal reflections; above this area there is considerably more freedom of choice, depending primarily on the size and extent of the lesions. It is important to realize that good preoperative management and skillful work at the table will ensure that 70 to 80 percent of all cases can receive either extirpative or palliative surgical therapy with an operative mortality under 10 percent; the operative mortality is somewhat higher for lesions in the left colon. On the other hand, the survival rate for tumors of the left colon which can be resected is slightly higher than for right colon cancers. There has been an impressive improvement in the 5-year survivals since 1930; in 1960 approximately half of all patients who could be resected were expected to survive this length of time. Of the 20 to 30 percent who are first seen with extensive lymphatic or perineural spread, a few will survive 5 years without surgical therapy. When patients without any evidence of lymphatic or distant spread of cancer are subjected to radical operations, the 5-year survival in some series has been as high as 80 percent. It is important that palliative surgical attempts not be discouraged, as the symptomatic relief they bring may allow the patient to live in comfort the shortened terminal months of his life.

Discussion of the complications of surgical therapy and the management of colostomies can be found in surgical texts.

OBSTRUCTION OF THE COLON AND RECTUM

Chronic colonic obstruction has been discussed above in the sections dealing with its principal causes—tumors, diverticulitis, and megacolon. Additional disorders which may present as chronic large-bowel obstruction are strictures resulting from inflammatory processes (ulcerative colitis, lymphogranuloma venereum, perirectal abscess), from pelvic disease (endometriosis, tumors), from traumatic scarring (either postoperative or crushing), or from radiation necrosis secondary to treatment of pelvic cancer.

The presenting symptoms in all cases are similar, the diagnosis is made clinically and radiologically, and the treatment is surgical.

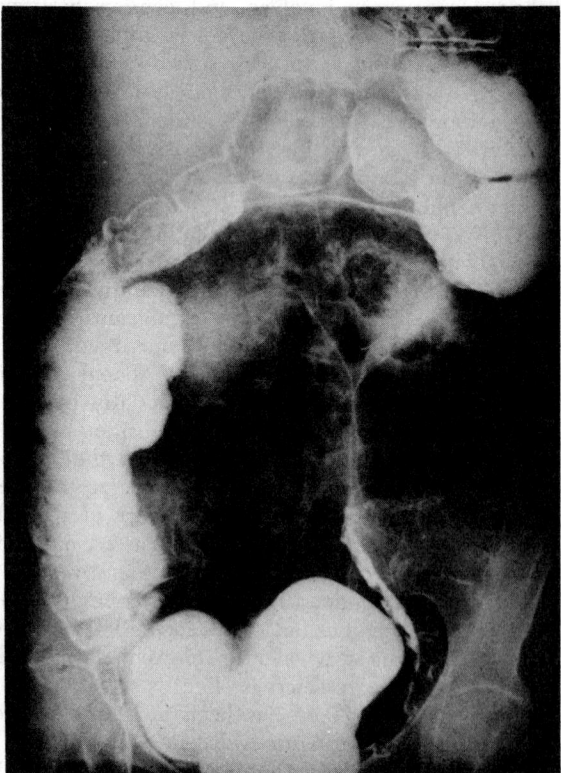

Fig. 320-8. Volvulus of the sigmoid.

Acute colonic obstruction has been discussed briefly in Chap. 318. Whereas acute small-bowel obstruction is more often due to mechanical and vascular causes, colonic obstruction occurring suddenly is statistically most often a result of neoplastic disease; other major causes of this process in adults are volvulus, diverticulitis, and intussusception.

Volvulus is a twisting of a portion of the colon on its mesentery, with trapping of air in the affected segment and progressive circulatory embarrassment as a result of the compression of the vascular pedicle to the segment. The two areas of colon most subject to this complication are the cecum and the sigmoid. *Cecal volvulus* is due to abnormal fixation of the cecum, associated with malrotation of the right colon. Severe volvulus of the cecum is uncommon except in Sweden; in the United States it accounts for less than 0.2 percent of all adult intestinal obstruction. Minor degrees of volvulus leading to recurrent right lower quadrant pain may be more common, since it is thought that 10 to 15 percent of the population have right colons sufficiently mobile to permit at least some degree of volvulus. The *symptoms* of acute cecal volvulus are severe, continuous right lower quandrant abdominal pain, followed by vomiting, constipation, and rapid intestinal distension. Treatment is surgical.

Sigmoid volvulus is more common than cecal volvulus and is especially common among persons of Eastern European ancestry. It is predominantly a disease of elderly persons with chronic constipation who eat food containing much roughage. The symptoms are usually those of increasing constipation for a few days preceding the first attack of hypogastric pain; this pain is usually colicky and discontinuous for a few hours but then becomes more severe and unremitting, as vascular supply to the twisted loop is throttled. The twisted loop enlarges enormously, rising up in the midline of the lower part of the abdomen to produce the characteristic radiologic picture (Fig. 320-8). In contrast to acute small-bowel obstruction, vomiting is rarely encountered; shock is generally absent unless gangrene and perforation of the loop have supervened.

Treatment is decompression. Although occasionally this can be done by a tube inserted via the sigmoidoscope, most of these patients require laparotomy, with decompression under direct vision, and whatever other extirpative surgical means are deemed necessary. Since sigmoid volvulus is known to recur in the same patient, it is probably wisest to resect the entire twisted loop at the time of operation.

Intussusception is the term applied to the invagination of one segment of intestine into another. *Primary intussusception,* which occurs without antecedent cause, is rarely seen after the third year of life; in infants it is a common cause of rectal bleeding *Secondary intussusception* is seen at all ages and anywhere in the gut, from esophagogastric junction to rectum. It usually occurs when an intraluminal neoplasm, benign or malignant, bulges out into the lumen, often buckling the wall from which it arises, and is propelled caudad by peristaltic activity. The tumor acts as the leading portion of the full thickness of the intestinal wall, producing a partial or complete obstruction to the propulsion of intestinal contents. The doubling over of the entire thickness of the gut wall leads to impairment of blood supply and eventual gangrene. In patients given anticoagulants, a small hemorrhage into the wall of the intestine may lead to a similar episode, *anticoagulant ileus*.

Symptoms are those of sudden abdominal pain and distension, with passage of blood-tinged rectal discharge. Low-lying intussusceptions may be felt on rectal examination, but usually a careful barium enema reveals the site and the characteristic "coiled-spring" appearance produced when the barium outlines the space between the intussuscepted bowel and the outer intussuscipiens.

Treatment is surgical removal of the underlying abnormality, or withdrawal of anticoagulants and supportive tube decompression.

Subacute and Chronic Colonic Obstruction

Much more difficult to identify are the insidious forms of subacute obstruction of the large bowel, which usually present as (1) intermittent lower abdominal pain of the colicky type, (2) gradually progressive constipation, (3) distension, or (4) a combination of these. The failure of the patient to complain actively or to appear very ill makes it easy for the physician to overlook the possible cecal twist or the obstructing tumor in the left colon. Very often it is the additional impetus provided by a fecal impaction which converts the vague symptoms into those of a definite closed-loop obstruction, with marked distension of the cecal area; in the elderly patient the distended bowel may rupture and produce an acute peritonitis, treatment of which uncovers the underlying tumor, diverticulitis, or volvulus.

Diagnostic aids consist of abdominal palpation and auscultation, which may identify markedly different patterns during the several days of such an episode, and digital examination, which may disclose an impaction, or an intussuscepting tumor, or blood on the stool. Roentgen examination is important in demonstrating on the open film unusual gas collections which define an obstruction and on the barium enema a definite obstacle to the passage of barium (Fig. 320-9). *Treatment* is that of the underlying lesion and is therefore usually surgical.

ACUTE NECROTIZING (MEMBRANOUS) ENTEROCOLITIS

This severe necrotizing lesion of large and small intestine has been known under a variety of names. It almost always occurs in association with a massive insult to the circulation (myocardial infarction with shock) in the otherwise well patient, in debilitated elderly patients who suffer mechanical trauma or undergo surgical therapy, and more recently in severely ill patients receiving antibiotic therapy.

The pathologic features are those of a coagulative necrosis of the mucosa of the small and large intestine; thrombosed capillaries and venules underlie the necrosis;

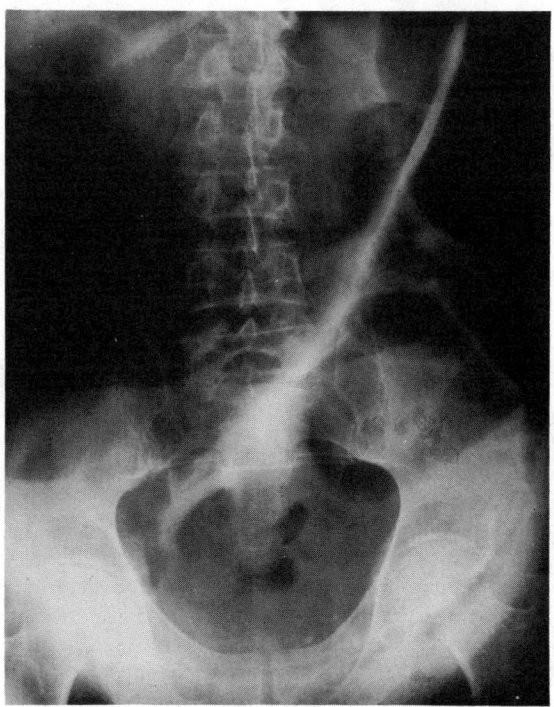

Fig. 320-9. Enormous dilatation of the cecum secondary to sigmoid cancer.

a pseudomembrane may be present in patchy distribution. Staphylococci may be found in large quantities but are not necessary for the diagnosis.

Symptoms are those of severe shock, accompanied by variable degrees of abdominal distension, high fever, and diarrhea. If the condition follows an operation, it usually occurs between the third and fifth postoperative days. The stools often contain whitish collections of exudate and staphylococci; the latter may be cultured by rectal swab if no stool is passed.

Treatment is that of shock, with special emphasis on blood, plasma, and adrenal steroids. If staphylococci are isolated from the stools, erythromycin or vancomycin is given in large doses. If no staphylococci are cultured, most authorities advise the use of polyvalent serum against clostridia. The case fatality rate is extremely high despite these measures, and intensive medical and nursing care is critical.

ANORECTAL PROBLEMS

Complaints centered in this area are among the most common and most troublesome encountered by the physician. Because of failure to understand the anatomy and function of perianal skin, anal sphincters, lower rectal mucosa, and levator muscles, many misdiagnoses are made, and therapy based on these misconceptions prolongs or even aggravates the difficulties. There is no way in which the physician can move with assurance in evaluating these complaints unless he learns the anatomy and constantly performs careful and thorough physical examinations directed to an appreciation of the disturbed physiology.

Fistulas and Abscesses

These septic disorders may be the first signs of primary colitis, enteritis, or diverticulitis, as previously discussed, or may be complications of surgical procedures employed for these or other conditions. *Fistula in ano*, a tract leading from the rectal lumen to the perianal skin, usually results from local anal crypt abscesses; fewer than 5 percent of such lesions found in medical practice in the United States are due to tuberculosis or cancer. The fistula is a chronically inflamed tube made up of fibrous tissue surrounding granulation tissue, the lumen of which may be difficult to demonstrate. *Perirectal abscesses* often represent the tracking down into the anal area of purulent material escaping from the rectosigmoid; diverticulitis, enteritis, or colitis may be the source. Previous anal or rectal surgical therapy may be causal. *Fistulas* between the rectum and vagina and between the rectum and bladder represent serious complications of granulomatous, septic, or malignant disorders and require that the patient be hospitalized for definitive diagnostic and therapeutic procedures.

Anal Lesions

These lesions comprise a wide variety of distressing inflammatory, traumatic, and neoplastic disorders. *Anal fissures* represent superficial erosions of the anal canal epithelium which can heal rapidly with conservative therapy. *Anal ulcers* are more chronic and deep and give symptoms largely as the result of painful spasm of the external anal sphincter during and after defecation. Bleeding may occur with either fissure or ulcer; healing of the ulcer often is associated with a hypertrophied anal papilla and some degrees of anal contracture. Crypt abscesses may produce pain early and should be treated promptly.

Hemorrhoids

The internal hemorrhoidal plexus of veins is located in the submucosal space above the valves of Morgagni; the anal canal separates it from the external hemorrhoidal venous plexus, but the two spaces communicate under the anal canal, the submucosa of which is attached to underlying tissue to form the interhemorrhoidal depression. Whenever the internal hemorrhoidal plexus is enlarged, there is associated increase in supporting tissue mass, and the resultant venous swelling is called an *internal hemorrhoid*. When veins in the external hemorrhoidal plexus become enlarged or thrombosed, the resultant bluish mass is called an *external hemorrhoid*.

Both types of hemorrhoids are very common and are associated with increased hydrostatic pressure in the portal venous system, characteristically noted during pregnancy, straining at stool, chronic liver disease, and sudden increases of intraabdominal pressure, or with local factors associated with diarrhea, tumors, or incomplete evacuation of feces. When internal hemorrhoids enlarge, pain is not a usual feature until the situation is complicated by thrombosis, infection, or erosion of the overlying mucosal surface. Most persons complain of bright-red blood on the toilet tissue or coating the stool, with a feeling of vague disquiet about the state of their anus. The discomfort is increased when the hemorrhoidal enlargement becomes great or prolapses through the anus; prolapse is often accompanied by edema and sphincteric spasm. Prolapse if not treated usually becomes chronic as the muscularis stays stretched, and the patient complains of constant soiling of underclothing with very little pain. Prolapsed hemorrhoids may become infected or thrombosed; the overlying mucous membrane may bleed profusely as the result of the trauma of defecation.

External hemorrhoids, lying as they do under the skin, are quite often painful, particularly if there is a sudden increase in their mass. These episodes result in a tender blue swelling at the anal verge due to thrombosis of a vein in the extrenal plexus and need not be associated with enlargement of the internal veins. Since the thrombus usually lies at the level of the sphincteric muscles, anal spasm often occurs.

The diagnosis of internal and external hemorrhoids is made by inspection, digital examination, and direct vision through the anoscope and proctoscope. Since such lesions are very common, they must not be regarded as the cause of rectal bleeding or chronic hypochromic anemia until a thorough investigation has been made of the more proximal gastrointestinal tract. Acute blood loss to shock levels can more certainly be attributed to internal hemorrhoids seen to be bleeding actively than can lesser degrees of chronic anemia in the presence of large but not definitely bleeding hemorrhoids.

Most hemorroids respond to conservative therapy, employing sitz baths or other forms of moist heat, compresses, suppositories, medications to soften the stool, and bed rest. Internal hemorrhoids which remain permanently prolapsed are best treated by surgical means; milder degrees of prolapse or enlargement with pruritus ani or intermittent bleeding can be successfully handled by the injection of sclerosing solutions. External hemorrhoids which become acutely thrombosed are treated by incision, extraction of the clot, and compressing the incised area following clot removal. No surgical procedure should be carried out in the presence of acute inflammation of the anus, ulcerative proctitis, or ulcerative colitis, and both proctoscopy and barium enema should always be performed before a patient is subjected to hemorrhoidectomy.

REFERENCES

Ackerman, L. V., and J. S. Spratt, Jr.: Do Adenomatous Polyps Become Cancer?, Gastroenterology, 44:905, 1963.

Brown, D. B., and W. F. Toomey: Diverticular Disease of the Colon, Brit. J. Surg., 47:485, 1960.

Kay, A. W., R. I. Richards, and A. J. Watson: Acute Necrotizing (Pseudomembranous) Enterocolitis, Brit. J. Surg., 46: 45, 1958.

Kirsner, J. B., J. A. Rider, H. C. Moeller, W. L. Palmer, and S. S. Gold: Polyps of the Colon and Rectum, Gastroenterology, 39:178, 1960.

Lennard-Jones, J. E., H. E. Lockhart-Mummery, and B. C. Morson: Clinical and Pathological Differentiation of Crohn's Disease and Proctocolitis, Gastroenterology, 54: 1162, 1968.

Lockhart-Mummery, H. E., and B. C. Morson: Crohn's Disease of the Large Intestine, Gut, 5:493, 1964.

——, C. E. Dukes, and H. S. R. Bussey: Multiple Congenital Polyposis, Brit. J. Surg., 43:476, 1956.

Marston, A., M. T. Pheils, M. L. Thomas, and B. C. Morson: Ischaemic Colitis, Gut, 7:1, 1966.

Morson, B. C.: Precancerous Lesions in the Colon and Rectum, J.A.M.A., 179:104, 1962.

Roth, J. A.: Ulcerative Colitis, chap. 69, in "Gastroenterology," 2d ed., vol. 2, H. L. Bockus (Ed.), Philadelphia, W. B. Saunders Company, 1964.

Swenson, O.: Hirschsprung's Disease (Aganglionic Megacolon), New Engl. J. Med., 260:272, 1959.

Wynder, E. L., and T. Shigematsu: Environmental Factors of Cancer of the Colon and Rectum, Cancer, 20:1520, 1967.

321 DISEASES OF THE PERITONEUM AND MESENTERY

Kurt J. Isselbacher

ACUTE PERITONITIS

Acute peritonitis is by definition an inflammatory process of the peritoneum that may appear in both acute and chronic forms. In the acute form the motor activity of the intestine is decreased, and the intestinal lumen becomes distended with gas and fluid. Fluid accumulates as a result of obstruction to the free passage of the 7 or 8 liters normally excreted daily into the lumen and absorbed from the distal small bowel and colon. While acute peritonitis is usually of bacterial origin, frequently one finds peritonitis may result from entry into the abdominal cavity of blood, urine, bile, or pancreatic juice.

CLINICAL PICTURE OF ACUTE PERITONITIS. This will usually consist of increasing diffuse abdominal pain, distension, nausea and vomiting, inability to pass feces or flatus, fever, hypotension, tachycardia, thirst, and oliguria. On physical examination the patient appears acutely ill, febrile, and with a variable degree of abdominal distension. The abdomen is usually acutely tender and tympanitic, often with rebound tenderness. Peristalsis may be present initially but usually disappears as the illness progresses. Hypotension is common, as is leukocytosis, which often is greater than 20,000 cells per cu mm. X-ray examination of the abdomen shows dilatation of the large and small bowel with edema of the small-bowel wall as evidenced by the distance between adjacent loops of gas-filled small intestine. Paracentesis is valuable in determining the nature of the exudate as well as whether

bacteria can be demonstrated or cultured. Lead, colic, gastric crises, and acute porphyria may cause severe abdominal symptoms that resemble the picture of acute peritonitis.

SYSTEMIC EFFECTS OF PERITONITIS. Spreading and progressive peritonitis usually results in an increased demand on the circulatory system, because the exudation of fluid leads to a reduction in the effective circulating blood volume. Some of the fluid is lost into the peritoneal cavity and the rest into the intestinal lumen.

With severe peritonitis respiratory demands are increased, and elevation of the diaphragm reduces ventilatory capacity and respiratory exchange. There is usually an increase in adrenal activity with increased production of glucocorticoids and aldosterone resulting in potassium loss and sodium retention. Catecholamines may be liberated in increased amounts, and the resulting peripheral vasoconstriction with increased peripheral resistance results in decreased organ perfusion usually affecting renal and cardiac function.

TREATMENT. Therapy depends primarily on early removal of the primary sources of peritoneal contamination, restoration of plasma volume, replacement of fluids and electrolytes through the common maintenance of adequate pulmonary function, and cardiac output plus the use of appropriate antibiotic therapy. The most common organisms in peritonitis are *Escherichia coli, Klebsiella, Aerobacter,* and enterococci. The appropriate antibiotics for each of these are noted in Chaps. 139, 144, and 148.

SECONDARY PERITONITIS

This term applies to the disease generally referred to as *peritonitis*. It may be due to entry of bacteria into the peritoneal cavity from a perforation in the gastrointestinal tract or from an external penetrating wound. It may be secondary to severe chemical reactions from the release of pancreatic enzymes, the digestive juices of the upper gastrointestinal tract, or bile as a result of injury or perforation of the intestine or biliary tract.

The most common causes of bacterial peritonitis are appendicitis, perforations associated with diverticulitis, peptic ulcer, gangrenous gallbladder, and gangrenous obstruction of the small bowel from adhesive bands, incarcerated hernia, or volvulus. Any lesion leading to the escape of intestinal bacteria may be a source, including a perforating carcinoma, foreign body, and ulcerative colitis. The peritoneal cavity is remarkably resistant to contamination, and unless continuing contamination occurs, the disease process becomes localized.

Gonococcal Peritonitis

This usually involves an extension of gonococcal infection from a primary focus in the female reproductive tract. The signs of inflammation usually are limited to the pelvis, but there may be findings of a mild generalized peritonitis. Occasionally the patient has right upper quadrant pain and tenderness caused by "violin string adhesions" above the liver. These are considered to be pathognomonic of invasion of the peritoneal cavity by gonococci (see Chap. 143).

Tuberculous Peritonitis

See Chap. 174.

PSEUDOMYXOMA PERITONEI

This is a rare condition resulting from rupture of a mucocele of the appendix or of a mucinous ovarian cyst. The abdomen becomes filled with masses of jellylike material. Occasionally, with removal of the mucocele or the ovarian cyst and most of the myxomatous material, a cure may ensue. In other cases, however, the mucoid material recurs, leading to progressive wasting and eventual death. Colloid carcinoma arising from the stomach or colon with peritoneal implants may resemble pseudomyxoma at laparotomy. The course of this type of highly malignant tumor is one of rapid cachexia and early death. The diagnosis can usually be made by the appearance of many highly malignant cells in the peritoneal implants.

CANCER OF THE PERITONEUM

Aside from mesothelioma, which appears uniquely associated with asbestosis but is otherwise very rare, cancer of the peritoneum is usually secondary to a neoplasm within the abdomen most commonly of the stomach and ovary. Invariably this type of metastatic malignancy is associated with progressive ascites with a high specific gravity and high protein content, often with large numbers of red cells or even gross blood. The diagnosis is established by demonstrating malignant cells in the fluid. The clinical progress of this malignant spread can sometimes be arrested by installations of radioactive gold, nitrogen mustard, or chloroquine.

BENIGN PAROXYSMAL PERITONITIS

See Chap. 256, Familial Mediterranean Fever (Familial Paroxysmal Peritonitis).

PNEUMATOSIS CYSTOIDES INTESTINALES

This is a condition in which multiple gas-filled blebs or cysts accumulate in the intestinal wall beneath the serosal surface of the bowel. The exact source of the gas has not been explained satisfactorily. In some instances, this disease is associated with specific ulceration of the intestinal mucosa, in particular peptic ulcer with outlet obstruction. Cysts in the wall of the small bowel are seen as an occasional complication of mesenteric vascular occlusion. In the large bowel, these cysts are usually benign, may be seen with a variety of other disorders, and usually disappear with time.

There are no specific physical findings secondary to the pneumatosis, and the diagnosis is made either by x-ray or at laporotomy. Occasionally the subserosal cysts may rupture, resulting in pneumoperitoneum.

CHYLOUS "PERITONITIS," OR ASCITES

This term refers to the accumulation of chyle (intestinal lymph) in the peritoneal cavity. The condition is sometimes associated with chylothorax. The fluid in the peritoneal cavity appears milky or creamy because of the presence of fat. This fat may be demonstrated microscopically by staining with Sudan III and may be diminished chemically by acidification of the fluid followed by extraction with ether. Many conditions may be associated with the cloudy or milky-appearing peritoneal fluid. The gross appearance is usually due to the presence of protein and desquamated cells. The turbidity of this fluid will not be removed with the ether but will clear with addition of alkali to the fluid.

The causes of chylous peritonitis include (1) penetrating or nonpenetrating trauma that damages the main duct in the lymphatic system within the abdomen, (2) intestinal obstruction, if it is associated with rupture of a major lymphatic channel, (3) congenital lymphangiectasia, or (4) malignant disease or tuberculous infection that obstructs the intestinal lymphatics.

The sudden accumulation of chyle in the peritoneal cavity often results in abdominal pain, signs of peritoneal irritation, and leukocytosis. These symptoms gradually subside leaving the patient with a distended but nontender fluid-filled abdomen. The roentgenographic technique of lymphangiography is of value in determining the location of the leak or site of obstruction to the lymphatic channels. The course depends upon the underlying etiologic factors.

REFERENCES

Burack, W. R., and R. M. Hollister: Tuberculous Peritonitis: A Study of Forty-seven Cases Encountered by a General Medical Unit in Twenty-five Years, Am. J. Med., 28:510, 1960.

Berner, C., et al.: Diagnostic Probabilities in Patients with Conspicuous Ascites, Arch. Intern. Med., 113:687, 1964.

Conn, H. O.: Spontaneous Peritonitis and Bacteremia in Laennec's Cirrhosis Caused by Enteric Organisms: A Relatively Common but Rarely Recognized Syndrome, Ann. Intern. Med., 60:568, 1964.

Doub, H. P., and J. J. Shea: Pneumatosis Cystoides Intestinalis, J.A.M.A., 172:1238, 1960.

Harley, J. B., A. S. Glushein, and E. R. Fisher: Eosinophilic Peritonitis, Ann. Intern. Med., 51:301, 1959.

Meigs, J. V., and J. W. Cass: Fibroma of the Ovary with Ascites and Hydrothorax: With a Report of Seven Cases, Am. J. Obstet. Gynecol., 33:249, 1937.

Siegal, S.: Familial Paroxysmal Polyserositis, Am. J. Med., 36:893, 1964.

Section 6

Disorders of the Hepatobiliary System

322 APPROACH TO THE PATIENT WITH LIVER DISEASE

Kurt J. Isselbacher

GENERAL CONSIDERATIONS

While disease of the liver or biliary tract may be directly responsible for the symptoms that bring the patient to the physician, not infrequently examination for nonhepatic complaints may provide the clues to otherwise asymptomatic or occult hepatobiliary disease. Liver function studies and other diagnostic procedures such as biopsy (as discussed in Chap. 324) are crucial, but much valuable information as to the possible nature and extent of liver disease can be obtained by a carefully elicited history and thorough physical examination.

IMPORTANCE OF CLINICAL HISTORY. Since laboratory tests often do not establish the specific cause of liver disease, the history is of the greatest significance. *Family history* is important with respect to jaundice, anemia, splenectomy, or cholecystectomy; a positive history may be helpful in diagnosing hemolytic anemia, congenital or familial hyperbilirubinemia, or gallstones. In Wilson's disease (hepatolenticular degeneration), there may be a family history of tremor or neurologic abnormalities. *Occupation* should be reviewed in detail, and *environmental factors* need to be examined. Note should be made of any contact with rats possibly carrying Weil's disease and for exposure to toxins such as carbon tetrachloride or beryllium. The patient should be asked about travel to other countries, especially to areas where hepatitis may be endemic. A careful and discrete questioning regarding alcohol intake is important in most patients. Since the alcoholic often denies or understates the amounts consumed, it is desirable to check the validity of the history with close friends or relatives of the patient.

Contact with jaundiced patients should be noted, especially in hospitals, schools, or the military where viral hepatitis is frequent. If the patient has had any *injections* in the previous 6 months, serum hepatitis may be the underlying disease. Injections include blood tests, blood or plasma transfusions, tattooing, and dental treatment. The patient should be asked about narcotics, hallucinogens, or stimulant *drugs* taken parenterally as well as about agents taken orally such as chlorpromazine or contraceptive drugs known to affect liver function.

A previous history of indigestion, fat intolerance, and right upper quadrant pain suggests cholelithiasis or choledocholithiasis Jaundice following shortly after operation on the biliary tract suggests residual stone, that which occurs within 6 months suggests serum hepatitis, and that occurring after 1 or more years may be due to stricture of the duct. Postoperative jaundice may be due to the anesthetic, especially multiple uses of halothane, or the impaired hepatic excretory function resulting from relative hypoxia of liver cells in the operative or postoperative period.

The *onset of the illness* should be noted. The relatively abrupt onset of nausea, anorexia, and aversion to smoking followed by progressive jaundice suggests infectious hepatitis. A gradual development of jaundice associated with pruritus suggests cholestasis. Jaundice associated with fever and chills makes cholangitis and extrahepatic biliary obstruction a likely possibility.

The patient with hepatitis generally feels ill, and dark urine and light stools occur before the appearance of scleral or skin icterus. In cholestatic jaundice, the patient may feel relatively well and complain only of symptoms due to the obstruction, such as pruritus.

PHYSICAL EXAMINATION. The general appearance should be noted. Pallor indicative of anemia may be a reflection of hemolysis, cirrhosis, or neoplasm. Significant cachexia, especially of the extremities, may be due to cancer or active cirrhosis. If the patient is jaundiced, the color of the jaundice should be observed; with hemolysis the jaundice is a mild *yellow,* with parenchymal disease, more of an *orange* color, and with prolonged biliary obstruction, a *deep-greenish* hue. In the alcoholic one should look for stigmata of cirrhosis such as parotid gland enlargement, Dupuytren's contracture, gynecomastia, and diminished axillary or pubic hair.

The *skin examination* may reveal ecchymoses due to prothrombin deficiency or purpura due to thrombocytopenia. *Palmar erythema* or *spider angiomata* may reflect acute or chronic liver disease. Spider angiomata are usually found above the umbilicus and especially on the face, neck, shoulders, forearms, and dorsum of the hands. In chronic cholestasis, *scratch marks, finger clubbing,* and *xanthoma* of the eyelids and extensor surfaces may be found. *A slate color* to the skin due to increased melanin should suggest the presence of hemochromatosis.

Evaluation of the *mental state* and *neurologic function* is important. Slight deterioration of the intellect and minimal personality changes may suggest hepatocellular disease or the presence of portal-systemic venous shunts, but care must be taken to exclude other causes such as primary or metastatic brain tumors. The presence of flapping tremor of the hands (asterixis) may be found in association with portal-systemic encephalopathy or impending hepatic coma.

Abdominal examination may reveal ascites, which together with dilated periumbilical veins, suggests cirrhosis and extensive portal collateral circulation. A very large nodular and rock-hard liver suggests the presence of hepatoma or hepatic metastases. A small liver may indicate cirrhosis (especially postnecrotic); a small liver which diminishes in size suggests severe hepatitis or massive hepatic necrosis. In the alcoholic, fatty infiltration and cirrhosis often produces a uniform enlargement of the liver. The liver edge is tender in hepatitis, in congestive heart failure, and occasionally in malignant disease and with alcoholism (especially "florid cirrhosis" or "alcoholic hepatitis").

A palpable and sometimes visibly enlarged gallbladder (Courvoisier's sign) suggests extrahepatic biliary obstruction often due to pancreatic cancer. A tender gallbladder and positive Murphy's sign suggests cholelithiasis or choledocholithiasis. A palpable spleen may indicate hepatitis; significant splenomegaly may be a reflection of portal hypertension.

DIAGNOSTIC PROCEDURES. These are reviewed in Chap. 324. For the proper evaluation of liver and biliary tract diseases chemical and biochemical tests of blood, urine, and stool are essential, and liver biopsy is often needed to help determine the nature of the liver disease. In addition, peritoneoscopy and special radiologic techniques such as cholangiography, angiography, and scintiscans of the liver may be employed. In the problem case, laparotomy should be performed. The exploration should be thorough, and if the diagnosis remains in doubt, should include operative liver biopsy and direct operative cholangiography or angiography.

CLASSIFICATION OF LIVER DISEASE

There has been a problem in the classification of liver disease, especially the spectrum of chronic liver disease. The problems of terminology and classification stem to a large degree from the fact that in many types of parenchymal disease, the etiology and pathogenetic mechanism is obscure. As a consequence, one finds an abundance of labels and names applied to hepatic disorders. Some individuals use the term *hepatitis* to imply viral infection, others simply to connote evidence of liver cell inflammation. One finds ambiguity in the use of the words acute, subacute, and chronic. *Chronicity* should refer to continuing or recurrent disease (i.e., duration). *Activity* should refer to evidence of the presence or perpetuation of liver cell injury; this is most readily identified on biopsy by the degree of hepatocellular necrosis and by serum transaminase elevations.

Because of the difficulties involved in defining the etiology of many types of liver disease, in most instances the process is best defined and described by an examination of the morphologic character of the lesion. Therefore, a *morphologic classification* of liver disease, as outlined in Table 322-1, appears at present more practical than one based on etiology.

Table 322-1. CLASSIFICATION OF LIVER DISEASE

I. Parenchymal
  A. Hepatitis
    1. Viral
    2. Drug-induced or toxic
    3. Chronic active (lupoid, plasma cell)
    4. Associated with systematic infections (e.g., leptospirosis, schistosomiasis)
    5. Granulomatous (e.g., sarcoidosis, tuberculosis)
  B. Cirrhosis
    1. Laennec's (portal, nutritional, "alcoholic")
    2. Postnecrotic
    3. Biliary
    4. Wilson's disease (hepatolenticular degeneration)
    5. Hemochromatosis
    6. Rare types (e.g., with galactosemia, cystic fibrosis of pancreas)
  C. Infiltrations
    1. Glycogen
    2. Fat (neutral fat, cholesterol, gangliosides, cerebrosides)
    3. Amyloid
    4. Lymphoma, leukemia
  D. Space-occupying lesions
    1. Hepatoma, metastatic tumor
    2. Abscess (pyogenic, amebic)
    3. Cysts (polycystic disease, Echinococcus)
    4. Gummas
  E. Functional disorders associated with jaundice
    1. Gilbert's syndrome
    2. Crigler-Najjar syndrome
    3. Dubin-Johnson and Rotor syndromes
    4. Cholestasis of pregnancy and benign recurrent cholestasis
II. Hepatobiliary
  A. Extrahepatic biliary obstruction (by stone, stricture, or tumor)
  B. Cholangitis
III. Vascular
  A. Chronic passive congestion and cardiac cirrhosis
  B. Hepatic vein thrombosis
  C. Portal vein thrombosis
  D. Pylephlebitis

REFERENCES

Schiff, L.: "Diseases of the Liver," 3d ed., Philadelphia, J. B. Lippincott Company, 1969.

Sherlock, S.: "Diseases of the Liver and Biliary System," 4th ed., Philadelphia, F. A. Davis Company, 1968.

323 DERANGEMENTS OF HEPATIC METABOLISM

David H. Alpers and
Kurt J. Isselbacher

The liver is an organ with a variety of metabolic functions, both synthetic and degradative. Although there are three major cell types which make up the liver—the hepatocyte, biliary epithelial cell, and Kupffer cell—most metabolic functions are carried out by the hepatocyte. Several observations are pertinent to derangements in liver function when the liver is damaged: (1) in view of its large reserve capacity, mild to sometimes moderate injury often may not be accurately reflected by changes of its synthetic or degradative activity; (2) some functions of the liver are much more sensitive to injury than others, and hence derangements may be found in some liver functions (and function tests) and not in others; (3) there is *no one single test* or procedure which effectively measures the total function of the liver. Therefore proper understanding of the metabolic responses of the liver to injury (or the effect of partial hepatectomy, for example) depends on a comprehension of the many known functions of the liver. Some of these are discussed below.

PROTEIN SYNTHESIS

The liver actively synthesizes many proteins, but of these *albumin* is quantitatively the most important. The body contains about 5 Gm albumin per kg body weight, and in the normal adult the daily albumin production by the hepatic endoplasmic reticulum is about 200 mg per kg. The half-life of serum albumin is 14 to 17 days. The liver is the only organ which synthesizes albumin. The rate of synthesis is limited and can be doubled only under conditions of excessive albumin loss or destruction. Once albumin is synthesized, it is transported from the rough endoplasmic reticulum to the smooth endoplasmic reticulum and the Golgi apparatus and from there to the hepatic sinusoids. During liver injury changes may occur in the actual synthesis of albumin or in its intracellular transport and release. When the liver is damaged, synthesis or release of albumin is usually affected more than catabolism, but in view of its half-life, several weeks may elapse before a pronounced decrease in serum albumin levels occur. In general, albumin catabolism (which also occurs in other tissues such as the gastrointestinal tract) tends to continue at a relatively constant rate, even in the presence of liver injury.

Other proteins produed by the liver include many of the blood-clotting factors: fibrinogen, prothrombin, and factors V, VII, and X. All of them have a half-life shorter than that of albumin, varying from 6 hr (factor VII) to 20 hr (prothrombin). Therefore when fresh blood is administered, the prothrombin level will be elevated only transiently, while more significant increases in serum albumin will result. Unlike albumin, not all globulins are synthesized by the hepatocytes; much of the α- and β-globulins are produced by liver cells, but normally most γ-globulins are synthesized by reticuloendothelial cells lining the sinusoids and in the spleen and bone marrow. In addition, infiltrating plasma cells and lymphocytes may be of importance in some forms of liver disease associated with hyperglobulinemia (such as chronic active hepatitis and primary biliary cirrhosis). The production and localization of γ-globulins in the liver in

these conditions can be detected by immunofluorescence techniques but probably account for only a portion of the γ-globulin production.

ENZYMES

In view of the many chemical reactions carried out by the liver, this organ contains thousands of protein catalysts or enzymes. Some are unique to the liver, while many others also are found in nonhepatic tissues. The leakage of enzymes out of liver cells into the bloodstream occurs with liver injury, and measurements of these serum enzymes are useful tests of abnormal liver function. When increased serum levels of enzymes such as the transaminases are found, several points must be kept in mind: (1) leakage of enzymes out of the liver cell occurs not only with *necrosis* but also with changes in *cell permeability* which may be produced by ischemia or hypoxia; (2) there is *no direct quantitative correlation* between the amount of liver cell injury and the height of serum enzyme levels, although in general, higher levels are found more frequently in more severe injury; (3) if the serum enzymes are measured sometime *after* the acute insult or injury, the initial rise may have been missed, and thus normal or *low* serum enzyme levels may be found as a consequence of decreased functioning liver cell mass.

In liver disease some enzymes may increase in the blood not primarily because of changes in cell permeability but actually as a result of *increased enzyme synthesis* in the liver. This is often the case when serum *alkaline phosphatase* levels are elevated with liver or biliary tract disease and obstruction of a hepatic duct can be shown to lead to increased synthesis of this enzyme. Alkaline phosphatase is also present in tissues such as bone, intestine, kidney, and placenta, and a variety of techniques are now available to distinguish these various alkaline phosphatase *isoenzymes*. For example, electrophoresis may be used to separate some of these isoenzymes; heat treatment tends to inactivate the bone alkaline phosphatase; L-phenylalanine selectively inhibits the intestinal enzyme. Another approach useful to determine whether an elevated alkaline phosphatase level reflects hepatic disease is to measure a related enzyme, *5'-nucleotidase*, which is elaborated by hepatic canalicular microvilli and is not found in bone.

Finally, because many of the routinely used serum enzyme assays are not specific for liver tissue, caution must be used in interpreting an elevated level, especially if it occurs as an isolated abnormality. Transaminase levels may be elevated during in vivo or in vitro hemolysis, reflecting the liberation of erythrocyte enzyme. Lactic dehydrogenase (LDH) is found in red cells, platelets, lung, myocardium, and skeletal muscle, and an elevated serum level may not correlate well with liver cell damage but may reflect the liberation of the enzyme from another tissue. The various LDH isoenzymes may be separated or identified by techniques such as starch electrophoresis. There are five different LDH isoenzymes;

LDH-5 is present in liver and hence will tend to be increased in the serum with liver injury.

AMINO ACID METABOLISM

The liver is the major site of amino acid metabolism in the body. Amino acids are derived either from the intestine or from other tissues as a result of protein breakdown or direct amino acid synthesis and reach the liver via the bloodstream. In the liver they are subject to anabolic (i.e., protein synthesis) or degradative processes. Catabolism or degradation of amino acids in the liver involves two major reactions: One of these is *oxidative deamination,* resulting in the formation of a keto acid and ammonia. This reaction is catalyzed by L-amino acid oxidases, with but two exceptions: glycine oxidation is catalyzed by glycine oxidase and glutamic acid oxidation by glutamic dehydrogenase.

Transamination, the process by which the amino group of an amino acid is transferred to a keto acid, is a far more important mechanism. The two major enzymes are the glutamic-oxalacetic acid and the glutamic-pyruvic transaminases. As a result, amino acids are able to enter the citric acid cycle to function in the intermediary metabolism of carbohydrates and lipids (see Chap. 75). Conversely, by transamination amino acids may be synthesized from keto acids. When the liver is acutely and severely damaged (e.g., in massive hepatic necrosis), utilization of amino acids by the liver is impaired, free amino acid levels in the blood increase, and an "overflow" type of aminoaciduria occurs.

Urea synthesis occurs primarily in the liver and involves the participation of four amino acids: ornithine, citrulline, arginine, and aspartic acid. By this process ammonia is rapidly removed and detoxified. The steps of the urea (Krebs-Henseleit) cycle are shown in Fig. 323-1. Because all of enzymes of the urea cycle reside in the liver, in the presence of severe liver damage urea synthesis may be depressed, and blood urea nitrogen (BUN) levels may fall significantly. In the absence of severe liver damage most of the free NH_3 is formed in the intestinal

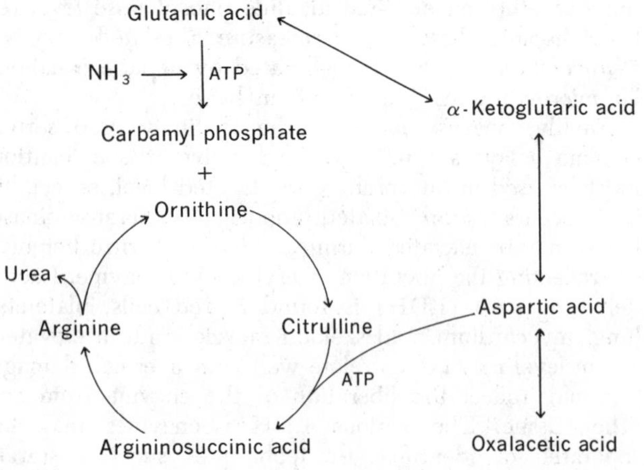

tract, primarily in the colon. Normally, approximately 25 percent of blood urea is excreted into the intestine, and NH_3 is produced by the action of bacterial ureases or from bleeding into the intestinal tract. Protein from the diet serves as a major source of ammonia because of the normal digestion of protein to amino acids and the subsequent deamination by bacterial enzymes. The ammonia formed in this manner enters the portal vein and is then detoxified in the liver by being converted to urea.

The four principal mechanisms leading to an increased blood NH_3 level in chronic liver disease are illustrated in Fig. 323-2. (1) If hepatic function is significantly depressed, *decreased urea synthesis* may occur with reduced removal of NH_3. (2) If portal hypertension accompanies cirrhosis, venous anastomoses will develop between the portal vein and systemic venous channels, and these *portal-systemic shunts* will allow NH_3 to escape hepatic detoxification, leading to elevated blood ammonia levels. (3) If there is *excessive nitrogenous material* in the intestine (from bleeding or dietary protein), excessive amounts of NH_3 will be formed by bacterial deamination of amino acids. (4) If metabolic alkalosis and hypokalemia accompany hepatic decompensation, there may be increased *renal NH_3 production* from glutamine by the action of glutaminase, leading to increased peripheral blood levels, because the NH_3 concentration in the renal veins is inversely proportional to the amount excreted in the urine.

Two additional factors are probably of importance in determining whether or not a given NH_3 level in the blood will be injurious to the tissues. First, NH_3 is removed from the blood by a variety of tissues, including brain, lungs, and muscle, and the degree of utilization is affected by the presence of AV shunts, which often occur in chronic liver disease. Second, the more alkaline the blood pH, the more toxic a given level of NH_3 is likely to be. At 37°C the pK of NH_3 is 8.9—i.e., close enough to the pH of blood so that small changes of blood pH might affect the NH_4^+/NH_3 ratio. Because *un-ionized NH_3 crosses membranes more readily than ionized NH_4^+ ions,* alkalosis favors the entry of ammonia into the brain by shifting the equilibrium of the following reaction to the right:

$$NH_4^+ + OH \rightleftarrows NH_3 + HOH$$

Alkalosis then, not only increases the peripheral blood levels of NH_3 by renal mechanisms but also increases tissues levels by its effect on the diffusion of NH_3 ions.

LIPID METABOLISM

Approximately 5 percent of the normal liver weight is due to fat, including phospholipids, triglycerides, fatty acids, cholesterol, and cholesterol esters. The liver is active in the synthesis of lipids, especially triglycerides. While some remain in the liver, most triglycerides are excreted into the bloodstream in the form of lipoproteins. The major steps in hepatic fatty acid and triglyceride metabolism are shown in Fig. 323-3.

Fig. 323-1. The chemical steps of the urea (Krebs-Henseleit) cycle.

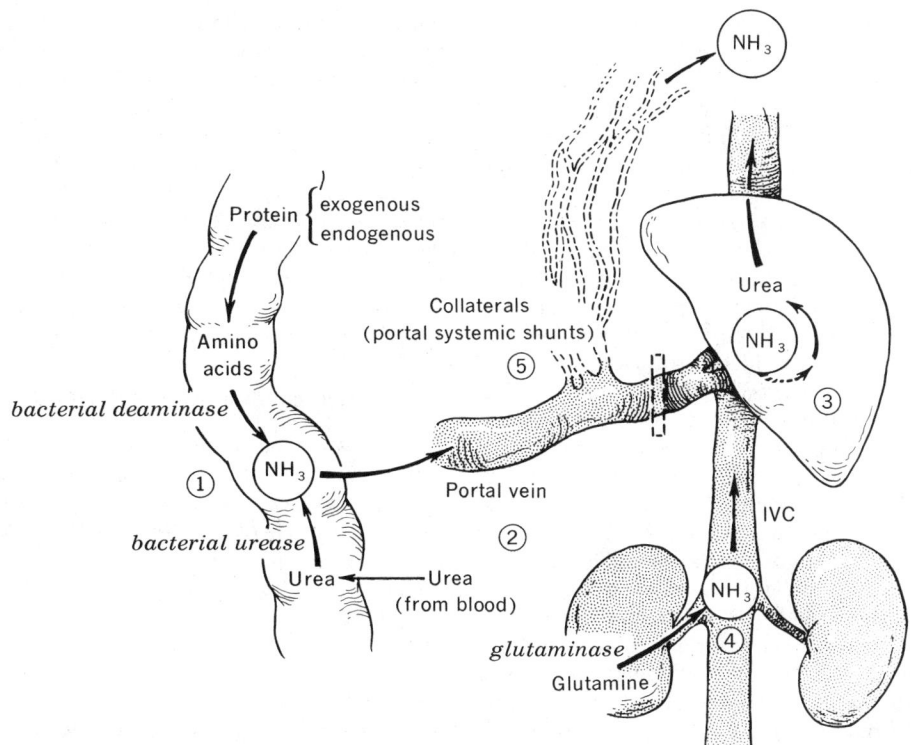

Fig. 323-2. Major factors (steps 1 to 4) influencing the level of blood ammonia. In cirrhosis with portal hypertension, venous collaterals allow ammonia to bypass the liver (5), allowing for the entry of ammonia into the systemic circulation (portal-systemic shunting).

Under normal conditions, most of the *fatty acids* taken up by the liver and *esterified to triglyceride* are derived from adipose tissue or the diet. Some fatty acids (especially saturated ones) are synthesized in the liver from acetate. The fatty acids may then be converted enzymatically to triglyceride, esterified with cholesterol, incorporated into phospholipids, or oxidized to CO_2 or ketone bodies. Most of the triglyceride is produced for export and in order to be secreted must be converted to *lipoproteins* by combining with relatively specific apoprotein moieties. Thus, protein synthesis is important for the release and secretion of triglyceride from the liver.

Studies on the production of a fatty liver have shown that singly or in combination one or more of these steps depicted numerically in Fig. 323-3 may lead to excessive hepatic triglyceride accumulation and hence a fatty liver. *Increased influx* of fatty acids (1) such as may occur with drugs producing lipid mobilization from adipose tissue or in diabetic ketosis may lead to a fatty liver. Similarly *increased levels of fatty acids in the liver,* either from enhanced fatty acid synthesis (2), or decreased oxidation (3), may lead to increased triglyceride formation. In some instances there may also be *increases* in the specific *enzymes* involved in fatty acid esterification to triglyceride (4). Finally, since release of triglyceride involves the formation of lipoproteins, lipid accumulation may occur because of *decreased protein synthesis* (5), *impaired interaction* of triglyceride with *apoprotein* (6), or *secretion* of lipoproteins from the liver (7).

In the case of *fatty livers* produced by toxins such as carbon tetrachloride, phosphorus, and ethionine and antibiotics like tetracycline, the major mechanism for lipid accumulation appears to be *impaired protein synthesis*.

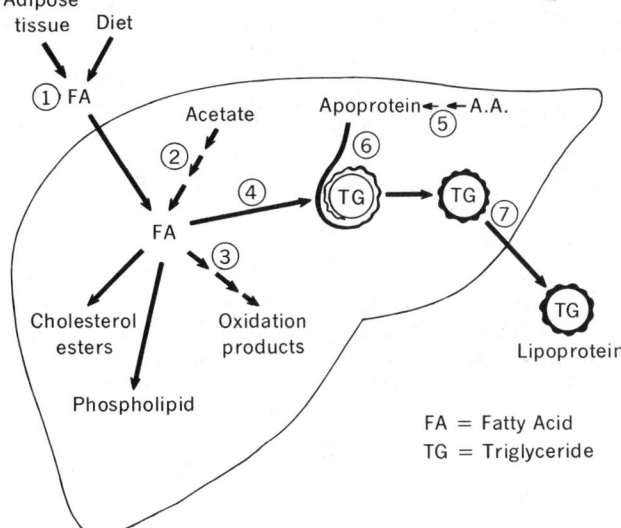

Fig. 323-3. Factors in the uptake and esterification of fatty acids to triglyceride by the liver including the formation and release of triglyceride as lipoprotein. The numbers refer to steps, which, if altered, may result in increased liver triglyceride (i.e., fatty liver).

Alcohol is perhaps the most common agent leading to a fatty liver, but the mechanism whereby alcohol leads to increased liver triglyceride is less clear. Alcohol administration, depending on dose or duration, may affect any of the seven steps shown in Fig. 323-3, and the primary factor for the production of the alcohol-induced fatty liver still remains to be determined.

Cholesterol synthesis is also carried out by the liver, and most of the body cholesterol is derived from the liver and intestine. The liver is also the only organ which converts cholesterol to bile salts, the major catabolites of cholesterol. In the plasma cholesterol exists either *free* or combined with fatty acids in the form of *cholesterol esters;* both are found in association with lipoproteins. The plasma and liver also contain an enzyme (cholesterol acyl transferase) important in the conversion of free cholesterol to its esterified form. Free cholesterol exchanges readily between tissues, and thus changes in plasma cholesterol levels reflect changes in total body cholesterol. However, changes in cholesterol esters may reflect, at least in part, hepatic damage.

Cholesterol is synthesized from 2-carbon precursors such as acetate. One of the key intermediate reactions involves the conversion of hydroxymethylglutaryl CoA to mevalonic acid. In the liver, dietary cholesterol appears to act as an "end-product inhibitor" and decreases *de novo* synthesis by inhibiting this key reaction.

Severe liver injury often leads to a decrease in total serum cholesterol levels, including both free and esterified fractions. This may be a reflection of decreased cholesterol and cholesterol ester synthesis, decreased production of the lipoprotein carriers, or both. In *cholestasis* (intra- or extrahepatic) *total serum cholesterol often increases* strikingly, but the cholesterol ester level increases to a much lesser extent, with the result that there is a *decrease* in the *ester fraction* (i.e., ester/total). This may be due to the fact that bile salts, which are increased in the plasma in cholestasis, appear to inhibit the plasma cholesterol-esterifying enzyme.

CARBOHYDRATE METABOLISM

Glucose is stored in the liver in the form of glycogen, and the latter accounts for 5 to 7 percent of the normal liver weight. Persons with cirrhosis tend to have less glycogen than normal, probably because of a reduced liver cell mass, and in the alcoholic decreased glucose intake is often an added factor. The blood glucose level represents a balance between tissue uptake and hepatic glucose production, which in turn is dependent on dietary glucose, glycogen reserves, and gluconeogenesis from precursors such as amino acids (see Chap. 75).

Hypoglycemia may be seen in severe liver damage and usually is due to decreased gluconeogenesis. This may occur with acute alcohol ingestion, especially when hepatic glycogen stores are depleted, because of the inhibition of gluconeogenesis by alcohol. Some hepatomas are associated with hypoglycemia, but the mechanism for this is unclear; a few cases have been reported with increased insulinlike activity in the plasma. *Hyperglycemia* and *impaired glucose tolerance* may occur in cirrhosis. This is often associated with increased plasma insulin levels during the glucose tolerance test, suggesting that the diabetes in these cases of chronic liver disease is due to insulin resistance.

Galactose is metabolized primarily by the liver, and *impaired galactose tolerance* occurs in liver disease. The galactose tolerance test was once used to evaluate liver function but is employed rarely now. Fructose is also largely metabolized by the liver, and considerations similar to those concerning galactose apply.

DETOXIFICATION MECHANISMS

The liver plays a key role in the detoxification of many substances, both exogenous (e.g., drugs) and endogenous (e.g., hormones). This is accomplished by two mechanisms: First, the *liver converts water-insoluble substances to water-soluble derivatives,* so that they can be excreted into the bile or urine and eliminated from the body. This is accomplished by *conjugation* with glucuronic acid, sulfate, etc. Second, the liver *inactivates* compounds by reduction, oxidation, or hydroxylation.

Hormones, such as the estrogens and corticosteroids, are an important class of compounds normally inactivated by the liver. In the case of corticosteroids and aldosterone, the liver first inactivates them by reduction to their tetrahydro derivatives and then conjugates them, mostly with glucuronic acid, so that they may be excreted in bile and urine. Estrogens, such as estradiol, may be converted to estriol and estrone and then conjugated with glucuronic acid or sulfate. Abnormalities in estrogen metabolism have often been considered the cause of spider angiomas, gynecomastia, loss of axillary or pubic hair, and testicular atrophy. However, there is not a good direct correlation between plasma or urine estrogen levels and these clinical features.

Estrogens also act directly on the liver by impairing hepatic secretory activity. Estradiol and related estrogens, such as those present in contraceptive pills, interfere with Bromsulphalein (BSP) excretion and may also elevate the plasma alkaline phosphatase level in some patients (see Chap. 325). Related steroids such as etiocholanolone and pregnanediol have also been shown to stimulate the activity of δ-aminolevulinic acid (ALA) synthetase leading to porphyrinuria. Since these steroids exert these effects only in their free (i.e., nonglucuronide) form, the increased hepatic levels of δ-aminolevulinic acid synthetase in patients with Laennec's cirrhosis may be due to the effect of gonadal steroids.

Drugs are another important class of compounds inactivated by the liver. The impairment of morphine conjugation or inactivation of barbituates (by side-chain oxidation) in the liver is an important factor in the increased effectiveness or toxicity of these drugs in hepatic disease. All the barbituates, except phenobarbital and barbital, are primarily metabolized in the liver and should be used with caution in hepatic disease. Moreover, many other sedatives (Librium, paraldehyde) are metabolized largely by the liver, and their effect may be markedly prolonged in a patient with hepatic failure.

REFERENCES

Goodman, DeW. S.: Cholesterol Metabolism and the Liver, Med. Clinics N. Am., 47:649, 1963.

Isselbacher, K. J., and N. J. Greenberger: Metabolic Effects of Alcohol on the Liver, New Engl. J. Med., 270:351, 1964.

Kappas, A.: Biologic Actions of Some Natural Steroids on the Liver, New Engl. J. Med., 278:378, 1968.

Zieve, L., Pathogenesis of Hepatic Coma, Arch. Intern. Med., 118:211, 1966.

Zimmerman, H. J., Serum Enzymes in the Diagnosis of Hepatic Disease, Gastroenterology, 46:613, 1964.

324 DIAGNOSTIC PROCEDURES IN LIVER DISEASE

Kurt J. Isselbacher
and William A. Tisdale

Prompt recognition of liver disease and determination of its nature and extent require an understanding of the physiologic bases of a wide variety of techniques that assess liver function. Since no "battery" of tests is universally applicable, those most appropriate to a given clinical problem must be selected, their potential value and risk considered, and the results interpreted in relation to the clinical findings.

LIVER FUNCTION TESTS

Many liver function tests are based on a wide variety of biochemical reactions, such that the clinician can select combinations of tests that often measure different aspects of hepatic function. Many tests, however, are still empiric and semiquantitative, and no single test is universally helpful in diagnosis. Some methods are too sensitive and lack diagnostic specificity, others are affected by nonhepatic factors, and many simply do not measure any true physiologic function of the liver.

The physician concerned with clinical liver disease should be guided by several practical principles: (1) The tests selected should assess different parameters of liver function. (2) Liver function tests should be used *serially* in order to evaluate the evolution or course of the disease. (3) All such tests should be interpreted within the total clinical context with the recognition that any laboratory test may be fallible. The discussion that follows deals with representative and commonly used tests and should be read in conjunction with Chaps. 45 and 323.

SERUM BILIRUBIN (See Chaps. 45 and 325). Spectrophotometric determinations of serum bilirubin in the clinical laboratory measure two pigment fractions: (1) the water-soluble conjugated fraction that reacts *directly* with diazo reagent and consists largely of bilirubin diglucuronide, and (2) the lipid-soluble *indirect-reaction* fraction that represents primarily free, or unconjugated, bilirubin. The serum of normal adults contains less than 0.25 mg direct-reacting bilirubin per 100 ml and 1 mg total bilirubin or less per 100 ml serum. As noted in Chap. 45, absolute levels of the bilirubin fractions in jaundiced patients may be less helpful than the ratio of conjugated to total pigment in classifying the type of jaundice. Since the serum bilirubin levels are determined to a great extent by metabolic functions of the liver, serial measurements of the two fractions are often helpful in monitoring the course of most types of hepatobiliary disease. Simple inspection of the serum and use of the icterus index are not satisfactory or reliable.

URINE BILIRUBIN. Clinically significant concentrations of urine bilirubin are measured by the Harrison spot test or the Ictotest R tablet method and appear only with an increase of the ultrafilterable portion of the serum conjugated bilirubin. The demonstration of bilirubinuria indicates an elevation of conjugated serum pigment levels above a "threshold" of about 0.4 mg per 100 ml. The presence of bilirubinuria suggests underlying hepatocellular or obstructive biliary tract disease. Bilirubinuria may often be detected before overt jaundice has appeared.

URINE UROBILINOGEN. Semiquantitative measurement of urobilinogen in a freshly collected 2-hr urine specimen by the Watson method (normal values 0.2 to 1.2 units) may serve as a practical index of liver function. Interpretation of results is often difficult in diseases that are characterized by both liver cell damage, which decreases the extraction of urobilinogen from the portal blood and increases urobilinogen excretion, and cholestasis, which decreases the enteric production of urobilinogen and reduces its urinary excretion. In addition, alteration of intestinal flora by broad-spectrum antibiotics or the presence of a portacaval shunt may result in significant changes of urine urobilinogen. This test is most helpful when used *serially* to evaluate the completeness of bile duct obstruction or to document the return of liver function toward normal after acute hepatic injury.

BROMSULPHALEIN (BSP) EXCRETION. Several dyes, including BSP (a phenolphthalein derivative), indocyanine green, and radioactive rose bengal, have been used to assess hepatic excretory function. The BSP test is at present the most widely used and useful. BSP is taken up rapidly by liver cells, concentrated and stored within the cytoplasm, and conjugated enzymatically with glutathione. Both free BSP and BSP-glutathione are secreted into the bile, since conjugation is *not* obligatory for biliary secretion. In diseases that produce hepatic cell dysfunction or impaired bile secretion, significant quantities of conjugated BSP may escape excretion and reenter the bloodstream. Although it was once considered to be a simple index of liver blood flow and excretory competence, the clearance of BSP from the blood depends also on the rate of hepatic uptake, storage capacity, conjugating activity, and an overall blood-to-bile transfer maximum. However, the techniques that measure these different parameters of BSP metabolism are not routine diagnostic tools.

The BSP test is simple, quantitative, and sensitive but notably *nonspecific*. A standard amount (5 mg per kg body weight) of BSP dye is injected carefully into a vein, a blood sample is withdrawn 45 min later from another venous site, and an alkalinized serum sample is analyzed for total BSP concentration. The result is expressed as the percentage of injected dye retained in the circulation. In normal adults, less than 5 percent of the test dose remains in the serum at 45 min. BSP retention increases with aging.

Despite its simplicity and sensitivity, the BSP test is often difficult to interpret. Abnormal retention may reflect the *presence* of liver cell damage or loss, as in hepatitis or cirrhosis, but not be a direct measure of the *extent* of parenchymal disease. Many diverse processes such as partial bile duct obstruction, focal intrahepatic duct obstruction by tumor, and cholestasis may produce BSP retention. Decreased hepatic blood flow as in shock or congestive heart failure results in marked BSP retention. The BSP test is therefore a sensitive index of *overall* liver cell function and is most helpful in the detection of focal or minimal hepatobiliary disease and in the study of anicteric patients.

A few practical aspects of the BSP test should be noted: (1) The dye is a local tissue irritant, and extravasation during injection produces painful inflammation and necrosis. (2) Anaphylactic reactions occur, but they are rare. (3) Gross obesity and fluid retention make calculation of an appropriate dose difficult, and results are often falsely high because of abnormal dye distribution. (4) Fever and certain drugs (notably the gallbladder dye iopanoic acid [Telapaque] and the synthetic androgen norethandrolone) may produce BSP retention without apparent liver cell damage. (5) The test has little value in patients with significant jaundice, since retention will occur regardless of the nature of the underlying disease.

FLOCCULATION AND TURBIDITY TESTS. A number of empirical flocculation and turbidity tests have been used to detect quantitative or qualitative changes in the serum proteins of patients with hepatobiliary disease. In general, increased levels of γ-globulins and decreased albumin concentration, both common features of hepatocellular disease, alter the stability of the colloidal solutions and produce positive reactions. These tests, which are nonspecific and affected by many nonhepatic factors, have been replaced in large part by chemical determinations of albumin and globulin concentrations and by protein electrophoretic methods.

SERUM ENZYME ASSAYS. Measurements of many serum enzymes have been used in an attempt to quantitate liver damage or to distinguish between hepatocellular (i.e., functional) and mechanical cholestasis. No specific or truly diagnostic test has been devised to solve either problem, but the enzymatic liver function tests described

below have proved helpful in the clinical study of many hepatobiliary diseases.

Alkaline Phosphatase. Human serum contains alkaline phosphatase, an enzyme which hydrolyzes synthetic phosphate esters at pH 9. As indicated in Chap. 323, this enzyme is produced by many tissues, especially bone, intestine, liver, and placenta, and is excreted in the bile. In normal serum, most of the enzyme is derived from bone. In hepatobiliary disease, isoenzyme fractionation studies indicate an increased release of the hepatic enzyme into the bloodstream with an additional increase often the result of secretion of enzyme into the bile. In general, in the absence of bone disease and of pregnancy, an elevated serum alkaline phosphatase level reflects impaired hepatic excretory function.

Several methods of comparable accuracy and sensitivity are available to measure alkaline phosphatase activity. The most widely used are the Bodansky (normal: 1.5 to 4.5 units) and the King-Armstrong methods (normal: 4 to 13 units). Growing children and women in late pregnancy have serum levels that may be twice those of men and of women not in late pregnancy.

Slight to moderate increases in alkaline phosphatase (6 to 10 Bodansky units) occur in many patients with parenchymal disorders usch as hepatitis and cirrhosis, and transient increases have been reported in virtually all types of liver disease. The most striking and persistent increases in activity, however, occur in diseases associated with cholestasis. Over 80 percent of patients with malignant biliary obstruction have phosphatase values in the range of 15 to 30 Bodansky units; about 60 percent of those with benign obstruction have levels above 15 Bodansky units, and most with intrahepatic cholestasis have values above 12 Bodansky units. Extremely high values may be associated with biliary obstruction complicated by cholangitis or tumor invasion of the liver. Two features of this test make it especially useful in cases of obscure liver disease: First, increases in serum alkaline phosphatase may precede elevations of the serum bilirubin level in obstructive biliary disease. Second, focal hepatic lesions (for example, granulomas, inflammatory infiltrates, and tumor metastases) may produce elevation of alkaline phosphatase level with little other evidence of liver dysfunction. Since bone is a source of the enzyme, extensive Paget's disease, bony metastases and other diseases associated with increased osteoblastic activity may produce high levels of alkaline phosphatase in the absence of liver disease.

5′-Nucleotidase and Alcohol Dehydrogenase. Other serum enzyme assays have been proposed as sensitive indicators of cholestasis. For example, the level of *5′-nucleotidase*, an enzyme not affected by the presence of bone disease, is usually elevated in obstructive biliary disease. However, elevations are seen also in patients with various hepatocellular diseases, and in general the alkaline phosphatase is a more sensitive measure of impaired bile excretion. *Serum alcohol dehydrogenase*, an enzyme derived almost exclusively from liver cells, is increased in most diseases with significant intrahepatic bile stasis and hepatocellular necrosis. However, occasionally increases of this enzyme may be found in the serum in cases of extrahepatic biliary obstruction.

Transaminases. Assays of many serum enzymes have been proposed as measures of hepatocellular damage. Of these, the serum glutamic-oxaloacetic (GOT) and glutamic-pyruvic (GPT) transaminases have proved to be the most practical. GOT occurs in all body tissues, especially in heart, liver, and skeletal muscle. GPT is present primarily in the liver and to a lesser extent in kidney and skeletal muscle. Although many studies have shown that the height and duration of serum enzyme elevations parallel the extent of liver cell damage (i.e., necrosis or altered cell permeability), precise quantitative correlations cannot be made in most clinical conditions (Chap. 323). Normal serum contains less than 40 Karmen units of GOT and less than 30 Karmen units of GPT.

In the absence of acute necrosis or ischemia of other tissues, such as the myocardium, high serum GOT and GPT levels suggest liver cell damage with extensive acute hepatic necrosis as in severe viral hepatitis, and serum levels of 1,000 to 3,000 units may be found. Less severe necrosis produces transient levels of 500 to 1,000 units. Mild chronic or focal liver diseases (for example, subclinical or anicteric viral hepatitis, Laennec's cirrhosis, granulomatous infiltrations, and tumor invasion) may be associated with transaminase levels of 50 to 200 units. With intrahepatic or extrahepatic cholestasis (in the absence of hepatic cell necrosis) GOT and GPT levels usually are not significantly elevated and rarely exceed 300 units.

Serial determinations of GOT and GPT are helpful in following the course of a patient with hepatobiliary disease, especially when one is dealing with liver cell necrosis. Caution is needed in the interpretation of abnormal levels. Serum transaminases may *decrease* in some patients with fulminant hepatitis, presumably because of previous excessive loss of enzyme from the liver. Laennec's cirrhosis and postnecrotic cirrhosis may be associated with only slight transaminase elevations.

Lactic Dehydrogenase (LDH). Lactic dehydrogenase, a glycolytic enzyme that catalyses the interconversion of pyruvate and lactate, is present in all body tissues, the myocardium, liver, skeletal muscle, kidney, and erythrocytes containing the largest amounts. The enzyme present in normal serum (42 to 98 Wacker units per ml) is derived from several tissue sources and can be separated by electrophoresis and other techniques into five isoenzymes. Moderate elevations of LDH levels are common in acute viral hepatitis and in cirrhosis; biliary tract disease may produce slight elevations. High serum levels may be found in metastatic carcinoma of the liver.

SERUM PROTEINS. Albumin, prothrombin, fibrinogen, and several other serum proteins are synthesized exclusively by liver cells, and extensive liver damage may lead to decreased blood levels of these proteins. Serum immunoglobulins, produced by lymphocytes and plasma cells, vary widely in concentration in hepatobiliary disease and reflect inflammatory or immune responses rather than liver cell dysfunction. Thus, analyses of the various serum proteins may provide helpful insights into the nature and extent of liver disease. As noted in Chap. 323, however, many nonhepatic factors also affect the metabolism of these proteins.

Albumin and Globulins. Total concentrations of serum albumin (normally 3.5 to 5 Gm per 100 ml) and globulin (normally 2 to 3.5 Gm per 100 ml) may be determined chemically. The level of each should be evaluated separately, because the *albumin/globulin, or A/G, ratio* has no physiologic significance. The concentrations of α_1-, α_2-, β-, and γ-globulins are usually measured by electrophoretic methods.

Hypoalbuminemia may occur in subacute and massive hepatic necrosis, chronic active hepatitis, cirrhosis, and other disorders with significant destruction or replacement of liver cells. The serum albumin level also serves as a useful guide to prognosis and therapy in these diseases. *Hyperglobulinemia* suggests the presence of chronic inflammatory disorders such as cirrhosis and chronic active hepatitis. Neoplastic and inflammatory diseases of the liver may produce increased levels of α_2-globulins, and some patients with bile duct obstruction have high β-globulin levels (see Chap. 113).

Immunoglobulins. Immunoelectrophoretic and immunodiffusion techniques permit the semiquantitative assay of the various immunoglobulin fractions, IgG, IgA, IgM, and IgD. Nonspecific immunoglobulin abnormalities occur in a variety of acute and chronic liver diseases. All three major immunoglobulin fractions may be increased slightly in the course of acute viral hepatitis. Increased concentrations of IgA and IgG are common in Laennec's cirrhosis, striking elevations of IgG levels are characteristic of chronic active hepatitis, and high levels of IgM may be seen in primary biliary cirrhosis. None of these changes, however, appear specific or diagnostic.

Clotting Factors. The serum activities of most clotting factors may be estimated by special tests, but direct determinations of fibrinogen and of the one-stage prothrombin time (which reflects activities of prothrombin, fibrinogen, and factors, V, VII, and IX) are the most useful.

Prolongation of the one-stage prothrombin time may occur in severe hepatitis or cirrhosis and in patients with chronic bile duct obstruction. A single abnormal prothrombin determination should not be interpreted as a sign of liver cell failure, because intestinal malabsorption of vitamin K may produce reductions in prothrombin levels. However, the persistence of an abnormal prothrombin time 24 and 48 hr after parenteral injections of vitamin K_1 (10 mg per day) suggests liver cell damage.

BLOOD LIPIDS. Determination of serum total cholesterol (normal: 130 to 230 mg per 100 ml) and cholesterol esters (normal: 50 to 70 percent of total cholesterol) has been a traditional liver function test, but the practical and physiologic interpretations of changes in these lipids are difficult (see Chap. 323). Empirically, acute or chronic diffuse liver disease often results in decreased total values and a decrease in the ester fraction; cholestasis, whether functional or mechanical, characteristically produces moderate to extreme elevations of the total cholesterol level but with a decrease in the percent esterified.

RADIOLOGIC PROCEDURES

ABDOMINAL ROENTGENOGRAM. Films of the upper abdomen and lower thorax rarely provide accurate estimates of liver size and shape, but gross hepatomegaly and hepatic masses that elevate or distort the diaphragm may be detected. Plain films of the abdomen may reveal calcific densities in the gallbladder, biliary tree, pancreas, or liver (as echinococcal cysts, hemangioma, or, rarely, a metastatic tumor mass).

BARIUM STUDIES OF THE GASTROINTESTINAL TRACT. An upper gastrointestinal series should be performed in cases of suspected portal hypertension, because esophagogastric varices can be demonstrated with about 70 to 90 percent accuracy when they are present. Enlargement of the left lobe of the liver (as with tumor, abscess, or cirrhosis) may displace the barium-filled stomach laterally and posteriorly.

CHOLECYSTOGRAPHY AND CHOLANGIOGRAPHY. The *oral cholecystogram* provides limited information in most patients with overt hepatobiliary disease, because parenchymal dysfunction and impaired bile excretion lead to decreased excretion of the contrast material and hence nonvisualization of the gallbladder. As stated above, iopanoic acid (Telapaque) may produce transient BSP retention in the absence of liver disease.

An *intravenous cholangiogram* may permit demonstration of the intrahepatic and extrahepatic bile ducts and the localization of obstructing lesions of the major ducts. Even faint visualization of a normal-sized biliary tree may be helpful in the differential diagnosis of obstructive jaundice. However, as with the oral cholecystography, liver dysfunction and moderate cholestasis may prevent adequate secretion of dye to permit visualization on x-ray.

Percutaneous transhepatic cholangiography is sometimes used to distinguish between mechanical biliary obstruction and intrahepatic cholestasis. This approach may be useful when decreased liver function precludes the use of intravenous cholangiography. With experience and proper precautions, dilated major ducts proximal to an obstructing lesion can be cannulated and visualized with dye in 75 to 90 percent of cases, whereas the normal or small ducts associated with intrahepatic cholestasis are rarely demonstrated. This procedure should be carried out in cooperation with a surgeon, because when a dilated duct is punctured and visualized, exploration of the biliary system should be carried out within four hours to avoid bile peritonitis. *Operative cholangiography* should be performed at the time of laparotomy in all cases of obscure obstructive jaundice, presumed biliary cirrhosis, or biliary tract stricture.

ANGIOGRAPHY. Visualization of the major branches and the overall arborization pattern of the hepatic artery may be obtained by selective catheterization and perfusion of the celiac artery, i.e., *celiac axis angiography*. This technique is relatively safe and may help to demonstrate primary or secondary tumor masses in the liver. Dilatation of the hepatic artery, "tumor blushes," and arteriovenous shunting are typical findings in such cases.

Percutaneous splenoportography, often performed in conjunction with portal vein manometry, provides an accurate, safe, and helpful means of demonstrating the size, patency, and collateral branching of the portal vein and its tributaries. Radiopaque dye is injected through a needle or catheter inserted into the spleen under local anesthesia. Serial films may demonstrate (1) dilated and tortuous splenic or portal veins distal to an obstruction, (2) venous obstruction by tumor or clot, (3) reflux of dye into the mesenteric or coronary veins in cases of portal hypertension, (4) extensive portal-systemic collateral flow throughout the abdomen and into esophagogastric varices, or (5) distortion of the intrahepatic portal vessels in various types of liver disease. The morbidity associated with this procedure is low and consists of transient local pain, occasional extravasation of dye or blood, and rarely anaphylactic reactions.

RADIOISOTOPE LIVER SCANS (Scintiscans). Hepatic scintiscans are performed by the intravenous injection of gamma-emitting isotopes that are extracted selectively by the liver, followed by external radiation scanning of the upper abdomen. [198]Colloidal gold ([198]Au is concentrated within Kupffer cells, whereas noncolloidal ^{131}I-labeled rose bengal is extracted by liver cells and excreted rapidly into the bile. [99]Technetium has a short half-life, is taken up by Kupffer cells, and gives a clear scan; the splenic uptake is greater than for colloidal gold. Hepatic scintiscans are useful for demonstrating the size and shape of the liver and for delineating intrahepatic or perihepatic masses. In addition, study of the excretion phase of rose bengal scans may help to differentiate intrahepatic cholestasis from low biliary tract obstruction.

Hepatic scanning should be regarded as a supplement to other methods of evaluating liver function, and its indications and limitations must be emphasized. Although tumor nodules larger than 3 cm in diameter can be demonstrated in about 80 percent of cases, false negative scans occur in about 20 percent of most series of metastatic cancer of the liver, because many hepatic metastases are too small to be detected by this method. Abscesses and cysts may be outlined with accuracy, but nonopaque areas may result from parenchymal disorders such as cirrhosis.

OTHER DIAGNOSTIC PROCEDURES

PORTAL AND HEPATIC VEIN MANOMETRY. Measurement of the splenic pulp pressure (a reliable reflection of the actual portal venous pressure) by *percutaneous portal manometry* and estimation of the wedged hepatic venous pressure (WHVP—an approximation of the postsinusoidal intrahepatic venous pressure) by *hepatic vein catheterization* are useful in the study of patients with known or presumed portal hypertension. While determination of the WHVP is not a routine procedure, the demonstration of a normal or slightly elevated WHVP in a patient with proved portal hypertension serves to localize the obstruction to the extrahepatic portion of the portal vein, the portal inflow system (as in schistosomiasis), or the presinusoidal vessels (as in some cases of fatty liver or myelofibrosis). Splenic pulp pressures greater than 25 to 30 cm of saline solution indicate significant portal hypertension.

PERCUTANEOUS NEEDLE BIOPSY OF THE LIVER. Percutaneous needle biopsy is a safe, simple, and often invaluable method of diagnosing liver disease. Although the needle biopsy sample is small, *diffuse parenchymal disorders* such as cirrhosis, hepatitis, and drug reactions may be diagnosed with remarkable accuracy. In *disseminated focal diseases* (such as granulomas or tumor infiltrates) serial sections may demonstrate the lesion. Culture of portions of the liver tissue may aid in the diagnosis of *infections* such as salmonellosis, brucellosis, or tuberculosis.

The biopsy may be performed under local anesthesia with the Menghini (aspiration) or the Vim-Silverman (cutting) needle using either the transpleural or subcostal approach. If the operator is skillful and the patient is carefully selected, morbidity should be low and limited to occasional postbiopsy pain or vasovagal reactions.

Some of the major indications for needle biopsy are (1) unexplained hepatomegaly or hepatosplenomegaly, (2) cholestasis of uncertain cause, (3) persistently abnormal liver function tests, (4) suspected systemic diseases or infiltrative diseases such as sarcoidosis or miliary tuberculosis, (5) fevers of unknown origin (in which culture of liver tissue may be helpful), and (6) suspected primary or metastatic liver tumor.

Needle biopsy should not be performed if (1) the patient is not able to cooperate, (2) clinical or laboratory evidence indicates impaired hemostasis (for example, the one-stage prothrombin time is greater than 50 percent of control, thrombocytopenia or purpura are present, or the bleeding time is prolonged), (3) there is infection of the right pleural space or septic cholangitis, (4) profound anemia, or (5) compatible blood is not available for transfusion in case of hemorrhage. Amyloidosis and carcinoma of the liver may increase the hazard of postbiopsy hemorrhage. Although biopsy in mechanical biliary obstruction may lead occasionally to the escape of bile and localized bile peritonitis, this complication is uncommon.

PERITONEOSCOPY. The serosal lining, liver, gallbladder, spleen, and other abdominal organs can be visualized with minimum discomfort and hazard by a skilled operator and often permits immediate diagnosis by inspection or directed needle biopsy. Peritoneoscopy is useful in the study of debilitated patients and in those with hepatomegaly, unexplained ascites, or abdominal masses.

LAPAROTOMY. When the most thorough clinical, laboratory, and biopsy studies fail to define the precise nature of hepatobiliary disease on occasion, the physician may need to advise exploratory laparotomy as the definitive diagnostic step. The medicosurgical team should be prepared to obtain full benefit from this direct approach, using biopsy, culture, cholangiography, and angiography as required.

REFERENCES

LIVER FUNCTION TESTS

Bradley, S. E.: The Circulation and the Liver, Gastroenterology, 44:403, 1963.

Discombe, G.: Flocculation Tests, Lancet, 1:1005, 1959.

Feizi, T.: Immunoglobulins in Chronic Liver Disease, Gut, 9:193, 1968.

Posen, S.: Alkaline Phosphatase, Ann. Intern. Med., 67:183, 1967.

Schoenfeld, L. J.: Sulfobromophthalein Transport and Metabolism, Gastroenterology, 48:530, 1965.

Walker, G., and D. Doniach: Antibodies and Immunoglobulins in Liver Disease, Gut, 9:266, 1968.

RADIOLOGIC AND OTHER DIAGNOSTIC PROCEDURES

Atkinson, M., and S. Sherlock: Intrasplenic Pressure as an Index of the Portal Venous Pressure, Lancet, 1:1325, 1954.

Baggenstoss, A. H.: Morphologic and Etiologic Diagnosis from Hepatic Biopsies without Clinical Data, Medicine, 45:435, 1966.

Conn, H. O., J. R. Mitchell, and M. G. Brodoff: Comparison of Radiologic and Esophogoscopic Diagnosis of Esophageal Varices, New Engl. J. Med., 265:160, 1961.

McAfee, J. G., R. G. Ause, and H. N. Wagner: Diagnostic Value of Scintillation Scanning of the Liver, Arch. Intern. Med., 116:25, 1965.

Ruzicka, R. F.: Radiologic Methods in Liver Diseases, in "Progress in Liver Diseases," vol. II, H. Popper and F. Schaffner (Eds.), New York, Grune & Stratton, Inc., 1965.

325   DISTURBANCES OF BILIRUBIN METABOLISM

Kurt J. Isselbacher

The normal metabolism of bilirubin and the approach to the patient with jaundice have been presented in Chap. 45. With a consideration of these pathways, the disorders of bilirubin metabolism can be divided into four major categories, namely, those due to (1) increased pigment production, (2) reduced hepatic uptake of bilirubin, (3) impaired hepatic conjugation, and (4) decreased excretion of the conjugated pigment from the liver into bile. The first three of these disorders are associated with predominantly unconjugated hyperbilirubinemia (i.e., more than 80 percent of serum bilirubin is unconjugated, or indirect-reacting). The fourth group, defective excretion, is associated with predominantly conjugated hyperbilirubinemia (i.e., more than 50 percent of serum bilirubin is conjugated, or direct-reacting) and with bilirubinuria.

DISORDERS CAUSING PREDOMINANTLY UNCONJUGATED HYPERBILIRUBINEMIA

Overproduction of Bilirubin

INCREASED DESTRUCTION OF CIRCULATING ERYTHRO-CYTES (Intravascular and Extravascular Hemolysis). In disorders associated with hemolysis, most commonly the hemolytic anemias, the rate of bilirubin production is increased and may even exceed the amount that can be removed by a normal liver. The resulting jaundice is primarily an unconjugated hyperbilirubinemia. There is often also a small but definite increase in the serum conjugated bilirubin, when the amount of bilirubin glucuronide formed exceeds the amount that the liver can excrete (see Chap. 45). If there is significant anemia or if other adverse factors are operative (e.g., fever, sepsis, hypoxemia, or vascular collapse), the ability of the liver to handle the pigment load will be compromised, and the degree of jaundice will be greater.

The clinical and diagnostic features of the various hemolytic anemias are described in Chap. 338. The presence of reticulocytosis, shortened red cell survival, and increased fecal urobilinogen, in the absence of clinical and laboratory evidence of liver disease, strongly suggest hemolysis and overproduction of bilirubin as the cause of the jaundice. It is obvious, however, that in some cases (e.g., cirrhosis, tumors, and sepsis), hemolysis *plus* deranged liver function may be present. In most cases of uncomplicated hemolytic states, the mean serum bilirubin level will be in the range of 3 to 5 mg per 100 ml; rarely, levels up to 10 mg may be seen.

Jaundice due to increased pigment production may also be seen as a consequence of tissue infarction (e.g., pulmonary infarcts) and large collections of blood in tissues (e.g., leakage from blood vessels after catheterization studies, rupture of an aortic aneurysm). If hypotension and hypoxia also supervene, jaundice is usually more pronounced, and the resulting impairment of liver function may also lead to a significant increase in the serum conjugated bilirubin level (see Postoperative Intrahepatic Cholestasis, below.)

With the exception of early infancy, elevations of serum unconjugated bilirubin levels are not generally harmful per se, and the prognosis is that of the hemolytic process itself. However, in the neonatal state and infancy, unconjugated bilirubin levels above 20 mg per 100 ml may lead to *kernicterus* due to bilirubin deposition in the lipid-rich basal ganglions (see Chap. 363). Chronic overproduction of bilirubin may result in the formation of gallstones composed predominantly of bilirubin ("pigment stones"). In this situation, all the potential complications of calculus disease of the biliary tract (Chap. 332) may be superimposed on the chronic hemolytic state which produced it.

INCREASED PRODUCTION OF BILIRUBIN FROM SOURCES OTHER THAN CIRCULATING ERYTHROCYTES. As indicated in Chap. 45, about 15 to 20 percent of the circulating bilirubin is normally derived from sources other than the destruction of circulating red cells. This represents the so-called "early-labeled fraction" and includes the synthesis of bilirubin from nonhemoglobin heme in the liver and from hemoglobin heme in the marrow.

In some conditions, jaundice results from an increased destruction of red cells or red cell precursors in the marrow—a process referred to as *ineffective erythropoiesis* (see Chaps. 45 and 61). In patients with thalassemia, pernicious anemia, and congenital erythropoietic porphyria, such an increased rate of formation of the early-labeled bilirubin fraction has been demonstrated. It is possible that some cases of unexplained unconjugated hyperbilirubinemia may be caused by an increased hepatic production of bilirubin from nonhemoglobin heme, but this phenomenon has not yet been demonstrated clinically.

Impaired Hepatic Uptake of Bilirubin

DRUGS. While numerous drugs might theoretically interfere with uptake of bilirubin by the liver, only one agent has been definitely shown to influence this process: *flavaspidic acid,* an active ingredient of male fern extract used in the treatment of tapeworm infestation, may cause unconjugated hyperbilirubinemia, as well as impairment of Bromsulphalein (BSP) clearance, during its administration. The jaundice readily subsides following treatment. The manner by which flavaspidic acid interferes with hepatic bilirubin uptake is unclear. The jaundice which may occur with *novobiocin* and the iodinated agent *bunamiodyl* is due in part to an interference in bilirubin uptake.

GILBERT'S DISEASE (Constitutional Hepatic Dysfunction; Familial Nonhemolytic Jaundice). Since the original report by Gilbert in 1907, there have been increasing reports of patients with this disorder characterized by unexplained mild, chronic elevations of the indirect-reacting bilirubin level in the serum. The patient with Gilbert's disease may show jaundice in the neonatal period, but more often it is first detected after the second decade. The patient often is unaware of jaundice until physical or laboratory examination reveals a mild or low-grade hyperbilirubinemia, usually ranging from 1.2 to 3 mg per 100 ml and rarely higher than 5 mg per 100 ml. The jaundice is chronic, and the degree of icterus fluctuates. It is often noted after stress or trauma. It may be first noticed following surgical therapy, infection, excessive exertion, or alcohol ingestion. While there may be a history of fatigue or asthenia, one can frequently ascribe these symptoms to the associated disorder which brings the patient to the physician. Liver function tests are normal (except for occasional slight increases in BSP retention), and liver histology shows no specific changes.

There are no specific tests for this disease, and *the diagnosis is one of exclusion* in a patient with unconjugated hyperbilirubinemia in whom occult or compensated hemolysis has been excluded. The underlying defect is considered to be due to impaired bilirubin uptake, but in some patients with more pronounced jaundice (i.e., bilirubin levels greater than 5 mg) impaired conjugation may also exist.

Often, cases of unconjugated hyperbilirubinemia are initially called Gilbert's disease because *overt* hemolysis has not been detected. However, in many instances, subsequent studies with more sensitive techniques (e.g., ^{51}Cr red cell labeling) do reveal *occult* hemolysis or ineffective erythropoiesis. Thus, many cases labeled "Gilbert's disease" may in fact be patients with mild or compensated hemolytic states. In view of this and other factors, it should be emphasized that since there is no specific diagnostic test, Gilbert's disease probably is not a single disease entity.

POSTHEPATITIS HYPERBILIRUBINEMIA. Some patients, after recovering from an attack of acute viral hepatitis, are found several months or years later to have a mild unconjugated hyperbilirubinemia. The histologic features of the liver are normal, and the bilirubin increase is of the same order of magnitude as in Gilbert's disease. Except for a history compatible with a prior attack of viral hepatitis, *these patients have no unique features to distinguish them from patients with Gilbert's disease;* in fact, they probably belong to this same broad disease group. It is important to reassure the patient that the mild unconjugated hyperbilirubinemia is of no clinical consequence and is not an indication that chronic liver disease has supervened.

Impaired Bilirubin Conjugation (Decreased Activity of Bilirubin Glucuronyl Transferase)

NEONATAL JAUNDICE (Physiologic Jaundice of the Newborn). Almost every infant exhibits some transient unconjugated hyperbilirubinemia between the second and fifth days of life. While during gestation the placenta serves to clear bilirubin from the fetus, after birth the infant must detoxify the pigments himself. However, at this stage the hepatic enzyme system is still "immature" and inadequate for the task. As a result, unconjugated bilirubinemia develops, usually not exceeding 5 mg per 100 ml serum. The activity of glucuronyl transferase increases within several days to 2 weeks after birth, and concomitantly the serum bilirubin returns to normal. In the premature infant the glucuronyl transferase activity is less, and the neonatal jaundice may be more pronounced. In infants with a superimposed hemolytic process (e.g., erythroblastosis), the excessive pigment load leads to more pronounced jaundice, and bilirubin levels may exceed 20 mg per 100 ml serum. It should be emphasized that neonatal jaundice is not present at the time of delivery; if jaundice is present at birth, other causes must be considered.

According to Arias, certain cytoplasmic proteins of the hepatocytes are involved in the normal binding of bilirubin and drugs by the liver. In experimental animals a so-called Y protein which appears to bind bilirubin is low in the neonatal state and increases with age. It has been proposed that deficiency of this protein may contribute to neonatal jaundice.

An additional facet of the "immature" liver is a concomitant defect in the excretion of *conjugated* bilirubin. Rarely this defect persists beyond the time needed for the development of adequate glucuronide conjugation and may explain the occasional presence of conjugated hyperbilirubinemia in infants with erythroblastosis (*inspissated-bile syndrome*).

CONGENITAL DEFICIENCY OF GLUCURONYL TRANSFERASE (Crigler-Najjar Syndrome; Congenital Nonhemolytic Jaundice). This disorder is due to a hereditary deficiency of glucuronyl transferase. The patients are usually jaundiced within a few days of birth, and serum unconjugated bilirubin reaches levels of 18 to 45 mg per 100 ml. Survival to adulthood is rare if the bilirubin levels exceed 20 mg per 100 ml. At these high levels, the unconjugated pigment with its special affinity for lipids is deposited in the basal ganglions, leading to kernicterus and death within the first few years of life. This genetic disorder appears to be inherited as an autosomal recessive. A strain of rats (Gunn rat) has a similar hereditary defect and is widely used as an experimental model of the Crigler-Najjar syndrome.

The diagnosis can be made by direct demonstration of the enzyme defect on liver tissue obtained by biopsy. Indirect measurements include evidence of impaired urinary excretion of glucuronides following the oral administration of drugs such as menthol or N-acetyl-*p*-aminophenol. Routine liver function tests show no abnormality, and liver histologic characteristics are normal. Because of the defective excretion of bilirubin into bile, urobilinogen excretion in urine and feces is low. The fact that patients with this syndrome do not show a continuing increase in serum bilirubin, despite continuous bilirubin production from hemoglobin, suggests that some alternative metabolic pathways may compensate in part for the defect in the conjugating mechanism. There is no effective treatment for maintaining the serum bilirubin at low enough levels to avoid some neurologic damage. Reduction of the serum bilirubin can be achieved by exchange transfusion, but such a lowering serves only as a temporary therapeutic measure. In some cases, transient lowering of the serum bilirubin level has been achieved with phenobarbitol administration, but the long-term benefits of such treatment remain to be determined.

Since the description of the Crigler-Najjar syndrome in 1952, a less severe form and a genetic variant of this syndrome has been described. In such patients, serum bilirubin levels are lower (ranging from 6 to 18 mg per 100 ml), jaundice may not appear until adolescence or adult life, and neurologic complications are uncommon. It is possible that such patients have a *partial deficiency of glucuronyl transferase,* and while no conjugate is detectable in plasma, some is present in gallbladder bile and duodenal aspirates. Phenobarbitol seems to be effective in lowering the serum bilirubin level in these patients. The exact relationship of these patients to those with the more typical Crigler-Najjar syndrome and those classified as having Gilbert's disease remains to be determined.

ACQUIRED DEFICIENCY OF GLUCURONYL TRANSFERASE. As with any enzyme, glucuronyl transferase is susceptible to inhibition by a variety of agents, and because of the decreased activity of the enyme in neonatal state, such inhibition may be more evident at that time. Neonatal jaundice may be pronounced or prolonged in infants treated with *drugs* such as chloramphenicol or novobiocin or with *vitamin K*. In some breast-fed infants jaundice has been ascribed to the presence of pregnane-3β,20α-diol, in *breast milk*. This hormone is a good inhibitor of glucuronyl transferase, and when the infant is removed from the breast, the "breast-milk jaundice" subsides.

Hypothyroidism delays the normal "maturation" of glucuronyl transferase. In cretins, neonatal jaundice may be prolonged for weeks or months. In fact, the presence of prolonged unconjugated hyperbilirubinemia after birth may be a clue to an underlying hypothyroidism.

In the infant, as well as in the adult, *liver cell damage* leads to impairment in glucuronide conjugation as a result of decreased transferase activity. However, since excretion is the rate-limiting step in bilirubin metabolism and since this step is always interfered with to a greater extent than conjugation in parenchymal liver disease, the pigment which accumulates in the blood is predominantly conjugated.

DISORDERS CAUSING PREDOMINANTLY CONJUGATED HYPERBILIRUBINEMIA

In most cases of jaundice due to primary liver disease, the plasma exhibits elevated levels of both conjugated and unconjugated bilirubin, and urine contains bilirubin. The relative proportions of the two pigments are highly variable. In many familial hepatic abnormalities (described below) and in some forms of drug-induced liver injury, the jaundice is almost entirely due to conjugated hyperbilirubinemia, 60 to 80 percent of the serum bilirubin giving a direct van den Bergh reaction. Such a pigment pattern is also seen with extrahepatic biliary obstruction.

In jaundice associated with diffuse liver cell damage as in hepatitis and cirrhosis, the conjugated bilirubin levels may be somewhat less than in the above cholestatic syndromes, with the direct-reacting values ranging from 40 to 70 percent of the total serum bilirubin. However, the pattern is quite variable, and in all of the above hepatic disorders, once the serum bilirubin components have been measured, repeated fractionation during the course of the disease is of little diagnostic or prognostic value. The main purpose of the initial fractionation should be to distinguish hepatic parenchymal disease from the disorders associated with predominantly unconjugated hyperbilirubinemia.

Familial Defects in Hepatic Excretory Function

DUBIN-JOHNSON SYNDROME (Chronic Idiopathic Jaundice). This disorder is characterized by a mild, chronic hyperbilirubinemia and the frequent presence of a *dark pigment in the liver cells*. The hyperbilirubinemia, which may begin at any age, is predominantly of the conjugated type, with total serum levels usually ranging from 3 to 10 mg per 100 ml. The patient may by asymptomatic or have vague constitutional or gastrointestinal symptoms. Not infrequently the liver is slightly enlarged; in about one-fourth of the cases there is mild hepatic tenderness. Oral and intravenous cholangiography usually fails to visualize the biliary tract. Liver function tests are variably affected, but BSP excretion is consistently diminished. In performing the BSP test, the serum level falls at 30 and 45 min, but then the *BSP may increase again* at 90 and 120 min. The increase is primarily in conjugated BSP, and this temporal pattern, while not specific, is characteristic of this disorder. In the liver the striking feature is the presence of a brown or black pigment in the hepatocytes. This nonbilirubin pigment, initially considered a lipofuscin, appears to be a melanin polymer.

The Dubin-Johnson syndrome is believed to be an inherited and familial disorder of hepatic excretory function. There is impaired excretion of many metabolites, including conjugated bilirubin, BSP, and iodinated dyes. Oral contraceptive agents may accentuate hyperbilirubinemia or may produce jaundice for the first time.

Features of cholestasis such as pruritus or steatorrhea are usually lacking, and serum alkaline phosphatase levels are *not* elevated. Impairment in the excretion of epinephrine metabolites may account for the accumulation of the melanin pigments. The overall prognosis of the disorder is excellent. It appears to be inherited as an autosomal dominant, affecting both sexes in many ethnic groups.

Rotor syndrome is similar in most respects to the Dubin-Johnson syndrome. However, *there is no pigment in the liver cells,* and the gallbladder is usually visualized on cholecystography. The BSP excretion pattern is similar to that seen in the Dubin-Johnson syndrome. The fact that in members of a family with chronic idiopathic jaundice one may find some with hepatic pigment and some without strongly suggests that the Rotor and Dubin-Johnson syndromes are genetically related variants.

BENIGN FAMILIAL RECURRENT CHOLESTASIS. This is a relatively rare syndrome characterized by recurrent attacks of pruritus and jaundice. During an attack the serum alkaline phosphatase level is markedly elevated, and liver biopsy shows the morphologic features of cholestasis. However, at laparotomy, biliary obstruction is not found, and operative cholangiography reveals a patent and apparently normal bilary tree. Remissions are the rule, and at such times hepatic function tests and liver morphologic features are usually normal. The cause of the disorder is unknown; cirrhosis does not develop, and disorder is benign. A congenital origin has been postulated based on the early age of onset and familial incidence.

RECURRENT JAUNDICE OF PREGNANCY (Intrahepatic Cholestasis of Pregnancy). During a normal pregnancy some changes in liver function occur, especially during the last trimester. Usually these consist of slight increases in BSP retention and of serum alkaline phosphatase. This mild increase in alkaline phosphatase during pregnancy is normally of placental rather than hepatic origin. Bilirubin increases never exceed 2 mg per 100 ml serum and usually are hardly detectable.

In a small number of pregnant patients an intrahepatic cholestasis may appear. This usually occurs in the third trimester but may develop any time after the seventh week of gestation. The clinical features consist primarily of pruritis and jaundice. Serum bilirubin levels are usually less than 6 mg and rarely higher than 8 mg per 100 ml. The serum alkaline phosphatase and cholesterol levels are elevated significantly, while other liver function tests are only mildly deranged. Histologically the liver shows varying degrees of cholestasis but only a few parenchymal cell changes. The clinical and laboratory abnormalities subside promptly after delivery and are usually completely normal within 7 to 14 days.

This condition has been seen more frequently in Scandinavia and Europe than in the United States. Since steroid hormones and specifically estrogens can induce changes in hepatic excretory function in normal individuals (see Chap. 323), these patients probably have an increased susceptibility or sensitivity to the hepatic effects of estrogenic and progestational hormones. The intrahepatic cholestasis is usually termed *recurrent*, since the syndrome often (but not always) reappears in subsequent pregnancies. The process is benign and self-limited, and treatment is usually not needed, but cholestyramine administration will diminish the pruritis. This disorder must be distinguished from the many other causes of jaundice not unique to pregancy such as viral hepatitis. It must also be distinguished from the idiopathic *acute fatty liver of pregnancy* and the *tetracycline-induced* fatty liver. The latter two conditions are rare, occur in the last trimester, and have a high fatality rate; however, in these disorders there is evidence of diffuse parenchymal damage and not just cholestasis.

Acquired Defects of Hepatic Excretory Function

DRUG-INDUCED CHOLESTASIS. A condition entirely analogous to the intrahepatic cholestasis of pregnancy may occur in some women following the use of oral contraceptive agents. A significant number of individuals using these drugs show mild increases in BSP retention, and even more have decreased BSP excretory capacity as measured by infusion tests. In some mild cholestatic jaundice may occur, liver function returns to normal when the drugs are withdrawn, and chronic liver disease does not appear to result. It is relevant that one-third of the reported patients with jaundice due to oral contraceptives also have a history of recurrent intrahepatic cholestasis of pregnancy.

The nature of these changes produced by the natural and synthetic female sex hormones is very similar to those resulting from the administration of certain testosterone analogues, especially those with α-substitutions at the 17 position of the steroid nucleus. These agents (such as methyltestosterone and norethandrolone) commonly cause BSP retention and less commonly cause jaundice or significant changes in other liver functions. However, unlike the female hormones, these agents have been implicated as a cause of chronic liver disease, especially biliary cirrhosis.

Because of these phenomena, synthetic steroid sex hormones should not be used in patients with liver disease. Conversely, in individuals using these agents the appearance of jaundice or abnormalities in transaminase or alkaline phosphatase contraindicates their further use. However, mild to moderate increases in BSP retention alone are probably not of clinical significance, although liver function tests should be carried out periodically.

As is discussed in detail in Chap. 326, there are many drugs which may produce not simply cholestasis but liver injury resembling acute hepatitis or cholestatic hepatitis. In contrast to the jaundice produced by the steroid hormones the clinical features are those of fever, rash, arthralgia, and eosinophilia with the liver showing a pronounced inflammatory reaction. These features suggest that such reactions are *allergic* or *toxic* in nature and therefore differ from the effects caused by the steroid hormones, which probably represent an exaggerated response by the liver to the normal action of these hormones.

POSTOPERATIVE INTRAHEPATIC CHOLESTASIS. Mild or transient jaundice may be observed on occasion following a variety of surgical procedures. Usually the jaundice is mild and persists for only a few days; often it can be ascribed to hemolysis or decreased liver function as a result of the stress of surgical therapy. However, on occasion one may see a pattern resembling obstructive jaundice, with total serum bilirubin levels ranging from 10 to 40 mg per 100 ml and alkaline phosphatase levels from 15 to 40 Bodansky units. This picture may be seen when there has been (1) massive loss of blood into tissues together with (2) hypotension or shock. In such patients blood loss has been followed by massive blood replacement, with often 20 to 40 units of blood being administered. While the clinical picture of cholestatic jaundice may suggest extrahepatic obstruction, the biliary tree can be shown to be patent, and histologic examination of the liver usually shows only mild cholestasis.

The cause of this type of postoperative cholestatic jaundice is uncertain. However, in all likelihood it reflects (1) increased pigment load due to (a) resorption and destruction of blood in tissues and (b) shortened survival of transfused red cells, (2) decreased liver function due to hypoxemia resulting from hypotension, and (3) decreased renal bilirubin excretion due to varying degrees of tubular necrosis as result of shock. This diagnostic possibility must be considered in the postoperative patient with marked cholestatic jaundice. The course of the jaundice is self-limited and will subside if the other systemic complications do not predominate and lead to death.

HEPATITIS AND CIRRHOSIS. These disorders, which are discussed in detail in Chaps. 326 to 328, constitute the most common disorders associated with jaundice. As has been stated previously, when the liver cell is damaged, as in viral hepatitis, there is often impairment in all three major hepatic phases of bilirubin metabolism, namely,

Table 325-1. LABORATORY FEATURES IN ICTERIC STATES

Bilirubin disorder	Bilirubin			Urobilinogen		Comments
	Serum		Urine	Urine	Stool	
	Unconjugated	Conjugated				
Overproduction: Hemolysis (intra- and extravascular)	↑	N	0	↑	↑↑	Splenomegaly; normal RBC survival; normoblasts in marrow.
Ineffective erythropoiesis	↑	N	0	↑	↑↑	
Defective uptake Gilbert's Posthepatitic hyperbilirubinemia Some drugs	↑	N	0	N-↓	N-↓	Normal liver biopsy; normal RBC survival; direct/total bilirubin < 20%.
Defective conjugation Congenital nonhemolytic Neonatal jaundice Drug inhibition (pregnanediol, chloramphenicol, vitamin K)	↑	Low	0	↓	↓	Genetic deficiency or absence of glucuronyl transferase. Delay in enzyme development. Of importance in neonatal period.
Defective excretion: Intrahepatic obstruction: Familial syndrome Dubin-Johnson	↑	↑↑	+	Variable	↓	Abnormal BSP curve, hepatic lipochrome pigment (melanin).
Rotor syndrome						Same, but no liver pigment.
Drugs (e.g., chlorpromazine, methyltestosterone)	↑	↑↑	+	↓	↓	↑ Alkaline phosphatase but other usually normal.
Benign recurrent cholestasis	↑	↑↑	+	↓	↓	↑ Alkaline phosphatase.
Idiopathic jaundice of pregnancy (3d trimester)	↑	↑↑	+	↓	↓	↑ Alkaline phosphatase in afflicted subjects may be reproduced or exacerbated by estrogens or progesterone.
Hepatitis (see below) Extrahepatic obstruction (tumors, stone, stricture of bile duct):						↑↑ Alkaline phosphatase (often > 15 Bodansky units).
Partial	↑	↑↑	+	N-↓	↓	
Complete	↑	↑↑	+	0	0	
Hepato cellular disease:* Hepatitis	↑	↑↑	+	↑	↓	Direct/total bilirubin > 20%; liver biopsy important for diagnosis.
During obstructive phase	↑	↑↑	+	↓-0	↓	
Cirrhosis: same as hepatitis						

* Note that in hepatic cellular disease there is generally an interference in all pathways of bilirubin metabolism (i.e., impaired uptake, conjugation, and excretion).

uptake, conjugation, and excretion. Since the excretory step is one which is rate-limiting and most readily affected by injury, significant amounts of conjugated bilirubin reenter the systemic circulation. There are also usually lesser increases in the serum unconjugated bilirubin. The latter is probably a reflection of the impaired uptake and conjugation and in part due to the shortened red cell life span often found in liver disease. In most patients with hepatitis and cirrhosis, the total serum bilirubin levels tend not to exceed 50 mg per 100 ml, but on rare occasions levels of up to 90 or 95 mg per 100 ml have been described.

Extrahepatic Biliary Obstruction

Anatomic or mechanical obstruction of the bile ducts is most commonly due to stones, tumors, or strictures. The clinical picture is quite similar to that of intrahepatic cholestasis with pronounced elevation of the alkaline phosphatase level. Usually, but not always, fever, pain and chills may be present. While the amount of direct-reacting (conjugated) bilirubin predominates in the serum, the amount of the total serum bilirubin which is direct-reacting is variable (60 to 80 percent) and of no real diagnostic or prognostic significance. In contrast to hepatitis and cirrhosis the serum bilirubin level often tends to plateau and rarely exceeds levels of 35 mg per 100 ml. The reason for this plateau is not clear but may be related to renal excretion of conjugated bilirubin or alternative pathways of bilirubin catabolism in obstructive jaundice.

REFERENCES

Benign Familial Recurrent Cholestasis

Schapiro, R. H., and K. J. Isselbacher: Benign Recurrent Intrahepatic Cholestasis, New Engl. J. Med., 268:708, 1963.

Summerskill, W. H. J., and J. M. Walshe: Benign Recurrent Intrahepatic Obstructive Jaundice, Lancet, 2:686, 1959.

Dubin-Johnson and Rotor Syndromes

Arias, I. M.: Studies of Chronic Familial Non-hemolytic Jaundice with Conjugated Bilirubin in the Serum, with and without an Unidentified Pigment in Liver Cells, Am. J. Med., 31:510, 1961.

Dubin, I. N.: Chronic Idiopathic Jaundice: A Review of Fifty Cases, Am. J. Med., 24:268, 1958.

Schiff, L., B. H. Billing, and Y. Oikawa: Familial Nonhemolytic Jaundice with Conjugated Bilirubin in the Serum, New Engl. J. Med., 260:1315, 1959.

Gilbert's Disease

Arias, I. M.: Chronic Unconjugated Hyperbilirubinemia without Overt Signs of Hemolysis in Adolescents and Adults, J. Clin. Invest., 41:2233, 1962.

Foulk, W. T., H. R. Butt, C. A. Own, F. F. Whitcomb, and H. L. Mason: Constitutional Hepatic Dysfunction (Gilbert's Disease): Its Natural History and Related Syndromes, Medicine, 38:25, 1959.

Powell, L. W., E. Hemingway, B. H. Billing, and S. Sherlock: Idiopathic Unconjugated Hyperbilirubinemia (Gilbert's Syndrome), New Engl. J. Med., 277:1108, 1967.

Neonatal Jaundice

Arias, I. M., L. Gartner, S. Seifter, and M. Furman: Prolonged Neonatal Unconjugated Hyperbilirubinemia with Breast Feeding and a Steroid Pregnane-3 (Alpha), 20 (Beta) Diol, in Maternal Milk That Inhibits Glucuronide Formation in Vitro, J. Clin. Invest., 42:913, 1963.

Levi, A. J., Z. Gatmaitan, and I. M. Arias: Deficiency of Hepatic Organic Anion-binding Protein as a Possible Cause of Non-haemolytic Unconjugated Hyperbilirubinaemia in the Newborn, Lancet, 2:139, 1969.

Childs, B., and V. A. Najjar: Familial Nonhemolytic Jaundice with Kernicterus: Report of Two Cases without Neurologic Damage, Pediatrics, 18:369, 1956.

Postoperative Cholestasis

Kantrowitz, P. A., W. A. Jones, N. J. Greenberger, and K. J. Isselbacher: Severe Postoperative Hyperbilirubinemia Simulating Obstructive Jaundice, New Engl. J. Med., 276:591, 1967.

Schmid, M., M. L. Hefti, R. Gattiker, H. J. Kistler, and A. Senning: Benign Postoperative Intrahepatic Cholestasis, New Engl. J. Med., 272:545, 1965.

Recurrent Jaundice of Pregnancy

Boake, W. C., S. G. Schade, J. F. Morrissey, and F. Schaffner: Intrahepatic Cholestatic Jaundice of Pregnancy Followed by Enovid-induced Cholestatic Jaundice, Ann. Intern. Med., 63:302, 1965.

Haemmerli, U. P.: Jaundice during Pregnancy, with Special Emphasis on Recurrent Jaundice during Pregnancy and Its Differential Diagnosis, Acta Med. Scand. Suppl. 444, 1966.

326 ACUTE HEPATITIS
Raymond S. Koff and Kurt J. Isselbacher

ACUTE VIRAL HEPATITIS

Acute viral hepatitis is a systemic infectious disease affecting predominantly the liver. It occurs in two epidemiologically distinct but clinically similar forms—infectious hepatitis (IH) and serum hepatitis (SH). Both forms are characterized pathologically by hepatic cell necrosis and clinically by a sequence of a grippe like prodrome, jaundice, and subsequent recovery. It is clear that many cases are mild with no overt clinical symptoms and are recognized or suspected only by the presence of abnormal liver function tests.

PROPERTIES AND ETIOLOGY OF THE HEPATITIS VIRUSES

Transmission studies in human volunteers have indicated that the infectious agents of IH and SH are viruses, and although the precise size of the IH virus is unknown, the SH virus has been postulated, on the basis of filtration studies, to be less than 26 mμ in diameter. Both agents resist freezing for months and are not destroyed by heating at 56°C for ½ hr. The SH virus is inactivated by heating at 60°C for 10 hr, and the IH virus is probably also susceptible to such treatment. Both viruses are resistant to ether. The IH virus remains infective after exposure to chlorine (1 part per million).

A number of "candidate" viruses have been isolated and propagated in tissue culture, but none has yet been confirmed as "the" hepatitis virus. Multiple serologic studies have revealed the presence of circulating antigens (hepatitis associated antigens) in patients with acute viral hepatitis transiently during the incubation period or early acute phase. One antigen, referred to as Australia antigen, has been demonstrated, by immunodiffusion and complement fixation techniques in the sera of approximately 25 to 65 percent of patients with suspected IH and 50 to 98 percent of patients with probable SH. This antigen is infrequent (0.1 to 7 percent) in normal populations in the U.S. and Europe, but it has been found to have a prevalence of 3 to 25 percent in some tropical countries and in patients with Down's syndrome and lepromatous leprosy. It is not clear whether such persons with persistent circulating antigen are carriers or have chronic anicteric hepatitis. The antigen has been localized to nuclei of hepatic cells by direct immunofluorescence, and electron microscopic examination of preparations of antigen have shown viruslike particles about 22 mμ in diameter. It has been suggested, *but not proven*, that Australia antigen may be serum hepatitis virus or one of its antigenic subunits, perhaps sharing an antigen with IH virus.

EPIDEMIOLOGY

The incubation period of IH varies between 15 to 60 days, irrespective of route of inoculation, and in most epidemics averages about 30 days. The incubation period of SH is longer, with a range of 60 to 180 days. As shown in Table 326-1, viremia occurs during the incubation

Table 326-1. COMPARISON OF EPIDEMIOLOGIC FEATURES OF INFECTIOUS HEPATITIS (IH) AND SERUM HEPATITIS (SH)

Feature	IH	SH
Incubation period	15–60 days	60–180 days
Route of infection:		
Oral	+	rare*
Parenteral	+	+
Presence of viremia during:		
Incubation period	+	+
Acute phase	+	+
Convalescence	rare	rare†
Presence of virus in feces during:		
Incubation period	+	rare†
Acute phase	+	rare†
Convalescence	rare	?

* Moderately contagious in one experimental study
† Probably rare; only limited data available

period and the early phase of the illness of both IH and SH; namely, 2 to 3 weeks before the onset of jaundice in IH and as early as 3 months before jaundice in SH. The duration of viremia is less clear. Viremia was not demonstrated 1 month after the onset of IH or during con-

valescence from SH in volunteer studies. In one recent study approximately 50 percent of mentally retarded children infected with SH virus had persistent circulating hepatitis associated antigen for as long as 3 years. Persistent viremia in previously healthy adults, however, is probably rare with either infection. Excretion of virus into the urine or nasopharyngeal secretions has not been conclusively demonstrated in IH or SH. Fecal excretion of virus in IH has been shown during the last 2 weeks of the incubation period and during the first few days of the acute phase of illness, regardless of the route of inoculation. Fecal shedding of virus after the disappearance of jaundice is extremely rare.

In contrast to IH virus, the early volunteer studies did not reveal fecal excretion of SH virus after parenteral transmission of SH; similarly, SH could not be transmitted by oral administration of serum or blood from patients with the acute disease. Subsequent observations, however, have suggested that fecal excretion of SH virus and transmission of SH by the fecal-oral route may occur. The frequency of such transmission is not known, although it is probably rare except in unusual circumstances (e.g., closed institutions with extremely poor sanitary standards).

Homologous immunity has been shown for both IH and SH under experimental conditions, more convincingly for IH than SH. It is not clear whether immunity is complete or lifelong, since reinfections have been well documented. However, second attacks may be due to different antigenic strains of virus. Heterologous immunity has not been demonstrated.

IH is a disease primarily of children and young adults; SH has no specific age preponderance. While no seasonal variation in the incidence of SH has been noted, in temperate climates the incidence of IH rises in late autumn, peaks in the winter, and drops in late spring and through the summer. Both IH and SH are worldwide in distribution. Cycles of 5 to 10 years between peak hepatitis epidemic years have been observed in North America and Europe and apparently reflect variations in the incidence of IH rather than SH.

Fecal-oral transmission, primarily by person-to-person contact, is the most common mode of spread of IH. A gradual build-up of cases, peak distribution in young children, familial aggregations, and geographic proximity of cases are typical of person-to-person transmission. History of recent contact with jaundiced persons or known hepatitis cases is found in at least 20 to 30 percent of patients in whom person-to-person transmission occurs. In addition, exposure to children and adults with anicteric infections or to asymptomatic carriers probably represents a significant source of infection. Estimates of the ratio of icteric to anicteric cases of IH have ranged from 1:1 for adults to 1:10 in children.

No convincing evidence of a respiratory route of infection or a role for arthropods as mechanical vectors of hepatitis is available. Careful epidemiologic studies have shown that a significant risk of hepatitis exists for animal handlers in contact with newly imported nonhuman primates and have suggested that these species may act occasionally as carriers of IH virus and may, in fact, be susceptible to human hepatitis virus infection.

Extensive outbreaks of IH have been traced to contaminated water, milk, and to the ingestion of other foods, including uncooked clams and oysters. Such common-source epidemics of IH more frequently affect adults than children, and the occurrence of a large number of cases in adults during an epidemic (especially in the summer) is suggestive of common-source rather than person-to-person spread.

Parenteral transmission is the predominant mode of spread of SH and an important source of IH. Virus has been transmitted in as little as 0.00004 ml of blood. Contamination of needles, syringes, lancets, and tattooing instruments has been associated with outbreaks of SH. Epidemics of either IH and SH have been associated with multidose syringe practices and traced to the use of contaminated hypodermic or infusion equipment. The sharing of needles among drug addicts has been responsible for sporadic cases as well as epidemics of hepatitis.

Transfusion-associated hepatitis may be either IH or SH, and the two are differentiated at present only by length of the incubation period. IH is probably as frequent a complication of transfusion as SH. The risk of posttransfusion hepatitis increases almost linearly with the number of units of blood transfused and is closely related to standards of donor selection. The incidence of clinically apparent hepatitis following transfusion has been variably reported between 0.3 to 9 cases per 1,000 units transfused, or 0.5 to 13 cases per 100 patients transfused. The risk of *anicteric hepatitis* following transfusion may be 3 to 10 times greater than that of *clinical hepatitis* with jaundice. The risk of viral hepatitis after transfusion of blood derivatives is dependent upon the methods by which these products are processed (Table

Table 326-2. HAZARD OF HEPATITIS FROM BLOOD PRODUCTS

Average risk—single donor products
  Whole blood
  Packed red cells
  Single donor plasma, fresh-frozen or aged
  Single donor platelet or antihemophilic factor concentrates
High risk—multiple donor products
  Pooled plasma, ultraviolet-irradiated or stored at 31.6°C or
    room temperature for 6 months
  Fibrinogen
  Antihemophilic factor concentrates
*No risk—multiple donor products, adequately treated**
  Human albumin
  Plasma protein fraction
  Gamma globulin
  Hyperimmune gamma globulin

  * Treatment refers to heating at 60°C for 10 hr or cold ethanol fractionation (method of Cohn).

326-2). Unfortunately no effective method has been found for the inactivation of the virus in whole blood.

PATHOLOGY

The characteristic morphologic lesions of IH and SH are identical and consist of a combination of hepatic cell necrosis and regenerative activity, a diffuse mononuclear inflammatory reaction, hyperplasia of Kupffer cells, and variable bile stasis. During the late incubation and acute prodromal phase of the disease, liver cell plates are disrupted, although the reticulin framework of the hepatic lobule is preserved. Liver cell damage is evident in the form of diffuse areas of hepatic cell degeneration and necrosis, with hepatic cell dropout, ballooning of cells, and acidophilic (Councilman-like) bodies. Nuclear size and staining is variable, and inclusion bodies are not seen. Liver cell regeneration is suggested by numerous mitotic figures, multinucleated cells, thick parenchymal plates, and cytoplasmic basophilia. So-called "rosette" or "pseudoglandular" hepatic cell formation may be seen occasionally. Mononuclear cell infiltrates are present in the portal zones and in areas of lobular necrosis. Polymorphonuclear cells and eosinophils comprise only a minor fraction of the inflammatory reaction. Kupffer cells appear prominent and often contain abundant yellow-brown (lipofuscin) pigment. Ductular proliferation is common. Bile stasis, in the form of bile plugs or thrombi in dilated bile canaliculi and bile droplets within parenchymal and Kupffer cells, is variable in extent, occasionally resembling that produced by mechanical bile-duct obstruction. Fatty infiltration is not a feature of viral hepatitis but rarely may be present during the late convalescent phase in mild form. The morphologic lesions of anicteric viral hepatitis are qualitatively identical to those described above, but quantitatively are usually more subtle. Limited electron microscopic studies of biopsy material from patients with acute viral hepatitis have shown disruption and dilation of the endoplasmic reticulum, enlarged mitochrondria, and prominent, vacuolated lysosomes. Focal dilatation of the bile canaliculi may be seen with loss of microvillous configuration. No characteristic viral inclusions or particles have been identified unequivocally.

CLINICAL FEATURES OF TYPICAL ACUTE VIRAL HEPATITIS

PRODROMAL PHASE. In most patients with acute viral hepatitis, the onset of jaundice is preceded by nonspecific constitutional and gastrointestinal symptoms. From 2 to 14 days before the appearance of jaundice, the patient abruptly develops anorexia, fatigue, malaise, and lassitude. This may be followed or accompanied by nausea, vomiting, diarrhea, and occasionally arthralgia. Loss of appetite may be striking and often includes a positive aversion for food. Distaste for cigarettes is another common and curious symptom. Right upper quadrant or epigastric discomfort, described as either a sense of fullness or pain, is common. Fever between 100 to 104°F and symptoms of a "flulike" illness, with cough, coryza, pharyngitis, myalgias, and photophobia are frequent with IH and less common with SH, which usually begins insidiously. However, when parenterally transmitted, IH may begin insidiously and usually without fever. Occasionally urticaria, skin rashes, angioneurotic edema, and rarely, polyarthritis may be noted during the prodromal phase.

In 1 to 4 days before the onset of jaundice, the urine darkens because of bilirubinuria, and often the stool color lightens. Pruritus may be a prominent symptom at this stage, but is usually transient. The clinical disease may be very mild in some patients, and overt jaundice may not be present at any time (anicteric cases). Physical findings may be minimal in the early prodromal phase, but hepatic enlargement and tenderness are present in most patients.

ICTERIC PHASE. Once jaundice appears, the clinical features of IH and SH are identical. The prodromal gastrointestinal symptoms usually decrease in severity within a few days, and fever subsides promptly. The jaundice usually reaches a maximum between the first and second week and decreases steadily thereafter. The duration of jaundice is variable but lasts less than 6 to 8 weeks in typical cases. Weight loss of 5 to 10 lb during the late prodromal and early icteric phase is common. The stools, which may have been clay-colored with the development of icterus, become darker again as the jaundice subsides.

Physical findings in the icteric phase include hepatic enlargement and tenderness. The liver begins to decrease in size and tenderness 1 to 2 weeks after the onset of jaundice and returns to normal size over a number of weeks. Posterior cervical lymphadenopathy and splenomegaly are present in about 20 percent of cases. Rarely, a few spider angiomas appear during the icteric phase and then disappear during convalescence.

RECOVERY PHASE. Immediately following the subsidence of jaundice, the patient usually feels well, but recovery is seldom complete at this stage. The liver may still be enlarged and mildly tender, and abnormalities of hepatic function are still evident. Fatigue is often a prominent symptom. The duration of this posticteric phase varies from 2 to 6 weeks but may be longer in some instances. Full clinical and biochemical recovery is to be expected within 3 to 4 months in most cases. Rarely the disease may run a mild but prolonged course, with hepatomegaly and intermittently abnormal liver function studies persisting for 1 to 2 years. In some patients circulating hepatitis associated antigen has been demonstrated during periods of hepatic dysfunction. Liver biopsy in these cases of "delayed convalescence" or "persistent hepatitis" discloses portal mononuclear infiltration and minimal hepatic cell necrosis without evidence of cirrhosis. Despite the delayed convalescence of these patients, full recovery usually occurs.

The *mortality of acute viral hepatitis* appears to depend in part on the mode of transmission. Patients with IH contracted via the fecal-oral route have a *case fatality rate of 0.1 to 0.4* percent. In contrast, parenterally transmitted IH (e.g., posttransfusion hepatitis with icterus) and SH have a *case fatality rate of 10 to 12 percent.* Increasing age, debility, the presence of malignancy, and possibly pregnancy have adverse effects on survival. Anicteric disease is rarely fatal.

LABORATORY FEATURES

No distinction can be made between IH and SH by laboratory tests. During the preicteric phase, the leukocyte count is usually within the normal range, but mild leukopenia may be seen. Neutropenia and lymphopenia are transient, followed by a relative lymphocytosis. Atypical lymphocytosis varying between 2 to 20 percent is common during the acute phase; these so-called "virocytes" are indistinguishable from the atypical lymphocytes of infectious mononucleosis. The heterophile agglutination test may be positive, but guinea pig kidney cell adsorption removes the antibody from hepatitis sera. Although unusual, mild reticulocytosis and slight hemolysis have been reported. As a rule, anemia is not a feature of viral hepatitis.

During the initial prodromal phase of illness the first detectable abnormality is a *progressive elevation of the serum transaminase* levels. Both serum glutamic oxaloacetic transaminase (SGOT) and serum glutamic pyruvic transaminase (SGPT) may be elevated 7 to 14 days prior to the onset of jaundice, reflecting hepatic cell necrosis and altered cell permeability with enzyme leakage into the blood. In general, the SGPT levels are higher than SGOT values at all stages of the disease. The actual serum transaminase levels are variable, but peak SPGT values between 400 and 3,000 units are typical of acute viral hepatitis. The laboratory diagnosis of anicteric hepatitis is often based solely on transaminase elevations, although the serum conjugated bilirubin may be mildly elevated despite the absence of clinical jaundice. Bromsulphalein (BSP) retention can be observed commonly before the onset of scleral icterus and in anicteric cases. When jaundice appears, the serum bilirubin is usually above 3 mg per 100 ml and typically reaches 5 to 20 mg per 100 ml. Higher levels or a progressive, erratic rise later in the course may indicate more severe disease. Serum alkaline phosphatase may be normal or only mildly elevated to levels of 5 to 15 Bodansky units. The cephalin-cholesterol flocculation test may become positive in the preicteric phase, followed by a positive thymol turbidity test. By the time scleral icterus appears, the majority of patients have positive flocculation tests. Urine urobilinogen may increase in the preicteric phase and then decline with the appearance of acholic stools, with a secondary rise when normal stool color returns later in the course of the illness. The total serum protein levels may remain near normal, but in some patients a slight decrease in the serum albumin occurs. Serum globulin levels may be mildly elevated due to an increase in the gamma-globulin fraction. Protein immunoelectrophoresis reveals that IgG and IgM levels are elevated, while IgA is slightly increased or normal.

During the icteric phase serum cholesterol may be normal or slightly low, with a decrease in the cholesterol ester fraction. The prothrombin activity may be moderately decreased during the period of jaundice but rarely produces clinical bleeding problems.

In a few patients mild and transient steatorrhea has been noted as well as slight microscopic hematuria and minimal proteinuria.

VARIANTS AND OTHER CLINICAL FORMS OF ACUTE VIRAL HEPATITIS (FIG. 326-1)

ANICTERIC HEPATITIS. Although the above description of acute viral hepatitis with jaundice serves as a prototype of the clinical expression of hepatitis virus infection, *many patients with acute viral hepatitis do not show clinical jaundice* (i.e., they have anicteric hepatitis). In children anicteric infection is the rule rather than the exception, and unexplained fever and symptoms of an upper respiratory infection or gastroenteritis may be the initial or only feature of viral hepatitis. In adults with anicteric acute viral hepatitis a prodrome may or may not be present, but it is usually less prominent than in hepatitis with jaundice. Fever, gastrointestinal symptoms, and anorexia and malaise, if present, are usually quite mild and short-lived. Hepatomegaly and mild hepatic tenderness are the only signs of liver disease in these patients, but may be absent in some cases. Helpful laboratory studies include the presence of elevated serum transaminase levels, BSP retention, and minimal conjugated hyperbilirubinemia. The course of the disease is frequently short, and rapid subsidence of symptoms with early improvement of liver function abnormalities is common. In the absence of a local epidemic, *the diagnosis of anicteric viral hepatitis may be very difficult* unless there is a high index of suspicion.

CHOLESTATIC HEPATITIS. Less than 5 percent of patients with either IH or SH may have a clinical course resembling that of bile duct obstruction, with severe pruritus and prolonged jaundice with acholic stools. Despite the pruritus and deep jaundice, these patients generally feel well and improve in time, although a number of weeks may be necessary for the jaundice to clear. Liver function studies, in these instances, reveal hyperbilirubinemia in the range of 20 to 30 mg per 100 ml, and the alkaline phosphatase may be 10 to 30 Bodansky units. Serum transaminase values are elevated, often exceeding 300 units. Liver biopsy reveals a striking degree of bile stasis, hepatic cell necrosis of variable severity, and an unusual number of polymorphonuclear leukocytes in the portal zone infiltrates.

SUBMASSIVE HEPATIC NECROSIS. This appears to be an extremely uncommon variant of acute viral hepatitis, although the evidence linking submassive hepatic necrosis to acute viral hepatitis is chiefly circumstantial. The prodromal and early acute phase may be quite similar to that of typical acute viral hepatitis, but the preicteric phase is usually longer than two weeks. Once jaundice is present, *the course of the illness is clearly different from that of typical acute viral hepatitis.* The patient continues to feel ill, and weakness and vomiting may persist. The serum bilirubin level may still be increasing after 2 weeks, and although it may fluctuate, the bilirubin tends

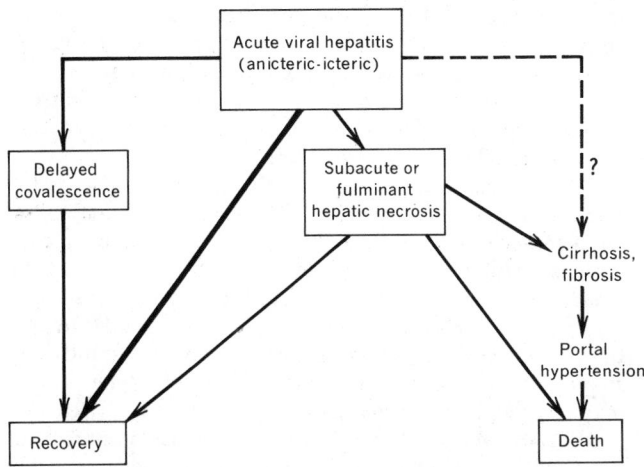

Fig. 326-1. Scheme showing possible sequelae of acute viral hepatitis.

gradually to plateau at levels greater than 20 mg per 100 ml. In contrast to typical viral hepatitis, transaminase levels remain elevated for many weeks. Hepatosplenomegaly persists, and spider angiomas and palmar erythema may be prominent. Hypoalbuminemia, hyperglobulinemia, and hypoprothrombinemia are often striking, and signs of fluid retention, portal hypertension, and hepatic encephalopathy may develop.

Liver tissue from patients with submassive hepatic necrosis reveals extensive zones of confluent liver cell necrosis with an inflammatory infiltrate of variable extent. The distinguishing morphologic feature is the presence of bands of cell dropout with reticulin collapse bridging adjacent portal triads and central veins. After many weeks or months of illness, some patients experience complete clinical recovery with either minimal fibrosis or no residual abnormality on liver biopsy. Another and possibly larger group of patients with submassive necrosis may progress to chronic liver disease (i.e., cirrhosis); in some patients, after months or years of illness, death may result from liver failure, variceal hemorrhage, or intercurrent sepsis.

It must be emphasized that submassive hepatic necrosis following hepatitis virus infection appears to be distinct from chronic active hepatitis with postnecrotic cirrhosis, a disease or diseases of unknown etiology. However, the presence of circulating hepatitis associated antigen in some patients during active phases of submassive hepatic necrosis and chronic active hepatitis suggests that hepatitis virus may be etiologically implicated in both diseases, at least in some patients (see Chap. 327).

MASSIVE HEPATIC NECROSIS (FULMINANT HEPATITIS, ACUTE YELLOW ATROPHY). Sudden shrinking of the liver, as determined by palpation and percussion, over a period of hours or days is an ominous sign of fulminant and often fatal hepatitis. The development of hepatic coma and a rapid decrease in liver size is associated with a case fatality rate of 60 to 90 percent. The interval between the onset of illness and death is usually less than

2 weeks. Profound depression of the serum prothrombin activity with overt bleeding is common prior to death. Transaminase levels, while previously high, may be only moderately elevated or near normal at the time of death. Severe hypoglycemia is an occasional feature. Hypotension and renal failure are common.

The striking feature at postmortem examination is the finding of a small, soft liver. Histologic examination reveals massive necrosis and drop out of liver cells of most lobules. The reticulin framework of the liver may be preserved, but characteristically there is collapse and condensation wherever necrosis has occurred. In patients who recover, hepatic fibrosis may be found subsequently on liver biopsy, although rarely liver biopsy may be completely normal.

EXTRAHEPATIC COMPLICATIONS. Acute pancreatitis, myocarditis, and atypical pneumonia have been reported infrequently in viral hepatitis, and the association with hepatitis may be merely fortuitous. However, viral invasion of these organs during the period of viremia is possible. Similarly, neurologic abnormalities other than hepatic encephalopathy, such as acute myelitis, aseptic meningitis, and peripheral neuritis, have been reported very rarely. In a small number of patients, pancytopenia may occur during the convalescent phase.

DIFFERENTIAL DIAGNOSIS

In the preicteric phase (or in anicteric cases) viral hepatitis may closely resemble other viral acute infectious diseases. Gastroenteritis and influenza may be considered, but hepatitis can usually be distinguished by the presence of liver enlargement and tenderness, transaminase elevations, and the subsequent course. Infectious mononucleosis with hepatitis may be clinically indistinguishable from viral hepatitis. However, large tender lymph nodes, pharyngitis, and splenomegaly are much more common in infectious mononucleosis. Eventually the differential heterophile agglutination or EB virus antibody test will provide the answer.

During the icteric phase, other infectious diseases to be considered include dengue fever, Q fever, and yellow fever, and these may be excluded by geographic and epidemiologic considerations. Leptospiral liver involvement is usually accompanied by severe myalgia, conjunctivitis, evidence of renal damage, and often, leukocytosis. Drug and toxic injury may result in jaundice, and abnormalities of liver function and histology in drug-induced hepatitis may closely resemble those of viral hepatitis. The presence of fatty change and zonal necrosis on liver biopsy suggests toxic injury, and a careful documentation of all exogenous drugs and occupational toxin exposures is necessary. Similarly "alcoholic hepatitis" must be considered, but usually the serum transaminases are not as markedly elevated, other stigmata of alcoholism may be present, and the finding of fatty infiltration, a neutrophilic inflammatory reaction and alcoholic hyaline on liver biopsy would be consistent with alcohol-induced disease rather than viral injury. Chronic liver disease may present with jaundice; however, the physical findings of cirrhosis may be present and helpful in excluding viral

hepatitis. The absence of recurrent fever, chills, and right upper quadrant pain is helpful in excluding acute cholangitis or cholecystitis. Extrahepatic bile duct obstruction due to choledocholithiasis or pancreatic carcinoma may resemble cholestatic hepatitis. Radiologic studies including duodenograms and intravenous cholangiography and percutaneous cholangiography will aid in diagnosis.

The patient with viral hepatitis does not tolerate major surgery well during the acute phase. Therefore, a number of procedures, including percutaneous liver biopsy, may be necessary to exclude the possibility of viral hepatitis prior to exploratory laparotomy in the diagnosis of surgical jaundice.

MANAGEMENT

TYPICAL ACUTE VIRAL HEPATITIS. There is no specific treatment. Hospitalization may be required for diagnosis, for clinically severe illness, atypical variants, and for those with posttransfusion hepatitis because of the high mortality. Although acute viral hepatitis tends to be self-limited, the extreme variability in the severity and course of viral hepatitis has resulted in a clinical impression that enforced and prolonged bed rest is essential to rapid recovery without residual chronic hepatic disease. It has been clearly shown, however, in young, previously healthy men, that strict bed rest has no advantage over a program with 1 hr of absolute rest after each meal. Furthermore, the incidence of cirrhosis was not increased 10 years later in patients treated with this rest program. However, regardless of age, most patients with severe symptoms will feel better with restricted physical activity and will desire bed or chair rest. A high-caloric balanced diet should be encouraged.

Intravenous feeding is necessary in the acute stage if the patient has persistent vomiting and cannot maintain oral intake. In previously well-nourished patients there is no evidence that dietary supplements are needed. If hepatic precoma develops, protein intake should be reduced and an oral, nonabsorbable antibiotic, such as neomycin, should be prescribed.

Drugs capable of producing adverse hepatic reactions or those metabolized primarily by the liver should be used with caution. There is no indication for systemic antibiotics. In an occasional patient pruritus may be severe, and the use of the bile-salt-sequestering resin, cholestyramine, will usually alleviate this symptom. Although administration of prednisone or other corticosteroids undoubtedly increases the appetite and sense of well-being in some patients with viral hepatitis and may also lower serum bilirubin levels, there is no evidence that these agents shorten significantly the convalescent phase or alter significantly the morphologic features of hepatitis. These drugs are usually reserved for patients with submassive hepatic necrosis or fulminant hepatitis.

Rigid isolation of the patient with hepatitis is not warranted. However, both patient and hospital staff must be reminded of proper hygienic practices, including careful washing of one's hands after examining the patient. A private room and bathroom to minimize inadvertent fecal spread is desirable.

Patients may be discharged from the hospital after the serum bilirubin has fallen below 2.0 mg per 100 ml and when other signs or symptoms indicate that the illness is waning. Abnormality of flocculation tests or mild elevation of SGOT or SGPT should not be considered contraindications to the gradual resumption of normal activity. Mild SGPT elevation may persist for as long as 10 to 24 months in some patients and has no prognostic significance.

SUBACUTE AND MASSIVE HEPATIC NECROSIS. While corticosteroids are not indicated in the treatment of typical viral hepatitis, they are occasionally prescribed in patients with submassive hepatic necrosis and fulminant hepatitis. Massive doses of corticosteroids often are given when liver function deteriorates progressively, when the course is prolonged with deepening jaundice, or when hepatic encephalopathy develops during the course of illness. The effectiveness of steroids in reversing serious hepatitis has not yet been established. Similarly the role of immunosuppressive agents in the treatment of these diseases is not clear. The goal of treatment of fulminant hepatitis is to support the patient by maintenance of fluid balance, support of the circulation, control of bleeding, and correction of hypoglycemia until liver cell regeneration and repair occurs. Protein intake is usually restricted, and oral neomycin is administered. In some cases exchange transfusion of whole blood, human cross-circulation, and porcine liver cross-perfusion have resulted in lightening of hepatic coma, but only rarely in survival. Human liver transplantation has been suggested, but technical difficulties have precluded its widespread use.

PREVENTION

INFECTIOUS HEPATITIS. Because virus is excreted for as long as 2 weeks before the onset of jaundice and usually before the diagnosis of hepatitis is suspected, the benefit of isolation or quarantine measures is limited. Spread of disease by the anicteric or subclinical case further compounds this difficulty.

It is generally agreed that 0.01 ml of gamma-globulin per pound body weight given intramuscularly early in the incubation period will prevent symptoms and jaundice in exposed contacts. Instead, these individuals probably develop subclinical infection with serum transaminase elevations, followed by immunity. Gamma-globulin administration is indicated for intimate contacts (adults and children who are household members). Pregnant women and elderly or debilitated patients, in whom the disease may be more severe, should receive gamma-globulin prophylaxis even if exposure is casual. While larger doses of gamma globulin (0.05 to 0.06 ml per lb) may provide a modifying effect for longer periods (perhaps up to 4 months), they are not more effective than the lower dosage in acute epidemic situations. The larger dose is recommended for individuals who are traveling in areas in which hepatitis is endemic and who require protection for more than 2 to 3 months.

PARENTERALLY TRANSMITTED INFECTIOUS AND SERUM HEPATITIS. The use of disposable hypodermic equipment is desirable, and multidose syringe techniques must be avoided. Sterile blood products should be substituted for whole blood when possible, and blood transfusions should be given only when essential. The cornerstone of establishing minimal hepatitis levels rests upon careful blood procurement programs that avoid drug addicts, patients with a past history of transfusion or hepatitis, and donors of questionable reliability. The screening of donors with liver function tests has proved to be of limited value because of a high frequency of both false-positive and false-negative results. The efficacy of serologic identification of circulating hepatitis associated antigens in donor blood is currently under evaluation.

Small doses of gamma-globulin are ineffective in modifying posttransfusion hepatitis. Larger doses, in the range of 10 ml, given within a week of transfusion and 30 days later, have provided conflicting results. The definitive role of gamma-globulin prophylaxis in SH is not known.

RELAPSES OR RECURRENCES AND SEQUELAE

Approximately 5 percent of patients with viral hepatitis have an exacerbation of the disease within 6 months of the onset. This is manifested by a recurrence of the initial symptoms, elevated transaminase levels, and in some patients, jaundice. Characteristically the recurrence is clinically milder than the initial episode. No distinction, however, between relapse and recurrent infection can be made. Only in special circumstances such as the addict who is reexposed and in whom two or more recurrences may follow is there a suggestion of repeated infection. These recurrences or relapses do not alter the prognosis, and residual liver disease has not occurred. Treatment is similar to that of the original episode.

POSTHEPATITIS HYPERBILIRUBINEMIA. In a small number of patients, mild unconjugated hyperbilirubinemia may persist for weeks, months, and occasionally, years. No evidence of chronic liver disease or abnormal histology is evident on liver biopsy (See Chap. 325).

POSTHEPATITIS SYNDROME. Postviral infection asthenia, malaise, and other vague symptoms may occur for 6 to 12 months following hepatitis in some patients. These symptoms have no functional significance and require no treatment other than reassurance. Liver function tests are completely normal, and liver biopsy usually shows no evidence of active hepatic disease.

POSTNECROTIC CIRRHOSIS. There is still considerable debate as to whether typical acute viral hepatitis may lead to postnecrotic cirrhosis. Although an occasional patient with postnecrotic cirrhosis gives a history of an episode of antecedent jaundice, the identity or nature of such an episode will remain obscure until serologic tests for hepatitis viruses are available in these patients. Prospective follow-up of a large number of patients with acute viral hepatitis has not revealed an increased incidence of cirrhosis. However, as stated above, if patients with subacute or fulminant hepatic necrosis survive, a scarred and cirrhotic liver may be found.

TOXIC AND DRUG-INDUCED HEPATITIS

Liver injury may follow the inhalation, ingestion, or parenteral administration of a number of chemical agents. These include industrial toxins (e.g., carbon tetrachloride, yellow phosphorus), the toxic cyclic peptides of *Amanita phalloides* (mushroom poisoning), or more commonly, pharmacologic agents used in medical therapy. It is essential that any patient presenting with jaundice or impaired liver function be carefully questioned about exposure to chemicals used in work or at home and drugs taken by prescription or home remedies bought "over the counter." In general, two major types of chemical hepatitis have been recognized: (1) *"direct toxic"* and (2) *"hypersensitivity."*

As shown in Table 326-3, *toxic hepatitis* is one which *occurs with predictable regularity* in individuals exposed to the offending agent and is dose-dependent. The latent period between exposure and liver injury is usually short (often several hours), although clinical manifestations may be delayed for 24 to 48 hr. Agents producing toxic hepatitis are generally systemic poisons, and liver injury is only one facet of the toxicity. In certain instances, particularly when the toxin is ingested, gastrointestinal symptoms may be more prominent, and liver injury may go unrecognized until jaundice appears. The direct hepatotoxins result in morphologic abnormalities which are reasonably characteristic and reproducible for each toxin. For example, carbon tetrachloride and chloroform characteristically produce a centrilobular zonal necrosis, whereas yellow phosphorus poisoning typically results in periportal injury. *Amanita phalloides* toxin usually produces massive hepatic necrosis.

Drug *hypersensitivity* reactions lead to a morphologic pattern that is more *variable;* a single agent is often capable of inciting a variety of lesions, although certain patterns tend to predominate. In contrast to toxic hepatitis, the occurrence of hypersensitivity hepatitis in those exposed to the agent is *unpredictable*, the response is *not dose-dependent*, and *may occur at any time* during or after exposure to the drug. Immunologic evidence of classic hypersensitivity mechanisms (i.e., the demonstration of specific circulating or tissue-fixing antibodies) in drug-induced hepatoxicity is not available. However, extra-

hepatic clinical manifestations of hypersensitivity are common and include arthralgias, rashes, fever, leukocytosis, and eosinophilia. Depending on the agent involved, hypersensitivity hepatitis may result in a clinical picture indistinguishable from viral hepatitis (e.g., halothane) or may simulate extrahepatic bile duct obstruction (e.g., chlorpromazine). In some cases there may be features of both cholestasis and hepatocellular damage.

These major differences between toxic and hypersensitivity hepatitis do not permit a classification of all adverse hepatic drug reactions. For example, substituted testosterone derivatives, such as methyl testosterone, regularly result in impairment of hepatic function and occasionally in jaundice when given in large doses, but they do not produce necrosis or fatty change in lower species and differ from the agents producing hypersensitivity hepatitis because manifestations of hypersensitivity are absent.

Because viral hepatitis is necessarily a presumptive diagnosis, and many adverse drug reactions produce a clinicopathologic picture resembling it, the establishment of an etiologic relationship between the use of a drug and subsequent liver injury may be most difficult. The relation is most convincing when the frequency of hepatic impairment following administration of the specific agent is high, when the latent period between the start of therapy and impaired function is short, and when rechallenge, after an asymptomatic period, results in a recurrence of signs, symptoms, and morphologic and biochemical abnormalities. Rechallenge is often ethically unfeasible, and documentation of adverse hepatic reactions must often await the collection of other clinical cases.

Treatment of toxic and drug-induced hepatic disease is largely supportive and does not differ from that for acute viral hepatitis. Withdrawal of the suspected agent is indicated at the first sign of an adverse reaction. In the case of the direct toxins, liver involvement should not divert attention from renal or other organ involvement which may prove a greater threat to survival than the liver disease. In Table 326-4, several classes of chemical agents are listed together with examples of the pattern of liver injury produced by them.

The following are the patterns of adverse hepatic reactions for some prototypic agents:

Table 326-3. SOME FEATURES OF TOXIC AND DRUG-INDUCED HEPATIC INJURY

Features	Type of hepatic reaction			
	Direct toxic effect (e.g., carbon tetrachloride)	Hypersensitivity		Other (e.g., methyltestosterone)
		(e.g., halothane)	(e.g., chlorpromazine)	
Predictable and dose related toxicity	+	0	0	+
Latent period	Short	Variable	Variable	Variable
Arthralgia, fever, rash, eosinophilia	0	+	+	0
Liver morphology	Necrosis, fatty infiltration	Similar to viral hepatitis	Cholestasis *with* portal inflammation	Cholestasis *without* portal inflammation

Table 326-4. PRINCIPAL ALTERATIONS OF HEPATIC
MORPHOLOGY PRODUCED BY SOME COMMONLY USED
DRUGS AND CHEMICALS

Principal morphologic change	Class of agent	Example
Cholestasis	Anabolic	Methyl testosterone
	Antithyroid	Methimazole
	Chemotherapeutic	Para-amino salicylic acid*
	Oral contraceptive	Norethynodrel with mestranol (Enovid)
	Oral hypoglycemic	Chlorpropamide
	Tranquilizer	Chlorpromazine
Hepatitis	Anesthetic	Halothane
	Anticonvulsant	Diphenylhydantoin
	Chemotherapeutic	Sulfonamides†
	Diuretic	Chlorothiazide
Toxic	Hydrocarbon	Carbon tetrachloride
	Metal	Phosphorus
	Mushroom	*Amanita phalloides*

* Occasionally associated with hepatitis.
† Occasionally associated with cholestasis.

CARBON TETRACHLORIDE HEPATOTOXICITY (Direct toxin). Poisoning may result from inhalation, accidental or purposeful ingestion, or possibly by skin absorption. Initial clinical manifestations include headache, dizziness, drowsiness, nausea, vomiting, and vasomotor collapse. Liver injury may be evident 1 to 4 days following intoxication, with jaundice and hepatomegaly, and serum transaminase levels may be markedly elevated. The striking pathologic features are centrilobular hepatic necrosis and diffuse fatty infiltration. Renal injury may be evident concomitantly or shortly thereafter, with azotemia, albuminuria, and oliguria progressing to anuria. Fatalities during the first week are usually due to liver injury, while deaths later in the course are usually the result of renal damage. When recovery occurs, it is complete by 4 to 6 weeks. Residual liver or renal disease has not been clearly demonstrated following a single acute exposure.

HALOTHANE HEPATOTOXICITY (Hypersensitivity reaction). Halothane, a nonexplosive fluorinated hydrocarbon anesthetic agent, structurally similar to chloroform, has been reported to result in severe hepatic necrosis in a small number of individuals, many of whom have previously been exposed to this agent. The failure to produce similar hepatic lesions in animals, the rarity of the hepatic impairment in humans, and the delayed appearance of hepatic injury suggests that halothane is not a direct hepatotoxin, but may be a sensitizing agent. Fever, moderate leukocytosis, and eosinophilia may occur in the first week following halothane administration. Jaundice usually is noted 7 to 10 days after exposure, but occasionally may be seen as long as 30 days later. Nausea and vomiting may precede the onset of jaundice. Hepatomegaly is often mild, but liver tenderness is common. Liver function tests are consistent with parenchymal cell damage, with elevated levels of SGOT. The pathologic changes seen at autopsy have been indistinguishable from massive hepatic necrosis due to viral hepatitis. The case fatality rate of halothane hepatitis is not known but may be close to 40 percent in cases with severe liver involvement. It is strongly suggested that patients in whom unexplained spiking fever or jaundice develops after halothane anesthesia not receive this agent again. Because cross-reactions between halothane and methoxyflurane have been reported, the latter anesthetic should probably not be used after halothane reactions.

CHLORPROMAZINE HEPATOTOXICITY (Cholestatic hypersensitivity reaction. About 1 percent of patients receiving chlorpromazine develop intrahepatic cholestasis with jaundice after 1 to 4 weeks of treatment. In rare instances, jaundice has been reported after a single exposure. Anicteric reactions are probably quite frequent. The onset may be abrupt with fever, rash, arthralgias, lymphadenopathy, nausea, vomiting, and epigastric or right upper quadrant pain. Pruritus may precede the appearance of jaundice, dark urine, and light stools. Eosinophilia with or without mild leukocytosis may be present, and conjugated hyperbilirubinemia, moderately elevated serum alkaline phosphatase, and mildly elevated serum transaminase levels of 100 to 200 are noted. Liver biopsy reveals bile stasis, bile plugs in dilated bile canaliculi, and a dense portal infiltrate of polymorphonuclear, eosinophilic, and mononuclear leukocytes. Occasionally, scattered foci of hepatic parenchymal necrosis may be evident. Jaundice and pruritus usually subside within a few weeks following cessation of therapy, without sequelae, and fatalities are extremely rare. Cholestyramine may be of value in relieving severe pruritus. In a small number of patients, jaundice is prolonged for several months to years, and a picture of primary biliary cirrhosis may develop.

METHYLTESTOSTERONE HEPATOTOXICITY (Cholestatic reaction). The administration of methyl testosterone, a C-17 substituted C-19 steroid, results in significant BSP retention in a high proportion of patients. In some patients cholestatic jaundice may develop with elevation of the serum alkaline phosphatase. Extrahepatic manifestations of hypersensitivity are absent. On liver biopsy, cholestasis is present with bile plugs in dilated canaliculi, and striking bile staining of liver cells. Feathery degeneration (microvesiculation) of hepatic parenchymal cells may be present, but in contrast to chlorpromazine, portal inflammation is absent. The lesion is reversible on withdrawal of the agent, and sequelae have not been reported. Fatal cases are extremely rare.

REFERENCES

Acute Viral Hepatitis

Blumberg, B. S., A. I. Sutnick, and W. T. London: Australia Antigen and Hepatitis, J.A.M.A., 207:1895, 1969.

Chalmers, T. C., R. D. Eckhardt, W. E. Reynolds, J. G. Cigarroa, Jr., N. Deane, R. W. Reifenstein, C. W. Smith, and C. S. Davidson: The Treatment of Acute Infectious Hepatitis: Controlled Studies of the Effects of Diet, Rest and Physical Reconditioning on the Acute Course of the

Disease and on the Incidence of Relapses and Residual Abnormalities, J. Clin. Invest., 34:1163, 1955.

Giles, J. P., R. W. McCollum, L. W. Berndtson, Jr., and S. Krugman: Viral Hepatitis: Australia/SH Antigen and Willowbrook MS-2 Strain, New Engl. J. Med., 281:119, 1969.

Hirshman, R. J., N. R. Shulman, L. F. Barker, and K. O. Smith: Virus-like Particles in Hepatitis, J.A.M.A., 208: 1667, 1969.

Koff, R. S., and K. J. Isselbacher: Changing Concepts in the Epidemiology of Viral Hepatitis: New Engl. J. Med., 278:1371, 1968.

——, G. F. Grady, T. C. Chalmers, W. J. Mosley, B. L. Swartz, and the Boston Inter-hospital Liver Group: Viral Hepatitis in a Group of Boston Hospitals. III. Importance of Exposure to Shell-fish in a Non-epidemic Period, New Engl. J. Med., 276:703, 1967.

Krugman, S., J. P. Giles, and J. Hammond: Infectious Hepatitis, Evidence for Two Distinctive Clinical, Epidemiological and Immunological Types of Infection, J.A.M.A., 200:365, 1967.

Netzger, D. M., and T. C. Chalmers: The Treatment of Acute Infectious Hepatitis. Ten-year Follow-up Study of the Effects of Diet and Rest, Am. J. Med., 35:299, 1963.

Toxic and Drug-induced Liver Disease

Klatskin, G.: Toxic and Drug-induced Hepatitis, pp. 498–601 in L. Schiff, "Diseases of the Liver," 3rd ed., Philadelphia, J. B. Lippincott Company, 1969.

Summary of the National Halothane Study, Possible Association between Halothane Anesthesia and Post-operative Hepatic Necrosis, J.A.M.A., 197:775, 1966.

Zimmerman, H. J.: Clinical and Laboratory Manifestations of Hepatotoxicity, Ann. N.Y. Acad. Sci., 104:954, 1963.

——: The Spectrum of Hepatotoxicity, Perspectives Biol. Med., 12:135, 1968.

327   CHRONIC ACTIVE HEPATITIS

*William A. Tisdale and
Kurt J. Isselbacher*

DEFINITION. The generic term *chronic hepatitis* has been applied in the past to a diverse group of disorders having clinical and pathologic evidence of prolonged diffuse liver cell damage and hepatic inflammation. Precise classification of these forms of liver disease has been difficult, for the medical literature contains many confusing descriptive synonyms, and the cause of the hepatitis in most cases has not been determined. *Chronic active hepatitis* is a persistent, usually progressive, destructive, and inflammatory disease of the liver often associated with immune disorders. It may be found together with postnecrotic cirrhosis, and rather than constituting a separate disease entity, the cirrhosis in all likelihood represents an advanced stage of the chronic active hepatitis.

The syndrome of chronic active hepatitis has been described under various titles. Since the disease often occurs in young individuals, especially women, the terms *chronic liver disease in young women, chronic liver disease in young people,* or active *juvenile cirrhosis* have been used. *Lupoid hepatitis* is another designation emphasizing the frequent occurrence of positive lupus erythematosus (LE) cells in the blood. *Plasma cell hepatitis* stresses the prominence of increased plasma cells in the liver, a finding which usually correlates directly with the degree of hypergammaglobulinemia in these patients. None of these names is satisfactory, and because of the variability of sex, age, and pathologic features in this disorder the term chronic active hepatitis is perhaps the most appropriate until the exact etiology is established.

ETIOLOGY. The cause of chronic active hepatitis is unknown. Viral hepatitis, disordered immunity, and endocrine abnormalities have received most attention in the search for the cause of chronic active hepatitis. The clinical illness may occasionally begin abruptly with features resembling acute viral hepatitis, and several cases have developed following blood transfusions or intimate contact with hepatitis patients. Biopsy specimens obtained early in the course of the clinical disease may in fact show some histologic features similar to those seen in viral hepatitis. Experimental studies with the canine hepatitis virus suggest that in partially immune animals a progressive hepatitis develops, a fact that may prove to have a clinical counterpart in chronic active hepatitis.

As indicated in Chap. 326, the so-called Australia antigen appears to be closely associated or identical with the virus of serum hepatitis. Usually, in acute infectious hepatitis, the antigen is present transiently, disappearing within 2 to 3 weeks after the onset of symptoms. However, in some patients with persistence of antigen in the serum, liver biopsies have shown evidence of chronic hepatitis. In several studies of chronic active hepatitis, 10 to 25 percent of patients have had Australia antigen present in the serum. These data support the concept that at least in some cases persistent infection with hepatitis virus may be important in the pathogenesis of chronic active hepatitis.

Immunologic abnormalities are frequently present in patients with chronic active hepatitis and suggest that disorders of immune responses may also play a role in its pathogenesis. Hypergammaglobulinemia, with striking increase in the serum IgG fraction, is present in over 50 percent of cases, and infiltrates of mononuclear cells which produce immunoglobulins are abundant in liver biopsy specimens. High titers of circulating antinuclear and anti-smooth muscle antibodies have been detected in patients with chronic active hepatitis, but cytotoxic antibodies directed specifically against liver cells have not been demonstrated. The frequent occurrence of "rheumatic" clinical features, the occasional finding of allergic vasculitis in the skin, kidneys, and other extrahepatic tissues, and the presence of positive LE cell tests in some patients have suggested an etiologic relationship between chronic active hepatitis and other diseases characterized by altered immunity. The remarkable predominance of this disease in young women and the high frequency of menstrual disorders suggest that endrocrine factors play an important role.

LIVER PATHOLOGY. Liver biopsy specimens, even early in the clinical course of disease, usually show a combination of active hepatocellular damage, inflammation, and fibrosis. This finding, together with the sampling error inherent in needle biopsies, often make it difficult to distinguish the stage of chronic active hepatitis from that of postnecrotic cirrhosis with active hepatitis.

Liver cell damage is most striking around portal triads. The degenerating cells are variable in size, appearing swollen with bizarre nuclei, or, less often, shrunken with pyknotic nuclei. The Councilman-like bodies often found in active viral hepatitis are not a prominent feature. Individual cells and clumps of cells become separated from lobular remnants by a very cellular *mesenchymal reaction*. Clusters of lymphocytes, plasma cells, reticuloendothelial cells, and fibroblasts are prominent within triads and along zones of liver cell degeneration ("piecemeal," or "aggressive," necrosis). Lymphoid follicles may be prominent in portal triads, and other inflammatory cells are scattered throughout intact lobules. *Fibrosis* starts in the portal zones and extends in to areas of active cell degeneration. As time progresses, the cellular infiltration decreases, the fibrous bands become denser, and regenerating nodules expand, the end result being a postnecrotic cirrhosis.

CLINICAL FEATURES. Chronic active hepatitis is typically a disorder of young people, 75 percent of the cases occurring in women. The disease, however, may be found in other age groups and in men.

The *onset of illness is usually insidious.* Malaise, weakness, low-grade fever, and anorexia may be present for weeks, after which jaundice appears. In a few patients the onset of symptoms is abrupt, resembling the icteric phases of acute viral hepatitis. Others experience arthralgia, polyarthritis, pleurisy, or symptoms of ulcerative colitis for weeks or months before the liver disease becomes apparent. In females, amenorrhea is very common.

Early in the clinical course of the disease, patients may appear healthy, may be slightly to moderately icteric, and may have spider angiomas or other signs of chronic liver disease. Low-grade fever is often present. The liver is usually moderately enlarged and firm, and splenomegaly is present in about two-thirds of cases. Signs of cirrhosis appear as the disease progresses, but even on initial examination ascites and prominent abdominal collateral veins may be evident, pointing to the existence of an underlying postnecrotic cirrhosis.

Extrahepatic Features. Many patients have some rheumatic symptoms and signs in the course of the illness. Arthralgia and nondeforming polyarthritis of the fingers and large joints occur in over half the cases. Patients may develop serositis, such as pleuritis or pericarditis. Skin lesions are frequent and include facial acne, striae of the legs and abdomen, purpura, erythematous maculopapular rashes of the face or hands, and urticaria. Ulcerative colitis may appear before or after the disease is diagnosed. Renal involvement is rarely clinically important but may be manifested by transient hematuria or the nephrotic syndrome. Uncommon systemic features have included convulsions, strokes, diffuse pulmonary fibrosis, chronic thyroiditis and intermittent episodes of hemolytic anemia.

Laboratory Findings. Moderate anemia, slight to moderate leukopenia, and thrombocytopenia are often present. Albuminuria and microscopic hematuria may be present during periods of increased activity of the disease. Liver function tests are usually grossly abnormal but may not correlate with the clinical or pathologic findings. Conjugated hyperbilirubinemia is usually present, total serum bilirubin levels ranging between 3 and 10 mg per 100 ml for months or even years. BSP retention is the rule, and flocculation tests are usually positive. Although serum transaminase levels may exceed 2,000 units, values of 100 to 300 units are more common.

A striking laboratory feature is hypergammaglobulinemia, which may antedate other signs of chronic liver disease for months or years. Many serologic abnormalities may be found. LE cell tests are positive in about 20 percent of cases, usually in those with fever and arthralgia. Tests for serum antinuclear factors and rheumatoid factors are often positive, and false positive serologic tests for syphilis may occur. About 70 percent of patients have circulating immunoglobulins that react with smooth muscle fibers. By contrast the mitochondrial immunofluorescent antibody test is usually negative.

The course of chronic active hepatitis is variable, but in most patients signs of postnecrotic cirrhosis develop within a period of 2 to 5 years after clinical onset. Ascites and edema appear gradually, and the "rheumatic" manifestations tend to decrease. Most patients die in hepatic coma precipitated by variceal hemorrhage or intercurrent infection, the total duration of illness ranging between 2 and 10 years. A few patients have entered prolonged clinical remission, and in these instances repeat liver biopsies have demonstrated only minimal hepatic scarring.

DIAGNOSIS. The diagnosis of chronic active hepatitis should be considered in patients, especially children and adolescents, who have chronic hepatocellular disease, hypergammaglobulinemia, and systemic features such as arthritis, skin rash, or ulcerative colitis. Support for confirmation of this diagnosis can then be obtained by needle biopsy of the liver. Because of its diverse clinical and serologic manifestations, chronic active hepatitis may be confused with a wide variety of other diseases. Persistent acute viral hepatitis (i.e., delayed convalescence), drug-induced hepatitis, and other types of cirrhosis, such as Wilson's disease, must be considered. Chronic active hepatitis with prominent systemic features may be confused with rheumatoid arthritis, systemic lupus erythematosus (SLE), or other inflammatory connective tissue diseases. In these instances, evidence of liver cell damage found by biopsy or biochemical tests will often establish the proper diagnosis. On occasion, however, it may be difficult to distinguish chronic active hepatitis from disseminated lupus erythematosus with hepatic dysfunction. The extreme γ-globulin changes, positive smooth muscle antibody tests, and relative sparing of the heart and kidneys favor the diagnosis of chronic active hepatitis rather than SLE. Some features suggesting chronic inflammatory disease of the liver are seen in leukemia or lymphoma and need to be considered in the differential diagnosis.

TREATMENT. Since specific treatment is not available, the essential elements include drug therapy to suppress or modify the disease, treatment of the complications of cirrhosis, and general supportive measures. *Bed rest* seems to alleviate the malaise and fatigability of acute exacerbations, but prolonged bed rest is of little value. If the hepatitis is active, as evidenced by serum transaminase increases and persistent clinical symptoms, and if no major contraindications to steroid therapy are apparent, a trial of *corticosteroids* is indicated. Prednisone may be given initially in high doses, such as 60 mg daily for 1 or 2 weeks. The doses are then tapered weekly in 5- to 10-mg steps until a daily maintenance dose of 15 to 20 mg is reached. Recurrence of clinical symptoms or deterioration in liver function, especially increases in serum transaminases or rising γ-globulin levels, may necessitate a brief return to higher doses. Most patients experience relief of symptoms on this regimen, and jaundice decreases, but studies of steroid-treated patients have *not* shown reduced hepatic scarring or a significant increase in longevity. Side effects are numerous, and it is often difficult to discontinue therapy without exacerbation of symptoms.

Immunosuppressive therapy, designed to control immunologic factors that may contribute to the progression of disease, has been effective in many patients. Azathioprine, in doses of 50 to 150 mg daily, or 6-mercaptopurine, given in initial doses of 0.5 to 1.5 mg per kg body weight daily, may induce clinical and chemical remission after a phase of deepening jaundice. They may be especially useful in patients who respond only partly to corticosteroids. On occasion, the usefulness of these drugs is limited by bone marrow depression, frequent intercurrent infections, or the appearance of drug resistance. Nausea, deepening jaundice, or signs of marrow suppression may require a decrease in drug dose. Both corticosteroid and immunosuppressive therapy are most effective in controlling the active hepatic manifestations. Neither regimen appears to affect the long-term survival rate or to prevent the development of postnecrotic cirrhosis.

Ascites and edema, hemorrhage from esophogeal varices, and bouts of hepatic coma may respond to appropriate measures until a stage of hepatic insufficiency is reached. Pregnancy is rare in young women with the menstrual disorders of chronic active hepatitis, but a few patients have tolerated one or more pregnancies without obvious deleterious effect on either mother or fetus.

REFERENCES

Doniach, D., I. M. Roitt, J. G. Walker and S. Sherlock: Tissue Antibodies in Primary Biliary Cirrhosis, Active Chronic (Lupoid) Cirrhosis, Cryptogenic Cirrhosis and Other Liver Diseases and Their Clinical Implications, Clin. Exp. Immunology, 1:237, 1966.

Mackay, I. R. and I. Wood: The Course and Treatment of Lupoid Hepatitis, Gastroenterology, 45:4, 1963.

Maclachlan, M. J., G. P. Rodnan, W. M. Cooper and R. H. Fennell: Chronic Active ("Lupoid") Hepatitis, Ann. Int. Med., 62:425, 1965.

Mistilis, S. P. and C. R. B. Blackburn: The Treatment of Active Chronic Hepatitis with 6-Mercaptopurine and Azothioprine., Aust. Ann. Med., 16:305, 1967.

Schaffner, F. and F. Klion: Chronic Hepatitis, Ann. Rev. Med., 19:25, 1968.

Sherlock, S.: Diseases of the Liver, Philadelphia, F. A. Davis Co., Fourth Edition, 1968.

Willocx, R. G. and K. J. Isselbacher: Chronic Liver Disease in Young People, Amer. J. Med., 30:185, 1961.

Wright, R., R. W. McCollum, and G. Klatskin: Australia Antigen in Acute and Chronic Liver Disease, Lancet, 2:117, 1969.

328 CIRRHOSIS

William A. Tisdale and Kurt J. Isselbacher

DEFINITION

MORPHOLOGIC. Cirrhosis is a generic term that includes all forms of chronic diffuse liver disease characterized by significant loss of liver cells, collapse and fibrosis of the supporting reticulin network with distortion of the vascular bed, and nodular regeneration of the remaining liver cell masses. The basic causative element of this complex lesion is diffuse liver cell death; the network of scars, the regenerating cell masses, and the changes in hepatic circulation develop secondarily. Less constant pathologic features of most types of cirrhosis include intralobular or portal inflammation, focal or widespread bile stasis, and proliferation of ductular cells.

CLINICAL AND FUNCTIONAL. The morphologic elements of cirrhosis often have dramatic clinical counterparts. Progressive loss of liver cells may produce jaundice, ascites and edema, central nervous system dysfunction, cachexia, and death—the syndrome of hepatic insufficiency. The advancing fibrosis leads to distortion of the intrahepatic vasculature, which in turn contributes to the development of portal venous hypertension with resultant esophageal and gastric varices and splenomegaly. Nodular regeneration often leads to distortion of liver shape and compression of intrahepatic venous and lymphatic radicles, which may result in ascites and portal hypertension. No clinical, etiologic, or morphologic classification of cirrhosis is satisfactory at present. Clinical signs and symptoms may not reflect accurately the extent and precise nature of the cirrhotic process; the etiology and many types of cirrhosis remains uncertain or unknown; pathologic patterns may represent nonspecific hepatic responses to many different forms of liver cell injury. However, in spite of these limitations, it is possible to categorize most cases of cirrhosis clinically, adding qualifying morphologic or etiologic terms when possible. Most types of cirrhosis can be classified as follows: (1) Laennec's, (2) postnecrotic, (3) biliary (either primary or secondary), (4) hemochromatosis, (5) cardiac or congestive, or (6) rare and nonspecific cirrhosis.

LAENNEC'S CIRRHOSIS

Definition

This form of cirrhosis, the most common variety encountered in North America and many parts of western Europe, is characterized by diffuse fine scarring, a fairly uniform loss of liver cells associated with fatty infiltration or active cell degeneration, and small (often less than lobule-sized) islands of preserved or regenerating parenchyma. These changes occur at a "unilobular" level and involve the entire liver in the same manner. The terms *alcoholic, portal,* and *fatty cirrhosis* have also been used to describe this type of chronic liver disease. However, each of these has misleading implications; alcoholism is not always a factor in the pathogenesis of Laennec's cirrhosis, the fibrosis and scarring may not be centered about the portal triads, and cirrhosis may develop in the absence of significant fatty infiltration of liver cells.

Etiology

Many epidemiologic studies have implicated *chronic alcoholism* as a major cause of Laennec's cirrhosis: between 15 and 20 percent of chronic alcoholic patients in the United States have clinical or morphologic evidence of cirrhosis; about 75 percent of patients with Laennec's cirrhosis admit to heavy drinking; the Prohibition era led to a temporary but distinct decline in deaths due to cirrhosis. Experimental studies of both normal and alcoholic subjects have shown that ethanol (in moderate to large doses) produces liver dysfunction and fatty infiltration (Chap. 323) despite the ingestion of a well-balanced diet. However, there is still no definite evidence that alcohol *by itself* leads to cirrhosis.

Most chronic alcoholics consume protein- and vitamin-poor diets, many develop other clinical syndromes clearly related to faulty nutrition (exemplified by folate deficiency or Wernicke's syndrome), and treatment of cirrhotic patients with protein-rich diets often produces clinical and morphologic improvement. For these and other reasons, absolute or relative *malnutrition* is regarded as a contributing factor to the evolution of cirrhosis. Although malnutrition per se does not lead to Laennec's cirrhosis, a reasonable concept, based on much circumstantial evidence, is that a combination of *chronic alcohol ingestion plus impaired nutrition* leads to liver cell damage and Laennec's cirrhosis.

Intercurrent bacterial *infections* are common in cirrhotic patients and seem, on occasion, to accelerate the course of the disease. There is, however, no firm data to implicate overt or latent infection in the pathogenesis of Laennec's cirrhosis. Icteric or anicteric subacute hepa-

titis, presumably of viral origin, may lead to the development of a finely nodular cirrhosis resembling Laennec's cirrhosis in its general morphology, perhaps explaining the frequent reports of portal cirrhosis in nonalcoholic patients in England. Serial biopsies in these cases do not show many of the characteristic histologic features of progressive alcoholic cirrhosis (see below), and such cases may represent variants of postnecrotic cirrhosis.

No *metabolic defect* has been identified in cirrhotic patients or their families that would suggest a unique "susceptibility" to ethanol or its toxic effects. It is clear, nonetheless, that individual tolerance to ethanol and its capacity to induce cirrhosis vary widely and that a true biological predisposition to ethanol-induced liver diseases may exist.

Pathology and Pathogenesis

In the early stages of Laennec's cirrhosis the liver is enlarged, yellow, greasy, and firm. The parenchymal cells are usually diffusely abnormal, and many are distended by cytoplasmic fat vacuoles, which disappear with therapy and recur promptly after resumption of alcohol ingestion. A characteristic cytologic feature of active Laennec's cirrhosis is the *Mallory body* or *alcoholic hyalin*. These beadlike clumps of perinuclear eosinophilic material are found in damaged cells and consist of swollen and fragmented cell organelles. An abundance of Mallory bodies usually indicates significant hepatic damage in association with alcohol ingestion. Except for Indian childhood cirrhosis, the Mallory body is not found in other nonalcoholic varieties of finely nodular cirrhosis. As the liver disease advances and hepatocytes are destroyed, weblike *septums of connective tissue appear in periportal zones* and in other areas of active cell degeneration. These fibrous septums become denser and more confluent, connecting portal triads and central veins. The fine connective tissue network contains small vessels, lymphatics, and other remnants of portal triads and surrounds small masses of liver cells. These lobular remnants undergo regeneration and form nodules. Some of the connective tissue septums may become broad as more liver cells are lost, reaching proportions that justify the use of the term "postnecrotic scarring" in some areas. Inflammation is usually mononuclear, inconspicuous, and concentrated within portal triads and areas of active liver cell damage. Bile stasis is usually minimal and transient, but may be a prominent morphologic feature during acute exacerbations of the disease. As the fatty infiltration subsides and the liver cell mass diminishes, the liver shrinks in size, acquires a finely nodular (hobnail) appearance, and becomes hard.

Laennec's cirrhosis is basically a progressive disease, but appropriate therapy and strict avoidance of alcohol may arrest the disease at most stages and permit repair and functional improvement. Continued loss of liver cells by fatty degeneration and focal necrosis, however, results in progressive stromal collapse, fibrosis, and vascular distortion. Although regeneration occurs within the small remnants of parenchyma, cell loss eventually exceeds replacement, the liver cell mass dwindles, and a phase of irreversible, or end-stage, cirrhosis is reached.

The terms *florid cirrhosis* and *alcoholic hepatitis* refer to active alcoholic liver disease characterized by numerous Mallory bodies, neutrophilic exudate, and central sclerosis of supporting reticulin resulting from liver cell loss. These elements may be found at any stage of progressive liver disease in the alcoholic, suggesting that the terms have no specific clinicopathologic meaning.

Clinical Features

SIGNS AND SYMPTOMS. Men are affected more frequently than women, but this sex difference has decreased steadily in recent years as drinking habits have changed in many Western countries. Although the average age of onset of symptoms is about fifty years, Laennec's cirrhosis may be found in alcoholic patients in the third or fourth decade of life.

Advanced Laennec's cirrhosis may be clinically silent, and about 10 percent of cases are discovered incidentally at laparotomy or autopsy. Typically, however, after 5 to 15 years of alcoholic excess, evidence of progressive liver dysfunction, fluid retention, and portal hypertension appears. Over a period of weeks or months, the patient notes gradually increasing weakness and fatigability, anorexia, slight weight loss, jaundice, intermittent ankle edema, and increasing abdominal girth due to ascites. A firm and enlarged liver may be the only sign of disease, but additional typical findings include muscle wasting, jaundice, arterial "spider" angiomas, palmar erythema, splenomegaly, and ascites. Loss of body hair, gynecomastia and testicular atrophy (in the male), parotid gland enlargement, purpura, clubbing of the fingers, Dupuytren's contractures, and diffuse hyperpigmentation of the skin are common but less important clinical signs. Low-grade fever without shaking chills is frequent in patients with active disease.

Jaundice and other signs of hepatic dysfunction may subside with therapy, but continued alcoholic excess and poor dietary habits lead to further episodes of hepatic decompensation. Acute acceleration of alcoholic liver damage may follow protracted drinking bouts. Fever, nausea and vomiting, deepening jaundice, hepatic precoma, and ascites may occur rapidly in association with widespread liver cell loss and inflammation. Although some patients die during the acute exacerbations, most recover after several weeks. A few patients experience one or more transient episodes of cholestatic jaundice during the course of alcoholic liver disease. Clinical and laboratory studies may suggest the diagnosis of mechanical biliary obstruction, but liver biopsy and the response to conservative therapy usually support the diagnosis of intrahepatic cholestasis. Over a period of 3 to 5 years, the cirrhotic patient becomes emaciated, weak, and chronically jaundiced, and ascites and signs of portal hypertension become increasingly prominent. Most patients with advanced cirrhosis die in hepatic coma (see page 1557), often precipitated by hemorrhage from esophageal varices or intercurrent infection. Acute and chronic

pancreatitis and peptic ulceration occur with greater frequency in cirrhotic patients than in normal subjects. Gram-negative bacteremia, acute bacterial peritonitis, and hepatoma are uncommon complications.

LABORATORY FEATURES. Leukopenia and thrombocytopenia, probably related to hypersplenism, are quite common; significant leukocytosis usually indicates associated infection or florid cirrhosis. Moderate anemia is common and may result from a combination of gastrointestinal blood loss, folic acid deficiency, a shortened red cell survival secondary to enlargement of the spleen, or the suppressive effects of alcohol on erythropoiesis. Acute episodes of nonimmune hemolysis associated with hyperlipemia (hyperlipidemic hemolytic anemia of Zieve) may contribute to the anemia in some patients. Depending on the extent of liver cell damage, liver function tests reveal an increase in both total and direct-reacting serum bilirubin fractions, BSP retention, slight to moderate elevations of the serum alkaline phosphatase, and minor changes in serum transaminases. Serum albumin levels are frequently depressed. Serum gammaglobulin concentrations are slightly and sometimes moderately elevated, especially when there is active disease. Serum levels of the major immunoglobulins are often increased, the most consistent abnormality being an elevation of IgG. If the cirrhosis is severe, profound hypoprothrombinemia may develop.

A diabetic type of impaired glucose tolerance may be demonstrated. However, clinical diabetes mellitus is uncommon, and the defect in glucose metabolism, thought to be the result of endogenous insulin resistance, may be transient. Low or low-normal blood urea nitrogen levels are seen in some patients with cirrhosis and malnutrition. For this reason, the plasma creatinine is a more accurate index of renal function. Hyponatremia, usually moderate in degree, is frequent in cirrhotic patients with ascites and edema.

Diagnosis

Laennec's cirrhosis should be strongly suspected in patients with a history of prolonged or excessive alcohol intake, physical findings of hepatomegaly, and other signs of chronic liver disease plus laboratory evidence of hepatic dysfunction. If there are no contraindications, most patients should have a needle biopsy of the liver to confirm the diagnosis as well as to determine the stage of the disease process. The physician must also keep in mind that when the course of an otherwise stable cirrhotic changes without obvious explanation, complicating conditions such as occult bleeding, hepatoma, and portal vein thrombosis should be sought.

Prognosis

Both retrospective and prospective studies of the natural history of Laennec's cirrhosis show that early, vigorous and meticulous medical care will prolong life, decrease morbidity, and delay or prevent the appearance of certain complications. Patients who abstain from alcohol and consume nutritious diets have a 5-year survival rate of about 60 percent, whereas those who continue to drink have a 40 percent 5-year survival rate. This generalization must be qualified by the fact that mortality rates are higher for those who develop one of the major complications of cirrhosis, and the 5-year survival after onset of either ascites or jaundice is reduced to about 33 percent. Massive variceal hemorrhage continues to be a major direct or contributing cause of death despite improvements in the medical and surgical treatment of portal hypertension. Over 80 percent of patients are dead within 5 years of their first episode of bleeding from esophageal varices.

Treatment

Laennec's cirrhosis is a serious chronic illness that usually requires prolonged medical supervision and management. In most instances it is desirable to hospitalize the patient for initial study and assessment of his response to therapy as well as for dietary and medical instruction.

In the absence of signs of impending hepatic coma, a *diet* containing at least 1 Gm protein per kg body weight and 2,000 to 3,000 cal per day should be prescribed. Because the patient with active cirrhosis is often anorectic or nauseated, these dietary aims may be achieved by offering the patient three or four small meals with supplemental feedings of eggnog or ice cream. Vitamin supplements, in the form of multivitamin capsules, may be given, but there is no rationale for the clinical use of lipotropic agents. The patient should understand clearly that neither nutritious diet nor added vitamins will protect his liver against the effects of further alcohol. *Alcohol should be absolutely forbidden.*

Minimal ascites and edema may disappear with bed rest alone, but more persistent fluid retention should be treated with a combination of *salt restriction,* utilizing diets that contain 200 to 500 mg of sodium, and *water restriction,* limiting fluid intake to volumes that equal the measured fluid loss of the prior day. It is often desirable to avoid the stringent dietary control needed to keep sodium intake below 500 mg, so that *diuretic agents* may be added. Mercuhydrin may induce a mild diuresis, but chlorothiazide (1.0 to 2.0 Gm) and spironolactone (100 to 200 mg) are more effective in mobilizing ascites and edema. Attempts at diuresis should be cautious, and special care must be taken to avoid potassium depletion or hyponatremia. Vigorous diuresis with agents such as furosemide and ethacrynic acid is especially hazardous in severely ill patients, and precise measurements of fluid balance and renal function are essential. Infusions of *salt-poor albumin* may produce a temporary rise in colloid osmotic pressure and induce diuresis, but repeated infusions may lead to elevations of portal vein pressure and variceal hemorrhage. *Therapeutic paracentesis* is indicated rarely because the hazards of protein loss and adverse circulatory responses (hypovolemia and hyponatremia) more than counterbalance the temporary relief of abdominal distention.

Confusion, drowsiness, or other signs of impending *hepatic coma* should be treated by prompt decrease in protein intake to levels of 20 to 30 Gm daily or less. A careful search for gastrointestinal hemorrhage should be made, including the aspiration of gastric contents, and appropriate therapy to control bleeding should be instituted (see page 1556). All drugs, especially diuretics and sedatives, should be omitted and any electrolyte imbalance corrected promptly (see Hepatic Coma, page 1557).

Anemia should be characterized and corrected by appropriate means. Blood transfusions should be given only for specific indications, because expansion of blood volume is hazardous in the presence of esophageal varices.

Fever, especially when low-grade and unaccompanied by chills or other signs of infection, may be only a manifestation of active cirrhosis. However, the presence of hectic or persistent fever or shaking chills requires a vigorous search for septic processes, especially urinary tract infection, pneumonia, and gram-negative bacteremias.

Renal failure may develop in patients with advanced and decompensated cirrhosis, and often appears after paracentesis, too-vigorous diuresis, a bout of gastrointestinal hemorrhage, hypotension, or hepatic coma. The cause of this complication is unknown, but structural abnormalities of the kidney are minimal, and functional changes suggest that decreased "effective" renal blood flow is often the major defect. Oliguria, normal urine sediment, decreasing ability to concentrate urine, and rising levels of serum creatinine are typical features of this syndrome. Treatment is usually unsuccessful, but correction of hypotension or hypovolemia may improve renal function. Infusions of 50 to 100 Gm of human serum albumin may transiently improve glomerular filtration rate and urine output in patients with slight impairment of renal function.

Adrenal steroids and androgens have been used to produce a sense of well-being and to stimulate appetite in acutely ill cirrhotic patients. They seem to have no specific benefits, however, and are rarely useful.

POSTNECROTIC CIRRHOSIS
Definition

This form of chronic liver disease, the most common type of cirrhosis on a worldwide basis, is characterized morphologically by (1) confluent, often massive loss of liver cells, (2) stromal collapse and fibrosis that produce broad bands of connective tissue containing the remains of many triads, and (3) irregular, often large nodules of intact or regenerating parenchyma. This pattern, which may vary considerably in extent and severity, results from an overall but unequal injury to the liver. As with other forms of cirrhosis, the appearance of advanced postnecrotic disease offers little insight into the original or potentiating causes of the liver cell damage.

The terms *toxic cirrhosis, coarsely nodular cirrhosis, posthepatitic cirrhosis, cryptogenic cirrhosis, multilobular cirrhosis,* and *healed yellow atrophy* are synonymous with postnecrotic cirrhosis.

Etiology

The precise cause of most cases of postnecrotic cirrhosis is unknown. In the United States, about one-quarter of patients with biopsy-proven postnecrotic cirrhosis give a history of recent or past jaundice compatible with *viral hepatitis;* other cases of established postnecrotic cirrhosis may possibly result from anicteric or inapparent subacute viral hepatitis. The inability to recover specific causative agents and the lack of diagnostic serologic tests, however, make these cause-and-effect relationships presumptive at present. *Chronic active hepatitis (of unknown cause)* (Chap. 327) terminates in a pattern of postnecrotic cirrhosis in most instances. A small percentage of cases stems from documented *intoxications* with industrial chemicals (e.g., phosphorus), poisons (e.g., *Amanita phalloides* toxins), or drugs (chloroform, iproniazid). Finally, certain *infections* (for example, brucellosis), *parasitic infestations* (clonorchiasis), *metabolic disorders* (hepatolenticular degeneration), and *advanced alcoholic liver disease* may produce confluent cell loss and result in postnecrotic cirrhosis.

Pathology and Pathogenesis

Typically, the postnecrotic liver is small, grossly distorted in shape, and composed of nodules of liver cells separated by dense, wide sunken scars. Microscopically, the established lesion includes (1) large islands of parenchymal cells with rounded (inactive) or ragged (active "piecemeal necrosis") margins; (2) interdigitating broad to thin fibrous septums containing distorted vessels, lymphatics, and bile ducts derived from many portal areas; and (3) prominent mononuclear inflammatory infiltrates, often in the form of follicles or clusters.

Current evidence suggests that infectious, toxic, metabolic, or nutritional factors initiate the postnecrotic process. The destruction appears to progress as the result of similar repeated or persistent insults or possibly on the basis of "autoimmune" liver cell injury.

Clinical Features

Postnecrotic cirrhosis should be suspected in nonalcoholic patients, especially those in the younger age group, with evidence of chronic liver disease.

SIGNS AND SYMPTOMS. Like those with Laennec's cirrhosis, a few patients with postnecrotic disease may have little clinical evidence of advanced cirrhosis, the diagnosis being made at operation or postmortem examination or by a needle biopsy performed to investigate asymptomatic hepatosplenomegaly. About 25 percent of patients present with signs and symptoms suggesting active hepatitis, but often with atypical features such as prolonged illness, intense and protracted jaundice, ascites, or manifestations of portal hypertension. Still others have bouts of upper abdominal pain, the sudden onset of unexplained ascites, episodes of hepatic precoma, or massive variceal hemorrhage as the major or initial clinical feature. The general signs and symptoms of postnecrotic cirrhosis resemble those described in Laennec's cirrhosis and reflect the loss of liver cell reserve, advancing portal hypertension, and disorders of salt and water metabolism. In general, however, patients with postnecrotic cirrhosis show less wasting and more persistent jaundice early in their clinical illness than do patients with Laennec's cirrhosis. A few patients experience migratory polyarthritis or protracted itching in the clinical course of otherwise typical postnecrotic cirrhosis. About 15 percent of cases are complicated by the development of hepatoma.

LABORATORY FEATURES. The results of hematologic and liver function tests resemble those seen in Laennec's cirrhosis, but protracted and dramatic hyperbilirubinemia, persistent moderate elevations of serum transaminases, and hypergammaglobulinemia (3 to 4 Gm per 100 ml serum) may be clues to the existence of postnecrotic cirrhosis.

Diagnosis and Prognosis

Postnecrotic cirrhosis should be suspected in young persons and nonalcoholic adults with signs and symptoms of cirrhosis. Most laboratory and radiologic studies are nondiagnostic, and needle or operative liver biopsy are the definitive diagnostic procedures. About 75 percent of cases of postnecrotic cirrhosis tend to progress despite supportive therapy and terminate in death after 1 to 5 years from exsanguinating variceal hemorrhage, hepatic coma, or superimposed hepatoma.

Treatment

Because the primary cause of this disease is rarely detectable or treatable, long-term care must include appropriate rest, control of ascites (page 1556), avoidance of drugs or excessive protein intake that may induce hepatic coma (page 1557), prompt treatment of infections, and surgical treatment of portal hypertension (page 1554) if variceal hemorrhage occurs.

BILIARY CIRRHOSIS
Definition

The term *biliary cirrhosis* refers to patients with clinical and chemical signs of chronic impairment of bile excretion and morphologic evidence of progressive liver destruction centered about the intrahepatic bile ducts. Major clinical concomitants of impaired bile excretion include protracted itching; progressive and prolonged jaundice with dark urine; steatorrhea; the development of cutaneous xanthelasmas and xanthomas; hepatomegaly; laboratory findings of marked elevations of serum alkaline phosphatase, cholesterol, and other lipid fractions; and slowly progressive decline of health. Morphologically, most forms of biliary cirrhosis evolve from chronic inflammatory lesions of the periportal liver cells, ductules, and interlobular ducts, and true cirrhosis represents a late and often nonspecific phase.

Etiology

Biliary cirrhosis can be classified either as "primary," in which case the process is related to chronic intra-hepatic cholestasis, or "secondary," indicating that the major cause is related to obstruction of the common bile duct or its large branches.

The etiology of *primary biliary cirrhosis* is still un-known, but there are a number of theories that are cur-rently being considered about the pathogenesis of this unique disease. The nearly exclusive (over 90 percent) occurrence of this disorder in adult, often middle-age, women strongly suggests an endocrine contribution. The occasional onset of primary biliary cirrhosis following a bout of atypical (so-called "cholangiolitic") hepatitis has led to speculation that viral destruction of liver and duct cells initiates the disease process. Although no drug has produced a picture of *typical* progressive biliary cirrhosis in humans or experimental animals, the oc-casional appearance of many elements of the syndrome in patients treated with phenothiazines suggests that drug hypersensitivity may be one etiologic factor. While hepatic copper levels have been found to be elevated, the relationship of this abnormality to the disease process is still unknown.

It is increasingly clear that primary biliary cirrhosis is associated with a remarkable number of specific and non-specific immunologic features.

1. Elevated serum levels of IgM are seen in about 80 percent of patients with primary biliary cirrhosis, but this abnormality is nonspecific and occurs occasionally in patients with mechanical bile duct obstruction.

2. Immunofluorescent studies have demonstrated a circulating antibody that reacts with the cytoplasm of bile ductular cells in 75 percent of patients with primary biliary cirrhosis. It is tempting to postulate "autodestruc-tion" of ductular cells by this mechanism, but similar antibody changes have occurred in many patients with simple viral hepatitis.

3. Periductal lymphocytes in liver biopsy specimens from patients with primary biliary cirrhosis have been shown to form IgM immunoglobulins, again raising the possibility of self-perpetuating immune disease.

4. The most promising diagnostic and investigative lead has been provided by the demonstration of a circulating antibody (IgG) in the serum of most pa-tients with primary biliary cirrhosis that reacts with mitochondria-rich cells. These antibodies have been de-tected in over 80 percent of patients with primary biliary cirrhosis but only rarely in other forms of liver disease. These observations suggest strongly that dis-ordered immune responses play a major role in the initiation or progression of the chronic hepatic lesion of biliary cirrhosis, but the exact mechanisms involved are unclear.

Finally, the long-standing concept that lipid deposits in the liver and biliary tract produce hepatic damage (so-called "xanthomatosis biliary cirrhosis") is incorrect because the generalized xanthomatosis is the result rather than the cause of the hepatic disease.

Most instances of *secondary biliary cirrhosis* result from long-standing partial or total obstruction of the common bile duct or its major branches. In adults, chronic bile duct obstruction by postoperative strictures or by gallstones, usually with superimposed infectious cholangitis, is the most common cause of this type of biliary cirrhosis. Tumors of the pancreas, biliary tree, or gallbladder that produce obstruction of the common bile duct occasionally induce cirrhosis but only rarely permit survival to this stage. A few patients with the peculiar pericholangitis of ulcerative colitis or with idi-opathic sclerosing cholangitis develop secondary biliary cirrhosis. Congenital atresia of the intra- or extrahepatic bile duct system, a relatively common anomaly, induces rapidly advancing periportal fibrosis in infants; most cases are inoperable and eventually fatal. In neither acquired nor congenital biliary obstruction is the exact pathogenesis of the cirrhotic process understood. Simple pressure effects, local toxicity of bile constituents, and secondary infection alone do not explain the mor-phologic events satisfactorily.

Pathology and Pathogenesis

The earliest recognizable lesion of *primary biliary cirrhosis* might be termed "chronic nonsuppurative chol-angitis," a diffuse necrotizing and inflammatory process centered about the portal triads. This is characterized by destruction of ductular and portal duct cells infiltration with acute and chronic inflammatory cells, local fibro-blastic reaction, and variable bile stasis. Progression of this process over a period of months to years (usually 3 to 5 years) leads to loss of liver cells, the formation of pseudolobules, expansion of periportal fibrosis into a network of connective tissue scars, with apparent loss of interlobular ducts and the development of true cir-rhosis. End-stage primary biliary cirrhosis may be in-distinguishable from postnecrotic cirrhosis in its gross and microscopic appearance.

Unrelieved obstruction of the extrahepatic bile ducts leads to (1) centrilobular bile stasis, cell degeneration, and focal areas of necrosis; (2) proliferation and dilata-tion of the portal ducts and ductules; (3) sterile or infected cholangitis with accumulation of polymorpho-nuclear infiltrates around bile ducts; and (4) progressive expansion of portal tracts by edema and fibrosis. Bile may collect in the peripheral areas of necrosis to form "bile lakes." While patients may tolerate biliary obstruc-tion for several years without the appearance of irrevers-ible secondary biliary cirrhosis, eventually a finely nodu-lar cirrhosis develops with isolated bile-stained pseu-dolobules surrounded by dense connective tissue septums. In both primary and secondary biliary cirrhosis, the liver is initially enlarged and greenish-yellow in appearance, but evolves to a smaller, firmer, more coarsely nodular organ as the disease progresses.

Clinical Features

SIGNS AND SYMPTOMS. Although not diagnostic, the early clinical course of *primary biliary cirrhosis* is quite characteristic. Typically, the patient is a young or middle-aged woman who develops persistent generalized itching (the earliest symptom in about 50 percent of cases), intermittent and then continuous dark urine, pale stools and jaundice, and gradual darkening (melanosis) of the exposed areas of the skin. In contrast to many other forms of cirrhosis, there are few early signs of liver cell failure and hepatic fibrosis, and most of the features reflect impaired bile excretion. Steatorrhea with associated malabsorption of lipid-soluble vitamins often produces purpura, diarrhea, and osteomalacia; the latter may be manifested by backache and bone pain. Protracted elevation of serum lipids, especially cholesterol, leads to the deposit of yellowish plaques or nodules in the subcutaneous tissues in the form of periorbital xanthelasmas and xanthomas over joints, in skin folds, and at sites of trauma. Over a period of months to years, the itching, jaundice, and hyperpigmentation slowly increase. At that time the pruritus and skin lipid deposits may decrease, ascites and edema usually appear, and signs of liver cell failure and portal hypertension supervene. Most patients die within 5 to 7 years from the first signs of the illness. Death usually is due to hepatic insufficiency that is often precipitated by variceal bleeding, intercurrent infection, or surgical procedures.

Physical examination may be entirely normal in the early phase of the disease when pruritis is the sole complaint. In addition, however, there may be jaundice of varying intensity, hyperpigmentation of exposed and irritated skin, xanthelasmas and xanthomas, moderate to striking hepatomegaly, splenomegaly, and clubbing of the fingers. Fever and chills are distinctly rare and usually indicate mechanical biliary obstruction or other associated diseases. Muscle wasting, spider angiomas, palmar erythema, ascites and edema, and the bony tenderness of osteomalacia appear in advanced stages of the disease.

Patients who develop *secondary biliary cirrhosis* usually have a long-standing history and give evidence of previous biliary tract disease. Pain varies in type. There may be right upper quadrant pain due to stretching of the liver capsule or due to disease in the gallbladder or bile duct. Signs and symptoms of true cirrhosis appear slowly; ascites and massive upper gastrointestinal hemorrhage usually occur with the end-stage of the disease.

LABORATORY FEATURES. The major chemical abnormalities of evolving biliary cirrhosis result from impaired bile excretion. Late in the course of the illness, evidence of failing liver cell function develops. There is usually conjugated hyperbilirubinemia, and total bilirubin concentrations range from 3 to 20 mg per 100 ml serum. In the final stages, bilirubin levels may exceed 50 mg per 100 ml. Serum alkaline phosphatase levels are usually dramatically elevated, and transaminase levels rarely exceed 150 to 200 units. Nonspecific increases in alpha-2, beta-, and gamma- (IgM) globulins are noted. Hyperlipemia is common in early biliary cirrhosis, with the most striking elevations being in the phospholipid and free cholesterol fractions. Serum bile salts (especially trihydroxy) are increased, and the elevations correlate reasonably well with the intensity of itching. Hypoprothrombinemia and mild to moderate steatorrhea are common. The mitochondrial antibody test is positive in most cases of primary but not secondary biliary cirrhosis.

Diagnosis

Biliary cirrhosis should be considered in any patient with signs, symptoms, and laboratory evidence of protracted obstruction to bile flow. The major diagnostic challenge, regardless of the duration of symptoms, is to exclude remediable causes of mechanical bile duct obstruction before permanent liver damage has occurred. Although patients with transient drug reactions and hepatitis may require only careful observation, those with chronic unexplained obstruction after study by liver biopsy and cholangiography (intravenous or percutaneous) will in most instances require laparotomy with thorough exploration and direct visualization of the biliary system. A positive mitochondrial antibody test is strong presumptive evidence of primary biliary cirrhosis. Clinical and biopsy studies usually suffice to diagnose uncommon causes of cholestatic jaundice such as hemochromatosis, postnecrotic cirrhosis, and fatty liver.

Treatment

Complete correction of any mechanical obstruction to bile flow is the most important step in the prevention and therapy of *secondary biliary cirrhosis*. The patient with well-documented *primary biliary cirrhosis*, a chronic and incurable disease, requires prolonged medical therapy with careful attention to the many complications of itching, malabsorption, fluid retention, portal hypertension, and late-stage hepatic insufficiency. A reasonably balanced, high-caloric *diet* is usually adequate, but some patients report relief of bothersome diarrhea when fat intake is decreased below 30 to 40 Gm per day. *Itching* is often extremely distressing to the patient and is refractory to most forms of therapy. Local skin cooling, topical menthol lotions, careful sedation, and antihistamine therapy may provide some relief. Systemic corticosteroids and various synthetic androgen compounds may decrease itching without altering the course of the disease. The bile salt-sequestering resin *cholestyramine* usually relieves itching when given in doses of 8 to 12 Gm daily. The *fat-soluble vitamins D, A, and K* should be given by parenteral injection at regular intervals to help prevent or correct osteomalacia and hypoprothrombinemia. Salt restriction and judicious use of oral diuretic agents usually prevent disabling ascites and edema. The occurrence of esophagogastric variceal hemorrhage may require a portacaval shunt.

HEMOCHROMATOSIS
See Chap. 107

CARDIAC CIRRHOSIS
Definition

As with other types of cirrhosis, the term *cardiac cirrhosis* has both morphologic and etiologic connotations. Structurally, it refers to a combination of chronic, destructive centrilobular vascular congestion, progressive atrophy of central liver cell plates, fibrosis that involves central and then portal zones, and limited regenerative and inflammatory reactions. The name implies that cardiac disease, notably congestive heart failure, is the basic cause. In actual fact, heart failure rarely leads to cirrhosis, and most instances of *true* cardiac cirrhosis result from uncommon disorders of the venae cavae, pericardium, or tricuspid valve. Thus, cardiac cirrhosis is a relatively rare cause of chronic liver disease.

Etiology

Excluding primary diseases of the hepatic venules veno-occlusive disease) and major hepatic veins (Budd-Chiari syndrome), only cardiovascular disorders that produce prolonged or recurrent hypertension of the cavae and right atrium can be listed as causes of cardiac cirrhosis; these include mitral or tricuspid valvular disease, prolonged constrictive pericarditis, and decompensated cor pulmonale.

Pathology and Pathogenesis

The acutely congested liver is swollen, tense with blood and edema fluid, and dark-colored. Chronic congestion leads to thickening of the capsule and increasing fine trabeculation, occasionally with prominent centrilobular stellate or bandlike scars. Many patients with known chronic hepatic congestion have both a finely and coarsely nodular cirrhosis at autopsy, suggesting that factors other than simple passive congestion have contributed to the process.

Clinical Features

The demonstration of slight jaundice, a firm and somewhat enlarged liver, and ascites in a patient with valvular heart disease, constrictive pericarditis, or cor pulmonale *of long duration* (usually more than 10 years) should suggest the presence of cardiac cirrhosis. In cases of marked tricuspid insufficiency, the liver often is pulsatile, but this feature disappears as cirrhosis develops. Variceal bleeding and coma are uncommon and are usually overshadowed by cachexia, fluid retention, and circulatory derangements. Splenomegaly may result from simple passive congestion and does not necessarily indicate the presence of cirrhosis.

Liver function tests are usually abnormal. Conjugated hyperbilirubinemia, BSP retention, hypoalbuminemia, increased transaminase levels, and mild elevations of serum alkaline phosphatase are the most common abnormalities.

Diagnosis

The enlarged and chronically congested liver, whether mildly scarred or actually cirrhotic, is usually recognized clinically. It is rarely necessary to establish the diagnosis with certainty, but needle biopsy provides a safe and direct approach.

Treatment

Prevention or treatment of cardiac cirrhosis depends on proper diagnosis and therapy of the underlying cardiovascular disorder. If constrictive pericarditis is present and pericardectomy is possible, the prognosis for the liver is good. Within 6 to 12 months liver function may improve, and the fibrous bands become narrower and avascular.

RARE AND NONSPECIFIC TYPES OF CIRRHOSIS

Neither clinical, etiologic, nor morphologic classifications of cirrhosis encompass all cases. The efficiency of detection and study of patients with cirrhosis varies widely throughout the world, but unexpected and unexplained cirrhosis accounts for about 10 percent of cases of this chronic liver disease seen at autopsy. Equally important, many patients with cirrhosis are "classified" improperly during life. A small and unrepresentative biopsy specimen from a patient with a poor history often accounts for the errors in diagnosis.

Cirrhosis may be found in association with the following diseases:

1. *Metabolic disorders:* galactosemia, diabetes mellitus, glycogen storage diseases, hereditary tyrosinemia, and the Fanconi syndrome
2. *Infectious diseases:* brucellosis, schistosomiasis, clonorchiasis, neonatal cytomegalovirus, and toxoplasma infections
3. *Infiltrative diseases:* as sarcoidosis
4. *Gastrointestinal disorders:* ulcerative colitis and cystic fibrosis of the pancreas
5. *Chemical intoxications:* pyrrolidizine alkaloids (veno-occlusive disease)

NONCIRRHOTIC FIBROSIS OF THE LIVER

Several diseases, either congenital or acquired, may produce localized or generalized hepatic fibrosis. The clinical manifestations in such cases may suggest on occasion the diagnosis of true cirrhosis, but the absence of clinical and functional evidence of hepatocellular damage, the lack of nodular regenerative activity, and the localized nature of the scarring usually serve to distinguish these conditions from true cirrhosis.

Schistosomiasis (See also Chap. 250)

The ova of *Schistosoma mansoni* elicit granulomatous and fibrotic reactions along the portal tracts, the result of a delayed hypersensitivity reaction or of a nonspecific foreign-body host response. The characteristic hepatic lesion of schistosomiasis is, therefore, noncirrhotic portal ("pipestem") fibrosis which produces progressive occlusion of the portal venules with resultant presinusoidal portal hypertension. True cirrhosis may be present in some cases, but nutritional deficiencies and other factors contribute to this process. Clinically, the signs of portal hypertension predominate. The liver and spleen are moderately enlarged. Hepatocellular function is usually normal, but BSP retention and elevation of serum alkaline phosphatase may be noted. Jaundice is uncommon.

Congenital Hepatic Fibrosis

This disorder is a variant of polycystic disease of the liver, which is congenital and, in some instances, familial. Typically, the patient is young, has no history or signs of hepatocellular disease, and presents with unexplained hepatosplenomegaly or hemorrhage from esophagogastric varices due to portal hypertension. Surgical correction of the portal hypertension may permit long-term survival, and progressive liver failure is rare. The biopsy findings are distinctive: normal masses of liver parenchyma are separated by mature fibrous bands containing networks of bile ducts. The cellular damage, inflammation, and nodular regeneration of cirrhosis are notably absent.

Hepatic Fibrosis Associated with Hereditary Hemorrhagic Telangiectasia (See Also Chap. 347)

Although patients with hemorrhagic telangiectasia may develop posttransfusion viral hepatitis or various forms of cirrhosis, many have multiple asymptomatic telangiectases of the liver and other viscera. In the liver, the telangiectases appear as scattered stellate blood-filled lesions surrounded by patchy areas of fibrosis. Rarely, these may be extensive and confluent, giving a coarsely nodular appearance to the liver and leading to the development of portal hypertension. Liver biopsy is contraindicated in these patients.

MAJOR SEQUELAE OF CIRRHOSIS

Patients with any form of cirrhosis, with its progressive loss of liver cell function and advancing distortion of intrahepatic vasculature, are threatened by three major hazards: *portal hypertension* and its complications of variceal hemorrhage and splenomegaly, disabling *fluid retention* in the form of ascites and edema, and *hepatic coma*. These sequelae of cirrhosis are important because no fewer than one-third of deaths in patients with Laennec's cirrhosis are related to variceal hemorrhage, ascites occurs in 60 to 85 percent of cases of advanced cirrhosis,

and about 50 percent of patients with cirrhosis die in hepatic coma. Other complications or superimposed conditions include portal vein thrombosis and hepatoma (especially in postnecrotic cirrhosis and hemochromatosis).

Portal Hypertension

DEFINITION. The normal adult liver is perfused by about 1,500 ml of blood per min, 60 to 75 percent by way of the portal vein. A balance among portal vein and hepatic artery inflows, hepatic vein outflow, and vascular resistance maintains a fairly constant low pressure within the portal system. Constriction of any major portion of the portal-hepatic venous bed with consequent increase in resistance to blood flow may lead to rising portal venous pressures despite the development of extensive but inefficient collateral channels. All forms of cirrhosis, many infiltrative disorders of the liver, and many nonhepatic diseases that produce obstruction of the hepatic veins or portal vein may be complicated by portal hypertension. Portal hypertension may be defined as persistent portal pressure in excess of 25 to 30 cm of saline, with sluggish flow in major venous trunks, evolution of numerous portal-systemic venous collaterals, and passive congestion of the spleen and other viscera.

PATHOGENESIS. As summarized in Table 328-1, portal

Table 328-1. FACTORS IN THE PATHOGENESIS OF PORTAL HYPERTENSION

I. Increased vascular resistance
   A. Intrahepatic
      1. Cirrhosis
      2. Infiltrations (e.g., tumors, sarcoidosis)
      3. Polycystic disease
      4. Schistosomiasis
   B. Portal vein
      1. Thrombosis
      2. Tumor
      3. Infection (pylephlebitis)
   C. Hepatic veins
      1. Thrombosis (Budd-Chiari syndrome)
      2. Veno-occlusive disease
II. Sustained high splanchnic inflow
   A. Splenomegaly
   B. Diffuse AV shunts(?)
   C. Major AV fistulae
III. Inadequate decompression via venous collaterals
   A. Esophageal
   B. Retroperitoneal
   C. Periumbilical
   D. Hemorrhoidal

hypertension results from a combination of *increased resistance to flow, sustained high splanchnic inflow,* and *inadequate collateral decompression.* With few exceptions, however, the primary factor in the development of portal hypertension is *obstruction* of the portal vein, the intrahepatic venous bed, or, rarely the hepatic veins.

Most cases of portal hypertension in the United States are caused by *cirrhosis,* which produces mechanical obstruction of portal venules ("presinusoidal block") and hepatic venules ("postsinusoidal block") by fibrosis, thrombosis, and nodular regeneration. Most clinical studies suggest that 30 to 60 percent of patients with cirrhosis have significant portal hypertension. The second most common cause of portal hypertension is *mechanical obstruction* of the extrahepatic portal vein, usually the result of thrombosis or tumor invasion. *Occlusion of the major hepatic veins* (Budd-Chiari syndrome) or their small intrahepatic branches (as in veno-occlusive disease) may lead to portal hypertension. About 5 to 10 percent of patients with the portal hypertension of cirrhosis have associated *portal vein thrombosis,* an important consideration in planning corrective vascular surgery. Finally, a small but significant number of patients with sustained portal hypertension have patent portal veins and no evidence of cirrhosis or other primary liver disease. Limited studies suggest that minimal sclerosis of the intrahepatic portal venules and, in some instances, associated high hepatic blood flow account for this picture (which may represent the now-discredited Banti's syndrome).

CLINICAL FEATURES. Many patients with portal hypertension of intra- or extrahepatic origin have symptoms or signs related only to the primary disease, and portal hypertension is tolerated without incident for years. Three major clinical consequences of portal hypertension may, however, lead to its recognition: (1) The development of extensive *portal-systemic venous collaterals,* with gastrointestinal hemorrhage; (2) the appearance of *congestive splenomegaly* with hypersplenism; and (3) the onset of episodic stupor or *portal-systemic encephalopathy.*

The *development of collateral channels* between the portal and systemic venous beds is the most characteristic consequence of portal hypertension. Major sites of collateral flow involve dilated veins around the rectum (hemorrhoids), cardioesophageal junction (esophago-gastric varices), and retroperitoneal space and the falciform ligament of the liver (periumbilical or abdominal wall collaterals). Although hemorrhoids bleed frequently and varices of the bowel rupture occasionally, massive hemorrhage from thin-walled varices in the upper stomach and lower esophagous is the most devastating complication of portal hypertension. Variceal bleeding occurs without obvious precipitating cause and presents usually as painless massive hematemesis or melena. Abdominal wall collaterals are helpful clinical signs of portal hypertension and appear as slightly tortuous epigastric vessels that radiate from the umbilicus towards the xiphoid and rib margins. Extreme prominence of these collaterals (so-called *caput Medusae*) is rare. Vascular bruits may be heard over the upper abdomen, the so-called Cruveilhier-Baumgarten syndrome. *Palpable splenomegaly,* the result of passive congestion, fibrosis, and siderosis, is present in most patients with significant and long-standing portal hypertension. Splenic enlargement is usually moderate in degree, but may occasionally reach massive proportions. The absence of a large spleen is not, however, convincing evidence against portal hypertension, and splenic size correlates poorly with the level of portal pressure. As noted in Chap. 350, splenic enlargement may be accompanied by abnormal sequestration and destruction of the circulating blood cells (hypersplenism). Patients with portal hypertension and extensive portal-systemic venous shunting, whether spontaneous or surgical, may experience repeated bouts of *portal-systemic encephalopathy* or *hepatic coma.* These episodes are often precipitated by gastrointestinal hemorrhage.

DIAGNOSIS. Portal hypertension should be suspected in all patients with cirrhosis or other chronic hepatic diseases, in those with unexplained splenomegaly, and in all patients with massive upper gastrointestinal hemorrhage not clearly due to peptic ulcer or intestinal neoplasm. Three diagnostic questions should be answered in these cases. (1) Is portal hypertension present? (2) Is the underlying cause hepatic or extrahepatic? (3) If gastrointestinal hemorrhage has occurred, is a ruptured esophogeal varix the source? The combination of prominent abdominal collateral veins, an enlarged spleen with pancytopenia, and ancillary signs of cirrhosis suggests portal hypertension. One may also obtain a direct measurement of the portal venous pressure by splenic puncture and visualize the portal system by splenoportography (Chap. 324). If no occlusion of the splenoportal trunk is demonstrated by x-ray examination and clinical or laboratory evidence suggests associated liver disease, needle biopsy of the liver should be carried out to define the precise nature of the hepatic lesion. A careful barium swallow with cinefluoroscopy of the esophagus and stomach may demonstrate varices with reasonable certainty (60 to 80 percent) and serves to exclude other lesions as possible sources of bleeding. If the condition of the patient permits, esophagoscopy should be carried out promptly during or after a bout of hematemesis, affording a direct view of the varices and of the bleeding site itself.

TREATMENT. General. Vigorous treatment of patients with fatty liver, early Laennec's cirrhosis, chronic active hepatitis, and other liver disease may lead to a fall in portal pressure and to the disappearance of varices. As a rule, however, portal hypertension caused by established cirrhosis or portal vein occlusion persists, and variceal hemorrhage remains a grave threat. No precise prognosis can be made in individual cases, but clinical studies suggest that over 30 percent of patients with cirrhosis and varices experience a major hemorrhage within 5 years and have an overall mortality of 60 to 80 percent. In contrast, the patient with normal liver function and variceal hemorrhage secondary to portal vein block tolerates episodes of hemorrhage relatively well. Despite technical improvements in surgical methods of portal vein decompression, it seems wise to reserve portacaval shunts for patients who bleed from varices. Limited studies have shown little justification for prophylactic portacaval anastomosis. Several methods of portacaval and splenorenal anastomosis are used, most produce satisfactory decreases in portal pressure, and recurrent variceal hemorrhage is distinctly rare.

Acute Variceal Hemorrhage. Prompt and effective care of the patient with massive hematemesis or melena from a ruptured varix requires coordinated medical-surgical efforts. The basic elements of management include the following:

Quantitative replacement of blood loss is essential to prevent further deterioration of liver function. It is often advisable to use freshly donated blood if massive replacement therapy is required. *Demonstration of esophageal varices, location of the actual bleeding site,* and *exclusion of other causes of gastrointestinal hemorrhage* by endoscopy or radiography are critical. It should not be assumed that known cirrhotics with proven or probable varices are bleeding from the varices, because about one-third of these patients have other potential bleeding sites in the upper gastrointestinal tract. In view of this fact, an "aggressive approach" to diagnosis is clearly indicated.

Temporary control of variceal bleeding may be achieved by vasopressin infusions, gastric cooling, or balloon tamponade. Infusion of 10 to 20 units of vasopressin over a 15- to 30-min period may lead to temporary decrease in variceal hemorrhage by lowering splanchnic blood flow and portal pressure. Transient decreases in cardiac output and effects of this agent on smooth muscles may make the use of vasopressin hazardous to patients with ischemic heart disease. Although the infusions may be repeated every 2 to 4 hr, the effects diminish with time. Insertion and inflation of a gastric cooling balloon has been used but demands special apparatus and careful monitoring to detect rebleeding or aspiration of esophageal contents. The Sengstaken tube or a modified single-balloon tube may be inserted into the stomach, inflated, and attached to traction to provide local compression of the submucosal veins. Although often effective in producing temporary control of massive hemorrhage, this device is difficult to place accurately and is uncomfortable for the patient, and its use is often complicated by rebleeding, esophageal erosions, airway obstruction, or aspiration. Both cooling balloons and Sengstaken tube must be regarded as temporizing measures that should, in most instances, be used to prepare the patient for definitive surgery. Active steps must be taken to *prevent or treat impending hepatic coma* (see page 1557).

Evaluation of liver function and *assessment of operative risk* are important but difficult. No clinical signs or battery of liver function tests can predict accurately the immediate postoperative morbidity and mortality. The severity and "activity" of cirrhosis as judged by needle-biopsy specimen provide the most accurate guide to immediate prognosis. In general, however, patients with compensated or stable cirrhosis have a much more favorable outlook than those with deepening jaundice, ascites, or signs of precoma. Careful dietary and diuretic therapy for 2 or 3 weeks may permit considerable recovery of liver function in the patient with active Laennec's cirrhosis.

In many patients, *semiemergency or elective shunt surgery* may be advisable. The results of many large clinical series indicate that the immediate and long-term mortality depends largely on the hepatic reserve of the patient, because variceal bleeding rarely recurs if a satisfactory portacaval shunt has been established. The type of surgical shunt procedure (i.e., portacaval or splenorenal) often depends on the experience and judgment of the surgeon. Portal decompression itself may correct the pancytopenia of hypersplenism. In infants and in other patients with extensive portal vein disease, effective portal-systemic shunts may be constructed, using other branches of the portal vein and the trunk of the inferior cava. Late complications in patients with functioning portacaval shunts include hepatic coma (15 to 20 percent), peptic ulceration (10 to 15 percent), slight unconjugated hyperbilirubinemia, and, rarely, accumulation of iron within the cirrhotic liver.

Ascites (See Also Chap. 46)

DEFINITION. Ascites, the accumulation of abnormal volumes of fluid within the peritoneal cavity, is a frequent manifestation of cirrhosis and other types of diffuse parenchymal liver disease. The development of ascites is often accompanied by hemodilution, edema, and oliguria. These and other clinical findings reflect the complex abnormalities of electrolyte, water, and protein metabolism that may complicate severe liver disease and other disturbances of the hepatic circulation.

PATHOGENESIS. Ascites is usually demonstrable clinically when 500 ml or more of fluid has accumulated in the peritoneal cavity. It results from disturbances of both local and systemic mechanisms that regulate the passage of fluid and solutes across vascular and serosal membranes. The *local or intraabdominal factors* favoring ascites formation in cirrhosis include the following:

1. *Portal vein hypertension.* Uncomplicated chronic portal hypertension of the extrahepatic type usually is not associated with ascites. However, clinical and experimental studies suggest that portal hypertension plays an important "permissive" role in ascites formation, because the addition of salt retention or hypoalbuminemia usually produces ascites.

2. *Obstruction to hepatic vein radicles.* Postsinusoidal block or diffuse block of the hepatic venous system (by cirrhosis, infiltration disease, or thrombi) leads to ascites formation.

3. *Elevated intrahepatic pressure.* This alteration is typically present in most types of cirrhosis.

4. *Increased flow of hepatic lymph.* Cirrhotic patients with persistent ascites have marked increases in the volume of thoracic duct lymph, and decompression of the thoracic duct (by cannulation or fistula) reduces the ascites. These and other observations suggest that alterations in intrahepatic and hilar lymph flow play a role in the pathogenesis of ascites in cirrhosis.

The most important *systemic factors* include the following:

1. *Increased sodium retention.* Although the exact

mechanism by which hepatic disease initiates increased production of aldosterone is unclear, patients with cirrhosis and ascites have striking secondary aldosteronism and consequently marked sodium retention.

2. *Impaired water excretion.* Patients with ascites have delayed excretion of water loads, a phenomenon thought to be the result of disordered antidiuretic hormone metabolism. This concept is unproven, but many patients have been shown to have decreased renal free water clearance.

3. *Decreased plasma colloid osmotic pressure.* Impaired synthesis of albumin, the serum protein that determines the colloid osmotic pressure, is a major consequence of hepatocellular damage and poor nutrition. In addition, abnormal albumin catabolism and loss of albumin into the intestinal lumen may be present and contribute to the hypoalbuminemia.

DIAGNOSIS. When clinical examination suggests the presence of ascites, a careful and atraumatic aspiration of 50 to 100 ml of fluid from a flank or low midline site should be attempted. Even in the most typical cases of cirrhosis, a sample of ascitic fluid should be examined for its appearance, color, cell count, presence of microorganisms, protein content, and, when appropriate, presence of malignant cells.

TREATMENT. With rare exceptions, ascites produced by diffuse liver disease disappears as the underlying process resolves. Therefore, the *major therapeutic objective is to improve liver function.* In addition, dietary and drug therapy designed to control the local and systemic factors involved in ascites production may be required. These regimens are usually successful if the patient is cooperative and the underlying hepatic disease is not far advanced. Sodium retention may be minimized by the use of a *low sodium diet* (less than 500 mg sodium per day). *Drug therapy* should include diuretic agents that antagonize the action of aldosterone, such as spironolactones, and agents that decrease proximal renal tubular absorption of sodium, such as chlorothiazide. Hypokalemia should be avoided. The abnormal water retention is best treated by *fluid restriction* during phases of active ascites formation.

Infusions of *mannitol* may induce transient osmotic diuresis and the administration of *salt-poor albumin* may produce temporary elevations of the plasma colloid osmotic pressure, but neither method is especially effective or practical. Both agents are distributed rapidly within the vascular and ascitic fluid spaces, and the effective increase in water transport from the abdomen into the plasma and then to the kidney is short-lived. In addition, repeated infusions of osmotically active substances may lead to significant elevations of portal venous pressure and therefore increase the hazard of variceal hemorrhage.

"*Therapeutic*" *paracentesis* should be avoided because major hemodynamic changes, altered renal function, and significant protein loss are likely to occur. The intravenous infusion of ascitic fluid removed by paracentesis, while theoretically avoiding some of these complications, has limited usefulness in clinical practice. *Surgical procedures* designed to overcome intractable ascites are rarely required. However, since the creation of a portacaval shunt for treatment of variceal hemorrhage often leads to loss of ascites, such surgery has been carried out in the rare case with "intractable ascites."

Hepatic Coma

DEFINITION. Hepatic coma (hepatocerebral intoxication, portal-systemic encephalopathy) is a complex syndrome characterized by disturbances in consciousness, fluctuating neurologic signs, asterixis or "flapping tremor," and distinctive electroencephalographic changes. This metabolic disorder of the nervous system may appear in the course of acute or chronic hepatocellular disease or as a complication of portal-systemic venous shunting. It may be *acute* and self-limiting or *chronic* and progressive.

DIAGNOSIS. The recognition of hepatic coma depends on four major elements. (1) The patient should have evidence of advanced hepatocellular disease, extensive portal-systemic collateral shunts, or both. The liver disease may be acute and massive, as in toxic or fulminant viral hepatitis, or chronic and advanced, as in cirrhosis. The portal-systemic venous shunts, which must permit a significant portion of the portal blood to bypass the liver, may be either *spontaneous* (e.g., naturally developing collaterals) or *surgical* (e.g., large portacaval anastomoses). Most patients who develop hepatic coma have, in fact, elements of both liver disease and portal-systemic shunting. (2) Disturbances of awareness and mentation are characteristic, and forgetfulness and confusion progress to stupor and finally to deep coma. (3) Mental changes are accompanied by shifting combinations of neurologic signs, which include rigidity, hyperreflexia, extensor plantor signs, and, terminally, seizures. A peculiar "flapping tremor" (more correctly termed asterixis), a nonrhythmic lapse in position of extremities, head, and trunk, is often seen in precoma and in advancing hepatic coma but may disappear as the patient lapses into an unresponsive state. This neurologic picture is nonspecific, however, and is encountered also in patients with uremia, ventilatory failure, and other forms of metabolic brain disease. (4) Most patients with the clinical features of hepatic coma have characteristic symmetrical, high-voltage, slow-wave (2 to 5 cps) patterns on the electroencephalogram. *Fetor hepaticus,* a unique musty odor of the breath and urine, may be noted in patients with hepatic coma and also those with an extensive collateral circulation. Several clinical variants of the "classic" syndrome of hepatic coma have been recognized. *Chronic progressive hepatocerebral degeneration,* which may develop in patients with stable liver disease or with portacaval anastamoses, is characterized by a slow decline in intellectual function, cerebellar ataxia, tremor, and choreoathetosis. Isolated signs of *myelopathy,* including spasticity and hyperreflexia of the legs, may antedate the other elements of hepatic coma by several months. Both of these conditions must be distinguished from other nonhepatic causes of deranged nervous system function, as well as from Wilson's disease.

PATHOGENESIS. No single biochemical or physiologic defect has been shown to be the actual cause of hepatic coma. Most studies have shown that hepatic coma and its associated disorders of cerebral function result from (1) the shunting of portal blood directly into the systemic circulation, so that the blood largely bypasses the liver; and (2) severe hepatocellular damage and dysfunction. Both circumstances have a common result: nitrogenous substances absorbed from the intestines are not metabolized by the liver before reaching the cerebral circulation. Ammonia is one such compound, and many patients with hepatic coma have elevated systemic arterial and venous blood levels of ammonia, so-called *ammonia intoxication.* Hyperammonemia is most often found in patients with portal-systemic venous shunting and in hepatic cell failure.

Undoubtedly, "toxic" substances other than ammonia are involved in the genesis of hepatic coma. The administration of methionine to patients with portal-systemic shunts has been shown to precipitate stupor or coma in the absence of hyperammonemia. The liver is believed to produce substances that are essential for normal brain metabolism, and in liver failure these may be reduced. Experimental studies have shown that administration of cytidine and uridine delays the onset of hepatic coma in hepatectomized animals, but these observations have not been confirmed in human studies. Decreased cerebral oxygen uptake and impaired intermediary metabolism of glucose in the brain are common but nonspecific features of hepatic coma.

Most patients with recurrent or progressive forms of hepatic coma have distinctive bandlike cerebral cortical necrosis with glial hyperplasia. These findings suggest that the syndrome may progress from a functional to a structural or irreversible phase.

TREATMENT. Early recognition and prompt treatment of progressive hepatic coma are essential because patients in profound coma respond poorly to all forms of therapy and are vulnerable to the added hazards of coma itself. Slight confusion, deterioration in self-care and handwriting, unusual somnolence, and asterixis should be sought for. It may be desirable to grade or classify the stages of hepatic coma since this is often helpful in charting the course of the illness and gauging the effects of therapy. One useful classification is based on the severity of mental and neurologic signs, and ranges from grade I (slight apathy or euphoria with or without objective neurologic signs) to grade V (true coma).

Treatment of the primary liver disease should be instituted whenever possible. In all cases, caloric intake should be maintained at a level of 2000 to 3000 cal per day, and this is best achieved by slow administration of 20 percent glucose solutions through a small nasogastric tube or a plastic catheter placed in a large vein. Attempts should be made to reduce levels of ammonia and other nitrogenous substances in the blood. Protein should be excluded from the diet for 2 or 3 days; laxatives such as magnesium citrate, 30 to 50 cc by mouth, should be administered, and a nonabsorbable antibiotic such as neomycin should be given in doses of 8 to 12 Gm orally per day to minimize intestinal production and absorption of ammonia; metabolic alkalosis and hypokalemia should be corrected; bleeding into the gastrointestinal tract should be controlled or minimized by appropriate means.

Factors or conditions that may complicate or potentiate coma should be corrected. These include anemia, systemic infections, alkalosis, hyponatremia, hypokalemia, and hypoglycemia. Opiates, sedatives, and diuretic agents should be avoided if possible.

Exchange blood transfusion has been introduced as a method of possibly saving some patients with hepatic coma due to massive hepatic necrosis. Other approaches under investigation include heterologous liver perfusion, cross circulation, and hepatic homotransplantation.

Chronic encephalopathy or *episodic coma* may respond to combinations of prolonged protein restriction (30 to 40 Gm per day) and small (2 to 4 Gm) daily doses of neomycin. Rarely, patients who are incapacitated by chronic neuropsychiatric symptoms may require surgical procedures that are designed to "isolate" the colon and thereby reduce ammonia production. Ileosigmoidostomy and colonic exclusion have been effective in some cases.

REFERENCES

Laennec's and Postnecrotic Cirrhosis

Baggenstoss, A. H.: Postnecrotic Cirrhosis: Morphology, Etiology and Pathogenesis, in H. Popper and F. Schaffer (Eds.), "Progress in Liver Diseases," Vol. I, New York, Grune and Stratton, Inc., 1961.

Leevy, C. M.: Clinical Diagnosis, Evaluation and Treatment of Liver Disease in Alcoholics, Fed. Proc., 26:1474, 1967.

MacDonald, R. A., and G. K. Mallory: The Natural History of Postnecrotic Cirrhosis, Am. J. Med., 24:334, 1958.

Powell, W. J., and G. Klatskin: Duration of Survival in Patients with Laennec's Cirrhosis, Am. J. Med., 44:406, 1968.

Shear, L., J. Kleinerman, and G. J. Gabuzda: Renal Failure in Patients with Cirrhosis of the Liver. I. Clinical and Pathologic Characteristics, Am. J. Med., 39:184, 1965.

Stone, W. D., N. R. K. Islam and A. Paton: The Natural History of Cirrhosis, Quart. J. Med., 37:119, 1968.

Biliary and Other Types of Cirrhosis

Carter, R. A. and S. Shaldon: The Liver and Schistosomiasis, Lancet, 2:1003, 1959.

Datta, D. V. and S. Sherlock: Cholestyramine for Long-term Relief of Pruritus Complicating Intrahepatic Cholestasis, Gastroenterology, 50:323, 1966.

Doniach, D., I. M. Roitt, J. G. Walker, and S. Sherlock: Tissue Antibodies in Primary Biliary Cirrhosis, Active Chronic (Lupoid) Hepatitis, Cryptogenic Cirrhosis and Other Liver Diseases and Their Clinical Implications, Clin. J. Immunol., 1:237, 1966.

Kanter, F. S., and G. Klatskin: Serological Diagnosis of Primary Biliary Cirrhosis: A Potential Clue to Pathogenesis. Trans. Assoc. Am. Physicians, 80:267, 1967.

Kerr, D. N. S., C. V. Harrison, S. Sherlock and R. N. Walker: Congenital Hepatic Fibrosis, Quart. J. Med., 30:91, 1961.

Paronetto, F., F. Schaffner and H. Popper: Immunocytochemical and Serologic Observations in Primary Biliary Cirrhosis, New Engl. J. Med., 271:1123, 1964.

Sherlock, S.: Primary Biliary Cirrhosis (Chronic Intrahepatic Obstructive Jaundice), Gastroenterology, 37:574, 1959.

Portal Hypertension and Ascites

Baker, L. A., C. Smith, and G. Lieberman: The Natural History of Esophageal Varices, Am. J. Med., 26:228, 1959.

Conn, H. O., and W. W. Lindenmuth: Prophylactic Portacaval Anastamosis in Cirrhotic Patients with Esophageal Varices, New Engl. J. Med., 279:725, 1968.

Mikkelsen, W. P., H. A. Edmondson, R. L. Peters, A. G. Redeker, and T. B. Reynolds: Extra- and Intrahepatic Portal Hypertension without Cirrhosis, Ann. Surg., 162:602, 1965.

Sherlock, S., and S. Shaldon: The Etiology and Management of Ascites in Patients with Hepatic Cirrhosis: A Review, Gut, 4:95, 1963.

Hepatic Coma

Adams, R. D.: The Encephalopathy of Portacaval Shunt (Eck Fistula), in H. Popper and F. Schaffner (Eds.): "Progress in Liver Diseases," Vol. II, New York, Grune and Stratton, Inc., 1965.

Gabuzda, G. J.: Ammonium Metabolism and Hepatic Coma, Gastroenterology, 53:806, 1967.

Victor, M., R. D. Adams, and M. Cole: The Acquired (Non-Wilsonian) Type of Chronic Hepatocerebral Degeneration, Medicine, 44:345, 1965.

Zieve, L.: Pathogenesis of Hepatic Coma, Arch. Intern. Med., 118:211, 1966.

329 TUMORS OF THE LIVER
William A. Tisdale
and Kurt J. Isselbacher

PRIMARY CARCINOMA

Carcinomas arising within the liver may be of liver cell (hepatoma), duct cell (cholangioma), or mixed origin. In most series hepatomas account for 80 to 90 percent. There is, however, little purpose in distinguishing between the two types, since both may be found in different parts of the same tumor and the clinical course is the same.

INCIDENCE AND EPIDEMIOLOGY. Primary liver cancers account for only 1 to 2 percent of malignant tumors in North and South America and in Europe. However, in parts of Africa and Asia they comprise 20 to 30 percent of all malignant conditions. Liver carcinoma is two to four times more frequent in men than in women, with the peak incidence occurring in the fifth and sixth decades of life.

The actual cause of hepatic cancer is unknown, but three observations are noteworthy: (1) about 75 percent of hepatomas and 20 to 50 percent of cholangiomas are found in association with cirrhosis; (2) hepatomas occur in 10 to 15 percent of cases of postnecrotic cirrhosis and hemochromatosis but are relatively uncommon develop-

ments in patients with Laennec's cirrhosis; (3) certain known hepatic carcinogens, such as aflatoxins, are present in foodstuffs in some parts of the world, such as Africa and Asia where one also finds a very high incidence of hepatoma.

CLINICAL FEATURES. Hepatic cancers often may escape clinical recognition during life. This is because they often occur in patients with an underlying cirrhosis and the patient's symptoms and signs may initially simply suggest a progression of the underlying liver disease. There are other clinical features often associated with hepatic carcinoma which should alert the clinician to the diagnosis: (1) pain, usually moderate in degree and localized to the upper abdomen or the right side of the chest, is a major complaint in more than half the cases; (2) profound weakness and weight loss are quite common; (3) tense ascites, often with rapid onset, is common, and the fluid is bloody in about 20 percent of the cases; (4) persistent fever unrelated to sepsis occurs in about 40 to 50 percent of cases; and (5) an enlarged or enlarging liver, often with palpable masses, is noted in over one-half of the cases. The presence of a friction rub over the liver should strongly suggest the presence of an underlying tumor. There are also rare metabolic features of hepatomas such as hypoglycemia, erythrocythemia, endocrine changes, such as precocious puberty, acquired porphyria, hypercalcemia, and dysglobulinemia.

Anemia, leukocytosis, moderate Bromsulphalein (BSP) retention, and elevated alkaline phosphatase levels are common laboratory findings.

DIAGNOSIS. The clinical features outlined above should suggest the possibility of primary carcinoma of the liver. Liver scintiscans may document the presence of one or more hepatic masses but unfortunately may not distinguish between primary and metastatic liver tumors and cannot prove the existence of a solitary and possibly resectable lesion. Celiac axis angiography may show distortion of vessels or "tumor blushes," but this technique may not distinguish primary cancer from metastatic disease; occasionally cirrhosis may produce a similar radiologic picture (except for the blushes).

A unique "fetal" alpha-1 globulin is found in a certain percentage of cases with hepatoma. The protein is detected immunologically by the double-gel diffusion technique. Its presence is diagnostic, and it does not occur in other forms of chronic liver disease or other types of malignancy (except occasionally in embryonal teratoblastomas). It has been found in the serum of 50 to 80 percent of hepatoma patients in Africa, but of white patients, only 25 to 30 percent have shown a positive test.

Needle biopsy of the liver is helpful, especially if the biopsy is taken in the area of a palpable nodule. False negatives may occur if the liver biopsy is simply performed in a routine manner using the intercostal approach. Cytologic examination of ascitic fluid rarely affords a specific diagnosis. For these reasons peritoneoscopy or laparotomy with open liver biosy is often required. This direct approach has the additional advantage of selecting the rare patients who are suitable for partial hepatectomy.

The course of the disease is usually rapid, and most patients die within 6 to 12 months from gastrointestinal hemorrhage, hepatic failure, or infection.

MANAGEMENT. If the patient is young, is in good general health, and has no obvious extrahepatic involvement, solitary hepatic lesions may be excised or partial hepatectomy carried out. Chemotherapy, particularly by regional perfusion of the hepatic artery, must be considered but is usually not helpful. It is possible that in the future liver transplantation may prove to be of value.

BENIGN TUMORS OF THE LIVER

These tumors are very rare. Hemangiomas, single or multiple, are the most common of the benign tumors. They are usually single and small but occasionally may be multiple or large. Clinically a vascular hum may be heard over the tumor in the liver. Needle liver biopsy is contraindicated if the diagnosis is suspected. Splenic venography, celiac arteriography, and scintillation scanning show a filling defect in the liver. Treatment is not usually indicated, and attempts at surgical removal are associated with difficulties, and if the tumor is diagnosed at laparotomy, it is best not to remove it.

Other benign tumors include hamartomas, adenomas, and benign cholangiomas.

METASTATIC TUMORS OF THE LIVER

Metastatic malignant tumors of the liver are common in clinical practice, probably ranking second only to cirrhosis as a cause of fatal liver disease. In the United States the incidence of metastatic carcinoma is at least twenty times greater than that of primary carcinoma. Hepatic metastases have been reported at autopsies in 30 to 50 percent of patients dying from malignant disease.

PATHOGENESIS. The liver is uniquely vulnerable to invasion by tumor cells. Its size, its high rate of blood flow, and the double perfusion by hepatic artery and portal vein combine to make it the most common site of metastases except for lymph nodes. In addition experimental studies suggest that local tissue factors appear to support the growth of metastatic implants. Virtually all types of neoplasms except those primary in the brain may metastasize to the liver. The most common primary tumors are those of the gastrointestinal tract, lung, or breast, melanomas, and lymphoma. Less common are metastases from tumors of the thyroid, prostate, and skin.

CLINICAL FEATURES. Most patients with metastatic malignancy of the liver present with (1) symptoms referable only to the primary tumor, asymptomatic hepatic involvement being discovered in the course of clinical evaluation; (2) nonspecific systemic symptoms of weakness, weight loss, fever, sweats, and loss of appetite; or (3) localizing features that indicate active hepatic disease—notably, abdominal pain, ascites, or jaundice.

Most patients with significant metastatic liver involvement have suggestive clinical signs: about two-thirds have hepatic enlargement; many have localized induration or tenderness of the liver (although palpable nodules are uncommon); signs of portal hypertension

may be present; a friction rub may be found in about 10 percent of cases, usually over tender areas of the liver. Jaundice occurs in 25 percent but is rarely an early or prominent feature.

Liver function changes are frequent but often nonspecific, reflecting the effects of fever, wasting, and therapy as well as neoplastic liver damage. Increased serum alkaline phosphatase, moderate to marked BSP retention, and moderate elevation of transaminase levels are most common. Two of these three tests are abnormal in about 80 percent of cases.

DIAGNOSIS. Evidence of metastatic invasion of the liver should be sought actively in any patient with a primary malignancy, especially of the lung, gastrointestinal tract, or breast, before therapy is undertaken. Serial studies of liver function and hepatic scintiscans may provide presumptive answers, but needle biopsy of the liver is usually indicated, affording positive diagnoses in 60 to 80 percent of cases with established metastases. Serial sectioning of specimens and repeat biopsies may increase the diagnostic yield by 10 to 15 percent. Liver biopsy may, on occasion, be the first and only proof of widespread malignancy when the primary tumor is occult.

TREATMENT. Most metastatic carcinomas respond poorly to all forms of treatment, which is usually palliative. Surgical removal of a large metastasis is occasionally feasible. Systemic chemotherapy using such drugs as methotrexate and fluorouracil may be resorted to and in some cases would appear to prolong life by a matter of several months. Metastases of the primary tumors from the colon and rectum seem more responsive to such chemotherapy than others.

REFERENCES

Alpert, M. E., J. Uriel, and B. deNechaud: Alpha-1 Fetoglobulin in the Diagnosis of Human Hepatoma, New Eng. J. Med., 278:984, 1968.

Alpert, M. E., and C. S. Davidson: Mycotoxins: A Possible Cause of Primary Carcinoma of the Liver, Am. J. Med., 46:325, 1969.

Fenster, L. F., and G. Klatskin: Manifestations of Metastatic Tumors of the Liver: A Study of 81 Patients Subjected to Needle Biopsy, Am. J. Med., 31:238, 1961.

MacDonald, R. A.: Primary Carcinoma of the Liver: A Clinicopathologic Study of 108 Cases, Arch. Intern. Med., 99:266, 1957.

Schonfeld, A., D. Babbott, and K. Gundersen: Hypoglycemia and Polycythemia Associated with Primary Hepatoma, New Engl. J. Med., 265:231, 1961.

Sherlock, S.: Hepatic Tumors, chap. 25, in "Diseases of the Liver," 4th ed., Philadelphia, F. A. Davis Company, 1968.

330 SUPPURATIVE DISEASE OF THE LIVER

William A. Tisdale

Suppurative diseases of the liver include isolated or disseminated microabscesses or macroabscesses of bacterial, fungous, or amebic origin. The infecting agents, single or multiple, reach the liver by way of the portal vein, hepatic artery or bile ducts, or, less often, by direct trauma or extension from adjacent structures. Such suppurative conditions are amazingly rare in clinical practice in view of the frequent occurrence of transient bacteremias, biliary obstruction, and abdominal infections. This resistance to sepsis reflects the unique capacity of the liver to trap and destroy organisms. Changes in the pattern of suppurative diseases of the liver in recent years are the result of the widespread use of antibiotics, improved surgical techniques, and the increasing incidence of abdominal trauma.

PYOGENIC (NONAMEBIC) LIVER ABSCESS

Many septic processes may be complicated by self-limited and undiagnosed microabscesses of the liver, necropsy examination of livers from patients dying with bacteremic states often showing multiple tiny foci of bacteria, cell loss, and inflammation. Some focal lesions tend to progress to gross liver abscesses on occasion and produce distinctive clinical features.

ETIOLOGY. Infected obstruction of the biliary tract accounts for 30 percent of abscesses, sepsis in organs drained by the portal vein (especially perforated viscera, infected surgical wounds, and colonic disease) for 15 to 20 percent, and general septicemia for approximately 20 percent. A few abscesses arise from penetrating trauma, from blunt trauma with secondary infection, or by extension from contiguous abscesses. A significant number of liver abscesses have no obvious associated or primary lesion, most of these probably resulting from cryptic bowel infections. Multiple abscesses are present in about two-thirds of cases. The infecting agents are usually multiple (70 percent of cases), but the etiologic agents cannot be identified with certainty in other instances. Coliform bacteria, staphylococci, other gram-negative organisms, and streptococci, in order of decreasing incidence, are the most common infecting organisms.

CLINICAL FEATURES. Signs of the associated septic or traumatic process may obscure those of liver abscess. However, persistent, often hectic fever, sweats and chills (recurrent with multiple abscesses), followed by aching pain over the liver, dramatic weight loss, nausea and vomiting, tender enlargement of the liver, and, on occasion, slight jaundice are characteristic of evolving abscesses. Leukocytosis, often in the range of 16,000 to 25,000 cells per cu mm, and nonspecific changes in liver function are common. Elevation and decreased movement of the diaphragm are usually noted on radiologic examination. Liver scans will help localize large lesions but should not be considered absolute guides to diagnosis or treatment.

MANAGEMENT. Proved or probable pyogenic liver abscesses should be treated vigorously by medical and surgical means. Blood, wound exudates, or T-tube drainage fluids should be cultured aerobically and anaerobically in an attempt to identify the infecting organisms and to determine their antibiotic sensitivity. Empiric treatment with bactericidal antibiotics effective against both gram-positive and gram-negative organisms should be instituted until specific pathogenic organisms have been isolated. In most cases the combination of a penicillinase-resistant penicillin (e.g., methicillin, 6 to 12 Gm intravenously daily) and kanamycin (1 to 2 Gm intramuscularly daily) are satisfactory. It must be emphasized that antibiotics alone are not enough and well-established abscesses, after they are localized, must be drained surgically. Simple aspiration is not sufficient. Multiple drainage may be needed.

AMEBIC ABSCESS

Although less common in North America than pyogenic liver abscess, "hepatitis" (cellulitis) and abscesses due to *Endamoeba histolytica* occur throughout the world, complicating symptomatic intestinal amebiasis in 10 percent of cases. More often, however, clinical evidence of evolving amebic abscess appears without antecedent intestinal symptoms. Most abscesses are single and occur in the right lobe of the liver.

The clinical presentation is often more gradual and less dramatic than that of pyogenic abscess, but the signs, symptoms, and laboratory features are similar. Amebic abscesses often produce anterior and medial elevations of the right diaphragm by x-ray. The most reliable and helpful serologic aid in the detection of extraintestinal amebiasis is the indirect hemagglutination test.

The trophozoites of *E. histolytica* are rarely demonstrated by stool examination and sigmoidoscopy in patients with amebic liver abscesses. For this reason, if the diagnosis is suggested by the clinical features and a positive indirect hemagglutination test, antiamebic therapy should be instituted. The combination of emetine (60 mg subcutaneously daily for 10 days) and chloroquine (1 Gm orally daily for 2 days and 0.5 Gm daily for 20 days) usually produces a prompt remission and obviates the need for surgical drainage of most abscesses (see Chap. 136).

REFERENCES

Cronin, K.: Pyogenic Abscess of the Liver, Gut, 2:52, 1961.

Lamont, N. M., and N. R. Pooler: Hepatic Amebiasis, Quart., J. Med., 27:389, 1958.

Milgram, E. A., G. R. Healty, and I. G. Kagan: Studies on the Use of the Indirect Hemagglutination Test in the Diagnosis of Amebiasis, Gastroenterology, 50:645, 1966.

Sheehy, T. W., L. F. Parmley, G. S. Johnston, and H. W. Boyce: Resolution Time of an Amebic Abscess, Gastroenterology, 55:26, 1968.

Stokes, J. F.: Cryptogenic Liver Abscess, Lancet, 1:355, 1960.

331 INFILTRATIVE AND METABOLIC DISEASES AFFECTING THE LIVER

Kurt J. Isselbacher and
William A. Tisdale

Many disseminated, systemic, or metabolic diseases involve the liver in a diffuse manner by the infiltration of abnormal cells or the accumulation of chemical substances or metabolites. Although infiltrative diseases may vary widely in their etiology and extrahepatic manifestations, the findings in the liver may be quite similar. Generalized enlargement and firmness of the liver, gradual and nonspecific deterioration of liver function, and, less often, signs of portal hypertension or ascites formation are typical features of this group of diseases. Differential diagnosis by clinical means may be difficult on occasion, but the diffusely infiltrated liver provides an excellent source of tissue for diagnostic and investigative purposes.

The infiltrative process may involve one or more of the structural components of the liver: the hepatocytes, the Kupffer cells and other elements of the reticuloendothelial system, the interstitial tissue, or the blood vessels.

LIPID INFILTRATIONS

Fatty Liver

Slight to moderate enlargement of the liver due to diffuse infiltration of liver cells by neutral fat (triglyceride) is a common clinical and pathologic finding. Although minimal fatty changes are often transient and have no clinical significance, persistent or extensive fatty infiltration may produce dysfunction and symptoms that require careful evaluation.

ETIOLOGY. The major causes of fatty liver encountered in clinical practice depend on the age, geographic location, and metabolic-nutritional status of the patient population. *Chronic alcoholism* is the most common cause of fatty liver in this country and other countries with a high alcohol intake. Over three-quarters of patients in most series are heavy drinkers, and the severity of fatty involvement seems roughly proportional to the duration and degree of alcoholic excess. *Protein malnutrition*, especially in infancy and early childhood, accounts for most cases of severe fatty liver in the tropical zones of Africa, South America, and Asia. The hepatic changes may be associated with other clinical and pathologic features of kwashiorkor. Patients with adult-onset *diabetes mellitus*, especially those who are overweight and have poorly controlled disease, may have fatty livers. *Obesity* is commonly associated with fatty infiltration of the liver, which often recedes as weight reduction occurs. In many *chronic illnesses*, especially those complicated by impaired nutrition or malabsorption, increased fat is found in liver cells. Thus, patients with ulcerative colitis, chronic pancreatitis, or protracted heart failure frequently have moderately fatty livers at the time of death.

Acute fatty changes, often associated with clinical symptoms and overt liver cell necrosis, may be produced by a number of *hepatotoxic agents*. Carbon tetrachloride intoxication, DDT poisoning, and ingestion of substances containing yellow phosphorus result in severe fatty liver changes. Acute and prolonged alcohol ingestion may also be considered in this category, since it may be associated with a rapidly enlarging and fat-laden liver. Two types of acute fatty liver deserve special comment: *Acute fatty liver of pregnancy*, a rare but often fatal condition seen during the third trimester of pregnancy, is characterized by nausea, vomiting, and abdominal pain, renal failure, and coma. *Massive tetracycline therapy*, in amounts of 3 to 12 Gm administered intravenously, has resulted in acute fatty liver and fatal hepatic coma in some pregnant patients.

PATHOGENESIS. The hepatic lipid deposits, which consist largely of triglycerides and lesser amounts of phospholipid and cholesterol, appear as vacuoles of varying size within the cytoplasm of liver cells. In extreme cases, every liver cell is involved, and lipids comprise up to 30 to 40 percent of the total liver weight.

The biochemical mechanisms leading to hepatic triglyceride accumulation have been described in Chap. 323. Fatty infiltration has been produced in experimental animals by a variety of toxic agents and drugs, such as alcohol, carbon tetrachloride, and orotic acid. Dietary deficiencies, such as choline deficiency, readily lead to increased fat in the liver in the rat. However, with few exceptions these experimental studies cannot be used directly to explain the pathogenesis of fatty liver in clinical disease. Moderate doses of ethanol may produce both acute and chronic fatty changes in human subjects, probably by its direct effects on hepatic triglyceride and fatty acid metabolism (Chap. 323). Protein deficiency seems to account for the fatty liver of kwashiorkor and impaired protein synthesis for the fat accumulation following tetracycline and carbon tetrachloride administration. In diabetes mellitus and in starvation, increased mobilization of fatty acids from adipose tissue may be involved.

CLINICAL FEATURES. A majority of patients with moderate to severe fatty livers have no symptoms. Massive fatty infiltration, especially if it is rapid in onset, may be associated with abdominal pain and anorexia. A firm and generally enlarged liver is present in most cases. Jaundice with features of cholestasis occurs in some alcoholic patients after bouts of heavy drinking.

Bromsulphalein (BSP) retention, hyperbilirubinemia, and elevated levels of serum alkaline phosphatase are characteristic of the acute "obstructive," or cholestatic, phase of alcoholic fatty liver disease. These latter changes may be recurrent, and hence causes of extrahepatic biliary obstruction have to be excluded.

Correction of the underlying nutritional or metabolic disorders leads in most instances to mobilization of the excess liver fat and to complete clinical recovery. Signs of cirrhosis may develop in patients with persistently fatty livers and chronic alcoholism. *There is, however, no evidence that a fatty liver per se leads to cirrhosis.* Sudden death from intercurrent infection or fat embolization to the lungs has been reported.

DIAGNOSIS. The findings of a firm, nontender, and generally enlarged liver with minimal hepatic dysfunction in a patient with chronic alcoholism, malnutrition, poorly controlled diabetes mellitus, or obesity should suggest a fatty liver. Needle biopsy of the liver will demonstrate the increased fat content and possibly the underlying primary disorder.

MANAGEMENT. Attention to nutritional factors, removal of alcohol or offending toxins, and correction of any associated metabolic disorders usually produce recovery. There appears to be no clinical rationale for the use of lipotropic agents such as choline. When indicated, attention should be directed to abstinence from alcohol, careful control of diabetes, weight loss, or correction of intestinal absorptive defects.

Fatty Liver with Encephalopathy (Reye's Syndrome)

This acute illness has been described in children up to twelve years of age. It is characterized by vomiting, progressive central nervous system damage, signs of hepatic injury, and hypoglycemia, and morphologically by extensive fatty vacuolization of the liver and renal tubules. The cause is unknown, although viral and toxic agents have been implicated. Cases have been reported from several countries, infants and children of either sex are affected, and familial occurrences have been described. In fatal cases, the liver is enlarged and yellow, with striking diffuse fatty microvacuolization of cells. Peripheral zonal hepatic necrosis has also been present in some cases. Fatty changes of the renal tubular cells and marked edema and neuronal degeneration of the brain are the major extrahepatic changes.

The onset seems to begin and often follows an upper respiratory tract infection in a previously healthy child. Within 1 to 3 days persistent vomiting occurs together with stupor, which usually progresses rapidly to coma. The liver is enlarged, but *jaundice and clinical signs of hepatic failure are characteristically absent or minimal.* Marked increase in serum transaminase, hypoglycemia, metabolic acidosis, and azotemia are the major findings. Death from cerebral damage occurs in most patients after 2 or 3 days. However, a few children have recovered following the administration of large quantities of glucose and the use of general supportive therapy.

The cause is unknown. Since the disease appears typically to follow apparent upper respiratory tract infections (and in some cases in association with chickenpox), virologic studies have been carried out. Isolations from stool and tissues have included Coxsackie virus, reovirus, ECHO virus 11, and adenovirus type 3, but the presence of these agents may have been coincidental rather than causal.

The condition bears some resemblance to the "vomiting sickness" of Jamaica, in which hypoglycemia and vomiting follow the ingestion of unripe akee fruit containing a hypoglycemic agent (hypoglycin). In this disease the liver contains increased fat but also periportal hepatic necrosis.

Niemann-Pick Disease (See Chap. 350)

This rare heritable disorder, found mainly in Jewish infants, is characterized by the accumulation of sphingomyelin and cholesterol in reticuloendothelial cells of the liver, spleen, marrow, and brain. Hepatomegaly and splenomegaly are present, but jaundice and other evi-

dence of hepatic dysfunction are rare. The liver shows clusters of lipid-filled foamy Kupffer cells. Diagnosis is made by lipid analysis of the tissue.

Gaucher's Disease (See Chap. 350)

Accumulations of large reticuloendothelial cells containing glucocerebrosides (Gaucher cells) in the liver and spleen account for the characteristic moderate to massive hepatosplenomegaly. Rarely, ascites or portal hypertension is produced by compression of the intrahepatic vasculature. The diagnosis may be made readily by liver biopsy and demonstration of the Gaucher cells.

Wolman's Disease

This is a rare familial lipoidosis that affects infants, producing hepatosplenomegaly and stippled calcification of the adrenal glands. Liver biopsy specimens show clusters of foam cells (reticuloendothelial cells filled with cholesterol ester and triglycerides), hepatocytes containing fat, and patchy fibrosis.

Other rare disorders of lipid metabolism may be associated with hepatomegaly and increased fat in the liver. These include abetalipoproteinemia (Chap. 113), Tangier disease (Chap. 113), and Fabry's disease (Chap. 113).

HEPATIC GLYCOGEN ACCUMULATION

Diabetic Glycogenosis

Hepatic enlargement caused by distension of liver cells with glycogen is present in some poorly controlled and often juvenile diabetic patients. Ketoacidosis and vigorous insulin therapy may further enhance hepatic enlargement and glycogen deposition. In the absence of cirrhosis, the hepatomegaly usually decreases with careful control of the diabetes.

Glycogen Storage Disease (See Chap. 111)

The normal liver contains 1 to 5 percent glycogen (by weight). In type I, II, and VI hereditary glycogen storage disease increased amounts of glycogen (and fat) are found. Types III and IV are associated with derangements of glycogen structure, and cirrhosis may be present. Enzymatic and chemical analysis of liver tissue is usually needed for diagnosis.

GALACTOSEMIA (See Chap. 112)

Hepatic changes are common in patients with unrecognized or untreated galactosemia. In the early weeks of life fatty infiltration and cholestasis may be noted in acutely ill infants. If the disease goes unrecognized for months or years, cirrhosis may develop.

OTHER INFILTRATIVE DISEASES

Hurler's Syndrome (See Chap. 399)

This is an uncommon hereditary disease characterized by the widespread tissue deposition of mucopolysaccharide (chondroitin sulfate B and heparin sulfate) in many tissues. The liver is frequently enlarged and firm. Microscopically, Kupffer cells and other macrophages are enlarged and filled with metachromatic granular material. Cirrhosis may be a late complication.

Mastocytosis (See Chap. 400)

Systemic hyperplasia of mast cells, which contain histamine, heparin, and other biologically active substances, frequently leads to the development of hepatosplenomegaly, even in the absence of the skin lesions of urticaria pigmentosa. Liver function is typically normal; in a few instances liver biopsy has shown dense portal tract infiltration by polygonal cells that contain metachromatic granules on staining with toluidine blue.

RETICULOENDOTHELIAL DISORDERS
(See Chaps. 350 and 351)

Moderate to massive hepatomegaly and splenomegaly occur frequently in the various types of leukemia and lymphoma. Jaundice, when present, is usually slight and results from hemolysis. Deep and protracted jaundice is distinctly rare and is caused by obstruction of the intrahepatic or extrahepatic bile ducts by tumor. Liver biopsy specimens reveal portal and sinusoidal infiltrates in most cases of leukemia, but the diagnosis should not be based on hepatic changes alone, for the cellular pattern may be mixed and nonspecific. Liver biopsy may afford a tissue diagnosis in patients with lymphoma or Hodgkin's disease, but the biopsy needle may miss tumor nodules on occasion, and the cellular infiltrates may show a nondiagnostic pattern.

Myeloid metaplasia and other myeloproliferative disorders associated with extramedullary hematopoiesis produce hepatomegaly which may reach huge proportions, especially following splenectomy. BSP retention is the most common functional change. Ascites and portal hypertension, apparently caused by diffuse involvement of portal venules and lymphatics, are rare complications.

GRANULOMATOUS INFILTRATIONS

Systemic granulomatous diseases, including sarcoidosis, miliary tuberculosis, histoplasmosis, brucellosis, schistosomiasis, berylliosis, and drug reactions, produce focal infiltrative hepatic lesions with great regularity. In addition, isolated granulomas of no diagnostic importance may be found occasionally in biopsy specimens in patients with various forms of cirrhosis and hepatitis. The liver infiltrated by granulomas may be slightly enlarged and firm, but hepatic dysfunction is usually limited to BSP retention and increased serum alkaline phosphatase levels. In a few patients with sarcoidosis or brucellosis portal hypertension may develop, and extensive postnecrotic scarring or postnecrotic cirrhosis may follow healing of the granulomatous lesions.

Needle biopsy of the liver reveals granulomas in these conditions with great frequency, often providing the first definite evidence of a systemic or disseminated granulomatous disease. In patients with sarcoidosis, having neither clinical nor laboratory indications of hepatic involvement, needle biopsy is positive in about 80 percent of cases. Portions of the biopsy specimen should be cultured if infections such as brucellosis or tuberculosis are suspected, but special stains rarely demonstrate the infecting organism. Serial sections of the biopsy specimen should be examined if granulomas are not apparent. Individual granulomas are rarely specific in their microscopic appearance, and final diagnosis usually requires other clinical, laboratory, or histologic data.

AMYLOIDOSIS (See Chap. 114)

Systemic amyloidosis, whether primary and idiopathic, familial, or secondary to chronic inflammatory or neoplastic diseases, often involves the liver. Grossly, the liver infiltrated with amyloid is enlarged and pale and rubbery in consistency. Microscopically, the birefringent amyloid deposits appear as homogeneous waxy material within the space of Disse, often being concentrated in the periportal areas with atrophy of adjacent liver cell plates. Selective involvement of the walls of blood vessels, especially of the hepatic arterioles, may be a striking feature of primary amyloidosis. With this possible exception, however, the hepatic lesions are the same in all forms of amyloidosis and are present in 60 to 90 percent of cases.

An enlarged and firm liver is found in about 60 percent of patients, and ascites occurs in advanced stages of the disease in about 20 percent of cases. Jaundice, portal hypertension, and other signs of chronic liver disease are usually absent. Liver function changes, although frequent, correlate poorly with the extent of liver infiltration. Hypoalbuminemia, BSP retention, and elevated serum alkaline phosphatase levels are common.

The presumptive diagnosis of hepatic amyloidosis is often made after examination of biopsy material obtained from other organs. The frequency and diffuse nature of liver involvement by the amyloid infiltrate, however, make needle biopsy a valuable diagnostic procedure. However, bleeding has been described after liver biopsy in some patients, and the procedure must therefore be used with caution.

REFERENCES

Gonnella, J. S., and A. I. Lipsen: Mastocytosis Manifested by Hepatosplenomegaly, New Engl. J. Med., 271:533, 1964.

Guckian, J. C., and J. E. Parry: Granulomatous Hepatitis, Ann. Intern. Med., 65:1081, 1966.

Klatskin, G., and R. Yessner: Hepatic Manifestations of Sarcoidosis and Other Granulomatous Diseases, Yale J. Biol. Med., 23:207, 1950.

Isselbacher, K. J., and D. H. Alpers: Fatty Liver: Clinical and

Biochemical Aspects, in "Diseases of the Liver," 3d ed., L. Schiff (Ed.), Philadelphia, J. B. Lippincott Company, 1969.

Levine, R. A.: Amyloid Disease of the Liver, Am. J. Med., 33:349, 1962.

Reye, R. D. K., G. Morgan, and J. Baral: Encephalopathy and Fatty Degeneration of the Viscera: A Disease Entity of Childhood, Lancet, 2:749, 1963.

Smetana, H. F., and E. Olen: Hereditary Galactose Disease, Am. J. Clin. Pathol., 38:3, 1962.

332 DISEASES OF THE GALLBLADDER AND BILE DUCTS

Americo A. Abbruzzese and Philip J. Snodgrass

THE PHYSIOLOGY OF THE BILIARY SYSTEM AND THE CHEMISTRY OF BILE

Bile formation begins at the microvilli of the bile capillaries, which are formed by the apposition of the cell membranes of the hepatocytes. By a process of active transport, conjugated bile salts, free cholesterol, phospholipids, and conjugated bilirubin are secreted into the lumens of the bile capillaries. Water, sodium, potassium, and chloride are also added to bile by the liver cells. Beginning at the terminal plate of the liver cords, the epithelial cells of the bile ducts contribute water, sodium, and bicarbonate to the bile. In the fasting state the sphincter of Oddi is closed most of the time, and bile passes into the gallbladder, where sodium and chloride are reabsorbed by a process of active transport and water is absorbed along with the sodium chloride, resulting in a fivefold to tenfold concentration of the remaining constituents of bile. Bicarbonate is also reabsorbed within the gallbladder, so that the pH of hepatic bile (7.5 to 7.7) is reduced to a pH range of 5.6 to 7. The daily volume of bile secretion in man averages 600 to 800 ml.

When food is ingested, cephalic vagal stimulation increases bile flow, and when acid and gastric contents, in particular fat, reach the duodenum, the hormonal phase of bile secretion and gallbladder contraction begin. *Secretin* is released from the duodenal mucosa and stimulates the bile duct epithelium to release water and bicarbonate, much as secretin stimulates the ductal cells of the pancreas. Simultaneously, *cholecystokinin*, a hormone which is identical to pancreozymin, is released from the duodenal mucosa and stimulates the gallbladder to contract and the sphincter of Oddi to relax. Such agents as fat or cholecystokinin which empty the gallbladder are called *cholecystogogues*. The bile salts which enter the small intestine are 95 percent reabsorbed in the ileum and return by an enterohepatic circulation to the liver to be excreted again into the bile. Bile salts are the most potent of *choleretics* (agents which increase bile flow). After a fatty meal, 4 to 8 Gm bile salts is excreted into the duodenum; since this is twice the bile salt pool within the liver, the bile salts circulate twice with each meal.

Once the gallbladder has contracted, hepatic bile is excreted steadily into the duodenum until the neural and hormonal stimuli cease with completion of eating and gastric emptying. The sphincter of Oddi then closes, and the gallbladder resumes the concentration and storage of bile. Representative figures for the composition of hepatic and gallbladder bile are summarized in Table 332-1.

Table 332-1. THE COMPOSITION OF HEPATIC AND GALLBLADDER BILE

Constituent	Hepatic bile, percent	Gallbladder bile, percent
Water	97	89
Solids	3	11
Bile salts	0.2–2.0	6
Bilirubin	0.02–0.07	2.5
Cholesterol	0.06–0.16	0.2–0.4
Phospholipids	0.04	0.1–0.4
Neutral fat	0.12	0.3–1.2
Inorganic salts	1.0	0.8

The primary bile acids are synthesized from cholesterol in the hepatic cells; cholic acid (the $3,7,12\text{-}\alpha\text{-hydroxy}$ form) and chenodeoxycholic acid (the $3,7\text{-}\alpha\text{-hydroxy}$ form) are the predominant products in man. These bile acids are then conjugated with glycine or taurine to form *bile salts* (glycocholate, taurocholate, glycochenodeoxycholate, and taurochenodeoxycholate). Compared to bile acids, bile salts are more soluble at an acid pH, better micelle formers in bile and in the intestinal lumen, and better activators of pancreatic lipases. Secondary bile salts are formed in the intestinal lumen by bacterial dehydroxylation of primary bile salts; glycodeoxycholates and taurodeoxycholates ($3,12\text{-}\alpha\text{-hydroxy}$ forms) account for 20 percent of the human bile salt pool.

Bile salts are *amphipathic* (liking both oil and water), i.e., molecules with a polar, hydrophilic surface and a nonpolar, *hydrophobic* surface. Above a critical concentration and temperature they form aggregates of a molecular weight of 16,000 to 40,000, called *micelles*, with their lipid-soluble surfaces facing each other and the hydrophilic hydroxyl groups exposed to the water phase. Such colloidal aggregates in water are clear to the eye. These bile salt micelles are able to take up insoluble amphipaths like cholesterol and hydrated or swelling amphipaths like lecithin to form *mixed micelles*. A phase diagram can be constructed, indicating the amounts of cholesterol which will remain solubilized in micelles at various bile salt and lecithin concentrations when the water phase is held at 90 percent, as in gallbladder bile. Over a wide range of bile salt and lecithin concentrations the maximal amount of cholesterol which can be solubilized is 4 percent by weight; any excess cholesterol is present in crystalline form.

The formation of micelles explains the fact that gallbladder bile is isosmolar with plasma, yet contains very high concentrations of bile salts and sodium. The aggregation of bile salts in micelles reduces their osmotic effectiveness, and, in addition, micelles bind sodium and potassium, removing them from the ionic, osmotically active state. The sodium ion activity in gallbladder bile, measured with a sodium-sensitive electrode, is 148 to 186 mM per liter, whereas the sodium content is 220 to 340 mM per liter. The other ionic constituents of bile are listed in Table 332-2. Bile also contains small amounts of plasma

Table 332-2. THE IONIC CONSTITUENTS OF BILE

Constituent	Hepatic bile, mM/liter	Gallbladder bile, mM/liter
Na^+	174	220–340
K^+	6.6	6–10
Cl^-	55–107	1–10
HCO_3^-	34–65	0–17
Bile salts	28–42	290–340
Ca^{++}	6	25–32
Mg^{++}	0.5	
Osmolality	299 mOsm/liter	299 mOsm/liter

proteins and mucoproteins. Certain dyes and drugs are excreted in the bile and are therefore diagnostically useful; examples are conjugated Bromsulphalein (BSP) or indocyanine green, and iodinated phthalein dyes used to visualize the gallbladder and biliary tree.

SYMPTOMATOLOGY

The primary symptoms of extrahepatic biliary tract disease, pain and jaundice, are caused by obstruction and inflammation. Fever and chills can occur with biliary disorders, even in the absence of pain and jaundice. Nausea and vomiting are reflex phenomena which occasionally dominate the clinical picture. Dyspepsia, flatulence, bloating, and fatty food intolerance have long been considered "the inaugural symptoms of gallbladder disease" (Moynihan, 1908), but the preeminence of these symptoms as hallmarks of gallbladder disease has been undermined by controlled studies. Dyspeptic symptoms are encountered more frequently in patients with normal cholecystograms than in those with abnormal cholecystograms, and patients with histories of fatty food intolerance experience no symptoms when fed meals high in concealed fat. Thus the association of dyspepsia and gallstones seems fortuitous, while fatty food intolerance appears to be a subjective bias rather than a characteristic symptom of biliary tract disease.

PAIN. The alimentary canal develops from midline endodermal cells, and pain emanating from its derivative organs is felt at various levels of the midline. Visceral pain represents a tonic response to the sudden distension of a hollow viscus, the pain fibers being conveyed to the spinal cord along with sympathetic afferents. In the conscious patient gradual elevation of pressure within the common bile duct evokes only vague discomfort, but abrupt elevation of pressure, to identical levels, causes severe epigastric pain. This particular pain has been traditionally called biliary "colic" and is caused by sudden obstruction of the biliary outflow system by stone or spasm. The pattern of biliary colic differs from the paroxysms of pain caused by violent peristalsis of the gut. Intestinal colic waxes to an agonizing peak and then wanes only to recur at intervals of 5 to 10 min. In contrast, biliary colic is abrupt in onset and reaches a level of maximal intensity which may last for several hours. The attack abates as suddenly as it began, leaving a residual soreness. The pain is not intensified by moving about; most patients are restless and may pace the floor.

The most common cause of biliary colic is a gallstone suddenly wedged into the cystic duct. The pain is felt predominantly in the epigastrium but often radiates along the costal margin to the right hypochondrium and inferior angle of the right scapula. Less usual sites of referral are the right shoulder or neck and the left upper quadrant of the abdomen. Tenderness or rigidity, localized to an area overlying the gallbladder, is caused by inflammation of the contiguous parietal peritoneum. In approximately 5 percent of cases with gallbladder disease, inflammation is, as far as can be determined, the sole cause of pain (acalculous cholecystitis).

Sudden and brief occlusion of the distal common bile duct produces acute epigastric pain. However, abrupt and protracted obstruction (calculus) may produce a more complex pain response. As the entire biliary tree distends proximal to the obstruction, additional visceral and somatic sensory receptors are stimulated, causing, in addition to epigastric pain, pain in the right upper quadrant, the right shoulder and neck, or the inferior angle of the right scapula. Gradual stenosis of the common duct is painless: the early pain of carcinoma of the head of the pancreas is due to perineural tumor infiltration and is not caused by the raised intraductal biliary pressure.

JAUNDICE. Mechanical blockage of the common bile duct is followed by jaundice, although there may be a variable lag period before both conjugated and unconjugated bilirubin increase in the blood and tissues. The variability of the interval between obstruction and jaundice depends on the state of the gallbladder mucosa and the distensibility of the gallbladder and bile ducts. Normal gallbladder mucosa can concentrate bile tenfold by absorbing water and electrolytes. When an otherwise normal biliary system is obstructed, these factors stabilize ductal pressure for hours despite the steady flow of hepatic bile into a closed system. Eventually the rate of absorption falls behind that of secretion, the biliary tree becomes maximally distended, and intraductal pressure rises. At a pressure of 23 mm Hg hepatic bile flow is suppressed, and conjugated bilirubin regurgitates into the blood. The rise in the unconjugated serum bilirubin level probably represents impaired uptake into the liver cells. Jaundice may not occur until several days after the block. However, when the gallbladder is absent or diseased, obstruction precipitates these events sooner, and scleral icterus appears within 24 hr.

Common duct stones (choledocholithiasis) occasionally cause persistent jaundice. More commonly, a stone acts as a ball valve, creating intermittent obstruction and a fluctuating bilirubin. An unexplained hyperbilirubinemia (rarely over 5 mg per 100 ml) accompanies some cases of acute cholecystitis without common duct calculi or pancreatitis.

Obstructive jaundice may produce secondary effects such as pruritus, steatorrhea, and bleeding tendencies. Although a good correlation has not been established between the serum level of bile salts and pruritus, bile salts do accumulate on the skin in obstruction and are thought to cause the itching. Steatorrhea and poor hemostasis are due to the exclusion of bile salts from the small bowel. Since conjugated bile salts are essential for the normal digestion and absorption of lipids, their absence causes excessive loss of fat and the fat-soluble vitamins A, D, E, and K in feces. The loss of vitamins A, D, and E are of little clinical consequence unless the obstruction is of long duration (biliary cirrhosis). However, vitamin K deficiency develops rapidly, within 1 to 3 weeks, depressing the synthesis of prothrombin (factor II), proconvertin (factor VII), Christmas factor (factor IX), and Stuart factor (factor X).

FEVER AND CHILLS. Fever is a common symptom of acute cholecystitis but is uncommon in the chronic form. The presence of fever may be due to sterile, obstructive inflammation in some patients, but infection may play a major role in most cases of acute cholecystitis, as bacteria are cultured from 75 percent of the gallbladder specimens or bile. Cultures are positive in less than 50 percent of patients with chronic cholecystitis. Chills and fever represent bacteremia and are usually associated with complications of biliary tract disease such as choledocholithiasis, strictures, and fistulas. When accompanied by pain in the right hypochrondrium, with or without hyperbilirubinemia, fever and chills suggest cholangitis. This pattern suggests that a combination of infection plus incomplete biliary stasis results in cholangitis.

Cancers which obstruct the common bile duct rarely lead to clinical cholangitis, and bile cultures from such patients are usually negative. The reasons for this useful differential fact are unclear, because all cancers for some time will produce only partial ductal obstruction. Partial (stones) or remitting obstruction (some cases of ampullary carcinoma) is occasionally complicated by cholangitis.

BLEEDING. Hemorrhage into the biliary passages (hemobilia) is rare, dramatic, and sometimes lethal. The diagnostic triad is right upper quadrant pain, obstructive jaundice (secondary to clots in the biliary tree), and gastrointestinal bleeding. This typical presentation may be altered by massive bleeding or by slow intermittent blood loss. The biliary system is such an unusual source of gastrointestinal hemorrhage that a diagnosis of hemobilia is seldom made preoperatively; it should be suspected when other causes of bleeding have been eliminated by investigation and exploration. A wide variety of diseases produce hemobilia, most commonly ruptured aneurysms of the hepatic artery or its branches, tumors and inflammatory diseases of the biliary system, trauma (including T-tube pressure necrosis or liver biopsy),

choledocholithiasis, and rarely cholecystitis, with or without stones.

BILIARY TRACT RADIOLOGY

In November, 1923, the gallbladder was opacified for the first time by Graham and Cole using an intravenous iodinated phthalein dye. Prior to this, the diagnosis of gallbladder disease depended entirely upon the demonstration of radiopaque calculi, calcium deposits in the gallbladder wall, and milk of calcium bile or gas within the biliary ducts. Although only one in five gallstones contains enough calcium to be visible on plain abdominal films, oral cholecystography identifies 70 percent of all gallstones. In an additional 20 to 28 percent, nonvisualization of the gallbladder is presumptive evidence of disease. Nonvisualization is defined as failure of the gallbladder to opacify following a second dose of contrast medium. The overall accuracy of oral cholecystography, proved in the operating room, is 90 to 98 percent. Only 3 percent of nonfunctioning gallbladders are normal at operation, and less than 2 percent of gallbladders, normal by cholecystogram, contain stones.

This high level of accuracy requires that certain conditions be satisfied: intestinal motility and absorption must be normal, hepatocellular function must be adequate to excrete the dye, and the serum bilirubin must not be rising or greater than 3 mg per 100 ml. Thirty percent of the nonvisualizing and sixty-four percent of the poorly concentrating gallbladders will opacify normally following the second dose. Small stones may be obscured if the gallbladder still concentrates the dye normally; upright or lateral spot films should be done to avoid this error (Fig. 332-1). A fatty meal, given if stones are not obvious, stimulates gallbladder evacuation and enhances the detection of low-density stones obscured by a heavy concentration of dye. "Failure to contract" or poor concentration of dye has little diagnostic significance. As purer preparations of cholecystokinin become available, a better correlation between contractile function and disease should be possible.

Despite its value in diagnosing gallbladder disease, oral cholecystography yields little information about the hepatic ductal system. Common or hepatic duct stones are present in 15 percent of all patients with cholelithiasis but are identified in only 2 percent by oral cholecystography. In 1953, the availability of sodium iodipamide made possible *intravenous cholangiography*. The larger biliary channels opacify in 10 to 30 min, reaching maximal concentrations at 30 to 40 min, provided liver function is normal. A maximally opacified common duct, with an unimpeded flow of dye into the duodenum, decreases in radiodensity within 60 min. Partial obstruction of the common duct prevents normal emptying and prolongs maximum opacification up to 2 hr. The normal common duct diameter is variable; values greater than 9 to 10 mm are considered abnormal, yet one out of four patients with stones has a common duct less than 10 mm in diameter. The common duct dilates very little (approximately 1 mm) after

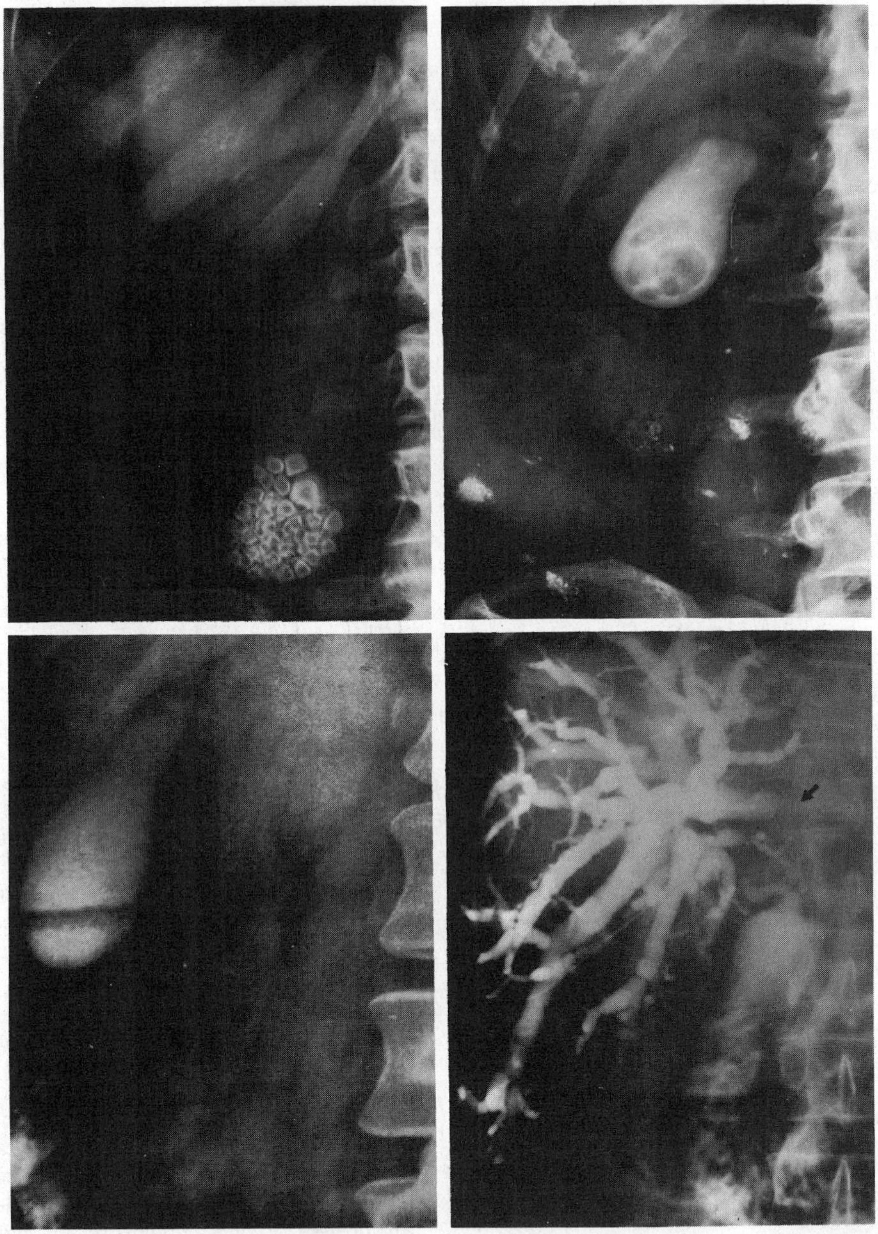

Fig. 332-1. Contrast studies of the biliary tract. *Upper left*, cholelithiasis. Multiple radiopaque stones in a gallbladder with impaired concentrating ability. *Upper right*, cholelithiasis. Nonopaque stones of varying sizes are shown as negative shadows within a gallbladder outlined by concentrated dye. *Lower left*, cholelithiasis. Numerous small stones are grouped in a layer near the bottom of the gallbladder. This picture was taken with the patient standing. Small stones such as these are dispersed when the patient is in a horizontal position and may be difficult to see. *Lower right*, percutaneous transhepatic cholangiogram. The needle, seen in the center of the figure, has punctured a dilated bile duct, and the injected contrast medium shows marked distension of the bile ducts in the right lobe of the liver but no filling of the left lobe. This was due to a bile duct carcinoma which completely blocked the left main hepatic duct and partially occluded the right main duct (*black arrow*), allowing a small amount of dye to enter the duodenum (*lower right*) and the gallbladder, which overlies the duodenal bulb.

cholecystectomy, but a more accurate correlation between duct size and pathologic changes can be obtained if the preoperative dimensions of the common duct are available for comparison. Adverse reactions to intravenous cholangiography include nausea, vomiting, hypotension, and rare anaphylactic reactions. The procedure should be reserved for patients with previous cholecystectomies, nonvisualizing oral cholecystograms, and acute conditions of the upper abdomen.

A third method for exploring the biliary system is

operative cholangiography. The procedure involves the introduction of contrast substance into the gallbladder, cystic duct, or common duct at operation, followed by radiography. Operative cholangiography has been practiced for nearly 40 years, but there is still disagreement that it adds diagnostic accuracy to palpation and probing of the common duct. Stones in the hepatic ducts, however, are best detected with this method.

Finally, *percutaneous transhepatic cholangiography* helps to distinguish extrahepatic from intrahepatic obstruction. A needle is inserted into the liver, and upon entering a dilated intrahepatic duct, bile is drained through a flexible polyethylene catheter and radiopaque dye injected to define the biliary anatomy. (Fig. 332-1). If, after several hepatic punctures, a dilated duct is not entered, the jaundice is assumed to be of hepatocellular origin and a possibly harmful exploration deferred. Percutaneous cholangiography should be performed only on good surgical candidates, because bleeding and/or bile peritonitis forces immediate intervention in 5 percent of patients.

BILIARY TRACT MANOMETRY

Biliary radiomanometry is a diagnostic technique combining simultaneous pressure readings and contrast roentgenographic studies of the gallbladder and bile ducts, and is commonly done during biliary surgical procedures in many European and Latin American countries. Its proponents point out that although cholangiography provides excellent morphologic detail, it is unable to detect motor dysfunction of the ducts or sphincter. Because operative fluoroscopy is impractical, intraluminal manometric pressure curves are substituted. The fact that these pressures are recorded during anesthesia and surgical manipulation of the ducts raises doubt as to their physiologic significance.

GALLSTONES

ETIOLOGY. There is no generally accepted view of the pathogenesis of gallstones. The causes commonly invoked are infection, stasis, and metabolic disturbances in bilirubin, bile salt, cholesterol, or phospholipid excretion. The stone-forming potential of infection has been ascribed to inflammatory injury of the gallbladder mucosa with a loss from the bile of cholesterol-stabilizing bile salts and lecithin. Bacterial growth in bile may increase its glucuronidase activity and hydrolyze bilirubin glucuronide, allowing insoluble calcium bilirubinate to form the nucleus for stone formation. Mucosal damage may also produce proteinaceous debris to serve as a nidus. Stasis as a factor in stone genesis was stressed by Aschoff, who regarded it as "the essential and common cause of all gallstone formation," somehow altering the physicochemical equilibrium of bile so that cholesterol, calcium salts, and bile pigments precipitate.

The principal stone-forming constituents of bile are cholesterol, calcium bilirubinate, and calcium carbonate. Traditionally, gallstones have been classified as pure (10 percent), mixed (80 percent), and combined (10 percent), with the implication that "pure" gallstones are a product of a metabolic derangement or of excessive bilirubin excretion while mixed stones are caused by infection. Modern analytical techniques do not disclose one dominant substance in the center of gallstones but a mixed core of cholesterol, bilirubin, and protein, suggesting a common cause. However, once the nucleus has been established, gallstones grow by accretion, and their final composition reflects the predominant bile constituents at the moment of crystallization. For example, in chronic hemolytic anemias, the stones contain mainly calcium bilirubinate.

The deposition of cholesterol on stones probably results from excessive concentrations of cholesterol or deficient concentrations of bile salts and lecithin which allow cholesterol to crystallize out of the mixed micelles. Bile from gallbladders containing cholesterol stones contains concentrations of these three constituents, which lie outside the micellar zone in phase diagrams. Moreover, vertebrate species whose bile always contains concentrations of bile salts, lecithin, and cholesterol which are optimal for micelle formation do not show spontaneous cholelithiasis. Hamster bile composition, like human bile, lies close to the zone of cholesterol crystallization, and in this species gallstones are induced by simple dietary manipulations.

PREVALENCE. Although autopsy data do not show the true prevalence of gallstones in the population at large, they indicate that approximately 10 percent of adults have gallstones. The age-adjusted prevalence rises to 30 percent in the seventh decade. The aphorism "forty, female, fertile, and fat" may describe certain patients, but it does not characterize a typical gallstone patient. Above twenty years of age, stones are more frequent in women than in men, but the sex difference becomes progressively less after the age of fifty. There is no clear evidence that pregnancy predisposes to the formation of gallstones, but in patients with gallstones symptoms are more likely to develop during pregnancy. When obese, normal-weight, and thin patients are compared, the frequency of gallstones does not differ. Diabetics, at autopsy, have a greater incidence of stones (2:1) than nondiabetics.

SYMPTOMS AND SIGNS. Gallstones may be silent (50 percent) or give rise to excruciating pain, chills, and fever. In between these extremes are a multitude of nonspecific abdominal disturbances which may represent coexisting disease rather than symptomatic gallstones per se. Right upper quadrant pain or tenderness and jaundice are the most clinically useful expressions of cholelithiasis.

DIAGNOSIS. The characteristic manifestation of gallstones is biliary colic. The simplest and most rewarding test of gallbladder function is an oral cholecystogram, provided the necessary criteria are fulfilled. If this and other roentgenologic techniques do not elucidate the diagnosis, some clinicians find duodenal drainage useful. The recovery of cholesterol crystals or, to a lesser degree, bilirubinate granules is important supportive evidence of cholecystic disease in the symptomatic, nonjaundiced patient with a normal BSP excretion.

COURSE AND INDICATIONS FOR SURGICAL TREATMENT. The most important complications of gallstones are acute and chronic cholecystitis. Choledocholithiasis, cholangitis, hepatic abscesses, biliary cirrhosis, empyema, fistulous communication to adjacent viscera, and gallstone ileus are less common hazards.

Biliary colic, with or without associated complications, is an indication for cholecystectomy, the cure rate approaching 90 percent. Patients can live a normal life and eat a normal diet without a gallbladder. Medical management of symptomatic gallstones is unsatisfactory, because low fat diets and anticholinergic drugs do not prevent recurrent attacks. However, therapeutic recommendations for patients with chronic, intermittent "digestive symptoms" who are found to harbor gallstones require deliberation. In many, symptoms will not respond to cholecystectomy despite the presence of stones. As a rule, surgical treatment for cholelithiasis is more likely to benefit patients with "digestive symptoms" and a calculous, nonvisualizing gallbladder than similar patients with a normally opacified gallbladder containing stones. Therefore, a search for coexisting disease which might be responsible for the "digestive symptoms" is mandatory before proceeding to cholecystectomy.

The management of the "silent" gallstone has been debated for one hundred years. Statistics pointing out the various complications of surgically untreated gallstones are compiled from symptomatic patients who have refused surgical treatment. Unfortunately, there are no prospective studies of patients with truly silent and surgically untreated stones. Until such information becomes available, silent stones in patients over sixty should be treated conservatively, since the risks of elective surgical treatment beyond this age exceed the risks of developing complications of the gallstones. If and when biliary colic develops, cholecystectomy is indicated. Diabetics with silent stones are an exception to this policy: diabetics and nondiabetics tolerate elective cholecystectomy equally well, but the morbidity and mortality of emergency cholecystectomy is greater in diabetics.

Although 75 to 80 percent of all primary gallbladder cancers have associated gallstones, less than 3 percent of stone-bearing gallbladders have associated cancers. Nevertheless, there is statistical evidence suggesting that prophylactic removal of asymptomatic stones in patients under forty-five years may prevent cancer. Above age sixty-five, the surgical mortality exceeds the risk of succumbing to cancer.

ACUTE CHOLECYSTITIS

Acute cholecystitis is associated with a gallstone impacted in the cystic duct in 90 to 95 percent of cases. Sudden distension of the gallbladder compromises its blood supply and lymphatic drainage, and commensal bacteria which normally inhabit calculous gallbladders proliferate. Except for the rare patient with *Salmonella*

typhosa infection, the cause of acute cholecystitis without gallstones (acalculous cholecystitis) is obscure.

SYMPTOMS AND SIGNS. Severe right upper quadrant pain, nausea, vomiting, fever, and minimal icterus suggest the diagnosis. However, the pain can be mild, sensed only as an epigastric distress, often relieved by vomiting. If pain radiates to the shoulder or subscapular region, the diagnosis is strengthened. Severe epigastric pain with overt jaundice suggests the complication of choledocholithiasis. Fever is found in over two-thirds of the patients. Local signs include muscle guarding or tenderness in the gallbladder area with discomfort on fist percussion over the liver. A tender mass comprising the swollen gallbladder and adherent omentum is palpable in approximately 50 percent of cases.

LABORATORY FINDINGS AND X-RAYS. The leukocyte count is elevated over a wide range of values, depending on the inflammatory reaction. Low-grade hyperbilirubinemia, increased serum alkaline phosphatase activity, and retention of BSP are often found. Serum glutamic transaminase and lactic dehydrogenase activities are occasionally increased; marked, transient increases in both enzymes suggest common duct stones. Oral cholecystography is of little diagnostic value during the acute attack.

DIAGNOSIS. Pain and tenderness in the right upper quadrant are the most frequent and important diagnostic clues to acute cholecystitis, and a past history of similar disturbances makes the diagnosis nearly certain. The differential diagnosis should include, in decreasing order of the frequency with which they simulate cholecystitis: myocardial infarction, perforated or penetrating ulcer, pancreatitis, right lower lobe pneumonia, intestinal obstruction, and acute right kidney disease. X-rays of the chest and abdomen, electrocardiograms, serum amylase or lipase determinations, and urinalysis will exclude, in the majority of patients, many of the differential diseases mentioned. Intravenous cholangiography has been used to differentiate between acute cholecystitis and pancreatitis. Opacification of the common duct without gallbladder filling favors cholecystitis, whereas opacification of the biliary ducts and gallbladder excludes cholecystitis. However, impaired excretion of the dye and no visualization is common in both diseases. Cancers of the gallbladders and bile ducts have no clinical features which distinguish them from benign gallbladder diseases.

COURSE. Most patients with acute cholecystitis have a complete remission of symptoms within 1 to 4 days, but in approximately 40 percent, if surgically untreated, complications develop. These include gangrene, perforation, empyema, peritonitis, pancreatitis, pylephlebitis, and cholangitis. In the aged patient, cholecystitis is a particularly dangerous disease, because fever and leukocytosis may occur with minimal clinical or chemical evidence of gallbladder disease.

CHRONIC CHOLECYSTITIS

Repeated attacks of mild to severe acute cholecystitis merit the clinical diagnosis of chronic cholecystitis.

Pathologically, the gallbladder mucosa and smooth muscle are partly replaced by fibrous tissue, and biochemically the ability to concentrate bile is impaired. The symptoms are similar to the acute form and range from biliary colic to indolent right upper quadrant and epigastric distress. Low-grade fever and hyperbilirubinemia are common. The diagnosis is confined by failure of the gallbladder to opacify after two doses of contrast medium. At operation, 95 percent of these gallballaders are sclerotic and contain stones. Cholecystectomy will cure 9 out of 10 patients with this clinical presentation. Patients with chronic, vague abdominal discomfort and dyspeptic symptoms are often thought to have chronic cholecystitis despite roentgenographic evidence of a normally functioning gallbladder. Their surgical specimens may show minor mucosal abnormalities, but the patients usually obtain no relief from their symptoms.

CHOLEDOCHOLITHIASIS

Calculi usually reach the bile ducts by expulsion from the gallbladder. This organ can generate an impressive force even in the presence of disease, as illustrated by the phenomenon of disappearing gallstones: 40 or more stones, demonstrated radiographically to be filling the gallbladder and the cystic and common ducts, have been completely disgorged from the biliary tree following typical biliary colic. The incidence of unsuspected common duct stones during routine cholecystectomy, for either acute or chronic disease, is 6 to 26 percent, the figure increasing with age. Common duct stones without concomitant stones in the gallbladder or occurring years after cholecystectomy are not rare. These stones are attributed to common duct stasis. When stasis and increased pressure persist, particularly with stricture or stone impaction high above the ampulla, stone formation may involve the hepatic duct and its branches.

SYMPTOMS AND SIGNS. The symptoms of choledocholithiasis are pain, jaundice, fever, and chills. The pain is steady, is localized to the epigastrium, often radiates to the back and right hypochondrium, and is associated with vomiting. Common duct stones rarely cause persistent obstruction; the jaundice is usually transient and mild, and frequently is missed entirely. Twenty percent of patients with choledocholithiasis have no pain and twenty-five percent no documentation of jaundice. Spiking fevers indicate cholangitis. The most frequently identified organisms are of enteric origin (*Escherichia coli* and *Streptococcus faecalis*). Intermittent fever, chills, and sweats, without pain or clinical jaundice, describes Charcot's hepatic fever. This presentation of common duct stones may be a serious diagnostic problem, because many of the patients maintain relatively good health in the interval between febrile episodes.

Physical signs of common duct stones include jaundice and upper abdominal tenderness. A history of cholecystectomy and common duct exploration does not exclude common duct stones; the frequency of residual calculi is an alarming 10 percent. While most gallbladders associated with choledochal stones are fibrotic and unable to dilate, a distended (but not always palpable) gallbladder occurs with 20 percent of obstructing common duct stones. Intravenous cholangiography will directly identify common duct stones in 50 to 60 percent of cases. When delayed emptying or dilatation of the common duct are included as indirect signs of stones, cholangiography detects 90 percent of cases.

LABORATORY FINDINGS AND X-RAYS. The laboratory features of choledocholithiasis may include leukocytosis, elevated levels of serum bilirubin, alkaline phosphatase, glutamic transaminase, and amylase, and BSP retention. The true incidence with which these biochemical alterations accompany common duct stones is uncertain, since the changes may be fleeting. The transaminases usually do not exceed 300 units. BSP retention is the most sensitive indicator of choledochal calculi but is not as specific for obstruction as the alkaline phosphatase. Striking increases in alkaline phosphatase can occur with minimal increases in bilirubin. One out of four patients will present with an elevated amylase level, presumably due to passage through, or impaction of, a stone in the ampulla of Vater, causing pancreatic edema and occasional hemorrhagic necrosis.

DIAGNOSIS. Common duct stones may be present without clinical, chemical, or radiologic clues to their existence. These asymptomatic cases may progress to suppurative cholangitis, which is often lethal in older patients. A painless common duct stone with jaundice must be differentiated from malignant disease and various forms of hepatitis. Intravenous cholangiography is of little value when the serum bilirubin is rising. If the disease is hepatitis, exploration increases its mortality. Percutaneous transhepatic cholangiography is useful in this situation; failure to enter a dilated duct after five hepatic punctures is presumptive evidence of hepatocellular disease. Liver biopsy may be attempted later.

GALLSTONE ILEUS

Intestinal obstruction secondary to a gallstone is an unusual complication of cholelithiasis and accounts for 2 percent of all small-bowel obstructions. The stone usually lodges at the terminal ileum, the narrowest portion of the normal gut, but stones can become impacted in the pylorus, duodenum, jejunum, or colon. The pathophysiology involves repeated episodes of acute cholecystitis, adhesions to adjacent hollow viscera, and the opening of a cholecystoenteric fistula. Most fistulas develop between the gallbladder and duodenum, but communications into the stomach and colon can occur. Stones less than 3 cm in diameter usually pass through the gut spontaneously.

Gallstone ileus is a disease of the elderly. Early symptoms may be vague and transient, because of intermittent obstruction. Even when the classic symptoms of intestinal obstruction are present, there is often delay before the urgency of the situation is appreciated. The average mortality is 30 percent. Helpful in the diagnosis of gallstone ileus is a history of cholecystitis, abdominal films showing intestinal obstruction with a radiopaque density in the lower abdomen, or x-ray evidence of a changing level of obstruction. Air outlining the biliary tree, in the absence of previous biliary surgical treatment, is virtually pathognomonic of a cholecystoenteric fistula. Meticulous surgical exploration is necessary to exclude additional stones; the recurrence rate of gallstone ileus is 10 to 15 percent.

HYDROPS, EMPYEMA, AND ABSCESS

A gallstone wedged into the cystic duct will cause hydrops or empyema in some 15 percent of cases. In both conditions, the gallbladder becomes distended to several times its normal volume. The trapped bile is sterile in the case of hydrops and infected in empyema. A curious and rare sequela of cystic duct obstruction is the deposition of milk of calcium bile within the gallbladder. It is of clinical importance, because the homogenous distribution of calcium salts produces a shadow compatible with a normal dye-filled gallbladder. Frank perforation of the gallbladder causing generalized peritonitis occurs in less than 1 percent of patients with acute cholecystitis. The omentum and serosa of contiguous viscera localize the perforation early, often producing a palpable mass and a friction rub. Cholecystostomy or cholecystectomy are indicated, depending on the clinical situation.

TREATMENT OF GALLSTONES AND THEIR COMPLICATIONS

Symptomatic cholelithiasis is a surgical disease. The internist's role is to alleviate symptoms and prepare the patient for surgical treatment. Morphine is commonly used to relieve biliary colic despite the fact that it increases intrabiliary pressure. Combined with atropine, the spasmogenic effect of morphine on the sphincter of Oddi is nullified. Meperidine, contrary to earlier opinion, shares with morphine the capacity to produce sphincter spasm. Gastric aspiration is indicated to reduce vomiting and distension and to avoid stimulation of gallbladder contraction by cholecystokinin. Less acutely ill patients respond to analgesics, sedation, and bed rest. Cholangitis should be treated with antibiotics effective in gram-negative infections.

Although intolerance to fats is not related to a specific disease, the restriction of fat in patients with documented gallstones is rational. Cholecystokinin, liberated by fat entering the duodenum, causes a vigorous gallbladder contraction which may precipitate biliary colic. Gastric acid or peptones also liberate cholecystokinin, but fat causes the most prolonged release of the hormone.

The following general rules apply to the surgical management of biliary tract diseases:

1. Acute cholecystitis is ideally treated by cholecystectomy, but the timing of the operation is controversial. Many physicians favor intervention within the first 48 hr. Conservatives, citing the predisposition to traumatic bile duct injury in edematous cholecystitis, wait 1 to 3 weeks unless the patient deteriorates.

It is prudent not to attempt cholecystectomy with impending perforation or necrosis of the gallbladder. In this situation, as in the debilitated patient with acute cholecystitis, simple gallbladder drainage (cholecystostomy) may be lifesaving. Cholecystostomy is also indicated when, at surgical dissection, inflammation obscures vital structures. Fifty percent of these patients who survive over 2 years will eventually need cholecystectomy.

2. If jaundice is the presenting symptom, diagnosis is more difficult, and clinical observation for 1 to 3 weeks may be necessary. Jaundice per se seldom requires immediate exploration unless cholangitis is suspected. The liver will tolerate uninfected obstruction for 6 weeks before fibrosis develops.

3. The decision to explore the common duct is based on the following criteria: a history of jaundice or pancreatitis, palpable ductal stones, gallbladder gravel or calculi smaller than the diameter of the cystic duct, and a dilated common duct. The frequency with which choledochostomy is performed varies from 7 to 42 percent, reflecting individual interpretation of these criteria. Stones are found in approximately half of the common ducts explored. Theoretically, with a combination of history, laboratory data, preoperative cholangiography, and the surgeon's evaluation at operation, exploration will be positive in 93 percent of cases, will miss stones in 2 percent and will be unnecessary in only 5 percent. Following choledochostomy, a T tube is left in the common duct draining bile to the exterior of the body. The tube also serves for postoperative cholangiography and is pulled out after 12 days.

POSTCHOLECYSTECTOMY SYNDROME

The postcholecystectomy syndrome describes a group of symptoms of variable severity and cause which follow removal of the gallbladder. Much confusion is associated with this entity, because it is used loosely to cover symptoms unrelated to gallbladder disease. It is a misnomer in many patients who complain of the same symptoms they had prior to cholecystectomy. Analysis of these patients reveals that, in the majority, the indications for cholecystectomy were not clear. Symptoms in this group are commonly due to extrabiliary causes: hiatus hernia, ulcer diathesis, chronic pancreatitis, or functional colonic disorders. However, there are patients with bona fide indications for cholecystectomy whose symptoms continue postoperatively as well as some who develop new symptoms referable to the biliary tract. This group is most representative of the postcholecystectomy syndrome. Symptoms are usually due to incomplete surgical measures (residual choledocholithiasis, cystic duct and gallbladder remnants, overlooked malignancy, biliary fistula) or surgical trauma (bile duct strictures, stenosis of the sphincter of Oddi). The postcholecystectomy syndrome is "often disregarded by the surgeon, recognized by the physician, battled with by the general practitioner and must prove such a bitter disappointment to the patient" (Mallet-Guy, 1956).

STRICTURE

Stricture is the most common complication of operative damage to the extrahepatic ducts. In a series of 1,600 biliary strictures, 96 percent were related to trauma during biliary surgical procedures. One out of 300 to 500 cholecystectomies results in a stricture, with fatal sequelae in about 30 percent of cases. Factors which predispose to these injuries are anatomic abnormalities and surgical treatment during the edematous or late fibrotic phase of cholecystitis. The repair of a stricture often entails a series of difficult reconstructive operations, and some patients remain permanently disabled by secondary liver damage.

Postoperative jaundice or a biliary fistula suggests bile duct injury. Jaundice is the most common finding, evident within the first postoperative week. An external fistula should be suspected if the wound continues to discharge bile after 7 days. Spontaneous internal choledochoduodenal fistulas may leave the patient entirely asymptomatic, but few function adequately. Fever, chills, and varying degrees of jaundice soon appear. Early recognition and repair offer a good prognosis.

BILIARY CIRRHOSIS (See Also Chap. 328)

Biliary cirrhosis, secondary to chronic choledocholithiasis or bile duct stricture, is a disastrous complication of gallstones, usually resulting from lack of recognition or failure of therapy by the physician, or neglect by the patient. While hepatic fibrosis develops as early as 2 months after complete obstruction, even in the absence of significant infection, its progression can generally be stopped and reversed by relief of the obstruction at this early stage. With continuing obstruction and particularly with infection, pruritus, jaundice, steatorrhea, and portal hypertension progressively afflict the patient. Treatment of pruritus is difficult: local applications are of little value; antihistamines help some patients; methyltestosterone or norethandrolone suppress itching but may aggravate the hyperbilirubinemia; cholestyramine, an anion exchange resin, interrupts the enterohepatic circulation of bile salts and improves pruritus but aggravates steatorrhea by further reducing the bile salt concentration in the gut lumen. Calcium supplements and intramuscular vitamin D and K may be necessary.

OTHER DISEASES

Biliary Dyskinesia

Under normal circumstances, food entering the duodenum stimulates the release of a mucosal hormone, cholecystokinin, which causes contraction of the gallbladder, relaxation of the sphincter of Oddi, and a smoothly integrated evacuation of bile from the biliary tree. The concept that pain may arise from a purely motor derangement has been postulated since 1887, when Oddi stated that interference with the coordination of biliary kinetics, i.e., contraction of a gallbladder against a tonic sphincter, could result in pain, jaundice, or both. Since then a vast literature has accumulated concerning "biliary distress" without demonstrable organic lesions in the extrahepatic system. Biliary dyskinesia includes three different kinds of motor dysfunction: disturbances in evacuation (dyskinesia), disorders of tone (dystonia), and disturbances of coordination (dyssynergia).

Biliary dyskinesia can be compared to the spastic colon syndrome, as both conditions share a negative clinical and laboratory evaluation. However, they differ in that many patients with biliary dyskinesia undergo surgical procedures based on operative biliary dynamics, including sphincterotomy, choledochoduodenostomy, vagotomy, or splanchnicectomy. Few patients benefit from these procedures, and a lack of correlation among symptoms, pressure studies, and surgical results has evoked skepticism in the United States and Great Britain regarding biliary dyskinesia as a disease entity.

SYMPTOMS, SIGNS, AND DIAGNOSIS. The clinical manifestations of biliary dyskinesia may run the gamut of traditional symptoms of acute or chronic cholecystitis with the exception that fever, chills, and leukocytosis are rarely noted. The patients are usually anxious females whose symptoms correlate well with emotional tension, situational stress, and fatigue. Their past histories often include investigations for nausea, headaches, giddiness, diarrhea, or constipation. Comprehensive evaluation of liver and pancreatic function together with conventional roentgenographic studies of the biliary system reveal no abnormalities. The following are used by enthusiasts to evaluate these patients: (1) pain, indistinguishable from biliary colic, precipitated by morphine, is taken as evidence of sphincter dysfunction; (2) timed duodenal drainage compares the appearance, volume, and duration of flow of various bile fractions (gallbladder versus hepatic bile); (3) cinecholecystography is used to compare structure and function of the biliary tree; (4) operative radiomanometry is considered in many areas of the world as a definitive investigation.

TREATMENT. The management of patients suspected of biliary dyskinesia requires careful assessment of the symptoms in relation to food, alcohol, chronic intake of medications, and tensions. Reassurance, phenothiazines, sedation, analgesics, and anticholinergics, alone or in combination, should be tried on an empirical basis.

Primary Sclerosing Cholangitis

This is a rare entity involving the extrahepatic biliary ducts, producing progressive biliary cirrhosis. It may appear alone or associated with ulcerative colitis, regional enteritis, gallstones, or other fibrotic processes such as periureteral or pulmonary fibrosis. The presenting symptoms are those of biliary obstruction. A definitive diagnosis is possible only at exploration. Attempts at both medical and surgical treatment have provided, at best, only temporary relief.

Cancer of the Gallbladder

Primary cancer of the gallbladder is predominantly a disease of older women. In gallbladder operations it has been recorded with a frequency of 0.2 to 5 percent, the higher figure occurring in patients over sixty-five. A causal relationship between gallstones and cancer of the gallbladder is not established. Carcinoma of the gallbladder is insidious; persistent right upper quadrant pain with weight loss and anorexia should alert the clinician. A common physical finding is a hard mass associated with the liver. Jaundice is usually a terminal event, due to obstruction of the common duct or metastasis to the liver. Five-year survival is less than 3 percent, regardless of treatment.

Cancer of the Bile Ducts

Carcinoma of the bile ducts is also a disease of old age but is more prevalent in males. It is encountered in 1 of every 1,000 biliary tract operations, the common duct most often being involved. Although the jaundice of ampullary carcinoma sometimes fluctuates because necrotic tumor sloughs into the duodenum, the jaundice of bile duct carcinoma is unremitting. Contrary to the poor results of radical surgical treatment with other biliary tract carcinomas, ampullary carcinoma has a five-year survival rate of 40 percent. Approximately one-third of the patients with ampullary or bile duct cancer have a palpable gallbladder and two-thirds an enlarged liver. Percutaneous cholangiography is the most useful procedure available, often localizing the lesion for operation.

Congenital Abnormalities

Congenital abnormalities of the gallbladder include complete absence of the viscus, anomalous structure such as double gallbladder, and unusual position within the liver. The bile ducts are also subject to numerous congenital defects, among which atresia and cystic dilatation are the most prominent. Surgeons must be wary of many normal variations of the biliary tree and blood vessels.

Unusual Infections

Cholecystitis due to *Salmonella typhosa* still accounts for some typhoid carriers. Patients with salmonellosis and gallstones should undergo cholecystectomy after antibiotic treatment of the salmonella infection. Tuberculosis, syphilis, actinomycosis, and septic emboli are very infrequent causes of biliary tract infection. The characteristic lesions of periarteritis nodosa are sometimes prominent in the walls of the gallbladder, which may not fill on cholecystography.

Ascaris worms, liver flukes, and *echinococcus cysts* may cause biliary obstruction with cholangitis and jaundice.

Small *polypoid masses* are occasionally found in the gallbladder, but their clinical significance is controversial. Many of these polyps are merely mucosal prominences containing localized cholesterol deposits; some are hamartomas, and rarely true adenomatous growths occur. The lesions cannot be held responsible for symptoms. That the adenomatous polyps progress to cancer is an unproved assertion used by those who insist on cholecystectomy whenever a polyp is discovered radiologically in the gallbladder. Adenomyomatosis is the solitary, segmental, or diffuse proliferation of surface gallbladder epithelium with the formation of either ducts, crypts, or diverticula (Rokitansky-Aschoff sinuses). It is a congenital lesion and is without clinical significance.

Traumatic Rupture of the Gallbladder

Traumatic rupture of the gallbladder with bile peritonitis may be a complication of abdominal injuries.

REFERENCES

Cooley, R. N.: The Diagnostic Accuracy of Radiologic Studies of the Biliary Tract, Small Intestines and Colon, Am. J. Med. Sci., 246:610, 1963.

Davenport, H. W.: "Physiology of the Digestive Tract," 2d ed., Chicago, The Year Book Medical Publishers, Inc., 1966.

Donaldson, R. M.: Diet and Gastrointestinal Disorders, Gastroenterology, 52:897, 1967.

Dynamics of the Common Duct, Lancet, 1:236, 1968.

Flemma, R. J., L. M. Flint, S. Osterhout, W. W. Shingleton: Bacteriologic Studies of Biliary Tract Infection, Ann. Surg., 166:563, 1967.

Hofmann, A. F., and D. M. Small: Detergent Properties of Bile Salts: Correlation with Physiological Function, Ann. Rev. Med., 18:333, 1967.

Kune, G. A.: The Elusive Common Bile Duct Stone, Med. J. Aust. 1:254, 1966.

Newman, H. F., and J. D. Northrup: The Autopsy Incidence of Gallstones, Surg. Gynecol. Obstet. (Internat. Abstr. Surg.), 109:1, 1959.

Zollinger, R. M., E. T. Boles, and G. B. Crawford: The Diagnosis and Management of Biliary-tract Disease, New Engl. J. Med., 252:203, 1955.

Section 7

Disorders of the Pancreas

333 APPROACH TO THE DIAGNOSIS OF PANCREATIC DISEASE

Philip J. Snodgrass

The discussion in Chap. 334 indicates that diseases of the pancreas are characterized by a wide spectrum of possible symptoms and signs and a lack of stereotyped clinical patterns. Thus a so-called "classic case" is the exception rather than the rule for acute or chronic pancreatitis or pancreatic carcinoma. Diagnosis is difficult, because pancreatic pain is usually nonspecific in character and radiation, and the retroperitoneal position of the gland makes it inaccessible to physical examination. Roentgenographic studies offer less diagnostic aid than they do in diseases of other abdominal organs, so that laboratory tests must be relied upon to a greater extent than in other abdominal diseases in order to detect or confirm the presence of pancreatic pathologic changes. Based on the considerations discussed in Chap. 334, an operational approach to the differential diagnosis of acute and chronic pancreatitis and pancreatic cancer will be described. This brief summary should serve as a practical guide to the evaluation of these patients.

Acute pancreatitis should be considered in the differential diagnosis of any acute abdominal emergency. Unless another diagnosis is obvious, determination of serum amylase activity pays excellent dividends as a screening test in the patient with acute abdominal or back pain. An activity greater than 180 Somogyi units per 100 ml serum raises the question of pancreatic involvement, and a value over 500 units makes pancreatitis highly likely. Other major abdominal emergencies that may also be associated with an elevated serum amylase level are perforated peptic ulcer, acute cholecystitis, and obstruction or infarction of bowel. Although the serum amylase level rarely exceeds 500 units in these diseases, the separation of such entities from pancreatitis occasionally can be very difficult. Prompt abdominal x-rays are necessary to look for free peritoneal air, pancreatic calcifications, or opaque gallstones. A peritoneal tap with a short-bevel intravenous needle in the midlateral quadrants will often yield a cloudy yellow to "prune juice" type of fluid with an amylase level higher than the serum activity. In acute pancreatitis, bile is not detected in the fluid as in a perforated duodenal ulcer, and bacteria are not seen on direct Gram stain of the fluid as in bowel infarction, although both these entities can be associated with peritoneal fluid very high in amylase.

If the differential findings listed in Table 334-1 do not suggest another diagnosis, prompt treatment for pancreatitis should be instituted. The appropriate measures consist of nasogastric suction, plasma and electrolyte replacement, and meperidine for pain. Surgical intervention should be avoided unless perforation, strangulation, or necrosis of gut cannot be ruled out.

Confirmation of the diagnosis of *chronic pancreatitis* during painful episodes requires increases in serum or urinary amylase or serum lipase activities. During quiescent periods, stimulation with secretin and pancreozymin will result in increases in the serum amylase or lipase activities in 50 percent or more of patients whose acinar tissue is not destroyed. When exocrine insufficiency is suspected, the simplest screening procedure is macroscopic inspection of the stool for gross fat and microscopic examination of a stool emulsion, looking for undigested meat fibers and for increased numbers of fat globules after Sudan IV staining. Quantitative proof of steatorrhea should be obtained by chemical fat analysis of a 3-day stool collection on a known fat intake. Pancreatic insufficiency as the cause of steatorrhea is implied by a normal D-xylose absorption test or a normal small-bowel pattern after a barium meal.

A secretin test is the most precise and accurate method of measuring exocrine functional capacity. The greatest experience has been gathered using the method of Dreiling: a double lumen tube is passed into the stomach and duodenum under fluoroscopic control, and duodenal contents are collected uncontaminated by gastric juice. Secretin is given as a single intravenous dose of 1 to 2 clinical units per kg body weight. Then four 20-min collections are obtained by intermittent suction, and the bicarbonate concentrations are measured. The usual response in chronic pancreatitis is a decreased bicarbonate concentration in a normal volume of pancreatic juice. The maximum bicarbonate concentration discriminates best between normal subjects and patients with proved chronic pancreatitis, can be measured accurately in any laboratory, and does not require complete volume recovery.

A logical sequence of diagnostic procedures when *pancreatic carcinoma* is suspected would be (1) serum and urinary amylase measurements, (2) an upper gastrointestinal barium study, (3) a glucose tolerance test if the patient is not already diabetic, and (4) if icterus is present, liver function tests designed to separate obstructive from hepatocellular jaundice. If these studies are consistent with the diagnosis of pancreatic tumor, it may be visualized by a selective celiac arteriogram or by a selenomethionine scan. The diagnosis of pancreatic cancer can be confirmed only by surgical exploration.

334 DISEASES OF THE PANCREAS
Philip J. Snodgrass

BIOCHEMISTRY AND PHYSIOLOGY OF THE EXOCRINE PANCREAS

ENZYME SYNTHESIS AND SECRETION. The human exocrine pancreas synthesizes and secretes more protein per gram of tissue than any other organ. Pancreatic juice contains 6 to 12 Gm digestive enzymes in an average daily volume of 2,500 ml. The proteolytic enzymes are secreted as the inactive precursors (zymogens) trypsinogen, chymotrypsinogen, proelastase, and procarboxypeptidases A and B. When trypsinogen enters the duodenum, it is activated by enterokinase, an enzyme from duodenal mucosa which cleaves one unique lysine-isoleucine bond of trypsinogen. This limited proteolysis releases an N-terminal hexapeptide and allows the molecule to refold, forming the active site of trypsin. Trypsin is critical to the activation process, because autocatalytically it activates other trypsinogen molecules and in addition activates the other zymogens to produce chymotrypsin, elastase, and carboxypeptidases A and B. These five proteases, along with a less well-characterized prolinase, hydrolyze the dietary proteins to dipeptides and amino acids by the time the proteins reach the upper jejunum.

The reserve capacity of the pancreas is tremendous; 90 percent of a dog's pancreas must be removed before protein digestion is impaired. The zymogens are synthesized in the acinar cells of the pancreas, where the proteins are assembled on ribosomes attached to the membranes of the rough-surfaced endoplasmic reticulum. The enzyme proteins are secreted into the tubules of the endoplasmic reticulum and travel through this tubular system to the Golgi apparatus, where the proteins are enclosed in lipoprotein membranes and are condensed into zymogen granules which accummulate at the apex of the cells. The zymogen granules are secreted into the ductal lumen by fusion of their lipoprotein membranes with the membrane of the cell, and their release is initiated by the peptide hormone pancreozymin or by vagal stimulation. The protective mechanisms which prevent autodigestion of the pancreas by these proteases are the synthesis of the enzymes as inactive zymogens; investment in lipiprotein membranes within the cell; the synthesis of two trypsin inhibitors, one being present in the gland and the other secreted into pancreatic juice; and the presence of trypsin and other protease inhibitors in the α_1- and α_2- globulin fractions of plasma. The trypsin inhibitor in human pancreatic juice acts reversibly, allowing free trypsin to be released in the intestinal lumen.

Pancreatic juice contains a ribonuclease and a deoxyribonuclease, but they are not secreted as zymogens. α-Amylase splits starch to limit dextrins and disaccharides, principally maltose. The fat-splitting enzymes are lipase, phospholipases A and B, and cholesterol esterase. Pancreatic juice also contains a nonspecific esterase which cleaves water-soluble esters of fatty acids. Conjugated bile salts are important in digestion of lipids; when bile is excluded from the gut, 60 percent of ingested triglycerides are lost in the stool, whereas only 40 percent are lost when bile is present but pancreatic juice is diverted. Bile salts emulsify triglycerides and thereby stimulate lipase which functions at water-lipid interfaces, and they also shift the pH optimum of lipase to 6.5, the pH of the jejunal contents. Bile salts function as direct activators of the phospholipases, cholesterol esterases, and the nonspecific esterase. Pancreozymin has two functions, one to release zymogen granules and the other, as cholecystokinin, to empty the gallbladder and to relax the sphincter of Oddi. The content of the diet modifies the enzyme content of the pancreatic juice in animals: a high starch diet results in a high amylase content and a high protein content in increased amounts of chymotrypsinogen and trypsinogen.

WATER AND BICARBONATE SECRETION. Water, bicarbonate, and electrolytes are secreted into pancreatic juice by the centroacinar and the ductal cells of the pancreas. Water and bicarbonate output is stimulated by secretin, a peptide hormone whose 27 amino acid sequence has been established by Jorpes and Mutt and is closely homologous to glucagon. Secretin, like glucagon, can release insulin from the beta cells of the islets of Langerhans. In addition, secretin stimulates the biliary epithelium to add water and bicarbonate to bile. The human pancreas produces 1,500 to 4,000 ml juice a day which is isosmotic with plasma and contains the following electrolytes: Na^+, 140 mEq per liter; K^+, 6 mEq per liter; Ca^{++}, 1.7 mEq per liter; Mg^{++}, 0.7 mEq per liter, and HCO_3^-, which varies from 27 mEq per liter in the resting state to a maximum of 140 mEq per liter during maximum secretin stimulation.

The pH varies directly with the bicarbonate concentration, ranging from 7.5 to 8.5, and chloride concentration varies inversely with bicarbonate. The bicarbonate output of 7 to 18 Gm per day is sufficient to neutralize gastric acid production, resulting in a pH in the distal duodenum near 7, which is close to the optimal pH for the function of the various pancreatic enzymes. In the Zollinger-Ellison syndrome, where the parietal cells secrete an overwhelming amount of acid, pancreatic bicarbonate is not able to neutralize the acid, and the pH of the duodenum and jejunum falls to 3 to 5, leading to ulcerations, impaired digestion, and diarrhea. Secretin is released from the duodenal mucosal cells when acid and the products of gastric digestion enter the duodenum; it acts in a feedback manner to inhibit gastrin-stimulated acid production. Since pancreozymin inhibits gastric motility, these two hormones account for most of the activity ascribed to the postulated hormone enterogastrone. Although acid is the strongest stimulus of pancreatic secretion, fat causes the most prolonged stimulation, peptides and digested proteins are intermediary in effect, and carbohydrate is the weakest stimulant. Low doses of pancreozymin stimulate and high doses inhibit gastric acid secretion, whereas gastrin stimulates the release of pancreatic enzymes. These phenomena are probably related to their chemical structures, because the five

C-terminal amino acids of pancreozymin are identical to those of gastrin. Although vagotomy reduces the tendency of the antrum to release gastrin, pancreatic secretion continues unimpaired in the vagotomized human being. Apparently vagal stimuli only reinforce the hormonal phase of pancreatic secretion.

PANCREATIC FUNCTION TESTS

These tests are based on the biochemistry and physiology of the pancreas and depend upon analyzing the blood, the intestinal contents, or both for pancreatic secretory products. Normally there is an exocrine-endocrine partition of pancreatic enzyme secretion wherein a small fraction of the secretory enzymes enter the lymphatics and plasma. When functioning acinar cells secrete into a ductal system which is blocked by stricture, stone, or tumor, an increased regurgitation of the enzymes occurs. In the serum of normal adults amylase activity varies from 60 to 180 Somogyi units per 100 ml serum and lipase activity from 0 to 1.5 Cherry-Crandall units per ml serum. Isoenzymes of α-amylase are detected in the γ-globulin fraction of human serum using electrophoretic methods; one isoenzyme is derived from pancreas, one from salivary glands, and one probably from the liver.

The pancreatic isoenzyme level is elevated specifically in acute pancreatitis. A few patients are known who have a high amylase activity in the serum and a low level in the urine, and show no evidence of pancreatic disease. Their amylase appears to be bound to plasma globulins, forming complexes too large to be excreted in the urine. The presence of protease inhibitors in plasma makes the assay of serum trypsin, chymotrypsin, elastase, etc., difficult to carry out and to interpret. The trypsin inhibitor capacity of plasma is sufficient to inactivate 0.9 mg crystalline trypsin per ml plasma, but if trypsin is assayed using synthetic ester substrates, a low level of activity can be detected in normal plasma, because trypsin bound to the α_2-macroglobulin inhibitor still has esterase activity but cannot hydrolyze protein substrates. In acute pancreatitis, there is increased activity of a serum protease which hydrolyzes benzoyl arginine amide; this arginine amidase activity correlates well with serum amylase. Serum lipase, when measured by methods which require 12 to 24 hr of incubation, was thought to be less sensitive than amylase in detecting pancreatitis, but improved rapid methods indicate that the serum amylase and lipase parallel each other closely during pancreatitis.

Latent pancreatic disease causing a partial secretory block may sometimes be brought to light by "evocative" tests. When the normal pancreas is stimulated by intravenous secretin and pancreozymin, the serum levels of amylase and lipase change but little, but in early cases of pancreatic cancer or chronic inflammation where functioning acini secrete against an obstruction, pancreatic stimulation may produce serum enzyme activities which exceed resting levels by 100 percent or more. If the gland is extensively destroyed, stimulation of pancreatic secretion is incapable of causing increased serum enzyme activities; in such cases extensive pancreatic damage is revealed by a diabetic glucose tolerance test and abnormal secretory responses on duodenal intubation.

Because the normal renal clearance of plasma amylase is 1 to 4 ml per min, the measurement of urine amylase activity reflects changes in serum amylase. The normal 24-hr output varies from 800 to 6,000 Somogyi units, and values above 15,000 units usually indicate acute pancreatitis. A 2-hr collection of urine allows this test to be used in the emergency diagnosis of acute or relapsing pancreatitis; an excretion of more than 300 units per hr is abnormal, and more than 1,000 units per hr is usual in acute pancreatitis. If renal failure is not present and circumstances permit an accurate urine collection, the 2-hr urine amylase test is said to be abnormal more often and for a longer time period than the serum amylase or lipase activities. Although the serum amylase activity is often increased in acute renal failure and in some cases of chronic renal failure, the situation can be differentiated from acute pancreatitis by measuring the urinary amylase. In acute pancreatitis both the serum and urine amylase activities are increased, while in renal failure only the serum amylase level is above normal.

Direct measurement of pancreatic secretion is accomplished by quantitative collection of duodenal contents after stimulation with secretin alone or in combination with pancreozymin. A double-lumen tube is passed into the duodenum, and the proximal part is used to remove gastric contents which interfere with bicarbonate and enzyme measurements. Results vary with the secretin preparations used and with the various doses employed. Using an augmented dose of highly purified secretin, 2 clinical units per kg body weight given intravenously, Hartley and his associates report the lower limits of normal to be 1.8 ml juice/kg body weight/hr, a maximum bicarbonate concentration of at least 82 mEq/liter, and a bicarbonate output of 6.2 mEq/hr. The most reproducible measurement with the highest level of discrimination between normal persons and patients with chronic pancreatitis appears to be the maximum bicarbonate concentration after secretin. Interpretation of volume and bicarbonate in the duodenum is obscured by secretin stimulation of bile flow, which can itself reach bicarbonate levels of 40 to 50 mEq per liter. When pancreozymin is given in addition to secretin, the output of amylase, lipase, or trypsin in the subsequent 10 to 20 min occasionally is reduced in chronic pancreatitis when the maximum bicarbonate concentration is still normal. Pancreozymin preparations are rather impure, leading to occasional side effects, and optimal doses have not been defined. Pancreozymin tests present further problems because the enzymes are more difficult to measure, quantitative collections of duodenal juice are necessary, and severe protein malabsorption can result in secondary deficiencies of pancreatic enzymes.

Pancreatic function can also be tested by instilling a test meal containing carbohydrate, protein, and fat into the duodenum and relying on the endogenous release of secretin and pancreozymin. The maximal concentrations of trypsin, amylase, or lipase are measured, avoiding the need for complete recoveries of pancreatic juice. However, the results in chronic pancreatitis appear to be less accurate than those using maximal bicarbonate concentrations. Early in the course of pancreatic disease exocrine function may be retained to the extent that duodenal intubation studies are within normal limits. At this point in the spectrum of disease the serum evocative tests offer the greatest chance of detecting pancreatic disease. As the pancreatic reserve is progressively impaired, more patients will show an abnormal result on duodenal intubation studies, and fewer will show a response to the evocative test. The accuracy of these tests is a function of the type of patient studied as well as the stimuli and collection methods employed.

Indirect evidence of pancreatic exocrine function can be obtained by various tests of absorption and digestion. When pancreatic insufficiency is advanced, microscopic examination of the stool shows abundant neutral fat droplets when stained with Sudan IV, and a lesser amount of fatty acids which are detected by heating the stool with Sudan IV and acetic acid. Moreover, undigested meat fibers with sharp edges indicate lack of pancreatic proteases. When enzyme output is abnormal, the administration of lipids, proteins, or starch which require digestion before absorption is often followed by a subnormal appearance in the blood of the products of their digestion. For example, ^{131}I-labeled triolein may be poorly absorbed in maldigestion as well as malabsorption states, but absorption of ^{131}I-oleic acid is more normal when the pancreas rather than the intestine is at fault. Supplements of oral pancreatic extracts should restore absorption of ^{131}I-triolein to normal in pancreatic insufficiency. In general, such tests are rather insensitive in mild exocrine insufficiency. Intestinal biopsies are usually normal, and D-xylose absorption is relatively unaffected by pancreatic insufficiency. Although abnormal glucose metabolism is a frequent manifestation of chronic pancreatic disease, evidence of impaired glucose tolerance is obviously not specific for pancreatic disease because of the high incidence of genetic diabetes in the population. When exocrine pancreatic insufficiency is suspected, the only way to settle the issue is to demonstrate impaired output of bicarbonate or enzymes into the duodenum after stimulation with hormones or test meals.

ACUTE PANCREATITIS

The pathologic spectrum of acute pancreatitis varies from pancreatic edema, to edema with fat necrosis, to necrosis with variable degrees of hemorrhage. The mortality rate is proportional to the severity of the pathologic process and is 5 to 10 percent in pancreatic edema, 20 to 30 percent in partial necrosis, and 50 to 80 percent in total hemorrhagic necrosis of the gland. The clinical manifestations vary widely, reflecting the severity of the pathologic process.

ETIOLOGY. Acute pancreatitis occurs in patients with alcoholism, gallstones, and peptic ulcer; occasionally it occurs as a complication of pregnancy, mumps, drugs such as steroids or chlorothiazide, or diffuse vascular disease such as periarteritis nodosa, or as a result of atheromatous embolism to the pancreatic arterial tree. Metabolic disorders associated with an increased incidence of acute pancreatitis are essential hyperlipemia and hyperparathyroidism. The mechanism for the increased incidence of acute pancreatitis in patients with hyperparathyroidism is unknown. The common denominator seems to be hypercalcemia, because the calcium concentration of pancreatic juice reflects the ionized portion of plasma calcium and pancreatitis has been observed in other hypercalcemic states such as multiple myeloma and sarcoidosis. Genetic disorders associated with pancreatitis include a hereditary form of pancreatitis associated with a renal tubular defect in the reabsorption of lysine and cystine. Trauma is a relatively frequent cause of pancreatitis and may be due to a blunt injury such as a blow to the abdomen by a steering wheel, a penetrating injury from a bullet or knife wound, inadvertent trauma from surgical procedures in the upper abdomen, or rarely electric shock. Approximately 20 percent of patients with acute pancreatitis appearently have no underlying or predisposing disease.

The pathogenesis of pancreatitis presumably depends on intrapancreatic activation of proteolytic and lipolytic enzymes with consequent digestion of pancreatic tissue and blood vessels. This pancreatic autodigestion usually develops in two situations: (1) when pancreatic secretion is blocked either by a lesion of a major duct or by diffuse blockage of many ductules and functioning acinar tissue is still secreting distal to the block or (2) when acinar tissue is exposed to direct injury by toxins, ischemia, inflammation, or trauma.

Experimentally, pancreatitis can be caused by obstruction of the main pancreatic ducts and stimulation of secretion, by creation of a closed duodenal loop, and by injection of bile, trypsin, bacteria, or combinations of these into the pancreatic duct. Reflux of bile into the pancreatic duct has been postulated as the cause of pancreatitis in the rare patient in whom a stone becomes impacted in the ampulla of Vater and a common channel exists between the common bile duct and the pancreatic duct, as it does in about 60 percent of human beings. When a stone is not found, reflux of bile is often ascribed to spasm or fibrosis of the sphincter of Oddi. Arguments against the common channel theory are as follows: reflux of bile into the pancreatic ducts can occur without untoward effects, the secretory pressure of the pancreas normally exceeds that of the biliary system, and fatal cases of pancreatitis have been documented in patients who have no common channel. Reflux of duodenal contents into the pancreatic ducts is postulated as the etiologic factor when the pancreatic duct empties separately from the bile duct.

There is an increased incidence of acute pancreatitis in patients with gallstones, even without evidence of common duct calculi. Removal of the gallstones usually cures this type of recurrent acute pancreatitis, but the mechanism for the relationship remains obscure. Direct injury of acinar tissue appears to be responsible for the pancreatitis that follows pancreatic trauma or a penetrating peptic ulcer. The mechanism by which alcoholism produces pancreatitis is uncertain: ethanol does not affect pancreatic function directly, but it does induce an increase in gastrin release and in gastric secretion, which increase pancreatic secretion. It is postulated that a duodenitis results from alcoholism, causing edema or spasm of the sphincter of Oddi; recurrent stimulation of secretion against obstruction are thought to result in pancreatic edema and fibrosis. Chronic pancreatitis in alcoholics may be partly a deficiency disease, because chronic pancreatic fibrosis characterizes the protein deficiency disease kwashiorkor and degenerative lesions can be induced in the pancreas of rats exposed to the methionine antagonist ethionine.

INCIDENCE. Except for individuals with hereditary pancreatitis or hyperlipemia or the occasional patient seen after abdominal trauma or with an ascaris in the duct of Wirsung, pancreatitis is rare in children. It affects adults of any age and has an incidence of about 27 per 100,000 population. As might be anticipated from the prevalence of predisposing disorders, pancreatitis associated with alcoholism, duodenal ulcer, or trauma is much more frequent in men than in women. The percentage of cases of acute pancreatitis associated with alcoholism or gallbladder disease varies greatly with the locale; for example, the rate due to alcoholism is high in the United States and France, but gallbladder disease accounts for most of the pancreatitis seen in England.

SYMPTOMS. Severe upper abdominal pain is the outstanding symptom of pancreatitis. The location of the pain is determined by the retroperitoneal position of the pancreas and corresponds roughly in location to the position of the lesion; lesions of the tail of the pancreas cause pain in the left upper quadrant, those in the body are perceived in the epigastrium, and diseases of the head in the epigastrium or right upper quadrant. A high percentage of pancreatic lesions cause pain referred to the back at the T_{10} to L_2 level. Patients with pancreatic pain occasionally obtain relief in a characteristic position by sitting with the trunk flexed, the knees drawn up, and the forearms folded across the abdomen to exert pressure upon it. The degree of pain varies with the severity of the pancreatic injury, but in most cases it is of such intensity that the patient demands analgesics. Centered initially in the upper midabdomen, the steady, boring pain usually diffuses to the back, chest, or lower abdomen. Nausea and vomiting, abdominal distension, and constipation are frequent complaints.

PHYSICAL EXAMINATION. The patient is distressed, anxious, and restless. Mottled skin, cold sweaty extremities, tachycardia, and shock are hallmarks of severe pancreatitis. Fever is not usually present initially but rises to 100 to 102°F within the first few days. Tenderness, voluntary resistance, and spasm in the upper abdomen are present to a variable degree, but in contrast to the intense pain these signs may be unimpressive. A board-like abdomen as is seen in a perforated peptic ulcer is unusual. Various degrees of ileus occur, but some patients continue to have bowel sounds in spite of severe pain. Ten percent of patients have gastrointestinal bleeding, usually from ulcerations of the stomach, duodenum, or colon. Acute pancreatitis can produce rales in the lower lobes, pleuritis with a friction rub, or signs of pleural effusions, the changes being more common on the left side.

LABORATORY DATA. Urinary output is depressed if there is hypotension and a decrease in circulating plasma volume, and acute tubular necrosis is not uncommon when shock is severe. The white cell count ranges from 8,000 to 20,000 with an increased percentage of polymorphonuclear leukocytes; occasionally there are leukemoid reactions with the white cell count as high as 50,000. The more severe cases show hemoconcentration with hematocrit values sometimes exceeding 60 percent. Plasma loss is due to tremendous subcapsular and peripancreatic edema and later to the diffuse "peritoneal burn" that results from intraabdominal enzymatic digestion. Transient hyperglycemia is common and is attributed to islet cell damage and the patient's marked adrenal response to stress. Mild jaundice may be detected within 1 to 3 days of onset in 25 percent of the cases.

The activity of the pancreatic enzymes in the blood provides the most helpful laboratory information. Within 8 hr of onset, serum amylase values rise in 90 percent of cases, and the values usually exceed 250 Somogyi units. Levels above 500 units are strongly suggestive of acute pancreatitis. After 48 hr, even in the presence of clinical evidence of continuing pancreatitis, the amylase values tend to return to normal. When massive hemorrhagic infarction of the pancreas occurs (pancreatic apoplexy), the amylase level may not rise at all. Serum lipase activity increases in parallel with the amylase but is prone to subside more slowly over a period of days. In patients with fat necrosis, blood calcium levels fall and remain depressed for 1 to 9 days. The initial fall is presumably due to precipitation of calcium soaps, from fatty acids liberated by lipolytic destruction of the abdominal and retroperitoneal fat. The persistent depression of serum calcium is unexplained. Frank or latent tetany may be seen in patients who develop hypocalcemia; tetany that persists after restoration of calcium to a normal level occasionally has been associated with a low serum magnesium concentration. In patients with clinical evidence of pancreatic necrosis, a normal serum calcium level provides a clue to underlying hyperparathyroidism.

Occasionally lipemic serum is seen the first day or two after an episode of acute pancreatitis and is due predominantly to increased numbers of chylomicrons. There is evidence that an inhibitor of lipoprotein lipase appears in the plasma during acute pancreatitis, and this could account for the chylomicronemia. Electrocardiograms can be abnormal in acute pancreatitis with transient S-T–segment depressions and T-wave changes due either to hypotension and myocardial ischemia or rarely to inflammatory changes in the pericardium. If shock is persistent in older patients, myocardial infarction may result.

X-RAY. Abdominal films may reveal moderately distended gas-filled loops of intestine; paralytic ileus particularly affects the duodenum, the jejunum near the pancreas ("sentinal loops"), and occasionally the transverse colon. Calcifications in the region of the pancreas are diagnostic of previous pancreatitis. Later, abdominal films may show a generalized haziness due to ascites and a loss of psoas shadows due to retroperitoneal edema and hemorrhage. Chest films often reveal elevation of the left side of the diaphragm and fluid in the left side of the chest which if tapped has an amylase activity higher than that in serum. Though rarely necessary, a barium meal usually demonstrates delayed gastric emptying and enlargement of the duodenal loop due to edema of the head of the pancreas. Intravenous cholangiography is of little help in differential diagnosis, because a nonvisualizing gallbladder often occurs with pancreatitis, as it does with cholecystitis, and the common duct may be dilated because of edema in the head of the pancreas.

COURSE. Pancreatic edema usually subsides in 2 or 3 days, and patients are feeling well and eating normally in 1 week. Acute necrotizing pancreatitis causes a prolonged illness in which hyperglycemia, hypocalcemia, persistent ileus, and collections of necrotic debris in and around the pancreas develop. Suppurative pancreatitis usually occurs in the second or third week, when bacteria invade the necrotic collections, and is associated with a secondary rise in temperature and white cell count. In cases where pancreatic apoplexy occurs, the patient may die suddenly. The major cause of death in the first few days is refractory hypotension. One reason for this may be massive hemorrhage, due to digestion of the walls of major blood vessels, but in addition to losses of blood and plasma, hypotension may be aggravated by the release of kinins from the pancreas into the lymphatics and plasma. Kallikrein, an enzyme plentiful in the pancreas, catalyses the release from a plasma α_2-globulin of the vasoactive peptides kallidin and bradykinin. These are potent vasodilators and mediate an inflammatory response, causing migration of leukocytes, increased capillary permeability, pain, and smooth muscle stimulation. Trypsin also can produce bradykinin directly from the α_2-globulin substrate (kallidinogen). These vasoactive peptides have been demonstrated in plasma, lymph, and in peritoneal fluid both in experimental and in human pancreatitis.

Fat necrosis is commonly seen in the pancreas and the peripancreatic tissues, often involves the omentum and mesenteric fat, and occasionally extends to the perinephric and retroperitoneal fat. Rarely fat necrosis involves the pleura, pericardium, mediastinum, bone marrow, skin, and even the brain. The mechanism for disseminated fat necrosis is not certain; it has been attributed to the action of lipolytic enzymes circulating in lymphatics or blood and has also been postulated to result from emboli of necrotic fat entering the circulation. Peritoneal fluid often accumulates in acute pancreatitis;

in milder cases it is a "beef broth" type of fluid, high in amylase activity, often containing gross or microscopic fat globules. In hemorrhagic necrosis, the fluid is turbid and bloody and accumulates in volumes ranging from 500 to 2,000 ml. The fluid contains many polymorphonuclear leukocytes but shows no bacteria on Gram stain and usually contains no bile.

Hemorrhagic phenomena may become obvious 3 to 6 days after onset by a blue-green-brown discoloration in the flanks (Grey Turner's sign) due to the seeping of blood to the abdominal wall by retroperitoneal routes. Rarely blood dissects beneath the anterior abdominal muscles, resulting in a bluish discoloration around the umbilicus (Cullen's sign). Digestion of hemoglobin results in the release of the heme moiety, which is oxidized and binds to serum albumin to form methemalbumin. Simple methods are available for measuring methemalbumin, and its appearance in a patient with a clinical picture of pancreatitis is good evidence for hemorrhagic necrosis. Abnormalities in the blood-clotting system occasionally occur in severe pancreatitis; these changes are postulated to result from a local release of trypsin in excess of its inhibitors, because free trypsin is able to convert prothrombin to thrombin, fibrinogen to fibrin, and plasminogen to plasmin. In rare cases there is evidence of diffuse intravascular coagulation with consumption of clotting factors leading to a generalized bleeding tendency.

By the second or third week, abscesses or pseudocysts may complicate pancreatitis. Abscesses occur as collections within the pancreas and pseudocysts as collections outside the pancreas, but both contain pancreatic secretions, necrotic debris, and inflammatory cells. These collections may become infected by staphylococci, by coliform organisms, or even by gas-forming anaerobes, and surgical intervention to drain the collections is necessary. Occasionally acute pancreatitis is characterized by recurrent pain, ileus, and inflammation, leading to death from wasting and sepsis.

DIFFERENTIAL DIAGNOSIS. Any severe pain in the abdomen or back should suggest pancreatitis. A history of previous attacks of pain is obtained often but is not specific for pancreatitis. If pancreatitis is suspected, the diagnosis can be established by the measurement of pancreatic enzymes in the blood, by exclusion of conditions most likely to simulate pancreatitis, and by the course of the disease. In considering the differential diagnoses (Table 334-1), it should be remembered that coronary occlusion and biliary colic are twenty times as common as acute pancreatitis, that perforated ulcer is three times as common, that mesenteric vascular occlusion is less common, and dissecting aneurysm is rare. One of the most difficult problems of differential diagnosis occurs in the patient who has either perforation of a peptic ulcer or obstruction or infarction of gut with leakage of intestinal contents into the peritoneal cavity. In these situations the pancreatic enzymes are absorbed via lymphatics into the blood, resulting in increased amylase activities and a picture which may closely mimic acute pancreatitis. Peritoneal fluid containing more than 7,000

Table 334-1. DIFFERENTIAL DIAGNOSIS OF ACUTE PANCREATITIS*

Disease	History	Physical examination	Laboratory findings
Acute pancreatitis	Sudden onset, often with immediate maximal development of pain Past or recent history of gallstones, alcoholism, peptic ulcer, dietary debauch, trauma, or upper abdominal surgical procedures	Abdominal findings moderate as compared to violence of pain. Tenderness extends to left of epigastrium. Abdominal distension moderate or absent. Peristaltic noises diminished or absent. Shock and cyanosis may be striking. Patient may be restless.	Elevation of amylase in serum and urine. Hypocalcemia in severe cases. Paracentesis: evidence of fat necrosis, sometimes sanguineous fluid, high amylase levels. X-ray may show fluid at base of left pleural cavity.
Perforated viscus, especially peptic ulcer ...	History of ulcer	Boardlike spasm and tenderness in epigastrium. Patient fears movement and jarring; shock rare.	X-ray shows free intraperitoneal air.
Mesenteric vascular occlusion..........	Elderly patient with cardiovascular disease or recent operation Development of pain may be gradual	....	WBC over 20,000. Paracentesis: sanguineous fluid. Stool may contain blood.
Acute intestinal obstruction........	Intermittent colic with relative comfort between pains Past history of abdominal operation or of inguinal or femoral hernia	Abdominal distension with loud peristalsis. Shock rare. Patient moves around with colic.	X-ray of abdomen shows characteristics of mechanical obstruction.
Biliary colic	Pain more right-sided, more gradual in onset, and less prostrating than that of pancreatitis	Tenderness maximal on right side of abdomen.	
Coronary occlusion ...	Pain usually maximal in chest, neck, or arms	Relatively few abdominal findings. Shock and restlessness often present.	Electrocardiographic abnormalities.
Dissecting aneurysm of aorta	....	Impaired femoral pulsations. Shock and restlessness often present.	Hematuria.

* The points listed are, if present, important guides toward the correct diagnosis, but they are not invariable features of the diseases under which they are grouped.

Somogyi units of amylase is characteristic of acute pancreatitis, but other acute intestinal emergencies such as perforated peptic ulcer may give ascitic fluid amylases as high as 4,800 units. When bowel is perforated, the peritoneal fluid usually contains bile or bacteria, and abdominal films often show air under the diaphragm on upright films. Acute cholecystitis may be accompanied by increases in amylase activity and can be confused with acute pancreatitis. Because a perforated, obstructed, or infarcted viscus requires early operative intervention, a laparotomy should be done whenever these diagnoses cannot be clearly differentiated from acute pancreatitis. In contrast to previous beliefs, mortality from pancreatitis is not increased greatly by a diagnostic laparotomy.

TREATMENT. The rationale of therapy is (1) to maintain an adequate circulating blood volume, (2) to keep pancreatic secretory activity at a minimum, and (3) to prevent potential and to treat actual complications.

Direct surgical attack with drainage of the necrotic areas of the pancreas has been generally abandoned as ineffective and incurs the risk of external pancreatic fistula. Surgeons who believe that pancreatitis is caused by bile reflux favor drainage of the gallbladder in the hope of achieving decompression, but no controlled studies have been done to indicate that this operation alters the course of established pancreatitis. Shock and hemoconcentration are treated with plasma or human serum albumin and electrolyte solutions, using the hematocrit, central venous pressure, and urine output as indices of adequate volume replacement. Whole blood usually is required in hemorrhagic pancreatitis. Meperidine or pentazocine are recommended for pain rather than opiates, because they cause less spasm of the sphincter of Oddi, but these often prove inadequate. In some patients, morphine or its derivatives may have to be used. Nothing is given by mouth, and constant gastric suction is employed to reduce intestinal distension and stimulation of pancreatic secretion by acid entering the duodenum. Placing of the nasogastric tube with radiologic monitoring is necessary in order to achieve complete collection of gastric juice, and nasogastric suction is continued until intestinal activity returns to normal. When shock is controlled, water, electrolytes, and glucose are given intravenously to meet daily nutritional needs, and insulin may be needed to control glucosuria. Because secondary infection of necrotic tissue, of partially obstructed biliary passages, and of atelectatic lung accounts for much of the late mortality in pancreatitis, appropriate antibiotic therapy of *established* infection is crucial. Prophylactic antibiotic therapy is often employed, but adequately controlled studies showing that it reduces mortality are lacking.

Other, less well-established measures may be used. Anticholinergics in full parenteral doses (e.g., 30 mg propantheline bromide) can be given every 6 to 8 hr to inhibit the vagal stimuli of pancreatic secretion, but these obscure interpretation of the pulse rate and tend to dry secretions, leading to further pulmonary problems, and their value in the successful management of pan-

creatitis is questionable. Numerous case reports assert that ACTH or parenterally administered adrenal glucocorticoids may help in the desperate case of acute pancreatitis, but these reports are difficult to evaluate, because no controlled studies have been done and acute pancreatitis can occur as a complication of adrenocortical therapy. Paravertebral, splanchnic, or epidural procaine block sometimes relieve pain dramatically, but these are rarely necessary. Hypocalcemia should be treated by slow intravenous injections of calcium gluconate, 10 ml of a 10% solution every 4 hr. The amounts needed are determined by the patient's clinical response and the serum calcium level. A polypeptide (Trasylol) extracted from beef parotid gland has been employed extensively in Europe to treat acute pancreatitis, because it is a potent kallikrein and trypsin inhibitor. Experimental pancreatitis responds to this inhibitor, but the agent must be given before or at the onset of the pancreatitis. This time factor may account for the lack of significant objective improvement in mortality and morbidity observed in the few controlled clinical trials.

As the patient improves, food may be given slowly, beginning with carbohydrate, which stimulates the pancreas least, and gradually adding protein and minimal amounts of fat. Recrudescence of symptoms may occur with food and signals the need for drainage of obstructing pancreatic collections or pseudocysts.

PSEUDOCYSTS

When collections of pancreatic juice and cellular debris break through the capsule of the pancreas, pseudocysts may form which are lined by fibroblasts and the serosal surfaces of adjacent organ structures. Usually located in the middle or left upper abdomen, the cysts occur in the lesser peritoneal sac, between the stomach and colon, between the stomach and the liver, or between the leaves of the transverse mesocolon. The pseudocysts may fluctuate in size or form tremendous masses that create symptoms by pushing the duodenum to the right, the stomach forward (Fig. 334-1), the left diaphragm upward, and the transverse colon downward. Aching distress rather than acute pain is the usual presenting complaint, and the pseudocysts are tender and usually readily palpable. The most common time for these to form is 3 to 4 weeks after a bout of acute pancreatitis. Signs of fluid or atelectasis at the left lung base are common. Barium contrast studies establish the location of the mass and exclude lesions of the gastrointestinal tract and kidneys. Jaundice occurs in 10 percent of cases, and occasionally a persistently increased serum amylase activity is a clue to a pseudocyst.

The principal differential diagnosis is upper abdominal neoplasm, particularly of the pancreas. If an attack consistent with pancreatitis has occurred within weeks or months, the history is helpful, but in approximately one out of three pseudocysts the initiating bout of pancreatitis is atypical and goes unrecognized. In these instances the existence of conditions predisposing to pancreatitis such as gallstones, alcoholism, duodenal ulcer, or trauma

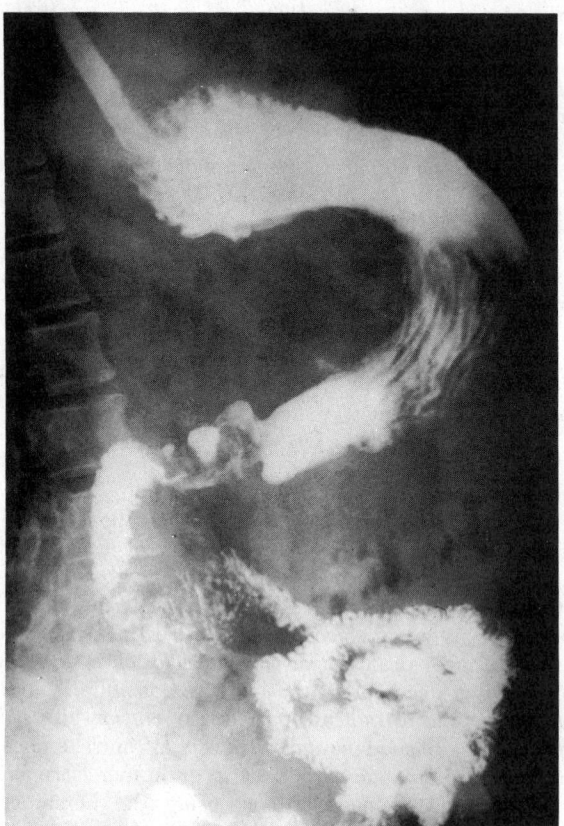

Fig. 334-1. Pancreatic pseudocyst. In this lateral view the body of the stomach appears to be pushed forward by a large mass between it and the spine. The cause of the pseudocyst is well known—a large penetrating duodenal ulcer.

provides a basis for suspecting a pseudocyst. Pseudocysts endanger life by rupturing into the peritoneal or pleural cavities, or by dissecting into the mediastinum, into the retroperitoneum, or even up into the neck. Therapy consists of external or internal drainage of the cyst; the lowest mortality and morbidity accompanies anastostomosis of the cyst wall to the stomach or to a loop of small bowel.

CHRONIC PANCREATITIS

Chronic pancreatitis is manifested by as broad a spectrum of clinical symptoms of varying severity as acute pancreatitis. The chronic relapsing form of the disease may be initiated by a severe attack of acute pancreatitis, but in the majority of patients it begins insidiously with mild recurrent bouts of abdominal pain. The most typical pattern resembles recurrent acute edematous pancreatitis. A persistent form of chronic pancreatitis without acute exacerbations is characterized by almost constant abdominal and back pain, and contrasts sharply with the pattern in a small number of patients in whom exocrine insufficiency and diabetes develop without any episodes of pain. In half of all cases, calcific deposits form in the ducts, the parenchyma, or both (Fig. 334-2); calcareous pancreatitis is particularly common when the cause is chronic alcoholism.

The same histopathologic changes occur in all clinical types but vary in extent and severity and consist of the following: replacement of acinar cells by fibrous tissue; foci of inflammation, edema, and necrosis; metaplasia and dilatation of the ductal system; variable deposits of calcium salts; and relative preservation of the islets of Langerhans. In some patients the pathologic process is limited to the head of the pancreas, in others it is a patchy process throughout the gland, and in its most extensive state the pancreas is reduced to a fibrous mass with multiple areas of stricture and dilatation of the ductal system. The formation of pseudocysts or abscesses is an occasional complication of any form of chronic pancreatitis. Chronic pancreatitis, like the acute variety, is associated primarily with alcoholism and gallstones and less often with ulcer, trauma, or metabolic disturbances. A diffuse fibrosis without inflammation or clinical symptoms occurs in hemochromatosis and in protein malnutrition.

Early in the disease, bouts of pain occur with minimal impairment of exocrine function. As inflammation and resulting fibrosis continue, pancreatic insufficiency gradually develops. When enzymatic secretion becomes inadequate, digestion is impaired, large amounts of fat and undigested protein are lost in the stool, and weight loss is severe. An increased incidence of duodenal ulceration has been attributed to the lack of bicarbonate secretion, but there is also evidence that the obstructed pancreas produces a gastric secretagogue. Careful questioning reveals that the stools are bulky, light, and greasy in appearance, and tend to float, all indications of steatorrhea. A characteristic of the stools which is uncommon in malabsorption syndromes is the presence of oil droplets. Although the absorption of vitamin D and K is impaired,

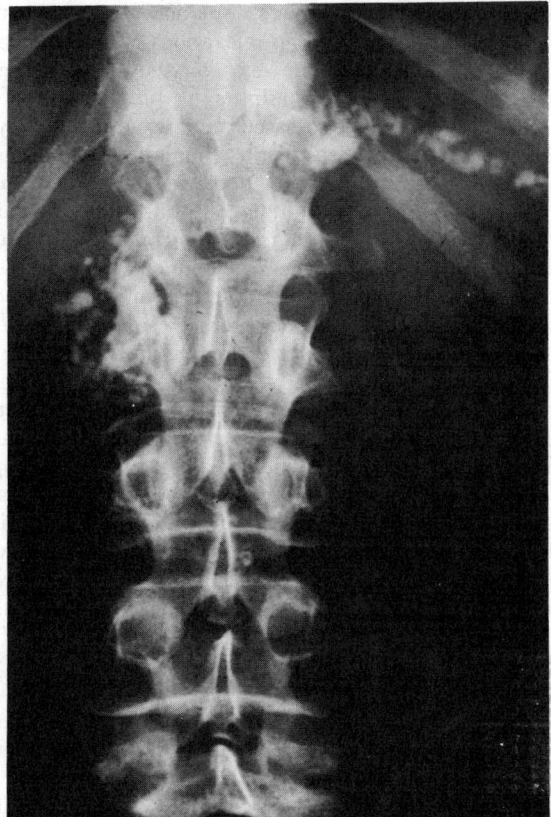

Fig. 334-2. Chronic relapsing pancreatitis. In this film of the upper abdomen the entire pancreas is shown outlined by extensive calcific deposits.

tetany and purpura as occur in sprue are unusual. Frank diabetes occurs in 10 percent of cases and is a sign of advanced disease, but impaired glucose tolerance is found earlier and in a higher percentage of patients. Increased absorption of iron occurs in some patients with pancreatic insufficiency leading to hemosiderosis of the liver; the mechanism for the occasional hyperabsorption of iron is unknown.

DIAGNOSIS. Chronic pancreatitis is a good diagnostic possibility in all patients having recurrent upper abdominal pain especially if (1) the pain or tenderness extends to the left of the midline, (2) alcoholism or gallstones are present, and (3) more common abdominal disorders have been excluded. The disease may explain mild recurrent jaundice, diabetes mellitus without a family history, or vague symptoms of indigestion, particularly if these phenomena are accompanied by recurrent low-grade fever and a persistently elevated sedimentation rate. If pancreatic calcification is seen on abdominal films, the diagnosis is obvious, but specially positioned oblique or lateral views may be necessary to demonstrate small calcareous deposits in the region of the pancreas. Before the acinar cells are greatly reduced in number, a diagnosis is confirmed most efficiently by repeated serum or urine amylase determinations taken within 8 to 12 hr of episodes of pain or by serum amylase and lipase responses to secretin and pancreozymin stimulation. As more acinar and ductal cells are destroyed, elevations of serum or urinary amylase levels become less frequent, and patients begin to show abnormal outputs of bicarbonate after secretin stimulation or decreased amylase, lipase, or trypsin secretion after pancreozymin stimulation. The abnormality in response to secretin or pancreozymin stimulation is *qualitative*. The volume output usually remains normal, while the concentrations of bicarbonate and enzymes in the pancreatic juice are reduced. This pattern contrasts with the *quantitative* defect seen when tumors obstruct the head of the pancreas, resulting in a decreased volume but normal bicarbonate and enzyme concentrations.

Interpretation of duodenal drainage tests in patients with severe malabsorption syndromes is difficult, because in these patients protein deficiency eventually develops, and then they may show evidence of secondary pancreatic insufficiency due to the lack of essential amino acids. Another problem is that patients with chronic liver disease will show a diminished concentration of bicarbonate after secretin stimulation, primarily due to dilution with a large amount of bile; the hourly output of bicarbonate is normal in chronic liver disease without pancreatic disease.

TREATMENT. The consequences of pancreatic insufficiency can be controlled with moderate success by dietary restriction of fats and by the oral administration of 10 to 20 Gm of potent pancreatic extracts daily. Balance studies indicate that the most effective way to administer these extracts is in doses of 1 to 2 Gm every few hours during the day. Supplements containing medium-chain triglycerides are useful, because this form of fat is well absorbed without lipolysis. Control of pain in chronic pancreatitis is often unsatisfactory, and many patients become addicted to narcotics. Low fat diets, anticholinergics, and antacids given in the hope of controlling gastric acidity and lessening the stimuli for pancreatic secretion are inconsistently effective.

Surgical treatment is most successful if a responsible biliary tract abnormality such as stones can be corrected. A direct attack on obstructions within the pancreatic ducts requires their demonstration by injection of radiopaque dye into the main duct after opening the duodenum and the ampulla. When strictures or stones involve primarily the head of the pancreas and the ductal system has become dilated distally, reverse drainage can be established by resecting the pancreatic tail and anastomosing the duct to a loop of jejunum. If the entire ductal system is involved with strictures and stones, it is sometimes necessary to split the gland longitudinally, opening the main pancreatic duct, and sewing a Roux-en-Y loop of jejunum over the pancreas. Once the gland has been destroyed functionally and the patient has developed intractable pain, the best symptomatic results have been obtained by a 95 percent resection of the pancreas, leaving a small cuff of gland along the duodenal loop; this maneuver avoids the more major procedure of a pancreaticoduodenectomy (Whipple procedure). Vagotomy,

subtotal gastrectomy to reduce gastric secretion, or cutting of a normal sphincter of Oddi have produced erratic results. Bilateral sympathectomy and splanchnicectomy may be used to relieve pain, but relief is often temporary.

FIBROCYSTIC DISEASE

Many organ systems are affected by this disorder of infancy and childhood, which is transmitted as an autosomal recessive trait: (1) The pancreatic acini are replaced by fibrotic tissue, multiple cysts, inspissated mucus, and eventually fat. The clinical manifestations of the consequent pancreatic insufficiency are malnutrition and bulky, greasy stools due to steatorrhea and creatorrhea. (2) In the newborn infant a thick meconium, presumably viscous because pancreatic digestion is absent, may cause meconium ileus. Later, the child may develop fecal impaction, rectal prolapse, and intussusception. (3) The mucous glands of the entire gastrointestinal tract may show this inspissation, so that the diagnosis can be made by rectal biopsy. (4) In a few cases, the smaller hepatic biliary channels are plugged, with the consequent development of cirrhosis and portal hypertension. The gallbladder often contains gelatinous material and is hypoplastic. (5) The sweat and saliva contain high concentrations of sodium and chloride; in hot weather this abnormality may cause acute salt depletion and at times death. (6) The most disabling obstructive pathologic changes affect the lungs, so that chronic bronchitis and emphysema develop and the patient is susceptible to bronchopneumonia.

The cause is obscure. One hypothesis holds that the abnormally viscid mucus blocks small tubular structures in the various organs involved. This concept of "mucoviscidosis," however, does not explain the abnormal composition of sweat, because sweat glands secrete no mucus. The diagnosis is made on the basis of the clinical picture, deficiency of pancreatic enzymes, and high levels of sweat electrolytes. Various methods of inducing sweating allow the sodium or chloride concentration to be measured; 99 percent of children with the disease will have a sweat chloride concentration exceeding 50 mEq per liter. Lack of digestion by stool of gelatin on an x-ray film is a useful screening test for trypsin deficiency in the first four years of life.

Treatment consists of pancreatic substitution therapy; a high calorie, high protein, low fat diet; water-miscible forms of vitamins A, D, and K; liberal use of salt; appropriate antibiotics for acute pulmonary infections and prophylactic broad-spectrum antibiotics; postural drainage; mist tents; and expectorants.

Because of an increasingly long survival of moderately severe cases and because of failure to recognize mild cases in childhood, adult fibrocystic disease may be more prevalent than appreciated heretofore. Some young adults regarded as having "idiopathic" pancreatitis, chronic bronchitis and emphysema, or hepatic cirrhosis may in fact be the victims of cystic fibrosis. Because sweat sodium and chloride concentrations increase normally with age, the diagnosis in adults is difficult to prove and rests on a positive family history and characteristic changes in mucous glands.

CANCER OF THE PANCREAS

INCIDENCE. Cancer of the pancreas predominantly affects patients over forty, attacks men twice as frequently as women, and accounts for about 1 in 20 deaths due to cancer. It is now seen as often as gastric cancer and one-third as often as colonic and rectal cancer in men and women. Diabetic patients are believed to have an increased susceptibility to the disease.

SYMPTOMS. Weight loss, pain, and unremitting jaundice are the outstanding symptoms. Digestive disorders, including anorexia, nausea, loose stools, or, more commonly, constipation, are prevalent. The site of the lesion, however, to a great extent influences the character of the symptoms, their time of onset, and their correct interpretation. Considering the total course of all types of pancreatic cancer, jaundice occurs less frequently than weight loss or pain, but diagnostically it is the most im-

portant symptom. Jaundice points specifically to the biliary passages, and lesions near the ampulla of Vater give early warning before extensive growth or metastasis has taken place. The course and intensity of the jaundice depend on the degree of biliary obstruction (Table 334-2). Itching is an associated symptom in three-fourths of the patients with jaundice, and may antedate clinical icterus in some patients.

Literally painless jaundice characterizes cancer in the head of the pancreas in only a few cases. More frequently, the patient has vague abdominal distress and fullness, which may be made either worse or better by eating. The severe pain of cancer in the body or tail may, however, be diagnostic; it bores through to the midback when the patient lies supine, and he obtains relief only by standing or by sitting hunched up with arms clasped about the knees. A number of patients with cancer of the pancreas complain of depression and a sense of impending doom before the onset of abdominal pain; this occurs in cancer of the pancreas to a much greater degree than in other abdominal neoplasms.

PHYSICAL EXAMINATION. Physical examination may re-

Table 334-2. CLINICAL FEATURES AND LABORATORY FINDINGS IN CANCER OF THE BILE DUCTS AND PANCREAS*

Clinical feature	Cancer of ampulla of Vater	Cancer of bile ducts	Cancer of head of pancreas	Cancer of body and tail of pancreas
Pain	Absent—60% Moderate—40%	Absent—40% Moderate to severe—60%	Absent to mild—15% Moderate to severe—85%	Almost invariably present. Agonizing and boring. Often worse in back and accentuated when patient is supine.
Jaundice: Onset	Early	Early	Variable	Late to terminal.
Character	Progressive and marked—80% Fluctuating—20%	Progressive and marked—90% Fluctuating—10%	Progressive and marked	Mild to moderate.
Weight loss before onset of jaundice†	None to mild	None to moderate	Occasionally none, but often 10 to 20 lb	Marked, 10 to 60 lb.
Fever and chills	20%	10%	None	May have low-grade fever. No chills.
Hepatomegaly	None to slight	Slight in some cases, but may be extreme	Moderate Marked only if metastases present	None to marked. Size depends on degree of metastatic involvement.
Enlarged gallbladder palpable or visible	50%	20%	50%	0.
Splenomegaly	None	None	None	Occasional.
Bile in stools and urobilinogen in urine	Absent—80% Fluctuating—20%	Absent—90% Fluctuating—10%	Absent	Present.
Occult blood in stools	82%	15%		Rare.

* Because of their anatomic proximity, advanced cancers of the ampulla of Vater, the bile ducts, and the pancreatic head at times cannot be distinguished clinically.

† All these cancers cause impressive weight loss sooner or later.

veal nothing except jaundice and the excoriations of scratching. In spite of biliary obstruction, hepatic enlargement is not striking unless the liver is involved by metastases. Protecting the liver from back pressure, the gallbladder is enlarged in nearly all malignant obstructions of the common duct but can be palpated in only half the cases. A definite finding of an enlarged, nontender gallbladder in a jaundiced patient without biliary colic may, therefore, be taken as a reliable sign of malignant choledochal obstruction (Courvoisier's law). No diagnostic inference is warranted if the gallbladder is not palpable. Unfortunately, by the time the diagnosis is suspected, the liver is often involved by metastases, or positive nodes are present in the left supraclavicular area. The spleen may be enlarged secondary to malignant invasion and thrombosis of the splenic vein.

LABORATORY DATA. The urine, blood, and feces of nonicteric patients are often normal. Those with icterus have persistent and progressive bilirubinemia and choluria. The stools may be greasy, "abundant, of a pultaceous consistence, very deficient in bile, and most dreadfully foetid" (Richard Bright, 1838). In at least half the cases, however, the clay-colored stools are not grossly fatty and are more like putty than butter. Because bile salts are necessary for the absorption of vitamin K, hypoprothrombinemia develops with prolonged biliary obstruction.

Pancreatic tumors lead to ductal obstruction and occasionally to local areas of pancreatitis. The serum amylase and lipase activities are abnormal in only 10 percent of cases, but the 1-hr urine amylase excretion is reported to be increased in as many as 27 percent. Lesions in the head of the pancreas, blocking the larger ducts, result in a diminished volume of pancreatic juice after secretin stimulation, although the bicarbonate concentration is often normal. Glucose tolerance tests or intravenous tolbutamide tests are abnormal in 50 to 70 percent of cases, but the patient's age or antecedent diabetes partly accounts for this finding. Because ampullary cancers tend to ulcerate and form fistulas between the biliary and alimentary tracts, the serum bilirubin may fluctuate, occult blood is often found in the stools, and bouts of cholangitis may occur (Table 334-2), all of which are less likely in carcinoma of the head of the pancreas.

COURSE. Pancreatic cancer leads to death by inanition, biliary obstruction, local extension, or distant metastases. By direct extension, the cancer may invade the liver, spleen, stomach, duodenum, colon, portal venous system, or peritoneum. Invasion of the gut or development of varices following malignant occlusion of the portal vein can cause moderate to severe gastrointestinal blood loss. Peritoneal seeding or, very rarely, portal obstruction is responsible for ascites. Metastatic lesions develop in the regional lymph nodes, liver, lungs, mediastinal and cervical lymph nodes, and bone.

DIAGNOSIS. In jaundiced patients, cancer of the head of the pancreas must be differentiated from liver disease, common duct stones, and ampullary or bile duct carcinomas. Liver function tests tend to show regurgitation jaundice and normal hepatocellular function in uncomplicated extrahepatic obstructions. Favoring pancreatic

cancer is a gradual onset of symptoms in elderly patients without antecedent acute malaise, intermittent colicky pains, or chills and fever. If itching is noticed before jaundice, mechanical obstruction of the biliary passages is likely. In early cases, before the diagnosis is made obvious by massive or metastatic growth, cancer is suggested by finding an enlarged gallbladder and a slightly enlarged, nontender liver and by the absence of stigmas of liver disease such as spider angiomas, dilated abdominal veins, and splenomegaly.

Common duct stones rarely cause complete and unremitting biliary obstruction; light-colored stools which contain urobilin or urobilinogen are unusual in pancreatic tumors and suggest stones or ampullary carcinoma. Radiologic procedures may show the effect of the pancreatic lesion on other organs. Changes in the mucosa or configuration of the duodenal loop or stomach may sometimes appear early, but secondary gastrointestinal abnormalities are usually signs of advanced disease. Greater detail of the duodenal loop and its mucosa can be brought out by administering 60 mg Pro-Banthine intramuscularly to induce atony of the duodenum, followed by infusion of barium through a duodenal tube (hypotonic duodenography). Selective celiac arteriography occasionally identifies a tumor stain but more commonly demonstrates narrowing of pancreatic vessels due to encroachment by tumor or displacement of vessels by a mass. Percutaneous cholangiography can confirm that there is an obstruction of the common duct in the region of the head of the pancreas, but the differential between stone and tumor still must be settled by surgical exploration.

Because the pancreas avidly takes up circulating amino acids and transforms them into secretory proteins, it has become possible to scan the pancreas as one does the thyroid, looking for nonfunctioning areas involved by tumor. ^{75}Selenium, a gamma-emitting isotope which can be substituted for the sulfur atom of methionine, is incorporated into proteins, as is the natural amino acid, and allows external scanning of the gland. Uptake of selenomethionine by the liver often obscures the pancreatic outline, but the liver signals can be subtracted if prior scanning of the liver with radioactive colloidal gold is done. This procedure is particularly useful in tumors of the body or tail of the pancreas and has permitted the detection of pancreatic tumors as small as 2 cm in diameter.

When the patient is not jaundiced, early diagnosis is difficult. Persistent pain and progressive weight loss with negative radiologic studies of the alimentary, renal, and biliary passages should raise the suspicion of pancreatic cancer. In patients with ascites, the character of the fluid and its cellular content often permit the diagnosis of cancer, but differential diagnosis from ovarian, gastric, or primary hepatic cancer is not easy. In expert hands, duodenal drainage after secretin stimulation will yield abnormal cells in 40 percent of patients with cancer of the pancreas or bile ducts.

TREATMENT. Resection of cancers of the pancreas is usually undertaken only for those involving the head of the gland, because tumors of the body and tail are rarely detected before metastases have occurred. Out of every 100 patients presenting to a physician with cancer of the head of the pancreas, only about 15 to 20 are suitable for resection at the time of exploration. Resection of the head of the pancreas and duodenum, anastomosis of the bile duct and pancreatic duct to the jejunum, combined with a subtotal gastrectomy (Whipple procedure) entail a 15 to 20 percent mortality. Eventually only 1 to 2 patients out of the original 100 patients survive 5 years, a testimony to this tumor's tendency for early lymphatic and blood vessel invasion. In jaundiced patients palliative anastomosis of the gallbladder to the intestinal tract affords relief from intolerable itching but does not prolong life. Radiotherapy and chemotherapy are notoriously ineffective in ductal carcinomas of the pancreas.

OTHER CONDITIONS. The islets of Langerhans are also a source of benign and malignant tumors, some of which have the remarkable propensity of producing hormonally mediated clinical syndromes. The insulin-secreting beta cell tumors are discussed in Chap. 96. Non-beta cell tumors or islet cell hyperplasia may be associated with gastric hypersecretion and unusually placed and intractable peptic ulcer disease (the Zollinger-Ellison syndrome). A hormone remarkably like gastrin has been extracted from these tumors and seems to account for the gastric secretory stimulation. Other patients with non-beta cell tumors present a syndrome of severe diarrhea and hypokalemia not associated with gastric hypersecretion. This has lead to the postulate of another pancreatic hormone derived from the non-beta cells. Adenomatous involvement of other endocrine glands, in particular the parathyroid, adrenal, and pituitary glands, is seen in a fourth of these patients, and usually there is a familial tendency to the disorder. This subject is discussed in detail in Chap. 314.

Ectopically placed pancreatic tissue may be found in the gastrointestinal tract, in Meckel's diverticulum, and various other areas. Nearly all pancreatic rests discovered in adults, however, occur in the distal stomach and duodenum. Unusual pancreatic neoplasms are cystadenomas, cystadenocarcinomas, and hemangiomas.

REFERENCES

Blumenthal, H. T., and J. G. Probstein: "Pancreatitis: A Clinical-Pathologic Correlation," Springfield, Ill., Charles C Thomas, Publisher, 1959.

Burton, P., E. M. Hammond, A. A. Harper, H. T. Howat, J. E. Scott, and H. Varley: Serum Amylase and Serum Lipase Levels in Man after Administration of Secretin and Pancreozymin, Gut, 1:125, 1960.

DeReuck, A. V. S., and M. P. Camerson (Eds.): "The Exocrine Pancreas, Normal and Abnormal Functions," Ciba Foundation Symposium, London, J. & A. Churchill Ltd., 1962.

Di Sant'Agnese, P. A., and R. C. Talamo: Pathogenesis and Physiopathology of Cystic Fibrosis of the Pancreas, New Engl. J. Med., 277:1287, 1967.

FitzGerald, O., P. FitzGerald, and J. P. McMullin: Chronic Pancreatitis, Rev. Surg., 21:77, 1964.

Gross, J. B., and M. W. Comfort: Hereditary Pancreatitis: Report on Additional Families, Gastroenterology, 32:829, 1957.

Hartley, R. C., E. E. Gambill, G. W. Engstrom, and W. H. J. Summerskill: Pancreatic Exocrine Function: Comparison of Responses to Augmented Secretin Stimulus, Augmented Pancreozymin Stimulus, and Test Meal in Health and Disease, Am. J. Dig. Dis., 11:27, 1966.

Howard, J. M., and G. L. Jordan, Jr.: "Surgical Diseases of the Pancreas," Philadelphia, J. B. Lippincott Company, 1960.

Jorpes, J. E.: Memorial Lecture: The Isolation and Chemistry of Secretin and Cholecystokinin, Gastroenterology, 55:157, 1968.

Section 8

Disorders of the Hematopoietic System

INTRODUCTION

M. M. Wintrobe

The hematopoietic system includes the circulating blood, the bone marrow, the spleen, and the lymph nodes, supplemented by the reticuloendothelial cells scattered about the body. The liver, through the presence in it of reticuloendothelial cells as well as by reason of other functions, is also intimately concerned in blood formation and destruction.

Since the blood and its constituents are so intimately related to the body as a whole, much will be found concerning the blood in various chapters in this book. In regard to the red blood corpuscles, attention is called especially to Chap. 61, Pallor and Anemia, where the synthesis and the destruction of hemoglobin and the classification, pathogenesis, and management of anemia are considered, as well as the symptoms and methods of study of a patient with anemia. The platelets, the phenomenon of coagulation, and the various ways in which bleeding is produced receive attention in Chap. 62, Bleeding. Alterations in leukocytes in various circumstances and the functions and kinetics of the white blood cells are discussed in Chap. 64. The significance of enlargement of the lymph nodes and of the spleen is described in Chap. 63.

In the present section, disorders of the hematopoietic system will be considered. It is evident that such disorders make themselves known in a variety of ways. They may be such that discovering their cause may tax the acumen of even the most discerning physician. In the main, however, they are characterized in part or whole by symptoms and signs such as pallor, cyanosis, jaundice, bleeding, or enlargement of the lymph nodes or spleen. A thorough understanding of these manifestations of disease is a prerequisite to the correct differentiation as well as the effective treatment of the disorders of the hematopoietic system.

The *approach* to the patient suspected of having a hematopoietic disorder is discussed, therefore, in Part Three under headings such as Pallor and Anemia, Bleeding, and Enlargement of Lymph Nodes and Spleen. Although in the following pages, descriptions of the various recognized disorders of the hematopoietic system will be found and their treatment discussed, it is urged that the reader confronted with a problem, for example, of anemia, first study Chap. 61; he will find there a discussion of anemias in general and will thereby be able to make his way more readily through the pages that follow or, for that matter, through other sections in this volume. The same is true, in principle, if the problem is one of bleeding, or lymph node enlargement, or splenomegaly.

335 POSTHEMORRHAGIC ANEMIA
M. M. Wintrobe

Anemia resulting from blood loss may have developed acutely because of the rapid loss of a large quantity of blood, or it may have come about very gradually over a period of many months or even years. Obviously there are also many possible variations between these two extremes. The causes of posthemorrhagic anemia are numerous, and the manifestations differ widely, the latter depending in part on the nature of the underlying disorder and in part on the quantity and speed of the blood loss. It is convenient to consider acute and chronic posthemorrhagic anemias separately, because their manifestations and, in certain respects, their treatment differ so greatly. It should be realized, however, that these two syndromes represent two extremes which depend, in the main, on the same underlying defect.

ACUTE POSTHEMORRHAGIC ANEMIA

ETIOLOGY. Trauma, the bleeding of a peptic ulcer, the rupture of an ectopic pregnancy, and hemorrhage in connection with hemophilia or thrombocytopenic purpura are examples of the widely varied possible causes of acute blood loss. They indicate that the blood loss may be external and recognizable at once, or internal and, consequently, sometimes not readily discovered.

SYMPTOMATOLOGY. The rapid loss of blood leads to reduction in blood volume, and the clinical manifestations are mainly circulatory. If the blood loss is great, "acute posthemorrhagic shock" develops (see Chap. 320). If the hemorrhage is visible to the patient, whether the amount of blood lost is great or small, symptoms may arise from the psychic effect of such bleeding. Generally speaking, symptoms are likely to appear sooner and are more pronounced in relation to the amount of blood lost when the bleeding is external than when it is not recognizable by the patient. The manifestations of anemia in general have been discussed already (Chap. 61). In addition, the symptoms of the underlying disorder may be present as well.

BLOOD PICTURE. Polymorphonuclear leukocytosis, with the leukocyte count rising even to 20,000 per cu mm, and an increase in the number of platelets are the first discernible changes. A few metamyelocytes and an occasional myelocyte may be seen in the differential count. Because the blood vessels of the skin and muscles constrict in response to the need to maintain the blood supply of the vital organs, because plasma is lost as well as red cells, and because restoration of plasma is slow the volume of packed red cells or hemoglobin level will not adequately reflect the true degree of blood loss. In the course of the succeeding 24 to 48 hr, however, fluid passes into the blood stream and anemia becomes apparent. At the same time, the bone marrow is stimulated and reticulocytes begin to increase in 1 or 2 days, reach a peak of 5 to 15 percent in 4 to 7 days, and, in the absence of continued bleeding, reach normal levels in about 10 days. At the same time as reticulocytosis occurs, polychromatophilia develops and even nucleated red cells may be seen. Since immature red cells are larger than older ones, the anemia may become macrocytic temporarily. The leukocyte count should return to normal in 3 or 4 days. A persistent reticulocytosis, forming a plateau-like curve, suggests that bleeding is continuing, for cessation of hemorrhage is marked by quick restoration of physiologic balance, with rapid regression of the signs of stimulated hematopoiesis. If the iron stores of the body are good and the blood loss has not been extreme, iron deficiency does not occur and hypochromia is slight or absent. When the drain on iron is greater than can be readily replenished, iron deficiency begins.

Very severe blood loss, of a degree which requires replacement with 5,000 ml or more of blood per 24 hr, is associated with thrombocytopenia.

When the acute hemorrhage is internal, destruction of the blood and absorption of the products may lead to an increased excretion of urobilinogen in the urine and stools, and, rarely, even slight bilirubinemia may be found. Bowel hemorrhage is often associated with an increase in the blood urea nitrogen level; this increase is due both to temporary impairment of renal function (prerenal azotemia, Chap. 301) and to absorption of large amounts of protein.

DIAGNOSIS. When acute hemorrhage is not evident, such signs as pallor, faintness, restlessness, sweating, and palpitation should lead to a search for hemorrhage. If the subject is recumbent, much blood may be lost before these signs appear. They can be brought out by tilting the patient to the erect position. Late signs of acute blood loss are air hunger, thirst, and a falling blood pressure.

PROGNOSIS. The amount and rapidity of the blood loss, the acuteness of the physician in discovering it, the availability of blood for transfusion, and the accessibility of the site of bleeding are the important considerations.

TREATMENT. Stopping of the hemorrhage, combating shock, and restoring the blood volume to normal are the essentials. Transfusions of whole blood are best, but human plasma or albumin, a plasma expander such as dextran, 0.9 percent sodium chloride in water, or 5 percent glucose in 0.9 percent sodium chloride, may be used, in that order of preference, while blood is being matched. In civilian practice it is now rarely necessary or justifiable to resort to unmatched universal donor blood. Speed in restoration of blood volume is more important than whether plasma or whole blood is used.

Other medical or surgical procedures depend on the cause of the hemorrhage. Rest and quiet, induced by morphine if necessary and not otherwise contraindicated, are important. Following the acute phase, a high protein diet should be provided. Whether or not iron is given depends on the extent to which the iron stores are thought to have been drained and the degree to which this loss has been counteracted by blood transfusion. Other supplements are not necessary.

CHRONIC POSTHEMORRHAGIC ANEMIA

This refers to that state in which blood loss has produced a chronic anemia and a deficiency of substances necessary for blood formation has developed. Although the factors essential for erythropoiesis are many, the chief deficiency resulting from chronic blood loss is that of iron. The manifestations of chronic posthemorrhagic anemia can therefore be discussed in the chapter which follows.

336 IRON-DEFICIENCY ANEMIA AND OTHER HYPOCHROMIC MICROCYTIC ANEMIAS

M. M. Wintrobe and G. R. Lee

IRON-DEFICIENCY ANEMIA

INCIDENCE. In the United States as many as 64 percent of infants, 13 percent of adult women, and 58 percent of pregnant women are iron-deficient. In other parts of the world, such as Great Britain, this type of anemia is still more common, and in Asia, the Middle East, and in some parts of Africa and of Central and

South America this anemia is not only very prevalent but may be very severe. An understanding of iron metabolism provides the explanations for these facts.

IRON METABOLISM. Iron is normally obtained by digestion of food. The newborn infant starts with a supply derived from the mother, but as growth occurs, dietary sources are necessary to meet the demands of the ever-expanding vascular space. In the female, with the onset of menarche, iron is needed to make up for the loss of blood; later, the demands of pregnancy exceed the saving due to amenorrhea.

The body of a normal adult contains approximately 2 to 6 Gm iron. One-half to two-thirds of this amount is found in hemoglobin, and about 3 mg circulates in the plasma as transferrin. Only a very small proportion of the total body iron is present in myoglobin and the heme enzymes (0.15 Gm). The remainder (1.2 to 1.5 Gm) represents a reserve which can be called upon for hemoglobin production and is stored in the liver, spleen, and bone marrow as ferritin and hemosiderin.

The average adult diet in the United States provides about 12 to 15 mg iron per day. Heavy meat eaters may get 20 mg. However, only 5 to 10 percent of this amount (0.6 to 1.5 mg) is absorbed. When there is increased need for iron, absorption may be more efficient (10 to 20 percent). Ingested iron is reduced to the ferrous form in the stomach and intestine. Absorption is most efficient in the duodenum and upper part of the small intestine. Iron is transported through the mucosal cell but the exact mechanism is still uncertain. The absorbed iron is then bound by plasma transferrin, a β_1-globulin, and transported to the bone marrow for hemoglobin synthesis. The normal plasma iron level is 60 to 190 μg per 100 ml, but the turnover is rapid so that 25 to 40 mg iron is transported in the plasma per day.

Conservation is the characteristic feature of iron metabolism. The iron derived from the breakdown of hemoglobin joins the body pool and is used again and again. Loss of iron from the body is minimal: probably no more than 0.5 to 1 mg per day in feces, urine, and sweat. Most of this amount is contained in cells desquamated from mucosal surfaces or the skin. Some iron is lost in bile. It has been claimed that in tropical climates the dermal loss of iron is great, perhaps several milligrams per day, but this is disputed. In women, the greatest normal cause of iron loss is menstruation. A normal woman loses 3 to 80 mg iron during a normal period, thus averaging 0.5 to 1 mg per day. The net loss of iron during a normal pregnancy is about 400 to 500 mg; i.e., an average of about 1.5 mg per day. During lactation the average loss is about 0.5 mg per day.

It follows that, in a temperate climate, the *requirement* for iron in a normal man or postmenopausal woman is 0.5 to 1 mg per day. For menstruating women it is 1 to 2 mg per day. During pregnancy 2.0 to 2.5 mg per day is required. The iron requirement for growth during infancy and childhood varies with the rapidity of growth at different periods. During the first year of life the need may be as high as 1 mg per day, but averages 0.6 mg; during childhood the average is about 1.0 to 1.5 mg per day. However, for the adolescent girl another 0.5 to 1.0 mg must be added to allow for menstrual loss.

CAUSES OF IRON DEFICIENCY. From this review of the iron economy of the body, it follows that children, female adolescents, and women in their reproductive years, are most in danger of developing iron deficiency. However, any circumstance which leads to a greater demand on the iron stores of the body than can be met results in iron deficiency. The possible factors leading to iron deficiency are (1) insufficient iron in the diet, (2) impaired absorption, (3) increased requirements, and (4) loss of blood. In many instances, more than one of these factors is responsible for the resulting deficiency.

Other than in infants and in rapidly growing children, *chronic loss of blood* by hemorrhage is by far the most common factor in the development of iron deficiency. Excessive menstruation and occult bleeding from the gastrointestinal tract (peptic ulcer, hookworm infection, esophageal varices, etc.) are the most common types of bleeding which may result in iron deficiency, since excessive menstrual loss is but an exaggeration of a physiologic process and gastrointestinal bleeding may pass unnoticed for a long time. A woman may lose as much as 200 ml blood during each menstrual period and not be aware that the loss is excessive. In an adult male, the discovery of iron-deficiency anemia should cause a diligent search for a source of bleeding, and this is most likely to be found in the gastrointestinal tract.

On the other hand, *decreased assimilation* of iron, whether from dietary deficiency of iron or from impaired absorption, or both, is rarely an important cause of iron deficiency unless the iron stores are already poor, demands for iron (as by rapid growth or frequent pregnancies) are great, or blood loss has occurred. Diets high in cereal content and low in animal protein and in green vegetables are relatively poor sources of iron. Furthermore, the nature of the diet itself, other than its iron content, influences the assimilation of iron. Thus a high level of calcium in the diet diminishes the formation of insoluble iron phosphates and favors absorption of iron, but excess calcium impairs iron assimilation, probably because of the consequent high pH. Again, the phytic acid content of some cereals interferes with the absorption of iron. Ascorbic acid favors iron assimilation, probably by promoting the reduction of ferric iron in food to the ferrous form. Protection against dietary iron deficiency is being provided in the United States and elsewhere by fortifying flour, bread, and infant cereals with iron, but the influence of long-established cultural practices, food faddism, and generally poor dietary habits is hard to overcome.

The gastric hydrochloric acid favors ionization and thus absorption; yet many persons are found in whom achlorhydria has existed for years without iron deficiency developing. Nevertheless, iron deficiency develops ultimately after total or partial gastrectomy in the absence of evidence of bleeding. Likewise, chronic diarrhea prevents efficient absorption, and in steatorrhea iron absorption has been shown to be impaired. Not only is the absorption of dietary iron inefficient in these situations, but increased absorption in response to need, which occurs normally, does not take place.

Nevertheless, since the normal loss of iron from the body is relatively small, none of these circumstances of impaired iron assimilation is likely to be an important cause of iron deficiency unless blood loss or increased needs have developed. The high requirements for iron in infants, children, and adolescents, and in premenopausal women, have been outlined above.

The syndrome of *chlorosis,* the "green sickness" of the last century and before, was probably no more than iron deficiency in adolescent girls in whom dietary iron was insufficient to meet the needs for growth and menstruation. Likewise the *chronic hypochromic anemia* of women thirty to forty-five years of age represents the ultimate combined effect of chronic loss of blood, frequent pregnancies, and poor diet in an individual whose iron deficiency may have had its beginning in adolescence. It is of interest that in many of these patients certain constitutional features similar to those encountered in pernicious anemia have been observed, such as early graying of the hair and achlorhydria.

SYMPTOMATOLOGY. Iron deficiency develops insidiously, and, depending on the personality of the patient and the cause of the deficiency and its severity, the accompanying clinical manifestations may range from few, if any, complaints to those common to all chronic anemias, such as increasing fatigability, headache, anorexia or capricious appetite, heartburn, palpitation, dyspnea, edema about the ankles, neuralgic pains, vasomotor disturbances, or numbness and tingling. It is evident that such symptoms also are found in the absence of anemia. Attempts to relate some of these manifestations to deficiencies of cellular iron metalloenzymes have not been successful.

Sore tongue, sore mouth, angular stomatitis, or dysphagia may occur in an occasional patient who is iron-deficient. The *Plummer-Vinson syndrome* is characterized by the feeling of food sticking in the throat, and in some cases a stricture at the mouth of the esophagus has been demonstrated, the opening being partially closed by a thin, mucous web which has been demonstrated roentgenographically and is easily ruptured by the passage of an endoscope.

Menstrual disturbances are common—menorrhagia, irregularity of flow, or even amenorrhea.

In the fully developed state, the clinical picture is striking: a tired, lifeless appearance; pallor; inelastic and often dry and wrinkled skin, sometimes with a brownish hue; dry and often scanty hair; and pearly white scleras are found. In many cases, some degree of papillary atrophy of the tongue, slight cardiac enlargement, functional systolic murmurs, a slightly enlarged liver, and a palpable spleen are discernible. When the deficiency is severe, the nails may be flattened, longitudinally ridged, or even concave (koilonychia), and may break easily. Findings on neurologic examination are nearly always normal.

BLOOD PICTURE. When significant anemia is present, a good blood smear will reveal thin, pale red corpuscles poorly filled with hemoglobin. In severe cases these may be mere rings. Tiny microcytes, "target-like" cells, elliptic cells, and bizarre poikilocytes also are found, as well as a certain proportion of normally filled corpuscles. The red corpuscle count may be normal or nearly so, or even greater than normal, while the hemoglobin and volume of packed red corpuscles are greatly reduced. The anemia is hypochromic and microcytic. The hypochromia is more significant than the microcytosis, although the latter may be extreme [mean corpuscular volume (MCV) even 55 to 70 cuμ]. Reticulocytes are usually normal in number but may increase temporarily following an acute episode of blood loss. The leukocyte count is normal or slightly reduced, and a slight thrombocytopenia may exist.

The *bone marrow* is hyperplastic and contains relatively increased numbers of normoblasts.

Gastric analysis reveals achlorhydria in two-thirds of patients after a test meal of alcohol and in half the patients after histamine. The augmented histamine test has shown true achlorhydria in 16 percent. Superficial gastritis or moderate atrophy has been demonstrated by gastric mucosal biopsy in many instances. Iron therapy may be associated with return of free hydrochloric acid secretion, especially in younger persons, but in many patients neither the secretory nor the morphologic changes are relieved.

DIAGNOSIS. Before significant anemia will occur, the iron stores must be depleted. Consequently, in equivocal instances, when the blood picture is not clear-cut or the anemia is not sufficiently severe to produce the classical picture, it is useful to measure the serum iron and the quantity of iron-binding protein. Although the serum iron is reduced both in iron deficiency and in association with chronic disorders (Chap. 340), in the latter the iron-binding capacity falls below normal while in the former it is increased (greater than 450 μg per 100 ml).

An additional useful procedure is the examination of the bone marrow after staining for iron. In iron-deficient subjects, no stainable iron will be visible, whereas marrow iron is normal or increased in the anemia of chronic disorders. If neither serum iron determinations nor bone marrow iron stains are available, a therapeutic trial of iron may aid in establishing the diagnosis. The clearest results from therapeutic trials are obtained when the anemia is severe and when there are no complicating illnesses to prevent an adequate response. If such a trial is to be made, it is helpful if serial observations of the reticulocyte count are made during the first 10 days of therapy. A significant reticulocytosis occurring 7 to 10 days after the onset of iron administration indicates a response. In a therapeutic trial period of 3 to 4 weeks, under such circumstances hemoglobin should increase an average of 0.2 Gm or more per day.

Iron deficiency is not the only cause of hypochromic microcytic anemia, even though it is the most common one. Other microcytic hypochromic anemias will be discussed in the next section.

TREATMENT. True iron deficiency can be relieved by the administration of iron, but this alone does not suffice; it is imperative to seek and, if possible, to correct the cause. Here the onus rests heavily with the physician, since effective iron therapy alone will satisfy the patient temporarily, but the opportunity to cure a malignant neoplasm (e.g., carcinoma of the cecum) or some other treatable condition may be lost if the cause is not discovered.

Contrary to the blandishments of the pharmaceutical manufacturers and their agents, nothing better has been devised for the correction of iron deficiency than ferrous sulfate. The addition of other minerals such as cobalt or copper, combination with vitamins, or the introduction of devices to improve absorption has accomplished nothing other than to increase the cost of therapy to the patient. Ferrous sulfate (300 mg of hydrated ferrous sulfate or 200 mg of the exsiccated salt), 3 or 4 tablets per day, is the optimal amount, but the dose should be increased gradually (1 tablet the first day, 2 the second, etc.) because tolerance for iron is thereby built up and fewer gastrointestinal side effects develop. It is easier, furthermore, to take iron when the stomach contains food.

The administration of ferrous sulfate is followed by a reticulocyte response, and hemoglobin regeneration ensues. Three tablets of $FeSO_4$ per day will provide about 35 mg of iron if about 20 percent is absorbed. Treatment for at least 6 months is needed in most cases if the body stores are to be replenished.

It is rare that parenteral therapy is required. When iron is absorbed poorly, as in *some* cases of steatorrhea, or when disease such as regional ileitis, ulcerative colitis, iliostomy, or colostomy prevents its use, iron-dextran or iron-sorbitol citric acid complex may be given intramuscularly. The first dose should be limited to 50 mg, because reactions, sometimes severe, occur. By repeated injections, a total of 1.5 to 2.0 Gm may be given in this way.

Transfusion of blood is rarely if ever needed, and free hydrochloric acid is not required, even if achlorhydria is present, because an excess of ferrous iron is prescribed and it is mainly the absorption of ferric rather than ferrous iron which is enhanced by the presence of acid.

OTHER HYPOCHROMIC MICROCYTIC ANEMIAS

Although iron deficiency is by far the most common cause of hypochromic, microcytic anemia, other causes (Table 61-3, II) should be considered. *Thalassemia* (Chap. 339) results in hypochromia and microcytosis with little or no anemia in the heterozygous, or "minor," form and causes severe hypochromic, microcytic anemia with features of hemolysis in the homozygous, or "major," form.

The *anemia of chronic disorders* (Chap. 340) usually is normocytic and normochromic. Occasionally, when the condition is of long standing, modest hypochromia and even microcytosis are observed. An incorrect diagnosis of iron deficiency may be made, not only because of the morphologic changes, but because the serum iron concentration may be reduced. In contrast to iron deficiency, however, the iron-binding capacity is normal or reduced, and iron is found in appropriately stained bone marrow specimens.

SIDEROBLASTIC ANEMIAS. These anemias (Table 336-1) are a group of uncommon disorders in which circulating hypochromic, microcytic erythrocytes are found in association with increased amounts of iron in developing normoblasts (*sideroblasts*). *Sideroblasts* are best detected in bone marrow aspirates stained with the Prussian blue reaction. In normal subjects, one to three small, blue granules may be seen in as many as 90 percent of normoblasts. In patients with sideroblastic anemias, both the size and the number of these iron-containing granules are increased. In some of the cells, the granules tend to form a ring around the nucleus (ringed sideroblasts). By electron microscopy, abnormal sideroblasts are characterized by extensive mitochondrial iron deposits. In contrast, visible nonheme iron in normal erythroblasts is found in the cytoplasm in the form of ferritin.

Table 336-1. THE SIDEROBLASTIC ANEMIAS

I. Congenital
   A. Pyridoxine-responsive
   B. Other congenital forms, including "anemia hypochromica sideroachrestica hereditaria"
II. Acquired
   A. Idiopathic
     1. Pyridoxine-responsive
     2. "Refractory" sideroblastic anemia
     3. "Preleukemia"
   B. Symptomatic
     1. Malignancies
     2. Chronic inflammatory diseases
     3. Certain drugs and toxins (isoniazid, cycloserine)

Sideroblastic anemias are characterized further by an increased serum iron concentration with complete or nearly complete saturation of the iron-binding protein. Reticuloendothelial iron stores also are markedly increased, and deposition of iron in parenchymatous organs is common. The latter may be severe enough to cause hyperpigmentation of the skin and impaired function of the liver, pancreas, and heart. Hepatosplenomegaly may be found on examination. The leukocyte and platelet counts are usually normal but may be slightly reduced.

Kinetic studies often reveal "ineffective erythropoiesis": plasma iron turnover is increased, but red cell iron utilization is impaired. Red cell survival is normal or only slightly reduced, and the reticulocyte count is normal. Nevertheless, there may be modest "indirect" hyperbilirubinemia and increased fecal urobilinogen excretion.

Sideroblastic anemias may be divided into two categories, congenital and acquired (Table 336-1). Further subdivision may be made on the basis of the effect of pyridoxine (vitamin B_6) therapy. In some patients, the administration of pyridoxine induces reticulocytosis and an increase in blood hemoglobin concentration. However, it is unlikely that correction of a pyridoxine-deficient state accounts for the improvement since (1) the amount of pyridoxine required greatly exceeds the estimated daily nutritional requirement; (2) the response is usually incomplete—the anemia is not completely relieved and morphologic abnormalities in the erythrocytes persist; (3) prompt relapse occurs when therapy is discontinued; and (4) no neurologic signs of vitamin B_6 deficiency are found.

Most of the patients with congenital, *pyridoxine-responsive sideroblastic anemia* have been males, and an X-linked hereditary pattern has been demonstrated in several families. In some of the reported patients, the free erythrocyte protoporphyrin content was reduced prior to institution of pyridoxine therapy and became normal or increased with treatment. Since pyridoxal phosphate is a cofactor for the enzymatic synthesis of delta-aminolevulinic acid (Chap. 61), it has been suggested that the genetic defect lies in this enzyme system.

A congenital form of sideroblastic anemia which does not respond to pyridoxine (*anemia hypochromica sideroachrestica hereditaria*) also appears to be inherited as an X-linked trait. In patients with this disorder, the free erythrocyte coproporphyrin is markedly increased and the free erythrocyte protoporphyrin is reduced. This finding suggests a deficiency in the enzyme coproporphyrinogen oxidase (Chap. 61).

Other cases of congenital sideroblastic anemia have been reported which do not fall into either of the above two categories. In one such family the microcytic, hypochromic cells were shown to be Xg^a-positive. There appear to be serveral different kinds of abnormality in hemoglobin synthesis which result in congenital sideroblastic anemia.

The *idiopathic, acquired sideroblastic anemias* usually are found in middle-aged or elderly subjects. In these disorders, the proportion of hypochromic erythrocytes is small, as a rule, so that the mean corpuscular hemoglobin concentration (MCHC) is not abnormal; however, a careful examination of the blood smear will detect the abnormal erythrocytes ("partial hypochromia"). The pathogenesis is not known. In a few of these patients, the anemia is partially relieved by the administration of pyridoxine, but in the majority this does not occur.

Myeloblastic leukemia has been observed as a terminal event in some cases of acquired sideroblastic anemia. This has led some investigators to regard the illness as a stage in the development of leukemia (i.e., "preleukemia"). There are no reliable figures regarding the frequency of this complication, nor are there reliable means for predicting its occurrence.

Symptomatic or secondary sideroblastic anemia has been observed in association with certain underlying illnesses. These include malignancies, such as Hodgkin's disease, multiple myeloma, and carcinoma of the prostate, and chronic inflammatory diseases, e.g., rheumatoid arthritis. Certain drugs (isoniazid, cycloserine, pyrazinamide) have been reported to induce sideroblastic anemia, apparently by interfering with vitamin B_6 metabolism. The drug-induced syndromes may be corrected by administering pyridoxine or by withdrawing the offending agent.

Treatment. Management of patients with sideroblastic

anemia requires a series of therapeutic trials. All such patients should be given pyridoxine in a dose of 50 to 200 mg per day for about 2 months. If no response occurs, further pyridoxine therapy is of no value. Some patients who do not respond to pyridoxine will improve when given adrenal corticosteroids, androgens, or a combination of the two. These agents may be employed in a regimen similar to that used in aplastic anemia (Chap. 341). Since the ultimate prognosis often is related to the degree of iron-loading, it follows that iron-containing medications are contraindicated, and blood transfusions should be kept to a minimum. It is rarely necessary to maintain the volume of packed red cells at more than about 25 ml/100 ml.

REFERENCES

Bothwell, T. H., and C. A. Finch: "Iron Metabolism," Boston, Little, Brown and Company, 1962.

Harris, J. W., and D. L. Horrigan: "Pyridoxine Responsive Anemia—Prototype and Variations on the Theme, *in* R. S. Harris, J. A. Loraine, and I. G. Wool (Eds.), "Vitamins and Hormones," New York, Academic Press Inc. 22:721–753, 1964.

Lee, G. R. et al.: Hereditary X-linked Sideroblastic Anemia, Blood, 32:59, 1968.

MacGibbon, B. H., and D. L. Mollin: Sideroblastic Anemia in Man: Observations on Seventy Cases, Brit. J. Hematol. 11:59, 1965.

Wintrobe, M. M.: "Clinical Hematology," 6th ed., pp. 777–782, Philadelphia, Lea & Febiger, 1967.

337 PERNICIOUS ANEMIA AND OTHER MEGALOBLASTIC ANEMIAS

M. M. Wintrobe and G. R. Lee

It was pointed out in an earlier chapter (Chap. 61) that anemia characterized by an increase above normal in the mean corpuscular volume may be due (1) to the presence of large numbers of immature red corpuscles, i.e., *"nonmegaloblastic macrocytic anemias"* (see Table 337-1); or (2) to a qualitative alteration in erythropoiesis which results in the formation of an abnormal erythrocyte precursor, the megaloblast, from which are derived abnormally large red blood cells. The clinical differentiation of these two types of anemia is easy. The treatment of one differs greatly from the treatment of the other. The *megaloblastic anemias* are the subject of the present discussion.

Pernicious anemia may be considered to be the prototype of this group of anemias. Not only is it of great historical importance, but it remains the most common cause of megaloblastic anemia in temperate zones. Moreover, many aspects of the symptomatology, laboratory picture, and pathologic physiology of pernicious anemia apply as well to other types of megaloblastic anemia. A

thorough understanding of pernicious anemia, therefore, forms a logical foundation upon which understanding of other disorders within this group can be built. For these reasons, pernicious anemia will be discussed initially. This will be followed by a discussion of the etiology, pathologic physiology, diagnosis, and therapy of the entire group of megaloblastic anemias.

PERNICIOUS ANEMIA

Pernicious anemia is characterized by megaloblastic anemia, achylia gastrica, and neurologic damage. It may be classed as a "conditioned" deficiency, in that it arises as the result of failure of the gastric fundus to secrete amounts of "intrinsic factor" sufficient to ensure intestinal absorption of vitamin B_{12}.

INCIDENCE. This is the most prevalent form of vitamin B_{12} deficiency in North America and Europe. In developing and tropical countries, pernicious anemia is uncommon but certain other forms of megaloblastic anemia are abundant.

Both sexes are affected equally. Pernicious anemia is rare in persons under the age of thirty, and its incidence increases with age. An exception is **juvenile pernicious anemia,** a very rare form observed in children, which differs from that seen in adults in that gastric atrophy and achylia gastrica are not observed.

Adult pernicious anemia most commonly affects persons of northern European extraction and is much less common in Orientals and Negroes. Perhaps because of this racial distribution, a typical somatotype is said to characterize the patient with pernicious anemia: many of the patients are found to be of "large and bulky frame," with prematurely gray hair and blue, widely set eyes. However, there are many exceptions to this generalization.

HISTORY. Although pernicious anemia was described at least as early as 1823 by Combe, it was the picture given by Thomas Addison in 1855 and the comprehensive description by Biermer in 1872 which drew attention to what was then an ultimately fatal (therefore "pernicious") anemia. Subsequent developments have completely changed the prognosis. In 1926, Minot and Murphy, by applying to man the pioneering investigations of Whipple and his associates, demonstrated that when massive amounts (½ lb per day) of fresh liver were given by mouth, patients with pernicious anemia experienced a remission of the illness.

Castle, in 1929, elucidated the role of the stomach in the pathogenesis of the disease. It had been observed previously that pernicious anemia is almost invariably accompanied by a greatly reduced total volume of gastric secretions (achylia) and by the absence of hydrochloric acid in these secretions. Castle demonstrated a more significant abnormality of gastric secretion; namely, the lack of an "intrinsic factor" which normally acts on an "extrinsic factor," present in beef muscle and other foods. The two factors were regarded as combining to form an "anti-pernicious anemia principle" which was stored in the liver.

The subsequent isolation of vitamin B_{12} and the demonstration of its therapeutic efficacy in pernicious anemia clarified some of the puzzling aspects of the pathogenesis of the disease. It is now apparent that the effect of liver observed by Minot and Murphy is accounted for by the high vitamin B_{12} content of liver, and that vitamin B_{12} is identical both with "extrinsic factor" and the "antipernicious anemia principle." "Intrinsic factor," a thermolabile glycoprotein, is required for absorption of the vitamin.

CLINICAL DESCRIPTION. The onset of the disease generally is insidious. In many instances at least two of the diagnostic triad of symptoms are encountered; namely, weakness, sore tongue, and numbness and tingling in the extremities. However, other complaints may overshadow these, and the presenting clinical picture may suggest some disorder of the digestive tract because of anorexia, diarrhea, and various other gastrointestinal symptoms; it may simulate cardiac dysfunction of the anginal or the congestive failure type; or one may be led to search for some malignant neoplasm or an obscure infection. In some instances the neural involvement is so pronounced that a primary neurologic disease is considered. Even renal or genitourinary disease or a mental disorder may be simulated.

The degree of soreness of the tongue varies greatly, and the involvement may be complete or patchy. The tongue may be "beefy" red when the symptoms are pronounced and is less red and smooth when they subside. The gastrointestinal symptoms also vary greatly. However, one consistent finding in relapse is anorexia. Symptoms referable to the circulatory system include dyspnea, palpitation, sensations of extra beats, weakness, vertigo, tinnitus, and precordial pain. Since pernicious anemia often appears for the first time in the older age groups, it may be difficult to determine to what extent anemia or the degenerative changes of old age have contributed to the development of heart failure.

Pallor; a flabby rather than wasted appearance; a slight or pronounced yellowish color of the skin together with faint icterus of the sclera; a tongue which is often glazed in appearance and sometimes is red and sore; a rapid pulse with slight cardiac enlargement and often precordial hemic murmurs; in many, a spleen which is just palpable; and often a slightly enlarged liver are the chief findings outside the nervous system. In the nervous system, loss of vibratory sense in the lower extremities (not necessarily symmetric), incoordination of the lower extremities, loss of finer coordination of the fingers, signs suggestive of lateral as well as posterior spinal cord involvement, and evidence of peripheral nerve degeneration are the most common findings and may be present in all degrees from slight or none to extensive involvement. Positive Babinski response, positive Romberg's sign, disturbed position sense, spasticity, increased or diminished reflexes, and sphincter disturbances may be encountered. Minor mental disturbances (irritability, memory disturbances, mild depression) or more serious mental symptoms may develop.

LABORATORY FINDINGS. Blood. The anemia is usually more severe than the complaints and physical examination would lead one to suspect. In the blood smear, macrocytes, often oval in shape, are characteristically seen (Fig. 337-1), but there is actually a great range in the size of the cells, and in addition, many bizarre-shaped corpuscles are found (poikilocytosis). Since the abnormally large cells predominate, the mean corpuscular volume is found to be greater than normal and ranges between 100 and 160 cu μ. There is a corresponding increase in the hemoglobin content of the red corpuscles (mean corpuscular hemoglobin), so that the concentration of hemoglobin in the corpuscles (mean corpuscular hemoglobin concentration) is normal. The red corpuscles in pernicious anemia and in other macrocytic anemias are not "hyperchromic," but, being thicker as well as larger in diameter than normal corpuscles, they appear to be supersaturated with hemoglobin, as one looks at them through a microscope. Some degree of diffuse polychromatophilia as well as basophilic stippling is found, and occasional nucleated red corpuscles may be encountered. The most striking changes, described in classic cases, are observed only when the anemia is very severe. Since the anemia is macrocytic, the red corpuscle count is reduced more than proportionately as compared with the hemoglobin or the volume of packed red corpuscles. Reticulocytes are usually within normal limits in untreated patients or, at most, are not greater than 3 or 4 percent.

Hypersegmentation of the nuclei of neutrophilic leukocytes is one of the earliest and most consistent blood findings in patients with pernicious anemia (Fig. 337-1C). Hypersegmentation is best detected by enumerating the nuclear segments in 100 consecutive neutrophils and calculating the average number of segments per cell. The normal range is 2.9 to 3.5. Other leukocyte abnormalities also are common in pernicious anemia in relapse. The neutrophils may be exceptionally large, and giant metamyelocytes are particularly characteristic. There usually is mild to moderate neutropenia; at times eosinophilia is

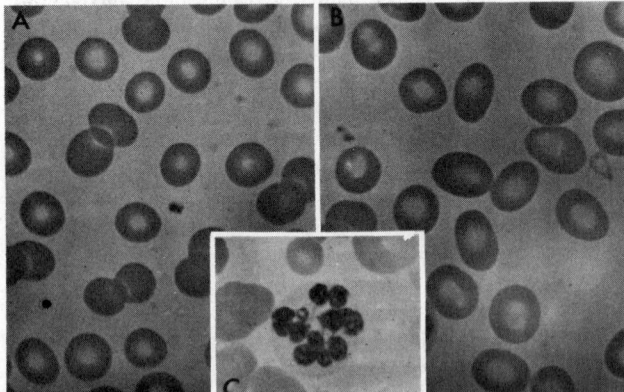

Fig. 337-1. The blood smear in megaloblastic anemia. A. Normal blood smear for comparison. B. Pernicious anemia. Most of the erythrocytes are large, oval, and well filled with hemoglobin. C. Pernicious anemia. Striking hypersegmentation of a neutrophilic leukocyte.

found, and an occasional myelocyte may be seen on the blood smear.

Platelets generally are reduced in number and may be large and bizarre in appearance. In exceptional cases, purpura is observed.

Bone Marrow. The bone marrow is red and is found to be crowded with cells. Cells of the red series make up 30 to 50 percent, rather than about 20 percent, of the cells of the marrow. The degree of hyperplasia and the degree of immaturity of the cells are roughly proportional to the severity of the anemia. The nucleated red corpuscles ("megaloblasts") differ from those found in other types of anemia in several respects. They are exceptionally large, and, more significantly, the nuclear chromatin is fine and sievelike, unlike the relatively coarse and "lumpy" material seen in normoblasts. The cytoplasm of these cells may be polychromatophilic or orthochromatic, and in a few is basophilic. Many abnormal mitotic figures may be present. At the same time, extraordinarily large leukocytes may be found in the marrow; in particular, large metamyelocytes may be seen with bizarre-shaped nuclei and peculiarly staining or vacuolated cytoplasm. Megakaryocytes may be reduced in number and may be morphologically abnormal.

Other Laboratory Findings. With very rare exceptions, histamine-fast achlorhydria is found in patients with pernicious anemia. In addition, the total volume of the gastric secretion and its enzyme content are markedly reduced. Mild hyperbilirubinemia due to an increase in the unconjugated or "indirect" fraction is not uncommon. Furthermore, the urobilinogen content of urine and feces is greater than normal. The urinary excretion of methylmalonic acid (p. 1596) is markedly increased.

PATHOLOGY. The significant findings are in the alimentary tract, the bone marrow, and the nervous system. The tongue usually appears smooth, and the papillae may be absent. Atrophy of the gastric mucosa may be striking, particularly in the fundus, where the parietal and chief cells are usually absent. The findings in the bone marrow have been described above.

In the nervous system, degenerative changes are found in the dorsal and lateral columns and, in more advanced cases, in the peripheral nerves. The earliest abnormality is loss of the myelin sheath, followed by degeneration of the axone and, finally, by death of the neurone. With appropriate therapy, all but the last are reversible.

Appropriate staining reveals the liver, spleen, and kidneys to be abnormally laden with iron. In the liver, this is found in the periphery of the lobules and in the Kupffer cells. There also may be fatty degeneration in the central cells of the lobules of the liver. The heavy deposit of iron is the consequence of the fault in red blood cell formation which leads to the development of anemia; when active blood regeneration follows therapy, the iron is used in blood formation.

PATHOLOGIC PHYSIOLOGY OF MEGALOBLASTIC ANEMIA

The megaloblast is a morphologic expression of a metabolic defect, namely, disordered synthesis of deoxy-

ribonucleic acid (DNA). Both vitamin B_{12} and folic acid are essential to DNA synthesis. A deficiency of one or both vitamins is the underlying abnormality in the overwhelming majority of patients with megaloblastic anemia.

Vitamin B_{12}, a reddish compound possessing a cobalt-containing tetrapyrrolic ring, is synthesized by certain microorganisms and is principally available to man in the flesh of animals having access to bacterial products. Efficient absorption of dietary vitamin B_{12} ("extrinsic factor") requires its interaction with a thermolabile glycoprotein with a molecular weight of about 70,000 ("intrinsic factor"), secreted in the gastric fundus. This substance has an unusually strong binding affinity for vitamin B_{12}. By attaching to specific receptors on the intestinal wall, intrinsic factor facilitates absorption of vitamin B_{12} by the ileum. In the presence of intrinsic factor, about 70 percent of ingested vitamin B_{12} is absorbed; less than 2 percent is absorbed in its absence.

Normally, after a delay of several hours in the gut wall, the vitamin B_{12} brought there through the intermediation of intrinsic factor is carried through the bloodstream by a specific protein carrier. The serum concentration of vitamin B_{12} in normal subjects is 200 to 900 $\mu\mu g$ per ml. The total body vitamin B_{12} content in the normal adult is about 5,000 μg (range, 2,000 to 10,000 μg), of which 1,700 μg is stored in the liver. Since biochemical evidence of deficiency is not seen until the total body content drops to less than 500 μg, the surplus of 4,500 μg constitutes a large storage pool. The average daily requirement for vitamin B_{12} in the normal adult is approximately 2.5 μg, but the requirement no doubt is increased during periods of rapid growth and in pregnancy. It has been postulated that the requirement is also increased in hemolytic anemias, in thyrotoxicosis, and even in infection.

The exact *role of vitamin B_{12} in DNA synthesis* is not certain, but it is clear that it is related to certain functions of folic acid. It is probable that in deficient subjects the vitamin B_{12}-dependent synthesis of methionine is blocked. As a result, folate, which is normally converted to tetrahydrofolate during methionine synthesis, becomes "trapped" as N^5-methyl tetrahydrofolate. By this mechanism a relative deficiency of other folate coenzymes develops, including N^5, N^{10}-methenyl tetrahydrofolate, a cofactor essential for the synthesis of the DNA precursor, thymidylic acid. Another step in DNA synthesis which may be vitamin B_{12}-dependent is the conversion of uridylic acid to deoxyuridylic acid.

The term **folic acid** has been used to denote either a single chemical substance (pteroylglutamic acid, PGA) or a whole group of unconjugated, conjugated, or formylated compounds owing their activity to the PGA radical, but the term *folate* or *folacin* (Chap. 85) is preferable for the latter, the term folic acid being used to refer to PGA only. Folates are synthesized by higher plants as well as by microorganisms, and are found in many vegetables, as well as in liver. About 90 percent of natural folic acid is found in conjugated form and must be split off by intestinal conjugases for absorption to occur. A normal balanced diet may contain 1.0 to 2.0 mg folic acid, but little is known about the efficiency of absorption of natural folates. The daily requirement in normal adults is about 50 μg (0.05 mg) per day, but may be as high as 300 μg per day in certain stressful situations, such as pregnancy. Destruction by cooking or loss by aqueous extraction may greatly reduce the amount of folate derived from the diet. Synthetic PGA is absorbed readily and rapidly throughout the small intestine. The serum contains 5 to 20 ng (nanograms) of folate per ml in normal subjects. Body stores of folic acid and its derivatives are less substantial than those of vitamin B_{12}. The estimated storage pool of 5 to 10 mg may be depleted after only several months of dietary deprivation.

After absorption, folates are reduced through specific liver enzymes to tetrahydrofolic acid, which is capable of accepting single-carbon fragments such as formyl, methyl, and formimino radicals. N^5-Formyltetrahydrofolate (folinic acid, "citrovorum factor"), N^5-methyl tetrahydrofolate, and N^5, N^{10}-methenyltetrahydrofolate are among the metabolites that are produced. In these forms folic acid acts as a carbon-transfer agent and as a coenzyme in the synthesis of nucleoprotein. It is essential for the synthesis of carbons 2 and 8 in purines, as well as for the synthesis of thymidylic acid from deoxyuridylic acid.

The alteration in DNA synthesis induced by deficiency of vitamin B_{12} or folate affects many of the tissues of the body, but is especially evident in the hematopoietic system. Before a cell can divide, it must precisely double its DNA content. When DNA synthesis is impaired, cell division is retarded. This is manifest morphologically in an alteration in the nuclear pattern of the red blood cell and an increase in its total size. The abnormal nuclear pattern in the **megaloblast** presumably results from the prolonged time between cell divisions, allowing for a greater degree of dispersion of nuclear material. Cytoplasmic processes are unaffected; consequently, hemoglobin formation proceeds normally and cell size increases. The maturation of granulocytes and megakaryocytes also is altered, accounting for the presence of giant metamyelocytes in the bone marrow and *hypersegmented polymorphonuclear leukocytes* in the blood. Cell division in nonerythropoietic tissues also is affected; in the mouth, stomach, and vagina, giant epithelial cells have been demonstrated.

The disordered metabolism of the erythrocytes which characterizes the megaloblastic macrocytic anemias is also manifested by erythroid hyperplasia in the bone marrow. This may be attributed, in part, to the fact that erythropoiesis is ineffective; i.e., many of the red corpuscle precursors, being imperfect, probably are destroyed in the marrow or very shortly after they have been released into the circulation. When red blood cell survival is measured it is found to be mildly shortened; however, the usual techniques for labeling red blood cells do not detect cells which are destroyed in the marrow and, therefore, do not appraise accurately the magnitude of the ineffective erythropoiesis. Ineffective erythropoie-

sis also accounts for the increased serum bilirubin and increased urobilinogen excretion that so often are found in these disorders. When radioactive glycine is fed to patients with megaloblastic anemia, a disproportionate amount appears in the so-called "early-labeled" bile pigments, indicating that much of the pigment is derived from a very short-lived population of erythrocytes.

The **neurologic damage** seen in some forms of megaloblastic anemia appears to be related specifically to deficiency of vitamin B_{12}, rather than of folic acid, and therefore probably is not related to the disordered synthesis of DNA. It is known that vitamin B_{12} is required for the enzymatic conversion of methylmalonyl coenzyme A to succinyl coenzyme A, a step in the catabolism of propionic acid; thus, excessive amounts of methylmalonic acid appear in the urine of vitamin B_{12}-deficient subjects, a phenomenon which forms the basis for a sensitive test of vitamin B_{12} deficiency. It has been suggested that retention of propionic acid catabolites may be responsible for the neurologic changes found in vitamin B_{12}-deficient subjects.

In pernicious anemia, vitamin B_{12} deficiency is conditioned by lack of intrinsic factor. In other forms of megaloblastic anemia, deficiency is produced in other ways, as will be discussed in the next section. The relatively high familial incidence of pernicious anemia suggests that the defect in intrinsic factor secretion may be genetically determined. In careful *family studies*, between 8 and 30 percent of patients with pernicious anemia have been found to have relatives with the disease. An even greater incidence of achlorhydria, gastric atrophy, and partial defects in vitamin B_{12} absorption has been observed in relatives of patients with pernicious anemia. Still more striking is the evidence for an hereditary basis of the form of pernicious anemia found in childhood. A number of pairs of siblings have been reported with this illness, including at least one set of monozygotic twins. It has been suggested that juvenile pernicious anemia represents the homozygous form of adult pernicious anemia. However, the absence of gastric atrophy and achylia gastrica in these children may indicate that it is a distinct entity.

Several observations suggest that pernicious anemia is produced by *autoantibodies* directed against the gastric mucosa and that the tendency to form such antibodies may be genetically determined. Antibodies directed against gastric parietal cells are found in 90 percent of patients with pernicious anemia. Similar antibodies are detected in most patients with atrophic gastritis without pernicious anemia, but are uncommon in normal subjects. A second type of antibody, one which reacts directly with intrinsic factor, is found in as many as 60 percent of patients with pernicious anemia but not in other patients with gastric atrophy. The incidence of both types of antibody is greater in relatives of patients with pernicious anemia than in the general population. Still other observations have been made which have been cited as reasons for considering pernicious anemia as representing an autoimmune disorder. Thus, pernicious anemia has been observed to be associated with autoimmune disorders of the thyroid more frequently than would be expected on the basis of chance alone. In addition, the chronic inflammatory lesions of the stomach in patients with pernicious anemia resemble those in the thyroid in patients with Hashimoto's thyroiditis. Furthermore, administration of adrenocorticosteroids may improve vitamin B_{12} absorption and induce hematologic improvement in pernicious anemia. Nevertheless, despite the above observations, a cause and effect relationship between the autoimmune phenomena and the gastric lesions in pernicious anemia remains to be demonstrated. It is possible that the antibodies are the consequence of a genetically determined defect in the gastric mucosa, rather than its cause.

MEGALOBLASTIC MACROCYTIC ANEMIAS OTHER THAN PERNICIOUS ANEMIA

Dietary deficiency of folate, of vitamin B_{12}, or of both; impaired absorption of these vitamins; increased requirements; or faulty metabolism may singly or in combination produce this type of anemia. Probably because of its less-efficient storage, folate deficiency is relatively common among the malnourished. In contrast, even in the strictest vegetarians ("vegans") vitamin B_{12} deficiency of a degree sufficient to produce megaloblastic anemia is very rare. Pure folate deficiency with macrocytic anemia has been produced experimentally in swine, but dietary deficiency of vitamin B_{12} alone has not resulted in macrocytic anemia.

The various forms of megaloblastic anemia are listed in Table 337-1, where those due to vitamin B_{12} deficiency and to folic acid deficiency are listed separately. However, a number of conditions are found under both categories. This can be accounted for, in part, by the intimate relationship of these two vitamins in metabolism, as discussed earlier. Deficiency of one affects the need for and metabolism of the other. This explains why, in a disorder such as pernicious anemia, when the specific fault is inability to absorb vitamin B_{12} efficiently from the diet, a hematologic response, albeit temporary or incomplete, follows administration of folic acid. Actually the propensity of an individual to develop a deficiency of these vitamins depends on many factors. Thus, in a person with imperfect means for absorption of vitamin B_{12}, the development of deficiency will depend on the degree and duration of intrinsic factor deficiency (e.g., lifetime or only since the performance of a gastrectomy), on intestinal factors influencing its absorption or permitting its utilization or destruction, or on altered metabolic requirements. Furthermore, other factors being equal, folic acid deficiency is likely to develop more readily than lack of vitamin B_{12} because storage of folic acid is less efficient than that of vitamin B_{12}.

The hematologic manifestations of *folic acid deficiency* are the same as those of vitamin B_{12} deficiency. The gastrointestinal manifestations are similar but tend to be more widespread and more severe than those of pernicious anemia. Thus diarrhea is usually present and may be accompanied by distension, meteorism, flatulence,

and the roentgenographic picture of sprue. Cheilosis and glossitis are common, and ulcerative stomatitis, pharyngitis, esophagitis with dysphagia, and perirectal and peroneal weeping and ulcerations may appear. However, neurologic abnormalities like those seen in pernicious anemia do not occur.

Certain syndromes may now be discussed separately.

NUTRITIONAL MACROCYTIC ANEMIA. This term refers to macrocytic anemia arising from dietary deficiency, as distinguished from deficiency resulting from lack of intrinsic factor or from faulty absorption. Since such anemia has been seen most often in the tropics, *tropical macrocytic anemia* is a synonym. The condition is particularly common in pregnant women. Weakness, shortness of breath, sore mouth, sore tongue, diarrhea, and edema are common complaints. In contrast to the condition found in pernicious anemia, achlorhydria is no more common in nutritional macrocytic anemia than in the population in general, and degenerative changes in the nervous system are practically never found. The blood picture and bone marrow are indistinguishable from those of pernicious anemia. Tropical macrocytic anemia probably is not a single clinical entity. In many patients the anemia has been relieved by the administration of yeast, Marmite (autolyzed yeast), or liver. In some cases a good hematopoietic response has followed the administration of folic acid, and in a few patients a good response to vitamin B_{12} and even to oral penicillin has been reported. That some form of dietary deficiency is the cause of this disorder is indicated by the observation that it does not recur if the diet is satisfactory.

Nutritional macrocytic anemia is uncommon in the temperate zones. Some of the instances of macrocytic anemia seen in *pellagra* may be accounted for by a lack of vitamin B_{12} in the diet. In other instances faulty absorption is important, and in many patients both mechanisms play a role. In *malabsorption syndromes,* as described elsewhere (Chap. 316), inadequate absorption is the main cause for the development of macrocytic anemia. In Great Britain, in particular, occult idiopathic steatorrhea with insignificant alimentary symptoms but accompanied by megaloblastic macrocytic anemia is not uncommon. The latter usually responds much better to the administration of folic acid than to vitamin B_{12}. A specific, selective vitamin B_{12} malabsorption disease beginning in infancy and childhood, *familial* in occurrence, and characterized by **relapsing megaloblastic anemia and proteinuria** has been described in Norway.

FOLLOWING SURGERY. Following *total gastrectomy* or extensive damage to gastric mucosa as, for example, by ingestion of corrosive agents, megaloblastic anemia may develop because the source of intrinsic factor has been removed. In such patients the absorption of orally administered vitamin B_{12} is impaired. Following *partial gastrectomy* the incidence of megaloblastic anemia is very much lower than after total gastrectomy, although iron-deficiency anemia is relatively common. The macrocytic anemia seen in association with *intestinal strictures, diverticuli, anastomoses,* and *"blind loops"* has been attributed to impaired absorption, but since good hema-

Table 337-1. CLASSIFICATION OF MACROCYTIC ANEMIAS

Type of anemia	Condition	Probable pathogenesis
Nonmegaloblastic macrocytic anemias*	Acute posthemorrhagic anemia	Presence in blood of many immature erythrocytes
	Hemolytic anemia	Presence in blood of many immature erythrocytes
	Aplastic anemia	Unknown
	Hypothyroidism	Unknown
	Liver disease	Unknown
Megaloblastic macrocytic anemias: Vitamin B_{12} deficiency............	Pernicious anemia†	Deficiency of gastric intrinsic factor
	Gastrectomy	Removal of source of intrinsic factor
	Intestinal disease (sprue, steatorrhea, etc.)	Intestinal malabsorption
	Selective vitamin B_{12} malabsorption	Hereditary defect
	Surgical and mechanical disorders (resection of small intestine, intestinal strictures, diverticuli, anastomoses and "blind loops")	Intestinal malabsorption, competition for vitamin B_{12}
	Fish tapeworm anemia	Competition for vitamin B_{12}
	Nutritional macrocytic anemia	Nutritional deficiency of animal or bacterial products
	Pregnancy, thyrotoxicosis(?)	Deranged metabolism (?)
Folate deficiency.................	Nutritional macrocytic anemia	Nutritional deficiency of vegetables and liver
	Intestinal disease (sprue, steatorrhea, celiac disease)	Intestinal malabsorption
	Megaloblastic anemia of pregnancy	Increased requirements and nutritional deficiency
	Megaloblastic anemia of infancy, some cases of scurvy	Increased requirements and nutritional deficiency
	Surgical and mechanical disorders (resection of small intestine, intestinal strictures, diverticuli, anastomoses, and "blind loops")	Intestinal malabsorption, competition for folic acid (?)
	Amethopterin or 6-MP therapy	Metabolic antagonism
	Anticonvulsant drugs	Metabolic antagonism, low stores
	Hemolytic anemias and other conditions with marrow hyperplasia	Increased demands, low stores
	"Achrestic" anemia and "refractory megaloblastic anemia"	Uncertain. Nutritional deficiencies and deranged metabolism (?)
	Miscellaneous (liver disease)	Impaired utilization (?)
Hereditary deficiency..............	Orotic aciduria	Enzyme deficiency

* In practice, the most common cause of what appears to be macrocytic anemia is laboratory error, most often in red corpuscle counting.

† Pernicious anemia is distinguished from the other conditions listed in that achlorhydria is always present and neurologic changes may occur.

topoietic responses have been observed when tetracyclines were given, it seems plausible that the anemia is caused by the colonization of the small intestine by large masses of bacteria which in some way divert folic acid or vitamin B_{12} from the host.

IN FISH TAPEWORM INFESTATION. True megaloblastic macrocytic anemia is seen, in Finland especially, in persons harboring the tapeworm, *Diphyllobothrium latum.* The anemia is attributable to competition between the worm and the intrinsic factor of the host for vitamin B_{12}. However, genetic factors also may be important in the pathogenesis, since instances have been reported in which the incidence of megaloblastic anemia was higher in family members than in other individuals living in the same house.

IN PREGNANCY. Megaloblastic anemia may be observed during the third trimester of pregnancy. In most cases it appears to be due to folate deficiency occurring as the result of a marginal diet and the demands of the developing fetus. The syndrome is most common in geographic areas where nutritional macrocytic anemia is observed. Occasionally, however, it is encountered in temperate zones, and historical evidence of dietary inadequacy may be difficult to elicit. Even in such cases, the serum folate level is reduced and a response to the administration of folate may be expected. Exceptional cases have been reported in which vitamin B_{12} appeared to be the deficient nutrient.

IN SCURVY AND IN INFANCY. Ascorbic acid may be involved in the stabilization of reduced folic acid. Occasionally patients with scurvy develop a folic acid deficiency which may be partially conditioned by the deficiency of ascorbic acid. The megaloblastic anemia of infancy, which appears sometimes in infants fed on unsupplemented dried milk formulas, probably reflects such a mixed deficiency of folic acid and ascorbic acid.

DURING ADMINISTRATION OF ANTIMETABOLITES. One of the toxic effects of methotrexate and 6-mercaptopurine, used in the treatment of leukemia, is the production of megaloblastic anemia. Interference with the metabolism of folic acid appears to be the explanation for the development of such anemia in a small proportion of patients receiving *anticonvulsant* drugs, such as diphenylhydantoin sodium, primidone, and barbital derivatives, although the possible coexistence of some degree of folic acid deficiency in the individuals affected must be considered to be likely.

IN PRESENCE OF EXCESSIVE DEMANDS. In rare instances of very active hematopoiesis, especially in hemolytic anemias, the hemoglobinopathies, and myelofibrosis, megaloblastic anemia has been observed, presumably because the demands for building materials exceeded those available in persons whose stores of these substances were marginal.

IN LIVER DISEASE. Macrocytic anemia occurs in a variable number of patients with chronic liver disease, and in a few it is megaloblastic. Because of the detergent effects of retained bile salts, erythrocyte membrane lipids may become altered, and an increase in membrane area results. This phenomenon may account for nonmegaloblastic macrocytosis in certain patients with liver disease. No wholly satisfactory explanation for the occasional case of megaloblastic anemia has been found. It is conceivable that the requirements for folic acid and vitamin B_{12} may be increased or their storage or utilization impaired, or that other factors are involved.

IN HYPOTHYROIDISM. Macrocytic anemia is sometimes seen in hypothyroidism, but the bone marrow is usually hypoplastic and normoblastic, and desiccated thyroid, not liver extract, vitamin B_{12}, or pteroylglutamic acid, is effective in relieving the anemia. Defective intestinal absorption of vitamin B_{12}, uninfluenced by intrinsic factor, has been demonstrated in some cases.

MISCELLANEOUS DISORDERS. In patients such as those described at one time as having *achrestic anemia* and *refractory megaloblastic anemia*, because they failed to respond to liver therapy, there may be impaired metabolism of folic acid or complex deficiencies of folic acid, ascorbic acid, choline, or perhaps other substances essential for the metabolic steps which result in normal erythropoiesis. **Megaloblastic anemia with orotic aciduria** has been described in which there was an inborn defect in the conversion of orotic to orotidylic acid. In *erythremic myelosis* ("DiGuglielmo's syndrome"), megaloblastic changes have been described, but giant multinucleated red blood cells with chromatin differing from that of megaloblasts are more characteristic.

DIAGNOSIS

Optimum therapy in macrocytic anemia is completely dependent on accurate diagnosis. In nonmegaloblastic anemias, therapy with folic acid or vitamin B_{12} is valueless. In megaloblastic anemias, correction of the underlying fault, if possible, and in any event selection of the proper vitamin are of critical importance. For example, if folic acid is given to a patient with pernicious anemia, transient hematologic improvement may be observed but neurologic lesions may appear and progress.

THE CLINICAL SETTING. When megaloblastic anemia is found together with neurologic symptoms in an elderly subject with a history of an adequate diet, pernicious anemia is the most likely diagnosis. The detection of neurologic disease is of great diagnostic help, since it occurs only in vitamin B_{12} deficiency; however, only a small proportion of patients exhibit such findings. The demonstration of achylia gastrica supports a diagnosis of pernicious anemia. This impression may be further confirmed by means of a Schilling test. Megaloblastic anemia in an infant, a pregnant woman, or an alcoholic suggests folate deficiency, and confirmation may be sought by the determination of serum vitamin content. A careful history should reveal exposure to the drugs associated with megaloblastic anemia, or uncover symptoms of malabsorption.

LABORATORY EVIDENCE OF SPECIFIC VITAMIN DEFICIENCY. When the clinical setting is complex, it is helpful to determine whether there is a deficiency of vitamin B_{12} or of folate. Two relatively simple, *indirect tests* are available for this purpose. Excessive **urinary excretion of methylmalonic acid** is a sensitive and relatively specific test for vitamin B_{12} deficiency. The **histidine loading test,** which consists of measurement of urinary formiminoglutamic acid (**FIGlu**) after the oral administration of histidine, is a sensitive test for folate deficiency; however, abnormal values also have been observed in some patients with severe vitamin B_{12} deficiency.

More direct evidence for specific vitamin deficiency consists of the determination of serum vitamin levels. Serum vitamin B_{12} concentration may be determined by means of a **microbiologic bioassay** system employing *Euglena gracilis* or by a simpler technique based on radioisotope dilution and coated charcoal. The normal range is 200 to 900 $\mu\mu g$ per ml, and values less than 100 $\mu\mu g$ per ml may be considered diagnostic of vitamin B_{12} deficiency. A microbiologic assay for folate is available which employs *Lactobacillus casei* as the test organism. The normal serum concentration ranges from 6 to 21 $m\mu g$ per ml; values of 4 $m\mu g$ per ml or less are diagnostic of folate deficiency.

Because of the technical problems associated with

Serum iron, μg/100 ml	140	180		8		42
Serum folate, mμg/ml	24.7	26 22	19.5	21	17.4	15.3
Serum vit. B$_{12}$, $\mu\mu$g/ml	24	30 26	86	258	571	348

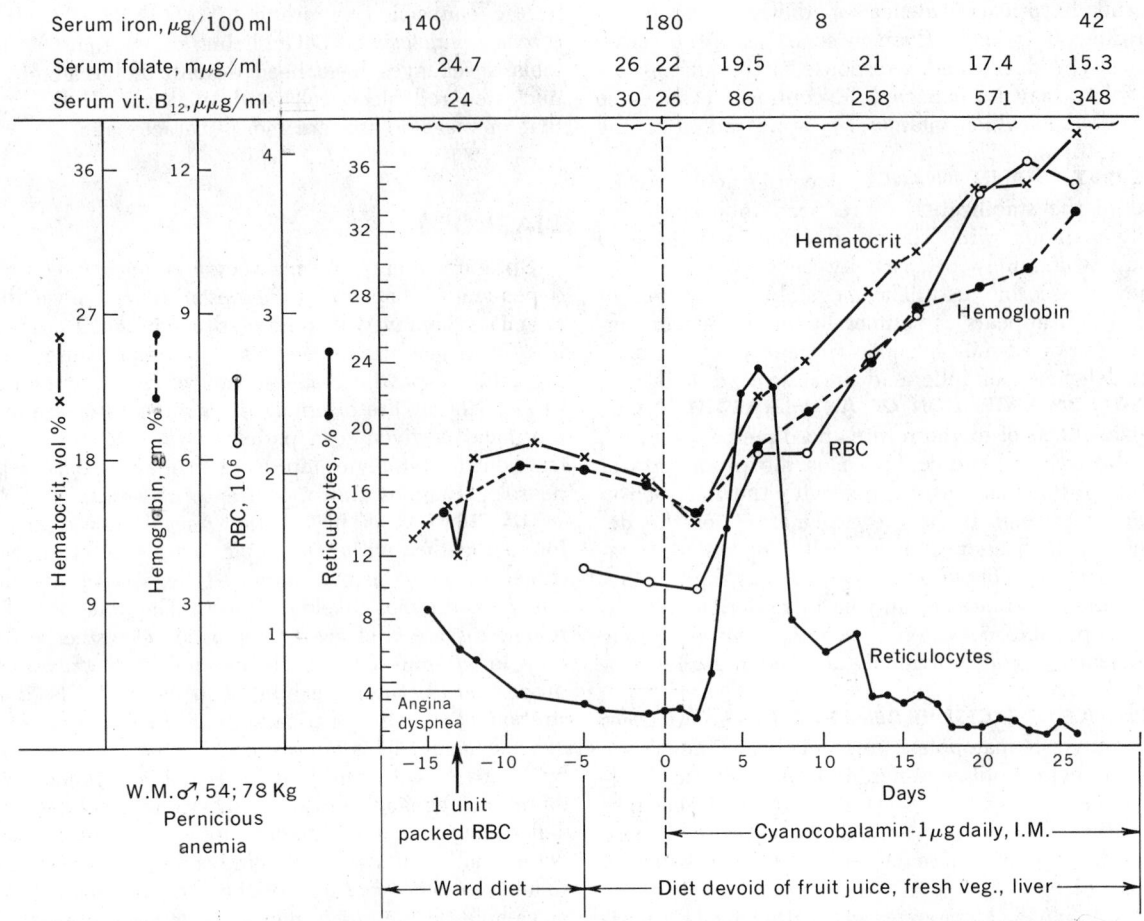

Fig. 337-2. The response to a minimal effective dose of vitamin B$_{12}$ (cyanocobalamin, 1 μg per day) in a patient with pernicious anemia. The earliest change is an increase in the reticulocyte count, which usually reaches a peak 5 to 7 days after therapy is begun. (*Courtesy of Dr. Victor Herbert, New Engl. J. Med., 268:368, 1963.*)

microbiologic assays, they are not generally available. The indirect tests are much simpler, but they, too, are not available in most routine clinical laboratories. For this reason, clinicians often must depend on **therapeutic trials** to establish the diagnosis. In performing a therapeutic trial, it is important to employ minimal effective doses, since larger doses may induce nonspecific responses. The minimal effective dose of vitamin B$_{12}$ is 1 μg per day; in the case of folate, it is 100 μg per day. During a trial, after a 5- to 10-day period of observation, one of these vitamins is administered parenterally. Reticulocyte counts should be performed daily during the control and trial periods, and the volume of packed red blood cells and hemoglobin should be determined at 5-day intervals. A response is detected when a significant reticulocytosis occurs 5 to 10 days after the onset of therapy, and reduction in the degree of anemia should follow. A typical response to minimal doses of vitamin B$_{12}$ is illustrated in Fig. 337-2.

The Schilling Test. The discovery of vitamin B$_{12}$ and the fact that the cobalt contained therein can be labeled radioactively have provided methods whereby the absorption of this vitamin can be measured. They offer a means by which defective absorption of the vitamin from the gastrointestinal tract can be demonstrated even in the absence of anemia. This is useful in treated cases of pernicious anemia, and to some extent is helpful in distinguishing pernicious anemia from other disorders of vitamin B$_{12}$ absorption. Several different techniques are available, but the most commonly used one, the Schilling test, depends on measurement of the excretion of the administered radioactive material in the urine. When radioactive vitamin B$_{12}$ is given by mouth to persons who can absorb it, radioactivity will appear in the urine if the person is simultaneously given a very large amount (1,000 μg) of nonradioactive vitamin B$_{12}$ intramuscularly. Normal individuals have been found to excrete 5 to 40 percent of the orally administered radioactivity in the urine in the next 48 hr if an oral dose of 2.0 μg is used. Patients with pernicious anemia excrete less than 5 percent under these conditions. In them, the simultaneous oral administration of intrinsic factor and radioactive vitamin results in increased excretion. In contrast, although excretion is also reduced in patients with one of the malabsorption syndromes (Chap. 316), no improvement occurs when intrinsic factor is added.

MANAGEMENT AND PROGNOSIS

PERNICIOUS ANEMIA AND OTHER VITAMIN B$_{12}$ DEFICIENCY STATES. With appropriate therapy it is now possible to restore the blood to normal and to promote a return of the general nutrition to normal. If changes are present in the nervous system, their advance can at least be halted, and in those cases in which death of nerve cells has not occurred, the neurologic lesions are reversible. The danger in pernicious anemia arises from failure to continue therapy and from complications and intercurrent conditions. In a chronic ailment like pernicious anemia, other diseases develop in the course of time. Among these, carcinoma of the stomach is particularly noteworthy, since the incidence of this disease in patients with pernicious anemia is more than three times as great as in other individuals. When changes in the nervous system exist, particularly if they involve the urinary sphincter, infection may occur. The existence of infection at the time of relapse may seriously interfere with the response to therapy.

Treatment, insofar as the blood changes are concerned, is extremely simple. The administration of an adequate amount of vitamin B$_{12}$ is followed by a reticulocyte response which reaches its maximum 5 to 7 or 8 days following initiation of therapy (Fig. 337-2). This is succeeded, as the reticulocyte count falls to normal, by a rapid disappearance of anemia and by the production of cells of normal size and shape. The leukocyte and the platelet counts likewise return to normal, bilirubinemia disappears, and the increased quantities of urobilinogen in the urine and stools are reduced to the normal range. The gastric achlorhydria persists.

Effective treatment may produce subjective improvement within 48 hr, and evidence of a change is often noted by the patient before the reticulocytes increase in number. He will experience a gain in appetite and a sense of well-being. Tongue symptoms, if present, disappear promptly. On the other hand, neural symptoms do not change quickly. Although the blood usually becomes normal in the course of 2 months from the beginning of treatment, the neurologic symptoms may still be present. However, those of milder intensity are likely to decrease or disappear.

The most efficient means of treatment is by the intramuscular injection of vitamin B$_{12}$. Intravenous therapy is effective but unnecessary. The effects of vitamin B$_{12}$ in pernicious anemia are very much more pronounced when the vitamin is given parenterally than when it is taken orally (60 to 100 times). Of the several forms of the vitamin that are available, hydroxycobalamin appears to be the most efficient, since a smaller proportion of the injected dose is lost in the urine. However, cyanocobalamin is quite satisfactory. The minimal effective intramuscular dose of vitamin B$_{12}$ is 1 μg or more daily. Larger amounts, up to 80 μg or more daily, produce greater effects, the mean response being roughly proportional to the logarithm of the dose. As larger doses are given, however, a greater proportion is promptly excreted.

For a patient in relapse, between 1,000 and 5,000 μg vitamin B$_{12}$ is given, since the substance is needed not only to produce a remission but to replenish the greatly depleted body stores. However, this is best administered in divided doses in the course of the first 2 weeks or more of therapy; otherwise, much of the vitamin will be excreted before it can be used or stored, as already indicated. An injection of 100 μg is a satisfactory amount to be given at one time. If possible, reticulocytes should be counted daily in order that the effectiveness of therapy, or lack of response, may be demonstrated early. An increased quantity of red blood cells, as measured by the volume of packed red blood cells, is not usually detectable before 10 days.

In pernicious anemia and in other conditions in which vitamin B$_{12}$ deficiency has developed because of an irreversible defect in absorption, lifelong **maintenance therapy** is required. The amount necessary may be calculated on the basis of approximately 2.5 μg vitamin B$_{12}$ for each day, but this does not need to be given at intervals shorter than a month or two; i.e., 100μg is injected intramuscularly every 30 days. Even longer intervals (up to 3 months) between injections are possible if hydroxycobalamin is used. Oral therapy with liver extract or vitamin B$_{12}$-intrinsic factor combinations is inconvenient, since daily intake is necessary. Only when the patient has some idiosyncrasy, or when sensitivity to the parenteral administration of vitamin B$_{12}$ cannot be overcome otherwise, is oral therapy justified. Then 200 to 1,000 μg vitamin B$_{12}$ orally every day is preferable to the use of vitamin B$_{12}$-intrinsic factor combinations or liver extracts. Folic acid, in doses which greatly exceed the normal daily requirement, induces a hematopoietic response in pernicious anemia. However, while the administration of vitamin B$_{12}$ relieves or prevents the advancement of the neurologic manifestations of pernicious anemia, these may appear and progress when only folic acid is given (see Chap. 85).

The diet should be such as to restore the patient to a state of normal nutrition and to maintain this state, but it need not contain any unusual foods.

Transfusion is rarely, if ever, required in pernicious anemia, since a physiologic response can be achieved in 48 to 72 hr if vitamin B$_{12}$ is given parenterally. Since the patient's anemia has developed gradually, he has become adjusted to it. When the cardiovascular system is imperfect, transfusion, by producing a sudden increase in blood volume, may sometimes be harmful and may precipitate acute cardiac failure with pulmonary edema. Iron is not needed as an adjunct except when iron deficiency exists as well. Supplementary therapy with various vitamins is likewise unnecessary. These can be and should be furnished in the diet in the form of food.

Particularly when changes in the nervous system exist, confinement to bed should be as brief as possible and the patient should be encouraged to use his limbs even when lying in bed. In addition, passive movement, massage, and dry heat are valuable for improving the tone of the muscles. Physiotherapy may permit adjustment to permanent damage resulting from the neurologic changes.

The development of an intercurrent disease, particularly infection, calls for an increase in the amount of vitamin B_{12} therapy, since requirements under such conditions seem to be increased.

FOLATE DEFICIENCY. The above comments regarding general supportive care and the use of blood transfusions apply equally well to the patient with folate deficiency. Repletion of folate stores may be accomplished by the oral administration of 5 to 15 mg per day of folic acid (pteroylglutamic acid). Rarely is there any need for parenteral therapy, even in patients in whom absorption is defective. Apparently, these large doses can circumvent the barrier to absorption. For antagonist-produced folic acid deficiencies, larger doses, as much as 100 to 200 mg per day, may be required. Folinic acid (citrovorum factor) may have some advantage in such situations, since conversion of folic to folinic acid may be one of the reactions that is blocked.

REFERENCES

Barness, L. A.: Vitamin B_{12} Deficiency with Emphasis on Methylmalonic Acid as a Diagnostic Aid, Am. J. Clin. Nutr. 20:573, 1967.

Doniach, D., and I. M. Roitt: An Evaluation of Gastric and Thyroid Autoimmunity in Relation to Hematologic Disorders, Seminars Hematol., 1:313, 1964.

Gough, K. R., A. E. Read, C. F. McCarthy, and A. H. Waters: Megaloblastic Anemia Due to Nutritional Deficiency of Folic Acid, Quart. J. Med., 32:243, 1963.

Herbert, V.: Megaloblastic Anemias—Mechanisms and Management, Disease-a-month, August, 1965.

Johns, D. G., and J. R. Bertino: Folates and Megaloblastic Anemia: A Review, Clin. Pharmacol. Therap., 6:372, 1965.

Lindenbaum, J., and F. A. Klipstein: Folic Acid Deficiency in Sickle Cell Anemia, New Engl. J. Med., 269:875, 1963.

Paulk, E. A., Jr., and W. E. Farrar, Jr.: Diverticulosis of the Small Intestine and Megaloblastic Anemia, Am. J. Med., 37:473, 1964.

Reynolds, E. H., G. Milner, D. M. Matthews, and I. Chanarin: Anticonvulsant Therapy, Megaloblastic Erythropoiesis and Folic Acid, Quart. J. Med., 35:521, 1966.

Spurling, C. L., M. S. Sacks, and R. M. Jiji: Juvenile Pernicious Anemia, New Engl. J. Med., 271:995, 1964.

Wintrobe, M. M.: "Clinical Hematology," 6th ed., Philadelphia, Lea & Febiger, 1967.

338 HEMOLYTIC ANEMIAS

Arthur Haut and
Maxwell M. Wintrobe

DEFINITION. Shortening of the "life span" of the red corpuscles is the essential feature of a hemolytic anemia. As outlined in an earlier chapter (Chap. 61), however, shortened erythrocytic life span characterizes a large variety of anemias. Therefore, to this criterion of hemolytic anemia must be added that of greatly accelerated destruction of mature red corpuscles.

PATHOGENESIS

The formation and destruction of hemoglobin were discussed earlier (Chap. 61), as were the pathogenesis and manifestations of various types of anemia. The causes of increased red blood cell destruction may be separated into three main groups: (1) those which depend mainly on an intrinsic defect of the red corpuscle, (2) those which are extracorpuscular in origin, and (3) those in which both an intrinsic corpuscular defect *plus* an extracorpuscular factor bring about hemolysis (see the accompanying classification).

CLASSIFICATION OF HEMOLYTIC DISORDERS

I. Intrinsic erythrocytic defects
  A. Congenital
    1. Hereditary deficiency of enzymes of the Embden-Meyerhof pathway (anaerobic glycolysis)
      a. Pyruvate kinase
      b. Triosephosphate isomerase
      c. Hexokinase
      d. Glucosephosphate isomerase
      e. Phosphoglycerate kinase
      f. 2,3-Diphosphoglycerate mutase
    2. Abnormalities of the phosphogluconate oxidative pathway ("hexosemonophosphate shunt")
      a. Glucose 6-phosphate dehydrogenase deficiency (Caucasian type)
      b. Glutathione reductase deficiency
      c. Deficiency of reduced glutathione
      d. Glutathione peroxidase deficiency
    3. Unknown mechanisms, associated with:
      a. Erythropoietic porphyria
      b. Erythrocytic inclusion bodies and pigmenturia (dipyrroles?)
    4. Hereditary elliptocytosis
    5. Qualitative abnormalities of globin peptides (hemoglobinopathies S, C, etc.)
    6. Quantitative abnormality in globin peptide synthesis (thalassemia syndromes)
  B. Acquired: vitamin B_{12} deficiency
II. Intrinsic erythrocytic defect *plus* an extraerythrocytic factor*
  A. Congenital
    1. Hereditary spherocytosis [spleen]
    2. Glucose 6-phosphate dehydrogenase deficiency ("primaquine-sensitive" type)
      [*a.* Certain drugs: (1) primaquine, pamaquine, (2) nitrofurantoin, (3) vitamin K substitutes, (4) sulfonamides, (5) para-aminosalicylic acid, (6) naphthalene, (7) sulfones, (8) phenacetin, acetanilid, acetylsalicylic acid, (9) probenecid]
      [*b.* Vegetable poison: fava bean (*Vicia fava*)]
  B. Acquired
    1. Paroxysmal nocturnal hemoglobinuria [normal plasma, complement]
III. Extraerythrocytic factors
  A. Agents extraneous to the patient
    1. Transfused incompatible erythrocytes
      a. Isoagglutinins anti-A and anti-B
      b. Isoagglutinins anti-Rh, Kell, Duffy, etc. ("intragroup" transfusion reactions)
    2. Hemolytic disease of the newborn

3. Chemical agents and drugs
   a. Related to size of dose: (1) phenylhydrazine, (2) toluene, (3) trinitrotoluene, (4) benzene, (5) acetanilid, (6) phenacetin, (7) aniline, (8) methyl chloride, (9) arsine, (10) lead
   b. Secondary immunohemolytic anemia, due to (1) haptene type: penicillin; (2) "innocent bystander" reaction: stibophen, quinidine, quinine, phenacetin; (3) alpha-methyl-dopa type
4. Infectious agents
   a. Malaria (blackwater fever)
   b. Bartonella (Oroya fever)
   c. Septicemia: *Clostridium welchii, Vibrio comma* (cholera), rarely others
   d. Viruses (atypical pneumonia, infectious mononucleosis)
5. Physical agents
   a. Heat: severe thermal burns
   b. Intravascular trauma
      (1) Aortic valve disease
      (2) Valve prostheses
      (3) Microangiopathic (malignant hypertension, cancer)
   c. Gamma irradiation
6. Vegetable poison: castor bean (ricin)
7. Animal poisons
   a. Snake venoms (lecithinase)
   b. Brown-spider venom (*Loxoceles recluses*)
B. Conditions developing within the body, with and without demonstrable "autoantibodies"
  1. Idiopathic acquired hemolytic anemias ("Coombs-positive")
  2. Secondary or "symptomatic" hemolytic anemias, associated with:
   a. Hodgkin's disease
   b. Chronic lymphocytic leukemia, lymphosarcoma
   c. Disseminated lupus erythematosus
   d. Metastatic carcinomatosis
   e. Sarcoidosis; myelofibrosis, myeloid metaplasia
   f. Liver disease; ovarian tumors
   g. Thrombotic thrombocytopenic purpura
   h. Renal cortical necrosis ("hemolytic-uremic syndrome")
  3. Paroxysmal cold hemoglobinuria

* Extraerythrocytic factor, shown in [brackets]

Phagocytosis, agglutinins and hemolysins, osmotic lysis, mechanical factors, and sequestration with erythrostasis condition or cause the destruction of red corpuscles. Intrinsic defects of erythrocyte metabolism predispose to the three last-named pathways of erythrocytic destruction. The importance of *phagocytosis* in the pathogenesis of hemolysis is not clear. Various types of *hemagglutinins* and *hemolysins* have been described (p. 1607). Immune hemolysins are not found free in the serum except in disorders which require special conditions for their maximum effect. Thus in paroxysmal cold hemoglobinuria (p. 1620), a fall in temperature is required for maximum activity of the hemolytic system. In most instances immune hemagglutinins remain attached to the red corpuscle. The *Coombs test* serves to demonstrate such factors (p. 1607).

The importance of *mechanical factors* is indicated by the fact that the osmotic and mechanical fragilities of the red corpuscles increase when the corpuscles are placed in natural or artificial immune serums in which hemolysins and agglutinins are present. Similar changes in fragility have been observed in association with hemolytic agents, such as saponin, or physical factors, such as heat. It is a plausible hypothesis that mechanical trauma is the ultimate mechanism whereby cell destruction occurs under normal circumstances and in many varieties of hemolytic anemia. *Osmotic lysis*, usually determined by the familiar hypotonic saline fragility test, probably does not operate in vivo except perhaps in the spleen under certain conditions. It has been shown that nearly spherical cells, strongly agglutinated cells, and those with weakened cell membranes are abnormally susceptible to mechanical destruction. In certain cases of acquired hemolytic anemia, increased mechanical fragility has been observed when osmotic fragility was normal. The increased mechanical fragility of sickled masses of erythrocytes may contribute to the increased red corpuscle destruction in sickle-cell anemia (Chap. 339).

Sequestration, by the *spleen*, plays an important part in hemolytic anemias when spherocytes are in the circulation. The spleen appears to have the property of selectively detaining and removing spheroidal cells, as distinguished from normal erythrocytes. This is equally true for the spleen of a patient with hereditary spherocytosis and for a normal spleen or one from a patient with another hematologic disorder but free of a hemolytic process.

Sequestration in the *spleen* and also in the *liver* plays an important role in acquired hemolytic anemias. In sequestering sensitized red corpuscles from the circulation, the spleen behaves as a highly proficient, passive filter. Thus, when sensitized red corpuscles are injected into the circulation of normal subjects, they are agglutinated by the plasma globulins, following which they are sequestered in the spleen and are hemolyzed within a few minutes. The speed of the hemolysis is such as to suggest the presence of a preformed lysin; leukocytes may be involved in this lytic process. In reactions involving "complete" antibodies (as when red corpuscles are injected into normal subjects hyperimmunized against them), sequestration and destruction occur in the liver to a greater extent than in the spleen. This is in contrast to the fate of sensitized corpuscles coated with "incomplete" antibodies described above.

Once spherocytes are mechanically trapped by the spleen, other mechanisms may bring about their destruction. The term *erythrostasis* has been applied to the processes to which red corpuscles are subjected when denied free access to fresh plasma. Erythrostasis in the sinusoids of the spleen may lead to depletion of glucose and other energy-yielding substrates. In the absence of these substrates, ATP accumulation ceases and the ATP-dependent sodium pump fails. This results in a lag of sodium efflux from red corpuscles and a net gain of sodium and water, which, in turn, could result in hemolysis not unlike the "osmotic hemolysis" of in vitro tests.

Following tagging of red corpuscles with ^{51}Cr, the relative importance of the spleen and liver in the hemolytic process can be estimated by comparing the radioactivity over the spleen with that over the heart and liver.

CLINICAL MANIFESTATIONS

Whether or not anemia develops and what the clinical manifestations may be depend on (1) the rate at which the increased breakdown of red corpuscles is occurring; (2) the ability of the bone marrow to make up for the shortened survival of the red corpuscles by increasing red blood cell production; (3) the capacity of the liver to extract from the plasma the increased quantity of bilirubin resulting from the breakdown of the red blood cells; (4) the quantity of haptoglobin available to bind the free hemoglobin and to prevent its escape through the kidneys; (5) the nature and manifestations of the disorder responsible for the reduced corpuscular life span; and (6) the occurrence of certain complications, such as gallstones or cholestasis, resulting from the increased formation of bilirubin. In certain instances, sudden depression of erythropoiesis takes place and a relatively stable state of balance between production and destruction may be upset. In this event, severe anemia develops suddenly (*hyporegenerative crisis*).

Jaundice is a sign common to all forms of hemolytic anemia, but its degree may be such that it is barely perceptible (when it is often overlooked, especially in yellowish incandescent illumination) or striking. Other symptoms may be entirely absent. Thus patients with hereditary spherocytosis are "more yellow than sick" except when a hyporegenerative crisis occurs.

In chronic hemolytic anemia of any cause, *splenomegaly* is common and the liver also may be enlarged. Complications such as cholelithiasis, due to bilirubin stones, or chronic leg ulcers may develop.

In some instances, there may be slowly progressive *anemia* and gradually increasing jaundice. The anemia may become profound, but if there has been time for cardiovascular adjustment (Chap. 61), there may be few manifestations. The age of the patient and underlying cardiopulmonary disease will affect the degree of this adjustment.

On the other hand, the onset of hemolytic anemia may be heralded by a severe, shaking chill followed by high fever, malaise, headache, and pain in the back, abdomen, or limbs. The abdominal pain may be so severe and may be accompanied by such marked muscular rigidity and spasm as to simulate an acute condition requiring surgery. Hemoglobin and methemoglobin in the urine may render it a dark color. If the hemolysis is rapid and severe enough, profound prostration and shock, accompanied by anuria and oliguria, may ensue. Jaundice develops rapidly. Weakness, palpitation, dyspnea, tachycardia, cyanosis, cardiac enlargement, hemic murmurs, vertigo, faintness, and other manifestations of rapidly developing anemia (Chap. 335) then appear. In certain types of acute hemolytic reactions, urticaria, vascular disturbances

suggesting Raynaud's phenomenon, and thrombosis and gangrene may be present (Chap. 278).

All grades of hemolytic anemia, from such acute fulminating disorders of several days' duration to extremely benign conditions of many years' standing, may be encountered. A chronic, congenital acquired hemolytic anemia may be interrupted by acute exacerbations.

It is possible for the survival of red corpuscles to be reduced to 20 days or less without development of anemia. Such a compensated state may be maintained for long periods of time. On the other hand, especially in association with an acute infection, sudden depression of erythropoiesis may take place. In such hyporegenerative crises the reticulocyte count falls, anemia develops rapidly, and the bone marrow may show hypoplasia. In other instances of reticulocytopenia, the maturation of the red blood cells may seem to be arrested, and megaloblasts have been demonstrated in some cases. In these instances, it is assumed that a relative deficiency of folic acid has developed, in which the demands of accelerated erythropoiesis are not met from the available dietary sources. Supplementary amounts of folic acid then allow restoration of erythropoiesis.

HEMATOLOGIC MANIFESTATIONS

The hematologic manifestations which accompany acute blood destruction consist of an initial phase of rapid destruction of red corpuscles and a second phase of rapid blood regeneration. These two phases usually overlap, especially when the hemolytic stimulus acts over a prolonged period of time.

The *anemia* may be mild or severe, depending on the intensity and duration of the hemolytic process. It is usually normocytic but may be macrocytic, especially during the stage of rapid regeneration when many relatively immature cells and reticulocytes, which are larger than mature erythrocytes, are present. It is not uncommon to find 10 to 25 percent reticulocytes in chronic cases, and as many as 60 percent or even more in acute cases. Polychromatophilia, stippling, nucleated red blood corpuscles, and Howell-Jolly bodies are usually present. There generally is marked variation in the size of the cells (anisocytosis), but there may be little variation in their shape (poikilocytosis). *Spherocytes* may be numerous, or *schistocytes* (irregularly shaped, "fractured red blood cells") may be found. In sickle-cell anemia and in elliptocytosis the characteristically shaped cells are present.

Stimulation of the *leukopoietic tissues*, in proportion to the severity of the hemolytic process, is the rule. Leukocytosis and a "shift to the left," with metamyelocytes, myelocytes, and even, rarely, myeloblasts in the circulation, accompany the accelerated erythropoiesis. *Platelets* may also increase in number, and large, bizarre forms may appear. In a minority of cases, however, such as certain cases of acquired hemolytic anemias with demonstrable "autoantibodies," and especially in paroxysmal nocturnal hemoglobinuria, leukopenia and thrombocytopenia may be present.

The *bone marrow* is hyperplastic. There is a great increase in the number of normoblasts and a consequent reduction in the myeloid-leukocyte/erythrocyte ratio from the normal 4:1 or 5:1 to about 1:1 or even less. The normoblasts are chiefly polychromatophilic and orthochromatic forms; as a rule there are proportionately not many pronormoblasts or basophilic normoblasts, although they may appear prominent because of the quantitative increase in erythroblastic elements. Megaloblasts, so characteristic of pernicious anemia and related macrocytic anemias, are not present unless a relative folic acid deficiency supervenes, as mentioned earlier.

PIGMENT METABOLISM

When the degree and rate of blood destruction are very great, hemoglobin is liberated into the plasma and, if the hemoglobin-binding capacity of the plasma (haptoglobin, hemopexin, Chap. 61) is exceeded, free hemoglobin is excreted by the kidneys and hemoglobinuria results. However, *red urine* must not be assumed to be necessarily indicative of hemoglobinuria. It may also be produced by intact red corpuscles (hematuria) or by myoglobinuria (both of which also give a positive guaiac or benzidine reaction), or by uroporphyrinuria. Microscopic and spectroscopic examination of the urine will usually suffice to reveal the cause of the abnormal color. Under certain circumstances, hematin (Chap. 61) may be released. Porphyrinuria can be recognized by the salmon-pink fluorescence in ultraviolet light of the porphyrins extracted into dilute hydrochloric acid or into organic solvents.

More often, blood destruction is less rapid. In such cases hemoglobinemia and hemoglobinuria are not found and there is only an increase in the plasma icterus index, serum bilirubin, and urobilinogen excretion in the urine and feces.

The *stools* assume a dark color, and increased quantities of urobilinogen may be found in the stool and urine (Chap. 61). The fecal urobilinogen may be increased when the urine urobilinogen and the bilirubin in the blood are not significantly greater than normal. Fecal urobilinogen determinations are of limited value, however, because (1) the bowel is incompletely evacuated, (2) urobilinogen is partially reabsorbed from the gut, (3) the heme of red corpuscles is not the only source of bile pigment, and (4) the measurement of urobilinogen does not include all oxidation products of heme degradation. Nevertheless, a threefold or greater increase in the daily fecal urobilinogen excretion, as estimated from analysis of random 10-Gm stool collections on two successive days, compared with that anticipated from an individual with the same degree of anemia but having a normal red blood cell survival, provides helpful evidence of excessive destruction of red corpuscles. Although the quantity of urobilinogen in the urine is related to the rate of blood destruction, it is so readily affected by liver function and by renal function, that this seemingly simple and aesthetically more acceptable approach to estimating urobilinogen production is not recommended.

The quantity of bilirubin in the plasma may rise as high as 10 mg per 100 ml. The reaction is indirect, but some increase in direct or "1-min" bilirubin (bilirubin glucuronide) may also occur. The intensity of the bilirubinemia depends not only on the extent of the blood destruction but also on the capacity of the liver to remove the pigment from the bloodstream and excrete it in the bile. A normally functioning liver is capable of excreting large quantities of bilirubin, but it is assumed that as anemia and consequent hypoxemia develop, the functional capacity of the liver becomes impaired and conjugated bilirubin accumulates in the bloodstream.

CLASSIFICATION

As stated above, hemolytic anemias are conveniently classified as due to intrinsic defects of the red corpuscles or to extracorpuscular influences acting alone or in concert (see Classification of Hemolytic Disorders, earlier in this chapter). In the main, those associated with intrinsic erythrocytic defects are familial and hereditary.

This classification is useful in considering therapy. When the disorder is attributed to a *congenital* intrinsic erythrocytic defect, usually little can be done to alter the rate of red blood cell destruction; when the lesion is *acquired*, it may be reversed. When there is a significant extracorpuscular factor as well as an intrinsic defect (category II in the Classification of Hemolytic Disorders), even though the inherited intrinsic defect may be unalterable, eliminating the extracorpuscular cofactor will allow some relief of hemolysis; and, conversely, addition of the cofactor will aggravate hemolysis in a previously stable situation. The patients in the first two groups will not destroy transfused, compatible normal erythrocytes at an excessive rate. The third category identifies patients who will hemolyze transfused red blood cells as readily as their own. Treatment for this group requires alteration of extracorpuscular factors.

The category *hereditary nonspherocytic hemolytic anemia* is now used only as a provisional description when evaluating a patient. The term encompasses all but hereditary spherocytosis among the hereditary disorders listed in the classification. Present-day knowledge of precise defects of the Embden-Meyerhof and phosophogluconic oxidative pathways provides a better basis for identifying cases of hemolytic anemia which previously could be classed only by the terms hereditary and nonspherocytic.

DIAGNOSIS

The first step is to *suspect* that a hemolytic process may be present. The most common clues are (1) reticulocytosis, sustained for weeks or longer without relief of anemia; (2) persistent reticulocytosis in the absence of anemia; (3) rapid aggravation of anemia, with or without accompanying reticulocytosis; (4) acholuric jaundice; and (5) unexplained splenomegaly in the presence of anemia.

In all the situations just named, both *overt and covert blood loss must be excluded* before hemolysis can be said to be present. Reticulocytosis per se is not evidence of hemolysis, but rather of accelerated erythropoiesis. When it persists, it may be deduced that abnormal blood destruction (or blood loss) is occurring only *if* the expected result of accelerated production, i.e., a rise in the volume of packed red blood cells, does not occur. The absence of reticulocytosis does not weigh against the occurrence of excessively rapid red blood cell destruction, but merely indicates that erythropoiesis is not accelerated.

The rate of red blood cell destruction can be estimated, when the degree of anemia is not changing, by measuring the survival time of the patient's red blood cells after tagging them with radioactive chromiun (^{51}Cr), or di-isopropylfluorophosphate (^{32}DFP), as discussed below (p. 1608). If compatible normal donor cells are tagged in a similar fashion and disappear from the patient's circulation at a rapid rate, a hemolytic disorder has been demonstrated; in addition, this fact proves that the cause of the excessive destruction must reside outside the patient's own red blood cells; i.e., an extracorpuscular factor is operating to produce hemolysis.

Tagging of the red corpuscles is most useful when the volume of packed red blood cells is constant and when a series of reticulocyte counts does not indicate whether erythropoiesis is accelerated or not. If sustained reticulocytosis of 7 percent or more is found and persistent blood loss has been excluded, the radioisotope test is not necessary to determine the presence of hemolysis. If the volume of packed red blood cells is rising or falling at the time the test is to be conducted, the results of red blood cell tagging may be erroneous and misleading.

If objective evidence of hemolysis has been found, the second step in diagnosis is to identify the particular cause of the hemolytic disease.

Certain additional tests have been devised which help in determining the nature of the underlying disorder and point to the precise diagnostic classification. These are discussed below. The several screening tests and specific diagnostic tests that are used to identify the individual hemolytic disorders are without value in the diagnosis of anemias other than hemolytic anemias, and they should not be carried out unless it has been clearly established that a hemolytic disorder is present. To do otherwise, may subject the patient to needless discomfort, inconvenience, delay in diagnosis, and expense.

OSMOTIC FRAGILITY TEST. Spherocytes will characteristically hemolyze in solutions of higher tonicity than will normal red corpuscles. Usually defibrinated blood and solutions of sodium chloride are used, the latter buffered to pH 7.4 with sodium (or potassium) phosphate. The test generally is positive in hereditary spherocytosis, and is sometimes positive in autoimmune hemolytic anemia if "acquired" spherocytes are present. It is usually negative in other forms of hemolytic anemia. If the test is negative but spherocytosis is suspected, the sensitivity of the test can be increased by incubating the

defibrinated blood under aseptic conditions at 37°C for 24 hr before adding it to the saline solutions. Under such conditions the fragility of normal corpuscles is increased slightly while that of corpuscles from patients with hereditary spherocytosis is increased markedly. The plotted curves of increased hemolysis are symmetric. In contrast, in hemolytic anemias without spherocytes, an asymmetric increase in osmotic fragility is more likely to be observed after incubation. In thalassemia, in which leptocytes are present, and less consistently in some of the hemoglobinopathies, osmotic fragility is decreased (Chap. 339).

A *simple screening test* to detect spherocytes and leptocytes by their abnormal osmotic fragility in solutions osmotically equivalent to 0.50 percent and 0.21 percent sodium chloride (about 170 and 70 mOsM, respectively) can be performed by adding 0.02 ml of capillary or anticoagulated venous blood to three centrifuge tubes. The first tube should also contain 4.0 isotonic (0.85 percent) sodium chloride; the second, 2.3 ml isotonic sodium chloride and 1.7 ml distilled water; and the third tube, 1.0 ml isotonic sodium chloride and 3.0 ml distilled water. After mixing by inversion and then centrifuging the tubes, there should be no hemolysis in the first tube, which serves as a control; hemolysis in the second tube only if spherocytes are present; and complete hemolysis in the third tube except when leptocytes are present, in which case erythrocytes containing hemoglobin will be seen at the bottom of the tube.

AUTOHEMOLYSIS. This test measures the amount of hemolysis which occurs spontaneously in sterile defibrinated blood incubated for 24 and 48 hr at 37°C. Increased autohemolysis is found in certain hemolytic disorders, and characteristic alteration of this response by the addition of glucose or adenosinetriphosphate (ATP) has been described (Table 338-1). Normally, 0.05 to 0.5 percent hemolysis occurs at 24 hr and 0.4 to 4.5 percent at 48 hr, as indicated in the Table. If glucose is present in a final concentration of about 5 mg per ml, then hemolysis of normal red corpuscles is not more than 0.4 percent at both 24 and 48 hr.

In hereditary spherocytosis, autohemolysis is considerably increased, but it is kept at normal levels, or nearly so, by the prior addition of glucose, or of ATP in a final concentration of about 12 mg per ml.

The test is also of value in recognizing certain of the hemolytic anemias due to deficiency of enzymes of the Emden-Meyerhof pathway or the phosphogluconate oxidative pathway. Thus, in glucose 6-phosphate dehydrogenase deficiency, there is a moderate increase in autohemolysis above normal, and this is only partially prevented by the addition of glucose. This is the type I autohemolysis of Selwyn and Dacie. In pyruvate kinase deficiency, autohemolysis is greatly increased; the addition of glucose is not protective, but ATP is protective. This is the type II autohemolysis. In triosephosphate isomerase deficiency, as in hereditary spherocytosis, both glucose and ATP are protective.

In autoimmune hemolytic anemias with spherocytosis, the autohemolysis may be increased but the effect of

Table 338-1. DIAGNOSTIC PATTERNS OF
AUTOHEMOLYSIS TESTS

Disorder	Hemolysis after 24 & 48 hr incubation at 37°C		
	No additive	Glucose added*	ATP added*
Normal	(0.05–0.5%/0.4–4.5%) 0/0 to +	(0.4%) 0	(0.4%) 0
Hereditary spherocytosis Triosephosphate isomerase deficiency	++	0	0
Glucose 6-phosphate dehydrogenase deficiency Hexokinase deficiency Glucose phosphate isomerase deficiency Phosphoglycerate kinase deficiency Hereditary elliptocytosis	++ or +++	+	+
Pyruvate kinase deficiency	++++	++++	+

* See text for quantities of additives.

Note: Zero and plus signs refer to degree of increase of hemolysis after 24 and 48 hr as compared with the tabulated normal values.

adding glucose is variable. In hereditary elliptocytosis, there may be type I autohemolysis.

SEROLOGIC TESTS. If presumptive tests are negative for *warm hemolysins* and *cold hemolysins,* and for hemolysis in *acidified serum,* the latter being characteristic of erythrocytes from patients with paroxysmal nocturnal hemoglobinuria, the diagnoses associated with these types of hemolysis may be excluded with little further laboratory investigation. When one of these tests is positive, the appropriate complete test must be carried out with suitable controls, in order to identify correctly the basis for the observed hemolysis. For example, if the presumptive test for a cold hemolysin is positive, the complete Donath-Landsteiner test should be carried out.

A *simple presumptive test* is performed by placing 0.05 ml of washed red corpuscles from freshly defibrinated blood in each of three test tubes containing 0.5 ml serum. The first is incubated for 1 to 2 hr at body temperature and then centrifuged. If hemoglobin is present in the supernatant serum, the presence of a *warm hemolysin* is suggested. The second tube is chilled for 20 min in cracked ice, then incubated for 1 hr and centrifuged. If the result is positive, a *cold hemolysin* is probably present. The test tube should be examined before it has been warmed. If only cold agglutinins are

present and no hemolysins, the red corpuscles agglutinate in the cold but fail to hemolyze when the tube is warmed, the clumps disappearing instead. When cold agglutinins are present, care must be taken not to shake the cells too much while they are agglutinated in the cold, since they may hemolyze and give a false reaction to the cold hemolysin test. The blood placed in the third tube is acidified with 0.05 ml of 0.2 N HCl. If hemolysis is apparent after incubation for 1 hr and subsequent centrifugation, the complete acidified-serum test for paroxysmal nocturnal hemoglobinuria (Ham's test) should be performed.

The *"direct" Coombs antiglobulin test* is carried out by mixing the patient's washed red blood cells with serum from rabbits immunized to human gamma-globulin, and examining the mixture for agglutination. It serves to demonstrate the presence of "incomplete" antibodies, i.e., those which are attached at some points on the surface of the red corpuscles and require a completing substance, such as antihuman globulin, to cause agglutination. A positive result is found in cases of acquired hemolytic anemia due to antibodies; in the type of paroxysmal cold hemoglobinuria associated with syphilis (p. 1620); and sometimes in hemolytic anemia associated with various physical or chemical agents, and also when isoimmunization has occurred, as in hemolytic disease of the newborn and in patients with hemolytic anemia due to intrinsic erythrocytic lesions who have received many transfusions. The test is negative in hereditary spherocytosis and in other forms of hemolytic anemia due to intrinsic erythrocytic lesions, including paroxysmal nocturnal hemoglobinuria.

The *"indirect" Coombs test* permits detection of antibodies in the patient's serum. In the indirect test, antihuman globulin serum is mixed with normal group O, Rh-positive, and Rh-negative red corpuscles which have been incubated in the patient's serum. If agglutination occurs with both Rh-positive and Rh-negative cells, Rh antibodies may be excluded and the conclusion drawn that circulating antibodies are present.

In performing the Coombs test it is important that potent antiserum be used and adequate controls carried out. False negative results may occur if the red corpuscles have not been washed sufficiently or as a result of a prozone reaction due to inadequate dilution of the serum. Cold hemagglutinins may cause a false positive reaction.

The detailed elucidation of a case of hemolytic anemia of the antibody type will often require the use of still other procedures, but these, in the main, are quite simple. They include (1) the setting up of agglutination tests at various temperatures and in several media, such as isotonic sodium chloride solution, bovine albumin solution, or polyvinylpyrrolidone (PVP), which are helpful in demonstrating and characterizing the agglutinin, and (2) the treatment of the red corpuscles with proteolytic enzymes, such as papain and trypsin, which renders them more susceptible to the demonstration of antibodies. For the antibody tests it is necessary in some instances to use the patient's own red corpuscles rather than any available group O red corpuscles, as is often the practice.

In other cases, the activity of certain erythrocytic enzymes is important in elucidating the nature of the hemolytic disorder. In certain hemolytic anemias *Heinz bodies* are common. These are intracorpuscular structures which probably represent denatured globin derived from hemoglobin in the course of an irreversible reaction with a toxic substance. They appear as refractile, irregularly shaped bodies often lying at or close to the periphery of the red blood cell, and sometimes are attached to the outer surface of the cell. They range in size from minute particles to bodies up to 3 μ in size. Several bodies may be present in the same cell, but the largest ones usually appear singly. They are not visible in blood films stained with Wright's stain, since the bodies and the surrounding hemoglobin stain the same pink color, but they can be stained supravitally with crystal violet. Heinz bodies can be produced in normal blood by mixing it with acetylphenylhydrazine, but a great many more develop in "primaquine-sensitive" (p. 1616) red blood cells. They also are observed in hemolytic anemias unrelated to exposure to recognized toxic agents ("inclusion body" anemia, "hereditary Heinz-body anemia," unstable hemoglobin anemias, Chap. 339).

SUCROSE TEST. This three-tube screening test depends on the enhanced hemolysis of complement-dependent systems in isotonic solutions of low ionic strength. One-half milliliter oxalated or citrated (but not EDTA-anticoagulated) blood is added to 4.5 ml isotonic (10 percent) sucrose. As controls, in place of sucrose, tube 2 contains isotonic NaCl or NaCl–sodium phosphate buffer (pH 7.4), and tube 3 contains distilled water. These controls are designed to measure hemolysis unrelated to the low ionic strength of the sucrose test solution, and to measure complete hemolysis, respectively. After inversion, the tubes must stand at room temperature for about 30 min for hemolysis to occur; they are then centrifuged. Hemolysis in the supernatant solution of tube 1 is presumptive evidence of paroxysmal nocturnal hemoglobinuria (PNH). In PNH there should be little or no hemolysis in tube 2. Quantitation of hemolysis can be achieved by measuring the absorbance at 540 nm (nanameters, mμ) of the supernatant from tube 1 (sucrose solution) and dividing this by the absorbance of the supernatant from tube 3, both values having been first reduced by the absorbance of the supernatant from tube 2. Disorders other than PNH may give a positive result; a negative test is acceptable evidence against the diagnosis of PNH.

RED BLOOD CELL SURVIVAL TESTS. The principles and limitations of these widely used tests should be borne in mind whenever their use is contemplated. Radioactive chromium (^{51}Cr), as sodium chromate, and radioactive diisopropylfluorophosphate (^{32}DFP) are used to tag red corpuscles and to measure their survival in vivo. The techniques are equally applicable to the patient's red corpuscles and to those of a healthy donor and therefore can distinguish between intrinsic erythrocytic defects and extraerythrocytic causes for hemolysis.

^{51}Cr is not an ideal cell label because it elutes from normal red corpuscles at a rate which approximates 1 percent daily. Hence, loss of the isotope from the circulation does not necessarily mean loss of the red blood cell with which it had been associated. It has been assumed that the same elution rate also applies to abnormal erythrocytes, but this may not be the case. Normally, half the isotope leaves the circulation ($T\frac{1}{2}$) in about 29 days. This contrasts with the actual survival time of normal red corpuscles of 120 days; i.e., an actual $T\frac{1}{2}$ of 60 days. The gamma radiation of ^{51}Cr is sufficiently penetrating to allow body-surface counting over the liver and spleen to measure isotope localization.

^{32}DFP binds irreversibly to the erythrocytic cholinesterase and, because it is not eluted from the red corpuscle, is a better label. However, the beta radiation of ^{32}P does not allow body-surface counting.

In the most commonly employed autotransfusion techniques, these procedures actually measure the rate of replacement of tagged red corpuscles by unlabeled, new corpuscles, rather than the "survival time" of the tagged corpuscles. Thus they indirectly measure red corpuscle production, rather than destruction. The amount of isotope present is measured as the "specific activity," which is isotope concentration per unit volume of blood. This may be recorded as a certain number of counts per minute (cpm) or disintegrations per second (dps) *per* milliliter packed red corpuscles or per unit volume of whole blood.

The effect of varying red corpuscle replacement rates on the apparent change in isotope "specific activity" is illustrated in Fig. 338-1. Only when the patient is in hematologic equilibrium (Fig. 338-1b), will the rate of fall of specific activity in the circulation be interpretable with reference to the normal situation. When the rate of red corpuscle production is *less than* the rate of red corpuscle destruction (Fig. 338-1a), the recorded rate of change of isotope specific activity will be less than that anticipated from the rate of red blood cell destruction alone. If red corpuscle production were zero, were it not for the rate of elution of the isotope from the red corpuscles, the specific activity would be unchanged with time, and the apparent $T\frac{1}{2}$ would be indefinitely long. On the other hand, when the rate of red corpuscle production *exceeds* the rate of corpuscle destruction, the specific activity will fall faster than that attributable to the rate of red corpuscle destruction and equivalent replacement, and the $T\frac{1}{2}$ *will be shortened. Abnormally short values for the $T\frac{1}{2}$ could be obtained when red blood cell survival is in fact normal but the volume of packed red blood cells is rising because of transfusion or any one of a number of causes unrelated to active hemolysis.* It is because the $T\frac{1}{2}$ is altered in an inverse relationship to changes from the normal balance of red corpuscle production and destruction that red blood cell survival tests become difficult to interpret if performed in patients in whom there is a significant rise or fall in the volume of packed red blood cells during the period that the test is carried out.

In cross-transfusion experiments, when a small volume of labeled red corpuscles with an *intrinsic defect* is given to a *normal recipient* (differing from the usual procedure of labeling and autotransfusing the patient's own cells),

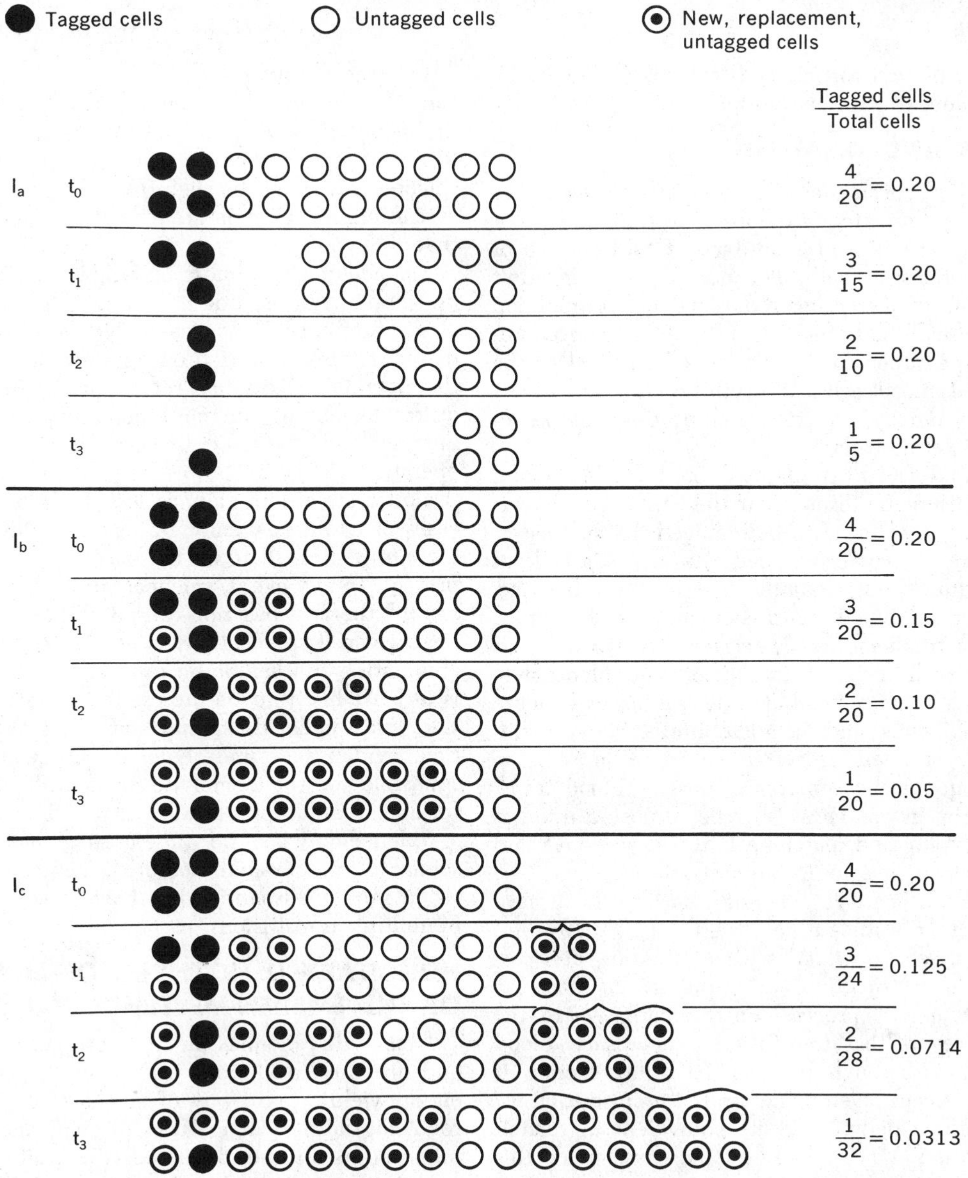

Fig. 338-1. Diagram to illustrate effect of varying red corpuscle replacement rates on the apparent changes in isotope specific activity of a patient's red corpuscles tagged with radioactive chromium (^{51}Cr). Anemia is progressing in 1a, hematologic equilibrium is illustrated in 1b, and in 1c erythrocyte production exceeds destruction.

In 1a, at time t_0 four tagged corpuscles and sixteen untagged corpuscles are illustrated. At time t_1, after the lapse of an interval t, one-fourth of the red blood cells have left the circulation, *the same proportion being derived from the tagged and untagged cells*, so that three tagged cells and twelve untagged cells remain. New corpuscles have not replaced those lost; i.e., anemia has progressed during the period of observation. The ratio of tagged cells to total cells remains at 1:5. At t_2 another tagged corpuscle and four additional untagged corpuscles have been lost: once again the ratio of tagged cells to total cells remains 1:5. At t_3 one tagged cell and four untagged cells remain and the ratio, or "specific activity," stays unchanged.

In 1b, new untagged corpuscles have replaced those which have been lost from the circulation. At t_1, one tagged corpuscle and four untagged corpuscles have been lost from the circulation but have been replaced by the same number, five, of new, untagged corpuscles. The ratio of tagged corpuscles to total corpuscles has fallen from 4:20 to 3:20, a decline from 0.20 to a value of 0.15 when expressed as a decimal. This process continues at t_2, so that the ratio falls to 2:20, or 0.10 when expressed as a decimal. Here, in contrast to the situation in 1a, the specific activity of isotope in the circulation has decreased as tagged corpuscles are lost. The effect may be seen to reflect the production of new, untagged corpuscles and their entrance into the circulation.

In 1c, at t_1, the one tagged corpuscle and four untagged corpuscles which had been lost from the circulation have been replaced by five new corpuscles, as in 1b, *plus* an additional four untagged, new corpuscles. Thus, the ratio of tagged corpuscles to total corpuscles has fallen to 3:24, a value of 0.125. This process is continued at t_2, causing the ratio ("specific activity") to fall to 2:28, or 0.0714 when expressed as a decimal.

the survival of the red corpuscles is measured directly by the disappearance of the radioisotope.

PROGNOSIS AND TREATMENT

Useful therapy of hemolytic anemia requires either (1) decreasing the rate of corpuscular destruction, or (2) increasing the rate of manufacture and release of new red corpuscles, or both. The bone marrow in adult man is capable of increasing red blood cell production at least six- to eightfold, and a healthy *bone marrow* approaches compensation for the decreased survival of the circulating red blood cells. If erythropoiesis already is accelerated maximally, effective therapy depends on reducing the rate of destruction.

Prognosis and treatment depend on the nature and cause of the hemolytic disorder. If the causative agent is a parasite or chemical, it must be removed. In such cases, no other therapy may be needed. An acute attack of hemolysis requires rest, maintenance of fluid balance, and relief of pain. Blood transfusion may be dangerous if the cause of the hemolysis is extracorpuscular and has not been removed, because the introduced blood may also be destroyed. Yet, when blood destruction is so acute that hemoglobinemia and hemoglobinuria are present, the possibility of death from circulatory collapse is so great that frequent and sometimes massive blood transfusions must be given. However, the utmost caution is necessary in typing and matching both the patient's and the donor's blood and in its administration.

In the acquired hemolytic anemias, both in the "symptomatic" and in the idiopathic varieties (p. 1619) and especially in cases associated with antibodies, *corticosteroids* provide an effective and rapid means for controlling the hemolytic process. Furthermore, where the anemia is so severe that transfusion is necessary, blood can be given with much less chance of a reaction if steroids have been given. The oral administration of 40 mg prednisone daily, or of its equivalent in related compounds, often suffices, but in some cases twice this amount, or even more, may need to be given at first. Methyl prednisolone or dexamethasone may be given by the intravenous route as the sodium succinate derivative when the patient is unable to take oral medication. It is preferred over hydrocortisone, which may also be given intravenously, because of the potentially dangerous salt-retaining effect of hydrocortisone when large doses are used. The most alarming manifestations of the hemolytic process usually subside within a few days, and then intravenous therapy may be replaced by oral administration of corticosteroids, and the dose may be reduced gradually. Patients vary widely in the amount of these hormones required to control the hemolysis and for maintenance therapy. In some, therapy may be discontinued entirely after several months, but in others it must be continued for years. When corticosteroids are employed for prolonged periods, careful consideration should be given to minimizing the undesirable side effects and the potential complications such as peptic ulcer, diabetes mellitus, osteoporosis, tuberculosis, and other infections (Chap. 92).

In cases of "symptomatic" hemolytic anemia of known cause, treatment of the underlying disorder may relieve the hemolytic anemia as well. When this does not occur, a trial of steroid therapy is justified. In certain instances splenectomy may be helpful, especially if leukopenia and thrombocytopenia are also present and the picture is that of "hypersplenism."

Splenectomy is almost invariably beneficial in hereditary spherocytosis, but it is much less successful in the other hereditary forms of hemolytic anemia. Furthermore, if splenectomy is carried out in an acute hemolytic phase, the operative mortality rate is high. In idiopathic acquired hemolytic anemia, therefore, corticosteroid hormones should be used first, at least in preparation for operation.

Corticosteroid therapy is less likely to be effective in cases of acquired hemolytic anemia without demonstrable antibodies than in those in which antibodies are present. In any event, splenectomy is advisable whenever steroid therapy has not caused the hemolysis to disappear. Even if splenectomy is not successful in completely eliminating the hemolytic process, corticosteroid therapy is at least likely to be more effective than before operation, and smaller doses may suffice. At the time of operation, evidence of underlying disease which may be responsible for the hemolytic anemia should be searched for and treated appropriately if found.

Splenectomy is of no value in sickle-cell anemia, thalassemia, or paroxysmal nocturnal hemoglobinuria except when immune isoantibodies have developed as a result of multiple transfusions.

HEREDITARY DEFICIENCIES OF ENZYMES OF THE EMBDEN-MEYERHOF PATHWAY

Hemolytic anemias in this category are congenital and are due to "inborn errors" in the main glycolytic, energy-yielding pathway of erythrocytes. They have the following additional features in common: (1) They are inherited as an autosomal recessive trait. (2) Hemolytic anemia occurs in homozygotes, who are necessarily deficient in the particular enzyme, whereas heterozygotes possess intermediate quantities of the specifically affected enzymes but are free of hemolytic disease. (3) In homozygotes, slight or even moderate macrocytosis occurs and some irregularly crenated erythrocytes and spicule forms are present. (4) Spherocytes are absent. (5) Hemolysis and anemia persist after splenectomy, although some benefit may result from the operation. (6) During in vitro incubation, the erythrocytes tend to lose potassium rather than, as in the case of hereditary spherocytosis, gain sodium.

The degree of anemia and of the hemolytic process itself varies not only among the different enzyme lesions represented in the group, but even among patients with the same enzyme deficiency. In these disorders glycolysis in mature erythrocytes is abnormal and red corpuscle survival may be extremely brief. However, reticulocytes are produced in large numbers in response to the anemia, and these immature corpuscles, in contrast to mature erythrocytes, contain mitochondria. These organelles provide an alternate pathway from which to derive energy: oxidative phosphorylation. As long as the young erythrocyte in the circulation retains this metabolic capability, it can survive despite its inborn error in the Embden-Meyerhof pathway. However, as it matures it is destined to an early death, the timing of which depends on the site and severity of the enzymatic lesion in the glycolytic

pathway. In turn, the location and severity of the lesion determine the severity of the hemolytic process and the resultant clinical syndrome.

PYRUVATE KINASE DEFICIENCY. This disorder, first described by Valentine et al. in 1961, is the most common cause of hemolytic anemia among the identifiable enzyme lesions of the Embden-Meyerhof pathway (Fig. 338-2).

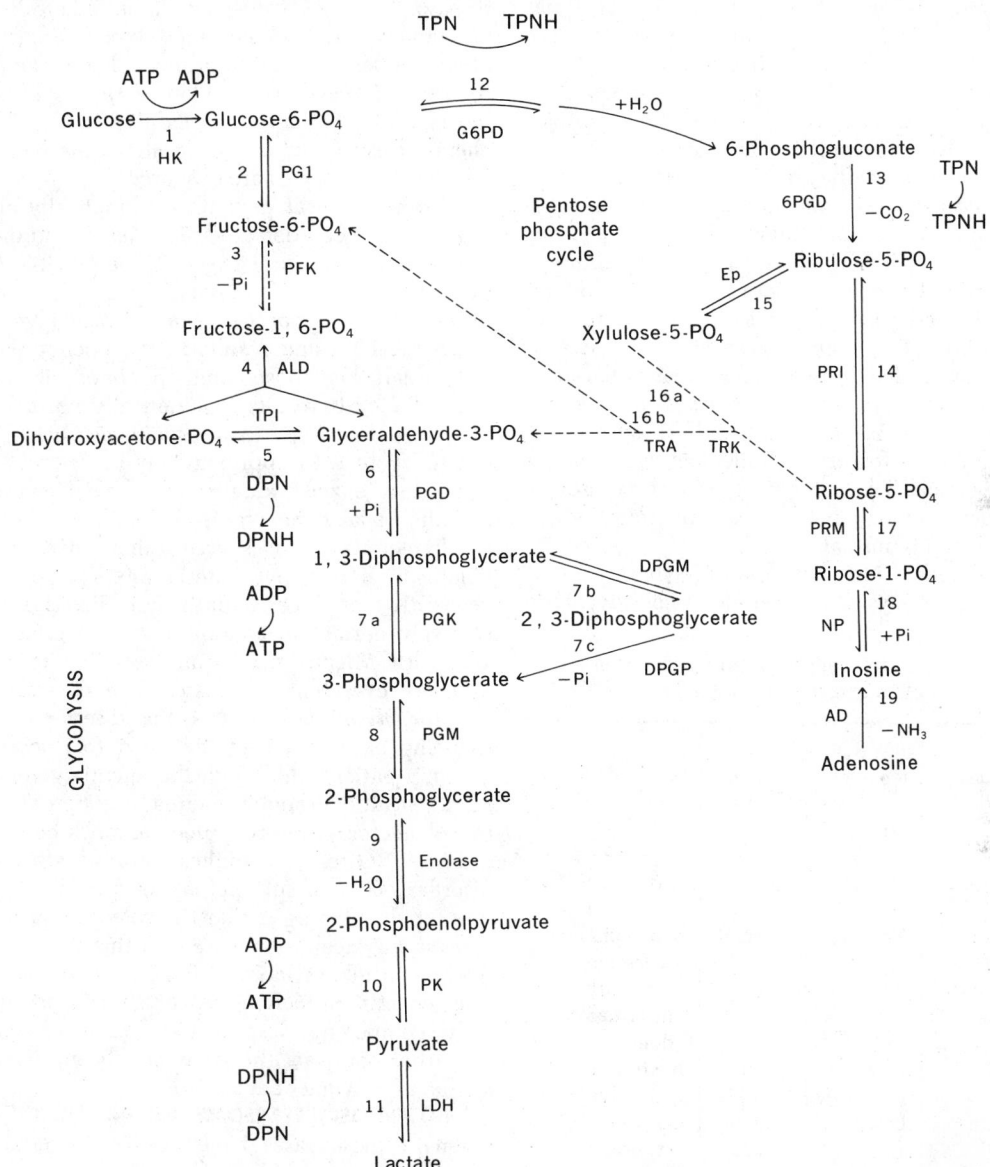

Fig. 338-2. Pathways for the metabolic breakdown of glucose in the red corpuscle and some of the enzymes involved. The various reactions are numbered in sequence: Embden-Meyerhof pathway, 1-11; phosphogluconate oxidative pathway (pentose phosphate shunt), 12-15.

The interrupted lines indicate that some steps have been omitted.

HK refers to hexokinase; PGI, phosphoglucose isomerase; PFK, phosphofructokinase; ALD, aldolase; TPI, triosephosphate isomerase; PGD, phosphoglyceraldehyde dehydrogenase (glyceraldehyde phosphate dehydrogenase): PGK, phosphoglyceric acid kinase; PGM, phosphoglyceromutase; DPGM, diphosphoglyceratemutase; DPGP, diphosphoglycerate phosphatase; PK, pyruvate kinase; LDH, lactic dehydrogenase; G6PD, glucose 6-phosphate dehydrogenase; 6PGD, 6-phosphogluconic dehydrogenase; PRI, phosphoribose isomerase; Ep, epimerase; TRK, transketolase; TRA, transaldolase; AD, adenosine deaminase; NP, nucleoside phosphorylase; PRM, phosphoribomutase. (*From Wintrobe, Clinical Hematology, 6th ed.*, Philadelphia, Lea & Febiger, 1967.)

At least 100 proved cases have been reported. It may be considered the prototype of the inherited enzyme deficiency disorders.

The disease has most frequently been reported in people of Northern European extraction, but it has also been found in other Europeans and people of Oriental, African, and still other racial groups. Most cases are discovered in infancy or early childhood. In some patients, marked anemia is found in the newborn period. In rare instances, in a seemingly healthy adult relative of a patient, the disorder is mild and fully compensated. Most patients, however, have the characteristic symptoms and signs of chronic hemolytic disorders (p. 1604). Despite the severity of the hemolytic process, survival to adult life is common and women have tolerated pregnancy without unusual complications.

The anemia is moderately severe, and the volume of packed red corpuscles may be between 15 and 35 ml per 100 ml. The red corpuscles are normochromic and slightly macrocytic; the slight macrocytosis reflects at least in part the reticulocytosis. Poikilocytosis is variable, and irregularly contracted red corpuscles or marked spicule formation may be seen, although these are not specific morphologic features. Reticulocytosis ranges from 5 to 45 percent. The autohemolysis test (p. 1606) is increased above normal, but the osmotic fragility (p. 1606) of fresh blood is normal.

In clinically affected individuals, all of whom are homozygotes, specific assays of the red blood cell glycolytic enzymes show very low levels of erythrocyte pyruvate kinase (PK) (Fig. 338-2, reaction 10), although the exact values obtained for the enzyme do not correlate well with the clinical severity of the disease. The activity of other glycolytic enzymes is normal or greater than normal, because reticulocytes are rich in many of these enzymes. Heterozygotes are free of anemia and hemolytic disease. Their PK values are intermediate between those of homozygotes and normal subjects. Some overlap between values in homozygotes and heterozygotes has been reported. Leukocytes and other tissues of homozygotes have normal PK activity (Table 338-2). The exact biochemical events which bring about the hemolysis of the affected erythrocytes are obscure.

In rare, atypical pedigrees a kinetically abnormal isoenzyme has been detected. This has led to the hypothesis that the occurrence of two of three possible genes affecting erythrocytic PK activity, PK_1, PK_1^A, and PK_2, determines the phenotype. The normal genotype is designated PK_1PK_1, and results in the phenotypically normal individual. The most common abnormal gene is designated PK_1^A. It results in kinetically normal but quantitatively deficient pyruvate kinase activity. The common heterozygote with approximately half-normal PK activity but normal enzyme kinetics may be designated $PK_1PK_1^A$, and the usual homozygote, $PK_1^APK_1^A$. The homozygote is characterized by severe quantitative deficiency of kinetically normal pyruvate kinase. The second abnormal gene, PK_2, produces a pathologic PK isoenzyme, quantitatively normal in amount but with abnormal kinetics and with Michaelis constants relative to phosphoenolpyruvate over tenfold greater than controls.

Splenectomy ameliorates the disease in most cases, reducing or eliminating the need for blood transfusion in many patients, although the anemia generally persists. Paradoxically, although anemia may be partially relieved by splenectomy, the reticulocytosis has been found to be increased. Often, the highest reticulocyte counts in this disorder occur in splenectomized patients. One explanation for this finding is that the spleen sequesters reticulocytes to an exceptional extent in this disease. Removal of the spleen allows more reticulocytes to circulate, and as they contain mitochondrial enzymes and are metabolically competent despite the lesion of the Embden-Meyerhof pathway, they temporarily survive and account for the improvement achieved.

TRIOSEPHOSPHATE ISOMERASE DEFICIENCY. Since 1965, seven of these cases have been discovered. Hemolytic anemia became evident in the first month of life. In addition, severe, progressive, neuromuscular disease characterized by spasticity and later by generalized flaccidity, with impaired neuromuscular development resulting in the inability or loss of the ability to stand, sit, or hold the head erect, was present. The disorder has been observed in individuals of French-Negro ancestry and of English-Caucasian ancestry. Heterozygotes are clinically well, and have about half the normal activity of erythrocytic triosephosphate isomerase. In homozygotes, erythrocytic triosephosphate isomerase activity (Fig. 338-2, reaction 5) is about 10 percent (or less) of the values found in nor-

Table 338-2. SOME FEATURES OF INHERITED RED BLOOD CELL ENZYME DISORDERS

RBC enzyme deficiency	WBC enzyme concentration	Other tissues	Mode of transmission
Pyruvate kinase.....	Normal	Normal	Autosomal recessive
Hexokinase..........	Normal	Normal	Autosomal recessive
Glucose 6-phosphate dehydrogenase	Variable*	Low†	X-linked; intermediate dominance
Triosephosphate isomerase	Low	Low‡	Autosomal recessive
Glucosephosphate isomerase	Low	Low in plasma	Autosomal recessive
Phosphoglycerate kinase	Low	. . .	X-chromosome linked
Glutathione reductase	Low	§	Autosomal dominant

* Sometimes low in affected Caucasians; normal in Negroes.

† Enzyme activity also low in ocular lenses and in platelets, liver, and other organs.

‡ Enzyme activity low in muscle, serum, and spinal fluid; this disorder is accompanied by a progressive neurologic disease.

§ May be accompanied by neutropenia or thrombocytopenia and neurologic disease.

mal persons; in addition, leukocytes, muscle, cerebrospinal fluid, and serum are deficient in the enzyme (Table 338-2). Elevated activity of several of the other erythrocytic enzymes is attributed to the presence of reticulocytes.

The usual features of chronic hemolytic anemia are present. The hemoglobin concentration may be from 5.5 to 10.5 Gm per 100 ml, and reticulocytes number about 15 percent. The autohemolysis test is abnormal (Table 338-1), but the osmotic fragility of fresh blood is normal.

Five of seven patients died prior to the age of five years; two were alive with severe generalized disease at four and one-half and five years of age. Deaths were attributable to the chronic hemolytic anemia, neuromuscular disorder, and infections, and possibly to cardiac involvement. The effect of splenectomy has not been reported.

Triosephosphate isomerase represents the only known means whereby dihydroxyacetone phosphate formed from 6-carbon compounds may be further metabolized by the Embden-Meyerhof pathway. A block at this step had been anticipated to result in an accumulation of dihydroxyacetone phosphate and a loss of that half of the three carbon moieties, this resulting in a decline in the rate of ATP synthesis (Fig. 338-2, reactions 7a and 10). However, measurements have revealed an increase in the rate of glucose utilization even greater than that generally observed in patients with similar elevations of the reticulocyte count, and only small decreases in ATP levels. The amount of lactate formed from glucose has not been deficient. Thus, a compensatory pathway, most likely the phosphogluconate oxidative pathway, appears to be activated in affected red corpuscles. Dihydroxyacetone phosphate accumulated in affected red corpuscles, but the paucity of other metabolic abnormalities leaves the biochemical mechanism for the striking clinical abnormalities unexplained.

HEXOKINASE DEFICIENCY. Congenital hemolytic anemia in an eleven-year-old girl was attributed to erythrocytic hexokinase deficiency. Hepatomegaly, jaundice, and anemia were present from birth. Osmotic fragility was markedly increased after incubation for 24 hr at 37°C, and the autohemolysis test was abnormal (Table 338-1). The anemia was partially relieved by splenectomy, and the osmotic fragility became normal. Postsplenectomy blood smears showed darkly staining red corpuscles, some bearing spicules, rare target cells, and rare spherocytes.

The patient had less than normal erythrocytic hexokinase (HK) (Fig. 338-2, reaction 1), despite persistent reticulocytosis, which ordinarily results in high HK values. In her brother, free of hemolytic disease, the levels of HK were even lower, whereas both parents had intermediate values. From a study of the family members it appeared likely that the patient is homozygous for a defective gene, the disorder being transmitted, like the other enzymopathies in this group, as an autosomal recessive trait. The significance of the strikingly reduced HK value in the hematologically and clinically normal sibling is not clear. In sharp contrast to the low HK values in the proposita, all other erythrocytic enzyme activities were normal or increased, conforming with the experience in other specific enzymopathies.

Hexokinase is strategically located at the first step in glycolysis, and in vitro it has the lowest activity of any of the glycolytic enzymes of the erythrocytes. Many consider HK as rate-limiting in glycolysis, and since there is no known substitute for its activity, it represents a critical step in energy production for the mature erythrocyte. The patient's red corpuscles utilized fructose and glucose at rates below those of normal cell populations and far below those of samples with comparable numbers of reticulocytes. The leukocytes were unaffected (Table 338-2).

GLUCOSEPHOSPHATE ISOMERASE DEFICIENCY. Four patients, in two unrelated Caucasian families, have been described in whom erythrocytic glucosephosphate isomerase (GPI) activity averaged about one-fifth of mean normal values. Leukocyte GPI was similarly affected. Other erythrocytic glycolytic enzymes were normal or increased in value, probably because of concomitant reticulocytosis. There were severe congenital hemolytic anemia and splenomegaly. Spherocytes were absent, the osmotic fragility of fresh blood was normal, and only slight abnormality was found after incubation at 37°C for 24 hr. The autohemolysis test was abnormal (Table 338-1). Splenectomy reduced the need for blood transfusions, but anemia persisted.

Parents of the affected patients and their unaffected siblings lacked clinical evidence of hemolytic disease. Their erythrocytic GPI activity was about one-half of normal values. The disorder was deduced to be transmitted as an autosomal recessive trait (Table 338-2).

Erythrocytic GPI reversibly catalyzes the interconversion of glucose 6-phosphate and fructose 6-phosphate, the second step in the Emden-Meyerhof pathway of anaerobic glycolysis (Fig. 338-2, reaction 2). In the reticulocyte-rich blood of affected patients, total metabolism of glucose to lactate is greater than normal and partial compensation for the inborn error is accomplished through bypassing the deficient enzyme step via the phosphogluconate oxidative pathway. How the enzymatic lesion results in premature hemolysis of erythrocytes is unknown. The erythrocytic GPI patterns were electrophoretically dissimilar in the two pedigrees, suggesting that in some cases two abnormal genes may interact to produce the lesion.

OTHER CAUSES. Chronic hemolytic anemia associated with neurologic disease and behavioral disturbances has been reported in two young boys of a single pedigree. The red corpuscles and leukocytes of both patients were found to be severely deficient in *phosphoglycerate kinase* (PGK) (reaction 7a, Fig. 338-2). The characteristic clinical and hematologic findings of chronic hemolytic anemia were present. Spherocytes were absent. Osmotic fragility was normal, but the autohemolysis test was not. It seems probable that the disorder is transmitted as an X-chromosome–linked disease. Severely affected males have been tentatively designated as hemizygotes. Females with hemolytic anemia and females who clearly transmitted the disorder were designated as heterozygotes in the pedigree studied. The propositus, an eleven-year-old Chinese boy, was partially improved by splenectomy, but moderate anemia and hemolysis persisted. Female heterozygotes were less severely affected. The enzyme PGK catalyzes the interconversion of 1,3-diphosphoglycerate and 3-phosphoglycerate (3-PG). ATP is generated in the forward reaction, in which 3-PG is the product; in the backward reaction, ADP is formed from ATP. The generation of ATP in the forward reaction may be by-passed if triose is metabolized via 2,3-diphosphoglycerate (2,3-DPG) through the Rapoport-Luebering shunt. Interference in the Embden-Meyerhof anaerobic pathway, with reduction in the synthesis of erythrocytic ATP, is presumed to be the mechanism resulting in hemolysis.

Chronic hemolytic anemia associated with deficiency of **2,3-DPG mutase** (Fig. 338-2, reaction 7b) has been recorded in several pedigrees, illustrating different clinical manifestations and different patterns of inheritance. In one, autosomal recessive inheritance was indicated. The enzyme deficiency was associated with low 2,3-DPG content of red corpuscles but a normal glycolytic rate. It has been postulated that the profound decrease in 2,3-DPG was rate-limiting for the monophosphoglycerate mutase reaction, wherein 2,3-DPG serves as a catalyst in the conversion of 3-PG to 2-phosphoglycerate in the main line of the Embden-Meyerhof pathway.

Congenital hemolytic anemia in a 24-year-old man was associated with half-normal activity of erythrocytic *phosphofructokinase* in the propositus and in two preceding generations.

Additional instances of all the syndromes described no doubt will be discovered in time.

Abnormalities of the Phosphogluconate Oxidative Pathway

Although only 10 percent of the glucose in mature red blood cells is metabolized via the phosphogluconate oxidative pathway, enzymatic abnormalities in this "shunt" may result in chronic hemolytic anemia or, alternatively, in acute hemolytic anemia following administration of certain drugs or chemicals. The exact biochemical mechanism which results in hemolysis in these disorders is not clear, although failure to defend normal concentrations of intraerythrocytic and membrane reduced thiol compounds appears to be a critical factor common to the several lesions discussed below.

GLUCOSE 6-PHOSPHATE DEHYDROGENASE DEFICIENCY (Caucasian Type). It has been estimated that 100 million or more persons of all races throughout the world are affected by glucose 6-phosphate dehydrogenase (G6PD) (Fig. 338-2, reaction 12) deficiency. The frequency of the disorder varies from 1 to 36 percent among different Caucasian population groups, and is especially frequent in peoples of the Mediterranean littoral.

In Caucasians, the disorder may differ from that in Negroes. *Chronic hemolysis* and *anemia* may be present in occasional patients even in the absence of drugs and other extracorpuscular factors which induce hemolysis and anemia in affected Negroes (p. 1616). This must be borne in mind in the differential diagnosis of chronic hemolytic anemias (Table 338-1).

G6PD deficiency has also been reported to be more severe in Caucasians and Orientals than in Negroes; the former may have even greater hemolytic sensitivity to primaquine and related compounds and even to acetylsalicylic acid (aspirin), than do affected Negroes. Furthermore, ingestion of fava beans may induce a severe hemolytic episode in G6PD-deficient Caucasians, but not in G6PD-deficient Negroes, indicating a role for still another extracorpuscular factor in favism.

The normal enzyme, designated (B+), is found in the majority of Caucasians and Negroes. The common variant found in many G6PD-deficient Mediterranean persons is called (B−), and it has abnormal kinetics with reference to G6P and galactose 6-phosphate. The G6PD enzyme of the Negro-type deficiency is designated (A−) and is probably structurally different from the less-common normal variant (A+), also found in Negroes. The more rapid inactivation of (A−) in the aging red corpuscle results in the G6PD deficiency of the mixed-age population of red corpuscles. The (A+) enzyme differs from the most common isozyme (B+), by a single amino acid: asparagine is replaced by aspartic acid.

Except as noted above, the features of the Caucasian type of G6PD deficiency are similar to the more thoroughly studied examples of this disorder in Negroes (Table 338-2), discussed later in this chapter (p. 1616).

Glutathione reductase deficiency has been found in 47 cases of chronic hemolytic anemia and in an additional 14 cases without hematologic disorder. It is transmitted as an autosomal dominant trait. Patients are susceptible to acceleration of hemolysis induced by the same drugs that have been implicated in the "primaquine-sensitive" type of hemolytic anemia associated with glucose 6-phosphate dehydrogenase deficiency (see Classification of Hemolytic Disorders at start of chapter). Neutropenia, thrombocytopenia, or pancytopenia has been induced in many cases by those drugs, or by chloroquine, chloramphenicol, phenylbutazone (Butazolidin), phenprocoumon (Marcumar), nitrolacker, or thallium. The usual findings common to chronic hemolytic anemias were present in most cases, but reticulocytosis was absent in some of the patients with pancytopenia. Glutathione reductase enables the regeneration of reduced glutathione (GSH) from oxidized glutathione. Although the enzyme activity of the red corpuscles of patients with this disorder was half the normal, erythrocytic reduced glutathione content was normal or increased; nevertheless, GSH stability (p. 1617) was abnormal in some cases, and the Heinz body test was abnormal in all cases. The activity of erythrocytic G6PD and other enzymes was normal or increased.

A well-compensated hemolytic anemia without spherocytosis but with susceptibility to hemolysis induced by primaquine or fava beans has been described in individuals with virtually complete **GSH deficiency**. The disorder is transmitted as an autosomal recessive trait. The defect appears to lie in the failure of attachment of glycine to glutamyl cysteine in the enzymatic synthesis of glutathione. Small amounts of chromate which are perfectly acceptable for red blood cell survival studies in other disorders (1 mM per liter of red corpuscles) have a markedly adverse affect on the in vivo viability of glutathione-deficient red corpuscles.

A compensated hemolytic disorder in newborn infants, associated with hyperbilirubinemia and increased susceptibility of red corpuscles to Heinz body formation in vitro, has been ascribed to *erythrocytic glutathione peroxidase deficiency.* The syndrome was self-limited, and evidence of hemolysis disappeared by three months of age. Affected infants have been found to have 40 percent less erythrocytic glutathione peroxidase activity than that found in the red corpuscles of normal infants; when both their parents were tested, one of the pair was found to have a slight reduction in activity of that enzyme. The significance of these observations is unclear, although for some time it has been suspected that deficiency of glutathione peroxidase might result in increased susceptibility to Heinz body formation and drug-induced hemolytic anemia.

OTHER INTRINSIC ERYTHROCYTIC DEFECTS

Hemolytic anemia may be associated with *congenital erythropoietic uroporphyria* (Chap. 108) and *protoporphyria.* Considerable improvement may follow splenectomy.

Elliptical red corpuscles may be present in small numbers in the blood of some individuals. In about 0.04 percent of the population, as many as 50 to 90 percent of the red corpuscles may be elliptical or oval in shape. This condition, known as *hereditary elliptocytosis,* is inherited as an autosomal dominant trait, but there is wide variation in gene penetrance or expression. In most instances, the disorder seems harmless, but occasionally a compensated hemolytic disease may be present, or an overt hemolytic anemia may result. In the very rare homozygous state, severe hemolytic anemia occurs. Splenomegaly is relatively common, and sequestration of the red corpuscles has been observed. Splenectomy has been found to relieve the hemolytic anemia in many cases, but the morphologic abnormality, whose basis is unknown, has persisted.

Often grouped together are those congenital hemolytic anemias associated with qualitative or quantitative abnormalities in the synthesis of the globin peptide moieties. These result in the *hemoglobinopathies* and *thalassemia* syndromes, respectively (Chap. 339).

The anemia of vitamin B_{12} deficiency exhibits features of a hemolytic disorder, apparently because of an acquired, intrinsic erythrocytic defect (Chap. 337).

HEMOLYTIC ANEMIAS RESULTING FROM THE COMBINED EFFECTS OF AN INTRINSIC ERYTHROCYTIC DEFECT *PLUS* AN EXTRAERYTHROCYTIC FACTOR

Recognition of the role of the extraerythrocytic factor in sustaining the hemolytic process in these disorders provides an approach to treatment which is not possible in those congenital hemolytic anemias due to an intrinsic erythrocytic defect *alone.* In the present group, removal or addition of the extraerythrocytic factor may result in relief or aggravation, respectively, of the hemolytic process.

Hereditary Spherocytosis (Chronic Acholuric Jaundice, Spherocytic Anemia, Chronic Familial Icterus, Congenital Hemolytic Jaundice)

This disorder, long considered the prototype of hemolytic anemias due to intrinsic erythrocytic defects, actually differs from most of that group by virtue of the crucial role played by the spleen in the pathogenesis of the anemia. In this disorder, removal of the spleen—the extraerythrocytic factor—relieves the anemia even though the intrinsic erythrocytic defect persists.

DEFINITION. This is a familial and hereditary disorder characterized by a variable degree of hemolytic anemia and jaundice, spherocytosis, and increased osmotic fragility of the red corpuscles.

HISTORY. During the early part of the present century, this familial disorder was clearly defined, becoming known as the type of Chauffard and Minkowski, and was distinguished from the acquired form described by Hayem and Widal.

ETIOLOGY. Transmitted as an autosomal dominant trait and especially common in people of northern European stock, this disorder is due to an inherited defect of the red corpuscles, which tend to be more spherical than normal as they age in the circulation. Spherocytes are especially subject to removal and destruction by the spleen (p. 1603). The corpuscular abnormality is related to excessive permeability of the red blood cell membrane to the ingress of sodium ion. As increased amounts of sodium gain access to the interior of the cell, the ATPase mechanism is stimulated, increasing the outward pumping rate of sodium ion and at the same time requiring an increased rate of glycolysis for replenishment of ATP. The abnormality is aggravated by *erythrostasis* in the spleen (p. 1603). It is not known whether the hyperpermeability of the membrane is the immediate result of a structural abnormality in the membrane proteins or lipids. It is now believed that the total and relative amounts of the various membrane lipids are normal. The stability of the membrane lipid components in hereditary spherocytosis and the nature of the membrane protein components in all erythrocytes are unresolved questions.

PATHOLOGY. The spleen is always enlarged, often weighing 1,000 to 1,500 Gm. The pulp and, to a lesser extent, the sinuses are greatly congested. Depending on the degree of anemia and the extent of blood destruction, hyperplasia and even metaplasia of the bone marrow occur, and deposits of iron pigment are found in the liver, kidneys, and even lymph nodes.

SYMPTOMS. Jaundice and splenomegaly are the most common manifestations; they may pass unnoticed for many years. A persistent sallow appearance, rather than obvious jaundice, may be present. Symptoms of anemia are usually absent or mild. At any time from birth to late adult life attention may be drawn to the disorder by the *crise de déglobulization,* which is characterized by fever, lassitude, palpitation, and shortness of breath or even by violent abdominal pain, vomiting, and anorexia. Rather than being episodes of increased blood destruction, as had always been assumed, these crises have been found to be associated with sudden, temporary reduction, or even cessation of blood formation (p. 1604). Since the life span of the red corpuscles in this hemolytic disease is very brief, anemia develops rapidly under these circumstances.

The liver may or may not be enlarged. Other developmental anomalies are often present. Chronic leg ulcers may be found, and striation and thickening of the frontal and parietal bones of the skull may be seen on roentgenographic examination. Cholelithiasis is a frequent complication, and symptoms of this complication may first bring the patient to the physician.

The anemia is usually moderate in degree but may be very mild or severe. It is normocytic or microcytic in type, but not hypochromic. When severe and associated with marked reticulocytosis, it may be macrocytic. There is little poikilocytosis, but small, deeply staining red corpuscles without central pallor (spherocytes) are usually plentiful, scattered among the cells of normal size. Polychromatophilia and normoblasts may be seen in the blood smear. The leukocytes may be normal in number, or increased, and the same is true of the platelets. Reticulocytes are characteristically increased in number, most often accounting for 5 to 20 percent of the erythrocytes.

Increased osmotic fragility of the red corpuscles is characteristic (p. 1606). Hemolysis, beginning at 220 mOsm, equivalent to about 0.64 percent saline solution, is not unusual. It may be complete at the point where hemolysis of healthy erythrocytes normally begins; i.e., about 150 mOsm, equivalent to about 0.44 percent saline.

Hyperbilirubinemia of the "indirect" type, consisting almost entirely of nonconjugated bilirubin, produces "acholuric jaundice," i.e., jaundice without bilirubin in the urine. There is an increased quantity of urobilinogen in the stools and in the urine, as is characteristic of hemolytic disorders.

DIAGNOSIS. Splenomegaly, acholuric jaundice, spherocytosis, reticulocytosis, and an increase of osmotic fragility and of autohemolysis, the latter prevented by the prior addition of glucose (Table 338-1), are characteristic findings in affected patients. Examination of other, even asymptomatic family members for the very same features is most valuable in establishing the diagnosis of *hereditary* spherocytosis in the patient at hand. The failure to find historical evidence of anemia or jaundice in other family members is an unreliable criterion for excluding relatives who may potentially be involved, and should not be a deterrent in seeking further evidence by physical and laboratory examination. Moreover, the absence of evidence of the disease in both parents of a patient does not necessarily exclude the diagnosis of hereditary spherocytosis. About 20 to 25 percent of cases are sporadic, probably the result of incomplete penetrance in the parent or of the occurrence of new cases through genetic mutation.

The Coombs test is negative except in occasional cases. In these it is likely that a superimposed acquired immunohemolytic process has developed. When the picture is not entirely typical, a careful study must be made to rule out other types of hemolytic anemia.

TREATMENT. During a "crisis," many blood transfusions may need to be give to avoid a very serious degree of anemia. As the lesion is intrinsic to the patient's erythrocytes, transfused red corpuscles survive normally in the patient's circulation, and the beneficial effects of the transfusions should persist until the patient recovers his usual degree of accelerated erythropoiesis and hematologic equilibrium. In the longer view, splenectomy remains the best treatment.

This is the one disorder in which *splenectomy* is associated with consistently satisfactory results. Although remissions may develop without splenectomy and latent periods of many years' duration may occur, as illustrated by the occasional diagnosis of patients after the age of forty or fifty years, permanent spontaneous recovery does not take place. The risk of hyporegenerative crises and serious anemia, progressive cholelithiasis, and the consequent risk of carcinoma of the gall bladder is always present. Splenectomy is usually deferred in infancy because of possible lowered resistance to infection when splenectomy is performed prior to two years of age. It is best performed as an elective procedure when the patient is otherwise in good health. At operation, a careful search should be made for accessory spleens, and those which are found should be removed. After splenectomy, anemia, jaundice, and reticulocytosis disappear. The spherocytosis as well as the increased osmotic fragility of the red blood cells persists, because the abnormal cells remain in the circulation as they are no longer subject to removal by the spleen. Should such red blood cells be transfused into a recipient with an intact spleen, they would be promptly removed from the circulation.

Glucose 6-phosphate Dehydrogenase Deficiency (Primaquine-sensitive Type)

From 10 to 14 percent of American Negroes and a variable percentage of individuals of other races (Orientals, also Causasians of Mediterranean background, Sephardic Jews, Iranians, and especially Sardinians), who are otherwise free of hemolytic disease and anemia, respond to the administration of amounts of primaquine and certain other compounds (see Classification, early in this chapter) which are innocuous to other individuals, with an abrupt hemolytic episode characterized by dark urine, marked anemia, jaundice, and reticulocytosis. The acute hemolytic phase ends spontaneously in about a week even if the drug is continued, and the anemia is gradually relieved, though reticulocytosis may persist for a while. In these individuals, the drug sensitivity has been shown to be associated with the X chromosome—linked transmission of an incompletely dominant gene, resulting in erythrocytic glucose 6-phosphate dehydrogenase (G6PD) deficiency (Table 338-2). The disorder is generally fully expressed in affected males, who are designated hemizygotes; in heterozygous females penetrance may vary from virtually indetectable to fully expressed enzyme deficiency, a phenomenon explained at least in part by the X chromosome mosaicism resulting from random X inactivation as hypothesized by Lyon. G6PD is concerned with the regeneration of NADPH, which, in turn, is required in the regeneration of reduced glutathione (GSH) from oxidized glutathione (GSSG). Primaquine and other redox compounds oxidize GSH and stimulate the phosphogluconate oxidative pathway (Fig. 338-2, reactions 12-15). When these compounds act in the case of G6PD deficiency, there is a rapid fall in erythrocytic GSH concentration and Heinz bodies form in red corpuscles. Hemolysis follows, but the exact biochemical mechanism by which this is brought about remains obscure. Structurally and kinetically aberrant forms of the enzyme have been discovered (p. 1614).

Because of the prevalence of the condition among certain population groups, it is worthwhile testing for G6PD deficiency in individuals at high risk before prescribing drugs capable of inducing the hemolytic reaction. Several simple screening tests are available, including a *spot test* which must be read under ultraviolet light, the methemoglobin reduction test, and the brilliant cresyl-blue reduction test. These will detect the fully expressed cases in males and females and most but not all of the intermediate cases occurring in heterozygous females. *Heinz bodies* (p. 1608) are readily formed when blood of G6PD-deficient patients is incubated with acetylphenylhydrazine.

If compounds capable of inducing hemolysis are not given to G6PD-deficient individuals, they will usually escape without a hemolytic episode even though the intrinsic erythrocytic defect is present. This is because the abnormality usually has no significant deleterious effect on the individual or on the red corpuscle life span in the absence of the offending chemical agent. In some cases, acute illnesses, such as infectious hepatitis and pneumonia, may be accompanied by a hemolytic episode even in the absence of known offending drugs.

Chronic Hemolytic Anemia with Paroxysmal Nocturnal Hemoglobinuria and Perpetual Hemosiderinuria (Marchiafava-Micheli Syndrome)

This is a rare disorder usually referred to as "paroxysmal nocturnal hemoglobinuria," or PNH. In this disorder, in addition to an intrinsic erythrocytic defect, an extracorpuscular factor is present in normal plasma, and, therefore, in most patients the hemolytic process is aggravated by transfusion of whole blood because of the normal plasma contained therein.

CLINICAL FEATURES. This disease occurs most com-

monly during the third or fourth decade and is characterized by hemolytic anemia and hemoglobinemia, the latter increasing during sleep. Hemoglobinuria, consequently, is most likely to be observed after sleep. The urine is usually brown or reddish brown. The symptoms are those of long-standing anemia, but there may be abdominal, lumbar, or substernal pain, which often ushers in an attack of hemoglobinuria. The findings, similar to those in other hemolytic anemias, include splenomegaly and well-marked anemia. The osmotic fragility of the red corpuscles is normal, and spherocytosis is not characteristic. There may be hemoglobinemia even when there is no hemoglobinuria. The urine contains increased amounts of urobilinogen as well as hemoglobin and hemosiderin. The urinary iron loss may amount to 10 mg daily, and iron-deficiency anemia may develop. Hemosiderin can often be demonstrated in leukocytes or epithelial cells of the urine. Leukopenia is usual and may be marked, and there may be thrombocytopenia as well. Indeed, this is one of the few types of severe hemolytic anemia which is accompanied by pancytopenia, and may lead to an erroneous diagnosis of aplastic anemia because of failure to consider the possibility of PNH.

PATHOGENESIS. The fault resides in the red corpuscles, which are unusually susceptible to hemolysis by subcomponents of the third component of complement (C'3a). This occurs without the prior intervention of antibody attachment to the red blood cell, nor the sequential attachment of C'1,4,2, as usually occurs in immune hemolysis. The difference between normal human red blood cells and PNH erythrocytes appears to involve the number of, and accessibility of, membrane sites concerned with the attachment of C'3a. By electron microscopy, abnormally coarse granularity and large surface pits have been seen on the membranes of PNH red blood cells, findings which may relate to their susceptibility to hemolysis. In distinction from immune hemolysis, in which the early stages of the C' sequence occur on the surface of the red blood cell and are mediated by the antibody coat, the C'-dependent hemolysis of PNH erythrocytes is preceded by the C' sequence in the serum surrounding the erythrocyte. It is these early phases which are dependent upon Mg^{++}. The increased sensitivity of complement-dependent hemolytic systems at an acid pH, and in isotonic media of low ionic strength, are exploited in the acidified-serum test (Ham's test) and the sucrose test for PNH (p. 1608). In contradistinction to the majority of hemolytic diseases due to intrinsic erythrocytic defects, the PNH lesion appears to be acquired rather than hereditary or congenital.

The mechanism by which the hemolytic system is activated during sleep is obscure. The degree of hemoglobinemia increases after administration of acid salts and may be inhibited temporarily by alkalinization, but this is not an effective approach to treatment.

DIAGNOSIS. In addition to the findings of intermittent hemoglobinemia and hemoglobinuria, perpetual hemosiderinuria, and other findings characteristic of hemolytic anemia, there is pancytopenia, a positive acidified-serum test, a positive sucrose screening test, a low leukocyte alkaline phosphatase score, and abnormally low erythrocyte acetylcholinesterase. In some instances, patients with negative tests for PNH and a seemingly established diagnosis of aplastic anemia, have been found to have positive tests for PNH months or years later.

TREATMENT. This is purely symptomatic. Splenectomy is of no value as a rule. The intensity of the hemolytic process varies; crises of severe anemia may occur. Transfusion of whole blood, packed red blood cells, or plasma usually precipitates hemolytic crises, probably because of the additional complement which is provided. Saline-washed red corpuscles can be given with impunity, and only these should be administered if transfusion is required. Iron deficiency may complicate the picture, but iron salts or iron-dextran complex for parenteral administration should be given with caution because of the number of reports of aggravation of the hemolytic process by the iron. The starting dose should be reduced to $\frac{1}{10}$ or $\frac{1}{20}$ of the usual daily dose. The potent androgens, fluoxymesterone and oxymetholone, given in daily doses of 0.5 to 1.0 and 0.5 to 1.5 mg per kg body weight, respectively, have brought about reduction in hemoglobinuria and partial or complete relief of anemia in a number of cases. Relapses have occurred if the androgen was abruptly withdrawn. A trial of one of these drugs for 3 months or longer, seems warranted, especially for the more severely affected patients. Although thrombocytopenia is common, purpuric or hemorrhagic manifestations are unusual; in fact, thrombotic complications are not infrequent. It has been reported that the anticoagulant dicoumarin (Dicumarol) impedes hemolytic activity in this disease; it has also been employed to prevent thrombotic complications. Heparin should be avoided, since it is thought to accelerate hemolysis. Infections are frequent in these patients, partly, perhaps, because of the associated leukopenia. Great care must be taken to differentiate the abdominal pain which may accompany an acute hemolytic crisis from a true surgical emergency, because needless abdominal operations may only further aggravate the hemolysis and lead to serious deterioration in the patient's condition. The prognosis varies greatly. Although a fatal termination may ensue in several years, in some cases the disorder has been compatible with life for many years and has even been known to disappear.

HEMOLYTIC ANEMIA DUE TO EXTRAERYTHROCYTIC FACTORS
Agents Extraneous to the Patient

The naturally occurring isoagglutinins α and β cause hemolysis when incompatible blood is given by transfusion. Proper cross-matching technique and identification of the blood of donors and of recipients of transfusions will avoid such disasters. When hemolytic transfusion reactions take place in spite of A, B, and O blood group compatibility, they are attributable in most instances to the development of anti-Rh (D) agglutinins. Next in frequency are the Kell antigen and antibody.

Other blood groups are only rarely involved (Chap. 342).

Erythroblastosis fetalis (*hemolytic disease of the newborn*) is due to the action of immune isoantibodies which enter the fetal circulation from the mother, via the placenta. The mother becomes immunized by an antigen which is lacking in her own red blood cells but is present in fetal red blood cells (which escape into her circulation) carrying a "foreign" antigen inherited from the father; or she may have been immunized by transfusion with blood containing erythrocyte antigens dissimilar to hers but similar to those of the fetus; or immunization may have been brought about by heterogenetic stimuli such as tetanus toxoid or vaccine containing group A substance. Spherocytosis and hyperbilirubinemia are prominent; the direct Coombs test is strongly positive when the condition is due to Rh, Kell, Kidd, and Duffy blood group systems; the test is weakly positive or even negative when erythroblastosis is due to anti-A.

ABO incompatibility is the most common cause of hemolytic disease of the newborn, the mother usually being of blood group O, and the iso-antibody anti-A$_2$. Rh incompatibility is, nowadays, a less-frequent cause of erythroblastosis, especially among Negroes, in whom the Rh-negative characteristic occurs only half as frequently as in Caucasians. The lower incidence is explained also by the fact that the Rh erythroblastotic child is more likely the result of the second or later pregnancy, whereas in the case of ABO incompatibility about half of the cases occur in the first pregnancy. Both medical alertness and family planning have acted to limit the number of pregnancies in which Rh incompatibility is known to exist, for the disease is likely to be more serious in such cases than when it is due to ABO incompatibility.

Certain chemical agents and drugs may produce hemolysis as a consequence of their usual pharmacologic activity, and in these instances (see Classification, early in this chapter, group III, A,3), the effect is related to the size of the dose.

Three *types of immunohemolytic anemia* secondary to drug administration have been identified. The *haptene type* is exemplified by the development of hemolytic anemia with an anti-gamma G type of positive direct Coombs reaction (and a negative anti-C' Coombs reaction) following the administration of penicillin in the range of 20 million units daily. The drug is firmly bound to the red corpuscle, perhaps through covalent linkage of a degradation product, benzylpenicilloyl. Anti-penicillin antibodies responsible for the hemolytic anemia and the positive Coombs test are present in the serum and red blood cell eluate. The antibodies react only with penicillin-coated red corpuscles, not with normal uncoated corpuscles, thereby distinguishing this condition from the autoimmune type of hemolytic anemia (p. 1619).

In the *"innocent bystander" type* of drug-induced hemolytic anemia, produced by quinine and stibophen, the red corpuscle is injured by the binding to its membrane of a drug-antibody complex formed in the plasma. The complex activates the complement mechanism at the cell membrane, heavily coating the cell with complement and producing a positive anti-C' Coombs reaction. These red corpuscles may lyse or may be removed from the circulation by the reticuloendothelial system. Meanwhile, the drug-antibody complex dissociates from the damaged red corpuscle to injure others. The relatively small number of complexes present accounts for the negative anti-gamma G Coombs reaction in this type of immunohemolytic anemia.

The *alpha-methyl-dopa type* of immunohemolytic anemia differs from the two preceding types in that the Coombs reaction is of the anti-gamma G type but the antibodies react not with the drug or drug-coated corpuscles, but with antigens, usually of the Rh system, of the patient's own red corpuscles, or other normal red corpuscles. The phenomenon appears to be that of a cross reaction in which an exogenous agent may induce the production of an antibody that reacts with the host's own erythrocytic antigens. From 10 to 20 percent of patients treated with alpha-methyl-dopa develop a positive Coombs test, but hemolytic anemia follows in only about 1 percent of these patients. Withdrawal of the drug results in a gradual reversal of this process. The antibody induced by alpha-methyl-dopa possesses all the characteristics of typical "warm antibody," the kind seen in Rh sensitization and in patients with severe "autoimmune" hemolytic anemia. The latter should always be considered as possible examples of drug-induced disease and should be studied carefully for an etiologic agent which can be eliminated, thereby permitting reversal of the process.

Infectious agents (Classification, group III, A,4) may produce hemolytic anemia by direct attack or infestation of the red corpuscles, or through the production of toxin or, as in the case of mycoplasma infection, by a type of cross reaction similar to the response to alpha-methyl-dopa described above. In the case of mycoplasma, a cold antibody, usually reactive with the I antigen of the red corpuscles, results.

A number of *physical agents* produce hemolytic anemia (Classification, group III, A,6). Among them is the mechanical trauma produced by the impact of red corpuscles on prosthetic heart valves. This results in random destruction of red corpuscles of all ages, appearance of fragmented and so-called "helmet" cells in the circulation, and, because of intravascular hemolysis, a significant loss of iron in the form of hemosiderin in the urine, leading to iron deficiency anemia.

In addition to the exogenous agents discussed above, there are *endogenous causes* for extraerythrocytic mechanisms which produce hemolytic anemia.

Secondary ("Symptomatic") Hemolytic Anemias

These types of anemia may be associated with a variety of disorders. The most common ones are listed in the Classification group III, B,2. In addition to the manifestations of hemolytic anemia, which may or may not be associated with autoantibodies of the type described above, there will be symptoms and signs of the underlying disorder, which are often not readily apparent and must be sought out carefully. In younger women, the possibility of disseminated lupus erythematosus should be considered, while in older patients, chronic lymphocytic leukemia or lymphosarcoma is a frequent cause of an immune type of hemolytic anemia. In many cases, the course of the hemolytic disease may be chronic and mild. In others, e.g., lupus erythematosus or chronic lymphocytic leukemia, the hemolytic anemia may be the predominating clinical feature. In such cases, treatment must be directed toward both the underlying disorder and the hemolytic process. Particularly in the case of lymphomas, where therapy might entail the use of agents which suppress erythropoiesis, control of the hemolytic process should be achieved early because reduction in the rate of red corpuscle regeneration might be expected to result in aggravation of the anemia if the hemolytic disorder is severe.

A great proportion of hemolytic anemias due to endogenous causes, including the secondary or so-called "symptomatic" hemolytic anemias already mentioned, are due to the production of "autoantibodies." Frequently, the Coombs test is positive (anti-gamma G reagent), indicating the presence of erythrocyte-bound antibodies, but no associated disease or causative agent is found. Such instances, diagnosed as "idiopathic" Coombs-positive hemolytic anemia, or idiopathic autoimmune hemolytic anemia, are diagnoses by exclusion.

Idiopathic Autoimmune Hemolytic Anemia

Whether the antibodies are the consequence of *auto-immunization* against red corpuscles or only represent erythrocyte-coating substances is disputed. The presence of other abnormalities of globulin synthesis, namely, anticomplementary substances, hypergammaglobulinemia, cryoglobulinemia, and antibodies against lipid antigens giving rise to false positive serologic tests for syphilis (Wassermann, Kahn, and VDRL) suggest that this is part of a generalized disturbance in immune systems.

The autoantibodies found in acquired hemolytic anemia may be nonspecific and react with human red blood cells without relation to any known blood group antigens. In some cases, however, the autoantibodies have a high degree of specificity, directed against various Rh antigens (anti-C, anti-D, anti-c, anti-e) and more rarely, against other blood groups, such as Kell, B, and O. Both specific and nonspecific antibodies may be found in the same patient. Furthermore, there is considerable variation from one patient to the next, in the temperature requirements, specificity, chemical nature, and in vitro reactions of the antibodies. "Warm" antibodies react well at 37°C and are not potentiated at lower temperatures. They usually are gamma G globulins, but nongamma G globulins or mixtures of both types have been found in some cases. Most commonly, these are "incomplete antibodies," i.e., they coat normal erythrocytes and may be detected by antiglobulin serum but do not cause agglutination in a saline medium, nor do they cause hemolysis. The fixation of these antibodies to red corpuscles is not inhibited by previous heat inactivation of the patient's serum at 56°C, to destroy complement, and it is only slightly increased by acidification of the serum to pH 7 or 6.5. "Cold" antibodies are markedly potentiated by reducing the temperature of the in vitro test system below 37°C. These antibodies are usually of the 19S, gamma M globulin type. They may act as agglutinating antibodies and under certain circumstances may fix complement and also bring about hemolysis.

The mechanism whereby hemolysis is initiated in vivo is not entirely clear because most of the autoantibodies encountered are not hemolytic in vitro. In a small proportion of cases, following the antigen-antibody reaction on the red blood cell membrane, the complement fixation sequence (C′1,4,2,3) ensues and defects appear in the membrane surface, representing holes of about 103 Å diameter, which may be visualized by electron microscopy. The nature of the reaction by which complement produces the holes in the lipid layer of the cell membrane is unknown. Lysis need not be by direct loss of hemoglobin through the hole, since excess water or ion transfer can cause the red corpuscle to reach the critical hemolytic volume at which the membrane becomes permeable to hemoglobin. In many cases, complement is not bound to the cell membrane, and in these cases another explanation has been offered. Red corpuscles coated with gamma G antibody may become adherent to receptor sites of monocytes and macrophages in vivo, and then sphere. This may well be the first step by the fixed tissue macrophages of the reticuloendothelial system in trapping and destroying red corpuscles coated with "incomplete" antibodies.

The *clinical manifestations* range from insidious and chronic anemia to an acute, severe, and fulminating illness. Remissions and exacerbations may occur spontaneously. The hematologic and clinical features are similar to those of other hemolytic anemias (p. 1604). Spherocytosis is usually not prominent, but it may be marked during periods of brisk hemolysis, and at such times the osmotic fragility and mechanical fragility of the red corpuscles are increased. Because the hemolytic system is dependent on extraerythrocytic factors, even normal transfused red blood cells will be hemolyzed, at a rate equivalent to that of the patient's red blood cells, and may also become spherocytes with abnormal osmotic fragility. If reticulocytosis is great, the anemia is likely to be macrocytic. In some cases when a thin film of oxalated blood is examined with the unaided eye, or under low-power magnification, a granular appearance is seen, attributable to the agglutination of the red corpuscles in the plasma. Sometimes, this may be detected when blood is first drawn from the patient by venipuncture; it can be observed along the inside of the glass container after mixing the blood with the dry anticoagulant, thus providing an early clue to the diagnosis. The direct Coombs test and the indirect Coombs test detect the globulin attached to the cell surface and the "autoantibodies" in the patient's serum, respectively. Tests for warm and cold hemolysins and cold agglutinins

need also be performed (p. 1607). *Treatment* was described earlier (p. 1610).

Paroxysmal Cold Hemoglobinuria

This is an uncommon disorder characterized by the sudden passage of hemoglobin in the urine, following local or general exposure to cold. Aching and pain in the back, legs, or abdomen, and other symptoms of acute hemolysis, such as a chill, fever, and malaise, are associated with the passage of dark-brownish urine. Other findings are those characteristic of acute hemolytic anemia. Symptoms may appear at any time from a few minutes to 7 or 8 hr following exposure.

Donath and Landsteiner showed that the hemoglobinuria is due to the sudden intravascular hemolysis of blood as the result of the action of an autohemolysin contained in the patient's blood. The hemolysin unites with the red corpuscles only at a low temperature, but destruction of the cells occurs only after the temperature of the blood has returned to normal body temperature. Appropriate screening and detailed tests have been devised to demonstrate this cold hemolysin (p. 1607), which has been found to be a complement-fixing 7S antibody. At the time of hemolytic attacks produced by chilling, strongly positive direct antiglobulin (Coombs) reactions have been observed, but these become negative after the attacks. Paroxysmal cold hemoglobinuria typically is a manifestation of congenital syphilis, and thorough antisyphilitic therapy ends the clinical manifestations.

A number of cases have been described, however, in which indications of syphilis were lacking even though, in some of the cases, the Wassermann reaction was positive. Since false positive Wassermann and Kahn reactions are not uncommon in acquired hemolytic anemia of the autoantibody type, it appears that paroxysmal cold hemoglobinuria is not exclusively a manifestation of syphilis and that some of the cases regarded as typically of syphilitic origin may well have been examples of autoimmune hemolytic disease of the cold-antibody type.

March hemoglobinuria is not likely to be confused with any of the conditions described above, because the symptoms usually are trivial, jaundice is unusual, and anemia does not develop. The condition is characterized by the passage of dark urine following prolonged walking or running. The amount of blood which is hemolyzed probably is small, and the condition is benign. Its cause is obscure.

REFERENCES

Beutler, E.: "Hereditary Disorders of Erythrocyte Metabolism," New York, Grune & Stratton, Inc., 1968.

Croft, J. D., Jr., S. N. Swisher, Jr., B. C. Gilliland, R. F. Bakemeier, J. P. Leddy, and R. I. Weed: Coombs'-test Positivity Induced by Drugs, Ann. Int. Med., 68:176, 1968.

Hartmann, R. C., D. E. Jenkins, Jr., L. C. McKee, and R. M. Heyssel: Paroxysmal Nocturnal Hemoglobinuria: Clinical and Laboratory Studies Relating to Iron Metabolism and Therapy with Androgen and Iron, Medicine, 45:331, 1966.

Jandl, J. H.: Mechanisms of Antibody-induced Red Cell Destruction, Ser. Haematol., 9:35, 1965.

——: Symposium on Disorders of the Red Cell, Am. J. Med., 40:657, 1966.

Wintrobe, M. M.: "Clinical Hematology," 6th ed., Philadelphia, Lea & Febiger, 1967.

Yachnin, S.: The Hemolysis of Red Cells from Patients with Paroxysmal Nocturnal Hemoglobinuria by Partially Purified Subcomponents of the Third Complement Component, J. Clin. Invest., 44:1534, 1965.

339 THE HEMOGLOBINOPATHIES AND THALASSEMIAS

Arthur Haut and
Maxwell M. Wintrobe

NORMAL AND ABNORMAL HEMOGLOBINS

The fact that a molecular abnormality in a single protein may produce serious ill effects and can be identified by simple, readily applicable procedures was discovered as the result of investigations concerning the nature of an hereditary, hemolytic anemia which causes serious illness in the Negro and is characterized by sickling of the red cells in vitro when they are deprived of oxygen. The elaboration of electrophoretic methods and the application of more complex techniques led to the discovery that hemoglobin is not a single homogeneous protein and that quantitative and qualitative differences in the various hemoglobins are inherited abnormalities which may produce few or no clinical changes or may cause serious ill health. These investigations have enriched our understanding not only of the pathogenesis of human disease but also of genetics and anthropology (Chap. 4). One of the abnormal hemoglobins, the sickle-cell anomaly, is believed to have conferred on its carriers increased ability to resist malarial infections.

About 97 percent of the hemoglobin in the red corpuscles of normal human adults is termed *Hemoglobin A* (Hb A) and consists of two pairs of coiled polypeptide chains: two α chains, each comprised of 141 amino acids, and two β chains, each made up of 146 amino acids. Hence, the designation, Hb $\alpha_2^A\beta_2^A$ or, more simply, Hb $\alpha_2\beta_2$. The minor fraction of the hemoglobin of normal adult erythrocytes is Hb A_2 and comprises 2.54 ± 0.35 percent of the total hemoglobin present. It possesses a different second set of polypeptide chains, δ chains in place of β chains, and is designated $\alpha_2^A\delta_2^{A_2}$. In fetal life, a different hemoglobin is present and progressively decreases in amount during infancy. Like Hb A_2, fetal hemoglobin (Hb F) possesses a pair of the same α chains as in Hb A, but the second set is different. Hb F

is therefore designated $\alpha_2^A\gamma_2^F$. Amino acid substitutions, occurring in the α, β, γ, and δ polypeptide chains, are transmitted as hereditable traits. The genetic control of production of α, β, γ, and δ chains is mediated via autosomal alleles. It is thought that α and β chain production is controlled by genes located on separate chromosomes. Those for the control of synthesis of β, γ, and δ chains are thought to be located in close proximity to one another on the same chromosome. Each parent contributes one member of an allelic pair of genes (Fig. 339-1). Thus a normal genotype would be α/α, β/β. Mutant genes may appear in the heterozygous or homozygous state, depending on the genotypes of the parents. However, only one allele can be inherited from each parent.

With the exception of Hb C_{Harlem}, only a single amino acid substitution has been found in each of the abnormal hemoglobins studied. In many instances, the exact location and nature of the amino acid substitution has been identified. If an α chain abnormality occurs, both the major hemoglobin component and the minor components (A_2, F) will be affected because they all incorporate α chains. Both α and β chain abnormalities may be present in the same individual, and each is inherited and transmitted separately. In addition to these qualitative differences in hemoglobin peptides, in certain hematologic disorders quantitative alterations in the percentages of the normal hemoglobin peptides have been found. Furthermore, complete deletion of a pair of chains may occur. Thus, Hb H is made up of four β chains (β_4), and Hb Bart's consists of four γ chains (γ_4).

Most abnormal hemoglobins are not sufficiently affected to alter their function, and therefore no clinical sequelae ensue. They have been discovered by chance alone. In other instances, either the oxygen affinity, solubility, stability or other characteristics are affected, and a clinical syndrome results. A classification based on the functional consequence of the abnormality is presented in Table 339-1.

NOMENCLATURE. The abnormal hemoglobins at first were identified serially by alphabetic letters because they were discovered by their individual electrophoretic mobility at alkaline pH. As the list grew longer and abnormal hemoglobins with the same electrophoretic mobility but certain other different characteristics were found, the geographic area where the abnormal hemoglobin was discovered was indicated as well; thus, Hb $G_{San José}$, Hb $G_{Philadelphia}$. When the exact amino acid sequence structure of the normal hemoglobins was determined, and as the nature and position of the amino acid difference in the abnormal hemoglobin was identified, it became possible to indicate the nature of the abnormality in a simple way. Thus Hb S (sickle-cell hemoglobin) is Hb $\alpha_2^A\beta_2^{6\ val}$. This means that the α chains in Hb S are normal, as in A hemoglobin, but in the β chains the sixth amino acid, which a diagram of the normal amino acid constitution of the β chain indicates is glutamic acid, has been replaced by valine. The genotype of the heterozygous state would indicate that this abnormality

Table 339-1. CLASSIFICATION OF THE DISORDERS
OF GLOBIN SYNTHESIS

I. Qualitative abnormalities of the globin peptides
   (amino acid substitutions or deletions)
   A. With clinical sequelae
      1. Abnormal heme-oxygen interaction
         (a) Diminished oxygen binding
             i) Fe^{++} heme
                Hemoglobin Kansas
             ii) Fe^{+++} heme
                Methemoglobins: M_{Boston}, $M_{Iwate (Kankakee)}$,
                   $M_{Hyde Park}$, $M_{Saskatoon (Chicago)}$, $M_{Milwaukee-1}$
         (b) Increased oxygen affinity
             Hemoglobins: Yakima, H^1, Bart's[2],
                Chesapeake, $J_{Capetown}$, Ypsi, Ranier, Hiroshima
      2. Normal heme-oxygen interaction
         (a) Readily precipitating (forms Heinz bodies)
             Hemoglobins: Bibba, Freiburg[3], Genova,
                Gun Hill[4], H^1, Hammersmith, Köln, Sabine,
                Santa Ana, Seattle, Sinai, St. Mary, Sydney,
                Ube I, Zürich
         (b) Aggregating and interacting
             Hemoglobins: S[5], C, I[5], D_{Punjab}, C_{Harlem}[5]
         (c) Other abnormal features
             Hemoglobin Lepore
   B. Not accompanied by clinical or physiologic sequelae
      (Hemoglobins: B_2, J, K, L, N, O, P, Q, and others)
II. Quantitative abnormality of globin peptide synthesis
   A. Diminished synthesis
      1. α chain: α thalassemia
      2. β chain: β thalassemia
   B. Increased synthesis
      1. γ chain
         (a) Hereditary persistence of fetal hemoglobin
             ("High F" gene)
         (b) Acquired in association with various anemias
      2. $β^J$

[1] Composed of four normal β chains; α chains absent. Forms inclusion bodies in addition to Heinz bodies; has both increased oxygen affinity and is unstable.
[2] Composed of four normal γ chains; α chains absent.
[3] Also a methemoglobin.
[4] β chain lacks a heme group, and five amino acids are deleted.
[5] These hemoglobins "sickle" erythrocytes.

is present in only one of the chromosomes governing β chains, whereas in the homozygous state, both chromosomes would code for this abnormality (Fig. 339-1).

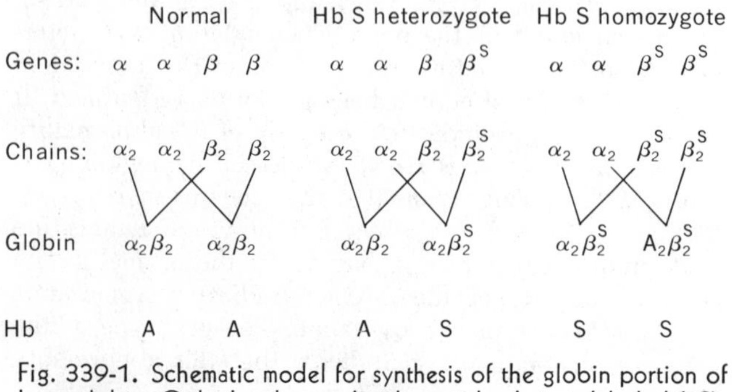

Fig. 339-1. Schematic model for synthesis of the globin portion of hemoglobin. Only the abnormal polypeptide chain is labeled (βS).

The hemoglobin disorders are referred to as *hemoglobinopathies* when they are related to qualitative differences in hemoglobin. These have been called *traits* when heterozygous, and *diseases* when homozygous, because as a rule the trait is harmless, whereas the homozygous state may have deleterious effects. Thalassemia, on the other hand, is thought to be due to the inheritance of a subnormal rate of synthesis of one or the other of the normal hemoglobin peptides and consequently is designated separately. Mixtures of abnormal hemoglobins and combinations of abnormal hemoglobins and thalassemia, due to double heterozygosity for different genes for controlling hemoglobin synthesis, also have been identified (see Table 339-2). Hemoglobinopathies may also occur in combination with other anomalies of the red cell which are inherited independently; viz., hereditary spherocytosis (Chap. 338).

HEMOGLOBINS WITH AMINO ACID SUBSTITUTIONS OR DELETIONS

The hemoglobin peptide chains are in part straight and in part in helical arrays. Straight chain sections of the amino acids occur at the amino and carboxy terminals and also alternately between the eight *helical* arrays of amino acids. The helices are identified by consecutive letters from A through H. The helices and the normal tertiary structure may be disrupted by amino acid substitutions, thereby interfering with oxygen binding, stability, or other properties of the protein.

Decreased Oxygen Affinity

A reduction in the percent saturation of hemoglobin occurring at various values for P_{O_2}, or decreased oxygen-binding capacity (diminished capacity of hemoglobin to reversibly combine with O_2 at any value of P_{O_2}), or both, result when certain amino acid substitutions occur (Table 339-2) in the α or β chain peptides about the critical regions of the crevice (E, F helices) where the heme prosthetic group is located (Table 339-1, A, 1, a). Affected individuals are *cyanotic*, but they generally are asymptomatic. Their hemoglobin has a *decreased oxygen saturation* at normal levels of Pa_{O_2} if considered with reference to the total number of heme groups present per mole hemoglobin. Erythrocytosis is usually absent. Only heterozygotes have been discovered. It is thought that the homozygous condition would be lethal in utero for want of oxygen delivery to fetal tissues. Distinctive absorption spectra and characteristic electrophoretic mobility of the oxidized hemolysates allow the presumptive diagnosis of these hemoglobins. Other features of the syndrome and its differential diagnoses are described in Chap. 344.

Hemoglobin *Kansas* is unique in this group because it maintains all of its iron atoms in the ferrous (Fe^{++}) state. It has a distinctive spectral absorption pattern and is chromatographically and electrophoretically distinguishable from normal Hb A even though it has a neutral amino acid substitution. In the "methemoglobin M" disorders, the iron atoms in the hemes of the abnormal chains are stable in the ferric (Fe+++) state, and the affected half of the molecule is incapable of the normal reversible association with oxygen. In four types of methemoglobin M, the altered function of the hemoglobin is attributed to substitution of *tyrosine* for one of the *histidines* of the globin peptides. Histidines are normally found at the points of the normal covalent linkage between the heme and globin and also close to the sixth coordination position and only oxygen-binding site of the iron atom of heme. In Hb M$_{Milwaukee-1}$, the substitution is different but it also occurs in the E helix. The profound changes in the physiologic function of these hemoglobins are the result of a single amino acid substitution and in turn reflect single mutations in the triplet base codon of the gene. Thus, the amino acid substitution *His → Tyr* would be the result of the codon change CAC → UAC.

Search for these abnormal hemoglobins is important in the evaluation of cyanotic patients who have normal Pa_{O_2}. Treatment is not ordinarily required for these conditions. Measures designed to reverse methemoglobinemia of other causes would not be helpful here. As in other hemoglobinopathies, transfusions may be employed as a temporary measure in the face of acute complicating illnesses.

Increased Oxygen Affinity

The converse of the lesion just described results from other amino acid substitutions in the regions near the F and G helices. These abnormal hemoglobins fail to release oxygen in the normal manner despite the low oxygen tension in the tissue capillaries. Their oxygen dissociation curve is hyperbolic rather than sigmoidal.

Hb *Yakima*, Hb *Kempsey*, and Hb *Ypsi* result from different substitutions at the same (ninety-ninth) residue in the β chain. Hb *Ranier* and Hb *Hiroshima* are also due to substitutions in the β chain, but near its carboxy terminus. However, in Hb *Chesapeake* and Hb J$_{Capetown}$, the substitutions occur in the α chain, at the ninety-second residue. Erythrocytosis occurs in all but the last named of these disorders. Some patients have been erroneously diagnosed as erythremia (Chap. 343). Increased erythropoietin excretion, presumably due to tissue anoxia, was found when the elevated volume of packed red cells in the patient with Hb Ranier was reduced by phlebotomy. Tissue anoxia may also be the cause of the erythrocytosis in the other disorders of this group. For this reason, phlebotomies or other measures to reduce the red cell mass are not advised.

Unstable Hemoglobins

READILY SUSCEPTIBLE TO PRECIPITATION. Certain amino acid substitutions, mainly in the β chain and sometimes involving the same sites as those already mentioned, produce unstable hemoglobins which are denatured prematurely in vivo or in vitro and result in *hemolytic disease, erythrocytic inclusion bodies,* and sometimes pig-

menturia. In this group (Table 339-1, 1A, 2a), hemolytic anemia may occur in heterozygotes even though less than half of the hemoglobin in each corpuscle is abnormal. In contrast, as described below, in conditions such as Hb S and Hb C, heterozygotes are usually asymptomatic, and only the homozygous state results in hemolytic anemia.

Many of the cases of hemolytic anemia with red cell inclusion bodies (Table 338-1) are included in this category. In some cases, Heinz bodies (Chap. 338) occur only after exposure to certain chemicals or after splenectomy; in others, they are found at all times. Some patients are free of anemia because the hemolytic disorder is fully compensated unless certain drugs are administered; others have a chronic hemolytic anemia.

Heterozygotes for Hb *Zürich* develop overt hemolysis, anemia, and Heinz bodies in their erythrocytes after administration of sulfonamides or primaquine and related oxyquinolones. In this disorder, the same amino acid residue is affected as in methemoglobin M$_{Saskatoon}$ (β 63), but a different amino acid has been substituted (Table 339-2). Hb *Sydney* is another unstable hemoglobin associated with chronic hemolysis. The same residue that is abnormal in methemoglobin M$_{Milwaukee-1}$ is affected here (β 67) but, again, with a different substitution. Hb *Freiburg* has the properties of both an unstable hemoglobin and a methemoglobin: affected individuals are cyanotic and have hemolytic anemia. Hemoglobin *Gun Hill* is unique because five amino acids are deleted from the β chain and this peptide lacks heme groups—necessarily reducing its oxygen-carrying capacity. A compensated hemolytic anemia and splenomegaly have been described in these cases. Hb *Hammersmith* results in a severe chronic hemolytic anemia, and Hb *Köln* results in chronic hemolysis with anemia provoked by minor infections. These examples point out the value of examining for an abnormal hemoglobin by electrophoresis and testing for hemoglobin stability at 50 to 60°C when an otherwise unexplained hemolytic anemia is encountered. This is especially important if red cell inclusions are demonstrated or pigmenturia is present, or if the anemia appears to be drug-related and a red cell enzymopathy is not found. Treatment is not fully satisfactory, except in the case of Hb Zürich where if the inciting drugs are not given, anemia may be avoided. In other diseases with chronic hemolysis, some benefit has resulted from splenectomy. Knowledge of the correct diagnosis avoids inappropriate treatment, such as corticosteroid hormones, which might be harmful and offer no potential benefit.

Aggregating and Interacting Hemoglobins

Sickle hemoglobin (Hb S), was the first of the abnormal hemoglobins to be recognized. It was electrophoretically separated from Hb A, and was shown to be the product of a single, identifiable, amino acid substitution. The studies of Pauling, Itano, and later, Ingram, opened a whole new field of investigation: that of molecular biology. Sickle hemoglobin gained its name from the sicklelike shape assumed by some of the red cells containing it when the oxygen tension was lowered (**Fig.**

Table 339-2. CHARACTERISTICS OF SOME HEMOGLOBINOPATHIES

Condition	Manifestations			Hemoglobin		
	Syndrome	Anemia	RBC morphology	Peptide chains[1]		Pathologic physiology
				α	β	
Heterozygous						
Hb Yakima	Erythrocytosis	No	Normal	Normal	99 Asp → His	
Hb Kempsey	Erythrocytosis	No	Normal	Normal	99 Asp → Asn	Increased
Hb Ypsi	Erythrocytosis	No	Normal	Normal	99 Asp → ?	
Hb Chesapeake	Erythrocytosis	No	Normal	92 Arg → Leu	Normal	oxygen
Hb J Capetown	None	No	Normal	92 Arg → Glu	Normal	
Hb Ranier	Erythrocytosis	No	Normal	Normal	145 Tyr → His	affinity
Hb Hiroshima	Erythrocytosis	No	Normal	Normal	143 His → Asp	
Hb Kansas	Cyanosis	No	Normal	Normal	102 Asn → Thr	Decreased
Hb M Boston	Cyanosis	No	Normal	58 His → Tyr	Normal	oxygen
Hb M Iwate	Cyanosis	No	Normal	87 His → Tyr	Normal	affinity[3]
Hb M Saskatoon	Cyanosis	No	Normal	Normal	63 His → Tyr	Methemoglobin
Hb M Hyde Park	Cyanosis	No	Normal	Normal	92 His → Tyr	Methemoglobin
Hb M Milwaukee-1	Cyanosis	No	Normal	Normal	67 Val → Glu	Methemoglobin
Hb Freiburg	Cyanosis	Hemolytic	Inclusion bodies	Normal	23 Val → 0	Unstable Hb
Hb Zürich	Sensitive to sulfonamide	Hemolytic	Inclusion bodies	Normal	63 His → Arg	Unstable Hb
Hb Köln	Chronic hemolysis	Severe	Inclusion bodies	Normal	98 Val → Met	Unstable Hb
Hb Genova	Chronic hemolysis	Severe	Inclusion bodies	Normal	28 Leu → Pro	Unstable Hb
Hb Hammersmith	Chronic hemolysis	Severe	Inclusion bodies	Normal	42 Phe → Ser	Unstable Hb
Hb H	Mild		Inclusion bodies[5]	None	β₄ Tetramer	Unstable Hb[5]
Hb Gun Hill	Chronic hemolysis	No	Normochromic[6] inclusions[4]	Normal	91–95 → 0	β chains lack heme[6]
Hb Santa Ana	Chronic hemolysis	Severe		Normal	138 Leu → Pro	Unstable Hb
Hb Sydney	Chronic hemolysis	Slight	Normochromic inclusions[8]	Normal	67 Val → Ala	Unstable Hb
Hb Sabine	Chronic hemolysis	Severe	Inclusions	Normal	91 Leu → Pro	Unstable Hb[9]
Hb Bibba	Chronic hemolysis	Severe	Heinz bodies	136 Leu → Pro	Normal	Unstable Hb[10]
Hb Sinai	Hemolysis, thrombocytopenia, splenomegaly	Variable	Normal	47 Asp → His	Normal	Unstable Hb[11]
Hb S	Asymptomatic	No		Normal	6 Glu → Val	Sickles
Hb C	Asymptomatic	No	Target cells	Normal	6 Glu → Lys	
Hb C Harlem[7]	Asymptomatic	No	Occasional target cells	Normal	6 Glu → Val also 73 Asp → Asn	Sickles
Hb D Punjab	Asymptomatic	No	Normal	Normal	121 Glu → Gln	
Hb I	Asymptomatic	No	Normal	16 Lys → Glu	Normal	Sickles[12]
Doubly heterozygous						
Hb SC	Hemolysis, pain, infarction	Marked	Many target cells	Normal Normal	6 Glu → Val and[13] 6 Glu → Lys	Sickles
Hb SD	Hemolysis, pain, infarction	Marked	Target Cells	Normal Normal	6 Glu → Val and[13] 121 Glu → Gln	Sickles
Hb Memphis/S	Hemolysis, pain, infarction	Marked	Target cells	23 Glu → Gln Normal	6 Glu → Val and[13] 6 Glu → Val	Sickles
Hb G Philadelphia/S	Hemolysis, pain, infarction	Marked	Target cells	68 Asn → Lys Normal	6 Glu → Val and[13] 6 Glu → Val	Sickles
Hb S-thalassemia	Chronic hemolysis	Severe	Target cells	Normal	6 Glu → Val	Sickles

Table 339-2. CHARACTERISTICS OF SOME HEMOGLOBINOPATHIES (Continued)

| Condition | Syndrome | Anemia | RBC morphology | Peptide chains[1] | | Pathologic physiology |
				α	β	
Homozygous						
Hb SS	Hemolysis, pain, infarction	Marked	Target cells	Normal	6 Glu → Val	Sickles
Hb CC	Arthralgia, splenomegaly, hemolysis	Mild	Many target cells	Normal	6 Glu → Lys	Crystals[14]
Hb EE	Slight	Mild	Target cells Microcytosis	Normal	26 Glu → Lys	

[1] The number and name of the replaced residue is followed (→) by its replacement. Abbreviations for amino acid residues: *Ala*, alanyl; *Arg*, arginyl; *Asn*, asparaginyl; *Asp*, aspartyl; *Gln*, glutaminyl; *Glu*, glutamyl; *Gly*, glycyl; *His*, histadyl; *Leu*, leucyl; *Lys*, lysyl; *Phe*, phenylalanyl; *Tyr*, tyrosyl; *Val*, valyl; *Met*, methionyl.

[2] Some cases of methemoglobinemia have been accompanied by mild erythrocytosis.

[3] Also, methemoglobinemia with decreased oxygen binding capacity.

[4] After incubation with brilliant cresyl blue.

[5] Also, high oxygen affinity.

[6] MCHC low because β chains lack heme; normochromic appearance on stained smear indicates normal concentration of protein component of hemoglobin in the red cells.

[7] Probably the same as Hb C_{Georgetown}.

[8] After 50°C or 48 hr at 37°C.

[9] Also deficient in heme-groups.

[10] 12% methemoglobin also present.

[11] Precipitated at 60°C.

[12] In 4% metabisulfite, rather than 2% as with Hb S.

[13] There are two types of abnormal hemoglobin molecules present in these conditions; single molecules do not contain two different kinds of β (or α) chains.

[14] Intraerythrocytic hemoglobin crystals have been seen.

339-2). The sickling phenomenon is explained by physical events in solutions of Hb S as the oxygen tension is reduced. At a concentration of approximately 20 gm per 100 ml, molecular aggregation of Hb S occurs, as evidenced by increasing viscosity and gelling. At higher concentrations, the deoxygenated Hb S forms rigid, regular structures: birefringent tactoids with parallel alignment of long chains of the molecules. These tactoids are responsible for the peculiar shape of the sickled red cell. The phenomenon is reversible upon reoxygenation, but repeated cycles within the intact red corpuscle result in loss of some of the substance of the sickled cell and, eventually, to hemolysis. At the molecular level, the tactoids are attributed to an interlocking between the α chains of one molecule and the abnormal β chains of the next. In Hb S, the substitution of the hydrophobic *valyl* for the hydrophilic *glutamyl* at β 6, allows that part of the β chain to stabilize in a ring formation through hydrophobic bonding between the normal N terminal valyl and the anomalous valyl at position number 6. The ring thus formed in the β chain fits into the complementary region in an α chain. Deoxygenation increases the distance between the β chains, and this is thought to facilitate the fit between the complementary sites of adjacent molecules; reoxygenation diminishes the distance between β chains and disrupts the interlock, dissolving

the tactoid and reversing the sickling. Tactoid formation is also disrupted by cooling to low temperatures, which decreases ring formation; the same effect results from reaction with propane gas, which forms stronger hydrophobic bonds with the critical valyls than the latter do to each other. These observations and the electron micrographs of "microtubules" formed by the longitudinal array of Hb S molecules support the hypothesis.

The extent to which sickling occurs depends upon the oxygen tension, the concentration of Hb S within the red corpuscle, the amount of Hb F, and the type and amount of any other hemoglobin present in the same cells which contain the Hb S. The proportion of Hb S in the blood of heterozygous individuals (sickle-cell trait) has been found to vary from 20 to 45 percent, whereas the amount in the blood of homozygotes (sickle-cell anemia) has ranged from 76 to 100 percent. These variations have been explained on the ground that the expression of the Hb S gene may be under the modifying influence of other genetic factors; the lower and higher proportions of Hb S are a familial characteristic. In the homozygous condition, the amount of sickling which occurs at moderate oxygen tensions and the associated clinical syndrome are far greater than in the case of the simple heterozygote. In the individual who is doubly heterozygous for two abnormal hemoglobins, the relationship between the concentration of Hb S within the cell, oxygen tension, sickling, and the severity of the clinical syndrome varies with the degree of physical interaction between the hemoglobin types within the cell. Hb F interacts least, and patients heterozygous for both Hb S and persistence of fetal hemoglobin (high F gene) have less sickling and relatively few symptoms despite the high proportion (70 percent) of Hb S in their red corpuscles. The combination of Hb C and Hb S results in greater interaction than between Hb A and Hb S, and the syndrome associated with the former (*Hb SC disease*) is intermediate in severity between sickle trait (Hb AS) and sickle-cell anemia (Hb SS). Hb D$_{Punjab}$ interacts most with Hb S, and its clinical syndrome (*Hb SD disease*) is also more severe than that of the other doubly heterozygous conditions. The coexistence of a gene for β thalassemia and one for Hb S can reduce the proportion of Hb A present so that it becomes the minor rather than the major component. The result is a higher concentration of Hb S within the red corpuscles and a more severe syndrome than would otherwise be the case for a simple heterozygote (Hb AS). The hybrid *Hemoglobin Memphis/S* is composed of the α chains of Hb Memphis ($\alpha_2^{23\ Glu \rightarrow Gln}\ \beta_2^A$) and the β chains of Hb S. Blood from individuals homozygous for Hb S but heterozygous for Hb Memphis contained 50 percent Hb S and 50 percent Hb Memphis/S. When deoxygenated, it was markedly less viscous than blood from patients with Hb S alone. Higher concentrations of the isolated, deoxygenated Hb Memphis/S were required for comparable increases in viscosity than were required for isolated Hb S. Thus, alteration in the interaction between the α and β chains seems to affect the sickling process. The clinical syndrome of patients with Hb Memphis/S is less severe

than that of patients homozygous for Hb S without the additional abnormality. On the other hand, in a similar situation with simultaneous homozygosity for Hb S and heterozygosity for Hb G$_{Philadelphia}$, an α chain variant, a moderately severe syndrome characteristic for sickle-cell anemia is found; 63 percent of the hemoglobin is Hb S and 36 percent is of a hybrid type—Hb G$_{Philadelphia}$/S ($\alpha_2^{68\ Asn \rightarrow Lys}\ \beta_2^{\ Glu \rightarrow Val}$).

An unusual variant of the Hb S structure is Hb C$_{Harlem}$. This hemoglobin was first identified by the letter "C" to indicate that it had the same electrophoretic mobility at pH 8.6 as did Hb C (and therefore probably two fewer negative charges at that pH than does Hb A). It has since been shown to have the same substitution at β 6 as does Hb S (accounting for one unit charge difference) and, in addition, it has a second amino acid substitution—being unique in this regard—further along the same β chain (Table 339-2). The first substitution accounts for the ability of this Hb C to sickle, while the second accounts for the additional charge difference and hence the "Hb C-like" mobility of this sickling hemoglobin. Compared with Hb S, the Hb C$_{Harlem}$ requires a higher concentration for equivalent change in viscosity upon deoxygenation. The molecular basis for the aggregation of Hb I, which sickles erythrocytes exposed to 4 percent metabisulfite, when it is present in 70 percent concentration, is not evident. The disorder is benign. In some individuals with only Hb C, crystal-like structures

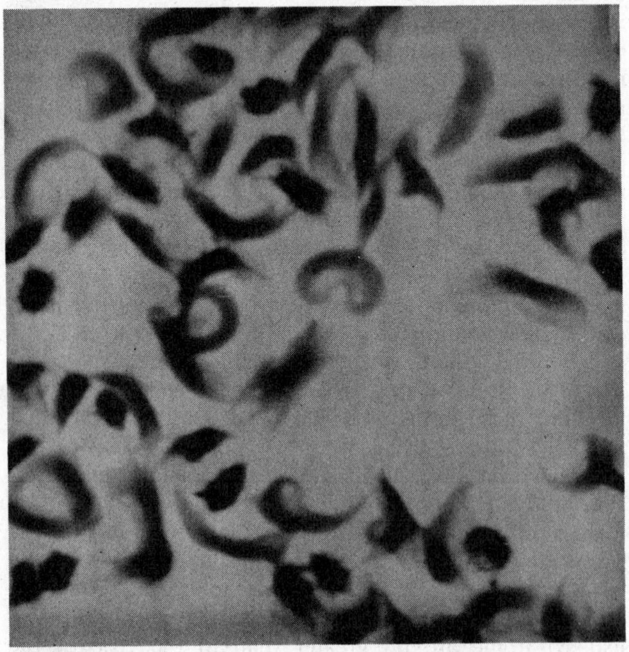

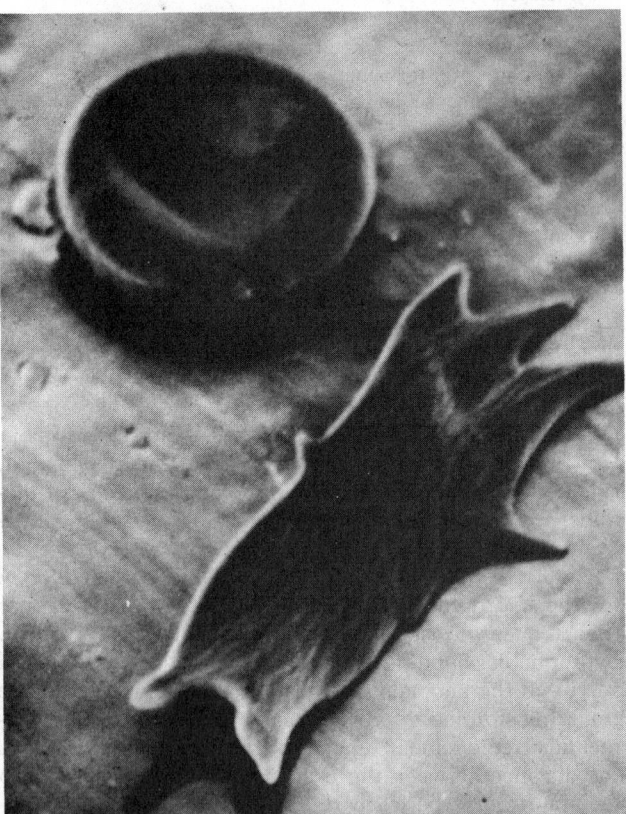

Fig. 339-2A. Sickled red corpuscles from a patient with sickle-cell anemia (formalin-fixed after sickling, ×1050). (*M. M. Wintrobe: Clinical Hematology, 1967, 6th ed., Philadelphia, Lea & Febiger.*)

Fig. 339-2B. Sickled erythrocyte, seen by the scanning electron microscope. (*Courtesy of Dr. Fernando Padilla.*)

may be seen within the red cells; these are more evident after mixing the blood with 3 percent sodium chloride. Intraerythrocytic crystals are prominent in individuals with both *hemoglobins S and C* coexisting in the same red corpuscles (*Hb SC disease*)

CLINICAL SYNDROMES

In most instances no illness is associated with the inheritance of an abnormal hemoglobin from only one parent. This applies to Hbs B₂, J, K, L, N, O, P, and Q, among others. Consequently, the *heterozygous* forms in many cases are of interest and value chiefly for genetic and anthropologic reasons. They can be recognized by simple paper electrophoresis or other similar techniques. The abnormal hemoglobins may manifest anodal mobility on electrophoresis at pH 8.6 which is slower or faster than that of Hb A. Some of these are represented in Fig. 339-3. Hemoglobins having the same electrophoretic mobility at pH 8.6 may actually have distinct primary structures. Thus there are nine hemoglobins "D" and nine hemoglobins "G."

Those abnormal hemoglobins with altered heme-oxygen reactivity and the readily precipitating (unstable) hemoglobins produce recognizable clinical syndromes even though they constitute less than half of the hemoglobin and the patients are only heterozygous for the abnormal gene.

Other abnormal hemoglobins which produce anemia and serious disease in patients who are homozygous for the responsible gene, may be innocuous in the heterozygous state. *Hemoglobin C trait* and *sickle-cell trait*, are examples. The phenotype *Hb AS* is rarely the cause of clinical problems. When a person with the sickle-cell trait is exposed to extremely low oxygen tension, as in high-altitude flying in unpressurized aircraft, or inadvertently, under general anesthesia, intravascular sickling may occur in the spleen, cerebral vessels, or lungs, and thrombotic phenomena or infarction may result. Hyposthenuria and idiopathic hematuria, probably the result of hemorrhage from the renal papillae, have also been noted in *sickle-cell trait*. Though usually brief, the hematuria may last many weeks and may be recurrent often enough to result in a significant loss of iron. It must be differentiated from other, more serious causes of hematuria. Awareness of this complication may avoid premature surgical intervention for some patients.

The phenotype *Hb AC* is asymptomatic and free of anemia. Target cells are found on the blood smears. It occurs in about 2.5 percent of American Negroes. Its incidence is highest in the Gold Coast of Africa.

Hemoglobin E is frequent among the peoples of Southeast Asia (13 to 35 percent), and *Hb H* is frequent among the Chinese and also other racial groups. Hb H (β₄) is an unstable hemoglobin and has a high oxygen affinity (Table 339-2). Hb H is abnormal only in the sense that it is composed only of normal β chains and lacks α chains entirely. Patients with Hb H disease are thought to be doubly heterozygous for two types of α-thalassemia genes. One of these genes (alpha-1) se-

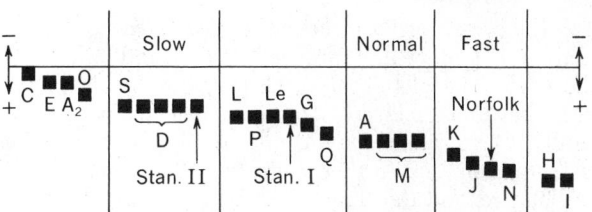

Fig. 339-3. Relative mobilities of normal and abnormal hemoglobins on paper electrophoresis at pH 8.6. The mobility of hemoglobin M (Chap. 344) is similar to that of normal hemoglobin (hemoglobin A). Other hemoglobins can be classified as *slow* (e.g., hemoglobin S; this group includes the D hemoglobins and Stanleyville II), *very slow* (e.g., hemoglobin C; this group includes the normal hemoglobin A₂ as well as the abnormal hemoglobins E and O), or *moderately slow* [(e.g., the G hemoglobins; this includes L, P, Q, Lepore (Le), and Stanleyville I)]. In addition, there are *fast* hemoglobins with electrophoretic mobilities faster than that of hemoglobin A. These include H, I, J, K, N, Norfolk, and Hopkins-1 and Hopkins-2. (Wintrobe: "Clinical Hematology," 6th ed., Philadelphia, Lea & Febiger, 1967.)

verely, or moderately, depresses α-chain synthesis as in the usual α-thalassemia heterozygote; the other (alpha-2) may be so mild in its effect that when present alone, as in one of the patient's parents, its expression may escape detection. Less than half of the hemoglobin in affected red corpuscles is Hb H. There is slight or moderate hemolytic anemia with hypochromic red corpuscles, and the clinical manifestations suggest thalassemia. The spontaneous denaturation of Hb H within intact erythrocytes is accelerated in vitro by redox compounds, and spherical inclusion bodies are formed, which stain with vital dyes. *Bart's hemoglobin*, a γ₄ tetramer, is the fetal hemoglobin analogue of Hb H. It occurs in the newborn affected with Hb H.

SICKLE-CELL ANEMIA, OTHER HOMOZYGOUS ABNORMAL HEMOGLOBIN STATES, AND COMBINATIONS THEREOF

DEFINITION. Sickle-cell anemia is a chronic, hereditary, hemolytic disease which is due to the inheritance from each parent of a gene for Hb S. The red corpuscles lack Hb A; when they are deprived of oxygen, they assume sickle and other bizarre, but mainly crescentic, shapes.

PATHOGENESIS. The sickled cell is a hemoglobin tactoid, thinly veiled and somewhat distorted by the cell membrane. In the homozygous individual the erythrocytes contain sufficient Hb S to sickle even when within the physiologic range of oxygen tensions. When sickled red corpuscles become trapped in the smaller vessels, erythrostasis occurs. Deoxygenation and reduced pH favor further sickling and further increase in blood viscosity. Plugs or masses of sickled erythrocytes become solid enough to occlude vessels, and thrombosis and infarction readily follow. A vicious cycle leading to more sickling develops. Among the clinical consequences are the painful "crises" which characterize this disorder, impaired circulation ultimately resulting in the formation of chronic leg ulcers, infarction, and later, marked shrinkage of the spleen (*autosplenectomy*), hepatomegaly, aseptic necrosis of bone, hematuria, priapism, pulmonary infarction, and central nervous system and other complications. The picture of shock may develop in patients with the abdominal crisis of sickle-cell anemia because capillary hypoxemia may result in plasma loss, hemoconcentration, and further stagnation. Shock may also be cardiogenic, and the clinical picture then resembles myocardial infarction or acute myocarditis. Bone pain may be due to distension of the intramedullary cavity by the vascular engorgement. In some cases there may be focal infarction of bone and of marrow. It is possible that the irregular sclerosis visible in roentgenograms of the long bones is due to healing of such infarcted areas with scarring and subsequent osteoid deposition. Other changes in the bones may perhaps be the result of marrow hyperplasia compensatory to the increased blood destruction.

After stasis, when red cells are released into free circulation, a certain proportion, having been fixed in irreversible sickled form have also become more fragile in terms of mechanical trauma. Consequently, they are more than normally susceptible to destruction by the trauma associated with circulation. Even when sickling is reversed by reoxygenation, there may be loss of part of the filamentous portions of the cell substance as the cell resumes its discoid shape. This process also leads toward hemolysis.

CLINICAL MANIFESTATIONS. This disorder is almost entirely confined to Negroes. The normal fetal hemoglobin which is present at birth lacks the abnormal β chain characteristic of Hb S. In infancy, as β chain synthesis replaces γ chain synthesis, Hb F is replaced by Hb S. The clinical manifestations develop as the proportion of Hb S within the red corpuscles rises. For reasons not fully understood, the time of onset of symptoms may vary widely. The course is that of a chronic, hemolytic anemia which is interrupted by periods of increased weakness, episodes of aching pain in the joints or elsewhere in the extremities, especially in the hands and feet (dactylitis), chest pain with accompanying electrocardiographic changes; or sudden attacks of severe abdominal pain which have often been mistaken for perforated peptic ulcer, intestinal obstruction, or some other abdominal emergency.

The victims of sickle-cell anemia are often poorly developed, and there may be some degree of retardation of secondary sex characteristics. Frequently the extremities are disproportionately long and thin. There may be bony deformities of various types. The scleras are icteric. Short, dark-red, comma-shaped or corkscrew-like vascular segments, seemingly isolated from other vessels, may be seen if the lower bulbar conjunctivas are examined with the +40 diopter lens of the ophthalmoscope. These are found in most patients with sickle-cell anemia, rarely in patients with Hb SC disease, and not at all in individuals with the sickle trait or in normal persons. Tortuous, irregularly dilated vessels frequently can be seen in the ocular fundi. There may be slight general lymph node enlargement, but splenomegaly is rare in the adult. The heart may be enlarged, and the cardiac signs may closely

simulate those of mitral stenosis or mitral regurgitation while the peripheral findings resemble those of aortic insufficiency.

Impaired ability to concentrate urine is common in both sickle-cell anemia and the sickle trait. Limitation in free water reabsorption has been ascribed to a failure to maintain a high solute concentration in the medullary interstitium. Indirect evidence attributes the latter to an increased renal medullary blood flow and to dilated and tortuous medullary blood vessels which distort spatial relationships and thereby decrease the efficiency of the countercurrent exchange system. The low oxygen tension and hyperosmolality of the renal medulla, which could result in sickling of erythrocytes passing through that area, may also play a role. The relative importance of these explanations is unclear, for the sodium pump in the ascending loop is anaerobic and there is no direct measure of medullary blood flow.

In many instances chronic leg ulcers are found over the internal or external malleoli. Roentgenograms may reveal radial striation in the skull, osteoporosis in the vertebral bodies, or areas of increased density or of aseptic necrosis resulting from infarction.

The anemia is usually severe and may be normocytic or macrocytic. The volume of packed red corpuscles is commonly 20 ml per 100 ml or less. Oval, cigar-shaped, sickled, or other bizarre forms of red corpuscles may be seen in the stained blood smear. The sickling is brought out clearly in wet films of blood which are examined under a cover glass sealed with petrolatum. In patients with sickle-cell anemia the typical sickled and oat-shaped forms with elongated, pointed filaments appear within a few hours. When only the sickle-cell trait exists, 24 hr is often required to produce this change, and only a proportion rather than practically all of the cells are affected. If reducing agents, such as 2% sodium metabisulfite are used, the characteristic forms appear promptly.

In sickle-cell anemia, reticulocytosis, polychromatophilia, normoblasts, leukocytosis with "shift to the left" in the myeloid series, and an increase in platelets are found on the blood smear. Hyperbilirubinemia and increased urobilinogen in the urine and stools also occur. Osmotic fragility is decreased. The bone marrow shows striking normoblastic hyperplasia. Occasionally, megaloblasts may be found. These are due to a superimposed deficiency of folic acid. The gap between the increased demands of the hyperplastic marrow and the relatively limited supply of that vitamin in the diet of the often impoverished Negro with sickle-cell anemia is increased by the custom of boiling "greens" for many hours, further lowering the folic acid content of the food.

Hyporegenerative crises with reticulocytopenia may develop, especially following infections, as in other hemolytic anemias (Chap. 338). Infections of the respiratory tract are frequent, as are osteomyelitis and bacteremia, particularly with *Salmonella*. Cerebral vascular accidents occur, and severe renal insufficiency is frequent in the third decade and later. Pregnancy is not associated with excessive hazard, but there is increased morbidity and fetal loss.

DIAGNOSIS. Sickle-cell anemia is often mistaken for some other disease. Rheumatic fever, myocarditis, peptic ulcer, renal or biliary calculus, osteomyelitis, and various neurologic disorders may be simulated. Suspicion is raised by the finding of a hemolytic anemia and the demonstration of sickling. Ultimately, the diagnosis rests upon the finding of only Hb S in the patient's erythrocytes. The Hb SS phenotype is indistinguishable from Hb SD disease if the hemoglobin electrophoresis is carried out at only pH 8.6. It may also be simulated by the simultaneous presence of heterozygosity for Hb AS and also for β thalassemia. However, Hb SD may be distinguished from Hb SS by electrophoresis at pH 6.2, and both conditions may be identified by appropriate studies of family members. Hb D does not sickle red corpuscles. Performance of both the sickle test and Hb electrophoresis, on the parents of the patient, will permit the correct identification of the AS and AD phenotypes.

In distinguishing persons with the sickle-cell trait who may also have another disorder accompanied by anemia from those who have sickle-cell anemia, it must be kept in mind that individuals with sickle-cell trait may develop any type of anemia (e.g., iron deficiency anemia), while sickle-cell anemia is always hemolytic. The proportions of target cells present, the finding of intraerythrocytic crystals, or the demonstration of inclusion bodies in the red corpuscles give clues concerning disorders resulting from combinations of the gene for Hb S with the genes for other abnormal hemoglobins or with the thalassemia gene. Study of the blood smears, paper electrophoresis of hemoglobin, and the alkali denaturation method for the demonstration of Hb F are simple and essential procedures which should be employed.

Homozygous *Hb C disease* is relatively rare. The hemolytic anemia is usually mild, and patients are rarely disabled. Mild icterus and moderate splenomegaly may be found. The blood contains as many as 80 percent *target cells.*

The *combination of hemoglobin C with S hemoglobin* is accompanied by sickling of the red corpuscles as well as by a hemolytic syndrome similar to sickle-cell anemia. It differs in that the hemolytic anemia is milder, target cells are more plentiful in the blood, and there is slowly progressive splenomegaly. It is very probable that most of the cases formerly reported as forms of sickle-cell anemia intermediate between the asymptomatic carrier state and the homozygous classical disease actually were cases simultaneously heterozygous for S and C hemoglobin. The correct diagnosis may be made by electrophoresis of the patient's hemoglobin. Hb S and Hb C are found; Hb A is absent. In individuals with *Hb SC* disease, mortality in pregnancy has been relatively high as the result of hemorrhagic and thrombotic complications. Aseptic necrosis of bone, particularly of the head of the femur, is common.

Hemoglobin SD disease is another combination found in the United States. The manifestations are less severe than in most cases of sickle-cell anemia, but differentiation may be difficult unless electrophoretic and family studies are carried out. Cases have been reported in Caucasians who have no evidence of Negro lineage. This may have been the disorder in some of the cases previously considered to have been sickle-cell anemia in Caucasians. In addition to Hb S, Hb D$_{\text{Punjab}}$ is present in all the red corpuscles. Hb A is lacking because the gene to produce β^A chains has been replaced in both chromosomes. The volume of packed red corpuscles is often in the range of 20 to 30 ml per 100 ml blood, and reticulocytes number 10 to 40 percent. The spleen is not enlarged.

Hemoglobin E disease, the homozygous condition for Hb E, is characterized as a rule by mild microcytosis, normochromic anemia, and minimal signs of hemolytic anemia. Target cells are plentiful. The spleen is normal in size or only slightly enlarged.

TREATMENT AND PROGNOSIS. Because these abnormal hemoglobin syndromes represent inherited anomalies, no treatment other than symptomatic therapy can be provided; no means has been devised whereby the abnormal state might be altered. A number of the conditions are asymptomatic. Sickle-cell anemia, however, is ultimately fatal, often before the age of thirty. Death may result from intercurrent infection, renal or cardiac failure, thrombosis or hemorrhage involving vital tissues, or it may follow one of the abdominal crises. Blood transfusions may be of value in abdominal crises with shock or in aplastic crises which accompany serious infections. In the interim between acute crises, the patient usually is adjusted to the chronic, severe, hemolytic anemia, and transfusions in that situation will only create the additional risks of homologous serum jaundice, transfusion reactions (Chap. 342) and, ultimately, hemosiderosis. Folic acid is useful only if megaloblastic transformation of the marrow has occurred (Chap. 338). Iron, vitamin B$_{12}$, and other antianemia agents, are of no value. Splenectomy also has no place in therapy. In acute crises, it is important to maintain adequate hydration and electrolyte balance, correcting acidosis if it occurs. Pain may be relieved through anodynes. One should search for infections which would respond to antibiotic therapy. There are no "specific" agents to reverse sickling in vivo or infarction.

QUANTITATIVE ABNORMALITY IN GLOBIN PEPTIDE SYNTHESIS

Thalassemia and the Thalassemia Syndromes

DEFINITION. The term *thalassemia* refers to a group of genetically determined diseases which are caused by partial or complete interference in the synthesis of one of the normal hemoglobin peptide chains. They are characterized by the presence of unusually thin red corpuscles (leptocytes), microcytosis, hypochromia, various degrees of anemia, and when the anemia is severe, numerous nucleated red corpuscles in the blood.

HISTORY. Cooley and Lee (1925) described a chronic progressive anemia commencing early in life that was associated with a characteristic mongoloid facies, splenomegaly, and a familial and racial incidence (*Cooley's* *anemia*). Later it became clear that this severe and fatal disease was the *homozygous* form of a disorder which is also seen in milder form at all ages as the *heterozygous* state (*thalassemia minor*). In the *homozygous* condition (*thalassemia major; Cooley's anemia*), there is a drastic abnormality in the synthesis of normal hemoglobin. These conditions have also been known as *erythroblastic anemia* and *hereditary leptocytosis*.

Those first discovered to be affected were chiefly of Italian, Greek, Syrian, or Armenian parentage; that is, individuals whose ancestors lived in countries bordering the Mediterranean. In certain communities of Italians, the anomaly has been observed in as many as 20 percent of those examined. Once called *Mediterranean anemia*, this disorder is now known to occur throughout the world and in all racial groups. A high incidence occurs in Thailand and elsewhere in the Far East. The range of severity is now recognized to be much broader than defined by the two categories, thalassemia minor and thalassemia major. Furthermore, a number of distinct, though related, biochemical lesions have been described for the different types of the disorder.

PATHOGENESIS. Although there is a disturbance in iron metabolism and heme synthesis in thalassemia, the primary defect is in the *rate of hemoglobin synthesis*. The selective deficiency in the rate of amino acid incorporation was first demonstrated in β chains during their synthesis on polyribosomes obtained from reticulocytes of patients with the common clinical forms of thalassemia major and minor. Synthesis of α, δ, and γ chains was not affected. The gene products, the affected peptides, are *qualitatively normal* and therein are distinct from the hemoglobinopathies; they only are quantitatively deficient (Table 339-1).

When the genetic anomaly depresses only β chain synthesis, the disorder is termed β *thalassemia*. This type comprises over 90 percent of all thalassemia and is expressed in both heterozygous and homozygous forms. Corresponding lesions, selectively depressing synthesis of α chains or δ chains result in α thalassemia and δ thalassemia, respectively. A less common variant of β thalassemia is termed ($\delta\beta$) thalassemia because both δ and β chain synthesis is suppressed but α and γ chain synthesis is not; as a consequence Hb F concentrations are usually considerably elevated. Whether a regulator gene mutation, modulator gene mutation, or other mechanism is concerned in effecting this quantitative disorder of peptide synthesis is not known.

In β *thalassemia*, in *heterozygotes*, the production of δ chains is increased to 0.26 picograms (pg) from a normal of 0.18 pg of δ chains, per δ gene per red corpuscle. This, together with the reduced production of Hb A resulting from deficient synthesis of β chains, produces a characteristic *increase in the proportion of Hb $A_2\delta_2$* (5.11 ± 1.36 percent, as compared with the normal of 2.54 ± 0.35 percent). Hb F is usually normal or only slightly elevated. In the *homozygous* state, there may be nearly complete absence of Hb A, for want of β chains, and the hemoglobin which is present in the hypochromic red corpuscles is mainly Hb F. The Hb F is distributed

in an irregular fashion, from cell to cell, in contrast to the situation in hereditary persistence of Hb F, when its distribution is quite uniform. Hb A_2 is normal in most patients but is elevated in some. The excess of α chains precipitates, in part as inclusion bodies. These may be seen by phase contrast microscopy or after methyl violet vital stain of red corpuscles or normoblasts. The means by which defective peptide synthesis results in leptocytes and target cells, rather than simple microcytosis or morphology exactly like that of iron deficiency anemia, is not understood.

In 5 to 10 percent of persons carrying the thalassemia trait, Hb A_2 levels are normal or low. Most of these are patients with α *thalassemia*, or rarely ($\delta\beta$) or even δ thalassemias. Since α chains are common to Hbs A, A_2, and F, synthesis of all of these hemoglobins is affected. In fetal life, excess of γ chains leads to formation of Bart's Hb (γ_4), and when β chain synthesis begins, the β_4 tetramer, Hb H, forms. The homozygous form of α thalassemia results in intrauterine fetal death or severe hydrops fetalis. Complete absence of α chains has been demonstrated in such cases; essentially only γ_4 tetramers were present as the hemoglobin.

LEPORE HEMOGLOBIN. This is the product of abnormal crossover and fusion of the δ and β genes (Fig. 4-16B) and has an abnormal electrophoretic mobility, similar to that of Hb S. In the heterozygous state it comprises about 9 percent of the hemoglobin, but its presence results in a mild thalassemia-like disorder with the characteristic morphologic alterations of the red corpuscles. Hb A_2 is normal or decreased. In the homozygous state and in individuals doubly heterozygous for both Lepore hemoglobin and thalassemia, the effect on hemoglobin synthesis, and the clinical result, are the same as in thalassemia major or somewhat less severe. In these cases, Hb F is the principal hemoglobin component and Hb$_{Lepore}$ comprises only a small proportion of the total pigment. Hb$_{Lepore}$ seems to be inherited as a single gene, resulting in the synthesis of an abnormal hemoglobin and depression of normal β chain synthesis.

PATHOLOGY. The most significant findings are pronounced medullary and extramedullary myeloid hyperplasia; the effects of such changes on the bones; and deposits of iron-containing pigment in the enlarged spleen, liver, pancreas, and other tissues.

CLINICAL SYNDROMES. Thalassemia Major. Thalassemia major develops insidiously within the first year or two of life, perhaps starting at birth. There is marked pallor and great enlargement of the spleen and even of the liver. The child often has a mongoloid appearance. Roentgenograms reveal great thickening of the diploë of the skull, with perpendicular striation, increase in the medullary portion of the long bones and thinning of the cortex, and other changes attributable to the extreme hyperplasia of the bone marrow. Anemia is severe, hypochromic, and microcytic; the red corpuscles are very thin and contain very little hemoglobin pigment. The peculiar distribution of hemoglobin in the cells gives them the "bull's eye" appearance of targets. Hence the name *target-cell anemia*. The red corpuscles are unusually resistant to hemolysis in hypotonic saline solutions. Normoblasts in the circulation, as well as polychromatophilia, basophilic stippling, Howell-Jolly bodies, and moderate reticulocytosis (19,000 to 25,000 per cu mm) with a "shift to the left," reflects the myeloid hyperactivity of the bone marrow. There is usually slight or moderate hyperbilirubinemia, with a corresponding increase in the urobilinogen content of the urine and stool. Serum iron levels are high. Hemoglobin F values may be elevated, even to a level of 90 percent or more. The concentration of hemoglobin A_2, relative to the total hemoglobin pigment, is within normal limits.

Thalassemia Minor. Thalassemia minor is usually asymptomatic and may pass entirely unnoticed; painstaking examination may be necessary to reveal any abnormality. Slight anemia or splenic enlargement, microcytosis and hypochromia, target cells, poikilocytosis out of proportion to the existent anemia, basophilic stippling of the red corpuscles, decreased fragility in hypotonic saline, and hyperbilirubinemia are some of the signs which, singly or in various combinations, mark this disorder. In other patients, pallor, fatigue, or routine examination of the blood, as during pregnancy, may lead to the discovery of moderate anemia. The volume of packed red corpuscles may be 30 to 35 ml per 100 ml in women and 35 to 40 ml per 100 ml in men. Serum iron levels are normal. In a number of patients, a history may be obtained of protracted, ineffectual treatment with iron, even parenteral iron, because the hypochromic appearance of the red corpuscles has suggested iron deficiency. Roentgenographic changes in the bones similar to those found in thalassemia major, though less pronounced, may be observed.

Thalassemia intermedia is a clinical descriptive term referable to cases which are more severe than thalassemia minor, yet less serious than thalassemia major. It has been used with reference to both homozygous and heterozygous conditions. Some examples are also heterozygous for a qualitatively abnormal hemoglobin.

The term *thalassemia minima* has been applied to instances in which clinical manifestations are very slight. Additional designations and clinical subdivisions have been proposed for other variations of the clinical picture because such a wide range is observed. Little is to be gained from such an extended clinical classification, however. *Microdrepanocytic disease* is the name given to the simultaneous heterozygosity for sickle-cell and thalassemia genes which results in a chronic hemolytic anemia with some of the characteristics of both sickle-cell disease and thalassemia. It is more commonly called *sickle-thalassemia disease* (see above).

DIAGNOSIS. The morphologic features of the red corpuscles are most important. The finding of hypochromic red corpuscles and only a slight reduction of the mean corpuscular hemoglobin concentration (MCHC) together with a greater reduction in the mean corpuscular volume (MCV) than would be estimated by judging from the corpuscular diameters on the blood smear, should suggest the possibility of leptocytosis and, hence, *thalassemia minor*. The other characteristic morphologic features were

mentioned above. The serum iron and marrow iron stores are normal or increased and the total serum iron-binding capacity is normal. These are important points in differentiating this condition from iron deficiency anemia. If the Hb A_2 concentration is increased, as determined by electrophoresis on starch block or starch gel or, less commonly, by chromatography on ion exchange cellulose, there is strong evidence to support the diagnosis of β thalassemia. If the Hb A_2 is not increased, one may be dealing with α, δ, or ($\delta\beta$) thalassemia, or a nonthalassemic disorder. Examination of family members often resolves uncertain cases by demonstrating the hereditary nature of the disorder.

The various forms of congenital hemolytic anemia, as well as plumbism, pyridoxine-responsive anemia, and various acquired forms of "refractory" anemia, must be distinguished from thalassemia. The hemoglobinopathies which may be associated with thalassemia, and the Lepore hemoglobin which may mimic thalassemia, are inherited independently of one another. These may be distinguished from "pure" thalassemia by hemoglobin electrophoresis. The Hb F content should be measured by the alkali denaturation technique or electrophoresis on agar gel. Thalassemia minor and minima have occasionally been confused with polycythemia vera because the erythrocyte count may be greater than normal. However, in thalassemia the hemoglobin concentration and volume of packed red cells are usually slightly below the average normal values because the red corpuscles are microcytic and hypochromic. In polycythemia, if the red corpuscles are hypochromic, the serum iron would be low rather than normal or high as is the case of thalassemia.

The *homozygous* forms of thalassemia rarely present a problem in diagnosis because the physical signs and the blood examination are usually quite characteristic. Both parents of the affected child usually show clear evidence of β thalassemia minor if that is the nature of the abnormality. However, in some instances it may be difficult or impossible to diagnose the α thalassemia heterozygote.

PROGNOSIS. The homozygous form of thalassemia is usually fatal, and those affected do not generally reach adulthood. The prognosis is more grave the earlier the disease becomes manifest. Less severe forms are compatible with longer life. The heterozygous form may have no influence whatever on life span.

TREATMENT. This is the most common form of human hypochromic microcytic anemia which does not respond to iron therapy. In fact, iron stores are often excessive. Hemosiderosis and even hemochromatosis have been described. Treatment with iron, either by the oral or parenteral route, is contraindicated unless iron deficiency, the result of a separate disease process, is specifically shown to be present (see Chap. 336). Multiagent "antianemia preparations," even those sold as "ethical drugs" and available only by prescription, are of no value. In rare instances, when megaloblastic changes occur in the bone marrow as a result of relative folic acid deficiency, 0.1 to 1 mg of folic acid orally, daily, for 1 month, will overcome that component of the anemia and replenish the liver stores of the vitamin. Splenectomy is of no value except where the spleen is cumbersome because of its size or when a superimposed acquired hemolytic anemia develops as the result of repeated transfusions.

REFERENCES

Bank, A., A. S. Braverman, J. V. O'Donnell, and P. A. Marks: Absolute Rates of Globin Chain Synthesis in Thalassemia, Blood, 31:226, 1968.

Beale, D., and H. Lehmann: Abnormal Haemoglobins and the Genetic Code, Nature, 207:259, 1965.

Bonaventura, J., and A. Riggs: Hemoglobin Kansas, a Human Hemoglobin with a Neutral Amino Acid Substitution and an Abnormal Oxygen Equilibrium, J. Biol. Chem., 243:980, 1968.

Comings, D. E., and A. G. Motulsky: Absence of Cis Delta Chain Synthesis in ($\delta\beta$) Thalassemia (F-thalassemia), Blood, 28:54, 1966.

Ingram, V. M.: "The Hemoglobins in Genetics and Evolution," New York, Columbia University Press, 1963.

Ranney, H. M., R. L. Nagel, P. Heller, and L. Udem: Oxygen Equilibrium of Hemoglobin M$_{Hyde\ Park}$, Biochim. Biophys. Acta, 160:112, 1968.

Reed, C. S., R. Hampson, S. Gordon, R. T. Jones, M. J. Novy, B. Brimhall, M. J. Edwards, and R. D. Koler: Erythrocytosis Secondary to Increased Oxygen Affinity of a Mutant Hemoglobin, Hemoglobin Kempsey, Blood, 31:623, 1968.

Wintrobe, M. M.: "Clinical Hematology," 6th ed., Philadelphia, Lea & Febiger, 1967.

Zuckerkandl, E.: The Evolution of Hemoglobin, Sci. Am., 212:110, 1965.

340 ANEMIA ASSOCIATED WITH CHRONIC SYSTEMIC DISEASE

G. R. Lee and M. M. Wintrobe

Anemia is found commonly in association with a wide variety of chronic diseases. These include long-standing infections; noninfectious inflammatory diseases, such as rheumatoid arthritis; malignancies; renal insufficiency; hepatic disease; and certain endocrine-deficiency states. The anemias of infection, rheumatoid arthritis, and cancer appear to be related in that they are accompanied by a characteristic disturbance of iron metabolism manifested by hypoferremia and reticuloendothelial siderosis.

In this chapter, the use of the term *anemia of chronic disorders* will be confined to those situations in which this disturbance of iron metabolism occurs regularly. While it is recognized that this terminology is not entirely satisfactory, as yet no alternative has found general acceptance. The anemias of renal insufficiency, hepatic disease, and endocrine deficiency are not characteristically accompanied by hypoferremia. The anemia of renal disease will be discussed below. The anemias of hepatic disease and endocrine deficiency have been considered in Chap. 61.

ANEMIA OF CHRONIC DISORDERS

CLINICAL DESCRIPTION. Anemia associated with hypoferremia and reticuloendothelial siderosis has been found in almost any inflammatory illness which lasts several months or longer. Examples are subacute bacterial endocarditis, tuberculosis, empyema, chronic fungal infections, lung abscess, pyelonephritis, rheumatoid arthritis, rheumatic fever, and other collagen diseases. This type of anemia may also occur in malignant disorders, including Hodgkin's disease, leukemia, and carcinoma of the lung, but it must be distinguished from the "myelophthisic" type of anemia that occurs with extensive bone marrow invasion (see below).

In most clinical circumstances, the anemia of chronic disorders becomes established during the first 2 months of illness and thereafter does not progress unless the underlying disease becomes worse. The anemia tends to be mild to moderate in severity; rarely is the blood hemoglobin concentration found to be less than 9 Gm per 100 ml. There is a rough correlation between the degree of anemia and the severity of the underlying disease. For example, in one study of patients with rheumatoid arthritis the mean blood hemoglobin concentration was 13.2 Gm per 100 ml in females with "slightly active" disease and 11.3 and 9.6 Gm per 100 ml in males and females, respectively, with "very active" disease. This moderate degree of slowly developing anemia rarely produces significant symptoms.

The erythrocytes are usually normocytic and normochromic; occasionally they are hypochromic, and only rarely are they both hypochromic and microcytic. In other respects, the red cells are morphologically normal, with little variation in size and shape and with no polychromatophilia or stippling.

Kinetic studies indicate that the anemia results from an inability of the bone marrow to compensate for a mild to moderate decrease in erythrocyte life span. These kinetic alterations are subtle, and significant deviations from normal in the reticulocyte count, serum bilirubin, or stool or urine urobilinogen are uncommon.

When studies of iron metabolism are performed, the serum iron is found to be reduced and the total serum iron-binding capacity is normal or reduced. Reticuloendothelial iron stores are increased and sideroblast iron is decreased. The free erythrocyte protoporphyrin is increased.

PATHOGENESIS. Cross-transfusion studies indicate that the shortened erythrocyte life span is due to an extracorpuscular mechanism rather than to a defect in the red cell itself, but the nature of the extracorpuscular factor or factors is unknown. The failure of the bone marrow to increase red cell production to a level sufficient to compensate for the increased destruction is not well understood. The cellularity of the marrow is normal or increased; furthermore, it can respond to erythropoietin and to measures which stimulate erythropoietin production, such as hypoxia, hemorrhage, and cobalt administration. These observations suggest that, for reasons unknown, the production of erythropoietin in the anemia of chronic disorders is not as great as would normally be expected with the given degree of anemia.

The designation *thesauric hypoferremic anemia* epitomizes the paradoxical association of hypoferremia with increased iron stores, phenomena which suggest that a barrier exists to the normal flow of iron from reticuloendothelial cells to plasma. Studies of hemoglobin or red cell iron "reutilization" with labeled iron have supported this suggestion. Neither the nature of the barrier nor the way in which it is produced is known.

TREATMENT. Therapeutic measures should be directed at the underlying chronic illness. The anemia will subside spontaneously if such measures are successful. None of the usual forms of antianemia therapy, such as vitamin B_{12} or iron, is effective. Cobalt chloride has been shown to stimulate red cell production in this type of anemia and to cause the volume of packed cells to increase. However, cobalt therapy is not recommended, since no particular benefits accrue to the patient from the increased number of red cells, and also because the gastrointestinal toxicity of cobalt may be significant. Sometimes, if anemia becomes severe (hemoglobin less than 7 Gm per 100 ml), blood transfusions may be necessary, but these should be used sparingly.

ANEMIA IN MALIGNANT DISEASE

Malignant disease is not necessarily accompanied by anemia. When it is, a number of etiologic factors must be considered. In carcinoma involving the gastrointestinal tract, *blood loss* is the most common cause of anemia. Depending on the amount lost and the duration of the process, the anemia may be that of acute blood loss (Chap. 335) or of iron deficiency (Chap. 336). In other malignancies, including the lymphomas, leukemias, and metastatic carcinomas, the *anemia of chronic disorders* (see above) may be observed.

Hodgkin's disease, multiple myeloma, and carcinoma of the kidneys, breast, prostate, thyroid and lungs, in particular, may invade the bone marrow, and in such an event, *myelophthisic anemia* may develop. This type of anemia is usually accompanied by alterations in leukocytes and platelets. Thus, there may be pancytopenia (Chap. 341), or a leukemoid picture, marked by leukocytosis and myeloid immaturity, may result. Sometimes these changes are accompanied by the appearance of nucleated red cells in the circulation; the term *leukoerythroblastic anemia* appropriately describes such an association. Morphologic alterations in the erythrocytes may be extreme, and wide variations in shape and size are common. In addition, polychromatophilia, coarse stippling, and a modest reticulocytosis may be observed. The last is thought to result from the premature release of reticulocytes from marrow ("shift" reticulocytosis) rather than from an increase in production of red cells.

Therapeutic measures should be directed at the underlying disease. When palliative therapy with radiation or chemotherapeutic agents is effective, partial relief of the anemia may be observed. On the other hand, adverse effects of therapy may lead to an increase in the degree of anemia. Thus, serial determinations of the volume of packed red cells, in conjunction with other hematologic measures and evidence of tumor activity, serve as useful guides to management.

ANEMIA OF RENAL INSUFFICIENCY

Anemia is found in association with uremia regardless of the nature of the underlying renal disease. In some cases, the symptoms of anemia constitute the patient's presenting complaints. A crude correlation exists between the degree of anemia and the degree of renal insufficiency. It has been observed that, on the average, the blood hemoglobin concentration decreases 1.8 Gm per 100 ml for each increase of 50 mg per 100 ml in the blood urea nitrogen. However, there are wide individual variations around this mean value. Increases in the blood urea nitrogen beyond 250 mg are accompanied by no further increase in the severity of the anemia.

Like the anemia of chronic disorders, the anemia of renal insufficiency is characterized kinetically by a shortened red cell survival and a subnormal marrow response. Two kinetic patterns have been described that differ from one another according to which of these abnormalities predominates. The more common pattern is that found in the *hypoproliferative anemia* of renal disease in which reduced red cell production predominates. The less common *hemolytic anemia* of renal disease is more severe and is characterized by a markedly shortened red cell life span.

The hypoproliferative anemia of renal disease is classified morphologically as normocytic and normochromic. Morphologic changes in erythrocytes on blood smear are minor, and the reticulocyte count is normal. In the hemolytic anemia of renal disease, there may be macrocytosis, reticulocytosis, polychromatophilia, stippling, anisocytosis, poikilocytosis, and the appearance of normoblasts in the circulation. Particularly characteristic is the presence of so-called "burr cells"—distorted or fragmented red cells with peripheral, sharp projections. The occurrence of such cells may be related to disease of the small blood vessels (*microangiopathic hemolytic anemia*). They are also seen, for example, in thrombotic thrombocytopenic purpura (Chap. 345).

The pathogenesis of the anemia of renal disease has been discussed elsewhere (Chap. 61).

As in the anemia of chronic disorders, cobalt administration may induce reticulocytosis, but the disadvantages of such therapy outweigh the benefits. Therapy should be directed at the underlying renal disease, and in those few situations in which adequate renal function can be reestablished the anemia will be relieved. In patients treated with long-term dialysis (Chap. 301), increased erythropoiesis has been observed as the patient's general condition has improved.

REFERENCES

Adamson, J. W., J. Eschbach, and C. A. Finch: The Kidney and Erythropoiesis, Am. J. Med., 44:725, 1968.

Cartwright, G. E.: The Anemia of Chronic Disorders, Seminars in Hematology, 3:351, 1966.

341 BONE MARROW FAILURE

M. M. Wintrobe and T. C. Bithell

Some degree of bone marrow insufficiency or failure is present in many varieties of anemia, not only in those which result from infection and chronic systemic disease (Chap. 340) or disseminated cancer, but also in those which are associated with deficiency of essential substance (vitamin B_{12}, folic acid) (Chaps. 336 and 337), abnormalities of heme or globin synthesis (the sideroblastic anemias, Chap. 336, the hemoglobinopathies, Chap. 339), and even accelerated destruction of erythrocytes (the hemolytic disorders, Chap. 338). However, the term is generally used more specifically to refer to those disorders, to be discussed in this chapter (Tables 341-1), in which marrow failure is the primary pathogenetic feature and is not the result of the aforementioned processes. In these disorders, the marrow is unable to produce sufficient cells to replace those normally utilized, and usually there is a reduction in the number of erythrocytes, platelets, and leukocytes (*pancytopenia*). In most cases, the precursor cells in the marrow also are reduced in number (*marrow hypoplasia or aplasia*), fat having replaced the blood-forming tissue. However, the morphologic appearance of the marrow may not correlate well with its functional capacity, and pancytopenia may sometimes be associated with a normally cellular or even a hypercellular marrow. As a consequence, the term *aplastic anemia*, traditionally used with reference to disorders characterized by a hypoplastic bone marrow, is applied here in a functional sense and includes all forms of primary bone marrow failure associated with pancytopenia, irrespective of the morphologic appearance of the marrow. The term *pure red cell aplasia* refers to cases in which only the red corpuscles and their precursors are affected, the white cells, platelets, and their marrow precursors being normal.

APLASTIC ANEMIA

ETIOLOGY AND PATHOGENESIS. In approximately half of the cases of aplastic anemia, no etiologic agent is apparent. Such "idiopathic cases" are most common in adolescents or young adults, and their pathogenesis is obscure. The rare Fanconi syndrome appears in young children and is associated with chromosomal aberrations, being inherited as an autosomal recessive trait in many cases.

Another large category is comprised of cases associated with exposure to various *chemical agents or to ionizing irradiation*. These agents may be divided into two groups (Table 341-1): namely, (1) those which regularly produce marrow hypoplasia or aplasia if a sufficient dose is given (*the myelosuppressive agents*); and (2) those which are only occasionally associated with such a change, i.e., which presumably depend on *idiosyncracy*. Agents in the first category have been or are used in the chemotherapy of leukemia, the lymphomas, and other tumors. Aplasia or hypoplasia of the marrow represents a predictable pharmacologic effect which generally depends on the dose of such agents administered. However, the bone marrow findings and the extent to which the three blood elements are affected vary considerably, and the pancytopenia and acellular marrow of classical aplastic anemia in some instances may be only the ultimate result of a series of stepwise changes. Benzene, for example, not only may produce aplastic anemia but also can be associated with a "regenerative" blood picture including even a leukemoid reaction, and the bone marrow may be hyperplastic rather than acellular. Likewise, internal irradiation produced by the ingestion of radium by radium-dial painters was associated with macrocytic anemia, nucleated red cells in the peripheral blood, and marrow hyperplasia. Both irradiation and benzene may produce chromosomal abnormalities, and both have been implicated in the production of leukemia.

Even less clearly understood are cases of aplastic anemia which are associated with the administration of usually innocuous drugs. The evidence that these drugs are etiologic is only circumstantial, since aplastic anemia has been observed only in a small proportion of those exposed, e.g., 1 of 25,000 individuals given quinacrin (Atabrine). However, in the case of those drugs with definite toxic potentiality (Table 341-1), a sufficient number of cases has been reported to make it seem very likely that the development of aplastic anemia was caused by exposure to the drug. Of particular note is *chloramphenicol*. Although the incidence of aplastic anemia in association with this antibiotic is very low in terms of its widespread use, this drug has so frequently been associated with this dyscrasia that there is little doubt of its etiologic role. Aplastic anemia associated with those drugs listed as probably toxic is even less common. However, even the most widely used and innocuous of drugs, such as aspirin, streptomycin, and tripelennamine, may be associated with serious bone marrow failure in rare susceptible individuals.

The mechanism by which these drugs produce aplastic anemia is obscure. Marrow aplasia is unrelated to a pharmacologic effect of the drug and is usually not dose-related, often developing after prolonged or intermittent administration of small doses and even long after the drug has been stopped. Reticulocytopenia, vacuolization of bone marrow normoblasts, and mild pancytopenia have been demonstrated in many patients receiving chloramphenicol. However, aplastic anemia has not developed in such individuals, and these findings may represent reversible suppression of bone marrow function unrelated to the pathogenesis of aplastic anemia. Most of the evidence favors the hypothesis that drug-induced aplastic anemia represents an idiosyncratic reaction in susceptible individuals, but attempts to demonstrate hypersensitivity in the sense of an antigen-antibody reaction have not been successful. It has been suggested that this idiosyncracy may reside in an intrinsic, possibly hereditary abnormality in the precursor cells of the marrow, such as an enzyme deficiency, analogous to that which conditions certain drug-induced hemolytic anemias

Table 341-1. APLASTIC OR HYPOPLASTIC ANEMIAS

Disorders Characterized by Primary Bone Marrow Failure

I. Aplastic anemia
  A. "Idiopathic"
  B. The Fanconi syndrome
  C. In association with chemical or physical agents
    1. Agents which predictably produce marrow hypoplasia
      a. Ionizing irradiation (x-rays, radioactive isotopes)
      b. Benzene and derivatives (toluene, TNT)
      c. Cytostatic agents (alkylating and antimitotic agents, antimetabolites)
      d. Other toxic agents (inorganic arsenic)
    2. Drugs which occasionally produce marrow hypoplasia as an idiosyncratic effect
      a. Of "definite" toxic potentiality; chloramphenicol, phenylbutazone, mephenytoin (Mesantoin), gold compounds, quinacrin (Atabrine), organic arsenicals, potassium perchlorate
      b. Of "probable" toxic potentiality; trimethadione, tolbutamide, carbutamide, diphenylhydantoin (Dilantin), sulfamethoxypyridizine (Kynex), acetazolamide (Diamox), sulfisoxazole (Gantrisin), insecticides [gamma benzene hexachloride, chlordane, chlorphenothane (DDT)]
II. "Pure" red cell hypoplasia
  A. "Idiopathic"
  B. Congenital (the Blackfan-Diamond syndrome)
  C. In association with tumors of the thymus
  D. Drugs
  E. Transient "aregenerative crises" in infections and hemolytic disorders

(Chap. 338). As yet there is little experimental evidence to support this concept.

In most cases, *pure red cell aplasia* appears to be idiopathic. A congenital form has been described in infants (the *Blackfan-Diamond syndrome*), and drugs such as chloramphenicol and diphenylhydantoin may produce a similar picture. Erythroid hypoplasia also may develop transiently during the course of various infections and hemolytic disorders (*aregenerative "crisis," acute erythroblastopenia*) and for longer in association with tumors of the thymus. There is indirect evidence to suggest that pure red cell aplasia is the result of an autoimmune process in some cases, but in the majority the pathogenesis is obscure.

CLINICAL MANIFESTATIONS. As a rule, the onset of aplastic anemia is insidious. The symptoms are attributable to anemia, or the effects of thrombocytopenia or of neutropenia may dominate the clinical picture. Progressive weakness, fatigability, and a "waxy" pallor are commonly seen. Mild purpura is usually the first bleeding manifestation and frequently is an early sign, but hemorrhage from the nose, gums, vagina, gastrointestinal tract, or into the retina may occur. Infection is common later in the course of the disorder. Indolent ulcerations in the mouth or pharynx, around the nose, rectum, or vagina are common, as are recurrent systemic infections.

Patients with aplastic anemia may carry on without serious trouble for months with very low leukocyte and platelet counts, but complications eventually develop, and in some cases serious bleeding or fulminant infection may appear suddenly, e.g., subarachnoid hemorrhage or septicemia. Such complications may suggest an explosive onset of the disease. Weight loss is unusual, and there is no sternal tenderness, hepatomegaly, or splenomegaly. Fever and lymphadenopathy, if present, are usually the result of infection.

After many transfusions, hemosiderosis (Chap. 342) develops, and then the spleen may become just palpable and the liver moderately enlarged. Bronzing of the skin may produce a misleading "healthy" picture, but examination of the nail beds and mucous membranes will reveal the true picture.

Fanconi's syndrome usually develops in the first decade of life, but in contrast to congenital pure red cell aplasia, is uncommon in neonates. This disorder is associated with a variety of congenital defects (bone abnormalities, particularly of the forearms and thumbs, microcephaly, hypogenitalism, genitourinary tract abnormalities) and a generalized olive-brown pigmentation of the skin.

LABORATORY DIAGNOSIS. The *peripheral blood* usually reveals pancytopenia with absolute neutropenia, the majority of the leukocytes being normal lymphocytes. The anemia usually is normocytic, sometimes macrocytic; the red cells vary little in size and shape, and polychromatophilia, basophilic stippling, and other evidences of accelerated red cell production are absent. The reticulocyte count is very low or zero. In pure red cell aplasia, however, these signs of red cell production sometimes may be seen.

Bone marrow examination is essential and can be done safely in spite of the thrombocytopenia and neutropenia if careful aseptic technique is used and if gentle pressure is maintained over the puncture site. In classical aplastic anemia, the marrow aspirate is composed mainly of erythrocytes and lymphocytes. In cases in which the marrow is not hypoplastic, various abnormalities may be seen, including megaloblastic changes in the erythroid precursors and a picture suggesting "arrest of maturation" of the granulocyte precursors. Immature granulocytes (myeloblasts, promyelocytes) are usually normal in number. Stainable iron is abundant, but "ringed" sideroblasts are not seen.

A dry tap should not lead to the assumption that the marrow is aplastic. Puncture at another site may yield marrow, and it is well to obtain an adequate specimen by means of biopsy with the Jensen needle or by open trephine biopsy.

Tests of *blood coagulation* usually are normal, but the bleeding time is prolonged, the tourniquet test positive, and clot retraction impaired as a result of thrombocytopenia. Although moderate shortening of the red cell life span may be demonstrated by *isotopic techniques*, this is of little significance, and other evidence of accelerated red cell destruction, such as indirect bilirubinemia or elevated fecal urobilinogen, is lacking. Ferrokinetic studies will reveal slow plasma iron turnover and poor tracer iron utilization for hemoglobin synthesis, but such measurements may be difficult to interpret and are not needed to establish a diagnosis. The *serum iron* usually is elevated and the total *iron binding capacity* is moderately reduced. The *fetal hemoglobin* may be elevated.

DIFFERENTIAL DIAGNOSIS. The diagnosis of aplastic anemia should be one of exclusion, for pancytopenia alone is not indicative of bone marrow failure. The causes of pancytopenia are many (Table 341-2), and appropriate steps must be taken to rule them out. Early acute myeloblastic leukemia (Chap. 348), disseminated tuberculosis (Chap. 174), and paroxysmal nocturnal hemoglobinuria (PNH) (Chap. 338), in particular, may simulate bone marrow failure, and the last may actually represent a stage of or be a sequel to aplastic anemia. The presence of nucleated red cells or polychromatophilia in the blood smear, immature leukocytes, or large morphologically abnormal platelets suggest "myeloproliferative" or myelophthisic disease (Chap. 340) rather than aplastic anemia.

Table 341-2. CAUSES OF PANCYTOPENIA

I. The hypoplastic or aplastic anemias (Table 341-1)
II. "Aleukemic," leukopenic, or subleukemic leukemia (Chap. 348)
III. Myelophthisic "anemias" (Chap. 340)
    A. Metastatic carcinoma in bone marrow
    B. Multiple myeloma, other dysproteinemias (Chap. 349)
    C. Myelofibrosis
    D. Osteopetrosis (Marble bone disease)
IV. Disorders involving the spleen—"hypersplenism"
    A. Lymphomas (Chap. 351)
    B. Congestive splenomegaly (Chap. 350)
    C. Infiltrative (Gaucher's disease, Niemann-Pick disease, Letterer-Siwe disease, Chap. 350)
    D. Infections (kala azar, miliary tuberculosis, syphilis)
    E. Of unknown etiology [Sarcoidosis (Chap. 254), "primary" hypersplenism (Chap. 350)]
V. Disorders due to deficiency of essential substances (pernicious anemia and other megaloblastic macrocytic anemias, Chap. 337)
VI. Paroxysmal nocturnal hemoglobinuria (rarely) (Chap. 338)

SOURCE: Adapted from M. M. Wintrobe, "Clinical Hematology," 6th ed., Philadelphia, Lea & Febiger, 1967.

The presence of splenomegaly, sternal tenderness, hyperglobulinemia, or lymphadenopathy should arouse suspicion that one is not dealing with aplastic anemia. In multiple myeloma and the other dysproteinemias, metastatic carcinoma, Gaucher's disease, and acute leukemia, the diagnosis may often be made by a careful examination of the bone marrow. If an enlarged lymph node is accessible, it may be advisable to examine it microscopically. Numerous other studies may be required in the search for the underlying disorder, e.g., roentgenograms of the bones and chest, serum protein electrophoresis, and PNH test.

The diagnosis of idiopathic aplastic anemia requires that exposure to chemicals be excluded. This is difficult, due to the prevalence of potentially toxic substances in the environment, and the physician must maintain an unusually high "index of suspicion" regarding chemical exposure, e.g., benzene in industry; solvents, insecticides, and hair dyes in the home; and various medications, including presumably innocuous drugs.

When there is pure red cell aplasia, one must avoid overlooking a causative chronic infection, systemic disease, or drug. Thymomas are rare, usually asymptomatic, and may be demonstrable radiologically. In some cases of the Blackfan-Diamond syndrome, splenic and hepatic enlargement and even generalized lymphadenopathy have been described.

TREATMENT. The mainstays in the treatment of aplastic anemia are good general supportive care, the judicious use of transfusions, steroid therapy, and in certain circumstances, splenectomy.

Supportive care is aimed at the removal of possible etiologic factors and the prevention and treatment of the complications of pancytopenia. Exposure to potentially toxic agents should be absolutely eliminated, even if the evidence is only circumstantial, which is usually the case. Antibiotics should not be used prophylactically when there is neutropenia, since this will favor the emergence of resistant bacteria and fungi and more will be lost than gained. It is better to be alert to the development of an infection and to identify the causative organisms, thus permitting specific therapy. Intramuscular and subcutaneous injections should be avoided if possible, and when performed, should be carried out with careful antisepsis. Mouth hygeine is very important, and wounds and abrasions of the mucous membranes and skin should be guarded against. "Reverse isolation" should be employed when patients with severe neutropenia are hospitalized.

Blood transfusions should be held to a minimum, since they may be required for many years. Hemosiderosis will develop ultimately, and sensitization to minor blood groups, leukocytes, and platelets may occur. These patients tolerate hemoglobin levels of 9 Gm per 100 ml and even lower levels quite satisfactorily. Blood selected for transfusion should be as type-specific and as fresh as possible. Platelet concentrates are valuable in the treatment of life-threatening hemorrhage.

Among the numerous agents which have been used to stimulate marrow function, only adrenocorticosteroids and androgenic hormones deserve mention. Hematinics such as vitamin B_{12}, folic acid, iron, and crude liver extract are valueless in the treatment of aplastic anemia. Cobalt is usually ineffective, and bone marrow transplantation still is in the experimental stage. A combination of corticosteroids (prednisone, 20 to 40 mg daily) and androgenic hormones (testosterone enanthate, 50 to 600 mg in sesame oil given intramuscularly every week to once in 3 weeks, oxymetholone, 2 to 4 mg/kg/day, or methyltestosterone linguets, 1 to 2 mg/kg/day) generally is more effective and in children has less propensity to produce side effects than either hormone alone. In many cases this regimen will result in a significant improvement in marrow function, and rarely, may be curative. However, the response is usually slow and therapy must often be continued for many months. Corticosteroids alone usually are disappointing, but may decrease transfusion requirements in some patients. Steroid therapy appears to be most effective in children; good results have been obtained in the Fanconi syndrome and in congenital red cell aplasia, but treatment usually must be maintained indefinitely.

Splenectomy may be of significant benefit in a few carefully selected patients with aplastic anemia. These include patients in whom there is evidence of accelerated destruction of red cells by the spleen (a "regenerative" blood picture, decreased survival of ^{51}Cr-labeled erythrocytes with splenic "sequestration" of labeled cells, splenomegaly), patients with unusually high transfusion requirements, and those with long-standing aplastic anemia and evidence of persisting marrow function. Splenectomy is seldom of value in the Fanconi syndrome or in congenital red cell aplasia and is rarely curative in the other forms, but it often will decrease transfusion requirements, and may reduce the dose of steroids required to maintain the patient. In red cell aplasia associated with thymomas, removal of the tumor is indicated but is without effect in many cases.

PROGNOSIS. Death usually results from infection or hemorrhage. Spontaneous remission may occur in about 20 percent of patients with congenital red cell aplasia and in a few cases due to toxic agents where the cause has been recognized and further exposure eliminated. About 50 percent of patients live a year or more, and approximately 25 percent live 3 years or more.

REFERENCES

Bithell, T. C., and M. M. Wintrobe: Drug-induced aplastic anemia, Seminars in Hematology IV: 194, 1967.

Diamond, L. K., and N. T. Shahidi: Treatment of aplastic anemia in children, Seminars in Hematology IV:278, 1967.

Loeb, V., Jr., C. V. Moore, and R. Dubach: The Physiologic Evaluation and Management of Chronic Bone Marrow Failure, Am. J. Med., 15:499, 1953.

Scott, J. L., G. E. Cartwright, and M. M. Wintrobe: Acquired Aplastic Anemia: An Analysis of Thirty-Nine Cases and Review of the Pertinent Literature, Medicine, 38:119, 1959.

342 BLOOD TRANSFUSION AND TRANSFUSION REACTIONS

M. M. Wintrobe and J. Foerster

INDICATIONS FOR BLOOD TRANSFUSION

FOR THE RESTORATION OF BLOOD VOLUME. By far the most important and most frequent indication for the use of *whole blood transfusions* is the restoration of an adequate blood volume after hemorrhage, trauma, or burns.

The extent to which blood may be lost when hemorrhage occurs within a viscus or a muscle mass frequently is underestimated. Likewise, it is not easy to judge the degree of plasma loss or red cell hemolysis after a severe burn. Arterial hypotension, when present, is indicative of massive blood loss, perhaps exceeding 30 percent of the patient's total blood volume, although this sign may be absent initially because of compensating vasoconstriction. Under such circumstances other signs of peripheral circulatory failure, such as cold, clammy skin, reduction in pulse pressure, tachycardia, and reduced urinary output, offer valuable clues. Because acute blood loss leads to proportionately reduced plasma and red cell volumes, measurements of hemoglobin concentration taken shortly after the bleeding episode do not reflect the extent of blood loss, as the development of "anemia" depends on the eventual restoration of the plasma volume. Indeed, hemoconcentration may initially be thought to be present in patients suffering from severe burns because of their inordinate plasma depletion. Nevertheless, red cell loss usually is sufficiently extensive to make whole blood transfusion, rather than plasma replacement, the initial therapy of choice. Direct measurements of intravascular red cell and plasma volumes by radioisotope or dye dilution techniques may be helpful if the many variables which affect these measurements are given adequate consideration.

MANAGEMENT OF ANEMIA. In the management of anemia other than that due to the acute loss of blood, transfusions are commonly used more frequently than is necessary or desirable. The discovery of such anemia calls for careful study to determine its cause, rather than the automatic administration of blood. Thus, there is no justification for blood transfusion in iron-deficiency anemias or in the macrocytic anemias with megaloblastic bone marrow unless the anemia is extremely severe or emergency surgical measures must be carried out. The patient who has such an anemia has become adjusted to it, and the sudden increase in intravascular volume produced by transfusion may indeed precipitate serious complications such as acute cardiac failure. A predictable and safe response can usually be achieved by correcting the deficiency responsible for the anemia. Again, in anemia associated with infection or in the management of the anemia of leukemia, Hodgkin's disease, or other disorders, the treatment of the underlying condition, whenever possible, is preferable to blood transfusion. Even in the management of aplastic anemia or other forms of anemia for which no specific therapy is available, *it is better to give only enough transfusions to maintain the hemoglobin at a level consistent with reasonable activity.* Thereby the risks accompanying transfusion therapy are reduced, and the accumulation of iron in the tissues is minimized. Such patients often are maintained quite satisfactorily at hematocrit levels of 30 to 35 ml per 100 ml blood, or even less. Patients with anemia due to chronic renal disease do best at hematocrit levels of 25 to 30 percent; at lower levels renal blood flow usually is decreased sufficiently to further increase nitrogen retention.

In patients suffering from acute acquired hemolytic anemias, and particularly when these are mediated by antibodies, transfusion must be approached with caution, since the transfused cells may be destroyed as readily as those of the recipient. In addition, serum antibodies make cross matching more difficult and thereby increase the hazards of isoimmunization. Consequently, it is wise to defer transfusion in the hope that the patient may reach a balance between red cell destruction and formation. Blood transfusions are better reserved for situations where the anemia is developing rapidly or where the danger of death or serious ill effects from shock is greater than the potential hazards of transfusion. In the more chronic forms of hemolytic anemia, where the hemolytic process has reached a state of equilibrium, transfusion therapy usually offers little for the patient.

BLOOD COMPONENT THERAPY. Whole blood transfusions, plasma, or plasma fractions can provide *specific clotting factors* which may be lacking in certain patients, such as the antihemophilic factors (VIII, IX), prothrombin, factors V and VII, and fibrinogen (Chaps. 62 and 346). Fresh normal plasma is capable of restoring all clotting factors, and its use is mandatory for supplying the labile clotting factors V and VIII. Stored plasma is an adequate source of prothrombin, factors VII, IX, X, and fibrinogen.

When indicated, whole blood, plasma, or albumin can be used to *restore the colloid osmotic pressure* of plasma to physiologic levels in some cases of hypoproteinemia. Thus, intravenous injections of salt-poor human serum albumin sometimes are valuable in certain patients with hepatic cirrhosis, the nephrotic syndrome, idiopathic hypoproteinemia, and the edema of malnutrition.

The use of isolated cellular components is rapidly increasing in popularity. The administration of *packed red blood cells* finds particularly wide application in situations where an increased red cell mass is the sole aim of therapy and has the advantage of reduced volume, which is of considerable importance in patients with limited cardiac reserve. In addition, the amount of transfused sodium and citrate is greatly reduced. The removal of the buffy layer from such cellular preparations has the added advantage of decreasing the incidence of febrile and other more serious reactions due to leukocyte isosensitization.

The use of *platelet transfusions* is of some value in the treatment of patients with thrombocytopenia due to aplastic anemia, leukemia, or chemotherapy, and the procedure may indeed be lifesaving. The platelets have to be isolated from freshly drawn blood and are administered in the form of acid concentrates or platelet-rich plasma. Isoimmunization usually develops only after transfusion of large numbers of platelets over extended periods of time. Approximately 30 percent of the injected platelets have been found in the circulation 1 hr after transfusion, but the yield is smaller in patients with fever or infection. The half-life of transfused platelets is approximately 36 to 48 hr, thus making frequent transfusions necessary.

Transfusions of *white blood cells* from normal donors or from patients with chronic myelocytic leukemia have been employed, perhaps with some success, in attempts to control infections in leukopenic patients. However, only 5 to 10 percent of transfused granulocytes can be recovered in the circulation, and their life span is very abbreviated. In addition, the large number of cells required for effective therapy makes widespread use of granulocyte transfusions impractical at this time.

EXCHANGE TRANSFUSION. The removal of blood possessing pathogenic properties and its replacement with normal blood constitute valuable procedures under special circumstances, most notably in certain cases of erythroblastosis fetalis (Chap. 338).

USE OF BLOOD SUBSTITUTES. Although the transfusion of whole blood is usually the best and most direct approach to the restoration of a depleted blood volume, blood substitutes must sometimes be employed in emergencies. Of these, plasma is the best, and in the dry form it can be transported easily and kept ready at hand, but the danger of transmitting the virus of homologous serum hepatitis is so great that the use of pooled plasma cannot be recommended. Next in order of effectiveness is serum albumin, which has a physiologic effect closely approaching that of plasma. However, it is very expensive. For this and other reasons, much attention has been given to the development of "plasma expanders," substances of such physicochemical properties that they will overcome the disparity between the capacity of the circulatory system and the circulating blood volume that exists in shock. Of these, the gelatins possess the fewest theoretical disadvantages, but dextran, a biosynthetic polysaccharide, has been found to be more practical and very effective. Normal saline solution administered in adequate quantities also appears to be an adequate temporary plasma expander. It should be borne in mind that plasma expanders should be employed only for acute emergencies and are not intended for chronic use.

RISKS INHERENT IN BLOOD TRANSFUSION

Risks inherent in transfusion therapy may be classified under several categories: (1) febrile and allergic reactions; (2) complications caused by overloading of the circulation; (3) reactions due to incompatibility; (4) risks, other than circulatory, associated with massive transfusions; and (5) miscellaneous ill effects, such as the transmission of infections, especially serum hepatitis, thrombophlebitis, air and fat embolism, and transfusion siderosis.

(1) *Simple febrile reactions* are observed in a considerable number of patients. A chill and subsequent fever usually occur within an hour after the transfusion, although the reaction may occasionally be delayed for as long as 24 hr. Headache, nausea, and vomiting may occur, but in most cases the reaction is mild and short-lived. Improperly prepared diluting fluids, soluble toxic substances derived from tubing, and small amounts of bacterial protein are among the causes of such febrile reactions. With improvements in transfusion technology

there have been fewer reactions. The reaction rate increases with the number of previous transfusions. Occasionally patients develop cold antibodies and react with a chill if the blood is given without warming.

Table 342-1. TRANSFUSION REACTIONS

Type	Cause	Incidence, %
Pyrogenic......	Bacterial pyrogens	1.8–2.9
Febrile.........	Leukoagglutinins	
Urticarial.......	Sensitivity (?)	0.8–1.1
Serum sickness..	Unknown	Rare
Hemolytic......	Mismatching of blood	0.1–0.5
Isosensitization..	Repeated transfusions and in pregnancy	Not rare
Circulatory overload	Injudicious augmentation of blood volume	Not rare
Infectious......	Grossly contaminated blood	Rare
Transmission of disease	Homologous serum jaundice, syphilis, malaria	0.45–1.0
Air embolism...	Entry of air into vein via tubing	Rare
"Cold reaction".	Cold agglutinins (?)	Not rare
Hypocalcemia...	Exchange transfusions	Not rare
Hemorrhagic diathesis	Massive transfusions, etc.	Rare (?)
Fat embolism...	Transfusion via bone marrow	Rare
Plasma sensitivity	Heat-labile plasma factor	In paroxysmal nocturnal hemoglobinuria

Allergic reactions, characterized simply by urticaria or occasionally by swelling of lymph nodes, sore throat, joint pains, fever and eosinophilia, occur in at least 1 percent of cases. They may develop some days after the transfusion. Angioneurotic edema and asthma also have been observed. These reactions sometimes are due to transfer of reagins to which the patient is sensitive. Such a transfer is less likely to occur if blood is drawn from donors who have fasted for several hours.

Patients with multiple transfusions usually develop leukocyte isoantibodies. The reactions mediated by these antibodies bear a striking resemblance to those caused by bacterial pyrogens and are sometimes severe and even life-threatening. Complete leukoagglutinins are found in a majority of patients who experience chills and a rise in temperature in connection with blood transfusions, but only in very few patients without these symptoms. The administration of buffy coat–poor blood usually prevents or minimizes these reactions.

(2) The administration of excessively large quantities of blood, or smaller amounts given rapidly, can cause circulatory failure, particularly in patients with preexisting heart disease. Symptoms of failure usually develop between 1 and 24 hr after transfusion, and death may result from pulmonary edema. Sudden overloading of the cardiovascular system can be minimized by the use of packed red cells and by the slow administration of blood. In patients with cardiac failure, the rate of infusion should not exceed 1 ml blood/lb body weight/hr and should often be slower than this. Only when there has been acute and severe hemorrhage does blood need to be given quickly. Measurement of the patient's venous pressure before transfusion provides a useful guide to the probability of inducing cardiac failure, which is likely if the pretransfusion venous pressure is above normal. Continuous central venous pressure monitoring is a useful aid, as it gives the earliest possible warning of a dangerous increase in venous pressure.

(3) The administration of incompatible blood is usually associated with the early and abrupt onset of symptoms such as chills and fever. If the transfusion is stopped immediately, no serious harm may result. Other manifestations include restlessness, anxiety, flushing of the face, precordial oppression and pain, an increase in pulse and respiratory rate, generalized tingling sensations, and pain in the back and thighs. Nausea and vomiting may follow and may be accompanied by signs of peripheral circulatory failure, including cold, clammy skin, a failing pulse, severe hypotension, and cyanosis. Acute renal failure frequently is associated with prolonged shock. Occasionally a hemorrhagic diathesis develops secondary to intravascular coagulation, which in turn is triggered by the release of thromboplastic substances from lysed red cells. The mortality rate of hemolytic transfusion reactions approaches 50 percent.

Human error resulting in the administration of ABO incompatible blood is the chief cause of transfusion reactions due to blood group incompatibility. Occasionally, the presence of weak A_2 or A_2B agglutinogens in the donor's blood has caused errors in typing. Sometimes a "universal" group O donor has extraordinarily high titers of anti-A and anti-B agglutinins, which may lead to lysis of the recipient's own red cells. The weak subgroups of A, such as A_x, may also be associated with hemolytic transfusion reactions.

Of the various components of the Rh-Hr system, anti-D (anti-Rh_0 is by far the most common antibody causing reactions, and anti-D plus anti-C (anti-Rh_1) is another frequent cause. Anti-c (anti-hr'), anti-E (anti-rh″) and anti-D plus anti-E (anti-Rh_2) are not rare, but other antibodies involving this system are found in less than 1 percent of cases.

(4) Reactions associated with massive blood transfusions include hyperkalemia (Chap. 296) due to leakage of potassium from red cells during storage and citrate toxicity related to the infusion of massive quantities of anticoagulants derived from multiple transfusions. In addition, a hemorrhagic diathesis frequently develops, presumably due to the replacement of the patient's blood by old blood lacking platelets and labile clotting factors.

(5) Miscellaneous ill effects of transfusions. Infections such as syphilis, malaria, and hepatitis are sometimes transmitted by transfusion. In addition, the blood may become infected during handling and storage. Thrombophlebitis may present a serious problem, particularly with prolonged intravenous placement of polyethylene

tubing. Air embolism occasionally results when blood is administered under pressure. Hemosiderosis closely resembling hemochromatosis (Chap. 107) follows the administration of large numbers of transfusions.

PRECAUTIONS IN BLOOD TRANSFUSION. In view of the many hazards inherent in the transfusion of blood, it is a good general principle to err on the side of giving too few rather than too many transfusions. In most situations this is but a palliative form of therapy, although sometimes a necessary and valuable one. However, as stated earlier, when dealing with hemorrhagic or traumatic shock, it is better to give more rather than less blood than is thought to be needed.

Except in an emergency, it is always wise to give the first 50 ml of blood slowly and under the scrutiny of a doctor or nurse. In addition, it is well, whenever possible, to wait at least 15 min in order to determine whether a reaction will occur. Fatal transfusion reactions have occurred only when more than 300 ml of blood was given. It is unwise to use blood for transfusion which has been brought to room temperature, cooled, and then rewarmed, since the likelihood of an infectious reaction is thereby increased.

DIAGNOSIS OF TRANSFUSION REACTIONS. The cardinal signs and symptoms of transfusion reactions have been discussed above. It should be stressed, however, that in patients under anesthesia, the only signs of a serious reaction may be increasing tachycardia, shock, and bleeding.

Group A, B, or AB incompatibility produces intravascular hemolysis, whereas Rh, Lewis, Kell, and Duffy incompatibilities usually cause extravascular hemolysis only. Under these circumstances, there may be no detectable hemoglobinemia or hemoglobinuria, although indirect hyperbilirubinemia will eventually develop. With intravascular hemolysis the plasma becomes pink, red, or dark red, and hemoglobinuria will occur, depending on the amount of blood destroyed. Leukopenia and thrombocytopenia may also be seen, as well as a deficiency of

Table 342-2. ABNORMALITIES TO BE LOOKED FOR IN SUSPECTED HEMOLYTIC TRANSFUSION REACTION

1. Free hemoglobin in plasma. Visible if >50 mg/100 ml. Should be present immediately.
2. Bilirubinemia. Increase of more than 0.5 mg over pretransfusion value. Maximal in 3 to 6 hr.
3. Hemoglobinuria (if plasma Hb >150 mg/ml). Urine may be red or black.
4. Methemalbuminemia (Schumm's test). Present after 6 to 48 hr.
5. Reduced haptoglobin levels; especially useful in mild reactions.
6. Agglutination of red cells from donor bag by serum of patient's blood *drawn before start of transfusion* (not the serum so labeled in the blood bank).
7. Bacteria in smear of donor blood, if contaminated.

SOURCE: M. M. Wintrobe, "Clinical Hematology," 6th ed., Philadelphia, Lea & Febiger, 1967.

N.B. All blood samples to be drawn with extreme care to avoid hemolysis.

fibrinogen, prothrombin, and labile clotting factors. Increased levels of fibrinolysins are sometimes detected.

Laboratory tests which should be carried out in the investigation of a suspected case of hemolytic transfusion reaction (Table 342-2) include the examination of the blood and urine of the patient for hemoglobinemia, bilirubinemia, and urinary pigments, and a rigorous serologic review of recipient and donor bloods, including reexamination of a pretransfusion sample of the patient's blood, the pilot tube of the blood that was cross matched for the recipient, and the blood which was actually given. Saline, serum, and antiglobulin typing and matching tests should be carried out on the collected blood specimens, and the blood and urine of the recipient should be reexamined repeatedly for the late appearance of signs of increased blood destruction and for the appearance of antibodies which may not be detectable at first. The blood and urine should be watched closely to detect developing azotemia. The administered blood should also be examined for bacteria, which should include a search for anaerobic organisms and cold saprophytes, in addition to the examination for routine organisms.

A detailed discussion of the therapy of transfusion reactions is to be found in the references listed below. The treatment of acute renal failure, the most serious consequence of a hemolytic transfusion reaction, is discussed elsewhere (Chap. 300).

REFERENCES

Mollison, P. L.: "Blood Transfusion in Clinical Medicine," 4th ed., Philadelphia, F. A. Davis Company, 1967.

Wintrobe, M. M.: "Clinical Hematology," 6th ed., Philadelphia, Lea & Febiger, 1967.

343 ERYTHREMIA (POLYCYTHEMIA RUBRA VERA)

M. M. Wintrobe and Arthur Haut

DEFINITION. Erythremia, also known as Vaquez's or Osler's disease or splenomegalic polycythemia, is a disease of unknown cause, insidious onset, and slow, chronic course. It is characterized by a striking absolute increase in the quantity of circulating red corpuscles and, often, by evidence of increased production of myeloid leukocytes and even of platelets. Splenomegaly and a red "cyanosis" of the skin, as well as increase in the viscosity of the blood and in the total volume of the blood, are additional features of this disorder.

HISTORY. Vaquez in 1892 described a case of polycythemia which he had originally attributed to congenital heart disease. Osler gave a more complete description in 1903.

ETIOLOGY AND PATHOGENESIS. In an earlier chapter (Chap. 33) various forms of polycythemia were discussed. The disease erythremia differs from other forms of polycythemia in that none of the circumstances or disorders known to be associated regularly, or even occasionally, with polycythemia can be found; significant oxygen unsaturation of the blood is lacking, and in most cases splenomegaly, leukocytosis due to an increased number of granulocytes, and other signs suggesting myeloid hyperplasia, including thrombocytosis, are present. These features suggest a close relationship to the various so-called "myeloproliferative" disorders, especially chronic myelocytic leukemia. In erythremia, as distinct from hypoxic poylcythemias, the urinary erythropoietin excretion has been found to be clearly less than normal, possibly due to a shut-off of erythropoietin output. It rises to normal values when the volume of packed red cells is reduced to normal limits by venesections.

Most commonly, erythremia appears in middle or later life. In very rare instances, polycythemia of unknown cause has been seen in children; equally rarely, it appears as a familial disorder. Such cases have not been characterized by signs of generalized myeloid hyperplasia and are probably unrelated to the classical disorder described by Vaquez and by Osler. The incidence of the disease is high in Jews and low in Negroes. Men are somewhat more often affected than women.

PATHOLOGY AND PATHOLOGIC PHYSIOLOGY. The striking pathologic changes are those related to the increase in total blood volume. All the organs are engorged with blood, the veins stand out like "bunches of thick worms," and there may be thromboses or anemic infarcts. The bone marrow is dark red and very cellular. Microscopically, this is found in most instances to be due to hyperplasia of all the marrow elements. In some patients the percentage of normoblasts is increased, in others the proportions of myelocytes and myeloblasts or of basophilic and eosinophilic cells may be greater than normal.

The spleen is enlarged, chiefly from hyperplasia of the pulp and distension with blood. Infarcts are common. There may be foci of extramedullary blood formation in the spleen, the liver, and occasionally elsewhere as well. Cirrhosis of the liver has been observed in a number of instances.

The relative quantity of red cells per unit of blood causes a great increase in blood viscosity, and this, probably, is responsible for many of the clinical manifestations. Although cardiac output and work, pulmonary functions, and the arterial saturation of the blood are normal, the circulatory minute volume is reduced, and the velocity of blood flow is greatly lowered. The resulting visceral stasis, together with the thrombocytosis, may explain the high incidence of intravascular thrombosis seen in this disorder. The existence of a hemostatic defect has been postulated mainly because of the excessive bleeding which may be associated with minor injuries or at operations. This can be explained in part by the physical distension of the vascular bed. Decreased platelet factor 3 activity and excessive friability of the blood clot have been reported.

SYMPTOMATOLOGY. The onset is insidious and the progress gradual. Headache, dizziness, ringing in the ears, or visual disturbances; dyspnea, lassitude, or weakness; skin or mucous membrane hemorrhages; pruritis,

especially after a hot shower or bath; a sense of weight in the abdomen because of the enlarged spleen; or irritability, depression, forgetfulness, or vague symptoms suggesting neurasthenia are complaints encountered in many patients. Various gastrointestinal symptoms, such as fullness, belching, or constipation, may be present, or symptoms of peptic ulcer may be found. Sometimes the symptoms are those attributable to increased metabolism: lassitude, increased sweating, and loss of weight. Swelling and pain in the extremities may be very troublesome. In still other patients the symptoms are so insignificant that the polycythemia is discovered only accidentally.

The face is a deep red rather than truly cyanotic. The color is most noticeable in the lips, cheeks, tip of the nose, ears, and neck. The distal portions of the extremities may be more truly cyanotic, since the highly viscous blood circulates more sluggishly there than is normal. Ecchymoses are common, and epistaxis and bleeding of the gums are frequently encountered. Cardiac abnormality is unusual, but vascular disturbances, including venous thromboses, coronary thrombosis, and cerebrovascular accidents, are common. The blood pressure is more often normal than elevated. Enlargement of the liver is frequent, and splenomegaly is found in at least 75 percent of cases. The spleen may be just palpable, or it may extend even to the pelvic brim.

Blood. The volume of packed red cells may be 55 to 83 ml per 100 ml whole blood. Unless hemorrhage has occurred or venesections have been performed, there is a corresponding increase in hemoglobin concentration. The numbers of erythrocytes, which may reach 7 to 10 million cells per cu mm, may be increased out of proportion to the volume of packed red corpuscles if iron reserves are limited or frank iron deficiency is present. The volume of packed white cells and platelets, i.e., the buffy coat which is seen on carefully examining the hematocrit, is also increased and may be from 1.5 to several ml per 100 ml blood, signifying the presence of leukocytosis, thrombocytosis, or both. On the blood smear, the individual red corpuscles appear normal, although occasional polychromatophilia or basophilic stippling may be noted. The finding of nucleated red corpuscles and the appearance of small numbers of myelocytes and even earlier forms in the blood give a clue to the hyperplastic state of the bone marrow; leukocytosis, occasionally of marked degree (60,000 leukocytes per cu mm), due to an increase of the granulocytes, and high platelet counts, which are often present, give further evidence of overactivity. Basophilic and eosinophilic leukocytes are more numerous than normal. The percentage of reticulocytes is not increased unless there has been recent bleeding. Leukocyte alkaline phosphatase is generally high, therein distinguishing erythremia from erythrocytosis and chronic myelocytic leukemia, but it may be normal, and only rarely has it been found to be low. The osmotic fragility of the red corpuscles is not significantly altered. There may be some evidence of increased blood destruction in the form of slight bilirubinemia and increased excretion of urobilinogen. The viscosity of the blood is greatly increased, even five- to tenfold. The thick, sticky blood may be slow to coagulate, and the clot may not retract. However, bleeding and clotting times are usually normal.

The total blood volume is substantially increased (150 to 300 percent of normal). This may be attributed to the increase in red corpuscle mass, but it does not entirely reflect the full magnitude of the latter, since the plasma volume is most often decreased, particularly in cases with the greater volume of packed red cells.

Other Laboratory Findings. These include increased basal metabolic rate in many instances; normal, increased, or reduced gastric secretion, even achlorhydria; occasionally, increased serum uric acid level and, sometimes, increased endogenous uric acid excretion; and normal urine or slight proteinuria. Blood histamine is increased in proportion to the number of circulating basophils. Erythrocyte glutamic oxalacetic transaminase, glucose 6-phosphate dehydrogenase, and hexokinase have been found to be increased, suggesting that the mean red corpuscle age is less than normal. In untreated erythremia, the plasma iron turnover often is greater than normal due to a shortening of the half time for plasma iron disappearance. This ferrokinetic feature, sometimes considered to be a differentiating point between erythremia and erythrocytosis, can be attributed to depleted iron stores and can be changed toward normal by iron repletion. A regularly occurring chromosomal anomaly has not been seen in erythremia, although aneuploidy, translocations, and deletions have been found; the last, in some cases, perhaps are the result of antecedent treatment with radioactive phosphorus.

DIAGNOSIS. The symptoms in erythremia may suggest a variety of disorders, but once the blood has been examined, the problem is to differentiate secondary forms of polycythemia (*erythrocytosis*) from the "primary" disorder (*erythremia*). The discovery of an increased volume of packed white corpuscles and platelets in the hematocrit tube, in addition to the increased volume of packed red corpuscles, and the absence of a bluish cyanosis and hypoxemia immediately favor the diagnosis of erythremia. Splenomegaly is very unusual in erythrocytosis, even when the erythrocyte count is very much increased. In erythrocytosis one rarely finds persistent neutrophilic leukocytosis, immature granulocytes, basophilia, eosinophilia, thrombocytosis, or an increase in the neutrophil alkaline phosphatase. Normoblasts are much more common in the blood in erythremia than in erythrocytosis, but in the latter, hypoxemia may lead to their appearance in the circulation.

Finding an increase in the volume of packed red corpuscles, the hemoglobin concentration, or the erythrocyte count, does not of itself allow one to conclude that there is an increase in the total body red corpuscle mass. Those findings could also result from a decrease in the body plasma volume without alteration in the red corpuscle mass, a situation termed *relative polycythemia*. Such instances are most often recognized by the associated clinical circumstances which have resulted in a reduction in plasma volume, e.g., fulminant diarrhea, protracted vomiting, extensive burns of the body surface, and other situations resulting in extraordinary fluid losses and dehydration. Some patients with persistent, unexplained elevation of values for the concentration of erythrocytes in the blood are found to have a normal red corpuscle mass on measurement of their blood volume. Such instances, often occurring in a heavily built, middle-aged, and sometimes hypertensive male, have been termed *stress erythrocytosis*. The term *Gaisbock's syndrome* sometimes is used in referring to patients with hypertension and polycythemia without splenomegaly, but it is confusing and misleading and should not be used.

Measurement of the red corpuscle mass differentiates relative polycythemia from absolute polycythemia, but it does not distinguish the absolute forms from one another, since an increased red corpuscle mass occurs both in erythremia and erythrocytosis (secondary polycythemia).

The blood volume and red corpuscle mass may be readily determined by using, for example, the dilution principle and injecting a measured small volume of the patient's own red corpuscles tagged with radioactive chromium (^{51}Cr). Predicted values for healthy persons, based on studies of 201 men and 101 women, are given in the Appendix. Height, weight, and body surface area are recognized as having bearing on the predicted values. The influence of age, lean body mass, and muscularity, though important, is less well understood. For some patients, especially those with the less common body proportions, the base of reference is important in evaluating the measured red corpuscle mass. Calculation of the red corpuscle mass per unit of body weight, per unit of body surface area, or per unit of lean body mass, sometimes results in different interpretations regarding the normality or abnormality of the value obtained. One should be aware of this possibility and not place too much reliance on the measured red corpuscle mass alone but rather give consideration to all of the clinical and laboratory findings. In equivocal cases, it is better to make additional observations at a later date in order to establish a sounder foundation before making a diagnosis.

Measurement of arterial oxygen saturation is useful in differentiating erythrocytosis due to cardiac or pulmonary disease, for in the latter, oxygen saturation is altered more or less in inverse proportion to the degree of polycythemia, whereas in erythremia it is normal or nearly normal. Other clinical features and laboratory procedures helpful in differentiating various forms of cyanosis and polycythemia are discussed elsewhere (Chaps. 33, 339 and 344). Attention should also be given to other possible causes of erythrocytosis: renal carcinoma, adenoma, cysts, hydronephrosis; cerebellar hemangioblastoma; adrenocortical carcinoma or hyperplasia, pheochromocytoma; ovarian carcinoma, uterine fibroids; hepatoma; familial erythrocytosis; or increased oxygen affinity (p. 1623). Not to be overlooked are patients with erythremia who present with anemia due to evident or occult blood loss. Careful attention to leukocyte, platelet, and erythrocyte morphology on the blood smear, measurement of the neutrophil alkaline phosphatase, and sometimes even resort to bone marrow biopsy will avoid confusion between "anemic erythremia" and myelofibrosis or chronic myelocytic leukemia. A normal serum vitamin B_{12} concentration and absence of the Ph^1 chromosome, would further diminish the likelihood of leukemia.

Unfortunately, some patients do not present all the classical features of erythremia, and since many are advanced in years, cardiac or pulmonary disease may be present as well. In approximately 20 percent of cases leukocyte and platelet counts are within normal limits, and in about 25 percent of patients the spleen is not palpable. The finding of papilledema or of another abdominal mass may be helpful, but even the demonstration of a renal lesion does not in itself prove that it is the cause of the polycythemia. In some cases great judgment is needed in making the differentiation. One must be patient in equivocal cases; for example, those without leukocyte or platelet increases and without apparent cause. Additional observations after there has been some opportunity for evolution of the disease may resolve the question of whether or not a given instance represents true erythremia.

COURSE AND COMPLICATIONS. Barring the development of serious complications, the course of erythremia, adequately treated, is chronic, and the disorder is often compatible with many years of life. The median duration is over 14 years from onset. The standard deviation is more than 6½ years, and thus, the survival of patients clearly varies widely. The most dangerous complications are vascular: thrombosis or hemorrhage. Therapy, by keeping the red corpuscle mass at a nearly normal level, can effectively reduce blood viscosity, and thus, serves to reduce the likelihood of such vascular accidents. Intercurrent infections, especially of the respiratory tract, may be troublesome, and bronchitis and emphysema may develop. Peptic ulcer and hypertension are frequent complications; less often, gout and cirrhosis of the liver occur. The development of typical chronic myelocytic leukemia in a number of cases of erythremia has given support to the view that there may be a close relationship between these two disorders. Acute leukemia occurs in about 10 percent of cases treated with radioactive phosphorus. This fact does not necessarily connote a bad result from such therapy, as the median survival of erythremia patients dying with acute leukemia is not less than that of patients treated with radiation but not developing leukemia, and it is superior to that of patients treated with some modality other than radiation. Concerning the occurrence of leukemia, the relative importance of the cumulative dose of the radioisotope, the duration of erythremia in a given patient, and the inherent predisposition toward acute leukemia in those patients, is still unclear.

TREATMENT. Treatment is symptomatic, since the cause of erythremia is unknown. When the diagnosis is not clear, it is best not to embark on treatment with radioisotopes or chemotherapy, although these are appropriate for the overt cases, as detailed below; venesections may be prescribed if these make the patient feel better, but it must be realized that they may compromise the value of subsequent diagnostic efforts by measurement of the blood volume.

In established cases of erythremia, symptomatic relief is best achieved by reducing the red corpuscle mass to something approaching normal. This is most quickly accomplished by *venesection*. Approximately a pint of blood is removed twice a week or even more often, care being taken to assure normal hydration so that the plasma volume may be expanded promptly. The procedure is repeated until the volume of packed red corpuscles approaches normal. Then the procedure may need to be repeated only once a month or less often. In emergency situations, multiple phlebotomies can be performed in a shorter time by returning the patient's own plasma to him after each venesection, thus rapidly reducing blood viscosity without the hazards of reduced systemic blood flow which result from acute, substantial reductions in blood volume.

Once the volume of packed red corpuscles has been reduced to normal values by venesections, recurrence of polycythemia can eventually be prevented by induction of iron deficiency if repeated phlebotomies become necessary. Erythropoiesis can also be inhibited by irradiation or by chemotherapy. The effects of irradiation are slow to appear, however. The intravenous injection of *radioactive phosphorus* (^{32}P) is more satisfactory than roentgen therapy. Although ^{32}P may be incorporated in bone, placing this agent in a strategic position, its biologic effect probably results from its incorporation into DNA and ATP, where the effect of radiation at close range and the conversion of radioactive ^{32}P into stable ^{32}S by radioactive decay may critically affect molecular reactions. Three to 5 mc ^{32}P is given at first. After 10 to 12 weeks, if symptomatic and hematologic improvement are inadequate, a second, usually smaller dose is administered. Sometimes another venesection or two may be needed. Subsequent therapy is "titrated" according to need, but intervals between injections should not be shorter than 10 weeks, and leukocyte and platelet counts should be included in the blood examinations as guides in avoiding marrow hypoplasia from overdosage. Remissions of 6 to 10 months are common, but much longer ones are not unusual. By combining the use of venesections and the conservative use of ^{32}P, the danger of the patient's developing leukemia may be minimized.

Although agents such as chlorambucil and busulfan have been shown to be effective in the treatment of erythremia, they require more frequent examinations of the patient's blood than is the case with radioactive phosphorus. Furthermore, alkylating agents are mutagenic and can produce chromosomal derangement. It remains to be seen whether their long-term use will result in a lower rate of occurrence of acute leukemia than is now the case, or whether survival will be equivalent to that achieved with radioactive phosphorus.

REFERENCES

Abilgaard, C. F., J. Cornet, and I. Schulman: Primary Erythrocytosis, J. Pediat., 63:1072, 1963.

Lawrence, J. H., N. I. Berlin, and R. L. Huff: The Nature and Treatment of Polycythemia, Medicine, 32:323, 1953; Am. J. Med. Sci., 233:268, 1957.

Modan, B., and A. M. Lilienfeld: Polycythemia Vera and Leukemia—The Role of Radiation Treatment, Medicine (Balt.), 44:305, 1965.

Osgood, E. E.: Polycythemia Vera: Age Relationships and Survival, Blood, 26:243, 1965.

Wintrobe, M. M.: "Clinical Hematology," 6th ed., Philadelphia, Lea & Febiger, 1967.

344 METHEMOGLOBINEMIA AND SULFHEMOGLOBINEMIA

George E. Cartwright

METHEMOGLOBINEMIA

The iron in the hemoglobin molecule is normally in the reduced or ferrous state (Fe^{++}), whether bound to oxygen or carbon dioxide or unbound. When reduced hemoglobin is oxidized, the iron is converted to the ferric state (Fe^{3+}) and methemoglobin is formed.

$$2HbFe^{++} + H_2O_2 \rightleftharpoons 2HbFe^{3+} OH$$

Methemoglobin is formed continuously in the erythrocyte and exists in equilibrium with reduced hemoglobin. Normally about 99 percent of the hemoglobin is in the reduced state and only 1 percent is oxidized. Since methemoglobin is incapable of binding oxygen or carbon dioxide, erythrocytes must of necessity possess mechanisms for maintaining hemoglobin in the reduced state. These mechanisms require energy and, therefore, are dependent on the metabolism of glucose.

The first mechanism employs reduced nicotinamide adenine dinucleotide ($NADH_2$) ("DPNH"), formed from the oxidation of glucose, as the electron donor. Methemoglobin is reduced by $NADH_2$ in the presence of the $NADH_2$-dependent enzyme, methemoglobin reductase (diaphorase enzyme) (MR-E).

$$1/2 \text{ glucose} + NAD \rightarrow \text{pyruvate} + NADH_2$$

$$NADH_2 + HbFe^{3+} \xrightarrow{\text{MR-E}} NAD + HbFe^{++}$$

A second mechanism for reducing hemoglobin is provided by the generation of reduced nicotinamide adenine dinucleotide phosphate ($NADPH_2$) ("TPNH"). When glucose 6-phosphate (G-6-P) is metabolized to 6-phosphogluconate (6-PG) by glucose 6-phosphate dehydrogenase (G-6-PD) in the first step in the pentose-phosphate pathway, $NADPH_2$ is produced. Methemoglobin is then reduced by the $NADPH_2$-dependent enzyme methemoglobin reductase (MR-E) in the presence of a cofactor (CoF). Methylene blue can substitute for the cofactor in the electron transfer system, and the activity of this pathway is enhanced greatly by the addition of methylene blue (MB).

$$G-6-P + NADP \xrightarrow{\text{G-6-PD}} 6-PG + NADPH_2$$

$$NADPH_2 + HbFe^{3+} \xrightarrow[\text{CoF or MB}]{\text{MR-E}} NADP + HbFe^{++}$$

A third mechanism for maintaining hemoglobin in the reduced state is through the glutathione pathway. $NADPH_2$ in the presence of glutathione reductase (GR), reduces oxidized glutathione (GSSG) to reduced glutathione (GSH). Reduced glutathione, in the presence of glutathione peroxidase (GP), is capable of destroying oxidant compounds such as hydrogen peroxide (H_2O_2) which have the capability of oxidizing hemoglobin.

$$NADPH_2 + GSSG \xrightarrow{\text{GR}} NADP + GSH$$

$$GSH + H_2O_2 \xrightarrow{\text{GP}} GSSG + H_2O$$

Under physiologic conditions, it is the $NADH_2$-dependent pathway which plays the major part in methemoglobin reduction. When the cells are exposed to excess oxidant compounds, the $NADPH_2$-dependent pathway, the glutathione pathway, and catalase, in addition to the $NADH_2$-dependent pathway, all play a significant part in regulating the levels of methemoglobin in erythrocytes.

ETIOLOGY. The known causes of methemoglobinemia are listed in Table 344-1. Methemoglobinemia may be either inherited or acquired.

Hereditary methemoglobinemia due to a deficiency of the $NADH_2$-dependent methemoglobin reductase enzyme (diaphorase) is transmitted as an autosomal recessive trait. Individuals heterozygous for the trait have about half the normal level of the diaphorase enzyme and are asymptomatic; 98 to 99 percent of the hemoglobin is in the reduced state. Individuals homozygous for the trait are completely lacking in the erythrocyte enzyme and are cyanotic from birth; 5 to 60 percent of the hemoglobin is present as methemoglobin. The rate at which methemoglobin is reduced is greatly impaired. The disease is manifest at birth, and life expectancy is probably not affected adversely in most cases. Mental retardation and other manifestations of central-nervous-system involvement have been observed in some patients. Whether this is coincidental or related to the disease has not been established.

Several families with methemoglobinemia have been described in which the disease appeared to be inherited as an autosomal dominant and in which no abnormality could be detected in the hemoglobin molecule. The biochemical lesion in these families has not been defined. Patients with a hereditary deficiency of erythrocyte $NADPH_2$-dependent methemoglobin reductase and with a "deficiency" of erythrocyte glutathione have been described, but in neither of these conditions has methemoglobinemia been found.

Hereditary methemoglobinemia associated with an abnormal hemoglobin (HbM) is transmitted as an autosomal dominant trait. At least 12 different M hemoglobins have been described. Those which have been fully characterized are listed in Table 344-1. In these diseases, the formation of methemoglobin is due to decreased oxygen affinity or binding capacity, as discussed earlier (Chap. 339), not to a slow rate of methemoglobin reduction. The hemoglobin Ms with an α chain anomaly are associated with cyanosis, which is present at birth. The

Table 344-1. CAUSES OF METHEMOGLOBINEMIA

I. Hereditary
   A. Enzymatic
      1. NADH$_2$-methemoglobin reductase deficiency (recessive)
      2. ? Others
   B. Hemoglobin M disease (dominant)
      1. HbM$_{Boston}$ ($\alpha_2{}^{58\ tyr}\beta_2$)
      2. HbM$_{Iwate}$* ($\alpha_2{}^{87\ tyr}\beta_2$)
      3. HbM$_{Milwaukee-1}$ ($\alpha_2\beta_2{}^{67\ glu}$)
      4. HbM$_{Hyde\ Park}$ ($\alpha_2\beta_2{}^{92\ tyr}$)
      5. HbM$_{Saskatoon}$† ($\alpha_2\beta_2{}^{63\ tyr}$)
      6. HbM$_{Freiburg}$ ($\alpha_2\beta_2{}^{23\ val\rightarrow0}$)

II. Acquired
   A. Nitrites
   B. Nitrates
   C. Chlorates
   D. Quinones
   E. Aminobenzenes
   F. Nitrobenzenes
   G. Nitrotoluenes

* Identical to HbM$_{Kankakee}$
† Identical to HbM$_{Emory,\ Kurume,\ and\ Chicago}$

patients are otherwise asymptomatic and life expectancy is not impaired. In patients with a β chain anomaly, cyanosis is absent at birth; it does not appear until HbF disappears; and it is frequently accompanied by a mild hemolytic anemia and splenomegaly.

Acquired (secondary) methemoglobinemia is more common than hereditary methemoglobinemia and is caused by contact with certain drugs and chemicals (Table 344-1). These agents preferentially oxidize hemoglobin and, in sufficient amounts, overcome the normal reducing mechanism of the *erythrocytes.* When exposure to the offending drug ceases, the methemoglobin is rapidly converted to the reduced compound and the cyanosis disappears.

Nitrates after ingestion may be converted to nitrites by intestinal bacteria, and after absorption from the intestine they produce methemoglobin. Cases of methemoglobinemia due to nitrates or nitrites have been reported following the use of bismuth subnitrates or of ammonia or potassium nitrate, from the therapeutic use of amyl nitrite or nitroglycerin, from food high in nitrates, in infants drinking well water high in nitrates, from the inhalation of nitrous gases by arc welders, and from corning syrup. Aniline dyes may produce methemoglobinemia by penetration of the intact skin. Contact with dyed blankets, laundry marks on diapers, and freshly dyed shoes has produced methemoglobinemia. The ingestion by children of certain red wax crayons containing *p*-nitroaniline has resulted in methemoglobinemia. The commonly dispensed analgesic and antipyretic drugs, acetanilid and phenacetin, are aniline derivatives and have frequently been found responsible for methemoglobinemia. Certain sulfonamides, such as sulfanilamide, Prontosil, sulfathiazole, and sulfapyridine, but not sulfadiazine or sulfamerazine, produce the condition.

Enterogenous cyanosis is a term used to refer to a clinical syndrome now rarely mentioned, which was characterized by attacks of cyanosis, headache, abdominal pain with either diarrhea or constipation, dyspnea, dizziness, collapse, and syncope. It was thought that the gastrointestinal disease caused abnormal production and absorption of nitrites. In the blood of these individuals, sulfhemoglobinemia was present frequently, together with methemoglobinemia. Since many of these patients were taking aniline derivatives for headache, there appears to be no need for differentiating these cases from other examples of acquired methemoglobinemia and sulfhemoglobinemia.

CLINICAL MANIFESTATIONS. When as little as 1.5 Gm methemoglobin is present in 100 ml blood, recognizable cyanosis results. In contrast, as discussed earlier (Chap. 33), about 5 Gm reduced hemoglobin must be present before a comparable degree of cyanosis occurs. Since methemoglobin is incapable of combining with oxygen, the symptoms of methemoglobinemia are attributable to the hypoxia produced by the lowered oxygen capacity of the blood. The severity of the symptoms is related to the quantity of methemoglobin present, the rapidity with which the methemoglobinemia develops, and the capacity of the individual's cardiorespiratory and hematopoietic systems to adjust to the hypoxia. In general, levels of less than 20 percent methemoglobin are usually not associated with symptoms. At levels of 20 to 50 percent, fatigue, weakness, dyspnea, tachycardia, headaches, and dizziness may occur. Only rarely is enough methemoglobin present to cause coma and death.

DIAGNOSIS. Methemoglobinemia should be suspected in any patient with cyanosis, particularly if physical examination fails to reveal evidence of cardiovascular or pulmonary disease and if the cyanosis is not promptly relieved by oxygen therapy. If blood withdrawn from the vein shows the characteristic chocolate-brown coloration, the diagnosis of an abnormal pigment is almost certain, especially if the color remains after shaking the blood in air.

A family history of cyanosis suggests the hereditary form of the disease; a recent history of exposure to drugs or chemicals suggests the acquired form. The inherited forms which are due to enzymic causes can be differentiated only by specific and elaborate techniques. The diagnosis of the hemoglobin M disorders can be established by starch block electrophoresis (pH 7.0 to 7.2) of hemolysates and by spectrophotometric absorption analysis.

Methemoglobin (other than M hemoglobins) may be differentiated from sulfhemoglobin by examining a 1:10 or 1:100 aqueous dilution of blood in a hand spectroscope. The absorption band of methemoglobin (630 mμ) may be confused with that of sulfhemoglobin (618 mμ), but on the addition of 2 or 3 drops of 5 percent potassium cyanide the band due to methemoglobin disappears, whereas the sulfhemoglobin band is unchanged. The addition of hydrogen peroxide causes dissolution of the sulfhemoglobin band, but not of the methemoglobin band.

TREATMENT. It is not necessary to treat most patients with *hereditary* methemoglobinemia. However, therapy may be required in the severe cases or in the milder cases for the relief of minor symptoms or for cosmetic purposes. The reducing agent ascorbic acid may be given daily by mouth in an amount of 100 to 500 mg. Methylene blue accelerates the reduction of methemoglobin and is effective in a daily dose of 100 to 300 mg by mouth. These agents are of no value in alleviating the cyanosis due to hemoglobin M.

In most patients with mild *drug-induced* methemoglobinemia no therapy is necessary other than removal of the offending agent, since the methemoglobin is reduced rapidly as a result of the intact normal reconversion mechanism. In those patients in whom therapy is necessary, methylene blue, 1 to 2 mg per kg body weight given intravenously over a 5-min period in a 1 percent solution, is the agent of choice. If cyanosis has not disappeared within an hour, a second dose of 2 mg per kg body weight should be given. The total dose should not exceed 7 mg per kg, since toxic effects such as dyspnea, precordial pain, restlessness, apprehension, a sense of oppression, and fibrillar tremors may occur.

SULFHEMOGLOBINEMIA

Sulfhemoglobin is a hemoglobin derivative of unknown composition which is not found in erythrocytes under normal circumstances. Once it has formed it cannot be converted to hemoglobin. The abnormal derivative remains in the erythrocytes until they are destroyed.

Sulfhemoglobinemia may result when one of the oxidizing drugs listed in Table 344-1 has been taken. Phenacetin (A.P.C., Empirin Compound, Stanback) and acetanilid (Bromo Seltzer) are the drugs found most frequently to be the causative agents. Constipation is present in at least half the patients.

Sulfhemoglobin is inert as an oxygen carrier, and when it is present intense cyanosis results. Somewhat less than 0.5 Gm sulfhemoglobin per 100 ml blood causes a degree of cyanosis equal to that of 1.5 Gm methemoglobin or 5 Gm reduced hemoglobin. Although the concentration of sulfhemoglobin may be found to be as high as 10 Gm per 100 ml, the life of the patient is not endangered and symptoms which can be attributed to the sulfhemoglobinemia are rarely present. Since many of the patients in whom sulfhemoglobinemia develops are neurotic or are taking drugs for a chronic headache or constipation, the symptoms which can be elicited are probably not attributable to the sulfhemoglobinemia. Symptoms of bromide intoxication frequently complicate the clinical picture in those ingesting Bromo Seltzer. Once formed, there is no way of removing the sulfhemoglobin except by phlebotomy. In time the affected red corpuscles wear out and are destroyed. Treatment requires interdiction of the offending drug and correction of the intestinal conditions associated with the disorder.

Rare cases of acquired hemolytic anemia with paroxysmal sulfhemoglobinemia and methemoglobinemia have been reported, and there is one reported instance of congenital sulfhemoglobinemia.

REFERENCES

Beutler, E.: "Hereditary Disorders of Erythrocyte Metabolism," New York, Grune and Stratton, Inc., 1968.

Finch, C. A.: Methemoglobinemia and Sulfhemoglobinemia, New Engl. J. Med. 239:470, 1948.

Jaffé, E. R., and P. Heller: Methemoglobinemia in Man, Progr. Hematol., 4:48, 1964.

Scott, E. M.: The Relation of Diaphorase of Human Erythrocytes to Inheritance of Methemoglobinemia, J. Clin. Invest. 39:1176, 1960.

Shibata, S., T. Miyaji, I. Iuchi, Y. Ohba, and K. Yamamoto: Hemoglobin M's of the Japanese, Bull. Yamaguchi Med. Sch. 14:141, 1967.

345   THE PURPURAS
T. C. Bithell and M. M. Wintrobe

The term *purpura* refers to extravasations of blood into the skin or mucous membranes. Purpura is but one manifestation of abnormal bleeding (Chap. 62) and is characteristic of the numerous disorders of the vascular and platelet phases of hemostasis. These disorders may conveniently be divided into those characterized by a significant reduction in the number of platelets (thrombocytopenic purpuras, Table 345-1) and the nonthrombocytopenic varieties (Table 345-2) in which the platelets are normal in number, bleeding being the result either of qualitative abnormalities of platelet function or of vascular disorders.

Thrombocytopenia is the most common cause of purpura. It may be produced by various chemical or physical agents, or may accompany certain infections or a variety of systemic disorders ("symptomatic thrombocytopenic purpura"). In many cases, thrombocytopenia is idiopathic; i.e., no etiologic factor is apparent.

IDIOPATHIC THROMBOCYTOPENIC PURPURA

Idiopathic thrombocytopenic purpura (ITP, purpura hemorrhagica) occurs most frequently in children, young adults, and premenopausal women. It is somewhat more common in females than in males, and often develops following an acute infection.

ETIOLOGY AND PATHOGENESIS. Although the pathogenesis of ITP is unclear, there is accumulating evidence that in most cases an autoimmune process is responsible for accelerated platelet destruction. Evidence for this hypothesis is provided by the following observations: (1) Platelets disappear from the circulation of patients with ITP with extraordinary rapidity. (2) This is the result of a process extrinsic to the platelet, since normal isologous platelets survive no longer than those of the patient. (3) Platelet destruction is the result of a passively transferable humoral substance, because the plasma of patients with this disease produces thrombocytopenia when in-

Table 345-1. CLASSIFICATION OF
THROMBOCYTOPENIC PURPURAS

I. "Primary" varieties
  A. Idiopathic thrombocytopenic purpura (ITP)
  B. Hereditary and congenital forms: Wiskott-Aldrich syndrome, May-Hegglin anomaly, amegakaryocytic thrombocytopenia, others
II. "Secondary" varieties
  A. Due to chemical or physical agents
    1. Agents commonly associated with generalized bone marrow suppression (Table 341-1)
    2. Agents not commonly associated with generalized bone marrow suppression or demonstrable platelet antibodies: aminopyrine, amobarbital, aspirin, chlorpheniramine, chlorpromazine, chlorpropamide, codeine, amphetamines, digitalis, digoxin, erythromycin, penicillin, phenacetin, phenobarbital, prednisone, prochlorperazine, reserpine, streptomycin, sulfadiazine, ristocetin, promethazine, tetracyclines
    3. Agents which may provoke platelet antibodies: quinidine, quinine, allylisopropylcarbamide (Sedormid) and congeners, chlorothiazides, digitoxin, acetazolamide (Diamox), antazoline, diphenylhydantoin, hydroxychloroquin, novobiocin, stibophen, various sulfonamides
  B. In association with various systemic disorders
    1. Blood disorders
      a. Those often characterized by pancytopenia (Table 341-2)
      b. Acquired autoimmune hemolytic anemia
      c. Thrombotic thrombocytopenic purpura
      d. The defibrination syndrome (Chap. 346)
    2. Infections: viral (measles, rubella, infectious mononucleosis, others), rickettsial (typhus), subacute bacterial endocarditis; also in acute fulminant bacterial infections* (meningococcemia, gram-negative septicemia, purpura "fulminans")
    3. Miscellaneous disorders: collagen vascular disease, sarcoidosis, azotemia, others
    4. Anaphylactic reactions*: heat stroke, massive burns, insect and snake bites
  C. Miscellaneous
    1. Due to isoimmunization by platelet antigens
      a. Following blood transfusions
      b. Fetal-maternal incompatibility
    2. Following massive blood transfusions
    3. As a complication of extracorporeal circulatory devices, hypothermic anesthesia
    4. In association with hemangioendotheliomas

  * In many such cases, thrombocytopenia may represent a facet of the defibrination syndrome (Chap. 346).

Table 345-2. CLASSIFICATION OF
NONTHROMBOCYTOPENIC PURPURAS

I. Vascular purpuras
  A. Allergic purpura (Henoch-Schönlein purpura)
  B. Chemical agents: iodides, belladonna, atropine, quinine, procaine penicillin, bismuth, mercury, copaiba, phenacetin, salicylic acid, merbaphen, chloral hydrate and other hypnotics
  C. Infections: subacute bacterial endocarditis, meningococcemia, staphylococcemia, typhoid fever, rheumatic fever, scarlet fever, smallpox, measles, diphtheria, Rocky Mountain spotted fever
  D. Chronic diseases: renal, cardiac, hepatic; hemochromatosis, Cushing's syndrome, polycythemia vera, generalized amyloidosis, blood-borne carcinoma emboli
  E. Disorders of connective tissue: Ehlers-Danlos syndrome, epidermolysis bullosa, pseudoxanthoma elasticum, osteogenesis imperfecta, "senile" and "cachectic" purpura
  F. Skin disorders: pigmentary, annular, telangiectatic purpura
  G. Scurvy
  H. Miscellaneous: autoerythrocyte sensitization; simple vascular purpura (purpura simplex, "Devil's pinches") hereditary purpura simplex
II. Disorders of platelet function
  A. Thrombasthenia (Glanzmann's disease) and related disorders
  B. Aspirin and other drugs
  C. The "thrombocytopathies"
    1. Hereditary
    2. Acquired: the myeloproliferative disorders (Chap. 350), azotemia, the dysglobulinemias (Chap. 349), liver disease, others
  D. Miscellaneous: hemorrhagic thrombocythemia

tiveness of splenectomy in ITP are consistent with the autoimmune hypothesis, and there is considerable direct evidence that the spleen acts as a sequestering site for damaged platelets. Moreover, the observed changes in the megakaryocytes, previously attributed to a suppressive or injurious effect of the spleen, may reflect only the result of accelerated platelet destruction, since comparable abnormalities are found in the marrow of normal animals rendered thrombocytopenic by plasmapheresis.

The demonstration of platelet antibodies in ITP by serologic methods has proved difficult, and the nature of the "immunizing event" remains almost totally obscure. It is likely that reported positive platelet agglutination and antiglobulin tests represent artifact, or isoantibodies produced by transfusion; even the most sensitive complement fixation techniques have failed to demonstrate platelet antibodies in most cases. Nevertheless, these negative results do not provide strong evidence against the autoimmune hypothesis. Rather, they probably reflect the exquisite sensitivity of the platelet to immunologic injury. This is clearly illustrated by the well-defined drug-induced platelet antibodies, discussed below, which may produce marked thrombocytopenia when they are present even in amounts which are undetectable by the most sensitive serologic tests.

jected into normal recipients. This effect closely resembles that produced by plasma containing clearly defined platelet antibodies. (4) Pregnant women with ITP will frequently give birth to thrombocytopenic infants even though their thrombocytopenia is in remission following splenectomy. (5) In most cases, the "thrombocytopenic factor" in plasma is identifiable as a 7-S gamma-globulin. The bone marrow findings and the therapeutic effec-

In addition to thrombocytopenia, a defect in the vascular endothelium probably exists in ITP because hemorrhage in this disorder is not always closely correlated with the platelet count. It is possible that in some cases autoantibodies may damage the megakaryocyte and the vascular endothelium, as well as the platelet.

There is much to suggest that ITP is a syndrome which may arise in a number of different ways. Although an immunologic mechanism explains most of the observed facts and is probably present in many cases, it is possible that in some instances the underlying cause may be splenic dysfunction which leads to excessive platelet sequestration, or that there may be metabolic aberrations leading to deficiency of factors necessary for platelet production, or that still unrecognized mechanisms are operative.

CLINICAL MANIFESTATIONS. ITP provides the prototype of purpuric bleeding. The *lesions* may range from the size of a pinpoint or slightly larger (petechiae) to much bigger areas (ecchymoses). Mucosal hemorrhage is common and sometimes severe, epistaxis and menorrhagia are particularly frequent. Menorrhagia may be the chief complaint and the only prominent clinical sign. Bleeding may occur into any tissue and from any orifice, and slow continuous oozing is frequently noted following surgical procedures or injuries, in contrast to the rapid and voluminous posttraumatic bleeding seen in the coagulation disorders.

Fever of mild degree may be present in acute cases. The spleen may extend a fingerbreadth below the costal margin but usually is not palpable. There is no lymphadenopathy, hepatomegaly, or sternal tenderness.

ITP may begin abruptly and disappear just as suddenly; alternatively its manifestations may seem to have been present a long time. The bleeding may be mild with only a few inconspicuous petechiae; or it may be severe and lead to serious blood loss or to hemorrhage into vital areas, such as the brain or the diaphragm. All variations between these extremes may be encountered.

LABORATORY DIAGNOSIS. Examination of the **blood** may reveal anemia, which is proportional to the amount of blood lost. If there has been significant acute bleeding, signs of accelerated erythropoiesis (reticulocytosis, polychromatophilia, even occasional nucleated red blood cells) and a moderate leukocytosis with slight "shift to the left" will be found. In some chronic cases, lymphocytosis has been observed. The few platelets which may be seen in the blood smear often are morphologically abnormal: giant, minute, or deeply stained forms.

In the **bone marrow,** the number of megakaryocytes is normal or may even be increased. Immature and morphologically abnormal megakaryocytes may be seen, and, in contrast to the normal picture, few or no platelets are found about their margins. However, these findings are not diagnostic of ITP, and the primary value of bone marrow examination in this disorder is to exclude the common causes of secondary thrombocytopenia; e.g., acute leukemia, myelophthisic processes, etc.

The bleeding time is prolonged, whereas the prothrom-

bin time, partial thromboplastin time, and other *tests of blood coagulation* are normal. Thrombocytopenia may be confirmed by a positive tourniquet test, impaired clot retraction, and an abnormal prothrombin consumption test, but these studies are rarely required in the diagnosis of thrombocytopenia.

DIFFERENTIAL DIAGNOSIS. The diagnosis of ITP is one of exclusion, and the numerous other causes of thrombocytopenia must be considered (Table 345-1). The history, physical examination, and bone marrow aspirate will serve to rule out many of these conditions. Lymphadenopathy, hepatosplenomegaly, and sternal tenderness, as well as anemia out of proportion to the blood loss, even in the absence of striking changes in the leukocytes, should suggest leukemia. Persistent leukopenia suggests leukemia, aplastic anemia, "hypersplenism," or disseminated lupus erythematosus; the last-named disorder may be characterized by persistent thrombocytopenia for months or years before other characteristic manifestations appear. Purpuric lesions must be differentiated from telangiectases and small angiomas (Table 347-1).

Although rarely, a prolonged bleeding time may be found in various coagulation disorders, including hemophilia (Chap. 346), von Willebrand's disease, and various disorders of platelet function. The platelet count is normal in all these disorders, which may be further distinguished from ITP by various ancillary tests (Chaps. 62, 346).

TREATMENT. Measures which are of proved value in the treatment of ITP include the administration of adrenocorticosteroids, splenectomy, and general supportive care.

Supportive therapy, in addition to appropriate nursing care, includes transfusions if blood loss has been severe, and iron if indicated. Platelet transfusions, in the form of fresh blood, platelet-rich plasma, or platelet concentrates, usually produce only transient improvement in ITP, because of the short platelet lifespan in this disorder. Nevertheless, they may be valuable in the preparation of the patient for surgery if bleeding is severe, or in the treatment of life-threatening hemorrhage—e.g., subarachnoid bleeding.

An initial period of supportive therapy is usually recommended because spontaneous remissions are common, especially in children. Remissions may be complete and permanent, and are particularly likely to occur if the onset has been acute and there is no history of previous hemorrhagic manifestations. Unfortunately the danger of bleeding into a vital organ such as the brain makes the waiting period a trying one. Recurrences are twice as common in females as in males. A more or less chronic course, punctuated perhaps by more acute phases, is more often seen in adolescents and adults but occurs at all ages.

The use of **corticosteroids** is often associated with a decrease in the severity of bleeding phenomena, and the thrombocytopenia may decrease or disappear, but these effects usually are temporary. As a consequence, these hormones are used mainly in the management of hemorrhagic emergencies and in the preoperative preparation of patients for splenectomy. Those which can be given orally are preferred. In general 20 to 60 mg prednisone is given per day, in divided doses.

Splenectomy results in "cure" in at least two-thirds of patients. Following splenectomy the platelet count may increase rapidly and to abnormally high levels, or, more often, it may rise gradually. In the bone marrow the previously abnormal megakaryocytes in most instances soon appear to be quite normal again and are seen to be surrounded by platelets. Even when splenectomy is not followed by complete recovery, considerable improvement may be expected, since bleeding often ceases even though the platelet count may not have increased greatly.

Splenectomy is *indicated* (1) in those cases of idiopathic thrombocytopenic purpura in which spontaneous remission has not occurred after six or more months' observation and the clinical manifestations are moderate or severe; (2) in patients who appear to respond to steroid therapy but require relatively large doses to maintain a clinical state devoid of serious hemorrhage; (3) in the rare patient whose growth and development or social or economic status are seriously impaired by bleeding; and (4) in women in the later stages of pregnancy, if the condition is severe and if other measures have failed.

The operation is *not indicated* (1) early in the first episode of ITP, especially in children, since spontaneous recovery is common; (2) in most cases of secondary thrombocytopenia; (3) in neonates, since recovery usually takes place naturally; (4) in cases in which the diagnosis has not been established clearly; (5) in the hereditary and congenital thrombocytopenias, discussed below; and, according to some authorities, (6) in acute fulminating cases, when the surgical mortality rate is particularly high. However, others consider this to be an indication for emergency splenectomy, and the question must be considered unsettled. Claims that splenectomy causes "dissemination" of unrecognized lupus erythematosus and increases the hazard of infection have not been substantiated.

THE HEREDITARY AND CONGENITAL THROMBOCYTOPENIAS

These are relatively rare. In the **Wiskott-Aldrich syndrome** (Chap. 69), thrombocytopenia is associated with recurrent infections and a fatal termination in early life. **Amegakaryocytic thrombocytopenia** is characterized by total aplasia of the bone marrow precursors as well as by various congenital abnormalities such as agenesis of the radii. Thrombocytopenia is one feature of the **May-Hegglin anomaly** (Chap. 64). Other varieties of hereditary thrombocytopenia have been described, some of which are characterized by strikingly large and morphologically abnormal platelets and appear to be related to the thrombocytopathies.

THE SECONDARY THROMBOCYTOPENIAS
Thrombocytopenia Due to Chemical and Physical Agents

Chemical and physical agents are common causes of secondary thrombocytopenia (Table 345-1). Those which are commonly associated with generalized bone marrow suppression are summarized in Table 341-1 and are discussed in Chap. 341. In some cases, such drugs may be associated with isolated thrombocytopenia in the absence of evidence of bone marrow suppression, which suggests that the drug may selectively suppress the megakaryocyte by a mechanism similar to that which produces aplastic anemia. Numerous other drugs have been associated with thrombocytopenia but have not been implicated in the production of aplastic anemia (Table 345-1, II, A, 2). As in the case of aplastic anemia, the evidence implicating all the afore-mentioned drugs is circumstantial, and thrombocytopenia appears to be an uncommon manifestation of individual idiosyncracy.

In the case of drugs which produce thrombocytopenia as the result of **platelet antibodies** (Table 345-1, II, A, 3), the pathogenesis is more clear. Commonly used drugs in this group are quinidine, quinine, and the chlorothiazides. The antibodies may be demonstrated by various serologic techniques, including platelet agglutination, complement fixation, and antiglobulin tests, but the mechanisms by which such ordinarily innocuous drugs provoke platelet antibodies are as yet unclear. Most evidence suggests that the drug acts as a hapten, and that the antibody is not directed against an intrinsic platelet antigen. These observations have led to the hypothesis (the "innocent bystander" hypothesis) that the platelet suffers immunologic injury as the result of its "spongelike" tendency to adsorb drug-antibody complexes. Platelet antibodies have also been reported in association with many of the drugs listed in group II, A, 2, but the serologic evidence is unconvincing.

In the antibody-dependent thrombocytopenias, fulminant bleeding may develop rapidly when a sensitized person receives the offending drug, and the platelet count will usually rise promptly when the drug is stopped; the effect of discontinuing the drug is less predictable in cases in which an antibody cannot be clearly demonstrated. Splenectomy is usually contraindicated, and therapeutic measures should be restricted to the prohibition of potentially toxic agents and to supportive care.

"Symptomatic" Thrombocytopenias

The numerous disorders of which thrombocytopenia may be a symptom are listed in Table 345-1, II, B. Those usually characterized by *pancytopenia* are discussed in detail elsewhere (Chap. 341). Numerous other disorders, which span the entire field of medicine, may be associated with thrombocytopenia, but a detailed discussion of each is beyond the scope of the present section.

Infectious diseases, ranging from mild viral exanthemas to serious rickettsial infections, are common causes of thrombocytopenia. Serious bleeding may be associated with various fulminant bacterial infections ("purpura fulminans")—e.g., fulminating meningococcemia, Waterhouse-Friderichsen syndrome (Chap. 142), and gram-negative septicemia (Chap. 134). In these disorders, and in the bleeding which may follow various anaphylactic reactions, heat stroke, massive burns, and snake bites, thrombocytopenia appears to be but one facet of a more generalized bleeding diathesis which may be related to the defibrination syndrome.

Thrombocytopenia is common in *uremia,* may complicate surgical procedures in which *extracorporeal circulatory devices* or hypothermic anesthesia are used, and may follow massive transfusions of stored blood. In these cases, thrombocytopenia is seldom severe and bleeding is usually mild. A more serious form of *posttransfusion thrombocytopenia* results from isoimmunization by various platelet antigens. Fetal isoimmunization by maternal platelets is responsible for some cases of neonatal thrombocytopenia. Thrombocytopenia in association with *hemangioendotheliomas* is relatively uncommon but is of unusual interest in that these vascular tumors appear to act as abnormal sequestering sites for platelets.

Thrombotic thrombocytopenic purpura usually is a fulminating disorder with fever, hemolytic anemia, migratory neurologic signs and symptoms, and renal involvement. The basic lesion is a vasculitis in which fibrin, erythrocytes, and platelets are entrapped. Occlusions are found in terminal arterioles and capillaries of all organs of the body.

The *treatment* of "symptomatic" thrombocytopenia should be directed at the cause. Steroid therapy may be beneficial in a few cases, and splenectomy may be helpful in secondary forms of thrombocytopenic purpura in which the cause cannot be treated or removed but in which the bleeding manifestations are severe, such as some cases of Gaucher's disease. If there is serious bleeding, platelet transfusions, usually in the form of platelet concentrates, are a valuable adjunct in the management of some patients with secondary thrombocytopenia.

THE NONTHROMBOCYTOPENIC PURPURAS

A wide variety of disorders may produce purpura but are not accompanied by thrombocytopenia (Table 345-2). These disorders fall into two broad categories; the vascular disorders, and the qualitative abnormalities of platelet function.

The Vascular Purpuras

These disorders are poorly understood, and in general seldom lead to serious blood loss. Results of laboratory tests of hemostasis and blood coagulation usually are normal, and the diagnosis must usually be made from the associated clinical findings, which are often characteristic.

ALLERGIC PURPURA

ETIOLOGY AND PATHOGENESIS. This disorder, also called Henoch-Schönlein purpura, is characterized by effusions of blood and plasma into the subcutaneous, submucous, and subserous tissues. The pathogenesis is obscure, although there is much indirect evidence to suggest an allergic basis. It is presumed that an antigen-antibody reaction occurs which damages the vascular endothelium. The resulting perivascular inflammation and serosanguineous extravasations produce, in addition to purpura, various localized and constitutional symptoms. However, only in a minority of cases has an allergen been demonstrated. In some instances this appears to have been bacterial (streptococci, typhoid vaccine), and considerable epidemiologic evidence suggests a close relationship between allergic purpura and acute glomerulonephritis. Sometimes an article of food (milk, eggs, pork, strawberries, etc.) appears to have been the responsible allergen; rarely hypersensitivity to cold has been implicated.

CLINICAL MANIFESTATIONS. This disorder is more common in children and young adults than in older persons. The *skin lesions* are variable in appearance, but purpura is usually associated with one or more of the common manifestations of allergy, such as erythema or urticaria. The lesions are usually located on the extremities, and may appear in crops. In contrast to most other purpuric lesions, they may be accompanied by itching or paresthesias. Necrotic areas, bullae, or ulcers may develop, and submucosal lesions may lead to external hemorrhage such as epistaxis or melena; serious blood loss is uncommon.

Effusions into the joints or viscera may produce various *localized symptoms.* Thus, there may be concomitant joint pain and swelling (**Schönlein's purpura**) or crises of abdominal pain (**Henoch's purpura**). In the latter form, serohemorrhagic effusion into the intestinal wall may lead to intussusception. The renal lesion consists of a glomerulitis and may result in hematuria, proteinuria, and profound though usually temporary disturbances of renal function. *Constitutional symptoms* such as fever and malaise are present in many cases.

DIAGNOSIS. The skin lesions of allergic purpura often are characteristic, and this disorder should be suspected whenever erythematous or urticarial lesions are associated with purpura. When accessible lesions are present, the diagnosis may be confirmed by skin biopsy. Serious diagnostic difficulties may arise when purpura is not obvious or is absent altogether. For example, bouts of abdominal pain accompanied by fever, leukocytosis, or melena cannot be readily distinguished from acute abdominal conditions which call for surgical intervention. Hematuria may be a prominent symptom when the kidney is involved, and is readily mistaken for acute poststreptococcal glomerulonephritis. Similarly, when joint symptoms predominate, it is easy to confuse the disease with rheumatic fever.

Examination of the *blood* may reveal modest neutrophilia or eosinophilia. Tests of hemostasis and blood coagulation usually are normal.

TREATMENT AND PROGNOSIS. The results of corticosteroid therapy have been equivocal or disappointing, and treatment is purely symptomatic. If an etiologic agent is discovered or suspected, further exposure should be eliminated.

Allergic purpura usually is self-limited. Individual attacks last from 1 to 6 weeks, during which the clinical manifestations may wax and wane in intensity, extent, or nature. Recurrences at intervals of months or years are not unusual, however, and in a significant proportion of patients, renal involvement may become chronic.

MISCELLANEOUS VASCULAR PURPURA

A multiplicity of **drugs** may lead to striking, generalized purpuric eruptions, which subside when administration of the drug is discontinued. The pathogenesis of drug-induced vascular purpura is unclear, but the disorder is thought to be the result of an allergic reaction. **Infectious processes** too numerous to list may result in vascular purpura, presumably because of capillary damage. Various hemostatic abnormalities other than vascular injury may be present in many of these cases. The purpuric manifestations of vascular injury should be distinguished from the embolic phenomena that also occur in some of these disorders, such as subacute bacterial endocarditis.

In **chronic renal disease** with azotemia, purpura of the skin and mucous membranes as well as large subcutaneous extravasations or hemorrhages into the internal organs may be found. Purpura in *acute glomerulonephritis,* on the other hand, usually is discrete and petechial and is likely to involve only the skin of dependent portions of the body. The purpura of renal disease is probably due to the combined effects of thrombocytopenia, abnormalities of platelet function, and certain coagulation abnormalities (Chap. 346). Hemorrhagic manifestations have also been noted in cases of hemochromatosis, primary amyloidosis, and polycythemia vera.

Mild purpura occasionally results from atrophy of the subcutaneous tissue ("purpura cachectica" and "purpura senilis"), skin fragility (Cushing's syndrome), hyperlaxity of the skin (Ehlers-Danlos syndrome), or degeneration of elastic tissue or collagen (pseudoxanthoma elasticum). Various *dermatologic conditions* may be associated with cutaneous hemorrhagic manifestations. These include annular telangiectatic purpura (Majocchi's disease), angioma serpiginosum, Shamberg's disease, and pigmented purpuric lichenoid dermatitis.

Scurvy (Chap. 82) may be associated with serious bleeding manifestations, including gingival bleeding and hemorrhage into the subcutaneous tissues, muscles, and skin, where the distribution of petechiae around hair follicles is characteristic. Subperiosteal hemorrhages may also occur in children. The bleeding in scurvy is attributed to a defect in the intercellular cement of small blood vessels, and promptly ceases after the administration of ascorbic acid or other antiscorbutic substances.

Autoerythrocyte sensitization is an uncommon disorder characterized by spontaneous painful ecchymoses surrounded by erythema and edema. Often heralded by prodromal stinging or burning, the lesions may enlarge progressively and are commonly associated with headache, nausea, and vomiting. These ecchymoses can be produced by the intradermal injection of a small volume of autologous red blood cells or their stroma, and in a clinically similar disorder by the intradermal injection of deoxyribonucleic acid. This condition is frequently associated with striking psychoneurotic symptoms, and it has been thought that the bleeding may be psychosomatic in origin.

Purpura simplex is a term generally applied to instances of mild purpuric skin manifestations in otherwise healthy persons. This appears to be particularly common in women ("Devil's pinches"); a hereditary form also has been described.

DISORDERS OF PLATELET FUNCTION

The disorders of platelet function are characterized by a prolonged bleeding time and frequently by morphologically abnormal platelets. The platelet count and results of various tests of blood coagulation usually are normal. Numerous varieties have been reported, but only a few have been adequately characterized, and despite intensive study, these disorders remain poorly understood.

THROMBASTHENIA (GLANZMANN'S DISEASE). This refers to a group of hereditary disorders of platelet function characterized by defective clot retraction and by the failure of the platelets to adhere to glass or aggregate in the presence of ADP or collagen fibers. The platelets of affected persons reveal various ultrastructural abnormalities, and in some cases deficiencies in the content of various enzymes, ATP, and platelet-bound fibrinogen have been demonstrated. In contrast to most nonthrombocytopenic purpuras, bleeding in this disorder may be serious and incapacitating, and postoperative hemorrhage is a significant hazard. Treatment includes hemostatics or styptics, and blood transfusion when necessary. Transfusion of normal isologous platelets may be a valuable therapeutic adjunct.

A mild, possibly hereditary bleeding disorder (the "Portsmouth syndrome") has been described in which **platelet aggregation by collagen fibers is defective,** although ADP aggregation and clot retraction are normal. An apparently identical abnormality in platelet function is produced by *aspirin,* which may be a common and frequently unrecognized cause of mild purpuric bleeding.

Less clearly characterized are the **"thrombocytopathies,"** in which there is thought to be an abnormality in the amount or coagulant activity of platelet phospholipids (platelet factor 3). In some cases, this may result in abnormal prothrombin consumption, or in defective thromboplastic function of the platelets as measured in the thromboplastin generation test, but techniques for the study of this aspect of platelet function are imperfect. The platelets often are large and morphologically abnormal, but ADP and collagen-induced aggregation and clot retraction are usually normal. Hereditary forms are rare, but acquired "thrombocytopathies" have been described in patients with the dysglobulinemias (Chap. 349), uremia, liver disease, and the "myeloproliferative" disorders (Chap. 350). The hemostatic defect in these cases is frequently compounded by thrombocytopenia, deficient platelet aggregation, and various coagulation abnormalities, but bleeding generally is mild, and treatment consists of supportive care and therapy directed at the underlying disorder.

Hemorrhagic thrombocythemia is an uncommon condition, possibly related to the "myeloproliferative" disorders (Chap. 350), which is characterized by greatly excessive numbers of platelets, and is clinically manifested by the paradox of recurrent bleeding and thrombosis. Splenomegaly and marked leukocytosis may be present.

REFERENCES

Carpenter, A. F., M. M. Wintrobe, E. A. Fuller, A. Haut, and G. E. Cartwright: Treatment of Idiopathic Thrombocytopenic Purpura, J.A.M.A., 171:1911, 1959.

Horowitz, H. I., and R. L. Nachman: Drug Purpura, Seminars Hematol., 2:287, 1965.

Ratnoff, O. D.: "Bleeding Syndromes," Springfield, Ill., Charles C Thomas, Publisher, 1960.

Shulman, N. R., V. J. Marder, and R. J. Weinrach: Similarities between Known Antiplatelet Antibodies and the Factor Responsible for Thrombocytopenia in Idiopathic Purpura, Ann. N.Y. Acad. Sci., 124:499, 1965.

Wintrobe, M. M.: "Clinical Hematology," 6th ed., Lea & Febiger, Philadelphia, 1967.

Zucker, M. B., and A. Lundberg: Platelet Transfusions, Anesthesiology, 27:385, 1966.

346 DISORDERS OF BLOOD COAGULATION

T. C. Bithell and M. M. Wintrobe

A classification of the disorders of blood coagulation is presented in Table 346-1. The *hereditary disorders* are rare but are the result of the deficiency of a single factor and consequently are relatively well understood. The clinical picture is dominated by profuse and often life-threatening hemorrhage from trivial injuries and is characterized by certain hemorrhagic manifestations which begin in childhood and persist throughout life. In contrast, *the acquired coagulation disorders* are common, but usually result in deficiencies of several coagulation factors, and platelet and vascular abnormalities often are present as well. The clinical picture frequently is dominated by signs and symptoms of an underlying disease, and bleeding, with few exceptions, is seldom as severe as that encountered in the hereditary forms.

Table 346-1. A CLASSIFICATION OF DISORDERS OF BLOOD COAGULATION

I. Inherited disorders
  A. Sex-linked recessive traits
    1. Factor VIII deficiency (classical hemophilia)
    2. Factor IX deficiency (Christmas disease)
  B. Autosomal recessive traits
    1. Factor XI deficiency (PTA deficiency)
    2. Prothrombin deficiency
    3. Factor V deficiency (Parahemophilia)
    4. Factor VII deficiency
    5. Factor X deficiency
    6. Fibrinogen deficiency (hereditary afibrinogenemia)
    7. Factor XII deficiency (Hageman trait)
    8. Factor XIII deficiency
  C. Autosomal dominant traits
    1. Von Willebrand's disease (pseudohemophilia, vascular hemophilia)
    2. Congenital dysfibrinogenemia
II. Acquired disorders
  A. Deficiencies of vitamin K–dependent coagulation factors
    1. Liver disease
    2. Drugs (coumarins, indanediones, salicylates, broad-spectrum antibiotics)
    3. Hemorrhagic disease of the newborn
    4. Biliary tract obstruction
    5. Malabsorption syndromes (sprue, celiac disease)
    6. Dietary deficiency
  B. Accelerated destruction of coagulation factors
    1. The "defibrination" syndrome
      a. Disseminated intravascular coagulation
      b. Abnormal fibrinolysis
  C. Abnormal inhibitors of coagulation
    1. Inhibitors of specific coagulation factors
    2. "Antithromboplastins"
    3. Antithrombins
  D. Miscellaneous coagulation disorders
    1. Liver disease
    2. Uremia
    3. Disorders of the hematopoietic system
      a. Leukemia, acute and chronic
      b. Polycythemia vera
      c. Myelofibrosis
    4. The dysproteinemias (multiple myeloma, hyperglobulinemia, macroglobulinemia)

THE HEREDITARY COAGULATION DISORDERS

Etiology and Pathogenesis

The hereditary nature of hemophilia was recognized in antiquity. Most evidence suggests that the genetic abnormality alters the biosynthesis of a single protein which is essential in the coagulation phase of hemostasis. Because most methods for the study of the coagulation factors measure only their biologic activity, it is difficult to distinguish between a deficiency of the requisite protein, i.e., a quantitative disorder, and qualitative aberrations in its structure which alter its function. Hereditary bleeding diatheses due to such qualitative abnormalities of fibrinogen (the congenital dysfibrinogenemias) and factor IX (B_m or B^+ variant of Christmas disease) have recently been described. For the same reason, it is also difficult to exclude the possibility that the disorder is the result of a genetically conditioned excess of an inhibitory substance. It has been hypothesized, for example, that factor VIII deficiency results from such a mechanism, although there is considerable evidence to the contrary.

Incidence

The hereditary coagulation disorders are relatively rare, the *absolute incidence* averaging only 1 in 20,000 persons. However, the economic and psychosocial consequences of these disorders are far more important than their statistical frequency would suggest.

The *relative incidence* of the various forms varies, depending on the particular population studied. In most large series, factor VIII deficiency (classical hemophilia) comprises approximately 80 percent, factor IX deficiency (Christmas disease) approximately 13 percent, factor XI deficiency (PTA deficiency) approximately 6 percent, and the remainder, which are exceedingly rare, total 1 percent. There is evidence for the existence of several additional hereditary coagulation disorders which have not yet been recognized in the International nomenclature.

Genetics

The mode of inheritance of the various hereditary coagulation disorders is seen in Table 346-1, and the details of the various genetic mechanisms involved are discussed at length elsewhere (Chap. 4). The genetics of factor VIII deficiency and factor IX deficiency is virtually identical, and provides a classical example of *sex-linked recessive inheritance* (Chap. 4, Fig. 4-11). In such disorders, the defective gene is located on the X chromosome and produces only an asymptomatic carrier state in females because of the presence of a normal allele. Since males lack a normal allele, the defect is manifest as clinical hemophilia. The Y chromosome is normal, and as a result, the affected male will not transmit the disorder to his sons, but all of his daughters will be carriers of the trait. Such female carriers will transmit the disorder to one-half of their sons and the carrier state to one-half of their daughters. The carrier state cannot exist in normal males.

Thus, for practical purposes, the genetic abnormality in factor VIII and factor IX deficiency is carried by both sexes but affects only males. The exception to this generalization, *hemophilia in the female,* is very rare, but may occur as the result of a mating between a carrier female and an affected male, a mating between a carrier female and an unaffected male who introduces a newly mutant gene, or from an abnormal complement of chromosomes.

The regularity with which the abnormal gene is suppressed by the normal allele in female carriers is somewhat variable due to the *phenomenon of X chromosome inactivation* (Chap. 4). As a result, many carrier females will have slightly lower blood levels of the deficient factor than the normal population. The detection of such carriers in the laboratory is of great practical importance, but in the case of factor VIII, the deficiency is slight and difficult to detect with presently available methods. Female carriers of factor IX deficiency have more clear-cut deficiencies and can be more readily detected. A mild bleeding diathesis may be present in an occasional carrier female.

Approximately 25 percent of patients with hereditary coagulation disorders give a negative family history, an observation which has been ascribed to an unusually high mutation rate for the responsible gene. Consequently, although the occurrence of abnormal bleeding in family members, particularly if it occurs in a characteristic pattern, may be of great help in diagnosis, *a negative family history does not exclude a hereditary coagulation disorder.*

The mode of inheritance of the disorders listed in Table 346-1 as autosomal recessive traits is not firmly established because of their extreme rarity and because of the inherent difficulty in distinguishing between a dominant trait with variable penetrance and a recessive or "intermediate" trait. In the case of the only common variety, i.e., factor XI deficiency, the study of several large kindreds has led to conflicting conclusions, the results suggesting an incompletely recessive trait in some, while others were more compatible with an autosomal dominant trait.

Clinical Picture

The hereditary coagulation disorders produce quite similar signs and symptoms regardless of the particular factor which is deficient. Consequently, their clinical picture can conveniently be described in terms of that encountered in the commonest forms, i.e., in factor VIII and IX deficiency, citing at the same time important differences between this prototype and less common forms.

Undoubtedly the most dramatic manifestation of the hereditary coagulation disorders is exsanguinating hemorrhage from a *traumatic injury.* However, the most characteristic bleeding manifestations, such as hemarthrosis, often develop without significant trauma, and their frequency and severity are generally proportional to the blood levels of the deficient factor. For example, in the case of factor VIII, *severe deficiency* (factor VIII levels 0 to 1 percent of normal) is clinically manifest by repeated and severe hemarthroses which almost invariably eventuate in crippling. Hemarthrosis is uncommon, however, *in mild factor VIII deficiency* (factor VIII levels 4 to 25 percent of normal), although serious bleeding may follow surgery or traumatic injuries. A comparable correlation between the clinical picture and blood levels of the deficient factor can be made in the other coagulation disorders, although information is more limited. Most are associated with less severe bleeding manifestations than is the case in either factor VIII or IX deficiency. This is particularly true of factor XI deficiency, in which the bleeding is considerably milder, and serious hemorrhage usually occurs only after trauma or surgery.

Factor XII deficiency (Hageman trait) is not associated with a significant hemorrhagic diathesis, despite gross abnormalities in the various tests of blood coagulation. This apparent paradox is of great theoretical interest, but for practical purposes factor XII deficiency remains a laboratory curiosity.

Hemarthrosis. Hemarthrosis is the most common, the most painful, and the most physically, economically, and psychiatrically debilitating feature of the hereditary coagulation disorders. The knee joint is most commonly affected, the elbow and the ankle are next in frequency, and the shoulder, wrist, and hip joints are less commonly involved. The earliest symptom is pain, which results from the distension of the joint with blood. If untreated, this may progress until the subchondral and synovial vessels become ischemic. Physical examination reveals muscle spasm and limitation of motion of the affected joint, which is usually held in a position of flexion. The affected joint may be warm and grossly distended and discolored, but in chronically damaged joints external evidence of bleeding may be minimal or absent. Hemorrhage into the periarticular structures is a common complicating feature.

The joint may regain normal function following the first episodes of hemarthrosis, but with each recurrence the synovia become progressively more thickened and vascular. Together with the weakening and imbalance of the periarticular supporting structures, this predisposes the joint to recurrent episodes of bleeding. Repeated bouts of subchondral and synovial ischemia produce a progressive loss of hyaline cartilage, subchondral bone necrosis, cyst and osteophyte formation, and ultimately, ankylosis of the joint. Hemarthrosis has been described in all hereditary coagulation disorders where sufficient data are available, with the curious exception of factor V deficiency.

Patients with coagulation disorders may not bleed abnormally from small cuts, e.g., razor nicks, and the onset of bleeding is frequently delayed for several hours following significant trauma (*delayed bleeding*). These phenomena probably reflect the hemostatic efficacy of the platelet thrombus in small wounds and its temporary value in larger injuries. *Petechiae,* characteristic of disorders of vessels and platelets, are rare in the coagulation disorders, but ecchymoses and *subcutaneous hematomas* are common, often large, and characteristically dissect deeper structures. Such dissecting hematomas may spread to involve an entire limb and produce serious consequences from the compression of vital structures, e.g., ischemic contracture of the forearm, femoral nerve palsy as a result of bleeding into the psoas sheath. Bleeding into the tongue, throat, or neck is especially dangerous, and may compromise the airway with surprising rapidity.

Internal soft tissue hemorrhages may create serious diagnostic problems. Bleeding into the retroperitoneal space or the psoas sheath may mimic acute appendicitis, and hemorrhage into the intestinal wall may be confused with bowel obstruction.

Gastrointestinal bleeding is not uncommon in the hereditary coagulation disorders. The source of bleeding is usually in the upper gastrointestinal tract, and in the majority of cases when bleeding is persistent or recurrent, is found to originate from some organic lesion, e.g., peptic ulcer, gastritis. To the contrary, *hematuria,* although more common, is seldom the result of pathology in the genitourinary tract. *Menorrhagia* is common in the autosomal traits. Bleeding into the *central nervous system* is relatively rare, unless it is the result of significant trauma. Bleeding from the *umbilical cord* is uncommon in all of the hereditary coagulation disorders, with the exception of afibrinogenemia and factor XIII deficiency, disorders which may also be associated with defective *wound healing.* Intraocular hemorrhage is uncommon, but the orbit is frequently involved.

Laboratory Diagnosis

In a previous chapter (Chap. 62) it was emphasized that most hemorrhagic disorders can be detected and categorized by four "primary" screening tests (Table 62-4). In addition, the results of the partial thromboplastin (PTT) and the prothrombin time localize the abnormality to either the intrinsic, extrinsic, or common pathways of coagulation (Fig. 62-3), and together with the bleeding time separate the hereditary coagulation disorders into five categories (Table 346-2A,B,C,D, and E). When interpreted in terms of the relative incidence of the various disorders (Column 4), and when supplemented by simple ancillary tests such as the clotting time, the prothrombin consumption test, and the thrombin time (Column 5), a reasonably accurate "presumptive" diagnosis of the hereditary coagulation disorders can usually be made without special equipment or reagents. More elaborate confirmatory tests are usually required for a definitive diagnosis (Column 6).

A *prolonged PTT and a normal prothrombin time* (Table 346-2A) suggest a defect in the *intrinsic* pathway of coagulation (Chap. 62, Fig. 62-3), i.e., a deficiency of factor VIII, IX, XI, or XII. Together, these disorders comprise over 95 percent of all hereditary coagulation disorders. Factor XII deficiency can be readily excluded, since it is not associated with significant bleeding.

Among the ancillary tests, the results of the clotting time and the prothrombin consumption test vary depending on the severity of the deficiency. These tests should never be relied upon to exclude a coagulation disorder, since both will usually be normal in mildly affected persons. This point deserves emphasis both because the diagnosis of hemophilia is often erroneously equated with a prolonged clotting time and also because the most serious diagnostic errors are usually made in the case of the mildly affected patient. Such patients may have an

Table 346-2. LABORATORY DIAGNOSIS OF THE HEREDITARY COAGULATION DISORDERS

[1] "Primary" screening tests			[2] "Presumptive" diagnosis	[3] Probable deficiency	[4] Relative incidence, %	[5] Ancillary tests			[6] Confirmatory tests
Partial thromboplastin time	Prothrombin time	Bleeding time				Clotting time	Prothrombin consumption test	Thrombin time	
A. Prolonged	Normal	Normal[1]	Defect in *intrinsic* pathway	VIII	80	Prolonged[2]	Abnormal[2]	Normal	Presumptive correction tests Thromboplastin generation test Specific assays
				IX	13				
				XI	6				
				XII	?	Prolonged[2]	Abnormal[2]	Normal	Significant bleeding absent
B. Prolonged	Prolonged	Normal	Defect in *common* pathway	Fibrinogen	<1	Prolonged[2]	Normal	Abnormal	Fi test, specific assay
				Prothrombin	<1	Prolonged[2]	—	Normal	Presumptive correction tests
				V	<1	Prolonged[2]	Abnormal[2]	Normal	Thromboplastin generation test
				X	<1	Prolonged[2]	Abnormal[2]	Normal	Specific assays
c. Normal	Prolonged	Normal	Defect in *extrinsic* pathway	VII	<1	Normal	Normal	Normal	Specific assay
D. Prolonged	Normal	Prolonged	"Hybrid" defect	VW disease	Common ?	Normal[3]	Normal[3]	Normal	Factor VIII assay; "new" factor VIII synthesis following plasma infusion; platelet adhesiveness tests
E. Normal	Normal	Normal		XIII others	<1	Normal	Normal	Normal	Clot solubility test for factor XIII

The platelet count, clot retraction, whole blood clot lysis time, and euglobulin lysis time are normal in all uncomplicated hereditary coagulation disorders.

[1] In severe deficiencies, a prolonged bleeding time and a positive tourniquet test are occasionally found.

[2] The coagulation time and the prothrombin consumption test are abnormal only in severe deficiencies.

[3] The coagulation time and prothrombin consumption test are usually normal unless the factor VIII deficiency is severe.

equivocal bleeding history and a normal clotting time but nonetheless may develop serious and unexpected bleeding following traumatic injuries or surgery.

Among the confirmatory tests which serve to distinguish between deficiencies of factors VIII, IX, and XI (Table 346-2, Column 6), various "presumptive" mixing techniques are the simplest. The *thromboplastin generation test* is a relatively elaborate, but more definitive, method.

The bleeding time is rarely prolonged in patients with severe deficiencies of any of the coagulation factors. In factor VIII deficiency, this may lead to confusion with von Willebrand's disease, and the more elaborate confirmatory tests for this disorder may be required (Table 346-2, Column 6).

A prolonged PTT and a prolonged prothrombin time (Table 346-2B) suggest the presence of a defect in the *common* pathway of coagulation which may result from a deficiency of factor V, X, prothrombin, or fibrinogen. Deficiencies of these factors are present in many of the most common acquired coagulation disorders, but hereditary forms are exceedingly rare. Consequently, *the presence of a prolonged prothrombin time strongly suggests the presence of an acquired coagulation disorder.* Hereditary afibrinogenemia can be excluded by the Fi test and the thrombin time, and the erythrocyte sedimentation rate is markedly reduced in this disorder. The thrombin time usually is prolonged in the congenital dysfibrinogenemias. Deficiencies of factors V, X, and prothrombin can be distinguished from one another by simple correction tests and by the thromboplastin generation test.

Factor VII deficiency is very rare and is the only disorder characterized by a *prolonged prothrombin time and a normal PTT* (Table 346-2C). Since factor VII is essential only in the tissue-activated *extrinsic* pathway of coagulation, this diagnosis can be confirmed by the presence of a normal clotting time, prothrombin consumption test, and thromboplastin generation test.

The coagulation tests listed in Table 346-2 may be normal in the case of the mild or partial forms of von Willebrand's disease, to be discussed, and in mild factor XI deficiency. Specialized techniques are required for the laboratory diagnosis of these disorders.

All coagulation tests will be normal in factor XIII deficiency (Table 346-2E). In this disorder, the fibrin polymers are not cross-linked by stable covalent bonds, and the clot will dissolve in solvents such as urea (the clot solubility test).

Therapy

Various styptics, drugs, and hormones have periodically been advocated for the treatment of the hereditary coagulation disorders. These include vitamin K, rutin, corticosteroids, and more recently, extracts of peanuts. None of these remedies are of proven value. Topical hemostatics (thrombin, fibrin-foam) may be of temporary value in small injuries. However, *replacement therapy,* i.e., the intravenous infusion of the deficient coagulation factor in the form of normal blood or blood products, remains the only reliable method of treatment.

Concentrated preparations of fibrinogen and factor VIII are now generally available, but with these exceptions, replacement therapy at present requires the use of *plasma.* Stored plasma is usually adequate except in the case of factor V deficiency, factor VIII deficiency, and von Willebrand's disease, where fresh or fresh frozen plasma is preferable.

Concentrated factor VIII, prepared commercially by various fractionation methods, e.g., glycine precipitation, or by the technique of cryoprecipitation is now generally available. Cryoprecipitation depends on the observation that the small amount of protein which precipitates in fresh frozen plasma thawed at 4°C is rich in factor VIII. Such *cryoprecipitates* can be prepared and stored in most routine blood banks. Concentrates avoid the problems of circulatory overload, and may produce fewer adverse effects in some patients, e.g., urticarial or febrile reactions (Chap. 342), but plasma is usually effective in the treatment of *"minor" bleeding* due to factor VIII deficiency, e.g., hemarthrosis, hematomas. In the case of *"major" bleeding,* e.g., soft-tissue bleeding in vital areas, traumatic injuries, surgery, concentrates are indicated, since adequate blood levels of factor VIII can seldom be attained with plasma.

It must be emphasized that the replacement therapy of major bleeding must be individualized. Thus, in most instances minor bleeding will respond to a single large daily dose of therapeutic material, whereas major bleeding requires more frequent administration, the exact regimen depending on whether the patient is mildly or severely affected, the site of bleeding, the presence of complicating factors, e.g., external blood loss, and the biologic half-life of the deficient factor. For example, therapeutic material should be administered three to four times a day in the case of factor VIII deficiency, because the in vivo half-life of this substance is short (10 to 18 hr). In the case of fibrinogen, prothrombin, and factor XIII, one course per day is usually effective, since the in vivo half-life of these factors is 3 to 5 days. The other factors, e.g., V, IX, X, and XI, occupy an intermediate position, and two to three courses per day are recommended. Replacement therapy of factor VII deficiency is difficult, since the in vivo half-life of this factor is very short (4 to 5 hr). A concentrate which is rich in factors VII, IX, X, and prothrombin has been made available and may provide the first satisfactory means of treating factor VII deficiency.

Therapy should always be initiated promptly and continued for 2 to 3 days after bleeding stops. Experience has taught that the two commonest mistakes in replacement therapy of the coagulation disorders are to "start too late and stop too soon."

All patients with *hemarthrosis* should receive prompt and adequate replacement therapy, since only in this manner can the permanent disability which results from repeated joint bleeding be minimized. Supportive therapy includes immobilization, packing of the joint in ice, and the administration of analgesics. Addicting narcotics should be avoided, and aspirin is contraindicated, since this drug may produce gastric erosions and gastrointestinal bleeding and may also provoke or aggravate hemorrhagic episodes by means of a poorly understood effect on platelet function. *Arthrocentesis* is usually unnecessary, but may be of significant benefit when the joint is severely distended or when resolution of the hemarthrosis is delayed despite adequate replacement therapy. Early ambulation and careful *physiotherapy* aimed at restoring full range of motion to the joint should be instituted as soon as the acute stage of hemarthrosis has resolved.

Special attention should be given to the preventive *dental care* of patients with hereditary coagulation disorders, so as to minimize the hazards, complications, and expense of operative dental procedures. Although deciduous teeth may be shed without significant difficulty, the extraction of even a single permanent tooth requires adequate replacement therapy. Multiple extractions save time and expense but create a major bleeding hazard, and should be carried out only in a hospital. Bleeding tooth sockets, particularly the third molar, should never be sutured, since this may lead to extension of bleeding into the neck.

VON WILLEBRAND'S DISEASE

Von Willebrand's disease (pseudohemophilia, vascular hemophilia) occupies a unique position among the hereditary coagulation disorders in that it is characterized by a deficiency of factor VIII and a prolonged bleeding time, the latter suggesting an additional abnormality in the vascular or platelet phases of hemostasis.

Accurate figures concerning the incidence of this disorder are lacking. However, in some areas it seems to be second only to classical hemophilia in frequency.

There is now general agreement that von Willebrand's disease is inherited as an autosomal dominant trait, but the mechanism by which the genetic abnormality produces the "dual" or "hybrid" hemostatic defect which characterizes this disease is uncertain. Most evidence is compatible with the hypothesis that the autosomal abnormality results in the deficiency of a single plasma factor (the *anti-VW factor*) which is essential for normal platelet or vascular function and is also required for normal factor VIII biosynthesis. This theory is based on the observation that in patients with this disorder, the infusion of normal plasma produces a gradual and sustained rise in the factor VIII level over a 24-to-48-hr period. This cannot be attributed to the factor VIII present in the infused plasma, since comparable results are obtained with factor VIII–deficient plasma. This phenomenon, termed *new factor VIII synthesis*, is presumably the result of anti-VW factor present in the administered plasma which stimulates previously deficient factor VIII biosynthesis for a time and is a valuable but cumbersome confirmatory test for von Willebrand's disease.

Both the bleeding manifestations and the laboratory findings in von Willebrand's disease are consistent with the hybrid nature of the disorder. Thus, although the *clinical picture* is usually dominated by cutaneous and mucosal bleeding characteristic of a "purpuric" disorder, symptoms suggesting a superimposed coagulation defect, e.g., hemarthrosis, dissecting intramuscular hematomas, and serious posttraumatic hemorrhage, occur in severely affected patients.

The bleeding time and the PTT are usually prolonged (Table 346-2D), with the latter reflecting a slight to moderate reduction in factor VIII. The prolonged bleeding time is the result of a poorly understood abnormality in the rate or efficiency with which a stable platelet thrombus is formed. Various tests of platelet adhesion and aggregation have been devised to measure this process more directly, but are as yet imperfect. The coagulation time and prothrombin consumption test are usually normal in von Willebrand's disease unless the factor VIII deficiency is severe.

Perplexing features of this disorder are the tendency of the laboratory abnormalities to fluctuate from time to time and the frequency of mild or partial forms of the disorder. It has been suggested, not unreasonably, that von Willebrand's disease is a syndrome rather than a specific entity.

TREATMENT. Von Willebrand's disease should be treated in essentially the same manner as factor VIII deficiency. Unfortunately, the clinical response, particularly in the case of mucosal bleeding, such as gastrointestinal hemorrhage and menorrhagia, is unpredictable and often transient. Cryoprecipitates or fresh plasma may be preferable to commercial factor VIII concentrates in the treatment of mucosal bleeding. Since the factor VIII levels attained by replacement therapy may be supplemented by "new" factor VIII synthesized by the recipient, prophylactic therapy should be initiated 1 to 2 days before surgery.

THE ACQUIRED COAGULATION DISORDERS

Deficiencies of the Vitamin K–dependent Coagulation Factors

Four coagulation factors, i.e., factors VII, IX, X, and prothrombin, are synthesized in the liver by a process which requires vitamin K (Chap. 85). A combined deficiency of these *vitamin K–dependent coagulation factors* develops in diverse clinical situations and is probably the most common of all coagulation disorders (Fig. 346-1).

Liver disease is the most frequent cause of this complex coagulation defect. Here, the hepatic cells cannot synthesize the required coagulation factors despite the presence of adequate amounts of vitamin K. Various additional hemostatic abnormalities are frequently present in severe liver disease. These abnormalities commonly include a deficiency of factor V and, rarely, a deficiency of fibrinogen, both of which are synthesized in the liver but are not vitamin K–dependent. Thrombocytopenia may be present in as many as 50 percent of patients with severe liver disease, and the defibrination syndrome, discussed below, may develop in some cases. The bleeding manifestations in liver disease are usually chronic and include bleeding into the skin and mucosa, recurrent epistaxis, gastrointestinal bleeding, and protracted hemorrhage following minor surgical procedures, e.g., liver biopsy.

Bleeding is a common complication of therapy with *coumarinlike drugs*. Hematuria and epistaxis are particularly common, and may develop while the prothrombin time is within the "therapeutic range." Self-intoxication with these drugs is not uncommon in psychotic and neurotic individuals. Salicylates may antagonize the hepatic biosynthesis of the vitamin K–dependent coagulation factors, but this per se rarely produces abnormal bleeding.

Hemorrhagic disease of the newborn is the result of vitamin K deficiency in the neonate (Chap. 85) and is no longer commonly seen in this country. The pathogenesis of the disorder is complex, but the most important factors appear to be a sterile gut, prematurity, maternal

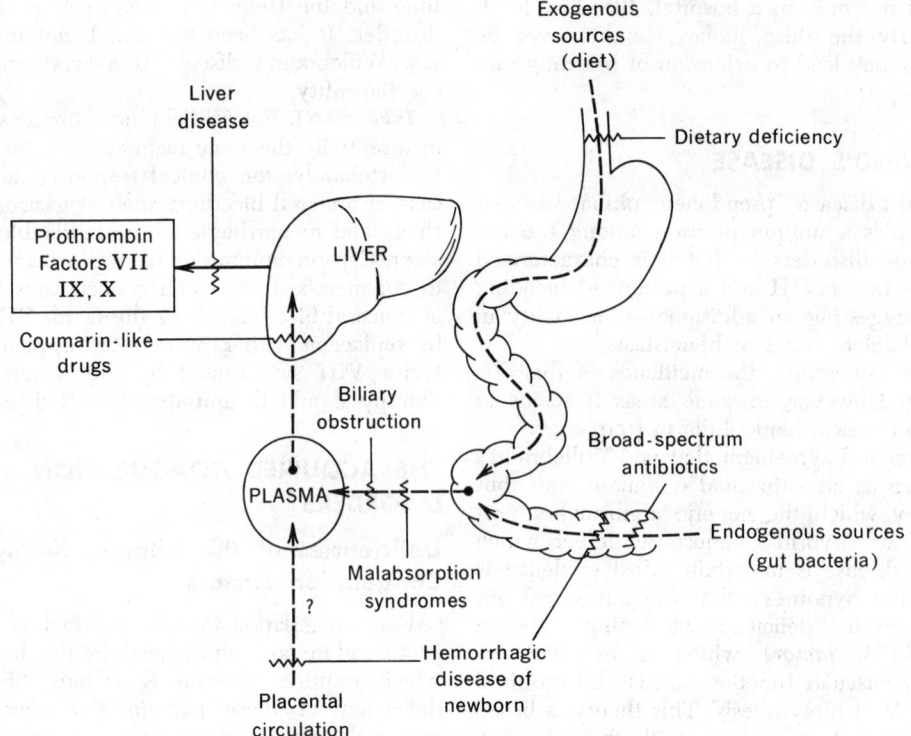

Fig. 346-1. Causes of deficiencies of the vitamin K–dependent coagulation factors. The pathway by which vitamin K is normally transported is illustrated by dashed lines.

deficiency of vitamin K, and blood loss or other obstetrical complications at birth. Petechiae are rare, but ecchymoses and mucosal bleeding, hematomas of the scalp, melena, and bleeding from the umbilical cord are commonly seen, the last in contrast to the commoner hereditary coagulation disorders.

Vitamin K (Chap. 85) is a fat-soluble substance and is absorbed only in the presence of bile salts. Consequently, deficiencies of the vitamin K–dependent coagulation factors may develop in *biliary tract obstruction.* Sprue, coeliac disease, and other *malabsorption syndromes* also produce this abnormality, as does the sterilization of the gut by the prolonged administration of *broad-spectrum antibiotics.*

The *laboratory findings* in deficiencies of the vitamin K–dependent coagulation factors are basically the same, regardless of the etiology, and are reflected in the screening tests by a prolongation of both the prothrombin time and the partial thromboplastin time. Except in the case of liver disease, the coagulation abnormalities will respond specifically and rapidly to the parenteral administration of vitamin K.

The Defibrination Syndrome

This is one of the most serious of the acquired coagulation disorders. It arises in diverse clinical situations and is characterized by an exceedingly complex hemostatic defect which results from the accelerated destruction or consumption of various coagulation factors and of

platelets. In addition, substances which impair various hemostatic functions are present. The pathogenesis of this syndrome involves two seemingly opposed processes, i.e., pathologic proteolysis and disseminated intravascular coagulation (Fig. 346-2).

The activation of the fibrinolytic enzyme, plasmin, in amounts which exceed the capacity of the antiplasmins (Chap. 62, Fig. 62-2) leads to the *pathologic proteolysis* of fibrinogen and other coagulation factors (factors V, VIII, and prothrombin). Deficiencies of these factors result if this process proceeds more rapidly than the rate at which they are repleted. Even when insufficient to deplete coagulation factors in the general circulation, the persistent or recurrent activation of plasmin produces bleeding, presumably as the result of the dissolution of hemostatically important fibrin "plugs" and the production of *fibrinogen degradation products.* The latter are protein fragments derived from the partial proteolysis of fibrinogen and fibrin. They act as inhibitors of thrombin, interfere with normal fibrin polymerization, and impair platelet aggregation. Pathologic proteolysis thus leads to impaired hemostasis by means of three interdependent processes, i.e., fibrinolysis, the production of inhibitory fibrinogen degradation products, and the depletion of essential coagulation factors in the severe case.

The entry of thromboplastic substances into the general circulation appears to be the initiating cause of *disseminated intravascular coagulation.* Coagulation proceeds in vivo much as in vitro; i.e., fibrinogen and the consumable coagulation factors (factors V, VIII, and prothrombin) are utilized, and the platelets are depleted (Fig. 346-2). In severe cases, the plasma becomes much like serum.

The *clinical picture* of the defibrination syndrome is usually characterized by the sudden onset of hemorrhage, which is often of serious proportions and is frequently associated with profound circulatory collapse. The predominant bleeding manifestations relate to the underlying disorder. Thus, in obstetrical accidents, profuse vaginal bleeding is seen, and in postsurgical defibrination syndromes, uncontrollable bleeding from the incision is usually the first sign. In severe cases, bleeding from all bodily orifices, venipuncture sites, and into the skin and mucosa develops. In others, e.g., disseminated carcinoma, bleeding into the skin and mucosa may be chronic and persistent, and in such patients a premonitory stage of "hypercoagulability" clinically manifested as a thromboembolic diathesis, may be seen.

The *diagnosis* of the full-blown defibrination syndrome is relatively easy. All of the screening tests of coagulation will be grossly abnormal, the fibrinogen level will be low, and reductions in other coagulation factors of variable degree will usually be found. The *thrombin time* is a valuable ancillary screening test in these disorders, since it is sensitive not only to the level of fibrinogen but also to the presence of fibrinogen degradation products. The definition of the basic pathogenetic process is much more difficult, since both intravascular coagulation and pathologic proteolysis produce a similar hemostatic defect in the severe case, and intravascular coagulation often produces compensatory activation of fibrinolysis.

The most reliable *laboratory criteria* are the presence of thrombocytopenia, which is rarely marked in pathologic proteolysis, and the severity of the coagulation defect, which is often relatively mild in pathologic proteolysis in contrast to intravascular coagulation, where the blood is often incoagulable. Rapid clot lysis and a shortened euglobulin lysis time may be present in either case, but these two tests are rarely as markedly or persistently abnormal in intravascular coagulation as in pathologic proteolysis.

Knowledge of the disorder which produces the defibrination syndrome may be helpful (Fig. 346-2). In those cases which develop as a complication of pregnancy, such as abruptio placentae and amniotic fluid embolism, and in those associated with septicemia, such as the Waterhouse-Friderichsen syndrome and endotoxin "shock," disseminated intravascular coagulation is presently thought to be the major factor. Pathologic proteolysis is frequently the initiating cause in liver disease, following surgery employing extracorporeal circulatory devices, and in prostatic and pancreatic carcinoma, although disseminated cancer may also produce intravascular coagulation. Evidence suggests that pathologic proteolysis is seldom the sole initiating cause of the defibrination syndrome, and in many cases it is probable that both pathologic proteolysis and disseminated intravascular coagulation are of pathogenetic importance.

TREATMENT. Management of the defibrination syndrome must be individualized, and adequate laboratory support is essential, since this syndrome often creates a serious therapeutic dilemma. Enzyme inhibitors such as epsilon-aminocaproic acid (EACA) often are effective in the treatment of pathologic proteolysis, but are contraindicated in intravascular coagulation, since they may favor the development of disseminated thrombosis. Despite the seeming paradox of treating a bleeding disorder with an

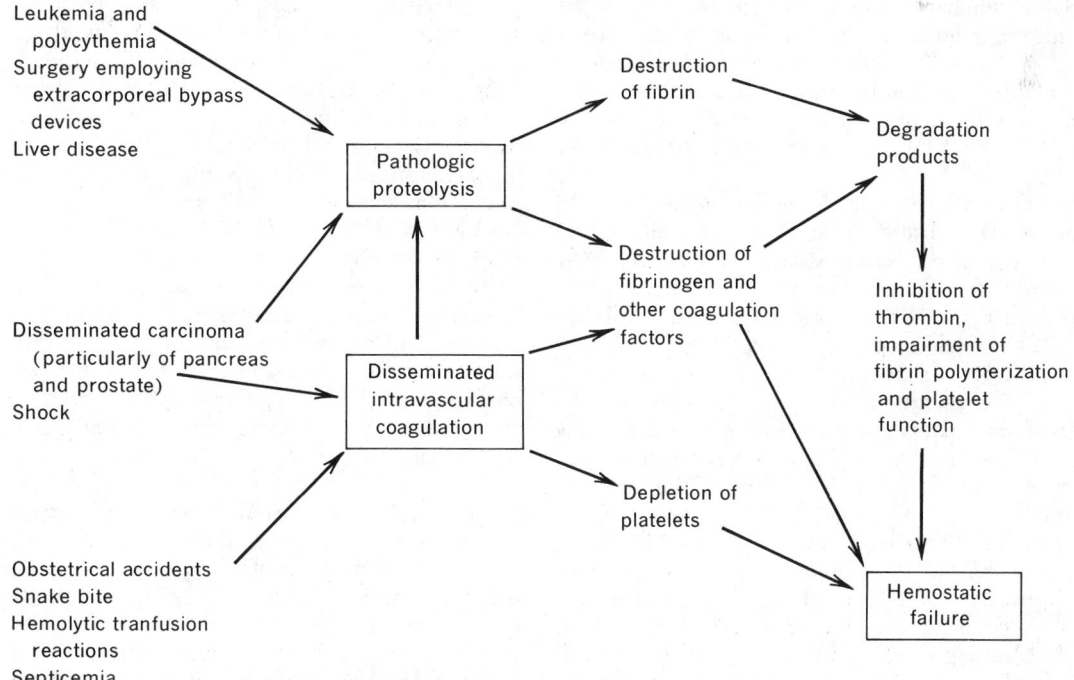

Fig. 346-2. The pathogenesis of the defibrination syndrome.

anticoagulant, intravascular coagulation should be treated with heparin. Replacement therapy is usually disappointing unless the basic pathologic process is arrested.

Acquired Inhibitors of Coagulation (The "Circulating Anticoagulants")

The acquired inhibitors of coagulation factors are uncommon and poorly understood, but may produce serious bleeding. One variety impairs coagulation by inactivating various individual coagulation factors. Such inhibitors are usually directed against factor VIII and most commonly develop in patients with factor VIII deficiency, where they produce a marked resistance to replacement therapy. Such *specific inhibitors of factor VIII* may also develop as a complication of pregnancy, in association with various collagen vascular diseases, and in elderly persons without obvious underlying disease. The circumstances under which these inhibitors develop suggest the presence of an autoimmune process, and indirect evidence is accumulating which suggests that such inhibitors are indeed antibodies to factor VIII. The *clinical picture* and *laboratory findings* resemble those of a specific deficiency of the factor against which the inhibitor is directed. In the case of the inhibitors of factor VIII, the severe case is indistinguishable from severe classical hemophilia (Table 346-2). Inhibitors which inactivate fibrinogen and factors V, VII, IX, XI, XII, and XIII in a similar manner have been described.

Other inhibitors apparently antagonize various active intermediates in coagulation rather than specific coagulation factors. Among these, the so-called *"antithromboplastins"* appear to be the most common. They usually develop in association with collagen vascular diseases, particularly disseminated lupus erythematosus, and act by inhibiting an intermediate in prothrombinase formation, possibly factor Xa. The clinical and laboratory picture resembles hemophilia, but in contrast to hemophilia and the aforementioned disorders due to specific inhibitors of factor VIII, the prothrombin time usually is prolonged.

Increased amounts of *antithrombins* may be found in the plasma in many disorders, and may be contributory factors in various complex hemostatic defects, e.g., liver disease, the defibrination syndrome. Antithrombins alone seldom produce significant bleeding. Of uncertain validity are reports of heparinlike anticoagulants.

Specialized tests are required for the demonstration of inhibitors of coagulation. They are all based on the principle that, in contrast to disorders due to deficiency of an essential factor, the addition of control plasma to inhibitor-containing plasma fails to correct the coagulation abnormalities.

Therapy of bleeding caused by acquired inhibitors of coagulation is difficult. In some cases, corticosteroids, immunosuppressive therapy, and exchange transfusion have been effective. In the case of specific inhibitors of factor VIII, bleeding can usually be stopped by the administration of factor VIII concentrates, but heroic doses often are required.

Miscellaneous Acquired Coagulation Disorders

Coagulation abnormalities may be encountered in virtually any serious chronic disease, e.g., uremia, various hematologic disorders (leukemia, polycythemia vera, myelofibrosis), and the dysproteinemias. These are discussed elsewhere (Chap. 345), since purpura is often the predominating bleeding manifestation, and the platelet and vascular abnormalities usually overshadow the coagulation defects. Although calcium is essential for normal blood coagulation, hypocalcemia per se, even if severe, does not produce abnormal bleeding.

REFERENCES

Biggs, R., and R. G. MacFarlane: "Treatment of Hemophilia and Other Coagulation Disorders." Philadelphia, F. A. Davis Company, 1966.

Shulman, N. R., D. H. Cowan, E. P. Libre, S. P. Watkins, and V. J. Marder: The Physiologic Basis for Therapy of Classic Hemophilia (Factor VIII Deficiency) and Related Disorders, Ann. Intern. Med., 57:856, 1967.

Wintrobe, M. M.: "Clinical Hematology." 6th ed., Philadelphia, Lea & Febiger, 1967.

347 HEREDITARY HEMORRHAGIC TELANGIECTASIA

M. M. Wintrobe and T. C. Bithell

This disorder is an hereditary vascular abnormality characterized by widespread telangiectases in the skin and mucous membranes. *Histologically*, there is diffuse involvement of small veins and capillaries, which are dilated, tortuous, and extremely thin, often consisting only of an endothelial layer. As a consequence, vascular support is poor and the contractility of the affected vessels is diminished. The disorder is inherited as an autosomal dominant trait by both sexes.

CLINICAL MANIFESTATIONS. The *lesions* range from pinpoint to about 3 mm in diameter, are round and bright red or violaceous in color, and characteristically blanch on pressure. They are most commonly found on the lips, tongue, and ears, and on the palmar and plantar surfaces of the fingers and toes. Although the lesions may be found in childhood, they usually increase in number and size as age advances, and in elderly patients some may become spiderlike.

The symptoms are a result of bleeding and the consequent anemia and usually become progressively more severe as age advances. Severe iron-deficiency anemia (Chap. 336) may develop. In general, telangiectases of the skin are less likely to bleed than are those of the mucous membranes. Trivial trauma may nevertheless produce profuse bleeding from superficial lesions, but significant postoperative bleeding is uncommon. Epistaxis is especially common, but bleeding may originate from

Table 347-1. DIFFERENTIATION OF "PURPURIC" AND TELANGIECTATIC LESIONS AND SMALL ANGIOMAS

Disorder	Appearance	Distribution	Duration; effect of pressure
Hereditary hemorrhagic telangiectases	Usually flat and round; red to purple, pinpoint to 3 mm in size	Centrifugal (face, lips, tongue, ears, nasal mucosa, palmar and plantar surfaces of hands and feet)	Permanent; blanch
Petechiae............	Flat, purple, of variable size and shape	Anywhere; most common in dependent areas	Appear and disappear in crops; do not blanch
Cherry angiomata......	Elevated, nodular, bright red, 1–3 mm in diameter	Chest and abdomen	Permanent; do not blanch
Spider telangiectases...	Flat or slightly raised with characteristic spider "legs"; bright red, 2–5 mm in size	Chest, clavicles, face, upper extremities	Permanent; blanch; "legs" fill from center
Angiokeratoma CDU...	Flat to slightly raised; dark red to blueblack; pinpoint to pinhead in size; associated with cornlike lesions and subcutaneous nodules	Centripetal (mainly chest and abdomen, umbilicus); in groups	Permanent; few blanch

telangiectases wherever they are: the face, tongue, lips, respiratory, or urinary tracts. Gastrointestinal bleeding is one of the most serious manifestations and is common after middle age. Involvement of various visceral vessels may produce symptoms. Pulmonary arteriovenous fistulas have been reported in a number of cases and may lead to hemoptyses, recurrent pulmonary infections, or significant cardiovascular symptoms (Chap. 263).

DIAGNOSIS. In the presence of the characteristic lesions and a typical family history, the diagnosis of hereditary hemorrhagic telangiectasia is not difficult. In cases in which externally visible lesions are lacking or are overlooked, perplexing diagnostic problems may result. This disorder should always be remembered in recurrent or intractable gastrointestinal bleeding of obscure etiology. In such cases, visceral angiography may be helpful in diagnosis. *Laboratory* tests of blood coagulation and hemostasis are usually entirely normal.

The lesions must be differentiated from purpuric lesions (Chap. 345), spider telangiectases of liver disease, senile cherry hemangiomas, and the rare *angiokeratoma corporis diffusum universale* (CDU) (Fabry) (Table 347-1). The last is a disorder of glycolipid metabolism resulting from an inherited deficiency of a ceramide trihexoside-cleaving enzyme. It is characterized by widespread involvement of the media of blood vessels, including the renal and pulmonary vasculature.

TREATMENT. There is no effective treatment for this disorder. Blood transfusions and the administration of iron may be indicated for the relief of anemia. Local measures to control the bleeding include nasal packs and the use of topical hemostatic agents and styptics, e.g., Gelfoam, thrombin. Electrocoagulation may be of temporary value in the case of accessible lesions of the skin or mucosa, but satellite lesions usually reappear nearby.

REFERENCES

Bagdade, John D., et al.: Fabry's Disease, Lab. Invest., 18: 681, 1968.

Wintrobe, M. M.: "Clinical Hematology," 6th ed., Philadelphia, Lea & Febiger, 1967.

348 THE LEUKEMIAS
Dane R. Boggs and M. M. Wintrobe

DEFINITION. Leukemia is a disease characterized by an abnormally large number of a specific type of leukocyte within the body in the absence of a demonstrable cause. Types of leukemia are differentiated according to the leukocytic system involved and on the basis of cell maturity. Depending on the type of leukemia and the efficacy of the therapy employed, patients may die within a few days of diagnosis or live for decades. With rare exceptions, all types of leukemia are eventually fatal.

HISTORY. Knowledge of leukemia can be traced to the period from 1839 to 1845 when Donné made the first microscopic observations, and Craigie, Bennett, and Virchow distinguished the clinical entity. Virchow recognized that the cells involved were leukocytes and distinguished a lymphatic and a splenic form. After Ehrlich's blood-staining methods were developed, Neumann, in 1891, identified the latter as myelocytic. Acute leukemia was described by von Friedreich in 1857, and Naegeli distinguished between lymphoblastic and myeloblastic leukemia in 1900.

Useful, palliative therapy for the chronic leukemias came with development of therapeutic x-ray equipment in the 1920s. However, until folic acid antagonist and adrenal glucocorticosteroid therapy became available in 1948 and 1949, no therapy was of appreciable benefit in the acute leukemias. In the search for a cure there is encouragement in the fact that at the present time a few patients with acute leukemia are alive who have been in remission for from 5 to 15 years. However, for practical purposes, leukemia still is incurable and, while research into its etiology holds promise, the pace of progress toward prevention or cure remains slow.

CLASSIFICATION. The leukemias are usually classified as acute or chronic and are further categorized according to the predominant cell involved. Actually, the terms acute and chronic have lost some of their prognostic implications because of present therapeutic regimens. Patients with acute lymphoblastic leukemia may live longer than some patients with chronic myelocytic leukemia. Nonetheless, the terms acute and chronic are still applicable, since in the former the illness usually is acute in onset, while in chronic leukemia the onset usually is insidious. A variety of clinical features help to distinguish the various forms of leukemia, but final diagnosis is based on microscopic examination of the blood and/or bone marrow.

Two common forms of leukemia arise from the lymphocytic system of cells: *acute lymphoblastic leukemia* and *chronic lymphocytic leukemia*. The lymphoblast, a large cell with homogeneous and rather granular chromatin, is the most common cell in acute lymphoblastic leukemia, while the small lymphocyte, with its nucleus of densely clumped chromatin, is the common cell in the chronic form. Plasma cells may be closely related to the lymphocytic system and when multiple myeloma is complicated by the release of large numbers of myeloma or plasma cells into the blood, the patient is considered to have *plasma cell leukemia* (see Chap. 349). Patients with lymphosarcoma may develop marked lymphocytosis or lymphoblastosis in the blood (*lymphosarcoma cell leukemia*), and when this occurs, the disease may be indistinguishable from that of patients with lymphocytic or lymphoblastic leukemia.

There are two common forms of leukemia involving the granulocytic cell system: *acute myeloblastic leukemia* and *chronic myelocytic leukemia*, as well as a wide variety of variants and/or subtypes of the granulocytic leukemias. In chronic myelocytic leukemia the entire spectrum of the neutrophilic series from myeloblast to segmented neutrophil is present in abnormally large numbers, and eosinophils and basophils usually are increased as well. Acute myeloblastic leukemia is characterized by an increase in myeloblasts, but with a hiatus of maturation beyond this point. Many patients who otherwise are virtually indistinguishable from patients with acute myeloblastic leukemia have cells with some morphologic features suggesting monocytes (*myelomonoblastic leukemia*); still others show a predominance of promyelocytes (*promyelocytic leukemia*). For purposes of clinical management patients with acute myeloblastic, myelomonoblastic, and promyelocytic leukemia can be considered as the same.

Other rare forms of leukemia include *eosinophilic leukemia*, which takes two forms. One mimics chronic myelocytic leukemia in clinical manifestations, whereas the other is more acute and cardiac manifestations are a cardinal feature. *Basophilic leukemia* has been described. Some patients with myeloblastic leukemia form prominent solid tumors composed of myeloblastic tissue. When their cut surface is exposed to air these tumors turn green because of their content of myeloperoxidase; they have been termed *chloromas*. In the bone marrow of patients with myeloblastic leukemia, bizarre erythroblasts which bear some resemblance to megaloblasts may be found. In a few patients, such changes in red cells may precede and/or overshadow the myeloblastic hyperplasia. Occasionally, such a patient with anemia and a hyperplastic "megaloblastoid" marrow has died without myeloblastosis. Patients with the above type of erythroid changes have been classified as having the *di Guglielmo* syndrome (*erythroleukemia*, erythremic myelosis).

Still other rare forms of leukemia do not easily fit into variant patterns of the lymphocytic and granulocytic cell systems. *Monocytic leukemia*, in which the cells are without appreciable myeloblastic features, is occasionally observed. In a clinically acute form the cells are usually very large and bizarre ("Schilling-type" leukemia). In another form which follows a more chronic course, the monocytes are more or less normal in appearance. In patients with congenital or acquired urticaria pigmentosa (Chap. 400) increased numbers of mast cells are found in various tissues and organs. Such patients occasionally develop blood mastocytosis (*mast cell leukemia*). Patients with idiopathic thrombocytosis and megakaryocytic hyperplasia of the bone marrow sometimes have been referred to as having *megakaryocytic leukemia*. These patients eventually develop a clinical picture compatible with myeloid metaplasia or myelofibrosis.

INCIDENCE, AGE, AND SEX DISTRIBUTION. The incidence of leukemia in the United States is approximately 6 per 100,000. Leukemia incidence was reported to be increasing steadily until approximately 1955 but has since stabilized.

The incidence of the various types of leukemia differs according to age. Acute myeloblastic leukemia and chronic myelocytic leukemia may occur at any age, although they are found most commonly in young adults. Chronic lymphocytic leukemia does not occur in children and is uncommon under the age of forty. Acute lymphoblastic leukemia is primarily a disease of children, although it occurs with decreasing frequency throughout life. Most series suggest that acute lymphoblastic leukemia is the most common of these diseases, followed in order of decreasing frequency by acute myeloblastic leukemia, chronic myelocytic leukemia, and chronic lymphocytic leukemia. Leukemia is the most common form of cancer in children but constitutes only 3.6 percent of deaths due to cancer in the general population.

In all types of leukemia, a slight predominance of male patients is found (approximately 3:2) and in chronic lymphocytic leukemia males predominate 2:1.

ETIOLOGY. The etiology of leukemia is unknown, although certain contributing factors have been recognized.

Ionizing irradiation in relatively large doses is a predisposing factor in the development of acute myeloblastic and chronic myelocytic leukemia, but there is little evidence to suggest that it plays a role in lymphoid leukemias. Survivors of Hiroshima and Nagasaki, pioneering radiologists, and patients given therapeutic irradiation have all developed granulocytic leukemia with uncommon frequency. Whether there is a "threshold" of irradiation dose below which there is no attendant increase in risk of developing leukemia or whether any exposure carries a slightly increased risk is uncertain.

Chemical leukemogens are recognized, and they are typified by benzol. Certain drugs, such as phenylbutazone, also are suspected as contributing factors in the development of leukemia. Acute myeloblastic and chronic myelocytic leukemia have been the usual types of leukemia following such exposure or therapy.

Genetic influences are suggested by certain observations. Patients with Down's syndrome, characterized by trisomy of chromosome 21, develop acute myeloblastic leukemia at least three times as frequently as do normal children. Instances of familial leukemia are rare but have been reported frequently enough in chronic lymphocytic leukemia to arouse suspicion of a genetic factor in this disease. Concordance of acute leukemia is significantly more frequent in monozygotic than in fraternal twins. Chronic myelocytic leukemia is characterized by deletion of the short arms of chromosome 21 (Philadelphia chromosome, Ph^1) in myelocytic, erythrocytic, and megakaryocytic cells, but since this abnormality is not present in lymphocytes or buccal mucosal cells, it would appear to be an acquired rather than an inherited abnormality. Chronic lymphocytic leukemia is rare in the Orient, but whether this represents a racial or environmental factor is not clear.

Many other factors, such as trauma, bacterial infections, and psychological influences, have been suggested as contributing factors in the development of leukemia, but the evidence supporting these suggestions is questionable.

Murine leukemia and that of a number of other mammals as well as of fowls have been demonstrated to be etiologically related to a *virus*. In certain instances the virus has been shown to be inherited and may be passed in mothers' milk as well. The incidence of leukemia in mice known to carry the virus varies from one strain to another, and the incidence can be increased or the age at which leukemia develops can be influenced by irradiation and by a variety of other leukemogenic agents. These observations suggest that the presence of a virus is essential to the development of leukemia, but that environmental and genetic factors may modify the frequency with which leukemia develops in its presence. There is suggestive but not definitive evidence that human leukemia may be caused by a virus.

CELLULAR PROLIFERATION PATTERNS. In the acute leukemias and in chronic myelocytic leukemia, studies with radioactive cell labels and of uric acid excretion suggest that an abnormally large number of leukocytes are produced and destroyed each day. An excessive rate of total cell production appears to be an essential part of these diseases. However, such evidence presently is lacking in chronic lymphocytic leukemia. In none of the leukemias has a shortened cellular generation time been demonstrated, and indeed, the percentage of potentially proliferating cells which are engaged in active DNA synthesis may be decreased. Thus, the overproduction of cells reflects a marked expansion of a potentially proliferating compartment of cells. However, the rate of self-replication of individual cells within this compartment is normal or even subnormal. The life span of leukemic cells may be abnormally long, which may contribute significantly to cellular accumulation in the disease.

The failure of cells in acute leukemia to mature normally is generally assumed to represent a cellular defect rather than a defect in extracellular factors regulating growth. In chronic myelocytic leukemia, the presence of the Philadelphia chromosome in myelocytic and erythrocytic precursors as well as in megakaryocytes suggests that the primary cellular defect in this disease lies in a stem cell which is pluripotential for these three systems of cells.

The mechanism which prevents the release of large numbers of immature cells to the blood in normal subjects apparently is intact in certain patients with acute leukemia and in a few patients observed very early in the course of chronic myelocytic leukemia. *Aleukemic leukemia* refers to those cases of acute leukemia in which no "blasts" are found in the blood. Leukopenia is seen in such cases as a rule, since the number of normal leukocytes usually is decreased. Patients with acute leukemia with blasts in the blood, but with a normal total leukocyte count have been termed *subleukemic*.

CLINICAL MANIFESTATIONS

The various types of leukemia are characterized by different signs, symptoms, and complications, but have certain features in common as well. Clinical manifestations can usually be related to one or more of the following factors: (1) formation of masses composed largely of leukemic cells (splenomegaly, lymphadenopathy, meningeal infiltration, bone pain, etc.); (2) reduced numbers of normal blood cells (thrombocytopenia with resultant hemorrhage, anemia with resultant fatigue, and neutropenia with resultant bacterial infection); (3) other specific problems (excess uric acid production with gout and/or uric acid nephropathy, failure to produce circulating antibodies in chronic lymphocytic leukemia with attendant bacterial infection); or (4) poorly understood manifestations, such as fever and weight loss.

CHRONIC MYELOCYTIC LEUKEMIA. The onset is insidious, and the first symptom usually is mild fatigue or a mass in the left side of the abdomen. At the time of diagnosis, physical abnormalities usually are limited to a palpable spleen and a small area of tenderness over the body of the sternum. Fever may be present occasionally, and some weight loss may have been noted. The diagnosis cannot be made with certainty unless blood neutrophils are increased. In a few patients with less than 50,000 neutrophils per cu mm there may be few or no immature neutrophilic leukocytes in the blood, but in most cases the entire spectrum of neutrophils from myeloblasts to segmented neutrophils is represented in the blood. Most patients have more than 100,000 neutrophilic cells per cu mm in the blood at the time of diagnosis, and the count may exceed 1 million. Examination of the marrow is of no diagnostic help but usually discloses that the barrier to release of immature cells is not completely destroyed, since the proportion of immature cells is higher in the marrow than in the blood. Until blastic crisis supervenes, it is the well-differentiated neutrophilic myelocytes and later forms which are found in the blood, and segmented neutrophils predominate. Basophils and eosinophils usually are increased in proportion or even out of proportion to the increase in neutrophilic cells. Monocytes may be normal or increased while lymphocytes usually are normal in absolute number. The severity of the disease is usually reflected by the height of the leukocyte count, and the count tends to increase as the disease progresses. Most patients are mildly anemic at the time of diagnosis, and anemia becomes severe in the terminal phase. Platelets often are increased at the time of diagnosis, and thrombocytopenia rarely develops spontaneously in the absence of a blastic crisis.

The most common cause of death in chronic myelocytic leukemia is the development of a phase which is heralded by an increasing percentage of myeloblasts in blood and marrow (*blastic crisis*). When this develops, the clinical picture approximates that of patients with acute myeloblastic leukemia.

ACUTE MYELOBLASTIC LEUKEMIA. Rapidly developing fatigue and a general sense of poor health, often accompanied by hemorrhagic manifestations and fever with or without bacterial infection, bring the patient to a physician. Physical examination usually discloses pallor, hepatosplenomegaly, sternal tenderness and petechiae, less often ecchymoses. An occasional patient has no demonstrable physical findings. The number of blasts in the blood ranges from none to more than a million. In approximately 40 percent of cases the total leukocyte count is not increased at the time of diagnosis. Normal blood leukocytes are almost always decreased, although an occasional patient has basophilia or eosinophilia. Anemia is present in more than 90 percent of patients at diagnosis and rapidly becomes more severe as the disease advances. Thrombocytopenia is present in most patients and bleeding from the nose or elsewhere is common. Death is usually due to bacterial infection or to hemorrhage.

The course of patients with myelomonocytic or promyelocytic leukemia is similar to that of patients with myeloblastic leukemia, except that in myelomonocytic leukemia, gum infiltration is more commonly present, while in promyelocytic leukemia, hemorrhage due to hypofibrinogenemia may occur.

ACUTE LYMPHOBLASTIC LEUKEMIA. The above description of the "typical" patient with acute myeloblastic leukemia also is valid for many patients with acute lymphoblastic leukemia. However, patients with this disease do differ from the former in certain clinical manifestations. Presentation with bone and joint pain is much more common in lymphoblastic leukemia. Whether this reflects the youth of the population affected, as compared to the older age of most of those with myeloblastic leukemia, or is due to a difference in the diseases is uncer-

tain. Infiltration of the meninges causing symptoms of increased intracranial pressure is a common manifestation of lymphoblastic leukemia. Lymph node enlargement may be present in myeloblastic leukemia, but lymph nodes are more commonly palpable and may be larger in lymphoblastic leukemia. Splenomegaly and hepatomegaly tend to be more prominent in lymphoblastic leukemia. The number of blasts in the blood and the severity of anemia, thrombocytopenia, and neutropenia are similar in the two diseases.

As will be discussed later, the most dramatic difference between the two diseases is the frequency of therapeutically induced remissions in lymphoblastic leukemia, as compared to the distressing resistance to therapy in myeloblastic leukemia. Bleeding and infection are the common modes of death in lymphoblastic leukemia.

CHRONIC LYMPHOCYTIC LEUKEMIA. This disease is so insidious in onset that in approximately one-fourth of patients it is discovered in an asymptomatic stage during a routine examination or during examination for unrelated disease. A vague sense of not feeling well, often accompanied by a specific complaint of fatigue is the most common presenting symptom, although presentation with a bacterial infection or because of an enlarged node is not uncommon. On physical examination, most patients have enlarged lymph nodes. A palpable spleen is the next most common physical sign (three-fourths of patients), and one-fourth have hepatomegaly. Sternal tenderness is less common than in other forms of leukemia. An increase in blood lymphocytes is a necessary diagnostic feature, and patients with bone marrow infiltration without increased blood lymphocytes are classified as having lymphosarcoma (Chap. 351). Leukocyte counts generally are not as high as in patients with chronic myelocytic leukemia, being in two-third of cases less than 100,000 lymphocytes per cu mm. Although a cursory look at a blood smear of a patient with chronic lymphocytic leukemia may suggest that he has no blood leukocytes except small lymphocytes, careful differential counts reveal that normal absolute numbers of neutrophils, eosinophils, monocytes, and basophils are usually present in untreated patients. Mild anemia is common, as is mild thrombocytopenia. However, except when hemolytic anemia supervenes or complications of cytotoxic therapy are induced, most patients do not develop severe anemia or thrombocytopenia for some years.

Since chronic lymphocytic leukemia is primarily a disease of old age, many patients die of causes apparently unrelated to leukemia. The most common complication and the usual cause of leukemia-related death is bacterial infection.

MANIFESTATIONS OF INFILTRATION WITH LEUKEMIC CELLS

The presence of excessive numbers of leukocytes is assumed to be directly or indirectly responsible for the manifestations of leukemia.

Splenomegaly is the most common physical manifestation of the leukemias. At diagnosis a palpable spleen is present in almost all patients with chronic myelocytic leukemia, in about 85 percent of patients with acute lymphoblastic leukemia, 75 percent of those with chronic lymphocytic leukemia, and 60 percent of those with acute myeloblastic leukemia. The relative size of the spleen in the different forms of leukemia tends to parallel this frequency. *Hepatomegaly* is detectable in approximately half of all patients at diagnosis. Enlarged *lymph nodes* are common at the time of diagnosis in chronic lympho- cytic leukemia (80 percent) and acute lymphoblastic leukemia (75 percent). While enlarged nodes may be found in myeloblastic and myelocytic leukemia, they generally are smaller. Cervical nodes are most commonly involved, although nodes in any area may be enlarged. Unless the patient notices the mass, none of these infiltra- tions lead to symptoms or organ failure. Splenic infarcts may produce pain, and splenic rupture is very occasion- ally reported, but neither of these events has any ap- parent relationship to the size of the spleen. Liver func- tion test are likely to be normal even in patients with markedly enlarged, infiltrated livers. These observations suggest that the leukemic cells are not "invasive" in the sense that the cells of many carcinomas are invasive, since in general, they tend not to destroy the function of the organs that they infiltrate.

Almost any organ or area of the body has been reported as being infiltrated by leukemic cells, but infiltrations other than those noted above which are most likely to produce symptoms and signs are those of the central nervous system, kidneys, lungs, bones, and skin.

Serious problems with *central-nervous-system infiltra- tion* can occur with any of the leukemias but are common only in the acute leukemias. In approximately one-fourth of patients with lymphoblastic leukemia, the leptome- ninges are infiltrated to a degree that a symptomatic in- crease in intracrannial pressure is produced. This com- plication is less frequent in myeloblastic leukemia and rare in other varieties. Headache, nausea and vomiting, stiff neck, seizures, blurred vision, and cranial nerve palsy are the attendant symptoms. Papilledema is a common finding. Examination of the spinal fluid usually reveals increased pressure and increased cell content (identifi- able as blasts with proper methods), and protein often is elevated and sugar decreased. If the patient still is responsive to corticosteroids, this therapy will often reverse the process, but intrathecal methotrexate, 0.2 mg per kg body weight, repeated at weekly intervals until the spinal fluid is normal, is the treatment of choice. Irradiation of the entire brain area is efficacious but in- duces alopecia. Most of the commonly employed anti- leukemia drugs do not enter the spinal fluid, and pre- sumably for this reason, this complication may develop in patients who otherwise are in complete remission.

Intracerebral infiltration is a cause of death in perhaps 10 percent of patients with myeloblastic leukemia and in an occasional patient with lymphoblastic leukemia. In such patients there appears to be a sudden spurt of growth of leukemic cells. The number of blasts in the blood begins to increase exponentially, and "leukostatic" lesions of rapidly growing cells occlude cerebral vessels. Cerebral hemorrhage accompanies rupture of these ves-

sels as the leukemic mass expands and large intracerebral hemorrhages with grossly visible solid leukemic tumors in their center are found at autopsy.

Infiltration of spinal meninges, compression of the spinal cord by leukemic tumors, and involvement of peripheral nerves are observed occasionally.

Renal enlargement is found with some frequency in the acute leukemias if routine radiographic studies are made, but this rarely results in renal failure. Most renal problems in all types of leukemia are referable to uric acid excess, hemorrhage, infection, or unrelated processes. Parenchymal *pulmonary* lung infiltration of serious degree is uncommon in any of the leukemias and almost never occurs in chronic lymphocytic leukemia. When parenchy- mal pulmonary infiltration arises in the acute leukemias, it is usually diffuse in nature and can be distinguished from pulmonary infection only by its failure to disappear after appropriate antibiotic therapy. Mediastinal or hilar lymph node enlargement and/or pleural effusions are the usual intrathoracic manifestations of leukemic in- filtration. A variety of radiologically demonstrable *bone lesions* are described in all forms of leukemia, but only patients with lymphoblastic leukemia commonly develop pain from such lesions. Pathologic fractures are extremely rare. Bone lesions which may produce excruciating pain are bone infarcts (which may not be demonstrable radio- graphically), infiltration raising the periosteum, and dis- crete circumscribed radiolucent lesions.

Skin infiltration with leukemic cells is rarely a serious symptomatic problem but is observed in a small percent- age of patients with any type of leukemia. Such infiltrates usually are circumscribed raised tumors which may be red or purplish in color. They rarely ulcerate or cause pain, but they may itch. An occasional patient with chronic lymphocytic leukemia may develop a very pru- ritic generalized infiltration of the skin, and at times, this may precede blood lymphocytosis. Such patients have been said to have lymphocytes which contain more PAS- staining material than lymphocytes of other patients with chronic lymphocytic leukemia (*Sézary syndrome*). Skin lesions in patients with leukemia not due to infiltration by leukemic cells have been termed leukemids.

The treatment of choice for localized, troublesome infiltration with leukemic cells, if accessible, is x-ray therapy. A relatively small dose of x-ray will usually eradicate a local infiltrate.

MANIFESTATIONS DUE TO A REDUCTION IN NORMAL HEMATOPOIETIC CELLS. Reduced numbers of normal cells are responsible for many of the symptoms and signs and constitute the usual cause of death. It has been assumed that thrombocytopenia, neutropenia, and anemia are due to decreased cell production, although other kinetic changes in these cell systems may play a role as well. The reason for the reduced production of normal cells is not clear. The obvious explanations, crowding out by leukemic cells or competition for nutrients, appear un- likely for a variety of reasons. It now seems clear that erythrocytes, neutrophils, megakaryocytes, and perhaps even lymphocytes share common pluripotential stem cells. An attractive hypothesis is that the primary defect in leukemia is in a stem cell and that the regulatory function for differentiating into various normal cells is disturbed, leukemic cells being produced instead.

Anemia. Decreased erythrocyte production is accompanied by a reduction in reticulocytes, and the erythrocytes usually are normocytic and normochromic. An occasional nucleated erythrocyte is not uncommon in patients with acute myeloblastic or chronic myelocytic leukemia, and may be seen in acute lymphoblastic and even chronic lymphocytic leukemia if anemia is severe. In myeloblastic leukemias with "megaloblastoid" marrows, large macrocytes may predominate and large numbers of erythroblasts may be observed in the blood. A modest reduction in red cell survival often is detectable in isotope-labeling studies, but frank hemolytic anemia with hyperbilirubinemia is rare in all types of leukemia except chronic lymphocytic leukemia. In that disease approximately 20 percent of patients may develop severe hemolysis. This complication occurs suddenly at any time during the course of the disease. The Coombs test usually becomes positive, and consequently, the accelerated red cell destruction is assumed to be an autoimmune phenomenon. This anemia usually responds to corticosteroid therapy, although an occasional patient requires splenectomy.

Anemia other than the rare hemolytic anemia is relieved by appropriate treatment of the leukemic process. The indications for transfusion are those which apply to any anemic patient and are discussed in Chap. 342.

Hemorrhage usually is related to thrombocytopenia. In an occasional patient, generally with acute promyelocytic leukemia, hemorrhage is due to hypofibrinogenemia or other nonthrombocytopenic causes. Life-threatening hemorrhage rarely develops unless the platelet count is less than 20,000 per cu mm, but in patients with less than 50,000 platelets ecchymoses usually and, less often, petechiae are present. Bleeding from almost any site or organ may be observed, but the most common forms of fatal or life-threatening hemorhage are intracranial and intraintestinal. Fatal gastrointestinal hemorrhage is more common in lymphoblastic than in myeloblastic leukemia. Intracranial hemorrhage due to thrombocytopenia is usually subarachnoid. Most instances of intracerebral hemorrhage are related to leukemic infiltration.

Decreased production is the probable cause of thrombocytopenia in most patients with leukemia, but an occasional patient with chronic lymphocytic leukemia develops severe thrombocytopenia in the presence of large numbers of megakaryocytes in the bone marrow. In this circumstance, steroid therapy and/or splenectomy usually is effective. In most thrombocytopenic patients there is no effective means of inducing increased platelet production except by inducing a remission in the leukemia by specific therapy.

Thrombocytopenic hemorrhage can be interrupted or prevented by administration of enough platelet transfusions. Since platelets cannot be stored for transfusion, fresh whole blood or fresh platelet concentrates must be used. The number of platelets which must be transfused to raise the platelet count above the danger level depends upon the size of the patient. Platelets from as much as 5 liters of blood may be required to stop hemorrhage in an adult. Since the life span of platelets in the blood is only about 10 days and that of transfused platelets usually shorter, the effect of platelet transfusion is quickly dissipated. However, in treatment centers where platelets are regularly administered prophylactically to thrombocytopenic patients, hemorrhage has become a less frequent cause of death in leukemia than it once was. The repeated use of a single platelet donor, coupled with in vitro tests for platelet compatibility, can reduce the frequency of formation of significant levels of antiplatelet antibodies by the patient.

Fever and infection are common problems in all types of leukemia, although bacterial infection is not particularly common in chronic myelocytic leukemia until blastic crisis supervenes. Fever in chronic lymphocytic leukemia is almost always due to infection, but in other forms of leukemia fever often occurs in the absence of infection as an intrinsic part of the disease. However, in any febrile leukemic patient an intensive search for infection, including blood and urine cultures, should be carried out before concluding that the fever is noninfectious. A "therapeutic trial" of antibiotics is not advisable in the absence of overt infection. Antibiotic-induced changes in the bacterial flora of the patient permit growth of antibiotic-resistant types of infection. Prophylactic antibiotic therapy should not be considered in these diseases for the same reason.

The frequent bacterial infections which develop in leukemia are explainable on the basis of neutropenia or of failure to form circulating antibodies in response to an antigenic challenge. Failure to form antibodies generally is limited to chronic lymphocytic leukemia and is often reflected by hypogammaglobulinemia. Cytotoxic drug therapy may impair antibody response in any of the leukemias. Neutropenia is present in most patients with active acute leukemia and is a frequent complication of cytotioxic therapy in any of the leukemias.

The impaired resistance of the leukemic patient leads not only to frequent infections but also to infections of unusual severity. Bacterial infections spread with startling rapidity, and bacteremia is frequent. In patients who have not recently received antibiotics, the organisms responsible for infection usually are pneumococci, streptococci, staphylococci, or *E. coli.* However, when a second infection follows closely on the heels of the first (superinfection), unusual organisms such as *Pseudomonas, Candida,* or *Aspergillus* are more frequently encountered. Most infections in patients with leukemia appear to arise from the patients' microbial flora, so that the alteration of the flora induced by antibiotics dictates to some degree the type of infection which is encountered. Almost all of the rare organisms have been reported as causes of infection in leukemia, and organisms which are ordinarily nonpathogenic may assume a pathogenic role in such patients.

Therapy of infection in patients with leukemia must be swiftly and aggressively applied, and antibiotics should be as specific as possible for the offending organism.

Prompt surgical drainage of abscesses is advisable, as is scrupulous local care of skin infections. Antiinfectious therapy is, at best, a delaying action unless specific antileukemic therapy leads to general improvement in the disease. As long as the defects in host defense persist, antibiotic control of one infection is usually followed with distressing rapidity by infection with another organism.

Excessive production of uric acid reflects the rate of cell turnover in the leukemias. Elevated serum and urine urate levels are common in all leukemias except chronic lymphocytic leukemia. Therapy with cytotoxic agents increases the rate of urate production. Gout may develop, but the most distressing complication of excess urate production is precipitation of urate crystals in renal collecting tubules. Anuria may develop in this circumstance.

If anuria follows institution of cytotoxic therapy, spontaneous recovery is the rule if proper fluid management is followed, although an occasional patient requires dialysis. If oliguria or anuria develops without relation to cytotoxic therapy then more vigorous management is indicated. The xanthine oxidase inhibitor, allopurinol, blocks the conversion of hypoxanthine to uric acid, thereby reducing the excessive urate load. Its prophylactic use will prevent uric acid nephropathy. Alkalinization of the urine increases urate solubility and should be used in oliguric patients. Antigout drugs such as Benemid (*p*-di-*n*-propylsulfamylbenzoic acid) are contraindicated because they increase the concentration of urates in the collecting tubules.

DIFFERENTIAL DIAGNOSIS

The symptoms and signs of the leukemias are found in many other diseases, but diagnostic difficulty should occur only in relation to those diseases in which the leukocytic changes observed in the leukemias are approximated (*leukemoid reactions*). Other instances of diagnostic confusion are due to inadequate attention to examination of the blood.

In the presence of certain infections (e.g., pneumococcal, meningococcal, tuberculosis), in a few patients with malignancy, especially if metastasizing, and following the use of certain toxic drugs, a picture mimicking that of chronic myelocytic leukemia may be observed. In most such patients, although leukocytosis is present, there are far fewer myelocytes and more older neutrophils in the blood than in chronic myelocytic leukemia. More reliable differentiating points are the absence of increased basophils and eosinophils in leukemoid reactions, the normal or high, rather than low, leukocyte alkaline phosphatase, and the absence of the Philadelphia chromosome. Neutrophils from more than 90 percent of patients with chronic myelocytic leukemia show an abnormally reduced staining reaction for alkaline phosphatase. The presence of the Philadelphia chromosome in neutrophil precursors is for all practical purposes pathognomonic for chronic myelocytic leukemia, although its absence does not rule out the disease, since a few patients with seemingly typical chronic myelocytic leukemia do not show this finding. Certain findings suggesting *myelofibrosis* or *polycy-*

themia vera may cause confusion and make it impossible to clearly categorize the patient. In the absence of a low alkaline phosphatase score and the Philadelphia chromosome, one should hesitate to make a diagnosis of chronic myelocytic leukemia in such cases.

Infectious mononucleosis may be mistaken for acute leukemia, but this diagnostic confusion reflects lack of experience in examining blood smears. Antibody studies also will be helpful (Chap. 255). Certain infections (e.g., pertussis, infectious lymphocytosis) may be associated with transient increases in numbers of small lymphocytes in the blood, but there are no causes of a marked and sustained increase in small lymphocytes in the blood other than chronic lymphocytic leukemia. Certain types of tumor cells in the bone marrow, such as those from neuroblastoma, may be confused with lymphoblasts. There are reports of patients with tuberculosis in whom a "leukemoid reaction" mimicking acute myeloblastic leukemia was observed. It is not certain whether these represented a leukemoid reaction or the association of myeloblastic leukemia and tuberculosis. As the neutrophil system recovers from drug-induced hypoplasia, the immaturity of bone marrow cells may temporarily suggest myeloblastic or myelocytic leukemia.

There is real difficulty in *distinguishing lymphoblastic leukemia and myeloblastic leukemia* in patients in whom the blasts are very immature. The clinical differences between the diseases which were outlined previously may be of some help in this distinction. The most reliable method for distinguishing lymphoblasts from myeloblasts is a difference in nuclear chromatin discernible on properly prepared and stained thin smears of blood or bone marrow. The nuclear chromatin of myeloblasts is very fine or reticular and the nuclear membrane is thin and of uniform thickness, while some clumping of chromatin and irregularities of thickness of nuclear membrane are found in lymphoblasts. Special stains may be of some value, but no single stain provides infallible differentiation between lymphoblasts and myeloblasts. Myeloblasts stain with the peroxidase stain if they contain specific granules, but when enough cells stain with peroxidase to be of great diagnostic benefit, the myeloid character of the leukemia usually should be discernible on Wright's stained smears. Sudan black stain is of the same significance as peroxidase stain. Mature neutrophils in myeloblastic leukemia are likely to take up less alkaline phosphatase stain than normal neutrophils, while these cells take up more than normal amounts of the dye in many lymphoblastic leukemias. Lymphoblasts are more likely to stain with PAS than are myeloblasts.

Preleukemia represents a form of leukemia which can be distinguished from aplastic anemia or normocytic normochromic anemia of nonleukemic cause only by observation. When first seen, these patients are anemic, granulocytopenia may be present, platelets may be abnormally high or low, and bone marrow examination is nondiagnostic. After weeks, months, or even in an occasional patient, years, myeloblastic leukemia develops. Whether such patients represent a very early stage of the leukemic process or whether their initial syndrome is a different disease which predisposes to the development of leukemia is unknown.

TREATMENT

While the cure of leukemia is an objective which has not been assuredly attained in any patient to date, it is well established that its treatment reduces morbidity and prolongs life in the acute leukemias. Appropriate management also is very important in the chronic leukemias. To provide the patient a maximum of comfort and happiness, whether or not cure will ever be possible, should be the physician's aim. To do this a sound understanding of medicine as a whole is necessary, in addition to familiarity with the various forms of leukemia and the pros and cons of the available therapeutic agents. He must be able to give wise counsel and should be prepared to discuss the many questions which arise as the result of the advice of well-intentioned but usually poorly informed friends and neighbors or the false hopes engendered by premature statements appearing in the various news media. The desperate desire to secure help and the wish for a miracle drug must be treated sympathetically. Kindness, thoughtfulness, and wisdom are as important in therapy as the therapeutic agents themselves. Reassurance, if founded on understanding and good care, is a most valuable therapeutic agent.

Hospitalization, visits to the physician or hospital, and needle punctures should be held to the minimum consistent with good care. The patient should be encouraged to maintain normal activities, whether these be play, going to school, housework, or breadwinning. The therapy which is chosen should be the simplest as well as the cheapest that is consistent with effective management.

The goals of therapy are accomplished through the use of antileukemic therapy which attempts to reduce and control the growth of the total mass of leukemic cells, and the employment of adjunctive therapy which is aimed at controlling complications such as infection, hemorrhage, the formation of troublesome localized leukemic tumors, hemolytic anemia, or uric acid nephropathy. Adjunctive therapy was discussed earlier in relationship to the common complications and forms as important a part of the management of the patient as does antileukemic therapy. The principles of adjunctive therapy which were outlined previously are applicable to all types of leukemia, but more specific antileukemic therapy differs for the four common leukemias and will be discussed separately for each type.

CHRONIC MYELOCYTIC LEUKEMIA. *Busulfan* is the treatment of choice, although radioactive phosphorus and x-ray to the spleen are effective modes of therapy also. Although it is unclear whether therapy prolongs the life of patients with chronic myelocytic leukemia, there is no question that therapy provides excellent and often prolonged symptomatic relief. The severity of this disease is reflected in the height of the leukocyte count, and patients with more than 50,000 leukocytes per cu mm blood may be symptomatic. This figure can be used as a rough guide to the need to begin antileukemic therapy in chronic myelocytic leukemia.

Busulfan (Myleran) is given in oral doses of 4 mg daily and is continued until the leukocyte count is reduced to 10,000 per cu mm. Most patients with active chronic myelocytic leukemia are mildly anemic, and as the leukocyte count decreases, the anemia usually is corrected. Sternal tenderness usually disappears, and the spleen shrinks in response to therapy. However, some evidence of disease persists in most patients, such as a small but palpable spleen, persistent basophilic leukocytosis, or an occasional immature myeloid cell in the blood. The duration of therapy required to bring the leukocyte count to normal depends primarily upon the height of the leukocyte count when therapy was begun. The curve of leukocyte decrease is an exponential function, so that the leukocyte count is reduced by one-half at fairly predictable intervals. In most patients approximately 2 months of continuous therapy will be required to accomplish these objectives.

Toxic reactions to busulfan that require interruption of the above type of therapeutic course are unusual. A few patients develop gastric discomfort, but the most serious complications are thrombocytopenia and leukopenia. If either develops, therapy with the drug should be discontinued. After many courses of busulfan or after prolonged maintenance therapy, patients commonly develop hyperpigmentation of the skin and a few develop interstitial pulmonary fibrosis, amenorrhea, testicular atrophy, gynecomastia, or a syndrome mimicking adrenal insufficiency.

If therapy is interrupted when the leukocyte count reaches normal levels, months and occasionally a year or more elapse before the patient again becomes symptomatic. When the leukocyte count increases to 50,000 or more per cu mm, busulfan therapy is resumed. Repeated remissions can be induced in this way. The duration of remission tends to become shorter with each successive course of the drug, but this is not always the case.

An alternative to repetitive, interrupted courses of busulfan is to reduce the dosage of the drug when the leukocyte count reaches normal levels with the hope of maintaining the leukocyte count within normal limits. Nothing is gained by this, however. Such maintenance therapy should be reserved for patients in whom the duration of unmaintained remissions has become distressingly short. Interrupted therapy requires fewer visits to the physician during remission than does maintenance therapy, and the incidence of the various toxic complications of the drug probably is lower with intermittent than with continuous busulfan administration.

The development of a progressive increase in the proportion of myeloblasts in blood and bone marrow (blastic crisis) signals the end of busulfan responsiveness, and at this point treatment is similar to that for acute myeloblastic leukemia.

CHRONIC LYMPHOCYTIC LEUKEMIA. The indications for therapy and the beneficial effects of antileukemic therapy are not clear in this disease. Corticosteroid therapy and a variety of alkylating agents, such as cyclophosphamide or chlorambucil, administration of radioactive phosphorus, or irradiation of the spleen will reduce the mass of lymphoid tissue, but the overall benefit is unclear. The most common serious complication and the major cause of death in chronic lymphocytic leukemia is bacterial infection. As outlined previously, this is usually due to inability to form circulating antibodies and often is reflected in hypogammaglobulinemia. There is no evidence that any of the above modes of therapy benefit the antibody-forming mechanism, whereas the likelihood of serious infection may be enhanced by superimposing or accentuating neutropenia by the use of one of these agents. However, some patients report that they feel better after a course of therapy, and at present, hematologic opinion ranges from recommending no therapy except when specific indications, such as anemia, develop to the recommendation that the leukocyte count should be kept within normal limits as much of the time as possible.

If severe anemia (usually but not invariably an overtly hemolytic anemia) or severe thrombocytopenia develops in chronic lymphocytic leukemia, *corticosteroid therapy* is indicated. In most such patients, prompt improvement is induced by administration of 20 to 40 mg prednisone per day, or more. As soon as the anemia and/or the thrombocytopenia is corrected, the drug dosage should be gradually tapered and stopped as soon as possible. If large doses of prednisone are required to maintain the improvement, splenectomy should be considered. The risk of long-term prednisone therapy may outweigh the risk of splenectomy, and in many patients splenectomy will relieve the hemolytic anemia or thrombocytopenia sufficiently to make prednisone therapy unnecessary.

In addition to its salutary effect upon anemia and thrombocytopenia, corticosteroid therapy is markedly lymphocytolytic. The blood lymphocyte count rises initially, but then it decreases and a rapid reduction in the size of enlarged lymph nodes, spleen, and liver takes place. However, these advantages are outweighed by the frequency of bacterial infections which often are associated with long-continued corticosteroid therapy. Consequently, such treatment cannot be recommended for the routine management of this disease.

Therapy with an *alkylating agent* such as chlorambucil will lead to a reduction in blood lymphocyte levels and in the size of enlarged organs and lymph nodes. In some patients anemia is improved. However, anemia, thrombocytopenia, and neutropenia may become more severe during therapy and often fail to return to pretreatment levels when therapy is stopped. Hence, chlorambucil, if used, should be employed in modest dosage (0.1 mg/kg/day) and packed red cell volume, leukocytes, and platelets should be checked at frequent intervals.

ACUTE LYMPHOBLASTIC LEUKEMIA. In the last 20 years a true revolution in therapy has occurred in this disease, leading to a marked prolongation in survival. With proper management at least one complete remission can be induced in almost all patients and as many as three successive complete remissions are not unusual. The drugs which are of proven benefit in this disease are listed in Table 348-1 and are divided into drugs which are useful in inducing a remission and those which are useful both in inducing and maintaining a remission. Corticosteroids and vincristine will induce remission, but the duration of the induced remission is not prolonged by continuing these drugs once a complete remission has been induced. Methotrexate (a folic acid antagonist) and 6-mercaptopurine prolong the duration of remission if administered on a continuous basis during remission. Whether cyclophosphamide will maintain, as well as induce, remissions is not entirely clear.

Table 348-1. CHEMOTHERAPEUTIC AGENTS OF PROVEN EFFECTIVENESS IN THE TREATMENT OF ACUTE LYMPHOBLASTIC LEUKEMIA

Agent	Useful in:		Rate of remission induction, %	Average duration of remission, months
	Inducing remission	Maintaining remission		
Prednisone........	Yes	No	60	
Vincristine........	Yes	No	50	
6-Mercaptopurine..	Yes	Yes	40	6
Methotrexate......	Yes	Yes	20	12*
Cyclophosphamide.	Yes	Yes?	20	3

* When administered as a twice weekly dose; if given daily, duration is only about 3 months.

In inducing remissions with a single drug, *prednisone,* 40 mg per day, is probably the drug of choice due to the frequency of remission and its lower toxicity in comparison to the other drugs. Maximum improvement is achieved within 6 weeks after the start of therapy. At this point the drug should be tapered rapidly and then discontinued. Half of the patients who achieve a complete remission with the first course of prednisone will respond to a second course, but a steady reduction in number of responders is seen with subsequent courses. *Vincristine,* 0.1 mg per kg, given intravenously at weekly intervals is effective in inducing remission but has very serious toxic effects. After 3 or 4 doses, deep tendon reflexes disappear in many patients, and unless the drug is discontinued, neurologic toxicity may progress until the patient is paralyzed. However, some patients can be brought into remission before neurologic toxicity supervenes. *Methotrexate* and 6-*mercaptopurine* can be used singly as remission-inducing drugs but are more commonly used to induce remission in combination with other drugs or are used to maintain remissions induced with prednisone or vincristine.

If more than one of the remission-inducing drugs is given, the frequency of remission increases (80 percent with prednisone and 6-mercaptopurine, 90 percent with prednisone and vincristine), but so does the toxicity. If *combined therapy* is used, prednisone in combination with one of the other drugs is preferred because the toxic effects of the two drugs used will be qualitatively different. Small groups of patients treated experimentally with prednisone, vincristine, methotrexate, and 6-mercaptopurine (VAMP) administered in combination to induce remission, and patients treated by other combinations of drugs, have remained in remission, unmaintained by drug therapy during remission, for much longer than have patients treated by any of the drugs administered alone. However, toxicity is severe and necessitates hospitalization and intensive supportive care. Hence, the role of such regimen in the general management of this disease remains to be determined.

For maintenance therapy after remission has been induced, methotrexate, 6-mercaptopurine, and perhaps, cyclophosphamide are useful. Methotrexate may be administered daily by mouth, but the duration of remission is longer if it is given orally in a dose of from 15 to 30 mg per square meter of body surface twice each week. A daily dose of 6-mercaptopurine is given orally in the amount of 2.5 mg per kg. Therapy is continued at full dosage until relapse occurs or until toxicity supervenes. If hematologic toxicity, gastrointestinal side effects, or oral ulceration develop, the drug should be discontinued until toxicity disappears and then be cautiously restarted, often at a somewhat reduced dose. Liver disease is an occasional side effect of both methotrexate and 6-mercaptopurine therapy. This is an indication for permanent discontinuation of the offending drug. If relapse occurs while the patient is receiving 6-mercaptopurine or methotrexate, the usefulness of this drug is ended, but if relapse occurs after the drug has been discontinued, a later trial with that agent is warranted. Attempts to delay the onset of drug resistance by alternating maintenance drugs during remission appear to be unsuccessful.

The exact method of therapy that one adopts for a patient with lymphoblastic leukemia is probably not too important. One should attempt to induce successive remissions and maintain each for as long as possible.

ACUTE MYELOBLASTIC LEUKEMIA. This disease and its common variants, myelomonoblastic leukemia and promyelocytic leukemia are very resistant to therapy. Of the agents listed in Table 348-1, only 6-mercaptopurine is of proven effectiveness in acute myeloblastic leukemia. Whether the other agents have no salutary effect whatever or whether they are of some slight benefit, particularly if combined with 6-mercaptopurine, is an open question.

A dose of 2.5 mg per kg 6-mercaptopurine is administered daily by mouth. If remission occurs (one-fourth of patients), some improvement will be evident within 8 weeks of beginning therapy. If improvement takes place, the drug should be continued until the patient relapses. Only 15 percent of patients achieve a complete remission with 6-mercaptopurine, but when remissions do occur, they tend to be longer than remissions in lymphoblastic leukemia.

DEVELOPMENT OF NEW DRUGS IN THE TREATMENT OF LEUKEMIA. A number of new drugs are being tested. Drugs which appear promising in treating leukemia in experimental animals are studied for unexpected toxicity in patients with carcinoma for whom no therapy of proven benefit is available. If not too toxic, they are then tried in the treatment of patients with leukemia whose disease is resistant to drugs of known usefulness. Unfortunately, a number of drugs which appeared promising in animal test systems have had little antileukemic effect in man. Others have been so toxic that an adequate test for antileukemic effect is impossible. The majority of internists and hematologists should await a complete and full investigation of any new drug by the leukemia research centers before contemplating its use. Initial reports of new drugs may be somewhat misleading. For instance, the initial trial of methylglyoxalbisguanylhydrazone (methyl GAG) suggested that a greater proportion of patients with myeloblastic leukemia would respond to this drug than to 6-mercaptopurine. Later experience did not substantiate the usefulness of methyl GAG, and its toxicity was found to be so great that it has not assumed a useful role in therapy of leukemia.

Preliminary studies suggest that there are four new drugs which may prove useful in treating leukemia, L-*asparaginase*, cytosine arabinoside, daunomycin, and hydroxyurea. L-asparaginase is an impurse enzyme preparation derived from such sources as *E. coli* which has distinct antileukemic properties. In experimental systems its antitumor activity correlates with reduction in levels of asparagine in serum and tumor tissue. Preliminary studies suggest that this agent is reasonably effective in inducing good remissions in acute lymphoblastic leukemia and is remarkably free of toxicity. Remissions have been short, however, and as yet it is unclear whether it will be useful in maintaining remission. *Cytosine arabinoside* is a synthetic, abnormal nucleoside which can induce remission in both myeloblastic and lymphoblastic leukemia. Remission rates suggest that it is at least as good a drug as 6-MP in the former disease.

Daunomycin, an antibiotic, has severe, delayed, and unpredictable toxic effects upon hematologic and myocardial tissue but will induce remissions in acute lymphoblastic and myeloblastic leukemia. Since it is very toxic and is primarily of benefit only early in the disease, its usefulness is in doubt. *Hydroxyurea*, a drug which has been known for 100 years, has been shown to induce remissions in chronic myelocytic leukemia.

DURATION OF SURVIVAL AND FACTORS INFLUENCING SURVIVAL

A statistically demonstrable prolongation of life has attended therapy in acute lymphoblastic and acute myeloblastic leukemia, but such a lengthening of survival is not certain in chronic myelocytic and chronic lymphocytic leukemia. The natural history of chronic lymphocytic leukemia is much longer than that of the other forms of leukemia. Patients in whom the diagnosis was made before symptoms developed lived an average of 10 years, and survival for 2 and 3 decades has been reported.

Analysis of a series of patients presenting with all degrees of severity at the time of diagnosis showed that more than half such patients with chronic lymphocytic leukemia lived more than 5 years from diagnosis. Patients with chronic myelocytic leukemia rarely live as long as 10 years, and blastic crisis usually signals the end of the disease within 3 to 4 years of diagnosis.

The survival of patients with the acute leukemias averaged but 3 months from diagnosis before the present drugs became available, and survival for more than a year was exceptional. Now the average duration of life is steadily increasing in acute lymphoblastic leukemia, being 1½ years or better in recent reports. A slight but significant prolongation of life has been observed in acute myeloblastic leukemia, attributable primarily to the few patients who respond favorably to therapy.

The duration of survival in acute lymphoblastic and acute myeloblastic leukemia depends primarily upon the number and duration of remissions. However, there are other prognostic factors in these diseases which help in predicting the duration of remissions and the duration of life. Patients in whom the total leukocyte count is low, few blasts are present in the blood, and sternal tenderness is absent, and who do not have serious hemorrhagic problems at the time of diagnosis tend to live longer than patients who do not present these findings. In patients with chronic lymphocytic leukemia the duration of life from diagnosis is shortened by the presence of any of the parameters of active disease and is inversely related to their severity.

REFERENCES

Boggs, D. R., M. M. Wintrobe, and G. E. Cartwright: The Acute Leukemias, Medicine, 41:163, 1962.

——, S. A. Sofferman, M. M. Wintrobe, and G. E. Cartwright: Factors Influencing the Duration of Survival of Patients with Chronic Lymphocytic Leukemia, Am. J. Med., 40:243, 1966.

——, and E. Frei, III: Clinical Studies of Fever and Infection in Cancer, Cancer, 13:1240, 1960.

Dameshek, W., and F. Gunz: "Leukemia," 2d ed., New York, Grune & Stratton, Inc., 1964.

Freireich, E. J., et al.: The Effect of 6-Mercaptopurine on the Duration of Steroid-induced Remissions in Acute Leukemia: A Model for Evaluation of Other Potentially Useful Therapy, Blood, 21:699, 1963.

——, and E. Frei, III: Recent Advances in Acute Leukemia, Progr. Hematol., 4:187, 1964.

Haut, A., W. S. Abbott, M. M. Wintrobe, and G. E. Cartwright: Busulfan in the Treatment of Chronic Myelocytic Leukemia: The Effect of Long Term Intermittent Therapy, Blood, 17:1, 1961.

Karon, M., et al.: The Role of Vincristine in the Treatment of Childhood Acute Leukemia, Clin. Pharmacol. and Therap., 7:332, 1966.

Osgood, E. E.: Treatment of Chronic Leukemias, J. Nucl. Med., 5:139, 1964.

Sutow, W. W., M. P. Sullivan, and G. Taylor: Status of Present Treatment for Acute Leukemia in Children, Cancer Res., 25:1481, 1965.

Wintrobe, M. M.: "Clinical Hematology," 6th ed., Philadelphia, Lea & Febiger, 1967.

349 MULTIPLE MYELOMA AND OTHER PLASMA CELL DYSCRASIAS

J. Foerster and M. M. Wintrobe

DEFINITION. The general category of plasma cell dyscrasias includes a number of disorders which share two basic characteristics: (1) the uncontrolled proliferation of cells normally involved in antibody production; and (2) the synthesis and secretion by these cells of a structurally homogeneous gamma-globulin and/or its constituent polypeptide subunits. The structure and function of these proteins and their normal immunoglobulin counterparts have been dealt with elsewhere (Chap. 70).

ETIOLOGY. The etiologic factors underlying the genesis of plasma cell dyscrasias remain obscure. Possible clues have come from studies of spontaneous and adjuvant-induced plasma cell tumors in inbred strains of mice, and these emphasize the interdependence of genetic and carcinogenic factors. The occasional association of multiple myeloma with chromosomal abnormalities in man and the rare familial occurrence of plasma cell dyscrasias similarly have drawn attention to possible genetic influences, but the likelihood of chance coincidence cannot be excluded.

The factors responsible for the excessive production of abnormal proteins (M-components) also are unknown, but it seems likely that the amount produced by an individual patient is a direct function of the number of abnormal cells present at a given time in the course of the disease. However, the unbalanced synthesis of constituent polypeptides, notably light chains and portions of heavy chains, may reflect abnormalities in structural or regulatory genes.

CLASSIFICATION. Among the plasma cell dyscrasias, several clinical patterns are recognized which may be classified as follows:

1. Multiple myeloma
2. Waldenström's macroglobulinemia
3. Heavy chain disease
4. Monoclonal gammopathy of unknown significance

The association of monoclonal gammopathy with lymphomas; nonreticular neoplasms (particularly those involving the colon); "myeloproliferative disorders," such as polycythemia vera, myelofibrosis, and chronic myelocytic leukemia; and Gaucher's disease has been reported. Because no causal relationships have been discovered in any of these combinations (with the possible exception of lymphomas which are derived from tissues normally engaged in immunologic responses), it is thought best to classify the protein abnormalities found in association with these disorders as monoclonal gammopathies of un-known significance. A more detailed classification does not seem warranted.

MULTIPLE MYELOMA

DEFINITION. Multiple myeloma is a neoplasm of plasma cells, with characteristic bony lesions, replacement of marrow by tumor tissue, and pathologic manifestations occasioned by the overproduction of myeloma proteins and their constituent polypeptide chains.

CLINICAL MANIFESTATIONS. It is well recognized that the clinically apparent stage of multiple myeloma usually is preceded by an asymptomatic period of variable dura-tion. A few instances of asymptomatic myeloma lasting for nearly 2 decades have been recorded. During this time an elevated erythrocyte sedimentation rate, a gamma-globulin spike on serum electrophoresis, or un-explained proteinuria may be the only manifestations of the disease. As the illness progresses, weakness, weight loss, and recurrent bacterial infections become prominent features and are followed by symptoms re-sulting from skeletal lesions and the development of chronic renal disease.

Increased *susceptibility to infection,* particularly in the form of recurrent bacterial pneumonias, is an extremely common finding and probably constitutes a major cause of death. There is a markedly impaired capacity for normal antibody production, sometimes associated with an increased rate of immunoglobulin catabolism, which is reflected in abnormally low concentrations of normal immunoglobulins of all classes. Defective cell-mediated immune responses also have been recognized.

The *skeletal lesions* are mainly confined to areas of red marrow and come to light because of a swelling, local tenderness, unrelenting pain, or a pathologic fracture. On roentgenograms the areas of involvement may appear as multiple "punched-out" osteolytic lesions, diffuse mot-tling, or generalized rarefactions. Occasionally, the first manifestation may be a solitary tumor. On the other hand, in a large number of patients, bony lesions are never recognized.

Chronic renal failure frequently becomes a prominent feature of the disease and is the end result of a number of interrelated factors. Of major importance is the glo-merular filtration of large quantities of light chains, a portion of which is actively reabsorbed by the proximal tubules (Chap. 70). In the majority of patients cellular degeneration and the appearance of proteinacious inclu-sion bodies occur in association with this process, lead-ing to a severe general impairment of tubular function. In addition, specific tubular reabsorption defects, in-cluding the adult Fanconi syndrome, have been de-scribed. The other major pathogenic effect of the ab-normal proteins is related to their incorporation into large hyaline casts which may form along the entire length of the tubule and may eventually lead to ob-struction, distension, and ultimate destruction of the whole nephron.

Other factors appear to be of equal importance in the genesis of chronic renal failure. Hypercalcemia due to bony destruction and immobilization may lead to all the manifestations of hypercalcemic nephropathy (Chap. 307), while hyperuricemia due to rapid cellular turn-over, frequently aggravated by therapy, results in the deposition of uric acid crystals in the distal tubules, collecting ducts, and ureters. In addition, renal amyloi-dosis is found in a considerable number of patients with multiple myeloma.

Acute renal failure is usually due to a sudden aggrava-tion of chronic renal disease by dehydration or other insults. Intravenous pyelography sometimes is associated with acute renal shutdown, presumably because of fluid restriction required in preparation for this procedure. Of equal importance may be the capacity of some contrast media to precipitate light chains in acid urine.

Involvement of the *nervous system* by multiple mye-loma is largely a function of its proximity to skeletal structures. Root compression is common, as is paraplegia due to compression of the spinal cord. Occasionally, cranial nerves may also become involved by tumor tis-sue. Root symptoms and peripheral neuropathies due to infiltration of these structures by amyloid have been described, as have occasional instances of polyneuropathy and proximal myopathy in the absence of direct invasion of these structures by amyloid.

Hypercalcemic encephalopathy is a potentially fatal complication of multiple myeloma and should be promptly identified because of its favorable response to therapy (Chap. 90).

Amyloidosis is a recognized complication of multiple myeloma. In addition to renal and neurologic involve-ment, amyloid deposits in the heart may lead to heart failure or arrythmias, and macroglossia and the carpal tunnel syndrome may be present.

The clinical manifestations of plasma cell dyscrasias are in most cases *not* related to the mere presence of an abnormal serum protein. Occasionally, however, clinical manifestations result which reflect the specific physico-chemical properties of the M-component in question. For example, 5 to 10 percent of all patients with myeloma have cryoglobulins (Chap. 70), although not more than a third of these ever become symptomatic, even in the winter. Another group of M-type globulins has the specific property of complexing with other proteins, such as clotting factors, leading to or aggravating an already existing hemorrhagic diathesis. This type of protein-protein complexing has been shown to involve fibrinogen, prothrombin, or Factors V, VII, or VIII.

LABORATORY FINDINGS. Anemia is usually moderate in degree and is normocytic in type. The many factors involved in its genesis include bone marrow replacement, chronic renal disease, decreased red cell survival, chronic infection, and the effects of therapy. The blood smear may show marked tendency to rouleau formation. Poly-chromatophilia, stippling, and normoblasts may be seen. A marked elevation of the erythrocyte sedimentation rate is found in most cases and is often an early clue to the presence of the disease. In the presence of cryoglobulins this may be temperature dependent.

The *bone marrow* usually contains myeloma cells, but their number may range from 3 to 96 percent. The cells frequently occur in clumps or sheets. Sometimes large forms with two or three nuclei may be seen. The individual myeloma cell is moderately large (15 to 30 μ), round or oval, and contains a round nucleus with chromatin that is finer than that of the mature plasma cell and does not show the typical wheel-spoke arrangement. It may contain one or two nucleoli. When Wright's or similar stains are used, the abundant cytoplasmic RNA is responsible for the cell's bright blue color. The perinuclear clear zone, so characteristic of mature plasma cells, often is not seen in myeloma cells. Mitotic figures are sometimes observed, and acidophil cytoplasmic inclusions (Russell bodies) also are described.

Hyperproteinemia due to the presence of an abnormal gamma globulin (M-component) is found in the majority of patients, although about 20 percent of all cases of multiple myeloma show no detectable abnormality in serum proteins. The distribution of various immunoglobulin classes among myeloma proteins is roughly proportional to the concentration of their normal counterparts in the serum. Nearly two-thirds of all myeloma proteins are γG globulins, and the incidence of γA myelomas is less than half that of the γG variety. The abnormal proteins show a similar predominance of κ over λ chains. A few γD myelomas and one case of a γE myeloma have been described. Most patients without serum gamma-globulin spikes excrete L chains in the urine. When renal disease becomes severe enough to substantially affect the clearance of the light chains, they may also appear as a homogeneous spike on serum electrophoresis.

The serum protein abnormalities usually are documented first by paper electrophoresis and then are identified further by immunoelectrophoretic methods. For diagnostic purposes, the contour of electrophoretic patterns is of greater importance than the height of an individual spike; tall, narrow, sharply defined peaks reflect the presence of a detectable quantity of a structurally homogeneous protein and are characteristic of multiple myeloma.

The presence of light chains in the urine is detected best by electrophoresis, which typically reveals an M-component with γ to α_2 mobility present in a concentration greater than that of albumin. The light chains may have the thermal properties of a *Bence-Jones protein* (precipitation at 50 to 60°C and resolubilization at 90 to 100°C). The incidence of positive reactions for Bence-Jones protein is maximal if the pH of the urine is carefully adjusted to 4.5 to 5.0 at all times.

The serum creatinine frequently is elevated because of renal failure. Hypercalcemia due to bone resorption and secondary hyperparathyroidism can be pronounced, and levels of 16 mg per 100 ml are not unusual. The inorganic phosphorus levels are usually normal or elevated and serum alkaline phosphatase activity is normal. Serum uric acid levels often are elevated, because of rapid cellular turnover, but poor renal function also plays a role.

DIAGNOSIS. The bone marrow findings, the typical serum and urinary protein abnormalities, and the characteristic skeletal lesions usually make the diagnosis self-evident. Difficulties may arise when the proper examinations are not carried out in patients with unexplained back pain, recurrent bacterial infections, obscure anemia, or renal failure in the absence of hypertension, retinal changes, or edema. When bony lesions represent the initial finding, they must be differentiated from those of hyperparathyroidism and some cases of metastatic malignancy, especially carcinoma of the breast. When a serum electrophoretic spike is the initial finding in the absence of skeletal lesions, it becomes necessary to consider other causes of monoclonal gammopathies. The differentiation between monoclonal gammopathies and disorders characterized by broad elevations of all gamma-globulins usually presents no special problems.

PROGNOSIS. The prognosis is unfavorable; the median survival is about 1½ years from the time of diagnosis. Only a few patients survive longer than 3 years. The prognosis does not appear to depend on the presence of the abnormal serum protein or on the type of myeloma protein found, but more probably is related primarily to the time at which the diagnosis is made. Asymptomatic cases are recognized now because of greatly simplified methods of diagnosis, and these patients can be expected to survive longer than the average. The patient's clinical status at the time of diagnosis probably provides the best index of prognosis, and significantly shorter survival can be expected in patients with a poor physical performance status, in those with a hemoglobin level of less than 9 Gm per 100 ml, and in those with uremia and hypercalcemia. There is suggestive evidence that patients treated with alkylating agents survive longer than those not receiving this type of therapy, but good statistics are too meager for conclusions to be drawn.

TREATMENT. General Measures. There is little doubt that the patient's comfort and productive life span can be influenced by treatment. Mobilization is a prime objective and often can be achieved by a combination of analgesics, supportive splints, and irradiation of local lesions to alleviate pain and to prevent fractures. Proper hydration must be maintained to prevent renal complications, particularly hypercalcemia and hyperuricemia. Allopurinol is helpful in the control of hyperuricemia (Chap. 106) and steroids in the treatment of hypercalcemia and its complications (Chap. 90). Plasmapheresis is of limited value in multiple myeloma, but is of benefit in the hyperviscosity syndromes (Chap. 70), which are rare in this disease.

Chemotherapy is the treatment of choice. Two alkylating agents, melphalan and cyclophosphamide, hold the greatest promise and are perhaps equally effective. Continuous therapy with dosages sufficient to produce significant leukopenia and/or thrombocytopenia result in considerable improvement in the majority of patients. Criteria for improvement include a significant decrease in marrow myeloma cells and serum M-component levels, an increase in normal immunoglobulin levels and a rise in hemoglobin values. More impressive is the rapid decrease in bone pain and the concomitantly improved performance status reported in a majority of patients treated with effective doses of melphalan. The result of therapy on skeletal lesions is less encouraging. Even after prolonged treatment, actual regression and recalcification of lesions is seen in very few patients, although temporary cessation of further bony destruction may be observed.

Melphalan may be administered in doses of 2 to 4 mg daily. *Cyclophosphamid* is given in daily oral doses of 1 to 4 mg/kg. The patient's leukocyte and platelet counts must be monitored carefully during therapy, lest bone marrow depression become too severe. Leukocyte counts of 2,000 to 2,500 per cu mm usually are considered safe lower limits. Patients with azotemia should not be given more than half the recommended dose until their response to the drug can be assessed. An objective response to therapy may not be seen for 2 to 3 months.

Intermittant therapy with melphalan (0.25 mg/kg/day for 4 days every 6 weeks) in combination with prednisone (1.0 mg/kg in a single dose three times a week) may be superior to continuous drug therapy.

Irradiation is the treatment of choice for the individual bone lesions which frequently become troublesome because of pain, pathologic fractures, or involvement of adjacent structures. It is necessary to restrict the field of therapy and the total dose administered in order to spare the bone marrow. The objectives of x-ray therapy usually are limited and pain relief may be noted with less than 500 r. Seldom are therapeutic doses of more than 1,500 r required. Under careful supervision x-ray therapy may be used in conjunction with chemotherapy.

MACROGLOBULINEMIA

DEFINITION. Primary or Waldenström's macroglobulinemia is defined as a neoplastic plasma cell dyscrasia specifically involving cells which normally synthesize γM macroglobulins and which produce large quantities of an electrophoretically homogeneous protein. The physicochemical properties of this protein are responsible for some of the manifestations of the disease.

CLINICAL MANIFESTATIONS. Waldenströms macroglobulinemia usually is a disease of the elderly. The disorder frequently is mild and is compatible with prolonged survival. Symptoms of vague ill health, weakness, and weight loss are common and may precede the more serious manifestations of recurrent infections, mucosal bleeding, and anemia by many years. In contrast to multiple myeloma, skeletal lesions are very rare, and the clinical features most closely resemble those of a lymphoma, with prominent lymphadenopathy and hepatosplenomegaly.

Symptoms and signs are related to the specific physicochemical properties of some macroglobulins; i.e., their ability to precipitate or gel on cooling, their capacity for increasing serum viscosity at body temperature, and their ability to participate in protein-protein interactions.

When a macroglobulin has the properties of a *cryoglobulin*, the clinical manifestations are those of cold sensitivity, Raynaud's phenomena, and peripheral vascular occlusion precipitated by cold. Patients suffering from the *hyperviscosity syndrome* (Chap. 70) frequently complain of weakness, fatigability, and anorexia. On examination they have dilated retinal veins with areas of localized narrowing, giving these vessels a "link sausage" appearance and leading to visual impairment, fundal hemorrhages, and exudates. Neurologic manifestations ranging from transient paresis to coma are the result of intracerebral vascular occlusion due to hyperviscosity. Similar changes in small vessels elsewhere may result in progressive peripheral neuropathies and myelopathies. *Protein-protein interactions* involve chiefly clotting factors and platelets, and may lead to considerable bleeding from the gastrointestinal tract and other organs.

In some patients with macroglobulinemia the M-protein appears to have the properties of a *cold agglutinin* with antibody specificity for the I-antigen of red cells (Chap. 70). At temperatures below 30°C, these antibodies bind to red cells and fix complement. Varying degrees of hemolysis may be seen, depending on the degree of exposure, the antibody titer, and the specific properties of the individual antibody (Chap. 338).

Amyloidosis has been observed in a few cases of macroglobulinemia and usually is of the secondary variety, involving chiefly the liver, spleen, and other parenchymal organs.

LABORATORY FINDINGS. Anemia due to inadequate production, decreased survival, and bleeding is found in over 80 percent of all cases. Cold agglutinins may be present, and the Coombs test may be positive. Neutropenia and thrombocytopenia occur, and a relative lymphocytosis is the rule. The erythrocyte sedimentation rate is usually markedly elevated, and a characteristic M-component is found on serum electrophoresis (Chap. 70). Cryoglobulins, when present, are easily detected by cooling. Serum viscosity is readily measured and serves as a useful index to the progress of the disease or its therapy. Bence-Jones proteinuria is seen occasionally.

DIAGNOSIS. The salient diagnostic features have been outlined above. The bone marrow is characteristically packed with small lymphoid cells more closely resembling lymphocytes than plasma cells. Many naked nuclei and a considerable number of mast cells also are seen. Similar cells are found in lymph nodes and aspirates of liver and spleen.

PROGNOSIS AND THERAPY. Both very malignant and extremely benign forms of macroglobulinemia are found, and survival after diagnosis ranges from several months to 12 years. The average life expectancy is about 3.5 years.

The serious manifestations of increased serum viscosity, bleeding diathesis, and severe depression of the bone marrow constitute the main indications for therapy. The most acute problems are usually those related to hyperviscosity. Because more than 70 percent of the macroglobulins are found in the intravascular compartment and the rate of macroglobulin synthesis is fixed, plasmapheresis is an extremely effective means of controlling symptoms of hyperviscosity on an emergency or even a long-range basis. The administration of alkylating agents such as chlorambucil or cyclophosphamide constitutes the method of choice for long-range therapy. Dosage schedules similar to those used in chronic lymphocytic leukemia (Chap. 348) seem to be adequate. In this way, many patients are maintained in remission.

HEAVY CHAIN DISEASE

Heavy chain disease, first described by Franklin in 1963, is a plasma cell dyscrasia characterized by the production of large amounts of a relatively homogeneous polypeptide closely related to the Fc fragment obtained by papain cleavage of nomral γG globulins. Only a few cases have been described.

Weakness and weight loss are common complaints, and marked susceptibility to infection is a characteristic feature. Transient, though sometimes severe, palatal edema and erythema, similar to that seen in infectious mononucleosis, have been noted in some patients. The physical findings of adenopathy and hepatosplenomegaly suggest a lymphoma. Lytic lesions of bones, the hallmark of multiple myeloma, have not been described.

Anemia usually is moderate, and relative lymphocytosis, eosinophilia, and moderate thrombocytopenia have been noted. The lymphocytes sometimes are atypical or plasmacytoid. Atypical or immature plasma cells and lymphocytes are the dominant cellular elements in bone marrow aspirates and lymph node sections, although reticulum cells and eosinophils are seen frequently Hyperuricemia has been described in all cases.

The serum concentration of the abnormal protein has ranged between 0.3 and 4.3 Gm per 100 ml and is usually associated with a considerable decrease in the concentration of normal immunoglobulins. The M-component has a sedimentation coefficient of 3.6 to 3.9, which corresponds to the sedimentation coefficient of Fc fragments produced by papain digestion of γG. The antigenic characteristics of the abnormal protein also correspond to those of its normal Fc counterpart.

Proteinuria appears to be a universal feature and may be the first finding to focus attention on the possibility of an underlying plasma cell dyscrasia. The urinary protein is not an L chain of the Bence-Jones type, but rather has the same electrophoretic and antigenic characteristics as the abnormal constituent in serum. The amount of protein excreted may vary from 50 mg to 15 Gm per day.

Survival from the onset of symptoms has ranged from 4 months to several years. Short-lived remissions with hematologic improvement have been described after irradiation of spleen and lymph nodes. Alkylating agents apparently are effective in temporarily reducing adenopathy and hepatosplenomegaly, but adequate trials have not been carried out.

MONOCLONAL GAMMOPATHY OF UNKNOWN SIGNIFICANCE

Benign, Essential, Monoclonal Gammopathy, Dysimmunoglobulinemia

The introduction of serum electrophoretic procedures as routine diagnostic tools has led to the discovery of many patients with typical M-components in their serum but without other signs or symptoms referable to this finding. Although some patients with this abnormality have been observed for many years without developing evidence of myeloma, macroglobulinemia, or other serious disease, a few have developed typical myeloma after asymptomatic periods as long as 2 decades. Whether all monoclonal gammopathies of this type represent early stages of one of the more virulent plasma cell dyscrasias is unanswered.

Although mild anemia and susceptibility to infection have been described in some patients with monoclonal gammopathy of unknown significance, this is the exception rather than the rule, and serious complications, such as renal disease, hyperviscosity syndromes, and the effects of protein-protein interactions, have not been reported. The hyperglobulinemia is usually moderate in degree and is extremely stable over many years. These monoclonal gammopathies are most commonly seen in the elderly, and have been reported with increasing frequency in people over seventy.

Sometimes monoclonal gammopathies are seen in patients suffering from chronic disorders such as nonreticular neoplasms, "myeloproliferative disorders," and chronic infections. These patients are usually elderly and the association is most likely coincidental. Where it has been possible to remove nonreticular neoplasms by apparently curative procedures, the serum protein abnormality has persisted in all instances.

Despite the eventual appearance of multiple myeloma in some patients with monoclonal gammopathies, therapy with alkylating agents does not appear to be warranted.

REFERENCES

Alexanian, R., et al.: Treatment for Multiple Myeloma, JAMA, 208:1680, 1969.

Carbone, P. P., L. E. Kellerhouse, and E. A. Gehan: Plasmacytic Myeloma, Am. J. Med., 42:937, 1967.

Fahey, J. L.: Serum Protein Disorders Causing Clinical Symptoms in Malignant Neoplastic Disease, J. Chron. Dis., 16:703, 1963.

Franklin, E. C., T. Lowenstein, B. Bigelow, and M. Meltzer: Heavy Chain Disease—A New Disorder of Serum Gamma Globulins, Am. J. Med., 37:332, 1964.

Osserman, E. F.: Plasma Cell Myeloma II. Clinical Aspects. New Engl. J. Med., 261:952 and 1006, 1959.

——: Plasma Cell Myeloma: Gamma Globulin Synthesis and Structure, Medicine, 42:357, 1963.

Waldenström, J.: Macroglobulinemia, Advan. Metab. Disor., 2:115, 1965.

Wintrobe, M. M.: "Clinical Hematology," 6th ed., Philadelphia, Lea & Febiger, 1967.

350 DISEASES OF THE SPLEEN AND RETICULOENDOTHELIAL SYSTEM

M. M. Wintrobe and D. R. Boggs

The functions of the spleen were outlined in an earlier chapter (Chap. 63). Disorders of the spleen most frequently produce enlargement of this organ. The significance of splenic enlargement and the differential diagnosis of splenomegaly were discussed in Chap. 63. Here several disorders which involve the spleen will be described which have not been discussed hitherto.

Congenital anomalies of the spleen may take various forms. Instead of being a single organ, the spleen may be subdivided into numerous small spleens, or a spleen of normal size and shape may be accompanied by an accessory spleen, or more than one. Rarely, the spleen assumes a retroperitoneal position and may force the left kidney downward. A *movable* spleen may be found in any part of the abdomen. If its pedicle becomes twisted, there may be sudden pain, enlargement, and signs of shock, as well as fever and vomiting if the torsion has developed acutely. Less severe symptoms occur if the process is more gradual.

Rupture of the spleen may occur following trauma, particularly if the spleen is diseased. Malaria, typhoid fever, leukemia, and infectious mononucleosis are among the diseases in which this has been observed. Agonizing abdominal pain or pain in the left scapular region, together with signs of internal hemorrhage, characterize this catastrophe. When subcapsular hemorrhage develops with the original trauma, rupture may be delayed for a few hours. Anemia develops rapidly, and leukocytosis occurs. Prompt surgical treatment is imperative. After traumatic rupture autotransplantation of splenic tissue (*splenosis*) sometimes occurs.

Infarction of the spleen may be sterile, in which event it is followed eventually by fibrosis and shrinkage. This has been observed as a complication of leukemia, as well as in sickle-cell anemia and the sickle-cell trait, and in sickle-cell–hemoglobin C disease. A septic infarct may terminate with the formation of an abscess. The most common symptom of infarction is pain. Careful examination will reveal a friction rub. Unless an abscess forms, necessitating surgical intervention, sedation and abdominal support to impair movement of the spleen suffice.

Aneurysms of the splenic artery are rare but may cause vague, crampy pain in the left upper part of the abdomen and even splenic enlargement. Occasionally the aneurysm is palpable and a bruit may be heard. Found predominantly in women and most frequently after middle age, rupture has been reported during pregnancy.

Congenital absence of the spleen may be suspected when Howell-Jolly bodies, occasional nucleated red cells, target cells, decreased osmotic fragility, siderocytosis, leukocytosis, and a variable degree of thrombocytosis are found in the absence of a discoverable cause and particularly when there is associated congenital heart or intestinal malformation.

CHRONIC CONGESTIVE SPLENOMEGALY

DEFINITION. This syndrome, also called *Banti's syndrome* or *splenic anemia*, is characterized by splenic enlargement, leukopenia, anemia and often thrombocytopenia, a tendency to gastric hemorrhage, and, in many cases, cirrhotic changes in the liver.

HISTORY. The term *splenic anemia* was originally used (1866) to refer to cases of anemia with splenomegaly which were not frank leukemia. Banti, in 1882 and subsequently, described a form of splenomegaly of unknown cause associated in its earliest stages with leukopenia, asthenia, and occasional hemorrhagic episodes. In the intermediary stage, hepatic enlargement occurred, as well as urobilinuria and a dirty-brownish discoloration of the skin. The final stage consisted of liver atrophy and ascites.

ETIOLOGY. Banti described the spleen as being characterized by conspicuous thickening of the fibrillar reticulum in the Malpighian corpuscles and red pulp ("fibroadenie"). These changes originated around the central artery of the follicle. In his opinion, the spleen was the primary seat of the disease. Later work showed that these changes are not specific and can be encountered particularly when there is increased venous pressure in the portal bed. That there is portal hypertension has been demonstrated by measurement (225 to 500 mm, or more, of water), and now most students of this syndrome consider the portal hypertension to be due to intrahepatic causes such as Laennec's cirrhosis or schistosomiasis, or to extrahepatic factors. Thus the designation *chronic congestive splenomegaly* has arisen. Cirrhosis of the liver, cavernous transformation of the portal vein, portal vein and splenic vein thrombosis, or variants in the anatomy of the venous pattern have been found in as many as 60 percent of the cases. Rarer causes are compression from pancreatic fibrosis or tumor or from an aneurysm of the splenic artery.

The hematologic changes observed in the Banti syndrome are attributable to the unequal distribution of the cells of the blood in the splenic vascular bed and the remaining parts of the circulation resulting from stasis of the portal circulation. Following splenectomy the blood values usually return to normal.

PATHOLOGY. The spleen weighs 600 to 1,200 Gm as a rule, but may weigh as much as 5,000 Gm. At first one finds an increase in the reticulum, cellular hyperplastic pulp, degenerative changes in the follicular arterioles, and congestion. Later the follicles become smaller, while fibrosis of the reticulum, trabeculae, and capsule increases. Periarterial hemorrhages and siderotic nodules deposited in the fibrous tissue around the arterioles are found in many instances.

SYMPTOMS. The symptoms are primarily those of the

underlying conditions and include all the various manifestations of hepatic failure or of congestive heart failure when these conditions are responsible for congestive splenomegaly. However, in a few patients, the initial symptoms may direct attention to the spleen itself. In such patients, the symptoms of anemia may be prominent, or a large mass in the left upper quadrant of the abdomen may be noted. In other instances the disorder may be announced explosively by the occurrence of a gastric hemorrhage.

The anemia is normocytic and moderate in degree unless hemorrhage has occurred, when it may be microcytic and hypochromic. In cases with long-standing and severe liver disease the anemia may be macrocytic. Leukopenia is found consistently, and thrombocytopenia is observed frequently. The bone marrow may show no abnormality, or slight myeloid hyperplasia may be present.

DIAGNOSIS. Other conditions leading to pancytopenia (Chap. 64) must be excluded, as well as the various causes of splenomegaly (Chap. 63). Even when gastrointestinal hemorrhage has occurred, the diagnosis should be made only after other possibilities have been excluded. Thus, a "silent" peptic ulcer may produce hypochromic microcytic anemia with slight splenic enlargement. Hookworm infection may produce chronic hypochromic anemia with moderate splenomegaly. Liver function should be studied in suspected cases, and esophageal varices should be looked for. Liver biopsy, roentgenographic examination with barium, and endoscopic study of the esophagus may be required. If liver function is good and other conditions have been excluded, portal or splenic vein thrombosis should be suspected. If a block is suspected, its site should be determined, if possible, by portal venography. Congestive splenomegaly due to extrahepatic causes is more likely to be found in patients below the age of eighteen than in older patients.

PROGNOSIS AND TREATMENT. In general, the large spleen and the associated hematologic abnormalities pose less of a threat to these patients than does hepatic failure or bleeding from gastric or esophageal varices. Splenectomy often leads to improvement or correction of anemia, neutropenia, and thrombocytopenia but is of little value in relieving portal hypertension. Therefore splenectomy as the sole surgical measure should be limited to such rare causes of congestive splenomegaly as splenic vein thrombosis or aneurysm of the splenic artery. In other circumstances, splenectomy should rarely be considered except in conjunction with a shunting operation designed to relieve the increased portal pressure. Portacaval shunt is usually preferred because of the large size of the vessels involved. If a large-caliber splenic vein is available or when the portal vein is obliterated, splenectomy and splenorenal shunts are recommended.

The risks of surgery in these patients are substantial, and surgical intervention is advocated only (1) in cases in which there is severe bleeding from the upper part of the intestine and in which the portal hypertension is due to extrahepatic block; and (2) in cases of portal

hypertension associated with cirrhosis of the liver where ascites and icterus are minimal or absent and there is a reasonable degree of hepatic reserve.

HYPERSPLENISM

The concept that the spleen may produce disease as the result of an exaggeration of its normal functions is based on the observation that anemia, leukopenia, or thrombocytopenia, or combinations of these manifestations, whether in association with specific disease entities or idiopathic, and usually in association with splenomegaly, may disappear following splenectomy. When the above-mentioned hematologic manifestations accompany recognizable disease entities the hypersplenism is "secondary;" otherwise it is "primary." According to this concept, the destructive potential of the spleen has increased or, in other cases, its hypothetic inhibitory effect on the bone marrow has become exaggerated. "Autoimmune" acquired hemolytic anemia and idiopathic thrombocytopenic purpura are examples of conditions which some investigators would classify as forms of hypersplenism. Although a helpful concept, use of the term has led to loose thinking and careless diagnosis. As outlined earlier (Chap. 63), the functions of the spleen are poorly understood.

"BIG SPLEEN SYNDROME." Well-marked splenomegaly accompanying a variety of diseases, such as lupus erythematosus, sarcoidosis, malignant lymphoma, chronic lymphocytic leukemia, myelofibrosis, and Gaucher's disease may be associated with moderate or marked anemia, together with moderate reticulocytosis (5 to 10 percent) and erythroid hyperplasia of the bone marrow. Overt signs of exaggerated blood destruction are not necessarily present. Counts over the spleen following tagging of the patient's own red cells with ^{51}Cr may indicate increased radioactivity there. In such cases there also may be leukopenia (due mainly to granulocytopenia) and thrombocytopenia. In other cases the granulocytopenia is the most prominent manifestation, as in Felty's syndrome and in kala-azar. Splenectomy has been observed in some of these cases to be associated with disappearance of the hematologic manifestations in whole or in part.

Thrombocytopenia in association with splenomegaly probably indicates that an increased proportion of the total body platelet pool is sequestered in the spleen, without a reduction in the size of the total platelet pool. Anemia accompanying splenomegaly may also be explained in part by increased splenic sequestration of red cells, but also is due, in part, to an increase in plasma volume. However, an increased rate of destruction of normal red cells may contribute to the anemia. As noted in Chap. 63, most red cells move rapidly through a normal spleen. Studies employing red cells labeled with radioactive chromium indicate not only increased splenic sequestration, but also a very slow splenic transit time for a portion of the sequestered cells. These slowly circulating, closely packed, sequestered red cells may have insufficient glucose available for glycolytic energy production and, as a consequence, suffer membrane damage and destruction.

MYELOFIBROSIS

DEFINITION. This term refers to a disorder characterized by splenomegaly, often of great proportion, together with varying degrees of fibrosis or osteosclerosis of the marrow cavity. Extramedullary blood formation is found in the spleen. *Agnogenic myeloid metaplasia, myeloid megakaryocytic hepatosplenomegaly,* and *chronic nonleukemic myelosis* are among the other names which have been used for this syndrome.

ETIOLOGY AND PATHOGENESIS. Most instances are idiopathic, and while the idiopathic form may occur at any age, most patients are more than fifty years of age. Both sexes are affected in approximately equal proportion. Occasionally myelofibrosis has developed following what has appeared to be typical chronic myelocytic leukemia, but sometimes the converse has been observed; namely, marked myeloid leukocytosis and other changes typical of chronic myelocytic leukemia have developed in patients whose findings previously had suggested myelofibrosis. A similar paradoxic relationship to polycythemia vera has been observed. Such cases have led to elaboration of the concept of *myeloproliferative disorders.* By this term, it is implied that myeloid leukemia, acute and chronic, polycythemia vera, myelofibrosis, and even "essential thrombocythemia" and the di Guglielmo syndrome (Chap. 348) result from overgrowth of all or some of the types of cells which are normally formed in the bone marrow and can be produced in sites where extramedullary blood formation occurs, such as the spleen. It is argued that one or more of the marrow elements may be produced in excess and that the bone marrow, initially hyperplastic, ultimately becomes fibrotic. The overlapping of the clinical and hematologic manifestations of these diseases which is seen occasionally gives support to the concept, but in the great majority of cases the manifestations and course of the various disorders named above are sufficiently distinct to permit a more specific diagnosis. Since the nature of the fundamental disturbance in these conditions is unknown and may be similar or quite different, the value of the term *myeloproliferative disorder* may be questioned. However, it does give comfort to those who gain security from having a name.

Myelofibrosis may follow chronic exposure to benzene and carbon tetrachloride, phosphorus poisoning, or irradiation exposure, as observed in radium-dial painters and atomic bomb survivors. Patients with tuberculosis and with carcinoma have developed a myelofibrosis-like syndrome, seemingly as a complication of their primary disease.

The pathogenesis of the anemia in myelofibrosis was discussed earlier (Chap. 61). It must be presumed that blood formation in this disease is not confined to the spleen, as was once assumed, since splenectomy has been carried out in some cases without serious aggravation of the disease resulting.

PATHOLOGY. The fibrosis is irregular and may be interspersed with fatty areas or even with marrow hyperplasia. It tends to be greatest in the flat bones and in time may become more pronounced. In certain patients, marrow fibrosis may be difficult to demonstrate in the early stages of disease. In such patients marrow aspirates are usually quite cellular and often contain increased numbers of megakaryocytes. The spleen tends to increase in size and may become huge. Extramedullary hematopoiesis is prominent, especially in the pulp, but areas of fibrosis and infarction may be found as well. Myeloid metaplasia may also be present in the liver, lymph nodes, kidneys, perirenal fat, or other sites.

CLINICAL MANIFESTATIONS. Weakness, fatigue, and ultimately, an awareness of a left-upper-quadrant mass are the usual complaints. Weight loss, sometimes anorexia, and episodes of abdominal pain from splenic infarction and perisplenitis, as well as pallor and gradual enlargement of the liver, ensue. Less commonly there may be arthralgia, bone pain, intolerance to heat, fever, and dependent edema, and even ascites and gastrointestinal hemorrhage.

Normal and even high hemoglobin values early in the course of the disease are followed by the development of anemia, which may become severe. Marked poikilocytosis is a feature, and some investigators consider "teardrop" poikilocytes characteristic. Polychromatophilia, occasional normoblasts, and reticulocytosis are additional features of the blood smear. Leukocytosis, with some shift to the left, is the rule, but the leukocyte count may be normal or low. In contrast to chronic myelocytic leukemia, the leukocytes stain heavily with the alkaline phosphatase stain in most, but not all, patients. Thrombocytosis and the presence of large and bizarre platelets are common, but ultimately, thrombocytopenia may occur. Serum uric acid usually is elevated.

DIAGNOSIS. The dry tap on marrow examination contrasts with the finding in chronic myelocytic leukemia, as does the usual finding of increased leukocyte alkaline phosphatase. Trephine biopsy confirms the inactive state of the marrow. With one exception, the Philadelphia chromosome abnormality which is common in chronic myelocytic leukemia has not been observed in marrow cells from patients with myelofibrosis. Roentgenographic evidence of myelofibrosis or osteosclerosis is found only in about 40 percent of the cases. Other causes of splenomegaly should be ruled out, as discussed elsewhere (Chap. 63).

PROGNOSIS AND TREATMENT. The course is slow but is likely to be progressive. The great majority of patients survive 3 to 5 years, a few even 10 years or longer. Transfusion may be needed if the anemia is severe but should be held to a minimum. Busulfan, 2 to 4 mg per day, may reduce the leukocyte count, size of the spleen, and the transfusion requirement but must be used cautiously to avoid serious depression of hematopoietic activity. Large doses of androgenic hormone (testosterone enanthate, 400 to 600 mg intramuscularly once a week) may relieve the anemia, but thrombocytopenia, if present, is less likely to be affected. If the transfusion requirement is very great, evidence of excessive splenic destruction should be sought by external counting over the spleen and liver following ^{51}Cr tagging of the red cells. Irradiation over the spleen to reduce its size is of limited value. When increased blood destruction is very troublesome and not relieved by other measures, as described above, splenectomy may be found to reduce the transfusion needs.

Death is usually due to infection, hemorrhage, or thrombosis, and a few patients die with a picture closely resembling acute myeloblastic leukemia.

GAUCHER'S DISEASE

DEFINITION. This is a rare, chronic familial disorder in which cerebrosides accumulate in reticuloendothelial cells. It is characterized by marked splenomegaly and often also by skin pigmentation, pingueculae of the scleras, and bone lesions. In infants progressive neurologic disturbances occur and are usually associated with a rapidly fatal course.

ETIOLOGY, MORBID ANATOMY, AND PATHOGENESIS. The disease may develop at any age. There is no clear sex predilection, but an unusual proportion of cases have occurred in Jewish families. However, other Caucasians, Negroes, and Orientals may be affected. Apparently a hereditable disorder, there nevertheless is uncertainty about the mode of inheritance. The observation that in many instances the mode of inheritance was mendelian recessive whereas in others it was dominant has led to the suggestion that more than one defect may be responsible for the disorder which ultimately becomes manifest. The clinical pattern is very similar in all affected members of any sibship.

The characteristic finding is widespread reticulum cell hyperplasia, these cells being filled with large amounts of glucocerebrosides. Although the exact metabolic defect has not been demonstrated, it would appear that there may be a specific deficiency of a hydrolase enzyme which is responsible for cleaving glucocerebroside. Cerebrosides which are normally present in tissues other than the brain are predominantly glucocerebrosides and appear to be identical to those found in Gaucher's cells. Thus, the disease may represent failure of a normal pattern of breakdown of glucocerebrosides. The reticulum cell hyperplasia may represent a compensatory response designed to provide storage space for this substance.

The cells are distinctive, being 20 to 80 μ in diameter, round, oval, or spindle-shaped, and possessing one or more small, eccentrically placed nuclei. The cytoplasm shows numerous wavy fibrillae, best seen on supravital preparations with the aid of phase microscopy. The cells are found in the spleen, bone marrow, lymph nodes, and liver. The spleen may weigh as much as several thousand grams.

Gaucher's cells are found throughout the body, and infiltration of the lungs, kidneys, thymus, tonsils, thyroid, adrenals, and lymphoid tissue of the intestinal tract has been described. They are scattered diffusely throughout the marrow and, in some areas, form tumorlike accumulations which may expand and erode the cortex, thereby producing lesions demonstrable radiographically.

In infants ganglion cell destruction, glial proliferation, and demyelination may be found in the brain although abnormal cerebroside content has not been demonstrated.

CLINICAL MANIFESTATIONS. Manifestations may appear at any age. Gaucher's disease has been recognized as early as the first week of life and as late as seventy-nine years of age. When it appears within the first 6 months of life, however, the course is relatively acute. Splenomegaly may be the first sign, but this is followed quickly by neurologic deficits which often include extraocular palsies and retroflexion of the head as the disease progresses to a fatal course within 1 to 2 years.

In the majority of cases, usually those appearing after six months of age, the progression is slow and there is little or no evidence of neurologic involvement. Splenomegaly, attended by mechanical discomfort, may be the only outstanding manifestation. Infarction or rupture of the spleen is uncommon. The liver may be enlarged, but the lymph nodes are usually not palpable. Pain in the limbs, due to involvement of bone by expanding marrow elements, is common. Pathologic fractures may occur. Roentgenographic changes are visible, the development of a radiolucent area in the lower end of the femur in the contour of an Erlenmeyer flask being a typical lesion. A hemorrhagic tendency secondary to thrombocytopenia is common and may be the presenting sign. Yellow-brown pingueculae on the conjunctiva on either side of the cornea and similar pigmentation on the exposed areas of the skin may be seen in adults.

In practically every case plasma acid phosphatase activity is increased when measured with phenylphosphate as substrate. In contrast to the prostatic enzyme, the acid phosphatase activity is not inhibited by L-tartrate. Other blood findings, as in other splenic disorders, include moderate anemia, leukopenia, and thrombocytopenia. Plasma cerebroside levels may be elevated in patients following splenectomy.

DIAGNOSIS. Diagnosis can be made by sternal or splenic puncture, which will reveal the characteristic cells. Phase microscopy of supravital marrow preparations reveals these unique cells to best advantage. Confirmation by tissue lipid analyses showing accumulation of glucocerebrosides is desirable.

TREATMENT AND PROGNOSIS. Although the disease coincidentally involves other parts of the reticuloendothelial system, splenectomy is worthwhile if the spleen is very large and thereby causes discomfort, or if there are serious symptoms attributable to the blood changes. Bone pain may respond to steroid therapy or to radiation. In infants the prognosis is not good, but patients who have survived to adolescence may live for many years even if splenectomy is not performed.

NIEMANN–PICK DISEASE

DEFINITION. This is a rare familial disorder, first described in 1914, in which sphingomyelin (ceramidephosphoryl-choline) and cholesterol accumulate in reticuloendothelial cells throughout the body. Hepatomegaly and retarded nervous and physical development are usually observed within the first 6 months of life, and death from inanition or intercurrent infection usually occurs within 1 to 3 years.

ETIOLOGY AND PATHOGENESIS. The disease is apparently inherited as a simple mendelian recessive trait, both sexes being equally involved. The disease has not been observed in more than one generation in a single pedigree. Over half the reported cases have been in Jews, but many other ethnic groups have been involved. Inbreeding may be the cause of the high incidence among the groups involved.

The characteristic "foam cells" are reticuloendothelial cells, 20 to 90 μ in diameter, and are so filled with vacuoles that they have a mulberry appearance. The nucleus is small and is placed excentrically but may be multiple. The vacuoles have a faint bluish hue with Wright's stain, are periodic acid–Schiff positive, and stain with Sudan III and other fat stains. Although these properties are not specific for sphingomyelin, it is assumed that this substance is contained in the vacuoles. These cells may be found everywhere but are especially prominent in the spleen, liver, lymph nodes, and bone marrow. Such tissues contain increased amounts of sphingomyelin, even ten- to fortyfold, increased cholesterol, and moderately increased non-sphingosine-containing phospholipids. These findings have led to the hypothesis that the underlying defect is a fault in sphingomyelin metabolism, perhaps a deficiency of sphingomyelinase.

Swelling, vacuolization, and degeneration of Nissl substance are found in the ganglion cells of the nervous system. There are also demyelination, scarring and fibrosis, and proliferation of glial cells which become converted to foam cells. In the retina destruction of ganglion cells in the surrounding area may leave a grayish background, against which the macula stands out as a "cherry-red spot." Although the anatomic changes in the nervous system resemble closely those in Tay-Sachs disease (Chap. 364), these two diseases are distinctly separate entities.

CLINICAL MANIFESTATIONS. The earliest sign usually is a poor feeding pattern in infants. In addition to hepatosplenomegaly there may be generalized lymphadenopathy, infiltrative lesions in the lung visible by x-ray, xanthomatous or infiltrative lesions of the skin, and skin pigmentation. Nutrition is poor and physical development is retarded. A relentless and widely varied pattern of neurologic disturbances follows (Chap. 364) until a nearly vegetative state is reached before death, which occurs in 1 to 3 years. However, in a few instances, the disease may develop more slowly and changes may be present for years in the absence of neurologic signs. Affected children may live to late adolescence and occasionally may reach adulthood. The cherry-red spot, which is seen in only about one-half the cases, may cause visual impairment.

Anemia and thrombocytopenia are usually moderate in degree. The leukocyte count usually is normal but may be increased or low. The lymphocytes and monocytes may show some vacuolization, but adequate histochemical studies of their contents have not been made.

Roentgenography may reveal diffuse miliary pulmonary mottling. Trabecular coarseness is demonstrable in the long bones, as well as widening and prominence of the medullary cavities and undermineralization.

DIAGNOSIS. There are no characteristic laboratory tests. Slight hyperlipemia is common, but plasma sphingomyelin levels are normal. The appearance of the foam cells, usually obtained by marrow aspiration, affords a tentative diagnosis. Biopsy of rectal mucosa showing changes in the ganglion cells of the myenteric plexus may also be helpful. A positive Smith-Dietrich stain is usually obtained, but specific histochemical tests for sphingomyelin are not available. Similar clinical and morphologic findings have been obtained in one family in which the stored lipid was a lipid phosphatide other than sphingomyelin. Diagnosis is made by lipid analysis of involved tissues. Cells from bone marrow propagated in tissue culture also contain excessive sphingomyelin, and such cells may be examined for confirmation when sufficient biopsy material is not available otherwise.

TREATMENT. There is no specific therapy, but x-ray therapy may be helpful in control of infiltrative skin lesions. Splenectomy is of little value.

HISTIOCYTOSIS X

Pathologic lesions containing common features in various degrees have led to the grouping of *Letterer-Siwe disease, Hand-Schüller-Christian disease,* and *eosinophilic granuloma* under a single heading, *histiocytosis X.* The common denominator is a distinctive, inflammatory histiocytosis. Reticuloendothelial proliferation and hyperplasia and granulomatous changes, featuring eosinophils and giant cells, are followed by the conversion of reticulum cells and histiocytes to foam cells or xanthomas containing cholesterol and its esters. Ultimately fibrosis may occur. The similarity in pathologic picture does not prove etiologic identity, however, and the relationship of these disorders to one another must as yet be considered unproved.

These three disorders differ in the sites of involvement and the predominating stage of tissue reaction. In these conditions, lipid accumulation is a secondary and inconsistent feature, and there is no clear-cut tendency for familial involvement. The nature of the underlying defect is unknown.

LETTERER–SIWE DISEASE

This has been observed most often in infants and young children, is variable in duration (a few weeks to several years), and has usually proved fatal. There is evidence of a wasting disorder, with enlargement of the spleen and liver, generalized lymphadenopathy, a hemorrhagic diathesis, especially petechiae and purpura, skeletal lesions, progressive anemia, and cutaneous manifestations. The last consist of discrete, yellowish-brown maculopapular lesions, or papules with a red border and yellow center. They are scattered over the face and trunk particularly, but may be found in the scalp and elsewhere. Whitish macules over the palate and tongue and weeping erosions in the axillas and other moist areas may develop. There may be a low-grade, persistent spiking fever. Diffuse histiocytic proliferation may occur in the lungs. Localized bone destruction may occur, especially in the calvarium.

Diagnosis is made by biopsy of bone or lymph nodes. The course is relatively acute, and secondary precipitation of cholesterol esters in histiocytes to form foam cells usually does not occur. *Treatment* involves supportive care, irradiation of the skin lesions and other areas of involvement, and antimicrobial therapy for secondary infections, as they occur. The disease is usually fatal, termination often being similar to that of acute leukemia. Steroid therapy or vinblastine (Chap. 348) may be helpful. Rarely, recovery occurs or a more chronic picture develops, as seen in Schüller-Christian disease.

HAND–SCHÜLLER–CHRISTIAN DISEASE

This may represent in chronic form the same disorder which, in acute or subacute form, presents the picture of Letterer-Siwe disease. Occurring predominantly in children, Schüller-Christian disease may also be found in adults, rarely in older persons. The pathologic feature is a histiocytic granuloma. The histiocytosis or granulomatosis may or may not be accompanied by intense eosinophilic reaction; the characteristic lipogranuloma is now thought to be the late phase in the evolution of the histiocytic lesion. The histiocytes contain so much cholesterol that they have the appearance of foam cells. The granulomas are found in bones, especially the skull, and in skin and viscera. Thereby the characteristic triad, rarely observed together in the same patient, of exophthalmos, diabetes insipidus, and defects in the membranous bones is produced. In the scalp soft-tissue nodules overlying the cranial defects may be palpated.

Xanthoma disseminatum is a cutaneous manifestation that may or may not be associated with bone and visceral lesions. The yellowish-brown maculopapular lesions are most frequently scattered over the face, especially the eyes and mouth, trunk and perineum, and in the axillae. They may occur in the mouth. Histologically they reveal foam cells and intensive histiocytic proliferation with or without eosinophils. The lesions are not painful but tend to recur when removed surgically. Fibrotic lesions associated with extracellular lipid deposits located under the tongue and in the pharynx and larynx, so-called *lipid proteinosis*, may represent an end stage of xanthoma disseminatum.

Visceral lesions may occur in the liver, spleen, kidneys, perirenal fat, walls of the larger blood vessels, brain, and lungs. There may be diffuse pulmonary infiltration, but more often it is perihilar or central. Hepatosplenomegaly and lymph node enlargement are usually modest and anemia is usually mild, but pancytopenia may occur. Although tissue cholesterol may be many times greater than normal, the plasma cholesterol level is normal.

Growth may be retarded and puberty delayed. Otitis media is a common complication. The course waxes and wanes irregularly, and spontaneous remissions occur. The skeletal lesions may respond to x-ray, but widespread radiation of chronic relapsing lesions usually produces more harmful side effects than benefit. Large doses of steroid may reverse all manifestations of the disease temporarily and can produce remissions of at least several years' duration. Vinblastine (Chap. 348) may have some value. From 15 to 30 percent of cases terminate fatally, but complete recovery may occur. Diabetes insipidus is likely to persist, however, and pulmonary lesions may produce alveolo-capillary block, pulmonary insufficiency, or right-sided heart failure. Rarely the disease becomes more acute, then resembling Letterer-Siwe disease.

EOSINOPHILIC GRANULOMA

This is the most benign of these conditions. It is characterized by single or multiple granulomas and osteolytic lesions with no discernible associated visceral involvement. Found in infants, children, and young adults, eosinophilic granuloma occasionally is seen at a later age. The condition is somewhat more common in males than in females and is rare in Negroes. The eosinophilic and histiocytic proliferation begins in the bone marrow but gradually erodes the cortex until the bone expands. Roentgenologically lytic lesions can be demonstrated within the medullary cavity, about 1 to 4 cm in diameter and with borders less distinct than those of bone cysts. In patients over the age of twenty years the lesions are found almost exclusively in the flat bones. At an earlier age they may also be present in long bones, especially the femur or humerus. The swellings may be silent, or there may be pain and swelling at the site of involvement. Rarely there is mild fever, but usually there are no constitutional symptoms. Pathologic fractures may occur. The blood is normal. Eosinophilia is unusual.

The granulomas may remain unchanged for years, but eventually, at least in some patients, fibrosis develops, eosinophils disappear, and the histiocytes become lipophages. Solitary granulomas are best treated by curettement or excision. Irradiation is reserved for lesions that are inaccessible to such therapy. The results are usually good, and the prognosis is excellent.

When multiple lesions occur, and especially when they are extraosseous, the distinction from milder forms of Schüller-Christian disease is unclear, and perhaps unimportant.

REFERENCES

Avery, Mary Ellen, J. G. McAfee, and Harriet G. Guild: The Course and Prognosis of Reticuloendotheliosis (Eosinophilic Granuloma, Schüller-Christian Disease and Letterer-Siwe Disease), Am. J. Med., 22:636, 1957.

Avioli, L. V., J. T. Lasersohn, and J. M. LoPresti: Histiocytosis X (Schüller-Christian Disease): A Clinicopathological Survey, Review of Ten Patients and the Results of Prednisone Therapy, Medicine, 42:119, 1963.

Crocker, A. C., and S. Farber: Niemann-Pick Disease, Medicine, 37:1, 1958; Am. J. Clin. Nutrition, 9:63, 1961.

Fredrickson, D. S.: in "The Metabolic Basis of Inherited Disease," 2d ed., J. B. Stanbury, J. B. Wyngaarden, and

D. S. Fredrickson (Eds.), New York, McGraw-Hill Book Company, 1966.

Lichtenstein, L.: Histiocytosis X: Integration of Eosinophilic Granuloma of Bone, "Letterer-Siwe Disease," and "Schüller-Christian Disease" as Related Manifestations of a Single Nosologic Entity, A.M.A. Arch. Pathol., 56:84, 1953.

MacPherson, A. I. S.: Assessment of the Results of Surgical Treatment in Portal Hypertension, Gastroenterology, 38: 142, 1960.

Medoff, A. S., and E. D. Bayrd: Gaucher's Disease in 29 Cases: Hematologic Complications and Effect of Splenectomy, Ann. Internal Med., 40:481, 1954.

Motulsky, A. G., F. Casserd, E. R. Giblett, G. O. Broun, Jr., and C. A. Finch: Anemia and the Spleen, New Eng. J. Med., 259:1164 and 1215, 1958.

Pitcock, J. A., E. H. Reinhard, B. Justus, and R. S. Mendelsohn: A Clinical and Pathological Study of Seventy Cases of Myelofibrosis, Ann. Internal Med., 57:73, 1962.

Rousselot, L. M., A. H. Moreno, and W. F. Panke: Studies on Portal Hypertension: IV. The Clinical and Physiopathologic Significance of Self-established (Non-surgical) Portal Systemic Venous Shunts, Ann. Surg., 150:384, 1959.

Sbarbaro, J. L., and K. C. Francis: Eosinophilic Granuloma of Bone, J.A.M.A., 178:706, 1961.

Williams, A. W., W. G. Dunnington, and S. J. Berte: Pulmonary Eosinophilic Granuloma: A Clinical and Pathological Discussion, Ann. Internal Med., 54:30, 1961.

Wintrobe, M. M.: "Clinical Hematology," 6th ed., Philadelphia, Lea & Febiger, 1967.

351 HODGKIN'S DISEASE AND OTHER "LYMPHOMAS"

M. M. Wintrobe and D. R. Boggs

In an earlier chapter (Chap. 63) the causes of lymph node enlargement were discussed and their differential diagnosis was considered. In this section the clinical manifestations of Hodgkin's disease and of other conditions chiefly affecting lymph nodes ("lymphomas"), such as lymphosarcoma, will be described. These disorders will be considered under one heading because their clinical manifestations are very similar.

DEFINITION. Hodgkin's disease, lymphosarcoma, giant follicular lymphoblastoma (lymphoma), and reticulum cell sarcoma are included in this group. They are characterized by painless, progressive enlargement of lymphoid tissue. Lymphadenopathy is a characteristic feature, and the spleen is frequently enlarged. Cachexia, anemia, and, in many instances, fever usually are late symptoms.

HISTORY. A disorder affecting the "absorbent glands and spleen" was described by Hodgkin in 1832. *Lymphoblastoma, malignant lymphogranuloma,* and many other terms were used in referring to the disease in subsequent descriptions. The picture of lymphosarcoma was described by Kundrat in 1893; Brill, Baehr, and Rosenthal

differentiated giant follicular lymphoblastoma in 1925. Roulet (1932) separated reticulum cell sarcoma from the general group of malignant diseases of lymphoid tissue. Some pathologists differentiate still other groups or call these groups by other names; others seek to avoid fine separations.

CLASSIFICATION. Clinically these disorders vary considerably in severity. Histologically they show marked differences, but these differences are not necessarily correlated with the clinical picture. They have been classified in various ways on histologic grounds. One of the most simple is that which differentiates those conditions with a simple histologic pattern from those with more complex patterns. In the first category are reticulum cell sarcoma and lymphosarcoma. The proliferating cells tend to encroach upon, obscure, and finally replace the architecture of the lymph node. The histologic pattern of Hodgkin's disease is more complex. Lymphocytes, plasma cells, granulocytes (eosinophilic and neutrophilic), monocytes, fibroblasts, and giant cells make up the picture. The giant Reed-Sternberg cells, 10 to 40 μ in diameter, are possessed of abundant cytoplasm, a multilobed nucleus or multiple nuclei, and prominent nucleoli. A variable amount of fibrosis may be present, and the lymph node architecture is often lost. In giant follicular lymphoma the striking feature is the presence of multiple, follicle-like nodules of various sizes. Other types of "lymphoma," difficult to classify, are observed from time to time.

ETIOLOGY. Hodgkin's disease forms about one-third to one-half of all cases of this group. It affects a younger age group than the other conditions, being most common in the second and third decades. However, no age is immune. Males are more frequently affected than females.

The cause of these disorders is unknown. There may not even be the common denominator of neoplastic growth to unite them, for many investigators have considered Hodgkin's disease to be an infectious granuloma. Efforts to transmit the disease to animals have failed, however, and attempts to incriminate various organisms, including the tubercle bacillus (human and avian), diphtheroid bacilli, and *Brucella* organisms, have not succeeded. There is much speculative interest in the possibility of a viral etiology of all the lymphomas and in the likelihood that an altered immune system is involved, particularly in Hodgkin's disease.

SYMPTOMS. In most cases lymph node enlargement, usually cervical, is the first symptom to attract attention. This may be bilateral but is more often unilateral. More rarely the axillary or the inguinal nodes are the first to enlarge. The nodes are discrete and movable at first; only later do they become matted together and fixed. As a rule, they are painless and not tender, and the overlying skin is normal. However, when they have developed rapidly or when nerves are infiltrated as well, they may be painful. This is true in Hodgkin's disease especially. The size of the nodes ranges from that of a pea to that of a large orange. There is a resilient firmness in most instances, but the growth of connective tissue may make the nodes of Hodgkin's disease harder in the course of time. Occasionally the nodes in the axillary or inguinal regions may become secondarily inflamed and even break down.

After an interval varying from months to years, evidence appears of lymph node involvement elsewhere. In most patients, spread of disease from the original site appears first in the contiguous lymph node area. Superficial nodes which may be affected include the supraclavicular, axillary, inguinal, subpectoral, brachial, or femoral. A common site, also, is the mediastinum, to which such symptoms as cough, dyspnea, stridor, or dysphagia should attract attention. Splenomegaly develops in more than half the cases of Hodgkin's disease and of giant follicular lymphoma; it appears less frequently in the other forms. The liver is often palpable. Ultimately cachexia develops and weight loss occurs.

The mode of onset of these disorders may vary greatly, however. The manifestations may arise first in the mediastinum, the lungs, the digestive tract, the genitourinary tract, the bones, and rarely, the nervous system. Infiltration of the lungs, atelectasis, or pleural effusion may occur. With obstruction of lacteals, the effusion may become chylous. Extranodal primary sites include the tonsils, nasopharynx, stomach, rectum, and spleen. In the gastrointestinal tract the tumor may be far advanced before it is first discovered. Colicky pain, loss of weight, anemia, a palpable tumor, and obstruction are signs produced by lymphosarcoma of the small intestine. The lacteals may be involved so extensively that fat absorption is impaired and steatorrhea results. When the retroperitoneal nodes are the chief ones to enlarge, the diagnosis may be very difficult to make and the chief symptoms may be fever, pain, and loss of weight. Diffuse involvement of the liver and, in Hodgkin's disease, fibrosis of the portal triads, may produce jaundice; more rarely, the latter is due to obstruction of bile flow by nodes at the hilum. Hematuria, pyuria, or pain is found when the genitourinary tract is involved. Localized pain and tenderness, spontaneous fractures, and neurologic changes due to extension into the spinal canal from vertebral lesions are the most common manifestations of bone involvement. Areas of rarefaction may be demonstrable in roentgenograms, although symptoms may be present long before roentgenographic signs become evident. Subperiosteal infiltration may occur, or the bone marrow involvement may be extensive. Of cutaneous manifestations, pruritus is the most frequent; it is encountered particularly in Hodgkin's disease. Brownish skin pigmentation, herpes zoster, and nodules produced by infiltration by the specific cells are among other skin manifestations which may be encountered. Single or multiple nodules may be found in the breast. Symptoms and signs may also develop which are secondary to swellings producing pressure in various areas.

Constitutional symptoms may appear early in Hodgkin's disease, but they occur late in the other lymph node disorders. Hodgkin's disease, in particular, may produce a great variety of manifestations, so that, in addition to the localized form, which is much the most common, a generalized type, an acute type with death in a few weeks or months, a "larval" or abdominal form, and a splenomegalic type have been described.

Fever is common in Hodgkin's disease, although the well-known Pel-Ebstein type of fever is actually uncommon, appearing no oftener than in 16 percent of cases. This form of fever consists of febrile periods of several days' to several weeks' duration in which the temperature remains at levels of approximately 102 to 104°F, alternating with periods of weeks to even months during which there is no fever whatever.

Blood Picture. The greatest degree of variation is found in the blood picture associated with these disorders. There may be no changes whatever. On the other hand, there may be profound anemia as well as striking changes in the leukocytes and platelets. In Hodgkin's disease, change in the blood occur relatively early. The anemia in Hodgkin's disease is usually only moderate in degree and normocytic in type; very occasionally, hemolytic anemia develops. The total leukocyte count in Hodgkin's disease may be slightly or moderately increased, it may be normal, or there may be leukopenia. Sometimes the leukocyte count may exceed 25,000 per cu mm. The differential count may show neutrophilia, relative and absolute lymphocytopenia, monocytosis, or eosinophilia. All these changes may be present at the same time, or none of them may be present. Eosinophilia, which is mentioned frequently as characteristic of Hodgkin's disease and which may sometimes be very pronounced, is found only in about 20 percent of cases. An absolute increase in the number of lymphocytes suggests some disease other than Hodgkin's. Neutropenia suggests extensive bone marrow or splenic involvement.

The leukocyte picture in the other forms of disease chiefly affecting lymph nodes is more frequently normal than in Hodgkin's disease. Relative and even absolute lymphocytosis may be seen. The lymphocytes may be of normal types, but unusual forms and "tumor cells" (Chap. 348) have been described. Monocytes may be increased in number, and young forms may be seen, but a consistent and characteristic picture has not been described.

The platelet count may be increased in Hodgkin's disease, and large, bizarre forms may be seen. It is more common, however, to find the platelet count normal. In some instances thrombocytopenia is present; this usually occurs when leukopenia is found as well. The presence of thrombocytopenia suggests extensive bone marrow or splenic involvement and is usually, although not necessarily, a grave sign.

Bone Marrow Picture. As would be expected from this description of the blood findings, changes in the bone marrow are not characteristic and are seldom helpful except in rare cases of so-called "bone marrow Hodgkin's," in which there is extensive involvement of the bone marrow. Reed-Sternberg cells have been demonstrated in the bone marrow in a few cases of Hodgkin's disease. Lymphocytosis may be found in the bone marrow in some cases of lymphosarcoma. Such cases raise serious doubt as to whether there is any true difference between them and chronic lymphocytic leukemia.

Immune mechanism. Response to antigenic challenge with production of circulating antibody is usually normal except in certain patients with lymphosarcoma. These patients may have reduced serum gamma-globulin and reduced production of circulating antibodies similar to patients with chronic lymphocytic leukemia (Chap. 348).

Many patients with Hodgkin's disease have impaired delayed hypersensitivity, as evidenced by lack of reaction to injection of skin test antigens, such as tuberculin, and abnormally long survival of tissue homografts. Patients with impaired delayed hypersensivity responses are more likely to be lymphopenic, to have a pathologic picture of "lymphocyte depletion" in involved lymph nodes, and to be in a more advanced clinical stage than are those with normal responses.

DIAGNOSIS. The differential diagnosis of lymph node enlargement was discussed in Chap. 63. Cases in which there is little or no enlargement of the superficial lymph nodes present the most difficult problem in diagnosis, for then a variety of inflammatory and neoplastic disorders of the mediastinum, lungs, gastrointestinal tract, or liver must be considered, and the possible presence of chronic infections such as brucellosis must be ruled out. Hodgkin's disease, in particular, may produce such varied manifestations that this disorder must be kept in mind almost whenever diagnosis is obscure. This disease is particularly suggested by such symptoms as relapsing fever, loss of weight, and splenic or hepatic enlargement, together with anemia, neutrophilia, and lymphopenia.

COURSE AND PROGNOSIS. The most important factor which seems to determine the course of these disorders is their inherent character. Cases of Hodgkin's disease and of lymphosarcoma are known to have run a chronic course for many years. In other instances the course is rapid and progression occurs in spite of therapy. The average survival time from the onset of symptoms in lymphosarcoma and reticulum cell sarcoma is approximately 2 years, but variations range from a few months to 10 years or longer. About 25 percent of patients have survived 5 years or longer. The median survival of the writers' cases of Hodgkin's disease was 43 months, but 35 percent survived for 5 years after the onset of symptoms. Pregnancy is not unusual in young women with Hodgkin's disease and seems to exert no deleterious effect. In giant follicular lymphoma a median survival of 72 months has been reported, with more than 50 percent surviving longer than 5 years.

In general, cases with the most favorable outlook are those in which only one accessible lymph node group is affected and where evidence of systemic involvement such as fever, loss of weight, increased sedimentation rate, and changes in the blood are lacking.

Clinical staging is of value in determining the prognosis and the type of treatment which should be employed. In addition to a careful medical history, physical examination, examination of the blood, and chest x-ray,

proper staging requires a roentgenologic survey of the bones, liver function tests, and a lymphangiogram of abdominal lymph nodes (Chap. 63) as part of the initial examination of most patients.

The staging classification for Hodgkin's disease adopted by a 1965 symposium in Rye, New York is as follows:

Stage I: Disease limited to one anatomic region or to two contiguous anatomic regions on the same side of the diaphragm

Stage II: Disease in more than two anatomic regions or in two noncontiguous regions on the same side of the diaphragm

Stage III: Disease on both sides of the diaphragm, but not extending beyond the involvement of lymph nodes, spleen and/or Waldeyer's ring

Stage IV: Involvement of the bone marrow, lung parenchyma, pleura, liver, bone, skin, kidneys, gastrointestinal tract, or any tissue or organ other than lymph nodes, spleen, or Waldeyer's ring

All stages are classified as *A* or *B* to indicate the absence or presence, respectively, of systemic symptoms. The following documented symptoms, otherwise unexplained, are significant: (1) fever; (2) night sweats; and (3) pruritus. Hodgkin's disease limited to nonlymphoid organs is excluded from this classification.

The *histologic type* of Hodgkin's disease, in addition to clinical staging, is of some prognostic value. Lukes and Butler, improving on an earlier classification by Jackson and Parker, were able to classify most cases on a continuum of pathologic appearance ranging from those with lymphocyte predominance to those with lymphocyte depletion. The extreme range of "lymphocyte predominance" corresponds to the morphologic classification of "paragranuloma" and that of extreme "lymphocyte depletion" to "sarcoma" in the classification of Jackson and Parker. In the presence of lymphocyte depletion the cellular pattern is dominated by reticulum cells and Reed-Sternberg cells or by diffuse fibrosis. Cases falling between lymphocyte predominance and depletion are spoken of as having "mixed cellularity." In addition, certain cases did not fit into this continuum, but rather were classed as "nodular sclerosis." This group was characterized by prominent trabecular bands of dense collagenous tissue and by Reed-Sternberg cells with relatively small nuclei and prominent, pale cytoplasm. Lymphocyte predominance and nodular sclerosis were found to have favorable prognostic implication, lymphocyte depletion unfavorable, and mixed cellularity intermediate.

The best survival rates can be expected for patients in stages I and IIA and the poorest in stages III and IV. With intensive irradiation therapy, 48 percent of patients with Hodgkin's disease in stages I and IIA survived 10 years or longer in Peters' series, but only 2.4 percent of patients in stage III fared this well. Their median survival was 11 months, as compared with 7 years for stages I and IIA. In Hodgkin's disease leukopenia or marked leukocytosis, anemia before therapy is begun, and skin infiltration are bad prognostic signs, but pruritus may be associated with relatively good survival. In the last analysis, however, a therapeutic trial should be attempted, for a prolonged remission may sometimes be encountered even in cases in which the general examination suggests a hopeless prognosis.

Terminally, patients with these diseases are plagued with severe anemia and great susceptibility to infection. Antibody production is impaired, and dormant tuberculosis may become active. This is especially true in patients who are receiving adrenocorticosteroids. Fungal and antibiotic-resistant infections may also present very serious therapeutic problems. Secondary amyloidosis is a rare complication of Hodgkin's disease.

TREATMENT. Surgical excision, irradiation, and chemotherapy all have their place in the treatment of these disorders. In general, it may be stated that irradiation is useful in localized disease, chemotherapy is useful in widespread disease, and surgery's usefulness is limited to diagnostic biopsy and a few specialized situations. In certain circumstances combined radiation and chemotherapy is of benefit.

In patients with localized disease (stages I and II) the theoretic goal of therapy should be to "cure" the disease while in the remainder therapy is directed primarily toward palliation. For practical purposes "curative" therapy is attempted with irradiation and palliative therapy is with either chemotherapy or irradiation.

The hope that Hodgkin's disease can be cured was spurred by the experience of Peters in employing intensive irradiation in patients with localized disease. *Cure* as used in Hodgkin's disease is difficult to define. In patients treated for localized disease the incidence of recurrence is reduced with each succeeding disease free year. Analysis of series of such patients has suggested that if no recurrence develops by 10 to 15 years, life expectancy is the same as that of the normal population. Recurrences after 10 years are unusual, but their existence makes it difficult to denote a finite disease-free period of time which constitutes a cure.

Surgical excision of localized, apparently solitary lymphomas should be limited to situations in which such surgery represents excisional biopsy. Radiotherapy of localized masses is reported to produce a higher "cure" rate than is surgical excision, even when widespread radical excision is employed. Surgical excision is also useful in treating localized masses whose quick removal is necessary to relieve organ dysfunction, as in a patient with paraparesis from a tumor compressing the spinal cord.

Radiation therapy is the treatment of choice for patients presenting with stage I or II disease (approximately one-third of patients with Hodgkin's disease and giant follicular lymphoma and a lesser proportion of patients with lymphosarcoma and reticulum cell sarcoma). The recommended tumor dose is 4,000 rad, delivered in about 1 month's time. With this dosage fewer than 5 percent of patients have developed a recurrence at the irradiated site, while with decreasing doses such recurrences become increasingly frequent. This dose of irradiation cannot be delivered safely unless equipment with

energy in the millions of electron volts range is employed (linear accelerator, betatron, or telecobalt-therapy apparatus).

As stated earlier, the most common pattern of spread from clinically involved areas appears to be from one to another contiguous group of lymph nodes. Because of the likelihood that undetectable spread of disease has already occurred in areas adjacent to obviously involved nodes, "prophylactic" irradiation of areas adjacent to the proven tumor is commonly administered. If the involved area is cervical or supraclavicular (the most common site for localized involvement) irradiation is given to axillary and mediastinal areas as well, and if the mediastinum is involved, the upper abdomen is treated as well. Similarly, if inguinal nodes are the primary site of disease, the entire pelvis and para-aortic abdominal area is treated.

With proper supravoltage equipment, skin damage is minimal with this type of irradiation therapy. However, this dose of irradiation can produce irreparable damage to such organs as the bone marrow, lungs, heart, and liver. Thus meticulously constructed, individually designed shields must be employed to protect as much of each vital organ as is possible.

A number of radiotherapy research centers are presently attempting "curative" therapy in stage IIIA and a few are even studying the results of such therapy in stages IIIB and IV. Thus, whether chemotherapy or radiotherapy is the treatment of choice in stage III is unsettled. However, there is little disagreement that chemotherapy is the treatment of choice in stage IV and most would consider chemotherapy the treatment of choice in stage IIIB.

The effect of irradiation may be dramatic, with large masses melting away in the course of a week. Pressure symptoms may disappear; fever and pruritus, if present, may be relieved; and pain caused by bone involvement may be alleviated. Pulmonary lesions may decrease in size, and pleural effusions may clear up. Anemia may disappear, and the leukocyte count, if elevated, may drop to normal. Primary reticulum cell sarcoma of bone is especially radiosensitive. In other cases, irradiation is less effective, in some instances being of scarcely any benefit. Prediction in advance as to the likelihood of benefit from therapy is often difficult. In general, the more chronic and slowly growing forms respond best to therapy. Remission following treatment may last but a few weeks or may persist for years. In some cases such improvement can be achieved many times by additional therapy.

For *chemotherapy,* nitrogen mustard, chlorambucil, cyclophosphamide, vinblastine, and adrenocorticosteroids are of established value. Procarbazine, a methylhydrazine derivative, appears quite active against Hodgkin's disease in preliminary trials and another new agent, methyl bisguanylhydrazone may also prove useful in this disease.

The action of *nitrogen mustard* in these disorders is similar to that of irradiation. Chemotherapy may be preferable to irradiation in patients who present with stage III or stage IV disease. Patients relapsing after irradiation often respond well to nitrogen mustard even when their tumor has apparently become "radioresistant." The results of treatment may be dramatic. Fever often disappears promptly, enlarged nodes or other masses decrease in size, and anemia, if present, also is alleviated. Abnormalities in the leukocytes may revert toward normal, although the immediate effect, noticeable within 5 to 14 days following the first dose of nitrogen mustard, may be leukopenia and an increase of anemia. Because of its bone marrow—depressing effect, it is preferable to allow 8 to 12 weeks between courses of nitrogen mustard therapy. Thrombocytopenia, if present at the initiation of therapy, is less likely to be relieved by treatment.

Nitrogen mustard [methyl-bis(β-chloroethyl) amine hydrochloride, HN2] is given intravenously in doses ranging from 0.1 to 0.3 mg per kg body weight per injection each day. As much as 0.6 mg per kg may be given in a course of therapy, but the usual amount is 0.4 mg per kg. In lymphosarcoma it is wise to give no more than 0.2 mg per kg until the patient's sensitivity to the drug has been determined. The drug is available in vials containing 10 mg. To prevent thrombosis, an intravenous infusion of normal saline solution is first introduced, and when this is flowing freely, 10 ml saline solution is added to the vial containing the mustard. The drug dissolves readily. The appropriate dose is then withdrawn and injected through the rubber tubing of the saline infusion. Nausea and even vomiting may follow several hours after injection of the drug, but are usually of shorter duration, even though sometimes more intense, than in irradiation sickness. The nausea and vomiting can be allayed or prevented by giving chlorpromazine in three 20- to 30-mg doses, 6 and 4 hr before and at the time of the injection.

The discovery of other chemotherapeutic agents has reduced the comparative importance of nitrogen mustard in the treatment of the various forms of leukemia and the lymphomas, with the exception of Hodgkin's disease.

Chlorambucil and *cyclophosphamide* have modes of action and a spectrum of antitumor activity very similar to nitrogen mustard. They have the advantage of consistent absorption from the intestinal tract, so they can be taken by mouth. Chlorambucil is usually given as a daily dose of 0.1 mg per kg of body weight, and cyclophosphamide as a daily dose of 100 mg per day, although some patients, particularly those with Hodgkin's disease, tolerate larger doses. Antitumor response to such daily oral therapy is slower than that observed with nitrogen mustard, but toxicity is also of more gradual onset and thus more easily controlled. Hematopoietic depression and gastrointestinal toxicity are the most common side effects, although hair loss and hemorrhagic cystitis are also not infrequent effects of cyclophosphamide.

The periwinkle alkaloid, *vinblastine*, also has value in the treatment of Hodgkin's disease, especially in patients refractory to other forms of therapy. Initially 0.10 to 0.15 mg per kg body weight is given intravenously for 1, 2, or 3 days. Alternatively, several days' rest are allowed between injections. If tolerated, the dose can be increased by increments of 0.05 mg per kg. The therapeutic dose is that quantity which produces mild leukopenia. In addition to gastrointestinal disturbances, as with other chemotherapeutic agents, neurologic changes may be produced (mental depression, paresthesias, loss of deep tendon reflexes, headache). Excessive doses may produce permanent central nervous system damage.

The *adrenocorticosteroids* are useful in these disorders, when frank hemolytic anemia is present. These agents may decrease anemia even in the absence of overt signs of increased blood destruction. Reduction in the size of lymph nodes may also occur, and fever may be reduced, with appetite and sense of well-being improved. Bleeding manifestations may be diminished. These effects, however, are not likely to be long lasting, especially in Hodgkin's disease, and the dangers of prolonged steroid therapy, including the development of disseminated tuberculosis and widespread fungal infections, must be kept in mind. The doses used, in terms of prednisone, range from 20 to 40 mg per day, but sometimes even more is needed to achieve an effect. If increased blood destruction requires large amounts of adrenocorticosteroids for its control, splenectomy may greatly reduce the need for steroids. This operation is less likely to be helpful when leukopenia and thrombocytopenia are severe and troublesome, but it may deserve a trial.

When an alkylating agent or vinblastine is used in previously untreated patients with Hodgkin's disease, the majority of patients improve significantly, and approximately one-fourth enjoy a complete remission. The duration of cyclophosphamide- and vinblastine-induced remissions is prolonged significantly by continuing the drug as maintenance therapy after remission is induced. Administering more than one drug at a time increases the remission rate. By combining drugs in which toxic effects are somewhat dissimilar, an 80 percent complete remission rate has been achieved in a relatively small series of patients with stage III and IV Hodgkin's disease. The use of cyclophosphamide, methotrexate, vincristine, and prednisone in combination or the use of nitrogen mustard, vincristine, procarbazine, and prednisone in combination has not resulted in prohibitive toxicity and may induce not only frequent but quite prolonged remission.

In general it may be said that chemotherapy should be used (1) in disease so widespread that irradiation is impractical, (2) as an adjunct to irradition therapy, and (3) when irradiation has lost its therapeutic effectiveness.

In addition to these measures, general supportive and symptomatic therapy will be required in individual cases, as discussed in Chap. 348.

REFERENCES

Aisenberg, A. C.: Hodgkin's Disease-Prognosis, Treatment and Etiologic and Immunologic Considerations, New Engl. J. Med., 270:508, 565 and 617, 1964.

Kaplan, H. S.: Clinical Evaluation and Radiotherapeutic Management of Hodgkin's Disease and the Malignant Lymphomas, New Engl. J. Med., 278:892, 1968.

Lukes, R. J., et al.: Natural History of Hodgkin's Disease as Related to Its Pathologic Picture, Cancer, 19:317, 1966.

Perry, S., et al.: Hodgkin's Disease, Ann. Int. Med., 67:424, 1967.

Peters, M. V., et al.: Natural History of Hodgkin's Disease as Related to Staging, Cancer, 19:308, 1966.

Rosenberg, S. A., et al.: Lymphosarcoma, A Review of 1269 Cases, Medicine, 40:31, 1961.

——: Report of the Committee on the Staging of Hodgkin's Disease, Cancer Res., 26:part 1, 1310, 1965.

Wintrobe, M. M.: "Clinical Hematology," 6th ed., Philadelphia, Lea & Febiger, 1967.

Section 9

Disorders of the Nervous System

352 APPROACH TO THE PATIENT WITH NEUROLOGIC AND PSYCHIATRIC DISEASE

Raymond D. Adams

Neurology is often regarded as one of the most difficult and exacting specialties of medicine. The student coming to the neurology clinic for the first time tends to be easily discouraged by what he sees. Already he is somewhat intimidated by the complexity of the nervous system through his brief contact with neuroanatomy, neurophysiology, and neuropathology, and often has a defeatist attitude. The ritual he then witnesses, of putting the patient through a series of maneuvers designed to evoke certain mysterious signs named after famous neurologists or called by unpronounceable terms, does not reassure him. In fact it often appears to conceal the very intellectual processes by which neurologic diagnosis is attained. Moreover, the student has had no training in the many special tests which are used, such as the lumbar puncture and cerebrospinal fluid examination and the electroencephalographic, pneumoencephalographic, and arteriographic examinations, and he does not know how to interpret the results of such tests when they are given him. Neurologic textbooks only confirm his fears as he reads the details of the countless rare diseases of the nervous system.

THE CLINICAL METHOD

The author believes that many of the student's difficulties with neurology may be overcome by proper instruction in the basic principles of clinical medicine. First and foremost he must know and acquire facility in use of the *clinical method*. Without a clear comprehension of this method he is virtually as helpless with a new problem as would be the botanist or chemist who attempted to do research without having an understanding of the scientific method.

The importance of the clinical method stands out more clearly in the study of neurologic diseases than in certain other fields of medicine, but the following remarks nevertheless have universal application. The solution of any clinical problem is reached by a series of inferences and deductions, each an attempt to explain an item in the history of an illness or a physical finding. Diagnosis is the mental act of selecting the one explanation most compatible with all the facts of clinical observation. Probably no two minds function exactly alike in this process, and indeed one physician may not reason the same way on two different clinical problems. Yet an analysis of the clinical method used will show that it generally consists of an orderly series of steps, as follows:

1. The essential clinical data are secured by history and physical examination.

2. Those clinical data which are considered relevant to the current problem are interpreted and translated in terms of anatomy and physiology. Certain complexes of symptoms and signs are recognized as having a meaningful relationship. This may be called *syndrome diagnosis*.

3. From these data the physician is able to determine the anatomic localization that best explains these findings. This may be called the *anatomic diagnosis*.

4. The course of the illness, the associated medical findings, and the accessory laboratory data are then ascertained.

5. Finally the *etiologic diagnosis* is deduced from these data and from the location of the disease process.

The elicitation of accurate and reliable data concerning the disordered functioning of the nervous system is the first step in diagnosis. If these data are incorrect, the diagnosis will surely be erroneous. The taking of the history and the performance of the physical examination, then, are the primary and fundamental steps in diagnosis. Where there is disagreement as to the diagnosis it will often be discovered that the source of the difficulty is an uncertainty as to the significant items in the history or physical examination. Repeated examination may be necessary in order to establish them beyond doubt. This is why it is said that the second examination is the most helpful diagnostic test in a difficult case.

Different disease processes may cause identical symptoms, which is understandable from the fact that several diseases may involve the same parts of the nervous system. For example, a spastic paraplegia may result from spinal cord tumor, syphilitic meningomyelitis, or multiple sclerosis. Conversely, one disease may cause several different symptoms. Despite the almost infinite number of possible combinations of symptoms and signs, a few occur with greater frequency than others in a given disease, and indeed some do not occur at all; and these can be recognized as the characteristic symptom complexes or syndromes. The experienced clinical worker acquires the habit of attempting to categorize every clinical case by placing it under one or another syndrome. In doing so he more or less determines the anatomic basis of the illness in question and at the same time narrows the range of possible etiologic factors.

The final diagnosis must state the locality of the disease as well as its nature and, to be complete, should express the degree of functional impairment as well. Anatomic diagnosis has precedence over etiologic diagnosis. To seek the cause of a disease without first ascertaining the part or parts of the nervous system affected would be analogous in internal medicine to an attempt at etiologic diagnosis without knowledge of whether the disease involved the lungs, stomach, or kidneys.

The study of neurology should always proceed from the general to the specific. The student must learn the identity and differential diagnosis of the common syndromes before the details of individual diseases. It should be kept clearly in mind, however, that syndromes are not diseases but rather abstractions set up by clinical workers in order to facilitate the diagnosis of disease. The inherent danger in the method is that it may inculcate a rigidity of thinking and keep one from conceiving of diseases in new relationships.

TAKING THE HISTORY

Skill in taking a clear, meaningful history of an illness is the mark of an able clinician. In fact, this faculty more than any other distinguishes the competent from the incompetent clinical worker. The following three points about history taking in neurology deserve comment.

1. Special care must be exercised to avoid suggesting to the patient the symptoms that one seeks. The clinical interview is a bipersonal engagement, and the conduct of the examiner has a great influence on the patient. Psychiatrists have talked and written about this so much that the repetition may seem tedious, but it is evident that many of the conflicting histories presented on ward rounds can be traced to leading questions that have suggested to the patient the symptoms that the examiner expects to find or to an unconscious distortion of the patient's story. Errors and inconsistency in recording the history are as often the fault of the physician as of the patient. Here the practice of making bedside notes is particularly to be recommended. Considerable experience may be necessary to keep a suggestible and highly circumstantial patient on the subject of his illness, and of course discreet questions are always necessary to draw out certain important points.

2. The mode of onset and the course of the illness are of paramount importance. Often the nature of the disease process can be decided by these facts alone. One must know how each symptom began and progressed from the onset of the illness to the present. If the patient cannot supply this information, it may be necessary to judge the course of the symptoms by what he was able to do at different times, i.e., how far he could walk, whether he could carry on his work, etc., or by changes in the clinical findings between successive examinations. Following a case and allowing time for a disease to evolve, a method relied upon by all astute physicians, takes advantage of the latter procedure.

3. Since neurologic diseases often derange the patient's mind, it is necessary in every case to decide by assessment of the mental status and the circumstances under which symptoms occurred whether or not he is competent to give the story of his own illness. If not, the history must be obtained from an outside source such as a relative, friend, or employer. The nature of certain illnesses, such as a convulsion, obviously precludes the patient's knowledge of all the details of that part of his illness. In general, students and some physicians, as well, tend to be careless in the estimation of the mental capacities of their patients. An attempt is sometimes made to take a history from a patient who is feeble-minded or so confused that he has no idea why he is in a doctor's office or a hospital, or from one who could not possibly have been aware of the details of the illness.

THE NEUROLOGIC EXAMINATION

The neurologic examination begins always with the history. The manner in which the patient tells the story of his illness may betray lack of coherence or confusion in thinking, defection of memory, faultiness of judgment, or difficulty in comprehending or in expressing ideas. Observation of such matters is an essential part of the examination of every medical case and provides information as to the adequacy of cerebral function. Usually this type of information can be obtained without embarrassment to the patient. The physician should maintain the same objective attitude toward the verbal responses of his patient and the thoughts expressed as he does in auscultation of the chest. A common error is to pass over inconsistencies in history and inaccuracies about dates and symptoms as being unimportant, only to discover later that these are the major symptoms of the illness.

The remainder of the neurologic examination should be performed as a part of the general physical examination, not as a special procedure, to be done later if indicated. It should always be carried out in an orderly, systematic manner, proceeding from the examination of the cranial nerves, to the upper extremities, trunk, and lower extremities, in order to avoid omissions. The cranial nerves can be tested along with the examination of the eyes, ears, nose, and throat. The arms should be examined after the cervical structures and before the heart and lungs, and the legs before the pelvic and rectal examination. Gait and station should be observed at some time during the procedure, usually before or after the rest of the examination.

The thoroughness of the examination of the nervous system must of necessity depend on the type of clinical problem presented by the patient. To spend a half-hour testing motor and sensory function in a patient seeking treatment for a sprained ankle is pointless and uneconomical. Furthermore, the procedure must be varied according to the condition of the patient. If he is comatose, obviously many tests cannot be done; infants and small children and psychotic patients must be examined in special ways. The following comments about the examination procedure apply to these particular clinical circumstances.

THE AVERAGE MEDICAL OR SURGICAL PATIENT WITHOUT NEUROLOGIC SYMPTOMS. Brevity is desirable in the neurologic examination, but any test that is undertaken should be done well and recorded accurately on the patient's chart. In the examination of the cranial nerves, the pupil size, reaction to light, ocular movements, visual acuity and auditory acuity (by question), movements of face, jaw, palate, and tongue should be scrutinized. Observing the bare, outstretched arms for atrophy, weakness, tremor, or abnormal movements, inquiring about strength and subjective sensory disturbances, and tapping the supinator, biceps, and triceps tendons to evoke reflexes are usually sufficient for the upper extremities. The abdominal reflexes should be tested when the abdomen is examined. Inspection of the legs as the feet, toes, and knees are actively flexed and extended, elicitation of the knee and ankle jerks, and stroking the lateral border of the foot for the plantar reflexes complete the essential part of the neurologic examination. The only sensory tests that should be attempted are vibration and position in the fingers, ankles, and feet. Coordination may be tested by watching the patient place his finger on the tip of his nose and run the heel up and down the front of his leg. This entire procedure does not add more than 3 or 4 min to the physical examination. The routine performance of these few simple tests may offer clues as to the presence of diseases of which the patient is not aware. For example, by finding Argyll Robertson pupils, absent tendon reflexes, and diminished vibratory and position sense in the legs the physician is alerted to the possibility of the gastric crises of tabes when there are no other symptoms of neurosyphilis.

An accurate record of the results of these tests should be kept. Even if the tests are negative and do not aid in understanding the present illness, they may be of use in accurately dating the later development of a neurologic disease.

PATIENTS WHO PRESENT SYMPTOMS OF A DISEASE OF THE NERVOUS SYSTEM. Several monographs have been written on the neurologic examination of such patients. For a full account of the methods the reader is referred to the books of Denny-Brown, Monrad-Krohn, Wartenberg, and DeJong, each of whom approaches the subject from a special point of view. A large number of tests have been devised, and it is not proposed to review

them. Many are of doubtful value and should not be taught to students of neurology. Merely to perform all these tests on any one patient would require several hours, and probably in many instances would not make the examiner any the wiser. The danger with all clinical tests is that the student and physician may regard them as the inscrutable symbols of disease rather than as ways of uncovering disordered functioning of the nervous system. In general the tests which provide the most useful information are few in number and relatively simple. The student should be taught to do these few tests well and to understand their meaning. The entire examination procedure should never require more than 15 or 20 min, because if it does, the patience of both examiner and patient is likely to be exhausted and the results become inaccurate.

Testing of Cerebral Function. Cerebral function is tested in detail only if there is a reason to suspect some defect from the patient's behavior during the general examination. Questions should then be directed toward determining orientation in time and place and insight into the current medical problem. Attention, speed of response, ability to give relevant answers to simple questions, and in general the capacity for sustained mental effort, all lend themselves to straightforward observation. Useful bedside tests of attention, memory, and clarity of thought are the repetition of a series of digits in forward or reverse order, serial subtraction of 7's from 100, the recall of the names of three objects after an interval of 3 min, and the solution of simple problems and riddles. Day-to-day recollection of the medical procedures and incidents in the hospital is an excellent test of memory. Other tests can be devised for the same purpose. Often the examiner can obtain a better idea of the clearness of the patient's sensorium and the soundness of his intellect by giving him a few tests and noting the manner in which he deals with them than by relying on a crude score of a formal intelligence or achievement test (see Chap. 31).

If there is any suggestion of aphasia, a record of the patient's spontaneous speech should be made. In addition, accuracy in the naming of objects, in the execution of spoken commands, and the ability to read and write should also be noted (see Chap. 29).

Testing the Cranial Nerves. The function of the cranial nerves must be investigated more fully than in the previous examination procedure. Tests of smell are carried out only if one suspects a lesion in the anterior fossa, and then it usually suffices to determine whether odors are perceived in each nostril. In every case of brain disease the visual fields should be outlined by a perimeter and scotomas should be sought on the Bjerrum screen. The careful use of a small white test object in a confrontation test of the visual fields is a useful method and should suffice in cases of spinal cord and peripheral nerve disease. It may at times, however, reveal or localize a scotoma more accurately than the use of the Bjerrum screen. Pupil size and reactivity to light and on accommodation and range of ocular movements should next be observed.

Sensation over the face should be tested with a pin

and wisp of cotton, and the corneal reflexes should be tried. Facial movements should be observed as the patient speaks and smiles, for a slight weakness may be more evident then than during voluntary movement. Audiograms and special tests of auditory recruitment and labyrinthine tests are needed if there is any suspicion of disease of the eighth nerve. The vocal cords should be inspected in cases of medullary disease, especially when there is hoarseness. Corneal and pharyngeal reflexes are usually of value only if there is a difference on the two sides; bilateral absence of gag and corneal reflexes is seldom significant. Inspection of the protruded tongue is helpful; atrophy, fibrillation, weakness, and instability of posture may be seen. Deviation of the protruded tongue to one or the other side as a solitary finding may usually be disregarded. Articulation and the pronunciation of words should be noted. The jaw jerk and buccal and sucking reflexes should be elicited, particularly if there is suspicion of dysphagia or dysarthria (see Chap. 29).

Tests and Motor Function. In the assessment of motor function the student must remind himself that observations of the speed and strength of movements, of muscle bulk, and of tone and coordination are usually more informative than the tendon reflexes. It is essential to have the limbs fully exposed and to watch the patient maintain the arms in the outstretched position; to perform simple tasks, such as touching first the examiner's finger and then his own nose; to make rapid alternating movements that necessitate sudden acceleration and deceleration and changes in direction; and to do simple tasks such as buttoning clothes, opening a safety pin, or handling common tools. Estimates of the strength of leg muscles with the patient in bed are often unreliable; there may seem to be no weakness even though the patient cannot step up on a chair or arise from a squatting position. Running the heel down the front of the other shin, and alternately touching the examiner's finger with the toe, then the opposite knee with the heel is the only test of coordination that can be carried out in bed. The maintenance of both arms or both legs against gravity is a useful test; the weak one, tiring first, soon begins to sag. Also, abnormalities of movement and posture and tremors may appear (see Chap. 22).

Tests of Reflex Function. A large variety of tests of reflex function have been devised. There are 20 or 30 special tests that can be performed on the foot alone. Most of them can be disregarded for all practical purposes; it is recommended that only the stroking of the outer part of the sole or lateral surface of the foot be used. If the plantar reflex is extensor, the other tests are superfluous; if it is equivocal or flexor in type, the other tests cannot be taken as substitutes. When the examiner is in doubt as to the nature of the response, an involuntary flexion of the leg at the hip, knee, and ankle after a series of pinpricks is a valuable confirmation of an extensor plantar reflex. The Hoffmann reflex in the hand, better called the "finger jerk," is merely a tendon reflex and is not equivalent to the Babinski sign. The biceps, triceps, and supinator or radial-periosteal reflexes, the knee and ankle reflexes, and the cutaneous abdominal and plantar reflexes permit an adequate sampling of reflex activity of the spinal cord.

Testing of Sensory Function. The testing of sensory function is undoubtedly the most difficult part of the neurologic examination. If the findings are to be reliable, it should be reserved for the end of the examination procedure and not prolonged for more than a few minutes. Usually an explanation of the purpose of the test should be given; yet too much discussion of it with a meticulous, introspective patient may encourage the reporting of useless minor variations of stimulus intensity. It is well to ask whether or not stimuli on opposite sides of the body feel the same, not whether they feel different. If the patient is highly suggestible, in which case sensory tests are unreliable, differences that demand further investigation will not then be reported.

The skin surface of the body is large, and it is not necessary to examine all areas. A quick survey of the face, neck, arms, trunk, and legs with a pin takes only a few seconds. One is of course usually seeking differences between the two sides of the body, a level below which sensation is lost, or a zone of relative or absolute anesthesia. Regions of sensory deficit can then be tested more carefully and mapped out. Hyperesthetic zones are usually not much help in diagnosis (more often than not an area appears to be hyperesthetic because of faulty technique); nevertheless they may call attention in some patients to areas of peripheral sensory disturbance. Variations in the sensory findings from one examination to another reflect differences in technique of examination as well as inconsistency in the responses of the patient.

Light touch, pain, temperature, and vibratory and position sense should be examined systematically in every neurologic case. Stereognosis, tactile localization, two-point discrimination, and the recognition of numbers written on the skin afford the means of evaluating cutaneous perception. If the patient is an unreliable witness, only a few tests such as those for position and vibratory sense in the fingers and toes, pinprick in hands, trunk, and feet, and stereognostic sense in hands are worthwhile (see Chap. 25).

Testing and Gait Stance. No examination is complete without seeing the patient on his feet and walking. An ataxia of gait may be the only neurologic abnormality, as in certain cases of cerebellar tumor. Stance, posture, and lack of certain highly automatic adaptive movements may provide the most definite clues in an early case of paralysis agitans (see Chap. 21).

THE COMATOSE PATIENT. Although subject to obvious limitations, examination of the stuporous or comatose patient may yield considerable information concerning the function of the nervous system. The special techniques involved have been presented in Chap. 26, Coma and Related Disturbances of Consciousness.

The demonstration of signs of focal cerebral or brain stem disease or of meningeal irritation is of aid in the differential diagnosis of the diseases which cause coma and which are the basis of the three syndromes outlined in Chap. 26.

THE PSYCHIATRIC PATIENT. One is compelled in the examination of psychiatric patients to rely less on the cooperation of the patient and to be unusually critical of his statements and opinions. The depressed patient, for example, may declare that his limbs are weak or useless when actually there is little or no diminution in muscular power; or the psychopathic patient may feign paralysis. The opposite is sometimes true—that the most psychotic patient may make accurate observations of his own symptoms, only to have them ignored because the attending physician has been in the habit of disregarding his complaints.

If the patient will speak and cooperate to the slightest degree, much may be learned as to the functional integrity of different parts of the nervous system. Aphasia can, in nearly every instance, be diagnosed by the manner in which the patient uses words in phrases and sentences, or responds to spoken or written commands. Often it is possible to determine whether there are hallucinations, defective memory, or other symptoms of recognizable brain disease merely by watching and listening to the patient. The visual fields can often be tested with fair accuracy by observing the patient's response to a moving stimulus or threat in all four quadrants of the fields. The tests of cranial nerve, motor, and reflex function in the legs, already outlined for the examination of the stuporous and comatose patient, can be carried out even better if minimal cooperation is obtained from the patient. It must be remembered, however, that the neurologic examination is never complete unless the patient will speak and carry out the usual tests. On numerous occasions mute and resistive patients judged to be schizophrenic have had some widespread cerebral disease such as hypoxic or hypoglycemic encephalopathy, a brain tumor, a vascular lesion, or extensive demyelinative lesions.

INFANTS AND SMALL CHILDREN. The reader is referred to the methods of examination outlined in the monographs of Gesell, André-Thomas, and Paine. The techniques of appraising nervous function in infants and small children are necessarily different from those used in the adult.

IMPORTANCE OF A WORKING KNOWLEDGE OF NEUROANATOMY AND NEUROPHYSIOLOGY

Once the technique of obtaining reliable clinical data is mastered, the student may find himself handicapped in the interpretation of the findings by a lack of facility in neuroanatomy and neurophysiology. These are highly complex subjects, and to acquire a practical working knowledge of them is time-consuming. Fortunately these subjects are taught well in most schools, and those principles which are immediately applicable to the clinical neurologic problem are to be found in most textbooks.

DIFFERENTIAL DIAGNOSIS

The differential diagnosis of the cause of a clinical syndrome requires knowledge of an entirely different order.

One must be conversant with the clinical details and the course and natural history of the more common disease entities. Many of these facts are simple and well known and can be found in any standard textbook on neurology. For instance, the distinguishing characteristics of vascular disease of the brain are its sudden onset and, if death does not occur, the subsequent improvement in the patient's neurologic status. Similarly, insidious onset and slow progression over a period of months or years, often punctuated by convulsions, are typical of brain tumor.

The findings in the general medical examination are of importance; the fallacy of studying nervous symptoms and disregarding the general medical findings must be obvious. To illustrate: low-grade fever, anemia, heart murmur, and splenomegaly indicate that in a case of unexplained apoplexy subacute bacterial endocarditis with embolic occlusion of a brain artery is the most likely cause. Pleocytosis in the cerebrospinal fluid with elevated protein level, abnormal gold sol, and a positive Wassermann test reaction establish a syphilitic etiology in a patient with symptoms of apoplexy, a progressive dementia, or blindness.

The anatomic diagnosis may suggest the cause of a disease. Thus when a unilateral Horner's syndrome, cerebellar ataxia, paralysis of a vocal cord, and analgesia of the face are combined with loss of pain and temperature sensation in the opposite arm, trunk, and leg, an occlusion of the posterior inferior cerebellar artery is suggested, because all the involved structures lie within the territory of this artery. In a sense the anatomic diagnosis determines and limits the possible disease entities. If the signs point to disease of the peripheral nerves, it is not necessary to consider the causes of disease of the spinal cord. Some signs themselves are almost specific, e.g., Argyll Robertson pupils for neurosyphilis or oculogyric crises for postencephalitic parkinsonism.

If one adheres faithfully to the method of making these clinical observations, and to the interpretations and methods of reasoning, neurologic diagnosis becomes relatively simple. In nearly every case it will be possible to reach an anatomic diagnosis. The cause of the disease may prove more elusive. Even the most experienced neurologist is unable to ascertain the cause of many neurologic syndromes.

THE PURPOSE OF THE CLINICAL METHOD OF NEUROLOGY

Finally, a word about the main purposes of the clinical method of neurology. Actually, diagnosis accomplishes two purposes: (1) it enables the physician to decide on the proper method of treating the ailing patient; (2) it serves as an essential method in the scientific study of the disease by permitting the identification and segregation of clinical phenomena. The medical profession is primarily concerned with the prevention and cure of illness, and all our knowledge is applied to this well-defined end. The practical physician applies himself to the diagnosis of diseases for which he has an effective treatment. Each of the treatable causes of a given syndrome must be carefully considered and excluded by clinical and laboratory methods. In the study of a case of disease of the spinal cord one must take special care to diagnose a tumor, subacute combined degeneration, spinal syphilis, or epidural abscess, for these are treatable spinal cord diseases. Failure to recognize amyotrophic lateral sclerosis is a less serious error as far as the patient is concerned. The failure to diagnose one case of chronic subdural hematoma is more serious than the incorrect diagnosis of several cases of brain tumor.

One cannot agree with those who hold that neurologic diagnosis is merely an intellectual pastime. It is true that means are available for treating only a few of the many diseases known to affect the nervous system. But there is no doubt that the first step in the scientific study of a disease process is the identification of it in the living patient. Until this is achieved it is impossible to apply adequately the "master method of controlled experiment." The clinical method of neurology thus serves both the physician in the practical diagnosis and treatment of a patient and the clinical scientist who seeks the ultimate cause of the disease. Finally, accurate diagnosis permits prognosis, which is advantageous to both the physician and the patient.

CLINICAL CLASSIFICATION OF DISEASES OF THE NERVOUS SYSTEM

The most informative and logical classification of the several hundred diseases to which the human nervous system is subject should be based on cause, mechanism, and established pathologic change. Unfortunately, this is not possible because of lack of data. But to resort to such a classification in this book, even if the data were available, would have certain disadvantages, for it would presuppose on the part of the student or physician a sufficient knowledge of each of these diseases so that they could be recognized at the bedside. Given such knowledge, the details could then be sought, under the appropriate heading, in a medical encyclopedia. As has been stated earlier, the plan of this book, which tries to conform to the logical steps of the clinical method, assumes that the physician proceeds in his study of a given patient from cardinal symptoms to the diagnostic syndrome and finally to the group of diseases most likely to underlie that syndrome. Syndromic diagnosis is an intermediary step which must precede the recognition of a disease, and it is the one most easily attained by clinical study alone. For the student of clinical medicine it seems more logical, therefore, to classify the diseases of the nervous system in relationship to the most common syndrome(s) by which they express themselves.

Using this approach, we would suggest that most diseases of the nervous system declare themselves and demand medical attention because of the development of one of the following disorders. The chapters to which the reader is referred for an account of the diseases most likely to cause the syndrome in question are noted after each of the subdivisions of this purely clinical classification.

1. Stroke (Chap. 357)
2. Convulsion or faint (Chap. 368; see also Chaps. 24, 28)
3. Cranial or spinal injury (Chaps. 356 and 358)
4. Fever, headache, and stiff neck (Chap. 360)
5. Major disorders of consciousness (Chaps. 358, 363, 368; see also Chap. 26)
6. Sensory and motor paralysis of a pattern indicative of *peripheral nerve disease* (Chaps. 354, 356; see also Chaps. 21, 24, 25—*spinal root or spinal tract disease*)
7. Major impairment of intellectual functions (Chap. 364); dementia (see also Chaps. 22, 31)
8. Special cerebral deficits—speech, calculation, thinking, visual function (Chaps. 357, 359, 364; see also Chaps. 30, 31)
9. Special disorder of cranial nerves, vision, hearing, facial movement, swallowing, voice, etc. (Chap. 365; see also Chaps. 23 and 24)
10. Disorder of gait and motility beginning in childhood (Chap. 365; see also Chap. 21)
11. Headache, vomiting, and signs of increased intracranial pressure (Chap. 359)
12. Chronic disorder of coordination, movement, or posture and the presence of tremor (Chap. 364; see also Chap. 359)
13. Failure in mental development (Chap. 365)
14. Abnormalities of cranial and spinal formation (Chap. 365)
15. Recurrent headache (Chaps. 10 and 367; see also Chap. 359)
16. Recurrent vertigo (Chap. 355; see also Chap. 23)
17. Uncontrollable drowsiness (Chap. 366; see also Chap. 27)
18. Nervousness, anxiety, depression (Chaps. 369, 371; see also Chap. 18)
19. Chronic fatigue (Chaps. 369, 371; see also Chap. 19)
20. Queer behavior (Chaps. 370, 372)

REFERENCES

André-Thomas, Yves Chesin, and Saint-Anne Dargassies: "The Neurological Examination of the Infant," London, National Spastics Society, 1960.

DeJong, Russell N.: "Neurologic Examination: Including the Fundamentals of Neuroanatomy and Neurophysiology," New York, Paul B. Hoeber, Inc., 1950.

Denny-Brown, D.: "Handbook of Neurology and Case Recording," Cambridge, Mass., Harvard University Press, 1942.

Gesell, A., and C. S. Amatruda: "Developmental Diagnosis," New York, Paul B. Hoeber, Inc., 1941.

Monrad-Krohn, G. H., and Refsum, S.: "The Clinical Examination of the Nervous System, 12th ed., New York, Paul B. Hoeber, Inc., 1964.

Paine, R. S. and Opfré T. E.: Neurologic Examination of Children, The Spastics Society of Medical Education and Information, W. Heinemann Medical Books, Ltd., London, 1966.

353 DIAGNOSTIC METHODS IN NEUROLOGY

Raymond D. Adams and
Robert R. Young

The strict analysis and interpretation of the data elicited by a careful history and examination may prove to be adequate for diagnosis; special laboratory tests can then do no more than corroborate the initial impression. But it more often happens that the final conclusion as to the nature of the disease is not reached by simple case study. The possibilities are reduced to two or three, but the correct one cannot be determined. Under these circumstances, one resorts to the laboratory tests outlined below.

It must be stressed that laboratory procedures should follow rather than precede clinical case study, except in emergencies when the disease threatens life, and time does not allow detailed clinical observation. Laboratory procedures are but a part of the clinical method outlined in Chap. 352. They should be undertaken only for the specific purpose of obtaining certain otherwise unavailable data which should shed light on the clinical problem. The procedures are costly, occasionally dangerous, usually require hospitalization, may be painful unless done with skill, and are misleading if not done competently. Part of the clinical training of every young neurologic physician is to master each of these special procedures and to learn to interpret the results correctly. Some of the more simple tests may be utilized by the general physician or internist.

LUMBAR PUNCTURE AND EXAMINATION OF CEREBROSPINAL FLUID

The information yielded by the cerebrospinal fluid (CSF) is often of crucial importance. Every physician must, therefore, be familiar with the technique of lumbar puncture and the methods of examining the CSF.

It must be assumed that the medical student and physician possess a certain general knowledge of the anatomy and physiology of the CSF, for limitations of space do not allow discussion of these subjects here.

INDICATIONS FOR LUMBAR PUNCTURE

1. To obtain pressure measurements and at times to relieve elevated intracranial pressure by withdrawing CSF.

2. To secure a sample of CSF for cellular, chemical, and bacteriologic examination.

3. To administer therapeutic substances—spinal anesthetics, antibiotics, etc.

4. To inject air, as in pneumoencephalography, or a radiopaque substance (Pantopaque) as in myelography.

Lumbar puncture is contraindicated if the CSF pressure is high, as shown by headache and papilledema, for it increases the possibility of a fatal cerebellar or tentorial pressure cone. However, if it seems important, in a given case of suspected increased intracranial pressure, to have the information yielded by CSF examination, the lumbar puncture may be performed with a fine-bore (No. 22 or 24) needle as the last part of the clinical study.

Cisternal puncture, although safe in the hands of the expert, is too risky a procedure to entrust to inexperienced house officers or students. The lumbar puncture is to be preferred except in obvious instances of spinal block requiring a sample of cisternal fluid or myelography above the lesion.

Experience with diagnostic neurologic problems teaches the importance of meticulous technique. The procedure should be done under sterile conditions. If procaine is used in and beneath the skin, it should be painless. Failure to enter the lumbar subarachnoid space after two or three trials can usually be corrected by doing the puncture with the patient in the sitting position and then assisting him to lie on his side for pressure measurements and fluid removal. The "dry tap" is more often due to an improperly placed needle than to a pathologic obliteration of subarachnoid space by compressive lesion of the spinal cord or chronic adhesive arachnoiditis. A bloody tap, due to transfixion of a meningeal vessel, may result in hopeless confusion, as regards diagnosis, if it is falsely interpreted as indicating subarachnoid hemorrhage.

Examination Procedures

Once the lumbar puncture is successful, some or all of the following aspects of the CSF should be studied: (1) pressure and rough "dynamics," (2) Queckenstedt's test, (3) gross appearance of CSF, (4) number and type of cells and microorganisms present, (5) protein, sugar, colloidal gold reaction, and in special instances, analysis of pigments, (6) exfoliative cytology using millipore filters, (7) Wassermann reaction and appropriate serologic precipitation reactions, (8) protein immunoelectrophoresis, and (9) bacteriologic cultures and virus isolation. See Appendix for normal values of CSF.

RADIOLOGIC EXAMINATION OF SKULL AND SPINE

Plain x-rays of the skull or spinal column, according to the nature of the symptoms, constitute an indispensable part of the thorough study of traumatic and neoplastic diseases and less often of infectious or metabolic ones. The procedure is relatively simple, and the findings are interpretable by most general radiologists. Space does not permit a discussion or an illustration of such common findings as fractures, bone erosion, intracerebral calcifications, premature closure or separation of sutures, or alterations of skull configuration.

Of much greater value in neurology and neurosurgery are three special radiologic procedures which now permit the visualization of all parts of the brain and spinal cord and their vessels.

1. *Angiography.* Introduced by Egas Moniz, this procedure has been developed over the last 30 years to the point where it is a relatively safe and extremely valuable method in the diagnosis of tumors, abscesses, intracranial

hemorrhages, and occluded arteries. Following local anesthesia, a needle or cannula can be placed percutaneously into the lumen of any of the larger arteries of the neck; or, a catheter can also be threaded into these vessels after being introduced into the brachial or femoral artery in a retrograde fashion, to cannulate any of the major cervical vessels. In these ways radiopaque contrast media can be injected to visualize the arch of the aorta, the origins of carotid and vertebral systems, and their extent through the neck into the cranial cavity. There, cerebral arteries down to about 1-mm lumen diameter may be seen as well as small veins of comparable size and vascular abnormalities (angiomas, aneurysms), occluded arteries, delayed circulation from occlusion of dural sinuses and veins, and displacement of vessels by mass lesions can often be shown with clarity.

2. *Pneumoencephalography* and *Ventriculography*. In recent years, the injection of air into the lumbar subarachnoid space with the patient in the sitting position has largely replaced the direct injection of air into the ventricles (ventriculography). Pneumoencephalography permits visualization in considerable detail of the size and position of the ventricles, the subarachnoid space (upper spinal and cerebral), and, indirectly, the structures which lie between the ventricles and the meninges. Hydrocephalus, mass lesions which displace or deform the ventricles, and atrophic states of the cerebrum are revealed by this technique.

3. Pantopaque *myelography* (and ventriculography). By injecting 5 to 15 ml Pantopaque through a lumbar puncture needle and then tipping the patient on a tilt table, the entire spinal subarachnoid space may be visualized. The procedure is almost as harmless as the lumbar puncture, provided that the Pantopaque is afterwards removed through the lumbar puncture needle. Ruptured lumbar and cervical disks and spinal cord tumors can be diagnosed accurately. Intraventricular injection of Pantopaque is occasionally done to visualize the third and fourth ventricles and the aqueduct of Sylvius in tumors of the posterior fossa, for instance, when air does not enter from below. In some clinics air has been used instead of Pantopaque to visualize masses within the spinal canal but is less accurate and more painful.

ELECTROMYOGRAPHY (EMG) AND ELECTROENCEPHALOGRAPHY (EEG)

The electromyographic examination is utilized to supplement the clinical study of many patients with neurologic diseases, especially those which affect the neuromuscular apparatus, and also of many medical patients with more primary or secondary diseases of the skeletal musculature. This technique will be described in relation to muscle diseases (see Chap. 374).

The electroencephalographic examination is part of the clinical study of the neurologic patient suspected of having a cerebral disease; it is also used in the evaluation of the nervous effects of many medical diseases.

The modern EEG laboratory uses commercially built apparatus capable of recording from many areas over the scalp at the same time. The usual console model electroencephalograph has from 8 to 16 or more separate amplifying and recording units. The amplified brain rhythms of frequency range of 0.5 to 30 cps are strong enough to move an ink-writing pen, which reproduces the wave form of the brain discharges on paper moving at a standard speed of 3 cm (1¼ in.) per sec (cf. standard ECG paper speed of 2.5 cm (1 in.) per sec). The resulting electroencephalogram appears as a number of parallel, wavy lines, as many as there are units, or "channels." Electrodes, which usually are solder or silver disks 0.5 cm in diameter, are placed over the scalp by means of adhesive material such as bentonite or collodion, using ordinary ECG paste under the electrode to make contact with the scalp. Patients are usually examined while seated with their eyes closed and relaxed in a comfortable chair or lying on a bed. The procedure is entirely painless and takes ½ to 1¼ hr. The ordinary EEG, therefore, represents the electrical activity recorded, under restricted circumstances usually during the waking state, from several parts of the brain during an almost infinitesimal segment of the person's life.

In addition to the resting record, a number of so-called "activating" procedures are usually carried out:

1. The patient is requested to breathe deeply 20 times a minute for 3 min. The resulting alkalosis may uncover or activate characteristic seizure patterns or other abnormalities.

2. A very powerful flashing light, such as a stroboscope, is placed over the patient's eyes and flashed at frequencies from 1 to 20 per second. This is done with the patient's eyes opened and closed, and the occipital leads may then show abnormal or localizing discharges.

3. The patient is allowed to fall into natural sleep or is given sedative drugs by mouth or by vein to produce sleep, and the EEG is recorded. The first two procedures are more commonly employed, but sleep is extremely helpful in bringing out abnormalities, especially where seizures are concerned, and all too often is omitted from study.

4. Small amounts of Metrazol (100 mg per min) may be given intravenously alone, or during the flashing of the light, to see if the threshold for Metrazol-activating discharges is lower than normal. Other activating agents, such as sounds or insulin are not as useful or safe. The purpose of this procedure is to produce diagnostically useful abnormalities without actually inducing convulsions.

The EEG record (electroencephalogram) consists of 50 to 100 pages, each 12 in. long and representing 10 sec time. These are obtained by a technician who is primarily responsible for the entire procedure, including notation of movements and noise responsible for artifacts and successive modifications of technique based upon what the record shows. She provides the electroencephalographer with the record which he attempts to interpret in the absence of the patient. These records are studied in the same careful manner as x-rays or electrocardiograms, and competent analysis requires knowledge of the limitations and artifacts produced by the technique, the apparatus, or the movements of the patient.

Certain preparations are necessary if electroencephalography is to be most useful. The patient should not be sedated and should not have been for a long time without food, for both sedative drugs and relative hypoglycemia modify the normal EEG pattern. The same may be said of mental concentration, extreme nervousness, or anxiety, which tend to suppress the normal alpha rhythm. When dealing with patients suspected of having epilepsy who are already being treated for it, most physicians prefer to have the first EEG made while the patient continues to receive drugs. If it is normal, and if the referring physician and the electroencephalographer agree, the test can be repeated 24 hr after withdrawal of anticonvulsants because it is well known that they reduce the incidence of abnormal interictal records in patients with proven epilepsy. It is unusual for seizures to begin during this short interval, though it may happen; longer periods without therapy are hazardous. Any special activating procedures can usually be worked out in advance with the electroencephalographer. In patients with suspected tumors, it is helpful to request a definite localization study and to indicate the suspected site.

TYPES OF NORMAL RECORDINGS. The normal electroencephalographic record in adults is usually easy to identify. The pattern shows symmetric 8 to 12 per sec, 50 μv sinusoidal *alpha* waves in both occipital and parietal regions. These waves wax and wane spontaneously and disappear promptly when the patient opens his eyes or fixes his attention on something (Fig. 353-1A). The frontal part of the normal record shows waves of lower amplitude, 10 to 20 mV, and faster rhythm, 18 to 24 per sec, which are called *beta* waves and are also symmetric on the two sides. Slow waves, spikes, or other unusual patterns are absent in a normal record. When the normal subject falls asleep, the rhythm slows in a symmetric, characteristic way; if the sleep is induced by barbiturates, an increase in the fast frontal frequencies is seen and is considered to be a normal change (Fig. 353-1B).

The record of the normal adult is not activated by the flashing light, although it is quite usual to see an occipital response to each flash. This is called the normal *evoked response,* or photic "driving." The arrival of the visual stimulus in the calcarine part of the occipital lobe (just under the midoccipital protuberance in man) occurs 20 to 30 msec after the flash of light. In animals it has been shown that this event produces in the cortex an extremely brief spike discharge, only a few milliseconds long and only 50 mV in amplitude when recorded from the surface. With the scalp electrodes 2 cm away from the brain and with the ink-writing oscillograph, which cannot follow or record discharges of such brief duration, this primary evoked response is not seen in the EEG. The primary response, however, secondarily activates a great many more neurones, which communicate with cells in the thalamus, with other areas in the cortex, and with the reticular formation in the brainstem, which discharges in turn

reverberate back to the occipital cortex. This latter discharge is some 60 to 80 msec long and 200 mV or more in amplitude. It is called the secondary *evoked response* and can be seen in the EEG of 90 percent of all subjects, even in the presence of the background of the regular brain waves. It appears some 50 or 60 msec after the primary response, the total latency between the flash and the secondary evoked response (Fig. 353-1C) being 70 to 90 msec.

The clinical utility of this evoked occipital response has increased the scope of electroencephalography in several ways: (1) one can be reasonably sure that a person with such a response can see, or at least perceive, the light and that a patient with such a response who claims to be totally blind is suffering from hysteria or is malingering; (2) when this evoked response is absent on one side of the head but present on the other, there is physiologic evidence of a lesion that is interfering with normal transmission between the optic decussation and the occipital lobe on this side, and the presence of hemianopsia may be implied; (3) when the flashing light causes the occipital response to spread all over the cortex and activate abnormal waves, there is evidence of a lowered seizure threshold. Actual seizure patterns may be produced in the EEG if the activation procedure is continued, or if the sensitivity is still greater, frank myoclonic jerks of face or arms, or rarely, major convulsions.

Overbreathing usually does not change the record in the normal adult. Metrazol has little effect on normal persons when less than 500 mg (in patients who weigh 150 lb) is injected at the rate of 100 mg per min. Children and adolescents are more sensitive to all the activating agents mentioned, and a different set of standards has to be applied to them. It is customary for children to develop slow activity (3 to 4 per sec) during the middle and latter part of overbreathing. This promptly disappears within a minute after the hyperventilation has stopped. Here it should be noted that the frequency of the dominant rhythms in infants is normally about 3 per sec, and they are very irregular. There is a gradual steady increase in frequency of these occipital rhythms with maturation, and so by the age of twelve to fourteen years, normal 9 to 10 per sec alpha is the dominant pattern in most children. Electroencephalographers agree that children's and infants' records are difficult to interpret because the wide range of normal values at each age makes rigid classification, using frequency criteria for instance, impossible. Nevertheless, asymmetric records, or records with seizure patterns, are clearly abnormal in children of any age.

TYPES OF ABNORMAL RECORDINGS. The most pathologic finding of all is the disappearance of the EEG pattern and its replacement by a flat line. This means that the electrical activity of the entire cortical mantle is absent. Acute intoxication with anesthetic levels of drugs, such as barbiturates, can produce this sort of isoelectric EEG. However, in the absence of CNS depressants or hypothermia, a flat record which persists, all over the head, long enough to be recorded in the routine laboratory, is a result of cerebral hypoxia or ischemia. Such a patient, without EEG activity, reflexes, spontaneous respiration, or muscular activity of any kind for 24 hr, is said to be in "irreversible coma." The brain of such patients is largely necrotic. There is no chance for neurologic recovery, and the patient may be considered dead, despite the preservation of vegetative (cardiovascular) functions supported by mechanical means, such as respirators.

Localized regions of such flattening may also occur when there is a large area of softening or an extensive surface tumor or clot lying between the cerebral cortex and the electrodes. With such a finding, the localization

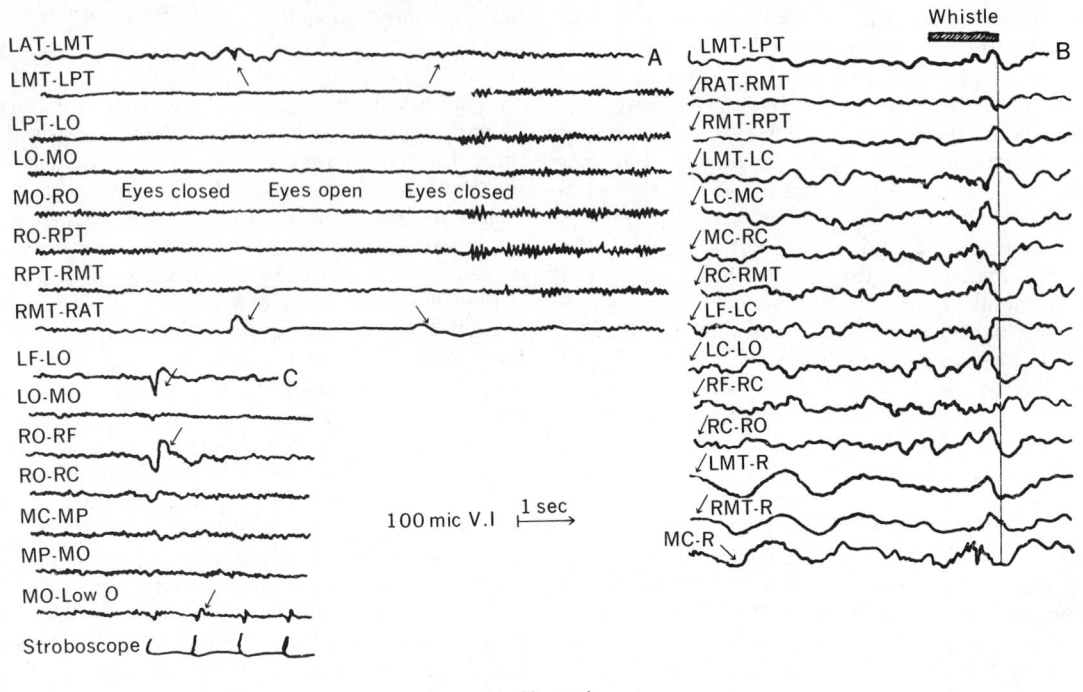

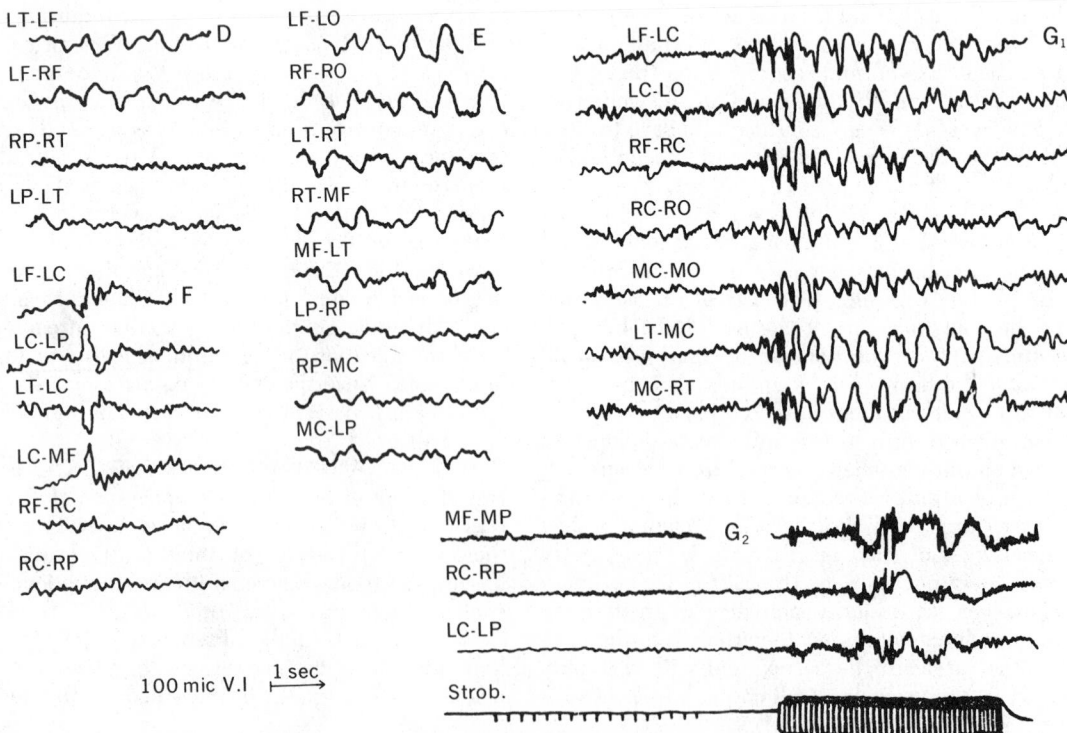

of the abnormality is precise, but of course the nature of the lesion cannot be ascertained. Most such lesions, however, are too small, relative to the recording arrangement, to be visible, and the EEG may then record abnormal waves arising from functional, though deranged, brain at the borders of the lesion.

These abnormal waves are best defined as slower and of higher amplitude than normal. Those which are less than 4 per sec with amplitude from 50 to 350 mV are called *delta* waves (Fig. 353-1*D, E*), and the higher-voltage faster waves are known as *spikes* or *sharp waves* (Fig. 353-1*F*). These fast and slow waves may be combined, and when a series of them suddenly interrupts relatively normal EEG patterns, they are highly suggestive of epilepsy. The ones associated with *petit mal* spells are 3 per sec spike and wave complexes that characteristically appear in all leads of the electroencephalogram at the same time and disappear equally suddenly at the end of the seizure (Fig. 353-1*G*). This has led to the theoretical localization of a pacemaker for the petit mal discharge in the thalamus or some deep gray structures ("centrencephalon") but such clinical and experimental evidence as exists tends to refute this hypothesis.

NEUROLOGIC CONDITIONS WITH ABNORMAL EEGs. In the following groups of neurologic disorders, the EEG may be of considerable help in reaching the correct diagnosis. In others, as will be mentioned, it is of little or of questionable value.

Epilepsy. All types of generalized epileptic seizure (grand mal and petit mal) are associated with some abnormality in the EEG provided it is being recorded at the time. The EEG is also usually abnormal during the more restricted types of seizures activity (psychomotor, myoclonic, Jacksonian). One exception is certain deep temporal lobe foci where the discharge fails to reach the scalp in sufficient amplitude to be seen against the background activity of the normal EEG, particularly if there is a strong alpha rhythm. If in these exceptional cases an anterior temporal electrode, which is most free of occipital alpha frequencies, does not show such a discharge from the depths, a nasopharyngeal lead will usually pick it up, especially during sleep. In perhaps 2 to 5 percent

of cases, the only way in which this deep activity can be sampled is by opening the skull and inserting an electrode into the substance of the brain. Some electroencephalographers are enthusiastic about the possible uses of depth electrodes and feel that a great deal of information about temporal lobe epilepsy can be obtained by this technique. Certainly most neurologists would be unwilling to allow depth electrode recordings to be made on any of their patients except the few who are having an operation on the brain. Although it is true that a rare patient with temporal lobe epilepsy and a normal EEG at the time of a seizure may be erroneously labeled as hysteric from the EEG alone, the clinical state itself is of help. Other exceptions in which, on occasion, no EEG abnormality may be recorded during a seizure include certain focal seizures (sensory, Jacksonian, myoclonic, and *epilepsia partialis continua*). This presumably means the neuronal discharge is too deep, discrete, or asynchronous to be transmitted by volume conduction and recorded via the EEG electrode which is some 2 cm from the cortex. Some of the different types of seizure patterns are shown in Fig. 353-1*D, E,* and *F*. The petit mal, myoclonic jerk, and grand mal patterns correlate closely with the clinical seizure type.

A fact of importance is that between seizures approximately 20 percent of all epileptic patients show a normal pattern, and it is for this reason that activation procedures are necessary. Moreover, though the records of as many as another 40 percent of epileptic patients are abnormal between seizures, the abnormality is nonspecific, and therefore the diagnosis of epilepsy can be made only by the correct interpretation of the EEG abnormality in relation to the clinical data.

Brain Tumor, Abscess, and Subdural Hematoma. Clinically significant intracranial space-occupying lesions are characteristically associated with abnormalities in the EEG, depending on their type and location, in up to 90 percent of patients. In addition to diffuse changes, to be described below, the classical abnormalities are focal or localized slow wave (usually delta) or occasionally, seizure activity. As a rule, those with the more rapidly expanding lesions (abscess, glioblastoma, some metastases)

Fig. 353-1. Abbreviations used in illustrations: R—right; L—left; F—frontal; C—central (motor area); T—temporal; P—parietal; O—occipital; A—anterior; M—mid; R—reference or inactive lead (such as nose, both ears, or midpost neck); mic V.—microvolt; sec—second; Strob.—stroboscope.

A. 8-channel record; normal subject with eyes open and closed. Note symmetry on the two sides and disappearance of alpha when eyes are open. Arrows show artifact in anterior temporal region from the eye movement.

B. A strip of 15-channel recording; subject asleep. Note slow waves, absence of normal alpha, and symmetry on the two sides. Block on first line shows whistle and evoked response in all leads. The small arrows indicate the channel for each electrode pair.

C. Normal subject, showing flash in eye and the evoked response in occipital area. It is seen only in low occipital lead. Arrows show eye movement in frontal leads.

D. Abnormal; brain tumor. Left frontal region showing slow delta waves.

E. Abnormal; head injury. Showing slow delta 3 per sec, and 5-per-sec theta both sides.

F. Abnormal; epilepsy (seizure pattern). Focal type with spike and slow-wave focus left temporal region occurring spontaneously.

G. Abnormal; epilepsy (seizure pattern). (1) Petit mal type, showing 3-per-sec spike and wave (activated by overbreathing). (2) Myoclonic jerk, short seizure activated by 15-per-sec stroboscope flash, but not by 5-per-sec flash.

have the greatest frequency of EEG abnormalities (90 to 95 percent). More slowly growing tumors (meningioma) often produce no change in the EEG, though they may be very evident clinically. The EEG abnormality has the correct lateralization in as many as 70 percent of patients with subdural hematomas and supratentorial tumors or abscesses. Therefore, when a patient in whom one of these conditions is suspected has a normal EEG, there are 9 chances to 1 against its presence. Thus both the positive and negative values of the EEG in such situations may be helpful, particularly when integrated with the other laboratory and clinical findings.

Cerebrovascular Diseases. Both the diffuse and localized EEG changes produced by cerebral infarcts and intracranial hemorrhage depend on their location and size rather than their type. The EEG has not been shown to be useful in the differential diagnosis of the various forms of vascular disease. Large hemispheral lesions, associated acutely with depressed levels of consciousness, produce widespread, diffuse slow wave activity of a nonspecific type as is seen with stupor or coma from any cause. The EEG is of little lateralizing value in acute subarachnoid hemorrhage, for example, and though a few very large infarctions betray themselves by ipsilaterally depressed EEG activity, most are not associated with asymmetrical abnormalities acutely. Resolution begins after a few days, cerebral edema subsides, and focal activity may then be seen (slow wave activity or suppression of normal background rhythms). Smaller infarctions are associated with focal abnormalities acutely which lateralize the lesion well but do not localize it precisely. In contrast with tumors, further resolution occurs and after 3 to 6 months, roughly 50 percent of patients with cerebrovascular accidents have a normal EEG despite the persistence of clinical abnormalities. Once this occurs, the prognosis for further recovery is poor. Perhaps half of these patients have had normal EEGs even when they were first recorded in the week or two following the ictus. This is often true with discrete lesions, especially small, deep ones, which have the best prognosis. The same may be said for patients with mild and short-lived EEG abnormalities. Large lesions of diencephalon or midbrain produce bilaterally synchronous slow waves, but, interestingly, those of pons and medulla may be associated with normal or near normal EEGs despite profound and catastrophic clinical changes.

Brain Injury. Cerebral concussion in animals is accompanied by a transitory disturbance in brain waves, but in man this is usually over before a recording can be made. Cerebral contusion or laceration produces EEG changes similar to those described for cerebrovascular disease. Diffuse changes often give way to focal ones, especially if the lesions are on the lateral or superior surface of the brain, and these in turn usually disappear over a period of weeks or months. Sharp waves or spikes sometimes emerge as the focal slow wave abnormality resolves, and may precede the occurrence of posttraumatic epilepsy (Fig. 353-1F). Following head injury, therefore, serial EEGs may be of prognostic value as regards the

prospect of epilepsy. They may also aid, as mentioned above, in evaluating patients for subdural hematoma.

Diseases Which Cause Coma and States of Impaired Consciousness. The EEG is abnormal in almost all conditions in which there is some impairment of consciousness (cf. brainstem infarctions above). In general, the more profound the change in consciousness, the more abnormal the EEG recording. In such situations the slow waves (delta) are bilateral, of high amplitude, and tend to be more conspicuous over the frontal regions (see Fig. 353-1E). This pertains to such differing conditions as acute meningitis or encephalitis, severe disorders of electrolyte and water balance, uremia, diabetic coma, liver coma, or impairment of consciousness accompanying the large cerebral lesions discussed above. In hepatic coma, the degree of abnormality in the EEG corresponds with the degree of confusion, stupor, or coma. Moreover, paroxysms of bilaterally synchronous wave and spike or "triphasic waves" are characteristic. Diffuse degenerative diseases (e.g., Alzheimer's disease and senile dementia) affecting the cerebral cortex are accompanied by relatively slight degrees of diffuse, slow wave abnormality in the theta (4 to 7 cps) range as described for Alzheimer's disease below. Certainly more rapidly progressive ones, such as subacute inclusion body encephalitis, Jakob-Creutzfeld disease, and to a lesser extent, the cerebral lipidoses have, in addition, very characteristic EEG changes consisting of paroxysms of delta waves and spikes. Slow waves without spikes reflect widespread disease of white matter, e.g. leukodystrophies. Even in situations where the EEG abnormality is not specific or diagnostic, it is useful in emphasizing the presence of structural or biochemical abnormalities of the brain. A normal EEG in a patient who is apathetic, slow, depressed, or forgetful is a point in favor of the diagnosis of an affective disorder or schizophrenia.

An EEG may also assist the physician in caring for a comatose patient when the pertinent history is unavailable. It may point to such otherwise unexpected causes as hepatic encephalopathy (bilaterally synchronous triphasic waves), intoxication with barbiturates or tranquilizers (excess fast activity), clinically inapparent continuous epileptic discharges, a large space-occupying lesion, or diffuse anoxia-ischemia.

Other Diseases of the Cerebrum. There are many disorders of nervous function that cause little or no alteration in the EEG. Multiple sclerosis and other demyelinating diseases are examples, though as many as 50 percent of *advanced* cases will have an abnormal record. Delirium tremens and Wernicke-Korsakoff disease, despite the dramatic nature of the clinical picture, cause little or no change in the EEG. Some degree of slowing usually accompanies confusional states which we have designated elsewhere as hypokinetic delirium (see Chap. 30). Interestingly, neuroses and psychoses, such as manic-depressive disorders or schizophrenia, and hallucinogenic drugs such as LSD, and the majority of cases of mental retardation cause no important modification of the normal record or are associated with minor nonspecific abnormalities. The EEG has not assisted us in the understanding of these disorders.

SPECIAL APPLICATIONS OF THE EEG. Because the EEG provides information about the status and function of the cerebrum, it is useful as a monitor in the operating room to ensure the presence of a viable brain during the increasingly extensive procedures of modern cardiovascular surgery. EEG apparatus has been available for some time now for indicating the level of anesthesia, and such simple equipment may be used by the anesthetist to monitor both the cardiac and cerebral status of *all* patients during surgical anesthesia.

In the neurosurgical operating room the EEG can be recorded from the exposed brain (*electrocorticogram*), and seizure patterns can be localized more precisely than from the scalp. Resections of such abnormal tissue have helped more than 50 percent of the patients with focal epilepsy who have undergone such procedures.

The routine EEG can be of value in the diagnosis of hysterical blindness, as stated above. Similarly, a response evoked by noise during light sleep can be of help in confirming the presence of hearing in a patient who feigns total deafness (Fig. 353-1*B*). These responses may also be useful in evaluating hearing and vision in infants.

In many subjects, however, the visual and auditory evoked responses are too small to be visible in the mélange of baseline noise and background activity of the routine EEG. Averaging techniques (largely computerized) may then be used to record them. This interesting new field of electroencephalography so far has proven to be useful clinically only in the evaluation of hearing in children and, to a lesser extent, in the study of vision.

CLINICAL VALUE OF MINOR EEG ABNORMALITIES. The gross EEG abnormalities discussed above are, by themselves, clearly and definitely abnormal and of obvious clinical significance. Any formulation of the patient's clinical status should consider and attempt to account for them. They include seizure discharge, generalized and extreme slowing, definite slow waves with a clear-cut asymmetry or a focus, and absence of normal rhythms. Certain other findings are of more doubtful significance and represent lesser degrees of abnormality which form a continuum between the undoubtedly abnormal and the completely normal. These records, which comprise such activity as 14 and 6 per sec positive spikes, scattered 5 to 6 per sec slowing, voltage asymmetries and moderate "breakdown" with hyperventilation or strobe, are termed borderline and are the most difficult to interpret. Ideally, the patient's physician should interpret the EEG himself just as he does the tests for cerebellar function or tendon reflexes. The EEG findings placed thus in the clinical context would be weighted appropriately but, unfortunately, this is not always technically possible. The physician then depends upon the report he receives in which the EEG is usually categorized as "normal" or "abnormal." Such categorization in borderline records is difficult, arbitrary, and often meaningless. It is important, therefore, for the physician to realize the clinical value of minor EEG abnormalities which may be meaningful

only if correlated with certain clinical phenomena. Whereas borderline deviations in an otherwise entirely normal person have no clinical significance, the same EEG findings, when associated with certain clinical signs and symptoms, even if they too are of minimal severity, become important. For example, a thirty-four-year-old woman with a history of tension headaches since age fourteen is under neurologic study because of insomnia, weight loss, and an increase in the frequency of her headaches. The neurologic examination, spinal fluid, and x-rays of skull are all within normal limits. The EEG shows a clear-cut reduction of voltage in the left occipito-parietal area and less alpha than the same area on the right side. The finding of such an asymmetry in the brain wave has no clinical significance in this case and should be disregarded. On the other hand, this same finding in a thirty-two-year-old man who was rendered unconscious in an automobile accident 9 days before and who shows slight awkwardness in his right hand and a continuous dull headache with a lack of usual alertness, now carries considerable diagnostic meaning. It points to the left hemisphere, which might show contusion or the presence of a subdural hematoma.

In conclusion, the electroencephalogram, like the electromyogram and the electrocardiogram, is part of the clinical findings and is meaningful only in relation to the clinical status of the patient at the time that it was taken.

PSYCHOMETRY, PERIMETRY, AUDIOMETRY, AND TESTS OF LABYRINTHINE FUNCTION

These methods, drawn largely from the field of physiologic psychology, are of utility in quantitating and in defining the nature of the psychic or sensory deficits produced by disease of the nervous system. Limitations of space do not permit a description of them here. The precise indications for doing these tests are (1) to obtain confirmation of a functional disorder in particular parts of the nervous system and to ascertain its nature; (2) to quantitate the disorder in order to determine, by subsequent examinations, the natural course of the underlying illness.

CONCLUDING REMARKS

Many of the procedures outlined here are highly technical and require special apparatus and carefully trained technicians. If the referring physician has never worked with these techniques, he must depend on the results of the technicians and also on their interpretations. Frequently he overestimates the power and objectivity of the special laboratory procedures and abdicates his role as the responsible physician by placing undue reliance upon them. This practice is to be discouraged. No one is better able to judge the significance of an abnormal laboratory datum in an abstruse clinical problem than a well-trained experienced clinician. Therefore, it behooves every physician, using these several laboratory procedures, to find out enough about them so that he will know their limitations and the reliability of the data which they provide.

REFERENCES

Berger, H.: Über das Elektrenkephalogramm des Menschen, Arch. Psychiat. Nervenkr., 87:527, 1929.

Gibbs, F. A., and E. L. Gibbs: "Atlas of Electroencephalography," 2d ed., vol. 1–3, Reading, Mass., Addison-Wesley Publishing Company, Inc., 1950–1964.

Hess, R.: "EEG Handbook," Sandoz Monographs, Switzerland, Sandoz Ltd., Basle, 1966.

Hill, D., and G. Parr (Eds.): "Electroencephalography: A Symposium on Its Various Aspects," 2d ed., New York, The Macmillan Company, 1963.

Kiloh, L. G., and J. W. Osselton: "Clinical Electroencephalography," 2d ed., London, Butterworth and Co. (Publishers), Ltd., 1966.

Schwab, R. S.: "Electroencephalography in Clinical Practice," Philadelphia, W. B. Saunders Company, 1951.

Taveras, J. M., and E. H. Wood: "Diagnostic Neuroradiology," Baltimore, The Williams & Wilkins Company, 1964.

354 DISEASES OF THE PERIPHERAL NERVOUS SYSTEM

Raymond D. Adams and
Arthur K. Asbury

Disease of the peripheral nervous system stands as one of the most difficult subjects in neurology. Since the structure and function of this system is relatively simple, one might suppose that our knowledge of its diseases would be complete. Such is not the case. At present a suitable explanation cannot be offered in as many as half the patients who enter a general hospital with a disease of the peripheral nervous system; nor have the pathologic changes been fully determined in any one of them. Moreover, the physiologic basis of many of the symptoms of peripheral nerve disease continues to elude experts in the field.

With these rather discouraging remarks behind us, we shall attempt to present a distillate of our personal experience that may be of value to the reader.

GENERAL CONSIDERATIONS

It is well to have clearly in mind the extent of the peripheral nervous system and the scope of the possible pathogenetic mechanisms whereby it can be affected.

The peripheral nervous system (PNS) includes all nervous structures lying outside the piarachnoid membrane of the spinal cord and brain stem, with the exception of the optic nerves and olfactory bulbs, which are special extensions of the brain. The parts of it within the spinal canal and cranial cavity and attached to the ventral and dorsal surfaces of the cord and ventrolateral

surface of the brain stem are the *spinal* and *cranial nerve roots* respectively. The dorsal roots (sensory) containing afferent fibers (the central axonal processes of the dorsal root ganglion cells) extend for a variable distance into the posterior columns (funiculi) of the spinal cord. The efferent ventral roots, composed of the emerging axones of anterior and lateral horn cells, finally terminate on muscle fibers or in sympathetic or parasympathetic ganglions. Traversing, as they do, the subarachnoid space, and lacking an epineural and in part a perineural sheath, the cranial and spinal roots are bathed by CSF, the lumbosacral roots presenting the longest exposure. The vast extent of the peripheral ramification of cranial and spinal nerves is noteworthy, as are their thick protective sheaths of perineurium and epineurium and their unique vascular supply through longitudinal arrays of richly anastomosing nutrient arterial branches. Sensory endings, freely branching or corpuscular, are the site of termination of the peripheral axones of dorsal root ganglion cells. Sympathetic afferent fibers, arising on blood vessels and in viscera, and the sympathetic and parasympathetic ganglions, with their rami communicantes and peripheral extent, complete this system. Segments of myelin, special extensions of Schwann cell plasma membrane, cover the axone but always maintain an independent though symbiotic relationship to it.

These many anatomic features reveal the possible pathways and mechanisms of peripheral nerve disease. Pathogenic processes directed at the anterior or lateral horn cells of the spinal cord, the nerve cells of dorsal root ganglions, or the nerve cells of sympathetic or parasympathetic ganglions would reflect themselves secondarily in degeneration of axones and myelin sheaths of the peripheral nerve fibers of these cells. Disease processes involving the oligodendrocytes or astrocytes in the ventral or dorsal columns (funiculi) of the spinal cord, wherein lie the axones of anterior horn cells or dorsal root ganglion cells, could also affect the function and structure of the peripheral nervous system. A pathologic process in the leptomeninges and CSF could damage the exposed anterior and posterior roots; perhaps it would damage the latter differently from the former because of their intimate relationship to groups of specialized arachnoidal cells (villi) where CSF is absorbed. Pathogenic processes such as amyloidosis confined to the various components of connective tissue might affect the peripheral nerves which lie enveloped within their sheaths. Diffuse or localized arterial diseases could theoretically injure nerves by narrowing or obliterating the nutrient arteries, thus curtailing their blood supply. Noxious agents with special affinities for the Schwann cells or their membranes which compose the myelin sheaths cause demyelination of peripheral nerves. Finally one might suppose that axoplasm of either motor or sensory nerve fibers or their peripheral endings and end organs might each have their particular liabilities to disease.

All this is theoretical and somewhat speculative. At present we can cite examples of diseases which are based on only a few of these potential disease pathways, e.g., diphtheria toxin, which acts directly on the membranes of the Schwann cells near the dorsal root ganglions and adjacent nerves; polyarteritis nodosa, which causes occlusion of nutrient arteries; tabes dorsalis, in which there is a treponemal meningoradiculitis of lumbosacral segments. But analogous anatomic possibilities doubtless are implicated in other diseases whose mechanisms remain to be divulged.

Pathologically we know the diseases of the PNS to have certain qualities in common. Degeneration of medullated nerve fibers (myelin sheaths and axis cylinders) is a feature of all of them, though it varies in degree and as to site of primary damage. However, the myelin sheaths themselves are the most susceptible element of nerve, for they may degenerate as part of a primary process involving the Schwann cells or some component of myelin itself or secondarily to axonal or nerve cell destruction. When the myelin sheath alone disintegrates, the highly structured lipoprotein disintegrates into fine particles, which are then converted through the action of histiocytes (macrophages) into cholesterol esters and removed via the bloodstream. Breakdown of axones causes fragmentation of myelin into blocks or ovoids in which lie fragments of axones. This is a feature typical of Wallerian degeneration. Focal myelin sheath degeneration is called *segmental demyelination.* Degeneration of both axone and myelin sheath may occur either distal to axonal interruption (Wallerian degeneration) or as a "dying back" phenomenon in more diffuse, metabolically determined polyneuropathies (axonal degeneration). In segmental demyelination, recovery may be rapid, because the intact axone need only become remyelinated over denuded segments to become functional once more. In contrast, with Wallerian or axonal degeneration, recovery is slower, often requiring months to a year or more, because the axone must regenerate and reconnect to its peripheral ending before function returns.

Aside from difference in pathologic pathway and the effects of disease on parenchymal elements of nerve, the various forms of polyneuropathy are distinguished by other characteristics of the lesions and by the topography of the nerve fiber changes. In fact these are the only available criteria for "differential diagnosis." In acute idiopathic polyneuritis and infectious mononucleosis, infiltrations of lymphocytes, plasma cells, and mononuclears in the spinal roots, sensory and sympathetic ganglions and nerves and a frequent perivenous location of myelin destruction characterize the disease. In polyarteritis nodosa with polyneuropathy, "necrotizing panarteritis" with occlusion and focal infarction of nerve and, less often, rupture and hemorrhage are the dominant findings. In amyloid polyneuropathy, it is the deposits of this foreign material in the walls of vessels and connective tissue sheaths secondarily affecting the nerve fibers either by compression or ischemia that are the basis of diagnosis. In diphtheritic polyneuropathy, the aforementioned location in and around the roots and sensory ganglions, the purely demyelinative character of the nerve fiber change, and the lack of inflammatory reaction permit its identification under the microscope. Other polyneuropathies (carcinomatous, myelomatous, porphyric, arsenical, ure-

mic) are topographically symmetrical but are not presently distinguishable from one another by histopathologic means. They await more definitive study. The least is known about the familial types of polyneuropathy. Although genetic factor can be envisaged, the biochemical mechanisms are just beginning to be recognized.

Concerning the causes of pathogenetic mechanisms and pathology of the mononeuropathies, even less is known. Compression, producing local or segmental ischemia, violent stretch, laceration from penetrating injuries are understandable, and the pathologic changes they cause have been reproduced in animals. Of localized infections of single nerves only leprosy, sarcoid, and zoster represent identifiable disease states. For the larger number of acute lesions the pathology has yet to be defined, since they are benign, reversible states usually, which allow no opportunity for postmortem examination.

Table 354-1. PRINCIPAL CAUSES OF
PERIPHERAL NEUROPATHY

I. Poisons
    A. Metals: arsenic, lead, mercury, antimony, bismuth, copper, phosphorus, thallium
    B. Drugs: Nitrofurantoin and related nitrofurazones, isoniazid, thalidomide, vincristine, diphenylhydantoin, stilbamidine, tetraethyl-thuram disulfide
    C. Organic substances: carbon monoxide, carbon disulfide, trichloroethylene, methyl alcohol, triorthocresylphosphate, immune serums, benzene and derivatives, acrylamide, organophosphorus compounds
II. Deficiency states and metabolic disorders
    A. Chronic alcoholism, beriberi, pellagra, subacute combined degeneration, pregnancy, chronic gastrointestinal disease, carcinoma of lung, diabetes mellitus, porphyria, amyloidosis, multiple myeloma, macroglobulinemia, uremia, hypoglycemia, lupus erythematosus
III. Specific inflammatory states and infections
    A. Acute idiopathic polyneuritis (acute febrile polyneuritis of Osler, Landry-Guillain-Barré syndrome)
    B. Polyneuropathy, complicating acute or chronic infection: diphtheria, Boeck's sarcoid, infectious mononucleosis
    C. Local infection of nerves: leprosy
IV. Vascular disease: polyarteritis nodosa, arteriosclerosis, diabetes mellitus
V. Genetically determined disorders: progressive hypertrophic polyneuropathy, peroneal muscular atrophy, and others
VI. Polyneuropathy of obscure origin: chronic progressive or recurrent polyneuropathy

The clinician is usually faced with two problems: (1) to establish the existence of disease of the peripheral nervous system; (2) to ascertain its nature and the possibilities of treatment. When muscular weakness, areflexia, atrophy, and sensory loss are demonstrable and conform to the region of distribution of one or many nerves, this is not difficult. The tendency for these diseases to affect the feet and lower legs more than the proximal parts, and the legs more than the arms, the frequent sparing of the trunk, the escape of vesical and anal sphincters, phenomena which probably reflect involvement of the largest and longest nerves, already commented upon in Chaps. 21 and 25, are relatively certain clues to diagnosis. But at times pain or dysesthesias may be the major symptoms, and the other subjective and objective neurologic findings are more difficult to put in evidence. Or the disorder

PRINCIPAL NEUROPATHIC SYNDROMES

I. Syndrome of acute ascending motor paralysis with variable disturbance of sensory function
   A. Acute idiopathic polyneuritis (Landry-Guillain-Barré syndrome)
   B. Infectious mononucleosis and polyneuritis
   C. Hepatitis and polyneuritis
   D. Diphtheritic polyneuropathy
   E. Porphyric polyneuropathy
   F. Toxic polyneuropathies (triorthocresyl-phosphate poisoning, Jamaica ginger)
II. Syndrome of subacute sensorimotor paralysis
   A. Symmetric polyneuropathies
      1. Alcoholic polyneuropathy and beriberi
      2. Arsenic polyneuropathy
      3. Lead polyneuropathy
      4. Nitrofurantoin and other intoxications
   B. Asymmetric polyneuropathies
      1. Diabetic
      2. Polyarteritis nodosa
      3. Subacute idiopathic polyneuritis
      4. Sarcoidosis
III. Syndrome of chronic sensorimotor polyneuropathy
   A. Acquired
      1. Carcinoma, myeloma, and other malignancy
      2. Paraproteinemias
      3. Uremia
      4. Beriberi
      5. Diabetes
      6. Connective tissue diseases
      7. Amyloidosis
      8. Leprosy
   B. Genetically determined disorders
      1. Peroneal muscular atrophy (Charcot-Marie-Tooth disease)
      2. Hypertrophic polyneuropathy (Dejerine-Sottas disease)
      3. Portuguese amyloidosis (Andrade's disease) and other types
      4. Heredopathia atactica polyneuritiformis (Refsum's disease)
      5. Abetalipoprotienemia
      6. Tangier disease
      7. Metachromatic leukodystrophy
IV. Syndrome of chronic relapsing polyneuropathy
   A. Idiopathic polyneuritis
   B. Porphyria
   C. Beriberi or intoxications
V. Syndrome of mono- or multiple neuropathy
   A. Pressure palsies
   B. Traumatic neuropathies
   C. Idiopathic-brachial and sciatic neuritis
   D. Serum neuritis
   E. Zoster
   F. Tumor invasion with neuropathy
   G. Leprosy
   H. Paratubercular (polyneuritis cranialis multiplex)

may be purely motor, raising a question of myopathy or dystrophy or anterior horn cell disease; again, only paresthesias, ataxia, and sensory loss are found, suggesting as alternative possibilities a disease of the posterior roots or the posterior columns of the spinal cord. Under these circumstances one must resort to a number of useful laboratory tests, such as (1) measurement of nerve conduction velocity (lowered in chronic nerve disease but not in spinal cord or muscle diseases); (2) electromyography, which distinguishes disorders of muscle due to primary disease (myopathy), denervation, and neuromuscular blockage; (3) CSF examination (increase in protein and sometimes in cells with radicular and meningeal diseases); and (4) nerve (sural nerve) and muscle biopsy.

Taking advantage of all available clinical and laboratory techniques and knowledge of the natural course of illnesses, the physician will find it helpful to be familiar with the following peripheral nerve syndromes. Stated another way, whenever one of the following syndromes can be identified, one is justified in considering any one of the several diseases of the peripheral nerve system listed in the following classification.

SYNDROMES OF PERIPHERAL NERVE DISEASE

Acute Ascending Motor Paralysis with Retained Sphincteric Functions and Variable Sensory Loss

This condition is also called the *Landry-Guillain-Barré syndrome*. Most of the severe, rapidly advancing (over a period of days) polyneuropathies fall into this category. Muscular weakness begins as a rule in the feet and legs (more or less symmetrically), and as the days pass it quickly ascends to involve the trunk, arms, and finally the cranial muscles (facial diplegia, dysarthria, dysphagia, dysphonia). Tingling paresthesias usually attend the weakness, and there may or may not be demonstrable loss of vibratory and position sense. The tendon reflexes disappear as the weakness becomes pronounced, and the plantar reflexes are at all times flexor or absent. The sphincters rarely are deranged and if so, are not so for more than a few days. As the paralysis ascends, the patient, at first able to walk though perhaps somewhat ataxic because of loss of position sense or spinocerebellar function, soon becomes bedfast, and further involvement of trunk and arm muscles will render him more or less helpless. Paralysis of intercostal muscles and diaphragm occur frequently, necessitating respiratory assistance. Dysphagia and inability to raise the laryngeal secretions require laryngotomy, which facilitates their removal, assures a clear airway, and permits the use of positive-pressure respiratory aids. Death occurs in approximately 20 percent of these cases, a fact which indicates the seriousness of the disease and the importance of treating the patient in a hospital where there is a trained respiratory team. Usually, however, the disease stabilizes within 2 to 3 weeks, i.e., the paralysis does not progress further. Many of our fatalities have taken place in the first 3 weeks, but a few patients have succumbed later, usually from complications of severe, respiratory paralysis (pneumonitis, bronchial plugs, atelectasis, anoxic encephalopathy) or autonomic paralysis.

A variant of the syndrome consists of a paralysis which begins in the arms or cranial muscles and pursues a descending course, again causing a rapidly advancing paralysis sufficient to prevent locomotion and effective motion of limbs and to cause respiratory paralysis. Rarely, a syndrome made up of a total ophthalmoplegia with severe ataxia of movement of the limbs has been observed (cf. Fisher).

Only minor differences separate (1) acute idiopathic polyneuritis of Landry-Guillain-Barré, (2) acute infectious mononucleosis, (3) porphyria, (4) diphtheritic polyneuropathy, (5) acute idiopathic hepatitis, (6) polyarteritis nodosa, (7) other toxic polyneuropathies, the diseases which induce this syndrome.

ACUTE IDIOPATHIC POLYNEURITIS OF LANDRY-GUILLAIN-BARRÉ. This disease seems to occur at all seasons, as if it is an endemic process, and it affects children and adults of all ages and both sexes. Its cause is unknown; all attempts to isolate a virus or microbial agent have failed. A mild respiratory or gastrointestinal infection has preceded the neuritic symptoms by 1 to 3 weeks in approximately half the patients, and a surgical procedure in another 10 percent.

The principal symptoms of peripheral nerve involvement conform to the general description given above. The weakness, which advances over a period of days, involves proximal as well as distal limb and also trunk muscles. Pain is exceptional; paresthesias (tingling and numbness) are frequent but are occasionally absent throughout the illness. The enfeeblement of muscle is so acute that it is not attended by atrophy, though hypotonia and areflexia are obvious. There is usually tenderness on deep pressure or squeezing of muscles. At an early stage the arms may be spared or their muscles may be less weakened than the leg muscles. Facial diplegia, the most frequent type of cranial muscle paralysis, usually comes later, after the arms are affected. However, other cranial nerves (ocular, bulbar) are often affected. When retention of urine occurs, it seldom requires catheterization for more than a few days.

The temperature is usually normal, and lymphadenopathy and splenomegaly do not occur. Electrocardiogram alterations of minor degree have often been reported. The CSF is under normal pressure and is acellular; elevations of protein level are found in most cases, but the values on the first lumbar puncture early in the disease are usually normal or only "slightly raised." In about 10 percent of patients a pleocytosis of 10 to 50 (rarely to 200 cells per ml, predominantly lymphocytes and mononuclear cells) is found. The white cell count and differential count tend to fall within normal limits. The pathologic changes in fatal cases have had a consistent pattern and form. When the disease was fatal within a few days, perivascular, lymphocytic infiltrates have been found. Later the diagnostic inflammatory cell infiltrates and perivenous demyelination are combined with Gombault segmental myelin degeneration and some Wallerian degeneration. Inflammation of roots accounts, evidently, for the CSF changes. Infiltrates in liver, spleen, lymph nodes, heart, and other organs are occasionally found and reflect the systemic nature of the disease.

The differential diagnosis includes poliomyelitis (distinguished usually by epidemic occurrence, meningeal symptoms, and pure areflexic paralysis) and acute myelitis (marked by sensorimotor paralysis below a given spinal level and sphincteric paralysis). The forms of polyneuropathy described below must also be differentiated from this syndrome.

The treatment most widely employed consists of corticosteroids in full doses (45 to 60 mg Meticorten per day for several weeks) with low salt diet and precautions against peptic ulceration of stomach and duodenum. Respiratory assistance is given when the vital capacity falls below 800 to 1,000 ml, and tracheostomy is usually performed at this time, especially if the patient has difficulty in removing secretions from the pharynx and tracheobronchial tree. Careful tracheal toilet, treatment of bronchial and pulmonary infections by the use of an appropriate antibiotic, and support of the blood pressure in the face of hypotension by vasopressor agents complete the therapeutic regimen. The best results are obtained by an efficient respiratory unit skilled in maintaining adequacy of ventilation and of cerebral circulation. Under the most ideal conditions the mortality is reduced from 20 to less than 5 percent.

Once recovery begins, physiotherapy (passive-movement positioning of limbs and later mild resistance exercises) should be given. Decision to discontinue respiratory aid and to close the tracheostomy are based on the degree of recovery of the patient's respiratory mechanism.

Prognosis for complete recovery is good. More than 90 percent of these patients are restored to normal function; the remaining have some mild weakness or reflex loss. Speed of recovery varies. Usually it takes place within a few weeks or months, but if nerves have degenerated, their regeneration may require 6 to 18 months.

INFECTIOUS MONONUCLEOSIS WITH POLYNEURITIS. Three neurologic syndromes have been described with this disease: (1) ascending sensorimotor paralysis, identical with that of the Landry-Guillain-Barré syndrome, (2) aseptic meningitis, (3) meningoencephalitis. All three appear during the midphase of the infection. The polyneuritis varies in severity and has rarely been fatal. The few autopsied cases have shown heavy infiltrations of lymphocytes, monocytes, and plasma cells in the nerves, roots, and meninges. The CSF contains as many as several hundred mononuclear cells, and the protein level is raised. The diagnosis is suggested by the other typical physical and laboratory findings in this disease (see Chap. 255).

INFECTIOUS HEPATITIS WITH POLYNEURITIS. Jaundice accompanied or followed by signs of disease of the peripheral nerves occurs most frequently as a complication of alcoholism and nutritional deficiency but has also been observed in familial amyloidosis. In our experience with this syndrome, the polyneuritis has followed the jaundice by several days or a few weeks and has the same relation to it as to respiratory or intestinal infections. Usually the diagnosis of the type of hepatitis has remained unclear. There is no basis for believing it is homologous serum hepatitis or infectious mononucleosis. It may be only that the mild interstitial hepatitis found in many fatal cases of acute idiopathic polyneuritis is more marked than usual. Recovery from the hepatitis has been the rule.

DIPHTHERITIC POLYNEUROPATHY. Typical diphtheria (see Chap. 169) follows pharyngeal and laryngeal infections. Local action of the exotoxin may paralyze pharyngeal and laryngeal muscles within a few days and may also cause blurring of vision due to loss of accommodation. But these and other cranial nerve symptoms may be overlooked. The first signs of the disease, coming 4 to 8 weeks later, are then an acute to subacute weakness of limbs with paresthesias and distal loss of vibratory and position sense. The weakness characteristically involves all four extremities at the same time or may descend from arms to legs. After a few days to a week or more the patient may be unable to stand or walk, and occasionally the paralysis is so severe and extensive as to impair respiration. The CSF protein level is usually elevated (50 to 200 mg per ml). After the pharyngeal infection is controlled, death in diphtheria is due usually to myocardiopathy or to polyneuropathy with respiratory paralysis.

Postmortem examination discloses a demyelination without inflammatory reaction of spinal roots, sensory ganglions, and adjacent spinal nerves. Axis cylinders, anterior horn cells, peripheral nerves distally, and muscle fibers remain normal.

The disease should be considered in all cases of acute polyneuropathy. Throat culture may demonstrate the Corynebacterium many weeks after the throat infection has subsided. Usually the history of nasal voice, dysphagia,blurred vision, and numb lips with a throat infection several weeks before provides the clue to the diagnosis. The ECG may be abnormal at the time of the polyneuritis. Occasionally the polyneuropathy has followed a local wound infection with *Corynebacterium.* Titers of antitoxin in the blood and a positive Schick test reaction have usually not been helpful (see Treatment, Chap. 169).

The prognosis for full recovery is excellent, once respiratory paralysis is circumvented.

PORPHYRIC POLYNEUROPATHY. As was stated in Chap. 108 (Porphyrins and Porphyria), a severe, rapidly advancing, more or less symmetric polyneuropathy with or without psychosis (nervousness, confusion) and convulsions may occur in the course of acute intermittent porphyria. The neuropathy may affect principally the motor or both the sensory and motor nerves; it may begin in the feet and legs and ascend, or it may begin in the arms and later spread to the trunk and legs. Often it is predominantly proximal in distribution. The CSF protein level is usually normal.

The course of the polyneuropathy is variable. If the disease is mild, it may be quite transitory, with regression of symptoms in a few weeks. If severe, it may rapidly progress to a fatal issue in a few days, the advance occurring without warning; or it may progress in a saltatory fashion over a period of weeks, finally resulting in a severe sensorimotor paralysis that may regress only over a period of months. Disorder of the central nervous system is more likely to precede the acute severe forms of neuropathy, but it may not appear at all.

The pathologic changes in the peripheral nervous system vary according to the stage of the illness at which death occurs. If the patient dies in the first few days, the myelinated fibers may appear entirely normal, despite an almost complete paralysis. If symptoms had been present for weeks, a severe degeneration of both the axones and myelin sheaths often is found in most of the peripheral nerves. No inflammatory reaction, vascular lesion, or other change distinguishes this form of neuropathy; it resembles that of alcoholism, uremia, etc.

See Chap. 108 for a discussion of treatment.

The prognosis for ultimate recovery is excellent, though relapse of the porphyria may result in further involvement of the peripheral nervous system (see Relapsing Polyneuropathy, below).

POLYARTERITIS NODOSA WITH POLYNEUROPATHY. Occasionally this form of neuropathy develops as rapidly as acute idiopathic polyneuritis. Most of the cases evolve more slowly, however, and the syndrome has been either symmetric or asymmetric in its distribution. For this reason the description will be given in the next section. At times a muscle biopsy may be needed to distinguish this acute form from acute idiopathic polyneuritis.

OTHER TOXIC POLYNEUROPATHIES THAT MAY CAUSE PARALYSIS IN A FEW DAYS. An example is triorthocresyl phosphate intoxication, in which the purely motor paralysis ultimately proves to be due to involvement of upper and lower motor neurones (see Chap. 117 for discussion of other chemical agents). The acute stages are accompanied by an encephalopathy with delirium and coma. Stilbamidine, used in the treatment of kala-azar and multiple myeloma, produces a purely sensory neuropathy predominating in the trigeminal nerves.

Subacute Sensorimotor Paralysis, Usually Beginning in the Feet and Legs and Later Involving Hands and Arms

OF SYMMETRIC DISTRIBUTION. Reference is made here to a neurologic disorder that develops over a period of a few weeks and pursues a variable course. Pain, hypersensitivity of skin, tenderness of muscles, and a mixture of dysesthesias and paresthesias are often prominent features of this clinical state. A purely symmetric syndrome of this type usually proves to be due to alcoholism, vitamin B deficiency (beriberi), arsenic, lead, Furadantin, or isoniazid therapy.

Alcoholic Polyneuropathy and Beriberi (See Chap. 81). All data point to a common nutritional factor for both these diseases, though it remains unclear whether the deficiency is one of thiamine, pyridoxine, pantothenic acid, or of several of the B vitamins. We have not been able to define a form of polyneuropathy due solely to the direct effect of alcohol.

In North America and Western Europe this form of polyneuropathy is rarely observed in the nonalcoholic person. Pure starvation does not produce it, the ideal conditions being a vitamin B deficiency in the face of a relatively high carbohydrate consumption. Of course, eccentricity of diet, gastrointestinal disorders, sprue, rice diet for hypertension, while neglecting to give vitamin supplements, all may create the circumstances for such a neuropathy.

After several months (approximately 3) of dietary inadequacy, numbness, tingling, and tenderness of the feet appear and are accompanied by weakness of the more distal muscles of the lower extremities, spreading within a few days to the calves and later the thighs. The leg muscles are always affected before the thighs, and foot drop, accompanied by weakness of the plantar flexors, is the first stage of the motor paresis. Involvement of the thighs is indicated by difficulty in arising from a squatting position. The tendon reflexes (ankle and knee jerks) are abolished, the skin and muscles are tender, and vibratory, and position and touch senses are diminished to a variable degree, increasing as one proceeds distally. The nerves supplying the muscles and skin of the trunk are usually spared, and as the disease progresses, numbness and sensitivity of the fingers, hands, and forearms, weakness of hand grip, and wrist drop are next to appear. Cranial structures are always spared unless Wernicke's disease is conjoined, in which instance there will be bilateral abducens and lateral gaze palsy and nystagmus, as well as cerebellar ataxia of gait, confusion, and memory defect (Korsakoff's psychosis). If pellagra or nutritional myelopathy also occur, signs of retrobulbar neuropathy, deafness, and pyramidal tract signs may be found resembling subacute combined degeneration.

This form of neuropathy produces a manifest sensorimotor disorder, which demands medical attention in only about half the patients in whom the diagnosis can be made. Once started, the syndrome often progresses over a period of days and weeks until the patient becomes confined to bed. But many alcoholics come to the physician with only a subclinical neuropathy (thin leg muscles, questionable sensory disorder over the shins and feet, and reduced or absent tendon reflexes). They give no history of having had a subacute symptomatic polyneuropathy. If untreated, the symptomatic form may progress over weeks and months to a severe atrophy of leg muscles, the polyneuropathy then becoming chronic. Edema is not infrequent (wet beriberi) and is due to dependency of limbs and stasis, more than to coincidental myocardial involvement.

Alcoholic Laennec's cirrhosis and a nutritional anemia may coexist. No other medical findings except weight loss are present. The CSF is normal in nearly all the cases (rarely is the protein elevated).

The pathologic changes of the neuropathy have not been fully described. The primary change encountered is axonal degeneration with destruction of both axis cylinder and myelin sheath, but variable amounts of segmental demyelination may also occur. Cursory studies show the most pronounced lesions to be in the distal parts of the longest and largest medullated fibers in the crural and, to a lesser extent, the brachial nerves. Vagi, phrenic, and trunk nerves are implicated only in the more advanced and fatal cases. Anterior horn cells and sensory ganglion cells undergo chromatolysis indicating axonal damage. Exceptionally, spinal roots and posterior columns of the spinal cord have shown degenerative changes. Recovery awaits remyelination and regeneration.

The disease process is invariably arrested by adequate diet, and the amount of B vitamins in the average food ration of the American public will be curative, though there is no harm in supplementing the diet with B vitamins (see Chap. 81). Positioning and splinting paralyzed limbs to prevent undue stretching and passive motion to prevent contracture are important. Occasionally pain and tenderness are so severe as to require analgesic medication. The pain may be of a burning type (causalgic) with excessive perspiration and only slight weakness and reflex changes. This latter, called the *burning foot syndrome*, has been ascribed to pantothenic acid deficiency, but we have not been able to prove its relationship to this vitamin or to separate it clearly from the usual alcoholic neuropathy. Cooling lotions, Darvon, aspirin, and codeine are needed. Sometimes sympathetic blocking agents are helpful. The pain subsides after some few weeks.

The prognosis for full functional recovery is good, but if the paralysis is complete one may anticipate a period of invalidism for 6 months or more. Vitamins do not hasten recovery. The tendon reflexes may remain absent or diminished. Fatalities have usually been the result of coincidental beriberi, heart disease, or cirrhosis rather than of the polyneuropathy. Vitamin supplements will prevent the polyneuropathy.

Arsenical Polyneuropathy. Nerve involvement from chronic arsenical poisoning is relatively infrequent. The symptoms develop rather slowly over a period of weeks and have the same sensory and motor distribution as was described in beriberi. The condition may be preceded by mental disturbances, convulsions, confusion, and coma, i.e., arsenical encephalopathy. Diagnosis is based on the subacute course of the polyneuropathy coupled with symptoms of gastrointestinal disorder, anemia, jaundice, brownish cutaneous pigmentation, hyperkeratosis of palms and soles, and white transverse banding of nails (Mees lines).

See Chap. 117 for diagnostic tests and treatment.

Poisoning due to mercury, thallium, antimony, and Furadantin may produce a similar picture; the first three of these intoxications respond to British anti-lewisite (BAL).

Lead Neuropathy. Lead neuropathy occurs following chronic exposure to lead, and its most characteristic feature is the predominantly motor affection involving mainly the upper extremities. The radial nerves are most frequently involved, producing wrist and finger drop with few or no sensory manifestations. Less commonly, weakness of the proximal shoulder-girdle muscle occurs, and in the lower extremities foot drop may appear. Clinically the paralyzed muscles are those which are most used. Important associated findings are anemia, basophilic stippling of red blood cells, lead line along the gingival margins, colicky abdominal pain, and constipation. Neuropathy occurs usually in adults and is infrequent in children. In contrast, lead encephalopathy, manifested by increased intracranial pressure, convulsions, blindness, and coma, occur almost exclusively in children. The diagnosis of lead neuropathy is established by the history of lead exposure, the characteristic motor involvement, the associated medical findings, and increased urinary excretion of lead. Treatment consists of withdrawal from exposure to lead and measures to eliminate lead from the blood stream (see Chap. 117). The prognosis for recovery of motor power is good, although in chronic cases recovery may be slow.

Nitrofurantoin Neuropathy. The earliest symptoms of nitrofurantoin neurotoxicity are tingling dysesthesias of the toes and feet, followed shortly by similar sensations in the fingers. If the offending agent is not discontinued, this may progress to a severe, sensorimotor, distal, symmetrical polyneuropathy. Usually neuropathic symptoms appear only after the drug has been administered in high dosage for several weeks or months, but rare patients have experienced dysesthesias after brief periods. Patients with chronic renal failure and azotemia are particularly prone to neurotoxicity with nitrofurantoin, presumably because of diminished excretion in the urine and consequent high tissue levels of the drug. To make matters more difficult, the uremic state itself may be responsible for a clinically similar polyneuropathy, so that the distinction between uremic polyneuropathy and nitrofurantoin neuropathy in the presence of chronic renal failure may be impossible.

Subacute Asymmetric Polyneuropathies. The most notable examples of this syndrome are diabetes mellitus, polyarteritis nodosa, and a more or less obscure form of idiopathic polyneuritis. Rarely, sarcoidosis presents in this fashion.

Diabetic Neuropathy. Only about 15 percent of patients with diabetes mellitus have both symptoms and signs of neuropathy, but nearly 50 percent either complain of neuropathic symptoms or exhibit slowing of nerve conduction velocity. Neuropathy is most common in older diabetics over fifty years of age, is uncommon under thirty years of age, and is rare in childhood diabetes.

A number of clinical syndromes have been delineated as follows: (1) diabetic ophthalmoplegia (described in Chap. 24); (2) acute mononeuropathy; (3) painful, asymmetric mononeuropathy multiplex, which may pursue an acute, subacute, or chronic course and which usually recovers; (4) distal, symmetric, primarily sensory polyneuropathy, affecting feet and legs more than hands in a chronic, slowly progressive manner; and (5) an autonomic neuropathy involving bowel, bladder, and circulatory reflexes. This latter type often coexists with other varieties of diabetic neuropathy.

The acute mononeuropathy involves most commonly the femoral or sciatic nerves and is presumably due to occlusion of vessels supplying the nerve. The outlook for recovery is good.

Painful, asymmetric mononeuropathy multiplex tends to occur in older patients with mild or unrecognized diabetes. Pain often begins in the low back or hip and spreads to thigh and knee on one side. It usually has a deep, burning character with superimposed, tearing, lancinating jabs and a propensity to become most severe at night. Muscle weakness and atrophy is usually most evident in pelvic girdle and thigh, although the distal muscles may not be spared. The upper extremities are usually spared. Sensory loss for position, vibration, touch, and pain is not generally severe, and may conform to either a multiple nerve or root distribution, or to both. The vesical and anal sphincters may be involved, and the knee jerk is often lost on the affected side. When the clinical picture is dominated by lancinating pain and sensory ataxia, with only slight weakness and bowel and bladder derangements, it resembles that of tabes dorsalis so closely that the condition goes by the name of *diabetic tabes.*

Recovery from this type of neuropathy is the rule, although months and even years are often required. There is a tendency for the same syndrome to recur after a lapse of months or years in the opposite lower extremity.

✱The distal, symmetric, primarily sensory form is the most common type of diabetic neuropathy. Numbness and tingling with relatively little pain are the main symptoms and are usually confined to the feet and lower legs. The ankle jerks are rarely preserved. Trophic changes in the form of deep ulcerations and neuropathic joints are occasionally encountered, presumably due to severe denervation of skin and joints. Muscle weakness is usually mild, but in some cases a crural weakness with only minor sensory disturbance may predominate.

Pathologically, severe nerve fiber loss is a prominent finding in this form of neuropathy. In addition, evidence of segmental demyelination and remyelination of remaining axons is apparent in teased nerve fiber preparations. Since myelin is formed from the cell membranes of Schwann cells, one may infer that the Schwann cell is a primary target of the pathologic process in the distal, symmetric type of diabetic neuropathy. Whether the nerve fiber loss is explained by this same process remains uncertain. The blood vessels in these nerves do not appear abnormal.

Symptoms of autonomic involvement include impairment of sweating and vascular reflexes, nocturnal diarrhea, atonic bladder, sexual impotence, and occasionally postural hypotension. The basis for this type of nerve damage is unknown.

In all forms of diabetic neuropathy, the CSF protein may be elevated (50 to 200 mg), and similar increases may be seen in diabetics with no clinical evidence of neuropathy. An explanation for this phenomenon has not been discovered.

The only known treatment is meticulous regulation of the diabetes mellitus along the lines described in Chap. 94. Maintenance of the blood sugar level in a relatively normal range is desirable, for there is some evidence that uncontrolled hyperglycemia is harmful. Vitamin supplements may have some merits, but no clear results have been obtained. Improvement and eventual recovery may be expected over a period of months, but during that time the management of the painful forms of neuropathy may be trying, because analgesic medication is required and one is faced with the possibility of drug addiction.

Polyarteritis Nodosa with Polyneuropathy. Involvement of the intraneural vessels happens in perhaps as many as 90 percent of cases (autopsy figures), but a symptomatic form of neuropathy develops in only 10 to 20 percent. Yet such involvement may be the principal clue to the diagnosis of the underlying disease when, up to that time, the main components of the clinical picture—abdominal pain, hematuria, fever, eosinophilia, hypertension, vague limb pains, and possibly asthma—have not fully declared themselves.

As was stated above, the polyneuropathy may develop acutely and be diffuse and more or less symmetric in distribution, but more often it is subacute, multiple, and asymmetric, i.e., a mononeuropathy multiplex. Both spinal and cranial nerves may be affected. No two cases are identical. The CSF protein level is usually normal. Muscle biopsy, taken near the motor point so as to include nerve, is useful in corroborating the clinical impression in the majority of cases.

Fatal issue is the rule. Corticosteroid therapy has not been successful in most cases. Spontaneous remission and therapeutic arrest are known, however, and a healed or healing form has been observed at autopsy, death having been due to other causes (see Chap. 391).

Subacute Asymmetric Idiopathic Polyneuritis. A few patients who consult the physician with an illness which at first glance has all the appearance of acute idiopathic polyneuritis will continue to become worse over a period of weeks or months. Some have an extremely high CSF protein level (600 to 1,500 mg), with a virtual Froin CSF syndrome (xanthochromia and spontaneous clotting). The higher concentration of protein fluids may induce headache, papilledema, and high CSF pressure, possibly because of the osmotic effect of the protein in increasing CSF volume. As the months pass, some symptoms improve as others appear. Ultimately most patients recover, though late fatality is known to occur; corticosteroids in full doses have proved to be beneficial in the majority of cases but may have to be continued over a period of months.

The pathology of these subacute forms has not been defined, nor is their relationship to the acute varieties of idiopathic polyneuritis settled.

Sarcoidosis. Another cause of subacute or chronic polyneuropathy, sarcoidosis, is discussed in Chap. 254. It may be associated with signs of central nervous system involvement (stalk of the pituitary with diabetes insipidus and the cerebellum with ataxia) or with lesions in muscles (polymyositis).

Chronic Progressive Atrophy of Muscle with Sensory Loss

In this syndrome weakness and muscular atrophy tend to progress over a period of months or years. The time of onset is often uncertain. In infants the condition is often mistaken for muscular dystrophy or infantile muscular atrophy until sensory tests become possible. In the developing child whose musculature naturally increases in power and volume, it may be difficult to decide whether or not the disease is progressive. Ataxia of limbs may be pronounced at a stage when sensory loss exceeds paresis. The atrophy of muscle and trophic changes in the skin are more marked than in the acute and subacute forms of polyneuropathy, which is why the syndrome must be differentiated from the other forms of severe muscular atrophy, i.e., motor system disease, muscular dystrophy (distal type), and syringomyelia. In some cases the distribution is quite asymmetric, e.g., in leprosy, or only a few of the nerves of the legs may be involved, e.g., in familial perforating ulcer. The feet and hands may be extremely wasted and subject to painless injuries, loss of digits, and Charcot's joints (Morvan's syndrome), while proximal structures are sound. In the majority of cases symmetry of pattern is the rule. The CSF protein level may remain elevated over a period of years.

Two main categories of disease are known to present with this syndrome, one acquired, the other familial. The familial analgesic varieties such as the perforating ulcer syndrome, Tangier disease, and amyloidosis cause little weakness or loss of reflexes and leave all forms of sensation except pain and temperature relatively intact. Most of the acquired forms are of obscure cause and mechanism.

CARCINOMATOUS AND MYELOMATOUS POLYNEUROPATHY. A slowly developing symmetric sensory or sensorimotor polyneuropathy may accompany the development of a carcinoma or multiple myeloma. Severe weakness, atrophy, ataxia, and sensory loss of the limbs may advance to the point where the patient is confined to a wheelchair or bed; and all this happens months or even a year or more before a small malignant tumor is found. The CSF protein level is often moderately elevated. This form of polyneuropathy has occurred most frequently with carcinoma of the lung but actually has been joined to every tumor. It may accompany either a solitary plasmocytoma of bone or multiple myeloma and in a few instances has been seen in macroglobulinemia without tumor formation. Thus polyneuropathy must be added to polymyositis or dermatomyositis, with which it is frequently conjoined as a nonspecific neurologic complication of malignant tumor growths. A peculiar type of myasthenia, spinocerebellar degeneration (particularly with carcinoma of the ovary), and multifocal leukoencephalopathy, the other neurologic complications of neoplasia, may coexist. The pathology of the neuropathy has been incompletely defined. The only known therapy consists of removing or controlling the tumor growth, which has resulted at times in improvement. Corticosteroid therapy has helped some patients.

Paraproteinemia. (See Chaps. 68 and 349.) More than a dozen patients with chronic neuropathies have been seen on our wards in recent years in whom no associated metabolic disturbance other than an abnormality of the immunoglobulins was found. In general, three protein abnormalities have occurred: (1) isolated macroglobulinemia (IgM); (2) diffuse increase in all three immunoglobulins (IgM, IgG, and IgA), and (3) a specific disorder of (IgA) immunoglobulin in ataxia-telangiectasis (see Chap. 365). In the latter disease, peripheral nerve dysfunction is evidenced by hyporeflexia, decreased nerve conduction velocities, and severe nerve fiber loss on sural nerve biopsy. In macroglobulinemia and diffuse immunoglobulinemia (not to be confused with multiple myeloma), the neuropathies have been chronic, some exquisitely so, relatively mild, and occasionally asymmetrical and distributed in a multiple nerve trunk pattern. Either prednisone or chlorambucil have at times led to reversal of neuropathy, although recovery has usually been incomplete.

UREMIC POLYNEUROPATHY. Some uremic patients whose renal impairment is chronic will develop a slowly progressive sensorimotor paralysis of the legs and then of the arms. Almost as frequently, the polyneuropathy has developed subacutely. Muscle atrophy, areflexia, and distal distribution in the limbs of neurologic defect leave little doubt of the peripheral nerve character of the disorder. Improvement has been observed after treatment on the artificial kidney, and recovery is the rule after successful renal transplantation. The CSF protein level may be moderately elevated (50 to 150 mg per ml). The pathology is that of a nondescript degeneration of large medullated fibers in nerves and spinal roots. There is no evidence of polyarteritis nodosa. Axis cylinders also degenerate with the expected chromatolysis of their neurones. Amyloid deposit in the nerve has not been found; there is no evidence of vitamin deficiency or of diabetes during life and no sign of polyarteritis nodosa at autopsy. The neuropathy has been observed with all types of chronic kidney disease.

BERIBERI. In all the regions of the world where nutrition is borderline and treatment for an evolving beriberi may of necessity be delayed or even impossible to obtain, the motor paralysis and atrophy of the legs and, to a lesser extent, thighs and arms, may reach an extreme degree. Thus this disease, though subacute in its evolution, becomes a frequent cause of chronic polyneuropathy. Uncontrolled diabetes may behave similarly.

CHRONIC POLYNEUROPATHY WITH CONNECTIVE TISSUE DISEASES. In a clinic where many patients with connective tissue disease are being studied, occasional examples of either subacute or chronic polyneuropathy or a mononeuropathy have appeared. The latter are usually related to rheumatoid arthritis and are difficult to distinguish from pressure palsies. The polyneuropathy is diffuse,

often symmetric, and variably painful. Little is known of its cause, mechanism, or pathology. Some of the most extremely painful polyneuropathies we have seen, extending over long periods of time, have had only minimal sensory loss, weakness, or reflex change in some part of the body, and the diagnosis has been difficult. An unexpected rise in CSF protein level or electromyographic evidence of denervation may sometimes prove to be important leads. Occasionally a chronic symmetric polyneuropathy may accompany lupus erythematosus. It probably is due to a small vessel arteritis. Perhaps more of the obscure polyneuropathies fall in this group of connective tissue diseases than is presently realized (see Chaps. 386, 391, 392).

AMYLCIDOSIS WITH CHRONIC POLYNEUROPATHY. As pointed out in Chap. 114, primary amyloidosis may occur as a sporadic or a familial disease, the latter being particularly common in Portugal and Brazil. The polyneuropathy usually begins in middle adult life, is often severe, and is usually preceded by gastrointestinal symptoms (anorexia, indigestion, diarrhea). Sensory and motor nerve fibers are affected. Symmetry of involvement is the rule. The tongue may be enlarged and weak, and ocular muscles may be paretic. Cerebrospinal fluid protein level is elevated. The diagnosis is suggested by the clinical picture, the polyneuropathy being combined with hepatomegaly (often jaundice), anemia, cardiac enlargement, and EEG change. The nerves are probably enlarged in some patients. Restricted syndromes (eye muscles, tongue, etc.) are known.

LEPROUS POLYNEURITIS. This is the classic example of an infectious neuritis, for the inflammatory reaction in the nerve is evoked by the leprous bacillus. In the early stages of the disease, the neuropathic process is restricted. The nerves most involved are ulnar, greater auricular, tibial, supraorbital, and peroneal. As a rule the condition is painless. The symptoms are principally those of sensory loss or paresis. Anesthesia permits unrecognized injury, infections, trophic changes, and loss of digits. The nerves may be palpably enlarged and beaded.

Diagnosis depends on character of clinical picture, skin and nerve changes often being associated.

See Chap. 175 for diagnostic tests and therapy.

GENETICALLY DETERMINED NEUROPATHIES. Two chronic familial polyneuropathies (peroneal muscular atrophy and progressive hypertrophic polyneuropathy) have been recognized for many years, but in neither has an associated metabolic disturbance been discovered. More recently, several other genetically determined neuropathies have been described (Refsum's disease, abetalipoproteinemia, metachromatic leukodystrophy, Tangier disease) with which a known metabolic disorder is associated. Familial amyloidosis with neuropathy also belongs to the group and is discussed above.

Peroneal Muscular Atrophy (Charcot-Marie-Tooth Disease). This is a hereditary disease with onset during adolescence or adult years. There is chronic degeneration of peripheral nerves and roots, resulting in distal muscle atrophy, beginning in the feet and legs and later involving the hands. Early symptoms are muscular wasting and weakness affecting the extensor and abductor muscles of the feet and producing an equinovarus deformity. Later, all muscles below the middle third of the thigh may be affected, resulting in a "stork leg" appearance of the legs. After a period of years, atrophy of hand and forearm muscles develops. The wasting never extends above the elbows or above the middle third of the thighs. The feet are short and arched, sometimes with perforating ulcers. Pain, paresthesias, and cramps are common. The sensory disorder is usually rather slight and in some instances cannot be detected at all. When it is present, there is impairment of position and vibratory sensation in the feet, and touch and pain sensation are lost in the feet. Reflexes are absent in the involved limbs. The progression of the illness is very slow, and it may arrest at any stage (see Chap. 364 for more complete descriptions).

Progressive Hypertrophic Polyneuropathy (Dejerine-Sottas Disease). This type of neuropathy is uncommon and is frequently familial. It begins usually in childhood and is slowly progressive. Pain and paresthesias in the feet are early symptoms, followed by development of symmetric weakness and wasting of the distal portion of the limbs. Sensation is impaired in a distal distribution, and the tendon reflexes are absent. Miotic pupils, nystagmus, and kyphoscoliosis have been observed in some cases. Other patients present with a recurrent polyneuropathy enlargement of the peripheral nerves because of hypertrophy and proliferation of the cells of Schwann and fibroblasts. Hypertrophic changes in nerve are not specific for this condition, but may also occur diffusely in Refsum's disease (see below), relapsing polyneuropathy and Andrade's amyloidosis, or in a single nerve or multifocal distribution, and possibly in diabetes mellitus. Palpable thickening of the ulnar and peroneal nerves may be conspicuous. In the absence of palpable enlargement of nerves, the diagnosis can be established by biopsy of a cutaneous nerve. The treatment is symptomatic.

Chronic Polyneuropathy with Ichthyosis, Deafness, and Retinitis Pigmentosa (Refsum's Disease). This rare, genetically determined disorder begins in childhood or early adolescence, and the polyneuropathy is sensorimotor, distal, and symmetrical in distribution, affecting legs more than arms. Although the nerves may not be enlarged clinically, hypertrophic changes with "onion-bulb" formation are an unfailing pathologic feature. The metabolic defect has been shown to be tissue accumulation of phytanic acid, a tetra-methylated 16-carbon fatty acid, due to inability to oxidize this substance to pristanic acid. The relationship between this biochemical lesion and the polyneuropathy remains uncertain.

Abetalipoproteinemia (Bassen-Kornzweig Syndrome; Acanthocytosis; See Chap. 113). The clinical manifestations of this unusual syndrome include (1) near absence of betalipoprotein in the serum; (2) retinitis pigmentosa; (3) acanthocytosis of the red blood cells; and (4) a chronic, progressive neurologic deficit, usually beginning in childhood. Extreme proprioceptive sensory loss, ataxia, and areflexia are the most constant features, although muscular weakness and atrophy, kyphoscoliosis, and cor-

ticospinal signs may also be encountered. The main burden of the neurologic disorder falls upon the peripheral nervous system, but the relationship between the neuropathy and the deficiency of betalipoprotein remains unknown.

Tangier Disease (See Chap. 113). In this rare familial disorder, which is marked by alpha$_1$ lipoprotein deficiency, two of six reported cases have had neuropathic symptoms and signs of a relapsing nature and denervation atrophy of muscle.

Metachromatic Leukodystrophy (See Chap. 364). Massive sulfatide accumulation throughout the central and peripheral nervous system, and to a lesser extent in other organs, occurs in this disorder, apparently because of congenital absence of the degradative enzyme, sulfatase. The abnormality is transmitted as an autosomal recessive trait. Progressive cerebral deterioration is the most obvious clinical aspect, but hyporeflexia, muscular atrophy, and diminished nerve conduction velocity indicate a neuropathic element. Metachromatically staining granules accumulate in the cytoplasm of Schwann cells in all peripheral nerves, as well as in central white matter. Sural biopsy may be used to establish the diagnosis, even early in the course of the illness.

Relapsing Polyneuropathy

Two diseases most regularly take this form: porphyria, in which the attacks recur because of the administration of barbiturates or spontaneous relapses, and idiopathic polyneuritis. The latter has no proven cause. Enlargement of nerves may occur, so that it is probable that some patients with hypertrophic polyneuropathy may fall into this category. Amyloidosis may also cause palpable enlargement of nerves, but by an obviously different mechanism.

Mononeuropathy or Multiple Neuropathy

This group of diseases differs in that one or a few of the nerves are involved in the disease process. The diagnosis rests on the finding of motor, reflex, or sensory changes confined to the territory of the nerve and the presence of other data pointing to its causation. A part of a plexus may also be involved. One variety, mononeuropathy multiplex, which has already been discussed, is due to leprosy, sarcoid, diabetes, and polyarteritis nodosa.

THE COMMON BRACHIAL AND CRURAL MONONEUROPATHIES

BRACHIAL PALSIES. The fifth to eighth cervical and first thoracic spinal nerves innervate the muscles of the shoulder girdles and upper extremities. The brachial plexus is formed by components of these nerves, and lesions of the nerves or their branches result in characteristic palsies. The following are the brachial palsies most likely to be observed on the medical wards of a hospital.

Long Thoracic Nerve. This nerve is derived from the fifth, sixth, and seventh cervical nerves and supplies the serratus magnus muscle. Paralysis of the serratus magnus muscle results in inability to raise the arm over the head from a forward position, and there is winging of the medial border of the scapula on pushing forward against resistance. It is injured most commonly by pressure on the shoulder, from either a sudden blow or prolonged pressure from carrying heavy weights. It is also involved at times in diabetic patients and as a manifestation of brachial and serum neuritides and in other idiopathic forms of neuritis (pleurodynia, Coxsackie disease).

Suprascapular Nerve. This nerve is derived from the fifth and sixth cervical nerves and supplies the supra- and infraspinatus muscles. Lesions may be diagnosed by the presence of weakness of abduction and external rotation of the arm and atrophy of the supra- and infraspinatus muscles. The nerve may be injured by blows on top of the shoulder and fracture-dislocations of the shoulder joint.

Upper Brachial Plexus Paralysis. This is due to injury to the fifth cervical nerve, caused most commonly by forceful separation of the head and shoulder during difficult delivery or by pressure in the supraclavicular region during anesthesia. The muscles affected are the biceps, deltoid, brachialis anticus, supinator longus, supra- and infraspinatus, and rhomboids. The arm hangs at the side, internally rotated, with the elbow extended. The forearm is pronated. Hand motion is unaffected. The prognosis for spontaneous recovery is generally good, especially in cases of birth injury. This condition as a result of birth injury (Erb-Duchenne brachial plexus palsy) is discussed in Chaps. 21 and 365.

Lower Brachial Plexus Paralysis. This is due to injury to the eighth cervical and first thoracic roots as a result of traction on the abducted arm in falls, during operation, and with tumors of the apex of the lung (superior sulcus or Pancoast's syndrome). Injury may occur during birth (Dejerine-Klumpke brachial plexus injury). There is paralysis and wasting of the small muscles of the hand and a characteristic claw-hand deformity. Sensory loss is limited to the ulnar border of the hand and inner side of forearm, and there may be an associated paralysis of the cervical sympathetic nerve with a Horner's syndrome if the Ti motor root is involved.

Lesions of the Cords of the Brachial Plexus. The outer and inner cords are most commonly affected. Dislocation of the head of the humerus, pressure of the cervical ribs, and stab wounds are the most frequent causes. Injury to the outer cord results in paralysis of the biceps and coracobrachialis muscles and all muscles supplied by the median nerve except the intrinsic hand muscles. There is some loss of sensation over the radial aspects of the forearm. Involvement of the inner cord, as may occur in compression by the cervical rib, results in paralysis of the muscles supplied by the ulnar nerve together with the median-innervated intrinsic muscles of the hand and sensory loss over the ulnar aspect of the hand and forearm.

Axillary Nerve. This nerve arises from the posterior cord of the brachial plexus and supplies the teres minor and deltoid muscles. It may be involved in injuries resulting from fractures of the neck of the humerus, serum neuritis, brachial neuritis, or as a part of a disease of unknown cause. The anatomic localization depends on the recognition of a paralysis of abduction of the arm, wasting of the deltoid muscle, and slight impairment of sensation over the outer aspect of the shoulder.

Musculocutaneous Nerve. This nerve is derived from the fifth and sixth cervical nerves and is a branch of the outer cord of the brachial plexus. It innervates the biceps and brachialis anticus muscles. Lesions of the nerve result in weakness of elbow flexion. Rarely is it injured alone.

Radial Nerve. This nerve is derived from the fifth to eighth cervical nerves and is the termination of the posterior cord of the brachial plexus. It innervates the triceps muscle and the supinator and extensor muscles of the forehand and hand. Complete radial paralysis results in inability to extend the elbow, paralysis of supination of the forearm, and complete wrist and finger drop. Sensation is impaired over the posterior aspect of the forearm and a small area over the radial aspect of the dorsum of the hand. The nerve may be injured in the axilla, for example in "crutch" palsy, but most commonly traumatism occurs in the lower arm where the nerve winds around the humerus. Common types of injury at this site are fractures and pressure palsies incurred during sleep.

Median Nerve. This nerve is derived from the sixth cervical to the first thoracic root and is formed by the union of two heads from the inner and outer cords of the brachial plexus. It innervates the pronators of the forearm, long finger flexors, and abductor and opponens muscles of the thumb and is a sensory nerve to the palmar aspect of the hand. Complete median nerve paralysis results in wasting of the affected muscles and inability to pronate the forearm or deviate the hand in an ulnar direction, paralysis of flexion of the index finger and terminal phalanx of the thumb, weakness of flexion of the remaining fingers, weakness of abduction and opposition of the thumb, and sensory impairment over the radial two-thirds of the palmar aspect of the hand and over the distal phalanges of the dorsum of the index and third fingers. The nerve may be injured in the axilla by shoulder dislocation and in any part of its course by laceration, stab, or gunshot wounds. The wrist is the most common site of external injury. Compression of the nerve at the wrist (carpal tunnel syndrome) may occur secondary to prolonged occupational pressure or local infiltration, for example, by a thickening of connective tissue and deposit of amyloid with multiple myeloma. Other systemic diseases associated with carpal tunnel syndrome are acromegaly and hypothyroidism. Incomplete lesions of the median nerve between the axilla and wrist may result in *causalgia*.

Ulnar Nerve. This nerve is derived from the eighth cervical and first thoracic roots. It innervates the ulnar flexor of the wrist, the inner half of the deep finger flexors, the adductors and abductors of the fingers, the adductor of the thumb, the two medial lumbricals, and muscles of the hypothenar eminence. It is the sensory nerve to the fifth and ulnar half of the fourth fingers and the ulnar border of the hand. Complete ulnar paralysis results in a characteristic claw-hand deformity owing to wasting of the small hand muscles and hyperextension of the fingers at the metacarpophalangeal joints and flexion at the interphalangeal joints. The flexion deformity is most pronounced in the fourth and fifth fingers. Sensory loss occurs over the fifth finger, the ulnar aspect of the fourth finger, and the ulnar border of the palm. The ulnar nerve is most commonly injured at the elbow because of fracture or dislocation involving the joint. *Delayed ulnar palsy* may occur many years after an injury to the elbow joint which has resulted in a cubitus valgus deformity of the joint. Because of the deformity, the nerve is stretched in its course over the ulnar condyle. The superficial location of the nerve at the elbow makes it a common site of pressure palsy. Prolonged pressure on the outer part of the palm may result in damage to the deep palmar branch of the ulnar nerve, causing weakness of small hand muscles but no sensory loss.

CRURAL PALSIES. The twelfth thoracic, first to fifth lumbar, and first, second, and third sacral spinal nerve roots compose the lumbosacral plexuses and innervate the muscles of the lower extremities and "saddle" region. The following are the common crural palsies.

Lateral Femoral Cutaneous Nerve. This nerve is derived from the second and third lumbar roots. It is a sensory nerve supplying the lateral aspect of the thigh. The nerve enters the thigh beneath the lateral end of the inguinal ligament and then enters the fascia lata, where it may become constricted. Compression of the nerve results in uncomfortable paresthesias along its cutaneous distribution and in sensory impairment. The condition is called *meralgia paresthetica* (mentioned below).

Obturator Nerve. This nerve is derived from the second, third, and fourth lumbar roots. It supplies the adductor muscles of the thigh, and injury to the nerve results in almost complete paralysis of adduction of the thigh. The nerve is most frequently injured during the course of a difficult labor and also as a result of dislocation of the hip or an obturator hernia. It may be affected in diabetes, polyarteritis nodosa, osteitis pubis, retroperitoneal carcinoma of the cervix of the uterus, and other tumors, etc.

Femoral Nerve. This nerve is derived from the second, third, and fourth lumbar roots. It supplies the iliacus, pectineus, sartorius, and quadriceps muscles and carries sensory impulses from the anteromedial aspect of the thigh and medial side of the lower leg. Following injury to the nerve, there is paralysis of extension of the knee, with wasting of the quadriceps muscle and also some weakness of hip flexion. The knee jerk is abolished. The nerve may be involved in fractures and dislocation of the hip and in fractured pelvis. It may be affected in diabetes, polyarteritis nodosa, and in retroperitoneal, pelvic, or abdominal lesions such as psoas abscess or tumor. Because of the femoral triangle, wounds in this region may be fatal.

Sciatic Nerve. This nerve is derived from the fourth and fifth lumbar and first, second, and third sacral roots. It provides the motor innervation of the hamstring mus-

cles and all those below the knee; and it carries sensory impulses from the posterior aspect of the thigh and posterior and lateral aspects of the leg and entire sole. In complete sciatic paralysis, the knee cannot be flexed and all muscles below the knee are paralyzed. The sciatic nerve is commonly injured in fractures of the pelvis or femur, in gunshot wounds of the buttock and thigh, and by the inadvertent injection of toxic substances such as paraldehyde. It may also be involved by pelvic tumors and in both diabetes mellitus and polyarteritis nodosa. Cryptogenic forms also occur and are actually more frequent than those with an identifiable cause. A ruptured lumbar disk often simulates sciatic neuropathy. Incomplete lesions of the sciatic nerve occasionally result in causalgia.

Common Peroneal Nerve. This nerve is one of the terminal divisions of the sciatic nerve in the popliteal fossa. It supplies the dorsiflexors of the foot and toes and everters of the foot and sensation to the dorsum of the foot and lateral aspect of the lower half of the leg. These functions are lost with lesions which completely interrupt the nerve. Pressure or sleep palsy is one of the most frequent types of injury, the compression being of that part of the nerve which passes over the head of the fibula. It is also commonly involved by fractures involving the upper end of the fibula and in diabetic neuropathy.

Tibial Nerve. This nerve is the other of the two terminal divisions of the sciatic nerve in the popliteal fossa. It supplies all the calf muscles and the flexors of the foot. Complete paralysis of the nerve results in a calcaneovalgus deformity of the foot, which no longer can be plantar-flexed. There is loss of sensation over the plantar aspect of the foot.

SOME OF THE DISEASES WHICH INVOLVE SINGLE NERVES OR PLEXUSES

INFECTIONS. In faucial diphtheria, selective involvement of the vagi and nerves to the ciliary muscles of the eye results in palatal paralysis and paralysis of accommodation. The palatal palsy occurs in the first 2 weeks of infection and the loss of accommodation about a week later. Both tend to improve rapidly. In cutaneous diphtheria, involvement of nerves locally results in paralysis of the muscles supplied by the spinal segment from which the infected region is innervated. In leprosy, granulomatous infection of multiple peripheral nerves usually takes place simultaneously, producing symptoms of polyneuritis rather than localized asymmetric neuritis, but the latter may be found in the early stages of leprous neuritis. Herpes zoster is a sensory neuritis of virus etiology, characterized by acute inflammation of one or more posterior root ganglions, spinal nerves, and roots and gray matter of the spinal cord. Lancinating pain and hyperalgesia over the skin surface supplied by affected roots occur for 3 or 4 days, followed by the appearance of a segmental herpetic eruption. If the inflammatory process spreads to involve adjacent motor roots of anterior horns of the cord, segmental motor weakness and wasting disappear. Paralysis of the oculomotor nerves may occur in conjunction with involvement of the Gasserian ganglion (ophthalmoplegic zoster). Facial paralysis may occur with involvement of the geniculate ganglion (Ramsay Hunt syndrome). Sarcoidosis may involve single or multiple peripheral nerves, producing asymmetric mononeuritis or polyneuritis. Unilateral or bilateral facial paralysis is common in association with parotitis and uveitis in sarcoidosis.

TRAUMA. External trauma may result in complete transection of a peripheral nerve or may impair conduction without interrupting the anatomic continuity of the involved nerve. Complete division of a mixed peripheral nerve results in paralysis and sensory loss corresponding to the region supplied by the damaged nerve. Recovery of function after complete division can take place only when the divided ends lie in apposition or have been sutured. Growth of nerve fibers from the center proceeds at a rate of 1 to 2 mm a day, and the recovery time can be estimated by the distance between the site of injury and the destination of the nerve. An early indication of regeneration is the presence of tingling sensation below the lesion (Tinel's sign) on tapping the nerve. Sensory recovery precedes the return of motor power. All forms of cutaneous sensation begin to return together. Appreciation of pain and temperature improves, but the stimuli are poorly localized for some time. Eventually there is recovery of the discriminative aspects of sensation, including localization of sensory stimuli, postural sense, recognition of slight differences in temperature, and appreciation of very light touch.

PRESSURE PALSIES AND ENTRAPMENT NEUROPATHIES. A period of prolonged compression of a nerve against an underlying bone results in temporary paralysis owing to local ischemia. Mild degrees of compression are followed by fairly rapid recovery. Severe compression, such as may occur during a bout of alcoholic intoxication, deep sleep, or anesthesia, may result in focal disintegration of myelin, damage to axis cylinders, and Wallerian degeneration of distal segments. Recovery may be rapid by reversal of functional disorder or slow awaiting regeneration. Common varieties of pressure palsy are radial nerve paralysis with wrist drop due to prolonged pressure against the back of the arm (Saturday night palsy), ulnar palsy due to repeated trauma to the nerve at the elbow, especially after an old fracture that changes the relation of the nerve to the bicipital groove, and peroneal nerve palsy with foot drop caused by compressing the nerve against the fibula, as in sitting with legs crossed or during obstetric procedures with legs in stirrups.

The entrapment neuropathies result from repeated compression of a nerve against bone or a point where it passes through a narrow space. Slowly the perineurium and epineurium thicken and strangulate the nerve with injury to some of its larger more peripheral fibers. Several unique syndromes are known: (1) median nerve entrapment in carpal tunnel (see above) and (2) *meralgia paresthetica*. This is a sensory neuropathy characterized by pain and paresthesia over the lateral aspect of the thigh because of compression of the lateral femoral cutaneous nerve in the fascia lata. Pressure on nerve

roots in the cervical and lumbar regions by *herniated intervertebral discs* results in pain, sensory impairment, and variable motor weakness corresponding to the area supplied by the involved root (see Chap. 13). Compression of the inner cord of the brachial plexus by a *cervical rib or by some other malformation of the thoracic outlet* (thoracic outlet syndrome) results in atrophy of small hand muscles and sensory loss in the ulnar nerve distribution. Usually the subclavian artery is compressed. When the median nerve is compressed at the wrist beneath the transverse carpal ligament (carpal tunnel syndrome), there are pain and paresthesias in the palmar surface of the hand and first three fingers, thenar atrophy, weakness in flexor of thumb and opponens muscle, and sensory impairment over the median nerve distribution.

TUMOR. Peripheral nerves may be compressed or invaded by primary or metastatic tumors arising in other tissues. Solitary tumors of nerve sheaths, or neuromas, commonly occur along the roots of spinal nerves, chiefly in the thoracic and lumbar regions. Compression of the nerve root and adjacent spinal cord may occur. Root compression causes pain referred to the distribution of the involved nerve, and there may be associated sensory impairment and motor weakness. Lymphomatosis and carcinomatosis of the cranial and spinal meninges may implicate single or multiple nerve roots. Tumor cells may be found in the cerebrospinal fluid. Solitary neuromas may involve any of the peripheral nerves, producing local pain and tenderness to palpation. Multiple neuromas occur in von Recklinghausen's disease and are associated with multiple congenital anomalies, as well as kyphoscoliosis, cutaneous pigmentation, and cutaneous fibromas. The treatment of solitary expanding nerve tumors of the limbs is wide excision with nerve graft or suture, if that is possible.

IDIOPATHIC NEUROPATHY. *Bell's palsy* is due to inflammation of the facial nerve in the fallopian canal as a result of an obscure, possibly infective process. Edema may play a part leading to compression of nerve fibers, with resulting acute unilateral paralysis of facial muscles (see Chap. 355).

Brachial neuritis is an acute affection of the brachial plexus, characterized by the acute or subacute onset of severe pain in the neck, arm, and hand, followed by moderate muscle weakness, slight impairment of sensation in the fingers and hand, numbness or hyperesthesia, and depressed reflexes in the involved arm. The pain is usually severe and constant and is aggravated by moving the arm or stretching the bachial plexus. Muscle wasting is rarely severe, but some cases of brachial neuritis, especially those described by the term *neuralgic amyotrophy*, may be followed by localized paralysis and atrophy of the shoulder girdle and arm muscles. Some of these have a familial incidence. Recovery slowly occurs over a period of several weeks to months. Symptomatic treatment, including complete rest of the involved arm and analgesics in the acute phase, followed by mild massage and exercise, usually suffices.

Sciatic neuritis causes pain in the lumbar region and behind the leg from buttock to ankle. The pain is aching or burning in quality and is aggravated by movement or straining. The sciatic nerve is tender to palpation or stretching. There may be slight weakness of the hamstrings and muscles below the knee. The ankle jerk is absent. Sensory impairment is usually slight. It is necessary to distinguish the symptoms of sciatic neuritis from those of sciatic compression. In compression (e.g., by tumor) the onset is more gradual, symptoms are progressive, muscle wasting is more conspicuous, the nerve is less tender to palpation, and sensory loss is greater. The course of sciatic neuritis is stationary at first, followed by slow improvement.

Serum neuritis develops several days after the onset of serum sickness. The fifth cervical nerve root is most commonly involved, with pain, paralysis, and atrophy corresponding to the distribution of the nerve. Occasionally the entire brachial plexus may be involved, and there is sometimes, but rarely, a generalized polyneuritis. The cause is not known but the condition is attributed to perineural edema, comparable to the urticaria of serum sickness, with compression of affected roots or nerves. Recovery is usually complete but may take weeks or months.

REFERENCES

Asbury, A. K., M. Victor, and R. D. Adams: Uremic Polyneuropathy, Arch. Neurol., 8:413, 1963.

Austin, J. H.: Observations on the Syndrome of Hypertrophic Neuritis, Medicine, 35:187, 1956.

Dyck, P. J.: Peripheral Neuropathy, Postgrad. Med., 41:279, 1967.

Fisher, C. M., and R. D. Adams: Diphtheritic Polyneuritis: A Pathological Study, J. Neuropathol. Exp. Neurol., 15: 243, 1956.

Haymaker, W., and J. W. Kernohan: The Landry-Guillain-Barré Syndrome, Medicine, 28:59, 1949.

Lovshin, L. L., and J. W. Kernohan: Peripheral Neuritis in Periarteritis Nodosa, Arch. Intern. Med., 82:321, 1948.

Raff, M. C., V. Sangalang, and A. K. Asbury: Ischemic Mononeuropathy Multiplex in Association with Diabetes Mellitus, Arch. Neurol., 18:487, 1968.

Thomas, P. K., and R. G. Lascelles: The Pathology of Diabetic Neuropathy, Quart. J. Med., 35:489, 1966.

355 DISEASES OF CRANIAL NERVES

Maurice Victor and Raymond D. Adams

The cranial nerves are susceptible to many diseases that rarely if ever affect the peripheral nerves, and for that reason alone they deserve to be considered separately. Reference has already been made to some of these diseases in Chap. 23, Vertigo and Disorders of Equilibrium and Gait, and in Chap. 24, Common Disturbances of Vision, Ocular Movement, and Hearing. But there the emphasis was on cardinal manifestations and the ways of demonstrating the disordered function. Here we are concerned with the principal syndromes involving those nerves and the diseases which cause them.

SYNDROME OF ANOSMIA AND AGEUSIA AND RELATED DISORDERS OF OLFACTION

The delicate filaments of the olfactory nerve, as they pass from the nasal mucous membrane through the cribriform plate of ethmoid bone to the olfactory bulbs, are easily damaged by diseases of the nasal mucosa, skull fractures, and meningeal lesions. If unilateral, *hyposmia* or *anosmia*, as the defect is called, will not be recognized by the patient. Bilateral anosmia, on the other hand, is a frequent complaint, and the patient is usually convinced that he has lost his sense of taste as well. This calls attention to the fact that much of taste is olfactory, and often it can be shown that the patient's ability to distinguish elementary taste sensations (sweet, sour, bitter, and salty) is intact. The olfactory defect can be verified readily enough by presenting the patient with a series of nonirritating olfactory stimuli (vanilla, lemon, cigarette, coffee, etc.), first in one nostril, then in the other, and asking him to distinguish between them. Ammonia and similar pungent substances should not be used because they stimulate the trigeminal nerve.

The sudden development of anosmia and impaired taste is related most often to a nasal infection. Little is known of its cause and nothing of its pathology. It may be transitory or permanent, and nothing can be done about it. In time the patient adjusts to the fact that the world no longer presents an interesting array of olfactory stimuli and that he no longer savors his food. These nerve filaments may be ruptured by head injury, especially if it is severe enough to cause fracture; the damage may be unilateral or bilateral and is usually permanent. Cranial surgery, especially if much CSF escapes while the patient is on his back so that the olfactory bulbs retract from ethnoid bones, subarachnoid hemorrhage, and chronic meningeal inflammation may have a similar effect.

The gradual development of anosmia should prompt an investigation of the anterior base of the skull. Meningiomas of the olfactory region may not only implicate the olfactory nerves but extend posteriorly to involve the optic nerves. Upward extension into the frontal lobes causes a lack of initiative (abulia), personality change (apathy, silliness, or witzelsucht), and forgetfulness. Large aneurysms of the anterior cerebral and anterior communicating arteries may produce a similar syndrome. Children with anterior meningoencephaloceles are usually anosmic and, in addition, may exhibit CSF rhinorrhea when the head is held in certain positions (demonstrated by examination of the fluid and by watching, under ultraviolet light, fluorescein issue from the nostrils after it has been instilled in the spinal subarachnoid space). Head injury, nasal injury, and hydrocephalus are more frequent causes of CSF rhinorrhea.

Parosmia, or perversion of the sense of smell, may occur with local nasal conditions such as empyema of the nasal sinuses. It may also be a troublesome symptom in middle-aged and elderly individuals who have depressive symptoms. Every article of food may have a horrid odor. Nothing is known of the basis of this state; there is no loss of discriminative sensation. Minor degrees of parosmia are not necessarily abnormal, for unpleasant odors have a way of lingering for several hours and of being reawakened by other olfactory stimuli, as every pathologist knows.

Olfactory hallucinations are always of central origin. As described in Chap. 28, a disagreeable odor may be the aura of a seizure. The evocative lesion is usually on the inferior and medial surface of one temporal lobe, in or near the uncus, and the seizure it produces is called *uncinate*. Schizophrenic patients sometimes complain of smelling disagreeable odors about themselves, which they believe cause other persons to shun them. These olfactory sensations rarely have the objectivity of a hallucination but are rather in the nature of a delusion. The sense of smell is demonstrably intact.

SYNDROME OF RETROBULBAR NEUROPATHY

The acute development of impaired vision in one eye or both eyes (in the latter case the eyes may be affected either simultaneously or successively) raises a number of interesting and troublesome problems. The most frequent clinical setting is one in which a child, adolescent, or young adult notes a rapid diminution of vision in one eye (as though a veil or haze covered every object seen). The diminution may progress to complete blindness. The optic disk and retina appear normal, but in some cases the optic disk is elevated or choked, and the disk margins are obscure and surrounded by hemorrhages (papilledema). Papillitis is distinguished from the papilledema of increased intracranial pressure by the effect on visual acuity. This is severely impaired in cases of papillitis, but relatively little affected by the high pressure of papilledema until late in the illness (although there may have been enlargement of the blind spot and slight constriction of the visual fields). In retrobulbar neuropathy after some few days or weeks the other eye may be similarly involved, the blindness then being complete except for slight peripheral vision. The pupillary light reflex is impaired. In a high percentage of patients, no cause can be found and after several more weeks there is spontaneous recovery. Vision may return to normal; occasionally a small scotoma is left. The optic disk later becomes slightly pale in many of the patients. The CSF may be normal or may contain 10 to 200 lymphocytes, and the protein level may be elevated.

About half of such patients will develop other symptoms and signs consistent with multiple sclerosis within 10 to 15 years, and even more will do so if the patients are observed for longer periods. Less is known about children with retrobulbar neuropathy, but the prognosis in them is probably similar to that in adults. Formerly the syndrome was blamed on sinusitis and treated as such, but Cushing long ago proved the error of this assumption. Sinus disease rarely affects vision except for an occasional mucocele which presses on an ocular or optic nerve. Regression of symptoms has been observed to accompany the administration of ACTH (45 units per day for 3 weeks) or Meticorten (45 mg per day for 3 weeks).

Simultaneous impairment of vision in the two eyes, with central or centrocecal scotomas, usually is due not to a demyelinative process but rather to a toxic or nutritional disorder. The former condition (so-called "tobacco-alcohol amblyopia") is observed most commonly in the chronic alcoholic patient. Impairment of visual acuity evolves over several days or weeks, and examination discloses bilateral, roughly symmetric central or centrocecal scotomas, the peripheral fields being intact. With appropriate treatment (nutritious diet and B vitamins), partial or complete recovery is possible, although some patients are left with a permanent defect in central vision and pallor of the temporal portions of the optic disks. The same disorder may be seen in nonalcoholic patients, under conditions of severe nutritional deprivation and in pernicious anemia. Impairment of vision due to methyl alcohol intoxication is more abrupt in onset and is characterized by large symmetric central scotomas, as well as by symptoms of systemic disease and acidosis (see Chap. 118). Treatment is directed mainly to correction of the acidosis.

Rarely amblyopia is due to cranial arteritis, some other vascular disease, or diabetes.

SYNDROME OF BITEMPORAL HEMIANOPIA

This type of visual disorder is usually related to a pituitary adenoma (ballooned sella shown in x-rays of the skull) but may also be due to craniopharyngiomas, saccular aneurysms of the circle of Willis, meningiomas of the tuberculum sellae (normal sella or thickened tuberculum by radiography), and rarely sarcoidosis, metastatic carcinoma, and Hand-Schüller-Christian disease. The lesion is always in the chiasm, involving the decussating nasal fibers from each retina.

SYNDROMES OF HOMONYMOUS HEMIANOPIA

See Chap. 24.

SYDROME OF VISUAL AGNOSIA

See Chap. 31.

SYNDROME OF OPHTHALMOPLEGIA

Rarely, children or adults may have one or more attacks of ocular palsy in conjunction with an otherwise typical migraine (*migrainous ophthalmoplegia*). The muscles innervated by either the oculomotor or the abducens nerve are affected. Presumably, intense vascular spasm in

Table 355-1. CRANIAL NERVE SYNDROMES

Site	Cranial nerves involved	Eponym	Usual cause
Sphenoidal fissure...........	III, IV, ophthalmic V, VI, sometimes II	....	Invasive tumors of sphenoid bone, aneurysms
Lateral wall of cavernous sinus	III, IV, ophthalmic V, VI, often with proptosis	Foix's syndrome	Aneurysms of cavernous sinus, cavernous sinus thrombosis, invasive tumors from sinuses and sella turcica
Petrosphenoidal space.......	II, III, IV, V, VI	Jacob's syndrome	Large tumors of middle cranial fossa
Apex of petrous bone........	V, VI	Gradenigo's syndrome	Petrositis, tumors of petrous bone
Internal auditory meatus....	VII, VIII	....	Tumors of petrous bone (dermoids, etc.), infectious processes
Pontocerebellar angle........	V, VII, VIII, and sometimes IX	....	Acoustic neuromas, meningiomas
Jugular foramen.............	IX, X, XI	Vernet's syndrome	Tumors and aneurysms
Posterior laterocondylar space	IX, X, XI, XII	Collet-Sicard syndrome	Tumors of parotid gland, carotid body, and secondary tumor
Posterior retroparotid space	IX, X, XI, XII, and Bernard-Horner syndrome	Villaret's syndrome	Tumors of parotid gland, carotid body, secondary tumor, lymph node tumors, tuberculous adenitis

branches of the ophthalmic artery causes a transitory ischemia of nerve. Arteriograms, done after the onset of the palsy, usually reveal no abnormality. Recovery is the rule.

The acute development of a sixth or third nerve palsy on one side is a relatively common occurrence in the adult. The pupil is usually spared. In more than half the patients so affected no cause can be assigned; fortunately, most of them recover in a few weeks to months. Other patients prove to have diabetes mellitus or, rarely, cranial arteritis; in these instances the disorder may be ascribed to vascular occlusion. Exophthalmic ophthalmoplegia and myasthenia gravis must always be ruled out.

The slow development of a complete ophthalmoplegia is most often due to an aneurysm, tumor, or inflammatory process in the cavernous sinus or at the superior orbital foramen (syndrome of Foix) (see Table 355-1).

Gaze palsies or mixed ophthalmoplegia and gaze palsies, due usually to vascular, demyelinative, or neoplastic processes in the brainstem, have already been discussed in Chap. 24.

SYNDROME OF FACIAL PAIN (TRIGEMINAL NEURALGIA, TIC DOULOUREUX)

The most striking disorder of the trigeminal nerve is tic douloureux. This occurs in middle-aged and elderly individuals and consists of excruciating paroxysms of pain in the lips, gums, or chin, and, very rarely, in the distribution of the ophthalmic division of the fifth nerve. The pain seldom lasts more than a few seconds or a minute or two but may be so intense that the patient winces, hence the term *tic*. The paroxysm recurs frequently, both day and night, for several weeks at a time. Another characteristic feature is the initiation of pain by obvious stimuli applied to certain areas on the face, lips, or

tongue, or by movement of these parts, the so-called "trigger zones." Sensory loss cannot be demonstrated in these cases. Kugelberg and Lindblom have studied the relationship between stimuli applied to the trigger zone and the pain paroxysm. They found that the adequate stimulus for precipitating an attack is touch and possibly tickle, rather than pain or temperature. Usually a spatial and temporal summation of impulses was necessary to trigger an attack, which was followed by a refractory period of up to 2 or 3 min. They suggest that the mechanism for the paroxysmal pain involves the nucleus of the spinal tract of the fifth nerve.

The diagnosis of this disorder must rest upon these strict clinical criteria, and the condition must be distinguished from other forms of facial and cephalic neuralgia and pain arising from diseases of the jaw, teeth, or sinuses. Tic douloureux is usually without assignable cause, although occasionally it is a manifestation of multiple sclerosis (may be bilateral) or of herpes zoster. Very rarely a tumor in the posterior fossa which has caused only an early irritative lesion in the nerve or its root may produce pain clinically indistinguishable from that of tic douloureux. Usually, however, space-occupying lesions, such as aneurysms, neurofibromas, or meningiomas, produce a loss of sensation.

The conventional treatment for tic douloureux is alcohol or phenol injection of the affected nerve at the foramen ovale and rotundum or section of the root of the trigeminal nerve between the ganglion and the brainstem. Stereotaxic electrolyte lesions have also been made. Antiepileptic drugs such as diphenylhydantoin (Dilantin) and 5-carbamyl-5H-dibenz (b,f)-azepine (Tegretol) have been found by some authors to shorten the duration of the attacks. Temporizing and using these drugs may permit a spontaneous remission to occur. Most of the patients with severe pain come to surgery.

Anesthesia and analgesia of the face may be induced by stilbamadine (in the treatment of kala-azar and multiple myeloma) and trichloracetic acid intoxication. Pain and itching may occur during recovery.

Tonic spasm of the masticatory muscles, known as *trismus,* is symptomatic of tetanus, although it may occur in hysteria, and lesser degrees may be associated with disease of the temporomaxillary joint, the teeth, and gums or may be a manifestation of encephalitis.

SYNDROME OF FACIAL PALSY (BELL'S PALSY) AND FACIAL SPASM

The seventh cranial nerve is mainly a motor nerve supplying all the muscles concerned with facial expression on one side. The sensory component is small (the nervus intermedius of Wrisberg); it conveys taste sensation from the anterior two-thirds of the tongue and probably cutaneous sensation from the anterior wall of the external auditory canal. The taste fibers originally traverse the lingual nerve (a branch of the mandibular) but then leave this nerve to join the chorda tympani. Secretomotor fibers innervate the lacrimal gland through the greater superficial petrosal nerve, and others travel to the sublingual and submaxillary glands via the chorda tympani.

Several other anatomic facts are worth remembering. The motor nucleus of the seventh nerve is anterior and lateral to the abducens nucleus, and in their intrapontine course the facial nerve fibers hook around the abducens nucleus before they emerge from the pons at a point just lateral to the corticospinal tract. After leaving the pons they enter the internal auditory meatus with the acoustic nerve. The facial nerve then bends sharply forward and downward around the anterior boundary of the vestibule of the inner ear. At this angle lies the sensory ganglion (named *geniculate* because of its close proximity to the genu). The nerve continues its course in its own bony channel, the facial canal, and makes its exit from the skull at the stylomastoid foramen. It then passes through the parotid gland and subdivides to supply the facial muscles, the stylomastoid, and the posterior belly of the digastric muscle. Within the facial canal, just distal to the geniculate ganglion, it gives off the branch to the sphenopalatine ganglion, i.e., the greater superficial petrosal nerve, and somewhat more distally it gives off a small branch to the stapedius and is joined by the chorda tympani.

A complete interruption of the facial nerve at the stylomastoid foramen paralyzes all muscles of facial expression. The corner of the mouth droops, the creases and skin folds are effaced, the forehead is unfurrowed, the palpebral fissure is widened, and the eyelids will not close. Upon attempted closure of the lids, the eye on the paralyzed side is seen to roll upward (Bell's phenomenon). The lower lid sags also, and the punctum falls away from the conjunctiva, permitting tears to spill over the cheek. Food collects between the teeth and lips, and saliva may dribble from the corner of the mouth. The patient complains of a heaviness or numbness in the face, but no sensory loss is demonstrable and taste is intact.

If the lesion is in the facial canal above the junction with the chorda tympani but below the geniculate ganglion, all the above symptoms occur and, in addition, taste is lost over the anterior two-thirds of the tongue on the same side. If the nerve to the stapedius is paralyzed, there is hyperacusis (painful sensitivity to loud sounds), and the sound produced by moving the jaw and facial muscles is no longer present in the ear on the affected side. If the geniculate ganglion or the motor root proximal to it is involved, lacrimation may be reduced. Lesions at this point may also affect the adjacent auditory nerve, causing deafness, tinnitus, or dizziness. Intrapontine lesions that paralyze the face usually affect the abducens nucleus and often the corticospinal tract.

If the peripheral facial paralysis has existed for some time and return of motor function has begun but is incomplete, a kind of contracture may appear. The palpebral fissure becomes narrowed and the nasolabial fold deepens. Attempts to move one group of facial muscles result in contraction of all of them (associated movements or synkinesis). Facial spasms develop and persist indefinitely, being initiated by every facial movement. This condition, called *facial spasms,* may also appear in adults who have never had a Bell's palsy. Presumably it is due to a benign constrictive lesion of the seventh nerve, which results in volleys of motor impulses spreading to all the muscles of facial expression. Anomalous regeneration of the seventh nerve fibers may result in other curious disorders. If fibers originally connected with the orbicularis oculi become connected with the orbicularis oris, closure of the lids may cause a retraction of the mouth; or if fibers originally connected with muscles of the face later come to innervate the lacrimal gland, anomalous tearing (crocodile tears) may occur with any activity of the facial muscles, such as eating (Bogorad's syndrome). With the passage of time, the face and even the tip of the nose become pulled to the unaffected side.

The most common disease affecting the facial nerve is Bell's palsy, presumably due to an inflammatory reaction in or around the nerve near the stylomastoid foramen. The onset is acute, and the paralysis may evolve over a few hours, although pain behind the ear may have been present for a day or two. Occasionally taste sensation is lost, and more rarely hyperacusis is present. In some cases there is mild pleocytosis in the cerebrospinal fluid. Fully 80 percent of patients recover within a few weeks. A reaction of degeneration at the end of 10 days indicates a long delay until regeneration occurs, and sometimes it is incomplete. Thus electromyography may be of value in distinguishing temporary conduction defects from a pathologic interruption in continuity of nerve fibers. Protection of the eye during sleep, massage of the weakened muscles, and a splint to prevent drooping of the lower part of the face are the measures generally employed in the management of such cases. The use of ACTH and the unroofing of the facial nerve in the facial canal have been tried in isolated cases, but the results are impossible to evaluate.

Tumors which invade the temporal bone (carotid body, cholesteatoma, dermoid) may produce a facial palsy, but the onset is insidious and the course progressive. The Ramsay Hunt syndrome, presumably due to herpes zoster of the geniculate ganglion, gives a severe facial palsy associated with a vesicular eruption in the external auditory canal and other parts of the cranial integument; often the eighth cranial nerve is affected as well. Acoustic neuromas frequently involve the facial nerve. Vascular lesions or tumors are the common forms of pontine disease which may cause facial palsy. Bilateral facial paralysis (facial diplegia) occurs in acute idiopathic polyneuritis and in a variety of sarcoidosis known as *uveoparotid fever* (*Heerfordt's syndrome*). *Melkersson's syndrome* refers to a rarely encountered triad of recurrent facial paralysis, recurrent—and eventually permanent—facial (particularly labial) edema, and less constantly, plication of the tongue. The cause is unknown. In the Far East leprosy may be the cause.

All these forms of nuclear or peripheral facial palsy must be distinguished from the supranuclear type. In the latter the frontalis and orbicularis oculi muscles are involved less than those of the lower part of the face, since the upper facial muscles, unlike the lower ones, receive upper motor neurone innervation from both hemispheres. In supranuclear lesions there may be a dissociation of emotional and voluntary facial movements, and often some degree of paralysis of the arm and leg or an aphasia (in dominant hemisphere lesions) is conjoined.

A curious disorder is the *facial hemiatrophy of Romberg*. It occurs mainly in females and is characterized by a disappearance of fat in the dermal and subcutaneous tissues on one side of the face. It usually begins in adolescence or early adult years and is slowly progressive. In its advanced form the face is gaunt and the skin is thin, wrinkled, and rather dark. The hair may turn white and fall out, and the sebaceous glands become atrophic. The muscles and bones are as a rule not involved. The condition is probably a form of lipodystrophy, and the localization within a dermatome indicates the operation of some neural factor of unknown nature.

The facial muscles on one side may be affected by irregular clonic contractions of varying degree (*facial hemispasm*). This condition may be due to an irritative lesion of the facial nerve (e.g., an acoustic neuroma) or may represent a transient or permanent sequela to a Bell's palsy. It may be caused by a plaque of multiple sclerosis. In the most common form, however, the cause and pathology are unknown. An involuntary recurrent spasm of both eyelids (blepharospasm) may occur in elderly persons as an isolated phenomenon or with varying degrees of spasm of the facial muscles. Relaxant and tranquilizing drugs are of little help, although in many cases this disorder may subside spontaneously. In very severe and persistent instances, the only effective treatment has been crushing of the facial nerve innervation of the orbicularis oculi muscles.

SYNDROME OF AURAL VERTIGO AND MÉNIÈRE'S DISEASE

Ménière's disease, or *Ménière's syndrome*, is the name applied to recurrent aural vertigo, accompanied by tinnitus and deafness. The latter symptoms may be absent during the initial attacks of vertigo, but they invariably assert themselves as the disease progresses and are increased in severity during an acute attack. With milder forms of the syndrome the patient may complain more of head discomfort and of difficulty in concentration than of vertigo and may be considered neurotic. Provided that deafness is not complete, the recruitment phenomenon can be demonstrated (see Chap. 24). Ménière's syndrome has its onset most frequently in the fifth decade of life, though young adults and the elderly are not spared. The pathologic changes in Ménière's syndrome are said to consist of a dilatation of the endolymphatic system which leads to a degeneration of the delicate vestibular and cochlear hair cells. The relation of these changes to paroxysmal disorder of labyrinthine function is unknown. During an acute attack, rest in bed is the most effective treatment, since the patient can usually find a position in which vertigo is minimal. Dimenhydrinate (Dramamine) or cyclizine (Marezine) in doses of 25 to 50 mg t.i.d. is useful in the more protracted cases. A low salt diet is still used in treatment, but its value is difficult to judge. Mild sedative and hypnotic drugs may help the anxious patient between attacks. Usually the deafness is progressive, and when it is complete, the vertiginous attacks cease. However, the course is variable, and if the attacks persist in a severe manner, permanent relief can be obtained by the administration of 10 to 12 Gm streptomycin in doses of 2 Gm per day or by surgical destruction of the labyrinth or section of the vestibular portion of the eighth nerve intracranially. Of course, the streptomycin effect is bilateral; hence it should not be used unless both sides are affected.

Another disorder of labyrinthine function is characterized by the occurrence of paroxysmal vertigo and nystagmus, with the assumption of certain critical positions of the head. This is the *positional vertigo of Barany*, of the so-called "benign paroxysmal type." A highly diagnostic feature of this disorder is the development of transient vertigo and rotary nystagmus when the patient rapidly assumes a supine or an upright position. The optimal position in which to bring out this disorder is to tip the patient backward with the head 30° below the level of the bed and rotated 30 to 45° to one side. On sitting up, the vertigo and nystagmus recur, but in the opposite direction. On repetition of the test, the response is characteristically reduced or entirely absent. Deafness only rarely accompanies this disorder, and the presence of mild ear infections or other labyrinthine disease can be detected in only a small proportion of cases. It is thought that positional nystagmus of the benign paroxysmal type is due to a lesion of the otolith apparatus which results in a qualitatively abnormal response to the positional stimulus.

There are many other causes of aural vertigo, such as purulent labyrinthitis complicating meningitis, serous labyrinthitis due to infection of the middle ear, "toxic labyrinthitis" due to drug intoxication (e.g., from alcohol, quinine, streptomycin, and salicylates), motion sickness, trauma, and hemorrhage into the internal ear. In these instances the attacks of vertigo tend to last longer than in the recurrent form, but in other respects the symptoms are similar. Streptomycin may damage the fine hair cells of the vestibular end organs and cause a permanent disorder of equilibrium.

There has been described a dramatic clinical syndrome, characterized by the abrupt onset of severe vertigo, nausea, and vomiting, without tinnitus or hearing loss. The vertigo persists for several days or weeks, and labyrinthine function is permanently ablated on one side. Occlusion of the labyrinthine division of the internal auditory artery would logically explain this syndrome, but so far postmortem confirmation of this idea has not been obtained. Nor is there any pathologic basis for the commonly held belief that spasm or arteriosclerotic changes in the labyrinthine blood vessels are responsible for vertigo.

Vertigo of vestibular nerve origin may occur with diseases that involve the nerve in the petrous bone or the cerebellopontine angle. Except that it is less severe and is less frequently paroxysmal, it has many of the characteristics of labyrinthine vertigo. The adjacent auditory division of the eighth cranial nerve may also be affected, which explains the frequent coincidence of tinnitus and deafness. The function of the eighth cranial nerve may be disturbed by tumors of the lateral recess (especially acoustic neuroma), as well as by meningeal inflammation in this region or, very rarely, by compression from an abnormal vessel.

Vestibular neuronitis and epidemic vertigo are the names that have been applied to a clinical syndrome which occurs mainly in young adults and is characterized by the abrupt onset of vertigo, nausea, and vomiting, without impairment of hearing. Otoscopic examination and tests of cochlear function disclose no abnormality, but the caloric responses are reduced, usually on both sides. The symptoms are benign, subsiding, as a rule, in 2 to 3 weeks. Although many of the reported cases have been associated with signs of systemic disease, and a few with signs of polyarteritis nodosa, the exact cause remains unknown. Similarly, the precise site of the lesion is not known, although it has been the subject of considerable speculation.

A particular variety of paroxysmal vertigo of childhood has been described by Basser. The attacks of vertigo occur in a setting of good health and are of sudden onset and brief duration. Pallor, sweating, and immobility are prominent manifestations, and occasionally vomiting and nystagmus occur. No relation to head posture or movement has been observed. The attacks are recurrent but tend to cease spontaneously after a period of several months or years. The outstanding abnormal finding is demonstrated by caloric testing, which shows impairment or loss of vestibular function, bilateral or unilateral, frequently persisting after the attacks have ceased. Cochlear function is unimpaired. The pathologic basis of this disorder has not been determined.

Cogan has described a peculiar syndrome in young adults, in which a nonsyphilitic interstitial keratitis is associated with vertigo, tinnitus, nystagmus, and rapidly progressive deafness. The prognosis for life and vision is good, but the deafness is usually permanent. The causation of Cogan's disease is not understood, although several patients later developed periarteritis nodosa.

The question of *viral infections of cranial nerves* is always raised by these acute palsies of the facial, trigeminal, and auditory nerves, especially when the affection is bilateral, involves several nerves in combination, or is associated with pleocytosis of CSF. Actually, the only proven virus etiology in this group of cases is that of herpes zoster, and search for this virus from cases of Bell's palsy or of vestibular neuronitis has not been rewarding. Since perceptive deafness, vertigo, and other cranial nerve palsies have been observed in conjunction with the parainfectious encephalomyelitis of varicella, measles, rubella, mumps, and scarlet fever and also with Landry-Guillain-Barré syndrome, an allergic etiology must be considered. Nothing is known of the pathology of the peripheral lesion or of the localization of a virus in the nervous system in these diseases. We have studied a number of cases of acute bilateral facial palsy, or facial palsy, numbness, and deafness or vertigo on one side and pleocytosis of CSF without succeeding in isolation of the causative agent. There is no treatment other than symptomatic; fortunately the prognosis for complete recovery is excellent.

SYNDROME OF DEAFNESS

See Chap. 24.

SYNDROME OF GLOSSOPHARYNGEAL NEURALGIA

Glossopharyngeal neuralgia is a syndrome which resembles trigeminal neuralgia in many respects. The pain is intense and paroxysmal; it originates in the throat, approximately in the tonsillar fossa. In some cases the pain is localized in the ear or may radiate from the throat to the ear, because of implication of the tympanic branch (Jacobson's nerve). Spasms of pain may be initiated by swallowing. There is no demonstrable sensory or motor deficit. A trial of Dilantin or Tegretol is the recommended therapy, but if this is unsuccessful, division of the nerve near the medulla is the treatment of choice.

Very rarely, herpes zoster may involve the glossopharyngeal nerve. One may occasionally observe a glossopharyngeal palsy in conjunction with vagus and accessory nerve involvement due to a tumor or aneurysm in the posterior fossa. Hoarseness due to vocal cord paralysis, some difficulty in swallowing, deviation of the soft palate to the sound side, anesthesia of the posterior wall of the pharynx, and weakness of the upper part of the trapezius and sternomastoid muscles comprise the syndrome (see Table 355-1, jugular foramen syndrome).

SYNDROME OF DYSPHAGIA AND DYSPHONIA

Complete interruption of the intracranial portion of one vagus nerve results in a characteristic paralysis. The soft palate droops and does not rise in phonation. There is loss of the gag reflex on the affected side, as well as of the "curtain movement" of the lateral wall of the pharynx, whereby the faucial pillars move medially as the palate rises in saying "ah." The voice is hoarse, often nasal, and the vocal cord lies immobile in an abducted or cadaveric position. There may also be loss of sensibility at the external auditory meatus and back of the pinna. Usually no change in visceral function can be demonstrated.

Complete bilateral paralysis is said to be incompatible with life, and this is probably true if the nuclei are involved in the medulla by poliomyelitis or some other disease. However, in the cervical region, both vagi have been blocked with procaine (Novocaine) for the treatment of intractable asthma, without mishap. The pharyngeal branches of both vagi may be affected in diphtheria; the voice has a nasal quality, and regurgitation of liquids through the nose occurs during the act of swallowing.

The vagus nerves, especially the left, are most often damaged as a result of thoracic disease. Aneurysm of the aortic arch, an enlarged left atrium, and tumors of the mediastinum and bronchi are much more frequent causes of an isolated vagus palsy than are intracranial disorders. The nerve may be implicated at the meningeal level by tumors and infectious processes and within the medulla by tumors and vascular lesions, e.g., the lateral medullary syndrome of Wallenberg, and by motor system disease. Herpes zoster may attack this nerve. Polymyositis and dermatomyositis, which cause hoarseness and dysphagia owing to direct involvement of laryngeal

and pharyngeal muscles, may be confused with disease of the vagus nerves.

When confronted with a case of laryngeal palsy, the physician must attempt to determine the site of the lesion. If it is intramedullary, there are usually other signs, such as ipsilateral cerebellar signs, loss of pain and temperature sensation over the ipsilateral face and contralateral arm and leg, and ipsilateral Bernard-Horner syndrome. If the lesion is extramedullary, the glossopharyngeal and spinal accessory nerves are frequently involved (jugular foramen syndrome). If it is extracranial in the posterior laterocondylar or retroparotid space, there may be a combination of ninth, tenth, eleventh, and twelfth cranial nerve palsies and Bernard-Horner syndrome. Combinations of these lower cranial nerve palsies are sometimes called the *syndrome of Collet-Sicard* and the *syndrome of Villaret,* respectively. If there is no sensory loss in the palate and pharynx, or no palatal weakness, the lesion is below the origin of the pharyngeal branches, which leave the vagus nerve high in the cervical region. The usual site of disease is then the mediastinum.

SYNDROME OF BULBAR PALSY

This syndrome is the result of weakness or paralysis of those muscles which are supplied by the bulb or medulla oblongata, namely the tongue, pharynx, larynx, sternomastoid, and upper trapezius. If development is rapid, as may happen in diphtheria or poliomyelitis, there is no time for muscle atrophy. The more chronic diseases, progressive

Table 355-2. BRAINSTEM SYNDROMES WHICH INVOLVE CRANIAL NERVES

Eponym	Site	Cranial nerves involved	Tracts and nuclei involved	Signs	Usual cause
Weber's syndrome........	Base of midbrain	III	Corticospinal tract	Oculomotor palsy with crossed hemiplegia	Vascular occlusion; tumor; aneurysm
Claude's syndrome.......	Tegmentum of midbrain	III	Red nucleus	Oculomotor palsy with contralateral cerebellar ataxia and tremor	Vascular occlusion; tumor; aneurysm
Benedikt's syndrome	Tegmentum of midbrain	III	Red nucleus and corticospinal tract	Oculomotor palsy with contralateral cerebellar ataxia, tremor, and pyramidal signs	Softening; hemorrhage; tuberculoma; tumor
Nothnagel's syndrome....	Tectum of midbrain	Unilateral or bilateral III	Superior cerebellar peduncles	Ocular palsies, paralysis of gaze, and cerebellar ataxia	Tumor
Parinaud's syndrome.....	Tectum of midbrain	Supranuclear co-ordinating mechanism for upward gaze	Superior colliculi	Paralysis of upward and sometimes downward gaze; fixed pupils; divergence of eyes	Pinealoma
Millard-Gubler syndrome and Raymond-Foville syndrome	Base of pons	VII and often VI	Corticospinal tract	Facial and abducens palsy and contralateral hemiplegia; sometimes palsy of gaze to side of lesion	Softening or tumor
Avellis's syndrome........	Tegmentum of medulla	X	Corticospinal tract Sometimes descending pupillary fibers, with Bernard-Horner syndrome	Paralysis of soft palate and vocal cord and contralateral hemiplegia	Softening or tumor
Jackson's syndrome......	Tegmentum of medulla	X, XII	Corticospinal tract	Avellis's syndrome plus ipsilateral tongue paralysis	Softening or tumor
Wallenberg's syndrome...	Tegmentum of medulla	Spinal V, IX, X, XI	Lateral spinothalamic tract Descending pupillodilator fibers Spinocerebellar and olivocerebellar tracts	Ipsilateral V, IX, X, XI palsy, Bernard-Horner syndrome, and cerebellar ataxia Contralateral loss of pain and temperature sense	Occlusion of posterior-inferior cerebellar artery

bulbar palsy (a form of motor system disease) or tumors or aneurysms of posterior fossa, result in marked wasting and fasciculation of the tongue, sternomastoid, and trapezius muscles. The condition must be distinguished from progressive muscular dystrophy and a restricted form of polymyositis which may be limited to neck muscles; these latter disorders seldom affect the tongue, however. It must also be differentiated from pseudobulbar palsy (see Chap. 21).

MULTIPLE CRANIAL NERVE PALSIES

As will be readily understood, several cranial nerves may be affected by the same disease process. One of the clinical problems that arise is whether the disease lies within or outside the brainstem. Lesions lying on the surface of the brainstem usually are featured by one or a succession of adjacent cranial nerve palsies and late and rather slight involvement of the long sensory and motor pathways and segmental structures lying within the brainstem. The opposite is true of the intramedullary, intrapontine, and intramesencephalic lesion. The extramedullary lesion is more likely to cause bone erosion or enlargement of the foramen of the axis (seen radiographically). The intramedullary lesion involving cranial nerves often produces a crossed sensory or motor paralysis (cranial nerve on one side, evidence of tract involvement on the other). In this way a number of distinctive syndromes to which eponyms have been attached are produced. These are listed in Table 355-1.

Involvement of multiple cranial nerves outside the brainstem is frequently the result of trauma (sudden onset), localized infections such as zoster (acute onset), granulomatous diseases (subacute onset), or tumors and saccular aneurysms (chronic development). Of the tumors, neurofibromas, meningiomas, cholesteatomas, carcinomas, and sarcomas have all been reported. The chordoma (see Chap. 359) may implicate a succession of lower cranial nerves. Owing to their anatomic relationships, the multiple cranial nerve palsies form a number of distinctive syndromes listed in Table 355-2.

From time to time one observes a benign form of multiple cranial nerve involvement on one or both sides of the face. The disease may recur over a period of years with variable degrees of recovery between attacks. Sarcoidosis is found to be the cause of some, and chronic glandular tuberculosis (scrofula), the cause of others. The condition is called *polyneuritis cranialis multiplex*. The malignant granuloma of the nasopharynx may also affect multiple cranial nerves, as do also nasopharyngeal tumors, platybasia, and adult Arnold-Chiari malformation. A purely motor disorder without atrophy raises the question always of myasthenia gravis (see Chap. 377).

REFERENCES

Brodal, A.: "The Cranial Nerves," Springfield, Ill., Charles C Thomas, Publisher, 1959.

Cogan, D. G.: "Neurology of the Ocular Muscles," 2d ed., Springfield, Ill., Charles C Thomas, Publisher, 1956.

——: "Neurology of the Visual System." Springfield, Ill., Charles C Thomas, Publisher, 1966.

Staff of Mayo Clinic: "Clinical Examinations in Neurology," 2d ed., Philadelphia, W. B. Saunders Company, 1963.

Wolfson, R. J. (Ed.), "The Vestibular System and Its Diseases," Philadelphia, University of Pennsylvania Press, 1966.

356 DISEASES OF THE SPINAL CORD

Raymond D. Adams

Diseases of the nervous system may at times limit themselves to the spinal cord and thereby produce a number of distinctive syndromes. Because of their frequency and gravity and the special difficulties attendant upon diagnosis, we have grouped these diseases in a special chapter under a series of relatively common syndromes.

THE SYNDROME OF GLOBAL PARALYSIS OF LEGS OR ALL EXTREMITIES DUE TO A MASSIVE TRANSVERSE LESION OF THE SPINAL CORD

This condition may best be considered in relation to trauma, one of the most frequent causes of it, but it also occurs with certain types of myelitis, infarction and hemorrhage in the spinal cord, and rapidly advancing compressive myelopathy.

(1) Injuries to Spine and Spinal Cord

Although injuries to the spinal cord may be the sole manifestation of a traumatic disease, it is seldom that the vertebral column is not harmed at the same time. Often there is an associated head injury, as is pointed out in Chap. 358.

A useful classification of spinal injuries is one which divides them into fracture-dislocations, pure fractures, and pure dislocations. The relative frequency of these types is about 3:1:1. Direct violence to the spine is an uncommon cause of vertebral disruption; except for stab and bullet wounds most spine injuries are the result of force *applied at a distance*. All three types of injury are produced by a similar mechanism, usually a vertical compression of the spinal column to which flexion is almost immediately added. Or, the neck is sharply extended. The two important variables in the mechanics of vertebral injury are the nature of the bones and the strength, direction, and point of impact of the force.

STRENGTH, DIRECTION, AND POINT OF IMPACT OF THE FORCE. If the injuring body striking the cranium is hard and the velocity is high, a skull fracture occurs, the elastic quality of the skull absorbing the force of the injury. If the injuring body is soft yet heavy, the spine and particularly its cervical portion will be the part injured. If the neck happens to be rigid and straight and the force is quickly applied to the head, the atlas and the odontoid process of the axis may break. If the force is not quickly applied and removed, an element of flexion occurs. Flexion movement plus a vertical force constitute the essential factors in fracture-dislocation or pure dislocation.

The other common mechanism of cord injury, sudden extension of the neck, is called the "whiplash injury." This is most frequent in the cervical region. It is especially frequent in civilian motor accidents and in forward falls. Cervical spondylosis adds to the hazard of spinal cord damage.

A special type of spine injury, occurring most often in military life, is that in which missiles of high velocity pass through the vertebral canal and destroy the spinal cord. In some cases they may strike the vertebral column without entering the spinal canal and agitate is so violently that the cord suffers injury. The term given the temporary spinal paralysis is *spinal concussion*. This condition may also be produced by violent falls flat on the back.

A study of 2,006 cases collected from the literature by Jefferson shows that most vertebral injuries occur at the first to second cervical, fourth to sixth cervical, and eleventh thoracic to second lumbar vertebras. Industrial accidents most often involve the dorsolumbar vertebrae. Accidents caused by falling, either in a sitting position or with head down as in diving accidents, affect the cervical region. In the author's neuropathologic material, which contains 26 cases, the usual circumstances of spinal injury were a state of alcoholic intoxication and a fall down a flight of stairs, automobile accidents, crushing industrial accidents, gunshot or stab wounds, and birth injury in that order of frequency. The majority of these fatal cases had fracture-dislocations or dislocations of the cervical spine.

MECHANISM OF SPINAL CORD INJURY

The spinal cord may escape injury even though there is vertebral dislocation, especially in regions where the spinal canal is large, i.e., in the cervical and lumbar regions. Rarely the spinal cord may be damaged without radiologic evidence of fracture or dislocation. One cannot easily determine the full extent of spinal injury by radiology or even at autopsy because of the difficulty in examining the vertebrae. By far the most satisfactory technique for demonstrating the degree of spine injury and the presence of a tearing of ligaments with dislocation is the x-ray, taken laterally, but one must be careful to avoid flexion or extension of the neck which may inflict further injury to the spinal cord. The most frequently established mechanism is a vertebral dislocation with or without fracture. The upper vertebras are displaced anteriorly, and there is a break in posterior longitudinal ligament and intervertebral disk. The spinal cord is most often subjected to a shearing force between the pedicles of the

vertebra above and the body and laminae of the vertebra below the dislocation.

When the cervical spine is sharply extended, especially in the presence of cervical spondylosis, the damage to the spinal cord is due to the sudden narrowing of the spinal canal. The spinal cord is caught between the lamina of the lower vertebra and higher one. Also, the ligamentum flavum may buckle and compress the cord. There may also be no x-ray evidence of the spinal lesion.

In direct trauma of the spine, as when it is struck in some part by a bullet, the means of spinal concussion is said to be *agitation*. This term has led to much confusion because it is not employed here in the usual sense of a transient interruption of neural function by trauma without perceptible structural change.

PATHOLOGY OF SPINAL CORD INJURY

As a result of squeezing or shearing of the cord, there is necrosis of gray matter and a variable amount of hemorrhage, chiefly in the more vascular gray matter. These changes are maximum at the point of injury and one or two segments above and below it. Rarely is the cord cut in two, and seldom is the piaarachnoid lacerated. The condition is best designated as *traumatic necrosis of the spinal cord*. As the lesion heals, it results in cavitation. Separation of such pathologic entities as hematomyelia, concussion, contusion, and hematorrhachis is rarely of value either clinically or pathologically.

As with most lesions, the total disease picture is compounded of an irreversible structural lesion and a disorder of function, each of which may vary in degree. The extent and permanence of the clinical manifestations are determined by the relative amounts of these two. An exception to this statement might be made for gunshot wounds of the vertebras. Here the explosive force of the missile may shatter myelinated fibers with maximal functional disturbance.

CLINICAL EFFECTS OF SPINAL CORD INJURY

The description of traumatic paraplegia by Riddock cannot be excelled. He divides the clinical picture into the two stages discussed below.

MUSCULAR FLACCIDITY OR "SPINAL SHOCK." The loss of function which is inflicted at the time of injury (fourth to fifth cervical vertebrae-quadriplegia; thoracic vertebrae-paraplegia, both with paralysis of bladder and bowel sphincters and loss of sensibility below the level corresponding to the spinal lesion) is accompanied by a complete or almost complete suppression of reflex activity of all spinal segments below the lesion. This condition is the so-called "spinal shock." The plantar reflexes are at first variable and may be absent, flexor, or extensor. The lower extremities lose heat if left uncovered and swell if dependent. Sweating is abolished. Cutaneous ulcerations may develop over bony prominences. Urine and feces are retained to the point where involuntary overflow or leakage results. Occasionally there is priapism because of venous congestion. A paralytic ileus may occur.

REFLEX ACTIVITY. If the lumbosacral segments are undamaged, spinal shock wears off in 2 to 3 weeks. The first sign of this is contraction of the hamstrings and flexion or extension of the toes on plantar stimulation. Then gentle and later strong involuntary flexor spasms make their appearance. Ankle jerks and then knee jerks return. Retention of urine and feces becomes less complete, and at irregular intervals urine is expelled by active contraction of the detrusor muscle. Reflex defecation and sweating also return. At times flexor spasms and later extensor spasms, with sweating and micturition, all occur after stimulation of the skin, viz., the *mass reflex*. This stage of reflex activity may last for years unless sepsis intervenes, in which case the state of spinal shock may return.

Less complete lesions of the spinal cord may result in little or no spinal shock or extensor spasm. Incomplete voluntary motor paralysis, a flaccid atrophic paralysis, variable sensory impairment in the arms, a spastic weakness of the legs, and a partial or complete Brown-Séquard syndrome are some of the resulting clinical pictures.

The final result may be permanent and complete disability, rarely consistent with survival for more than a short time (days to weeks), or a gradual improvement and complete or almost complete recovery may occur. Any residual symptoms after 6 months are likely to be permanent.

The level of the cord lesion can be determined by the clinical picture. A complete paralysis of arms and legs usually indicates a dislocation at the fourth to fifth cervical vertebrae. If the legs are paralyzed and the arms can be abducted and flexed, the dislocation is likely to be at the fifth to sixth cervical. Paralysis only of hands and of legs indicates the level of vertebral disorder to be the sixth to seventh cervical. When the motor paralysis involves muscles above the knees and sensory loss includes the twelfth thoracic dermatome, the site is the eleventh to twelfth thoracic. If the paralysis is below the knees and the first lumbar escapes, the lesion is at the twelfth thoracic, first lumbar vertebra. Prognosis for the latter group of patients, with preponderantly cauda equina lesions, is better than for those with injury to the eleventh to twelfth thoracic vertebrae. In all cases of spinal cord injury any elicitable movement or preserved sensation during the first 48 to 72 hrs gives a favorable prognosis for recovery.

TREATMENT

In general, the treatment for spinal cord injuries is conservative and symptomatic. The degree of injury can be lessened by assuring that no movement of cervical spine (especially flexion) is made from the moment of the accident. Corticosteroid therapy, as for brain swelling (Chap. 358), may reduce the swelling of spinal cord tissue. If the spinal cord injury is associated with dislocation of the vertebrae, traction on the neck is necessary to secure proper alignment. This is accomplished by a head halter attached through the head of the bed over a pulley to a weight of 10 to 15 lb. or, even better, the use of tongs which fasten onto the skull (Crutchfield). In thoracic crush injuries, hyperextension can be maintained by placing a narrow pillow under the affected area. Traction should be continued for 4 to 6 weeks, and then a brace may be substituted. Early fixation and traction of spine in some centers for the treatment of spinal cord injury have almost completely replaced decompression by laminectomy. The aftercare of patients with paraplegia and disturbance of vesical or rectal function is similar to that of patients with like symptoms from other causes. Decubitus ulceration can be prevented by special skin care. Tidal drainage is a valuable adjunct in preventing infection, stone formation, and contracture and in securing return of function. Daily enemas are usually the most effective means of controlling fecal incontinence. Physiotherapy, muscle reeducation, and the application of proper braces are all important in the rehabilitation of the patient. All this is best carried out in centers for rehabilitation of spine injuries.

(2) Myelitis

The spinal cord appears to be vulnerable to three types of inflammatory processes, all of which have been called *myelitic*. First there are the specific viral infections which tend to involve principally the gray matter (hence called poliomyelitic). Zoster and the three viruses of poliomyelitis are the most frequent examples. Secondly, all the subacute and chronic primary meningeal infections may induce damage, either on the spinal roots and outer surfaces of spinal cord, i.e., to the white matter of posterior, lateral, and anterior funiculi (meningoradiculitis and meningomyelitis). Syphilis offers the best known and most numerous examples of this category of inflammatory diseases, as in tabes dorsalis (which is essentially a treponemal lumbosacral meningoradiculitis) and syphilitic meningomyelitis. Meningeal vascular lesions are often added, resulting in myelomalacia. Tuberculous meningitis and fungous meningitis provide other examples. Thirdly, there is a group of primary inflammations of white matter, the leukomyelitides. Although the white (and gray) matter may be site of an infective inflammatory process (abscess, tuberculoma, gumma and parasitic inflammations), these are rare. Most of the leukomyelitides are of unknown cause. Three varieties have been delineated: (1) postinfectious myelitis, (2) demyelinative myelitis (acute or chronic relapsing multiple sclerosis), and (3) acute or subacute necrotizing myelitis. (For discussion of pathology, see Chap. 362).

Whereas any one of the above forms of chronic meningitis or leukomyelitis may induce the clinical picture of a tranverse cord lesion, this lesion is usually due to one of the demyelinative or necrotizing forms of myelitis. A painless (rarely painful) paraplegia, beginning simultaneously in both legs or more often first in one leg then the other, and in sacral segments ascends to the abdomen and thorax. Either sensory or motor symptoms may initiate the disease, but both are present as it progresses. Like all cord lesions with involvement of tracts, the loss of sensory and motor function involves all parts of the body below a certain level, and urinary retention and then overflow incontinence and obstipation are included. In only a few

471 6231

patients will vaccination against smallpox, or rabies inoculation, or a frank chickenpox or measles be found to have preceded the neurologic symptoms (days to 1 to 2 weeks); in all the rest, the illness develops without explanation. The conjunction of retrobulbar neuritis with the cord lesion is called neuromyelitis optica or Devic's disease. This is not a disease but a syndrome occurring in necrotizing myelitis (usual cause), multiple sclerosis, and postinfectious myelitis. If the spinal cord lesion is severe and paralysis is complete, spinal shock supervenes with the same flaccidity and areflexia of legs mentioned under spinal cord trauma. The CSF may be normal or may contain lymphocytes and mononuclears (numbering from 20 to 1,000 or more per ml), and the protein is sometimes raised. If the cord lesion swells there may be a dynamic block (positive Queckenstedt test). When the latter is found, it always suggests the possibility of an *epidural spinal abscess,* another important and treatable cause of the rapid development of a transverse cord lesion with spine ache and fever.

Treatment of the demyelinative and necrotizing myelitides consists of ACTH (40 units twice a day for a week, then once a day for 2 to 3 weeks) or Meticorten (45 mg per day for 3 weeks). Improvement usually occurs, but the relationship to therapy is uncertain. Except for patients with the postinfectious form of myelitis there is always danger of later progression or relapse. Prevention of decubitus ulceration, early catheterization and bladder care, and rehabilitation measures, the usual procedures in the management of the paraplegia patient, must also be employed.

(3) Spinal Epidural Abscess

Children or adults may be affected. An injury to the back, often trivial, at the time of a furunculosis or other skin infection or a bacteremia may permit seeding of the spinal epidural space or of vertebral body. The latter gives rise to osteomyelitis with extension to the epidural space. The suppurative process is accompanied at first only by fever and aching in the region of the spine and later by radicular pain. After several days or a few weeks there is a rapid onset and progression of paraplegia, sensory loss in the lower parts of the body, urinary and fecal retention, and sphincteric incontinence. Percussion of the spine elicits tenderness over the site of the infection. Examination reveals all the signs of transverse cord lesion with spinal shock. The CSF contains small numbers of cells (neutrophilic leucocytes and lymphocytes), and the protein is relatively high (100 to 400 mg per ml). More importantly there is a dynamic block (positive Queckenstedt test). If not treated surgically by laminectomy and drainage at the earliest possible moment, the spinal cord lesion, which is due to ischemia (compression mainly of veins), becomes irreversible. Emergency myelography must be used to determine the level of block and the operative site. Antibiotic therapy must also be given.

Another circumstance in which an acute spinal epidural abscess may develop is in a patient with some combination of chronic medical diseases in which a septicemia

occurs. Here the symptoms of spine disease may be minimal until the onset of the spinal cord lesion some weeks later. Staphylococci or some other organism may reach the epidural or subdural spinal space via a lumbar puncture needle or during epidural anesthesia. The localization is then over lumbar and sacral roots. Pain may be severe and neurologic symptomatology minimal.

Subacute pyogenic infections and granulomatous infections (tuberculosis, fungal) may also arise in the spinal epidural space causing symptoms and signs of disorder of spinal tracts at the level of the lesion. The clinical picture is less dramatic, and the diagnosis depends on the demonstration, in a patient with weakness and/or sensory loss or ataxia of the legs, of a partial or complete block by pantopaque myelography. The treatment depends on the nature of the underlying disease and the general condition of the patient (see Chap. 135).

(4) Infarction of Spinal Cord (Myelomalacia) and Hemorrhage (Hematomyelia)

Unlike the brain, the spinal cord is rarely the site of vascular disease. The spinal arteries are not susceptible to atherosclerosis, and emboli rarely lodge here. As was stated in relation to chronic meningeal infections, an endarteritis of surface arteries may lead to thrombosis with devastating ischemic necrosis of the spinal cord. Polyarteritis nodosa may have a similar effect though the nervous system localization in this disease is usually peripheral. Atherosclerotic thrombosis of the aorta or dissecting aortic aneurysms may cause myelomalacia by occluding nutrient arteries at cervical, thoracic, or lumbar levels. Paralysis during cardiac surgery, requiring clamping of the aorta for more than 30 min, and aortic arteriography may result in the syndrome. Sudden development of symptoms referable to spinal tract lesions (sensory or motor or both) always bespeaks an infarctive or hemorrhagic vascular lesion of the spinal cord. The onset of symptoms in such cases is more rapid than in the myelitides.

Hemorrhage into the spinal cord is rare. Aside from the aforementioned traumatic variety of hematomyelia, it is usually traceable to a vascular malformation or an hematologic disease.

THE SUBACUTE OR CHRONIC SYNDROMES OF SPINAL CORD DISEASE

These take several forms for the reason that the responsible diseases have a variety of different localizations in the tracts and gray matter. Most of the remaining diseases of the spinal cord may be grouped around the following syndromes.

Syndrome of Spastic Ataxic Paraparesis

The gradual development of ataxia and weakness of the legs is the common manifestation of several diseases. In late childhood or adolescence a syndrome of this type which begins insidiously and progresses steadily over a period of years usually indicates the existence of Friedreich's ataxia or one of its variants. In early adult life multiple sclerosis, syphilitic meningomyelitis, and chronic adhesive spinal arachnoiditis are the more frequent causes of it. And in middle and late years of life subacute combined degeneration, nutritional combined system disease, and cervical spondylosis reach their highest incidence.

(1) Friedreich's Ataxia

This classic form of hereditary ataxia, first clearly depicted by Nikolaus Friedreich of Heidelberg in 1863, forms a relatively distinct symptom complex which generally runs true to form, although it overlaps other heredodegenerative syndromes, particularly the chronic familial polyneuropathies and progressive optic atrophy (discussed in Chap. 364). In some families, the disorder occurs with dominant inheritance; more often it is a recessive trait.

CLINICAL ASPECTS. As with other progressive ataxias, the disorder first appears in the legs. Thus, the patient, previously healthy, begins to stagger and lurch in walking and is unsteady, often in a tremulous fashion, on standing. Clumsiness and intention tremor of the hands and arms appear later along with faulty articulation and abnormal rhythm (scanning) of speech. These symptoms usually result from changes in the cerebellum. The limbs, in addition to being ataxic, generally show considerable weakness. Examination usually discloses nystagmus and skeletal deformities: kyphoscoliosis, the basis of which is not certain, and a peculiar foreshortening and high arching of the feet (pes cavus) with cocking of the toes (sometimes called the "Friedreich foot" and best ascribed to atrophy and contractures of the musculature of the feet at a time when the bones of the feet are malleable). Typically, there is the unusual combination of total absence of tendon reflexes with extensor plantar reflexes (Babinski sign). This results from the presence of pyramidal tract degeneration together with peripheral neuropathy. The presence of a sensory neuropathy is further indicated by impairment of position and vibration sense in the extremities and, in some patients, by impairment of the sensations of pain, temperature, and light touch in a distal and roughly symmetrical distribution. The optic disks may be pale, indicating optic atrophy, although actual blindness is relatively rare. Some patients are of low intelligence or may become demented in the course of the disease. Survival beyond early adult life is rare, with death frequently the result of associated myocardial disease.

Occasionally very mild or fragmentary forms of the disorder (such as pes cavus and absent or hyperactive tendon reflexes) may be encountered with little if any disability or progression. Such abnormalities are most likely to be seen in other members of the family of a patient afflicted with the fully developed form of the disease.

PATHOLOGY. The principal changes are in the spinal cord and peripheral nerves; they are typical of a chronic degenerative process. In the cord the disease affects chiefly the sensory fibers of the posterior columns, the spinocerebellar tracts, and the corticospinal (pyramidal) tracts. Additional lesions of varying extent may be found in the brainstem and in the cerebellum itself although the latter structure occasionally is intact. Involvement of other parts of the central nervous system at higher levels occasionally occurs. In the peripheral nerves the lesions vary likewise in severity and extent. They resemble those encountered in the chronic peripheral neuropathies described in Chap. 354. In addition to the neuropathologic changes, there is in some cases a peculiar form of myocardial degeneration resulting in thickening and fibrosis of the myocardium. There are no other associated visceral lesions.

DIFFERENTIAL DIAGNOSIS. The classic form of Friedreich's ataxia is readily recognizable and cannot easily be confused with other conditions. It is to be expected, however, that variations in the clinical manifestations may occur because of the variable pathologic changes. One particularly well-known variant was described in 1926 by Levy and Roussy in which the muscle wasting of the legs is severe and is combined with areflexia, sensory ataxia, and tremor. There have been reports of Friedreich's ataxia in some members of a family and of the Levy-Roussy syndrome in others. Familial spastic paraplegia with or without optic atrophy (Behr's syndrome) is another closely related disease. In the absence of a family history, and with atypical clinical findings, further diagnostic studies to exclude tumor, chronic basal meningitis, intoxication, or congenital malformation will be necessary.

No treatment is known. Physical medicine and rehabilitation measures are of little value in cerebellar ataxia.

(2) Multiple Sclerosis

Probably an ataxic paraparesis ranks as the most common manifestation of an established form of multiple sclerosis. Asymmetric involvement of limbs and signs of cerebral, optic nerve, brainstem, and cerebellum manifestations provide important information for the diagnosis of this disease. Nevertheless, purely spinal involvement may occur, no lesions being found outside of the spinal cord even at autopsy. See Chap. 362 for further details.

(3) Syphilitic Meningomyelitis

Here as in multiple sclerosis the degree of alteration of vibratory and position sense and ataxia is variable. Some patients, such as Erb described with primary lateral sclerosis, have almost pure pyramidal spasticity and weakness of the legs requiring differentiation from motor system disease and familial spastic paraplegia. In others sensory ataxia and posterior column signs predominate. The confirmation of diagnosis depends on the finding of a positive Wassermann reaction in the CSF, but a late and advancing form of the disease may appear with a negative CSF in a known syphilitic patient. See Chap. 177 for a discussion of pathology and treatment.

(4) Subacute Combined Degeneration of the Spinal Cord and Brain Due to B12 Deficiency and Syndrome of Nutritional Combined System Disease-Strachan Syndrome

These two forms of the more treatable diseases of the spinal cord are fully described in Chap. 363, Metabolic and Nutritional Disorders of the Brain.

Progressive spastic or spastic-ataxic paraparesis may also develop in conjunction with hepatic decompensation.

(5) Cervical Spondylosis

Osteophytic overgrowth in the cervical spinal canal during the late years of life encroaches upon the spinal cord, narrowing it and compressing the spinal cord or impairing its circulation by occlusion of nutrient radicular arteries. Stiff neck, cervical pain, numbness, and weakness or atrophy of hands are combined with ataxia, spastic weakness of legs, or an ataxic paraparesis. X-rays disclose the bony overgrowth, which can be confirmed by myelography. The CSF protein may be elevated and the Queckenstedt test may be positive. Immobilization of the head with a cervical collar has resulted in relief of symptoms in some cases. Decompressive laminectomy with cutting of denticulate ligaments has halted the disease in the majority of instances and has often permitted some degree of recession of symptoms. An anterior approach, permitting removal of osteophytes, has given better results.

SYNDROME OF SPASTIC PARAPARESIS WITH OR WITHOUT CERVICOBRACHIAL AMYOTROPHY

Although a few such cases are traced to multiple sclerosis, syringomyelia, cervical pachymeningitis, or cervical meningomyelitis, the purely motor syndrome is nearly always traceable to amyotrophic lateral sclerosis. Paralysis, atrophy, and fascicular twitching of hands and arms are joined with spastic weakness and hyperreflexia in legs with Babinski signs (see Chap. 364). Cervical spondylosis and high cervical tumors must also be considered in the differential diagnosis.

SYNDROME OF SEGMENTAL SENSORY DISSOCIATION WITH BRACHIAL MUSCULAR ATROPHY (SYRINGOMYELIC SYNDROME)

This syndrome is most often ascribable to a syringomyelia, but examples have been found in patients with intramedullary cord tumors, traumatic myelopathy, postradiation myelopathy, syphilitic cervical pachymeningitis, cervical spondylosis, extramedullary tumors, or high cervical canal and necrotizing myelitis. For a description of syringomyelia, see Chap. 365. Developmental Abnormalities.

OTHER SYNDROMES CAUSING ASYMMETRIC WEAKNESS OF LEGS. Sensory Loss (Ataxia) and Sphincteric Disturbances

Here a miscellany of diseases (vascular malformations, chronic adhesive arachnoiditis following spinal anasthesia, and infections and metabolic and nutritional diseases, etc.) would have to be considered, but only spinal cord tumor will be discussed.

(1) SPINAL CORD TUMORS

Growths and other space-occupying lesions within the spinal canal can be conveniently divided into two groups: (1) those which arise within the substance of the spinal cord and invade and destroy tracts and central gray structures (intramedullary) and those which arise outside the spinal cord (extramedullary) from the vertebral bodies and epidural tissues (extradural), and the meninges, or roots (intradural). The relative frequency of spinal tumors in these different locations in a general hospital is about 5 percent intramedullary, 40 percent intradural-extramedullary, and 55 percent extradural. The percentages of extradural lesions in a general hospital population is usually higher than in most neurosurgical series (e.g., Elsberg's figures of 10, 67, and 16 percent respectively), which often do not include many of the lymphomas, metastatic carcinomas, etc., most of which are extradural.

The cellular origin of the intramedullary gliomas has been mentioned in the section on intracerebral tumors. The proportions of the different cell types differ, however. Kernohan, who has had one of the largest series of pathologic cases, found all the gliomas represented in the spinal cord. Ependymoma was noted to make up 40 percent of the cases, and the remainder were more or less evenly distributed among astrocytomas, glioblastomas, oligodendrogliomas, ganglioneuromas, medulloblastomas, hemangiomas, and hemangioblastomas. The hemangioma is the common source of spontaneous hematomyelia, and the hemangioblastoma may give rise to a syringomyelia.

SYMPTOMATOLOGY. Patients with spinal cord tumor are likely to manifest one of two clinical pictures: either a purely sensorimotor spinal tract and rarely a syringomyelic syndrome or a radicular-spinal syndrome, nearly always painful.

(a) COMPRESSION OF SENSORIMOTOR SPINAL TRACTS. The predominant clinical syndrome relates to spinal cord compression. With intraspinal tumors, the onset of the compressive symptoms is usually gradual over a period of weeks and months, and the course is progressive. The initial disturbance is likely to be motor, and often the distribution is asymmetric. With cervical lesions the order of motor impairment is first the arm, then the leg, and finally the opposite arm. With thoracic lesions one leg usually becomes weak and stiff before the other one. Subjective sensory symptoms (tingling paresthesias) of the spinal tract type take the same pattern. Pain and temperature are more likely to be affected than touch, vibration, and position senses and are contralateral to the maximum motor weakness (Brown-Séquard syndrome). Nevertheless the posterior columns are also frequently involved. The bladder and bowel usually become paralyzed coincident with motor paralysis of the legs. If the compression is relieved, there is recovery from these sensory-motor symptoms in the reverse order of their affection. The first part affected is the last to recover, and sensory symptoms disappear before motor.

(b) COMPRESSIVE–IRRITATIVE RADICULAR SYMPTOMS. This syndrome of spinal cord compression is often combined with radicular pain, i.e., pain in the distribution of a spinal root. It is described as knifelike or as merely a dull ache with superimposed sharp pains which are intensified by cough, sneeze, or strain and radiation in a distal direction, i.e., away from the spine. Segmental sensory changes (parethesias, hyperalgesia, impairment of pain and touch) or motor disturbances (spasm, cramp, twitching, atrophy, fascicular twitching, and loss of tendon reflex) and an ache in the spine are the usual manifestations of a compressive-irritative lesion of roots. Tenderness of spinous processes over the growth is found in half the patients. These segmental changes, particularly the sensory ones, often precede the signs of spinal cord compression by months or years if the lesion is benign. Sphincter disturbances usually appear late.

The clinical findings upon examination are (1) spastic weakness of the legs, in one leg more than in the other, with thoracolumbar lesions, and of the arms and legs with cervical lesions, (2) a sensory level for pain on the trunk below which pain sense is reduced or lost, (3) posterior column signs, and (4) a spastic bladder under weak voluntary control.

The diagnosis is established by x-rays of the spine (erosion of vertebras, widened spinal canal), lumbar puncture, and electromyography to demonstrate the fasciculations resulting from involvement of motor roots. The most important diagnostic test of all is pantopaque myelography for the direct visualization of the compressive lesion, but such necessary procedures, including lumbar puncture, may occasionally exacerbate the symptoms and signs.

(c) SPECIAL SPINAL SYNDROMES. Unusual clinical syndromes may be found in patients with tumors near the foramen magnum. They may produce a quadriparesis with pains in the back of the head and stiff neck, a weakness and atrophy of the hands and dorsal neck muscles, and either bizarre sensory changes or no sensory loss whatsoever. Lesions of the tenth, eleventh, and twelfth thoracic and the first lumbar vertebrae may result in a curious syndrome of mixed cauda equina and spinal cord symptoms. *Lesions of the cauda equina* alone, always difficult to separate from diseases of the plexus and multiple nerves, are usually attended in the early stages with pain which is variously combined with an asymmetric, atrophic, areflexic paralysis, radicular sensory loss, and later sphincteric disorder. This must be distinguished from *tumors of the conus medullaris* (lower sacral segments of spinal cord) in which there are early disturbances of sphincters of the bladder and bowel, back pain, hypesthesia, and anesthesia over the sacral dermatomes, a lax anal sphincter with loss of anal and bulbocavernosus reflexes, and sometimes weakness of lower leg muscles. A Babinski sign means that the spinal cord is involved above the fifth lumbar segment.

PATHOLOGY, ANATOMY, AND PHYSIOLOGY. Peculiarities of anatomic structure are decisive factors in determining the symptomatology of tumor growths. The structure of the spine was described in Chap. 13, Pain in the Back and Neck. Epidural growths arise from hematogenous deposits or tumors which extend from the vertebral bodies or from extraspinal spaces through intervertebral foramena.

Intramedullary growths both invade as well as compress and distort fasciculi in the adjacent white matter. As the cord enlarges from the tumor growing within it or is compressed from a tumor growing without, the free space around the cord is consumed and the cerebrospinal fluid below the lesion becomes isolated or loculated from the rest of the so-called "circulating cerebrospinal fluid" above. This can be demonstrated by a positive Queckenstedt test (Chap. 353), Froin's syndrome, and interruption of the flow of pantopaque in the subarachnoid space (myelogram).

DIFFERENTIAL DIAGNOSIS. Several problems may arise in the diagnosis of patients with spinal cord tumors. In the early stages spinal tumor must be distinguished from other diseases which cause pain over certain segments of the body, i.e., those affecting the gall bladder, kidney, stomach and intestinal tract, pleura, etc. Here the localization of the pain to a dermatome, its intensification by effort, segmental sensory changes, and minor alterations of motor, reflex, or sensory function in the legs will usually provide the clues to the compressive-irritative radicular lesion. Examination of the cerebrospinal fluid, x-ray of the spine, and myelography will settle the diagnosis in most instances.

If symptoms and signs of disorder of sensory and motor tracts of the spinal cord are present, there is still the problem of locating the segmental level of the lesion. At first the sensory and motor deficiencies may be more pronounced in those parts of the body farthest removed from the lesion, i.e., in feet or lumbosacral segments. Later these sensory and motor levels may ascend, but at any time they may continue to be far below the lesion. Of greatest help in determining the level of the lesion are the locality of the root pains and atrophic paralysis and lastly the upper level of hypalgesia. Again, myelography is necessary to locate the exact level of the cord compression. If localization of the cord lesion in terms of spinal segments has been established, there is still the problem of ascertaining the vertebral localization, for the two do not correspond (see Chap. 21 for a statement of the relationship of spinal segment to vertebras).

Once vertebral and segmental levels are settled, there is still the necessity of determining whether the lesion is neoplastic and extradural, intradural-extramedullary, or intramedullary. This is important from the standpoint of etiologic diagnosis. If there is a visible or palpable spinal deformity or x-ray evidence of vertebral destruction, one may confidently assume an extradural localization. Without x-ray changes one still suspects extradural lesion if root pain developed early and is bilateral, spine ache is prominent, and percussion tenderness is marked, if motor symptoms below the lesions precede sensory changes, and sphincter disturbances are late. To distinguish between intradural-extramedullary and intramedullary lesions is almost impossible. Radicular pain, asymmetry of signs of motor and sensory tract involvement, and early cerebrospinal fluid blockage (positive Queckenstedt test and high protein) favor the extramedullary localization. With extradural lesions one must differentiate between ruptures of disk, spondylosis (hypertrophic spurring and osteophyte formation in cervical spinal canal), tuberculous caries, other pyogenic, fungous, or syphilitic granulomatous lesions, secondary carcinoma, or lymphoma. With intradural-extramedullary lesions, meningioma, neurofibroma, meningeal carcinomatosis, cholesteatoma, teratomatous cyst, or meningomyelitic process is most likely. Intramedullary lesions are usually gliomas or vascular malformations. A negative Queckenstedt test, normal or relatively low protein in cerebrospinal fluid, and a negative myelogram will serve to rule out intraspinal tumors or granulomatous lesions in most instances.

TREATMENT. This varies with the nature of the lesion and the clinical condition of the patient. Intradural-extramedullary tumor should be removed. Laminectomy, decompression, marsupialization of cysts, and x-ray therapy is the treatment of intramedullary gliomas. Extradural malignant growths are best managed by the use of opiates for pain, x-ray therapy, endocrine therapy (for carcinoma of breast and prostate), or nitrogen mustard treatment (for certain lymphomas). Sometimes laminectomy and decompression are necessary for diagnosis and prevention of irreversible compressive effects and infarction of the spinal cord. With tuberculous caries, immobilization of the spine in hyperextension and streptomycin therapy are indicated, and laminectomy should be reserved for exceptional cases with complete and irreversible spinal block. Immobilization of the neck and later the use of a collar (Thomas or other) is the treatment of choice in spondylosis. Only in a rapidly advancing compressive spinal cord syndrome in a relatively young person should there be a laminectomy and cutting of the denticulate ligaments.

In conclusion, it is always well to remind oneself that of the more than 30 diseases of the spinal cord there are available effective means of treating only a few—extramedullary spinal cord tumors, syphilis (meningomyelitis and tabes), epidural granulomas (pyogenic, tuberculous, fungous), subacute combined degeneration, and nutritional myelopathy. The physician's major responsibility is to determine whether or not his patient has one of the treatable diseases.

INJURIES TO SPINAL ROOTS, PLEXUSES, AND PERIPHERAL NERVES

Discussions of these subjects will be found in Chaps. 13 and 353.

REFERENCES

Brock, S. (Ed.): "Injuries of the Brain and Spinal Cord and Their Coverings," 3d ed., Baltimore, The Williams & Wilkins Company, 1949, p. 71.

Elsberg, C. A.: "Tumors of the Spinal Cord," London, Paul B. Hoeber, 1925.

Kernohan, J. W., H. W. Wolkman, and A. W. Adson: Intramedullary Tumors of the Spinal Cord, Arch. Neurol, Psychiat., 25:679, 1931.

Kuhn, W. G., Jr.: Care and Rehabilitation of Patients with Injuries to the Spinal Cord and Cauda Equina: Preliminary Report on 113 Cases, J. Neurosurg., 4:40, 1947.

Prather, G. C., and F. H. Mayfield: "Injuries of the Spinal Cord," Springfield, Ill., Charles C Thomas, Publisher, 1953.

Seddon, H. J.: Pott's Paraplegia: Prognosis and Treatment, Brit. J. Surg., 22:769, 1934–35.

Wyburn-Mason, R.: "Vascular Abnormalities and Tumors of the Spinal Cord," London, Kimpton, 1943.

357 CEREBROVASCULAR DISEASES

C. Miller Fisher, Jay P. Mohr, and Raymond D. Adams

Vascular diseases of the nervous system rank first in frequency amongst all the neurologic diseases. The recognition of this fact and of the need of careful investigation of the causes and mechanisms of these diseases has aroused increasing interest in this subject in the past few years, and for the first time the common "stroke" is being made the object of systematic study. Furthermore, it is evident to all who work in this field of medicine that the cerebrovascular diseases provide one of the best approaches to the study of neurology since they comprise about 50 percent of all neurologic hospital admissions to adult wards. In the past the neurologist, in attempting to learn the secrets of the function of the human brain, has depended heavily on the focal ischemic lesion, and there is no reason to doubt that cerebrovascular diseases will continue to offer instructive examples of disorders of nervous function, the assiduous study of which will be well repaid.

The term *cerebrovascular disease* is intended here to denote any disease in which one or more of the blood vessels of the brain are primarily implicated in a pathologic process. By pathologic process is meant any abnormality of the vessel wall, an occlusion by thrombus or embolus, rupture of a vessel, a failure of cerebral blood flow due to a fall in blood pressure, a change in the caliber of the lumen, altered permeability of the vascular wall, or increased viscosity or other quality of the blood. The pathologic process within the vessel may be described not only according to its grosser aspects—thrombosis, embolism, rupture of a vessel, etc.—but also in terms of the more basic vascular disorder, i.e., atherosclerosis, hypertensive arteriosclerosis, arteritis, trauma, aneurysm, developmental malformation, etc. Furthermore, in classifying cerebrovascular diseases it is not sufficient to consider only the primary vascular lesion; equal weight must be given the resulting parenchymal changes in the brain. These latter are of two types, ischemia with or without infarction, and hemorrhage. Aside from these the vascular lesion is silent, the only exceptions being the local pressure effects of an aneurysm, vascular headache (migraine, hypertension, arteritis), and occasionally increased intracranial pressure as in hypertensive encephalopathy and venous thrombosis.

Brain tissue is dependent for its existence on the moment-to-moment supply of oxygenated blood. In Stokes-Adams attacks unconsciousness occurs within 10 sec of cardiac arrest. In animal experiments the stoppage of blood flow for longer than 3 min produces irreversible damage. When brain tissue is deprived of blood and oxygen, it undergoes ischemic necrosis (infarction) and is destroyed. Obstruction of the nutrient artery by thrombus or embolus is the usual cause, but failure of the systemic circulation and hypotension, if severe and prolonged enough, can also produce infarction. Cerebral infarcts vary greatly in the amount of congestion and hemorrhage found within the softened tissue. Some infarcts are strikingly pallid (pale infarction); others show mild congestion (dilatation of vessels and some extravasation of red blood cells); and still others show an extensive scattering of petechial hemorrhages throughout the damaged gray matter (red infarction). Thrombotic infarcts are usually pale, while embolic infarcts are sometimes pale, sometimes red; i.e., red infarction is usually a sign of embolism. The reason for the different coloration of softenings is not known, although one hypothesis attributes it to the fragmentation and the migration of embolic material from its original site of arrest, the movement distally allowing blood to enter the part of the infarct lying more proximally.

A hemorrhage consists of an extravasation of blood into the parenchyma or the subarachnoid space or both. The blood, once the leakage stops, is slowly resorbed over a period of weeks and months. Damage to the brain results from the pressure of the mass of blood on the surrounding tissue combined with physical disruption of the region directly involved.

In classifying cerebrovascular disease it is most practical from the clinical viewpoint to preserve the three classical divisions, thrombosis, embolism, and hemorrhage, listing the causes of each in the corresponding section. These three make up the majority of strokes. The method has some disadvantages in not providing a precise niche for disorders such as reversible ischemia, hypertensive encephalopathy, venous thrombosis, etc. These latter will be discussed separately.

THE STROKE SYNDROME

The clinical picture resulting from vascular disease is in most instances so distinctive that the diagnosis is more readily made than any other in the realm of neurology.

The cardinal feature is the *stroke,* a term which connotes the sudden and dramatic development of a focal neurologic deficit. In its severest form, the patient falls hemiplegic and even unconscious—an event so striking as to deserve its own separate designation, namely, apoplexy, stroke, shock, or cerebrovascular accident. In its mildest form, it may consist of only a trivial neurologic disorder insufficient to disturb the customary activities of the patient or to demand medical attention.

Undoubtedly, the most characteristic feature is the sequence of events which may be called the *temporal profile* of the stroke. It is the suddenness with which the neurologic deficit develops that especially stamps the disorder as vascular. The speed of evolution, though variable, depending on the cause, is comparatively rapid, and the deficit appears in a matter of seconds, minutes, hours, or at most a few days. When a thrombotic stroke develops over a period of several days, it usually progresses in a stepwise fashion, i.e., in a series of sudden changes, rather than smoothly. A slow, gradual downhill course over a period of several days to a few weeks or more indicates that the process is probably not vascular in nature. Later in the course of the illness, if the attack is not fatal, stabilization occurs, followed by some degree of recovery. Not infrequently an extensive deficit reverses itself dramatically within a few hours or a day. More often, however, the improvement is gradual, taking place over weeks and months.

It must not be supposed that every neurologic abnormality in patients with cerebrovascular disease can be related by the patient or his family to a stroke. Often the exact date of onset of a given symptom cannot be remembered. One has the impression that some of the vascular incidents, especially in the hypertensive patient, are so mild that they do not attract notice until their cumulative effects become manifest as a neurologic deficit of indeterminate date. Furthermore, patients with lesions in the right (nondominant) parietal region often have anosognosia and cannot be depended upon to give any of the important details of their illness. In dominant hemispheral lesions, aphasia hampers history taking.

The neurologic deficit in a stoke depends, of course, on the location of the infarct or hemorrhage in the brain and the size of the lesion. Hemiplegia is the classical sign of vascular disease and occurs chiefly with massive lesions of either cerebral hemisphere, but it also occurs with lesions of the brainstem. In the most serious cases of hemorrhage, the patient literally falls in his tracks, paralyzed on one side, and soon passes into deep coma and dies within a few hours. In other cases, more commonly in infarction, the patient may have a pure motor hemiplegia but remains alert and without other deficit, and from the beginning it is obvious that he will survive his illness whether or not neurologic recovery occurs. A stroke, however, may give rise to many manifestations other than a hemiplegia, e.g., numbness, sensory deficit, dysphasia, blindness, diplopia, dizziness, dysarthria, etc. In the following paragraphs these manifestations will be emphasized equally with hemiplegia.

To summarize briefly, it might be said that the stroke

syndrome is the common denominator of all cerebrovascular diseases and is recognized chiefly by its temporal profile and characteristic focal neurologic deficit.

In practice, however, the diagnosis of cerebrovascular disease is usually supported by the entire constellation of clinical features. Often the patient is elderly and arterial hypertension is present. There may be evidence of vascular disease at other sites, e.g., heart, lower limbs, and aorta; or the patient may have diabetes mellitus and thereby be predisposed to atherosclerosis. A source of emboli may be present (atrial fibrillation, myocardial infarction, subacute bacterial endocarditis, etc.). Many strokes are preceded by transient warning episodes of weakness, numbness, dizziness, etc., and these attacks, if they are nonconvulsive in nature, should always suggest thrombotic cerebrovascular disease. The neurologic signs may occur in certain combinations having a neurovascular relationship; i.e., they may depend on structures which lie within a given vascular territory, as in the lateral medullary syndrome, and thus suggest occlusive vascular disease. And last but not least, the presence of blood in the cerebrospinal fluid in nontraumatic illness signifies that the process is vascular, and diagnostic deductions can proceed from that vantage point.

CEREBRAL THROMBOSIS

Of these many causes, thrombosis with atherosclerosis accounts for the overwhelming majority of cases seen clinically. Several other (hypotension, cerebral herniation, with ruptured aneurysm) are conveniently included here although they are really examples of infarction without actual thrombosis.

Thrombosis with Atherosclerosis

Atherosclerosis in the arteries of the brain is similar to that elsewhere in the body. The atheromatous plaques tend to form at branchings and curves. The severity of the process runs parallel to but is somewhat less severe than that of other arteries—aorta, lower limbs, and heart. Thrombosis is most likely to occur where the plaque narrows the lumen to the greatest degree. The most common sites of thrombosis are the internal carotid artery at the carotid sinus in the neck, at the main bifurcation of the middle cerebral artery, in the vertebral and basilar arteries in the region of their junction, in the posterior cerebral artery as it winds round the cerebral peduncle, and in the anterior cerebral artery as it curves upward over the corpus callosum. Occlusion of the common carotid, brachiocephalic, or subclavian arteries in the upper thorax occasionally is responsible for cerebral ischemia, and the vertebral arteries may be narrowed at their origins from the subclavian. Hypertension aggravates the atherosclerotic process and leads to deposition of atheromatous material in smaller vessels (1 mm and less), and thrombosis will then occur in the penetrating branches of the middle, posterior cerebral, and basilar arteries, producing small infarcts, called *lacunes*, in the internal capsule, central white matter, deeper parts of

Table 357-1. CAUSES OF CEREBRAL THROMBOSIS

I. *Atherosclerosis*
II. *Ruptured saccular aneurysm*
III. Cerebral thrombophlebitis: secondary to infection of ear, paranasal sinus, face, etc.; with meningitis and subdural empyema; debilitating states, post-partum, postoperative, cardiac failure, hematologic disease (polycythemia, sickle-cell disease), and of undetermined cause
IV. Arteritis
   A. Meningovascular syphilis, arteritis secondary to pyogenic and tuberculous meningitis, rare types [typhus, schistosomiasis mansoni, malaria (?), trichinosis (?), mucormycosis, etc.]
   B. Connective tissue diseases: polyarteritis (necrotizing, granulomatous, allergic, Wegner's), temporal arteritis, Takayasu's disease, granulomatous arteritis of aorta, lupus erythematosus
V. Hematologic disorders: polycythemia, sickle-cell disease, thrombotic thrombocytopenic purpura, etc.
VI. Trauma to carotid
VII. Dissecting aortic aneurysm
VIII. Systemic hypotension: "simple faint," acute blood loss, myocardial infarction, Stokes-Adams syndrome, traumatic and surgical shock, sensitive carotid sinus, severe postural hypotension
IX. Complications of arteriography
X. Migrainous aura with persistent deficit
XI. With tentorial, foramen magnum, and subfalcial herniation
XII. Hypoxia
XIII. Miscellaneous types: radioactive or x-ray radiation, lateral pressure of intracerebral hematoma, unexplained middle cerebral infarction in closed head injury, pressure of unruptured saccular aneurysm, mural thrombus in fusiform aneurysm, local dissection of carotid or middle cerebral artery, complication of contraceptive medication
XIV. Undetermined cause as in childhood

the basal ganglions, and brainstem. In hypertension the cerebellar and ophthalmic arteries also are liable to involvement. It is extremely rare for the cerebral arteries to be significantly affected beyond their first major branching; i.e., thrombotic occlusion over the convexities seldom occurs. The details of the process by which thrombosis becomes superimposed on atherosclerosis are poorly understood, and according to the encrustation theory, the two processes are closely related.

The effect of atherosclerotic thrombosis on the brain is not easy to predict accurately, and this is also true of embolic occlusion. If the obstruction lies proximal to the circle of Willis, collateral flow via the circle may be and often is adequate to prevent infarction. In occlusion of the internal carotid artery in the neck anastomotic flow may pass along the external carotid artery and retrograde in the ophthalmic artery or other smaller external-internal connections. In vertebral artery blockage low in the neck blood may reach the upper part of the vertebral artery via the deep cervical, thyrocervical, or occipital arteries. If the occlusion is distal to the circle of Willis, i.e., in the stem of one of the cerebral or cerebellar arteries, a series of subarachnoid interarterial anastomoses that join many of the branches of the major cerebral arteries end-to-end may carry sufficient blood into the compromised territory to prevent or lessen the ischemic damage (Fig. 357-4). There is a capillary anastomotic system between adjacent brain arteries, and although it appears always to be the source of some collateral supply, it is probably inconsequential. The collateral flow is occasionally so great that a major arterial trunk can be entirely occluded without visible damage to the parenchyma. In other cases, occlusion may lead to softening throughout a vast area which extends to the outermost boundaries of the territory nourished by the affected vessel. In between these two extremes there are countless variations in the size, shape, and completeness of an infarct, depending on factors such as the availability of collateral flow, the speed of occlusion (time for compensation), and the level of the systemic blood pressure. These factors and possibly others such as hypoxia and altered physical state of the blood may also at times operate adversely to produce ischemia in the territory of partially occluded vessels.

The actual state of the arterial lumen during the period when the stroke is evolving varies from case to case, and the spectrum of pathologic changes is not yet fully known. Judging from arteriographic and surgical findings in the carotid and vertebral arteries in the neck, it is likely that when prodromal transient ischemic attacks are occurring, atherosclerosis and superimposed thrombus only incompletely occlude the affected artery; blood flow for reasons not yet understood is intermittent in the territory distal to the stenosis. Or the main vessel is totally occluded while a compensating collateral channel is stenotic. By the time the neurologic deficit persists and is advancing, the superimposed thrombus will in the majority of cases have progressed to block completely the main vessel of supply. When the stroke becomes fully established, complete occlusion is the rule. It is common to find more than one vessel affected by stenosis or occlusion, and then it is especially difficult to decipher the interplay of hemodynamic factors leading to symptoms, transitory or persistent. It must be pointed out, too, that it is by no means uncommon for stenosis or occlusion of the carotid and vertebral arteries to be "silent" or nearly so.

CLINICAL PICTURE. In general, the evolution of the total clinical picture in cerebral thrombosis is much more variable than in embolism and hemorrhage. In approximately 80 percent of cases, the main part of the stroke (paralysis or other deficit) is preceded by minor signs or by one or more transient, warning ischemic attacks, which in a sense herald the oncoming vascular catastrophe. *A history of such prodromal episodes is of paramount importance in establishing the diagnosis of cerebral thrombosis.* Such episodes may precede embolism and intracerebral hemorrhage, but this is extremely uncommon. Transient warning attacks in carotid-middle cerebral disease consist of mono- or hemiplegia, mono- or hemiparesthesia, blindness in one eye, speech disturbance, confusion, etc., and in the vertebral-basilar system, of dizziness, diplopia, numbness, impaired vision

in one or both visual fields, dark vision, dysarthria, headache, etc. The attacks last from a few seconds up to 8 hr or so and the final stroke may be preceded by hundreds of attacks or by only a single one. The stroke may come within a day of the first one or may be delayed for weeks or even months, and sometimes the attacks die away without leading to a stroke. When these minor ischemic attacks are not part of the picture, one must depend on other factors in identifying the cerebrovascular process as one of cerebral thrombosis.

The main part of the thrombotic stroke, whether or not it is preceded by warning attacks, develops in one of several ways. There may be but a single attack, the whole illness developing in a few hours. The patient may awaken in the morning with a full-blown paralysis (or other deficit) or have it come on shortly after arising, perhaps while eating breakfast. Another pattern is for the stroke, once it commences, to have a stuttering intermittent progression in the next several hours or days. Or a partial stroke may develop, and after the patient has improved for several hours a full paralysis may develop. Again, after one or more fleeting episodes, there may be a longer-lasting attack, succeeded in a day or two by the occurrence of a complete and permanent paralysis. The affection may involve several parts of the body simultaneously or, as not infrequently happens, one part, such as a limb or one side of the face, is first paralyzed and the other parts become involved serially in steplike fashion until the stroke is fully developed. This may take several days or weeks, during which time there may be improvement and superimposed transient episodes of worsening. All these various modes of development bespeak cerebral thrombosis, and the whole process may be referred to as *thrombosis in evolution*. It might be commented that in the transitory attacks and the abrupt episodes of progression we are really witnessing the temporal profile of the stroke syndrome in miniature. The principle of intermittency seems to characterize the thrombotic process from the beginning to the end. In thrombotic strokes either the onset or progression of the stroke is particularly common during sleep or shortly after arising (60 percent of cases). Occasionally a thrombotic stroke comes on in what appears to be a slow, gradual fashion, but in most of these cases careful inquiry will reveal an uneven or saltatory progression, and actually there are only a few cases—these are usually pure motor hemiplegia—in which it can be said that the evolution of the thrombotic stroke was truly gradual over a period of several days. Table 357-2 shows the way in which the clinical picture developed in 125 cases of cerebral thrombosis diagnosed clinically, for the most part.

Headache, although absent in the majority of cases, is not uncommon in cerebral thrombosis, generally being on one side in the front part of the head in occlusion of the carotid system and at the back of the head or in the forehead in basilar disease. The headache is usually not so violent as in cases of intracranial hemorrhage. Its cause is unknown. Presumably it is related in some way to the disease process within the vessel, since it may antedate

Table 357-2. DEVELOPMENT OF THE CLINICAL PICTURE
IN 125 CASES OF CEREBRAL THROMBOSIS

Clinical development	No. of cases	Percentage
Transient ischemic attacks progressing to a persistent neurologic deficit, major or minor................................	53	42
Stepwise development of a stroke, with or without transient ischemic attacks......	23	18
Stroke developing as a single event.......	21	17
Abrupt (hours), with or without fluctuations...............................	*14*	
Slow, gradual (a few days), with or without minor fluctuations..............	*7*	
Transient ischemic attacks only..........	17	14
Development of a limited stroke followed by transient ischemic attacks..........	11	9

the other symptoms of the stroke. Stiffness of the neck rarely occurs with cerebral infarction.

Hypertension, an important aggravating factor in atherosclerosis, is more often present than not. Diabetes is not uncommon. Often there is evidence of vascular disease elsewhere, e.g., angina pectoris, electrocardiographic abnormality, myocardial infarction, absence of one or several peripheral pulses in the lower limbs, or intermittent claudication. The retinal arteries may show uniform or focal narrowing, increase and irregularity of the light reflex, or displacement of the veins, but these alterations cannot be correlated with cerebral atherosclerosis, and thus fundoscopic examination is at present of little or no help in assessing the state of the intracranial arteries. The patient, although usually elderly, is not invariably so, and persons in the fourth decade or even younger may be stricken.

The *specific neurologic abnormality* depends on the location and size of the infarct or the focus of ischemia. The territory of any vessel, large or small, deep or superficial, may be involved. The carotid and basilar systems are approximately equally affected. In involvement of the carotid system, *unilateral* signs predominate: hemiplegia, hemihypesthesia, hemianopia, aphasia, and agnosia. In basilar disease, one more commonly finds *bilateral* signs, motor and/or sensory, in combination with a disturbance of cranial nerves, cerebellum, or other structures localized in or related to the brainstem. In order that carotid occlusion cause bilateral signs, the vessels to both hemispheres would have to be affected at the same time (bilateral carotid occlusion) or one carotid have been occluded silently in the past, neither a common event. It is important therefore to determine if the signs and symptoms indicate unilateral or bilateral lesions.

In order to understand the particular groupings of neurologic symptoms and signs, the student must be familiar with certain points of neurovascular anatomy which will now be presented. The clinical syndrome associated with occlusion of each of the cerebral and

cerebellar arteries will then become clear. It has already been pointed out that, because of differences in collateral blood flow, speed of occlusion, etc., the ischemic effect of occlusion at any one site is highly variable. Therefore the clinical picture resulting from the occlusion of any particular artery differs from one patient to another; partial syndromes are in the majority. The following descriptions apply particularly to infarction and ischemia due to thrombosis or embolism. Although hemorrhage within these vascular territories may give rise to many of the same effects, the total clinical picture is apt to differ, because in its deep extension the hemorrhage may involve the territory of more than one vessel. Also it displaces tissues and causes an increase in intracranial pressure.

VASCULAR ISCHEMIC SYNDROMES. Middle Cerebral Artery. The middle cerebral artery through its cortical branches supplies the lateral surface of the hemisphere except for the frontal pole, a strip along the superomedial border irrigated by the anterior cerebral, and the lowest temporal convolutions, which are in the territory of the posterior cerebral artery.

Its area includes the cortex and white matter of the lateral and inferior aspects of the frontal lobe, the motor cortex (areas 4 and 6, the centers for contraversive eye movements, and in the dominant hemisphere the motor speech area of Broca), the cortex and white matter of the lateral parietal lobe (sensory cortex, angular and supramarginal convolutions), the lateral and superior parts of the temporal lobe, and the insula. The penetrating branches of the middle cerebral artery supply the putamen, outer globus pallidus, the posterior limb of the internal capsule above the plane of the upper border of the globus pallidus, the adjacent part of the corona radiata, the body of the caudate nucleus, and the superior and lateral portion of the head of the caudate nucleus (Fig. 357-1).

The middle cerebral territory is the region most frequently affected in embolic and thrombotic cerebrovascular disease. The artery may be occluded in its stem,[1] blocking the mouths of the penetrating vessels as well as the flow to the superficial (cortical) vessels, or its major branches can be involved individually. The classical picture of total superficial and deep middle cerebral infarction is a contralateral hemiplegia, hemianesthesia, and homonymous hemianopia (Fig. 357-2). If the dominant hemisphere is involved, global or total sensorimotor aphasia also is present. If the nondominant hemisphere is affected, speech is spared but apractognosia of the minor hemisphere is added to the clinical syndrome (see

---

[1] The term *stem* refers to the section of artery lying between the origin of the middle cerebral and the first major branching. The stem of the anterior cerebral artery lies between its origin and the junction with the anterior communicating artery. The stem of the posterior cerebral stretches from its origin to the posterior communicating artery. The stem of the internal carotid artery extends from the region of the clinoid process to the bifurcation into the middle and anterior cerebral arteries.

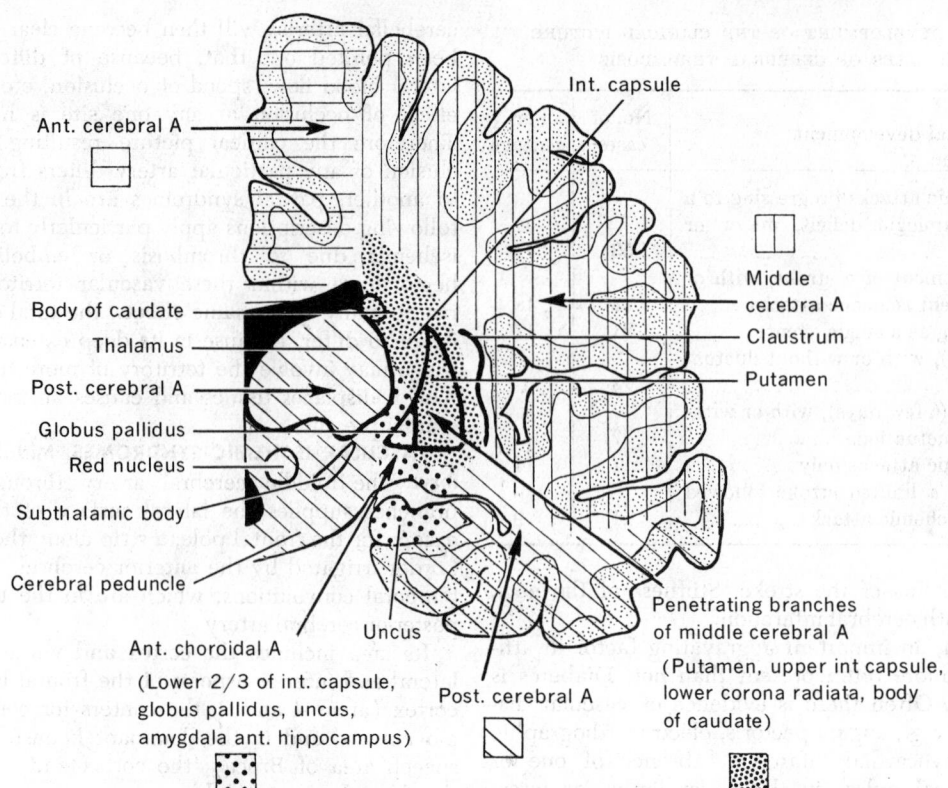

Fig. 357-1. Diagram of a cross section of cerebral hemisphere to show the deep and superficial territories of the major cerebral vessels.

below). When collateral circulation limits the ischemia to a part of the territory, only some of the symptoms and signs listed in Fig. 357-2 will occur.

Thrombotic occlusion of the stem of the middle cerebral artery is relatively uncommon compared with embolic. When the circulation falters, ischemic threat first appears in the distal reaches of the middle cerebral territory, but collateral flow from the anterior cerebral artery through the subarachnoid interarterial anastomoses will compensate. Depending on the effectiveness of this influx, the area of infarction is more or less limited, with the production of partial middle cerebral syndromes of varied severity. Infarcts from embolic occlusion tend to be more extensive.

An embolus may enter any of the middle cerebral branches, producing a corresponding partial deficit. It may block predominantly either the superior or inferior division of the middle cerebral (Fig. 357-2) with involvement, on the one hand, of the arteries or motor part of the hemisphere (superior division) or, on the other hand, the posterior or sensory part of the hemisphere (inferior division). Selective involvement of the posterior part of the hemisphere, e.g., receptive aphasia without paralysis, is a reliable sign of embolic occlusion of the inferior division of the middle cerebral artery. A similar complimentary rule for the superior division, i.e., a motor-sensory deficit in the limbs and a speech disorder without receptive aphasia, is almost as reliable, but

anterior cerebral and internal carotid artery occlusion occasionally also produces this picture.

Lacunar State in Middle Cerebral Territory and Other Vascular Fields. Hypertension combined with atherosclerosis results in thrombotic occlusion of individual penetrating branches running to the internal capsule and putamen, resulting in lacunes 2 to 15 mm in extent. When they involve the internal capsule, a pure motor hemiplegia results, recovery from which is often nearly complete. In the thalamus or above they are manifested by a pure hemisensory defect (see p. 147); in the midbrain the common syndrome is hemiparesis with cerebellar ataxia on the same side as the weakness; in the pons the most frequent syndrome is dysarthria with a clumsy hand (see p. 118) or a pure hemiplegia. Other syndromes such as pure hemiballismus will be defined. In all, the neurologic syndrome develops abruptly without change in state of consciousness. Multiple lacunes involving the corticospinal and corticobulbar motor tracts cause the clinical picture of "pseudobulbar palsy" (more appropriately called *bipyramidal palsy*), featuring bilateral upper motor neurone signs, viz., spasticity, increased tendon reflexes, Babinski sign, dysarthria, and dysphagia. Spasms of excessive crying or laughing, marché-à-petit-pas, and mental impairment are also part of the picture. Lacunes are sometimes said to be the basis of so-called "arteriosclerotic parkinsonism," but proof that such an entity exists is wanting.

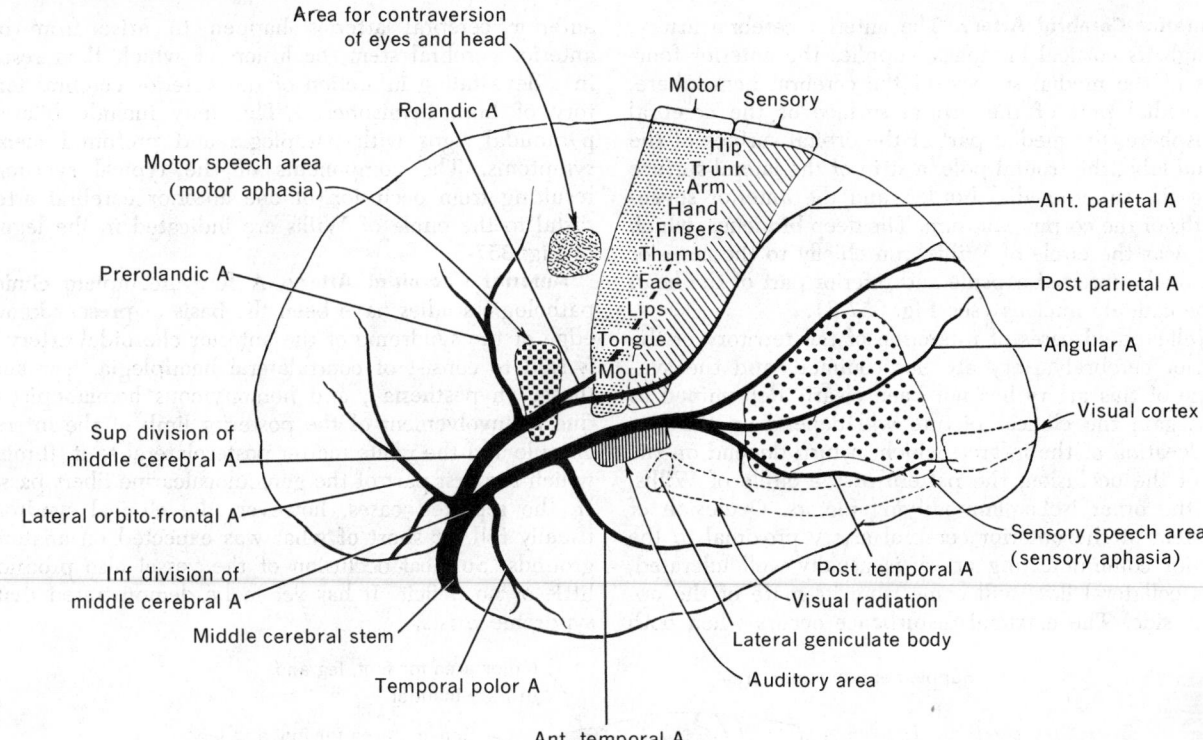

Fig. 357-2. Diagram of the lateral aspect of the cerebral hemisphere showing the branches and distribution of the middle cerebral artery and the principal regions of cerebral localization. Below is a list of the clinical manifestations produced by infarction in the territory of the middle cerebral artery and the corresponding regions of cerebral damage. In each case the signs and symptoms are separated from the anatomic area by a colon (:).

Paralysis of the contralateral face, arm, and leg: Somatic motor area for face and arm and the fibers descending from the leg area to enter the corona radiata.

Sensory impairment over the contralateral face, arm, and leg (pinprick, cotton touch, vibration, position, two-point discrimination, stereognosis, tactile localization, barognosis, cutaneographia): Somatic sensory system corresponding to motor involvement described above.

Motor aphasia: Motor speech area of the dominant hemisphere.

Sensory aphasia [word deafness, anomia, jargon speech, sensory agraphia, acalculia, alexia, finger agnosia, right-left confusion (the last four comprise the Gerstmann syndrome)]: Amusia, Sensory speech area and parietooccipital cortex of the dominant hemisphere.

Ideational apraxia: Sensory speech area (parietal portion).

Apractognosia of the minor hemisphere (amorphosynthesis), anosognosia, hemiasomatognosia, unilateral neglect, agnosia for the left half of external space, dressing "apraxia," constructional "apraxia," distortion of visual coordinates, inaccurate localization in the half field, impaired ability to judge distance, upside-down reading, visual illusions (e.g., it may appear that another person walks through a table): Nondominant supersensory zone (area corresponding to speech area in dominant hemisphere). Loss of topographic memory is usually due to a nondominant lesion, occasionally to a dominant one.

Homonymous hemianopia (often homonymous inferior quadrantanopia): Optic radiation deep to second temporal convolution.

Paralysis of conjugate gaze to the opposite side: Frontal contraversive field or fibers projecting therefrom.

Avoidance reaction of opposite limbs: Parietal lobe lesion.

Miscellaneous: Frontal ataxia due (?) to lesion of frontopontine tract, loss or impairment of optokinetic nystagmus due to lesion of supramarginal or angular gyrus; disturbance of caloric nystagmus due to posterior temporal lobe lesion; limb-kinetic apraxia (?) related to premotor cortical damage; asymbolia for pain due to lesion of dominant parietal lobe; intellectual deterioration, mirror movement, Cheyne-Stokes respiration, contralateral hyperhidrosis, occasionally mydriasis: the localization of the responsible lesions for the last five is not known. Acute lesions of the nondominant hemisphere may cause some degree of amnesia and confabulation mimicking Korsakoff's syndrome.

Capsular hemiplegia: This results usually from a softening of the upper portion of the posterior limb of the internal capsule and the adjacent corona radiata. Motor paralysis is the chief sign, and dysphasia, homonymous hemianopia, and significant sensory loss seldom occur in the syndrome.

Anterior Cerebral Artery. The anterior cerebral artery, through its cortical branches, supplies the anterior four-fifths of the medial surface of the cerebral hemisphere, the medial part of the orbital surface of the cerebral hemisphere, the medial part of the orbital surface of the frontal lobe, the frontal pole, a strip of the lateral surface along the superomedial border, and the anterior seven-eighths of the corpus callosum. The deep branches, which arise near the circle of Willis, run chiefly to the anterior limb of the internal capsule and inferior part of the head of the caudate nucleus (see Fig. 357-3).

Well-studied cases of infarction of the territory of the anterior cerebral artery are not common, and the syndrome of this artery has not been clearly determined as yet. Again the clinical picture will depend on the size and location of the infarct, which in turn depend on the site of the occlusion, the pattern of the circle of Willis, and the other ischemia-modifying factors. Occlusion of the stem of the anterior cerebral artery proximal to the anterior communicating artery is usually well tolerated, since collateral flow will come from its mate of the opposite side. The maximal disturbance occurs when both anterior cerebral arteries happen to arise from one anterior cerebral stem, occlusion of which then results in a devastating infarction of the anterior cerebral territory of both hemispheres. This may include bilateral pyramidal signs with paraplegia and profound mental symptoms. The components of the typical syndrome resulting from occlusion of one anterior cerebral artery distal to the circle of Willis are indicated in the legend of Fig. 357-3.

Anterior Choroidal Artery. A few incomplete clinico-pathologic studies have been the basis of present knowledge of the syndrome of the anterior choroidal artery. It is said to consist of contralateral hemiplegia, hemianesthesia (hypesthesia), and homonymous hemianopia, all due to involvement of the posterior limb of the internal capsule and the white matter posterolateral to it, through which the first part of the geniculocalcarine fibers passes. In the reported cases, however, the clinical syndrome usually fell far short of what was expected on anatomic grounds. Surgical occlusion of the vessel also produced little or no deficit. It has yet to be demonstrated that a syndrome exists.

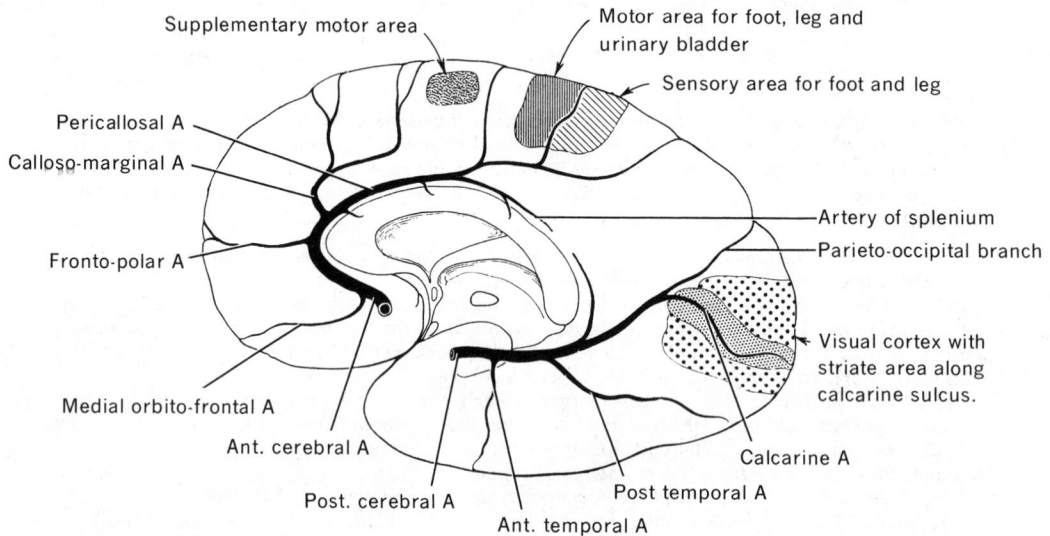

Fig. 357-3. Diagram of the medial aspect of the cerebral hemisphere to show the branches and distribution of the anterior cerebral artery and the principal regions of cerebral localization. Below is a list of the clinical manifestations produced by infarction in the territory of the anterior cerebral artery and the corresponding regions of cerebral damage. In each case signs and symptoms are separated from the anatomic area by a colon (:).

Paralysis of opposite foot and leg: motor leg area.
A lesser degree of paresis of opposite arm: involvement of arm area of cortex or fibers descending to corona radiata therefrom.
Cortical sensory loss over toes, foot, and leg: sensory area for foot and leg.
Unwitting urinary incontinence: sensorimotor area in paracentral lobule.
Contralateral grasp reflex, sucking reflex, gegenhalten (paratonic rigidity), "frontal tremor": medial surface of the posterior frontal lobe (?) supplementary motor area.
Abulia (akinetic mutism) slowness, delay, intermittent interruption, lack of spontaneity, whispering, motor inaction, reflex distraction to sights and sounds: uncertain localization—probably inferomedial lesion near subcallosum. Impairment of gait and stance (gait apraxia): frontal cortex near leg motor area. Mental impairment (perseveration) and dysmemory: localization unknown.
Miscellaneous: dyspraxia of left limbs due to involvement of corpus callosum; tactile aphasia in left limbs due to lesion of corpus callosum, frontal ataxia (the occurrence of such a disorder mimicking cerebellar ataxia is disputed) has not been reported with vascular lesions; cerebral paraplegia may be due to bilateral anterior cerebral artery occlusion. (Note: aphasia and hemianopia do not occur.)

Internal Carotid Artery. The clinical picture of occlusion of the internal carotid artery is very variable. Not infrequently occlusion is completely asymptomatic, while in other cases it produces a devastating massive infarction which leads to death in a few days. Between these two extremes lies every shade of variation. As a rule, the infarct involves some part of the middle cerebral territory, but when the anterior communicating artery is very small, the ipsilateral anterior cerebral territory may be affected too, in which case the anterior part of the hemisphere (the frontal lobe) bears the brunt of the insult, while the region posterior to the Rolandic fissure tends to be spared. When both anterior cerebral arteries arise from a common stem on one side, infarction may involve the anterior cerebral territory bilaterally. The posterior cerebral artery also may be supplied from the internal carotid rather than from the basilar artery, in which case its territory, too, may be softened, and thus the entire hemisphere and even part of the other may be involved. Not infrequently the tissue in the territory of the anterior choroidal artery is also infarcted. When one carotid has been asymptomatically occluded at a previous time, occlusion of the other can result in bilateral hemispheric infarction.

In symptomatic occlusion of the internal carotid artery, when the deficit is advanced, the picture usually resembles that of middle cerebral occlusion with a contralateral hemiplegia, and hemihypesthesia and aphasia, when the dominant hemisphere is involved. When the anterior cerebral territory is also involved, the clinical picture will include some or all of the features already mentioned under anterior cerebral territory. Patients with infarction in the combined territories of the middle and anterior cerebral arteries are much less responsive than those with lesions in only one territory, and often they are in a stupor.

When the circulation in one carotid is compromised and collateral flow is restricted, it is the most distal or terminal parts of the middle and anterior and at times the posterior cerebral territories that suffer first and most. This gives rise to a *watershed* or *border-zone* configuration of infarction in which the contiguous distal fields of each vessel are selectively involved. When well developed, the zone of damage forms an elongated strip of variable width extending from the frontal pole to the occipital. Therefore carotid infarcts of less than maximal extent tend to be located distally rather than proximally in the Sylvian region. Likewise it is in this most vulnerable region that transient ischemic attack symptoms are liable to arise in carotid stenosis, taking the form of weakness or paresthesias in the upper extremity and, if more extensive, in the face and tongue. The relative sparing of the posterior part of the hemisphere is reflected in a low incidence of homonymous hemianopia.

In addition to supplying the brain, the internal carotid artery supplies the optic nerve and retina via the ophthalmic artery (Fig. 357-4). Transient monocular blindness occurs intermittently as a warning symptom prior to the onset of the stroke in almost 25 percent of cases of symptomatic carotid occlusion. However the picture of central retinal artery occlusion rarely develops at the time of the stroke.

Whereas most cerebral vessels are inaccessible within the skull and topical diagnosis is made only by inference, in carotid occlusion more direct diagnostic tests are available. Pulsation may be reduced or absent in the internal or common carotid arteries in the neck, in the external carotid branch in front of the ear, or in the internal carotid artery when palpated in the pharynx. Severe stenosis within the carotid sinus due to an atherosclerotic plaque—with or without superimposed thrombus—may give rise to a local bruit, which can be an important finding in assessing the carotid circulation. Occasionally the murmur results from stenosis at the mouth of the external carotid artery and can then be misleading. Stenosis of the carotid sinus with an accompanying murmur may be present bilaterally. Murmurs may occur lower in the neck along the common carotid arteries, or subclavians. Propagation distally of an aortic valvular murmur must be distinguished from carotid bruits. Pressure in the central retinal artery is usually reduced on the side of carotid occlusion or severe stenosis, and a pressure difference in the two eyes on careful ophthalmodynamometry will point strongly to carotid occlusion. Dilated collateral channels coursing over the forehead may also suggest carotid occlusion. Retinal embolism, either of shining white or plain type, may point to carotid disease. An additional sign of carotid occlusion is the presence on the *opposite* side of an intracranial murmur, heard best by placing the bell of the stethoscope over the eyeball. The murmur is presumably due to augmented blood flow through the remaining patent vessel. Headache associated with cerebral thrombosis or embolism in the carotid artery is situated just above the eyebrow, while in the middle cerebral artery, it is usually more lateral, at the temple. Another test consists of compressing the patent opposite carotid artery in the neck, precipitating unconsciousness, seizures, or an electroencephalographic change, but such a maneuver cannot be recommended for routine use.

The common carotid arteries may be occluded at their origin, as in "pulseless disease" or the *aortic arch syndrome*. The neurologic symptoms and signs of carotid occlusion, just discussed, may or may not be present, depending on the adequacy of the circle of Willis and of the vertebral-basilar system. The following manifestations, for the most part nonneurologic, have been reported in the aortic arch syndrome: absence of pulsation in carotid and radial arteries, faintness on arising from the horizontal position, recurrent loss of consciousness, headache, neck pain, paresthesias of various parts of the body, transient blindness (unilateral or bilateral), dimness of vision with exercise, premature cataracts, retinal atrophy and pigmentation, atrophy of the iris, leukomas, peripapillary arteriovenous anastomoses, optic atrophy, claudication of the jaw muscles, perforation of the nasal septum, saddle-nose deformity, trophic ulceration of the face, facial atrophy (unilateral or bilateral), indolent infections of the face, abnormal facial pigmentation, and loss of hair. This condition was originally de-

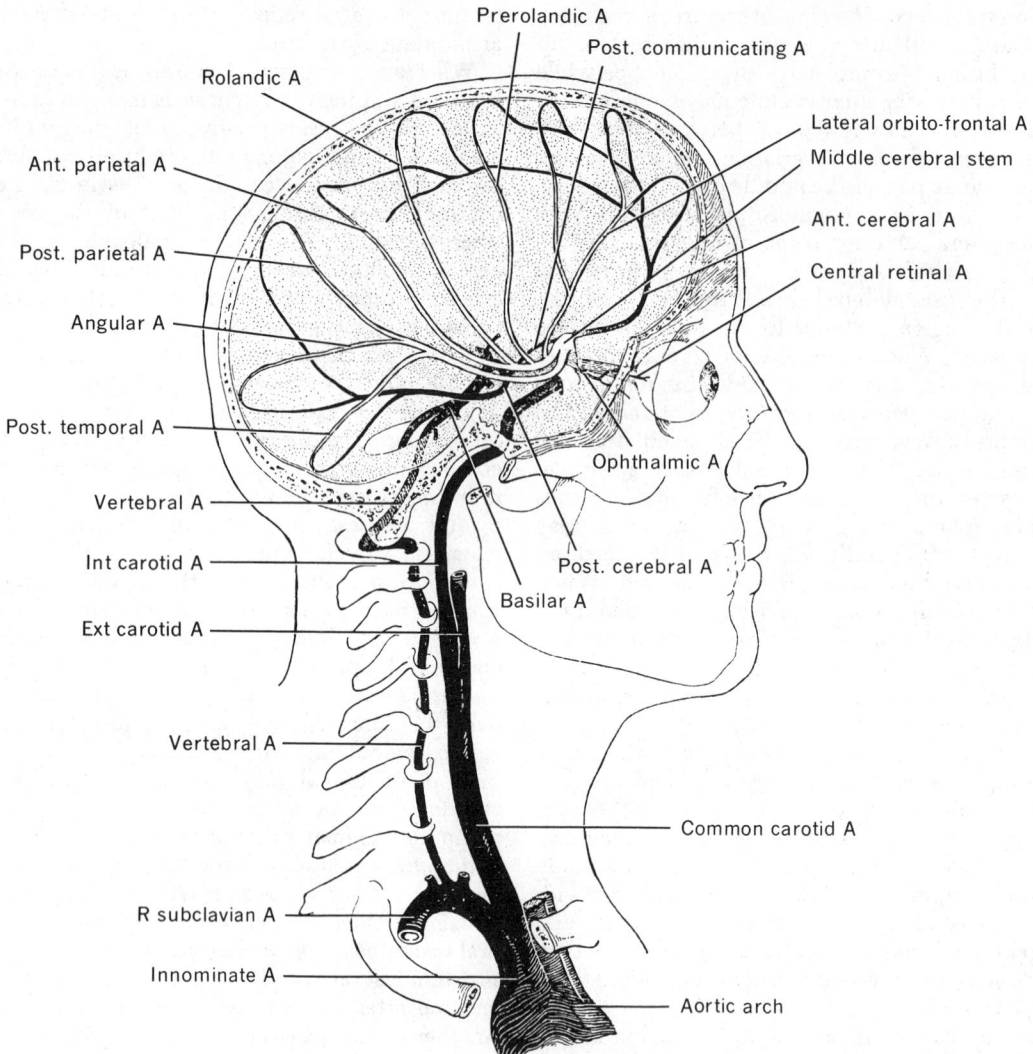

Fig. 357-4. Drawing to illustrate the arrangement of the major arteries carrying blood from the heart to the brain (only the right side is shown). The posterior communicating artery connects the internal carotid and the posterior cerebral arteries, forming an important anastomosis between the carotid and basilar systems. Further distally, the subarachnoid interarterial anastomoses which link the middle cerebral with the anterior and posterior cerebral arteries are shown. The ophthalmic and central retinal arteries have been included to remind the student that observations and measurements of the retinal circulation provide information concerning the carotid circulation.

scribed in Japan, particularly in young women who were found to be suffering from a granulomatous arteritis involving all three major trunks arising from the aortic arch (Takayasu's disease, see Chap. 277). An incomplete aortic arch syndrome consisting of various combinations of carotid, subclavian, or innominate occlusion or stenosis is not uncommon. The majority of the cases of pulseless disease in the United States and Europe, both the partial and the complete syndrome, have been due to severe atherosclerosis, which has often been mistakenly called *Buerger's disease*.

VERTEBRAL-BASILAR POSTERIOR CEREBRAL SYSTEM. Posterior Cerebral Artery. In 71 percent of cases both posterior cerebral arteries arise from the basilar artery; in 22 percent one comes from the basilar and one from the internal carotid artery; and in 7 percent both come from the internal carotid. The terminal or cortical branches of this vessel supply the undersurface of the temporal and occipital lobes, as well as the entire medial surface of the occipital lobe including the visual area (areas 17, 18, and 19). From the more proximal part of the artery between its origin at the bifurcation of the basilar artery and the cortical distribution many important branches arise.

The interpeduncular branches arising near its origin penetrate the brainstem to supply the red nucleus, subthalamic nucleus of Luys, substantia nigra, the most medial part of the cerebral peduncle, the oculomotor nucleus, the reticular substance of the midbrain, the decussation of the superior cerebellar peduncles, rubro-thalamic tract, medial longitudinal fasciculus, and the medial lemniscus. The thalamoperforating branches also arise here and pass to the inferior medial and anterior parts of the thalamus. Branches arising serially along the parent vessel as it encircles the midbrain supply the cerebral peduncle, lateral part of the medial lemniscus, corpora quadrigemina, pineal gland, lateral geniculate bodies, choroid plexus, and hippocampus. The thalamo-geniculate branches supply the pulvinar and the lateral nuclei of the thalamus (Fig. 357-5).

Again the clinical picture resulting from occlusion will depend on the site of the obstruction, the ischemia-modifying factors, and the site and size of the resultant infarct. Occlusion proximal to the posterior communicating artery may be tolerated if collateral flow via that vessel is adequate; however, the penetrating branches arising from the stem of the posterior cerebral artery may be occluded at their mouths. Even distal to the posterior communicating artery, occlusion may cause no damage if collateral flow via the subarachnoid interarterial anastomoses is sufficient.

Classically, occlusion of the cortical or superficial branches of the posterior cerebral artery gives rise to a contralateral homonymous hemianopia because of involvement of the primary visual area in the calcarine region. This syndrome and the effects of branch occlusions are listed in Fig. 357-5.

Bilateral lesions of the occipital lobes, if extensive, cause total blindness of the cortical type, because of a bilateral homonymous hemianopia. The pupillary reflexes are retained, and funduscopically the optic nerves are not atrophic, unlike the situation in disease of the optic nerves. Often the patient is unaware of the blindness and may in fact deny it when questioned specifically (see p. 136). More commonly the bilateral lesions are incomplete and a sector of the visual field is left intact. When the remnant is very restricted, vision may fluctuate greatly from moment to moment, suggesting hysteria. In small calcarine lesions there may be loss of central vision only (bilateral homonymous central scotomas); on the other hand, in larger calcarine lesions, only central vision may be spared, and vision is likened to looking through a narrow pipe (gun-barrel vision). With bilateral lesions, there is usually a loss of memory, the severity of which varies from case to case. There may or may not be the various cortical disturbances described under unilateral lesions.

When occlusion of the *posterior cerebral artery* occurs more proximally (one might speak of anterior syndromes), the clinical picture will comprise signs of damage to thalamus, cerebral peduncle, midbrain, and subthalamus, and possibly, in addition, the manifestations just described (hemianopia, etc.), depending on the collateral inflow of blood. Best known is the *thalamic syndrome* of Dejerine and Roussy, which results from infarction of the region of the sensory nucleus in the posterolateral part of the thalamus (supplied by the thalamogeniculate vessel). The lesion may be so small

as to be overlooked on pathologic examination. The central feature is a sensory loss on the opposite side of the body, usually affecting deep and superficial sensation (pain, temperature, touch, proprioception); or rarely, it may be of the dissociated type, either pain and temperature or vibratory and position sense being affected while the other sensory modalities are relatively spared. It may take a monoplegic pattern. Sometimes there develops later an associated intractable agonizing pain in the affected parts of the body (thalamic pain), occurring spontaneously and augmented by all types of stimulation of the affected parts. However, this spontaneous pain is often entirely missing, whereas hyperpathia is common (see p. 147). Distortion of taste is not infrequent. In the motor sphere there may be a mild evanescent hemiparesis, and in some patients the affected limbs show hemiballismus, choreoathetosis, incoordination, intention tremor, asynergy, cramplike spasms, and a postural abnormality of the hand (see Chap. 22). The mind is usually spared.

Occlusion of the stem of the posterior cerebral artery may lead to a hemiplegia owing to infarction of the cerebral peduncle, but this is uncommon. Occlusion of the thalamoperforate branches which originate from the most medial part of the posterior cerebral stem gives rise to several different syndromes, depending on the branches involved: (1) a superior syndrome in which the upper part of the red nucleus or dentatothalamic tract is involved, producing on the opposite side of the body a gross ataxia (see Chap. 23); (2) an inferior syndrome (Claude's syndrome), in which a third-nerve palsy and contralateral cerebellar signs are combined; (3) Weber's syndrome, i.e., a third-nerve palsy combined with a contralateral hemiplegia (see Chap. 355); (4) *hemiballismus,* which probably arises also from an occlusion of the branch of the posterior cerebral artery running to the subthalamic nucleus of Luys; (5) Parinaud's syndrome, paralysis of conjugate vertical gaze which results from damage to the region of the posterior commissure; (6) peduncular hallucinosis (visual hallucinations of brightly colored scenes and objects) has been observed in occlusion of the posterior cerebral artery, but the site of the lesion has not been determined. More often an intracerebral hemorrhage is responsible. Finally, (7) extensive infarction of the upper part of the midbrain results in deep coma, bipyramidal signs, and "decerebrate rigidity" (reflex extensor posture).

Lacunar infarction in the posterolateral thalamus causes a pure sensory or paresthetic stroke consisting of numbness and sensory loss in the face, arm, and leg on one side.

Vertebral Artery. The vertebral arteries are the chief arteries of the medulla, and each supplies the lower three-fourths of the pyramid, the medial lemniscus, all or nearly all of the retro-olivary region (the lateral medullary region), the restiform body, and the postero-inferior part of the cerebellar hemisphere (see Fig. 357-6). The relative size of the vertebral arteries varies a good deal, and in approximately 10 percent of cases, one vessel is so small that the other can be considered the only artery of supply to the brainstem. In this case,

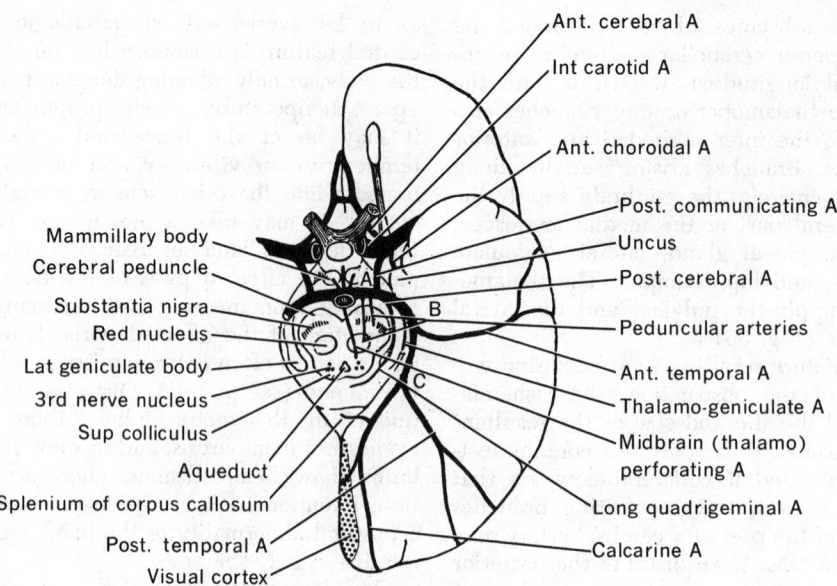

Fig. 357-5. Diagram of the inferior aspect of the brain to show the branches and distribution of the posterior cerebral artery and the principal anatomic structures. Below is a list of the clinical manifestations produced by infarction in the territory of the posterior cerebral artery and the corresponding regions of damage. In each case the signs and symptoms are separated from the anatomic area by a colon (:)

Peripheral territory

Homonymous hemianopia (often upper quadrantic): Calcarine cortex or optic radiation nearby. Hemiachromatopsia may be present. Macular or central vision tends to be preserved because occipital polar striate is spared.

Bilateral homonymous hemianopia, cortical blindness, unawareness or denial of blindness; tactile naming, achromatopsia, failure to see to-and-fro movements, inability to perceive objects not centrally located, apraxia of ocular movements, inability to count or enumerate objects, tendency to run into things which the patient sees and tries to avoid: Bilateral occipital lobe with possibly the parietal lobe involved also. Verbal dyslexia without agraphia, color anomia: Dominant calcarine lesion of posterior part of corpus callosum.

Memory defect: Hippocampal lesion bilaterally or the dominant side only; or involvement of hippocampal system at another level (mammillary bodies, psalterium).

Topographic disorientation and prosopagnosia: Usually with lesions of nondominant, calcarine and lingual gyri. Simultanagnosia, perseveration: Dominant visual cortex.

Unformed visual hallucinations, peduncular hallucinosis, metamorphopsia, teleopsia, illusory visual spread, irreminiscence, paliopsia, distortion of outlines, central photophobia: Calcarine cortex. Complex hallucinations, usually nondominant.

Central territory

Thalamic syndrome—sensory loss (all modalities), spontaneous pain and dysesthesias, choreoathetosis, intention tremor, spasms of hand, mild hemiparesis: Posteroventral nucleus of thalamus in territory of thalamogeniculate artery. Involvement of the adjacent subthalamic body or its afferent tracts results in hemiballismus and choreoathetosis.

Thalamoperforate syndrome—(a) superior, crossed cerebellar ataxia; (b) inferior, crossed cerebellar ataxia with ipsilateral third nerve palsy (Claude's syndrome): Dentatothalamic tract and issuing third nerve.

Weber's syndrome—third nerve palsy and contralateral hemiplegia: Third nerve and cerebral peduncle.

Contralateral hemiplegia: Cerebral peduncle.

Paralysis or paresis of vertical eye movement, skew deviation, sluggish pupillary responses to light, slight miosis and ptosis (retraction nystagmus and "tucking" of the eyelids may be associated): Supranuclear fibers to third nerve, interstitial nucleus of Cajal, nucleus of Darkschewitsch, and posterior commissure.

Contralateral rhythmic, ataxic action tremor; rhythmic postural or "holding" tremor (rubral tremor): Dentatothalamic tract (?) after decussation. The site of the lesion is actually unknown.

Decerebrate attacks: Damage to motor tracts of upper brain stem.

Resting tremor or tremor not easily abolished by relaxation has been omitted because of the uncertainty of its occurrence in the posterior cerebral artery syndrome.

Peduncular hallucinosis may occur in thalamic-subthalamic ischemic lesions, but the exact location of the lesion is unknown.

if collateral inflow from the carotid system via the circle of Willis is unavailable, occlusion would be equivalent to occlusion of the basilar artery or bilateral occlusion of the vertebral arteries. The posterior inferior cerebellar artery is usually a branch of the vertebral artery, but not infrequently it has a common origin with the anterior inferior cerebellar artery from the basilar artery. It is necessary to keep these anatomic variations in mind when visualizing the effects of vertebral artery occlusion.

The results of vertebral occlusion are quite variable. When there are two good-sized vertebral arteries, occlusion on one side occurs not infrequently without any recognizable symptoms and signs or pathologic changes. If the subclavian artery is blocked proximal to the origin of the vertebral artery, exercise of the arm on that side may draw blood from the vertebral-basilar system into the arm, sometimes resulting in the symptoms of basilar insufficiency. Fisher has called this the "subclavian steal" syndrome. If the occlusion of the vertebral artery is so situated as to block the mouth of one or more arteries supplying the lateral medulla, the lateral medullary syndrome may be precipitated, and this is probably the most common picture in vertebral occlusion (see below). When the branch to the anterior spinal artery is blocked, collateral influx from the spinal artery branch of the opposite side is usually sufficient to prevent infarction. If the branch to the pyramid is occluded, that part of the corticospinal tract may be infarcted unless collateral flow is adequate. Also, any of these branches may become occluded in its course after leaving the vertebral artery and may produce similar effects. Rarely, occlusion of the vertebral artery or one of its medial branches produces an infarct which involves the medullary pyramid, the medial lemniscus, and the emergent hypoglossal fibers [contralateral paralysis of arm and leg (face spared), contralateral loss of position and vibration sense, and ipsilateral paralysis and atrophy of the tongue]. This is the medial medullary syndrome (see Fig. 357-6D). Vertebral occlusion can also lead to symptoms by blocking the posterior inferior cerebellar artery. Occlusion of the vertebral arteries low in the neck is usually compensated for by anastomotic flow to the upper part of the vertebral arteries via the thyrocervical, deep cervical, and occipital arteries, or an influx from the anterior part of the circle of Willis may occur.

The *posterior inferior cerebellar artery* supplies the inferior portion of the lateral medullary region, the restiform body, and the inferior surface of the cerebellar hemisphere. It may be occluded at its mouth, i.e., by thrombosis of the vertebral artery, or anywhere along its course. Some patients tolerate obstruction of the vessel with little or no ill effect; in others an extensive infarct results in the cerebellum and/or the posterolateral medulla. It should be pointed out that the various cerebellar arteries are connected to their neighbors by subarachnoid interarterial anastomoses, in the same way as the main arteries of the cerebrum, and the potential for collateral flow to a compromised territory is excellent.

The clinical picture resulting from occlusion of the posterior inferior cerebellar artery is variable. Often no

serious damage results. Occasionally the *lateral medullary syndrome* may be evoked through blockage of flow along the inferior artery of the lateral medulla. Although occlusion of the posterior inferior cerebellar artery is usually stated to be the cause of the lateral medullary syndrome, this appears to be true in only a very small minority of patients; more careful studies show that in 8 out of 10 cases the vertebral artery is occluded, and in the other 2 either the posterior inferior cerebellar artery is occluded or no arterial occlusion is found. Infarction in the posterior medullary region causes ipsilateral cerebellar ataxia and rarely hiccup. The symptoms associated with infarction of the inferior part of the cerebellum have not been clearly determined, but they also probably include ataxia.

The *lateral medullary syndrome* is produced by infarction of a small wedge of lateral medulla lying posteriorly to the inferior olivary nucleus (see Fig. 357-6D). The classical syndrome consists of the symptoms and signs listed below the figure. This syndrome, one of the most striking in neurology, is almost always due to infarction.

Basilar Artery. The basilar artery supplies not only the pons and upper part of the cerebellum but also in most cases the tissue in both posterior cerebral territories. Occlusion may occur in the trunk of the basilar artery or in any one of its branches.

The branches of the basilar artery may be conveniently grouped as follows: (1) paramedian, seven to ten in number, supplying a wedge of pons on either side of the midline; (2) the short circumferential branches, five to seven in number, supplying the lateral two-thirds of the pons and the middle and superior cerebellar peduncles; and (3) the long circumferential, two in number on each side running laterally across the pons to reach the cerebellar hemispheres (the superior cerebellar artery and the anterior inferior cerebellar artery).

Occlusion of the basilar artery evokes a vast array of clinical manifestations reflecting involvement of a large number of structures [corticospinal and corticobulbar tracts, cerebellum, middle and superior cerebellar peduncles, medial and lateral lemnisci, spinothalamic tracts, medial longitudinal fasciculi, pontine nuclei, vestibular and cochlear nuclei, descending hypothalamospinal sympathetic fibers, the upper medulla, and the third, fourth, fifth, sixth, seventh, and eighth cranial nerves (including the nuclei, the segment within the brainstem, and the peripheral nerve itself) (see Fig. 357-6).

The picture of basilar occlusion due to thrombosis may arise in several ways: (1) occlusion in the basilar artery itself, usually in the lower third at the site of an atherosclerotic plaque; (2) occlusion of both vertebral arteries, with closure of the second amounting to basilar obstruction; (3) occlusion of a single vertebral artery, when there is only one of good size. It must be emphasized that thrombosis may involve only a branch of the basilar artery rather than the trunk, and this is the most common cause of basilar symptoms. When the obstruction is embolic, the embolus usually lodges at the upper bifurcation of the basilar or in one of the posterior cerebral arteries, since if it is small enough to pass through the

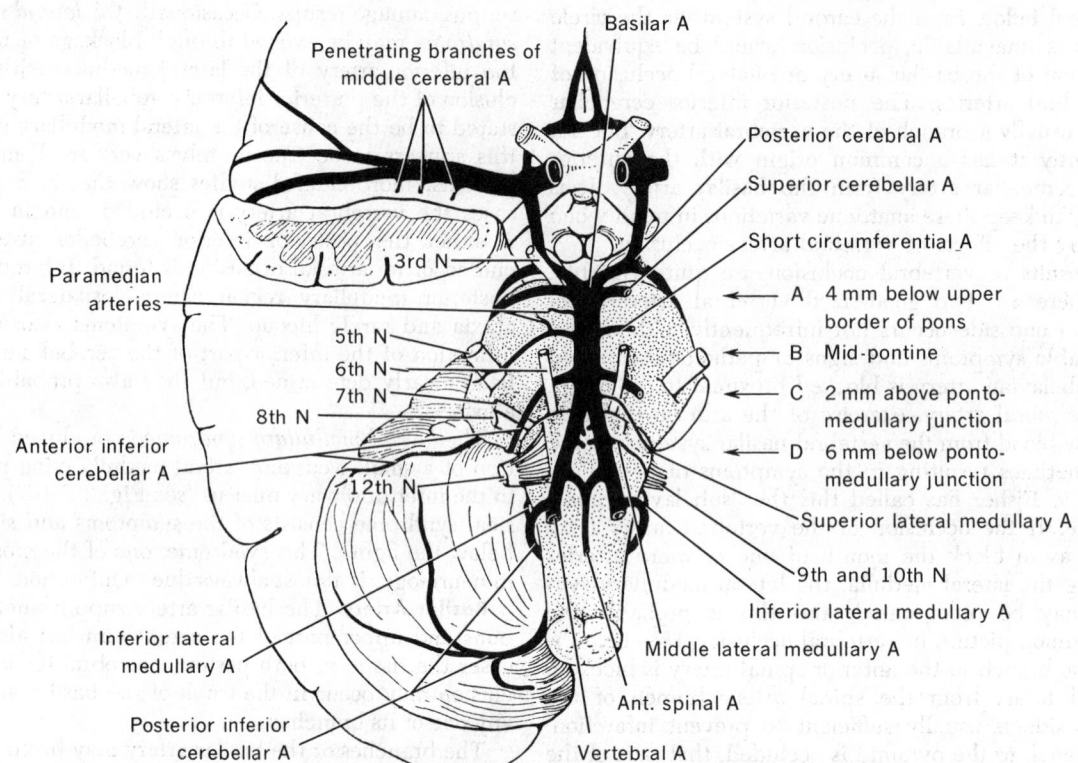

Fig. 357-6. Diagram of the brainstem showing the principal vessels of the vertebral-basilar system. The letters and arrows on the right indicate the levels of the four cross sections A, B, C, and D which follow. Although typical vascular syndromes of the pons and medulla have been designated by sharply outlined shaded areas, the student must appreciate that since satisfactory clinicopathologic studies are far from numerous, the diagrams are not necessarily accurate nor do they always represent established fact. The great frequency with which infarcts fail to produce a well-recognized syndrome and the special tendency for syndromes to merge with one another must be emphasized.

vertebral artery, it should easily traverse the length of the basilar artery, which is usually of greater diameter than either vertebral artery.

The composition of the complete basilar syndrome is given in Fig. 357-6D. In the presence of the full syndrome, it is usually not difficult to make the correct diagnosis. The aim should be, however, to recognize basilar insufficiency long before the stage of total deficit has been reached. The early manifestations occur in many combinations, and it would be difficult to list all the possibilities.

In regard to occlusion of individual basilar branches, the main signs of thrombosis of the *superior cerebellar artery* are severe ipsilateral cerebellar ataxia (middle and/or superior cerebellar peduncles), nausea and vomiting, slurred speech, and loss of pain and temperature over the extremities, body, and face of the opposite side (spinothalamic tract). Partial deafness, a static tremor of the ipsilateral upper extremity, Horner's syndrome, and bulbar myoclonus have also been reported. In occlusion of the *anterior inferior cerebellar artery* the extent of the infarct is extremely variable. The size of this artery and the territory it supplies vary inversely with that of the posterior inferior cerebellar artery. The principal findings

are ipsilateral cerebellar ataxia (middle cerebellar peduncle), Horner's syndrome, ipsilateral deafness, whirling dizziness, nystagmus, tinnitus, nausea, vomiting, and paresis of conjugate lateral gaze. Pain and temperature sensation may be lost on the opposite side of the body. If the occlusion is close to the origin of the artery, the corticospinal fibers may also be involved, producing a hemiplegia. Occlusion of the *artery to the retro-olivary space* will produce the lateral medullary syndrome. Occlusion of a *paramedian branch* will result in infarction of the corticospinal fibers, the adjacent pontine nuclei, and the pontocerebellar fibers on one side of the pons. If the infarct extends deeply to reach the tegmentum, as it occasionally does, paralysis of conjugate lateral gaze and a contralateral sensory deficit will result. Occlusion of smaller branches in patients with hypertension and atherosclerosis results in small infarcts (lacunes), which cause a pure motor hemiparesis and dysarthria, and which in the long run contribute to the lacunar state and the syndrome of pseudobulbar palsy.

One of the hallmarks of a brainstem lesion is *bilateral* motor and sensory signs. Within the brainstem, tracts descending to and ascending from each side of the body either cross each other or run in close proximity, in contrast to the cerebral hemispheres where the motor and sensory tracts subserving the two sides of the body are distantly separated.

Other cardinal brainstem signs are a "crossed" cranial nerve and long tract deficit or peripheral involvement of the cranial nerves 3 to 12. Although it is correct to emphasize that bilateralism of a lesion strongly suggests

brainstem involvement, it must be pointed out with equal force that in many instances of infarction within the basilar territory the lesion is limited to one side, bespeaking occlusion of a basilar branch rather than of the main trunk.

In the diagnosis of disease of the brainstem it is impossible from motor signs alone to distinguish a hemi-

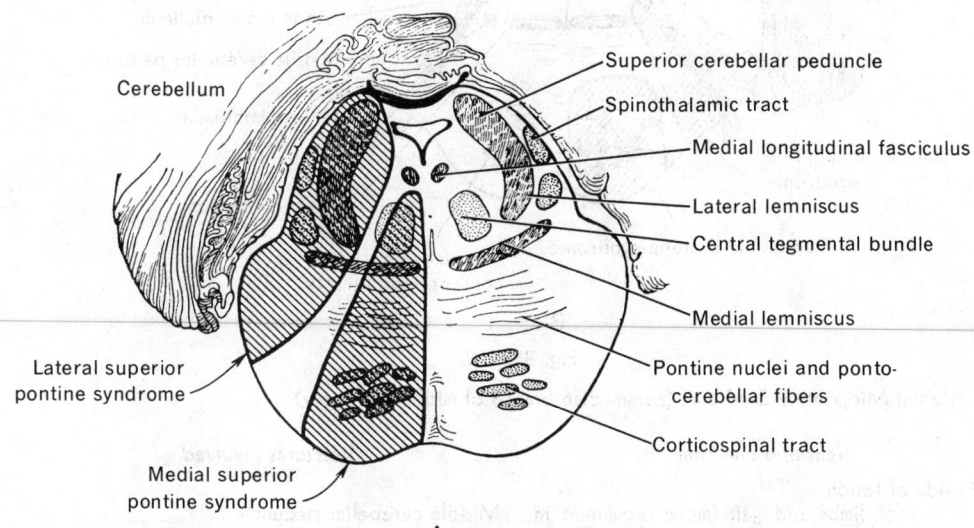

Fig. 357-6A.

1. Medial Superior Pontine Syndrome (paramedian branches of upper basilar artery)

Signs and symptoms	Structures involved
On side of lesion	
Cerebellar ataxia (probably)	Superior and/or middle cerebellar peduncle
Internuclear ophthalmoplegia	Medial longitudinal fasciculus
Myoclonic syndrome, palate, pharynx, vocal cords, respiratory apparatus, face, oculomotor apparatus, etc.	Localization uncertain—central tegmental bundle (?), dentate projection (?), inferior olivary nucleus (?).
On side opposite lesion	
Paralysis of face, arm, and leg	Corticobulbar and corticospinal tract
Rarely touch, vibration, and position are affected	Medial lemniscus

2. Lateral Superior Pontine Syndrome (syndrome of superior cerebellar artery)

Signs and symptoms	Structures involved
On side of lesion	
Ataxia of limbs and gait, falling to side of lesion	Middle and superior cerebellar peduncles, superior surface of cerebellum, dentate nucleus
Dizziness, nausea, vomiting	Vestibular nucleus
Horizontal nystagmus	Vestibular nucleus
Paresis of conjugate gaze (ipsilateral)	Uncertain
Loss of optokinetic nystagmus	Uncertain
Skew deviation	Uncertain
Miosis, ptosis, decreased sweating over face (Horner's syndrome)	Descending sympathetic fibers
Static tremor reported in one case	Dentate nucleus (?), superior cerebellar peduncle (?)
On side opposite lesion	
Impaired pain and thermal sense on face, limbs, and trunk	Spinothalamic tract
Impaired touch, vibration, and position sense, more in leg than arm	Medial lemniscus (lateral portion)
(There is a tendency to incongruity of pain and touch deficits.)	

(The bracket to the right of "Vestibular nucleus / Vestibular nucleus / Uncertain / Uncertain / Uncertain" reads: Territory of descending branch to middle cerebellar peduncle from superior cerebellar artery)

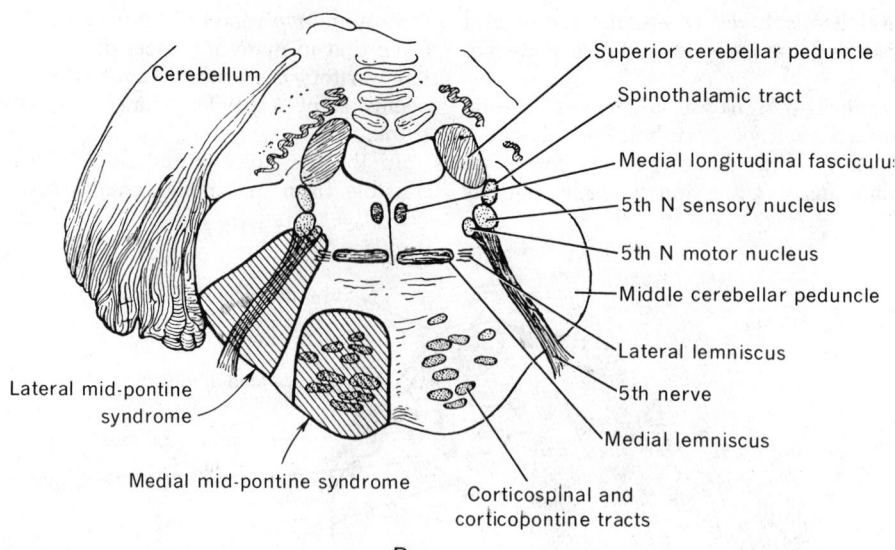

B

Fig. 357-6B.

1. Medial Midpontine Syndrome (paramedian branch of midbasilar artery)

Signs and symptoms	*Structures involved*
On side of lesion	
Ataxia of limbs and gait (more prominent in bilateral involvement)	Middle cerebellar peduncle
On side opposite lesion	
Paralysis of face, arm, and leg	Corticobulbar and corticospinal tract
Deviation of eyes	
Variable impaired touch and proprioception when lesion extends posteriorly. Usually the syndrome is purely motor	Medial lemniscus

2. Lateral Midpontine Syndrome (short circumferential artery)

On side of lesion	
Ataxia of limbs	Middle cerebellar peduncle
Paralysis of muscles of mastication	Motor fibers or nucleus of fifth nerve
Impaired sensation over side of face	Sensory fibers or nucleus of fifth nerve

plegia of pontine origin from one of cerebral origin, and we are dependent on coexisting phenomena. In a lower brainstem hemiplegia the eyes may move more easily to the side of the paralysis just opposite to the supratentorial lesions. In brainstem lesions, as in cerebral, a flaccid paralysis gives way to spasticity in the following days, weeks, or months, and there is no satisfactory explanation for the variability in this period of delay. The pattern of sensory disturbance may be helpful in localization. A dissociated sensory deficit over the face or one-half the body usually indicates a lesion within the brainstem, while a sensory loss over one side of the body involving all modalities with no suggestion of dissociation in any region indicates a lesion at the thalamic level or higher. When position sense, two-point discrimination, and tactile localization are affected relatively more than pain, temperature, and tactile sense, a cortical lesion is suggested; the converse suggests a brainstem location. When both motor and sensory manifestations are bilateral, it is almost unequivocal evidence that the lesion lies infratentorially.

When hemiplegia or hemiparesis and sensory loss are coextensive, the lesion lies supratentorially. Additional manifestations which point unequivocally to a brainstem site are whirling dizziness, diplopia, cerebellar ataxia, Horner's syndrome, and deafness. The several brainstem syndromes illustrate the important point that the cerebellar system, spinothalamic tract, trigeminal nucleus, and sympathetic fibers can be involved at different levels, and neighborhood phenomena must be used in order to identify the exact level.

Lacunar infarction in the pons may cause a pure motor hemiparesis or the dysarthria–clumsy-hand syndrome (dysarthria, facial weakness, slight impairment of the hand). Pontine lacunes are particularly associated with pseudobulbar emotional lability.

A myriad of eponymic brainstem syndromes, e.g., Weber, Claude, Benedict, Foville, Raymond-Cestan, Millard-Gubler, already mentioned in Chap. 355, have been described in relation to brainstem lesions. In their classical descriptions most of these syndromes relate to tumors and other nonvascular diseases, and only occasionally is one of them encountered in association with vascular disease. The diagnosis of vascular disorders in this region of the brain is not greatly facilitated by these

syndromes, and it is preferable to memorize the neuroanatomy of the brainstem.

The great desirability of being able to categorize brainstem vascular cases with accuracy need hardly be

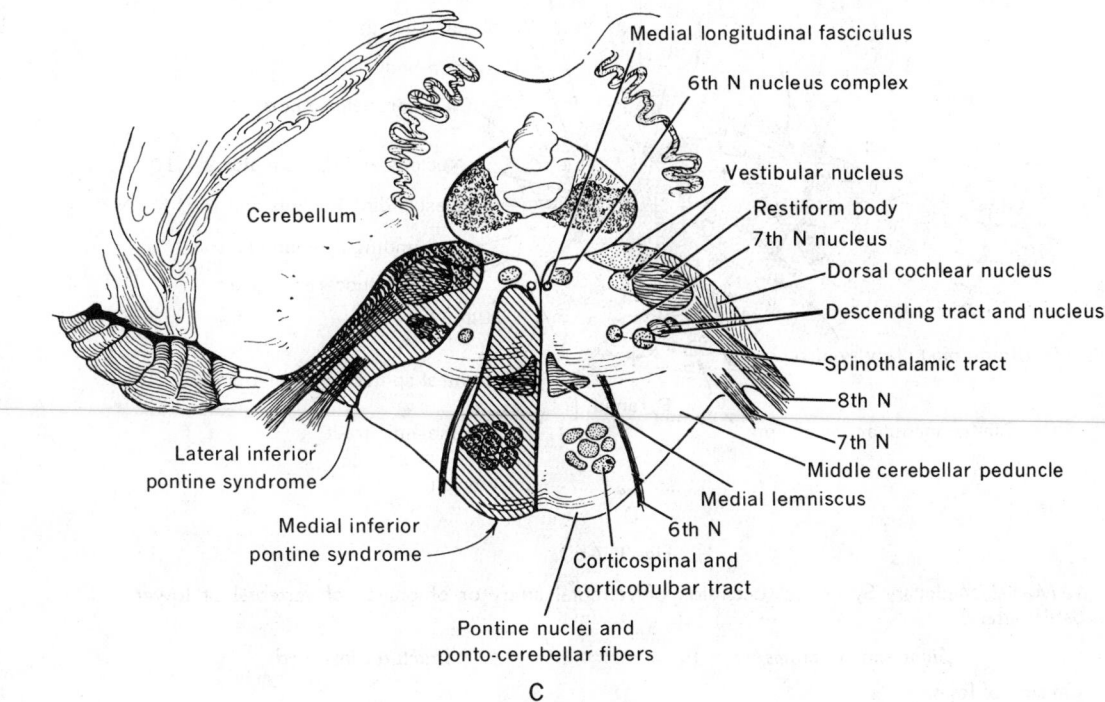

C

Fig. 357-6C.

1. Medial Inferior Pontine Syndrome (occlusion of paramedian branch of basilar artery)

Signs and symptoms	*Structures involved*
On side of lesion	
Paralysis of conjugate gaze to side of lesion (preservation of convergence)	"Center" for conjugate lateral gaze
Nystagmus	Vestibular nucleus
Ataxia of limbs and gait	Middle cerebellar peduncle (?)
Diplopia on lateral gaze	Abducens nerve
On side opposite lesion	
Paralysis of face, arm, and leg	Corticobulbar and corticospinal tract in lower pons
Impaired tactile and proprioceptive sense over half of the body	Medial lemniscus

2. Lateral Inferior Pontine Syndrome (occlusion of anterior inferior cerebellar artery)

On side of lesion	
Horizontal and vertical nystagmus, vertigo, nausea, vomiting, oscillopsia	Vestibular nerve or nucleus
Facial paralysis	Seventh nerve
Paralysis of conjugate gaze to side of lesion	"Center" for conjugate lateral gaze
Deafness, tinnitus	Auditory nerve or cochlear nucleus
Crossed diplopia	Uncertain
Ataxia	Middle cerebellar peduncle and cerebellar hemisphere
Impaired sensation over face	Descending tract and nucleus fifth nerve
On side opposite lesion	
Impaired pain and thermal sense over half the body (may include face)	Spinothalamic tract

3. Total Unilateral Inferior Pontine Syndrome (occlusion of anterior inferior cerebellar artery). Lateral and medial syndromes combined.

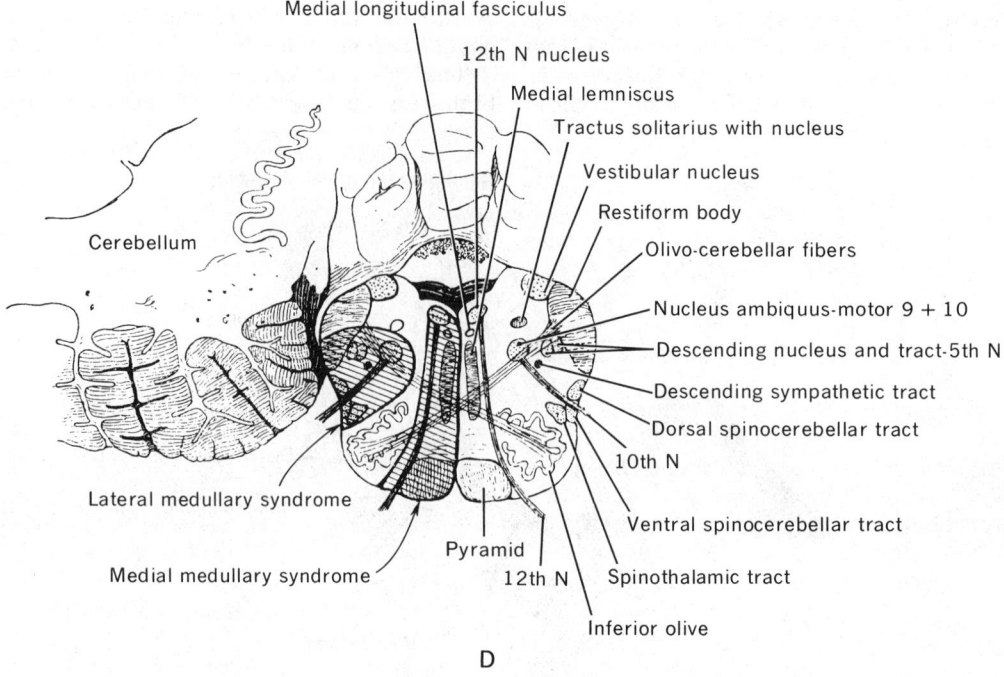

D

Fig. 357-6D.

1. Medial Medullary Syndrome (occlusion of vertebral artery or of branch of vertebral or lower basilar artery)

Signs and symptoms	Structures involved
On side of lesion	
Paralysis with atrophy of half the tongue	Issuing twelfth nerve
On side opposite lesion	
Paralysis of arm and leg sparing face	Pyramidal tract
Impaired tactile and proprioceptive sense over half the body	Medial lemniscus

2. Lateral Medullary Syndrome (occlusion of any of five vessels may be responsible—vertebral, posterior inferior cerebellar, or superior, middle, or inferior lateral medullary arteries)

Signs and symptoms	Structures involved
On side of lesion	
Pain, numbness, impaired sensation over half the face	Descending tract and nucleus fifth nerve
Ataxia of limbs, falling to side of lesion	Uncertain—restiform body, cerebellar hemisphere, olivocerebellar fibers, spinocerebellar tract (?)
Vertigo, nausea, vomiting	Vestibular nucleus
Nystagmus, diplopia, oscillopsia	Vestibular nucleus
Horner's syndrome (miosis, ptosis, decreased sweating)	Descending sympathetic tract
Dysphagia, hoarseness, paralysis of palate, paralysis of vocal cord, diminished gag reflex	Issuing fibers ninth and tenth nerves
Loss of taste	Nucleus and tractus solitarius
Numbness of ipsilateral arm, trunk, or leg	Cuneate and gracile nuclei
Hiccup	Uncertain
On side opposite lesion	
Impaired pain and thermal sense over half the body, sometimes face	Spinothalamic tract

3. Total Unilateral Medullary Syndrome (occlusion of vertebral artery.) Combination of medial and lateral syndromes.

4. Lateral Pontomedullary Syndrome (occlusion of vertebral artery). Combination of lateral medullary and lateral inferior pontine syndromes.

5. Basilar Artery Syndrome (the syndrome of the lone vertebral artery is equivalent). A combination of the various brainstem syndromes plus those arising in the posterior cerebral artery distribution. The clinical picture comprises bilateral long-tract signs (sensory and motor) with cerebellar and peripheral cranial nerve abnormalities.

mentioned. An analysis of the authors' experience with a large number of these cases shows that too often it has been impossible to either designate the vessel involved or fit the clinical picture to an eponym. It seems more practical, therefore, to classify the cases according to the topography of the lesions within the brainstem, and for this purpose the classification shown in Fig. 357-6 was drawn up. There are some twelve syndromes in all, eight being medial and lateral lesions at four different levels of the brainstem—upper pons, midpons, lower pons, and midmedulla. Three are combinations of two or more of these eight syndromes, and the final one represents a full brainstem infarction. The principal syndromes are full basilar, lateral medullary, anterior inferior cerebellar artery, superior cerebellar, medial pontine, pontomedullary, and medial medullary, in that order. Possibly division of the pons into three levels is excessive, and two would have sufficed. The medial superior pontine syndrome is very rare. However, a list has been useful in cataloging day-to-day clinical cases.

LABORATORY. The cerebrospinal fluid pressure is normal in patients with cerebral thrombosis, unless the infarct is large and associated with severe swelling of the damaged tissue. Cerebral thrombosis never causes blood in the spinal fluid, which is "crystal clear" unless the infarct is especially congested, when a very faint xanthochromia (1 to 2 on a scale of 10) may occur. A slight increase in the leukocytes of the spinal fluid (3 to 8 polymorphonuclears) is common in the first few days of the illness. Rarely, and for unexplained reasons, a brisk, transient pleocytosis (400 to 2,000 polymorphonuclears per cu mm) occurs on about the third day. A persistent increase in the number of white blood cells of the cerebrospinal fluid suggests the presence of chronic meningitis (syphilis, tuberculosis, torula), granulomatous arteritis, septic embolism, cerebral thrombophlebitis, or a nonvascular process. The total amount of protein may be normal, but frequently it is raised to 50 to 80 mg per 100 ml. Rarely is it over 100, in which case some other diagnosis should be seriously considered. A Wassermann or some other specific test for syphilis is still routinely made in many clinics but can be dispensed with unless the rest of the clinical and laboratory picture points toward neurosyphilis. A positive test in a bloody fluid is not valid, since syphilitic reagin may have been carried into the fluid by the contaminating blood. Skull x-rays are not remarkable, and the pineal gland will not be shifted unless severe cerebral swelling has occurred, in which case the patient will usually be stuporous or comatose. Reference has already been made to the use of ophthalmodynamometry in the diagnosis of carotid obstruction.

The electroencephalogram is still of limited value in indicating infarction or distinguishing it from hemorrhage and from nonvascular conditions. In cerebral infarction the electrical activity may be found to be of a slightly slower frequency and lower voltage than normal. High-voltage slow waves (3 to 5 per sec) are evidence in favor of hemorrhage or tumor. The pneumoencephalogram may be normal or show local swelling in the acute stages of arterial occlusion, but in the healed stages local ventricular dilatation may occur at the site of tissue loss due to infarction. This procedure is not recommended as a diagnostic laboratory test in patients with occlusive cerebrovascular disease because of the danger of precipitating progression of the neurologic syndrome, due to the hypotensive state which so often attends the introduction of air. Carotid arteriography will demonstrate the blocked artery if it is in the carotid or in the proximal parts of the middle cerebral or anterior cerebral stems. To detect occlusion in the proximal parts of the common carotid or vertebral arteries or the innominate and subclavian trunks, injection into the subclavian or the arch of the aorta is necessary. Arteriography provides essential information about cerebral hemodynamics. It is not without risk, and in patients with vessels narrowed by atherosclerosis the infarction may be extended. It should be used when the diagnosis of vascular disease is uncertain, when vascular surgery may be possible, or when anticoagulant therapy is contemplated in an indefinite case. Radioactive concentration studies (e.g., technesium or arsenic scan) used for the detection of tumor, abscess, etc. often show a mildly positive picture over infarcts. Scintillation counting over the two sides of the skull after the intravenous injection of radioactive material may provide a comparative index of circulation in the two carotid systems.

COURSE AND PROGNOSIS. When the patient is seen early in the course of cerebral thrombosis, it is extremely difficult to give an *immediate prognosis*. Where does the patient stand in the stroke process when first examined? Is worsening to be anticipated or not? No rules have yet been laid down which allow one to predict the course. A mild paralysis today may become a disastrous hemi-

Signs and symptoms	Structures involved
Paralysis or weakness of all extremities, plus all bulbar musculature	Corticobulbar and corticospinal tracts bilaterally
Diplopia, paralysis of conjugate lateral and/or vertical gaze, internuclear ophthalmoplegia, horizontal and/or vertical nystagmus	Ocular motor nerves, apparatus for conjugate gaze, medial longitudinal fasciculus, vestibular apparatus
Blindness, impaired vision, various visual field defects	Visual cortex
Bilateral cerebellar ataxia	Cerebellar peduncles and the cerebellar hemispheres
Coma	Tegmentum of midbrain, thalami
Sensation may be strikingly intact in the presence of almost total paralysis. Sensory loss may be syringomyelic or the reverse or involve all modalities	Medial lemniscus, spinothalamic tracts or thalamic nuclei

plegia tomorrow, or the patient's condition may only worsen temporarily for a day or two. In basilar artery occlusion, dizziness and dysphagia may progress in a few days to total paralysis and deep coma. The course of the deficit is so often progressive that a pessimistic attitude on the part of the physician is justified in what appears to be a mild case.

Progression of the stroke is probably due to increasing stenosis of the involved artery by mural thrombus or to extension of the thrombus along the artery to block side branches and hinder anastomotic flow. In the basilar artery, thrombus may gradually build up along its entire length. In the carotid system, thrombus at times propagates distally from the site of origin in the neck to the intracranial supraclinoid portion, and possibly into the anterior cerebral artery, preventing collateral flow from the opposite side. In middle cerebral occlusion, retrograde thrombosis may occur back to the mouth of the anterior cerebral, perhaps secondarily infarcting the territory of that vessel. Some of the ischemia-modifying factors already referred to probably also play a part in the progression.

Several other circumstances influence the *immediate prognosis* in cerebral thrombosis. In the case of large infarcts, swelling of the infarcted tissue may occur, tentorial herniation follow, and the patient die in 2 to 4 days. Milder degrees of swelling and increased intracranial pressure, though causing an apparent progression for 2 to 3 days, may not prove fatal. In extensive basilar infarction associated with deep coma, the patient seldom lives for more than a few days. If coma or stupor is present in a case from the beginning, survival may be largely determined by the success in keeping the airway clear and maintaining fluid and electrolyte balance (see Chap. 26). Respiratory and urinary infections are constant dangers, and once they begin, there is usually a rapid decline in the patient's condition as his temperature rises.

As for the *eventual, or long-term, prognosis* of the neurologic deficit, there are too many possibilities to recount them in detail. In the introduction it was pointed out that improvement is the rule if the patient survives. Lacunar infarcts with a pure motor hemiparesis fare very well. In the case of small infarcts, recovery may start within hours or a day or two, and restoration may be complete. In cases of severe deficit there may be no significant recovery whatsoever, and after months of assiduous efforts at rehabilitation, the patient may remain bereft of speech, with the upper extremity still totally useless and the lower extremity serving only as an uncertain prop in attempting to walk. Between these two extremes there is every degree of recovery. It is safe to say that the longer the delay before movement begins, the poorer the prognosis becomes. If recovery is not started in 1 or 2 weeks, the outlook is gloomy both for motor activity and speech, and in general it may be said that whatever motor paralysis remains after 5 to 6 months will probably be permanent. Aphasia, dysarthria, and cerebellar ataxia may improve for a year or longer, and sensory improvement has been detected for up to 2 years. A hemianopia which has

not cleared in a few weeks will usually remain permanently, although reading and color discrimination may continue to improve. Lateral medullary infarction might be regarded as an exception to the above rule, for difficulty in swallowing may be protracted (4 to 7 weeks), and yet relatively normal function may be restored finally.

Characteristically, the paralyzed muscles are flaccid in the first days or weeks following a stroke, and the tendon reflexes may be unchanged, slightly increased, or decreased. Gradually spasticity develops, and the tendon reflexes become brisker. The arm tends to assume a flexed adducted posture, whereas the leg is usually extended and adducted. Function is rarely if ever restored after the slow evolution of spasticity. Conversely, the early development of spasticity in the hand, or the appearance of a grasp reflex, and other postural reactions may presage a favorable outcome. Bowel and bladder control usually returns and sphincteric disorders persist only in patients with the most severe hemiplegia or bilateral motor deficit. Not uncommonly the hemiplegic limbs are at first tender and ache on manipulation, interfering with the physical therapy program. Nevertheless, physiotherapy should be initiated early in order to prevent contracture of muscles at shoulder, elbow, wrist, knuckles, knee, and ankle, a frequent complication and often the source of pain and added disability, particularly in relation to the shoulder. An annoying, unsteady, "dizzy" feeling in the head often persists after damage to the vestibular system in brainstem infarcts.

Recurrent cerebral (epileptic) seizures are a complication in some 20 percent of cases of infarction in which the cerebral cortex has been involved. They are infrequent during the evolution of a thrombotic stroke and usually appear within a few weeks or months. The occurrence of a seizure followed by postictal (Todd's) paralysis must not be construed as extension of an infarct.

Many patients complain of fatigability and are depressed. The explanation of these symptoms is uncertain; psychologic factors may be important. Only a few patients become serious *behavior problems* or are psychotic after a stroke, but paranoid trends, ill temper, stubbornness, and peevishness are common.

Finally, in regard to prognosis, it must be mentioned that having had one thrombotic stroke, the patient is in danger in the ensuing months and years of suffering delayed progression of his deficit or having a stroke at another site. The latter is especially true in hypertension.

TREATMENT OF CEREBRAL THROMBOSIS. The treatment of cerebrovascular disease and strokes may be divided into four parts: (1) general medical management in the acute phase, (2) measures to restore the circulation and arrest the pathologic process, (3) physical therapy and rehabilitation, (4) preventive measures against strokes and vascular disease.

General Medical Management in the Acute Phase. In essence, this is the care of the comatose or helpless patient (see Chap. 26).

Measures to Restore the Circulation and Arrest the Pathologic Process. Once a thrombotic stroke has developed fully, no therapy so far devised is of any value in restoring the cerebral tissue or its function. *To be effective, therapy must be preventive.* The diagnosis of thrombosis must be made at the earliest possible stage and the full catastrophe circumvented by every means. It will be appreciated, therefore, that all the measures used in combating a stroke in so far as they are designed to alleviate, check, or prevent the cerebral ischemic process are really preventive in nature. They will be instituted at various stages of the process—when only transient ischemic attacks are occurring or at any point in the progression of a thrombosis-in-evolution or when almost the full neurologic deficit has appeared. Even when persistent signs and symptoms have appeared, it is conceivable that some of the tissues affected, particularly at the edges of the infarct or islands within, have not been irreversibly damaged and will survive if blood flow can be increased.

The following therapeutic methods are being tried at present or have been tried in the recent past:

Medical Measures to Improve the Blood Supply to the Brain. Clinical observation indicates that strokes and ischemic attacks in many cases develop when the patient gets up from his bed, particularly in the morning or postoperatively. On the assumption that decrease in the cerebral circulation resulting from the upright position can aggravate cerebral ischemia, it is recommended that patients with a stroke as the result of ischemic infarction should remain horizontal in bed for 7 to 10 days initially and that, when ambulation starts, special attention should be given to preservation of the systemic circulation (avoid standing quietly for prolonged periods, sit with the feet up, etc.). Elevating the foot of the bed 14 in. or more in the acute stage may be beneficial. It is of great importance that the systemic blood pressure be maintained (correction of blood loss, use of Levophed in myocardial infarction with vascular collapse, avoidance of autonomic blocking agents, etc.). Injections of epinephrine have been recommended as a means of raising the systemic blood pressure above the usual levels. Although this enhances cerebral blood flow and might be beneficial, a systematic trial in thrombotic cases has not been undertaken. Anemia must be corrected. Polycythemia, if severe, may slow the circulation locally and must be treated.

Anticoagulation. According to present reports, anticoagulant therapy prevents transient ischemic attacks and postpones the arrival of an impending stroke whether the carotid or vertebral system is involved. Anticoagulants also halt the advance of a progressive thrombotic stroke, but not in all cases. In assessing anticoagulant therapy one faces the question of where in the course of the stroke the patient stands when he is first examined. Will his course be benign or disastrous? There are no reliable rules for prediction at the present time. Anticoagulants are not of value in the fully developed stroke. Whether when given for a prolonged period of time they prevent the recurrence of a thrombotic stroke is still under study, but the incidence of severe hemorrhagic complications appears to limit their value in these cases.

When *anticoagulant therapy* is instituted in thrombotic cases, heparin is used intravenously in a dose of approximately 50 mg every 4 hr in cases with a progressing stroke or with transient ischemic attacks occurring more than once in 2 days. Heparin therapy is maintained for 1 to 3 weeks, when Coumadin therapy is instituted and continued well-regulated for 1 year or more. Coumadin therapy can be used alone from the beginning when transient ischemic attacks are infrequent. Anticoagulant therapy is not recommended in lacunar strokes unless they are at the stage of frequent transient ischemic attacks.

The use of anticoagulant drugs makes an accurate clinical diagnosis imperative. Intracranial hemorrhage must be ruled out by relying primarily on examination of the cerebrospinal fluid; it is to be remembered, however, that a clear fluid does not necessarily exclude hemorrhage (see p. 1757). A control prothrombin concentration and coagulation time are desirable before therapy is started, but if this is not feasible, the initial doses of anticoagulant drugs can usually be given safely if there is no evidence of active bleeding anywhere in the body. The question whether or not severe hypertension is a contraindication to anticoagulant therapy has not been accurately answered. There is no reliable evidence that complications are more frequent in the presence of hypertension if the prothrombin activity is maintained at 25 percent or higher, and therefore the authors have not withheld anticoagulant therapy in these patients; however, when the diastolic blood pressure is in the range of 130 mm Hg or more, an attempt is made at the same time to lower the pressure gradually with hypotensive agents, exercising care not to prejudice further the circulation in the region of the infarct by too great a reduction in the systemic pressure. It is preferable to avoid reduction of the blood pressure in the 2-week period immediately following a thrombotic stroke.

Anticoagulant therapy is relatively safe provided the prothrombin concentration is determined regularly (once a day, for the first 10 days, thence thrice a week, and finally every week or 10 days) at a laboratory using reliable methods. Therapy can be prolonged for months and years, and only occasionally is it necessary to interrupt treatment because of unexplained disturbances of coagulation. Coumadin overdosage will cause hemorrhage from the kidney, nose, bowel, skin, or into muscle, as well as subdurally and into brain. Although most of these accidents are not serious, vitamin K_1 should be administered immediately.

Surgery. In recent years surgical management of the arterial obstruction in the neck and thorax has been used with increasing frequency, employing thromboendarterectomy or bypass grafts. The region of the carotid sinus is most frequently amenable to such therapy, but operation must be carried out at the stage of carotid stenosis rather than during total occlusion; otherwise secondary clot will have formed in the distal reaches of the artery, whence removal is impossible. Other sites suitable for surgical management include the common carotid, innominate, and subclavian arteries. Operation on the vertebral artery at its origin has not proved beneficial. Before operation the existence of the lesion and its extent must be determined by arteriography. Surgery is undertaken at the stage of transient ischemic attacks or early in the course of thrombosis-in-evolution. When total infarction has occurred, surgery will be ineffective even though patency of the vessel is restored. Surgery is not without risk, and its place in the treatment of cerebrovascular diseases has not been fully determined. In only a small minority of the total number of thrombotic strokes are the lesions so situated that surgery becomes feasible.

Cerebral Vasodilators. Despite experimental evidence that these agents increase the cerebral blood flow, as measured by the nitrous oxide method, they have not proved beneficial in careful studies in human stroke cases at the stage of transient ischemic attacks, thrombosis-in-evolution, or in the established stroke. This is true of nicotinic acid, Priscoline, alcohol, papaverine, and inhalation of 5% carbon dioxide. A few clinical trials have indicated that histamine, aminophylline, acetazolamide, and intraarterial papaverine have some merit. In opposition to the use of these methods is the suggestion that vasodilators are harmful rather than beneficial, since by lowering the systemic blood pressure they reduce the intracranial anastomotic flow.

Thrombolytic Agents. Fibrinolysin and profibrinolysin activator have not proved helpful in cases of transient ischemia, thrombosis-in-evolution, and the established stroke.

Physical Therapy and Rehabilitation. Beginning within a few days, the joints of the paralyzed limbs should be passively carried through a full range of movement fifty times a day. Contracture (and periarthritis) must be avoided, especially at the shoulder, elbow, and ankle. Pain, soreness, and aching in the paralyzed limbs may temporarily interfere with exercises. The patient can be placed in a chair after 1 week or so, depending on the severity of his illness. Nearly all hemiplegics can learn to walk again to some extent, usually within a 3- to 6-month period, and this should be a primary aim in rehabilitation. A short or long leg brace is often required. Speech therapy is of questionable value but should be tried. At least it is of value in improving the morale of the patient. Physical therapy seems not to benefit patients with cerebellar ataxia. As the hemiplegic patient improves, and if mentality is preserved, instruction in the activities of daily living, using various special devices, can assist him in becoming at least partially independent in the home.

General Preventive Measures Against Strokes and Vascular Disease. Avoiding Situations in Which Strokes Are Likely to Occur. (1) Particular care should be taken to maintain the systemic blood pressure, oxygenation, and intracranial blood flow during surgical procedures, especially in elderly patients; (2) hypotensive agents, whether given therapeutically or for diagnostic procedures, should be administered with care; (3) in the elderly patient in whom deep sleep might help to precipitate cerebral ischemia, oversedation should be avoided; (4) systemic hypotension, severe anemia, and polycythemia should be

treated promptly; (5) rapid diuresis may be contraindicated.

Factors Which Determine Ultimate Outcome. The ultimate solution of the problem of cerebrovascular disease lies in more fundamental fields. Atherosclerosis and hypertension must be prevented or alleviated (see Chap. 275 for proxphylaxis of atherosclerosis and Chap. 276 for the treatment of hypertension).

TRANSIENT ISCHEMIC ATTACKS OF CEREBRAL ORIGIN

It has already been pointed out that when transient ischemic attacks precede a stroke, they almost always stamp the process as thrombotic. Furthermore, neuropathologic studies indicate that these attacks are linked almost exclusively to atherosclerotic thrombosis. They belong, therefore, under the heading of cerebral thrombosis, but they are discussed separately here because of their importance clinically and therapeutically. Occasionally the development of cerebral embolism is associated with a few transient ischemic attacks and, rarely, cerebral hemorrhage.

In recent years increasing attention has been directed to these attacks, with the purpose of averting the threatening stroke by administering anticoagulant drugs or performing surgical endarterectomy at the stage of prodromal symptoms. There would seem to be little doubt that they are due to transient focal ischemia, and they might be referred to as temporary strokes which fortunately reverse themselves. Corresponding to the higher incidence of atherosclerosis in hypertension and in the male population, about two-thirds of all patients with transient ischemic attacks are men and/or hypertensive.

CLINICAL PICTURE. Thrombosis of virtually any cerebral or cerebellar artery, deep or superficial, can be associated with transient ischemic attacks, e.g., common carotid, internal carotid, middle cerebral, anterior cerebral, ophthalmic, vertebral, basilar, posterior cerebral, the cerebellar arteries, and the penetrating branches to the deep structures of the basal ganglions and brainstem. If the posterior cerebral arteries are included in the vertebral-basilar system, ischemic episodes are slightly more common in that system than in the carotid. Transient ischemic attacks can occur by themselves, or they may precede, accompany, or follow the development of a stroke. So far, it has not been possible to distinguish the early cases destined to do well from those in which a full-blown stroke will develop.

Transient ischemic attacks last a few seconds up to 12 hr, the most common duration being a few seconds up to 5 to 10 min. It is uncommon for recurrent discrete attacks to last more than 30 min. There may be only a few attacks or several hundred. Between attacks, the neurologic examination may disclose no abnormalities. A stroke may ensue after the second episode or may be postponed until hundreds of attacks have occurred over a period of weeks or months. Not infrequently the attacks gradually cease and no important paralysis occurs, a fact which makes any form of therapy difficult to evaluate.

The neurologic features of the transient episode indicate the territory or artery involved and are fragments borrowed from the stroke which often is approaching. In the carotid system ischemia occurs foremost in the distal middle cerebral territory at the watershed region, producing weakness or numbness of the opposite hand and arm. However, many different combinations may be seen: face and lips, or lips and fingers, fingers alone, hand and foot, etc. Other manifestations include transient monocular blindness or blurring of vision, aphasia, difficulty in calculation and other temporo-parieto-occipital disturbances (when the dominant hemisphere is involved), confusion, veering to one side, headache, and occasionally jerking or twitching mimicking a focal epileptic seizure. Lack of pulsation in the carotid artery in the neck or pharynx, reduced pressure in the appropriate central retinal artery, and a carotid bruit in the neck indicate carotid disease.

The clinical picture in the vertebral-basilar system is exceedingly diverse, since so much motor and sensory traffic is sustained by the blood carried in these vessels. Occurring in the most varied combinations, the following manifestations in their approximate order of frequency may be recognized: dizziness, diplopia (vertical or horizontal); dysarthria; weakness of part or all of one side of the body, or both sides; headaches; staggering gait; veering to one side; numbness of part or all of one side, or both sides, or crossed numbness (one side of face and opposite limbs); a feeling of cross-eyedness; dark vision, blurred vision; tunnel vision; partial or complete blindness; scintillating scotomas; pupillary change; ptosis; paralysis of gaze; speechlessness; and dysphagia. Less common symptoms include noise or pounding in the ear or in the head, head or face pain, peculiar head sensations, vomiting, hiccups, memory lapse, confused behavior, drowsiness, unconsciousness (rare), impaired hearing, deafness, a feeling of movement of a part, hemiballismus, peduncular hallucinosis, forced deviation of the eyes, sweating, and facial redness.

It is not always easy to identify the territory affected. However, the occurrence of monocular blindness with or without contralateral weakness or numbness always points to the carotid system, as does receptive or sensory aphasia. The hallmarks of vertebral-basilar involvement are bilateral weakness and/or numbness, i.e., a disturbance of the long motor or sensory tracts bilaterally.

The attacks may all take approximately the same pattern or they may vary considerably in detail, although maintaining the same basic pattern. For example, weakness or numbness may involve fingers and face in some episodes and fingers only in others; or dizziness alone may occur in some attacks, while in others diplopia is added to the picture. In basilar artery disease each side of the body may be affected alternately. All the involved parts may be affected simultaneously, or a definite march or spread from one region to another can occur in a period of 10 to 60 sec, or even a few minutes; e.g., numbness may spread from the hand to the face, or the reverse. The individual attack may cease abruptly or fade gradually.

MECHANISM. The onset of attacks in some patients is clearly related to standing up after lying or sitting. In general, attacks are likely to occur when the patient is up and around rather than lying down, but in many cases the episodes bear no relation to position or activity. They have been encountered in relation to exercise, exertion, emotional outbursts of anger or joy, and during bouts of coughing. Transient symptoms present on awakening from sleep usually indicate that a stroke is in the offing.

Ophthalmoscopic observations of the retinal vessels made during episodes of transient monocular blindness show either arrest of the blood flow in the retinal arteries and breaking up of the venous column to form "boxcar" pattern or white material temporarily blocking the retinal arteries. This indicates that in ischemic attacks a temporary, complete or relatively complete cessation of blood flow occurs locally, possibly with associated microembolism. Currently, recurrent ischemia is widely held to be the result of platelet emboli from sites of atherothrombosis, but proof is lacking. In the past, transient ischemic attacks have been attributed to cerebral vasospasm or to transient episodes of systemic arterial hypotension with resulting compromise of the intracranial circulation. Neither of these factors has been established. Although dropping the blood pressure to 90 or even 80 mm Hg by tilting the patient upright on a tilt table may cause electroencephalographic changes, it has not in the authors' experience reproduced the attacks. Vasodilator drugs have been without effect. There is good evidence that the attacks are abolished by anticoagulant drugs, but the mechanism of this is not known. Whatever their exact cause, they are closely related to vascular stenosis due to atherosclerosis and thrombosis. A proper recognition of the transient ischemic episode is of importance, since the use of anticoagulant drugs may prove of value in warding off an oncoming stroke.

DIFFERENTIAL DIAGNOSIS. The following conditions must be differentiated: cerebral seizures (epileptic seizures), Ménière's syndrome, migraine accompaniments, Stokes-Adams attacks, hypersensitive carotid sinus reflex, transient global amnesia, insulin reactions, attacks of anxiety and depression, akinetic falling spells of the aged, and recurrent cerebral embolism.

Frank motor *convulsions* rarely if ever occur in ischemic attacks. The patient may report a feeling of movement, distortion, drawing, jumping, or jerking, but an isolated frank focal seizure has not been encountered. On the other hand, a cerebral seizure rarely displays as its own manifestation a temporary paralysis of a limb or of one side of the body. Unconsciousness is rare in ischemic attacks, and its occurrence even in only a few attacks indicates another diagnosis (seizure, Stokes-Adams attack, etc.). Incontinence of bowel and bladder, tongue biting, cyanosis, and residual sleepiness or muscle soreness are indicative of a seizure rather than an ischemic episode. In the sensory sphere, the distinction between ischemic episodes and seizures is less clear, for numbness or scintillating visual phenomena are seen in both conditions, and therefore in making a differentiation one must rely on the presence of associated phenomena (dizziness, diplopia, etc.). When numbness appears simultaneously in face, hand, and leg, i.e., when there is no "march," ischemia rather than a seizure is probably responsible. When a sensory march occurs, the pace of it may serve to distinguish the two in exceptional cases, for the numbness spreads from one part to another in a few seconds in a seizure and often over a period of many minutes in a few of the ischemic episodes.

Dizziness associated with brainstem ischemia is less likely to have a clear rotatory component than that seen in Ménière's syndrome or labyrinthitis. In making a diagnosis, however, one depends on the presence of associated symptoms and signs. It is a simple matter to decide that the dizziness is of central origin when there are other evidences of brainstem involvement, by history or by neurologic examination: diplopia, dysarthria, cerebellar ataxia, vertical nystagmus, persistent horizontal nystagmus, numbness, weakness, dysphagia, etc. On the other hand, the isolated presence of the triad—recurrent dizziness, tinnitus, and chronic deafness (i.e., signs of both auditory and vestibular involvement)—is almost certain evidence of Ménière's syndrome. In the early stages the pictures at times resemble each other closely, however, and only an especially thorough search will reveal signs indicating that the disorder is due to ischemia of the brainstem. Tinnitus of a constant hissing or ringing type is a rare complaint in brainstem vascular disease. When dizziness is the sole symptom in an elderly person, it is often impossible to make an accurate diagnosis, and only after observing the patient for a period of time will the nature of the underlying disease be disclosed. Finally, it must be remembered that since both basilar artery disease and Ménière's syndrome are common conditions, the two may coexist.

The visual, sensory, and motor phenomena which precede the headache (or occur in its absence) in some cases of migraine bear a close resemblance to ischemic manifestations, but since migraine originates in early life, its differentiation from ischemic attacks does not ordinarily pose a problem. An important point is that migrainous accompaniments in 75 percent of cases develop gradually over a period of 5 to 10 min, marching across the affected region, whereas transient ischemic phenomena rarely do this. When vascular disease has its onset in the twenties or thirties, the two may be confused until the history is carefully taken. A migrainous accompaniment may return after a headache-free interval of 10 to 20 years. It is not rare for migrainous accompaniments to appear for the first time in the forties or fifties. Still more important, periodic headaches may be inobvious, leading to a denial of migraine. Headache, at times of great intensity, can accompany cerebral thrombosis, and in an elderly person the occurrence for the first time of periodic headache associated with numbness or weakness should suggest atherothrombosis rather than migraine. *Stokes-Adams attacks* and *hypersensitivity* of the *carotid sinus*

reflex cause "collapsing spells" with unconsciousness, confusion, pallor, sweating and jerking, but almost never do they produce focal neurologic manifestations such as numbness, weakness, diplopia, etc. Difficulty in differentiation of these conditions will arise only when the clinical details of the episode are not available, and usually a careful minute-by-minute description of the attack will enable the physician to make the correct diagnosis. Only in an occasional case of basilar artery insufficiency will an ischemic episode result in unconsciousness, usually accompanied by other symptoms such as weakness, numbness, blindness, or dysarthria. In akinetic falling spells of the aged, the patient falls unconscious without convulsive movements, color change, or alteration in pulse, blood pressure, or respiration. Within a few seconds or a minute or two consciousness is restored.

Occasionally ischemic attacks may be confused with tussive syncope, multiple sclerosis, ulnar neuropathy, carpal tunnel syndrome, overhydration (hyponatremia), cataplexy with narcolepsy, brachial discomfort with hiatus hernia, cervical disk disease, severe postural hypotension, unusual symptoms in angina pectoris, recurrent pulmonary embolism, etc.

Cerebral embolism is frequently suggested as an explanation for recurrent cerebrovascular episodes. However, this seems unlikely if all the attacks are of approximately identical pattern, for successive emboli coming from a distance could not be expected to enter the same arterial branch. Moreover, one would expect the involved cerebral tissue to be at least partially damaged, leaving some residual signs. When only a single transient episode has occurred, the factor of recurrence does not assist in the diagnosis, and cerebral embolism must then be strongly considered. Single transitory episodes and multiple episodes of different pattern must be clearly distinguished from recurrent attacks *of the same pattern*.

TREATMENT. The therapy of transient ischemic attacks has already been discussed under cerebral thrombosis (p. 1747), where it was pointed out that anticoagulants or surgical endarterectomy usually stop the attacks and prevent indefinitely the onset of a threatening stroke. Surgery must be seriously considered in carotid and subclavian cases. In many patients the attacks cease spontaneously, and anticoagulant therapy can be withheld if the episodes are few and spaced at long intervals. In nonsurgical cases, however, anticoagulants are indicated if the attacks are becoming more frequent, more severe, or of longer duration, or if each attack no longer clears away completely, and a persistent neurologic deficit is accumulating.

Other measures that have been recommended include administration of phenobarbital, papaverine, or nicotinic acid, inhalation of 5% carbon dioxide, breathing into a paper bag, and stellate block or cervical sympathectomy, but none of these has proved effective under careful clinical testing. On several occasions the authors have been impressed with the salutary effect of having the patient stop smoking cigarettes. For the more general therapeutic measures applicable in these cases, see pp. 1746–1748.

OTHER CAUSES OF CEREBRAL THROMBOSIS (Infarction)

It will be seen from the list at the beginning of this chapter that there are a few causes of cerebral thrombosis other than atherosclerosis. There are fewer still that are important in the stroke picture. In some of those included, the mechanism is ischemia without actual thrombosis.

Venous thrombosis is a rather uncommon condition and rarely mimics a cerebrovascular stroke. Arising in relation to extracranial and intracranial sepsis, surgical operations, parturition, and chronic wasting illnesses, particularly in children, it can cause a relatively mild neurologic illness with raised intracranial pressure, headache, visual obscurations, and focal seizures, or on the other hand, it can lead to extensive cerebral infarction and hemorrhage, with grave neurologic manifestations and death.

Systemic hypotension usually results in unconsciousness (syncope) without focal motor and sensory signs. But if the state of vascular collapse persists for a sufficient length of time, ischemia distal to the point of stenosis, may result. Infarction will occur in the watershed or borderzone regions of the cerebrum and cerebellum. It has already been mentioned that transient ischemic attacks and persistent strokes often develop under circumstances which suggest that a fall of the systemic blood pressure was the precipitating factor. Hypotension occurs in "simple faint," acute blood loss, myocardial infarction, Stokes-Adams syndrome, traumatic and surgical shock, cardiac arrest or anesthetic accident during surgery, hypersensitivity of the carotid sinus reflex, and in the several types of postural hypotension [idiopathic, postsympathectomy, tabetic, diabetic, with autonomic blocking agents, with reserpine (Serpasil), and on getting up and around after surgical operations].

Arteriography occasionally causes cerebral infarction. In some cases this is the result of cerebral thrombosis, but the pathogenesis of other cases requires further study. *Arteritis* is no longer a common cause of cerebral thrombosis, at least in North America, owing to the present satisfactory treatment of syphilis. Necrotizing or granulomatous arteritis, whether limited to the cerebral vessels or occurring as part of a polyarteritis, usually produces a series of small ischemic deficits in brain, optic nerve, or spinal cord, and only rarely mimics a stroke. Idiopathic giant-cell arteritis involving the large arteries arising from the aortic arch is a rare cause of unilateral or bilateral carotid occlusion but must be kept in mind. It appears to be much more common in young women in Japan, the aforementioned Takayasu's syndrome or "pulseless disease." Cranial arteritis or temporal arteritis is usually limited to the extracranial arteries except for the small vessels supplying the optic and oculomotor nerves. Unfortunately, in over 50 percent of cases permanent blindness or a severe impairment of vision results. The process usually involves the internal or common carotid arteries, but rarely causes a stroke (Chap. 394). Occasionally vertebral-basilar ischemia is reported.

Polycythemia is stated to be a cause of cerebral thrombosis, but further study of the matter is required. *Thrombotic thrombocytopenic purpura* usually leads to multiple small infarcts and fluctuating changing neurologic symptoms, but it is capable of causing infarcts several centimeters in diameter. Sickle-cell disease is associated with obstruction of small arteries, including the cerebral. A *dissecting aortic aneurysm* may involve the large vessels arising from the arch and result in carotid occlusion and hemiplegia, a concomitant fall in systemic blood pressure probably contributing to the picture. *Carotid occlusion* may be the result of direct *trauma* to the neck, or it may be precipitated by a "closed head injury," sometimes of a seemingly trivial nature. *Hypoxia* usually produces a diffuse destruction of neurones rather than frank infarction, but bilateral softening of the globus pallidus is a classical feature. *Tentorial and subfalcial herniation* and sometimes a cerebellar pressure cone can cause infarction by compression of the posterior cerebral, anterior cerebral, and inferior cerebellar arteries, respectively. Under the rare types of infarction, it should be mentioned that carotid occlusion has been described following tonsillectomy, in association with *cavernous sinus thrombophlebitis*, and the trigeminal ganglionitis of herpes zoster. Also, a previously transient and harmless migrainous aura can be transformed into a persistent deficit, presumably because of infarction as the result of excessive ischemia. This complication most frequently takes the form of a homonymous hemianopia. Contraceptive therapy with progestin-estrogen combinations can cause cerebral infarction with or without vascular occlusion. Finally, a category for *cerebral infarction of undetermined cause* is included, for it must be admitted that in some cases even at neuropathologic examination it is impossible to determine the exact cause of an infarct.

Omitted here is *Binswanger's chronic progressive subcortical encephalitis*, a rare disease of cerebral white matter tentatively attributed by Binswanger to atherosclerosis. The status of the disease is uncertain at present, and further investigation of the problem is warranted before the disease can be accepted as a separate entity.

CEREBRAL EMBOLISM

In most cases of cerebral embolism, the embolic material consists of a fragment which has broken away from a thrombus within the heart. Embolism due to fat, tumor cells, or air is a rare occurrence and seldom enters into the differential diagnosis of strokes. The embolus usually becomes arrested at a bifurcation or other site of narrowing of the lumen. Ischemic infarction usually follows and is pale, red, or mixed; red infarction, as pointed out earlier, nearly always indicates embolism. Any region of the brain may be affected, but the territory of the middle cerebral artery is most frequently involved. The two hemispheres are approximately equally affected. Large embolic masses will block larger vessels (sometimes the carotids in the neck), while tiny fragments may reach vessels as small as 0.2 mm, in which case the resultant infarct might be so small as almost to escape detection at autopsy. The exact behavior of embolic material is not fully understood. Often, it remains arrested and plugs the lumen solidly, but in many cases it breaks up into fragments which enter smaller vessels and disappear completely, so that careful pathologic examination fails to reveal their final location. The anatomic diagnosis must then be made by inference, e.g., the absence of a vascular occlusion at the proper site to explain the infarct, the absence of atherosclerosis or other cause for

Table 357-3. CAUSES OF CEREBRAL EMBOLISM

  I. Cardiac origin
      A. Atrial fibrillation and other arrhythmias (with rheumatic, atherosclerotic, hypertensive, or congenital heart disease
      B. Myocardial infarction with mural thrombus
      C. Acute and subacute bacterial endocarditis
      D. Heart disease without arrhythmia or mural thrombus (mitral stenosis, etc.)
      E. Complications of cardiac surgery
      F. Valve prostheses
      G. Nonbacterial thrombotic (marantic) endocardial vegetations
      H. Paradoxical embolism with congenital heart disease
      I. Trichinosis
 II. Noncardiac origin
      A. Atherosclerosis of aorta and carotid arteries (mural thrombus, atheromatous material)
      B. From sites of cerebral artery thrombosis (basilar, vertebral, middle cerebral)
      C. Thrombus in pulmonary veins
      D. Fat
      E. Tumor
      F. Air
      G. Complications of neck and thoracic surgery
III. Undetermined origin

thrombosis in the cerebral vessel, a ready source of embolus, infarcts in other organs such as kidney and spleen, the occurrence of hemorrhagic infarction, and last, but not least, the clinical history.

Because of the rapidity with which occlusion develops in embolism, there is not much time for collateral influx to become established. Thus sparing of territory distal to the site of occlusion is not so common as in thrombosis. However, all the ischemia-modifying factors mentioned under thrombosis are still operative and will influence the size, shape, and severity of the infarct.

Brain embolism is essentially a manifestation of heart disease. Many kinds of heart disease can be associated with embolism. The commonest direct cause is *chronic atrial fibrillation* due to atherosclerotic or rheumatic heart disease, the source of the embolus being mural thrombus deposited within the atrial appendage. Atrial fibrillation due to other types of heart disease can, of course, also lead to embolism, e.g., hypertensive, congenital, thyrotoxic, or syphilitic. Embolism probably occurs also during paroxysmal atrial fibrillation or flutter, but there is need for further exact documentation of such cases. *Mural thrombus* deposited on the damaged endocardium overlying a myocardial infarct is the second most frequent

source of cerebral emboli. Emboli can also arise from atrial thrombus associated with severe mitral stenosis without atrial fibrillation. *Cardiac surgery*, especially valvoplasty, may disseminate fragments of thrombus or particles of a calcified valve leaflet. Mitral and aortic valve prostheses are associated with embolism in 70 percent of cases. Subendocardial fibroelastosis, idiopathic myocardial hypertrophy, cardiac tumors, and cardiac lesions in trichinosis are rare causes of embolism.

The *vegetations of acute and subacute bacterial endocarditis,* being infected, give rise to septic embolism, which results in several different pathologic pictures in the brain. In some cases the infarcts (they are usually multiple) do not differ from those due to bland emboli; in others, tiny septic infarcts develop, or as in acute bacterial endocarditis, there may be miliary abscesses into which a small amount of hemorrhage may occur (focal embolic encephalitis) and even meningitis. Mycotic aneurysm, now seen infrequently, is another complication of septic embolism and may be a source of intracerebral or subarachnoid hemorrhage.

Marantic or nonbacterial endocarditis occasionally causes cerebral embolism and can produce a most baffling clinical picture, especially when associated, as it often is, with carcinomatosis. Paradoxic embolism can occur when an abnormal communication exists between the right and left sides of the heart, or when both ventricles communicate with the aorta. Thus embolic material arising in the veins of the lower extremity or, indeed, anywhere in the systemic venous tree may, particularly in conditions of pulmonary hypertension, bypass the pulmonary circulation and reach the cerebral vessels.

The following sources of embolic material are less frequent or more difficult to prove: (1) Mural thrombus, deposited upon ulcerated atheroma in the arch of the aorta or in the carotid arteries, may break loose and find its way into brain arteries. Massage of the carotid sinus, a favorite site for atherosclerosis, may dislodge mural thrombus, with the production of a hemiplegia. This is one of the reasons why carotid massage should always be carried out gently. (2) Atheromatous material may be washed out of a large plaque in the aorta or carotid arteries and carried distally into the branches of the cerebral tree. (3) The pulmonary veins are a source of cerebral emboli, as indicated by the occurrence of cerebral abscesses in association with pulmonary suppurative processes and by the high incidence of carcinoma of the brain secondary to pulmonary deposits. (4) Surgery of the neck and thorax can be complicated by cerebral embolism. A rare type is that which follows thyroidectomy, in which thrombosis in the stump of the superior thyroid artery extends proximally until a section of it, protruding into the lumen of the carotid, is carried away into the cerebral arteries.

Cerebral embolism must always have occurred when secondary tumor is deposited in the brain, and cerebral embolism regularly accompanies septicemia. However, it is rare for a mass of tumor cells or bacteria to be large enough to occlude a cerebral artery and produce the picture of a stroke. Nevertheless tumor embolism has been reported secondary to cardiac myomyxomas and occasionally with other tumors. It must be distinguished from the marantic endocarditis and embolism which occasionally complicate carcinomatosis. Embolism in the course of septicemia usually means that a vegetative endocarditis is present with thrombus formation. Cerebral fat embolism is usually related to trauma. As a rule, the emboli are minute and widely dispersed, giving rise to multiple petechial hemorrhages in white matter; accordingly the clinical picture is usually not focal, as in a stroke. Cerebral air embolism is a rare complication of criminal abortion or of cervical and thoracic operations and was formerly encountered as a complication of pneumothorax therapy.

Not infrequently at autopsy the diagnosis of cerebral embolism is made with full justification without finding a source. The same is true of embolism elsewhere in the body. Possibly the routine search for a thrombotic nidus is not sufficiently thorough, and small thrombi in the atrial appendage, the pulmonary veins, or the endocardium between the papillary muscles of the heart may be overlooked. Nevertheless, in some cases studied most carefully, no source of embolic material has been discovered.

CLINICAL PICTURE. Of all strokes, those due to cerebral embolism develop most rapidly. "Like a bolt out of the blue," the full-blown picture evolves within several seconds or a minute, exemplifying most strikingly the temporal profile of a stroke. The neurologic deficit nearly always comes in a single sudden attack, only rarely in stuttering fashion. As a rule, there are no warning episodes whatsoever. This statement is possibly too stringent, for in occasional cases a transient episode may precede the final arrival of the stroke. However, any emphasis on these exceptions is misleading. The embolus strikes at any time of the day or night. Getting up to go to the bathroom is a time of danger. When the stroke occurs during sleep, its exact mode of development will not be known.

The neurologic picture will depend on the artery involved and where the obstruction lies. The syndromes related to each cerebrovascular territory are the same as those outlined under thrombosis (see pp. 1731–1746). A large embolus may plug the internal carotid artery or the stem of the middle cerebral artery, producing a severe hemiplegia. More often the embolus is smaller and passes into one of the branches of the middle cerebral artery, producing a strikingly focal disorder: motor aphasia, a monoplegia (or part thereof), a receptive type of aphasia with little or no motor paralysis, or a sensorimotor paralysis with little or no involvement of the supersensory zone. In fact, most patients diagnosed as having middle cerebral artery thrombosis prove to have emboli in the middle cerebral artery (or an atherosclerotic thrombosis of the carotid artery). It is important to realize that an embolus in its passage along an artery may produce a severe neurologic deficit which is only temporary and which clears up almost as quickly as it came, as the embolus finally passes into a small branch supplying a relatively silent part of the hemisphere. In other words, embolism is one of the causes of a single evanescent stroke, and a common one. Also it can give rise to multiple transient attacks of differing pattern. It has already been pointed out that recurrent transient ischemic attacks of the same pattern are not likely to be embolic, since successive emboli would hardly lodge at identical sites. Embolic material entering the vertebral-basilar system occasionally lodges in the vertebral artery just below its union with the basilar, but more often it traverses the vertebral and also the basilar, which is larger, and is not held up until it reaches the upper bifurcation. If arrested here, it abruptly produces deep coma and total paralysis. More often the embolus enters one, or both, of the posterior cerebral arteries and, by infarcting the visual cortex, causes a unilateral or bilateral homonymous hemianopia. Embolic infarction of the undersurface of the cerebellum is common, whereas embolic material rarely enters the penetrating branches of the pons.

The general neurologic disturbance associated with embolic strokes is not significantly different from that seen in thrombotic cases, and the reader is referred to the description of the changes in consciousness, respiration, etc., on p. 1746. Again the patient may have a most devastating hemiplegia and yet be alert. Headache is not uncommon.

Although the abruptness with which the stroke develops and the lack of prodromal symptoms point strongly to embolism, it is the total clinical picture upon which the diagnosis is based. If hemorrhage is ruled out, there remains only thrombosis to be excluded. The presence of atrial fibrillation, a history of myocardial infarction (recent or in the preceding months), or the occurrence of embolism to other regions of the body all support the diagnosis of embolism. Embolism merits the most careful consideration in young persons in whom atherosclerosis is rather unlikely. Not infrequently the first sign of myocardial infarction is the occurrence of embolism; therefore, it is advisable that *an electrocardiogram be made in all patients with cerebrovascular stroke of uncertain origin.*

Acute and subacute bacterial endocarditis do not usually present as a stroke due to infarction, although this happens occasionally. The signs of endocarditis, anemia, splenomegaly, and often a pleocytosis in the cerebrospinal fluid should point to the correct diagnosis.

The diagnosis of the other causes of cerebral embolism —cardiac surgery, neck surgery, pulmonary vein thrombosis, marantic endocarditis, paradoxic embolism, tumor, fat, and air—need not be enlarged upon here.

LABORATORY FINDINGS. The description under thrombosis (p. 1745) applies for the most part to embolism except insofar as hemorrhagic infarction and septic embolism (focal embolic encephalitis) are concerned. Cerebral embolism in some 30 percent of cases produces a hemorrhagic infarct, which in most instances does not cause the cerebrospinal fluid to be bloody. However, in some excessively hemorrhagic infarcts, the fluid may be grossly bloody and contain as high as 10,000 or more red cells per cu mm. In the milder cases of hemorrhagic infarction, a slight xanthochromia (grade 1 to 3 on the scale of 1 to 10) may appear after a few days. The possibility that an embolic infarct is unusually bloody underlines the danger of administering anticoagulants routinely without a careful examination of the cerebrospinal fluid in cases of cerebral embolism. Also, it is the single exception to the rule that blood in the spinal fluid is unequivocal evidence that the stroke is due primarily to a hemorrhage.

In septic embolism resulting from subacute bacterial endocarditis the white blood cells in the cerebrospinal fluid may be increased, usually numbering up to 200 per cu mm and occasionally reaching several hundred; the proportion of lymphocytes and polymorphonuclears varies with the acuteness of the septic process. There may also be several hundred or more red blood cells, and a faint xanthochromia is often present. The protein values are elevated, and the sugar content is within normal limits. No bacteria are seen or obtained by culture. In acute bacterial endocarditis there may be either the cerebrospinal fluid formula of subacute endocarditis or a frank purulent meningitis.

COURSE AND PROGNOSIS. The remarks made concerning the *immediate prognosis* in cerebral thrombosis apply as well here. As a rule, all but the most aggravated cases survive the initial insult. Massive brainstem infarction as a result of basilar embolism is almost always fatal. The *eventual prognosis* as to survival is determined by the occurrence of further emboli and the gravity of the underlying illness—cardiac failure, rheumatic heart disease, myocardial infarction, bacterial endocarditis, malignant growth, etc. The threat of an early recurrence of embolism is very real, and it is not uncommon to have the second embolus strike within a few days or weeks of the first. The urgency of anticoagulant therapy is thereby emphasized. The *eventual prognosis* regarding the neurologic deficit is not different from that given for cerebral thrombosis (p. 1745). The fact that an embolic episode may last only minutes or hours before clearing up should be stressed, especially in estimating the effect of any therapeutic measure.

TREATMENT. The first three phases of therapy—(1) general medical management in the acute phase, (2) measures directed to restoring the circulation, and (3) rehabilitation—are much the same as described under cerebral thrombosis (see p. 1746). Attempted embolectomy at the bifurcation of the common carotid artery has usually failed but should be considered. If pulsation in the temporal artery in front of the ear is present, it means the embolus is not at that bifurcation but has passed up into the internal carotid system, and embolectomy will probably be unsuccessful. The same is true of embolectomy of the middle cerebral artery. Fibrinolysin therapy has not been effective. In the field of prophylaxis there is strong evidence that the use of long-term anticoagulant therapy is effective in the prevention of embolism in cases of atrial fibrillation, myocardial infarction, and valve prosthesis. After cerebral embolism has occurred, the question arises as to the necessity of delaying anticoagulant therapy for several days to avoid precipitating bleeding into a hemorrhagic infarct. It is the authors' practice always to perform a lumbar puncture first in order to rule out gross hemorrhage from the infarct. If the cerebrospinal fluid is clear, the authors proceed with anticoagulant therapy, since there is the constant danger of another embolus breaking away from the heart. We have not encountered a case in which the use of anticoagulant drugs has seemed to increase the degree of hemorrhage within a hemorrhagic infarct, and indications are that such therapy is relatively safe. Rare exceptions to this statement may be expected. The use of anticoagulant therapy in patients with acute myocardial infarction, including those judged to be in the "good risk" category, is advisable. In cerebral embolism associated with subacute bacterial endocarditis, anticoagulant therapy is usually held to be contraindicated because of the danger of intracranial bleeding, but this viewpoint is not well founded. Nevertheless caution is advisable in this matter, and it is preferable to rely on a rapid sterilization of the bloodstream.

Valvoplasty and amputation of the atrial appendage have substantially reduced the incidence of embolism in rheumatic heart disease. The need for special care in preventing emboli from entering the carotid arteries during the performance of cardiac valvoplasty is appreciated by all thoracic surgeons.

INTRACRANIAL HEMORRHAGE

Although more than a dozen causes of intracranial hemorrhage have been listed, the first two, hypertensive intracerebral hemorrhage and ruptured saccular aneurysm, are much more important than the others and account for most of the hemorrhages which give rise to the clinical picture of a stroke. Duret hemorrhages, hypertensive encephalopathy, and idiopathic brain purpura will not simulate a stroke and are included only for the sake of completeness.

Hypertensive Intracerebral Hemorrhage

Hypertensive intracerebral hemorrhage is the ordinary, well-recognized brain hemorrhage. Although sometimes the levels of blood pressure are only in the range of 160 to 170/90, in most cases they are much higher. Hypertensive hemorrhage occurs within brain tissue, and rupture of the arteries lying in the subarachnoid space is practically unknown, apart from aneurysm. It is a mistake to think of hypertensive hemorrhage as arising from the large arteries at the base of the brain. The extravasation which results from rupture of an artery forms a roughly circular or oval mass, which disrupts the tissue as the bleeding continues and it grows in volume. Adjacent brain tissue is displaced and compressed. If the hemorrhage is large, midline structures are displaced to the opposite side and vital centers are compromised, leading to coma and death. Rupture or seepage into the ventricular system usually occurs, and the spinal fluid becomes bloody in more than 90 percent of cases. A hemorrhage of this type almost never ruptures directly into the subarachnoid space through the cerebral cortex, and the blood reaches the subarachnoid spinal fluid via the ventricular system. When the hemorrhage is small and placed at a distance from the ventricles, the cerebrospinal fluid may remain clear even on repeated examinations.

Extravasated blood undergoes a series of changes beginning with phagocytosis at the outer rim producing a brown-orange zone of hemosiderin-filled macrophages. The mass gradually decreases in size, and after a period of some 2 to 6 months, only an orange-stained cleft is left at the site of the hemorrhage.

Hemorrhages might be classified as massive, small, slit, and petechial. "Massive" refers to huge hemorrhages several centimeters in diameter; "small" to those 1 to 2 cm in diameter; "slit" applies to a special type of hypertensive hemorrhage which lies subcortically at the junction of white and gray matter and which in the healing stage becomes narrowed to a long, thin, orange cavity.

In order of frequency, the most common sites for hypertensive hemorrhage are (1) the putamen and adjacent internal capsule (50 percent of cases), (2) thalamus, (3) cerebellar hemisphere, (4) pons, and (5) various parts of the central white matter (frontal lobe, corona radiata, etc., probably extensions from the putamen). The vessel involved is usually a penetrating artery. The nature of the vascular lesion which leads to arterial rupture is not known, and indeed, the site of the rupture has not been reliably identified. Atherosclerosis is held by many to be a factor, but there is no proof for this view, and hemorrhages are encountered in the absence of

Table 357-4. CAUSES OF INTRACRANIAL HEMORRHAGE
(Including Intracerebral, Subarachnoid, Ventricular, and Rarely Subdural)

1. *Hypertensive and intracerebral hemorrhage*
2. *Ruptured saccular aneurysm*
3. *Ruptured angioma*
4. Trauma including posttraumatic delayed apoplexy
5. Hemorrhagic disorders: leukemia, aplastic anemia, thrombopenic purpura, liver disease, complication of anticoagulant therapy, hyperfibrinolysis, hypofibrinogenemia, hemophilia, Christmas disease
6. Undetermined cause (normal blood pressure and no angioma)
7. Hemorrhage into primary and secondary brain tumors
8. Septic embolism, mycotic aneurysm
9. With hemorrhagic infarction, arterial or venous
10. Hypertensive encephalopathy
11. Idiopathic brain purpura
12. Secondary brainstem hemorrhage
13. With inflammatory disease of the arteries and veins
14. Miscellaneous rare types: after vasopressor drugs, upon exertion, during arteriography, during painful urologic examination, as a late complication of early-life carotid occlusion, complication of carotid-cavernous arteriovenous fistula, with anoxemia, migraine, teratomatous malformations. (Acute inclusion body encephalitis produces xanthochromia and up to 2,000 red blood cells or more in the cerebrospinal fluid; acute necrotizing hemorrhagic encephalopathy may be associated with up to 100 red blood cells in the cerebrospinal fluid; tularemia and snake venom poisoning may cause bloody cerebrospinal fluid.)

grossly visible atherosclerosis. Small aneurysmal dilatations were reported by Charcot and Bouchard to be the basis for the rupture. Hyalinosis and necrotizing change in the small arteries due to hypertension have also been described as the precursor of hemorrhage; this cannot at the moment be affirmed or denied. Another hypothesis attributes the hemorrhage to a confluence of myriads of smaller diapedetic hemorrhages rather than a single extravasation, but this is entirely without grounds and represents a confusion of hemorrhagic infarction and massive hemorrhage.

CLINICAL PICTURE. The clinical picture conforms accurately to the temporal profile of a cerebrovascular stroke; namely, it has an abrupt onset and rather rapid evolution. The stroke usually evolves gradually and steadily over an appreciable length of time, taking minutes, hours, or occasionally days (average of 1 to 24 hr) to reach its peak, depending on the speed of bleeding. Usually there are no recognizable warning or prodromal symptoms. Often the patient has been well, and headache, dizziness, and epistaxis have not occurred with any consistency as prodromal symptoms. There is no sex or age predilection except that the younger are usually spared. However, average age of occurrence is less than in thrombotic infarction. In the great majority of cases, the hemorrhage comes on while the patient is up and active, and onset during sleep is a rarity. Hypertension is maintained early in the course of the stroke or may even rise higher, so that the existence of hypertension will be easily established when the patient is first examined. Hypertension is usually of the "essential" type, but other causes must always be considered—renal disease, toxemia of pregnancy, pheochromocytoma, ACTH overdosage, injection of excessive amounts of epinephrine, and rarely, violent exertion or an intense emotional experience. Cardiomegaly is usually present.

There is usually only one episode of hemorrhage, and recurrence of bleeding from the same site, as occurs in cases of saccular aneurysm, is not encountered. Once bleeding has become arrested, rebleeding in the near future, i.e., after the first few days, is not to be anticipated. When blood is spilled into the tissues, it is removed only slowly, over a period of weeks and months, during which time symptoms and signs persist. Hence the neurologic deficit is never transitory in intracerebral hemorrhage, as it so often is in thrombosis and embolism, and, for the same reason, rapid fluctuations in the neurologic deficit from one examination to another are not to be expected.

The neurologic signs and symptoms vary with the site and size of the extravasation. The most common picture is that associated with a *putaminal hemorrhage*, in which the adjacent internal capsule is implicated. The patient complains of something going awry within the head. In a few minutes the face sags on one side, speech becomes slurred or aphasic, the arm and leg gradually weaken, and the eyes tend to deviate away from the side of the paretic limbs. A carefully taken history often reveals that these events occurred gradually over a period of 5 to 30 min. This type of evolution is virtually diagnostic of intracerebral bleeding. Gradually the paralysis worsens, the affected limbs become flaccid, pinprick is not appreciated, a Babinski sign appears, speaking becomes impossible, and confusion gives way to stupor. In the worst cases, signs of upper brainstem compression appear—coma, Babinski sign bilaterally, deep, irregular, or intermittent respiration, dilated fixed pupils, and occasionally decerebrate rigidity.

Thalamic hemorrhage of moderate size also produces a hemiplegia or hemiparesis via pressure on the adjacent internal capsule. The sensory deficit equals or outstrips the motor weakness. Dysphasia may be present with lesions of the dominant side and apractognosia on the nondominant. A homonymous field defect if present usually clears in a few days. Thalamic hemorrhage by virtue of its extension medially and into the subthalamus causes a series of ocular disturbances, including paralysis of vertical gaze, forced deviation of the eyes downward, inequality of pupils, with absence of light reaction, skew deviation with the eye opposite the hemorrhage being displaced downward and medially, ipsilateral ptosis and miosis, absence of convergence, an assortment of lateral gaze abnormalities (paresis or pseudoparesis of the sixth nerve), retraction nystagmus, and tucking of the eyelids. Another unusual sign is so-called "peduncular hallucinosis." Neck retraction may be prominent. Hemorrhage into the nondominant thalamus is liable to produce mutism.

In *pontine hemorrhage*, deep coma ensues in a few minutes, and the clinical picture includes total paralysis, prominent decerebrate rigidity, and small (1 mm) pupils that react to light. Lateral eye movements, evoked by head turning or irritation of the ears with ice water, are impaired. The cerebrospinal fluid will be sanguineous. Death usually occurs within a few hours, but there are rare exceptions where consciousness is retained and the clinical manifestations indicate a lesion in the tegmentum of the pons, e.g., disturbances of lateral ocular movements, crossed sensory or motor disturbances, small pupils, cranial nerve palsies, and bilateral signs of pyramidal tract involvement.

Cerebellar hemorrhage usually develops over a period of several hours, and loss of consciousness at the onset is almost unknown. Repeated vomiting is a hallmark of cerebellar hemorrhage, along with inability to walk or stand, occipital headache, and vertigo. There is a paresis of conjugate lateral gaze of the eyes, forced deviation of the eyes to the opposite side, or an ipsilateral sixth nerve weakness. In the most acute phase of the illness there may be little or no evidence of cerebellar disease, and only a minority of cases show nystagmus or cerebellar ataxia of the limbs, although these signs must always be sought. Other ocular signs include "ocular bobbing," blepharospasm, involuntary closure of one eye, skew deviation, and maintenance of vertical eye movements including small pupils which continue to react until very late in the illness and exhibit slight inequality. A mild ipsilateral facial weakness and a diminished corneal reflex are common. Dysarthria and dysphagia may be prominent. Contralateral hemiplegia and facial weakness do not occur. Occasionally at the onset there is a quadriplegia with preservation of consciousness or a spastic paraparesis. The plantar reflexes are flexor early, extensor late. As the hours pass, the patient becomes stuporous, then comatose as a result of brainstem compression.

It will be noted that in the localization of intracerebral hemorrhages, ocular signs are important. In putaminal hemorrhage the eyes are deviated to the side opposite the paralysis; in thalamic hemorrhage the eyes are deviated downward and the pupils may be unreactive; in pontine hemorrhage the eyeballs are fixed and the pupils tiny and reactive; and in cerebellar hemorrhage the eyes are deviated laterally in the absence of paralysis.

At each of the above sites the hemorrhage is usually massive, and the patient survives only a few hours or a few days, succumbing as a result of secondary brainstem insult. Rarely does a patient survive once deep stupor supervenes, although in some cases he may linger in an unresponsive state for a week or two. In some 30 percent of cases, however, the hemorrhage is less extensive and survival is possible, hemorrhage into the thalamus especially tending to be somewhat smaller than putaminal or cerebellar hemorrhage.

A *severe headache* is often considered to be a constant accompaniment of intracerebral hemorrhage, and in many cases it is prominent and a helpful diagnostic point. Nonetheless in almost 50 percent of our cases headache has been absent or insignificant. *Nuchal rigidity* is frequently found, but again it is so often absent that failure to find it must by no means detract from the diagnosis. If the neck becomes stiff, it will become supple again as coma deepens. *Vomiting* occurs once or twice at the onset of intracerebral hemorrhage, and repeated *vomiting* should suggest a cerebellar location. *Coma* is said to be a sign of cerebral hemorrhage, and it is more frequent in hemorrhage than in infarction, but of equal importance is the fact that the patient often is far from comatose and may even be alert and responding accurately when first seen. This is true with grossly bloody spinal fluid, and thus the adage that hemorrhage into the ventricular system always precipitates coma is quite incorrect. Only if bleeding into the ventricles is massive will coma result. *Cerebral seizures*, usually focal, occur in some 10 percent of cases of supratentorial hemorrhage in the first few days, especially as the result of a subcortical "slit" hemorrhage. The fundi often show hypertensive changes in the arteries, and rarely fresh preretinal (subhyaloid) hemorrhages occur, the latter being much more common in ruptured aneurysm or angioma. Severe hypertension accompanied by papilledema need by no means be present for cerebral hemorrhage to occur.

Many of the less precisely localized neurologic manifestations described under cerebral thrombosis are also encountered in intracerebral hemorrhage, including coma, stupor, drowsiness, confusion, Cheyne-Stokes respiration, grasping and sucking reflexes, incontinence of bowel and bladder, and unilateral and bilateral extensor rigidity.

Although the proper interpretation of this array of clinical data allows the correct diagnosis to be established in most cases, the examination of the cerebrospinal fluid for blood is the single most important step in the detection of intracranial bleeding.

LABORATORY FINDINGS. Any urinary abnormalities will for the most part reflect coexisting renal disease, although transient glucosuria has been reported to result specifically from intracranial hemorrhage. The white blood cell count often rises to 15,000 to 20,000, a higher figure than in thrombosis. The sedimentation rate is elevated. In cases of massive hemorrhage, the cerebrospinal fluid is often under increased pressure, but in almost half of our cases readings under 200 mm were obtained. The fluid is usually grossly bloody, although not so bloody as in ruptured saccular aneurysm (the count ranging from a few thousand cells up to 1 million). In smaller hemorrhages into central structures the cerebrospinal fluid contains a lesser amount of blood, and in occasional cases of intracerebral hemorrhage, particularly in those of the "slit" type, between cortex and white matter, it remains free of blood and clear of xanthochromia in repeated taps. In these latter cases, slight xanthochromia may appear after a few days to a week. At times the spinal fluid may be clear grossly but contain some 200 to 400 red cells, and it is then difficult to decide if this represents intracranial bleeding or a traumatic tap. These details are mentioned because they are of great importance in the essential task of making an accurate diagnosis of the type of stroke prior to the use of therapeutic measures such as anticoagulant drugs, surgical exploration, hypothermia, etc. A *traumatic bloody spinal tap* greatly complicates the diagnostic problem. In a bloody tap the pressure tends to be low, the fluid that first flows from the needle is more bloody than that which comes later (third tube less bloody than the first), the fluid often clots in the test tube, and xanthochromia is either absent or at most present only in proportion to the amount of serum bilirubin admixed with the fluid. Bloody fluid due to cerebral hemorrhage is often under increased pressure, there is an even admixture of blood in all samples, the cerebrospinal fluid will not clot, and if more than 8 to 12 hr has elapsed since the hemorrhage, a definite xanthochromia will be present in the supernatant fluid after centrifugation, which should always be carried out if there is any question of the reliability of the tap. However, the presence of xanthochromia after centrifugation may be due to the bilirubin contained in the blood spilled by a traumatic tap and therefore is not an infallible index of subarachnoid or brain hemorrhage. The white blood cells of the cerebrospinal fluid are accounted for by the amount of hemorrhage, and their ratio to red cells is usually the same as in the circulating blood. After hemolysis of red blood cells, the white cell count may be disproportionately increased. Sometimes after a questionably traumatic tap it is worthwhile to perform immediately another puncture at a higher level.

Lumbar puncture is not completely innocuous, since temporal lobe or cerebellar herniation may be aggravated in cases of massive supratentorial hemorrhage or softening and in cerebellar hemorrhage. Despite this danger, the procedure is necessary if specific therapeutic measures are contemplated or if any doubt exists as to the diagnosis of cerebrovascular disease. X-ray of the skull early in the stroke sometimes shows a shift of the cal-cified pineal gland to the side of the cranium opposite the lesion, a change not seen in infarction. The electroencephalogram does not show a typical or diagnostic pattern, but high-voltage, slow waves are the most common finding with hemorrhage into the cerebral hemisphere. X-ray of the chest will often show cardiomegaly.

COURSE AND PROGNOSIS. The immediate prognosis is grave, some 70 to 75 percent of patients dying in 1 to 30 days. Either the hemorrhage extends into the ventricular system, or temporal lobe herniation and midbrain compression occur. Sometimes the hemorrhage appears to seep gradually into vital centers. Gastric erosion and gastrointestinal hemorrhage of neurogenic origin may occur at any time within the first week or two. When the hemorrhage is smaller, survival is possible, and the restitution of motor function, speech, etc., can be excellent, since, in contrast to infarction, the hemorrhage has to some extent pushed brain tissue aside instead of destroying it. Function may be slow to return, because extravasated blood is slow to be resorbed or removed from the tissues. Since rebleeding from the same site is unlikely, the patient may live for many years. In some instances of medium-sized cerebral and cerebellar hemorrhages, the patient survives and his condition gradually stabilizes, but definite papilledema appears after several days of increased intracranial pressure. This does not mean that the hemorrhage is increasing in size or swelling, only that papilledema is slow to develop. Healed scars impinging on the cortex are liable to be epileptogenic.

TREATMENT. *The general medical management of the comatose, apoplectic patient is the same as that outlined under thrombosis* and in Chap. 26. Measures to stem the hemorrhage and restore the integrity of damaged tissue have been relatively ineffective up to the present. *Surgical removal of the clot* in the acute stage, either by evacuation or aspiration, has seldom proved successful except in patients with a hemorrhage lying near the surface and who are not comatose. The prospect that acute cerebellar hemorrhage may be amenable to surgical therapy is being explored. In the smaller hemorrhages that reach a subacute stage, papilledema may appear, and this in many instances has dictated unnecessary surgical evacuation of the hemorrhage when the patient's condition stabilized. The prognosis in hemorrhage into the cerebral hemisphere is probably little altered by surgery; the outlook for cerebellar cases seems to have improved. Attempts to halt the hemorrhage by lowering the systemic blood pressure through the use of autonomic blocking agents have not been effective, and in many instances the inadvertent occurrence of disastrously low levels of blood pressure has complicated the illness. Artificial hypothermia has been used sporadically, but there are insufficient data to permit appraisal of this procedure. Intermittent compression of the ipsilateral carotid in the neck may be beneficial in acute putaminal cases.

The *only preventive measure* is lowering the blood pressure in cases of essential hypertension by every possible means. If ACTH or one of the adrenal steroids is being given, toxicity must be watched for. When hypotension threatens during surgical procedures, injections of excessive amounts of epinephrine or ephedrine must be avoided. Toxemia of pregnancy must be detected early.

Ruptured Saccular Aneurysm

This is the fourth most frequent of the cerebrovascular disorders after thrombosis, along with atherosclerosis, embolism, and hypertensive intracerebral hemorrhage. Saccular aneurysms take the form of small, thin-walled blisters protruding from the arteries of the circle of Willis or the major branches arising therefrom. These saccules or *berries,* as they have been called, are located for the most part at bifurcations and branchings and are presumed to be the result of developmental defects in the media and elastica. A small number of aneurysms have been attributed to incomplete involution of embryonic vessels. Owing to the local weakness, the intima bulges outward, covered by adventitia; the sac gradually enlarges, until finally dissolution of the wall and rupture occur. Saccular aneurysms vary in size from tiny nubbins 2 mm in diameter up to spherical masses 2 or 3 cm in diameter, averaging 8 to 10 mm. Aneurysms vary greatly in form: some are round and connected to the parent artery by a narrower stalk; others are broad-based without a stalk; and still others are narrow cylinders. The site of rupture is always the dome of the aneurysm, which may present one or more secondary sacculations. In routine autopsies the incidence of ruptured aneurysms is 1.8 percent, of unruptured aneurysms, 2.0 percent.

Saccular aneurysms are rare in childhood, even at routine postmortem examination, and increase in frequency to reach their highest plateau of incidence between thirty-five and sixty-five years. Therefore, they are not congenitally formed anomalies but develop over the years on the basis of a developmental arterial defect. There is an increased incidence of congenital polycystic disease of the kidney and of coarctation of the aorta in association with

saccular aneurysm. Hypertension is more frequently present than in the average population, but aneurysms occur in persons with normal blood pressure. Atherosclerosis, although present in the walls of about 50 percent of aneurysms, probably plays no part in their formation or enlargement.

From 85 to 90 percent of saccular aneurysms lie on the anterior part of the circle of Willis. The four most common sites are (1) in relation to the anterior communicating artery, (2) at the origin of the posterior communicating artery from the stem of the internal carotid, (3) at the first major bifurcation of the middle cerebral artery, and (4) at the bifurcation of the internal carotid into middle and anterior cerebral arteries (see Fig. 357-7). Other sites include the internal carotid in the cavernous sinus, at the origin of the ophthalmic artery, at the junction of the posterior communicating artery with the posterior cerebral, at the bifurcaation of the basilar artery, and at the origins of the three cerebellar arteries. In 8 percent of cases there is more than one aneurysm, and they may be situated unilaterally or bilaterally.

Several types of aneurysm other than saccular occur, e.g., mycotic, fusiform, diffuse, and globular. The last three are named for their predominant morphologic aspects and consist of enlargement or dilatation of the entire circumference of the involved vessels, usually the internal carotid, vertebral, or basilar arteries. Frequently showing atherosclerotic deposition in their walls, they are often referred to as arteriosclerotic, but most likely they are at least partly developmental in nature. They press on neighboring structures or become occluded by thrombosis and rupture only infrequently.

CLINICAL PICTURE. Prior to rupture, saccular aneurysms are usually asymptomatic and rarely cause even headache. Occasionally, large aneurysms immediately distal to the cavernous sinus may compress the optic nerves or chiasm, third nerve, hypothalamus, or pituitary

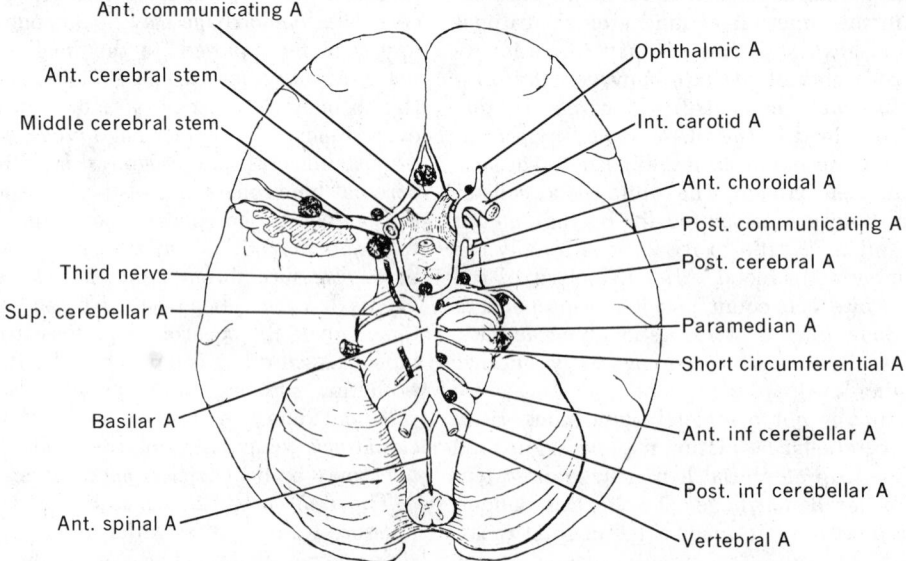

Fig. 357-7. Diagram of the circle of Willis to show the principal sites of saccular aneurysm. Approximately 90 percent of aneurysms are on the anterior half of the circle.

gland. In the posterior fossa, one or more of the cranial nerves may be compressed adjacent to the brainstem.

When rupture occurs, blood under high pressure is discharged into the subarachnoid space (the circle of Willis lies in the subarachnoid space), and the resulting clinical events fall into one of three patterns: (1) the patient may be stricken with an excruciating generalized headache and fall unconscious almost immediately; (2) headache may develop as in (1), but the patient remains relatively lucid; (3) consciousness may be lost quickly without any preceding complaint. Focal convulsive seizures or decerebrate rigidity occur at the onset of hemorrhage in about 10 percent of patients. If the hemorrhage is massive, a fatal issue may ensue in a matter of minutes, hours, or a day or two, deep coma persisting in association with irregular respiration, attacks of extensor rigidity, and finally respiratory arrest and circulatory collapse. In these rapidly fatal cases, the blood has usually dissected intracerebrally and entered the ventricular system. Death occasionally occurs within 5 min, and ruptured aneurysm must be considered in the differential diagnosis of sudden death.

In mild cases, consciousness, if lost, may be regained within a few minutes as the blood diffuses through the subarachnoid space, but a residuum of confusion and amnesia persists for a day or two, accompanied by severe headache and stiff neck. It is not uncommon for drowsiness and confusion to last 10 days or longer. If the hemorrhage is confined to the subarachnoid space, there are few or no lateralizing neurologic signs.

In most patients there are no warning symptoms; in some, however, minor leakage from the aneurysm sometimes precedes devastating rupture by a few days or weeks, headache being the chief sign of such an event. Aneurysmal rupture usually occurs while the patient is active rather than during sleep, and in many instances sexual intercourse or other exertion precipitates the ictus.

Gross lateralizing signs in the form of hemiplegia, hemiparesis, or aphasia are absent in the majority of cases, but can occur and are due to an intracerebral clot or infarction in the territory of the involved artery. The aneurysm may rupture partly into the subarachnoid space and partly into brain tissue (subarachnoid-cerebral hemorrhage) and even reach the ventricular system (subarachnoid-cerebrovascular hemorrhage), rendering the patient stuporous or comatose. The initial neurologic deficit may clear in a matter of days, indicating that hemorrhage into tissues was not responsible for the focal signs. The pathogenesis of such manifestations is not fully understood, but a transitory fall in pressure in the circulation distal to the aneurysm is postulated. Transient deficits, still more evanescent, are not uncommon; paresis or aphasia, for example, may be present only for a few minutes or so after the onset of bleeding, constituting a reliable telltale of ruptured aneurysm. A delayed hemiplegia or other deficit may occur a few days after rupture. This is attributable to focal narrowing of a large artery at the base, usually interpreted as vasospasm resulting from the presence of extravasated blood. Areas of ischemic necrosis of tissue in the territory of the vessel bearing the aneurysm, usually without thrombosis of the vessel, may be found postmortem.

Although in most patients the neurologic manifestations do not point to the exact site of the aneurysm, in many instances there are clues to the localization. For example: (1) Third nerve palsy (ptosis, diplopia, mydriasis, and oculomotor paralysis) usually indicates an aneurysm at the junction of the posterior communicating artery and the internal carotid stem. The third nerve passes immediately lateral to this point. (2) Transient paresis of one or both of the lower limbs at the onset of the hemorrhage is suggestive of an anterior communicating aneurysm which has interfered with the circulation in the anterior cerebral arteries, causing ischemia of the motor areas for the lower extremities. (3) Hemiparesis or aphasia often points to an aneurysm at the bifurcation of the middle cerebral artery which has critically reduced the circulation in the middle cerebral system. (4) Unilateral blindness or amblyopia indicates an aneurysm which lies anteromedially in the circle of Willis (at the origin of the ophthalmic artery, at the bifurcation of the internal carotid artery, or in the anterior communicating region). (5) A state of retained consciousness with akinetic mutism or abulia favors an aneurysm of the anterior communicating artery which has caused ischemia of or hemorrhage into one or both of the frontal lobes, hypothalamus, or corpus callosum. (6) The side on which the aneurysm lies may be indicated by a unilateral preponderance of headache or preretinal hemorrhages, by the occurrence of monocular pain, or by the lateralization of an intracranial sound heard at the time of rupture of the aneurysm. Sixth nerve palsy, unilateral or bilateral, results from the presence of subarachnoid blood and raised intracranial pressure and is seldom of localizing value. Other neurologic signs which have relatively little localizing value include sucking and grasping reflexes, choreoathetosis, and extensor rigidity.

In summary, the clinical sequence of sudden violent headache, collapse, brief unconsciousness and confusion, combined with an absence of prodromal symptoms and a paucity of lateralizing signs is diagnostic of a ruptured saccular aneurysm.

Other clinical data may be of assistance in reaching a correct diagnosis. Nuchal rigidity is usually present. Examination of the fundi not infrequently reveals smooth-surfaced, sharply outlined collections of blood which cover the retinal vessels—the so-called "preretinal" or "subhyaloid" hemorrhages. These are usually a sign of ruptured aneurysm or angioma but can occur in hypertensive hemorrhage and cranial trauma. Bilateral Babinski signs are found in the early days following rupture. The patient may appear to be normally alert, when impairment of memory and confabulation are found on more careful testing. A fever with the temperature rising to 102°F is common in the first week. The escaping blood occasionally enters the subdural space and produces a subdural hematoma, evacuation of which may be lifesaving. Aneurysmal rupture may complicate pregnancy, but pregnancy is not associated with an increased incidence of aneurysmal rupture. Spontaneous intracranial bleeding with normal blood pressure should always suggest ruptured aneurysm, ruptured angioma, or hemorrhage into a cerebral tumor.

LABORATORY FINDINGS. Any urinary abnormality is usually due to concomitant renal disease. Rarely diabetes insipidus occurs. A leukocytosis of 15,000 to 18,000 is common. The cerebrospinal fluid is usually extremely bloody, with red cell counts reaching to 1 million per cu mm or higher. When the hemorrhage is very slight, there may be only a few thousand cells. It is unlikely that an aneurysm can rupture entirely into brain tissue without some leakage of blood into the subarachnoid fluid, and therefore the diagnosis of ruptured saccular aneurysm must never be made unless blood is present in the spinal fluid. Only expanding saccular aneurysms which either compress the optic nerves, chiasm, cranial nerves, or brainstem or lie within the cavernous sinus produce symptoms without hemorrhage. Usually deep xanthochromia is found after centrifugation. The cerebrospinal fluid is under greatly increased pressure, as high as 1,000 mm (see p. 1757 regarding traumatic tap). The white blood cells in the spinal fluid are usually present in the same proportion to red blood cells as in the circulating blood, but in some patients within 48 hr a brisk leukocytosis appears, reaching 2,000 to 3,000 cells per cu mm.

X-rays of the skull are usually negative, though in a few patients one or both of the anterior clinoid processes show erosion by the pressure of an adjacent aneurysm, or calcification has occurred in the region of a previous hemorrhage. A calcified pineal gland may be displaced by an intracerebral or subdural clot.

Carotid and vertebral angiography, using Hypaque, will demonstrate the aneurysm in some 85 percent of patients in whom aneurysm appears to be the correct diagnosis on clinical grounds, i.e., in cases of so-called "spontaneous subarachnoid hemorrhage."

Acute subarachnoid hemorrhage may be associated with electrocardiographic abnormalities suggestive of myocardial ischemia. The electroencephalogram is of little help in localizing the lesion unless a gross neurologic deficit is present, in which case the lateralization is probably already evident clinically. The abnormality usually consists of slow waves.

COURSE AND PROGNOSIS. The outstanding characteristic of this condition is the tendency for the hemorrhage to recur. This threat colors all prognostications, and unfortunately there appears to be no way of determining reliably which cases will rebleed. The cause of the intermittency of bleeding is not understood.

Patients with the typical clinical picture of spontaneous subarachnoid hemorrhage but in whom the angiogram shows no aneurysm or angioma have a better prognosis than those in whom the lesion is demonstrated.

McKissock et al. found that the patient's state of consciousness at the time of arteriography was the best single criterion of prognosis. Using their data as representative of any large medical center, it can be shown that of every 100 patients coming to arteriography, 17 will be stuporous or comatose, and 83 will appear to be recovering

from the ictus. At the end of the next 6 months, of the first 17, 7 will have died from the original hemorrhage and 7 more will have had a fatal recurrence, making a total of 14 deaths and 3 survivors. Of the other 83, one will have died of the original hemorrhage and 52 will have had a recurrence, of which 33 will have died, making a total of 34 deaths and 49 survivors. Thus, of the total of 100, at the end of 6 months, 8 will have died of the original hemorrhage, 59 more will have had a recurrence, with 40 deaths, making a total of 48 deaths and 52 survivors. The gravity of the illness is immediately apparent. In regard to the recurrence of bleeding, it was found that of every 50 patients seen on the first day of the illness, 5 will rebleed in the first week (all fatal), 8 in the second week (5 fatal), 6 in the third and fourth weeks (4 fatal), and 2 in the next 4 weeks (2 fatal), making a total of 21 recurrences in 8 weeks (16 fatal). Rerupture did not occur in the first 2 days; thereafter it occurred at a steady rate for the next 19 days and tapered off abruptly.

Of the survivors in the first group, all but one returned to work, and in the second group, 36 went back to full work, 12 were partly disabled, and 4 were totally disabled. The disability was due to paralysis, mental deterioration, or epilepsy.

TREATMENT. General medical management in the acute stage is similar to that described under cerebral thrombosis (p. 1746). Any specific medical measures are based on the assumption that decreasing the arterial blood pressure is the most reasonable way of arresting the hemorrhage and preventing recurrence. Absolute bed rest for 4 to 8 weeks is prescribed, with the head of the bed raised some 15 to 20°. Straining during bowel movement is forbidden, and laxatives or gentle enemas are administered. Coughing and all forms of exertion are avoided. The patient is fed. The duration of the period of bed rest is empirical and not founded on any reliable clinical observations or the formation of scar tissue around aneurysms. Sedatives (barbiturates) and analgesics (opiates, acetylsalicylic acid) are important in aiding relaxation. Hypotensive agents (Reserpine, Aldomet) are used to bring hypertensive blood pressures to normal. In the presence of severe hypertension, blocking agents may be cautiously used to lower the blood pressure to 160/100, great care being exercised not to precipitate excessive hypotension and cerebral infarction. Drug therapy is usually not very effective in lowering the blood pressure of normotensive patients confined to bed. Promazine intramuscularly is used to control nausea and vomiting. Dilantin or phenobarbital may be prescribed to prevent cerebral seizures.

The place of repeated drainage of the cerebrospinal fluid by lumbar puncture is still uncertain, although several workers have concluded that it does not affect the outcome of the illness. At present, one lumbar puncture is usually carried out for diagnostic purposes, and thereafter it is performed only for the relief of intractable headache, to detect recurrence of bleeding, or to measure the intracranial pressure prior to surgery.

In maintaining fluid balance, intravenous fluids should

be used sparingly and in the proper electrolyte combination (a mixture of equal parts of 5% glucose in water and normal saline solution or balanced electrolytes) in order to minimize the danger of aggravating brain swelling. Any abnormality of concentration of electrolytes in the blood must be corrected. If diabetes insipidus has occurred, it should be treated with Pitressin. Vitamins C and K have been recommended routinely, but there is no evidence that they are beneficial. Disorders of blood coagulation should be amended. Body hypothermia for 2 to 5 days in the stage of acute hemorrhage has been used with uncertain efficacy. Intravenous hypertonic urea or Mannitol may be effective in temporarily reducing the intracranial pressure.

After resting in bed for 6 weeks, the patient is gradually allowed to resume activity and may return to work in 4 months. It seems logical to advise that heavy labor not be resumed.

SURGICAL THERAPY. Apart from occasionally evacuating an associated intracerebral clot, surgical treatment is for the most part directed to the prevention of recurrence of the hemorrhage. The procedures are either *extracranial* (ligation of the common carotid in the neck) or *intracranial* (resection of the aneurysm; ligation of the neck of the aneurysm; wrapping or tamponade of the aneurysmal sac by muscle, fascia, plastic coating, or arterial graft; trapping the aneurysm; ligation of the main vessel proximal to the aneurysm). Occasionally extracranial and intracranial procedures are combined. Because of the high operative mortality if surgery is undertaken early, operation has usually been delayed until the patient's condition has stabilized following the first hemorrhage. During the waiting period, however, the patient is likely to suffer a further hemorrhage, and in an effort to intervene before this happens neurosurgeons are now attempting to operate much earlier than formerly, sometimes using hypothermia and hypotension during surgery. Before treatment is undertaken, the site, size, and form of the aneurysm must be determined by angiography. At the same time the pattern of the anterior half of the circle of Willis is noted, as it may influence the choice of operative procedure. It has been demonstrated that surgical treatment improves upon the natural outlook for aneurysms at the posterior communicating artery and the bifurcation of the middle cerebral artery. The mortality for anterior communicating aneurysms remains unchanged. After aneurysmal rupture a chronic obstructive or communicating hydrocephalus may develop, causing persistent stupor, which is relieved by ventriculoatrial shunting.

OTHER CAUSES OF INTRACRANIAL HEMORRHAGE

An *angioma,* or hemangioma, consists of a tangle of abnormal vessels forming an abnormal communication between the arterial and venous systems, really an arteriovenous fistula. It is a developmental abnormality, not a neoplasm, but the constituent vessels enlarge with growth and the passage of time. Angiomas vary in size from a small blemish a few millimeters in diameter lying in the cortex to a huge mass of tortuous channels comprising an arteriovenous shunt of sufficient magnitude to raise the cardiac output. Hypertrophic dilated arterial "feeders" approach the main lesion, disappear below the cortex, and break up into a network of thin-walled blood vessels which connect directly with draining veins. The latter often form huge, dilated, pulsating channels, carrying away arterial blood. The blood vessels forming the tangle interposed between arteries and veins are usually abnormally thin and do not have the normal structure of arteries or veins. Angiomas occur in all parts of the brain, brainstem, and spinal cord, but the larger ones are more frequently found in the posterior half of the hemispheres, commonly forming a wedge-shaped lesion extending from the cortex to the ventricular lining.

Angiomas predominate in males over females about 2:1. They may occur in more than one member of a family in the same or successive generations. Although the lesion is present from birth, the onset of complaints is most common between the ages of ten and thirty, but occasionally it is delayed as late as the fifties. The chief clinical features are epileptic seizures and cerebral or cerebral-subarachnoid hemorrhage occurring in a child or young adult. In 50 percent the first manifestation is a seizure, in 20 percent an intracerebral hemorrhage with hemiplegia, and in 20 percent a typical subarachnoid hemorrhage. The seizure pattern depends on the site of the lesion; when focal motor in type the seizure may be followed by a temporary postictal paralysis. When hemorrhage occurs, blood may enter the subarachnoid space almost exclusively, producing a picture identical with that of ruptured saccular aneurysm, but since the angioma lies within the cerebral tissue, the bleeding is more likely to be partly intracerebral, causing hemiparesis, hemiplegia, or death. Before rupture, chronic nondescript headache is a frequent complaint. Occasionally typical migraine with accompaniments is associated, but this is probably a coincidence. Huge angiomas may produce a slowly progressive neurologic deficit because of depletion of blood from adjacent brain tissue. Proptosis has been encountered. When the vein of Galen is involved, hydrocephalus may result. Not infrequently one or both carotid arteries pulsate unusually forcefully in the neck. A systolic bruit heard over the carotid in the neck, the mastoid process, or the eyeballs in young adults is almost pathognomonic of angioma. The patient should be exercised in order to bring out a bruit if none is present at rest. A bruit may be heard over a spinal angioma of large size. The blood pressure may be raised or normal, and it is axiomatic that the occurrence of intracranial bleeding with normal blood pressure should lead to the suspicion of an angioma, ruptured saccular aneurysm, or hemorrhage into a tumor. The eye grounds may reveal a retinal vascular abnormality. Preretinal hemorrhages may be found after hemorrhage has occurred. X-ray of the skull occasionally shows crescentic linear calcification in the vicinity of larger angiomas. Pneumoencephalography may show the picture of an expanding lesion combined with cerebral atrophy, a combination typical of angioma. Arteriography is necessary to establish the diagnosis with certainty and will demonstrate angiomas larger than 5 mm in diameter. Small angiomas may be obscured by the resulting hemorrhage, and even at autopsy a careful microscopic search may be necessary to find them.

Most angiomas bleed sooner or later. The first hemorrhage may be fatal, but in more than 90 percent of cases bleeding stops, and the patient survives. Recurrence of hemorrhage with a fatal outcome is a constant danger. In recent years it has been the practice of neurosurgeons to perform a block dissection of angiomas of suitable size and location.

Although *intracranial bleeding due to head trauma* does not rightfully fall within the scope of the stroke problem, it must be mentioned here because of the great frequency with which it enters into the differential diagnosis, especially in cases in which the history is inadequate or the patient falls and injures himself at the onset of the stroke. *Acute extradural* and *acute subdural hemorrhage* must always be considered in the patient who under unknown circumstances has rather abruptly developed a neurologic deficit such as hemiparesis or confusion, whether the spinal fluid is bloody or not. In *chronic subdural hemorrhage,* which can occur without known trauma, the indefinite picture of drowsiness, confusion, and mild hemiparesis may be erroneously attributed to a stroke, especially in elderly persons. These three conditions must be constantly kept in mind, since failure to make the correct diagnosis deprives the patient of lifesaving surgical intervention. There should be no hesitation in carrying out arteriography or placing diagnostic burr holes in all patients in whom subdural hemorrhage cannot be excluded on clinical grounds. *Cerebral contusion and laceration* may be a cause of subarachnoid hemorrhage, and if the patient has fallen and struck his head at the time of the onset of the stroke, it may be difficult or impossible to decide if the red blood cells in the cerebrospinal fluid are due to a cerebrovascular stroke or to cerebral contusion. Trauma may also cause *acute* or *delayed intracerebral hemorrhage, acute intracerebellar hemorrhage, acute infratentorial subdural hemorrhage, acute brain swelling,* and on rare occasions, extensive *focal infarction* of undetermined pathogenesis.

Several *hemorrhagic hematologic disorders* are not infrequently complicated by hemorrhage into the brain. The most frequent of these are leukemia, aplastic anemia, and thrombocytopenic purpura. As a rule this complication signals a fatal issue. Any part of the brain may be involved, and not infrequently the lesions are multiple. Usually there is already evidence of abnormal bleeding elsewhere (skin, mucous membranes, kidney) by the time cerebral hemorrhage occurs. Intracranial bleeding is a complication of anticoagulant therapy.

Hemorrhages of undetermined origin are of importance, since both clinically and pathologically hemorrhages are found in which the blood pressure is normal and neither an aneurysm nor angioma can be demonstrated. In some postmortem cases a careful microscopic search discloses a small angioma in the cerebral tissue at one side of the hemorrhage, and on this basis it is suspected that in other cases, too, an overlooked angioma may have been the cause of the extravasation of blood. Primary intraventricular hemorrhage, a rare event, is at times due to angioma or neoplasm of the choroid plexus, which may not have been seen by the prosector.

Hemorrhage into primary and secondary brain tumors is not rare, and when it is the first manifestation of the neoplasm, the correct diagnosis may be extremely obscure. Chorionepithelioma, melanotic carcinoma, renal cell carcinoma, bronchogenic carcinoma, pituitary adenoma, glioblastoma multiforme, and medulloblastoma may present in this way. Careful inquiry will usually disclose the fact that signs of a neurologic disorder compatible with intracranial tumor growth have preceded the onset of hemorrhage. Examination clinically and by x-ray may reveal evidence of intracranial tumor or of secondary tumor deposits in other organs. A chest film will frequently show metastatic or primary neoplasm and should be performed in all cases of obscure intracerebral hemorrhage.

Septic embolism may lead to massive fatal intracranial bleeding via a *mycotic aneurysm.* Any part of the circulatory tree may be involved, but usually the aneurysm lies at a branching or forking of a small vessel (about 0.5 mm in diameter) within the subarachnoid space.

On infrequent occasions bleeding within an area of *hemorrhagic infarction* as a result of cerebral embolism or venous thrombosis reaches major proportions, forming an intracerebral hematoma, and the cerebrospinal fluid becomes bloody.

Hypertensive encephalopathy may in its most advanced stage result in intracerebral hemorrhages, which can vary in size from petechial to massive.

Idiopathic brain purpura, or hemorrhagic encephalitis, consists of multiple petechial hemorrhages scattered throughout the white matter of the brain. The picture is that of a diffuse cerebral disease. There is never blood in the spinal fluid, and the condition should never be confused with a typical stroke.

Brainstem hemorrhages secondary to temporal lobe herniation are extremely common but never present as a cerebrovascular stroke.

Inflammatory disease of arteries and veins, especially polyarteritis nodosa and lupus erythematosus, occasionally cause hemorrhage into the nervous system. In polyarteritis rupture of a vessel may occur on the basis of a concomitant hypertension or local vascular disease. In lupus erythematosus—if it can be included in the arteritides—hemorrhage is attributable to hypertension or disease of the vascular wall of undetermined nature. Bleeding nearly always occurs into the parenchyma rather than the subarachnoid space.

The rarer types of hemorrhage listed in the classification are self-explanatory.

Hemorrhages of *intraspinal* origin may be the result of angiomas, hematomyelia, bleeding into tumors, subdural extravasation (trauma, anticoagulants, spontaneous) and circulatory changes around benign tumors.

HYPERTENSIVE ENCEPHALOPATHY

This term refers to an acute syndrome in which severe hypertension is associated with headache, nausea, vomiting, convulsions, confusion, stupor, and coma. Focal or lateralizing neurologic signs, either transitory or lasting, are rare and always suggest some other form of vascular disease (hemorrhage, embolism, or atherosclerotic thrombosis). By the time the neurologic manifestations appear, the hypertension has usually reached the malignant stage, with retinal hemorrhages, exudates, papilledema (*hypertensive retinopathy* grade IV), and evidence of renal and cardiac disease. In many but not all of the cases, the cerebrospinal fluid pressure and the protein values are both elevated, the latter sometimes to over 100 mg per 100 ml. The hypertension may be essential or due to chronic renal disease, acute glomerulonephritis, acute toxemia of pregnancy, pheochromocytoma, Cushing's syndrome or ACTH toxicity. Lowering of the blood pressure with hypotensive drugs may reverse the picture in a day or two. If the hypertension cannot be controlled, the outcome is fatal. Neuropathologic examination may reveal a rather normal-looking brain, but usually cerebral swelling and/or hemorrhages of various sizes from massive to petechial will be found. A cerebellar pressure cone may cause fatality, and in some instances the event was seemingly encouraged by a lumbar puncture. Microscopically there are in addition to small hemorrhages clusters of glial cells, necrosis of arterioles, and minute cerebral infarcts.

The term *hypertensive encephalopathy* should be reserved for the above syndrome and not used to refer to chronic recurrent headaches, dizziness, epileptic seizures, recurrent transient ischemic attacks, or small strokes which often occur in association with high blood pressure. For further discussion, see pp. 1256 and 1262.

INFLAMMATORY DISEASES OF BRAIN ARTERIES

Inflammatory diseases of the vessels of the brain have been mentioned on several occasions in the preceding paragraphs, and here they are reviewed and discussed briefly.

Meningovascular syphilis, formerly one of the most frequent causes of occlusive vascular disease in patients of all ages, has become a rarity since the introduction of penicillin therapy (see Chap. 177).

Tuberculous meningitis, fungous meningitis, and the subacute forms of bacterial meningitis (influenzal bacillus, staphylococcus, pneumococcus) may also be accompanied by vascular disorders of the occlusive type, in either the cerebral arteries or veins. Occasionally in tuberculous meningitis a stroke may be the first clinical sign of meningitis; more often it develops after the meningeal symptoms are established.

Typhus, schistosomiasis mansoni, mucormycosis, malaria, and *trichinosis* are rare types of infective inflammatory diseases of the arteries and, unlike the above, are not secondary to meningeal inflammation. In typhus and other rickettsial diseases, capillary and arteriolar changes and perivascular inflammatory cells are found in the brain, and presumably they underlie the convulsions, acute psychoses, and coma which reflect the central nervous system involvement. The internal carotid artery may be occluded in diabetic patients during orbital and cavernous sinus infections with mucormycosis. In trichinosis the sudden onset of convulsions, aphasia, hemiplegia, and coma may either accompany or, as happens more often, follow the systemic and muscular symptoms. The cause of the cerebral symptoms has not been established. Parasites have been found in the brain; in one of our cases the cerebral lesions were produced by bland emboli arising in the heart and related to a severe myocarditis. Malaria of the malignant or falciparum variety is frequently attended by a clinical state known as "cerebral malaria" in which convulsions and coma and sometimes focal symptoms appear to be due to blockage of capillaries and precapillaries by masses of parasitized red blood corpuscles.

The *arteritides of obscure origin* include polyarteritis nodosa, disseminated lupus erythematosus, granulomatous arteritis, giant-cell arteritis, temporal (cranial) arteritis, and rheumatic arteritis (see Chap. 394).

Lupus erythematosus causes cerebral symptoms in over 50 percent of cases. Seizures and psychoses are common. Small cerebral infarcts lead to widespread focal deficits. Accompanying hypertension may precipitate hemorrhage or hypertensive encephalopathy, or endocarditis may cause cerebral embolism.

Temporal arteritis (cranial arteritis) is an uncommon affliction of elderly persons in which the external carotid system, particularly the temporal branches, is the seat of a subacute granulomatous inflammation with an exudate of lymphocytes, monocytes, neutrophilic leukocytes, and giant cells. Usually the most severely affected parts of the artery become thrombosed. Headache or head pain is the chief complaint. Systemic manifestations include anorexia, loss of weight, malaise, and polymyalgia rheumatica. The inflammatory nature of the illness is indicated by some one or several of the following: fever, slight leukocytosis, increased sedimentation rate, and anemia. Occlusion of branches of the ophthalmic artery results in blindness in one or both eyes in over 25 percent of patients, and occasionally an ophthalmoplegia due to involvement of ocular nerves occurs. An arteritis of the aorta and its major branches, including carotid, subclavian, coronary, and femoral arteries, is found at postmortem examination. Significant inflammatory involvement of intracranial arteries is rare, but strokes occur occasionally, on the basis of internal carotid, middle cerebral, or vertebral occlusion. The diagnosis depends on the finding of a tender thrombosed or thickened cranial artery and the demonstration of the lesion in a biopsy. Meticorten and ACTH bring striking subjective relief and prevent blindness. See Chap. 391 for further discussion.

Another type of *giant-cell arteritis,* which occurs in younger people, is described in Chaps. 392 and 394.

Thromboangiitis obliterans of cerebral vessels (Winiwarter-Buerger disease) has not been included in the foregoing list. Despite the large amount of literature on the subject, the pathology is so dubious that it does not merit further exposition. All the patients that the authors have studied proved to have had either atherosclerosis of the carotid or cerebral arteries with "stasis thrombosis" of more distant cerebral branches. Buerger's disease of the legs has an equally uncertain status.

DIFFERENTIATION OF CEREBROVASCULAR DISEASE FROM OTHER NEUROLOGIC ILLNESSES

It has already been stated that the diagnosis of a vascular lesion rests solely on recognition of the stroke syndrome and that without evidence of this the diagnosis must always be in doubt. Three useful criteria in the identification of the stroke have already been emphasized: (1) the tempo of the clinical syndrome, (2) evidence of focal brain disease, and (3) the clinical setting. The temporal profile can usually be defined by means of a clear history of premonitory phenomena, the mode of the onset, and the evolution of the neurologic disturbance taken in relationship to the medical status at the time of examination. If these data are lacking, the course may still be determined by extending the period of observation for a few more days or weeks. An inadequate history is probably the most frequent cause of diagnostic errors.

Few other neurologic illnesses mimic cerebrovascular disease. When the details of the history are missing, however, subdural hematoma, brain tumor, brain abscess, and senile dementia may lead to diagnostic difficulties. The reader should refer to Chaps. 353, 359, and 364 for further discussion of differential diagnosis.

REFERENCES

Fields, W. S.: "Pathogenesis and Treatment of Cerebrovascular Disease," Springfield, Ill., Charles C Thomas, Publisher, 1961.

Kubik, C. S., and R. D. Adams: Occlusion of Basilar Artery—Clinical and Pathologic Study, Brain, 69:73, 1946.

Walton, J.: "Subarachnoid Hemorrhage," Edinburgh, E. and S. Livingstone, Ltd., 1956.

358 TRAUMATIC DISEASES OF THE BRAIN

Karl-Erik Aström, Henri vander Eecken, and Raymond D. Adams

Head injury, which is the basis of some of the most frequent and serious neurologic disorders in these times of high-velocity transport and mechanization in industry, poses many problems to the practicing physician. To deal with head injuries effectively demands a knowledge of the clinical manifestations as well as a sound grasp of fundamental physiologic mechanisms. The physician must stand prepared at all times, for he may at any moment be summoned to render aid or to assess the clinical status of a person who has suffered an injury of the head or spine. The present chapter undertakes to review the salient facts concerning these injuries of the nervous system and to outline an approach to these problems that has been useful to the authors.

PHYSIOLOGIC AND PATHOLOGIC CONSIDERATIONS

The very language with which certain types of head injury are discussed divulges a number of misconceptions that have been inherited from previous generations of physicians. Words have crept into medical vocabulary and have often been retained long after the ideas for which they stood have been refuted—clear evidence of the disadvantage of prematurely adopting explanatory rather than descriptive terms. The word *concussion*, for example, implies the violent shaking and agitation of an organ or the functional impairment which results therefrom. Yet despite numerous experiments to demonstrate these physical changes within the nerve cells (vibration effects, formation of intracellular vacuoles, etc.), no confirmation of their existence has been possible. Similarly the word *contusion*, meaning a bruising or crushing without interruption of physical continuity, is applied rather indiscriminately to a variety of clinical states, some of which could not depend on a pathologic change of this type, e.g., "minor contusion state or syndrome"—an expression introduced by Wilfred Trotter, who was himself most critical of words that "embalm a fallacious theory."

In all attempts to analyze the mechanism of brain damage in head injury one fact stands preeminent—that there must be the sudden application of a physical force of considerable magnitude to the head. Unless the head is struck, the brain suffers no injury—except in the rare and somewhat controversial cases of crush injury to the chest or explosive injury with raised intrapulmonary pressure. A second fact, also susceptible of easy verification, is that the size of the area on the skull over which the force is exerted is of importance. High-velocity missiles destroy a small part of the skull and penetrate the cranial cavity without significant displacement of the head or brain; and heavy, crushing injuries which result from the skull being compressed between two converging objects may crush the brain. In these two circumstances it is interesting to note that the patient may suffer severe and often fatal injury without immediate loss of consciousness. Hemorrhage, destruction of brain tissue, and, if the patient survives for a time, meningitis or abscess, are the principal pathologic changes created by injuries of this type. They offer little difficulty to understanding.

The common civilian injury is one in which a rapidly moving blunt object strikes the head or the head is flung against a hard surface. Injuries of this type, often termed *blunt head injuries*, are remarkable in two respects: (1) they almost always induce at least a temporary loss of consciousness; (2) even though the skull is not penetrated and fragments of bone are not driven into its cavity, the brain may suffer gross damage, i.e., contusion, laceration, hemorrhage, swelling, herniation, etc. Clinicians as well as experimental physiologists have sought a theory which would bring into plausible form all gross neuropathologic changes, the skull fracture and the transient paralysis of nervous function (concussion) or prolonged coma, so often observed in fatal cases. It may be said that a comprehensive theory, acceptable to all workers in this field, has not been developed as yet.

The relation of skull fracture to injury of the cerebral tissues has been viewed in changing perspective through the entire history of this subject. In earliest times fractures dominated the thinking of the medical profession, and cerebral lesions were regarded as secondary. Later it became known that the skull, although rigid, is still flexible enough to yield to a severe blow without fracture. Therefore, the presence of a fracture, although a rough measure of the violence to which the brain has been exposed, is not an infallible index. Even in fatal head injury autopsy may reveal an intact skull in some 20 to 30 percent of cases. Also many patients suffer skull fractures without serious or prolonged disorder of cerebral function.

The modern trend is to be interested more in the presence or absence of brain injury than in the fracture of the skull itself. Nevertheless fractures cannot be dismissed without a few comments, for they assume importance in indicating the site and possible severity of brain damage, in providing an explanation for cranial nerve palsies, and in affording potential pathways for the ingress of bacteria and air or the egress of cerebrospinal fluid.

The existence of a basal skull fracture may be indicated by signs of cranial nerve damage. Cranial nerves which are particularly liable to injury are the olfactory, optic, oculomotor, first and second branches of the trigeminal, the facial, and the auditory. Anosmia and an apparent loss of taste (actually a loss of perception of aromatic flavors, elementary tastes—salt, sweet, bitter, sour—being retained) are frequent sequelae of head injury, especially of falls on the back of the head. In the majority of cases the anosmia is permanent or the patient may have some perversion of smell (parosmia). The anosmia may be unilateral and not noticed by the patient. The mechanism of these disturbances is believed to be displacement of the brain and tearing of the olfactory nerve filaments. A fracture in or near the sella may tear the stalk of the pituitary gland, with resulting diabetes insipidus. A fracture of sphenoid bone may lacerate the optic nerve, with complete blindness from the beginning. The pupil is dilated and unreactive to a direct light stimulus but still takes part in the consensual reflex. The optic disk becomes pale, i.e., atrophic, after an interval of several weeks. Partial injuries may result in a troublesome blurring of vision. Injury to the eighth cranial nerve with petrosal fractures causes loss of hearing and/or dizziness, immediately after injury. The deafness due to nerve injury must be distinguished from that caused by rupture of the eardrum or the presence of blood in the middle ear, and

the vertigo, from posttraumatic giddiness. In oculomotor nerve injury there is a divergent squint, with loss of internal and vertical movement of the eye and a fixed, dilated pupil. Diplopia only on looking down suggests trochlear nerve affection. Direct injury of the facial nerve by a basal fracture may be present immediately after the injury or may be delayed, coming on after several days. This delayed form is usually transitory, and its mechanism is not known. It may be misinterpreted as an important progression of the traumatic intracranial lesion. Injury to the ophthalmic or maxillary divisions of the trigeminal nerve may be the result either of a basal fracture across the middle cranial fossa or of a direct extracranial injury to the branches of the nerves. Numbness and paresthesias over the area of skin supplied by the nerve or a troublesome neuralgia are the sequelae of these injuries.

If the skin is lacerated over the skull fracture and the underlying meninges are torn, or if the fracture passes through the posterior wall of a nasal sinus, bacteria or air may enter the cranial cavity with resulting meningitis, abscess, and aerocele. Cerebrospinal fluid may also leak into the sinus and present as a watery discharge from the nose (cerebrospinal fluid rhinorrhea). Persistence of the rhinorrhea or the occurrence of episodes of recurrent meningitis (headache, convulsions, fever, and stiff neck with pleocytosis and sometimes bacteria) are often indications for a repair of the torn dura mater over the fissure. Depressed fractures are of significance only if the underlying dura is lacerated by spicules of bone or the brain is compressed.

Much has been written about the mechanism of coma in closed or blunt head injury. Two facts concerning this condition stand out clearly: (1) it bears only an indefinite relationship to skull fracture; (2) the optimal conditions for its production are those in which there is some change in the momentum of the head; i.e., movement is suddenly imparted to it by a blow, or its movement is suddenly arrested. Striking the stationary head of an experimental animal will cause a loss of brainstem reflexes only if the head was free to move, not if it is clamped in one position (Denny-Brown and Russell). This finding alone would stand in refutation of such theories of concussion as a wave of high intracranial pressure due to the indentation of the skull or a subsequent wave of negative pressure (Kahn, Ward, and Clark), cerebral anemia (Trotter), shattering of the myelinated fibers of cerebral white matter (Strich and Symonds), or a general vibration or agitation transmitted via the skull. The speed of acceleration or deceleration of the head necessary for this concussive effect must exceed 28 ft per sec. The initial action of the blunt injury of this type is to excite the nervous system (the "stars" that one sees with a minor injury, the gasp of the animal); and this is followed by transient paralysis of cerebral function, i.e., abolition of consciousness, suppression of reflexes, arrest of respiration, etc. The means whereby the latter effects are produced is not known. Equally obscure is the site of injury, whether diffuse in the cerebral cortex (Denny-Brown and Meyer) or in the diencephalon and midbrain.

In fatal cases of severe head injury, where this concussive injury must also have existed, the brain is almost invariably bruised or lacerated, and often there is hemorrhage, either meningeal or intracerebral. The observation of these gross pathologic findings had led to the widely prevalent view that head injuries are largely matters of bruises and hemorrhages and of urgent operations. That this can hardly be the case is suggested by the fact that some patients survive head injuries almost as severe as the fatal ones and yet make an excellent recovery. At autopsy years later old contusions (*plaques jaunes*) and hemorrhages of approximately the same distribution and extent as those observed in some of the immediately fatal cases are found. One can only conclude, therefore, that most of the immediate symptoms of severe head injury, both general and localized, depend on invisible and highly reversible changes in the brain, probably of the same nature as those which underlie concussion. Nevertheless these bruises, lacerations, hemorrhages, and localized swellings of tissues cannot be disregarded, because they are probably responsible for many of the fatalities that occur 12 to 72 hr or more after the injury. Of these lesions the most important are the surface bruising of the brain beneath the point of impact (*coup* injury) and the more extensive lacerations and contusions on the opposite side of the brain (*contrecoup* injuries). The inertia of the brain, which causes it to be flung against the side of the skull that was struck and to be pulled away from the contralateral side, has been invoked to explain these coup-contrecoup contusions. This theory has been further elaborated by Holburn, who points out that the brain is roughly spherical and that all movements of the head describe an arc with its axis centered where skull is attached to spine. Sudden changes in the momentum of the head, therefore, induce a swirling motion to the brain, which may then suffer injury against all rough, bony prominences (wings of sphenoid bones, petrous parts of temporal bones, rough surfaces of orbital and frontal bones).

CLINICAL MANIFESTATIONS OF HEAD INJURY

The physician upon being called to see a patient who has had a head injury will generally find him in one of three clinical conditions; each, as Trotter, Symonds, and Rowbotham have pointed out, must be dealt with differently. It is usually possible to place the patient in one of these three categories by assessing the mental and general neurologic status when he is first seen and at intervals of time after the accident.

PATIENTS WHO ARE CONSCIOUS OR ARE RAPIDLY REGAINING MENTAL CLARITY WHEN FIRST SEEN (MINOR HEAD INJURY). The typical example is a patient who was rendered unconscious by a knock on the head and then regained his senses within seconds, minutes, or hours. Roughly two degrees of disturbance of consciousness may have occurred. First, there is the patient who was never unconscious at all. He was observed to have struck his head and was stunned or "saw stars." By all criteria his head injury was insignificant when judged in terms of life and death and severe brain damage, though in exceptional cases there is always the possibility of skull fracture or epidural or subdural hematoma. Nevertheless, a troublesome group of symptoms may have developed at once or within a few days. The patient may begin to complain of a headache, dizziness, loss of confidence in himself, inability to concentrate, nervousness, poor sleep, fatigue, and depression. The headache is of a pressing, aching type and is characteristically worsened by any physical and mental effort, stooping, and excitement. No clue is provided as to the mechanism of these symptoms. The possibility that they represent a traumatic or compensation neurosis is suggested because of their purely subjective nature, the lack of abnormal neurologic signs, and the absence of change in cerebrospinal fluid or alteration of the EEG. In recent years a better appreciation of the constancy of this clinical syndrome has favored the view first put forward by William Trotter that it is the direct physical effect of injury, incorrectly designated by him *minor cerebral contusion* state. The severity of these symptoms is not clearly related to the severity of the head injury. Their persistence constitutes a most vexatious therapeutic problem.

If consciousness was temporarily abolished, the patient is said to have suffered a *concussion*, defined by Trotter as "an essentially transient state due to head injury which is instantaneous in onset, manifests widespread symptoms of a purely paralytic kind, does not as such comprise any evidence of structural cerebral injury and is nearly always followed by amnesia for the actual moment of the impact." The patient, if observed immediately after the injury, shows a complete paralysis of nervous function. In a few instances death has occurred at this time, from respiratory arrest or cardiac arrhythmia, and no lesion was found at postmortem examination. However, the usual sequelae is for the pulse and respiration (if they were depressed or arrested) to return at once and for muscle tone, reflexes, voluntary movement, and mental clarity to be regained within a few minutes. Only an amnesia for the accident and the events that immediately preceded (retrograde amnesia) and followed it (anterograde amnesia) will remain. Thereafter the patient may suffer the same headaches, giddiness, and nervousness described above.

These relatively trivial head injuries may rarely be followed by a number of other puzzling features, all of which indicate the occurrence of some process in addition to concussion: (1) *Delayed traumatic collapse:* following an accident a few patients, after walking about and seeming to be mentally normal, will turn pale and fall unconscious for a few minutes. This is a vasomotor syncopal attack and is probably related to injury, pain, and emotional upset. Rarely does the patient exhibit any focal or lateralizing neurologic signs. The suggestion that this represents medullary edema is hardly tenable. (2) *Immediate traumatic paraplegia:* with falls on top of the head, which may injure the motor areas for the lower extremities, both legs may become temporarily weak and numb, sometimes with bilateral Babinski signs and sphincteric incontinence. Concussion of the cervical spinal cord is another possible mechanism of the paraplegia. (3) *Immediate hemiplegia or monoplegia:* these conditions may develop immediately after a minor injury, with or without blood in the cerebrospinal fluid, and are commonly attributed to a relatively circumscript injury with minimal concussion or a direct contusion or laceration of the underlying brain (cerebrospinal fluid is then sanguineous). (4) *Immediate traumatic epilepsy:* a series of focal seizures may occur with a minor bruise of the cortex and may be followed by a postepileptic paralysis of short duration. (5) *Delayed hemiplegia* or *monoplegia:* an "interval" paralysis in cases of minor or major injury usually signifies an epidural hemorrhage, a subdural hemorrhage or hygroma, arterial thrombosis, spreading venous thrombosis, or intracerebral hemorrhage. (6) *Acute drowsiness, confusion,* and *headache* or *coma,* due presumably to localized and generalized traumatic brain edema; children who have concussions are especially liable to headache, drowsiness, and vomiting, which may have its onset some hours after the injury. In these children infusions and clyses of water and 5 percent glucose are particularly dangerous; such treatment may prove fatal, owing to a water intoxication and severe brain swelling. Apparently an excessive output of antidiuretic hormone and water retention occur under these circumstances. (7) *Posttraumatic nervous instability* (see below).

PATIENTS WHO ARE AND HAVE BEEN UNCONSCIOUS SINCE THE TIME OF THE ACCIDENT (MAJOR HEAD INJURY). **The Clinical State.** In this group, which includes the patients with the more severe head injuries, the outlook is obviously less favorable and one is concerned at first for their life. However, within this group there is still a wide variation in the severity of the traumatic brain disease. A certain number of patients die at once or within a few minutes, and it may be assumed that the direct injury to the brain or some other organ was incompatible with life. Other patients in this group recover consciousness rapidly after several hours, but a few remain deeply comatose for days or even weeks. If the pupils dilate and become fixed and all brainstem reflex mechanisms, including the maintenance of respiration, are paralyzed and remain so over a period of hours (EEG usually isoelectric as described on p. 1805), the outlook is hopeless. The mortality rate in those who reach a hospital in coma has been approximately 20 percent, and most of them die within the first 12 to 24 hr. Of those alive after 24 hr, the mortality is 7 to 8 percent, and after 48 hr the figure falls to 1 percent.

In the patient whose prognosis is favorable, the coma is less deep; i.e., he is confused, stuporous, or semicomatose (see Chap. 26). For a time he may be restless and difficult to control. The reflexes are normal, as are pulse, blood pressure, and respiration. He is able to swallow and may or may not speak. There are no obvious neurologic signs. In contrast, those patients whose illness will end fatally may be moribund from the beginning. Their coma is profound. The limbs may be flaccid and without reflexes. The corneal and pharyngeal (gag)

reflexes are absent. The pupils are small and unreactive to light, or dilated and fixed, or unequal. The ocular axes are divergent or askew. The jaw sags, the tongue falls back in the throat, saliva drools from the mouth, and swallowing is obviously lost. There may be surgical shock at first for a brief period, with the usual findings of pale and moist skin, weak and rapid pulse, subnormal temperature, and a blood pressure that is difficult to obtain. Within a few hours, however, the temperature usually rises, and this may continue until death. The breathing may be stertorous and later feeble and irregular. The state of consciousness and the temperature chart provide information of great value in appraising the status of the patient. An ascending pulse rate, possibly interspersed by short periods in which there is a bounding, slow pulse, and rising temperature or a combination of fast pulse and subnormal temperature, is a sign of grave prognosis.

In the group of patients whose outlook is less bleak, deep coma soon gives way to semicoma. The blood pressure stabilizes, and the temperature and pulse, having risen to 101 to 102°F and 100 to 110 per min, respectively, remain at these levels. Muscular tone is regained in the limbs, and the tendon reflexes are present. This is a critical period, for a sudden rise in temperature, cyanosis, and increasing respiratory difficulty may result in a fatal issue. Once the patient regains full consciousness sufficiently to respond to a spoken command, the physician no longer needs to be concerned about survival and may begin to think about the possibility of focal brain damage and prospects for recovery. There is still a substantial risk in the first 2 or 3 weeks, however, from pneumonia, meningitis, or epidural and subdural hemorrhage, which may intervene and impair the chances of survival. It is often said that death during the first 12 hr is the result of the direct injury of the brain; that which occurs later is usually the result of some complication of cranial trauma (intracerebral or subarachnoid hemorrhage, herniation of the temporal lobe, localized or generalized edema, epidural or subdural hemorrhage, meningitis, pneumonia).

There is another group of patients to which some reference must be made for they represent difficult problems in diagnosis and therapy. Here a known or evident head injury is not followed by deep or lasting coma, but instead the patient is awake and able to respond upon arrival at the hospital. Yet as the hours pass it is apparent that his condition is deteriorating, and within a day or two he lapses into coma. A sanguineous cerebrospinal fluid under slightly elevated pressure attests to the existence of contusion. The progressive nature of the illness suggests intracerebral, epidural, or subdural hemorrhage; yet at postmortem examination only contusion, localized edema (sometimes generalized), and temporal lobe pressure cone are found to be the basis of the clinical syndrome. The point to remember is that consciousness may return early, i.e., within minutes or hours, after a head injury severe enough seriously to contuse the brain and to lead to death, after some few days.

The course of clinical events in those who survive the first 24 to 48 hr is much like that in patients with brief concussion, except that it is likely to be more prolonged, so that one may witness all the varying stages of recovery in slow motion. As coma lessens, the patient opens his eyes; he may pause in his restless activity and seem to listen to what is said. He reacts briskly to painful stimuli applied to the face, passive manipulations of the head, and pinching the inner surface of the arms and legs. Moaning and groaning are the first vocal activities to return; their absence in patients who are beginning to respond always suggests aphasia. Restlessness, irritability, and hyperactivity may assume such proportions that the patient must be restrained. For example, he may resist all attempts to help him, struggle against restraints, yell, talk incessantly and without sense, strike at everyone near the bed, etc. This state, sometimes loosely called *traumatic delirium,* may last hours or days but eventually is replaced by a more quiet confusional state. Then the patient will begin to speak, unless the injury has caused a lack of impulse to act (abulia) or incapacity for speech (aphasia); and he is variably able to engage in conversation. But his thinking processes are slow and inefficient, and his thoughts are likely to be incoherent. Often he cannot understand the purposes of his splints, bandages, catheters, etc., and will remove them even when asked repeatedly not to do so. Movements and reactions to stimuli are more or less automatic. Memory is obviously faulty. As confusion lessens, there may be a brief period when mental function is nearly normal; yet later there will be little or no memory of what transpired. From a close study of this clinical sequence it is obvious that the capacity to form, retain, and reproduce new experiences is one of the best tests of the mental status. Not until the patient reaches the stage of continuous anterograde memory will he regard himself as fully normal. In looking back upon this period he can recall only a few events and has the impression that he was unconscious all this time. Retrograde amnesia for the accident and for the events which preceded it, which often extends over a period of minutes, hours, or even days, is another invariable accompaniment of severe head injury. This period of retrograde memory defect shortens as convalescence proceeds.

Focal and lateralizing neurologic symptoms and signs, as would be anticipated, will be observed with notable frequency in this group of patients. These abnormalities are presumably related to hemorrhage and contusion; and in as much as they are usually engrafted on a severe concussive injury, they become manifest as consciousness is regained. Local injury to the brain without a disturbance of consciousness occurs exceptionally, and then more often with the penetration of the skull with missiles or a direct glancing blow by a relatively small object (golf ball, stone), and sometimes with depressed fractures. Of the focal symptoms, hemiparesis is probably the most frequent. The weakness in the arm and leg may be evidenced even during coma by the hypotonia, the less frequent movement of the limbs, inequality of tendon reflexes, and a more persistent Babinski sign on one side. Complete hemiplegia is rarely observed. Hemihypesthesia, although occasionally found, is less common,

possibly because sensory tests are difficult to interpret until mental clarity is regained. Homonymous hemianopia is not at all infrequent and may present early as an inattentiveness to visual stimuli on one side. Aphasia, usually of mixed type, may be noted in a number of cases. A series of focal seizures may occur within a few days of the time of injury and, as said before, is probably due to cortical contusion. Such seizures usually cease after a few days and do not necessarily signify that epilepsy is to be a sequel to the trauma. Diabetes insipidus, disturbances of sleep (reversal of rhythm, somnolence, later narcolepsy), diplopia, heteronymous visual field defects, gastrointestinal hemorrhage, amenorrhea, and impotence in the male indicate damage to the hypothalamus and walls of the third ventricle. Midbrain or diffuse cerebral lesions are evidenced by ocular palsies, protracted coma (weeks, months, or years), decerebrate rigidity, crossed ocular-limb paralyses, bilateral Babinski signs, and later dysarthria, ataxia of limbs on one side, and sensory disturbances.

Laboratory Findings. In this group of patients with severe head injury there is a high incidence of skull fracture. The cerebrospinal fluid is usually sanguineous (red blood cells usually 100,000 per cu mm or less) and under elevated pressure (between 200 and 300 mm) in the majority of patients. The prognosis is distinctly less good in those with more than 100,000 red cells per cu mm and pressures in excess of 300 mm. Nevertheless death may occur in patients who have no skull fracture, a subnormal intracranial pressure, and relatively clear cerebrospinal fluid. The electroencephalogram regularly shows focal and diffuse abnormalities.

Neuropathologic Findings. In patients who die during the first few hours or days after a severe head injury, hemorrhage and necrosis of tissue will frequently be observed. In 50 consecutive autopsies summarized in Rowbotham's excellent monograph, only 2 showed no macroscopic change. Lacerations of cerebral cortex (28 percent), surface contusions (48 percent), subarachnoid hemorrhage (72 percent), acute subdural hemorrhage (16 percent), and extradural hemorrhage (20 percent) were the usual findings. As a rule, several of these pathologic changes were found in the same case. Skull fractures were discovered in 72 percent.

PATIENTS WHO ARE UNCONSCIOUS WHEN FIRST SEEN BUT WHO ARE SAID TO HAVE BEEN CONSCIOUS AFTER THE ACCIDENT (PRESENCE OF LUCID INTERVAL). This group of patients is smaller than the other two but is of great importance because it includes many who are in urgent need of surgical treatment. The initial coma may have been brief or there may have been none at all, in which instance one might conclude that there was neither concussion nor contusion. The following conditions must be considered in every case of this type.

Acute Epidural Hemorrhage. This condition is due as a rule to a temporal or parietal fracture with laceration of the middle meningeal artery and vein. Less often there is a tear in a dural venous sinus. The injury, even when it fractures the skull, may not have produced coma. A typical example is a child who has fallen from a bicycle or a swing or has suffered a hard blow to the head in a fight and was only momentarily unconscious. A few hours or a day or two later (exceptionally the interval may be as long as several days or a week, especially with venous bleeding), he develops headache of increasing severity, vomiting, drowsiness, confusion, seizures (which may be one-sided), hemiparesis, with slightly increased tendon reflexes and Babinski sign. As coma develops, the hemiparesis with Babinski sign may give way to spastic limbs, and Babinski signs bilaterally. There may be aphasia. Respirations become deeper and stertorous, then shallow and irregular, and finally stop. The pulse is often slow (below 60) and bounding, with a concomitant rise in systolic blood pressure. The pupil may dilate on the side of hematoma. The cerebrospinal fluid is usually under increased pressure, though normal and subnormal pressures do not exclude the possibility of an epidural hematoma. The fluid may be clear or sanguineous, depending on whether or not there is an associated contusion, laceration, or subarachnoid hemorrhage. Death, which is almost invariable if the clot is not removed surgically, comes at the end of a comatose period, rarely if ever in a conscious patient, and is due to respiratory arrest. The visualization of a fracture line across the groove of the middle meningeal artery and a knowledge of the side of the head struck (the clot is usually on that side) are of aid in diagnosis and of lateralization of the lesion. The surgical procedure is placement of several burr holes (a single one may miss the clot), drainage, identification of the bleeding vessel, and ligation. The operative results are excellent, except in the cases with extended fractures and laceration of the dural venous sinuses, in which instance the epidural hematoma may be bilateral rather than unilateral, as it ordinarily is. If coma, bilateral Babinski signs, spasticity, or decerebrate rigidity supervene before operation, the prognosis for life becomes poor. This usually means that a temporal lobe herniation and crushing of the midbrain have already occurred.

Acute and Chronic Subdural Hematoma. The problems created by the acute and chronic subdural hematoma are so different that they must be discussed separately. In *acute subdural hematomas,* which may be unilateral or bilateral, the latent interval is usually longer than in epidural hemorrhage—many days or 1 to 2 weeks. Headaches, drowsiness, sometimes agitation, slowness in thinking, and confusion, all of which progressively worsen, are the most frequent symptoms. Focal or lateralizing signs (hemiplegia) are late and tend to be less prominent than the disturbance of consciousness. Frequently the acute subdural hematoma is combined with cerebral contusion and laceration, so that the clinical effects of these several lesions are difficult to distinguish; and there are some patients in whom it is impossible before operation to state whether the surface clot is epidural or subdural in location. The treatment is bilateral temporal burr holes, and this is also one of the most certain diagnostic procedures. The surgical results are less certain than in chronic subdural hematoma. If the clot that is found is too small to explain the symptoms, the surgeon usually

proceeds to do a right subtemporal decompression. Exceptionally the subdural hematoma forms in the posterior fossa and gives rise to headache, vomiting, pupillary inequality, dysphagia, cranial nerve palsies, ataxia of trunk and gait, and stiff neck in some combination.

In chronic hematoma, the traumatic etiology is less clear. The head injury, especially in the elderly person, may be trivial (striking the head against the branch of a tree, or on the mantel of a fireplace during a faint, etc.), and it may have been forgotten completely. A period of weeks then follows when headaches (not invariable), giddiness, slowness in thinking, confusion, exaggeration of certain personality traits, and rarely a seizure or two are the main symptoms. The initial impression may be that the patient has a brain tumor, a drug intoxication, or a depressive, senile, or other psychosis. As with acute subdural hematoma, the disturbance of consciousness (drowsiness, inattentiveness, incoherence of thought, stupor, or coma) is more prominent than focal or lateralizing signs. The latter usually consist of hemiparesis and rarely of an aphasic disturbance. Hemianesthesia and homonymous hemianopia are seldom observed, probably because the anatomic structures subserving these functions are deep and not easily compressed (in the case of the geniculocalcarine pathway) and sensory changes are likely to be overlooked in a stuporous, confused patient. Hemiplegia, i.e., complete paralysis of one arm and leg, is usually indicative of an intracerebral lesion rather than of a compressive surface lesion. Another important feature of the hemiparesis is that it may be contralateral or ipsilateral, depending on whether or not herniation of the temporal lobe through the notch of the tentorium into the posterior fossa and compression of the contralateral cerebral peduncle are present; if they are present, pyramidal signs are then ipsilateral to the clot or bilateral. As the condition progresses, the patient becomes comatose but often with striking fluctuations of awareness. The ipsilateral pupil dilates (Hutchinson's pupillary sign), owing, it is believed, to direct pressure of the herniating temporal lobe upon the oculomotor nerve. The dilated pupil and ptotic eyelid are more reliable indications of the side of the hematoma than the hemiparesis, though they, too, can be misleading in certain cases. Convulsions are usually seen only in alcoholics or patients with a contusion and cannot be regarded as a cardinal sign of subdural hematoma, even though they are not infrequent. Roentgenograms of the skull are usually negative except for a shift of a calcified pineal to one side or an occasional unexpected fracture line. The electroencephalogram is usually bilaterally abnormal, sometimes with reduced voltage or electrical silence over the subdural hematoma and high-voltage slow waves over the opposite sides because of the damping effects of the clot and displacement of the brain respectively. The branches of the middle cerebral artery are separated from the skull and displaced contralaterally in an arteriogram. The cerebrospinal fluid may be clear, bloody, or xanthochromic, depending on the presence or absence of recent or old contusion and subarachnoid hemorrhage, and the pressure may be elevated, normal, or subnormal.

Of all these diagnostic procedures, arteriography and direct burr hole exploration are the most reliable.

The acute, rapidly evolving subdural hematomas are due to tearing or bridging veins and direct compression of the brain by an expanding clot of fresh blood. Unlike the epidural arterial hemorrhage, which is progressive, the bleeding is usually arrested by the rising intracranial pressure. The chronic subdural hematoma is believed to cause symptoms by becoming encysted by fibrous membranes (pseudomembranes) which grow from the dura. In its encysted state, as red corpuscles hemolyze and blood proteins disintegrate, the osmotic pressure rises and fluid enters the hematoma, with the result that the hematoma enlarges and the compressive effects increase. Severe cerebral compression and displacement with temporal lobe—tentorial herniation are the usual causes of death. Treatment consists of placing burr holes and evacuating the clot before deep coma has developed.

Subdural hygromas (collections of blood and cerebrospinal fluid in the subdural space) may also form after an injury, as well as after meningitis (in an infant) and pneumoencephalography (see Chap. 360). It is said that a tear of the arachnoid permits the accumulation of cerebrospinal fluid into the subdural space, where it becomes trapped. The patient may complain of severe headache, drowsiness, and confusion, which are relieved when the subdural fluid is drained.

Cerebral Hemorrhage (Immediate and Delayed). Acute, massive brain hemorrhages are more frequent in elderly than in young patients and are usually fatal within a few hours. The clinical picture is similar to that of hypertensive brain hemorrhage (deepening coma with hemiplegia, a dilating pupil, bilateral Babinski signs, stertorous and irregular respirations). Indeed the problem that cannot be solved even at postmortem examination is whether the patient had a hemorrhagic type of stroke and then fell, or a fall that caused the head injury and hemorrhage. If the bleeding is slow, there may be an interval of 2 to 3 days between injury and the symptoms of the oncoming hemorrhage. Coma or confusion, if present from the time of the injury, may obscure the signs of the intracerebral hemorrhage. Craniotomy with evacuation of the clot has given a successful result in a few cases.

TRAUMATIC OCCLUSION OF CAROTID ARTERY. In this relatively rare form of cranial trauma, though most dramatic when it occurs, the patient is usually young, athletic, and the mechanism of the injury unclear. An accident on the playing field of seemingly trivial type is followed after an interval of hours or days by a massive hemiplegia, hemianesthesia, homonymous hemianopia, and, if left-sided, aphasia. Occlusion is demonstrable by arteriography. Hemorrhage into the wall of the common or internal carotid artery has been found in a few patients. (See Chap. 357)

REPEATED CONCUSSION (PUNCH DRUNK). The cumulative effects of repeated injuries, observed almost exclusively in professional boxers, constitute a type of head injury difficult to classify for it has never been well-studied pathologically. It is a common observation that after a number of years in the ring, pugilists often become forgetful, slow in thinking, and slightly dysarthric. Their movements are stiff and uncertain, especially those involving the legs, there is an unsteadiness of gait, and occasionally involuntary movements. The plantar reflexes may be extensor on one side or both sides. The electroencephalogram shows slow waves of theta and sometimes of delta type. The anatomic basis of this disease is unknown. The postulation of showers of petechial hemorrhages from repeated blows on the jaw should not be given credence until demonstrated pathologically. The brain is atrophied, and a pneumoencephalogram will reveal dilated lateral ventricles. The findings of diffuse degeneration of the cerebral white matter have been demonstrated in rabbits and monkeys which have been subjected to repeated concussions (Jakob) and offer a more acceptable possibility. Low pressure hydrocephalus is another possibility.

SEQUELAE OF SEVERE HEAD INJURY

The signs of focal brain disease, whether due to open and penetrating or closed head injuries, tend always to ameliorate as the months pass. A hemiplegia is often reduced to a minimal hemiparesis or ineptitude of voluntary motor function with exaggerated reflexes and an equivocal Babinski sign on that side, and aphasia improves to become a stuttering or hesitant paraphasia which is not disabling except in a professional worker, speaker, or writer. Many of the signs of brain stem disease improve, often to an astonishing degree.

PROTRACTED TRAUMATIC COMA AND PSEUDO-COMA. Of particular interest is the outcome of those rare conditions in which the patient remains comatose for weeks or months or even years. The authors have examined the brains of nearly a dozen cases of this type, and nearly all have shown numerous foci of hemorrhage and ischemic necrosis in the midbrain and subthalamus, especially in the tegmentum and tectum. They were probably due in most instances to temporal lobe herniation and midbrain compression, for one could see where one side of the base and tegmentum had been indented by the free edge of the tentorium. In others there may have been direct injury to the midbrain and pons, with numerous small hemorrhages. Presumably these pathologic changes are not constant, for scattered lesions in the cerebral cortex (contusions of the summits of convolutions, ischemia with necrosis in the depths of sulci) and a remarkable diffuse degeneration of cerebral white matter have also been observed in cases of this type (Strich). These patients, while comatose (i.e., unreceptive to stimuli and unresponsive) or in a state of pseudocoma (receptive and capable of signaling by blinking their eyes but otherwise unresponsive), usually exhibit a variety of neurologic abnormalities: unequal pupils; dilated, fixed pupil and oculomotor palsy on one side and hemiplegia on the other; disturbances of gaze; bilateral pyramidal paralysis with Babinski signs; extensor postures of arm and leg on one side and flexed arm and extended leg on the other; brain stem attacks (extension of limbs, increased respiration, blood pressure, and sweating on stimulation of any kind); and involuntary movements (tremor, chorea, athetosis). Some remain in this reduced mental state until death (after nearly 10 years in one of the author's cases, but usually after a few months or a year or two). The majority, however, may regain enough function to leave the hospital; not a few, surprising as it may seem, are restored to full alertness and adequate mental function. Residual weakness of limbs, slurred speech, ocular palsies, ataxia of an arm or leg, or involuntary movements are frequent. During convalescence, language mechanisms may be found disturbed in various ways, i.e. mutism, akinesia or adynamia (lack of volition or impulse to speak or move), dysarthria, and, if there are contusions of the cortex of the dominant hemisphere, an aphasia as well. Any one or a combination of these abnormalities may be present.

EPILEPSY. Posttraumatic epilepsy, which occurs in 20 to 40 percent of patients, is one of the most dreaded complications of head injury. Its basis is nearly always a contusion or laceration of the cortex. The likelihood of epilepsy is said to be greater in parietal and posterior frontal lesions, but it may arise from lesions in any area of the cerebral cortex. The incidence of epilepsy is much greater in "open" than in "closed" head injuries. Indeed, in cases of pure concussion without contusion or laceration, seizures are not much more frequent than in the general population. The interval between head injury and the first seizure averages about 9 months, but it may be much longer, i.e., many years, particularly in children. The longer the interval, the less certain one is of its relationship to the traumatic incident. There is a slightly greater tendency for those patients who had seizures at the time of head injury to become subject to recurrent seizures later. The seizures are always of focal character, or grand mal; petit mal is rarely if ever due to trauma. The significance of the different patterns of focal seizures, which vary according to the location of the lesion, has been worked out in detail by Penfield and his associates (see Chap. 28) and by Russell et al. The frequency of seizures in any given patient varies widely; some patients have only a few, others many, with episodes of status epilepticus. The electroencephalogram is of value in diagnosis; a focus of spike or sharp waves is the characteristic finding. Usually the seizures can be controlled by anticonvulsant medications, and only the recalcitrant cases are likely to require excision of the epileptic focus. The surgical results vary according to the methods of selection and technique of operation. Seizures are abolished in approximately 50 percent of cases by excision of the focus. They tend to decrease in frequency as the years pass, and some patients (an estimated 10 to 30 percent) stop having them.

IMPAIRMENT OF MENTAL FUNCTION. Fortunately this is a rare sequela to head trauma. Although mental function may be disturbed by focal lesions which produce dysphasia, agnosia, apraxia, etc., intellectual functions and memory are usually preserved.

POSTTRAUMATIC NERVOUS INSTABILITY. Undoubtedly the most troublesome sequela of head injury is that alluded to above in the discussion of the first group of cases under Clinical Manifestations—*headache, giddiness,* and *nervous instability.* This has been called the *postconcussional syndrome* or the *minor contusion syndrome* (Trotter), or *posttraumatic vasomotor neurosis* (Friedmann). All these terms are objectionable on the grounds that they suggest an explanatory hypothesis, as yet unproved. Headache is the central symptom, usually, at times localized to the part struck. It is variously described as an aching, throbbing, pounding, stabbing, pressing pain and is remarkable for its variability. The intensification of symptoms by mental and physical effort, straining, stooping, and emotional excitement has already been mentioned. Rest and quiet may relieve them. Thus the headache becomes a major obstacle to convalescence, which demands always a resumption of normal activities. The dizziness is usually not a true vertigo but a giddiness. The patient feels suddenly unsteady, dazed, weak, or faint. However, a certain number of patients report symptoms which suggest a labyrinthine disorder. For example, objects in the environment are said to move momentarily, and looking upward or to the side may cause a sense of unbalance. Labyrinthine tests may show either hypo- or hyperreactivity, or the results may prove to be normal. The data are usually so indefinite that it is impossible to state whether or not the labyrinth and vestibular mechanisms have been injured. Exceptionally, vertigo is accompanied by diminished excitability of both the labyrinth and the cochlea, and one may assume the existence of direct injury to the nerve or end organ. The giddy patient usually is intolerant of noise, emotional excitement, and crowds. Tenseness, restlessness, inability to concentrate, a feeling of nervousness, fatigue, worry, apprehension, and an inability to tolerate the usual amount of alcohol complete the clinical picture. In contrast to the multiple subjective symptoms, detailed tests of intellectual functions and memory show little or no impairment. This syndrome, once established, may persist for months or even years, but usually the symptoms lessen as time passes. Strangely, it is almost unknown in children. Its intensity and duration are augmented by compensation problems and litigation, suggesting a psychopathologic process.

EXTRAPYRAMIDAL AND CEREBELLAR DISORDERS. The question of *posttraumatic Parkinson's syndrome* has been discussed many times, usually with the general conclusion that a true traumatic parkinsonism does not exist. Most patients have merely had paralysis agitans or postencephalitic Parkinson's disease brought to light by head injury. Cerebellar ataxia is a rare consequence of cranial trauma. When present, it is frequently unilateral and due to injury of the superior cerebellar peduncle. An ataxia of gait may reflect a communicating hydrocephalus.

POSTTRAUMATIC HYDROCEPHALUS. These not infrequent examples of posttraumatic hydrocephalus exhibit intermittent headaches, vomiting, confusion, and drowsiness, and autopsy has demonstrated an adhesive basilar meningitis, attributed to subarachnoid or ventricular hemorrhage. Later, mental dullness, apathy, and psychomotor retardation are the principal manifestations. The CSF pressure may then have fallen to a normal level (low-pressure hydrocephalus). Since symptoms like these have been observed occasionally after the rupture of a saccular aneurysm with massive subarachnoid hemorrhage, due presumably to blocking of the aqueduct and fourth ventricle by blood clot, this mechanism has also been suggested as a possible explanation of traumatic hydrocephalus in patients with cerebral confusion. Response to ventriculo-atrial shunt may be dramatic.

POSTTRAUMATIC PSYCHIATRIC DISORDERS. In contrast to nervousness and nervous instability, which are common sequelae of injuries of all types, posttraumatic psychoses are relatively infrequent. The most distressing psychiatric syndromes have been suspiciousness and paranoid delusions, unaccountable outbursts of violent temper, sometimes with homicidal or suicidal tendencies, progressive hyperactivity, delirium, and mania, and episodes of bizarre behavior with subsequent amnesia, reminiscent of temporal lobe seizures. Alcoholism may provoke some of these behavioral abnormalities. Some of these illnesses are undoubtedly due to residual brain damage in individuals of peculiar personality makeup. However, attempts to account for psychoses of this type by reference to constitutional peculiarities and predisposition, laid bare, so to speak, by head injury, have not been convincing.

CLINICAL APPROACH TO THE PATIENT WHO HAS SUFFERED HEAD INJURY; SUGGESTED PLAN FOR MANAGEMENT

The physician who undertakes to treat the "head injury case" must at all times bear in mind that assiduous attention to detail may prove to be lifesaving, and that accurate documentation of all diagnostic findings and therapy is desirable if the medical data are later to be used in the arbitration of insurance claims, worker's unemployment compensation, etc. The suggestions which follow can do no more than serve as guides, for every patient presents a combination of problems that the physician has not encountered before and may not observe again in identical form.

Exact data concerning the patient's medical status before the accident (previous illnesses, work and social record, emotional stability), the nature and precise circumstances of the accident, the duration of retrograde and anterograde amnesia, and all that transpired afterward should be obtained and recorded. Verbatim statements should be written down whenever possible.

The treatment problems presented by each of the three groups of clinical cases discussed above are as follows.

MINOR HEAD INJURY. In this group are included patients who (1) were never unconscious at any time, (2) were briefly unconscious at the time of the first examination, (3) are rapidly regaining consciousness.

Circumstances dictate how each case is managed. If the injury was trivial and the scalp was not lacerated, and if the patient is entirely clear mentally, little or nothing need be done. When the patient is unable to give an accurate account of what has happened and appears still to be somewhat confused or incoherent, he should be compelled to lie down or at least remain in one place. It often happens that the confusion is not detected and the patient is permitted to resume activity while still acting in an irrational manner. He may get into his car and attempt to drive, only to have another accident; or if he is an athlete he may continue to play a game and make a series of errors.

When a conscious or nearly conscious patient is admitted to a general hospital, it is tempting to let him go his way. Experience teaches caution, however. A complete examination, with the patient fully undressed, should be carried out. It is well, if there is any likelihood of litigation, to obtain x-rays of the skull and an electroencephalogram. Whether to perform a lumbar puncture will usually depend on how serious the injury was, on the prominence of posttraumatic headache, etc. A simple fracture without involvement of paranasal sinuses requires no special treatment but is believed to contraindicate vigorous athletic activities for several months or a year.

PATIENTS WHO ARE UNCONSCIOUS WHEN FIRST SEEN. If the physician arrives on the scene of the accident, a hurried examination should be made before the patient is moved in order to determine whether there is dangerous hemorrhage from a laceration of the scalp or other parts of the body and whether there is a likelihood of a fracture-dislocation of the cervical spine, which is occasionally associated with head injury. If the patient is in shock, with cold clammy skin and feeble pulse, he should be covered with warm blankets. In moving an individual with a potential cervical spine injury, the spine should be kept straight at all times and flexion of the neck should be avoided. This can best be done by placing sand bags or firm pillows on either side of the head and warning everyone against neck flexion. An even safer method is to place the patient on a stretcher face down and arrange pillows to assure a clear airway. Bleeding from the scalp can usually be controlled with a firm pad unless an artery is divided, and then a suture becomes necessary.

In the hospital, where all such patients should be taken, the first steps should be to control shock. This can usually be done by the application of warmth, keeping the head low, and leaving the patient alone for a few minutes. The shock will usually come under control in a few minutes with or without vasopressor drugs or transfusions. Persistent shock is rare in head injury and always raises the suspicion of a ruptured viscera with internal bleeding, extensive fractures, or traumatism of the cervical spinal cord. A quick survey will enable one to estimate the depth of coma, size of pupils, and presence of obvious fractures; and if shock is not present, or after the blood pressure has stabilized, a more detailed examination can be performed. The skull should be carefully inspected and palpated. The hair should be cut off around the scalp wound. A bogginess of the temporal or postauricular region (Battle's sign), bleeding from the nose or ear, extensive conjunctival edema, and hemorrhage are useful signs of underlying skull fracture. However, it should be remembered that rupture of the eardrum or a blow on the nose may also cause bleeding from the ear and nose, respectively. Fractures of the orbital bones may cause displacement of the eye, with resulting diplopia, and fracture of the jaws, disalignment of the teeth, and great discomfort on attempting to open the mouth. Careful notes should be made regarding temperature, pulse, blood pressure, state of consciousness, pupil size, ocular movements, corneal reflexes, facial movements during grimace, swallowing, tone of limb muscles, movements of limbs, predominant postures, and reflexes. Vital signs and consciousness should be checked and recorded by the nurse or physician every 2 hr. A proper airway must be maintained. The best position for the patient is semisupine, with the head on a pillow and turned to one side. If urine is retained and the bladder distended, a catheter should be inserted and kept there. If coma persists for more than 48 to 72 hr, a nasal tube should be passed and fluids and nourishment given by that route. Intravenous fluids should be administered slowly and not in excessive amounts; even hypertonic glucose may increase oncoming pulmonary and cerebral edema, the danger of the latter being especially great in children. Lumbar puncture should be done as soon as practicable for diagnostic purposes (immediately if bacterial meningitis is suspected), and if the pressure is elevated it should be lowered to 100 to 150 mm. The practice of daily lumbar punctures has its advocates and its opponents. The authors have tended to use them only if the pressure is elevated and the patient's condition is not improving. Hypertonic solutions intravenously are of therapeutic value. One hundred milliliters of hypertonic urea, or if not available, 50 to 100 ml of 25 percent mannitol may be injected intravenously in an attempt to lower CSF pressure. Recently corticosteroid, e.g., Decadron (16 to 48 mg per day), have been strikingly effective in reducing brain swelling and permitting vital signs to stabilize. X-rays of skull and other parts should be taken after the first day or two, unless there is a suspicion of an epidural hemorrhage, in which case they should be made at once, to visualize a crack across the course of the middle meningeal artery. Restlessness is controlled by sodium phenobarbital or paraldehyde, but only if careful nursing does not quiet the patient and permit him to sleep for a few hours at a time.

Once the patient has regained consciousness, the danger of suffocation, aspiration pneumonia, thrombophlebitis, and pulmonary embolism has usually passed, and therapy can proceed along the lines indicated for the first group.

It is often stated that death from head injury during the first 12 to 24 hr is the direct effect of primary brain injury and cannot be prevented. The advisability of any surgical procedure during the period is much debated. If the patient survives for one, two, or more days and remains in coma, the control of brain swelling and hemorrhage by surgical means must be considered. Should the condition of the patient then begin to deteriorate (pulse rising, temperature subnormal or rising, state of consciousness worsening, hemiplegia more obvious, plantar reflexes more clearly extensor), a decision must be made concerning an epidural or subdural hemorrhage and of increasing brain edema with temporal lobe herniation. Rowbotham, who has had a large experience with cases of this type, recommends a right-sided temporal decompression and two inspection burr holes in the left, one at the Sylvian point and one at the parietal eminence, for some of these patients. In his opinion the indications for surgery are (1) retrogression following a period of improvement, which cannot be controlled by lumbar puncture and oral and rectal hypertonic solutions of intravenous dehydration measures; (2) decerebrate rigidity which has its onset after an interval of 24 hr (early decerebrate rigidity implies primary brainstem injury) if meningitis is ruled out; (3) a dilated fixed pupil on one side, with no improvement after 12 hr; (4) prolonged unconsciousness associated with persistently high cerebrospinal fluid pressure. Not all neurologists and neurosurgeons are agreed on the value of surgical decompression, but certainly the removal of a large epidural or subdural hemorrhage, which cannot be diagnosed easily in the comatose patient, may be a lifesaving procedure.

In recent years a striking reduction in the mortality of these acute head injuries has been obtained by the application of intensive care together with the free use of tracheostomy. Many of the comatose patients who would otherwise have succumbed to respiratory obstruction, pulmonary infections, or dehydration are thereby saved. Also, greater efforts to evacuate intracranial hematomas as soon as possible seems to have helped. The mortality rate of a group of patients in a state of decerebrate rigidity is reduced by 50 percent, and the total mortality of all hospitalized patients has fallen from about 10 to 3.5 percent. Survivors may be left permanently disabled, but a surprising number, the percentage increasing up to 7 years, return to productive work.

The treatment of the patient with protracted coma has been outlined in Chap. 26. Every patient presents special problems which must be dealt with individually.

PATIENTS WHO TEMPORARILY RECOVERED CONSCIOUSNESS (LUCID INTERVAL) AND THEN BECAME STUPOROUS OR COMATOSE. The treatment is that of epidural, subdural, and delayed cerebral hemorrhage. This has already been discussed.

GENERAL CONVALESCENCE

A head injury carries dire import to most lay individuals, who often fear for their mind and are concerned about their capacity to resume their place in society. In former times, therapeutic measures often involved long discussions of the seriousness of the injury, protracted bed rest, and inactivity, all of which served only to engender greater anxiety. Even worse, these measures were not of proved value. It is now widely acknowledged that the patient does better if his physician tends to minimize the seriousness of his head injury and to reassure him that he will recover. Early rehabilitation should be encouraged. It may safely begin as soon as the cerebrospinal fluid becomes clear, usually within a few weeks at the most, except of course in the rare cases of protracted coma.

Posttraumatic headache, dizziness, and nervousness are the most difficult symptoms; an optimistic prognosis and the institution of a program of graded mental and physical activities to the point of tolerance stand the best chance of restoring the patient to a useful life. The patient should be told that he must expect a certain amount of headache and should carry on in spite of it. Meprobamate, 200 mg t.i.d., is useful for anxiety, and a non-habit-forming analgesic medication should be given for the more severe headaches (Empirin or aspirin). Insomnia may require a barbiturate medication or chloral hydrate at first, but these drugs should be discontinued as soon as possible. Any litigation that may be involved should be settled within 6 to 9 months. To delay settlement usually works against the best interests of the patient. The severity of his injury can be ascertained within this period of time, and a longer period of observation only enhances his worries and fears and reduces his motivation to return to work.

The prognosis of head injury, in good hands, is influenced by several variables. Elderly patients often remain disabled, especially when compensation is involved. Young and middle-aged adults do better if they are not entitled to compensation (Russell's figures: 70 percent of patients with compensation benefits back at work in 18 months; 83 percent of those without compensation working at the end of this period). Russell also pointed out that the severity of the injury as measured by the duration of traumatic amnesia was a factor. If the period of amnesia was less than 1 hr, 95 percent of patients were back at work within 2 months; if longer than 24 hr, only 80 percent had returned to work within 6 months. About 60 percent, however, still had symptoms at the end of 2 months, and 40 percent at the end of 18 months. Of the most severely injured (those comatose for several days), many will remain permanently disabled. However, recovery is always better than one expects, and the motor impairment, aphasia, and dementia tend to clear. Improvement may continue over a period of 5 or more years. Children seem to recover more completely than adults. Rehabilitation centers are of great help in restoring morale and reeducating the patient.

(For discussion of traumatism of spinal cord, nerve roots, and peripheral nerves, see Chaps. 356, 361, and 354.)

REFERENCES

Brock, S. (Ed.): "Injuries of the Brain and Spinal Cord and Their Coverings," 3d ed., p. 71, Baltimore, The Williams & Wilkins Company, 1949.

Merritt, H. H.: Diagnostic Considerations in Patients with Head Injury, Res. Publ., Assoc. Res. Nervous Mental Disease, 24:379, 1943.

Munro, D.: "The Treatment of Injuries to the Nervous System," Philadelphia, W. B. Saunders Company, 1952.

Rowbotham, G. F.: "Acute Injuries of the Head," 4th ed. Baltimore, The Williams & Wilkins Company, 1964.

359   NEOPLASTIC DISEASE OF THE BRAIN

Henry deF. Webster and Raymond D. Adams

Tumors of the central nervous system play a very important part in neurologic medicine and occupy a distinct field by themselves. It may be said of them generally that they occur in great variety; produce neurologic symptoms because of size, location, and invasive qualities; usually destroy the tissues in which they are situated and displace those around them; are a frequent cause of increased intracranial pressure; and are often lethal.

For the student of medicine the most important facts to know are that (1) many types of tumor occur in the cranial cavity and spinal canal and that certain ones are much more frequent than others (see Table 359-1); (2)

Table 359-1. INCIDENCE OF INTRACRANIAL AND INTRASPINAL TUMORS AT BOSTON CITY HOSPITAL, 1900–1930

Total no. of autopsies		10,592
Total no. of tumors		1,458
Tumors of other organs	1,270	
Intracranial and intraspinal tumors	188 (12.7%)	
Gliomas	81 (43.1%)	
Pituitary adenomas	6 (3.2%)	
Sheath tumors	22 (11.7%)	
Meningioma .. 18		
Acoustic neuroma.... 4		
Metastatic tumors	29 (15.4%)	
Blood vessel tumors	6 (3.0%)	
Congenital tumors	8 (4.3%)	
Granulomas	19 (10.1%)	
Spinal cord tumors	4 (2.1%)	
Unclassified	13 (7.1%)	

some of these tumors, such as the craniopharyngioma, meningioma, and schwannoma, have a disposition to grow in certain parts of the cranial cavity; (3) their growth rates vary, some like the glioblastoma being highly malignant and invasive, others like the meningioma being benign and compressive. These pathologic peculiarities are important for they have valuable clinical correlations, providing the explanation of slowly or rapidly progressive clinical states, excellent or poor prognosis after surgical excision, etc. It is for these reasons that the clinician is encouraged to learn a histologic classification and to think always in terms of particular types of intracranial and intraspinal tumors.

The one place where these pathologic-clinical correlations tend to fail is in the glioma group of tumors, i.e., astrocytoma-glioblastoma series, and this is regrettable because tumors of this type are so common. Often these gliomas are of mixed cell type. For example, one part of the tumor may be a typical astrocytoma and another an oligodendrocytoma. Also the degree of differentiation or its opposite, the degree of anaplasia, varies from one part of the tumor to another. As would be expected with such heterogeneous growths, a biopsy sample is often misleading with reference to the expected clinical behavior of the tumor. For example, the clinician may be led to believe that a tumor which in a biopsy is composed of astrocytes is benign, whereas actually the main mass of it still in the brain is a glioblastoma; or a small nodule of glioblastoma in an excised specimen may suggest a hopeless prognosis when actually the remainder of the tumor in the brain is a well-differentiated astrocytoma.

TYPES OF BRAIN TUMORS AND THEIR INCIDENCE

Most of the available statistics on the different types of tumors of the central nervous system have been collected in special neurosurgical clinics and are somewhat misleading, for they fail to reveal their natural incidence in an unselected population. The figures in Table 359-1, compiled by Peer, are thus rather exceptional, for they avoid this error of selection and represent the natural incidence of these tumors in postmortem material during the period 1900–1930, at a time when very little neurosurgery was being performed in the hospital from which they were taken (Boston City Hospital).

These data reveal that the central nervous system and its enveloping tissues are fruitful soil for tumor growth and, further, that the bulk of these tumors are gliomas, metastatic tumors, and meningiomas. The increasing rarity of gummas and tuberculomas, noted in all pathologic material from the United States during the past 2 decades, leads to the belief that far fewer than 10 percent of intracranial growths are of granulomatous nature; and the rising age of the population and the increasing frequency of all types of tumors would probably raise the figures for secondary tumors. Of the gliomas, approximately half are glioblastoma multiforme, and the remainder are divided between astrocytoma, oligodendroglioma, ependymoma, medulloblastoma, and undiagnosed gliomas. All statistics show the peak age incidence to be the fifth decade of life, with a fairly symmetric curve which reflects the lessening incidence at the extremes of age—infancy and the senescence. In children, tumors of the posterior fossa (medulloblastomas, ependymomas, and gliomas) predominate; in adults, supratentorial tumors (glioblastomas, meningiomas, and metastatic carcinomas) are more frequent. Males appear to be more susceptible to intrinsic tumors of the brain (gliomas) than females, the ratio being 2:1. In contrast the meningioma occurs more frequently in elderly women.

INTRACRANIAL TUMORS

PATHOPHYSIOLOGY. The cranium, according to the Monro-Kellie law, contains three elements—nervous tissue, blood, and cerebrospinal fluid—the total bulk of which must always be constant. Any increase in the volume of the brain, for example, can take place only at the expense of one of the other elements; and a diminished volume of brain (as in cerebral atrophy) is compensated by an increase in the amount of cerebrospinal fluid. Another noteworthy fact is that the cerebrospinal fluid pressure, while reflecting the volume of the intracranial mass, is largely maintained by the pressure under which the blood is delivered to the skull. In profound shock the cerebrospinal fluid pressure falls, and at death it is zero.

When a tumor or other space-occupying mass forms in the cranial cavity, the volume of cerebrospinal fluid within the subarachnoid and ventricular spaces is reduced and the cerebrospinal fluid is displaced into the spinal and perioptic subarachnoid spaces. Soon, however, the limits of these adjustments are surpassed, and the pressure throughout the ventricles and in all parts of the subarachnoid space rises. Presumably the veins in the cerebral tissues adjacent to the tumor are compressed, with resulting increase in venous pressure locally—the conditions necessary for *regional swelling*, or *edema*. Inasmuch as any general increase in venous pressure results in retarded absorption of cerebrospinal fluid and an increase in its volume, the pressure in the subarachnoid space and veins is nearly the same at all times. If the rise in cerebrospinal fluid pressure is slow, the stasis of blood resulting from this elevated venous pressure can be compensated for by vasodilatation of arteries and arterioles, and cerebral circulation is unimpaired. If the rise is rapid and to high levels approaching diastolic blood pressure, the blood pressure must rise, usually the systolic more than the diastolic, in order to maintain cerebral blood flow. As a rule this is accompanied by a slow, bounding pulse. Under these conditions, the velocity of cerebral blood flow again approaches normal. Presumably these circulatory reflexes, which result in the rise of blood pressure and bradycardia, are initiated by venous stasis and accumulation of carbon dioxide in the vasomotor center in the medulla oblongata. The respiratory centers also become affected, for increases in intracranial pressure usually cause an irregularity and finally a cessation of respiration.

These changes in blood pressure, pulse, and respiration are of importance in the clinic, for they may afford valuable clues as to the existence of increased intracranial pressure. Not less valuable is the papilledema, or "choked disk," that can be seen with an ophthalmoscope in the optic fundi of most patients who have elevated intracranial pressure of more than a few days' standing. The papilledema is best accounted for by the high pressure in the subarachnoid space surrounding the optic nerves.

Raised intracranial pressure due to a mass or enlargement of the ventricles (blockage of cerebrospinal fluid circulation), when severe, causes obtundation of cerebral function. This is manifested clinically by a number of characteristic symptoms and electroencephalographically by diffuse slowing of the electrical activity of the cortex. The rate of cerebral blood flow is slowed.

Another extremely important anatomic fact is that the closed cranial "box" is subdivided into fairly rigid compartments by two infoldings of dura mater, one the falx, which lies between the two cerebral hemispheres, and the other the tentorium, which separates the cerebellum from the occipital lobes. These anatomic arrangements and the opening at the base of the skull through which the spinal cord and medulla are joined leave three important apertures, the foramen magnum, the tentorial opening or "notch," and the subfalcial or supracallosal space. A tumor growth in one compartment, say the right middle cranial fossa, raises the pressure in that compartment more than in the others, and either brain or tumor tissue tends to be displaced along lines of least resistance, i.e., through the subfalcial space to the left half of the cranial cavity and through the tentorial opening into the posterior fossa on the right side. These brain displacements are exceedingly dangerous and contribute, as a rule, to the death of the patient in most cases of intracranial tumor, abscess, trauma, and subdural and epidural hemorrhage. The temporal lobe–tentorial hernia is said to stretch the ipsilateral oculomotor nerve (Hutchinson's pupil—a dilated pupil on the side of a lesion, and also a drooping eyelid); to displace and compress the midbrain with resulting stupor or coma, bilateral pyramidal signs (often greater on the side of the hernia), decerebrate postures of extension of all four extremities, and perhaps irregularity and final arrest of respiration; and to distort and partially block the aqueduct of Sylvius and to narrow the perimesencephalic subarachnoid space with resulting hydrocephalus and rising intracranial pressure. Also, the posterior cerebral arteries may be occluded on one side or both sides, with infarction of the occipital lobes. The cerebellar-foramen magnum pressure cone (herniation of cerebellar tonsils), in which the cerebellar tissue or tumor mass is displaced into the cervical spinal canal with compression of the medulla oblongata, results in tilting or altered posture of the head, dilated pupils, impairment of consciousness, and death due to respiratory arrest. The physiologic and clinical effects of subfalcial herniation are not known.

A knowledge of these effects of elevated intracranial pressure and of the herniations and displacements of tissue is necessary if one is to understand the clinical behavior of intracranial growths. Symptoms and signs of brain tumor depend not only on the invasion and destruction of important nervous structures but also on these pressure phenomena.

CLINICAL AND PATHOLOGIC CHARACTERISTICS. It may be said at the very outset that tumors of the brain may exist with hardly any symptoms. Often only a slight deficiency in mental power, a slowness in comprehension, or a loss of capacity in sustaining continuous mental activity suggests any deviation from normal health.

Specific signs that would lead to a suspicion of any real cerebral disease may be wholly wanting. In some patients, on the other hand, there is evidence of cerebral disease in the form of a seizure or some other dramatic symptom, but the evidence is not clear enough to warrant the diagnosis of a cerebral tumor. In a third group, the existence of a new growth in the brain may be determined with much probability by the presence of signs of elevated intracranial pressure, but there are no symptoms which disclose localization of the growth. Lastly, the symptoms may be so clear and definite as to make it probable not only that there is a new growth within the cranium but that it is located in one particular region. In fact these localized growths may create unique tumor syndromes, unlike those of any other disease.

These are the plain facts of clinical observation; in the further exposition of this subject, therefore, all intracranial tumors are considered in relation to the common clinical circumstances in which they are likely to be encountered, as follows:

1. The patient whose presenting symptom is either a decline in general mental ability or a seizure.

2. The patient with unmistakable evidence of raised intracranial pressure.

3. Specific intracranial tumor syndromes.

THE PATIENT WITH GENERAL SYMPTOMS OF CEREBRAL DISEASE OR A SEIZURE AS THE MAIN COMPLAINT. In general practice or on the wards of the hospital, these are the patients who give the most trouble in diagnosis and about whom decisions are often made with a great degree of uncertainty. Their symptoms are general, as a rule, and not until some time has elapsed will signs of focal brain disease be added; and when they do, they are not always of accurate localizing value. Altered psychic function, headache, giddiness, and seizures comprise the usual symptoms in this group of patients.

As pointed out by Knapp, some *change in mental function* may be found in nearly every patient of this type, but it may be necessary to obtain the observations of a person who knows the patient intimately to learn of it. A lack of power of persistent application to the tasks of the day, an undue irritability, emotional lability, a "peculiar inertia," faulty insight, forgetfulness, inability to retain impressions, indifference to common social practices, lack of initiative and spontaneity, all of which may be attributable to worry, anxiety, or depression, are the usual symptoms. Much of this behavior is accepted by the patient with forbearance, and if he has any complaint it is of being weak, tired, dizzy (nonrotational), or "queer in the head." Inordinate drowsiness, a remarkable equanimity, and stoicism may be prominent findings. These symptoms become more persistent and obtrusive with the passage of time. Usually within a few weeks or months the drowsiness and mental dullness increase. Then a curious inertia and lack of spontaneity become even more conspicuous and are evident during the interview. The patient seems strangely indifferent to the questions of the examiner. A long pause precedes each reply, and at times he may not bother to respond at all. Or at the very moment when the examiner has decided that the patient has not heard the question and prepares to repeat it, an appropriate, sensible answer is given, usually in relatively few words. The responses are often much more intelligent than would be expected from the torpid mental state. There are, in addition, patients who are confused or demented (see Chap. 30). The dullness and somnolence may gradually increase, and finally, as increased intracranial pressure supervenes, they end in coma.

Mental symptoms of this type cannot be ascribed to disease in any particular part of the brain. S. A. K. Wilson has expressed the opinion that tumors are most likely to be accompanied by intellectual disturbance when they interfere with large association fiber systems such as the corpus callosum, inferior and superior longitudinal fasciculi, etc.; growths limited to the cortex and subcortical white matter are less likely to affect the mind. The drowsiness, torpor, inertia, lack of spontaneity, and general restriction of mental horizon are usually related to increased intracranial pressure and are unrelated to the site and nature of the lesion.

The *headaches* in the "tumor patient" may vary exceedingly. In some the pain is slight, temporary, and dull in character; in others it may be severe and unendurable, being either dull or sharp, but as a rule transitory or intermittent. If there are any characteristics of the headache, it would be its nocturnal occurrence, its presence on first awakening, and its deep nonpulsatile quality. However, these are not specific attributes, since migraine, hypertensive vascular headaches, etc., may also begin early in the morning on first awakening. The patient does not always complain of the pain even when it is present, and often he betrays its existence by placing his hand on his forehead and looking distressed.

The mechanism of the headache is not known. In the majority of instances, the intracranial pressure is normal during the first weeks when the headache is present, and one can attribute it only to distortion or alteration of blood vessels in or around the tumor. Later the headache appears to be related to rises in intracranial pressure. The location of the headache bears some relation to the situation of the growth. Tumors above the tentorium cause headache on the side of and in the vicinity of the tumor, usually in the orbital, frontal, temporal, or parietal regions. Tumors in the posterior fossa usually cause ipsilateral retroauricular or occipital headache. With elevated intracranial pressure, bifrontal and bioccipital headache is the rule, regardless of the location of the tumor.

Vomiting appears in about one-third of the patients with tumor syndromes of this type and usually accompanies the headache. It is more frequent with tumors of the posterior fossa. Some patients may vomit unexpectedly and forcibly, without preceding nausea (projectile vomiting), but others suffer both nausea and great pain. Usually the vomiting is not related to the ingestion of food, often occurring before breakfast.

No less frequent is the complaint of *giddiness* or *dizziness*. As a rule it is not described with accuracy and consists of a more or less confused sensation in the head, coupled with feelings of strangeness and insecurity when the head position is altered.

One or more generalized *convulsions* is the other major symptom which calls attention to the existence of cerebral tumor. Their frequency in various statistical analyses is 20 to 50 percent of all patients with cerebral tumors. The onset of a seizure during adult years and the existence of a localizing aura are always suggestive of tumor. The localizing significance of seizure patterns has already been discussed (see Chap. 28). The seizures may occur once or many times and may precede other symptoms for as long as 10 years or more in cases of astrocytoma or meningioma.

The management of patients who present any one of the aforementioned symptoms requires brief discussion. The physician is well advised, whenever he encounters any clinical problem of this type, to consider the possibility of a cerebral tumor in its early stages. A careful inquiry should then be made concerning the rest of the symptoms of this complex. In other words, if either a recurrent headache, of a type which the patient recognizes as different from his customary headaches, or a seizure, appearing for the first time, has occurred, there is indication for a careful review of the patient's general behavior. In obtaining further data, one must rely heavily on the observations of other members of the family. A thorough neurologic examination with careful inspection of optic fundi, a test of visual fields, motor, reflex, and sensory functions in the limbs, alertness, memory, facility in language (speaking, reading, writing, and understanding the spoken word), calculation, and tests of visuospatial orientation must follow. Sooner or later other regional or localizing symptoms and signs will be discovered, and it is only by repeated examinations that one will note the earliest stages of a hemiparesis, aphasia, visual field defect, hemianesthesia, etc. (For the interpretation of these localizing symptoms and signs the reader is referred to Chaps. 21, 25, 30.) Unmistakable signs of increased intracranial pressure may become manifest and establish the diagnosis of tumor with reasonable certainty (see Astrocytoma, below).

The necessity of performing confirmatory diagnostic tests will be realized sooner or later, and the decision as to the appropriate time for doing them requires balanced clinical judgment. Since many of the symptoms described above are in no way specific, one should rely on repeated and thorough examinations and should not proceed too quickly to expensive and difficult diagnostic tests. Watchful waiting without unduly alarming the patient is the best plan for a certain period. As more of the clinical picture unfolds, however, there comes a time when x-rays of the skull and chest (always done to help rule out metastatic carcinoma), lumbar puncture (for pressure, cells, protein, and Wassermann reaction), and localizing electroencephalogram should be made, preferably by admitting the patient to a hospital. Perimetry, audiograms, vestibular tests, and psychometric tests are also helpful in the study of many of these patients. Pneumoencephalography and carotid arteriography are reserved in most medical neurologic clinics for those in whom the total clinical syndrome is already strongly suggestive of tumor. These procedures are too costly and hazardous to be used routinely in every "tumor suspect."

TUMORS WHICH TEND TO PRODUCE GENERAL CEREBRAL SYMPTOMS OR SEIZURES. The following tumors are most likely to produce initial convulsions or a vague syndrome of headache, giddiness, vomiting, dull or stuporous state, and psychic changes: glioblastoma multiforme, astrocytoma, oligodendroglioma, metastatic carcinoma, meningioma, and primary reticulum cell sarcoma of the cerebrum.

Glioblastoma Multiforme. In all statistic analyses of surgical and postmortem material, glioblastoma multiforme is responsible for more than 25 percent of intracranial gliomas and for more than 90 percent of gliomas of the cerebral hemispheres in adults. Approximately 20 to 30 percent of the cerebral tumors are bilateral, occupy more than one lobe of a hemisphere, or show multicentric foci of growth. Although predominantly cerebral in location, similar tumors may be observed in the brainstem, cerebellum, or spinal cord. The peak incidence is in middle adult life, but no age group is spared.

The glioblastoma is a highly malignant tumor which infiltrates the brain extensively and may attain enormous size. It may extend to the meningeal surface or the ventricular wall, which probably accounts for the elevation of protein level (often over 100 mg per 100 ml) in many cases and sometimes a pleocytosis of 10 to 100 cells or more, mostly lymphocytes. The tumor has a variegated appearance, being a mottled gray, red, orange, or brown, depending on the degree of necrosis and whether hemorrhage is recent or old. It is highly vascular, and in an arteriogram one can often see a network of abnormal vessels, mistaken at times for a hemangioma, and the displacement of normal vessels which may result from any "mass lesion." Some part of one lateral ventricle is often distorted, and both lateral and third ventricles are displaced contralaterally, which may be demonstrated by pneumoencephalography or ventriculography. The vessels in the tumor are excessively permeable to ^{32}P, radioactive arsenic, mercury, which is the basis for radioactive scanning techniques. Calcification and cavity formation are not prominent. The characteristic microscopic pathologic findings are great cellularity with pleomorphism of cells and hyperchromatism of nuclei; identifiable astrocytes with fibrils in combination with astroblasts, tumor giant cells, and cells in mitosis; a curious neoplastic proliferation of the cells of small vessels (adventitial and endothelial); necrosis, pseudopalisading of viable cells, hemorrhage, and thrombosis of vessels. Temporal lobe–tentorial herniation, midbrain compression, midbrain and pontine hemorrhages, and increased intracranial pressure are usually the immediate causes of death.

Clinically the diffuse cerebral symptoms and seizures (present in 30 to 40 percent of cases) usually give way to a more definite frontal, temporal, parietooccipital, or callosal syndrome in a few weeks or months. Seldom, however, do the symptoms and signs point to one lobe,

and often one is satisfied to be able to specify the region of the hemisphere which is involved.

Astrocytoma. The astrocytoma may occur anywhere in the brain or spinal cord. Favored sites are cerebrum, cerebellum, thalamus, optic chiasm, and pons. It is a slowly growing tumor of infiltrative character with a marked tendency to undergo some type of degeneration, with the formation of large cavities or pseudocysts. In some instances much of the tumor may be composed of a pseudocyst surrounded by a thin border of astrocytic tissue, and the only sizable mass of tumor tissue may be a mural nodule. Others of these tumors are noncavitating, grayish-white, firm, and relatively avascular, almost indistinguishable from normal white matter, with which they may merge imperceptibly. Calcium deposits may occur in parts of the tumor and may be seen in a plain x-ray of the skull. The cerebrospinal fluid is acellular, the only abnormality being the increased pressure and elevated protein level in some cases. The tumor by its mass may distort the lateral and third ventricles (seen in pneumoencephalogram or ventriculogram) and may be seen to displace the anterior and middle cerebral arteries in a carotid arteriogram. Microscopically the tumor tissue is composed of well-differentiated astrocytes of fibrillary, protoplasmic, or transitional type.

The majority of cerebral astrocytomas undergo malignant degeneration and present as mixed astrocytomas and glioblastomas.

The astrocytoma may cause trivial symptoms for a long period of time. Seizures, headaches, and bizarre mental symptoms may be present for several years, in a few instances more than 10, before the diagnosis is made. The average survival period after the first symptom is 67 months in cerebral growths and 89 months in cerebellar ones. The cystic astrocytoma of the cerebellum is particularly benign, and some patients are alive and well as long as 20 years after part of the cyst was excised. In such cases, of course, accuracy of the original diagnosis of neoplasm is always open to question. The astrocytoma of the pons, optic nerves, and chiasm will be discussed in more detail later on in this chapter.

Oligodendrocytoma. The oligodendrocytoma is a relatively rare cerebral tumor (5 to 10 percent of gliomas) and is usually slow in its rate of growth (average span of evolution is 66 months). It is generally a soft solid tumor, rarely cystic or hemorrhagic, and through its tendency to calcify (spherules and particles of calcium in microscopic sections) often casts a shadow in the roentgenogram of the skull. Microscopically it is composed of small round cells with spherical nuclei and cytoplasm that stains poorly, forming a halo around the nucleus. Seizures are uncommon, and generalized or focal cerebral symptoms may be present for a long time before the mass of the tumor declares its presence by increased intracranial pressure.

Ependymoma and Ependymoblastoma. Although occasionally this tumor presents as a solitary mass in a cerebral hemisphere in adults, presumably arising from the ependymal wall of the lateral ventricle, its most distinctive form is a papillary growth filling the fourth ventricle of children. It will be discussed further on pp. 1834 and 1835.

The treatment of all forms of glioma of the cerebral hemispheres is partial excision, if feasible, after surgical biopsy. Opinion is divided as to whether x-radiation is beneficial. In many cases the diagnosis of glioblastoma multiforme can now be made from clinical, arteriographic, radioactive isotope, and EEG, and one is justified, at least in some cases, in withholding surgery. The control of intracranial pressure is maintained by the use of Decadron.

Meningioma (Arachnoidal Fibroblastoma and Endothelioma). This is a benign tumor composed of specialized arachnoidal lining cells, arising usually in places where there are arachnoidal villi. Since these clusters of arachnoidal cells penetrate the dura in the vicinity of the venous sinuses, they often appear to originate from the dura itself, hence the old term *dural endothelioma*. Grossly the tumors are firm, gray-white, lobulated, bulbous, or plaquelike masses which indent or compress but do not invade brain tissue. Many of them are highly vascular. In size they are variable; some are only a centimeter or two in size and are turned up as incidental findings at autopsy. Others, usually those which have produced symptoms, have attained a size of 3 to 4 cm or more. The cellular composition permits easy identification. The cells are of uniform type and have the peculiar disposition to encircle one another and to form characteristic whorls and psammoma bodies. The common sites of these tumors are the olfactory groove, tuberculum sellae, parasagittal region, Sylvian fissure, cerebellopontine angle, and spinal canal. Inasmuch as they lie on the surface of the brain in or next to the dura, changes in the skull are frequent. The skull may be eroded over the tumor, and the diploic vessels, which provide part of the blood supply of the tumor, dilate and are usually prominent in an x-ray. Or the tumor cells may invade the bone and stimulate osteoblastic activity, as a consequence of which a bony bulge may be seen and felt, or an endostosis is visualized on the inner table of the skull in an x-ray. The meningioma must be listed with metastatic carcinoma and the true cholesteatoma of the skull as the three tumors most likely to cause a visible cranial boss in relation to cerebral symptoms (*benign, exotoses are neurologically asymptomatic*). Offering a broad vascular meningeal surface as they do, these tumors often elevate the protein level of the cerebrospinal fluid. Their striking vascularity accounts for a characteristic "blush" seen in arteriograms; and the excessive permeability of the vessels, as well as the superficial location of the tumors, makes them ideal subjects for localization with radioactive isotopes. The displacement without invasion of cerebral tissue probably explains the interruption locally of normal alpha frequencies in the electroencephalogram with sharp waves or theta waves, in contrast to the delta waves so often found in infiltrative gliomas. Multiple meningiomas may be found, particularly in cases of neurofibromatosis.

These tumors may be found at any age but are more frequent in advanced years, especially in women.

Metastatic Carcinoma. Of the secondary tumors of the brain only metastatic carcinoma will be discussed here because the other tumors that metastasize to the brain are decidedly rare. Carcinomas reach the brain by hematogenous spread. Probably 35 to 40 percent come from the lung, and approximately 15 percent each from the breast, gastrointestinal tract (usually colon or rectum), and kidney. Melanotic carcinoma of the skin, carcinoma of the stomach, gallbladder, liver, thyroid, testicle, uterus, ovary, etc., account for the remainder, no one of them usually being responsible for more than 3 or 4 percent of secondary tumors of the brain. Carcinoma of the prostate, esophagus, oropharynx, or skin (except for melanocarcinoma) rarely if ever is disseminated in the brain. In more than 75 percent of cases the metastases are multiple and are scattered through both the cerebrum and cerebellum, often near the surface and involving white matter, cortex, and meninges. The hypernephroma and thyroid carcinoma have a greater tendency to form solitary metastases than other tumors, and as with the chorioepithelioma and some lung tumors, the metastases are likely to be hemorrhagic. The tumor tissue generally has all the gross and microscopic features of any carcinomatous implant and excites rather little glial reaction but much edema.

The usual clinical picture in metastatic carcinoma of the brain has already been described under Glioblastoma Multiforme. However, a number of other rather striking clinical neurologic syndromes also occur. One that is particularly difficult to diagnose is a widespread *carcinomatous meningoencephalopathy* with headache, nervousness, depressed mood, trembling, mental confusion, and forgetfulness, the whole picture looking very much like that of general paresis. Carcinomatosis of the cerebellum with headache, dizziness, and ataxia, the ataxia being brought out only by having the patient walk, is another difficult condition to diagnose during life. Such patients may be regarded as hysterical until sudden death due to a cerebellar pressure cone terminates the illness. Here the metastases may be more or less limited to the midline structures of the cerebellum. Symptoms and signs referable to one or several cranial and spinal nerve roots may be combined with headache and confusion in widespread *carcinomatosis of the craniospinal meninges* (carcinomatous meningitis). Usually the cerebrospinal fluid contains a few white blood cells (lymphocytes) and an elevated protein level. Tumor cells can often be identified in Papanicolaou stains of cerebrospinal fluid sediment, and if many are present in the meninges, the sugar values may be subnormal, even as low as zero.

When the syndromes due to these several varieties of metastatic tumor are fully developed, diagnosis is relatively easy. If only headache and vomiting are present, a common error is to explain these symptoms on a psychologic basis. One should make a psychiatric diagnosis only if the patient has the standard symptoms of the mental illnesses (see p. 1884). A lumbar puncture, a chest x-ray (positive in 75 percent of cases of metastatic tumor of brain), sedimentation rate (increased in metastatic carcinoma but not glioblastoma), and other x-rays (gastrointestinal series, barium enema, and pyelograms if symptoms point to these organs) are advisable. The inflammatory neurologic syndromes which accompany carcinoma but which are not due to tumor invasion of the central nervous system, polyneuritis (especially with carcinoma of the lung), polymyositis, and spinocerebellar degeneration (ovarian and other carcinomas) should also be kept in mind.

TUMORS OF INFECTIVE ORIGIN (GRANULOMAS AND PARASITIC CYSTS). Tuberculoma is much less frequent in the United States than it was 20 years ago, and gumma has become almost nonexistent. In fact a patient with serologic syphilis and a positive Wassermann reaction of the cerebrospinal fluid has a greater chance of having two diseases, a cerebral tumor and asymptomatic neurosyphilis, than a gumma. The tuberculoma may occur in any part of the brain, but in children it is more likely to develop in the posterior fossa, i.e., in the cerebellum or brainstem, than in the cerebrum. Often there are a small number of cells and an increased protein content in the cerebrospinal fluid because the lesion frequently lies contiguous to the meninges; and it may at any time give rise to a tuberculous meningitis with typical cerebrospinal fluid formula (50 to 300 cells, increased amount of protein, decreased sugar content, and decreased chloride content).

In South America tuberculoma and gumma are much more frequent, and one can usually depend on evidence of disease in other parts of the body, especially the lungs, and characteristic changes in the cerebrospinal fluid (see Chap. 353) to indicate the nature of the lesion. In addition, cysticercus cellulosae and hydatid cysts are common lesions and should always be suspected when seizures, increased intracranial pressure, or diffuse cerebral symptoms develop in the adult. X-rays of the skull and skeletal muscles (e.g., thigh) may reveal characteristic calcific deposits in cysticercosis. Torula and other fungous granulomas and *Schistosoma japonicum* infection may also present as space-occupying cerebral lesions.

PATIENTS WITH UNMISTAKABLE SIGNS OF INCREASED INTRACRANIAL PRESSURE WHEN FIRST SEEN. A certain number of patients show all the characteristic symptoms and signs of increased intracranial pressure (periodic bifrontal and bioccipital headaches which awaken the patient during the night or are present upon awakening, vomiting that may or may not be expected and may or may not be projectile, mental torpor, and papilledema) when first seen. The physician confronted with this clinical problem is forced to take immediate action, for the condition is potentially dangerous. A critical rise in intracranial hypertension may occur at any time and result in coma, respiratory arrest, and death. Admission to a hospital with neurosurgical service is therefore usually urgent. Nevertheless all the medical aspects of the patient's problem should first be worked out.

Three questions demand immediate answers: (1) Does the patient have a space-occupying intracranial lesion? (2) Where in the cranial cavity is it situated? (3) What is its nature? With respect to the first question it is well to keep in mind that a number of medical conditions may simulate an intracranial growth that causes only the general symptoms of increased intracranial pressure. These are (1) "pseudotumor cerebri," (2) hypertensive encephalopathy, (3) chronic pulmonary disease with hypercapnia and hypoxia, (4) chronic meningitis or adhesive arachnoiditis and/or aqueductal stenosis, (5) thrombosis of cerebral veins and dural sinuses, (6) Addison's disease, hypoparathyroidism, (7) excessive vitamin A and chloromycetin therapy in children, and (8) withdrawal from corticosteroid therapy in children. Several of these conditions have been discussed elsewhere in this book, and it is sufficient to mention them briefly; others have not been considered before and will be discussed in detail.

Pseudotumor Syndromes. In the condition of *pseudotumor cerebri* (meningeal hydrops) the patient, more often than not a child or young woman, complains of headaches of some weeks' standing and when first examined is found to have papilledema or choked disk, with slightly constricted visual fields and enlarged blind spots. Other neurologic signs, with the occasional exception of a vague dizziness, diplopia due to a slight abducens weakness, or paresthesias of some part of the body, are conspicuously absent, and the patient appears remarkably "bright" and well. The cerebrospinal fluid is acellular with normal protein content, a ventriculogram reveals small or normal-sized ventricles, and an arteriogram reveals patency and normal position of arteries and veins, including the superior sagittal and lateral sinuses. With the use of corticosteroid drugs (Decadron, 6 to 12 mg every 6 hr) and daily, then biweekly, then weekly lumbar punctures to lower the cerebrospinal fluid pressure, most of the patients gradually recover over a period of weeks to months. Extremely high cerebrospinal fluid pressure with episodes of cloudy vision (obscurations) may herald the onset of blindness and require a right subtemporal decompression as an emergency measure. The cause of the condition is unknown.

Extreme hypertension (diastolic pressures of 120 mm or over), retinal arteriolar changes with hemorrhages and exudates in the periphery of the optic fundi, signs of renal disease, and headache, convulsions, confusion, stupor, or coma are the basis of the diagnosis of *hypertensive encephalopathy* (see p. 1763). *Chronic emphysema or other lung disease*, with cyanosis, dyspnea, cough, signs of cor pulmonale with right-sided congestive heart failure and secondary polycythemia, may be attended by bilateral papilledema, elevated cerebrospinal fluid pressure, high venous pressure, severe headache, drowsiness, stupor, or coma and a peculiar lapse in the posture of the outstretched limbs and other contracted skeletal muscles (flapping movements or asterixis similar to the flap in impending liver coma). The finding of an elevated P_{CO_2} and diminished arterial oxygen concentration substantiate the diagnosis. *Chronic meningitis or adhesive arachnoiditis* due to chronic fibrosing meningeal diseases such as syphilis, postspinal anesthesia arachnoiditis, and cryptogenic meningeal diseases may be attended by headache, papilledema, seizures, blindness, paraplegia, or quadriplegia. The cerebrospinal fluid protein level may be normal or elevated, with or without a "dynamic block"; and the lateral, third and fourth ventricles are enlarged in the ventriculogram. Syphilis and the other chronic meningitides may also cause *aqueductal stenosis* owing to a proliferative gliotic ependymitis, with enlargement of the lateral and third ventricles (see Chap. 177). *Thrombosis of the jugular veins and of the lateral and posterior parts of the superior sagittal sinus* may result in increased intracranial pressure, with otherwise normal cerebrospinal fluid and usually small ventricles (see Chap. 360). No explanation can be given for the papilledema with headache, drowsiness, and confusion and elevated cerebrospinal fluid pressure observed in conjunction with *Addison's disease,* corticosteroid withdrawal, vitamin A overdosage, and also in rare cases, hypoparathyroidism. The mechanism is not known; usually the ventricles are of normal size.

"TRUE AND FALSE LOCALIZING SIGNS." If the clinical findings permit the exclusion of the aforementioned conditions, there is reasonable certainty that the patient has an intracranial growth. The problem then is to search for signs that will localize the lesion. In doing this, several pitfalls must be avoided. One common source of error is to place undue reliance on a sign which proves to have no localizing value whatsoever. With experience in this field one comes to distrust any symptom or sign which develops late, after headache and increased intracranial pressure have been established, for it often turns out to be a "false localizing sign." Under these circumstances drowsiness, slowness in response, inattentiveness, and emotional blunting can be found as often with cerebellar as with cerebral growths. Ataxia of gait, urinary incontinence, and psychomotor retardation may occur as part of a communicating hydrocephalus from any cause. Unilateral or bilateral abducens palsy is another common false localizing sign, and reference has already been made to the drooping eyelid, dilated pupil, ipsilateral hemiparesis and bilateral Babinski signs, and coma in temporal lobe herniation. Jacksonian and generalized seizures and ipsilateral or bilateral pyramidal signs may be observed in the advanced stages of a cerebellar tumor. Early and sometimes relatively slight focal signs that may be easily overlooked are sometimes the most reliable guides to the localization of the tumor. Examples are a mild weakness or stiffness and hyperreflexia of an arm and leg in a frontal tumor; ataxia of gait (but not of limbs) and head tilt in cerebellar tumors; paralysis of upward gaze with the Argyll Robertson pupillary phenomenon in pinealomas; pale optic disks and chiasmal field defects in craniopharyngiomas; and homonymous visual inattentiveness and sensory extinction (see Chaps. 24 and 25) in posterior cerebral tumors.

TUMORS WHICH TEND TO PRODUCE ELEVATED INTRACRANIAL PRESSURE WITHOUT CONSPICUOUS LOCALIZING SIGNS. The tumors most likely to cause increased intracranial pressure with few or no focal or lateralizing signs

are medulloblastoma, ependymoma of the fourth ventricle, hemangioblastoma, pinealoma, colloid cysts of the third ventricle, gliomas of tegmentum of the midbrain blocking the aqueduct, and craniopharyngioma. In addition, in some of the cerebral gliomas discussed above, particularly those of the corpus callosum and frontal lobes, increased intracranial pressure may precede focal cerebral signs.

Medulloblastoma. This is a rapidly growing tumor which arises in the posterior part of the vermis of children. The midline part of the cerebellum may be invaded and completely destroyed. The tumor also fills the fourth ventricle and compresses the medulla. The tonsils of the cerebellum are forced down into the cervical spinal canal (cerebellar pressure cone) in fatal cases. Seedings of the tumor may be seen on the walls of the third and lateral ventricles, on the meningeal surfaces of the brain, and around the spinal cord. The tumor is solid, reddish gray in color, and poorly demarcated from the adjacent brain tissue. It is very cellular, and the cells are small, closely packed with little cytoplasm, many mitoses, and scant stroma, and have a tendency to form clusters or pseudorosettes. As already stated, these cells resemble the "indifferent cells" which may be observed in the embryonic or fetal brain and are thought to be capable of differentiation into either glial cells or neuroblasts. Bailey and Cushing introduced the name *medulloblastoma* in 1925. Although medulloblasts as such have not been described in the fetal or adult human brain and the cell type is not known for certain, the term is retained if for no other reason than its familiarity. In adults a somewhat similar neuroblastoma of less malignant character may arise in the cerebral hemisphere.

The clinical picture is distinctive. Typically, the patient, a child of five to ten years, becomes listless, vomits repeatedly, and has a morning headache. The first diagnosis which suggests itself may be gastrointestinal disease or abdominal migraine. Soon, however, a stumbling gait, frequent falls, and a squint lead to a neurologic examination and the discovery of papilledema. Ataxia of the limbs may be absent at all times. Decerebrate attacks (tonic cerebellar fits) may occur in the late stages of the disease. The tumor is highly radiosensitive, and surgery with x-ray treatment may prolong life for several years. Recent trials of intrathecal Methotrexate and vincristine have yielded promising results in some cases.

Ependymoma and Papilloma of the Fourth Ventricle. This tumor also arises from the walls of the fourth ventricle in children. It is a firm, whitish lobulated growth composed of small cells arranged in the form of small rosettes around vessels or central clear areas and containing blepharoplasts in their cytoplasm. The clinical syndrome is much like that of the medulloblastoma except for the absence of ataxia of gait. The tumor is not very sensitive to x-ray, and surgical removal offers the only hope of survival. Prolongation of life is sometimes attained through ventriculoatrial shunting of CSF. The papilloma or papillary adenocarcinoma of the choroid plexus of the fourth ventricle gives rise to a similar syndrome but tends to occur later in life.

Hemangioblastoma of the Cerebellum. The disease of Lindau is described in Chap. 365. Dizziness, ataxia of gait or of the limbs on one side, symptoms and signs of increased intracranial pressure, and in some instances a retinal angioma (von Hippel's disease) and polycythemia constitute the neurologic syndrome. Familial incidence is well known. Craniotomy with opening of the cerebellar cyst and excision of the mural hemangioblastomatous nodule may be curative.

Pinealoma. This may be either a teratoma or a glioma of the pineal gland. The teratoma is a firm, discrete noninvasive mass which usually reaches 3 to 4 cm in greatest diameter. It compresses the superior colliculi and sometimes the superior surface of the cerebellum, with narrowing of the aqueduct of Sylvius. Often it extends anteriorly into the third ventricle and may then compress the hypothalamus. Microscopically it is composed of large, spherical epithelial cells (much like those of a seminoma), separated by a network of reticular connective tissue which contains many lymphocytes. The gliomas have the usual morphologic characteristics of an astrocytoma of varying degrees of malignancy. Children, adolescents, and young adults, either male or female, may be affected. In some cases the clinical syndrome consists solely of symptoms and signs of increased intracranial pressure, and the diagnosis can be made only by a ventriculogram which reveals the tumor. The most characteristic localizing signs, however, are inability to look upward (Parinaud's syndrome), and slightly dilated pupils which react on accommodation but not to light. Sometimes an ataxia of the limbs, choreic movements, or spastic weakness appears in the later stages of the illness. A Torkildsen ventriculocisterna magna shunt of cerebrospinal fluid and x-ray therapy have been remarkably successful in controlling the symptoms. Attempts at surgical removal of the tumor have usually proved fatal (see also Chap. 100).

Colloid (Paraphyseal) Cyst of the Third Ventricle. This is a papillomatous structure always situated in the anterior extremity of the third ventricle between the interventricular foramens and attached to the roof of the ventricle. Usually it is about a centimeter in diameter, is oval or round with a smooth external surface, and is filled with a glairy colloid material. The wall is composed of a layer of epithelial cells surrounded by a capsule of fibrous connective tissue. These benign cysts may exist for long periods of time; they produce neurologic symptoms by blocking the third ventricle and causing an obstructive hydrocephalus. This tumor should be suspected when the following clinical syndromes are found: dementia with or without headache, intermittent severe bifrontal-biooccipital headaches, sometimes modified by posture (ball valve obstruction of the third ventricle), crises of headache with obtundation, "frontal lobe" incontinence, unsteadiness of gait, bilateral paresthesias, dim vision, and weakness of legs with sudden falls. The treatment is surgical excision, but recently, satisfactory results have been obtained by ventriculoatrial shunt of CSF, leaving the benign growth untouched.

Craniopharyngioma (Suprasellar or Rathke's Pouch Cyst, Hypophyseal Duct Tumors, Adamantinomas, Ameloblastomas). This is a benign congenital or "rest cell" tumor. By the time it has grown to a diameter of 3 to 4 cm it is almost always cystic. Usually it lies above the sella turcica, depressing the optic chiasm and extending up into the third ventricle. Less often it is subdiaphragmatic, i.e., within the sella, where it compresses the pituitary body, erodes one part of the wall of the sella or a clinoid process but seldom balloons the sella like a pituitary adenoma. The tumor is oval, round, or lobulated and has a smooth surface. The wall of the cyst and the solid parts of the tumor consist of cords and whorls of epithelial cells, often with intercellular bridges and keratohyalin, separated by a loose network of stellate cells. The cyst contains dark albuminous fluid and cholesterol crystals. Calcium deposits are found in nearly all of them and can be seen in plain x-rays of the suprasellar region in about 40 percent of cases. The sella beneath the tumor tends to be flattened and enlarged. This is more often a tumor of children than of adults, but patients of all ages may be seen with it. In children, adiposity, delayed or infantile physical and sexual development (Froehlich's syndrome or Lorain syndrome—see Chap. 87), headaches, vomiting, dim vision with chiasmal field defects (see Chap. 24), optic atrophy, or papilledema comprise the clinical picture. In adults, waning libido, amenorrhea, slight spastic weakness of the legs, headache without papilledema, and mental dullness and confusion are often found. Later drowsiness, diabetes insipidus, and disturbances of temperature regulation may occur, indicating hypothalamic involvement.

In the differential diagnosis of these several tumor syndromes a careful clinical analysis is often more important than laboratory procedures. Arteriography and electroencephalography are not so helpful as in cerebral tumors. The tests which, though somewhat hazardous, are likely to give the most useful information are the air ventriculogram or a combined ventriculogram-pneumoencephalogram and the Pantopaque ventriculogram (injection of radiopaque fluid). Modern neurosurgical techniques reinforced by corticosteroid therapy before and after surgery and careful control of temperature and water balance postoperatively permit complete excision of the tumor in the majority of cases.

In certain marginal states of hydrocephalus benefit may accrue from the administration of acetazolamide (Diamox) in doses of 250 mg 3 or 4 times a day. Surgical shunting of CSF has given the best results, however.

PATIENTS WITH SYMPTOMS AND SIGNS OF A SLOWLY PROGRESSIVE LESION IN A PARTICULAR REGION OF THE CRANIAL CAVITY. In this group of conditions general cerebral symptoms and the signs of increased intracranial pressure occur late or not at all. The physician arrives at the correct diagnosis by being able to make an anatomic or regional diagnosis from a set of neurologic findings and by reasoning that the etiology must be neoplastic because of the slowly progressive nature of the illness. Special x-rays of the skull, cerebrospinal fluid examination, and, depending on the location of the disease, either pneumoencephalography or arteriography will usually confirm the clinical impression.

The following tumors produce unique syndromes usually diagnostic of a special type of tumor.

Acoustic Neurofibroma or Neurinoma. This slowly growing benign tumor may occur as a solitary lesion or as a part of the syndrome of neurofibromatosis. By the time of operation the tumor has usually attained a size of 4 to 6 cm in diameter. It arises from the extramedullary part of the eighth cranial nerve, usually within the internal auditory meatus, where the intracranial part of the nerve first acquires the histologic character of a peripheral nerve, i.e., has Schwann cells and fibroblasts. The space in which it lies is the cerebellopontine angle, i.e., between the cerebellum, pons, and medulla posteriorly, the petrous pyramid anteriorly, and the tentorium above. The internal auditory meatus is usually enlarged (visible in x-rays), the middle cerebellar peduncle and the anterolateral part of the cerebellum are depressed, and the trigeminal, facial, glossopharyngeal, and vagus nerves are displaced and stretched over the surface of the growth. The fourth ventricle is deformed, displaced, and narrowed (visible in a pneumoencephalogram), and there is hydrocephalic enlargement of the aqueduct and of the third and lateral ventricle in the late stages. The tumor is vascular, and the surrounding cerebrospinal fluid has a high protein content (cerebrospinal fluid protein of 300 mg per 100 ml or over is not infrequent). The microscopic picture is that of a typical neurofibroma (axis cylinders mixed with masses of fibrous connective tissue in interlacing strands, palisaded nuclei, and mononuclear giant cells without mitoses). The typical clinical syndrome, which usually occurs in adult men or women, consists of tinnitus, deafness, and rotational vertigo (seldom in discrete attacks as in Ménière's syndrome, Chap. 355) of several years' standing, followed by stiff neck and postauricular or suboccipital pain, spasms and twitching or slight weakness of the face, paresthesias or pain in the face, dysphonia and dysphagia, and homolateral cerebellar ataxia of the arm and leg. Headache, vomiting, and choked disk are late findings. Variations of this syndrome are numerous. Early in its development only progressive deafness, tinnitus, and vague vertigo may be present, and the abnormal audiogram, impaired vestibular function, elevated cerebrospinal fluid protein level, widened internal auditory meatus, and obliteration of the lateral recess of the fourth ventricle in a pneumoencephalogram must be depended upon for diagnosis. Dementia may later be the presenting syndrome, and the deaf ear may be overlooked. Unilateral cerebellar ataxia and dizziness may predominate, and definite signs of involvement of the fifth, seventh, and eighth cranial nerves may not be found. The only treatment is surgical excision.

The *trigeminal* or *gasserian ganglion neurinoma* and *meningioma* of the *cerebellopontine angle* may be indistinguishable from an acoustic neurinoma. They should always be considered if early tinnitus and deafness and

an unresponsive labyrinth ("dead labyrinth") are not the initial symptoms of the cerebellopontine angle syndrome. A true *cholesteatoma of the temporal bone* may simulate this clinical picture, but usually the facial weakness is early and severe, the ear is deaf, and labyrinthine function is absent, whereas the other cranial nerve signs, cerebellar ataxia, and increased intracranial pressure are absent. The *tumor of the glomus jugulare* (a flat ovoid body, found in the adventitia of the jugular bulb, immediately below the floor of the middle ear and near the ramus tympanicus of the ninth cranial nerve) may, like the acoustic neurofibroma, basal meningioma, metastatic cancer, syphilitic meningitis, neurofibroma of other cranial nerves, and vascular malformation, cause unilateral lower cranial nerve palsies (see Chap. 355). It is a purplish-red, highly vascular tumor composed of large epithelioid cells in an alveolar pattern and an abundant capillary network. Partial deafness, facial palsy, dysphagia, and unilateral atrophy of the tongue, combined with a vascular polyp in the auditory meatus and a palpable mass below and anterior to the mastoid eminence, often with a bruit, comprise the syndrome. The jugular foramen is eroded (visible by x-ray), and the cerebrospinal fluid protein level may be elevated. Women are affected more than men, and the peak incidence is during middle adult life. The tumor grows slowly over a period of many years, sometimes 10 or more. The treatment is x-ray radiation. Surgical excision has usually been unsuccessful.

The Pituitary Adenomas. These tumors, which are so common, particularly in late adult life, often are discovered when a patient begins to complain of a visual disturbance. A unilateral or bilateral temporal hemianopsia progressing to blindness, with optic atrophy, is the usual finding and with x-ray evidence of an expanded sella turcica leads to a diagnosis of pituitary adenoma. As the growth enlarges and extends laterally, an oculomotor palsy is occasionally seen, and large suprasellar extensions may involve the hypothalamus or temporal lobe. If there are signs of acromegaly, one may assume that an eosinophilic adenoma is present; if not, and signs of pituitary insufficiency are present (amenorrhea without "hot flashes," sexual impotence, etc.—see Chap. 87), the tumor is usually a chromophobe adenoma. Basophilic adenomas, one of the causes of Cushing's syndrome, rarely if ever produce enlargement of the sella or visual symptoms. The diagnosis is made from the endocrine picture (see Chap. 87). The cerebrospinal fluid is usually under normal pressure, and protein level is elevated only in exceptional cases. Other conditions may rarely expand the sella (craniopharyngioma, carotid aneurysm), and there are also rather wide normal variations in its size. Hence the diagnosis of pituitary adenoma should not be made because of minor enlargements in the absence of neighborhood neurologic signs. In doubtful cases a pneumoencephalogram permits visualization of the suprasellar extension of the tumor. Treatment is x-ray radiation and, if vision is threatened despite x-ray therapy, either transnasal or transfrontal surgical excision. More recently excellent results have been obtained with proton-beam bombardment. Replacement endocrine therapy is also needed.

Meningioma of the Sphenoid Ridge. This tumor arises from arachnoid cap cells over the lesser wing of the sphenoidal bone. As it increases in size, it may expand medially to encroach on structures in the wall of the cavernous sinus, anteriorly to invade the orbit, or laterally to erode or invade the temporal bone. Most prominent among the symptoms are a slowly developing unilateral exophthalmos, slight bulging of the bone in the temporal region, and roentgenologic evidence of thickening or erosion of the lesser wing of the sphenoid bone. Variants of the clinical syndrome include oculomotor palsy or syndrome of Foix (p. 1715), blindness in one eye with optic atrophy, anosmia (and sometimes the Kennedy syndrome—see below), mental changes, uncinate fits, and increased intracranial pressure. Sarcomas arising from the skull bones, metastatic carcinoma, orbitoethmoidal osteoma, tumors of the optic nerve, and angiomas of the orbit must be considered in the differential diagnosis. Auscultation of the skull, x-ray of the skull, and carotid arteriography are helpful in differentiating these lesions.

Meningioma of the Olfactory Groove. This tumor is a growth derived from arachnoidal cap cells along the cribriform plate. The diagnosis depends on the finding of ipsilateral or bilateral anosmia, ipsilateral or bilateral blindness, often with optic atrophy on one side and papilledema without atrophy on the other (Kennedy syndrome), and mental changes. The tumors may reach enormous size before coming to the attention of the physician. The anosmia, if unilateral, is rarely if ever reported by the patient. The unilateral visual disturbance may consist of a slowly developing unilateral central scotoma. Confusion, forgetfulness, inappropriate jocularity (witzelsucht) are the usual psychic disturbances. The patient is indifferent to or jokes about blindness. Usually there are x-ray changes along the cribriform plate and an extremely high cerebrospiral fluid protein level (200 to 400 mg).

Glioma of the Brainstem. Astrocytomas of the brainstem (formerly called "bipolar spongioblastomas") are slow-growing, firm, white infiltrating growths which insinuate themselves between tracts and nuclei. They produce a variable clinical picture, depending on their exact location in the medulla, pons, and midbrain (see Chaps. 23 and 24 for syndromes). The characteristic features, in the early stages, are signs of crossed motor or sensory disturbances, which always indicate brainstem disease, and, as the lesion advances, an orderly succession of new signs due to involvement of neighboring structures, and finally signs of bilateral disease in the brainstem. Headache, vomiting, and papilledema occur late. The course is slowly progressive over years unless some part of the tumor becomes more malignant (glioblastoma multiforme), in which instance the illness may terminate fatally within months. The main clinical problem is to differentiate between this disease, multiple sclerosis, and vascular malformations of the pons. Pneumoencephalography to visualize the fourth ventricle and aqueduct and occasionally vertebral arteriography are helpful in diagnosis. The treatment is x-ray radiation and if intracranial pressure is increased, a Torkildsen ventriculocisterna magna shunt.

Glioma of the Optic Nerves and Chiasm. This tumor is often found in patients with von Recklinghausen's disease and, like the glioma of the brainstem, arises most frequently during the period of childhood and adolescence. The initial symptoms are dimness of vision with constricted fields, bizarre bilateral field defects of homonymous, heteronymous, sometimes bitemporal type, blindness, and optic atrophy with or without papilledema. Hypothalamic signs (infantilism, adiposity, polyuria, somnolence, and genital atrophy) are common. X-rays reveal an enlargement of the optic foramen. With this finding and the lack of ballooning of the sella or suprasellar calcification, pituitary adenoma, Hand-Schüller-Christian disease, and craniopharyngioma can be excluded. The treatment is surgical excision or x-ray, depending on the exact location.

Chordoma. This is a soft, jellylike gray-pink growth composed of cords or masses of large cells with granules of glycogen in their cytoplasm and often multiple nuclei and intercellular mucoid material. They are locally invasive but do not metastasize. Any part of the vertebral column or the base of the cranium are the most common sites, especially the base of the skull (from physaliphora ecchondrosis) or the lumbosacral region (giving rise to a cauda equina syndrome). Those in the base of the skull create a remarkable clinical picture in which all or any combination of cranial nerve palsies from the second to twelfth on one side or both sides are combined with a retropharyngeal mass and erosion of the clivus of sphenoid bone and the occiput. It is one of the five tumors that may present both as an intracranial and as an extracranial mass. (The other four are the meningioma, neurofibroma, glomus jugulare tumor, and carcinoma of sinuses or pharynx.) The treatment is x-ray therapy.

NASOPHARYNGEAL GROWTHS WHICH ERODE THE BASE OF THE SKULL. These are rather common in a general hospital and arise from the mucous membrane of the paranasal sinuses or the nasopharynx near the eustachian tube, i.e., the fossa of Rosenmueller (*transitional cell carcinoma, Schmincke tumor*). In addition to symptoms of nasopharyngeal or sinus disease, which may not be prominent, facial pain and numbness (trigeminal), abducens palsy (sixth cranial nerve), and other cranial nerve palsies may occur. Diagnosis depends on inspection and biopsy of a nasopharyngeal mass, biopsy of an involved cervical gland, and x-ray evidence of erosion of the base of the skull. The treatment is x-ray therapy.

PROGNOSIS. The prognosis of intracranial tumor is influenced by the nature of the growth, its location, and other factors. As a general rule, unless an operation is performed almost all intracranial tumors end fatally. Death in most instances is preceded by a critical rise in intracranial pressure and tentorial or foramen magnum herniation. The more malignant tumors, such as the glioblastoma multiforme, medulloblastoma, and metastatic carcinoma, end fatally within a year, as a rule, whereas the slowly growing meningiomas and astrocytomas often permit survival for many years.

The prospects for recovery after surgery depend largely on the type of tumor. With meningiomas and acoustic neurofibromas, if completely excised, there may be a complete cure. In gliomas the outlook is more bleak. Cure is rare, for seldom can complete excision be accomplished. Nevertheless with the slow-growing gliomas, partial excision, the marsupialization of a cyst, and the relief of increased intracranial pressure by long-term corticosteroid therapy may lead to improvement and resumption of a useful life for many years. With metastatic growth the outlook is dismal, though if there are no metastases in other organs and the cerebral deposit appears to be solitary, operation has occasionally resulted in temporary recovery for a few months or a year or two.

CONCLUSIONS. The physician's responsibilities in this field of intracranial tumors are (1) diagnosis—he must separate the tumor cases from all the others which pass through his hands; (2) exclusion of the possibility that the intracranial mass is part of a general disease which would contraindicate surgery, i.e., metastatic carcinoma, syphilis, tuberculosis, parasitic infection, etc.; (3) exclusion of the several pseudotumor syndromes; (4) maintenance of the patient in the best possible condition, until surgery can be undertaken (fluids, electrolytes, corticosteroid therapy, etc.); (5) assisting the surgeon in the postoperative medical management. In inoperable cases the objectives are to maintain the morale of the family and patient as long as possible and to provide intelligent supportive therapy.

In general, although the results of therapy are frequently disappointing, there are always the few dramatic successes that serve as a perpetual stimulus to the physician, and so it is always with the next patient that he hopes to achieve a cure.

(For tumors of spinal cord and nerves, see Chaps. 354, 355, and 356.)

REFERENCES

Bailey, P.: "Intracranial Tumors," 2d ed., Springfield, Ill., Charles C Thomas, Publisher, 1948.

——, D. N. Buchanan, and P. C. Bucy: "Intracranial Tumors in Infancy and Childhood," Chicago, University of Chicago Press, 1939.

—— and H. Cushing: "A Classification of the Tumors of the Glioma Group upon a Histogenic Basis with a Correlated Study of Prognosis," Philadelphia, J. B. Lippincott, 1926.

Peers, J. H.: Occurrence of Tumors of Central Nervous System in Routine Autopsies, Am. J. Pathol., 12:911, 1936.

360 PYOGENIC INFECTIONS OF THE CENTRAL NERVOUS SYSTEM

Maria Z. Salam and Fuad Sabra

The incidence of all intracranial suppurative infections has been significantly reduced since the introduction of sulfonamide drugs and antibiotics. No longer does one find wards full of patients with mastoid and sinus infections, which pose the constant threat of intracranial extension; and serious pulmonary infections, another source of hematogenous inflammation in the cranial cavity, have diminished. Nevertheless bacterial infections of the nervous system are by no means rare, and when they do occur they offer such grave problems in diagnosis that a separate chapter for their consideration seems advisable.

Ordinary bacterial meningitis (leptomeningitis) is without question the most common of this group of disorders, developing as it does at any period of life but with particular frequency in the young and old. Although this disease is now amenable to effective therapy, delay in diagnosis may result in death or grave and permanent injury to the brain. It ranks sixth among the causes of death in children one to fourteen years of age. Every physician, therefore, must be competent in the recognition of this disease, i.e., in the methods used in diagnosis, in the interpretation of the neurologic complications, and in treatment.

There are in addition several other less frequent states, such as brain abscess, subdural empyema, and thrombophlebitis, which raise problems of a different nature. At times they challenge the diagnostic ingenuity of the physician, but their gratifying response to therapy once again prompts us to have a detailed knowledge of their clinical features.

PATHOGENESIS OF INTRACRANIAL SUPPURATION

All pyogenic infections of the cranial contents originate in one of two ways, by hematogenous spread, namely, emboli of bacteria or of infected thrombi, or by extension from surface structures (ears, paranasal sinuses, osteomyelitic foci in skull, penetrating cranial injuries, or congenital sinus tracts).

Concerning the hematogenous pathway surprisingly little is known, for human autopsy material seldom divulges information on this point, and animal experimentation (injecting virulent bacteria into the bloodstream) has yielded somewhat contradictory results. In pneumonia, bacteremia seems to be a common forerunner of meningitis; in chronic pulmonary diseases, septic thrombi have been seen in veins in the lung and as emboli in the small arteries of the brain; in acute and subacute bacterial endocarditis, bacterial emboli are found in cerebral and meningeal arteries. The ideal sites of lodgment of these emboli for the production of meningitis, whether in choroid plexuses or in meningeal or superficial cerebral vessels, have not been ascertained.

With respect to the formation of brain abscess, the experimental data inform us that the cerebral tissues are resistant to infection. Direct injection of virulent bacteria into the brain of an animal seldom results in abscess formation. In fact this condition has been successfully produced only by injecting the culture medium with the bacteria or by first causing necrosis of the tissue and then inoculating it with bacteria. In human beings infarction of brain tissue by arterial occlusion (embolism) or venous occlusion (thrombophlebitis) appears to be the common and perhaps necessary antecedent.

The cranial epidural and subdural spaces evidently are rarely the site of blood-borne infection, in contrast to the spinal epidural space, where this happens not infrequently.

Cranial bones and the dura mater, which serves essentially as the inner periosteum of the skull, protect the cranial cavity against the ingress of bacteria. But this protective mechanism may fail if suppuration occurs in the middle ear, mastoid cells, or frontal, ethmoid, and sphenoid sinuses. Two pathways have been demonstrated in postmortem material.

1. Infected thrombi may form in diploic veins and spread along these vessels into the dural sinuses (into which they flow) and from there in retrograde fashion along the meningeal veins into the brain.

2. An osteomyelitic focus may form, with erosion of the inner table of bone and invasion of the dura, subdural space, piarachnoid, and even the brain substance. Each of these pathways may be visualized in some fatal cases of epidural abscess, subdural empyema, leptomeningitis, cranial venous sinusitis and meningeal thrombophlebitis, and brain abscess. However, in many cases coming to autopsy one cannot determine the pathway.

Hematogenous infections during bacteremias usually permit a single type of virulent organism to gain entry to the cranial cavity (meningococcus, pneumococcus, influenza bacillus, staphylococcus, or streptococcus). In contrast, septic cerebral emboli from chronic lung infections, congenital heart disease with brain abscess, and extension from ear or sinus infections often infect with multiple types of organisms, e.g., staphylococcus, fusiform bacillus, oral spirochetal organisms, resulting in "mixed infections" which offer rather more complex problems in therapy. Not infrequently, when active suppuration has occurred, the demonstration of the causative organism, even from the pus of an abscess, may be unsuccessful.

BACTERIAL MENINGITIS (LEPTOMENINGITIS)

This condition consists essentially of an inflammation of the piarachnoid and the fluid residing in the space which it encloses and also of the ventricles of the brain. Since the subarachnoid space is continuous around the brain and spinal cord and the optic nerves, an infective agent gaining entry to any one part of it may extend immediately to all of it, even its most remote recesses, i.e., meningitis is always cerebrospinal. It also reaches the ventricles, either directly or by reflux through the basal foramens of Magendie and Luschka.

The effect of bacteria or other organisms in the subarachnoid space is to cause an inflammatory reaction in the pia and arachnoid and in the CSF; in the pyogenic forms, pus accumulates in this space. The infective agent or its toxin, if allowed sufficient time to act, injures those structures which lie within the subarachnoid space (cranial and spinal roots) and adjacent to it (pial arteries and veins, underlying cerebral and cerebellar cortices, subpial white matter of the spinal cord, peripheral fibers of optic nerves, ependymal lining of ventricles, and subependymal tissues). In addition purulent material may interfere with the flow of CSF from the ventricles or along the subarachnoid space over the brainstem, with resulting obstructive or communicating hydrocephalus, respectively. Although the outer arachnoidal membrane proves to be a remarkably effective barrier to the extension of infection, nevertheless some reaction of the cranial subdural space and even the inner surface of the dura and spinal epidural space may occur. This happens more often in infants (subdural effusions) than in adults.

The most immediate clinical effects of acute subarachnoid suppuration, distinguishing it from infections in other parts of the body, are severe headache, generalized convulsions, drowsiness, stupor, or coma. The one clinical sign of importance is stiffness of the neck (resistance to passive movement) on forward bending. The Kernig and Brudzinski signs are of the same nature but less reliable. The basis of these symptoms and signs is explained below. Any circumstance which prolongs the meningitis should increase the risk of injury to all the enumerated structures; this fact accounts for many features of the clinical picture in the subacute and chronic varieties of meningeal infection. The potential pathologic-clinical relations of acute, subacute, and chronic meningitis are summarized as follows:

I. In acute meningitis
  A. Pure piarachnoiditis; headache, stiff neck, and Kernig and Brudzinski signs. These signs depend on activation of protective, flexor reflexes which shorten the spine and immobilize it (extension of neck and flexion of hips and knees reduce stretch on inflamed spinal structures; all the clinical signs of meningitis, it will be noted, demonstrate activation of these postural reflexes).
  B. Subpial toxic encephalopathy (tissue beneath pia not penetrated by bacteria, hence (?) toxic change): confusion, stupor, coma, and convulsions (cerebral infarction due to cortical vein thrombosis may underlie this syndrome in some cases).
  C. Inflammatory or vascular involvement of cranial nerve roots: ocular palsies, facial weakness (exception is direct involvement of eighth nerve and cochlea with ear infections), or other conditions. N.B., deafness may be due either to middle ear infection or to extension of meningeal infection to the inner ear.
  D. Thrombosis of meningeal veins: focal convulsions, focal cerebral defects such as hemiparesis, aphasia (rarely prominent), etc., which usually appear only after the first week or two of meningeal infection.
  E. Ependymitis, choroidal plexitis, if doubtful there are any recognizable clinical effects aside from those of the associated hydrocephalus.
II. In more subacute and chronic forms of meningitis
  A. Obstructive or communicating hydrocephalus, due at first to purulent exudate around the base of the brain, later to meningeal fibrosis and rarely to aqueductal stenosis: variable degrees of impairment of consciousness, decorticate postures (arms flexed, legs extended),

impaired grasp and sucking reflexes, and sphincteric incontinence. Later, enlarging head, in a child. In the mildest form, only psychomotor retardation, unsteadiness of gait, and incontinence. CSF pressure in adult may be elevated; or, if the ventricles are greatly enlarged, it may seem to fall within limits of normal.

B. Subdural effusion and empyema with sterile and infected effusions: impaired alertness, refusal to eat and vomiting, immobility, bulging fontanels, and persistence of fever despite clearing of CSF. In infants the effusion causes an exaggerated transillumination. With subdural empyema: fever is more pronounced, CSF is under increased pressure, and there are one-sided convulsions, hemiplegia, etc. (If fever is present but CSF pressure is normal and one-sided cerebral signs are clearly in evidence, thrombophlebitis is the leading possibility.)

C. Extensive venous or arterial infarction: unilateral or bilateral hemiplegia, decorticate or decerebrate rigidity, cortical blindness, stupor or coma with or without seizures.

III. Late effects or sequelae

A. Meningeal fibrosis around optic nerves, or spinal cord and roots: blindness, spastic paraparesis with sensory loss in the lower segments of the body, respectively.

B. Severe cerebral damage: dementia, stupor or coma, and paralysis.

C. Persistent hydrocephalus in the child: with blindness, arrest of all mental activity, bilateral spastic hemiplegia

These general remarks about leptomeningitis apply more or less to all forms of the disease, the acute suppurative and the lymphocytic types (see Chap. 204, Pathogenesis of Viral Diseases), the subacute tuberculous and fungous types, and the more chronic syphilitic type. The longer the infection persists, the more numerous and prominent become the late complications; this is why they are so pronounced in subacute influenzal bacillus meningitis or tuberculous meningitis (especially when these infections have been refractory to treatment) and in chronic fungous or syphilitic meningitis. In the latter the neurologic syndromes deriving from meningitis are so remarkable that they receive special names such as tabes dorsalis or general paresis, but the basic process is still the same.

Thus, meningitis may be broadly viewed as a pathologic process which exerts its effects to a variable degree on all parts of the cerebrospinal neuraxis with which the fluid is in contact.

Since in this chapter we are considering only pyogenic infections, the lymphocytic (aseptic), tuberculous, fungous, and syphilitic types of inflammation will not be discussed further.

TYPES OF BACTERIAL MENINGITIS. *Diplococcus pneumoniae, Hemophilus influenzae,* and *Neisseria meningitidis* account for approximately 70 percent of all cases of meningitis found in a general hospital; the rare types make up the remainder. *Diplococcus pneumoniae* is the most frequent present-day pathogen when all age groups are considered, *H. influenzae* ranks as the foremost meningeal pathogen in the pediatric age bracket.

The pathogenic agent is identified eight to nine times out of ten by culture of CSF; smears of the sediment and gram staining are less reliable, especially if there has been pretreatment with an antibiotic. In smear preparations of the CSF our most common error has been to mistake *H. influenzae* for diplococci. In 5 to 10 percent of cases no organism is obtained either by culture or by smear, even though the CSF formula suggests a bacterial meningitis. Treatment must be directed to the latter, using broad-spectrum antibiotics, though it must be conceded that ECHO 9 virus infections may simulate bacterial meningitis.

SPECIAL CLINICAL FEATURES OF THE DIFFERENT TYPES OF BACTERIAL MENINGITIS. Meningococcus. Meningococcal meningitis is the only type that often occurs in epidemics. It may be preceded by high fever and skin eruption due to meningococcemia. The meningeal infection is hematogenous. Headache, drowsiness, and stiff neck are the principal symptoms. Convulsions occur in some patients. Evolution usually is rapid, especially with some of the more virulent organisms, which may result in the Waterhouse-Friderichsen syndrome, in which circulatory collapse and death may occur within hours of onset of illness, even before treatment can be given. In diagnosis the petechial skin eruption is important, but ECHO 9 viral infections and staphylococcus endocarditis may also produce an eruption. Usually the meningeal infection responds quickly to therapy, with prompt regression of fever, signs of meningeal irritation, and all other neurologic disorders. Few of the late neurologic complications are now observed if therapy (penicillin G, or chloramphenicol if patient is allergic to penicillin) is prompt and adequate; they still occur if insufficient treatment permits prolongation of the infection.

Pneumococcus. Pneumococcal meningitis is next in importance and may develop as a complication of an ear infection (or sinusitis or skull fracture, especially with CSF rhinorrhea) or with pneumonia. Other predisposing conditions are: head trauma, CSF rhinorrhea, immune globulin deficiency, postsplenectomy, and sickle-cell disease. Patients are usually stuporous or comatose by their arrival at a hospital, and they may exhibit questionable signs of focal cerebral disorder. Stiff neck and back on forward bending and Kernig and Brudzinski signs are present in nearly all patients. Early in the infection the CSF may be swarming with diplococci with relatively little cellular reaction. Response to therapy (penicillin G, or erythromycin if patient is allergic to penicillin) is less rapid than in meningococcal meningitis; the confusion and stupor, often with a mild degree of aphasic disorder or a Babinski sign and questionable hemiparesis, may persist for several days after the temperature has fallen and the CSF has begun to clear. This is still one of the most malignant types of meningitis in children and elderly adults.

Influenza Bacillus. Meningitis produced by the influenza bacillus in children (most frequent in the first 2 to 3 years of life—90 percent before 5 years of age) has often resulted in severe cerebral damage because of delay in diagnosis (development may be insidious) and slowness of response to therapy. In the newborn infant, irritability, somnolence, vomiting, episodes of cyanosis, and depressed activity should alert one to the diagnosis even in the absence of fever and stiff neck. In later infancy, vomiting, fever, bulging fontanels, convulsions, and drowsiness or stupor may occur without stiff neck. In later childhood and adult life, the symptoms are similar to those in pneumococcal meningitis. Attention should be called to the serious neurologic deficits that result from this infection. Like pneumococcal meningitis, there may be an ear infection, but it is not always certain whether or not it is the source of the meningitis, since there is usually septicemia as well. Prompt treatment with chloramphenicol or ampicillin has saved the life of over 90 percent of children and prevented serious complications.

Staphylococcus aureus, Streptococcus, Escherichia coli, Pyocyaneus, Aerobacter aerogenes, and Other Odd Types of Meningitis. Meningitis caused by the first two of these agents often develops as a complication of ear and sinus disease or as a part of a septicemia. *Escherichia coli, Klebsiella, Proteus vulgaris, Hemophilus influenzae,* and *Listeria* are the most frequent types of neonatal meningitis. Their occurrence is favored by difficulty in parturition and prematurity. Other types of meningitis arise under usual conditions, e.g., in infants with meningomyelocele or hydrocephalus, postnatal infections, postlumbar puncture, or postspinal anesthesia. *Pseudomonas* is the usual cause of meningitis in the burned child.

RECURRENT BACTERIAL MENINGITIS. Three categories of disease are associated with recurrent bacterial infections of the subarachnoid space: (1) persistent parameningeal suppurative focus in the ears, paranasal sinuses, or skull; (2) gross anatomic defects, congenital (dermal sinuses, meningomyelocele, or meningoencephalocele) or traumatic, usually with CSF rhinorrhea; (3) impaired immunity to bacterial infections. In addition there is a condition known as Mollaret's recurrent meningitis, characterized by recurrent febrile attacks, malaise, headache, meningeal signs, and a CSF containing several thousand neutrophilic leukocytes per milliliter but with normal sugar values and only slightly elevated protein content. An unidentified virus has been isolated from one case. Spontaneous remission is the rule.

The therapy of recurrent bacterial meningitis must be directed to the offending organism, but in addition the pathway must be sought and eradicated if possible.

GENERAL REMARKS ON THERAPY. The specific sulfonamide or antibiotic favored for each form of bacterial meningitis is listed in Table 135-1 and discussed in the appropriate chapters. These agents have greatly reduced the mortality rate (to less than 8 percent, exclusive of newborn infants, in whom it is still 85 percent), though the neurologic sequelae such as epilepsy, blindness, spastic weakness, cranial nerve palsies, and deafness are increasing (18 percent in some series). The latter are probably due to delay in diagnosis and/or improper choice of drugs. Extremely high intrathecal pressures (>450 mm) are treated with intravenous urea or mannitol and dexamethazone, as described in Chap. 359. The argument

over intravenous versus intrathecal administration continues, but time has proved that once an effective medication is at hand, the parenteral route is adequate. Only in exceptional cases of pneumococcal and influenzal bacillus meningitis, tuberculosis, and cryptococcosis, where response to therapy may be inadequate, is the question any longer raised.

Each of the neurologic complications of bacterial meningitis requires special management. Generalized seizures are usually controlled by parenteral administration of Dilantin or sodium phenobarbital. Focal motor seizures may prove to be resistant, however, and for them paraldehyde by rectum or intravenously has been more effective than some of the other anticonvulsants. The therapy of thrombophlebitis is uncertain, and results obtained to date are difficult to assess. Although one hesitates to use anticoagulants in the face of incompletely controlled infection, yet favorable results from this treatment have been reported in small groups of patients (e.g., those with cavernous sinus thrombophlebitis). Subdural empyema demands burr holes in the temporal region for purposes of diagnosis and surgical drainage. Subdural effusions usually can be removed by repeated aspirations through the lateral border of the anterior fontanel, since they rarely occur after the age of two years; but some of the persistent ones have required craniotomy and surgical removal. Patients with communicating and obstructive hydrocephalus should be observed until it is clear that the head enlargement continues to progress over a period of weeks or months. Then an atrioventricular shunt should be performed.

PROGNOSIS. Children who make a prompt response to therapy usually recover and develop normally thereafter. But a distressingly large number will be found to have severe sequelae. (One out of ten children with an acquired form of mental retardation will have had bacterial meningitis as its cause.) Their prognosis is poor. Often it is necessary to send them to a home for the mentally retarded, once it is clear (after 1 to 2 years) that the neurologic deficits are irreversible. Adults usually recover completely, and after a week or two even the most careful testing uncovers no neurologic or psychiatric abnormalities.

ACUTE SUBDURAL EMPYEMA "SUBDURAL ABSCESS"

Here the clinical manifestations relate to a suppurative process which lies in the cranial subdural space, usually on one side, and covers the inner surface of the dura and outer membrane of the arachnoid. The proper term for the condition is not "abscess" but *empyema,* which means suppuration in a preformed space.

In all our cases the infection had gained entry to the subdural space from a paranasal sinus (usually frontal or ethmoidal) or, less often, from the mastoid cells. In two instances only had the subdural space been infected by extension of bacteria from the bloodstream or a brain abscess. In infants the cranial subdural space may be invaded by bacteria during the course of a meningitis (e.g., influenza bacillus).

In brief, the usual history consists of symptoms of chronic sinusitis or mastoiditis, recently reactivated, with evidence of local pain and arrest of/or increase in purulent nasal or aural discharge. Generalized headache and fever are the first signs of intracranial spread; they are followed rapidly by unilateral motor seizures, hemiplegia, hemianesthesia, hemianopia, and aphasia (with involvement of the dominant hemisphere). Stupor or coma accompanies the advance in cerebral symptoms. The condition progresses with alarming rapidity, usually over a few days or a week (unlike the more slowly developing abscess). Fever is always present, and the neck is stiff. The CSF is under increased pressure (usually 200 to 400) with raised white cell count (50 to 1,000) of both neutrophilic leukocytes and lymphocytes, elevated protein content (100 to 300 mg per ml), but normal sugar values. The diagnosis can now be confirmed relatively easily by carotid arteriography, which discloses inward displacement of meningeal vessels and contralateral shift of the anterior cerebral arteries. A temporal burr hole with exposure of the dura demonstrates pus under increased pressure, which can then be drained through enlarged burr holes or a craniotomy. This procedure and appropriate antibiotic therapy may be lifesaving. Without surgery most patients with these diseases will die, usually within 7 to 14 days, often while the unsuspecting surgeon is waiting for a better localization of an assumed cerebral abscess (common mistaken diagnosis). Several of our treated patients have made a surprisingly good recovery from their focal neurologic disorder within a few months.

PATHOLOGY. Unilateral subdural pus, often mistakenly called meningitis, depresses the underlying cerebral hemisphere. The arachnoid, when cleared of exudate, is cloudy, and thrombosis of meningeal veins may be seen. Microscopic study demonstrates various degrees of organization of the exudate on the inner surface of the dura, and infiltration of the underlying pia with small numbers of neutrophilic leukocytes, lymphocytes, and mononuclear cells. The cerebral veins, particularly their outer parts, are thrombosed. The superficial layers of the cerebral cortex will have undergone ischemic (infarct) necrosis, which finding probably accounts for the unilateral seizures and signs of disordered cerebral function. Temporal lobe pressure cone will have terminated the illness in most of the fatal cases.

DIFFERENTIAL DIAGNOSIS. The four conditions that need to be distinguished from subdural empyema are cerebral thrombophlebitis, brain abscess, acute hemorrhagic leukoencephalitis, and acute hemorrhagic viral (inclusion body) encephalitis (see Chap. 361 for useful guides in their separation).

EXTRADURAL ABSCESS

This condition is almost invariably connected with an osteomyelitic process in a cranial bone which originates from an infection in an ear or a paranasal sinus. Pus and granulation tissue accumulate on the outer surface of the dura, separating it from the cranial bone.

Symptomatically there are only the local effects of the inflammatory process; frontal or auricular pain, purulent discharge from sinus or ear, and fever and local tenderness are the only signs noted on examination. Sometimes a slight stiffness of the neck is noted. Localizing neurologic signs are usually absent. Exceptionally, a fifth and sixth cranial nerve palsy appears with infections of the petrous part of the temporal bone (petrositis with Gradenigo's syndrome) or a focal seizure of unexplained cause may occur. The CSF is usually clear and under normal pressure, but it may contain a few lymphocytes and neutrophilic leukocytes (20 to 100 per ml) and slightly raised protein level. The treatment consists of antibiotic medication and surgical drainage; the management does not differ essentially from that of the primary sinusitis or mastoiditis from which the extradural infection has arisen.

SPINAL EPIDURAL ABSCESS

This type of abscess possesses clinical features all its own and constitutes an important neurologic and neurosurgical emergency. The symptoms and signs being entirely spinal, it is discussed in Chap. 356, Diseases of the Spinal Cord.

INTRACRANIAL THROMBOPHLEBITIS

The lateral cavernous and superior longitudinal sinuses are the common sites. Evidence of centripetal infection from the middle ear and mastoid cells, the paranasal sinuses, and the skin around the upper lip, nose, and eyes, can usually be demonstrated. Fever tends to be high and intermittent.

In *lateral sinus thrombophlebitis*, which usually follows chronic mastoiditis, earache and mastoid tenderness are followed over a period of days or weeks by generalized headache and papilledema. As a rule there are no other neurologic signs. Pulmonary embolism may occur but usually is asymptomatic. As a diagnostic aid, compression of the jugular veins separately, during the Queckenstedt maneuver, will demonstrate a failure of rise in CSF pressure ipsilaterally (Tobey-Ayer test). When the intracranial pressure is greatly elevated, the suspicion of cerebellar or cerebral abscess is raised, but the syndrome differs with respect to a lack of cerebellar or other neurologic signs (especially nystagmus to side of lesion and ataxia of arm and leg, the common findings in cerebellar abscess).

Cavernous sinus thrombophlebitis secondary to oculonasal infections presents characteristically with orbital edema, chemosis, venous congestion, and evidence of III, IV, and ophthalmic V and VI cranial nerve palsies. Later spread through the circular sinus to the opposite cavernous sinus results in bilateralization of symptoms. The CSF is usually normal unless there is an associated meningitis or subdural empyema. The only effective therapy in the fulminant anterior variety of disease, to which the above description applies, has been one of the antibiotics or sulfonamide drugs; anticoagulants have been used in some instances. The value of the latter has not been settled. The posterior part of the cavernous sinus may be infected via the superior and inferior petrosal veins without the occurrence of orbital edema or ophthalmoplegia. Mucormycosis may cause a similar clinical picture in the diabetic patient.

Thrombophlebitis of the superior longitudinal sinus may develop without symptoms. Usually, however, it is associated with unilateral convulsions and hemiplegia, first on one side of the body, then on the other, because of extension into the superior cerebral veins. The paralysis may be predominantly monoplegic (leg). Headache, papilledema, and increased intracranial pressure may accompany these signs. The diagnosis can be corroborated by the slowing of circulation and the failure of the superior sagittal sinus to fill during the late stage of the carotid arteriogram. Treatment consists of use of broad-spectrum antibiotics and temporization until the thrombus recanalizes.

All types of thrombophlebitis, especially those related to ear and paranasal sinus infection, may be complicated by other forms of intracranial suppurative infection, i.e., bacterial meningitis, subdural empyema, or brain abscess. Therapy in such patients must be individualized. The initiating focus should be brought under control, but to eradicate it surgically once intracranial extension has occurred (except possibly with cranial epidural infection) is to court disaster. A better plan is to treat the intracranial disease and to decide, after it has been eradicated, whether further surgery on the ear or sinus is necessary. In complicated cases the treatment of bacterial meningitis, which is often fatal, usually takes precedence over the surgically treated diseases (brain abscess and subdural empyema), but this rule is not hard and fast.

Aseptic thrombosis of intracranial venous sinuses, particularly the internal and superior longitudinal, may also develop after sinus and ear infections. One form, which may give rise to an obscure increased intracranial pressure because of occlusion of one lateral and superior sagittal sinus, has been called *otitic hydrocephalus* by Symonds. However, the term lacks precision because venous occlusion does not lead to ventricular enlargement and when the latter has followed an ear infection, it has been due to chronic meningitis. The more usual conditions which may be accompanied by aseptic thrombosis are postpartum and postoperative states (when platelet counts and fibrinogen levels rise), congenital heart disease, marasmus in infants, and sickle-cell anemia and primary or secondary polycythemia (see Chap. 343).

BRAIN ABSCESS

Most of the focal suppurative processes forming within the brain are linked to chronic ear and sinus or pulmonary infections. Approximately 40 percent of all brain abscesses are secondary to disease of the middle ear and mastoid cells, and of these, about one-third arise in the anterolateral part of the cerebellar hemisphere, the re-

mainder lying above the tegmen tympani in the middle and inferior part of the temporal lobe. Frontal sinusitis accounts for roughly 10 percent of the cases, the abscess being almost invariably situated in the anterior and inferior part of the frontal lobe. Of the remaining 50 percent of cases, a small portion are due to penetrating wounds and the remainder are metastatic. Of the latter, about half are traceable to a primary septic focus in the lung (usually bronchiectasis, empyema, or lung abscess), and in the others, the source of infection may be in the skin, bone (distinct osteomyelitic focus), or the heart. In some 5 to 10 percent of cases the source cannot be ascertained.

Brain abscesses are particularly frequent with congenital heart disease in which there is a right-to-left shunt (e.g., tetralogy of Fallot) and other types of septal defect with pulmonary arteriovenous shunts. They may also complicate arteriovenous vascular abnormalities of the lung. In the traumatic cases the site of the abscess will clearly depend on the area which has been injured. The metastatic abscesses are most likely to occur in the distal territory of the middle cerebral arteries, beginning at the junction of gray and white matter. In contrast to the otogenic and rhinogenic abscesses, they may be multiple.

Curiously enough, bacterial endocarditis rarely gives rise to brain abscess. Instead, the picture is one of focal embolic encephalitis with or without signs of embolic vascular disease (see Chap. 357). In the subacute form of endocarditis the emboli are sterile and cause only infarction, miliary foci of tissue necrosis, focal meningeal inflammation, and rarely mycotic aneurysms (CSF may contain a mixture of neutrophilic leukocytes, lymphocytes, and red blood corpuscles; the protein level may be elevated, but cultures are sterile and sugar values remain normal). In the acute form of bacterial endocarditis, miliary abscesses and purulent meningitis may develop, or there may be infarcts and meningeal or cerebral hemorrhages. Probably the larger symptomatic abscess does not have time to form, before the infection is suppressed by antibiotic medication or takes the life of the patient.

The infective agent varies from case to case. Though almost any one of the common pyogenic organisms may cause a cerebral abscess, the most frequent are streptococci, pneumococci, and staphylococci. As mentioned above, abscesses secondary to infections of the lung and those arising in relation to congenital cyanotic heart disease are likely to have a mixed bacterial flora (anaerobic streptococcus, fusiform bacillus, and oral spirochetes, etc.). Less often organisms such as *E. coli*, actinomyces, or even *Endamoeba histolytica* may be responsible.

CLINICAL MANIFESTATIONS. In patients who harbor chronic ear, sinus, or pulmonary infection a recent reactivation of the infection has usually preceded the onset of cerebral symptoms. The invasion of the cranial cavity by the infective process may be asymptomatic but in approximately half the cases is attended by a convulsion, a transitory focal neurologic disorder (cerebral embolus), or a syndrome of generalized headache, stiff neck, and CSF reaction (pleocytosis and increased protein but sterile fluid and normal sugar values). The latter raises suspicion of meningitis. These early symptoms may subside or appear to respond reassuringly to antibiotic medication. Then as days or even weeks pass, recurrent headache, slowness in mentation, further focal or generalized convulsions, and manifest signs of increased intracranial pressure announce the presence of an inflammatory mass in the brain. Usually the general symptoms of infection are less conspicuous than one might expect. In the phase of invasion and suppurative encephalitis there may be pyrexia, but as the abscess becomes encapsulated the temperature returns to normal. And, if the invasion stage of cerebral infection was not recognized, the clinical picture does not differ from that of a brain tumor. The CSF pressure in the established stage of the abscess is usually elevated, and except in a few of the deep metastatic cerebral abscesses, it nearly always reveals a pleocytosis 25 to 300 cells per ml (neutrophils and lymphocytes) and a rather high protein level (75 to 300 mg per 100 ml). A focal neurologic disorder also appears as the signs of increased pressure develop; these disorders vary with the location of the abscess, as follows:

Temporal Lobe Abscess. If the abscess lies in the dominant hemisphere, a dysphasia, which is often the "nominal" or "amnestic" type (in which the patient cannot name objects), usually occurs. A homonymous upper quadrantic field defect is the most frequent cerebral disorder, being due to involvement of the inferior portion of the optic radiation. Contralateral facial weakness is usually present, but motor or sensory defect in the limbs is minimal.

Cerebellar Abscess. Headache in the postauricular or suboccipital region is usually the first symptom and must be separated from symptoms of the ear disease itself. Coarse nystagmus to the side of the lesion and a cerebellar ataxia of the ipsilateral arm and leg then develop. The latter, though present in most patients, may be difficult to demonstrate if the patient is very ill. As a rule the signs of increased intracranial pressure are more prominent than those of cerebellar deficit. Mild pyramidal signs and evidence of brain stem compression (the latter, ipsilateral; the former, ipsilateral or contralateral) may be present late in the illness.

Frontal Lobe Abscess. Headache, drowsiness, inattention, and general impairment of mental function are prominent. Hemiparesis with unilateral motor seizures and motor or expressive dysphasia (dominant hemisphere) are the most frequent neurologic signs.

Aside from the CSF changes, the EEG demonstrates a focal slow-wave (delta) abnormality over a cerebral abscess, and may be used to follow the development or regression (after therapy) of abscess. Arteriography gives evidence of a cerebral mass by showing displacement of anterior, middle, or posterior cerebral arteries; and pneumoencephalography or ventriculography discloses deformation of ventricles. Radioactive isotopes localize as well in an inflammatory process as in a meningioma.

In all forms of brain abscess the illness, if not recognized and treated, is terminated either by the development of a tentorial or foramen magnum pressure cone or by rupture and flooding of the ventricle by pus (ventricular empyema). Rarely the abscess becomes heavily encapsulated and passes into a chronic stage, which may continue to be mildly symptomatic over a period of a year or more.

PATHOLOGY. Localized inflammatory necrosis and edema and septic thrombosis of vessels represent an early reaction to bacterial invasion of the brain (suppurative encephalitis). This is followed within a few weeks by encapsulation of the liquefied brain and of accumulated pus. The abscess capsule consists of fibroblasts and newly formed vessels (granulation tissue), and it increases in thickness over a period of weeks. The meninges adjacent to the abscess, especially near the point of entry of infection, are infiltrated by neutrophils, lymphocytes, and plasma cells.

DIAGNOSIS. The diagnosis of a brain abscess depends on (1) a demonstrated source of infection in ear, sinus, or lung; or the presence of right-to-left congenital cardiac shunt; (2) evidence of increased intracranial pressure; (3) focal cerebral or cerebellar signs; (4) an inflammatory reaction in the CSF (increase in number of cells and amount of protein in more than 80 percent of patients).

When all these signs are present and the clinical state has a time course extending over a period of weeks, the diagnosis is relatively easy. If no source of infection is present and there are only the symptoms and signs of a mass lesion, the condition must be differentiated from a malignant tumor, subdural hematoma, or granuloma. Sometimes only surgical exploration will settle the diagnosis. When the inflammatory nature of the intracranial process is established (source of infection, reaction of CSF), brain abscess must be distinguished from subdural empyema, thrombophlebitis, necrotizing viral encephalitis, and acute hemorrhagic leukoencephalitis (see Chap. 362). Here the CSF is of help as shown in Table 360-1.

Treatment. During the stage of acute suppurative encephalitis, to carry out an intracranial operation accomplishes little, probably causing only additional swelling of the brain tissue and a wider dissemination of the inflammatory process. At this stage intensive broad-spectrum antibiotic medication (choice decided by sensitivity of the organism to various antibiotics) and the control by intravenous urea or mannitol of excessively increased intracranial pressure (if patient's condition is threatened by such increase) are preferable. At times this medical program suppresses what appears to be an early abscess, with full recovery taking place. However, surgical intervention is required in the majority of patients. Occasionally deepening coma and the threat of brain herniation forces one to operate in the acute stage, but usually it is possible to wait until the inflammatory process has localized. The usual methods of treatment are unroofing the abscess and drainage, if it is superficial, and aspiration of the pus and installation of bacitracin or other antibiotics or total excision, if the abscess is encapsulated and accessible. These procedures have reduced the mortality from more than 50 to 10 percent or less. The least satisfactory results are obtained

Table 360-1. CEREBROSPINAL FLUID IN THE SUPPURATIVE INTRACRANIAL DISEASES
AND OTHERS WITH WHICH THEY MAY BE CONFUSED

	Pressure	WBC	Protein	Sugar	Bacteria
Bacterial meningitis	180–500	500–25,000	100–500 mg	<40	+
Subdural empyema	200–400	20–300	100–500	>40	0
Brain abscess	200–500	0–500	100–500	>40	0
Epidural abscess	Normal	0–200	30–150	>40	0
Bacterial endocarditis					
Acute	Normal	100–10,000	100–500	>40	+ or 0
Subacute	Normal	10–500	30–150	>40	0
Acute necrotizing hemorrhagic leukoencephalitis	Normal or elevated	20–2,000	50–500	>40	0
Acute inclusion body encephalitis	Normal	20–500	50–150	>40	0
Thrombophlebitis	Normal or elevated	0–100 (RBC in some)	50–100	>40	0

in metastatic abscesses, particularly if they are multiple. Variable neurologic deficits are left in about 30 percent of the surviving patients. Of these, one of the most troublesome has been focal epilepsy. In patients with congenital heart disease, if the cerebral abscess is successfully treated, an anatomic correction of the cardiac anomaly is indicated to prevent recurrences.

REFERENCES

Adams, R. D., and C. J. Kubik: The Effects of Influenzal Meningitis on the Nervous System, N.Y. State J. Med., 47:2676, 1947.

Haggerty, R. J., and M. Ziai: Acute Bacterial Meningitis in Children, Pediatrics, 25:742, 1960.

Kerr, F. W., R. B. King, and J. N. Neagher: Brain Abscess: A Study of 47 Consecutive Cases, J.A.M.A., 168:868, 1958.

Kubik, C. S., and R. D. Adams: Subdural Empyema, Brain, 66:18, 1943.

McKay, R. J., F. D. Ingraham, and D. D. Matson: Subdural Fluid, Complicating Bacterial Meningitis, J.A.M.A., 152:387, 1953.

361 VIRAL INFECTIONS OF THE NERVOUS SYSTEM: ASEPTIC MENINGITIS AND ENCEPHALITIS

*Byron Kakulas and
Raymond D. Adams*

More than 40 viruses are known to be capable of causing infection and symptomatic injury to the nervous system. In many instances the neurologic manifestations appear during the course of a generalized disease with its own peculiarities and easy identification, such as mumps, chickenpox, or pleurodynia. But it may happen that overt evidences of the infection are limited to the nervous system, and the resulting syndrome can be either relatively stereotyped or highly varied. If the latter condition prevails, clinical diagnosis may be difficult and one must, perforce, turn to laborious and complicated laboratory procedures for the identification of the causative agent, i.e., to ascertain the nature of the disease. But these diagnostic methods are not always successful, and even the most experienced laboratories have failed to establish the cause of the disease in as many as 30 to 50 percent of cases.

Those viruses which affect the nervous system primarily are said to be neurotropic. There are a considerable number of them, and their clinical manifestations are diverse, as might be expected. However, four clinical syndromes recur with regularity, and should be familiar to all students of medicine. These are the syndromes of (1) poliomyelitis, almost invariably a result of infection by one of the polioviruses; (2) zoster ganglionitis; (3) aseptic, or nonsuppurative, or "lymphocytic" meningitis; (4) encephalitis or meningoencephalitis. The first and second of these (poliomyelitis and herpes zoster) are discussed in Chaps. 216 and 225, the third and fourth are described below.

THE SYNDROME OF ASEPTIC MENINGITIS

The term *aseptic meningitis* was first introduced by Wallgren in 1925 to designate what was thought to be a specific disease, but it is now applied to a symptom complex that can be produced by any one of several dozen infective agents, the majority of which are viral. In bold outline the syndrome consists of fever, signs of meningeal irritation, and an abnormal cerebrospinal fluid (CSF).

Headache, out of proportion to that often associated with febrile states, ranks as the most frequent symptom in this group of diseases. A variable degree of drowsiness, confusion, or stupor, or rarely coma, may occur, but as a rule the derangement of consciousness tends to be relatively mild. Stiffness of the neck and spine on forward bending attest to the presence of meningeal irritation, but at first it may be so slight as to pass unnoticed. Here the Kernig and Brudzinski signs help very little, for they are often absent in the presence of a manifest viral meningitis. Frank neurologic signs of other types are infrequent; an isolated strabismus and diplopia, vague weakness, pain or paresthesias in an extremity, a slight inequality of reflexes, or a wavering Babinski sign are elicited only exceptionally. The meningitis may be asymptomatic.

The CSF findings consist of pleocytosis (mainly mononuclear except in the initial stage when a proportion of the cells are neutrophilic leukocytes) and bacteriologic sterility. The protein level is usually normal or slightly elevated. The concentration of glucose in the CSF is normal; this is important because a low sugar value in an infection which evokes a lymphocytic or mononuclear pleocytosis usually signifies tuberculous (Chap. 174), or mycotic (Chap. 176) meningitis, or rarely metastatic carcinoma, lymphoma, or sarcoid of the meninges. Since the CSF glucose level may be normal in the early stages of tuberculosis or crytococcosis, this determination should be repeated at intervals until the diagnosis is established or the patient is definitely convalescent.

Viral Infections that are Predominantly Meningeal

The majority of cases of aseptic meningitis are accounted for by nonparalytic poliomyelitis (Chap. 216), Coxsackie viruses (Chaps. 210 and 211), ECHO viruses (Chap. 212), mumps (Chap. 231), and lymphocytic choriomeningitis (LCM) (Chap. 215). Indeed these viral infections together with leptospirosis comprise about 95 percent of all cases of aseptic meningitis of established etiology. But in every series of cases published from virus isolation centers as many as one-fourth or more of them have an indeterminate cause.

Of the rarer types of aseptic meningitis one should mention the milder forms of postvaccinal meningoencephalitis or the meningoencephalitis which follows measles (Chap. 220), rubella (Chap. 221), chickenpox (Chap. 224), and prophylactic treatment of rabies (Chap. 217). Here the diagnosis is made on the history of the recent infection (usually within a few days or a week) or inoculation (usually within a few weeks).

Herpes simplex (Chap. 226) and the arthropod-borne (arbor) encephalitis viruses (Chap. 218) are responsible for a small proportion of cases of aseptic meningitis. Infections by arbor viruses are likely to be encountered in epidemics along with cases of frank encephalitis and tend to occur in certain geographic areas, points which facilitate early clinical recognition, though specific identification of the virus may still be difficult.

Neurologic manifestations, including the syndrome of aseptic meningitis, may appear in the course of syphilis (Chap. 177), influenza (Chap. 208), infectious mononucleosis (Chap. 255), psittacosis (Chap. 209), lymphogranuloma (Chap. 229), Rift Valley fever and encephalomyocarditis, Q fever, Behçet's disease, Vogt-Koyanagi disease, Harada's disease, Mollaret's recurrent meningitis, and other of the viral agents mentioned in Chap. 239.

The icteric stage of infectious hepatitis (Chap. 326) rarely is preceded by mild meningitis, the nature of which is evident when the jaundice appears. Among diseases of possible or probable viral causation, infectious mononucleosis (Chap. 255) sometimes produces what appears

to be a primary meningitis; and rarely a primary atypical pneumonia (Chap. 207) is complicated by aseptic meningitis or other neurologic disorder.

Differential Diagnosis of the Infective and Noninfective Forms of Lymphocytic Meningitis

Clinical distinctions between the many forms of aseptic meningitis cannot be made with a high degree of reliability, but useful leads can be obtained by careful attention to certain details of history and physical examination. The *season* during which the illnesses occur may be helpful. Enteroviral infections (poliomyelitis, Coxsackie, and ECHO) are diseases of midsummer and early fall, August and September usually being the peak months. The arthropod-borne diseases also occur in summer and fall (coinciding with the population of insect vectors), and though leptospirosis may appear at any season, its incidence in the United States shows a striking peak in August. Mumps and infectious mononucleosis are diseases of late winter and spring. Lymphocytic meningitis is particularly common in late fall and winter, presumably because field mice enter dwellings at this time. A definite past history of mumps aids in excluding the disease, second attacks being unusual. A preceding upper respiratory infection of a week's duration suggests LCM. Sore throat, lymphadenopathy, and rash point to infectious mononucleosis or ECHO infection. Severe back and leg pain occur in poliomyelitis, leptospirosis, and trichinosis. Aseptic meningitis during pregnancy is likely to be poliomyelitis. Exposure to such animals as mice (LCM), dogs, rats, or swine (leptospirosis) may give a hint as to diagnosis. A skin rash favors the presence of infectious mononucleosis, ECHO viral infections, and leptospirosis (often a transient, blotchy erythema). Icterus suggests infectious mononucleosis or viral hepatitis; it is not present in pure meningeal leptospirosis. Conjunctival suffusion is common in leptospirosis and may be seen in trichinosis. Slight tenderness and swelling of salivary glands and testes may be the only signs of mumps. Pulmonary infiltrates suggest LCM, infectious mononucleosis, psittacosis, or leptospirosis.

Aside from viral isolation, few laboratory tests are helpful. The peripheral leukocyte count is often normal, but leukopenia may be present. However it accompanies so many of the diseases responsible for aseptic meningitis (infectious mononucleosis, Colorado tick fever, LCM, lupus erythematosis, etc.) that rarely is it a useful finding. Eosinophilia should suggest a parasitic infection, and occasionally infectious mononucleosis may be identified by the blood smear. Lymphocytic choriomeningitis produces the most intense pleocytosis in the CSF (counts above 1,000 cells per ml are almost always due to this disease), and mumps gives an almost pure lymphocytic pleocytosis. Serologic tests on the CSF should be interpreted with caution because inflammation of many types can produce a false positive reaction; infectious mononucleosis and lupus erythematosus often evoke biologic false positive serum tests for syphilis. Liver function tests are abnormal in many patients with infectious mononucleosis and in anicteric hepatitis; hepatic abnormalities are not regularly present in the other entities under consideration.

Three other categories of disease may cause an apparently sterile, predominantly lymphocytic or mononuclear reaction in the leptomeninges; bacterial infections lying adjacent to the meninges; specific infections or parainfectious diseases in which the organism is difficult to isolate; and neoplastic invasion (usually lymphoma or carcinoma). The recognition of these is of great importance, since they require vigorous antibiotic therapy or some other form of treatment (syphilis, tuberculosis, cryptococcosis).

With respect to pyogenic infections in which the CSF does not show a purulent meningitis and is sterile, it must be remembered that antibiotic therapy given in inadequate dosage during a systemic or pulmonary infection may suppress a coexistent meningitis to the point where mononuclear cells predominate, glucose level is normal, and organisms are not detected in the CSF. A mistaken diagnosis of aseptic meningitis may then be made when the CSF is examined. The true state of affairs becomes evident only when the patient worsens and bacteria again appear. Careful attention to the history of recent antimicrobial therapy sometimes permits recognition of these cases before serious symptoms recur. A smouldering paranasal sinusitis or mastoiditis may produce a similar CSF change because of intracranial extension (epidural or subdural infection). Or a brain abscess, the localizing signs of which are obscure, may deceive the clinician into making a diagnosis of aseptic meningitis (see Chap. 360).

In the second group of diseases, acute syphilitic meningitis is of importance and may be symptomatic or asymptomatic. In former times it was likely to develop as a neurorecurrence after inadequate arsenic therapy, but now it may be merely the first manifestation of a florid syphilitic infection (see Chap. 177). Tuberculous meningitis often masquerades as an innocent aseptic meningitis; the diagnosis may at first be difficult because the tubercle bacillus is hard to see in stained smears, and cultures and guinea pig inoculations require considerable time. Similarly the cryptococcus may not be diagnosed for the reason that the organisms, may be present in such low number as to be overlooked in smears.

Children with scarlet fever or streptococcus pharyngitis rarely have been noted to develop meningeal signs and pleocytosis, the result of a sterile "serous" inflammation that does not involve invasion of the meninges by visible organisms. The same is true of subacute bacterial endocarditis.

In the third group, leukemias and lymphomas are the most conspicuous source of neoplastic meningeal reactions. In children with myelogenous leukemia, a leukemic meningitis with cell counts numbering into the thousands occurs not infrequently in the late stages of the illness. In adults a pleocytosis with lymphocyte or lymphoblast counts reaching as high as 4,000 per ml of fluid may complicate lymphocytic and lymphoblastic lymphomas with or without leukemia. The sugar values may fall to 0, and the protein level is elevated.

In carcinomatous "meningitis" (in breast, stomach, lung, melanoma, or other organ) great numbers of cells may extend through the leptomeninges, involving cranial and spinal nerve roots, and produce a picture of meningoradiculitis with low sugar values. Millipore filter preparations usually permit identification of the tumor cells.

Finally, in a number of other subacute or chronic infections of obscure origin, probably viral, the CSF formula corresponds to that of aseptic meningitis. These are (1) Behçet's disease, distinguished clinically by the triad of genital ulceration, uveitis, and involvement of central nervous system (cranial nerve palsies, seizures, mental disturbance, aphasia, hemiparesis, cerebellar ataxia); (2) Vogt-Koyanagi and Harada's diseases with various combinations of uveitis, depigmentation of hair and skin around the eyes, loss of eyelashes, dysacusis and deafness; (3) Mollaret's recurrent meningitis (cf. p. 1788); and allergic or hypersensitivity meningitis, described by Barrett and Thies, occurring in the course of serum sickness and diseases of connective tissue such as lupus erythematosus.

In summary, though clinical findings, season occurrence, and laboratory tests can sometimes enable the physician to direct further diagnostic efforts along specific lines, they may not be conclusive. Most important is to keep in mind always the possibility of tuberculosis, cryptococcosis, syphilis, inadequately treated pyogenic meningitis, and brain abscess, all of which may simulate aseptic meningitis. These diseases offer more pressing diagnostic problems, for they may take the life of the patient if they are not diagnosed and treated. In contrast, the various forms of aseptic viral meningitis are usually self-limiting and benign.

THE SYNDROME OF ENCEPHALITIS

From the above discussion it is evident that the separation of the clinical syndrome of aseptic meningitis and encephalitis is not always easy, because in some patients with the former condition a nonspecific drowsiness or confusion may be present when in fact there is no evidence of an inflammatory reaction in the substance of the brain. Conversely, in some patients with encephalitis the cerebral involvement may be so mild as to escape notice and only the meningeal symptoms and CSF abnormality may be manifest. These facts make it difficult to place complete reliance on statistical data about the relative incidence of encephalitis collected in surveys from various virus laboratories. It is our impression that many cases of mumps and LCM are little more than examples of intense meningitis. They rarely have caused death with postmortem demonstration of cerebral lesions, and surviving patients seldom have residual signs.

The core of the encephalitis syndrome is an acute illness with evidence of meningeal involvement, added to which are various combinations of the following symptoms and signs: convulsions, confusion, stupor, or coma; aphasia or mutism; hemiparesis with asymmetry of tendon reflexes and Babinski signs; involuntary movements, ataxia, and myoclonic jerks; nystagmus, ocular palsies, and facial weakness. Some one or other of these groups of findings predominate in certain types of encephalitis, as will be pointed out below, but always the clinical diagnosis in the setting of a febrile aseptic meningitis rests on the demonstration of focal derangement of the function of the cerebrum, brainstem, or cerebellum. The illnesses produced by these viral agents vary in duration but are usually measured in terms of weeks or, exceptionally, months. Death occurs in 5 to 20 percent of patients with viral encephalitis. Residual signs such as mental deterioration, amnestic defect, personality change, and hemiparesis are seen in about 20 percent of patients. This overall figure fails to reflect, however, the wide variation in the incidence of late changes that follow infection by different viruses. For example, neurologic sequelae have been observed in 80 to 90 percent of patients with Eastern equine encephalitis and in only 5 to 10 percent of those with Western equine infections.

Table 361-1. VIRAL CAUSES OF ENCEPHALITIS

Disease	Page Reference
Eastern equine	980
Western equine	980
Venezuelan equine (rare)	981
St. Louis	982
Japanese B	981
Murray Valley (Australian X disease)	979
Ilheus	979
Russian tick-borne complex:	
Russian spring-summer	979
Louping ill (rare)	979
Kyasanur Forest disease (rare)	979
Central European	979
Diphasic milk fever	979
West Nile fever (rare)	979
Colorado tick fever (rare	979
Encephalitis lethargica (von Economo)	1796
Rabies	976
Polioencephalitis	968
Coxsackie (rare)	965
Herpes simplex	996
Lymphocytic choriomeningitis (rare)	967
Mumps (rare)	1007
Cat-scratch disease (rare)	1005
Psittacosis (rare)	959
Influenza (rare)	956
Lymphogranuloma venereum (rare)	1004
Primary atypical pneumonia (rare)	954
Infectious hepatitis (rare)	1535
Encephalomyocarditis (Columbia-SK: Mengo, etc.)	1025
Postinfectious or postvaccinal demyelinating Encephalitis	1797
Vaccinia	991
Rabies	976
Varicella	993
Rubeola	985
Rubella	987
Exanthem subitum	989
Smallpox	990
Dengue	1014
Yellow fever	1012

ETIOLOGY. Whereas numerous virus, bacterial, fungus, and parasitic agents are listed as causes of the encephalitis syndrome, only the viral ones are being considered here, for reference is usually being made to them when the term *encephalitis* is used. The number of viral infections or postviral allergic reactions is large (see Table 361-1), and one might suppose that clinical problems would be infinitely complex. However, those forms of viral encephalitis that occur with sufficient frequency to be of diagnostic importance are relatively few, and they tend to have geographic and seasonal incidence. In the United States, Eastern and Western equine encephalitis (Chap. 218) have been observed mainly in California; there have been only two recognized outbreaks of Eastern equine encephalitis in New England, each in the early autumn. St. Louis encephalitis (Chap. 218), another arthropod-borne late-summer encephalitis, has rarely been encountered in Eastern United States. Japanese B encephalitis, Russian spring-summer, and Murray Valley encephalitis (Australian X disease) (Chap. 218) are virtually unknown in the United States. Epidemic (lethargic) encephalitis has not been observed in the acute form in the United States or Western Europe since 1930, through patients with residual symptoms (Parkinson's syndrome) are still to be seen in neurology clinics.

In addition to the viruses that primarily exert their effects on the central nervous system, there is another large group of them in which cerebral involvement is an unusual complication in the course of a well-defined clinical illness. These diseases (also listed in Table 361-1) are fully described on the pages referred to in the table.

ACUTE ARTHROPOD FORMS OF ENCEPHALITIS

Eastern equine encephalitis may be considered representative of a whole group of acutely devastating viral diseases of cerebral gray and white matter. A brief interval after exposure, the victim, usually a child, becomes febrile and then within hours or a few days convulses and lapses into coma with manifest hemiplegia. The CSF pressure is often elevated, heavy in cell content (up to 2,000 to 3,000, with a large proportion of neutrophilic leukocytes) with elevated protein values. In as many as 25 to 50 percent of cases, depending on the epidemic, death terminates the illness within 1 or a few days, and at autopsy there is extensive inflammatory necrosis of large portions of one or both cerebral hemispheres. Survivors slowly recover, but many are left with residual focal cerebral deficits. The disease is nonprogressive after the first few days.

Western equine encephalitis, St. Louis, North Dakota, and Japanese B encephalitis differ from this picture in their relatively slower rate of attack and progression and their more protracted course, as pointed out in Chap. 218, but still the principal symptoms are cerebral in type.

Rabies stands apart because it is distinguished by a relatively long latent period (months) after the bite of the rabid animal, during which the virus multiples in neurones, and by the predominance of dysphagia (hence salivation), throat spasms induced by attempts to swallow water (hence hydrophobia), dysarthria, numbness of face, and facial spasms to which are added a confusional psychosis. The localization indicates the intensive involvement of the tegmental medullary nuclei in the rabid form of the disease (paralytic form is due to spinal cord affection) (see Chap. 217).

Encephalitis Lethargica (von Economo's Disease, Sleeping Sickness)

This disease first occurred in the wake of the pandemic of influenza during and for about 10 years after World War I. No disease like it can be found in medical annals before 1914. Although the viral agent was never identified, the clinical and pathologic features were typical of viral infection. The principal symptoms were pronounced somnolence, from which the disease takes its name, and ophthalmoplegia. A small number of patients were overly active rather than somnolent, and such patients often had also a disorder of movement in the form either of chorea or myoclonus. Headache, insomnia, dizziness, fatigability, or frank confusional psychosis were not infrequent. In contrast, paralysis (hemiplegia), cortical sensory loss, aphasia, disorders of hearing or vision, and convulsions were virtually unknown. The onset was acute or subacute, and the symptoms persisted for several weeks. Lymphocytic pleocytosis was found in half the patients, together with variable elevation of protein level. More than 20 percent of the victims died within a few weeks. A high proportion of the survivors developed within months or years (sometimes after an interval as long as 25 years) the syndrome of parkinsonism (see Chaps. 22 and 364). In fact, this is the only form of encephalitis known to cause an immediate or delayed extrapyramidal syndrome of this type. Myoclonus, dystonia, bulimia, obesity, reversal of sleep pattern, and in children a psychopathic personality with compulsive behavior were other distressing sequelae.

The pathology was typical of a neurotropic viral infection (nerve cell destruction, and neuronophagia, perivascular cuffing with lymphocytes and mononuclear cells, and meningeal infiltrations of similar cells) localized principally to the region of the midbrain, subthalamus, and hypothalamus. In the patients who die years later of Parkinson's syndrome, fibrillary changes in the nerve cells of substantia nigra, oculomotor, and adjacent nuclei; destruction of nerve cells; and gliosis are the only findings.

No new cases have been seen in the United States and Western Europe since 1930. The only treatment available for the survivors consists of antiparkinsonism drugs and surgery, as outlined in Chap. 364.

ACUTE AND SUBACUTE INCLUSION BODY ENCEPHALITIS

First described by Dawson in 1939 and extensively studied by van Bogaert, in both subacute and chronic forms, this disease (more likely group of diseases) is the only one which occurs sporadically throughout the year and in patients of all ages and in all parts of the world. Whereas herpes simplex has been isolated from many of the acute cases and rubeola virus from subacute sclerosing ones, no causative agent has been found in others. Identity of etiology has been claimed by Haymaker on the basis of the pathology, particularly the large intranuclear (Cowdry type B) inclusion bodies in the astrocytes, oligodendrocytes, and nerve cells, but the evidence now is clearly against this unitary concept.

Nothing is known of the incubation period of these diseases. In acute encephalitis rarely has there been herpetic lesions of the skin or mucous membranes. A febrile onset and convulsions, confusion, hallucinations, stupor, or coma have been the usual initial symptoms. The picture evolves over a period of days or weeks, and the confusional psychosis shows elements of delirium or Korsakoff's amnestic state, the latter being more evident as the weeks pass. Age at onset has varied from childhood to the most advanced years ($>$ sixty to seventy years in several of our patients). The CSF has shown a pleocytosis and increased protein content in most of the patients. The virus has been isolated from the brain (biopsy, autopsy) and CSF in only a few patients, and a rising titer of neutralizing antibodies has been demonstated in others. The mortality rate is high (30 percent), and many of the survivors have been left with the most severe mental sequelae in the form of a complete Korsakoff's psychosis or global dementia. Prognosis is not hopeless, however, for a few patients have recovered to the point where they can resume an independent life.

The subacute and chronically progressive forms of inclusion body encephalitis have affected children and adolescents for the most part. Widespread myelin destruction in the cerebral hemispheres with gliosis (sclerosing encephalitis) is combined with focal lesions of the brainstem. The clinical picture is that of a slowly evolving mental deterioration (dementia) associated with myoclonic jerks, falling spells, and cerebellar ataxia. The CSF may contain no cells, but the protein level may be elevated particularly the γ-globulin fraction (first zone gold sol curve). High levels of neutralizing antibody to measles virus have been found in serum and CSF, but this infective agent has been isolated from the brain tissue only once. It is still uncertain as to whether this virus has been seen in electron microscopic sections of the brain. The course of the disease is progressive, death usually occurring within a few months or years.

The pathology of the acute inclusion body encephalitis is marked by an intense hemorrhagic necrosis of the medial and inferior parts of the temporal lobes, and the orbital parts of the frontal ones. This distribution of lesion is so characteristic that the diagnosis can be made by simple inspection. The subacute sclerosing form involves the cerebral cortex and white matter of both hemispheres. Destruction of nerve cells, neuronophagia, and perivenous cuffing by lymphocytes and mononuclear cells indicate the viral nature of the infection. Degeneration of medullated fibers (myelin and axis cylinders) occurs in the white matter and is accompanied by perivascular cuffing and fibrous gliosis. The inclusion bodies in nerve and glial cells may be difficult to find. Treatment with some of the new antiviral agents is being tried.

The diagnosis may be difficult. The acute inclusion body encephalities must be distinguished from acute hemorrhagic leukoencephalitis (see p. 1799), acute subdural empyema, acute cerebral abscess, thrombophlebitis, and septic embolism (see p. 1789). The subacute to chronic variety simulates the childhood and adolescent dementing diseases such as lipid storage disease (see Chap. 364) and Schilder's disease (see Chap. 362).

CHRONIC "SLOW" VIRAL ENCEPHALITIS

The idea that viral infections may lead to chronic disease, especially of the nervous system, has been entertained for half a century but only recently has received firm support from the following observations: (1) the demonstration of a slowly progressive noninflammatory degeneration of nigral neurones long after an attack of encephalitis lethargica; (2) the discovery in Iceland and England of a chronic viral degenerative disease of white matter in sheep (Visna and scrapie); (3) the finding of inclusion bodies in the most chronic cases of sclerosing encephalitis and the EM demonstration of viral particles in multifocal leukoencephalopathy; (4) the transmission of Kuru to chimpanzees by Gajdusek and Gibbs; and (5) late onset of motor system disease after poliomyelitis. Claims have also been made for a viral causation of multiple sclerosis by Schubladze, of amyotrophic lateral sclerosis by Zilber, of epilepsia partialis continua and Vilynisk encephalomyelitis by Chumakov, and of Jakob-Creutzfeldt's disease by Gajdusek, but the evidence is questionable. From these observations has emerged the concept of the "slow viruses," the common features of which are: long period of latency (months or years); protracted progression of illness after onset of symptoms; limitation of infections to a single host species; and localization of noninflammatory degenerative lesions in a single organ or tissue system.

These slow viruses so perfectly simulate a purely degenerative disease that views of all the major degenerative diseases of white and gray matter of the brain are being altered. One of the most exciting prospects in medical neurology is thus unfolding before us. Some of these slow virus effects are discussed at greater length in Chap. 219.

There is presently no known treatment for any of these diseases.

OTHER CAUSES OF ENCEPHALITIS

The most important nonviral diagnostic possibilities to be considered in a patient with the syndrome of encephalitis are syphilis (Chap. 177), pertussis (Chap. 152), leptospirosis (Chap. 181), relapsing fever (Chap. 182), epidemic typhus (Chap. 199), scrub typhus (Chap. 200), Rocky Mountain spotted fever (Chap. 195), trypanosomiasis (Chap. 243), toxoplasmosis (Chap. 244), cerebral malaria (Chap. 241), trichinosis (Chap. 247), schistosomiasis (Chap. 250), and cysticercosis (Chap. 252).

REFERENCES

Von Economo, C.: "Encephalitis Lethargica," New York, Oxford University Press, 1931.
"Current Topics in Microbiology and Immunology," Vol. 40, Berlin, Springer-Verlag OHG, 1967.

362 MULTIPLE SCLEROSIS AND OTHER DEMYELINATING DISEASES

David C. Poskanzer and
Raymond D. Adams

A large and important group of neurologic disorders are termed the *demyelinating diseases* because they share the common pathologic feature of foci of degeneration, involving the myelin sheath of nerves. These foci vary in size, shape, distribution, and rate of development in the different illnesses. The axis cylinder often suffers damage, as does the myelin sheath, but the destruction of myelin is considered the primary change.

Because no clear etiology has been ascertained for this group of diseases and a wide variety of etiologic theories have been proposed, including infective, metabolic, allergic, and vascular ones, a classification must be based on a combination of clinical and pathologic factors. It is, of course, possible that the process of demyelination may have several different causes and may be a common manifestation of different diseases. Although intermediate and transitional cases exist among the various demyelinating diseases, four syndromes can be clearly distinguished on the basis of history, clinical examination, and pathologic findings.

1. Acute disseminated encephalomyelitis (including postinfectious and postvaccinial encephalomyelitis)
2. Acute necrotizing hemorrhagic leukoencephalitis
3. Multiple sclerosis
4. Diffuse cerebral sclerosis

ACUTE DISSEMINATED ENCEPHALOMYELITIS

Acute disseminated encephalomyelitis may be defined as an acute encephalitic or myelitic process of variable course and severity, characterized by symptoms indicating damage chiefly to the white matter of the brain or spinal cord and pathologically by perivascular cellular infiltration and perivenous demyelination.

An acute encephalitis, myelitis, or encephalomyelitis of this type may occur concurrently or follow shortly upon the exanthem of measles, smallpox, chickenpox, and rubella. A similar demyelinating illness with multiple perivascular foci of demyelination occurs following vaccination against rabies and against smallpox. Some cases clinically and pathologically indistinguishable from these two categories of acute disseminated encephalomyelitis appear to develop without any clearly defined preceding illness or vaccination. The disease has grave significance because of the substantial death rate and the high frequency of persistent neurologic defects in patients who recover. The etiology of the process is unclear, but it is generally thought to represent a form of hypersensitivity. A laboratory model for the disease, the experimental allergic encephalomyelitis of animals, can be produced by innoculating the animals with a combination of brain tissue and adjuvants.

PATHOLOGY. There are no distinctive changes on naked-eye examination of the brain. Microscopically, the white matter shows innumerable small zones of demyelination from 0.1 to 1 mm in diameter, which invariably surround small and medium-sized veins. The axis cylinders are more or less intact. There is a perivascular infiltration with lymphocytes, histiocytes, and plasma cells. Meningeal infiltration is another invariable feature but is rarely marked.

Postvaccinial Encephalomyelitis. A severe demyelinating illness may occur following vaccination against rabies, with an incidence reported between 1 in a 1,000 and 1 in 4,000 persons vaccinated. The lesion is presumably due to sensitization of brain tissue contained in the vaccine. The use of killed duck embryo vaccine which is free of nerve tissue has apparently substantially reduced the incidence of the encephalomyelitic complications of rabies vaccination.

Encephalomyelitis following vaccination against smallpox has been known since 1860 but appears to have occurred only in isolated instances until 1922, when a real epidemic of postvaccinial encephalomyelitis was first recognized. The disease usually begins in the tenth to twelfth day after vaccination, though it may appear at any time between the second and twenty-fifth days. The mortality rate is high, between 30 and 50 percent, but varies among epidemics. If recovery occurs, it is usually complete. A typical estimate of incidence is 1 in 5,000 vaccinated. The disease occurs much more frequently after primary vaccination than after revaccination, perhaps as much as twentyfold. It is practically unknown in infants vaccinated before the age of one year, and it is believed that the earlier the child is vaccinated, the more favorable are his chances of avoiding this complication. The occurrence of the disease, as might be expected, parallels an increase in the number of persons vaccinated when smallpox threatens, but there is good evidence that the incidence of postvaccinial encephalomyelitis varies considerably from time to time and from one place to another. The source of material used for the vaccination seems to have no bearing on its occurrence.

The onset of the illness is generally abrupt, with headache, drowsiness, fever, and vomiting. There may be stiffness of the neck and other signs of meningeal irritation. Convulsions are occasionally seen. Soon afterward, signs of spinal cord involvement usually appear, with flaccid paralysis generally involving all four limbs, though hemiplegia may occur. Tendon reflexes disappear, and

the plantar responses become extensor. Sphincter control is generally lost, and sensory loss, though variable, may be extensive and severe. Nystagmus, ocular palsies, and pupillary changes give evidence of brainstem involvement. Stupor and deepening coma may occur. The onset of coma and evidence of brainstem involvement indicate a rapid worsening of prognosis. Despite the general features of the typical case, variations are common. One patient may suffer a predominantly encephalitic illness with convulsions and coma and little evidence of cord damage, another may have a hemiplegia, or a pure transverse myelitis may occur without headache, neck stiffness, or clouding of consciousness. The site of vaccination has no influence on the neurologic syndrome, and the florid skin lesions in the form of a generalized vaccinia or erythematous rash does not increase the likelihood of neuroparalytic accident. Spinal fluid almost invariably shows an increase in protein and lymphocytes, but in rare cases it is normal.

The association of the neurologic disorder with vaccination or innoculation usually leaves the diagnosis in little doubt, and the characteristic combination of encephalitic and myelitic features will help to distinguish the condition from meningitis, virus encephalitis, and poliomyelitis. Rarely, an atypical case may mimic any one of these disorders. On occasion, the disease may suggest involvement of nerve roots and peripheral nerves and be indistinguishable from idiopathic polyneuritis (Guillain-Barré syndrome).

Improvement involving recovery of consciousness and regression of neurologic signs may be surprisingly complete. A significant proportion of patients may show residual neurologic signs, intellectual impairment, and psychoneurotic sequelae many years after the illness, however.

Postinfectious Encephalomyelitis. This syndrome is often referred to as parainfectious encephalomyelitis because of its onset prior to, in association with, or after the rash of measles or other exanthem.

Clinically evident neurologic complications occur in between 1 in 800 and 1 in 1,000 cases of measles. A measles epidemic in a large city may well include 100,000 cases and will therefore result in a substantial number of neurologic complications. The mortality rate among cases with such complications ranges from 10 to 20 percent, and about 50 percent of the victims are left with persistent neurologic damage. The rate of neurologic complications may in fact be considerably higher than is apparent clinically. A high rate of abnormalities in the spinal fluid and in the electroencephalogram is observed in the studies of children with measles. Patients without clinically apparent neurologic residua may undergo significant and sometimes permanent changes in behavior. The neurologic complications of measles alone provide adequate justification for the prevention of the disease through the use of vaccine.

Following smallpox the incidence of neurologic complications is approximately 2.5 cases out of 1,000. The occurrence of encephalomyelitis complicating chickenpox is less common and that complicating rubella is quite rare. An acute demyelinating process probably occurs in association with mumps, but the clinical picture is complicated by the presence of a true viral encephalomyelitis in mumps and often cannot be differentiated from a postinfectious process in the living patient.

The syndrome generally begins 2 to 4 days after the rash. The most common clinical picture is one dominated by convulsions and deepening coma. Less commonly, the patient may develop hemiplegia, show evidence of cerebellar disease, or occasionally develop a transverse myelitis or polyradiculitis. Chorea and athetoid movements are also seen infrequently. In many cases the disease is much less severe and the patient suffers transient encephalitic illness with headaches, confusion, and signs of meningeal irritation. It is not entirely clear that all the neurologic complications described are truly encephalomyelitic; in some cases cerebrovascular disease, particularly thrombophlebitis, acute toxic encephalopathy or hypoxic encephalopathy may be responsible.

Neurologic complications of chickenpox appear to be more benign, and there is some question as to whether a true postinfectious encephalomyelitis actually occurs following chickenpox. Cerebellar signs are more commonly seen following this illness than following measles. The cerebrospinal fluid as in postvaccinial encephalomyelitis contains lymphocytes and elevated protein.

PREVENTION AND TREATMENT. Primary vaccination in infancy is a specific preventive measure for postvaccinial encephalomyelitis, since persons not vaccinated at that time will almost certainly be vaccinated at a later age when the risk of encephalomyelitis is considerably higher.

The use of killed duck embryo vaccine may well have largely eliminated the occurrence of post-rabies-vaccination encephalomyelitis. Measles vaccine may have eliminated the largest group of the postinfectious encephalomyelitides.

The use of ACTH or high-potency steroids appears to be the treatment of choice, though controlled trials of this treatment have not been carried out. The steroids appear to be effective in controlling the manifestations of experimental allergic encephalomyelitis in animals.

ACUTE NECROTIZING HEMORRHAGIC ENCEPHALOMYELITIS

In a small number of patients dying from a fulminating encephalopathic illness, certain distinctive pathologic features may be found. On section of the brain, the white matter of one or both hemispheres is seen to be destroyed almost to the point of liquefaction. The involved tissue is pink or yellowish gray and flecked with multiple small hemorrhages. Sometimes similar changes are localized to the brainstem or spinal cord. On histologic examination one finds widespread necrosis of small blood vessels, necrosis of brain tissue around the vessels with intense cellular infiltration, multiple small hemorrhages, and a violent inflammatory reaction in the meninges. The pathologic picture resembles that of disseminated encephalo-

myelitis in its perivascular distribution with the added feature of more widespread necrosis leading to diffuse sclerosis and a tendency to congregate into large foci in the cerebral hemispheres.

The clinical course of the illness resembles that of acute disseminated encephalomyelitis save for its apoplectiform onset and rapidity of progress, leading often to death within 48 hr; it is also true that neurologic signs are frequently unilateral or purely bulbar in type, reflecting the localized nature of the pathologic process. It is probable that certain patients showing an explosive myelitic illness are suffering from a necrotizing myelitis of similar type, but pathologic evidence in support of this view has been difficult to obtain. The cerebrospinal fluid examination discloses a more intense reaction than in other demyelinating diseases. Often a polymorphonuclear pleocytosis of up to several thousand cells and a considerable increase in amount of protein are detected.

The etiology of this condition remains obscure, but the resemblance to the other demyelinating diseases should be noted, a resemblance which is strengthened by the fact that certain patients showing the typically fulminating clinical picture have recovered, some completely, others with neurologic sequelae of variable severity. Acute encephalitis due to herpes simplex or other viruses also figures in the differential diagnosis. The points of similarity to other demyelinative diseases are sufficient to suggest that steroid drugs should be used in such cases; in several personally observed patients, we have had the impression that they produced a favorable result.

MULTIPLE SCLEROSIS

Multiple sclerosis, referred to in the British Commonwealth as *disseminated sclerosis* and among French-speaking physicians as *sclérose en plaque*, is one of the most common chronic neurologic diseases. It is characterized clinically by remissions and recurrences extending over a period of many years. Though pleomorphic in its clinical presentation, the picture is determined by the location of foci of demyelination which tend to have a predilection for certain portions of the nervous system. The result is a group of symptom complexes which can often be readily diagnosed.

Classical features include impairment of vision, nystagmus, dysarthria, intention tremor, ataxia, impairment of perception of position and vibratory senses, bladder dysfunction, paraplegia, and alteration in emotional responses. For purposes of diagnosis, it is generally required that both evidence of more than one discrete lesion and a history of exacerbation and remission be present.

Diagnosis is particularly difficult in the early years of the disease. Long latent periods between a minor initial episode which may not even come to medical attention, and the development of subsequent symptoms are responsible for a lag, often of many years, between actual onset and final diagnosis. In most cases, there are relapses interspersed with periods of remission, but in other cases (as many as half of the total number) the disease presents as an intermittently or steadily progressive illness.

PATHOLOGY. Macroscopically, the brain before being sectioned generally shows no evidence of disease, but the surface of the spinal cord may feel uneven. On section, numerous scattered lesions are seen which are slightly depressed and which, by virtue of their pinkish gray appearance (due to loss of myelin) stand out in contrast to the surrounding white matter. The lesions may vary in diameter from less than 1 mm to several centimeters: they affect principally the white matter of brain and spinal cord and do not extend beyond the root entry zone of brainstem and spinal cord. They also encroach frequently on cerebral gray matter but do not destroy nerve cells. The lesions appear to have a predilection for elongate structures where myelin abuts pial veins, hence the frequent involvement of spinal cord and the optic nerves and chiasm. They are frequently seen in the paraventricular areas of the brain in relation to the veins in the walls of the lateral ventricles.

The histologic appearance depends on the age of the lesion. Relatively recent lesions show a predominantly perivenous distribution of the demyelination with sparing of axis cylinders, degeneration of oligodendroglia, neuroglial reaction, and perivascular infiltration with mononuclear cells. Later large numbers of microglial phagocytes infiltrate the lesion, and astrocytes in and around it increase in number and size. A long-standing lesion, on the other hand, will show thickly matted, relatively acellular fibroglial tissue, with only occasional perivascular macrophages; in such a lesion intact axis cylinders may still be discovered, but many are destroyed, and this in turn leads to descending and ascending degeneration of long-fiber tracts. All gradations of pathologic change between these two extremes may be found in lesions of variegated size and shape.

ETIOLOGY. The cause or causes of multiple sclerosis remain undetermined. A number of epidemiologic facts have been clearly established, however, which must eventually be incorporated in any etiologic hypothesis. The disease has been shown to be rare between the equator and latitudes 30 and 35 degrees north and south. It becomes more common with increasing latitude thereafter. For example, the prevalence of multiple sclerosis is six times as great in Winnipeg, Mannitoba as in New Orleans, Louisiana. An exception to the geographic pattern appears to exist in Japan, where the prevalence rates are uniform and extremely low. Several studies indicate that a person who migrates from a high risk to a low risk zone carries the high risk of multiple sclerosis with him, even though the disease may not become apparent until 20 years after migration. This pattern has been demonstrated both in South Africa and in Israel.

An increase in familial occurrence of multiple sclerosis has long been recognized. The disease is about eight times more common in immediate relatives (parents and sibs) than in patients in the general population. Twin studies have failed, however, to corroborate a genetic predisposition, and within families with more than one affected member, no consistent genetic pattern is evident. There is a tendency to consider all diseases with an increased familial incidence, such as multiple sclerosis, as hereditary. Instances of the same condition in several members of the family may actually reflect common exposure to a similar environmental factor, however. For example, paralytic poliomyelitis is eight times as common in immediate family members than the general population.

The age distribution of the disease follows a normal distribution with a mean between thirty and thirty-five. There is virtually no other disease that has an age at onset similar to that of multiple sclerosis. Women seem to have a higher prevalence and incidence than do men.

Several studies have now demonstrated a shift toward higher socioeconomic groups in the general pattern of distribution of the disease in the population.

PRECIPITATING FACTORS. A variety of events occurring immediately before the onset of illness have been regarded as precipitating factors in relation to multiple sclerosis. These include various types of infection, emotional trauma, injury, and pregnancy. Though there seems to be a definite increase in number of exacerbations during the pregnancy year, other traumatic factors during the course of the illness, including lumbar puncture and surgical procedures, have not been shown to be of statistical significance.

At the present time two etiologic theories, which are not necessarily exclusive of one another, are receiving the most attention. These include the possibility that multiple sclerosis is caused by an infection early in life with a long incubation period, as might be expected among the so-called "slow virus" infections, an example of which is Kuru. The other theory stresses the possibility of autoimmunity to one's own neurologic tissue. At the moment there is no direct confirmation of either theory. The data favoring an infectious etiology with a long incubation period is epidemiologic; that supporting the autoimmune hypothesis cannot be investigated in the absence of an animal model of multiple sclerosis.

CLINICAL MANIFESTATIONS. About 40 percent of patients with multiple sclerosis have an episode of optic neuritis as their initial symptom. The syndrome is one of rapid onset over a period of several days of partial or total loss of vision in one eye, often associated with pain on movement of the eye. Characteristically, a scotoma will be present involving macular vision, but a wide variety of field defects can occur. Some patients will develop bilateral optic neuritis simultaneously or within a few days to weeks. In about half of the patients, if serial examination is carried out some evidence of inflammation or elevation of the optic nerve, termed *optic papillitis,* will be seen. The occurrence of papillitis depends on the proximity of the demyelinating lesion to the nerve head. It should be recalled that the optic nerve is in fact a tract of the brain, because demyelinating lesions in multiple sclerosis are known not to occur outside the central nervous system. Of patients with optic neuritis about one-third recover completely, one-third will show considerable improvement, one-third will show no evidence of improvement whatever. As in most acute exacerbations of demyelinating disease, improvement in the majority of cases will have begun within 2 weeks of the onset of neurologic damage. Much longer periods of up to months may elapse, however, during which improvement in neurologic function may occur. It should be noted that only about 40 percent of patients who develop optic neuritis will go on to have other lesions of multiple sclerosis. It is unclear at this time whether optic neuritis when it occurs alone and is not followed by other evidence of demyelinating disease is a subclass of multiple sclerosis with only a single lesion or a manifestation of other disease processes. No other etiology for optic neuritis has been established at this time.

The remaining 60 percent of patients with multiple sclerosis will present with some evidence of a lesion of the spinal cord or brainstem. The frequency of involvement of the posterior columns of the cord is responsible for the commonly related symptoms of tingling of the extremities and the tight bandlike sensations around trunk or limbs, characteristic of dysfunction of the posterior columns. Diplopia may be a common presenting complaint as a result of brainstem lesions. These lesions may cause an internuclear ophthalmoplegia due to involvement of the medial longitudinal fasciculus and characterized by inability to adduct one or the other eye on lateral gaze in either direction or by nystagmus present to a greater degree in the abducting than the adducting eye. An internuclear ophthalmoplegia, when present bilaterally, is virtually diagnostic of multiple sclerosis. Other manifestations of brainstem involvement include transient facial anesthesia and vertigo and vomiting because of affection of the vestibular connections. The occurrence of tic douloureux in a young person should immediately bring to mind the diagnosis of multiple sclerosis due to involvement of the descending tract of the fifth cranial nerve.

Nystagmus and cerebellar ataxia, with or without weakness and spasticity of the limbs, represent another common syndrome and reflect involvement of the cerebellar and corticospinal tracts and their connections. The ataxia of cerebellar type can be recognized by scanning speech, tremors and titubation of head, intention tremors of arms and legs, and incoordination of voluntary movements. It may be mixed with sensory ataxia from involvement of the posterior columns of the spinal cord. Ultimately spinal cord involvement becomes predominant in most advanced cases. It is a common aphorism that the patient with multiple sclerosis presents with symptoms in one leg and signs in both. The patient will complain of weakness, ataxia, or sensory loss in one lower extremity and have evidence of bilateral corticospinal-tract disease manifested by Babinski signs in both lower extremities.

Symptoms of bladder dysfunction including hesitancy, urgency, frequency, and incontinence occur commonly with spinal cord involvement. In males, these symptoms are often associated with impotence, a symptom which the patient will not often report unless specifically questioned in this regard. About 5 percent of patients with multiple sclerosis over the course of their disease will have a seizure, presumably as the result of involvement of subcortical connections, with demyelinating lesions.

It has often been pointed out that patients with multiple sclerosis develop euphoria, a pathologic cheerfulness which seems inappropriate in relation to their obvious neurologic deficit. This syndrome, the result of lesions of the white matter, probably of the frontal lobes, is often associated with other signs of cerebral impairment. There are, however, an equal number of patients who are depressed, irritable, short tempered, and have deficits such as loss of memory because of lesions in other locations.

CLINICAL COURSE. The symptoms described above may occur individually or in combination during exacerbations. Some patients will have a series of exacerbations of the disease, each with complete remission. Often such exacerbations may be severe enough to cause total quadriplegia or even coma. Most patients will have a series of exacerbations, each followed by a remission or stabilization and leaving in its wake some evidence of permanent neurologic deficit upon which succeeding acute manifestations are superimposed. After a period of years some patients who have had a series of acute exacerbations tend to develop an inexorably progressing downhill course. When the initial course of the disease is steadily progressive and the lesion is limited to the spinal cord, diagnosis is particularly difficult. Such cases tend to occur among the older patient group. It has been suggested that this syndrome be considered a special subclass of multiple sclerosis.

CEREBROSPINAL FLUID. In a small number of cases, particularly the acute ones, there may be a slight mononuclear pleocytosis in the spinal fluid. This pleocytosis is in fact the only way in which activity of the disease may be measured. None of the other laboratory tests aid in measuring the activity or inactivity of the disease.

The proportion of gamma-globulin in the spinal fluid appears to be altered in multiple sclerosis, while the protein content is usually normal. The alteration in distribution of globulins may be demonstrated by an abnormality of the colloidal gold curve, usually a first-zone abnormality, but occasionally midzone in type, in the presence of a negative Wassermann reaction. When gamma-globulin content is measured directly, it is abnormal in about 60 percent of the patients with multiple sclerosis. The gamma-globulin abnormality, however, tends to reflect the duration of the disease, and therefore is usually abnormal in the established case rather than in an initial exacerbation when an abnormal laboratory test would be helpful in establishing the diagnosis.

Some patients with demyelinating disease will have elevations of spinal fluid protein but a spinal fluid protein in excess of 100 mg per 100 ml is so uncommon in multiple sclerosis that another diagnosis should be entertained.

Acute Multiple Sclerosis. Occasionally, multiple sclerosis runs an acute or subacute course leading to death in weeks or months. Alternatively, an acute course may develop rapidly, then remit partially or completely to be followed by characteristic relapses. In some of these cases, the onset is marked by headache, vomiting, delirium, and by a succession of symptoms indicating severe involvement of the brainstem or the brain, optic nerves, and spinal cord. In the so-called "cerebral" cases, there may be mental changes, convulsions, aphasia, hemianopia, and variable long-tract signs; the spinal type may show the picture of transverse myelitis. These forms of the disease are uncommon and are difficult to distinguish from disseminated encephalomyelitis with which we tend to group them. They differ pathologically in the larger size of lesions, being more like those of multiple sclerosis.

Neuromyelitis Optica Syndrome. This disorder, referred to as *Devic's disease,* is said to represent a combination of bilateral optic neuritis and transverse myelitis. Attempts to clinically define patients with this combination of symptoms have failed to provide any data of prognostic value. Perhaps it is best to consider neuromyelitis optica as a particular form of multiple sclerosis. Pathologic studies of fatal cases, particularly those in which cavitation of white matter is found, have revealed a more acute and uniformly destructive process than is often seen in multiple sclerosis, however.

DIAGNOSIS. In the characteristic case with evidence of wide dissemination of the lesions throughout the nervous system, the diagnosis of multiple sclerosis is in little doubt. It is an excellent clinical rule that the disease should not be diagnosed when all the patient's symptoms and signs can be explained by a single lesion. Disseminated encephalomyelitis is a self-limited, monophasic disease and stupor and coma occur only rarely in multiple sclerosis. The other acute manifestations may mimic labyrinthitis, meningovascular syphilis, and encephalitis.

Confusion may occasionally arise with the hereditary ataxias, which are generally distinguished by their familial incidence and other associated genetic traits and by their stereotyped clinical pattern. Amyotrophic lateral sclerosis and subacute combined degeneration may occasionally be mimicked by demyelinating disease, but muscle wasting and fasciculations will identify the former, and the latter can be confirmed by a low level of vitamin B_{12} in the serum, the presence of megaloblasts in the bone marrow, the anemia present in most cases and the absence of acid in the gastric secretions.

Patients with a progressive spastic paraplegia should be carefully evaluated for the presence of intrathecal neoplasm or cervical spondylosis. Radicular pain at some point in the illness is a frequent manifestation of neoplasm and is rare in multiple sclerosis, and muscle wasting due to anterior horn or spinal root involvement as is sometimes seen in spondylosis is almost unknown in multiple sclerosis. The occurrence of nystagmus in association with other neurologic symptoms should be carefully evaluated. A common cause of nystagmus is the ingestion of barbiturates or diphenylhydantoin. The possibility that an anxious patient with another neurologic lesion has taken a barbiturate to aid him in sleep should never be disregarded when nystagmus in association with evidence of a lesion elsewhere might establish a diagnosis of multiple sclerosis.

Basilar impression of the skull, or platybasia, should also be considered in the differential diagnosis, but patients with these conditions have a characteristic shortening of the neck, and careful radiographs of the base of the skull will be diagnostic. Occasional tumors of the posterior fossa have been misdiagnosed as multiple sclerosis because of the affection of a wide variety of neurologic systems in the brainstem.

Careful clinical appraisal will usually lead to accurate diagnosis, but the label "multiple sclerosis" should not be placed upon a patient until the evidence is unequivocal. Such a diagnosis will explain almost any subsequent neurologic event, and attention may be directed away from the possibility of another perhaps treatable disease.

PROGNOSIS. The duration of the disease is exceedingly variable. Though some patients die within a few months, the average duration of the disease is in excess of 20 years. At the end of 20 years, between a quarter and a third of patients are still actively carrying out their work.

The final state of the bedridden, incontinent patient, racked by painful flexor spasms of the lower limbs and febrile episodes of intercurrent infection from bedsores is one of the most distressing in medicine.

TREATMENT. A large number of remedies have been tried in the treatment of multiple sclerosis and many have thought to have been successful because of the remitting nature of the disease. Only the use of adrenocortical stimulating hormone (ACTH) has withstood evaluation in reasonably controlled trials of exacerbations of both optic neuritis and exacerbations of multiple sclerosis. A substantial group of patients, however, fail to respond to this treatment in the acute exacerbation. A rigorously controlled cooperative study of the value of ACTH in multiple sclerosis is now being carried out. There is also data to suggest that the long-term use of ACTH in small doses on alternating days may reduce the frequency of recurrences.

ACTH has been generally preferred over the corticosteroids in the treatment of multiple sclerosis because the initial trials and control studies have been carried out with it. A variety of dosage regimes have been employed. It seems important that a high dose be used initially to be effective. We give ACTH intramuscularly in a dose of 40 units of gel every 12 hr for a period of 7 to 10 days. The dose is then reduced by 10 units every 3 days. Many patients who show improvement on this therapy, continue to improve or maintain their previous improvement even though the medication is gradually reduced and discontinued. Other patients begin to have a recurrence of symptoms as the dose is gradually reduced and are often maintained on small doses of ACTH (20 to 40 units) every other day for a period of several months. Because of the risk of potassium depletion, the patients are given potassium supplement in a dose of 60 mEq a day. Euphoria and depression may be severe enough to terminate medication, and a tranquilizer may be necessary because of the complaints of difficulty sleeping and nervousness. The occurrence of peripheral edema due to sodium retention can be treated with mild diuretics and salt restriction. Gastrointestinal bleeding and the activation of tuberculosis should be considered as possible complications of the treatment. Hirsuitism and acne cannot be prevented but disappear when the medication is stopped.

The importance of an understanding and sympathetic physician cannot be overemphasized in the care of patients with a chronic debilitating neurologic disease of this kind. Some patients consider the uncertainty of prognosis worse than true disability. General support can be rendered by providing bedrest, in acute exacerbations, prevention of excessive fatigue, and meticulous attention to the prevention of bedsores in the disabled patient by the use of alternating pressure mattresses, silicone gel pads, and other special devices. The use of belladonna alkaloids and bethanechol chloride in the treatment of bladder dysfunction can be helpful. Antibiotics and acidifying drugs to treat and suppress urinary tract infections should also be employed. In patients with disorders of bowel function a program of bowel training can often be successfully undertaken. Injections of dilute solutions of phenol either into peripheral nerves or intrathecally for relief of spasticity and flexor spasms have been of value.

DIFFUSE CEREBRAL SCLEROSIS

In 1912 Schilder first called attention to a disease causing progressive massive demyelination of the white matter often beginning in one or both occipital or temporal lobes. It has been referred to as *Schilder's disease* or *encephalitis periaxialis diffusa.* Since that time, many other cases have been described, some resembling Schilder's original description, others differing with respect to familial occurrence and widespread symmetric destruction and gliosis of the white matter, often with metachromatic bodies and globoid bodies representing catabolic products of myelin.

The diffuse types of cerebral sclerosis constitute a group of entities, including the globoid body leukodystrophy of Krabbe, sudanophilic leukodystrophy, and the metachromatic leukodystrophy of Greenfield, which may involve peripheral nerves as well as central nervous system tissue. For the moment, they are a group of diseases with unknown etiology occurring sporadically, though occasionally running in families, characterized clinically by progressive visual failure, mental deterioration, and spastic paralysis and pathologically by massive demyelination of the white matter of the cerebral hemispheres. Each entity is unquestionably a specific inherited biochemical defect in the metabolism of myelin proteolipids. The causes of these diseases for the moment are unknown, and there is no treatment. For further discussion see appropriate heading under degenerative nervous diseases (Chap. 364).

REFERENCES

Adams, R. D., and C. S. Kubik: The Morbid Anatomy of the Demyelinative Diseases, Am. J. Med., 12:510, 1952.

McAlpine, D., C. E. Lumsden, and E. D. Acheson: "Multiple Sclerosis," Edinburgh and London, E. & S. Livingstone, 1965.

Poskanzer, D. C.: Epidemiological Evidence for a Viral Etiol-ogy for Multiple Sclerosis, pp. 55–63, "Slow, Latent, and Temperate Virus Infections," U. S. Department of Health, Education, and Welfare, NINDB Monograph No. 2, 1965.

Wolf, A., E. A. Kabat, and A. E. Bezer: The Pathology of Acute Disseminated Encephalomyelitis Produced Experimentally in the Rhesus Monkey and Its Resemblance to Human Demyelinative Disease, J. Neuropathol. Exp. Neurol., 6:333, 1947.

363 METABOLIC AND NUTRITIONAL DISEASES OF THE NERVOUS SYSTEM

Hugo Moser, Maurice Victor, and Raymond D. Adams

Each of these categories of diseases is based on intricate and often unique biochemical changes within the nervous system, and for this reason they are described here in one chapter, even though their causes and pathogeneses are different.

METABOLIC DISEASES OF THE NERVOUS SYSTEM

One large group of metabolic diseases of the nervous system is related to a demonstrable fault in general metabolism, the latter traceable to a disease of the heart and circulation, lungs, liver, kidneys, and endocrine glands. Acute hypoxia, hypercapnia, acute hepatic stupor or coma, uremia, hypoglycemia with hyperosmolarity, hyponatremia, hypo- and hyperkalemia, acidosis (diabetic, uremic, and other), Addison's disease, Cushing's syndrome, hyper- and hypothyroidism, and hypoparathyroidism are the most typical examples. A second group comprises disorders of the nervous system and other organ systems in which a metabolic abnormality affects both the brain and other organs. Here reference is made to such conditions as gargoylism, the lipidoses, hepatolenticular degeneration, porphyria, galactosemia, glycogen storage disease, several of the syndromes of aminoaciduria with mental defect, and the serum lipoprotein abnormalities. Many of these diseases are familial, as are others of still a third group which encompasses cerebral disorders of assumed metabolic origin in which no evidence of disease in other viscera or in blood can presently be evoked. Representative of this third class of disease are the leukodystrophies, some of the lipid storage diseases, Friedreich's ataxia, dystonia musculorum deformans, Jakob-Creutzfeldt-Heidenhain's disease, and many others discussed in the chapter on degenerative diseases. It requires no imagination to see that only a thin veil of ignorance separates the diseases of this third category from those called degenerative (see Chap. 364).

A classification of the above type provides a conceptual locus for all the known varieties of metabolic nervous disease and ultimately will bring them into orderly relationship to the chemistry of the nervous system. However, it leaves the clinician without a practical approach to the subject until he has been able to reach a diagnosis. Only then is it possible to turn to the relevant published literature for detailed information concerning

Table 363-1. CLASSIFICATION OF METABOLIC DISEASES
OF THE NERVOUS SYSTEM

I. Metabolic diseases presenting as a syndrome of episodic confusion, stupor, or coma.
   A. Hypoxia
   B. Hypercapnia
   C. Hypoglycemia
   D. Hyperglycemia
   E. Acidosis (including ketotic hyperglycinemia and isovaleric and methylmalonic aciduria)
   F. Uremia
   G. Hypo- and hypernatremia and hypo- and hyperkalemia
   H. Hepatic failure and Eck fistula
   I. Addison's disease
   J. Maple syrup urine disease (in infants)
   K. Argininosuccinic aminoaciduria, hyperglycinemia, citrullinemia, hyperammonemia, isovaleric acidemia (in children), and methylmalonic aciduria
II. Metabolic diseases presenting as progressive extrapyramidal syndrome
   A. Acquired and familial hepatocerebral degeneration
   B. Kernicterus
   C. Fahr's disease
   D. Lesch-Nyhan's hyperuricemia
III. Metabolic diseases presenting as progressive cerebellar ataxia.
   A. Lipid storage diseases
   B. Ataxia telangiectasia
   C. Bassen-Kornsweig disease
   D. Argininosuccinic aciduria and Hartnup's disease
   E. Cerebrotendinous xanthomatosis
      (Friedreich's ataxia and the familial cerebellar ataxias, the degenerative diseases from which the above must be differentiated, will ultimately be brought into this category.)
IV. Metabolic diseases presenting as polyneuropathy.
   A. Refsum's disease
   B. Porphyria
   C. Tangier disease
   D. Macro- and cryoglobulinemias
   E. Some cases of Bassen-Kornsweig syndrome and ataxia telangiectasia
      (Probably Charcot-Marie Tooth peroneal muscular atrophy, Dejerine-Sottas hypertrophic polyneuropathy, and other of the chronic familial degenerative diseases of the peripheral nervous system will eventually fall into this group.)
V. Metabolic diseases presenting as mental retardation.
   A. Phenylketonuria
   B. Milder forms of maple syrup urine disease
   C. Homocystinuria
   D. Galactosemia
   E. Histidinemia, cystathioninuria, argininosuccinic aciduria, hyperlysinemia, citrullinemia, hyperammonemia, isovaleric acidemia, carnosinemia, hyperalininemia, methylmalonic aciduria, sulfituria, hyperglycinemia, hypervalinemia, hydroxyprolinemia, Lowe's syndrome of oculocerebrorenal syndrome (see Table 102-1).

Table 363-1. CLASSIFICATION OF METABOLIC DISEASES
OF THE NERVOUS SYSTEM (*continued*)

VI. Metabolic disorders associated with dementia.
   A. Hypothyroidism
   B. Cushing's disease
   C. Hypoparathyroidism and Fahr's syndrome
      (Lipid storage diseases and leukodystrophies will eventually fall into this category.)

his patient. More helpful, it would seem, would be a classification in which diseases with similar clinical manifestations are grouped together. Final diagnosis would depend then on the differentiation by a combination of clinical and laboratory methods of the several diseases subsumed in a single syndrome. Such is the scheme which follows.

Only a few of these many diseases will be considered in detail here, and the reader is referred to other sections of the book for the definitive discussion of the metabolic aberration and its main clinical expression, if generalized. Also, in attempting to classify any given patient, reference should be made to the syndromes listed in Chaps. 364 and 365.

Syndrome of Impaired Consciousness

The general character of these types of derangement has been described in detail in Chap. 26, and it was there stated that a metabolic disorder of the brain should be considered when there was an acute disturbance of consciousness without localizing or lateralizing signs and without change in the cerebrospinal fluid. Intoxication with alcohol or other drugs enters prominently in the differential diagnosis, as do nutritional disorders due to lack of B vitamins.

ACUTE HYPOXIC ENCEPHALOPATHY. The mechanism of cerebral damage from hypoxia has already been described in Chap. 26. But, it is important for the clinician to realize that a hypoxic or ischemic accident (the two are virtually indistinguishable neurologically) encountered in the emergency room or on the wards of a general hospital is one of the more frequent complications of many diseases, causing death or, even worse, permanent coma or mental enfeeblement. The medical situations which most often have led to this have been strangulation (vomitus or blood in bronchi, surgical pack, sponge, or foreign body in trachea); respiratory-cardiac arrest during inhalation, spinal, or intravenous anesthesia; cardiac disease with arrest; any disease which causes paralysis of respiratory muscles, such as poliomyelitis or acute idiopathic polyneuritis; and central nervous system disease (cerebrovascular lesions, hypoxic encephalopathies in children, epilepsy, or respiratory arrest). Carbon monoxide intoxication has similar effects.

Mild hypoxia induces only inattentiveness, poor judgment, and motor incoordination and has no lasting effects if corrected. Severe hypoxia causes coma within less than a minute, but again recovery will be complete if breathing, oxygenation of blood, and cardiac action are restored within 3 to 5 min. Periods of hypoxia with coma that exceed 5 to 6 min usually result in serious and permanent injury to the brain, particularly in those parts most susceptible to injury because of the marginal efficiency of their circulation (globus pallidus, cerebral cortex, especially that of the hippocampus and parieto-occipital regions, and cerebellar cortex). However, it is difficult to judge the degree of hypoxia accurately, since slight heart action or an imperceptible blood pressure may serve to maintain some degree of circulation. Hence some individuals have made an excellent recovery after alleged cerebral hypoxia of 8 to 10 min or longer. *An important clinical rule is that degrees of hypoxia which do not at any time abolish consciousness rarely if ever cause permanent damage to the nervous system.*

The patient who has suffered a serious hypoxic episode may be breathing normally and have good color and normal heart action when first seen. The hypoxic crisis has already terminated. Yet he may be profoundly comatose with dilated, fixed pupils, eyes slightly divergent and roving from side to side, the limbs inert, and tendon reflexes diminished or absent. Within a few minutes after cardiac action and breathing have been restored, generalized convulsions and also isolated or grouped twitches of muscles (myoclonus) supervene. If the damage is severe, coma persists and decerebrate postures may be present or occur upon pinching the limbs, and bilateral Babinski signs can also be evoked. In the first 24 to 48 hr death may terminate this state, in a setting of rising temperature, deepening coma, and circulatory collapse. If the patient survives this period, he usually begins to respond in varying degrees. A period of restlessness and chaotic movement, sometimes clearly revealing ataxia, and myoclonic jerks or choreoathetosis may then appear and endure for variable periods of time.

The most severe degree of hypoxia, often complicated by circulatory collapse (ischemia), is manifested by complete unreceptiveness and unresponsiveness with abolition of all brain stem reflexes. Natural respiration cannot be sustained. No electrical activity is seen in the patient's electroencephalogram (it is isoelectric). This is called the brain death syndrome. At autopsy nearly all the cerebral, cerebellar, and brain stem structures are found to have been destroyed.

When this syndrome of cerebral death occurs, the outlook for recovery is hopeless, and one must consider the advisability of discontinuing all supportive measures (respiratory aid, vasopressor agents, etc.). Such victims often become donors of vital organs. However, one must exercise caution in reaching the conclusion of irreversible brain damage unless the evidence of hypoxia and ischemia is definite, for anesthesia, drug intoxication, and hypothermia may also cause deep coma and an isoelectric electroencephalogram.

When improvement takes place, as it usually does in the less damaged patients, consciousness may be regained and then confusion, visual agnosia, or any one of several types of abnormal movement (action or intention myoclonus, extrapyramidal rigidity, choreoathetosis) becomes manifest. Some of these patients quickly pass through this acute hypoxic phase and proceed to make a full recovery; others are left with some disabling syndrome. Seizures may or may not continue to be a problem. One unexplained phenomenon is an initial improvement for 1 to 2 days followed by a relapse, further progression of the neurologic syndrome, and death after 1 to 2 weeks. In some instances this delayed hypoxic relapse has been found associated with a widespread cerebral demyelination.

The permanent neurologic sequelae, which may be classed as the *posthypoxic syndromes,* are *dementia* with or without extrapyramidal signs, *visual agnosia, parkinsonian syndrome, choreoathetosis, cerebellar ataxia,* and *intention or action myoclonus.*

The essential mechanism in hypoxic encephalopathy is a lack of oxygen and an arrest of all aerobic metabolic processes necessary for the Krebs tricarboxylic cycle and the hydrogen transport system. Neurones are injured to such a degree they cannot survive. The phenomenon of delayed progression is not understood but may be due to the blockage or exhaustion of some enzymatic process during the period when brain metabolism is restored or even increased (as in hyperthermia).

Diagnosis depends on (1) the history of the hypoxic event and evidence of reduced oxygenation of arterial blood or CO intoxication (the latter is indicated by its cherry red color or spectroscopic band only for a few minutes to hours after the episode), blood pressures below 70 systolic, or cardiac arrest; (2) the typical sequences of events outlined above after a possible hypoxic episode has terminated. Renal damage (anuria) and injury to the myocardium may also have occurred, and evidence of such provides corroborative evidence of hypoxia.

Treatment is mainly the prevention of a critical degree of hypoxic injury. After the physician quickly secures a clear airway, artificial respiration, external thoracic cardiac massage and open-chest surgery, and the use of a cardiac defibrillator or pacemaker all have their place, and every second counts in their prompt utilization. Once cardiac and pulmonary function are restored, there is some evidence from the work of Blalock and his associates that reducing cerebral metabolic requirements by continuous hypothermia for 48 to 72 hr may prevent the delayed worsening referred to above. Oxygen may be of value during the first hours and days, but it is probably of little use after the blood becomes well oxygenated. Dexamethazone in doses of 8 to 12 mg every 6 hr helps combat brain swelling. Seizures should be controlled by intramuscular sodium hydantoin (Dilantin), 100 mg every 6 hr, or sodium phenobarbital, 120 mg every 4 hr by mouth or stomach tube or four times a day parenterally. If severe, continuous and unresponsive to drugs, controlled respiration and curare may be helpful. Often the seizures cease after 1 to 2 days. If they persist, they are often myoclonic, and Mebaral, 500 mg per day, or phenobarbital, 300 mg per day, in several divided doses may be useful in their control.

HYPERCAPNIA (AND HYPOXIA) IN PULMONARY DISEASE. Chronic emphysema, chronic fibrosing lung disease, and in some instances a seeming inadequacy of the respiratory center (Chap. 280) lead to respiratory acidosis, with an elevation of P_{CO_2} and a reduction in arterial P_{O_2}. Secondary polycythemia, cor pulmonale, and heart failure often accompany these diseases of the lungs, and pulmonary infection may be superimposed. The clinical syndrome is comprised of an action tremor and a coarse twitching of all muscles sustained in a state of contraction (termed *asterixis*), *headache, papilledema, mental dullness, drowsiness, confusion,* and *coma.*

The cerebrospinal fluid is under increased pressure. P_{CO_2} may exceed 75 mm Hg, and the oxygen content of arterial blood ranges from 85 percent to as low as 40 percent. The mechanism of cerebral damage is said to be CO_2 narcosis, but the biochemical details are not known. The danger of administering morphine, which depresses the respiratory center, or the inhalation of oxygen, which removes the sole stimulus to the respiratory center, is now widely recognized; many patients so treated in the past have lapsed into coma (CO_2 narcosis) and have died.

Forced ventilation with an intermittent positive-pressure device, inhalation of oxygen if hypoxia is severe, the treatment of heart failure with digitalis and diuretic measures, venesection to reduce the viscosity of the blood, and antibiotics to combat pulmonary infection has been the most effective program of therapy and has often resulted in a surprising degree of improvement that may be maintained for months or years. If coma should persist, the arterial O_2 level should be rechecked; it may be critically reduced. Or the pH of CSF may be very low, in the range of 7.15 to 7.25. In CO_2 narcosis the correction of the acidosis of blood is easier than CSF, which tends to lag.

Unlike pure hypoxic encephalopathy, prolonged coma due to hypercapnia is exceptional. The papilledema and the jerky, intermittent postures or asterixis (the latter characteristic only of liver failure, hypercapnia, uremia, and rarely, other metabolic disorders) are features of diagnostic import. The syndrome is apt to be mistaken for brain tumor, a confusional psychosis of nondescript type, or a disease causing chorea or myoclonus. In the latter instance it must be distinguished from a chronic extrapyramidal syndrome, as outlined below.

HYPOGLYCEMIC ENCEPHALOPATHY. This condition has been discussed in Chaps. 26 and 96. It is a rather frequent cause of profound coma, episodic confusion, and convulsions and merits separate consideration as a metabolic disorder of brain function. The essential biochemical datum is a blood sugar level of less than 25 to 30 mg per 100 ml, lasting 1 to 2 hr, and leading to exhaustion of the store of cerebral glucose and glycogen. Within this brief span of time, as cerebral oxidation proceeds without exogenous glucose, the structural components of neurones i.e., lipid and protein substances are metabolized and irreversible damage occurs.

Clinically the most common situations in which severe hypoglycemia develops are (1) accidental or deliberate overdose of insulin or of one of the oral antidiabetic agents, (2) insulin therapy in schizophrenia, (3) an islet cell insulin-secreting tumor of the pancreas, (4) rarely, following an alcoholic debauch or some form of acute liver disease (acute nonicteric hepatoencephalopathy of childhood), (5) glycogen storage disease in infancy, (6) an idiopathic state in the neonatal period. In functional hyperinsulinism the hypoglycemia is rarely of sufficient severity or duration to damage the central nervous system.

The clinical picture has already been sketched. The initial symptoms, as the level of blood glucose descends, are nervousness, hunger, and cold, and these gradually give way to confusion, drowsiness, and occasionally excitement or overactivity. In the next stage forced sucking, grasping, motor restlessness, muscular spasms, and finally decerebrate rigidity occur in that sequence. Myoclonic twitching and convulsions may develop in some patients but are by no means the rule. Deepening coma is attended by dilatation of pupils, pale skin, shallow respiration, slow heart, and hypotonicity of limb musculature—the so-called "medullary phase" of hypoglycemia. Should glucose be administered before this medullary phase appears, the patient is restored to normalcy, retracing the aforementioned steps in reverse order. However, once this medullary phase is reached, and particularly if it persists for a time before the hypoglycemia is corrected by intravenous glucose or spontaneously by the so-called "gluconeogenic activities" of the adrenal glands and liver, recovery is delayed for a period of days or weeks and may be incomplete. Although the lowering of blood sugar is equally severe in both instances, a huge dose of insulin with intense hypoglycemia, even of relatively brief duration (30 to 60 min), is more dangerous than smaller ones, possibly because it impairs or exhausts essential enzymes. This condition cannot then be overcome by large quantities of glucose intravenously. The cerebral cortex suffers major damage; cortical nerve cells degenerate and are replaced by microgliacytes and astrocytes. But, the distribution of lesions is not quite the same as in hypoxic encephalopathy.

The major difference, clinically, between hypoglycemia and hypoxia lies in the clinical setting of the illness and the mode of evolution of the neurologic disorder. Hypoglycemia usually unfolds more slowly over a period of 30 to 60 min rather than suddenly within seconds or a few minutes. The recovery phase and sequelae of the two conditions bear close resemblance and may not be easily differentiated. Recurrent hypoglycemia, as with an islet cell tumor, may masquerade for some time as a recurrent confusional psychosis or convulsive illness, and diagnosis awaits a period of demonstrably low blood sugar or hyperinsulinism.

The correction of the hypoglycemia at the earliest moment is the obvious therapy. It is not known whether hypothermia or other measures will increase the tolerance or safety period in hypoglycemia or alter the outcome.

HEPATIC STUPOR AND COMA. Chronic hepatic insufficiency with portacaval shunting of blood is often punctuated by episodes of mental dullness, drowsiness, confusion, stupor or coma, "flapping tremor" of outstretched limbs, or intermittency of sustained postures (asterixis).

This condition has been described fully in Chap. 328. Less widely known is the fact that a pure portal-systemic shunt (Eck fistula) may be attended by a similar clinical picture. Also, there are a number of hereditary diseases of childhood which may lead to episodic coma with or without seizures. A special type of acute nonicteric hepatoencephalopathy, first described by Raye and his associates, occurs in children, presenting a picture of an acute toxic encephalopathy.

In many patients the syndrome does not advance beyond the stage of flapping and confusion with mild electroencephalographic changes. In this mild form it must be distinguished from the acute confusional psychoses or hypokinetic delirium and, if a disorder of posture and movement is prominent, from extrapyramidal syndromes.

Reducing the protein intake, ridding the intestinal tract of blood, suppressing the bacterial action on protein in the intestinal tract with neomycin or kanamycin, and the administration of sodium glutamate intravenously, which sometimes lowers the NH_3 levels of the blood, have been found to restore many of these patients to a relatively normal state. Should these therapeutic measures not control NH_3 production, death is inevitable.

Although the biochemical mechanism is not fully understood, the most plausible hypothesis is that the levels of blood NH_3 are elevated because the diseased or bypassed liver fails to convert it into urea; glucose metabolism of the brain at the Krebs cycle stage is disturbed by withdrawal of alpha ketoglutarate from the metabolic pool as the cerebral tissues attempt to remove the NH_3 formed *in situ*. Also the quantity of ATP is decreased.

In acute hepatitis, delirious, confusional, and comatose states also occur but their mechanisms are still obscure. NH_3 may be elevated but usually not to a degree that would be expected to affect central nervous system function.

OTHER METABOLIC ENCEPHALOPATHIES. Limitations of space permit only brief reference to other important metabolic disturbances of the brain. *Metabolic acidosis,* such as that due to diabetes mellitus or renal failure, produces the typical drowsiness, stupor, and coma with dry skin and Kussmaul breathing described in Chap. 94. Acidosis in infancy and childhood may occur in the course of hyperammonemia, isovaleric acidemia, maple syrup urine disease, hyperglycinemia, etc. There is no recognizable neuropathologic change. High-voltage, slow electrical activity predominates in the electroencephalogram, and correction of the acidosis restores nervous function to a normal level, provided coma has not persisted for too long a time, in which instance death supervenes. Extreme degrees of hyperosmolarity of the blood may develop in the course of diabetes mellitus (blood glucose > 400 mg) and in childhood in hypernatremic dehydration, resulting in both instances in convulsions, tremulous movements, and coma. Hyponatremia, usually with water intoxication, is another cause of infantile episodic coma. *Uremic encephalopathy* is poorly understood because of the existence of two neurologic syndromes, one of hypertensive encephalopathy, the other a somnolent twitching-convulsive syndrome (uremic twitching) which is highly characteristic of renal failure but still of obscure cause (see Chap. 301). Encephalopathy due to *Addison's disease* (adrenal insufficiency) may be attended by episodic confusion, stupor, or coma without special identifying features. Its basis remains unclear. Hypotension and diminished cerebral circulation and hypoglycemia are the principal hypotheses presently being entertained, and measures which correct these conditions appear to have been beneficial in some instances. Brain atrophy from whatever cause, if complicated by a febrile state, may result in coma.

A point not previously emphasized is that an episode of stupor or coma with or without convulsions in infancy and childhood may be the first medical datum to suggest an hereditary metabolic disease. In the case of maple syrup urine disease the first episode within the first week or two of life may prove fatal, and the physician's only role would be to watch for biochemical evidence of the disease in the next child; but milder forms also occur and induce a stupor or coma periodically or in conjunction with each infection which the child has. If the disease passes unrecognized, he becomes more and more retarded. Isovaleric acidosis, methylmalonic aciduria, and the ketotic form of hyperglycinemia may result in a comatose state due to acidosis.

Syndrome of Extrapyramidal Tremor, Rigidity, Dystonia, and Choreoathetosis (See Chap. 22)

Unlike the group of diseases which cause episodic coma, only a few of which are genetic in origin, the diseases which cause progressive extrapyramidal syndrome (and the other syndromes which follow—cerebellar ataxia, polyneuropathy, and mental retardation) are frequently hereditary. As was pointed out in Chap. 22, the patient is usually normal at birth and the neurologic disorder becomes manifest in childhood and adolescence after its biochemical basis has existed for months or years. This fact tells us that the injury of the nervous system is often a secondary phenomenon. The complexity of structure, organization, and slow development of the nervous system accounts for the delayed onset and wide diversity of syndromes. But other organs do not altogether escape, and they may show manifest dysfunction early, which facts are important from the diagnostic point of view, for prevention of the neurologic syndrome looms as a possibility, providing the biochemical abnormality can be detected early and controlled. This requires screening programs for the study of blood and urine; the laboratory data instead of a complaint or clinical sign become the cardinal manifestations of disease, a theme which was elaborated in the introduction to Part Three of Section 10. Physicians and pediatricians must join in their efforts in case finding and employ biochemical screening techniques and cytologic studies of the blood and other tissues of the adult and child (including amniotic fluid studies during the first and second trimesters of pregnancy). These diagnostic tests, new ones of which are being introduced every few months, will be described in connection with special diseases.

The outstanding examples of a progressive nonhereditary and hereditary extrapyramidal syndrome are the von Woerkam and the Wilson-Westphal-Strumpell hepatocerebral degenerations. In the *acquired* hepatocerebral degeneration, any type of chronic liver cirrhosis or Eck fistula may give rise to the *episodic stupor* and *coma,* mentioned above, and to a *slowly evolving faciocervical choreoathetosis* and *cerebellar ataxia* of *limbs*. Rarely a progressive spinal spastic paraplegia is added to the clinical picture (primary hepatic degeneration of pyramidal tracts of spinal cord) (Chap. 328). Neuronal loss and hyperplasia of protoplasmic astrocytes are formed in basal ganglia, cerebral, and cerebellar cortices. Ceruloplasmin levels in blood and copper excretion in urine are normal. Control of the hyperammonemia, which usually attends this disease, is beneficial. In the familial hepatocerebral degeneration the syndrome is exclusively extrapyramidal. During adolescence and in early adult life a tremor of one or both arms or a slowly developing extrapyramidal rigidity of trunk and limbs, resembling Parkinson's disease or choreoathetosis, introduces the disease, and evidence of liver disorder is difficult to discern. However, a cirrhosis of subacute, recurrent hypertrophic type invariably precedes the onset of the neurologic abnormality, and more importantly, there is a stage when a deficiency of ceruloplasmin and an abnormality of copper transport exist without evidence of malfunction of either liver or brain, as was pointed out in Chap. 110. In the late and relatively irreversible neurologic stages of the disease the clinical picture assumes a more striking form, consisting of rigidity, flexion dystonia, tremors, dysarthria, and dysphagia and cerebellar ataxia. Personality change and intellectual impairment appear at some point in the course of the illness and terminate in dementia or even as akinetic mutism. But, unlike the acquired hepatocerebral degeneration, episodic coma is rare. Easy substantiation of the diagnosis in the late phases of the disease is secured by the finding of the corneal (Kayser-Fleisher) rings of golden-brown copper pigment (see Plate 4). The neuropathologic changes consist of cavitation or shrinkage of the lenticular nuclei (hence Wilson's term *hepatolenticular* degeneration), neuronal loss in basal ganglia and cerebellar nuclei, and hyperplasia of protoplasmic astrocytes in these parts and the cerebral cortex. Brain and liver copper are increased. Liver cirrhosis, which always precedes the encephalopathy, is due to the copper deposition. The differential diagnosis includes consideration of the acquired forms of liver disease and degenerative diseases such as juvenile Parkinson's syndrome, Hallervorden-Spatz disease, or a late variety of lipid storage disease.

At an earlier period of life (late childhood) the gradual development of progressive rigidity, dystonia, and choreoathetosis, progressing over a period of 5 to 15 years, should suggest Hallervorden-Spatz disease (see Chap. 364). Surely it too represents an inborn error of metabolism, affecting only the cerebrum, where degenerative changes in basal ganglia are accompanied by deposit of organic ferruginous compounds. However, there is no systemic disturbance of iron metabolism.

In hypoparathyroidism, seizures and tetany tend to occur at some interval of time after the level of ionized calcium in the blood is lowered. In exceptional cases athetosis of an arm or leg may appear later (announcing the onset of a slowly progressive extrapyramidal syndrome which may in its complete form simulate Parkinson's disease), a cerebellar ataxia, or athetosis. Radiographs of the skull reveal deposits of calcium within the lenticular nuclei and dentate regions of the cerebellum. Postmortem examination discloses calcium salt in the walls of small vessels and as isolated rods or spherules, not unlike those seen in lesser degree in some normal elderly individuals. Measures which elevate serum calcium may halt the progress of the extrapyramidal syndrome and at the same time suppress the seizures and tetany. A similar picture of calcium deposits, severe enough to cause a mild progressive choreoathetosis, may be observed without any change in levels of serum Ca, in which instance it is called Fahr's syndrome. Some of our patients have also been mentally retarded.

Choreoathetosis, becoming manifest within the first year of life and persisting into adulthood, stands as a well-known sequela to hypoxia at birth and also to kernicterus. The latter is a complication of a neonatal Rh or ABO blood incompatibility (erythroblastosis fetalis) which usually develops in the 3 to 5 days of postnatal life and is due to serum bilirubin levels in excess of 25 mg per 100 ml. The acute rise of bilirubin, occasioned by hemolysis and immaturity of the glucuronide pathway of the liver, destroys neurones in the subthalamic nuclei of Luys, the globus pallidi, and certain other brainstem nuclei. Lesions in the latter structures account for deafness and ocular gaze disorder. Exchange transfusions of female blood or other measures to lower serum bilirubin or to bind it have greatly reduced the incidence of this frequently fatal or permanently disabling neurologic condition.

There are obviously other conditions in childhood which give rise to rigidity and athetosis, but the cause of most of them cannot presently be ascertained. One new entity has recently been isolated—*Lesch-Nyan syndrome* of hyperuricemia and hyperuricosuria due to a deficiency of hypoxanthine-guanide phosphoribosyl transferase. Feeblemindedness and a compulsive self-mutilation are other characteristics of it.

Syndrome of Cerebellar Ataxia (See Chaps. 22 and 23)

As was stated above, signs of cerebellar disease, slowly becoming apparent during adult life, may be the first manifestation of acquired hepatocerebral degeneration. The speech becomes slurred (more than scanning or explosive), the gait mildly ataxic, and the limbs slow and clumsy or tremulous. Clues as to the nature of the difficulty are usually provided by the episodic coma and cirrhosis or Eck fistulation. Later a faciocervicotrunkal choreoathetosis and dementia are added.

Young children who develop a cerebellar ataxia with or without a choreoathetosis, apraxia of ocular movements, delayed mental development, and recurrent sinopulmonary infections may later be found to have telangiectasia of ears and conjunctivas. Familial incidence and deficiency of a gamma-globulin (IgA) are other features that help to identify the disease before the telangiectasia appears; the relationship of the latter to the pathogenesis remains unclear.

Cerebellar ataxia may also present as the dominant neurologic syndrome in the more slowly evolving lipid storage diseases. It also constitutes one of the features of Bassen-Kornsweig's disease, cerebrotendinous xanthomatosis, and rarely, of Refsum's disease (See Chaps. 113, 364, and 365).

Episodic cerebellar ataxia with or without seizures demarcates a special clinical state peculiar to childhood when it is traceable to Hartnup's disease and argininosuccinic aminoaciduria. In the former condition there are skin lesions not unlike those of pellagra. The ataxia may appear after a seizure and last several days. Mental retardation may be added.

Syndrome of Subacute or Chronic Polyneuropathy (See Chap. 354)

An acute or slowly progressive sensorimotor polyneuropathy of varying severity, afflicting several members of a family, has come to be recognized as another of the common clinical denominators of a number of diseases. In recent years several metabolic aberrations have been discovered. The best-known member of the group is porphyric polyneuropathy. Attacks of the disease are related in some obscure manner to increased urinary excretion of coproporphyrin I and III, and an increase in d-aminolevulinic acid. The importance of barbiturates in provoking an outbreak of the disease has been amply verified (see Chap. 108 for details of the metabolic abnormality).

In *Refsum's syndrome* the polyneuropathy which appears slowly during childhood is distinguished from the other familial polyneuropathies by an associated ichthyosis or xerodermia, nerve deafness, and pigmentary degeneration of the retina. Levels of phytenic acid in the blood are increased, but the role of this substance in the metabolism of nerve fibers is unclear (see Chap. 113 for further details of biochemical abnormality and Chap. 354 for more complete statement of clinical picture). Dietary reduction in phytenic acid has been beneficial. *Tangier disease* is another chronic familial polyneuropathy, recently isolated by Fredrickson and colleagues, associated with a deficiency of beta lipoprotein content of the blood; and in Bassen-Kornsweig disease, where deficient absorption of cholesterol and other lipids from the intestinal

tract has been noted, the peripheral nerves also degenerate (Chaps. 113 and 365). Another separable group of polyneuropathies are associated with cryoglobulinemia and macroglobulinemia (1g M increase) (Waldenström's disease).

Syndrome of Mental Subnormality in Child or Adult

Among the patients in an institution for the mentally retarded who are most severely affected but yet retain normal facial and somatic features and relatively intact motility and sensation, one finds a small percentage (estimated at 1 to 5) who suffer from any one of the inborn errors of metabolism listed in Table 363-2. The largest number of these are disorders of amino acids. A few of the more common types are described in Chap. 102. The clinical picture is relatively monotonous. Apart from the delay in psychosensorimotor development, beginning in infancy, these patients show few other distinctive abnormalities. A mild spasticity or chorea may be observed, but this is exceptional, unlike the cases of congenital malformation of the brain and "birth injuries"; and gross deformities of face, eyes, ears, jaw, etc., so common in the chromosomal anomalies, are also lacking. The details of the syndrome are described further in Chaps. 31 and 365. The guidelines to these inborn errors of metabolism are laboratory tests described in the introduction to Part Three, Section 10, as "cardinal laboratory manifestations." A number of the laboratory tests are very simple, require only a small quantity of the patient's urine, and can be performed in the physician's office. These include the ferric chloride test (positive in phenylketonuria, maple syrup urine disease, and histidinemia), the dinitrophenylhydrazine test for ketones (positive in phenylketonuria, maple syrup urine disease, and tyrosinosis), tests for reducing sugar but not the enzymatic assay for glucose (galactosemia, pentosuria, fructose intolerance), the nitroprusside test (homocystinuria, cystinuria), and the Berry spot test (for disorders of polysaccharide metabolism). In the adult or older child these simple tests will almost always permit detection of the disorders mentioned. In newborn infants, however, more refined techniques are frequently needed. Other recommended tests include study of blood and urinary amino acids by paper chromatography and/or high voltage electrophoresis and measurement of blood ammonia concentration 2 to 4 hr after eating a meal containing 1 Gm protein per kg body weight (normally, this should be less than 70 μg per 100 ml). Special tests to be considered under certain circumstances (see Table 363-2) include measurement of serum uric acid, calcium, cholesterol, and ceruloplasmin.

These methods of "metabolic screening" are being refined in a number of centers; semiautomated techniques should make it possible to perform a large number of pertinent tests on small samples of blood or urine at reasonable cost.

Table 363-2. INBORN ERRORS OF METABOLISM WHICH CAUSE NEUROLOGIC SYMPTOMS IN ADULTS OR OLDER CHILDREN

Disease	Mental subnormality	Extra-pyramidal syndrome	Intermittent coma	Convulsions	Cerebellar syndrome	Peripheral neuropathy	Spastic paralysis	Somatic abnormalities	Laboratory tests	
									Blood	Urine
Phenylketonuria	90%	–	–	25%	–	–	–	Eczema—20% diminished rejuvenation	Phenylalanine < 15 mg per 100 ml	Phenylpyruvic acid present; Ferric chloride test positive
Maple syrup urine disease (intermittent form)	Present except in intermittent form	–	+	50%	–	–	Except in intermittent form	Maple syrup odor	Elevated leucine, valine, isoleucine	Branched chain keto acids present; Ferric chloride test positive
Homocystinuria	60%	–	–	10–30%	–	–	+ Due to infarcts	Dislocated lenses, malar flush long, thin extremities, genu valgum	Methionine increases	Cyanide nitroprusside test positive; Homocystine increases
Hyperglycinemia	+	–	+ (In ketotic form) 20%	+	–	–	+	–	Glycine increases	Glycine increases
Argininosuccinic aciduria	95%	–	–	70%	30%	–	–	Short, stubby hair (trichorrhexis nodosa), 60%	Ammonia (postprandial) increases	Argininosuccinic acid present
Histidinemia	About 50%	–	–	–	–	–	–	–	Histidine increases	Imidazolepyruvic acid present; Ferric chloride test positive
Hartnup's disease	20%	–	–	–	45%	–	–	Pellagralike rash (75%)		Monoamino monocarboxylic in excess; Amino acids and indoles in excess
Hurler's syndrome	+	–	–	–	–	–	–	Cloudy cornea, small stature, lumbar gibbus, large liver and spleen, gargoyle facies, hydrocephalus	Alder-Reilly granules in leukocytes	Polysaccharides increase (Chondroitin sulfate B, Heparitin sulfate)
Hunter's syndrome	Variable	–	–	–	–	–	–	Resemble Hurler's but less severe. No corneal clouding or lumbar gibbus	Same as Hurler's	Same as Hurler's
Sanfilippo syndrome	+	–	–	–	–	–	–	"Coarse" features, moderately small stature, moderate joint stiffness		Polysaccharides increase (Heparitin sulfate)
Wilson's disease	+	+	–	Up to 50%	+	–	–	Kayser-Fleischer ring, cirrhosis of the liver	Ceruloplasmin decreases	Aminoaciduria
Hallevorden–Spatz syndrome	++	++	–	–	–	–	+	–		
Lesch–Nyhan syndrome	++	–	–	–	–	–	+	Self-mutilation, kidney stones, tophi	Uric acid increases; Hypoxanthine-guanine phosphoribosyltransferase absent; Phosphoribosyltransferase present	Uric acid increases
Metachromatic leukodystrophy	+ (late)	Rarely	–	–	+	+	+	Mild "cherry red spot" in macula		Sulfatides increases; Arylsulfatase A. decreases
Refsum's disease	–	–	–	–	+	+	–	Retinitis pigmentosa, ichthyosis	Phytenic acid increases	
Bassen–Kornzweig syndrome	–	Rarely	–	–	+	+	–	Retinitis pigmentosa	Acanthocytes, low density lipoproteins absent	
Tangier disease	–	–	–	–	–	+	–	Large tonsils with yellow or orange discoloration, occasionally large spleen	Absent, high density lipoprotein	
Cerebrotendinous xanthomatosis	+	–	–	+	+	–	+	tendon xanthomata, cataracts	High cholesterol (30–50%)	
Lipidoses Juvenile (Spielmeyer-Vogt) and adult (Kuf's)	+	–	–	+	+	+	+	Pigmentary degeneration of retina		
Acute intermittent porphyria	–	–	–	+	–	+	–	–		Porphobilinogen increases
Ataxia telangiectasia	–	Rarely	–	–	+	+	–	Telangiectasia on conjunctiva and other characteristic areas	Gamma IgA immunoglobu in decrease (80%)	

Syndrome of Progressive Dementia with or without Spastic Paralysis (See also Chap. 31)

In many of the inborn errors of metabolism, such as phenylketonuria, damage to the nervous system occurs during the first few years of life, but after that no further deterioration occurs, and in fact to a limited degree, maturation and development may proceed, but at a retarded rate. In certain other disorders, however, the function of the nervous system may be relatively normal during the first few years and then become progressively impaired. The clearest example of this is metachromatic leukodystrophy (sulfatide lipidosis), which allows normal development for the first 2 to 3 years and then a progressive gait disturbance, due to a mild involvement of peripheral nerves and more severe affection of pyramidal and cerebellar systems, all in conjunction with a deterioration of intellect. The course may be so slow that if the history is not evaluated carefully, this disease is mistaken for "cerebral palsy" or some static defect in the nervous system resulting from birth injury. The onset is usually early childhood, but in a small number of patients symptoms do not begin until adolescence or adult years, and in this "late onset" type, the initial symptoms are apt to be in the mental or emotional sphere. Diagnosis depends upon demonstration of a deficiency or complete absence of arylsulfatase A activity and excessive sulfatide excretion in the urine. The juvenile (Batten-Spielmeyer-Vogt) and adult (Kuf's) form of lipid storage disease may also give rise to a clinical syndrome, characterized by seizures, dementia, ataxia, visual loss, and progressive paralysis. The biochemical basis of these disorders is not understood, and clinical diagnosis is difficult. The demonstration of lipid storage in the neurones of the rectal mucosa is the most useful laboratory aid.

NUTRITIONAL DISEASES OF THE NERVOUS SYSTEM

The general principles of deficiency disease have been presented in Chap. 77, and the reader should review them as an introduction to this discussion of deficiency disease of the nervous system. The term *deficiency* is used here in its strictest sense, to designate those diseases or syndromes which result from the lack of an essential nutrient in the diet or from a conditioning factor which increases the need for that nutrient. The neurologic diseases which comprise this category are the following:

1. Pellagra
2. Wernicke's disease and Korsakoff's psychosis (also alcoholic cerebellar degeneration)
3. Nutritional polyneuropathy
4. Strachan's syndrome
5. Subacute combined degeneration of the spinal cord due to B_{12} deficiency
6. Nutritional retrobulbar neuropathy or amblyopia

Before discussing each of these disorders, some general remarks, applicable to all of them, may suitably be made. Of the known vitamin deficiencies only those of the B group are of importance in neurologic disease. A lack of the other known vitamins does not appear to have any effect on the brain, spinal cord, peripheral nerves, or muscles of man. Thiamine chloride, nicotinic acid, pyridoxine, pantothenic acid, and riboflavin all play a role in carbohydrate metabolism, upon which the central nervous system depends for its principal source of energy. These vitamins are essentially coenzymes mainly in the Krebs citric acid cycle. Vitamin B_{12} is also of importance, but little is known of its mode of action.

Except for subacute combined degeneration of the spinal cord (vitamin B_{12} deficiency) and certain components of Wernicke's disease (vitamin B_1 deficiency), it is not possible to relate the clinical deficiency syndromes in man to a lack of single vitamins. For example, polyneuropathy may result from one of several vitamin deficiencies (thiamine chloride, pyridoxine (vitamin B_6), pantothenic acid, and probably vitamin B_{12}. Moreover, such syndromes as pellagra and beriberi are often the result of a simultaneous deficiency of multiple vitamins.

With the exception of subacute combined degeneration of the cord, these syndromes are rarely seen in pure form. In patients with nutritional disease, it is usual for both the central and peripheral nervous systems to be involved, a combination found in few other circumstances. Also, the examination of these patients frequently discloses nonneurologic signs of malnutrition such as general wasting lesions of the skin and mucous membranes and circulatory abnormalities. In general, however, one should think of the possibility of a nutritional disease if a patient presents himself with a neurologic illness that conforms to one of the following syndromes:

1. A subacute confusional delirious or amnestic state
2. A symmetrical subacute sensorimotor polyneuropathy
3. A symmetrical subacute posterolateral degeneration of the spinal cord
4. Subacute bilateral degeneration of optic nerves

Throughout the world the nutritional disorders of the nervous system are most often observed in the alcoholic population of the large urban centers. The role of alcohol is mainly to displace food in the diet, but it also increases the demand for B vitamins, which are necessary to metabolize the carbohydrate furnished by alcohol itself.

Subacute Confusional Delirious or Amnestic Syndrome (See Chap. 30)

PELLAGRA. This disease has already been described in Chap. 80. This discussion is concerned only with the neurologic manifestations, which in themselves are extremely diverse. Pellagra is essentially an encephalopathy, although involvement of other parts of the nervous system may occur. The early mental symptoms may be mistaken for those of a psychoneurosis. Insomnia, fatigue, nervousness, irritability, and feelings of depression are then the common complaints. However, careful examination, especially as the disease advances, will reveal slowing and inefficiency of mental processes and impairment of memory. Sometimes an acute confusional psychosis combined with changing rigidity of the limbs, grasping and sucking reflexes, and Babinski signs dominates the clinical picture. Pellagra not only may produce insanity but occasionally may result from it because of the anorexia and refusal of food that accompany certain mental illnesses. The manifestations of spinal cord involvement have not been clearly delineated, perhaps because the mental state of the patients has precluded accurate testing. In general, they are referable to both the posterior and the lateral columns, predominantly the former. Neuropathic signs are frequent and are often difficult to distinguish from affection of the posterior columns. Other manifestations such as tremors, extrapyramidal rigidity, sucking and grasping reflexes, and coma have often been included in the pellagrous syndrome, as have various disorders of the special senses.

Pathologic Changes. The distinctive neuropathologic changes in pellagra are most readily discerned in the large cells of the motor cortex, the cells of Betz, which appear swollen and rounded with eccentric nuclei and loss of the Nissl particles. This change was first described by Adolf Meyer as *central neuritis* and is frequently referred to as *axonal reaction* because of the similarity to the nerve cell change which occurs in the anterior horn cells when their axones are severed. The central neuritis of pellagra is probably not dependent on injury to the axones of the Betz cells, but it appears to represent a primary affection of the whole motor cell. The spinal cord lesions take the form of a symmetric degeneration of the dorsal columns, especially of Goll, and to a lesser extent of the pyramidal tracts. The posterior column degeneration affects a specific system of fibers and is secondary to the degeneration of the posterior roots. The nature of the pyramidal tract lesion in pellagra is not known; one can only speculate that this change is secondary to the pyramidal cell degeneration.

A *spastic paretic syndrome,* apart from the other symptoms and signs of pellagra, may be a rare manifestation of deficiency disease. The chief clinical signs are spastic weakness of the legs with absent abdominal and increased tendon reflexes, clonus, and extensor plantar responses. These signs are usually accompanied by other signs of nutritional deficiency, such as Wernicke's disease and retrobulbar and peripheral neuropathy. Spastic weakness of the legs has also been observed in conjunction with chronic liver disease.

WERNICKE'S DISEASE. In 1881, Carl Wernicke described an illness of sudden onset, characterized by mental disturbance, paralysis of eye movements, and ataxic gait. Swelling of the optic discs with retinal hemorrhages was also said to be present, and in all three of his patients there was a progressive depression of the state of consciousness and death. A fatal outcome was at one time regarded as a universal feature of this disease. Wernicke described focal vascular lesions, primarily affecting the gray matter around the third and fourth ventricles and aqueduct of Sylvius. He regarded the disease as inflammatory in nature and suggested the name *acute superior hemorrhagic polioencephalitis.*

Since Wernicke's time, views regarding this disease have undergone considerable modification, clinically, pathologically, and etiologically.

Symptoms and Signs. The crux of the clinical picture is the ocular disturbance, and the clinical diagnosis of Wernicke's disease can hardly be made without it. The ocular disturbance consists of weakness or paralysis of the external recti, nystagmus, both horizontal and vertical, and various palsies of conjugate gaze. These signs show a considerable diversity. The paralysis of conjugate movement varies from merely a nystagmus on extreme gaze in one direction to a complete loss of ocular movement in that direction. Vertical movements may be affected, though abnormalities of horizontal movement are commoner. Paralysis of downward gaze and internuclear ophthalmoplegia are less usual manifestations. Next to nystagmus, one most frequently encounters a lateral rectus muscle weakness or paralysis. The sixth nerve palsy is always bilateral, though not always symmetric, and is accompanied by diplopia and internal strabismus. With complete paralysis nystagmus is absent, but it becomes evident as the weakness improves. In advanced stages of the disease there may be a complete loss of ocular movement, and the pupils, which ordinarily are spared, may become miotic and nonreacting. Other ocular disturbances such as ptosis, retrobulbar neuropathy, retinal hemorrhages, and involvement of the near-far focusing mechanism are decidedly rare, although they do occur on occasion. The authors have never observed papilledema in this disease.

The ataxia affects stance and gait predominantly. In its severest form, the patient is unable to stand or walk without support. The mildest degree of ataxia may be brought out only by special tests, such as heel-to-toe walking. In contrast to the gross disorder of locomotion is the relative infrequency of a clear-cut intention tremor. When present, it affects the legs more than the arms. Scanning speech is present only in isolated instances. The ataxia of gait is cerebellar in origin, but it is often mistakenly attributed to a polyneuropathy. It is indistinguishable from alcoholic cerebellar degeneration (Chap. 118), which is also a deficiency disease in all probability.

Symptoms of deranged mental function are found in over 80 percent of patients and take one of several forms. (1) A small proportion of patients show the symptoms of delirium tremens or its variants, i.e., hallucinations and other disorders of sense perception, confusion, agitation, and autonomic overactivity. The symptoms are usually mild and evanescent in nature and may clear without specific treatment. (2) The majority of patients are apathetic, listless, and severely confused. Unconsciousness as part of the initial episode is distinctly rare, but mild drowsiness is common. The patient's mental state is best described as one of disinterest or indifference. His spontaneous speech is minimal, and he is inattentive and cannot concentrate on the simplest tasks. Many questions directed to him go unanswered, or he may suspend conversation in the middle of a sentence to turn over and sleep. He is readily roused from this state, however. Whatever questions the patient answers betray disorientation in time and place, misidentification of those around him, and an inability to grasp the meaning of his illness or immediate situation. Many of his remarks are irrational and show no consistency from one moment to another. Under these circumstances a proper evaluation of intellectual function is seldom possible. (3) Some patients, from the time they are first seen, show a disorder of retentive memory and other cognitive functions characteristic of *Korsakoff's psychosis*. In this syndrome, which may occasionally manifest itself in the absence of the ocular and ataxic signs, the disorder of retentive memory is impaired out of all proportion to other cognitive function. Hand in hand with the disorder of past memory is a persistent inability to acquire new information and skills, i.e., to make "new memories." Although the retrograde and anterograde amnesia are the dominant features of Korsakoff's psychosis, other perceptual and conceptual functions, which depend little on memory, are impaired to a minor degree. As a rule, patients with this disorder have only limited insight into their disability, and they tend to be apathetic and inert. Fabrication (confabulation) of real or imagined events of recent past is widely regarded as a specific symptom of Korsakoff's psychosis, but it is found in many other confusional states as well. Although confabulation is frequently present in the early stages of Korsakoff's psychosis, it is not discerned in all the patients and is characteristically absent in the chronic stages of the disease.

The outcome of Korsakoff's psychosis varies. In approximately one-quarter of patients complete or almost complete recovery occurs. More commonly there is slow and incomplete recovery over a year or longer. Depending on the severity of the residual symptoms, the patient may or may not be able to lead an independent existence out of a hospital. The residual mental state is usually one in which the patient shows large gaps in memory and the inability to sort out events in their proper temporal sequence. If the patient is seen for the first time during this stage, the diagnosis of "alcoholic deteriorated state" or "organic brain syndrome due to alcohol" is commonly made.

The symptoms of Wernicke's disease may all appear simultaneously and rather acutely, but more frequently the ophthalmoplegia and ataxia precede the mental signs by a few days or 1 to 2 weeks. The patient may also show other stigmata of malnutrition, the most frequent of which is polyneuropathy. The signs of neuropathy are usually slight and could not account for the disordered gait. Nevertheless, in a small proportion the neuropathy is so severe that stance and gait cannot be tested. Occasionally, amblyopia or spinal spastic ataxia may be added to the clinical picture. The advanced stages of beriberi heart disease are rarely observed in Wernicke's disease, although indications of disordered cardiovascular func-

tion, such as tachycardia, exertional dyspnea, postural hypotension, and minor electrocardiographic abnormalities, are common. Occasionally the patient may die suddenly, the mode of death suggesting "cardiovascular collapse." It has been shown that Wernicke's disease is characterized by a state of high cardiac output which is out of proportion to the oxygen consumption. This is probably due to an abnormal state of vasodilatation, which in turn may be related specifically to thiamine deficiency. Death occurs in about 15 percent of hospitalized patients and is usually due to the complications of cirrhosis of the liver or to infection.

Pathologic Changes. Postmortem examination reveals symmetrically located lesions in the paraventricular regions of the thalamus and hypothalamus, the mammillary bodies, the periaqueductal region of the midbrain, the floor of the fourth ventricle, and the anterior lobe of the cerebellum, particularly the vermis. The lesions are invariably found in the mammillary bodies and less consistently in the other areas. Microscopically the principal change consists of varying degrees of necrosis of parenchymal structures. Many nerve cells and fibers are destroyed; others remain intact and are seen against a background of reactive glial elements, both astrocytes and microgliacytes. The blood vessels are prominent, owing to adventitial and endothelial proliferation. Hemorrhagic lesions, as the original name suggests, are present in only a small proportion of cases. When present, they give the appearance of being of recent origin. The oculomotor nuclei and the medial longitudinal fasciculi are involved only to a mild degree, which is consistent with the rapid clinical improvement in oculomotor function.

Etiology. Wernicke's disease is no longer regarded as inflammatory in nature or the result of the neurotoxic effects of alcohol. Nutritional deficiency is now established as the causal factor. Outbreaks have been encountered in prisoner-of-war camps, and occasional cases have been reported in wasting diseases of varied origin where alcohol played no part. The specific nutritional factor in most, if not all, of the symptomatology of Wernicke's disease is thiamine. The experimental evidence for this statement, both in animals and in man, is quite convincing. The marked sensitivity of the ophthalmoplegia to the administration of thiamine accounts for the rapid disappearance of this sign following the ingestion of one or two meals. The quality of prompt reversibility suggests that these symptoms are due to a biochemical abnormality and not to structural change. On the other hand, the memory loss responds slowly or not at all, suggesting that this symptom is the result of structural changes, presumably in the medial dorsal nuclei of the thalamus and mammillary bodies.

THE UNITY OF WERNICKE'S ENCEPHALOPATHY AND KORSAKOFF'S PSYCHOSIS. Several allusions have already been made to the relationship between these two syndromes. Clinically, the majority of patients with Wernicke's disease show signs of Korsakoff's psychosis either from the time they are first seen or following recovery from the initial state of apathy and drowsiness. Conversely, the vast majority of patients with an amnestic-confabulatory psychosis show the stigmata of Wernicke's disease (slight nystagmus and ataxia) even years after the onset of the illness. The pathologic changes in the brain are very much the same whether the patient dies in the acute stages of Wernicke's disease or in the chronic phase of the illness when the ocular palsies have cleared and the amnestic symptoms predominate. It would appear that *in the nutritionally deficient alcoholic patient,* Wernicke's disease and Korsakoff's psychosis represent but different facets of the same disease process.

Treatment of the Wernicke-Korsakoff Syndrome. Wernicke's disease represents a medical emergency, and its recognition demands the immediate administration of thiamine. A delay of a few hours may be crucial in determining whether the patient who presents only ocular and ataxic signs will be prevented from developing mental signs and whether the patient with early Korsakoff's changes will be restored to a state of mental competency. Although 2 to 3 mg thiamine are sufficient to modify the ocular signs, much larger doses are usually employed—50 mg intravenously and 50 mg intramuscularly, the latter dose being repeated each day until the patient resumes a normal diet. The other B vitamins may be given by mouth in the dosages outlined in Chap. 76. If the patient cannot or will not eat, parenteral feeding and administration of B vitamins become necessary.

A particular danger attends the treatment of the severely depleted alcoholic patient with intravenous glucose solution. This solution may exhaust the patient's last reserve of B vitamins and either precipitate Wernicke's disease, where it was not present before, or cause a rapid worsening of the athiaminotic state with circulatory collapse and death. For this reason, B vitamins must be added in all cases requiring parenteral glucose. If signs of cardiac weakness are betrayed by pulmonary edema, feeble heart sounds, tachycardia, and low blood pressure, rapid digitalization should be undertaken. Since these patients are confused and forgetful, they must be supervised continually, preferably on a medical ward.

A special problem in management arises when the patient recovers from the acute phase of the illness and the amnestic psychosis becomes prominent. The disposition of the patient to family, nursing home or mental institution should be undertaken on the basis of the severity of the mental illness as well as the existing family and social circumstances.

Syndrome of Subacute and Chronic Symmetrical Sensorimotor Polyneuropathy (See Chap. 354)

NUTRITIONAL POLYNEUROPATHY (NEURITIC BERIBERI). For the definitive discussion of this disease the reader should turn to Chap. 81. Here only a few additional remarks will be made about the clinical subtleties of it.

Symptoms and Signs. The symptomatology of nutritional polyneuropathy is remarkably diverse. In fact, many patients are asymptomatic. Only on examination will thinness of the leg muscles and loss or depression of the knee and ankle jerks or of the ankle jerks alone be detected. Less frequently, calf tenderness, somewhat diminished muscle power in the feet and legs, or a patchy blunting of pain and touch sensation over the feet and shins are also found.

Patients with the manifest form of polyneuropathy report a variety of symptoms consisting of weakness, paresthesias, and sometimes pain. The symptoms are usually insidious and slowly progressive over a period of a few weeks or months, although at times there may be a rapid progression of the weakness. In a very small group the transition from an asymptomatic state to one of virtual paralysis occurs in a matter of several days. The symptoms are at first referred to the distal portions of the limbs and progress proximally if the illness remains untreated. The legs are affected earlier than the arms and practically always more severely. Motor and sensory symptoms tend to occur concomitantly although the patient may complain much more of one than the other. Usually weakness constitutes the source of disability. Sensory symptoms may, however, be troublesome; they consist mainly of numbness, prickly feelings, coldness, deadness, tenderness of the calf and plantar musculature, or unusual sensitivity to contact. In a minority of patients, pain and paresthesias constitute the chief complaints. The pain may take the form of a dull constant ache in the feet or sometimes the entire leg; often the pains are sharp and lancinating, momentary in duration, similar to the lightning pains of tabes dorsalis. Complaints of coldness are common, but they are purely subjective, the feet feeling either warm or cold to touch. Much more distressing and incapacitating are the "burning" feelings and sensations of heat; usually these affect the soles of the feet and less frequently the dorsal aspects of the feet as well. These feelings fluctuate in intensity or may be clearly intermittent in nature. Characteristically, a patient afflicted with pain and paresthesias suffers not one but all of the sensory symptoms enumerated. The painful symptoms are made much worse by light pressure or by a contactual stimulus. In severe cases the patient cannot bear to have the bedclothes touch his feet or to touch an eating utensil. Because of these dysesthesias, he may be unable or unwilling to walk, despite the preservation of motor power.

The examination reveals varying degrees of motor, reflex, and sensory loss. As the symptoms would suggest, the signs are symmetric, usually more prominent in the distal portions of the limbs, and often confined to the legs. The weakness varies greatly in degree. It may be evident only with muscular exertion, or it may take the form of a foot and wrist drop or even of a complete paralysis of the limb. The deep reflexes in the legs are almost universally lost even with the mildest degrees of weakness. In the arms the tendon reflexes may occasionally be retained despite serious loss of power in the hands. In a small number of patients, particularly those with pain and paresthesias, the reflexes may be brisk. The sensory loss usually involves all the modalities. Although one cannot adequately equate touch, pain, temperature, and vibratory and position sense, some patients show an impairment or loss of one modality out of proportion to the others. There is no sharp border between normal and impaired sensation; the sensory loss, which is most profound distally, shades off gradually, the transition to normal sensation occurring over a long vertical extent of the limb.

As a rule, only the limbs are affected, and the abdominal, thoracic, and bulbar musculature are intact. In some instances of Oriental beriberi, sensory loss has reportedly involved the face and abdomen as well. Tinnitus, vertigo, nerve deafness, aphonia due to vocal cord paralysis (particularly in infants) and retrobulbar neuropathy may also complicate beriberi in rare instances. The relation of this latter group of disturbances to beriberi has been a point of contention that cannot be settled with finality since the specific cause of neither is known. Far more frequently, these disturbances are engrafted on the syndrome of ataxia and burning, tender feet and are, therefore, appropriately considered as a part of Strachan's syndrome. .

The *spinal fluid* in the nutritional neuropathies and in Wernicke-Korsakoff disease is usually normal although rare cases show a modest elevation of the protein content. Normal spinal fluid findings may be helpful in distinguishing the rapidly evolving form of nutritional polyneuropathy from infectious polyneuritis.

Recovery is invariably a slow process. In the mildest cases there may be considerable restoration of motor power in a few weeks; in the severest forms several weeks may pass before the first signs of recovery become manifest and up to a year before the patient is able to walk unaided. Recovery in severely affected patients is often incomplete, and they may be left with some weakness of the feet and an absence of the knee and ankle jerks. Contractures may develop because of inadequate physiotherapy and greatly prolong convalescence.

The "Burning Feet" Syndrome. The term *burning feet* is frequently applied to a state in which pain in the extremities is the outstanding symptom and in which the advanced signs of neuropathy may be absent. It was the subject of many reports from the prisoner-of-war and internment camps of the Far East. The pain was variously described as tingling, burning, aching, shooting, cramplike, or resembling the lightning pains of tabes. The pain was often very severe; it was greatest at night and interfered with sleep. Some patients gained relief from the application of cold; others only from movement. The presence of associated neuritic signs was a variable matter. In some patients, wasting, dropped foot, reflex loss, and sensory changes were completely wanting; in a significant proportion of patients the tendon reflexes were exaggerated but without clonus or extensor plantar responses. However, in other patients, the painful feet were but one stage in the evolution of a peripheral neuropathy characterized by tenderness of the calves, reflex and sensory loss, and ataxia and complicated in many cases by retrobulbar neuropathy.

As has been mentioned, pain is the outstanding symptom in a relatively small number of patients with alcoholic polyneuropathy. These patients do not constitute a distinct group in terms of their neurologic signs. In some cases the pain and dysesthesia may be associated with a severe degree of motor, reflex, and sensory loss. In others the weakness may be slight or absent, and in rare instances reflexes may be retained. However, in all cases there is some degree of sensory loss, even where the slightest stimulus appears intolerable. The term *hyperesthetic* is not well chosen to describe such cases since it implies a heightened receptiveness of the nervous system or an increased response of the receptors to tactile and painful stimuli. Actually, there is an underlying sensory deficit, i.e., an elevated threshold to various stimuli; once the stimulus is perceived, however, it may have a severely painful or unpleasant quality (hyperpathia). The term *burning* is also not particularly applicable, considering the wide variety of symptoms in addition to thermal dysesthesias. Because of this, as well as the fact that the hands may be involved, the term *acrodysesthesias*, or *painful extremities*, seems preferable.

The specific deficiency responsible for the dysesthesias has not been clearly established. The pathophysiology is likewise unknown. Spillane suggests that this affection represents an early stage of the nutritional disturbance in the nerves to the lower limbs. He draws an analogy to the burning pain produced by the interruption of the circulation of the limbs. The authors have been impressed by the similarity of the pain to causalgia and in several patients have succeeded in abolishing it for several hours to days by paravertebral sympathetic block. These observations require confirmation.

Syndrome of Subacute Posterolateral Degeneration of Spinal Cord (See Chap. 356)

STRACHAN'S SYNDROME. Beginning with the report of Strachan in 1888 and culminating in the recent observations among prisoners of war and civilian internees, there has appeared a large number of reports concerning a nutritional disorder of the nervous system which cannot be forced into the boundaries of the classical syndromes described above. Strachan was the first to describe this syndrome, although he did not recognize its nutritional etiology. .

Strachan's syndrome is essentially a disorder of the peripheral and optic nerves. Clinically, sensory symptoms and signs dominate the picture; in this respect the syndrome differs from beriberi. Paresthesias of the extremities, face, and trunk, painful "hyperesthesia" of the feet, loss of superficial and deep sensation, and ataxia are the common manifestations. On the other hand, foot drop and muscle weakness occur very rarely. A frequently associated disorder is failing vision, which may go on to complete blindness and pallor of the optic disks. In general, deafness and vertigo are rare complications, but in some outbreaks these symptoms were so common as to earn the epithet "camp dizziness." Along with the neurologic signs there may be varying degrees of stomatoglossitis, corneal degeneration, and genital dermatitis. These mucocutaneous lesions are often spoken of together as the *orogenital syndrome* and are quite distinct from those of pellagra.

There have been only a few pathologic studies of this syndrome. Aside from the damage to the papillomacular bundle in the optic nerve, the most consistent abnormality has been a loss of medullated fibers in each column of Goll adjacent to the midline. This indicates a systematized degeneration of the central process of the bipolar sensory neurone of the lumbosacral spinal ganglions. The fact that the primary sensory neurone is the chief site of disease is consistent with the predominant sensory symptomatology.

Patients with this syndrome are occasionally found amongst the alcoholic population of the United States. It may also accompany chronic liver disease and nontropical sprue or occur as an inexplicable illness in late adult life.

SUBACUTE COMBINED DEGENERATION OF THE SPINAL CORD AND BRAIN DUE TO B$_{12}$ DEFICIENCY (See Chap. 337).

Subacute combined degeneration of the spinal cord, the neurologic component of pernicious anemia, is due to vitamin B$_{12}$ deficiency but is clearly different from the other nutritional disorders. The disease results not from the lack of vitamin B$_{12}$ in the food but from the inability to transfer minute amounts of this nutrient across the intestinal mucosa. Such "starvation in the midst of plenty" has been called *conditioned deficiency disease* because the condition depends on the lack of an intrinsic factor in the gastric secretion. The general features of pernicious anemia are fully discussed in Chap. 337; here only the neurologic manifestations will be considered.

Clinical Manifestations. Symptoms of nervous system disease are present in the large majority of patients with pernicious anemia. The patient first notices general weakness and paresthesias consisting of tingling, "pins and needles" feelings, or other vaguely described sensations. The paresthesias tend to be constant, to progress steadily, and to be the source of much distress. They are localized in the distal parts of all four limbs in a symmetric distribution, the lower extremities usually being involved before the upper ones. As the illness progresses, stiffness and weakness of the limbs, especially the legs, develop, which combined with a defect in postural sensation produce a weak, unsteady gait and awkwardness of the limbs. If the disease remains untreated, an ataxic paraplegia with variable degrees of spasticity and incoordination may develop.

Early in the course of the illness, when only paresthesias are present, there may be no objective signs. Later, the neurologic examination discloses a disorder of the posterior and lateral columns of the spinal cord, predominantly of the former. Loss of vibration sense is by far the most consistent sign; it is more pronounced in the legs than in the arms, and frequently it extends over the trunk. Position sense is involved somewhat less frequently. The motor signs include loss of power, spasticity, changes in the tendon reflexes, clonus, and extensor plantar responses. These signs are usually limited to the legs. At first the patellar and Achilles reflexes are found to be diminished in activity as frequently as they are increased, and they may even be absent. With treatment the reflexes may return to normal or become hyperactive. The gait at first is predominantly ataxic, later ataxic and spastic.

Isolated instances of loss of superficial sensation below a segmental level on the trunk do occur, implicating the spinothalamic tracts, but such a finding should always suggest the possibility of some other disease of the spinal cord. The defect of cutaneous sensation may take the form of a mild blunting of touch, pain, and temperature sensation over the limbs in a distal distribution, but such a finding is also uncommon.

The nervous system involvement in subacute combined degeneration is characteristically, though not always, entirely symmetric. A definite asymmetry of motor or sensory findings maintained over a period of weeks or months should always cast doubt on the diagnosis of subacute combined degeneration of the spinal cord.

Mental signs are frequent, ranging from irritability, apathy, somnolence, suspiciousness, emotional instability to a marked confusional or depressive psychosis, or intellectual deterioration. Signs of visual impairment are distinctly rare; when present, they take the form of centrocecal scotomata. If involvement of the optic nerve is severe, optic atrophy may occur.

Neuropathologic Changes. The pathologic process takes the form of diffuse, although uneven, degeneration of the white matter. There are multiple foci of spongy degeneration, often in relation to small blood vessels. The myelin sheaths and the axis cylinders are both affected, the former perhaps earlier and to a greater extent than the latter. There is relatively little fibrous gliosis in the early lesions, but in the older treated cases gliosis is pronounced. The changes begin in the posterior columns of the thoracic cord and spread from this region up and down the cord, as well as forward into the lateral columns. The lesions are not limited to specific systems of fibers within the posterior and lateral funiculi but are scattered irregularly through the latter.

Treatment. The treatment of subacute combined degeneration of the cord differs in no way from the treatment of the other manifestations of pernicious anemia. Theoretically, 1 μg of parenterally administered vitamin B$_{12}$ is adequate, but in practice much larger doses are used.

The most important factor influencing *response* to treatment is the duration of the disease. Recovery may be complete if therapy is instituted within a few weeks of the onset of symptoms. For this reason subacute combined degeneration represents a medical emergency. If symptoms have been present for longer than a month or two, only partial recovery can be expected, and in longstanding cases the best that can be expected is arrest of progression.

The chief obstacle to *early diagnosis* is the lack of parallelism between the hematologic and neurologic signs. This is particularly the case in patients who have received folic acid, which serves to maintain a hematologic remission for an indefinite period while the neurologic signs worsen, often to an irreversible stage. Under these circumstances the most reliable diagnostic procedure is the Schilling test (Chap. 337).

Syndrome of Bilateral Retrobulbar Neuropathy (Nutritional Amblyopia) (See Chaps. 24, 355, and 364)

This term refers to the visual failure which occurs in nutritional disease and which is not due to a lesion of the cornea or other parts of the eye concerned with refraction. The optic nerve lesion consists of a degeneration of myelinated fibers more or less confined to the zone of the papillomacular bundle.

Clinically the characteristic symptom is a blurring of vision for near and distant objects, usually developing gradually over a period of several weeks. Examination discloses a reduction in visual acuity, the presence of central and centrocecal scotomata, larger for red than for white test objects. A mild pallor of the temporal portion of the optic disk and retinal hemorrhages may be seen occasionally. These changes are always bilateral and more or less symmetrical. Untreated, the disease may progress to irreversible optic atrophy. With nutritious diet and vitamin supplements, improvement occurs in all instances, though to a variable extent.

Deficiency amblyopia was particularly prevalent during World War II in the prisoner-of-war and civilian interment camps of the Far East. Although it had previously been described in association with beriberi and pellagra, the peak incidence did not coincide with that of either of these syndromes but with the syndrome of mucocutaneous lesions in the orogenital regions and "burning feet." In this country, many, if not all, of the cases of retrobulbar neuropathy attributed to the toxic effects of alcohol or tobacco are probably of nutritional origin. Retrobulbar neuropathy may occur as the only manifestation of deficiency, but far more frequently it is combined with other nutritional syndromes, such as peripheral neuropathy and the Wernicke-Korsakoff syndrome.

Although the nutritional origin of this type of amblyopia seems established, the specific nutrient responsible is uncertain. Isolated reports have implicated riboflavin, thiamine, and vitamin B_{12}, but the evidence provided is inconclusive. Since a specific nutritional deficiency can rarely be determined in this disorder, treatment consists of the administration of a balanced diet and supplementary B vitamins and interdiction of alcohol, where this is a factor.

REFERENCES

Courville, C. B.: "Cerebral Anoxia," Los Angeles, San Lucas Press, 1953.

Himwich, H. E.: "Brain Metabolism and Cerebral Disorders," Baltimore, The William & Wilkins Company, 1951.

Merritt, H. H., and C. C. Hare (Eds.): Metabolic and Toxic Diseases of the Nervous System, vol. 32, Research Publications of the Association for Research in Nervous and Mental Disease, Baltimore, The Williams & Wilkins Company, 1953.

Spillane, J. D.: "Nutritional Disorders of the Nervous System," Baltimore, The Williams & Wilkins Company, 1947.

Victor, M., and R. D. Adams: The Effect of Alcohol on the Nervous System, in Metabolic and Toxic Diseases of the Nervous System, vol. 32, Research Publications of the Association for Research in Nervous and Mental Disease, Baltimore, The Williams & Wilkins Company, 1953.

364 DEGENERATIVE DISEASES OF THE NERVOUS SYSTEM

(Including Parkinson's Disease)

Edward P. Richardson, Jr.,
Ansgar Torvik, and
Raymond D. Adams

The term *degenerative* as applied to diseases of the nervous system is used to designate a group of disorders in which there is gradual, generally symmetric, relentlessly progressive wasting away of structural elements of the nervous system, for reasons still unknown. Many of the conditions so designated depend on abnormal genetic factors and thus appear in more than one member of the same family; this general group of diseases is therefore frequently referred to as heredodegenerative. A number of other conditions, not apparently differing in any fundamental way from the hereditary disorders, occur only sporadically, i.e., as isolated instances in a given family. Sir William Gowers in 1902 suggested the now-familiar term *abiotrophy*, by which he meant that diseases of this class were the result of "defective vital endurance" of the structures affected, leading to their premature death. This term, of course, tells nothing of the true nature of the defects. It is to be assumed that the basis for these diseases must be found in some disorder of the metabolism of the parts involved.

Within relatively recent times there has been some elucidation of the nature of a number of nervous disorders which, in their symmetric distribution and gradually progressive course, resemble the class of diseases under discussion.

The large group of the degenerative diseases of the nervous system manifest themselves by a number of syndromes distinguished by their clinical and pathologic features. Nevertheless, there are certain aspects common to all, the recognition of which can assist the clinician in arriving at the diagnosis of a disorder of this class. Some of these are summarized in the following paragraphs.

GENERAL CONSIDERATIONS. It is a characteristic of the degenerative diseases that they begin insidiously and run a gradually progressive course which may extend over many years. The earliest changes may be so slight that it is frequently impossible to assign any precise time of onset. As with other gradually developing conditions, the patient or his family may give a history implying an abrupt appearance of disability. This is particularly likely to occur if there has been an injury, or if some other dramatic event has taken place in the patient's life, to which illness might conceivably be related. In such a case, skillful taking of the history may bring out that the patient or family has suddenly become aware of a condition which had, in fact, already been present for some time but had passed unnoticed. Whether or not trauma or other stress may bring on or aggravate one of the degenerative diseases is still a question that cannot be answered with certainty. It would seem highly improbable from all that is known. In any event, it must be kept in mind that the disease processes under discussion by their very nature develop spontaneously without relationship to external factors.

The family history is of great importance, but one cannot always be immediately satisfied with that obtained on first contact with the patient. One reason for this is that patients or their relatives may be ashamed to disclose that a neurologic disease occurs in the family. Another is that it may not be realized that an illness is hereditary when other members of the family have a much less severe form of the disorder than the patient and have themselves been unaware of the abnormality— as not infrequently occurs in the hereditary ataxias and related conditions. Moreover, in modern Western families the small sibships may prevent even well-established hereditary diseases from expressing themselves. It must, of course, be remembered that familial occurrence of a disease does not always mean that it is hereditary; it may indicate instead that more than one member of a family has been exposed to the same infectious or toxic agent.

Another significant feature of the degenerative nervous diseases is that in general their ceaselessly progressive course is uninfluenced by all medical or surgical measures. Dealing with a case of this kind is often, therefore, an anguishing experience for all concerned. Yet symptoms can often be alleviated by wise and skillful management, and the physician's kindly interest may be of great help to a patient even when curative measures cannot be offered.

The bilaterally symmetric distribution of the changes brought about by these diseases has already been mentioned. This feature alone may serve to distinguish conditions in this group from many other diseases of the nervous system. At the same time, it should be pointed out that, in the earliest stages, greater involvement on one side or in one limb is not uncommon. Sooner or later, however, despite the asymmetric beginning, the inherently symmetric nature of the process asserts itself.

A striking feature of a number of disorders of this class is the almost selective involvement of anatomically or physiologically related systems of neurones. This is clearly exemplified in amyotrophic lateral sclerosis, in which the process is almost entirely limited to cortical and spinal motor neurones, and in the cases of progressive ataxia, in which the Purkinje cells of the cerebellum are alone

affected. Many other examples could be cited (e.g., Friedreich's ataxia) in which certain neuronal systems disintegrate, leaving others perfectly intact. An important group of the degenerative diseases has therefore been called "system diseases" ("progressive cerebrospinal system atrophies"—Spatz), and many of these are strongly hereditary. It must be realized, however, that selective involvement of neuronal systems is not exclusively a property of the degenerative group, since several disease processes of known cause have similarly circumscribed effects on the nervous system. Diphtheria toxin, for instance, selectively attacks the myelin of the peripheral nerves, and triorthocresyl phosphate affects particularly the corticospinal tracts in the spinal cord as well as the peripheral nerves. Another example is the special vulnerability of the Purkinje cells of the cerebellum to hyperthermia. On the other hand, several of the conditions included among the degenerative diseases are characterized by pathologic changes that are diffuse and unselective. These exceptions nevertheless do not detract from the importance of affection of particular neuronal systems as a distinguishing feature of many of the diseases under discussion.

Typically, the pathologic process in the nervous system is one of slow involution of nerve cell bodies or their prolongations as nerve fibers, unaccompanied by any intense tissue reaction or cellular response. The cerebrospinal fluid, therefore, shows little if any change—at most a slight elevation of protein, without abnormalities in pressure, cell count, or in other constituents. Moreover, since these diseases invariably result in tissue loss, rather than in new tissue formation (as with neoplasms or inflammation), x-ray visualization of the ventricular system or subarachnoid space shows either no change or an enlargement of these compartments. These negative laboratory findings thus help to distinguish the degenerative disorders from the other large classes of progressive disease of the nervous system—tumor and infections.

CLASSIFICATION. Since etiologic classification is impossible, subdivision of the degenerative diseases into individual syndromes rests on descriptive criteria, based largely on pathologic anatomy but to some extent on clinical aspects as well. In the terms used to designate many of these syndromes, the names of a number of distinguished neurologists and neuropathologists are commemorated. A useful way of keeping in mind the various disease states is to group them according to the outstanding clinical features that may be found in an actual case. The following classification, intended to be of practical help to the physician, is based on such a plan.

CLASSIFICATION OF THE DEGENERATIVE DISEASES
OF THE NERVOUS SYSTEM

I. Syndrome in which progressive dementia is an outstanding feature, in the absence of other prominent neurologic signs
   A. Diffuse cerebral atrophy
      1. Senile dementia
      2. Alzheimer's disease
   B. Circumscribed cerebral atrophy (Pick's disease)

SYNDROMES IN WHICH PROGRESSIVE DEMENTIA ALONE PREDOMINATES

In the disease entities about to be discussed, the clinical picture is dominated by gradual loss of intellectual capacities, i.e., by dementia. Other neurologic abnormalities, except in the terminal stages, are absent or relatively insignificant. (For further discussion of dementia, including its clinical evaluation, Chap. 31 should be consulted.)

Diffuse Cerebral Atrophy: Senile Dementia; Alzheimer's Disease

Some degree of shrinkage in size and weight of the brain, i.e., "atrophy," has been shown to be the inevitable accompaniment of advancing age. In many instances, this is of no clinical significance, and there are many very old people who remain alert and perceptive, with keen intellect, to the end. Nevertheless, severe degrees of diffuse cerebral atrophy are as a general rule associated with some evidence of dementia. When these changes occur in old age (and the definition of when old age begins is largely subjective), it is usual to speak of *senile dementia*. That this is a fairly frequent condition is common experience. Much more infrequent is a pathologically identical progressive dementia with diffuse brain atrophy coming on well before the senile period—a presenile dementia. This condition, classically described in 1906 by Alois Alzheimer, has since become generally known as *Alzheimer's disease*. The distinction between the two conditions is purely clinical: pathologically, they differ only in that the characteristic abnormalities tend to be more severe and widespread in cases beginning at an earlier age than at the senile period.

PATHOLOGY. The brain presents a generally shrunken appearance, with atrophy of the convolutions and symmetric enlargement of the lateral and third ventricles. Frequently, these changes are especially pronounced in the frontal and temporal lobes. Microscopically, there is widespread loss of nerve cells, most apparent in the cerebral cortex, but often present likewise in the basal ganglions, with secondary glial proliferation. In addition, two types of lesion give this disease process its distinctive character: (1) microscopic deposits of amorphous material, scattered throughout the cerebral cortex and most easily seen with silver staining methods—the so-called "senile plaques"; (2) the Alzheimer fibrillary change in nerve cells. This striking abnormality consists of the presence within the cytoplasm, of thick fiberlike strands of silver staining material, often in the form of loops, coils, or tangled masses.

CLINICAL ASPECTS. Although Alzheimer's disease has been described as occurring during every age period, it is most frequently a disease of the later decades of life. A number of well-documented familial cases have been recorded, but there is not sufficient evidence to indicate that this is truly a hereditary disorder. Most of the cases actually seen in practice are sporadic. The onset is insidious and subtle, with changes most noticeable first in memory for recent happenings and in overall judgment of situations. Emotional disturbances such as depression or anxiety states, or odd, unpredictable quirks of behavior, may be salient features in the early stages. Progression is very slow and gradual, and unless the condition is earlier brought to a close by the effects of advanced age, it may smolder on for some 10 to 15 years.

In the milder cases, including those of the senile period, the noteworthy features are those of simple dementia, as described in Chap. 31. More unusual disorders of thought and intellect, including aphasia, apraxia-like disturbances, and abnormalities of space perception, may be seen in the more severe forms such as occur in the presenile group. Not infrequently, the patient walks in a shuffling manner with short steps, and there is a generalized stiffness of the musculature with slowness and awkwardness of all movements; these abnormalities have been attributed to involvement of the basal ganglions. Neurologic examination characteristically discloses no other significant findings. Additional investigative procedures, including the usual blood and cerebrospinal fluid determinations and electroencephalography, do not yield any conclusive or pertinent data. The enlargement of the ventricular system and subarachnoid space resulting from the diffuse brain atrophy can be demonstrated by pneumoencephalography; otherwise, no characteristic roentgenographic findings are seen. During the course of the illness, occasional convulsive seizures may occur, but they do not always accompany the disorder. Terminally, a state of total helplessness is reached, and the patient dies from intercurrent disease. Usually, long before the end, institutional care is necessary.

DIFFERENTIAL DIAGNOSIS. Several disease states for which effective treatment is available may give rise to progressive intellectual deterioration closely resembling what may be seen with the diffuse cerebral atrophy above described. It is imperative that these be looked for. Specific examples include chronic subdural hematoma, chronic "normal pressure" hydrocephalus, frontal meningioma, bromide intoxication, myxedema, pernicious anemia (vitamin B_{12} deficiency), and neurosyphilis. Various other forms of intoxication, infection, metabolic disorder, or neoplasm may have to be considered. Thus, in addition to careful clinical assessment, and whatever laboratory investigations may be indicated to exclude the various possibilities listed above, special procedures such as pneumoencephalography or carotid angiography may be necessary. Vascular disease of the brain is often included in the differential diagnosis, but dementia on the basis of cerebrovascular disorders characteristically progresses in a halting or stepwise fashion, whereas progression in senile dementia or Alzheimer's disease is gradual and steady.

No specific therapy is known. The management should be along the lines of that described in Chap. 31 for the delirious and demented patient.

Pick's Disease (Circumscribed Cerebral Atrophy)

This remarkable form of cerebral disease characterized by the circumscription of the atrophy, a lobar sclerosis, was first described in a series of publications by Arnold Pick in Prague, around the turn of the past century. In the differential diagnosis of dementia in the presenile period, it is often mentioned in the same breath with Alzheimer's disease. It is, however, an extremely rare condition as compared with diffuse cerebral atrophy of the Alzheimer type.

PATHOLOGY. So striking are the gross pathologic changes in the brain that in typical cases the diagnosis can be made at a glance. One sees severe atrophy of the anterior portions of the frontal and temporal lobes, and there is a curiously sharp line of demarcation between the atrophied portions and the remainder of the brain, which appears normal or nearly so. In some cases, the frontal atrophy is more prominent; in others, the temporal lobes are more severely involved; in general, both regions are affected. Characteristically, there likewise are atrophic changes in a number of subcortical structures: caudate nucleus, putamen, thalamus, and substantia nigra, and in the descending frontopontine fiber system. In the diseased regions, there is local destruction of central and convolutional white matter out of proportion to the degree of loss of nerve cell bodies in corresponding areas of the cortex. A noteworthy histologic feature of this condition is the occurrence of numerous swollen "ballooned-out" nerve cells in the atrophic regions, a finding which has been interpreted as an axonal reaction or retrograde cell change secondary to the degenerative process in the periphery. Another frequent cell nerve change is the presence of spherical intracytoplasmic inclusions that stain deeply with silver impregnation methods; the significance of these is unknown.

CLINICAL ASPECTS. There is no satisfactory way of differentiating between Alzheimer's and Pick's disease during life, nor is this of any practical importance. Familial occurrence is on record in a number of instances. Progression is slow and relentless, the average duration of Pick's disease being about 7 years.

DIFFERENTIAL DIAGNOSIS. The considerations noted above with respect to Alzheimer's disease apply to Pick's disease as well.

SYNDROME COMBINING DEMENTIA WITH OTHER NEUROLOGIC SIGNS

Huntington's Chorea (Chronic Progressive Hereditary Chorea)

This condition, which genetically follows the pattern of a mendelian dominant trait, was classically described in 1872 by George Huntington, who, with his father and grandfather, both physicians, observed cases in members of a family living near their home on Long Island. Unmistakable in its typical form, the affliction combines progressive dementia with bizarre involuntary movements and odd postures. Atypical cases have also been recognized (see below), but in general the disorder runs true to form.

PATHOLOGY. The brain has a generally atrophic appearance, especially noticeable in the frontal lobes. Particularly characteristic is severe bilateral atrophy of the caudate nucleus, which becomes flattened and concave instead of projecting as a convex rounded eminence into the anterior horn of the lateral ventricle. The putamen, likewise, is shrunken, although not to the same extent as the caudate nucleus. The globus pallidus is generally involved to some degree, but less severely than the caudate nucleus and putamen. Microscopically, the affected regions show severe nerve cell loss with reactive glial changes.

CLINICAL ASPECTS. This distressing condition generally makes its appearance in early to middle adult years. Its typical hereditary nature has been emphasized, but it is not at all rare for sporadic cases to occur. The involuntary movements (bizarre grimacing, respiratory irregularity, faulty articulation of speech, and irregular, arrhythmic, unpatterned movements of the limbs, imparting to the gait a peculiar dancing quality) tend to be less quick and more athetoid than in Sydenham's chorea (see Chap. 22). A few reported cases which on genealogic and pathologic grounds must be classified with Huntington's chorea have shown progressive rigidity, rather than choreiform movements. As a general rule, dementia runs parallel with the motor disorder. Occasionally it may appear before or after chorea; very rarely it may be lacking altogether. The advance of the disease is slow. There is increasing disability because of both involuntary movements and mental changes, terminated after many years by death from intercurrent infection or, not rarely, by suicide.

DIFFERENTIAL DIAGNOSIS. There is no difficulty in the recognition of typical cases. The relatively late onset, the slowly progressive course, the prominent dementia, and lack of association with rheumatic fever, help to exclude Sydenham's chorea. Hepatolenticular degeneration (Wilson's disease) may display clinical abnormalities resembling those of Huntington's chorea, but the specific changes characteristic of that disorder, including liver disease, corneal Kayser-Fleischer rings, and typical biochemical abnormalities (increased copper excretion, aminoaciduria), are absent in Huntington's chorea. Sporadic cases of choreiform movements beginning in middle or late life may present a difficult problem in exact diagnosis. The occasional cases of violent choreiform movements produced by vascular lesions, classically in the subthalamic region, are characterized by sudden onset, unilateral distribution (hemiballismus), and a tendency to improve after a period of initial severity. Virus encephalitis may occasionally be associated with choreiform movements; acute development, fever, and pleocytosis in the cerebrospinal fluid help in recognizing such cases. Phenothiazine drugs may induce generalized chorea, but without dementia. Although it occurs rarely, self-limited chorea may appear in older persons without identifiable cause.

TREATMENT. It is impossible to halt the progress of this disease by any of the suggested forms of treatment. Chlorpromazine has been proposed as a means of controlling the chorea but has not been successful in the authors' hands.

Cerebrocerebellar Degeneration

The progressive cerebellar degenerations of late life, and some cases of spinocerebellar degeneration, may be accompanied by significant dementia, the pathologic basis for which is not always easily demonstrated. These disorders are dealt with more fully below in the section devoted to conditions manifested by ataxia.

Creutzfeldt-Jakob Disease (Subacute Spongiform Encephalopathy)

H. G. Creutzfeldt (1920) and A. M. Jakob (1921, 1923) described a diffuse disorder of the central nervous system of adults that was characterized clinically by progressive dementia, spasticity or rigidity, and ataxia and pathologically by neuronal degeneration in the cerebral cortex, basal ganglia, and spinal cord. These reports have subsequently given rise to the concept that there is a clinicopathological entity combining dementia with prominent motor impairment (including progressive weakness with muscular atrophy in some instances) and very widespread neuropathological changes to which the name *Creutzfeldt-Jakob* (or *Jakob-Creutzfeldt*) *disease* is applicable. This term is now firmly established in the nomenclature of neurologic diseases; its precise definition and limitations, however, remain uncertain.

Meanwhile, there has been increasing awareness of the existence of another distinctive cerebral disease of rapid evolution, in which profound dementia is combined with ataxia and diffuse myoclonic jerks. The major neuropathologic changes in this disorder are in the cerebral and cerebellar cortex; the outstanding features of the lesions are widespread neuronal loss and gliosis accompanied by a striking vacuolation or spongy state of the affected regions. These changes, both clinical and pathologic, occur so regularly and with such remarkable uniformity from case to case that there can be no doubt that they form a distinct nosologic entity. This disease state has come in recent years to be designated as "subacute spongiform encephalopathy." At the same time, because of some features in common with what Creutzfeldt and Jakob had earlier described, it has frequently been referred to as Creutzfeldt-Jakob disease. It seems to us hardly likely, however, that subacute spongiform encephalopathy and the somewhat ill-defined syndrome of Creutzfeldt and Jakob, previously referred to, can truly be the same disease. Pending further knowledge, at any rate, we believe that they should be kept distinct from one another, or at least that when "Creutzfeldt-Jakob disease" is spoken of, it should be clearly stated whether subacute spongiform encephalopathy is meant, or the slower progressive dementia with signs of pyramidal and extrapyramidal dysfunction. Preciseness in definition of these states is of greater importance now than before, because recent evidence suggests that subacute spongiform encephalopathy may be due to a transmissible agent (Gibbs et al., 1968).

PATHOLOGY. In subacute spongiform encephalopathy, as already indicated, the disease affects principally the cerebral and cerebellar cortex, generally in a diffuse fashion, although in some cases the occipitoparietal regions are almost exclusively involved, as in those described by Heidenhain (1929). The degeneration and disappearance of nerve cells is associated with extensive astroglial proliferation; ultrastructural studies have shown that the microscopic vacuoles which give the tissue its typically spongy appearance are located within the cytoplasmic processes of glial cells. Despite the possibility referred to above that the disease may be the result of an infection, the lesions show no evidence of an inflammatory reaction.

In the cases that conform to what Creutzfeldt and Jakob described, the disease process in the cerebral cortex is more focal than in spongiform encephalopathy, the Rolandic regions being chiefly affected, and there is more extensive involvement of the basal ganglia. Furthermore, the spinal cord typically shows some loss of anterior horn cells and degeneration of the corticospinal tracts in a manner reminiscent of amyotrophic lateral sclerosis, a condition that is discussed in a later section of this chapter.

CLINICAL ASPECTS. Subacute spongiform encephalopathy is in most cases a disease of late middle age, although it can occur in young adults and very possibly in children as well.

In the early stages, a great variety of clinical manifestations may be seen, but those most frequently observed are changes in behavior, emotional responses, memory, and reasoning, together with abnormalities of vision such as peculiar distortions of the appearance of objects or actual impairment of visual acuity. The disease characteristically progresses with great rapidity, so that obvious deterioration may be seen from week to week. Sooner or later, in all cases, sudden myoclonic contractions of various muscle groups appear, perhaps unilaterally at first, but later becoming generalized. These generally are brought on by sudden sensory stimuli of all sorts, but they occur spontaneously as well, particularly in the late stages. Sudden jerks of individual fingers are typical. Ataxia and dysarthria are likewise prominent. Hallucinations, confusion, delusional ideas, and other evidences of delirium are frequently seen as the disease progresses. These changes gradually give way to stupor and coma, but the myoclonic contractions may continue to the end. In all cases, the electroencephalogram shows distinctive abnormalities, especially when the disease is fully developed. The total course of the illness is generally less than a year from onset; it may be confined to a few weeks or months. The outcome is invariably fatal, with death from intercurrent infection. Investigations of blood and cerebrospinal fluid consistently show no significant findings.

When the cases of subacute spongiform encephalopathy are set apart as a distinct group, the remaining cases that have been classified as Creutzfeldt-Jakob disease have as their outstanding features progressive dementia and spastic weakness of the limbs coming on in late middle age and progressing to death within a year or two. Other neurologic abnormalities that have been described include generalized rigidity, inexpressiveness ("masking") of the face, ataxia, convulsions, and muscular atrophy. Cases of this kind are the ones to which *Creutzfeldt-Jakob disease* is most applicable, if this name is to be used at all. On the whole, though, it would be preferable if complex or unclassifiable cases of diffuse degenerative disease of the nervous system were given descriptive names, rather than being grouped under what gives the impression of being a specific diagnostic

term. At any rate, if the eponym is to be retained, those using it should make entirely clear what syndrome they are applying it to.

DIFFERENTIAL DIAGNOSIS. In the earliest stages, the mental changes may be misinterpreted as an atypical or unusually intense emotional reaction to environmental factors or as one of the major psychoses. Intoxication, as with bromides or other central nervous system depressants, or infection, such as neurosyphilis, may have to be considered, but none of these is likely to produce so dramatic a clinical picture. In its fully developed form, the only other disease process that resembles it is subacute sclerosing panencephalitis (SSPE) (see Chap. 361), but this is chiefly a disease of children or young adults, rather than middle age or the presenile period. The cerebrospinal fluid regularly shows elevation of gamma-globulin (IgG) in SSPE, however, whereas it is normal in subacute spongiform encephalopathy. Cerebral lipidosis in children or young adults (see below) can result in a similar combination of myoclonus and dementia, but in such cases there are retinal changes that do not occur in any of the varieties of Creutzfeldt-Jakob disease.

No treatment is known.

Lipidoses of the Nervous System

The conditions to be considered here differ from other degenerative disorders in that the underlying biochemical abnormality is better defined. They are characterized by a more or less widespread derangement of lipid metabolism, which results in abnormal accumulations of lipids in the cytoplasm of cells of the nervous system and often of other organs as well. (For information relating to the problem of the lipidoses in general, Chaps. 113 and 365 should be consulted.) This process leads to abnormal function and, eventually, to death of the affected nerve cells. There is ample evidence for hereditary transmission of these disorders, the basis for which must consist of genetically determined abnormalities of enzyme systems concerned with intracellular lipid metabolism. This group of diseases is currently the subject of much intensive biochemical and ultrastructural investigation, which has contributed significantly to identifying the lipids involved and in more precise description of the metabolic derangement, although much has yet to be learned regarding the enzymopathies themselves.

SPECIAL CLINICAL TYPES. The forms of lipidoses which affect the nervous system exclusively are often classified together as *amaurotic family idiocy*. This term emphasizes the important hereditary aspect, but it is not entirely satisfactory, since it can be correctly applied only to cases occurring in infancy. In the older child and adult, blindness (amaurosis) may never develop, and "idiocy," strictly speaking, implies defective intelligence existing from earliest infancy. Another name frequently given to this group of lipidoses is *cerebromacular degeneration*, but it is accurate only for infantile cases and for patients with the combination of cerebral lesions and degeneration of the macular part of the retina.

Within the group of diseases designated as amaurotic family idiocy, the following varieties are generally distinguished.

Tay-Sachs Disease. This is the classic form of amaurotic family idiocy occurring in infants, almost exclusively in Jewish families. It is characterized by extremely widespread neuronal involvement (see Chap. 113 for further details).

Late Infantile Form (Jansky-Bielschowsky). This variety, which is rare, begins at a somewhat later age than Tay-Sachs disease (age three to four) and has a more chronic course. It is biochemically and pathologically (by electron microscopy) distinguishable from both Tay-Sachs disease and juvenile amaurotic idiocy, but has features in common with both.

Juvenile Form (Spielmeyer-Vogt-Batten). This form of lipidosis is not confined to patients of Jewish parentage. Clinically, the onset is between the ages of five to ten, and the course is relatively prolonged, with death at the time of adolescence or early adulthood. The retinal lesions typically take the form of pigmentary degeneration (retinitis pigmentosa). The intraneuronal accumulations differ considerably from those encountered in infantile amaurotic idiocy of Tay-Sachs and Jansky-Bielschowsky types both under light and electron microscopy, although, in common with these disorders, they have the histochemical properties of a glycolipid. Their chemical composition has not as yet been successfully determined.

Adult Form (Kuf's). This is an extremely rare disorder with a very prolonged course. In all essential respects, it is identical to the juvenile form, except that retinal lesions may be completely absent.

GENERALIZED LIPIDOSES WITH CNS INVOLVEMENT. In addition to the group of lipidoses exclusively affecting the nervous system, there are a number of more generalized disorders of lipid metabolism in which the nervous system participates.

Generalized Gangliosidosis. Two rare forms of generalized lipidosis in infants have lately been recognized, both of them characterized by abnormal accumulations of gangliosides in many organs in addition to the nervous system. One of them closely resembles Tay-Sachs disease in that the substance that accumulates abnormally is the same monoganglioside (GM2 in the Svennerholm classification) that is present in excess in the neurones in Tay-Sachs disease. This is generally referred to as *Tay-Sachs disease with visceral involvement.* The other, termed *generalized gangliosidosis,* is characterized by excessive amounts of GM1 ganglioside.

Niemann-Pick Disease. This disease has already been discussed in Chap. 113. The typical accumulation of large amounts of lipid in macrophages (reticuloendothelial cells) in many organs, including particularly the liver and spleen, is accompanied by lipidosis of the nervous system, similar to that occurring in the various forms of amaurotic family idiocy. The lipid involved here is mainly sphingomyelin.

Hunter-Hurler Syndrome (Gargoylism). This disorder, often called gargoylism because of the bizarre facial appearance of patients afflicted with the disease, belongs to the group of mucopolysaccharidoses, in which there are abnormalities of connective tissue in many organs. In the Hunter-Hurler variety, mental retardation is a prominent clinical feature, and there are striking intraneuronal accumulations of lipid (ganglioside) resembling those found in amaurotic family idiocy.

For further information Chap. 399 should be consulted.

Gaucher's Disease. This generalized metabolic disorder of childhood, already described in Chap. 113, resembles Niemann-Pick disease in many respects, inasmuch as it likewise is characterized by extensive lipid accumulations in various organs, especially the spleen, liver, and bone marrow. The nervous system, however, is much less regularly affected; it may be entirely normal in cases occurring in late childhood or adult life, although it usually is involved in infants.

CLINICAL ASPECTS. The majority of cases of lipidosis occur in infancy and childhood, after a period of normal development. Motor regression, disinterest, and loss of visual capacity are the leading features and are well covered by the term amaurotic family idiocy. At certain phases the limbs become enfeebled with exaggerated reflexes. The fundal change "cherry-red spots" at maculae, surrounded by a gray halo, gives the diagnosis. Its absence suggests "spongy degeneration" in which progressive blindness is combined with psychomotor regression (see below); excessive startle to sound (auditory myoclonus) is another characteristic finding. Later the child becomes decerebrate and dies in 2 to 3 yrs. In patients with onset later in life cerebellar ataxia, epilepsy, and myoclonic dementia give the diagnosis especially when associated with atypical retinitis pigmentosa. In the late childhood and adult forms choreoathetosis and dementia may be conjoined and retinae are normal. (See Chaps. 365 and 399 for differential diagnosis.)

Leukodystrophy (Degenerative Diffuse Cerebral Sclerosis)

This rare group of conditions, in which familial incidence has frequently been observed, is characterized by a widespread disintegration of white matter in association with a remarkable sparing of the nerve cell bodies in the gray matter. There is thus a superficial resemblance to Schilder's disease ("encephalitis periaxialis diffusa"), which is best considered as an unusual variant of multiple sclerosis; in fact, the leukodystrophies have frequently been grouped together as *familial Schilder's disease.* The best evidence at present indicates, however, that the leukodystrophies represent disorders of the metabolism of the myelin sheath lipids, and thus are related to the neuronal lipidoses previously discussed. The leukodystrophies can be further classified on the basis of pathologic and biochemical differences into a number of subtypes, some of which are considered below.

PATHOLOGY. The distinguishing feature is diffuse, symmetric breakdown of the white matter of the cerebral hemispheres, in which, as a rule, axones suffer damage to approximately the same degree as the myelin sheaths. Also characteristic is the presence, within the devastated regions, of lipid breakdown products of myelin which show distinct histochemical differences from the familiar lipid products met within all the other disease processes destroying myelin, such as infarction, traumatic necrosis, secondary fiber tract degeneration, demyelinative lesions in multiple sclerosis or Schilder's disease, and so on. The relative intactness of the nerve cell bodies forms a striking contrast to the extensive white matter lesions.

VARIETIES OF LEUKODYSTROPHY

Metachromatic Leukodystrophy. This is now known to be a genetically determined metabolic disorder of sphingolipid metabolism in which cerebroside sulfate (sulfatide) accumulates excessively in many organs, especially brain and kidneys, because of deficient activity of a sulfuric acid esterase, perhaps arylsulfatase A. Since neutral cerebrosides and sulfatides are among the chief lipid components of myelin, all myelin-containing parts of the nervous system, both central and peripheral, are affected in this disease. The metabolic abnormality is well tolerated by other organs, as far as their functional integrity is concerned, but in the nervous system the excessive accumulation of sulfatides leads to disintegration of myelin at all levels. Sulfatides have the property of altering the absorption spectrum of dyes such as toluidine blue and cresyl violet, so that in their presence the color obtained is purple or red or even brown instead of the expected blue or violet—a phenomenon known as *metachromasia*. The name *metachromatic leukodystrophy* comes from the fact that the diseased cerebral white matter stains intensely metachromatically because of the large amounts of phagocytosed sulfatide that accompany the breakdown of the myelin. Metachromatic material indicative of sulfatide can also be readily demonstrated postmortem in kidney tubule cells, Kupffer cells of the liver, and in other organs, unaccompanied by any evidence of tissue damage. In the gallbladder the sulfatide deposits apparently do lead to destructive tissue changes, with the result that nonfunctioning of the gallbladder on radiographic examination is one of the manifestations of the disease.

The disease is mostly seen in infants and young children, but it occasionally occurs in adults, including a few of fairly advanced age.

Krabbe's Form of Leukodystrophy. In this variety, first described by Knud Krabbe in 1916 as a familial disorder of infants, the lipid breakdown products also are atypical as compared with those occurring in most pathologic processes which destroy myelin. They differ histochemically from the metachromatic material just described in several ways, including absence of metachromasia. Typical of this disorder is the presence of unusual multinucleated phagocytic cells resembling foreign-body giant cells, within which the lipid breakdown products are contained; these are the so-called "globoid cells." In this disease, the biochemical abnormality is less well defined than in metachromatic leukodystrophy, although the diseased white matter contains a relative increase of galactocerebrosides, which are the chief component of the phagocytosed material in the globoid cells.

Spongy Degeneration of the Nervous System (Van Boegaert-Bertrand; Canavan). This rare inherited disease of infants is generally classified with the leukodystrophies because the cerebral white matter is the chief site of pathologic changes. Characteristic of the disease is a fine-meshed spongy cavitation of the tissue associated with breakdown of myelin in some regions and, probably, failure of myelination in others. This spongy state is apparently the result of a large increase of water, some of which is within the myelin sheaths, producing their disruption. The pathologic findings suggest failure of regulation of intracellular fluid balance, perhaps mainly affecting glial cells, but the biochemical and enzymatic defects that underlie this disease have not yet been identified.

Late-life Leukodystrophy. In recent years, a few cases have been described of a very chronic form of white matter degeneration occurring in the presenile period, in which the atypical lipid products most closely resemble the lipofuscins, the "wear and tear" lipid pigment of advancing age. This is an extremely rare condition, about which very little so far is known.

Pelizaeus-Merzbacher Disease. In this condition, which is characterized clinically by a pronounced familial tendency and a very chronic course, the white matter lesions are patchy and irregular, rather than evenly distributed as in the other forms of leukodystrophy. Furthermore, there is relative sparing of axones. Another distinguishing feature of this disorder is that the breakdown products of the myelin, although very sparse (as would be expected from the prolonged course), are of the usual sort regularly seen with myelin destruction, rather than being atypical as in metachromatic leukodystrophy. What has been called *sudanophilic leukodystrophy* may well be identical with Pelizaeus-Merzbacher disease. The underlying basis for the lesions is still wholly unknown.

CLINICAL ASPECTS. The symptoms and signs in all the forms of leukodystrophy are mainly those of a progressive dementia, often associated in the early stages with weakness and unsteadiness of gait. Likewise prominent are spasticity and exaggeration of tendon reflexes, referable to the destructive lesions in the corticospinal motor system. Generalized convulsive seizures may occur but are infrequent. In metachromatic leukodystrophy there is at first spastic weakness of limbs, but because of later involvement of the peripheral nervous system, muscle-stretch reflexes are lost. As opposed to the neuronal lipidoses and other diseases principally affecting the nerve cell bodies in the gray matter, paralysis and other functional deficits are generally more prominent in the leukodystrophies than abnormal movements or seizure-like activity. On the whole, though, clinical phenomena do not serve to differentiate leukodystrophy clearly from other forms of diffuse progressive cerebral disease. As the biochemical abnormalities underlying the leukodystrophies become better understood, however, positive recognition of these disorders during life will be possible. This has already occurred with metachromatic leukodystrophy in that the metabolic disorder results in excretion of abnormal amounts of sulfatide which can be recognized in the urine by a reliable biochemical test. Biopsy of a peripheral nerve has often been used to establish the diagnosis of this disease, since the characteristic metachromatic material is easily demonstrable thereby even in the early stages, but recent studies have shown that the operative procedure of even so simple a biopsy as this can now be circumvented because of the possibility of demonstrating sulfatide excess in circulating leukocytes.

In the other varieties of leukodystrophy, there are as yet no reliable biochemical tests whereby the diagnosis can be made during life. The disease can generally be identified in a brain biopsy, but this is a procedure which is justifiable only under very rare circumstances—such as genetic counseling, or a carefully thought out research project in which a specimen of fresh tissue might lead to some new insight with an otherwise hopeless disease.

DIFFERENTIAL DIAGNOSIS. Familial occurrence, signs referable to a disorder of long projection and associative fiber systems, and relative lack of convulsive manifestations may suggest the diagnosis during life. Otherwise, the identification of these conditions requires pathologic examination, except insofar as it may be possible to identify some of these diseases by appropriate biochemical tests.

Progressive Familial Myoclonic Epilepsy (Unverricht-Lundborg-Lafora Disease)

This rare disorder forms a distinct clinicopathologic syndrome characterized by recessive heredity. Typically, it appears in adolescence or early adult life, beginning with generalized convulsive seizures, which are followed after an interval of years by myoclonic jerks of increasing frequency and severity and progressive dementia, with death within 5–10 yrs. The pathologic features suggest a disorder of nerve cell metabolism, the nature of which remains unidentified.

PATHOLOGY. In many of the cases on record, distinctive intracytoplasmic inclusion bodies within nerve cells may be found at all levels in the central nervous system, although they are most frequent in the cerebral cortex, dentate nucleus of the cerebellum, substantia nigra, and thalamus. These bodies, which have the histochemical properties of a complex carbohydrate, were initially described by Gonzalo Lafora (1911) and are generally known as Lafora bodies. Material with similar staining properties has also been found in heart-muscle fibers and in liver cells in several cases.

CLINICAL ASPECTS. The onset in most cases is at about the time of puberty. The convulsive seizures, with which the disorder usually begins, are in no way distinctive. The myoclonic jerks are sudden, asymmetric or symmetric brief contractions of muscle groups of the limbs, face, and trunk, occurring arrhythmically and unpredictably, usually with sufficient force to displace the parts affected. They characteristically are provoked by all sorts of stimuli, but occur spontaneously as well. The sudden contractions may interfere seriously with willed movements, or may cause the patient to fall abruptly.

The disorder progresses gradually, running a course over several years, with terminal stages characterized by profound dementia and total helplessness. Treatment with anticonvulsant medication may relieve the generalized convulsive seizures and reduce the frequency of the myoclonic jerks, but has no effect on the dementia.

DIFFERENTIAL DIAGNOSIS. Other forms of progressive familial dementia with myoclonus may have to be considered. These are discussed above in the descriptions of Jakob-Creutzfeldt disease and the lipidoses. There is in addition a more benign form of myoclonic epilepsy which begins in childhood or adolescence and permits survival to middle age or longer. There are no distinctive pathologic changes—only nonspecific degenerative lesions. In Unverricht myoclonic epilepsy, convulsive seizures are more prominent than in the other disorders mentioned. The diagnosis of these different forms of myoclonus is based on clinical picture and course of illness. All forms of treament have hitherto been ineffective.

Hallervorden-Spatz Disease

This unusual disorder, often familial, is associated with a rather variable clinical picture in which abnormalities of posture and muscle tone, involuntary movements, and progressive dementia predominate. Pathologically, there are characteristic abnormalities in the basal ganglions, suggesting a localized disorder of metabolism. The features of the condition were classically described in an affected family by Hallervorden and Spatz (1922).

PATHOLOGY. Distinctive for this condition is the accumulation of large amounts of pigmented material in the globus pallidus and zona reticulata of the substantia nigra, resulting in grossly visible brownish discoloration of these regions. Microscopically, there are irregular pigmented, ferruginous concretions and granules of varying brownish or greenish hues, depending on the stains used. There is no systemic disorder of iron metabolism. Nerve cell loss occurs in these regions and likewise to some extent in the cerebral cortex, although it generally is not so severe as in other forms of degenerative brain disease and is overshadowed by the pigmentary disorder in the basal ganglions. Another feature of the disease is focal swelling of axons in a scattered distribution throughout the brain, including regions which otherwise appear to be normal.

CLINICAL ASPECTS. The disorder typically makes its appearance in childhood or adolescence, with abnormalities in muscle tone and movements such as rigidity and choreoathetosis. Abnormal postures of the trunk characteristic of torsion spasm (dystonia) may be seen. Cerebellar ataxia and myoclonus are also present in some instances; or the clinical picture may be reminiscent of parkinsonism. Speech becomes indistinct, and there is progressive intellectual impairment. Eventually, the involuntary movements give way to increasing generalized rigidity, and death comes as a rule about 10 years after onset.

DIFFERENTIAL DIAGNOSIS. No feature of the clinical picture serves to distinguish this particular disorder from other conditions showing dementia with extrapyramidal motor abnormalities. Hepatolenticular degeneration must be excluded by appropriate laboratory tests. The clearly progressive course sets this condition apart from clinically similar abnormalities resulting from accidents or illnesses at birth or in the neonatal period. There is at present no effective treatment for the disease. A recent (unpublished) attempt at using a chelating agent (deferoxamine mesylate) in one case led to no definite benefit.

Familial Hepatolenticular Degeneration (Wilson's Disease)

This condition is discussed in Chap. 110.

Acquired Hepatocerebral Degeneration

This condition is discussed in Chap. 363.

EXTRAPYRAMIDAL SYNDROMES OF ABNORMAL POSTURES OR INVOLUNTARY MOVEMENTS

Paralysis Agitans (Parkinson's Disease)

This by no means rare condition was named and classically described by James Parkinson in 1817. His remarkably complete account gives this definition

Involuntary tremulous motion, with lessened muscular power, in parts not in action and even when supported; with a propensity to bend the trunk forward, and to pass from a walking to a running pace, the senses and intellects being uninjured.

Typically, paralysis agitans is a disorder of middle or late life, with very gradual progression and a prolonged course. Although it has been seen to occur in families (the estimated familial incidence is 5 percent), it usually is sporadic. It is well recognized, however, that the epidemic encephalitis of von Economo, which occurred in a worldwide distribution in the years following World War I, was followed by a syndrome clinically indistinguishable from paralysis agitans. It is usual in such instances to speak of postencephalitic parkinsonism, whereas the term Parkinson's disease should be reserved for true paralysis agitans of unknown cause. Paralysis agitans bears no consistent relationship to any known disease process such as arteriosclerosis, trauma, or intoxication, although such conditions have often been invoked as etiologically significant and may at times produce somewhat similar clinical manifestations.

PATHOLOGY. Despite the general medical familiarity with the condition and an extensive literature on the subject, it cannot be said that the pathologic changes of paralysis agitans are yet fully understood. The only regularly observed changes have been in the aggregates of melanin-containing nerve cells in the brainstem (substantia nigra, locus caeruleus, dorsal motor nucleus of the vagus), where varying degrees of nerve cell loss with reactive gliosis, most pronounced in the substantia nigra, along with distinctive eosinophilic intracytoplasmic inclusions (Lewy bodies, after their description by F. H. Lewy in 1913) are a consistent finding. Changes have also been described in other structures of the basal ganglions, but they are not clearly different in nature or degree from what may be encountered in other patients of similar age without extrapyramidal motor disorders. The histopathological evidence therefore suggests that paralysis agitans can be considered as belonging with the system diseases, the affected system being that of the pigmented nuclei of the brainstem. Significantly, extensive lesions in these same pigmented nuclei characterize the pathologic findings in postencephalitic parkinsonism in which Lewy bodies typically are absent. Recent biochemical studies, which show a decrease of dopamine in the caudate nucleus and putamen—an alteration consistently found on experimental ablation of the substantia nigra—lend further support to the idea that Parkinson's disease is indeed a disorder of a particular neuronal system.

CLINICAL ASPECTS. In its fully developed form, this disorder cannot be mistaken for any other. The stooped posture, the stiffness and slowness of movement, the rigidity of facial expression, and the rhythmic tremor of the limbs which subsides on active willed movement or complete relaxation are familiar to every clinician. Although symmetric in the later stages, the disorder typically begins asymmetrically, e.g., as a slight tremor of the fingers of one hand or in one leg. Also typical is more or less general stiffness of the musculature so that even where tremor is inapparent, the disease may betray itself by a somewhat staring and immobile facial expression, a monotonous voice, a general slowness of all motor activity, and a curious lack of the little spontaneous movements of postural change that are so characteristic of the normal individual. When tremor is minimal, patients often are able to alleviate it by resting their hands on a table or the arms of a chair or by keeping them in their pockets. The tremor, although fluctuating from moment to moment in amplitude, characterizes the later course. The tremor is generally most pronounced in the hands but may involve also the legs (and thus secondarily the trunk), lips, tongue, and neck muscles, and is easily seen in the eyelids when they are lightly closed. There is no total paralysis, although general enfeeblement of voluntary movement is characteristic of the fully developed disorder. Together with the stooped attitude, there is the typical "festinating" gait, whereby the patient, prevented by the abnormality of postural tone from making the appropriate reflex adjustments required for effective walking, progresses with quick shuffling steps at an accelerating pace as if to catch up with his center of gravity. Clinical examination of the tendon and plantar reflexes discloses no abnormalities. There are no sensory changes, although deep aching in joints and muscles is common. Eventually, the patient may become so incapacitated by rigidity and tremor as to be helpless in caring for himself. It has often been observed, however, that even severely disabled patients may under great emotional stress perform complex motor acts quickly and efficiently in a manner that ordinarily would be impossible for them. Thus, a patient may be able to jump up and run out of a burning building on hearing the call of "Fire"—only to be helpless as before once the crisis is past. Although the temporary alleviation under extreme provocation can never be long maintained, it is nevertheless true that the severity of the symptoms is considerably influenced by emotional factors, being aggravated by anxiety, tension, and unhappiness, and minimal when the patient is in a contented frame of mind. Despite the inherently progressive nature of the condition, much can be achieved with good medical management, and patients may continue for years to live effective, happy lives in spite of this affliction. Intellectual deterioration is not a consistent feature of paralysis agitans, but it must be conceded that in very advanced stages of the condition dementia may be encountered.

DIFFERENTIAL DIAGNOSIS. In typical cases, this is not difficult. The extrapyramidal syndromes associated with most diseases of known cause or established nature such as cerebral vascular disease, cerebral hypoxia (including carbon monoxide asphyxia), or metallic poisoning differ from paralysis agitans in a number of respects, such as atypical behavior or tremor, presence of signs of pyramidal tract deficit, or early onset of dementia. The differentiation from postencephalitic parkinsonism may be impossible; a clear history of an attack of epidemic encephalitis (prolonged somnolence, disturbance of consciousness, diplopia) and relatively early age of onset of the disorder and the presence of tics, localized spasms, and oculogyric crises may be the only clues to this diagnosis. In recent years, a neurologic disorder strikingly similar to Parkinson's disease has been seen following the prolonged administration of large amounts of reserpine and phenothiazine drugs, which subsides on withdrawal of the offending drug—a matter of considerable theoretic and practical importance. Parkinsonism is rarely, if ever, produced by cerebral neoplasms.

TREATMENT. Although there is no treatment that is known to halt or reverse the neuronal degeneration that presumably underlies Parkinson's disease, methods are now available which can bring about a considerable degree of relief from symptoms in many patients. An important part of any therapeutic program is the maintenance of optimum general health and neuromuscular efficiency by planned programs of exercise, activity, and rest; expert physical therapy may be of great help in achieving these ends. In addition, the patient often needs much emotional support in meeting the stress of the illness, in comprehending its nature, and in carrying on courageously in spite of it. Along with these general supportive measures, which are applicable to many chronic illnesses, patients generally require a carefully thought out program of treatment specifically aimed at counteracting the pathophysiologic disorder that produces their disabilities. This treatment can be medical (with drugs) or surgical, or a combination of both. Experience over many years has shown that the drugs that are most

beneficial in the symptomatic treatment of Parkinson's disease are anticholinergic agents related to atropine. Several synthetic preparations of this kind are now available, including trihexyphenidyl (Artane), cycrimine (Pagitane), procyclidine (Kemadrin), biperiden (Akineton), and benztropine methanesulfonate (Cogentine), among others. Whereas these drugs differ little from one another in their overall effectiveness in large groups of patients, an individual patient may respond better to one of them than to another, and occasionally after a patient has received one of these medications for a prolonged period, change to another one may be attended by some additional improvement—perhaps only from the psychologic effect of a change in regimen. In order to obtain maximum benefit from the use of these drugs, they should be given in gradually increasing dosage to the point where toxic side effects begin to appear. These side effects are those expected from anticholinergic agents: dryness of the mouth (which can be beneficial when drooling of saliva is a problem), blurring of vision from pupillary mydriasis (for which corrective spectacle lenses may be indicated), constipation, and sometimes urinary retention (especially with prostatism). Mental slowing, confusional states, hallucinations, and impairment of memory, especially in patients with already impaired mental functioning, can occur as troublesome toxic effects of these drugs and may sharply limit their usefulness under these circumstances. The optimum dosage level for a patient is when the greatest relief from tremor and rigidity is achieved within the limits of tolerable side effects. This may occur with trihexyphenidyl, for example, within a range of 6 to 20 mg daily in divided doses, or in a sustained-release capsule. With any of these drugs, a dosage level is reached when a further increase serves only to precipitate severe toxic effects with no further alleviation of the symptoms of the disease. The dose must then, of course, be reduced. It is possible, nevertheless, once maximum benefit from one of the anticholinergic agents has been achieved, to then add one of the antihistaminic drugs such as diphenhydramine (Benadryl) or phenindamine (Thephorin). These drugs have some ameliorating effect on the motor derangement, but it is insufficient for them to be used as the primary therapeutic agent. However, an antihistamine in combination with an anticholinergic drug can give better results in many patients than either one alone. Drowsiness is the chief side effect of the antihistamines, and this in turn can be combated with one of the analeptics such as dextroamphetamine (Dexedrine). From what has been said, it is clear that the drugs to be used, and how much, vary from patient to patient: what is inadequate for one is too much for another. The patients who can be expected to benefit the most from treatment with classic anti-Parkinson drugs are those with relatively mild disease in whom relief from the symptoms is sufficient to warrant tolerance of some side effects. In those more severely affected, the relief is partial at best, and as the disease advances, eventually a degree of incapacity is reached which is not significantly responsive to even the most carefully planned regimen of medications. Even so, there is no doubt that for a significant period the patient's effectiveness and well-being can be considerably enhanced by the wise use of these drugs. An important note of warning must be provided at this point: Under no circumstances should a medication program with anticholinergic agents be stopped suddenly. If this happens, the patient is likely to become totally immobilized and incapacitated by an abrupt and severe increase of tremor and rigidity.

To the list of anti-Parkinson drugs must now be added L-dihydroxyphenylalamine (L-dopa). The theoretical basis for the use of this compound is the decrease of catecholamines in extrapyramidal motor centers, already referred to, that has been found to be characteristic of Parkinson's disease. At the present moment, L-dopa is still on experimental trial, but current reports indicate that its effects in a majority of patients, even those with far-advanced stages of the disease, are far better than anything that has ever been obtained by other drugs. This new agent is not without serious toxic effects, so that it undoubtedly will not be universally applicable, but it surely will turn out to be a powerful force in the struggle against the disease. At present the most efficacious program of medical therapy consists of 3 to 6 gms of L-dopa in six divided doses plus 2–4 mg of Artane and 10 to 20 mg of ethopropazine (Parsidol) thrice daily.

Another important advance in the attempt to relieve the symptoms of Parkinson's disease has been the recent development of stereotoxic surgery. This involves the placement of precisely localized focal lesions in the central nuclei of the brain, either in the globus pallidus or ventrolateral thalamus, contralateral to the side of the body chiefly affected. The best results occur in patients who are relatively young and in good general health with sound mentality, in whom tremor or rigidity are the predominant symptoms, rather than akinesia, which is not relieved by any surgical procedure. Opinions among neurosurgeons still differ as to the best way of making the lesion, and studies are still in progress as to what its ideal location should be. Needless to say, when a patient is being referred for surgical treatment, a neurosurgeon with special competence in these complex techniques should be selected. The most successful surgical results of all are obtained in patients in whom the tremor and rigidity are mainly unilateral; under these circumstances the motor abnormalities can be reversed almost to the extent of achieving a normal state. Involvement of both sides of the body is not necessarily a contraindication to operation; to liberate the limbs on one side from tremor or rigidity may enable the patient to carry out many activities effectively that would otherwise be denied to him. Bilateral operations (first on one side and then on the other) have been extremely successful in some patients, but the risks of physical or mental crippling as a result of the surgical procedures are considerably greater than with the unilateral operation. As already indicated, akinesia does not respond to surgical measures. This is true of some of the other distressing aspects of Parkinson's disease, such as weakness of the voice and the abnormalities of posture and gait

that are independent of rigidity as such. Successful surgical treatment does not halt the advance of the disease itself, but it does reverse some of the symptoms to the extent of bringing the patient back to a more nearly normal level of motor performance, so that he obtains some 5 years more or less of reprieve from its effects. Eventually, however, the akinetic aspects of the disease assert themselves, finally bringing about severe incapacity if the patient lives long enough. In the meantime, medical treatment, and, in a few carefully selected cases, reoperation, can defer as long as possible this stage of total invalidism.

Dystonia Musculorum Deformans (Torsion Spasm)

This is a clinical term, denoting a state characterized by slow, nonrhythmic, involuntary movements which produce abnormal, at times bizarre, postures of the trunk and limbs. With passage of time, these postures tend to become more or less fixed. Underlying the clinical disorder may be any of several pathologic conditions, such as the residual lesions of epidemic encephalitis, the pigmented deposits of Hallervorden-Spatz disease (described above), hepatolenticular degeneration (Wilson's disease), or the scars of cerebral birth injury in the broad sense, or kernicterus. In addition, there are a few rare cases with relatively early onset and progressive course and, in some instances, familial occurrence.

PATHOLOGY. Until lately, very few cases of dystonia musculorum deformans not due to one of the definable disease processes indicated above had been adequately studied neuropathologically. Reported results from the few that had been examined led to uncertainty as to what the pathologic-anatomic basis of the clinical state might be, although it was generally assumed that the basal ganglia were diseased. A careful study by Zeman and Dyken in 1967, which included comparison of the findings in patients with the disease with control material, demonstrated that there is, in fact, no definable neuronal or other histologically demonstrable disease process to which the clinical abnormalities can reasonably be attributed. These negative findings, which are perhaps surprising, must not be interpreted as indicating that there is "no disease" in the brain, but rather that the pathologic state is not one that can be disclosed by the usual histopathologic techniques.

CLINICAL ASPECTS. The motor abnormalities are described in Chap. 22. In the early stages, the involuntary muscular contractions are intermittent and variable in location and severity, but typically interfere with motor performance by superimposing an unwanted posture upon parts in use. One leg may briefly be pulled into a flexed or extended position or one shoulder elevated. Later the neck and thoracic muscles pull, and grimacing may occur. Progression may be relatively rapid in cases with onset during early childhood, but is slow in those beginning in late childhood or adult life. The end result is extreme disability, with grossly distorted postures of the trunk and contractures of the limbs. Affection of face and tongue muscles results in faulty articulation of speech, which eventually becomes incomprehensible. The tendon and plantar reflexes, which can be assessed only during moments of relaxation of the affected parts, are characteristically normal.

Dementia is not a necessary accompaniment of the condition, except perhaps in the terminal stages; but with severe derangement of all available methods of communication, an adequate evaluation of mental capacity may be impossible.

Spasmodic torticollis (see Chap. 22) may well be a form of dystonia, but it typically does not progress to involve the musculature generally. However, torticollis may be an early symptom in cases which later show the typical generalized motor abnormalities.

DIFFERENTIAL DIAGNOSIS. Hepatolenticular degeneration should be seriously considered in any case presenting these motor symptoms, and appropriate measures should be undertaken for its investigation (see Chap. 110). The progressive course, and possibly the family history, differentiate the degenerative group from the "symptomatic" dystonias resulting from infections or metabolic disorders occurring at birth or later.

TREATMENT. This is most unsatisfactory. Dystonia is notoriously unresponsive to drug therapy, although antispasmodic drugs such as those used for parkinsonism should be tried. Neurosurgical treatment of the sort used for Parkinson's disease has been sufficiently promising to be worth serious consideration in every case, especially if the patient is young.

SYNDROMES OF SLOWLY DEVELOPING ATAXIA

The conditions about to be considered are distinguished clinically by progressive unsteadiness in standing and walking, along with more or less impaired coordination of other motor acts. Pathologically, they are characterized by degeneration of the cerebellum and/or its related fiber systems, and thus constitute classic examples of the system diseases. Although sporadic instances occur, hereditary transmission is an outstanding feature in many cases; thus, this group of disorders is often referred to as the *hereditary ataxias*. Their subdivision into more or less separate entities is largely arbitrary, with pathologic changes of varying distribution underlying clinically indistinguishable symptom complexes. Furthermore, there is considerable overlapping with other forms of hereditary nervous disease, so that in a given case a remarkable combination of defects may be encountered. These facts have led to the idea that in the ataxias there is a group of closely related genetically determined abnormalities which may occur together in an almost infinite series of combinations, so that it is not possible to separate well-defined disease pictures. Nevertheless, certain constellations of symptoms and pathologic findings occur with sufficient regularity to warrant their separation for purposes of discussion. The classification about to be given is not entirely satisfactory but is designed to be of practical help to the physician confronted with a case.

Cerebellar Degenerations

To be discussed are the forms of progressive ataxia which are associated with pathologic changes predominantly in the cerebellum. These include both hereditary and sporadic cases and comprise, in addition, the rather rare subacute spinocerebellar degeneration associated with the presence of carcinoma of various types elsewhere in the body. The hereditary and sporadic forms of cerebellar degeneration resemble one another so closely that, for the purposes of the present discussion, they will all be referred to as "hereditary cerebellar degeneration." Most cases are seen in adults, with the onset occurring in middle life.

PATHOLOGY. In hereditary cerebellar degeneration the cerebellum is obviously atrophied. In one group of cases, these changes are chiefly localized to the superior vermis and adjacent parts of the cerebellar cortex, whereas in an even larger group, the entire cerebellar cortex is affected. Microscopically there is loss of nerve cells principally affecting the Purkinje cells, although the granule cells are often involved as well. In most cases, there is an associated atrophy of nerve cells in the inferior olivary nuclei in a distribution dependent on the location and extent of the changes in the cerebellar cortex. It no longer seems justifiable to separate the cases with associated olivary degeneration from the rest and to designate them as "cerebello-olivary degeneration," as has been done in the past. In *olivopontocerebellar degeneration*, there are extensive degenerative changes in the pontine nuclei, middle cerebellar peduncles, and olivary nuclei. In addition changes in the cerebellar cortex such as have been noted above may or may not be present. In all varieties of cerebellar degeneration, affection of other neuronal systems—as, for instance, the cerebral cortex and basal ganglions—may be encountered. In some cases, there are changes in the dentate and roof nuclei of the cerebellum and their projections in the superior cerebellar peduncles (*dentatorubral atrophy*), but these are always found in association with more diffuse cerebellar or spinocerebellar degeneration. *Carcinomatous cerebellar (spinocerebellar) degeneration* is characterized by extensive cell loss in all parts of the cerebellar cortex, often associated with inflammatory (lymphocytic) infiltrations in the perivascular and subarachnoid spaces. In addition there are degenerative changes in the long-fiber tracts of the spinal cord. These lesions do not depend on the presence of tumor implants anywhere in the nervous system or its coverings, but rather are thought to be due to an obscure infectious (? metabolic) process somehow resulting from the presence of carcinoma.

CLINICAL ASPECTS. In the hereditary form of cerebellar degeneration the abnormality appears first in the legs, resulting in unsteadiness of stance and gait of the peculiar wavering, lurching character so typical of cerebellar ataxia (see Chap. 22). This has been correlated with the localization of changes in the superior vermis of the cerebellum and adjacent parts of the cerebellar cortex. With more extensive cerebellar involvement, a disturbance in articulation and rhythm of speech occurs that may progress to total incomprehensibility, and the arms likewise become ataxic. There may be nystagmus, but it is often absent. Where there is affection of other neuronal systems, additional neurologic abnormalities, such as exaggerated tendon reflexes, extensor plantar responses, rigidity, tremor, and dementia, may be encountered (*cerebrocerebellar degeneration*). Progression is gradual and slow, being measured in decades, and may not necessarily shorten life. There is no specific treatment available for any of the progressive ataxias, although encouragement and gait training may enable a patient to overcome his disability to some extent. We have not been able to differentiate a cortical parenchymatous from the olivoponto cerebellar degeneration clinically. Both diseases are familial; there is a greater tendency for other extrapyramidal and pyramidal symptoms to appear in the latter.

In the cases associated with carcinoma, the tempo of evolution of the process is relatively rapid, with severe disability coming on within a period of months. Vertigo, diplopia, and nausea may be prominent. In an occasional patient, the neurologic symptoms have appeared before there was any obvious evidence of carcinoma. In contrast to the consistently normal cerebrospinal fluid findings in the forms of cerebellar degeneration noted above, the cerebrospinal fluid may show increased lymphocytes and protein in the carcinomatous spinocerebellar degeneration.

DIFFERENTIAL DIAGNOSIS. The slow but relentless progression in the absence of abnormalities in the cerebrospinal fluid distinguishes the hereditary group from other forms of cerebellar ataxia such as may occur with neoplastic, infectious, or demyelinative disease, with drug intoxications (e.g., barbiturates), or with hyperpyrexia. The degenerative disorders under discussion tend to occur in a setting of otherwise good general health; this, together with the other clinical differences, distinguishes them from alcoholic cerebellar ataxia of deficiency disease, with or without Wernicke-Korsakoff syndrome. Alcoholic cerebellar degeneration usually develops rapidly, and then may remain more or less stationary for the remainder of the patient's life (Chap. 363). The form of spinocerebellar degeneration associated with carcinoma may be distinguished from direct carcinomatous involvement of the nervous system by the symmetry of the findings and the absence of increased intracranial pressure.

Hereditary Ataxia of Pierre Marie

This designation has been applied to cases of hereditary progressive ataxia with onset in early adulthood. Considerable doubt has been raised as to the validity of retaining the concept of Marie's hereditary ataxia, because pathologically this is by no means a uniform group. When Pierre Marie wrote about the subject in 1893, Friedreich's ataxia (see Chap. 356) had relatively recently become recognized as a distinct entity. Marie pointed out, on the basis of case reports in the literature, that there were other cases of hereditary ataxia, of later onset, which could not be fitted into Friedreich's description. He offered the suggestion that the cerebellum itself was the major site of disease in these cases. Subsequent pathologic examination of the cases he reviewed have shown that he was partly in error in this supposition; nevertheless, following his report, the concept of Marie's ataxia has appeared repeatedly in the writings on hereditary ataxia. Cases that might be classified with this group either are indistinguishable from those discussed above under the cerebellar degenerations or are variants of Friedreich's ataxia.

SYNDROME OF MUSCULAR WEAKNESS AND WASTING, WITHOUT SENSORY CHANGES

Motor System Disease

This general term is used to designate a progressive disorder of motor neurones in the cerebral cortex, brainstem, and spinal cord, manifested clinically by muscular weakness, with muscle atrophy and spasticity with exaggeration of tendon reflexes in varying combinations. It is a disease of middle life, generally appearing in the fifth or sixth decades. Customarily a subdivision is made on the basis of the particular grouping of symptoms and signs observed. Thus, the most frequent form, in which muscular atrophy and hyperreflexia are combined, is called *amyotrophic lateral sclerosis*. Rather more rare are the cases in which weakness and atrophy alone exist without clinical evidence of corticospinal tract dysfunction; for these, the term *progressive muscular atrophy* is used. Where the disorder affects predominantly the musculature innervated by the cranial nerves, it is usual to speak of *progressive bulbar palsy*. Very rarely, the clinical state is dominated by spasticity and hyperreflexia without obvious muscular wasting; such cases are classed as *primary lateral sclerosis*. There is no reason to believe that these subgroupings are anything other than clinical variants of the same disease process, which is another classic example of a system disease. Most cases are sporadic, but occasionally this disorder occurs in families in a manner suggesting genetic transmission.

PATHOLOGY. There are widespread selective atrophy and loss of motor nerve cells at all levels of the central nervous system, including the Betz cells in the motor areas of the cerebral cortex. Some evidence of disease in the corticospinal motor system is usually found pathologically, even when physical signs referable to such changes were not observed during life. The atrophy of fibers in skeletal muscles is typically that due to loss of motor innervation.

CLINICAL ASPECTS. The disease begins insidiously and may be well advanced before the patient is aware of it. Although often asymmetric initially, the weakness and muscular wasting gradually become symmetric and widespread. Classically, the disorder becomes first evident in the small muscles of the hands, but it may begin in one or both of the legs, or in muscles supplied by cranial nerves. Vague feelings of discomfort in the muscles, tightness, numbness (without objective sensory changes), and recurrent cramps may be early symptoms. The progressive atrophy of the musculature is accompanied by widespread visible fascicular twitchings of groups of muscle fibers, a classic feature that can be related to degeneration of the motor nerve cells supplying the involved muscles. Despite extensive involvement of skeletal muscles generally, sphincter control remains intact. Sooner or later the disease affects muscles supplied by the brainstem, resulting in weakness, atrophy, and fasciculations in the tongue and facial musculature associated with dysarthria and impairment of chewing or swallowing. The functions of the ocular muscles, oddly enough, are invariably spared. In most cases, the weakness and muscular wasting are accompanied by exaggeration of tendon reflexes, extensor plantar reflexes and spasticity, to a degree dependent on the severity of degeneration in the corticospinal (pyramidal) motor system. Affection of corticobulbar fibers results in manifestations of pseudobulbar palsy such as involuntary weeping or laughter, exaggerated reflex movements of the facial muscles or expression, and sucking reflexes. Progression is unhalting and relatively rapid, leading to extensive paralysis, with death from respiratory weakness or aspiration pneumonia, generally within about 2 to 5 years or more from onset. Intelligence and awareness are typically preserved to the end.

DIFFERENTIAL DIAGNOSIS. Spinal cord compression from tumors in the cervical region or from cervical spondylosis with osteophytes projecting into the vertebral canal can at times give rise to weakness, wasting, and fasciculations in the upper limbs and spasticity in the legs, thus closely resembling amyotrophic lateral sclerosis. The absence of cranial nerve involvement may be helpful in differentiation, although some compressive lesions at the foramen magnum may implicate the twelfth cranial (hypoglossal) nerve, with resulting affection of the tongue. Absence of pain or of sensory changes, normal function of bowels and bladder, normal roentgenographic studies of the spine, and absence of changes in the composition of dynamics of the cerebrospinal fluid are all points in favor of motor system disease and against spinal cord compression. Where doubt exists, contrast myelography should be performed and the cervical region should be visualized.

Chronic inflammatory disorders of the meninges and spinal cord, exemplified by syphilitic meningomyelitis or some cases of adhesive arachnoiditis, may have to be considered. These conditions can readily be recognized by cerebrospinal fluid changes and, if necessary, by abnormal myelographic findings. Nutritional myelopathy can be excluded by history and on other clinical grounds.

Although fasciculations are a prominent feature of motor system disease, they are not, in the absence of weakness, muscle atrophy, or loss of tendon reflexes, valid signs of it, for they may occur in a variety of metabolic or toxic disorders (e.g., thyrotoxicosis, salt depletion) as well as in otherwise healthy individuals. Careful clinical evaluation suffices in such instances to exclude serious neurologic disease.

Progressive weakness from intrinsic disease of muscle (myopathy, polymyositis) may occasionally be difficult to distinguish from progressive muscular atrophy of the type under discussion; yet the differentiation is important from the standpoint of prognosis or treatment. Under such circumstances, the diagnosis can be made by muscle biopsy and electromyography.

There is no known treatment for any form of motor system disease.

Infantile Muscular Atrophy (Werdnig and Hoffmann), Amyotonia Congenita (Oppenheim)

The form of progressive muscular atrophy described by Werdnig and Hoffmann is a disease of infants and young children, typically afflicting several members of a family. Pathologically, it closely resembles the adult disease described above. Amyotonia congenita is a purely clinical term, used to designate abnormal laxness of somatic musculature observed at birth or in early infancy; it may occur in a number of different pathologic processes, including Werdnig-Hoffmann disease. For further details of these conditions, Chap. 365 should be consulted.

Hereditary Spastic Paraplegia

This very rare disorder is characterized by weakness and spasticity of the legs, with early onset (childhood or adolescence) and slow progression. Later the arms may be affected, but usually to a lesser degree. The pathologic changes closely resemble those of Friedreich's ataxia, and there is reason now to believe that this condition is in fact an incomplete form of Friedreich's disease in which spastic weakness overshadows minimal or absent ataxia and sensory changes. The diagnosis is made by the family history and by excluding other possible causes of bilateral spastic weakness of the limbs. The relationship to Friedreich's ataxia is further confirmed by the occurrence of pes cavus and optic atrophy in some cases. One group of patients also has progressive dementia. The combination of optic atrophy and spastic paraparesis beginning in childhood is called Behr's syndrome.

SYNDROMES COMBINING WEAKNESS AND WASTING WITH SENSORY CHANGES

Progressive Neural Muscular Atrophy

The degenerative disorders characterized by progressive weakness and wasting of skeletal muscles combined with sensory changes are chronic diseases of peripheral nerves, often occurring as hereditary conditions. Although clinical and pathologic subvarieties exist, there is no sharp dividing line between them, and they are best considered together under the designation given above, in which the term *neural* emphasizes the peripheral nerve affection. As already pointed out above, chronic peripheral neuropathy is an associated disorder in some of the hereditary ataxias and is regularly encountered in the classic form of Friedreich's ataxia. An additional connecting link with other genetically determined nervous diseases is the occurrence of progressive optic atrophy or pigmentary degeneration of the retina in some cases. Common to all is for the peripheral neuropathy to begin distally and to progress in a centripetal fashion and for the feet and legs to become first affected, with involvement of the hands and more proximal parts only after a considerable interval.

The variety most usually seen is that generally called *peroneal muscular atrophy* (*Charcot-Marie-Tooth disease*), a name which draws attention to the changes in the lower legs, although the disorder affects far more than the peroneal group of nerves. This condition was first clearly differentiated from other forms of muscular atrophy by Charcot and Marie in France, and independently by H. H. Tooth in England, in 1886. In rare cases which are otherwise similar, there is a remarkable palpable thickening of peripheral nerve trunks. Such cases are generally designated as *hypertrophic interstitial neuropathy* (*of Dejerine and Sottas*, the French neurologists who, in 1893, first described the condition clinically and pathologically). In a few cases, there are pronounced trophic and vasomotor abnormalities of the affected parts, chiefly the feet, which may lead to chronic, poorly healing, perforating ulcers on the ball of the foot, among other abnormalities (*familial neurovascular dystrophy*, Wadulla, 1949, Krücke, 1955; *hereditary sensory neuropathy*, Denny-Brown, 1951). Probably related is the unusual condition described by Refsum (1946) and called by him *heredopathia atactica polyneuritiformis*, in which peripheral neuropathy and ataxia are associated with progressive nerve deafness, retinitis pigmentosa, and a high cerebrospinal fluid protein, and possibly familial amyloid polyneuropathy (for further details, see Chap. 354).

PATHOLOGY. The lesions are typical of a chronic multiple peripheral neuropathy with secondary atrophic changes in muscles. The degenerative process in the nerve fibers is associated with abortive regenerative phenomena and with proliferation of connective tissue and Schwann cells which, in the hypertrophic variety, may reach extreme degrees. In the central nervous system, there are varying degrees of overlap with the lesions found in the various forms of hereditary ataxia already discussed.

CLINICAL ASPECTS. The disorder usually begins in childhood and progresses very slowly. In the classic cases of peroneal muscular atrophy, the combination of pes cavus with extreme atrophy of the anterior tibial and calf muscles ("stork legs") and wasting of the lower thigh musculature (giving an appearance like an "inverted champagne bottle") presents a striking picture. There is total absence of deep reflexes, and sensation is altered as described in Chap. 356 on Friedreich's ataxia. The possibility of combinations with other hereditary neurologic syndromes has already been pointed out. Although death in a state of extreme debility in early adult life is common, progression in some cases may be extremely slow and may lead to very little disability. Measurements of

phytenic acid, alpha and betalipoproteins, cholesterol, and gamma globulins in the serum serve to distinguish some of the recently discovered metabolic neuropathies.

DIFFERENTIAL DIAGNOSIS. It may be necessary to consider various other forms of chronic polyneuropathy (toxic, metabolic, nutritional), described in Chap. 354. The familial incidence, early onset, very slow progression, and absence (usually) of significant blood and cerebrospinal fluid changes, except for increased amount of protein in some patients, are generally sufficient for the accurate recognition of the hereditary neuropathies under discussion. In occasional sporadic or atypical cases, biopsy of muscle and of a small cutaneous nerve twig (most conveniently the sural cutaneous nerve) will be necessary.

TREATMENT. Although no specific treatment is available, patients whose disease is of slow progression and in whom conditions are otherwise favorable may be greatly helped by measures to ensure a stable walking surface, such as corrective shoes, braces to prevent foot drop, and even orthopedic procedures to stabilize the joints.

SYNDROME OF PROGRESSIVE VISUAL LOSS

As already stated in previous sections, progressive impairment or loss of vision, due to degenerative changes in the visual system (retinas and optic nerves), may be an accompaniment of morbid processes affecting the nervous system diffusely—in particular, the nervous system lipidoses and the hereditary ataxias. Occasionally, however, the peripheral visual system is the major, or only, site of disease. In such cases, the disorders are strongly hereditary. For detailed discussion of these conditions, standard reference works on ophthalmology should be consulted. Nevertheless, two entities, because of their close relationship with other degenerative diseases of the nervous system, warrant some discussion here.

Hereditary Optic Atrophy (Leber)

This rare condition is characterized by the relatively rapid development of bilateral blindness with optic atrophy, coming on in early adult life. It was first thoroughly described by Leber in 1871. Typically, it occurs as a sex-linked recessive trait, chiefly affecting men; but it likewise may be seen in women.

PATHOLOGY. In the only recorded case with autopsy, the changes occurred primarily in the ganglion cells of the retina, with secondary degeneration in optic nerve fibers. Because of the limited examination in this case, it is not known whether there were lesions in other parts of the nervous system.

CLINICAL ASPECTS. The condition often begins asymmetrically, with blurring of vision in one eye followed in days or weeks by similar affection of the other eye. Vision then deteriorates rapidly over ensuing weeks or months, generally with eventual total blindness as a result, although arrest before this stage has been seen, or even a little improvement after initial steady progression. In the early stages, examination of the visual fields shows large central scotomas. The optic disks may be normal at first, or may be swollen (optic neuritis); later the appearance is typically that of optic atrophy, with pale, clearly outlined disks.

DIFFERENTIAL DIAGNOSIS. Multiple sclerosis may at times act in a manner identical to that just described, but without a definite hereditary background and with a much better outlook for improvement of vision. Toxic or nutritional amblyopia can generally be excluded by history and associated clinical findings. In some cases it may be necessary to eliminate the possibility of a tumor compressing the chiasmal region and optic nerves, although some evidence of bitemporal defects would be then expected, rather than bilateral central scotomas alone. In addition to careful roentgenograms of the skull and cerebrospinal fluid examination, pneumoencephalographic visualization of the chiasmal region may be indicated in cases of serious doubt. Early onset of optic atrophy with spastic paralysis of legs (Behr's disease) should also be distinguishable on clinical grounds.

Pigmentary Degeneration of the Retina (Retinitis Pigmentosa)

This may at times occur as a relatively independent disorder, although it is often associated with other abnormalities, of which cataracts, deafness, and mental deficiency are outstanding. It is strongly hereditary, chiefly as a recessive trait, although dominant inheritance has been seen. Pigmentary degeneration of the retina is one of the features of the Laurence-Moon-Biedl syndrome. Special varieties of the condition also accompany some cases of neuronal lipidosis or hereditary neuropathy as already noted.

PATHOLOGY. The principal lesion is a degeneration of the rods and cones, associated with displacement of melanin-containing cells from the pigment epithelium into more superficial parts of the retina. Other retinal structures are relatively intact.

CLINICAL ASPECTS. The disorder typically begins in childhood, first as night blindness. The visual fields become concentrically narrowed from the periphery to the center, until eventually (by adolescence, or perhaps not until middle age) very little useful vision remains. Ophthalmoscopic examination may be normal at first, but generally discloses irregular patches of dark pigment in the periphery of the retina. When cataracts are likewise present, as sometimes is the case, visual acuity may be significantly improved by their removal. The frequent association of the retinal lesions with other neurological abnormalities has been mentioned in previous paragraphs.

DIFFERENTIAL DIAGNOSIS. Chorioretinitis from other causes (e.g., syphilis) may present a similar ophthalmoscopic appearance and should be excluded. The hereditary background and the progressive course, with night blindness and peripheral constriction of the visual fields, may lead to the diagnosis even in the rare cases where pigmentary deposits in the retina are absent. The slowly progressive or relatively stationary tapeto retinal degenerations of childhood can be distinguished clinically and by electroretinogram. In most instances, the opinion of a qualified ophthalmologist must be obtained.

REFERENCES

Blackwood, W., W. H. McMenemey, A. Meyer, R. M. Norman, and D. S. Russell: "Greenfield's Neuropathology," Baltimore, The Williams & Wilkins Company, 1963.

Collins, G. H., R. R. Cowden, and A. H. Nevis: Myoclonus Epilepsy with Lafora Bodies, Arch. Pathol., 86:239, 1968.

Cotzias, G. C., P. S. Papavasiliou, and R. Gellene: Modification of Parkinsonism: Chronic Treatment with L-Dopa, New Engl. J. Med., 280:337, 1969.

Gibbs, C. J., Jr., et al.: Creutzfeldt-Jakob Disease (Spongiform Encephalopathy): Transmission to the Chimpanzee, Science, 161:388, 1968.

Kirschbaum, W. R.: "Jakob-Creutzfeldt Disease," New York, American Elsevier Publishing Company, Inc., 1968.

Rozdilsky, B., J. N. Cumings, and A. F. Huston: Hallervorden-Spatz Disease, Acta Neuropathol. (Berlin) 10:1, 1968.

Selby, G.: Stereotactic Surgery for the Relief of Parkinson's Disease, J. Neurol. Sci., 5:315, 1967.

Yahr, M. D., and R. C. Duvoisin: Medical Therapy of Parkinsonism, Mod. Treat., 5:283, 1968.

Zeman, W., and P. Dyken: Dystonia Musculorum Deformans. Clinical, Genetic and Pathoanatomical Studies, Psychiat. Neurol. Neurochir., 70:77, 1967.

365 DEVELOPMENTAL ABNORMALITIES

Philip R. Dodge and Raymond D. Adams

The human nervous system is subject to a variety of developmental abnormalities which may be traced to genetic faults or to diseases acquired in utero, at birth, or during the early years of life. Some of these conditions are manifest at birth; others may be recognized only in late infancy and early childhood, after some degree of maturation is attained. Together these diseases comprise a large segment of pediatric neurology, and to discuss them fully it would be necessary to touch upon the entire field of nervous disease in infancy and childhood. However, in a textbook of medicine, limitations of space preclude a presentation of pediatric disease, and for this reason only those conditions which are likely later to come to the attention of the internist and general physician are considered.

MAJOR PROBLEMS OF PEDIATRIC NEUROLOGY

The diseases included in this chapter differ from most of those acquired in late childhood, adolescence, and adult life in that they are likely to cause (1) deformity of the skull, spine, and limbs, (2) delayed or abnormal motor and speech development, (3) or mental retardation. The corollary of this axiom is that when any one of these abnormalities is observed in the adult there is a strong probability of a disease of the nervous system that had its onset before birth or during infancy or early childhood. Understanding fully the significance of these three types of clinical disorder will enable the student or physician to deal effectively with the majority of patients who suffer from developmental abnormalities. For this reason this chapter is devoted to an exposition of these topics. In addition, certain seizure problems peculiar to the pediatric age group deserve consideration here.

Malformations of the Cranium, Spine, and Limbs

A congenital abnormality may be defined as a structural deformity of some tissue or organ of the body, which is present at birth. It may be "gross or microscopic, on the surface of the body or within it, familial or sporadic, hereditary or nonhereditary, single or multiple" (Warkany).

Estimates as to the incidence of congenital abnormalities of the nervous system vary substantially, depending upon the definition adopted by the reporter and the time in life when the survey was made. Malpas found a congenital malformation of the nervous system in approximately 1 percent of 13,000 births, and McIntosh and his associates give a figure of 1.3 percent of total births, 7.2 percent of stillbirths, 6.1 percent of infants dying in the first days of life, and 1.1 percent of live births. Malformations of the central nervous system are of importance in stillbirth and infantile mortality. They cause 76 percent of all fetal deaths and 39 percent of deaths in the first year of life, according to Record and McKeown. As was pointed out by Murphy, the nervous system is involved in 60 percent of all patients with congenital malformations.

General understanding of these malformations has been advanced by experimental teratology, a branch of biology that seeks the causes of abnormalities of structural development. In the progeny of animals possessing certain abnormal genes, developmental abnormalities can be predicted in ratios that agree with established genetic laws. Equally predictable results have been obtained by subjecting the embryo or fetus, under controlled conditions, to certain environmental stresses. X-ray, hypoxia, deficient diet, viral infections, and toxic substances have been shown to induce a variety of defects in the central nervous system, depending on the stage of embryogenesis at which the noxious agent is applied to the pregnant animal. These genetically and environmentally determined malformations serve as experimental models which can be investigated to great advantage.

In human beings four categories of disease have genetic implications. First there are chromosomal abnormalities (of obscure origin) which are associated with a failure in normal development of the brain as well as of other organs. Examples are mongolism with a trisomy of the 21–22 pair of chromosomes (also two other trisomies —of 13–15 and 17–18), Turner's syndrome, and Klinefelter's syndrome. The second group comprises those biochemical diseases in which a single abnormal gene, inherited usually as an autosomal recessive trait, results in a biochemical disturbance that blights the development of the brain or other organs, if not corrected. Examples are galactosemia and phenylpyruvic oligophrenia. The third group includes diseases inherited as dominant traits such as neurofibromatosis (of von Recklinghausen), craniofacial dysostosis (Crouzon), and tuberous sclerosis. In these there are no well-defined biochemical changes. In another group are placed those individuals whose genetic inheritance has varied sufficiently from the mean of the population as to place them in an inferior status intellectually and physically. Here, as well as in the first group, multiple factors must operate, and the effects of environmental, or exogenous, agencies are difficult to separate from genetic, endogenous ones. Examples of a defect of the nervous system due to the action of a noxious agent during human development are less numerous. Exposure to roentgen radiation during the first trimester of pregnancy is said to produce microcephaly and mental defect. Maternal infection with German measles (rubella) during the first trimester of pregnancy may result in mental defect, deafness, cataracts, and heart disease in the newborn. Toxoplasmosis, cytomegalic inclusion disease, and syphilis may damage the fetal nervous system in the latter half of the period of intrauterine life. Isoimmunization by Rh and ABO blood factors may affect the nervous system during the first days of postnatal life, leaving in its wake a permanent mental defect, choreoathetosis, and deafness. Lastly, and least well understood, dietary deficiency, especially of protein, during critical phases of brain development may lead to subnormality.

ABNORMALITIES OF THE HEAD

Alterations in the size and shape of the head, when observed in the adult, can usually be traced to infancy. At least three separate factors are operative: (1) the growth thrust of the developing brain and the intracranial pressure, (2) the time at which the suture lines close, (3) the existence of external pressures against the skull. In addition a depressed fracture, cephalohematoma, craniocele, or tumor may cause a localized cephalic deformity.

It is the constant outward pressure of the developing brain which under normal circumstances causes the head to enlarge rapidly in the first months and years of life. Any disease which destroys a substantial portion of the cerebral hemispheres in infancy will usually result in microcephaly. Excessive intracranial pressure, as from hydrocephalus or chronic subdural hematomas, will enlarge the head to an abnormal degree. Focal lesions, e.g., destruction of one hemisphere, result in smallness of the skull on that side, just as a unilateral subdural hematoma enlarges it. Regarding premature closure of the sutures (synostosis), it should be noted that this may occur without abnormality of the brain. If all sutures close, cranial expansion is prevented; or if some sutures close and others remain open, enlargement will occur only at the latter sites, and the skull then becomes deformed. A flattening of one side of the head (plagiocephaly) often is found in defective or sick infants who lie in one position for prolonged periods of time. The weight of the head against the bed prevents part of the skull from expanding, but the cranial capacity is usually undiminished.

MACROCRANIA (Enlargement of the Head). A general enlargement of the head must be distinguished from a misshapen head; i.e., one that is enlarged in one direction only. Three different conditions must be considered in the differential diagnosis—infantile hydrocephalus, infantile chronic subdural hematoma, and macroencephaly.

Hydrocephalus. This, the most frequent cause of increased size of the head, is the only condition in which there may be enormous enlargement. The majority of severely hydrocephalic infants die within a few months or years and are not seen by internists, but a few linger on. Sometimes the hydrocephalus becomes arrested and there is long-term survival.

Hydrocephalus due to congenital causes may appear years after birth. If the sutures have already closed (after the twelfth year), the head cannot enlarge and the hydrocephalus is occult, resulting in compression and atrophy of the cerebrum. Increased intracranial pressure with papilledema, vomiting, and mental dullness are then the usual signs.

The most frequent causes of hydrocephalus are:

1. Arnold-Chiari malformation with spina bifida and meningomyelocele.

2. Atresia or stenosis of the aqueduct of Sylvius with obstructive hydrocephalus and a small, normal-appearing posterior fossa. This may be an inherited abnormality, an accompaniment of an Arnold-Chiari malformation or of neurofibromatosis, or the result of a chronic meningo-ependymal inflammation.

3. Atresia of the foramens of Luschka and Magendie (Dandy-Walker syndrome) with obstructive hydrocephalus and enlargement of the posterior fossa. Here the basal foramens fail to form or are sealed off, and the cerebrospinal fluid cannot enter the subarachnoid space.

4. Chronic meningitis with communicating or obstructive hydrocephalus. This is due to obliteration of the subarachnoid space over the brainstem and/or obstruction of the foramens of Luschka and Magendie. The meningitis may be due to syphilis, toxoplasmosis, or a chronic pyogenic or other infection, or may follow subarachnoid hemorrhage. Often the cause cannot be ascertained.

5. A tumor of the fourth ventricle (medulloblastoma, ependymoma, or teratoma), of the third ventricle (craniopharyngioma), or of the pineal body (teratoma) may result in obstructive hydrocephalus (see Chap. 359).

6. Other conditions such as hypertrophy of the choroid plexuses and achondroplastic dwarfism with hydrocephalus, while rare, are the most obscure.

Subdural Hematoma and Effusion in Infancy. This is a not infrequent cause of a symmetric enlargement of the skull. It may occur in several circumstances: (1) trauma to the head at birth or later, (2) with bleeding diseases or in poorly nourished, sickly infants, some of whom are said to have had scurvy, (3) in association with pyogenic meningitis, and (4) secondary to encephaloclastic disease processes with brain atrophy or, rarely, the result of rapid shrinkage due to an episode of hypertonicity of blood. In acute subdural hematoma the symptoms are the same as those described in Chap. 358, Traumatic Diseases of the Brain, with the exception that focal seizures on the contralateral side of the body are more frequent. Whether the seizures are due to the subdural collection of fluid or to associated cortical injury is not known. In the chronic subdural hematoma of infancy the initial symptoms are usually failure to thrive, irritability, vomiting, and a reduced level of responsiveness. Later the cranium enlarges, symmetrically as a rule, even though the subdural hematoma is unilateral. X-ray films of the skull even years later will reveal that a characteristic enlargement of the middle cranial fossa has occurred, followed later, after resorption or removal of the clot, by thickening of the skull and enlargement of the frontal and ethmoidal sinuses (Davidoff and Dyke).

Macrocephaly is also associated with a certain small group of patients with idiopathic mental retardation and increased stature.

Macroencephaly. This is a rare cause of enlargement of the head. The brain is malformed and greatly increased in size; specimens weighing over 2,500 Gm have been recorded (normal is 1,350 to 1,550 Gm). Mental retardation, feebleness of movement, and enlargement of the head with small ventricles are the criteria for clinical diagnosis. Macroencephaly is characteristically found in the late stage of Tay-Sachs disease, gargoylism, spongy degeneration of the brain (Canavan), some cases of achondroplastic dwarfism, and the leukodystrophy associated with hyaline bodies.

The *diagnosis* of hydrocephalus and its differentiation from macroencephaly and subdural hematoma is usually established by inserting a needle through the lateral border of the anterior fontanel and aspirating the subdural space. If negative, air can be injected into the spinal subarachnoid space (pneumoencephalography); this will rule in or out subdural hematoma. The lumbar injection of air should be preferred, for punctures of the ventricle in the hydrocephalic brain may lead to focal injury and formation of diverticulae. If the cortical mantle is thin or the subarachnoid space dilated, cerebrospinal fluid may be obtained and mistaken for subdural fluid. The latter is usually xanthochromic, with a total protein content of 300 to 2,000 mg per 100 ml. In the older child or adult, carotid arteriography and, if positive, burr holes and craniotomy are indicated. Macroencephaly is distinguished by the small lateral and third ventricles. The entrance into the ventricles of air that has been introduced into the lumbar subarachnoid space, or the passage of a dye such as phenolsulfonphthalein, injected into the lateral ventricles, to the lumbar subarachnoid space, is of help in determining whether the hydrocephalus is due to an obstruction in the ventricular system (*obstructive hydrocephalus*) or is *nonobstructive* (also called *communicating hydrocephalus*). The latter is usually due to obliteration of subarachnoid space over the medulla, pons, and midbrain by a fibrosing meningitis. Thrombosis of the superior sagittal sinus may cause headache and elevated intracranial pressure but usually does not result in expansion of the ventricles.

The *treatment* of these conditions is becoming more effective with the improvement of one-way valves. If the hydrocephalus has stabilized, i.e., if the head is no longer enlarging, no treatment should be undertaken. If the head is large and the patient is mentally enfeebled or has other serious malformations, surgical therapy is ill-advised. If the hydrocephalus is suspected of being progressive, one may give acetozolamide, 250 mg t.i.d., and measure the circumference of the head each week to see if it is under control. If not, and if the patient's neurologic status is good, operative treatment is indicated. Ventriculoatriostomy, in which the cerebrospinal fluid is shunted from occipital (or frontal) horn of lateral ventricle of the brain to right atrium of the heart by a tube with a one-way valve, is applicable to the treatment of all types of hydrocephalus and has largely replaced other forms of surgical treatment. In certain instances of obstructive hydrocephalus, the Torkildsen procedure (short-circuiting the fluid through a tube from the occipital horn of the lateral ventricle to the cisterna magna) may be used. The treatment of chronic subdural effusion is repeated percutaneous aspiration by needle; in some cases the membranes enclosing the subdural hematoma must be removed at a later stage. Nothing can be done about macroencephaly.

SPECIAL DEFORMITIES OF THE SKULL. The usual cause of a severely misshapen head in the child, adolescent, or adult is cranial dysostosis or synostosis, of one or several cranial sutures. The most plausible explanation of it is that the mesenchymal tissues which form the cranial bones are defective, the premature ossification being secondary. The occasional association of cranial synostosis with syndactylism (Apert's syndrome) has been cited in support of this hypothesis. The developmental defect and synostosis are believed to date from intrauterine life. Closure of the sagittal suture results in an elongated, dolichocephalic head, to which the term *scaphocephaly* is applied. When the coronal suture fuses prematurely, the growth is restricted in the anteroposterior diameter, and only lateral and, to a lesser extent, vertical enlargement may occur. This condition is called *brachycephaly* (wide skull) or *acrobrachycephaly*. Synostosis of all sutures leaves the cranium small but usually with the greatest growth in the vertical direction, the so-called *oxycephaly* or *turrencephaly*. *Plagiocephaly* refers to an asymmetric deformity of the skull which may be due to synostosis of a single coronal suture or to the application of some external force. *Crouzon's craniofacial dysostosis scaphocephaly* is associated with a "beak nose." This condition is inherited as a mendelian dominant. In *Apert's syndrome* webbed or "mitten" fingers and toes are combined with acrobrachycephaly. *Hypertelorism*, as described by Greig in 1924, is a rare deformity characterized by wide separation of the eyes and a flat, retracted bridge of the nose. Mental retardation frequently accompanies this deformity and Apert's syndrome. The primary abnormality in hypertelorism has usually been ascribed to an abnormally large lesser wing of the sphenoid bone. In several instances a dominant mode of inheritance has been found.

More often than not there are no related neurologic symptoms and signs referable to craniosynostosis. If all sutures are stenosed, a gradual increase in intracranial pressure may occur during the most active growth period of the brain. In these patients the orbits are shallow and the eyes bulge. Headache, divergent strabismus, papilledema, optic atrophy and later blindness, nystagmus, mental retardation, and behavioral abnormalities are the most striking clinical manifestations. In roentgenograms of the skull one observes the primary suture involvement, prominence of convolutional markings, and a depression and smallness of the sella turcica.

In the absence of increased intracranial pressure, the diagnosis of premature closure of the sutures should always raise the suspicion of defective growth of the brain (see below, Microcephaly). If it is recognized during the early months of life, prophylactic surgery is indicated for craniostenosis. The major indication is usually cosmetic, but occasionally it is carried out to relieve the increased intracranial pressure.

MICROCEPHALY. This term is used to designate any condition in which there is an abnormally small head. An occipitofrontal circumference of less than 19 in. after the age of ten years is given as the dividing line between normal and abnormal. Microcephaly is accompanied by a reduction in the mass of the brain, and two types of pathologic change have been reported. There is one form in which the growth disturbance appears to be the sole factor; the brain, except for its smallness, has a normal appearance. This is called *microcephaly vera*. The other is a focal arrest of growth due either to embryonal failure in development of a part of the cerebral hemisphere (*schizencephaly*) or to an acquired disease which has resulted in destruction of one, or both, of the cerebral hemispheres (*encephaloclastic microcephaly*).

Microcephaly vera may occur in several members of one generation of a family and can often be linked to a recessive gene. The head tends to be extraordinarily small, usually measuring 15 in. or less in circumference. It is usually of symmetric shape and, owing to the lack of frontal prominence, resembles the skull of a monkey. The ears are large and often malformed. The neurologic picture varies. All patients show simple mental retardation of moderate or severe degree. Seizures and quadriparesis have been described in some patients, but in the authors' experience are much less frequent than in the other forms of microcephaly. Those patients with focal arrest of growth or destruction of cerebral tissue, *schizencephaly*, and *encephaloclastic microcephaly* exhibit a wide variety of clinical findings. The mental state in the most severe cases is usually that of an idiot, and all cerebral functions fail to develop. The cerebral hemispheres may have a relatively simple form or may be represented only by membranes filled with clear or yellowish fluid (*hydranencephaly*). In others, in which the cerebral defect is restricted to one cerebral hemisphere or part of a hemisphere, there may be hemiplegia with a small arm and leg, gross hemianesthesia, homonymous hemianopia, and seizures, with lesser degrees of mental backwardness. The skull on the side of the damaged hemisphere is smaller, and in roentgenograms the frontoparietal bones are thick, the middle fossa is shallow, and the paranasal sinuses are enlarged.

ABNORMALITIES OF THE SPINE OF NEUROLOGIC SIGNIFICANCE

A remarkable variety of neurologic syndromes is associated with abnormality of the vertebral column. Some of these, such as hemivertebra, platybasia, fusion of the atlas and occiput or of vertebras (Klippel-Feil syndrome), or congenital dislocation of the atlas, are the consequence of a malformation of the spine itself, and the enclosed spinal cord may or may not be involved. Others, such as spina bifida occulta, spinal meningocele or myelomeningocele, or dysraphism, involve the whole neural tube, including spinal cord, investing meninges, vertebral bodies, and even the overlying skin and subcutaneous tissues.

In many of these patients the neurologic defect which appears in infancy does not shorten life; in others it may be recognized only during adult life.

PRIMARY MALFORMATIONS OF VERTEBRAS. These are most frequent in the cervico-occipital region.

The Klippel-Feil Deformity. This abnormality consists of maldevelopment and fusion of two or more cervical vertebras, resulting in a short neck of limited mobility. The hairline is low, often at the level of the first thoracic vertebra. There may or may not be associated neurologic symptoms or signs. The importance of the spinal deformity lies in its frequent association with other abnormalities, especially platybasia and syringomyelia, the symptoms of which may not become manifest until adolescence or adult life.

Platybasia (Basilar Impression). In this maldevelopment of the base of the skull there is invagination of the occiput and upper cervical spine into the posterior fossa. Often the foramen magnum itself is imperfectly developed or the atlas and occiput are fused. The exact teratogenesis of this anomaly is uncertain. It may in some instances be asymptomatic, but frequently there is "crowding," distortion, or compression of the spinal cord, medulla, and cranial and spinal nerves. The resulting clinical picture is variable. Symptoms may be present from early life or may begin in late childhood, adolescence, or even adult years. Early symptoms, in patients old enough to give a history, consist of "dizzy" or "weak" spells; occipital neuralgia; transient paresthesias in the occipital region, neck, or arm; double vision; facial paresthesias and deafness; cerebellar ataxia; and spastic weakness of the legs. The symptoms may at first be intermittent and at any time in the course of the illness may be aggravated by straining, moving the head, or placing the head and neck in certain positions. Inspection alone provides a clue to diagnosis. The whole configuration of the head and neck is unnatural. The neck is short; the ears and hairline are low; neck movements are obviously re-

stricted; and the normal cervical lordosis is lost or greatly exaggerated, sometimes to the extent that the occiput lies almost on the upper dorsal spine and shoulders.

Instability of the junction of axis on atlas (atlantoaxial dislocation) may cause compression of the spinal cord. This may also occur as a consequence of rheumatoid arthritis, other debilitating diseases, and trauma (tear of ligaments which bind the odontoid process to the body of C_1). The treatment is surgical.

Platybasia and these related anomalies of the spine should be suspected in all cases presenting progressive cerebellar, brainstem, and cervical cord syndromes. Many of these patients have been diagnosed as having multiple sclerosis. The clinical suspicion of platybasia and other spine anomalies can be confirmed by a true lateral roentgenogram of the skull. In such a projection the extension of a line drawn from the hard palate and posterior border of the foramen magnum (Chamberlain's line) and another through the spine and body of the first cervical vertebra (Bull's line), instead of being more or less parallel as they normally are, intersect when extended. The relation of cervical vertebras is also seen. An acquired form of platybasia occurs with rickets and Paget's disease. It is usually asymptomatic but sometimes involves the lower cranial nerves.

The Arnold-Chiari Malformation. This condition, in which medulla and inferior-posterior portions of the cerebellar hemispheres project caudally through the foramen magnum, often to the level of the second cervical vertebra, has already been mentioned as a cause of hydrocephalus. When present, it is nearly always associated with a spinal meningocele or myelomeningocele, and often there are deformities of the cervical spine and cervico-occipital junction. The symptoms of hydrocephalus dominate the clinical picture in infants; but in milder cases, there may develop during adolescence or adult years any one of the several syndromes already described under platybasia. When platybasia and the Arnold-Chiari malformation coexist, it is generally impossible to decide which of the two is responsible for the clinical findings.

Methods of treatment of platybasia and the Arnold-Chiari malformation have not been entirely satisfactory. If clinical progression is slight or uncertain, it is probably advisable to do nothing. If progression is certain and disability is increasing, upper cervical laminectomy and enlargement of the foramen magnum are indicated. Sometimes these procedures halt the course of the illness or result in improvement. The surgical procedure must be done cautiously, however, for extensive manipulation of these structures may aggravate the symptoms or even cause death.

Malformations Associated with a Defect in Closure of the Neural Arch. Many deformities along the posterior surface of the body are accompanied by an abnormality in the formation of the posterior aspect of the neural arch and closure of the primitive neural tube. The entire neural canal, including the cranium, may fail to close (*craniorhachischisis totalis*), or there may be only a minute defect in one or more of the vertebral arches, demonstrable by roentgenograms (*spina bifida occulta*). The latter is said to occur in one-quarter of the population. It has been estimated that in approximately 1 of every 900 births there is a serious closure defect in the spine or, more rarely, in the cranium.

Defects of this type may be found at any point along the neuraxis. They are most frequent in the lumbosacral and cranial regions, less so in the cervical, and rare in the thoracic region. The character of the abnormality varies. There may be an outpouching of neural elements (nerve root and cord) through a defect in mesenchymal tissue and skin (*myelomenigocele*); less often, actually in less than one-fifth of all cases, only a thin-walled cyst composed of meninges and containing no neural tissue can be found. The cranial defect similarly may consist of an encephalocele with evagination of cerebral tissue and meninges through a midline defect in the membranous bones of the skull. These are most often occipital in location, though a few may be frontal, presenting either anteriorly or inferiorly into the nasal cavity. Probably the most astonishing cranial defect of all, and one nearly as frequent as the myelomeningocele, is *anencephaly*. In this condition there is a gross defect or absence of the membranous bones of the skull; the cerebral hemispheres and corpus striatum are also absent, and the remainder of the brain is grossly malformed. Patients with severe defects of this type usually do not survive for more than a few hours or days after birth.

Meningocele and Myelomeningocele. Meningocele may exist alone and unaccompanied by any symptoms or signs. Myelomeningocele, in contrast, is associated with some dysfunction of those nervous structures that lie within the wall of the sac. The signs may be minimal, limited to sensorimotor dysfunction of a few segments, or pronounced, with total paraplegia and incontinence of urine and feces.

Sinus Tracts and Congenital Cysts. These are often indicated by a small dimple in the skin or by a tuft of hairs along the posterior surface of the body in the midline. These signs occur most often in the lumbosacral and occipital regions and are thought to represent failure of closure of the anterior or posterior neuropores. (The pilonidal sinus, in the opinion of the authors, should not be included in this group.) Small *sinus tracts* may exist at these points and are of clinical importance because they frequently connect with the central nervous system or its coverings and are not uncommonly associated with dermoid cysts at the central end of the tract. These cysts most often occur in the cerebellum or in the lumbosacral regions, and the sinus tracts which connect them to the skin provide free access for bacteria and are often a source of *abscess* and *recurrent meningitis*. Evidence of such tracts should be sought in every instance of meningitis in children and adolescents, especially when infection has recurred.

There are, in addition, other *congenital cysts* and *tumors* which may produce progressive symptoms and signs by compressing the spinal cord or by implicating nerve roots.

Diastematomyelia. This is another unusual abnormality of the spinal cord. Here a bony spicule or ridge protrudes into the spinal canal from the body of one of the thoracic or upper lumbar vertebras. If the bony abnormality is in the thoracic region, there will be duplication of, or splitting of, the spinal cord (diplomyelia); with growth it leads to a "traction myelopathy." It is of significance only during childhood and will not be discussed further.

All these spinal abnormalities are of particular interest to internists when they begin to produce symptoms for the first time in an adolescent or adult. Several clinical syndromes have been delineated: (1) Progressive spastic weakness of the legs during late childhood or adolescence in a patient known to have had a meningocele or myelomeningocele. Presumably the spinal cord, which is securely attached to the lumbar vertebras, is stretched during the period of rapid lengthening of the vertebral column. (2) An acute cauda equina syndrome following some unusual activity or incident, e.g., rowing or a fall in a sitting position, in patients who have had an asymptomatic or symptomatic spina bifida or meningocele. The implicated sensory and motor roots are believed to be injured by sudden or repeated stretching. Weakness of bladder control, impotence (in the male), numbness of feet and legs, or foot-drop comprise the clinical syndrome. (3) Progressive cauda equina syndrome in the lumbosacral region. (4) Syringomyelia.

Syringomyelia. This term refers to a cavity (Greek *syrinx* meaning "pipe" or "tube"). The cavity occupies the central parts of the spinal cord in the cervical region but may extend upward into the medulla oblongata (syringobulbia) or downward into thoracic or even lumbar segments. In approximately 15 percent of cases studied postmortem, an intramedullary tumor (hemangioblastoma or glioma) has been found in or near some part of the syrinx. The syrinx is independent of the central canal and replaces the gray matter of the posterior or anterior horns of the spinal cord and also interrupts the crossing pain and temperature fibers in the anterior commissure in several successive cord segments. The cavity is lined with astrocytic glia and thick-walled blood vessels. It may enlarge the spinal cord and even widen the interpedicular spaces, but the cerebrospinal fluid in the cavity always has a relatively low protein level. The cause is unknown. Familial incidence is rare. A blastomatous formation akin to tuberous sclerosis or central von Recklinghausen's disease but with tendency for the abnormal tissue to cavitate is one explanation. A hydromyelia, sometimes associated with hydrocephalus, appears more plausible. Elevated pressure of CSF within the spinal canal may widen it, and this condition and the associated bony abnormalities lead to necrosis of the spinal cord and the formation of central cavities.

The clinical triad upon which the diagnosis is based consists of (1) segmental sensory loss or dissociation (loss of pain and temperature sense and preservation of sense of touch) over neck, shoulders, and arms, (2) amyotrophy, and (3) thoracic scoliosis. Symptoms usually begin in late childhood, adolescence, or adult life and progress irregularly, often being arrested for long periods of time. The segmental sensory loss or dissociation and amyotrophy are caused by cavitation of the gray matter of the ventral commissure and anterior horns, respectively. Analgesia and thermanesthesia account for severe painless ulcers, injuries, and burns so often sustained by patients with syringomyelia; Charcot joints, also common in this disease, result from injury of the denervated joint tissue. Areflexia without atrophy may be due to involvement of the afferent limb of the reflex arc; destruction of anterior horn cells is probably the more frequent cause, particularly if accompanied by muscle atrophy. A useful clinical rule is that a neurologic disease which leaves all deep tendon reflexes in the arms intact is probably not syringomyelia. A Horner's syndrome on the affected side may result from involvement of cells of the intermedial lateral cell column of the eighth cervical to first thoracic segments of the spinal cord. Pyramidal tract signs in the legs tend to appear late in the course of the disease and are attributable to extension of the syrinx into the lateral columns of the cord, the decussation of corticospinal tracts at the first cervical segment, or compression of these tracts by a distended syrinx. If the cavity enlarges the spinal cord, a spinal subarachnoid block may result, and prolonged pressure may cause widening of the spinal canal and erosion of pedicles. The kyphoscoliosis, which may antedate other evidence of disease by several years, is thought to result from weakness due to asymmetric involvement of anterior horns in the thoracic region.

A syrinx in the brainstem (syringobulbia) usually extends into the lateral tegmentum of the medulla, being so placed as to result in nystagmus and sensory impairment over one or both sides of the face. Unilateral palatal and vocal cord paralysis as well as weakness and atrophy of one side of the tongue are other clinical signs which call attention to lesions at this level of the neuraxis.

The association of cavitation of the spinal cord with myelomeningocele (so-called "myelodysplasia"), Arnold-Chiari malformation, platybasia, and other congenital defects about the cervicocranial junction has been commented on in previous sections.

The treatment of syringomyelia is unsatisfactory. The fact that the disease process may remain stationary for some months or years before progressing makes evaluation of any mode of therapy difficult. Decompression of a distended syrinx up to the foramen magnum may alleviate temporarily those symptoms and signs resulting from local compression of ascending and descending spinal tracts, but relief is seldom lasting. Reducing the pressure within the cavity by opening it or making a ventriculosubarachnoid shunt has given unpredictable results. The effects of x-ray treatment, based on the belief that symptoms result from a gliomatous malformation of the cord which subsequently cavitates, have been difficult to evaluate. It is worth a trial.

MALFORMATIONS OF THE EXTREMITIES

A variety of primary skeletal defects, such as absence

of or increase in number of digits or extremities, fusion or webbing of digits (syndactylism), and deformity of digits or limbs or abnormalities of size have neurologic import, for they tend to be associated with malformations of the central nervous system. For example, *syndactylism* is frequently combined with oxycephaly (Apert's syndrome). In *mongolism* the fifth digit is usually short and curved (clinodactylia), the hands are broad and simian like, and there is usually only a single transverse crease in the palm. In arachnodactyly the digits are long and tapering, a condition frequently linked to disease of the aorta and congenital heart disease and to dislocation of the lens (cf. Marfan's syndrome, Chap. 395).

Absence of extremities (amelia) has an established relationship to exposure during embryonic life to thalidamide. Shortening of all the extremities with normal growth of the trunk is characteristic of achondroplasia. In gargoylism and Morquio's syndrome both the trunk and the limbs are short and deformed and joint motion is limited. Thus dwarfism may be importantly linked in this condition with a neurologic abnormality, just as it is in cretinism, mongolism, gargoylism, and Morquio's disease. The sufferers from these and several other neurologic diseases in which growth is stunted may be referred to collectively as "amented midgets"; and since many of them reach adult years, they must be treated by general practitioners, internists, and surgeons for other diseases which develop during this age period. The most exciting developments in this field involve some of the disorders of mucopolysaccharide metabolism (see Chap. 399). The internist must be able to distinguish these many types of genetic achondroplasia (Morquio's syndrome, Turner's syndrome, gargoylism, Down's syndrome, Seckel's bird-headed, and other dwarfs with facial and cranial abnormalities) from endocrine dwarfism.

In some cases the deformity of the extremities is the direct consequence of a congenital neuromuscular defect. In fact, this happens so often that whenever deformities of the limbs are known to have begun early in life, one should at once evaluate the status of the nervous system. In most cases of *clubfoot* (talipes equinovarus), no abnormality of the nervous system can be ascertained. In a few, however, the deformity results from paralysis of the anterior tibial and peroneal muscles due to a primary defect in the anterior horn cells of the lumbosacral segments of the spinal cord. The contracture of calf muscles is secondary to their unapposed activity. Widespread weakness and contractures of many limb muscles may cause extensive deformities (*arthrogryposis multiplex* or *amyoplasia congenita*). This syndrome may also be the result of any one of several other primary neural or muscular diseases such as congenital absence of muscles, muscular dystrophy, and rarely may result from infantile motor neurone disease (congenital absence of anterior horn cells and *Werdnig-Hoffmann infantile muscular atrophy*). Reconstructive surgery and the techniques of physical medicine may permit a certain measure of rehabilitation in those patients with nonprogressive diseases. However, severe mental defect, which is frequent in these conditions, tends to discourage elaborate programs of therapy.

BIRTHMARKS AND ASSOCIATED NEUROLOGIC CONDITIONS

A number of neurologic abnormalities are combined with congenital defects of skin or retina, explained usually by their common ectodermal origin. The terms *congenital ectodermal dysplasias, congenital neurocutaneous syndromes,* or *phacomatoses* (Greek *phakos,* lentil mole or freckle) are used frequently to designate this general class of disorders. The major syndromes include *neurofibromatosis, tuberous sclerosis, encephalotrigeminal syndrome,* and rarely the *cerebelloretinal hemangioblastomatosis.* Another variant of the latter is the *myelocutaneous* (Klippel-Trelauney) *syndrome,* in which a vascular malformation of spinal cord and meninges is associated with a vascular nevus within the area of skin innervated by the involved spinal segments. Recently it has been suggested that *ataxia telangiectasia* be included with this group of conditions.

NEUROFIBROMATOSIS (VON RECKLINGHAUSEN'S DISEASE). This is an inherited disease (mendelian dominant) in which spots of increased skin pigmentation are combined with multiple neurofibromas. The pigmented spots are irregular in shape with relatively even borders, vary in size from a few millimeters to several centimeters, and are of brownish-coffee color (*café-au-lait*). They are most prominent over the trunk, in the axillae (axillary freckles) and about the pelvis. Similar lesions occur in individuals without neurofibromatosis but in such instances are generally smaller than 2 cm in diameter and fewer than 5 in number. The tumors arise from the neurilemmal sheath (Schwann cells) and fibroblasts of the peripheral nerve. They are usually multiple and vary in size from minute lesions to large tumors several centimeters in diameter. The majority are smoothly rounded or lobulated, soft or firm, and can sometimes be seen or felt along the course of a peripheral nerve. Often they sink into the subcutaneous fat on gentle pressure. Like the pigmented lesions, the tumors are more frequent over the trunk than on the extremities. The pigmented areas, due to giant melanosomes in pigment epithelial cells, become increasingly apparent with age; the tumors of nerve sheaths are often not demonstrable early in life. Most of the tumors in neurofibromatosis are asymptomatic; but occasionally, if they attain a large size or occupy an unusual position, they may produce symptoms by pressing upon contiguous structures. Tumors of the spinal nerve roots may compress the spinal cord and at the same time extend through the intervertebral foramens to form a large mass in the posterior mediastinum (dumbbell tumors). Acoustic neurinomas, usually bilateral in patients with neurofibromatosis, may produce deafness and symptoms and signs of a cerebellopontine angle tumor. Other histopathologic types of tumor (meningioma, glioma) are encountered more frequently in neurofibromatosis than in the general population. Diffuse overgrowth of Schwann cells and fibroblasts may also occur giving rise to plexiform neuromas. They may cause hideous deformities often with overgrowth of underlying bone. Bone cysts may also form. Most of these tumors are rare in infancy and childhood, though pontine glioma and glioma of the optic nerve are exceptions to this clinical rule. The latter condition should always be considered in the differential diagnosis of unilateral (rarely bilateral) blindness, proptosis, and extraocular muscle paralysis in childhood, especially if there are signs of von Recklinghausen's disease. Enlargement of the optic foramens, demonstrable by roentgenogram, is a valuable aid in diagnosis. Pulsating exophthalmos may result from congenital absence of part of the sphenoid bone. Pheochromocytoma is an infrequent accompaniment of the disease. In about 5 to 10 percent of cases of neurofibromatosis one of the tumors will become sarcomatous.

Fibrous dysplasia, congenital vertebral anomalies, local gigantism of an extremity, subperiosteal bone cysts, and pseudoarthrosis of the tibia may be associated with neurofibromatosis. Any of these can lead to scoliosis, a common skeletal deformity in children with this disease, so that neurofibromatosis must be added to the list of neurogenic kyphoscolioses (the others are syringomyelia, Friedreich's ataxia, and poliomyelitis). Stenosis of the aqueduct with obstructive hydrocephalus is at times observed in neurofibromatosis. Mental retardation is common in families with von Recklinghausen's disease. This has recently been related to developmental abnormalities of the cerebral cortex. Spina bifida, hypospadias, glaucoma, and elephantiasis are occasionally seen.

About one-third of cases of neurofibromatosis are discovered accidentally on routine examination, there being no complaints. Another third come seeking advice about the cosmetic aspects of the disease and the remainder present with neurologic syndromes. There is no treatment for the disease other than excision of symptomatic tumors.

TUBEROUS SCLEROSIS (BOURNEVILLE'S DISEASE). This curious disease, of dominant inheritance, is manifested by the clinical triad of convulsive seizures, progressive mental deficiency, and adenoma sebaceum. The latter are fine, wartlike lesions predominantly in a butterfly distribution over the cheeks and forehead. The individual adenomas vary in size from 0.1 to 1.0 cm and are elevated and pinkish or pinkish-yellow in color. In addition, the skin over the lower back may be thick, rough, and of yellowish color (sharkskin patch, shagreen). Actually the earliest lesions are foliate light spots ("white spots") over the trunk, which are seen most clearly under ultraviolet light (Wood's lamp). If distinguished from avascular nevi and vitiligo, they are highly diagnostic and may provide the earliest clue to mental retardation or infantile epilepsy. The mental deficiency may be relatively stationary or progressive. The seizures are usually generalized but may be focal. Retinal tumors, optic atrophy, cataracts and hyperoncomas, syndactylism, spina bifida, and other visible malformations may be conjoined.

The lesions of the skin are pathologically fibromas and not true adenomas. Some are rather vascular and suggest telangiectasia. The brain lesions consist of areas of malformed cortex with extensive astrogliosis and a curious mixture of glioblasts and monster nerve cells. Calcification may or may not be present. Masses of subependymal glial tissue account for nodules which project into and form the "candle gutterings" on the walls of the ventricles that are often seen in pneumograms. In Bourneville's original case, death was due to rhabdomyoma of the heart. This lesion has been combined in some cases with vascular malformations of kidney, liver, adrenal glands, and pancreas.

The diagnosis is aided by roentgenograms of the skull. Calcified nodules occur particularly in the temporal lobe. The center of the nodule tends to be more densely radiopaque than the periphery. The electroencephalogram is usually abnormal but without specific pattern. The cerebrospinal fluid may be normal; rarely the total protein level is elevated.

The only treatment is symptomatic. The prognosis for life beyond the third decade is poor. Death may be due to seizures, associated tumors or intercurrent diseases.

CEREBELLORETINAL HEMANGIOBLASTOMATOSIS (LINDAU'S AND VON HIPPEL'S DISEASE). This condition is discussed here though the skin is seldom involved. As the name implies, the syndrome consists of a vascular malformation of the retina and cerebellum. The retinal lesion usually has the characteristics of a malformation; the cerebellar lesion consists of a slowly growing cystic tumor. The clinical symptoms and signs consist of progressive cerebellar ataxia, headache, and papilledema. Polycythemia, possibly related to the production of erythropoitin, has been observed in many cases and has in a few instances disappeared after excision of the tumor. Rarely do these tumors appear before adolescence. Some cases are familial.

This condition is often associated with malformation of other organs, especially with visceral tumors. Angiomas of the liver, cysts of the pancreas and kidneys, and tumors of the epididymis and kidney, which have been the cause of death in some cases, are the major parts of the syndrome. Pheochromocytomas have been described in this and in other of the phakomatoses. Syringomyelia has been observed in a few cases, and if a careful search is made, a hemangioblastoma can often be found in relation to the syrinx at some level.

The cerebellar hemangioblastoma demands surgical treatment, and if the nodule of tumor is found in the wall of the cyst and is excised, the results can be excellent; if inoperable, X-radiation should be tried.

ENCEPHALOTRIGEMINAL SYNDROME (STURGE-WEBER-DIMITRI DISEASE). This curious disease consists of capillary or cavernous hemangiomas within the cutaneous distribution of the trigeminal nerve and of a predominantly venous hemangioma of the leptomeninges. If the skin lesion is within the area of supply of the ophthalmic division of the trigeminal nerve, the occipital lobes are more commonly involved, whereas a facial nevus is more often associated with involvement of the parietal and frontal lobes. The intracranial or cutaneous lesion may occur separately.

Pathologically, in addition to the large number of abnormal blood vessels in the meninges, the cortex is destroyed, and in some cases a band of calcium develops within the lesion. This band, following the convolutional pattern as it does, is responsible for the characteristic roentgenographic picture.

The first neurologic symptom is usually a focal seizure on the side opposite the skin lesion. Transient postictal (Todd's) paralysis or permanent paralysis may follow the seizure. Sensorimotor paralysis or permanent visual field defect, the most frequent findings, may be either of insidious onset with slow progression or apoplectic. Hemorrhage into the meninges has been reported, but this must be a rare event. Possibly occlusion of cortical vessels will, in certain instances, be responsible for neurologic deficits. Blindness in the eye on the side of the nevus is frequent and is nearly always due to glaucoma. Most patients with this malformation survive for many years, often with residual mental and other neurologic defects.

The lesions are usually too extensive to be treated surgically, though hemispherectomy has been advised by some surgeons. Anticonvulsant medication is indicated, but the seizures may be difficult to control.

Hemangioma of trunk or upper or lower extremity may be associated with a spinal cord vascular malformation. The extremity may be hypertrophied. The cord lesion may bleed or infarct the nervous tissue producing a sensorimotor paralysis.

ATAXIA TELANGIECTASIA. Only recognized as a disease entity recently, this condition has attracted considerable interest. Inherited as a recessive trait, the disease is characterized neurologically by a progressive cerebellar ataxia, apraxia of ocular movement, and choreoathetosis beginning during the early years of life. Telangiectasis of bulbar conjunctivas and skin, especially about the ears, neck, and in flexor creases at the elbows and knees, appear somewhat later. Recurring pulmonary and sinus infections have been prominent in many cases, and a deficiency in the IgA globulins and defective delayed hypersensitivity are found. The associated pathologic changes consist of an extensive loss of Purkinje cells of the cerebellum and degeneration of neurones in other parts of the basal ganglia. The changes in the latter and in the spinal nerves have not been adequately characterized. Dysplasia of the thymus has been well documented, and death usually occurs by the second or third decade of life from infection or a reticuloendothelial tumor.

Abnormalities of Motor Function (Cerebral Palsy)

In this category of neurologic defect a major disturbance of motor function, usually nonprogressive, has been present since infancy or childhood. The popular term for these conditions is *cerebral palsy*. The name is not altogether appropriate, nor is such a crude classification of nervous disorders particularly useful from the viewpoint of the physician, because it results in a collocation of diseases of widely differing etiologic and anatomic types. The hereditary and acquired, the intrauterine, natal, and postnatal diseases lose their identity. Nevertheless, the term has been adopted as a slogan for fund-raising societies and for a major rehabilitation movement throughout the United States, and it will not soon disappear from medical terminology.

CLINICAL APPROACH TO MOTOR DISTURBANCES WHICH HAVE DEVELOPED IN INFANCY OR CHILDHOOD

Motor abnormalities which have their onset early in life are so numerous and diverse that it is necessary to acquire some knowledge of the motor system in order to interpret them. It is helpful to attempt to categorize a given case according to the extent and nature of the abnormality.

These motor abnormalities of infancy and childhood are relatively frequent, and many of the affected children reach adult years.

SPECIAL TYPES

INFANTILE SPASTIC AND RIGID PARALYSES. The pattern of paralysis or rigidity is important, for it provides information as to the etiology and possible pathogenetic mechanism.

Cerebral Spastic Diplegia (Little's Disease). In 1862 Little called attention to the concurrence of "Abnormal Parturition, Difficult Labours, Premature Birth, and Asphyxia Neonatorum" and of a spastic weakness that affected legs more than arms. He emphasized the prenatal or natal origin, the diplegic (legs more than arms) distribution of the paralysis, and the nonprogressive course. Little was of the opinion that asphyxia caused the cerebral damage, but the present view is that it represents a syndrome of multiple causes and of diverse pathology.

S. A. K. Wilson distinguishes three types: the paraplegic, diplegic, and the generalized and pseudobulbar. These differ from one another only in respect to the severity of affection of the arms and bulbar musculature. Pure paraplegias and pure pseudobulbar cases are relatively rare. Usually all four extremities are involved, the legs much more than the arms. As a rule the nervous system damage is recognized at birth or soon thereafter by some abnormality of breathing, sucking and swallowing, color of mucous membranes, or responsiveness. These latter signs may indicate either a congenital defect of the nervous system or birth injury. The stiff, awkward movements of the legs, maintained in an extended, adducted posture, attract attention at this time or in the ensuing weeks. Seizures occur in some cases, and it is not uncommon to observe a delay in all the normal developmental sequences, especially those which depend on the motor system. Once walking is attempted, the characteristic stance and gait become manifest. The legs are advanced stiffly in short steps, each describing part of the arc of a circle; adduction is often so strong as to lead to actual crossing (scissors gait) with lower legs slightly splayed out and the feet flexed and turned in, the heels no longer touching the ground. The legs tend to be short and small, but the muscles are not markedly atrophic, as

in infantile muscular atrophy and dystrophy. Passive manipulation of the limbs reveals marked spasticity in the extensors and adductors and also slight shortening of calf muscles. The hands and arms may be little if at all affected, but in many cases there is awkwardness and stiffness of the fingers and in a few, pronounced weakness and spasticity. Speech may be well articulated or noticeably slurred, and often the face is set in a spastic smile. The deep tendon reflexes are exaggerated, those in the legs more than in the arms, and the plantar reflexes are extensor. Usually there is no disturbance of sphincteric function, though delay in acquiring voluntary function is usual. Athetotic postures and movements of the face, tongue, and hands are present in some cases and may actually conceal the pyramidal weakness. Ataxic and hypotonic forms also exist. The mentality ranges from normal to idiocy.

Surprisingly little information has been obtained concerning the cause, mechanism, and morbid anatomy of this syndrome. Most of the children are full term, but a higher incidence of spastic diplegia is known to be associated with prematurity. Only exceptionally are the Apgar scores of vital function in the first minutes and hours after birth reduced. The claim that physical birth injury is responsible has been challenged, and the existence of an antenatal lesion in some cases can no longer be doubted. Clinical study is handicapped by the fact that some of the infarcts of the cerebral cortex and white matter may occur in utero when the fetus cannot be tested, and the possibility of silent injuries to the nonfunctioning cerebrum.

INFANTILE HEMIPLEGIA. In this not uncommon condition of infancy and childhood, a functional difference between the two sides may be noticed at birth or during the first 6 to 12 months of life. Acquired forms following an infection or thrombosis of cerebral arteries or veins usually develop later. The parents may be the first to notice that movements of prehension and exploration are carried out with only one arm. The affection of the leg is usually recognized later, i.e., during the first attempt to walk.

Mental defect may be associated with infantile hemiplegia but is much more common with cerebral diplegia and with bilateral hemiplegia. Convulsions occur in 35 to 50 percent of children with congenital hemiplegia. They may commence at any time of life but more often in infancy or early childhood, if the disease was congenital. If the hemiplegia was acquired during infancy, seizures often accompany the onset. They may be generalized but are frequently unilateral and limited to the hemiplegic side. Often, after a series of seizures, the affected side will be weak for several hours or longer (Todd's paralysis).

Double Hemiplegia. This term is applied to bilateral weakness of face, arms, and legs. The arms are severely affected, in contrast to their minimal affection in cerebral diplegia.

Quadriplegic States. Differing from bilateral hemiplegias in that the bulbar musculature is not involved, this condition is relatively rare but may result from a bilateral cerebral lesion. However, a spastic quadriplegia should always alert one to the possibility of a high cervical cord lesion. Although this may occasionally result from cysts, tumors, and other malformations, it is usually produced in the infant by a fracture-dislocation of the cervical spine, incurred during a difficult breech delivery.

Similarly in *paraplegia* with weakness or paralysis limited to the legs, the lesion may be cerebral or spinal. Sphincter disturbances and a definite loss of somatic sensation below a certain level on the trunk should always favor a spinal localization. Congenital cysts, tumors, and diastematomyelia are more frequently found in cases of paraplegia than of quadriplegia.

The *etiology, pathogenesis,* and *morbid anatomy* of infantile cerebral hemiplegia, bilateral hemiplegia, and quadriplegia are not well understood. Birth injury has been invoked as a leading cause, and there is no doubt that prolonged labor, delay in breathing, bulging fontanel, bloody cerebrospinal fluid, and periods of apnea and cyanosis occur with greater frequency in a series of hemiplegic infants than in any other group of infants. Also birth injury is more frequent in hemiplegic than in diplegic cases. The mechanism of the injury is not known.

CONGENITAL EXTRAPYRAMIDAL SYNDROMES IN INFANCY AND CHILDHOOD. The spastic and rigid cerebral diplegias discussed above shade almost imperceptibly into the extrapyramidal syndromes. Many such cases can be found in every cerebral palsy clinic, and they appear from time to time in adult medical clinics. Pyramidal tract signs may be completely absent, and the inexperienced student, familiar only with the pure cerebral spastic diplegia syndrome, is always puzzled as to their classification. Some extrapyramidal cases of this type undoubtedly are attributable to the same pathologic processes as cerebral spastic diplegia and attest to the diverse clinical manifestations of these states; others represent separate diseases such as erythroblastosis fetalis with kernicterus. In the interest of being able to state accurately the probable pathologic basis and future course of these illnesses, it is desirable to separate the extrapyramidal syndromes due to prenatal and natal diseases, which usually become manifest during the first year of life, from the acquired postnatal syndromes such as familial athetosis, dystonia musculorum deformans, and cerebellar ataxia. The latter have been discussed in Chap. 364, Degenerative Diseases of the Nervous System.

Congenital Choreoathetosis (Double Athetosis). Probably the most frequent representative of this group, this condition is like the spastic states in that it may not be recognized at birth but only after several months have elapsed. The nature of chorea and athetosis has been discussed in Chap. 22, Tremor, Chorea, and Other Abnormalities of Movement and Posture. All combinations of chorea, athetosis, hemiballismus, and even dystonia may be found in a single case, or one or another type of movement disorder may predominate. However, in all instances there is a defect in voluntary movement.

Choreoathetosis in infants and children varies in severity. In some the disorder is so mild that the abnormal movements are misinterpreted as restlessness or the "fidgets"; in others every voluntary act is rendered ineffective by these involuntary movements, leaving the patient nearly helpless. The tongue may extrude itself from the mouth with constant drooling, and the face is contorted in a never-ending series of grimaces. Speech is slurred, inarticulate, and punctuated by grunts and unpleasant throat sounds. The hands and arms are engaged in a constant play of writhing, twisting movements, and all attempts to use the limbs result in a slow, spreading spasm of the entire limb or all the musculature (intention spasm). Bizarre postures may be assumed. The arms may be carried in a flexed or extended position in front of or behind the body, and the legs may be extended. The feet may be deformed; walking on the heels or side of the foot is more common than the "toe walking" of the cerebral diplegic. Movements may also be ataxic, and tremors are not uncommon. A retardation of motor development is the rule in these cases. Upright posture and walking may, in fact, never be acquired or may be delayed until the age of three to five years in severe cases; only in the most severe cases is locomotion impossible. Tonic neck reflexes or fragments thereof are commonly noted. The tendon reflexes are not consistently abnormal; plantar reflexes are characteristically flexor, though they may be difficult to interpret because of the continuous play of flexion and extension of the toes. The various sensory pathways usually function normally.

It is because of the motor and speech impairment that patients are many times erroneously classified as mentally defective. No doubt in some patients this evaluation is correct, but others retain adequate intellectual function and can be educated. With growth and development new postures and new motor capacities are acquired. The less severely affected patients can make successful occupational adjustments. However, the severely handicapped patients, even with the help of rehabilitation clinics and corrective orthopedic operations, rarely achieve a degree of motor control that will permit them to lead an independent existence. One sees these unfortunate individuals in public places bobbing and weaving as they walk along.

The most frequently observed pathologic change in the brain has been a curious whitish, marblelike appearance of the shrunken putamen, thalamus, and cerebral cortex. These whitish strands represent foci of nerve cell destruction and gliosis with a peculiar condensation or formation of myelinated fibers (hypermyelination). Oscar and Cecile Vogt, who first described this condition, called it *état marbré* or *status marmoratus*. They attributed it to neonatal asphyxia, but the hypoxic factor is far from established.

The *neurologic sequelae of kernicterus* are of importance here and are encountered not infrequently in adults. It is true that the majority of infants who suffer this disease die within the first week or two of life, and those who survive are mentally retarded, deaf, and totally unable to sit, stand, or walk, so that the tendency is always to put them in homes for the feebleminded. It is only the exceptional patient, obviously less damaged, who is mentally normal or at most only slightly backward. These are the ones who exhibit a variety of motor disorders as they grow older, the most frequent being mild ataxia or choreoathetosis, which involves the face and arms. A few have also shown rigid limbs and a picture not too different from that of cerebral spastic diplegia with involuntary movements. Kernicterus should always be suspected if an extrapyramidal syndrome is accompanied by bilateral deafness and ocular palsies. The neuropathology in these milder surviving cases consists of nerve cell loss and gliosis in the subthalamic nucleus of Luys, the globus pallidus, thalamus, and oculomotor and cochlear nuclei. No one explanation of the neurologic lesion has been accepted. Elsewhere we have postulated severe liver damage and hyperbilirubinemia as a cause of the brain disease, but this hypothesis is unproved. Others attribute the brain damage to hypoxia.

CONGENITAL ATAXIA. The combination of cerebral diplegia with cerebellar ataxia has already been mentioned. In these patients difficulty in standing and walking cannot be attributed to spasticity or paralysis. Incoordination similar to that seen in cerebellar disease and hypotonia are the principal findings. The motor defect may be so great that the child is never able to sit or stand; the muscles are of normal size, and voluntary movements, though weak, are possible in all the limbs. In less severe cases sitting, standing, and walking are merely delayed, and with advancing years cerebellar ataxia and tremor become manifest. Relative improvement may occur as the child grows older. The tendon reflexes are present and the plantar reflexes are either flexor or extensor. Many of these patients suffer a degree of amentia and retardation of speech development that results in their placement in homes for the feebleminded. In relatively few of the recorded cases have the pathologic changes of this condition been studied. Aplasia or hypoplasia of the cerebellum has been reported only a few times. Radiation of the abdomen of a parturient woman during the first trimester of pregnancy is said to have resulted in cerebellar hypoplasia in a few cases. A cerebral and cerebellar lesion may coexist with congenital ataxia which is the reason for its classification as cerebrocerebellar diplegia.

Aside from the congenital ataxias, some of which are cerebellar and others probably of cerebral type, there are other forms of childhood ataxia which have an acute onset and which persist during adolescence and adult life. Batten has written informatively on this subject, calling those forms the acute cerebellar ataxias of childhood. Some are sequelae of an infection (a postinfectious encephalitis, especially postvaricella), and a few may be due to virus infections which affect the cerebellum more than other parts of the nervous system. Hyperthermia, with temperatures over 106°F, may result in extensive destruction of Purkinje cells and ataxia. Some of these patients with cerebellar ataxia have other more prominent neurologic disturbances such as opsoclonus, lightning-like jerks of eyes, and trunkal myoclonus (see Chap. 22). This syndrome may occur as an infectious "encephalitis" or without explanation. In the latter instance the motor disorder may be permanent. ACTH, surprisingly, may suppress the jerks. Cerebellar tumors and demyelinative and lipid storage diseases also occur at this age and may at times give rise to a more slowly evolving cerebellar ataxia. Labyrinthine injury resulting from streptomycin therapy and polyneuritis or mumps are the common causes of noncerebellar ataxia, which must be differentiated from the above condition.

The hereditary ataxias are likely to begin at a later age and are progressive. They are discussed in Chap. 364.

In all these congenital diseases of the brain, once the symptoms and signs are well established, there is no progression of the illness. In fact, with further maturation and training there may be improvement. The clinical course thus distinguishes this whole group of diseases from those of delayed onset and progressive course (see Schilder's disease, lipid storage diseases, congenital neurosyphilis, and toxoplasmosis).

THE FLACCID PARALYSES OF INFANCY AND CHILDHOOD. The cerebral form, first described by Foerster and called *cerebral atonic diplegia*, has already been mentioned in connection with congenital cerebellar ataxia. It can usually be distinguished from spinal and peripheral nerve paralysis by the retention of postural reflexes (flexion of the legs at the knee and hip when the patient is lifted by placing the hands in the axillae), the preservation of tendon reflexes, and the failure of mental development.

The syndrome of *infantile muscular atrophy* (Werdnig-Hoffmann disease) is the leading example of the category of infantile spinal muscular atrophies. These little patients are usually brought to the clinic by their parents because of a difficulty with feeding and a delay of motor development. About half of them are said to have been normal at birth and during the first weeks of life. Others have been slack, feeble infants from the day they were born and even before, since some mothers recall a weakness also of fetal movement. Slowness in feeding, frequent choking, constant drooling, recurrent respiratory infections due to weak respiratory movements, and aspiration of milk are troublesome in early life. As a rule, the patient prefers a supine posture; his motor deficit is manifested by an inability to maintain the head in stable balance and also by the absence of the usual movements of the trunk. The arms tend to be kept at the sides and flexed at the elbows, bringing the hands over the chest. The legs are characteristically abducted and flexed at the hips and knees so that the soles of the feet oppose one another ("frog posture"). When the infant is pulled to a sitting position, the head lolls and all but the most feeble support reactions in the legs are absent. Despite this profound weakness, all muscle groups are capable of feeble movement until late in the course of the illness. The tendon reflexes are invariably absent in those cases in which the disease begins before birth or during the early months of life. Rarely the tendon reflexes may be preserved, if the disease has an onset at a later age. A remarkable action tremor of the arms may then be observed. Atrophy of muscle is obscured by subcutaneous fat tissues ("puppy fat"), and fascicular twitches, though detectable in an electromyogram, are invisible to the naked eye except in the tongue. In contrast to their feeble movements, these patients usually are attractive, with bright, sparkling eyes and lively countenance, which attest to normal brain development. All sensory functions are likewise retained. The illness progresses slowly over a period of months or a few years, and few of these patients survive until puberty. Several members of a sibship may suffer the same illness, but the antecedents do not, the pattern of inheritance usually being autosomal recessive. In biopsy material or at autopsy the muscles are thin and the majority of their fibers are atrophic, preserving their fetal dimensions as though improperly innervated or denervated. The anterior horn cells in the spinal cord and brainstem have disappeared or are in process of degenerating and are replaced by fibrous astrocytes. There is no known treatment for the disease.

Of interest in internal medicine has been the discovery that milder forms of familial progressive motor system disease may begin in later childhood, adolescence, or adult life and their advance is more slow. Spasticity, indicative of pyramidal tract involvement, is a feature of some of them. These cases must be distinguished from the acquired forms of motor system disease (see Chaps. 21 and 364).

A few patients suspected of having infantile muscular atrophy prove with the passage of time to be merely rather inactive, "slack" children, and motor development occurs later but at a slower rate. A few may remain rather weak with thin musculature. Such cases fall into the vague category of *amyotonia congenita* described by Oppenheim, Brandt, and others, or into the group called *benign congenital hypotonia* (Walton) or *benign congenital myopathy* (Turner). Most recently Shy and his associates have found several other myopathologic changes in certain families; they have called these "central core disease" and "rod-body myopathy," pleoconial and megaconial and myotubular myopathies (see Chap. 376). Probably other types of myopathy will also be discovered as causes of this syndrome of congenital hypotonia. Muscle biopsy reveals a definite abnormality in only a few of the cases, and the electromyogram is often normal. Polymyositis and acute idiopathic polyneuritis may rarely manifest themselves as a syndrome of amyotonia congenita.

Infantile muscular dystrophy and lipid and glycogen storage diseases may also produce a clinical picture of progressive atrophy and enfeeblement of muscles. The diagnosis of *glycogen storage* disease (the Pompé form of the original von Gierke's disease) should be entertained when the syndrome of infantile muscular atrophy is associated with clinical enlargement of heart, liver, or spleen. The motor disturbance in this condition may be related in some way to the abnormal deposits of glycogen found in skeletal muscle, though it is more likely due to the degeneration of the anterior horn cells of the spinal cord, which are distended with glycogen and

other substances. Lipid storage disease of *Tay-Sachs* and the variants which occur later in life may also cause thinness of limb musculature, feebleness of movement, and diminution or loss of tendon reflexes. Regression of mental development, blindness, and macular degeneration, which are almost always present to some degree, should leave little doubt as to the nature of the illness. Also muscular dystrophy, either familial or nonfamilial, may begin during fetal life or during infancy and childhood. There is obvious palsy of the limbs, with proximal and trunk muscles more involved than distal ones. Contractures are frequent, with a leg or arm held in a curious abducted or extended posture. This state of contracture of the limbs in infants is called *arthrogryposis,* already referred to above, under Malformations of the Extremities. It may be caused by either a primary muscular disease or a defect of the central nervous system.

Brachial plexus palsies, well-known complications of dystocia, usually result from forcible extraction of the fetus by downward traction on the shoulder in a breech presentation, or from traction and tipping of the head in a shoulder presentation. The effects of such injuries are lifelong, and their early onset in adults is betrayed by the inadequate osseous development of the affected limb. The upper brachial plexus and roots of the fifth cervical or the lower plexus and roots of the seventh and eighth cervical and first thoracic nerves suffer the brunt of the injury. Sometimes the entire plexus is involved. The upper plexus injuries (*Erb's plexus syndrome*) are estimated to be twenty times more frequent than lower (*Klumpke's plexus syndrome*), according to Ford, who has examined more than 200 cases of this type (see Chap. 354).

Facial paralysis, due to injury of the facial nerve immediately distal to its exit from the stylomastoid foramen by the application of forceps, is another common peripheral nerve affection in the newborn. The failure of one eye to close and the difficulty in suckling make this condition easy to recognize. It must be distinguished from congenital facial paralysis or facial diplegia usually with weakness of the abducens muscles (*Moebius's syndrome*). In most cases of facial paralysis function is recovered after a few weeks; in some the paralysis is permanent and may account for an asymmetry observed in later life (see Chap. 355).

The Retarded Child or Adult (Feeblemindedness)

Mental retardation has been commented upon in the discussion of many of the craniospinal malformations and in the several varieties of cerebral palsy. However, it may also occur as the only neurologic abnormality and must therefore be discussed separately.

To the pediatrician the clinical problem of mental retardation is one of the most difficult, and to the parents it is one of the most dreadful of all conditions. The intelligent father and mother are alert to every sign of possible brain injury, and often they become alarmed about trivial deviations from their standard of normal development. Slowness in sitting, standing, walking, delay in speech, or difficulty in accomplishing toilet training may be seized upon as an indication of feeblemindedness, and indeed, they often are. The internist and general physician are apt to see only the milder noninstitutionalized patients who reach adolescence and adult years and then develop other diseases. It is also noteworthy that the majority of individuals now residing in institutions for the care of the feebleminded are of adult age.

The primary responsibility of the physician in cases of this type is to determine whether there is unmistakable evidence of maldevelopment or some ongoing disease of

Table 365-1. CLINICAL CLASSIFICATION OF THE VARIETIES OF NONPROGRESSIVE MENTAL RETARDATION

I. Mental defect with associated developmental abnormalities in nonnervous structures
    A. Those affecting cranioskeletal structures
        1. Microcephaly   6. Gargoylism
        2. Macrocephaly   7. Mongolian idiocy
        3. Hydrocephalus   8. Cretinism
        4. Craniostenosis   9. Cleidocranial dysostosis
        5. Morquio's disease 10. Achondroplasia
    B. Those affecting nonskeletal structures
        1. Phacomatoses (tuberous sclerosis, von Recklinghausen's disease, Sturge-Weber syndrome, etc.)
        2. Gonadal dysgenesis (Turner syndrome)
        3. Klinefelter's syndrome
        4. Myotonic dystrophy
        5. Ectodermal dysplasia
        6. Congenital heart disease
        7. Deafness and congenital heart disease following maternal rubella
II. Mental defect without developmental anomalies in nonnervous structures, but with focal cerebral and other neurologic abnormalities[1]
    A. Cerebral spastic diplegia with or without involuntary movements (rarely associated ichthyosis)
    B. Cerebral hemiplegia, unilateral or bilateral
    C. Congenital choreoathetosis or ataxia
        1. Kernicterus
        2. Status marmoratus (hypoxia?)
    D. Congenital atonic diplegia
    E. Rarely with other inherited neuromuscular abnormalities (muscular dystrophy, Friedreich's ataxia, etc.)
III. Mental defect without signs of other developmental abnormality or neurologic disorder
    A. Simple mental retardation
    B. Kernicterus (some cases)
    C. Hypoxia (some cases)
    D. Heller's disease, variably progressive, may affect nonnervous structures
    E. Mental defect associated with inborn errors of metabolism (e.g., galactosemia, phenylketonuria, hypothyroidism, maple syrup urine disease, etc.) (See p. 1810)
    F. Congenital infections (e.g., cytomegalic inclusion disease, syphilis, toxoplasmosis, etc.)

[1]A number of progressive neurologic diseases—chronic subdural hematoma, lipidoses, and cerebral scleroses—may be confused with these static defects.

the brain. Difficulties relating to the uncertainty in evaluating cerebral function during early infancy have already been discussed. From experience one learns that successive examinations, over a period of months or years, may be required in order to evaluate the infant's or child's capacity for mental development. Above all, the physician should not permit himself to be forced into a hasty or premature judgment. Deafness, blindness, congenital speech defects (word deafness and word blindness), and motor defects must be searched for with particular care, for they may account for an apparent delay in mental development by interfering with the learning processes. Emotional privation and neglect may also lead to some degree of backwardness. It is now known, however, that mental retardation of significant degree cannot be explained in this way (see Chap. 7).

The student confronted with a backward infant is likely to be rather bewildered by the vast array of developmental abnormalities and diseases which may affect the brain at an early age and prevent normal mental development. There are more than 150 of them. It becomes necessary to acquire a way of thinking about these problems. The authors' bedside approach has been to attempt to categorize each case according to the scheme presented in Table 365-1. This can be done by obtaining the necessary clinical data—a careful history, in order to determine whether or not the condition is progressive, and a physical examination in which one searches for evidences of cranial, skeletal, ectodermal, cardiac, and other developmental abnormalities. Once a case is categorized, it is less difficult to decide which of several diseases is present.

CLINICAL CHARACTERISTICS. As an aid to the general physician who must undertake the diagnosis and management of backward children, the following comments may be of some value. Mental retardation manifests itself most obviously in the spheres of motor, language, social, and intellectual development. The severely retarded child at idiot level with an intelligence quotient (IQ) of less than 20 and unable to look after himself often does not sit up, walk, or stand, and if any one of these motor activities is acquired, it appears late and is imperfectly performed. Language is not mastered, or at most only a few words are understood and uttered. The patient is continuously idle and can only vocalize in meaningless ways. He does not engage with people and objects around him nor does he make known his needs for water, food, excretion, etc. He does nothing for himself and exhibits only primitive emotional reactions. Physical growth is usually retarded; nutrition may be poor, and susceptibility to respiratory infections is common. Sphincteric control may never be accomplished. A variety of physical deformities are common in this group, and they always suggest that the brain disease began in the antenatal period, because of either a genetic disorder or a disease which occurred during the first 12 weeks of pregnancy. Affections of the nervous system which have their onset later in life are usually not attended by bodily disfigurement.

If the mental defect is less pronounced, with the IQ 20

to 50 (i.e., imbecile), or 50 to 70 (i.e., moron), and if specific motor defects do not coexist, then sitting, walking, and speech are acquired but only after a delay, in many cases. The existence of a cerebral defect may be noted for the first time when the child fails to speak normally during the second and third years of life and seems not to be able to learn the usual household tasks and play activities as well as other children. However, delay in language development must not by itself be taken as a mark of mental retardation, for many bright children who are obviously intelligent and who show remarkable talent in communicating by gesture are slow in talking. Toilet training also may be difficult to accomplish in the retarded child, but again it may be delayed in an otherwise normal child because of incorrect parental attitudes and emotional problems. The appearance of these retarded children is revealing, for many have a dull, apathetic appearance, and their motor activity may be either reduced or excessive. Some are very docile and affectionate; others display a curious inquisitiveness, irritability, and destructiveness. The most extreme degree of this overactivity is seen in the patient with "organic driveness," a term introduced by Eugene Kahn to designate the incessantly moving, incorrigible child who strikes at or bites every person or object which thwarts him in any way and who demolishes every object which he can reach. Some of these children seem strangely impervious to injury, and neither reward nor punishment influences them. This organic driveness is perhaps more commonly observed in acquired postnatal encephalitis than with congenital diseases. Rhythmic rocking, rolling, head banging, and bouncing movements are common in retarded children and may be performed hour after hour, often to the accompaniment of bleating sounds, squeals, and other ejaculations. Here the abnormality is not the appearance of rhythmic movements of the body, which are observed at one period in the development of many normal children, but their persistence. Music may encourage rhythmic movement and gives pleasure to many retarded children.

The least severely retarded child (IQ 50 to 70) grows and develops in many ways not different from normal, and he can be taught useful occupational skills. A few of these persons can work under careful supervision. All scholastic pursuits are relatively unsuccessful, and vocational training is of more value than other types of education.

SPECIAL VARIETIES OF MENTAL RETARDATION. Several of the special types of mental retardation are being discussed in this and other chapters (see Lipidoses and Cerebral Sclerosis, in Chap. 113). In the following pages are presented only those with special features.

Mongolism (Down's Syndrome). This is a unique condition, and although accounting for only about 1 percent of all mental defectives, it is the reason for one-third to one-half the admissions to state schools. Mental retardation which varies from mild to severe, a curious facial configuration, and a dwarfed physical stature constitute a clinical triad. Many of the stigmas of mongolism can be recognized in the neonatal period. The head tends

to be small and oval, with the forehead sloping. The ears are set low on the scalp and are oval with small lobules. The eyes slant slightly upward and outward owing to the presence of an epicanthal fold, which covers the medial angle of the palpebral fissure. The bridge of the nose is generally absent or poorly developed, and the crest of the nose is small. The mouth tends to hang open, and the tongue is usually enlarged, heavily fissured, and protruding. Gray-white specks of depigmentation are seen in the iris (Brushfield's spots). The little fingers are often short and curved, owing to a hypoplastic middle phalanx. The hands are broad and simianlike, with a single transverse palmar crease. A number of other characteristic dermal markings are noted in fingers and toes. Lenticular opacities and congenital heart lesions (septal defects) are found in some cases. At birth the mongoloid child is of average size, but at later periods of life he is characteristically small. Benda estimates that the average adult person with mongolism, of whom there are many, never exceeds the stature of a ten-year-old boy. The resemblance to the Oriental is at most superficial; in fact the differences are so striking that it is quite easy to recognize the condition in those of Oriental heritage.

The mortality rate is high in the first years of life, death usually being due to respiratory infections, interventricular cardiac lesion with failure, or leukemia. Of the mongoloid patients who survive to puberty, many live to advanced years, coming then under the care of the internist.

Older mothers are more apt to have mongoloid babies than are young mothers. The mean age of the mother at the time of birth of the mongoloid child is thirty-seven. It is thought by some workers that a genetic factor is responsible, but familial incidence is rare. Aside from having a rather rounded shape, which conforms to that of the skull, a subnormal weight, and a relatively simple convolutional pattern, with particular smallness of the frontal lobes and superior temporal convolutions, the brain of the mongolian idiot shows no abnormalities. Trisomy of chromosome pair 21–22 or translocation of parts of these chromosomes has been found consistently in patients with Down's syndrome and are in some uncertain way responsible for the disorder.

Cretinism. This is due to congenital deficiency of thyroid secretion and is distinguished from myxedema, a form of hypothyroidism acquired later in life (see Chap. 89).

Gargoylism (Hunter-Hurler Disease). This condition is discussed in Chap. 113.

Osteochondrodystrophy (Morquio's Disease). Sometimes confused with gargoylism, this is a nonprogressive osseous disorder with a cranial appearance similar to that of gargoylism. Most patients have a normal mind, although a few have a stationary mental defect. No visceral lesions have been observed. The primary defect is believed to be one of the chondroblasts. Recent evidence suggests that some cases of Morquio's disease represent a special type of mucopolysaccharidosis.

Phenylketonuria (Phenylpyruvic Oligophrenia). This condition is discussed in Chap. 101.

Galactosemia. Another congenital metabolic disease, galactosemia is transmitted by a single, autosomal recessive gene. It is characterized clinically by mental defect, cataract, nausea, vomiting, hepatomegaly, jaundice, and the excretion of large quantities of galactose in the urine. The biochemical defect is discussed in Chap. 112.

Anhidrotic Ectodermal Dysplasia. This is a congenital disorder in which there are anhidrosis, defects in salivation, lacrimation, sparse hair, and faulty dentition. Heat intolerance with paroxysmal fever, unrelated to infection, may occur. Several of the patients with reported cases have been feebleminded. A sex-linked inheritance pattern has been reported. The neuropathologic basis for this disease is unknown. There is no treatment.

Heller's Disease (Dementia Infantilis). This condition is of uncertain status. Neurologists and some psychiatrists look upon it as a cerebral disease of undetermined cause. Other psychiatrists believe it to be a form of precocious schizophrenia. As a rule, the onset is before the third year of life. At this age, usually without previous illness, a change in character is noted. Irritability, negativism, disobedience, and outbursts of unprovoked temper become manifest. Restlessness and destructiveness are other prominent symptoms. Toys with which the child had played normally are now senselessly destroyed. Within a few months there is complete loss of speech and also failure in the understanding of words. Grimacing and ticlike movements appear, but motor and sensory functions are preserved. Continence of sphincters is lost. The mental regression continues to a stage of idiocy, but all through the illness the patient continues to give an impression of greater intelligence than do most feebleminded individuals. Many patients of this type reach adult life but remain in institutions. The pathology of this disorder is uncertain, although in a few cases a neuronal lipidosis has been found.

Autism, in which an infant or small child is mute, socially detached, preoccupied with whirling toys, and rigidly insistent on sameness of environment, is a closely related condition (see Chap. 7).

Simple Mental Retardation. Although presented last, this category includes the great bulk of children with mental defect of indeterminate etiology who exhibit neither craniovertebral nor neurologic abnormality. The degree of mental impairment tends to be mild (moron, feebleminded, educable) or moderate (imbecile, trainable). Penrose found that this group of aments comprised 25 percent of 1,280 institutionalized children, and of course those who are in institutions represent only the more severely damaged individuals in our society. The physical appearance of these children or adults is usually not strikingly abnormal; yet many of the aforementioned characteristics of the mentally retarded individual are to be observed. Seizures occur in a significant number, being several times more frequent than in a normal population. Within the limits of their intelligence, the success of these individuals in learning to look after themselves is often determined by the effectiveness of their teachers and the suitability of the environment in which they are placed. The brighter ones can profit to some extent from

formal education. Those less well endowed may be trained to care for their personal wants and needs and may profit from a limited amount of manual training. Special schools and classes are of great help. Later in life, supervised work situations are possible solutions to their occupational needs.

Society, in the final analysis, determines the eventual disposition of these unfortunates. Many of them, being not unattractive and giving less trouble than many other defective children, may adjust to foster families and live in a community. They need protection, for they are easily led astray and may commit infractions of the law, usually of a minor sort. Sexual offenses are common in the girls. Institutionalization is required when family and society cannot or do not wish to look after them. Reproductivity is frequently impaired in those with severe mental defects but may be distressingly undisturbed in many of the less defective individuals.

The problem of eugenics assumes great importance. This type of mental defect is often seen in families in which one or both parents are dull or retarded. The term *familial* may be applied to this group. However, the majority of cases are sporadic. Probably multiple etiologic factors may lead to simple mental retardation. The pathologic change is variable, ranging from "no demonstrable lesion" to several different gross and microscopic abnormalities.

MANAGEMENT OF THE RETARDED CHILD AND HIS PARENTS. It is an unpleasant task to inform parents that their child is abnormal in any respect, and many, if not most, parents find it difficult to accept a mental defect without much self-recrimination and feelings of guilt. To give an honest statement of the degree of the child's retardation and, on the basis of the nature of the problem, some professional estimate of the likelihood of future growth and development, once one is sure of the status and potentialities of the child, requires tact and sympathetic understanding. The family must eventually be told to what extent the child is likely to be trainable or educable. Obviously this can often be no more than an educated guess, and if there is still reasonable doubt about the future, this fact should be so stated. In general it should be possible to give at least a rough approximation of the child's capabilities and likely attainments. Frequently the parents themselves are well aware of the child's limitations, and then a useful technique is to ask the parents to estimate the nature of the problem. The physician is in this way informed of the degree of their insight and their general attitudes. He may then agree with them or may amplify and clarify any misconceptions.

The parents will want to know the probable cause of the defect and the likelihood of subsequent children being affected. In most instances the answer to the second question will depend on the etiology. If the abnormality is determined by known genetic factors, as in congenital microcephaly, phenylpyruvic oligophrenia, or tuberous sclerosis, there is of course a strong likelihood of other children being abnormal. If on the other hand the abnormality is due to specific environmental influences peculiar to the pregnancy, as in the case of maternal rubella, excessive radiation to the pelvis, or premature placental separation, the prospects of having other normal children are good. Unfortunately in the great majority of cases the etiology will not be certain, and advice must be tendered cautiously. It is quite clear from the studies of Penrose, Halperin, and others that the chance of parents of normal intelligence with one defective child having other subnormal children is greater than that of the general population. If one or both parents is of less than normal intelligence, or if there is consanguinity in the parents, then the risk is considerably greater.

Special Paroxysmal Disorders of Nervous Function in Infancy and Childhood

The convulsive disorders have been discussed in Chap. 28, Convulsions, and all that was said there applies to infants and children as well as adults. An important point to remember is that epilepsy is much more of a problem in children's medicine than of adult medicine. Varieties of seizure are seen in infants and children which never occur later in life or are followed by other types of seizures. Many special problems are raised, and these must be known and properly interpreted by the physician, who may see the patient at a more advanced age.

The incidence of convulsions is known to be high in infancy and early childhood, and seizures at that age may have an altogether different significance than in the adult. All the seizure patterns that may be witnessed in the adult may also occur in infancy and childhood—i.e., focal motor and Jacksonian as well as petit mal and psychomotor seizures—but certain ones appear only at this age. These are the petit mal and its variants and massive myoclonus (infantile flexor or extensor spasms). Then, too, there are other types of spells, unique to infancy and childhood, which must be distinguished from convulsions, i.e., breath-holding spells and the congestive attacks that accompany congenital heart disease.

Seizures have different meanings at different periods of infancy and childhood. A series of seizures that occurred during the neonatal period must always be regarded as an omen of cerebral damage. It may have been due to cerebral injury or hypoxemia with unresponsiveness, pallor, periods of apnea, bulging fontanel, and grossly bloody cerebrospinal fluid. Hypoglycemia, hypocalcemia, and pyridoxine deficiency are other causes of neonatal fits which may be correctable. Or seizure may reflect a congenital brain disease, sometimes of such major proportions as to have prevented further development, or it may have been so slight as not to disturb the normal maturation processes. Actually very little is known of the import of seizures at this period with reference to prognosis for mental development. A single outburst of seizures in a previously healthy infant occurring in conjunction with any illness may not continue beyond this period of life. Presumably they are an expression of the low convulsive threshold of the infantile nervous system. However, they may signify the onset of a fatal process such as acute toxic encephalopathy, thrombosis of the superior sagittal sinus or cerebral veins, meningitis, brain hemorrhage from an angioma, or massive arterial infarction. Idiopathic epilepsy also begins during infancy and childhood and may interfere relatively little with normal development. Brain tumors are an infrequent cause of seizures during infancy and childhood.

FEBRILE FITS

Certain infants and children are disposed to convulsions with fever. Lennox estimates that approximately 2 percent of all children have one or more convulsions with fever at one time or another during infancy or childhood. In some 20 percent of these cases it can be decided in retrospect that fever has served merely to precipitate a seizure in an individual who has suffered a cerebral disease or who has idiopathic epilepsy. Such individuals will continue to have seizures, unassociated with fever. In the other 80 percent of cases, seizures occur only during febrile episodes and never recur beyond early childhood. The reason for this low seizure threshold in the infantile brain is unknown, but a family history of similar febrile fits in other members of the family can be obtained in about 50 percent of cases.

From the history it can usually be learned that febrile convulsions have occurred between the ages of one and three years; only a few cases are seen earlier or later—up until the age of seven or eight years. Any febrile illness may have been provocative, but usually a rapid ascent of temperature to 103°F. or higher was responsible. The seizures themselves are generalized and of short duration and may have occurred singly or in a cluster of two or three. The postictal coma is of short duration. No record of focal or lateralizing neurologic signs can be obtained. The cerebrospinal fluid is clear and acellular, and the amount of total protein is normal. The electroencephalogram is diffusely abnormal, with theta and delta waves predominating in all leads immediately after the seizure, with rapid return to normal at the termination of the illness. After the illness there should be no residual signs of brain disease.

It must be remembered that there are certain sources of error in the diagnosis of febrile convulsions. The fever may have been caused by convulsions, as so often happens in idiopathic epilepsy, especially with status epilepticus. Some primary inflammatory disease of the brain or meninges may have been responsible for both fever and convulsions. Meningitis, for example, may have begun in this way but would probably have ended fatally if not diagnosed and treated.

MASSIVE MYOCLONUS

This syndrome, known also by the names *infantile muscular spasm, Blitzkrampf, myoclonic seizure,* "salaam fit," "flexor spasm," and "jackknife seizure," has been recognized recently and should be known to general physicians and internists because they may see the patient long after the seizures have stopped. In essence, it is a sudden synchronous contraction of many muscle groups. Contraction of flexor muscles usually predominates, and there is a sudden flexion of trunk, neck, and extremities, often accompanied by a cry or occasionally by a laugh. In some patients there is a combination of flexor and extensor movements, and least often the contraction of extensor muscles predominates, with a straightening of the body and a fall backward. The spasm itself is usually momentary, but often recurs once or several times, with each spasm separated from the next by an interval of a few seconds. There may be only a few spasms in a cluster or upward of a hundred or more in a series. They are especially frequent as the patient is falling off to sleep or upon awakening. The patient may fall, if he is standing at the time of the spasm. Sensory precipitation by handling, feeding, noise, and fever have been noted.

Massive myoclonic spasms usually begin during the first few months of life and tend to disappear or to be replaced by other seizure patterns between the second and third years of age. Massive myoclonus has been observed in a number of clinical states including tuberous sclerosis, following severe trauma, with congenital malformations, mongolism, and disorders of amino acid metabolism such as phenylketonuria and maple syrup urine disease. The frequent association of mental retardation (in 90 percent of the cases) and the consistent diffusely abnormal electroencephalogram with bursts of high-voltage slow waves, referred to as *hypsarrhythmia* by Gibbs, suggest a diffuse neuronal pathology of obscure type for the majority of patients. It is of interest that the seizures may become less frequent as the dementia progresses.

The treatment of the seizures is difficult. Some patients respond dramatically to the first drug tried but soon become resistant to it. Several authors have reported recently that treatment with adrenocorticotropic hormone is beneficial, especially if it is begun in the first 2 to 3 weeks of the illness.

"BREATH-HOLDING SPELLS"

This is a special type of attack peculiar to young children. Anger or a mild injury is the precipitating factor. The patient begins to cry or scream. After a few moments he suddenly stops breathing and remains apneic for many seconds to as long as a minute. During this period there is a color change from an initial redness to cyanosis, presumably as the result of hypoxia. If this persists for a short period, the patient suddenly becomes limp and is unresponsive for some seconds. Convulsive twitching may occur, but rarely is there a sustained convulsion. The whole attack is over in one to a few minutes. The child may then be drowsy and sleep for a short while thereafter or may be at once as alert as before. Such attacks usually begin late in the first year of life and rarely occur after the third year. They are outgrown, so to speak. The mechanism is unclear; in breath holding the infant may perform the Valsalva maneuver and then faint, as in tussive syncope. In the "pallid" form a cardiac arrhythmia or asystole appears to underlie the disorder. This variety may persist into adult life.

Apnea may be observed as a fragment of a generalized seizure, and must be differentiated from breath holding.

The sequence of events is so characteristic in breath holding that the diagnosis is usually not difficult.

CONGESTIVE ATTACKS WITH CONGENITAL CARDIAC AND PULMONARY DISEASE

This condition has been described only recently and is of importance in the histories of cases of congenital heart disease. Cyanotic infants and children with gravely limited cardiopulmonary function may, upon some unusual exertion or excitement or while crying, momentarily lose consciousness and twitch a few times. Presumably the spell depends on hypoxia or inadequacy of cerebral blood flow. It must be distinguished from seizures which occur with a higher than normal frequency in patients with congenital heart disease.

CONCLUSION

A knowledge of these special neurologic problems of infancy and childhood is of value to the student, as well as to the general physician or internist; it enables him to understand the nature of such illnesses when they are encountered in adults and permits better evaluation of their possible relationship to any new illness. Also, the habit of making observations on the level of native intellectual endowment is of importance. The histories given by patients with neurologic problems must always be carefully checked against an outside source; in planning for therapy one must always enlist the aid of the responsible member of the family or, if the patient is institutionalized, of the nurse or attendant. Finally, problems in eugenics are likely to arise, and the physician is often asked to advise the family or health agencies in the community on such matters. Accurate diagnosis and a carefully established genealogy usually permit a separation of a genetic from an acquired disease and are of some value in predicting the occurrence of such diseases in the progeny of the afflicted individual.

REFERENCES

Ford, F. R.: "Diseases of the Nervous System in Infancy, Childhood and Adolescence," 4th ed., Springfield, Ill., Charles C Thomas, Publisher, 1960.

366 NARCOLEPSY AND CATAPLEXY

Raymond D. Adams

This clinical entity has long been known to the medical profession. Westphal described attacks of uncontrollable natural sleep in 1877, and Gélineau gave it the name *narcolepsy* in 1880. But it was not until 1916 that Henneberg called attention to the common association of temporary paralysis of cranial muscles and limbs during laughter or other emotional states (cataplexy). Paralysis during the period of falling asleep (hypnopompic) and paralysis at the time of awakening (hypnogogic), the so-called "sleep paralyses," were added to the syndrome by Wilson in 1916; episodic diplopia was included by Levin in 1943.

CLINICAL STATE. The above tetrad of symptoms appears to be not infrequent, as shown by the fact that several hundred cases were observed in the Mayo Clinic over a period of years. Males are affected more often than females. As a rule the condition begins in late childhood, adolescence, or early adult life, and narcolepsy is the presenting symptom. The essential disorder is one of uncontrollable sleepiness. Several times a day, usually while sitting in class, the subject is assailed by an uncontrollable desire to sleep. His eyes close, his muscles relax, his breathing deepens slightly, and he has all the appearances of a person who is dozing. A noise, a touch, or even the cessation of the lecturer's voice are enough to awaken him, and he may feel momentarily refreshed. Often the impulse to sleep is so frequent and insistent that a student so afflicted will never remain awake for a single period in class. Somnolence may occur in unusual situations, as while standing or carrying on a conversation.

Approximately 70 percent of these patients, if questioned carefully, will admit to having cataplexy. Reference is made here to the curious circumstance that hearty laughter, more rarely excitement, sadness, or anger, will cause the patient's head to fall forward, his jaws to drop open, his knees to buckle, even with falling to the ground, all with perfect preservation of consciousness but inability to move. The attack lasts only a minute or two. Much less frequent are the sleep paralyses and episodic diplopia. The narcolepsy does not alter the nocturnal sleep pattern.

Once the condition begins, it usually continues over most of adult life, perhaps becoming less frequent with age. No other neurologic abnormality is associated with it, nor does one later develop. All investigative procedures usually yield negative results, and one has only the patient's description or the observed phenomena on which to make a diagnosis.

CAUSE AND PATHOGENESIS. The cause of the condition is unknown. Attempts to impute it to encephalitis lethargica carry little conviction, since the disease long antedated the outbreak of this infection. It bears no relationship to epilepsy or migraine. A psychogenesis has been offered, but the relevance of the psychologic observations remains open to question. No autopsies in which the brain was thoroughly examined have been reported. Rarely, a narcoleptic state may accompany multiple sclerosis, idiopathic epilepsy, cerebral trauma, or a craniopharyngioma.

In recent years much interest has centered on the nature of the sleep and its EEG pattern. In many patients the normal sequence of slow wave and rapid eye movement (REM) sleep is altered, and in an attack the REM is predominant. It is associated sometimes with peculiar dreamlike or hallucinatory experiences.

The greatest difficulty in diagnosis relates to the problem of separating narcolepsy from the normal sleep pattern. Many sedentary, obese adults doze readily after breakfast, if unoccupied, or after dinner, during a game of bridge, or in the theater. But characteristic of narcolepsy is the irresistible urge to sleep under unusual circumstances (such as standing up) and the tendency of the sleep to recur many times a day. When cataplexy is conjoined, diagnosis becomes virtually certain. Excessive somnolence, easily mistaken for idiopathic narcolepsy, may attend obesity and hypercapnia, heart failure, hypothyroidism, excessive use of barbiturates and alcohol, etc.

TREATMENT. There is no therapy which will control all the symptoms. The narcolepsy responds best to (1) strategically placed naps (during lunch hour, before or after dinner, etc.) and (2) the use of analeptic drugs [amphetamine sulfate (Dexedrine), methylphenidate (Ritalin) or pipradol (Meratran)]. The time of medication should be adjusted to the study or work habits of the patient. The usual dose of amphetamine varies from 5 to 10 mg given three to five times a day. This is ordinarily well tolerated and does not cause wakefulness at night. The dose of Ritalin is 10 to 20 mg thrice daily, and of Meratran, 2.5 to 5.0 mg twice or thrice daily. These drugs have rather little effect on cataplexy, but fortunately this is less frequent and can be controlled by avoidance of emotional situations. Rarely it is so severe and easily provoked as to be disabling, a state for which no treatment has been successful (Chap. 27).

REFERENCES

Brock, S., and B. Wiesel: The Narcoleptic-cataplectic Syndrome, J. Nervous Mental Disease, 94:700, 1941.

Levin, M.: The Pathogenesis of Narcolepsy, J. Neurol. Psychopathol., 14:1, 1933.

Wilson, S. A. K.: The Narcolepsies, Brain, 51:63, 1928.

367 MIGRAINE

Raymond D. Adams
and John F. Griffith

The term *migraine* refers to periodic, hemicranial, throbbing headaches which begin in childhood, adolescence, or early adult life and continue to recur with diminishing frequency during advancing years.

Two closely related clinical syndromes have been identified. The first is called "classic" or "typical" migraine, the second "common" or "atypical." The typical syndrome is ushered in by a disturbance of neurologic function (hemianopsia or central blindness, hemiparesthetic disturbance, slight speech abnormality or aphasia, or hemiparesis) followed in a few minutes by hemicranial headache, nausea, and vomiting, all of which last for hours or as long as a day or two. The other is characterized by an unheralded onset of hemicranial or generalized headache with or without nausea and vomiting but following the same temporal pattern. Both headache syndromes respond to ergot preparations, if administered early in the attack. Their genetic nature is evidenced by concurrence in several members of the family of the same and successive generations in 60 to 80 percent of cases; but inheritance is somewhat less clear in the atypical than the typical variety, perhaps because diagnosis is less certain.

Classic migraine presents such a dramatic and at times confusing sequence of events that it merits further description. On awakening in the morning, or at any time of day, the patient may have a sense of vague premonition of an attack. Then abruptly there is a disturbance of vision consisting usually of bright spots or dazzling zigzag lines which give way within minutes to scotomatous defects; usually they are bilateral and often of homonymous and congruent pattern (corresponding parts of the field of vision of each eye). Soon thereafter, numbness and tingling of lips, face, hand (on one or both sides), slight confusion of thinking, weakness of an arm or leg, mild aphasia, dizziness and uncertainty of gait, drowsiness, or confusion (rarely coma) are added to the clinical picture. Only one or a few of these neurologic phenomena are present in any given patient and they tend to occur in the same combination in each attack. They last 5 to 15 min, and if the weakness or numbness spreads from one part of the body to another or one symptom follows another, it does so slowly in a period of minutes (not in seconds as in a convulsion). Just as inexplicably as they come they soon begin to recede, and within minutes they are followed by a unilateral throbbing headache which slowly increases in intensity. At its peak, in an hour or so, nausea and vomiting may occur. The headache lasts hours or a day or two and is always the most unpleasant feature of the illness.

Much variation occurs. When this "sick headache" as it is called, is most severe, the patient is forced to lie down and to shun light and noise. Milder forms, especially if partially controlled by medication, do not force withdrawal from accustomed activities. Any one of the three principal components—neurologic derangement, headache, or vomiting—may be absent. Particularly with advancing age there is a tendency for the headache and vomiting to become less severe, finally leaving only the neurologic abnormality. The neurologic symptomatology is also subject to variation. Although visual disturbances are far and again the most common manifestation, they differ in detail from patient to patient; numbness and tingling of the lips and fingers of one hand are probably next in frequency, with transient aphasia or a thickness of speech following in that order. A relatively rare syndrome of vertigo, staggering, drowsiness, and stupor has been delineated by Bickerstaff and called *basilar artery migraine*. Also, he has reported the loss of consciousness at the onset, especially in migrainous young women. Recurrent unilateral headaches associated with extraocular muscle palsies have been called *ophthalmoplegic migraine*. A transient third nerve palsy with associated ptosis of one eyelid is the usual picture; rarely, the abducens nerve is affected and lateral movement is impaired. Disturbances of the mind may appear—a strange excitement, an unaccountable irritability or depression, or

a slight mental confusion, which is the more common. The headache, though typically hemicranial (the word *migraine* is said to be derived from *megrim*, meaning hemicrania) may be frontal, temporal, or generalized. In children abdominal pain and vomiting may accompany the headache (abdominal migraine). The attacks, instead of beginning in childhood and recurring in the usual fashion every few weeks or months with diminishing frequency in middle and late adult years, may begin in adult life or even middle age or suddenly increase in frequency during menopause or when hypertension and vascular disease develop. The neurologic symptoms, instead of being transitory, may leave a permanent deficit (e.g., a homonymous visual field defect) reminiscent of an ischemic stroke. The use of hormones to prevent pregnancy has increased the frequency and severity of migraine and in several reported instances has resulted in a stroke.

Between attacks the migrainous patient is essentially normal. For a time when psychosomatic medicine was much in vogue, there was much insistence on a migrainous personality characterized by tenseness, rigidity in thinking, meticulousness, and perfection. The migrainous attack was said to occur often during the letdown period, after many days of hard work or stress. But, further personality analyses have not borne out these ideas, and the temporal relations between headache and the day's activities have not been consistent. Moreover, the fact that the headaches may begin in early childhood, when the personality is relatively amorphous, would argue against this idea. During an attack, the electroencephalogram reveals a nonspecific slowing of wave frequencies in one-third to one-half of all patients. Carotid arteriograms show arterial constriction at the onset of the headache, and the cerebral circulation is found to be slowed by blood flow studies early in the attack and speeded up once headache begins. Migraine is frequent, estimated at 5 percent of general population and females are slightly more susceptible to migraine than males, and there is a tendency for the headaches to occur during the period of premenstrual tension and fluid retention. The migrainous attacks usually cease during pregnancy. Reserpine treatment and estrogens and progesterone may increase their frequency. A few patients have linked their attacks to certain articles of diet, such as chocolate. There is no clear relationship, despite many statements to the contrary, between migraine and vascular malformations of the brain and psychoneurosis. The relationship to epilepsy is less clear; convulsions are slightly increased in frequency in the migrainous patient and his relatives.

PATHOGENESIS. Over a century ago Parry observed that the headache of migraine could be relieved temporarily by compressing the common carotid artery in the neck on the same side. Many physicians have since noted prominence of the temporal artery during the headache and occasionally even a mild edema or flush of the temple and cheek on that side. Graham and Wolff were the first to measure the pulsation of the temporal arteries on the side of the headache and found it to be increased during the headache. Further, as the pulsation decreased, either spontaneously or after the administration of ergotamine, the headache disappeared. Vasoconstriction was early postulated as the basis of the neurologic symptoms; it has been confirmed in at least one chance carotid arteriogram and has been inferred from prompt abolition of the visual or neurologic disorder upon administration of nitrites. Thus the vascular theory of migraine came to be accepted, supported further by surgical observations, that the extracranial arteries can be a source of pain. However, it is quite apparent that the theory does not explain why the intracranial and extracranial arteries should periodically undergo spasm and dilatation in the migrainous individual, nor does it account for the nausea and vomiting (infrequent in all other headaches except those due to tumor) or the tenderness and swelling of the temporal vessels and surrounding tissues. In fact it has even been questioned as to whether the pain could be due merely to the increased pulsatile activity of the vessels.

A new hypothesis has been put forth by Sicuteri and his colleagues—that the observed vasospasm and later hyperemic pulsations are induced by a release of amines such as norepinephrine and epinephrine and serotonin in individuals whose vessels are peculiarly sensitive. These substances are known to be powerful vasoconstrictors. It was found that some migraine patients during their attack excrete increased amounts of the terminal metabolites of the catecholamines, particularly 5-hydroxyindoleacetic acid, (5-HIAA) derived from serotonin, and of vanilomandelic acid (VMA), a product of norepinephrine and epinephrine. Lance and his coworkers found a corresponding reduction in serotonin levels in the blood. Other observations in line with this are that (1) reserpine, which reduces the level of serotonin in platelets, brain, and other tissues, may provoke migraine; (2) the injection of serotonin gives partial or complete relief of headache, and (3) a serotonin antagonist, methysergide, wholly prevents attacks. However, it is still difficult to reconcile these data with the finding of Chapman et al. that a heat-stable polypeptide with some of the properties of bradykinin (one of the plasma kinins) not only can be aspirated from the edematous subcutaneous tissue, but if reinjected at another site will cause increased capillary permeability, pain, and lowered skin threshold in the overlying skin. Its algogenic action is potentiated by serotonin. Whether this substance, called *neurokinin,* escapes secondarily during the phase of vasodilatation or initiates the vasodilatation is not known. While this humoral amine theory is incomplete, and several of the findings need verification, nonetheless it does promise clarification of the migraine syndrome and possibly other forms of vascular headache.

DIAGNOSIS. Typical migraine should occasion no difficulty in diagnosis if the above facts are kept in mind and if a good history is obtained. That is possible, as a rule, for migraine patients tend to be intelligent.

The real difficulties come from three sources: (1) ignorance of the fact that a progressively unfolding neurologic syndrome may be migrainous in origin; (2) lack of appreciation that the neurologic disorder may occur without headache; (3) lack of awareness that recurrent headaches, which may be an isolated phenomenon, may take many forms, some of which may prove difficult to distinguish from the other common types of headache described in Chap. 10.

Some of these problems merit further elaboration because of their practical importance, as follows:

The neurologic part of the migraine syndrome may resemble focal epilepsy, the clinical picture of a vascular malformation such as an angioma or aneurysm, or some other vascular disease such as a thrombotic or embolic stroke. Here it is the pace of the neurologic symptoms of migraine more than their character that reliably distinguishes the condition from epilepsy. The clinical profile of the aura of epilepsy is measured in seconds, for it depends on spreading neural excitation, in contrast to the slow progression of migraine, which is based on spreading vascular spasm.

Ophthalmoplegic migraine will always suggest a carotid aneurysm, but in relatively few cases has carotid arteriography revealed such an abnormality. Despite many claims that hemicranial painful attacks invariably on the same side of the head (unlike migraine) should raise the question of a vascular malformation, Bull and his associates at the National Hospital, London, in a large series of cases, have not been able to confirm this by arteriography. Of course focal epilepsy, protracted headache, stiff neck and bloody CSF, a persistent neurologic deficit, and cranial bruit would be indicative of a vascular type of headache associated with angioma or aneurysm. Only in the earlier stages, when periodic throbbing headache is the sole symptom, might it be confused with true migraine.

Attacks indistinguishable from epilepsy may also appear in association with hypertensive and the cerebral arteriosclerotic vascular diseases of late life. Here one is aided by late age of onset, more persistent and frequent headaches, and the evidence of vascular disease of heart, lower extremities, and brain.

A special problem relates to paroxysms of throbbing headache, not hemicranial in distribution, not preceded by a neurologic aura, and not accounted for by other known cause. Are they examples of atypical, or common, migraine? Unfortunately, since diagnosis depends on the interpretation of the patient's description of symptoms and since there is as yet no biologically valid confirmatory laboratory test, the controversy as to where migraine begins and ends is of the armchair type. Favoring the diagnosis of migraine are lifelong history, childhood onset, positive family history, and response of the headache to ergot derivatives.

A variety of episodic attacks have been described as migraine equivalents: attacks of abdominal pain with nausea, vomiting and diarrhea; pain localized in the thorax, pelvis, and extremities; bouts of fever; transient disturbances in mood (psychic equivalents); recurrent nocturnal orbital (cluster) headache, or migrainous neuralgia (see Chap. 10). The only advantage of considering such attacks as migrainous is that it protects some patients from unnecessary diagnostic procedures and surgical intervention. But, it may also prevent necessary surgery. One should not prejudge the issue by adopting the term migraine for which there is presently no scientific justification and which serves here as a rather threadbare cloak for ignorance.

From all this discussion the reader should be left with the idea that the migraine syndromes are rather larger and more protean than the rigid stereotyped descriptions we have given would suggest. In these days of complicated diagnostic procedures it is tempting to take x-rays of the skull and perform arteriography and electroencephalography on every patient. Such tests are expensive and sometimes dangerous. A conservative approach would lead to temporization, reserving a single lateral skull film or EEG for the exceptional case.

TREATMENT. Migraine may require no treatment at all, other than an explanation of its nature to the patient and a reassurance that it will do him no harm. Some patients know, or allege to know, that certain acts induce attacks, and it is obvious enough that they should be urged to avoid these acts, if possible. In certain persons it has been claimed that the correction of a refractive error, an elimination diet, or psychotherapy for some personality disorder has relieved their migraine. However, this is so exceptional that cause and effect relationship must be doubted, in view of the variability of the disease itself.

Treatment of the neurologic aura is rarely required because of its brevity. Yet this is the time to initiate treatment of the oncoming headache. If many of the headaches are mild, the patient may already have learned that 0.6 Gm acetylsalicylic acid and possibly 5 mg Dexedrine will suffice to control the pain so he can carry on. More severe attacks respond only to ergot preparations (ergotamine and dihydroergotamine). In such patients the attack can be cut short by the intravenous injection of 1 mg dihydroergotamine methane sulfate or 0.5 mg ergotamine tartrate, the former being less likely to induce vomiting. The injection should be repeated in 30 min, if necessary. When administered early (within 30 to 60 min of onset) some 90 percent of patients will be relieved of the headache. Oral medication in the form of three 1-mg tablets, to be held under the tongue until dissolved, and repeated in 2-mg doses every half hour until the headache is relieved or a total of 9 mg is taken, is almost as effective. Caffeine, 100 mg with 1 mg of ergotamine (Cafergot), is a useful combination when taken in the form of a tablet (two at onset of headache and a third in half an hour) or as a rectal suppository (2 mg ergotamine and 100 mg caffeine) if vomiting prevents oral administration.

Because of the danger of prolonged vascular spasm in patients who have vascular disease or are pregnant, ergot preparations must be used cautiously, if at all. Even in healthy individuals more than 10 to 15 mg ergotamine per week is risky. For the frequent atypical migraine headaches, some of which respond poorly to ergot, one should prescribe a preparation containing 150 mg of acetylsalicylic acid, 160 mg of acetophenetidin and Dexedrine, 5 mg, and phenobarbital, 30 mg. This can be repeated once or twice in a severe attack. Once the head-ache has become intense ergot is of little help, and one must resort to codeine sulphate, 30 mg, or meperidine (Demerol), 50 mg, as the only means of terminating the pain.

In individuals with frequent migrainous attacks (1 to 3 times a week) efforts at prevention are worthwhile. Some success has been obtained with preparations of ergot, 0.5 mg, atropine, 0.3 mg, and phenobarbital, 15 mg (Bellergol) twice or three times a day for a few weeks. ACTH (40 units per day) or prednisone (45 mg per day for 3 to 4 weeks) have also been helpful in some difficult refractory patients. Recently methysergide (Sansert) in a dose of 6 to 8 mg per day given for several weeks or months has proved to be most promising in reducing the frequency of or abolishing attacks. The main contraindication has been retroperitoneal fibrosis; this complication has been reported in several dozen cases, when the patient has been treated continuously for more than six months.

All experienced physicians appreciate the importance of helping the patient rearrange his schedule so as to control his tensions and hard-driving ways of living, so often a feature of many migrainous patients. There is no one way of accomplishing this, but in general, long and costly psychotherapy has not been helpful, or at least one can say there is no substantial data as to its value.

REFERENCES

Chapman, L. F.: A Humoral Agent Implicated in Vascular Headache of the Migraine Type, Arch. Neurol. 3:223, 1960.

Graham, J. R., and H. G. Wolff: The Mechanism of the Migraine Headache and the Action of Ergotamine Tartrate, Arch. Neurol. Psychiat., 39:737, 1938.

Lance, J. W., and H. Hintzenberger: The Control of Cranial Arteries by Humoral Mechanism and Its Relation to the Migraine Syndrome, Headache, 7:93, 1967.

Parry, C. H.: Collections from the Unpublished Medical Writings of the late Caleb Hillier Parry, vol. 1, London, Underwood's, 1825.

Sicuteri, F.: Vasoneuroactive Substances and Their Implication in Vascular Pain, chap. 2 in "Research and Clinical Studies of Headache," Friedman (Ed.), Baltimore, Williams & Wilkins, 1967.

Smith, R.: Background of Migraine, New York, Springer Publishing Co., Inc., 1967.

368 IDIOPATHIC EPILEPSY
Raymond D. Adams

In Chap. 28 the general problem of convulsive disorders and their medical implications were presented in detail. The common seizure patterns, their underlying cerebral anatomy and physiologic mechanism, and the relevant biochemical changes, not too well known to be sure, were described. The high frequency of epileptic lesions in the cerebral cortex and the failure of demonstrated lesions in other parts of the nervous system to be associated in the typical convulsive disorders was stressed. With respect to the possible causes of seizures it was pointed out that they differ according to the age of the patient at the time of their onset. In the adult who begins to have a convulsive disorder the cause is likely to be discovered sooner or later; but in the infant or child, or the adult who has had seizures since childhood, our success is limited and the greater number of cases fall into the category of idiopathic epilepsy. It is about this latter group, which makes up the majority of patients seen by the medical profession, especially during the first three decades of life, that the following remarks are made.

Many physicians will find it curious, indeed almost comic, that neurology should be concerned with the treatment of an important entity when it has little or no idea of its cause. Perhaps they would suggest that it would be worthwhile to try to do some research on problems such as these and learn something about them before making them the subjects of book chapters. As a matter of fact the very nature of the human nervous system and this particular manifestation of the nervous disease have defied analysis. In the development of such a complex structure as the brain a minor disturbance may occur and be expressed by a seizure tendency. During the long intrauterine period a noxious factor might injure the brain without betraying itself by other symptom or sign. And we know that in infancy and childhood, diseases of the brain may masquerade as a relatively trivial infection, etc. To make the problem more difficult seizures have a way of occurring not at the time of a cerebral insult but months or years later when the disease has become inactive. Thus, it is possible for the cerebrum of man to harbor one or more potentially epileptic lesions of indeterminate type; and they are usually nonprogressive. Since epilepsy is rarely fatal the only chance at pathologic study may come years after the onset of the responsible disease, when all distinguishing marks have vanished; and if the lesions are small and unobtrusive only special cytologic methods, i.e., serial sections of the whole cerebrum, might reveal their residual effects.

The fact that a group of idiopathic epileptic disorders is set apart from all convulsive states of known cause should not discourage one from attempting a complete diagnosis in every patient, namely (1) to obtain knowledge of the existence of the convulsive state, (2) to ascertain the cause of the cortical lesion, and (3) to determine its localization. But in the younger subject, whose brain is more disposed to seizure activity than that of an older person, and in whom stationary lesions are more frequent, the pursuit of causation tends to be less vigorous.

THE CLINICAL STATE. Idiopathic epilepsy tends to express itself with maximal frequency at two periods in life, between the ages of two and five years and around puberty. More often than not the first seizure is generalized, though a series of petit mal, "staring spells," may precede its appearance. Up to this moment development may have been normal, and a neurologic examination is

likely to disclose no other abnormality. Although the seizures may be either of generalized motor type (51 percent of cases) or petit mal (8 percent) in the beginning, as the years pass and the seizures continue, approximately 40 percent of patients will have both these types or psychomotor seizures in addition. The latter are also frequent in pure form. See Chap. 28 for further description of seizures.

The severity of the convulsive state varies from a single attack every several years to many per day. If the generalized seizures are at all frequent they pose a constant threat of injury or social embarrassment, often preventing the further education of the child or gainful occupation of the adult. Of the milder form of disorder, however, sufficient medical control may be achieved so that there is no interference with the normal life activities. In enlightened communities no longer is an intelligent epileptic stigmatized by teachers or employers, and virtually all patients without other neurologic abnormalities can find their place in society. Probably those cases with evidences of mental retardation, character changes, hemiparesis, etc., should be removed from the category of idiopathic epilepsy.

The common diagnostic procedures performed in the interval between seizures are usually uninformative, i.e., CSF is normal, x-rays of skull are normal, pneumoencephalogram and arteriograms where they have been done are negative. Only the electroencephalogram will demonstrate an abnormality in 60 to 75 percent of cases, either a generalized paroxysmal 3-per-sec spike-slow wave complex (dart-dome), sharp waves, or some other alterations (see Ch. 353).

PROGNOSIS. Without doubt the appearance of a convulsion poses a serious problem for the patient, his family, and his physician. There is first of all the possibility of its being the initial manifestation of a neurologic disease which will take the life of the patient (e.g., infiltrating glioma). But even if the convulsion is due to a stationary, healed lesion, life expectancy is slightly reduced owing to the danger of injury or rarely, unexplained death. If seizures are frequent or difficult to control, mentation may be altered; the patient is dull, vague, querulous, and illogically argumentative. If seizures are infrequent and the EEG relatively normal between attacks, prognoses for successful schooling, occupational adjustment, and marriage are excellent. Mental deterioration, fortunately, occurs rarely, contrary to lay opinion, and when it becomes evident over a few weeks one must suspect (1) wrong initial diagnosis (not idiopathic epilepsy but seizures due to some defineable cerebral disease), (2) drug intoxication from anticonvulsant medication, (3) recurrent subclinical seizures, (4) subdural hematoma resulting from head injury.

TREATMENT. The treatment of epilepsy of all types can be divided into three parts: the removal of causative and precipitating factors, the regulation of physical and mental hygiene, and the use of anticonvulsant drugs.

The Removal of Causative and Precipitating Factors. Infections of the central nervous system, such as the meningitides and syphilis, that may give rise to convulsive seizures should be treated by appropriate measures. The same may be said of hyponatremia, hypocalcemia, or other conditions. Disturbances of the endocrine system resulting from adenomas of the pancreas or hypoparathyroidism require surgery and appropriate replacement therapy, respectively. Of course, these remarks do not appy to idiopathic epilepsy.

Whenever convulsive seizures are associated with a surgically removable lesion of the brain, such as tumor or abscess, removal of such a lesion is usually indicated. It must be remembered, however, that convulsive seizures will be relieved in only about 50 percent of cases of meningioma of the brain and in a much smaller percentage of cases of glioma or abscess of the brain. In such cases, further treatment with drugs is necessary.

Surgery has also been advocated for the removal of cortical scars secondary to cerebral trauma, of vascular lesions, and birth injuries on the assumption that such scars are surrounded by irritable foci which act as a trigger mechanism for the seizures. Reduction in the frequency of seizures has been reported as a sequel to these operations by a number of neurosurgeons. This treatment should be limited to the group of patients with focal attacks which do not respond to medical therapy. In addition, such lesions should be excised only by neurosurgeons who have facilities for the adequate localization of the lesion. Medical treatment will still be required for most of these patients after operation.

Patients with infantile hemiplegia and convulsive seizures that have not responded to anticonvulsant therapy have been subjected to a radical neurosurgical procedure, the complete removal of the cerebral hemisphere involved. Good results have been reported in a few of these cases, but it is hardly a treatment which is of great promise.

The anterior tip of the temporal lobe and the amygdaloid nuclei have been removed or destroyed by stereotaxis in patients with psychomotor seizures who have failed to respond to medical therapy and in whom it was possible to demonstrate a temporal lobe focus by electroencephalography. Favorable results have been reported for this procedure by some neurosurgeons.

Physical and Mental Hygiene. The epileptic patient should have a wholesome, regular diet consisting of simple foods with an abundance of vegetables and fresh fruits. Excessive quantities of alcoholic beverages of any sort are ill-advised. Constipation can be a troublesome symptom and should be avoided by the establishment of regular bowel habits. This can be developed by training and the use of mild laxatives when necessary.

The patient should be encouraged to maintain regular hours of sleep. Physical activity is desirable, and a moderate amount of physical exercise should be recommended. With proper safeguards, even the more dangerous sports, such as horseback riding and swimming, may be permitted. The uncontrolled epileptic patient, however, should not be allowed to drive an automobile or operate unguarded machinery.

Simple, superficial psychotherapy will frequently prevent or help overcome feelings of inferiority and self-consciousness present in many epileptic patients. Both the patient and his family will benefit from such therapy, and a proper family attitude should be established. Oversolicitude and overprotection should be discouraged. It is important to emphasize that the patient should be allowed to live as normal a life as possible.

Every effort should be made to keep children in school, and adults should be encouraged to work. Many communities have vocational rehabilitation centers, and advantage should be taken of such facilities. Patients should be encouraged to participate in available recreational activities, such as movies, dancing, and parties.

The Use of Anticonvulsant Drugs. Success in the management of patients with epilepsy depends on the ability of the physician to prevent the occurrence of seizures. Approximately 75 percent of patients with convulsive seizures can have their attacks controlled or reduced in frequency by the use of anticonvulsant drugs. Although these drugs are not a cure for epilepsy, their use is the most important step in the treatment of patients with convulsive disorders.

For a long time the bromides and phenobarbital were the only two drugs available for the medical treatment of epilepsy. Recently, however, many new compounds have appeared. The search for a more effective anticonvulsant is constantly going on, and new compounds are being given therapeutic trials in many clinics.

The drugs commonly used at present in the treatment of patients with convulsive seizures are the barbiturates, hydantoins, oxazolidinediones, and, to a lesser extent, the acetylureas and bromides. The available products which have been given a thorough clinical trial and their daily dosages are given below:

General Principles. Certain drugs are more effective in one type of seizure than in another, and it is necessary to use the proper drugs in the optimum dosages for the different types of seizures. If satisfactory results are not obtained with one of the drugs, the others should be tried, but frequent shifting of drugs is not advisable, and each should be given an adequate trial before another is substituted. In some patients a combination of two or more drugs will produce better results than one alone.

Intelligent management of drugs depends on having the patients chart daily their medication and the number, time, and circumstances of their seizures. Ideally such a base line should be established before medication is begun, since each patient tends to have his own pattern of seizures, but often this is impractical. Changes in medication should be made only when a given program is shown to be inadequate. As shown by Buchthal and his associates, frequent measurements of blood levels of diphenylhydantoin and barbiturate are useful. For Dilantin, the therapeutic level is 10 to 15 μg per ml, and one-half of patients have side effects at 30 or more μg per ml. These consist of ataxia, slurred speech, staggering, nystagmus, diplopia, mental dullness, forgetfulness, and confusion. Coma occurs when the level exceeds 50 μg. Clinical and electroencephalographic improvement were not noted be-

Table 368-1. ANTICONVULSANT MEDICATIONS*

Generic name	Trade name	Total daily dose per kg body wt; and usual adult dose	Principal therapeutic purposes
Phenobarbital	Luminal	1–5 mg; 60–200 mg	Major seizures; partial seizures; psycho-motor seizures; and petit mal
Diphenylhydantoin	Dilantin	4–7 mg; 200–500 mg	Major seizures; psychomotor seizures; partial epilepsy
Primidone	Mysoline	10–25 mg; 750–1,500 mg	Major seizures; psychomotor seizures; partial epilepsy
Ethosuximide	Zarontin	20–30 mg; 1,000–1,500 mg	Petit mal
Trimethadione	Tridione	10–25 mg; 500–1,250 mg	Petit mal
Paramethadione	Paradione	10–25 mg; 500–1,250 mg	Petit mal
Mephenytoin	Mesantoin	7–12 mg; 300–600 mg	Major seizures; psychomotor seizures; focal epilepsy
Mephobarbital	Mebaral	2.5–10 mg; 200–500 mg	Same as phenobarbital; myoclonic epilepsy
Methsuximide	Celontin	10–20 mg; 500–1,000 mg	Petit mal
Acetazolamide	Diamox	5–15 mg; 250–750 mg	Petit mal; infantile spasms; major seizures
Nitrazepan	Mogadon	0.15–2 mg; 10–100 mg	Infantile spasms; myoclonic epilepsy
Ethotoin	Peganone	10–20 mg; 500–1,000 mg	Major seizures; focal seizures
ACTH		40–60 units per day	Infantile spasms

* Children usually need larger doses than adults, if dose is calculated according to body weight. Excessive drowsiness can often be counteracted by dextroamphetamine (Dexedrine), methamphetamine (Desoxyn), or methylphenidate (Ritalin).

low 10 μg per ml. The therapeutic level for phenobarbital is probably about 15 to 20 μg per ml, though the range has not yet been exactly determined. Side effects appear in patients on long-term treatment at 25 μg per ml.

When changing medication, the dosage of the new drug should be gradually increased to an optimum level at the same time as the dosage of the old drug is gradually decreased. The sudden withdrawal of a drug may lead to status epilepticus, even though a new drug is substituted. Once an anticonvulsant or a combination of anticonvulsants is found to be effective, its use should be maintained for a period of years.

The therapeutic dose for any patient must be determined to some extent by trial and error. Not uncommonly a drug is discarded as being ineffective, whereas in reality a slightly increased dosage would have led to a complete disappearance of all the attacks. It is, however, inadvisable to administer a drug to the point where the patient is so dull and stupid that he is more incapacitated by the toxic effects than by the seizures. It is highly doubtful whether the prolonged administration of anticonvulsant medication is a factor in the development of the mental deterioration that occurs in a small percentage of the patients with convulsive seizures. However, there is some evidence that chronic Dilantin intoxication can lead to cerebellar degeneration (loss of Purkinje cells) and to polyneuropathy. It is not uncommon to note an improvement in the mental faculties of some patients following control of the seizures by the use of anticonvulsant drugs. The recent claim of pulmonary fibrosis after prolonged Dilantin therapy seems to be unfounded. An antifoliate effect on blood serum and a reduction of protein-bound iodine (without lowering of the BMR) have been reported.

Indications for Use of Specific Drugs. Grand Mal Seizures. For those patients with infrequent grand mal seizures (from one to four per year), phenobarbital can be tried first because of its high therapeutic index and its relatively low toxicity. When the seizures are more frequent, Dilantin is the drug of choice. A combination of Dilantin (0.3 to 0.4 Gm) and phenobarbital (0.1 to 0.2 Gm) is more often effective than either of the drugs used alone. When these drugs are used in combination, a full therapeutic dose of each drug must be given. Occasionally, Mesantoin or a combination of this drug with the Dilantin or Mysoline will succeed where Dilantin alone has failed. Only rarely will bromides or a combination of bromides and phenobarbital or Dilantin prove to be more effective.

The toxic effects of phenobarbital, which are drowsiness and mental dullness, nystagmus, and staggering, should be used as indications of excess dosage. Only skin eruption is a contraindication to its further use; otherwise these symptoms can be controlled by reducing the dose. Dilantin almost always leads to hirsutism, hypertrophy of gums, and as was stated above, ataxia, stupor, or coma. If skin rashes and other hypersensitivity phenomena (polyarteritis) occur, discontinuation of the medication is necessary. Reduction of dose controls the other symptoms.

Psychomotor Attacks. Drugs effective in the treatment of grand mal seizures are effective in the treatment of patients with psychomotor attacks. Dilantin, 300 to 400 mg per day, and Mysoline, 750 to 1,000 mg per day, have given the best results. The results on the whole are not as good as in grand mal epilepsy.

Petit Mal Attacks. As a rule, drugs effective in the treatment of grand mal and psychomotor seizures are relatively ineffective in the treatment of patients with petit mal attacks. Zarontin, 750 to 1,500 mg per day, has been most successful and has the advantage over trimethadione (Tridione), paramethadione (Paradione), and phenisuximide (Milontin) in producing less side effects. It is wise to begin with a single dose of 250 mg per day and increase it every week until therapeutic effect is achieved. Toxic symptoms to Tridione and Paradione are skin eruptions and photophobia. Aplastic anemia has been reported, hence monthly blood counts during the first year are indicated. Methylphenylsuccinamide (Celontin), (adult dose 0.3 Gm three or four times a day) and acetazolamide (Diamox) (adult dose 0.25 to 0.75 Gm per day) have been useful in controlling difficult cases of petit mal and massive myoclonus in children.

Minor Seizures and Focal Attacks. The same drugs effective in the treatment of grand mal and psychomotor seizures are effective against minor seizures and focal attacks. Minor seizures, which appear in patients whose grand mal attacks have been controlled, can occasionally be checked by simply increasing the dose of the drug or drugs that the patient is already taking. If the minor attacks are very infrequent and nonincapacitating, no great effort need be made to treat them.

Petit Mal Plus Other Types. When patients are subject to petit mal seizures as well as grand mal or psychomotor seizures, they should receive Zarontin plus diphenylhydantoin sodium, phenobarbital, or Mesantoin. The treatment of the special types of convulsions in infancy and childhood is discussed in Chap. 365.

Myoclonic Epilepsy. Mebaral (0.2 to 0.5 Gm) and phenobarbital (0.1 to 0.2 Gm) have been the most effective agents in this type of seizure. The treatment of massive myoclonus in infants, which depends on either ACTH or a combination of Mogadon and Diamox, is discussed in Chap. 365.

Status Epilepticus. Recurrent convulsions at a frequency which does not allow consciousness to be regained in the interval between seizures (status epilepticus) probably constitute the most serious therapeutic problem. Most patients who die of epilepsy do so because of uncontrolled recurrent seizures or an injury sustained as a result of seizure. Rising temperature, circulatory collapse, and lower nephron nephrosis is a sequence of events which may be encountered in fatal cases.

It must be conceded that at present no known drug will safely control all recurrent convulsions. This is not surprising, for there are many causes of convulsions and not all cases are alike. Clinical experience teaches that in some patients the convulsive tendency is so overwhelming that no amount of anticonvulsant medication, even deep ether anesthesia, will prevent recurrence of seizures. In others the liability to recurrent convulsions lasts only a few hours or at most a few days, regardless of whether anticonvulsant medication is given. The real hazard in treating resistant recurrent convulsions is that consciousness and vital functions may be suppressed to a degree incompatible with life. The risk of deep coma without convulsions is greater than semicoma or stupor with an occasional convulsion.

The following medications have been recommended for recurrent convulsions with brain disease and for status epilepticus.

1. Sodium phenobarbital in doses of 0.3 to 0.4 Gm intramuscularly and a repeated dose of 0.1 to 0.2 every 2 hr until a maximum of 0.8 to 1.0 Gm per 24 hr is reached.

2. Diphenylhydantoin sodium (Dilantin) in doses of 0.4 to 0.5 Gm per day orally (through stomach tube) or intravenously. This is usually given morning, noon, late afternoon, and evening.

3. Trimethadione (Tridione) in doses of 1.0 to 2.0 Gm intravenously.

4. Paraldehyde intravenously in doses of 1.0 to 8.0 ml paraldehyde per 15 lb body weight. Some physicians inject it intramuscularly in doses of 10.0 to 15.0 ml, but there is danger of sensorimotor paralysis if the drug is injected in the vicinity of a peripheral nerve.

5. Thiopental (Sodium Pentothal) in doses of 0.3 to 0.6 Gm intravenously or intramuscularly.

6. Tribromoethanol (Avertin) by rectum in doses of 25 mg per kg body weight and followed by 10 to 15 mg per kg body weight at 15- to 30-min intervals as indicated by the response of the patient.

7. Ether by inhalation.

Recently, diazepam (Valium) in intravenous doses of 5 to 10 mg repeated every few hours (to a maximum of 50 mg per 24 hr) has proven to be one of the most effective means of controlling status epilepticus.

These many treatments attest that no one of them is altogether satisfactory. The author has had the most success with the following program. When the patient is first seen, an intramuscular injection of 0.3 Gm sodium phenobarbital is given. Diphenylhydantoin sodium, 0.1 to 0.2 Gm, is then administered intravenously or through a stomach tube and additional amounts are added later to a total of 0.5 Gm per day. If seizures continue for the next 2 hours 0.2 Gm sodium phenobarbital is again injected. If the seizures continue for the next 1 to 2 hr, 0.2 Gm sodium phenobarbital is again injected. If the seizures cease for an hour or two and then recur, this amount of barbiturate may be given in repeated doses up to a total amount of 1.0 Gm per 24 hr. If the seizures are not controlled by the diphenylhydantoin and the first two injections of phenobarbital, 10 mg of Valium may be injected intravenously. If seizures continue, all medication except diphenylhydantoin sodium should be discontinued, and either a light ether anesthesia or a light Pentothal anesthesia up to 0.5 Gm intravenously, should be tried. Should the seizures continue despite all these medications, one is justified in the assumption that the convulsive tendency is so strong that it cannot be checked by reasonable quantities of anticonvulsants. One then depends entirely on diphenylhydantoin sodium 0.5 Gm and sodium phenobarbital 0.4 Gm per day. For infants and children, correspondingly smaller doses should be administered. For special types of recurrent seizures such as those associated with brain abscess, subdural empyema, or thrombophlebitis, paraldehyde is highly effective. The dose is 4.0 to 8.0 ml injected intramuscularly, taking care to avoid nerves, and it may be repeated every 3 to 4 hr.

Hyperthermia, which occurs in most cases of severe status epilepticus, must be controlled by the measures outlined in Chap. 16.

REFERENCES

Lennox, W., and M. Lennox: "Epilepsy and Related Disorders," Boston, Little, Brown and Company, 1960.

Penfield, W., and H. Jasper: "Epilepsy and Functional Anatomy of the Human Brain," Boston, Little, Brown and Company, 1954.

Yahr, M. D.: "Anticonvulsants—Clinical Considerations," ARNMD, vol. 37, pp. 57–71, Baltimore, The Williams & Wilkins Company, 1959.

Section 10

Psychiatric Disorders

369　INTRODUCTION TO PSYCHIATRIC DISEASES. THE PSYCHONEUROSES: ANXIETY NEUROSIS AND PSYCHASTHENIA

Raymond D. Adams

In the introduction to the section on Alterations of Nervous Function (Chap. 17) the argument was propounded that many of the diagnostic categories of neurosis and psychosis are psychogenically determined reaction patterns and not specific diseases, each with a definable cause, mechanism, distinctive symptomatology, course, and treatment. The major types of psychoneurosis, it is argued, are but the principal clusterings of symptoms, never to occur in pure form. Every patient is different, and his symptoms present themselves in every conceivable combination. Diagnosis, therefore, is deemphasized, and instead one searches for clues as to the underlying psychopathology.

Although not wishing to dispute the psychoanalytic point of view, the author finds the psychogenetic approach so diffuse and imprecise as to leave the average medical student and physician without any frame of reference; and seldom can the student orient himself in this broad field of psychiatry. For this reason the editors have decided to present the principal psychiatric entities as separate illnesses or complications of medical diseases, stressing practical diagnostic criteria based on simple observation. These chapters will be found to prepare the physician for the majority of mental illnesses and to indicate at what point expert psychiatric opinion should be requested.

The practicing physician or internist must assume primary responsibility for patients with the following psychiatric problems: (1) *Functional Illnesses,* a term which covers four types of nervous disorder—(*a*) acute anxiety and hysterical conversion reactions, (*b*) psychosomatic reactions, (*c*) hypochondriasis, (*d*) malingering and other psychopathic behavior. Next in order of frequency are (2) *Acute Psychoses,* which take one of five forms as a rule—(*a*) delirium, (*b*) other acute clouded and confusional states, (*c*) acute schizophrenic or pseudoschizophrenic reaction (exhaustion, endocrine, and postpartum psychoses), (*d*) beclouded dementias, and (*e*) other behavioral syndromes. (3) *Suicide,* representing (*a*) a situational reaction or reactive depression, (*b*) true endogenous depression, (*c*) hysterical reaction, (*d*) acute psychotic episode. (4) The *Alcoholic Patient* and (5) *Dementia* or *Amentia.* Once the nature of the psychiatric problem is ascertained, psychiatric consultation should be requested, but with the knowledge that many patients will object and some, usually those with neuroses, psychosomatic complaints, and hypochondriasis, will refuse to see the psychiatrist.

Of the four conditions listed under the heading of "functional illnesses" only the acute anxiety and hysterical conversion reactions belong clearly and unequivocally in the domain of psychiatry. Often in his first confrontation with such patients the internist may intentionally or inadvertently have alleviated the anxiety or eradicated the somatic symptom of hysteria (paralysis, blindness, aphonia, seizure). Malingering by a psychopathic personality is always distinguished from hysteria with difficulty. Psychosomatic illnesses and hypochondriasis fall in the twilight zones of medicine. Nearly always a physical illness lurks in the background, and the request for a psychiatric consultation to relieve undue tension, oversolicitude, and preoccupation with personal illness is seldom rewarding. Clinical diagnosis proceeds along the lines specified in Chap. 370, and educational guidance and a carefully contrived rearrangement of the patient's daily activities usually prove more helpful than formal psychiatric intervention, to which objection is usually raised.

The acute psychosis is so dramatic and reveals its true

nature so readily that the internist does well to admit the patient on a general hospital service and then to ascertain its type, as outlined in Chaps. 18 and 30. Formerly it was the practice to send such patients directly to specialized psychiatric hospitals. But now, with the easy availability of calming and sedating drugs, they can be managed in general hospitals where facilities for all types of medical care may be obtained. Since many of these illnesses, especially deliria and acute confusional states, may terminate in 2 to 3 weeks, the stigma attached to incarceration in an "insane asylum" is avoided. Even the acute schizophrenic reaction can be controlled until it is decided whether the illness necessitates a protracted stay in a psychiatric hospital.

The suicidal patient poses a combined medical and psychiatric problem. Self-inflicted wounds require surgical attention, and overdose of drugs, respiratory aid and other measures as outlined in Chap. 26. Then must come the analysis of the underlying illness and prevention of another suicidal attempt. In actuality few patients, even psychotic ones, immediately repeat their efforts at self-annihilation. It is in the months ahead that suicidal risk rises again to high proportions in the truly depressive psychoses. Of importance is to determine whether the suicide was merely an incident resulting from a violent argument or a histrionic display in a hysterical state, for repetition of suicide in such individuals is rare. From the descriptions (Chaps. 18, 370, 371) of the four common conditions which provoke suicide, their differentiation is not difficult, but the physician should reinforce his opinion by psychiatric consultation, if possible. Preferably the psychiatrist should be introduced soon after the patient's arrival and have the first of a series of interviews before defensive rationalizations have been built-up. He should also share in making the decision concerning future treatment.

The diagnosis and treatment of the alcoholic patient always seems extremely easy, and instead of objecting to psychiatric consultation, he rather welcomes it. Experience teaches that if this is done while the patient is still "hung over" and bothered by withdrawal symptoms, his vows to abstain forever and to enter a therapeutic contract are ephemeral. Far more helpful are a series of interviews with the physician or psychiatrist when the patient has recovered but is still in the hospital, in which the dangers of alcoholism and the nasty social implications of continual inebriety are emphasized (see Chap. 118).

The demented, so-called "arteriosclerotic" patient now comes increasingly under medical surveillance because his nervous disorder may be due to several correctable pathologic processes (see Chap. 30). According to the circumstances, the help of a neurologist or psychiatrist may be sought in carrying out some of the diagnostic studies and planning future care.

METHODS OF CLINICAL STUDY

In psychiatric medicine one proceeds in a case study by employing the conventional methods of history and examination, as described in Chap. 30. However, inasmuch as the nervous disorder is more complex than that of many others under consideration in neurologic medicine and is expressed in more abstruse ways as a behavioral disturbance with prominent subjective aspects, the history must be extended almost to the point of a biography and the details checked for accuracy against those given by parent or spouse. The physician's office and hospital room impose severe restrictions on both the range and variety of effective stimuli and the behavioral display. An adequate examination requires not only prolonged observations but also study during social interaction with meaningful people in the patient's life. The many components of behavior, as described in Chap. 30, should be systematically reviewed during the "mental status" evaluation.

Psychologic tests must be used in many of the patients in order to quantitate the disorder and provide a basis for determining in the future the natural course of the illness. Many psychiatrists favor the so-called "projection tests" (Rorschach, thematic apperception, etc.) which give some hint of the affective reactions to complex stimuli.

Electroencephalography, CSF examination, cranial x-rays, and pneumoencephalography are resorted to in many of the more serious mental diseases. Measurement of catecholamines and other agents related to norepinephrine and acetylcholine metabolism are of limited value in diagnosis.

THE PSYCHONEUROSES

From a simple descriptive point of view the psychoneuroses include seven clinical syndromes: (1) fatigue, or neurasthenia, as it was formerly called; (2) simple nervousness, anxiety neurosis, and neurocirculatory asthenia; (3) phobic neurosis; (4) obsessive compulsive neurosis (also called psychasthenia); (5) hysteria; (6) hypochondriasis; and (7) reactive depression. Although they are easily identifiable and separable, if presenting in pure form, experience will show that many patients exhibit symptoms which belong to more than one of these categories and, hence, must be considered as having "mixed psychoneuroses."

The causes and the exact mechanisms of symptoms produced in these many syndromes are unknown. It is a generally accepted proposition that all involve maladjustment in interpersonal (social) relations; in other words, they may be psychogenic. But the more penetrating students of psychiatry do not dismiss lightly the possibility of genetic or obscure biochemical factors. For example, certain types of aggressive behavior are known to be inherited as a mendelian dominant trait, and introversion is also heritable. Even Freud, the most emphatic exponent of the psychogenic etiology, underscored the importance of heredity, constitution, and the possibility of endocrine abnormalities. There is also general acceptance of the idea that the psychoneuroses need not be and usually are not disabling; i.e., they are "partial reactions" in an otherwise healthy person, not "total reactions," as in the psychoses.

According to Finesinger and Cobb, patients with psychoneuroses may be studied advantageously from the following points of view. (1) *Verbal accounts* given by the patient. Here reference is made to the patient's statements concerning his feelings, fantasies, and ideas. These are believed to provide the best clues to diagnosis. Supplementary data concerning the emerging patterns of thought may be secured by the free association of ideas, a method widely employed in psychoanalysis. Unfortunately, information of this type, although of great theoretical interest, has not been used for the critical testing of the original postulates of the psychoanalytic school. (2) *Motor behavior* (besides the verbal accounts), such as visible facial expressions and other acts which denote worry, tension, restlessness, excitement, or their opposites. These activities involve the cerebrospinal nervous system. (3) *Visceral reactions*. These depend on the autonomic nervous system, which controls the activities of smooth muscle and glands. Derangements in this sphere express themselves during emotion as combinations of rapid heartbeat, accelerated respiration, intestinal and bladder contractions, pupillary dilatation, sweating, flushing, pallor, etc. Four major emotional states—rage, fear, love, and sorrow—may thus be differentiated. (4) *Reactions to environmental stimuli*, past or present. The patient's symptoms are examined in relation to stimulus situation. Here the remarkable feature is that in the psychoneuroses the emotional reaction is not consonant with the manifest external or professed internal stimuli. Anxiety under the circumstances of a potentially threatening situation is, of course, an understandably normal reaction, but in the neurotic person a similar reaction occurs without evident cause. It is the contention of many experienced psychiatrists that the stimulus situation is there and may be discovered only by the free association of psychoanalysis or by the exploration of biographic details, i.e., remembered (conscious) and forgotten (subconscious) experiences. Or in the language of the behaviorist or reflexologist, the inexplicable emotion may be regarded as a conditioned response to an inapparent or forgotten fragment of an emotionally charged experience. Therapy in either instance logically consists of making these connections known to the patient (abreaction) and interrupting the conditioned reaction by negative conditioning. The symptoms then become natural, meaningful, and tolerable. Unfortunately, there are no accurate data as to the efficacy of these modes of therapy.

Each of the major types of psychoneurotic reaction will be described in the following chapters. In the remainder of this chapter the anxiety state, a syndrome common to many psychiatric and medical diseases, will be discussed in detail.

THE ANXIETY STATES

As indicated in Chap. 18 anxiety is not a disease *sui generis* or the manifestation of a single psychiatric illness. Instead it stands as a syndrome which may occur in relatively pure and uncomplicated form, as in anxiety neurosis, or in association with other psychic or physical disorders, as in hysteria, psychasthenia, depression, schizophrenia, and delirium tremens.

INCIDENCE OF ANXIETY STATE (AND OTHER PSYCHIATRIC SYNDROMES) IN A GENERAL HOSPITAL. As a clinical syndrome the anxiety state outranks all other general medical problems requiring diagnosis in a hospital, though probably it is less frequent than depression. In 1,000 successive psychiatric consultations in a large diagnostic clinic it was noted that approximately 25 percent of patients suffered from an anxiety state and that 50 percent expressed some degree of depressive mood. In contrast, frank hysteria occurred much less frequently (5 percent), and all the other psychiatric syndromes (mixed psychoneuroses, obsessive-compulsive neuroses, compensation neuroses, psychopathic personality, paranoia, manic-depressive psychoses, the schizophrenias, alcoholic psychoses, and psychoses with brain disease) comprised not more than 10 percent of the total number.

The relatively pure anxiety states may occur in an acute or chronic form.

Acute Anxiety Neurosis

This illness may arise in otherwise healthy adults and exist as the major part of a relatively pure syndrome. Its onset may be abrupt, in the form of a frank anxiety attack, or it may develop gradually as a nervous state of increasing severity, punctuated later by anxiety attacks. The attacks may be solitary or recurrent.

The predominant feature of the illness is the anxiety attack. It usually begins with a distressing presentiment of disaster or a sense of imminent dissolution. The patient feels that he will lose his mind or die (angor animi). Angor animi is manifested by such expressions as "I am dying," "This is the end," "Oh, my God, I am going." This is followed within a few seconds or minutes by palpitation, difficulty in breathing, tightness in the throat, a feeling of smothering or suffocating; trembling, sweating, and giddiness. Hyperventilation may be pronounced, and as a consequence paresthesias of the lips and fingers and even carpopedal spasms may occur. Sometimes there is a sense of unreality or a feeling that one cannot move or is in a trance. The visceral symptoms point to a disorder of function in organs supplied by the vagus nerves. Indeed Gowers was so impressed with this fact that he called spells of this type *vasovagal attacks,* and Nothnagel referred to them as *angina pectoris vasomotoria.*

Such attacks come on most often when the patient is in a crowd. He feels pent-up, oppressed, unable to breathe, and tries to leave as quickly as possible. Other provocative situations are small, closed rooms, elevators, tunnels, and subway cars. Some attacks begin when the patient is alone in his own home or walking down the street. They may occur at night and awaken him from a sound sleep. At times they appear to be induced by a troublesome dream. A particular situation may invariably provoke an anxiety attack.

Except in minor details, all the attacks are alike in any one individual. Their duration varies from a few minutes to an hour. Immediately following an attack, distressing weakness to the point of exhaustion may become apparent and persist for several hours or days. Between attacks, except for being upset over such an alarming experience, the patient may feel well, though often he complains of being tired, "nervous," and preoccupied with a fear of further attacks. Attacks of this type may occur once or several times a day. Many patients believe that they are having a heart attack and call their physician, regardless of the hour. Some physicians have reported that anxiety attacks are the most frequent cause of emergency calls at night. An illness of this type may be self-limiting; in fact, many patients recover without ever seeing a physician, according to Ross. In such cases often the severe form becomes chronic and demands medical attention.

Chronic Anxiety Neurosis and Neurocirculatory Asthenia

An individual who develops this syndrome may have been healthy before the onset of symptoms, or he may have been anxious in the past and may have had acute attacks of anxiety. From the history alone, two general categories of patients may be differentiated: those who give convincing evidence of good health, nervous stability, and ability to do muscular work and to engage actively in athletics without fatigue prior to the onset of illness; and those who have had a lifelong illness with symptoms of poor exercise tolerance, inability ever to do hard work, tenseness, "nervousness," and intolerance to crowds. Patients in the former group suffer from a chronic anxiety neurosis; those in the latter group have chronic neurocirculatory asthenia.

The onset of chronic anxiety neurosis is rare before the age of eighteen or after thirty-five to forty; the mean age of onset in Cohen's series was twenty-five. The illness is twice as frequent in women as in men. The course is variable. Most often there are periods of several weeks' duration when the symptoms are so severe as to interrupt the patient's activities. These may be separated by periods of partial or complete remission. There is a high familial incidence of this illness, but the explanation of this fact is not known.

In addition to a typical anxiety attack, or many of them, the patient usually complains of fatigue, restlessness, tenseness, apprehension, and "nervousness" developing over a period of weeks. Pressure headaches, often described as a bandlike sensation encircling the head, and palpitation are other prominent and troublesome symptoms. The physician, finding little or nothing by objective examination, often attributes the fatigue and other symptoms to low blood pressure or anemia, and prescribes a tonic or vitamins. The patient, on learning that no evidence of structural disease was found on examination, may be reassured for a few days, but as his symptoms return, he is again assailed by doubts concerning his health. Anxiety attacks are usually the reason for such patients' seeking medical aid for the first time.

The relative frequency of 20 different symptoms that comprise the syndrome of acute anxiety neurosis has been tabulated by Cohen and by Miles and Cobb. Nervousness, apprehension, palpitation, and breathlessness head the list; while trembling, fatigue on effort, chest pain, dizziness, sweating, and headache occurred in more than 50 percent of cases. Paresthesias, sighing, smothering, vascular throbbing, nightmares, anorexia, pain radiating to the left arm, fatigue on minor exertion, depression, and syncope were less frequent. Concerning the smothering, the patient usually remarks, "I can't get enough air," "I have to fight for my breath." The chest pain consists of a feeling of pressure or aching, usually in the precordium, and rarely is of a darting or stabbing nature. The dizziness is of the type referred to as giddiness (see Chap. 23). Faintness is frequent; actual syncope is uncommon. Nevertheless, the patient's fear of fainting may cause him to seek the quiet of his own home and to shun people. The appetite is poor, and digestive complaints, e.g., nausea, epigastric pressure, a sensation of abdominal fluttering, are not infrequent.

The physical examination usually yields relatively little of positive value. Cohen, in one of the most thorough and objective reports on this condition, has noted only (1) slight and inconstant tachycardia, (2) slight tachypnea, (3) sighing respirations, (4) flushed face and neck, (5) tremor of the outstretched fingers, and (6) brisk tendon reflexes. The results of standard clinical laboratory procedures—i.e., blood cell counts, urinalysis, blood sugar tests, nonprotein nitrogen determination, basal metabolic rate, electrocardiogram, and electroencephalogram—are within normal limits.

Neurocirculatory asthenia (also called effort syndrome, irritable heart, soldier's heart, DaCosta's syndrome, nervous heart, vasomotor neurosis, chronic vasomotor instability, cardiac neurosis), in contrast, is a chronic, perhaps lifelong illness, which manifests itself by excessive fatigability, palpitation, and dyspnea on slight exertion. It usually becomes apparent during adolescence and interferes with the physical activity of the patient, particularly in his participation in vigorous games. Nervousness, tenseness, and the other symptoms listed for the acute anxiety state, including frank anxiety attacks, also occur in chronic neurocirculatory asthenia.

Patients with neurocirculatory asthenia frequently consult cardiologists because of the suspicion that they suffer from heart disease, and indeed many such cases are mistakenly diagnosed as mild rheumatic heart disease because of the chance finding of a systolic murmur or an unexplained tachycardia.

Many of these individuals make a satisfactory adjustment to their illness by limiting their activities. In times of war, when they are inducted into the army, their nervous instability and cardiopulmonary symptoms are so prominent as to render them unfit for active duty. In this respect, it is of interest that all the more important studies of neurocirculatory asthenia have been undertaken during a war.

The physical findings are the same as those of the chronic anxiety state. Occasionally there is a slight systolic murmur and the T waves may be flattened in leads I and II. Approximately half the children of patients with neurocirculatory asthenia have been found to suffer from the same syndrome. A 20-year follow-up on 173 cases by Wheeler, White, Reed, and Cohen showed that the symptoms were still present in 88 percent of the patients but only 15 percent had had moderate to severe disability from them.

Most of the patients were able to work and enjoy a normal family and social life. Psychosomatic illnesses or other types of psychoneurosis had not developed.

CAUSE AND MECHANISM OF THE CLINICAL STATE (See Chap. 18).

DIAGNOSIS. This subject was discussed in Chap. 18 where the difficulties in distinguishing anxiety from other diseases which persistently or intermittently activate the autonomic nervous system, thyroid, and pituitary glands were stressed.

Once the diagnosis of anxiety state, with or without anxiety attacks, has been established with reasonable certainty, the next problem is to determine its significance. Is it but a manifestation of a more serious illness such as schizophrenia or a depressive psychosis? Is it combined with other neurotic symptoms such as phobic obsessive-compulsive neurosis or hysteria? Is it merely an expression of fear or anger due to some event that has recently occurred to upset the affairs of the patient, or is it a chronic lifelong illness? Is it a reaction to the development of an organic brain disease?

In order to answer these questions the physician must make pointed inquiry as to the presence of mood depression, distortion of logical thinking and inappropriateness of affect, hysterical symptoms, obsessions, compulsions, phobias, and dementia. It is helpful to bear in mind that anxiety states that develop for the first time after the thirty-fifth year of life almost invariably prove to be agitated depressions or the result of brain disease. See Table 372-2 for differential diagnosis. See also Chaps. 271 (coronary heart disease), 89 (thyrotoxicosis) 93 (pheochromocytoma), 72 (bronchial asthma), 98 (menopause).

MANAGEMENT AND TREATMENT. There is rather little available information as to the effectiveness of different methods of treatment in anxiety neurosis and neurocirculatory asthenia. The few published reports suggest that supportive medical care, simple psychotherapy, deep psychotherapy such as psychoanalysis, and institutional psychiatric therapy, all give results that are roughly comparable, i.e., they produce improvement in about 50 to 70 percent of cases. Many psychiatrists are of the opinion that frequent psychotherapeutic interviews have produced the highest percentage of cures, but this conclusion cannot be drawn from the published data.

Adequate examination and detailed case study as performed in a hospital are an important part of therapy. The patient should be reassured that there is no other serious medical disease. He should be told firmly and convincingly that he is suffering from a nervous disorder from which he will recover. His illness should not be passed off as imaginary. Many physicians encourage their patients to give up smoking because this tends to aggravate the pulmonary and vasomotor symptoms; but if smoking appears to relieve the tension, they probably should not be deprived of this support. If the patient is extremely irritable and upset, a trial of sedatives is indicated. Barbital in doses of 0.3 Gm b.i.d. or phenobarbital 0.032 Gm. t.i.d. should be given for 2 or 3 weeks. During the past few years encouraging results in controlling anxiety have been obtained by the authors with the use of meprobamate in doses of 200 to 400 mg or methaminodiazepoxide (Librium), 5 to 10 mg, four times a day. Tonics and vitamins are sometimes of value as supportive measures. However, since there is no serious medical disease, and in order to be consistent, it is well to avoid the use of all medication and encourage the patient to resume his activities. If anxiety symptoms recur he should be urged to be as tolerant of them as possible. Obvious sources of anxiety should be avoided. The hyperventilation symptoms which occur in the last part of the anxiety attack can to some degree be voluntarily controlled and this is often reassuring to the patient, for he then knows that he is the master of at least part of his attacks.

These few simple measures will relieve symptoms in about half or more of the cases, particularly the more acute ones in which fear of disease is paramount. Chronic and severe cases should be referred to a psychiatrist, if one is available. Psychotherapy should probably not be prolonged. Some of the more experienced psychoanalysts, including Freud, have stated that psychoanalysis is not indicated for this condition.

Chronic neurocirculatory asthenia is best managed as any other chronic incurable medical ailment. The patient is given every possible assistance in adjusting to his disability.

PSYCHASTHENIA (Obsessive-compulsive Neurosis, Phobic Neurosis, Obsessive-compulsive-ruminative State)

The terms *psychasthenia* and *neurasthenia* have quite different meanings in psychiatry. The former refers to an illness characterized by obsessions, morbid fears, and doubts. It will be discussed in some detail below. The latter term had wide popularity in the nineteenth century and is now obsolete. It referred to a state in which the major symptoms were chronic fatigability, lack of endurance, backache, and headache. Upon further study most patients with this type of condition proved to be suffering from anxiety neurosis, neurocirculatory asthenia, a depressive psychosis, or hysteria. There seems now to be no need for this diagnostic category.

Psychasthenia in its fully developed form is a relatively rare condition, probably occurring in not more than 0.5 percent of the population for whom psychiatric consultation is sought in a diagnostic clinic. Lesser degrees of it, manifest as excessive hand washing and other irrational habits or rigid, obsessional thinking, are much more frequent, and it may interfere with the therapy and management of medical disease.

Psychasthenia is discussed in this chapter on anxiety

because anxiety is a prominent feature in the majority of patients.

This type of neurosis, like many others, usually develops during adolescence or early adult years, and females and males are both affected, the former somewhat more frequently. The beginning of the illness is gradual in most cases and no date can be assigned to it, but in others its onset may be precipitated by some unusual event in the personal life of the patient with which he is unable to cope.

The outstanding characteristics of the illness are *obsessions, phobias, compulsions,* and *anxiety.* Westphal, who was the first to make a study of obsessions, concluded that anxiety is always secondary to the obsession, but this opinion appears to be too absolute, for in some cases anxiety precedes the obsession. Rosanoff and others are inclined to the view that obsessions and anxiety are "two manifestations of the same fundamental psychic disorder."

An *obsession* may be defined as an imperative idea which persists in the patient's mind despite his desire to be rid of it. It is like a tune "running in the head," which every normal person has experienced from time to time. Often these thoughts are unpleasant, and some of them are frightening. Obsessions are of various forms. The most common are the *intellectual obsessions,* in which the mind of the patient is occupied either by some abstract or concrete idea—a word, an object, or image of a scene; *impulsive obsessions,* in which the mind is dominated by an impulse to kill oneself, to stab one's children, or to perform some other objectionable act; *inhibiting obsessions,* in which every act must be ruminated upon and analyzed before it is carried out—a state aptly called "doubting mania." Every effort of will or deliberate attempt at distraction fails to rid the patient of the obsessive thought. It engulfs his mind; it renders him miserable and inefficient. Probably the most disturbing of these obsessions are the impulsive ones, in which the patient is constantly struggling with the fear that he will put his terrible thought into execution. Even as he tells of his obsession he seeks reassurance that he will not yield to it. Fortunately, such patients rarely obey their fatal impulses.

Phobias are similar to obsessions. In fact they are really obsessive fears. The most common phobias are those of open places, closed places, high places, dirt, traveling, syphilis or other venereal disease, cancer, insanity, or death.

Compulsions are the third feature of the illness. These are single acts or series of acts which the patient feels he must carry out in order to put his mind at ease or to relieve his nervousness. Examples are repeatedly checking the locks on the doors or the gas jets, adjusting articles of clothing, repeated hand washing, wiping with a clean handkerchief objects which have been touched, etc.

Certain motor disturbances of an apparently less meaningful nature are also present in many cases. Usually they involve a small group of muscles and are of limited extent. They consist of repetitive movements of the shoulders, arms, hands, and certain of the facial muscles, i.e., habit spasms, also called *tics.* Their outstanding feature, unlike other involuntary movements, is that they take place only with accompanying consciousness.

In all these phobias, obsessions, compulsions, and motor agitations the patient recognizes the absurdity of his behavior, yet is incapable of controlling himself, much as he desires to do so. He suffers a curious feeling of insufficiency or incompetency in being unable to expel these troublesome thoughts.

The majority of these patients are tense, nervous, and apprehensive. They may complain of typical anxiety attacks. After the condition has persisted for a time they may become discouraged or depressed over their helplessness in escaping from their obsessions and compulsions. This distraught emotional state is usually inconstant and is often related to the fear that an idea may eventuate in reality. Fatigue, anorexia, and general lack of interest, which are often present, are probably related to the anxiety and depression. In other respects the patients do not deviate from normal.

CAUSE AND MECHANISM. Janet expounded the theory that the very domination of the mind by these disturbing thoughts indicates a defect in what is commonly called willpower. It was his impression that such individuals really differ from the normal person in that they have less power of mental inhibition and that the processes of attention do not function normally, which is why distracting and irrelevant thoughts cannot be eliminated. Indecisiveness is believed to be another common manifestation of this weakness. For all these fundamental defects Janet has suggested the term *psychasthenia,* and by this he vaguely implies a genetic origin but offers no further evidence on this point.

The psychoanalysts have offered a theory in terms of their familiar postulates concerning the human psyche. To them the psychasthenic behavior is the result of the imperfect repression of some disagreeable wish. They conceive of this wish as having an ideational as well as an emotional, or affective content. The latter is the attached libido. If the whole of the disagreeable wish is completely repressed, the energy of the affect may be converted into a physical symptom such as hysterical paralysis or anesthesia (conversion hysteria). If repression is imperfect or incomplete so that only the ideational content is thrust out of the mind, the energy of the affect may then be converted into fear with a resultant phobia, or displaced to another idea which then becomes an obsession or compulsion. The puzzling persistence of the idea or fear is, for them, due to the emotional energy of another idea, which cannot be recalled except by the aid of free association.

Janet's and Freud's theories are not incompatible. Janet has described the condition of the psychasthenic mental state, and Freud has described the conditions which bring about each specific psychasthenic phenomenon. To the neurologist, however, both theories appear to be only partial explanations. One rather expects that some more basic defect, as yet unexplained, must allow these irrational ideas or compulsions to dominate the mind.

DIAGNOSIS. Since the prevailing emotional state in patients with psychasthenia is one of anxiety and depression, it is necessary to distinguish between this condition, anxiety neurosis, and depressive psychosis. There are important differences between them, and they can be distinguished rather easily in most instances. In psychasthenia the depression tends to be evanescent and closely related to the obsessive thinking. As the latter improves the depression lightens. In uncomplicated anxiety states, although baseless fears are not uncommon, they are never so persistent or so disabling as in psychasthenia; and the indecisiveness, compulsive actions, and habit spasms are lacking. Schizophrenia must be considered when an adolescent or young adult begins to harbor peculiar ideas, but then the mental status almost invariably reveals the other disturbances in affectivity, thought, and attention, which are described in Chap. 372.

TREATMENT. The treatment of these rare forms of psychoneurosis is probably best left to psychiatrists, or at least there should be a trial of psychotherapy in most cases. Whereas a few spectacular improvements are said to have been accomplished by psychoanalysis, for the most part the results which have been obtained in a series of patients have never been reported. Presumably the outlook for recovery is poor. In exceptionally severe cases electroconvulsive and insulin shock therapy has been undertaken as a last resort, with some degree of success. The former has proved effective when a strong depressive element colors the clinical picture. Tranquilizing drugs are just now being tried, and appear to be effective in some patients.

REFERENCES

See end of Chap. 372.

370 HYSTERIA AND PSYCHOPATHIC PERSONALITY
(With Remarks on Malingering)
Raymond D. Adams

HYSTERIA

CLINICAL DESCRIPTION. The so-called "classic" form of hysteria without doubt predominates in women, as confirmed in all contemporary clinical studies. Hope, who collected statistical data on the incidence of neuroses, has not observed a typical case of hysteria in a man in more than 10 years. During this period, in which several thousand psychiatric cases were seen in consultation, the diagnosis of female hysteria was made 813 times. There were, however, eight male cases with an illness that bore some resemblance to the classic form of hysteria, but they differed in one important respect—a tangible, material compensation factor was present in each.

From this, however, it must not be assumed that a neurosis in which compensation factors are prominent is limited to men, for one sees it in many women as well. One must conclude that classical hysteria is exceedingly rare in males and that women are as likely to develop a psychosomatic illness in which a tangible financial gain is a factor as are men.

Because of this and other important differences between the two forms of disease, each is presented separately on the following pages, one under the heading of hysteria, the other as compensation neurosis.

"Classic" Hysteria. By a careful review of the history of any given case it can usually be learned that the disease had its onset at the time of puberty or adolescent years. A few cases may appear to begin before puberty, at the age of eight or nine up to fourteen years, but before this period of life it is so rare that it should seldom be considered as a diagnostic possibility. Once established, hysteria often appears to be a lifelong illness or type of reaction, and symptoms continue to occur intermittently, though with lessening frequency, throughout adult years even to an advanced age. There are, no doubt, cases of lesser severity which exhibit symptoms only once or a few times, just as there are lesser degrees of all conditions. The patient may be seen for the first time during the middle period of life or later, and the earlier history may not at first be obtained. Careful probing, however, will almost invariably reveal that the earliest manifestations of this illness had appeared before the age of twenty-five years.

Other interesting and valuable data are also brought to light by a careful past history. During late childhood and adolescence the normal activities of the patient, including education, have usually been interrupted by periods of illness. Sometimes diseases such as rheumatic fever or tuberculosis were suspected. Later in life, problems in work adjustment and marriage are frequent. There is a notably high incidence of marital incompatibility, separation, and divorce. The patient's life history is punctuated with symptoms and illnesses which do not conform to recognizable patterns of medical and surgical disease. For these, many forms of therapy, including surgical operations, have been performed. Rarely has adult life been reached without at least one abdominal operation, usually done because of pain, persistent nausea, and vomiting, or generalized weakness. The indications for the surgical procedure have usually been unclear, and further, the same symptoms or others have recurred to complicate the convalescence. The biographies of these patients are also replete with disorders which center about menstrual, sexual, and procreative functions. Menstrual periods may be painfully prostrating, irregular, or excessive. Sexual intercourse may be painful, unpleasant, or unsatisfactory. Pregnancies may be difficult; the usual vomiting of the first trimester may persist all through the gestational period, with weight loss and prostration; labor may be severe and prolonged, and all manner of unpredictable complications are said to occur during and after parturition.

Hysteria is, then, rarely a monosymptomatic disease.

Expressed another way, the only forms which can be diagnosed with any degree of assurance are polysymptomatic, involving almost every organ system. The only limit to their variation and pleomorphism is the limit of the patient's ability to produce them by an effort of will (conscious or unconscious). Accordingly, symptoms and signs which are beyond volitional control cannot be accepted as manifestations of hysteria. A list of the most frequent symptoms, all statistically significant, which were elicited during a study of 50 unmistakable cases of female hysteria and compared with a control group of 50 healthy women of the same age who were working regularly in a factory and who appeared to have no recognizable psychiatric illness (Cohen, Robins, et al.) include the following: headache, blurred vision, lump in the throat, loss of voice, dyspnea, palpitation, anxiety attacks, anorexia, nausea and vomiting, abdominal pain, food dyscrasia, sexual indifference, painful intercourse, paresthesias, dizzy spells, nervousness, and easy crying.

The examination of the female hysteric patient demonstrates a number of useful findings, mostly in the sphere of mental status. The personality disorder may best be characterized as one of "emotional immaturity and emotional instability," to use a phrase from the text book of Mayer-Gross, Slater, and Roth. The patient's response to questions regarding the chief complaint usually arouses suspicion of hysteria. A vague reply or the narration of a series of incidents or problems, many of which prove to have little or no relevance to the question, follows. However, unlike the situation in a psychotic illness, general insight is more or less intact, and there is no evidence of hallucinations, delusions, disturbance in logical thinking, or loss of appreciation of the reality of the situation. The manner of the patient is often amiable and even ingratiating. The description of symptoms tends to be dramatic and exaggerated and does not necessarily accord with the facts as elicited from other members of the family; yet at the same time a rather casual emotional reaction is manifested. The patient may insist that everything in her life is quite normal and controlled, when, in fact, her medical record is chequered with disorders of dramatic behavior and unexplained illness. This calm attitude toward a turbulent illness is so common that it has been singled out as an important characteristic which the French call *la belle indifférence*. Other patients, however, are obviously tense and anxious, and frank anxiety attacks are reported by many of them. Also, "any attempt at disproving the somatic nature of the complaints meets with anxiety and dramatic protest." Memory defects (amnesic gaps) are usually demonstrated while the history is being taken; the patient appears to have forgotten important segments of the history, particularly those which related to the development of her symptoms (Lindemann).

There are no characteristic physical findings. Although many writers have commented on the rather youthful, girlish appearance and coquettish manner of many of the patients, this by no means characterizes all of them. The so-called "stigmas" of hysteria, i.e., corneal anesthesia, absence of gag reflex, spots of pain and tenderness over the scalp, sternum, breasts, lower ribs, and ovaries, are often suggested by the examiner and are too inconsistent to be of much help in diagnosis.

Special Hysterical Syndromes. A few hysterical syndromes recur with great regularity, and every physician may expect to encounter them. They constitute some of the most puzzling diagnostic problems in medicine.

Hysterical Pain. This may involve any part of the body; generalized or localized headache, "atypical facial neuralgia," abdominal pain, back pain with camptocormia are the most frequent and most troublesome to the clinician. Here the greatest source of error is to mistake the pain of osteomyelitis, metastatic carcinoma, or brain tumor, before other symptoms have developed, for a manifestation of hysteria. In many of these patients the response to analgesic drugs has been unusual, and not a few of them are suspected of or may be suffering from drug addiction. They may respond to a placebo as though it were a potent drug, but it should be pointed out that this is a notoriously unreliable means of distinguishing hysterical pain from that of other diseases. The most helpful diagnostic features are inability of the patient to give a clear, concise description of the type of pain, its location, and other features; the dramatic elaborations of its intensity and effects; its persistence, either continuous or intermittent, for long periods of time; the lack of conformation to other pain syndromes; the absence of other diseases which could account for pain; the assumption of bizarre attitudes and postures; the coexistence of other hysterical symptoms.

Hysterical Vomiting. This is often combined with pain and tenderness in the lower abdominal quadrants and results in many unnecessary appendectomies and the removal of pelvic organs in adolescent girls and young women. The vomiting is somewhat unusual, in that it often occurs after a meal, leaving the patient hungry and ready to eat again; it may be induced by unpleasant circumstances. Some of these patients can vomit on command, regurgitating food from the stomach like a ruminant animal. Vomiting may persist for weeks with no cause being found. Weight loss may occur but seldom to the degree anticipated. The usual first trimester vomiting of pregnancy may continue throughout the entire 9 months, and occasionally pregnancy will be interrupted because of it. Anorexia may be another prominent symptom.

Hysterical Seizures and Other Psychical States, e.g., Trances and Fugues. These conditions seem to be less frequent than in the days of Charcot, when *la grande attaque d'hystérie* was often exhibited before medical audiences. Nevertheless they do occur and must be distinguished from convulsive seizures and catalepsy. To witness an attack is of great assistance in diagnosis. The lack of aura, initiating cry, hurtful fall, and incontinence, the presence of peculiar movements such as grimacing, squirming, biting, striking at or resisting those who offer assistance, the retention of consciousness during a motor seizure which involves both sides of the body, the long duration of the seizure and abrupt termination by strong sensory stimulation are all typical of the hysterical attack. Sometimes hyperventilation will initiate an attack and is therefore a useful maneuver in the hospital or clinic. Both epilepsy and hysteria may be combined in the same patient, in which instance the resulting illness invariably causes difficulty in diagnosis. Hysterical trances or fugues, in which the patient wanders about for hours or days and carries out complex acts, may also simulate temporal lobe epilepsy, epilepsy equivalent, or any of the conditions which lead to confusional psychosis or stupor. Here the most reliable point of differentiation comes from observation of the patient, who, if hysterical, is likely to indicate a degree of alertness and promptness of response not seen in confusional states. After the episode is past, an interview with the patient under the influence of hypnosis, strong suggestion, Pentothal, or scopolamine will often bring to light memories of what happened during the episode. This will exclude the possibility of an epileptic fugue.

Hysterical Paralyses and Tremors. Hysterical palsies usually involve an arm, a leg, one side of the body, or both legs. If the affected limb can be moved at all, muscle action is weak, and often the strength of voluntary movement is in proportion to the resistance offered. Movements are characteristically slow, tentative, and poorly sustained. One can feel agonist and antagonist muscles contracting simultaneously. When the resistance is suddenly withdrawn, there is no follow-through, as with normal movements. The muscular tone in the affected limbs is usually normal, but rigidity may sometimes be found. Walking may be impossible, there may be a veritable astasia-abasia, or the gait may be bizarre (see Chap. 23). This discrepancy between the ability to walk and to move the legs is, of course, not unique to hysteria; it also occurs in frontal lobe apraxia and in ataxia from midline cerebellar lesions. If the limb has been held in a rigid posture for a long time, contractures may set in. The features of hysterical tremor are described in Chap. 22 and need not be repeated here. The tendon reflexes are always normal, but with hysterical anesthesia of one-half the body, the abdominal and plantar reflexes may be suppressed on the affected side. Anethesia or hypesthesia is almost always inadvertently induced by the examining physician. Seldom is sensory loss a spontaneous complaint of the patient, though the symptoms of "numbness" and paresthesias are not uncommon. The sensory loss may involve one or more limbs below a sharp line (stocking and glove distribution) or may involve one-half the body. Touch, pain, taste, smell, vision, and hearing may all be affected on that side, which is an anatomic impossibility from a single lesion.

Hysterical Amnesia, Somnambulism, and Pseudodementia (Ganser's Syndrome). Patients brought to a hospital in a state of amnesia are usually hysterical or psychopathic. Usually after a few hours or days, with encouragement they divulge their whole life history. The epileptic patient or the victim of a concussion or acute confusional psychosis does not come to a hospital asking for help in establishing his identity. Moreover, the complete loss of memory for all previous life experiences by a patient who is otherwise able to comport himself normally is not observed in any other condition.

In Ganser's syndrome, which usually occurs in psychopathic males involved in a crime, the patient pretends to have lost his mind or to have become insane. He acts in the way he believes an insane or feeble-minded person should act. He may babble and give silly and obviously incorrect answers to every question asked of him. Usually his behavior is obviously an act.

Unexplained Hyperpyrexia. Among the sporadic cases of unexplained fever which turn up in every diagnostic clinic, there are always a few hysterical patients. Although our clinical material is not large, the authors have been impressed with the number of student nurses, nurses, and nursing aides among them. Some of these patients will be found to have no fever if the nurse or doctor checks the temperature. Others have oral temperatures of 99 to 100°F, which must be regarded as normal for some individuals. Finally, there are a few well-documented cases of verified hyperpyrexia, said to be of psychogenic origin. In these the possibility of some obscure hypothalamic disorder cannot be excluded. Diagnosis is assisted by a longitudinal history and the elicitation of the other symptoms of hysteria.

Dermatitis Factitia (Hysterical Dermatoneurosis). This condition is seen more often in the psychopathic than in the hysteric patient. The skin eruptions induced by the patient are characterized by erythema, ulcerations, gangrene, and variable degrees of dermatitis. Usually a caustic or irritant chemical or a sharp instrument such as a nail file has been used. The lesions are most commonly observed on parts of the body accessible to the right hand, i.e., right side of the face, neck, anterior trunk, anterior surface of left arm. They are multiple, sharply outlined, appear at variable intervals of time, and do not conform to any of the standard dermatologic diseases. They resist all treatment until protected from the continued manipulations of the patient and then they heal promptly.

Hysteria with an Important Factor of Compensation. As stated before, hysteria in men is most often encountered in patients who serve the military, in veterans' hospitals, and in places where injured civilian workers are treated. As in the classic form of hysteria described above, multiple symptoms are noted in the majority of cases. Furthermore, many of the symptoms are the same as those listed under female hysteria, i.e., headache, nervousness, irritability, pain in the back and extremities, dizziness, dyspnea, palpitation, nausea, vomiting, paresthesias, blurred vision, anxiety attacks, depression, faints, amnesia, loss of libido, and trance states. A tangible gain from the illness may easily be discovered by simple questioning. This is usually in the form of monetary compensation, which, surprisingly enough, is often less than the patient could earn if he returned to work. Another interesting feature is the frequency with which the patient expresses extreme dissatisfaction with the medical care given him;

he is often frankly hostile toward the physicians and nurses. Descriptions of symptoms tend to be lengthy and circumstantial, and the patient fails to give details which are necessary in diagnosis. Many of these patients have already been subjected to an excessive number of hospitalizations when first seen, and rather dramatic mishaps may have occurred in carrying out diagnostic and therapeutic procedures. The majority have been suspected of and many accused of malingering by at least one physician in the past, which may be responsible for the aggressive behavior and uncooperative attitude of some of the patients. In fact compensation hysteria, as pointed out below, is at times indistinguishable from malingering. The diagnosis of hysteria in the male probably should be made with great caution unless some obvious compensation factor is present.

Women who suffer injury while at work or are involved in auto accidents may exhibit these same symptoms and signs. Individuals with hysterical personalities may also be excessively disposed to accidents. This is one of the causes of the *accident-prone syndrome.*

CAUSE AND PATHOGENESIS. Over the years, from the time when hysteria was first recognized, many theories and hypotheses have been advanced, purporting to explain its cause and mechanism. Up to the present, none has been validated. The student is referred to any of the current textbooks of psychiatry for an account of the psychopathologic explanations offered by Charcot, Babinski, Janet, and Freud.

DIAGNOSIS. The method of diagnosis subject to the least error is that employed in medicine generally, i.e., an informative history (obtained from the patient himself as well as from sources other than the patient) and a physical and mental status examination (see Table 372-2). The elicitation of the attributes of a neurotic character by interview and special so-called "projective" tests (Rorschach and Thematic Apperception Tests), methods popular with dynamic psychiatrists, may be helpful but are by no means infallible. Even evidence of extreme suggestibility and the tendency to dramatize symptoms cannot be taken as absolute criteria of the disease, for they may appear under certain conditions in nonhysterical individuals. The psychiatrist obtains help from an analysis of the character of the patient, but this is not likely to be of use to physicians who are not versed in special psychiatric techniques. A longitudinal history, the manner and attitude of the patient, and the absence of symptoms and signs of other medical and surgical disease probably will permit the accurate diagnosis of the majority of cases.

TREATMENT. The treatment of hysteria may be considered from two aspects: the correction of the long-standing basic personality defect, and the removal of the recently acquired physical symptoms.

Since the main defect in thinking and in character development in the hysteric patient may be profound, little or nothing can be done about it at present in the most severe cases. Psychoanalysts have attempted to modify it by long-term reeducation, but their results are unavailable and there are no control studies for the few reports of therapeutic success. One has the impression that in many cases the underlying illness is so pervasive that nothing can be accomplished except to grant that the patient is inadequate in certain respects and requires medical support. Many psychiatrists, for this reason, are inclined to regard the female hysteric with a life-long history of ill health as having a severe psychopathy. In other less severe cases and especially in those in whom the hysterical symptoms have appeared under the pressure of a major crisis, psychotherapy appears to have been helpful and the patients have been able thereafter to resume their places in society.

The acute outbreak of symptoms can usually be controlled by persuasion. Here the best tactic is to treat the patient as though he has had an illness and is now in the process of recovering. The earlier this is done after the development of symptoms, the more likely they are to be eradicated. In chronic cases strong pressure to get out of bed and resume function must be applied. Compensation neuroses are often quite difficult to treat, and a settlement of claims may be necessary before the symptoms are relieved.

The following therapeutic principles should be observed in the average case of hysteria where expert psychiatric opinion is not available or in severe cases where previous psychiatric treatment has failed.

1. Hysteria must be treated as a tangible, definite illness. The patient should never be told, "There is nothing wrong with you," or "It's just your imagination." This at once alienates her, and she almost invariably terminates her relations with the physician. The patient should not be dismissed as a malingerer or a faker of illness.

2. Simple understandable language should be employed in interviews with these patients; abstruse psychologic terms should be avoided. It is unnecessary to employ the term *hysteria* in discussions with these patients or their families, since it conveys a derogatory connotation which the physician should not imply.

3. The care of the patient should be entrusted to one physician.

4. All indicated examinations and laboratory procedures for the investigation of the chief complaints should be conducted before actual treatment is begun. Once the treatment is started, one should avoid, if possible, rechecking or repeating laboratory or examination procedures.

5. Persuasion and suggestion, both direct and indirect, should be employed in the treatment of patients. Illustratively, the patients should be encouraged, told that they are better, urged to resume work or household duties and to continue participation in routine activities. Symptoms should be ignored and medication should be withheld.

6. There should be several personal interviews in which the patient is permitted to direct the discussion. He should be assured of the privacy of the interview, of the impersonal, "morally neutral" position of the physician, and of the advantages of "thinking things out more thoroughly." Any questions which the patient asks should be answered truthfully in accordance with the physician's knowledge, in simple, direct terms.

7. Every illness in such patients should be evaluated as a possible manifestation of hysteria. The possibility of other diseases must not be overlooked. Surgical procedures should be used only if strict criteria of surgical disease are satisfied.

How successful this program will be over a long period of time is not known. The eradication of some recently acquired hysterical symptom is relatively easy. The real test of therapy is, however, whether it assists the patient to a satisfactory adjustment to family and to daily activities, prevents unnecessary medical treatments and operations, and makes possible the prompt diagnosis of any medical or surgical disease, which may strike a hysteric patient just as it does any other person.

PSYCHOPATHIC PERSONALITY
(Constitutional Psychopathic Inferiority, C.P.I.)

Aside from those patients who suffer from psychoneuroses, epilepsy, psychoses, and feeblemindedness, there still remains a large number who do not fit any of these categories but are still incapable of making a satisfactory adjustment to civilized society. This rather heterogeneous group includes drug addicts, many habitual criminals, the chronically unemployed, and those who are more or less constantly under the care of social welfare agencies. The majority come from the lower strata of society where lack of parental discipline, neglect, etc. are frequent. Only a small segment of this group, those who develop symptoms and signs suggestive of disease, ever come to the attention of the medical profession. However, all of them, those with as well as those without symptoms, seem in some manner to be lacking an essential trait which permits a normal, stable adjustment to life. As a consequence, they remain social misfits.

The group of these patients which displays behavioral disturbances for which medical advice is sought in general hospitals is not large. Only 33 were found among 10,039 patients examined by the Psychiatric Service of the New England Center Hospital over an 8-year period. However, in large municipal hospitals and in military service and veterans' hospitals the number of cases is much greater.

CLINICAL DESCRIPTION. This disorder becomes manifest early in life, and both sexes are equally susceptible. However, recognition before the age of twenty-one is difficult because one depends for diagnosis largely on evidence of protracted behavioral disturbances over many years. The common turbulent emotional outbreaks during adolescence are particularly difficult to assess in this respect. Experienced physicians know that many boys and girls who appear destined for a life-long psychopathy settle down and become stable citizens, once adulthood is reached.

The most distinctive feature of the constitutional psychopath is his *impulsivity*. He seems unable to control his impulse to any act which provides immediate gratification of his urges and instinctual drives. Without any apparent concern he will withdraw from a team, quit a job, aban-

don his family, seek financial gain regardless of the means, drink excessively, or be sexually promiscuous. When brought to task for his misdemeanor he appears sorry and may persuade others that he will reform, only to repeat the same act or some other one equally irresponsible when the occasion arises. This *inability to profit from experience* despite adequate intelligence and a proved capacity to learn in school is another noteworthy feature. These defects result in an apparent inability to conform to the moral and ethical standards of his social group; hence he is classed as a "moral imbecile."

The complaints and somatic symptoms which bring these individuals to a general hospital are multiple and varied. Like the hysteric, they have amnesias, trances, fits, paralyses, gait disturbances, unexplained prostration, alleged hemorrhage, unexplained fever, etc. Psychotic episodes may also occur but are remarkably brief as a rule. They tend to develop at the time of some crisis or during an episode of heavy drinking or drug addiction and consist of outbursts of uncontrollable temper, fits of depression with feeble attempts at suicide, and unsystematized delusions and hallucinations. Often they clear up within 2 or 3 days after the patient enters a mental hospital. Their reckless impulsivity predisposes some of these patients to accidents (accident-prone syndrome).

At the time of examination the manner and attitude of the patient are especially informative. He is engaging, talkative, and very persuasive, often convincing the physician and family of the correctness of his position and arousing their sympathy. He may be courteous, ingratiating, and flattering to those around him. On the other hand some such patients are irritable and irascible and may be provoked to anger by some triviality. Only when his story is checked against that of the family does one begin to realize that the present episode has followed a pattern of behavior which has created endless problems over a period of years. Furthermore it is then apparent that the patient himself has no real insight into his condition and is inclined to blame his plight on ill luck, various injustices perpetrated by others, or destiny. Even when caught rubbing his thermometer on the bed sheet to feign the fever of some infectious disease, or when found picking his gums to produce an impression of obscure gastrointestinal bleeding, he appears totally uninterested and leaves the hospital saying he is sorry that the doctors did not believe him.

In recent years it has been discovered that a number of these patients have minor electroencephalographic abnormalities, some of clearly paroxysmal type compatible with epilepsy, and others, nonspecific and diffuse. Also psychologic tests may in some instances reveal findings of the type seen in patients with brain disease.

CAUSE AND PATHOGENESIS. For such a heterogeneous group of behavioral disorders as this represents, one would hardly expect to find a common etiologic factor or mechanism. The word *constitutional* is deplorably ambiguous, for it refers both to genetic factors and to those which result from unfavorable environmental influence. All diseases, in this sense, are constitutional. Yet the term will probably continue to be used until it is possible to separate the particular entities which it presently embraces and to find their cause and mechanism.

Two general theories have been elaborated to account for these aberrations in behavior: (1) character neurosis, (2) structural disease of the nervous system. According to the theory of character neurosis, the abnormal nervous and mental processes are due to psychogenic factors which operated in early life. Here one is on treacherous ground, for little evidence has been forthcoming in favor of this idea, and critics of the theory maintain that the adverse effect of psychologic factors is the result of an intrinsic brain disease rather than the cause of the illness. Adherents of the concept of neurologic disease refer to the remarkable variety of behavioral changes, often limited to emotional control and character structure, which followed in the wake of the great epidemic of lethargic encephalitis after World War I, and also to the rather high incidence of electroencephalographic abnormalities. Here again evidence is wanting, for no thorough neuropathologic studies have been made. A final opinion on this matter cannot be expressed at this time. One can only say that the problems involved in such cases are at present beyond the realm of scientific knowledge.

DIAGNOSIS. The key to diagnosis is the evidence by well-documented history of a long-enduring behavior disturbance in which impulsive actions, inadequate self-discipline, weak inhibition, faulty judgment, and the failure to learn by experience have led to a series of immoral and unethical actions (see Table 372-2). In addition, there are the physical symptoms of the type seen in the malingerer and hysteric. Finally the mercurial affective response, varying from a nonchalant, persuasive manner or boastfulness to open hostility, and the utter lack of insight complete the picture.

Alcoholic psychoses, schizophrenia, and manic-depressive psychosis must at times be differentiated, and this is usually possible when all the data of the history and mental examination are at hand. Needless to say, however, some of these individuals do develop frank alcoholic psychoses or have epilepsy, particularly of the temporal lobe type. Such cases can easily be confused with hysteria because of their multiple spurious somatic symptoms. The differentiation is usually not difficult if it is remembered that the number of symptoms is much greater in the hysteric than in the psychopath and, in the cases of male hysteria, the possibility of material gain is more obvious. Hysterical stigmas are not prominent and are certainly less impressive than the tendency of these patients to "put on an act." The defect in the psychopath shows most clearly in his inability to make a satisfactory adjustment to school, to work, and to marriage. Lastly, unethical or immoral conduct is peculiar to the psychopath. When alcoholism is added to a psychopathic personality state, the resulting psychoses differ in no way from those occurring in other individuals.

TREATMENT. The early recognition of psychopathic personality with proper instruction of the family as to the serious nature of the illness may save much expense and embarrassment. Unfortunately many of these individuals are so nearly normal that the possibility of mental disease may not be considered. As yet no treatment has emerged which has modified the behavior of these patients. Reeducation and both superficial and "deep" psychotherapy are of little value because of the inability of these patients to profit by experience.

MALINGERING

This problem frequently arises in connection with both hysteria and psychopathic personality, and the physician should know how to deal with it. It is rarely a medical diagnosis, except under the rare circumstances in which a patient is caught in the act of producing a sign of disease or confesses to have done so. The term *malingering* means to consciously and deliberately feign an illness or disability in order to attain a desired goal. It would be correct to say that it does not present as an isolated phenomenon and that whenever it occurs it must be interpreted as a sign of serious personality disturbance, often one which prevents effective work or military combat, though noteworthy exceptions to this statement can be found.

The relationship between hysteria and malingering is nebulous to say the least. Certainly there is a close similarity in the two conditions and there may be great difficulty in establishing a clinical differentiation. Jones and Llewellyn have observed:

"Nothing . . . resembles malingering more than hysteria; nothing hysteria more than malingering. In both alike we are confronted with the same discrepancy between fact and statement, objective sign and subjective symptom—the outward aspect of health seemingly giving the lie to all the alleged functional disabilities. We may examine the hysterical person and the malingerer, using the same tests, and get precisely the same results in one case as the other."

The main points of difference between the two conditions which are cited by most authors are (1) the conscious or unconscious quality of the motivation, being always more or less unconscious in the hysteric and more or less conscious in the malingerer; (2) the influence of persuasion, which is usually effective in hysteria and not in the malingerer; (3) the attitude of the patient, the hysteric appearing more genuinely ill and inviting examination, the malingerer not.

The tendency of the psychopath to malinger has already been mentioned. Most of the more obvious cases of malingering which the authors have seen have been psychopaths, and for this reason comment on this phenomenon is made in relationship to this disease.

One observes in the malingerer pain, hyperesthesia, anesthesia, limping gait, tremor, contracture, paralysis, amaurosis, deafness, stuttering, mutism, amnesia, epileptiform seizures and fugues, unexplained gastrointestinal bleeding, pains and unexplained skin lesions, in short, almost the same array of symptoms and signs as in the psychopath and the compensation hysteric. Indeed the line between the two, especially between the malingerer and the "compensation hysteric," is too ambiguous to be of clinical value. Probably the medical profession has placed too great a reliance on degree of conscious awareness of deception. In such "weak-minded," unstable, and morally defective individuals, the words *conscious, unconscious,* and *deception* are too vague and subjective to serve as useful guides in practical work.

REFERENCES

See end of Chap. 372.

371 MANIC-DEPRESSIVE PSYCHOSIS, INVOLUTIONAL MELANCHOLIA, AND HYPOCHONDRIASIS

Raymond D. Adams

Each term in the title of this chapter stands for a highly distinctive clinical state which will receive separate description in the following pages. Nevertheless, they bear close relationship to one another, which is the justification for considering them as a related group of diseases. Depression is the most important member of the group and, as pointed out in Chap. 18, is the most frequent of all major psychiatric illnesses, accounting for an estimated 50 percent of all psychiatric illnesses and 12 percent of all medical admissions to a hospital for diagnosis.

Some illnesses of this type take the form of a relatively pure, uncomplicated depression. Others are mixed with anxiety and agitation and, because of their tendency to occur for the first time in the middle and late years of life, have been called involutional melancholia. Some are clearly reactions to real or imaginary life situations and, if persistent and troublesome, are regarded as *neurotic depressions. Mania* is less frequent than depression and may develop as a relatively pure clinical state, or it may be preceded or followed by episodes of depression, in which instance the illness is called *manic-depressive psychosis;* Lastly, there are not a few mild depressions which masquerade as *hypochondriasis;* although this psychiatric syndrome may rarely occur as a manifestation of a protracted and obstinate neurosis, it will not prove misleading to think of it always in relation to depression.

Aside from the prevalence of depression, mania, and hypochondriasis, physicians should be well acquainted with these symptom complexes for several reasons. One of the paramount dangers is suicide, which may be attempted and successfully executed, often before the depressive symptoms have been recognized, i.e., while the patient is being treated for "low blood pressure," "nerves," "emotional problems," and "chronic infection," or even before he has sought medical care. Prompt diagnosis may therefore prevent a tragedy. Furthermore, the syndrome of endogenous or involutional depression can often be treated successfully, and the patient may thus be spared a prolonged and disagreeable illness.

The symptoms common to this entire group of illnesses, because of their frequent occurrence in medical practice, were presented as constituting one of the cardinal manifestations of disease (see Chap. 18). The point was made in the introduction to the section on Psychiatric Diseases that the physician must assume the responsibility for recognizing the depressed state and distinguishing it from a number of other medical and psychiatric conditions. It was further suggested that the existence of this depressive syndrome, depending on its clinical context, should suggest a number of possible diseases, each of which requires a special mode of management. These may be classified as follows:

I. Reactive depressions
   A. In association with medical disease
   B. In association with current emotional problems
II. Depression in association with psychoneuroses
III. Depression as a concomitant of demonstrable neurologic diseases
IV. True or uncomplicated depression
   A. Manic-depressive psychosis—depressed state
   B. Involutional melancholia

In subdividing the true or uncomplicated depressions into manic-depressive psychosis (depressed phase) and involutional melancholia, the authors do not intend to imply that they represent distinct disease entities. They may indeed represent the same disease occurring at different periods of life. They are separated in this classification out of deference to time-honored psychiatric teaching, and because such a separation appears to be useful in treatment.

REACTIVE DEPRESSION

This term is used to denote a depressive syndrome precipitated by physical or emotional factors which in themselves could conceivably sadden the average person. Though some authorities, namely, Kraepelin, Kretschmer, and Bleuler, tend to minimize the importance of reactive features in the production of depression, it is certain that one encounters the depressive reaction after a physical or emotional disturbance in individuals whose basic temperament does not conform to that of the manic-depressive group.

Depression in Association with Medical Disease

Depression in patients with serious medical disease does not appear to differ from idiopathic depression. The patients exhibit the same depressed mood, pessimistic ideational content, and agitation or slowing of psychomotor activity. Their thought content centers on the physical disease from which they suffer and the incapacity induced by it. Great concern is expressed because of the change in life pattern imposed by the disease. Chronic, debilitating, incapacitating illnesses such as Ménière's disease, arthritis, diabetes mellitus, pernicious anemia, tuberculosis, and malignancy are the ones upon which the depressive reaction is most frequently engrafted. Physical examination and appropriate laboratory studies demonstrate the typical findings of these diseases. A careful history may reveal that the symptoms of the physical disease may have antedated the depressive reaction by many months. The prognosis for recovery from the depressive syndrome is largely determined by the prognosis of the physical disease with which it is associated. If the latter can be successfully treated and the patient's normal life pattern restored, there may be a concomitant disappearance of the depressive symptoms. In many cases, however, the depression outlasts the medical disease and must be treated as a separate illness. Conversely, if the medical disease is incurable, the likelihood of the depression responding to treatment is poor.

Depression in Association with Emotional Problems

Depression as a reaction to various emotional disturbances such as the death of relatives or loved ones, serious financial reverses, marital problems, unrequited love, or a series of stressful environmental impacts is qualitatively identical with that encountered in the previously described circumstances. However, quantitatively it is often less severe than the depression of manic-depressive psychosis or involutional melancholia. The discussion of the particular emotional factor with which the depressive reaction is associated brings forth an outburst of sadness and weeping. Conversely, when the conversation is diverted from the patient's emotional problems to neutral topics, a surprising elevation of the mood with a lightening of the depression becomes almost immediately apparent. Usually these patients do not have hallucinations or delusions. Weight loss is infrequent. Suicide is not so common in this group as in the true depressions. From the history it is clearly evident that the existence of the emotional problem antedated the appearance of the depressive reaction. Recovery from the depression usually occurs. The length of time that the depressive reaction exists before recovery ensues is determined largely by the patient's ability to resolve the emotional problem with which it is associated.

PSYCHONEUROTIC DEPRESSION

Depressive symptoms in psychoneurotic individuals unquestionably do occur. It may be difficult to decide whether they are a part of the psychoneurosis with a particular psychodynamic mechanism or an independent illness. In anxiety neurosis, hysteria, and psychasthenia, saddening or depression of mood is usually transitory, lasting only a few minutes or a few hours and rarely longer than a day or two. It bears direct temporal relationship to the incapacity induced by the psychoneurosis or to the exacerbations of symptoms of the psychoneurosis. On the other hand the author has encountered clear-cut depressive episodes of varying duration occurring in patients who have had the symptoms of chronic neurocirculatory asthenia or hysteria for many years preceding the onset of the depression. The occurrence of a typical involutional depression late in life in patients who have had anxiety neurosis or hysteria for many years has also been witnessed. In each of these circumstances the previous existence of the psychoneurosis in no way altered the natural course of the depression. It seems probable that such patients have two illnesses, i.e., psychoneurosis and depression.

DEPRESSION AS A CONCOMITANT OF DEMONSTRABLE NEUROLOGIC DISEASE

Depression as one of the early manifestations of organic disease of the brain is readily recognized by the cardinal symptoms of depressed mood and pessimistic ideational content associated with psychomotor retardation or agitation, in conjunction with dementia and other neurologic abnormalities. At times the depressive reaction may be so marked as to obscure the basic neurologic aspects of the clinical picture. In milder forms only an inexplicable fatigability and disinterest in customary activities demarcates the depressive reaction. A careful history of change in established behavior patterns, defective judgment, and moral lapses, and the observation of marked lability of affect, distractibility of attention, impairment of memory (especially for recent events), disorientation in time and space, a depleted fund of knowledge, a reduction in general comprehension, and perseveration in speech, action, and thought are the usual distinguishing features. Positive neurologic findings as described in Chap. 30 are demonstrable in many cases. The occurrence of the depressive reaction in these disorders is considered by some authorities to represent an exaggeration of the previous personality pattern; i.e., the depressed patient is said to have had a premorbid temperament of the cyclothymic type. The outlook for recovery from the depression in these cases is to a large extent dependent upon the prognosis of the coexistent neurologic disease. In general it is unfavorable.

TRUE OR UNCOMPLICATED DEPRESSION

Manic-Depressive Psychosis and Endogenous Depression

True depression occurs most often in individuals who suffer a curious illness known as manic-depressive psychosis. This disease has been known to the medical profession since the appearance of the first article on the subject by Falret in 1854. Later Baillarger, Kahlbaum, and Kraepelin described the disease more fully.

CAUSE AND MECHANISM. "A taint from the side of the family," Kraepelin's idea of the cause of manic-depressive insanity, has received ample corroboration from recent genetic studies. These disclose an incidence of 20 to 25 percent in other members of the biologic family and 66 to 96 percent in the identical twin, even wher the latter was raised by a foster family. A greater frequency in females has suggested to some investigators a sex-linked genetic possibility. The disease is believed to express itself also through body habitus which tends toward rounded obesity and large body structure (a mixture of endomorphic and heavy mesomorphic habitus according to the classification of Sheldon). The inherited trait is believed to direct the structurization of personality during the formative years, along obsessive-compulsive lines (Abraham), excessive development of ego (Freud), rigidity, conventionalism, excessive competitiveness, and insensitivity to the feelings of others (Cohen).

The medium by which gene alters function has been sought in an endocrine disorder without success. Recently, however, the discovery that iproniazid, an antidepressant agent, increases the quantity of epinephrine in the brain by inhibiting monoamine oxidase, and imipramine (another antidepressant) has a similar effect by another mechanism has given new stimulus to chemical theories. This is in line with another earlier observation that reserpine can produce depression, an effect that can be counteracted by dopamine, a precursor to catecholamine. From these studies one can conclude, as does Kety, that this evidence supports "the concept that certain biogenic amines, especially the catecholamines, in particular areas of the brain play important roles in mediating normal and abnormal affective states." Therapeutic agents such as drugs and electroshock are capable of increasing the synthesis, release, or otherwise enhancing the effective concentration of norepinephrine and possibly other amines.

Manic-depressive psychosis, as the name implies, consists of episodes of mania or depression or both. *Mania,* which has not been described in previous sections of this book, is undoubtedly one of the most dramatic of all psychiatric illnesses. Within days or weeks a reasonably well-balanced individual may develop uncontrollable enthusiasm. In *hypomania,* the mildest form of the illness, it is not always easy to decide whether the patient is mentally sick or merely acting peculiarly because of some change in the circumstances of his work or family life; often some unusual event may appear to have affected him unduly. First it may be noticed that the patient is attracting more attention than ordinarily. The routine of daily living is suddenly broken. Facial expression is more gay and animated; dress is less restrained or eccentric in some way. All actions and reactions are more brisk. Conversation is louder, and there is a tendency to talk excessively and to be argumentative. The handwriting is larger and suggestive of haste and impatience. The mind is more active, and ideas come more freely, sometimes with the result that the patient is more witty and socially more agreeable than usual. New theories which solve the most abstruse problems come to mind; new enterprises may be enthusiastically undertaken without due deliberation and then abandoned a few days later, only to be replaced by others. The patient is physically more active. He is restless, paces the floor, moves from one place to another, sleeps rather little, and has an almost inexhaustible energy. Friends or members of the family, realizing that something may be wrong, that the patient needs supervision, soon become weary and perplexed with his noisy, changeable ways. Another disturbing symptom is a loss of inhibitions and deviation from customary standards of conduct. The patient may be less discreet than formerly; he thinks nothing of discussing personal or family problems before strangers. If opposed, he may be irritable and argumentative.

As these symptoms become more prominent, the family may seek medical help; often this is prompted by some act which upsets the family or the community. It may be an assault upon someone who has criticized or disagreed with the patient, or some deviation from moral standards, such as excessive sexual indulgence or alcoholism. The patient has relatively little insight, as a rule, and may resist attempts at treatment or hospitalization. To make matters more difficult, he is plausible at this stage and has a ready and often coherent explanation for his actions. There is no clouding of consciousness or forgetfulness. The physician seeing the patient for a short time may note only the extreme restlessness and overactivity as being at all peculiar.

Acute mania is a more severe degree of hypomania. At this stage the abnormality of the patient's behavior is abnormal beyond question. Ideas now flow rapidly, one suggesting another and another, the connecting threads being very loose. This is termed *flight of ideas.* The associations are usually obvious and the coherence superficial, unlike those of the schizophrenic. Motor activity likewise increases until finally there is at times almost a frenzy of excitement. The stream of thought and activity may be difficult to interrupt; yet at any time there may be a pause, and momentarily the patient is able to recognize his physician and his whereabouts and to make a sensible remark. Hallucinations may occur but are transitory, and delusions, if present, are usually changeable and poorly elaborated. The mood is merry, gay, but interrupted by periods of irritability and anger. Memory and intellectual functions are impossible to examine accurately, but there is nothing to suggest that they are disordered. Judgment and insight are limited or absent.

In *hyperacute* or *delirious mania* the patient is completely uncontrollable. He paces the floor and, if restrained, struggles constantly and tosses about. Speech is completely incoherent and his utterances make no sense at all. The patient gives no thought to his actions, exposes himself unabashedly, is careless in his habits, and is totally uncooperative. There are auditory and visual hallucinations, suspicions, and delusions.

Manic illnesses of this type may last for weeks or months, but in the majority of instances the symptoms gradually subside. A few patients pass into a stage of chronic mania which may persist indefinitely. After an acute or hyperacute mania terminates, there is usually little or no memory for the details of what has happened.

At all stages of mania *the elated mood* and *increase in psychomotor activity* are the evident and characteristic qualities of the illness. In the hypomanic state the clarity of the sensorium distinguishes it from a mild delirium. Acute and hyperacute mania, however, in which orientation, thinking, and judgment are deranged, are at times almost impossible to distinguish from delirium or from an excited schizophrenic state unless one knows the background of the illness and the early symptoms.

Transitional phases between pure manic excitement and pure depression are not too infrequent. Here the rather difficult diagnosis is usually established by the fact that the patient is known to have manic-depressive psychosis and then begins to exhibit a mixture of the symptoms of both phases of the illness. These "mixed states," as originally described by Kraepelin, may take the form of a maniacal stupor, agitated depression, nonproductive mania, depression with flight of ideas, and akinetic mania.

In depression the clinical picture is the converse of mania. There is simple retardation with slowing of both mental and physical functions and depression of mood. The milder forms may masquerade as hypochondriasis, but the more severe ones are easily recognized. *Depressive stupor,* in which the patient remains in bed, refuses to speak, and has to be fed and urged to attend to bladder and bowels is the most severe grade of depression. The patient's thoughts are pessimistic, and he has no interest in anything. Delusions are usually present. Psychomotor retardation is so marked that the patient may take no notice of objects and people around him. Consciousness appears befogged. Fortunately depressive stupor and maniacal delirium are rare and are not likely to be encountered by the physician in general practice.

The different phases of manic-depressive psychosis may succeed each other in the same individual; or a patient may be subject only to recurrent attacks of depression separated by periods of normalcy. But depression is approximately ten times more frequent than mania. These latter cases are called *endogenous depression.* An attack of depression may be replaced by one of mania, or a manic episode may be followed by a depressive episode. The duration of these episodes is subject to extraordinary variations; they may last from a few weeks to a year or more. As a rule, however, depressive patients are more subject to recurring depressions than to mania, and the same may be said for the manic patient. After a single attack of depression, the chance of recurrence is 9 out of 10.

In manic-depressive insanity the prognosis is relatively good. A young person nearly always recovers from an individual attack. There is no evidence to suggest that repeated attacks ever lead to dementia. For this we have the authority of Kraepelin, who wrote, "Usually all morbid manifestations completely disappear but where that is not the case, only a rather slight, peculiar psychic weakness develops, which is just as common to the types here taken together as it is different from dementias in diseases of other kinds." (See Table 372-2 for differential diagnosis.)

Involutional Melancholia

This is likely to occur in individuals whose temperaments are characterized by rigidity, overscrupulousness, overconscientiousness, meticulousness, and high ethical standards. They have usually been very active, busy, and hardworking and may have performed a dull, uninteresting job in a methodical fashion. Shortly before the actual onset of the illness, there is usually a precipitating or exciting factor such as an illness which temporarily changes the patient's life pattern, the breaking up of his home, a change in family relationships, business problems, or the death of a relative.

Involutional melancholia is more common in women than in men, the ratio being about 3:2. The age range of onset is stated arbitrarily in the literature as being between forty and fifty-five years in women and between fifty and sixty-five years in men. However, we have encountered involutional depression in classic form occurring as early as thirty-two years of age in women and forty-two years of age in men, and as late as sixty-eight years in women and eighty-one years in men. Because of the occurrence of these depressions in the age epoch picturesquely referred to as the "involutional period," and because of their association with the symptoms of the menopause in women, attempts have been made to relate them to the endocrinologic change of the climacterium. However, the most careful workers in this field have failed to establish this mechanism, and attempts at therapy with varying doses of androgenic, estrogenic, and progestational substances both orally and parenterally have failed to effect any change in the natural course of the illness.

In its fully developed form the clinical picture of involutional melancholia is that of an agitated depression. The mood is anxious, apprehensive, despondent, and dejected, and there is often an undercurrent of irritability. Instead of exhibiting a paucity of ideas and retardation of speech, many of these patients are communicative and talk a great deal. The content of their utterances is repetitious and monotonous. Moreover, if the patient's speech is interrupted by a question, it is usually answered tersely and to the point, following which there is immediately a return to his complaints, with much rumination and a repetition of the same phrases again and again. The patient's state of dependence is evidenced by his frequent visits to the physician for reassurance. Ideas with a depressive coloring, self-recrimination and self-depreciation, somatic preoccupations with fears regarding the existence of incurable disease, nihilistic delusions, suicidal preoccupations, fatigue, anorexia, and insomnia comprise the clinical picture. In their motor excitement the patients walk about wringing their hands, plucking at their apparel, and generally tormenting themselves and those about them by continually lamenting their fate. These patients are mentally clear as to their surroundings, perceive accurately, and are well oriented. In its mildest form the clinical picture is characterized by tenseness, anxiety, apprehension, uneasiness, self-concern, fatigue, insomnia, and anxiousness with or without prominent delusion formation, and lesser degrees of depression.

Often patients with an agitated depression have any one or several of the cardiovascular, genitourinary, or other diseases common to this age group. These associated diseases, strangely enough, may be ignored by the patient and are only discovered on routine physical examination. A common mistake is to confuse the symptoms of depression with those of some other organic disease and to expect the depressive symptoms to disappear when the latter is treated.

The prognosis was poor before the advent of modern therapy.

TREATMENT. In the management of the true depressions, i.e., manic-depressive psychosis (depressed phase) and involutional depression, the first question to be considered by the physician is whether to treat the patient himself or refer him to a psychiatrist. Mild or moderately severe depressions can, in many instances, be safely managed by competent general practitioners who are aware of the dangers inherent in the disease. The chief risk is suicide, particularly in the early stages of the depression, sometimes before the symptoms are fully recognized, and in the late stages, just as the symptoms are subsiding. The patient may commit suicide after having denied even the thought of such action. His relatives must therefore understand the nature of the illness and guard against such an eventuality by constant supervision. However, the maintenance of this supervision must be tactful and unobtrusive so that the patient does not get the idea that he is being "spied upon," "watched," or "policed" and thus have the suicidal impulse accentuated by inadvertent harmful suggestion. Failing to secure such cooperation from the relatives, the physician should refuse to accept responsibility for the management of the patient.

The treatment should consist of psychotherapy and pharmacotherapy. The psychotherapy employed should consist of reassurance, education as to the nature and course of the illness, and helping the patient find the positive values in his life situation. The patient should be told that his illness is not a serious one, and the self-limited quality should be emphasized. In patients who have had a previous depressive illness, the recovery from that episode should be dwelt upon and used as a point of reassurance in the present illness. The physician should not say, "There is nothing wrong with you," or that the symptoms are imaginary. Instead he should state that though real and distressing, the symptoms do not have their basis in demonstrable structural disease. The expressed belief of the patient or his relatives that he "should fight this thing off," or "It's up to me, I'll just have to snap myself out of it," should not be encouraged. He should be told not to force himself into activities which are repellent but to resume them as he improves. A helpful point in management is to work out a daily program which includes mild exercise, physical therapy, rest, simple diet, and a few activities which the patient is likely to enjoy. This gives him and his family a tangible approach to the problem. At the outset, interviews in which these psychotherapeutic principles are employed should be conducted once or twice weekly. As the patient improves he should be urged, at first cautiously and within the limits of symptomatic tolerance, to increase the range of his activities until his normal routine is reestablished. It is estimated that about 50 percent of patients improve or recover from psychotherapy alone.

Along with psychotherapy, drugs should be employed. It was shown by Lindemann in 1931 and later by other workers that Sodium Amytal, employed in nonhypnotic doses, is an effective antidepressant and produces at least temporary amelioration of depressive symptoms. When it is employed in conjunction with amphetamine, a synergistic effect occurs. The dose found to be effective in mildly and moderately depressed patients is Sodium Amytal, 0.12 to 0.20 Gm (amobarbital) t.i.d. in conjunction with dextroamphetamine (Dexedrine), 5 to 10 mg b.i.d. daily. As a synergist for Sodium Amytal, Benzedrine Sulfate works equally as well as Dexedrine Sulfate. However, the latter drug is preferable because it does not elevate the blood pressure. Since the depressive reaction is characteristically worse in the morning, the medication is given upon arising and after the midday meal. In patients in whom anorexia and weight loss are prominent, it is better to prescribe the medicine after breakfast as well as after the midday meal, since the Dexedrine sulfate may increase the anorexia. If the beneficial effects produced by the medicine wane late in the afternoon, a third dose can be given. However, it is inadvisable to give Dexedrine after 6 P.M. unless a strong sedative is prescribed upon retiring, because it may interfere with sleep. There is considerable individual variation, and the dose here prescribed may have to be adjusted to secure optimal benefit. If the patient becomes torpid, drowsy, or somnolent 20 to 30 min after taking the medicine, the Dexedrine should be increased to 12.5 mg. On the other hand, if apprehension, tenseness, or palpitation supervenes 20 to 30 min after the medicine has been taken, the Dexedrine should be reduced to 5 mg. At times it is not necessary to employ nocturnal sedation, since the patient may sleep well on the regimen outlined. If nocturnal sedation is necessary because of insomnia, a barbiturate preparation should not be used, since additional amounts of barbiturates decrease the patient's tolerance to the beneficial effects of Sodium Amytal. Chloral hydrate, 1 to 2 Gm, or paraldehyde, 8 to 10 ml, is usually efficacious.

In the past several years a great many drugs collectively known as "tranquilizers" have been employed in the treatment of various psychiatric illnesses. In some instances, however, when slight to moderate improvement has occurred on the drug regimen described in the preceding paragraph, a greater amelioration of symptoms has been obtained when chlorpromazine, in doses of 10 to 25 mg; meprobamate, in doses of 200 to 400 mg; or Librium, 5 to 10 mg at 10 A.M., 2 P.M., and 6 P.M. has been added.

The most interesting new development in the therapy of depressive disease has been the introduction of a series of drugs classed as monoamine oxidase inhibitors, such as iproniazid (Marsalid), isocarboxazid (Marplan), phenelzine (Nardil), or as tricyclic compounds, such as imipramine (Tofranil) and amitryptyline (Elavil). Tofranil has had the most thorough evaluation and, when given in a dosage of 75 to 400 mg per day, starting with 25 mg t.i.d. and increasing slowly until a good result is obtained (usually the effect does not become evident for 7 to 10 days), there has been a considerable degree of success. The advantage is that there is no interruption of experiential continuity such as occurs with electroshock therapy, and there is ease of administration, lower cost, and possibility of continuous supportive psychotherapy. If it is not successful, Elavil in a dose of 75 to 150 mg per day or Marplan, 10 to 30 mg per day, should be tried. The author's experience would indicate that these drugs along with the barbiturate sedatives and analeptic drugs are less successful than electroshock therapy. Tryptophane in a dose of 50 mg twice or three times a day has recently received a favorable report. Lithium carbonate 300 to 600 mg per day in divided doses has proven to be the best means of controlling mania and of preventing recurrent attacks.

With the tricyclic antidepressants the blood pressure should be followed carefully, since postural hypotension may be a problem. Ephedrine sulfate, 40 mg b.i.d. or t.i.d., may counteract it. Dryness of mouth, dysuria, and urinary retention, other side effects of Tofranil, can be combated with pyridoxine hydrochloride, 25 mg two to four times a day. Great caution must be exercised in the use of these drugs, particularly of chlorpromazine, since jaundice, resulting from interstitial hepatitis, and leukopenia may develop. Another complication observed by Campbell is a blood picture resembling chronic granulocytic leukemia or myeloid metaplasia. In most instances, however, these complications disappear when chlorpromazine is discontinued. Hypotension is another troublesome symptom but is not apt to occur unless oral doses of chlorpromazine exceed 20 to 50 mg daily.

Reserpine should not be employed in the treatment of the depressive syndrome because it may produce depressive symptoms in patients who have shown no evidence of depression preceding its usage. Because of the tendency of reserpine to produce depressive symptoms, it occurred to the author to employ it in the treatment of the manic phase of manic-depressive psychosis. Although controlled data have not been secured, it is the clinical impression that the manic phase of this illness may respond to oral doses of 0.5 to 1.0 mg three to four times a day or parenterally in a dose of 2.5 mg twice a day.

Whenever possible, the custody and administration of the medicine should be assigned to a responsible member of the family. When this cannot be done, the total amount of medicine prescribed at a given time should be small so as to avoid the tragedy of self-inflicted harm should the patient, in a suicidal attempt, take all the medicine in his possession.

If the mild or moderately depressed patient fails to show signs of improvement after a satisfactory trial period of 2 to 3 weeks on this combined conservative regimen, he should then be referred to a psychiatrist for treatment. The delay imposed by trial of conservative treatment, though it be unsuccessful, does not prevent the patient from responding favorably to treatment carried out by a psychiatrist.

All severe depressions, as soon as the diagnosis is rea-sonably certain, should be referred to the psychiatrist for treatment. In most instances severely depressed patients should be admitted to a psychiatric hospital where electroshock therapy and appropriate medical measures to ensure adequate nutrition and elimination can be provided. There must be facilities for the prevention of self-inflicted injury. These measures are augmented by appropriate occupational, recreational, and physical therapy. Electroshock therapy appears to have had its greatest success in the treatment of involutional depression and the depressed phase of manic-depressive psychosis. Although carefully controlled experiments cast some doubt upon the efficacy of electric shock therapy in terminating an individual depressive episode or preventing recurrences, nevertheless it is the author's clinical impression that it does indeed favorably influence the course of the individual depressive episode. This type of treatment should be given by a psychiatrist.

Neurosurgical treatment in the form of prefrontal and other types of lobotomy have been introduced in recent years. If they are to be used at all they should be reserved only for those severe and chronic cases which have failed over a period of many years to improve on all other methods of therapy.

Patients with reactive depressions in association with emotional problems require psychotherapy, which is often quite time-consuming and beyond the scope of the average general practitioner. In a patient with long-standing psychoneurosis and a complicating depression, the latter should be treated by the measures outlined for uncomplicated depressions.

HYPOCHONDRIASIS

The status of hypochondriasis as a psychiatric illness has changed over the years. Originally it was believed to be a particular form of mental illness of the same general category as hysteria; current psychiatric opinion now favors the view presented by Bleuler that it is a symptom complex which may occur in psychoneuroses, schizophrenia, manic-depressive psychosis, or involutional depression.

The author's experience has led him to believe that hypochondriasis is usually a manifestation of a mild depression, and for this reason it is classified with the depressions. However, there are a few patients in every medical clinic, quite rare to be sure, in whom hypochondriasis appears to have persisted for long periods of time without other attendant psychiatric symptoms. This illness should probably then be classified as a psychoneurosis.

Hypochondriasis (so-named because the symptoms usually relate to the subcostal viscera) *is a condition in which the patient is unjustifiably preoccupied with the functions of his own body and with matters of health.* The main clinical characteristics of this illness are (1) the great number and variety of symptoms and complaints, all seemingly without foundation, and (2) the patient's peculiar attitude and reaction to his symptoms. There may be some complaints referable to every organ of the body, but those which occur most frequently are referable to the abdominal and pelvic viscera. Rectal pain, dryness or mucus and other abnormalities of the stool, difficulty in swallowing, epigastric distress, bloating, belching, abdominal cramps, fullness and pressure in the genital organs, frequency of urination and dysuria, nasal discomfort, difficulty in breathing, fatigue, backache, chest pains, and insomnia are some of the complaints. As regards the patient's attitude and reaction to the symptoms, it is to be noted that in his mind they represent manifestations of disease. Often no amount of argument or of negative examinations and laboratory tests will persuade him that he is wrong. The pervasive influence of these symptoms is revealed by the patient's manner of discussing them. He is overtalkative and dominates the interview with an endless description of his ailments. The pressure of speech may be so great that the examiner finds it difficult to interrupt its flow in his quest for specific information. The descriptions may be vague and the language rather bizarre, but in many instances they are meticulous, detailed, and repetitious. The patient speaks of his symptoms with great familiarity, as though they have been subjects of careful study, and it is evident that he has been so much engrossed with them that they have interfered with his work and social activities. It is impossible usually to divert the conversation to any other topic. Physical examination may disclose no abnormality or only a number of relatively unimportant signs of unrelated diseases. The same may be said of the neurologic examination.

The nature of the illness of which hypochondriasis is a part is revealed by other psychiatric symptoms. In the few cases of relatively pure uncomplicated hypochondriasis which the author has seen, the habit of self-observation and worry about health can often be traced to childhood or adolescence and may have begun during some protracted period of ill health, such as rheumatic fever, tuberculosis, or osteomyelitis, at that time. Sometimes the parents had evinced a similar concern over health problems. Rigid habits of eating, dress, elimination, and elaborate measures to avoid infections may have been inculcated by the parents and maintained throughout life. Other neurotic symptoms may have appeared during adult years. The patient shows no evidence of depression, distortion of "reality appreciation," delusions, or hallucinations.

Far more common than the above picture is that in which the hypochondriasis has developed in the middle or late years of adult life in a setting of mild depression. The latter may be obscured by the hypochondriasis unless one makes pointed inquiry about the patient's mood, affect, energy output, interests, and capacity for work and enjoyment.

The appearance of bizarre somatic symptoms in adolescence should always raise in the physician's mind the possibility of schizophrenia, the diagnosis of which is made by obtaining evidence of the typical disorder of affect, thinking, and attention described in Chapter 372.

The cause of hypochondriasis must be as varied and uncertain as that of the neuroses and psychoses of which

it is a part. Current theories of the rare lifelong forms of hypochondriasis are for the most part psychologic. It has been proposed that the patient is merely imitating the patterns observed in his parents, or that he uses the symptoms unconsciously in order to obtain indefinitely the privileges of being ill and receiving attention and affection. Feelings of insecurity, parental oversolicitude, fear of punishment, unhappiness in the home or school are emphasized in some formulations of the psychologic problem.

The treatment of uncomplicated hypochondriasis is extremely difficult. If it is part of a disabling neurotic state the problem is best managed by a psychiatrist. For the innumerable elderly adults with mild hypochondriacal symptoms who are among the most faithful attendants of every outpatient clinic, the management should be by general physicians. Reassurance, sympathetic evaluation of symptoms, a program which includes symptomatic measures, regularly scheduled periods of work and rest, encouragement to carry on normal activities despite symptoms enable many of these patients to carry on with reasonable comfort. Sodium Amytal, Dexedrine, and similar drugs should be used as outlined above if depressive symptoms coexist.

REFERENCES

See end of Chap. 372.

372 SCHIZOPHRENIA, PARANOIA, PUERPERAL AND ENDOCRINE PSYCHOSES

Raymond D. Adams

SCHIZOPHRENIA (Dementia Praecox)

Definition. Schizophrenia is the most serious unsolved disease in American society, according to "Medical Research: A Midcentury Survey," and is a disease or group of diseases in which there is a slow, steady deterioration of the personality. It begins usually during adolescence and early adult life and involves particularly the affective life—thinking, conduct, and the depth of insight. The cause is unknown, and no definable neuropathologic changes have been established. A hereditary factor operates in at least a certain proportion of cases.

HISTORICAL BACKGROUND. Morel, Kahlbaum, Hecker, and Kraepelin wrote the earliest descriptions of the disease. Kraepelin not only separated the disorder from manic-depressive psychosis but also observed that the several different syndromes of hebephrenia, catatonia, and paranoid psychosis were but varieties of this one pathologic process. Bleuler considered the disease misnamed *dementia praecox* because many cases instead of being "precocious" had their onset later in life and the term *dementia* did not adequately characterize the fundamental disorder. He declared the main abnormality to be a dissociation of emotional experience and overt behavior, for which the term *schizophrenia* was proposed.

CAUSE AND MECHANISM. Part of the difficulty in theorizing about this condition relates to imprecision in the definition of it. Bleuler contends that schizophrenia is not a disease process but rather a disposition in the direction of psychic life due to not one but many causes. It is a syndrome, so to speak. Batchelor and many others dispute this point of view, arguing that there is a "nuclear syndrome" which must be the clinical manifestation of a single disease with a single cause. The latter concede that there are a variety of other illnesses such as amphetamine psychosis, cortisone psychosis, alcoholic hallucinosis, and the psychosis of temporal lobe epilepsy which may simulate true schizophrenia (the schizophreniform psychoses) but that these can and should be separated on the basis of premorbid personality, mode of onset, character of clinical picture, natural course, and response to therapy. The paranoid form of schizophrenia, in particular, they believe to represent a different illness, more closely related to paranoia and depression than to the nuclear schizophrenic illness. Also acute undifferentiated schizophrenia seems to differ from all other types.

If one assumes the nuclear group of schizophrenias to be comprised of a chronic, lifelong illness that may first declare itself in childhood, adolescence, or early adult life by symptoms of vagueness and inattentiveness, illogical thoughts and delusional thinking, hallucinations, bizarre hypochondriacal complaints, feelings of passivity and influence, the incongruity of affect, its genetic aspects loom up importantly. Kallman pointed out in 1952 that "no analysis of a statistically representative group of blood relatives of schizophrenic and manic-depressive patients has so far been completed in any country without showing a significant increase in the expectancy rate for either psychosis." The expectancy rate for schizophrenia in the general population is between 0.7 and 0.9 percent. The genetic data which he presents may be summarized as follows: 11 percent of 5,000 siblings of schizophrenic patients were found to be suffering from the same disease; in 90 sets of fraternal twins, one of whom had schizophrenia, the disease occurred in the second twin in 11 percent of cases—the same incidence as in nontwin siblings; in 62 sets of identical, or monozygotic, twins, however, the disease occurred in the second twin in 68 percent of cases.

Unfortunately other studies of the genetic aspects of schizophrenia have given rather variable results. For example, the concordance rate in monozygotic twins has varied from 6 to 86 percent, but some of these were open to the criticism that they were not always controlled for essential variables. In more recent studies the figure has been from 40 to 60 percent. One of the more interesting lines of support for the genetic origin has come from the Copenhagen study of Kety and his associates, where a 10 percent prevalence of schizophrenia was found in the close biologic relatives of schizophrenics who had been separated from their biologic families in the first month of life and raised by individuals not biologically related to them. The prevalence of schizophrenia and related disorder, in the families that raised them, was not greater than in the general population, and the same was true of adopted children of families who had not had schizophrenia. The fact that these findings applied only to chronic undifferentiated and pseudoneurotic types of schizophrenia and not to the acute undifferentiated variety would suggest that the latter is a different disease. The close similarity of the pseudoneurotic and chronic schizophrenia informs us that the disease is a spectrum of malfunction which includes in the mildest form subtle personality and character disorders.

The manner in which a genetic factor can operate an interval of time after birth to produce this disease has never been determined. Obviously a genetic mechanism cannot transmit mental experience but can only transmit the capacity for having mental experiences. A variety of hypotheses have been advanced, but all are as yet unproved. Kety's formulation is the most reasonable one— that what is genetically transmitted is a polygenic predisposition which by interaction with as yet unspecified environmental factors can lead to a phenotype of varying intensity of illness. The reader should refer to textbooks of psychiatry for further information concerning these hypotheses.

INCIDENCE. Strecker estimated that at least 30,000 individuals develop this disease each year in the United States alone, an occurrence rate of about 25 per 100,000, which is not too different from that of tuberculosis. According to Mayer-Gross, Roth, and Slater, values of expectation in the general population range from 40 to 80 per 100,000.

CLINICAL MANIFESTATIONS. The illness declares itself largely by certain abnormalities of affectivity and thinking which are most clearly demonstrated by an examination of the mental functions of the patient. The medical history has not always been helpful in the author's experience. It is true, as stated above, that in the majority of cases the family will report a long-standing inability to form warm and satisfactory contacts with people and a tendency to shun activities of an "outgoing" nature, especially with members of the opposite sex, a disposition to indulge largely in solitary pursuits and daydreaming, all of which are special behavioral abnormalities of the introverted, schizoid, or dystonic type of personality. However, other patients have shown no prepsychotic behavioral abnormality whatsoever.

PRIMARY SIGNS. The more specific and characteristic signs unique to schizophrenia are (1) disturbances in affect, (2) disturbances in thought processes and associations, (3) disturbances in attention. These along with disturbance of activity were the basic features set forth by Bleuler, who derived the name from his concept of the disease—a splitting of personality. The initiative is split into a variety of potential activities, resulting often in total inactivity or catatonia; the individual is split off from reality; the thoughts and associations are split away from their appropriate affective content. The detachment from reality is called autism and results in ambivalence which expresses itself in affectivity and initiative. In terms of easy remembrance, schizophrenia, then, may be described as a disease of "four As": association, affect, autism, and ambivalence.

The secondary signs include hallucinations, delusions, muteness, catatonia, and negativism. Unfortunately, full agreement as to what is primary and secondary has never been reached. Schneider, one of the leading psychiatrists in Germany, includes amongst symptoms of the first order of importance: "the hearing of one's own thoughts, feelings of unreality, depersonalization, auditory hallucinations, somatic hallucinations, the feeling of one's thoughts being controlled by some outside agency (passivity feelings), the extension of one's thoughts to others." Symptoms of second order are other types of hallucinations, perplexity, and alterations of or lack of affect. In the view of another authority, "asthenia of psychic activity" stands as the central disorder. Until there is better understanding of the basic pathologic process, there would seem to be no possibility, except in terms of frequency, to separate primary and secondary effects. Any given clinical constellation of symptoms gains in specificity with the number of abnormalities included within it, but also the absence of other major nervous derangements such as clouding of sensorium, impairment of learning and memory, aphasia, acalculia, and visual-spatial disorientation are equally denominative features. Every component of the schizophrenic complex may sometime appear as an expression of other organic neurologic diseases.

Inappropriate or Inadequate Affect. In many though not all patients with schizophrenia, the affect, or outward expression of emotion, is bland, rigid, inappropriate, or ambivalent. Personal events of serious importance are discussed in a casual manner without any outward show of emotional concern, i.e., *inadequate* or *bland affect*. The patient may discuss the death of a near-relative, the dinner menu, and his admission to the hospital with the same apparent feeling and affect; i.e., the affect is rigid. He may relate that he has been pursued by his enemies or is at the moment about to be killed by a secret machine and, instead of expressing fear and anxiety, he appears faintly amused; i.e., emotional response is inappropriate. A friendly or unfriendly act on the part of a member of the family may fail to excite any response. He appears to be neither pleased nor displeased.

Disturbances in Thinking and Ideational Associations. In the patient's spontaneous utterances and in his replies to questions one finds that his thinking about any given topic is apt to be illogical, tangential, and irrelevant. When asked why he came to the hospital the patient may reply, "My brother brought me"; "The doctor suggested it"; "The ambulance brought me"; or "It was the hospital nearest my house." All these statements may have been true, but in each instance there had been a conspicuous behavioral change which had caused the family great concern and had led to the patient's commitment. The reason given for admission offered by the patient must thus be considered clearly "peripheral" or tangential. Inappropriate explanations may be offered. A patient seen tearing his shirt to shreds said that he was doing it because it was raining outside—an example of

illogical association. In conversation, seemingly unrelated and impertinent items may be brought up and even given as answers to direct questions, Such disturbances in thinking are called *associational irrelevancies*.

Not infrequently ideas that would at first appear illogical or irrelevant are actually quite sensible on further analysis. The lack of coherence is often, and may be in nearly all such instances, the result of *associational gaps* or *associational condensation*. In the former the patient makes a series of statements without supplying the connecting details, which he appears to consider unnecessary. One of the authors' patients stated that her present trouble was due to "speech and financial matters"; only after careful questioning was it learned that there had been a heavy financial loss because of poor crops on the farm and that she believed the neighbors to be speaking disparagingly of her and her family. These beliefs were reported to the sheriff who, upon finding them completely fallacious, sent her to a hospital for examination. Another patient said he came to the hospital because "First come best." This proved on further inquiry to indicate a series of ideas that an older brother whom he believed to be persecuting him was always favored by his family. The problem finally came to medical attention when he assaulted the brother with a knife because he had borrowed one of the patient's neckties. Probably this process of associational condensation accounts for some of the neologisms that appear in the speech and writing of schizophrenic patients.

The essence of the thinking disorder in schizophrenia is a failure to respect the usual cause-and-effect relationships and the usual method of drawing conclusions from factual evidence. The thinking is not rambling, incoherent, and chaotic, as in confusional psychoses, but instead appears to be directed inexplicably into certain devious channels. One often has the impression that with time and patient questioning some logical thread could eventually be followed through the disconnected, irrelevant, and distorted ideas; but, communication being limited, this is usually not possible.

Disturbances in Attention. Often there are lapses in "selective" attention or a preoccupation with certain ideas, and at these times the patient may ignore the questions of the examiner. Later he may respond alertly and focus his attention on the problem at hand and in fact may indicate that he heard the examiner's earlier questions even though he did not reply to them. At this stage he may be highly distractible and all sensory impressions crowd equally in upon his mind and tax his powers of assimilation. He fails to screen out irrelevant material. In the later stages of the illness he appears continuously preoccupied and it is impossible to attract or to hold his attention even momentarily. Yet, this disorder is quite different from that which occurs in the delirious or confused patient, where clouding of sensorium is the main feature.

Secondary Signs. The term *secondary* denotes those signs which appear to derive from the afore-mentioned disorders of thinking, emotion, and attention. The most important of these are delusions, hallucinations, rigidity, resistiveness, negativism, and mannerisms. Although not unique to schizophrenia, they occur with sufficient frequency to be of importance, and at times they appear to dominate the clinical picture.

Delusions. These false beliefs in schizophrenic patients are frequently of the *paranoid type*. The paranoid delusion has two components, a grandiose idea of one's own importance and an "idea of persecution." The patient may rationalize his delusion in several ways. Believing himself to be an important person and observing his signal lack of success in competitive life, he assumes that he suffers the fate of many prominent people, that of being persecuted by jealous rivals. Or, conscious of his own inadequacies, he continuously projects the blame on others. In addition, the schizophrenic patient suffers *somatic delusions,* usually beliefs that some part of his body is deteriorating or diseased, and *nihilistic delusions,* in which he denies the existence of himself and of everyone and everything around him. These delusions are related to the primary disorders of thinking but may at times be the most striking feature of the illness.

Hallucinations. Hallucinations are also a prominent symptom in schizophrenia. They may be auditory, visual, olfactory, or tactile. Unlike the hallucinations of delirium, they are usually rather ambiguous psychic phenomena, not always well enough described so that one can be sure of the sensory modality involved; and seldom are they projected into extracorporeal space. The patient admits to hearing voices but often does not state whence they come. In addition, sensory *misinterpretations* also occur. If two individuals are seen talking together, the patient assumes that he is the subject of their conversation and that they are making derogatory remarks about him. A casual gesture, a peculiar odor, an unusual sound are all interpreted as being intended to annoy him. These are called *ideas of reference.* Another unusual and closely related symptom is that in which the patient feels that his thoughts and actions are being controlled by some person or outside agency; these are called *ideas of influence,* or "passivity feelings."

Catatonia, Resistiveness, and Negativism. These are closely related phenomena. The catatonic patient lies immobile and is mute. He may permit himself to be dressed and led about or will sit or stand in one position for hours or days. No effort is made to eat or drink or even to empty the bladder and bowels for long periods of time. There may be incontinence and utter neglect of toilet and dress. This state of speechlessness and motionlessness suggests the possibility of aphasia or anarthria with paralysis, but it is ordinarily recognized for what it is by the lack of pathologic reflexes and the occasional normal movement or speech. Although the limbs may be supple, often attempts at passive movement demonstrate rigidity, which on closer observation suggests a deliberate or willed *resistiveness.* An extreme degree of resistiveness is *negativism,* in which the patient makes an action opposite to the one requested. When asked to open the eyes, he closes them tightly; if requested to protrude the tongue he clenches his jaw; and if told to sit down, he

will stand up. These phenomena of immobility, rigidity, resistiveness, and negativism are known collectively as catatonia. The term *stupor* is often added, even though there is no important disorder of consciousness and the patient is able to recount accurately all that transpired during the period of unresponsiveness.

Stereotypy of Utterance and Movement, Bizarre Mannerisms, Grimaces. The schizophrenic patient may utter certain words or expressions over and over again. This is termed *echolalia.* Certain movements may be repeated incessantly. The face may be set in a silly expression. Stereotyped, relatively automatic rituals may be reproduced again and again, seemingly dictated by some impulse and without regard as to their appropriateness.

Other Physical Findings. In contrast to these important behavioral abnormalities, other objective neurologic signs are conspicuously absent. Certain difficulties in the interpretation of neurologic findings are encountered when contractures have developed in limbs that have been held in one position for a long time. The extremities then may be edematous and cyanotic, and the tendon reflexes are difficult to elicit. Pinprick or painful stimulation may fail to evoke response from certain areas of the body. Blood pressure is low and the heart is small. The circulation time may be reduced. One is also impressed, when a group of these patients are gathered together, with the peculiar appearance and dysplastic physique of many of them. However, these abnormalities do not compose a recognizable clinical syndrome.

THE COMPOSITE CLINICAL PICTURE AND NATURAL COURSE OF SCHIZOPHRENIA. In a large proportion of cases the disease develops slowly and insidiously over a period of months and years during late childhood and adolescence. If the patient is examined at this stage it may be difficult to ascertain the nature of the illness. One may observe only that the patient is vague, suggestible, rather apathetic, and uninterested in his daily affairs. In reply to questions, he says repeatedly that he does not know the answer or does not care. He may be excessively preoccupied with his health, a rather unnatural state in adolescents. Often there is an appearance of mild depression. The physician who first examines the patient is apt to make a diagnosis of "nervousness," psychoneurosis, or some obscure medical disease.

The psychiatric nature of the illness becomes evident, as a rule, when the patient expresses overtly some delusional idea or becomes excited and begins to hallucinate. This may be precipitated by an infectious disease or an operation, or may seemingly result from worry or guilt over some problem that has arisen in the home or at school. A scene follows in which the patient attempts to escape, to seclude himself, or to assault someone whom he blames for his predicament. Exceptionally, and this is particularly true of the catatonic syndrome, the illness develops acutely, no antecedent symptoms having been known. This clinical state is recognized at once as being the result of a psychiatric illness. Once a diagnosis of schizophrenia is reached, it is usually not difficult to distinguish the special form of the disease.

Formerly it was asserted that schizophrenia was a hopeless and incurable disease, but now it is viewed with less pessimism. Some patients make a fairly prompt recovery within a few weeks and remain well thereafter. Of course, one never knows whether the diagnosis was correct, but at least the patient had shown some of the typical clinical signs. The remission rate is estimated to be 11 to 20 percent, but these figures are not applicable to all cases since they are obtained from a study of discharge rates from psychiatric hospitals and include the more severe cases, all of which were treated in some way, even if the treatment amounted to no more than hospitalization. The remissions may be complete or partial. In the latter state the patient leaves the hospital and returns to work but carries on at a reduced level of efficiency and continues to have minor symptoms. Factors said to influence the outcome favorably are early age of onset, a catatonic form of illness, acute development of symptoms, and retention of relatively normal affectivity. The temporary improvement seen in some cases following an intravenous injection of Sodium Amytal is said to favor the possibility of a good prognosis. Of those patients who recover, some will later relapse.

Ordinarily the mental illness, once it has developed, progresses for a time and then becomes more or less stationary. Many of the active symptoms of the progressive period subside, and the patient settles down to a custodial existence for the remainder of his life. In this fixed, chronic stage he is often classed as demented or deteriorated. However, the dementia, even in the most advanced stages, differs from that of general paresis and certain other organic brain diseases. If one can allow sufficient time to observe and to interview the patient, he may say or do something which indicates that he is and has been aware of what is going on around him and can also remember recent happenings. Other patients will remain mute, and of course there is no way of judging the quality of their mental activity. Another difference from degenerative brain disease is the potential reversibility of the process, with resumption of adequate psychic function. This phenomenon, admittedly rare in the late stages of the illness, is one of the reasons for calling schizophrenia a "functional psychosis."

Death may occur rarely during a period of intense excitement and excessive psychomotor activity which has lasted several days, and usually no explanation for it is found at autopsy. As a rule, however, the schizophrenic patient lives for many years and eventually dies of some other disease. As he is neglectful of health and nutrition, his age at death is apt to be younger than that of the general population. The coincidence of schizophrenia and of tuberculosis is high.

SPECIAL TYPES OF SCHIZOPHRENIA. The following subtypes are recognized: (1) simple, (2) hebephrenic, (3) catatonic, (4) chronic undifferentiated, (5) pseudoneurotic, (6) schizoaffective, (7) childhood, (8) paranoid, and (9) acute undifferentiated. Of these the physician should be familiar with the paranoid and catatonic varieties, since they may have an acute onset at times while the patient is in the hospital for some other illness. The simple and hebephrenic forms are usually seen in the population of patients found in a mental hospital. The essential features of each type are listed below.

Simple. This form, the most difficult to diagnose, is manifested chiefly by blunting of affect, a reduction in interests, and an impoverishment of social relationships. Often the patient appears simply to have adjusted at a lower psychobiologic level. Apathy and indifference mark all his behavior and are rarely accompanied by delusions or hallucinations. The onset is often so insidious that one hardly can decide when the patient who is regarded as eccentric began to be psychotic. Once the symptoms develop, they may gradually increase in severity over long periods, usually ending with apparent mental deterioration. This condition must be distinguished from the schizoid personality, in which abnormal character traits seem not to interfere with education and work.

Hebephrenic. This is characterized by shallow, inappropriate affect, unpredictable giggling, silly behavior and mannerisms, delusions that are often of a somatic nature, hallucinations, and regressive behavior.

Catatonic. Motor abnormalities such as stupor, mutism, negativism, and waxy flexibility or excessive activity and excitement are characteristic. The patient may improve or regress to a more or less vegetative state in which he remains for long periods of time.

Chronic Undifferentiated and Pseudoneurotic. With the passage of time many of the distinguishing features of the special types of schizophrenia are lost, and the patients, regardless of the original form of their illness, begin more and more to resemble one another. By then elements of all the types can be observed in various constellations. Vagueness of thought, irrational concern about the problems of the world, about health, general disorganization of activities, inability to study, to work or even to carry out the essential actions in personal care, remoteness, and suspiciousness are the dominating features and most disabling aspects of the illness. In some of the patients the symptoms at all times lack the definite character of those described above and resemble more those of some of the nervous and anxiety states, viz., *pseudoneurotic*. Yet they differ in their extreme chronicity and the less clear-cut nature of the syndrome. Only when viewed in longitudinal profile is it realized that the course of the illness is essentially that of chronic schizophrenia.

The presence of numerous neurotic symptoms including anxiety attacks, gross hysterical symptoms, somatic preoccupation, phobias, obsessions, and compulsions occurring in a patient with a few cardinal symptoms of schizophrenia distinguishes the condition as the pseudoneurotic form of the disease.

Schizoaffective. This category is intended for those cases showing significant admixtures of schizophrenic and manic-depressive reactions. The mental content may be predominantly schizophrenic, with pronounced elation or depression; or predominantly affective changes may be complicated by schizophrenic-like thinking or bizarre behavior. The "prepsychotic personality" may be at variance with the predominant trend of the illness. On prolonged observation, such cases usually prove to be schizophrenic. In some instances at least it is probable that the patient has both schizophrenia and manic-depressive psychosis.

Childhood Form. The schizophrenic reactions occurring before puberty are placed in this category. The clinical picture may differ from schizophrenic reactions in other age periods because of the immaturity and plasticity of the patient at the time of onset of the reaction. Psychotic reactions in children manifesting primarily autism (tendency to preoccupation with dreams, fantasies, and ruminations) are sometimes classified here. Cases of this type are at present often classified as *Heller's syndrome*. Their relationship to schizophrenia is dubious.

Paranoid. Here delusions of persecution, ideas of reference, and auditory hallucinations, which may have begun acutely with much fear and apprehension or gradually, come to be accepted with greater complacency and inappropriateness of mood. The acute onset may have begun at a time of withdrawal from chronic alcoholism (see Chap. 118). Eventually thinking becomes less realistic and the hallucinations are less definite and no longer projected externally. The behavior is unpredictable with aggressiveness and a prevailing attitude of hostility in some. Others show excessive concern about religion, and related ideas may be the basis of their delusions of persecution or omnipotence. As was stated above, the lack of family history, the lack of premorbid schizoid traits, the later age of onset, and in the acute cases the initial character of the clinical picture all tend to set this disease apart from the other forms of schizophrenia.

Acute Undifferentiated Psychoses. Amongst adolescents and young adults a wide variety of symptoms which resemble schizophrenia may appear as an acute illness. Attention may be called to the patient's plight by his unexpected assault on someone who is an imagined persecutor, a dramatic attempt at suicide, or an outburst of frenzied excitement. Examination discloses confusion of thinking and turmoil of emotion, ideas of reference, a dreamlike state, or catatonia. There may have been prodromal symptoms for some weeks. Excitement or depression of mood may be present. Hallucinations are prominent. The symptoms often subside in a few weeks, and many of these patients recover and remain well. A few lapse into one of the chronic schizophrenic states. European psychiatrists have been reluctant to follow the tendency of American psychiatrists to call this illness schizophrenic. As pointed out above, the disease underlying it differs from chronic undifferentiated and the other types of schizophrenia in that it shows little tendency to occur in other members of the family.

Patients with any of the above conditions may improve sufficiently to be able to get along in the community, yet continue to show recognizable residual symptoms in thinking and affectivity. Such cases are classed as *schizophrenia, residual type*.

DIFFERENTIAL DIAGNOSIS. Already it has been pointed

out that the schizoid or mildly schizophrenic individual is often considered nervous, eccentric, or psychoneurotic. At this early stage the disturbances in thinking and affect so characteristic of schizophrenia are not recognized. The illness presented by the acutely excited or "stuporous" schizophrenic must be distinguished from mania, severe depression, acute confusional psychoses and delirium, and some of the endocrine psychoses. Here a common source of error in the very disturbed, speechless patient is to misdiagnose a rapidly advancing brain disease as schizophrenia. The author has seen hypoxic encephalopathy, encephalitis, lipid-storage disease, Schilder's disease, brain tumor, and epileptic psychoses all mistaken for schizophrenia. The usual source of error has been that the patient was mute and resistive, and because of muteness, it was impossible to evaluate thinking and emotional reactions. Chronic alcoholic hallucinosis and paranoid schizophrenia are easily confused. In fact the author has not been able to separate them except by the knowledge of their mode of onset and the history of prolonged alcoholism before the illness. The deteriorated schizophrenic must be distinguished from the patient with true dementia. Schizophrenic patients who exhibit rigid attitudes and postures must be differentiated from those who suffer basal ganglion diseases. (See Table 372-2 for differential diagnosis.)

Many of the above errors can be avoided if one insists that at least three of the following mental signs—disturbance of affect, disturbance of insight, disturbance in ideational association, perceptual disorders, and abnormality in subject-object differentiation—be present. If these signs alone are manifested, a diagnosis of *simple schizophrenia* is justified. If in addition the patient has persecutory delusions, grandiose ideas, and hallucinations, a more specific diagnosis of paranoid schizophrenia is assured. The addition of negativism, resistiveness, rigidity, and apparent "stupor" categorizes the case as one of catatonic schizophrenia; while the conjunction of mannerisms, inappropriate laughter, giggling, and immature emotional development places it in the group of hebephrenic schizophrenia. Finally, it is only proper to say that until such time as some reliable and incontrovertible test for schizophrenia is developed, diagnosis will always be uncertain in many cases.

TREATMENT AND MANAGEMENT. The management of the schizophrenic patient is difficult, and in most instances it is best to refer him to a psychiatrist. Mild cases may be cared for by a general physician, and undoubtedly many of them are under a mistaken diagnosis. However, once the patient has had a frankly psychotic episode, hospitalization is usually necessary, and some advantage to the patient and his family accrues from establishing a relationship with a psychiatrist who has had experience with this type of case.

Several new methods of therapy have been introduced in recent years. They have been difficult to evaluate because of uncertainty as to the natural course of the illness. The most important have been custodial treatment and psychotherapy, insulin coma, electric or Metrazol therapy, lobotomy, chlorpromazine and other phenothiazines, monoamine oxidase inhibitors, and other new drugs collectively termed *tranquilizers*.

The choice of drugs depends on the characteristics of the presenting syndrome. Excitement, agitation, and restlessness, if mild, are controllable by barbiturates, chloral hydrate, or paraldehyde. If severe, the phenothiazines are indicated, usually in high dosage: chlorpromazine, 600 to 1,200 mg per day; thioridazine, 400 to 600 mg per day; trifluoperazine, 20 to 50 mg. If the acute reaction is marked by disturbances of thought and perception, phenothiazines, especially those of the piperazine group, are given. Apathy and withdrawal, stupor or catatonia are treated by trifluoperazine, 5 to 15 mg, or butaperazine, 20 to 60 mg. Imipramine, 200 to 300 mg per day, or anticholinergic agents such as procyclidine, 5 to 20 mg, or benztropine, 2 to 4 mg, will help counteract the sedative effects of chlorpromazine. The actions of these medications are difficult to evaluate, and the physician would be well advised to call on psychiatric consultants in their management.

The results obtained by these methods are summarized in Table 372-1.

Table 372-1. EFFECTS OF VARIOUS TYPES OF THERAPY EMPLOYED IN SCHIZOPHRENIA

Type of therapy	No. of patients	Complete remission and social remission, %
Custodial and supportive treatment..	11,080	19
Convulsive therapy...............	7,357	29
Insulin coma....................	9,433	43
Lobotomy......................	1,211	18
Chlorpromazine.................	1,517	34
Reserpine......................	897	22

From these data it is obvious that schizophrenia is a serious disease and one for which there is no specific therapy. The older methods of prolonged institutional or custodial care have resulted in fewer remissions than vigorous supportive treatment in a more natural hospital environment. The tranquilizing drugs are opening a new field of therapy and may provide fresh insight into the nature of the basic process.

PARANOIA AND PARANOID REACTIONS

Already it has been pointed out that suspiciousness and distrustfulness are distortions of thinking which may occur as symptoms of several clinical syndromes, particularly depressive psychosis and schizophrenia and sometimes in dementing diseases. More important from the viewpoint of the general physician is the not-infrequent occurrence of an acute paranoid syndrome during the course of a focal or systemic infection, or following an operation. This condition has also been observed in military personnel who suffer extreme fatigue (combat psychosis). Only upon the closest examination will it be noted that these patients are not perfectly oriented as to their present surroundings, are unable to recollect the details of all that has happened in the preceding days, are disorganized in their activities, and sleep relatively little. These facts, once established, enable one to recognize the illness as an example of either an acute confusional psychosis or a mild delirium, and proper use of sedation and careful nursing usually result in a gratifying recovery within a few weeks. Certainly these several different conditions should always come to mind whenever ideas of self-reference and delusions of persecution are observed.

There is, however, another group of illnesses, relatively rare to be sure, in which an elaborate, systematized delusion of persecution develops insidiously in middle or late adult life and is not accompanied by any other psychical abnormality. Such individuals are said to be suffering from a strange malady called *paranoia*. Limitations of space do not permit further discussion of this condition. The interested reader should refer to one of the textbooks of psychiatry.

PUERPERAL OR POST-PARTUM PSYCHOSIS

This psychosis is difficult to classify. It resembles in some respects either schizophrenia or manic-depressive psychosis but also has features peculiar to delirium and the acute confusional psychoses. It is mentioned here with schizophrenia because this is the condition with which it is most likely to be confused in clinical medicine. Depression may also occur as a post-partum state and requires treatment along the lines discussed in Chap. 371. Most of these postpartum illnesses are self-terminating, but the danger of suicide during the illness demands prompt diagnosis and early treatment.

THE ENDOCRINE PSYCHOSES

One of the most provocative discoveries in the field of psychiatry in contemporary times is that relatively normal individuals may become psychotic when they develop hyper- or hypothyroidism, Cushing's disease, or adrenal insufficiency, or receive therapeutic doses of ACTH. If these conditions were no more than examples of drug-induced psychosis, they would be interesting enough. The fact is, however, that they differ considerably from the usual toxic delirium or confusional state. The syndrome, reminiscent of puerperal psychosis and some cases of "combat psychosis" seen during World War II, comprises features that are suggestive of a manic-depressive psychosis or schizophrenia on the one hand and of the confusional psychoses on the other. These endocrine psychoses have far-reaching medical significance, for they provide experimental models of psychoses that can be created by the manipulation of metabolic factors.

Table 372-2. DIFFERENTIAL DIAGNOSIS OF MAJOR PSYCHIATRIC SYNDROMES

Syndrome	Mental status examination	Physical examination
Anxiety neuroses....	Restless Tense Anxious Sighing respirations Voluble	Few abnormal physical findings, including: High resting pulse rate Respiratory rate over 20 Tremor of fingers Hyperactive tendon reflexes
Hysteria...........	Overtalkative Friendly, ingratiating manner Emotional response—casual, objective, indifferent, or anxious Chief complaint—nonspecific, multiple, or irrelevant Symptoms described in dramatic, histrionic fashion	Weakness or paralysis of arm and leg or both legs Hemianesthesia, aphonia, blindness
Psychasthenia......	Affect appropriate Motor activity—restless, tense, and anxious Vasomotor overactivity—blushing and sweating Associations—direct and to the point Mental content—obsessions, compulsions, and phobias No formal thought disorder Evidence of concern or depression of mood in relation to symptoms	No objective physical findings Facial and respiratory or other tics but usually no other abnormal physical findings
Depression........	Facial expression—plaintive, troubled, or anguished Mood—depressed, discouraged, "blue," "unhappy," "low in spirits," "glum," "morbid" Speech—retarded to point of mutism or push of speech with restricted content Motor activity—decreased to point of stupor or accelerated to point of agitation Content—pessimistic thoughts; fear of cancer or other serious disease, self-depreciation, self-accusation, feeling of inferiority or guilt, somatic delusions, e.g., "rotting," "blood dried up" Suicidal preoccupation or attempts Abstract judgment colored by depressed mood Personal judgment present or absent Nihilistic delusions and hallucinations consistent with morbid mood in severe cases Thought processes, mood, and affect parallel	Signs of neglect and dehydration may be present in cases of severe depression Weight loss, severe constipation
Mania............	Mood—happy, elated, exalted—"feel good," "best ever" Stream of speech—rapid, digressible, with flight of ideas Motor activity—increased, great activity, may be increased to point of incessant activity Affect—mercurial, rapidly changing through euphoria, exaltation, irritability, and violent anger Content—consistent with elevated mood and may embrace overconfidence, exaggerated self-esteem, and delusions of grandeur Unsystematized paranoid delusions may occur Impairment of judgment or insight	Signs of dehydration may be present
Dementia.........	Change in personality (by history) Intellectual impairment Disturbances in orientation Defective intellectual capacity and grasp Disturbance in clarity of thinking Memory impairment, particularly for recent events Distractibility of attention Perseveration in speech, actions, and thoughts Blunting of moral and ethical standards (by history) Lability of emotional response, vacillating from depression, elation, or irritability to violent anger	Signs consistent with basic disease process Dysarthria Aphasic disturbances Sphincter disturbances Signs of focal brain disease are evidenced by pyramidal, extrapyramidal, or cranial nerve disturbance

Table 372-2. DIFFERENTIAL DIAGNOSIS OF MAJOR PSYCHIATRIC SYNDROMES (*Continued*)

Syndrome	Mental status examination	Physical examination

Delirium...........	Facial expression perplexed, bewildered
	Clouding of sensorium
	Attention—distractible and poorly sustained; span increased (increased vigil)
	Perceptual disturbance—illusions, hallucinations (visual, auditory, or olfactory)
	Delusions—dictated by perceptual impairment
	Affect parallels perceptual content and is usually apprehensive, anxious, or fearful
	Upon recovery there is amnesia for the illness
		Autonomic overactivity
		  Flushed face
		  Rapid pulse
		  Fever
		  Sweating
		  Dilated pupils
		Usually no focal neurologic signs
		
		Tremor of extremities

Primary mental confusion	Facial expression—perplexed Confusion in relationship to external stimuli Attention—detached, preoccupied—span restricted (decreased vigil) Perceptual disturbance—illusions and hallucinations Delusions—consistent with perceptual disturbance Affect—concerned or fearful Motor activity usually slowed—may be retarded to point of stupor	Consistent with disease process, or exogenous, noxious agent responsible for condition
Schizophrenia.......	Disturbance in affect—bland, rigid, or inappropriate Disturbance in associations—vague, tangential, irrelevant, or neologistic Impairment of insight—nil Thought processes—shallow, illogical, or fragmented Feeling—occasionally tense and anxious but usually phlegmatic, dull, or apathetic Delusions—paranoid, somatic, nihilistic, ideas of influence and reference Hallucinations—visual, auditory, olfactory—usually not vivid Emotional response does not parallel thought processes	There are no physical signs directly related to the disease process
Psychopathic personality	History of poor social adjustment, poor work record, civilian arrests, suicidal attempts, proved theft, chronic alcoholism, and failure to advance in army or civilian life Usual reason for referral—behavioral disturbances and/or multiple somatic complaints Examination—voluble, plausible, friendly, and oversolicitous—tendency to explain away difficulties in terms of misfortune or a fault of others Longitudinal history reveals conspicuous inability to profit by experience	There are no physical signs directly related to the disease process
Post-partum psychosis	Onset 4 to 10 days following delivery Facial expression—somber, dejected, puzzled, or bewildered Emotional reaction—depressed Attention—preoccupied Awareness—restricted or perplexed. Depersonalization or derealization may be present Motor activity—increased to point of agitation or decreased to point of stupor Speech stream shows blocking and paucity of ideas Hallucinations and delusions Retrograde amnesia may be present Insight lacking Confusion	Physical signs present are those of the normal post-partum state, viz., breast engorgement, subinvolution of the uterus, and lochia. In many cases there is evidence of dehydration, shown by dryness of lips, mucous membranes, and skin

ACTH and Cortisone Psychoses

This psychiatric syndrome is now occurring far less frequently than when these hormones were first introduced into medicine. Presumably the products are now more refined and there are more reliable data as to safe dosage. The psychosis usually develops over a period of a few days after the patient has received the hormone for a week or more. The features are extremely variable. Some of the patients become elated, euphoric, excited, and talkative, as though under pressure to speak, while others are mute. Thinking may be confused, illogical, tangential, and incoherent. Hallucinations and sensory misinterpretations may appear. The prevailing emotional response varies from apathy to anxiety and panic, depression, or elation. Although mental confusion is not prominent, the state of awareness is not altogether normal, and at times the patient is frankly beclouded, confused, and bewildered. In the motor sphere there may be incessant activity or immobility, resistiveness, and even negativism verging on catatonia. Clouding of the sensorium, disorientation, and confusion, the hallmarks of deliria and the confusional psychoses, have not been prominent in the ACTH and cortisone psychoses. Once established, these psychoses have lasted for several weeks and recovery has been complete. Usually the hormone was stopped as soon as the diagnosis was established.

The mechanism of this psychosis is not known. From the few available studies it has been learned that the occurrence of the psychosis is not related to the premorbid personality. Although the dosage of ACTH or cortisone has usually been high, there has been no exact correlation between dose level and the occurrence, severity, and duration of the psychosis. The mental disturbance appears unrelated to the rapidity and intensity of the therapeutic response to ACTH and cortisone.

Thyroid Psychoses

A great deal has been said and written about the pervasive effects of abnormal thyroid function on all organs, including the neuromuscular apparatus and central nervous system. These effects are discussed in the chapters on endocrine disease.

The hyperthyroid patient often shows minor changes in his emotions and mentation. Restlessness, irritability, apprehension, emotional liability, and even at times agitation may occur. Either of two trends may be observed in the relatively rare psychotic thyroid patient. There may be mania with its characteristic increase in psychomotor activity, overtalkativeness, flight of ideas; or depression with its somber mood, weeping, and agitation. Visual and auditory hallucinations are present in both groups of cases. The clinical picture is seldom clear. Usually the psychiatrist finds something more than simple mania or agitated depression, usually some clouding of the sensorium with perplexity and confusion suggestive of delirium. The condition is said to be related to the premorbid personality, some personality types being more vulnerable, but this point is disputed. The condition is not directly related to the level of the basal metabolic rate. Careful studies of cerebral blood flow and cerebral metabolism during and after the psychosis have not been done. Treatment of hyperthyroidism does not result in prompt arrest of the psychic disorder, but usually recovery takes place over a period of months. One must distinguish this illness from other types of recurrent psychosis which happen to coincide with or be precipitated by hyperthyroidism.

With myxedema there is also a characteristic slowness and thickness of speech, mental dullness, listlessness and apathy, drowsiness, irritability, and sometimes suspiciousness. The patient may sleep most of the day and night. This encephalopathy can usually be distinguished from depression by the lack of definite melancholia and the presence of a memory disturbance, particularly for recent events. Definite slowing occurs in the EEG. Hypothermia may be prominent. The cerebrospinal fluid total protein is usually elevated. Reduced cerebral blood flow and cerebral metabolism have been found, and with improvement on therapy these functions are restored to normal.

Other Endocrine Psychoses

Mental aberrations have been observed in Cushing's disease and Addison's disease. They are rare, and because of limitations of space the reader is referred to the current medical literature for references on the subject.

REFERENCES

Carter, A. B.: The Prognoses of Certain Hysterical Symptoms, Brit. Med. J., 1:1076, 1949.

Cohen, M. E.: Neurocirculatory Asthenia: Anxiety Neurosis, Neurasthenia, Effort Syndrome, Cardiac Neuroses, Med. Clinics N. Am., 33:1343, 1949.

——, E. Robins, J. J. Purtell, M. W. Altman, and D. E. Reid: Excessive Surgery in Hysteria, J.A.M.A., 151:977, 1953.

Freedman, A. M., and H. I. Kaplan: "Comprehensive Textbook of Psychiatry," Baltimore, The Williams & Wilkins Company, 1967, chap. 15.6, p. 661, Schizophrenia VI by M. Fink and T. M. Itil.

Freud, S.: "Selected Papers on Hysteria and Other Psychoneuroses," translated by A. A. Brill, Nervous and Mental Disease Monograph Series No. 4, 1920.

Huston, P. E., and M. Locher: Involutional Psychosis: Course When Untreated and When Treated with Electric Shock, Arch. Neurol. Psychiat., 59:385, 1948.

Janet, P.: "The Major Symptoms of Hysteria," New York, The Macmillan Company, 1907.

Jones, A. B., and L. J. Llewellyn: "Malingering," New York, McGraw-Hill Book Company, 1917.

Kahn, E.: "Psychopathic Personalities," New Haven, Yale University Press, 1931.

Lamson, E. T., F. Elmadjian, J. M. Hope, G. Pincus, and D. Jorjorian: Aldosterone Excretion of Normal, Schizophrenic and Psychoneurotic Subjects, abstracted in J. Clin. Endocrinol. Metab., 16:954, 1956.

Lindemann, E.: Psychological Changes in Normal and Abnormal Individuals under the Influence of Sodium Amytal, Am. J. Psychiat., 11:1080, 1932.

——: Hysteria as a Problem in a General Hospital, Med. Clinics N. Am., 22:591, 1938.

Mayer-Gross, W., E. Slater, and M. Roth: "Clinical Psychiatry," London, Cassell & Co., Ltd., 1960.

Purtell, J. J., E. Robins, and M. E. Cohen: Observations in Clinical Aspects of Hysteria, J.A.M.A., 146:902, 1951.

Robins, E., J. J. Purtell, and M. E. Cohen: Hysteria in Men, New Engl. J. Med., 246:677, 1942.

Rosanoff, A. J.: "Manual of Psychiatry," New York, John Wiley & Sons, Inc., 1920.

Shands, H. C., J. E. Finesinger, and A. L. Watkins: Clinical Studies of Fatigue States, Arch. Neurol. Psychiat., 60: 210, 1949.

Venning, E. H., I. Dyrenfurth, and J. C. Beck: Effect of Anxiety upon Aldosterone Excretion in Man, J. Clinics Endocrinol. Metab., 17:1005, 1957.

Wheeler, E. O., P. D. White, E. W. Reed, and M. E. Cohen: Neurocirculatory Asthenia, J.A.M.A., 142:878, 1950.

Section 11

Diseases of Striated Muscle

373 CLINICAL MYOLOGY AND CLASSIFICATION OF MUSCLE DISEASES

Jean Rebeiz, Maria Z. Salam, and Raymond D. Adams

The muscle fiber has been more thoroughly studied than any other cell of the human or animal body, but until comparatively recent times little had been learned of the diseases to which it is subject. However, clinicians, pathologists, and biochemists are now beginning to concentrate on the conditions which impair its function and imperil its survival, and even in the period of time which has elapsed since the first edition of this book, several monographs devoted exclusively to diseases of muscle have appeared.

GENERAL CONSIDERATIONS. The striated muscle tissue constitutes the principal organ of locomotion as well as a vast metabolic reservoir. Disposed in more than 600 separate muscles, this tissue comprises as much as 40 percent of the weight of adult man. Intricacy of structure undoubtedly accounts for its diverse susceptibilities to disease, and for this reason reference to the following anatomic characteristics provides an appropriate introduction to this chapter.

A single muscle is composed of thousands of fibers which course for variable distances along its longitudinal axis. Some fibers extend the entire length of the muscle; others are joined end to end by connective tissue. Each fiber is a relatively large and complex multinucleated cell varying in length from a few millimeters to several centimeters (34 cm in the human sartorius muscle) and in diameter from 10 to 100 μ. Although the fiber represents an indivisible anatomic and physiologic unit, disease may affect only one part of it, leaving the remainder to atrophy, degenerate, or regenerate depending on the nature and severity of the disease. The nuclei of each cell, which are oriented parallel to the longitudinal axis of the fiber and number into the thousands lie beneath the cytoplasmic membrane (true sarcolemma), and hence are called "sarcolemmal." The cytoplasm (sarcoplasm) of the cell is abundant and contains myofibrils and various other organelles such as mitochondria, microsomes, and endoplasmic reticulum. The myofibrils in turn are composed of longitudinally oriented interdigitating filaments (myofilaments) of contractile proteins (actin and myosin). Droplets of stored fat, glycogen, various proteins, many enzymes, and myoglobin, the latter imparting the red color to muscle, have been identified within the sarcoplasm or its organelles.

The individual muscle fibers are enveloped by delicate strands of connective tissue (endomysium) which provide for their support and permit unity of action. The blood vessels, of which there may be several for each fiber, and nerve filaments lie within the endomysium. Similar reticular tissue and sheets of collagen (perimysium) bind together groups or fascicles of fibers and surround the entire muscle (epimysium). These latter connective tissue tunics are also richly and variably vascularized, different types of muscle having different arrangements of arteries and veins; and fat cells (lipocytes) are embedded within the interstices. The muscle fibers are attached at their ends to tendon fibers, which in turn connect with the skeleton. By this means contraction maintains posture and effects movement.

Other notable characteristics of muscle are its natural mode of activation, i.e., innervation, by nerve and the necessity of intact nerve supply for the maintenance of its nutrition. Each muscle fiber receives a nerve twig from a motor nerve cell in the anterior horn of the spinal cord or nucleus of a cranial nerve, which joins it at a point called the neuromuscular junction (also called motor end-plate). And, as was pointed out in Chap. 21, groups of muscle fibers with a common innervation from one anterior horn cell constitute the "motor unit" which is the basic physiologic unit in all reflex, postural, and voluntary activity. Acetylcholine and cholinesterase, which play a special role in neuromuscular transmission, are concentrated at this junction zone. In addition to the motor nerves there are two types of sensory receptors (proprioceptors), the muscle spindles and Golgi tendon organs, which participate in reflexes; and finally there are free nerve endings which subserve pain sensation.

It would be a mistake to predicate that apparent similarity of structure renders all muscles equally susceptible to disease. In point of fact, no disease affects all muscles in the body and each disease has as one of its features a unique topography within the musculature. These topographic differences between diseases provide incontrovertible evidence of unique structural qualities, not presently disclosed by the light microscope. One factor may relate simply to fiber size. Consider, for example, the large diameter and length of the fibers of the glutei and paravertebral muscles in comparison to the ocular muscles. Again, the number of fibers composing a motor unit may be of significance in explaining selective vulnerability; e.g., in the ocular muscles they contain only 6 to 10 muscle fibers, whereas in the gastrocnemius, as many as 1,800 fibers. Allusion has already been made to individual differences in vascular patterns of supply, permitting some muscles to withstand the effects of hypoxia or vascular occlusion better than others. Subtle metabolic differences between fibers within any one muscle have been revealed by enzyme studies, the larger fibers being richer in glycolytic and poorer in oxidative enzymes than the small fibers. Doubtless other differences will be discovered.

These anatomic and biochemical qualities inform us of some of the possibilities of pathogenesis of myopathic disease. Thus, one may envisage causative agents which affect each of the different components of sarcoplasm, namely, an enzyme, an essential substrate, the filamentous proteins, the endoplasmic reticulum, or the sarcolemma itself. Again, the endomysial connective tissue could be the primary pathway in disease, since it so closely invests the muscle. Inadequacy of blood supply in relation to the metabolic requirement of oxygen by active muscle, or frank ischemia from vascular occlusion could be postulated as another mechanism of disease. Finally, the nerve or its cell of origin in the spinal cord is known to bear the brunt of certain pathologic processes, leaving the muscle fibers to wither, and thus reflecting the unique trophic influence of nerve on muscle.

Normal muscle possesses a limited capacity to regenerate, a point often forgotten. Acute destructive processes of the muscle fiber, e.g., inflammatory, metabolic, and certain other diseases, are usually followed by fairly complete restoration of the muscle cells, providing the endomysial sheaths of connective tissue have not been disturbed. Unfortunately many pathologic processes of muscle are chronic and unrelenting and destroy completely the muscle fibers. Under such conditions any regenerative activity fails to keep pace with the disease, and the loss of muscle fibers is permanent.

CLINICAL MANIFESTATIONS OF MUSCLE DISEASE (CLINICAL MYOLOGY)

Considering the large number and diversity of diseases of striated muscles, it would appear that they exceed the number of symptoms and signs by which they express themselves clinically. Different diseases thus must share certain common symptoms and even syndromes. To avoid excessive repetition in the description of individual diseases there is some advantage to discussing in one place all the clinical manifestations, a subject which we propose to call *clinical myology*.

Weakness and Paralysis

Reduced strength of contraction, reflected in diminished power of single contractions [peak or power factor (PF) in performance] or of repeated contractions [endurance factor (EF)], stands as the indubitable sign of muscle disease. Fatigability per se less reliably denotes muscle affection, since it is most often due to some psychic aberration linked to anxiety and depression or to systemic illness. It is noteworthy that slight weakness of muscle may be present, even though PF, because of crudeness of clinical measurement and lack of quantitation and the uncertainty of gaining the patient's full cooperation, may seem to reveal no definite diminution in power. Theoretically, with milder degrees of weakness, a diminution in EF elicited in a series of timed contractions against a fixed resistance (ergogram) may more reliably demonstrate the disorder than does PF. Furthermore, sustained or repeated maximal muscle contraction over a given period of time evinces optimally the myasthenic reaction, i.e. a rapid failure of contraction, with the power being restored within minutes by rest. This, in fact, in combination with a restoration of power, i.e., disappearance of the myasthenic state, by neostigmine and edrophonium (Tensilon) and a worsening of it by small doses of curare (see Chap. 377), stands as the most valid diagnostic criterion of the various forms of myasthenia gravis.

QUALITATIVE CHANGES IN THE CONTRACTILE PROCESS

In addition, there are other qualities of muscular contraction and relaxation that may be evoked by observing, during one or a series of maximal actions of a group of muscles, the speed and efficiency of contraction and relaxation. Slow waves of contraction in a muscle like the quadriceps may be seen on change in posture (contraction myoedema) in hypothyroidism. Here it is often associated with percussion myoedema, and slowness of tendon reflex. Slowness in relaxation is another indication of a thyroid deficiency state, accounting for the complaints of uncomfortable tightness and firmness of proximal limb muscles.

A prolonged failure of relaxation with after-discharge is a characteristic of myotonia, as in the diseases congenital myotonia (of Thomsen) and dystrophic myotonia (of Steinert). But a true myotonia, with its long electrical discharges of action potentials, unlike the electrically silent myoedema and contracture (see below), requires strong contraction for its elicitation, is more evident after a period of relaxation, and tends to disappear with repeated contractions. (See Chap. 374.) This persistence of contraction is demonstrable upon tapping a muscle (percussion myotonia), a phenomenon easily distinguished from the electrically silent local bulge (myoedema) induced by a sharp tap of a muscle in the myxedematous or cachectic patient.

Increase in power in a series of several voluntary contractions in the absence of myotonia is a feature of the inverse myasthenic syndrome of small-cell carcinoma of the lung. It, too, has its electromyographic equivalent —a rapid increase in the voltage of a series of action potentials (see Chap. 374).

The effect of cold on muscle contraction may also prove informative; either paresis or myotonia, lasting for a few minutes, may be evoked or enhanced by cold in the paramyotonia of von Eulenberg.

Myotonia and myoedema must be distinguished from the recruitment and spread of involuntary spasm induced by strong and repeated contractions of limb muscles in patients with mild or *localized tetanus,* which is not a phenomenon of muscle but is due to an abolition of inhibitory spinal mechanisms.

The repeated contraction of forearm and leg muscles after the application of a tourniquet (above arterial pressure) to the proximal part of a limb will often elicit latent tetany. The latter state must be separated from ordinary cramp by its special mode of development, duration, its enhancement by hyperventilation, the presence of accompanying tingling, prickling paresthesias, and also from true contracture.

In *true contracture* a group of muscles, after a series of strong contractions, may remain shortened for many minutes, unable to relax because of failure of the metabolic mechanism necessary for relaxation; and the muscle in this shortened state remains electrically silent in the electromyogram, in contrast to the tremendous high-voltage, rapid discharges observed with cramp, tetanus, and tetany. Such contracture occurs in McArdle's phosphorylase deficiency, where it is aggravated by arterial occlusion, but it has been seen by the authors in another disease, as yet undefined, where the tourniquet has no effect and phosphorylase seems to be present in adequate amounts, at least as judged by histochemical stains. The latter may be due to a phosphofructokinase defect. (See Chap. 111).

Pseudocontracture (myostatic contracture), which inevitably follows all conditions which occasion prolonged fixation and complete inactivity of the normally innervated muscle, is another common disorder. But here the shortened state of the muscle, which may persist for days or weeks, has no established anatomic, physiologic, or chemical basis. It is distinguished from *ankylosis* by the springy nature of the resistance coincident with increased tautness of muscle and tendon during passive motion, and from *Volkmann's contracture* where there is evident fibrosis of muscle and the surrounding tissues due to ischemic injury, usually after a fracture of forearm.

TOPOGRAPHY OF PARALYSIS: PATTERNS OF PARALYSIS

As was stated above, in the majority of the diseases under consideration, some of the muscles are affected and others are spared and each one exhibits its own pattern. Moreover, the topography or distribution of involvement tends to follow the same pattern in all patients with the same disease. Thus, determination of the topography of muscular involvement becomes another of the most valid diagnostic attributes of a disease, ranking next in importance after altered quantity and quality of contraction. In myasthenia gravis it is the ocular, pharyngeal, laryngeal, facial, masseter, and lingual muscles that are affected in that order, either exclusively or in conjunction with a milder involvement of trunk and limb muscles. In *familial periodic paralysis* limb and trunk muscle involvement is disproportionately more severe than that of cranial muscles, though in the worst attacks all muscles except diaphragm and heart may be weakened. In the majority of the muscular dystrophies and diffuse forms of idiopathic polymyositis, the proximal and trunk muscles are affected and the distal limb muscles and facial muscles are relatively spared. There is, however, a rare form of distal dystrophy in adults where the forearm and hand and foot and leg muscles become weak and atrophic, resulting in a clinical picture that bears a close resemblance to that produced by the common varieties of chronic polyneuropathy (e.g., Charcot-Marie-Tooth peroneal muscular atrophy). Restricted types of dystrophy, exophthalmic ophthalmoplegia, and polymyositis may involve only ocular, oculopharyngeal, or cervical muscles. These and other topographic patterns of muscle disorder will be described more fully in the following chapters.

VOLUMETRIC CHANGES IN MUSCLE

Altered volume of muscular mass stands as another feature of disease which may be evidenced in all except the most obese patient. There are, of course, innate differences in muscle development, a greater salience of muscle in the male than in the female, and differences due to use and disuse. Greatly increased size and strength of muscles (hypertrophia musculorum vera) may be observed in *congenital myotonia* (circus freaks with phenomenal muscular development often have this disease), in rare instances of a pathologic cramp syndrome, in some patients destined to develop muscular dystrophy, and in deLange's syndrome of congenital athetosis with feeblemindedness. Muscle enlargement in progressive muscular dystrophy more often takes the form of pseudohypertrophy, where increased size is accompanied by weakness. Here large and small fibers are mixed with fat cells which have replaced many of the degenerated muscle fibers. Other muscles are atrophied in the same patient. Cachexia, malnutrition, and lipodystrophy tend to reduce muscle bulk without significantly reducing power of contraction (pseudoatrophy). Denervation due to lesions of peripheral nerve or spinal cord, which if complete leads to a loss of bulk up to 75 percent of the original volume within 3 months, is invariably attended by paralysis. The most severe degrees of atrophy usually signify denervation or dystrophy.

TWITCHES, SPASMS, CRAMPS, AND CONTRACTURE

Fascicular twitches during rest, if pronounced and combined with muscular weakness and atrophy, usually signify motor neurone disease (amyotrophic lateral sclerosis, progressive muscular atrophy, or progressive bulbar palsy); but they may be seen in lesser degree in other diseases of gray matter of spinal cord (e.g., syringomyelia or tumor), in lesions of anterior roots (e.g., ruptured intervertebral disk), and in peripheral neuropathies. Widespread fascicular twitches spreading in a wavelike pattern along the entire length of a muscle with associated weakness progressing to complete flaccid paralysis within minutes form the striking clinical picture of organic phosphate insecticide poisoning. The same sequence evolving at a slightly slower pace may occur in poliomyelitis. Fasciculations during contraction indicate, instead, a state in which the muscle is excessively irritable, often for reasons that are not known, or in a condition which leaves muscle with some paralyzed motor units, so that during contraction small and large units are not enlisted smoothly. One may observe this latter phenomenon years after a poliomyelitis has left a muscle weakened. *Benign fasciculations*, a common finding in otherwise normal individuals, can usually be distinguished by the lack of muscular weakness and atrophy; and *myokymia* is a rare form of the condition in which innumerable twitchings impart a rippling appearance to the muscle.

Cramps at rest or with movement (action cramps) are frequently reported in motor system disease, tetany, and dehydration after excessive sweating and salt loss and other metabolic diseases (uremia, hypocalcemia, and hypomagnesemia), but there is a benign form (idiopathic cramp syndrome), in which no other neuromuscular disturbance can be found. Here cramp may be induced by every strong contraction, thereby greatly limiting physical activity. The disorder responds at least partially to quinine sulfate in oral doses of 0.2 to 0.3 Gm twice or thrice daily. A particularly malignant and progressive form of painful spasm is known as the *stiff man syndrome;* this appears to be an obscure disease of the central nervous system. Continuous spasm, with no demonstrable disorder of a neuromuscular level, intensified by the action of muscles, is a common manifestation of tetanus and also follows the bite of the black widow spider.

PALPABLE ABNORMALITIES OF MUSCLE

Altered structure and function of muscle are not accurately revealed by palpation. Of course, the difference between the firm hypertrophied muscle of a well-conditioned athlete and the slack muscle of a sedentary person is as apparent to the palpating finger as to the eye. And the persistent contraction in myxedema, contracture, tetanus, cramp, etc., is easily felt. In muscular dystrophy the muscles are said to have a "doughy" or "elastic" feel, but this is difficult to judge. In the Pompé type of glycogen storage disease attention may be attracted to the musculature by an unnatural firmness and increase in bulk. The swollen, edematous weak muscles in acute paroxysmal myoglobinuria or severe polymyositis may feel taut and firm but are usually not tender. Areas of tenseness in muscles which otherwise function normally, a state called *myogelosis*, may be found in patients with fibrositis or fibromyositis, and their nature has not been divulged by biopsy.

A mass developing in one part of a muscle, or throughout a muscle, poses a special clinical problem. It may, if chronic, be a tumor (rhabdomyosarcoma, angioma, metastatic carcinoma, or desmoid) or a granulomatous inflammation (sarcoid, tuberculoma, or mycosis). Hard masses are usually calcium (myocalcinosis) or bone deposit (myositis ossificans). If a muscle mass develops rapidly, hemorrhage, either spontaneous or traumatic, must be considered. A ruptured tendon may take this form but always causes a bulge which, for obvious reasons, becomes manifest on contraction, and the muscle exhibits a diminished power of contraction.

TENDON (STRETCH) REFLEXES

The tendon reflexes are altered in the majority of muscle diseases, particularly those which involve peripheral nerves. In muscular dystrophy and polymyositis they tend to be reduced in proportion to the reduction in muscular power. In the myopathy of hypothyroidism, in which the contractile process is slowed, there is a characteristic prolongation of the tendon reflex and the opposite condition of quickening and brevity of the tendon reflex may be less reliably demonstrated in hyperthyroidism.

MUSCLE PAIN

Pain localized to a group of muscles is extremely severe in wry neck, fibrositis and fibromyositis, acute brachial neuritis, radiculitis, Bornholm's disease, or pleurodynia, but little is known of its cause in any of these diseases. In contrast, the established forms of muscle disease, even the most serious ones such as polymyositis, are usually painless. In the latter condition, if pain is present, it usually indicates coincident involvement of connective tissues and joint structures. Tenderness of muscle is a variable state normally, and it tends to be more definite in polyneuritis, poliomyelitis, and polyarteritis nodosa than in polymyositis and in the various forms of dystrophy and other myopathies where there is usually no increase in the sensitivity of muscle tissue.

DIAGNOSIS OF MUSCLE DISEASE

These various clinical phenomena, along with certain laboratory data including muscle biopsy, when integrated with information concerning the natural course of the pathologic process, enable one to diagnose relatively easily most of the diseases of muscle.

The clinical recognition of myopathic diseases is facilitated, as a rule, by a prior knowledge of a few syndromes. The following ones recur with regularity, and their identification and proper analysis in terms of common underlying diseases are indicated. Diagnostic accuracy will be aided by an intelligent use of the laboratory methods described in Chap. 374.

We have grouped in the following classification all the common diseases around their manifest syndromes.

SYNDROMIC CLASSIFICATION OF MUSCLE DISEASES

I. Acute (days) or subacute (weeks) paralytic disorders of muscle (may cause weakness or paralysis)
   A. Primary diseases of muscle
      1. Rarely fulminant myasthenia gravis
      2. Polymyositis and dermatomyositis
      3. Alcoholic polymyopathy
      4. Acute paroxysmal myoglobinuria
        (*Note:* first attack of episodic weakness may enter into differential diagnosis; see below)
      5. Botulism
      6. Organophosphate poisoning
      See also: Acute spinal or peripheral nerve diseases (denervation paralysis where paralysis is often severe and widespread and atrophy may or may not be present).
       a. Poliomyelitis
       b. Acute idiopathic polyneuritis, or other forms of polyneuropathy (porphyria, beriberi, etc.)
       c. Rarely polyarteritis nodosa with polyneuropathy and other neuropathy

II. Chronic (i.e., months to years) paralytic disorders of muscle (weakness usually with severe atrophy)
   A. Progressive muscular dystrophy
      1. Duchenne type
      2. Facioscapulohumeral type (Landouzy-Déjerine)
      3. Limb girdle type (Erb's)
      4. Distal type (Gowers', Welander's)
      5. Myotonic dystrophy (Steinert's disease)
      6. Progressive ophthalmoplegic or oculopharyngeal type
   B. Chronic polymyositis
      See also the progressive muscular atrophies and other forms of motor system disease (amyotrophic lateral sclerosis, progressive bulbar palsy) and infantile muscular atrophy (Werdnig-Hoffman disease) as well as chronic neural muscular atrophies such as: peroneal muscular atrophy (Charcot-Marie-Tooth), hypertrophic polyneuritis (Déjerine-Sottas), amyloid polyneuropathy, chronic nutritional, arsenical, leprous, and other polyneuropathy
   C. Chronic thyrotoxic and other myopathies
   D. Chronic slowly progressive or relatively stationary polymyopathies
      1. Central core disease
      2. Nemelline myopathy
      3. Pleoconial, megaconial and myotubular polymyopathies
      4. Glycogen storage disease
      5. Congenital benign hypotonia and congenital universal hypoplasia of muscle

III. Episodic weakness of muscle
   A. Myasthenia gravis
   B. Symptomatic myasthenia of other types
      1. With lupus erythematosus disseminatus
      2. With polymyositis
      3. With rheumatoid arthritis
      4. With nonthymic carcinoma
   C. Familial periodic paralysis
   D. Hereditary adynamia [normokalemic periodic paralysis (Gamstorp's)]
   E. Paramyotonia congenita (von Eulenberg's)
   F. Hyper- and hypokalemia (including primary hyperaldosteronism)
   G. Acute thyrotoxic myopathy (also thyrotoxic periodic paralysis)

IV. Stiffness, soreness, involuntary spasm, and cramp
   A. Congenital myotonia (Thomsen's disease) paramyotonia congenita and myotonic dystrophy
   B. Tetanus
   C. Tetany
   D. Black widow spider bite
   E. Hypothyroidism with pseudomyotonia (Debré-Semelaigne and Hoffmann syndromes)
   F. Myopathy resulting from myophosphorylase deficiency (McArdle's syndrome) and other forms of contracture
   G. Contracture with Addison's disease
   H. Idiopathic cramp syndrome

V. Myalgic states
   A. Connective tissue diseases (rheumatoid arthritis, menopausal arthritis, lupus erythematosus, polyarteritis nodosa, scleroderma, polymyositis)
   B. Localized fibrositis or fibromyositis
   C. Many forms of polyneuritis
   D. Trichinosis
   E. Myopathy of myoglobinuria and McArdle's syndrome
   F. Myopathy with hypoglycemia
   G. Bornholm's disease
   H. Anterior tibial syndrome

VI. Localized muscle mass(es)
   A. Rupture of a muscle
   B. Muscle hemorrhage
   C. Muscle tumor
      1. Rhabdomyosarcoma
      2. Desmoid
      3. Angioma
      4. Metastatic nodules
   D. Localized idiopathic myopathy
   E. Localized and generalized myositis ossificans
   F. Fibrositis (myogelosis)
   G. Granulomatous infections
      1. Sarcoidosis
      2. Tuberculosis
   H. Pyogenic abscess

374 LABORATORY AIDS IN THE DIAGNOSIS OF NEUROMUSCULAR DISEASES

*Leonard W. Jarcho and
Raymond D. Adams*

Clinical suspicion of neuromuscular disease now finds ready confirmation in the laboratory. Absolute proof of diagnosis, however, is rarely forthcoming from this source. All laboratory data must be evaluated in the light of clinical findings based on broad knowledge of muscle disease.

BIOCHEMISTRY OF NEUROMUSCULAR DISEASE

The biochemical tests presently in use fall into two categories: measurement of serum electrolytes and enzymes; detection of myoglobin and abnormal amounts of creatine and creatinine in the urine. Current research on sarcoplasm promises even more valuable microchemical analysis of bits of muscle taken at biopsy.

CHANGES IN SERUM ELECTROLYTES AND THEIR EFFECTS ON NEUROMUSCULAR EXCITABILITY. The concentration of electrolytes and their fluxes in relation to neuromuscular activity were brilliantly elucidated and expounded by Hodgkin and Huxley. They are now known to be the basis of the electrical events of nerve impulse conduction and muscle fiber contraction.

In the resting state all nerve and muscle fibers are *polarized,* i.e., the interior of the cell is negative to the outside surface. With one electrode inserted into the fiber and another on the surface, a voltmeter will record a potential difference of 50 to 100 mv. This *resting membrane potential* is related to the unequal distribution of potassium on the two sides of the membrane, the interior of the cell being much richer in this ion. When the fiber responds to stimulation or injury, there are rapid leakage of potassium to the outside and corresponding inward migration of sodium. The membrane potential falls to zero, and the area of cell surface affected is said to be *depolarized.* For a fraction of a millisecond polarization is opposite to that of the resting state, and the surface is negative to the interior. This surface negativity spreads along the fiber as a wave of electrical charge, preceded at all points by the flux of K and Na ions. Recorded at usual speeds, it appears as a sharp wave, the *action potential.* Clearly these events, the hallmarks of all excitable tissues, are modified by the concentration of K and Na ions in extracellular fluids and inside the cells. Other ions, particularly Ca and Mg, are also influential.

The *neuromuscular junction* (motor end-plate) has properties of special importance. Here a terminal motor nerve twig indents the surface of the muscle fiber which it innervates. The membranes of the two cells, the neurilemma and the sarcolemma, remain separated by a thin cleft. Across this space acetylcholine is discharged, liberated from presynaptic vesicles in the terminal nerve filaments by the arrival of the *nerve action potential.* The specialized area of muscle membrane which forms the distal portion of the end-plate reacts to the presence of acetylcholine by local depolarization, the *end-plate potential.* If this surface negativity is large enough to reach threshold, the neighboring area of muscle membrane is depolarized and a *muscle action potential* is propagated over the surface of the sarcolemma. The electrical change is probably distributed from the surface of the muscle fiber inward to all the myofibrils via the endoplasmic reticulum. Within a millisecond the contractile proteins (myofilaments) of the entire fiber shorten. This mechanical change lasts a great deal longer than the action potential. A second electrical wave can therefore arrive before the muscle fiber has relaxed and might therefore have no effect. Nerve impulses arriving at a frquency of 25 to 30 per sec result in a series of completely fused muscle twitches or prolonged contraction (tetanus). The mechanical event can thus be smoothed into a continuous process, but the electrical variation remains a series of peaks of negativity, separated by plateaus during part of which the membrane is in its resting polarized state. This *repolarization* after passage of an action potential is necessary, if the membrane is to be capable of transmitting a second volley. At the end-plate repolarization is possible only if acetylcholine is removed, a process achieved by the enzyme cholinesterase. If this enzyme fails or if acetylcholine is formed in excessive amount, the end-plate remains depolarized and cannot respond to further nerve impulses. *Anticholinesterases* such as neostigmine (Prostigmine), pyridostigmine (Mestinon), edrophonium (Tensilon), physostigmine (Eserine), diisopropyl fluorophosphate (DFP), tetraethylpyrophosphate (TEPP), and several of the "nerve gases" act in this way to paralyze muscle. These *depolarizing blocking agents* paralyze by maintaining the end-plate in a depolarized state, so that it is not tripped off by the arrival of further nerve impulses. Extracts of curare and the quaternary ammonium ions, the so-called "competitive blocking agents," paralyze muscle in a different way by occupying receptor sites at the end-plate and preventing the access of acetylcholine.

Biochemical disturbances may account not only for impairment of neuromuscular processes, resulting in weakness or paralysis, but also for their enhancement, reflected in excessive irritability. In the latter case "spontaneous" discharges may occur, or a single nerve impulse may set off a train of action potentials in nerve or muscle. The common cramps of calf and foot muscles (painful, sustained, involuntary contractions with motor unit discharges at frequencies up to 300 per sec) are apparently due to increased excitability of the peripheral parts of the motor nerve. Hypocalcemia and hyponatremia predispose to cramps, as does the unaccustomed use of a muscle. Quinine, procaine amide, and warmth tend to prevent them.

The manner in which the muscle action potential initiates the contractile process has not been fully determined. The energy for this process is derived from the action of adenosine triphosphate (ATP) on the special muscle proteins, actin and myosin. The change in shape of these protein molecules results in shortening of the myofilaments and hence the myofibrils and whole fiber. The phosphate bonds of ATP supply the energy for this process and they must be replenished constantly, a reaction which involves interchanges with phosphocreatine. Myoglobin, another important muscle protein, plays a part in the transfer of oxygen, and a series of oxidative enzymes is involved in this exchange. Many glycolytic and other enzymes (transaminases, aldolase, phospho-creatine kinase) are implicated in the metabolic activity of muscle, the most active phases of which appear to be required for the restoration of the contracted fiber to the relaxed state.

To summarize, the muscle fiber, which is totally dependent on nerve for its stimulus to normal contraction, many be paralyzed in a number of ways. There may be failure of nerve to conduct an impulse, insufficiency of acetylcholine to depolarize the muscle cell, inaccessibility of the motor end-plate to normally released acetylcholine because of the presence of a competing substance, or excess of a depolarizing substance preventing repolarization of the end-plate. Finally the sarcolemmal membrane itself may fail to distribute the muscle impulse throughout the fiber. Similarly, fascicular twitching, cramps, and muscle spasms may be due to excessive activity at a number of points in the neuromuscular apparatus. There may be unstable polarization of the nerve fiber, as in tetany, or unexplained hyperirritability of the motor neurone, as in amyotrophic lateral sclerosis. The level of the threshold at which the sarcolemma is depolarized may be reduced, or a change may occur within the muscle fiber itself, which, once shortened, may have insufficient energy for restoration to a relaxed state (contracture).

When the musculature is acutely and diffusely weakened, or when twitchings, spasms, and cramps occur, serum electrolytes should be studied. They reflect extracellular levels, and the ECG (see Chap. 260) may betray alterations in intracellular content in cardiac muscle, which tend to parallel those in skeletal muscle. If the plasma level of *potassium falls below 2.5 mEq or rises above 7 mEq per liter,* weakness of extremity and trunk muscles results. When the concentration reaches 2 mEq or 9 mEq there is almost invariably flaccid paralysis of these muscles and later of the respiratory ones as well, only those of cranium, e.g., extraocular, tending to be spared. In addition the tendon reflexes are diminished or absent. The reaction of muscle to percussion is also reduced or abolished, which suggests impairment of transmission not only in nerve and at neuromuscular junction, but also along the sarcolemmal membranes themselves. A rise or fall in *the plasma concentration of sodium* causes generalized lassitude and muscular weakness, presumably because of the depolarizing action of the sodium in nerve and muscle. Sodium loss may result in muscle cramps, as does also hypocalcemia and hypoxia. *Hypocalcemia* of 7 mg per 100 ml or less (as in rickets or hypoparathyroidism) or relative reduction in the proportion of ionized calcium (as in hyperventilation) causes increased irritability and spontaneous discharge of sensory and motor nerve fibers as well as muscle fibers. The sensory manifestations are tingling and prickling in fingers, lips, tongue, and feet; the motor manifestations consist of spasms of distal musculature and face (tetany), laryngospasm with stridulous breathing, and at times convulsions. In latent tetany the unstable polarization of nerve fibers can be demonstrated by tapping the facial nerve be-

hind or over the ramus of the mandible (Chvostek's test) or compressing the circulation to proximal parts of the nerves in the arm with a tourniquet (Trousseau's sign). Frequent repetitive and finally spontaneous discharges appear in the electromyogram (EMG). *Hypercalcemia* above 12 mg per 100 ml (as in vitamin D intoxication, hyperparathyroidism, and carcinomatosis) causes reduction in excitability of nerve and muscle fibers and release of acetylcholine. *Reduction in the plasma concentration of magnesium* results in muscle spasm and convulsions; and an *increase in magnesium levels* leads to muscle weakness and depression of central nervous function (confusion). The weakness in muscle is said to be due mainly to reduced release of acetylcholine plus inhibition of the depolarizing action of acetylcholine at the motor end-plate.

CHANGES IN THE SERUM LEVELS OF ENZYMES ORIGINATING IN THE MUSCLE CELLS. In all diseases which cause extensive damage to striated muscle fibers, intracellular enzymes leak out of the fiber and enter the blood. Those which are now being measured in most hospital laboratories are the transaminases, aldolase and lactic acid dehydrogenase. But, as is noted in Chap. 324, high concentrations of these enzymes are found in heart muscle and liver cells; hence raised serum values may be due to myocardial infarction or hepatitis, as well as to the necrobiotic diseases of striated muscle (polymyositis, muscle trauma, muscle infarction, Meyer-Betz paroxysmal myoglobinuria, and the more rapidly advancing muscular dystrophies). For the serum levels to be interpretable, one must have evidence of the integrity of heart and liver. Phosphocreatine kinase (creatine kinase), on the other hand, though present in heart and brain, is found in highest concentration in striated muscle. The normal level is 1 to 2 units (according to new system of grading, this is 10 to 50 units) with an upper limit of 3.5 to 4.0. In patients with degenerative lesions of striated muscle it may exceed 1,000. Even more interesting is its rise in some patients with progressive muscular dystrophy before there is enough destruction of fiber to be clinically manifest. Moreover, the unaffected female carriers of the trait in Duchenne's pseudohypertrophic form may now be identified because they show slight elevations of serum creatine kinase level. All workers are agreed that alterations of serum enzyme levels are nonspecific for dystrophy, since they occur in all types of disease which destroy the muscle fiber. Moreover, in the more slowly evolving types of dystrophy, such as that of Landouzy-Déjerine, the serum levels of creatine kinase may be normal. As would be expected, the values are normal in all forms of denervation paralysis and muscular dystrophy.

ENDOCRINOPATHIES. In a number of disorders of endocrine glands muscle weakness may be a prominent feature, and occasionally it becomes even a chief complaint. While these diseases are discussed in detail elsewhere (Chaps. 377 and 378), it should be noted that such weakness, local or generalized, acute or chronic, may occur in the absence of changes in serum electrolytes or enzymes. Specific hormone assays are then necessary for diagnosis.

This is particularly true of thyrotoxicosis, where severe muscle paresis may appear without the classical signs of Graves' disease.

MYOGLOBINURIA. The red pigment, myoglobin, is responsible for much of the color of muscle. It is an iron-protein compound present in the sarcoplasm of striated skeletal and cardiac fibers. Of the total body hematin compounds, about 25 percent is in muscle, the remainder in red corpuscles and other cells. Destruction of striated muscle, regardless of the process, liberates myoglobin. Because of its relatively small size, the molecule filters through the glomerulus and appears in the urine, imparting to it a burgundy-red color. The serum is effectively cleared and retains its normal color. In contrast, hemolysis of red corpuscles frees hemoglobin, coloring both serum and urine because of the high renal threshold. Myoglobinuria should thus be suspected when the urine is deep red and the serum normal in color. As in hemoglobinuria the guaiac and benzidine tests are positive and the final demonstration depends on spectroscopic analysis, which shows an absorption band at 581 μ. The urine does not fluoresce, as it does in porphyria. Myoglobin appears in the urine in the following conditions: spontaneous myoglobinuria of unknown cause, e.g., Meyer-Betz paroxysmal myoglobinuria; as a result of crushing or infarction of muscles; in rare cases of polymyositis, alcoholic and other myopathies such as McArdle's disease; following extreme muscular activity; after the ingestion of certain toxic substances (from fish poisoned by waste products, as in Haff's disease).

CREATINURIA. Creatine, an amino acid, is a prominent constituent of striated muscle tissue. It may be ingested (exogenous creatine) but is also synthesized in the liver from glycine, arginine, and methionine. It is delivered to the skeletal muscles, which contain the largest amount of this compound of any organ (150 mg per 100 Gm fresh weight muscle tissue). Creatinine, the anhydride of creatine, is a degradation product which is excreted in the urine. The creatinine content of muscles is low (about 5 mg per 100 ml), since it diffuses readily through the sarcolemma. Normal male serum contains 0.2 to 0.6 mg per 100 ml of creatine; the female, 0.4 to 0.9 mg. Creatinine serum levels range from 0.8 to 1.4 mg and are increased only in serious renal disease. Adult 24-hr urine excretion of creatine averages from 60 to 150 mg in normal males and 100 to 300 mg in females. Creatinine excretion is remarkably constant at 1.0 to 1.6 Gm. In diseases such as progressive muscular dystrophy there are decrease in creatinine excretion, increase in creatine excretion, and hypercreatinemia. The creatine content of the muscle fiber is diminished. The same alterations occur in neurogenic atrophy, and with reduction in muscle mass in polymyositis, hyperthyroidism, Addison's disease, and male eunuchoidism. Ingestion of 1 to 3 Gm creatine will not significantly raise its level in blood or urine in a normal person, for his muscles are not saturated; but in an individual with a reduced muscle mass, creatinemia and creatinuria result. This type of creatine tolerance test thus merely indicates reduction in functional muscle mass.

PHYSIOLOGY OF NEUROMUSCULAR ACTIVITY

Electromyography

The earliest studies of neuromuscular function involved the effects of electric stimuli. It was discovered long ago that muscle responds to current, especially if it is applied to the motor point where the nerve enters. Furthermore, the quicker impulse of faradic current is normally more effective than the galvanic, and this relation is reversed after denervation (Erb's reaction of degeneration). Lapicque related intensity of current to strength of contraction in his term *chronaxie,* now largely supplanted by the plotting of strength-duration curves.

Functional organization of movement was clarified by Sherrington, who introduced the important concept of the *motor unit:* a motor neurone, its axone, and all the muscle fibers which it innervates. All movement, posture, and reflex activity are now interpreted in terms of the organization and integration of large numbers of these motor units by spinal and supraspinal mechanisms. Strength of muscle contraction can be reduced to the number of motor units enlisted at a given time, and the speed of contraction, to the rate of their recruitment. Tendon reflex is caused by a volley of sensory impulses from stretch receptors in muscle which briefly activate a group of the large (alpha) motor nerve cells. Effectiveness of movement is related to the manner in which motor units of different muscles are activated and inhibited in reciprocal relationships. Coordination of movements, posture, and automatic movements such as walking and running are understandable in terms of more complex spinal integrations of muscles. Paralysis represents the reverse, an inactivation of motor units or whole muscles, complete only upon severance of the peripheral motor innervation and followed then by extreme atrophy of muscle fibers, fibrillation, and unusual sensitivity to acetylcholine.

The electric currents given off by nerve and muscle had been discovered as early as 1794 by Galvani. Yet the systematic recording of these currents as a measure of the structural and functional status of muscle lagged behind other electrical techniques such as electrocardiography and electroencephalography. The reasons are largely two, one anatomic, the other technical. The heart and brain, though exceedingly complex, are single organs and their total electrical output can be sampled effectively for clinical purposes from a relatively limited number of electrode positions. The striated muscles, on the other hand, are numerous and scattered and in some instances of large size. As a result no small series of leads will give an average picture of their electrical activity. They must be tested laboriously, one at a time, because disease may be spread irregularly through many of them, so that normal findings in one area do not exclude the possibility of pathologic phenomena close by. These anatomic difficulties pose the technical problem of finding suitable electrode systems for both electroneurography and electromyography. External plate electrodes, such as those used in electrocardiography and electroencephalography, will pick up potentials representing the chance summation of many units, giving only an average picture. A more detailed physiologic analysis requires needle electrodes, which register the activity of only a small number of motor units or muscle fibers.

Three types of needle electrodes are in general use: unipolar, bipolar, and concentric. All three are made of fine wire or hypodermic needle tubing coated with insulating material so as to leave at the tip only a few microns of bare, conducting metal. In the unipolar application a single needle is used, the other electrode being a diffuse skin lead. Bipolar electrodes consist of two needles, separated by a distance of 2 mm or less for most uses. A concentric electrode may be made from a hypodermic needle by inserting a shellacked wire in the lumen, so that one lead encircles the other. The potential forms seen with these three types are not identical. Most satisfactorily explained according to current theory are the records obtained with bipolar needles. Such electrodes pick up the action potentials of those few muscle fibers which lie in the immediate vicinity of their bare tips. If the needles are oriented in the long axis of the muscle fibers, the action potential reaches first one, then the other. The electrode on the active, or depolarized, portion of the fiber becomes negative to its mate, and the recording instrument is deflected from the base line. By convention, the negative potential is recorded as an upward deflection (Fig. 374-1). As the potential propagates farther along the muscle fiber, it reaches a point equidistant from the two electrodes, and the record returns to base line. When the action potential reaches the second electrode, a deflection opposite to the first is inscribed. Thus a diphasic potential is recorded. Because of the extreme rapidity of these events, the inertia-free cathode ray oscillograph (CRO) is the preferred recording instrument for electromyography.

MOTOR UNIT ACTIVITY

The simple diphasic potential discussed above should theoretically result from the activity of a single muscle fiber. In healthy muscle single fibers do not act alone. Normally, excitation arrives via the motor nerves. Within a motor unit the fibers are not necessarily of uniform diameter, length, or shape, and their spatial orientation with regard to the electrodes will vary. Normal muscle activated through its nerve therefore produces rather complex potentials, presumably the result of summation of single-fiber potentials of varying characteristics. Some of the factors involved in producing the wave forms seen in normal muscle have been demonstrated in animal experiments, but the limits of normal variation are not yet well defined.

THE NORMAL ELECTROMYOGRAM (EMG)

Normal muscle is electrically silent when it is at rest. Once insertion activity following placement of the needles has died down, the electrodes record no propagated

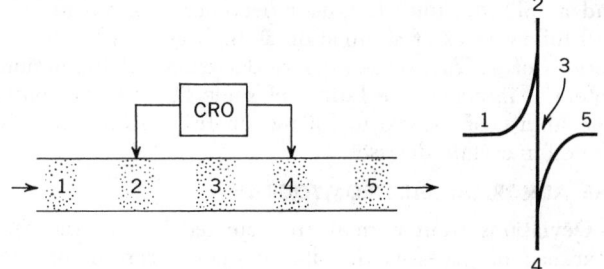

Fig. 374-1. The active (shaded) area is negative to all other points on the fiber surface. It is shown at five points in its course (from left to right) along the fiber. At each point, the correspondingly numbered portion of the diphasic potential is inscribed on the face of the cathoderay oscillograph (CRO).

action potentials. In very tense individuals it may take considerable training to reach this point of complete relaxation, for properly placed electrodes will record minimal activity of which the person is not conscious. If now the muscle is voluntarily contracted, action potentials appear on the CRO screen. Slowly graded contraction allows one to observe the manner in which force is normally accumulated (Fig. 374-2 C). As contraction begins, the potential of one motor unit appears. It will be relatively constant in the form characteristic for its own motor unit, and it will differ slightly from the potentials of other units in number of phases, shape, duration, amplitude, and rate of repetition. A slight increase in the voluntary force exerted results in a speeding up of this rate to a critical level, when a second unit is "recruited" and its potential also appears on the screen. If contraction is maintained at this minimum level, the record is indistinguishable from that of "fasciculation," which is also the activity of a few motor units, except that in the latter activity is involuntary and continues at rest. As the strength of contraction is increased, more motor units enter the picture, and their potentials begin to overlie each other. There results a disorderly crowd of action potentials of all sizes and shapes. Individual potentials of motor units can no longer be distinguished. The maximal amplitude of oscillation is many millivolts. Obviously, a weak muscle with few contracting fibers will produce a smaller total potential than normal. However, unless reduction in output is sufficient to break up the *interference pattern* just described, so that individual motor unit potentials become identifiable, we have no certain evidence of abnormality. As long as a muscle is held actively contracted, the interference pattern continues. Gradual relaxation will show a gradual dropping out of motor units, until only a few are left firing, then one, then none.

Skeletal muscle may also be artificially stimulated to contract. In man the usual method is the application of electric shocks to the skin overlying a motor nerve. With proper stimulating conditions there will be one response for each shock. The form of this response will depend upon the number of motor units activated and the number sampled by the recording electrodes. If repeated shocks are given, each response will have the same form and amplitude, until fatigue supervenes. Normal muscle will follow rates of stimulation as high as 25 per sec for periods of at least 60 sec before decrement of the action potential indicates the failure of some fibers to respond. The ability of muscle to follow repetitive stimulation is altered in certain diseases.

THE ABNORMAL ELECTROMYOGRAM

Deviations from normal are detected in (1) the appearance of excessive irritability upon insertion of the recording needle; (2) the occurrence of "spontaneous" activity during relaxation (fibrillation and fasciculation); (3) alteration in size and duration of action potentials recorded during graded single or successive voluntary or electrically induced muscular contractions; (4) the demonstration of special phenomena such as myotonia or coupling (tetany), or electrical silence during obvious shortening of the muscle (contracture).

IRRITABILITY ON NEEDLE INSERTION. At the moment the needle is placed in the muscle there is usually a brief burst of action potentials which cease once the needle is stable, providing it is not in a position to irritate a motor nerve fiber. Myotonic muscle is extremely irritable; chains of insertion activity may be prolonged and recur at the slightest movement of the needle. This is also true of conditions which dispose to muscle cramp.

"SPONTANEOUS ACTIVITY" DURING COMPLETE RELAXATION. Relaxed muscle is normally electrically silent. Incomplete relaxation may be attended by flurries of action potentials which subside when the limb is repositioned to relieve involuntary tension. Persistent firing of motor units or of single fibers, known respectively as fasciculation and fibrillation, is then abnormal.

Fibrillation. The two phenomena of fibrillation and fasciculation have often been confused with each other.

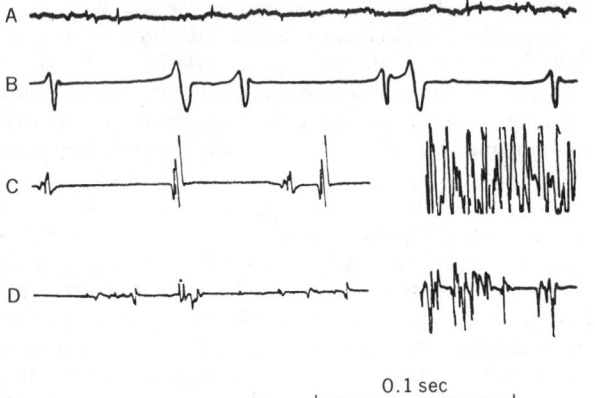

0.1 sec

Fig. 374-2. Electromyographic patterns. *A.* Fibrillation. Tibialis anterior, 11 years after gunshot wound of nerve. Totally random potentials of 1 to 2 msec in duration and maximum amplitude of about 0.1 mv. *B.* Fasciculation. Amyotrophic lateral sclerosis. Potentials of two units, each firing with its own fairly regular rhythm. Maximum amplitude of about 3 mv. *C.* Normal muscle. Contraction starts gently with two motor units (amplitudes of about 1 and 3 mv). Right-hand record shows "interference activity." *D.* Muscular dystrophy. Contraction starts with several units of abnormally low voltage (maximum of about 0.3 mv) and bizarre form. Maximal effort is insufficient to maintain "interference" pattern.

Fasciculation, defined in detail in the next paragraph, consists of synchronous contraction of *groups of muscle fibers* integrated by a single axone into a motor unit. Fibrillation is the contraction of *single muscle fibers*, enabled to appear only when destruction of their axone has disintegrated the motor unit.

When a motor neurone is destroyed by disease, or when its axone is severed, the distal part of the axone degenerates, a process which takes several days. The muscle fibers formerly innervated by the branches of the dead axone, viz., the motor unit, are disconnected from the nervous system. For reasons which are still obscure, 8 to 12 days after death of the axone the denervated fibers develop spontaneous activity, i.e., even while no effort is being made by the patient to contract the muscle, action potentials are generated along the surface of the denervated muscle fibers. Each fiber fires at its own rate and without relation to the activity of its fellows. There results a totally random conglomeration of diphasic potentials (Fig. 374-2A), among which it is occasionally possible to pick out by some unusual characteristic that of a particular fiber. This activity is termed *fibrillation*. Fibrillary potentials have a duration of 1 to 2 milliseconds (msec). They rarely exceed 200 μv in amplitude, but much smaller ones will be recorded from fibers relatively distant from the electrodes. When potentials of this sort are observed in resting muscle, it may be concluded that some of the fibers are denervated. Diseases such as poliomyelitis, which cause necrosis of motor axones, or injuries of peripheral nerves or anterior spinal roots, frequently produce only partial denervation of the involved muscles. In such muscles, one electrode placement may pick up fibrillation at rest in denervated fibers and normal potentials during activity from nearby healthy fibers. Fibrillation continues until the muscle fiber is reinnervated by the outgrowth of new axones from the central nervous system, or until the fiber is replaced by connective tissue. This phenomenon has been observed for several years after poliomyelitis.

Since the action potentials of motor units normally accompany contraction in muscle, it is not surprising to find that fibrillating muscle also is mechanically as well as electrically active. In the tongue, where the epithelium is thin and wet, faint shimmering motions may be seen as the fibers contract. Elsewhere in the body the isolated contraction of single fibers is ordinarily not of sufficient strength to be visible through the skin. Visible twitchings, sometimes loosely called fibrillation in the clinic, are usually fasciculation.

Fasciculation. Fasciculation is the spontaneous, involuntary contraction of motor units, singly or in groups. Since a relatively large number of muscle fibers contracts in synchrony, visible dimpling or twitching of the skin occurs, though ordinarily not enough power is exerted to move a joint. The form of the accompanying potential varies, presumably because it is made up of the summed activity of variable numbers of fibers of slightly differing characteristics. Commonly, it will have three to five phases, a duration of 8 to 10 msec (somewhat less in the facial muscles), and an amplitude of several millivolts (Fig. 374-2*B*). The pattern tends to repeat at a fairly regular rate, indicating a rhythmic activation of the fibers by the responsible axones.

Traditionally, fasciculation occurs in chronic, slowly advancing, destructive disease of the anterior horn cells such as amyotrophic lateral sclerosis and progressive spinal muscular atrophy. It has been reported in the early stages of poliomyelitis, less commonly than in the chronic diseases mentioned, perhaps because the affected cells die too rapidly. In all these cases the damaged neurone seems to be "irritated" by the disease process. It fires repetitively and, in so doing, trips off activity in all the muscle fibers that it innervates. It has been shown that fasciculation may also follow peripheral nerve lesions, giving way to fibrillation upon death of the axone. More important is the fact that fasciculation occurs occasionally in many normal persons, constantly in some, so that it need not be evidence of disease at all. Shivering, induced by low temperature, and the twitchings associated with depressed serum calcium levels are also forms of fasciculation. Finally, as was said, when needle electrodes are inserted into normal muscles, the mechanical irritation which they produce may cause the activation of a few fibers.

ABNORMALITIES IN SIZE AND DURATION OF ACTION POTENTIALS. Giant Action Potentials in Partially Denervated Muscle.

If the total motor nerve supply to a muscle is physically interrupted, there is at first no electrical activity and later fibrillation, which persists as long as muscle tissue remains. Partial denervation reduces the number of action potentials appearing during contraction. Those which remain increase in amplitude, sometimes to two to three times normal size. These giant potentials are believed to be generated by motor units containing more than the usual number of muscle fibers. Presumably new nerve twigs have sprouted from the undamaged axones reinnervating previously denervated fibers and adding them to their own motor units. Thus incomplete "interference pattern," giant action potentials, fibrillation potentials, and the small number of motor units in action relative to strength of contraction are the characteristic EMG features of partial denervation.

Reduced Size and Duration of Action Potentials.

The presence of large numbers of low-voltage, short-duration action potentials (often a rich interference pattern in a weak muscle) is characteristic of the muscular dystrophies and myopathies. The duration of the action potential may remain normal (8 to 10 msec) while amplitude is reduced. The obvious explanation is that a disease process has destroyed scattered fibers within a motor unit, reducing its population. This phenomenon occurs in all forms of progressive muscular dystrophy and, unfortunately, does not distinguish the types, nor separate them from polymyositis, dermatomyositis, and other chronic myopathies. In the myositides, however, fibrillation potentials may also be seen, presumably because of the destruction of terminal nerve twigs by the inflammatory process. When destruction of all the muscle fibers is completed, *electrical activity ceases.*

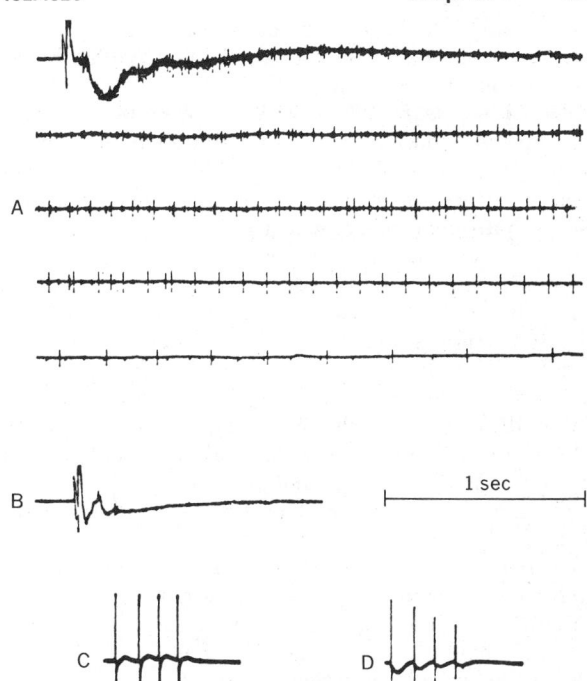

Fig. 374-3. Myotonia and myasthenia. *A.* Myotonia congenita (Thomsen's disease). The five lines are a continuous record of activity in the biceps brachii following a tap on the tendon. The initial response is within normal limits, but it is followed by a prolonged burst of rapid activity, gradually subsiding over a period of many seconds or minutes. *B* Same electrode placement as in (*A*). Response to the fifth of a series of tendon taps. "Warm-up" has occurred, and the characteristic prolonged myotonic activity is no longer evident. *C.* Response of normal muscle to shocks applied to the motor nerve at a rate of approximately 3 per sec. At this rate of stimulation the amplitude of the first response is maintained throughout the series of four shocks. *D.* Myasthenia gravis. Same conditions as in (*C*). The first potential is of normal amplitude, but as stimulation continues, the response falls off and may eventually reach zero if stimulation continues. (*Records C and D courtesy of Dr. David Grob, Department of Medicine, Johns Hopkins Hospital.*)

Progressive Reduction or Augmentation of Action Potentials in Successive Contractions.

In certain disorders the initial motor unit potentials are normal whether contraction is induced voluntarily or by electric stimuli applied to the nerve. After a few shocks at rates as low as 1 to 10 per sec, the amplitude of the potentials falls off and may reach zero, while normal muscles follow the electrical stimuli with little decrement over a minute or two at rates as high as 40 to 50 per sec. This phenomenon is characteristic of the several varieties of *myasthenia gravis*. It is remarkably similar to the partial block at the neuromuscular junction produced by curare and, like it, may be relieved by neostigmine. Similar but less definite decline of the action potentials with repetitive stimulation may occur in poliomyelitis. It is thus possible that there may be damage elsewhere than in the nerve cells in this disease. In some cases of carcinoma of the lung and sarcoidosis with muscular weakness the opposite condition may be observed. If electrical stimulation through nerve is rapid (20 to 30 per sec), action potentials may be small with the first muscular contraction and increase in voltage with each successive one until a more nearly normal state is attained. Neostigmine has no effect on this phenomenon.

SPECIAL ABNORMALITIES OF EMG. Myotonia. In myotonic muscle, contraction persists despite voluntary attempts at relaxation. The symptom occurs in several hereditary diseases, myotonia congenita (Thomsen's disease), dystrophia myotonica (Steinert's disease), and normokalemic periodic paralysis (von Eulenberg's paramyotonia), appearing in myotonic dystrophy in combination with a definite pattern of muscle wasting and certain other stigmas (see Chap. 377). Minor forms occur sporadically under other circumstances. The characteristic electrical picture is seen during voluntary contraction or direct stimulation of the muscle, either electrically or by a blow. The motor unit potential appears entirely normal, but it is not followed by the silence which normally occurs on relaxation. Instead there is a burst of rapid activity, which may take as long as several minutes to subside (Fig. 374-3A). Some of the potentials of this prolonged discharge have the duration, amplitude, and form of single-fiber activity, while others appear to have the characteristics of motor unit potentials. If the muscle is activated repeatedly at short intervals, the late discharge becomes briefer and briefer and eventually disappears (Fig. 374-3A), and the patient finds that he can relax the exercised muscle at will. This phenomenon has been called *warm-up*. Although there is evidence of abnormal reflex patterns in myotonia, the characteristic repetitive discharge does not arise in the nervous system, for it is not blocked by curare.

High-frequency coupling of action potentials, indicating instability of the polarization of the nerve fiber, occurs in tetany.

Contracture, pseudomyotonia of hypothyroidism, percussion and contraction myoedema, and percussion fasciculation have no electrical counterpart (EMG is silent). This aspect of these phenomena is important in their definition.

STATISTICAL ANALYSIS

In electrocardiography it is frequently possible to decide that a single complex is abnormal because its measurements lie outside of well-established limits for the lead under consideration. For reasons discussed above, it is often difficult to make this decision in the case of an individual motor unit potential in skeletal muscle. As a result, attempts have been made to establish curves of frequency distribution for various parameters, such as duration and amplitude of potentials. It has been found that duration varies in different normal muscles and that it tends to increase with age. In the dystrophies a normal distribution of durations occurs, while some types of myositis show a shift of the curve toward shorter durations. Muscles weakened as a result of disease of neurones tend to produce prolonged potentials. In poliomyelitis there is evidence that more pronounced prolongation forebodes poor functional recovery. The meaning of all these findings is still obscure. Further research is necessary before electrical abnormalities can be correlated with other pathologic findings.

Electroneurography

Disease of peripheral nerve may produce the electromyographic evidences of denervation discussed above. More direct observations of neural function can be made by the measurement of conduction velocity.

CONDUCTION VELOCITY OF NERVE

Data of considerable clinical interest may be obtained by determining conduction velocity in peripheral nerve. Any accessible nerve is stimulated through the skin while the resulting muscle action potential is recorded with appropriate electrodes. Conduction time is measured from the shock artefact to the onset of the response. A second stimulus is then applied to another point along the nerve, and the new conduction time is measured. The distance between the two points of stimulation divided by the difference in conduction times gives a measure of velocity of propagation of the nerve action potential. When studies are carried out in this manner, the calculated velocities are those of the largest motor fibers. In normal adults the range is between 45 and 75 meters per sec. Lower values are recorded in infants and in the aged. Conduction in afferent fibers may be measured by stimulating the skin and recording the time taken for an impulse to reach a certain point along a nerve.

Conduction velocity measured in this manner may be markedly reduced in acute or chronic peripheral neuropathies of whatever etiology. The technique has been found clinically useful in differentiating lesions of peripheral nerve from central lesions and from primary muscle disease. It may give objective evidence at an early stage of disorders otherwise manifested only by indefinite sensory findings.

Biopsy Myopathology

Muscle biopsy can be of great diagnostic value, but both surgical and microscopic techniques must be exacting. The muscle chosen for study should be easily accessible, and there should be evidence that it has been affected but not totally destroyed by the disease in question. Muscle biopsy is indicated (1) to attempt to differentiate among neuropathic atrophy, dystrophy, metabolic myopathy, and polymyositis; (2) to support the diagnosis of diffuse diseases of connective tissue and blood vessels (e.g., polyarteritis nodosa, lupus), or special infections (e.g., trichinosis, toxoplasmosis); (3) for diagnosis of metabolic diseases involving muscle (e.g., glycogen storage disease) and the special myopathies (rod body and central core myopathies); (4) in the scientific study of disorders of neuromuscular transmission (e.g., myasthenia gravis, periodic paralysis), usually by a combination of histochemical techniques and methylene blue staining of nerve endings. In most instances it is possible to distinguish histologically among the effects of denervation, the dystrophies and other necrotizing myopathies, special disfigurative myopathies, and polymyositis.

As a rule the biopsy procedure requires no more than a cleanly excised $1.0 \times 1.0 \times 2.0$ cm block of muscle, which is then fixed in 10 percent neutral formalin, embedded in paraffin, and cross and longitudinal sections stained by H and E, phosphotungstic acid hematoxylin, or Mallory trichrome methods. Special techniques may be applied if it is desirable to visualize special qualities of a disease, such as the methylene blue–cholinesterase technique for nerve endings and myoneural junctions (method of Coërs and Wolff) or histochemical stain for enzyme content of muscle fibers (phosphorylase in McArdle's disease, etc.). Electron microscopy can also be performed on carefully selected blocks of tissue fixed in gluteraldehyde. All these latter are of interest to research workers and are available only in centers where muscle diseases are under investigation.

THE USE OF LABORATORY TESTS IN THE STUDY OF MUSCLE DISEASE

The results of none of the diagnostic laboratory procedures described above may be taken as infallible indices of specific diseases of muscle. Each procedure is subject to technical error and the findings to misinterpretation. A biopsy specimen may be excised from an unaffected muscle or portion of a muscle and be negative in the face of clinical evidence of obvious disease; or rough excision and improper fixation and staining may produce artefacts which the unwary may misinterpret as marks of disease when in fact the muscle is microscopically normal. Similarly, EMG study may fail to record fibrillations in obviously denervated muscle, or a few fasciculations may be seen in an otherwise typical dystrophic process. As in the study of all disease, laboratory data have important significance only if viewed against the background of the clinical findings.

REFERENCES

Adams, R. D., D. Denny-Brown, and C. M. Pearson: "Diseases of Muscle: A Study in Pathology, 2d ed., New York, Paul B. Hoeber, Inc., 1962.
——, L. M. Eaton, and G. M. Shy: "Neuromuscular Disorders," Baltimore, The Williams & Wilkins Company, 1960.
Walton, J. N.: "Disorders of Voluntary Muscle," 2d ed., Boston, Little, Brown and Company, 1969.

375 ACUTE AND SUBACUTE MYOPATHIC PARALYSIS

Frank H. Tyler and
Raymond D. Adams

As was remarked in Chap. 22, sudden paralysis of skeletal muscles in a limb or sector of the body, developing over a period of minutes or hours, can usually be traced to a vascular disorder of spinal cord or brain, and rarely to a myelitis or encephalitis. Acute paralysis developing in the course of days (1 to 14) is usually due to poliomyelitis or acute idiopathic polyneuritis (Landry-Guillain-Barré syndrome) and rarely another form of polyneuropathy (porphyria, polyarteritis). The primary diseases of muscle, by contrast, rarely cause a rapidly developing widespread paralysis. Instead, their course is usually subacute (2 to several weeks) or chronic. The only exceptions that the authors have observed are rare cases of myasthenia gravis in which the evolution of the disease to a severe and incapacitating paresis has been over 2 or 3 days, in rare cases of polymyositis, and in some of the cases of acute thyrotoxic myopathy which we have suspected of being a combination of myasthenia gravis and hyperthyroidism. In some of the cases of paroxysmal myoglobinuria, a moderately severe weakness of the limbs has appeared within a few hours of physical exertion, but usually the clinical picture has been at once complicated by renal damage and anuria. Occasionally an attack of myoglobinuria has followed an infection and has led to severe paralysis of trunk and limb muscles within a few days to 2 or 3 weeks. A pronounced, rapidly developing paralysis of the limbs and respiratory and cranial musculature may occur after the bite of certain species of ticks (tick-bite paralysis); and botulism causes a fulminant paralysis of ocular and other cranial muscles, leading to respiratory failure and death in a few hours or days (see Chap. 171). The initial attack of periodic paralysis or of hyper- or hypopotassemia must also enter the differential diagnosis of the acute muscle paralysis. The clinical analysis of these acute syndromes is aided by certain laboratory data such as the electrocardiogram, serum potassium level, sodium and chloride values, serum enzymes such as creatine phosphokinase, and protein-bound iodine measurement; and the cerebrospinal fluid may be of great help. The response to neostigmine or edrophonium (Tensilon) (Chap. 377) aids in the diagnosis of acute myasthenia gravis.

The two principal categories of subacute myopathy are dermatomyositis (polymyositis if there is no skin involvement) and polymyopathy due to metabolic diseases.

DERMATOMYOSITIS AND POLYMYOSITIS

DEFINITION. These are relatively common diseases which affect primarily the striated muscle, skin, and other connective tissues of the body. The term used varies according to the distribution of the pathologic process. If restricted clinically to the striated muscles, the disease is called polymyositis; if the skin is involved, it is designated as dermatomyositis; and if other connective tissues are implicated, the term of choice is dermatomyositis with rheumatoid arthritis, rheumatic fever, lupus erythematosus, or scleroderma.

HISTORY. Polymyositis has been known since the original descriptions by Wagner in 1863 and 1887, and the dermatomyositis form was first reported by Unverricht in 1887. The literature since that time and a general statement of present knowledge are found in the monographs of Walton and Adams in 1958 and Walton in 1969.

ETIOLOGY. The cause of the disease is unknown. All attempts to isolate an infective agent have been unsuccessful. In one recent observation virus particles were seen in muscle cells. The finding has not been corroborated. Its close association with diseases of connective tissue suggests a common etiology or pathogenesis, possibly an autoallergic inflammation. The clinical grouping of patients in this category is not overly precise and probably results in the inclusion of other diseases of noninflammatory type, namely, metabolic myopathies.

CLINICAL MANIFESTATIONS. This type of muscle disease tends to appear in several clinical settings, as follows.

Polymyositis. A subacute symmetric weakness of proximal limb and trunk muscles without dermatitis or with minimal skin lesions. The onset is usually insidious and the course slowly progressive over a period of several weeks or months. The disease may develop at almost any age (one to eighty years) and in either sex. The majority of patients range from thirty to sixty years of age, and females outnumber males 2:1. A respiratory or obscure systemic infection may precede the muscle weakness, but in many patients the first symptoms develop during excellent health. The patient first becomes aware of a painless weakness of the proximal limb muscles, especially hips and thighs, and acts such as arising from a squatting or kneeling position, climbing or descending stairs, walking, putting an object on a high shelf, or combing the hair become increasingly difficult. In restricted forms of the disease only the neck muscles or quadriceps may be involved. Pain of aching variety, in buttocks, joints, and calves, is experienced in only a small percentage of cases (15 percent) and usually indicates a combination of polymyositis and arthritis or other connective tissue disease. The weakness progresses over a period of weeks and months. When the patient is first seen, the facial, anterior, and posterior neck muscles (head may loll), the pharyngeal and laryngeal muscles (dysphagia and dysphonia), all the trunk, the girdle muscles of shoulders and hips, upper arms, and the thighs are usually involved. Ocular muscles are almost never affected; the forearm, hand, leg, and foot muscles are spared in all but about 25 percent of cases. The muscles are usually not tender, and atrophy and reduction in tendon reflexes, though present, are not so pronounced as in denervation diseases. When reflexes are disproportionately reduced, one must think of carcinomatosis with polymyositis and neuritis. The skin and mucous membranes and joints are unchanged. In a recent review of our cases of polymyositis and dermatomyositis a surprising number of cardiac abnormalities were observed. Most were relatively minor EKG changes, but several had arrythmias of significance. Among the fatal cases about half showed clinical evidence of severe cardiac disease and had myocardial fiber necrosis at autopsy, usually with only modest inflammatory response. As a rule, evidence of systemic infection is absent. Exceptionally there is low-grade fever, especially if joint pain coexists, and a spot or a few spots of dermatitis may be present at one stage of the illness.

Dermatomyositis. The skin changes may precede, accompany, or follow the muscle syndrome and take the form of a localized or diffuse erythema, maculopapular eruption, scaling eczematoid dermatitis, or even an exfoliative dermatitis. Of particular importance is the occurrence of a lilac-colored (heliotrope) change in the skin over the bridge of the nose, cheeks, forehead, and around the fingernails. Itching may be troublesome in some cases. The skin lesions are restricted and unimportant in some cases, consisting, as mentioned, of only a patch or more of dermatitis. Periorbital and perioral edema is frequent, particularly in more fulminating episodes. Signs of other connective tissue disease are more frequent (one-third to one-half of all patients) than in examples of pure polymyositis. The limb weakness is usually proximal but may be diffuse, i.e., distal and proximal, just as in polymyositis. Raynaud's phenomenon is reported in nearly a third of the patients. Others will develop a mild form of scleroderma. Esophageal weakness may be demonstrated by fluoroscopy in approximately 30 percent of all patients. The superior constrictors are involved almost universally, but careful analysis by cinefluorography may be required to demonstrate the abnormality.

Connective Tissue Diseases with Polymyositis or Dermatomyositis. This combination involves rheumatic fever, rheumatoid arthritis, scleroderma, or lupus erythematosus where there is greater muscular weakness and atrophy than can be accounted for by the original disease. Inasmuch as pain in arthritis may limit motion, result in atrophy, and impair the power of voluntary movement, the diagnosis is not easy, and sometimes reliance must be put on muscle biopsy, urinary excretion of creatine and creatinine, and measurements of muscle enzymes in the serum. Malaise, aches, and pains may be the only symptoms in the early stages of the disease. Sjögren's syndrome of keratitis desiccans, swelling and diminished secretion of salivary glands, and xerostomia and rheumatoid arthritis may accompany polymyositis (see Chap. 394).

Carcinoma with Polymyositis or Dermatomyositis. This syndrome is placed in a separate category, although the muscle and skin changes are indistinguishable from those in the above forms of the disease. Approximately 10 percent of all adults, especially the elderly, who have polymyositis or dermatomyositis are found to have a carcinoma or some other tumor. Some cases of thymoma are accompanied by polymyositis. The incidence of this neoplastic syndrome is slightly higher in men than in women. Over 1,000 examples have been reported in the literature, being linked most often with bronchogenic carcinoma. The tumors, however, have occurred in every organ of the body. The muscle and skin tissues show no evidence of tumor cells. The polymyositis may antedate the clinical manifestations of the malignancy by 1 to 2 years. The relationship is not understood.

LABORATORY FINDINGS. Regardless of the clinical associations, in all forms of polymyositis the creatine excretion in the urine is moderately elevated in most cases and creatinine excretion is low. The serum levels of the several types of transaminase and other tissue enzymes such as creatine phosphokinase and aldolase are elevated. Serum α_2- and γ-globulin values may be raised. Tests for circulating rheumatoid factor (latex fixation and sensitized sheep cell procedure) are positive in less than half the cases. Myoglobin is occasionally found in the urine when the muscle affection is acute and severe. The sedimentation rate may be normal or elevated. Lupus erythematosus preparations of blood smears are negative, as a rule. The electromyogram reveals a typical "myopathic pattern," i.e., many abnormally brief action potentials of low voltage and, in addition, numerous fibrillation potentials and salvos of pseudomyotonic activity (see Chap. 374). The electrocardiogram has been abnormal in a few of the authors' cases. The muscle biopsy, if taken from an affected muscle, usually demonstrates the typical pathologic changes of the disease.

PATHOLOGY. The principal changes in muscle tissue consist of widespread destruction of muscle fibers, with all the expected cellular reaction thereto (myophages and fibroblastic proliferation), and infiltrates of inflammatory cells (lymphocytes, mononuclear leukocytes, plasma cells, and rare neutrophilic leukocytes). Evidences of regenerative activity in the form of proliferating sarcolemmal nuclei, basophilic (ribonucleic acid–rich) sarcoplasm, and new myofibrils are almost invariable. Many of the residual muscle fibers are small, with increased numbers of sarcolemmal nuclei. Either the degeneration of muscle fibers or the infiltrations of inflammatory cells may predominate in any given biopsy specimen, though at autopsy both types of change are in evidence. There are also inflammatory changes in the skin and other organs, but these are discussed in Chaps. 400 and 393.

DIAGNOSIS. Patients with a pure polymyositis are often suspected of having progressive muscular dystrophy because of the similar distribution of weakness (proximal and trunk muscles). Unlike dystrophy, however, the development is much more rapid, individuals may be affected at all ages (one rarely sees a dystrophy begin after thirty years of age), and the laryngeal, pharyngeal, neck muscles, and esophagus are usually involved. It must be conceded, however, that in some patients, especially children, it is virtually impossible even with biopsy to distinguish a chronic polymyositis from a rapidly advancing dystrophy.

A few patients with poly- or dermatomyositis and malignancy will exhibit signs of one of the other paraneoplastic syndromes (polyneuritis, subacute cerebellar degeneration, combined system disease, or multifocal leukoencephalopathy). A peculiar type of inverse myasthenia has also been reported, especially with small-cell carcinomas of the lung (oat cell, squamous cell). A sense of stiffness and pain on motion in these latter patients may be mistaken for rheumatoid arthritis.

The painful varieties of the polymyositis must be separated from early connective tissue disease. If the latter is not established, it may be impossible to reach a correct diagnosis even after all the laboratory data have been obtained. Such patients may be classified as hysteric,

neurotic, or depressed or may be suspected of having some metabolic disease.

Trichinosis may be confused with idiopathic polymyositis, especially if the history of pork ingestion is not obtained. The high eosinophil counts in the blood, the relatively slight weakness of limbs, the conjunctival edema, the ocular and lingual weakness, the symptoms of cerebral involvement (hemiplegia, aphasia, coma, etc.), the positive skin reaction to trichinae antigen, and the muscle biopsy establish the diagnosis in most cases.

TREATMENT. The various measures which have been suggested are of uncertain value. Our most gratifying results have been obtained by a program which consists of (1) prednisone, 40 to 60 mg per day for a month, gradual reduction in steps of 5 mg, and finally 1 mg every week over the period of a year; (2) acetylsalicyclic acid 2.9 Gm every 4 hr except during the night (blood levels of 20 to 30 mg per 100 ml); and (3) physiotherapy—gentle massage, passive movement, and then "resistance exercises" as the evidences of activity (elevated sedimentation rate and high serum enzyme values) subside. Vitamin E or alpha-tocopherol has been used with doubtful benefit. Oral penicillin should be taken most of the year (200,000 units twice a day) to prevent streptococcal infections.

Elderly patients in particular should be reexamined every few weeks for malignancy. If found, it should be excised, if possible, or treated by x-ray or chemical agents. The muscle weakness may disappear if the tumor is eradicated. Response to corticosteroids may occur in patients with polymyositis associated with tumor.

PROGNOSIS. Only a few of the patients will die, usually with some pulmonary, renal, or cardiac complication. The majority improve upon therapy, and in fact, the muscle weakness may lessen even in those patients with an advancing malignancy. A few patients recover completely, but more often some weakness of the shoulders and hips, usually not disabling, remains at the conclusion of treatment. Relapse may occur at any time up to 1 to 15 years or more. Corticosteroids should not be discontinued too soon, for the relapse which may follow is more difficult to treat than the original symptoms of the disease. Acetylsalicylic acid and penicillin may possibly reduce the likelihood of the relapse.

Sarcoid Polymyopathy. In the medical literature there are some 25 or so cases of a subacutely progressive polymyositis involving proximal limb and trunk muscles, in which biopsy has demonstrated a noncaseating granulomatous involvement of muscle. In all other respects the patients are indistinguishable from those with the idiopathic polymyositis described above. Most of them have not shown many of the other characteristic manifestations of sarcoid (see Chap. 254), and it is only proper to inquire as to whether the finding of a few Langhans'-type giant cells in the muscle is a sufficient basis for the diagnosis of sarcoid. The writers are skeptical of this entity, but the problem is presently unresolved. Response to cortocosteroid therapy is not different from that of idiopathic polymyositis.

Polymyopathy with Hypokalemic Periodic Paralysis. A rare complication of *familial periodic paralysis* (see Chap.

377) takes the form of a subacute or chronic persistent weakness of thigh and pelvic musculature. Onset may be in middle adult years, long after a troublesome adolescent periodic paralysis has ameliorated or ceased altogether. Biopsy reveals the extreme degrees of vacuolization and hydropia so characteristic of this form of periodic paralysis, and muscle fiber degeneration may be consequent to it. Slight increase in muscle enzymes in serum and a myopathic EMG substantiate the diagnosis already indicated by the sequence of clinical events. Administration of potassium (4.0 to 5.0 Gm orally per day), which alleviates or suppresses the periodic paralysis may be beneficial.

METABOLIC DISEASES OF MUSCLE

The boundaries of this category of disease cannot be sharply drawn at this time. With advance in knowledge it is probable that many diseases presently classified as degenerative, and possibly some labeled as polymyositic, will be linked to specific defects in enzymes within the muscle cells. Limitations in space permit the description of only a few representative forms of the better known metabolic myopathies.

Thyroid Myopathies

During the past two decades several myopathic diseases related to alterations in thyroid function have been recognized. These are (1) chronic thyrotoxic myopathy, (2) exophthalmic ophthalmoplegia (infiltrative ophthalmopathy), (3) myasthenia gravis associated with toxic diffuse goiter or with hypothyroidism, (4) periodic paralysis associated with toxic diffuse goiter, and (5) muscle hypertrophy and slow muscle contraction and relaxation associated with myxedema and cretinism. Although not frequent, several examples of each of these diseases may be seen in a single year in any large general hospital.

Chronic thyrotoxic myopathy is a disease characterized by progressive weakness and atrophy of skeletal musculature, occurring in conjunction with overt or covert (masked) hyperthyroidism. The muscular disorder may reach proportions such as to suggest progressive muscular atrophy (motor system disease). It is estimated that the middle-aged patient is most likely to suffer from this complication of hyperthyroidism and that men are more susceptible than women. The onset is insidious, the weakness progresses over weeks and months, and exophthalmos need not be present. The pelvic girdle and thigh muscles are weakened more than others (Basedow's paraplegia), though all are affected to some extent, even bulbar and rarely ocular muscles. However, the shoulder and hand muscles are the ones which show the most conspicuous atrophy. Tremor and coarse twitching during contraction may occur, but the authors have not seen fasciculations at rest or true fibrillations (in the electromyogram). The tendon reflexes are normal or lively. Creatine excretion in the urine is increased, and tolerance to ingested creatine diminished, but the degree of it has not correlated with the degree of weakness. Serum enzyme levels are not elevated. Electromyograms have disclosed no definite abnormality, and biopsies of muscle, except for slight volumetric reduction in fibers, have been normal. Injections of neostigmine have no effect. Muscle power and bulk are gradually restored when thyroid function is reduced to normal levels.

Exophthalmic ophthalmoplegia is a weakness of external ocular muscles (pupillary and ciliary muscles are always spared) which is conjoined with exophthalmos in Graves' disease. The exophthalmos varies in degree, being sometimes absent at an early age of the disease, and is not in itself responsible for the weakness. Both the ocular weakness and exophthalmos may precede the hyperthyroidism or follow the effective treatment of it. The ocular palsy may occasionally be unilateral, especially in the beginning. Many of the fibers of the eye muscles in biopsies and in autopsy material have degenerated, and infiltrations of lymphocytes, mononuclear leukocytes, and lipocytes are present; hence the term *infiltrative ophthalmopathy*. All external eye muscles may be affected, often one more than others, accounting for strabismus and diplopia; upward movements are usually limited to the greatest degree. Prostigmine has no effect. The condition often runs a self-limited course like the exophthalmos itself, and therapy is difficult to evaluate. Certainly the maintenance of a euthyroid state is desirable (see Chap. 89 for treatment of hyperthyroidism). If the exophthalmos reaches a degree which threatens injury of the cornea, the operation of unroofing the orbits, introduced by Naffziger, is indicated.

In patients with marked periorbital and conjunctival edema high dose corticosteroids (about 80 mg prednisone per day) may give partial control of the ophthalmic problem including the extraocular muscle weakness. Because of the toxicity of the corticoid, it should be reserved for patients who would otherwise require surgical intervention. However, in a number of patients it has been possible to carry them over the crisis and avoid the trauma and risks of surgery.

Thyrotoxic periodic paralysis resembles the familial periodic paralysis (described below) and consists of attacks of mild to severe weakness of limb and trunk muscles, usually with sparing of those of the cranium, which develops in a few minutes or hours and lasts part of a day or longer. In some series as many as half of the cases of periodic paralysis have been in individuals who suffered from hyperthyroidism. Unlike what has been found in typical hypokalemic periodic paralysis, a family history is not obtained. In most cases the serum potassium levels have been low during the attacks and the administration of several grams of KCl has terminated the attack. Treatment of the hyperthyroidism abolishes the symptomatic manifestations of the muscular disorder.

Myasthenia gravis in typical neostigmine-responsive form may accompany hyper- or hypothyroidism. In hyperthyroidism the typical weakness and poorly sustained contraction of the aforementioned chronic thyrotoxic myopathy are added to the myasthenia, without appearing to affect the response to or requirement for neostigmine. In contrast, hypothyroidism, even of mild degrees, seems to aggravate the myasthenia gravis, greatly increasing the need for neostigmine and at times inducing a myasthenic crisis. Thyroxin is beneficial and, with respect to myasthenia, restores the patient to his status before the onset of the thyroid insufficiency. However, the myasthenia gravis (described in Chap. 377) is independent of thyroid disease. Each disease must be treated separately.

Hypothyroidism, whether in the form of myxedema or cretinism, is often accompanied by a series of changes in skeletal muscle consisting of increased volume, stiffness, and slowness of contraction. Action myospasm and percussion myoedema along with the slowness of tendon reflexes assist the examiner in making a bedside diagnosis (see Chap. 89). These changes probably account for the large tongue and typical dysarthria of this disease. The clinical syndrome simulates hypertrophia musculorum vera and myotonia congenita. Cretinism manifesting these muscle symptoms is known as *Debré-Semelaigne syndrome,* and myxedema with a similar muscle picture is called *Hoffmann's syndrome.* In neither of these two syndromes is there real evidence of myotonia by either clinical test or electromyogram, and muscle biopsies have revealed only large fibers. In the rare condition where myotonia and hypothyroidism coexist, the myotonia appears to be accentuated by the hypothyroidism. Creatinine excretion is reduced, creatine tolerance is increased, and transaminase values in the serum are normal. The administration of thyroxin corrects the abnormality of muscle.

The effect of thyroid secretion on the muscle fiber in all these myopathies is still a matter of conjecture. Clinical data indicate that this hormone influences in some manner the contractile process without interfering in any way with the transmission of impulses in the peripheral nerves or across the myoneural junctions. In hyperthyroidism this functional disorder enhances the speed of the contractile process and reduces its duration, the net effect being a weakening, an excess fatigability, and a loss of endurance in muscle action. In hypothyroidism the converse of these changes occurs.

The thyroid hormone also acts on the central nervous system, and in some syndromes such as myxedema and the acute toxic encephalopathy and myopathy of hyperthyroidism it is possible to observe the effects of both a neurologic and a muscular disorder.

Alcoholic Polymyopathy with Cardiopathy

Occasionally in alcoholics during a severe drinking bout one observes the rapid development of universal muscle weakness over a period of a few days. At the onset muscle pain and cramps are common. It may reach such proportions as to render the patient bedfast, and biopsy reveals extensive segmental necrosis of sarcoplasm. All the limb and trunk muscles may be affected; there is no record of it extending to ocular and other cranial muscles. Myonecrosis is reflected by high levels of muscle enzymes. Myoglobin may appear in the urine, leading to renal failure. Signs of cardiac enlargement and decompensation accompany the polymyopathy in some instances. Most patients recover within a few weeks, but relapse in another spree of drinking has been noted. Restoration of motor power is attendant upon regeneration but may be complicated by polyneuropathy in other syndromes of neuromuscular disability associated with alcoholism.

First observed in Swedish alcoholics, this condition has appeared in American clinics; and Perkoff and his associates find some evidence that it is due to a transient suppression of myophosphorylase during bouts of alcoholism. It is too frequent (in milder degrees) to represent an inborn error of metabolism. Some cases formerly described as beriberi cardiopathy may fall in this group.

Cortisone Myopathy

The widespread use of adrenal corticosteroids in recent years has brought to light a new muscle disease, probably not dissimilar to that which has been noted in rabbits receiving cortisone. The proximal limb and girdle musculature becomes extremely weak, to the point where it is difficult to elevate the arms and to arise from a sitting, squatting, or kneeling position, and walking itself may be hampered. The electromyogram shows the myopathic pattern of small but abundant action potentials and also fibrillations; in biopsies there is evidence of scattered atrophic and a few degenerating and regenerating muscle fibers without infiltrates of inflammatory cells. The serum creatine kinase and aldolase levels are raised, and there is a creatinuria. Discontinuation of corticosteroid administration leads to recovery within a few weeks. The dose levels of corticosteroid have frequently been high and sustained over a period of months, but there is only a poor correlation between total dose and severity of myopathy. Improvement upon lowering the dose has been reported. Corticosteroid preparations containing fluorine are said to have been particularly culpable, but all corticosteroids may produce the disorder. A similar myopathy occurs regularly in patients who suffer from Cushing's syndrome. The mechanism of the muscle disease is unknown.

Myopathy and Myoglobinuria

In any disease that results in rapid destruction of striated muscle fibers, myoglobin and other muscle proteins may enter the bloodstream and appear in the urine. The latter is dark red or burgundy-colored, much like the urine in hemoglobinuria. However, in hemoglobinuria the serum initially is pink because hemoglobin but not myoglobin is bound to haptoglobin. This complex is not excreted in the urine. The complex of hemoglobin-haptoglobin is removed from the blood plasma over a period of hours, and if hemolysis continues, the haptoglobin may be depleted so that hemoglobinuria is present without grossly evident hemoglobinemia. Differentiation of the two pigments in urine is difficult. There are very small differences on spectroscopic examination, but both are rapidly degraded to other compounds, such as hematin, with differing spectra. Thus great care must be taken with such procedures.

When myoglobinuria is severe, renal damage may ensue and lead to anuria. The mechanism of the renal damage is not clear; probably it is not simply a mechanical obstruction of tubules by precipitated myoglobin. Alkalinization of the urine by the ingestion of sodium bicarbonate is said to protect the kidney by preventing the formation of myoglobin casts, but it is of doubtful value, and the sodium may actually be harmful if anuria has already developed. Therapy is the same as in the anuria which follows surgical shock (see Chap. 300).

The following conditions may give rise to myoglobinuria:

1. Crush injury to a limb.
2. Strain or excessive use of muscles, especially the pretibial muscles which are confined in the tight pretibial compartment (pretibial syndrome).
3. Extensive infarction as in occlusion of the main artery of a limb or a subcutaneous infusion into the lower leg (with resultant swelling and probable ischemia).
4. Polymyositis.
5. Haff disease, which results from eating fish poisoned by toxic resinous acids derived from cellulose. This was first reported in the bay (Haff) of Königsberg, Germany.
6. Alcoholic polymyopathy.
7. Familial myoglobinuria (Meyer-Betz disease) occurs in families with or without a diffuse chronic myopathy or dystrophy. The attack of myoglobinuria may be precipitated by strenuous exertion or possibly by an infection. Weakness, stiffness, and tenderness or swelling of muscles are the principal symptoms and vary in intensity. The muscle fibers are later found in various stages of degeneration and regeneration. The degree of renal injury usually determines the outcome. No therapy is known except that of complete inactivity and measures which assist return of renal function. Some patients will be shown to have a lifelong disposition to attacks of myoglobinuria; hence physical activity must be curtailed and exertion avoided. In others there may be but a single attack with complete or nearly complete recovery. Nothing is known of the precise mechanism by which the muscle fibers are damaged, but presumably an enzymatic defect of the muscle fibers reduces the tolerance of the muscle to maximal activity (a fault in anaerobic metabolism?). It is probable that more than one disease is presently included in this category.
8. Extreme hyperthemia, especially with convulsions.

Other Metabolic Myopathies

A progressive areflexic muscular atrophy giving rise to a syndrome of infantile muscular atrophy, or slack child, has been recorded in two of the five established forms of glycogen storage disease (see Chap. 111).

A syndrome of painful muscles and generalized weakness has been reported in hypoglycemia (see Chap. 111).

In hyperparathyroidism and osteomalacia resulting from renal tubular acidosis (a form of Milkman's syndrome), muscular weakness, fatigability, atrophy, and discomfort after exercise have been noted. The tendon reflexes are normal or hyperactive.

A contracture of hamstring muscles which prevents upright stance has been found several times in patients with Addison's disease. Biopsy has revealed normal muscle tissue; the electromyogram is normal; and the tendon reflexes are retained.

A primary defect of phosphorylase has been established as the cause of another condition known as McArdle's syndrome. This is a chronic familial myopathy with weakness, stiffness, and discomfort in the muscles following exercise. Therefore it is more likely to be considered in connection with the myalgic and muscle stiffness syndromes (Chap. 378).

Central core disease, described by Shy and McGee in 1956, is a familial, nonprogressive polymyopathy which manifests itself by hypotonia and delay in locomotion in childhood and thinness and slight weakness of proximal muscles. The tendon reflexes are preserved. Muscle biopsy has shown large fibers with a conglomerate core of central fibrils which are devoid of both oxidative and phosphorylase enzymes. Recently *nemeline* or *rod body, pleoconial, megaconial,* and *myotubular polymyopathies* presenting a similar clinical picture, have been recorded by Engel and Shy.

REFERENCES

Walton, J. N. and R. D. Adams: "Polymyositis," Edinburgh and London, E. and S. Livingstone, Ltd., 1955.

376 PROGRESSIVE MUSCULAR ATROPHY AND PARALYSIS

Frank H. Tyler and
Raymond D. Adams

As intimated in the clinical classification (Chap. 373), one of the major causes of the syndrome of progressive weakness and wasting of the musculature of the limbs and trunk is muscular dystrophy. This category of disease can usually be differentiated from the familial or nonfamilial varieties of neuropathy by the pattern of the muscle involvement (usually proximal in the dystrophies and distal in most of the neuropathies), by the absence of sensory disturbances, the less severe reduction of tendon reflexes, the normal cerebrospinal fluid, the characteristic electromyogram, and the findings in a muscle biopsy. It can usually be distinguished from spinal muscular atrophy, exemplified in the adult by motor system disease and in the infant by Werdnig-Hoffmann muscular atrophy, by the proximal and symmetric pattern of muscle involvement (total lack of pattern in motor system disease and asymmetry of involvement in the muscles of forearms and hands or feet and legs), lack of coarse fasciculations, and the characteristic electromyogram and biopsy changes. These two forms of chronic muscular atrophy due to diseases of the nervous system are described in Chaps. 21 and 364 and will not be discussed further in this section.

THE MUSCULAR DYSTROPHIES

HISTORY AND TERMINOLOGY. Progressive muscular dystrophy (*dystrophia musculorum progressiva*) was described by several prominent physicians in the middle and latter half of the nineteenth century. The many names used since that time to designate types of this condition have been a source of confusion. Duchenne reported a group of young patients, mostly males, with muscular enlargement as well as atrophy; this disease has since been referred to as *pseudohypertrophic muscular dystrophy*. Leyden and Möbius called attention to a clinically similar group in which, however, muscular enlargement was lacking. Thus arose the name *simple atrophic* type. Landouzy and Déjerine described muscular dystrophy of the facial, pectoral, and shoulder girdle muscles, which they called the *facioscapulohumeral* type; and Erb reported a condition of limb-girdle dystrophy and little or no facial involvement, which he termed *juvenile dystrophy*. Recently, Walton and others have insisted on the distinction between "limb-girdle dystrophy" and facioscapulohumeral dystrophy because the former has earlier onset and lack of typical dominant inheritance as well as the lack of facial involvement. A number of other syndromes have been described, but as they are rare and, in some cases, of doubtful relationship to the more typical disorders, they will not be considered here.

It is now generally agreed that all these groups represent the end stage of more than one disease process. Clinical and genetic evidence permits the separation of at least six syndromes: Duchenne (pseudohypertrophic), facioscapulohumeral, limb-girdle, distal ocular, and myotonic dystrophy. The criteria for each group are mode of inheritance, age of onset, rate of progression, localization of initial involvement, morphologic changes, and associated dystrophy of other organs (eye, testicles, skin, brain). Nearly all patients with typical dystrophic muscle disease fit well into one of these syndromes. It should be emphasized that other much rarer types do exist, but description of their characteristics is beyond the scope of this discussion.

CAUSES AND PATHOGENESIS. The cause of muscular dystrophy is an abnormality of genes. Although in many instances a family history cannot be obtained by direct questioning, in more than 40 to 50 percent of cases other affected individuals are found on careful examination of the members of the pedigree. Other considerations lead to the conclusion that the disease may be caused either by a previously latent recessive trait or by the occurrence of a mutation. Although it is quite possible that the same clinical manifestations may occur occasionally as the result of a nongenetic mechanism, the occurrence of the genetic pattern in the majority of instances must be included in any concept of the mechanism of these disorders.

By analogy with the other known genetic disorders, it must be presumed that some abnormality in the intracellular metabolism of the muscle fibers is caused by the genetic abnormality. This could be a modified or absent enzyme system within the muscle cell or some defect in the muscle metabolism resulting from inability to absorb or to metabolize normally a substance vital to muscle function.

The occurrence of creatinuria in patients with muscular dystrophy has led to extensive study of creatine synthesis as the basis of the metabolic anomaly. Although there is some evidence of both increased synthesis and imperfect control of normal synthesis, the significance of this to the fundamental anomaly is as yet unknown. Many other metabolic systems in the muscle are under investigation or have been investigated in the past. As yet no clear-cut mechanism by which the observed chemical changes could lead to the muscular damage has been proposed.

The pattern of development of muscular atrophy is remarkably similar from one patient to another with the same type of dystrophy. Within a local group of muscles, it has been suggested that the affection bears a relationship to their order of development in the embryo; those muscles which appear earliest manifest the first and most severe weakness and atrophy. Even when one part of the muscle develops earlier than another, the atrophy follows this order. Thus, the upper fibers of the trapezius muscle form very early, at the same time as the muscles innervated by the cranial nerves. The lower fibers of the pectoral muscle are among the earliest of girdle muscles to develop; and the disease always involves the lower part of this muscle most severely. On the other hand, the variation in severity of the disease in different patients and variation in area of initial involvement in the various types make the possibility of this embryologic factor an incomplete explanation of the process. Some other differences (probably biochemical) between muscles are probably being revealed by these diseases.

As in other genetically determined metabolic disorders, it is probable that a single enzymatic abnormality underlies the entire disease process and accounts for all its manifestations, even in such a disease as myotonic dystrophy in which many systems are involved. Only continued search at the basic level of metabolic processes will lead to an understanding of the pathogenesis of these disorders.

CHILDHOOD TYPE OF DUCHENNE'S PSEUDOHYPERTROPHIC PELVIFEMORAL MUSCULAR DYSTROPHY

Although several of the different varieties of muscular dystrophy begin in infancy and childhood (myotonic dystrophy, fascioscapulohumeral dystrophy), the most frequent and dreaded form in this age period is that first described by Duchenne.

The Duchenne type has been subdivided into three distinct categories as follows: (1) severe, sex-linked recessive form; (2) mild, sex-linked recessive form; (3)

mild autosomal recessive form. These occur, according to Walton, Milhorat, and others, in a ratio of 27:3:5 respectively.

The severe sex-linked variety, which has been the most thoroughly studied, may begin in fetal life and is not infrequently (in nearly half the cases) manifest during the second and third years of life, thus interfering with the beginning of locomotion. More often such children are normal at birth and their early muscular and other development is normal. Onset after ten years of age would place the case in the second category of milder disease.

Females may transmit the disease but do not suffer from it, as a rule. The carrier female may be identified (with about 80 percent accuracy) by the creatine kinase test on serum (which is slightly elevated), muscle biopsy (slight dystrophic changes), and a slightly myopathic electromyogram.

The most frequent initial complaints relate to the early involvement of pelvifemoral muscles resulting in frequent falls, difficulty in rising from the floor or climbing stairs, awkward, peculiar gait, and inability to run properly. Muscle weakness often is not recognized initially by the family. The onset is insidious, and the course is slowly progressive over months and years. Later, shoulder girdle and trunk muscles become affected, and usually the child becomes confined to chair or bed before the age of ten years. Fatality is frequent during the second decade of life owing to obesity and kyphoscoliosis, sudden cardiac failure, and pulmonary infection.

When the patient is examined, the findings naturally vary with the stage of the disease, but early the calves and sometimes the quadriceps and deltoid muscles are unusually large and firm even though weak, i.e., pseudohypertrophy. The weakness is evidenced by a typical waddling gait (weak glutei), a curious manner of "climbing up one's legs" (weak extensors of hip and spine), and winging of scapulae on elevation of arms. The abdomen is protuberant because of weak abdominal muscles and an exaggerated lordosis is required to maintain balance. Facial muscles are entirely spared or affected late in the course of the illness. More specifically one may find weakness of the iliopsoas, quadriceps, gluteus, and anterior tibial muscles in the lower extremities and later of the serrati, pectorals, latissimi, biceps, and brachioradialis muscles in the upper extremities. The forearm and hand muscles and the gastrocnemius and foot muscles retain good power until late in the illness. Early in the disease the tendon reflexes in the arms are preserved, and even at a late stage it is usually possible to obtain ankle reflexes. The neurologic findings are otherwise within normal limits.

Cardiac involvement is commonly observed in the late stages of the disease, manifest as tachycardia and also by signs of decompensation. Prolongation of the P-R interval, slurring of the QRS complex, bundle branch block, and elevation or depression of the S-T segments are seen in the ECG. The shafts of long bones are thin (disuse atrophy). Intelligence is usually normal, though for large groups of patients with Duchenne's dystrophy it is estimated to be 10 percent below that of the general population. Mental retardation, when present, tends to be proportional to the severity of the muscular dystrophy. It is nonprogressive.

The mild sex-linked variety and the less definite autosomal recessive form differ from the above only in later age of onset, slower progression (permitting survival into adult years), and less frequent fatality.

The Leyden-Möbius pelvicrural atrophic dystrophy is probably a variety of either Duchenne's or Erb's limb-girdle dystrophy.

FACIOSCAPULOHUMERAL TYPE OF LANDOUZY-DÉJERINE

This disease is inherited as an autosomal dominant disorder with complete penetrance. This, plus the fact that affected persons are often not incapacitated during the childbearing period, accounts for the high familial incidence and also high prevalence in a community.

Facioscapulohumeral dystrophy often begins later than the Duchenne type, though we have seen mild facial weakness at two to three years of age. The average age of onset is thirteen years but ranges between nine and twenty years. A few patients even beyond fifty years of age are found on close examination to have the disorder, although they have not recognized their disability. As this implies, the degree of involvement may be extremely slight; other patients, however, are significantly incapacitated before the age of twenty.

The pattern of muscular involvement differs from that of other dystrophies, as is indicated by the name. Weakness of facial muscles is nearly always present. All the facial muscles are involved in the process, but the orbicularis oris may show a weakness which results in abnormal movements and inability to pucker the mouth or whistle normally. There are weaknesses of the orbicularis oculi and diffuse flattening of the face; and asymmetric movements, particularly about the mouth, are extremely characteristic. The diagnosis may be suspected after watching the patient's face while he gives his history. The facial weakness may be the earliest change.

Usually, however, it is weakness of the muscles of the pectoral girdle and winging of the scapulae which bring the patient to the physician. In contrast, the pelvifemoral muscles are strong and there is no pseudohypertrophy. These patients cannot raise their arms above their heads, but they frequently maintain normal strength in the forearms and hands until an advanced age.

The axial and pelvic musculature becomes involved later in the disease, and the tibial and peroneal groups may also become weak and atrophic.

The same complications and associated abnormalities as were described in childhood dystrophy will eventually occur, but there are fewer associated congenital anomalies; and heart disease due to dystrophy and severe scoliosis is extremely rare. The average patient lives out a normal life span, becoming completely incapacitated only very late in life.

LABORATORY DATA. Laboratory examinations yield no abnormalities except creatinuria, which is usually not so marked as in childhood dystrophy, and creatinine excretion is not so greatly reduced as in childhood dystrophy. Some patients, particularly those with minimal involvement, may have relatively insignificant creatinuria. The serum enzyme levels are raised only slightly if at all.

LIMB-GIRDLE DYSTROPHY OF ERB

This form of muscular dystrophy is characterized by occurrence in either sex; onset during the second and third decades of life; transmission as an autosomal recessive trait and, in rare instances, as a dominant one; primary involvement of the muscles of either the shoulder girdle or the pelvic girdle, usually with spread to the other after a variable period of time; pseudohypertrophy in calves and other muscles in only a small proportion of cases. The course of the illness is variable, but usually the rate of progression is slow, and severe disability does not occur until the disease has been present for 20 or more years. Facial muscles are spared. *Formes frustes* are known, one type being limited to the quadriceps muscles.

The purity of this entity has been much debated. It evidently overlaps clinically with the third subvariety of Duchenne's dystrophy and with Landouzy-Déjerine dystrophy. The muscles involved are essentially the same as in Duchenne's dystrophy. Cardiac impairment is rare, and the range of intelligence, like that of the Landouzy-Déjerine groups, is normal.

LABORATORY FINDINGS. These are the same as in Landouzy-Déjerine dystrophy.

DISTAL TYPE OF DSYTROPHY

Gowers and Spiller many years ago and Welander more recently have called attention to patients with slowly progressive atrophy of the muscles of the hands and feet. In these patients muscle biopsy has shown the characteristic lesions of muscular dystrophy. The disorder apparently begins in middle adult life (average age, forty-seven years) and is slowly progressive but produces only moderate disability. Welander was able to show the existence of an autosomal dominant transmission of the trait in some of the families which she studied. The disorder must be unusual, for the authors have observed only two such patients in Boston and Salt Lake City over a period of years. It should be noted that the cardinal manifestation of this disorder, i.e., atrophy and weakness of the lower leg and hand muscles, is characteristic of peroneal muscular atrophy. This latter disease is also a genetically determined disorder of autosomal dominant inheritance in which the patients usually develop more severe atrophy and weakness with minimal sensory loss in the lower leg, the forearm, and hand, in contrast to the distal type of dystrophy. This and other

features of neuropathy, such as delayed conduction velocity of peripheral nerves, prove to be useful in differential diagnosis.

Biemond and more recently Magee and DeJong have observed a distal form of dystrophy in children.

MYOTONIC DYSTROPHY

DEFINITION. Myotonic dystrophy (myotonia dystrophica, myotonia atrophica, Steinert's disease) is a hereditary disease characterized by myotonia, muscular wasting of a characteristic pattern, cataracts, testicular atrophy, and frontal baldness.

CLINICAL PATTERN. The myotonia in the early years may be more prominent than the other manifestations. Although the disease usually begins in early adult life it may be observed in infancy and childhood. Myotonia, as was stated in Chap. 373, consists of an inability to relax a muscle normally after its contraction and is the result of repetitive discharge of the contractile mechanism of the fiber. It is a symptom which may be seen in an occasional patient with any of several other neuromuscular disorders. Most characteristically it is demonstrable in the adductors of the thumb, forearm muscles, and tongue. The patient's inability to let go after shaking hands may give the clue to the proper diagnosis. This difficulty tends to disappear after repetitive motion. Idiomuscular contractions elicited by direct percussion of the muscle are also delayed in relaxation. This latter sign (percussion myotonia) may be present when the grasp response and other clinical evidence of myotonia are not found. The muscular atrophy which develops is in some respects similar to that in the diseases described above. A different type of facial involvement occurs, however. In general the patient exhibits a rather dull, expressionless facies, with ptosis of the eyelids due to weakness of levator muscles. The forehead is furrowed as a compensatory effort on the part of the frontalis muscle to overcome the ptosis. The latter may become so severe that the patient must tip his head back to see straight ahead. Closure of the eyes (orbicularis oculi) is also weak, a combination with ptosis which is invariably myopathic. The "dystrophic" facial movements of the facioscapulohumeral dystrophy do not occur. The voice becomes nasal and expressionless. Atrophy of the temporalis muscles is usually severe. Atrophy of the sternocleidomastoids is disproportionately marked; the other muscles of the anterior part of the neck may be so atrophic that the trachea is seen immediately beneath the skin. Extreme difficulty in flexing the neck, with moderately strong extension, is explained by the preservation of the spinalis group of muscles. The long flexors and extensors of the fingers are involved. In the lower extremities the weakness begins in the anterior tibial group but soon spreads to the peronei and gastrocnemii and later to the quadriceps and hamstrings. The tendon reflexes are reduced, and contractures may occur late in the illness.

These patients, whether male or female, also develop progressive *alopecia*, usually frontal, at an early age.

Testicular atrophy with androgenic deficiency usually develops in males. The latter are frequently sterile and sometimes impotent. In some patients, gynecomastia and elevated gonadotropin excretion are found. Testicular biopsy may show peritubular fibrosis. Thus, all the clinical characteristics of Klinefelter's syndrome may be present. However, the nuclei of skin or bone marrow cells only rarely have been shown to have "sex chromatin mass" (one individual with myotonic dystrophy has had a sex chromosome complement of XXY); and the majority of patients are of the usual male XY sex chromosome constitution. Ovarian deficiency occasionally develops in females. This is seldom severe enough to interfere with the menstrual pattern or fertility. The lens opacities of myotonic dystrophy are of two types. The first consists of fine dustlike subcapsular deposits which frequently appear scintillating and colored under the slit lamp but often cannot be seen with the ordinary ophthalmoscope. This type of opacity is virtually always present in patients with other signs of the disorder. Its appearance is so characteristic as to be virtually diagnostic. The second type of cataract is like the usual senile cataract and seldom appears except in elderly patients, being of little diagnostic usefulness. *Blepharoconjunctivitis* is an extremely common finding, even in patients with little weakness of facial muscles, and is universal in advanced cases. The disease affects the gastrointestinal tract, causing in particular weakness and dilatation of the esophagus.

Neurologic examination reveals no sensory or other motor abnormalities. Mental retardation is a common finding in these patients or in their siblings. The brain weight in such cases is reduced below normal levels by more than 200 Gm, and there is an abnormality of cortical lamination. *Dystrophic heart disease* is also a frequent aspect, as it is in childhood dystrophy (contrasting with the facioscapulohumeral type), but because it usually occurs at an advanced age and presents no specific features, it is difficult to differentiate from other types of heart disease common in elderly persons.

Among all the dystrophies the myotonic variety is the most variable. Rarely a patient may exhibit only one of the features, such as myotonia or the characteristic cataracts; and in many cases one or more of the dystrophic features may be missing. Nonetheless diagnosis is seldom difficult on physical examination alone if care is taken to look for the features described. The diagnosis is obvious in patients who have significant disability from their myotonic dystrophy.

Two rare but distinct diseases are closely related to myotonic dystrophica and need mention in order that they may not be confused with it: *myotonia congenita* (*Thomsen's disease*), a familial disorder of dominant inheritance in which there is lifelong myotonia, which is most severe following rest, excitement, or anxiety, but without the other manifestations of myotonia dystrophica; and *paramyotonia congenita*, an even rarer disorder, in which myotonia along with episodic weakness occurs only following exposure to cold. The latter is also familial, of dominant inheritance, of lifelong duration, and benign in character. It is genetically separate from both the other myotonias. Both these disorders respond to quinine, as described below.

Myotonia dystrophica is inherited as a typical mendelian dominant trait, but certain members of a given line may manifest only one or two of the usual group of findings. Myotonia is the most common finding on physical examination, while cataracts are often mentioned in family histories. Care must be used, however, in the evaluation of this evidence, because cataracts of other etiology may occur in the nondystrophic line and lead to confusion. Search by history and examination for other features of the syndrome in individuals with cataract will usually prevent such errors.

Routine laboratory data are of no aid in making the diagnosis. Creatinuria is irregular and frequently absent. The characteristic afterpotentials of myotonia can be demonstrated electromyographically and may be useful where clinical demonstration of myotonia is difficult. In addition, the electromyogram shows the usual myopathic pattern of many low-voltage, brief action potentials of myopathy.

Jequier has reported hyperostosis frontalis interna. The sella turcica is often small. The 17-ketosteroid levels in urine are low.

RESTRICTED DYSTROPHIES

Progressive Ophthalmoplegia and Oculopharyngeal Dystrophy

Isolated dystrophic involvement of the extraocular muscles is another relatively rare form of muscle dystrophy. The disorder usually appears in adult life and must be differentiated from other causes of ophthalmoplegia. A progressive external ophthalmoplegia (sparing of pupils and muscles of accommodation), ptosis, and sometimes weakness of orbicularis oculi, extending over a period of years, represent the typical clinical syndrome. Isolated involvement of other cranial or spinal muscles may be conjoined. Affection of eye muscles is a relatively uncommon feature of the other forms of muscular dystrophy. Similarity of the histologic findings on biopsy to other varieties of dystrophy has been the means of establishing the myopathic character of this disorder.

Hayes, Adams, and Victor have observed several patients with a progressive dysphagia developing in late life (beyond fifty years of age). The disease appeared to be inherited as a mendelian dominant trait. Each individual complained of increasing difficulty in swallowing and inanition. Temporal atrophy and ptosis were seen in some individuals. Biopsy of temporal muscles and electromyograms were compatible with muscular dystrophy, not with denervation as E. W. Taylor had previously supposed.

LABORATORY DATA. Apart from the ECG abnormalities already mentioned, the electrical reactions of skeletal muscle are reduced and the EMG exhibits the characteristic pattern of low voltage and brief action potentials. Excretion of creatine in the urine is increased, and that of creatinine is decreased. Levels of transaminases, aldolase, and creatine kinase are elevated in the serum. The creatine kinase, the most sensitive and specific of these tests, may be raised (>4.0 or, by the new standard, 50 units) even before the disease is recognized clinically, and it is also slightly elevated in the normal female carriers of this trait.

PATHOLOGY OF THE MUSCULAR DYSTROPHIES

The atrophic muscles appear white or fatty, a change frequently described as "fish flesh," and the diagnosis may be suspected from the gross appearance. Microscopically, probably the most important change is necrosis of single fibers. Some of the remaining ones are enlarged, and many others are atrophic; the sarcolemmal nuclei are increased in number, forming chains and appearing centrally in the fibers. Other fibers within a microscopic field may appear entirely normal. The distribution of involved muscle fibers is entirely random, quite unlike the pattern of "group atrophy" of spinal and neural atrophic diseases. The damaged and atrophic fibers ultimately disappear and are progressively replaced by fibrous tissue and fat cells.

The lesions are similar in all types of dystrophy. Myotonic dystrophy differs in that there are spiral annulets of myofibrils, zones of sarcoplasm free of myofibrils, and unusually prominent "rowing" of nuclei in addition to the usual dystrophic changes. In the very advanced cases, in which all muscle fibers have disappeared, it may be difficult to recognize the tissue as muscle. The peripheral nervous system and spinal cord are unchanged, although in the late stages of the disease there may be a secondary loss of nerve cells and fibers.

Other biochemical studies have been undertaken, but the significance of the results is uncertain. To summarize, there is a lowering of the intramuscular enzymes involved in the glycolytic systems (with the exception of hexokinase and lactic dehydrogenase); normal oxidative enzymes and metabolism (cytochrome oxidases succinoxidase, succinic dehydrogenase remain proportional to residual muscle substance); diminished total body potassium, but always in proportion to residual muscle mass; increased excretion of all amino acids in urine; change of myoglobin pattern, especially in Duchenne's dystrophy, to a fetal type (probably a regenerative phenomenon). None of these changes is specifically related to the dystrophic process.

Under the electron microscope the earliest changes are fragmentation and dissolution of myofilaments, together with abnormalities in the structure and organization of endoplasmic reticulum and mitochondria. In myotonic dystrophy myofilamentous loss tends to be subsarcolemmal, with nuclear increase.

TREATMENT OF THE MUSCULAR DYSTROPHIES

There is no treatment for any of the dystrophies of muscle, and the physician is forced to stand helplessly and witness the spectacle of unrelenting progressive paralysis. The various preparations recently recommended such as vitamin E, inositol, anabolic steroids, amino acid and protein supplements to diet, and most recently, Levadosin and digitalis preparations have not yet been shown to have beneficial effect.

Quinine has a mild curarelike action at the motor endplate and thus relieves the myotonia. Although symptomatic relief of the myotonia is usually achieved, the drug has no effect on the progress of the muscle atrophy or other degenerative aspects of the disease. The usual dose is 0.3 to 0.6 Gm orally, repeated as needed about every 6 hr. Mild toxic symptoms such as tinnitus may develop before enough quinine has been given to obtain satisfactory relief of the myotonia. Some patients find the side effects more distressing than the myotonia and prefer not to take quinine except on special occasions when the myotonia is troublesome in a particular activity. Procaine amide and diphenylhydantoin are also effective but only occasionally useful.

Surgical management of the cataracts when they are mature is indicated.

Androgens may be administered and provide symptomatic benefit when deficiency is apparent, but a relation of the hormone to the pathogenesis of the disease is not established.

Two factors are of importance in the management of these patients—avoidance of prolonged bed rest and inactivity, and encouragement of the patient to maintain as full and normal a life as possible. These measures help to prevent the rapid worsening associated with inactivity and to conserve a healthy attitude of mind. Obesity should be avoided; this may require careful attention to diet.

CHRONIC, SLOWLY PROGRESSIVE, OR RELATIVELY STATIONARY MYOPATHIES (OTHER THAN MUSCULAR DYSTROPHY)

Central core myopathy (Shy and Magee); nemeline myopathy (Engel and Shy); pleoconial, megaconial, and myotubular polymyopathies; McArdle's phosphorylase deficiency; some cases of familial periodic paralysis; and familial paroxysmal myoglobinuria are examples of diseases in which a congenital thinning and weakness of muscles progresses slowly over a long period of time. Many of the children have been categorized as floppy or hypotonic. In each instance the basic pathologic process induces a distinctive alteration (disfiguration) of the muscle fibers and the increasing weakness is due to a mild necrobiosis of individual muscle fibers, leading ultimately to their disappearance. Diagnosis, as a rule, depends on some other attribute, either clinical or pathologic or an associated episodic disorder of function. If the latter, the disease must be considered in another context, as indicated in the clinical classification in Chap. 373.

Central core disease and nemeline myopathy are rare familial affections of muscle beginning in childhood. In the former, each striated muscle fiber is marked by a core of hyaline appearance; in the latter, myriads of rod-like structures resembling bacilli collect in aggregates beneath the sarcolemma. In both diseases thinness of proximal limb and trunk muscles imparts a myopathic aspect to the patient's bodily configuration. Progression of the disease is so slow that in childhood it is more than counterbalanced by the natural growth and development of the musculature. In pleoconial and megaconial myopathy, these fibers are observed to contain unusually large or altered mitochondria or central tubes. Diagnosis depends on biopsy.

Paroxysmal (familial) myoglobinuria, McArdle's disease, and familial periodic paralysis are described in Chaps. 375 and 377. In most patients muscular power and bulk are preserved between attacks of myoglobinuria, contracture, or weakness; however, if the attacks are frequent and severe, necrosis of muscle fibers will occur and result in a gradual loss of fibers (numerical reduction).

REFERENCES

Tyler, F. H., and F. E. Stephens: Studies in Disorders of Muscle: II. Clinical Manifestations and Inheritance in Facioscapulohumeral Dystrophy in a Large Family, Ann. Intern. Med., 32:640, 1950.

Walton, J. N.: "Disorders of Voluntary Muscle," 2d ed., Boston, Little, Brown and Company, 1969.

—— and F. J. Nattrass: On the Classification, Natural History and Treatment of the Myopathies, Brain, 77:169, 1954.

377 EPISODIC MUSCULAR WEAKNESS

Raymond D. Adams

Characteristic of most of the muscular diseases included in this chapter is the episodic nature of the weakness, the patient being normal or only slightly weak between attacks, and the evident disorder of neuromuscular transmission or of muscle membrane excitability (see Chap. 374).

The diseases listed under Episodic Weakness in the classification in Chap. 373 should be considered when a patient with an apparently intact nervous system and relatively normal-appearing muscles complains of episodic or fluctuating weakness or paralysis.

In myasthenia gravis and thyrotoxic myopathy with myasthenia or periodic paralysis, some degree of weakness is persistent at all times but is made worse by activity. Exhaustion and fatigability with drug intoxication (organophosphates, phenothiazine drugs, barbiturates, and bromides), neurasthenia, depression, and other states of excess fatigability can be separated as a rule on clinical grounds (see Chap. 20).

MYASTHENIA GRAVIS

DEFINITION. The disease, first described in 1672 by Thomas Willis and later by Goldflam and Jolly, is characterized by weakness and easy fatigability; it most frequently affects the facial, oculomotor, laryngeal, pharyngeal, and respiratory muscles. Partial recovery with rest and after the administration of anticholinesterase drugs is often an important feature.

CLINICAL PATTERN. Myasthenia gravis occurs at all ages and in both sexes, but females are affected twice as often as males. The period of highest incidence is in the third decade of life. No significant familial occurrence has been noted.

The onset may be insidious, but is often subacute and rarely acute, being precipitated by infection or emotional upset. Weakness of ocular muscles with drooping of the eyelids, which may be unilateral at first, occurs in 90 percent of cases. Diplopia due to unequal weakness of the ocular muscles is usually the first symptom; it is often transient and intermittent, but may persist and at times causes complete paresis of ocular movement. The pupils are never affected. Facial and pharyngeal muscles are weakened in 70 percent of cases. The facial involvement gives rise to a smooth, relatively immobile facies. The smile has an unnatural appearance in that the lips elevate but do not retract; it resembles a snarl. The tongue may be weak and is bilaterally furrowed, the so-called "trident tongue."

Weakness of the laryngeal and pharyngeal muscles may be the initial symptom in a smaller number of patients. Choking and aspiration of food are then common and obvious symptoms. As a result of paresis of palatal muscles, fluids may be regurgitated through the nose when swallowing is attempted. The involvement of tongue, laryngeal, and facial muscles results in abnormal speech of a rather feeble "mushy" type, and the voice has a nasal quality; if the patient continues to talk for a short time, the abnormality becomes more severe to the point where speech becomes unintelligible. This is in striking contrast to the psychoneurotic patient, who also complains of weakness but can talk interminably without change in voice or enunciation. Affection of masseter muscles may prevent closure of the mouth, and the patient habitually holds his hand under his jaw.

A generalized weakness of skeletal muscles is also present in advanced cases of myasthenia gravis but seldom occurs in the absence of involvement of muscles innervated by cranial nerves. As in other myopathies, the proximal or girdle muscles, especially those of the shoulder girdle, are most severely affected. In the most advanced or severe stages, weakness may be universal.

Easy fatigability and relatively prompt, partial recovery after rest are quite typical, and a history of this phenomenon can be elicited in most cases. Also it may be characteristically demonstrated by having the patient perform a repetitive long-sustained motion with an involved muscle or group of muscles. As the disease process becomes more severe and of longer duration, the weakness also tends to be more extensive. There are no other neurologic abnormalities in the average patient.

The disease may be aggravated to a variable extent by a number of factors. The most frequent of these are infections of the upper part of the respiratory tract, excitement, general fatigue, loss of sleep, menstruation, high carbohydrate meals, and the intake of alcohol. Medications which increase the neural and muscular block, such as curare, quinine, and quarternary ammonium compounds and hypothyroidism may add to the myasthenia, resulting in more severe paralysis, and should be avoided or treated.

Muscular atrophy is not seen in the great majority of patients but may be present, particularly if the process has been of long duration. It is most frequently seen in a few muscles, such as the temporal masseter, cervical, and proximal shoulder girdle muscles. Exceptionally a degenerating process in one muscle or a few muscles accounts for weakness. The tendon reflexes are preserved even with severe myasthenia. Stiffness and paresthesias of face or hands are frequent complaints, but usually there is no evidence of sensory impairment. The external vesical and anal sphincters may be weakened, with stress incontinence.

Approximately 8 to 10 percent of myasthenic patients have a small-celled tumor of the thymus gland. Macrocytic anemia has been reported in a few patients. Thyrotoxicosis, polymyositis, rheumatoid arthritis, and lupus erythematosus may occur in conjunction with myasthenia gravis, and there is a special variety which accompanies malignant tumors.

The illness usually develops over a few weeks (exceptionally in a few days); it may advance irregularly or remain at the same level of severity for a long time. Remissions, partial or complete, occur in about half the patients, usually in the first few years. There may also be relapses, completely unpredictable as to time of occurrence or severity, and they usually reproduce the initial syndrome.

The life of the patient with severe myasthenia is endangered by progression of paralysis. Fatality most frequently occurs in the first year of the disease and again in the period between the fourth and seventh years. If the disease has been present for 10 years or more, it usually remains benign. Respiratory infections are a threat and should be treated by appropriate sulfonamides and antibiotics. Some female patients have a reduced fertility, but pregnancy does occur and may be followed by a normal delivery. Remissions and occasionally relapses have accompanied pregnancy. The offspring may exhibit a mild or severe *myasthenia* at birth which may threaten their lives. This type of neonatal myasthenia lasts only a few weeks, and spontaneous recovery is the rule. Later in childhood the usual variety of myasthenia may develop.

Respiratory insufficiency may come on quite abruptly or may be insidiously progressive. This is the complication that commonly terminates life. Fatal accessions of profound weakness may be evoked by an overdose of neostigmine.

PATHOLOGY. Collections of small round cells, presumably lymphocytes, are seen among the muscle fibers and around the small blood vessels in a majority of cases. Other organs may also show similar cellular infiltrations. Single muscle fibers or groups of fibers in a state of degeneration have been found in a few muscles in about half the fatal cases. There is no lack of acetylcholine or cholinesterase at myoneural junctions in histochemical stains, but two groups of investigators have noted that the motor end-plates are abnormally thin and unbranched. The latter have been examined under the electron microscope by Zacks, who observed a patchy decrease in electron density of the muscle membrane within the end-plate zone. The thymic tumors have been of both lymphoblastic and epithelial types. They are more frequent in elderly patients. The tumor, whether called benign or malignant, remains confined to the mediastinum. In the nontumor cases, the thymus shows hyperplasia of lymph follicles, according to Castleman and Norris.

PATHOGENESIS. The disease is believed to be the result of a specific functional abnormality at the *neuromyal junction*. Normally, acetylcholine, released at this junction, facilitates the passage of impulses across from nerve terminals to the muscle fiber. Cholinesterase is normally present and hydrolyzes the acetylcholine; physostigmine and neostigmine antagonize cholinesterase. The block in neuromuscular transmission is evidenced in the electromyogram (Chap. 374) as a progressive decline in the voltage of action potentials. The exact nature of the block has eluded all investigators. It is not corrected by acetylcholine given intrarterially. Curare, quinine, or the quarternary ammonium compounds, which normally impair transmission across the neuromyal junction or over the surface of the muscle fiber, act in unusually small dosages to enhance the weakness in myasthenic patients. A circulating curarelike factor has never been demonstrated in the blood, and exchange transfusions of blood from normal patients have been of no value. A faulty catabolism of acetylcholine has also been postulated.

Recently antinuclear, anti-end-plate, and antimuscle antibodies have been demonstrated in some cases, and the possibility has been suggested that one of these antibodies inhibits the action of either acetylcholine or cholinesterase, more likely the latter, at receptor sites on the muscle fibers.

DIAGNOSIS. The diagnosis usually is made without difficulty if one carefully evaluates the history and thinks of the disease. The characteristic pattern of *myasthenic fatigability* is easy to demonstrate by having the patient make some repetitive or sustained movement, such as looking up toward the ceiling for 2 to 3 min. The eyelids progressively droop until they cover the iris. Strength returns to the levator palpebrae muscles after a few minutes of rest. Intramuscular injection of 0.5 to 2.0 mg neostigmine usually results in prompt relief of the muscular weakness, which is evident both to the patient and to the physician. When the larger doses of neostigmine are used, it is important to administer about 1 mg atropine prior to the neostigmine in order to minimize the parasympathomimetic effects of the neostigmine. Many times a patient who is unable to sit up, speak, or swallow will in the course of 5 to 15 min after neostigmine administration regain strength in a dramatic fashion. Occasionally patients with localized ocular palsies do not respond promptly to neostigmine, but then the effect is nearly always obvious in other groups of muscles. Edrophonium chloride (Tensilon) is very similar in its action to neostigmine. For diagnostic testing it has the advantage that the response to an intravenous injection is always instantaneous and the action is dissipated within a few minutes. The usual dose is 10 mg. Also, severe side reactions are uncommon, making it unnecessary to administer atropine except in patients with asthma or cardiac disease. Although the short duration of action of this drug makes it unsatisfactory for maintenance therapy, in a myasthenic crisis it may be given by continuous intravenous drip. Another use is to determine if the weakness which develops in a myasthenic patient on neostigmine or similar therapy is the result of an exacerbation of the myasthenia gravis or of overtreatment with neostigmine or related compounds, which of themselves may cause weakness. If the weakness is due to the latter, 5 or 10 mg edrophonium administered intravenously, briefly worsens the patient's condition. If, on the other hand, improvement ensues, higher doses of neostigmine or other longer-acting agent can be given safely. Curare must be used cautiously in patients with myasthenia and should be limited to the unusual circumstance in which the diagnosis seems improbable but needs to be more effectively ruled out (see Chap. 374). The weakness of thyrotoxic myopathy and motor system disease and the tiredness of neurasthenia which are sometimes confused with myasthenia gravis do not show the fluctuations of myasthenia gravis nor respond to neostigmine. Such patients develop large numbers of fasciculations after neostigmine, as do many normal persons. In thyrotoxicosis, however, a typical myasthenia may occur and be added to the thyroid myopathy, and, as was stated above, hypothyroidism, if present, actually enhances myasthenic weakness (see Chap. 89).

TREATMENT. The management of these patients is divided into two parts: the treatment of acute episodes of severe paralysis and the long-term management. Neostigmine is by far the most useful drug during acute attacks and should be given parenterally in doses of 1 mg and in multiples of this amount until the desired degree of improvement has been attained. The side reactions are gastrointestinal and uterine cramps, which may be partially controlled by the simultaneous administration of atropine.

Other problems which must be taken care of during the acute episode are to protect the patient from hypostatic pneumonia and other infections and to watch for impaired respiratory exchange with resulting cyanosis and respiratory acidosis due to failure of respiratory excretion of normal amounts of carbon dioxide. At times a respirator for maintaining respiratory exchange may be lifesaving. If these complications are prevented, most patients experience a remission after a few weeks or months. Some recover completely. Others, as time goes on, relapse, and a slow general trend toward increasing severity of the disease may become apparent.

Mild cases may require no special medical attention except during relapse. In the slightly more severe case, neostigmine in oral doses of 15 mg every 2 or 3 hr, or multiples of this dose, as needed, is the most useful medication and may be quite effective. Over a period of months or years, the dosage may have to be increased progressively, and the cost becomes nearly prohibitive for some families. The maximal effect of neostigmine given orally appears in half an hour and decreases rapidly after that time. If the patient becomes resistant to this medication, Mestinon bromide (60 mg is equivalent to 15 mg neostigmine) may be substituted, tablet for tablet. Mytelase chloride (5 to 7.5 mg is equivalent to 15 mg neostigmine) may also be tried, beginning always with a small dose of 5.0 mg every 2 hr and increasing to tolerance and to maximum therapeutic effect. All three of these drugs are available in syrup form (for tube feeding) and in delayed timespace tablets which have an effect for 3 to 12 hr.

Supplementing neostigmine with ephedrine (25 mg three times daily) and potassium salts (KCl, 25 percent aqueous solution in doses of 4 to 6 ml t.i.d.) may be of slight therapeutic value in certain cases particularly in relieving the weakness which occurs between doses of neostigmine. The possible usefulness of these agents must be investigated for each patient. Many anticholinesterase agents other than neostigmine have been investigated in an attempt to find an agent with more prolonged action and fewer side effects. Of these, pyridostigmine (Mestinon) is probably the best and does have a more prolonged period of activity. Ambenonium (Mysuran) is also said to be effective in some patients. The most severe and chronic forms of myasthenia gravis do not respond to any of these drugs, and the patient is forced to live a miserable existence in and out of a respirator. The mortality rate in such patients is high.

Variation in the intensity of the disease at different times makes evaluation of any type of management extremely difficult. The statement is nowhere better demonstrated than in attempting to assess the results of thymectomy and radiation of the thymus. Dramatic and apparently permanent cures have been effected by these measures, particularly excision of the thymus, in as many as 30 to 40 percent of cases; the majority of patients continue to have symptoms of myasthenia after thymectomy. Some proponents of the procedure believe that only early, chronically active but not too severe cases should be selected for operation. One authority has noted particularly beneficial effects of thymectomy in young women. However, it should be noted that these are the patients in whom spontaneous remissions are most frequent. The postoperative management of these patients is difficult (see books by Osserman and by Viets and Schwab if it is to be undertaken); it requires oxygen, a respirator, an aspirator, and excellent nursing. Preferably the patients should spend the postoperative period in a special care unit with a trained team of nurses and physicians. Parenterally administered neostigmine should be used in place of oral medication. Intravenous prostigmine (1 mg being equivalent to 15 mg of the oral dose) may be given during and after surgery in 1 liter of 5% glucose and water or normal saline solution over a 4-hr period. The adequacy of treatment may be checked by the response to Tensilon. Because of the unpredictability of remissions, the relatively few examples of striking improvement, and the great danger to the patient, thymectomy cannot be recommended as a routine procedure.

Thymomas usually respond to x-ray therapy, and the associated myasthenia improves.

Symptomatic Myasthenia Gravis

Typical myasthenia gravis has been reported most frequently in conjunction with thyroid disease. Eaton has shown that hyperthyroidism adds its typical muscle weakness to the myasthenia without increasing the requirement of anticholinesterase drugs. Hypothyroidism if present makes the myasthenia worse, and the latter improves as the thyroid deficiency is treated. A few of our patients with lupus erythematosus and polymyositis have had myasthenia gravis. Perhaps the most interesting form is that special one which accompanies the small-cell carcinoma of the lung. Weakness in these patients is usually in the pelvic, thigh, and shoulder-arm muscles and is accompanied by aching and stiffness. Contrary to what happens in true myasthenia gravis, ocular and bulbar muscles are usually spared. Initial movements are weak, and strength improves with each of the first several contractions. The reason for this is seen in the electromyogram, where low-voltage action potentials increase in amplitude with rapid frequencies of neuromuscular stimulation (20 to 30 per sec) and diminish in amplitude with low frequencies (1 to 2 per sec). Neostigmine has little effect on the weakness; tubocurarine and decamethonium make it worse, even when very small doses, easily tolerated by the normal person, are given. Muscle biopsies have shown degeneration of end-plates, according to McDermott. The condition may precede the appearance of the malignant tumor by as long as 2 years, but not all patients develop a tumor. The same peculiar muscle disorder has been observed by Shy in sarcoidosis.

EPISODIC MYASTHENIA OF OTHER TYPES

At least four different muscle syndromes of recurrent muscle weakness have now been identified: (1) familial periodic paralysis, (2) hyperthyroidism with periodic paralysis; (3) congenital paramyotonia (von Eulenberg's), and (4) hereditary periodic adynamia (Gamstorp's). In each of these conditions the patient may develop over a period of a few hours a disorder of skeletal muscles which may vary from weakness to total paralysis and which subsides and disappears completely after a few hours or days. Differences between them are small, but the latter two appear to share, in some instances at least, a mild degree of restricted myotonia. The syndrome must be differentiated from cataplexy (always of seconds or a few minutes' duration, precipitated by strong emo-

tion and conjoined with narcolepsy [see p. 1850]), from syncope (the physical weakness is always combined with impairment of consciousness [see p. 106]), from hydrocephalic attacks with limb weakness (headache and signs of increased intracranial pressure [see p. 1780]), and from "drop seizures," one of the varieties of epilepsy (see petit mal triad and myoclonus, p. 164).

Familial Periodic Paralysis

CLINICAL PATTERN. Familial periodic paralysis is a very rare disorder which occurs in certain families, usually being inherited as a mendelian dominant trait. The clinical story is striking. The patients are normal except for well-demarcated episodes in which intense weakness or complete paralysis of limb and trunk muscles develops. The attacks begin in early life and may come at varying intervals throughout life, being more frequent in adolescence or early adult life.

A single attack may last from a few minutes to several days, the average duration being 12 to 48 hr. The attacks in many patients have a periodicity and duration characteristic for that individual or family. During the episode there are marked hypotonia of the affected muscles and hyperextensibility of the joints. The tendon reflexes are absent or greatly reduced but return to normal as strength and tone return. The muscles are refractory to electric stimulation. The facial, pharyngeal, thoracic, and diaphragmatic muscles are affected only in very severe cases, but respiratory embarrassment and death have been reported.

The attacks are precipitated by several factors, such as violent exercise or a large high carbohydrate meal. Attacks often begin during sleep or are present on awakening. Profuse diaphoresis may precede the attack. Usually no definite precipitating cause can be discovered.

In the average patient there is no evidence of progressive muscular disease, and physical examination of a patient between attacks frequently demonstrates no abnormality. Exceptionally some degree of weakness, usually mild, persists after the termination of the attack and is cumulative in successive attacks.

PATHOGENESIS. During the attack the *serum potassium level* drops sharply. This apparently results from the sudden passage of potassium into the cells of the body, because the urinary excretion of potassium falls at the same time. The intracellular potassium of muscle has been demonstrated to rise during attacks. The relation to excess carbohydrate intake has frequently been noticed; there are a fall in serum potassium level and a rise in intracellular muscle and liver potassium levels during rapid glycogen storage. However, the timing of the two events is frequently not similar. The initial potassium changes are observed in all individuals during the first few hours after carbohydrate ingestion, while the paralysis in periodic paralysis is frequently delayed by 8 to 12 hr and is associated with a second series of changes in potassium levels. Thus the mechanism of the metabolic anomaly is not entirely clear. Biopsies of muscle taken during the attacks of paralysis reveal sarcoplasmic vacuolization.

Hyperthyroidism with Periodic Paralysis

See Chaps. 89 and 375.

Congenital Paramyotonia (von Eulenberg's Disease)

The principal feature of this disease is stiffness (myotonia), weakness, or paralysis which follows exposure to cold. It is inherited as a mendelian dominant trait. At first only the myotonic features of this disease were described, and it was always regarded as a variant of congenital myotonia (Thomsen's syndrome). Shy has called attention to the fact, known for a long time, that in some cases there are attacks of weakness similar to those of periodic paralysis. The latter may or may not be related to cold. It is of interest that the serum potassium level is not reduced in attacks and in fact the administration of potassium may induce an attack, in which respect it differs from the usual variety of familial periodic paralysis. In this way it is similar to if not identical with Gamstorp's *adynamia episodica hereditaria* (see below). The resting potential of muscle fibers during attacks is diminished. The myotonia of von Eulenberg's syndrome may be limited to the eyelids or tongue.

The relationship between myotonia congenita, myotonia dystrophica, paramyotonia congenita, adynamia episodica hereditaria, and familial periodic paralysis is close and remains somewhat controversial.

Adynamia Episodica Hereditaria (Gamstorp's Disease)

This is a hereditary disease (mendelian dominant) characterized by periods of weakness or paralysis of skeletal muscle not unlike that described in familial periodic paralysis. The onset is between the ages of five and ten years. The attacks, which may last for one to many hours, tend to occur during rest after physical exertion, particularly if the patient is wet, cold, or hungry. Tingling of lips, fingers, and toes may occur at the onset of attacks. Weakness varies in degree. Respiratory embarrassment has not been noted. Between attacks the patient is symptom-free, though in a few cases mild weakness persists, as in the family of Tyler.

Serum potassium level rises transiently during the attack, and in the electrocardiogram the T waves are high and peaked. The amount of urinary potassium does not increase before or during attacks. Administration of 2 to 5 Gm KGL induces an attack. Glucose tends to prevent this phenomenon. Reducing the serum K below a certain level, which varies from patient to patient, has been effective in preventing attacks.

This condition is worse during puberty; after this period the prognosis is good both for survival (no fatal cases) and for effective work.

Hyperaldosteronism and Other Alterations of Potassium Metabolism

Another syndrome of potassium depletion recognized recently has been called *primary hyperaldosteronism, Conn's syndrome,* or potassium-losing nephritis. This disorder results in marked hypopotassemia, with episodes of paralysis similar to those of periodic paralysis. Tetany, polyuria, hypertension, and other manifestations, not found in the hereditary cases, are commonly present. Most of the patients have adrenal tumors which secrete aldosterone and possibly other steroids. (See Chap. 92.) Care should be taken to distinguish this disease from familial periodic paralysis.

The same clinical picture may be observed in patients with other disorders when serum potassium is depleted, as in severe diarrhea or in overtreatment of a patient with Addison's disease with deoxycorticosterone; the plasma potassium levels observed are usually lower than those found during attacks of familial periodic paralysis.

Extreme hypokalemia is also accompanied by muscular weakness or paralysis (see Chap. 376).

TREATMENT OF PERIODIC PARALYSIS

Episodes of familial periodic paralysis with hypokalemia are treated by the oral administration of potassium salts in doses of 2 to 8 Gm until the attack is relieved. In the rare instance when acute respiratory or pharyngeal paralysis appears, it may be necessary, to give potassium intravenously. Great care should be observed in its use, for it may be quite toxic if administered too rapidly. Normal renal function, sufficient fluids to maintain a good urine volume, and slow administration are the most important precautions which should be taken in giving potassium salts intravenously. In patients with periodic paralysis who have frequent episodes, attacks may be prevented by giving 4 to 8 Gm potassium chloride in divided doses per day by mouth. In the flaccid paralysis which results from von Eulenberg's paramyotonia and adynamia episodica hereditaria with hyperkalemia, potassium is of course contraindicated. Diuril, on the other hand, will prevent attacks by keeping the potassium levels below a critical point.

REFERENCES

Grob, D.: Course and Management of Myasthenia Gravis, J.A.M.A., 153:529, 1953.
—— and A. McG. Harvey: Abnormalities in Neuromuscular Transmission, with Special Reference to Myasthenia Gravis, Am. J. Med., 15:695, 1953.
Osserman, K. E.: "Myasthenia Gravis," New York, Grune & Stratton, Inc., 1958.
Talbott, John H.: Periodic Paralysis: A Clinical Syndrome, Medicine, 20:85, 1941.
Viets, Henry R.: Myasthenia Gravis, New Engl. J. Med., 251:97, 141, 1954.
—— and R. S. Schwab: "Myasthenia Gravis," New York, Grune & Stratton, Inc., 1958.

378 OTHER MAJOR MUSCLE SYNDROMES

Raymond D. Adams

These are the other syndromes by which diseases of muscle declare themselves clinically.

THE STIFFNESS SYNDROMES ASSOCIATED WITH CONGENITAL DISEASES OF MUSCLE

In some of the primary diseases of muscle (in contrast to the neurologic diseases attended by spasticity and rigidity) passive movement may evoke no abnormality even though myotonia is present and hampers strong voluntary movements. However, if the myotonia is diffuse and lifelong, it may persist most of the time. This is particularly true of congenital myotonia or Thomsen's disease in which there is often a positive family history. On the other hand, if the stiffness and slowness of movement are acquired during childhood or adult life, are diffuse in distribution, and are not accompanied by reflex changes, or evidence of myotonia, three conditions suggest themselves—hypothyroidism, some form of congenital myopathy, and the "stiff-man syndrome." Hypothyroidism, McArdle's syndrome, and central core disease of Shy et al. have already been discussed. The stiff-man syndrome is a rare condition seen in only a few adults by Henry Woltman and others, and its cause has not been established. It may be attended by violent and painful spasms, sometimes localized to one muscle group but more often diffuse. Over a period of years, it progresses to involve all the skeletal muscles to the point where the patient is completely disabled. Examples of this have been observed in pseudohypoparathyroidism, but in other instances serum calcium levels, including ionized calcium, are normal. Spasms of pain, general stiffness, and slowness of movement, particularly in the legs may occasionally be observed in patients with osteoporosis and osteomalacia. The symptoms may improve on vitamin D therapy (see Chap. 381).

Tetanus and tetany, discussed in Chaps. 90 and 374 need only be mentioned in passing. In tetanus the spasm is of acute onset, beginning some days after a wound, may be generalized or localized, is increased by muscular activity and excitement, and lasts for several weeks to months. It is superimposed on a background of muscle stiffness especially in the masseter (trismus) and trunk muscles. In tetany the spasms are always intermittent and are localized principally in the hands and feet, i.e., carpopedal spasms. They are accompanied by prickling and tingling, positive Chvostek's and Trousseau's signs, and a characteristic electromyogram change (see Chap. 374). Extreme spasm localized mainly to the trunk muscles which assume boardlike rigidity may arise as the consequence of the bite of the black widow spider. And finally, several of the newer phenothiazine compounds acting on the brain may also produce an acute rigidity of muscles but usually with attendant tremors of the jaw and limbs, dystonic postures, weakness of muscles, and sometimes syncope or confusion, in various combinations. These latter phenomena should permit easy distinction from myotonia, tetanus, and tetany.

CONGENITAL MYOTONIA (Thomsen's Disease)

DEFINITION. This is a hereditary disease in which a difficulty in initiating movement is combined with slowness of relaxation. Originally described by Julius Thomsen, who suffered from the disease himself, later descriptions by Strumpell, Erb, and Westphal served to establish its nosologic position as a lifelong, familial disease. Erb provided the first description of its pathology and called attention to two additional unique features, muscular excitability and hypertrophy.

CLINICAL MANIFESTATIONS. The disease begins in the first years of life (usually by the age of six to eight years) and persists throughout its span. The disorder appears to be transmitted as an autosomal dominant trait. However, the patient frequently fails to give a family history, and myotonia may be difficult to demonstrate clinically in some individuals who nonetheless have typical electrical myotonia. It may be present in a milder subclinical degree early in life and interfere with learning to stand and walk. However, its chief feature, myotonia, is seldom demonstrable before the end of the first months or even the first 1 to 2 years of life unless unusually severe, and it becomes more intense at adolescence (in myotonia dystrophica, myotonia usually is milder and has a later onset). Muscular hypertrophy may also be noted during the early years of life. The typical slowness of contraction and persistence of contraction upon attempted relaxation is best provoked by strong voluntary movements after a period of inactivity, but it may be induced by electrical stimulation or by percussion. It is most prominent in the legs, where the first movements of walking or running after a period of rest are slow and stiff. It is also present in the hands and arms and even the face and eye muscles. With repetition of the contraction, the movement characteristically becomes more facile and rapid and relaxation more prompt, until both are normal. Clinically this slowness of relaxation is most easily demonstrated in the forearm and hand muscles and in the orbicularis oculi during voluntary effort. Percussion myotonia, which may be evoked in any of these muscles and in the tongue, consists of a persistent contraction, for half a minute or more, of a segment of a muscle which has been tapped. Myotonia does not accompany the tendon reflex, but it may alter the abdominal and cremasteric reflexes. The muscles being repeatedly involved in these strong contractions are hypertrophied, though Patterson and Maas call attention to the development of a mild dystrophic change in some cases. Cataract, temporal baldness, testicular atrophy, and muscle weakness and wasting do not occur in Thomsen's disease. When present, they always signify myotonic dystrophy.

LABORATORY DATA. The only metabolic abnormality is a mild creatine intolerance and increased urinary excretion in some patients. The electromyogram is characteristic (see Chap. 374) in that voluntary attempts to arrest muscle contraction are followed by a persistence of action potentials for several seconds. The biopsy of muscle reveals little or nothing of interest except large fibers with occasional rows of central sarcolemnal nuclei.

TREATMENT. Quinine sulfate 0.3 to 0.6 Gm three times daily reduces or relieves the myotonia, but often patients dislike it because of side effects (tinnitus, etc.). Procaine amide in doses of 250 to 500 mg orally three times daily is said to be superior to quinine.

PROGNOSIS. The disease remains unchanged throughout the patient's life. The later development of dystrophy must be exceptional.

Paramyotonia Congenita (von Eulenberg's)

This rare disease, already discussed, is one in which slowness and stiffness of movement are most clearly evoked by cold. The myotonia tends to be rather mild and is often restricted to the hands and tongue or facial muscles (eyelids). The aforementioned episodes of weakness may also be induced by cold but may occur spontaneously. The myotonia is seldom of sufficient intensity to require treatment (see Chap. 376).

Debré-Semelaigne and Hoffmann Syndromes in Hypothyroidism

These conditions were described in Chap 375 on myopathy due to thyroid disease. The principal findings are relatively large muscles and slowness of movement. Myotonia and paramyotonia do not occur. The diagnosis of this muscular disorder usually offers no difficulty, for the other symptoms of deficient thyroid function (cretinism and myxedema) are fairly obvious, as a rule. The delayed tendon reflex, found in no other disease, is a useful clinical test.

Muscle Cramps

Everyone has experienced muscle cramps. They are common in the feet and legs especially at night when the limbs are cool, particularly after there has been some unusual exertion during the day. A strong movement tends to initiate the cramp; the muscle becomes hard and painful, and relief can be obtained only by massaging and stretching of the offending muscle. The electromyogram shows a continuous burst of action potentials of abnormally high frequency and voltage. Patients may also use the word cramp to describe other sensations, pains usually, but without spasm. A few questions in these instances should enable the examiner to ascertain that reference is being made to a different order of phenomena, a dysesthesia.

The most common variety of pathologic cramping is that which occurs during physical activity, e.g., in the legs while walking, so-called intermittent claudication, and it indicates a serious impairment of circulation in the extremity. It contrasts to cramps at rest which have not this meaning at all. A severe, persistent tendency to cramp in many of the muscles of the body may appear in the following conditions: (1) salt loss from excessive sweating or diarrhea, e.g., cholera; (2) tetany from whatever cause; (3) motor system diseases; (4) *a benign generalized cramp syndrome* in which painful spasms and fasciculations, both of obscure origin, are the only manifestations. The underlying pathophysiology of all varieties of cramp is hyperexcitability of the motor nerve fiber or the membrane of the muscle fiber. Typical of both levels of disorder is enhancement by ischemia. The treatment is to correct any existing alteration of electrolytes such as sodium chloride depletion from excess sweating. In the benign cramping syndrome, quinine sulfate 0.3 to 0.6 Gm t.i.d. by mouth has been beneficial in some cases, and procaine amide orally in a dose of 0.5 Gm one to three times a day has recently been introduced as a therapeutic agent.

A type of muscle spasm with slow relaxation, differing from cramp by its electrical silence, has recently been traced by Brody to a decrease in the relaxation factor.

MYALGIC STATES

Diffuse muscle pain, which merges with malaise, is a frequent expression of a large variety of systemic infections, e.g., influenza, brucellosis, dengue, Colorado tick fever, glanders, measles, malaria, relapsing fever, rheumatic fever (cf. growing pains), salmonellosis, toxoplasmosis, trichinosis, tularemia, and Weil's disease. When this pain is remarkably intense and especially if localized to one group of muscles, the most likely diagnostic possibility is epidemic myalgia (also designated as pleurodynia, devil's grip, painful neck, and Bornholm's disease). Poliomyelitis also may be accompanied by intense pain at the onset of neurologic involvements, and later the paralyzed muscles may ache. Herpes zoster is another well-known cause of segmental pain. Nothing is known of the pathologic basis for the pains of either pleurodynia or poliomyelitis. Inflammation in spinal nerves and dorsal root ganglia, which may precede the vesicular skin eruption by as long as 72 to 96 hr, is the cause of the segmental pain in herpes zoster. The muscle tissue has been little studied by pathologists, and random biopsies have proved to be relatively uninformative in all these diseases.

Fibromyositis and myogelosis (see Chap. 394). One would suppose that by definition fibrositis or fibromyositis would represent an inflammation of the fibrous tissues of the muscles, fascia, aponeuroses, and probably nerves as well. Unfortunately, the pathologic changes remain obscure. Only the clinical facts are at hand: a muscle or group of muscles become painful and tender after exposure to cold, dampness, minor trauma, or for no reason that can be discerned. The neck and shoulders are the common sites. Firm, tender zones, sometimes several centimeters in diameter, are found within the muscles, and palpation and active contraction or passive stretching of them increases the pain—points of diagnostic value. In Europe, following the descriptions by Lange and Schadé in 1921, the term *myogelosis* was applied to this condition, but it has never gained popularity in the United States. Usually the condition clears up in a few days, and local heat and massage are found to give comfort while symptoms are present. The condition is a "favorite" with physiotherapists and osteopaths who believe their maneuvers and adjustments to be helpful, as indeed they may. Rarely a similar syndrome is but the forerunner of what proves after some days, with the onset of neurologic signs, to be a radiculitis, brachial neuritis, or an outbreak of herpes zoster.

Diffuse muscular soreness and aching may at times be the initial symptoms in rheumatoid arthritis, preceding the signs of joint involvement by a period of weeks or months. The muscles are tender, but since this may be found in otherwise normal individuals, particularly women, it is difficult to interpret. Often the patient observes that aching pain occurs not at the time of activity but some hours or even a day or two later, resembling the discomfort following the excessive use of unconditioned muscles. However, a program of conditioning exercises does not alleviate the pain. An increased sedimentation rate, a positive latex-fixation test, or other of the laboratory aids listed in Chap. 386 may clarify the diagnosis. Muscle biopsy may reveal a nonspecific interstitial nodular myositis. Occasionally a localized weakness of muscle, a slightly reduced tendon reflex, or a zone of impaired cutaneous sensation within the territory of a nerve will indicate the existence of a disease of the peripheral nervous system—an interstitial polyneuritis—which can sometimes be confirmed by the finding of infiltrates of lymphocytes, mononuclear leukocytes, and plasma cells in a nerve or muscle biopsy.

In thin, asthenic adults who exhibit this rather ambiguous symptomatology without other abnormalities, the authors have found it difficult to exclude hysteria or other psychoneurosis or depression. In every such individual it is well to search for evidence of rheumatic state and brucellosis as well as the metabolic myopathy which accompanies hyperparathyroidism and renal tubular acidosis, hypoglycemia, the intrinsic phosphorylase defect (McArdle's syndrome), phosphofructokinase defect, and myoglobinuria before calling for a psychiatric consultant. Patients with these latter diseases often complain of soreness, stiffness, and lameness after any strenuous muscular effort.

The treatment for each of these conditions will be found in the appropriate section of the book.

LOCALIZED MUSCLE MASSES

Masses may be found in one or many muscles in a variety of clinical settings, and the clinical findings in each one have a different significance.

Muscle rupture giving rise to a large bulge upon contraction is usually caused by a violent strain attended by an audible snap and then a bulge which appears when the muscle contracts. A weakening in contractile power

and mild discomfort are usually noted by the patient. The biceps muscle is the one most often affected. Treatment is immediate surgical repair; if delayed, little can be done for the condition.

Hemorrhage into muscle may occur as a consequence of trauma, as a complication of the use of anticoagulants, in hematologic diseases, or after a minor trauma in a patient with Zenker's degeneration who is convalescing from typhoid fever or other infection.

Tumors include desmoid tumor (a benign massive growth of fibrous tissue in parturient women and after surgery), *rhabdomyosarcoma* (a highly malignant tumor with strong liability to local recurrence and metastasis), and *angioma.*

Thrombosis of arteries or, more often, of veins causes congestion and infarction of muscle.

Myositis ossificans refers to the deposit of bone within the substance of a muscle. Two types are recognized. One is a localized form which appears in a single muscle or group of muscles after trauma, and the other is a progressive, widespread ossifying process in many muscles of the body and entirely unrelated to trauma. In the localized traumatic form, after a single traumatic blow or the tear of a muscle or repeated minor trauma, a painful area, probably a herniation, develops in the muscles. It is gradually replaced by masses of solid cartilaginous consistency, and within 4 to 7 weeks' time a solid mass of bone can be felt and becomes visible in the x-ray. As would be expected, this most frequently happens in vigorous adult men, and the pectoralis major, biceps, brachii, or thigh muscles of militiamen, cavalrymen, and athletes are the usual sites of the abnormality. Symptoms tend to subside if the patient desists from the activity which produced the mass.

Generalized myositis ossificans is a disease of unknown origin and consists of bone formation within muscles of children, adolescents, or young adults. Only this latter disease need be discussed in any further detail here.

PATHOLOGY. The first stage is believed to be as an interstitial myositis or fibrositis. Biopsies of early indurated swellings have revealed extensive proliferation of interstitial connective tissue in which little inflammatory cell reaction is found. The adjacent muscle fibers become compressed by the connective tissue, which retracts and calcifies. Osteoid and cartilage formation occur at a later stage, developing in the connective tissue and enclosing intact muscle fibers.

CLINICAL MANIFESTATIONS. Nearly 75 percent of all reported cases have had congenital anomalies, the most frequent of which is a failure of development of the great toes or thumbs and less often other digits. The first symptom is often a firm swelling in a vertebral or cervical muscle. There is, in addition, a mild tenderness and a discomfort during muscle contraction, and the overlying skin may be reddened and slightly swollen. A trauma may have been recalled as the initiating factor, but as the months pass other muscles not injured in any recognizable way become similarly involved. At first x-rays reveal no important changes, but within 6 to 12 months calcium deposits are observed and one can feel stony-hard masses within the muscle. As the disease advances, limitation of movement, contractures, and deformities become increasingly evident, and occasionally the patient is converted into a virtual "stone man." Scoliosis, rigidity of spine, abnormal postures, and limited expansion of the thorax may ultimately occur.

DIAGNOSIS. The principal problem in diagnosis is to differentiate this condition from calcinosis universalis, which usually occurs in relationship to scleroderma or polymyositis. It is not clear whether a sharp dividing line can be drawn between the two conditions. In calcinosis universalis there is said to be calcinosis (calcium deposit) in the skin, subcutaneous tissues, and connective tissue sheaths around the muscles, whereas in myositis ossificans there is bone formation within the muscles. Probably the pathologic data are too meager to fully justify this distinction at present. Vitamin D calcinosis, resulting from the prolonged ingestion of large doses of vitamin D, may also produce widespread deposition of masses of calcium around muscles, joints, and subcutaneous tissue.

PROGNOSIS. The disease may undergo spontaneous remissions and exacerbations and may halt at a point where the patient is capable of adequate function, remaining in this state for years. If death is to occur, it is related to the enfeebled, debilitated, malnourished condition of the patient, the final illness often being a terminal pneumonia or other intercurrent infection.

TREATMENT. No medical treatment is of proved value. Excision of bony deposits may be undertaken if it is certain that they are causing particular trouble. Some of the calcium deposits in calcinosis universalis have disappeared under cortisone therapy, and because of the unclear relationship of this disease to generalized myositis ossificans, it is probably advisable to try this form of therapy, using the same plan as that described in the chapter on diseases of connective tissue (Chap. 394).

REFERENCES

Adams, R. D., D. Denny-Brown, and C. Pearson: "Diseases of Muscle," 2d ed., New York, Paul B. Hoeber, Inc., 1962.

——, L. M. Eaton, and G. M. Shy: "Neuromuscular Disorders," Baltimore, The Williams & Wilkins Company, 1961.

Walton,, J. N.: "Disorders of Voluntary Muscle," 2d ed., Boston, Little, Brown and Company, 1969.

Section 12

Disorders of Bone

379 METABOLIC BONE DISEASE: GENERAL CONSIDERATIONS

George Nichols, Jr.

The reader should refer to Chap. 83, "Vitamin Deficiency" for discussion of Rickets and Osteomalacia.

Although diseases of the skeletal system must have been known for centuries, thanks to the deformities and fractures which so often accompany them, their relationship to disturbances of calcium and phosphate metabolism and endocrine disease has been recognized only for the past 60 to 70 years. Even now information concerning the causes of these disorders is either absent or incomplete, and effective therapy is available for only a few. In order to understand the nature of metabolic bone disease, the physician must bear in mind something of the anatomy, chemistry, and physiology of the skeletal system. This is of special importance since many new concepts which are at considerable variance with "classic" teaching concerning skeletal metabolism are beginning to emerge. The purpose of this chapter is to review these concepts, indicating only in general terms their relation to the pathogenesis of metabolic bone disease as far as it is known. The detailed descriptions of individual metabolic bone diseases follow in later chapters.

Embryology

Bone, like other connective tissues, is derived embryonically from the mesenchyme. Two types are recognized: membranous bone, which develops between flat layers of collagenous tissue (skull, etc.), and endochondral bone, formed by replacement of a cartilaginous anlage. The latter form includes most of the skeleton and is the type of bone which is most rapidly formed. Long-bone growth through replacement of growing cartilage at the epiphyseal plate is a typical example.

Histology

By far the major part of the bulk and weight of bone is extracellular material. This material is composed of two phases—an organic phase, 95 percent of which consists of collagen fibers with a small amount of mucopolysaccharide, and a mineral phase which consists of innumerable exceedingly small crystals deposited on, between, and probably in the collagen fibers. It is this combination of a strong flexible fibrous protein matrix heavily impregnated with closely packed tiny mineral crystals which imparts the well-known physical characteristics of rigidity and elasticity to the bone (Chaps. 83, 380).

This heavily calcified extracellular material is entirely

encased in a layer of small cuboidal cells with large nuclei called *osteoblasts*. These, with their precursor cells and some collagen fibers, form the periosteum and endosteum. A variety of evidence suggests that at least some of the osteoblasts are engaged at all times in the synthesis of new organic bone matrix which is continuously being laid down around them. The biochemical steps involved in the synthesis of matrix by the osteoblasts and their control are being examined currently in several laboratories. It is becoming clear not only that these cells can synthesize both polysaccharide and collagen but also that O_2 and exogenous substrate (glucose, amino acids, or both) are required for collagen synthesis. Moreover, the rate of synthesis is profoundly affected by a variety of hormonal factors as well as by age. Although much remains to be done before metabolic bone disease can be described in terms of such observations, this approach promises to be fruitful in the future.

As the process of new matrix synthesis continues, the osteoblast seems to be entrapped in its own product and eventually becomes embedded in the substance of the bone. These entrapped cells, which assume an elongated oval shape, are then termed *osteocytes*. Although the morphologic characteristics of the cell change once it is buried and it apparently ceases to synthesize collagen (perhaps because of lack of O_2 or substrate), osteocytes normally continue viable, apparently deriving their nutrition through very fine canaliculi (Volkmann's canals) which interconnect the individual cells and the perivascular spaces of nutrient vessels. The precise function of the osteocyte and its role in skeletal metabolism remain unknown, although some reports (which will be discussed further below) suggest that they may be concerned with bone resorption under certain conditions.

In addition to osteoblasts and osteocytes, a third cell type—the characteristically multinucleated giant *osteoclast*—is found in bone. This cell is much less common in normal bone and is to be found only in areas where active bone resorption is taking place. Its close application to the surface of the calcified matrix in small surface indentations (Howship's lacunas) and the increased number of osteoclasts seen in bone undergoing rapid resorption both in vivo and in tissue culture, together with other evidence, have led to the belief that these cells are the ones which resorb bone. The unanswered question is whether they are the only cells possessing the necessary apparatus to perform this function.

Physical Chemistry

Basic calcium phosphate salts are to be found deposited on the collagenous organic matrix in two forms—as innumerable tiny needle-shaped crystals ($1,500 \times 50$ Å) and in what appear to be tiny hollow spheres of amorphous (noncrystalline) material. According to the most recent concepts, the amorphous material is the form in which calcium and phosphate are initially precipitated. This material then rearranges (probably quite rapidly) through processes of recrystallization into the crystalline form. The small size of the crystals and their shape result

in an enormous surface area/volume ratio in the mineral (about 150 acres for a 70-kg man)—a fact which accounts for the remarkable reactivity of the skeletal mineral stores. Recent crystallographic studies indicate that this salt is largely if not wholly of the hydroxyapatite series, but chemical analysis shows that it varies considerably in composition from the theoretical formula of $10Ca^{++} \cdot 6(PO_4)^{3-} \cdot 2(OH)^-$. Moreover, it contains significant amounts of Na^+, Mg^{++}, CO_3^{2-}, and citrate^{3-} ions, which, with the exception of Mg^{++}, appear capable of substituting for either Ca or P in the crystal structure itself, as well as being held in the hydration shell of the crystal or adsorbed on its surface. In addition, strontium (Sr), radium (Ra), plutonium (Pu), lead (Pb), fluoride (F), and other so-called "bone-seeking" ions may be readily incorporated into or bound on the crystal. Normally these are found only in trace amounts, if at all, and probably have little physiologic significance. However, when their radioactive isotopes are ingested (e.g., Sr^{90} from fallout or Ra from luminous paints), radiation damage to bone cells and malignant degeneration may occur, or in the case of F, the solubility characteristics of the mineral may be altered.

In order to appreciate how the *bone mineral* is formed and its relationship to the normal concentrations of Ca and P in the plasma, it is necessary to recall the physical states in which Ca and P exist in the blood. Of the total Ca in plasma in normal situations (10 mg per 100 ml), about 50 percent is present bound to plasma proteins and is not diffusible into the extravascular fluids, 5 percent is present in soluble and readily diffusible complexes with citrate (Ca-Cit.$^-$)HPO$_4$$^=$, SO$_4$$^=$, and perhaps other anions, and 45 percent is present as free Ca^{++} ions. We now know that the Ca ion is the biologically significant form and is the one whose concentration is closely defended by homeostatic mechanisms. Inorganic phosphate exists in two main forms at normal plasma pH (7.38 to 7.40)—H$_2$PO$_4$$^-$ and HPO$_4$$^=$, in the approximate ratio of 1:4. In addition, PO$_4$$^{3-}$ is present in small amounts. All three are readily diffusible.

It is well known that at pH 7.4 the Ca and P concentrations in water solution must be raised above the *solubility product* of CaHPO$_4$ (1×10^{-6}) before precipitation occurs. However, CaHPO$_4$ salt is not stable in water at pH 7.4, where it promptly rearranges into tricalcium phosphate or some closely related form, with the release of H$^+$ and PO$_4$$^{3-}$. Since the solubility product of such tricalcium phosphates is *much* lower (1×10^{-25}) than that of CaHPO$_4$, massive rapid precipitation occurs. Thus water solutions of Ca^{++} and PO$_4$$^{3-}$ with ion products between 1×10^{-6} and 1×10^{-25} are termed "metastable." The normal concentrations of Ca^{++}, HPO$_4$$^=$, and PO$_4$$^{3-}$ ions in plasma are such that their ion products, 0.8×10^{-6} and 1×10^{-23} for Ca $\times$ HPO$_4$ and Ca$_3$(PO$_4$)$_2$, respectively, fall into this metastable range.

The only ways in which precipitation of Ca-P salts from metastable solutions can be brought about are by seeding the solution with a crystal of *hydroxyapatite* or by introducing some other substance capable of forming the nucleus for crystal formation by binding one or the other of the ions and raising the local concentration. Work has shown that pure collagen fibers can nucleate calcium phosphate from metastable solutions, probably because of the binding of phosphate. Keratin (the organic matrix of dental enamel) seems to have this capacity, and perhaps degradation products of other proteins or polysaccharides share it, a fact which may be very important in pathologic calcium deposition. It is important to note that a variety of substances can inhibit nucleation and crystallization, presumably by blocking the required sites on the organic matrix or by binding one or another of the requisite ions. Such inhibitors have been found in normal urine and plasma and doubtless are present in normal soft tissues, all of which contain collagen. They probably play a role in the control of bone formation as well, but their nature and mode of action are as yet unknown.

One other fact of the physical chemistry of the mineral must be mentioned. Once nucleation and crystal formation have occurred, the very high $Ca^{++}PO_4^{3-}$ ion product in the interstitial fluid relative to hydroxyapatite causes very rapid growth of the new crystals. Such rapidly formed crystals contain many defects or "strains." These defects cause the newly formed crystal to be much more receptive to exchange with other ions, to be less dense, and to be more rapidly soluble. As time passes the cystals appear to undergo internal rearrangement and slow growth, during which the "strains" become less, the crystal packing becomes denser, and, as a result, the crystal becomes more stable and therefore less reactive and less rapidly soluble. It is of considerable interest that experiments suggest that in the presence of very small amounts of F, bone mineral crystals are larger and perhaps have fewer defects, i.e., are more stable—facts which may account for the beneficial effects of F on dental caries, etc.

New Bone Formation

On the basis of these data a general picture of new bone synthesis can be drawn. New collagen matrix is synthesized from suitable substrates by the osteoblast and laid down about it. When some inhibitor is removed or some process initiates nucleation, multitudinous submicroscopic crystal seeds or tiny accumulations of amorphous calcium phosphate salt suddenly form along the collagen fibers, drawing Ca and P ions from the bathing interstitial fluids and displacing the water in the matrix as they rearrange into crystals and grow. This process of calcification proceeds rapidly, so that 70 percent of the eventual burden of Ca-P salt is deposited in a matter of hours. After that, as days and weeks pass, the mineral gradually "matures," becoming more densely packed and less reactive until the maximum capacity for mineralization is reached, at which point the bone remains unchanged until removed by the processes of resorption.

Unlike the densely cellular soft tissues of the body or, indeed, the other supporting tissues, bone shares with skin and mucous membranes the characteristic of being continually destroyed and resynthesized throughout life. These two processes—new bone *accretion* and *resorption* of old bone—together are termed *remodeling*. Remodeling in the adult skeleton may be divided into two general types, depending on the type of bone involved, although the basic pattern of resorption of old well-established bone followed by replacement with new bone is the same in both types and is presumed to proceed through the same biochemical mechanisms.

In dense, cortical bone, such as the shaft of the femur, remodeling is carried out by the burrowing of new vascular channels through the compact bone, which is resorbed ahead of the advancing vessel in some manner not yet understood. The recent identification of an osteoclast at the advancing tip of each such resorption canal is an important new observation in this area. Once the new vascular channel has been made, osteoblasts appear (their source is being debated) around the wall of the vessel and begin to lay down concentric rings of new bone matrix which rapidly calcifies. As this process proceeds, the vascular channel is gradually reduced in diameter until the central vessel is reduced to the dimensions of a small capillary. These concentric layers of bone with their central vessel form the Haversian systems and give the name *Haversain remodeling* to this process.

The other type of remodeling occurs at bone surfaces, rather than in its depths. The surfaces involved may be the surfaces of the small trabeculae of the cancellous bone in the metaphysis of a long bone or a vertebral body, the periosteal and endosteal surfaces of the shaft of a long bone, or the surfaces of membranous bones such as the skull and scapulae. In this type of remodeling the osteoblasts in a microscopic area swell, become rounded, and separate from the surface of the calcified matrix. Eventually they become indistinguishable from other round cells in the bone marrow. In addition, adjacent osteocytes appear to undergo similar swelling, while the mineral and matrix around them are resorbed. Osteoclasts appear in increased numbers, and the calcified bony substance is eroded away. As in Haversian remodeling, once the resorption process has run its course, new osteoblasts differentiate, apparently from adjacent round cells, and begin to lay down new flat lamellae of bone to replace that which was removed. It is of great interest to note the close association of accretion and resorption which characterizes this process. Indeed, resorption invariably appears to stimulate accretion—a linkage which is of great importance in understanding bone disease, although its cause remains unknown.

The rate at which remodeling occurs appears to vary considerably, depending on the area of the skeleton under consideration and whether growth is going on. These variations, together with the type of bone involved, have a profound influence on the rate at which different areas of the skeleton turn over during life. For example, in a single bone such as the femur the trabecular bone in the distal metaphysis may turn over completely in a few months, while areas of the dense cortical bone of the mid-shaft may not turn over once in the life of the individual. In addition to these local factors, the overall rate of skeletal remodeling appears to be influenced by age, hormonal factors (such as parathyroid hormone), and disease. It should be noted that while percentage change in cellular remodeling activity may be the same for all the skeleton is a given disturbance, the degree to which this becomes manifest in increases or decreases of turnover will vary greatly, depending on the density of the bone involved, its cellularity, etc.

In addition to studies of new bone synthesis, biochemical investigations have begun to shed some new light on the mechanism of bone resorption. Of particular importance to an understanding of metabolic bone disease and disturbances of Ca and P metabolism are studies related to the mineral phase.

Level of Calcium^{++} Ion

In preceding paragraphs it was pointed out that the solubility characteristics of hydroxyapatite are such that the interstitial fluids and plasma are supersaturated with Ca^{++} and PO_4^{3-} ions at normal plasma pH. This fact requires either that the skeletal mineral be sealed off from the circulating fluids or that some mechanism exist which maintains levels of Ca ion in the interstitial fluid above those dictated by bone mineral solubility at pH 7.4. The ready exchange of Ca isotopes with bone mineral stores, as well as the rapidity with which externally induced plasma Ca concentration increases or decreases are repaired, has strongly favored the latter concept. It is now known that bone cells—presumably osteoblasts but perhaps osteocytes and osteoclasts as well—share with tumors, polymorphonuclear leukocytes, and some other cell types the ability to produce large quantities of organic acids from glucose even under aerobic conditions. The chief acid produced is lactic acid, but, in addition, significant amounts of citric and pyruvic acids are released. These observations, together with the close application of the osteoblasts and other cells to the surface of the bone matrix, have led to the so-called "acid theory" to explain the levels of Ca^{++} found in the circulation. According to this proposal, organic acids are produced sufficiently rapidly by the bone cells to maintain the pH at the interface between the calcified matrix and the inner surface of the osteoblasts at about 6.8—a pH at which bone mineral solubility has been shown to be sufficiently increased to maintain the same levels of Ca^{++} (and PO_4^{3-}) as are found in plasma.

Although considerable indirect evidence has been advanced in favor of this theory, direct proof has not been obtained, partly because of technical reasons. Moreover, despite its attractive simplicity, some observations (such as the precision with which bone resorption can be localized) are difficult to explain on this basis alone. This has led to the suggestion that some type of cellular transport mechanism may be involved—an idea which has just begun to have experimental support.

From the foregoing considerations, it is apparent that the concentration of Ca^{++} ion normally present in the interstitial fluid may be conceived as consisting of two fractions—one dependent on the physical solubility of the mineral phase and another dependent on the metabolic rate of the bone cells, especially the rate at which they elaborate organic acids. These two phenomena—bone mineral solubility and bone cell metabolism—may be seen to be *the two fundamental factors* most likely to control the level of Ca^{++} ion in the extracellular fluids. Moreover, it is apparent that they can operate *entirely independently of the overall state of Ca balance of the body or the rates at which bone matrix resorption and accretion are taking place.* Thus, hypercalcemia and hypocalcemia may be thought of as the result of disturbances in the physical solubility of the mineral, the metabolic production of acid by the bone cells, or both. Experimental confirmation of the several parts of this hypothesis is available from studies of the distribution of Ca between bone fragments and incubation media in vitro using both animal and human bone.

Collagenase

While the mechanisms involved in the solubilization of bone mineral and their relation to the homeostasis of Ca concentration have been under study for some time, fruitful investigations of the resorption of the organic matrix are far less advanced. However, an enzyme, collagenase, which is capable of breaking down collagen at neutral pH, and a variety of other hydrolytic enzymes active at acid pH have now been found in bone. These appear to be encased in the bone cells in intracellular particles (lysosomes) from which they can be released experimentally by physical or chemical forces. Precisely how these enzymes play their parts in bone resorption is not yet clear, but their total activities have been shown to increase after treatment of animals with parathyroid hormone. In one instance evidence has been advanced suggesting that impairment of the stability of the intracellular storage particle by a drug (heparin) may increase bone resorption.

Cardiovascular Considerations

It is apparent that the various biochemical and physiologic phenomena described above imply an intimate "contact" of bone with the rest of the organism and suggest the presence of an extensive circulation. It has been estimated that from 5 to 10 percent of the cardiac output at rest goes to the skeleton. Since some areas, such as cortical bone, are far less vascular than others, this implies a very high blood flow in some parts. Although O_2, glucose, amino acids, Ca, P, etc., are needed for bone synthesis, and an extensive and active circulation must be needed to remove cellular metabolic end products and the residues of bone resorption, little experimental work on the metabolic effects of impaired blood flow to bone has yet been done.

Hormonal Regulation

This brief review would be incomplete without some mention of the present state of information with regard to the action of hormones in bone, especially since the skeleton so often reflects disturbances in endocrine balance. As the clinical syndromes involved are described elsewhere in detail, these remarks will be confined to pertinent biochemical and physiologic aspects.

PARATHYROID. Of particular interest are recent studies of the action of parathyroid hormone, which for many years has been known to cause increased bone resorption. This hormone has now been shown to have several effects on bone cell metabolism. Following a single dose of parathyroid extract, O_2 consumption and collagen synthesis are reduced while acid production (both lactic and citric), collagenase activity, the synthesis and release of lysosomal acid hydrolases and polysaccharide turnover are increased. These changes are accompanied by the changes in cell structure typical of bone resorption. As parathyroid stimulation continues, new bone accretion becomes accelerated also, with the result that a state of increased turnover or remodeling ensues. Biochemically the metabolic pattern is typical of such a state—O_2 consumption and incorporation of substrate into new collagen are increased, as is the production of acid. Although these changes seem to be preceeded by increased rates of RNA synthesis, at least in some cells the identity of the metabolic steps involved in these changes is not yet known.

Nevertheless, the physiologic results can be predicted on the basis of current concepts. The increased acid production should cause a shift in steady state Ca equilibrium toward the interstitial fluid, tending to raise the Ca^{++} ion concentration in the circulation. The increased turnover rate of bone should create a less "mature" pool of bone mineral, with smaller, more defective, and therefore more easily solubilized crystals, thus enhancing this tendency. Experimental corroboration of these views has been obtained in both animals and man. It should be noted that these changes per se need not *necessarily* cause hypercalcemia or skeletal demineralization. The former can be profoundly influenced by extraskeletal factors; the latter is controlled by the state of calcium balance and the degree to which stimulation of resorption of matrix is met by secondary stimulation of new matrix synthesis.

OTHER HORMONES. Although the actions of other hormones on bone have been studied, much less is known about their modes of action. However, some observations pertinent to the present discussion should be mentioned. Cortisol and other glucocorticoids have been shown to inhibit protein synthesis in vitro in several connective tissues, including bone, and to stabilize lysosomal membranes, the former having potential importance in new bone matrix synthesis, the latter in its resorption. Thyroid hormone, too, seems to inhibit bone cell protein synthesis in vitro. The sex hormones have long been known to have skeletal effects. In addition to being involved in epiphyseal closure, both testosterone and estrogens are thought to exert anabolic influences on the skeleton, although the evidence for this in the case of testosterone is not clear. Estrogens can be shown to exert

either stimulatory effects on matrix synthesis or block bone resorption depending on the species.

Growth hormone, in addition to stimulating cartilage growth, increases amino acid uptake in animal bone. Glucocorticoids also appear to affect Ca metabolism and the Ca distribution both in the bone and between the skeleton and the circulation. The former effect seems to involve the cartilage of the growth plate, causing accumulations of Ca salts in this area as well as failure of normal growth. The latter effect appears to be opposite to that of parathyroid hormone and vitamin D and has been used as a diagnostic test. Neither mechanism is as yet understood.

VITAMIN D. Finally, two other factors influencing the bone and Ca equilibrium must be mentioned. Vitamin D, in addition to its well-known effects on Ca absorption in the gut, has now been shown to affect the skeleton as well. Its action with respect to Ca equilibrium and lactic acid production has been shown to resemble closely that of parathyroid hormone. It has been suggested, on the basis of biochemical experiments, that this vitamin is absolutely *required* for parathyroid hormone action on bone. Other investigators believe that the relationship is synergistic but independent. The proof of these propositions must await further work.

CALCITONIN. In addition to vitamin D, the recently discovered hypocalcemic factor "calcitonin," which seems to be elaborated by cells derived from the ultimobranchial body, must exert its action on the skeletal mechanisms supporting interstitial Ca^{++} ion concentrations, since no other system would be capable of sufficiently rapid response. Although clear evidence of suppression of bone resorption by calcitonin has been obtained, the precise locus of action and the identity of the cells and biochemical mechanisms involved remain to be discovered.

Summary

The foregoing review indicates that metabolic bone disease potentially may result from disorders of diverse origin in a variety of areas both intrinsic and extrinsic to the skeleton. For example, at the *bone cell level* the synthesis of new bone matrix might be disturbed in a variety of ways. Mechanisms for the synthesis of calcifiable collagen of normal strength might be lacking, excess inhibitors of nucleation might be present, or the mechanisms responsible for their removal might fail. Similarly, resorptive mechanisms might be disturbed: acid production might be increased or decreased, causing changes in Ca equilibrium and hyper- or hypocalcemia. These disturbances could occur with or without changes in the rate of production or release of the cathepsins needed to lyse and remove the recalcified organic matrix.

Disturbances of vascularity in the bone itself can create disease. Thus, accretion depends on an adequate supply of nutrients, including O_2, which would be decreased with local vascular occlusion (plugging of Haversian capillaries, etc.) or decreased flow secondary to muscle wasting, etc. On the opposite side of the coin, increased rates of vascular invasion, as seen in Paget's disease, create still another set of problems, characterized by excessive rates of remodeling.

Turning to factors extrinsic to the skeleton capable of causing bone disease, it is obvious that *nutritional disturbance,* including disorders of absorption and excretion of necessary substrates and vitamins, can markedly influence the intrinsic skeletal activity of accretion and resorption even though the cellular mechanisms per se may be quite normal.

Finally, hormonal imbalance, including the secretions of the adrenals, gonads, thyroid, and pituitary as well as the parathyroids, is capable of producing bone disease in two ways: through direct action on cellular mechanisms in the skeleton itself, and secondarily through effects on other organs of absorption and excretion and the general nutrition of the organism.

Thus, it is apparent that metabolic bone disease may be primary in the skeleton or secondary to many external forces. Although not enough is yet known to classify all bone disease in the terms attempted here, progress in this direction is being made. The relative simplicity of this approach and its promise in terms of improved understanding and better therapy make it seem a desirable goal for which to aim.

REFERENCES

Fourman, P., P. Royer, M. J. Levell, and D. B. Morgan: "Calcium Metabolism and the Bone," 2d ed., Oxford, Blackwell Scientific Publications, Ltd., 1968.

Gaillard, P. P., R. V. Talmage, and A. M. Budy (Eds.): "The Parathyroid Glands—Ultrastructure, Secretion, and Function," Chicago, The University of Chicago Press, 1965.

Griffith, G. C., G. Nichols, Jr., J. D. Asher, and B. Flanagan: Heparin Osteoporosis, J.A.M.A., 193:91, 1965.

Harris, W. H., and R. P. Heaney: Skeletal Renewal and Metabolic Bone Disease (Cont.), New Engl. J. Med., 280:253, 1969.

McLean, F. C., P. La Croix, and A. M. Budy (Eds.): "Radioisotopes and Bone," Philadelphia, F. A. Davis Company, 1962.

Schartum, S., and G. Nichols, Jr.: Calcium Metabolism of Bone *in vitro:* Influence of Bone Cellular Metabolism and Parathyroid Hormone, J. Clin. Invest., 40:2083, 1961.

Termine, J. D., and A. S. Posner: Amorphous Crystalline Interrelationships in Bone Mineral, Calcified Tissue Res., 1:8, 1967.

380 OSTEOPOROSIS
Clayton Rich

Definition

Osteoporosis is a chronic disorder of old people, more severe in women, in which there is a progressive decrease in bone mass and an increased incidence of fractures. The bone loss occurs predominantly because of increased resorption, a process which is present to a variable degree in the entire aging population. Except in a few cases where osteoporosis is secondary to some known chemical or physical cause, there is no one etiologic disturbance that we now can recognize and, except for the reduced quantity of bone and the consequences of decreased bone mass and strength, there are no distinguishing features between patients with osteoporosis and other patients of the same age. Therefore, the distinction between osteoporotic and normal patients appears to be a matter of degree; those in whom bone loss is moderate being classified as normal, whereas those in whom it is so severe as to have caused vertebral or other fractures or to be easily recognized on x-ray films, being classified as having osteoporosis. Thus, osteoporosis can be regarded as the most severe segment of a continuum of age-related bone loss which affects the entire population.

Age-Related Bone Loss

Numerous studies in which quantitative methods have been applied to evaluate bone mass in populations all show an increase in bone density during childhood and adolescence, reaching a plateau between twenty and thirty-five years of age and, thereafter, a gradual loss of bone with increasing age. The maximum bone mass achieved during adult life varies, being less in women than men, less on the average in Caucasians than Negroes, and less in hypogonadal and chronically malnourished than in normal subjects. The rate of bone loss, starting around thirty-five years of age, is extremely variable from person to person, but averages 20 to 30 percent for several long bones and 50 percent for the vertebral bodies during the next 4 decades, or 1 to 2 percent loss per year of the remaining bone mass throughout this period. Obviously, a very low bone mass at the age of sixty-five could result from failure to achieve a normal bone mass by the age of twenty, even though subsequent age-related bone loss was no greater than average, or could result from an accelerated rate of bone loss after age thirty-five, or both. Although cases of osteoporosis undoubtedly occur as a result of both of these processes, the one which appears to be the most significant is accelerated bone resorption. However, it is most likely that the lower incidence and milder course of osteoporosis in males than females and in Negroes than Caucasians is significant because of greater initial mass of the skeleton, so that, even after the same percentage reduction, enough bone is left so that fractures are less common. The difference between bone mass of men and women first becomes evident at adolescence and presumably is because of secretion of testosterone (accordingly, the most profound effect of hormones in determining osteoporosis may be during adolescence rather than senescence, as is usually thought).

Throughout life, there is continuous remodeling of bone due to osteoclastic resorption at vascular and endosteal surfaces, followed by osteoblastic bone formation, to fill in the resulting resorption cavities. These two processes seem closely linked, as if the stimulus to osteoclastic differentiation in some way also causes a stimulus to osteoblastic differentiation so that, under normal conditions, about 400 mg calcium is removed by bone resorption and a like amount deposited in new bone in adults each day, and under conditions where one rate is accelerated or decreased, as in hyper- or hypoparathyroidism, the other rate undergoes a like change, although not necessarily to the same degree.

Quantitative morphologic analysis of normal human bone shows that, with increasing age, the osteoclastic resorptive activity increases, so that osteoclasts are found acting along an increased fraction of the vascular and endosteal surfaces. Because this process is not accompanied by any corresponding increase in bone formation, there is a resulting loss of bone mass. Furthermore, there is a distinctive pattern to this resorption, which, in general, follows the surface/volume ratio in different bones. The trabeculae, which are composed of thin sheets of bone bordered by endosteum, have at least ten times the surface/volume ratio as does compact cortical bone, and therefore, a greater proportion of trabecular bone is lost than is cortical bone. That is why parts of the skeleton which bear weight or are subject to trauma, which are composed predominately of trabecular bone, such as the vertebral bodies and the distal radius, are so frequently fractured in osteoporosis.

Resorption also is accelerated at the endosteal surface of the tubular bones and at the vascular surfaces of Haversian systems nearest to the endosteum. Because of this and because formation is much less active at these sites, there is a progressive expansion of the medullary cavity and an increased porosity of the remaining, thinner cortex. Bone formation continues to occur at a very slow rate at the periosteum so that the long bones become wider, but have an increasingly thin and porous cortex, at the same time that the trabecular part of the skeleton is undergoing progressive resorption.

Coincident with these quantitative, age-related changes, there is an increase in the incidence of fractures within the general population. For example, it has been found, in independent studies carried out in Sweden and Scotland, that the rate of fracture of the proximal femur doubles in every 5-year period after the age of thirty-five to forty in both men and women. The incidence of all fractures in a large group of women over forty-five years old was found to be 35 per 1,000 subjects at risk per year. These fracture rates constitute an enormous public health problem; indeed, the consequence of fractures of the femur is a leading cause of hospitalization and a significant cause of death in women over seventy. It is obvious that decreased bone mass must contribute to this increased fracture rate; in fact, it is the only cause so far identified. However, the possibility of other changes, such as decreased tensile strength or decreased elasticity of bone occurring with age, have not so far been adequately studied.

The reason for age-related bone loss is unknown. The rate of loss remarkably parallels the loss of many other tissues, such as muscle and nephron, with age, and why this happens is not understood for any of these tissues. In addition to whatever contribution "age" may make, a number of experimental conditions cause identical or similar changes and appear to contribute to or influence the severity of the bone loss, but no one of them could remotely be considered a primary etiologic factor in a significant number of cases. These factors are immobilization, calcium and possibly other nutritional deficiencies, and deficiencies or excess of steroid hormones and are considered later because of their influence on the severity of osteoporosis.

OSTEOPOROSIS

Osteoporosis is distinguished from age-related bone loss on rather superficial grounds; either there is evidence of deformity of a vertebral body or fracture of other bone from minor trauma or the bones are so demineralized as to be readily recognized on routine diagnostic x-ray films. This latter criterion is arbitrary and will distinguish only the most severe cases, as it has been shown that demineralization of vertebral bodies cannot be appreciated on visual inspection from x-ray films until about one-third of the bone mass has been lost. It may be possible, by use of quantitative radiographic and photon absorption methods for measuring regional bone density, which will show a 5 to 10 percent change, to determine some level of bone density below which there is a significantly increased risk of vertebral or other fractures and thus achieve an operational distinction between osteoporosis, as a morbid process, and the rest of the population exhibiting age-related bone loss. Whether or not this can be done depends upon whether or not osteoporosis is, in fact, a quantitative disorder as presently seems likely, in which the only abnormality is a decreased amount of bone, with the remaining bone being qualitatively normal.

Incidence

Osteoporosis is a rare disease in young adults of either sex, but its incidence increases sharply in the fifth decade in women and about a decade later in men; by the eighth decade it is a relatively common disease found almost as often in men as in women. The incidence in hospitalized patients and hospital outpatients is about 20 percent in women and 5 percent in men fifty years old, but by the age of seventy the incidence in women and men has risen to about 30 and 20 percent, respectively.

Although most patients with osteoporosis appear to be otherwise healthy, it is of interest that the incidence of osteoporosis is higher in subjects with several chronic diseases than in the general population. These include patients with prolonged nutritional insufficiency of calcium or proteins (as often is found in chronic alcoholism), subjects with gonadal insufficiency or those treated with glucocorticoids, patients with rheumatoid disease (with or without steroid therapy), and persons with diabetes mellitus.

Etiology

Histologic and biochemical studies show several metabolic patterns in osteoporosis. Bone formation and matrix metabolism are usually normal or slightly reduced, but they are sometimes found to be accelerated; the rate of bone resorption is always disproportionately accelerated. This suggests that there may be different etiologic disturbances, all of which cause similar structural changes in bone and thereby lead to the clinical picture of osteoporosis. As already stated, osteoporosis does not appear to be sharply differentiated on clinical or morphologic grounds from the general condition of age-related bone loss. So far as can now be determined, those patients with the most severe bone loss, and therefore, osteoporosis, are simply those in whom the random grouping of the various factors which promote bone loss within the entire population have occurred to a particular degree. In addition to possible unknown primary etiologic abnormalities and some possible role of age, the severity of bone loss depends to a very significant degree upon the modifying influence of a number of factors, such as calcium and possibly other nutritional deficiencies, hormonal disturbances, and physical activity, as described below.

CALCIUM DEFICIENCY. Osteoporosis can be caused experimentally in animals by deficiency of dietary calcium and is relatively common in a number of states in which intake or absorption of calcium is diminished (malnutrition, alcoholism, Laennec's and biliary cirrhosis, and some patients with intestinal lactase deficiency, who do not tolerate lactose and, therefore, voluntarily restrict their intake of milk products). However, it has been shown that the intake of calcium by most osteoporotic subjects is adequate and, furthermore, that a majority of persons whose intake of calcium has been low throughout their lives never develop osteoporosis. Studies of intestinal absorption of calcium in osteoporosis are not conclusive but point to the likelihood that calcium absorption is normal in some, but definitely low in others, and in such patients, reduced absorptive efficiency may play an important etiologic role. Thus, calcium deficiency may be the primary cause in some cases and increase the severity in others, but it does not appear to be the usual cause of the disease.

OTHER DIETARY DEFICIENCIES. Combined osteoporosis and osteomalacia is found in some patients with intestinal absorptive defects. This can be produced in animals, where it is clear that deficiency of vitamin D causes the osteomalacia and deficiency of calcium causes osteoporosis.

In the past it has been assumed that, because phosphorus is much more plentiful in most food than calcium and because it is well absorbed from the human intestine, phosphate deficiency could not be a significant cause of osteoporosis. However, the striking effect of phosphate on reducing hypercalcemia, presumably by reducing bone resorption, recent reports of calcium and phosphate retention and clinical improvement of osteoporotic patients treated with phosphate, and some nutritional and tissue culture work which suggests that resorption may be inhibited by phosphate, have all stimulated a great deal of interest in the possible role of phosphorus in bone metabolism and osteoporosis. Conclusive evidence has not been brought forth, but certainly, phosphate deficiency or abnormality of phosphorus metabolism must be considered potentially very important.

Most patients who take an inadequate diet experience combined deficiencies of protein, vitamins, phosphorus, and calcium. Osteoporosis has been caused experimentally by diets deficient in protein, and it is probable that lack of protein, vitamins, and other nutrients contributes significantly to the osteoporosis of subjects with chronic diseases.

IMMOBILIZATION. Decreased osteoblastic and increased osteoclastic activity occur as a result of immobilization. This process can be acute and, if a large portion of the skeleton is immobilized (as after inflammatory or traumatic injury of the spinal cord), may lead to hypercalcuria and even hypercalcemia. There is generalized loss of skeletal mass of the immobilized part, but the intensity of loss may vary in different parts of a bone, leading to an appearance on x-ray films of patchy demineralization. This process is an important factor in the osteoporosis that develops in persons with rheumatoid and other chronic joint diseases. The same patchy appearance is often seen in x-rays of the bones of aged osteoporotic patients and probably indicates that immobilization has played an important secondary role in their disease.

GONADAL HORMONE INSUFFICIENCY. The concept that osteoporosis occurs primarily because of reduced gonadal function, with failure of the inhibitory effect of estrogens on osteoclastic activity (in postmenopausal women) and of androgens to promote connective tissue formation (in aged men) is supported by experimental work in lower mammals which shows that both androgens and estrogens promote bone mass and by clinical impressions that osteoporosis is accelerated at the time of menopause. However, there is no significant difference between the menstrual history or degree of estrogen deficiency between postmenopausal patients with osteoporosis and those without, which suggests that, although gonadal hormones have an important secondary influence on the severity of osteoporosis, their deficiency is not the primary cause of the disease. Similarly, there is no evidence that men with osteoporosis are deficient of testosterone or that they vary from other men of the same age in this respect.

Clinical Manifestations

The natural history of osteoporosis has not been studied adequately, and little is known of the prognosis of untreated patients. A few subjects have quite severe progressive disease, but in the majority, recognizable changes occur late in life. Even when compression fractures of the vertebrae are present, morbidity usually is slight. Symptoms appear to be less severe in old than in younger people. For example, 70 percent of elderly persons in nursing homes found by x-ray to have osteoporosis with vertebral compression fractures were asymptomatic and gave no history of ever having had back pain.

Back pain in osteoporosis is of two types: one is acute and severe, and the other, which can follow an acute episode, is more mild and chronic. It is important to remember that both types of pain usually resolve spontaneously and that they will generally be followed by months or years during which there are no symptoms. It is this intermittent character of untreated osteoporosis that makes an assessment of therapy based upon clinical response very hazardous.

The acute pain has sudden onset and is sharp, severe, and localized over a vertebra. It is made worse by motion and usually subsides gradually in 3 to 4 weeks, irrespective of treatment. This pain is associated with compression fractures of the vertebral bodies. However, pain frequently is not present in older subjects (presumably when vertebral deformation occurs slowly), and sometimes the fractures are not extensive enough to be apparent in x-ray films of the spine, so that this symptom does not correlate well with the progression of osteoporosis as documented radiologically. The other type of pain is milder, dull, and aching; often paraspinal but sometimes in the deep midline; may be present for months; usually occurs after the patient has been standing or sitting for some time, and is relieved by rest.

Physical manifestations occur as a result of fractures. The changes in the vertebra are collapse of the centrum, usually of the lower dorsal and lumbar bodies that support the greatest weight. Because the vertebral column remains supported posteriorly by the vertebral articulations, the result is kyphosis, with consequent limitation of chest mobility and loss of vertical height, but gibbous deformity and spinal cord injuries are uncommon. Other bones, particularly the distal radius, ribs, metacarpals, metatarsals, proximal femur, and pelvis may fracture following minor trauma. The signs, symptoms, and treatment are the same as for any other fractures and they heal normally, except insofar as mechanical weakness makes internal fixation difficult. Femoral fractures constitute the principal cause of serious morbidity contributed to by osteoporosis.

Diagnosis

The concentrations of calcium, phosphate, and phosphatase in blood are normal in subjects with osteoporosis. The x-ray findings are of generalized skeletal demineralization and vertebral compression fractures. X-ray signs that are occasionally useful in the recognition of skeletal demineralization include reduction of the width of the cortex of long bones, accentuated contrast between the end plates and centra of the vertebral bodies, accentuated vertical trabeculation of the centra, and localized or generalized concavity of the end plates.

A presumptive diagnosis of osteoporosis is made from the recognition of x-ray changes of skeletal demineralization or of vertebral compression fractures. However, because there are no specific signs, symptoms, or laboratory or x-ray findings in osteoporosis, a definite diagnosis can be made only by exclusion of other disorders that can lead to the same skeletal changes. Early age (in which osteoporosis is a rare cause of vertebral demineralization), fracture of the vertebral articular processes (leading to gibbous deformity or neurologic involvement), isolated compression fracture of the higher dorsal or cervical vertebra, and localized bone destruction and weight loss all militate against the diagnosis of osteoporosis and suggest malignancy.

Differential Diagnosis

The causes of skeletal demineralization (listed in Table 380-1) that must be excluded are (1) neoplastic proc-

Table 380-1. CAUSES OF GENERALIZED SKELETAL DEMINERALIZATION

I. Malignant states
   A. Malignant disorder of marrow elements (especially multiple myeloma)
   B. Carcinomatous infiltration of marrow
   C. Humoral action on bone from several tumors (with or without bone metastases)
II. Nonmalignant disorders of marrow
   A. Infiltration or hyperplasia
III. Metabolic bone diseases
   A. Hyperparathyroidism (primary or secondary)
   B. Osteomalacia
      1. Vitamin D deficiency
         a. Decreased production
         b. Decreased intake
         c. Decreased absorption (disorders of stomach, pancreas, biliary system, or small intestine)
      2. Vitamin D resistance
         a. Congenital
         b. Acquired (chronic uremia; occasionally toxic)
   C. Osteoporosis
      1. Primary osteoporosis (idiopathic, postmenopausal and senile)
      2. Secondary influences on primary osteoporosis
         a. Disuse or immobilization
         b. Calcium deficiency
         c. Gonadal insufficiency
         d. Glucocorticoid excess
         e. Malnutrition
      3. Secondary osteoporosis
         a. Immobilization
         b. Glucocorticoid excess
         c. Hyperthyroidism
         d. Acromegaly
         e. Gonadal insufficiency
      4. Associated with heritable disorders of connective tissue
         a. Osteogenesis imperfecta
   D. Other
      1. Scurvy
      2. Hypophosphatasia

esses, (2) marrow disorders, (3) hyperparathyroidism, (4) osteomalacia from vitamin D deficiency or vitamin D resistance (congenital or acquired, as in uremia), (5) secondary osteoporosis, and (6) heritable connective tissue disorders. In order to exclude neoplastic and marrow diseases, it should be shown that x-rays of the entire skeleton indicate no localized bone destruction; that the erythrocyte sedementation rate, peripheral blood cells, and plasma proteins are normal; and that there is no other evidence of malignant disease (particularly of multiple myeloma, which may simulate osteoporosis early on, also cancer of the kidney, thyroid, lung, breast, or prostate, which frequently metastasize to bone). To rule out metabolic bone diseases other than osteoporosis, the concentration of calcium, phosphorus, alkaline phosphatase, and urea in plasma must be normal and steatorrhea or renal tubular disorders absent. The various causes of secondary osteoporosis must be excluded by clinical and laboratory evaluation. Tests such as measurement of the protein-bound iodine and plasma cortisone concentration, marrow examination, or special radiologic procedures may often be indicated. Bone biopsies have heretofore been difficult to evaluate, but with standardization of sampling and histologic techniques and with experience in the interpretation of undecalcified sections, valuable information is gained, especially in differentiating osteoporosis from osteomalacia and in recognizing the combination of both.

Treatment

The objectives of treatment are to institute a lifelong program of appropriate physical activity, optimal nutrition, and treatment with pharmacologically active agents. It is most important to avoid immobilization. Since osteoporosis can be recognized on the basis of x-ray changes or pathologic fractures only after about one-third of the skeletal calcium has been lost, it must take years to develop, and it is not surprising that improvement in x-ray appearance is not readily seen, even after years of treatment. It might be expected that changes would be observed using the more precise quantitative methods for regional bone densitometry, but thus far, results generally have been inconclusive. The effects of treatment are difficult to evaluate because of the variable course of osteoporosis. Therefore, reliance has been placed chiefly on measurement of external balance based on the assumption that calcium retention indicates the formation of new bone. Several agents, all of which cause calcium retention in normal subjects, have been found to do the same in most patients with osteoporosis. This suggests that these agents may be helpful in managing the disease, but it does not justify the assumption that a deficiency of one or the other of them is the cause of osteoporosis.

The largest clinical experience has been accumulated in the treatment of postmenopausal women with *sex steroids*. Several times the physiologic dosage of estrogens or androgens has been shown to cause significant retention of calcium and phosphorus in about 80 percent of subjects during the first few weeks of treatment, but no studies have shown the effects of physiologic dosage and in the few studies carried out after several months of treatment, no change was found from the pretreatment results. As with other methods of treatment of osteoporosis, those with the severest disease (idiopathic osteoporosis) respond the least, or not at all.

Supplementation of *calcium intake* to a total of about 1,600 mg calcium per day also causes retention of calcium, presumably because of inhibition of parathyroid-regulated osteoclastic activity. However, the same tendency for reduced calcium retention with continued treatment is seen as with patients treated with estrogens, so that, after several months, a new steady state tends to develop. An analysis of bone formation and resorption, using ^{45}Ca kinetic methods, shows that the early retention of calcium during estrogen or calcium therapy is caused by a reduction of bone resorption, with the formation rate unchanged, but that, after several months of therapy, bone formation had also been reduced so that both rates were similarly depressed and no further calcium retention occurred. The best explanation for this is that there is some inherent relationship between bone resorption and bone formation which causes them usually to remain in balance.

Several other agents have been evaluated by metabolic studies and clinical trial. Prolonged retention of calcium has been observed during treatment of most osteoporotic subjects given a moderate dose of *sodium fluoride* (10 mg fluoride ion per day), an agent that has a complex action on bone. It reduces the solubility of bone crystals by converting them in part from hydroxyapatite to the larger, less chemically reactive fluorhydroxyapatite; accelerates bone turnover (formation and resorption), causes histologic changes of osteomalacia, and eventually will cause osteosclerosis in normal persons. Radiographic density studies have demonstrated an increase in bone mass of several osteoporotic patients treated with fluoride for 1 to 2 years. Although these results are promising, the action of fluoride on bone is so complex and so poorly understood that it should be considered highly experimental and used with caution.

As described above, several osteoporotic patients have had significant calcium retention and a good clinical response when treated with at least 1.5 Gm per day *phosphorus* (as phosphate). These results also are promising, but until a greater amount of experience has been gained, it is not possible to predict how regularly such results will be obtained and whether the initial degree of calcium retention will persist or, as with calcium and estrogen therapy, it will diminish during prolonged therapy.

Calcitonin, a hormone that inhibits bone resorption, is another agent that has great promise as a form of treatment for osteoporosis which also is undergoing experimental and clinical trial.

GENERAL MEASURES. Immobilization or inactivity causes disuse atrophy of bone and weakens the muscular support of the skeleton. Therefore, graded physical therapy should be directed at strengthening the back muscles but should avoid any sudden strain. The patient must be reassured that a brace is not necessary to strengthen a weakened back and that it will promote rather than prevent further trouble. When necessary for reasonable comfort, an elastic lumbosacral corset may be required in the daytime; during episodes of severe back pain, a rigid brace may be necessary but should be used as little as possible. Many patients will find relief from a hard mattress, often over a bed board. Appropriate analgesics should be given.

The *diet* should provide adequate proteins and vitamins, especially vitamin D, 1,000 to 2,000 units per day, and supplemental calcium and phosphorus. Calcium diphosphate tablets fortified with vitamin D are available, and four 0.5 Gm tablets given twice a day will provide 900 mg calcium, 700 mg phosphorus, and 2,700 units vitamin D. Otherwise, calcium gluconate or lactate may be given to supplement the dietary intake by 1.2 Gm calcium per day. The dose must be reduced if hypercalcuria occurs, but this is uncommon. Women may be treated with at least a physiologic amount of estrogen (1.25 to 2.50 mg conjugated estrogens per day or the equivalent) for 3 weeks each month. Such therapy has not increased the incidence of breast or uterine carcinoma and may have reduced it. Men should be given 400 mg of a depot form of testosterone per month or the equivalent of a less androgenic steroid for its anabolic effect. Although there is little evidence that bears on the point, combined treatment with androgens and estrogens may offer some additional advantage. However, few women tolerate androgenic steroids for long periods. Because the objective is to maintain adequate therapy for the rest of the patient's life, procedures that have undesirable side effects must be avoided.

Prophylaxis

In view of the clinical and laboratory evidence that calcium absorption decreases with age and the finding that many old persons refuse to ingest an adequate diet, it seems advisable that 700 to 800 mg calcium be taken each day as a supplement and that an optimal amount of vitamin D be given as a multivitamin tablet.

"SECONDARY" OSTEOPOROSIS

The basic rate of bone remodeling in secondary osteoporosis may be increased (as in hyperthyroidism and acromegaly), decreased (in Cushing's syndrome and chronic disuse atrophy), or normal, but in any case there is disproportionately increased bone resorption, which results in the same structural and clinical changes as in the primary disease. The diagnosis rests upon recognition of the underlying abnormality. Hyperthyroidism and Cushing's syndrome are particularly likely to be overlooked when their nonskeletal manifestations are inconspicuous.

Immobilization

In addition to its important influence upon the course of primary osteoporosis, immobilization is a state in which osteoporosis will always occur and therefore can be considered a definite cause of osteoporosis independent of any underlying metabolic abnormality.

Steroid-induced Osteoporosis (Chap. 92).

Rapidly progressive osteoporosis is present in 70 to 90 percent of patients with Cushing's syndrome, and a similarly high incidence of severe osteoporosis can be caused by treatment with glucocorticoids if a sufficiently high dose is given. Thus, glucocorticoids also are a definite cause of osteoporosis. However, it is probable that many patients who develop generalized skeletal demineralization from a moderate dose of glucocorticoids have underlying primary osteoporosis aggravated by steroid therapy and often, more significantly, by inactivity. For example, the incidence of generalized osteoporosis was found to be about 15 percent in a group of patients with rheumatoid disease, whether or not treated with steroids, but was most severe and more common in those with joint disease of the longest duration. Sex steroids have not been valuable in reducing the incidence of steroid-induced osteoporosis.

Gonadal Insufficiency (Chaps. 97 and 98)

The early onset of osteoporosis, and probably increased incidence, in castrates of either sex establishes that absence of these hormones adversely effect the course of osteoporosis. It is not clear whether or not gonadal insufficiency alone will cause the disease.

Hyperthyroidism (Chap. 89)

Calcium absorption is reduced, probably because of the rapid intestinal transit of food. The rate of turnover of bone, as well as other tissues, is accelerated, and there often is hypercalcuria; all contributing to a negative calcium balance and an increased incidence of osteoporosis. Mild hypercalcemia is found occasionally in thyrotoxicosis.

Acromegaly (Chap. 87)

As in hyperthyroidism, both bone growth and resorption are stimulated, and osteoporosis is a relatively common finding. This may result in part from redistribution of the original amount of bone mineral into an enlarged volume of bone. Several other factors appear to promote osteoporosis in patients with acromegaly; early in the disease some patients may have slightly hyperactive adrenal function, and diminished gonadal function is common late in the disease. Occasional patients have hyperparathyroidism.

Other Hormonal Agents

Although osteitis fibrosa and osteoporosis in other respects differ fundamentally, the two disorders have the common feature of increased bone resorption, though to different degrees. In each, osteoclastic activity is accelerated; but only slightly in osteoporosis, so that the changes cannot be appreciated by conventional histologic methods. In contrast, in hyperparathyroidism and some tumors, particularly of the kidney and lung, in which a substance which closely resembles parathyroid hormone is elaborated by the neoplastic tissue, there is greatly accelerated bone resorption, often leading to the recognizable histologic and x-ray changes of osteitis fibrosa. A few patients with hyperparathyroidism or malignant diseases are found to have osteoporosis rather than osteitis fibrosa.

On theoretical grounds, one could predict that calcitonin deficiency could cause osteoporosis. This intriguing and important possibility has not yet been adequately evaluated (Chap. 91).

REFERENCES

Fleisch, H., H. J. J. Blackwood, and M. Owen (Eds.): "Calcified Tissues," Berlin, Springer-Verlag OHG, 1965.

Heaney, R. P.: Editorial, A Unified Concept of Osteoporosis, Am. J. Med., 39:877, 1965.

Henneman, P. H., and S. Wallach: A Review of the Prolonged Use of Estrogen and Androgen in Postmenopausal and Senile Osteoporosis, A.M.A. Arch. Intern. Med., 100:715, 1957.

Smith, R. W., Jr., and J. Rezek: Epidemiologic Studies of Osteoporosis in Women of Puerto Rico and Southeastern Michigan with Special Reference to Age, Race, National Origin and to Other Related or Associated Findings, Clin. Orthop., 45:31, 1966.

Whedon, G. D.: "Osteoporosis in Clinical Endocrinology II," E. B. Astwood (Ed.), p. 349, New York, Grune & Stratton, Inc., 1968.

381 PAGET'S DISEASE OF BONE
Stephen M. Krane

Paget's disease of bone (osteitis deformans) is among the most common of the chronic skeletal diseases. It is in the strict sense a focal disease, although it may be occasionally widespread. The initial event seen histologically is excessive resorption of bone mediated by cells such as osteoclasts, associated with the replacement of normal marrow by vascular, fibrous connective tissue. At some stage in the disease, and to a variable degree, the resorbed bone is replaced by coarse-fibered, dense trabecular bone organized in haphazard fashion. In the process of formation, the irregular and often rapid deposition of new bone leads to an increase in the number of prominent, irregular cement lines which gives the bone its characteristic "mosaic" pattern. Some areas of bone may show evidence of both excessive resorption and the chaotic new bone formation.

Incidence

The incidence of Paget's disease is difficult to determine, since it is most often asymptomatic and is detected usually when roentgenograms are obtained for other reasons. However, it is probable that the disorder occurs with an incidence of greater than 3 percent in individuals over the age of forty. The disease has been reported only rarely in subjects below age thirty, although in retrospect some patients are able to date the onset of their disease to that period. The incidence also seems to increase with increasing age. However, it is of interest that in some areas of the world, such as India, Paget's disease is exceedingly rare.

Etiology

Almost a century after the original description of the disorder, and despite intensive study and widespread interest, the etiology of Paget's disease is unknown. No convincing evidence of endocrine abnormality has been produced. Although pagetic bone can be exceedingly vascular, out of proportion to any other disorder, it has not been established that the vascular abnormality is primary. The observations that some of the manifestations of the disease can be suppressed with the use of adrenal corticosteroids and salicylates are of interest, although not sufficient to support earlier hypotheses that an inflammatory process is the fundamental lesion.

Pathophysiology

The characteristic feature of Paget's disease is the increased resorption of bone accompanied by some increase in bone formation, which is usually adequate to compensate for the increase in resorption. However, during the course of the illness some imbalance between bone resorption and formation may occur. When resorption predominates (for example in the variant, *osteoporosis circumscripta*), the bones are brittle and soft and exceedingly vascular. This has been termed the *osteoporotic, osteolytic,* or *destructive phase* of the disease, where the external calcium balance may be negative. More commonly the excessive resorption is followed closely by formation of new pagetic bone (so-called "mixed" phase of the disease). The other extreme is characterized by progressive decrease in resorption rate, as activity of the disease decreases, eventually leading to hard, dense, less vascular bone (so-called "osteoplastic" or "sclerotic" phase) and a positive external calcium balance. Generally in Paget's disease the rate of bone formation is closely geared to that of bone resorption such that the magnitude of the increase in bone turnover is not reflected in the overall calcium balance. Techniques utilizing the analysis of disappearance rates of injected radioisotopes of calcium or strontium have shown that the rates of bone resorption and formation may be increased enormously in patients with active Paget's disease, occasionally more than twenty times normal. This increase in bone turnover correlates well with the increased levels of alkaline phosphatase in the plasma, which are higher in Paget's disease per unit of involved bone than in any other condition. Although bone resorption may be increased markedly, organic phosphate ions from the inorganic mineral phase of bone, reutilization of these ions for new bone formation, and presumably, feedback control of parathyroid hormone secretion, usually maintain the concentration of calcium ions in the plasma at normal levels. The concentration of phosphate in the plasma is normal or slightly elevated. When marked imbalance of bone formation and resorption occurs in favor of resorption, such as after prolonged immobilization or fractures, urinary calcium excretion may be increased, and rarely hypercalcemia may be encountered. Bone resorption involves the organic phase as well as the mineral phase. The organic matrix consists largely of collagen which has a high content of the amino acid hydroxyproline. Since hydroxyproline is not reutilized in collagen biosynthesis, some of the hydroxyproline released from matrix in resorption is excreted in the urine, mostly in the form of small peptides. In Paget's disease, therefore, it is not surprising that increased urinary excretion of these hydroxyproline peptides is regularly observed. The rate of urinary hydroxyproline excretion correlates well with the level of plasma alkaline phosphatase and the rate of bone turnover as measured by isotope techniques. In general, these three indices also correlate both with the extent and the activity of the disease. Rarely will isolated involvement of a small bone result in a markedly elevated phosphatase level.

Radiologic Changes

The radiologic findings in Paget's disease reflect the underlying pathology. Cystic or honeycombed radiolucency is characteristic of the lytic phase, whereas uniform increased density with "expansion" of the involved bone is characteristic of the sclerotic phase. Deformity with bowing is often seen in the long bones, which also may show dense, parallel trabeculations. Thickening of the cortex of the long bones is usually noted on the convex side of the curve. In the long bones the disease usually starts at one end and proceeds to the other, occasionally seen as a V-shaped advancing edge followed closely by the invasion of new pagetic bone. In the skull, the outer table is often thickened with irregular increases in bone density. One form of the disease, *osteoporosis circumscripta,* which describes the lesion in the skull, is characterized by rarefied cystlike defects, often with little evidence of new bone formation. Paget's disease is spotty in the extent of its involvement and often asymmetrical, and even in cases with the most widespread disease, some areas of some bones are completely spared. The pelvic bones are most commonly involved, followed by the femur, skull, tibia, lumbosacral spine, dorsal spine, clavicles, and ribs in that order. Small bones are not as frequently diseased, although typical pagetic bone has been described in the footplate removed during stapedectomy. Some of the changes in remodeling in pagetic bone may be related to the stresses produced by muscle pull or gravity, such as the characteristic lateral bowing of the femora or the anterior bowing of the tibiae.

Clinical Picture

The clinical presentation of patients with Paget's disease is extremely variable and is a function of the extent of the disease, the particular bones involved, and the presence of associated complications. Many patients are asymptomatic. In these individuals the disorder is discovered because of radiologic findings during the course of examination of the pelvis or spine for an unrelated disease or complaint, or because of the finding of an elevated level of plasma alkaline phosphatase. Other individuals may gradually become aware of a swelling or deformity of a long bone or develop a disturbance in gait due to unequal length of and change in the distribution of mechanical forces in the lower extremities. Enlargement of the skull is usually not noticed by the patient, who does not usually pay much attention to increasing hat size. However pain in the face and headache has been an initial complaint in some patients. Backache and pain in the lower extremities have been encountered frequently. The pain is usually dull, but occasionally shooting or knifelike pains are described. Pain in the lower extremities may be due to fractures, usually incomplete, which occur along the convex lateral surface of the femora or the anterior surface of the tibia. Pain may also be due to involvement of the hip joint resembling degenerative joint disease and characterized by narrowing of the joint space, bony lipping at the margin of the acetabulum, and deepening of the acetabulum. Angioid streaks of the retina have been observed in patients with Paget's disease. Hearing loss, usually of the nerve deafness type in patients with Paget's disease, is also common and is believed to be related to involvement of the temporal bone. More serious neurologic complications can result from overgrowth of pagetic bone at the base of the skull (platybasia) due to compression of the brainstem. Compression of the spinal cord and paraplegia has been observed, particularly with involvement of the middorsal spine. Pathologic fractures of vertebrae have also produced spinal cord lesions.

Complications

The increased vascularity of the bones involved with Paget's disease in the active, destructive phase is responsible for the increased warmth noted through the skin over such bones. When the disease is widespread, involving over one-third of the skeleton, the increased blood flow through the involved skeleton may be associated with *high cardiac output.* In the rare patient with Paget's disease at this stage so-called "high output heart failure" may result. However, heart disease in pagetic individuals is usually accounted for by the same conditions that occur in other patients of similar age. Pathologic fracture is a frequent complication in patients with Paget's disease, usually occurring in bones involved in the destructive phase of the disease. In the weight-bearing bones fractures are often incomplete, multiple, and on the convex side of the bone. They may occur spontaneously or follow only slight trauma and result in pain but heal spontaneously and result in no major disability. More serious fractures may also occur. Under these circumstances the fracture itself or immobilization accompanying the fracture may upset the delicate balance between bone formation and resorption in favor of resorption. At this stage the imbalance may be reflected in increases in urinary calcium excretion and in rare instances the serum calcium level may rise to dangerous levels.

There is no characteristic level of urinary calcium excretion in Paget's disease, although there is a tendency for calcium excretion to be higher at any point in the disease when the resorptive phase predominates. This may be a factor which accounts for the somewhat higher incidence of *urinary stone* in patients with Paget's disease, although many of the urinary calculi reported in such patients may be unrelated to the Pagetic process.

Sarcoma is the most dreaded complication of Paget's disease. Fortunately, the incidence is low, probably no greater than 1 to 2 percent, although higher incidence has been noted in some series which include many patients with polyostotic involvement. The sarcomas most frequently arise in the femur, humerus, skull, face, and pelvis, and rarely in the vertebra. In about 20 percent the tumors are multicentric. Histologically, they are usually osteosarcomas, although fibrosarcomas and chondrosarcomas have also been found. Increase in pain and swelling are the most common complaints which lead to recognition of the sarcomas. The level of alkaline phosphatase in the serum of the patients with sarcomas reflects the activity and extent of the Paget's disease, although in occasional patients an "explosive rise" of the phosphatase level may accompany the growth of the sarcoma. However, in some patients with limited involvement, phosphatase levels may be only slightly elevated and give no clue to the development of the malignant lesion. The prognosis is extremely poor following the development of sarcomas and ablative operative therapy is rarely curative.

As previously mentioned, immobilization of the patient with Paget's disease upsets the equilibrium between bone formation and resorption in favor of resorption. The increment in calcium released from bone and not reutilized in the formation of new bone may then be excreted in the urine. Rarely, under these circumstances, *hypercalcemia* may occur as well with resulting anorexia, nausea, vomiting, dehydration, renal insufficiency, and even death if untreated.

Therapy

There is no specific therapy of Paget's disease. Acetylsalicylic acid is an effective analgesic, and if it can be tolerated in large enough doses (3.6 to 4.0 Gm per day) for period of months or years, there may be some suppression of the disease activity, as shown by decreases in the level of alkaline phosphatase in the serum and decreased urinary excretion of hydroxyproline. Indo-

methacin, 25 mg t.i.d., may also relieve pain, especially in the presence of hip involvement. Corticosteroids will suppress the disease but only in large doses (greater than 60 mg per day of prednisone) which are usually not tolerated and, therefore, are not recommended. It is of interest, however, that the high cardiac output of some patients with Paget's disease may be reduced significantly after only a few days of such treatment. Although the use of sodium fluoride (10 mg fluoride ion) for greater than a year has produced amelioration of symptoms and decrease in the indices of activity of the disease, the use of this drug is still experimental. Orthopedic procedures also have a role in the management of selected cases. Mold arthroplasty may be helpful in the individual with severe hip involvement, and osteotomy is useful to correct marked bowing deformities. In patients with fractures or orthopedic procedures or in patients immobilized for any reason, determinations of urinary and serum calcium levels should be performed at intervals to anticipate the development of hypercalcuria and hypercalcemia. Early ambulation and adequate fluid intake are essential. Preparations of sodium phytate or inorganic phosphate to reduce hypercalcuria may also be useful under these circumstances (Fleet's Phospho-soda, 4 cc t.i.d.).

REFERENCES

Avioli, L., and M. Berman: Role of Magnesium Metabolism and the Effects of Fluoride Therapy in Paget's Disease of Bone, J. Clin. Endocrinol., 28:700, 1968.

Jaffe, H. L.: Paget's Disease of Bone, Arch. Pathol., 15:83, 1933.

McKenna, R. J., C. P. Schwinn, K. Y. Soong, and N. L. Higinbotham: Osteogenic Sarcoma Arising in Paget's Disease, Lancet, 17:42, 1964.

Nagant deDeuxchaisnes, C., and S. M. Krane: Paget's Disease of Bone: Clinical and Metabolic Observations, Medicine, 43:233, 1964.

Reifenstein, E. C., Jr., and F. Albright: Paget's Disease: Its Pathologic Physiology and the Importance of this in the Complications Arising from Fracture and Immobilization, New Engl. J. Med., 231:343, 1944.

Steinbach, H. L.: Some Roentgen Features of Paget's Disease, Am. J. Roentgenol., 86:950, 1961.

382　NEOPLASMS OF BONE
Stephen M. Krane

Histology

Primary neoplasms of the skeletal system reflect in their histologic characteristics the cellular and extracellular components of the skeleton. However, it is not always possible to prove that a tumor arises from the same type of tissue that it produces. The precursor cell of bone tissue is the osteoprogenitor cell which may be transformed by modulation into the specialized cells of bone tissue: the osteoblast, osteocyte, and osteoclast. These cells can also modulate back to the osteoprogenitor cell. In addition to the normal pathway of modulation, under certain conditions osteoprogenitor cells may be transformed into nonosteogenic cells such as chondroblasts and fibroblasts. Each of these cells can produce its characteristic extracellular matrix, and neoplasms arising from them may thus be recognized. Primary neoplasms of bone can arise also from hematopoietic, vascular, and neural elements.

Pathophysiology

Tumors in bone produce some resorption of normal skeletal tissue by (1) production of substance(s) that can lyse bone, (2) inducing modulation of cells of the osteogenic series into cells involved in the process of resorption, such as osteoclasts, and (3) interfering with blood supply. Tumors will also produce some reaction in surrounding bone and alter the normal contour. The epiphyseal plate, articular cartilage, cortex, and periosteum of bone often offer a barrier to the spread of neoplastic tissue. Alteration of the contour of the cortex is not due to "expansion" of this region but to remodeling of the bone in the area and formation of new bone with the new contour. Some tumors induce primarily an osteoplastic or sclerotic reaction in surrounding bone, which results in increased radiodensity. Primary neoplasms may appear as less radiopaque than surrounding bone or more radiopaque, depending upon the degree of calcification or ossification of the matrix and the density of the tissue. Bone tumors are recognized because of (1) the presence of a mass in the soft tissues, (2) deformity of a bone, (3) pain and tenderness, and (4) pathologic fractures. Tumors of bone may also be detected incidentally on roentgeongrams obtained for other clinical reasons.

There are numerous pitfalls in the clinical diagnosis and interpretation of histologic features of tumors of bone. Management of the patient therefore requires cooperation of experts in various disciplines. For example, the expert pathologist in interpreting the histologic appearance of a bone tumor will not do so without examining the roentgenogram of the tumor from that patient with the assistance of an experienced radiologist.

Benign Tumors

Tumors of bone may be considered as benign or malignant. The most common benign tumors are *osteochondromas* (exostoses) and chondromas (which may be multiple in Ollier's disease), benign giant-cell tumors, and fibromas. As a rule the benign tumors are not painful except for osteoid osteomas, benign chondroblastomas, and benign chondromyxoidfibroma. The usual clinical problem is that of slowly progressing mass and deformity. Treatment is usually accomplished by removal of the tumor and/or curettage and bone grafting.

Malignant Tumors

The most common malignant tumor of bone is multiple myeloma, which arises from hematopoietic cells. Reticulum cell sarcoma also may be a primary bone tumor. Malignant tumors of nonhematopoietic origin include chondrosarcomas, osteosarcomas, fibrosarcomas, Ewing's tumor, malignant giant-cell tumor, and chondromas. *Osteogenic sarcoma* arises presumably from the osteoprogenitor cell and usually contains some osteoid tissue at least in small foci. Some tumors in addition contain cartilaginous and fibrous elements as well as show a wide variation in their histopathology. They are most common in the second and third decade and are rare under the age of ten or over the age of forty years. When they do occur in older individuals, some predisposing cause is present such as Paget's disease or prior radiation therapy. In primary osteogenic sarcomas the lesions arise usually in the metaphyseal region of long bones, especially in the distal femur and the proximal tibia. The most common symptoms are pain and swelling present for weeks or months. The roentgenographic appearance is a function of the amount of ossification or calcification present. Tumors may be predominantly lytic or sclerotic but most often exhibit a combination of these processes. Destruction of the cortex of the bone is usually noted by the time the sarcoma is recognized. High plasma alkaline phosphatase levels are often present in those sarcomas that are predominantly osteogenic and the level of this activity parallels the course of the tumor. When lesions are adequately treated by amputation or radiation, the level of alkaline phosphatase falls, and when metastases appear, the level rises again, often reaching values higher than those present initially. When values are initially very high, the course is often rapidly fatal. Metastases occur primarily by the hematogenous route especially to the lung. Osteogenic sarcomas are relatively radio-resistant, and although some use radiotherapy as an adjacent to primary ablative treatment, i.e., amputation, the mortality is extremely high even when treatment is promptly instituted.

Chondrosarcomas are clinically distinguishable from osteogenic sarcomas. In contrast to the latter, chondrosarcomas arise usually in adulthood and old age, with the peak incidence in the fourth, fifth, and sixth decades. Most are located in the pelvic girdle, ribs, and upper ends of the femur and humerus and are rare in the distal portions of the extremities. Chondrosarcomas may also arise by malignant transformation of osteochondromas. As a rule chondrosarcomas are slow growing and slow to recur. Radiographically the lesions appear as destructive, with mottled increases in radiodensity which reflect the variable degree of calcification and even ossification. Radical excision is the treatment of choice.

Ewing's tumor is a malignant sarcoma composed of small round cells which occurs most frequently in the first 3 decades of life. Most are located in long bones in any portion, although any bone may be involved. Ewing's sarcoma is a highly malignant lesion with an extremely low incidence of cure whether by ablative surgery or irradiation.

Tumors Metastatic to Bone

The skeleton is one of the most common sites of metastases from carcinomas and sarcomas. Skeletal metastases may be relatively silent or may produce symptoms by the same mechanism that primary tumors do, i.e., pain, swelling, deformity of a bone, encroachment on hematopoietic tissue in the marrow, and pathologic fractures. In addition, rapidly lytic skeletal metastases can result in hypercalcemia and in some instances renal insufficiency secondary to the hypercalcemia. The bones involved most commonly are the vertebras, proximal femur, pelvis, ribs, sternum, and proximal humerus in that order of frequency.

Malignant cells reach the skeleton via the bloodstream. Those that survive may proliferate and distort the normal architecture, probably by production of substances which cause dissolution of the mineral phase and the organic matrix. Osteolysis may also result from stimulation of modulation of osteoclasts from osteoprogenitor cells in the surrounding bone. Parathyroid hormonlike polypeptides and osteolytic sterols are substances which may be formed by some malignant tumors. Examples of carcinomatous metastases which are usually predominantly osteolytic are those arising from thyroid, kidney, and lower bowel. Other tumors induce an osteoblastic response in which the new bone arises from skeletal cells and not the tumor itself. The resulting lesion may appear more dense than the surrounding tissue. Occasionally the increase in radiodensity is uniform, simulating osteosclerosis. Carcinoma of the prostate characteristically produces osteoblastic metastases. Carcinoma of the breast produces both osteolytic and osteoblastic metastases. As a rule, osteolytic metastases are the ones which produce hypercalcemia, hypercalcuria, and increased hyproxyprolinuria (reflecting matrix destruction) and are associated usually with normal or slightly increased levels of serum alkaline phosphatase. Osteoblastic metastases, on the other hand, are often accompanied by hyperphosphatasia and may even be associated with hypocalcemia. With some metastases (such as in carcinoma of the breast) there may be phases in which osteolysis predominates (with hypercalcuria, hypercalcemia, and normal alkaline phosphatase levels) alternating with phases in which alkaline phosphatase levels rise and the skeletal lesions become more sclerotic.

Treatment of skeletal metastases is usually palliative. In the case of slowly growing localized lesions such as in some instances of carcinoma of the thyroid or occasionally in carcinoma of the kidney, local radiation is useful to relieve pain or reduce compression of surrounding structures. Many patients, for example, with carcinomas of breast or prostate will survive for years even after extensive skeletal metastases are recognized. Castration and estrogen therapy will slow the progress of the lesions in patients with metastatic prostatic carcinoma. When patients with mammary cancer are treated with estrogens or androgens, the character of the reaction to the metastases may temporarily shift from a predominantly osteoplastic to a lytic phase with resultant hypercalcemia. It is also important to recognize that hypercalcemia in patients with malignant tumors is not due solely to skeletal metastases, although this is the most common situation. Production of parathyroid hormone-like polypeptides by extraskeletal neoplasms may also result in elevation of serum calcium levels. In the latter hypophosphatemia is often encountered whereas in the hypercalcemia associated with skeletal metastases serum phosphorous levels are normal or elevated. Hypercalcemia per se, whether spontaneous or induced by therapy, may produce symptoms such as anorexia, polyuria, polydipsia, depression, and eventually coma. In addition nephrocalcinosis can result from hypercalcemia and death may result from renal insufficiency. Treatment of hypercalcemia of any cause is discussed elsewhere (see Chap. 90).

REFERENCES

Baker, W. H.: Abnormalities in Calcium Metabolism in Malignancy; Effect of Hormone Therapy, Am. J. Med., 21: 714, 1956.

Dahlin, D. C.: "Bone Tumors," pp. 1–224, Springfield, Ill., Charles C Thomas, Publisher, 1957.

Jaffe, H. L.: "Tumors and Tumorous Conditions of the Bones and Joints," pp. 1–629, Philadelphia, Lea & Febiger, 1958.

Lafferty, F. W.: Pseudohyperparathyroidism, Medicine, 45: 247, 1966.

Lichtenstein, L.: "Bone Tumors," p. 411, St. Louis, The C. V. Mosby Company, 1965.

Ross, F. G. M.: Osteogenic Sarcoma, Brit. J. Radiol., 37:259, 1964.

383 HYPEROSTOSIS
Stephen M. Krane

A number of disease states have in common an increase in the mass of bone per unit volume (hyperostosis). Such increase in bone mass is detected radiologically as increase in the density of the bone, often associated with a variable degree of disturbance in the architecture of the tissue. The additional bone may be located at the periosteum, in the Haversian systems, or in the trabeculae of the cancellous regions. When immature bone of woven- or coarse-fibered type is laid down at the periosteum or trabecula, the spongy bone becomes more dense, with encroachment upon the medullary spaces. Such a response may be seen in areas adjacent to tumors or in association with infection. In some diseases the increase in bone mass may be spotty, as in osteopoikilosis, whereas in others most of the skeleton may be involved, such as in the malignant form of osteopetrosis in children. The mechanism of the increase in mass is usually not due to an abnormal increase in the ratio of mineral to matrix, except in some disorders such as osteopetrosis where islands of calcified cartilage may persist. (The mineral density of calcified cartilage is greater than that of bone.) In most of these disorders it is not possible to distinguish whether the increase in bone mass is due to excessive formation of new bone or decreased resorption of bone already formed. In some diseases such as in the osteosclerosis of renal insufficiency, although the bone mass may be increased, the new bone formed may be poorly mineralized, with widened osteoid seams. However, despite this defective mineralization of the trabeculae, the increased mass results in increased radiodensity.

A classification of hyperostosis is given in Table 383-1.

Table 383-1. CAUSES OF HYPEROSTOSIS

  I. Endocrine disorders
     A. Healing phase of osteitis fibrosa cystica
     B. Hypothyroidism
     C. Acromegaly
 II. Radiation osteitis
III. Chemical poisoning
     A. Fluoride
     B. Elemental phosphorus
     C. Beryllium
     D. Arsenic
     E. Vitamin A intoxication
     F. Lead
     G. Bismuth
 IV. Osteomalacic disorders
     A. Renal tubular osteomalacia (vitamin D resistance or phosphate diabetes)
     B. Chronic renal glomerular failure
  V. Osteosclerosis (localized) associated with chronic infection
 VI. Osteosclerotic phase of Paget's disease
VII. Osteosclerosis associated with carcinomatous metastases and with malignant lymphoma
VIII. Osteosclerosis of erythroblastosis fetalis
 IX. Unclassified diseases
     A. Osteopetrosis (marble bone disease of Albers-Schönberg)
     B. Pycnodysostosis
     C. Osteomyelosclerosis
     D. Hyperostosis corticalis generalisata
     E. Hyperostosis generalisata with pachydermia
     F. Progressive diaphyseal dysplasia (osteopathia hyperostotica multiplex infantilis; Camurati-Engelmann disease)
     G. Melorheostosis
     H. Osteopoikilosis
     I. Hyperostosis frontalis interna

Several of these conditions will be discussed in more detail in other chapters, although some general comments are pertinent. Bone that is denser than normal may be seen occasionally in the osteitis fibrosa associated with active hyperparathyroidism. Furthermore, when the hyperparathyroidism is successfully treated, bone resorption is decreased abruptly out of proportion to the rate of bone formation and may lead to the production of areas of bone of density greater than in surrounding skeleton, especially in the healing of brown tumors. In hypothyroidism, both the rates of bone formation and resorption may be decreased, but the balance may be in favor of formation, resulting in bones that are of increased density but with an architecture that is not disturbed. The occurrence of increased bone density in renal tubular abnormalities associated with osteomalacia has been appreciated only recently. The increased mass of bone, however, is associated with widened osteoid seams, similar to the findings in chronic renal glomerular insufficiency. In the vertebral bodies the bone appears denser in transverse bands at the upper and lower margins with a relatively radiolucent center. This "sandwich" appearance is similar to that seen in some patients with osteopetrosis and has been termed by the British the "rugger jersey sign."

Osteopetrosis

Osteopetrosis (marble bone disease of Albers-Schönberg) is a rare disease which in its severe form probably has an autosomal recessive form of inheritance. The so-called "malignant" variant starts in utero and progresses rapidly with marked anemia, hepatosplenomegaly, hydrocephalus, cranial nerve involvement, and death, often due to infection. A less fulminant form may be seen in which the anemia is not as severe, and neurologic abnormalities are not as frequent, but in which recurrent pathologic fractures are the main feature. Although the majority of cases are in infants and children, many are discovered first in adult life when roentgenograms are obtained because of fractures or unrelated diseases. There is no particular predilection for either sex.

The increased bone mass is generally thought to be due to a failure of normal remodeling of bone. Osteoclasts are decreased in number, and there is little evidence of bone resorption. Islands of calcified cartilage which have not been resorbed but are encased in bone may be seen. In addition to the defect in remodeling of calcified cartilage, there is also a defect in remodeling of bone resulting in thickened cortices and lack of funnelization of the metaphyses. Despite the density of the bone it is abnormal mechanically and fractures readily. Osteomalacia or rickets is usually seen in osteopetrosis in children.

The histologic changes are reflected in the roentgenograms, which reveal uniformly dense, sclerotic bone often without distinction between the cortical and cancellous regions. The long bones are usually involved with increased density along the entire shaft. Foci of increased density may be seen in the epiphyses corresponding to regions of unresorbed calcified cartilage. The metaphyses have a characteristic clubbed or splayed appearance. Horizontal bandings of increased density are seen in the long bones alternating with zones of decreased density, suggesting that the defect may be intermittent during periods of growth. The skull, pelvis, ribs, vertebra, and other bones may also be involved. The phalanges and the distal humerus may appear normal when the disease is not severe.

Encroachment upon the marrow cavity is associated with anemia of the myelophthisic type with foci of extramedullary hematopoiesis in liver, spleen, and lymph nodes, with enlargement of these organs. Neurologic abnormalities are associated with encroachment on cranial nerves, which may result in optic atrophy, nystagmus, papilledema, exophthalmos, and impairment of extraocular motility. Facial paralysis and deafness are frequent; trigeminal lesions and anosmia have also been described. In infants with severe disease, macrocephaly, hydrocephalus, and convulsions may occur. Infections such as osteomyelitis are frequent in these children.

Fractures are a common complication even with trivial trauma. Healing of such fractures is usually satisfactory although delayed union may occur. When the disease is first manifested in adult life, fractures may be the only clinical problem. Levels of calcium and alkaline phosphatase in the plasma are usually normal in adults, although in children hypophosphatemia and occasionally moderate hypocalcemia have been noted. The mechanism of the skeletal abnormality in osteopetrosis is not known. However, a process resembling osteopetrosis has been described in the so-called "gray-lethal" strain of mice. These animals also have an increased number of parafollicular cells in their thyroid glands and hypocalcemia. Since these cells produce thyrocalcitonin, a hormone that produces hypocalcemia and hypophosphatemia by decreasing bone resorption (see Chap. 91), the speculation has been offered that thyrocalcitonin production or release may be excessive in osteopetrosis. Attempts have been made to restrict calcium intake to stimulate bone resorption. Despite the extramedullary hematopoiesis that has been found in the spleen, splenectomy can occasionally decrease erythrocyte destruction in this organ and increase the life-span of the erythrocytes.

Pycnodysostosis

Pycnodysostosis is a disorder which resembles osteopetrosis but is a more benign condition not associated with hepatosplenomegaly, anemia, or cranial nerve involvement. In addition to a generalized increase in bone density, features of the disease include short stature, separated cranial sutures, hypoplasia of the mandible, persistence of deciduous teeth, and partial aplasia of the terminal phalanges. Longevity is not decreased, and the patient usually presents to the physician because of frequent fractures. Pycnodysostosis is inherited as a mendelian recessive trait. It has been suggested from karyotope analysis that the gene which determines this disorder is located on the short arm of a small accrocentric chromosome.

Osteomyelosclerosis

Osteomyelosclerosis is a disorder in which the marrow cells are replaced by diffuse fibroplasia, occasionally accompanied by osseous metaplasia. When the latter is prominent, increased skeletal density is seen on roentgenograms. Osteomyelosclerosis is probably a phase in the course of the myeloproliferative disorders and is characteristically accompanied by extramedullary hematopoiesis. A disease distinct from those described above has been termed *hyperostosis corticalis generalisata* (van Buchem's disease). It is characterized by osteosclerosis of the skull (base and calvarium), lower jaw, clavicles, and ribs, with hyperplasia of the diaphyseal cortex of the long and short bones. Alkaline phosphatase levels in the serum are elevated, and histologic observations have suggested that the process is due to increased formation of bone of normal structure. The major clinical manifestations are due to neural compression and consist of optic atrophy, facial paralysis, and perception deafness. In *hyperostosis generalisata with pachydermia* (Uehlinger), the sclerosis involves metaphyses, diaphyses, and epiphyses due to increased formation of subperiosteal spongy bone. Pain and swelling of joints and thickening of the skin of the lower arms are common.

Progressive Diaphyseal Dysplasia

A disorder in which a symmetrical osteosclerosis occurs, usually limited to the diaphyses of the long bones, especially the femurs and tibiae, has been termed *progressive diaphyseal dysplasia* (Camurati-Engelmann disease). The alkaline phosphatase levels are normal. Pain in the legs, fatigue, abnormal gait, and muscle wasting are the major manifestations.

Melorheostosis

Melorheostosis is a rare condition which begins usually in childhood, characterized by areas of sclerosis that appear in the bones of one limb. All segments of the bone may be involved, with the dense structures appearing as sclerotic areas which have a "flowing" distribution. The involved limb is often extremely painful.

Osteopoikilosis

Osteopoikilosis is a benign disorder usually discovered by chance and is not associated with symptoms. It is characterized by dense spots of trabecular bone less than a centimeter in diameter, usually of uniform density, that are located in the epiphyses and adjacent parts of the metaphyses. All bones may be involved except the skull, ribs, and vertebras.

Hyperostosis Frontalis Interna

Hyperostosis frontalis interna is an abnormality of the inner table of the frontal bones of the skull first described by Morgagni and consisting of smooth, rounded enostoses covered by dura and projecting into the cranial cavity. These enostoses are usually less than 1 cm at their greatest diameter and usually do not extend posteriorly beyond the coronal suture. The abnormality is found almost exclusively in women, who are frequently obese, hirsute, and who have a variety of neuropsychiatric complaints (Morgagni-Stewart-Morel syndrome). However, hyperostosis frontalis interna has also been seen in women with no obvious illness or particular associated disease. There is no good evidence that the finding in the skull is a manifestation of a generalized metabolic disorder.

REFERENCES

Collins, D. H., and O. G. Dodge: "Pathology of Bone," pp. 1–254, London, Butterworth & Co. (Publishers), Ltd., 1966.

Dent, C. E., J. M. Smellie, and L. Watson: Studies in Osteopetrosis, Arch. Dis. Child., 40:7, 1965.

Elmore, S. M., W. E. Nance, B. J. McGee, M. Engel-deMontmollin, and E. Engel: Pycnodysostosis, with a Familial Chromosome Anomaly, Am. J. Med., 40:273, 1966.

Follis, R. H., Jr.: A Survey of Bone Disease, Am. J. Med., 22:469, 1957.

Hinkel, C. L., and D. D. Beiler: Osteopetrosis in Adults, Am. J. Roentgenol., 74:46, 1955.

Van Buchem, F. S. P., H. N. Hadders, J. F. Hansen, and M. G. Woldring: Hyperostosis Corticalis Generalisata, Am. J. Med., 33:387, 1962.

384 OTHER DISORDERS OF BONE AND CARTILAGE

Stephen M. Krane

FIBROUS DYSPLASIA
(Albright's Syndrome)

Albright and his associates, in 1937, described a syndrome characterized by "osteitis fibrosa disseminata, areas of pigmentation and endocrine dysfunction, with precocious puberty in females." It was subsequently recognized that the bony lesions, called *fibrous dysplasia*, may occur in the absence of the other features of Albright's syndrome. The fundamental nature of the osseous disorder is unknown; the disease does not appear to be heritable. The frequency of the disease is approximately the same in both sexes.

Incidence

In approximately one-quarter of a large series of patients with fibrous dysplasia the skeletal lesions were monostotic in their distribution, whereas in the remainder polyostotic lesions were described. In the patients with solitary bone involvement the majority of the lesions were in craniofacial bones and ribs. Other features of the syndrome were usually absent in these subjects. In contrast, the polyostotic lesions occur in almost every bone occasionally including over 50 percent of the skeleton, although involvement of the lower extremities is espe-

cially frequent; whereas unilateral involvement is occasionally striking, bilateral involvement does occur. Approximately one-half of the females with the polyostotic form have abnormal pigmentation and sexual precocity. Abnormal pigmentation is also seen in about one-half of the males.

Pathology

The lesions of polyostotic fibrous dysplasia are of uniform reddish gray color and are finely gritty in texture. Microscopically they are composed of fibrous tissue having the appearance typical of fibromata embedded in which are areas of coarse fiber bone with wide osteoid seams. Cement lines are prominent. Mature lamellar bone does not form. Occasionally multiple islands of cartilage and fluid-filled cysts are present. The lesions of monostotic-fibrous dysplasia are similar to those in the polyostotic form except that the cartilage and fluid-filled cysts are not found.

Radiologic Changes

The roentgenographic appearance of the lesions is that of a radiolucent area with a smooth border, which typically is associated with focal thinning of the cortex of the bone. These lesions are not usually cysts in the strict sense, since they are not fluid-filled cavities. They occasionally appear multiloculate. The so-called *ground-glass appearance* reflects the content of the thin, calcified trabeculae of fiber bone. Frequently deformities are present such as coxa vara, shepherd's-crook deformity of the femur, bowing of the tibia, Harrison's grooves, and protusio acetabuli. Involvement of facial bones usually with lesions of increased radiodensity may give rise to a leonine appearance (leontiasis ossea) superficially resembling that seen in some patients with leprosy. Advanced skeletal age may be noted, which in females is correlated with sexual precocity but may also be seen in males without sexual precocity. Although the lesions tend to spare the epiphyseal regions before puberty, in older individuals fibrous dysplasia may develop in the epiphyses.

Clinical Picture

The clinical course is highly variable. Skeletal lesions are usually detected because of deformity or fractures. In some females sexual precocity is the presenting complaint, occasionally present years before the appearance of skeletal symptoms. Serum calcium and phosphorus values are usually normal. In approximately one-third of patients with polyostotic fibrous dysplasia, levels of serum alkaline phosphatase may be elevated in some instances to very high values. In some of these subjects, high cardiac output similar to that seen in extensive Paget's disease may be found. In general, patients with extensive involvement have widespread disease when symptoms first appear whereas with mild disease at the onset extensive disease does not usually develop.

The abnormal cutaneous pigmentation that is seen in

most patients with Albright's syndrome consists of isolated dark-brown to light-brown maculae which tend to remain on one side of the midline. The border is usually, although not always, irregular or jagged ("coast-of-Maine") in contrast to the smooth borders of the pigmented maculae of neurofibromatosis ("coast-of-California"). As a rule there are fewer than six of the lesions, which range in size from 1 cm to ones covering very large areas. When the lesions are present in the scalp, the overlying hair may be more deeply pigmented than that over the remainder of the scalp. There is a strong tendency for the pigmentation to be on the same side and often overlying the skeletal lesions.

The sexual precocity of unknown cause previously mentioned is usually restricted to females, although it has been described rarely in males. Premature vaginal bleeding and development of axillary and pubic hair and of breasts are the main features. In the few ovaries that have been examined histologically no ovulation was seen. Precocious sexuality is not limited to patients with cranial involvement, and although the characteristic pigmented maculae are usually found, this association is not invariable. Another abnormality that is present with high frequency is hyperthyroidism.

Although the lytic lesions of fibrous dysplasia resemble superficially the brown tumors of hyperparathyroidism, the age of the patient, normocalcemia, increased density of bone in the skull, and areas of cutaneous pigmentation identify the former condition. Neurofibroma may involve bone and produce cutaneous pigmentation as well as nodules in the skin. The pigmented maculae of neurofibromatosis are more numerous and more widely distributed than in fibrous dysplasia, usually have smooth borders, and tend to involve areas such as the axillary folds. Other lesions which may have a roentgenographic appearance similar to that of isolated fibrous dysplasia are unicameral bone cysts, aneurysmal bone cysts, and non-ossifying fibromata. So-called "leontiasis ossea" is most often due to fibrous dysplasia, although other causes of hyperostosis may also produce this appearance such as craniometaphyseal dysplasia, hyperphosphatasia, and in adults, Paget's disease.

Treatment

Fibrous dysplasia, when symptomatic, can be managed by a variety of orthopedic operative procedures such as osteotomy, curettage, and bone grafting. Indications for such procedures include progressive deformity, nonunion of fractures, and persistent pain unresponsive to conservative treatment.

DYSPLASIAS AND CHONDRODYSTROPHIES

A variety of diseases of bone and cartilage have been called dystrophies or dysplasias. Classification has been difficult, since the underlying defect is not usually known. It is possible that a biochemical lesion, for example, in the metabolism of the mucopolysaccharides, such as that demonstrated in the Hunter and Hurler syndromes, will also be found in a number of these disorders and permit more than a descriptive classification. However, a useful scheme has been proposed by Rubin based on the consideration of errors in modeling of bone and cartilage as departures from normal development (Table 384-1).

Table 384-1. PROPOSED CLASSIFICATION OF BONE DYSPLASIAS

I. Epiphyseal dysplasias
   A. Epiphyseal hypoplasias
      1. Failure of articular cartilage; spondyloepiphyseal dysplasia, congenita and tarda
      2. Failure of ossification of center: multiple epiphyseal dysplasia, congenita and tarda
   B. Epiphyseal hyperplasia
      1. Excess of articular cartilage: dysplasia epiphysalis hemimelica
II. Physeal dysplasias
   A. Cartilage hypoplasias
      1. Failure of proliferating cartilage: achondroplasia, congenita and tarda
      2. Failure of hypertrophic cartilage: metaphyseal dysostosis, congenita and tarda
   B. Cartilage hyperplasias
      1. Excess of proliferating cartilage: hyperchondroplasia
      2. Excess of hypertrophic cartilage: enchondromatosis
III. Metaphyseal dysplasias
   A. Metaphyseal hypoplasias
      1. Failure to form primary spongiosa: hypophosphatasia, congenita and tarda
      2. Failure to absorb primary spongiosa: osteopetrosis, congenita and tarda
      3. Failure to absorb secondary spongiosa: craniometaphyseal dysplasia, congenita and tarda
   B. Metaphyseal hyperplasia
      1. Excessive spongiosa: familial exostosis
IV. Diaphyseal dysplasias
   A. Diaphyseal hypoplasias
      1. Failure of periosteal bone formation: osteogenesis imperfecta, congenita and tarda
      2. Failure of endosteal bone formation: idiopathic osteoporosis
   B. Diaphyseal hyperplasias
      1. Excessive periosteal bone formation: Engelmann's disease
      2. Excessive periosteal bone formation: hyperphosphatasia

Pathologic processes in the skeletal dysplasias would be expressed as a deficiency (hypoplasia) or excess (hyperplasia) in relation to normal development. Several of the more common of these will be described.

Spondyloepiphyseal Dysplasia (Morquio-Brailsford's Disease)

This is an example of a disorder primarily affecting the epiphysis in the formation of the articular cartilage. This disorder is inherited as an autosomal recessive. In children with the disease, skeletal growth is retarded and the trunk is deformed. Radiologic examination reveals flattening of the vertebral bodies and irregular and deformed epiphyses. Identical skeletal abnormalities have been found in the so-called "Morquio-Ullrich's disease," in which corneal opacities and dental defects are prominent features. However, it is felt by many that the latter abnormalities would be found in all patients with the typical skeletal findings if careful examination were performed. Keratosulfate is excreted in the urine in excessive amounts, and it is likely that a disturbance in the metabolism of this polysaccharide is the underlying problem.

Achondroplasia

Achondroplasia is an example of a physeal dysplasia in which dwarfism results from decrease in the proliferation of cartilage in the growth plate. This disorder of unknown cause is among the more common types of dwarfism. Histologic sections through the growth plate show a thin zone of cartilage cells with absence of the normal columnar arrangement and zone of provisional calcification. Formation of the primary spongiosa is defective. However, formation and maturation of the secondary ossification centers and articular cartilage are not disturbed. Appositional growth at the metaphysis continues, with resulting flare in this region of the bone; intramembranous bone formation at the periosteum is normal. The result of abnormal proliferation at the growth plate, leaving other areas relatively unaffected in the tubular bones, is the production of short bones which are proportionately thick. However, the length of the spine is almost always normal. The appearance of short limbs with a normal trunk is characteristic accompanied by a large head, saddle nose, and an exaggerated lumbar lordosis. The disease is usually recognized at birth. Those who survive the period of infancy have normal mental and sexual development, and longevity may be unimpaired.

Enchondromatosis
(Dyschondroplasia, Ollier's Disease)

This is also a disorder affecting the growth plate in which the hypertrophic cartilage is not resorbed and ossified in a normal fashion. It results in masses of cartilage with disorderly arrangement of the chondrocytes showing variable proliferative and hypertrophic changes. These masses are located in the metaphyses in close association with the growth plate. The disorder is usually recognized in childhood by the appearance of deformities or retardation in growth. The most common sites of involvement are the ends of long bones, usually in that region where rate of growth is most marked. The pelvis is often involved, but bone such as ribs, sternum, and skull are seldom affected. There is also a tendency toward unilateral involvement. Chondrosarcoma develops rarely in the enchondromata. The association of enchondromatosis and cavernous hemangiomata in the soft tissues is known as Maffucci's syndrome.

Multiple exostoses (Diaphyseal Aclasis)

This disorder is probably best considered as an hereditary one of the metaphysis in which areas of the growth plate become displaced and are followed by formation of spongiosa in an abnormal position in relation to the shaft. Usually the growth of these exostoses ceases when growth of the adjacent plate ceases. The lesions may be solitary or multiple and are usually located in the metaphyseal areas of long bones with the apex of the exostosis directed toward the diaphysis. Often the lesions produce no symptoms, but occasionally interference with the function of a joint or tendon or compression of nerves may result. Dwarfing is seen occasionally. The metacarpals may be shortened, resembling that seen in Albright's hereditary osteodystrophy. Indeed, multiple exostoses are sometimes seen in patients with the pseudohypoparathyroid syndrome.

An exostosis may suddenly begin to enlarge long after growth should have ceased, and occasionally, chondrosarcomas develop at the site of an exostosis. Although the exact incidence of this complication is not known, estimates of as high as 7 to 11 percent have been made.

RELAPSING POLYCHONDRITIS

Relapsing polychondritis is an inflammatory disease of cartilaginous structures. The cause is unknown, and although it may occur as a separate entity, it is often associated with other disorders of connective tissue such as rheumatoid arthritis and systemic lupus erythematosus. It may occur at any age, and both sexes are equally affected. The course is commonly a relapsing one with attacks which last from a few days to several months occurring from several times a month to once in several years. The external ear and the cartilage of the nose are the common sites, but other cartilages may also be involved, including those of joints, trachea, larynx, bronchi, costal cartilage, and epiglottis. During an acute attack of a cartilaginous structure such as the ear, there is swelling, redness, pain, and tenderness. Fever and malaise are prominent systemic manifestations. Subsequently the ear may become softened and atrophic. Saddle-nose deformity may result from involvement of the nose; the joint disease resembles rheumatoid arthritis. Ocular involvement with episcleritis, iritis, and conjunctivitis is also seen. During acute attacks the erythrocyte sedimentation rate is usually elevated, and urinary excretion of acid mucopolysaccharides is increased. In the patients with involvement of the tracheobronchial tree respiratory obstruction may result in death if not treated promptly with tracheostomy.

Histologic sections from biopsy or necropsy material have shown diffuse destruction and alteration in the staining properties of the cartilage matrix, focal calcification, metaplastic bone formation, replacement of cartilage with fibrous tissue, and a variable, chronic inflammatory reaction. Salicylates may be helpful in the mild cases, although corticosteroids are indicated in patients with severe involvement. Initial dose of prednisone or its equivalent usually is 30 mg daily with gradual tapering as the clinical signs permit.

TIETZE'S SYNDROME
(Costochondral Syndrome)

Tietze's syndrome is a disorder of unknown cause which is characterized by painful tender swellings of the costochondral junctions. Individuals in the third and fourth decades are most commonly affected, and the disorder is rare before puberty and after the age of sixty. There is no predilection for either sex. Most patients have single episodes involving a single area, with the gradual or sudden onset of pain followed by swelling in the same area. The second costal cartilage on either side is the most common area but almost all of the costochondral articulations have been involved. In some individuals multiple areas are tender in an individual attack. On examination a firm, tender swelling is palpable without warmth or fluctuation. Fever and systemic symptoms are absent, and all laboratory examinations, including the erythrocyte sedimentation rate, are normal. Pain lasts from weeks to months, and swelling lasts for a longer period. When biopsies have been performed, the cartilage appears normal. The disorder is self-limited, and no treatment is indicated except for nerve block and local infiltration with corticosteroids only in those instances where pain is unbearable. The major interest in Tietze's syndrome is that the pain in the anterior chest region may mimic that of myocardial infarction or angina pectoris. Neoplasms and suppurative, rheumatoid, and gouty arthritis may all have to be considered in the differential diagnosis.

REFERENCES

Albright, F., A. M. Butler, and A. D. Hampton: Syndrome Characterized by Osteitis Fibrosa, Disseminate Areas of Pigmentation and Endocrine Dysfunction, with Precocious Puberty in Females. Report of Five Cases, New Engl. J. Med., 216:727, 1937.

Alterman, S. L., and A. L. Lieber: Albright's Hereditary Osteodystrophy. The Effect of Treatment during Adolescence, Ann. Intern. Med., 63:140, 1965.

Benedict, P. H.: Endocrine Features in Albright's Syndrome (Fibrous Dysplasia of Bone), Metabolism, 11:30, 1962.

——, G. Szabo, T. B. Fitzpatrick, and S. J. Sinesi: Melanotic Macules in Albright's Syndrome and in Neurofibromatosis, J.A.M.A., 209:72, 1968.

Burch, G. E., and N. P. dePasquale: Tietze's Disease, Geriatrics, 19:61, 1964.

Harris, W. H., H. R. Dudley, and R. J. Barry: The Natural History of Fibrous Dysplasia. An Orthopaedic, Pathological and Roentgenographic Study, J. Bone Joint Surg., 44A:207, 1962.

Kaye, R. L., and D. A. Sones: Relapsing Polychondritis. Clinical and Pathologic Features in Fourteen Cases, Ann. Intern. Med., 60:653, 1964.

Langer, L. O., Jr., and L. S. Carey: The Roentgenographic Features of the KS Mucopolysaccharidosis of Morquio (Morquio-Brailsford's Disease), Am. J. Roentgenol., 97:1, 1966.

Levey, G. S., and J. J. Calabro: Tietze's Syndrome: Report of Two Cases and Review of the Literature, Arthritis Rheumat., 5:261, 1962.

Rubin, P.: "Dynamic Classification of Bone Dysplasias," pp. 1–410, Chicago, Year Book Medical Publishers, Inc., 1964.

Section 13

Disorders of the Joints

385 APPROACH TO THE PATIENT WITH JOINT DISEASE

Lawrence E. Shulman

TERMINOLOGY. Terms used to designate abnormal conditions of the joints are numerous and ambiguous. *Rheumatism* is a generic designation for pain, stiffness, or deformity of joints, muscles, and related structures. The *rheumatic diseases* include a large group of musculoskeletal disorders characterized by alterations in articular structures (synovium, joint capsule, cartilage, and bone) or in connective tissue surrounding the joints, as in tendons. Because of the prominent involvement of the connective tissue in many of these disorders it has become the custom to designate them as *diseases of connective tissue*. The term *arthritis* is often used to denote any disorder of joints, although it should be restricted to inflammation of the joints. A joint disorder unaccompanied by grossly evident inflammation is frequently called an *arthropathy*. If pain, tenderness, or stiffness originates from a nonarticular structure, such as muscle, tendon, ligament, or bursa, the condition is often labeled *fibrositis*. Whenever possible, more specific terminology, such as *tendinitis* or *bursitis*, should be used.

PREVALENCE. Public health surveys show that more than 14 million persons in the United States suffer from some form of rheumatism, indicating that it is second only to nervous and mental diseases as a cause of chronic illness and disability. Of the 14 million people with rheumatic complaints, 45 percent have arthritis; over 10 percent are partially disabled; and almost 2 percent are completely disabled. More than half the disabled are under forty-five years of age. In other countries, the toll from rheumatic disease is even greater. In Great Britain, for example, half the population have nondisabling rheumatic symptoms, 7 percent are incapacitated for at least 1 day each year, and one-sixth of industrial absences are ascribed to rheumatism. In Switzerland, arthritis is responsible for 16 percent of all sickness reports to insurance companies, and the same proportion of total absence from work. Among the major categories of chronic disease, the rheumatic diseases cripple most and kill least. Much of the disability occurs in young people during the productive years of life.

CLASSIFICATION. A workable and logical classification of joint diseases cannot be constructed satisfactorily on etiologic grounds because the causes of so many disorders are unknown. Separation on the basis of pathologic change is helpful but may actually restrict knowledge because connective tissue can react to injury in only a limited number of ways. Differentiation on clinical grounds alone is similarly unsatisfactory, because widely divergent pathologic processes can give rise to the same clinical picture. Disorders classified as acute arthritides may become chronic, and chronic arthritides may begin acutely or have acute exacerbations.

Most classifications of joint diseases include etiologic, pathologic, and clinical factors. The American Rheumatism Association has now approved a detailed nomenclature, and its use is recommended. The accompanying outline is offered as a useful guide to differential diagnosis because it is based largely on pathogenetic features.

HISTORY. The *age* of the patient contributes to diagnosis but is less important than is commonly believed. In the elderly, arthritis is often assumed to be degenerative joint disease; in the young or middle-aged, rheumatoid arthritis. Actually, the probability of rheumatoid arthritis increases up to the age of fifty-five years, after which it remains stationary; conversely, degenerative joint disease may begin as early as the second decade.

Females are more likely to have Heberden's nodes (10:1), systemic lupus erythematosus (8:1), or peripheral rheumatoid arthritis (2:1), whereas ankylosing spondylitis is decidedly more common in men (9:1).

It is important to know the *occupation* and *avocations* of the arthritic patient. Injury at work or at play gives rise to such conditions as "housemaid's knee," "nurse's feet," "boxer's bursitis," "student's elbow," "baseball fingers," and "weaver's bottom." Trauma can also play an important role in the selection of the sites affected in degenerative joint disease.

Careful attention must also be paid to the *family history*. The family incidence of gout varies from 10 to 18 percent.

"Growing pains" in childhood may direct one's attention to rheumatic fever or juvenile rheumatoid arthritis. Repeated throat infections, especially if known to be of streptococcal origin, point to rheumatic fever. A history of unexplained fever, skin disorders, serositis, and hematologic abnormalities may suggest that the arthritis is merely one manifestation of a collagen disease. Urethritis may precede arthritis and conjunctivitis in Reiter's syndrome or gonorrhea. At times, renal calculi may appear before gouty arthritis. Nephritis may antedate arthralgia in systemic lupus erythematosus. Clearly, a history of trauma to a joint or arthritis in the remote past must be sought, because such an event may be related to the present rheumatoid illness.

CLASSIFICATION OF DISORDERS OF JOINTS

I. Arthritis caused by specific infection
   A. Pyogenic arthritis
      1. Staphylococcus
      2. Streptococcus
      3. Pneumococcus
      4. Gonococcus
      5. Meningococcus
      6. Salmonella
   B. Tuberculosis
      1. Arthritis
      2. Spondylitis (Pott's disease)
   C. Syphilis
      1. Congenital (Clutton's joints)
      2. Acquired (secondary or tertiary)
   D. Viral
      1. Rubella
      2. Mumps
   E. Less-common infectious arthritides
      1. Bacterial
      2. Rickettsial
      3. Fungal
      4. Parasitic
      5. Viral
II. Arthritis possibly caused by specific infection: Reiter's syndrome
III. Arthritis as a sequel to specific infection: rheumatic fever
IV. Arthritis caused by hypersensitivity to foreign agent
   A. Drug reactions
   B. Serum sickness
   C. Anaphylactoid purpura
V. Arthritis in widespread inflammatory disease, cause unknown
   A. Rheumatoid arthritis and variants
      1. Adult peripheral type
      2. Juvenile rheumatoid arthritis (Still's disease)
      3. Felty's syndrome
      4. Sjögren's syndrome
      5. Caplan's syndrome
   B. "Connective tissue" or "collagen" diseases
      1. Systemic lupus erythematosus
      2. Polyarteritis (periarteritis nodosa)
      3. Systemic sclerosis (scleroderma)
      4. Dermatomyositis, polymyositis
   C. Granulomatous reactions
      1. Sarcoidosis
      2. Erthyema nodosum
   D. Others
      1. Ankylosing spondylitis
      2. Psoriatic arthritis
      3. Arthritis of ulcerative colitis, regional ileitis, and Whipple's disease
      4. Familial Mediterranean fever
VI. Arthritis caused by metabolic or endocrine disorders

    A. Gout
    B. Hyperparathyroidism
    C. Ochronosis
    D. Acromegaly
    E. Hypothyroidism
    F. Agammaglobulinemia
    G. Hemophilia
    H. Hemoglobinopathies
    I. Hemochromatosis
    J. Gaucher's disease
    K. Scurvy

VII. Degenerative joint disease (osteoarthritis)
    A. Generalized
    B. Localized
      1. Hereditary (such as Heberden's nodes)
      2. Secondary to previous trauma or infection
      3. Secondary to faulty body mechanics

VIII. Arthritis caused by trauma to joints
    A. Direct trauma
    B. Internal mechanical derangement of joint

IX. Neurogenic arthropathy (Charcot's joint)
    A. Tabes dorsalis
    B. Syringomyelia
    C. Neuropathy of diabetes mellitus
    D. Peripheral nerve injuries
    E. Leprosy

X. Arthritis caused by bleeding into joints
    A. Direct trauma
    B. Disorders of blood coagulation: hemophilia and variants

XI. Neoplasms
    A. Synovioma
    B. Pigmented villonodular synovitis
    C. Giant-cell tumor of tendon sheath
    D. Leukemia
    E. Multiple myeloma
    F. Metastatic

XII. Hypertrophic osteoarthropathy

XIII. Arthritis secondary to lesions of bone
    A. Aseptic necrosis of bone
      1. Primary, of unknown cause
      2. Secondary to
        a. Trauma
        b. Vascular occlusion
    B. Neoplasms of bone
      1. Primary
      2. Metastatic to bone
    C. Osteochondromatosis
    D. Osteochondritis dissecans
    E. Endocrine diseases of bone

XIV. Miscellaneous
    A. Shoulder-hand syndrome
    B. Chondrocalcinosis (pseudogout)
    C. Relapsing polychondritis
    D. Behçet's syndrome
    E. Polymyalgia rheumatica
    F. Erythema multiforme
    G. Reticulohistiocytosis of joints
    H. Tietze's syndrome
    I. Psychogenic rheumatism (hysterical "arthritis")

XV. Para-articular conditions ("nonarticular rheumatism")
    A. "Fibrositis"
    B. Tendinitis and peritendinitis (bursitis)
    C. Tenosynovitis
    D. Tendon sheath cyst (ganglion)
    E. Myositis
    F. Neuritis
    G. Carpal tunnel syndrome
    H. Panniculitis
    I. Intervertebral disk syndromes

Meticulous inquiry into *events immediately preceding the onset* of arthritis may yield clues to diagnosis. An antecedent infection of an organ or of more than one, especially if accompanied by bacteremia, indicates that the arthritis may be infectious. Streptococcal tonsillitis or pharyngitis preceding the arthritis by 1 to 4 weeks strongly suggests rheumatic fever. Prior injections of penicillin or foreign protein, especially if accompanied by fever or urticaria, bring to mind the arthritis of serum sickness. Frequently, rheumatoid arthritis is preceded by overwork, emotional stress, or exposure to a cold, damp environment and is ushered in by constitutional symptoms such as feverishness, malaise, fatigability, anorexia, paresthesias, and weight loss. Constitutional symptoms are not characteristic of degenerative joint disease.

The *mode of onset* of the arthritis should be ascertained. A joint disorder may appear explosively (as in rheumatic fever), subacutely (as in rheumatoid arthritis), or insidiously (as in degenerative joint disease).

It is also important to obtain a full characterization of the patient's joint *pain.* The pain of acute gouty arthritis, for example, is constant and severe and is not influenced by position or time of day. In contrast, the discomfort in degenerative joint disease is usually transient, mild, and superficial; it emerges with attempted movement after a period of rest in one position and disappears readily after brief exercise. In contrast, the patient with rheumatoid arthritis complains of morning stiffness which disappears gradually only after an hour or more, whereas the pains in the affected joints may become more severe as the day progresses.

The patient should also be asked about the occurrence of other signs which reflect articular inflammation, namely, excessive *heat, discoloration of the skin, tenderness,* or *swelling* of the involved joint.

Valuable diagnostic information may come from ascertaining which joint was involved first, i.e., the proximal interphalangeal joint in rheumatoid arthritis, the sacroiliac in anklyosing spondylitis, the distal interphalangeal joint in degenerative joint disease, the great toe in gout, or the shoulder in bursitis. It is important to find out whether the arthritis is *migratory* and, if it is, the nature of its spread. In degenerative joint disease, for example, the sites of arthritic symptoms do not tend to change; whereas migration of the arthritis is characteristic of rheumatic fever (where it is rapid and transient) and of rheumatoid arthritis (where it tends to be slower and additive).

The *course of the disease* may provide additional diagnostic clues. Acute exacerbations with complete remissions are characteristic of the early stage of gout.

Overall progression with partial remissions is the most common course in rheumatoid arthritis; in degenerative joint disease, the illness is usually static or slowly progressive.

The presence and extent of *deformities* and the *functional capacity* of the patient may also aid in diagnosis. Some disorders, such as rheumatoid arthritis, are notoriously deforming and crippling; others, such as rheumatic fever, produce no residual articular disability.

The details of previous management and its effect should be recorded carefully. The daily dose and duration of drug administration are important, because the program may not have been sufficient to constitute a valid therapeutic trial.

PHYSICAL EXAMINATION. All accessible joints should be systematically and meticulously examined for heat or discoloration, swelling, tenderness, limitation of motion, deformity, and crepitation. The *temperature* and *color* of the skin proximal and distal to the joint should be compared with those over the joint. *Swelling* of the joint may result from one or more of the following: (1) the accumulation within the joint space of fluid, demonstrable by fluctuation, as in the "patellar click"; (2) thickening of the soft tissue (synovium, capsule, ligament, or adipose tissue); (3) localized periarticular effusion in a tendon sheath or bursa; (4) diffuse periarticular edema; or (5) bony enlargement, as in acromegaly, tumors of bone, or the osteophytes of degenerative joint disease. It is important to be sure that the joint is really enlarged, since muscle atrophy may give a false impression of joint size. The degree of *tenderness* should be recorded and subsequently interpreted with the help of the sensory examination and an evaluation of the emotional state of the patient.

Limitation of motion may result from (1) muscular spasm or guarding, (2) effusions large enough to distend the capsule, (3) fibrosis of the capsule, (4) fibrosis across the joint space from one synovial surface to another (fibrous ankylosis), (5) bony bridging across the space (bony ankylosis), or (6) various disorders of tendon, muscle, or nerve.

Crepitation, a grating feeling or noise, results from the rubbing together of opposing joint surfaces. The character of crepitation varies: fine, or "rubbing," in rheumatoid arthritis, where the abrasive surface is villous granulation tissue; coarse, or "crunching," from the osteophytes and disorganized cartilage in degenerative joint disease. Crepitation should be distinguished from "cracking" or "snapping," caused by tendons slipping over bony prominences.

A few *instruments* are available for quantifying disability of joints and related structures. Simplest, and perhaps most important, is a tape measure with which the circumference of large joints and certain muscle groups is recorded. It should also be used to measure the chest expansion in patients with ankylosing spondylitis. With a jeweler's ring sizer the size of the smaller joints of the fingers and toes can be determined. A dynamometer or a sphygmomanometer may be used to record grip strength. The range of motion of a joint can be measured with a goniometer. These instruments are especially useful in following the course of illness in studies designed to test the efficacy of a therapeutic agent.

The *functional capacity* of the patient should also be recorded carefully. Can he get out of bed, walk, or climb stairs? Can he comb his hair, tie his shoelaces, unscrew a bottle cap, or sweep the floor?

Organs other than the joints also deserve special attention in the physical examination of the patient with arthritis. These include skin, subcutaneous tissue, eyes, pharynx, lymph nodes, lungs, heart, liver, spleen, muscles, and nerves.

To illustrate, valuable clues to the diagnosis of the joint disorder come from abnormalities of the *skin.* Urticaria points to serum sickness. Petechiae and ecchymoses suggest meningococcemia or a defect of blood coagulation; a "butterfly rash" suggests systemic lupus erythematosus; and erythema marginatum points to rheumatic fever.

The patient complaining of arthritis of the hands may show nothing but diffuse swelling of the skin and subcutaneous tissue as in the early stages of scleroderma. *Subcutaneous nodules* are frequently encountered in patients with various forms of arthritis. Those occurring on the extensor surfaces of the forearms just distal to the elbows are thought to be the hallmark of rheumatoid arthritis, although sarcoid nodules or gouty tophi occasionally occur in the same location. A striking feature of rheumatoid nodules is their symmetry. The nodules in rheumatic fever are transient, less symmetric, softer, and not so frequently near joints; the distribution of those of polyarteritis nodosa and amyloidosis tends to be linear, along the course of affected arteries. The external ears should be carefully searched for gouty *tophi.* Tophi or nodules near joints are usually fixed to the periosteum or the joint capsule. Benign synovial cysts (ganglions) or fatty tumors (lipomas) should not be mistaken for nodules or tophi.

The *ocular examination* may yield useful information in differential diagnosis. Conjunctivitis suggests Reiter's syndrome; keratitis, Sjögren's syndrome or Clutton's joints; uveitis, ankylosing spondylitis or sarcoid; "cytoid bodies," systemic lupus erythematosus; and retinal arterial thromboses, polyarteritis nodosa.

Similar differential diagnostic analyses may be constructed for other extraarticular organs.

LABORATORY TESTS. After a careful history has been recorded and a thorough physical examination performed, the appropriate laboratory studies should be done. In rheumatoid arthritis, rheumatic fever, or sarcoid, anemia may be mild or moderate; in some patients with a collagen disease, it may be more severe. In rheumatoid arthritis, the anemia is typically hypochromic and normocytic, whereas in systemic lupus erythematosus, it is usually normochromic and normocytic but may be hemolytic. The white blood cell count is slightly elevated in serum sickness, rheumatic fever, some cases of active rheumatoid arthritis, certain infections, polyarteritis nodosa, and leukemia. Leukopenia is frequently found in tuberculous arthritis, systemic lupus erythematosus, and sarcoid and, by definition, is a feature of Felty's syndrome.

The erythrocyte *sedimentation rate* is an important laboratory determination in rheumatology. It is particularly useful in (1) the differential diagnosis of early arthritis; (2) estimating the activity of rheumatic fever or rheumatoid arthitis; and (3) determining by serial tests the course of the arthritis and the effect of therapy. The sedimentation rate is usually high in infectious arthritis, serum sickness, acute phases of rheumatic fever, rheumatoid arthritis and its variants, collagen disorders, and acute gouty arthritis. Normal values are recorded in degenerative joint disease, traumatic arthritis, neurogenic arthropathy, "fibrositis," and psychogenic rheumatism.

Serologic tests may also aid in diagnosis. One or more of the standard serologic tests for syphilis (STS) may not only indicate that the patient has one of the several rheumatic sequelae of this infection, but also may suggest the possibility of gonococcal arthritis. If the STS is positive, a more specific treponemal test should also be performed, because many patients with a false positive STS have some form of connective tissue disease. Streptococcal antibody tests help in the diagnosis of rheumatic fever and glomerulonephritis.

Rheumatoid factor tests may be very informative. The sheep cell agglutination test is positive in approximately 75 percent of patients with active peripheral rheumatoid arthritis and in over 90 percent of patients with subcutaneous nodules. It is not entirely specific, and positive tests may be found in patients with other connective tissue diseases and also unrelated disorders. The latex fixation test, especially the commercially available slide test, is even less specific for rheumatoid arthritis but is useful as a screening procedure.

Lupus erythematosus cell preparations should also be made in arthritic patients, especially those in whom the diagnosis is uncertain. The importance of this test becomes clear because arthralgia or arthritis is the presenting manifestation in one-third of patients with systemic lupus erythematosus. Other *antinuclear factor* tests may be useful in screening for certain rheumatic disorders, or in providing greater specificity for systemic lupus erythematosus, as is the case with anti-DNA antibodies.

The serum *complement* level aids in differential diagnosis and is reduced in active systemic lupus, in contrast to normal or elevated levels in other disorders.

Because the rheumatic manifestations of gout are so pleomorphic, all patients with joint complaints should have a blood *uric acid* determination.

Urinalysis and tests of renal function may help in difficult diagnostic situations by focusing attention on the possibilities of Reiter's syndrome, gout, one of the collagen disorders, or amyloidosis secondary to rheumatoid disease.

X-ray findings aid materially when interpreted in the light of clinical and other laboratory information. They should not be considered the final arbiter, however, because different types of arthritis may produce identical roentgenographic changes. Furthermore, even in obviously inflamed joints, the x-ray findings may be totally negative.

Bacteriologic, cytologic, and chemical examination of *synovial fluid* may provide further information of diagnostic and prognostic importance. Normal synovial fluid is scanty, clear, pale yellow, sticky, and relatively acellular. It is essentially a dialysate of plasma. The fluid, which helps to lubricate the articulating surfaces, contains mucin, a protein-polysaccharide complex similar to that found in the ground substance of connective tissue. On the addition of synovial fluid to dilute acetic acid, a tight ropy clot is formed (mucin clot test).

A proper examination of joint fluid should include all tests used in analysis of fluid from other body cavities, i.e., volume, appearance, specific gravity, pH, cell count (including differential count), and concentrations of protein and sugar (with comparative blood levels). Anaerobic and aerobic cultures should be planted immediately and Gram's stain of the centrifuged sediment should be examined. If tuberculosis is suspected, appropriate stains and cultures should be carried out. The mucin clot test should be performed. Because mucin is usually present, the diluting medium for white blood cell counts of joint fluid should consist of physiologic saline solution not acetic acid. Neither inclusion-containing cells nor synovial fluid enzymes have attained diagnostic significance.

Examination with the polarizing microscope may reveal the urate crystals of gout or the calcium pyrophosphate crystals of "pseudogout," either in the synovial fluid leukocytes or free in the fluid itself.

When all the above methods have failed to clarify the diagnostic problem, a synovial *biopsy* may prove useful. In performing biopsies, strict aseptic precautions should be observed. A method of securing punch biopsies of synovial membrane has been introduced, but its usefulness is somewhat limited by the small amount of tissue available for examination. Nevertheless, synovial biopsy can settle diagnostic problems by differentiating gout from rheumatoid arthritis (by revealing urate crystals), or rheumatoid from tuberculous arthritis (by demonstrating acid-fast bacilli). Moreover, biopsy findings have added to the knowledge of the rheumatic diseases by showing, for example, that diseases such as sarcoid and progressive systemic sclerosis (scleroderma) may involve the synovium.

REFERENCES

Bennett, P. H., and P. N. W. Wood (Eds.): "Population Studies of the Rheumatic Diseases," International Congress Series, Excerpta Medica Foundation, 1968.

Cohen, A. S. (Ed.): "Laboratory Diagnostic Procedures in the Rheumatic Diseases," Boston, Little Brown and Company, 1967.

Copeman, W. S. D. (Ed.): "Textbook of Rheumatic Diseases," 3d ed., Baltimore, The Williams & Wilkins Company, 1964.

Decker, J. L., A. J. Bollett, I. F. Duff, L. E. Shulman, and G. H. Stollerman: Primer on Rheumatic Diseases, J.A.M.A., 190:127, 425, 509, 741, 1964.

Dixon, A. S. (Ed.): "Progress in Clinical Rheumatology," Boston, Little Brown and Company, 1965.

Hollander, J. L. (Ed.): "Comroe's Arthritis and Allied Conditions," 7th ed., Philadelphia, Lea & Febiger, 1966.

Kellgren, J. H. (Ed.): "Epidemiology of Chronic Rheumatism," vol. 1, Philadelphia, F. A. Davis Company, 1963.

Rheumatism Reviews, First through Sixteenth: Ann. Intern. Med., vols. 8–15, 28, 39, 45, 50, 53, 56, 59, 61, 1935–1964; Seventeenth and Eighteenth: Arthritis & Rheum., vols. 7, 11, 1966, 1968.

Ropes, M. W., and W. Bauer: "Synovial Changes in Joint Disease," Cambridge, Harvard University Press, 1953.

386   RHEUMATOID DISEASE

Lawrence E. Shulman

DEFINITION. Rheumatoid arthritis (also *atrophic arthritis, chronic proliferative arthritis, chronic infectious arthritis*) is a systemic disorder of unknown cause in which symptoms and inflammatory change predominate in articular and related structures. The disease tends to be chronic and to produce characteristic, crippling deformities.

EPIDEMIOLOGY. According to several surveys in temperate countries, the incidence of rheumatoid arthritis among those fifteen years of age or older is approximately 1 percent for "definite" rheumatoid arthritis and 3 percent for "probable" rheumatoid arthritis. A large proportion of patients become incapacitated; in one study, 58 percent were unable to carry out their ordinary occupations or duties.

The disease may begin at any time from infancy through the ninth decade. In the United States the onset of the disease is most frequent in the fourth decade.

It is generally held that the disease is three times as common in women as in men, but this does not apply at all ages; in older patients, if more definite criteria such as roentgenographic changes are used, neither sex predominates. There is no racial predisposition.

Earlier studies seemed to show a familial tendency in rheumatoid arthritis, presumably on the basis of a genetically determined susceptibility. With improved methodology in family studies, however, the evidence for familial aggregation is less impressive.

Similarly, recent epidemiologic data cast doubt on the dictum that rheumatoid arthritis is more prevalent in cold, damp climates. Detailed studies in a climate chamber have shown that symptoms are more frequent and severe in an environment of high relative humidity and low barometric pressure.

PATHOLOGY. The histologic changes in the joints consist of edema, proliferation of capillaries, fibrosis, and infiltration first by polymorphonuclear leukocytes, then by lymphocytes and plasma cells. There are often areas of "fibrinoid" necrosis. Plasma cells in both synovial membranes and lymph nodes may contain rheumatoid factor.

The consequences are thickening and villous hypertrophy of the synovial membrane, destruction of cartilage and bone, and ankylosis. The layer of granulation tissue, called *pannus*, begins to invade and destroy cartilage. When subchondral granulation is extensive, bony trabeculae may be resorbed. Changes similar to those in the synovial membrane are also found in joint capsules, tendon sheaths, and bursae.

The distinctive *rheumatoid nodule* consists of granulation tissue and foci of fibrinoid necrosis surrounded by palisades of large mononuclear cells. Examination of nodules of recent onset suggests that the primary change is a vasculitis. Nodules are found mainly in the subcutaneous tissue but are occasionally seen in aorta or myocardium and in the lung, especially of coal miners with pulmonary fibrosis (Caplan's syndrome).

Secondary *amyloidosis* has been found at necropsy in 5 to 40 percent of severely affected individuals.

About 10 percent of patients with rheumatoid arthritis have *vasculitis* on muscle biopsy. A smaller proportion have widespread necrotizing *arteritis*.

PATHOGENESIS. It is generally believed that the lesions of the synovium in rheumatoid arthritis are related to immune phenomena in ways not fully understood. According to present concepts, an unidentified antigenic stimulus elicits antibody production by the plasma cells in the synovium. As the antigen-antibody complexes are formed, the antibody is altered, becomes foreign, and stimulates the production of rheumatoid factor by synovial plasma cells and regional lymph nodes. The antigen-antibody complexes may fix complement, and induce phagocytosis and lysosomal release. Lysosomal membranes in rheumatoid synovium are unusually fragile; the released enzymes give rise to tissue damage and inflammation.

Although serum complement in rheumatoid arthritis is normal or occasionally elevated, synovial fluid complement is reduced in active disease. This low synovial fluid complement is associated with anticomplementary activity and the presence of cryoproteins, and seems related more closely to antinuclear factors than to rheumatoid factors.

The role of rheumatoid factors is uncertain. They may, in fact, be protective (rather than pathogenetic) by having the capacity to localize the antigen-antibody complexes. When large amounts of rheumatoid factor are given by repeated transfusion to normal volunteers, no disease ensues. Also, patients with agammaglobulinemia, and little or no rheumatoid factor, have an unusually high incidence of rheumatoid arthritis.

The search for the responsible antigen(s) continues. Numerous attempts to identify a virus have been unsuccessful. Other microorganisms have been found on occasion in rheumatoid synovial fluid, but their specificity for this disease has not been confirmed. An altered protein-polysaccharide has been suggested as an initial antigenic stimulus.

Synovial cells from patients with rheumatoid arthritis grown in tissue culture produce a collagenase which may be responsible for the destruction of articular cartilage in rheumatoid arthritis. The amount of collagenase is related to both systemic activity and synovial cellularity.

CLINICAL FEATURES. In a few patients, the illness is acute and fulminating, with high fever, intense joint inflammation, and the rapid evolution of severe deformities. Ordinarily, however, mild deformities develop insidiously and with only moderate discomfort.

At the onset, symptoms are frequently nonrheumatic and consist of fatigability, anorexia, weight loss, and occasional fever. Only later does the patient notice evanescent aches and pains in muscles and joints.

The majority of patients seeks medical care after *joint pain*, swelling, redness, heat, or deformity has appeared. The knees, hands, and feet are the most common sites involved initially. Rheumatoid arthritis is characteristically polyarticular and migratory in an additive manner. Once affected, a joint tends to remain inflamed for weeks, months, or years. Symmetry of joint involvement is characteristic. Joint deformities are caused by intrinsic articular disease, shortening of tendons, and the muscle imbalance which results from involuntary splinting or from a true myositis. Ulnar deviation of the fingers is a hallmark of rheumatoid arthritis. Other deformities include "swan-neck" deformities of fingers and subluxations of various joints.

Rheumatoid arthritis may involve any diarthrodial joint, including the temporomandibular (impairing mastication), the cricoarytenoid of the larynx (with hoarseness or obstruction, sometimes demanding tracheostomy), and the joints of the cervical spine, with atlantoaxial subluxation threatening cervical cord compression.

The *skin*, especially that of the distal extremities, is cool, pale, and clammy, probably a consequence of digital arterial insufficiency, which has been shown by arteriography. Excessive sweating of palms and soles is characteristic. Over the fingers, the skin appears taut and shiny. Erythema of the hypothenar eminences, "liver palms," is a common finding. *Purpura* and splinter hemorrhages are the consequences of vasculitis.

Subcutaneous nodules, found in 10 to 30 percent of patients, are firm, nontender, round or ovoid masses varying from 2 mm to 2 cm in diameter. They are not fixed to overlying skin, but may be attached to underlying structures, and tend to occur over pressure points and near joints. The most common site is the extensor surface of the forearm just below the elbow. Patients with nodules generally have active, severe diseases. Nodules usually persist for months or years and may be confused with those of other diseases (gout, sarcoid, or xanthomatosis).

Muscle aching, tenderness, and stiffness occur early and are prominent throughout the course. Prolonged morning stiffness is a cardinal feature, important in diagnosis. Muscular atrophy and weakness may be striking.

Of the various *ocular lesions* in rheumatoid arthritis, the most common are keratoconjunctivitis sicca (see Sjögren's Syndrome, further on in this chapter) in 15 percent of patients, and anterior, nongranulomatous uveitis, seen in about 3 percent. Episcleritis and scleritis may also appear, sometimes as nodules; rarely these perforate the sclera and cause extrusion of the uveal tract, a condition called *scleromalacia perforans*.

During active phases of the disease, the lymph nodes may be enlarged to an extent to suggest lymphoma.

Clinical *heart disease* attributable to rheumatoid disease is unusual. This contrasts sharply with the high incidence of granulomatous and fibrotic cardiac lesions reported in postmortem examinations of patients with rheumatoid arthritis.

Other clinical features which are encountered in the course of rheumatoid arthritis include pleuritis (with or without effusion), pneumonitis, splenomegaly, peripheral neuropathy, chronic leg ulcers, Baker's cysts, and leg edema. *Pleural fluid glucose* concentration may be extremely low. *Pulmonary manifestations* include interstitial fibrosis, "honeycomb" lung, and nodules which may cavitate. The *polyneuropathy* and leg ulcers are usually associated with diffuse vasculitis and a poor prognosis. Baker's cysts may extend down to the gastrocnemius; they may rupture and cause calf pain simulating that of thrombophlebitis.

LABORATORY FINDINGS. A moderate normocytic, hypochromic anemia occurs in active rheumatoid arthritis. It does not usually respond to iron therapy, folic acid, or vitamin B_{12}, and splenectomy is ineffective. Transfusion is rarely indicated.

The peripheral leukocyte count is within normal limits in 80 percent of cases. A mild leukocytosis is common in early active disease; a mild leukopenia is sometimes found in older patients. The platelet count may be elevated.

The erythrocyte sedimentation rate is elevated during active disease and is valuable as a rough index of activity. Other nonspecific host factors which may be used to estimate disease activity include C-reactive protein and hyperglobulinemia, with elevations in the IgG, IgA, and IgM immunoglobulin fractions.

Serologic tests for *rheumatoid factor* are positive in 75 percent of adult patients with "classical" or "definite" rheumatoid arthritis, as defined by the criteria of the American Rheumatism Association. Because these tests are almost uniformly negative in rheumatic fever, gout, osteoarthritis, ankylosing spondylitis, and suppurative arthritis, they are useful in differential diagnosis and in clinical investigations, where comparability of groups of cases is required. The rheumatoid factor has prognostic significance: patients with consistently positive tests generally follow a progressively unfavorable course.

The rheumatoid factor is a macroglobulin (19S) with a molecular weight of about one million. It circulates in the plasma as a soluble complex (22S), combined with smaller γ-globulins (7S) of 160,000 mol wt.

Several serologic tests for rheumatoid factor are in common use, but the basic principle of all is the same: the test serum is added in serial dilutions to a suspension of particles which have been coated with a "sensitizing" substance. The particles may be sheep or human red blood cells, latex (a synthetic polystyrene), or bentonite (a natural clay). In the sheep cell agglutination test the red blood cells are coated with a subagglutinating dose of rabbit antiserum against sheep erythrocytes; in the latex or bentonite tests the inert particles are coated with aggregated human γ-globulin. The test is considered positive when the serum agglutinates sensitized sheep cells or bentonite particles in a dilution of 1:32 or higher, or latex particles in a dilution of 1:160 or higher. The latex fixation test is relatively easy to perform, more sensitive, and less specific than the sheep cell agglutination test.

The tests are infrequently positive before the sixth month of illness. They are positive in 95 percent of patients with subcutaneous nodules, and high titers are found in patients with splenomegaly, vasculitis, or neuropathy. Only 10 to 20 percent of those with juvenile rheumatoid arthritis have positive tests. The tests are sometimes positive in other connective tissue diseases (systemic lupus erythematosus and progressive systemic sclerosis) and seemingly unrelated conditions (subacute bacterial endocarditis, sarcoid, liver disease, leprosy). In random samples of the normal population the frequency of positive tests ranges from 1 to 5 percent, and increases with age.

Lupus erythematosus cells are found in 3 to 30 percent of patients with rheumatoid disease; *antinuclear antibodies* are found in 20 to 70 percent. Both organ-nonspecific and granulocyte-specific antinuclear factors are demonstrable.

The *synovial fluid* is turbid, its viscosity is reduced, and mucin clot formation is poor. There is a polymorphonuclear leukocytosis of 10,000 to 50,000 cells per cu mm.

Radiologic examination of the affected joints is helpful in diagnosis and in charting the course of rheumatoid arthritis. The earliest changes are subtle and consist of soft-tissue swelling, osteoporosis, periosteal elevation, erosions, and narrowing of joint space. Osteoporosis is at first juxtaarticular (paraepiphyseal) but becomes diffuse. Erosions at the joint margins are the most characteristic radiologic features of chronic rheumatoid arthritis. Narrowed joint space results from destruction of articular cartilage and is nonspecific.

DIAGNOSIS. In the patient who gives a history of prodromal symptoms, paresthesias, weight loss, and repeated episodes of acute migratory polyarthritis, and who has symmetric deforming arthritis with "subluxations," ulnar deviation, and subcutaneous nodules, the diagnosis of rheumatoid arthritis is easy. Difficulty arises in earlier stages when the clinical picture is that of an acute polyarthritis or merely monarticular disease.

Among the syndromes which can mimic rheumatoid arthritis in its early phases are rheumatic fever (Chap. 269), systemic lupus erythematosus (Chap. 392), and acute gout (Chap. 106). Reiter's syndrome (Chap. 390) may be differentiated from rheumatoid arthritis by (1) its prevalence in young men; (2) history of recent urethritis; (3) predominance of arthritis in the lower extremities; and (4) its mucocutaneous manifestations.

Degenerative joint disease is distinguished from rheumatoid arthritis by the presence of Heberden's nodes, involvement of the distal rather than the proximal interphalangeal joints, and the infrequent involvement of the wrist and metacarpophalangeal joints.

In the last analysis, the most helpful diagnostic aids are certain physical signs (sustained symmetric inflammatory polyarthritis, ulnar deviation, and subcutaneous nodules), positive test for rheumatoid factor, and characteristic roentgenographic abnormalities.

TREATMENT. General Measures. The physician should help the patient to develop a realistic outlook by telling him that much can be done to relieve pain and prevent crippling but that the course of his disease cannot be predicted with precision and that medical care may be required for months or years. Psychologic support may be needed frequently. Patients with rheumatoid arthritis are characterized as unaggressive, tense, depressed, and oversensitive.

A large intake of calcium and protein may combat or prevent osteoporosis, but this has not been proved. Some patients feel better in a warm, dry climate, but this is by no means curative, and personal considerations often mitigate against such a move.

Patients with acute polyarthritis and fever should be at bed rest. In milder cases, 8 to 10 hr of sleep at night, and brief rest periods during the day "are advisable." Patients should be encouraged to continue work as long as excessive fatigue or trauma to joints can be avoided.

Drugs. Pain must be relieved before active physical therapy can be undertaken. Drugs such as morphine and Demerol must be avoided because of the danger of addiction. Codeine may be used in unusual circumstances for brief periods.

Salicylates should be tried first; they are cheap and frequently achieve the desired result. Acetylsalicylic acid (aspirin) and buffered preparations are about equally effective. Enteric-coated salicylate tablets are advisable for those with gastrointestinal toxicity or peptic ulcers.

The initial dosage of aspirin in ambulatory patients is usually 2.4 Gm daily; this should be increased progressively until the desired response is achieved or side reactions supervene. Blood salicylate levels are often helpful in regulating therapy.

Salicylate therapy should be given the fullest possible trial before turning to other agents. When patients are not satisfactorily managed with salicylates and physical therapy, one may use antimalarials, gold, adrenocortical steroids, phenylbutazone, or indomethacin.

Phenylbutazone (Butazolidin) has had widespread clinical trial. It is more effective in ankylosing spondylitis and acute gout than in peripheral rheumatoid arthritis, but major clinical improvement has been reported in 25 to 40 percent of cases of rheumatoid disease, a figure approaching a placebo effect in some studies. The incidence of untoward reactions varies. In one series of 800 cases, side reactions appear in 40 percent of patients, and in 15 percent therapy with the drug had to be discontinued. Untoward reactions include agranulocytosis, hypoplastic or hemolytic anemia, thrombocytopenia, peptic ulceration, and retention of sodium and water. A dosage of no more than 300 to 400 mg daily is recommended, but hematopoietic disorders occur occasionally at this level. In view of the toxicity of phenylbutazone, it should not be given until other measures have failed, and it is contraindicated in patients with a history of allergy, peptic ulcer, cardiovascular disease, or renal disease. Many physicians believe that phenylbutazone has no real place in the treatment of rheumatoid arthritis. Certainly, failure to observe improvement within 7 to 10 days is indication for abandoning it.

Clinical reports on the efficacy of *indomethacin* in rheumatoid arthritis vary widely. Controlled therapeutic trials at tolerated doses, 50 to 100 mg per day, show little, if any, advantage over salicylates. Doses greater than 100 mg daily cause frequent side effects, especially nausea, heartburn, peptic ulcer, and headache, lightheadedness, and inability to concentrate.

Both *chloroquine phosphate* and *hydroxychloroquine sulfate* have been shown by "double-blind" therapeutic trials to have a significant antirheumatic effect. Improvement is slower and less dramatic than with steroid therapy. The drugs are administered orally, in dosage of 250 to 500 mg chloroquine or 200 to 400 mg hydroxychloroquine daily. Side reactions occur in up to 50 percent of patients. The rare, but irreversible, retinal degeneration has discouraged the long-term use of these agents.

Adrenocortical steroid therapy is of limited value in rheumatoid disease. After several years of experience with these agents, certain general conclusions may be drawn. (1) Prednisone, singled out for this discussion, is a potent, nonspecific, anti-inflammatory agent. (2) In the vast majority of patients prednisone in adequate dosage can induce rapid improvement in symptoms and signs, as shown by regression of fever, joint manifestations, enlarged lymph nodes, and nodules. Synovial fluid may revert to normal. (3) Anemia may not be corrected, the erythrocyte sedimentation rate may not be reduced to normal levels, and levels of rheumatoid factor may remain unaltered. (4) Some patients fail to improve. In many instances, this may be attributed to irreversible changes, severe contractures, or ankylosis which had taken place prior to therapy, or to insufficient dosage. (5) Subjective and functional improvement usually exceeds objective improvement. (6) Joint destruction, as shown by serial roentgenographic studies, usually progresses. (7) Prednisone therapy alone is insufficient and should be combined with the usual conservative program—rest, physical therapy, and salicylates.

The initial dose should be low, equivalent to 10 mg or less of prednisone, daily. After manipulation, a maintenance dose is determined, but every effort should be made to keep this at a minimum. Under any circumstances, gradual dose reduction should be carried out periodically at least every 6 months, in the hope that the patient may be entering a remission. In practice, complete withdrawal from corticosteroids has been difficult.

Complications of steroid therapy to which patients with rheumatoid arthritis are especially susceptible are (1) gastric and duodenal ulcers (more common in persons with untreated rheumatoid arthritis than in the general population); (2) osteoporosis and fractures, commonly of the thoracic and lumbar vertebral bodies, especially in postmenopausal women; (3) necrotizing arteritis (also

a feature of the untreated disease and resulting at times in neuropathy or leg ulcers); and (4) aseptic necrosis of the femoral or humeral head.

Intraarticular injections of suspensions of corticosteroid esters are useful when only one or two easily accessible joints are involved. The amount injected varies, depending on the size of the joints. In most cases substantial relief of pain and stiffness lasts for 1 or 2 weeks. The disadvantages of this mode of therapy are the brevity of the benefit and the danger of introducing infection into the joint.

Until the advent of adrenocortical steroid therapy, *gold compounds* were among the most popular agents in the treatment of rheumatoid arthritis. Significant improvement has been reported in 40 to 60 percent of patients given gold over a period of several months, and the improvement is characteristically gradual. Remissions after a single course (total dosage of 1.0 Gm) are usually temporary. The value of maintenance therapy has not been fully determined.

Several gold compounds are available; most of them contain approximately 50 percent of metallic gold, are water-soluble, and are given intramuscularly. The usual regimen consists of an initial test dose of 10 mg, a second injection of 25 mg 1 week later, and 50 mg weekly thereafter until a total dose of 1.0 Gm has been given. Maintenance therapy is usually 50 mg every second or third week.

Toxic reactions occur in as many as half the patients, vary in severity, but are rarely fatal.

Preliminary experiences with *immunosuppressive agents* have been favorable; controlled therapeutic trials are in progress. Intraarticular injections of an alkylating agent, triethylene thiophosphamide (Thiotepa) have given conflicting results.

Physical Therapy. A primary objective is prevention of loss or normal joint motion which ultimately leads to crippling. Therapeutic exercises, essentially nontiring movement to carry the joints through their normal range of motion daily, are prescribed.

Prevention of deformity requires attention to positioning in bed and to posture in general. Use of a board beneath the mattress prevents sagging. The patient should be encouraged to lie flat on his back when resting or sleeping, to use as small a pillow as possible under the head and neck, to avoid altogether the use of pillows under the knees, and to sit in a chair with a firm seat and straight back.

Graded *exercises* are given to increase or maintain muscle power. For bed patients, "muscle setting" (isometric contraction) is prescribed for the quadriceps and gluteals.

Heat will diminish pain and spasm and permit increased range of motion. A hot bath is effective, but hot compresses or a heat bulb may be used for one or two joints. The paraffin bath, which can be set up at home, is particularly effective for hands and wrists.

Diathermy, x-ray therapy, ultrasound, and massage have no place in the therapy of rheumatoid arthritis.

Canes and crutches are prescribed as assistive devices when it is necessary to reduce stress on the hip, knees, and feet. Splints and casts, properly applied, are useful, especially "gutter splints" or long leg cylinder casts worn at night to avoid flexion contractures.

Therapists can also give specific training to increase the patient's capacity to perform activities of daily living. In addition, appropriate devices, such as a long-handled shoehorn, a bathtub seat, and a built-up knife and fork can enable a patient to remain self-sufficient.

Surgical Therapy. Orthopedic surgeons have become interested in the surgical treatment of rheumatoid arthritis, particularly in the therapeutic and prophylactic value of synovectomy of the knee and other joints. In addition to synovectomy, operative procedures on the hands include arthroplasty, intrinsic and extrinsic release, tendon transfers, and decompression of medial and ulnar carpal tunnel syndromes. Controlled observations are difficult to obtain but have been initiated with respect to synovectomy.

VARIANTS OF RHEUMATOID ARTHRITIS

JUVENILE RHEUMATOID ARTHRITIS. Commonly called "Still's disease," this disorder begins in children before puberty and comprises 4 percent of all cases of rheumatoid arthritis. Most cases begin in early childhood, predominantly in girls.

Systemic symptoms and signs are severe. Fever rising daily to 105°F may continue for months. Lymphadenopathy occurs in 60 percent of cases and splenomegaly in 30 percent. A transient, recurrent rash, consisting of small, salmon-colored macular or maculopapular lesions, is seen in one-fourth of cases. Pericarditis, pleuritis, and pneumonitis are common, but subcutaneous nodules are relatively rare. The juvenile form tends to affect the larger joints, especially in the earlier stages, and cervical spondylitis, particularly between the second and third cervical vertebras, is common. Growth and development may be impaired. Involvement of the temporomandibular joint and impairment of mandibular growth produce a receding chin, which is characteristic of childhood rheumatoid arthritis. The leukocyte count is often as high as 50,000 per cu mm, and the usual tests for rheumatoid factor are positive in only 10 to 20 percent of patients.

Early in the disease, especially in its systemic form, differentiation from acute rheumatic fever or systemic lupus erythematosus may be difficult. In a third of cases, juvenile rheumatoid arthritis is monarticular (hip or knee) at the onset and tuberculous arthritis must be ruled out.

The natural history of juvenile rheumatoid arthritis has not been fully charted. The disease may be mild and may result in little deformity. Small joint involvement at the onset, the presence of rheumatoid factor, and occurrence at older ages indicate a poor prognosis. Disease activity may persist well into adult life. In such patients, the rheumatoid disease may simulate the adult form. In cases with prolonged and severe involvement, secondary amyloidosis may appear. Management is generally similar to that for adult rheumatoid arthritis. Particular attention should be paid to the proper alignment of joints and to the prevention of trauma.

FELTY'S SYNDROME. In 1924 Felty reported a series of five patients with febrile migratory polyarthritis, splenomegaly, and leukopenia. Subsequently, many other cases were described, and this triad has since borne his name. Other features include hyperpigmentation, leg ulcers, lymphadenopathy, and hepatomegaly. This syndrome is usually encountered in far-advanced rheumatoid disease, and its separation as a clinical entity may be unwarranted. The serum may contain unusually large amounts of rheumatoid factor. Lupus erythematosus (LE) cells and antinuclear antibodies occur more frequently than in rheumatoid arthritis in general. There may be anemia and thrombocytopenia, in addition to the neutropenia. The hematologic abnormalities respond to splenectomy, but the arthritis remains unaffected. The indications for splenectomy are repeated infections and refractory leg ulcers.

SJÖGREN'S SYNDROME. In 1933, Sjögren, a Swedish ophthalmologist, reported among patients with keratoconjunctivitis sicca (dry eyes) the additional findings of xerostomia (dry mouth), enlargement of the lacrimal and salivary glands, and in two-thirds of the cases, rheumatoid arthritis. Most patients are women; their mean age is fifty years.

In the fully developed case, the disorder involves virtually all the exocrine glands of the body. Keratoconjunctivitis sicca is recognized because of (1) stinging and grittiness of the eyes, (2) reduced lacrimal secretion as measured by the Schirmer test, (3) desquamation of corneal or conjunctival epithelium as demonstrated by rose-bengal staining, and (4) filamentary keratitis (slit-lamp examination). With xerostomia, there are dry mouth, decreased salivary flow, and an abnormal sialogram. The lacrimal and/or parotid glands are enlarged in one-half the cases. The mucosa of nose, pharynx, and larynx is often dry and atrophic, and patients may have dry cough, with tracheobronchitis, pneumonitis, and pleuritis. Involvement of the alimentary tract results in dysphagia, achlorhydria, or constipation. Many patients have atrophic vaginitis.

Half the patients have definite rheumatoid arthritis; a few, transitory polyarthritis. Felty's syndrome is encountered occasionally. Less frequently seen in Sjögren's syndrome are nonthrombocytopenic purpura, Raynaud's phenomenon, thyroid enlargement, lymphadenopathy, splenomegaly, hepatomegaly, focal myositis, arteritis, and peripheral neuropathy. Sjögren's syndrome has been associated with each of the collagen disorders (systemic lupus erythematosus, progressive systemic sclerosis, polyarteritis, and polymyositis) and with hyperglobulinemic purpura of Waldenström. Some patients develop a "pseudolymphoma" with vasculitis; and a few have had true lymphoma.

One-third have mild anemia, and leukopenia (with fewer than 4,000 leukocytes per cu mm) is also found in about a third of patients. The erythrocyte sedimentation rate is usually rapid. Most patients have hyperglobulinemia. Some have renal tubular acidosis. Tests for rheumatoid factor are positive in almost all patients, even in those without arthritis. Lupus erythematosus cells are found in 10 percent of patients; and antinuclear antibodies, in 70 percent. Cryoglobulinemia has been reported. There is an appreciable incidence of complement-fixing antibodies to suspensions of homogenates from various tissues; these antigens are neither organ-nor species-specific.

The salivary and lacrimal glands reveal massive infiltration with lymphocytes and plasma cells, as in the thyroid in Hashimoto's disease, atrophy of acini, proliferation of the duct-lining cells, and myoepithelial islands. This is the histologic picture of Mikulicz' disease, and on the basis of this and other evidence Morgan and Castleman in 1953 concluded that Sjögren's syndrome and primary Mikulicz' disease were the same. Muscle biopsy may reveal widespread acute or mild chronic focal myositis.

The etiology of Sjögren's syndrome is unknown. Because of the striking similarity of the histopathologic changes in the salivary and lacrimal glands to those in the thyroid gland in Hashimoto's disease, and in view of the abundance of abnormal serum factors and circulating antibodies to tissue components (including salivary duct cells), it is considered to be a disorder of abnormal immunologic behavior. Moreover, impaired lymphocyte transformation and delayed hypersensitivity have been described. This syndrome is more common than has been generally realized. Every effort should be made, however, to rule out other causes of salivary gland enlargement such as lymphoma, leukemia, tuberculosis, sarcoid, hepatic cirrhosis, and malnutrition (Chap. 231).

Most patients need no systemic therapy. Local measures, such as methylcellulose (artificial tears) for keratoconjunctivitis sicca, are often very beneficial; methylcellulose swab or spray may alleviate the xerostomia. Treatment of the arthritis is the same as for rheumatoid disease. In patients with severe parotid enlargement, the response to radiotherapy is often striking but these patients may be peculiarly liable to lymphoma. Surgical excision should be discouraged because of recurrences and the risk of injury to the facial nerve.

REFERENCES

Caplan's Syndrome

Caplan, A.: Certain Unusual Radiologic Appearance in the Chest of Coal Miners Suffering from Rheumatoid Arthritis, Thorax, 8:29, 1953.

Felty's Syndrome

Felty, A. R.: Chronic Arthritis in the Adult, Associated with Splenomegaly and Leucopenia, Bull. Johns Hopkins Hosp., 35:16, 1924.

Green, R. A., and V. L. Fromke: Splenectomy in Felty's Syndrome, Ann. Intern. Med., 64:1265, 1966.

Rheumatoid Arthritis

Duthie, J. J. R., P. E. Brown, L. H. Truelove, F. D. Barager, and A. J. Lawie: Course and Prognosis in Rheumatoid Arthritis, Ann. Rheum. Dis., 23:193, 1964.

Hamerman, D.: New Thoughts on the Pathogenesis of Rheumatoid Arthritis, Amer. J. Med., 40:1, 1966.

Hart, F. D., and E. Lewis-Faning: Gold Therapy in Rheumatoid Arthritis: Report of Multi-centre Controlled Trial, Ann. Rheum. Dis., 19:95, 1960.

Kellgren, J. H., and F. Bier: Radiologic Signs of Rheumatoid Arthritis, Ann. Rheum. Dis., 15:55, 1956.

Lamont-Havers, R. W. (Ed.): Conference on Immunologic Aspects of Rheumatoid Arthritis and Systemic Lupus Erythematosus, Arthritis Rheum., 6:401, 1963.

Lazarus, G. S., J. L. Decker, C. H. Oliver, J. R. Daniels, C. V. Multz, and H. M. Fullmer: Collagenolytic Activity of Synovium in Rheumatoid Arthritis, New Engl. J. Med., 279:914, 1968.

Ragan, C., and E. Farrington: Clinical Features of Rheumatoid Arthritis: Prognostic Indices, J.A.M.A., 181:663, 1962.

Ropes, M. W., G. A. Bennett, S. Cobb, R. Jacox, and R. A. Jessar: Diagnostic Criteria for Rheumatoid Arthritis, Bull. Rheum. Dis., 9:175, 1958 (revision).

Schmid, F. R., N. S. Cooper, M. Ziff, and C. McEwen: Arteritis in Rheumatoid Arthritis, Am. J. Med., 30:56, 1961.

Ziff, M.: Some Immunologic Aspects of the Connective Tissue Diseases, Ann. Rheum. Dis., 24:103, 1965.

Sjögren's Syndrome

Block, K. J., W. W. Buchanan, M. J. Wohl, and J. J. Bunim: Sjögren's Syndrome: A Clinical, Pathological, and Serological Study of Sixty-two Cases, Medicine, 44:187, 1965.

387 DEGENERATIVE JOINT DISEASE

Lawrence E. Shulman

DEFINITION. Degenerative joint disease (DJD), otherwise known as *osteoarthritis, hypertrophic arthritis,* or *senescent arthritis,* is a chronic disorder characterized pathologically by degeneration of articular cartilage and hypertrophy of bone, clinically by pain which appears with activity and subsides with rest, and by typical roentgenographic findings. DJD usually affects weight-bearing joints and the distal interphalangeal joints of the fingers. It may develop spontaneously with advancing age (primary osteoarthritis) or at an earlier age as a sequel to injury of various kinds. There are no systemic manfestations.

EPIDEMIOLOGY. Degenerative joint disease is worldwide. The fact that it is best known in temperate climates is probably a reflection of the longer life span of the populations in these areas.

Roentgenographic abnormalities usually do not appear until the third or fourth decade, but after the age of fifty, virtually everyone has some characteristic roentgenographic changes. Nevertheless, only a minority experience symptoms. Although this disorder is not as disabling as rheumatoid arthritis, it has economic importance. For example, an industrial survey showed that 14 percent of all patients with objective evidence of musculoskeletal disease had DJD. DJD is largely a disorder of middle and late life, and often appears in women at the time of the menopause. Most studies reveal that DJD is divided equally between the sexes, although for a variety of reasons (occupational, genetic, etc.) the distribution of joint involvement differs between sexes.

ETIOLOGY. Anatomic studies reveal that alterations in the articular cartilage characteristic of DJD begin to appear in the second decade and increase in frequency and severity with age. It is commonly held that these changes result from "wear and tear," i.e., from cumulative trauma. Although there is little doubt that repeated injury plays a role, the wear-and-tear concept does not explain the disease completely. The common involvement of the distal interphalangeal joints (Heberden's nodes) is an example. These joints are not exposed to more frequent or severe injury than the metacarpophalangeals, which are rarely involved in DJD. Necropsy studies have failed to uncover any difference in the incidence of this disorder between laborers and sedentary workers.

Heredity clearly plays a role in the pathogenesis of Heberden's nodes, which are ten times more common in women than in men. Stecher showed that they are inherited as a sex-influenced characteristic, dominant in the female and recessive in the male. The importance of heredity in the pathogenesis of DJD at other sites has not been demonstrated.

An excess of DJD is found in certain other diseases, notably acromegaly, hypothyroidism, diabetes mellitus, and hyperparathyroidism.

ANATOMIC CHANGES AND PATHOGENESIS. The initial change in DJD is degeneration of articular hyaline cartilage, which becomes inelastic, yellow, and opaque. Microscopically, the cartilage surface is made uneven by shallow linear furrows which later deepen into clefts, or fissures, running perpendicular to the surface of the cartilage. Later, fraying and ulceration lead to destruction. These changes can be produced in vitro by incubating normal human cartilage with hyaluronidase, papain, or lysosomal enzymes.

Where the articular cartilage becomes thin, the underlying calcified cartilage becomes thick and dense, and granulation tissue appears in subchondral bone, breaks through the cartilage, and reaches the joint space, This new bone thickens and becomes highly polished, a process that is called *eburnation*. Bony excrescences or spurs, called osteophytes, form at the joint margin.

The synovial membrane eventually becomes scarred; fibrous thickening and contraction of the joint capsule may be extensive late in the disease.

CLINICAL FEATURES. In the small proportion of patients with DJD who have symptoms, there is insidious onset of joint pain and stiffness. The pain is characteristically aching and mild; it appears with exercise of the part and abates with rest. The stiffness, or articular "jelling," develops after prolonged rest in a fixed position and disappears a few minutes after resuming activity (in contrast to that of rheumatoid arthritis, which may last for hours). Although the disorder is frequently progressive, it rarely causes the degree of discomfort and invalidism encountered in rheumatoid arthritis.

Objectively the joints may appear entirely normal, even in patients with symptoms. Joint enlargement, when present, is the result of secondary hypertrophy of bone. The enlarged joints feel hard and knobby, and there may be tenderness, but excessive warmth or erythema is rare. In the later stages, a grating sensation, or crepitus, may be felt on moving the affected joint. There are no diagnostic laboratory abnormalities or changes in the synovial fluid.

In the symptomatic patient, the *roentgenographic appearance* may be normal. Abnormalities include (roughly in order of advancing disease) unevenness and narrowing of the joint space; sharpening of articular margins; irregularity and widening of the surfaces; bony sclerosis, or eburnation; osteophytes, or marginal lipping; and bone cysts. Osteoporosis is not a feature of DJD; when it is present, other causes of arthritis should be sought.

The most commonly involved joints are those that bear weight (knees, hips, and lumbar spine), the cervical spine, and distal interphalangeal joints of the fingers (*Heberden's nodes*). Some patients with Heberden's nodes never develop joint disease elsewhere. Similar lesions at the proximal interphalangeal joints are called *Bouchard's nodes*. Involvement of the hips gives rise to the greatest disability. Cervical spine lesions are most common at the lower cervical articulations; they may cause neurologic symptoms and signs, as well as dysphagia if anterior spurring is pronounced.

Erosive osteoarthritis is a disease characterized by intense inflammation, erosions, and osteophytes of the proximal and distal interphalangeal joints and of the first carpometacarpal joints in middle-aged women. Histopathologically, in the acute inflammatory phase, the synovium reveals all the features of rheumatoid arthritis; in the chronic osteophytic phase, the cartilage shows all the changes of DJD. It is readily separated clinically from rheumatoid arthritis by the absence of systemic manifestations, prolonged morning stiffness, periarticular osteoporosis, tendon involvement, subcutaneous nodules, and rheumatoid factor. The sedimentation rate is normal or minimally elevated. Although subluxations and deformities may develop, the course is self-limited; only conservative management is recommended.

DIAGNOSIS. Since DJD and rheumatoid arthritis, the two most common forms of chronic joint disease in the middle-aged and the elderly, differ so widely in both prognosis and management, it is important to distinguish one disorder from the other. In virtually every instance, this is readily accomplished. In contrast to rheumatoid arthritis, DJD is confined to the joint structures and is not a systemic disease. There are no constitutional symptoms and signs and no laboratory abnormalities. The joints are not hot or red and there are no subcutaneous nodules. The sheep cell agglutination test is negative.

Even though roentgenographic changes of an affected joint may be those of DJD, the articular symptoms and signs may be caused by a coexistent joint disorder such as rheumatoid arthritis, chondrocalcinosis, or gout. In these cases, objective evidence of inflammation may have great diagnostic significance. Errors of overdiagnosis are commonly made in cases demonstrating osteophytosis of the spine, a condition that rarely gives rise to symptoms. In patients with back symptoms, some other process, such as a herniated nucleus pulposus, may be responsible. At any rate, if pain believed to be attributable to DJD is severe and fails to respond to the usual measures, other diseases such as metastatic tumor, multiple myeloma, and osteomyelitis should be considered.

TREATMENT. The most important feature in the care of the patient with DJD is to advise him that although his disease is annoying and at times uncomfortable, it is not serious and will not cause severe pain, disability, and crippling. Such reassurance spares the patient the anguish of thinking that he has "arthritis" and that "nothing can be done." Conservative measures, such as adequate rest of the involved joints, physical therapy, including corrective exercises, and analgesics such as salicylates, usually suffice. Attention should be directed toward eliminating or minimizing trauma. Obese patients should lose weight. Certain occupational adjustments may be made. Abdominal supports for lumbar spine disease aggravated by a sagging abdomen, and a Thomas collar or head traction for cervical spine involvement are other means of eliminating precipitating influences. Repeated intra-articular injections of hydrocortisone are beneficial only in those patients with a superimposed, nonspecific inflammatory response to fragmented cartilage or bone. The systemic use of potentially hazardous agents such as adrenocortical steroids or phenylbutazone is unjustified. Indomethacin is said to have special analgesic properties for DJD of the hip. Corrective orthopedic surgical methods may be needed for severely diseased hips or knees unresponsive to conservative management. Cup arthroplasty may improve function and reduce pain in patients with severe hip disease, especially if the disease is bilateral. Surgical removal of large osteophytic spurs at certain sites may be indicated.

REFERENCES

Barland, P, R. Janis, and J. Sandson: Immunofluorescent Studies of Human Atricular Cartilage, Ann. Rheum. Dis., 25:156, 1966.

Bennett, G. A., H. Waine, and W. Bauer: "Changes in the Knee Joint at Various Ages with Particular Reference to the Nature and Development of Degenerative Joint Disease," New York, The Commonwealth Fund, 1942.

Bunim, J. J.: Arthritis in the Elderly Patient (Osteoarthritis), Bull. N.Y. Acad. Med., 32:102, 1956.

Kellgren, J. H., and R. Moore: Generalized Osteoarthritis and Heberden's Nodes, Brit. Med. J., 1:181, 1952.

Peter, J. B., Pearson, C. M., and Marmor, L.: Erosive Osteoarthritis of the Hands, Arthritis Rheum., 9:365, 1966.

Sokoloff, L.: Biology of Degenerative Joint Disease, Perspect. Biol. Med., 7:94, 1963.

Stecher, R. M.: Heberden's Nodes: A Clinical Description of Osteoarthritis of the Finger Joints, Ann. Rheum. Dis., 14:1, 1955.

388 HYPERTROPHIC OSTEOARTHROPATHY

Lawrence E. Shulman

DEFINITION. This disorder, also known as *hypertrophic pulmonary osteoarthropathy*, *secondary hypertrophic osteoarthropathy*, and *Marie-Bamberger syndrome*, is characterized by (1) clubbing of the fingers and toes, (2) chronic periostitis with new bone formation at the distal ends of the long bones, and (3) arthritis. In the vast majority of cases, this syndrome is secondary to chronic disease elsewhere; in the remainder, it is hereditary or idiopathic. Because of its frequent association with diseases of the lung, the disorder is often called "hypertrophic pulmonary osteoarthropathy," but this is restrictive because the primary problem may be in the heart, liver, or gastrointestinal tract. Clubbing and osteoarthropathy may occur independently. The periostitis and arthritis are most frequently encountered in patients with intrathoracic diseases.

Formerly, chronic suppurative conditions, such as bronchiectasis, were the most common underlying diseases, but now pulmonary neoplasms head the list. Osteoarthropathy may appear several months before any other symptom or sign of bronchogenic carcinoma.

CLASSIFICATION. Hypertrophic osteoarthropathy usually occurs symmetrically. Usually all four extremities are involved, but only one extremity, more commonly an arm, may be affected. The syndrome is conveniently categorized by the location of the primary disease.

1. *Pulmonary.* Various pulmonary, pleural, and mediastinal disorders lead to this syndrome. It occurs in 5 to 10 percent of cases of bronchogenic carcinoma; it has a high incidence in pleural tumors but is rare in metastatic tumors in the lung. It also occurs in bronchiectasis, lung abscess, and empyema but is rare in tuberculosis. Arthropathy has occurred with Hodgkin's disease, aortic aneurysm, and other disorders of the mediastinum.

2. *Cardiac.* Hypertrophic osteoarthropathy occurs in cyanotic forms of congenital heart disease but is not seen in noncyanotic forms. It is sometimes present in subacute bacterial endocarditis.

3. *Hepatic.* The incidence of this syndrome is high in cholangiolitic or primary biliary cirrhosis, but much lower in obstructive biliary tract disease or portal and postnecrotic cirrhosis.

4. *Gastrointestinal.* Many of the intraabdominal conditions leading to osteoarthropathy are characterized by chronic diarrhea. They include ulcerative colitis, regional enteritis, amebic and bacillary dysentery, intestinal tuberculosis, polyposis of the colon, neoplasms, idiopathic steatorrhea, and rectal stricture from lymphogranuloma venereum.

5. *Miscellaneous.* Although it is very rare in spontaneous myxedema (and cretinism), several cases of osteoarthropathy have developed following thyroidectomy for Graves' disease with exophthalmos. Cases have been described in chronic urinary tract infections and syringomyelia.

The *hereditary* form of osteoarthropathy (*pachydermoperiostitis; Touraine-Solente-Gole syndrome*) is rare and is distinguished from the acquired form by remarkable thickening of the skin over the face and limbs, by little bone or joint pain, and by the absence of increased peripheral blood flow. It is inherited as an autosomal dominant trait with considerable variability in expressivity. It appears shortly after puberty, progresses for about 10 years, and remains stationary thereafter.

Many cases designated as *idiopathic* are examples of the hereditary form or of acquired disease in which the primary condition is unrecognized. A few cases of typical osteoarthropathy are, however, unexplainable. A syndrome of idiopathic periosteal hyperostosis with high fever and elevated serum IgG immunoglobulin occurs in children, with spontaneous gradual recovery.

Unilateral clubbing and osteoarthropathy are most commonly caused by aneurysm of the aorta, brachiocephalic, or subclavian arteries. Other causes are apical lung cancer, axillary tumors, subluxation of the shoulder, and brachial arteriovenous anastomoses.

PATHOLOGY. The basic lesion is chronic inflammation of periosteum, synovial membrane, joint capsule, and adjacent subcutaneous tissue. The periosteum early in the disease shows edema, vascularization, and round-cell infiltration and, at its inner margin, osteoid formation. Initially, only scattered foci of new bone appear; later, the distal segments may become completely encased by new bone.

The synovial membrane, articular capsule, and subcutaneous tissue about the affected bones and joints become thickened and chronically inflamed. There may be an intermittent hydrarthrosis. Rarely, the synovitis goes on to pannus formation, ankylosis, and degeneration of cartilage.

PATHOGENESIS. Theories advanced for the mechanism of osteoarthropathy include (1) chronic infection, (2) action of toxin absorbed from the primary focus, (3) capillary stasis caused by elevated venous pressure, (4) arterial hypoxemia, (5) local hypoxia, (6) action of local toxins formed as a result of circulatory disturbances, (7) anterior pituitary overactivity, (8) thyroid underactivity, and (9) the elaboration by pleural mesothelial cells of an osteoblast-stimulating substance. None of these hypotheses accounts for more than a small proportion of cases.

The first and only experimental reproduction of this condition was achieved by Mendlowitz and Leslie in the dog by anastomosing the left pulmonary artery to the left atrium, creating a situation similar to cyanotic congenital heart disease. As osteoarthropathy developed, the systemic cardiac output increased while the pulmonary blood flow remained normal. Cross-circulation experiments have shown that a humoral factor is not involved.

After resection of a lung abscess or tumor, symptoms and signs of osteoarthropathy frequently subside within a few days. The speed of improvement suggests that the alterations in the peripheral circulation are corrected rapidly, perhaps by interrupting an abnormal pulmonary-vascular reflex. This hypothesis is supported by several reports of prompt improvement in hypertrophic osteoarthropathy after dividing the vagus in patients with inoperable lung cancer. Thoracotomy alone is ineffective.

MANIFESTATIONS. In clubbing, there is a sensation of warmth or burning in the fingertips but pain is unusual. The first change is thickening about the nailbed, which can be detected by a reduction in the angle made by the nail and the dorsal plane of the distal phalanx, normally about 15°. Hyperhidrosis of the hands and feet is common.

Rheumatic complaints vary greatly in severity. Deep-seated burning pain and exquisite tenderness over the distal ends of the long bones are typical in acute and advanced cases. Over the affected bones and joints, the skin is dusky red, warm, and tender, and the subcutaneous tissue is thickened. The joints are swollen, and their mobility is restricted. Most commonly involved are the knees, ankles, wrists, elbows, and metacarpophalangeal joints. Rarely, there is slight fever.

In the early stages of clubbing, the terminal phalanges appear normal roentgenographically, but with advancing disease they reveal flaring of the ungual process and osteoporosis. The roentgenographic evidence of osteoarthropathy consists of periosteal thickening along the shafts of the long bones. This appears first and is thickest in the region of the distal epiphyses, especially at the point of musculotendinous insertion. The periosteal elevation spreads proximally as the disease progresses. Later, the cancellous portion of the involved bone becomes osteoporotic and the cortex becomes thin.

The course of hypertrophic osteoarthropathy reflects the activity of the underlying disease. In cases where it waxes and wanes with exacerbations and remissions of the primary process, the roentgenograms show a tree trunk–like layering of thin sheets of newly formed bone. In cases secondary to chronic suppuration, the osteoarthropathy emerges insidiously and is usually mild. In cases secondary to lung tumors, the clubbing and arthropathy may appear very suddenly. Articular symptoms and signs sometimes antedate clubbing of the fingers, but this is unusual.

DIAGNOSIS. When clubbing, arthritic symptoms, and periosteal proliferation by x-ray are all present, this syndrome is easily recognized. The patient in whom arthritic symptoms predominate is often thought to have rheumatoid arthritis or some other form of polyarthritis. In patients with erythema and superficial tenderness about the ankles, thrombophlebitis or cellulitis is a frequent diagnosis. Differentiation from acromegaly is usually not difficult. The diagnosis cannot rest on evidence of periosteal proliferation alone, because scurvy, syphilis, trauma, lymphangitis, varicose veins, and other conditions give rise to periosteal disorders.

TREATMENT. Therapeutic efforts in hypertrophic osteoarthropathy should be directed toward the elimination of the underlying condition or its amelioration. In cases where the osteoarthropathy is severe and a satisfactory attack on the primary disease is not possible, disabling symptoms have been relieved by analgesics, corticosteroid therapy, or intrathoracic vagotomy.

REFERENCES

Goldbloom, R. B., P. B. Stein, A. Eisen, J. B. McSheffrey, B. S. Brown, and F. W. Wigglesworth: Idiopathic Periosteal Hyperostosis with Dysproteinemia, New Engl. J. Med., 274:873, 1966.

Mendlowitz, M.: Clubbing and Hypertrophic Osteoarthropathy, Medicine, 21:269, 1942.

Rimoin, D. L.: Pachydermoperiostosis (Idiopathic Clubbing and Periostosis), New Engl. J. Med., 272:923, 1965.

Vogl, A., S. Blumenfeld, and L. B. Gutner: Diagnostic Significance of Pulmonary Hypertrophic Osteoarthropathy, Am. J. Med., 18:51, 1955.

389 NONARTICULAR RHEUMATISM

Lawrence E. Shulman

The patient complaining of "rheumatism" often is referring to symptoms resulting from dysfunction of tissues or structures near joints. These include tendons, bursae, bones, muscles, nerves, and adipose tissue. This heterogeneous group of extraarticular disorders is probably responsible for more rheumatic complaints than any one of the intrinsic joint disorders. Approximately 30 percent of patients who attend arthritis clinics in the United States have nonarticular rheumatism.

FIBROSITIS. This is a controversial term which Gowers introduced in 1904 to describe the chronic inflammation of fibrous tissue which he believed to be responsible for "lumbago." This concept was avidly adopted to explain aches and stiffness in various sites of the body, and "fibrositis" has become a wastebasket term to cover many forms of nonarticular rheumatism. In addition to stiffness and soreness, there are often tenderness and limitation of motion of the affected part. The presence of nodules has been overemphasized; in many instances, these are really fat hernias or lipomas. Frequent sites of pain are the lower part of the back, gluteal region, neck, shoulder, and chest. Fatigability is the only constitutional manifestation. Precipitating factors include viral or bacterial infections; trauma; overexposure to cold, dampness, or drafts; and more specific connective tissue disorders, such as bursitis or tenosynovitis. Many patients are middle-aged and seem depressed. Alternatively, "fibrositis" may be a phenomenon of aging. Bi-

opsies of "nodules" or tender areas almost never reveal evidence of inflammation. Most cases are not alleviated by salicylates or anti-inflammatory agents. The local application of heat or injection of an anesthetic is often of transient benefit.

TENOSYNOVITIS. Inflammation of tendons and tendon sheaths may be associated with various types of arthritis or may occur independently. It is more frequent in gonococcal than in other forms of arthritis, occurring in nearly half of all cases. Occasionally, gonococcal tenosynovitis occurs without arthritis. Tuberculous tenosynovitis is chronic and destructive. The most common site is the wrist. Tenosynovitis also occurs in rheumatoid arthritis, systemic lupus, and gout. Suppurative tenosynovitis is rare.

Nonspecific tenosynovitis is thought to be a consequence of single or repeated injuries incurred during movements demanding strength and speed. The wrist and ankle tendons and their sheaths are most commonly involved. If conservative therapy (immobilization, heat, and analgesics) fails, local injection of corticosteroid or surgical excision of the sheath may be indicated.

BURSITIS. This term is used loosely by patients to signify bilateral or unilateral shoulder pain, but bursitis may involve one of the 140 or more bursae in the body. A bursa is a closed sac lined with synovium and containing a small amount of synovial fluid. The most commonly affected deep bursae (those situated between bony prominences and muscle or tendon) include the subacromial, subgluteal, supratrochanteric, and Achilles. The most frequently involved superficial bursae (those situated between bony prominences and skin) are the olecranon and prepatellar. Subacromial bursitis is estimated to be the cause of shoulder pain in 80 percent of patients who do not have evidence of rheumatic disease elsewhere. Its numerous synonyms include *subdeltoid bursitis, calcific bursitis, calcific tendinitis, periarthritis of the shoulder,* and *Duplay's disease.* Increasing attention is now being given to bursitis elsewhere, especially in the hip region.

The pathogenesis of subacromial bursitis is obscure. It is generally held that acute or chronic trauma leads to rupture of a calcium "abscess" which has formed in the tendon of one of the short rotator shoulder muscles (supraspinatus, infraspinatus, teres minor, or subscapularis). Inflammation within and about the bursa is thought to be secondary to the tendinous necrosis and calcification.

In acute subacromial bursitis, agonizing pain appears suddenly in the region of the shoulder joint and is aggravated by motion, especially abduction. The pain often radiates into the neck or down the lateral aspect of the arm to the fingertips. There is exquisite tenderness over the greater tuberosity of the humerus. In approximately half the cases, roentgenograms of the shoulder reveal one or more calcific deposits over the greater tuberosity and localized atrophy of adjacent bone. The acute attack may subside completely or pass into a chronic phase, which is usually mild.

Adhesive capsulitis (also called *adhesive tendinitis, chronic adhesive bursitis*, or *"frozen shoulder"*) is distinguished from subacromial bursitis by a more insidious onset, less pain, and more stiffness. Dense adhesions form between the opposing surfaces of the subacromial bursa. Some investigators believe that the initial change is degeneration of the biceps tendon. It is thought to result from prolonged immobilization, senescence, or trauma. In advanced cases, the arm becomes locked at the side and the shoulder muscles atrophy.

Therapeutically, an attack of bursitis may require no more than rest, immobilization with slings or splints, physical therapy, and analgesic drugs. The local injection of procaine or hydrocortisone sometimes affords prompt relief. Aspiration or surgical removal of the calcific deposit is recommended if disability is persistent. In adhesive capsulitis, manipulation of the shoulder under anesthesia may become necessary, but it must be carried out with great care.

CARPAL TUNNEL SYNDROME. The carpal tunnel is formed dorsally and laterally by the bones of the wrist and ventrally by the transverse carpal ligament. The median nerve passes through this space, and encroachment upon the tunnel results in typical neurologic manifestations. Trauma, fibrous sclerosis of tendon sheaths, rheumatoid or other granulomatous inflammations, the edema before menses and during pregnancy, acromegaly, and amyloidosis are among the many causes of the syndrome. The disorder is especially frequent in middle-aged women.

There is severe burning pain, worse at night, of the first four digits, often bilaterally. The ability to abduct the thumb is impaired, and there is atrophy of the adductor pollicis brevis, with flattening of the thenar eminence. The pain may be elicited by hitting the median nerve at the wrist or by rapid wrist flexion. The diagnosis may be confirmed also by delayed nerve conduction to the branches of the median nerve distal to the wrist. There have been reports of similar involvement of the ulnar tunnel and of the tarsal tunnel with entrapment of the posterior tibial nerve.

Conservative measures (analgesics, splinting, local injections of anesthetic or corticosteroid) occasionally suffice. Surgical decompression, with release of the transverse ligament and debridement, is often eventually necessary and usually curative.

390 OTHER DISEASES AFFECTING THE JOINTS

Lawrence E. Shulman

REITER'S SYNDROME

DEFINITION. Reiter's syndrome (*Reiter's disease, venereal arthritis, infectious uroarthritis, idiopathic blennorrheal arthritis, arthritis urethritica*) is recognized strictly by the triad of arthritis, nongonococcal urethritis, and conjunctivitis. Many patients also have characteristic mucocutaneous manifestations. The complete triad (or tetrad) is not common, but incomplete forms such as arthritis and urethritis or conjunctivitis are frequent.

EPIDEMIOLOGY AND PATHOGENESIS. Reiter's syndrome is largely a disorder of young men, although it has been reported at all ages and in females. The incidence seems to be high in military populations.

In Britain and the United States the disease is generally considered to be of venereal origin. In Scandinavia, France, North Africa, and the Far East, the syndrome is frequently looked upon as a complication of bacillary dysentery. Support for this thesis was obtained from a Finnish report of 334 cases of Reiter's syndrome, occurring during an epidemic of dysentery caused by *Shigella flexneri;* and from an outbreak of 10 cases (2 percent) of Reiter's syndrome after an epidemic of 602 cases of Shigella dysentery aboard a U.S. Naval vessel. None of the 664 men without dysentery developed Reiter's syndrome.

Recent reports have also strongly implicated a Bedsonia (psittacossis-like) microorganism, that has been isolated from joints, urethra, and/or eyes of several patients with Reiter's syndrome. In many of these patients, serum antibody against a psittacosis antigen has been demonstrated by complement fixation. The pathogenetic role of Bedsonia remains to be elucidated. The information concerning mycoplasma as possible pathogens is conflicting. Classical Reiter's syndrome has also been associated with gonorrhea. It seems likely that several types of microorganisms with different portals of entry may induce Reiter's syndrome.

MANIFESTATIONS. The triad of Reiter's syndrome usually evolves over a 3- to 4-week period, although this varies from days to months. Urethritis usually appears first, followed by conjunctivitis and then by arthritis. In most cases, the arthritis is the most severe and prolonged of the manifestations. There may be fever (to 103°F), malaise, anorexia, or weight loss.

The initial attack is usually self-limited. The urethritis and conjunctivitis disappear after days or a few weeks, but the arthritis may last for months or years. Recurrences are almost the rule, as many as eight episodes having been recorded in a single individual.

The first attack of *arthritis* is likely to be explosive. Typically, it is a migratory polyarthritis with heat, tenderness, and swelling. The more commonly affected joints are, in order, the knees, ankles, metatarsophalangeal joints, and wrists. However, any peripheral joint may be involved, and the disease may be monarticular. Severe pain in one or both of the heels is a common complaint. Evidence of spondylitis, such as low-back pain and stiffness or tenderness over spinous processes, sometimes appears late in the disease. Subsequent attacks of arthritis tend to come on more slowly than the initial attack.

Although the *genitourinary involvement* is usually obvious, with dysuria and urethral discharge, it may be necessary to massage the prostate to establish the diagnosis. The urethral meatus is frequently red and edematous. At the same time there may be (1) nonbacterial cystitis manifested by frequency of urination, suprapubic pain, and terminal hematuria, (2) prostatitis, or (3) seminal vesiculitis. Urethral stricture is a rare complication.

The most common *ocular manifestation* is conjunctivitis, which usually starts in one eye, then spreads to the other. Photophobia, burning pain, and hyperemia may be intense; they subside in 1 to 2 weeks. Other ocular lesions are superficial keratitis, corneal ulcers, episcleritis, and iritis.

Mucocutaneous lesions are important diagnostically. They appear early in the disease and may precede other manifestations. The most common sites are the glans penis (80 percent), mouth (50 percent), and the soles and palms (30 percent). The penile lesions begin as small blebs, which coalesce into large patches with sharply defined borders ("balanitis circinata"); in the circumcised individual, these may be hyperkeratotic.

The *oral lesions,* on the palate, buccal mucosa, tongue, and pharynx, consist of small papules or vesicles which coalesce to form irregular gray patches demarcated by a red serpiginous border. They are painless.

The lesions on the soles and palms consist of *keratoderma blennorrhagicum,* beginning as hyperkeratotic red-purple papules, often in clusters, which may later coalesce. No microorganism has been recovered consistently from these lesions, and there is no evidence that they are the result of gonorrheal infection. *Hyperkeratoses* may cover the entire soles. Accumulation of keratotic material beneath the fingernails and toenails is also characteristic.

Aortic regurgitation, caused by focal medial necrosis at the root of the aorta and dilatation of the aortic ring, as in ankylosing spondylitis, has also been reported in Reiter's syndrome, as have conduction defects.

LABORATORY FINDINGS. There may be moderate anemia or neutrophilic leukocytosis of 10,000 to 20,000 per cu mm. The erythrocyte sedimentation rate is rapid and parallels the clinical course.

The characteristic *radiologic signs* consist of juxta-articular "fluffy" periosteal proliferation, periosteal thickening over calcaneal spurs, sacroileitis (often unilateral), and asymmetric syndesmophytes. Erosions at joint margins are also seen. Synovial fluid analysis may reveal a striking polymorphonuclear reaction.

DIAGNOSIS. It is important to distinguish Reiter's syndrome from gonococcal arthritis, which, strictly, should be diagnosed only by identifying gonococci. Many cases formerly considered to be gonorrheal arthritis were, in all likelihood, Reiter's syndrome. The distinction is important, because untreated gonococcal arthritis is often rapidly destructive. A relationship between "nonspecific" urethritis and Reiter's syndrome seems likely. Separation of Reiter's syndrome from rheumatoid arthritis or spondylitis is usually not difficult; on the other hand, Reiter's syndrome may resemble psoriatic arthritis closely because the cutaneous features of both are similar. The mucocutaneous lesions may also resemble erythema multiforme exudativum (Stevens-Johnson syndrome) or Behçet's syndrome.

TREATMENT. Treatment is purely symptomatic. Mild cases require only salicylates. Most severe cases usually respond to phenylbutazone or indomethacin. Corticosteroids are rarely needed.

ANKYLOSING SPONDYLITIS

DEFINITION AND ETIOLOGY. This disorder (also called *Marie-Strümpell arthritis* or *rheumatoid spondylitis*) is a chronic arthritis involving the spine, sacroiliac joints, and, in a minority of cases, peripheral joints. Contrary to earlier thinking, it is considered to be a disorder separate and distinct from rheumatoid arthritis for the following reasons. Ninety percent of patients with spondylitis are men, whereas 60 to 70 percent of those with rheumatoid arthritis are women. Spondylitis usually begins at a younger age; onset after thirty years of age is unusual. Subcutaneous nodules are absent in spondylitis. When peripheral joints are involved in spondylitis, the common sites are the shoulders, hips, and knees; in rheumatoid arthritis, fingers, wrists, toes, and ankles are most often affected. Rheumatoid factor tests are usually negative in spondylitis. Other points include the tendency for spondylitis to produce calcification of ligaments (absent in rheumatoid arthritis), to respond to x-ray therapy, and to fail to respond to gold. The role of inheritance is firmly established in spondylitis. It occurs in identical twins, and is twenty-two times more common among relatives of spondylitis patients than in the rest of the population. The disease may, in fact, be more closely related to Reiter's syndrome, enteritis, and psoriasis, in which significant proportions of patients develop sacroileitis and at times spondylitis at other sites.

PATHOLOGY. The basic lesion is synovitis, which usually begin in the sacroiliac joints. Synovitis of the spine is confined to the posterior intervertebral apophyseal joints, the true diarthrodeses of the vertebral column, and the costovertebral joints. Later the spinal ligaments become calcified. Demineralization of the vertebral bodies may appear during any phase of the disease. Bony bridges, *syndesmophytes,* are formed laterally and anteriorly. At autopsy, 6 percent of patients have amyloidosis.

CLINICAL FEATURES. Spondylitis usually begins insidiously, with stiffness of the back after inactivity, lumbar pain with radiation to buttock and thigh, and limitation of forward bending. Constitutional symptoms are usually mild or absent. Roentgenograms show squaring of the vertebrae, beginning in the lumbar region. Lumbar lordosis is lost, and, with involvement of the costovertebral joints, chest movement diminishes. Pain may be elicited by deep inspiration, coughing, or sneezing. As the spine fuses, it may be held erect, the so-called "poker spine," but more frequently, the result is dorsal kyphosis with the head fixed in forward displacement. Such patients run the risk of cervical cord compression. Peripheral joint involvement may either precede or follow spinal disease. In many instances it is brief and intermittent, but in one-fourth of patients it persists, characteristically in the shoulders and hips.

Approximately 3 percent of patients develop *aortitis*

and aortic regurgitation. Microscopically, focal necroses are seen in the media of the root of the aorta. These lesions may extend to involve the atrioventricular bundle, and cardiac *conduction defects* are not uncommon.

Nongranulomatous *uveitis* occurs in 20 to 30 percent of patients; it varies greatly in severity and duration. Scleromalacia perforans does not occur.

COURSE. Although the course of the disease is variable, the usual pattern is persistent activity for months or years, with pain, low-grade fever, weight loss, anemia, and a high sedimentation rate. As the spine fuses, pain disappears, on the average 10 years after onset. In contrast to patients with rheumatoid arthritis, most patients with spondylitis continue to lead relatively normal and productive lives; fewer than 10 percent become totally incapacitated. If clinically detectable aortic regurgitation develops, life expectancy is shortened.

TREATMENT. The general principles of management are the relief of pain and the preservation of the best possible skeletal function. For analgesia, salicylates in the fullest tolerable doses should be tried first. Phenylbutazone (Butazolidin) and indomethacin are both highly effective in ankylosing spondylitis, in sharp contrast to their results in rheumatoid arthritis. Corticosteroid therapy is rarely used, and should be reserved for patients with severe disease who can not tolerate other drugs. X-ray therapy affords pain relief but has been discarded because of a high incidence of leukemia after radiotherapy for spondylitis.

Special attention should be paid to keeping deformities to a minimum by seeing that fusion takes place in the optimal position. The patient should become "posture-conscious." He should use a bed board and a firm mattress, as well as a small pillow or no pillow at all to prevent kyphosis and neck flexion. A small pillow under the lumbar spine may preserve the normal lordosis. Exercises of the paravertebral, abdominal, and respiratory muscles designed to maintain a straight back and neck and to retain ventilatory sufficiency are useful. Chest expansion should be recorded serially. Muscle relaxants are usually not beneficial. Back braces may help to combat thoracic kyphosis. If extreme deformity develops, vertebral osteotomy may be indicated.

PSORIATIC ARTHRITIS

The incidence of arthritis is greater in patients with psoriasis than in the general population. In a minority of those with psoriasis and arthritis there is striking involvement of the interphalangeal joints, often with marked destruction and psoriatic changes in the adjacent nails. Some investigators consider this true "psoriatic arthropathy." In the majority of patients, the joint disease resembles rheumatoid arthritis. Several features, however, distinguish most cases from true rheumatoid arthritis: less symmetry, absence of subcutaneous nodules, high incidence of sacroiliac involvement, and negative tests for rheumatoid factor.

An entire finger may be affected, giving a sausage-like appearance; and roentgenograms of digital joints may show pencil-in-cup deformities.

The psoriasis usually antedates the arthritis by months or years, but they may appear simultaneously or the arthritis may come first. In general, there is little correlation between activity of skin lesions and that of the arthritis.

The principles and details of management are similar to those for rheumatoid arthritis except that antimalarials should be avoided because they may exacerbate psoriatic skin lesions. Contrary to some reports, oral triamcinolone has no advantage over other corticosteroids. Long-standing severe psoriasis with multilating arthritis may respond favorably to treatment with methotrexate and other immunosuppressive agents.

Many patients with active, extensive psoriasis have hyperuricemia, and a few develop clinical gout, which responds to the usual treatment.

ARTHRITIS AND GASTROINTESTINAL DISEASE

ULCERATIVE COLITIS. Rheumatic complaints occur in as many as half of all cases of ulcerative colitis. After degenerative joint disease, traumatic arthritis, rheumatic fever, and gout have been excluded, four groups remain: (1) "colitic arthritis," 10 to 20 percent of cases; (2) ankylosing spondylitis, 5 to 10 percent; (3) typical rheumatoid arthritis, 2 to 3 percent (an incidence approximating that in the general population), and (4) hypertrophic osteoarthropathy.

Colitic arthritis is an acute synovitis which is frequently monarticular; when polyarticular, it is often asymmetric. The joints involved are knee, ankle, elbow, and proximal interphalangeal joint, in order of decreasing frequency. Single attacks last a few weeks, but recurrence is the rule. Histologically, the synovitis is nonspecific. The arthritis usually accompanies exacerbations of long-standing colitis and is more common in patients with perianal suppuration, pseudopolyposis, or erythema nodosum. Features which help to distinguish colitic arthritis from rheumatoid arthritis are (1) younger age at onset; (2) absence of residual deformity; (3) absence of subcutaneous nodules or tendon sheath lesions; (4) paucity of radiologic changes; (5) negative tests for rheumatoid factor; and (6) an apparent cure after colectomy. Patients with rheumatoid arthritis rarely develop ulcerative colitis.

Spondylitis as a complication of colitis is seen equally in females and males. Symptoms may antedate by several years, coincide with, or follow the onset of colitis; they may persist after colectomy. In most patients, radiologic changes are confined to the sacroiliac joints. Many patients complain of low-back pain during attacks of colitis but have no objective evidence of spondylitis.

REGIONAL ENTERITIS. Both peripheral arthritis and spondylitis may complicate regional enteritis, the incidences being estimated at 2 to 6 percent and 1 to 2 percent, respectively. Most patients have ileocolitis (Crohn's disease). The distribution of the acute or subacute arthritis resembles that in ulcerative colitis, and the severity of the arthritis parallels the activity of the intestinal disease.

WHIPPLE'S DISEASE. This disorder, also known as intestinal lipodystrophy or lipogranulomatosis, is a systemic disease of middle-aged men, manifested by intermittent arthritis, weight loss, cutaneous hyperpigmentation, lymphadenopathy, abdominal pain, diarrhea, and intestinal malabsorption. Diagnosis may be made by finding periodic acid-Schiff (PAS)–positive particles in lymph node, jejunal, or rectal biopsy. By electron microscopy, bacilliform bodies have been found within and near macrophages.

The joint involvement, which usually antedates other manifestations by months or years, consists of a migratory polyarthralgia or polyarthritis affecting the larger joints. Articular recurrences accompany exacerbations of abdominal symptoms, but joint deformities do not develop. Ankylosing spondylitis may appear late in the disease. Curiously, histopathologic studies of synovium have failed to show the characteristic PAS-positive macrophages, and there is only a nonspecific synovitis with mononuclear cells.

CHONDROCALCINOSIS

This disease, also called "pseudogout," is a chronic arthritis with recurrent acute attacks. Examination of synovial fluid reveals crystals. The disorder is also recognized radiologically by characteristic linear calcifications.

During an acute attack *crystals* are seen both within and outside synovial fluid leukocytes, especially under polarized light. The crystals have been identified as calcium pyrophosphate dihydrate. Intraarticular injection of synthetic crystals reproduces the acute attack. The disease is considered to be a crystal-induced synovitis, closely resembling gout. Diseased cartilage is the presumed source of the crystals.

The disorder, however, differs from gout. Both sexes are equally affected. The most commonly involved joint is the knee: small joints are usually spared. Acute attacks may not respond to colchicine. Under polarized light, the crystals differ from those of gout, having the configuration of blunt rods or rhomboids and being only weakly and positively birefringent (in contrast to the strong negative birefringence of urate crystals).

Linear calcifications are seen by x-ray in fibrocartilage, as in the meniscus of the knee, symphysis pubis, and annulus fibrosus, and at times, in articular hyaline cartilage.

Chondrocalcinosis is encountered in, and perhaps associated with, degenerative joint disease, hemochromatosis, hyperparathyroidism, Wilson's disease, ochronosis, diabetes mellitus, and even gout.

Joint aspiration often gives significant relief. Acute attacks respond to phenylbutazone, and at times to salicylates or colchicine. If salicylates do not control the acute attack, phenylbutazone, which is very effective in this disorder, may be given.

RELAPSING POLYCHONDRITIS

In this rare disorder, the cartilages in various parts of the body undergo inflammation and dissolve. The basic defect is thought to be either a hypersensitivity to cartilage or an enzymatic chondrolysis, similar to that produced in rabbits by papain injections.

Clinically, the cartilages of the nose and ears are particularly susceptible, and these structures collapse. Other cartilaginous areas which become involved, but less frequently, include the middle ear, larynx, trachea, bronchi, costosternal articulations, intervertebral disks, and peripheral joints. Aortic valvular regurgitation and aneurysms of the ascending aorta are also found.

The disease is serious, with many deaths caused by collapse of the tracheobronchial tree. The initial experience with corticosteroids has been favorable.

POLYMYALGIA RHEUMATICA (See Chap. 394)

TIETZE'S SYNDROME

Also called *costochrondritis*, this disorder consists of severe parasternal pain, usually unilateral, over one or more of the upper four ribs. There are swelling and tenderness over the costochrondral junction, but curiously, biopsies of affected cartilages have revealed no abnormalities. Although the pain may last for weeks and months, it eventually disappears. The nature of the disorder is obscure.

PSYCHOGENIC RHEUMATISM

This term refers to the rheumatic manifestations of psychoneurosis, in which patients complain of stiffness, pain in joints, tendons, or muscles, and limitation of joint motion. In the United States Armed Forces during World War II, psychogenic rheumatism was thought to be the most common rheumatic disease; in the British forces such cases were labeled "fibrositis." Essential for this diagnosis are good general health, emotional instability, absence of objective joint changes clinically and radiologically, normal laboratory findings, vacillating complaints, and failure to respond to analgesics and physical therapy. Some investigators feel that a category of psychogenic rheumatism is unjustified and that there is probably some organic basis for the symptoms.

REFERENCES

Ankylosing Spondylitis

Blumberg, G., and C. Ragan: The Natural History of Rheumatoid Spondylitis, Medicine, 35:1, 1956.

Cruickshank, B.: Pathology of Ankylosing Spondylitis, Bull. Rheum. Dis., 10:211, 1960.

Chondrocalcinosis

McCarty, D. J., Jr., and R. A. Gatter: Pseudogout Syndrome (Articular Chondrocalcinosis), Bull. Rheum. Dis., 14: 331, 1964.

Psoriasis

Wright, V.: Psoriatic Arthritis: Comparative Radiographic Study of Rheumatoid Arthritis and Arthritis Associated with Psoriasis, Ann. Rheum. Dis., 20:123, 1961.

Reiter's Syndrome

Noer, H. R.: An "Experimental" Epidemic of Reiter's Syndrome, J.A.M.A., 197:693, 1966.

Weinberger, H. J., M. W. Ropes, J. P. Kulka, and W. Bauer: Reiter's Syndrome, Clinical and Pathological Observations: Long-term Study of 16 Cases, Medicine, 41:91, 1962.

Wright, V.: Arthritis Associated with Venereal Disease, Ann. Rheum. Dis., 22:77, 1963.

Relapsing Polychondritis

Dolan, D. L., G. B. Lemmon, Jr., and S. L. Teitelbaum:

Relapsing Polychondritis, Amer. J. Med., 41:285, 1966.

Pearson, C. M., H. M. Kline, and V. D. Newcomer: Relapsing Polychondritis, New Engl. J. Med., 263:51, 1960.

Tietze's Disease

Kayser, H. D.: Tietze's Syndrome: Review of Literature, Am. J. Med., 21:982, 1956.

Ulcerative Colitis

McEwen, C., C. Lingg, J. B. Kirsner, and J. A. Spencer: Arthritis Accompanying Ulcerative Colitis, Am. J. Med., 33:923, 1962.

Wright, V., and G. Watkinson: The Arthritis of Ulcerative Colitis, Brit. Med. J., 2:670, 1965.

Whipple's Disease

Caughey, D. E., and E. G. L. Bywaters: Arthritis of Whipple's Syndrome, Ann. Rheum. Dis., 22:327, 1963.

Farnan, P.: Whipple's Disease: The Clinical Aspects, Quart. J. Med. (New Series), 28:163, 1959.

Section 14

Disorders of Other Supporting Tissues

INTRODUCTION

Ivan L. Bennett, Jr.

This section contains descriptions of diseases whose manifestations are mainly attributable to damage of the body's "soft skeleton," the connective tissue. Generally, common or related causation is the basis for classification, and ideally, similarity in manifestations is the most useful clinical criterion for grouping diseases. Here, we are dealing for the most part with diseases of obscure origin. Furthermore, because injury to connective tissue can produce structural or functional abnormalities in almost any organ system or anatomic site, it is difficult to select a few predominant symptoms and signs from the diverse manifestations that may accompany such diseases and to rely on them as a logical starting point. If they are considered by the clinician as generalized disorders of connective tissue, however, they are less perplexing. For example, several genetically determined diseases, once looked upon as esoteric syndromes composed of a peculiar hodgepodge of unrelated abnormalities, are now known to be relatively common. When viewed as disorders of connective tissue, such associations as ectopia lentis, inguinal hernia, and aortic dissection in Marfan's syndrome or angioid streaks and melena in pseudoxanthoma elasticum are logical and expected.

In addition to the major "collagen vascular diseases," a few relatively unusual diseases of uncertain cause but closely related histologic manifestations are included: relapsing panniculitis, Wegener's granulomatosis, and scleredema. Rheumatic fever (Chap. 269) and acute hemorrhagic glomerulonephritis (Chap. 304) are discussed in another part of the book. Dermatomyositis (Chap. 375) has been included elsewhere with other diseases of muscle, and rheumatoid arthritis and its variants (Chap. 386) are described in the section on joint diseases and rheumatism.

391 POLYARTERITIS NODOSA

Philip A. Tumulty

DEFINITION. Polyarteritis nodosa is characterized by focal and diffuse inflammatory damage to blood vessels, especially small and medium arteries, which results in altered function of the organs involved. The disease runs a subacute or chronic course, and its clinical manifestations are often confusingly diverse.

INCIDENCE AND ETIOLOGY. Polyarteritis is relatively uncommon. It is most often seen in the fourth decade, although it has occurred in infants and the aged. The disease is two to three times more frequent in males than in females. There is no known racial or familial predisposition. The disease has been reported in an individual with macroglobulinemia and cryoglobulinemia who had inherited a chromosome translocation involving chromosomes 4 and 5.

Many possible causes have been considered, including specific infectious agents, "toxins," and neurogenic disturbances. Necrotizing arteritis morphologically similar to that of polyarteritis in man has been produced in rabbits by sensitization to proteins, and in rats by several procedures that induce hypertension.

In many cases of polyarteritis nodosa, the onset of symptoms has closely followed serum sickness or sensitivity reaction to drugs, including sulfonamides, iodides, penicillin, and thiouracil. The chronic administration of estrogens to rats is said to induce an arteritis, and the disease has been described in a female impersonator who took stilbestrol chronically. There is a close association between chronic bronchial asthma and polyarteritis. While the possibility of diverse etiologies cannot be excluded, it seems certain that hypersensitivity is one cause of the disease in man.

PATHOLOGY. The principal lesion is an inflammation of small and medium arteries, including the vasa vasorum. Veins and capillaries are sometimes involved. Necrosis and destruction of all coats are found. Involvement is usually segmental, and only a portion of the circumference of the artery may be attacked. Eosinophils are usually prominent in the acute lesions. The consequences of the injury vary; there may be rupture, healing with fibrosis, thrombosis with recanalization, or aneurysm formation. It is common to find lesions in all stages of inflammation and repair in biopsy or autopsy specimens; this is in keeping with the subacute or chronic intermittent clinical course. Granulomatous nodules that seem unrelated to vessels may occur in various organs or on serosal surfaces, and focal or diffuse glomerulonephritis is a frequent feature of the disease.

Arteritis is a feature of many diseases, including lupus erythematosus, rheumatoid arthritis, serum sickness, and rheumatic fever. Furthermore, arterial changes morphologically indistinguishable from those of polyarteritis may be found in the intestinal submucosa in some patients with uremia or at the periphery of necrotizing or suppurative bacterial lesions. Therefore, the presence of arteritis, especially in the absence of a prominent eosinophilic component in the inflammation, is not diagnostic of polyarteritis nodosa, and biopsy findings must be interpreted in light of the entire clinical picture. The relationship of polyarteritis nodosa to temporal arteritis, Wegener's granulomatosis, so-called "malignant rheumatoid disease," and other collagen-vascular disorders remains speculative. For diagnostic purposes, each of these various conditions has individual clinical characteristics, and until more is known, it is well to regard them as separate entities.

MANIFESTATIONS. The initial manifestations are so variable that there is no "typical" mode of onset. Symptoms sometimes appear abruptly in an individual who has previously been entirely well; more often, the initial symptoms seem to follow another illness. The primary incident may be some banal disorder like pulmonary infection or cholecystitis with apparent recovery, or a period of vague indisposition with the subsequent development of new manifestations and overt disability.

Disease of a single organ system, such as nephritis or neuritis, is not at all infrequent in polyarteritis, but initially the patient more often gives the impression that he is suffering from some subacute febrile disease, perhaps infectious in origin, without localizing signs. Frequent early complaints are weakness, myalgia, arthralgia, fatigability, anorexia, weight loss, headache, chilliness, and fever. There may be afebrile intervals, but patients usually continue to be unwell; a few patients never have fever. Drenching sweats are common, and disproportionate tachycardia is frequent.

The emphasis on the "triad" of fever, abdominal pain, and hypertension in a young man as being typical of polyarteritis is misleading. A majority of patients fails to show this picture. Early in its course, many of the "typical features" of polyarteritis may be absent, including hypertension, impressive urinary alterations, eosinophilia, and focal organ system changes and the patient is merely ill in a very general, nonspecific fashion.

Skin and Mucous Membranes. Cutaneous or subcutaneous nodules are an important diagnostic feature. They range from the size of a millet seed to that of a pea, occur singly or in crops, regress very quickly (repeated examination is mandatory), and may be located on any part of the body, including the soles, scalp, scrotum, penis, and tongue. Occasionally, they are pulsatile and clearly represent small aneurysms, but it is rare to find this type. The nodular lesions may be distributed linearly along vessels, and the overlying skin may be normal, reddened, or ulcerated. Only a minority of patients have these striking lesions.

Far more frequent are such nonspecific eruptions as urticaria, petechiae, purpura, hemorrhagic bullae, and erythematous rashes. Occasionally Raynaud's phenomenon is seen, and rarely, arterial involvement will simulate thromboangiitis obliterans with acrocyanosis and peripheral gangrene. *Livido racemosa*, arborescent red or purplish markings which fade into normal skin without sharp demarcation, is an unusual but diagnostically important cutaneous finding in polyarteritis. Mucosal lesions are rare. Localized or generalized edema of the face, trunk, or extremities may occur and sometimes is the earliest change.

Musculoskeletal. Weakness and atrophy of skeletal muscles, sometimes associated with marked tenderness, often constitute a prominent early feature, simulating other forms of polymyositis, a primary muscular atrophy, or trichinosis. Symmetric involvement of peripheral muscles is usual, but truncal muscles may be affected, sometimes leading to respiratory difficulties. Arthralgias are more common than arthritis, although deformities indistinguishable from rheumatoid disease occur, and rheumatoid factor may be present. Patients appearing to have classical chronic rheumatoid disease may eventually die from a diffuse arteritis. Whether or not this so-called "malignant rheumatoid disease" is a variant of classical polyarteritis nodosa remains obscure. Patients never treated with steroids have had this course, and these agents can not be incriminated as the cause of this syndrome.

Eyes. Ocular manifestations are common and may arise in any of four ways: (1) direct involvement of retinal vessels with exudation, hemorrhage, "cytoid" bodies, retinal detachment, arterial occlusion, papilledema, and optic atrophy; (2) exudative lesions such as scleritis, episcleritis, chemosis of the conjunctiva, necroses of the sclera, corneal ulcers, choroidal abnormalities, iritis, uveitis, keratitis; (3) cerebral arterial disease with extraocular palsy or pupillomotor disturbances and visual field defects; (4) hypertensive retinopathy. Pseudotumor of the orbit and Sjögren's syndrome are sometimes observed.

Lungs and Pleura. Pulmonary manifestations occur in about 25 percent of patients with polyarteritis. Histologic changes may be present without symptoms, and the roentgenographic findings and clinical manifestations are rarely diagnostic. The observed changes range from nodular opacities resembling miliary tuberculosis or carcinomatosis to confluent pneumonic consolidation, usually basilar or extending fanlike from the hilum. There may be cavitation if larger vessels are involved, and pulmonary infarcts or rupture of vessels may lead to hemoptysis. Lesions in the submucosal vessels may result in tracheobronchial ulceration, with cough and bloody sputum. Pneumothorax sometimes occurs. Apart from any parenchymal changes, diffuse pulmonary arteritis may result in pulmonary hypertension and its sequelae. Secondary bacterial or fungal infection may lead to pneumonitis or lung abscess.

The relationship of polyarteritis to bronchial asthma has been stressed. A history of typical asthmatic attacks may precede the onset of systemic arteritis by many years. Whether the asthma is of the ordinary atopic type or is a harbinger of pulmonary arteritis is not known.

An attempt has been made to characterize a group of patients with polyarteritis nodosa whose illness is primarily pulmonary. The individuals all have chronic pulmonary alterations of long standing, develop what appears to be a respiratory infection, and then are found to have high blood eosinophilia, numerous eosinophils in acute arteritic lesions, and many focal necrotic or granulomatous lesions unrelated to blood vessels in the liver, spleen, kidneys, lymph nodes, and heart. Patients regarded as having benign Loeffler's pneumonia recurrently over a period of years have ultimately developed a diffuse arteritic disease. Pleurisy occurs with or without effusion, which is occasionally bloody, and, at times, represents secondary infection.

Serial roentgenograms of the lungs may help in establishing a diagnosis of polyarteritis if they show regression of earlier lesions, appearance of new infiltrates, and, in general, continuous flux. The instability of the findings contrasts with those in lupus erythematosus, which are likely to remain stable for many months. Eosinophilia, frequently not prominent in polyarteritis, is said to be present in the majority of patients with pulmonary arteritis.

Cardiovascular. Episodes of pericarditis with or without small effusions are frequent; a massive bloody effusion with tamponade may result from a ruptured vessel. The myocardium is affected by coronary arteritis; rarely, the clinical picture may be dominated by coronary insufficiency and terminate with massive infarction. Focal granulomatous myocarditis is sometimes severe enough to produce congestive failure or conduction defects. With the onset of renal insufficiency and hypertension, cardiac enlargement and failure are even more likely. Warty, nonbacterial vegetations sometimes appear on the endocardium. They can be the nidus for bacterial endocarditis.

The concurrent existence of rheumatic heart disease and polyarteritis has been recognized for many years and is one of the bases of the argument that hypersensitivity is a common factor in the etiology of these two diseases.

Gastrointestinal. Abdominal pain, nausea, vomiting, diarrhea, and intestinal bleeding are often early manifestations. Features of "multisystem" disease are sometimes preceded by an episode of clinically uncomplicated appendicitis, cholecystitis, or pancreatitis. Later, confusing indications of systemic disease appear or abdominal pain continues. Recognition that the abdominal episode is associated with disease in other organs may lead to the correct diagnosis.

Depending on the extent and localization of vascular disease, many intraabdominal disturbances occur: focal pain; acute diffuse pain without findings at laparotomy; focal or diffuse, sometimes massive bleeding; intraabdominal hematomas mistaken for tumor, cyst, or aneurysm; perforation of a viscus, especially the gallbladder; mucosal ulcerations; infarction of the gut; subphrenic abscess; peritonitis; small-intestinal obstruction due to thickening and adhesions; malabsorption; intraabdominal hemorrhage.

A moderate degree of hepatomegaly is usual. Because the hepatic arterial and venous radicles may be involved in the disease, there may ensue enough vascular insufficiency to produce true infarction of the liver parenchyma. Indeed, polyarteritis is the most frequent cause of large hepatic infarcts. Pain, friction rubs, and jaundice signal massive infarction. Smaller foci of destruction heal with scarring, which, in a single biopsy specimen, may resemble cirrhosis. Granulomas may be scattered through the liver, producing a "granulomatous hepatitis." Pathologic studies have indicated that the liver is the fourth most commonly affected organ, and in a number of patients the presenting problem centers about liver dysfunction, including hepatomegaly, ascites, and jaundice, features which usually are attributed to hepatitis or cirrhosis. In some instances liver biopsy can provide the answer.

Polyarteritis may pose the differential diagnosis of an intraabdominal mass lesion, due to perihepatic, perisplenic, perirenal, or retroperitoneal hematomas resulting from rupture of an arteritic lesion. These hematomas may be huge, very tender, or pulsatile and often are mistaken for an abscess, tumor, cyst, or aneurysm.

Spleen and Lymph Nodes. Lymphadenopathy is not characteristic of polyarteritis. Mild splenic enlargement is present in about one-third of the cases. Rarely, splenic infarction or hemorrhage around the spleen has been observed; this may simulate a large tumor.

Genitourinary. Some type of renal involvement occurs in at least 80 percent of patients. Often, however, this does not become clinically evident until late in the disease; hence, the absence of hypertension or renal abnormalities should not be regarded as being incompatible with the diagnosis of polyarteritis, especially early in a patient's course.

Rupture of a renal artery can produce a large perirenal hematoma, which on several occasions has been mistaken for a tumor or cyst. Renal infarcts are not infrequent. However, focal or diffuse glomerulonephritis is by far the most important renal lesion in polyarteritis. It may be severe and progressive, may be accompanied by hypertension, and leads to death from uremia or congestive heart failure. Commonly the nephritic changes are not associated with hypertension, at least not initially. Several patients have been reported who developed acute nephritis following streptococcal infections, but who subsequently were found to have acute polyarteritis. The relationships between these events are not clear. Acute nephritis due to polyarteritis may not be associated with other evidence of a generalized arteritis and may appear to be primarily renal disease. Alternatively, arteritis may implicate different segments of the aorta and its major branches, including one or both renal arteries, which may result in unilateral renal hypertension. Hypertension sometimes fluctuates so strikingly that pheochromocytoma is suspected. Formation of an intrarenal arteriovenous fistula following needle biopsy of the kidney in patients with polyarteritis has been reported. Severe hypertension resulted, which responded to surgical therapy when the true nature of the lesion was recognized after a bruit was heard.

The vessels of the bladder may be affected, producing changes resembling those of "hemorrhagic cystitis." The testes and epididymis are frequently involved; testicular infarction with severe pain and subsequent atrophy is more frequent in polyarteritis nodosa than in any other disease.

Nervous System. Peripheral neuritis, a result of inflammation of nutrient vessels, is the most commonly encountered abnormality of nervous function and is often the first and most marked disability. Indeed, in any obscure illness, the appearance of neuritis should immediately call to mind the possibility of polyarteritis. In about half the affected patients, involvement is mononeural; in the others, a symmetric polyneuritis, more severe in the lower extremities, is seen. Severe pain is common, and the sensory deficit frequently exceeds the motor. Regression of the neuritis is characteristic.

Involvement of carotid, vertebral, meningeal, or deep cerebral vessels can lead to hemiplegia, transverse myelitis, convulsions, cerebellar dysfunction, extrapyramidal disorders, optic atrophy, or subarachnoid hemorrhage.

Cranial palsies are not common; the facial nerve is most frequently involved. Involvement of meningeal vessels may result in changes in the spinal fluid, suggesting aseptic or lymphocytic meningitis.

LABORATORY FINDINGS. Leukocytosis is the rule and often reaches 20,000 to 40,000 cells per cu mm. Mild eosinophilia occurs in 20 to 30 percent of cases, and strikingly elevated eosinophil counts are occasionally found. An increased platelet count (above 500,000 per cu mm) is common. The sedimentation rate is elevated; mild anemia, even in the absence of uremia, is frequent. It may be hemolytic and associated with a positive Coombs test. The urine may show protein, erythrocytes, leukocytes, and a variety of cellular and noncellular casts, a so-called "telescoped" sediment. False positive serologic tests for syphilis are found in a small number of cases, and many serum protein changes, including hyperglobulinemia, cryoglobulinemia, macroglobulinemia, as well as circulating anticoagulants have been reported. Rheumatoid factor may be present, as well as serum antibodies to cellular constituents. Serum complement is normal or increased, even in patients with renal involvement.

DIAGNOSIS. Abdominal pain, muscular aches, peripheral neuritis, evidence of renal disease, or hypertension in a setting of weight loss, fever, and leukocytosis are the predominant clinical features, but variation is endless. The process may run an acute, subacute, or chronic course over a period of months or years. Periods of remission of varying length may punctuate the indolent evolution of a bewildering array of seemingly unrelated disorders. Careful search for cutaneous nodules and repeated attempts to confirm the diagnosis by biopsy examination are essential. Skin or muscle is probably the best tissue for examination. Lymph nodes will rarely give the diagnosis. Testicular biopsy is worthwhile. Renal biopsy often shows glomerular disease, but the specific diagnosis of polyarteritis is difficult to establish on this basis. Liver biopsy is very unlikely to show the vascular lesion. It is important to take skin and muscle from an area which is tender or painful and is hence more likely to show inflammation. Because the demonstration of arteritis is the only method for establishing the diagnosis of polyarteritis, repeated biopsy examinations are in order. Recently, arteriography has been reported to be helpful in demonstrating aneurysms and/or zones of ischemic necrosis within the parenchyma of various organs. In contrast, congenital and degenerative aneurysms are said to be extraparenchymal in location.

PROGNOSIS. Spontaneous remissions may occur, and remissions may be induced with corticosteroid therapy. Complete recovery does occur. This is most likely to happen when the disease seems drug-induced or when significant vascular involvement is confined to the integument. The overall outlook, however, is not good, and most patients eventually die from the disease. The 5-year survival rate of treated patients is said to be 48 percent, contrasted with 13 percent of untreated persons. The occurrence of appreciable hypertension and renal disease early in the course worsens the outlook. Their development may be delayed by early institution of adequate treatment. Early death is generally due to renal failure, infarction of the heart or brain, congestive heart failure, or gastrointestinal bleeding.

TREATMENT. The long-term use of corticosteroids, as outlined in the section on systemic lupus erythematosus (Chap. 392) is the only present therapy of any value. Although these agents may result in further injury to tissues because of occlusion of vessels during healing, this may happen spontaneously, and there is no other choice. A dosage schedule of prednisone or its equivalent which suppresses all manifestations of the active inflammatory process should be adopted, and symptomatic improvement, absence of new lesions, betterment of renal alterations, and return of sedimentation rate to normal should result from treatment. The initial dosage should be high, in the range of 60 to 80 mg prednisone per day. Subsequent alterations in therapy must be planned stepwise, guided by clinical and laboratory evidence of the active inflammatory process. The dosage of prednisone should be reduced very gradually to the smallest daily maintenance which assures suppression of inflammation. Therapy may be required for months or even years. While the patient is receiving corticosteroids, adherence to a modified ulcer program is essential. Complicating bacterial, fungal, and other infections which occur not infrequently and are easily mistakenly attributed to the primary disease process, should be watched for carefully.

REFERENCES

Frohnert, P. P., and S. G. Sheps: Long Term Follow-up Study of Periarteritis Nodosa, Am. J. Med., 43:8, 1967.

Kimbrell, O. C., and J. A. Wheliss: Polyarteritis Nodosa Complicated by Bilateral Optic Neuropathy, J.A.M.A., 201: 139, 1967.

Lose, G. A.: The Natural History of Polyarteritis, Brit. Med. J., 2:1148, 1957.

Zeek, P. M.: Periarteritis Nodosa and Other Forms of Necrotizing Angiitis, New Engl. J. Med., 248:764, 1953.

392 SYSTEMIC LUPUS ERYTHEMATOSUS

Philip A. Tumulty

DEFINITION. Systemic lupus erythematosus (SLE) is a disease of unknown cause, a basic feature of which appears to be altered immune reactivity. It can affect any organ system, singly or in combinations. The course of SLE is often episodic, punctuated by periods of remission over a span of many years.

INCIDENCE AND ETIOLOGY. Systemic lupus erythematosus is not uncommon. Its incidence has been approxi-mated to that of the lymphomas. Females are affected six to eight times more frequently than males. A noteworthy peak of incidence occurs in females aged twenty to forty years.

The biologic hallmark of SLE is the presence in the serum of a wide variety of peculiar proteins having the characteristics of antibodies, which suggests that the basic disorder is an alteration in immune reactivity. Serum factors directed against erythrocytes, white blood cells, platelets, and clotting elements, as well as against kidney, heart, and liver tissues, and thyroglobulin have been demonstrated. The Wassermann reaction is frequently positive, and the so-called "rheumatoid factor" is found in approximately 20 percent of patients. The LE factor, which promotes phagocytosis of nucleoprotein, the "LE phenomenon," is the antibody most characteristic of the disease, but many patients also possess antinuclear antibodies which react with whole nuclei, nucleoprotein, deoxyribonucleic acid (DNA), and histone. Anticyto-plasmic factors have also been described. Similar factors are present in other disorders, including rheumatoid arthritis, scleroderma, Sjögren's syndrome, Hashimoto's thyroiditis, myasthenia gravis, and pernicious anemia, but SLE is notable for the occurrence of a profusion of these serum factors, quantitatively as well as qualitatively.

Serum abnormalities may antedate all other manifestations of SLE. Of a group of 192 asymptomatic individuals discovered to have a biologic false positive test for syphilis, 7 percent developed SLE while under observation, and 22 percent a collagen-like disorder. Most of these individuals were females.

Whether or not this altered immune reactivity is genetically transmitted is not known. There are reported instances of SLE in twins and other family members. Relatives of patients with SLE may have other diseases of the "immune" or collagen type, including scleroderma, rheumatoid arthritis, dermatomyositis, rheumatic fever, glomerulonephritis, Sjögren's syndrome, Hashimoto's thyroiditis, hypogammaglobulinemia, hemolytic anemia, and thrombocytopenia. Some family members who are asymptomatic are found to react positively for the various serum factors listed above.

It appears that symptomatic illness in these individuals with immunologic abnormalities can be triggered by a variety of stressful stimuli, including exposure to sun, drug ingestion, pregnancy, emotional reactions, and operative procedures.

The frequency of "overlap" syndromes, in which there is the simultaneous or sequential occurrence in the same patient of manifestations of several of the "connective tissue" or "immune disorders" suggests that underlying altered immune reactivity can express itself in many clinical pictures. This has led to the suggestion that the clinical entities such as SLE, rheumatoid arthritis, scleroderma, etc., may be not different diseases but different clinical expressions of the same basic disorder.

The relationship between drug reactions and SLE deserves comment. Whether drugs produce the disorder directly or merely unveil a latent immune abnormality is not clear. Often what appears to be a "primary" drug reaction is found to be another episode in the long course of SLE. In a study of 50 patients with "hydralazine-induced lupus," 74 percent had clinical or laboratory evidence indicating underlying SLE, and in a large number, one or more manifestations of a lupus-like state persisted or reappeared after the drug was halted. Among therapeutic agents known to be related to SLE are iodides, heavy metals, Dilantin, Tridione, isoniazid, Pronestyl, hydralazine, methyldopa, antibiotics, sulfonamides, and thiourea derivatives.

Whether the serum factors play a direct etiologic role in the lesions of SLE or are only biologic by-products of the disease is not known. The concentration of serum antinuclear factors often rises and the concentration of serum complement often falls when patients with SLE are actively ill, and these changes tend to reverse as the disease remits. There are many exceptions to these generalizations, and patients may die with SLE at a time when little serum antinuclear activity is detectable and serum complement is normal or high. Present evidence supports the idea that some serum factors can cause clinical manifestations (such as the anti-red blood cell factor in inducing hemolytic anemia) while others do not. The plugging of the glomeruli by antigen-antibody complexes has been demonstrated by immunofluorescent techniques.

A highly important but moot question is whether this disordered immune reactivity, or autoimmunity, plays a primary or secondary causal role. Are viral, bacterial, or other unknown agents the primary cause? The relationships of *Treponema pallidum* to the serologic and immunologic alterations of syphilis, the association between neoplasms and dermatomyositis, and the incitement of polyarteritis by drugs are just a few examples bearing on this question. A lupus-like disorder has appeared spontaneously in certain strains of dogs and mice, more often females. In one such family of mice, a filtrable virus-like agent has been recovered. Attention has centered about the thymus in SLE because of its role in immune phenomena (Chaps. 68 to 70). Histologic changes have been described in this organ in SLE similar to those seen in disturbances of the immunologic system. However, theymectomy in a small group of patients with SLE has not altered their course. A number of patients with SLE have eventually developed a lymphoma or lymphoblastic leukemia, leading to the speculation that tissues which are immunologically very active may be more prone to malignant change. A patient with SLE has been described who developed a malignant ovarian dysgerminoma. When this tumor was removed, all clinical and laboratory evidences of SLE disappeared.

PATHOLOGY. The typical histologic alterations are swelling of collagen, "fibrinoid" changes in the ground substance, and infiltration of polymorphonuclear leukocytes, plasma cells, and lymphocytes. These lesions have been observed in almost all structures of the body but are more often seen in the walls of small arteries and arterioles, the skin, spleen, glomeruli, endocardium, and serous membranes. Hematoxylin bodies, remnants of injured nuclei closely resembling the inclusions in LE cells,

sometimes occur in association with these lesions and are pathognomonic of SLE.

MANIFESTATIONS. The clinical characteristics of the disease are chronicity with periods of remission and activity and multi-organ system involvement. The course may be fulminant, with death occurring after a few weeks, but more often it is protracted over many years. During periods of activity, fever, malaise, weakness, anorexia, and weight loss are common. Mild activity may occur with a disarming dearth of constitutional signs, and the vagueness of the patient's complaints may lead to the false impression of psychoneurosis.

Skin and Mucous Membranes. Cutaneous lesions occur sometime in the course of SLE in 85 percent of patients. They may appear alone or with systemic manifestations and have been confused with lichen planus, seborrhea, sarcoidosis, psoriasis, scleroderma, erythema multiforme, dermatomyositis, eczema, acne rosacea, and drug reactions. Pleomorphic, erythematous, maculopapular eruptions, often symmetrical, appear most commonly on the face, neck, and extremities. The "typical" malar butterfly appears less often. Quite characteristic of lupus are vascularized lesions around the nail beds and the tips of the digits, with eventual thinning and atrophy of the skin in these locations. Patchy edema, blebs, and bullae, sometimes hemorrhagic, or small areas of ulceration may appear, and gangrene of the extremities may occur. In chronic lesions, the skin becomes thickened, scaly, and atrophic. Urticaria, altered pigmentation, and alopecia are common. Erythema nodosum and purpura are frequent. The mucous membranes are usually involved only during severe exacerbations of the disease, and show ulceration or hemorrhagic foci.

Biopsy of skin lesions is not too helpful in diagnosis, and the changes are not uncommonly nonspecific.

Raynaud's phenomenon sometimes precedes other evidences of SLE by several years, although this is more common in scleroderma.

Approximately 10 percent of patients with cutaneous "discoid lupus" eventually develop manifestations of SLE.

Lymphatics and Spleen. Lymphadenopathy, especially cervical and axillary, is sometimes so prominent that the diagnosis of lymphoma or tuberculous adenitis (which sometimes complicates SLE) is suggested. Splenomegaly is frequent but is rarely massive.

Musculoskeletal. It is unusual for SLE to occur without involvement of the joints, which is often the earliest and only abnormality, sometimes for a prolonged period. Acute migratory polyarthritis may simulate rheumatic fever closely in its dramatic response to salicylates and arthralgias without objective changes. Deforming arthropathy indistinguishable from rheumatoid arthritis is also seen. The concomitant occurrence of SLE and rheumatoid disease cannot be excluded, but deformities once considered to be characteristic of rheumatoid arthritis also occur in patients with unequivocal SLE. The joints may be the site of a complicating infection, most often due to staphylococcus, particularly if the patient is receiving corticosteroids. The physical changes associated with such an infection may be minimal, nonspecific, and easily mistaken for the basic disease. Diagnostic arthrocentesis is imperative.

Muscle atrophy and weakness may be so pronounced that patients may be suspected of having dermatomyositis or muscular dystrophy. At times, it is difficult or impossible to distinguish lupus from dermatomyositis even by histologic examination or muscle.

Aseptic necrosis of bone, particularly of the femoral head, has been noted in SLE, as well as in other members of this family of disorders. Though long-term steroid administration may play a role in its causation, it has developed in patients never given these agents. Pain in the hip, thigh, or knee may precede roentgenographic changes by many months.

Eyes. Nonspecific retinal hemorrhages and exudates are not rare, and conjunctivitis is common. More helpful diagnostically is the finding in 10 to 20 percent of patients of small, round or oval, white opacities adjacent to vessels in the central fundus. These *"cytoid bodies"* are believed to represent foci of retinal neural degeneration secondary to occlusion of small vessels, and may accompany any disorder in which this process occurs, including vasculitis, markedly increased intracranial pressure, very severe anemia, diabetes mellitus, sepsis, macroglobulinemia, and severe hypertension with arteriosclerosis.

Corneal involvement in SLE resulting in tearing, sticking pain, and foreign-body sensation is frequent.

Lungs and Pleura. Recurrent pleurisy is common. Effusions are usually small; massive hydrothorax should suggest a complicating infection such as tuberculosis.

Pulmonary infiltrates, especially in the basilar segments, may be a direct result of SLE, as may more extensive involvement which may mimic miliary tuberculosis or lymphangitic carcinomatosis, and lead to respiratory insufficiency or cor pulmonale. However, no pulmonary lesion in a patient with SLE should be accepted as primary lupus until complicating infection has been excluded. Such infections may be caused by a host of organisms, including pneumocystis carinii and nocardiosis. The infiltrates of SLE may persist without changes for many months. The finding by x-ray of the combination of plate areas of basilar atelectasis, elevation of the diaphragm, and pleuritis is suggestive but not diagnostic of SLE. Abnormal physical signs are not prominent. Pulmonary arteritis may result in hemoptysis, cavity formation, or lung abscess, if secondary infection occurs. If the arteritis is diffuse, pulmonary hypertension may ensue, even in the absence of obvious parenchymal changes.

Cardiovascular. Pericarditis is very frequent, and although tamponade has been observed, large effusions are unusual. Complicating bacterial pericarditis must be excluded.

Typical flat vegetations occur on the heart valves, especially the mitral. Unlike the lesions of rheumatic fever, which follow the line of valve closure, lupus vegetations are found under the valve leaflets, in the commissure. These so-called Libman-Sacks vegetations do not usually interfere with valve function, but rare instances of valvular stenosis or regurgitation attributable to SLE are known. The vegetations may form a nidus for bacterial endocarditis.

Myocarditis is not evident clinically in most patients, but it can produce congestive failure or various conduction abnormalities.

Lesions of the arteries, indistinguishable histologically from those of polyarteritis nodosa save for a paucity of eosinophils, are frequent in SLE. They can lead to malfunction of any organ during the course of the disease and are responsible for many puzzling clinical manifestations.

Gastrointestinal. Any portion of the esophagus, stomach, or intestine may be involved by infarcts or ulcerations, the majority of which are due to arterial changes. The result may be dysphagia and functional changes simulating scleroderma, massive hemorrhage, diarrhea, or focal abdominal pain. Malabsorption consequent to diffuse intestinal changes is seen but is rare. Mild hepatomegaly is frequent in SLE, but jaundice and overt evidence of disordered liver function are not common. Patients with chronic active hepatitis may have typical clinical and histologic alterations of SLE. This so-called "lupoid hepatitis" is discussed in Chap. 327.

Kidneys. Focal or diffuse glomerulonephritis, often with classic "wire-loop" changes, is present in the kidneys of a majority of patients who die with SLE. The deposition of complement and gamma-globulin on the basement membrane can be demonstrated by immunofluorescent techniques.

Episodes of acute nephritis, a typical nephrotic syndrome, and varying degrees of chronic renal impairment are very common. Microscopic hematuria, red blood cell casts, and proteinuria are the usual urinary findings, but occasional patients may show only pyuria without hematuria. It is not unusual for patients with relatively normal urine and adequate renal function, as measured by the usual tests, to show distinct histologic alterations in renal biopsy specimens. This tendency for abnormal urinary findings to appear late in the course of the renal lesion explains the apparent abruptness of the onset of renal failure in some individuals with SLE.

Recovery from episodes of acute nephritis is common, but the appearance of renal impairment of a significant degree is an ominous sign. However, sustained remissions may occur occasionally despite a pronounced degree of renal insufficiency, or nephrosis. In the absence of renal failure, persistent hypertension is unusual in uncomplicated SLE.

Complicating pyelonephritis is rather frequent in patients with SLE. Consequently, when urinary abnormalities are present, it is necessary to differentiate bacterial infection from SLE per se. Also, the nephrotic syndrome (due to renal vein thrombosis) and hypertension (due to unilateral vascular alterations) have been reported.

Central Nervous System. Many abnormalities may occur, but because they are produced by vascular lesions of varying extent and location, no typical pattern results. Psychotic episodes, convulsions, hemipareses, and transient cranial palsies are relatively common. Peripheral neuritis and spinal cord lesions are unusual. Epileptiform seizures in patients with SLE have often been mistaken initially for idiopathic epilepsy, and similarly, a definite diagnosis of SLE is made only after a patient has been treated for several episodes of psychotic behavior.

Several instances of the concomitance of SLE and of myasthenia gravis have been reported, and manifestations of SLE have appeared after thymectomy for this disorder.

Aseptic meningitis with fever, headache, and polymorphonuclear pleocytosis in the cerebrospinal fluid may occur in SLE, sometimes in the absence of other distinctive signs of this disease. Cryptococcosis and tuberculosis may complicate the course of SLE.

Generally, a significant disorder of the nervous system signifies a severe exacerbation of the disease and frequently demands intensive therapy.

Other Organs. Systemic lupus erythematosus frequently is associated with Sjögren's syndrome and Hashimoto's thyroiditis, suggesting that autoimmune mechanisms are important in the etiology of all three diseases. The concurrence of thrombotic thrombocytopenic purpura and SLE has been reported also.

LABORATORY FINDINGS. The peripheral leukocyte count is usually normal or depressed, although complicating bacterial infection may induce a brisk leukocytosis. Even with marked leukopenia, the differential count remains normal; appreciable neutropenia is not characteristic of SLE.

Moderate anemia is common. Hemolytic anemia may occur and may dominate the clinical course; the Coombs test is sometimes positive, and in such cases a primary hematologic disorder is often suspected initially.

Thrombocytopenia with purpura is a rather frequent presenting manifestation. Splenectomy has led to amelioration of the platelet deficiency in these patients. In one well-studied group of patients with "idiopathic" thrombocytopenic purpura, splenectomy was effective, but in subsequent years, other manifestations of SLE appeared. The spleens showed the typical "onion-peel" lesion of small arteries in every case. Systemic lupus erythematosus should be suspected in any patient with thrombocytopenia, and if splenectomy is done, a careful search for these diagnostic lesions is in order.

In a few patients, circulating anticoagulants (antibodies to clotting factors) have been demonstrated.

Immunoglobulin abnormalities are present in most patients with SLE. Serum globulin concentrations above 4.0 Gm per 100 ml occur in over 50 percent of cases. Electrophoresis reveals a heterogeneous increase of gamma-, beta$_2$-, and alpha-globulins. Macroglobulinemia and cryoglobulinemia infrequently occur at a quantitative level sufficient to produce clinical manifestations.

Approximately 80 percent of patients with SLE will eventually have a positive LE cell test. The cells are often present intermittently during the course of the disease.

Other immune reactions are gaining importance in establishing the diagnosis of SLE and in following the progress of the disease. Probably the most widely used newer method for detecting antinuclear factors employs immunofluorescence. The interpretation of antinuclear-factor (ANF) titers varies according to the method used. This test is usually more sensitive than the LE cell test and is positive in nearly all patients with active SLE. Serial ANF titers are of some value in managing patients, because the titers may vary according to the intensity and activity of the disease, but these relationships are not constant enough for complete reliance in planning therapy.

Serum complement is reduced in about 75 percent of patients with active SLE but may be normal or elevated. The reduction in complement correlates somewhat with the degree of activity, particularly if there is nephritis. Serum ANF titers usually vary inversely with complement. A low serum complement may be of help in distinguishing SLE from rheumatic fever, polyarteritis, dermatomyositis, rheumatoid arthritis, and various infections which are usually characterized by a normal or elevated serum complement level. However, reduced serum complement may also occur in serum sickness, acute glomerulonephritis, and the nephrotic syndrome.

Nonphagocytized masses of transformed nuclear material identical to the LE cell inclusion (ECM) are found in the absence of LE cells as well as with them. The full significance of such masses has not been determined, but it should not be disregarded. A significant number of patients initially found to have only ECM are subsequently found to have SLE or related disorders.

In addition to the search for LE cells, biopsy of skin, subcutaneous tissue, muscle, or lymph node is occasionally helpful in establishing the diagnosis.

DIAGNOSIS. It is often exceedingly difficult to make a clinical diagnosis of SLE because of the episodic involvement of many organ systems, singly or in combination, over a period of many years. If only one organ is involved, some monosystem disease such as arthritis or pleurisy may be diagnosed erroneously. The relationship between seemingly unrelated episodes of past illness may not be appreciated. Also, many of the commonly associated clinical manifestations such as fever, malaise, anorexia, and weakness are nonspecific. In attempting to make an accurate clinical diagnosis of SLE it is always necessary to interpret the presenting complaint (e.g., arthritis) in terms of the past history. For example, a history of a previous episode of pneumonia, an attack of pleurisy, and a skin eruption following sun exposure should give new meaning to a present complaint of arthritis, and lead to appropriate studies for SLE.

The following is a list of conditions not infrequently confused with SLE:

Rheumatic fever	Hemolytic or other obscure
Rheumatoid arthritis	anemias
Felty's syndrome	Leukopenia due to other
Various skin disorders	causes
Dermatitis medicamentosa	Virus pneumonia
Syphilis	Drug reaction
Idiopathic thrombocytope-	Septicemia
nic purpura	Dermatomyositis

Scleroderma

Chronic basilar pulmonary
   infection

Raynaud's syndrome

Tuberculosis

Trichinosis

Bacterial endocarditis

Lymphoma

Acute or chronic nephritis

Nephrosis

Ulcerative colitis

Meningitis

Cerebrovascular accident

Epilepsy

Psychosis

Functional illness

Sjögren's syndrome

Polyarteritis nodosa

Hepatitis

TREATMENT. No definitive curative therapy is known. However, with judicious management, the disease can often be controlled well enough for patients to lead active lives with a minimum of disability or discomfort.

General. Direct exposure to sunlight should be avoided. Also insofar as possible elective surgery, trauma, emotional stress, nonessential drugs, and serum products, including transfusions, all of which appear to be capable of triggering an exacerbation of SLE, are contraindicated. The role of pregnancy is not clearcut; in some patients it appears to activate the disease, most often in the first 8 weeks post partum; in others there is no effect. The severity and extent of illness must be balanced against the desire for a family.

For many patients, the unqualified term "lupus" has come to have as bad a connotation as "cancer" or "leukemia," and thoughtless use of it should be avoided. The patient's morale should be maintained during the course of SLE, which may encompass many years.

For reasons not clear, perhaps because of the dysproteinemia or adrenal steroid therapy, patients with SLE seem liable to bacterial and other infections, which they resist poorly. The therapeutic implications of realizing that all manifestations of illness in these patients are not necessarily directly attributable to SLE are obvious, because infection is a very common cause of the death in these patients.

Specific Measures. The drugs available for the treatment of SLE are nonspecific anti-inflammatory agents, and in formulating a therapeutic program, the safest, simplest, and cheapest should be selected. Selection should be based on a thorough evaluation of the patient's renal status, so that latent active nephritis requiring intensive treatment is not overlooked. An individual who feels well, has normal kidneys, but whose blood contains many LE cells requires no specific therapy, and there is no evidence that chronic administration of corticosteroids blocks later appearance of other manifestations of the disease. A patient with a recurrent eruption on the face and arms, occasional episodes of myalgia and arthralgia, and no active renal disease, is best treated with such general measures as adequate rest, salicylates, and local therapy for the rash.

Antimalarial drugs sometimes help discoid skin lesions, but their relative ineffectiveness and untoward side effects limit their usefulness. Irreversible retinal degeneration may result from the chronic use of chloroquine in dosage greater than 250 mg daily. Corneal opacities also occur but are usually reversible when therapy is discontinued.

Nausea, vomiting, anemia, and diarrhea are not uncommon reactions, and 10 to 15 percent of patients acquire a dermatitis.

Bed rest and salicylates alone may be highly effective in quieting the acute rheumatic manifestations of SLE. As in rheumatic fever, an adequate salicylate level must be maintained. If steroids have to be employed, the concomitant use of salicylates may enable the use of smaller maintenance dosages of the hormone.

Corticosteroid therapy should be reserved for those manifestations of SLE which cannot be brought readily under control by simpler measures. Indications include active renal disease, acute myocarditis, progressive or disfiguring eruptions, involvement of the nervous system, lupus pneumonitis, hemolytic anemia, thrombocytopenia, and marked fever and constitutional symptoms.

There is no evidence that any one of the corticosteroid compounds is superior, but prednisone has enjoyed widest usage. Chronic administration of some of the newer fluorinated compounds has been associated with excessive wasting of peripheral muscles and exaggeration of vascular lesions in a few instances.

In the belief that SLE is a disease of abnormal immune reactivity, various immunosuppressive agents are being employed, but results have been equivocal and the drugs are toxic.

Moderate dosages of prednisone are usually effective. An exception is the rare "lupus crisis," in which an overwhelming exacerbation of the disease is controlled only by massive doses of steroids. From 40 to 60 mg prednisone daily in four divided doses almost invariably brings about prompt subsidence of symptoms in SLE. As soon as fever, pain, and other manifestations are controlled, the dosage should be reduced very gradually until a maintenance level (usually 15 to 20 mg daily) is found. If the disease flares up, the dosage is increased again. Maintenance therapy may have to be continued for months or years, but in all patients the amount of steroid taken should be reduced cautiously at regular intervals to see if a lower dose will maintain them in remission. The key to success is gradual, planned reduction of dosage; precipitious withdrawal of steroids or abrupt lowering of the dosage should be avoided.

Very large dosages of steroids for a prolonged time have been advised in the treatment of lupus nephritis while the patient's progress is monitored by serial renal biopsies. Though at times this approach is advisable, in general, the moderate dosages outlined above are adequate.

There may be confusion between effects of SLE and of steroids upon the central nervous system, but SLE is associated with central-nervous-system manifestations only when other organ systems are involved; these patients will often improve when steroid dosage is increased.

A peptic ulcer regimen should be given patients who are receiving steroids for SLE.

PROGNOSIS. Because of previous failure to recognize the episodic recurrences in SLE, accurate information about the natural history of the disease is scanty. Similarly, definite evidence that steroids alter the duration of life is lacking. It appears that the duration of illness in SLE is a function of the varying severity of the disease, ranging from fulminant illness with death in a few weeks to reasonable good health for 15 or even 20 years despite occasional episodes of active disease.

A deciding factor in prognosis is the amount of irreversible renal damage. The outlook is not good once chronic renal impairment appears. The longer the interval without renal injury, the less likely it is that serious involvement of the kidneys will occur. It is probable that the control of inflammation by adrenal steroids can minimize renal damage and prolong life. In addition, antibiotics prevent many deaths from complicating infection.

REFERENCES

Alaroon-Segoria, D., K. G. Wakim, J. W. Worthington, and L. E. Ward: Clinical and Experimental Studies on the Hydralazine Syndrome and Its Relationship to Systemic Lupus Erythematosus, Medicine, 46:1, 1967.

Dubois, E.: Treatment of Systemic Lupus, Bull. Rheumatic. Dis., 18:477, 1967.

Gary, N. E., J. F. Maher, and G. E. Schreiner: Lupus Nephritis. Renal Function after Prolonged Survival, New Engl. J. Med., 276:73, 1967.

Harvey, A. M., L. E. Shulman, P. A. Tumulty, C. C. Conley, and E. H. Schoenrich: Systemic Lupus Erythematosus, Review of Literature and Clinical Analysis of 138 Cases, Medicine, 33:291, 1954.

Kunkel, H. G.: Mechanisms of Renal Injury in Systemic Lupus Erythematosus, Arthritis Rheumat., 9:725, 1966.

Townes, A. S.: Complement Levels in Disease, Johns Hopkins Med. J., 120:337, 1967.

393 SCLERODERMA
Philip A. Tumulty

DEFINITION. Scleroderma is a chronic disease of unknown cause characterized by diffuse sclerosis of the connective tissue of the integument and other organs. Although it occurs at almost any time of life, the majority of patients are between twenty and fifty years of age, and females are affected three times as frequently as males. Familial cases have been reported. Scleroderma is less common than systemic lupus erythematosus (SLE), but more common than polyarteritis or dermatomyositis.

PATHOLOGY AND ETIOLOGY. As in SLE, a variety of antibiodies may be found in the serum. Also, "clinical crossovers" are seen, in which features of scleroderma become blended with those of other members of the so-called "collagen-vascular" spectrum, including SLE, rheumatoid arthritis, and dermatomyositis. These findings suggest that immune mechanisms may be involved in causation. The prominent vasomotor reactivity of some patients and instances of apparent onset after injury to vessels or nerves have pointed to the importance of neurovascular

factors. Exposure to silica has been reported in some patients with scleroderma, and it has been questioned whether silica could be a stimulant to antibody production, but most patients have not been exposed to this material.

The amount of collagen in the dermis is not increased and the concentration of hydroxyproline is normal, although that of hexosamines is increased. There is no increased concentration of neutral or acid mucopolysaccharides. It has been suggested that patients with scleroderma have abnormal tryptophan metabolism which leads to overproduction of serotonin, resulting in inflammation and sclerosis. Family members of a patient with scleroderma were found to have abnormal tryptophan metabolism. Abnormal tryptophan metabolism has also been reported in patients with SLE, porphyria, and cancer, as well as in otherwise healthy persons. In three cases "virus particles" are said to have been seen in the muscles of patients with scleroderma when viewed with the electron microscope, and mitochondria were damaged. The significance of these observations is obscure.

The principal histologic change consists of swelling, hypertrophy, and condensation of collagen, with the formation of dense, compact connective tissue. Early, there is variable inflammation, but this rarely persists. In the skin, there are atrophy of the epidermis and appendages, increase or decrease in pigment, and often calcinosis. The walls of small arterial vessels undergo "fibrinoid" changes, and there may be occlusion and secondary ischemic alterations.

MANIFESTATIONS. Visceral scleroderma may precede all cutaneous alterations, or it may be associated with integumentary changes which are vague and nonspecific. These visceral abnormalities, which may dominate the patient's course, are readily attributed to other causes. In the early stages, the symptoms accompanying scleroderma may be very nondescript and the physical changes unimpressive, leading to the conclusion that the patient must have a functional illness. Scleroderma must be considered in the differential diagnosis of many frequently encountered disorders, including:

1. Fever of unknown origin (FUO) (rare)
2. Unexplained dyspnea, with a diffusion defect
3. Pulmonary fibrosis
4. Pulmonary hypertension—cor pulmonale
5. Pleuritis
6. Myocarditis
7. Pericarditis (hemorrhagic)
8. Endocarditis (infective, noninfective)
9. Malignant hypertension and uremia
10. Conduction defects
11. Dysphagia, epigastric distress, hiatus hernia
12. Malabsorption syndrome
13. Duodenal obstruction
14. Enterocolitis
15. Rheumatoid disease, SLE, dermatomyositis, polymyositis
16. Neurasthenia, hypochondriasis
17. Osler-Weber-Rendu disease

18. Raynaud's phenomenon
19. Skin changes involving edema, atrophy, sclerosis, altered pigmentation, calcinosis

Scleroderma may be classified as follows:

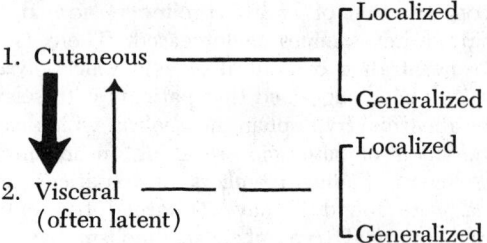

1. Cutaneous —————— Localized
                      Generalized

2. Visceral —————— Localized
   (often latent)   Generalized

Cutaneous alterations, which may be localized or generalized, usually precede clinically evident visceral changes, which may involve one or several of the organ systems. Less frequently, one or several of the organ systems may be affected by scleroderma in the complete absence of clinically detectable changes in the skin. A long time, sometimes years, may intervene between the appearance of clinically evident cutaneous scleroderma and recognized visceral involvement, or vice versa. The changes in the viscera may progress insidiously and may be overlooked; the reported incidence of visceral involvement is probably much too low. Likewise, visceral scleroderma probably precedes cutaneous scleroderma much more often than is appreciated. The long clinical latency of visceral involvement is a basic feature of this disease. For example, a patient on general examination appears to have scleroderma confined to his face, chest, and hands. Pulmonary diffusion studies may show a marked deficit, the glomerular filtration rate may be depressed, and the motility of the lower end of the esophagus may be abnormal.

Visceral changes may accompany localized as well as generalized cutaneous scleroderma. Finally, it is estimated that 5 percent of localized cutaneous scleroderma becomes generalized.

The clinical beginnings of scleroderma are often very subtle, suggesting neurasthenia, or they may indicate involvement of a single organ system. Common presentations are (1) weakness, weight loss, easy fatigability, neurasthenia, (2) vague musculoskeletal aching, (3) arthritis (rheumatoid), (4) Raynaud's phenomenon, (5) stiffness of hands, (6) altered pigmentation, (7) unexplained edema (localized or generalized), (8) thickening of skin (localized or generalized), (9) telangiectases, (10) loss of body hair, (11) dysphagia, heartburn, (12) dyspnea on exertion, (13) FUO, (14) renal insufficiency, hypertension (malignant), (15) right- or left-sided heart failure, (16) pleuritis, pericarditis.

Integument. The skin and subcutaneous tissues can be involved diffusely or focally. The focal form occurs as patches, often about the neck (morphea), as linear streaks sometimes following the course of nerves or blood vessels, or as sclerodactylia. Chronic edema may be the only early change. Alterations in pigment and vascular lesions such as telangiectasia of the skin or mucous membranes are common. These phenomena may appear very gradually or with dramatic suddenness. The arms, trunk, head, and legs are involved in sequence. The skin develops a waxy hardness and luster. The face becomes expressionless, and the nose, ears, and lips appear smaller, thinner, and sharper. If the process extends to the buccal mucosa, talking and swallowing may be difficult. The fingertips thicken and shorten, the overlying skin atrophies, and often, numerous tiny, painful, pitted ulcers appear. These heal with scarring or become chronic, with deposition of calcium and extrusion of chalky material. Subcutaneous calcification is sometimes diffuse. Axillary and pubic hair is usually lost, but except for atrophy, the nails are spared. Inability to sweat may cause discomfort.

The distinctive combination of calcinosis, Raynaud's phenomena, sclerodactylia, and telangiectasia is referred to as the "CRST syndrome." The telangiectases are not familial and they are generally not the source of major bleeding. The course of this syndrome is usually relatively benign, and visceral involvement often is confined to the gut. The occurrence of telangiectases in scleroderma emphasizes that an essential histologic change is a peculiar capillary structure, with unique marked blunting and clublike deformities of the terminal ends of the capillaries.

Gastrointestinal Tract. The principal pathologic alterations in the gastrointestinal tract are degeneration and atrophy of smooth muscle, with or without connective tissue replacement, and obliterative vascular lesions. Smooth-muscle atrophy is not necessarily related to vascular lesions, and its pathogenesis is not clear; an abnormality in the autonomic nervous system may be responsible. From a clinical standpoint, the muscle changes produce adynamic phenomena, with loss of propulsive power and dilatation of the bowel or esophagus. Secondary factors are esophagitis and alteration in intestinal flora, which may be important in malabsorption. Dysphagia, bloating, constipation, and even obstruction are common symptoms.

The obliterative vascular lesions may result in ulceration, perforation, infarction, abscess formation, and hemorrhage anywhere in the gut.

Table 393-1 summarizes the clinical manifestations resulting from these changes.

Table 393-1. THE GASTROINTESTINAL TRACT IN SCLERODERMA: CLINICAL MANIFESTATIONS

Esophagus	Duodenum-jejunum	Colon
Dysphagia	Bloating	Distension
Heartburn	Dyspepsia	Obstipation
Dyspepsia	Obstruction	Constipation
Esophagitis	Malabsorption	Diarrhea
Regurgitation	Ulceration	Ulceration
Hiatus hernia	Infarction	Infarction
Infarction	Perforation	Perforation
Perforation	Hemorrhage	Hemorrhage
Hemorrhage		

The order of frequency of involvement is the esophagus, duodenum, jejunum, and colon. The severity of visceral change is unrelated to the degree of dermal involvement.

The lower two-thirds of the esophagus becomes stiffened, wide, and patulous, with diminished or absent peristalsis. Reflux esophagitis with distal narrowing commonly follows. Although patients may complain of dysphagia or heartburn, striking functional derangement is often disclosed by appropriate x-ray studies in an individual who has had no symptoms; when scleroderma is suspected, the esophagus should be investigated. Changes in motility demonstrated by pressure tracings are characteristic. Similar functional derangements of the esophagus have been seen in patients with SLE and have also been described in women whose only other detectable abnormality was Raynaud's syndrome.

Liver. The liver is infrequently implicated, and where liver disease exists, a specific relationship to scleroderma is not certain. Obstructive jaundice due to extensive vascular and sclerosing lesions in the extrahepatic ducts has been described.

Lungs. Pulmonary fibrosis and pulmonary vascular obstruction are the major pulmonary abnormalities in scleroderma. The fibrotic changes may lead to the formation of cysts, emphysema, atelectasis, asthma, bronchiectasis, pneumonitis, or abscess. Vascular obstruction may result in pulmonary hypertension and cor pulmonale. Secondary factors playing roles of varying importance are fixation of the chest wall, pleural fibrosis, aspiration of gastric contents, complicating infection, and embolism.

There is no correlation between the extent of pulmonary fibrosis and the degree of pulmonary vascular obstruction, nor between the amount of change noted in roentgenograms of the chest and the actual extent of the fibrotic or vascular changes. One patient may have enough pulmonary hypertension to result in cor pulmonale and yet have clear lung fields, while another may have a snowstorm appearance of the lungs with normal pulmonary vascular resistance. Conversely, a patient may have disabling exertional dyspnea, and pulmonary function studies may show a marked diffusion defect, yet the chest roentgenogram may demonstrate little or no fibrosis, even though at postmortem examination considerable fibrotic change is observed.

Table 393-2, from Sachner, is a summary of the results of studies of pulmonary function in scleroderma. Diffusion defects are among the earliest physiologic abnormalities.

As in all collagen disorders, the lower portions of the lungs are affected to a greater degree than are the upper. Involvement may be patchy or diffuse, symmetric or asymmetric.

Pleurisy is common. If an effusion is very large or recurrent, a complicating infection and, in particular, tuberculosis, should be ruled out. Pleurisy may occur in the absence of any pulmonary vascular or fibrotic abnormalities, and may recur. Recurrent pneumothoraces have been reported.

Complicating pulmonary infections are common and

Table 393-2. PULMONARY FUNCTION TESTS IN SCLERODERMA

1. Alteration of viscoelastic properties of lung
   - a. Vital capacity . . . . Decreased
   - b. Residual volume . . . . Normal or decreased
   - c. Lung compliance . . . . Decreased
   - d. Airway resistance . . . . Decreased
   - e. Tissue resistance . . . . Increased
2. Diffusion and ventilation-perfusion disturbances
   - a. Diffusing capacity of lung . . . . Decreased
   - b. Venous admixture . . . . Increased
   - c. Physiologic dead space/tidal volume . . . . Increased
3. Pulmonary hypertension
   - a. Pulmonary arterial pressure . . . . Increased
   - b. Pulmonary blood flow . . . . Decreased
4. Normal function of chest bellows
   - a. Chest wall compliance . . . . Normal
   - b. Maximum pressures at mouth . . . . . Normal

SOURCE: From M. A. Sachner, Scleroderma, "Modern Medical Monographs," vol. 26, New York, Grune & Stratton, Inc., 1966.

depend on the degree of fibrosis, the ability to perform satisfactory pulmonary toilet, the tendency to aspiration pneumonia resulting from esophageal abnormalities, and the use of steroids. Often, it is impossible to determine whether an observed abnormality is due to scleroderma or to infection.

Patients with extensive scleroderma are subject to pulmonary embolism. The platelike areas of atelectasis in the basilar portions of the lungs, so typical of pulmonary infarction, are common in scleroderma.

In addition to pulmonary embolism and tuberculous pleurisy, many common pulmonary disorders may be confused with scleroderma of the lung, including fibrosis, focal or diffuse infiltrative processes, emphysema, and bronchiectasis.

The Heart. Though involvement of the pericardium and of the myocardium is not uncommon, pulmonary and/or systemic hypertension secondary to scleroderma of the lungs and kidneys are the major causes of heart failure.

Recurrent episodes of pericarditis are frequent, but constrictive pericarditis rarely results. Pericarditis may be dry, or there may be an effusion, which is sometimes large enough to produce tamponade or occasionally is hemorrhagic. Like the pleura, the pericardium may become infected by tuberculosis or other bacteria or fungi.

In the myocardium, scleroderma produces atrophy and degeneration of muscle fibers, which are replaced by dense collagenous tissue, highly vascular connective tissue, and interstitial edema. These changes may lead to conduction defects or to myocardial failure.

Fibrotic or calcific nodules are sometimes found along the line of valve closure, and stenosis and regurgitation of the mitral and aortic valves has been described. Infective endocarditis may be a complication. Panaortitis with aortic valvulitis due to scleroderma has been reported but must be very rare.

The Kidney. Characteristic histologic lesions in the kidney consist of striking intimal proliferation and fibrinoid necrosis of interlobular arteries, necrotizing glomerulitis, and cortical infarction. These lesions may exist focally for a long time without appreciable clinical evidence of renal abnormality. Some patients with scleroderma develop slowly progressive uremia over a period of many months. More often, renal failure appears abruptly, hypertension and uremia follow a malignant course, and the patient dies within weeks. There is nothing characteristic about renal function tests or the urinary sediment. Renal biopsy may be very helpful in diagnosis. Renal insufficiency is a grave prognostic sign in scleroderma and may dominate the patient's course, with little clinical evidence of scleroderma in other tissues.

It has been suggested that the administration of adrenal steroids increases the likelihood of abrupt renal failure, but sudden hypertension and uremia have occurred in many individuals with scleroderma who received no hormonal treatment.

The association of Raynaud's phenomenon and malignant hypertension in scleroderma suggests that vasopressor materials may be responsible for both renal and cutaneous manifestations.

Musculoskeletal. Polyarthralgia or arthritis is the earliest complaint and may simulate rheumatoid disease. The latex test may be positive. Involvement of the cricoarytenoid joints may lead to hoarseness. Fibrosis of the synovium may produce squeaking noises. Joint fluid is turbid. containing a moderate amount of protein and many polymorphonuclear cells. Avascularization may lead to disappearance of the phalanges, the ends of the radius and ulna, or the femoral heads. Thickening of the periodontal membrane may result in loosening of the teeth. The carpal tunnel syndrome has been described. Rib erosions, a radiographic feature of rheumatoid disease, are also noted in scleroderma. Rheumatoid nodules occur. Myositis that is clinically and histologically indistinguishable from dermatomyositis and SLE is not uncommon.

Central Nervous System. Focal vascular lesions in the brain, cord, or peripheral nerves may result in mental aberrations, convulsions, hemorrhage (sometimes subarachnoid), pareses, paralysis, and sensory changes.

Endocrine Glands. The adrenals, parathyroids, and gonads rarely show lesions, but Hashimoto's thyroiditis is occasionally present.

Other Organs. Moderate splenomegaly occurs, but lymph node enlargement is not a feature. Sjögren's syndrome sometimes accompanies scleroderma.

LABORATORY FINDINGS. None is diagnostic of scleroderma or specific for it. The hemogram is usually normal except for an elevated sedimentation rate. The concentration of serum gamma-globulins may be increased.

Biopsy of skin and muscle may be helpful in establishing the diagnosis, although several specimens may be needed if changes are mild.

COURSE. The disease may progress relentlessly, reach a plateau, or regress strikingly over a period of months and years. The visceral lesions seem less likely to undergo remission than do those in the skin. The eventual outcome is largely determined by the degree to which vital structures are damaged by scarring and obliterative vascular lesions. Death is usually due to aspiration pneumonia, pulmonary insufficiency, heart failure, uremia, or inanition secondary to gastrointestinal malfunction.

Presently available survival rates are inaccurate. Complicating infections are a major cause of morbidity and death. Though scleroderma usually progresses slowly, it may begin and advance with dramatic suddenness, and the patient may die in a few months.

There have been descriptions of the concurrence of scleroderma and malignant neoplasms, including those arising from the lung and gastrointestinal tract, adrenal gland, and breast. There have been several instances of carcinoid tumors.

TREATMENT. A number of agents are said to be of limited value, including dimethylsulfoxide (DMSO), ethylenediaminotetraacteic acid (EDTA), pyridoxine, reserpine, Potaba, penicillamine, and dextran infusions, but the results are not impressive and are limited largely to some loosening of tight skin and healing of digital ulcers. Evidence that any of these agents significantly affects the systemic changes is lacking.

Eradication of established sclerotic and atrophic changes is not to be expected, but steroids may halt and reverse the edematous inflammatory phase. From 40 to 60 mg daily of prednisone should be given initially in divided doses. Depending on clinical response, this dosage may be reduced gradually to a maintenance level of 15 to 20 mg daily and should be continued at this level until maximum regression has been achieved. Many months or years of continuous treatment may be required. These patients must be placed on a six-feeding, modified ulcer diet with antacids after meals and at bedtime.

Indomethacin, in dosage of 75 to 150 mg daily, has appeared to benefit some patients. Thyroid hormone has also seemed to help some patients when given in moderate dosages.

Esophagitis may be ameliorated by elevating the head of the bed and by administering antacids. Physiotherapy, including heat, massage, and passive motion, may be comforting and can prevent fixation of affected extremities.

REFERENCES

Rodnan, G. P., and T. Medsger, Jr.: Musculo-skeletal Involvement in Progressive Systemic Sclerosis (Scleroderma), Bull. Rheumatic Dis., 17:419, 1966.

Sachner, M. A.: Scleroderma, "Modern Medical Monographs," vol. 26, New York, Grune & Stratton, Inc., 1966.

Salen, G., F. Goldstein, and C. W. Wirts: Malabsorbption in Intestinal Scleroderma, Ann. Intern. Med., 64:834, 1966.

Schimke, R. N., C. H. Kirkpatrick, and M. H. Delp: The CRST Syndrome, Arch. Intern. Med., 119:365, 1967.

Tumulty, P. A.: Clinical Synopsis of Scleroderma, Simulator of Other Diseases, Johns Hopkins Med. J., 122:236, 1968.

Weaver, A. L., M. B. Divertie, and J. L. Titus: The Lung in Scleroderma, Proc. Staff Meetings Mayo Clinic, 42:754, 1967.

394 MISCELLANEOUS AND RARER DISORDERS OF CONNECTIVE TISSUE

Philip A. Tumulty

WEGENER'S GRANULOMATOSIS

DEFINITION. Wegener's granulomatosis is a syndrome of unknown cause characterized by necrotizing granulomatous lesions, generalized arteritis, and glomerulitis.

Individuals of any age may be affected, most commonly those in the fourth and fifth decades. Their past health has generally been good, with no unusual allergic background. The outcome of the untreated disease has been fatal in most instances, generally after 6 to 8 months, although occasionally the course is intermittent or subacute for several years. A localized, more benign form of the disorder may involve the lungs.

PATHOLOGY. There are three histologic alterations: (1) necrotizing granulomas in the upper and/or lower part of the respiratory tract, (2) focal inflammatory lesions of both arteries and veins, which are usually widely disseminated, (3) focal glomerulitis. Because similar changes occur in other hypersensitivity diseases, this process has been regarded as a manifestation of abnormal immune mechanisms. It is postulated that the initial lesion in the respiratory passages is a granulomatous infection of bacterial, viral, or other origin, and that the secondary lesions in the lungs, skin, and kidneys are the products of an autoimmune reaction to the injured tissues, as in drug hypersensitivity states. Whether Wegener's granulomatosis is a clinical variant of polyarteritis nodosa or a distinct entity is not known.

MANIFESTATIONS. Although any organ may be affected, the characteristic clinical triad consists of intractable rhinitis and sinusitis, nodular pulmonary lesions, and terminal uremia. The first symptoms are usually respiratory. The patient appears with rhinorrhea, sinusitis, nasal obstruction, epistaxis, cough, hemoptysis, pleurisy, or pneumonia. Otorrhea, sometimes progressing to deafness, hoarseness, and dysphagia, may occur. The gums may become painful and may ulcerate. Sometimes, however, the initial features are fever, weakness, malaise, and weight loss, and the respiratory disorder becomes prominent somewhat later. The course is usually relentlessly progressive. Ulceration and erosion of cartilage and bone may occur in the nasal passages and sinuses, resulting in saddle nose deformity. Eye involvement is common, either through orbital extension with exophthalmos, chemosis, exposure keratitis, and papillitis, or through focal ocular involvement with episcleritis, scleritis, corneal ulceration, conjunctivitis, uveitis, and retinitis with hemorrhages and cytoid bodies. Any portion of the lungs may be involved. The typical lesions are necrotizing granulomas which often appear as round opacities with central cavitation. At other times, bronchopneumonic patches or multiple nodular densities, which are often peribronchial, are seen. Secondary bacterial or fungal infections are common. Patients have been described with Wegener-like lesions, confined to the lungs or elsewhere, in which the progression was very slow or halted altogether.

The lesions of Wegener's granulomatosis are usually multiple, bilateral, and confined to the lower lung fields. They simulate primary or secondary tumors, or other granulomatous processes. Cavitation is common. Bizarre reticuloendothelial cells may be present and may resemble those in Hodgkin's disease. The real nature of the process may not be recognized unless typical vasculitis is observed.

Skin rashes, similar to those observed in polyarteritis, are common, as are polyarthritis and myositis. Typical skin changes consist of papules with necrotic centers having the appearance of papulonecrotic tuberculides, or papulovesicular lesions which are usually on the extremities, the fingers, elbows, knee joints, and buttocks. Pyoderma gangrenosum, petechiae, or multiform bullous and hemorrhagic exanthems occur. There is a tendency for the lesions to appear in operative scars.

Although any or all of the organ systems may be affected, pericarditis, myocarditis, and vascular lesions in the brain and cord and the peripheral and cranial nerves, resulting in a variety of neurologic abnormalities, are common.

In time, renal involvement becomes evident, with the appearance of protein, red blood cells, and red blood cell casts in the urine. Renal failure is sometimes rapid, and the patient dies in uremia in a matter of weeks.

The terminal phase may be dominated by uremia or by other effects of the generalized arteritis. High fever, arthritis, and hemorrhagic lesions of the skin and mucous membranes may be prominent.

Anemia and leukocytosis, occasionally with a mild eosinophilia, are common accompaniments. Hyperglobulinemia is frequent.

This syndrome is to be distinguished from other conditions in which vasculitis and granuloma formation may occur. Included among these disorders are syphilis, tuberculosis, fungal infections, sarcoidosis, lethal midline granuloma, and polyarteritis nodosa.

TREATMENT. Although the results have frequently been disappointing, adrenal steroid therapy has at times appeared to retard advancement of the disease and to induce a remission. Treatment with these agents should be begun as early as possible and should be continued with large dosages for a prolonged period, as outlined in Chap. 392. Premature cessation of steroids may induce an uncontrollable exacerbation of the disease. Imuran, nitrogen mustard, and chlorambucil have been effective in a few patients. Immunosuppressive therapy must be prolonged and may need to be combined with steroid administration. Secondary fungal and bacterial infections are a common complication of therapy.

TEMPORAL (GRANULOMATOUS) ARTERITIS

DEFINITION. Temporal arteritis, first described by Jonathan Hutchinson in 1890, is a clinical syndrome of unknown cause characterized by granulomatous inflammation of the temporal or occipital arteries, headache, blindness or lesser visual disturbances, and associated systemic reactions such as fever, malaise, and weight loss. It is but one of a wide variety of clinical expressions of a granulomatous arteritis which may implicate any branch or branches of the arterial tree, singly or in combination. Polymyalgia rheumatica is another clinical expression of the same process.

INCIDENCE AND ETIOLOGY. Males and females in the age group of fifty to eighty are equally affected. The relationship of temporal arteritis to Takayashu's disease, a form of granulomatous arteritis occurring in younger persons, especially females, is not well delineated. No familial or other predisposing factors are recognized, although occasionally the disease has seemed to follow respiratory infections. It is best regarded as the clinical complex resulting from predominantly carotid involvement by a granulomatous arteritis, which may be widespread or may remain focal. It is probably not a clinical variant of polyarteritis nodosa; its pathologic alterations and response to therapy with steroids are quite different from those of polyarteritis nodosa.

PATHOLOGY. The histologic alterations involve the entire arterial wall, particularly the media. Areas of necrosis are accompanied by diffuse infiltration of mononuclear cells. Giant cells are conspicuous. Characteristically, the elastic tissue is fragmented. The vessel may become thrombosed, but aneurysms are rare. The aorta and any of its branches may be affected, and to a lesser extent, veins, as well. These changes are often confined to a small segment, and are missed easily if adequate material is not obtained for biopsy study.

MANIFESTATIONS. Granulomatous arteritis may manifest itself with constitutional changes or with changes which are the product of obliterative arteritis. These are often very localized, as for example, the sudden loss of vision in one eye, and are frequently not recognized as being part of a general disease. The constitutional manifestations include fever, sweats, fatigue, weakness, weight loss, depression, anxiety, anorexia, arthralgias or arthritis, myalgias, headache, and anemia.

The nonspecific manifestations may dominate the patient's illness and may precede the appearance of any localized alterations for long periods. Hence, granulomatous arteritis must be considered in the differential diagnosis of many systemic disorders, including fever of unknown origin and anxious depressive states.

On the other hand, the constitutional accompaniments of granulomatous arteritis may be minimal and easily overlooked, and the dramatic changes induced by localized arterial obliteration may dominate the course of the disease.

The nature of the local manifestations is obviously dependent on which vessels are involved by the granulomatous process. When the temporal and/or occipital arteries are implicated, the following may appear: headache, which is often described as severe and throbbing; localized swelling, pain, and tenderness along the affected vessels; phantom fleeting tender spots in the scalp, retro-orbital pain, or pain in or behind the ears; pain in the face or in the tongue when eating solid foods; pain in the occiput or neck; facial pain, sore throat; swollen, painful, and weak tongue; intermittent claudication of the tongue (rarely progressing to gangrene), deafness, blindness, diplopia, and ptosis; and swelling at the angles of the jaw, suggesting mumps.

Involvement of the vertebral, carotid, and basilar arteries may result in convulsions and temporal lobe seizures, with hallucinations, vertigo, psychosis, and major or minor strokes. Myocardial infarction or angina pectoris may be the result of coronary artery involvement. Intermittent claudication in the arms or legs, or the aortic arch syndrome may result. The pulmonary artery may be obstructed, which may lead to ischemic changes in the lungs and pulmonary hypertension. Abdominal angina or acute mesenteric occlusion may occur. Obstruction of the renal arteries, which may be unilateral, may produce hypertension.

Of great importance are the visual complications as the result of changes in the carotid, ophthalmic, or retinal arteries. Although these changes are usually closely associated with the local manifestations of temporal arteritis, they occasionally precede it, or follow it after a period of prolonged remission. One eye or both eyes may be affected. There is no clear-cut relationship between the degree of involvement of the temporal or other arteries and the eyes. Ophthalmoplegias and transient diplopia may occur. Impairment of vision may be partial or complete, transient or permanent, and usually occurs in the first 10 months of the disease. There is usually some residual defect, but surprising recovery of vision may take place, even after as long as 5 days of total blindness. The loss of vision is often strikingly out of proportion to changes visible ophthalmoscopically. Papilledema, ischemic optic neuritis, closure of the retinal artery or its branches, hemorrhages, cotton wool spots, and segmental field defects are the changes most often seen, but the retina may look perfectly normal. The repeated episodes of transient loss of vision in older individuals may be confused with atherosclerotic blockage of the internal carotid arteries. Some degree of permanent loss of vision is said to occur in almost half the affected individuals, and 15 percent become blind.

This disorder mimics a host of other diseases common to this period of later life, including neuropsychiatric, degenerative, infectious, and collagen-vascular processes. Its earliest presentation is often so vague and bizarre that the patient is thought to have functional illness. Recently, temporal arteritis has been found, sometimes unexpectedly, in elderly individuals with so-called "polymyalgia rheumatica," a syndrome in which muscular soreness, weakness, and wasting become associated with weight loss and other constitutional signs. Also, initial presentation of temporal arteritis with severe polyneuropathy as the dominant feature is being recognized.

The disease may run its course in a few months or may persist for several years. The mortality rate is estimated at 10 to 15 percent. Death usually results from changes produced in the heart, great vessels, central nervous system, or kidneys by the arteritis. Pneumonitis and other infections commonly eventuate in the death of these elderly patients.

A mild leukocytosis with shift to the left, increased sedimentation rate, and moderate normocytic, normochromic anemia are common. There may be striking rouleaux formation of the red blood cells. Eosinophilia is not prominent. An abnormal serum electrophoretic pattern with hypergammaglobulinemia may be present.

The diagnosis is established by observing the histologic changes in an affected vessel. A biopsy of the temporal artery may give the answer even in the absence of symptoms and signs, but if possible, a clinically affected area should be sought.

TREATMENT. Adrenal corticosteroids have been highly effective in suppressing (though not eradicating) the inflammatory process and in relieving local and systemic manifestations, usually within a few days. The overall effectiveness of steroids has exceeded by far that generally observed in patients with classical polyarteritis nodosa. It is essential to institute adequate treatment before serious local obliterative vascular changes have occurred; early treatment is imperative in preventing blindness. Treatment may be required for many months. Recurrences are common if therapy is inadequate, and tapering of steroids should be gradual.

SCLEREDEMA

DEFINITION. Scleredema is a disease of unknown cause characterized by spreading swelling and induration of the skin and subcutaneous tissues. It occurs at any age, most commonly in childhood and young adulthood. It may be seen in the neonatal period. Females are twice as often affected as males. Three familial cases have been reported.

PATHOLOGY. Scleredema is a misnomer, because there is neither sclerosis nor edema. The chief histologic alteration is pronounced swelling of the collagen of the skin and subcutaneous tissues, with deposition between the bundles and about the vessels of a peculiar mucinous material. There is moderate infiltration by lymphocytes and plasma cells, but no intense inflammation. The process subsides without residuals.

Scleredema often follows respiratory bacterial or viral infections. In over 50 percent of cases, these infections have been streptococcal in origin.

Histochemical studies suggest the accumulation of a water-soluble mucopolysaccharide in and between the collagen fibers of the dermis. This material is either chondroitin sulfate A or hyaluronic acid. Such an accumulation of mucopolysaccharides in the dermis may be a function of excessive production or defective removal by fibroblasts, or both.

MANIFESTATIONS. Following the initial infection, there is usually an asymptomatic interval, lasting from a few days to 6 weeks. The disease begins with swelling and induration of the skin and subcutaneous tissues. The swelling does not pit, and the skin feels as though it had been infiltrated with wax. These changes may be preceded by a blotchy erythematous or livid rash and, at times, by a short period of malaise, low fever, and musculoskeletal aching. The swelling usually starts in the neck, spreading in turn to the face, scalp, shoulders, trunk, arms, and abdomen. The legs are less often involved, but hand and foot involvement occurs in 10 percent of affected individuals. The genitals are rarely affected. The face becomes masklike, and the patient appears "hidebound." Involvement of the eyelids may lead to pronounced chemosis, and the tongue and pharynx may be affected so extensively that dysarthria and dysphagia result. Additional features include sterile effusions in the pleura, pericardial, peritoneal or joint cavities, and muscle weakness. Histologic alterations in the viscera comparable to the changes in the skin have been described in one patient.

The swelling may spread rapidly and reach its maximum in a matter of days or a few weeks. Improvement generally begins after 3 to 6 months and continues for about 18 to 24 months. The areas of initial involvement, the face and the neck, often are the last to clear. Residual patches may persist for many years. Relapses are not common, but recurrence after a prolonged symptom-free period has been observed up to 40 years after the initial episode. These recurrences usually follow a course similar to that of the initial illness.

The white blood cell count is usually normal, as are the sedimentation rate and other laboratory studies. An elevated serum gamma-globulin level has been recorded in a few instances.

DIFFERENTIAL DIAGNOSIS. It is most important to distinguish this relatively benign disease from scleroderma (Chap. 393). Sometimes it is quite impossible to separate the two diseases on clinical grounds or even by biopsy examination, and the distinction becomes clear only from the clinical course. The following points are often helpful in differentiation: in scleredema the hands and feet are relatively unaffected, and although there may be mild thickening of the skin of the extremities, there is no atrophy or Raynaud's phenomenon, commonly noted in scleroderma. Furthermore, in scleredema there is no pigmentation or calcinosis of the skin, the process involutes completely without residua, and abnormalities in the esophagus, lungs, kidneys, or other viscera are rarely encountered. Dermatomyositis must also be differentiated. Less frequently confused with scleredema are myxedema, myxedema circumscripta, amyloidosis, sarcoidosis, lymphomatous infiltration, edema of other causes, and trichinosis.

TREATMENT. Therapy is difficult to evaluate because of the variable clinical course. Any infection should be eliminated. Physical therapy may be helpful. Adrenal steroids and thyroid hormone have not been effective, nor have pituitary extract, hyaluronidase, estradiol, fibrinolysins, pilocarpine, and thorium X.

RELAPSING FEBRILE NODULAR NONSUPPURATIVE PANNICULITIS (Weber-Christian Disease)

DEFINITION. Relapsing febrile nodular nonsuppurative panniculitis (Weber-Christian disease) is characterized by recurrent tender or painless inflammatory and necrotic nodules in the panniculus, fever, malaise, and other systemic manifestations. Its cause is unknown.

PATHOLOGY. The nodules consist of necrotic fatty tissue infiltrated with lymphocytes, plasma cells, and macrophages. Foreign-body giant cells are often present, and some vessels may show a perivasculitis. Healing occurs with scarring and atrophy, resulting in characteristic areas of depression in the skin. Similar alterations have also been noted in the fatty tissue in other parts of the body, including the epicardial, peripancreatic, periadrenal, perirenal, and mesenteric fat.

Some believe this is another disorder in which autoimmunity and hypersensitivity are important. It has been described in association with systemic lupus, rheumatoid arthritis, dermatomyositis, and sarcoid. Thyroiditis is said to accompany it at times, and leukoagglutinins have been reported.

MANIFESTATIONS. The disease usually occurs between the ages of twenty and fifty. Formerly regarded as primarily a disease of obese women, it is now known to affect men as well.

The illness commonly begins insidiously, with the appearance of subcutaneous nodules. These may occur on any part of the body but are usually confined to the thighs, buttocks, legs, abdomen, breasts, and arms. The lesions vary from 0.5 to more than 10 cm in diameter; they are usually very tender but in rare cases are painless. They are freely movable, and the overlying skin is usually red or violaceous, becoming brownish later.

With the appearance of the nodules, the patient generally develops chills, fever, malaise, nausea, and musculoskeletal aching. Splenomegaly and regional adenopathy are not rare. The nodules do not suppurate, but in some instances an oily liquid is extruded from them.

Panniculitis may involve the tissues in or about the joints, and may simulate arthritis. A roentgenogram of such a joint may show fat necrosis and may suggest the diagnosis. Areas of fat necrosis in the bone marrow may appear as punched-out lesions on roentgenograms, and may be interpreted as tumor or myeloma.

Isolated involvement of the adipose tissue of the mesentery of the small intestine may occur, resulting in abdominal pain with or without a palpable intraabdominal mass, usually in the left upper quadrant. The course is benign, and spontaneous recovery occurs.

A systemic type of Weber-Christian disease has been described, and it has been postulated that in healing, this process may lead to diffuse fibrosis of the sort hitherto ascribed to tumors, granulomatous infections, and Sansert. The fibrosis may be retroperitoneal, in the mediastinum, about the spleen, in the mesentery, the adipose tissue around the bowel, the pericardial area, around the urinary bladder, and in the bile ducts.

COURSE. The disease subsides spontaneously after days or weeks, only to recur weeks, months, or years later. The only residuals in the skin are concave or dimpled areas. These atrophic depressions are a characteristic and important diagnostic feature. Death due to the uncomplicated disease is unusual.

The white blood cell count may be moderately elevated, or there may be a leukopenia. Sometimes there is a mild anemia.

DIAGNOSIS. This disease must be distinguished from lipomatosis, adiposis dolorosa (Dercum's disease), erythema nodosum, erythema induratum, sarcoid, and insulin atrophy. It is early mistaken for thrombophlebitis in obese persons. Factitious lesions due to self-injection of milk have been mistaken for it. Panniculitis and fat necroses may be associated with neoplasm and inflammation of the pancreas. Evidence of pancreatic disease may be minimal or absent, and the condition may be mistaken for the idiopathic form of panniculitis.

TREATMENT. Present methods are unsatisfactory. Sulfonamides and antibiotics are of no benefit. In some cases, adrenal corticosteroids have produced transient symptomatic relief, with disappearance of fever and nodules, and should be tried.

REFERENCES

Scleredema

Greenberg, L. M., C. Geppert, H. G. Worthen, and R. A. Ford: Scleredema "Adultorum" in Children. Review of World Literature, Pediatrics, 32:1044, 1963.

Temporal (Granulomatous) Arteritis

Brok, M. I.: Articular and Vascular Manifestations of Polymyalgia Rheumatica, Ann. Rheumatic Dis., 26:103, 1967.

Cullen, J. F.: Occult Temporal Arteritis. A Common Cause of Blindness in Old Age, Brit. J. Ophthalmol., 51:513, 1967.

Fessel, W. J., and C. M. Dearson: Polymyalgia Rheumatica and Blindness, New Engl. J. Med., 276:1403, 1967.

Hamrin, B., and N. Jonsson: Involvement of Large Vessels in Polymyalgia Arteritica, Lancet, I:1193, 1965.

Harrison, M. J. G., and A. T. Bevan: Early Symptoms of Temporal Arteritis, Lancet, II:638, 1967.

Hunder, G. G., and S. G. Sheps: Intermittent Claudication and Polymyalgia Rheumatica. Association with Panarteritis, Arch. Intern. Med., 119:638, 1967.

Warrell, D. A., C. Godfrey, and E. G. J. Olsen: Giant Cell Arteritis with Peripheral Neuropathy, Lancet, I:1010, 1968.

Wilske, K. R., and L. A. Healey: Polymyalgia Rheumatica— Manifestation of Giant Cell Arteritis, Ann. Intern. Med., 66:77, 1967.

Weber-Christian Disease

Ackerman, A. B., D. T. Mosher, and H. A. Schwamm: Factitial Weber-Christian Syndrome, J.A.M.A., 198:731, 1966.

Arnold, H. A., and A. R. Bainsborough: Weber-Christian Disease with Visceral Involvement: Case Report and Review of the Literature, J. Can. Med. Assoc., 89:1138, 1963.

Harbrecht, P. J.: Variants of Retroperitoneal Fibrosis, Ann. Surg., 165:388, 1967.

Milner, R. D.: Systemic Weber-Christian Disease, J. Clin. Pathol., 18:150, 1965.

Mitchinson, M. J.: Systemic Idiopathic Fibrosis and Systemic

Weber-Christian Disease, J. Clin. Pathol., 18:645, 1965.

Roserstock, H. A.: Weber-Christian Disease. Report of a Case Documenting the Presence of Leukoagglutinins, J.A.M.A., 203:890, 1968.

Wegener's Granulomatosis

Bouroncle, B. A., E. J. Smith, and F. E. Cuppage: Treatment of Wegener's Granulomatosis with Imuran, Am. J. Med., 42:314, 1967.

Carrington, C. B., and A. A. Liebow: Limited Forms of Angiitis and Granulomatosis of Wegener's Type, Am. J. Med., 41:497, 1966.

Constantine, H., G. Desforges, and E. A. Gaensler: Noninfectious Necrotizing Granulomatosis of the Lung. Wegener's syndrome, Med. Thorac., 23:115, 1966.

Hollander, D., and R. T. Manning: The Use of Alklyating Agents in the Treatment of Wegener's granulomatosis, Ann. Intern. Med., 67:393, 1967.

Nielsen, K., I. Christiansen, and E. Jensen: Wegener's Granulomatosis. A Survey and Three Cases, Acta Med. Scand., 181:577, 1967.

Reed, W. B., A. K. Jensen, B. E. Konwaler, and D. Hunter: The Cutaneous Manifestations in Wegener's Granulomatosis, Acta Dermato-Venereol. (Stockholm), 43:250, 1963.

395 THE MARFAN SYNDROME

Victor A. McKusick

DEFINITION. Marfan's syndrome [synonyms: arachnodactyly, dolichostenomelia (long thin limbs), dystrophia mesodermalis congenita, typus Marfanis] is a heritable, generalized disorder of one element of connective tissue, clinically manifested by abnormalities of the eye (especially ectopia lentis), of the skeletal system (especially excessive length of the long bones), and of the cardiovascular system (especially diffuse and/or dissecting aneurysm of the ascending aorta).

CLINICAL MANIFESTATIONS. Skeleton. Characteristically, the tubular bones are excessively long, resulting in arachnodactyly and in anomalous proportions. Normally after puberty the ratio of upper segment (pubic symphysis to crown) to the lower segment (pubic symphysis to sole) is about 0.92 (SD = 0.04) in whites and 0.85 (SD = 0.03) in Negroes. Because of the excessively long lower segment, the ratio is usually lower in patients with Marfan's syndrome. The arm span exceeds the height. The patient with the Marfan syndrome is taller than the average for his age and family; however, the deviation from the normal skeletal proportion is of more specific diagnostic significance. Excessive longitudinal growth of ribs may result in outward displacement of the sternum (pigeon breast, pectus carinatum) or inward displacement (pectus excavatum, *Trichterbrust*). Redundant ligaments, tendons, and joint capsules result in loose-jointedness, hyperextensibility of joints, genu recurvatum (backward curvature of the legs at the knees),

flatfoot, kyphoscoliosis, and habitual dislocation of the hips, patella, clavicles, mandible, and other joints. Hernia occurs with increased frequency. In general, patients with the Marfan syndrome display a sparsity of subcutaneous fat (Fig. 395-1).

Eye. Ectopia lentis (subluxation of the lens, dislocated lens) is the ocular hallmark of Marfan's syndrome. Iridodonesis, tremor of the iris, is occasionally a clue to the presence of dislocated lenses. Occasionally the margin of a dislocated lens is visible through the undilated pupil, and occasionally the lens may be totally dislocated into the anterior chamber. To exclude minor subluxation, it is necessary to dilate the pupil maximally and perform a careful slit-lamp examination. Under these circumstances one sees in the severely affected person that the suspensory ligaments are redundant, attenuated, and fragmented.

Myopia, often of high grade, is usually present; a long orbit generally occurs as an integral part of the syndrome. Spontaneous detachment of the retina is frequent.

Cardiovascular System. The principal cardiovascular manifestation of Marfan's syndrome is a weakness of the aortic media such that the portion subject to greatest hemodynamic stress of certain types—the ascending aorta—tends to undergo progressive dilatation or acute dissection. The dilatation, beginning as early as the first or as late as the fifth decade, occurs first in the coronary sinuses. Profound aortic regurgitation may precede evidence of dilatation of the aorta on ordinary radiographic

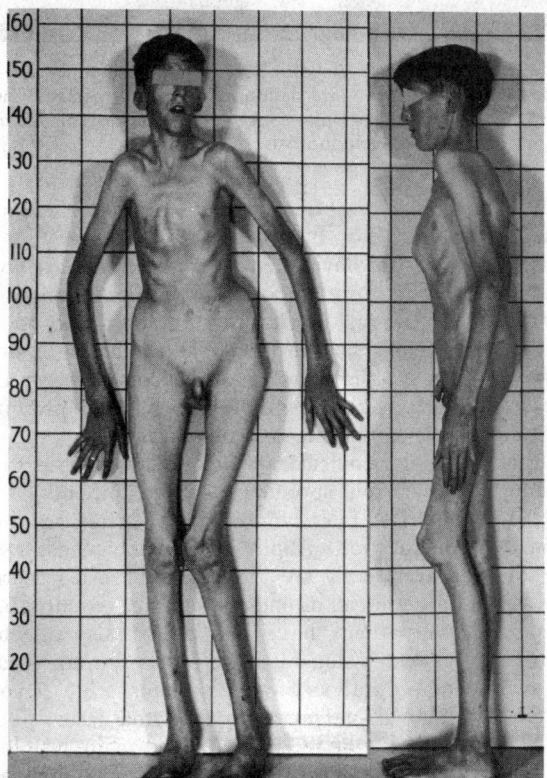

Fig. 395-1. Typical features of Marfan's syndrome in an eleven-year-old boy.

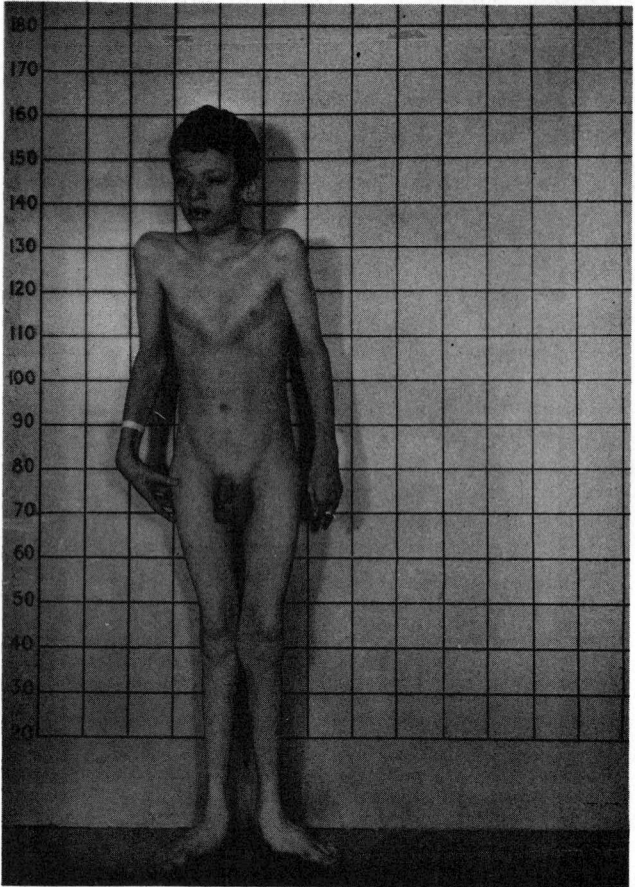

Fig. 395-2. An eleven-year-old boy with homocystinuria manifested by severe mental retardation, bilateral dislocated lenses, pectus carinatum, "rocker-bottom feet," genu valgum, spinal curvature, and generalized osteoporosis.

study. The clinical features of acute dissection are discussed in Chap. 277.

Less-common cardiovascular complications are bacterial endocarditis superimposed on minor changes of heart valves, "partial" mitral regurgitation due to redundant cusps and chordae tendineae producing systolic clicks and late systolic murmur, and incomplete coarctation of the aorta. Mitral regurgitation may be profound and functionally significant in some cases.

Other internal ramifications include cystic disease of the lung and recurrent spontaneous pneumothorax.

INHERITANCE. Marfan's syndrome is inherited as an autosomal dominant trait. About 15 percent of cases are sporadic and apparently are the result of fresh mutation occurring in a germ cell of one or the other parent; about 85 percent of patients have one parent also affected. Paternal age effect is demonstrable in the sporadic cases; the average age of fathers of such patients is 5 to 7 years higher than that of patients with inherited cases.

PATHOLOGY AND BASIC DEFECT. The main histologic abnormality is that of the aortic media. Probably in most cases normal at birth if examined by the usual techniques, it undergoes changes which in the mildest form are iden-

tical with Erdheim's cystic medial necrosis seen in other settings (Chap. 277). In its advanced form, there are loss of elastic fibers, scarring, hyperplasia of smooth muscle in large whorls, and dilatation of the vasa vasorum. What element of connective tissue is fundamentally defective is unknown. The elastic fiber is under suspicion.

DIFFERENTIAL DIAGNOSIS. Given cardiovascular and skeletal manifestations consistent with Marfan's syndrome, one cannot be certain of the diagnosis unless ectopia lentis, the most specific of the components of the syndrome, can be demonstrated, or unless close relatives display unmistakable evidence of the disease. Confusion results from the fact that there is wide variability in the clinical severity of this syndrome, and its individual components display some independence in their severity ("expressivity") or even in whether they are present at all ("penetration"). When the mutant gene for this syndrome occurs in pyknic stock, the affected person is likely to display less-impressive skeletal abnormalities. The patient must be judged against the background of his family.

The main condition to be distinguished from Marfan's syndrome is homocystinuria (Table 395-1), which is

Table 395-1. COMPARISON OF MARFAN'S SYNDROME AND HOMOCYSTINURIA

	Marfan's Syndrome	Homocystinuria
Skeleton...........	Arachnodactyly and loose-jointedness	Arachnodactyly less striking; reduced joint mobility
Deformity of anterior part of chest..	Frequent	Frequent
Scoliosis..........	Frequent	Frequent
Skin..............	Striae distensae frequent	Malar flush and livedo reticularis frequent
Ectopia lentis......	Present in about 70% of cases	Present in almost 100% of cases over 10 years old
Vascular disease....	Mainly aortic	Mainly thrombotic
Mental retardation.	Not a feature	Frequent (about ⅔ of cases)

identified by specific tests on the urine. Homocystinuria qualifies as a heritable disorder of connective tissue because of the ocular, skeletal, and cardiovascular features which simulate those of Marfan's syndrome. The features are ectopia lentis, chest deformity, scoliosis, generalized osteoporosis, recurrent thromboses in arteries and veins, and mental retardation. The patients tend to be tall and have chest deformity and scoliosis as in Marfan's syndrome, although usually none of these features is as extreme. Loose-jointedness is not impressive, and the fingers usually show reduced joint mobility (Fig. 395-2). Ectopia lentis is progressive and is demonstrable in the great majority of patients by the age of ten years. Generalized osteoporosis, with "codfish vertebrae" and proneness to fracture in severe cases, is present in some degree in all patients. Thrombosis in arteries and veins may occur at any age and at any site. Coronary artery occlusion, bilateral thrombosis of the internal carotid artery, and thrombosis of the inferior vena cava have been observed in children or teenagers with homocystinuria. Mental retardation in some degree occurs in about two-thirds of cases.

The diagnosis of homocystinuria rests on demonstration of homocystine in the urine. The cyanide nitroprusside test is positive for both cystine and homocystine. Further tests, such as high-voltage paper electrophoresis, permit the differentiation. Enzymatic confirmation is provided by demonstrating very low activity of cystathionine synthetase in liver biopsy material or in fibroblasts grown in culture from skin.

Like other Garrodian inborn errors of metabolism, homocystinuria is inherited as an autosomal recessive trait. The fundamental defect in homocystinuria is deficient activity of cystathionine synthetase, the enzyme which normally catalyzes the condensation of homocysteine and serine to form cystathionine. Ectopia lentis, osteoporosis, and skeletal deformity may result from interference of accumulated sulfhydryl groups with cross-linking in collagen. The mechanism of vascular thrombosis is obscure. The cause of mental retardation is also not understood, although intracranial thromboses undoubtedly contribute in many cases. Furthermore, the normal presence of cystathionine and cystathionine synthetase in brain and their absence from the brain of the homocystinuric suggest that deficiency of a substance synthesized distal to the enzyme block is involved in the mental retardation. The *Weill-Marchesani syndrome* is characterized by ectopia lentis, short stature, stiff joints, congenital pulmonic stenosis (in some cases), and autosomal recessive transmission.

TREATMENT. In some girls who are already very tall by the age of nine or ten, induction of precocious puberty with estrogen has been practiced with satisfactory results in terms of reducing the adult height attained. In markedly asthenic children and perhaps in adults with signs of aortic dilatation, anabolic steroids may have a place. In patients with early dilatation of the aorta (as signaled, for example, by the murmur of aortic regurgitation), reserpine or propanolol in subhypotensive doses may protect the aorta by reducing the abruptness of the ventricular ejection. The ascending aorta is being replaced with increasing success in patients with Marfan's syndrome.

Homocystinuria should be treated along the lines of phenylketonuria and galactosemia, in which pathologic effects of metabolites accumulating proximal to an enzyme block are averted by specific dietary restrictions; patients with homocystinuria are being treated with low methionine diet (supplemented by cystine, which in homocystinurics becomes an essential amino acid). The results are difficult to evaluate. Pyridoxine (vitamin B_6) is a coenzyme for cystathionine synthetase, and some patients seem to be benefited by the administration of this vitamin. In retarded patients, a trial in which cystine plus homoserine is given, is being performed in an attempt to synthesize cystathionine in a retrograde direction. Long-

term anticoagulants of the coumadin type are indicated in cases of recurrent thrombosis.

REFERENCES

McKusick, V. A.: "Heritable Disorders of Connective Tissue," 3d ed., St. Louis, The C. V. Mosby Company, 1966.

Schimke, R. N., V. A. McKusick, T. Huang, and A. D. Pollack: Homocystinuria: A Study of 38 Cases in 20 Families, J.A.M.A., 193:711, 1965.

396   THE EHLERS–DANLOS SYNDROME
Victor A. McKusick

DEFINITION. The Ehlers-Danlos syndrome (synonyms: cutis hyperelastica, "India rubber men," dermatorrhexis with dermatochalasis and arthrochalasis) is a heritable and generalized disorder of one element of connective tissue, clinically manifested by fragility and hyperelasticity of the skin and loose-jointedness.

CLINICAL MANIFESTATIONS. Characteristically, the skin can be stretched through an unusually great range, but returns promptly to its normal position on release. Later on, the skin may lose its elasticity, become truly cutis laxa, and hang in flabby folds or wrinkles. The skin is

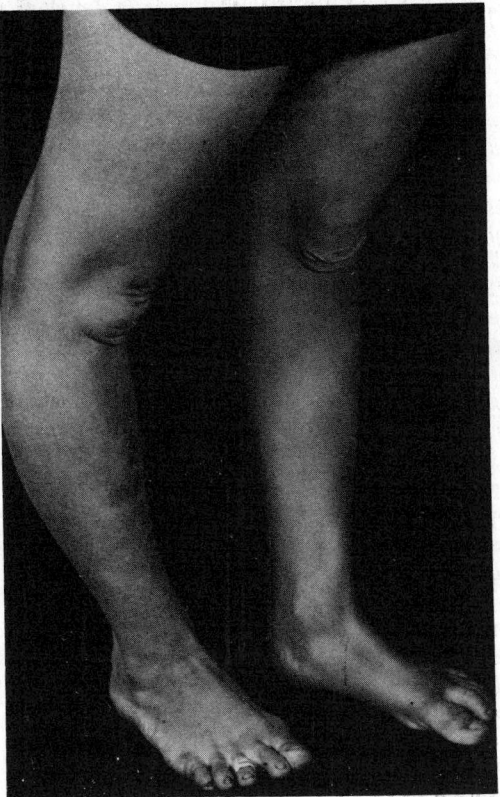

Fig. 396-1. The loose-jointedness and the "cigarette paper" scarring of the Ehlers-Danlos syndrome.

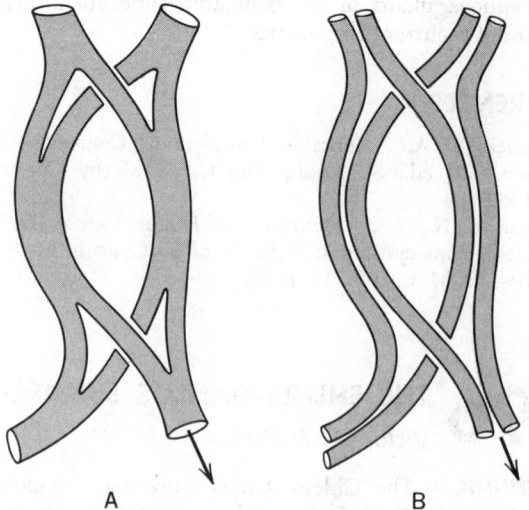

Fig. 396-2. Schematic representation of the postulated nature of the defect in the collagen basketry in the Ehlers-Danlos syndrome. A. Normal. B. Ehlers-Danlos syndrome. (After Jansen.)

fragile, so that minor trauma is likely to produce gaping, "fish-mouth" wounds which bleed little and hold sutures poorly. There is easy bruisability. Firm spherules up to about 1 cm in diameter develop subcutaneously, can be moved about through a considerable range, and can be demonstrated radiographically because of calcification. "Cigarette paper" scars develop over the knees, shins, etc. So-called "molluscoid pseudotumors" develop on the knees, ankles, and elbows as soft, poorly outlined swellings that may be several centimeters in diameter.

The loose-jointedness results in genu recurvatum, habitual dislocation of various joints, flatfoot, etc. Recurrent hydrarthrosis may result from the repeated trauma due to poor stabilization, especially in the knees (Fig. 396-1).

Internal ramifications include diaphragmatic hernia or eventration of the diaphragm, ectasia or diverticula of portions of the gastrointestinal and respiratory tracts, and spontaneous pneumothorax. Spontaneous rupture of the bowel is a rare complication.

INHERITANCE. The Ehlers-Danlos syndrome is usually inherited as an autosomal dominant condition. Genetic heterogeneity is likely in this disorder, and there are probably several fundamentally distinct entities with features justifying their designation as Ehlers-Danlos syndrome.

PATHOLOGY AND BASIC DEFECT. The basic defect appears to be abnormality in the way the collagen "wickerwork" is arranged such that excessive extensibility of collageneous structures is possible (Fig. 396-2). The normal elastic tissues appear to function in restoring structures to their normal position; the elastic fibers may, in fact, be hyperplastic, possibly in response to the repeated stimulus of extra stretching.

REFERENCE

McKusick, V. A.: "Heritable Disorders of Connective Tissue," 3d ed., St. Louis, The C. V. Mosby Company, 1966.

397 OSTEOGENESIS IMPERFECTA
Victor A. McKusick

DEFINITION. Osteogenesis imperfecta (synonyms: fragilitas ossium, osteopsathyrosis idiopathica, disease of Eddowes, Lobstein, van der Hoeve, Vrolik) is a heritable, generalized disorder of one element of connective tissue with clinical manifestations in the eye (blue scleras), ear (progressive deafness), skeleton (especially multiple fractures), joints (loose-jointedness), and skin. The nosography of this syndrome has been much confused because of this wide variability in its clinical expression. Osteogenesis imperfecta congenita and tarda have been separated. A further separation of the tarda type into levis and gravis forms has been suggested. A hereditary disease characterized by fragility of bones without blue scleras has been claimed as a separate entity and called specifically osteopsathyrosis idiopathica. Until there is convincing evidence to the contrary, however, the information available leads the author to maintain that all the several clinical pictures which have been described, and which go by separate names in many instances, are one and the same disease which has wide systemic ramifications and an exceedingly great range of clinical severity.

CLINICAL MANIFESTATIONS. Skeleton. Multiple fractures with trivial trauma are a main feature. Intrauterine fractures may permit antenatal diagnosis. Usually after puberty, the victim of this disease becomes less subject to fractures; susceptibility may return in later life, especially after the menopause in the female. Bowing of bones, porotic appearance on the roentgenogram without fracture, "codfish" or "hourglass" vertebras, platybasia (basilar impression of the skull) are all features. Dwarfism, with short legs and relatively large head, may be confused with achondroplasia. The calvarium tends to bulge laterally, and the head and face have a triangular configuration which often permits diagnosis from photographs alone.

Eye. The change in the sclera, which may be various shades of blue, is the only important ocular feature.

Ear. The deafness has the clinical features of conventional otosclerosis: variable age of onset, steady progression, and tendency to begin during pregnancy. The tympanic membrane may be blue like the sclera.

Joints. Loose-jointedness is one of the four cardinal features of the disease. It is responsible, at least in part, for the flatfoot, kyphoscoliosis, and habitual dislocation of joints. Weakness of ligaments and tendons responsible for the loose-jointedness sometimes results in rupture of tendons from relatively minor stress.

Others. Hernia is frequent. The teeth are characteristically small, misshapen, and bluish yellow. Kyphoscoliosis may lead in later life to cardiorespiratory complications.

INHERITANCE. Usually, osteogenesis imperfecta is clearly inherited as an autosomal dominant disorder. Some aspects of its genetics are still confused. Certain features, especially those concerning sporadic cases and the so-called congenital form, suggest a recessive mode of inheritance in some cases.

PATHOLOGY AND BASIC DEFECT. In the bones, peculiar basophilic-staining material is found in place of osteoid. In other tissues, there are a sparsity of collagen fibers and replacement by fibers with tinctorial and other characteristics of reticulin. There appears to be a generalized defect in maturation of collagen.

REFERENCES

McKusick, V. A.: "Heritable Disorders of Connective Tissue," 3d ed., St. Louis, The C. V. Mosby Company, 1966.

398 PSEUDOXANTHOMA ELASTICUM
Victor A. McKusick

DEFINITION. Pseudoxanthoma elasticum (synonyms: PXE, Groenblad-Strandberg syndrome) is a hereditary, generalized disorder of one element of connective tissue, resulting in premature breakdown of the skin in exposed areas, angioid streaks in the fundus oculi, and hemorrhage from arterial degeneration.

CLINICAL MANIFESTATIONS. Skin. In the second, third, or fourth decade of life, patients affected by PXE are likely to develop changes in the skin of the neck, axillas, inguinal areas, and periumbilical zone, consisting of thickening, grooving, and formation of yellowish, diamond-shaped, rectangular, or polygonal nodules (Fig. 398-1). The skin in involved areas becomes inelastic, lax, and redundant. In women, the changes in the neck may be cosmetically disturbing. The skin changes simulate those in actinic elastosis (senile elastosis, sun dermatosis), which differs from PXE, however, by lack of involvement in unexposed areas such as the axilla and groin and by the presence of changes on the hands.

Eye. Angioid streaks develop at a variable time, often as early as the second decade. They are brownish or gray and four or five times wider than the veins but resemble vessels in the manner in which they course over the fundus. Proliferative changes occur in the retina, with angioid streaks as points of origin. Hemorrhage contributes further to the ocular damage, which may progress to near-blindness.

Arterial Tree. Pulses may be weak or absent in the extremities. Calcification of arteries is often demonstrable by radiography early in life. Brachial arteriograms show characteristic occlusion of the radial and/or ulnar arteries, with blood supply to the hands through dilated interosseous arteries. Intermittent claudication and easy fatigability of the arms and legs occur. Many of the affected persons suffer from angina pectoris and hypertension. Recurrent gastrointestinal hemorrhage is the problem which most often brings the patient to the attention of the internist. Occasionally, some lesion such as peptic ulcer or hiatus hernia is discovered and the vascular disease of PXE is considered only an aggravating factor. More often, no such lesion is found. Hemorrhage from other sites— uterine, urinary, nasal, or subarachnoid—may occur.

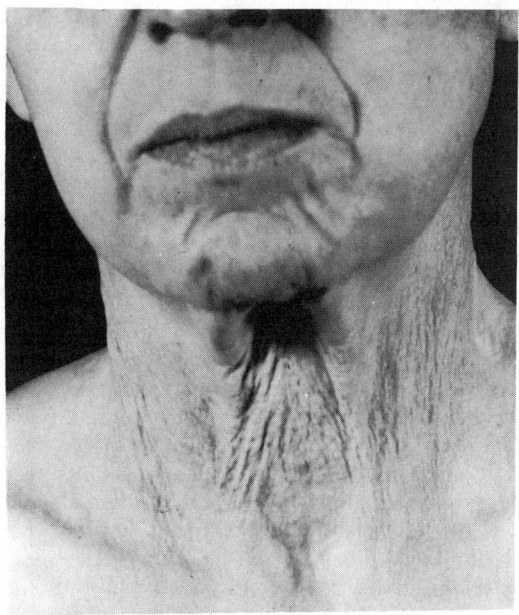

Fig. 398-1. The skin in pseudoxanthoma elasticum.

INHERITANCE. Pseudoxanthoma elasticum behaves genetically like an autosomal recessive trait.

PATHOLOGY AND BASIC DEFECT. The skin and media of arteries of intermediate and smaller size (and occasionally the endocardium and pericardium) become the site of markedly altered connective tissue fibers which are basophilic, have an affinity for calcium, and display the tinctorial characteristics of elastic fibers. In some areas, material of this description is reduced to amorphous or granular accumulations. The basis for angioid streaks appears to be basophilic change and subsequent crazing (cracking) of Bruch's membrane behind the retina. The earliest histologic change detectable involves the elastic fibers.

REFERENCE

Goodman, R. R., et al.: Pseudoxanthoma Elasticum: A Clinical and Histopathological Study, Medicine, 42:297, 1963.

399 THE GENETIC MUCOPOLYSACCHARIDOSES
Victor A. McKusick

More than eight distinct genetic disorders of mucopolysaccharide metabolism have been delineated by clinical, genetic, and biochemical and cell culture studies. Five of these are shown in Table 399-1 and are discussed in this chapter in some detail. More will undoubtedly be found. Six of the eight conditions (including all those in Table 399-1) show excessive excretion of mucopolysaccharide in the urine, and the pattern of excretion assists in their delineation. Cell culture techniques have been

Table 399-1. THE GENETIC MUCOPOLYSACCHARIDOSES

	MPS	Clinical	Genetic	Biochemical
I	(Hurler's syndrome).....	Early clouding of cornea, grave manifestations	Autosomal recessive	Chondroitin sulfate B
II	(Hunter's syndrome)....	No clouding of cornea, milder course	X-linked recessive	Heparitin sulfate Chondroitin sulfate B
III	(Sanfilippo's syndrome)..	Mild somatic, severe CNS effects	Autosomal recessive	Heparitin sulfate Heparitin sulfate
IV	(Morquio's syndrome)...	Severe bone changes of distinctive types, cloudy cornea, intellect ±, aortic regurgitation	Autosomal recessive	Keratosulfate
V	(Scheie's syndrome).....	Stiff joints, coarse facies, cloudy cornea, intellect ±, aortic regurgitation	Autosomal recessive	Chondroitin sulfate B

useful in establishing the nature of these conditions as mucopolysaccharidoses by demonstrating accumulation of mucopolysaccharides in the cytoplasm of the patient's cells, and in confirming the mode of inheritance by demonstrating mucopolysaccharides in the cytoplasm of both parents in autosomal recessive forms and in the mother only in the X-linked recessive form. All these conditions are inherited as recessive traits, and all but one are autosomal recessive. Presumably a specific enzyme defect concerned in degradation of mucopolysaccharide is present in each. Neurovisceral lipidosis, otherwise known as generalized gangliosidosis, shares features of both the mucopolysaccharidoses and the lipidoses. The enzymatic defect involves β-galactosidase. Since this enzyme is involved in a degradative function of both ganglioside and mucopolysaccharide, the combination of features is not unexpected.

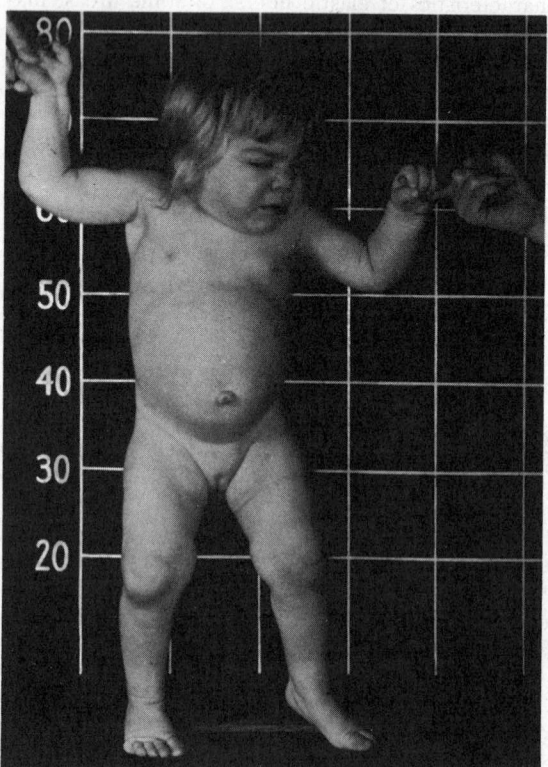

Fig. 399-1. Mucopolysaccharidosis I (Hurler's syndrome).

The designations used for the mucopolysaccharides in Table 399-1 are being replaced by other preferred terms: chondroitin sulfate B = dermatan sulfate; heparitin sulfate = heparan sulfate; keratosulfate = keratan sulfate. Although these terms may become generally used, it is unlikely that the alternative term for acid mucopolysaccharide, glycosaminoglycuronoglycan, will.

MUCOPOLYSACCHARIDOSIS I
(Hurler's Syndrome)

DEFINITION. Hurler's syndrome (Fig. 399-1) is the prototype of these disorders.

CLINICAL MANIFESTATIONS. The cardinal features are gross facies, dwarfism, lumbar gibbus and radiologic changes from involvement of the osseous skeleton, stiff joints including clawhand, corneal clouding, hepatosplenomegaly, cardiac disorders, and mental retardation. Clinically this is the severest of the mucopolysaccharidoses (MPS), usually leading to death in the first decade. The child usually seems normal at birth. The several manifestations appear in the first year or two and are progressive. There may be dyspnea, precordial pain, and congestive heart failure, and murmurs referable to any of the valves of the heart may occur. Death is attributable to cardiac causes or intercurrent respiratory infection.

INHERITANCE. Hurler's syndrome is an autosomal recessive condition.

PATHOLOGY AND BASIC DEFECT. As in all the mucopolysaccharidoses, metachromatically staining inclusions of mucopolysaccharide may be found in the circulating polymorphonuclear leukocytes (Reilly granulation) or lymphocytes and are most consistently seen in the clasmatocytes of the bone marrow. Cells of an inflammatory exudate and fibroblasts cultured from skin also show the mucopolysaccharide.

Connective tissue from many sites shows characteristic "gargoyle cells," which are probably fibroblasts distended with mucopolysaccharide. Collagenosis is stimulated. Material presumably identical to that in the fibroblasts "balloons" the neurones of the central nervous system, peripheral ganglions, and retina, the Kupffer and parenchymal cells of the liver, the reticulum cells of spleen and lymph nodes, and the epithelial cells of endocrine glands. Extensive intimal deposits of mucopolysaccharide are found in the aorta, pulmonary artery, and coronary arteries, resulting in "pseudoatherosclerosis." The heart valves become scarred and deformed. Involvement of the meninges results in internal hydrocephalus.

Two mucopolysaccharides are excreted in the urine and are identified in various organs: chondroitin sulfate B and heparitin sulfate.

MUCOPOLYSACCHARIDOSIS II
(Hunter's Syndrome)

DEFINITION. Hunter's syndrome (Fig. 399-2) differs from Hurler's syndrome in its milder course, lack of corneal clouding, and mode of inheritance.

CLINICAL MANIFESTATIONS. Grotesque facies, stiff joints, hepatosplenomegaly, and cardiac involvement occur as in MPS I. Lumbar gibbus and corneal clouding do not occur, and mental retardation is less severe and more slowly progressive. Survival to age sixty years has been observed. Progressive deafness is a consistent feature.

INHERITANCE. Hunter's syndrome is an X-linked recessive condition. Studies of cultures of fibroblast from skin of the parents of patients corroborate this by demonstrating accumulations of mucopolysaccharide in the cytoplasm of the mother's cells and not of the father's cells, in cases where the mother is a carrier. In some cases the disorder in the patient is the result of fresh mutation. Furthermore, Lyon's principle is well substantiated by the finding that about half the mother's fibroblasts show accumulations of mucopolysaccharide and that two classes of fibroblasts can be cloned, one of which is abnormal like the cells of the hemizygous-affected son and the other of which is normal.

PATHOLOGY AND BASIC DEFECT. Qualitatively the

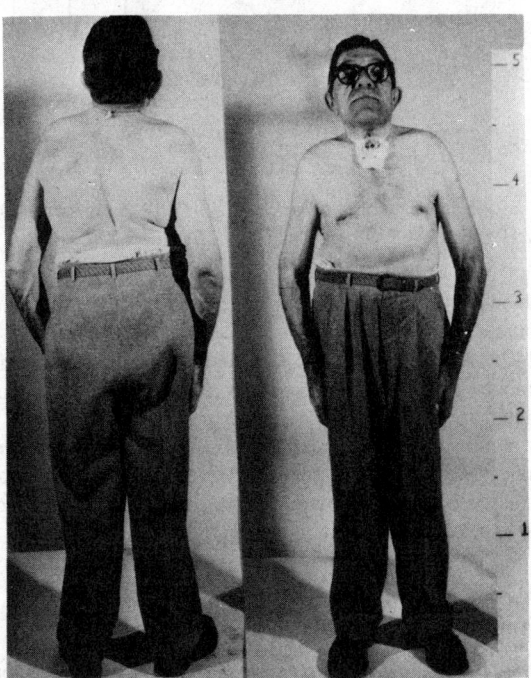

Fig. 399-2. Mucopolysaccharidosis II (Hunter's syndrome), in a forty-six-year-old man. (*Courtesy, Dr. John F. Murray and New England Journal of Medicine.*)

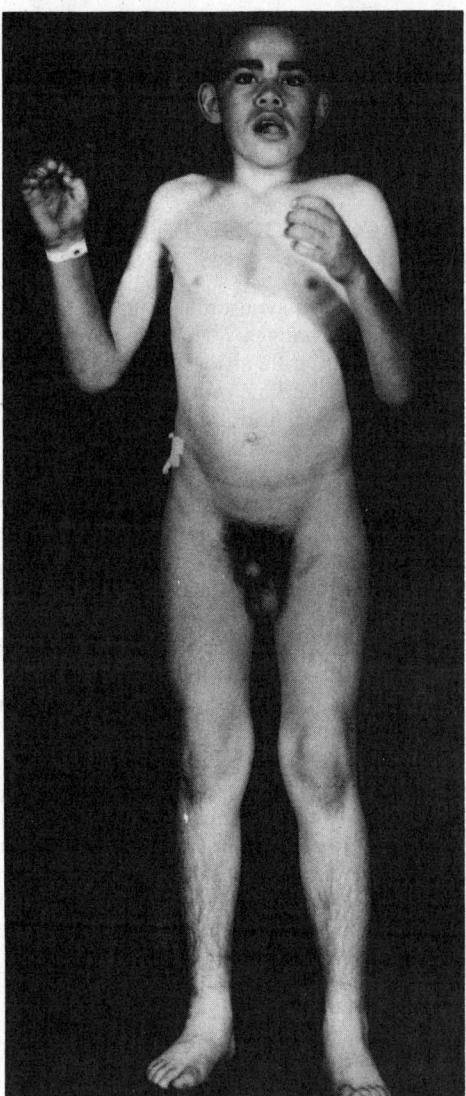

Fig. 399-3. Mucopolysaccharidosis III (Sanfilippo's syndrome).

changes are similar to those of MPS I. The same two mucopolysaccharides, chondroitin sulfate B and heparitin sulfate, are excreted in excess in the urine.

MUCOPOLYSACCHARIDOSIS III
(Sanfilippo's Syndrome)

DEFINITION. This syndrome (Fig. 399-3) is characterized by severe mental retardation with relatively mild somatic changes and characteristic mucopolysacchariduria.

CLINICAL MANIFESTATIONS. Agitation and progressive mental retardation first become evident at about five years of age and rapidly progress, with loss of speech and deterioration to imbecility by age fifteen. Gross facies, generalized hypertrichosis, hepatosplenomegaly, and stiff joints are less striking than in the other mucopolysaccharidoses. Corneal clouding does not occur. Skeletal

changes, in the spine for example, are minimal. The calvarium is markedly thickened.

INHERITANCE. Sanfilippo's syndrome is an autosomal
recessive condition.

PATHOLOGY AND BASIC DEFECT. Only heparitin sulfate
is excreted in the urine in large amounts.

MUCOPOLYSACCHARIDOSIS IV
(Morquio's Syndrome)

DEFINITION. Morquio's syndrome (Fig. 399-4) is characterized by skeletal changes (which in young children
are distinguished with difficulty from those of Hurler's
syndrome), corneal clouding, aortic regurgitation, and
distinctive mucopolysacchariduria. These patients have
been diagnosed as having the Morquio-Ullrich syndrome.
It is likely, however, that this is the disorder described
by Morquio and Brailsford and that many entities which
have been lumped under the Morquio designation are
different, e.g., multiple epiphyseal dysplasia.

CLINICAL MANIFESTATIONS. Flat vertebras, drastic hip
changes, generalized osteoporosis, and thoracic deformity, including sternal abnormality, are typical of the skeletal changes. The wrists are loose-jointed rather than stiff,
but contractures of the fingers occur. Hepatosplenomegaly
is only moderate. The skeletal features are evident early
and bring the patients to medical attention. By their teens
most patients have "steamy" corneas and aortic regurgitation. Evidence of spinal cord compression and cardiorespiratory symptoms are usually present by this stage.
Hypoplasia of the odontoid process of the second cervical
vertebra and subluxation of the first on the second cervical vertebra can lead to quadriplegia. Death occurs at
about twenty years of age in most patients.

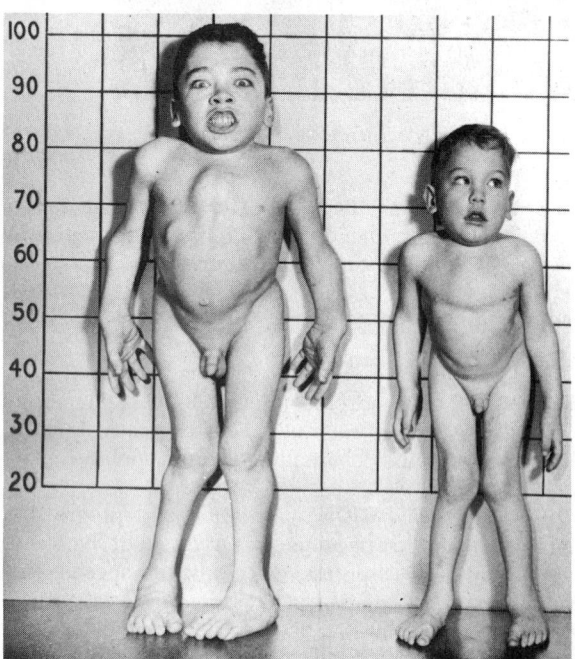

Fig. 399-4. Mucopolysaccharidosis IV (Morquio's syndrome).

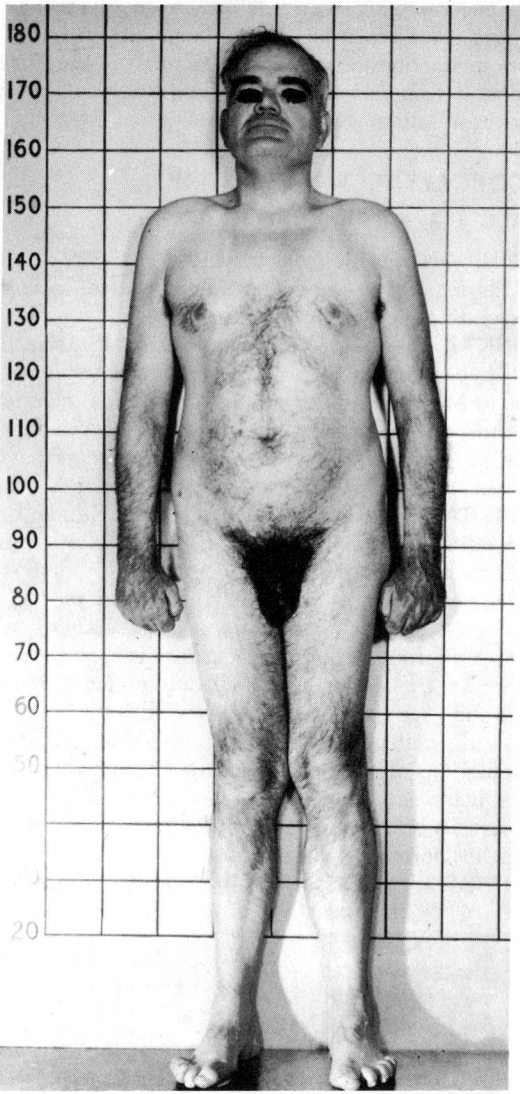

Fig. 399-5. Mucopolysaccharidosis V (Scheie's syndrome), in a
forty-six-year-old man.

INHERITANCE. Morquio's syndrome is an autosomal recessive disorder.

PATHOLOGY AND BASIC DEFECT. Keratosulfate is excreted in the urine in excessive amounts and is deposited
in macrophages and various parenchymal cells. A non-
keratosulfate-excreting type of Morquio's syndrome is
closely similar in many of its clinical manifestations
(which are milder, however) and is a mucopolysaccharidosis, as indicated by accumulations in fibroblasts.

MUCOPOLYSACCHARIDOSIS V
(Scheie's Syndrome)

DEFINITION. Scheie's syndrome is characterized particularly by stiff joints and clouding of the cornea, with
long survival and little impairment of intellect.

CLINICAL MANIFESTATIONS. By about ten years of age,

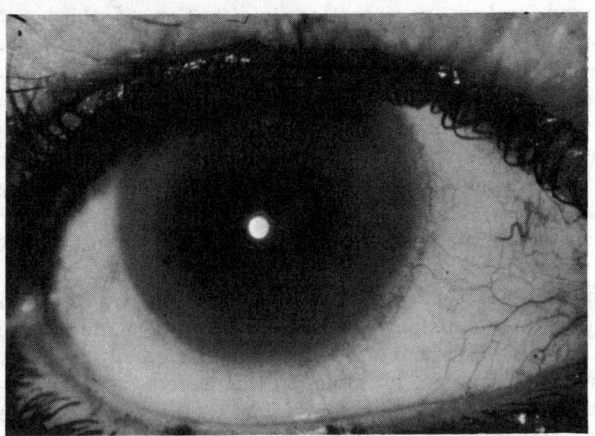

Fig. 399-6. Corneal clouding, greatest at periphery in mucopolysaccharidosis V.

stiff joints, especially in the hands and feet, are noted. The mouth is broad. Hypertrichosis is generalized (Fig. 399-5). Corneal clouding is first detected in the teens and is progressive, with greatest density in the peripheral portions (Fig. 399-6). Disability from stiffness of the fingers is aggravated by the carpal tunnel syndrome, manifested by atrophy of the thenar muscles and numbness in the distribution of the median nerve to the fingers. Intellect is impaired little if at all, but psychosis occurs in some cases. Aortic regurgitation is present in most of these patients by the third decade. Survival to age fifty years has been observed.

INHERITANCE. Scheie's syndrome is an autosomal recessive disorder.

PATHOLOGY AND BASIC DEFECT. Chondroitin sulfate B is excreted in the urine in excess. Collagenosis, e.g., in the fingers and carpal tunnel, appears to be induced by the primary disturbance in mucopolysaccharide metabolism.

REFERENCE

McKusick, V. A., et al.: The Genetic Mucopolysaccharidoses, Medicine, 44:445, 1965.

Section 15

Cutaneous Manifestations of Disease

400 DISEASES AFFECTING THE SKIN

Faye D. Arundell and
Eugene M. Farber

Since the skin is so readily visualized by the patient, trivial and important lesions alike cause concern. Passing disturbances which might remain completely unnoted in other organs attract attention to the skin. The physician must differentiate the trivial disturbances, certain common diseases which ordinarily affect only the skin, and cutaneous and subcutaneous changes which are more or less distinctive manifestations of systemic disease.

The physician familiar with the principles of applied anatomy, physiology, and chemistry of the skin and with the dozen-or-so chief patterns of disease which it presents will be able to classify over 90 percent of all dermatologic syndromes with reasonable accuracy and to treat most of them effectively. If, in the course of the initial examination, the skin lesions of a patient can be classified as representative of a common or uncommon disease, as banal or serious, as a local disturbance or a manifestation of systemic disease, much has been accomplished. Many diseases of the skin can be diagnosed with accuracy on inspection as surely as the pathologist recognizes a characteristic cytologic picture, provided the examination is adequate and complete. Others require further study, and all the resources of general medicine and of the laboratory may be needed.

Dermatologic diseases are encountered frequently by the general physician and by all medical specialists. It became clear from the enormous amount of skin disease among the United States Armed Forces during the Second World War, that any general physician practicing in a temperate zone will find that some 7 to 15 percent of his patients present as their chief complaint a disease affecting the skin. In warm, humid, tropical climates this incidence may rise to 25 percent or more. Under conditions of disaster and war, the skin of the affected population offers a particularly fertile field for microorganisms and parasites. In industry various dermatoses comprise 50 to 80 percent of occupational diseases.

DERMATITIS AND ECZEMA

Various types of acute and chronic dermatitis constitute over 50 percent of all dermatologic practice. Although the changes in the skin follow a basic pattern which is fairly constant, the factors which may initiate or prolong a dermatitis are numerous (Chap. 56).

The morphologic changes of acute and chronic dermatitis are clear-cut and not easily confused with other skin reactions. The signs of dermatitis, in the order of their evolution, are as follows: (1) erythema and swelling, (2) oozing and/or vesiculation, (3) crusting and scaling, (4) thickening and evidence of repeated excoriation, (5) hyperpigmentation, scratch papule formation, and lichenification. The first three changes are those of an acute dermatitis; the last two are seen only if the process persists for several weeks or longer. Although there is no entirely satisfactory classification which will include all variants of the dermatitis-eczema group of diseases, some categorization is useful. Separate classification of a particular group is justified and helpful if one or more of the following criteria are satisfied: it is a type in which a definite cause can be determined; it occurs in a fairly regular pattern which is helpful in determining the prognosis in the individual patient, gives clear indication for certain types of treatments, or indicates the need for further allergic and other medical studies. The following main groups exist.

CONTACT DERMATITIS. In determining the etiologic factors in a dermatitis suspected of being due to an external contactant, the localization of the lesions is often most informative. If the process is confined to exposed areas of the face, hands, and upper part of the chest, the probability is strong that something in the patient's environment is responsible. If the dermatitis is patchy or linear, it is probable that a plant or chemical substance is responsible. This may be either a primary irritant or a true allergic sensitizing agent. If the dermatitis is even and diffuse on exposed surfaces, the possibility of some airborne contactant must be considered, e.g., the vapor from bichloride, ragweed pollen, etc. However, photosensitivity, either from some systemic metabolic disturbance or induced by one of several drugs, e.g., sulfonamides, chlorothiazides, quinidine, dimethylchlortetracycline, and griseofulvin, must receive consideration. In both contact dermatitis and photosensitivity, the scalp is rarely involved.

A careful and extremely searching history is necessary in many cases of contact dermatitis in which the causative factor is not immediately apparent. The periodicity of the eruption, the distribution of lesions, and the relation of flare-ups to particular activities must be considered. Though the initial signs of dermatitis may appear within 24 hr after contact, the reaction may be delayed for 72 hr or more.

Occupational contact dermatitis is common and is the leading type of medical disability related to work. The range of sensitizers is great, and the precautions that must be taken in industry to avoid contact with certain chemicals, e.g., chromates or phenothiazines, must sometimes be elaborate.

The use of patch tests with suitable concentrations of suspected sensitizers is a useful method of study. It is not a procedure for the novice, however, because with primary irritants and strong sensitizers, marked reactions, including ulceration, may result if the concentration is too high.

Once allergic contact sensitization has been acquired, it is almost impossible to reverse it significantly by prolonged oral or parenteral administration of the compound. Many preparations designed to produce hyposensitization in persons sensitive to poison ivy are available; controlled studies have shown that they are of limited value. If further exposure can be prevented, the sensitivity tends to diminish over a period of years. Older individuals tend to have less severe contact sensitivity reactions.

In topical medicaments for the skin it is important not to apply sensitizing compounds which may later be administered systemically. Reactivity induced by repeated application commonly recurs, often in a more severe form, if the compound is later administered systemically. Many thousands of examples of this were seen when sulfonamide and penicillin-containing creams were in wide use. Novocain and chemically related compounds are another group to which systemic sensitization may be induced.

ATOPIC DERMATITIS. This exceedingly chronic dermatitis possesses distinctive features in respect to localization of lesions, personal and familial evidence of allergy, and a characteristic though often erratic course. In older children and adults the sites of principal involvement are the face, neck, and antecubital and popliteal spaces. However, in some patients the eczema may be much more widespread, or may be largely localized to a smaller area, such as the hands. Atopic dermatitis probably produces more chronic disability than any other disease in which the chief manifestations are in the skin. This, plus the fact that the affected patient frequently manifests other evidence of atopy, namely, asthma or hayfever, makes the disease of considerable medical importance. In addition, because corticosteroid therapy often is rapidly effective in relieving the inflammatory changes, the problem of untoward physiologic effects arising from prolonged therapy of this type given for atopic dermatitis is assuming increasing importance. Atopic dermatitis of and by itself is not fatal, but the suddenly developing complication of secondary infection by the virus either of herpes simplex or of vaccinia may sometimes lead to death.

SEBORRHEIC DERMATITIS. This form of dermatitis is distinguished by the localization of lesions, frequent association with evidence of sebaceous dysfunction, increased vulnerability to secondary bacterial infection, and a course which often is chronic. In widespread forms it may be very disabling. The sites of involvement are the scalp, eyebrows, face, and the presternal and interscapular regions. In more extensive cases, all the intertriginous areas may be involved, particularly in obese females. Secondary bacterial or monilial infection frequently is encountered.

NUMMULAR DERMATITIS. This type of dermatitis has a distinctive morphologic pattern (nummular, or coinlike). The lesions are frankly dermatitic, round, and vary from 2 to 4 cm in diameter. Low-grade secondary infection is common. The distribution is chiefly on the extensor surfaces of the extremities and the posterior shoulders and back, though any site may be affected. The dermatitis is most common in patients above middle age. It is seen more frequently in individuals with atopic backgrounds. The causative factors are poorly understood, but a psychosomatic component often is prominent. The lesions commonly recur at the same site, and the outlook for immediate cure of the disease is poor, though permanent remission may ordinarily be anticipated eventually.

LICHEN SIMPLEX CHRONICUS (circumscribed neurodermatitis). This is a very common condition in which the changes are due almost entirely to scratching and rubbing. The lesions usually are sharply circumscribed. Any site may be affected, but the common ones are the occipital region in women, the neck, and the lower legs. Many cases of vulvar and anal pruritus fall into the group of circumscribed neurodermatitis. The area involved becomes itchy, either as a result of some preceding irritation or, often, without any previous lesion. The scratch-itch-scratch cycle becomes firmly established. Psychosomatic factors often are prominent, and many patients indulge in scratching as a means of relieving nervous tension.

STASIS DERMATITIS. This is a type of dermatitis in which the basic etiologic factors are peripheral venous disease and tissue edema. It is important that prompt measures to control the dermatitis be undertaken before it has become severe and chronic. Stasis dermatitis is characterized by greatly increased vulnerability to primary irritants and sensitization reactions to topical medication.

CHRONIC DERMATITIS OF HANDS AND/OR FEET. This is a classification based entirely on the region involved, but it is justified because it designates such a common problem. The etiologic factors often are complex. Contact, atopic, and nummular dermatitis not infrequently are localized to the hands and feet.

MANAGEMENT

A definite diagnosis of the type of dermatitis should be established. Whenever possible the causative agent should be removed and underlying precipitating or aggravating factors should be properly managed (Chap. 56).

The *topical treatment* of dermatitis varies according to the stage of the eruption. The acute vesicular weeping phase is best treated with open wet compresses made with several layers of soft muslin without occlusive plastic coverings. The cloths are soaked in tepid plain tap water, wrung out, and applied to the affected areas for 20 to 30 min three times daily. The compresses must not be allowed to dry out while they are in contact with the skin. When secondary infection is present the following solutions are recommended as wet dressings: potassium permanganate 1:15,000; Burow's solution 1:200; silver nitrate 1:2,000. During the subacute and chronic stages, corticosteroid topical preparations are beneficial. Fluocinolone acetonide and triamcinolone acetonide lotions, creams, and ointments are available in concentrations of 0.01 to 0.2 percent. Corticosteroid lotions and creams should be applied frequently but sparingly during the subacute stage. In chronic dermatitis these creams and ointments may be covered by occlusive plastic dressings.

The systemic treatment of dermatitis is symptomatic.

Oral antihistamines such as diphenhydramine (Benadryl, 100 to 200 mg daily) and cyprohepatadine (Periactin, 8 to 16 mg daily) are effective antipruritics and sedatives. It may be necessary to use systemic corticosteroids in severe acute or generalized dermatitis. A short course of prednisone; namely, 40 mg by mouth the first day, with a gradual reduction of the dosage to termination within 7 to 10 days, is recommended in explosive contact dermatitis.

Dermatitis Herpetiformis

Dermatitis herpetiformis (Duhring's disease) is an uncommon, chronic disease characterized by recurrent bouts of a polymorphic eruption which is intensely pruritic.

The disease may appear at any age, though it is rare in children. It is more common in males than in females and usually appears in middle adult life. The eruption is extremely chronic and recurrent, and there are instances in which it persisted for as long as 40 years.

The typical lesion in dermatitis herpetiformis is a vesicle, and such lesions are commonly grouped, i.e., herpetiform. The base is erythematous, urticarial, or papular. The vesicles are most commonly 3 to 10 mm in diameter but occasionally may be much larger, resembling pemphigus or a bullous drug eruption. The lesions are symmetrically distributed on the elbows, knees, forearms, thighs, scapular areas, and the buttocks. However, any part of the skin surface may be involved.

Exacerbations of the eruption may be preceded for a few days by a general feeling of malaise, at times with a slight fever. Prior to the appearance of any visible skin lesions, violent pruritus and burning frequently develop.

Marked excoriation and occasional secondary infection are features of this disease. Hyperpigmentation and depigmentation of previously involved areas persist between attacks.

A diagnosis of dermatitis herpetiformis can be established by biopsy of a typical early lesion. The histologic changes are readily distinguished from those of pemphigus. Patients with the disease are frequently sensitive to iodides, either applied as a patch test or administered systemically.

Approximately two-thirds of patients with dermatitis herpetiformis show the characteristic changes of celiac sprue in the proximal small intestine. The mucosal changes are of limited extent, and overt manifestations of malabsorption are absent or mild. It appears that the skin and bowel changes are independent entities. Although the bowel changes respond to a gluten-free diet in the majority of patients, the cutaneous eruption is not influenced by this treatment.

The most effective *treatment* for dermatitis herpetiformis is sulfapyridine in a dose of 0.5 Gm three to four times daily. This compound has a specificity not shared by other sulfonamides. Unfortunately, treatment with this potentially toxic agent must ordinarily be continued for long periods of time, and every effort to find the lowest effective dose should be made. As alternate treatment diaminodiphenylsulfone (Avlosulfon), 50 to 100 mg daily, or salicylasosulfapyridine (Azulfidine), 2 to 4 Gm daily, may be tried. External treatment is relatively ineffective.

Herpes Gestationis

This disease seems to be a variant of dermatitis herpetiformis which occurs in women during the second half of pregnancy or in the early phases of the puerperium. The eruption shows exacerbations and partial remissions until the time of delivery or within weeks thereafter. It ordinarily disappears completely and does not return until a subsequent pregnancy. There is some evidence to indicate that women with herpes gestationis tend to abort or have a stillborn fetus. However, the disease is so rare that generalizations are hazardous. The treatment is similar to that for dermatitis herpetiformis.

ACNE

This is the classic stigma of adolescence, almost a normal physiologic reaction in the skin. Hereditary determinants condition the follicular orifice "target organ" response, namely comedones (blackheads), yet fundamentally the excitant is hormonal. At least 75 percent of both sexes show some evidence of acne at the age of puberty. There is no significant sex difference in incidence or severity. In some patients comedones may begin to develop at the age of nine or ten. The pustules, inflammatory papules, and cysts of acne may persist for a variable period of time, sometimes spanning the entire adolescent period and the twenties. The hormonal excitation of acne is androgenic. Eunuchs do not develop the disease. ACTH and testosterone injections in susceptible individuals of any age may produce acne.

The *histopathologic sequence of events* in acne is helpful in understanding the progression of the disease. The principal events are as follows:

1. Marked increase in the size and excretion of the sebaceous glands in response to androgenic hormones.

2. The formation of comedones (blackheads) and superficial cysts. These contain keratin, some lipids, and enormous numbers of Corynebacteria and *Staphylococcus albus*. Coagulase-positive *Staphylococcus aureus* is uncommon and inconstant if cultures from cysts are taken without surface contamination.

3. The rupture of cyst and follicular walls. This allows bacteria and irritating foreign material to escape into the dermis. The inflammation is intensified by the action of the bacteria on sebaceous contents to form very irritating free fatty acids.

4. The combination of enlarged follicles, progressive derangement of the epidermis, formation of new cysts, scar tissue replacement, and continuing chemical and bacterial inflammation. Under such circumstances acne may become self-perpetuating and may persist for many years.

The most serious syndrome related to acne is a triad of extensive cystic acne (*acne conglobata*), recurrent infection of the apocrine glands in the axillas and anogenital region (*hidradenitis suppurative*) (Chap. 139), and a persistent deep folliculitis of the scalp. Permanent cure of this syndrome is often impossible to achieve.

TREATMENT. Although the androgenic stimulus is basic to the development of the disease, there are no regularly effective means of combating acne from this etiologic standpoint. The main therapeutic attack on acne is through topical measures: (1) local therapy, which may help in relieving the plugging and rupture of the follicular orifice; (2) judicious drainage of purulent lesions by means which are least likely to produce scarring; and (3) combating infection with appropriate antibacterial measures. None of these measures is curative in the strict sense; all are palliative and serve only to keep the acne in check and to prevent undue scarring until the hormonal and, sometimes, emotional storm of adolescence has subsided.

The treatments used for acne are extraordinarily numerous. In assessing the value of some of them, attention should be paid to the associated factor of the passage of time in judging the true curative influence of a particular method. There are some methods, moreover, such as stringent restrictions of diet, and the use of x-ray therapy, which may have harmful effects if employed overzealously and without good medical judgment.

Preparations containing sulfur and resorcin undoubtedly are useful in mild acne, particularly if the lesions are superficial. They should be used to the point of producing a mild chapping effect. Regular removal of comedones is helpful. Drainage of frankly pustular lesions requires judgment. It should not be done too early in the course of the lesion but may promote more rapid healing if performed when the nodule is fully fluctuant and the infection is near the surface. Injection of an insoluble corticosteroid, e.g., triamcinolone acetate, into such lesions often is very helpful.

The restriction of foods and drugs is important in some patients with acne but should not be done on any routine basis. Iodides and bromides make acne worse. Foods such as chocolate and nuts so frequently cause exacerbations as to make routine elimination justifiable. From this point on, it is advisable to individualize dietary regulations. It should be kept in mind that in most patients with acne, juvenile growth is rapid and energy output high so that dietary restrictions must be advised with care and good reason.

Trauma to the skin may induce and perpetuate inflammatory acne lesions. Constant pinching, rubbing, and picking of the face may become a subconscious habit and lead to much scarring. Violent traumatic exercise, such as wrestling or football, sometimes produces inflammatory acne lesions, as does the rubbing of sweaters, dirty sweat shirts, or bacteria-laden shoulder pads and other gear.

In chronic severe acne antibacterial therapy is effective and justified. Such therapy must often be continued for long periods of time and should be initiated and supervised with good medical judgment. In general, broad-spectrum antibiotics should be given in full dosage initially to determine whether or not they will be effective. Then the dose may be reduced to the lowest level which appears to keep the condition under control. Because tetracyclines accumulate in pilosebaceous units, the maintenance dose may be as little as 250 mg daily.

Hormonal therapy of many types has been used in acne. Although such therapy may sometimes appear to be helpful, it should be used only on the basis of adequate endocrinologic study and supervision. The administration of orally effective contraceptive compounds (combinations of estrogen and progestins) has achieved a considerable vogue in the treatment of chronic acne in women. Diminution of the rate of sebum excretion is demonstrable in patients who receive the compound through three or four menstrual cycles. Early in the course of treatment some temporary flare-up of the acne may be noted.

Sunlight and vacation have a good effect on acne and may provide a striking demonstration of the inadequacies of previous treatment. In so-called "tropical acne," which occurs in a warm, humid environment, a widespread and severe pustular eruption may develop on the face and entire trunk. This type of acne usually occurs in persons who have evidenced acne previously, but sometimes is seen in those in whom there has been no previous sign of the disease. Treatment is futile until the patient can reside in a cool, dry environment.

The technique known as skin planing, surgical planing, or dermabrasion is useful for the treatment of acne scars in carefully selected patients. The most popular method involves freezing the skin with an ethyl chloride or Freon refrigerant spray, followed by mechanical removal of the epidermis and upper dermis by means of a high-speed rotary steel brush. The epidermis then regenerates rapidly from the numerous pilosebaceous and sweat gland units which remain.

SUPERFICIAL FUNGOUS INFECTIONS
(Ringworm)

The resident cutaneous flora is predominantly bacterial, but a single fungus genus, *Pityrosporum*, with two species, also is represented. *Pityrosporum ovale*, a yeastlike budding organism, occurs in abundance in the scalp and in areas of high sebaceous gland activity, but its etiologic relationship to dandruff or seborrheic dermatitis has never been proved. *Pityrosporum orbiculare*, though normally a skin resident, may play a part in the development of the common banal disease tinea versicolor. Spores of saprophytic mold fungi contaminate the cutaneous surface more or less continuously, but for the most part they remain dormant on the skin. Common weed fungi, such as species of *Penicillium* and *Aspergillus*, proliferate on diseased skin and have often been wrongly incriminated as the primary cause of cutaneous disease. Weed fungi are particularly likely to colonize necrotic ulcers, the inflamed ear canal, and disease of the subungual skin. Recovery of these fungi from such areas should not be interpreted as signifying pathogenicity.

The importance of the superficial fungi as a cause of many cutaneous diseases has been considerably exaggerated and has led to many unnecessary reactions from treatment by irritating so-called "fungicidal compounds." It is worthy of emphasis that inflammatory reactions on the feet are by no means always due to fungi, and even if a pathogenic fungus is recovered, it may be only a minor contributor to the inflammatory changes which may be present.

The superficial ringworm infections may be divided into two main groups: (1) the keratinolytic and (2) the nonkeratinolytic, a miscellaneous group. The distinctive property of the ringworm fungi is the possession of an enzyme which enables them to digest keratin. With this biochemical equipment, the nails can be disintegrated, hair dissolved, and the scaffolding of the stratum corneum, the keratinized cells, demolished. The matrix of the hair and nails is not attacked, nor the living epidermis itself. Except in unusual instances, there is no tendency for these fungi to invade living tissue, nor has any toxin been isolated. However, sensitization to ringworm fungi may be induced. This is seen most strikingly in inflammatory reactions occurring during the course of ringworm of the scalp or in some instances of acute inflammatory eruptions of the feet.

The ringworm fungi, or dermatophytes, are divided into three genera, *Trichophyton*, *Microsporum*, and *Epidermophyton*. At least one pathogenic ringworm organism (*Microsporum gypseum*) has been repeatedly isolated from the soil, which it presumably inhabits as a saprophyte. By and large, however, human infections are contracted either from infected animals or from other human beings. Certain species, the so-called "anthropophilic" organisms, show a distinct preference for human beings, occurring rarely or not at all in animals. The best example of this is the organism which commonly causes ringworm of the scalp, especially in urban areas, *Microsporum audouini*. The zoophilic ringworm fungi, on the other hand, are frequent pathogens of domestic animals, from which they may be transmitted to human beings. The anthropophilic species have the clinical peculiarity of causing relatively noninflammatory and often very persistent types of ringworm; the zoophilic organisms tend to incite short-lived inflammatory diseases in man.

The transmissibility of ringworm infections has been greatly overrated. Transmissibility can be demonstrated regularly only in certain types of ringworm infections of the scalp, occurring almost entirely in children. It is difficult to produce an infection with superficial ringworm fungi experimentally in man unless the epidermis has been severely injured. Familial infections with superficial ringworm fungi, with the exception of tinea capitis, are very uncommon. This is in contrast to some other infections, such as the virus of warts, in which infection of all members of the family living together is sometimes observed.

An important principle that provides much insight into certain peculiarities of the host-parasite relationship in ringworm infections is that if superficial ringworm infections become markedly inflammatory, there is a tendency toward spontaneous cure. Marked inflammation is incompatible with the continued proliferation of the fungus, because it is either desquamated along with other products in the wake of the inflammatory reaction or finds itself in an inhospitable environment owing to interference with normal keratin synthesis. The success of the ringworm parasite in entrenching itself on the surface depends on its not provoking much reaction in the host. This is particularly well seen in one of the most chronic of all common ringworm infections of adults, that due to *Trichophyton rubrum*, in which the inflammatory changes may be minimal, but in which the infection, once established, may persist for many years. On the other hand, when the parasite injures the host to the point of provoking a significant tissue reaction, it seals its own doom, and the infection is almost always short-lived. This type of spontaneous cure is the basis for a clinical rule that such lesions should be treated conservatively. Antifungal agents become superfluous and unnecessary; the treatment is essentially that which might be applied to an acute or chronic dermatitis of any type.

SPECIFIC TREATMENT. The clinical use of the antifungal antibiotic, griseofulvin, dates from 1958. Acquired resistance of fungi to the antibiotic does not yet seem to be a significant clinical problem.

Griseofulvin is highly active against all known species of *Trichophyton, Microsporum,* and *Epidermophyton.* It is not effective against *Candida albicans,* the organisms causing tinea versicolor or erythrasma, or the deep fungus pathogens. The antibiotic is fungistatic, not fungicidal.

Active material is concentrated in the stratum corneum, the hair, and the nails as these structures are formed and is transferred to the periphery at the same rate as the normal growth of the keratinous structure. It is clinically important to recognize that the antibiotic does not penetrate to infected dead keratinous structures, particularly nails and hairs, but is deposited only as new keratin is formed.

The average dose for adult patients is 1.0 Gm daily. Better absorption is obtained if the drug is taken with meals, especially those including some fat. In occasional patients, a lack of clinical response may dictate an increase in the dose to 2.0 Gm daily. Micronized preparations of griseofulvin are available in which the effective dose may be as low as 500 mg per day.

Toxic reactions resulting from therapeutic doses of griseofulvin in man include (1) gastrointestinal distress or loose stools, (2) headaches, (3) urticaria, and (4) an erythematous morbilliform eruption. All these reactions disappear promptly when drug therapy is stopped.

The most significant reactions to griseofulvin are those which occur in patients receiving more than one drug at the same time. The therapeutic activity of griseofulvin is decreased by treatment with phenobarbital, presumably by enzyme induction. The reduction of the pharmacologic activity of coumarin congeners which occurs in some patients in the presence of the simultaneous administration of griseofulvin may be potentially life-threatening. The enzymes induced by griseofulvin appear to increase the metabolic inactivation of warfarin, causing a fall in anticoagulant activity.

RINGWORM OF THE FEET

This is the most common type of ringworm infection. The majority of young American adult males probably acquire some fungous infection of the feet. Fungous infections of the feet are extremely rare in children and are not common in women.

The favorite sites of involvement in ringworm of the feet are the interdigital spaces, especially the third and fourth, the inner side of the arch, and the toenails. Scaling is a constant feature of subacute or chronic fungous infections of the feet. Inflammation in interdigital spaces may be variously caused by fungi, monilia, corynebacteria, or simple maceration, or it may be due to psoriasis or some other disease of the skin. The fungus most commonly cultured is *Trichophyton mentagrophytes.* The intertriginous involvement may remain chronic and localized or may sometimes show acute exacerbations, with the formation of vesicles and bullae extensively over the feet and with vesicular lesions elsewhere on the body, particularly the hands ("id" reaction).

Ringworm infections of the feet may persist as occasional patches of vesicles which tend to localize on the instep portion of the sole and on the heel and ball of the foot. In severe cases the entire sole may be involved. The process rarely extends to the dorsum of the foot. If the dorsal surface of the toes is involved, a contact dermatitis from applied medication or from footgear should be suspected.

During exacerbations of the vesicular type of ringworm infection, the lesions frequently fuse and contain a yellowish, gelatinous fluid. Vesicles on the sole may be so deep as to appear papular and may not rupture spontaneously.

The most chronic type of ringworm infection of the feet is caused by *T. rubrum.* This is frequently unilateral. It is characterized by diffuse scaling, often of a fine, branny character, by relative lack of inflammation, and by extreme chronicity. The process may become diffuse over the entire plantar surface and extend over the sides of the foot in a "moccasin" distribution. The condition is sometimes difficult to differentiate from ichthyosis, from a congenital keratosis, or from psoriasis.

Involvement of the toenails is almost inevitable in any long-standing fungous infection of the feet. This may be difficult to differentiate from the traumatic distortion which occurs inevitably in the toenails of older persons. It is probable that fungi in and under the nails are the chief source of what appear to be reinfections of other parts of the foot.

TREATMENT. Dryness is the most important single factor, especially in intertriginous involvement. A patient with subacute or chronic ringworm should be most meticulous and careful about drying the toes after bathing. The wearing of tight occlusive footgear should be avoided whenever possible, and during warm weather the wearing of sandal-type or aerated shoes is worthwhile. If there is excessive perspiration, the use of a nonabrasive foot powder is helpful; it may be found advisable to change the socks once or twice daily.

The actual treatment of the infection depends on the degree of inflammation. Vesicles and bullae should be opened. Tops of bullae should not be cut away completely because this exposes the underlying dermis. A shake lotion such as calamine may be used sparingly to advantage. Compresses or soaks with physiologic saline or Burow's solution are soothing and cleansing. Ointments should be used only after the process becomes less acute and should be applied at night rather than in the morning. It is of particular importance that evidence of secondary bacterial infection be watched for.

In subacute or chronic types of fungous infection, several preparations are useful. The newer antifungal agent, tolnaftate (Tinactin), has shown excellent results. If there is thickened skin on the soles or macerated debris between the toes, a preparation which will increase exfoliation should be prescribed. Between the toes, a preparation containing 3 percent salicylic acid and 6 percent benzoic acid in 70 percent propyl alcohol is useful. The same chemicals may be incorporated in an ointment-type base yielding a half-strength Whitfield's ointment.

A ringworm infection of the feet becomes of increased importance in patients with peripheral vascular disease or with diabetes. The scrupulousness of foot hygiene must be redoubled, and particular care should be taken not to use chemicals with possible cauterant effects on the skin because a very slowly healing ulcer may result.

MAJOCCHI'S GRANULOMA

This is a distinctive manifestation of ringworm infection in the form of a granulomatous folliculitis and perifolliculitis. It occurs most frequently in women who shave their legs and who have a diffuse *T. rubrum* infection of the feet. Indefinite and rather indistinct scaling patches develop on the lower half of the lower leg, and inflammatory nodules develop at the borders of these patches. The nodules rarely exceed a centimeter in diameter and are flat or only slightly elevated. If the lesion is observed early, it may be seen to be centered by a hair. The nodules are not pruritic and usually only slightly tender. They do not progress to suppuration and persist as long as 3 or 4 months. They may then become slowly absorbed or undergo necrosis and heal with a depressed scar. Histopathologic examination reveals a characteristic foreign-body granuloma; degenerating fungous elements may be demonstrated by the Hotchkiss-McManus method.

RINGWORM OF THE NAILS

Care must be taken not to confuse other nail dystrophies with a ringworm infection. The most common of these are psoriasis, chronic dermatitis of the distal phalanges, chronic paronychial infection, and arthritis involving the distal joint.

Griseofulvin is the recommended treatment for fungous infections of the fingernails. Because of the slow growth rate, it is necessary to administer the drug daily for periods of as long as 5 or 6 months in the treatment of fingernail infections. The toenail grows even more slowly. Clinical cure of toenail infections may require a period of treatment of eighteen months or longer; hence, griseofulvin is rarely recommended for treatment of ringworm of the toenails. Daily applications of topical antifungal solutions containing tolnaftate or undecylenic acid may control toenail infections.

RINGWORM OF THE GROIN

This is a common affliction, especially in males during the summer months. The characteristic lesions are seen in the crural folds and the upper inner thigh, usually with a scaling ring in the latter area. Several other conditions may be confused with ringworm of the groin, particularly psoriasis and seborrheic dermatitis. Anal and vulvar pruritus are uncommonly due to fungi, though *Candida* may sometimes play a role. In *Tinea cruris* it is particularly important not to use compounds which will produce any irritation. Tinactin solution applied twice daily is the treatment of choice.

RINGWORM OF THE BODY

Extensive ringworm infections of the trunk or extremities are uncommon in temperate climates, though they are seen with some frequency in the Tropics. In the presence of a ring-shaped, moderately inflamed lesion, the odds are generally in favor of some condition other than a fungous infection, e.g., pityriasis rosea, seborrheic dermatitis, or psoriasis. In those instances in which a proved extensive fungous infection of the skin of the trunk and extremities is observed in patients in temperate climates, patients should be subjected to careful study for systemic disease, particularly hematologic or diabetic.

RINGWORM OF THE HANDS

Though fungous infections of the hands are by no means rare, this diagnosis is made with too great frequency. The infection in this area has so much in common with infections of the feet that it need not be considered in any great detail. There are two main types: (1) the inflammatory vesicular and (2) the noninflammatory squamous. The former is uncommon in temperate climates, though dermatophytids associated with infections of the feet are common. *Trichophyton mentagrophytes* is the organism usually recoverable from the acute vesicular type. The course is one of spontaneous healing provided the hands are not subjected to constant chemical or traumatic irritation.

RINGWORM OF THE SCALP

Tinea capitis is predominantly a disease of children and will not be considered in detail here. It is caused by a variety of fungi. In cases which are transmitted from man to man, and in which the most common causative organism is *M. audouini*, the course without treatment is one of great chronicity; healing does not occur unless increased resistance of the host becomes evident in the form of inflammatory changes. Such a local response may become quite severe and produce the lesion called a *kerion*. This has the appearance of a bacterial infection and in time involutes spontaneously with cure of the ringworm infection, usually without permanent alopecia. In ringworm of the scalp acquired by children from animals, in which *M. canis* is the most common causative organism, the process is ordinarily inflammatory from the onset and is self-limited.

Treatment of tinea capitis with griseofulvin is remarkably effective. A single dose of 3 Gm often is curative.

Various fungi are capable of producing chronic infection of the scalp in adults. *Favus,* caused by *Trichophyton schoenleini,* is said to be relatively common in Eastern Europe but is rare in the United States. Another type of adult ringworm of the scalp, that due to *T. tonsurans,* occurs in Mexico, the Southwestern United States, and California. The condition resembles seborrheic dermatitis or psoriasis, and there usually is moderate to marked loss of hair. It cannot be detected easily because there is no fluorescence on Wood's light examination, as is the case with almost all ringworm infections in childhood. The proper diagnosis is made, in most cases, only if the clinical acuity of the examiner is high and if adequate mycologic studies are done.

ERYTHRASMA

Erythrasma was formerly regarded as a fungous disease but has now been shown to be bacterial. The causative organism is *Corynebacterium minutissimum.* The differentiation from ringworm is important in selecting the most effective type of therapy.

The infection is most common in the toe webs, but there is little in the morphologic appearance to differentiate it from a chronic fungous infection or intertrigo. There is scaling, fissuring, and slight maceration, usually confined to the third and fourth interspaces. The most characteristic type of erythrasma occurs in the genitocrural region. The lesions, large round patches, with even involvement throughout the patch, are principally found in the portions of the upper inner thigh coming in contact with the scrotum. The patches are initially pink and irregular, then become brown, with slight scaling. Erythrasma may involve the axillae, trunk, and proximal portions of the extremities quite widely. The lesions are well-defined scaling plaques which may be confused with tinea versicolor or psoriasis. A diagnosis of erythrasma is easily established if the lesions are examined with a Wood's light. This reveals a characteristic coral-red fluorescence.

The organism causing erythrasma is sensitive to broad-spectrum antibiotics, particularly erythromycin. Lesions on the body and proximal parts of the extremities respond promptly to such therapy, though recurrences sometimes are noted. Infection of the toe webs responds less satisfactorily, however, and topical treatment, as for a chronic fungous infection or intertrigo, may be necessary.

SKIN TUMORS

Primary and secondary tumors affecting the skin constitute an extraordinarily diverse group. This short sec-

tion describes only some of the most common and characteristic skin tumors.

HEMANGIOMAS

One of the most common skin tumors is the hemangioma. Some one-third of all newborn infants present this problem for evaluation. These lesions are best grouped into three classes for prognosis and therapy. The first is the *port-wine stain (nevus flammeus).* This lesion appears as a perfectly flat blue-red patch of variable size. It represents a diffuse telangiectasis of mature vessels in the dermis. No form of treatment is satisfactory. These lesions are of cosmetic significance only, so that potentially harmful or scarring modalities should not be employed. The parents should be acquainted with the fact that the lesions will probably neither extend nor fade. Efforts must be directed toward methods of obscuring the lesion if it is in a distressing location. Several commercially available cosmetic products are suitable for this.

The second major type of hemangioma is the *capillary angioma (strawberry mark).* This lesion is usually seen at birth, or shortly thereafter, may show considerable enlargement, and then undergoes spontaneous involution in a matter of months or years. The lesions are red to blue and consist of compressible vascular tumors. Over one-half are on the face. During the period of enlargement, the temptation to treat vigorously is strong, but it should be resisted in view of the excellent cosmetic appearance associated with spontaneous resolution. Rare exceptions are made in the case of a bleeding angioma, an extending ulcer, or interference with the function of an eye or body orifice, e.g., the urethra and anus. In such instances, one has a choice of treatments: local freezing, surgical excision, or electrocoagulation. The immature angioma is made up of vessels which may show sclerosing changes at any time. In two-thirds of the cases this occurs before the age of two years, but in some the involution is not complete until the child is older. The signs of disappearance are subtle at first, but later one sees white or gray islands appearing in the crimson lesions.

Mature angioma (cavernous hemangioma), the rarest form, shows no tendency to involution, nor is it radio-sensitive. The lesion is made up of adult-type arterial and venous channels, with numerous shunts. Much of the tumor is in the subcutaneous tissue, but parts may be raised in nodules or plaques. These lesions are distinguished from the immature type by the fact that they show no increase in size with age. The only definitive treatment is excision and grafting. Often such radical treatment is impractical and the lesion is best left alone.

PIGMENTED NEVI AND MELANOMAS

It is impossible to examine any single pigmented nevus (Fig. 400-1) and state positively that it will never undergo a malignant change. On the other hand, it is neither feasible nor justifiable to undertake wholesale excision of pigmented moles; some degree of clinical judgment must be exercised.

Pigmented nevi often are not manifest at birth but characteristically develop during infancy and childhood, and a few do not appear until adulthood. Nevi commonly appear first as macules. Histologic examination of these lesions shows clumps or aggregations of nevus cells at the epidermal-dermal junction. This type is known as a *junction nevus*. As the child becomes older, these macules may become thickened and slightly elevated, and the histologic picture changes, with cords or bands of nevus cells becoming aggregated in the dermis. This lesion is called a *compound nevus*. With the further passage of time, more elevation of the lesion occurs and the nevus cells aggregate entirely within the dermis. This is the *intradermal nevus,* a mature lesion which is almost always benign.

In children, a pigmented nevus may evolve rapidly, with cellular features of hyperplasia resembling a malignant melanoma of the adult. To this lesion the term *juvenile melanoma* has been applied. However, true malignant melanomas are rare in childhood.

The presence of pigment alone does not indicate that a papule or tumor of the skin is a melanocytic nevus. Certain entirely unrelated tumors, many of them benign, may show marked hyperpigmentation. The seborrheic keratosis, a very common lesion, is the best example of this. *Histiocytoma,* a common fibromatous lesion arising from the dermis (seen on the lower legs of women) may also be pigmented. Senile or actinic keratoses are sometimes dark, and pigmentation is frequent in basal cell epitheliomas.

Certain general considerations in the assessment of nevi apply to all morphologic types. A sudden change in the pigmentation, either to more marked pigmentation, to splotchy irregular character, or to fuzziness at the border of the lesion, must be regarded with suspicion, particularly in flat lesions.

The presence of fully developed, stiff hairs in the nevus is a reassuring sign. Although it is not an absolute dictum that hairy moles do not precede melanoma, it can be said that they almost never do. Such lesions often are traumatized by repeated pulling of the hair or during shaving.

A significant change in size of a pigmented nevus in adults must almost always be regarded as a basis for excision. The one exception to this is the common occurrence of acute or chronic follicular infection in hairy nevi, with tenderness and swelling. Such inflammatory changes are no cause for alarm, but if the mole becomes repeatedly infected, excision is advisable.

Ulceration and/or bleeding of previously quiescent moles are two signs of melanoma which are most commonly mentioned in cancer propaganda. These are late changes, however, and it is essential to recognize the more subtle prodromal changes in moles if melanoma is to be controlled.

PIGMENTED LESIONS OF THE MUCOUS MEMBRANES

Melanocytic nevi may involve the stratified epithelium of the mouth and mucocutaneous junction of the anus. Such lesions usually are flat and may be exceedingly difficult to interpret clinically. The decision is often crucial because melanoma arising in the mucous mem-

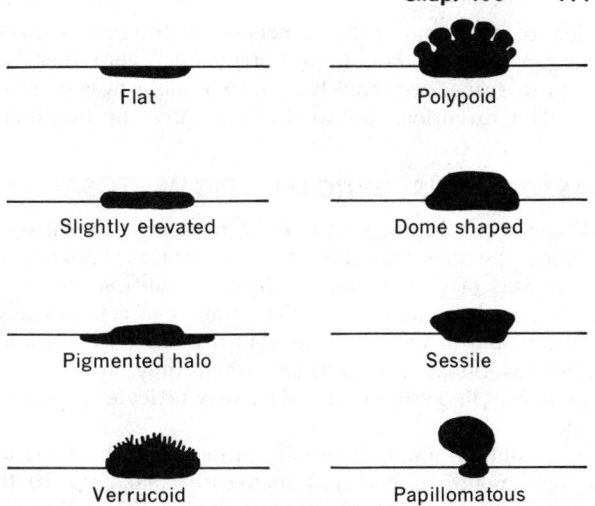

Fig. 400-1. Various morphologic patterns in pigmented nevi. The lesions in the left column are, in general, more likely to be junction nevi. (*After B. Shaffer, A.M.A. Arch. Dermatol., 72:120, 1955.*)

branes is rarely cured. Pigmentation of the mouth in Negroes is common and is ordinarily blotchy and fairly diffuse. Hyperpigmentation from chronic irritation, e.g., along the bite margin, is also common and need not be a cause for worry. In the Peutz-Jeghers syndrome, pigmented macules of the mouth, lips, and/or digits may be associated with intestinal polyposis. The most difficult lesions to interpret are freckles on the lips or dilated superficial blood vessels, usually veins (*venous lakes*), which are commonly blue-black and may become sclerosed. Although these latter lesions usually are recognizable, punch biopsy may occasionally be indicated.

CANCER OF THE SKIN

The majority of skin cancers arise in the epidermis and are known as *basal cell epitheliomas*. They are destructive tumors which present no immediate or direct threat to life, but if they are not removed completely they will progress relentlessly through the years, possibly killing by invasion into underlying structures. The typical basal cell epithelioma is recognizable as a discrete, pale, waxy nodule. However, the range of appearances is so great that histologic study of any suspicious growth or ulcer is essential. Crusted bleeding lesions, pearly borders, and telangiectasia, all suggest an epithelioma. The lesions may be of any size and may be multiple. Over 90 percent occur on the exposed areas, namely, the head and neck. Treatment may be surgical excision, curettage, electrocoagulation (the last two for small early lesions only), or x-ray. In every instance, however, tissue must be examined histologically.

Squamous cell carcinoma is the active, invasive metastasizing form of cancer of the epidermis. Such lesions commonly arise on the face and neck, one-third being located on the lower lip. These all are areas which are overexposed to sunlight or are sites of chronic irritation. Often the precancerous changes of leukoplakia and actinic keratoses are the warning signals. Complete eradication of all tumor cells is necessary. Surgery and/or roentgen therapy should be employed. Where there is reason to suspect regional lymph node metastasis or subcutaneous extension, radical dissection may be required.

MASTOCYTOSIS (URTICARIA PIGMENTOSA)

Overgrowth and aggregations of mast cells in the skin produce the condition known as urticaria pigmentosa. The lesions may be solitary nodules or multiple disseminated macules and papules. They are characteristically yellow to tan in color and develop urticarial wheals and sometimes bullae and purpura when they are rubbed vigorously. On occasion the lesions may urticate spontaneously.

The solitary tumor is usually observed at birth or in the first month of life, and such cases make up 10 to 15 percent of all cutaneous mastocytosis. The disseminated form of urticaria pigmentosa is also most common in infancy, 64 percent of all cases developing in the first 6 months of life.

Systemic involvement is found in 10 percent of cases. This form of the disease is eight times more common with adult onset of the disease as compared with children. In systemic disease the mast cell content is increased in any or all of the following organs: lymph nodes, bones, reticuloendothelial system, liver, and spleen. Such involvement usually is benign, but in one-third of cases it is malignant, resulting in leukemia and death. The prognosis for complete spontaneous recovery by puberty of solitary and of disseminated mastocytosis of childhood is good. Malignant systemic disease is rare in children, but it has been reported to occur.

SYSTEMIC MANIFESTATIONS OF CUTANEOUS DISEASES

In the vast majority of dermatologic diseases, even in extensive and severe ones, the skin is the only organ involved. However, no organ of the body is completely isolated in life. Both cutaneous manifestations of systemic diseases and systemic manifestations of predominantly skin diseases are recognized.

Psoriasis

Psoriasis is an inherited disease which is estimated to affect more than 4 million Americans. The prime manifestations of psoriasis are limited to the skin and nails, but about 10 percent of psoriatics develop arthritis. The classic skin lesion of psoriasis is a well-demarcated, red raised plaque topped by silvery scales. Tiny bleeding points appear on the surface when the silvery scale is scraped off. Coalescence of papules results in the large plaques and geographic outlines that are seen in adults.

The lesions of psoriasis are symmetrically distributed over the elbows, knees, and scalp. However, more widespread involvement of the extremities and trunk is common. *Guttate psoriasis* is characterized by the sudden onset of widespread symmetric teardrop-sized (guttate)

lesions. This type of psoriasis is frequently associated with overt or asymptomatic beta-hemolytic streptococcal infections of the throat in children. Appropriate antibiotic treatment of the infection usually results in improvement in the guttate psoriasis. The intertriginous areas, axillae, inguinal folds, perianal region, intergluteal cleft, and umbilicus are involved in the "inverse pattern" of psoriasis. Another common distribution is the "seborrheic pattern" with involvement of the eyebrows, central face, presternal area, and retroauricular folds. Sterile pustules may surmount psoriatic plaques on the palms and soles and may occur in a rare generalized pustular type of psoriasis. Any type of psoriasis may progress to an exfoliative dermatitis.

Subtle but highly specific changes occur in the fingernails and toenails. Multiple tiny "ice-pick" pits in the nail plates are almost diagnostic of psoriasis. Other nail changes, such as loosening and separation of the distal end of the nailplate, piling up of keratinous debris under the free edge of the nail, and opaque yellow areas in the nail, are suggestive of psoriasis in the absence of fungous infections of the nails.

Arthritis, the only recognized systemic disease associated with psoriasis, develops in approximately 10 percent of psoriatics. Cutaneous or nail lesions precede the arthritis in 64 percent of cases. Skin and joint manifestations begin simultaneously in 23 percent. There is a definite correlation between the severity of the skin, nail, and joint involvement. Exacerbations and remissions of the arthritis parallel those of the cutaneous lesions.

Many times the arthritis is indistinguishable from rheumatoid arthritis, but a distinctive type of *psoriatic arthritis* also occurs. The clinical features which characterize psoriatic arthritis are asymmetrical involvement of distal interphalangeal joints and severe destruction and mutilation of the affected joints. The disease destroys the distal interphalangeal joints, widens the joint spaces, and causes resorption or "whittling" of the tufts of the distal phalanges of the fingers and toes. Severe psoriatic arthritis may cause mushrooming of the small joints and arthritis mutilans. Sacroiliac involvement and bony ankylosis of the affected joints are common. The latex fixation test is negative in psoriatic arthritis. Elevation of serum uric acid secondary to widespread cutaneous disease is seen in 20 percent of patients with psoriasis and arthritis. Changes in serum proteins, mainly increases in the gamma-globulin fractions, occur in approximately 45 percent of cases of psoriatic arthritis.

The *management* of psoriatic arthritis is a special therapeutic problem. The antimalarial drugs are contraindicated, since they induce severe exacerbations of psoriasis which may proceed to generalized exfoliative erythroderma. Systemic corticosteroids have a beneficial effect on the skin and joint disease. However, when the corticosteroids are discontinued, a large proportion of patients exhibit a rebound phenomenon and develop more extensive and severe psoriasis than was present in the pretreatment state. Systemic corticosteroid therapy is justified in psoriasis only in disabling cases which cannot be controlled by any other means. Folic acid antagonists have a palliative effect on psoriasis and psoriatic arthritis. Because of systemic toxicity, their use is restricted to adults with severe resistant psoriasis. Because of the potential hazards of the treatment, the leukocyte count and renal and liver functions must be checked before instituting treatment and at regular intervals during treatment. Women of childbearing age should not receive folic acid antagonists.

Topical medications are the mainstay of the treatment of psoriasis. Only a few of the hundreds of therapeutic approaches to psoriasis which have been used through the years have withstood the test of time. None of these changes the individual's inherited tendency to develop psoriasis, but in most patients the disease can be completely controlled. Patients with psoriasis of moderate severity usually respond to simple methods of treatment, but more extensive disease requires a variety of treatments which are best managed by an experienced physician.

Tar and ultraviolet light, preferably in combination, still are the most beneficial, safest agents for the treatment for psoriasis. Patients with widespread involvement are treated in a hospital with an intensive daily regimen including repeated application of 1 to 5 percent crude coal tar ointment, and tar and oil baths before a single daily whole body exposure to increasing amounts of artificial ultraviolet light. Remissions of psoriasis usually persist for 5 to 18 months following 3 to 5 weeks of this intensive treatment. Modifications of this program using natural sunlight and more purified photosensitizing tar preparations (1 to 10 percent Wright's coal tar solution in a cream or lotion) are useful for ambulatory care. The small minority of psoriatics who are hypersensitive to ultraviolet light develop new lesions after light exposure and cannot be treated with this program.

Corticosteroid creams and lotions unquestionably are beneficial in psoriasis by virtue of their anti-inflammatory actions and their suppressive action on epidermal cell turnover rate, which is five to seven times faster than normal in psoriasis. The penetration and effectiveness of the corticosteroids is enhanced if they are applied under occlusive polyethylene dressings or injected directly into the lesions. Corticosteroids penetrate psoriatic lesions more readily than normal skin; therefore, the total amount applied to the skin each day must be controlled in order to prevent adrenal suppression. Scrubbing baths and vigorous tar shampoos help to remove scales and permit application of topical medications directly on the inflamed skin.

Pemphigus Vulgaris

Pemphigus vulgaris is an uncommon blistering disease involving epithelial surfaces of the skin, mouth, nose, pharynx, larynx, intestinal, and genitourinary tract. It is invariably fatal within months or years if adequate corticosteroid therapy is not instituted.

The eruption is characterized by the development of asymtomatic large flaccid bullae on apparently normal skin and mucous membranes. The initial lesions occur on surfaces which are subjected to constant friction and maceration, namely, the mouth, axillae, and inguinal regions. The fragile bullae rupture easily, especially on mucosal surfaces, forming painful raw denuded areas. The erosions enlarge peripherally and heal very slowly without any scarring except for postinflammatory hyperpigmentation.

Pemphigus attacks adults primarily, rarely adolescents, and never children. Since the initial lesions in many patients are confined to the mouth, pemphigus must be considered in the differential diagnosis of chronic oral erosions in all adults.

The natural course of pemphigus is one of gradual progression, occasional remissions, and inevitable recurrences. Hypoalbuminemia, electrolyte imbalance, anemia, and cachexia develop secondary to the loss of large amounts of protein, fluid, and blood from the denuded epithelial surfaces. Patients with oral involvement are unable to eat and maintain their nutrition. Serious toxicity, leukocytosis, and eosinophilia are present in severe cases. The erosions may be infected secondarily and this may be followed by septicemia.

The diagnosis of pemphigus is readily confirmed by skin biopsies and smears of the bullous lesions. *Acantholysis*, a characteristic change of the epidermal cells marked by disruption of intercellular connections, is the hallmark of pemphigus. Acantholytic cells are present in smears obtained from the bases of the bullae. The classification of the exact type of pemphigus depends on the level of the acantholytic process in the epidermis. The epidermal cells separate just above the basal cell layer in pemphigus vulgaris. The acantholytic clefts are present in the outer layers of the epidermis in the uncommon forms of pemphigus, namely pemphigus erythematosus, pemphigus foliaceus and Brazilian pemphigus. The serum of patients with pemphigus vulgaris contains an autoantibody which binds to the intercellular areas of human epidermis and of mouse esophageal epithelium.

The mortality rate of pemphigus vulgaris has been reduced from 100 percent to 50 percent with the advent of systemic corticosteroid therapy. This treatment is lifesaving if instituted early and in adequate doses. Expert medical management is necessary for preexisting conditions and for the inevitable side effects which are secondary to large doses of corticosteroids.

The initial dose of corticosteroids required to suppress pemphigus vulgaris is very large, usually in the range of 80 to 150 mg prednisone daily. Treatment should be commenced in a hospital under close supervision. The large initial dose must be continued for 6 to 8 weeks until no new lesions develop and all of the lesions are healed. The dose of corticosteroids may then be reduced, rapidly at first and then more slowly, to maintenance levels. A few patients have maintained remissions for several years. Most patients require small maintenance doses of corticosteroids indefinitely. Expert nursing care and a program similar to that used in extensive burns are necessary for the local treatment of the extensive areas of denuded skin until the disease is suppressed by the systemic therapy.

Mycosis Fungoides

Mycosis fungoides (ulcerative mushroomlike tumors) is a distinctive cutaneous lymphoma. The disease begins in the skin and remains confined to the skin for years. Its course is slowly progressive, marked by spontaneous remissions and relapses, and ends fatally. Before the advent of antibiotics, high energy electron beam therapy, potent topical corticosteroids, and topical and systemic chemotherapeutic agents, most patients with mycosis fungoides died of secondary sepsis. These newer palliative measures prolong the total duration of the disease, and 60 to 80 percent of patients with mycosis fungoides now living much longer than they once did, ultimately are found to have a systemic lymphoma, at least at autopsy. The associated systemic lymphomas which become manifest after years or decades of mycosis fungoides include lymphosarcoma, reticulum cell sarcoma, and Hodgkin's disease.

Mycosis fungoides evolves in three distinct phases any one of which may progress to exfoliative erythroderma.

Stage 1. Eczematous premycotic phase. The onset of the premycotic phase of mycosis fungoides is insidious and has a nonspecific histologic picture. The lesions are always pruritic, usually intensely so. Clinical suspicions of mycosis fungoides are aroused by the recurrent itchy, well-demarcated patches of chronic dermatitis.

Stage 2. Plaque stage. Well-demarcated, pruritic, raised, infiltrated plaques characterize the second stage. Eczematous patches and lymphadenopathy may be present. Skin biopsies of the infiltrated plaques reveal diagnostic changes of mycosis fungoides.

Stage 3. Tumor stage. The final stage of mycosis fungoides is characterized by multiple red-brown tumors which grow rapidly and usually ulcerate. Secondary bacterial infection and septicemia are common during the ulcerative episodes.

Treatment during any of the stages is palliative. Long-term remissions have been obtained with high-energy electron beam therapy.

CUTANEOUS MANIFESTATIONS OF SYSTEMIC DISEASE

The skin contains target organs for many hormones and an appreciable proportion of the vessels, connective tissue, and nerve fibers of the body. Genetic, metabolic, endocrine, vascular, neurologic, and allergic diseases often are accompanied by cutaneous changes. Many of these cutaneous changes are subtle; others are easily recognizable and diagnostic. Since many cutaneous signs and symptoms are reflections of the underlying systemic problems, adequate investigation and specific treatment must be directed towards the systemic lesion. Examples are the pathognomonic skin changes of pseudoxanthoma elasticum (Chap. 398), which precede the systemic lesions by many years.

ENDOCRINE AND METABOLIC DISEASES

The skin is influenced by many hormones. Darkening of the linea alba and nipples during pregnancy and the development of baldness in genetically predisposed men are striking physiologic end-organ responses to sex hormones. The early skin changes accompanying many endocrinopathies and metabolic diseases are subtle, but in some instances the histologic changes are diagnostic even in very early lesions.

NECROBIOSIS LIPOIDICA DIABETICORUM. A striking localized atrophy of the skin accompanied by lipid deposits occurs in diabetics. The diabetes may not be overt; a glucose tolerance test or cortisone GTT may be necessary to make this diagnosis. The lesions are asymptomatic and occur chiefly on the lower extremities. In 75 percent of patients the lesions are bilateral from the onset. The early lesions are flat red or yellow plaques which enlarge by peripheral extension to become large atrophic depressed areas with glazed-porcelain surfaces, yellow centers, and violet borders. Ulceration of the plaques, usually following minor trauma, occurs in one-third of the patients.

Skin biopsies of the lesions show a characteristic degeneration of collagen fibers, loss of elastic fibers, perivascular inflammation, and varying degrees of obliterative changes in small blood vessels. Extracellular deposits of lipids, chiefly cholesterol and phospholipids, are present in varying amounts in the center of the lesions.

Of patients with necrobiosis lipoidica diabeticorum 86 percent have diabetes mellitus when the cutaneous lesions appear or develop diabetes very shortly afterwards. One-half of the patients have other complications of diabetes such as retinopathy, nephropathy, or neuropathy. The cutaneous lesions may progress despite good therapeutic control of the diabetes. Corticosteroids, either injected intralesionally or applied topically and covered by polyethylene dressings, may halt the progression of individual lesions. In 17 percent of cases involution of the lesions occurs after many years of active progression of the disease.

PRETIBIAL MYXEDEMA. Circumscribed myxedema localized to the pretibial areas and feet is associated with or preceded by hyperthyroidism. Exophthalmus almost invariably accompanies pretibial myxedema. The cutaneous lesions appear within 3 years of thyroidectomy or therapy with thiouracil or radioactive iodine. Bilateral, edematous, nonpitting, red or tawny plaques and nodules with prominent hair follicles develop on the anterior aspects of the legs. The lesions are erythematous initially and become hard and waxy as they progress. Individual lesions may coalesce to create elephantiasis of the legs and feet. Skin biopsies of the involved areas reveal diagnostic dermal deposits of mucin containing large amounts of hyaluronic acid. Long-acting thyroid stimulator (LATS) (Chap. 89) is present in 90 to 100 percent of patients with pretibial myxedema, but its relationship to pretibial myxedema is not clear. The skin lesions respond to systemic, intralesionally injected and topically applied corticosteroids. Treatment with topical applications of highly concentrated 0.2 percent fluocinolone cream produces remission without undesirable systemic side effects.

GASTROINTESTINAL DISEASES

The skin and intestinal tract are involved simultaneously by similar pathologic processes affecting epithelial, mesodermal, and vascular tissues. Pemphigus, lichen planus, scleroderma, and anaphylactoid purpura are examples of diseases in which the oral and gastrointestinal changes may be the initial and most dramatic manifestations. The pathogenesis of other cutaneous diseases related to diseases of the intestinal tract, such as pyoderma gangrenosum with ulcerative colitis, is obscure.

Blue rubber-bleb nevus syndrome, hereditary hemorrhagic telangiectasia, pseudoxanthoma elasticum (Chap. 398), Peutz-Jeghers syndrome, and Gardner's syndrome are characterized by skin changes which are of diagnostic importance in obscure gastrointestinal bleeding. Soft, blue tumors of the skin of the trunk and arms are present at birth or appear in early life in the *blue rubber-bleb nevus syndrome*. Multiple cavernous hemangiomas on the mucosal surfaces are the source of the hemorrhages from the intestinal tract associated with the syndrome. Multiple localized dilatations of venules and capillaries of the nasal mucosa, tongue, palate, conjunctiva, larynx, lungs, and gastro-intestinal tract occur in *hereditary hemorrhagic telangiectasia* (Chap. 347). The development of the telangiectatic lesions in the skin often is delayed until later life in patients with this syndrome. Pigmented freckle-like macules of the skin around the mouth and on the tips of the fingers and toes appear in infancy in *Peutz-Jeghers syndrome* (Chap. 317) but fade or disappear at puberty. The pigmented macules on the lips, gums, palate and tongue persist throughout life. Recognition of the usual "freckles" of Peutz-Jeghers syndrome may clarify the diagnosis in patients with obscure intestonal bleeding or intussusception caused by hamartomatous polyps of the small intestine. Complete visualization of the colon and appropriate measures to prevent the development of malignant tumors in multiple polyposis are indicated in all patients with *Gardner's syndrome*. The multiple epidermal cysts, fibromas, lipomas, and osteomas of Gardner's syndrome appear in childhood, antedating the onset of gastrointestinal symptoms.

PYODERMA GANGRENOSUM.

Chronic, undermining, burrowing ulcers are a cutaneous manifestation of ulcerative colitis (Chap. 320). Although pyoderma gangrenosum is at times associated with other systemic diseases, such as arthritis and regional ileitis, the majority of large series report the association with ulcerative colitis in at least half the patients with pyoderma gangrenosum. Exacerbations and remissions of the cutaneous ulcers usually are synchronized with the activity of the underlying disease.

The early lesions are pustules, vesicles, boils, or inflammatory nodules. These lesions rapidly break down and produce creeping ulcers which spread peripherally. The advancing border is raised, purple-red, undermined, and surrounded by an erythematous halo. Segments of the border may advance at different rates forming irregular outlines, while the centers heal with characteristic flex-ible, thin, hairless scars. The ulcers may reach very large proportions covering almost the whole abdomen, trunk, or extremity.

The pathogenesis of the disease is obscure, but the original concept of symbiotic bacterial infection in the involved skin is no longer tenable. Some ulcers are sterile while others contain a variety of organisms. Pyoderma gangrenosum does not respond to cutaneous or systemic antibiotic therapy. Among the theories advanced to explain the condition are an autoimmune process, Schwartzman reaction, allergic reaction to gram-negative bacteria, or viral disease. Rejection of autografts, delayed hyperimmune response to autologous leukocytes, hypogammaglobulinemia, a tendency to basophilia in the cutaneous exudates in skin window studies, and paraproteinemia have been reported in patients with pyoderma gangrenosum. Injections of gamma-globulin, however, do not benefit the skin lesions. The only effective therapy for pyoderma gangrenosum is the adequate control of the ulcerative colitis, if that is present. Systemic corticosteroid therapy is uniformly beneficial in pyoderma gangrenosum.

MALIGNANT ATROPHIC PAPULOSIS.

This disease, affecting mainly young men, begins with a cutaneous phase and ends fatally with intestinal infarction, perforation, and peritonitis. The skin lesions are white infarcts with a highly characteristic appearance. Each lesion begins as a pale pink papule, develops a depressed crusted center, and heals in weeks or months, leaving porcelain-white atrophic scars. Active lesions resemble small doughnuts composed of raised pink rings around dead white centers. New lesions appear intermittently. From 3 weeks to 3 years following the onset of the cutaneous phase, other organs become involved. Multiple infarcts of the gastrointestinal tract are the most common systemic manifestations, but similar lesions may occur in the brain and heart. The pathologic process in the skin and other organs is a thrombosing fibrinoid end-angiitis affecting arterioles and veins.

SKIN MARKERS OF INTERNAL MALIGNANT NEOPLASMS

The cutaneous manifestations of malignant tumors, in addition to metastatic lesions, include changes ranging from nonspecific cachexia and pigmentation to diagnostic markers such as acanthosis nigricans. The skin changes may precede or coincide with the onset of symptoms of the internal malignancy. In most instances the pathophysiologic relationship between the dermatosis and the neoplasm is unknown. Several different mechanisms probably are involved, since the skin signs include epidermal, dermal, vascular, and neurologic changes (Table 400-1).

ACANTHOSIS NIGRICANS

Acanthosis nigricans *developing in adults* is the classic dermatosis associated with internal neoplasms. The eruption is a striking symmetrical hyperpigmented hyperkeratotic change in the epidermis of intertriginous areas. The axillae, anogenital region, umbilicus, breasts, and

Table 400-1. SKIN MARKERS OF INTERNAL NEOPLASMS

I. Epidermal manifestations
    A. Acanthosis nigricans
    B. Acquired ichthyosis
    C. Increased lanugo hair
    D. Exfoliative erythroderma
    E. Alopecia mucinosa
    F. Arsenical keratoses
    G. Bowen's disease
II. Dermal manifestations
    A. Dermatomyositis
    B. Amyloidosis
    C. Lichen myxedematosus
    D. Scleroderma (rarely)
III. Vascular manifestations
    A. Carcinoid syndrome
    B. Figurate erythema group reactions
    C. Chronic urticaria
IV. Neurologic manifestation
    A. Generalized pruritus
V. Blisters and vesicular eruptions
    A. Herpes zoster
    B. Pemphigoid
    C. Dermatitis herpetiformis

neck develop black or dark brown velvety or warty surfaces. The changes may involve more extensive areas of the skin and mucosal surfaces resulting in velvety thickening of the palms and soles and a warty overgrowth of the oral and anal mucosae.

Four types of acanthosis nigricans are recognized:

1. CONGENITAL. The skin changes appear in early infancy and have no systemic importance. Congenital acanthosis nigricans is not related to internal carcinomas.

2. JUVENILE. The onset of acanthosis nigricans at puberty is associated with significant endocrinologic diseases in more than one-third of cases. The endocrine disorders which are associated with this skin lesion include diabetes mellitus, lipoatrophic diabetes, gigantism, acromegaly, Stein-Leventhal syndrome, and Addison's disease.

3. PSEUDOACANTHOSIS NIGRICANS. Dark warty thickening of the skin folds may appear at any age in obese brunettes. The eruption is usually less extensive than the malignant type and never involves mucosal surfaces. Mild degrees of pseudoacanthosis nigricans disappear with weight reduction.

4. MALIGNANT ADULT ACANTHOSIS NIGRICANS. The onset of acanthosis nigricans in adults is highly significant in terms of associated malignancies. The eruption, which may precede the symptoms of the internal malignant neoplasm by several years, may reach extensive proportions, including involvement of the mouth. Various studies have shown that malignant acanthosis nigricans is associated with internal neoplasms in 100 percent of cases. The neoplasms invariably are adenocarcinomas, of which 90 percent are intraabdominal and 61 percent are gastric. The eruption improves and clears when the tumor is eradicated. Recurrences of the skin lesions accompany recurrent and metastatic adenocarcinoma.

DERMATOMYOSITIS

The onset of dermatomyositis (Chap. 375) in adults past the age of forty years is associated with internal neoplasms in 15 to 50 percent of cases. Childhood dermatomyositis is not associated with cancer. The classic features of dermatomyositis, namely heliotrope eyelids, facial edema, and erythema, atrophy, and edema of the skin over the extensor surfaces of the small joints of the hands and proximal muscle weakness, are the same whether or not a malignant neoplasm is present. A variety of neoplasms have been reported in association with dermatomyositis in adults, including carcinomas of the breast, prostate, intestinal tract, lung and bronchi, as well as lymphomas and melanomas. Adequate treatment of the neoplasm usually results in improvement of the associated dermatomyositis.

ERYTHEMA GROUP REACTIONS

Reactions of the cutaneous vasculature to a variety of stresses cover a spectrum ranging from simple erythema to urticarial lesions (erythema and edema), bullae, purpura, and hemorrhages. The erythema group of reactions are cutaneous symptom complexes that have been classified according to their morphology. It is of the utmost importance to recognize that these reactions are purely symptom complexes which always demand delineation of the underlying causes.

ERYTHEMA MULTIFORME

All of the changes mentioned above may be present simultaneously in erythema multiforme. The eruption is characterized by sudden onset, symmetrical distribution, and frequent, though not invariable, involvement of the mucous membranes, palms, and soles. Conjunctival involvement may lead to blindness. The lesions persist for days or weeks. Wheals, annular urticarial lesions and bullae and erosions occur in severe cases. Bullae may be absent, but multiringed "target" lesions, with or without central bullae, are diagnostic. Constitutional symptoms are absent or mild in most cases but *erythema multiforme exudativum,* a serious, potentially fatal variety, is accompanied by high fever, headache, prostration, and erosions of the mouth, nose, urethra, and vagina.

Erythema multiforme may be associated with or caused by any of the following:

1. Drug reactions: butazolidin, phenobarbital, sulfonamides, penicillin, antipyrine, quinine, antihistamines, arsenic, mercury
2. Viral infections
3. Bacterial infections
4. Mycoplasma infections
5. Deep mycoses
6. Malignant neoplasms

Elimination of the causative factor, oral antihistamines, and symptomatic treatment of the cutaneous and mucosal lesions often suffice for the milder types of erythema multiforme. The eruption tends to resolve spontaneously, but recurrences are not unusual. Severe erythema multiforme with constitutional symptoms and marked involvement of the mucosal surfaces of the mouth, eyes, and genitalia (Stevens-Johnson syndrome) demands prompt and intensive systemic corticosteroid therapy. The initial daily dose required by adults with severe erythema multiforme is 60 mg prednisone. Ophthalmologic consultation is mandatory for involvement of the eyes in order to prevent secondary bacterial infections, keratitis, iritis, uveitis, and blindness. Parenteral alimentation is necessary in patients with severe oral involvement.

ERYTHEMA NODOSUM

Erythema nodosum is another reaction pattern of the skin and subcutaneous tissues of diverse causation. The eruption is characterized by extremely tender, bright red nodules on the anterior surfaces of the lower legs. The nodules usually are bilateral and may involve the arms and trunk as well as the pretibial regions. Crops of nodules begin abruptly, resolve slowly by undergoing ecchymotic color changes, and heal spontaneously without ulceration, suppuration, or scarring. Mild constitutional symptoms consisting of fever, malaise, and arthralgia may occur. Biopsies of the lesions show characteristic panniculitis and perivascular inflammation.

Erythema nodosum is a symptom of an underlying infection, systemic illness, or drug reaction. It is seen in association with the following:

1. Drug reactions: sulfonamides, iodides, bromides, tetracyclines, oral contraceptives
2. Bacterial infections: streptococcal infections, scarlet fever, pharyngitis, tonsillitis, diphtheria, tuberculosis, leprosy, chancroid, meningococcemia
3. Mycotic infections: coccidioidomycosis, histoplasmosis, blastomycosis, trichophyton infections
4. Viral infections: lymphogranuloma venereum, cat-scratch fever
5. Systemic diseases: rheumatic fever, sarcoid, systemic lupus erythematosus, chronic ulcerative colitis, regional ileitis

The management of erythema nodosum centers on the detection and elimination or treatment of the underlying disease. Bed rest, analgesics, salicylates, and elastic support of the involved extremities are helpful symptomatic treatments. Since erythema nodosum is usually self-limited and resolves rapidly with treatment of the underlying disease, systemic corticosteroid therapy is rarely indicated. Corticosteroid therapy is contraindicated until the possibility of systemic infection is ruled out.

ERYTHEMA INDURATUM

This is another nodular eruption of the legs and is classified as a type of tuberculid. It is differentiated from erythema nodosum by virtue of a chronic indolent course, ulceration and scarring, localization to the calves of young women, and histologically, a tuberculoid granulomatous involvement of the subcutaneous fat. The tuberculin skin test usually is strongly positive in patients with erythema induratum, but no organisms are present in the skin lesions. The lesions promptly respond to systemic treatment with antituberculous drugs. (See Chap. 174)

GENERALIZED EXFOLIATIVE ERYTHRODERMA

This important reaction pattern of the skin is characterized by a universal erythema and generalized shedding (exfoliation). The whole cutaneous surface is red, thickened, and scaling. Severe pruritus and moderate to severe constitutional symptoms usually accompany the reaction. The universal vasodilatation of cutaneous vessels results in marked heat radiation from the skin. Because of the difficulty in maintaining the body core temperature, the patients shiver and chill in moderately cool environments. Moderate to complete anhidrosis, secondary to the cutaneous reaction, may cause febrile episodes induced by warm environmental temperatures. Marked dependent edema occurs secondary to the skin involvement. Hypoalbuminemia, as the result of the large amounts of protein shed in the exfoliative process, and high output cardiac failure, secondary to massive vasodilatation, contribute to the edema in some patients. Patients with exfoliative dermatitis are highly susceptible to furuncles, cellulitis, deep abscesses, and thrombophlebitis. Lymphadenopathy is present in all of the patients; hepatomegaly occurs in approximately 20 percent of them, but splenomegaly is present only in those patients in whom the cutaneous reaction is a manifestation of lymphomatous disease.

Although exfoliative erythroderma is most common in patients over forty years of age, it occurs in all age groups from infancy to old age. It is twice as common in men as in women. In the majority of patients the cutaneous reaction persists for 1 year or less, but in some cases the reaction persists or recurs for years or decades.

Exfoliative erythroderma is merely a symptom, not a disease entity. The underlying cause may be primary in the skin, a drug reaction, or a lymphoma of a cutaneous or systemic type. Approximately 10 percent of patients with exfoliative erythroderma have an associated lymphoma or leukemia. In another 10 percent, the erythroderma represents an adverse response to a drug. Hence, in all patients with exfoliative erythroderma the following conditions must be ruled out:

1. Lymphoma, leukemia, mycosis fungoides
2. Drug reactions
3. Primary skin diseases: psoriasis; eczematous dermatitis: atopic, stasis, contact, and seborrheic; rare dermatoses: pemphigus foliaceous, pityriasis rubra pilaris, congenital ichthyosiform erythroderma

Every patient with exfoliative dermatitis demands careful study. Biopsy of the skin, often with repetition at regular intervals if the diagnosis remains obscure, is mandatory. Studies of the bone marrow, biopsy of lymph nodes, and lymphangiograms are indicated when changes in the peripheral blood, splenomegaly, or unusual lymphadenopathy are present.

Symptomatic treatment, prompt recognition and treatment of systemic complications, and skilled nursing care are essential components of the management of exfoliative erythroderma. Covering the whole skin surface with inexpensive, nontoxic, bland, partially occlusive ointments reduces the heat loss from the skin. Petrolatum, vegetable oils, and a mixture of equal parts of water and Aquaphor usually are well tolerated and contribute significantly to the patient's comfort. The fact that these preparations are inexpensive is important, since a pound of ointment may suffice for only 1 to 2 days' treatment. The extensive application of materials containing phenol, tars, mercury, or salicylic acid that are absorbed through inflamed skin in potentially toxic amounts must be avoided. Topical corticosteroid preparations under occlusive dressings are not recommended because quantities sufficient to cause adrenal suppression are readily absorbed. The environmental temperature should be controlled to prevent chills and fevers. A high caloric, high protein diet with frequent feeding is essential. Oral antihistamines and sedatives usually are required to relieve the associated pruritus. Systemic corticosteroid therapy should be used only when all other methods fail to control the cutaneous reaction. Early recognition and prompt treatment of secondary infections, cardiac failure, electrolyte imbalance, and hypoproteinemia are essential.

REFERENCES

Abrahams, I., J. T. McCarthy, and S. L. Sanders: 101 Cases of Exfoliative Dermatitis, Arch. Dermatol., 87:96, 1963.

Arundell, F. D., R. D. Wilkinson, and J. R. Haserick: Dermatomyositis and Malignant Neoplasms in Adults: A Survey of 20 Years' Experience, Arch. Dermatol., 88:772, 1960.

Baer, R. L., and V. H. Witten: Selected Benign Pigmented Cutaneous Lesions, in "Year Book of Dermatology," Chicago, The Year Book Medical Publishers, Inc., 1958–1959.

Baker, H. M. B., D. N. Golding, and M. Thompson: Psoriasis and Arthritis, Ann. Intern. Med., 58:909, 1963.

Bluefarb, S. M.: "Cutaneous Manifestations of the Malignant Lymphomas," Springfield, Ill., Charles C Thomas, Publisher, 1960.

Burns, J. J.: Implications of Enzyme Induction for Drug Therapy, Am. J. Med., 37:327, 1964.

Butterworth, T., and L. P. Strean: "Clinical Genodermatology," Baltimore, The Williams & Wilkins Company, 1962.

Cullen, S. I., and P. M. Catalano: Griseofulvin-Warfarin Antagonism, J.A.M.A., 199:150, 1967.

Curth, H. O., and B. M. Aschner: Genetic Studies on Acanthosis Nigricans, Arch. Dermatol., 79:55, 1959.

Cyr, D. P., M. C. Geokas, and G. H. Worsley: Mycosis Fungoides: Hematologic Findings and Terminal Course, Arch. Dermatol., 94:558, 1966.

Degos, R.: Malignant Atrophic Papulosis: A Fatal Cutaneointestinal Syndrome, Brit. J. Dermatol., 66:304, 1954.

Eddy, D. D., and E. M. Farber: Pseudoxanthoma elasticum, Arch. Dermatol., 86:729, 1962.

Hildick-Smith, G., H. Blank, and I. Sarkany: "Fungus Diseases and Their Treatment," Boston, Little, Brown and Company, 1964.

Komisaruk, E.: Glucose Tolerance Test in Necrobiosis Lipoidica Diabeticorum, Arch. Dermatol., 90:208, 1964.

Kriss, J. P., V. Pleshakov, A. Rosenblum, and G. Sharp: Therapy with Occlusive Dressings of Pretibial Myxedema with Fluocinolone Acetonide, J. Clin. Endocrinol. Metab., 27:595, 1967.

Lever, W. F.: "Pemphigus and Pemphigoid," Springfield, Ill., Charles C Thomas, Publisher, 1965.

Muller, S. A., and R. K. Winkelman: Necrobiosis Lipoidica Diabeticorum. A Clinical and Pathological Investigation of 171 Cases, Arch. Dermatol., 93:272, 1966.

Perry, H. O., and L. A. Brunsting: Pyoderma Gangrenosum, Arch. Dermatol., 75:380, 1957.

Rook, A., D. S. Wilkinson, and F. J. Ebling: "Textbook of Dermatology," Philadelphia, F. A. Davis Company, 1968.

Spring, M.: Symposium: Cutaneous Manifestations of Systemic Disease, N.Y. State J. Med., 63: No. 21 and 22, 1963.

Vesey, C. M. R., and D. S. Wilkinson: Erythema Nodosum; a Study of Seventy Cases, Brit. J. Dermatol., 71:139, 1959.

Section 16
Disorders of the Eye

401 OCULAR MANIFESTATIONS OF SYSTEMIC DISEASE

Carl Kupfer

Because the tissues of the eye are, for the most part, transparent, the effects of systemic disease on ocular tissue can be observed directly, and in many instances their manifestations can be assessed when they cannot be readily viewed elsewhere. In a relatively small period of time during the physical examination, the entire sensorimotor system involved in visual perception can be studied (visual acuity) and the ocular structure, including optic nerve, retina, choroid, and their blood vessels, can be directly visualized (ophthalmoscopy).

In this chapter, the examination of the eye will be discussed from the standpoint of its usefulness as a part of the complete examination of the patient, and its bearing in relation to various systemic diseases will be considered.

MEASUREMENT OF VISUAL ACUITY

The determination of visual acuity is perhaps the single most important portion of the examination of the visual system. If visual acuity cannot be improved by refraction to 20/20, there is some defect in the sensory side of the visual system which must be defined and its etiology determined. The measurement of visual acuity utilizes the Snellen chart, which is based on letters subtending 5 min of arc at various distances from the eye. The letters at the top of the chart subtend 5 min of arc at a distance of 200 ft, while those near the bottom of the chart subtend 5 min of arc at 20 ft. Thus, if a patient can see only the letters at the top of the acuity chart, and the patient is 20 ft away from the chart, his vision is 20/200. If, on the other hand, he sees the letters at the bottom, his vision is 20/20. The measurement of visual acuity can be modified for small examining rooms by using acuity charts suitable for the shorter working distance.

In all cases, visual acuity should be measured with the patient wearing his eyeglasses, if he uses such glasses for driving or watching television. If the visual acuity is less than 20/20 with his glasses, there may be an additional refractive error; this possibility can be ruled out quite easily by having the patient look through a pinhole, with his glasses still on. A pinhole permits a small pencil of light to fall on the fovea without being refracted. The pinhole should provide an opening of about 2 mm in diameter. If the visual acuity is not improved to 20/20 with the pinhole, then there is some organic defect in the visual system which must be investigated further.

CLARITY OF THE MEDIA

Light entering the eye is focused on the outer layer of the retina, the rods, and cones. Consequently, the media (tissues and fluids) through which the light passes to reach the retina must be transparent. These media are the cornea, the aqueous humor of the anterior chamber, the lens, the vitreous humor within the vitreous cavity, and the retina itself. An opacity of these media in the visual axis will interfere with the focus of light on the rods and cones and decrease the visual acuity. The physician can make an objective determination of the clarity of the media in two ways; each depends upon the pupil being dilated to at least 6 mm in diameter.

Pupillary dilatation is accomplished by instilling one drop of 10 percent phenylephrine (Neo-Synephrine) in each eye after visual acuity, the pupillary response to light, and the intraocular pressure have been recorded. This is done preferably at the beginning of the physical examination, because the action of phenylephrine is not evident until about 20 min following instillation. If dilatation is not satisfactory, a second drop may be administered. An attack of angle-closure glaucoma may be precipitated by pupillary dilatation, but this occurs extremely infrequently when phenylephrine is used and can be relieved promptly by intensive instillation of 4 percent pilocarpine drops. A patient with a known history of glaucoma should have his pupils dilated only with the consent of his ophthalmologist. For all practical purposes, the benefits of routine dilatation of the pupils for adequate ophthalmoscopic examination far outweigh the risks. In addition, because phenylephrine is a short-acting mydriatic, not a cycloplegic, it will not interfere with reading or driving, and the pupil returns to normal size within 2 to 3 hr.

Following pupillary dilatation, the examiner first uses a +6 lens in the sighting aperture of the ophthalmoscope and illuminates the pupillary space from a distance of about 6 to 8 in. Normally, the entire pupillary area will have a uniform bright red reflex as the diffuse light is reflected back from the blood vessel–rich choroid beneath the retina. Any opacities in the media (vitreous, lens, anterior chamber, cornea) will be silhouetted against the red reflex and will appear dark gray or black. After this, by adjusting the lens of the ophthalmoscope, the examiner focuses on the optic nervehead as clearly as possible. If, through the 6-mm pupil, the optic nerve and retinal blood vessels are seen clearly, it may be assumed that there are no opacities in the media and strongly suggests that the visual acuity should be 20/20. When the nerve and vessels are just barely visible because of hazy media, a visual acuity of about 20/200 would be expected. If the media are crystal clear and the visual acuity has been recorded as less than 20/20, the cause of the decreased visual acuity must be located in the macular portion of the retina, the optic nerve, or farther back in the visual system.

THE ORBIT

Because the walls of the orbit are rigid, a volumetric increase in the contents of the orbit results in the eye being pushed forward. Exophthalmos per se does not usually cause limitation of extraocular movements unless the cranial nerves innervating the extraocular muscles are interrupted. In close approximation to the orbit is the frontal sinus above, sphenoidal sinus posteriorly, maxillary sinus below, and ethmoidal sinuses medially. For the most part, the orbit contains fat which, being compressible, permits the eye to be pushed back gently into the orbit for 5 mm or so. The extraocular muscles (except for the inferior oblique) have their origin at the apex of the orbit and form a small muscle cone as they insert onto the eye. Within this muscle cone runs the orbital portion of the optic nerve from the apex of the orbit to the eye. The optic nerve is somewhat longer than this distance and measures about 25 to 35 mm in length. This not only permits ample movement of the eyeball in all directions, but allows for exophthalmos of at least 10 mm or so without any stretch being exerted on the optic nerve.

In the presence of **exophthalmos** it is necessary to determine (1) the amount and direction of the exophthalmos, (2) the ease with which the eye can be reposited into the orbit, (3) whether a palpable mass is present in the orbit, and (4) the involvement of cranial nerves II to VI. (5) Certain additional diagnostic tests should be carried out, including x-ray examination of the bones of the orbit and adjacent sinuses, and studies of thyroid function (Chap. 89).

1. *Amount and direction of the exophthalmos.* The amount of exophthalmos is determined by means of a Hertel exophthalmometer which measures the distance from the lateral orbital rim to the apex of the cornea. Absolute values vary with the subject, but in the case of unilateral exophthalmos a difference of more than 2 mm between the two eyes is significant. The direction of exophthalmos is of some diagnostic importance. The most common cause of exophthalmos is an abnormality in anterior pituitary or hypothalamic function (Chap. 89). In this type of exophthalmos the eye is pushed straight forward. Dermoids or tumors of the lacrimal gland, arising in the upper outer quadrant of the orbit, tend to push the eye down and in, while a mucocele of the frontal sinus depresses the eye, and an osteoma or fibroma, arising usually in the upper inner quadrant, pushes the eye down and out.

2. *The presence of a palpable mass.* In general, if a mass is present within the orbit and is of sufficient size to produce a significant amount of exophthalmos, it usually can be palpated by sliding the little finger in the space between the eye and the orbital wall while the patient looks in the appropriate direction. In the absence of a palpable mass, surgical exploration usually is contraindicated unless there is other evidence of a tumor (i.e., roentgenographic changes).

3. *The ease with which the eyeball is reposited into the orbit.* Standing behind the patient, the physician presses the eyeball through the patient's closed lids and estimates the ease with which the eyeball can be reposited. Normally, this can be done rather easily. Increased resistance is characteristic of endocrine exophthalmos or of a mass in the orbit.

4. *Cranial nerve involvement.* The visual acuity of the eye should be tested as well as the extraocular movements and the corneal sensitivity. Because the cranial nerves subserving these functions pass through the muscle cone, a space-occupying mass at the apex of the orbit can interrupt all the cranial nerves directly, thereby producing a complete external ophthalmoplegia and loss of vision (**syndrome of the apex of the orbit**) (see Chaps. 24 and 355).

5. *Other diagnostic tests.* In all cases of exophthalmos, roentgenograms of the orbit with views of the superior orbital and optic foramens and sinuses should be made, to rule out optic nerve gliomas, meningiomas, lacrimal gland tumors that invade bone, and disease of the paranasal sinuses.

Since the most common cause of unilateral or bilateral exophthalmos is endocrine, appropriate tests of thyroid function (Chap. 89) are necessary in the presence of exophthalmos of unknown etiology. In patients whose symptoms may be limited to vague ocular discomfort and whose signs may be only slight lid retraction and minimal exophthalmos, it is not unusual for the protein-bound iodine test to be normal while the thyroid suppression test (Chap. 89) is abnormal. In addition, there often is increased resistance to repositing the eyeball into the orbit, suggesting decreased orbital resiliency. Other causes of exophthalmos related to systemic diseases are optic glioma in association with neurofibromatosis (von Recklinghausen's disease, Chap. 365), metastatic tumor (most common in carcinoma of the breast), lymphoma (Chap. 351), and Wegener's granulomatosis (Chap. 394).

THE CONJUNCTIVA AND SCLERA

The conjunctiva is the mucous membrane covering the inner surface of the lids (palpebral conjunctiva) and the outer surface of the sclera (bulbar conjunctiva). The sclera is a dense collagenous envelope of the eye itself which is continuous anteriorly with the cornea at the limbus, and is perforated posteriorly by the exit of the optic nerve from the eye. The conjunctiva and sclera can be examined simply with a hand light by lifting the upper and lower lids from the eye. In jaundice, these tissues are stained with the circulating bilirubin and appear yellow (Chap. 45). Markedly dilated bulbar conjunctival blood vessels in a patient who is ataxic should suggest ataxia-telangiectasia (Chap. 365). General diseases of mucous membranes, such as benign mucous membrane pemphigoid and erythema multiforme (Chap. 400), often involve the palpebral and bulbar conjunctiva, resulting in adhesions between these two structures. In osteogenesis imperfecta (Chap. 397), the sclera is particularly thin and allows the pigmented choroid beneath to be visualized more easily; this gives the appearance of blue sclera. In collagen vascular disease, particularly rheumatoid arthritis, there may be recurrent focal necrosis of the collagen of the sclera, which gradually causes thinning and occasionally perforation of the sclera (scleromalacia perforans, Chap. 386). Finally, often of concern to the patient but not of clinical significance, there is the frequent subconjunctival hemorrhage, discovered usually upon awakening in the morning. The hemorrhage slowly clears in 2 to 3 weeks without sequelae.

THE CORNEA

The cornea may be regarded as a collagen matrix containing mucopolysaccharides bounded by an epithelium on the anterior surface and by mesothelium on the posterior surface. The cornea is avascular and derives its nutrition by diffusion of metabolic substrates from blood vessels in the adjacent conjunctiva, from the tears anteriorly, and from the aqueous humor posteriorly. Consequently, the cornea may be regarded as an agar-diffusion plate into which certain constituents of the blood diffuse and can precipitate out of solution if the proper conditions exist. In hypercalcemia secondary to sarcoid (Chap. 254), hyperparathyroidism (Chap. 90), and vitamin D intoxication (Chap. 83), calcium phosphates and carbonates precipitate within the cornea, primarily beneath the epithelium, producing the **band keratopathy** seen in these conditions (Plate 6). If the calcium deposition interferes with vision, it can be removed by the topical application of ethylenediaminetetraacetic acid (EDTA). In a similar manner, cystine crystals are deposited within the cornea in cystinosis (Chap. 102), cholesterol esters in hypercholesterolemia (Chap. 113), chloroquine crystals in those patients receiving this drug for chronic discoid lupus or other reasons, and copper in hepatolenticular degeneration (Kayser-Fleischer ring, Chap. 110).

The cornea, being derived from surface ectoderm, may show lesions in association with dermatologic diseases. In acne rosacea, corneal ulceration with inflammatory cell infiltration and vascularization is not too uncommon. Herpes simplex infection of the skin or mucous membrane may be followed by corneal involvement (see below). Herpes zoster involving the ophthalmic division of the trigeminal nerve may be accompanied by inflammation with round opacities in the cornea and a secondary iridocyclitis requiring intensive ophthalmic treatment with topical atropine and corticosteroid drops. Finally, there is the group of mucocutaneous-ocular syndromes) Behçet's, p. 2005; Reiter's, Chap. 390; and Stevens-Johnson, Chap. 400) which often are accompanied by a keratitis. In addition, the cornea is exposed to external agents and often is traumatized and then secondarily infected. This often occurs in obtunded patients whose eyelids may remain partially open. The cornea can be protected by gently taping the eyelids so that they will be kept closed.

The most common cause of corneal infection leading to an opacity and decreased visual acuity is the herpes simplex virus (see Chap. 228). Involvement of the corneal epithelium is manifested as a characteristic dendritic ulcer, a linear opacity with short radiating lines. Secondary involvement of the corneal collagen appears as a round, grayish-white infiltrate, the so-called disciform keratitis. It is very important that the dendritic ulcer of the cornea *not* be treated with corticosteroids. Although this treatment initially will provide symptomatic relief, it may lead to corneal perforation. Similarly, bacterial or fungal ulcers of the cornea may lead to perforation and loss of the eye in the absence of appropriate antibiotics or antifungal therapy. Infections of the cornea always are a serious threat to vision and require immediate and specific treatment by an ophthalmologist.

AQUEOUS HUMOR

The aqueous humor is a relatively protein-free ultrafiltrate of the blood (similar to cerebrospinal fluid) which is produced continuously by the ciliary processes (similar to the choroid plexus) located behind the lens. The aqueous humor then passes anterior to the lens through the pupillary space, into the anterior chamber from which it leaves the eye by way of Schlemm's canal, a circumferential channel in the angle of the anterior chamber between the iris and the cornea. Schlemm's canal conveys the aqueous fluid into venous channels which drain into the cavernous sinus by way of the orbital veins.

If the resistance to the passage of aqueous humor out of the eye by way of Schlemm's canal becomes increased, then the intraocular pressure, which normally is about 15 mm Hg, becomes elevated; this elevation in intraocular pressure is referred to as **glaucoma**. About 90 percent of cases of glaucoma are the *wide-angle* type, in which the cause of increased resistance to outflow of aqueous fluid is unknown. An additional 5 percent are the *narrow-angle* type, in which the outflow is blocked by the iris when the pupil is dilated; e.g., with cycloplegic drugs such as atropine or homatropine. Mydriatics alone, such as 10 percent phenylephrine, usually do not elevate the intraocular pressure. The remaining 5 percent of cases of glaucoma are secondary to some disease process that blocks the outflow channels, such as inflammatory debris in uveitis or red blood cells following hemorrhage in the anterior chamber (*hyphema*) secondary to trauma. Glaucoma occurs in about 2 percent of persons over the age of forty and is asymptomatic for many years. It is characterized by loss of vision in the peripheral part of the field rather than in the central part. Therefore, decreased visual acuity is recognized late in its course. For these reasons, routine measurement of intraocular pressure in patients over the age of forty, using a Shiötz tonometer, should be included in every general medical examination before the pupil is dilated; this test can be performed by any physician. With the patient in the recumbent position on the examining table, a drop of local anesthetic is placed in each eye after the patient has been requested to look at a mark on the ceiling directly above him. The upper and lower lids are gently held away from the eye, and the tonometer is placed on the cornea so that the instrument is perfectly vertical. The scale reading is recorded, and the pressure in millimeters of mercury is obtained from the conversion chart supplied with the tonometer case.

Increased intraocular pressure may develop within 1 to 4 weeks following the use of topical preparations containing corticosteroids. If treatment with steroids is continued, the elevated pressure may eventually damage the optic nerve and lead to irreversible loss of visual field.

THE LENS

The lens is derived from surface ectoderm and, like the skin, grows continually throughout life. As new lens fibers are laid down on the surface of the lens, the underlying fibers are compressed and gradually form the nucleus. The lens is avascular and is bathed by the aqueous humor, depending completely on this substance for the delivery of necessary substrates and the removal of harmful metabolites. In this "organ culture" situation, the lens is quite responsive to changes in systemic metabolism. Because lens fibers are laid down continuously, systemic disease which affects the composition of the blood and, hence, the aqueous humor can affect the transparency of newly formed lens fibers, causing visible opacities (**cataract**). Thus, in hypoparathyroidism (Chap. 90), the low blood calcium level results in a low concentration of aqueous humor calcium. This affects adversely the permeability properties of the lens fiber membrane. The lens fibers being formed at such a time are opaque, and during each episode of hypocalcemia a band of opacification forms in the lens.

One of the major advances in the understanding of the metabolism of the lens has been the clarification of the etiology of cataracts in diabetes (Chap. 94) and galactosemia (Chap. 112). These so-called "sugar cataracts" occur with high sustained blood levels of either glucose or galactose (Chap. 112) in the respective cases. In diabetes, with increasing blood glucose, the aqueous humor glucose level increases and large amounts of glucose diffuse into the lens. Within the lens, an aldose reductase reduces the glucose to its sugar alcohol, sorbitol, which not only is metabolized very slowly, but diffuses out of the lens with great difficulty. Hence, a large amount of sorbitol can accumulate in the diabetic lens, bringing about an osmotic gradient with movement of water from aqueous humor into the lens fibers. This results in swelling of lens fibers and a change in the refractive properties of the lens. These diabetics develop blurred vision because of an induced myopia. Reduction in the blood glucose will reverse these changes. However, if the accumulation of sorbitol persists, irreversible cataractous changes secondary to liquefaction of lens fibers occur, and decreased visual acuity results. The pathogenesis of galactose cataracts is similar except that the accumulated sugar alcohol is dulcitol. Because of its embryologic derivation from surface ectoderm, the lens may become cataractous in diseases involving the skin, such as sclerodema and atopic dermatitis.

A large number of drugs can produce cataracts, mostly by unknown mechanisms. Historically one of the most notorious of these drugs was dinitrophenol, used for weight reduction during the 1930s. More recently, triparenol (Mer 29), chlorpromazine in high doses, and corticosteroids have been implicated, the last being particularly dangerous when applied topically, although cataracts also occur with appreciable frequency in patients receiving long-term oral corticosteroid therapy. When such medications are used, the status of the lens should be followed by repeated ophthalmic examinations.

Although the lens itself is derived from surface ectoderm, it is suspended by zonular fibers that are derived from mesoderm. Therefore, in mesodermal abnormalities such as Marfan's syndrome (Chap. 395) or homocystinuria (Chap. 102), the zonular fibers are weakened and finally rupture, allowing the lens to be dislocated (Plate 6). The iris is no longer supported by the anterior surface of the lens and appears tremulous on small eye movements (*iridodonesis*). Iridodonesis is pathognomonic of dislocation of the lens.

THE VITREOUS HUMOR

The vitreous humor fills the vitreous cavity, which is bounded by the lens anteriorly and the retina posteriorly. It consists almost entirely of water contained in a fragile network of collagen fibrils in which molecules of hy-

aluronic acid are trapped. Vitreous hemorrhage arises from rupture of a retinal blood vessel and appears to the patient as a shower of black or red dots. Depending on the extent of the hemorrhage, the examiner may notice no abnormality, or streaks and clumps of blood in the vitreous, or complete obscuration of the normal red reflex. In diabetes mellitus, vitreous hemorrhage commonly occurs from newly formed blood vessels and, together with the other effects of extraretinal or proliferative retinopathy, constitutes the leading cause for blindness among diabetics (Plate 7). In the absence of a predisposing cause such as diabetes, vitreous hemorrhage almost always occurs as the result of a tear in the retina which, if untreated, may lead to retinal detachment. Any change in the pattern of opacities in the media or the occurrence of flashing lights merits careful ophthalmologic scrutiny.

Asteroid hyalosis is the term applied to the deposition of calcium soaps within the vitreous. It is recognized by the spectacular appearance of glistening objects on ophthalmoscopic examination. This condition is usually unilateral, does not interfere with vision, and is associated with diabetes mellitus in one-fourth of cases.

THE CHOROID

The choroid lies beneath the retina and contains many melanocytes dispersed throughout a rich vascular bed. The nutrition of the outer layers of the retina depends on diffusion of metabolites from the underlying choroid. The choroid is part of the uveal tract, which is formed by the iris, ciliary body, and choroid. Inflammation of each of these structures is referred to as iritis, cyclitis, and choroiditis respectively. Inflammation of the entire uveal tract is called *uveitis*. Some systemic diseases have a predilection for some or all of the uveal tract, and when the choroid is the site of inflammation, very often the overlying retina also becomes involved in a chorioretinal lesion.

When **sarcoid** (Chap. 254) involves the choroid and retina, it takes the form of small white nodules, usually in the lower retina, often along the course of vessels (Plate 7). The nodules are small white granulomas which are about a tenth of a disk diameter in size. The appearance of these retinal nodules is pathognomonic of sarcoid. However, good pupillary dilatation is necessary for their visualization.

Toxoplasmosis (Chap. 244) appears primarily as a retinitis from which small pseudocysts containing the organism have been isolated. These are large (2 to 3 disk diameters), round, circumscribed areas of atrophy into which pigment cells have migrated and proliferated (Plate 7). Several lesions may be confluent with one another. Although scattered throughout the retina, they are usually seen about the central portion of the retina. These lesions are not pathognomonic for toxoplasmosis but should suggest this diagnosis in the face of uveitis and a positive Sabin's dye test.

A characteristic ophthalmoscopic picture has been described in patients who have lived at least 2 years in areas endemic for **histoplasmosis** (Chap. 188) and who have lung calcifications and a positive histoplasmin skin test. Scattered throughout the periphery of both retinas are multiple, small (one-fourth disk diameter), round chorioretinal lesions with a white atrophic center and scattered pigment. These patients complain of sudden decrease in visual acuity of one eye. On ophthalmoscopic examination, edema and hemorrhage, presumably from a leaking blood vessel in the underlying choroid, are seen in the macula (Plate 7). The leak can be demonstrated by injecting fluorescein intravenously. *Histoplasma capsulatum* has not been isolated from these lesions, but it has been presumed that they represent the result either of dissemination of the organism or of a hypersensitivity reaction. In none of these cases has active systemic disease been present; the complement fixation test has been negative. Treatment is required to prevent loss of central vision, a frequent complication either in one eye or in both. Oral corticosteroids appear to influence favorably the course of the disease.

THE RETINA

The retina is about 0.4 mm in thickness and is transparent. In all parts of the retina, there are three layers of cells, except in the center of the macula (the fovea), where only the outer receptor layer is present. Light traversing the media of the eye must pass through the entire thickness of the retina to reach the receptor layer of rods and cones which contain the visual pigment. The middle layer of cells to which the receptor layer connects is the bipolar cell layer, and this in turn connects with the innermost or ganglion cell layer. The axons of the ganglion cells make up the innermost portion of the retina, running parallel to the surface of the retina to reach the optic nervehead, where, as they pierce the lamina cribrosa to form the optic nerve, they acquire myelin sheaths. Because the retina is neuroectodermal in origin and the optic nerve embryologically is an outgrowth of the neural tube, the optic nerve is in fact a tract of the brain with pial septums and is supported by oligodendrocytes (not Schwann cells) and astrocytes. Thus, it is analogous to the spinothalamic or spinocerebellar tracts and as such can be involved in diseases which affect second-order neurones; e.g., heredonfamilial and degenerative disease (Chap. 362) (Schilder's disease, neuromyelitis optica, disseminated sclerosis, and Behr's hereditary cerebellar ataxia).

The *vascular supply* to the retina is from the central retinal artery, a branch of the ophthalmic artery, which, soon after entering the eye, divides into four arterioles supplying the four quadrants of the retina. The arterioles quickly form a capillary bed which is confined to the inner and middle portion of the retina wherein lie the bipolar cells and retinal ganglion cells and their axons of the nerve fiber layer. The outer portion of the retina, including the rods and cones and their cell bodies, is supplied from the underlying choroidal vascular bed. Consequently, obstruction of the central retinal artery will re-

sult in death of the ganglion cell layer and nerve fiber layer and loss of vision. Since the optic nerve consists of the axones of the ganglion cells, primary optic atrophy will result (Plate 6). On the other hand, interference with the nutrition of the outer retinal layer of rods and cones will, if involving the macular region, also result in decreased visual acuity but will not be accompanied by optic atrophy, since the ganglion cells and their axones remain intact.

Although the central retinal artery, while still in the optic nerve, has an internal elastic lamina, a media, and an adventitia, these structural components are lost when the artery has divided into branch vessels which have the characteristics of arterioles. Therefore the response of the retinal vasculature to atherosclerosis and hypertension is that of an arteriole rather than an artery.

The walls of the retinal vessels are transparent, and what is seen on ophthalmoscopy is the column of blood. In atherosclerosis (Chap. 357) the lumen is narrowed from thickening of the basement membrane and hyalinization of the wall, while in hypertension the lumen is narrowed from fibrous tissue replacement of the media. In both cases the column of blood is narrowed and there is increased light reflection from the thickened vessel wall, which has a different refractive index than the adjacent retinal tissue. Both processes may lead to increased tortuosity of the vessels, marked impression of the arteriole on the vein at crossings, and obliteration of segments of vessels. In general the hypertensive changes (Chap. 276), which include diffuse narrowing and tortuosity of the arteriolar tree, large cotton wool exudates, and papilledema, correlate well with the degree of hypertension and provide an index of intracranial involvement. The exudates, the so-called **cytoid bodies,** are caused by microinfarcts of capillaries of the nerve fiber layer which result in patches of edema in the nerve fiber. The atherosclerotic changes include the appearance of glistening white "plaques" on the arterial walls (Chap. 357) and localized venous distension distal to an obstruction by an atheromatous plaque compressing the vein at the arteriovenous junction. In both situations, deep and superficial hemorrhages and exudates are common.

Since the central retinal vein shares a common adventitia with the central retinal artery, atheromatous plaques in the latter are sometimes associated with thrombosis of this vein. The intravascular venous pressure must always exceed that of the intraocular pressure, which is about 15 mm Hg. If the rate of blood flow through the veins is decreased because of an increase in the intraocular pressure, which may occasionally equal or slightly exceed the venous pressure, stasis and occlusion may occur. If venous stasis is detected early, occlusion can occasionally be prevented by improving blood flow with anticoagulants or by lowering the intraocular pressure medically by the use of parasympathomimetic drugs (pilocarpine, anticholinesterases), sympathomimetic drugs (epinephrine), or carbonic anhydrase inhibitors (acetazoleamide).

Although the capillary bed per se cannot be visualized

with the ophthalmoscope, the capillary aneurysm in diabetes and the cotton wool exudates (secondary to microinfarcts of capillaries in the nerve fiber layer) characteristic of hypertension and collagen vascular disease can be seen.

The cells within the retina are architecturally oriented so that the outer layers of receptor cells and bipolar cells are situated at right angles to the surface of the retina while the inner ganglion cell and nerve fiber layer are laid parallel to the surface of the retina. Thus, if there is a hemorrhage in the deep capillary bed at the level of the bipolar cells, the hemorrhage will dissect the cell layer parallel to the direction of the cell processes and come to lie along these processes. When viewed with the ophthalmoscope, the hemorrhage will be seen "head on" and appear to be round and punctate. This is equally true for deep exudates, whether they be the result of transudation from the deep capillary bed (hypertension) or deposition of fatty esters (diabetes) in the outer cell layer. On the other hand, if the hemorrhage occurs from the capillary bed of the nerve fiber layer, it will dissect along the nerve fibers running parallel to the surface of the retina. When viewed with the ophthalmoscope, the hemorrhage will be seen to be spread out over a relatively large area and appear to be flame-shaped. Pre-retinal (subhyaloid) hemorrhages, due to subarachnoid hemorrhage secondary to ruptured saccular aneurysms and hemangiomas, are large and smoothly marginated, lie in front of the retina, and often demonstrate a fluid level.

Outer Layer

Degeneration of the outer receptor layer and adjacent pigment epithelium of the retina occurs usually as a manifest hereditary trait (**retinitis pigmentosa**), but involvement of these structures may appear also in a number of systemic diseases. This disease is manifested by night blindness at an early age, constriction of peripheral visual fields with preservation of central visual acuity until late in the disease, marked attenuation of the retinal arterioles, and bone spicule-like clumping of pigment scattered throughout the retina (Plate 6). Retinitis pigmentosa may be part of the Laurence-Moon-Biedl syndrome (Chap. 87), progressive external ophthalmoplegia, Bassen-Kornzweig disease (acanthocytosis and heredodegenerative neuromuscular disease with abetalipoproteinemia, Chap. 113) and Refsum's disease (chronic polyneuritis with accumulation of phytanic acid, Chap. 364). The outer retinal layer of cells is also selectively involved in the macular area in the Batten-Mayou type of cerebromacular degeneration, as well as in idiopathic senile macular degeneration. The latter is one of the main causes of visual loss in the elderly patient.

Beneath the pigment epithelium is a basement membrane, called *Bruch's membrane.* Small excrescences of this membrane are seen ophthalmoscopically as **drusen bodies,** small whitish spots deep to the retina. Breaks in Bruch's membrane with subsequent repair by fibrosis

give rise to **angioid streaks.** These occur in a number of systemic diseases, particularly pseudoxanthoma elasticum (Chap. 398), Paget's disease of bone (Chap. 382), sickle-cell disease (Chap. 339), hyperphosphatemia, and acromegaly (Chap. 87) (Plate 6). When the macular region is affected there may be a significant loss of visual acuity. Finally, this layer appears to be susceptible to a number of drugs such as the phenothiazines. The latter agents bind selectively to the melanin in the pigment epithelium, eventually with degeneration of the outer retinal layers. The dosages should be kept at minimal levels to prevent these changes, and all patients receiving these drugs should have frequent examinations of central visual fields using small color test objects.

Inner Layer and Optic Nerve

The *optic nervehead* (optic disk or papilla) is seen easily on ophthalmoscopy through the dilated pupil; it normally has a pink coloration. Adjacent to the edge of the nervehead are often seen either deposits of pigment or whitish crescents which represent the pulling away of the underlying vascular choroid from the edge of the nervehead. These are normal variations. Veins entering the nervehead normally pulsate, but an absence of pulsation usually has no clinical significance. The nervehead is about 1.5 mm in diameter, and the site of lesions or other anatomic loci is conveniently measured in terms of disk diameters away from the nervehead.

When **optic atrophy** is present, the nervehead no longer looks pink. There are two clinical types of optic atrophy: primary and secondary. If the pathologic process causes either degeneration of the ganglion cells in the retina or degeneration of their axons in the optic nerve beginning about 5 mm behind the nervehead, or in the chiasma or tract, then in time the nervehead will become white and slightly shrunken, with very distinct margins—*primary optic atrophy* (Plate 6). If, however, the pathologic process is at the optic nervehead within the first few millimeters of it, then, in time, there may be a reactive proliferation of glial tissue. The margins of the optic nervehead will then be obliterated, and the nervehead will appear gray—*secondary optic atrophy.* Primary optic atrophy is seen in occlusion of the central retinal artery and destruction of the optic nerve beyond the eye by tumor, etc. Secondary optic atrophy is seen following optic neuritis (papillitis) and long-standing papilledema.

A similar clinical differentiation is made as to the locus of an inflammatory process such as a demyelinating plaque. If the process is anywhere in the optic nerve posterior to the first few millimeters of optic nerve, the clinical picture is referred to as **retrobulbar neuritis.** If the inflammation is within the first few millimeters of optic nerve, the clinical picture is that of **optic neuritis** or papillitis. In the latter case, the inflammatory reaction and edema are visualized. The pathogenesis of these two lesions is identical. Since the optic nerve is about 40 to 50 mm long, the clinical picture of retrobulbar neuritis is much more frequent than that of optic neuritis. The long cylindric form of the optic nerve with medullated fibers lying next to pial venules renders the structure highly vulnerable to the pathogenetic mechanism of multiple sclerosis. In this respect it resembles the spinal cord, where a similar anatomic arrangement exists.

Inflammation of the optic nervehead (optic neuritis) may be indistinguishable ophthalmoscopically from **papilledema** due to increased intracranial pressure. In both cases, the edges of the nervehead are blurred in outline and elevated, and the veins are distended and without pulsations. Splinter hemorrhages are seen superficially in the swollen nerve fiber layer at the nervehead margin. In general, visual acuity and visual field are usually affected in optic neuritis and not in papilledema. However, in every case of suspected optic neuritis or papilledema, cerebrospinal fluid pressure should be measured. It is elevated in papilledema and normal in optic neuritis (Chap. 24).

Temporal to the nervehead, about 2 disk diameters, is the area of the *macula*. It is about 1.5 mm in diameter and lies in a region free of large vessels. In the center of the macula is the *fovea*. Since the fovea is a small depression in the retina, the light from the ophthalmoscope tends to be scattered from the sloping sides, causing a light reflection. However, the absence of this reflection is of no clinical significance. Lesions of the macula will almost always decrease visual acuity, for the fovea is the only portion of the retina that has the potential for 20/20 vision.

The axones of the macular ganglion cells collect in a compact bundle referred to as the papillomacular bundle; the bundle enters the optic nervehead on the temporal side, forming a wedge of tissue. Although the nerve fibers in this bundle spread throughout the optic nerve, they respond to inflammation within the optic nerve and to compression from without as a functional unit. When these fibers are affected by disease such as demyelination, visual acuity is usually impaired and there is a central scotoma in the visual field, suggesting that nerve conduction in the papillomacular bundle has been interrupted selectively. Irreversible damage of this bundle results in pallor of the temporal wedge of the optic nervehead (temporal pallor) (Plate 6).

OPTIC ATROPHY AND OPTIC (RETROBULBAR) NEURITIS

A diagnosis of optic atrophy requires a thorough work-up to establish the etiology. This includes the course of visual loss, associated symptoms, quantitative perimetric fields, and x-ray examination of the orbit and optic foramens. Although the most common cause of optic atrophy is an expanding lesion within the orbit or cranium, emphasis in this discussion will be placed on other causes more related to systemic disease.

Multiple sclerosis (Chap. 362) often affects the optic nerve. Although there usually is good recovery from the initial episode of inflammation, recurrent episodes lead eventually to optic atrophy, especially in the temporal portion of the optic nervehead, the papillomacular bundle (Plate 6).

Inflammatory processes that involve the optic nerves with eventual optic atrophy may be due to meningovascular syphilis (Chap. 177), Behçet's disease (recurrent ulcers of the eye, mouth, and genitalia, chronic uveitis, and recurring hypopyon), meningitis of bacterial, tuberculous, or fungal origin, and viral meningitis or encephalitis.

Optic neuritis may occur in diabetes (often in association with peripheral neuritis), in pernicious anemia and subacute combined degeneration, Paget's disease of bone, fibrous dysplasia (accompanied by decreased diameter of the optic foramens), or poor nutrition (probably the basis of tobacco-alcohol ambyopia). Poisons such as methyl alcohol (Chap. 116) will produce decreased visual acuity bilaterally within hours after ingestion, and primary optic atrophy follows in several weeks. Finally glaucoma must be considered as a cause of primary optic atrophy associated with deep excavation of the disk by the increased intraocular pressure. Deep cupping of the optic nervehead is seen ophthalmoscopically.

PAPILLEDEMA

Papilledema is a neurosurgical emergency requiring immediate hospitalization. Visual acuity usually is unimpaired, although after some weeks of high intracranial pressure it may be decreased markedly in a matter of days. The hallmarks of papilledema are the raised and blurred edges of the optic nervehead bilaterally, absent venous pulsations, dilated veins, and some splinter and flame-shaped hemorrhages near the nervehead (Plate 6). Normal visual acuity and lack of pain on eye movement differentiate it from optic neuritis or papillitis, but decreased visual acuity may occur in longstanding papilledema. Therefore, in every patient thought to have bilateral optic neuritis, intracranial pressure must be measured to establish the diagnosis definitely and to rule out the possibility of papilledema. A source of additional confusion is the fact that an optic nerve that is atrophic cannot develop the signs of papilledema with elevated intracranial pressure. Therefore a swollen optic nervehead on one side and optic atrophy on the other may be due either to papilledema with elevated intracranial pressure or to optic neuritis in the other eye.

Although an intracranial mass in the cranium blocking the circulation of cerebrospinal fluid leads to papilledema, there are many other less obvious causes such as emphysema, hypoparathyroidism, withdrawal from corticosteroids, meningeal hydrops, and diseases which markedly elevate the cerebrospinal fluid protein, such as intraspinal tumors and the Guillain-Barré syndrome.

RETINAL VASCULAR DISEASE

Vascular lesions may be arterial, venous, or capillary.

Arterial Lesions. Occlusion of the central retinal artery or its branches may be secondary to emboli, atheroma, ischemia, or inflammation.

Occlusion of the central retinal artery usually is caused by *emboli* from postrheumatic vegetations in younger patients or by atheromas in the carotid and ophthalmic arteries in older ones. Visual loss is sudden. The ophthalmoscopic appearance of occlusion of the central retinal artery during the first day or so is one of a whitish-gray retina and a cherry-red spot at the macula. Occasionally the embolus can be visualized and the blood column can be seen to be interrupted distal to the embolus. Within several days the arterial bed usually reopens and the edema subsides, so that within 1 to 2 weeks the retina may appear normal. After several weeks the optic nerve becomes pale, since the nerve fiber layer and the ganglion cell layer of the retina normally supplied by the central retinal artery undergo degeneration. Following occlusion of the central retinal artery, only light perception usually remains unless a cilioretinal artery is present. Since this vessel arises from the choroidal vascular bed, rather than the central retinal artery, that portion of the retina which it supplies (namely, a small area between the optic nervehead and the macula) will be preserved, and hand movements or counting of fingers will be possible. If the patient is seen within the first few minutes following an embolus to the central retinal artery, paracentesis of the anterior chamber using a small Bard-Parker No. 11 blade should be attempted in an effort to lower intraocular pressure immediately and allow the embolus to pass along to a smaller branch arteriole.

In the case of a branch artery occlusion, the retina will be gray and edematous only in the quadrant supplied by the branch artery, with the apex of the sector at the optic nervehead. Visual acuity is usually not affected, provided the macula is spared. A sector field defect will persist, however, corresponding to the involved portion of the retina.

When occlusion of the ophthalmic or central retinal artery is secondary to *atheroma*, the plaque and thrombus cannot be visualized. If the patient is seen within 10 to 15 min of the occlusion, some ophthalmologists attempt to relieve the secondary retinal vascular spasm by retrobulbar injection of local anesthetic or by superior cervical ganglion block, but it is doubtful if these measures are of any value. The ophthalmoscopic appearance during both the acute and late stages is indistinguishable from that following embolization of the central retinal artery.

A picture similar to that of occlusion of the central retinal artery may be caused by *ischemia* of the retina under conditions of general circulatory collapse, as in hemorrhage or in cardiorespiratory arrest. If the patient survives, the decreased visual acuity usually is noted several days later and may be accompanied by retinal edema and, still later, by primary optic atrophy.

A more common cause of *intermittent retinal ischemia* (**amaurosis fugax**) is carotid stenosis. The monocular blackouts or blindness in one eye may be accompanied by hemiplegia or hemisensory symptoms on the opposite side of the body (Chap. 357). The cause of this may be established by ophthalmodynamometry; the retinal artery pressure on one side is found to be significantly lower than that on the other side. During the amaurotic period,

one can see, by ophthalmoscopy, the arrest of retinal circulation.

The attacks of amaurosis may be relieved by treatment with anticoagulants or surgical endarterectomy. Ischemia of this type can also result from atheromatous plaques within the aortic arch and carotid arteries (aortic arch syndrome) and in Takuyasu's disease (Chaps. 277, 357). One of the most important causes of retinal arterial occlusive disease is temporal arteritis (giant-cell arteritis), which occurs only in elderly patients and is accompanied by decreased visual acuity, field defects, and a markedly elevated sedimentation rate. There may be pain and tenderness over the temporal artery, but this is not invariant. Ophthalmoscopic findings may be identical to those of central retinal artery occlusion secondary to an atheroma, or only edema of the optic nervehead may be revealed. The inflammation is usually located in the ophthalmic artery or the central retinal artery behind the lamina cribrosa and may follow headache, fever, and malaise by a period of weeks. If this diagnosis is suspected and the sedimentation rate is elevated, systemic corticosteroids (60 mg prednisolone daily) should be given immediately. Blindness in one eye or in both eyes develops in about half the patients with temporal arteritis. Consequently, early treatment is indicated, in order to attempt to prevent the arteritis from involving the second eye.

Venous Lesions. Occlusion of the central retinal vein occurs commonly in association with diabetes, glaucoma, and atheroma of the central retinal artery. Again visual acuity decreases rapidly, but unlike the ophthalmoscopic picture of central retinal artery occlusion, there is the typical "blood and thunder" appearance of dilated veins and numerous scattered hemorrhages of all shapes and sizes. When a branch of the central retinal vein is occluded, the retinal hemorrhages are confined to the appropriate quadrant(s) (Plate 7).

Preceding an occlusion of the retinal vein, one often sees venous stasis, characterized by dilatation of veins, a few retinal hemorrhages, and decreased blood flow through the veins. Venous stasis may go on to vein occlusion if not treated by anticoagulation and lowering of intraocular pressure. Venous stasis is characteristically seen in association with increased blood viscosity; e.g., in polycythemia, multiple myeloma, sickle-cell disease, macroglobulinemia of Waldenström, cryoglobulinemia, leukemia, and cystic fibrosis of the pancreas.

Capillary Lesions. Occlusive disease in capillaries is manifested by the appearance of cotton wool exudates in the nerve fiber layer of the retina. This occurs most commonly in hypertension and diabetes but is found also in collagen vascular disease (particularly lupus erythematosus), as well as in scleroderma, Hodgkin's disease, and multiple myeloma (Plate 7).

The most common disease of retinal capillaries is the *microangiopathy of diabetes mellitus,* in which round hemorrhages and exudates in the outer retinal layers and capillary microaneurysms are characteristically found.

These lesions are most marked in the central region of the retina surrounding the optic nervehead and macula. The round hemorrhages, exudates, and capillary aneurysms are *intraretinal* (Plate 7). At some point in time, retinal capillaries, especially at the nervehead but occasionally near the periphery, become dilated in clusters and proliferate anteriorly into the vitreous, along with other mesodermal elements, to form the characteristic picture of *extraretinal* or proliferative retinopathy (Plate 7). Vitreous hemorrhage is likely to result; when it does, the patient experiences a veil or cloud over the eyes, and in a matter of minutes there may be a marked decrease in visual acuity. The vitreous hemorrhage may clear completely, but with recurrent bleeding the vitreous contracts and the retina becomes detached. The intraretinal and extraretinal forms of diabetic retinopathy may exist independently or concurrently; the former is compatible with normal or somewhat reduced visual acuity for a long period of time, but the latter frequently leads to total blindness. Although pituitary ablation using various techniques has been tried in the treatment of diabetic retinopathy, no control series has demonstrated a statistically significant difference in prognosis between the treated and nontreated patients after 5 years.

REFERENCE

Cogan, David G.: "Neurology of the Visual System," Springfield, Ill., Charles C Thomas, Publisher, 1966.

APPENDIX

Laboratory Values of Clinical Importance

BODY FLUIDS AND OTHER MASS DATA

Body fluid, total volume: 56% (in obese) to 70% (lean) of body
  weight
  Intracellular: 30 to 40% of body weight
  Extracellular: 23 to 25% of body weight
Blood:
  Total volume: Male: 75 ml/kg body weight
    Female: 67 ml/kg body weight
  Plasma volume: Male: 44 ml/kg body weight
    Female: 43 ml/kg body weight
  Red cell volume: Male: 30 ml/kg body weight (1.15–1.21 L
    per sq m surface area)
    Female: 24 ml/kg body weight

$$\text{mEq (milliequivalent)} = \frac{\text{mg/100 ml} \times 10 \times \text{valence}}{\text{atomic weight}}$$

$$\text{mg/100 ml} = \frac{\text{mEq} \times \text{atomic weight}}{10 \times \text{valence}}$$

ASCITIC FLUID

See Chap. 46, p. 262.

Atomic Weights of Elements Commonly Encountered in Clinical Medicine

Calcium	40.08	Magnesium	24.32
Carbon	12.01	Nitrogen	14.008
Chlorine	35.46	Oxygen	16.00
Copper	63.54	Phosphorus	30.98
Hydrogen	1.008	Potassium	39.100
Iodine	126.91	Sodium	22.997
Iron	55.85	Sulfur	32.07

CEREBROSPINAL FLUID

Cells: <5 per cu mm, all lymphocytes
Pressure, initial (horizontal position): 70–200 mm water
Calcium*: 1.13–1.30 mEq/L
Chloride,* as Cl⁻: 118–127 mEq/L
Cholesterol: 0.06–0.22 mg/100 ml
Colloidal gold test: Not more than two in any tube
Creatinine: 0.4–1.5 mg/100 ml
Glucose*: 44–100 mg/100 ml

  * Since the cerebrospinal fluid concentrations are equilibrium values, measurement of blood plasma obtained at the same time is recommended.

pH*: 7.35–7.70
Magnesium (average)*: 0.82–1.08 mEq/L
Nonprotein nitrogen*: 12–30 mg/100 ml
Phosphorus (inorganic)*: 1.2–2.1 mg/100 ml
Potassium*: 2.18–3.38 mEq/L
Protein:
  (Total): 14–45 mg/100 ml
  Lumbar: 14–45 mg/100 ml
  Cisternal: 15 mg/100 ml
  Ventricular: 10 mg/100 ml
Sodium*: 217–237 mEq/L
Urea nitrogen*: 6–28 mg/100 ml

CHEMICAL CONSTITUENTS OF BLOOD **

(See also under Function Tests, especially Liver, and Metabolic and Endocrine)
Acetone, serum: 0.3–2.0 mg/100 ml
Albumin, serum: 4.0–5.2 Gm/100 ml
Aldolase, 0–8 IU/L
Alpha amino nitrogen, plasma: 3.0–5.5 mg/100 ml
Ammonia, whole blood, venous: 30–70 μg/100 ml
Amylase, whole blood (Somogyi): 60–180 units/100 ml; 0.8–3.2
  IU/L
Ascorbic acid, whole blood: 0.4–1.0 mg/100 ml
  Leukocytes: 25–40 mg/100 ml
Barbiturates, serum: 0
  "Potentially fatal" level (Schreiner)
    phenobarbital: approx. 8 mg/100 ml
    most short-acting barbiturates: 3.5 mg/100 ml
Base, total, serum: 145–155 mEq/L
Bilirubin, total, serum (Malloy-Evelyn): 0.3–1.0 mg/100 ml
  Direct, serum: 0.1–0.3 mg/100 ml
  Indirect, serum: 0.2–0.7 mg/100 ml
Bromides, serum: 0
  Toxic levels: above 17 mEq/L; 150 mg %
Calcium, ionized: 2.3–2.8 mEq/L; 4.5–5.6 mg/100 ml
Calcium, serum: 4.5–5.5 mEq/L; 9–11 mg/100 ml
Carbon dioxide–combining power, serum (sea level):
  21–28 mEq/L; 50–65 vol %
Carbon dioxide content, blood (sea level):
  21–30 mEq/L; 50–70 vol %
Carbon dioxide tension, arterial blood (sea level):
  42 ± 4 mm Hg
Carbon monoxide content, blood:
  Symptoms with over 20% saturation of hemoglobin
Carotenoids, serum: 100–200 μg/100 ml

  ** IU = International units.

Chlorides, serum (as Cl): 98–106 mEq/L;
 355–376 mg/100 ml
Cholesterol: Total, serum (Man-Peters method)
 (mean ± 1 SD): 194 ± 36 mg/100 ml
 Esters, serum: 100–180 mg/100 ml
Cholesterol ester fraction of total cholesterol, serum: 68–72%
Copper, serum (mean ± 1 SD): 114 ± 14 μg/100 ml
Corticoids, plasma (Porter-Silber) (mean ±1 SD):
 13 ± 6 μg/100 ml at 8:00 A.M.
Cortisol (competitive protein binding):
 14 ± 5 μg/100 ml at 8:00 A.M.
Creatinine, serum (Peters): 1–1.5 mg/100 ml
Dilantin, plasma:
 Therapeutic level, 10–20 μg/ml
 Toxic level, >20 μg/ml
Ethanol, blood:
 Marked intoxication, 0.3–0.4%
 Alcoholic stupor, 0.4–0.5%
 Coma, above 0.5%
Fat, neutral, serum: 150–250 mg/100 ml
Fatty acids, serum: 380–465 mg/100 ml
Fibrinogen, plasma: 0.2–0.4 Gm/100 ml
Globulins, serum: 1.3–2.7 Gm/100 ml
Glucose (fasting), blood (Nelson-Somogyi):
 60–90 mg/100 ml; plasma, 75–105 mg
Hemoglobin, blood (sea level):
 Males: 14–18 Gm/100 ml
 Females: 12–16 Gm/100 ml
Icterus index, serum: 4–6 units
Iodine
 See p. 450, Metabolic and Endocrine
Iron, serum, males and females (mean ± 1 SD):
 105 ± 25 μg/100 ml
Iron-binding capacity, serum (mean ± 1 SD):
 325 ± 37 μg/100 ml
 Saturation, percent: 20–45
Ketones, total: 0.5–1.5 mg/100 ml
Lactic acid, blood: 6–16 mg/100 ml
Lactic dehydrogenase, serum: 200–450 units/ml (Wrobleski)
 60–100 units/ml (Wacker); 25–100 IU/L
Lead, serum: <20 μg/100 ml
Lipase, serum (Cherry-Crandall): 1.5 ml N/20 NaOH (upper
 limit of normal). (However, values above 1.0 should be
 regarded with suspicion.)
Lipid phosphorus (Man-Peters) (mean ± 1 SD): 9.2 ± 1.4
 mg/100 ml
Lipids, total, serum: 500–600 mg/100 ml
Lipids, triglyceride, serum: 50–150 mg/100 ml
Magnesium, serum: 1.5–2.5 mEq/L; 2–3 mg/100 ml
Nitrogen, nonprotein, serum: 15–35 mg/100 ml
Nutrients, various; See Table 78–2, p. 399
Osmolality, serum: 285–295 mOsm/L
Oxygen capacity, blood: 18–22 vol %
Oxygen content: Arterial blood (sea level): 17–21 vol %
 Venous blood, arm (sea level): 10–16 vol %
Oxygen per cent saturation (sea level):
 Arterial blood: 97 vol %
 Venous blood, arm: 60–85 vol %
Oxygen tension, blood: 95–100 mm Hg
pH blood: 7.38–7.44
Phosphatase, acid, serum:
 Bessey-Lowry method: 0.10–0.63 units
 Bodansky method: 0.5–2.0 units

Fishman-Lerner (tartrate sensitive): <0.6 unit/100 ml (up to
 0.15/100 ml)
 Gutman method: 0.5–2.0 units
 International units: 0.2–1.8
 King-Armstrong method: 1.0–5.0 units
 Shinowara method: 0.0–1.1 units
Phosphatase, alkaline, serum:
 Bessey-Lowry method: 0.8–2.3 units (3.4–9)*
 Bodansky method: 2.0–4.5 units (3.0–13.0)*
 Gutman method: 3.0–10.0 units
 International units: 21–91 U/L at 37°C incubation
 King-Armstrong method: 5.0–13.0 units (10.0–20.0)*
 Shinowara method: 2.2–8.6 units
Phosphokinase, serum creatine (Hughes): 0.33–4.49 μM
 creatine/ml serum/hr at 37°C; 10–50 IU/L
Phospholipids, serum: 150–250 mg/100 ml
Phosphorus, inorganic, serum: 1–1.5 mEq/L; 3–4.5 mg/100 ml
Potassium, serum: 3.5–5.0 mEq/L; 13–19 mg/100 ml
Proteins, total, serum 6.5–8.0 Gm/100 ml
Proteins, electrophoretic fractions:

	Plasma, %	Serum, %	Serum, % (paper)
	(Tiselius)		
Albumin	55.2	58 ± 3	45–55
Globulins: α_1	5.3	5 ± 2	5–8
α_2	8.7	12 ± 3	8–13
β	13.4	11 ± 4	11–17
Fibrinogen:	6.5		
Globulins: γ_1 $\}$	11.0	2 ± 2 $\}$	15–25
γ_2		12 ± 3	

Salicylate, plasma: 0
 Therapeutic range: 20–25 mg/100 ml
 Toxic range: over 30 mg/100 ml
Serotonin, 5-hydroxyindole acetic acid (urinary metabolite):
 2–8 mg/24 hr
Sodium, serum: 137–142 mEq/L; 315–326 mg/100 ml
Steroids . . . See p. 2012 under Metabolic and Endocrine
Sulfates, inorganic, serum: 0.5–1.5 mg/100 ml
Transaminase, serum glutamic, oxalacetic (SGOT)
 (mean ± 1 SD): 22 ± 7 units/ml/min; 6–18 IU/L at
 25°C incubation
Transaminase, serum glutamic pyruvic (SGPT)
 (mean ± 1 SD): 16 ± 9 units/ml/min; 3–26 IU/L
Urea nitrogen, whole blood: 10–20 mg/100 ml
Uric acid, serum, enzymatic method (Praetorius)
 (mean ± 1 SD):
 Males: 5.0 ± 1.2 mg/100 ml
 Females: 3.8 ± 0.9 mg/100 ml
Uric acid, serum (Talbot): 2.5–5.0 mg/100 ml
Vitamin A, serum: 50–100 μg/100 ml
Zinc, serum: 120 ± 20 μg/100 ml

FUNCTION TESTS

Circulation

Cardiac output (Fick): 2.6–3.6 L/sq m/min
Circulation time: Arm to lung, ether: 4–8 sec

 * Values in brackets are those found in children

Arm to tongue, calcium gluconate: 12–18 sec
  Decholin: 10–16 sec
  Saccharin: 9–16 sec
Pressures, intracardiac and intraarterial:
  Aorta: Systole: 120 mm Hg
    Diastole: 80 mm Hg
  Atrium: Left (mean): 2–12 mm Hg
    Right (mean): 0–5 mm Hg
  Pulmonary artery: Systole: 20–30 mm Hg
    Diastole: 8–14 mm Hg
    Wedge (mean): 2–12 mm Hg
  Ventricle, left: Systole: 120 mm Hg
    Diastole: 2–12 mm Hg
  Ventricle, right: Systole: 25 mm Hg
    Diastole: 0–5 mm Hg
  Venous (antecubital): 70–140 mm H_2O

Gastrointestinal (see also Stool)

Absorption tests:
  d-Xylose absorption test:
    After an overnight fast, 25 Gm xylose is given in aqueous solution by mouth
    Urine collected for the following 5 hr should contain 5–8 Gm (or >20% of ingested dose)
    Serum xylose should be 25–40 mg/100 ml 1 hr after the oral dose
  Vitamin A absorption test:
    A fasting blood specimen is obtained and 200,000 units vitamin A in oil given by mouth. Serum vitamin A levels should rise to twice fasting level in 3 to 5 hr
Gastric Juice:
  Volume: 24 hr, 2–3L; nocturnal, 600–700 ml; basal, fasting 30–70 ml/hr
  Reaction: as pH, 1.6–1.8; titratable acidity of fasting juice, 15–35 mEq/hr
  Acid output:
    Basal: females   2.0 ± 1.8 mEq/hr
         males   3.0 ± 2.0 mEq/hr
    Maximal (after subcutaneous histamine acid phosphate 0.04 mg/kg, preceded by 50 mg phenergan; or histalog 1.7 mg/Kg, or gastrin 2.0 µg/Kg):
         females   16 ± 5 mEq/hr
         males   23 ± 5 mEq/hr
  Basal acid output/maximal acid output ratio: 0.6
  Tubeless gastric analysis with azure A dye: acid present if more than 0.6 mg dye is excreted in urine over a 2-hr period (CAUTION: A negative test is meaningless and requires performance of the ordinary test with a gastric tube.)
  Jejunal secretion, fasting: chloride, 80–140 mEq/L; HCO_3, 2–32 mEq/L; total base, 110–150 mEq/L.

Liver

Bromsulphalein (5 mg/kg body weight, IV):
  5% or less retention at end of 45 min
Cephalin-cholesterol flocculation: 0 or + at 48 hr

Cholinesterase (pseudocholinesterase), serum:
  0.5 pH units or over/hr
Galactose tolerance, after ingestion of 40 Gm:
  Excretion of not more than 3 Gm in urine in 5 hr
Prothrombin test: Increase of 15% or more in prothrombin concentration in blood in 24 hr after injection of synthetic vitamin K
Thymol turbidity: 0–4 units
Urobilinogen:
  Urine: Semiquantitative (2 hr): 0.5–1.5 units
    Quantitative: 1–3.5 mg/24 hr
  Stool: Semiquantitative (per 100 Gm): <350 units
    Quantitative: 40–280 mg/24 hr
Zinc sulfate turbidity: <4 units

Metabolic and Endocrine

Adrenal-pituitary function tests
  Adrenocortical inhibition test (Liddle) (See p. 490)
  Aldosterone, secretion rate, 50–250 µg/24 hr on low sodium diet
  Corticotropin (ACTH) response tests (See p. 489)
  Cortisol, secretion rate, 10–25 mg/24 hr
  Insulin tolerance test: Blood glucose usually falls to 50% of fasting level in 20–30 min and returns to normal levels in 90–120 min after I.V. administration of 0.1 unit crystalline insulin per kg body weight
  Metapyrone test (See p. 491)
Basal metabolic rate: −15% to +15% of mean standard
Catecholamines, urinary excretion (24 hr):
  Free catecholamines, epinephrine and norepinephrine, 100 µg.
  Metanephrine, normetanephrine, 1.3 mg.
  V.M.A., 6.0 mg.
Creatine tolerance test: 70% ingested creatine retained in adults
Estrogens, urinary (Brown method)
  Females (postpubertal, premenopausal)
    Estrone, 5–20; estradiol, 2–10; estriol, 5–30 µg/24 hr.
  Females (postmenopausal)
    Estrone, 0.3–2.4; estradiol, 0–1.4; estriol, 2.2–7.5 µg/24 hr.
  Males and prepubertal females
    Estrone, 0–5; estradiol, 0–5; estriol, 0–10 µg/24 hr.
Glucose tolerance test, oral: 100 Gm glucose or 1.75 Gm glucose/kg body weight. Blood sugar not more than 160 mg/100 ml "true glucose" (Somogyi-Nelson) after ½ hr; return to normal by 2 hr; sugar not present in any urine specimen
Hyperparathyroidism, tests for (See pp. 472, 473)
Iodine, butanol extractable: 3.2–6.5 µg/100 ml
Iodine, protein bound: 4.0–8.0 µg/100 ml
Iodine, radioactive (^{131}I), uptake: Range 15–45% in 24 hr; mean 35%
Iodine, total 5.5–9.5 µg/100 ml
Iodine, thyroxin (column method) (T_4I) 2.9–6.4 µg/100 ml
Resin T3 (Triosorb sponge) 25–35%
Thyroxine (binding displacement) 4–11 µg/100 ml
TSH test (See p. 451)
Renin test (See p. 491)
Tolbutamide test, and other tests for hypoglycemia (See 543, 544)

Plasma and Urine Steroids

	Plasma	Urine
17-hydroxycorticoids	7–25 μg/100 ml (8 a.m.)	1–10 mg/24 hr (Porter-Silber) 5–20 mg/24 hr (ketonic)
17-ketosteroids		6–18 mg/24 hr (male) 3–12 mg/24 hr (female)
Testosterone	0.37–1.0 μg/100 ml (male) 0–0.1 μg/100 ml (female)	47–156 μg/24 hr (male) 0–15 μg/24 hr (female)
Aldosterone	0.015 μg/100 ml	5–25 μg/24 hr

T_3 suppression test (Werner): Measure I^{131} neck uptake before and after one week of T_3 75 mg/day p.o. I^{131} uptake should decrease at least 50%

Triiodothyronine uptake, erythrocyte (RBC-T_3): 11.0%–17.0% (female); 11.8%–19.0% (male)

Triiodothyronine uptake, resin (Triosorb Abbott): 25%–35%

Pancreatic island function tests (see pp. 543–544)

Water loading test (Soffer): More than 50% excretion of a 1,500 ml water load in 5 hr

Metanephrine urinary excretion: up to 1 mg/24 hr volume

Pulmonary

RANGE OF NORMAL VALUES OF LUNG VOLUMES FOR SEATED SUBJECTS OF AVERAGE SIZE
(First value in each column is for shorter individual)*

	Age 20–39		Age 40–59		Age >60	
	Men	Women	Men	Women	Men	Women
Vital Capacity (L)	3.35–5.90	2.45–4.38	2.72–5.30	2.09–4.02	2.42–4.70	1.91–3.66
Residual Volume (L)	1.13–2.32	1.00–2.00	1.45–2.62	1.16–2.20	1.77–2.77	1.32–2.40
Total Lung Capacity (L)	4.80–7.92	3.61–6.18	4.50–7.62	3.41–6.02	4.35–7.32	3.31–5.86
$\frac{RV†}{TLC‡} \times 100$	20–30	26–33	30–36	33–39	36–43	39–42

* Height: Men, 62–72 in.; Women, 56–70 in.
† RV = Residual volume.
‡ TLC = Total lung capacity.

NORMAL SPIROMETRIC VALUES FOR STANDING SUBJECTS

	Men, age 20–39	Women, age 17–29	Men, age 40–59	Women, age 30–45	Men, age >60	Women, age 46–62
Forced expiratory volume in 1 sec (*FEV*, %)	>76	>80	>69	>81	>73	>76
Maximal midexpiratory flow (*MMF*, L/min)	143–414	111–322	103–395	121–332	91–283	107–250
Maximal breathing capacity (*MBC*, L/min)	135–200	75–135	110–175	68–121	90–135	58–105

PREDICTION FORMULAS FOR LUNG VOLUMES* AND SPIROMETRIC TESTS†

	Men			Women		
	Age, yr (A)	Height, cm (H)	Constant in the equation (C)	Age, yr (A)	Height, cm (H)	Constant in the equation (C)
Vital capacity, L	−0.031	+0.064	−5.335	−0.018	+0.052	−4.36
Residual volume, L	+0.017	+0.027	−3.447	+0.009	+0.032	−3.90
Total lung capacity, L	−0.015	+0.094	−9.167	−0.008	+0.079	−7.49
$\frac{RV‡}{TLC§} \times 100$	+0.343		+16.7	+0.0265		+21.7
Forced expiratory volume (FEV) in 1 sec, L	−0.028	+0.037	−1.59			
Maximum breathing capacity	−1.26	+1.34	−21.4	−0.7		+113

* Seated subjects; †Standing subjects.
‡ RV = Residual volume.
§ TLC = Total lung capacity.

To calculate the predicted value: (1) multiply the figure in column A by the patient's nearest age in years; (2) multiply the value in column H by height (cm); (3) add these two results algebraically; and finally, (4) add or subtract the constant listed in column C. A useful general rule is that a 20 percent deviation from the predicted value is probably significant.

Renal

Clearances (corrected to 1.73 sq m body surface area):
  Measures of glomerular filtration rate:
    Inulin clearance (C_I): Males: 124 ± 25.8 ml/min
      Females: 119 ± 12.8 ml/min
    Endogenous creatinine: 91–130 ml/min
      Urea: 60–100 ml/min
  Measures of effective renal plasma flow and tubular function:
    Para-aminohippuric acid (C_{PAH}):
      Males: 654 ± 163 ml/min
      Females: 594 ± 102 ml/min
    Tubular maximum for PAH, males and females:
      77.2 mg/min
    Diodrast: 600–800 ml/min;
      20–30% excretion in 15 min
Concentration and dilution test:
  Specific gravity of urine: After 12 hr fluid restriction: 1.025
    or more
  After 12 hr deliberate water intake: 1.003 or less
Phenolsulfonphthalein: After intravenous injection:
  Excretion in urine in 15 min: 25% or more
  Excretion in urine in 2 hr: 55–75%
  After intramuscular injection:
  Excretion in urine in 2 hr: 55–75%
  Protein excretion, urine
    Males, 0–60 mg/24 hrs.
    Females, 0–90 mg/24 hrs.

Specific gravity, maximal: 1.002–1.028
Tubular reabsorption phosphorus:
  79–94% of filtered load

HEMATOLOGIC EXAMINATIONS

(See also Chemical Constituents of Blood)

Bone Marrow (see Table 61-6, p. 315)

Erythrocytes and Hemoglobin (see table p. 2015)

Carboxyhemoglobin: Up to 5% of total
Fragility, osmotic: Slight hemolysis: 0.45–0.39%
  Complete hemolysis: 0.33–0.30%
Hemochromogens in plasma: 3–5 mg/100 ml
Hemoglobin, fetal: <2% of fetal
"Life span": Normal survival: 120 days
  Chromium, half-life ($T\frac{1}{2}$): 28 days
Methemoglobin: Up to 1.7% of total
Plasma iron turnover rate: 20–42 mg/24 hr (0.47 mg/kg)
Protoporphyrin, free erythrocyte (E.P.):
  20–38 μg/100 ml RBCs
Reticulocytes: 0.5–2.0% of red cells
Sedimentation rate: Westergren: <15 mm/1 hr
  Wintrobe: Male: 0–9 mm/1 hr
    Female: 0–20 mm/1 hr

NORMAL VALUES AT VARIOUS AGES

Age	Red cell count, millions/cu mm	Hemoglobin, Gm/100 ml	Vol. packed RBC, ml/100 ml	Corpuscular values			
				MCV, $cu\mu$	MCH, $\gamma\gamma$	MCHC, %	MCD, μ
Days 1–13........	5.1 ± 1.0*	19.5 ± 5.0*	54.0 ± 10.0*	106–98	38–33	36–34	8.6
Days 14–60......	4.7 ± 0.9	14.0 ± 3.3	42.0 ± 7.0	90	30	33	8.1
3 mon–10 yr.....	4.5 ± 0.7	12.2 ± 2.3	36.0 ± 5.0	80	27	34	7.7
11–15 yr.........	4.8	13.4	39.0	82	28	34	
Adults:							
Females........	4.8 ± 0.6	14.0 ± 2.0	42.0 ± 5.0	87 ± 5	29 ± 2	34 ± 2	7.5 ± 0.3
Males.........	5.4 ± 0.8	16.0 ± 2.0	47.0 ± 5.0	87 ± 5	29 ± 2	34 ± 2	7.5 ± 0.3

MCV = mean corpuscular volume. MCH = mean corpuscular hemoglobin. MCHC = mean corpuscular hemoglobin concentration. MCD = mean corpuscular diameter. (Wintrobe: "Clinical Hematology," 6th ed., Philadelphia, Lea & Febiger, 1967.)

* The range of values represents almost the extremes of observed variations (93 percent or more) at sea level. The blood values of healthy persons should fall well within these figures.

Leukocytes

NORMAL VALUES

	Percent	Average	Minimum	Maximum
Total number, per cu mm		7,000	4,300	10,000
Neutrophils:				
Juvenile and band..	0–17	520	100	2,100
Segmented........	25–69	3,000	1,100	6,050
Eosinophils..........	0–7	150	0	700
Basophils............	0–0.75	30	0	150
Lymphocytes........	21–49	2,500	1,500	4,000
Monocytes..........	3–7	430	200	950

Platelets and Coagulation

Platelets, per cu mm, Brecher-Cronkite method:
290,000 (140,000–440,000)
Bleeding time (Ivy method, 5-mm wound)
0.5–9.5 min
Clot retraction:
Qualitative: Apparent in 60 min, complete in <24 hr, usually <6 hr
Coagulation time (Lee-White):
Majority and range (glass tubes): 9–15 min, 2–19 min
Majority and range (siliconized tubes): 20–60 min
Whole clot lysis: >24 hr
Prothrombin time (Quick one stage): Comparable to normal control (with most thromboplastins, 11–16 sec)
Partial thromboplastin time (P.T.T.) (Nye–Brinkhous method): Comparable to normal control. With standard technique, 68–84 sec)

Schilling Test

Excretion in urine of orally administered radioactive vitamin B₁₂ following "flushing" parenteral injection of B₁₂: 8–40%

SEROUS FLUIDS (pleural, pericardial, peritoneal)

pH: 6.80–7.60
Specific gravity: 1.010–1.026
Protein:
Total: 0.30–4.10 Gm/100 ml
Albumin: 50.5–69.8%
Globulin: 29.5–45.8%
Fibrinogen: 0.3–4.5%

STOOL

Bulk: Wet weight: <197.5 Gm/day (mean 115 ± 41)
Dry weight: <66.4 Gm/day (mean 34 ± 16)
Fat, on diet containing at least 50 Gm fat: <7.0 Gm/day when measured on a 3-day (or longer) collection (mean 4.0 ± 1.5)
As percentage of dry weight:
<30.4 (mean 13.3 ± 8.07)
Coefficient of fat absorption: >93%
Fatty acid: Free: 1–10% of dry matter
Combined as soap: 0.5–12% of dry matter
Nitrogen: <1.7 Gm/day (mean 1.4 ± 0.2)
Protein content: Minimal
Water: Approximately 65%
Urobilinogen: 40–280 mg/24 hr
Coproporphyrin: 400–1,000 μg/24 hr

URINE

(See also Function Tests, Metabolic and Endocrine)
Acidity, titratable: 125–150 mEq/24 hr
α-Amino nitrogen: 0.4–1.0 Gm/24 hr
Ammonia: 30–50 mEq/24 hr
Amylase (Somogyi): 260–950 mg glucose/24 hr
Calcium, 10 mEq or 200 mg calcium diet:
<7.5 mEq/24 hr or <150 mg/24 hr
Copper: 0–25 μg/24 hr
Coproporphyrins (types I and III): 100–300 μg/24 hr
Creatine, as creatinine: Adult males: <50 mg/24 hr
Adult females: <100 mg/24 hr

Creatinine: 1.0–1.6 Gm/24 hr
D-Xylose excretion: 5–8 Gm/5 hr after oral dose of 25 Gm
Glucose, true (oxidase method): 50–300 mg/24 hr
Ketones, total (mean ± 1 SD): 50.5 ± 30.7 mg/24 hr

Lactic dehydrogenase: 560–2,050 units/8 hr plasma at 25°C
Lead: <0.08 μg/ml or <120 μg/24 hr
Protein: <50 mg/24 hr
Urobilinogen: 1–3.5 mg/24 hr

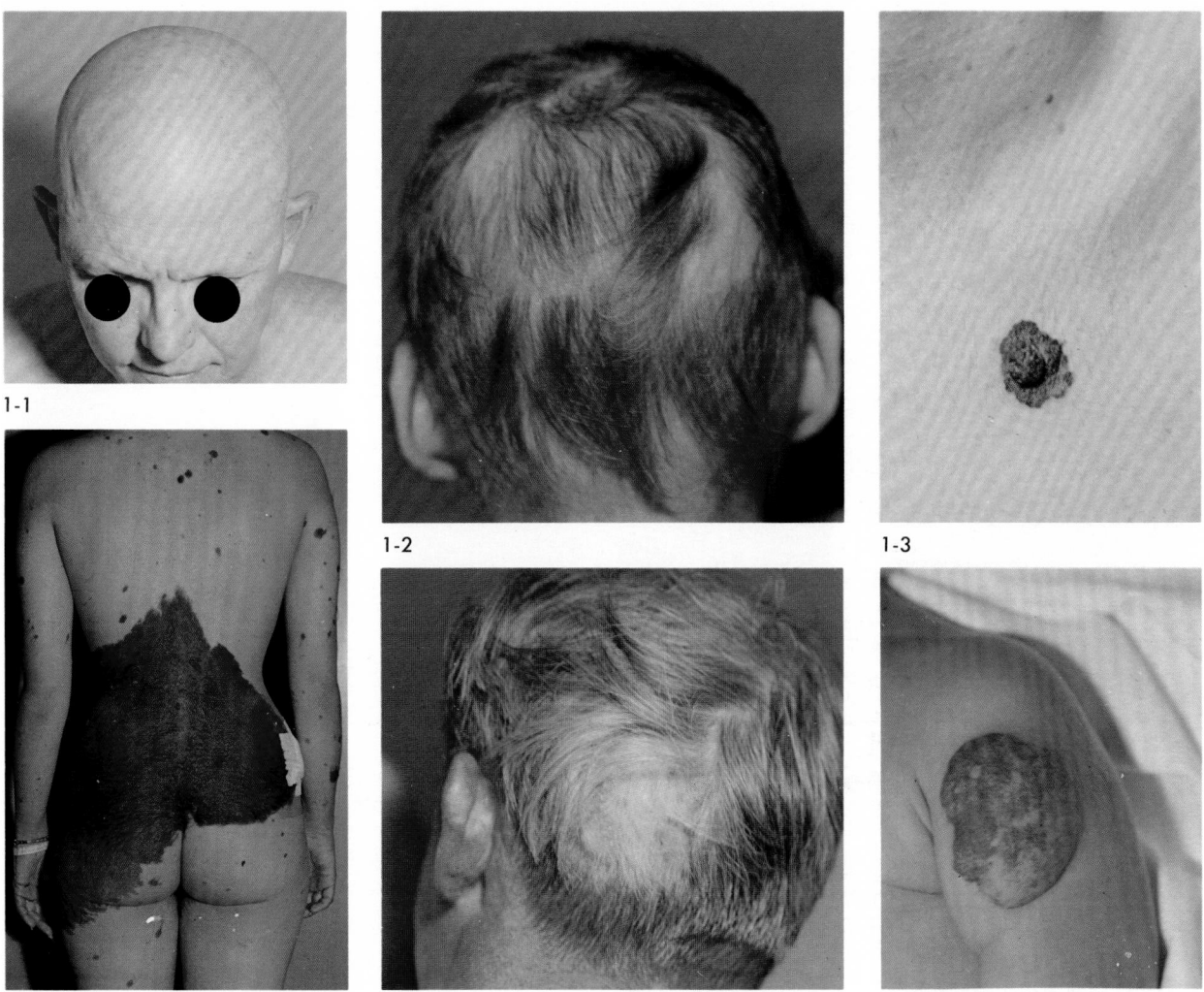

1-1 *Alopecia universalis.* There is complete loss of all scalp and body hair, eyebrows and eyelashes. The prognosis for regrowth when there is extensive involvement of this type is poor.   1-2 Transient *partial alopecia* following cancer chemotherapy with Methotrexate. The prognosis for regrowth is excellent.   1-3 *Malignant melanoma.* The dark raised central tumor is surrounded by splotchy irregular pigmentation.   1-4 Extensive *hairy pigmented nevus.* Such lesions are usually present at birth.   1-5 *Discoid lupus erythematosus* of the scalp causes erythema, atrophy, scarring and permanent alopecia.   1-6 *Strawberry hemangioma.* White sclerotic plaques within the crimson lesion indicate that spontaneous resolution is occurring.

Plate 1

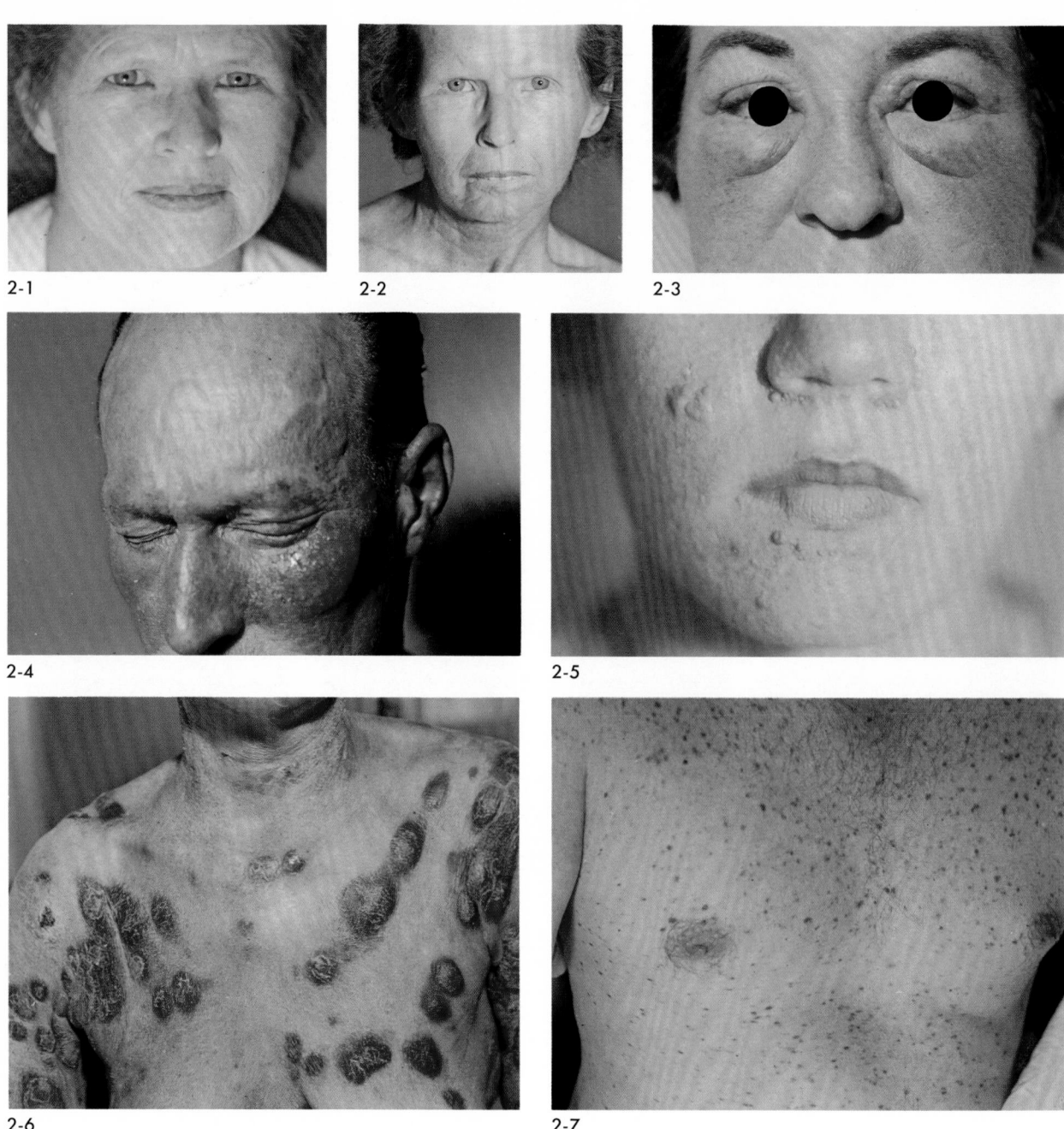

2-1 *Systemic scleroderma* in the early stages of the disease.   2-2 The same patient with systemic *scleroderma* 10 years later showing beaking of the nose, wrinkles around the mouth, hyperpigmentation, and waxy, bound-down skin. 2-3 *Dermatomyositis*. Heliotrope discoloration and edema of the eyelids are characteristic of the disease.   2-4 *Mycosis fungoides*. Well-demarcated raised plaques are present in the second stage of the disease.   2-5 Tumor stage of *mycosis fungoides*. Ulceration and secondary infection of the tumors is common.   2-6 *Adenoma sebaceum*, the skin lesions of tuberous sclerosis. The patient is mentally retarded and has epileptiform seizures.   2-7 *Urticaria pigmentosa*, brownred macules and papules become red raised wheals after they are rubbed.

Plate 2

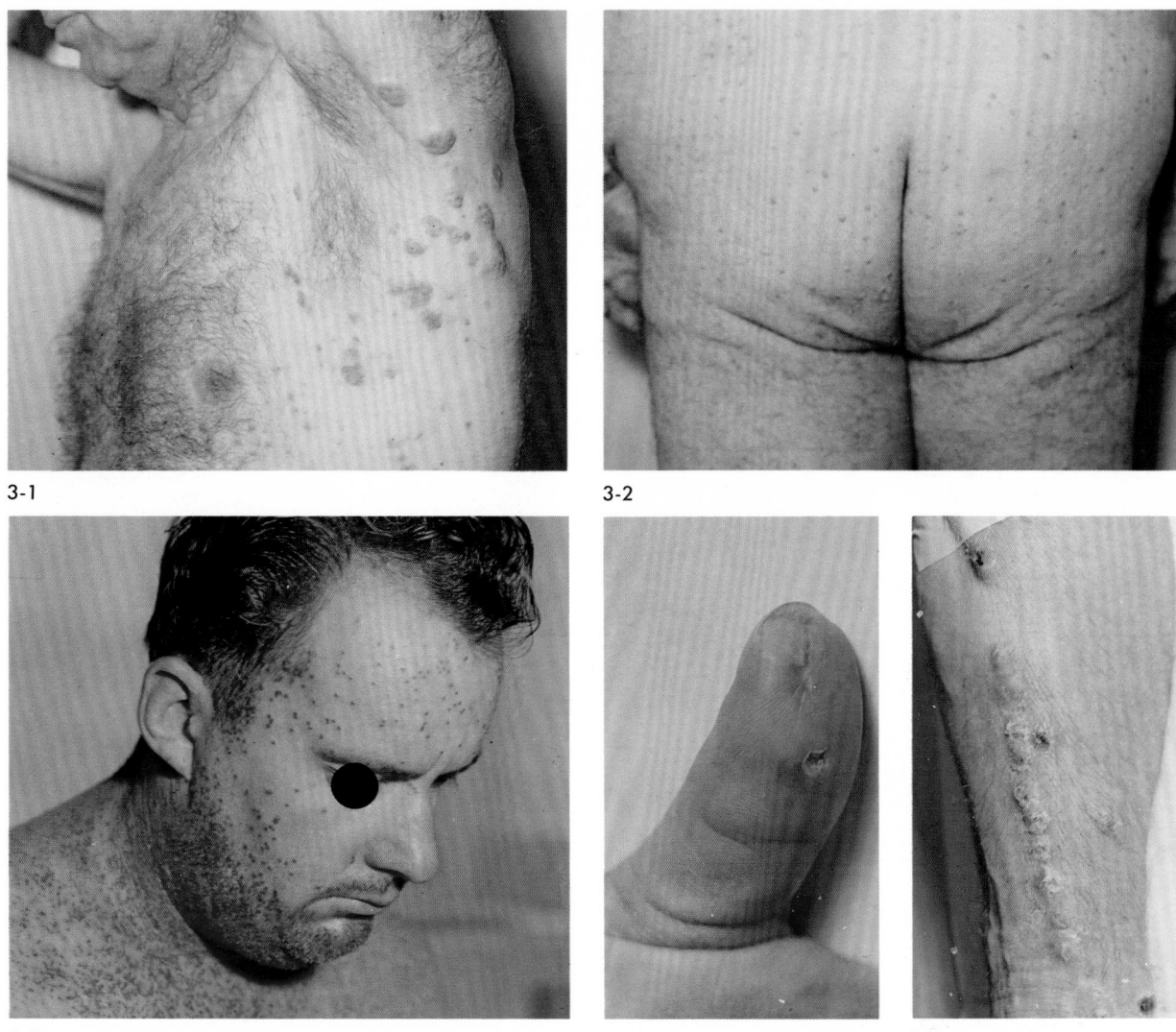

3-1
3-2
3-3
3-4
3-5

3-1 *Xanthomata* are yellow or orange nodules which accompany marked hyperlipemia. 3-2 The skin lesions of *eruptive xanthomatosis* are firm red or yellow papules. 3-3 *Eczema herpeticum* in a man with atopic dermatitis. The eruption is caused by the herpes simplex virus. 3-4 Ulcers of a thumb caused by vascular occlusion in *Buerger's disease*. 3-5 *Sporotrichosis* shows a primary inoculation complex pattern with multiple nodules along the wrist and forearm.

Plate 3

4-1 *Necrobiosis lipoidica diabeticorum;* the yellow atrophic pretibial lesions may ulcerate.   4-2 *Erythema nodosum;* the tender red pretibial nodules resolve without scarring.   4-3 *Erythema multiforme* commonly involves the palms with large bullae and diagnostic target lesions.   4-4 Large *urticarial plaques,* annular lesions, and target lesions may occur without bullae in *erythema multiforme.*   4-5 *Psoriatic arthritis* is usually accompanied by psoriasis of the hands and nails.   4-6 *Psoriasis* is characterized by well demarcated red plaques covered by silvery scales.

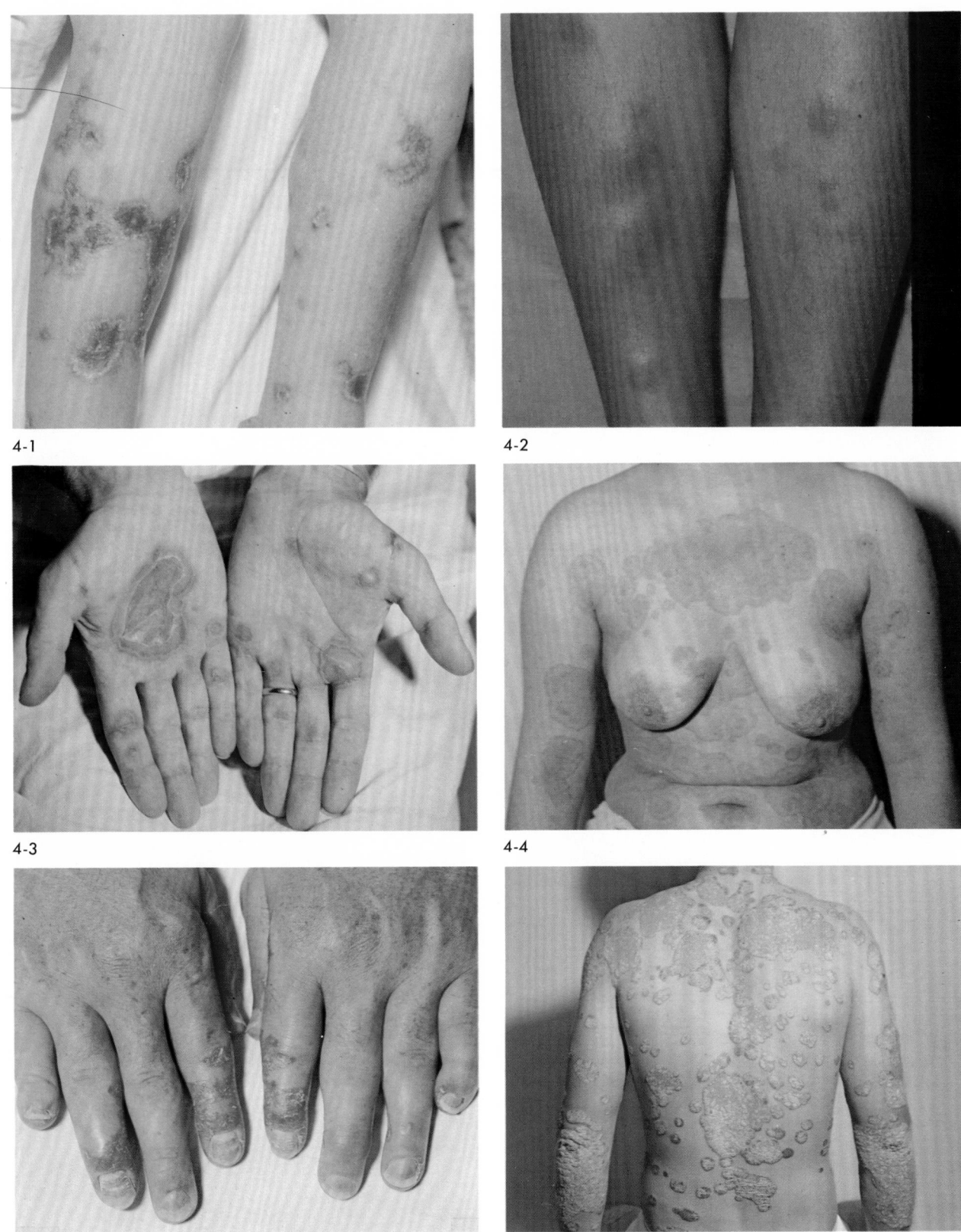

4-1

4-2

4-3

4-4

4-5

4-6

Plate 4

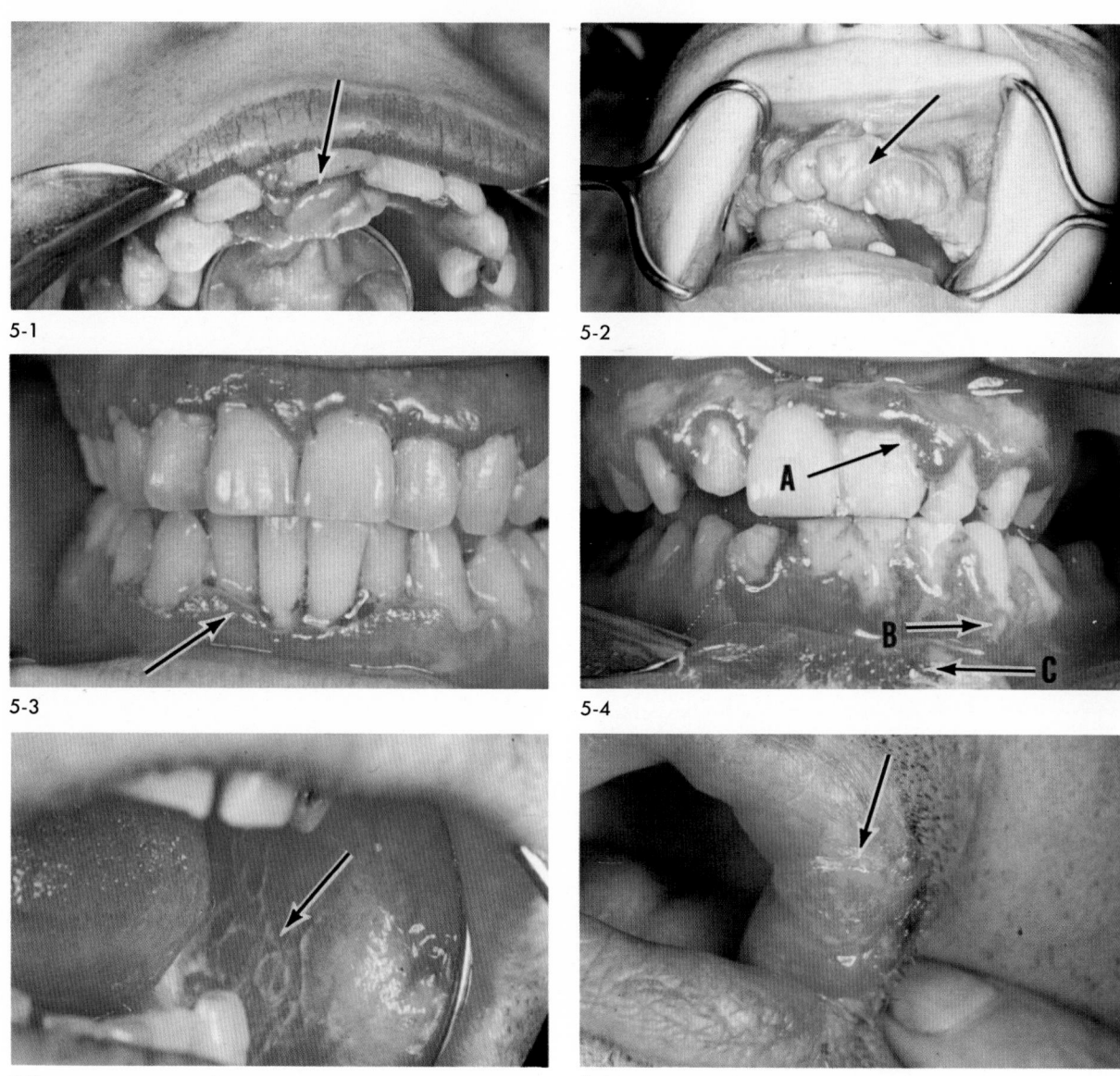

5-1 Pregnancy tumor—large growth derived from gingiva, occuring during pregnancy; tissue is very vascular; ordinarily, tumor will regress following parturition; 5-2 *Dilantin hyperplasia*—marked overgrowth of gingiva which almost completely covers anterior maxillary teeth. Severity of condition appears to be directly related to the dose of the drug used and the degree of laxness of oral hygiene procedures; 5-3 *Acute necrotizing ulcerative gingivitis*—a painful, necrotizing disease of the gingiva affecting the interdental papillae and marginal gingiva and leading to rapid destruction of tissue; responds dramatically to antibiotics; note greyish pseudo-membrane along margin of affected gingiva (arrow) which indicates that the process is active; 5-4 *Acute primary herpetic gingivostomatitis*—acute manifestation of primary infection with herpes simplex virus; oral signs include inflammation of marginal gingiva (A), aphthous ulcers on gingiva (B), buccal mucosa, tongue or palate, and crusted raw lesions on lips (C); condition is very painful, and is often confused with acute necrotizing ulcerative gingivitis; 5-5 *Lichen planus*—oral manifestations of lichen planus usually appear prior to the skin lesions and frequently take the form of elevated greyish-white lines arranged in a reticular pattern on the buccal mucosa (arrow). 5-6 *Carcinoma of the lip*—represents the most common malignant tumor of the oral mucous membrane; the lower lip is usually affected; note the raised indurated border surrounding the raw ulcer (arrow) and the crusting adjacent to the skin margin.

Plate 5

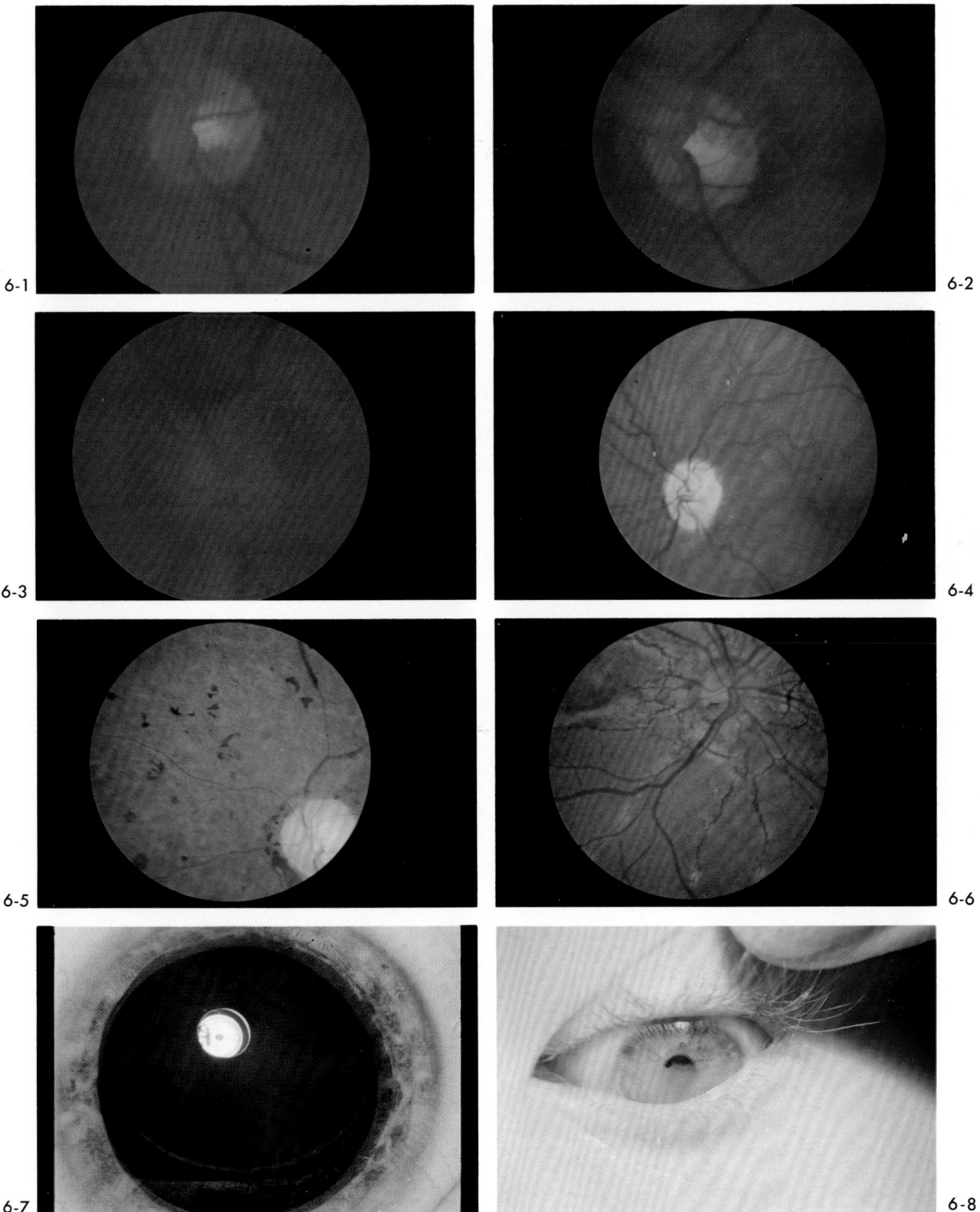

6-1 Normal optic nervehead, right eye   6-2 Temporal pallor, optic nervehead, left eye. Compare with normal right optic nerve figure 1.   6-3 Papilledema   6-4 Optic atrophy   6-5 Retinitis pigmentosa   6-6 Angioid streaks   6-7 Dislocation of crystalline lens   6-8 Band keratopathy.

Plate 6

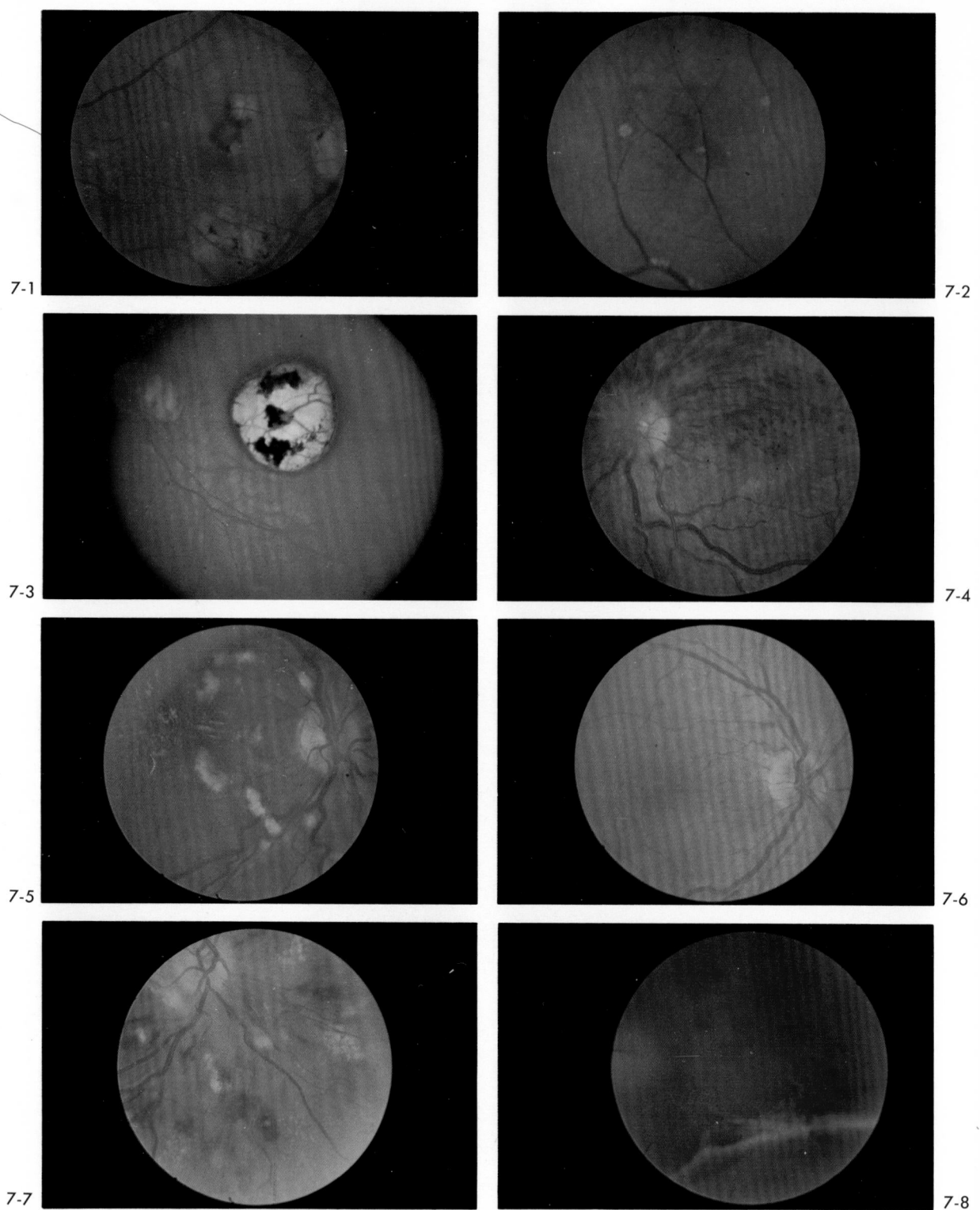

7-1 Histoplasmosis   7-2 Sarcoid   7-3 Toxoplasmosis   7-4 Occlusion of superior temporal vein with edema of macula   7-5 Hypertensive retinopathy   7-6 Early intra-retinal diabetic retinopathy   7-7 Advanced intra-retinal diabetic retinopathy   7-8 Advanced extra-retinal (proliferative) diabetic retinopathy.

Plate 7

Index

Index

Boldface page numbers refer to the principal discussion of a subject. Under a general category the subentries for specific conditions may refer to the principal discussion only, and more information will be found under the name of the condition. See muscle diseases and muscular dystrophy.